Mulholland & Greenfield's

SURGERY

SCIENTIFIC PRINCIPLES AND PRACTICE

EIGHTH EDITION

Mulholland & Greenfield's

SURGERY

SCIENTIFIC PRINCIPLES AND PRACTICE

EIGHTH EDITION

Justin B. Dimick, MD, MPH, FACS
Frederick A. Coller Distinguished Professor
Chair, Department of Surgery
University of Michigan Medical School
Ann Arbor, Michigan

Hasan B. Alam, MD, MBA, FACS
Loyal and Edith Davis Professor of Surgery, and
Professor of Cell & Developmental Biology
Chair, Department of Surgery
Northwestern University Feinberg School of Medicine
Surgeon-in-Chief, Northwestern Memorial Hospital
Chicago, Illinois

Timothy M. Pawlik, MD, PhD, MPH, MTS, MBA, FACS, MAMSE, FSSO
Professor and Chair
Department of Surgery
The Urban Meyer III and Shelley Meyer Chair for
Cancer Research
Surgeon-in-Chief
The Ohio State University Wexner Medical Center
Columbus, Ohio

Mary T. Hawn, MD, MPH, FACS
Emile Holman Professor and Chair of Surgery
Department of Surgery
Stanford University School of Medicine
Stanford, California

Julie Ann Sosa, MD, MA, FACS, MAMSE, FSSO
Leon Goldman, MD Distinguished Professor of Surgery
Chair, Department of Surgery
Professor, Department of Medicine
Affiliated Faculty, Philip R. Lee Institute for Health
Policy Studies
University of California San Francisco (UCSF)
San Francisco, California

Dawn M. Coleman, MD, FACS
Professor, Surgery
Chief, Division of Vascular and Endovascular Surgery
Duke University School of Medicine
Durham, North Carolina

Wolters Kluwer

Philadelphia • Baltimore • New York • London
Buenos Aires • Hong Kong • Sydney • Tokyo

Acquisitions Editor: Nicole Dernoski
Senior Development Editor: Ashley Fischer
Editorial Coordinator: Thirupura Sundari
Marketing Manager: Kirsten Watrud
Senior Production Project Manager: Alicia Jackson
Manager, Design & Graphic Arts: Stephen Druding
Manufacturing Coordinator: Lisa Bowling
Prepress Vendor: Aptara, Inc.

8th edition

9 8 7 6 5 4 3 2 1

Printed in Mexico

Cataloging-in-Publication Data available on request from the Publisher

ISBN: 978-1-9752-4355-5

shop.lww.com

QUADM0426

Preface

The editors are pleased to present the eighth edition of *Mulholland and Greenfield's Surgery: Scientific Principles & Practice*. The field of surgery has changed fundamentally in the years since the first edition of this text. Growth in the knowledge base of clinical surgery continues exponentially. Surgical practice has been transformed through scientific advancements and the introduction of new technology. The accelerating pace of scientific progress demands rapid adoption of new ideas into surgical therapy and a commitment to lifelong learning. Accordingly, the new edition of *Mulholland and Greenfield's Surgery* seeks to integrate new scientific knowledge with evolving changes in surgical care.

The eighth edition has many updates. First, the composition of the editorial team continues to evolve. Dr. Gilbert Upchurch, who provided excellent service as the editor for vascular surgery for several editions, stepped down. Dr. Dawn Coleman has agreed to join the editorial team. The expertise, energy, and vision of this great team of editors have resulted in a fantastic edition.

Second, we continue to make changes to the style, content, and authors. We have kept the vision of the text by integrating science and practice but have shortened the book by eliminating some chapters that can be accessed elsewhere and are less relevant to current practice. We also instructed authors to shorten chapters and consolidate information into easy-to-read tables.

On behalf of the editorial team, we hope that you find the eighth edition of *Mulholland and Greenfield's Surgery: Scientific Principles & Practice* to be an important part of your surgical library. We have carefully curated the content to serve your lifelong education goals and, ultimately, to improve the care of your patients.

Justin B. Dimick, MD, MPH, FACS

Contents

List of Algorithms

Contributors

Ali B. Abbasi, MD
Department of Surgery
UCSF School of Medicine
San Francisco, California

Ola Ahmed, MD, MMEd, PhD, FRCS
Fellow
Department of Abdominal Organ Transplantation and Hepatobiliary Surgery
Washington University School of Medicine
St. Louis, Missouri

Chiaka O. V. Akarichi, MD
Assistant Professor
Department of Surgery
UT Southwestern Medical School
Dallas, Texas

Hasan B. Alam, MD, MBA, FACS
Loyal and Edith Davis Professor of Surgery, and Professor of Cell & Developmental Biology
Chair, Department of Surgery
Northwestern University Feinberg School of Medicine
Surgeon-in-Chief, Northwestern Memorial Hospital
Chicago, Illinois

Omar Al-Nouri, DO, FACS
Associate Professor
Scripps Medical Group
La Jolla, California

Dean J. Arnaoutakis, MD, MBA
Associate Professor of Surgery and Vice Chair of Clinical Research
Department of Surgery
USF Health Morsani College of Medicine
Tampa, Florida

George J. Arnaoutakis, MD
Associate Professor and Chief
Division of Thoracic and Cardiovascular Surgery
The University of Texas at Austin Dell Medical School
Austin, Texas

Emre Arpali, MD, PhD
Associate Professor
Division of Transplant Surgery
Medical College of Wisconsin
Milwaukee, Wisconsin

Leah M. Backhus, MD, MPH, FACS
Thelma and Henry Doelger Professor of CV Surgery
Department of Cardiothoracic Surgery
Stanford University School of Medicine
Stanford, California

Andrea Badillo, MD
Professor of Surgery and Pediatrics
Division of Pediatric Surgery
Children's National Hospital
Washington, DC

Andrew J. Bauer, MD
Professor
Department of Pediatrics
Perelman School of Medicine at the University of Pennsylvania
Director, The Thyroid Center, Division of Endocrinology and Diabetes
The Children's Hospital of Philadelphia
Philadelphia, Pennsylvania

Joal D. Beane, MD
Assistant Professor of Surgery
Department of Surgery
The Ohio State University College of Medicine
Columbus, Ohio

Bradley D. Beasley, DPM, CWS
Podiatric Surgery Specialist
Department of Restoration Foot and Ankle
Restoration Foot and Ankle
Broken Arrow, Oklahoma

Robert J. Beaulieu, MD, MSE
Assistant Professor of Vascular Surgery
Department of Surgery
University of Michigan Medical School
Ann Harbor, Michigan

Mark F. Berry, MD
Mylavarapu Rogers Professor
Department of Cardiothoracic Surgery
Stanford University School of Medicine
Stanford, California

Marc G. Besselink, MD, MSc, PhD
Professor of Pancreatic and Hepatobiliary Surgery
Department of Surgery
Amsterdam UMC
Amsterdam, the Netherlands

Jacqueline J. Blank, MD, FACS
Assistant Professor of Surgery
Department of Trauma and Acute Care Surgery
Medical College of Wisconsin
Milwaukee, Wisconsin

Steven F. Bolling, MD
Professor of Cardiac Surgery
Department of Cardiac Surgery
University of Michigan Medical School
Ann Arbor, Michigan

Stefan A. W. Bouwense, MD, PhD
Surgeon
Department of Surgery
Maastricht UMC+
Maastricht, Limburg, The Netherlands

Alexandra Briggs, MD, FACS
Assistant Professor of Surgery
Dartmouth Hitchcock Medical Center
Geisel School of Medicine at Dartmouth
Lebanon, New Hampshire

Carlos V. R. Brown, MD
Professor of Surgery
Department of Surgery
The University of Texas at Austin Dell Medical School
Austin, Texas

Brandon R. Bruns, MD, MBA
Professor of Surgery
Department of Surgery
UT Southwestern Medical School
Dallas, Texas

Benjamin Bryner, MD
Assistant Professor of Surgery
Department of Surgery, Division of Cardiac Surgery
Northwestern University Feinberg School of Medicine
Chicago, Illinois

Errol L. Bush, MD, FACS
Associate Professor of Surgery
Surgical Director, Advanced Lung Disease and Lung Transplant Program
Department of Surgery, Division of Thoracic Surgery
Johns Hopkins Medicine
Baltimore, Maryland

Rebecca L. Buttar, MSc, MD
Fellow
Department of General Surgery
University of Calgary
Alberta, Canada

Andrew M. Cameron, MD, PhD
Director
Department of Surgery
Johns Hopkins Medicine
Baltimore, Maryland

Eric P. Cantey, MSc, MD
Assistant Professor of Medicine
Department of Cardiology
University of Michigan Medical School
Ann Harbor, Michigan

Tatiana C. P. Cardenas, MS, MD, FACS
Assistant Professor
Department of Surgery and Perioperative Care
The University of Texas at Austin Dell Medical School
Dell Seton Medical Center at the University of Texas
Austin, Texas

Alfred J. Casillan, MD, PhD
Instructor of Surgery
Division of Thoracic Surgery
The Johns Hopkins Hospital
Baltimore, Maryland

William C. Chiu, MD
Professor and Director
Surgical Critical Care Fellowship Program
Department of Surgery
University of Maryland School of Medicine
University of Maryland Medical Center
Baltimore, Maryland

Jordan M. Cloyd, MD
Associate Professor
Department of Surgery
The Ohio State University Comprehensive Cancer Center
Columbus, Ohio

Dawn M. Coleman, MD, FACS
Professor, Surgery
Chief, Division of Vascular and Endovascular Surgery
Duke University School of Medicine
Durham, North Carolina

Trevor D. Crafts, MD
Assistant Professor of Surgery
Department of Surgery
Rocky Mountain Regional VA Medical Center
Aurora, Colorado

Joseph Cuschieri, MD
Professor of Surgery and Laboratory Medicine
UCSF School of Medicine
Chief of Surgery and Trauma Medical Director
Zuckerberg San Francisco General Hospital
San Francisco, California

Donnele Daley, MD
Assistant Professor
Department of Surgery
University of Michigan Medical School
Ann Arbor, Michigan

Michael C. Dalsing, MD, MBA, FACS, DFSVS, DFAVF
Professor Emeritus
Department of Surgery, Division of Vascular Surgery
Indiana University School of Medicine
Indianapolis, Indiana

Kimberly A. Davis, MD, MBA
Professor
Division Chief, General Surgery, Trauma and Critical Care
Department of Surgery
Yale School of Medicine
New Haven, Connecticut

Aaron J. Dawes, MD, PhD
Assistant Professor
Department of Surgery
Stanford University School of Medicine
Stanford, California

Keith A. Delman, MD
Surgeon-in-Chief at Grady Memorial Hospital and Associate Chair
Department of Surgery
Emory University School of Medicine
Atlanta, Georgia

Marc de Moya, MD, MHPE, FACS
Professor and Chief of Acute Care Surgery
Department of Surgery
Medical College of Wisconsin
Milwaukee, Wisconsin

Ana C. De Roo, MD, MSc
Assistant Professor
Department of Surgery
University of Wisconsin School of Medicine and Public Health
Madison, Wisconsin

Justin B. Dimick, MD, MPH, FACS
Frederick A. Coller Distinguished Professor
Chair, Department of Surgery
University of Michigan Medical School
Ann Arbor, Michigan

Elijah Dixon, MD, MSc, BSc, FRCSC, FACS
Professor of Surgery and Oncology
Department of Surgery
University of Calgary
Calgary, Alberta, Canada

Georgiana Alina Dobri, MD
Associate Professor of Clinical Endocrinology and Neurosurgery
Department of Surgery
Weill Cornell Medicine
New York, New York

Lesly A. Dossett, MD, MPH
Maud T. Lane Research Professor for Cancer Quality Improvement
Chief, Division of Surgical Oncology
University of Michigan Medical School
Michigan Medicine
Ann Arbor, Michigan

Maria Bernadette Majella Doyle, MD, MBA, FRCSI, FACS
Executive Vice Chair
Department of Surgery
Professor of Surgery
Department of Abdominal Transplant
Washington University School of Medicine
St. Louis, Missouri

Ty B. Dunn, MD, MS
Professor
Department of Surgery
Medical College of Wisconsin
Milwaukee, Wisconsin

Chigozirim N. Ekeke, MD
Thoracic Surgeon
Department of Thoracic Surgery
University of Michigan Medical School
Michigan Medicine
Ann Arbor, Michigan

Kendal M. Endicott, MD, FACS
Director of Complex Aortic Surgery Program
Department of Vascular Surgery
Inova Health System
Falls Church, Virginia

Micaela M. Esquivel, MD
Clinical Associate Professor of Surgery
Department of Surgery
Stanford University School of Medicine
Stanford, California

Dalya M. Ferguson, MD, MS
Assistant Professor
Department of Surgery
McGovern Medical School at UTHealth Houston
Houston, Texas

Paula Ferrada, MD, FACS, FCCM, MAMSE
Professor
Department of Surgery
University of Virginia School of Medicine
Chair
Department of Surgery
Inova Fairfax Medical Campus
Medical Director, Perioperative Services IFMC
Division and System Chief for Trauma and Acute Care Surgery
Inova Healthcare System
Falls Church, Virginia

Sarah B. Fisher, MD, MS, BA
Assistant Professor
Department of Surgical Oncology
MD Anderson Cancer Center
Houston, Texas

James W. Fleshman, MD, FACS, FASCRS
Chair of Surgery
Professor
Michael E. DeBakey Department of Surgery
Baylor College of Medicine
Baylor University Medical Center
Dallas, Texas

Yuman Fong, MD
Chair and Professor
Department of Surgery
Professor of Experimental Therapeutics
Director of International Medicine
City of Hope
Duarte, California

Katherine A. Gallagher, MD
Professor of Surgery
Department of Surgery, Department of Microbiology and Immunology
University of Michigan Medical School
Ann Arbor, Michigan

Hiba Z. Ghandour, MD
Department of Surgery
Duke Congenital Heart Surgery Research and Training Laboratory
Duke University Hospital
Durham, North Carolina

Mira H. Ghneim, MD, MS, MPH
Assistant Professor
Department of Surgery, Program in Trauma
University of Maryland School of Medicine
R Adams Cowley Shock Trauma Center
Baltimore, Maryland

Brian F. Gilmore, MD
Assistant Professor of Surgery
Division of Vascular and Endovascular Surgery
Duke University School of Medicine
Durham, North Carolina

Ankush Gosain, MD, PhD, MBA, FACS, FAAP
C. Bruce Morton Professor of Surgery
Department of Surgery
University of Virginia School of Medicine
Surgeon-in-Chief
UVA Health Children's Hospital
Charlottesville, Virginia

Joshua C. Grimm, MD
Co-Director, Thoracic Aortic Surgery
Department of Cardiovascular and Thoracic Surgery
The University of Texas at Austin Dell Medical School
Austin, Texas

Gabriella Grisotti, MD, PhD
Fellow
Department of Surgery
UCSF School of Medicine
San Francisco, California

Elizabeth G. Grubbs, MD
Professor
Faculty Academic Development
MD Anderson Cancer Center
Houston, Texas

Andrew J. Gunderson, PhD
Assistant Professor
Department of Surgery
The Ohio State University College of Medicine
Columbus, Ohio

Jonathan W. Haft, MD
Professor
Department of Cardiac Surgery
University of Michigan Medical School
Ann Arbor, Michigan

Krista L. Haines, DO, MA
Assistant Professor of Surgery
Department of Surgery
Duke University School of Medicine
Duke University Hospital
Durham, North Carolina

Amy L. Halverson, MD, MHPE, FACS, FASCRS
Professor of Surgery
Department of Surgery
Northwestern University Feinberg School of Medicine
Chicago, Illinois

Barbara C. S. Hamilton, MD, MS
Assistant Professor of Cardiac Surgery
Department of Cardiac Surgery
University of Michigan Medical School
Ann Arbor, Michigan

Scott L. Hansen, MD
Professor and Chief of Plastic Surgery
Department of Surgery
UCSF School of Medicine
San Francisco, California

Daniel A. Hashimoto, MD, MSTR
Assistant Professor
Director of Penn Computer Assisted Surgery and Outcomes Laboratory
Departments of Surgery, Computer and Information Science
Perelman School of Medicine at the University of Pennsylvania
Philadelphia, Pennsylvania

Salila S. Hashmi, MD, FACS, FSSO
Clinical Assistant Professor
Department of Surgery
City of Hope Cancer Center Atlanta
Newnan, Georgia

Robert B. Hawkins II, MD, MSc
Assistant Professor
Department of Cardiac Surgery
University of Michigan Medical School
Ann Arbor, Michigan

Mary T. Hawn, MD, MPH, FACS
Emile Holman Professor and Chair of Surgery
Department of Surgery
Stanford University School of Medicine
Stanford, California

Jin He, MD, PhD
Associate Professor of Surgery
Department of Surgery
Johns Hopkins Medicine
Baltimore, Maryland

Holly L. Hedrick, MD
Professor of Surgery
Children's Hospital of Philadelphia, Perelman School of Medicine
Philadelphia, Pennsylvania

Peter K. Henke, MD
Professor of Surgery
Department of Surgery
University of Michigan Medical School
Ann Arbor, Michigan

Ryan Howard, MD, MS
Clinical Instructor of Surgery
Department of Surgery
University of Michigan Medical School
Ann Arbor, Michigan

Andrew M. Ibrahim, MD, MSc
George D. Zuidema Professor
Director, Center for Healthcare Outcomes and Policy
Vice Chair for Health Services Research
Department of Surgery
University of Michigan Medical School
Ann Arbor, Michigan

Kenji Inaba, MD, FRCSC, FACS
Professor of Surgery, Anesthesia, and Emergency Medicine
Vice Chair of Surgery
Chief of Trauma and Surgical Critical Care
Program Director of Surgical Residency
Keck School of Medicine of USC
LA General Medical Center
Los Angeles, California

Hope T. Jackson, MD, FACS
Associate Professor of Surgery and Clinical Track
Department of Surgery
University of Michigan Medical School
Ann Arbor, Michigan

Eric I. Jeng, MD, MBA, FACS, FACC, FCCP
Associate Professor of Surgery
Associate Director, Aortic Disease Center
Surgical Director, Bicuspid Valve Program
Surgical Director, Mechanical Circulator Support Program
Department of Surgery, Division of Cardiovascular Surgery
University of Florida College of Medicine
Gainesville, Florida

D. Rohan Jeyarajah, MD, FACS
Physician
Department of Surgery
Methodist Richardson Medical Center
Richardson, Texas

Adam P. Johnson, MD, MPH
Assistant Professor of Surgery
Division of Vascular and Endovascular Surgery
Duke University School of Medicine
Durham, North Carolina

Ashley W. Johnston, MD
Assistant Professor of Pediatric Urology
Department of Urology
Duke University School of Medicine
Durham, North Carolina

Bellal Joseph, MD
Martin Gluck Professor and Chief of Trauma Surgery
Executive Vice Chair of Surgery
Department of Surgery
University of Arizona College of Medicine
Tucson, Arizona

Jacob R. Joseph, MD
Clinical Associate Professor
Department of Neurosurgery
University of Michigan Medical School
Ann Arbor, Michigan

Gregory J. Jurkovich, MD, FACS
Distinguished Professor of Surgery
The Lloyd F. & Rosemargaret Donant Chair in Trauma Medicine
Vice Chair, Department of Surgery
UC Davis School of Medicine
UC Davis Health
Sacramento, California

Loay S. Kabbani, MD, MHSA
Program Director for the Vascular Surgery Fellowship
Henry Ford Health
Detroit, Michigan

Matthew F. Kalady, MD
Professor of Surgery
Chief of the Division of Colon and Rectal Surgery
Director of the James Colorectal Cancer Center
Director of the Clinical Cancer Genetics Program
Division of Colon and Rectal Surgery
Department of Surgery
The Ohio State Wexner Medical Center and the James Comprehensive Cancer Center
Columbus, Ohio

Lillian S. Kao, MD, MS
Professor and Chief of the Division of Acute Care Surgery
Department of Surgery
McGovern Medical School at UTHealth Houston
Houston, Texas

Ken Kazahaya, MD, MBA, FACS
Director of the Complex Pediatric Head and Neck Surgery Program
Division of Pediatric Otolaryngology
The Children's Hospital of Philadelphia
Philadelphia, Pennsylvania

Kaitlyn J. Kelly, MS, MAS
Associate Professor
Department of Surgery
University of Wisconsin School of Medicine and Public Health
Madison, Wisconsin

Sachin Kheterpal, MD, MBA
Professor of Anesthesiology
Department of Anesthesiology
University of Michigan Medical School
Ann Arbor, Michigan

Mary T. Killackey, MD, FACS
Chair and Professor
Department of Surgery
Tulane University School of Medicine
New Orleans, Louisiana

Joshua Kong, MD
Surgeon
Department of Hepatopancreaticobiliary Surgery
Methodist Richardson Medical Center
Richardson, Texas

Meera Kotagal, MD, MPH
Assistant Professor
Director of Trauma Services
Division of Pediatric General and Thoracic Surgery
Cincinnati Children's Hospital Medical Center
University of Cincinnati College of Medicine
Cincinnati, Ohio

Anai Kothari, MD, MS
Assistant Professor of Surgery
Department of Surgery, Division of Surgical Oncology
Medical College of Wisconsin
Milwaukee, Wisconsin

Olga Lavryk, MD, PhD
Surgeon
Department of Colorectal Surgery
Cleveland Clinic
Cleveland, Ohio

Katherin E. Leckie, MD, MS
Vascular Surgeon
Allina Health Minneapolis Heart Institute
Minneapolis, Minnesota

Hanmin Lee, MD
Professor
Chief, Pediatric Surgery
Department of Surgery
UCSF School of Medicine
San Francisco, California

Steven G. Leeds, MD, FACS
Assistant Professor
Division Chief of Minimally Invasive Surgery
Texas A&M University College of Medicine
Baylor University Medical Center
Dallas, Texas

Benjamin Levi, MD
Dr. Lee Hudson-Robert R. Penn Chair
Division Chief of General Surgery
Director at the Center for Organogenesis Regeneration & Trauma
Professor in Surgery at the UT Southwestern Medical School Medical Center
Department of Surgery
UT Southwestern Medical Center
Dallas, Texas

Jayme E. Locke, MD, MPH, FACS, FAST
Professor of Surgery
Arnold G. Diethelm MD Endowed Chair in Transplant Surgery
UAB Heersink School of Medicine
Birmingham, Alabama

Joann M. Lohr, MD, FACS, RUT, CWSP
Vascular Surgeon
William Jennings Dorn VA
Columbia, South Carolina

Chandler A. Long, MD
Associate Professor of Surgery
Department of Surgery, Division of Vascular Surgery
Duke University School of Medicine
Duke University Medical Center
Durham, North Carolina

Michael C. Lowe, MD, MA, FACS, FSSO
Associate Professor
Department of Surgery
Emory University School of Medicine
Atlanta, Georgia

Felix Y. Lui, MD
Associate Professor of Surgery
Section of General Surgery, Trauma and Surgical Critical Care
Yale School of Medicine
New Haven, Connecticut

Natalie S. Lui, MD
Assistant Professor
Department of Cardiothoracic Surgery
Stanford University School of Medicine
Stanford, California

Nicole Lunardi, MD, MSPH
Department of General Surgery
UT Southwestern Medical School
Dallas, Texas

Heather G. Lyu, MD, MBI
Assistant Professor
Department of Surgical Oncology
MD Anderson Cancer Center
Houston, Texas

Louis J. Magnotti, MS, MD
Professor of Surgery
Division of Trauma Surgical Critical Care, Burns, and Acute Care Surgery
University of Arizona College of Medicine—Tucson
Tucson, Arizona

Shishir K. Maithel, MD
Professor of Surgery
Division of Surgical Oncology
Department of Surgery
Winship Cancer Institute
Emory University School of Medicine
Atlanta, Georgia

Mahmoud B. Malas, MD, MHS, RPVI, FACS
Professor of Surgery
Department of Surgery
Division of Vascular and Endovascular Surgery
UC San Diego School of Medicine La Jolla, California

Kelly Michele Malloy, MD, MBA, FACS
Professor of Otolaryngology—Head and Neck Surgery
Chief Clinical Officer, Michigan Medicine
Director, Head and Neck Surgical Oncology & Microvascular Reconstruction Fellowship
University of Michigan Medical School
Ann Arbor, Michigan

Samuel P. Mandell, MD, MPH, FACS, FABA
Associate Professor, Medical Director, Parkland Burn Center
Department of Surgery
UT Southwestern Medical School
UT Southwestern Medical Center
Dallas, Texas

Julie A. Margenthaler, MD
Professor of Surgery
Department of Surgery
Washington University School of Medicine
St. Louis, Missouri

Peter T. Masiakos, MD, MS
Associate Professor of Surgery
Department of Pediatric Surgery
Harvard Medical School
Massachusetts General Hospital
Boston, Massachusetts

Michael R. Mathis, MD
Associate Professor
Department of Anesthesiology
University of Michigan Medical School
Ann Arbor, Michigan

Kazuhide Matsushima, MD
Associate Professor of Surgery
Department of Surgery
Keck School of Medicine of USC
Los Angeles, California

Robert E. Merritt, MD, MBA
Director of Thoracic Surgery
Department of Surgery
The Ohio State University Wexner Medical Center
Columbus, Ohio

Barbra S. Miller, MD
Clinical Professor of Surgery
Department of Surgery
The Ohio State University College of Medicine
Columbus, Ohio

Katherine A. Morgan, MD, FACS
Professor and Head, Pancreatic Surgery
Department of Surgery
NYU Grossman School of Medicine
NYU Langone Health
New York, New York

Courtney E. Morgan, MD
Associate Professor of Vascular Surgery
Department of Surgery
University of Wisconsin School of Medicine and Public Health
Madison, Wisconsin

Arden M. Morris, MD, MPH
Professor of Surgery
Stanford University School of Medicine
Stanford, California

Melanie S. Morris, MD, FACS, FASCRS
Professor
Vice Chair of Perioperative Services
Department of Surgery, Division of Gastrointestinal Surgery
UAB Heersink School of Medicine
Chief of General Surgery at Birmingham VA Hospital
Medical Quality Officer, Perioperative Services at UAB Hospital
Birmingham, Alabama

Anays Murillo, MD, MPH
Fellow
Boston University Chobanian & Avedisian School of Medicine
Boston Medical Center
Boston, Massachusetts

Lena M. Napolitano, MD, FACS, FCCP, MCCM
Massey Foundation Professor of Surgery
Department of Surgery
University of Michigan
Ann Arbor, Michigan

Erika Adams Newman, MD, FAAP, FACS
Chief, Section of Pediatric Surgery
Department of Surgery
University of Michigan Medical School
CS Mott Children's Hospital
Ann Arbor, Michigan

Valentine Nfongen Nfonsam, MD, MS, FACS, FASCRS
Professor and Executive Vice Chair
Department of Surgery
Morehouse School of Medicine
Atlanta, Georgia

Kristina J. Nicholson, MD, MSc
Assistant Professor
Department of Surgery
University of Pittsburgh School of Medicine
University of Pittsburgh Medical Center
Pittsburgh, Pennsylvania

Andrea T. Obi, MD
Associate Professor of Surgery
Department of Surgery, Division of Vascular Surgery
University of Michigan Medical School
Ann Arbor, Michigan

Robert W. O'Rourke, MD
William J. Fry Professor of Surgery
Department of Surgery
University of Michigan Medical School
Ann Arbor, Michigan

Douglas M. Overbey, MD, MPH
Surgeon
Department of Surgery
Duke University Medical Center
Durham, North Carolina

Emily A. Partridge, MD, PhD
Assistant Professor of Surgery
Division of Pediatric General, Thoracic and Fetal Surgery
Children's Hospital of Philadelphia
Philadelphia, Pennsylvania

Eric M. Pauli, MD, FACS, FASGE, FEBSAWS (Hon.)
David L. Nahrwold Professor of Surgery
Chief, Division of Minimally Invasive and Bariatric Surgery
Vice Chair, Clinical Affairs
Director of Abdominal Wall Surgery
Program Director, Abdominal Wall Surgery Fellowship
Department of Surgery
Penn State College of Medicine
Penn State Health
Hershey, Pennsylvania

Timothy M. Pawlik, MD, PhD, MPH, MTS, MBA, FACS, MAMSE, FSSO
Professor and Chair
Department of Surgery
The Urban Meyer III and Shelley Meyer Chair for Cancer Research
Surgeon-in-Chief
The Ohio State University Wexner Medical Center
Columbus, Ohio

Audrey C. Pendleton, MD
Assistant Professor of Surgery
Columbia University Medical Center
New York, New York

Joshua Person, MD
Assistant Professor
Department of Surgery
The University of Texas Medical Branch
Galveston, Texas

Robin T. Petroze, MD, MPH
Associate Professor
Department of Surgery, Section of Pediatric Surgery
University of Michigan Medical School
Ann Harbor, Michigan

Paul Picton, MBChB, MRCP, FRCA
David W. Learned Collegiate Professor of Anesthesiology
Department of Anesthesiology
University of Michigan Medical School
Ann Harbor, Michigan

Michael Pienta, MD, MS
Cardiothoracic Surgeon
Sentara Mid-Atlantic Cardiothoracic Surgeons
Norfolk, Virginia

George A. Poultsides, MD, MS
Professor, Chief of Surgical Oncology
Department of Surgery
Stanford University School of Medicine
Stanford, California

Eric Yates Pruitt, MD
Department of Surgery, Division of Thoracic and Cardiovascular Surgery
University of Florida Health
Gainesville, Florida

Krishnan Raghavendran, MBBS
Professor Division of Acute Care Surgery
Founding Director, Center for Global Surgery
Department of Surgery
University of Michigan Medical School
Ann Arbor, Michigan

Venkatakrishna Rajajee, MBBS
Director
Division of Neurocritical Care
Department of Neurosurgery
University of Michigan
Ann Harbor, Michigan

Benjamin I. Rapoport, MD, PhD
Assistant Professor of Neurosurgery
Icahn School of Medicine at Mount Sinai
New York, New York

Todd E. Rasmussen, MD
Professor of Surgery and Consultant in Vascular and Endovascular Surgery
Department of Surgery
Mayo Clinic
Rochester, Minnesota

Chandrajit P. Raut, MD, MSc
Richard E. Wilson Professor of Surgery in the Field of Surgical Oncology
Harvard Medical School
Chief, Division of Surgical Oncology
Brigham and Women's Hospital
Surgeon-in-Chief and Chair, Department of Surgery
Dana-Farber Cancer Institute
Boston, Massachusetts

Marissa Ray, MD
Fellow
Department of Surgery
University of Cincinnati College of Medicine
Cincinnati, Ohio

John E. Rectenwald, MD, MS
Chair, Division of Vascular Surgery
Department of Surgery
University of Wisconsin School of Medicine and Public Health
Madison, Wisconsin

Rishindra M. Reddy, MD, MBA
Endowed, Tenured José José Alvarez Research Professor in Thoracic Surgery
Department of Surgery
University of Michigan Medical School
Ann Arbor, Michigan

Jennifer L. Rickard, MD, MPH
Associate Professor
Department of Surgery
University of Minnesota Medical School
Minneapolis, Minnesota

Bradley A. Rittenhouse, MD
Surgeon
Division of Trauma
Brooke Army Medical Center
Fort Sam Houston, Texas

William P. Robinson III, MD, FACS, DFSVS
Professor and Chief
Division of Vascular Surgery
Southern Illinois School of Medicine
Springfield, Illinois

Christina L. Roland, MD, MS
Associate Professor of Surgery
Department of Surgical Oncology
MD Anderson Cancer Center
Houston, Texas

Jonathan C. Routh, MD, MPH
Paul H. Sherman Distinguished Associate Professor of Surgery, Pediatrics, and Population Health Sciences
Department of Urology
Duke University School of Medicine
Chief, Duke Center for Children's Surgery
Durham, North Carolina

Teviah E. Sachs, MD, MPH
Chief of Surgical Oncology
Boston University Chobanian & Avedisian School of Medicine
Boston Medical Center
Boston, Massachusetts

Joseph V. Sakran, MD, MPH, MPA, FACS
Executive Vice Chair of Surgery
Director of Clinical Operations of Surgery
Associate Professor of Surgery and Nursing
Department of Surgery Acute Care and Trauma Services
Johns Hopkins Medicine
Baltimore, Maryland

Benjamin Samstein, MD
Professor of Surgery
Chief of Liver Transplant and Hepatobiliary and Pancreatic Surgery
Weill Cornell Medicine
New York-Presbyterian Hospital
New York, New York

Naveen F. Sangji, MD, MPH
Assistant Professor of Surgery
Department of Acute Care Surgery
University of Michigan Medical School
Ann Arbor, Michigan

Mary Catherine Santos, MD, MSEd
Professor, Surgery and Pediatrics
Department of Surgery
Penn State College of Medicine
Penn State Health Milton S. Hershey Medical Center
Hershey, Pennsylvania

Hjalmar van Santvoort, MD, PhD
Professor of Pancreatic Surgery
Department of Surgery
St. Antonius Hospital Nieuwegein
Nieuwegein, The Netherlands

Thomas M. Scalea, MD, FACS, MCCM
Physician-in-Chief
R Adams Cowley Shock Trauma
University of Maryland School of Medicine
Baltimore, Maryland

Martin A. Schreiber, MD, FACS, FCCM
Adjunct Professor of Surgery
Department of Surgery
Uniformed Services University
Bethesda, Maryland

Theodore H. Schwartz, MD
Professor of Neurosurgery
Mount Sinai Hospital
Icahn School of Medicine
New York, New York

John W. Scott, MD, MPH
Associate Professor
Department of Surgery
University of Washington School of Medicine
Division of Trauma, Burn, and Critical Care Surgery
Harborview Medical Center
Seattle, Washington

Carolyn D. Seib, MD, MAS
Associate Professor
Department of Surgery
Stanford University School of Medicine
Stanford, California

Farris Serio, DO
Fellow
Department of Surgery
Oregon Health & Science University
Portland, Oregon

James Shadiow, PhD
Fellow
Department of Surgery
University of Michigan Medical School
Ann Arbor, Michigan

Jenny M. Shao, MD
Clinical Assistant Professor of Surgery
Department of Surgery
University of Michigan Medical School
Ann Arbor, Michigan

Kyle H. Sheetz, MD, MSc
Assistant Professor of Transplant Surgery
Department of Surgery
University of Michigan Medical School
Ann Arbor, Michigan

Alexander D. Shepard, MD
Senior Staff Surgeon
Department of Surgery
Division of Vascular Surgery
Henry Ford Hospital
Detroit, Michigan

Matthew J. Sideman, MD, DFSUS, FACS
Professor and Chief, Division of Vascular and Endovascular Surgery
Department of Surgery
UT Health San Antonio
San Antonio, Texas

Anaar E. Siletz, MD, PhD
Assistant Professor of Surgery
Department of Surgery
Keck School of Medicine of USC
Los Angeles General Medical Center
Los Angeles, California

Raymond Malcolm Smith, MD, FRCS, MB, CHB
Orthopedic Surgeon
Boston Medical Center—Brighton
Brighton, Massachusetts

Christopher J. Sonnenday, MD, MHS
The Darrell A. Campbell, Jr, MD Collegiate Professor of Transplant Surgery
Transplant Center Director, University of Michigan Health
Executive Vice Chair, Department of Surgery
University of Michigan Medical School
Ann Arbor, Michigan

David I. Soybel, MD
Professor of Surgery
Geisel School of Medicine at Dartmouth
Hanover, New Hampshire

Jason L. Sperry, MD, MPH
Professor of Surgery and Critical Care Medicine
Department of Surgery
University of Pittsburgh School of Medicine
Pittsburgh, Pennsylvania

Kristan L. Staudenmayer, MD, MS
Associate Professor of Surgery
Department of Surgery
Stanford University School of Medicine
Stanford, California

Scott R. Steele, MD, MBA
Chair, Department of Colorectal Surgery
President, Main Campus
Cleveland Clinic
Cleveland, Ohio

Emily Steinhagen, FACS, FASCRS, MD
Associate Professor of Surgery
Department of Surgery
Case Western Reserve University School of Medicine
University Hospitals Cleveland Medical Center
Cleveland, Ohio

Peter G. Stock, MD, PhD
Professor of Surgery
Department of Surgery, Transplant Division
UCSF School of Medicine
San Francisco, California

Chad K. Sudoko, MD
Fellow
Division of Pediatric Otolaryngology
The Children's Hospital of Philadelphia
Philadelphia, Pennsylvania

Kevin E. Taubman, MD
Adjunct Clinical Associate Professor of Surgery
Department of Surgery
Indiana University School of Medicine
Indianapolis, Indiana

Dana A. Telem, MD, MPH
Lazar J. Greenfield Professor of Surgery, Section Chief General Surgery
University of Michigan Medical School
Ann Arbor, Michigan

Samuel A. Tisherman, MD, FACS, FCCM
Professor
Department of Surgery and the Program in Trauma
University of Maryland School of Medicine
Baltimore, Maryland

Umberto Tosi, MD
Department of Neurological Surgery
Weill Cornell Medicine
New York, New York

Shahab Toursavadkohi, MD
Professor of Surgery
Department of Vascular Surgery
University of Maryland
Baltimore, Maryland

Marc D. Trust, MD, FACS
Assistant Professor
Department of Surgery and Perioperative Care
The University of Texas at Austin Dell Medical School
Austin, Texas

Susan Tsai, MD, MHS
Professor
Department of Surgery
The Ohio State University College of Medicine
Columbus, Ohio

Jennifer F. Tseng, MD, MPH
Professor of Surgery Emerita
Department of Surgery
Boston University Chobanian & Avedisian School of Medicine
Boston, Massachusetts

Kiara A. Tulla, MD
Assistant Professor
Department of Surgery, Division of Abdominal Transplant and HPB
Tulane School of Medicine
New Orleans, Los Angeles

Joseph W. Turek, MD, PhD, MBA
Chief, Pediatric Cardiac Surgery
Department of Cardiothoracic Surgery
Duke University Medical Center
Durham, North Carolina

Michael B. Ujiki, MD, FACS, FASGE, FAFS
Louis Biegler Chair of Surgery
Department of Surgery
Endeavor Health
Evanston, Illinois

Gilbert R. Upchurch Jr, MD, FACS
Edward M. Copeland and Ann and Ira Horowitz Chair of Surgery
Department of Surgery
University of Florida College of Medicine
Gainesville, Florida

Lars W. A. J. VanderBroeck, MD
Researcher
Department of Surgery
Maastricht UMC+
Maastricht, Limburg, The Netherlands

Seth A. Waits, MD
Surgical Director of Liver Transplantation
University of Michigan Medical School
Ann Arbor, Michigan

Thomas W. Wakefield, MD
Emeritus Professor of Vascular Surgery
Section of Vascular Surgery, Department of Surgery
University of Michigan Medical School
Ann Arbor, Michigan

John Patrick Walker, MD
Vice Chair of Operations, Surgical Director of Perioperative Services
Department of Surgery
The University of Texas Medical Branch
Galveston, Texas

Mitchell R. Weaver, MD
Vascular Surgeon
Department of Surgery
Henry Ford Hospital
Detroit, Michigan

Sharon Weber, MD, FACS
Division Chair, Surgical Oncology
Department of Surgery
University of Wisconsin School of Medicine and Public Health
Madison, Wisconsin

Alice C. Wei, MD, MSc, FRCSC, FACS
Attending Surgeon, Hepato-Pancreato-Biliary Service
Department of Surgery
Memorial Sloan Kettering Cancer Center
New York, New York

Russell N. Wesson, MBChB
Surgical Director of Liver Transplant
Division of Transplant Surgery
Department of Surgery
Johns Hopkins Medicine
Baltimore, Maryland

Elizabeth C. Wick, MD
Professor of Surgery
Department of Surgery
UCSF School of Medicine
San Francisco, California

Allison R. Wilcox, MD
Assistant Professor of Surgery
Department of Surgery
Dartmouth Hitchcock Medical Center
Geisel School of Medicine at Dartmouth
Lebanon, New Hampshire

Kibileri Williams, MBBS, MSc
Assistant Professor
Department of General and Thoracic Surgery
Children's National Hospital
Washington, DC

Paul E. Wise, MD, FACS, FASCRS
Professor of Surgery, Vice Chair for Education
Department of Surgery
Washington University School of Medicine
St. Louis, Missouri

Seth E. M. Wolf, MD
Fellow
Duke Congenital Heart Surgery Research and Training Laboratory
Durham, North Carolina

Sandra L. Wong, MD, MS
William P. Timmie Professor of Surgery
Dean
Department of Surgery
Emory University School of Medicine
Atlanta, Georgia

Sherry M. Wren, MD, FACS, FCS(ECSA), FISS
Professor of Surgery
Department of Surgery
Stanford University School of Medicine
Stanford, California

Part One Scientific Principles

1

Surgical Nutrition and Metabolism

Krista L. Haines

SCIENTIFIC PRINCIPLES

Key Points

1 In the absence of indirect calorimetry, critically ill patients should be provided nutritional support targeting 25 to 30 kcal/kg/d.

2 In the setting of sepsis, the basal metabolic rate (BMR) increases. Indirect Calorimetry is the gold standard for measuring energy expenditure in critically ill patients. When not available, total energy requirements need to be assessed, increasing energy requirements by 20% to 30% for mild or moderate infection and approximately 50% above basal levels in severe infection.

3 Assessment of nutritional status is key in the perioperative period. Malnutrition is associated with worse outcomes after injury or surgery.

4 There is no single laboratory biomarker that accurately reflects a patient's nutritional status.

5 A strong relation between protein depletion and postoperative complications has been demonstrated in nonseptic, nonimmunocompromised patients undergoing elective major gastrointestinal (GI) surgery.

6 Preoperative optimization with nutritional support is indicated in patients who are malnourished or at risk of becoming malnourished.

7 The maintenance of an intact brush border and intercellular tight junctions prevents the movement of toxic substances into the intestinal circulation and minimizes bacterial translocation. These functions may be affected in critical illness. Enteral nutrition helps restore them.

8 Critically ill patients should receive early enteral nutrition within 48 hours of intensive care unit admission. Nutritional support should prioritize the provision of adequate protein.

9 Routine monitoring of gastric residual volumes is not recommended. Postpyloric feeding can be used for patients at high risk of regurgitation or for patients with gastric feeding intolerance.

10 Enteral nutrition is preferable to parenteral nutrition in the presence of a functioning GI tract. However, recent guidelines note no significant differences in clinical outcomes between enteral and parenteral nutrition. When early enteral is not feasible, parenteral is effective with similar outcomes.

Surgery has a significant impact on the body, causing the release of stress hormones and is associated with a considerable inflammatory response. Nutritional support is needed to prevent and treat the catabolic state induced by surgery. Patients undergoing gastrointestinal (GI) procedures with evidence of malnutrition at baseline are more likely to suffer postoperative morbidity and mortality and require longer hospital stays than their well-nourished counterparts. It has been shown that poor nutritional status can detrimentally affect postoperative outcomes, and in a consensus review of Enhanced Recovery After Surgery (ERAS), it was recommended that patients receive carbohydrate loading 24 hours preoperatively and nutritional supplements from the day of surgery until oral intake is achieved.

In addition to patients undergoing elective surgery, severe injury and critical illness are associated with a hypermetabolic catabolic state that can increase energy expenditure dramatically and complicate resuscitation and recovery of the critically ill or severely injured patients. Nutritional support is an integral part of caring for critically ill surgical patients, and the Society of Critical Care Medicine (SCCM), the American Society for Parenteral and Enteral Nutrition (ASPEN), and the European Society for Clinical Nutrition and Metabolism (ESPEN) have made recommendations toward providing early, aggressive nutritional support that enables patients to preserve their immune function, maintain lean body mass, and minimize metabolic complications. This chapter addresses the areas of nutritional assessment and management of the surgical patient, reviewing key metabolic principles and providing an overview of pertinent literature.

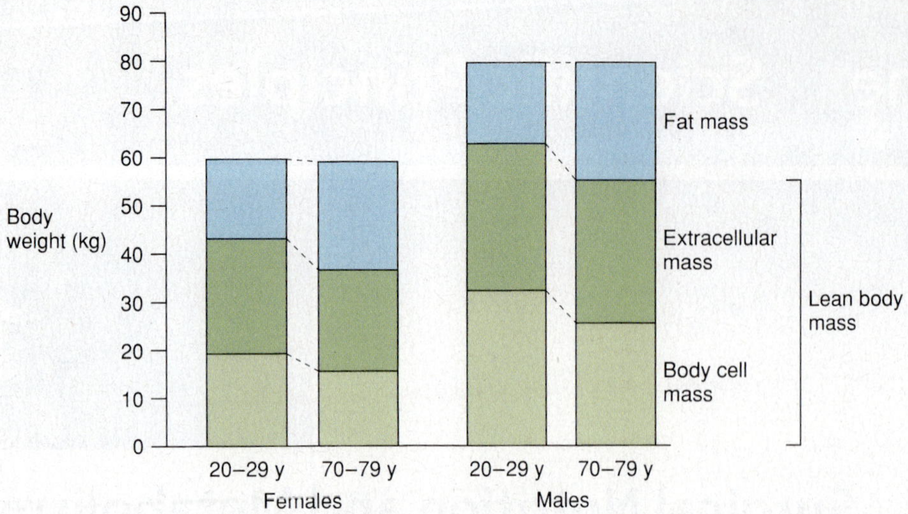

Figure 1.1. Body composition as a function of gender and age. (Data from Cohn SH, Vartsky D, Yasumura S, et al. Compartmental body composition based on total-body nitrogen, potassium, and calcium. *Am J Physiol-Endocrinol Metab*. 1980;239(6):E524–E530.)

BASIC METABOLIC PRINCIPLES

Body Composition

Total body mass is composed of aqueous and nonaqueous components, with the former constituting approximately 55% to 60% of total body mass (total body water [TBW]). Mineralized bone and adipose tissue make up the majority of the nonaqueous component. The relationship between total body mass and TBW is relatively constant for an individual and typically reflects the amount of body fat. Solid organs and muscles contain a higher proportion of water than bone and fat; therefore, young, lean males have a higher proportion of their total body mass as water than obese or elderly individuals. Obesity, older age, and female gender shift the body composition to a greater fat mass (**Fig. 1.1**).

The aqueous portion is divided into three functional fluid compartments: plasma (5% of body weight), interstitial or extracellular fluid (ECF; 15% of body weight), and intracellular fluid (ICF; 40% of body weight) (**Fig. 1.2**). In a typical 70-kg male, there are approximately 3.5 L of plasma, 10.5 L of interstitial fluid, and 28 L of intracellular volume while the remainder 28 kg represents the nonaqueous portion. The body cell mass constitutes the body's metabolic engine, while the extracellular component forms that supports the scaffolding for the body cell mass.

ENERGY AND SUBSTRATE METABOLISM

Measuring Energy Expenditure

In healthy individuals, total energy expenditure (TEE) reflects the activity of the fat-free mass (FFM), which primarily comprises organ systems that are highly metabolic, including the brain, heart, liver, and kidneys. More specifically, TEE is the combination of basal metabolic rate (BMR), physical activity, and thermogenesis secondary to nutritional intake. The measurement of energy expenditure (EE) poses a challenge for critically ill or surgical patients as this dynamic process changes over the course of the disease process and is often not accurately measured by predictive equations. TEE can be measured by direct calorimetry, which measures the total amount of heat produced by metabolic processes. However, direct calorimetry is expensive and not widely available. In contrast, indirect calorimetry (IC) is a more feasible option.

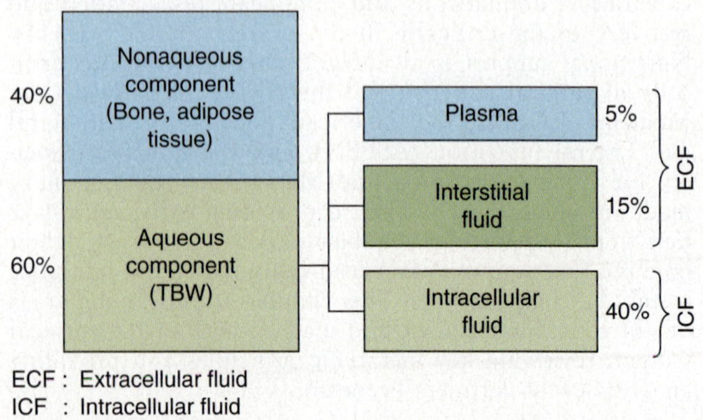

Figure 1.2. Aqueous and nonaqueous body composition.

Indirect Calorimetry

IC is the gold standard for accurately determining resting energy expenditure (REE) in critically ill patients, and its use has been linked to reduced mortality and improved clinical outcomes. By measuring oxygen consumption and carbon dioxide exhalation, IC calculates heat production and precisely assesses caloric needs. While historically hindered by bulky equipment and time-intensive calibration, advancements in modern IC devices now allow for more efficient and practical point-of-care testing. Accurate IC measurements require careful patient selection, particularly in intubated patients, where conditions such as stable hemodynamics, the absence of air leaks, and consistent ventilator settings are ideal. Newer IC machines are adaptable for both intubated and extubated patients, with guidelines recommending FiO_2 below 70%, positive end-expiratory pressure (PEEP) at or below 16 cm H_2O, and peak airway pressure at or below 30 cm H_2O for optimal accuracy. IC should be timed 4 hours before or after continuous renal replacement therapy (CRRT) and at least 4 hours after intermittent hemodialysis, with measurements delayed for 60 minutes following any procedures or medication adjustments. By adhering to these protocols, IC can provide precise and individualized caloric needs for critically ill patients.[1]

Energy Expenditure Fluctuates

EE in surgical and ICU patients fluctuates daily, complicated by injury and disease severity, nutritional status, and treatments, making caloric need predictions challenging.[2–5] Predictive formulas to calculate EE are inaccurate, and tissue injury accompanying major trauma further complicates estimating requirements.[2,4,5] Recent ICU nutrition guidelines recommend serial IC measurements, which may be the solution as it has been associated with improved clinical outcomes.[6–9]

Predictive Equations for Energy Expenditure

In most cases, EE is not measured but estimated based on all metabolic activities that occur within the FFM. There are >200 predictive equations developed for calculating EE that generally consider body weight, height, age, and gender. When applied to

Table 1.1. The Harris–Benedict Equation and Adjustment Using the Harris–Benedict Principle

Men	BMR = 88.362 + (13.397 × weight in kg) + (4.799 × height in cm) – (5.677 × age in years)
Women	BMR = 447.593 + (9.247 × weight in kg) + (3.098 × height in cm) – (4.330 × age in years)
Little to no exercise	Daily kilocalories needed = BMR × 1.2
Light exercise (1–3 d/wk)	Daily kilocalories needed = BMR × 1.375
Moderate exercise (3–5 d/wk)	Daily kilocalories needed = BMR × 1.55
Heavy exercise (6–7 d/wk)	Daily kilocalories needed = BMR × 1.725
Very heavy exercise (twice per day, extra heavy workouts)	Daily kilocalories needed = BMR × 1.9

Adapted from Roza AM, Shizgal HM. The Harris Benedict equation reevaluated: resting energy requirements and the body cell mass. *Am J Clin Nutr*. 1984;40(1):168–182.

critically ill or surgical patients, several equations will incorporate a stress factor to account for the increased metabolic state associated with illness or surgery. Several equations that predict basal EE and daily caloric requirements have been developed from the aforementioned variables, with the Harris–Benedict equation being among the most widely used (**Table 1.1**).

Nevertheless, studies indicate that predictive formulas used to calculate EE in ICU patients are accurate only 14% to 40% of the time, with an overall accuracy of 30% or less in acutely ill patients.[2,10–12] Additionally, the large tissue injuries further complicate and often render equations for estimating calorie and protein requirements inaccurate in surgical patients.[2,4,5]

Once the BMR has been calculated, minor adjustments based on exercise frequency and intensity can be made to estimate the daily caloric requirement for an adult to maintain current weight. The Mifflin–St. Jeor equation appears to be even more accurate in estimating BMR in healthy individuals.

$$\text{Men} \quad \text{BMR} = (10 \times \text{weight in kg}) + (6.25 \times \text{height in cm}) - (5 \times \text{age in years}) + 5$$

$$\text{Women} \quad \text{BMR} = (10 \times \text{weight in kg}) + (6.25 \times \text{height in cm}) - (5 \times \text{age in years}) - 161$$

The estimated BMR is adjusted upward for critically ill patients with highly inflammatory conditions. Not surprisingly, basal energy requirements increase significantly with an active inflammatory response but minimally after elective surgery. The largest increases in EE are seen in patients with severe polytrauma or major burns.[12] Based on expert consensus from SCCM and ASPEN, in the absence of IC, either a predictive equation should be used or critical ill patients should receive
1 25 to 30 kcal/kg/d.[5]

Predicting Caloric Need for Underweight and Obese Patients

IC is also the gold standard for estimating caloric needs in obese patients. When this is not available or feasible for critically ill obese patients, the Pennsylvania State University 2010 predictive equation is recommended with the Mifflin–St. Jeor equation as an alternative if the equation cannot be used.

Table 1.2. Fuel Reserves of a Healthy, 70-kg Adult Male

Energy Source	kg	kcal Value
Fat	14	125,000
Protein		
Skeletal muscle	6	24,000
Other	6	24,000
Glycogen		
Muscle	0.15	600
Liver	0.075	300
Free glucose	0.02	80

However, in general, predictive equations are less accurate for estimating the caloric needs of underweight and obese patients. Based on expert consensus, in the absence of IC, patients with body mass index (BMI) 30 to 50 should receive 11 to 14 kcal/kg (actual body weight)/d, and patients with BMI >50 should receive 22 to 25 kcal/kg (actual body weight)/d. For patients with a BMI of 30 to 40, 2.0 g/kg (ideal body weight)/d of protein should be provided, and patients with a BMI ≥40 should
2 be provided 2.5 g/kg (ideal body weight)/d of protein.

Body Fuels

Human metabolism is organized in such a way that fuel consumption occurs in a hierarchical way when more than one energy source is present, with excess stored for the postprandial or fasting period. In the postprandial state, the body contains fuel reserves that it can also mobilize in an orderly fashion as fasting is prolonged. The same fuel reserves are accessed during stress metabolism, although in a less orderly fashion (**Table 1.2**).

Fat is the body's largest energy reserve, providing 9 kcal/g when oxidized, with virtually limitless storage capacity. Protein is the second-largest energy store, yielding 4 kcal/g when oxidized. Unlike fat, protein serves both structural and functional roles, so severe protein loss can lead to significant functional impairments. During malnutrition, proteolysis releases amino acids for gluconeogenesis to produce glucose as fuel. Carbohydrate reserves, stored as glucose or glycogen in the liver, are minimal and can be depleted within 12 hours unless replenished, also yielding 4 kcal/g when used for energy (**Table 1.3**).

Carbohydrates

Carbohydrates are the primary fuel source for the human body, typically providing 45% to 60% of daily energy. Enteral carbohydrates yield about 4 kcal/g, while intravenous sources like dextrose offer slightly less at 3.4 kcal/g. Glucose, the main unit of carbohydrate metabolism, is derived from dietary carbohydrates through enzymatic processes starting in the oral cavity and continuing in the small intestine. Glucose absorption triggers insulin release, promoting anabolic activities like protein synthesis and glycogen storage. During stress, glucagon

Table 1.3. Energy Value of Various Energy Sources

Energy Source	Energy Value
Fat	9 kcal/g
Carbohydrates (enteral)	4 kcal/g
Carbohydrates (intravenous)	3.4 kcal/g
Protein	4 kcal/g

promotes the breakdown of glycogen, fat, and protein to meet heightened energy demands. Although carbohydrate digestion deficiencies are rare in surgical patients, those with conditions like celiac or Whipple disease may have impaired absorption. The central nervous system and blood cells rely on glucose, and during fasting, the body adapts by breaking down protein and converting fat into ketones. Stress further accelerates gluconeogenesis and glycogen breakdown, ensuring an abundant glucose supply for the body's inflammatory response.

Lipids

Lipids are the second most utilized energy source for the human body, contributing 35% to 45% of daily caloric intake, with each gram providing approximately 9 kcal. Upon entering the proximal small bowel, lipids trigger the release of cholecystokinin and secretin, prompting bile secretion from the gallbladder, essential for absorbing long-chain fatty acids, primarily in the distal ileum. Surgical resection of this area can lead to bile salt depletion and fat malabsorption. Lipids are classified by hydrocarbon chain length: short-chain fatty acids (2 to 5 carbons) fuel colonocytes and are absorbed in the colon; medium-chain fatty acids (6 to 9 carbons) are easier to digest, requiring no bile salts or lipase, and are absorbed directly into portal circulation; long-chain fatty acids (over 9 carbons), including essential linoleic and linolenic acids, need bile salts for emulsification, lipase for digestion, and micelles for transport, reaching the bloodstream via the lymphatic system. Insufficient intake of these essential fats can cause deficiency, preventable by ensuring they constitute 3% to 4% of daily calories. These fats are precursors to eicosanoids, crucial for the inflammatory response, and are stored as long-chain triglycerides due to their high-energy bonds.

Protein

Protein differs from carbohydrates and lipids by containing nitrogen, a critical structural component, with no inactive stores—only functional or structural proteins exist in the human body. Proteins, composed of amino acids, provide 4 kcal/g when used for energy. Dietary proteins are broken down into amino acids and peptides by gastric pepsin and pancreatic proteases, then absorbed mainly in the proximal GI tract. These amino acids are primarily sent to the liver for protein synthesis, with branched-chain amino acids (BCAAs) transported to muscles, and excess amino acids converted to glycogen or fatty acids. Intracellular proteins are also continuously recycled, with nitrogen excreted mainly through urine as urea. During amino acid metabolism, toxic ammonia is generated, transported safely to the viscera by glutamine and alanine, and converted to urea in the liver for excretion. Impaired kidney or liver function can lead to harmful ammonia accumulation, affecting the central nervous system.

Providing protein recommended for patients depends on 3
clinical conditions and comorbidities. SCCM and ASPEN recommend that critically ill patients receive 1.2 to 2.0 g/kg of protein per day, with burn patients and polytrauma patients having higher protein needs.

Vitamins

Vitamins A, D, E, and K are fat-soluble and absorbed in the small bowel with long-chain fatty acids. From there, they are transported to the liver (vitamins A and K) or the skin and subcutaneous tissue (vitamins D and E) for storage. Fat-soluble vitamins are required for normal immune function and play a significant role in wound healing. Daily vitamin A intake in patients on chronic corticosteroid regimens may counteract most of the steroid-mediated adverse effects of wound healing.

Vitamins B1 (thiamin), B2, B6, B12, vitamin C, niacin, folate, biotin, and pantothenic acid are water-soluble and absorbed in the proximal small bowel before being transferred to the liver for use or storage. These vitamins are essential for normal amino and nucleic acid metabolism. Deficiencies, particularly in vitamins B1, B9 (folate), and B12, can occur post-surgery. Thiamin is crucial for carbohydrate metabolism and gluconeogenesis, with deficiency often resulting from alcoholism, malabsorption (eg, after Roux-en-Y gastric bypass), decreased intake, or increased losses. Thiamin deficiency can lead to Wernicke encephalopathy, Wernicke–Korsakoff syndrome, and beriberi, which affect the central nervous system. Folate, vital for protein metabolism, can be deficient in individuals with alcoholism or poor nutritional intake, potentially leading to anemia and other complications. Folate supplementation is also critical during pregnancy to prevent neural tube defects due to increased demand for embryonic DNA synthesis.

Electrolytes and Trace Elements

Electrolytes, including sodium (Na^+), potassium (K^+), calcium (Ca^{2+}), magnesium (Mg^{2+}), and chloride (Cl^-), are critical for maintaining electrical and osmotic balance across plasma membranes. Sodium is the primary extracellular electrolyte, vital for volume homeostasis and blood pressure control, while potassium is a key intracellular cation involved in electrical conduction, muscular contraction, and biochemical reactions.

Trace elements, such as iron, iodine, zinc, chromium, copper, selenium, manganese, and molybdenum, are essential for various metabolic, immunologic, and healing functions. Iron is crucial for hemoglobin and mitochondrial function, with deficiencies leading to impaired cerebral, muscular, and immune system functions before anemia becomes apparent. Iodine is necessary for thyroid hormone production, and deficiencies can cause goiter and hypothyroidism. Zinc deficiency can lead to skin discoloration, neuritis, hair loss, and sensory alterations. Chromium deficiency, often seen with total parenteral nutrition (TPN), impairs glucose tolerance. Copper deficiency presents with microcytic anemia, abnormal skin keratinization, and, in severe cases, pancytopenia. Selenium deficiency, also common with prolonged TPN, can cause neuromuscular dysfunction and heart failure. Manganese deficiency manifests as weight loss, hair color changes, and hypolipidemia, while molybdenum deficiency is associated with hypomethioninemia, hypouricemia, and central nervous system dysfunction (**Table 1.4**).

NUTRITIONAL ASSESSMENT

Perioperative malnutrition is a key modifiable risk factor that independently predicts poor postoperative outcomes, including increased mortality, morbidity, length of stay, readmission rates, and hospital costs.[13,14] Thus, an accurate nutritional assessment is critical to identifying patients in need of nutritional support and determining the degree of nutritional support needed. Metabolism is altered to varying degrees by stress, namely, surgical injury, critical illness, infection, and physical trauma.

Subjective Global Assessment (SGA) is a commonly utilized tool for evaluating nutritional status in surgical patients, known for its reproducibility and correlation with clinical outcomes. SGA considers weight loss, nutritional intake changes, functional capacity, GI symptoms, and disease-related metabolic demands, coupled with a physical exam for edema, muscle wasting, and subcutaneous fat loss. Patients are classified as A (no malnutrition), B (moderate or indeterminate malnutrition), or C (severe malnutrition), though SGA provides limited insight into whether malnutrition is due to starvation or inflammation. Despite its widespread use, SGA may have limitations in critically ill patients, prompting ASPEN and SCCM to recommend alternative screening tools like the Nutritional Risk Screening (NRS 2002) and NUTrition Risk in the Critically Ill (NUTRIC) score. NRS 2002 evaluates hospital patients for malnutrition risk based on factors like weight loss, BMI, food intake, and disease severity, while the NUTRIC

Table 1.4. Summary of the Daily Requirements of Vitamins, Electrolytes, and Trace Elements in a Per Os Diet by Healthy Adults

Vitamins	
Retinol (vitamin A)	1000 mg
Thiamine (vitamin B_1)	1.4 mg
Riboflavin (vitamin B_2)	1.7 mg
Pyridoxine (vitamin B_6)	2.2 mg
Ascorbic acid (vitamin C)	60 mg
Niacin	20 mg
Folate	200 mg
Biotin	150 mg
Pantothenic acid	4–7 mg
Retinol (vitamin A)	1 mg
Vitamin D	5 mg
Vitamin E	10 mg
Vitamin K	75–150 mg
Electrolytes	
Sodium	90–150 mEq
Potassium	60–90 mEq
Calcium	1,300 mg
Magnesium	350 mg
Phosphorus	800 mg
Trace Elements	
Iron	10 mg
Iodine	150 mg
Zinc	15 mg
Chromium	5–200 mg
Copper	2–3 mg
Selenium	100 mg
Manganese	2.5–5 mg
Molybdenum	100–500 mg

score incorporates age, APACHE II and SOFA scores, comorbidities, and IL-6 levels, if available. The Global Leadership Initiative on Malnutrition (GLIM) introduced criteria in 2016 that are increasingly recognized globally. GLIM requires at least one phenotypic criterion (eg, nonvolitional weight loss, low BMI) and one etiologic criterion (eg, reduced food intake, inflammation) for diagnosing malnutrition. The GLIM criteria offer a comprehensive assessment, enhancing the ability to identify and treat malnutrition, particularly in patients with acute injuries or chronic illnesses. Subsequent studies have validated the GLIM criteria as a sensitive and specific tool for malnutrition assessment.

Anthropometric Measurements and Nutritional Indices

Anthropometric measurements have been used extensively to provide information regarding lean body mass, total fat stores, and overall nutritional health. Body composition studies aid in determining TBW, fat, and nitrogen. These anthropometric measurements can be easily performed at the bedside or in an ambulatory setting. They may include an individual's height and weight (which allows calculation of the BMI), triceps skinfold, mid-humeral circumference, and other body part summations. The BMI is widely used to measure overnutrition (a BMI of 25 to 29.9 suggests overweight status, whereas a BMI >30 defines obesity). The BMI is calculated from an individual's height and weight using the following formula:

$$\text{BMI} = \text{weight (kg)/height (m)}^2 = 703 * \text{weight (lb)/height (in)}^2$$

More advanced techniques and measurements include x-ray absorptiometry, which allows a more accurate assessment of total fat and lean body mass. Apart from the BMI, most anthropometric measurements are operator dependent, and skill and experience are essential to obtain accurate studies.

Sarcopenia

Sarcopenia is a condition characterized by a progressive loss of muscle mass, strength, and function in both obese and nonobese patients.[15] For hospitalized patients, sarcopenia is associated with increased length of stay and higher rates of complications, including urinary tract infections, wound infections, and reintubation. Despite the known risks associated with sarcopenia, the clinical diagnosis is often missed due to inadequate screening and failure to adhere to protocols.[16] Debate over a common definition of sarcopenia has hindered the development of standardized assessments and therapeutic interventions. Though sarcopenia is often described as a chronic disorder that afflicts the elderly, the condition can not only present acutely in patients but also begin as early as their 4th decade of life. However, the development of readily accessible, inexpensive, and objective techniques to aid in the clinical evaluation of sarcopenia has lagged behind interest in treating and managing the disease. Physical evaluations—such as grip strength, the 30-second sit-to-stand test, 4-m gait speed, and 6-minute walk distance—and screening and assessment tools like the Mini Nutritional Assessment are frequently used in the diagnosis of sarcopenia but are time intensive and require the patient's active participation, which may not be feasible in all clinical scenarios. In addition, radiologic tests, including computed tomography (CT), dual-energy x-ray absorptiometry (DXA), and ultrasound, are utilized for measurements of muscle mass.

Nutritional indices provide a means of risk stratification, objectively comparing individuals, and guiding nutritional support. The BMI is one of the most commonly utilized nutritional indices. It provides information on normal, overweight, or obese status and on the degree of protein–calorie malnutrition in underweight individuals.

Serum Protein Levels

An ideal biochemical marker of malnutrition would be highly sensitive and specific to nutrition intake. Although a single laboratory biomarker that could effectively describe a patient's nutritional status is lacking, numerous freely circulating serum 4 transport proteins have been used. The most commonly utilized ones are albumin, prealbumin, transferrin, and retinol-binding protein (RBP), each with its advantages and disadvantages. Many nutrition-unrelated parameters, most commonly inflammation, dilution secondary to large-volume resuscitation, and chronic liver failure, affect the levels of these serum markers. Although it is customary for markers of inflammation, usually the C-reactive protein, to be measured with biomarkers including prealbumin, limited data exist to support this practice.

Albumin

Albumin is a serum protein synthesized in the liver with a long half-life (approximately 20 days) and a relatively large total pool size. Only 5% of total body albumin is produced daily. Its main function is to carry molecules in the bloodstream and to help maintain intravascular oncotic pressure. Due to its large pool, long half-life, and relative slow turnover, it has been used as an indirect marker of protein intake, hepatic synthetic ability, and chronic nutritional status. Unfortunately, it is a negative acute-phase reactant, decreasing during the acute-phase response, and numerous nutrition-unrelated factors may affect its levels in either direction (**Tables 1.3 to 1.5**). Albumin is neither a sensitive nor specific marker for malnutrition, as patients with even severe starvation can have normal levels. In critical care, hypoalbuminemia more commonly reflects illness acuity, especially during the acute phase, due to its function as a negative acute-phase reactant, its redistribution to the interstitial space, and dilution secondary to large-volume resuscitation.

Prealbumin

Prealbumin, also known as transthyretin, is a visceral protein primarily synthesized by the liver and, to a lesser extent, by the choroid plexus in the central nervous system. Prealbumin's primary function is to transport thyroxin (T4) and retinol (vitamin A) in the bloodstream. Like albumin, prealbumin is a small component of the total body protein pool and is influenced by many of the same factors that affect serum albumin. However, prealbumin has a shorter half-life (2 to 3 days), making it more responsive to acute changes in nutrient intake. It is a negative acute-phase reactant, meaning its levels decrease during the acute inflammatory response. Therefore, rising prealbumin levels may indicate an improvement in nutritional status or the resolution of inflammation. Prealbumin is often measured alongside C-reactive protein, with low prealbumin and high C-reactive protein levels typically seen in inflammatory conditions rather than malnutrition.

Retinol-Binding Protein

The majority of RBP is present in the bloodstream in the form of retinol-circulating complex that includes prealbumin, retinol (vitamin A), and RBP. It is catabolized in the kidneys, and its levels may be elevated in end-stage renal failure. RBP is dependent on vitamin A and zinc, as low levels of these conutrients inhibit mobilization of RBP in the liver. To some extent, measuring the RBP provides the same information as measuring prealbumin. RBP is less commonly used as a marker of nutrition, as it has a short half-life (approximately 12 hours), levels are affected by renal failure, and the measurement assay is more costly.

Transferrin

Transferrin, has also been identified and used as a nutrition biomarker. It has a half-life between that of albumin and prealbumin (8 to 10 days) and plays a key role in iron transport, its levels are affected by iron status. Iron deficiency may lead to increased levels secondary to greater iron absorption. Under these circumstances, it may be a better marker of total iron-binding capacity, rather than malnutrition.

Nitrogen Balance

Nitrogen balance is a key marker for evaluating overall nutritional status, particularly in patients receiving nutritional support. It reflects whether protein intake and catabolism are balanced and is often assessed alongside trends in prealbumin levels. Nitrogen balance is calculated by subtracting the nitrogen excreted (primarily through urine) from the nitrogen intake over 24 hours. Intake is estimated by dividing total protein intake by 6.25, while output is typically measured as urine urea nitrogen (UUN), with additional adjustments to account for unmeasured losses. A nitrogen balance of −2 to +2 g/d indicates equilibrium and is generally the target in nutritional support. More negative balances suggest the need for increased protein intake, while more positive balances, although often indicative of anabolism in recovering patients, can also result from measurement errors in acutely ill patients. However, nitrogen balance assessment has limitations, including false-negative results in overfed patients, delayed re-equilibration after nutritional adjustments, and inaccuracies in patients with renal insufficiency or upper GI bleeding.

$$\text{Nitrogen balance (g/day)} = \text{Protein intake}/6.25 - (\text{TUN} + 2)$$

$$\text{Nitrogen balance (g/day)} = \text{Protein intake}/6.25 - (\text{UUN} + 2 + 3)$$

OVERFEEDING AND MALNUTRITION

Overfeeding

While adequate caloric intake is necessary to maintain weight and promote health, overprovision of calories can lead to overfeeding and obesity. Excess calories, especially as carbohydrates, can lead to increased CO_2 production (which may prolong ventilatory weaning), hyperglycemia (which can contribute to immunosuppression and increase the risk for infectious complications), lipogenesis (indicated by a respiratory

Table 1.5. Serum Proteins Used in Nutritional Status Assessment

Marker	Reference Range	Half-Life	Elevated in	Decreased in
Albumin	3–5 g/dL	14–20 d	Dehydration, marasmus, blood transfusions, and exogenous albumin administration	Aggressive resuscitation, ascites, eclampsia, liver failure, inflammatory states, nephrotic syndrome, protein-losing states, burns, trauma/postoperative states, kwashiorkor, cancer, collagen diseases, corticosteroid use, chronic bed rest, zinc deficiency, and pregnancy
Prealbumin	18–45 mg/dL	2–3 d	End-stage renal failure, corticosteroid use, and oral contraceptives	Postoperative states, hepatitis, liver failure, inflammatory states, dialysis, hyperthyroidism, pregnancy, and severe hyperglycemia
Retinol-binding protein	4–6 mg/dL	12 h	End-stage renal failure, diabetes, obesity, vitamin A overdose, corticosteroid use, and oral contraceptives	Postoperative states, hepatitis, liver failure, inflammatory states, and vitamin A deficiency
Transferrin	200–250 mg/dL	8–10 d	Iron deficiency, dehydration, pregnancy (third trimester), oral contraceptives, estrogens, chronic anemia, hepatitis, liver failure, hypoxia, and end-stage renal failure	Pernicious anemia, anemia of chronic disease, folate-deficiency anemia, aggressive resuscitation, chronic infectious states, iron overload, acute catabolic states, uremia, nephrotic syndrome, liver failure, kwashiorkor, old age, zinc deficiency, corticosteroids, and cancer

Adapted from Parrish CR. Serum proteins as markers of nutrition: what are we treating? *Pract Gastroenterol.* 2006;43(10):48–64.

quotient [RQ] > 1), and hepatic steatosis (which can interfere with normal liver function). Additionally, excessive nutritional support may lead to mineral or vitamin poisoning and severe electrolyte imbalances, with hypophosphatemia being the most common. To avoid overfeeding, specifically in critically ill patients with numerous active medical conditions, IC may be indicated to accurately estimate EE during the various stages of the disease.

Malnutrition

Starvation

During short fasting periods, insulin levels drop while glucagon levels rise, leading to glycogen breakdown in the liver to release glucose, typically depleting liver glycogen stores within 24 hours. Once carbohydrate stores are exhausted, the body relies on protein and fat degradation to meet caloric needs. Starvation downregulates insulin, causing muscle wasting as proteins break down to release amino acids like alanine and glutamine, which are then used for gluconeogenesis in the liver. The resulting glucose primarily supports the central nervous and hemopoietic systems. Gluconeogenesis requires energy, supplied by the oxidation of free fatty acids, which are released from triglycerides through hormone-sensitive lipase activation in fatty tissue, triggered by low insulin and high glucagon levels. Additionally, the body recycles energy sources through mechanisms like the Cori cycle, while BCAAs are secreted by the liver to provide energy for skeletal and cardiac muscles. Despite these adaptations, prolonged gluconeogenesis leads to significant lean body mass loss, potentially reaching fatal levels after around 4 weeks. After 7 to 10 days of starvation, the brain adapts to using ketones from fat as its primary energy source, leading to a decrease in BMR by up to 30%, and a slowdown in energy-intensive functions such as voluntary muscle activity and cardiac function.

Starvation versus Inflammation as the Cause of Malnutrition

Both starvation and the systemic inflammatory response result in lean body mass loss, which should indicate nutritional support. However, the two processes have key dissimilarities that differentiate one from the other. Starvation leads to progressive loss of both lean mass and body fat, preservation of serum
5 protein levels, and reversal of the metabolic response with feeding. The most common causes of starvation in surgical patients are functional and include nausea and emesis, ileus, dysphagia, and malabsorption. On the other hand, during a significant inflammatory response, the BMR increases significantly (both anabolism and catabolism) and becomes relatively insensitive to feeding, and levels of acute-phase proteins change. Inflammation may additionally worsen malnutrition by interfering with caloric intake acutely (anorexia of acute illness) or in the chronic state (cancer cachexia, **Table 1.6**).

Substrate Metabolism Changes during Stress

During the neuroendocrine response to stress, metabolism of commonly used nutritional substrates undergoes significant changes.

Altered Carbohydrate Metabolism

Hyperglycemia occurs commonly after injury, and its intensity generally reflects the severity of the stressor. During the ebb phase, insulin levels are low and glucose production is only minimally elevated. During the flow phase, hepatic gluconeogenesis occurs at a faster pace from peripheral tissue–released precursors and hyperglycemia persists, while insulin levels are normal or elevated. This phenomenon suggests relative insulin resistance.

Altered Protein Metabolism

After a major injury, nitrogen losses increase. These correlate to the extent of trauma and the injury victim's preexisting nutritional status. In patients not receiving nutrition, protein

Table 1.6. Metabolic Differences between the Response to Simple Starvation and Stress

	Simple Starvation	Stress/ Inflammation
Basal metabolic rate	–	++
Presence of mediators	–	+++
Major fuel oxidized	Fat	Mixed
Ketone body production	+++	±
Hepatic ureagenesis	+	+++
Negative nitrogen balance	+	+++
Gluconeogenesis	+	+++
Muscle proteolysis	+	+++
Hepatic protein synthesis	+	+++

breakdown exceeds synthesis, resulting in a negative balance. Providing exogenous calories is important to maintain a neutral nitrogen balance. Skeletal muscle is the chief source of the nitrogen lost in urine following extensive injury, and it appears that amino acid release from muscle is heavily skewed toward glucogenetic precursors (alanine and glutamine), even though these comprise less than 5% of muscle total protein.

In addition to skeletal muscle, the kidneys and the GI tract release alanine, which may be used for glucogenetic purposes, even though the majority enters metabolic pathways that favor the production of urea and ammonia to be excreted from the body.

Altered Lipid Metabolism

To support the increased metabolic rates after injury or elective surgery, triglycerides are released from adipose tissue for energy production. Glucose administration minimally affects this lipolysis, which appears to result from continuous neuroendocrine stimulation. Although mobilization and oxidation of free fatty acids are accelerated in injured subjects, ketone synthesis is minimal and occurs independently of protein catabolism. When severely injured patients remain unfed, their fat and protein stores become depleted rapidly, and the resultant malnutrition increases their susceptibility to infectious complications, multiple-organ system failure, sepsis, and ultimately death.

Stressor-Dependent Adjustments to the Metabolic Response

Response to Elective Surgery and Accidental Injury

One of the earliest consequences of major surgery is the rise in levels of circulating cortisol in response to a sudden release of adrenocorticotropic hormone (ACTH) from the anterior pituitary gland. This cortisol remains elevated for 24 to 48 hours after operation. Cortisol has generalized effects on tissue catabolism and mobilizes amino acids from skeletal muscle that provide substrates for wound healing and serve as precursors for the hepatic synthesis of acute-phase proteins or new glucose, as delineated earlier (**Fig. 1.3**). Associated with the activation of the adrenal cortex is stimulation of the adrenal medulla through the sympathetic nervous system, with release of epinephrine and norepinephrine. These circulating neurotransmitters play an important role not only in increasing vascular tone, which may be lessened from circulating cytokines, but also in promoting amino acid release from skeletal muscle, lipolysis in adipose tissue, and gluconeogenesis in the liver.

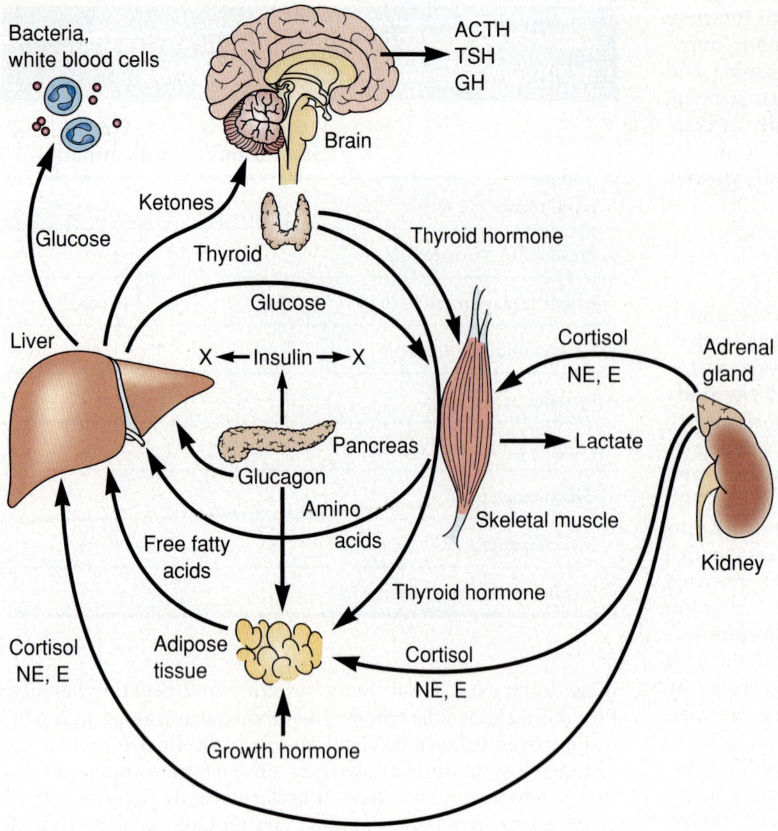

Figure 1.3. During sepsis, metabolism shifts to greater glucose synthesis and utilization, likely mirroring the greater metabolic needs of the pathogens and the mobilized host white blood cells.

The neuroendocrine response to surgical trauma alters mechanisms regulating salt and water excretion, leading to antidiuretic hormone (ADH) and aldosterone secretion, which promote water and sodium reabsorption in the renal tubules. This often results in weight gain from salt and water retention postsurgery, with edema occurring in surgical wounds due to local cytokine-induced increased vascular permeability. This edema typically resolves as the inflammatory response subsides, and diuresis begins 2 to 3 days postoperatively. Additionally, postoperative periods see increased glucagon release and decreased insulin levels, driven by heightened sympathetic activity. The adrenergic–corticoid phase, lasting 1 to 3 days, is marked by catabolism and may worsen with inadequate caloric intake. This is followed by the adrenergic–corticoid withdrawal phase and eventually an anabolic phase, which usually begins 3 to 6 days after major surgery, characterized by positive nitrogen balance and weight gain as protein synthesis and muscle strength return.

Whether controlled in surgery or accidental, the body's response to tissue trauma shares similarities but differs in magnitude. Accidental injuries occur in uncontrolled, contaminated environments, often leading to substantial and life-threatening volume loss, heightened pain, and a significant sympathetic response. In contrast, elective surgeries are performed in clean, controlled settings with measures to manage hydration, anxiety, and pain, resulting in a more moderate and generally better-tolerated physiologic response (**Table 1.7**).

Metabolic Adaptations to Sepsis

The metabolic changes following invasive infection are not dissimilar to those seen after elective surgery and accidental

Table 1.7. Differences between Elective Surgery and Accidental Injury

Insult	Elective Surgery	Accidental Injury
Tissue damage	Minimal and controlled, usually occurring in a clean environment; tissues are dissected with care along anatomic planes and reapproximated	Can be substantial; tissues torn in contaminated field. Debridement often necessary
Hypotension	Uncommon. Pre- and intraoperative hydration employed and volume status carefully monitored intraoperatively	May occur with significant blood loss and lead to shock. Fluid resuscitation often delayed
Pain, fear, and anxiety	Typically attenuated with perioperative analgesics and anxiolytics	Generally present in the first hours after trauma
Infectious complications	Relatively rare. Procedures take place in a sterile field, and preoperative administration of antibiotics is commonplace	More common due to contamination and tissue devitalization
Overall stress response	Controlled and of lesser magnitude. Starvation better tolerated	Controlled and proportional to the magnitude of the injury. Malnutrition poorly tolerated

trauma, although they are typically less predictable. Severe infection is characterized by fever, hypermetabolism, diminished protein economy, altered glucose dynamics, and accelerated lipolysis, much like the injured patient. Anorexia that commonly follows systemic infection is an added factor contributing to the loss of lean body mass.

Hypermetabolism and increased oxygen consumption are additional traits, with the latter reaching peak levels that may be 50% to 60% higher than baseline in severe sepsis. A portion of this metabolic acceleration can be attributed to the escalation in enzymatic reaction rates associated with fever. The BMR is estimated to rise by 10% to 13% for every 1 °C rise in central temperature. Glucose metabolism is increased to much greater levels in systemically infected subjects than in trauma victims. As an example, burn patients synthesize glucose at a rate approximately 50% above normal. If superinfection ensues, hepatic glucose production doubles and the additional glucose requirements appear to correlate with the bacterial burden and white blood cell activation (**Fig. 1.3**).

Increased proteolysis and nitrogen excretion leading to negative nitrogen balance, typically occur following invasive infection in a pattern that is similar to that described for injury. Visceral amino acid uptake is accelerated during sepsis, and this is matched by faster amino acid efflux from skeletal muscle. In infected burn patients, splanchnic amino acid uptake is amplified >50% above rates in uninfected burn victims with comparable injuries. These amino acids serve either as glucose precursors or as building blocks for acute-phase protein synthesis.

Fat is another major fuel utilized for energy in infected patients. Increased fat catabolism is particularly profound in patients during inadequate nutritional support or relative starvation periods. Among other reasons, lipolysis is accelerated by heightened sympathetic activity, and serum triglyceride levels reflect the balance between synthesis in the liver and storage in the peripheral adipose tissue. Marked hypertriglyceridemia has been associated with certain gram-negative infections, but frequently, triglyceride concentrations are normal or low, indicating enhanced utilization and clearance by other organs. Infected patients cannot convert fatty acids to ketones as efficiently in the liver, and do not adapt to starvation, as well as their fasted, unstressed counterparts. It is postulated that the low ketone state of infection is a consequence of hyperinsulinemia, which in turn follows insulin resistance in high-degree catabolic states.

Trace elements and electrolytes (zinc, iron, potassium, magnesium, and inorganic phosphate) typically follow alterations in nitrogen balance. Although the iron-binding capacity of transferrin typically remains unchanged in early infection, free iron cannot be found in the plasma of patients with severe pyrogenic infections. Similar changes are seen in zinc levels. These decreases cannot be totally accounted for by total body losses; rather, an accumulation of these elements appears to occur in the liver through not yet elucidated mechanisms. Unlike iron and zinc, serum copper levels generally rise, seemingly due to greater ceruloplasmin synthesis in the liver. Moreover, commonly observed in sepsis, most patients on CRRT exhibit micronutrient deficiencies.[17] This highlights the importance for clinicians to monitor serum copper, carnitine, and vitamin B6 deficiencies in this population.

Metabolic Response to Cancer and Acquired Immunodeficiency Syndrome

Patients with cancer and acquired immunodeficiency syndrome (AIDS) have similar metabolic states, characterized by chronic malnutrition, typically a result of anorexia and treatment side effects, and prolonged low-grade inflammatory changes. Cancers of the aerodigestive tract interfere with taste, swallowing, and/or digestion, precluding adequate caloric and/or protein intake. Supplementation with zinc and B vitamins may help taste-related symptoms, and soft mechanical diets may allow greater caloric intake in patients with swallowing difficulties or proximal GI tract malignancies. The aggressive management of nausea and vomiting may also afford greater interest in food.

Cancer- and AIDS-related cachexia is seen in the later stages of disseminated disease and represents a chronic catabolic state due to unrelenting inflammation that is difficult to reverse, even with adequate caloric and protein supplementation. Proinflammatory cytokines (TNF, IL-1, and IL-6) are constantly released in response to the tumor or an infectious source in AIDS, respectively, and lead to a chronic state of muscle wasting and fat loss. The cachexia of cancer and AIDS is difficult to manage, as removing the inflammatory stimulus can prove elusive. However, mitigation of the chronic, low-grade inflammatory response may be useful, as can aggressive early nutritional supplementation and appetite stimulants.

Age and Gender

Certain patterns in the metabolic response to surgical pathology that occur with aging can be attributed to alterations in body composition. Although weight remains roughly stable, fat mass tends to increase with age while lean body mass tends to decline. The loss of strength that accompanies immobility, starvation, and acute surgical illness may have significant consequences. Although the increased energy requirements after elective surgery occur essentially independent of age, the capacity of muscle to serve as a source of amino acids may be limited during acute surgical illness in the elderly, and muscle strength may rapidly become inadequate for respiratory function.

Older age is often associated with reduced muscle mass and an increased prevalence of cardiovascular and pulmonary diseases. The combination of decreased arterial compliance, lower baroreceptor sensitivity, and a blunted response to catecholamine surges can impair cardiovascular homeostasis during acute surgical illness, potentially leading to inadequate tissue oxygenation when demand is heightened.[18,19] Malnutrition exacerbates these issues by causing immune dysfunction, impaired wound healing, loss of muscle mass and strength, and other complications that prolong hospital stays and diminish quality of life. Studies have demonstrated that older adult trauma patients with malnutrition experience worse surgical outcomes, including higher mortality rates, more frequent complications, and longer hospital stays.[20,21] Consequently, personalized nutritional interventions aimed at treating malnutrition hold promise for improving recovery outcomes.[22]

Gender, in addition to age, may affect the body's ability to adapt to surgical stress. Observed differences in the metabolic response between men and women in general reflect differences in body composition. Lean body mass, as a proportion of total body weight, is lower in women than in men. This difference is thought to account for the lower net loss of nitrogen after major elective abdominal surgery in women. Women, in general, have approximately half the skeletal muscle mass of men of the same age. Therefore, young muscular men experience the greatest nitrogen losses during acute surgical illness, as opposed to elderly, sedentary women.

NUTRITIONAL SUPPORT

Nutritional Support in Elective Surgery

Perioperative nutrition is important for any patient undergoing an elective surgical procedure. Malnutrition and underfeeding are risk factors for perioperative complications. **Table 1.8** highlights the key aspects of perioperative care per the ESPEN. Patients undergoing major elective surgical procedures, particularly for cancers, should undergo nutritional screening as they are being prepared for surgery.

Most patients undergoing elective noncancer surgeries are adequately nourished and typically fast only for a few hours

Table 1.8. Key Aspects of Perioperative Care

- Integration of nutrition into the overall management of the patient
- Avoidance of long periods of preoperative fasting
- Reestablishment of oral feeding as early as possible after surgery
- Start of nutritional therapy early, as soon as a nutritional risk becomes apparent
- Metabolic control, eg, of blood glucose
- Reduction of factors that exacerbate stress-related catabolism or impair gastrointestinal function
- Minimized time on paralytic agents for ventilator management in the postoperative period
- Early mobilization to facilitate protein synthesis and muscle function

From Weimann A, Braga M, Carli F, et al. ESPEN guideline: clinical nutrition in surgery. *Clin Nutr.* 2017;36(3):623–650.

before the procedure. The outdated practice of making all patients NPO after midnight is no longer recommended, with most patients able to consume clear liquids up to 2 hours before anesthesia. Preoperative intake of carbohydrate-based liquids (CHO-loading) has been shown to reduce postoperative insulin resistance and hospital stay duration. Early oral intake after elective procedures is generally preferred and may help reduce the risk of postoperative ileus. Studies support the safety of resuming oral or enteral feeding early after GI surgery, particularly within 24 hours for major head, neck, or intestinal cancer surgeries. ERAS protocols, which include nutritional assessment and early postoperative enteral nutrition (EN), have become the standard of care in many surgical disciplines globally.

Preoperative malnutrition is a well-established risk factor for complications following elective surgery. Various definitions and diagnostic criteria exist, with one proposed criterion being a BMI < 18.5 kg/m² or a combination of weight loss >10% or >5% over 3 months, along with a reduced BMI or low fat-free mass index (FFMI). For patients identified as malnourished or those at high risk for delayed postoperative nutrition initiation, preoperative nutritional support may be
6 necessary. Standard high-protein feeding formulas are typically sufficient for most surgical patients, with the choice of product and volume tailored based on nutrition assessments. Most tube-feeding formulas are rich in water-soluble dietary fiber, a standard component of nutritional care in surgical patients. Adjustments can be made for specific conditions, such as cardiac or renal failure, or diabetes. Preoperative supplementation with balanced macronutrient and high-protein formulas is recommended for patients presenting for elective surgery who meet malnutrition criteria. This support should begin as early as possible, with a minimum of 2 to 4 weeks required to derive any benefit.

Nutritional Support in Critical Care

While resuscitation, bleeding control, and preservation of the vital body functions, such as maintenance of gas exchange and supporting of adequate cardiac output, remain immediate priorities for survival in any critically ill surgical patient, it is increasingly recognized that nutritional support is an integral part of the metabolic care of the critically ill, and aggressive pursuit of target energy requirements is associated with optimal wound healing, recovery, and rehabilitation (**Fig. 1.4**). Critically ill patients who are typically quite catabolic often have anorexia that can be adaptive or maladaptive and may be unable to be fed by mouth volitionally for extended periods. Severe malnutrition can complicate the hospital course and adversely affect outcomes. Numerous studies have demonstrated the association between energy deficit in critical illness and longer ICU stays, greater incidence of infectious complications, and even

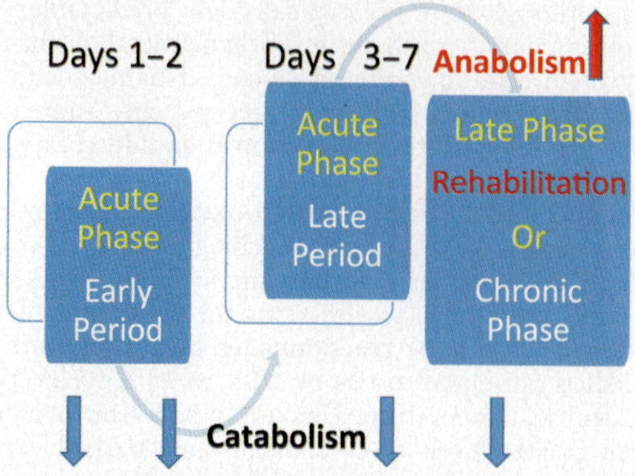

Figure 1.4. Description of the acute and late phases following infection/stress/injury. After injury, the acute phase is composed of an early period and a late period. Then the postacute phase can progress to convalescence and rehabilitation or chronicity and prolonged inflammatory and catabolic syndrome (PICS). (From Martindale RG, McClave SA, Vanek VW, et al. Guidelines for the provision and assessment of nutrition support therapy in the adult critically ill patient: Society of Critical Care Medicine and American Society for Parenteral and Enteral Nutrition: executive summary. *Crit Care Med.* 2009;37:1757–1761.)

mortality. The management of nutritional support in critically ill patients is largely guided by the ESPEN guideline on clinical nutrition in the ICU and the Guidelines for the Provision and Assessment of Nutrition Support Therapy in the Adult Critically Ill Patient from SCCM and ASPEN. **Table 1.9** summarizes the recommendations for nutritional support in critically ill patients from SCCM and ASPEN.

7 Upon admission to the ICU, some assessment of nutritional risk should be performed. The finding that enteral nutrients exert a trophic effect on the cellular integrity and function of the gut mucosa has provided the rationale for initiating enteral feedings early in the course of critical illness. In fact, evidence from multiple studies supports that critically ill patients who were fed earlier had better overall outcomes.

Table 1.9. Bundle Statements from the Society of Critical Care Medicine and American Society for Parenteral and Enteral Nutrition's Guidelines for the Provision and Assessment of Nutrition Support Therapy in the Adult Critically Ill Patient

- Assess patients on admission to the intensive care unit (ICU) for nutrition risk and calculate both energy and protein requirements to determine goals of nutrition therapy.
- Initiate enteral nutrition (EN) within 24–48 h following the onset of critical illness and admission to the ICU, and increase to goals over the first week of ICU stay.
- Take steps as needed to reduce risk of aspiration or improve tolerance to gastric feeding (use prokinetic agent, continuous infusion, chlorhexidine mouthwash, elevate the head of bed, and divert level of feeding in the gastrointestinal tract).
- Implement enteral feeding protocols with institution-specific strategies to promote delivery of EN.
- Do not use gastric residual volumes as part of routine care to monitor ICU patients receiving EN.
- Start parenteral nutrition early when EN is not feasible or sufficient in high-risk or poorly nourished patients.

From McClave SA, Taylor BE, Martindale RG, et al. Guidelines for the provision and assessment of nutrition support therapy in the adult critically ill patient: Society of Critical Care Medicine (SCCM) and American Society for Parenteral and Enteral Nutrition (A.S.P.E.N.). *JPEN J Parenter Enteral Nutr.* 2016;40(2):159–211.

Current recommendations are that critically ill patients
8 receive EN within 48 hours of ICU admission. Despite early enthusiasm for postpyloric feeds, it is now recognized that most patients can be fed safely into the stomach. If that fails, converting to postpyloric feeding via a nasojejunal tube is recommended. Routine monitoring of gastric residual volumes is no longer recommended. Interruptions in enteral feeding should be minimized to prevent inadequate nutrient delivery.

There is ongoing discussion in the literature regarding the optimal quantity and quality of nutritional support for critically ill patients. Current guidelines emphasize a comprehensive approach that considers the route, timing, and content of nutrition provided. The appropriate calorie intake via EN remains uncertain. A meta-analysis of randomized controlled trials comparing initial underfeeding to full feeding in acutely critically ill patients found no significant difference in overall mortality between the groups. However, a subgroup analysis indicated that patients who received more than one-third of their caloric requirements had significantly lower mortality. A recent multicenter, double-blind, randomized trial comparing energy-dense and routine EN also failed to demonstrate a mortality benefit with the use of an energy-dense formulation. There is increasing recognition that adequate protein provision may be more critical than achieving caloric goals via carbohydrate substrates. Current recommendations suggest providing 1.2 to 2.0 g/kg of actual body weight per day of protein, with potentially higher requirements in patients with burns or polytrauma. One universally accepted guideline is the avoidance of overfeeding, which should be a priority during the early phase of critical illness.

Another frequently asked question is whether it is safe to enterally feed patients who are requiring hemodynamic support with vasopressors. One randomized trial comparing EN to parenteral nutrition (PN) in patients requiring vasoactives did not demonstrate a reduction in mortality or the risk of secondary infections, but an increased risk of GI complications in enterally fed patients, including intestinal ischemia.

For years, PN was considered far inferior to EN. TPN has recently been shown to be safe in four recent randomized controlled trials. These trials show there is no association between early TPN use at ICU admission and risk of infection versus EN as had previously been hypothesized to exist. These data supporting the safety of early TPN use are thought to be due to better glucose control, improved focus on preventing central line infections, new lipid formulations, and other improvements in supportive care that have become ubiquitous.

The ESPEN and ASPEN/SCCM guidelines endorse using enteral over PN when possible. In patients who are severely mal-
7 nourished and cannot tolerate EN, preoperative PN is associated with fewer complications than in patients who were not provided with nutritional supplementation. In critically ill patients, if PN is to be used, the timing of when to initiate it is controversial. Current recommendations are for patients at high nutritional risk to have PN initiated as soon as possible.[5] For patients at low nutritional risk, currently ESPEN recommends starting PN after 2 days if patients aren't meeting their targeted EN, whereas ASPEN advises waiting until day 7. The most recent RCT in 2022 suggests supplemental PN is associated with reduced infections in patients undergoing abdominal surgery.[23]

Parenteral Nutrition Considerations

One significant downside of PN is the concern of disuse of gut enterocytes, which may exacerbate intestinal microflora translocation from the gut lumen to the mesenteric lymph circulation, worsening total bacterial load and stress, as well as cause a loss of gut mucosal immunity. Due to the high osmolarity of its content, PN must be delivered centrally to minimize the risk of venous sclerosis. Patients on PN therapy should be monitored regularly by measuring blood sugar, serum electrolytes, and liver function tests, as abnormalities in these laboratories are common. PN–related complications can be broadly categorized in **Table 1.10**.

Table 1.10. TPN-Related Complications

Complication	Etiology
Access-Related	
Pneumothorax	Air accumulation between the pleural leaflets from puncture/laceration
Carotid/Subclavian arterial injury	Accidental puncture of the adjacent arterial structure
Catheter malposition and arrhythmias	Tip of catheter may find its way into an unintended venous structure or the right atrium, causing arrhythmogenesis
Venous thrombosis	Thrombus formation in a major vein, due to alterations in blood flow and the presence of a foreign body
Metabolic	
Hyperglycemia	Excessive carbohydrate administration, glucose intolerance, or a combination of the two
Hypoglycemia	Sudden cessation of TPN, while insulin stimulation has not subsided
CO_2 retention	Carbohydrate calories in excess of energy requirements
Azotemia	Excessive protein administration with inadequate calories
Essential fatty acid deficiency	Inadequate essential fatty acid administration
Hypertriglyceridemia	Rapid fat infusion or decreased fat clearance
Hypophosphatemia and hypokalemia	Sudden full-strength nutritional restitution in a starved patient (refeeding syndrome)
Any electrolyte abnormality	Excess or inadequate electrolyte supplementation
Hemorrhagic diathesis	Vitamin K deficiency
Infectious	
Skin site cellulitis	Skin flora enters the subdermal/subcutaneous space
Pneumonia, other systemic infectious	High n-6 fatty acid content adversely affects immune function

Hyperglycemia

Hyperglycemia is common in surgical patients. Hyperglycemia is a well-recognized side effect of PN. Current guidelines recommend a target blood glucose range of 140 or 150 to 180 mg/dL. Most hyperglycemia can generally be controlled with subcutaneous or intravenous insulin administration if mild or moderate. Insulin can be added to PN once the daily insulin requirements have been calculated. It has been shown that stressed individuals can maximally oxidize up to 4 to 5 mg of glucose/kg/min. For a 70-kg man, this is equal to approximately 400 to 500 g/d (1600 to 2000 kcal/d). Therefore, it is common for patients to receive up to two-thirds of their daily caloric needs in carbohydrate form through PN. Excess glucose can result in hyperglycemia and glycosuria, and can be converted to fat and deposited in the liver. Glycosuria, with its osmotic load, can lead to osmotic diuresis, which can be misinterpreted as a sign of adequate resuscitation status or transition to the recovery phase, while the patient may be clinically worsening.

Fats

Fat is an important fuel for the critically ill, as stressed patients preferentially utilize endogenous fat as an energy source. Unlike traditional starvation, fat oxidation is only minimally affected by carbohydrate administration during stress, and glucose infusion above certain levels may lead to hepatic steatosis.

SCIENTIFIC PRINCIPLES

Lipid emulsions in PN serve as artificial chylomicrons, enabling the delivery of essential fatty acids and energy by bypassing normal digestive processes.[24] The inclusion of lipids in PN provides essential linoleic acid, inhibits lipogenesis from carbohydrates, and helps lower the RQ, which may benefit patients with CO_2 retention.

Fatty acids in lipids, classified by saturation, carbon length, and double bond location, play crucial roles in cell function and influence clinical outcomes in critically ill patients. Lipids also include emulsifiers, phytosterols, and alpha-tocopherols, which help reduce adverse effects like cholestasis and oxidative stress.[25] While Lipids are essential for nonprotein nutrition and modulating immune function, their formulation is controversial.[26,27] Soybean oil-based lipids, rich in omega-6 fatty acids, have been linked to increased inflammation, elevated liver enzymes, and higher infection risks in long-term PN users due to proinflammatory metabolite production.[25,28–33] Conversely, omega-3 fatty acids, found in fish oils, are associated with anti-inflammatory effects. Moreover, alternative lipid formulations combining soy, medium-chain triglycerides olive, and fish oils have been shown to reduce inflammation, improve antioxidant profiles, decrease cholestasis, and improve clinical outcomes compared to traditional soybean-based lipids.[34,35] Lower inflammatory lipid emulsions are recommended for daily use and should be initiated at the start of TPN therapy if other lipid-containing medications, such as propofol, are not being administered. These findings underscore the importance of optimizing lipid composition in PN to enhance surgical patient outcomes.

Electrolytes

The amounts of the various electrolytes provided to patients receiving PN vary, depending on volume status and preexisting electrolyte abnormalities. Careful monitoring of serum electrolyte levels is critical, especially during the acute phase of disease or in severely malnourished individuals, because as metabolism switches to the anabolic phase, potassium and phosphate can move rapidly into the intracellular compartment, leading to potentially fatal electrolyte abnormalities from refeeding syndrome. Vitamin and trace mineral levels, although not as life-threatening, should be monitored as well. The composition of a standard PN solution is shown in **Table 1.11**.

Table 1.11. Composition of a Standard Total Parenteral Nutrition Formulation

Volume		
10% Amino acid solution		500 mL
50% Dextrose solution		500 mL
Fat emulsion		—
Electrolytes + vitamins + minerals		~50 mL
Total volume		~1050 mL
Composition		
Amino acids		50 g
Dextrose		250 g
Total N		50/6.25 = 8 g
Dextrose kcal		250 g × 3.4 kcal/g = 840 kcal
mOsm/L		~2000
	Usual Concentration	**Range of Concentrations**
Electrolytes to Total Parenteral Nutrition Solutions		
Sodium (mEq/L)	60	0–150
Potassium (mEq/L)	40	0–80
Acetate (mEq/L)	50	50–150
Chloride (mEq/L)	50	0–150
Phosphate (mEq/L)	15	0–30
Calcium (mEq/L)[a]	4.5	0–20
Magnesium (mEq/L)	5	5–15

[a]Generally added as calcium gluconate or calcium chloride: one ampule of calcium gluconate = 1 g of calcium = 4.5 mEq.

Enteral Nutrition Considerations

EN is less expensive than PN and should be started early, within 48 hours, as previously discussed. The GI tract can be used for the administration of complex nutrients that cannot be provided as readily intravenously, such as polypeptides and fiber. Gut processing of many of these nutrients stimulates hepatic protein synthesis, while intravenous administration bypasses the portal circulation altogether. In addition to the systemic benefits of EN, enteral feedings afford significant local benefits to the gut mucosa itself. Enterocytes are being fed directly, and the absorptive surface of the mucosa is stimulated and maintained. Luminal nutrients, such as glutamine and short-chain fatty acids, fuel small bowel enterocytes and colonocytes, respectively. The trophic effects of luminal nutrition are well documented, even if small amounts of enteral feedings are provided; evidence suggests that earlier EN is preferable. An additional immunologic benefit of EN is that complex polypeptides and long-chain fatty acids stimulate the production of gut-derived immunoglobulin A, which is important in maintaining the mucosal immunity barrier. Luminal nutrients also help maintain a normal pH and flora, thus diminishing the risk of opportunistic bacterial overgrowth in the bowel.

Gastrointestinal Function

Although EN is generally the preferred method for nutritional support in malnourished patients or patients at risk for developing malnutrition, an intact and well-functioning GI tract is required. Postoperative ileus is frequent, reflects functional immobility of the GI tract, and is typically proportional to the amount of manipulation the bowel sustained during the surgical intervention. Contraindications to enteral feedings are usually relative or temporary and include short, obstructed, or perforated bowel, a GI tract in discontinuity, protracted vomiting, fistulas, or active GI ischemia. ESPEN and the European Society of Intensive Care Medicine endorse contraindications to EN and suggest withholding EN in critically ill patients with uncontrolled shock, uncontrolled hypoxemia and acidosis, uncontrolled upper GI bleeding, gastric aspirate >500 mL/6 h, bowel ischemia, bowel obstruction, abdominal compartment syndrome, and high-output fistula without distal feeding access. The ASPEN/SCCM recommendations are similar.

Complications of Enteral Nutrition

Despite the numerous benefits of EN, it is not completely free of complications. These can be categorized into access-related, functional, and metabolic and are summarized in **Table 1.12**. In general, these can be avoided with meticulous care while inserting and maintaining feeding tubes, considering using nasal bridles, ensuring head-of-bed elevation to minimize the risk of aspiration, using motility agents when gastric motility is suboptimal, closely monitoring patients' metabolic profile and adjusting content, or adding bulking agents if osmotic diarrhea develops.

Enteral Feeding Formulations

Enteral feedings are generally categorized into intact or polymeric, hydrolyzed or monomeric, or modular. With the intact or polymeric formulations, protein, carbohydrate, and lipid molecules exist in an unaltered form. Hydrolyzed or monomeric formulations contain predigested proteins, simple sugars, and medium-chain triglycerides. Modular feeds typically contain one type of fuel, carbohydrate, lipids, or fat, and can be combined to address each patient's specific needs. Despite previous enthusiasm for specialty feeds for a variety of disease states, current recommendations are for standard polymeric enteral

Table 1.12. Enteral Nutrition–Related Complications

Complication	Etiology
Access-Related	
Feeding tube malposition, clogging, and accidental removal	The feeding tube can be misplaced in the tracheobronchial tree; it can become clogged with dense tube feedings or inadequately crushed medications, or be accidentally removed
Oro/nasogastric or enteral tube perforation of the proximal gastrointestinal tract or tracheobronchial tree	Accidental puncture of the wall of the structure the feeding tube in placed into
Pressure ulcers at skin entry site and sinusitis	A foreign body is continuously pressing against healthy skin and increases risk of bacterial colonization of the nasal passages
Functional	
Nausea, vomiting, and abdominal distension	Usually due to delayed gastric emptying
Diarrhea	Usually polyfactorial, but high protein content and high osmolarity of enteral feedings are the most common culprits
Metabolic	
Electrolyte abnormalities	When enteral nutrition content is inadequate to cover daily needs. Hyperosmolarity may be a consequence when calorically dense enteral feedings are administered
Volume overload	From excess sodium and water loading, typically in patients with preexisting heart failure
Hyperglycemia	Less common than in patients receiving TPN but may manifest in patients with diabetes or impaired glucose tolerance or can herald sepsis

feeding formulas for medical patients. Postoperative surgical patients and patients with traumatic brain injury may benefit from immunomodulating enteral formulations, although the quality of evidence is low. Some of the most commonly used enteric feeding formulas and their metabolic characteristics are shown in **Table 1.13**.

Macro- and Micronutrient Selection

Protein

An additional topic of debate is whether the selection of specific macro- and micronutrients included in nutritional formulas, be it enteral or parenteral, can afford specific benefits to patients receiving them, depending on the underlying pathology. Gluconeogenesis from amino acids (glutamine and alanine) released from muscle protein breakdown cannot be fully suppressed with exogenous glucose and insulin administration due to the complex hormonal stress response the human body elicits during critical illness, which results in relative insulin resistance. It was postulated, therefore, that exogenous amino acid and oligopeptide infusion would help minimize lean body mass erosion. Therefore, the optimal protein to total energy ratio in critical illness was previously unknown. More recent studies in critically ill populations suggest that the provision of protein is more closely linked to the outcome than the provision of total energy in the form of carbohydrates and fats. In addition, the dose of protein required by critically ill patients appears to be higher than previously thought. At least two studies have demonstrated better outcomes when high-protein targets were met.

Glutamine

Glutamine, the most abundant nonessential amino acid, is primarily released through skeletal muscle proteolysis and plays a crucial role in hepatic gluconeogenesis during stress. Low glutamine levels are linked to poor outcomes in critical illness, result from muscle wasting, and are vital for immune cells, enterocytes, and hepatocytes. While early studies suggested glutamine supplementation might reduce infectious complications, hospital stays, and mortality, recent high-quality trials indicate that aggressive supplementation may increase mortality in patients with organ failure. Routine glutamine supplementation is not recommended but may be beneficial in cases of severe depletion or intestinal mucosa damage from chemo- or radiation therapy. Similarly, although arginine supplementation may lower infection risk and shorten hospital stays, there is no supporting evidence for its use during critical illness.

Micronutrients

Micronutrients consisting of electrolytes, vitamins, and trace elements are administered in critical illness to prevent deficiencies and associated complications. With repletion of micronutrient stores after starvation, refeeding syndrome can occur. Refeeding syndrome is associated with the reintroduction of feeding after a period of caloric deprivation and is characterized by hypophosphatemia. This can be life-threatening and present with lactic acidosis, cardiac arrhythmias, worsening respiratory failure, and even heart failure. Therefore, routine administration of physiologic doses of micronutrients during critical illness is warranted. Provision of therapeutic doses of trace elements (selenium, copper, zinc, and iron) and vitamins (E, C, and beta-carotene) with antioxidant activity has also been proposed; however, a recent randomized controlled trial failed to demonstrate a benefit. Selenium supplementation may also be beneficial in subjects with selenium deficiency, and the potential benefit is supported by a recent meta-analysis.

Nutritional Access

Parenteral Nutrition Access

Parenteral solutions are administered through a central venous catheter, generally inserted in the subclavian or internal jugular vein, or through peripherally inserted central catheters (PICCs) that are typically inserted via veins of the antecubital fossa with the tip in the atriocaval junction. Current recommendations are to choose the smallest device possible with the fewest number of lumens and always reserve one lumen to be dedicated to the PN administration. Peripheral parenteral nutrition (PPN) can be infused through peripheral venous cannulas. Peripheral intravenous feedings may be used for infusion of protein, lipid, and lower-concentration dextrose solutions. PPN is limited in caloric delivery due to the large volumes needed to meet daily demands, but it avoids central venous cannulation. It can be considered for short-term PN, for example, in the case of postoperative patients with ileus, which is expected to resolve in a few days.

Enteral Nutrition Access

In the acute phase of surgical illness, enteral feeding is commonly administered through oral or nasal enteric feeding tubes, which can be placed either in the stomach (gastric) or beyond the pylorus into the duodenum or proximal jejunum (postpyloric). Gastric feeding offers advantages such as providing a reservoir for bolus feedings, stimulating the biliary and pancreatic axis, and reducing the risk of diarrhea due to

Table 1.13. Commonly Used Enteral Nutrition Formulations

Product Name	Calories (per mL)	Protein (g/L)	Carbohydrates (g/L)	Fat (g/L)	Fiber (g/L)	Osmolality (mOsm/L)	Special Features
Tube Feeding Formulations							
Osmolite 1 Cal	1.06	44	144	35	0	300	Isotonic
Jevity 1.2 Cal	1.2	56	169	39	18	450	High protein with fiber
Jevity 1.5 Cal	1.5	64	50	50	22	525	Concentrated calories with fiber
Promote with Fiber	1	63	138	28	14	380	Very high protein with fiber
Nepro with Carb Steady	1.8	81	161	96	13	745	Renal formula
TwoCal HN	2	84	219	91	5	725	Calorie and protein dense
Vital AF 1.2 Cal	1.2	75	111	54	5	425	Peptide-based elemental with high protein
Vital high protein	1	88	112	23	0	353	Peptide-based elemental with high protein
Pivot 1.5 Cal	1.5	94	172	51	7.5	595	Immune support
Vivonex RTF	1	50	176	12	0	630	Elemental (amino acids)

Product Name	Calories	Protein (g)	Carbohydrates (g)	Fat (g)	Fiber (g)	% Water	Special Features
Oral Supplements[a]							
Ensure Plus (per 8 fl)	350	13	51	11	3	76	High calorie and high protein
Glucerna Shake (per 8 fl)	220	10	26	9	3	84	Diabetic formula
Ensure Clear (per 6.8 fl)	200	7	43	0	0	84	Clear liquid
Juven (per 24 g)	80	14 (amino acids)	8	0	0	n/a	Helps build lean body mass to support healing
Pro-Stat Sugar free (per 30 mL)	100	15	10	0	0	n/a	Protein
Nutrisource fiber (per 4 g)	15	0	4	0	3	n/a	Fiber

[a]Per amount noted in product name column.
Adapted from Boston University Medical Center's Nutrition Formulary, 2014.

the dilutional effect of gastric secretions on tube feeding osmolarity. However, it also poses a risk of aspiration, particularly in patients with altered mental status or those on neuromuscular blockade. In cases of gastric feeding intolerance, prokinetic agents are the first line of treatment, and if intolerance persists, the feeding tube may need to be advanced to a postpyloric
9 position. Nasoduodenal or nasojejunal tubes, although smaller and more comfortable for patients, are more prone to clogging, and their placement should be confirmed radiographically before feeding begins.

For patients requiring longer-term EN, especially those with chronically impaired mental status, dysphagia, or oropharyngeal or proximal GI tract pathology, transabdominal GI access is often necessary. This is traditionally provided through a Stamm gastrostomy, where a laparotomy incision is made to access the gastric lumen, and a feeding tube is secured in place.

Increasingly, these procedures are performed laparoscopically for a less invasive approach. Alternatively, percutaneous endoscopic gastrostomy (PEG) tubes can be inserted without the need for a laparotomy or general anesthesia, making them suitable for bedside insertion under endoscopic guidance. PEG placement involves transillumination of the gastric wall, followed by inserting and securing the feeding tube through a small abdominal incision.

In cases where prolonged small bowel feeding is anticipated, such as after major abdominal surgery, feeding jejunostomies may be considered. This involves elevating a loop of proximal small bowel, typically 20 to 40 cm distal to the ligament of Treitz, and securing it to the abdominal wall for direct feeding access. Jejunostomies can be performed laparoscopically or through a minimally invasive approach. Additionally, dual-lumen transgastric jejunal feeding tubes can be used, offering the benefits of small bowel feeding with the lower morbidity associated with gastrostomy. These tubes pass through percutaneously placed gastrostomy tubes, providing a versatile option for patients requiring both gastric and jejunal feeding access.

NUTRITIONAL CONSIDERATIONS IN SPECIAL POPULATIONS

Sepsis and Septic Shock

In the setting of severe inflammation and fever, such as that occurs with sepsis, the BMR increases. Total energy requirements need to be assessed, increasing energy requirements by 20% to 30% for mild or moderate infection and approximately 50% above basal levels in severe infection. Many of the recommendations about nutritional support in the setting of sepsis have been previously discussed. Based on expert consensus, the ASPEN/ESPEN/SCCM guidelines suggest that critically ill patients receive EN and, if not possible, parental nutrition within 24 to 48 hours as soon as the patient is hemodynamically stable. Initiation of EN while the patient is still in shock may aggravate impaired splanchnic perfusion. The NUTRIREA-2 study demonstrated an increase in GI complications when patients on vasoactive agents were fed enterally early in the course of septic shock. Provision of goal calories does not need to be achieved, but provision of goal protein has demonstrated benefit. Supplemental PN or PN alone is not recommended early in the course of sepsis and septic shock, but should be instituted if EN is not feasible once the patient is hemodynamically stable.

Acute Respiratory Failure

A common complication in surgical patients is respiratory failure requiring prolonged mechanical ventilation. The primary concern in these patients is ensuring adequate gas exchange, specifically the transport of oxygen and CO_2 across the capillary–alveolar membrane. Often, the need for ventilatory support arises from a pulmonary infection, which, combined with a postoperative state, contributes to hypermetabolism. This hypermetabolic state increases oxygen consumption, leading to greater CO_2 production as more substrate is oxidized to meet elevated energy demands. While nutritional support may take a backseat in mechanically ventilated patients, where the focus is on managing the underlying cause of respiratory insufficiency, it is important to consider the composition of nutritional support, as it can impact the weaning process, especially in those with chronic CO_2 retention. Although there was initial enthusiasm for enteral formulas high in fat and low in carbohydrates to reduce CO_2 production, this approach only reduces CO_2 in overfed patients. In cases of fluid overload, fluid restriction with energy-dense enteral feeds may be appropriate.

Acute Renal Failure

Renal failure affects the body's ability to clear the by-products of protein metabolism but does not change the catabolic rate or protein requirements. Therefore, a careful balance needs to be achieved between the need for protein and to limit uremia. When acute surgical stress is superimposed, consideration for potentially earlier or more aggressive renal support should be given so that the body is not restricted of protein, which is critical during the hypermetabolic phase of acute disease. Based on expert consensus, patients with acute renal failure should be placed on a standard enteral formulation, energy (25 to 30 kcal/kg/d) provision, with standard recommendations for protein (1.2 to 2 g/kg actual body weight per day). Only if significant electrolyte abnormalities develop a specialty formulation designed for renal failure should be utilized. In patients on renal replacement therapy, patients should receive increased protein, up to a maximum of 2.5 g/kg/d, and micronutrients monitored. Protein should not be restricted in patients with acute renal failure to avoid or delay initiating renal replacement therapy.

Acute Liver Failure

Patients with liver disease are often chronically malnourished, typically presenting with protein depletion yet an intolerance to protein due to the risk of encephalopathy with high nitrogen intake. Liver damage and portosystemic shunting can lead to imbalances in circulating amino acids, with an increased plasma ratio of aromatic to BCAAs. This imbalance favors the transport of aromatic amino acids across the blood–brain barrier, where they act as precursors for neurotransmitters that exacerbate encephalopathy and lethargy. Historically, protein restriction was employed to mitigate hepatic encephalopathy, but this approach can worsen nutritional status, decrease lean muscle mass, and paradoxically reduce ammonia elimination. Consequently, protein should not be restricted to manage hepatic encephalopathy. Additionally, solutions enriched in BCAAs and deficient in aromatic amino acids have not demonstrated significant benefits in patients receiving lactose and luminal-acting antibiotics treatment.

Complications of Gastrointestinal Surgery

After GI surgery, whether elective or emergent, complications such as anastomotic leaks and enteroatmospheric or enterocutaneous fistulae can complicate nutritional management. In critically ill patients with surgical complications after abdominal or esophageal surgery who are unable to eat orally, EN, rather than PN, should be utilized unless the patient is in discontinuity, has obstruction of the GI tract, or has abdominal compartment syndrome. GI cutaneous or GI atmospheric fistulas with high output (commonly defined as having output >400 mL/24 h) represent a classic indication for long-term PN. Oral intake in patients with such fistulas typically results in greater output, especially in fistulas involving the proximal GI tract, which can lead to dehydration and significant metabolic disturbances and adversely affect the ability of the fistula to heal. In the case of an unrepaired anastomotic leak or fistula, feeding access distal to the defect should be the goal to allow for EN. If distal feeding access is not achieved, PN is appropriate. PN has been shown to increase the spontaneous rate of closure of enterocutaneous fistulas by improving overall nutritional status in the host or improving perioperative outcomes in those requiring surgical therapy. Somatostatin and analogs have been used to aid with fistulous output and spontaneous closure with varying results. In patients treated via a damage control laparotomy approach or with an open abdomen, early EN is recommended if there is intestinal continuity. Additional protein supplementation may be appropriate due to the high protein loss of the exudate.

Burns

Burn victims often suffer from prolonged ileus, which encumbers enteral nutritional support. Even if the bowel is usable and patients are not on mechanical ventilation, they are frequently unable to consume adequate calories due to anorexia of severe injury, and extreme catabolism. Based on expert consensus, early (within 4 to 6 hours of injury) EN should be administered to all

burn patients to meet estimated energy needs. PN should only be reserved for those patients for whom EN is not feasible or not
10 tolerated. EN has been associated with fewer infections and improved survival when compared with PN. Patients with burns should also be provided protein in the range of 1.5 to 2 g/kg/d. IC is recommended to assess energy needs in burn patients with routine repeated measures.

Acute Pancreatitis

Mild pancreatitis is defined by the absence of organ failure and local complications, while moderate to severe acute pancreatitis is defined by transient organ failure. Differentiating patients with severe acute pancreatitis from those with mild severity helps identify those patients who will require early provision of nutrition therapy. ASPEN/SCCM recommends that the initial nutrition assessment in acute pancreatitis evaluates disease severity to guide nutritional therapy and that frequent reevaluation is performed. Patients with moderate to severe acute pancreatitis should have a nasal or oral enteric tube placed and EN with a standard polymeric formulation initiated at a low rate and advanced to goal as fluid volume resuscitation is completed. This is based on studies that have demonstrated benefits from early EN. PN should be initiated when EN is not tolerated.[36] Probiotics may be beneficial in patients with acute pancreatitis.

Trauma

Trauma patients have a high risk of developing septic complications and multiple organ failure. Early EN has been shown to reduce septic complications and organ failure rates when initiated within 24 hours. Both ASPEN/SCCM and ESPEN recommend early enteral feeding with a high-protein polymeric formulation in the immediate posttrauma once the patient is hemodynamically stable. Immunomodulating formulae may be considered in severely injured patients. For patients with traumatic brain injury, early feeding is associated with decreased infection rates and better outcomes.

Solid Organ Transplant

Malnutrition is a major factor influencing outcomes after transplantation. Candidates for solid organ transplantation should have regular assessments of their nutritional status, and if they meet criteria for malnutrition, oral nutritional supplements or even tube feeding is advised. Since there is often a long preoperative waiting period, there is time to try to replete patients nutritionally. In addition to malnutrition, obesity remains a significant metabolic risk factor for the outcome of patients undergoing organ transplantation. Despite some suggestions of the benefit of immunomodulating formulas in the literature, a consistent benefit has not been demonstrated. After solid organ transplantation, early intake, either orally or via a feeding tube, within 24 hours is recommended. No strong recommendations are made for the use of probiotics, PN, or omega-3 fatty acid provision. Long-term nutritional monitoring and counseling are recommended.

Bariatric Surgery

Bariatric patients pose a special challenge, as they are at an increased risk for several macro- (usually protein) and micronutrient deficiencies (most commonly vitamins D and B_{12}, calcium, iron, folic acid, zinc, and selenium). Nutritional support of the obese or postweight loss surgery patient is particularly complex because of the balance needed between minimizing overfeeding and avoiding the hypercatabolic state. There is widespread consensus that early oral nutrition after bariatric surgery is appropriate. Clinical practice guidelines recommend a preoperative assessment, including screening for malnutrition and deficiency in vitamins and trace elements. Early postoperative EN is advocated and protein supplementation to meet daily requirements of 60 g of protein per day. Standard oral supplements should be avoided in bariatric patients as they can cause dumping syndrome. Postoperative nutritional follow-up by a dedicated team is essential to monitor weight loss and prevent deficiencies of micronutrients. ERAS principles have been applied and appear to be beneficial in bariatric surgery. In case of a major complication requiring reoperation, recommendations are no different from those for patients undergoing any major abdominal surgery. Despite the excessive fat stores, critically ill postoperative bariatric patients should receive early and timely nutrition, as protein–calorie malnutrition does occur. Consideration for IC, which allows accurate estimation of the caloric requirements, is appropriate, and early involvement of a nutritionist is essential.

Geriatrics

Attention to appropriate nutritional support of the geriatric or frail patient is of paramount importance, both in the perioperative stage and in the ICU, given the multiple physiologic alterations seen in both frailty and older age. These alterations include greater fat to muscle mass ratio, decreased cardiac and pulmonary reserves, poor dentition, polypharmacy, and a high incidence of malnutrition. Malnutrition rates may be as high as 85% in nursing home residents. Compared to younger cohorts, elderly patients are more likely to have comorbid disease processes affecting their general nutritional status, including diabetes, cancers, cardiac, pulmonary, and renal insufficiency. Given that a certain degree of lean body mass loss is to be expected in this demographic, a higher protein intake (>1.5 g/kg/d) should be the goal preoperatively in the elderly undergoing elective surgery or early in the recovery phase after emergency procedure or acute surgical illness. As soon as they can tolerate an oral diet, all older adults should be prescribed high-protein supplements following surgery and not placed on clear liquid diets. Data shows that early oral nutrition supplements alone postoperatively improve the length of stay, but patients rarely receive them.

Obesity

Overweight and obese patients have become more prevalent in ICUs as the prevalence of obesity increases in the general population. Generally, an isocaloric high-protein diet can be administered to obese patients, preferentially guided by IC measurements and urinary nitrogen losses. Other common metabolic derangements include decreased glucose tolerance, altered lipid metabolism, lack of micronutrients, and decreased gut motility. Recommendations for early EN apply similarly to overweight and obese patients as to other critically ill and postoperative patients. High-protein hypocaloric feeding should be implemented to preserve lean muscle mass whenever feasible.

ACKNOWLEDGMENTS

We gratefully acknowledge the contributions of previous edition authors, Melissa H. Coleman and Deborah M. Stein, as portions of those chapters have been retained in this revision.

References

1. Wischmeyer PE, Molinger J, Haines K. Point-counterpoint: indirect calorimetry is essential for optimal nutrition therapy in the intensive care unit. *Nutr Clin Pract*. 2021;36(2):275–281.
2. Oshima T, Berger MM, De Waele E, et al. Indirect calorimetry in nutritional therapy. A position paper by the ICALIC study group. *Clin Nutr*. 2017;36(3):651–662.
3. Wischmeyer PE. Nutrition therapy in sepsis. *Crit Care Clin*. 2018;34(1):107–125.
4. Fraipont V, Preiser JC. Energy estimation and measurement in critically ill patients. *JPEN J Parenter Enteral Nutr*. 2013;37(6): 705–713.
5. Guttormsen AB, Pichard C. Determining energy requirements in the ICU. *Curr Opin Clin Nutr Metab Care*. 2014;17(2):171–176.
6. Singer P, Blaser AR, Berger MM, et al. ESPEN guideline on clinical nutrition in the intensive care unit. *Clin Nutr*. 2019;38(1):48–79.
7. McClave SA, Taylor BE, Martindale RG, et al. Guidelines for the provision and assessment of nutrition support therapy in the adult critically ill patient: Society of Critical Care Medicine (SCCM)

and American Society for Parenteral and Enteral Nutrition (A.S.P.E.N.). *JPEN J Parenter Enteral Nutr*. 2016;40(2):159–211.
8. Heidegger CP, Berger MM, Graf S, et al. Optimisation of energy provision with supplemental parenteral nutrition in critically ill patients: a randomised controlled clinical trial. *Lancet*. 2013;381(9864):385–393.
9. McClave SA, Martindale RG, Rice TW, Heyland DK. Feeding the critically ill patient. *Crit Care Med*. 2014;42(12):2600–2610.
10. Moonen HP, Hermans AJ, Bos AE, et al. Resting energy expenditure measured by indirect calorimetry in mechanically ventilated patients during ICU stay and post-ICU hospitalization: a prospective observational study. *J Crit Care*. 2023;78:154361.
11. Whittle J, Molinger J, MacLeod D, et al. Persistent hypermetabolism and longitudinal energy expenditure in critically ill patients with COVID-19. *Crit Care*. 2020;24(1):581.
12. Niederer LE, Miller H, Haines KL, et al. Prolonged progressive hypermetabolism during COVID-19 hospitalization undetected by common predictive energy equations. *Clin Nutr ESPEN*. 2021;45:341–350.
13. Vaid S, Bell T, Grim R, Ahuja V. Predicting risk of death in general surgery patients on the basis of preoperative variables using American College of Surgeons National Surgical Quality Improvement Program data. *Perm J*. 2012;16(4):10.
14. Martindale RG, McClave SA, Taylor B, Lawson CM. Perioperative nutrition: what is the current landscape? *JPEN J Parenter Enteral Nutr*. 2013;37:5S–20S.
15. Marzetti E, Calvani R, Tosato M, et al. Sarcopenia: an overview. *Aging Clin Exp Res*. 2017;29:11–17.
16. Guralnik JM, Cawthon PM, Bhasin S, et al. Limited physician knowledge of sarcopenia: a survey. *J Am Geriatr Soc*. 2023;71(5):1595–1602.
17. Fah M, Van Althuis LE, Ohnuma T, et al. Micronutrient deficiencies in critically ill patients receiving continuous renal replacement therapy. *Clin Nutr ESPEN*. 2022;50:247–254.
18. Spencer G. Projections of the Population of the United States, by Age, Sex, and Race: 1983 to 2080. *Current population reports*. 1984.
19. Mather M, Pollard K, Jacobsen LA. Reports America. Washington, DC: *Population Reference Bureau*. 2009:1–15.
20. Havens JM, Columbus AB, Seshadri AJ, et al. Malnutrition at intensive care unit admission predicts mortality in emergency general surgery patients. *JPEN J Parenter Enteral Nutr*. 2018;42(1):156–163.
21. Haines KL, Lao W, Nguyen BP, et al. Evaluation of malnutrition via modified GLIM criteria for in patients undergoing emergent gastrointestinal surgery. *Clin Nutr*. 2021;40(3):1367–1375.
22. Wischmeyer PE, Bear DE, Berger MM, et al. Personalized nutrition therapy in critical care: 10 expert recommendations. *Crit Care*. 2023;27(1):261.
23. Gao X, Liu Y, Zhang L, et al. Effect of early vs late supplemental parenteral nutrition in patients undergoing abdominal surgery: a randomized clinical trial. *JAMA Surg*. 2022;157(5):384–393.
24. Singer P. Advances in medical nutrition therapy: parenteral nutrition. *Nutrients*. 2020;12(3):717.
25. Raman M, Almutairdi A, Mulesa L, Alberda C, Beattie C, Gramlich L. Parenteral nutrition and lipids. *Nutrients*. 2017;9(4):388.
26. Berlana D. Parenteral Nutrition Overview. *Nutrients*. 2022;14(21):4480.
27. Boullata JI, Mirtallo JM, Sacks GS, et al. Parenteral nutrition compatibility and stability: a comprehensive review. *JPEN J Parenter Enteral Nutr*. 2022;46(2):273–299.
28. Calder PC, Jensen GL, Koletzko BV, Singer P, Wanten GJ. Lipid emulsions in parenteral nutrition of intensive care patients: current thinking and future directions. *Intensive Care Med*. 2010;36:735–749.
29. Calder PC. Rationale and use of n-3 fatty acids in artificial nutrition. *Proc Nutr Soc*. 2010;69(4):565–573.
30. Hayes BD, Gosselin S, Calello DP, et al. Systematic review of clinical adverse events reported after acute intravenous lipid emulsion administration. *Clin Toxicol (Phila)*. 2016;54(5):365–404.
31. Fischer GW, Hunter KW, Wilson SR, Mease AD. Diminished bacterial defences with intralipid. *Lancet*. 1980;2(8199):819–820.
32. Waitzberg DL, Bellinati-Pires R, Salgado MM, et al. Effect of total parenteral nutrition with different lipid emulsions of human monocyte and neutrophil functions. *Nutrition*. 1997;13(2):128–132.
33. Furukawa K, Yamamori H, Takagi K, et al. Influences of soybean oil emulsion on stress response and cell-mediated immune function in moderately or severely stressed patients. *Nutrition*. 2002;18(3):235–240.
34. Haines KL, Ohnuma T, Trujillo C, et al. Hospital change to mixed lipid emulsion from soybean oil-based lipid emulsion for parenteral nutrition in hospitalized and critically ill adults improves outcomes: a pre-post-comparative study. *Crit Care*. 2022;26(1):317.
35. Haines KL, Ohnuma T, Hornik CD, et al. Change to Mixed-Lipid Emulsion From Soybean Oil-Based Lipid Emulsion in Pediatric Patients. *JAMA Netw Open*. 2023;6(9):e2332389.
36. Wu P, Li L, Sun W. Efficacy comparisons of enteral nutrition and parenteral nutrition in patients with severe acute pancreatitis: a meta-analysis from randomized controlled trials. *Biosci Rep*. 2018;38(6):BSR20181515.

2

The Pathogenesis of Obesity and Metabolic Disease

Robert W. O'Rourke

Key Points

1 Obesity is a polygenic phenomenon; up to 70% of the propensity to obesity is due to genetic influences.

2 Epigenetics and environment interact with genetics to produce the obesity phenotype.

3 Control of food intake via satiety and hunger is a dominant mechanism of body weight regulation, but multiple other processes contribute.

4 The hypothalamic feeding center is a dominant central control site of energy homeostasis, with multiple afferent inputs and diverse efferent outputs involving all organ systems.

5 Bariatric surgery regulates body weight via multiple mechanisms that are qualitatively different from responses to nonsurgical weight loss.

6 Metabolic disease encompasses all organ systems with pleiotropic pathology.

7 Cell stress responses to chronic nutrient excess underlie the pathogenesis of metabolic disease.

8 Adipose tissue acts as a critical nutrient "buffer" to protect other tissues from nutrient excess; as adipose buffering capacity is overwhelmed, nutrient excess overflows to all tissues, causing metabolic disease.

GENETICS OF OBESITY

Metabolic Thrift, Genetics, and Epigenetics

The propensity toward an obese or lean body habitus is rooted in genetics. Evolutionary selection has hard-wired our species to be biased toward an obese phenotype—while rare single-nucleotide polymorphisms (SNPs) have been identified that predispose toward leanness,[1] the majority of SNPs associated with body weight predispose to overweight and obesity. The *thrifty gene hypothesis*, proposed by geneticist James Neel, posits that humans are predisposed to a *thrifty metabolism* by genes selected over eons of evolution in environments characterized by food scarcity.[2] These genes were adaptive in our ancient past but lead to a blossoming of obesity in our modern *obesogenic environment*. While competing theories exist (eg, predation release, genetic drift), Neel's hypothesis remains the basis of a modern understanding of obesity as a genetic phenomenon. *Quantitative analysis of twin studies*, in which phenotypic traits of thousands of twin pairs are analyzed using statistical methods based on Mendelian principles, consistently demonstrate that approximately 70% of the tendency to obe-
1 sity is due to genetics.[3] *Genome-wide association studies* (GWAS), involving sequencing thousands of genomes and correlating SNPs with phenotypic traits and disease, have identified thrifty genes postulated by Neel decades earlier. Many obesity SNPs lie in genes associated with body weight regulation. SNPs in the melanocortin 4 receptor gene, which regulates hypothalamic satiety and hunger responses, are implicated in 5% of cases of human obesity. Other obesity-associated SNPs lie in genes encoding leptin and its receptor, proopiomelanocortin (POMC), fat mass and obesity-associated (FTO) locus, ghrelin, neuropeptide Y, adiponectin, glucagon-like peptide-1 (GLP-1), and other genetic loci associated with satiety and hunger. Other SNPs lie in genes not clearly related to energy balance, including loci that regulate neural and limb development, DNA repair, and other cellular functions, testament to the fact that the processes that regulate energy homeostasis overlap with all aspects of physiology. The effect size of each individual SNP on the obesity phenotype is small, with hundreds of SNPs contributing to obesity, each with relatively small independent effects on BMI, ranging from as low as 0.04 kgm^{-2} to 0.35 kgm^{-2}. GWAS studies have so far identified over 1,100 genetic loci that independently correlate with human obesity.[4] Obesity is a complex polygenic phenotype.

While classical Watson–Crick–Franklin genetics has honed human metabolism over millennia, epigenetic regulation of the genome fine-tunes metabolic phenotype over shorter periods of time. The *thrifty phenotype hypothesis* was proposed by Hales and Barker in 1992 to explain the observation that infants born to malnourished mothers are at increased risk of adult obesity and metabolic disease compared to offspring born to the same mothers during well-nourished pregnancies.[5] The fetus was presumed to be responding to instability in environmental food resources by adjusting its phenotype toward a thrifty metabolism, a phenomenon termed *fetal programming*. A similar response was subsequently observed in fetuses born of mothers with obesity and diabetes. Excess or scarcity of nutrients may be interpreted similarly by the fetus as signs of unstable food resources, explaining the similar effect of maternal under- and over-nutrition on offspring metabolic phenotype. Subsequent research demonstrated that these effects are mediated by *epigenetic* mechanisms, covalent modification of the genome independent of changes in nucleotide base-pair sequence, including but not limited to DNA methylation, glycosylation, and histone modification, changes that persist for one or more generations and that exert pro-
2 found effects on gene expression. Epigenetic modification of the genome is widespread, occurs primarily during fetal development but extends into adulthood, and regulates normal developmental processes as well as pathologic responses. Epigenetics allows the fetus to respond in utero to environmental cues delivered by changes in maternal homeostasis, the "weather forecast" model. Epigenetic modifications in response to fetal under- and over-nutrition are demonstrated across species, play an important role in disease pathogenesis,

and suggest that intervention must occur early, prior to birth, to prevent adult obesity and metabolic disease.

Human Metabolic Diversity and Environment

The multiple thrifty SNPs in the human genome impart genetic heterogeneity that underlies the intrinsic variability of human body habitus and metabolism, with a wide range of body types from lean to obese, gynecoid and android obesity phenotypes, variability in age of onset, triggers, and severity of obesity, differences in response to weight loss interventions, as well as differences in satiety and hunger thresholds, metabolic rates,
3 and multiple specific metabolic functions. This *metabolic diversity* has allowed humans to adapt to a wide range of habitats. Multiple examples exist of human subpopulations whose genetic heritages are adaptive in native environments, but maladaptive in a modern obesogenic environment. Polynesians, for example, manifest a genetic propensity to obesity and insulin resistance that provided a selective advantage in the ancient South Pacific environment, but imparts a high risk for obesity and metabolic disease in our modern environment. Similar human subpopulations metabolically adapted to specific niche environments but at high risk for metabolic disease in industrialized society include Inuit Eskimos, Aboriginal Australians, and Pima Indians. Environment plays a critical role in the obesity phenotype. Modern environmental contributors include an excess of processed food and a structured *built environment* that discourages physical activity. Modern processed food is not only calorie dense but also highly palatable, stimulating central nervous system (CNS) reward centers and hunger/satiety circuits not designed for chronic stimulation, thus reinforcing overeating. Physical activity is markedly decreased in our modern environment. Paleolithic humans were estimated to have consumed 30% more calories than modern humans, but engaged in significantly higher levels of physical activity. Other factors also contribute, including disruption in Circadian rhythms, home temperature stability, and assortative mating patterns. An evolving field of environmental engineering has arisen to address these issues (**Fig. 2.1**).

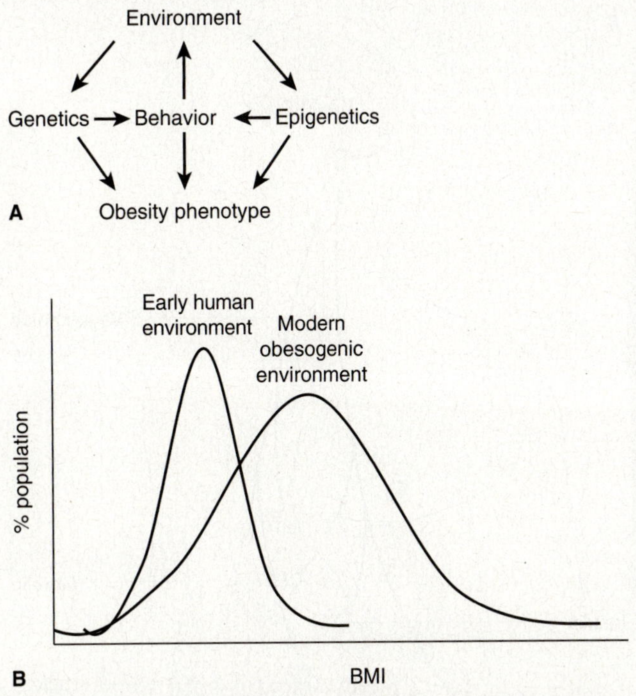

Figure 2.1. Interactions between environment and genetics dictate phenotype: **A:** Environment alters genetics over millennia, while the effects of environment on epigenetics take place over generations. In the case of humans, genetics dictates our behavior, which in turn has led us to create an obesogenic environment, creating a vicious cycle that exacerbates the obesity epidemic. **B:** The obesity phenotype blossoms in a modern obesogenic environment, with the population BMI curve broadening and shifting rightward, with an increase in median BMI. The increase in median BMI is relatively modest, but a substantially larger percentage of people populate overweight and obese BMI ranges. Of note, the schematic graphs shown are similar to those that describe the shift in US population National Health and Nutrition Examination Survey (NHANES) BMI data from 1970s to 2000s.

PHYSIOLOGY OF OBESITY

The Adipostat

Excess adipose tissue is the *sine qua non* of obesity, and human metabolism has evolved tightly regulated processes to optimize and defend adipose tissue stores. A dominant determinant of systemic metabolic homeostasis is the quantity of existent adipose tissue stores, the adequacy of which is determined by the
4 hypothalamic feeding center (HFC) in the mid-brain. The hypothalamus was first identified as a central locus of energy homeostasis as early as 1940, when hypothalamic ablation experiments in rats were observed to induce hyperphagia and obesity.[6] The HFC receives multiple afferent neural and hormonal inputs from all organ systems, including adipose tissue, and orchestrates a range of responses via efferent outputs that monitor and maintain adipose tissue stores, regulate all aspects of metabolism, and which together comprise the *adipostat*, the sum total of all processes that defend body weight. The amount of adipose tissue "deemed" adequate by the HFC varies among individuals and is dictated by multiple thrifty genes, which collectively determine the *adipostat set-point*. The hypothalamus of a lean person "considers" a lower amount of adipose tissue to be adequate, while the hypothalamus of a person with obesity requires higher levels of adipose tissue stores. Weight loss alerts the HFC to deviation from the adipostat set-point, which in turn triggers robust compensatory responses (eg, increased hunger, decreased satiety, decreased metabolic rate) that restore adipose tissue mass to baseline levels. HFC-mediated metabolic responses are characterized by tight regulation; deviation outside the range of these responses for more than limited periods of time is not possible based on conscious choice, but rather is controlled by the mid-brain, explaining the high failure rate of diet-induced weight loss, and the lack of efficacy of liposuction for weight loss. Bariatric surgery-induced weight loss is an exception to this rule, inducing poorly understood paradoxical responses that bypass the adipostat. Multiple physiologic mechanisms comprise the adipostat and regulate body weight. Most important in humans are the collective satiety and hunger systems that regulate food intake. Regulation of metabolic rate, adipocyte physiology, and the microbiome also contribute.

Satiety and Hunger

Regulation of food intake is the dominant mechanism by which humans control body weight. The hypothalamus integrates information regarding nutritional status, environment, and energy expenditure delivered by central and peripheral orexigenic and anorexigenic signals. The arcuate nucleus of the hypothalamus is a crucial site for integration of fasting and feeding signals. Two types of neurons with opposing actions on feeding behavior have been identified in the arcuate nucleus. Neurons that express POMC and cocaine and amphetamine-related transcript (CART) suppress food intake, reduce body weight, and increase energy expenditure. In contrast, orexigenic neurons produce neuropeptide Y and agouti gene–related transcript (AgRP), and act to stimulate food intake and reduce energy expenditure (**Fig. 2.2**). Of interest, separate signaling pathways within the HFC likely control homeostatic feeding behavior and nonhomeostatic hedonic feeding behavior, each with distinct afferent inputs and efferent outputs from other areas of the CNS. Hedonic feeding may override homeostatic feeding in response to stress and

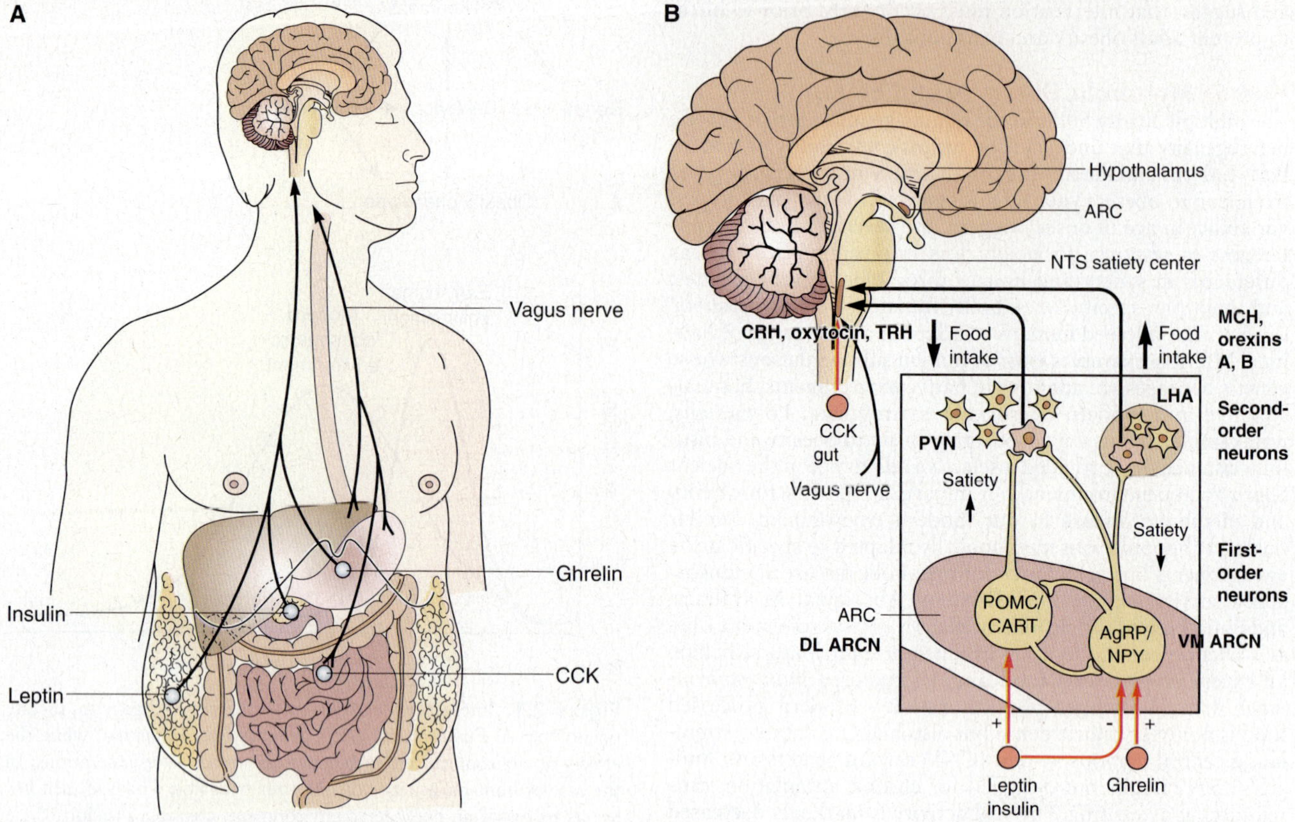

Figure 2.2. A simplified schematic of the hypothalamic feeding center and its primary afferent signals: Multiple hormones secreted by the gastrointestinal tract and adipose tissue act as afferent signals that regulate the arcuate nucleus (ARCN) within the hypothalamic feeding center. These signals impact first-order ARCN neurons, which in turn communicate with second-order paraventricular nucleus (PVN) and lateral hypothalamic area (LHA) neurons to coordinate behavioral and metabolic output. PVN signaling is primarily anorexigenic and catabolic, and is enhanced by leptin and insulin, while LHA signaling is primarily orexigenic and anabolic and inhibited by leptin and insulin. Higher-order anorexigenic PVN outputs include corticotropin-releasing hormone (CRH), oxytocin, and thyrotropin-releasing hormone (TRH); higher-order orexigenic LHA outputs include melanin-concentrating hormone (MCH) and orexins A and B. Both pathways negatively regulate the other. Other peripheral and central mediators stimulate first- and second-order neurons as well, including ghrelin, CCK, GLP-1, serotonin, endogenous cannabinoids, and norepinephrine.

emotion, an example, of how regulation of food intake interfaces with virtually all aspects of human behavior.

The Ob mouse, a mutant strain described in 1950, manifests an obese phenotype along with immune, endocrine, and reproductive abnormalities. In 1994, Jeffrey Friedman at the Rockefeller University identified an inactivating point mutation in the *Ob* gene in these mice responsible for their phenotype, and went on to characterize the protein product of this gene, termed leptin (Gr *leptos*, thin).[7] Leptin is a 16-kD hormone secreted by adipose tissue in response to feeding that binds receptors in the HFC and induces satiety. Leptin mediates communication between adipose tissue, gut, and brain that signals the status of adipose tissue stores, which in turn dictates food intake. As such, leptin is a paradigmatic adipokine, a hormone secreted by adipose tissue with direct effects on the hypothalamic adipostat, and an example of the complex interorgan communication that underlies weight regulation (**Fig. 2.3**). Friedman's discovery led to identification of rare humans with leptin mutations with an Ob phenotype that was reversed with administration of exogenous recombinant leptin. Excitement around this discovery was palpable, as leptin was thought to represent a "cure" for obesity. But this excitement collided with a growing understanding of the genetics of obesity, as leptin therapy was demonstrated to be ineffective in common human obesity, which was found to be not the result of a single leptin mutation, but rather a polygenic phenotype characterized by hypothalamic resistance to leptin satiety effects. Nonetheless, the discovery of leptin led to an explosion of research, with subsequent identification of multiple *adipokines*, including adiponectin, resistin, visfatin, fibroblast growth factor 21 (FGF21), dipeptidyl peptidase 4 (DPP-4), vaspin, and apelin. As research proceeded, other classes of molecules were identified with important roles in regulating body weight, including *gut hormones* and *cytokines*. Receptors for adipokines, gut peptides, and cytokines are widely expressed not only in the HFC and other areas of the CNS, but also by multiple peripheral tissues outside the CNS, exerting pleiotropic functions that include regulation of satiety and hunger, immune function, glucose homeostasis, lipid metabolism, and endocrine and reproductive functions (**Fig. 2.4**). This functional diversity speaks to the intimate association of energy homeostasis with all aspects of physiology.

Ghrelin is an orexigenic gut hormone expressed primarily by oxyntic glands in the fundus of the stomach but also by the hypothalamus. The ghrelin receptor, a member of the G protein–coupled receptor family, is widely distributed in central and peripheral tissues, including pituitary, hypothalamus, pancreas, stomach, and intestine. In humans, plasma acyl-ghrelin levels increase with fasting and decrease with feeding, and intravenous administration of ghrelin stimulates hunger and food intake. Ghrelin secretion is increased with diet-induced weight loss and reduced in obesity. Ghrelin antibodies and ghrelin receptor antagonists are under study as therapeutic agents. GLP-1 and gastric inhibitory peptide (aka glucose-dependent insulinotropic polypeptide, GIP) are gut hormones and canonical "incretins" (*discussed further below*) with diverse effects on multiple tissues, including regulation of satiety in the hypothalamus, metabolism in skeletal muscle, adipose tissue, and liver, and insulin secretion by the pancreas. Recent studies of GLP-1- and GIP-receptor agonists demonstrate weight loss

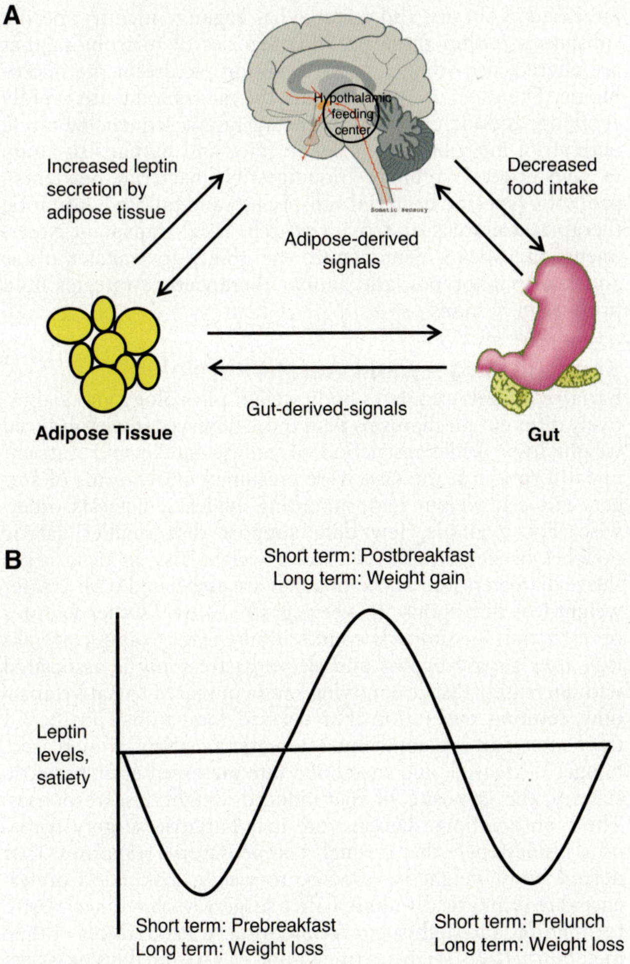

Figure 2.3. Leptin mediates communication between adipose tissue, gut, and brain: A: Signals from the gastrointestinal tract triggered by a meal circulate to adipose tissue and induce adipocyte leptin secretion. Leptin circulates to the hypothalamus, where it binds receptors in the arcuate nucleus to induce satiety, leading to decreased food intake. Leptin is one of many signals that mediates bidirectional communication between gut, adipose tissue, and brain. Other organ systems are also involved, including immune and reproductive systems and the liver. B: Leptin regulates allostatic control of short-term and long-term food intake. Postprandial leptin secretion induces satiety for a period of hours, after which leptin levels and satiety wane, prompting food intake. Similarly, leptin, along with other mediators of food intake, controls long-term weight regulation: diet-induced weight loss leads to decreased adipose tissue mass, reducing peak postprandial leptin levels, leading to decreased postprandial satiety and increased food intake at each subsequent meal until adipose tissue mass is restored to set-point levels. In this manner, leptin functions as a component of the adipostat. This allostatic control provides an explanation for rebound weight gain after diet-induced weight loss.

approaching that seen with bariatric surgery.[8] Multiple other gut hormones regulate food intake and other aspects of energy homeostasis, including insulin, amylin, oxyntomodulin, pancreatic polypeptide, and peptide YY.

In addition to immunoregulation, cytokines play an important role in the control of food intake. TNF-α, IL-6, and IL-β, for example, regulate food intake and energy expenditure in the context of cachexia and inflammatory states. Multiple mechanisms mediate the effects of cytokines, including direct effects on neurons in the hypothalamus, regulation of secretion of gut hormones (TNF-a and IL-6, eg, potentiate GLP-1 secretion by ileal L-cells), and effects on peripheral organs including but to limited to adipose tissue, pancreas, and skeletal muscle (TNF-a, eg, induces lipolysis in adipose tissue, and

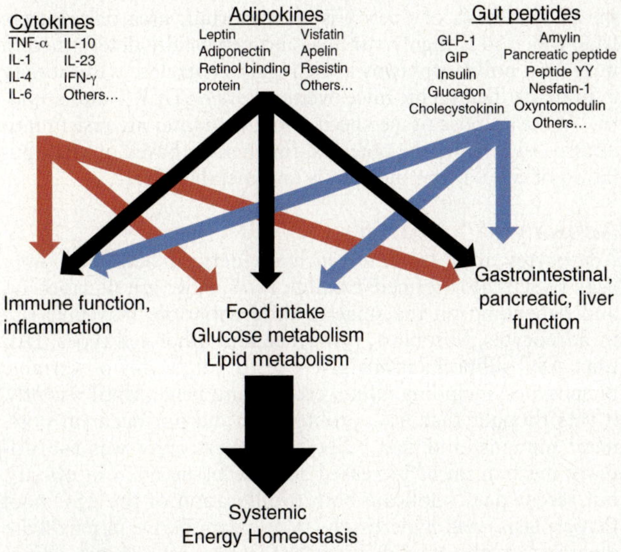

Figure 2.4. Primary peptide mediators of energy homeostasis: Cytokines, adipokines, and gut peptides regulate diverse aspects of metabolism to control global energy homeostasis. Each of these proteins has dominant functions within its primary family, but also demonstrates cross-regulatory functions in other domains. In addition, mediators participate in crosstalk at the level of cellular receptors and downstream intracellular signaling mediators. Shown are only partial lists of peptides and the physiologic functions they control.

induces insulin resistance in multiple cell types). Cytokines are secreted by macrophages and other immune cells at sites of sterile inflammation in multiple organs that result from chronic nutrient excess and exert their effects predominantly in a paracrine manner. Inflammation is a key response to nutrient excess (*discussed further below*), and the term "metainflammation" is used to describe the close link between chronic sterile inflammation and metabolism.

Metabolic Rate

In humans who lose weight with diet, total energy expenditure is decreased up to 20% beyond that expected by loss of fat and fat-free mass alone and is accompanied by a corresponding decrease in voluntary physical activity. Conversely, overfeeding and weight gain induce compensatory increases in total energy expenditure.[9] These compensatory changes in energy expenditure counteract caloric restriction and contribute to adipostat responses that defend adipose tissue mass. Importantly, studies in twin cohorts demonstrate a significant genetic component to variability in energy expenditure responses to overfeeding, suggesting that variability in metabolic rate responses to weight change contributes to the development of obesity in those at risk.[3] Differences in sympathetic nervous system activity contribute. Humans with obesity demonstrate decreased sympathetic nervous system activity, and higher levels of sympathetic nervous system activity predict successful diet-induced weight loss. Differences in endocrine responses also contribute, with humans with obesity manifesting differences in thyroid hormone and catecholamine balance associated with decreased metabolic rates.

Fundamental differences in energy utilization and thermogenesis at the cellular level also play an important role. Skeletal muscle energy utilization efficiency is increased in humans who achieve successful weight loss and decreased in those who gain weight, while humans with obesity manifest decreased skeletal muscle non–exercise-induced thermogenesis and diet-induced thermogenesis,[10] with differences in uncoupling protein (UCP) function implicated. UCP uncouple oxidative phosphorylation from electron transport in mitochondria, creating a proton leak that generates heat rather than ATP. The role of UCPs in the pathogenesis of obesity is an important area of research. UCP function is highly variable and genetically determined in mice, and polymorphisms in UCP genes correlate with obesity in humans. Transgenic mice over-expressing UCP-1 under control of the adipose tissue-specific AP2 promoter are resistant to obesity, suggesting the potential for therapy based on manipulation of cellular thermogenesis and metabolic rate.

Adipocyte Physiology

Adipocytes arise from mesenchyme-derived *adipocyte stem cells* (ASC), also termed *preadipocytes*. ASC are pluripotent, and depending on the stage of differentiation, may give rise to adipocytes, fibroblast, myocytes, and other cell types. Distinct ASC subpopulations give rise to adipocytes of variable phenotypes, including white, brown, and beige. Until recently, it was thought that ASC proliferation did not occur in postnatal humans, and that adipocyte hypertrophy was the primary mechanism of increased adipose tissue mass in obesity, but recent data implicate both proliferation of the ASC pool (hyperplasia) and hypertrophy. These data derive in part from ingenious methods studying incorporation of C14 into adipocyte DNA in individuals born before and after mid-20th century nuclear bomb testing, which raised environmental C14 levels.[11] Separate data demonstrate that adipocytes in human obesity manifest increased hypertrophic capacities, contributing to progressive obesity, and epigenetic programming has been implicated in these effects.[12]

Recent studies applying single-cell and single-nuclear sequencing to adipose tissue demonstrate marked heterogeneity in ASC and adipocytes, with metabolically beneficial and metabolically detrimental subpopulations. This diversity extends to other cell types within adipose tissue, with multiple distinct subpopulations of macrophages, T cells, endothelial cells, and other cell types, testament to the functional complexity of the adipose tissue organ. Combining these data with other advanced-omics analyses, including ATAC-Seq (Assay for Transposase-Accessible Chromatin with high-throughput sequencing), in vitro and in vivo lineage tracing of cell subpopulations, and spatial-omics technologies, are transforming our understanding of the cellular landscape of adipose tissue in health and disease, with the promise of targeting metabolically beneficial and metabolically detrimental cell subpopulations.[13]

The Microbiome

The microbiome plays an important role in energy homeostasis. Animals raised in germ-free environments manifest increased food intake, decreased body weight, and do not develop obesity and insulin resistance when fed a high-fat diet, demonstrating that gut microbiota contribute to nutrient digestion. Gut microbiota ferment non–host-digestible polysaccharides into monosaccharides and short-chain fatty acids that are absorbed by host enterocytes and colonocytes. Products of microbiota fermentation act not only as nutrients, but also regulate host metabolism: short-chain fatty acids induce satiety, mediated in part by increased secretion of GLP-1 and peptide YY and decreased secretion of ghrelin. Separate data demonstrate interactions between microbiota and adipose tissue, liver, skeletal muscle, and CNS. These effects are mediated by short-chain fatty acids, activation of toll-like receptors on host cells via lipopolysaccharide and other bacterial products, regulation of host systemic and cellular metabolism, and other diverse mechanisms.

Alterations in the microbiome contribute to obesity and metabolic disease. Germ-free mice, when colonized with stool from obese mice, gain more weight than mice colonized with stool from lean mice, demonstrating an obesity-specific microbiome. Obesity in mice and humans is associated with an increase in gram-negative gut bacteria, with a concomitant increase in lipopolysaccharide absorption from the gut, which has been postulated to contribute to inflammation and insulin resistance. The ratio of gut Firmicutes/Bacteroidetes species is increased in obesity, and research has begun to identify specific subspecies within these broad categories of microbiota that are altered, providing a high-resolution picture of the microbiome. The tools used to evaluate the microbiome are rapidly evolving, and include shotgun metagenomic sequencing along with stool microbiota transfer in mice and humans to study in vivo effects. Prebiotic (nondigestible bacterial nutrients), probiotic (specific bacterial subspecies), and tailored antibiotic therapies are areas of active research. Fecal transplant experiments in rodents demonstrate the ability to transfer obese and lean phenotypes, and similar therapeutic strategies hold promise in humans.

Bariatric Surgery and Weight Physiology

Bariatric surgery regulates body weight physiology via qualitatively different mechanisms than those observed in diet-induced
5 weight loss. While restriction of caloric intake and nutrient malabsorption in the past were presumed mechanisms of surgery-induced weight loss, mounting evidence suggests otherwise. For example, few data support that smaller gastric pouches or sleeves achieve greater weight loss; in fact, larger sleeve diameters and antral pouches are associated with greater weight loss in response to sleeve gastrectomy.[14] Other features of restriction are similarly counterintuitive: for example, weight loss after gastric bypass and sleeve gastrectomy is associated with increased gastric emptying rates compared to native anatomy, refuting the notion that delayed food transit in the GI tract after surgery contributes to satiety. Satiety is increased, hunger decreased, and metabolic rate increased after bariatric surgery, the opposite of diet-induced weight loss responses. These observations demonstrate that bariatric surgery somehow "sidesteps" the normal compensatory responses that defend body weight in response to weight loss. Food preferences are dramatically altered after surgery, with reduced desire for high-fat and high-sugar foods. Surgery also induces unique metabolic effects; diabetes often improves within days or weeks of gastric bypass, before substantial weight loss, the result of changes in gut hormone secretion secondary to altered intestinal anatomy. Observations in the early 20th century that an oral glucose load elicits a greater insulin response than an identical intravenous glucose load led to postulation of the existence of *incretins*, gut hormones secreted in response to a meal that potentiate insulin secretion and regulate systemic glucose metabolism. Subsequent research led to the discovery of GIP and GLP-1, incretin hormones secreted by duodenal K-cells and ileal L-cells, respectively in response to nutrient delivery to the small intestine. Incretins have diverse effects on glucose homeostasis, potentiating central insulin secretion and peripheral insulin sensitivity. The *foregut and hindgut hypotheses* have been proposed to explain this phenomenon: bypass of the alimentary stream from the stomach, duodenum, and proximal jejunum (foregut), and increased caloric delivery to the distal jejunum and ileum (hindgut), both the result of gastric bypass Roux-en-Y anatomy, regulate gut hormone secretion. Similarly, sleeve gastrectomy results in accelerated gastric emptying (possibly due to loss of receptive antral relaxation), and thus also increases caloric delivery to the ileum (hindgut). These anatomic changes alter secretion of gut hormones, including but not limited to GIP and GLP-1, resulting in improvement in glucose homeostasis. Evidence supports the hindgut hypothesis, including data demonstrating increased postprandial serum GLP-1 levels after gastric bypass.[15] While debate persists regarding the magnitude of these effects on diabetes remission after gastric bypass, an understanding of incretin physiology has led to the development of GLP-1 and GIP agonists as pharmacologic therapy for diabetes and weight loss independent of bariatric surgery, transforming pharmacotherapy for obesity.[8]

Gut anatomic derangements mediate additional changes. While data is conflicting, gastric bypass and sleeve gastrectomy are in some studies associated with decreased serum levels of the orexigenic hormone ghrelin, which is secreted from the gastric fundus, and may contribute to reduced hunger after surgery. Gastric bypass and sleeve gastrectomy are associated with increased secretion of peptide YY and oxyntomodulin, gut hormones secreted by ileal L-cells in response to feeding that induce satiety, inhibit gut motility, and are central mediators of the "ileal brake" mechanism.[15] Bariatric surgery alters bile acid metabolism, increasing serum levels of conjugated bile acids, which mediate diverse effects by binding bile acid receptors in multiple cell types (eg, Takeda G protein receptor 5 [TGR5], nuclear receptor farnesoid X receptor [FXR]), with beneficial effects on glucose and lipid metabolism. Bile acid-directed therapy through manipulation of TGR5 and FXR signaling is an active area of research. Bariatric surgery disrupts vagal and enteroenteric innervation of the gut and alters CNS satiety responses. Finally, bariatric surgery is associated with alterations in gut microbiota that contribute to weight loss and resolution of metabolic disease.

Summary

Satiety and hunger, metabolic rate, adipocyte physiology, and the microbiome are a few of many processes that regulate metabolism and are dysregulated in obesity. Differences in lipid and glucose metabolism, immune function, central and peripheral nervous system function, and multiple other processes contribute to the variability of the obesity phenotype and metabolic diversity in humans, driven by genetic polymorphisms selected over eons of evolution. The question is often posed, should obesity be considered a disease? Rather, obesity is better thought of as a phenotypic response to an environment that is radically different than that in which our species evolved, a phenotype that was adaptive and enhanced survival during our evolution, but has become maladaptive and blossoms in our modern obesogeic environment. An understanding of these genetic–environment interactions and the physiologic mechanisms of weight regulation will lead to novel therapy for obesity. Bariatric surgery provides a unique opportunity, as surgery-induced weight loss, unlike diet-induced weight loss, somehow bypasses the adipostat. An understanding of incretin physiology has led to the development of transformative GLP-1- and GIP-based pharmacotherapy. As further mechanisms of surgery-induced weight loss are deciphered, additional pharmacotherapy developed through "reverse-engineering" of bariatric surgery will emerge.

PATHOPHYSIOLOGY OF METABOLIC DISEASE

Obesity and Metabolic Disease

Obesity is associated with a range of pathology involving every organ system that is collectively referred to as metabolic disease. While underlying mechanisms are multiple, the root cause of metabolic disease is a failure of adipose tissue nutrient buffering capacity, leading to overflow of nutrients, metabolites, cytokines, and adipokines from adipose tissue to other tissues not as well-equipped to process nutrients. The effects of overflow differ depending on the target tissue, but the fundamental cellular responses to nutrient excess common to all tissues, adipose included, underlie the pathogenesis of metabolic disease.

Nutrient Excess

Energy homeostasis is the overriding goal of all biologic systems. Metabolism (Gr. *metabole*, change) may be defined as the sum-total of all chemical reactions and physiologic processes that regulate cellular and systemic energy homeostasis. At the cellular level, metabolic processes are fundamental to all metazoan life and are highly conserved across phyla; examples include the citric acid cycle and mitochondrial respiration, which utilize multiple enzymes, the structure and function of which are conserved from yeast to humans. At the systemic level, metabolic processes are central to maintaining homeostasis and interface with virtually every organ system and physiologic process. The basic substrates of metabolism are macronutrients, including fatty acids, amino acids, and carbohydrates, and their metabolites, along with micronutrients that catalyze reactions that synthesize and degrade macronutrients and higher-order macromolecules. Cellular nutrient flux provides substrate for macromolecule synthesis via anabolic metabolic processes, which are in turn degraded via catabolic metabolic processes. Maintaining the balance between anabolism and catabolism at cellular and systemic levels is of critical importance. Cancer, for example, may be viewed as a metabolic imbalance that favors cellular anabolism over catabolism. Cachexia, in contrast, may be considered a disorder that favors systemic catabolism over anabolism. The nutrient flux with which cells are constantly faced determines the balance between anabolism and catabolism and dictates organism-wide energy homeostasis. Nutrients are, like oxygen, high-energy–capacity molecules, capable of participating in energy-intensive, potentially damaging reactions. Cell physiology has therefore evolved to control exposure, flux, and sequestration of these high-energy molecules. These regulatory processes were evolutionarily selected to manage *transient* nutrient excess but are not well-adapted to *chronic* nutrient excess. Maladaptive responses to chronic nutrient excess underlie the pathogenesis of metabolic disease and occur in all cells, explaining the involvement of virtually every organ system in metabolic
6 disease. These processes include fundamental cell stress responses: *endoplasmic reticulum (ER) stress*, *oxidative stress*, and *inflammation*.

Cellular Responses to Nutrient Excess

The ER is a complex organelle present in all eukaryotic cells that orchestrates synthesis and intracellular transport of macromolecules. The rough ER, studded with ribosomes, is responsible for protein synthesis, while the smooth ER coordinates lipid and carbohydrate synthesis. The ER receives a constant influx of nutrients, which it sequesters and directs toward macromolecule synthesis or degradation, carefully metering cell nutrient exposure. In this capacity, the ER acts as a nutrient sensor, responding to changes in nutrient flux by balancing cell anabolism and catabolism. The ER also responds to hypoxia, toxins, electrolyte disturbances, and a host of other stimuli that alter cell homeostasis. Excess nutrient flux, like other forms of stress, leads to a series of stepwise ER responses collectively referred to as the *ER stress response*. The initial ER stress response to modest increases in nutrient flux induces increased expression of *chaperone proteins* involved in macromolecule synthesis to accommodate increased anabolism of excess nutrients. If nutrient excess persists beyond cellular processing capacity, the ER stress response progresses to activate the *unfolded protein response*, which downregulates global protein expression. If nutrient excess persists beyond the capacity of the ER to maintain proper protein synthesis, then the unfolded protein response progresses to induce cell *apoptosis*. The unfolded protein response thus protects cells from modest increases in nutrient flux and induces cell death in the face of extreme nutrient excess.

Macromolecule synthesis generates reactive oxygen species (ROS) (eg, superoxides, oxygen/hydroxyl free radicals, hydrogen peroxide) which, like nutrients, are highly energetic molecules capable of damaging cells. Cells have evolved multiple mechanisms to sequester ROS, which together comprise the *oxidative stress response*, including antioxidant enzymes (eg, superoxide dismutase, glutathione peroxidase, catalase), scavenging molecules (eg, ascorbic acid, urate, divalent ions), and the thioredoxin and glutaredoxin systems. The ER and mitochondria are primary cellular sites of control of oxidative stress. When nutrient flux, macromolecule synthesis, and ROS production exceed cellular antioxidant capacity, cells activate oxidative stress responses, which increase expression of antioxidant proteins, sequester ROS, and increase mitochondrial uncoupling, transiently reducing cellular ROS production.

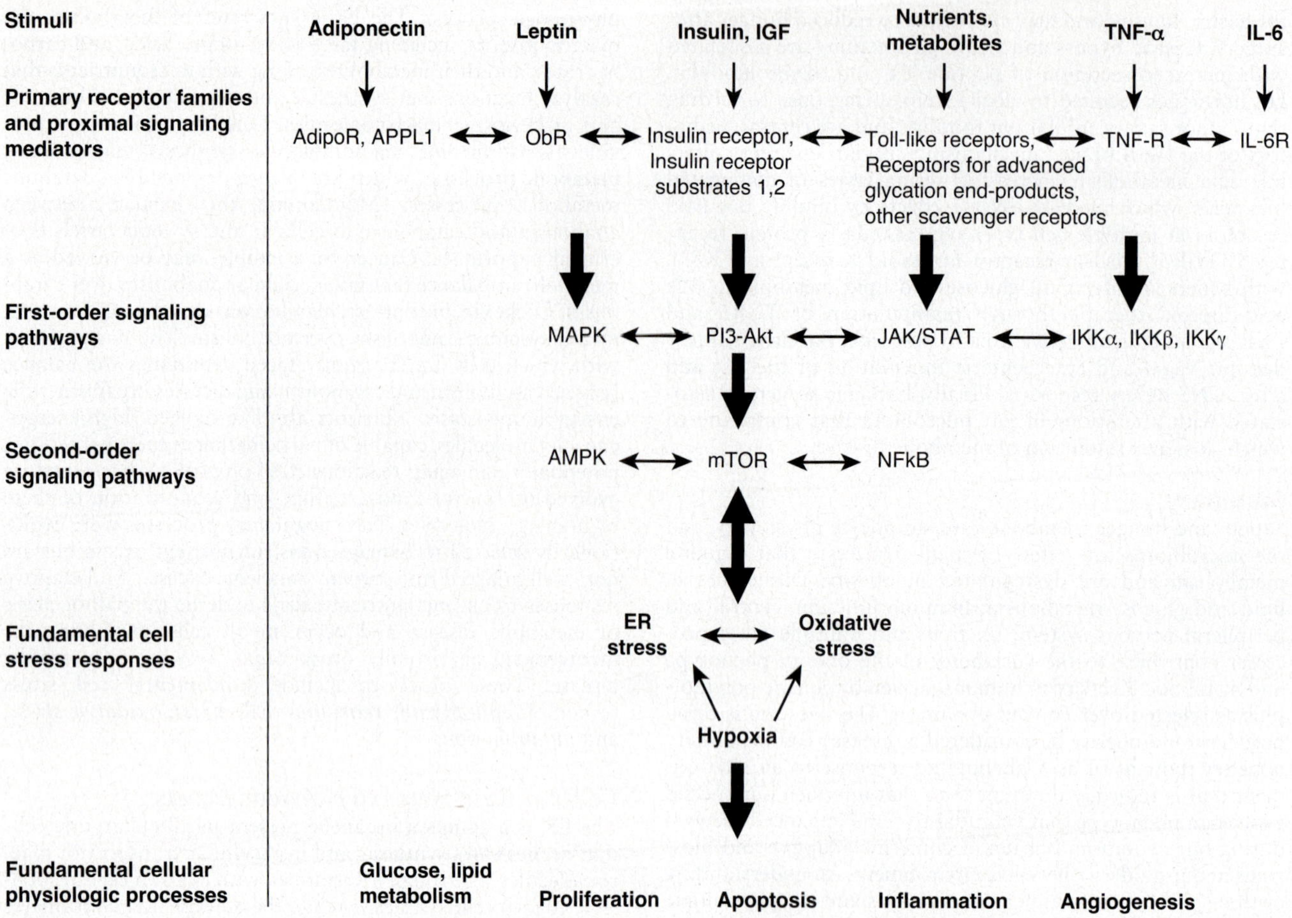

Figure 2.5. Highly simplified schematic of major cell signaling pathways that regulate energy homeostasis and cell stress responses: Primary stimuli for all cells include adipokines, insulin, IGF-1, nutrients and metabolites including free fatty acids, and their derivatives such as ceramide (which activate Toll like receptors, TLR), glucose, fructose, and advanced glycation end-products (which activate receptors for advanced glycation end-products, RAGE), and cytokines. Primary intracellular signaling nexus include mitogen-activated protein kinases (MAPK), PI3-Akt, JAK/STAT signaling mediators, AMP-activated protein kinase (AMPK), mammalian target of rapamycin (mTOR), and NFkB, all of which are linked to ER stress and oxidative stress responses. These pathways engage in highly redundant crosstalk via cross-reactivity of intracellular signaling mediators and induction of gene transcription and conspire to integrate multiple stimuli to regulate fundamental aspects of cell metabolism, survival, and death in response to nutrient availability and cell stressors such as hypoxia.

Oxidative stress responses overlap with ER stress responses, and if oxidative stress persists, the unfolded protein response is activated and leads to apoptosis.

Increased nutrient flux generates an *inflammatory response* designed to scavenge debris and byproducts from increased cell apoptosis and turnover that results from ER and oxidative stress. This sterile inflammatory response and its metabolic effects has been termed "metainflammation." Testament to the close relationship between metabolism and inflammation, inflammatory and metabolic mediators demonstrate functional overlap. For example, TNF-α and leptin, in addition to regulating inflammation and satiety respectively, each play reciprocal roles in regulating body weight and inflammation.[16,17] All satiety and hunger factors and inflammatory cytokines manifest dual immunoregulatory and metabolic functions. In addition, molecular byproducts of metabolism trigger inflammation. Free fatty acids are ligands for toll-like receptors, while advanced glycation end-products bind receptors for advanced glycation end-products (RAGE), which in turn activate innate immune cells, establishing a molecular link between metabolism and inflammation. Obesity is associated with a state of chronic systemic inflammation that plays a central role in the pathogenesis of metabolic disease. Serum cytokine levels are increased in obese animals and humans, and adipose tissue manifests a panleukocyte infiltrate, findings that directly correlate with the magnitude of obesity and severity of metabolic disease.

Cell stress responses potentiate one another. Fundamental cell signaling pathways, including PI3-Akt, MAPK, AMPK, mTOR, JAK-STAT, and NFκB, are triggered by multiple stimuli that are dysregulated in obesity, including adipokines, cytokines, growth factors, and nutrients and metabolites. These signaling pathways participate in crosstalk, establishing a vicious cycle that perpetuates cell stress in the face of chronic nutrient excess (**Fig. 2.5**). These processes are common to all cells and affect all tissues in late-stage obesity, explaining the diverse manifestations of systemic metabolic disease, but these
7 processes are initiated within adipose tissue.

Adipose Tissue Heterogeneity

Adipocytes reside in multiple discrete anatomic depots as well as within every organ and every tissue. Adipose tissue is more than simply a storage depot for lipid; only half the cells in adipose tissue are adipocytes, the remainder comprising the so-called stromovascular cell fraction, which consists of leukocytes, fibroblasts, endothelial cells, adipocyte stem cells, and other cell types. Adipose tissue is highly innervated with sympathetic and parasympathetic afferent and efferent fibers and has important immunoregulatory and endocrine functions. Adipose tissue participates in robust communication with the CNS and all peripheral organs, orchestrating responses to alterations in nutrient availability, systemic health and metabolism, ambient temperature, and a host of other stimuli. Adipose tissue is a central regulator of systemic energy homeostasis.

Hibernating bears accumulate substantial adipose tissue without developing inflammation or cell stress, while in some humans, excess subcutaneous adipose tissue appears to protect from metabolic disease. These examples demonstrate that adipose tissue phenotype is as important as quantity with respect to metabolic health. Adipose tissue may be broadly divided into white and brown phenotypes. White adipose tissue comprises the majority of adipose tissue in humans, is strongly associated with metabolic disease, and increases with obesity and age. White adipose tissue derives from mesodermal stem cells that migrate to sites of canonical anatomic depots in early embryonic development and proliferate to form defined depots in late fetal and early neonatal periods. White adipose tissue includes visceral and subcutaneous depots, which are further divided into omental, mesenteric, and retroperitoneal visceral subdepots, and deep and superficial subcutaneous subdepots, each with distinct functional characteristics. Brown adipose tissue, in contrast, comprises a minority of total adipose tissue in humans, less than 0.5% of total body weight, decreases with obesity and age, and has beneficial effects on metabolism, manifesting lower lipid storage capacity and higher levels of fatty acid oxidation and thermogenesis via expression of mitochondrial UCPs. Brown adipose tissue develops in rodents during gestation from precursor cells that also give rise to myocytes and form defined brown adipose tissue depots prior to birth. Brown adipose tissue in humans is most voluminous in the neonatal period, but positron emission tomography demonstrates cervical, supraclavicular, mediastinal, paraspinous, and perirenal brown adipose tissue in adult humans as well.[18] Recent data support that the dichotomy between white and brown adipose tissues is overly simplistic, and that adipocyte phenotype spans a spectrum. An intermediate phenotype, termed *"brite"* (brown-in-white) or "*beige adipocytes*," are found in white adipose tissue in rodents and humans. These cells manifest brown adipocyte functions and proliferate in response to cold stress and β-adrenergic stimuli, suggesting phenotypic plasticity. Clinical trials studying pharmacologic "browning" of adipocyte phenotype are in progress.

Adipose tissue is anatomically heterogeneous. Human obesity may be broadly classified into android and gynecoid phenotypes, defined by excess visceral and subcutaneous adipose tissue, respectively, with the former strongly associated with metabolic disease, while the latter is less associated with metabolic disease, and possibly protective. Surgical lipectomy of visceral adipose tissue but not subcutaneous adipose tissue in mice ameliorates diabetes.[19] Similar studies of visceral omentectomy in humans demonstrate conflicting and less robust results, likely due to more complex human adipose tissue depot anatomy, but excess visceral adipose tissue measured by waist circumference and imaging techniques nonetheless correlates strongly with metabolic disease. Mechanisms underlying the disproportionate effect of visceral adipose tissue on metabolic disease are multiple. Due to its abdominal location, visceral adipose tissue exerts a disproportionate effect on liver metabolism via portal overflow (*discussed below*). Intrinsic functional differences also contribute, as visceral adipose tissue manifests higher levels of inflammation, lipolysis, β-adrenergic receptor expression, steroid sensitivity, insulin resistance, and adipocyte proliferation and differentiation relative to subcutaneous adipose tissue.

Adipose Tissue Failure

Adipocytes are exquisitely well designed to manage high levels of nutrients. Hypertrophy is an early response of adipocytes to chronic nutrient excess in early obesity. Free fatty acids are absorbed by adipocytes through pinocytosis mediated by fatty acid–binding proteins, synthesized from glucose and glutamine via de novo lipogenesis, and stored in lipid droplets via a highly regulated process mediated by perilipin proteins. All cells are capable of storing lipid to some degree, but adipocytes have an extremely high lipid storage capacity, and are one of only a few cell types that can hypertrophy to diameters greater than 100 microns, the diffusion distance of oxygen. Adipocyte hypertrophy beyond this threshold establishes a state of cellular hypoxia. Decreased adipose tissue capillary density and blood flow in obesity exacerbates this hypoxic state, with broad effects on adipocyte metabolism, inducing insulin resistance, ER and oxidative stress, and inflammation. Targeting hypoxia-inducible factor-1α, a cellular hypoxia response protein, ameliorates murine metabolic disease, suggesting the possibility of hypoxia-based therapy.

Inflammation is a dominant feature of adipose tissue dysfunction and is directly linked to insulin resistance and dysregulation of lipid metabolism at tissue and systemic levels. Hypoxia induces adipocyte apoptosis and necrosis, which in turn recruits an inflammatory response to scavenge dead and dying adipocytes. Adipose tissue macrophages (ATM) are a central component of this response. ATM in obesity shifts from an M2 scavenging/remodeling phenotype to an inflammatory, diabetogenic phenotype.[20] While M1/M2 phenotypes are a useful paradigm, recent research single-cell sequencing data in mice and humans demonstrate substantial heterogeneity in ATM subpopulations with multiple overlapping phenotypes.[21] ATM expresses inflammatory cytokines, including TNF-α, IL-6, and IL-1, which induce insulin resistance and aberrations in glucose and lipid metabolism in adipocytes via multiple mechanisms. Induction of insulin resistance in other cell types by immune cells is an adaptive mechanism, designed to preferentially shunt glucose to activated immune cells during infection, a process that becomes maladaptive and perpetuates adipose tissue inflammation in obesity. Supporting a central role for ATM in metabolic disease, obese mice transgenically engineered to lack macrophage homing molecules in adipose tissue do not develop ATM infiltrates or diabetes. Agents that interfere with macrophage homing to adipose tissue show promise as a treatment for diabetes. Finally, adipose tissue inflammation involves more than macrophages, with a panleukocyte infiltrate that includes T-cells, B-cells, NK cells, NKT cells, and eosinophils. Therapy targeting these cell subpopulations is an area of active research.

As inflammation persists, adipose tissue undergoes fibrotic remodeling, with increased expression of matrix metalloproteases and collagens and increased extracellular matrix (ECM) turnover, further impairing adipose tissue function. Adipose tissue fibrosis limits adipocyte hypertrophy and lipid storage capacity, accelerating adipocyte stress. Obese collagen VI knockout mice demonstrate increased adipocyte hypertrophic capacity due to decreased fibrosis and are protected from systemic metabolic disease.[22] Other data demonstrate that ECM regulates adipocyte metabolism in disease and depot-specific manner, such that nondiabetic adipose tissue ECM can rescue dysfunctional diabetic adipocyte metabolism.[23] These observations speak to an important role of the adipose tissue ECM in regulating adipocyte metabolism (**Fig. 2.6**).

SYSTEMIC METABOLIC DISEASE

Adipose Tissue Overflow

Patients with rare congenital and acquired lipodystrophy syndromes who lack adipose tissue suffer from metabolic disease, including insulin resistance, hyperlipidemia, and hepatic steatosis, demonstrating that an absence of adipose tissue is as detrimental as its excess. In lipodystrophy and in obesity, adipose tissue nutrient buffering capacity is overwhelmed, in the former due to a lack of adipose tissue, and in the latter due to dysfunctional adipose tissue that results from chronic nutrient excess and cell stress. As obesity progresses and adipose tissue nutrient buffering capacity fails, nutrients *overflow* into the systemic circulation to other tissues not well adapted to

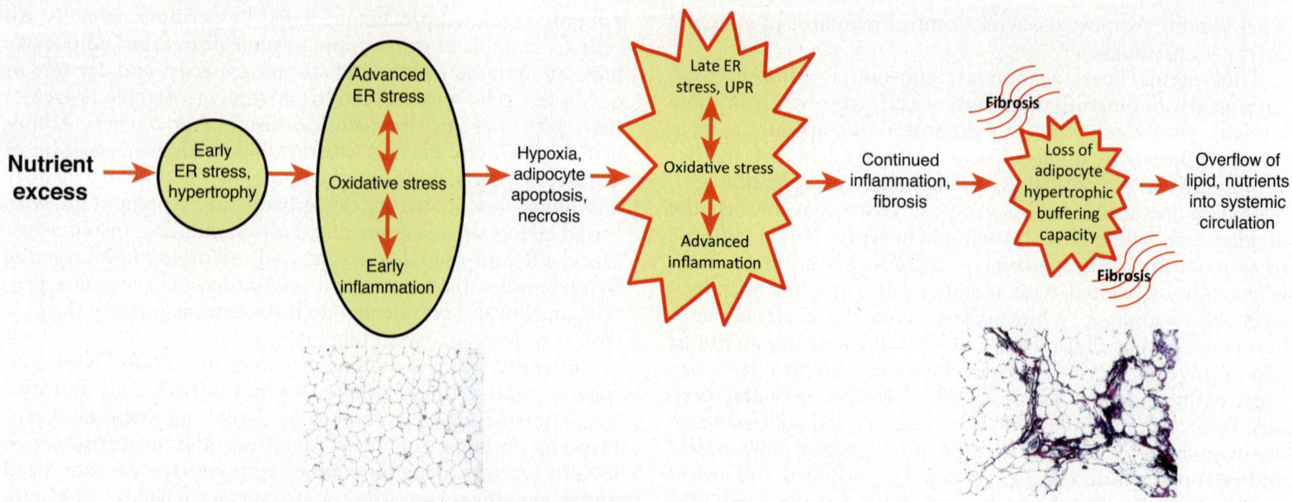

Figure 2.6. Nutrient excess and cell stress in adipocytes: Nutrient excess is an early signal that induces ER stress and hypertrophy in adipocytes. ER stress is tightly linked to oxidative stress and inflammation, and each of these processes induces and potentiates the others. As hypertrophy progresses, adipocyte diameter expands beyond the diffusion distance of oxygen, leading to cellular hypoxia, which exacerbates cell stress responses, leading to adipocyte apoptosis and necrosis via the unfolded protein response and other advanced cell stress responses. Adipocyte apoptosis and necrosis trigger the recruitment of an advanced inflammatory response designed to scavenge dead and dying adipocytes. This inflammatory response is associated with fibrotic tissue remodeling, which limits adipocyte hypertrophy and lipid buffering capacity of surviving adipocytes, leading to overflow of lipids, nutrients, metabolites, and inflammatory products from adipose tissue into the systemic circulation. Photomicrographs of human adipose tissue (from O'Rourke Laboratory) stained with Sirius Red, a collagen-avid dye, display nonfibrotic hypertrophied adipose tissue (**left**) and adipose tissue with advanced fibrotic changes (**right**).

manage nutrient excess. Cell stress responses, initially confined to adipose tissue, affect all tissues and cause systemic metabolic disease (Fig. 2.7).

8 In addition to its distinct functional phenotype, visceral adipose tissue contributes disproportionately to metabolic disease via direct anatomic communication with the liver via the portal venous system. *Portal overflow* of free fatty acids, nutrients and metabolites, and hormones and cytokines from visceral adipose tissue to the liver is an early step in metabolic disease progression. As obesity progresses, *peripheral overflow* extends beyond the liver to involve all tissues, including skeletal muscle, pancreas, vasculature, kidneys, lungs, and the CNS; inflammation and ER stress occur in the hypothalamus, causing aberrations in CNS efferent outputs that exacerbate obesity and metabolic disease. In essence, adipose tissue dysfunction "metastasizes" to other tissues. Nutrients and metabolites are central mediators of these systemic effects. Free fatty acids and their metabolites (eg, ceramides, diacylglycerols) cause systemic *lipotoxicity* by binding toll-like receptors and immunostimulatory scavenger receptors, inducing inflammation, insulin resistance, ER stress, and apoptosis. Metabolic products of glucose and fructose (eg, advanced glycation end-products, glucosamines), mediate similar effects. Cytokines and adipokines overflow from adipose tissue as well. TNF-α expressed by ATM and adipocytes exerts proinflammatory and diabetogenic effects. Leptin also promotes inflammation and regulates cellular glucose homeostasis. Expression of adiponectin, which attenuates inflammation and has beneficial effects on metabolism, is decreased in obesity as adipose tissue shifts toward a proinflammatory milieu.

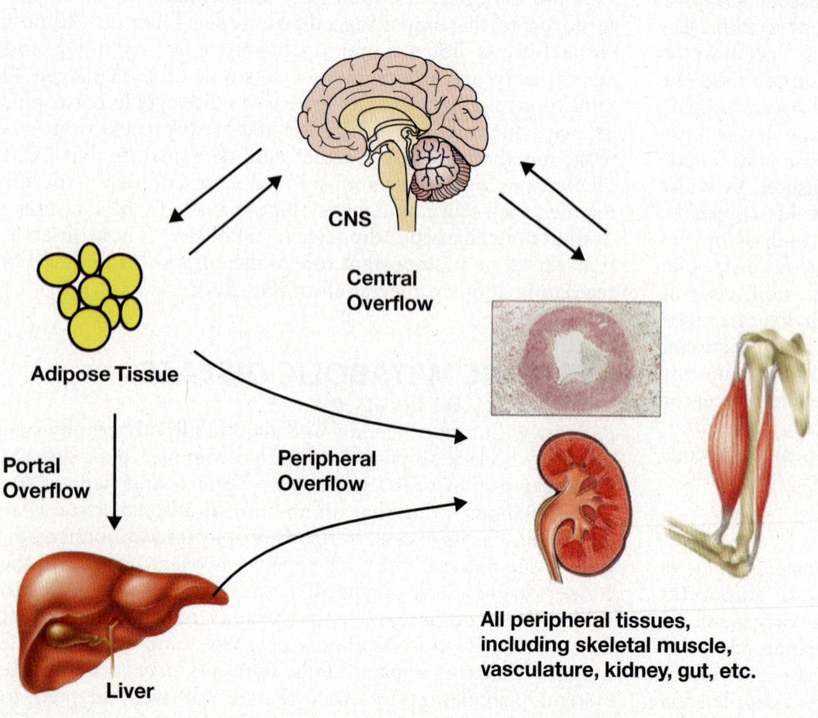

Figure 2.7. Adipose tissue overflow, interorgan communication, and systemic metabolic disease: As adipose tissue buffering capacity is overwhelmed, lipids, nutrients, cytokines, and adipokines overflow into the systemic circulation and cause systemic metabolic disease via the same cellular effects that initially unfold in adipocytes. Early overflow occurs via the portal system, which drains visceral adipose tissue venous effluent into the liver, which becomes the first site of systemic metabolic disease and an important secondary site of nutrient buffering via the development of hepatic steatosis. Overflow progresses to involve all peripheral tissues, inducing cell stress and disease in all organ systems. Overflow involves the central nervous system as well, as inflammation and cell stress have been documented in the hypothalamus in obesity, which in turn is thought to disturb peripheral metabolic function via alterations in CNS efferent signaling.

Liver Disease

The liver is the first organ affected by adipose tissue failure. Portal overflow induces hepatic steatosis, the result of an imbalance in delivery and export of hepatocyte lipid. Over 90% of patients with BMI >40 manifest hepatic steatosis, up to 30% of whom will develop steatohepatitis; 10% to 30% of those with steatohepatitis will develop cirrhosis. Race and genetic predispositions to steatohepatitis exist, with Asians and Hispanics at higher risk than Whites or Blacks. The term metabolic dysfunction-associated steatotic liver disease (MASLD, previously nonalcoholic fatty liver disease, NAFLD) is used to define diet-associated aberrations in hepatic lipid content and their resultant metabolic effects. Metabolic dysfunction-associated steatohepatitis (MASH, previously nonalcoholic steatohepatitis, NASH) defines MASLD that progresses to inflammation and fibrosis. Sources of hepatic lipid include dietary fats delivered from the gut as chylomicrons, lipids synthesized by hepatocytes via de novo lipogenesis, and free fatty acids delivered from adipose tissue, with the latter constituting over 60% of hepatic lipid delivery. Lipids are exported from the liver primarily in the form of very low-density lipoproteins (VLDL). Abnormalities in each of these aspects of hepatic lipid delivery and efflux have been identified in obesity. As lipid storage capacity is reached, hepatocytes undergo ER, oxidative, and inflammatory stress, causing steatohepatitis, a histologic entity characterized by Mallory bodies, hepatocyte ballooning and an inflammatory infiltrate consisting of macrophages (Kupffer cells) and other leukocytes. As in adipose tissue, TNF-α plays a central role in the hepatic inflammation; neutralization of TNF-α ameliorates steatohepatitis in mice and is under study as therapy in humans. Weight loss reverses steatosis and halts progression of steatohepatitis. Thyroid hormone receptor-β (THR-β), expressed at high levels by hepatocytes, regulates fatty acid metabolism. THR-β agonists reduce hepatic fibrosis and inflammation and represent a novel therapeutic option for MASH. Resmetirom, a THR-β agonist, is the first pharmacologic agent approved by the FDA for treatment of steatohepatitis.[24]

Diabetes

Insulin resistance is a central metabolic response of all cells to stress. Free fatty acids are important mediators of cellular insulin resistance. Insulin regulates not only glucose homeostasis in adipocytes, but also lipid metabolism, inhibiting lipolysis and free fatty acid release. Nutrient excess, with resultant ER and oxidative stress, induces insulin resistance in adipocytes, impairing glucose uptake, attenuating insulin's inhibitory effects on lipolysis, and increasing free fatty acid release by adipocytes. Free fatty acids in turn activate toll-like receptors on ATM, inducing inflammatory cytokine expression, including TNF-α. TNF-α induces insulin resistance by regulating expression and phosphorylation of genes involved in glucose homeostasis, including insulin receptor, insulin receptor substrates, the cell signaling nexus protein Akt, and glucose transporter molecules. TNF-α also promotes lipolysis, exacerbating free fatty acid release by adipocytes. While other mediators contribute, TNF-α provides an example of the vicious cycle in adipose tissue that contributes to worsening insulin resistance. As adipose tissue buffering capacity is overwhelmed, free fatty acids overflow into the systemic circulation, causing lipotoxicity, which contributes to insulin resistance in peripheral tissues. Skeletal muscle, responsible for 70% of systemic glucose utilization, is a dominant site of peripheral insulin resistance. Lipotoxicity triggers ER, oxidative, and inflammatory stress responses in skeletal muscle myocytes, along with increased macrophages and diabetogenic inflammatory cytokines, contributing to skeletal muscle insulin resistance. As fatty acid delivery to skeletal muscle and liver increases, energy production in these organs shifts from glucose utilization to fatty acid oxidation. Increased free fatty acid beta-oxidation leads to increased hepatic gluconeogenesis and reduced muscle glucose utilization, exacerbating hyperglycemia. The initial response of pancreatic beta cells to peripheral insulin resistance and hyperglycemia is a compensatory increase in insulin secretion, causing hyperinsulinemia, a pathognomonic feature of early type 2 diabetes. As disease progresses, lipotoxicity and cell stress responses eventually lead to pancreatic beta cell exhaustion, decreased insulin secretion, and hypoinsulinemia. Genetics plays an important role in type 2 diabetes: Asian, Black, and Hispanic race are associated with multiple diabetes-associated SNPs and increased disease risk. Worldwide incidence of diabetes is rapidly increasing and is an emerging health crisis.

Cancer

The incidences of almost all types of cancer increase in a dose-dependent manner with BMI, with risk ratios ranging from 2 to >6.[25] At the cellular level, energy homeostasis involves fundamental processes central to carcinogenesis, and signaling pathways activated by chronic over-nutrition promote cell proliferation. Chronic inflammation, characteristic of obesity and a risk factor for cancer, activates NFκB and other signaling pathways that increase production of ROS that contribute to oncogenic mutation and induce expression of inflammatory cytokines that act as cell mitogens. Over-nutrition in obesity predisposes to a state of chronic anabolism, with increased expression of growth factors including insulin, insulin-like growth factor-1, and leptin. Inflammation on a background of chronic anabolism creates an ideal milieu for carcinogenesis. Steroid metabolism is aberrant in obesity and adipose tissue is a source of estrogen, which may promote estrogen-responsive cancers. Epidemiologic data suggest that long-term metformin use is associated with decreased cancer incidence, suggesting the potential for metabolism-based cancer therapy. Adipocytes and adipocyte stem cells are important components of the tumor microenvironment, providing growth factors and energy substrates that promote tumor growth, and suggesting the possibility of adipocyte-targeted therapy for cancer.

SUMMARY

Obesity is associated with an increased risk of cardiovascular disease, including hypertension, atherosclerosis, and hyperlipidemia, the result of cell stress responses that afflict the vasculature. Allergy, atopy, and autoimmune diseases are increased in obesity due to alterations in immune and inflammatory function. While mechanical stress due to excess weight are contributing factors to sleep apnea, osteoarthritis, and gastroesophageal reflux disease, fundamental cell stress mechanisms, including inflammation, have also been implicated. The pansystemic nature of metabolic disease provides opportunity for developing therapy that will simultaneously treat multiple obesity-related pathologies.

References

1. Zillikens MC, Demissie S, Hsu YH, et al. Large meta-analysis of genome-wide association studies identifies five loci for lean body mass. *Nat Commun*. 2017;8(1):80.
2. Neel JV. Diabetes mellitus: a "thrifty" genotype rendered detrimental by "progress"? *Am J Hum Genet*. 1962;14(4):353–362.
3. Bouchard C, Tremblay A, Despres JP, et al. The response to long-term overfeeding in identical twins. *N Engl J Med*. 1990; 322:1477–1482.
4. Loos RJF, Yeo GSH. The genetics of obesity: from discovery to biology. *Nat Rev Genet*. 2022;23(2):120–133.
5. Hales CN, Barker DJ. Type 2 (non-insulin-dependent) diabetes mellitus: the thrifty phenotype hypothesis. *Diabetologia*. 1992; 35(7):595–601.

6. Hetherington AW, Ranson SW. Hypothalamic lesions and adiposity in the rat. *Anat Rec.* 1940;78:149–172.
7. Zhang Y, Proenca R, Maffei M, Barone M, Leopold L, Friedman JM. Positional cloning of the mouse obese gene and its human homologue. *Nature.* 1994;372(6505):425–432.
8. Jastreboff AM, Aronne LJ, Ahmad NN, et al. Tirzepatide once weekly for the treatment of obesity. *N Engl J Med.* 2022; 387(3):205–216.
9. Leibel RL, Rosenbaum M, Hirsch J. Changes in energy expenditure resulting from altered body weight. *N Engl J Med.* 1995; 332:621–628.
10. Levine JA, Eberhardt NL, Jensen MD. Role of nonexercise activity thermogenesis in resistance to fat gain in humans. *Science.* 1999; 283(5399):212–214.
11. Spalding KL, Arner E, Westermark PO, et al. Dynamics of fat cell turnover in humans. *Nature.* 2008;453(7196):783–787.
12. Parrillo L, Spinelli R, Costanzo M, et al. Epigenetic dysregulation of the homeobox A5 (HOXA5) Gene associates with subcutaneous adipocyte hypertrophy in human obesity. *Cells.* 2022;11(4):728.
13. Massier L, Jalkanen J, Elmastas M, et al. An integrated single cell and spatial transcriptomic map of human white adipose tissue. *Nat Commun.* 2023;14(1):1438.
14. Berger ER, Clements RH, Morton JM, et al. The impact of different surgical techniques on outcomes in laparoscopic sleeve gastrectomies: the first report from the Metabolic and Bariatric Surgery Accreditation and Quality Improvement Program (MBSAQIP). *Ann Surg* 2016;264(3):464–473.
15. Simoneau M, McKay B, Brooks E, Doucet É, Baillot A. Gut peptides before and following Roux-En-Y gastric bypass: a systematic review and meta-analysis. *Obes Rev.* 2024;25(5):e13702.
16. Hotamisligil GS, Shargill NS, Spiegelman BM. Adipose expression of tumor necrosis factor-alpha: direct role in obesity-linked insulin resistance. *Science.* 1993;259(5091):87–91.
17. Lord G, Matarese G, Howard J, Baker R, Blooms S, Lechler R. Leptin Modulates T-cell immune response and reverses starvation-induced immunosuppression. *Nature.* 1998;394:897–901.
18. Virtanen KA, Lidell ME, Orava J, et al. Functional brown adipose tissue in healthy adults. *N Engl J Med.* 2009;360: 1518–1525.
19. Shi H, Strader AD, Woods SC, Seeley RJ. The effect of fat removal on glucose tolerance is depot specific in male and female mice. *Am J Physiol Endocrinol Metab.* 2007;293(4):E1012–E1020.
20. Lumeng CN, Bodzin JL, Saltiel AR. Obesity induces a phenotypic switch in adipose tissue macrophage polarization. *J Clin Invest.* 2007;117:89–93.
21. Nance SA, Muir L, Lumeng C. Adipose tissue macrophages: Regulators of adipose tissue immunometabolism during obesity. *Mol Metab.* 2022;66:101642.
22. Khan T, Muise ES, Iyengar P, et al. Metabolic dysregulation and adipose tissue fibrosis: role of collagen VI. *Mol Cell Biol.* 2009;29(6):1575–1591.
23. Baker NA, Muir LA, Washabaugh AR, et al. Diabetes-specific regulation of adipocyte metabolism by the adipose tissue extracellular matrix. *J Clin Endo Metab.* 2017;102(3):1–12.
24. Harrison SA, Bedossa P, Guy CD, et al. MAESTRO-NASH Investigators. A Phase 3, randomized, controlled trial of resmetirom in NASH with liver fibrosis. *N Engl J Med.* 2024;390(6):497–509.
25. Calle EE, Rodriguez C, Walker-Thurmond K, Thun MJ. Overweight, obesity, and mortality from cancer in a prospectively studied cohort of U.S. adults. *N Engl J Med.* 2003;348(17):1625–1638.

3

Wound Healing

James Shadiow and Katherine A. Gallagher

SCIENTIFIC PRINCIPLES

Key Points

1 Wound healing is a complex process that involves four major phases: hemostasis, inflammation, proliferation, and remodeling.

2 Innate immune cells play a major role in the inflammatory phase of healing.

3 Macrophages are critical for the transition from the inflammatory to the proliferative phase.

4 Multiple factors can adversely impact healing including advanced age, poor nutrition, obesity, DM, steroids/chemotherapy.

The role of disease states including diabetes and cancer-related treatments including radiation, chemotherapy, and steroids negatively influence wound repair. Hence, a thorough understanding of the pathways/processes involved in both normal and pathologic healing is essential. Thus, a fundamental understanding of the wound-healing cascade is essential to surgical practice. Besides the controlled injury that occurs in elective surgery, all invasive surgical procedures cause soft tissue trauma regardless of the circumstances. All aspects of surgical care from patient selection, surgical instruments and technique, and postoperative management are needed to optimize tissue healing and avoid complications. In addition to surgical procedures, there is the growing problem of people suffering from chronic wounds, particularly in diabetes is on the rise. Nonhealing wounds affect about 10 million people in the United States, with persons 65 years and older accounting for the majority of these events. The development of new data regarding the normal and pathologic wound-healing responses both at the cellular levels and the biologic markers associated with healing will help develop new therapeutic strategies.

PHASES OF WOUND HEALING

1 Wound healing is a dynamic process that occurs in a programmed series of four phases: hemostasis, inflammation, proliferation, and remodeling.[1] These steps occur in a linear fashion under normal, nondiseased conditions. The timing of these four phases of wound repair is illustrated in **Figure 3.1** and the major cell types involved are shown in **Figure 3.2**.

Hemostasis

The hemostasis phase begins almost instantaneously after injury. The tissue response is mediated by: (1) blood leaking into the wound, (2) proteins stored in the ECM, and (3) locally resident surviving cells following injury.

Following injury, hemostasis occurs and is characterized by the recruitment of platelets and circulating coagulant factors to the wound site to initiate clotting, as shown in **Figure 3.3**.[2] Concurrent with platelet recruitment, injured cells release damage-signaling factors, which activate resident macrophages,[3–6] as well as damage-associated molecular patterns (DAMPs).[7] Together, these stimulate recruitment of polymorphonuclear neutrophils (PMNs) from the vasculature to defend against pathogens.[3,5,7] As platelets aggregate to the exposed collagen bed, they secrete cytokines and growth factors such as platelet-derived growth factors (PDGFs), that promote clotting and serve to further recruit PMNs.[8] Once PMNs begin to migrate to the wound, this initiates the inflammation stage.

The plasma membrane of each platelet contains specific receptors for collagen known as the glycoprotein Ia/IIa complex. When plasma membrane receptors come into contact with collagen of the ECM (type I) and the basement membrane of the vascular endothelium (type IV), platelets bind and anchor to the site. Simultaneously, platelet activation occurs, and the platelet changes from a rounded amorphous shape to a flattened configuration and discharges the contents stored in cytoplasmic granules in an event known as the platelet release reaction. These bioactive factors serve a dual purpose in hemostasis and wound healing. Platelet anchoring is strengthened by von Willebrand factor (vWF) released by damaged endothelium and activated platelets. Platelet binding is also characterized by rapid vascular restriction and the formulation of a stable fibrin clot. Platelets are the main cellular players in the first phase. Platelet-derived functions that achieve hemostasis include: adhesion, aggregation, and formation of a procoagulant surface that facilitates the

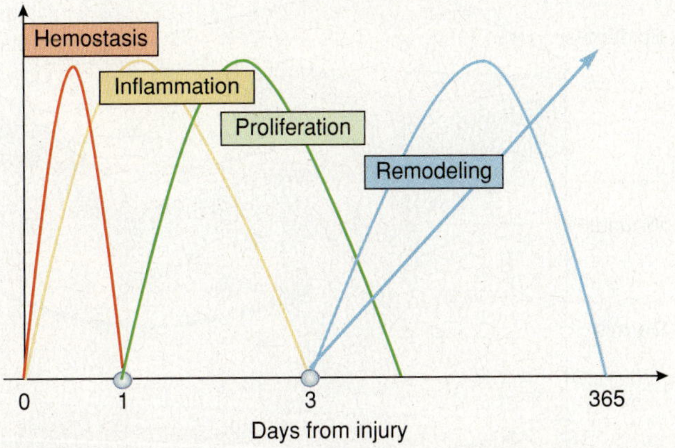

Figure 3.1. Four phases of wound healing: plotted against "Time" on the x-axis, the four phases shown in different colors occur sequentially, and overlap. Overall the total time period for completion is 1 year.

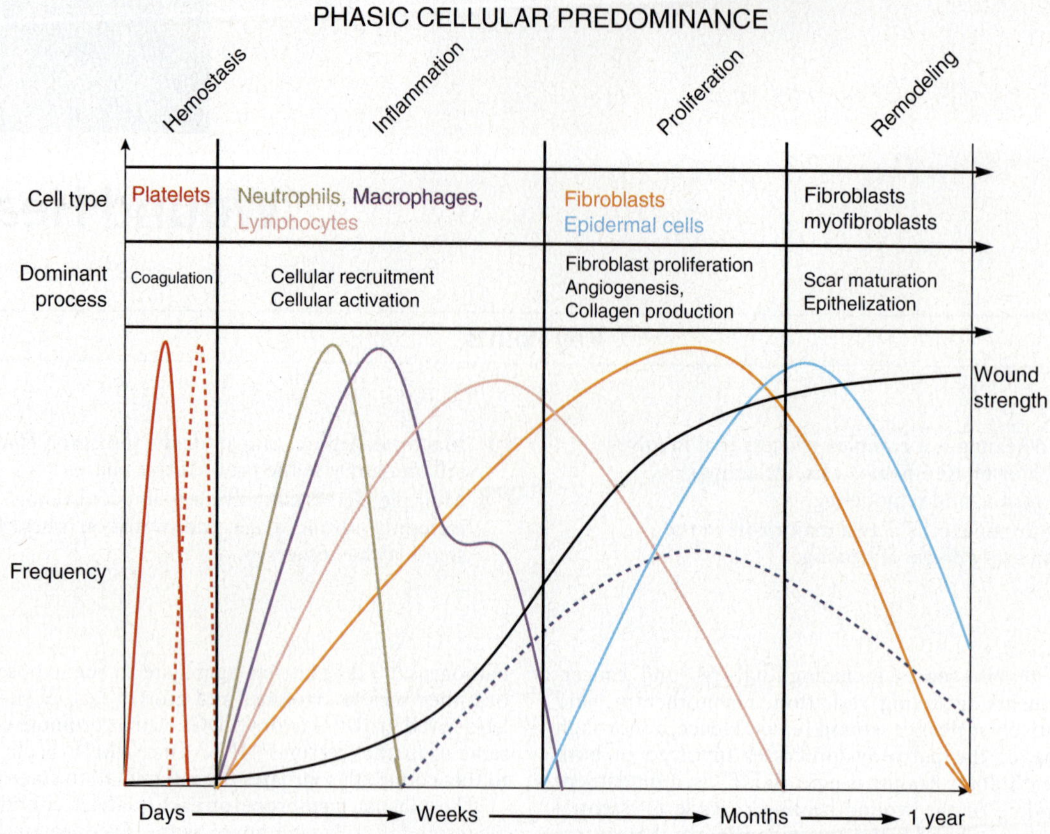

Figure 3.2. The dominant cells, physiologic process as well as the temporal distribution of the four phases of wound healing.

generation of thrombin and results in a fibrin plug. In addition, platelets express and release substances that promote tissue repair and influence future processes such as angiogenesis, inflammation, and the immune response. They contain large, secreted pools of biologically active proteins, including PDGF, transforming growth factor-β (TGF-β), and vascular endothelial growth factor (VEGF) as well as cytokines. The therapeutic use of platelets in a fibrin clot has a positive influence in clinical situations requiring rapid healing; dental implant surgery, orthopedic surgery, muscle and tendon repair, skin ulcers, hole repair in eye surgery and cardiac surgery are situations where the use of autologous platelets accelerates healing.

The growing platelet plug inside the vessel is stabilized by fibrin polymerized from circulating fibrinogen. The vascular response is mediated by local factors modulated by the systemic control of sympathetic nervous system. Vasoconstriction, mediated by catecholamines and prostaglandins (thromboxane and PGF 2α), normally is limited to the time required to achieve hemostasis. Vasodilation and alteration in capillary permeability soon follow mediated by histamine, prostaglandins (PGE2 and PGI2), VEGF released from resident interstitial mast cells, and damaged endothelium. This causes increased blood flow and controlled delivery of fluid, leukocytes, macrophages, and relevant plasma proteins to the wound environment which facilitates the inflammatory phase.

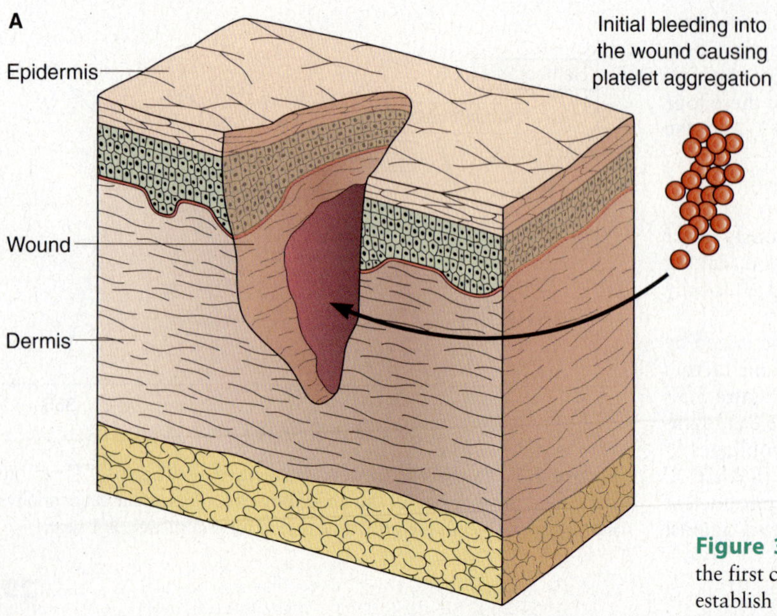

Figure 3.3. A: Diagrammatic wound-healing model. Platelets, the first cells to arrive at the wound are critical to create a clot and establish hemostasis.

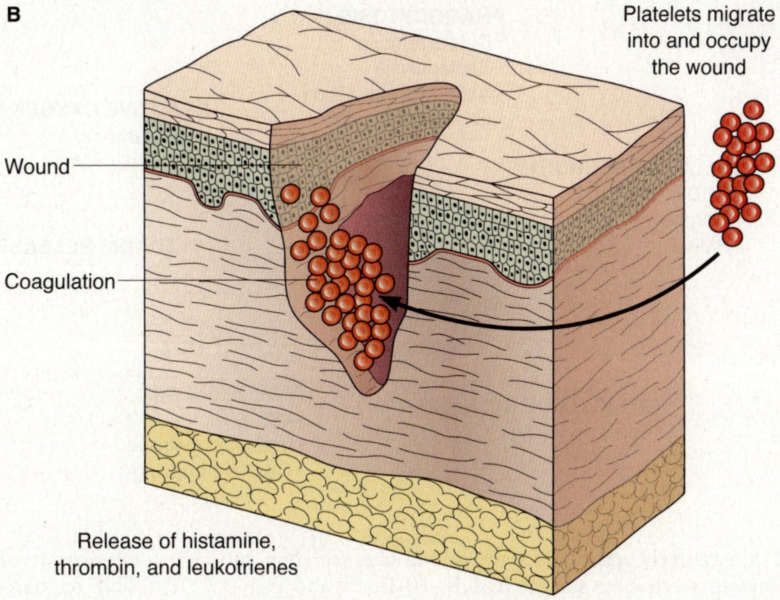

Figure 3.3 (*Continued*) B: Phase 1—Hemostasis.

Platelets release two factors with particular importance for wound healing: PDGF and TGF-β which in turn stimulate chemotaxis and proliferation of inflammatory cells.

Additionally, immediately after injury, the wound is hypoxic due to damage to the microcirculation. Hypoxia likely contributes to the preparation of the next phases of healing. Hypoxia increases keratinocyte migration, early angiogenesis, proliferation and clonal expansion of fibroblasts, and the transcription and synthesis of aforementioned growth factors and cytokines, including PDGF, VEGF, and TGF-β.

Inflammatory Phase

The second phase of healing involves inflammation (acute
2 then chronic) that begins following the hemostasis phase. The cells involved in this phase are mainly immune cells, as shown in **Figure 3.4.** Neutrophils (PMNs) dominate during the early part of the inflammation phase; however, their presence is
3 short lived as they start to wane after 24 to 48 hours.[9] PMNs set the stage for the appearance of macrophages, the most important cellular mediator of the inflammatory phase of wound healing (**Fig. 3.5**). Neutrophils release chemokines that are responsible for recruiting circulating monocytes from the peripheral blood to the wound site. Recruited monocytes that differentiate into macrophages and dendritic cells, along with F4/80+ resident tissue macrophages, carry out the critical steps of the inflammatory phase of wound healing.[10,11] However, the specific roles of recruited monocytes/macrophages, dendritic cells, and tissue macrophages in wound healing are unclear.[12] Wound macrophages initially display a "classical" activation state, indicated by expression of proinflammatory cytokines such as IL-12, IL-1β, IL-6, TNF-α, and iNOS.

Proinflammatory, or M1-like, macrophages work to clear debris, recruit additional inflammatory cells (**Fig. 3.6**), and promote tissue regenerative processes including angiogenesis. Stimulated macrophages produce high levels of proangiogenic factors like VEGF, contributing significantly to the wound angiogenic response downstream of inflammation.[13] Indeed, depletion studies in skin have shown that macrophages are a crucial source of the overall proangiogenic stimulus.[14,15] As the inflammatory phase progresses, macrophages phagocytose apoptotic cells in the wound and chemokines are released (eg, CXCL12), promoting the transition from a proinflammatory state to one promoting tissue repair and remodeling.[16,17] This occurs as the predominant macrophage phenotype in the wound transitions to

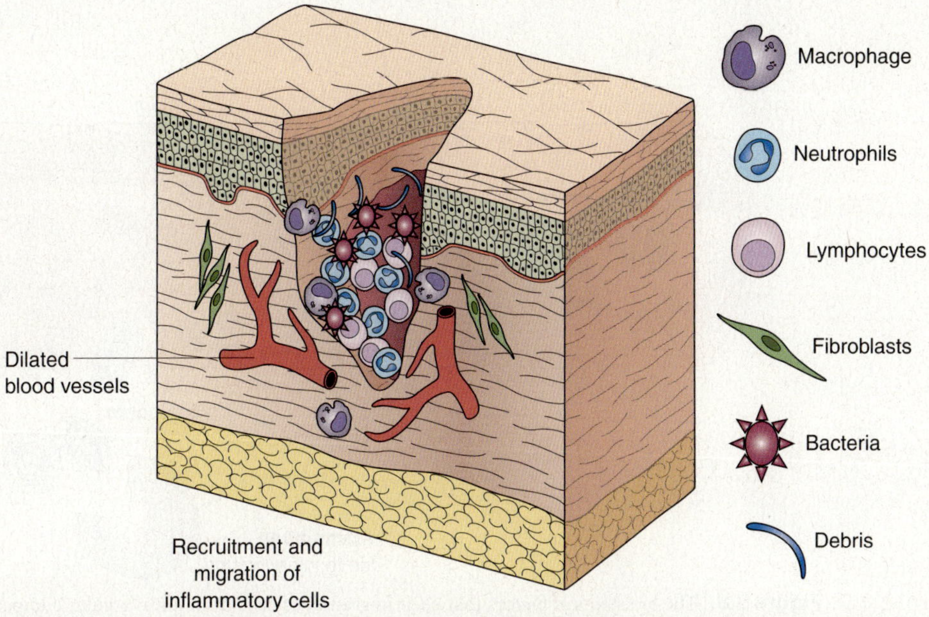

Figure 3.4. Phase 2—Inflammation.

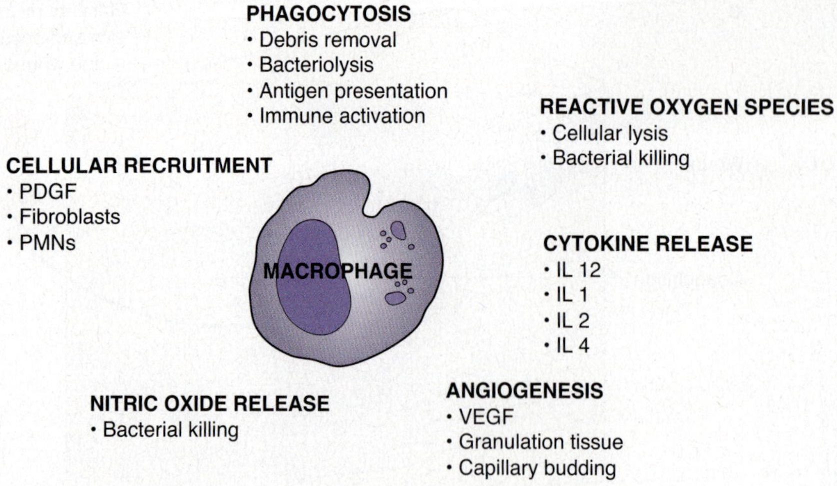

Figure 3.5. Macrophage functions.

an "alternatively activated" state, or M2-like, secreting anti-inflammatory cytokines such as IL-4, IL-10, IL-13, and TGF-β.[10,18] In vivo, macrophages exist along a spectrum and the distinct phenotypes seen in vitro (eg, M1, M2) are rarely seen.[10,19,20]

The mechanisms underlying monocyte–macrophage phenotype plasticity in vivo are complex but are under intense investigation. An early step in this transition of monocyte–macrophages from the proinflammatory to the anti-inflammatory phenotype, and thus the initiation of tissue repair, is the ingestion of apoptotic PMNs and other immune cells by monocyte–macrophages. Apoptotic neutrophils have been found to secrete a variety of signaling molecules, such as lysophosphatidylcholine, which attract monocyte–macrophages via the chemotaxis receptor G2A, causing subsequent engulfment of these cells.[21] As wound healing progresses, monocyte–macrophages show increased expression of MerTK, a cell-surface tyrosine kinase involved in phagocytosis of apoptotic cells; these MerTK^{+}Ly6C^{lo} monocyte–macrophages demonstrate the ability to produce VEGF and TGF-β.[22] Indeed, it appears that phagocytosis of these apoptotic cells triggers the release of these growth factors and augments other tissue repair processes. In one study, Voll et al.[23] demonstrated that coculture of LPS-activated monocyte–macrophages with apoptotic lymphocytes inhibited monocyte–macrophage expression of proinflammatory mediators such as TNF-α and increased release of anti-inflammatory cytokines. These findings were replicated in a subsequent study where human peripheral blood monocytes failed to upregulate expression of proinflammatory mediators IL-1β, IL-8, and TNF-α, but demonstrated increased TGF-β expression in monocyte–macrophages that engulfed apoptotic PMNs compared with naive monocyte–macrophages.[24]

In addition to the cellular and molecular mechanisms underlying monocyte–macrophage plasticity, the maturing field of epigenetics has become a new focus in the investigation of monocyte-macrophage–mediated inflammation. A number of epigenetic alterations have been associated with MΦ polarization.[25,26] Histone deacetylases (HDACs) are a group of epigenetic regulators associated with influencing monocyte–macrophage phenotype via alterations in chromatin conformation. For example, HDAC3 has been found to promote proinflammatory and inhibit anti-inflammatory monocyte–macrophage polarization.[27–29] In Mullican et al.,[28] mice lacking HDAC3 in monocyte–macrophages displayed a gene expression profile recapitulating in vitro M2 activation. Furthermore, a chromatin immunoprecipitation assay revealed localization of HDAC3 to a subset of sites bound by PU.1, a major determinant of the monocyte–macrophage epigenome.[30,31]

Epigenetic enzymes also play a role in monocyte–macrophage phenotype skewing in type 2 diabetes (T2D) and metabolic syndrome. Hyperlipidemia has been shown to induce DNA methylation and repress anti-inflammatory cytokines; similarly, a genome-wide analysis for promoter methylation in MΦs revealed hypomethylation of M1 genes and hypermethylation of M2 reparative genes.[32] DNA methyltransferase 3b has been found to promote M1 activation in

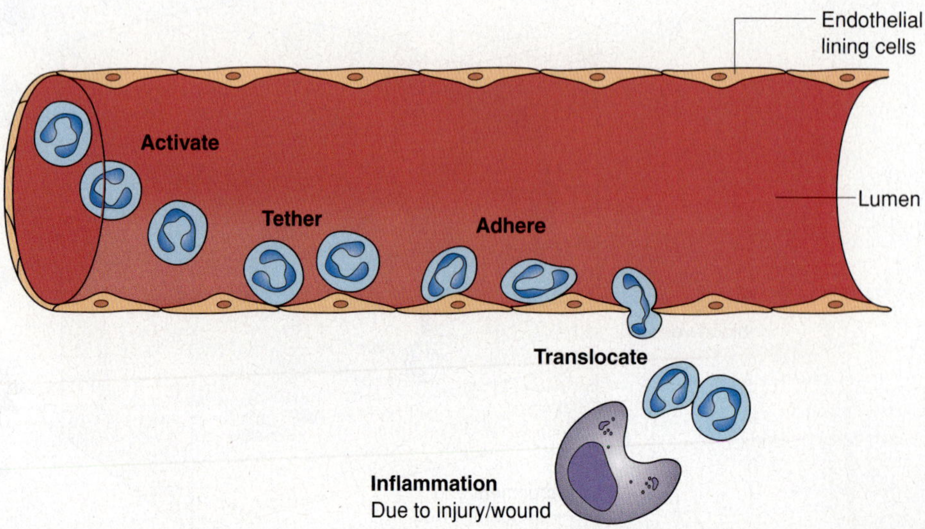

Figure 3.6. The biochemical factors that elicit migration of cells from intravascular compartment into the wound site.

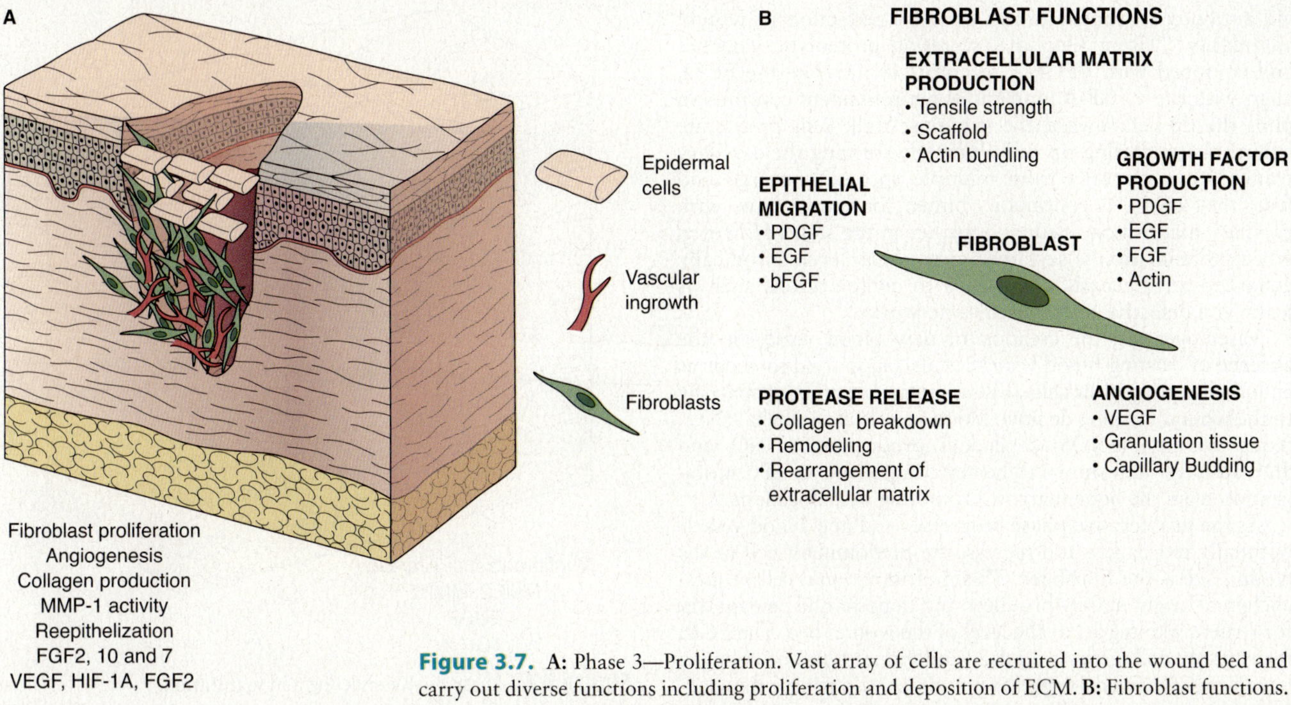

Figure 3.7. **A:** Phase 3—Proliferation. Vast array of cells are recruited into the wound bed and carry out diverse functions including proliferation and deposition of ECM. **B:** Fibroblast functions.

obese mice by DNA methylation of peroxisome proliferator–activated receptor γ1 promoter. Furthermore, knockdown of DNA methyltransferase 3b enhances M2 activation and suppresses the M1 response.[33]

Given the role of epigenetic factors in the systemic inflammatory milieu of T2D and metabolic syndrome, attention has recently turned to epigenetic alterations present within diabetic wounds. Alterations in histone methylation have been linked to impairments in diabetic wound healing. As mentioned previously, pathologic expression of IL-1β contributes to impaired wound healing.[34] In a study by Kimball et al.,[10] monocyte–macrophages isolated from wounds of a diet-induced obese mouse model of T2D expressed increased IL-1β after stimulation with LPS, and chromatin immunoprecipitation analysis revealed increased histone H3 lysine (H3K) 4 (H3K4; activation mark) and decreased H3K27 (repressive mark) methylation, suggesting an epigenetic mechanism underlying IL-1β expression. Another epigenetic event that strongly influences healing is decreased global methylation through a reduction of (H3K27) trimethylation.[35] Gallagher et al.[36] discovered that, in diet-induced obese mice, the IL-12 promoter exhibited increased demethylation of the repressive H3K27me3 mark in bone marrow progenitor cells, circulating blood monocytes and tissue monocyte–macrophages. This allowed increased expression of proinflammatory IL-12. Further, the histone demethylase enzyme JMJD3 was decreased at the IL-12 gene, suggesting that these monocyte–macrophages were epigenetically preprogrammed toward a proinflammatory phenotype, ultimately negatively impacting wound healing.[36]

MicroRNAs regulate gene expression and interact with epigenetic enzymes through a complicated feedback network. It has recently been demonstrated that hyperglycemia leads to changes in the microRNA signature in wound healing, and they have been found to play a role in the dysregulated inflammation of diabetic wounds.[37–39] For example, miR-125b epigenetically enhances monocyte–macrophage activation by increasing the responsiveness to IFN-γ and concurrently inhibits the reparative phenotype by targeting the M2 transcription factor IRF4.[40] Thus, although this field of study is in its relative infancy, there is great potential for continued exploration of the epigenetic mechanisms in inflammatory disease and diabetic wound healing.

Proliferation Phase

The subsequent proliferation phase is characterized by the recruitment and activation of keratinocytes and fibroblasts (**Fig. 3.7A**). During this phase, growth factors stimulate keratinocytes to reepithelialize the wound.[18] During this time, the provisional matrix established by platelets during hemostasis is replaced by granulation tissue, a new connective tissue with dense vascularization and fibroblast populations. Fibroblasts secrete proteinases and matrix metalloproteases (MMPs) to degrade the provisional matrix while simultaneously secreting collagen and other extracellular matrix (ECM) proteins into the granulation tissue (**Fig. 3.7B**).[41] Emerging evidence has also identified a distinct activated fibroblast subtype in several forms of tissue repair including wound healing. The FSP1+ fibroblast subset, which is distinct from the well-established, injury-activated αSMA+ myofibroblasts, appears to play a significant role in promoting angiogenesis and possibly regenerative wound healing through robust expression of *Vegfa*, *Vegfb*, and other proangiogenic factors, including *Grem1*, *Angpt1*, and *Fgf1*.[42]

The defining characteristic of the proliferative phase of healing is ECM production. The provisional ECM is a protein scaffold that stabilizes wound edges and provides a framework for migration of PMNs, macrophages, fibroblasts, and other cells into the wound from surrounding tissues. As the inflammatory phase slows, the proliferative phase begins and becomes dominant, and fibroblasts replace macrophages as the most numerous cell type. Like macrophages, fibroblasts are multifunctional. They are responsible for new tissue formation, collagen production, and the laying down of the ECM.

Simultaneously, angiogenesis occurs as new capillaries form, and blood vessels penetrate the provisional ECM sprouting from vessels of the surrounding uninjured tissues. Although angiogenesis is greatest during the proliferative stage giving rise to highly vascularized granulation, it is initiated immediately after tissue injury and is mediated throughout the wound-healing process. The steps of sprouting angiogenesis include enzymatic degradation of capillary basement membrane, endothelial cell (EC) proliferation, directed migration of ECs, tubulogenesis (EC tube formation), vessel fusion, vessel pruning, and pericyte stabilization.[43] An endothelial tip cell guides the developing capillary sprout through the ECM toward an angiogenic stimulus, the most well studied being VEGF-A. In murine wound models, neutralization of VEGF via antibody treatment causes a ~50% reduction in wound vascularity.[44] Using filopodia, secreting proteolytic enzymes and equipped with VEGF-A receptors to navigate the ECM, align with the VEGF-A gradient as actin filament contraction pulls the tip cell toward the stimulus. Stalk cells proliferate behind the migrating tip cell ultimately forming the capillary trunk. When tip cells from multiple sprouts converge and fuse, they create a continuous lumen for blood flow, with capillary maturation occurring further in the stage. However, when inflammation is sustained at the local level, chronically enhanced angiogenesis often leads to complications such as leaky and defective microvascular networks.[45]

Vasculogenesis, the creation of new blood vessels in the absence of existing blood vessels, is also supported to occur as endothelial progenitor cells (EPCs) migrate from bone marrow to the wound forming de novo blood vessels. Endothelial (NO) oxide synthase (eNOS)–dependent production of NO and SDF-1α have been shown to be key components of EPC mobilization from the bone marrow promoting vasculogenesis.[46]

As the proliferative phase progresses and new blood vessels optimally reorganize and regress, the predominant cell in the wound site is the fibroblast. This multifunctional cell of mesenchymal origin mainly produces and deposits the new matrix for structural integrity at the level of the wound bed. The ECM is primarily collagen. At least 23 individual types of collagen have been identified—type I is present mostly in scar tissues.[47] Fibroblasts produce collagen via their attachment to the cables of the provisional fibrin matrix.[48] During this process, there is an important step involving hydroxylation of proline and lysine residues.[49] The collagen molecule transforms itself into the classical triple helical structure and thereafter its nascent chains are modified through glycosylation[50]; this procollagen molecule is released into the extracellular space.[51] The hydroxyproline in collagen gives the molecule its stable helical conformation,[52] whereas fully hydroxylated collagen has higher stability, unhydroxylated forms are fragile, similar to collagen produced under anaerobic disease conditions or vitamin C–deficient states (scurvy), where in the collagen undergoes denaturation easily and can break.

Finally, collagen released into the extracellular space undergoes further processing by cleavage of the procollagen N- and C-terminal peptides. Cross-linking steps give collagen its strength and stability over time.[53]

As the proliferation stage concludes, vascular stabilization occurs involving Ang-1/Tie-2–dependent production of endothelial-secreted PDGF for the recruitment of smooth muscle cells and pericytes. PDGF deficiency results in poorly formed immature blood vessels.[54] Angiogenesis is then suppressed in the final stages of healing as tissue hypoxia is restored, inflammation subsides, growth factors decline, pericytes secrete inhibitory TGF-β, and endostatin from collagen XVIII inhibits vascular proliferation.

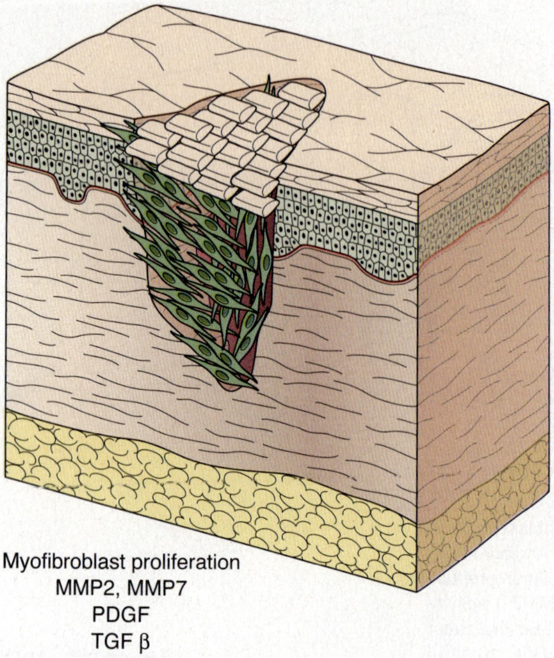

Figure 3.8. Phase 4—Remodeling and maturation.

Remodeling Phase

The final phase of wound healing is the remodeling phase and begins once granulation tissue is present (**Fig. 3.8**). Here, fibroblasts differentiate into contractile myofibroblasts that contract the wound and the collagen III deposited in the ECM during the proliferation phase is exchanged for collagen I which has a higher tensile strength.[55] Once healed, the site is mechanically functional but many structural components, for example, hair follicles, may not recover and the healed site has, at maximum, ~70% of the original tensile strength.[18]

The remodeling phase is characterized by continued synthesis and degradation of the ECM components trying to establish a new equilibrium—and the formation of an organized scar (**Fig. 3.9**). Collagen degradation occurs[56] via the action of specific collagenases that are secreted by various cells;

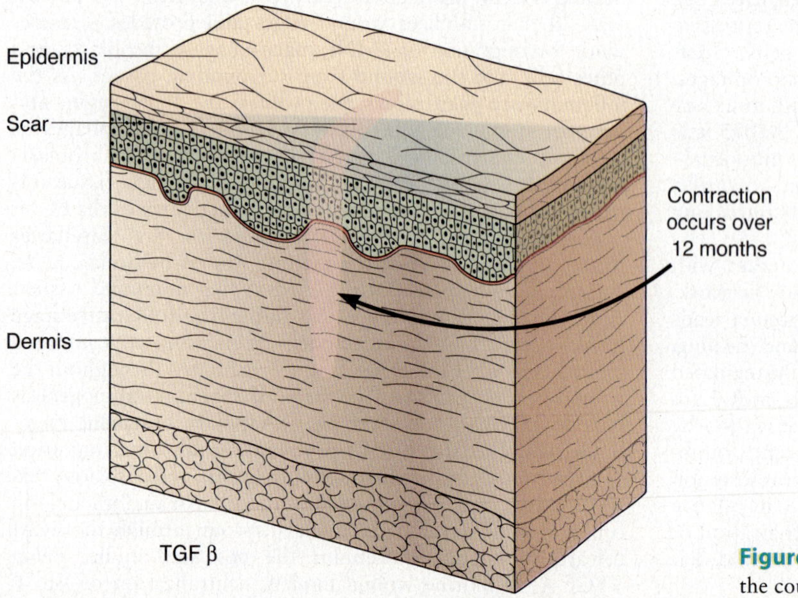

Figure 3.9. Contraction of scar—This process occurs over the course of 1 year.

fibroblasts, neutrophils, and macrophages each of which can cleave the collagen molecule at differing specific locations on all three chains and break it down to characteristic three-quarter and one-quarter pieces. These collagen fragments undergo further denaturation and digestion by other proteases. Several molecules including TGF-β play a major role in the remodeling phase.Figure 3.9. Effects of biofilm on wound healing.

Patterning newly vascularized tissue involves the selective regression of certain vessels and network maturation through branching and splitting by nonsprouting angiogenesis, known as intussusception.[57] Intussusception, where vessel lumens are divided internally by transcapillary tissue pillars, is not well understood, but Tie receptors are known to play a role.[58]

CLINICAL CONSIDERATIONS

Multiple clinical pathologies can impair wound healing.

Chronic Versus Acute Wounds

4 Wounds heal within a reasonable time of 4 to 6 weeks. Those that do not are termed chronic. As shown in **Table 3.1**, a variety of factors and disease conditions impair wound healing and result in chronic nonhealing wounds. Reasons that lead to chronicity instead of normal healing, are complex—but the salient points are detailed below. The most important concept is a persistent proinflammatory condition that paradoxically leads to increased degradation of matrix proteins and an unstable wound that is recalcitrant to healing.

Advanced Age and Gender

Many clinical and animal studies at the cellular and molecular level have examined age-related changes and delays in wound healing. It is commonly recognized that, in healthy older adults, the effect of aging causes a temporal delay in wound healing, but not an actual impairment in terms of the quality of healing.[59] Delayed wound healing in the aged is associated with an altered inflammatory response, such as delayed T-cell infiltration into the wound area with alterations in chemokine production and reduced macrophage–phagocytic capacity.[60] Overall, there are global differences in wound healing between young and aged individuals.

Sex hormones play a role in age-related wound-healing deficits. Compared with aged females, aged males have been shown to have delayed healing of acute wounds. A partial explanation for this is that the female estrogens (estrone and 17β-estradiol), male androgens (testosterone and 5α-dihydrotestosterone, DHT), and their steroid precursor dehydroepiandrosterone (DHEA), appear to have significant effects on the wound-healing process.[61] It was recently found that the differences in gene expression between elderly male and young human wounds are almost exclusively estrogen regulated.[62] Estrogen affects wound healing by regulating a variety of genes associated with regeneration, matrix production, protease inhibition, epidermal function, and genes primarily associated with inflammation.[63] Studies indicate that estrogen can improve the age-related impairment in healing in both men and women, while androgens regulate cutaneous wound healing negatively.

Several treatments to reduce the age-related impairment of healing have been studied. Interestingly, exercise has been reported to improve cutaneous wound healing in older adults as well as aged mice, and the improvement is associated with decreased levels of proinflammatory cytokines in the wound tissue. Improved healing response may also be due to an exercise-induced anti-inflammatory response in the wound.[64]

Table 3.1. Cellular and Biologic Events that Frame the Normal Wound-Healing Process

Phase	Cellular and Biophysiologic Events
Hemostasis	Vascular constriction Platelet aggregation, degranulation, and fibrin formation (thrombus)
Inflammation	Neutrophil infiltration Monocyte infiltration and differentiation to macrophage Lymphocyte infiltration
Proliferation	1. Reepithelialization 2. Angiogenesis 3. Collagen synthesis 4. ECM formation
Remodeling	1. Collagen remodeling 2. Vascular maturation and regression

ECM, extracellular matrix.

Nutrition

Malnutrition or specific nutrient deficiencies can have a profound impact on wound healing after trauma and surgery. Patients with nonhealing wounds and experiencing nutrition deficiency often require special nutrients, energy, carbohydrates, proteins, fat, vitamins, and mineral metabolism all can affect the healing process.[65]

Glutamine is the most abundant amino acid in plasma and is a major source of metabolic energy for rapidly proliferating cells such as fibroblasts, lymphocytes, epithelial cells, and macrophages, glutamine improves nitrogen balance and diminishes immunosuppression and plays a critical role in stimulating the early inflammatory phase of wound healing. Major surgery, trauma, and sepsis require supplementation of glutamine. Oral glutamine supplementation has been shown to improve wound-breaking strength and to increase levels of mature collagen.[66]

Lipids are used as nutritional support for surgical or critically ill patients to help meet energy demands and provide essential building blocks for wound healing and tissue repair. Polyunsaturated fatty acids (UFAs), consist mainly of two families, n-6 (omega-6 found in soybean oil) and n-3 (omega-3 found in fish oil). Although fish oil has been widely touted, effects of omega-3 fatty acids on wound healing are not conclusive. They have been reported to affect proinflammatory cytokine production, cell metabolism, gene expression, and angiogenesis in wound sites.[67]

Vitamins, Micronutrients, and Trace Elements

Vitamins C (L-ascorbic acid), A (retinol), and E (tocopherol) show potent antioxidant and anti-inflammatory effects. Vitamin C has many roles in wound healing and a deficiency in this vitamin has multiple effects on tissue repair. Vitamin C deficiencies result in impaired healing and have been linked to decreased collagen synthesis and fibroblast proliferation, decreased angiogenesis, and increased capillary fragility. Also, vitamin C deficiency leads to impaired immune response increased susceptibility to wound infection. Similarly, vitamin A deficiency leads to impaired wound healing. The biologic properties of vitamin A include antioxidant activity, increased fibroblast, proliferation, modulation of the cellular differentiation and proliferation, increased collagen and hyaluronate synthesis, and decreased MMP-mediated ECM degradation.[1]

Obesity

The prevalence of obesity continues to increase among adults, children, and adolescents in the United States, with more than 30% of adults and 15% of children and adolescents classified as obese in a recent study. Obesity is well known to increase the risk of many diseases and health conditions, which include coronary heart disease, T2D, cancer, hypertension, dyslipidemia, stroke, sleep apnea, respiratory problems, and impaired wound healing. Obese individuals frequently face wound complications, including skin-wound infection, dehiscence, hematoma and seroma formation, pressure ulcers, and venous ulcers.[68] An increased frequency of wound complications has been reported for obese individuals undergoing both bariatric and nonbariatric operations.[69] In particular, a higher rate of surgical site infection occurs in obese patients.

The function of adipose tissue used to be considered as primary caloric storage. However, more recent findings have documented that adipose tissue secretes a large variety of bioactive substances that are collectively named adipokines. Both adipocytes as well as resident macrophages in adipose tissue are known to produce bioactive molecules including cytokines, chemokines and hormone-like factors such as leptin, adiponectin, and resistin. Adipokines have a profound impact on the immune and inflammatory response.[70] The negative influence of adipokines on the systemic immune response seems likely to influence the healing process, although direct proof for this is lacking. Impaired peripheral blood mononuclear cell function, decreased lymphocyte proliferation, and altered peripheral cytokine levels have been reported in obesity. Importantly, many of the obesity-related changes in peripheral immune function are improved by weight loss.[71]

Diabetes Mellitus

Over 30 million people over the age of 18 in the United States have diabetes mellitus.[72] Additionally, another 86 million live with "prediabetes," a condition that can progress to T2D.[72] The overall prevalence of diabetes continues to increase, thereby contributing to increasingly high health care costs.[72] Diabetes-related health care expenditure was 548 billion USD in 2013, accounting for 11% of the total adult health care cost, and is projected to exceed 627 billion USD by 2035.[73] Further, it is estimated that approximately 7 million people go undiagnosed thus delaying disease treatment and management.[72] Nonhealing wounds that result in lower limb amputation, are among the most common complications associated with diabetes and account for more than 200 billion USD annually in health care costs and loss of productivity.[74] Importantly, amputation is associated with high mortality rates of 16.7% at 12 months and over 50% at 5 years, rates that are worse than many cancers.[75]

Impaired wound healing in diabetes is the result of a combination of factors that promote inflammation and disrupt epithelialization and wound closure. Although this process is complex, it has been shown that neutrophils and macrophages recruited to the site of the wound are critical components of the healing process.[76–78] During the normal healing process, macrophages are initially proinflammatory and then transition to an anti-inflammatory phenotype where they promote tissue repair and transition to the next phase of healing.[77,79,80] In diabetic wounds, however, this macrophage transition is altered, causing them to remain in a proinflammatory state and preventing wound resolution.[11,36,81,82] The factors driving the macrophage transition are not fully understood but recent evidence suggests that epigenetics plays a role in regulating macrophage function in both normal and diabetic wound healing.[36,83–86] These processes include DNA methylation of CpG islands, and methylation of histone tails.

Additionally, reepithelialization is delayed in diabetic wounds due to impaired keratinocyte and fibroblast function brought on by hyperglycemia and accumulation of advanced glycation end products (AGEs),[87–90] and epigenetic regulation has also been implicated in these processes.[91–93]

The etiology of nonhealing diabetic foot ulcerations is multifactorial due to a combination of peripheral neuropathy, peripheral artery disease, and altered immune function.[94] These factors work together to predispose the diabetic patient to ulceration and infection. Despite the cause of the wound, it is failure of the wound to heal that is responsible for considerable morbidity and mortality associated with diabetes. Neuropathic edema makes the diabetic foot susceptible to ulceration and infection[95] and ischemia resulting from occlusive arterial disease reduces blood flow,[96] both contributing to delayed healing in the diabetic wound. Additionally, recruitment of EPCs is impaired in diabetes due to reduced NO production which, ultimately, results in impaired angiogenesis.[46] However, the most direct effects on wound healing come from functional alterations in cells activated by the immune response, including platelets, macrophages, neutrophils, ECs, fibroblasts, and keratinocytes; all contributing to a failure to progress through the normal phases of wound healing.

Platelets

Platelets are key constituents of hemostasis and are responsible for some of the earliest events in response to injury, initially forming a platelet plug. As healing progresses, however, the clot must be degraded in order for reepithelialization to occur. Sustained high glucose and insulin resistance causes platelets to release high levels of fibrinogen and plasminogen activator inhibitor 1 (PAI-1), making them more adherent to the vascular endothelium and more likely to aggregate.[97,98] Additionally, under diabetic conditions, platelets have been shown to be less responsive to NO released from the vascular endothelium which normally reduces aggregation at the vessel wall.[99] Exacerbating this, defects in insulin signaling cause the vascular endothelium to produce less NO.[100,101] Thus, platelet dysfunction in diabetes contributes to development of microvascular disease that is well established in diabetic patients. Hence, in the setting of wound healing, the platelet phenotype induced by diabetes hinders wound healing by reducing coagulation during hemostasis.

Neutrophils

Neutrophils are important components during the inflammatory phase of wound healing, working to clear pathogens. However, sustained recruitment and activation of neutrophils are associated with chronic, nonhealing wounds.[102–104] In fact, it has previously been reported that depletion of neutrophils accelerates the rate of reepithelialization in sterile, nondiabetic and diabetic murine wounds.[105] Elevated levels of neutrophil-derived proteases are believed to contribute to persistent inflammation and delayed wound healing.[102,103] In addition to proteases, neutrophils release extracellular traps (NETs) composed of decondensed chromatin lined with cytotoxic proteins to kill microbes.[104] It has been shown that the protein responsible for NET formation, peptidyl deiminase 4 (PAD4), is elevated in neutrophils from diabetic mice and humans making them more susceptible to NETosis. Separately, NLRP3 and NETs production are elevated in human and rat diabetic wounds, with NETs triggering NLRP3 inflammasome activation and IL-1β release via the TLR-4/TLR-9/NF-κB signaling pathway and generating reactive oxygen species.[106] Alleviation of NLRP3 inflammasome activity beneficially regulated immune cell infiltration and accelerated wound healing in a diabetic rat model. Together these mechanisms illustrate the contribution of neutrophils for sustained inflammation in diabetic wounds.[104]

Monocytes/Macrophages

Monocytes are recruited to the wound site very early during the inflammatory phase where they differentiate into macrophages and dendritic cells. Despite the lack of clarity regarding the in vivo definition of these cells, there is substantial evidence that infiltrating monocytes/macrophages are critical for establishing the initial inflammatory phase as well as promoting the transition from a proinflammatory to anti-inflammatory environment.[36,77,79] In diabetic wounds this transition does not occur and macrophages remain in a persistent inflammatory state where they promote the destruction of the surrounding tissue both directly and indirectly by recruiting other proinflammatory immune cells.[36,107,108] It has been recently reported that Ly6C^{Hi} monocytes/macrophages, which have been shown to promote inflammation, normally transition to Ly6C^{Lo}, which are more regenerative; however, in diabetic wounds, a second wave of Ly6C^{Hi} macrophages are recruited during the reparative phase and fail to transition to the anti-inflammatory Ly6C^{Lo} cells contributing to a sustained proinflammatory environment.[10] Plasticity of macrophages may be largely due to alterations in epigenetic profiles and responses. In diabetic wound macrophages, JMJD3 is elevated, a histone demethylase regulating H3K27me3-mediated gene repression, regulated by IL-6 via the JAK1,3/STAT3 pathway which induces NF-κB by IL-6 via the JA and increased inflammatory macrophage gene expression. However, macrophage-specific nanoparticle inhibition of JMJD3 improves wound repair by reducing inflammatory cytokines.[109] Setdb2 also regulates macrophage plasticity during normal and pathologic wound repair via trimethylation of H3K9 at NF-κB binding sites on inflammatory cytokine gene promoters to suppress transcription, with its expression in wound macrophages regulated by interferon (IFN)-β.[110] However, in diabetic wounds, macrophages failed to exhibit a surge in IFN-β during the transition from the inflammatory phase. Consequently, these macrophages showed reduced recruitment of Setdb2 to inflammatory cytokine promoters, leading to unchecked transcription of inflammatory genes where only pharmacologic targeting of Setdb2 or the uric acid (UA) pathway improves wound healing.

Furthermore, it has been shown that hyperglycemia and formation of AGEs impede the phagocytic capacity of macrophages ability to clear apoptotic neutrophils thereby promoting a sustained proinflammatory state.[111,112] Since the transition from a pro- to anti-inflammatory state is partly stimulated by neutrophil clearance, this results in a higher number of proinflammatory macrophages present in the wound. Additionally, studies have shown that monocyte–macrophage infiltration is sustained in diabetic mouse models due to alterations in expression of P-selectin and macrophage chemoattractant protein 1 (MCP-1).[107]

Endothelial Cells

ECs line the luminal surface of blood vessels and are responsible for regulating vascular tone (ie, vasodilation, vasoconstriction), vascular permeability, and oxygen/nutritive diffusion.

The perturbation of angiogenesis in diabetic wounds is complex. Compared to wild-type mice, diabetic mice exhibit significantly decreased vessel surface area, branch junction number, total vessel length, and total branch number in their wounds, along with increased capillary permeability and decreased pericyte coverage.[113] Diabetic wounds also show significant disruptions in the expression of factors affecting vascular regrowth, maturation, and stability, including downregulation of VEGF-A, Sprouty2, PEDF, LRP6, Thrombospondin 1, CXCL10, CXCR3, PDGFR in wounds, along with Semaphorin3a, Neuropilin 1, Angiopoietin 2, NG2, and RGS5.

Vasodilation is regulated by expression of vasoactive factors such as eNOS.[114] Reduced eNOS expression and NO production are associated with diabetic peripheral neuropathy and peripheral artery disease and contribute to decreased peripheral blood flow which, in turn, slows wound healing.[115,116] Indeed, impaired wound healing and angiogenesis defects have been observed in eNOS$^{-/-}$ mice comparable to that of diabetic (*db/db*) mice.[117] Diabetic mouse wounds exhibit reduced or unproductive angiogenesis and significantly fewer vessels despite the presence of proangiogenic factors.[113] However, defective wound healing in the mouse model of diet-induced obesity has been overcome by modulating NO production via overexpression of eNOS. The beneficial effects of NO-dependent improvements in wound healing are likely due to proangiogenic effects as multiple reports witness experimental conditions that improve endothelial NO production in conjunction with increases in tube formation in vitro.[116,118,119]

Notch1 signaling regulates endothelial tip-stalk function. Notch1 is activated by hyperglycemia in diabetic skin and specifically impairs granulation development, proliferation, angiogenesis, and ultimately wound healing in diabetes.[120] Local inhibition of Notch1 signaling in experimental wounds markedly improves angiogenesis and healing in diabetic mice. However, it is unclear if the improvements stemming from inhibition of Notch signaling in vivo are endothelial dependent or contributed by keratinocytes and fibroblasts.

Additionally, EPCs are required for neovascularization of the wound and eNOS stimulates mobilization of EPCs from the bone marrow[46,121]; the observed decrease in eNOS during diabetes also contributes to impaired local angiogenesis. High glucose has been shown to impair the proliferation and function of early and late EPCs.[119] NO donor reversed the impairments, suggesting the role of NO-mediated mechanisms in hyperglycemia-caused EPC functional impairment.

Keratinocytes and Fibroblasts

Recently, the complex role type I IFNs play in keratinocytes in early normal and diabetic wound healing has been illustrated.[122] In diabetic conditions, decreased IFN-κ in wound keratinocytes impairs early inflammation, while the histone methyltransferase MLL1, upregulated after injury, regulates IFN-κ expression through an H3K4me3-mediated mechanism. Studies using a genetically engineered mouse model, and human tissues show that MLL1 controls IFN-κ expression in keratinocytes, and administering IFN-κ early after injury enhances diabetic tissue repair by boosting inflammation, collagen deposition, and reepithelialization.

However, most notably, the late phase of wound healing is carried out by keratinocytes and fibroblasts. In nonhealing diabetic wounds, a variety of alterations in keratinocyte function contribute to diminished epithelialization including defective keratinocyte migration and proliferation,[123,124] gap junction abnormalities,[125] chronic inflammation and infection,[107,126] reduced angiogenesis,[16,121] oxidative stress,[126] and abnormal expression of MMPs.[92,127,128] The mechanisms associated with these processes have been reviewed elsewhere.[129–131]

Alterations in fibroblast function also contribute to dysfunctional epithelialization and delayed healing in diabetic wounds. These are primarily involved with decreased proliferation, increased apoptosis, and impaired migration to the wound site.[89,90,132] Impaired wound healing in diabetes is strongly linked to disrupted fibroblast differentiation into myofibroblasts, interrupted myofibroblast activity, and insufficient extracellular matrix production.[133] Hyperglycemic conditions interfere with cytokine signaling pathways, such as the transforming growth factor-β pathway, affecting fibroblast differentiation and function, leading to a compromised microenvironment for myofibroblast formation and weakened wound contraction.

Together, crosstalk between the two cell types is important for reepithelialization and is dependent on a delicate balance between proinflammatory and anti-inflammatory cytokine expression in the wound.[134] Alterations in both keratinocytes and fibroblasts can be induced directly by hyperglycemia and AGE formation.[87,88,91,135,136]

In summary the impaired healing that occurs in individuals with diabetes, involves hypoxia, dysfunction in fibroblasts and epidermal cells, impaired angiogenesis and neovascularization, high levels of MMP, damage from reactive oxygen species and AGEs, decreased host immune resistance and neuropathy.

MEDICATIONS AND DIETARY SUPPLEMENTS

Glucocorticoid Steroids

Systemic glucocorticoids, which are frequently used as anti-inflammatory agents, are well known to inhibit wound repair via global anti-inflammatory effects and suppression of cellular wound responses, including fibroblast proliferation and collagen synthesis. Systemic steroids cause wounds to heal with incomplete granulation tissue and reduced wound contraction.[137] Glucocorticoids also inhibit production of HIF-1, a key transcriptional factor in healing wounds.[138] Beyond effects on repair itself, systemic corticosteroids may increase the risk of wound infection. While systemic corticosteroids inhibit wound repair, topical application produces quite different effects. Topical low-dosage corticosteroid treatment of chronic wounds has been found to accelerate wound healing, reduce pain and exudate, and suppress hypergranulation tissue formation in 79% of cases. While these positive effects are striking, careful monitoring is necessary to avoid a potential increased risk of infection with prolonged use.[139]

Peripheral Vascular Disease

Total disease prevalence based on objective testing has been evaluated in several epidemiologic studies and is in the range of 3% to 10%, increasing to 15% to 20% in persons over 70 years.[140] Peripheral vascular disease (PVD) is an independent risk factor for subsequent ulceration and limb loss in diabetes. It is present in 50% of patients with diabetic foot ulcer (DFU), a proportion that may be increasing. Those with DFU and peripheral arterial disease (PAD) are less likely to heal and more likely to require amputation compared to patients without PAD. It is therefore essential that PVD is identified in all patients with diabetes.

Patients with PVD commonly suffer from chronic toe and foot sores, cramping leg muscles when walking, or numbness, weakness or heaviness in the muscles. Other chronic PVD symptoms include:

- Numbness in the extremities
- Weakness and atrophy of calf muscles
- A feeling of coldness in legs or feet
- Changes in the color of the feet: feet will turn pale when elevated and turn dusky red when in the dependent position
- Hair loss over the dorsum of the feet, thickening toenails
- Painful ulcers and/or gangrene in tissue, typically in the toes

Traditional wound care algorithms include aggressive detection of PAD and treatment with revascularization for all patients with PVD and lower extremity wounds—in order to prevent limb amputation. This is covered in data in other chapters.

Cigarette Smoking

It is well known that smoking increases the risk of heart and vascular disease, stroke, chronic lung disease, and many kinds of cancers. Similarly, the negative effects of smoking on wound-healing outcomes have been known for a long time.[141] Postoperatively, patients who smoke show a delay in wound healing and an increase in a variety of complications such as infection, wound rupture, anastomotic leakage, wound and flap necrosis, epidermolysis, and a decrease in the tensile strength of wounds.[142]

Most studies have focused on the effects of nicotine, carbon monoxide, and hydrogen cyanide from smoke. Nicotine interferes with oxygen supply by inducing tissue ischemia, since nicotine can cause decreased tissue blood flow via vasoconstrictive effects.[143] Nicotine stimulates sympathetic nervous activity, resulting in the release of epinephrine, which causes peripheral vasoconstriction and decreased tissue blood perfusion. Nicotine also increases blood viscosity caused by decreasing fibrinolytic activity and augmentation of platelet adhesiveness. In addition to the effects of nicotine, carbon monoxide in cigarette smoke also causes tissue hypoxia. Carbon monoxide binds to hemoglobin with an affinity of 200 times greater than that of oxygen, resulting in a decreased fraction of oxygenated hemoglobin in the bloodstream. Hydrogen cyanide, another well-studied component of cigarette smoke, impairs cellular oxygen metabolism, leading to compromised oxygen consumption in the tissues. Beyond these direct tissue effects, smoking increases the individual's risk for atherosclerosis and chronic obstructive pulmonary disease, two conditions that might also lower tissue oxygen tension.[76,144]

Chemotherapy and Radiation

Chemotherapy Drugs

Most chemotherapeutic drugs are designed to inhibit cellular metabolism, rapid cell division, and angiogenesis and thus inhibit many of the pathways that are critical to appropriate wound repair. These medications inhibit DNA, RNA, or protein synthesis, resulting in decreased fibroplasia and neovascularization of wounds.[145] Chemotherapeutic drugs delay cell migration into the wound, decrease early wound matrix formation, lower collagen production, impair proliferation of fibroblasts, and inhibit contraction of wounds.[137] In addition, these agents weaken the immune functions of the patients, and thereby impede the inflammatory phase of healing and increase the risk of wound infection. Chemotherapy induces neutropenia, anemia, and thrombocytopenia, thus leaving wounds vulnerable to infection, causing less oxygen delivery to the wound, and also making patients vulnerable to excessive bleeding at the wound site.

Radiation

Radiation is one of the most commonly used therapies for the treatment of multiple types of human cancer.

References

1. Burgess C. Topical vitamins. *J Drugs Dermatol.* 2008;7(7 Suppl):s2–s6.
2. Nurden AT, Nurden P, Sanchez M, Andia I, Anitua E. Platelets and wound healing. *Front Biosci.* 2008;13:3532–3548.
3. Jaramillo M, Olivier M. Hydrogen peroxide induces murine macrophage chemokine gene transcription via extracellular signal-regulated kinase- and cyclic adenosine 5′-monophosphate (cAMP)-dependent pathways: involvement of NF-kappa B, activator protein 1, and cAMP response element binding protein. *J Immunol.* 2002;169(12):7026–7038.
4. Razzell W, Evans IR, Martin P, Wood W. Calcium flashes orchestrate the wound inflammatory response through DUOX activation and hydrogen peroxide release. *Curr Biol.* 2013;23(5):424–429.
5. Niethammer P, Grabher C, Look AT, Mitchison TJ. A tissue-scale gradient of hydrogen peroxide mediates rapid wound detection in zebrafish. *Nature.* 2009;459(7249):996–999.
6. Tang D, Kang R, Xiao W, et al. Nuclear heat shock protein 72 as a negative regulator of oxidative stress (hydrogen peroxide)-induced HMGB1 cytoplasmic translocation and release. *J Immunol.* 2007;178(11):7376–7384.
7. Rani M, Nicholson SE, Zhang Q, Schwacha MG. Damage-associated molecular patterns (DAMPs) released after burn are associated with inflammation and monocyte activation. *Burns.* 2017;43(2):297–303.
8. Barrientos S, Stojadinovic O, Golinko MS, Brem H, Tomic-Canic M. Growth factors and cytokines in wound healing. *Wound Repair Regen.* 2008;16(5):585–601.
9. Reinke JM, Sorg H. Wound repair and regeneration. *Eur Surg Res.* 2012;49(1):35–43.
10. Kimball A, Schaller M, Joshi A, et al. Ly6C^Hi blood monocyte/macrophage drive chronic inflammation and impair wound healing in diabetes mellitus. *Arterioscler Thromb Vasc Biol.* 2018;38(5):1102–1114.

11. Boniakowski AE, Kimball AS, Jacobs BN, Kunkel SL, Gallagher KA. Macrophage-mediated inflammation in normal and diabetic wound healing. *J Immunol.* 2017;199(1):17–24.
12. Olingy CE, San Emeterio CL, Ogle ME, et al. Non-classical monocytes are biased progenitors of wound healing macrophages during soft tissue injury. *Sci Rep.* 2017;7(1):447.
13. Spiller KL, Anfang RR, Spiller KJ, et al. The role of macrophage phenotype in vascularization of tissue engineering scaffolds. *Biomaterials.* 2014;35(15):4477–4488.
14. Goren I, Allmann N, Yogev N, et al. A transgenic mouse model of inducible macrophage depletion: effects of diphtheria toxin-driven lysozyme M-specific cell lineage ablation on wound inflammatory, angiogenic, and contractive processes. *Am J Pathol.* 2009;175(1): 132–147.
15. Lucas T, Waisman A, Ranjan R, et al. Differential roles of macrophages in diverse phases of skin repair. *J Immunol.* 2010; 184(7):3964–3977.
16. Hesketh M, Sahin KB, West ZE, Murray RZ. Macrophage phenotypes regulate scar formation and chronic wound healing. *Int J Mol Sci.* 2017;18(7):1545.
17. Vågesjö E, Öhnstedt E, Mortier A, et al. Accelerated wound healing in mice by on-site production and delivery of CXCL12 by transformed lactic acid bacteria. *Proc Natl Acad Sci U S A.* 2018;115(8):1895–1900.
18. Landen NX, Li D, Stahle M. Transition from inflammation to proliferation: a critical step during wound healing. *Cell Mol Life Sci.* 2016;73(20):3861–3885.
19. Martinez FO, Gordon S. The M1 and M2 paradigm of macrophage activation: time for reassessment. *F1000Prime Rep.* 2014; 6:13.
20. Martinez FO, Sica A, Mantovani A, Locati M. Macrophage activation and polarization. *Front Biosci.* 2008;13:453–461.
21. Peter C, Waibel M, Radu CG, et al. Migration to apoptotic "find-me" signals is mediated via the phagocyte receptor G2A. *J Biol Chem.* 2008;283(9):5296–5305.
22. Crane MJ, Daley JM, van Houtte O, Brancato SK, Henry WL Jr, Albina JE. The monocyte to macrophage transition in the murine sterile wound. *PLoS One.* 2014;9(1):e86660.
23. Voll RE, Herrmann M, Roth EA, Stach C, Kalden JR, Girkontaite I. Immunosuppressive effects of apoptotic cells. *Nature.* 1997;390(6658):350–351.
24. Fadok VA, Bratton DL, Konowal A, Freed PW, Westcott JY, Henson PM. Macrophages that have ingested apoptotic cells in vitro inhibit proinflammatory cytokine production through autocrine/paracrine mechanisms involving TGF-beta, PGE2, and PAF. *J Clin Invest.* 1998;101(4):890–898.
25. Van den Bossche J, Neele AE, Hoeksema MA, de Winther MP. Macrophage polarization: the epigenetic point of view. *Curr Opin Lipidol.* 2014;25(5):367–373.
26. Ivashkiv LB. Epigenetic regulation of macrophage polarization and function. *Trends Immunol.* 2013;34(5):216–223.
27. Chen X, Barozzi I, Termanini A, et al. Requirement for the histone deacetylase Hdac3 for the inflammatory gene expression program in macrophages. *Proc Natl Acad Sci U S A.* 2012;109(42): E2865–E2874.
28. Mullican SE, Gaddis CA, Alenghat T, et al. Histone deacetylase 3 is an epigenomic brake in macrophage alternative activation. *Genes Dev.* 2011;25(23):2480–2488.
29. Shakespear MR, Halili MA, Irvine KM, Fairlie DP, Sweet MJ. Histone deacetylases as regulators of inflammation and immunity. *Trends Immunol.* 2011;32(7):335–343.
30. Ghisletti S, Barozzi I, Mietton F, et al. Identification and characterization of enhancers controlling the inflammatory gene expression program in macrophages. *Immunity.* 2010;32(3):317–328.
31. Natoli G, Ghisletti S, Barozzi I. The genomic landscapes of inflammation. *Genes Dev.* 2011;25(2):101–106.
32. Babu M, Durga Devi T, Makinen P, et al. Differential promoter methylation of macrophage genes is associated with impaired vascular growth in ischemic muscles of hyperlipidemic and type 2 diabetic mice: genome-wide promoter methylation study. *Circ Res.* 2015; 117(3):289–299.
33. Yang X, Wang X, Liu D, Yu L, Xue B, Shi H. Epigenetic regulation of macrophage polarization by DNA methyltransferase 3b. *Mol Endocrinol.* 2014;28(4):565–574.
34. Mirza RE, Fang MM, Ennis WJ, Koh TJ. Blocking interleukin-1β induces a healing-associated wound macrophage phenotype and improves healing in type 2 diabetes. *Diabetes.* 2013;62(7): 2579–2587.
35. Lewis CJ, Mardaryev AN, Sharov AA, Fessing MY, Botchkarev VA. The epigenetic regulation of wound healing. *Adv Wound Care (New Rochelle).* 2014;3(7):468–475.
36. Gallagher KA, Joshi A, Carson WF, et al. Epigenetic changes in bone marrow progenitor cells influence the inflammatory phenotype and alter wound healing in type 2 diabetes. *Diabetes.* 2015;64(4):1420–1430.
37. Cheng Y, Zhang C. MicroRNA-21 in cardiovascular disease. *J Cardiovasc Transl Res.* 2010;3(3):251–255.
38. Kantharidis P, Wang B, Carew RM, Lan HY. Diabetes complications: the microRNA perspective. *Diabetes.* 2011;60(7):1832–1837.
39. Palmero EI, de Campos SG, Campos M, et al. Mechanisms and role of microRNA deregulation in cancer onset and progression. *Genet Mol Biol.* 2011;34(3):363–370.
40. Chaudhuri AA, So AY, Sinha N, et al. MicroRNA-125b potentiates macrophage activation. *J Immunol.* 2011;187(10):5062–5068.
41. Diegelmann RF, Evans MC. Wound healing: an overview of acute, fibrotic and delayed healing. *Front Biosci.* 2004;9:283–289.
42. Saraswati S, Marrow SMW, Watch LA, Young PP. Identification of a pro-angiogenic functional role for FSP1-positive fibroblast subtype in wound healing. *Nat Commun.* 2019;10(1):3027.
43. DiPietro LA. Angiogenesis and wound repair: when enough is enough. *J Leukoc Biol.* 2016;100(5):979–984.
44. Wilgus TA, Ferreira AM, Oberyszyn TM, Bergdall VK, Dipietro LA. Regulation of scar formation by vascular endothelial growth factor. *Lab Invest.* 2008;88(6):579–590.
45. Costa C, Incio J, Soares R. Angiogenesis and chronic inflammation: cause or consequence? *Angiogenesis.* 2007;10(3):149–166.
46. Gallagher KA, Liu ZJ, Xiao M, et al. Diabetic impairments in NO-mediated endothelial progenitor cell mobilization and homing are reversed by hyperoxia and SDF-1 alpha. *J Clin Invest.* 2007;117(5):1249–1259.
47. Prockop DJ, Kivirikko KI. Collagens: molecular biology, diseases, and potentials for therapy. *Annu Rev Biochem.* 1995;64:403–434.
48. Clark RA. Fibrin and wound healing. *Ann N Y Acad Sci.* 2001; 936:355–367.
49. Peterkofsky B. Ascorbate requirement for hydroxylation and secretion of procollagen: relationship to inhibition of collagen synthesis in scurvy. *Am J Clin Nutr.* 1991;54(6 Suppl):1135S–1140S.
50. Blumenkrantz N, Assad R, Peterkofsky B. Characterization of collagen hydroxylysyl glycosyltransferases as mainly intramembranous microsomal enzymes. *J Biol Chem.* 1984;259(2):854–859.
51. Prockop DJ, Sieron AL, Li SW. Procollagen N-proteinase and procollagen C-proteinase. Two unusual metalloproteinases that are essential for procollagen processing probably have important roles in development and cell signaling. *Matrix Biol.* 1998;16(7): 399–408.
52. Zanaboni G, Rossi A, Onana AM, Tenni R. Stability and networks of hydrogen bonds of the collagen triple helical structure: influence of pH and chaotropic nature of three anions. *Matrix Biol.* 2000;19(6):511–520.
53. Hornstra IK, Birge S, Starcher B, Bailey AJ, Mecham RP, Shapiro SD. Lysyl oxidase is required for vascular and diaphragmatic development in mice. *J Biol Chem.* 2003;278(16):14387–14393.
54. Onimaru M, Yonemitsu Y, Fujii T, et al. VEGF-C regulates lymphangiogenesis and capillary stability by regulation of PDGF-B. *Am J Physiol Heart Circ Physiol.* 2009;297(5):H1685–H1696.
55. Gabbiani G. The myofibroblast in wound healing and fibrocontractive diseases. *J Pathol.* 2003;200(4):500–503.
56. Parks WC. Matrix metalloproteinases in repair. *Wound Repair Regen.* 1999;7(6):423–432.
57. Djonov V, Schmid M, Tschanz SA, Burri PH. Intussusceptive angiogenesis: its role in embryonic vascular network formation. *Circ Res.* 2000;86(3):286–292.

58. Patan S. TIE1 and TIE2 receptor tyrosine kinases inversely regulate embryonic angiogenesis by the mechanism of intussusceptive microvascular growth. *Microvasc Res.* 1998;56(1):1–21.
59. Keylock KT, Vieira VJ, Wallig MA, DiPietro LA, Schrementi M, Woods JA. Exercise accelerates cutaneous wound healing and decreases wound inflammation in aged mice. *Am J Physiol Regul Integr Comp Physiol.* 2008;294(1):R179–R184.
60. Swift ME, Burns AL, Gray KL, DiPietro LA. Age-related alterations in the inflammatory response to dermal injury. *J Invest Dermatol.* 2001;117(5):1027–1035.
61. Gilliver SC, Ashworth JJ, Ashcroft GS. The hormonal regulation of cutaneous wound healing. *Clin Dermatol.* 2007;25(1):56–62.
62. Hardman MJ, Ashcroft GS. Estrogen, not intrinsic aging, is the major regulator of delayed human wound healing in the elderly. *Genome Biol.* 2008;9(5):R80.
63. Hardman MJ, Emmerson E, Campbell L, Ashcroft GS. Selective estrogen receptor modulators accelerate cutaneous wound healing in ovariectomized female mice. *Endocrinology.* 2008; 149(2):551–557.
64. Emery CF, Kiecolt-Glaser JK, Glaser R, Malarkey WB, Frid DJ. Exercise accelerates wound healing among healthy older adults: a preliminary investigation. *J Gerontol A Biol Sci Med Sci.* 2005; 60(11):1432–1436.
65. Arnold M, Barbul A. Nutrition and wound healing. *Plast Reconstr Surg.* 2006;117(7 Suppl):42S–58S.
66. da Costa MA, Campos AC, Coelho JC, de Barros AM, Matsumoto HM. Oral glutamine and the healing of colonic anastomoses in rats. *JPEN J Parenter Enteral Nutr.* 2003;27(3):182–185; discussion 185–186.
67. McDaniel JC, Belury M, Ahijevych K, Blakely W. Omega-3 fatty acids effect on wound healing. *Wound Repair Regen.* 2008;16(3): 337–345.
68. Wilson JA, Clark JJ. Obesity: impediment to postsurgical wound healing. *Adv Skin Wound Care.* 2004;17(8):426–435.
69. Momeni M, Hafezi F, Rahbar H, Karimi H. Effects of silicone gel on burn scars. *Burns.* 2009;35(1):70–74.
70. Calabro P, Yeh ET. Obesity, inflammation, and vascular disease: the role of the adipose tissue as an endocrine organ. *Subcell Biochem.* 2007;42:63–91.
71. de Mello VD, Kolehmainen M, Schwab U, et al. Effect of weight loss on cytokine messenger RNA expression in peripheral blood mononuclear cells of obese subjects with the metabolic syndrome. *Metabolism.* 2008;57(2):192–199.
72. Centers for Disease Control and Prevention. National Diabetes Statistics Report, 2017. 2017.
73. Guariguata L, Whiting D, Weil C, Unwin N. The International Diabetes Federation diabetes atlas methodology for estimating global and national prevalence of diabetes in adults. *Diabetes Res Clin Pract.* 2011;94(3):322–332.
74. Menke A, Casagrande S, Geiss L, Cowie CC. Prevalence of and trends in diabetes among adults in the United States, 1988–2012. *JAMA.* 2015;314(10):1021–1029.
75. Lamont P, Franklyn K, Rayman G, Boulton AJ. Update on the diabetic foot 2012: the 14th biennial Malvern Diabetic Foot Conference, May 9–11, 2012. *Int J Low Extrem Wounds.* 2013;12(1):71–75.
76. Theilgaard-Mönch K, Knudsen S, Follin P, Borregaard N. The transcriptional activation program of human neutrophils in skin lesions supports their important role in wound healing. *J Immunol.* 2004;172(12):7684–7693.
77. Wynn TA, Vannella KM. Macrophages in tissue repair, regeneration, and fibrosis. *Immunity.* 2016;44(3):450–462.
78. Maruyama K, Asai J, Ii M, Thorne T, Losordo DW, D'Amore PA. Decreased macrophage number and activation lead to reduced lymphatic vessel formation and contribute to impaired diabetic wound healing. *Am J Pathol.* 2007;170(4):1178–1191.
79. Willenborg S, Lucas T, van Loo G, et al. CCR2 recruits an inflammatory macrophage subpopulation critical for angiogenesis in tissue repair. *Blood.* 2012;120(3):613–625.
80. Italiani P, Boraschi D. From monocytes to M1/M2 macrophages: phenotypical vs. functional differentiation. *Front Immunol.* 2014;5:514.
81. Murray PJ, Allen JE, Biswas SK, et al. Macrophage activation and polarization: nomenclature and experimental guidelines. *Immunity.* 2014;41(1):14–20.
82. Sica A, Mantovani A. Macrophage plasticity and polarization: in vivo veritas. *J Clin Invest.* 2012;122(3):787–795.
83. Kimball AS, Joshi A, Carson WF IV, et al. The histone methyltransferase MLL1 directs macrophage-mediated inflammation in wound healing and is altered in a murine model of obesity and type 2 diabetes. *Diabetes.* 2017;66(9):2459–2471.
84. Wang X, Cao Q, Yu L, Shi H, Xue B, Shi H. Epigenetic regulation of macrophage polarization and inflammation by DNA methylation in obesity. *JCI Insight.* 2016;1(19):e87748.
85. Yan J, Tie G, Wang S, et al. Diabetes impairs wound healing by Dnmt1-dependent dysregulation of hematopoietic stem cells differentiation towards macrophages. *Nat Commun.* 2018; 9:33.
86. De Santa F, Totaro MG, Prosperini E, Notarbartolo S, Testa G, Natoli G. The histone H3 lysine-27 demethylase Jmjd3 links inflammation to inhibition of polycomb-mediated gene silencing. *Cell.* 2007;130(6):1083–1094.
87. Peppa M, Brem H, Ehrlich P, et al. Adverse effects of dietary glycotoxins on wound healing in genetically diabetic mice. *Diabetes.* 2003;52(11):2805–2813.
88. Zhu P, Yang C, Chen LH, Ren M, Lao GJ, Yan L. Impairment of human keratinocyte mobility and proliferation by advanced glycation end products-modified BSA. *Arch Dermatol Res.* 2011;303(5):339–350.
89. Lerman OZ, Galiano RD, Armour M, Levine JP, Gurtner GC. Cellular dysfunction in the diabetic fibroblast: impairment in migration, vascular endothelial growth factor production, and response to hypoxia. *Am J Pathol.* 2003;162(1):303–312.
90. Xuan YH, Huang BB, Tian HS, et al. High-glucose inhibits human fibroblast cell migration in wound healing via repression of bFGF-regulating JNK phosphorylation. *PLoS One.* 2014;9(9): e108182.
91. Zhang J, Yang C, Wang C, et al. AGE-induced keratinocyte MMP-9 expression is linked to TET2-mediated CpG demethylation. *Wound Repair Regen.* 2016;24(3):489–500.
92. Ling L, Ren M, Yang C, et al. Role of site-specific DNA demethylation in TNFalpha-induced MMP9 expression in keratinocytes. *J Mol Endocrinol.* 2013;50(3):279–290.
93. Park LK, Malone AG, Smith A, et al. Genome-wide DNA methylation analysis identifies a metabolic memory profile in patient-derived diabetic foot ulcer fibroblasts. *Epigenetics.* 2014; 9(10):1339–1349.
94. Dinh T, Tecilazich F, Kafanas A, et al. Mechanisms involved in the development and healing of diabetic foot ulceration. *Diabetes.* 2012;61(11):2937–2947.
95. Ward JD, Boulton AJ, Simms JM, Sandler DA, Knight G. Venous distension in the diabetic neuropathic foot (physical sign of arteriovenous shunting). *J R Soc Med.* 1983;76(12):1011–1014.
96. Rayman G, Williams SA, Spencer PD, Smaje LH, Wise PH, Tooke JE. Impaired microvascular hyperaemic response to minor skin trauma in type I diabetes. *Br Med J (Clin Res Ed).* 1986;292(6531): 1295–1298.
97. Undas A, Wiek I, Stêpien E, Zmudka K, Tracz W. Hyperglycemia is associated with enhanced thrombin formation, platelet activation, and fibrin clot resistance to lysis in patients with acute coronary syndrome. *Diabetes Care.* 2008;31(8):1590–1595.
98. Juhan-Vague I, Roul C, Alessi MC, Ardissone JP, Heim M, Vague P. Increased plasminogen activator inhibitor activity in non insulin dependent diabetic patients—relationship with plasma insulin. *Thromb Haemost.* 1989;61(3):370–373.
99. Förstermann U, Mügge A, Alheid U, Haverich A, Frölich JC. Selective attenuation of endothelium-mediated vasodilation in atherosclerotic human coronary arteries. *Circ Res.* 1988;62(2): 185–190.
100. Bucala R, Tracey KJ, Cerami A. Advanced glycosylation products quench nitric oxide and mediate defective endothelium-dependent vasodilatation in experimental diabetes. *J Clin Invest.* 1991;87(2):432–438.

101. Tessari P, Cecchet D, Cosma A, et al. Nitric oxide synthesis is reduced in subjects with type 2 diabetes and nephropathy. *Diabetes*. 2010;59(9):2152–2159.
102. Hanses F, Park S, Rich J, Lee JC. Reduced neutrophil apoptosis in diabetic mice during staphylococcal infection leads to prolonged Tnfalpha production and reduced neutrophil clearance. *PLoS One*. 2011;6(8):e23633.
103. Karima M, Kantarci A, Ohira T, et al. Enhanced superoxide release and elevated protein kinase C activity in neutrophils from diabetic patients: association with periodontitis. *J Leukoc Biol*. 2005;78(4):862–870.
104. Wong SL, Demers M, Martinod K, et al. Diabetes primes neutrophils to undergo NETosis, which impairs wound healing. *Nat Med*. 2015;21(7):815–819.
105. Opneja A, Kapoor S, Stavrou EX. Contribution of platelets, the coagulation and fibrinolytic systems to cutaneous wound healing. *Thromb Res*. 2019;179:56–63.
106. Liu D, Yang P, Gao M, et al. NLRP3 activation induced by neutrophil extracellular traps sustains inflammatory response in the diabetic wound. *Clin Sci (Lond)*. 2019;133(4):565–582.
107. Wetzler C, Kämpfer H, Stallmeyer B, Pfeilschifter J, Frank S. Large and sustained induction of chemokines during impaired wound healing in the genetically diabetic mouse: prolonged persistence of neutrophils and macrophages during the late phase of repair. *J Invest Dermatol*. 2000;115(2):245–253.
108. Loots MA, Lamme EN, Zeegelaar J, Mekkes JR, Bos JD, Middelkoop E. Differences in cellular infiltrate and extracellular matrix of chronic diabetic and venous ulcers versus acute wounds. *J Invest Dermatol*. 1998;111(5):850–857.
109. Audu CO, Melvin WJ, Joshi AD, et al. Macrophage-specific inhibition of the histone demethylase JMJD3 decreases STING and pathologic inflammation in diabetic wound repair. *Cell Mol Immunol*. 2022;19(11):1251–1262.
110. Kimball AS, Davis FM, denDekker A, et al. The histone methyltransferase setdb2 modulates macrophage phenotype and uric acid production in diabetic wound repair. *Immunity*. 2019;51(2):258–271.e5.
111. Friggeri A, Banerjee S, Biswas S, et al. Participation of the receptor for advanced glycation end products in efferocytosis. *J Immunol*. 2011;186(11):6191–6198.
112. He M, Kubo H, Morimoto K, et al. Receptor for advanced glycation end products binds to phosphatidylserine and assists in the clearance of apoptotic cells. *EMBO Rep*. 2011;12(4):358–364.
113. Okonkwo UA, Chen L, Ma D, et al. Compromised angiogenesis and vascular Integrity in impaired diabetic wound healing. *PLoS One*. 2020;15(4):e0231962.
114. Ignarro LJ, Buga GM, Wood KS, Byrns RE, Chaudhuri G. Endothelium-derived relaxing factor produced and released from artery and vein is nitric oxide. *Proc Natl Acad Sci. U S A*. 1987; 84(24):9265–9269.
115. Veves A, Akbari CM, Primavera J, et al. Endothelial dysfunction and the expression of endothelial nitric oxide synthetase in diabetic neuropathy, vascular disease, and foot ulceration. *Diabetes*. 1998;47(3):457–463.
116. Chen Z, Haus JM, Chen L, et al. Inhibition of CCL28/CCR10-mediated eNOS downregulation improves skin wound healing in the obesity-induced mouse model of type 2 diabetes. *Diabetes*. 2022;71(10):2166–2180.
117. Lee PC, Salyapongse AN, Bragdon GA, et al. Impaired wound healing and angiogenesis in eNOS-deficient mice. *Am J Physiol*. 1999;277(4):H1600–H1608.
118. Chen Z, Haus JM, Chen L, et al. CCL28-induced CCR10/eNOS interaction in angiogenesis and skin wound healing. *FASEB J*. 2020;34(4):5838–5850.
119. Chen YH, Lin SJ, Lin FY, et al. High glucose impairs early and late endothelial progenitor cells by modifying nitric oxide-related but not oxidative stress-mediated mechanisms. *Diabetes*. 2007;56(6):1559–1568.
120. Zheng X, Narayanan S, Sunkari VG, et al. Triggering of a Dll4-Notch1 loop impairs wound healing in diabetes. *Proc Natl Acad Sci U S A*. 2019;116(14):6985–6994.
121. Thum T, Fraccarollo D, Schultheiss M, et al. Endothelial nitric oxide synthase uncoupling impairs endothelial progenitor cell mobilization and function in diabetes. *Diabetes*. 2007;56(3):666–674.
122. Wolf SJ, Audu CO, Joshi A, et al. IFN-κ is critical for normal wound repair and is decreased in diabetic wounds. *JCI Insight*. 2022;7(9):e152765.
123. Lan CC, Liu IH, Fang AH, Wen CH, Wu CS. Hyperglycaemic conditions decrease cultured keratinocyte mobility: implications for impaired wound healing in patients with diabetes. *Br J Dermatol*. 2008;159(5):1103–1115.
124. Werner S, Breeden M, Hübner G, Greenhalgh DG, Longaker MT. Induction of keratinocyte growth factor expression is reduced and delayed during wound healing in the genetically diabetic mouse. *J Invest Dermatol*. 1994;103(4):469–473.
125. Pollok S, Pfeiffer AC, Lobmann R, et al. Connexin 43 mimetic peptide Gap27 reveals potential differences in the role of Cx43 in wound repair between diabetic and non-diabetic cells. *J Cell Mol Med*. 2011;15(4):861–873.
126. Lan CC, Wu CS, Huang SM, Wu IH, Chen GS. High-glucose environment enhanced oxidative stress and increased interleukin-8 secretion from keratinocytes: new insights into impaired diabetic wound healing. *Diabetes*. 2013;62(7):2530–2538.
127. Lu W, Li J, Ren M, et al. Role of the mevalonate pathway in specific CpG site demethylation on AGEs-induced MMP9 expression and activation in keratinocytes. *Mol Cell Endocrinol*. 2015;411:121–129.
128. Robert I, Aussems M, Keutgens A, et al. Matrix metalloproteinase-9 gene induction by a truncated oncogenic NF-kappaB2 protein involves the recruitment of MLL1 and MLL2 H3K4 histone methyltransferase complexes. *Oncogene*. 2009;28(13):1626–1638.
129. Kearon C, Akl EA, Ornelas J, et al. Antithrombotic therapy for VTE disease: CHEST Guideline and Expert Panel Report. *Chest*. 2016;149(2):315–352.
130. Usui ML, Mansbridge JN, Carter WG, Fujita M, Olerud JE. Keratinocyte migration, proliferation, and differentiation in chronic ulcers from patients with diabetes and normal wounds. *J Histochem Cytochem*. 2008;56(7):687–696.
131. Becker DL, Thrasivoulou C, Phillips AR. Connexins in wound healing; perspectives in diabetic patients. *Biochim Biophys Acta*. 2012;1818(8):2068–2675.
132. Desta T, Li J, Chino T, Graves DT. Altered fibroblast proliferation and apoptosis in diabetic gingival wounds. *J Dent Res*. 2010;89(6):609–614.
133. Wan R, Weissman JP, Grundman K, Lang L, Grybowski DJ, Galiano RD. Diabetic wound healing: the impact of diabetes on myofibroblast activity and its potential therapeutic treatments. *Wound Repair Regen*. 2021;29(4):573–581.
134. Werner S, Krieg T, Smola H. Keratinocyte-fibroblast interactions in wound healing. *J Invest Dermatol*. 2007;127(5):998–1008.
135. Alikhani Z, Alikhani M, Boyd CM, Nagao K, Trackman PC, Graves DT. Advanced glycation end products enhance expression of pro-apoptotic genes and stimulate fibroblast apoptosis through cytoplasmic and mitochondrial pathways. *J Biol Chem*. 2005;280(13):12087–12095.
136. Okano Y, Masaki H, Sakurai H. Dysfunction of dermal fibroblasts induced by advanced glycation end-products (AGEs) and the contribution of a nonspecific interaction with cell membrane and AGEs. *J Dermatol Sci*. 2002;29(3):171–180.
137. Franz MG, Steed DL, Robson MC. Optimizing healing of the acute wound by minimizing complications. *Curr Probl Surg*. 2007;44(11):691–763.
138. Wagner AE, Huck G, Stiehl DP, Jelkmann W, Hellwig-Bürgel T. Dexamethasone impairs hypoxia-inducible factor-1 function. *Biochem Biophys Res Commun*. 2008;372(2):336–340.
139. Hofman D, Moore K, Cooper R, Eagle M, Cooper S. Use of topical corticosteroids on chronic leg ulcers. *J Wound Care*. 2007; 16(5):227–230.
140. Selvin E, Erlinger TP. Prevalence of and risk factors for peripheral arterial disease in the United States: results from the National Health and Nutrition Examination Survey, 1999–2000. *Circulation*. 2004;110(6):738–743.

141. Siana JE, Rex S, Gottrup F. The effect of cigarette smoking on wound healing. *Scand J Plast Reconstr Surg Hand Surg.* 1989; 23(3):207–209.
142. Ahn C, Mulligan P, Salcido RS. Smoking-the bane of wound healing: biomedical interventions and social influences. *Adv Skin Wound Care.* 2008;21(5):227–236; quiz 237–238.
143. Sorensen LT, Jorgensen S, Petersen LJ, et al. Acute effects of nicotine and smoking on blood flow, tissue oxygen, and aerobe metabolism of the skin and subcutis. *J Surg Res.* 2009;152(2): 224–230.
144. Siasos G, Tsigkou V, Kokkou E, et al. Smoking and atherosclerosis: mechanisms of disease and new therapeutic approaches. *Curr Med Chem.* 2014;21(34):3936–3948.
145. Zimmerman-Pope N, Waldron DR, Barber DL, Forrester SD, Wilcke JR, Marini M. Effect of fenoldopam on renal function after nephrotomy in normal dogs. *Vet Surg.* 2003;32(6):566–573.

4

Cancer Immunology and Immunotherapy

Andrew J. Gunderson, Susan Tsai, and Joal D. Beane

Key Points

1. The immune system plays a dual role in cancer, either suppressing tumor progression or, paradoxically, supporting it through immunosuppressive tumor microenvironment (TME) adaptations. Advancements in understanding these mechanisms have driven the development of targeted immunotherapies.
2. Tumor-induced immunosuppression, immune checkpoint upregulation, and TME complexities, such as the presence of Tregs, myeloid-derived suppressor cells (MDSCs), and cancer-associated fibroblasts (CAFs), remain significant hurdles. Overcoming these barriers is critical to expand therapeutic efficacy.
3. The emergence of immune checkpoint inhibitors (eg, anti–PD-1/PD-L1, anticytotoxic T-lymphocyte–associated protein 4 [CTLA-4]) and adoptive cell therapies (chimeric antigen receptor [CAR-T] and tumor-infiltrating lymphocyte [TIL]) has transformed cancer care, offering durable responses in previously untreatable cancers.
4. Predictive biomarkers like tumor mutational burden (TMB), microsatellite instability (MSI), and programmed death ligand 1(PD-L1) expression, provide crucial insights for optimizing patient selection and improving immunotherapy outcomes.
5. The integration of immunotherapy with traditional cancer modalities (surgery, radiation, and chemotherapy) and innovations like oncolytic viral therapies and personalized cancer vaccines promise synergistic, multimodal treatment strategies, heralding a new era of oncology.

Cancer immunology has emerged as one of the most important fields within cellular and molecular immunology buoyed by seminal advancements over the past decade. One of the hallmarks of cancer is the presence of unrestrained proliferation and the ability to invade distant regions of the body.[1] In this context, the immune system plays a pivotal role, either by suppressing tumor growth or, in some cases, inadvertently facilitating its progression. The immune microenvironment surrounding a tumor is highly complex, consisting of a diverse population of immune cells, each with distinct functions. Certain cells, such as myeloid-derived suppressor cells (MDSCs) and regulatory T cells (Tregs) promote tumor progression through the expression of immunosuppressive molecules. These cells can weaken the immune system's ability to mount an effective response. In contrast, immune cells such as cytotoxic T lymphocytes (CTLs) and natural killer (NK) cells act as the body's primary defense against cancer, employing mechanisms that directly target and destroy tumor cells. Understanding how different components of the immune system function within the tumor microenvironment (TME) is crucial to determine antitumor responses and identifying potential therapeutic strategies. This chapter offers an overview of the immune system's role in cancer, highlighting key players within the TME and discussing some of the most widely used immune-based therapies in cancer treatment.

HISTORICAL CONTEXT OF IMMUNOTHERAPY

The use of bacterial or viral infections to enhance immune responses against cancer has a long history. In 1858, Rudolf Virchow first identified a link between tumors and inflammation, observing that neoplastic tissues were often infiltrated by leukocytes from the immune system.[2] This connection laid the groundwork for the concept of cancer immunotherapy. In the late 1800s, William Coley, a surgeon and often referred to as the father of immunotherapy, pioneered efforts to harness the immune system to treat cancer.[3] Generally regarded as one of the first systematic and documented clinical attempts at immunotherapy, Dr. Coley treated a patient with sarcoma with live and heat-killed formulations of *Streptococcus bacterium*. This hypothesis came from the circumstantial evidence that occasionally some cancer patients achieved tumor regressions following infection. "Coley's toxin" as the treatment came to be known, demonstrated some effectiveness in patients with sarcoma but the results were difficult to replicate by other clinicians due to the inconsistencies in bacterial formulations and the sometimes dangerous inflammatory side effects they would induce. Mechanistically it was thought that the induction of fever by the bacteria was required for the antitumor effect, lending credence to the powerful influence of inflammation on malignancies. While this approach provided an early proof of concept, the lack of understanding about its mechanisms and the associated infection risks limited its development. The idea of cancer immunotherapy reemerged in the 20th century, bolstered by new technologic advancements. In early 1900s, Paul Ehrlich suggested that the immune system could continuously eradicate cancerous cells in the body.[4] This theory was later refined by Lewis Thomas and Sir Frank Macfarlane Burnet, who proposed the "cancer immunosurveillance" hypothesis, stating that tumor-associated antigens (TAAs) are recognized and targeted by the immune system, similar to how the body rejects foreign tissue in grafts. Experimental support for this hypothesis grew with the development of mouse models and clinical observations of spontaneous cancer regression in patients with autoimmune diseases.

Further advances in molecular and biochemical techniques eventually confirmed that the immune system, particularly

T-Cell Activation in Cancer

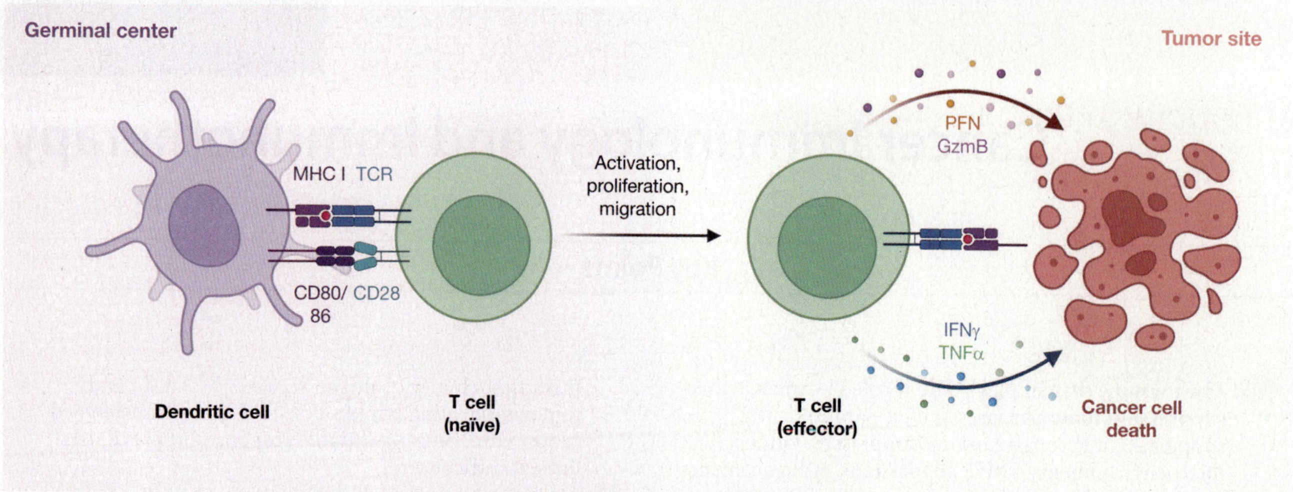

Figure 4.1. T-cell activation in cancer. Dendritic cells (DCs) present tumor-derived antigens on MHC class I molecules to the T-cell receptor (TCR) of naïve T cells, along with costimulatory signals through CD80/CD86 binding to CD28, leading to T-cell activation, proliferation, and migration. Activated effector T cells traffic to the tumor site, where they induce cancer cell death through perforin (PFN) and granzyme B (GzmB) release, as well as cytokine-mediated effects via interferon gamma (IFNγ) and tumor necrosis factor alpha (TNFα).

T cells, can recognize and attack cancer cells. This breakthrough laid the groundwork for modern cancer immunotherapy, which has since transformed oncology. Immunotherapies now extend survival for patients with otherwise rapidly fatal cancers and their use is expanding rapidly. As new therapeutic combinations and drug targets are identified, immunotherapy will continue to play an increasingly central role in cancer treatment in the years to come.

OVERVIEW OF TUMOR IMMUNOLOGY

The success of cancer immunotherapy has demonstrated that immune cells, particularly T cells, can be harnessed to eliminate tumor cells. Breakthroughs such as immune checkpoint inhibitors and adoptive T-cell therapies have demonstrated remarkable clinical efficacy, leading to durable responses in some patients, even with advanced or metastatic cancers. However, despite these achievements, only a subset of cancer patients currently derives meaningful and sustained benefits from immunotherapies. This limited response underscores the complexity of tumor-immune interactions and the need for deeper insights into the mechanisms at play.

A more comprehensive understanding of the biology of both innate and adaptive immune cells, as well as their intricate interactions with the TME, is crucial to advance the field. Innate immune cells, such as macrophages, dendritic cells (DCs), and NK cells, play pivotal roles in initiating and shaping the adaptive immune response, while adaptive immune cells, including T cells and B cells, directly mediate antigen-specific tumor eradication. Dysregulation of these processes within the TME, often driven by immune suppression, metabolic alterations, and stromal components, poses significant barriers to effective immunotherapy.

Elucidating these interactions will be instrumental in several key areas. First, it will enable the optimization of existing immunotherapies by identifying strategies to overcome resistance mechanisms and enhance response rates. Second, it will aid in the development of predictive biomarkers to better stratify patients, ensuring that therapies are tailored to those most likely to benefit. Finally, it will facilitate the discovery of novel therapeutic targets, including combinatory approaches that leverage multiple facets of the immune system or disrupt the immunosuppressive elements of the TME.

T Cells

T cells, or T lymphocytes, are a cornerstone of the adaptive immune system and play a critical role in recognizing and eliminating foreign or abnormal cells, including cancerous or pathogen-infected cells. These cells originate from hematopoietic stem cells in the bone marrow but mature in the thymus, where they undergo positive and negative selection to ensure self-tolerance and antigen specificity. The primary function of T cells is to mediate immune responses against specific antigens, a task accomplished through their T-cell receptor (TCR), which recognizes peptides presented by major histocompatibility complex (MHC) molecules on the surface of other cells. This specificity enables T cells to identify and eliminate threats such as intracellular pathogens and tumor cells with precision, setting them apart as critical effectors in cellular immunity.[5]

The ability of T cells to interact with MHC molecules is fundamental to their functionality. MHC class I molecules, expressed on virtually all nucleated cells, present intracellularly derived peptides to CD8+ CTLs. This allows CD8+ T cells to monitor and respond to internal cellular abnormalities, such as viral infections or oncogenic mutations. CD8+ CTLs recognize intracellular abnormalities, such as viral infections or oncogenic mutations, through peptide-MHC class I complexes on target cells. Upon recognition, CTLs induce apoptosis via the perforin–granzyme pathway, Fas-FasL interactions, and cytokine-mediated mechanisms, ensuring precise and efficient elimination of aberrant cells while minimizing collateral
1 damage (**Fig. 4.1**). Conversely, MHC class II molecules, primarily expressed on professional antigen-presenting cells (APCs) such as DCs, macrophages, and B cells, present extracellular antigens to CD4+ helper T cells. These interactions are pivotal in initiating and regulating immune responses, as CD4+ T cells coordinate the activation and function of other immune cells, including macrophages and B cells. This division of labor underscores the complexity and specialization within the T-cell population, enabling multifaceted responses to diverse immunologic challenges.

T cells are classified into several subsets based on their phenotypes and functions. CD8+ T cells are the immune system's primary executors of cytotoxicity, employing perforin and granzymes to induce apoptosis in target cells. In contrast, CD4+ T cells act as master regulators, producing cytokines that modulate the activity of other immune cells. Within the

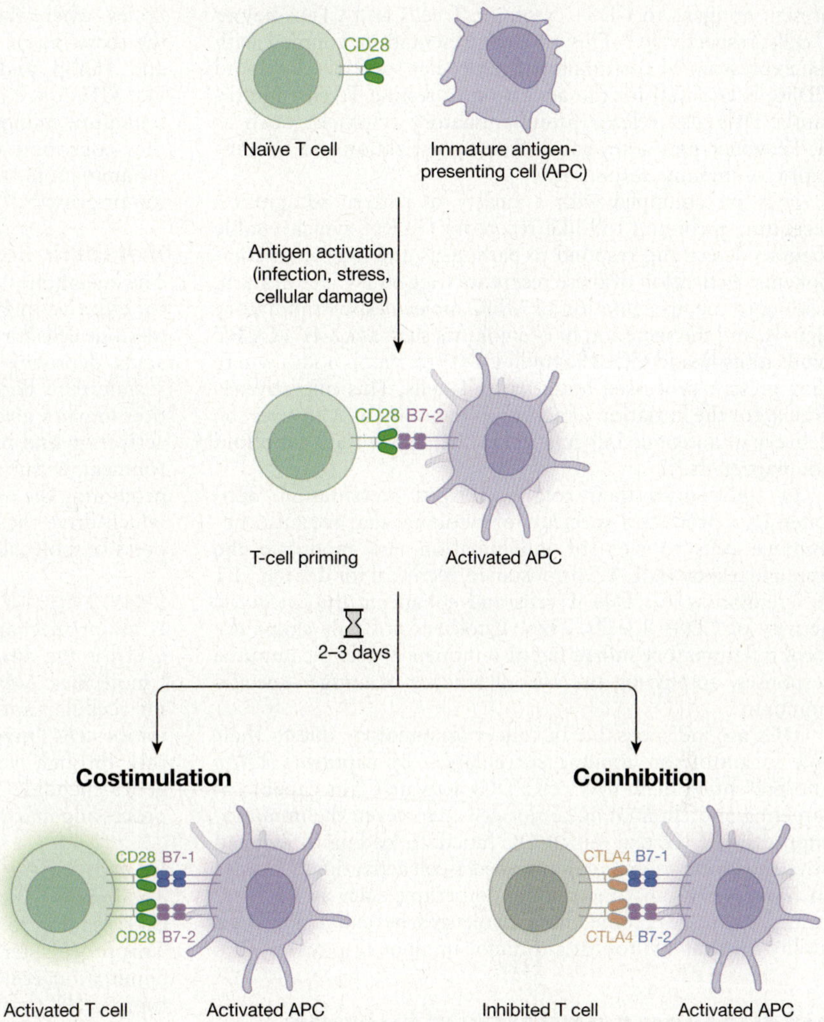

Figure 4.2. T-cell priming and cosignaling pathways. Naïve T cells are primed by antigen-presenting cells (APCs) following antigen activation caused by infection, stress, or cellular damage. This process involves the interaction of CD28 on T cells with B7-1 (CD80) or B7-2 (CD86) on APCs. Depending on the signaling pathway, costimulation (via CD28-B7 interaction) leads to T-cell activation, while coinhibition (via CTLA-4-B7 interaction) inhibits T-cell responses. These opposing signals determine whether the T cell becomes activated or suppressed, playing a critical role in immune regulation and tumor immunology.

CD4+ subset, helper T cells differentiate into specialized lineages, including Th1, Th2, Th17, and Tregs.[6] Th1 cells, for instance, are critical for antiviral and antitumor immunity, producing cytokines such as interferon-gamma (IFN-γ) to activate macrophages and enhance cytotoxic responses. Th2 cells facilitate B-cell activation and antibody production, while Th17 cells contribute to inflammatory responses. Tregs, on the other hand, play a suppressive role, maintaining immune homeostasis and preventing autoimmunity.[7] This diversity allows T cells to address a wide range of immunologic needs, from pathogen clearance to immune regulation.

The activation of T cells is a finely tuned process requiring two distinct signals to ensure specificity and prevent autoimmu-
1 nity (**Fig. 4.2**). Signal 1 involves the engagement of the TCR with an MHC-peptide complex, providing antigen-specific recognition. Signal 2 is a costimulatory signal delivered through interactions between molecules on APCs (eg, CD80/CD86) and receptors on T cells (eg, CD28). Together, these signals trigger clonal expansion and differentiation of T cells into effector and memory cells. Effector T cells migrate to sites of infection or tumor growth to mediate direct immune responses, while memory T cells provide long-term immunity by persisting and rapidly responding to subsequent exposures to the same antigen. Importantly, immune checkpoints such as cytotoxic T-lymphocyte–associated protein 4 (CTLA-4) and PD-1 act as brakes on T-cell activation, preventing overactivation and limiting autoimmunity.[8,9] These inhibitory pathways have become key therapeutic targets in cancer immunotherapy, with drugs like checkpoint inhibitors unleashing T cells to combat tumors effectively.

Although much emphasis on antitumor immunity has focused on adaptive immunity, effector cells of the innate immune response, NK cells, can act alone or in concert with adaptive immunity. NK cells can recognize and kill target cells without prior sensitization. These cells express activating and inhibitory cell-surface receptors and when their activating receptors are engaged without concomitant ligation of their inhibitory receptors, they can kill targets directly. NK cells have been traditionally viewed as providing the first line of defense against virally infected cells. NK cells can also interact with the adaptive immune system. They can modulate the function of APCs, promote Th1 responses, and potentially dampen autoimmune responses.

Antigen-Presenting Cells (APCs)

DCs are specialized professional APCs that play a pivotal role in bridging innate and adaptive immunity. Their primary function is to take up, process, and present antigens to T cells, thereby initiating and regulating immune responses. DCs are strategically distributed throughout the body, residing in lymphoid tissues, skin, and mucosal surfaces of various organs, where they serve as sentinels of the immune system. In their immature state, DCs circulate in peripheral tissues, equipped with a high capacity for antigen uptake and processing. Upon encountering an antigen, these cells undergo maturation, migrating to lymph nodes where they interact with T and B lymphocytes to activate adaptive immune responses.[10,11]

Immature DCs are highly efficient at capturing antigens through mechanisms such as phagocytosis, macropinocytosis, and receptor-mediated endocytosis. Once internalized, antigens are processed into peptide fragments and loaded onto MHC molecules for presentation to T cells. DCs express both MHC class I and MHC class II molecules, enabling them to present antigens to CD8+ cytotoxic T cells and CD4+ helper T cells, respectively.[11] This antigen presentation, coupled with the expression of costimulatory molecules such as CD80 and CD86, is essential for the activation of resting T cells. Importantly, DCs also release proinflammatory cytokines, such as IL-12, which play a key role in T-cell polarization and amplification of immune responses.

DCs are equipped with a variety of pattern recognition receptors, including toll-like receptors (TLRs), which enable them to detect and respond to pathogens and microbial components. Activation of these receptors triggers DC maturation, leading to the upregulation of MHC molecules, costimulatory signals, and the secretion of chemokines such as CCR7. CCR7 binds to its ligand CCL19, guiding DCs to lymph nodes where they present processed antigens to T cells. This migration is crucial for the initiation of adaptive immunity, as it ensures the delivery of antigenic information to the appropriate lymphoid compartments.[12]

In addition to their role in antigen presentation, activated DCs produce a spectrum of cytokines that recruit other immune cells to sites of inflammation and modulate the immune response. IL-12, for instance, is critical for driving Th1 differentiation in CD4+ T cells and enhancing the cytotoxic activity of CD8+ T cells. These cytokines not only shape the local inflammatory milieu but also influence systemic immune responses, amplifying the overall efficacy of antigen-specific immunity.

DCs are indispensable in cancer immunology due to their role in antitumor immune surveillance. By capturing TAAs and presenting them to T cells, DCs activate CTLs capable of targeting and eliminating tumor cells. However, the immunosuppressive TME can impair DC function, leading to reduced antigen presentation and diminished T-cell activation.[13] Efforts to harness DCs in cancer immunotherapy, such as DC vaccines, aim to overcome these challenges by enhancing their ability to stimulate robust antitumor immune responses.

MECHANISMS OF IMMUNE EVASION

Tumors have evolved a variety of mechanisms to evade immune detection and elimination, many of which are shaped by the TME which is a complex network of immune cells,
1 stromal cells, cytokines, and metabolic factors that collectively promote tumor survival and progression while suppressing effective antitumor immunity. These immune-evasion strategies often involve a combination of immunosuppressive signaling, recruitment of regulatory immune cells, metabolic reprogramming, and direct interference with antigen-
2 presentation pathways.

Immunosuppressive Cytokines and Molecules

Cytokines produced by innate and adaptive immune cells within the TME, such as type-1 and type-2 interferons (IFN-α/β and IFN-γ), can paradoxically enhance immune evasion. For example, these cytokines induce the expression of programmed death ligand 1 (PD-L1) on tumor cells, which engages the PD-1 receptor on T cells, leading to T-cell exhaustion and reduced effector activity.[14] Similarly, the enzyme indoleamine 2,3-dioxygenase (IDO) is upregulated in many tumors, catabolizing tryptophan into kynurenine, a metabolite that suppresses T-cell function and promotes Treg activity.[15] Vascular endothelial growth factor (VEGF), commonly secreted in response to hypoxia within the TME, not only promotes angiogenesis but also inhibits dendritic cell maturation and effector T-cell infiltration, further impairing antitumor responses.

Recruitment of Regulatory Immune Cells

The recruitment of immunosuppressive immune cells to the TME is another critical mechanism of immune evasion. Tregs are frequently enriched in the TME and tumor-draining lymph nodes, where they suppress effector T-cell responses through the secretion of immunosuppressive cytokines, such as IL-10 and TGF-β, and direct inhibitory interactions via molecules like CTLA-4.[7] Type 2 macrophages (M2 macrophages) and immature monocytes are also recruited to the TME, where they contribute to a wound-healing response that suppresses inflammation, facilitates tissue remodeling, and promotes tumor growth.[16]

Metabolic Reprogramming in the TME

The metabolic landscape of the TME is highly unfavorable for effective immune responses. Tumor cells often outcompete immune cells for essential nutrients, such as glucose and amino acids, depriving T cells of the metabolic resources needed to sustain their effector functions. For instance, glucose deprivation impairs glycolysis in T cells, a critical pathway for their activation and proliferation.[17] Furthermore, the hypoxic environment within tumors exacerbates immune dysfunction by promoting the expression of hypoxia-inducible factors (HIFs), which drive the production of VEGF and other immunosuppressive molecules.[18]

Downregulation of Antigen Presentation

A major mechanism by which tumors evade recognition by CTLs is the downregulation or complete loss of MHC class I molecules. MHC class I is essential for the presentation of intracellular antigens to CD8+ T cells, and its loss renders tumor cells "invisible" to these effector cells. Tumors achieve this through various mechanisms, including mutations in genes encoding MHC class I components, defects in antigen processing machinery, and epigenetic silencing.[19]

Immune Selection and Evolution

The immune system exerts strong selective pressure on tumor cells, leading to the emergence of immune-resistant variants. This process, termed "immunoediting," involves three phases: elimination, equilibrium, and escape. During the escape phase, tumor cells that have acquired immune-evasion mechanisms proliferate and dominate the tumor population. These mechanisms include increased expression of inhibitory ligands like PD-L1, recruitment of immunosuppressive cells, and metabolic reprogramming, as well as genetic alterations that reduce antigenicity or immunogenicity.[20]

TYPES OF IMMUNOTHERAPY

Cytokine Therapy

Cytokine therapy represents one of the earliest applications of immunotherapy in oncology, leveraging the immune-stimulating properties of proinflammatory cytokines to combat tumors. Following the discoveries of cytokines and advances in molecular biology, recombinant versions of interleukin-1 (IL-1), tumor necrosis factor alpha (TNF-α), interferons (IFNs), and interleukin-2 (IL-2) were developed and tested for their therapeutic potential. While these therapies yielded mixed results, they laid critical groundwork for modern immunotherapy approaches.

Interleukin-2 (IL-2)

IL-2, discovered in the 1970s as a T-cell growth factor, was pivotal in understanding immune cell activation. IL-2 plays a central role in the activation and proliferation of T cells and NK cells, making it a promising candidate for cancer therapy. Early studies demonstrated that IL-2 could sustain the growth of T cells in culture, facilitating research into T-cell biology. Recognizing its potential to enhance immune responses, researchers began investigating IL-2 as a therapeutic agent for cancer. Dr. Steven Rosenberg and the Surgery Branch at the National Cancer Institute (NCI) spearheaded efforts in the 1980s and 1990s to use high-dose IL-2 as a treatment for metastatic cancers.[21] Their pioneering work demonstrated that high-dose IL-2 could induce durable responses in patients with metastatic renal cell carcinoma (RCC) and metastatic melanoma. High-dose IL-2, administered at doses of 600,000 to 720,000 IU/kg intravenously, resulted in overall response rates of 15% to 20% for these cancers, with complete responses (CR) observed in a subset of patients. Remarkably, these responses often lasted many years, highlighting IL-2's potential for inducing long-term remission.

Despite its efficacy, high-dose IL-2 therapy is associated with significant toxicity, including vascular leak syndrome, hypotension, and organ dysfunction, which limit its broader application. Nevertheless, the U.S. Food and Drug Administration (FDA) approved IL-2 for metastatic RCC in 1992 and for metastatic melanoma in 1998. These approvals marked IL-2 as the first FDA-approved cancer immunotherapy, setting the stage for subsequent advances in the field.

Interferons (IFNs)

Interferons, particularly IFN-α, have also been extensively evaluated for their antitumor potential. IFNs exhibit potent antiviral, antiproliferative, and immune-stimulating effects. Preclinical studies demonstrated that IFN-α could directly inhibit tumor growth by inducing apoptosis and senescence while enhancing antitumor immunity by promoting DC maturation and T-cell cytotoxicity.

One of the earliest successes with IFN-α therapy was observed in hairy cell leukemia, in which patients treated with IFN-α achieved significant disease remission. This success spurred further exploration of IFN-α in other malignancies, particularly melanoma and RCC.[22] Clinical trials demonstrated that high-dose IFN-α could improve survival and reduce the risk of cancer recurrence when used as an adjuvant therapy after surgical resection of tumors. However, the benefits were tempered by significant toxicities, including flu-like symptoms, fatigue, and hematologic abnormalities, which limited its widespread use.

Challenges and Legacy

Despite initial promise, both IL-2 and IFN-α were eventually overshadowed by newer therapies, including targeted therapies and immune checkpoint inhibitors, which offered improved efficacy and reduced toxicity. Nonetheless, IL-2 and IFN-α remain important milestones in cancer immunotherapy, demonstrating the potential of cytokines to harness the immune system for therapeutic benefit. Importantly, these early cytokine therapies laid the foundation for subsequent developments, including engineered cytokines and combination therapies designed to enhance efficacy while minimizing adverse effects.[23]

Immune Checkpoint Blockade

Immune checkpoint inhibitors are currently the most widely used class of FDA-approved immunotherapy drugs, revolutionizing cancer treatment by reinvigorating T-cell–mediated
3 antitumor immunity. These therapies target inhibitory pathways, or "immune checkpoints," that tumors exploit to suppress immune responses. Checkpoint molecules such as programmed cell death protein 1 (PD-1) and CTLA-4 normally function to prevent autoimmunity and chronic inflammation by negatively regulating T-cell activity. However, tumors hijack these mechanisms, effectively silencing T cells and promoting immune evasion.

CTLA-4: Mechanism and Therapeutic Targeting

CTLA-4 is a checkpoint molecule expressed early during T-cell activation. It competes with CD28, the costimulatory receptor required for T-cell activation, by binding CD80/CD86 on APCs with higher affinity. This outcompetes CD28, raising the activation threshold and dampening T-cell responses. Genetic studies in mice revealed that CTLA-4 deficiency leads to severe lymphoproliferative disorders, underscoring its critical role in immune homeostasis.[24] Mechanistically, CTLA-4 predominantly regulates CD4+ T cells, particularly Tregs, which suppress effector T-cell activity.[25]

Therapeutic blockade of CTLA-4 with monoclonal antibodies such as ipilimumab enhances T-cell activity by preventing CTLA-4–mediated suppression and, in some cases, depleting Tregs within tumors. Pioneering work by Dr. Jim Allison demonstrated the efficacy of CTLA-4 blockade in preclinical models, leading to ipilimumab's FDA approval in 2011 for metastatic melanoma.[26] Clinical trials, such as the CheckMate 067 and EORTC 18071 studies, further established the efficacy of ipilimumab as monotherapy and in combination with anti–PD-1 antibodies, leading to its approval for high-risk melanoma and advanced RCC.[27,28]

PD-1 and PD-L1: Distinct Mechanisms of Suppression

PD-1, expressed on T cells after prolonged antigen exposure, mediates immune suppression in a temporally and mechanistically distinct manner from CTLA-4. PD-1 binds its ligands, PD-L1 and PD-L2, which are expressed by various immune and tumor cells. The interaction of PD-1 with PD-L1 initiates downstream signaling that recruits SHP2 phosphatases, inhibiting TCR and CD28 signaling pathways critical for T-cell activation. This creates a feedback loop where IFN-γ released by tumor-infiltrating lymphocytes (TILs) induces PD-L1 expression on tumor and APC surfaces, effectively silencing PD-1+ T cells.[29]

Unlike CTLA-4, PD-1 plays a central role in maintaining T-cell exhaustion—a differentiation state associated with chronic antigen exposure and reduced cytotoxic function. Therapeutic blockade of the PD-1/PD-L1 axis reactivates exhausted T cells, leading to robust antitumor responses. Agents such as nivolumab, pembrolizumab, atezolizumab, and durvalumab are FDA-approved for a range of cancers, including melanoma, non–small-cell lung cancer (NSCLC), and urothelial carcinoma, due to their superior response rates and
3 reduced toxicity compared to CTLA-4 inhibitors (**Table 4.1**).[30]

LAG3 and Emerging Checkpoints

Lymphocyte-activation gene 3 (LAG3) represents a newer checkpoint target. LAG3 binds MHC class II molecules, contributing to T-cell suppression by reducing cytokine production and T-cell proliferation. LAG3 expression often colocalizes with PD-1 on exhausted T cells, marking deeply suppressed phenotypes. Recent FDA approval of LAG3 inhibitors in combination with anti–PD-1 antibodies underscores the therapeutic potential in reversing immune suppression and enhancing effector T-cell activity.[31]

The Role of T-Cell Exhaustion and T-Stem Cells

Chronic antigen exposure drives T-cell exhaustion, a state characterized by terminal differentiation, impaired effector function, and epigenetic silencing of key immune response genes. Despite these limitations, subsets of PD-1+ T cells retain a stem-like phenotype (T-stem), which serves as progenitors for effector and exhausted T cells. Studies in tumor-bearing mice and cancer patients treated with anti–PD-1 therapy reveal that T-stem cells migrate from lymph nodes to tumors, where they replenish exhausted T-cell populations and sustain antitumor responses. T-stem cells are often localized in tumor-associated tertiary lymphoid structures (TLS) or antigen-presenting cell niches, which are associated with improved prognosis. Strategies to expand or enhance the function of T-stem cells could significantly improve immunotherapy outcomes. Research into the signaling pathways and transcriptional programs that maintain T–stem cell populations is ongoing and holds promise for developing novel therapeutic approaches.

Predicting Response to Immune Checkpoint Blockade

Predicting which patients will respond to immunotherapy
4 remains a complex and evolving field, given the variability

Table 4.1. Select Clinical Trials Utilizing PD-1 Checkpoint Inhibition

Cancer Indication	PD-1 Inhibitor	Key Clinical Trial(s)	Summary of Efficacy
Melanoma	Pembrolizumab	KEYNOTE-001[32]	Improved overall survival (OS) and progression-free survival (PFS) compared to standard therapy
Non–small-cell lung cancer	Pembrolizumab	KEYNOTE-189[33]	Improved OS and PFS in both first-line setting
Renal cell carcinoma	Nivolumab	CheckMate-205[34]	Superior OS (25.0 vs. 19.6 mo) compared to everolimus
Gastric cancer	Pembrolizumab	KEYNOTE-059[35]	ORR of 11.6%, 15.5% in PD-L1 positive advanced gastric cancer
Colorectal cancer (Microsatellite instability-high)	Pembrolizumab	KEYNOTE-164[36]	Increased PFS and OS in patients with MSI-H or mismatch repair-deficient colorectal cancer
Hepatocellular Carcinoma	Nivolumab	CheckMate-040[37]	Durable responses in patients with advanced HCC (median duration of 17 mo)

of patient responses to treatments like immune checkpoint inhibitors. While these therapies have revolutionized cancer treatment, only a subset of patients experience significant benefits. Identifying reliable biomarkers is crucial to predicting which patients will respond and to optimizing treatment strategies.

A robust preexisting T-cell infiltration within the TME is one of the strongest predictors of a positive response to immunotherapy. Tumors characterized by dense T-cell infiltration, often termed "hot" tumors, generally respond better to immune checkpoint inhibitors (**Fig. 4.3**).[38] The immunoscore, a quantitative measure of T-cell density in tumor samples using immunohistochemistry, has emerged as an independent prognostic marker for survival across many cancer types, irrespective of therapy.[39] However, not all T-cell infiltration patterns are equivalent. For example, in some tumors, T cells are confined to the stromal borders, unable to penetrate the cancer cell regions, reflecting an immune-excluded phenotype that is less favorable for therapy. In contrast, other tumors display TLS, which are organized lymphoid aggregates resembling lymph nodes and are predictive of better responses to checkpoint blockade.[40] TLS are associated with both improved survival

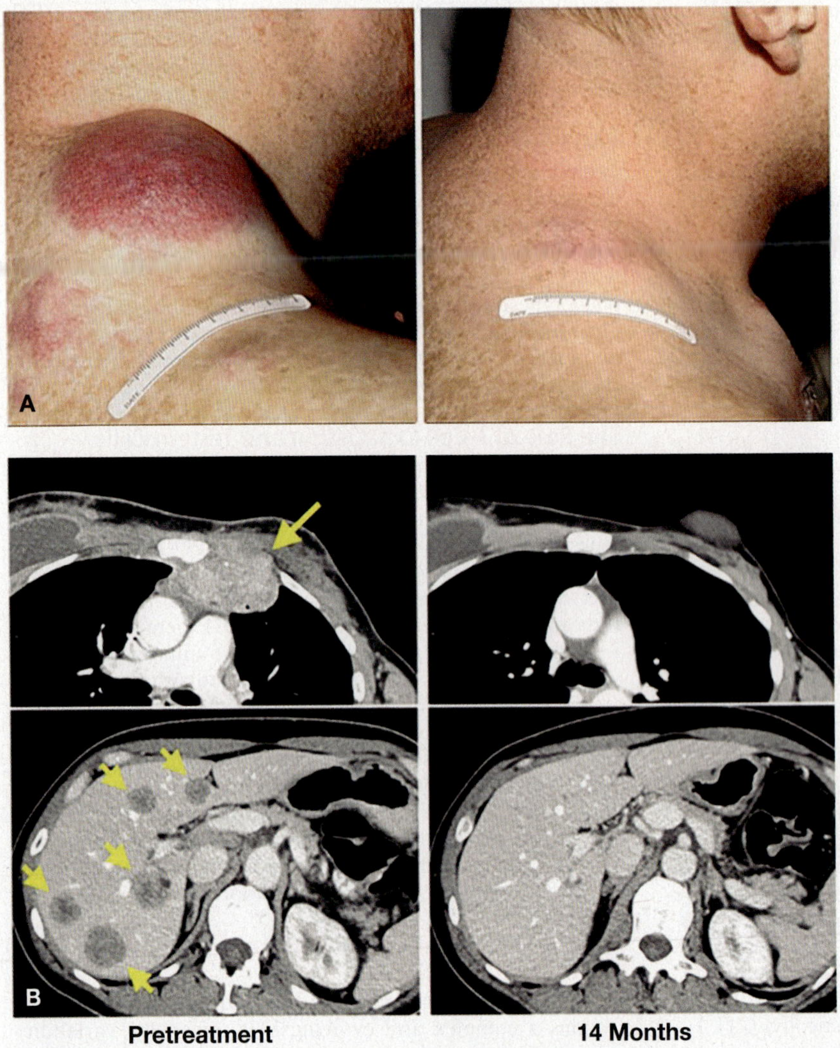

Figure 4.3. A: Before and after pictures of a patient with advanced melanoma who underwent treatment with TIL. Within 2 weeks of treatment, the large tumor had disappeared. **B:** Separate patient before (**left**) and 14 months after treatment (**right**) with TIL.

Table 4.2. Comparison of Types of Cellular Immunotherapy

Type of Adoptive T-Cell Therapy	Source of T Cells	Modification/ Expansion Process	Targeted Cancer Types	Key Features
Tumor-infiltrating lymphocytes (TIL) therapy	T cells isolated from the patient's tumor	T cells are expanded to large numbers in the laboratory	Primarily solid tumors, especially metastatic melanoma	TILs are naturally primed to recognize and attack the patient's specific cancer
Chimeric antigen receptor (CAR) T-cell therapy	T cells collected from the patient's blood	T cells are genetically engineered to express a CAR targeting a specific cancer antigen	Blood cancers such as acute lymphoblastic leukemia (ALL) and diffuse large B-cell lymphoma (DLBCL)	CAR T cells are highly effective in hematologic malignancies and can achieve high response rates
T-cell receptor (TCR) therapy	T cells collected from the patient's blood	T cells are modified to express specific TCRs recognizing cancer antigens	Solid tumors, including synovial sarcoma and certain melanomas	TCRs can target intracellular proteins presented by MHC, allowing broader application to solid tumors

and a more robust antitumor immune response, highlighting the interplay between cell-mediated and humoral immunity, particularly the role of tumor-reactive B cells in potentiating 3
antitumor activity.

Genomic biomarkers also play a critical role in predicting immunotherapy response, with tumor mutational burden (TMB) being one of the most clinically relevant. TMB quantifies the total number of mutations per megabase of tumor DNA, providing an indication of neoantigen availability. Higher TMB correlates with greater likelihood of T-cell recognition and response.[41] Patients with tumors exhibiting defects in DNA mismatch repair (dMMR) or microsatellite instability-high (MSI-high) status exhibit exceptionally high TMB. These tumors are often highly immunogenic and demonstrate excellent responses to PD-1 blockade, leading to the FDA's cancer-agnostic approval of pembrolizumab for patients with MSI-high or dMMR tumors.[36]

PD-L1 expression, a biomarker related to the PD-1/PD-L1 immune checkpoint pathway, is frequently assessed to predict responses to anti–PD-1/PD-L1 therapies. High PD-L1 expression on tumor cells has been associated with improved response rates to these therapies, yet many patients with low or undetectable PD-L1 expression also respond. This discrepancy highlights the complexity of PD-1/PD-L1 signaling and suggests that PD-L1 expression on immune cells within the TME or outside the tumor, such as in lymph nodes, may also play a significant role. Despite significant advancements, challenges remain in interpreting these biomarkers in clinical practice. Factors such as tumor heterogeneity, spatial distribution of immune cells, and dynamic changes in biomarker levels over time must be carefully considered. Multimodal approaches that combine genomic, immunologic, and systemic biomarkers offer the most comprehensive insights into patient responses, paving the way for more personalized and effective cancer immunotherapy.

Adoptive T-Cell Therapy

Adoptive T-cell therapy is a novel approach in cancer treatment that leverages the body's adaptive immune response to fight cancer by enhancing the antitumor capabilities of T cells. This immunotherapy strategy involves extracting immune cells from a cancer patient from either tumor tissue or peripheral blood, expanding and enhancing the antitumor properties of those cells ex vivo, and reinfusing them back into the patient. Autologous cell transfer is preferred to avoid graft versus host response but allogenic transfers are also utilized in certain contexts. There are three types of adoptive T-cell therapy based on the source of the T cells, how they are modified or expanded, and whether the specific receptors they express are endogenous or genetically engineered to express (**Table 4.2**).

Tumor-Infiltrating Lymphocyte (TIL) Therapy

Among the earliest and most extensively studied forms of ACT is TIL therapy. Developed in the 1980s by Dr. Steven Rosenberg at the NCI, TIL therapy involves isolating T cells that naturally infiltrate a patient's tumor, expanding these cells ex vivo, and reinfusing them into the patient. TILs are enriched with T cells that are naturally primed to recognize tumor-specific neoantigens, providing a highly specific and potent antitumor response. In TIL therapy, tumor fragments are cultured in high doses of interleukin-2 (IL-2), promoting the proliferation of tumor-reactive T cells. After selecting the most reactive T-cell clones, these cells are expanded to billions using agonist antibodies against CD3 and IL-2. Prior to reinfusion, patients undergo a lymphodepletion regimen with cyclophosphamide and fludarabine to optimize the cytokine milieu, facilitating TIL expansion and activity in vivo. Early trials in metastatic melanoma patients reported CR in 23% of cases, with some patients achieving durable remissions lasting years (**Fig. 4.4**).[42]

Recent clinical trials have demonstrated encouraging results with TIL therapy for advanced melanoma. In a pivotal study published in the *Journal of Clinical Oncology*, metastatic melanoma patients treated with TIL therapy achieved an objective response rate (ORR) of 56%, with durable responses in some cases lasting for years.[43] A Phase II trial further reported a 36% ORR, including 12% CR, highlighting TIL therapy's efficacy and safety. These findings led to the FDA's approval of TIL therapy for metastatic melanoma in early 2024.[44] Ongoing research aims to extend TIL therapy's success to other solid tumors, including cervical, ovarian, and NSCLC.[45]

Chimeric Antigen Receptor (CAR) T-Cell Therapy

CAR T-cell therapy involves genetically engineering T cells to express synthetic receptors that target specific proteins in cancer cells (**Fig. 4.5**). Unlike TIL therapy, CAR T cells do not rely on MHC-dependent antigen presentation, allowing them to target surface antigens directly. This therapy was pioneered by the NCI in the early 2010s, with the first clinical success reported in a patient with refractory B-cell lymphoma treated with CAR T cells targeting CD19.[46]

CAR T cells are engineered using a lentiviral construct encoding a single-chain variable fragment (scFv) from an antibody specific to a tumor antigen, coupled with intracellular

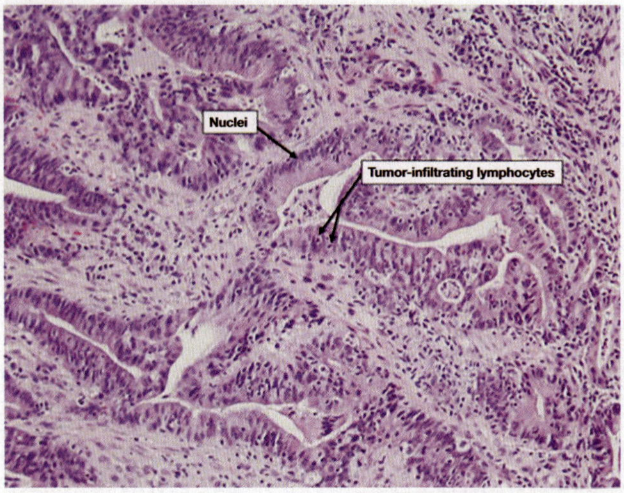

Figure 4.4. H&E slide of a colorectal tumor under a microscope, showing tumor-infiltrating lymphocytes (TIL) and cell nuclei in the tumor. Significant numbers of TIL are suggestive of an immunologically "hot" tumor.

signaling domains like CD3-zeta and costimulatory molecules such as 4-1BB or CD28. Upon infusion, these cells can recognize and kill cancer cells independent of MHC. Early trials demonstrated high efficacy in hematologic malignancies, with ORRs exceeding 80% in relapsed or refractory acute lymphoblastic leukemia (ALL) and complete remission in many patients.[47,48]

The FDA has approved several CAR T therapies, including tisagenlecleucel (Kymriah) for pediatric ALL, axicabtagene ciloleucel (Yescarta) for relapsed/refractory large B-cell lymphoma, and idecabtagene vicleucel (Abecma) for multiple myeloma. While CAR T therapy has revolutionized the treatment of blood cancers, translating its success to solid tumors remains challenging due to issues like antigen heterogeneity, T-cell infiltration barriers, and the immunosuppressive TME. Strategies such as multitargeted CARs, armored CAR T cells, and cytokine-secreting CARs are being investigated to overcome these obstacles.[49–51]

TCR Therapy

TCR therapy modifies T cells to express specific TCRs that recognize intracellular tumor antigens presented on MHC molecules. Unlike CAR T cells, TCR-engineered T cells can target intracellular proteins, broadening the range of potential cancer targets. However, TCR therapy requires precise matching of patient-specific MHC molecules, adding complexity to its application.

Early trials of TCR therapy have shown promise in solid tumors, such as synovial sarcoma and melanoma. For example, patients treated with NY-ESO-1 TCR-engineered T cells achieved an ORR of 50%, demonstrating the therapy's potential.[52] Advances in genomic sequencing and neoantigen identification are enabling the development of personalized TCR therapies tailored to individual patients, enhancing efficacy and specificity.[53]

Despite their success, ACT therapies face several challenges, including antigen loss, T-cell exhaustion, and immunosuppressive TME. Research is focusing on improving the persistence and functionality of adoptive T cells through strategies like combination therapies, next-generation CAR and TCR constructs, and stem-like T-cell populations. Clinical trials exploring the use of ACT in combination with immune checkpoint inhibitors, cytokine therapies, and conventional treatments are underway to maximize therapeutic outcomes.

Vaccine Therapy

In 1970, landmark experiments demonstrated that tumor-specific immunity could be induced in mice. Scientists demonstrated that inoculating naïve, inbred mice with methylcholanthrene (MCA)-induced sarcomas, followed by removal of the transplanted tumor, conferred protection against rechallenge with the same tumor. These preconditioned mice rejected subsequent inoculations with tumor cells derived from the same MCA sarcoma but remained susceptible to genetically distinct MCA sarcoma lines from other hosts. These findings provided the first evidence that the immune system could recognize tumors as nonself and eliminate them, even though they originated from self-tissues.[54] This discovery paved the way for understanding the immune system's role in tumor surveillance and control. It also spurred decades of research into harnessing the immune system to develop prophylactic and therapeutic cancer vaccines.

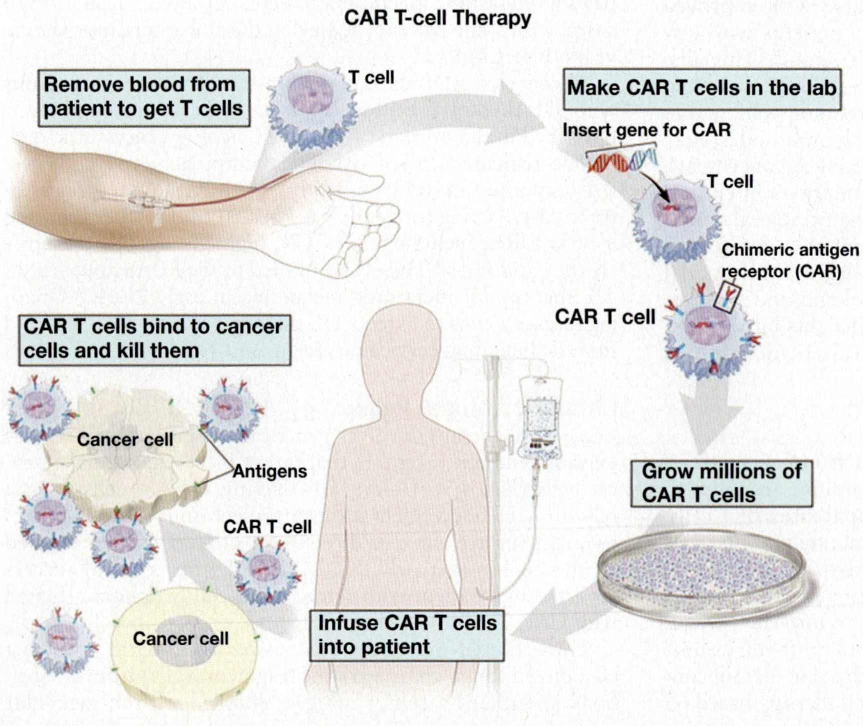

Figure 4.5. CAR T-cell therapy is a type of treatment in which a patient's T cells (a type of immune cell) are changed in the laboratory so they will bind to cancer cells and kill them. White blood cells, including the T cells, are removed by an apharesis machine that sends the rest of the blood back to the patient. Next, the gene for a special receptor called a chimeric antigen receptor (CAR) is inserted into the T cells in the laboratory. Millions of the CAR T cells are then grown in the laboratory and then given back to the patient by infusion where the CAR-T cells are able to bind to an antigen on the cancer cells and kill them. (© 2017 Terese Winslow LLC, U.S. Govt. has certain rights.)

Table 4.3. Summary of Current Vaccine Platforms

Vaccine Type	Description
Peptide-based vaccines	Use of predefined or patient-specific peptides derived from tumor antigens, combined with adjuvants to enhance immunogenicity.
mRNA vaccines	Liposome-encapsulated mRNA encoding tumor-specific antigens or oncogenic drivers; promising in personalized immunotherapy.
Whole tumor cell vaccines	Utilize irradiated autologous or allogeneic tumor cells engineered to express dendritic cell (DC) maturation factors to enhance immune responses.
Vector-based vaccines	Attenuated bacterial or viral vectors encoding tumor antigens; efficiently deliver antigens and stimulate robust immune responses.
DC vaccines	Direct transfer of ex vivo antigen-loaded dendritic cells to prime T-cell responses.

Tumor Antigens: Targets for Vaccination

Advances in immunology revealed that tumors express antigens that can be recognized by the immune system. These tumor antigens are broadly classified as tumor-specific antigens (TSA) that are neoantigens arising from nonsynonymous mutations, unique to individual tumors, or TAAs, which are nonmutated antigens overexpressed in tumors but expressed at low levels in normal tissues. Examples include gp96, WT1, MAGE, NY-ESO-1, tyrosinase, and carcinoembryonic antigen (CEA). While TAAs are shared among patients and theoretically easier to target, their self-derived nature often limits their immunogenicity due to central and peripheral tolerance. Conversely, TSAs, arising from somatic mutations, are highly immunogenic but unique to individual patients, necessitating personalized approaches. Prophylactic vaccines targeting oncogenic viral infections have demonstrated significant success in preventing virus-associated cancers. For example, the HPV vaccine (Gardasil), introduced in 2006, has led to a dramatic reduction in cervical cancer rates and other HPV-associated malignancies, including head and neck squamous cell carcinoma (HNSCC).[55] Similarly, ongoing efforts to target Epstein–Barr virus (EBV) antigens aim to reduce nasopharyngeal carcinoma and other EBV-driven cancers. In addition, technologic advancements, particularly in genomic sequencing, have led to the development of diverse vaccine platforms (**Table 4.3**).

Unlike prophylactic vaccines, therapeutic cancer vaccines face challenges, particularly in the presence of established tumors. Tumor-induced immunosuppression within the microenvironment, characterized by Tregs, MDSCs, and immune checkpoint molecules like PD-1 and CTLA-4, dampens vaccine efficacy. As a result, therapeutic vaccines may be most effective in the adjuvant setting in which they can prevent recurrence following surgical resection or remission induction. Promising strategies include combining vaccines with immune checkpoint inhibitors, oncolytic viruses, or adoptive cell therapies to overcome immunosuppression and enhance vaccine efficacy.

Oncolytic Viral Therapy

5 Oncolytic viral therapy leverages the natural infective and replicative properties of viruses, enhanced through genetic engineering, to selectively target and destroy cancer cells while activating immune responses within the TME. This dual mechanism of direct oncolysis and immune activation positions oncolytic viruses as a transformative approach in oncology, offering both cytotoxicity and immunomodulation.

T-VEC: A Benchmark in Oncolytic Therapy

The FDA approval of talimogene laherparepvec (T-VEC),[56] an oncolytic herpes simplex virus type-1 (HSV-1), for advanced melanoma marked a significant milestone. In the pivotal Phase III OPTiM trial, T-VEC demonstrated an ORR of 26.4%, with a CR rate of 10.8%, and a durable response rate (DRR) of 16.3% compared to 2.1% with the control treatment.[56] While overall survival (OS) improvements were not statistically significant, a trend favoring T-VEC (23.3 vs. 18.9 months) underscored its clinical potential. This approval established T-VEC as the first oncolytic virus available for patient care. Other oncolytic viruses, such as pelareorep and DNX-2401, are advancing the field. Pelareorep, an oncolytic reovirus, demonstrated synergy with paclitaxel in metastatic breast cancer, achieving an ORR of 58% compared to 31% with paclitaxel alone. Ongoing Phase III trials are investigating its combination with pembrolizumab to enhance antitumor immunity.

Cytotoxic Therapy and Immunogenic Cell Death

For decades, cancer treatment was defined by three foundational modalities: surgery, radiation, and chemotherapy. These were often used in combination to maximize patient outcomes. However, cytotoxic therapies alone rarely achieve durable cures, serving instead to attenuate tumor progression and prolong survival. Many patients with unresectable disease or postsurgical relapse required novel approaches to improve outcomes. The discovery that cytotoxic therapies could elicit immune responses through the induction of cell death provided a foundation for integrating immunotherapy into these traditional modalities. The induction of cell death via necrosis or programmed pathways, including apoptosis, ferroptosis, necroptosis, and pyroptosis, releases danger- and pattern-associated molecular patterns (DAMPs and PAMPs), such as HMGB1, calreticulin, ATP, and cyclic dinucleotides (CDN).[57,58] These molecules are sensed by innate immune cells, including macrophages and DCs, via TLRs and nucleic acid-sensing pathways, creating an adjuvant effect that enhances T-cell activation through cytokine production and antigen presentation.

Certain chemotherapeutics, such as anthracyclines, have superior immunostimulatory properties. These agents induce endoplasmic reticulum (ER) stress and autophagy in cancer cells, enhancing immune recognition. Chemotherapy efficacy in preclinical models is significantly reduced in immunodeficient animals lacking T cells, DCs, or interferon pathways.[59] Additionally, some chemotherapeutics indirectly support antitumor immunity by depleting immunosuppressive cells. For example, cyclophosphamide reduces Tregs, and paclitaxel, 5-fluorouracil, and gemcitabine deplete MDSCs. However, high doses of chemotherapy can suppress T-cell function, underscoring the need for fine-tuned regimens. Clinical trials combining chemotherapy with immune checkpoint inhibitors have demonstrated added survival benefits in cancers such as lung and breast cancer, resulting in the approval of combination therapies.[60,61]

Radiation therapy elicits immune responses distinct from chemotherapy by inducing DNA damage and double-strand breaks. This process releases micronuclei and CDNs, which activate the stimulator of interferon genes (STING) pathway.[62] STING activation promotes type-I interferon production, enhancing DC-mediated antigen presentation and fostering an M1-type inflammatory response that supports CD8+ T-cell activity.

Mouse models deficient in DCs or STING pathway components exhibit resistance to radiotherapy, underscoring the pathway's critical role in radiation efficacy.[63] Furthermore, exogenous STING agonists can enhance radiotherapy's effects in tumor-bearing mice.[64]

Table 4.4. Strategies to Overcome Tumor Immune Suppression

Target	Mechanism of Suppression	Therapeutic Strategies
TAMs	IL-10, TGF-β secretion; VEGF-mediated angiogenesis	CSF1R inhibitors, CD40 agonists, CCL2/CCR2 blockade
MDSCs	Nutrient depletion (arginase, iNOS); checkpoint expression	Gemcitabine, 5-FU, CXCR2 blockade, ATRA
Tregs	IL-10, TGF-β secretion; FoxP3+ immune suppression	CCR4 blockade, low-dose cyclophosphamide, anti–CTLA-4
CAFs	Matrix stiffness; recruitment of suppressive immune cells	TGF-β inhibitors, IL-1 blockade, CAF reprogramming

Overcoming Tumor-Induced Immunosuppression

Tumors employ diverse strategies to evade immune recognition and cytotoxicity. These mechanisms include both intrinsic pathways, such as immune checkpoint upregulation and
2 extrinsic pathways that mimic wound-healing processes. These extrinsic pathways involve recruitment of immunosuppressive cells and reprogramming of the TME to create an immune-tolerant niche. Overcoming these barriers is critical to enhance the efficacy of immunotherapy and is summarized in **Table 4.4**.

Intrinsic Mechanisms of Immune Suppression: Checkpoints

As discussed, tumors exploit immune checkpoint molecules such as PD-1/PD-L1 and CTLA-4 to suppress T-cell activity. These mechanisms, originally designed to prevent autoimmune damage, are co-opted by tumors to attenuate effector T-cell responses. Immune checkpoint blockade therapies targeting these pathways (eg, anti–PD-1, anti–CTLA-4) have revolutionized cancer treatment, but resistance and incomplete responses highlight the need to address additional suppressive factors in the TME.[8,9]

Extrinsic Mechanisms of Immune Suppression

Tumor-Associated Macrophages (TAMs)

TAMs are a predominant component of most solid tumors and play a pivotal role in immune evasion. TAMs are often polarized toward an M2-like phenotype, characterized by immunosuppressive and protumorigenic functions including angiogenesis with secretion of VEGF, matrix remodeling with deposition and modification of extracellular matrix (ECM) components, and T-cell suppression with expression of IL-10, TGF-β, and PD-L1. Mouse models deficient in macrophages exhibit reduced tumor growth, underscoring TAMs' critical role in tumor progression.[65] Therapies targeting TAMs aim to repolarize TAMs to an M1-like phenotype using agents such as CD40 agonists or TLR agonists, deplete TAMs using CSF1R inhibitors, which block macrophage recruitment or survival, and inhibit TAM recruitment through blockade of CCL2/CCR2 signaling.[66] While promising in preclinical models, these strategies face challenges in clinical translation due to incomplete TAM depletion and off-target effects.

Myeloid-Derived Suppressor Cells (MDSCs)

MDSCs are developmentally related to macrophages but remain in an immature state due to tumor-driven factors. MDSCs suppress T-cell responses through arginase-1 and iNOS production, depleting nutrients critical for T-cell function (eg, arginine), secretion of TGF-β and IL-10 to inhibit effector T-cell activity, and expression of immune checkpoint molecules, such as PD-L1.[67] Strategies to target MDSCs include depletion using gemcitabine or 5-fluorouracil, differentiation induction with agents such as all-trans retinoic acid (ATRA), or inhibiting recruitment through blockade of CXCR2 signaling. Despite promising preclinical results, translating these findings into effective clinical therapies remains challenging.

Tregs

Tregs are enriched in tumors and secondary lymphoid tissues, where they secrete IL-10 and TGF-β to suppress effector T-cell activity. Tumors exploit Tregs to maintain an immunosuppressive environment. Strategies to attenuate Treg activity include targeting Treg recruitment by blocking CCL22/CCR4 signaling, depleting Tregs using low-dose cyclophosphamide or anti–CTLA-4 antibodies, and inhibiting Treg function by targeting FoxP3 or CTLA-4.[68] However, selective Treg modulation without affecting normal immune regulation remains a significant hurdle.

Cancer-Associated Fibroblasts (CAFs)

CAFs are a heterogeneous population of fibroblasts in the TME with primarily protumorigenic functions. CAF subsets include myofibroblastic CAF, which is induced by TGF-β, these cells promote ECM deposition and stiffness, impeding T-cell infiltration, and inflammatory CAFs which are induced by IL-1 signaling, these cells secrete chemokines that recruit TAMs, MDSCs, and Tregs.[69] Emerging single-cell transcriptomic profiling has identified smaller subsets of immune-stimulating CAFs, offering potential therapeutic targets. Current approaches to modulate CAF activity include blocking TGF-β signaling to reduce matrix stiffness, targeting IL-1 signaling to inhibit iCAF recruitment of suppressive cells, and reprogramming CAFs to an antitumorigenic phenotypes.

SUMMARY

Cancer immunotherapy has revolutionized oncology, transformed the treatment landscape, and offered durable, long-term responses for many patients. Breakthroughs such as immune checkpoint inhibitors, adoptive cell therapies, cancer vaccines, and oncolytic viral therapies underscore the potential of harnessing the immune system to combat malignancies. While treatments like PD-1/PD-L1 and CTLA-4 inhibitors, CAR T cells, and TIL therapies have shown remarkable efficacy, challenges persist in expanding these benefits across diverse cancer types. Tumor-induced immunosuppression, immune escape mechanisms, and the complexity of the TME remain significant barriers. Biomarkers such as TMB, MSI, and PD-L1 expression have provided tools to optimize patient selection and treatment strategies, though further research is needed to refine their predictive power.

Looking forward, the integration of immunotherapy with traditional modalities like surgery, chemotherapy, and radiation promises to create synergistic, multimodal treatment approaches. Advancements in understanding the interplay between tumors and the immune system, coupled with novel strategies to overcome resistance, will likely expand the reach and efficacy of these therapies.

References

1. Hanahan D. Hallmarks of cancer: new dimensions. *Cancer Discov*. 2022;12(1):31–46.
2. Virchow R. Cellular pathology. As based upon physiological and pathological histology. Lecture XVI–Atheromatous affection of arteries. 1858. *Nutr Rev*. 1989;47(1):23–25.
3. Starnes CO. Coley's toxins in perspective. *Nature*. 1992; 357(6373):11–12.
4. Decker WK, da Silva RF, Sanabria MH, et al. Cancer immunotherapy: historical perspective of a clinical revolution and emerging preclinical animal models. *Front Immunol*. 2017;8:829.
5. Murphy K, Weaver C. Janeway's Immunobiology. 9th ed. Garland Science/Taylor & Francis Group, LLC; 2016:904.
6. Zhu J, Paul WE. CD4 T cells: fates, functions, and faults. *Blood*. 2008;112(5):1557–1569.
7. Sakaguchi S. Regulatory T cells: key controllers of immunologic self-tolerance. *Cell*. 2000;101(5):455–458.
8. Pardoll DM. The blockade of immune checkpoints in cancer immunotherapy. *Nat Rev Cancer*. 2012;12(4):252–264.
9. Sharma P, Allison JP. The future of immune checkpoint therapy. *Science*. 2015;348(6230):56–61.
10. Lanier LL. NK cell recognition. *Annu Rev Immunol*. 2005;23: 225–274.
11. Vivier E, Tomasello E, Baratin M, Walzer T, Ugolini S. Functions of natural killer cells. *Nat Immunol*. 2008;9(5):503–510.
12. Caligiuri MA. Human natural killer cells. *Blood*. 2008;112(3): 461–469.
13. Guillerey C, Huntington ND, Smyth MJ. Targeting natural killer cells in cancer immunotherapy. *Nat Immunol*. 2016;17(9): 1025–1036.
14. Dong H, Strome SE, Salomao DR, et al. Tumor-associated B7-H1 promotes T-cell apoptosis: a potential mechanism of immune evasion. *Nat Med*. 2002;8(8):793–800.
15. Munn DH, Mellor AL. IDO in the tumor microenvironment: inflammation, counter-regulation, and tolerance. *Trends Immunol*. 2016;37(3):193–207.
16. Noy R, Pollard JW. Tumor-associated macrophages: from mechanisms to therapy. *Immunity*. 2014;41(1):49–61.
17. Chang CH, Qiu J, O'Sullivan D, et al. Metabolic competition in the tumor microenvironment is a driver of cancer progression. *Cell*. 2015;162(6):1229–1241.
18. Rankin EB, Giaccia AJ. Hypoxic control of metastasis. *Science*. 2016;352(6282):175–180.
19. Garrido F, Aptsiauri N, Doorduijn EM, Garcia Lora AM, van Hall T. The urgent need to recover MHC class I in cancers for effective immunotherapy. *Curr Opin Immunol*. 2016;39:44–51.
20. Schreiber RD, Old LJ, Smyth MJ. Cancer immunoediting: integrating immunity's roles in cancer suppression and promotion. *Science*. 2011;331(6024):1565–1570.
21. Rosenberg SA, Lotze MT, Muul LM, et al. A progress report on the treatment of 157 patients with advanced cancer using lymphokine-activated killer cells and interleukin-2 or high-dose interleukin-2 alone. *N Engl J Med*. 1987;316(15):889–897.
22. Kirkwood JM, Ibrahim JG, Sondak VK, et al. High- and low-dose interferon alfa-2b in high-risk melanoma: first analysis of intergroup trial E1690/S9111/C9190. *J Clin Oncol*. 2000; 18(12):2444–2458.
23. Atkins MB. Interleukin-2: clinical applications. *Semin Oncol*. 2002;29(3 Suppl 7):12–17.
24. Tivol EA, Borriello F, Schweitzer AN, Lynch WP, Bluestone JA, Sharpe AH. Loss of CTLA-4 leads to massive lymphoproliferation and fatal multiorgan tissue destruction, revealing a critical negative regulatory role of CTLA-4. *Immunity*. 1995;3(5):541–547.
25. Wing K, Onishi Y, Prieto-Martin P, et al. CTLA-4 control over Foxp3+ regulatory T cell function. *Science*. 2008;322(5899): 271–275.
26. Leach DR, Krummel MF, Allison JP. Enhancement of antitumor immunity by CTLA-4 blockade. *Science*. 1996;271(5256):1734–1736.
27. Robert C, Schachter J, Long GV, et al. Pembrolizumab versus ipilimumab in advanced melanoma. *N Engl J Med*. 2015; 372(26):2521–2532.
28. Hodi FS, O'Day SJ, McDermott DF, et al. Improved survival with ipilimumab in patients with metastatic melanoma. *N Engl J Med*. 2010;363(8):711–723.
29. Freeman GJ, Long AJ, Iwai Y, et al. Engagement of the PD-1 immunoinhibitory receptor by a novel B7 family member leads to negative regulation of lymphocyte activation. *J Exp Med*. 2000;192(7):1027–1034.
30. Topalian SL, Hodi FS, Brahmer JR, et al. Safety, activity, and immune correlates of anti-PD-1 antibody in cancer. *N Engl J Med*. 2012;366(26):2443–2454.
31. Andrews LP, Yano H, Vignali DAA. Inhibitory receptors and ligands beyond PD-1, PD-L1 and CTLA-4: breakthroughs or backups. *Nat Immunol*. 2019;20(11):1425–1434.
32. Robert C, Long GV, Brady B, et al. Nivolumab in previously untreated melanoma without BRAF mutation. *N Engl J Med*. 2015;372(4):320–330.
33. Gandhi L, Rodriguez-Abreu D, Gadgeel S, et al. Pembrolizumab plus chemotherapy in metastatic non-small-cell lung cancer. *N Engl J Med*. 2018;378(22):2078–2092.
34. Motzer RJ, Escudier B, McDermott DF, et al. Nivolumab versus everolimus in advanced renal-cell carcinoma. *N Engl J Med*. 2015;373(19):1803–1813.
35. Fuchs CS, Doi T, Jang RW, et al. Safety and efficacy of pembrolizumab monotherapy in patients with previously treated advanced gastric and gastroesophageal junction cancer: phase 2 clinical KEYNOTE-059 trial. *JAMA Oncol*. 2018;4(5):e180013.
36. Le DT, Uram JN, Wang H, et al. PD-1 blockade in tumors with mismatch-repair deficiency. *N Engl J Med*. 2015;372(26):2509–2520.
37. El-Khoueiry AB, Sangro B, Yau T, et al. Nivolumab in patients with advanced hepatocellular carcinoma (CheckMate 040): an open-label, non-comparative, phase 1/2 dose escalation and expansion trial. *Lancet*. 2017;389(10088):2492–2502.
38. Galon J, Pagès F, Marincola FM, et al. The immune score as a new possible approach for the classification of cancer. *J Transl Med*. 2012;10:1.
39. Pages F, Mlecnik B, Marliot F, et al. International validation of the consensus Immunoscore for the classification of colon cancer: a prognostic and accuracy study. *Lancet*. 2018;391(10135):2128–2139.
40. Helmink BA, Reddy SM, Gao J, et al. B cells and tertiary lymphoid structures promote immunotherapy response. *Nature*. 2020;577(7791):549–555.
41. Rizvi NA, Hellmann MD, Snyder A, et al. Cancer immunology. Mutational landscape determines sensitivity to PD-1 blockade in non-small cell lung cancer. *Science*. 2015;348(6230):124–128.
42. Rosenberg SA, Yang JC, Sherry RM, et al. Durable complete responses in heavily pretreated patients with metastatic melanoma using T-cell transfer immunotherapy. *Clin Cancer Res*. 2011;17(13):4550–4557.
43. Sarnaik AA, Hamid O, Khushalani NI, et al. Lifileucel, a tumor-infiltrating lymphocyte therapy, in metastatic melanoma. *J Clin Oncol*. 2021;39(24):2656–2666.
44. Dudley ME, Wunderlich JR, Yang JC, et al. Adoptive cell transfer therapy following non-myeloablative but lymphodepleting chemotherapy for the treatment of patients with refractory metastatic melanoma. *J Clin Oncol*. 2005;23(10):2346–2357.
45. Stevanovic S, Pasetto A, Helman SR, et al. Landscape of immunogenic tumor antigens in successful immunotherapy of virally induced epithelial cancer. *Science*. 2017;356(6334):200–205.
46. Grupp SA, Kalos M, Barrett D, et al. Chimeric antigen receptor-modified T cells for acute lymphoid leukemia. *N Engl J Med*. 2013;368(16):1509–1518.
47. Maude SL, Frey N, Shaw PA, et al. Chimeric antigen receptor T cells for sustained remissions in leukemia. *N Engl J Med*. 2014;371(16):1507–1517.
48. Schuster SJ, Bishop MR, Tam CS, et al. Tisagenlecleucel in adult relapsed or refractory diffuse large B-cell lymphoma. *N Engl J Med*. 2019;380(1):45–56.
49. Park JH, Riviere I, Gonen M, et al. Long-term follow-up of CD19 CAR therapy in acute lymphoblastic leukemia. *N Engl J Med*. 2018;378(5):449–459.

50. Abramson JS, Palomba ML, Gordon LI, et al. Lisocabtagene maraleucel for patients with relapsed or refractory large B-cell lymphomas (TRANSCEND NHL 001): a multicentre seamless design study. *Lancet*. 2020;396(10254):839–852.
51. June CH, O'Connor RS, Kawalekar OU, Ghassemi S, Milone MC. CAR T cell immunotherapy for human cancer. *Science*. 2018;359(6382):1361–1365.
52. Robbins PF, Morgan RA, Feldman SA, et al. Tumor regression in patients with metastatic synovial cell sarcoma and melanoma using genetically engineered lymphocytes reactive with NY-ESO-1. *J Clin Oncol*. 2011;29(7):917–924.
53. Stronen E, Toebes M, Kelderman S, et al. Targeting of cancer neoantigens with donor-derived T cell receptor repertoires. *Science*. 2016;352(6291):1337–1341.
54. Prehn RT, Main JM. Immunity to methylcholanthrene-induced sarcomas. *J Natl Cancer Inst*. 1957;18(6):769–778.
55. Kjaer SK, Nygard M, Dillner J, et al. A 12-year follow-up on the long-term effectiveness of the quadrivalent human papillomavirus vaccine in 4 Nordic countries. *Clin Infect Dis*. 2018;66(3):339–345.
56. Andtbacka RH, Kaufman HL, Collichio F, et al. Talimogene laherparepvec improves durable response rate in patients with advanced melanoma. *J Clin Oncol*. 2015;33(25):2780–2788.
57. Krysko DV, Garg AD, Kaczmarek A, Krysko O, Agostinis P, Vandenabeele P. Immunogenic cell death and DAMPs in cancer therapy. *Nat Rev Cancer*. 2012;12(12):860–875.
58. Galluzzi L, Buque A, Kepp O, Zitvogel L, Kroemer G. Immunogenic cell death in cancer and infectious disease. *Nat Rev Immunol*. 2017;17(2):97–111.
59. Zitvogel L, Apetoh L, Ghiringhelli F, Andre F, Tesniere A, Kroemer G. The anticancer immune response: indispensable for therapeutic success? *J Clin Invest*. 2008;118(6):1991–2001.
60. Antonia SJ, Villegas A, Daniel D, et al. Durvalumab after chemoradiotherapy in stage III non-small-cell lung cancer. *N Engl J Med*. 2017;377(20):1919–1929.
61. Schmid P, Cortes J, Pusztai L, et al; KEYNOTE-522 Investigators. Pembrolizumab for early triple-negative breast cancer. *N Engl J Med*. 2020;382(9):810–821.
62. Woo SR, Fuertes MB, Corrales L, et al. STING-dependent cytosolic DNA sensing mediates innate immune recognition of immunogenic tumors. *Immunity*. 2014;41(5):830–842.
63. Deng L, Liang H, Xu M, et al. STING-dependent cytosolic DNA sensing promotes radiation-induced type I interferon-dependent antitumor immunity in immunogenic tumors. *Immunity*. 2014; 41(5):843–852.
64. Demaria S, Ng B, Devitt ML, et al. Ionizing radiation inhibition of distant untreated tumors (abscopal effect) is immune mediated. *Int J Radiat Oncol Biol Phys*. 2004;58(3):862–870.
65. Mantovani A, Marchesi F, Malesci A, Laghi L, Allavena P. Tumour-associated macrophages as treatment targets in oncology. *Nat Rev Clin Oncol*. 2017;14(7):399–416.
66. Ries CH, Cannarile MA, Hoves S, et al. Targeting tumor-associated macrophages with anti-CSF-1R antibody reveals a strategy for cancer therapy. *Cancer Cell*. 2014;25(6):846–859.
67. Gabrilovich DI, Ostrand-Rosenberg S, Bronte V. Coordinated regulation of myeloid cells by tumours. *Nat Rev Immunol*. 2012; 12(4):253–268.
68. Nishikawa H, Sakaguchi S. Regulatory T cells in tumor immunity. *Int J Cancer*. 2010;127(4):759–767.
69. Ohlund D, Handly-Santana A, Biffi G, et al. Distinct populations of inflammatory fibroblasts and myofibroblasts in pancreatic cancer. *J Exp Med*. 2017;214(3):579–596.

5

Hemostasis

Andrea T. Obi and Peter K. Henke

SCIENTIFIC PRINCIPLES

Key Points

1. During the time that thrombin forms, natural anticoagulant mechanisms oppose further thrombin formation and help to localize thrombin activity to areas of vascular injury. Just as thrombin generation is key to coagulation, antithrombin is the central anticoagulant protein.
2. The endothelial cell acts as a nonthrombogenic surface, and inflammation tips the balance to procoagulant state.
3. Thrombosis and inflammation are closely linked and may perpetuate each other. Leukocytes and chemokines are involved with normal DVT resolution. These essential inflammatory mechanisms may drive vein wall injury.
4. Both acquired and inherited factors contribute to pathologic thrombosis; often occurring together.
5. Factor VIII and IX deficiency states are involved in hemophilia A and B and von Willebrand disease.

BASIC CONSIDERATIONS

Coagulation is an essential homeostatic mechanism for survival and involves tightly controlled processes to maintain vascular integrity, including thrombosis localization, amplification, and neutralization. These coordinated steps occur at the vessel, cellular, and subcellular levels. Thrombosis, directly or indirectly, is the underlying leading cause of death in the world and is an essential part of surgery.

Platelets form the initial hemostatic plug after vascular injury and are locally activated and aggregation induced (**Fig. 5.1**). Platelet aggregation is mediated by receptors that are part of the mammalian integrin family. This family includes the β_1 family, mediating platelet interaction with cells, collagen, fibronectin, and laminin; the β_2 family, present on leukocytes mediating interactions between leukocytes and other cells important in inflammation; and the β_3 family (cytoadhesion), including the megakaryocyte-specific glycoprotein (Gp) IIb/IIIa receptor and the vitronectin (Vn) receptor present on platelets and other cells.[1] Platelet aggregation is mediated by GpIIb/IIIa, which binds fibrinogen, von Willebrand factor (vWF), fibronectin, Vn, and thrombospondin to activated platelets. These high-density receptors are hidden on inactivated platelets and become exposed on the surface of activated platelets.

Two platelet activation routes are thought to occur physiologically. Without direct vessel damage, platelet activation may occur via tissue factor (TF) deencryption and activation by protein disulfide isomerase (PDI), with factor VIIa generation and activation of platelets. Alternatively, subendothelial collagen may directly bind to GpVI and vWF, leading to platelet capture and activation. Of note, PDI inhibition can directly block experimental thrombus formation.

Once stimulated, activated platelets contract, with externalization of negatively charged procoagulant phospholipids, including phosphatidylserine and phosphatidylinositol (termed platelet factor 3). This allows the coagulation proteins to assemble on the surface membrane of platelets, accelerating the coagulation reaction. During platelet activation, granules release calcium and serotonin, and membranes are exposed that are rich in receptors for factors Va and VIIIa, as well as fibrinogen, vWF, and adenosine di phosphate (ADP), a potent activator of other platelets. vWF is responsible for platelet adhesion through binding to GpIb, whereas fibrinogen forms bridges between activated platelets by binding to GpIIb/IIIa on adjacent stimulated platelets. Platelets also release polyphosphates that activate factor XII and the intrinsic pathway.

While long thought to be a bystander in venous thrombosis (VT) as compared to the arterial system, the role of the platelet is now thought to play a critical role, as well as direct later inflammatory cell actions.[2] First, recent clinical trials suggest antiplatelet therapy may reduce recurrent venous thormboembolism (VTE).[3] Second, in stasis and nonstasis experimental murine VT, genetic deletion of vWF was associated with significantly reduced VT size and not restored with recombinant factor rVIII. Intravital microscopy also showed direct association of leukocytes and platelets in a growing acute thrombus. Consistently, platelets via $GpIb_2$, may promote VT by colocalizing leukocytes and coagulation factors at the site of injury or stasis in the vein.[4]

Once the platelet plug has formed, the stage is set for coagulation protein assembly (**Fig. 5.2**). Initiating agents for coagulation include subendothelial collagen and TF, usually from vascular injury.[1] There is also growing evidence that blood-borne TF associated with leukocytes, or circulating in soluble form, is also involved with venous thrombogenesis.[5] Leukocyte adhesion to platelets may trigger leukocyte activation, causing recruitment of blood-borne TF onto the surface of leukocytes associated with thrombus, or recruitment of TF-positive leukocytes onto the growing thrombus. TF, both blood borne and local, activates the extrinsic pathway of coagulation by complexing with activated factor VII (VIIa), activating factors IX and X to factors IXa and Xa. Factor Xa, activated factor V (Va), ionized calcium, and factor II (prothrombin) form on the platelet phospholipid surface to initiate the prothrombinase complex, which catalyzes the formation of thrombin faster than can be achieved with factor Xa alone.

Thrombin is central to coagulation and acts to cleave fibrinopeptide A (FPA) from the α chain of fibrinogen and fibrinopeptide B (FPB) from the β-chain. This leads to the release of fibrinopeptides and the formation of new fibrin monomers, which then cross-link, resulting in fibrin polymerization. Thrombin also activates factor XIII, which catalyzes

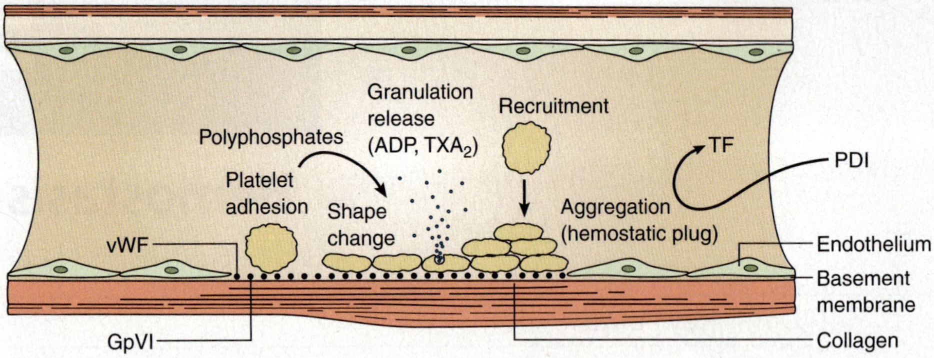

Figure 5.1. Primary hemostasis is achieved initially with a platelet aggregation as illustrated. Note that platelet adhesion, shape change, granule release, followed by recruitment, and the hemostatic plug at the area of subendothelial collagen (binds to GpVI) exposure are the initial events for thrombus formation. Platelets can also be activated by PDI with deencryption of TF.

the cross-linking of fibrin to make the clot firm, activates platelets and activates factors V and VIII, two nonenzymatic cofactors, to Va and VIIIa. This is important because only activated factors Va and VIIIa are involved in coagulation. Factor XIIIa also cross-links other plasma proteins, such as fibronectin and α_2-antitrypsin, resulting in their incorporation into the clot.

The intrinsic pathway of blood coagulation requires activation of factor XI to XIa. This may occur by both the contact activation system through activation of factor XII, plasma prekallikrein, and high–molecular-weight kininogen and, more importantly, through thrombin with negatively charged surfaces. Factor XIa activates factor XI autocatalytically and also catalyzes the conversion of factor IX to IXa. After activation, factor VIIIa dissociates from vWF and assembles with factors IXa and X. Factor IXa, factor X, ionized calcium, and thrombin-activated factor VIII (VIIIa) then assemble on the platelet surface in a complex called the *Xase complex* to catalyze the activation of factor X to Xa. Factor Xa then shunts into the prothrombinase complex for further amplification of thrombin formation.

The importance of a mechanism of factor XI activation independent of the contact activation system is apparent because patients deficient in those factors of the contact activation system, including factor XI, have abnormal prolongation in bleeding, whereas patients deficient in factor XII, prekallikrein, and high–molecular-weight kininogen do not. The contact activation system is the most important coagulation process involved in extracorporeal bypass circuits, including cardiopulmonary bypass and extracorporeal membrane oxygenation.

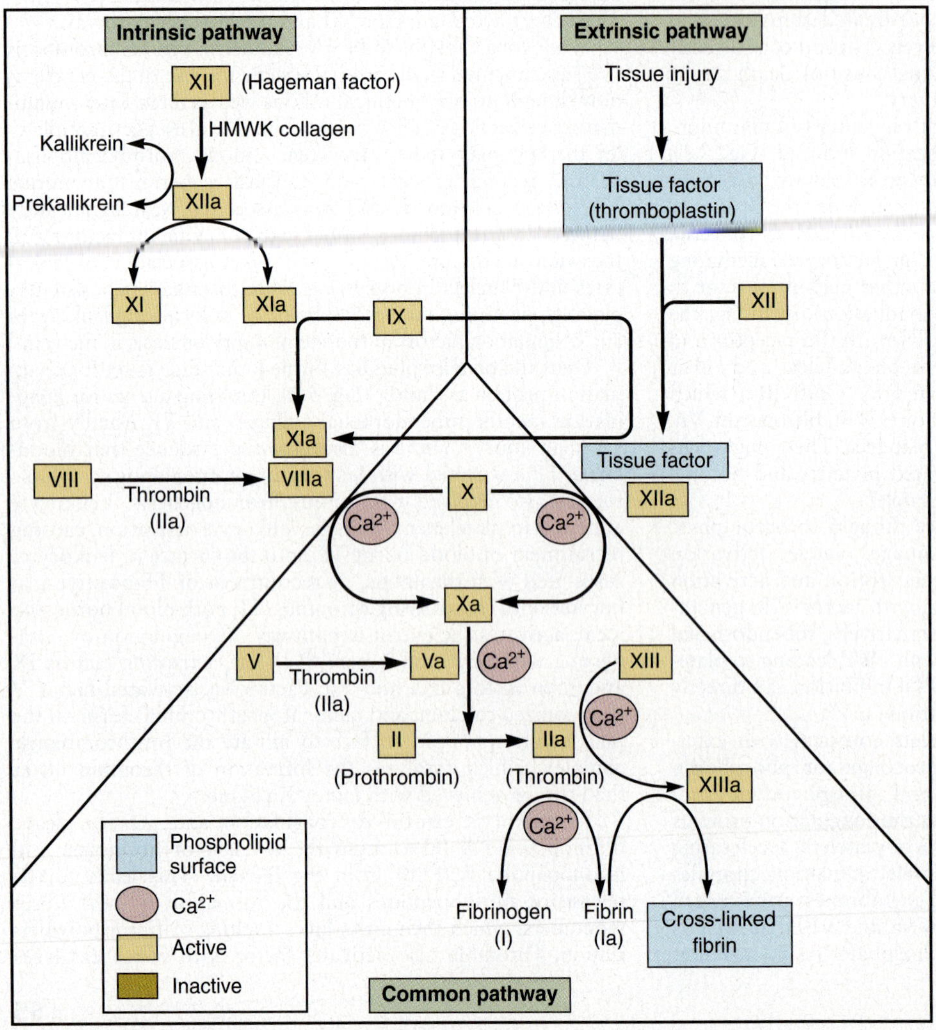

Figure 5.2. The classical pathway showing the interface between the intrinsic pathway, extrinsic pathway, and the common pathway is illustrated with the ultimate production of thrombin. This catalyzes fibrin from fibrinogen, and then cross-links the fibrin to form a stable clot. Antithrombin is a primary anticoagulant. Note antithrombin complexes with IIa to inhibit fibrin polymerization, as well as factor Xa, and inactivate factors Va and VIIIa.

NATURAL ANTICOAGULANT MECHANISMS

1 At the same time that thrombin forms, natural anticoagulant mechanisms oppose further thrombin formation and help to localize thrombin activity to areas of vascular injury.[6] Just as thrombin generation is key to coagulation, antithrombin (AT) is the central anticoagulant protein (**Fig. 5.2**). This Gp of 70-kD molecular weight binds to thrombin, preventing the removal of FPA and FPB from fibrinogen, prevents the activation of factors V and VIII, and inhibits the activation and aggregation of platelets. In addition, AT directly inhibits factors IXa, Xa, and XIa.

A second natural anticoagulant is activated protein C (APC), which inactivates factors Va and VIIIa, thus reducing the Xase and prothrombinase complex acceleration of the rate of thrombin formation. In the circulation, protein C is activated on endothelial cell surfaces by thrombin complexed with one of its receptors, thrombomodulin (TM). The formation of this thrombin–TM complex accelerates the activation of protein C compared with thrombin alone. Thrombin, at the same time, by binding to TM, loses its platelet-activating activity as well as its enzymatic activity for fibrinogen and factor V. Protein S is a cofactor for APC.

Another innate anticoagulant is tissue factor pathway inhibitor (TFPI). The protein binds to TF–VIIa complex, inhibiting the activation of factor X to Xa and the formation of the prothrombinase complex. A fourth natural anticoagulant is heparin cofactor II. Its concentration in plasma is estimated to be significantly less than that of AT, and its action is implicated primarily in the regulation of thrombin formation in extravascular tissues. Finally, thrombin is inactivated when it becomes incorporated into the clot.

FIBRINOLYSIS

In addition to natural anticoagulants such as proteins C and S, physiologic clot formation is balanced by a contained process of clot lysis, which prevents thrombus formation from proceeding outside of the injured area (**Fig. 5.3**). The central fibrinolytic enzyme is plasmin, a serine protease generated by the proteolytic cleavage of the proenzyme, plasminogen. Its main substrates include fibrin, fibrinogen, and other coagulation factors. Plasminogen, tissue plasminogen activator (tPA), and α_2-antiplasmin (α_2-AP) become incorporated into the fibrin clot as it forms. Plasminogen activators are serine proteases that activate plasminogen, by cleavage of a single arginine–valine peptide bond, to the enzyme plasmin. Plasminogen activation provides localized proteolytic activity. The major endogenous plasminogen activators include tPA and urokinase, and intrinsic factors, such as factor XII, prekallikrein, and high–molecular-weight kininogen. These later factors of the contact system are more important in clot lysis than thrombus formation. These enzymes may also liberate bradykinin from high–molecular-weight kininogen, resulting in an increase in vascular permeability, prostacyclin (PGI_2) liberation, and tPA secretion. Finally, APC has been found to proteolytically inactivate the inhibitor to tPA, thus promoting tPA activity and fibrinolysis. Thrombin promotes tPA release from endothelial cells as well as the production of plasminogen activator inhibitor (PAI-1) from endothelial cells.

Fibrin, when digested by plasmin, yields one molecule of fragment E and two molecules of fragment D. In physiologic clot formation, fragment D is released in dimeric form (D-dimer), and is a marker for fibrinolysis of formed clot. An elevated D-dimer level after treatment of deep vein thrombosis (DVT) is one biomarker that has been found to accurately predict an ongoing risk of recurrent VTE.[7]

Two primary inhibitors of plasmin are important. First, α_2-AP is released by endothelial cells and complexes with plasmin. In physiologic fibrinolysis, α_2-AP is bound to fibrin and excess plasmin is readily inactivated. In plasma, PAI-1 is the primary inhibitor of plasminogen activators. It is secreted in an active form from liver and endothelial cells and stabilized by binding to Vn. PAI-1 levels are elevated by hyperlipidemia.

In summary, coagulation is a balance of thrombus formation, inhibition of thrombus formation, and thrombus dissolution. The central mediators are TF, platelets, thrombin, and plasmin. Abnormalities in coagulation occur when one process—thrombus formation, thrombus inhibition, or fibrinolysis—overcomes the others and dominates the delicate balance.

ENDOTHELIUM AND HEMOSTASIS

2 Through its ability to express procoagulant and anticoagulant factors, vasoconstrictors, and vasodilators, as well as key cell adhesion molecules and cytokines, the endothelial cell is a key regulator of hemostasis (**Fig. 5.4**). The vascular endothelium maintains a vasodilatory and local fibrinolytic state in which coagulation, platelet adhesion and activation, and leukocyte activation are suppressed.

Vasodilatory endothelial products include adenosine, nitric oxide (NO), and PGI_2. A nonthrombogenic endothelial surface is maintained by four main mechanisms, including endothelial production of TM and subsequent activation of protein C, endothelial expression of surface heparan and dermatan sulfate, constitutive expression of TFPI by endothelium (which is markedly accelerated in response to heparin), and local production of tPA and urokinase plasminogen activator (uPA).[8] Finally, the elaboration of NO and interleukin (IL)-10 by the endothelium inhibits leukocyte adhesion and activation.

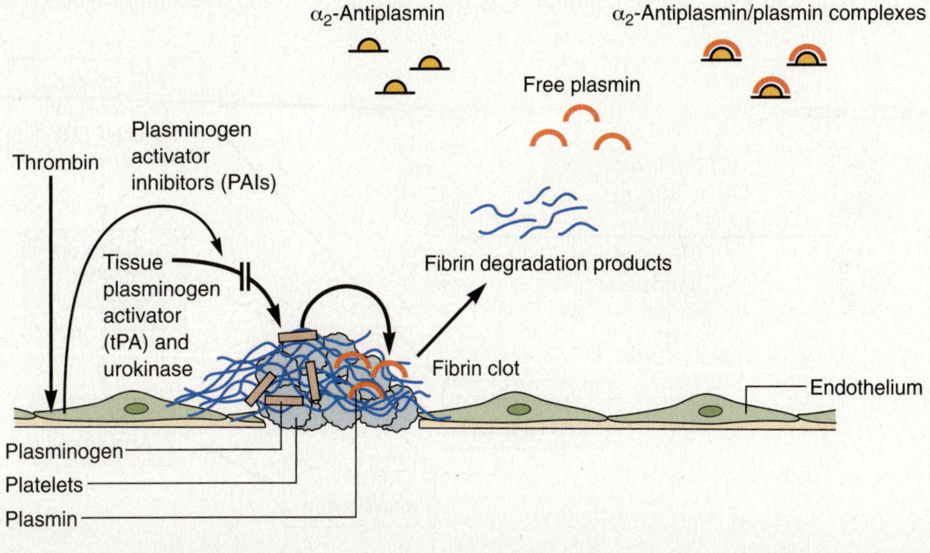

Figure 5.3. Hemostasis with thrombus production is a tight and intricate process that is locally confined. Balancing thrombus production are tissue plasmin activator and urokinase plasminogen activator which activate plasmin and cause thrombolysis. These are balanced by plasminogen activator inhibitor-1 and α_2-antiplasmin. Free plasmin is complexed rapidly. Fibrin degradation products, such as D-dimer, are produced.

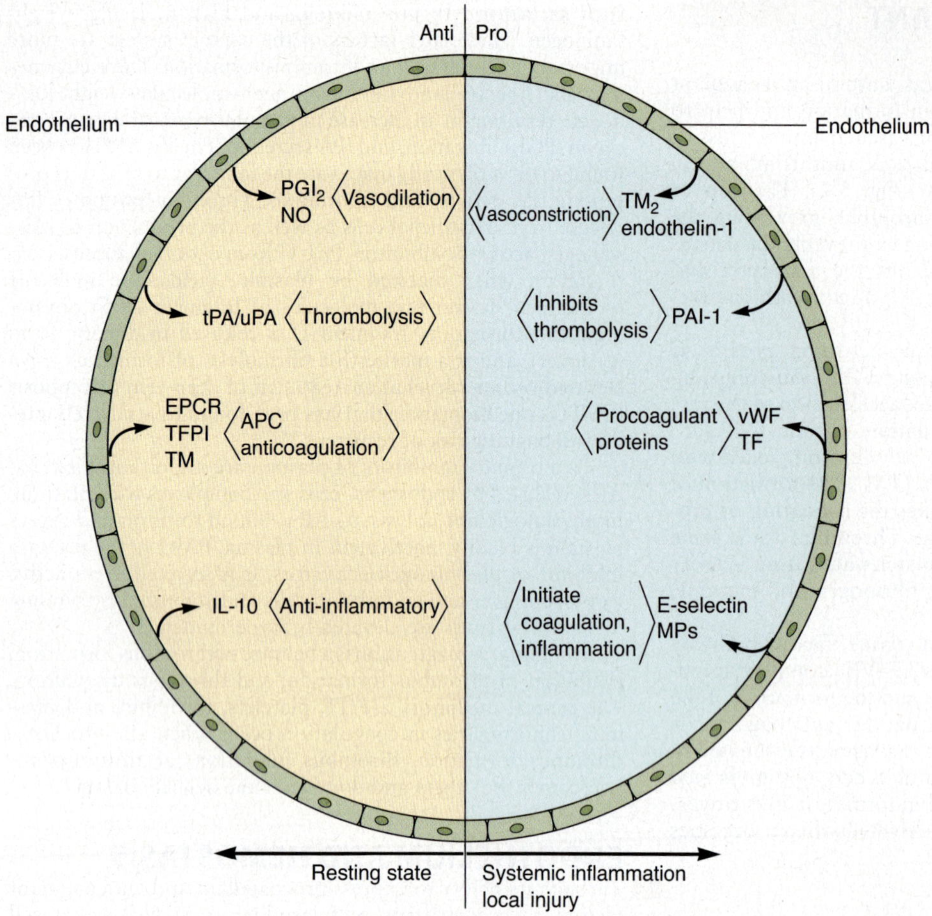

Figure 5.4. The endothelium is a primary interface allowing both anticoagulant functions in the resting state, with prostacyclin, NO, plasminogen activators, and thrombomodulin. Procoagulant proteins are expressed on activated endothelium including selectins, von Willebrand factor, TF, as well as PAI-1.

During states of endothelial disturbances such as injury, a prothrombotic and proinflammatory state of vasoconstriction is driven by the endothelial surface. Endothelial release of platelet-activating factor (PAF) and endothelin-1 promotes vasoconstriction. Endothelial cells increase production of vWF, TF, PAI-1, and factor V to augment thrombosis with exposure to prothrombotic stimuli. Finally, in response to endothelial injury, endothelial cells are activated, resulting in increased surface expression of cell adhesion molecules, promoting leukocyte adhesion and activation.

THROMBOSIS, INFLAMMATION, AND RESOLUTION

After VT, an acute to chronic inflammatory response occurs in the vein wall and thrombus progressing from thrombus amplification, to organization, and vein recanalization (often at the expense of vein wall fibrosis and vein valvular damage). Initially, there is an increase in neutrophils (PMN) in the vein wall followed by monocytes/macrophages. Cytokines, chemokines, and inflammatory factors (eg, tumor necrosis factor [TNF]) facilitate inflammation. The ultimate response of the vein wall depends on proinflammatory and anti-inflammatory mediator balance at the interface between the leukocyte, activated platelet, and endothelium.

Cell Adhesion Molecules

Selectins (P- and E-selectins, sP-sel, sE-sel) have been found to be intimately involved in thrombosis (**Fig. 5.5**). P selectin is the first upregulated Gp on activated platelets (α granules) and endothelial cells (Weibel–Palade bodies). They mediate the adhesion of leukocytes, platelets, and even cancer cells in

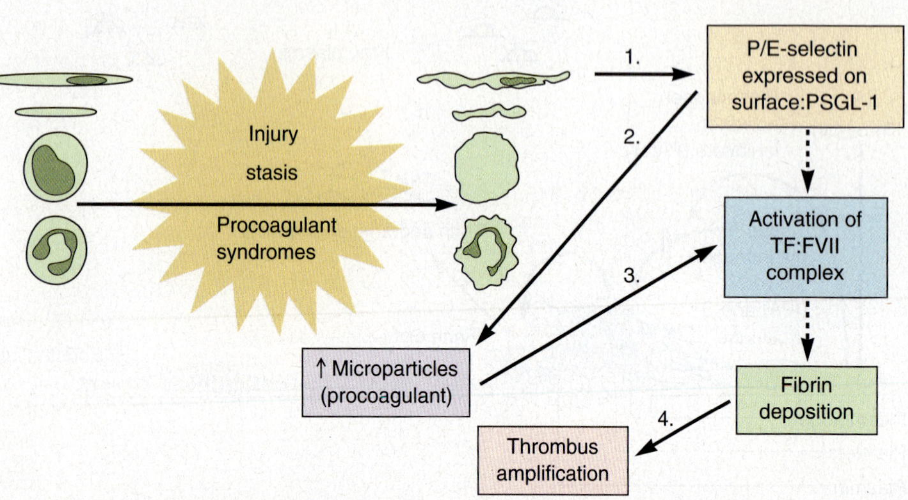

Figure 5.5. The interaction between stasis injury and procoagulant syndromes is represented by Virchow triad. Endothelial and vascular injuries cause leukocytes and platelets to express P- and E-selectins and the PSGL-1 receptor. Microparticles are released which express TF. This stimulates the coagulation pathway, fibrin production, and thrombus amplification.

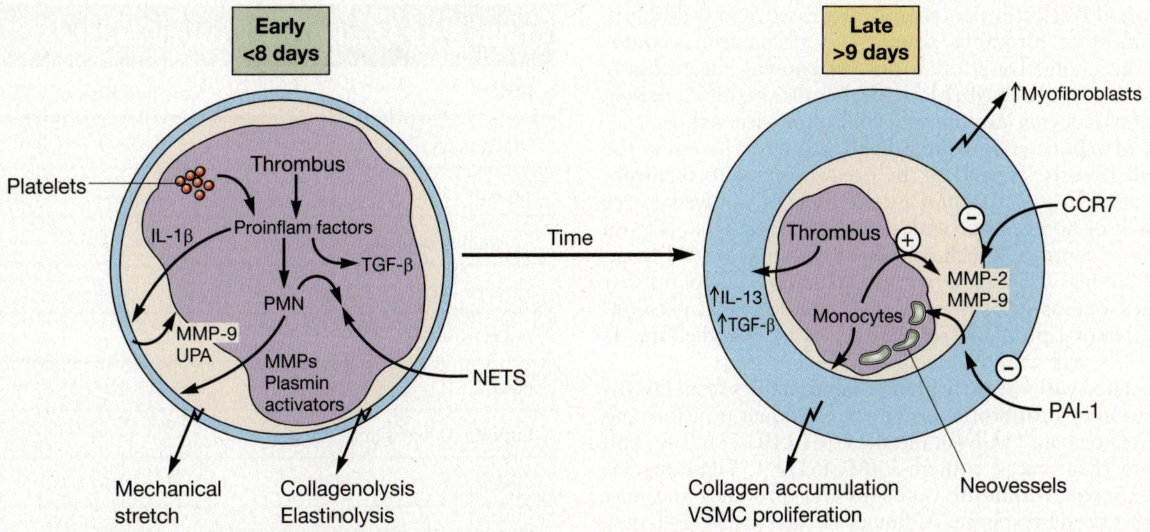

Figure 5.6. The proposed resolution mechanism involves both early thrombolysis with a large distending clot and then, over time, a fibrotic thrombus that resembles scar tissue as produced. Note proinflammatory factors, as well as neutrophils (releasing NETs), platelets, and MMP, are present early with subsequent vein wall injury related to collagenolysis and elastinolysis. Later, vascular smooth muscle cell proliferation appears to occur, with thrombus resolution with increased profibrotic growth factors such as IL-13 and TGF-β. This promotes collagen accumulation. Both PAI-1 and CCR7 are protective against fibrosis.

inflammation and thrombosis. sP-sel is released from activated platelets and endothelial cells and levels rise significantly during pathologic conditions.[9] The P-selectin receptor is P-selectin glycoprotein ligand-1 (PSGL-1). P-selectin: PSGL-1 interactions trigger the release of procoagulant microparticles (MPs) that support fibrin formation, thrombus growth, and increase monocyte TF expression.

sP-sel has been studied as a biomarker for DVT,[9] and combining sP-sel with Wells score (clinical pretest probability of DVT) establishes the diagnosis of DVT. An sP-sel (≥90 ng/mL) combined with Wells score (≥2) showed a better positive predictive value (PPV) (91%) than D-dimer (≥500 ng/mL) combined with Wells score (≥2), which was 69%. E-selectin, upregulated after P-selectin, is an important regulator of thrombus formation and fibrin content in a mouse VT model. Endotoxin-induced TF-mediated coagulation is enhanced in humans carrying the *S128R* E-selectin allele, and patients homozygous for the *S128R* E-selectin allele have an increased risk for VTE recurrence. E-selectin has been shown to be efficient at raising the affinity and avidity of two (CD18) integrins which support neutrophil trafficking to sites of acute inflammation and recruit platelets and red blood cells.

Other factors of importance to venous thrombogenesis include vWF, a factor that stabilizes procoagulant factor VIII to promote the initiation and formation of stable thrombus at the site of vascular inflammation and TF. TF activity is increased in cells treated with chemotherapy and in circulating MPs. Patients with cancer have elevated MPs, suggesting a role for TF in the pathogenesis of cancer-associated DVT.

Leukocytes and Thrombosis

Inflammatory cells are important to the process of thrombus recanalization and organization (**Fig. 5.6**).[10] Thrombus resolution resembles wound healing and involves profibrotic growth factors, collagen deposition, matrix metalloproteinase (MMP) expression, and activation. As the thrombus resolves, a number of proinflammatory factors are released into the local environment, including interleukin-1 beta (IL-1β) and tumor necrosis factor alpha (TNF-α).[11] The cellular sources of these different mediators are probably leukocytes and smooth muscle–like cells within the resolving thrombus and adjacent vein wall. The observation that leukocytes invade the thrombus in a specific sequence suggests their importance in the normal thrombus resolution.

The first cell type in the thrombus is the neutrophil (PMN). Although PMNs may cause vein wall injury, they are essential for early thrombus resolution by promoting both fibrinolysis and collagenolysis, based on a total stasis VT model. It is likely the timing of PMN influx and the amount of perithrombus blood flow that tip PMN activities toward thrombosis or
3 thrombolysis. Conversely, in a nonstasis VT model, PMNs promote thrombosis.[4] Through processes that also involve the initial activation of leukocytes and platelets, PMNs form neutrophil extracellular traps (NETs), which are extracellular fragments of DNA containing histones and antimicrobial proteins.[4,12] The NETs provide a scaffold for thrombus formation, are proinflammatory and prothrombotic. Consistently, circulating DNA was significantly elevated in DVT patients, compared with controls. Of interest was a significant positive correlation of circulating DNA with C-reactive protein, D-dimer, vWF, and the Wells score (all $P < .01$).[13]

The monocyte/macrophage is likely the most important cell for later DVT resolution.[10,11] Monocyte influx into the thrombus peaks at day 8 after thrombogenesis, and correlates with elevated MCP-1 levels, which has been associated with DVT resolution. Indeed, precedent exists in humans that the monocytic activation state may predict long-term DVT resolution.

Thrombi have been found to contain increasing amounts of both tPA and uPA activities as they resolve, and this activity is expressed by invading monocytes. For example, mice genetically deleted for uPA had impaired thrombus resolution with reduced monocyte infiltration at the margins of the thrombus, with few neovascular channels present.[14] Mice gene deleted for tPA, however, were not similarly affected, suggesting that uPA, not tPA, is responsible for this activity.

The local venous environment is by definition hypoxic. A major angiogenic growth factor is hypoxia-inducible factor-1 alpha (HIF-1α). Experimental data in a stasis model of VT suggest that thrombosis stimulates increased vein wall HIF-1α and that by exogenous stimulation of HIF-1α expression, thrombus recanalization was increased and associated with accelerated VT resolution. Thus, thrombus resolution is in part dependent on neovascularization.

Recent data linking inflammation to fibrosis demonstrate that inhibition of the inflammatory response can decrease vein wall fibrosis. In a rat model of stasis DVT, treated with either low–molecular-weight heparin (LMWH) or an oral inhibitor to P-selectin 2 days after establishment of thrombosis, inhibition of P-selectin significantly decreased vein wall injury (independent of thrombus size).[15] The mechanism accounting for this protective effect is not yet known, but probably does not involve leukocyte blockade, because no differences in influx of monocytes into the vein wall were observed.

Loss of venous endothelium likely also contributes to the vein wall fibrosis, as well as the predisposition to recurrent thrombosis. An experimental model of DVT showed lower expression of homeostatic endothelial genes such as NO and TM than in controls, which correlated with loss of vWF-positive cell luminal staining. Other investigators have found that prolonged venous stasis is associated with decreased plasminogen activators, probably related to loss of endothelium, as well as early vein wall dysfunction.

Associated with the early biomechanical injury from DVT is an elevation of profibrotic mediators, including transforming growth factor beta (TGF-β), interleukin-13 (IL-13), IL-6, and monocyte chemotactic protein-1 (MCP-1).[15,16] These mediators are present within the vein wall and thrombus and may drive the fibrotic response. Although exogenous MCP-1 may hasten DVT resolution, it promotes organ fibrosis in vivo. The profibrotic growth factor TGF-β is also present in the thrombus and is activated with normal thrombolysis. TGF-β may be a key mechanism promoting vein wall fibrosis.[17]

Late fibrosis has been observed in our mouse model of DVT, which demonstrated a significant increase in vein wall collagen after stasis thrombogenesis.[16] Based on experimental studies, elastinolysis and collagenolysis seem to occur early, as measured by an increase in vein wall stiffness, persisting through 14 days, and are accompanied by elevated MMP-2 and MMP-9 activities.[16] Correlating with this increase in fibrosis is altered procollagen I and III gene expression, as well as an increase in MMP-2 and MMP-9 gene expression and activity. Genetic deletion of MMP-2 or MMP-2/9 is associated with decreased midterm vein wall fibrosis, possibly by modulating vein wall elastin/collagen metabolism as well as monocyte influx. It has been demonstrated that decreasing inflammation with a selectin inhibitor or with neutralizing IL-6 can also decrease vein wall fibrosis.[15] Moreover, the thrombus size itself does not drive the vein wall injury response; rather, the mechanism of thrombosis seems more important.[16] Finally, PAI-1 overexpression is associated with decreased vein wall fibrosis, in part by decreased MMP-2/9 activity.

ARTERIAL VERSUS VENOUS THROMBOSIS

Thrombosis in the arterial system occurs somewhat differently than in the venous system. The elements required for the initiation of DVT were described by Virchow as stasis, endothelial injury, and hypercoagulability of the blood. In arterial circulation, endothelial vascular injury (whether acute or chronic) is key to thrombosis. This is most clearly demonstrated by the typical atherosclerotic plaque rupture. In advanced lesions, the lipid core of the plaque is rich in inflammatory cells, cholesterol crystals, and TF (generated by activated macrophages within the plaque). Plaque ulceration exposes highly thrombogenic lipids to the bloodstream, activating coagulation, platelet aggregation, and leading to the deposition of clot. Platelet deposition occurs at the apex of stenosis, the point of maximal shear force. The blood flow velocity itself regulates how quickly both thrombi form and dissolve.

A platelet-rich thrombus is observed in arterial thrombus, while in contrast, venous blood stasis and changes in its composition (leading to hypercoagulability) incite the formation of thrombus from local procoagulant events, including small endothelial disruptions at venous confluences, saccules, and valve pockets. Hypercoagulable states have classically been highly associated with VTE, but do play a role in cardiovascular disease as well. Moreover, HMG-CoA reductase inhibitors (statin) not only decrease atherothrombotic events but also incident VTE,[18] suggesting some common pathogenic pathways.

Table 5.1. Acquired Hypercoagulable States

Risk	Relative Risk of VTE
Malignancy	++++
Trauma	++
Indwelling catheters	+
Surgery	++++
Pregnancy	+
HRT/OC	+
Lupus anticoagulant	+++
Obesity	+
Postoperative infection	++++
IBD	+++
Prolonged immobility	++

HRT, hormone replacement therapy; IBD, inflammatory bowel disease; OC, oral contraceptive; +, low risk; ++, moderate risk; +++, high risk; ++++, very high risk.

PROCOAGULANT STATES

Acquired Procoagulant States

Most thrombotic clinical episodes have an identifiable cause, although environmental risks and genetic predispositions to thrombosis may account for many of the VTEs that manifest clinically.[19]

4 The most common risk factors for VTE are prior DVT, malignancy, immobility, intravenous catheters, increased age, major surgery, trauma, infections such as pneumonia and urinary tract infection, and certain chemotherapies (**Table 5.1**). Certain medications such as oral contraceptives and estrogen-based hormone replacement therapies also increase the risk of VTE.

Of primary importance to surgeons is how best to estimate perioperative VTE risk, and apply appropriate prophylaxis. This can be done with a screening form, such as that devised by Caprini. Essentially, this is a focused assessment of VTE risks related to current illnesses and history that may not be fully covered in the routine history and physical. The recommendations are also well detailed in the routinely updated American College of Chest Physicians VTE evidence-based guidelines. The higher the risk, the more intensive the prophylaxis should be. For example, an outpatient hernia patient may require no prophylaxis outside of early ambulation, whereas a hip replacement in an obese patient would be best treated with an antithrombotic as well as sequential compression devices on the lower extremities. However, all patients should be assessed for VTE risk.

Malignancy

Cancer represents an independent risk factor for the development of VTE, with a sixfold increased risk in cancer patients. Importantly, cancer patients undergoing surgical procedures have twice the risk of development of postoperative DVT. Highest rates of VTE are seen in pancreas, stomach, and lung cancer. The malignancy itself activates a procoagulant phenotype by expression of TF by malignant cells, release of TF-bearing MPs, and increased activation of NETs—the

Table 5.2. Diagnostic Criteria for Antiphospholipid Antibody Syndrome

Clinical Criteria (must have ≥1)	1. ≥1 clinical episode of, objectively confirmed, arterial, venous, or small vessel thrombosis 2. Pregnancy morbidity: ≥1 unexplained fetal death at ≥10-wk EGA; ≥1 premature birth (≤34th wk of gestation) due to eclampsia, severe preeclampsia, or placental insufficiency; ≥3 unexplained consecutive spontaneous abortions at <10-wk EGA
Laboratory Criteria (must have ≥1)	1. LA (+) ≥2 occasions, at least 12 wk apart, according to ISTH guidelines (prolonged PL-based clotting assay, lack of correction with 1:1 mix, and correction with excess PL) 2. ACLA and/or anti-β_2 glycoprotein-I antibody (medium or high immunoglobulin G [IgG] and/or IgM isotype titer ≥2 occasions, at least 12 wk apart using standardized ELISA assays)

ACLA, anticardiolipin antibody; EGA, estimated gestational age; ELISA, enzyme linked immunosorbent assay; ISTH, International Society of Thrombosis and Haemostasis; PL, phospholipid.

downstream effects of which have been outlined above. An extended duration of pharmacoprophylaxis—28 days—was found to be associated with a decreased incidence of DVT, and current guidelines recommend extended thromboprophylaxis in cancer patients after operative intervention.[20]

Inflammatory Bowel Disease

Since the first half of the last century, a link between inflammatory bowel disease (IBD) and VTE has been recognized. While there does appear some correlation between thrombosis and the inflammatory nature of the disease, the link between the inflammatory and coagulation cascades does not tell the whole story. A recent retrospective cohort study of the National Surgical Quality Improvement Program database demonstrated that the presence of IBD is an independent risk factor for postoperative VTE with an odds ratio of 2.

Trauma

As with other acquired prothrombotic states, the systemic inflammatory milieu is associated with VTE in trauma patients. Activation of inflammatory pathways through TNF-α with increased circulating TF and procoagulant MP induces a prothrombotic state. Incidence of VTE in trauma patients is around 2%, and this may be higher in patients with other risk factors, such as old age, obesity, and prolonged immobility after bone fractures. LMWH with application of pneumatic compression devices has been shown to be the preferred thromboprophylaxis in trauma patients, and this is reflected in anticoagulation (AC) guidelines. However, optimal dosing regimens are not well defined.

Lupus Anticoagulant/Antiphospholipid Syndrome (Antiphospholipid Antibody)

Antiphospholipid antibody (APLA) syndrome is a particularly virulent hypercoagulable state that results in both arterial thrombosis and VTE. For the diagnosis of antiphospholipid syndrome, both clinical and laboratory criteria are necessary (**Tables 5.2** and **5.3**). The prolongation in the activated partial

SCIENTIFIC PRINCIPLES

Table 5.3. Severity and Frequency of VTE due to Hypercoagulable States

	Frequency (%) VTE	Thrombotic Phenotype	Diagnostic and Therapeutic Considerations
High Risk for Thrombosis			
▪ AT deficiency	0.5–3	Venous >> arterial ▪ May have thrombosis at unusual sites ▪ Inherited cases become apparent by age 50 y ▪ Homozygous patients die in utero ▪ Can be acquired from liver or kidney disease, sepsis, DIC, or malnutrition	Suspect in patients who cannot be adequately anticoagulated on heparin Anticoagulation with direct thrombin inhibitors is recommended; alternatively, may administer FFP with heparin Lifelong anticoagulation recommended following the first VTE
▪ Protein C deficiency	3	Venous >> arterial ▪ Patients often present between ages 15 and 30 with VTE ▪ Homozygous patients die at birth from purpura fulminans ▪ Can be acquired from liver failure, DIC, and nephrotic syndrome	If asymptomatic heterozygote carriers, aggressive thromboprophylaxis is recommended in the perioperative period Lifelong anticoagulation is recommended following first episode of thrombosis Patients are at particular risk of warfarin-induced skin necrosis and must undergo bridging anticoagulation with heparin, LMWH, or direct thrombin inhibitor
▪ Protein S deficiency	3–6	Venous >> arterial ▪ Cofactor to protein C; deficiency results in clinical state identical to protein C deficiency ▪ Acquired deficiency can occur in liver disease, nephrotic syndrome, OCP use, pregnancy, and during breastfeeding	If asymptomatic heterozygote carriers, aggressive thromboprophylaxis is recommended in the perioperative period Lifelong anticoagulation is recommended following the first episode of thrombosis Patients are at particular risk of warfarin-induced skin necrosis and must undergo bridging anticoagulation with heparin, LMWH, or direct thrombin inhibitor

(*continued*)

Table 5.3. Severity and Frequency of VTE due to Hypercoagulable States (*Continued*)

	Frequency (%) VTE	Thrombotic Phenotype	Diagnostic and Therapeutic Considerations
▪ Antiphospholipid antibody syndrome	3–5	Venous > arterial ▪ Associated with thrombosis, fetal loss, stroke, MI, visceral infarction, extremity gangrene, and graft thrombosis ▪ May be induced by medications, cancer, and certain infections	Treatment is with warfarin followed by heparin; direct oral anticoagulants are associated with higher thrombosis risk For recurrent fetal loss, LMWH is recommended Anti-Xa levels should be used to monitor LMWH/heparin levels
Lower Risk for Thrombosis			
▪ Factor V Leiden (FVL)	20–60	Venous >> arterial ▪ Combined defects with protein C or S deficiency or prothrombin G20210A increase thrombotic risk	Diagnosis is made with a clot-based functional assay and genetic analysis to determine hetero- vs homozygosity Long-term anticoagulation is not necessary after first episode of thrombosis in a heterozygote, but is recommended after recurrent thrombosis
▪ Hyperhomocysteinemia	10	Arterial ~ venous ▪ Can be acquired via smoking, coffee consumption, diabetes, cancer, hypothyroidism, and low dietary levels of folate and vitamins B_6 or B_{12} ▪ Common medications that increase levels: metformin, methotrexate, theophylline, levodopa, and anticonvulsants	Diagnosis is made via fasting homocysteine levels or after a methionine oral loading regimen Treatment is through/by folate supplementation Anticoagulation choice and duration should not be influenced by diagnosis of hyperhomocysteinemia
▪ PT G20210A	4–6	Venous >> arterial ▪ Thrombosis risk is increased in combination with FVL and pregnancy ▪ Most prevalent in Caucasians	Long-term anticoagulation is recommended for patients with recurrent thrombosis or when diagnosed in conjunction with FVL
▪ Dysfibrinogenemia	1–3	Venous > arterial ▪ Common presentations include VTE and digit ischemia	Standard anticoagulation according to guidelines
▪ Dysplasminogenemia	<1	Arterial ~ venous	Standard anticoagulation according to guidelines
▪ Elevated factors VIII, IX, and XI	1	Venous > arterial Thrombosis risk is dose responsive, for example, factor VIII:C above the 90th percentile is associated with fivefold increased risk of VTE Acquired and environmental factors precipitate VTE	Diagnosis is with activity assays; however, factor VIII carrier is vWF which is an acute phase reactant and must be accounted for, usually by measuring ESR or CRP Standard anticoagulation according to guidelines

AT, antithrombin; DIC, Disseminated intravascular coagulation; ESR, erythrocyte sedimentation rate; HITTS, heparin-induced thrombocytopenia and thrombosis syndrome; LMWH, low–molecular-weight heparin; OCP, oral contraception; PAI-1, plasminogen activator inhibitor-1; VTE, venous thromboembolism.

thromboplastin time (aPTT) is strictly a laboratory phenomenon. The dilute Russell viper venom time confirms the presence of a lupus anticoagulant. There is imperfect agreement between diagnostic tests for this abnormality. Approximately 80% of patients with a prolonged aPTT will have a positive APLA, but only 10% to 50% of patients with a positive APLA will have a prolonged aPTT. Treatment of APLA syndrome can include standard AC, higher intensity AC, intravenous gamma globulin, complement inhibitors, and plasmapheresis.[21]

Hypercoagulability Testing

Clinical signs of possible thrombophilia include thrombosis at a young age (<40), unprovoked thrombosis, recurrent thrombosis, thrombosis at unusual locations such as the mesentery, CNS venous sinus, and portal vein, a family history of thrombosis, particularly unprovoked, severe, and in those <50 years of age. Testing for hereditary defects in patients with thrombosis with no family history has pros and cons. Testing may improve understanding of pathogenesis of thrombosis, identify and counsel affected family members, and obviate expensive diagnostic testing (eg, CT scans) looking for a malignancy. However, testing may result in patients being treated over aggressively or facing insurance implications.

In order to determine the efficacy of hypercoagulable testing, a multicenter international observational registry on clinical characteristics, treatment patterns, and outcome in consecutive patients with symptomatic, objectively confirmed acute VTE was done. In this study, 22,847 patients were enrolled and 4503 tested for thrombophilia. Of the total patient population, 8.4% had factor V Leiden, 6.8% had PTG20210A, and 3% had activated protein C resistance (APC-R). The authors concluded that for the low incidence and in accordance with the recommendations made by other authors and international bodies, "the undertaking of thrombophilia testing on patients with a first episode of VTE is not advisable."[22]

A hypercoagulable screen may include routine coagulation tests such as the aPTT and platelet count, AT activity and antigen assay, protein C antigen and activity levels, protein S antigen level, and mixing studies to identify a lupus anticoagulant (if indicated); APC-R assay and factor V Leiden gene analysis; prothrombin G20210A genetic analysis; homocysteine level; an APLA screen that includes anticardiolipin antibody; fibrinogen level; FVIII, FIX, and FXI levels and a functional plasminogen assay.

Inherited Procoagulant States

Defects with High Risk for Thrombosis

Inherited procoagulant states at high risk for thrombosis consist of AT III deficiency, protein C deficiency, and protein S deficiency. AT is a serine protease inhibitor (SERPIN) of thrombin, kallikrein, and factors Xa, IXa, VIIa, XIIa, and XIa. It is synthesized in the liver and has a half-life of 2.8 days. Protein C and its cofactor protein S are both vitamin K–dependent factors synthesized in the liver with half-lives of 4 to 6 hours and 12 to 14 hours, respectively. The majority of cases of protein C or protein S deficiency are inherited as autosomal dominant. Protein deficiency is divided into a type I deficiency (quantitative) and a type II deficiency (qualitative). Patients heterozygous for protein C deficiency usually have antigenic protein C levels less than 60% of normal. Protein S is a cofactor to protein C in inactivating FVa and FVIIIa, and is regulated by complement C4b-binding protein.

Defects with Lower Risk for Thrombosis

Resistance to APC (Factor V Leiden)

Resistance to APC has been reported to be present in 20% to 60% of cases of idiopathic VTE and is the most common underlying abnormality associated with VTE. This disorder is present in 1% to 2% of the general population. As a result of the substitution of a single amino acid, glutamine for arginine, at position 506 in the protein for factor V, caused by a nucleotide substitution of guanine for adenine at 1691 in factor V gene, hypercoagulability is conferred by resistance to inactivation of factor Va by APC. Factor V Leiden accounts for 90% of APC-R. As other mutations (eg, Hong Kong, Cambridge) can cause APC-R but are not necessarily captured on standard genetic testing, it is paramount that patients undergo both functional and genetic assessment.

Prothrombin G20210A Polymorphism

Prothrombin (factor II), a vitamin K–dependent factor synthesized in the liver, becomes thrombin when activated. A genetic polymorphism in the distal 3′ untranslated region of the gene for prothrombin, a transition from guanine to adenine at the 20210 nucleotide of the prothrombin gene, has been described in patients with VTE. This results in a normal prothrombin but at increased levels. This polymorphism confers an increased risk for VTE by 2.8-fold, is associated with 4% to 6% of patients with VTE, and is the second most common cause of hypercoagulability in Caucasians.

Hyperhomocysteinemia

Hyperhomocysteinemia has been a known risk factor for atherosclerosis and vascular disease for more than 25 years, though a direct cause-and-effect relationship has not been established. However, a meta-analysis suggests the risk of VTE to be 2.5-fold with elevated homocysteine levels. Two enzyme deficiencies, N^5,N^{10}-methylenetetrahydrofolate reductase (MTHFR) or cystathionine β synthase, are responsible for elevated homocysteine levels. Although mutations in these enzymes are not infrequent, the common polymorphism in MTHFR alone is not a factor in either the elevation of plasma homocysteine or thrombosis.

Other Disorders Associated with Thrombosis

Defective Fibrinolysis/Dysfibrinogenemia/Lipoprotein(a)

Abnormal plasminogens (dysplasminogenemias), although rare (<1%), have been described in cases of spontaneous arterial thrombosis or VTE. Both type I quantitative and type II qualitative deficiency states have been described. Numerous molecular defects have been classified. Defective thrombin binding or resistance to plasmin-mediated breakdown has been described. Although not clearly documented, defects in plasminogen activators, tPA or uPA, may incite thrombotic events. Elevated PAI-1 has been associated with DVT and myocardial infarction.

Lipoprotein(a), associated with low density lipoprotein (LDL), has both atherogenic and prothrombotic properties. It prevents plasminogen from binding to cells or fibrin and inhibits fibrinolysis. Elevated levels of lipoprotein(a) have been associated with VTE in childhood; it is a weak thrombotic risk factor in adults.

Abnormal Platelet Aggregation

It has been recognized for some time that there are patients who have thrombosis and may have hyperactive/hyperresponsive platelets but this entity is poorly defined. Diabetes mellitus, which is known to be associated with hyperactive platelets and hyperlipidemic states, may be a contributing factor. Although platelet aggregation assays may be helpful in making the diagnosis, these assays are not yet validated for this specific circumstance and, thus, the incidence and importance of platelets to thrombosis are not well known. Bleeding time measurements are not specific, and not recommended for making this diagnosis.

Standard anticoagulant treatment is recommended for this condition. Aspirin and the thienopyridine derivatives such as clopidogrel may be useful, but their utility is unknown.

Elevated Procoagulant Factors: VIII, IX, and XI

Elevated prothrombotic factors have only recently been associated with primary and recurrent VTE.

Disseminated Intravascular Coagulation and Sepsis-Induced Coagulopathy

DIC is a primary form of acute thrombosis. Causes of DIC include sepsis, trauma, pancreatitis, obstetric complications such as abruptio placentae or amniotic embolism, transplant rejection, malignant tumors, certain snake bites, hematologic malignancies, and hepatic failure. Coagulation in DIC is activated by the release of TF into the circulation causing unregulated activation of the coagulation cascade, leading to massive thrombin production and fibrin generation. Fibrinolysis then becomes activated as well, leading to bleeding in the later, hemorrhagic stages of the syndrome because of the consumption of clotting factors, depletion of fibrinogen, and unchecked plasmin activity. Laboratory values in DIC reveal a downtrend in platelet count—even within the normal range, decreased fibrinogen level, prolonged PT, and concomitant elevation in fibrin split products and the presence of a positive D-dimer test. The treatment of DIC requires treatment of the underlying condition. The need for platelet or plasma transfusion is based on the presence of hemorrhage, rather than on particular laboratory values.[23] Sepsis-induced coagulopathy (SIC) has been recently recognized as a distinct entity from DIC and is characterized by thrombocytopenia, elevated PT/INR, and organ failure. In contrast to DIC, patients with SIC have improved fibrinolysis from increased PAI-1 production.[24]

BLEEDING DISORDERS

Although the surgeon deals more often with procoagulant states than bleeding disorders, it is important to recognize these disorders when they occur.

Table 5.4. Common Bleeding Disorders

Disorder	Defect	Laboratory Values	Treatment
Hemophilia A	Sex-linked recessive deficiency of FVIII	Prolonged aPTT Decreased FVIII: ■ <2% severe deficiency ■ 2–5% moderate deficiency ■ >5% mild deficiency	FVIII concentrate Levels 80–100% needed for surgery/ life-threatening hemorrhage
Hemophilia B	Sex-linked recessive deficiency of FIX	Prolonged aPTT Decreased FIX: ■ <4% severe deficiency ■ 20–40% moderate deficiency	FVIX concentrate; Vitamin K Levels 80–100% needed for surgery/ life-threatening hemorrhage
Von Willebrand disease	Autosomal dominant or recessive	Prolonged platelet aggregation Decreased FVIII activity ± decreased vWF antigen Decreased ristocetin-induced platelet aggregation	Desmopressin acetate (DDAVP) (mild cases) vWF:FVIII concentrate ■ Levels ≥50% for major surgery/neuroaxial analgesia ■ Cryoprecipitate as alternative Antifibrinolytic agents

aPTT, activated partial thromboplastin time; FVIII, factor VIII; FIX, factor IX; vWF, von Willebrand factor.

Coagulation Factor Deficiency

5 Coagulation factor deficiency states are important causes of bleeding (**Table 5.4**) and the most common are factor VIII and IX deficiency states, termed hemophilia A and B, and type I von Willebrand disease (vWD). Hemophilia A incidence is approximately 1 in 5000 births. Clinical findings range from bleeding into joints and muscles, epistaxis, hematuria, and bleeding after minor trauma, to prolonged postoperative bleeding, retroperitoneal bleeding, and intramural bowel hemorrhage. The minimum level of factor VIII required for hemostasis is 30%, and spontaneous bleeding is uncommon with factor VIII levels greater than 5% to 10% of normal. Although the half-life of factor VIII is 2.9 days in normal subjects, the half-life of factor VIII concentrates is only 9 to 18 hours.[25] Acquired deficiency has been reported to occur with the development of antibodies to factor VIII after therapy. Inhibitor antibodies develop in approximately 10% to 15% of patients with hemophilia A, although the incidence of antibody formation may be much higher in previously untreated patients and in those with severe hemophilia A.

Factor IX deficiency (Christmas factor) is an inherited disorder but may also be acquired because of enhanced factor IX clearance in states such as the nephrotic syndrome, abnormal protein production in vitamin K deficiency, and acquired specific inhibitors to factor IX in various autoimmune diseases, such as SLE. It is clinically indistinguishable from hemophilia A, and laboratory screening tests reveal a prolonged aPTT, with other test results normal, although a greater proportion of patients have only mild or moderate deficiency.

Rare Factor Deficiencies

Other specific factor deficiencies are much less common and receive only a brief mention here. These include factors II, XI, V, VII, and X. These can be measured by serum assays, although this is not routinely available in many hospitals. The treatments are primarily FFP concentrates to give back the clotting factors.

Platelet Disorders

vWF causes platelet adhesion to collagen, initiating platelet plug formation. It also forms a complex with factor VIII in the blood. Produced in endothelial cells and megakaryocytes (compared with the liver for factor VIII), it has a circulating half-life of 6 to 20 hours. vWD, a deficiency of vWF, is the most common of the inherited coagulation disorder. Six different subtypes have been identified for their deficiency state. Variants include types I and III (quantitative decreases in normal-appearing vWF) and type II (qualitative abnormalities in structure and function of vWF). vWF deficiency is probably as common as hemophilia A, although the true incidence may surpass what is generally appreciated because many mild cases probably remain undiagnosed. Clinical manifestations include easy bruisability, mild-to-moderate epistaxis, gingival bleeding, menorrhagia, rare joint or muscle bleeding, prolonged bleeding following surgery, and subcutaneous bleeding. Spontaneous bleeding is not as common as in hemophilia A.

Desmopressin acetate (DDAVP) is available for the treatment of mild cases of type I and 2 vWD: about 80% of patients will respond with an increase in vWF ag and FVIII activity within 60 minutes. In other type II states and type III vWD, factor VIII concentrates are necessary. Recombinant factor VIII/vWF concentrates that avoid the infectious risks of transfusion are available.

Inherited defects of platelet receptors include defects of GpIIb/IIIa (Glanzmann thrombasthenia), characterized by impaired platelet binding to vWF, fibrinogen, and fibronectin. In patients with defects in GpIb (Bernard–Soulier syndrome), the absolute number of platelets is decreased, the platelets are larger, and platelet aggregation and adhesion are abnormal. Acquired deficits occur in uremia; both GpIb and GpIIb/IIIa receptors are defective, resulting in impaired adhesion and aggregation. Acquired deficits also occur in patients who previously received platelet transfusions and then acquired immune-mediated antiplatelet antibodies.

Abnormalities in Fibrinolysis

Abnormalities in fibrinolysis can also lead to bleeding disorders. Fibrinogen deficiency from inherited defects resulting in defective fibrin formation, polymerization, or crosslinking is characterized by prolonged TCT. Deficiency can also be acquired from consumption during DIC and from primary fibrinolytic states. A fibrinogen level of 100 mg/mL should be achieved to stop bleeding related to fibrinogen abnormalities.

Genetic or acquired deficiencies in α_2-AP may be associated with bleeding, whereas deficiencies in factor XIII (fibrin-stabilizing factor) may lead to highly lysable clot. α_2-AP deficiency is treated with ε-aminocaproic acid or tranexamic acid. Homozygous patients with factor XIII deficiency and less than 1% of normal plasma activity often show bleeding from the umbilical cord at birth, bleeding after trauma or surgery, and delayed bleeding 24 to 36 hours later. Screening test results include a shortened euglobulin lysis time. A specific assay for factor XIII activity exists. Treatment consists of FFP, cryoprecipitate, and factor XIII concentrates.

References

1. Golebiewska EM, Poole AW. Platelet secretion: from haemostasis to wound healing and beyond. *Blood Rev*. 2015;29(3):153–162.
2. Morrell CN, Aggrey AA, Chapman LM, Modjeski KL. Emerging roles for platelets as immune and inflammatory cells. *Blood*. 2014;123(18):2759–2767.
3. Brighton TA, Eikelboom JW, Mann K, et al. Low-dose aspirin for preventing recurrent venous thromboembolism. *N Engl J Med*. 2012;367(21):1979–1987.
4. von Brühl ML, Stark K, Steinhart A, et al. Monocytes, neutrophils, and platelets cooperate to initiate and propagate venous thrombosis in mice in vivo. *J Exp Med*. 2012;209(4):819–835.
5. Mackman N. New insights into the mechanisms of venous thrombosis. *J Clin Invest*. 2012;122(7):2331–2336.
6. Furie B, Furie BC. Mechanisms of thrombus formation. *N Engl J Med*. 2008;359(9):938–949.
7. Palareti G, Cosmi B, Legnani C, et al. D-dimer testing to determine the duration of anticoagulation therapy. *N Engl J Med*. 2006;355(17):1780–1789.
8. Aird WC. Phenotypic heterogeneity of the endothelium: II. Representative vascular beds. *Circ Res*. 2007;100(2):174–190.
9. Rectenwald JE, Myers DD Jr, Hawley AE, et al. D-dimer, P-selectin, and microparticles: novel markers to predict deep venous thrombosis. A pilot study. *Thromb Haemost*. 2005;94(6):1312–1317.
10. Wakefield TW, Myers DD, Henke PK. Mechanisms of venous thrombosis and resolution. *Arterioscler Thromb Vasc Biol*. 2008;28(3):387–391.
11. Saha P, Humphries J, Modarai B, et al. Leukocytes and the natural history of deep vein thrombosis: current concepts and future directions. *Arterioscler Thromb Vasc Biol*. 2011;31(3):506–512.
12. Fuchs TA, Brill A, Duerschmied D, et al. Extracellular DNA traps promote thrombosis. *Proc Natl Acad Sci USA*. 2010;107(36):15880–15885.
13. Diaz JA, Fuchs TA, Jackson TO, et al. Plasma DNA is elevated in patients with deep vein thrombosis. *J Vasc Surg Venous Lymphat Disord*. 2013;1(4):341–348.e1.
14. Singh I, Burnand KG, Collins M, et al. Failure of thrombus to resolve in urokinase-type plasminogen activator gene-knockout mice: rescue by normal bone marrow-derived cells. *Circulation*. 2003;107(6):869–875.
15. Myers DD Jr, Henke PK, Bedard PW, et al. Treatment with an oral small molecule inhibitor of P selectin (PSI-697) decreases vein wall injury in a rat stenosis model of venous thrombosis. *J Vasc Surg*. 2006;44(3):625–632.
16. Henke PK, Varma MR, Moaveni DK, et al. Fibrotic injury after experimental deep vein thrombosis is determined by the mechanism of thrombogenesis. *Thromb Haemost*. 2007;98(5):1045–1055.
17. Bochenek ML, Leidinger C, Rosinus NS, et al. Activated endothelial TGFβ1 signaling promotes venous thrombus nonresolution in mice via endothelin-1. *Circ Res*. 2020;126(2):162–181.
18. Glynn RJ, Danielson E, Fonseca FA, et al. A randomized trial of rosuvastatin in the prevention of venous thromboembolism. *N Engl J Med*. 2009;360(18):1851–1861.
19. Reitsma PH, Versteeg HH, Middeldorp S. Mechanistic view of risk factors for venous thromboembolism. *Arterioscler Thromb Vasc Biol*. 2012;32(3):563–568.
20. Stevens SM, Woller SC, Baumann Kreuziger L, et al. Executive summary: antithrombotic therapy for VTE disease: second update of the CHEST Guideline and Expert Panel Report. *Chest*. 2021;160(6):2247–2259.
21. Cohen H, Isenberg DA. How I treat anticoagulant-refractory thrombotic antiphospholipid syndrome. *Blood*. 2021;137(3):299–309.
22. Gabriel F, Portolés O, Labiós M, et al. Usefulness of thrombophilia testing in venous thromboembolic disease: findings from the RIETE registry. *Clin Appl Thromb Hemost*. 2013;19(1):42–47.
23. Levi M, Toh CH, Thachil J, Watson HG. Guidelines for the diagnosis and management of disseminated intravascular coagulation. British Committee for Standards in Haematology. *Br J Haematol*. 2009;145(1):24–33.
24. Iba T, Nisio MD, Levy JH, Kitamura N, Thachil J. New criteria for sepsis-induced coagulopathy (SIC) following the revised sepsis definition: a retrospective analysis of a nationwide survey. *BMJ Open*. 2017;7(9):e017046.
25. Coppola A, Di Capua M, Di Minno MN, et al. Treatment of hemophilia: a review of current advances and ongoing issues. *J Blood Med*. 2010;1:183–195.

6

Surgical Infections

Lena M. Napolitano

Key Points

1 Surgical infections include intra-abdominal infections (appendicitis, cholecystitis/cholangitis, diverticulitis, colitis including *Clostridium difficile* colitis, pancreatitis, and peritonitis), soft tissue infections (necrotizing and nonnecrotizing), surgical site infections (SSIs), and hospital-acquired infections (HAIs) that occur in surgical patients (pneumonia, central line–associated bloodstream infections [CLABSI], and catheter-associated urinary tract infections [CAUTIs]). Any of these surgical infections can result in sepsis or septic shock.

2 Early appropriate empiric broad-spectrum antimicrobial therapy, to cover all potential causative pathogens, is an important adjunct to source control in the treatment of surgical infections. Inappropriate antimicrobial therapy is associated with increased mortality.

3 A key concept in surgical infections is "*source control*," defined as any physical intervention to remove or eliminate a focus of invasive infection (drainage, debridement, and device removal) and to restore optimal anatomic function.

4 Pathogen identification and appropriate deescalation of antimicrobial therapy are of paramount importance in treatment of surgical infections, as increasing prevalence of multi–drug-resistant pathogens has been identified in both abdominal and skin surgical infections.

5 Complicated intra-abdominal infection (cIAI) extends beyond the hollow viscus of origin into the peritoneal space and is associated with either abscess formation or peritonitis. Recommendations for specific antimicrobial therapy for cIAI are based on whether the infection is "community acquired" or "health care associated."

6 In patients with intra-abdominal infections who have undergone an adequate source-control procedure, fixed-duration antibiotic therapy for 4 days is noninferior to longer duration antimicrobial therapy until resolution of physiologic abnormalities, with no difference in SSI, recurrent intra-abdominal infection, or death.

7 Fecal microbiota transplant (FMT) is now an accepted treatment for severe and fulminant *C. difficile* colitis. Two surgical procedures possibly indicated for *C. difficile* colitis treatment include (1) total abdominal colectomy (for peritonitis, colonic perforation, ischemia, necrosis, toxic megacolon with impending perforation, septic shock with organ failure) and (2) diverting loop ileostomy and intraoperative colonic lavage for toxin reduction with colonic preservation.

8 The initial treatment of infected pancreatic necrosis is percutaneous catheter or endoscopic drainage with additional drain placement as required.
Lack of clinical improvement of necrotizing infected pancreatitis with initial percutaneous drainage warrants consideration of minimally invasive techniques for pancreatic necrosectomy including video-assisted retroperitoneal debridement (VARD) or transluminal direct endoscopic necrosectomy (DEN).

9 Acute bacterial skin and skin structure infections are defined as bacterial infection of the skin with a lesion size area of at least 75 cm^2 (lesion size measured by the area of redness, edema, or induration), including cellulitis, wound infection, and abscess.

10 Early operative debridement is the major determinant of outcome in necrotizing soft tissue infections (NSTIs). Delayed definitive debridement remains the single most important risk factor for death.

1 Surgical infections include intra-abdominal infections (appendicitis, cholecystitis, diverticulitis, colitis, and pancreatitis), soft tissue infections (necrotizing and nonnecrotizing), surgical site infections (SSIs), and hospital-acquired infections (HAIs) that occur in surgical patients (pneumonia, central line–associated bloodstream infections [CLABSIs], and catheter-associated urinary tract infections [CAUTIs]).[1] Appropriate therapy of surgical infections to optimize patient outcomes includes four steps: (1) early diagnosis, (2) early initiation of appropriate empiric broad-spectrum antimicrobial therapy, (3) adequate source control (surgical or interventional radiology), and (4) pathogen identification and appropriate deescalation of antimicrobial therapy (**Table 6.1**).

The initial management of all surgical infections should include the initiation of early empiric antimicrobial therapy to cover all potential causative pathogens, since early and appropriate empiric antibiotic therapy improves patient outcomes and decreases mortality.[2] The choice of early empiric antimicrobial therapy is guided by the specific site of infection,

Table 6.1. Appropriate Therapy of Surgical Infections

1. Early diagnosis of surgical infection.
2. Early initiation of appropriate empiric broad-spectrum antimicrobial therapy.
3. Adequate source control.
4. Pathogen identification and appropriate deescalation of antimicrobial therapy.

Table 6.2. Hour-1 Bundle, Surviving Sepsis Campaign Guidelines 2021

1. Measure lactate level[a]
2. Obtain blood cultures before administering antibiotics
3. Administer broad-spectrum antibiotics to cover all potential causative pathogens within 1 h
4. Begin 30 mL/kg crystalloid for hypotension or lactate level ≥4 mmol/L
5. Apply vasopressors if hypotensive to maintain MAP ≥65 mm Hg

[a]Remeasure lactate if initial lactate is elevated (>2 mmol/L).
Adapted from Evans L, Rhodes A, Alhazzani W, et al. Surviving sepsis campaign: International Guidelines for Management of Sepsis and Septic Shock: 2021. *Crit Care Med.* 2021;49(11):e1063–e1143.

the common pathogens associated with that infection, and by local and regional antibiograms. The goal of antimicrobial therapy is to achieve antibiotic levels at the site of the infection that exceed the minimum inhibitory concentration of the microbial pathogens present.

EARLY USE OF APPROPRIATE BROAD-SPECTRUM ANTIMICROBIAL THERAPY

2 Early use of appropriate broad-spectrum antimicrobial therapy is an important adjunct to appropriate surgical management of surgical infections. Numerous studies have confirmed that inappropriate empiric antibiotics (ie, antibiotics that do not cover the causative pathogens) and delay in antibiotic administration are associated with increased mortality.[2] In patients who manifest sepsis or septic shock, every hour delay of antimicrobial therapy is associated with increased mortality. The Surviving Sepsis Guidelines recommend administration of IV antimicrobials within 1 hour for sepsis and septic shock (**Table 6.2**).[3]

SOURCE CONTROL

3 Source control is defined as any physical intervention to remove or eliminate a focus of invasive infection (drainage, debridement, and device removal) and to restore optimal anatomic function. Source control should be achieved as quickly as possible.[4] In surgical infections, antimicrobial agents are used in conjunction with adequate source control of the initial infection. Adequate source control can be accomplished by either surgical or percutaneous interventional radiologic techniques. A number of factors have been identified that predict failure of source control for intra-abdominal infections (**Table 6.3**).

Table 6.3. Clinical Factors Predicting Failure of "Source Control" for Intra-Abdominal Infection

Delay in the initial intervention (>24 h)
High severity of illness (APACHE [Acute Physiology and Chronic Health Evaluation] II score ≥15)
Advanced age
Comorbidity and degree of organ dysfunction
Low albumin level
Poor nutritional status
Degree of peritoneal involvement or diffuse peritonitis
Inability to achieve adequate drainage or debridement
Presence of malignancy

PATHOGEN IDENTIFICATION

4 Pathogen identification is extremely important, in part related to increased prevalence of multi–drug-resistant pathogens that are associated with surgical infections. Whenever possible, high-quality specimens should be obtained from source-control procedures for Gram stain and culture in order to identify causative pathogens and determine antimicrobial susceptibility of the bacterial isolates identified. This will enable appropriate deescalation of antimicrobial therapy from broad-spectrum therapy to directed potential single antimicrobial agent therapy.

INTRA-ABDOMINAL INFECTIONS

Classification

5 Complicated intra-abdominal infection (cIAI) extends beyond the hollow viscus of origin into the peritoneal space and is associated with either abscess formation or peritonitis. "Uncomplicated" intra-abdominal infection involves intramural inflammation of the gastrointestinal tract and has a substantial probability of progressing to cIAI if not adequately treated.

Diagnosis

Patients with cIAI present with abdominal pain and gastrointestinal symptoms. A comprehensive abdominal physical examination must be performed in these patients. If peritonitis is present, evaluation for emergent laparotomy without diagnostic studies is considered. If peritonitis is not present, recent evidence-based guidelines recommend that computed tomography (CT) scan of the abdomen and pelvis is the diagnostic imaging modality of choice to evaluate for cIAI and its source.[5]

Treatment

6 Early definitive source control (percutaneous or surgical) and appropriate empiric systemic antimicrobial therapy to cover all potential causative pathogens are the mainstays of treatment of cIAIs.[6] Successful source control is defined as complete, definitive resolution of infection by an index procedure that requires no further intervention.[4] The Surgical Infection Society 2024 Guidelines on the Management of Intra-Abdominal Infection recommend undertaking source control within 6 hours in higher-risk patient with associated septic shock, and within 12 hours, in lower-risk patients. For critically ill cIAI patients, abbreviated laparotomy with temporary abdominal closure may be required to facilitate more definitive source control, but timely abdominal closure is recommended as soon as possible.[5] Culture and susceptibility testing of the infection source should always be obtained for definitive pathogen identification and to guide antimicrobial therapy.[7]

In order to select appropriate empiric antimicrobial agents for use, cIAIs are further classified as "community-acquired" or "health care-associated or hospital-acquired."

Community-Acquired Complicated Intra-Abdominal Infection

For patients who have "community-acquired" cIAI, determination of whether the disease is "mild/moderate (appendicitis, mild diverticulitis)" or "severe (fecal peritonitis, perforated diverticulitis)" facilitates appropriate antimicrobial treatment. Patients with "severe" community-acquired cIAI should have antibiotics that cover *Pseudomonas* and *Enterococcus* pathogens, and both single-agent and combination-agent regimens are available for use. A number of antimicrobials are no longer recommended for use in community-acquired cIAI:

- Ampicillin/sulbactam is not recommended because of high resistance of *Escherichia coli* to this agent (B-II).
- Cefotetan and clindamycin are not recommended for use because of increasing resistance of the *Bacteroides fragilis* group to these agents (B-II).

- Because of the availability of less toxic agents demonstrated to be of at least equal efficacy, aminoglycosides are not recommended for routine use in community-acquired cIAI in adults (B-II).

Health Care–Associated Complicated Intra-Abdominal Infection

For patients with "health care–associated" cIAI, empiric antimicrobial agents with broad-spectrum activity are preferred. Specific antimicrobials are recommended based on whether the patient and/or institution have high risk for infection with multi–drug-resistant pathogens. Quinolone-resistant *E. coli* have become common in many communities, and quinolones should not be used unless hospital antibiograms confirm greater than 90% susceptibility of *E. coli* to quinolones. In patients with health care–associated cIAI, carbapenems are an excellent single-agent regimen for empiric treatment.

Duration of Antibiotics for Complicated Intra-Abdominal Infection

Duration of antibiotics for treatment of cIAI has long been controversial. The Study to Optimize Peritoneal Infection Therapy (STOP-IT) randomized trial examined the efficacy of short-course (4 days) antimicrobial therapy in patients with cIAIs who had undergone an adequate source-control procedure. Fixed-duration antibiotic therapy for 4 days was noninferior to longer duration antimicrobial therapy (until 2 days after resolution of fever, leukocytosis, and ileus), with no difference in the composite endpoints of SSI, recurrent intra-abdominal infection, or death.[8]

The STOP-IT trial had few ICU patients. The DURAPOP trial compared 8- versus 15-day antibiotic therapy for postoperative ICU patients ($n = 249$) with postoperative cIAI with adequate source control and adequate empiric antimicrobial therapy. No differences in 45-day mortality rate, ICU and hospital length of stay, reoperation rate, or emergence of MDR bacteria were identified, and 8-day antibiotic duration was recommended for ICU patients with cIAI.[9]

SPECIFIC INTRA-ABDOMINAL INFECTIONS

Appendicitis

Appendicitis is common with over 300,000 hospital discharges in the United States per year and a lifetime risk of almost 1 in 11 persons. Appendicitis is classified as *uncomplicated* (nonperforated, no abscess, or phlegmon) or *complicated* (perforated appendicitis, periappendicular abscess or peritonitis, defined as acute inflammation of the peritoneum secondary to infection of the appendix). Although ultrasound is recommended for diagnosis confirmation in children and CT imaging is recommended in adults, all diagnostic imaging (ultrasound, CT, and MRI) has significant limitations in discriminating between complicated and uncomplicated appendicitis.[10] The negative predictive value for complicated appendicitis for CT is high (93%), but its positive predictive value is 74%.

Although appendectomy provides definitive source control for the treatment of acute nonperforated appendicitis, with intravenous (IV) antibiotics administered preoperatively and repeat dosing intraoperatively if the surgery is prolonged, a number of controversies in diagnosis and management of appendicitis persist.[11]

Antibiotics Versus Appendectomy for Uncomplicated Appendicitis

In patients with uncomplicated appendicitis appendectomy is definitive source control and has historically been the standard of care. But a number of randomized trials have confirmed that acute uncomplicated appendicitis can be treated successfully with medical management (antibiotics alone) if a patient accepts the subsequent risk of recurrence. Nonoperative management is also ideal for patients who are high-risk surgical candidates.

In a 2022 systematic review and meta-analysis (eight randomized trials, 1995–2021), nonoperative treatment (antibiotics) was not statistically different in treatment success at 30 days or major complications versus operative treatment (appendectomy) for acute uncomplicated appendicitis.[12] But length of stay and recurrent appendicitis (median rate 18%) were significantly higher in the nonoperative management group. In a 2024 meta-analysis and trial sequential analysis comparing antibiotics versus appendectomy for uncomplicated appendicitis (eight randomized trials, $n = 3213$), no difference in complication rates was identified, but antibiotics had a reduced treatment efficacy (RR 0.80, 95% CI 0.71 to 0.90, $P < .00001$) and at 1 year, was successful in 540 out of 837 participants (64.6%, RR = 0.69, 95% CI 0.61 to 0.77, $P < .00001$). There was no difference in length of stay.[13]

The 2024 SAGES Guideline[14] suggests that adult and pediatric patients with uncomplicated or complicated appendicitis be managed operatively (conditional recommendation, low/very low certainty of evidence). In practice, a personalized approach including patient decision making regarding whether they prefer antibiotics or appendectomy for treatment of uncomplicated appendicitis is used, and a publicly available decision support tool called AppyOrNot (AppyOrNot.org) provides an educational video to assist patient decision making. The results of this informed patient decision-making process are now included in a treatment algorithm[15] for adult patients with acute appendicitis (**Algorithm 6.1**).

Oral Versus IV Versus No Antibiotics for Uncomplicated Appendicitis

Oral antibiotic monotherapy is an acceptable treatment alternative for uncomplicated acute appendicitis. The APPAC II multicenter randomized trial compared oral antibiotic monotherapy (7 days oral moxifloxacin) to combined IV and oral antibiotics (IV ertapenem 2 days and levofloxacin 5 days). One-year treatment success was over 70% in both groups.[16] At year 3, cumulative treatment success was 63.4% in the oral antibiotic monotherapy group and 65.2% in the IV/oral antibiotic group. No differences in the 3-year true recurrence rate of appendicitis (25.5% oral vs 25.8% oral/IV), overall complication rate (6.1% oral vs 7.3% oral/IV), or quality of life measures were identified.[17] These study results support potential outpatient management of acute uncomplicated appendicitis with oral antibiotics. The Surgical Infection Society 2024 Guidelines[5] recommend oral moxifloxacin for empiric therapy of lower-risk patients undergoing nonoperative management of acute uncomplicated appendicitis.

Since acute appendicitis is similar to diverticulitis, and antibiotics are no longer recommended in uncomplicated diverticulitis in healthy patients, some have recommended that uncomplicated appendicitis also does not require antibiotics. APPAC III was a small ($n = 72$) double-blind, placebo-controlled, superiority randomized trial in adults with CT-confirmed uncomplicated acute appendicitis which compared placebo to antibiotics (IV ertapenem followed by oral levofloxacin and metronidazole). The 10-day treatment success was not different (87% placebo vs 97% antibiotics).[18] A noninferiority trial of antibiotics versus placebo has been recommended.

Laparoscopic Versus Open Appendectomy

Appendectomy can be performed by laparoscopic or open approach. A Cochrane review of 85 randomized trials ($n = 9765$, 8520 adults; 1245 children) that compared laparoscopic versus open appendectomy reported that the laparoscopic approach had a higher rate of intra-abdominal abscess but was more favorable related to decreased pain intensity, decreased SSIs, decreased hospital length of stay, and decreased time to return to normal activity.[19] A short course (24 hours) of IV

Algorithm 6.1

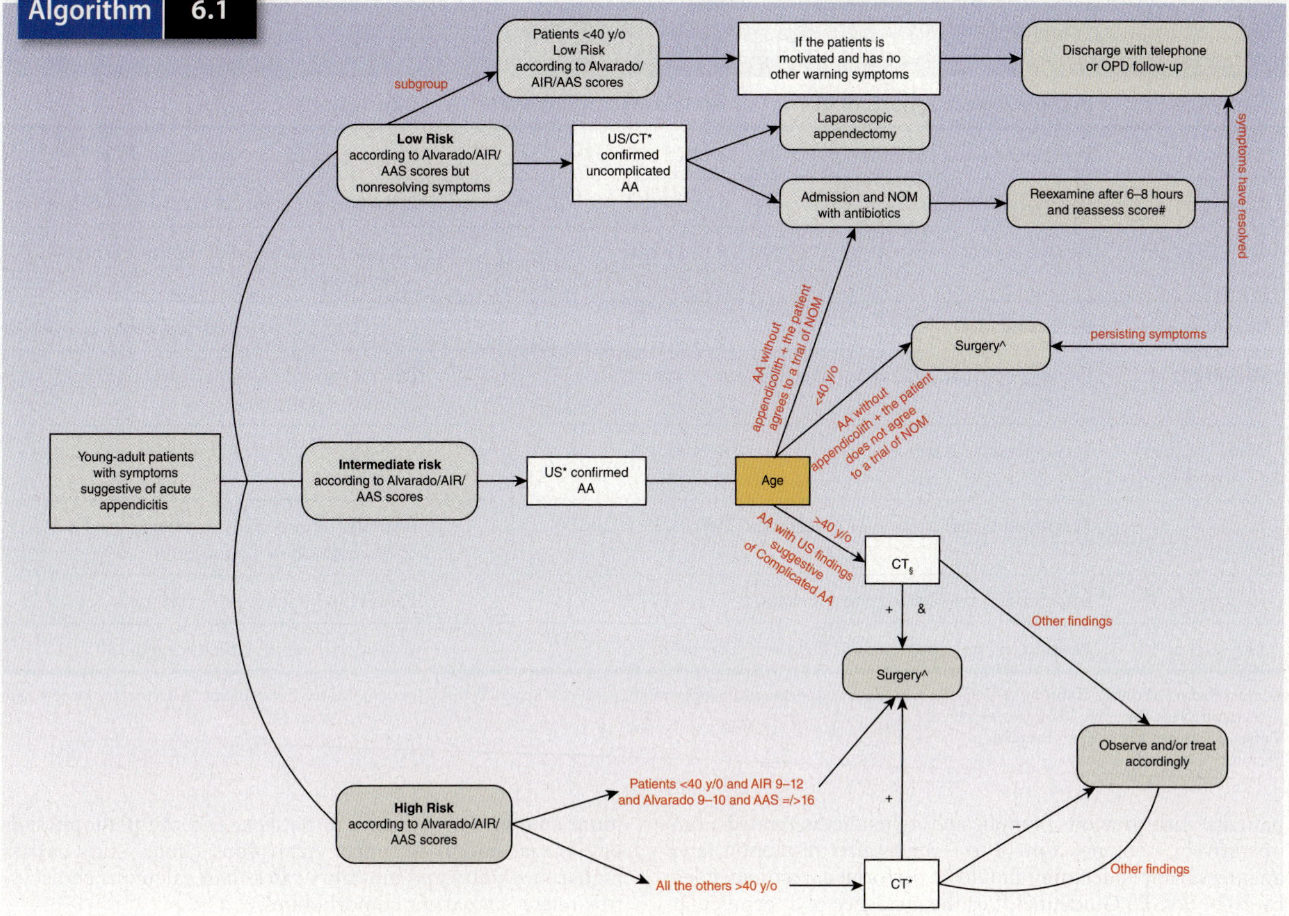

Algorithm 6.1. Practical WSES Algorithm for the diagnosis and treatment of adult patients with suspected acute appendicitis. *We recommend the routine use of a combination of clinical scores and US; consider use of CT scan if US inconclusive. If no improvements after observation and reassessment, consider US or CT based on age and probability of other diseases. ^Surgery is meant as lap appendectomy. In case of abscess or phlegmon on US/CT, consider also antibiotics + percutaneous drainage. &Patients >40 years with complicated appendicitis treated nonoperatively should undergo colonic screening and interval full-dose contrast-enhanced CT scan and interval appendectomy. Consider CT in patients >40 years with clinical/US signs of complicated AA. From Di Saverio S, Podda M, De Simone B, et al. Diagnosis and treatment of acute appendicitis: 2020 update of the WSES Jerusalem guidelines. *World J Emerg Surg*. 2020;15(1):27.

antibiotic therapy is recommended for patients with acute complicated appendicitis undergoing adequate source control by laparoscopic or open appendectomy.

Time to Appendectomy and Perforation Risk

It has long been thought that appendiceal luminal obstruction leads to appendiceal perforation without timely surgical intervention. This belief led to attempts to decrease time from presentation and diagnosis of acute appendicitis to operating room start time. With the advent of early appropriate empiric systemic antimicrobial therapy, this fundamental concept is no longer true. As discussed previously, in patients with uncomplicated appendicitis, antibiotic treatment alone does not lead to appendiceal perforation.

The PERFECT open-label multicenter randomized trial compared appendectomies scheduled within 8 or 24 hours in adult patients (n = 1803) with predicted uncomplicated acute appendicitis. Appendiceal perforation rate was similar between groups (8% vs 9%) and no significant differences in complications rates (7% vs 6%) were found, with no mortality.[20] A meta-analysis comparison (15 studies, n = 33,596) of daytime versus nighttime appendectomy reported no differences in postoperative mortality or complication rates, but the conversion to laparotomy was almost twofold higher among patients who underwent appendectomy during nighttime.[21] These data support postponing night-time appendectomy to daytime if possible.

Complicated Appendicitis: Abscess or Phlegmon Management

Appendiceal abscess or phlegmon account for up to 10% of complicated acute appendicitis cases. Current evidence and expert opinion supports initial nonoperative management with IV transitioned to oral antibiotics and percutaneous drainage, if possible, followed by interval appendectomy. Repeat CT imaging is recommended to confirm resolution of infection, and colonoscopy is recommended prior to interval appendectomy. A Cochrane systematic review of appendectomy timing (early vs delayed) for patients with appendiceal phlegmon or abscess included eight randomized trials (n = 828) and reported very low–certainty evidence with no clear advantage to either.[22] Surgeons must make individualized decisions regarding appendectomy timing in these cases and should consider the benefit of definitive infection source control versus the difficulty and complexity of the surgery required.

Interval Appendectomy After Initial Nonoperative Management

Interval appendectomy refers to appendectomy 6 to 12 weeks after the initial diagnosis of appendicitis. Importantly, in

Table 6.4. Overview of Published Studies Reporting Quantitative Data in Adult Patients Undergoing Interval Appendicectomy for Complicated Appendicitis (Abscess, Phlegmon, Perforation, Mass) and Incidence of Neoplasm

Reference	Preoperative diagnosis of IA	Neoplasm diagnosis after IA	Conclusions
Mallinen et al.	Periappendicular abscess	3 of 25 (12)	Consider IA in patients aged > 40 y
Carpenter et al.	Periappendicular abscess or perforation	5 of 18 (28)	Preoperative staging recommended before IA
Furman et al.	Periappendicular abscess or phlegmon	5 of 17 (29)	Consider IA in all adult patients, especially those aged ≥ 40 y
Wright et al.	Perforated appendicitis	11 of 89 (12)	Consider IA in patients aged ≥ 40 y
Al-Kurd et al.	Periappendicular abscess or phlegmon	6 of 106 (3.7)	Do not consider IA routinely; consider follow-up imaging
Mima et al.	Periappendicular abscess	4 of 47 (9)	Consider IA to rule out neoplasm in elderly patients
Son et al.	Periappendicular abscess or phlegmon	14 of 111 (12.6)	Consider IA, especially in patients aged ≥ 40 y; consider follow-up imaging
de Jonge et al.	Appendiceal mass (phlegmon ± abscess)	7 of 64 (11)	Fallow-up imaging recommended
Hayes et al.	Perforation, phlegmon, and/or abscess	36 of 402 (8.9)	Consider IA in all patients aged ≥30 y

Adapted from Peltrini R, Cantoni V, Green R, et al. Risk of appendiceal neoplasm after interval appendectomy for complicated appendicitis: A systematic review and meta-analysis. *Surgeon.* 2021;19(6):e549–e558.
Values in parentheses are percentages.
IA, interval appendicectomy.

patients with previous complicated appendicitis treated non-operatively, a colonoscopy (4 to 6 weeks after resolution) and an interval appendectomy should be performed (recommended by 2024 SAGES Guideline),[14] as the incidence of appendicular neoplasm is high (3% to 17%, pooled prevalence 11%) in adult patients with complicated appendicitis (**Table 6.4**).[23,24] Appendiceal mucinous neoplasms occurred in 43%, adenocarcinoma in 29%, neuroendocrine neoplasm in 21%, globet cell carcinoma in 13%, and adenoma or serrated lesions in 20% of cases.

Appendiceal neoplasm is rare in patients with uncomplicated appendicitis treated with antibiotics. In a review of 4962 patients with appendicitis (38% complicated, 62% uncomplicated) enrolled in four comparative studies, the overall incidence rate of neoplasm was 1.98% (3.29% complicated, 1.49% uncomplicated, OR 0.44, 95% CI 0.16 to 1.23; $P < .087$).[25] The most common appendiceal neoplasms in this study of majority uncomplicated appendicitis were neuroendocrine tumors (49.21%), nonmucinous adenocarcinoma (24.24%), mixed adenoneuroendocrine tumor (MANEC) (11.40%), and mucinous adenocarcinoma (4.44%). There was a significant difference between complicated and uncomplicated appendicitis in rates of adenocarcinoma (50% vs 13%), neuroendocrine tumor (NET) (31% vs 74%), and MANEC (19% vs 13%) ($P < .001$).

See also Chapter 68: Appendiceal Diseases.

Biliary Infections

Biliary infections include acute cholecystitis which may be calculous or acalculous, may include choledocholithiasis or not, and cholangitis.[26] Acute cholecystitis and ascending cholangitis are primary inflammations of the gallbladder and bile ducts, respectively, which are caused by infection and possible biliary obstruction.

Acute Cholecystitis

Acute cholecystitis is inflammation of the gallbladder, resulting from obstruction of the cystic duct and subsequent bacterial invasion and overgrowth. Cholelithiasis is the cause of cystic duct obstruction in more than 90% of cases of acute cholecystitis in the United States. Acalculous cholecystitis is more common in critically ill patients and the pathophysiology is transmural ischemia. Acalculous cholecystitis carries higher morbidity and mortality rates than calculous cholecystitis related to patient comorbidities.

The diagnosis of acute cholecystitis is made based on the common constellation of right upper quadrant tenderness, leukocytosis, and fever. Initial diagnostic imaging is right upper quadrant ultrasound to evaluate for gallstones, gallbladder wall thickening, and pericholecystic inflammation (median sensitivity 73%, specificity 83%). If ultrasound is inconclusive or is discordant with the clinical evaluation, then cholescintigraphy (99mTc-hepatobiliary iminodiacetic acid, hepatobiliary iminodiacetic acid scan (HIDA scan), median sensitivity/specificity 89%/67%) or contrast-enhanced CT scan imaging is recommended. The 2024 IDSA Guidelines suggest CT as the subsequent imaging modality if ultrasound is inconclusive due to its ability to identify complications and rule out other etiologies.[7] Magnetic resonance cholangiopancreatography (MRCP) is useful for evaluating concurrent choledocholithiasis and biliary tract abnormalities.

The Tokyo Guidelines classify severity grading for acute cholecystitis into Grade I (mild), II (moderate), and III (severe) based on clinical, laboratory, and imaging criteria, with higher severity grades associated with worse outcomes, prolonged hospital length of stay, and conversions to open surgery (**Table 6.5**).[27] Treatment recommendations are then based on severity classification and coexistent comorbidities and ASA classification (**Algorithm 6.2**).[28,29]

Early systemic antimicrobial treatment is indicated for acute cholecystitis to cover the causative pathogens, including aerobic, enteric, Gram-negative bacilli (ie, *E. coli*, Klebsiella, Enterobacter, and Proteus), and aerobic Gram-positive organisms (ie, Enterococcus and Streptococcus). Anaerobes are uncommon, identified in approximately 15% of isolates. Clostridial organisms can be identified in cases of emphysematous cholecystitis confirmed by identification of gas in the gallbladder wall.

For patients with acute cholecystitis who are not candidates for cholecystectomy related to comorbidities or surgical risk, three nonsurgical options for treatment are available: (1) percutaneous cholecystostomy tube, (2) endoscopic transpapillary drainage,

Table 6.5. Severity Grading for Acute Cholecystitis: Tokyo Guidelines 2018

Severity of Acute Cholecystitis		Treatment
Mild (Grade I)	Does not meet the criteria of "Grade II" or "Grade III" acute cholecystitis Also defined as acute cholecystitis in a healthy patient with no organ dysfunction and mild inflammatory changes in the gallbladder, making cholecystectomy a safe and low-risk operative procedure	Early laparoscopic cholecystectomy if the patient meets the criteria of CCI ≤5 and ASA-PS ≤2
Moderate (Grade II)	Acute cholecystitis associated with any one of the following conditions: ▪ Elevated WBC count (>18,000/mm^3) ▪ Palpable tender mass in the right upper abdominal quadrant ▪ Duration of complaints >72 h ▪ Marked local inflammation (gangrenous cholecystitis, pericholecystic abscess, hepatic abscess, biliary peritonitis, emphysematous cholecystitis)	Early laparoscopic cholecystectomy by experienced surgeons if the patient meets the criteria of CCI ≤5 and ASA-PS ≤2 If not, after medical treatment and/or gallbladder drainage, laparoscopic cholecystectomy would be indicated
Severe (Grade III)	Acute cholecystitis associated with dysfunction of any one of the following organs/systems: ▪ Cardiovascular dysfunction (hypotension requiring vasopressors) ▪ Neurologic dysfunction (decreased level of consciousness) ▪ Respiratory dysfunction (PaO_2/FiO_2 ratio <300) ▪ Renal dysfunction (oliguria, serum creatinine >2 mg/dL) ▪ Hepatic dysfunction (elevated PT/INR >1.5) ▪ Hematologic dysfunction (platelet count <100,000/mm^3)	Lap-C is indicated with strict criteria: favorable organ system failure, and negative predictive factors, with CCI ≤3 and ASA-PS ≤2 and who are being treated at an advanced center (where experienced surgeons practice) If the patient is not considered suitable for early surgery, early/urgent biliary drainage is recommended followed by delayed Lap-C once the patient's overall condition has improved.

CCI, Charlson comorbidity index; ASA-PS, American Society of Anesthesiologists physical status classification system.
Adapted from Yokoe M, Hata J, Takada T, et al. Tokyo Guidelines 2018: Diagnostic criteria and severity grading of acute cholecystitis (with videos). *J Hepatobiliary Pancreat Sci.* 2018;25:41–54; Okamoto K, Suzuki K, Takada T, et al. Tokyo Guidelines 2018: flowchart for the management of acute cholecystitis. *J Hepatobiliary Pancreat Sci.* 2018;25:55–72.

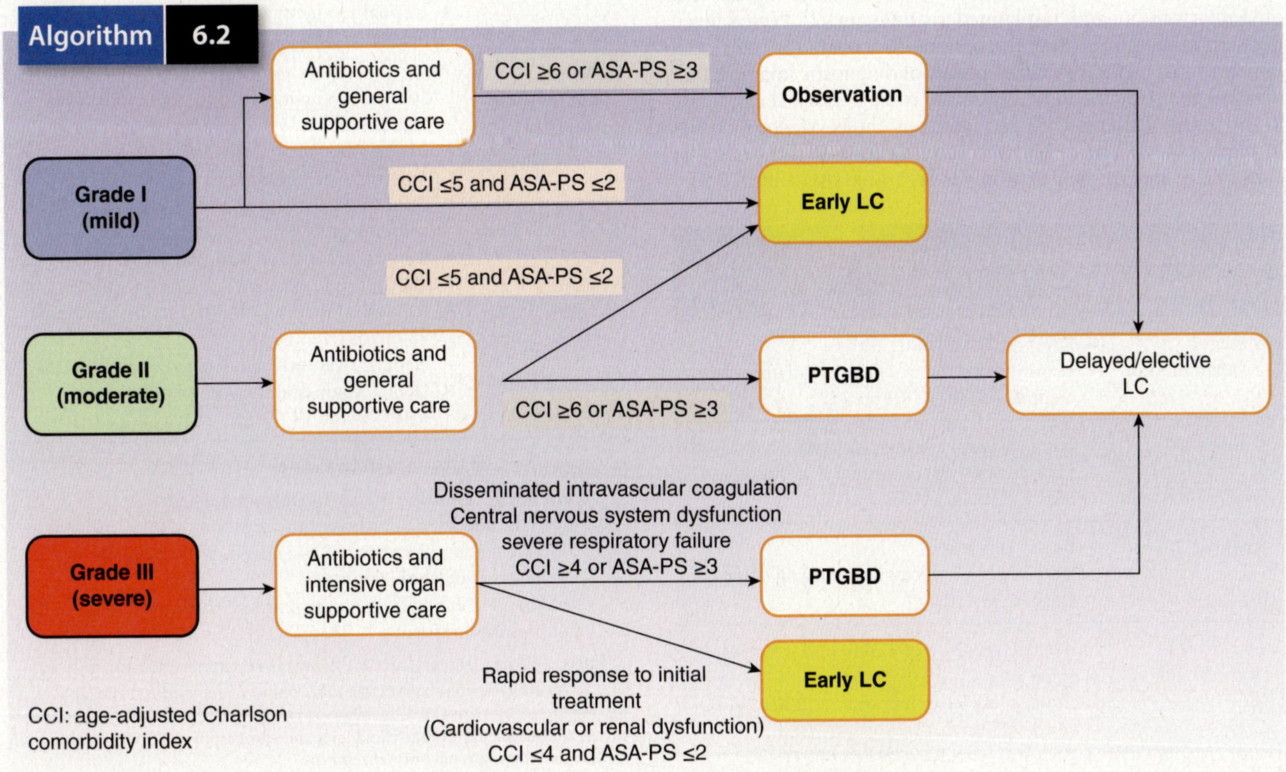

Algorithm 6.2. Simplified TG18 flowchart for the management of AC. All patients managed in a single flowchart based on the severity of AC grades and their comorbidities. LC, laparoscopic cholecystectomy; CCI, Charlson comorbidity index; ASA-PS, American Society of Anesthesiologists Physical Status classification system, PTGBD, Percutaneous transhepatic gallbladder drainage.

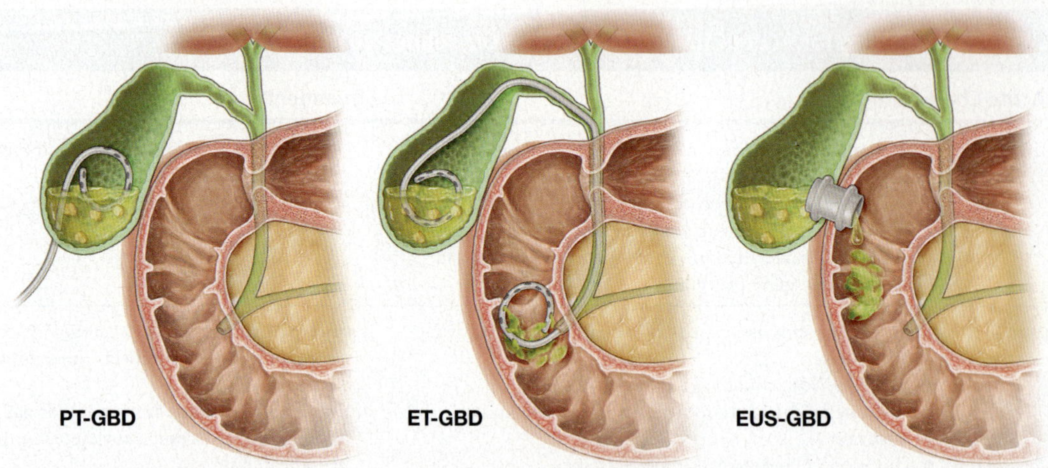

Figure 6.1. For patients with acute cholecystitis who are not candidates for cholecystectomy related to comorbidities or surgical risk, three non-surgical options for treatment are available: (1) percutaneous cholecystostomy tube (PT-GBD), (2) endoscopic transpapillary drainage (ET-GBD), and (3) endoscopic ultrasound-guided gallbladder drainage (EUS-GBD).

and (3) endoscopic ultrasound-guided gallbladder drainage (EUS-GBD) (**Fig. 6.1**). The DRAC-1 Trial[30] randomized 80 very high–risk surgical patients to percutaneous cholecystostomy tube or EUS-GBD and reported that EUS-GBD significantly reduced 1-year adverse events (25.6% vs 31 77.5%, $P < .001$), 30-day adverse events (12.8% vs 47.5%, $P = .010$), reinterventions after 30 days (2.6% vs 30%, $P = .001$), number of unplanned readmissions (15.4% vs 50%, $P = .002$), and recurrent cholecystitis (2.6% vs 20%, $P = .029$). The DRAC-1 Trial criteria definition of high risk for cholecystectomy included one of the following: Age ≥80 years old, ASA Grade 3 or higher, age-adjusted Charlson Comorbidity Index >5, or Karnofsky score <50.

In a systematic review and network meta-analysis (10 studies, $n = 1267$), EUS-GBD had the lowest risk of recurrent cholecystitis and percutaneous cholecystostomy had the highest risk of reintervention and unplanned readmissions.[31] Personalized decision making regarding the optimal procedure for individual patients must include a careful review of diagnostic imaging, and whether the patient can be optimized to be a surgical candidate in the future. Patients with percutaneous cholecystostomy tubes in place can also be considered for transition to EUS-GBD or endobiliary stent if their anatomy is favorable (**Algorithm 6.3**).

Table 6.6. Diagnosis of Cholangitis: Tokyo Guidelines 2018

Systemic inflammation	▪ Fever and/or shaking chills ▪ Laboratory data: evidence of inflammatory response (WBC, CRP, etc.)
Cholestasis	▪ Jaundice (total bilirubin ≥2 mg/dL) ▪ Laboratory data: abnormal liver function tests (ALP, GGT, AST, and ALT)
Imaging	▪ Biliary dilatation ▪ Evidence of the etiology on imaging (stricture, stone, stent, etc.)
Diagnosis of cholangitis	Suspected: presence of 1 item in A + 1 item in either B or C Definite: presence of 1 item in A, 1 item in B, and 1 item in C

ALP, alkaline phosphatase; ALT, alanine transaminase; AST, aspartate aminotransferase/aspartate transaminase; CRP, C-reactive protein; GGT, γ-glutamyl transferase; WBC, white blood cell.

Adapted from Kiriyama S, Kozaka K, Takada T, et al. Tokyo Guidelines 2018: diagnostic criteria and severity grading of acute cholangitis (with videos). *J Hepatobiliary Pancreat Sci*. 2018;25:17–30.

Table 6.7. Treatment of Acute Cholangitis by Severity Classification: Tokyo Guidelines 2018 Criteria

Severity of Acute Cholangitis

Mild (grade I)	Does not meet the criteria of "severe" or "moderate" acute cholangitis at time of initial diagnosis
Moderate (grade II)	Acute cholangitis associated with any two of the following conditions: ▪ Abnormal WBC (>12,000, <4000/mm³) ▪ High fever (≥39 °C) ▪ Age ≥75 y ▪ Hyperbilirubinemia (total bilirubin ≥5 mg/dL) ▪ Hypoalbuminemia (<lower limit of normal × 0.7)
Severe (grade III)	Acute cholangitis associated with the onset of dysfunction in at least one of the following organs/systems: ▪ Cardiovascular dysfunction (hypotension requiring vasopressors) ▪ Neurologic dysfunction (disturbance of consciousness) ▪ Respiratory dysfunction (PaO_2/FiO_2 ratio <300) ▪ Renal dysfunction (oliguria, serum creatinine >2 mg/dL) ▪ Hepatic dysfunction (elevated PT/INR >1.5) ▪ Hematologic dysfunction (platelet count <100,000/mm³)

Assessment of Urgency of Draining

Urgent biliary drainage (<24 h) is indicated when:

a. severe (grade III) acute cholangitis is present.
b. obstructive biliary stones are associated with severe or moderate acute cholangitis.
c. mild acute cholangitis is not responding to IV antibiotics and fluid resuscitation.

Early (but not urgent) ERCP (<72 h) is recommended for patients with mild acute cholangitis who respond to medical therapy.

ERCP, endoscopic retrograde cholangiopancreatography; PT/INR, prothrombin time and international normalized ratio.

Adapted from Kiriyama S, Kozaka K, Takada T, et al. Tokyo Guidelines 2018: diagnostic criteria and severity grading of acute cholangitis (with videos). *J Hepatobiliary Pancreat Sci*. 2018;25:17–30.

From Miura F, Okamoto K, Takada T, et al. Tokyo Guidelines 2018: initial management of acute biliary infection and flowchart for acute cholangitis. *J Hepatobiliary Pancreat Sci*. 2018;25:31–40.

Algorithm 6.3

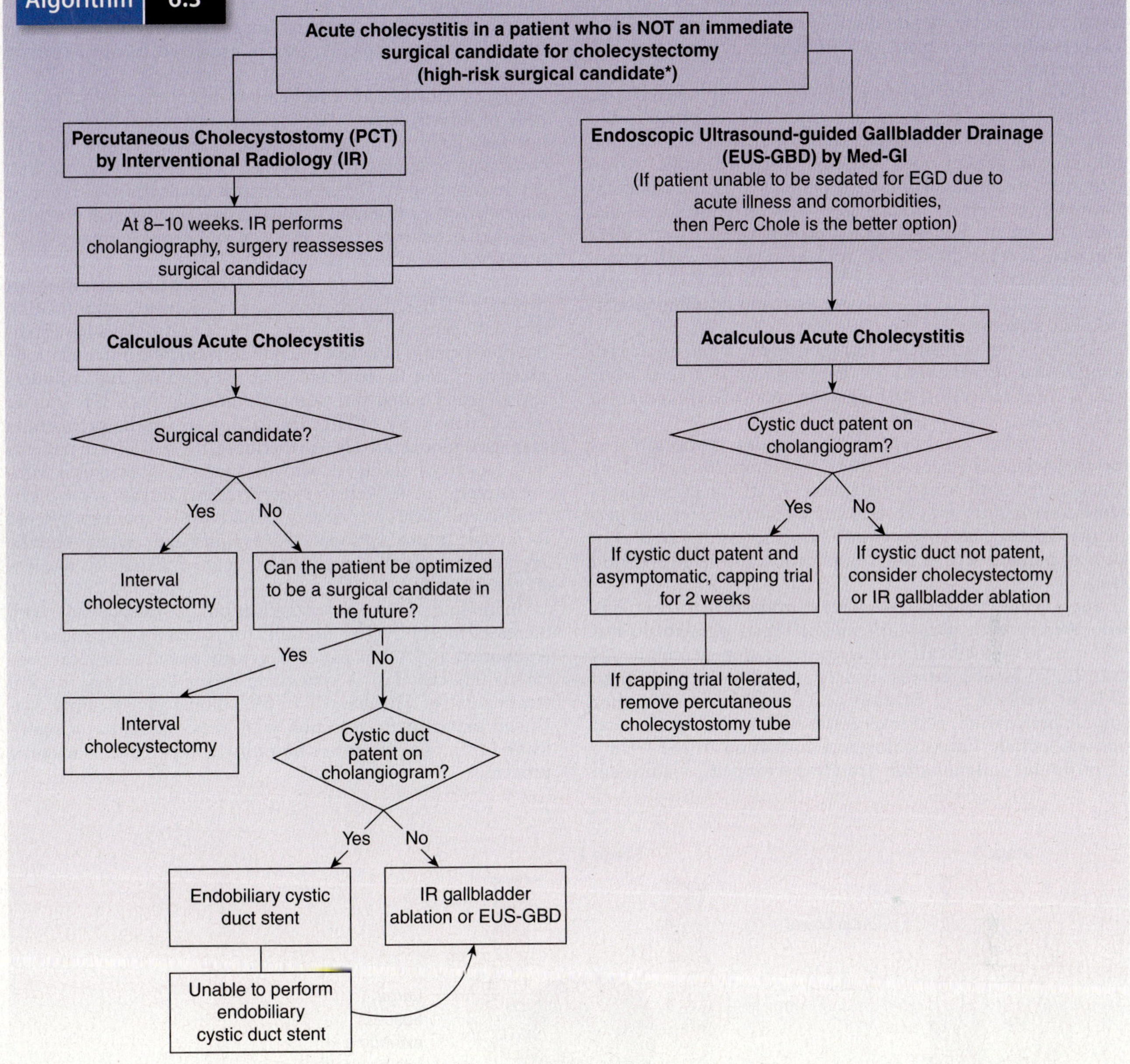

Algorithm 6.3. Nonsurgical management of acute cholecystitis. Management algorithm for patients older than 65 years with acute diverticulitis.[37]

Cholangitis

Cholangitis signs/symptoms include jaundice, fever, right upper quadrant tenderness, hyperbilirubinemia, and leukocytosis. Ultrasound confirms common bile duct dilation (>7 mm). Acute cholangitis has long been diagnosed on the basis of clinical signs of Charcot triad (jaundice, fever, right upper quadrant abdominal pain), which provides highly specific diagnostic criteria, but very low sensitivity (about 26%). Initial treatment includes IV antibiotics, fluid resuscitation, and analgesia, with fasting to enable emergency drainage if indicated. Appropriate evidence-based recommendations for diagnosis and treatment from the Tokyo Guidelines are provided in **Tables 6.6** and **6.7**.[32,33] For treatment recommendations, urgent biliary drainage (<24 hours) is indicated in severe cholangitis or when (1) obstructive biliary stones are associated with moderate–acute cholangitis or (2) mild–acute cholangitis is not responding to IV antibiotics and fluid resuscitation.

For patients with biliary infections, specific evidence-based guideline recommendations for antimicrobial treatment are based on specific patient populations. For patients undergoing cholecystectomy for acute cholecystitis with complete source control (ie, complete cholecystectomy), antimicrobial therapy should be discontinued within 24 hours of the operation, unless there is evidence of infection outside the wall of the gallbladder. For patients with gallbladder perforation or pericholecystic abscess, antimicrobial treatment should be continued until signs and symptoms of infection are resolved (normal white blood cell [WBC] count, no fever, abdominal findings resolved). For acute cholangitis, antimicrobial therapy should be continued for 4 to 7 days after source control is obtained.[34] See also Chapter 58: Calculous Biliary Disease.

Diverticulitis

Diverticulitis is a common intra-abdominal infection. Its pathophysiology is associated with altered gut motility, increased luminal pressure, and an altered colonic microenvironment. CT imaging with enteral and IV contrast is recommended to confirm the diagnosis. *Uncomplicated diverticulitis* involves thickening of the colon wall and pericolonic inflammatory changes. *Complicated diverticulitis* also includes the presence of abscess, peritonitis, obstruction, stricture, and/or fistula. Only 12% of patients with diverticulitis present with complicated disease.

Although antibiotics were previously recommended as first-line therapy for acute uncomplicated diverticulitis, a systematic review of 9 studies (2505 patients) reported no difference in patient outcomes comparing antibiotics to no antibiotics in immunocompetent patients with mild uncomplicated diverticulitis.[35] Guidelines[36] now recommend selected antibiotic use in patients with uncomplicated diverticulitis who have comorbidities or are frail, who present with refractory symptoms or vomiting, or who have a CRP >140 mg/L or WBC count $>15 \times 10^9$ cells per liter, and in immunocompromised patients.

Antibiotic treatment is recommended in patients with *complicated diverticulitis* or *uncomplicated diverticulitis* with a fluid collection or longer segment of inflammation on CT scan.

Antimicrobial treatment of diverticulitis is the same as for cIAI which is reviewed above. Antibiotic therapy alone is associated with a very high success rate for complicated acute diverticulitis with abscess size <4 cm diameter, and percutaneous drainage of abscesses >4 cm successfully resolve in 80% of patients with a low complication and reintervention rate.

Surgery for acute diverticulitis is indicated for patients who present with peritonitis and/or sepsis or who do not improve with medical management and/or percutaneous drainage of associated abscess/infection. Although less than 25% of patients will develop generalized peritonitis after colonic perforation, it is severe with high mortality. Surgical options include simple colostomy formation in the setting of profound inflammation (rarely performed), traditional sigmoid resection with colostomy (Hartmann procedure), and sigmoid resection with a primary colocolonic or colorectal anastomosis with or without a diverting loop ileostomy. Laparoscopic surgery is preferred to open surgery when possible.

Since recurrence after recovery from an uncomplicated episode of diverticulitis is rare and two or more recurrences are not associated with increased risk of complications, elective colectomy following two episodes of diverticulitis is no longer recommended. Decisions regarding surgical intervention and colectomy must therefore be based on individual potential risks and benefits of colon resection and patient-oriented goals of care.

Hinchey proposed a practical clinical classification of diverticulitis based on the severity of peritoneal contamination (**Fig. 6.2**) identified at operation.[37] The modified Hinchey classification includes Hinchey Ia (confined pericolic inflammation–phlegmon) and Ib (confined pericolic abscess), and considers classification based on radiologic imaging with CT scan as well. The majority of Hinchey Ib–II cases can be successfully managed nonoperatively. Furthermore, the majority of patients with Hinchey I–II disease who are successfully managed without surgery are unlikely to experience any further acute diverticulitis and therefore, surgery should not be routinely offered to avoid future episodes. A personalized patient-specific approach for elective surgery after acute diverticulitis resolves should be used.

Increasing Hinchey classification is associated with increased mortality. The mortality for patients with Hinchey III is reported as 6% but increases greatly to 35% for fecal peritonitis (Hinchey IV). A systematic review comparing surgical treatments for Hinchey III or IV colonic diverticulitis confirmed that primary resection with anastomosis has a significant advantage with lower mortality compared to Hartmann procedure.

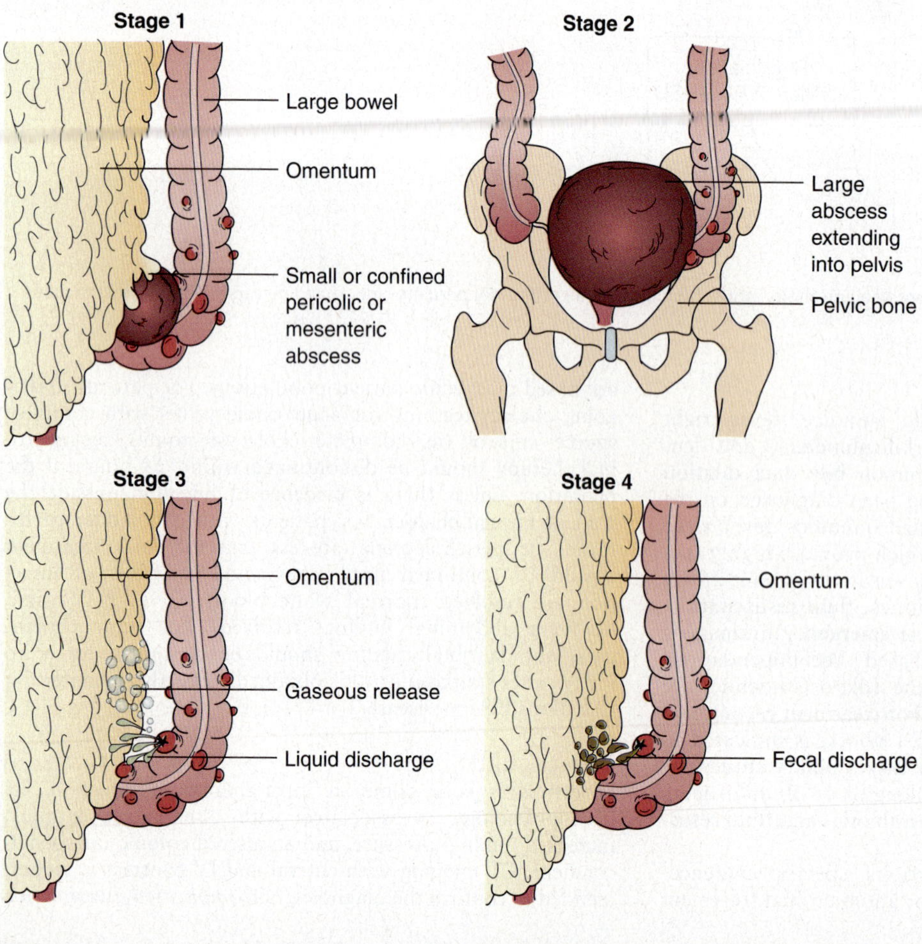

Figure 6.2. Hinchey classification scheme. Patients with stage 1 disease have small, confined, pericolic, or mesenteric abscesses, whereas those with stage 2 disease have larger abscesses, often confined to the pelvis. Stage 3 disease, or perforated diverticulitis, is present when a peridiverticular abscess has ruptured and caused purulent peritonitis. Rupture of an uninflamed and unobstructed diverticulum into the free peritoneal cavity with fetal contamination, the so-called free rupture, signifies stage 4 disease and carries the highest risk of an adverse outcome.

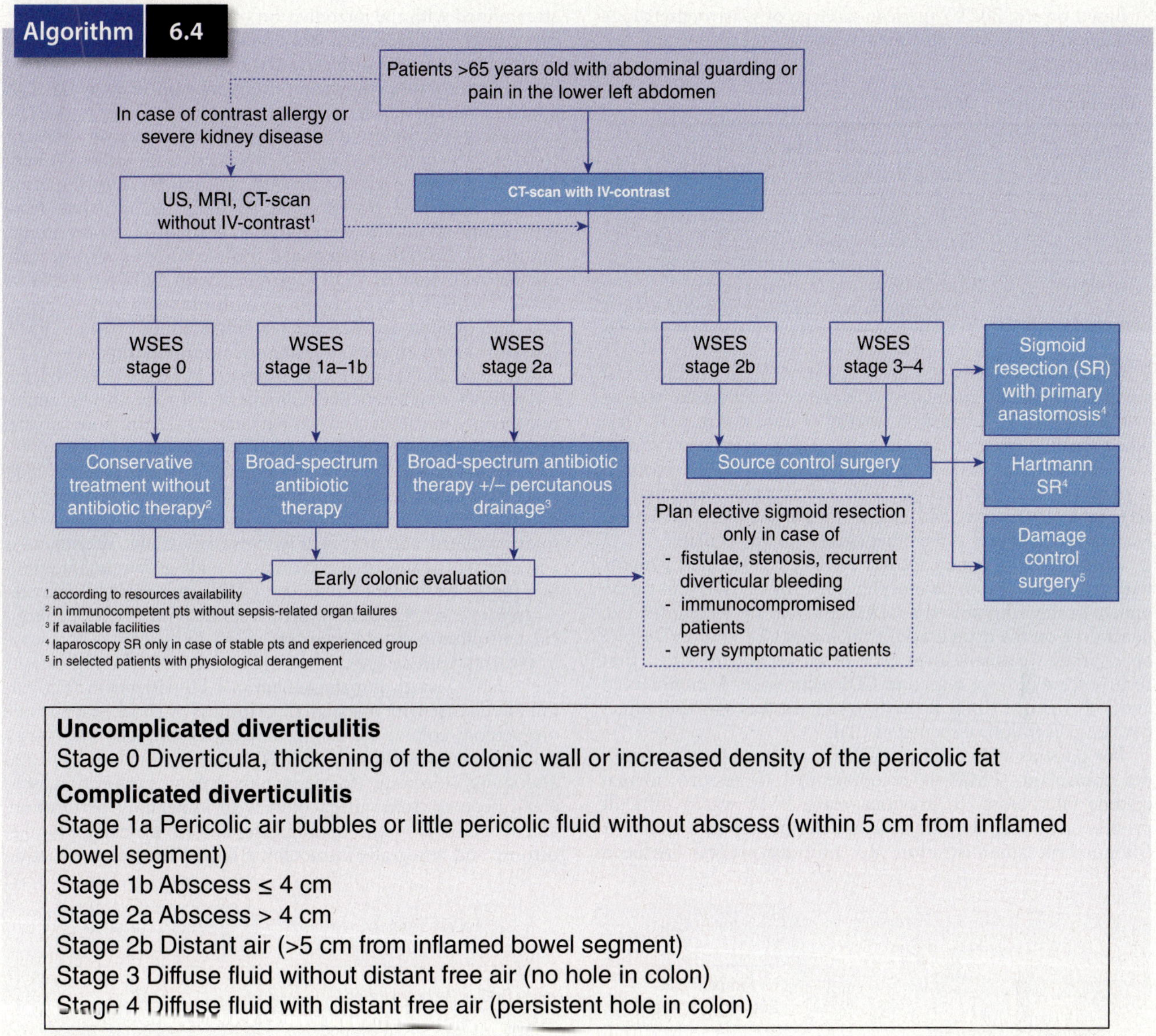

Algorithm 6.4. Acute- and late-phase management of patients with pancreatic necrosis. (Adapted from Baron TH, DiMaio CJ, Wang AY, Morgan KA. American Gastroenterological Association Clinical Practice Update: management of pancreatic necrosis. *Gastroenterology*. 2020;158(1):67–75.e1.)

The American Society of Colon and Rectal Surgeons Clinical Practice Guidelines[38] recommend the following for the treatment of left-sided colonic diverticulitis (**Algorithm 6.4**)

- Percutaneous drainage for abscess >3 cm in size (1B)
- Recommend elective surgery after complicated disease (eg, abscess, fistula, stricture, 1B)
- Colonoscopic evaluation to confirm diagnosis (0.7% to 11% risk of malignancy, 1C)
- Individualized decision for surgery in uncomplicated disease based on risk (1B)
- Urgent surgery if peritonitis or failure of medical treatment (15% to 30% of patients, 1C)
- Surgery not recommended just for young age at index presentation (1C)
- Laparoscopic lavage not recommended (1A)
- Complete sigmoid resection down to rectum for sigmoid diverticulitis (1C)
- Anastomosis (1B) and laparoscopic approach (1A) preferred if possible and safe

See also Chapter 66: Diverticular Disease.

Clostridioides Difficile Infection and Colitis

The incidence and severity of clostridioides difficile infection (CDI) has increased, particularly in surgical patients who have been exposed to prior antimicrobial therapy. There has been a substantial change in the management of CDI related to the emergence of the NAP1/BI/027 strain which is associated with higher toxin production and more severe forms of disease. CDI may be associated with mild-to-moderate diarrhea or colonic ileus and obstipation to severe colitis.[39]

Early diagnosis of CDI is imperative. Recommended testing includes two steps, using a glutamine dehydrogenase assay for the *Clostridium difficile* antigen, followed by enzyme immunoassay toxin testing. Polymerase chain reaction (PCR) confirmatory testing is used if the antigen is positive and toxin is negative. Radiologic testing is helpful, and CT may show colonic mucosal edema (thumbprinting or target sign), ascites, inflammation, and fat stranding and the "accordion sign" which indicates alternating edematous colonic haustra separated by transverse mucosal ridges filled with enteral contrast.

Based on the 2021 American College of Gastroenterology guidelines, CDI is now classified as nonsevere, severe, and fulminant disease:

Classification	Definition
Nonsevere	Leukocytosis with a WBC <15,000 cells/mL and a serum creatinine level ≤1.5 mg/dL
Severe	Leukocytosis with a WBC ≥15,000 cells/mL and a serum creatinine level >1.5 mg/dL
Fulminant	Criteria for severe infection, plus hypotension or shock, ileus or megacolon

Initial management of CDI is cessation of all antibiotics, if possible. National guidelines[40,41] have evidence-based recommendations for CDI based on severity of disease (**Fig. 6.3**). Oral fidaxomicin (a macrocyclic antibiotic with a narrow antimicrobial spectrum against *C. difficile*, staphylococci, and enterococci) is preferred first-line therapy, with vancomycin considered an acceptable alternative, and enteral metronidazole is no longer recommended except if the other agents are not available.

Recurrent CDI occurs in over 25% of CDI-treated patients within 30 days. When patients have recurrent CDI, oral fidaxomicin or tapering/pulsed dose vancomycin are recommended, depending on the drug used for the initial CDI course. Despite appropriate treatment, over 50% of these patients with a first recurrence will have a second CDI recurrence. A monoclonal antibody against toxin B (bezlotoxumab) was safe and effective for prevention of recurrent CDI.[42]

7 For patients with multiple CDI recurrences, fecal microbiota transplant (FMT) is recommended to restore normal colonic microbiota. In previous years, FMT was a difficult process, including identification of a donor and nasojejunal or colonoscopic administration. Recently, the process has been streamlined with the introduction of standardized frozen samples from commercialized stool banks. Frozen samples are just as effective as fresh samples, and the thawed prepackaged 150-mL live microbiota suspension (Rebyota, approved by US FDA 11/2022) can be administered by rectal enema[39] rather than by colonoscopy or nasojejunal routes. The efficacy and safety of Rebyota was confirmed in five prospective clinical trials with more than 1000 patients enrolled. An oral FMT formulation (Vowst, approved by US FDA 4/2023) includes live fecal microbiota spores to reestablish a normal gut microbiome, and the ECOSPOR randomized trials confirmed significantly greater reduction in CDI recurrence with VOWST (88% vs 60%).[43] FMT has been shown in multiple trials to have a success rate of 60% to 90% after a single administration. FMT has also shown efficacy in immunocompromised patients.

National clinical guidelines suggest FMT also be considered for patients with severe and fulminant CDI refractory to antibiotic therapy, in particular when patients are deemed poor surgical candidates (strong recommendation, low quality of evidence).[44,45] This is based on a recent meta-analysis which reported that FMT resulted in resolution of severe/fulminant CDI in 88% of patients.[46] These data confirm that this disease is pathogen- and toxin mediated, and treatment with normal colonic microbiota is very effective treatment. Based on these findings, surgical intervention for the treatment of fulminant CDI has markedly decreased.

In rare cases, CDI may warrant surgical intervention. Surgical consultation should occur very early in the course of disease in patients with severe and complicated CDI. The indications for potential surgical management of CDI patients include fulminant disease with associated peritonitis or shock states, toxic megacolon, colonic ischemia, or perforation. The two surgical procedures indicated for CDI treatment include (1) total abdominal colectomy (for peritonitis, colonic perforation, ischemia, necrosis, toxic megacolon with impending perforation, and septic shock with organ failure) and (2) diverting loop ileostomy and antegrade intracolonic lavage for toxin reduction

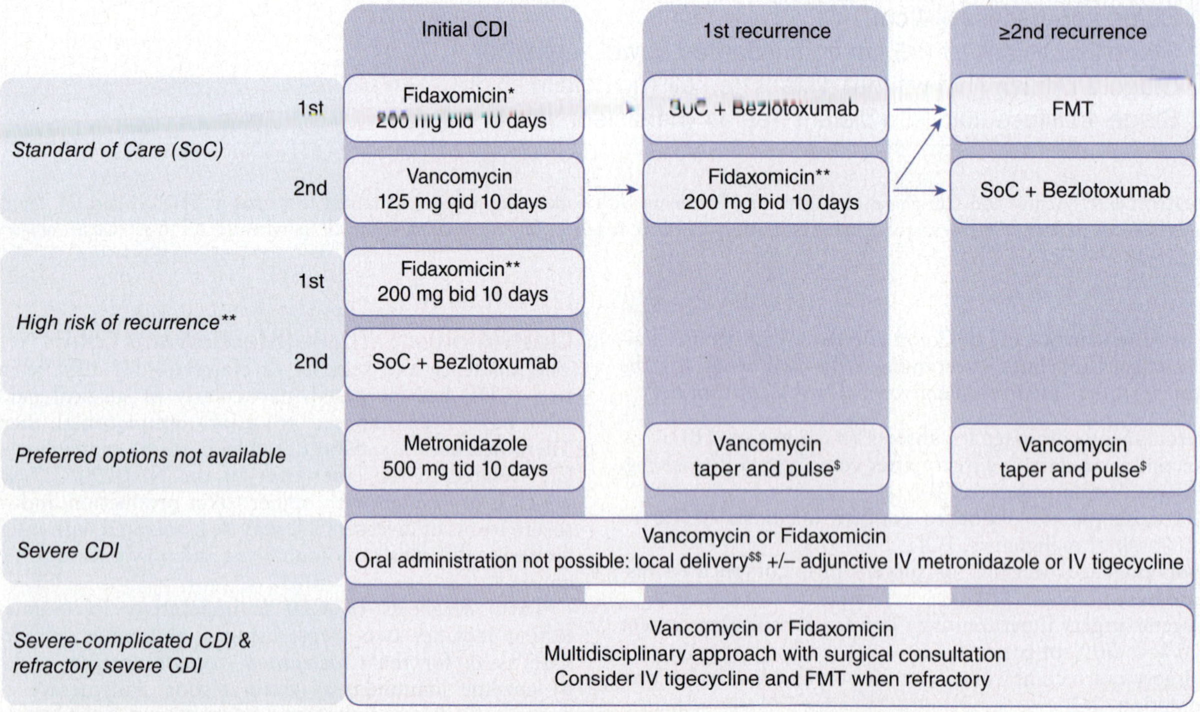

* Risk stratification for risk of recurrence may be applied for selective use of fidaxomicin in case of limited access or resources.

** Consider extended fidaxomicin: 200 mg bid on day 1–5, 200 mg q48h on day 7–25. Most important risk factor for recurrence is age >65–70 years. Additional risk factor(s) to consider are healthcare-associated CDI, prior hospitalizations ≤ 3 months, prior COI episode, continued non-CDI antibiotic use, and PPI therapy started during/after CDI diagnosis. The risk of recurrence is assumed higher with more risk factors present.

$ Vancomycin taper and pulse: 2 weeks 125 mg qid, followed by 1 week 125 mg bid, then 1 week 125 mg qd, then 1 week 125 mg q48h, and finally 125 mg q72h for 1 week.

$$ Rectal or nasoduodenal delivery

Figure 6.3. Current guidelines for treatment of *Clostridioides difficile* infection in adults. (Adapted from van Prehn J, Reigadas E, Vogelzang EH, et al; Guideline Committee of the European Study Group on Clostridioides difficile. European Society of Clinical Microbiology and Infectious Diseases: 2021 update on the treatment guidance document for Clostridioides difficile infection in adults. *Clin Microbiol Infect*. 2021;27(Suppl 2):S1–S21.)

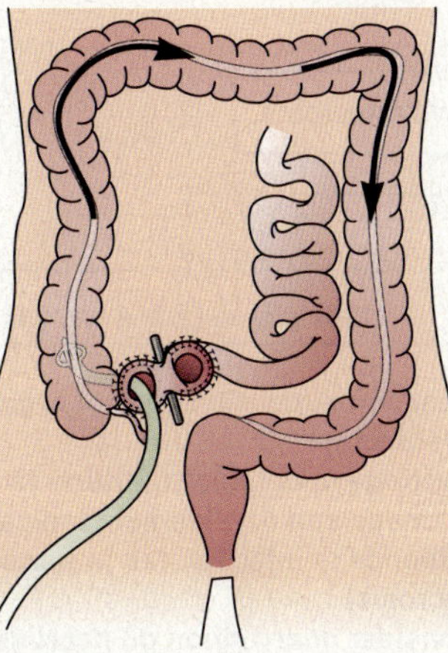

Figure 6.4. Diverting loop ileostomy with antegrade colonic irrigation for CDI. Before surgery is started:

1. Place the patient in lithotomy position with easy access to rectum.
2. Place a fluid collection bag (commonly used by urology) under the patient's rectum for drainage collection.
3. Place a rectal drainage tube (large Malecot catheter, large Foley catheter, #9 or #10 endotracheal tube, or other large catheter).
4. Have 8 L of warmed polyethylene glycol 3350/electrolyte solution (GoLYTELY; Braintree Laboratories) available in OR for intraoperative colonic irrigation, and dulcolax suppository.

Intraoperatively:

1. Ensure that the colon is viable and without perforation.
2. Create a loop ileostomy (laparoscopic or open).
3. Place a 24-Fr Malecot catheter into the efferent limb of the ileostomy and advance into the right colon through the ileocecal valve. Secure to skin with sutures.
4. Infuse 8 L of warmed polyethylene glycol 3350/electrolyte solution (GoLytely; Braintree Laboratories) into the 24-Fr Malecot catheter via the efferent limb of the ileostomy.
5. Once colonic lavage is completed, perform rectal examination to empty rectum, place dulcolax suppository in rectum to encourage colonic emptying.
6. Instill antegrade colonic enema with vancomycin (500 mg in 500 mL) via ileostomy efferent limb, continue postoperatively.

(Adapted from Neal MD, Alverdy JC, Hall DE, et al. Diverting loop ileostomy and colonic lavage: an alternative to total abdominal colectomy for the treatment of severe, complicated Clostridium difficile associated disease. *Ann Surg*. 2011;254:423–427; discussion 427–429.)

while preserving the colon (**Fig. 6.4**). A systematic review (3683 patients, 5 studies) of diverting loop ileostomy (20%) versus total abdominal colectomy (80%) for CDI[42] reported no difference in overall mortality rates (30%). No randomized studies have been published to date comparing these two options. The Surgical Infection Society Guidelines recommend that total abdominal colectomy be the procedure of choice for definitive therapy of fulminant nonperforated CDI, with colon preservation recommended in select patients with lower-severity disease, decreased comorbidities, and patient preference.[47]

Pancreatitis

Classification of acute pancreatitis is based on local disease (whether pancreatic necrosis is present or not, whether it is sterile or infected) and systemic determinants (whether organ failure is present or not, whether it is transient or persistent) of severity (**Fig. 6.5**). Early management requires goal-directed fluid resuscitation (with avoidance of overresuscitation and abdominal compartment syndrome), assessment of severity of pancreatitis, diagnostic CT imaging to assess for necrotizing pancreatitis, consideration of endoscopic retrograde cholangiopancreatography (ERCP) for biliary pancreatitis, and early enteral nutrition support. Antibiotic prophylaxis for severe acute or necrotizing pancreatitis is not recommended, as it is an inflammatory disorder initially.

Early aggressive fluid resuscitation was previously recommended for the management of acute pancreatitis to attempt to avoid transition to necrotizing pancreatitis. The WATERFALL (Early weight-based aggressive vs nonaggressive goal-directed

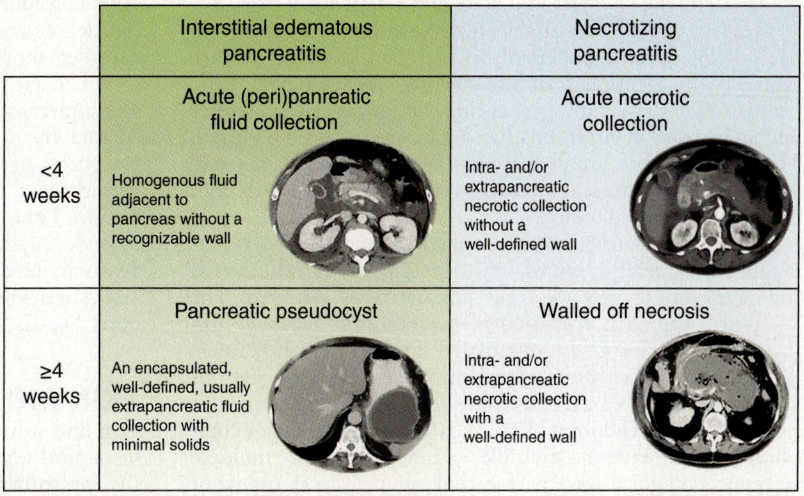

Figure 6.5. Classification of acute pancreatitis and associated fluid collections. Based on international consensus according to the Acute Pancreatitis Classification Working Group (revised Atlanta criteria). From: Trikudanathan G, Wolbrink DRJ, van Santvoort HC, Mallery S, Freeman M, Besselink MG. Current concepts in severe acute and necrotizing pancreatitis: an evidence-based approach. *Gastroenterology*. 2019;156(7):1994–2007.e3.

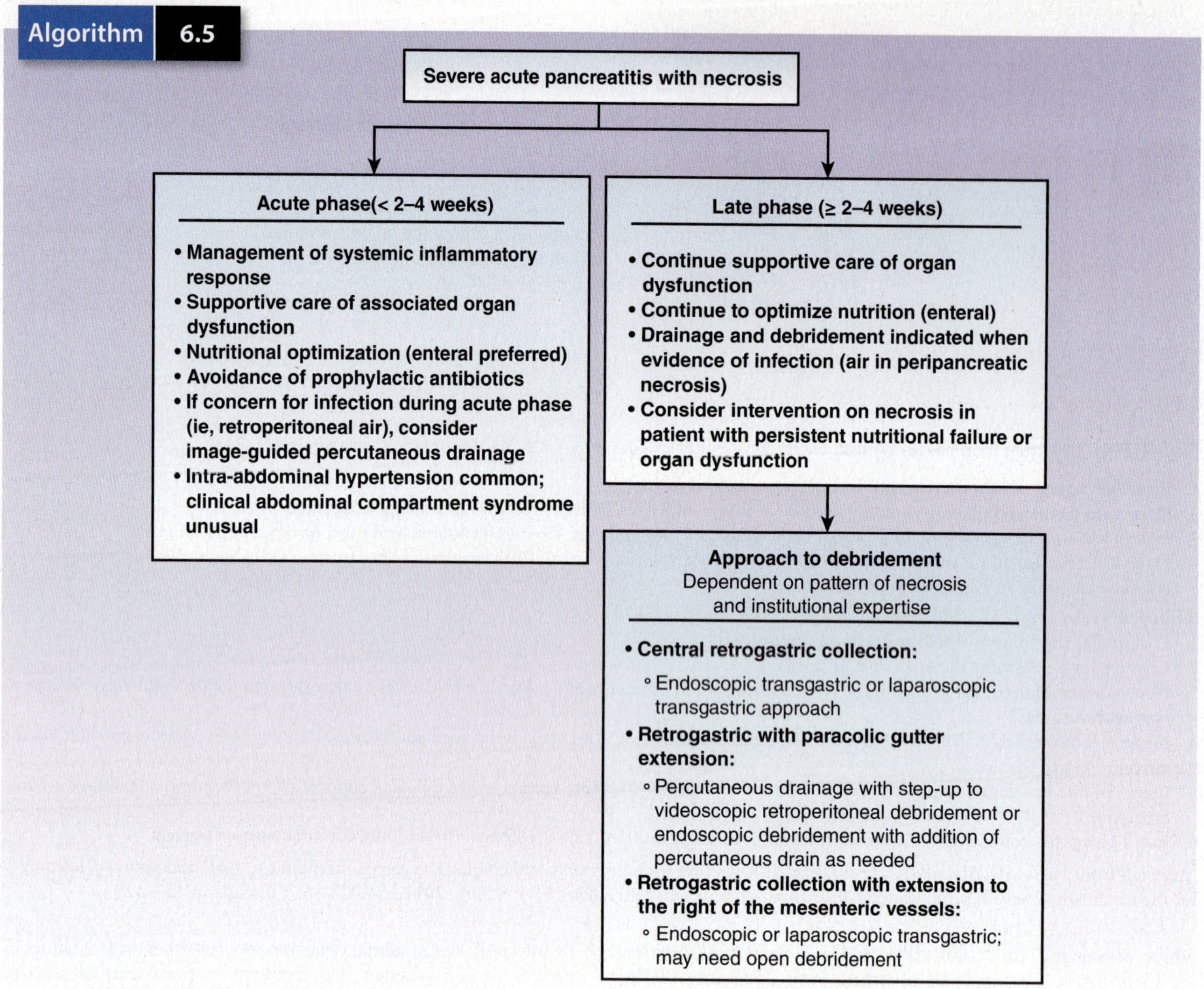

Algorithm 6.5. Algorithm for endoscopic and percutaneous management of walled-off pancreatic necrosis with indications for drainage and debridement (infection, severe symptoms). (Adapted from Baron TH, DiMaio CJ, Wang AY, Morgan KA. American Gastroenterological Association Clinical Practice Update: management of pancreatic necrosis. *Gastroenterology*. 2020;158(1):67–75.e1.)

fluid resuscitation in the early phase of acute pancreatitis) randomized trial confirmed that early aggressive fluid resuscitation did not result in any improvement in clinical outcomes. The trial was halted at the first interim safety analysis due to safety concerns, with development of fluid overload in 20.5% of the patients in the aggressive-resuscitation group (20 mL/kg IV crystalloid bolus and 3 mL/kg/h) versus 6.3% in the moderate-resuscitation group (10 mL/kg IV crystalloid bolus and 1.5 mL/kg/h).[48]

Necrotizing pancreatitis is high risk for progression to necrotizing *infected* pancreatitis. Therapeutic antibiotics are required for treatment of documented infected pancreatic necrosis. Causative pathogens include Gram-negative microbes and an increase in Gram-positive organisms has been reported. Therefore, empiric broad-spectrum IV antimicrobials are recommended with deescalation to pathogen-directed antibiotics once cultures are obtained.

8 The initial treatment of infected pancreatic necrosis is percutaneous catheter or endoscopic (transgastric/transduodenal) drainage with a second drain placement as required. The "step-up" approach consisted of percutaneous drainage followed, if necessary, by minimally invasive retroperitoneal necrosectomy. The minimally invasive step-up approach, as compared with open necrosectomy, reduced the rate of the primary composite endpoint (12% vs 50%, including major complications [new-onset multiple organ failure or multiple systemic complications, perforation of a visceral organ or enterocutaneous fistula, or bleeding] or death), but the mortality rate did not differ significantly between groups (19% vs 16%). The long-term follow-up of patients in the PANTER trial confirmed the step-up approach for necrotizing pancreatitis to be superior to open necrosectomy, without increased risk of reinterventions (**Algorithms 6.5 and 6.6**). Lack of clinical improvement after initial percutaneous drainage warrants consideration of minimally invasive techniques for pancreatic necrosectomy including video-assisted retroperitoneal debridement (VARD), minimally invasive retroperitoneal pancreatic necrosectomy (MIRP), or transluminal direct endoscopic necrosectomy (DEN). VARD and MIRP use the tract created by percutaneous drainage catheters as a guide for placement of a laparoscope into the retroperitoneum so that debridement and lavage can be performed under direct visualization. Long-term follow-up studies confirmed no difference to endoscopic versus surgical step-up approach in reducing death/major complications, but the endoscopic approach was associated with fewer pancreatic fistulas and fewer reinterventions. See also Chapter 50: Acute Pancreatitis.

SKIN AND SOFT TISSUE INFECTIONS

Skin and soft tissue infections (SSTIs) span a broad spectrum of clinical entities from limited cellulitis to rapidly progressive necrotizing soft tissue infection (NSTI), which may be

Algorithm 6.6

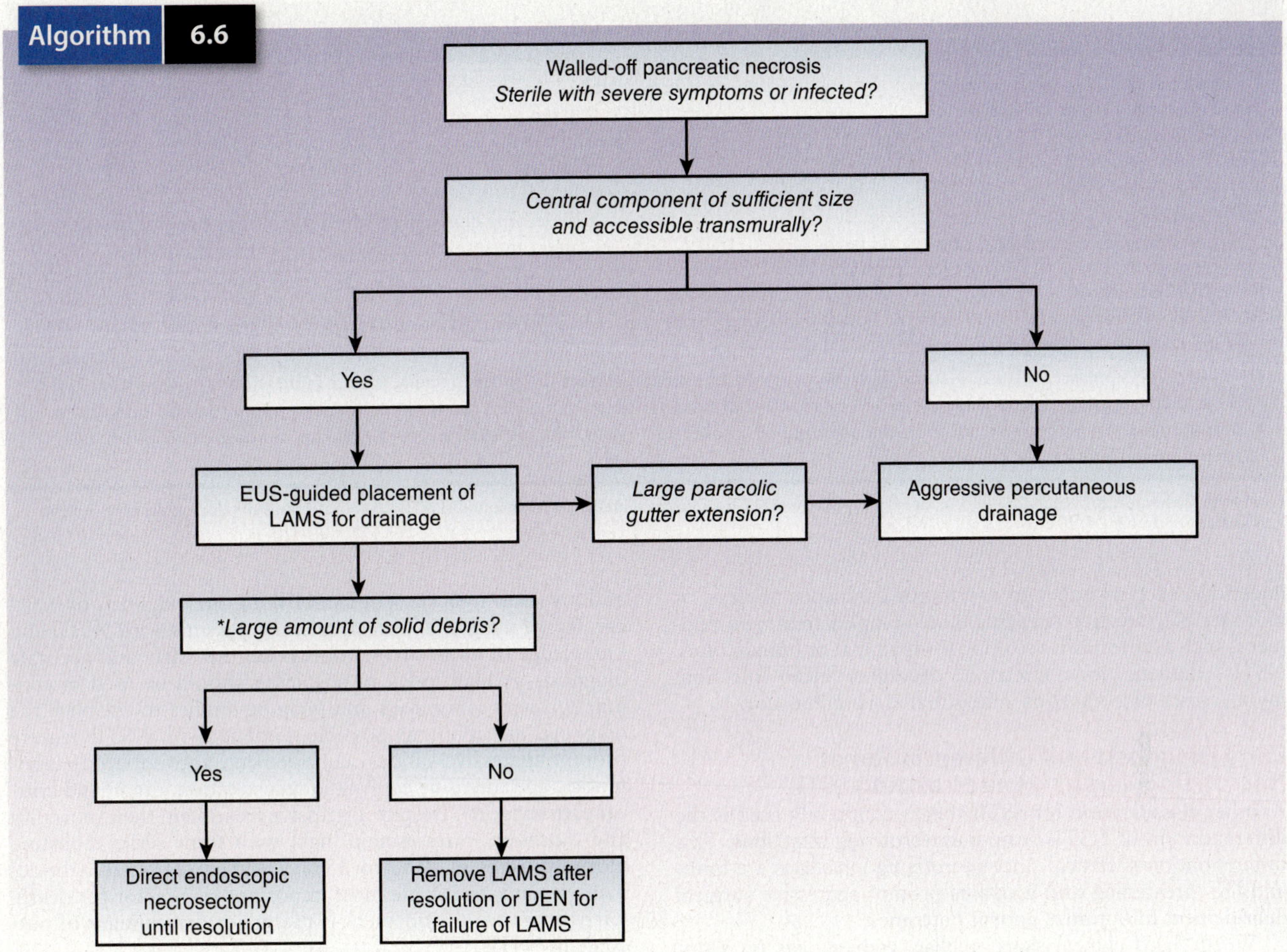

Algorithm 6.6. Flow diagram for approach to endoscopic management of walled-off pancreatic necrosis in a patient with a strong indication for drainage and/or debridement. (Adapted from Baron TH, DiMaio CJ, Wang AY, Morgan KA. American Gastroenterological Association Clinical Practice Update: management of pancreatic necrosis. *Gastroenterology*. 2020;158(1):67–75.e1.)

associated with septic shock or toxic shock syndrome and organ failure.[49] Methicillin-resistant *Staphylococcus aureus* (MRSA) has emerged as a common identifiable cause of severe SSTIs, therefore initiation of empiric anti-MRSA antimicrobials is warranted in all cases of severe SSTIs.

The complex interplay of environment, host, and pathogen is important to consider when evaluating SSTIs and planning therapy. The key to a successful outcome in caring for patients with severe SSTIs is (1) early diagnosis and differentiation of necrotizing versus nonnecrotizing SSTI, (2) early initiation of appropriate empiric broad-spectrum antimicrobial therapy with consideration of risk factors for specific pathogens, (3) "source control," that is, early aggressive surgical intervention for drainage of abscesses and debridement of NSTIs, and (4) pathogen identification and appropriate deescalation of antimicrobial therapy.

Classification of Skin and Soft Tissue Infections

The FDA previously classified SSTIs into two broad categories for the purpose of clinical trials evaluating new antimicrobials for the treatment of SSTIs: **uncomplicated** and **complicated** (**Table 6.8**). **Uncomplicated** SSTIs include superficial infections such as cellulitis, simple abscesses, impetigo, and furuncles. These infections can be treated by antibiotics and/or surgical incision for drainage of abscess alone. In contrast, **complicated** SSTIs include deep soft tissue infections that require significant 9 surgical intervention such as infected ulcers, infected burns, and major abscesses, and these patients also have significant underlying comorbidities, that is, disease states which complicate (and usually delay) response to treatment. Complicated SSTIs are a significant clinical problem, in part, related to the increasing resistance of infecting bacteria to current antibiotic therapies.

Uncomplicated Skin and Soft Tissue Infections

Uncomplicated SSTIs are associated with ***low*** risk for life- or limb-threatening infection. These patients can be treated with empiric antibiotic therapy according to likely pathogen and local resistance patterns.

Complicated Skin and Soft Tissue Infections

Complicated SSTIs are associated with ***high*** risk for life- or limb-threatening infection. In these patients, it is of paramount importance to initiate appropriate and adequate broad-spectrum initial empiric antimicrobial therapy with coverage for MRSA, and to consider the need for surgical intervention for abscess drainage or debridement.

Patients with complicated SSTIs require hospitalization for treatment. Specific circumstances that warrant hospitalization include the presence of tissue necrosis, sepsis, severe pain, altered mental status, immunocompromised state, and organ failure (respiratory, renal, and hepatic). SSTIs can lead to serious, potentially life-threatening local and systemic complications. The infections can progress rapidly, and early recognition and proper medical and surgical management is cornerstone of therapy.

The FDA changed the SSTI terminology and issued final guidance for the treatment of acute bacterial skin and skin structure infections (ABSSSIs). This guidance defined ABSSSI as cellulitis, erysipelas, wound infection, and major cutaneous abscess with the definitions outlined in **Table 6.8**. Unfortunately, this new guidance does not address less serious skin

Table 6.8. Comparison of Old and New Classification of SSTIs by FDA

▪ Uncomplicated ▪ Superficial infections, such as: ▪ simple abscesses ▪ impetiginous lesions ▪ furuncles ▪ cellulitis ▪ Can be treated by antibiotics or surgical incision alone	▪ Complicated ▪ Deep soft tissue, such as: ▪ infected ulcers ▪ infected burns ▪ major abscesses ▪ Significant underlying disease state which complicates response to treatment ▪ Requires significant surgical intervention and antimicrobials

New FDA Definition:

ABSSSI defined as bacterial infection of the skin with a lesion size area of at least 75 cm^2 (lesion size measured by the area of redness, edema, or induration), including the following:

- **Cellulitis/erysipelas:** A diffuse skin infection characterized by spreading areas of redness, edema, and/or induration.
- **Wound infection:** An infection characterized by purulent drainage from a wound with surrounding redness, edema, and/or induration.
- **Major cutaneous abscess:** An infection characterized by a collection of pus within the dermis or deeper that is accompanied by redness, edema, and/or induration.

From https://www.fda.gov/regulatory-information/search-fda-guidance-documents/acute-bacterial-skin-and-skin-structure-infections-developing-drugs-treatment. Accessed September 24, 2020.

infections, such as impetigo and minor cutaneous abscess, or more serious infections needing more complex treatment regimens, such as infections resulting from animal or human bites, NSTIs, diabetic foot infection, decubitus ulcer infection, myonecrosis, osteomyelitis, and ecthyma gangrenosum.

Early Diagnosis and Differentiation of Necrotizing Versus Nonnecrotizing SSTI

Another classification for SSTIs that is commonly used is the differentiation of **NSTIs** from **nonnecrotizing infections**. This differentiation is critical since necrotizing infections are limb- and life threatening and warrants prompt aggressive surgical debridement to optimize patient outcomes.

When "hard clinical signs" (bullae, crepitus, gas on x-ray, hypotension with SBP <90 mm Hg, or skin necrosis) of NSTI are present, establishing the diagnosis of NSTI is not difficult. However, hard signs of NSTIs are often absent on presentation, thus potentially delaying diagnosis and surgical intervention. CT imaging can be helpful, with a negative predictive value of 100% and a positive predictive value of 76% in diagnosing NSTI. If there is any question regarding the possible diagnosis of an NSTI, it is imperative to proceed with prompt surgical intervention and to be certain that the surgical incision is continued down to the fascial and muscle level to make a definitive diagnosis.

Early Initiation of Appropriate Empiric Broad-Spectrum Antimicrobial Therapy With Anti-MRSA Coverage and Consideration of Risk Factors for Specific Pathogens

Antimicrobial therapy is an essential element in the management of severe SSTIs. As in all serious life-threatening infections, it is important to initiate **early** and **appropriate** empiric antimicrobial therapy and include empiric coverage for MRSA in all patients with complicated or severe SSTIs.[50] It is well established that prompt appropriate treatment of hospitalized infections reduces mortality. Cultures should be obtained with any drainage or surgical procedure to determine the causative pathogens and adjust antimicrobial treatment. If patients have had prior SSTIs, it is mandatory to review any prior culture results, as that will assist in guidance of appropriate empiric antimicrobial therapy. This is particularly common in patients with recurrent MRSA SSTIs. Specific risk factors for other causative pathogens should also be considered when initiating empiric antibiotics for SSTIs. In patients with possible NSTI, empiric antitoxin antimicrobials should also be initiated (clindamycin, linezolid).

Necrotizing Soft Tissue Infections (NSTIs)

NSTIs are aggressive soft tissue infections that cause widespread necrosis, and can include necrotizing cellulitis, fasciitis, and myositis/myonecrosis. Establishing the diagnosis of NSTI can be the main challenge in treating patients with NSTI, and knowledge of all available tools is key for early and accurate diagnosis. A high index of suspicion should be used in conjunction with laboratory and imaging studies to establish the diagnosis as rapidly as possible. Patients with NSTIs require prompt aggressive surgical debridement, appropriate IV antibiotics, and intensive care (fluid resuscitation, organ and critical care support). Despite aggressive treatment, their mortality and morbidity rates remain high, with some series reporting mortality rates of 25% to 35%. Delayed definitive debridement remains the single most important risk factor for death.
10 Early operative debridement is the major determinant of outcome in NSTIs.

The laboratory risk indicator for necrotizing fasciitis (LRINEC) score is a diagnostic scoring system for distinguishing NSTIs from other severe soft tissue infections based on laboratory tests routinely performed for the evaluation of severe SSTIs (**Table 6.9**). The cutoff value for the LRINEC score was 6 points with a positive predictive value of 92% and negative predictive value of 96%. Patients with a LRINEC score of ≥6 should be carefully evaluated for NSTI.

Diagnostic Imaging in Necrotizing Soft Tissue Infections

NSTIs necessitate prompt aggressive surgical debridement for satisfactory treatment in addition to antimicrobial therapy. Because of the rapidly progressive and potentially fatal outcome of this condition, if imaging cannot be performed expeditiously, delaying treatment is not justified. Plain film findings may reveal extensive soft tissue gas. CT imaging can reveal asymmetric thickening of deep fascia in association with gas, and associated abscesses may also be present. MR imaging can also assist in the diagnosis of NSTIs. MR imaging has been documented to effectively differentiate between necrotizing and nonnecrotizing infections of the lower extremity and other areas of the body, but should not delay prompt surgical intervention in NSTIs management.

Microbiology of Necrotizing Soft Tissue Infections

Necrotizing fasciitis and myonecrosis are typically caused by infection with *group A streptococcus (GAS)*, *Clostridium perfringens*, or, most commonly, aerobic and anaerobic organisms as part of a polymicrobial infection that may include *S. aureus*. MRSA has recently been described as a predominant monomicrobial cause of necrotizing fasciitis. A retrospective review of patients presenting with necrotizing fasciitis indicated that MRSA was the most common pathogen, accounting for one-third of the organisms isolated.

Table 6.9. The Laboratory Risk Indicator for Necrotizing Fasciitis (LRINEC) Score

Variable, Units	Score
C-reactive protein, mg/L	
<150	0
≥150	4
Total white cell count, per mm^3	
<15	0
15–25	1
>25	2
Hemoglobin, g/dL	
>13.5	0
11–13.5	1
<11	2
Sodium, mmol/L	
≥135	0
≤135	2
Creatinine, μmol/L	
≤141	0
>141	2
Glucose, mmol/L	
≤10	0
>10	1

The maximum score is 13; a score ≥6 should raise the suspicion of necrotizing fasciitis and a score of ≥8 is strongly predictive of this disease.

NSTIs have been classified into two types, either polymicrobial (**type I**) or monomicrobial (**type II**). Polymicrobial infections are more common, due to both aerobic and anaerobic organisms, and commonly occur in the trunk and perineum. NSTIs that are monomicrobial in origin commonly occur in the limbs and are typically caused by infection with GAS, *C. perfringens*, or *S. aureus*. Increasingly, MRSA has been identified as the causative microbe in NSTIs, but a separate category for this NSTI does not currently exist. Given this finding, anti-MRSA empiric antimicrobial therapy should be initiated in all patients with NSTIs and pathogen-directed antimicrobial therapy should be considered once tissue culture results are available.

Uncommon microbiologic causes of NSTIs and primary sepsis include *Vibrio* and *Aeromonas* species, virulent Gram-negative bacteria, and members of the Vibrionaceae family that thrive in aquatic environments. These NSTIs are likely to occur in patients with hepatic disease, diabetes, and immunocompromised conditions. These organisms are found in warm sea waters and are often present in raw oysters, shellfish, and other seafood. The diagnosis of vibrio NSTIs should be suspected when a patient has the appropriate clinical findings and a history of contact with seawater or raw seafood. Early fasciotomy and culture-directed antimicrobial therapy should be aggressively performed in those patients with shock, leukopenia, severe hypoalbuminemia, and underlying chronic illness, especially a combination of hepatic dysfunction and diabetes mellitus. The rates of amputation and mortality are very high in these patients, and early definitive management is of paramount importance.

Pyomyositis

Myositis is a rare infection that may lead to serious and potentially life-threatening local and systemic complications. The infection can progress rapidly, and early recognition and proper medical and surgical management is therefore the cornerstone of therapy. With the increasing prevalence of community-associated MRSA as a pathogen in severe SSTIs, pyomyositis is more common than in past years. Myositis often occurs in muscle sites that have been compromised by injury, ischemia, malignancy, or surgery. The predominant pathogens are *S. aureus*, GAS, Gram-negative aerobic and facultative bacilli, and the indigenous aerobic and anaerobic cutaneous and mucous membranes local microflora.

CT scan imaging is a rapid and sensitive diagnostic test and commonly demonstrates diffuse enlargement of the involved muscle and may demonstrate the presence of fluid collections within the muscle suggesting the presence of abscesses. MRI is more sensitive in showing early inflammatory changes prior to development of abscesses in myositis. Percutaneous drainage or surgical exploration are warranted in order to treat pyomyositis, with concomitant appropriate IV antimicrobial therapy. Surgical intervention is required if there is potential concern for necrotizing myositis, in which case, fasciotomies and extremity amputation are sometimes necessary.

SURGICAL SITE INFECTIONS (SSIs)

Epidemiology

SSI is the leading nosocomial infection among surgical patients and the second most common nosocomial infection overall. In the United States, greater than 40 million inpatient and outpatient surgical procedures are performed each year and 2% to 5% are complicated by SSIs. SSIs result in increased length of stay and increased cost.

Definitions

SSIs are defined in three specific categories by the Centers for Disease Control and Prevention (CDC), including superficial incisional SSI, deep incisional SSI, and organ/space SSI (**Fig. 6.6** and **Table 6.10**), depending on the depth of the infection at the surgical incision site. In addition, the SSI must occur within 30 days after the operative procedure if no implant is left in place or within 1 year if implant is in place, and the infection appears to be related to the operative procedure. More specific criteria regarding these definitions are available in the CDC Guideline for Prevention of Surgical Site Infection.

Risk Factors for Surgical Site Infection

SSI risk is strongly associated with wound classification, with low risk for SSI in *clean* and *clean–contaminated* wound classes, and high risk for SSI in *contaminated* and *dirty–infected* wound classes. Three independent variables have been shown

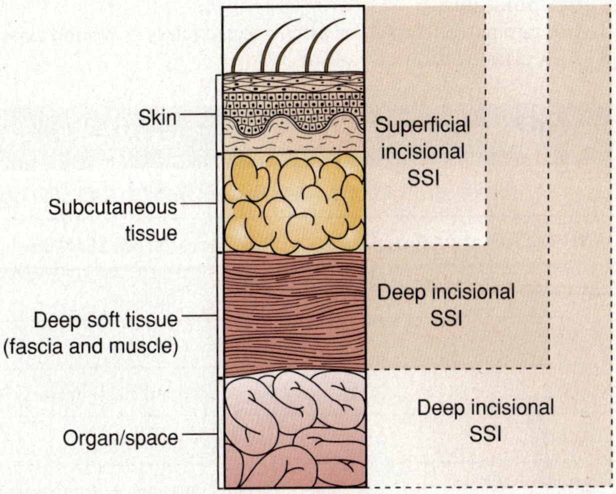

Figure 6.6. Surgical site infection (SSI) definitions by CDC. Cross-section of the abdominal depicted. **Superficial incisional SSI** involves only the skin and subcutaneous tissue layer of the incision. **Deep incisional SSI** involves deep soft tissues (eg, fascia and muscle layers) of the incision. **Organ/Space SSI** involves any part of the body, excluding the skin incision, fascia, or muscle layers, that is opened or manipulated during the operative procedure (eg, intra-abdominal abscess or thoracic empyema).

Table 6.10. CDC/NHSN Classification of Surgical Site Infections (SSIs)

Type of SSI	Definition
Superficial incisional	Infection occurs within 30 d after the operative procedure and involves only skin and subcutaneous tissue of the incision and patient Has at least one of the following: a. Purulent drainage from the superficial incision. b. Organisms isolated from an aseptically obtained culture of fluid or tissue from the superficial incision. c. At least one of the following signs or symptoms of infection: pain or tenderness, localized swelling, redness, or heat, and superficial incision is deliberately opened by surgeon and is culture positive or not cultured. A culture-negative finding does not meet this criterion d. Diagnosis of superficial incisional SSI by the surgeon or attending physician
Deep incisional	Infection occurs within 30 d after the operative procedure if no implant[a] is left in place or within 1 y if implant is in place and the infection appears to be related to the operative procedure and involves deep soft tissues (eg, fascial and muscle layers) of the incision, and patient has at least one of the following: a. Purulent drainage from the deep incision but not from the organ/space component of the surgical site. b. A deep incision spontaneously dehisces or is deliberately opened by a surgeon and is culture positive or not cultured when the patient has at least one of the following signs or symptoms: fever (38 °C), or localized pain or tenderness. A culture-negative finding does not meet this criterion c. An abscess or other evidence of infection involving the deep incision is found on direct examination, during reoperation, or by histopathologic or radiologic examination d. Diagnosis of a deep incisional SSI by a surgeon or attending physician

[a]Implant: A nonhuman-derived object, material, or tissue (eg, prosthetic heart valve, nonhuman vascular graft, mechanical heart, or hip prosthesis) that is permanently placed in a patient during an operative procedure and is not routinely manipulated for diagnostic or therapeutic purposes.
From Horan TC, Andrus M, Dudeck MA. CDC/NHSN surveillance definition of health care-associated infection and criteria for specific types of infections in the acute care setting. *Am J Infect Control.* 2008;36:309–332.

to be associated with SSI risk. The National Healthcare Safety Network (NHSN) SSI Risk Index for an individual patient includes an ASA score greater than 2, classification of wound as contaminated or dirty, and prolonged duration of operation.

NHSN SSI Risk Index and Standardized Mortality Ratio (SIR)

The NHSN SSI Risk index assigns surgical patients into categories based on the presence of three major risk factors. The patient's SSI risk category is simply the number of these factors present at the time of the operation.

1. Operation lasting more than the duration cut point hours, where the duration cut point is the approximate 75th percentile of the duration of surgery in minutes for the operative procedure
2. Contaminated (class 3) or dirty/infected (class 4) wound class
3. ASA classification of 3, 4, or 5

The laparoscopic surgical approach is associated with decreased SSI incidence, and a modified risk index (category 1 when procedure was performed with a laparoscope) has been created to address this approach.

The NHSN standardized infection ratio (SIR) is a summary measure used to track HAIs (HAIs) at a national, state, or local level over time. The SIR adjusts for various facility- and/or patient-level factors that contribute to SSI risk within each facility. The SIR compares the actual number of SSIs reported to the number that would be predicted, given the standard population (ie, NHSN baseline), adjusting for several risk factors that have been found to be significantly associated with differences in SSI incidence. A SIR >1.0 indicates that more SSIs were observed than predicted; conversely, a SIR <1.0 indicates that fewer SSIs were observed than predicted. SSI risk adjustment for SIR is variable, dependent on the operative procedure performed (**Table 6.11**).

Table 6.11. NHSN Uses Procedure Data for SSI Risk Adjustment

	Predictive Risk Factors from the All SSI Logistic Regression Model, Adults ≥18 years of age
NHSN Operative Procedure	**Risk Factor(s)-All SSI Model, Adults**
AAA	Procedure duration
AMP	Anesthesia, wound class, hospital bed size, age, procedure duration
APPY	Gender, wound class, hospital bed size, closure, procedure duration, BMI
AVSD	Procedure duration
BILI	Gender, emergency, trauma, wound class, hospital bed size, scope, age, procedure duration
BRST	ASA score, age, procedure duration, BMI
CARD	Emergency, medical school affiliation, age, procedure duration, BMI
CABG	Gender, diabetes, trauma, medical school affiliation, hospital bed size, age, procedure duration, BMI, age–gender interaction

Surgical Site Infection Prevention

Preventive measures for SSI include antimicrobial prophylaxis, sterilization methods, proper ventilation of operating rooms, use of barriers, no shaving, clipping if hair removal is required, proper surgical skin preparation and surgical techniques, maintenance of normothermia, glycemic control, and the provision of supplemental oxygen (**Table 6.12**).

Antimicrobial prophylaxis for SSI is most effective when provided 30 to 60 minutes prior to the initial surgical incision, allowing adequate blood and tissue concentrations at the time of skin incision. Risk of SSI increases when antimicrobial prophylaxis is given too early (more than 2 hours prior to skin incision) or too late (after skin incision). In addition, the correct antimicrobial must be administered to cover the potential causative pathogens, dependent on the surgical procedure performed.

Treatment of Surgical Site Infection

Once superficial or deep incisional SSI is diagnosed, "pathogen identification" is of paramount importance. In years past, the surgical incision was opened and dressing changes were initiated with no culture of the surgical site obtained. In today's era of multi–drug-resistant pathogens, a Gram stain and culture of the surgical site should always be obtained in order to

Table 6.12. Essential Practices to prevent Surgical Site Infections

Essential Practices for SSI Prevention	Quality of Evidence
1. Administer antimicrobial prophylaxis according to evidence-based standards and guidelines. HIGH	High
2. Use a combination of parenteral and oral antimicrobial prophylaxis prior to elective colorectal surgery to reduce the risk of SSI. (Quality of evidence: HIGH)	High
3. A. Decolonize surgical patients with an antistaphylococcal agent in the preoperative setting for orthopedic and cardiothoracic procedures. B. Decolonize surgical patients in other procedures at high risk of staphylococcal SSI, such as those involving prosthetic material.	A. High B. Low
4. Use antiseptic-containing preoperative vaginal preparation agents for patients undergoing cesarean delivery or hysterectomy.	Moderate
5. Do not remove hair at the operative site unless the presence of hair will interfere with the surgical procedure.	Moderate
6. Use alcohol-containing preoperative skin preparatory agents in combination with an antiseptic.	High
7. For procedures not requiring hypothermia, maintain normothermia (temperature >35.5 °C) during the perioperative period.	High
8. Use impervious plastic wound protectors for gastrointestinal and biliary tract surgery.	High
9. Perform intraoperative antiseptic wound lavage.	Moderate
10. Control blood-glucose level during the immediate postoperative period for all patients.	High
11. Use a checklist and/or bundle to ensure compliance with best practices to improve surgical patient safety.	High
12. Perform surveillance for SSI.	Moderate
13. Increase the efficiency of surveillance by utilizing automated data.	Moderate
14. Provide ongoing SSI rate feedback to surgical and perioperative personnel and leadership.	Moderate
15. Measure and provide feedback to HCP regarding rates of compliance with process measures.	Low
16. Educate surgeons and perioperative personnel about SSI prevention measures.	Low
17. Educate patients and their families about SSI prevention as appropriate.	Low
18. Implement policies and practices to reduce the risk of SSI for patients that align with applicable evidence-based standards, rules and regulations, and medical device manufacturer instructions for use.	Moderate
19. Observe and review operating room personnel and the environment of care in the operating room and in central sterile reprocessing.	Low
Additional approaches	
1. Perform an SSI risk assessment.	Low
2. Consider use of negative pressure dressings in patients who may benefit.	Moderate
3. Observe and review practices in the preoperative clinic, postanesthesia care unit, surgical intensive care unit, and/or surgical ward.	Moderate
4. Use antiseptic-impregnated sutures as a strategy to prevent SSI	Moderate

Adapted from Calderwood MS, Anderson DJ, Bratzler DW, et al. Strategies to prevent surgical site infections in acute-care hospitals: 2022 Update. *Infect Control Hosp Epidemiol*. 2023;44(5):695–720.

determine the optimal antimicrobial therapy that is required for SSI treatment.

SSI treatment includes four strategies for successful treatment: (1) early empiric antimicrobial therapy; (2) decision making regarding whether the surgical site should be opened; (3) pathogen identification; and (4) deescalation of antimicrobial therapy once culture results are available.

For organ/space SSI, "source control" and "pathogen identification" are both high priorities in order to achieve successful treatment. In the case of intra-abdominal abscess, source control can be provided by either interventional radiology percutaneous drainage or open surgical drainage of the abscess. Abscess fluid should be sent for Gram stain and culture, and empiric antimicrobial treatment should be deescalated once culture results are available.

References

1. Aubry ST, Napolitano LM. Management of common postoperative infections in the surgical intensive care unit. *Infect Dis Clin North Am.* 2022;36(4):839–859.
2. Zasowski EJ, Bassetti M, Blasi F, et al. A systematic review of the effect of delayed appropriate antibiotic treatment on the outcomes of patients with severe bacterial infections. *Chest.* 2020;158(3):929–938.
3. Evans L, Rhodes A, Alhazzani W, et al. Surviving sepsis campaign: International Guidelines for Management of Sepsis and Septic Shock 2021. *Crit Care Med.* 2021;49(11):e1063–e1143.
4. Coccolini F, Sartelli M, Sawyer R, et al. Source control in emergency general surgery: WSES, GAIS, SIS-E, SIS-A guidelines. *World J Emerg Surg.* 2023;18(1):41.
5. Huston JM, Barie PS, Dellinger EP, et al; Therapeutics and Guidelines Committee. The surgical infection society guidelines on the management of intra-abdominal infection: 2024 update. *Surg Infect (Larchmt).* 2024;25:419–435.
6. Sartelli M, Barie P, Agnoletti V, et al. Intra-abdominal infections survival guide: a position statement by the Global Alliance For Infections In Surgery. *World J Emerg Surg.* 2024;19(1):22.
7. Bonomo RA, Chow AW, Edwards MS, et al. 2024 Clinical Practice Guideline Update by the Infectious Diseases Society of America on complicated intra-abdominal infections: risk assessment, diagnostic imaging, and microbiological evaluation in adults, children, and pregnant people. *Clin Infect Dis.* 2024;79:S81–S87.
8. Sawyer RG, Claridge JA, Nathens AB, et al. Trial of short-course antimicrobial therapy for intraabdominal infection. *N Engl J Med.* 2015;372(21):1996–2005.
9. Montravers P, Tubach F, Lescot T, et al. Short-course antibiotic therapy for critically ill patients treated for postoperative intra-abdominal infection: the DURAPOP randomised clinical trial. *Intensive Care Med.* 2018;44:300–310.
10. Bom WJ, Bolmers MD, Gans SL, et al. Discriminating complicated from uncomplicated appendicitis by ultrasound imaging, computed tomography or magnetic resonance imaging: systematic review and meta-analysis of diagnostic accuracy. *BJS Open.* 2021;5(2):zraa030.
11. Dahiya DS, Akram H, Goyal A, et al. Controversies and future directions in management of acute appendicitis: an updated comprehensive review. *J Clin Med.* 2024;13(11):3034.
12. de Almeida Leite RM, Seo DJ, Gomez-Eslava B, et al. Nonoperative vs operative management of uncomplicated acute appendicitis: a systematic review and meta-analysis. *JAMA Surg.* 2022;157(9): 828–834.
13. Brucchi F, Bracchetti G, Fugazzola P, et al. A meta-analysis and trial sequential analysis comparing nonoperative versus operative management for uncomplicated appendicitis: a focus on randomized controlled trials. *World J Emerg Surg.* 2024;19(1):2.
14. Kumar SS, Collings AT, Lamm R, et al. SAGES guideline for the diagnosis and treatment of appendicitis. *Surg Endosc.* 2024;38: 2974–2994.
15. Di Saverio S, Podda M, De Simone B, et al. Diagnosis and treatment of acute appendicitis: 2020 update of the WSES Jerusalem guidelines. *World J Emerg Surg.* 2020;15(1):27.
16. Sippola S, Haijanen J, Grönroos J, et al. Effect of oral moxifloxacin vs intravenous ertapenem plus oral levofloxacin for treatment of uncomplicated acute appendicitis: the APPAC II randomized clinical trial. *JAMA.* 2021;325(4):353–362.
17. Selänne L, Haijanen J, Sippola S, et al. Three-year outcomes of oral antibiotics vs intravenous and oral antibiotics for uncomplicated acute appendicitis: a secondary analysis of the APPAC II randomized clinical trial. *JAMA Surg.* 2024;159(7):727–735.
18. Salminen P, Sippola S, Haijanen J, et al. Antibiotics versus placebo in adults with CT-confirmed uncomplicated acute appendicitis (APPAC III): randomized double-blind superiority trial. *Br J Surg.* 2022;109(6):503–509.
19. Jaschinski T, Mosch CG, Eikermann M, Neugebauer EA, Sauerland S. Laparoscopic versus open surgery for suspected appendicitis. *Cochrane Database Syst Rev.* 2018;11(11):CD001546.
20. Jalava K, Sallinen V, Lampela H, et al. Role of preoperative in-hospital delay on appendiceal perforation while awaiting appendicectomy (PERFECT): a Nordic, pragmatic, open-label, multicentre, non-inferiority, randomised controlled trial. *Lancet.* 2023; 402(10412):1552–1561.
21. Tang G, Wang J, Chen R, Zhang J, Zhou R. Daytime versus nighttime appendectomy in term of complications and clinical outcomes: a meta-analysis. *Int J Colorectal Dis.* 2024;39(1):131.
22. Zhou S, Cheng Y, Cheng N, Gong J, Tu B. Early versus delayed appendicectomy for appendiceal phlegmon or abscess. *Cochrane Database Syst Rev.* 2024;5(5):CD011670.
23. Peltrini R, Podda M, Di Saverio S, Bracale U, Corcione F. Interval appendicectomy for complicated appendicitis: do not let your guard down! *Br J Surg.* 2021;108(9):e288–e289.
24. Peltrini R, Cantoni V, Green R, et al. Risk of appendiceal neoplasm after interval appendectomy for complicated appendicitis: a systematic review and meta-analysis. *Surgeon.* 2021;19(6):e549–e558.
25. Solis-Pazmino P, Oka K, La K, et al. Incidence rate and histology of appendiceal neoplasms in complicated versus uncomplicated appendicitis: a meta-analysis and systematic review. *Langenbecks Arch Surg.* 2023;408(1):432.
26. Napolitano LM, Alam HB, Biesterveld BE, et al. *Evaluation and Management of Gallstone-Related Diseases in Non-Pregnant Adults [Internet].* Michigan Medicine University of Michigan; 2021. https://www.ncbi.nlm.nih.gov/books/NBK569245/
27. Yokoe M, Hata J, Takada T, et al. Tokyo Guidelines 2018: diagnostic criteria and severity grading of acute cholecystitis (with videos). *J Hepatobiliary Pancreat Sci.* 2018;25:41–54.
28. Okamoto K, Suzuki K, Takada T, et al. Tokyo Guidelines 2018: flowchart for the management of acute cholecystitis. *J Hepatobiliary Pancreat Sci.* 2018;25:55–72.
29. Mishima K, Fujiyama Y, Wakabayashi T, et al. Early laparoscopic cholecystectomy for acute cholecystitis following the Tokyo Guidelines 2018: a prospective single-center study of 201 consecutive cases. *Surg Endosc.* 2023;37:6051–6061.
30. Teoh AYB, Kitano M, Itoi T, et al. Endosonography-guided gallbladder drainage versus percutaneous cholecystostomy in very high-risk surgical patients with acute cholecystitis: an international randomised multicentre controlled superiority trial (DRAC 1). *Gut.* 2020;69(6):1085–1091.
31. Podboy A, Yuan J, Stave CD, Chan SM, Hwang JH, Teoh AYB. Comparison of EUS-guided endoscopic transpapillary and percutaneous gallbladder drainage for acute cholecystitis: a systematic review with network meta-analysis. *Gastrointest Endosc.* 2021;93(4):797–804.e1.
32. Kiriyama S, Kozaka K, Takada T, et al. Tokyo Guidelines 2018: diagnostic criteria and severity grading of acute cholangitis (with videos). *J Hepatobiliary Pancreat Sci.* 2018;25(1):17–30.
33. Miura F, Okamoto K, Takada T, et al. Tokyo Guidelines 2018: initial management of acute biliary infection and flowchart for acute cholangitis. *J Hepatobiliary Pancreat Sci.* 2018;25(1): 31–40.
34. Buckman SA, Mazuski JE. Review of the Tokyo guidelines 2018: antimicrobial therapy for acute cholangitis and cholecystitis. JAMA network clinical guideline synopsis. *JAMA Surg.* 2019;154(9): 873–874.

35. Au S, Aly EH. Treatment of uncomplicated acute diverticulitis without antibiotics: a systematic review and meta-analysis. *Dis Colon Rectum*. 2019;62(12):1533–1547.
36. Peery AF, Shaukat A, Strate LL. AGA clinical practice update on medical management of colonic diverticulitis: expert review. *Gastroenterology*. 2021;160(3):906–911.e1.
37. Fugazzola P, Ceresoli M, Coccolini F, et al. The WSES/SICG/ACOI/SICUT/AcEMC/SIFIPAC guidelines for diagnosis and treatment of acute left colonic diverticulitis in the elderly. *World J Emerg Surg*. 2022;17(1):5.
38. Hall J, Hardiman K, Lee S, et al. The American Society of Colon and Rectal Surgeons Clinical Practice guidelines for the treatment of left-sided colonic diverticulitis. *Dis Colon Rectum*. 2020;63(6):728–747.
39. Lee C, Louie T, Bancke L, et al. Safety of fecal microbiota, live-jslm (REBYOTA™) in individuals with recurrent *Clostridioides difficile* infection: data from five prospective clinical trials. *Therap Adv Gastroenterol*. 2023;16:17562848231174277.
40. Johnson S, Lavergne V, Skinner AM, et al. Clinical Practice Guideline by the Infectious Diseases Society of America (IDSA) and Society for Healthcare Epidemiology of America (SHEA): 2021 focused update guidelines on management of clostridioides difficile infection in adults. *Clin Infect Dis*. 2021;73(5):e1029–e1044.
41. Poylin V, Hawkins AT, Bhama AR, et al; Clinical Practice Guidelines Committee of The American Society of Colon and Rectal Surgeons. The American Society of Colon and Rectal Surgeons Clinical Practice Guidelines for the management of clostridioides difficile infection. *Dis Colon Rectum*. 2021;64(6):650–668.
42. Shellito AD, Russell MM. Diverting loop ileostomy for Clostridium difficile colitis: a systematic review and meta-analysis. *Am Surg*. 2020;86(10):1269–1276.
43. Jain N, Umar TP, Fahner AF, Gibietis V. Advancing therapeutics for recurrent clostridioides difficile infections: an overview of vowst's FDA approval and implications. *Gut Microbes*. 2023;15(1):2232137.
44. Kelly CR, Fischer M, Allegretti JR, et al. ACG Clinical Guidelines: prevention, diagnosis, and treatment of clostridioides difficile infections. *Am J Gastroenterol*. 2021;116(6):1124–1147.
45. Peery AF, Kelly CR, Kao D, et al; AGA Clinical Guidelines Committee. AGA Clinical Practice Guideline on fecal microbiota-based therapies for select gastrointestinal diseases. *Gastroenterology*. 2024;166(3):409–434.
46. Song YN, Yang DY, van Zanten SV, et al. FMT for severe or fulminant CDI: systematic review and meta-analysis. *J Can Assoc Gastroenterol*. 2022;5(1):1–11.
47. Forrester JD, Colling KP, Diaz JJ, et al. Surgical Infection Society Guidelines for total abdominal colectomy versus diverting loop ileostomy with antegrade intra-colonic lavage for the surgical management of severe or fulminant, non-perforated clostridioides difficile colitis. *Surg Infect (Larchmt)*. 2022;23(2):97–104.
48. de-Madaria E, Buxbaum JL, Maisonneuve P, et al; ERICA Consortium. Aggressive or moderate fluid resuscitation in acute pancreatitis. *N Engl J Med*. 2022;387(11):989–1000.
49. Sartelli M, Coccolini F, Kluger Y, et al. WSES/GAIS/WSIS/SIS-E/AAST global clinical pathways for patients with skin and soft tissue infections. *World J Emerg Surg*. 2022;17(1):3.
50. Worldwide Antimicrobial Resistance National/International Network Group (WARNING) Collaborators. Ten golden rules for optimal antibiotic use in hospital settings: the WARNING call to action. *World J Emerg Surg*. 2023;18(1):50.

7

Shock

Joseph Cuschieri

Key Points

1 Shock is a clinical syndrome that results from inadequate tissue perfusion.

2 Shock can be caused by hypovolemic, cardiogenic, extracardiac obstructive, and distributive conditions.

3 Hypovolemic shock due to ongoing fluid, blood, and/or plasma loss leads to progressive cardiovascular deterioration, ultimate hypotension, oliguria, confusion, irreversible cell injury, and death.

4 Cardiogenic shock results in decreased tissue perfusion due to intrinsic cardiac pump failure.

5 Extracardiac obstructive shock attenuates cardiac pump function due to external compression of inflow and outflow (tamponade, tension pneumothorax, etc.).

6 Septic and traumatic shock, forms of distributive shock, are systemic inflammatory responses to infection or tissue injury with cellular breakdown, producing severe hypotension requiring massive volume resuscitation and a high risk of multiple organ failure and death.

7 Complications of an episode of shock include ischemia–reperfusion injury from oxidant stress; potential secondary immunosuppression with enhanced nosocomial infection risk; hypothermia and coagulopathy; and multiple organ failure syndrome, including abdominal compartment syndrome (ACS).

8 Treatment of shock requires goal-directed appropriate volume resuscitation with the treatment of the underlying etiology and careful monitoring of the adequacy of end-organ perfusion to avoid under- and overresuscitation.

1 The concept of shock, first described by Cannon in 1929, refers to inadequate blood flow causing cellular hypoxia and subsequent dysfunction at both cellular and organ levels.[1] Blalock later identified the four major causes of shock: hematogenic, neurogenic, cardiogenic, and vasogenic. He also noted the significant third-space fluid loss following shock resuscitation, leading to a therapeutic focus on restoring intravascular volume and replacing the interstitial fluid with a balanced salt solution.[2] Shock can become irreversible and unresponsive to volume resuscitation, as Wiggers highlighted nearly a century ago.[3] Factors sustaining this shock state lead to progressive organ dysfunction and death despite temporary improvements.

Today, shock is classified into four groups—hypovolemic, cardiogenic, extracardiac obstructive, and distributive.[4] Early recognition and treatment are crucial to prevent irreversible shock caused by uncorrected critical oxygen delivery deficits. Future therapies are expected to move beyond basic recognition, fluid resuscitation, and cardiovascular support, focusing on understanding the events leading to organ damage and irreversibility. This chapter outlines these events, current therapeutic approaches, and future perspectives.

EVALUATION OF SHOCK

Recognizing and treating shock before the onset of decompensation is critical for patient outcomes. Assessment should include clinical appearance, hemodynamic measurements, physiologic responses, and biochemical analyses.

In many shock states, vasoconstriction leads to cool skin and poor capillary refill, while neurogenic or septic shock often presents with warm skin and good capillary refill. Hyperventilation is a common response to metabolic acidosis, and decreased cerebral blood flow with increased catecholamine levels can cause anxiety and restlessness. Continued shock may lead to lethargy, but true coma is rare unless there is complete cardiovascular collapse or severe hypoxia.

Initial hemodynamic assessment should evaluate the pulse rate and character, blood pressure, shock index, central venous pressure (CVP), cardiac function, and pulse pressure variation (PPV). Tachycardia is a normal response to volume loss. Narrowing pulse pressure indicates vasoconstriction's impact on diastolic blood pressure. Importantly, the shock index, calculated as heart rate divided by systolic blood pressure, is a useful tool for early detection of shock, assessing severity, and monitoring treatment response.[5] A normal shock index ranges from 0.5 to 0.7, with values above 0.7 indicating early shock. CVP reflects venous tone rather than true blood volume, and changes in CVP due to treatment or ongoing hemorrhage may be more informative than a single measurement, but this remains debatable. Pulmonary artery catheters (PACs) are no longer routinely used, with invasive monitoring using PPV and noninvasive measures like echocardiography preferred for assessing volume status and cardiac function.[6]

Urine output is a valuable measure of perfusion and volume status. A urinary catheter should be placed in patients being evaluated for shock, with hourly urine output targets of 0.5 to 1 mL/kg for adult patients, at least 1 mL/kg for most pediatric patients, and 1 to 2 mL/kg for patients younger than 2 years. Inadequate urine output in the setting of previous normal kidney function indicates inadequate perfusion and cellular hypoxia.

Shock induces a shift from aerobic to anaerobic metabolism, increasing lactate levels in the blood. Effective resuscitation reduces serum lactate levels, and the time to normalize lactate is a significant survival predictor.[7] The base deficit, reflecting the amount of base needed to return blood pH to 7.40, is categorized as normal (2 to –2), mild (–3 to –5), moderate (–6 to –9), and severe (> –10).[8] Normalizing base deficit with volume infusion indicates successful resuscitation, and its normalization time may have a greater prognostic value than lactate levels.[9] Severe base deficit abnormalities are linked to chronic critical illness (CCI), and early correction can improve outcomes.[10] Importantly, these biochemical changes occur even with compensated shock, making blood gas analysis, including base deficit and lactate, essential for all suspected shock cases. A lactate level of ≥4 mmol/L or a base deficit of ≥6 mEq/L should prompt a strong suspicion of shock.

Additional markers, such as central and mixed venous oxygen saturation, provide a global assessment of perfusion. Improvement toward normal values indicates successful resuscitation and can guide resuscitation efforts.

By combining clinical assessment, hemodynamic measurements, urine output, and biochemical markers, health care providers can effectively diagnose and manage shock, improving patient outcomes.

TYPES OF SHOCK

Although several different classifications for shock have been described, the most widely accepted classification of shock was proposed by Weil and Shubin in 1971.[4] This classification divides the shock syndrome into four distinct categories 2 (**Table 7.1**). Despite this separation, however, there is considerable overlap between the categories, with some patients

SCIENTIFIC PRINCIPLES

Table 7.1. Classification System and Causes of Shock

Classification	Etiology	Cause
Hypovolemic	Hemorrhagic	Trauma Gastrointestinal
	Nonhemorrhagic	Absolute fluid loss (renal, gastrointestinal) Redistributive or "third spacing"
Cardiogenic	Myocardial	Ischemia Infarction Contusion Cardiomyopathy Myocarditis Pharmacologic/toxic (beta blockers, calcium channel blockers, tricyclic antidepressants, anthracycline) Metabolic (hypophosphatemia, hypocalcemia, acidosis)
	Valve failure	Infection Injury Ruptured papillary muscle Stenosis
	Arrhythmias	Ischemia Pharmacologic/toxic Metabolic
Extracardiac Obstructive	Extrinsic compression	Mediastinal tumors
	Increased intrathoracic pressure	Tension pneumothorax Positive-pressure ventilation
	Intrinsic vascular flow obstruction	Pulmonary embolism Air embolism Tumors (myxoma) Proximal aortic dissection Aortic coarctation Acute pulmonary hypertension Tamponade Pericarditis
Distributive	SIRS related	Trauma Sepsis Pancreatitis Burns
	Anaphylactic/anaphylactoid	Drugs Venoms
	Neurogenic	Spinal cord injury
	Toxic/pharmacologic	Vasodilators Benzodiazepines
	Endocrine	Adrenal insufficiency Thyroid Myxedema

SIRS, systemic inflammatory response syndrome.

Table 7.2. Hemodynamic Patterns in Shock

Type	CO	SVR	PAOP	CVP	SvO_2
Hypovolemic	↓	↑	↓	↓	↓
Cardiogenic					
Left ventricular MI	↓	↑	↑	N, ↑	↓
Right ventricular MI	↓	↑	N, ↓	↑	↓
Extracardiac Obstructive					
Pericardial tamponade	↓	↑	↑	↑	↓
Pulmonary embolism	↓	↑	↑	↑	↓
Distributive					
Early	↑, N, ↓	↑, N, ↓	N	N, ↑	N, ↑
Early after fluid administration	↑	↓	N, ↑	N, ↑	↑, N, ↓
Late	↓	↑	N	N	↓

CO, cardiac output; CVP, central venous pressure; MI, myocardial infarction; N, normal; PAOP, pulmonary artery occlusion pressure; SvO_2, mixed venous oxygen saturation; SVR, systemic vascular resistance.

presenting with more than one factor at the same time. Given this overlap, it is helpful to evaluate the hemodynamic pattern to elucidate the etiology and appropriately manage the patient (**Table 7.2**).

3 Hypovolemic Shock

Hypovolemic shock is the most common form of shock encountered in surgical practice. It is characterized by a significant reduction in intravascular volume, preventing the heart from pumping sufficient blood to vital organs. This condition is typically due to blood loss, and evidence of shock requires a loss of more than 20% of circulating blood or plasma. The severity of symptoms varies with the amount and duration of fluid loss (**Table 7.3**).[11] Early identification and control of the source of blood loss is critically important. Resuscitation is an adjunct to hemorrhage control, but not a substitute. Strategies/tools for hemorrhage control depend upon the source (eg, embolization, surgical control, torniquet, aortic balloon), but it is important to make hemorrhage control a priority.

Class I: Mild hemorrhage (up to 15% blood volume). No significant changes in vital signs or capillary refill; minimal treatment required.

Class II: Moderate hemorrhage (15% to 30% blood volume). Symptoms include tachycardia, tachypnea, slightly reduced blood pressure, and delayed capillary refill. Usually treated with crystalloid solutions; some may require blood transfusion.

Class III: Severe hemorrhage (30% to 40% blood volume). Symptoms include marked tachycardia, hypotension, and mental status changes. Requires blood transfusion and crystalloids.

Class IV: Life-threatening hemorrhage (over 40% blood volume). Symptoms include severe hypotension and negligible urine output. Immediate transfusion and surgical intervention are often necessary.

Individual susceptibility to blood loss varies, influenced by factors like age, preexisting conditions, and medications. Plasma loss can also cause hypovolemic shock, typically presenting with hemoconcentration, elevated BUN and creatinine, and hypernatremia.

Cardiogenic Shock

Cardiogenic shock results from decreased cardiac output (CO) despite adequate intravascular volume, leading to tissue hypoperfusion. It arises from issues with the cardiac muscle, electrical conduction system, or valves, with anterior wall myocardial infarction being the most common cause. In surgical patients, it may be triggered by pulmonary embolism, myocardial contusion, or pulmonary hypertension.

Table 7.3. Classification of Hemorrhagic Shock

	Class I	Class II	Class III	Class IV
Blood Loss (mL)	Up to 750	750–1500	1500–2000	>2000
Blood Loss (%)	Up to 15	15–30	30–40	40
Heart Rate	<100	>100	>120	>140
Blood Pressure	Normal	Normal	Decreased	Decreased
Pulse Pressure	Normal	Decreased	Decreased	Decreased
Respiratory Rate	14–20	20–30	30–40	>35
Urine Output (mL/h)	>30	20–30	5–15	Minimal
Mental Status	Normal	Mildly anxious	Anxious and confused	Confused and lethargic
Fluid Replacement	Crystalloid	Crystalloid	Crystalloid and blood	Crystalloid and blood

Distinguishing cardiogenic shock from other types of shock can be challenging, particularly in geriatric patients where combined cardiogenic and hypovolemic shock is not uncommon. Symptoms of systemic hypoperfusion, typical of other shock causes, also appear in cardiogenic shock. Diagnosis can be aided by a history of cardiac disease, physical signs like pulmonary rales, cardiac murmurs, an S3 gallop, and jugular venous distention. Electrocardiograms can detect significant ischemia or other pathologies, chest radiographs might reveal bilateral pulmonary infiltrates indicative of cardiogenic edema, and cardiospecific serum tests (troponin I and creatine phosphokinase [CPK]) may indicate myocardial damage.

Manifestations of cardiogenic shock develop due to the failure of peripheral perfusion, the adrenergic response, and the heart's inability to handle blood returning from the lungs and periphery. In the absence of sepsis or tissue injury, the metabolic needs of peripheral tissues usually do not increase. Sympathetic-mediated constriction of the peripheral vasculature attempts to maintain central blood pressure and perfusion of cerebral and coronary circulations, making the clinical findings similar to those of hypovolemic shock.

Ineffective contractile activity of the heart's right or left side causes blood to accumulate in the respective venous circulations. Acute left ventricular myocardial infarction leads to shock when more than 40% of the left ventricle is involved, occurring in about 10% of Q-wave infarctions. Acute right ventricular myocardial infarction is rare, occurring in about 5% of inferior wall infarctions. Diagnosis and treatment of these infarctions differ significantly.[12]

In patients in shock, especially those with compromised cardiac function, mechanical ventilation should be considered. The work of breathing can be significant, particularly for agitated or distressed patients. Intubation and mechanical ventilation can reduce oxygen needs, allow for comfortable sedation, secure the airway, and optimize gas exchange. This can favorably shift the balance between myocardial oxygen needs and availability.

Cardiogenic shock tends to be self-perpetuating. Myocardial perfusion relies on the pressure gradient between the coronary artery and the left ventricle and the duration of diastole, both compromised by the hypotension and tachycardia characteristic of this condition. High-volume fluid resuscitation, sometimes necessary for other forms of shock, is poorly tolerated and likely to be detrimental to an individual with cardiogenic shock.

Extracardiac Obstructive Shock

4 A subset of patients with perceived evidence of cardiogenic shock do not have intrinsic cardiac disease but experience pump failure due to extrinsic compression that limits diastolic filling and CO. Conditions such as cardiac tamponade, tension pneumothorax, diaphragmatic herniation of abdominal viscera, mediastinal hematoma, aortic dissection, massive pulmonary embolism, and, occasionally, positive-pressure mechanical ventilation, can all precipitate shock by exerting constricting pressure on the myocardium. Prompt diagnosis and treatment are critical to improving outcomes, as untreated obstructive shock can quickly lead to organ failure and death.

Distributive Shock

5 Distributive shock occurs when there is inappropriate oxygen utilization, typically associated with systemic inflammatory response syndrome (SIRS). While SIRS is classically triggered by sepsis, it can also result from other immune processes including trauma, pancreatitis, and various types of tissue injuries. In addition, distributive shock can arise from noninflammatory causes, such as loss of vascular tone due to spinal cord injury, endocrine dysfunction, or anaphylaxis.

Septic Shock

6 Septic shock is defined as sepsis accompanied by hypotension that persists despite adequate fluid resuscitation.[13] It occur when bacterial products interact with immune system cells, leading to the release of mediators that cause circulatory disturbances and direct and indirect cell damage. Hemodynamic changes in septic shock can be categorized as early (warm or hyperdynamic) or late (cold or hypodynamic), primarily characterized by ventricular contractility and peripheral vasomotor impairment. These stages can be misclassified if not properly evaluated.

Early septic shock is marked by peripheral vasodilation, flushed and warm extremities, and a compensatory increase in CO. Although increased venous capacitance reduces venous return to the heart, CO is maintained through tachycardia and decreased afterload due to systemic vasodilation.

Late septic shock is characterized by impaired myocardial contractility due to local and systemic release of cardiac depressants, worsening peripheral perfusion, vasoconstriction, extremity mottling, oliguria, and hypotension. Peripheral oxygen utilization may be severely impaired by bacterial toxins, such as lipopolysaccharide (LPS), and the inflammatory products of the host's immune response, leading to metabolic dysfunction and acidosis despite high systemic oxygen delivery. This inappropriate oxygen utilization and systemic shunting cause confusion regarding the adequacy of resuscitation and lead to progressive cell death. Both systemic hypoperfusion and altered tissue metabolism create a vicious cycle that propagates the inflammatory response, resulting in progressive cellular injury.

Due to both volume deficits and cardiovascular dysfunction, persistent perfusion deficits are common and contribute to multiple organ failure and mortality. The fluid volume required for treatment may exceed that needed for other forms of shock due to persistent microvascular endothelial capillary leak. This profound leak can lead to extreme interstitial and total body fluid imbalances, potentially causing marked hypoxia and abdominal compartment syndrome (ACS).

Early resuscitation and cardiovascular support are crucial for treating septic shock, but equally important are early infection source control and appropriate antimicrobial administration. Studies have shown that even a few hours delay in initiating antimicrobial therapy significantly increases mortality.[14]

Traumatic Shock

The major contributor to shock after injury is hypovolemia due to hemorrhage. Even when hemorrhage ceases or is controlled, patients can continue to suffer loss of plasma volume into the interstitium of injured tissues and develop progressive hypovolemic shock. In addition, tissue injury evokes a broader, pathophysiologic, immunoinflammatory response and a potentially more devastating degree of shock than that produced by hypovolemia alone.

The degree to which direct tissue injury and an inflammatory response participate in the development and progression of traumatic shock distinguishes it from purely hypovolemic shock. Traumatic shock results from direct tissue or bony injury, resulting not only in hypovolemia caused by fluid and blood loss, but also in an immunologic and neuroendocrine response to tissue destruction and devitalization. This combined insult complicates what might otherwise be straightforward hemorrhagic shock by inducing a systemic response that utilizes many of the inflammatory mediators present in septic shock.[15] These mediators propagate and intensify the effects of the initial hypovolemia and make subsequent multiple organ failure far more likely than those that occur with hypovolemic shock alone.

Although this condition can lead to increased fluid requirements, common problems associated with this condition, such as rhabdomyolysis, should be aggressively evaluated and treated with optimal resuscitation. Additionally, common patient characteristics, such as morbid obesity, can alter traumatic shock resuscitation, resulting in delayed correction of metabolic acidosis and increased risk for organ dysfunction.[16]

Thus, initial management of the seriously injured requires the assurance of an airway, breathing, and circulation. Later management requires appropriate volume resuscitation and control of ongoing losses. Control of hemorrhage is a major concern and demands priority over attention to other injuries. After resuscitation and control of volume losses, efforts become necessary to minimize the potentially lethal post shock sequelae, including acute respiratory distress syndrome (ARDS), multiple organ dysfunction syndrome (MODS), and CCI.[10]

Emerging therapies aimed at modulating the immune response and enhancing tissue repair are underway, and provide hope in future treatment of both septic and traumatic shock.

Neurogenic Shock

Neurogenic shock is defined as the failure of the nervous system to provide effective peripheral vascular resistance, resulting in inadequate end-organ perfusion. Classic findings include warm, flushed, flaccid extremities, paraplegia, confusion, oliguria, and hypotension. Injury to the proximal spinal cord, which interrupts autonomic sympathetic vasomotor pathways, disrupts basal vasoconstrictor tone to peripheral veins and arterioles. This leads to profound vasodilation of all microvascular beds below the level of cord injury, diminishing venous return to the heart, reducing CO, and precipitating hypotension. Injuries at or above the 4th thoracic vertebrae may disrupt sympathetic innervation to the heart, resulting in significant bradycardia and decompensation.

Like the initial therapy for shock resulting from hypovolemia, treatment of the relative hypovolemia due to vasodilation of neurogenic shock requires intravenous volume resuscitation. Restoration of the pathologically expanded intravascular space improves preload and CO, and may reverse hypotension. However, maintaining adequate hemodynamics often requires vasopressor support to avoid the administration of excessive fluids. Monitoring cardiac preload should be considered to ensure adequate (but not excessive) filling volume, as loss of vasomotor capacity within the pulmonary circulation predisposes these patients to pulmonary edema. Since spinal cord injury is often associated with other traumatic injuries, the diagnosis of isolated neurogenic shock must be a process of exclusion.

Physiologic Response to Hypovolemia

Common to the majority of shock states is an initial decrease in circulating intravascular volume. This reduction is due directly to fluid loss or secondarily to fluid redistribution. This reduction in circulating fluid volume initiates both a rapid and sustained compensatory response. Within minutes, a rapid compensatory response occurs primarily due to adrenergic output. Sustained responses, in contrast, occur slower and result in intravascular fluid reabsorption and renal conservation of water and electrolytes (**Algorithm 7.1**).

Acute Response

Hypovolemia triggers the release of epinephrine and norepinephrine due to decreased signals from arterial baroreceptors, lasting up to 24 hours. This causes vasoconstriction, tachycardia, and increased myocardial contractility. Vasoconstriction in small veins and venules shifts blood to the central venous circulation, raising right-sided filling pressures, while pulmonary vasoconstriction enhances left-sided pressures. Simultaneously, blood is shunted to the heart and brain from the skin, kidneys, and viscera, boosting stroke volume (SV) and CO. This vasoconstriction affects arterioles, pre- and postcapillary sphincters, small veins, and venules, reducing hydrostatic pressure and leading to the reabsorption of interstitial fluid (water, sodium, chloride) into the vascular space. This process, known as transcapillary refill, helps restore blood volume.

Sustained Response

Sustained compensatory responses include the release of vasoactive hormones and fluid shifts from the interstitial and intracellular spaces to the intravascular compartment. Decreased renal blood flow, increased adrenergic activity, and compositional changes in tubular fluid lead to the secretion of renin from the juxtaglomerular complex. Renin promotes the formation and release of angiotensin I by the liver. Circulating angiotensin I is rapidly converted to angiotensin II by the lungs, which is the most potent known arterial and arteriolar vasoconstrictor. Angiotensin II also stimulates the release

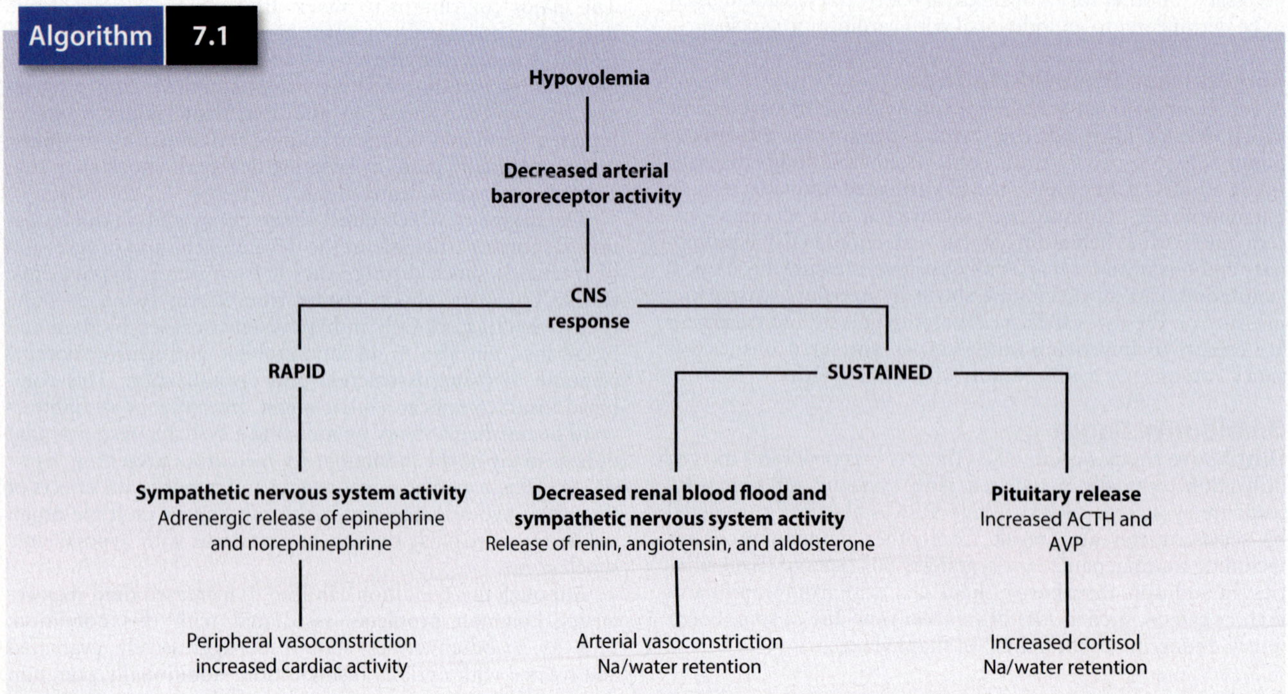

Algorithm 7.1. Neurohormonal response to hypovolemia. CNS, central nervous system; ACTH, adrenocorticotropic hormone; AVP, arginine vasopressin.

of pituitary adrenocorticotropic hormone (ACTH). Increased circulating levels of both angiotensin II and ACTH result in increased secretion of aldosterone. Consequently, sodium (Na^+) reabsorption occurs in the distal renal tubules in exchange for potassium (K^+) and hydrogen ions.

Additionally, hypovolemia and increased serum osmolarity reduce stimulation of arterial baroreceptors, leading to the release of arginine vasopressin (AVP) This hormone functions as a potent vasoconstrictor and increases water reabsorption of water by enhancing water permeability and passive Na^+ transport in the distal renal tubule. The combined effects of aldosterone and AVP are to decrease glomerular filtration and increase tubular reabsorption of salt and water, thereby replenishing intravascular volume deficits.

Finally, the increased release of the stress hormones (epinephrine, ACTH, cortisol, and glucagon) triggers glycogenolysis, lipolysis, and protein catabolism, causing a negative nitrogen balance and high extracellular glucose concentrations due to decreased insulin release and resistance. This leads to increased glucose utilization by insulin-independent tissues such as the brain and heart. In addition to glucose, products of anaerobic metabolism from hypoperfused cells accumulate in the extracellular compartment, inducing hyperosmolarity. This extracellular hyperosmolarity draws water from the intracellular space, increasing interstitial osmotic pressure, which in turn drives water, Na^+, and chloride across the capillary endothelium into the vascular space.

ORGAN-SPECIFIC COMPENSATORY RESPONSES TO SHOCK

Cardiac and Microvascular Response

Shock significantly affects cardiovascular physiology. Reduced SV results from a loss of preload, requiring neuroendocrine and renal compensatory responses, along with intravenous fluids, to increase ventricular end-diastolic volume and restore CO. However, myocardial contractility issues may arise, shifting the focus from preload to intrinsic myocardial dysfunction.

Microvascular perfusion is crucial in shock. The microvasculature, including arterioles and veins, responds to shock through sympathetic nerve-induced vasoconstriction or vasodilation. Venous blood volume serves as an autotransfusion reservoir, mobilized by α-adrenergic vasoconstriction. Vasoconstriction prioritizes the perfusion of critical organs like the central nervous system (CNS) and myocardium, while peripheral areas like skin, kidneys, muscles, and the splanchnic vascular beds receive less blood flow.

Endothelial capillary function is compromised in shock, leading to increased permeability. Circulating inflammatory mediators like TNF-α, IL-1, and nitric oxide contribute to endothelial capillary leaks. Restoring peripheral perfusion, removing infections, and supporting cardiopulmonary function are essential to reverse this condition.[17]

Neuroendocrine Response

The neuroendocrine response to shock involves the hypothalamus, autonomic nervous system, and secretory endocrine glands, aiming to restore tissue perfusion and manage metabolic substrates. Baroreceptors and chemoreceptors detect hypoxia, hypotension, or hypovolemia, triggering sympathetic vasoconstriction, which redistributes blood to vital organs. Reduced CO is countered by reflex tachycardia through the release of catecholamines and inhibition of cardiac vagal activity.

Catecholamines, cortisol, and glucagon induce hyperglycemia by promoting glycogenolysis and gluconeogenesis and reducing insulin release. Renal secretion of renin, stimulated by adrenergic activity and hypoperfusion, produces angiotensin II, which enhances vasoconstriction and aldosterone release. This leads to concentrated urine and maintains intravascular volume. Vasopressin further aids in water reabsorption and vasoconstriction.

Immunoinflammatory Response

Shock, especially septic or traumatic, triggers a systemic inflammatory response, involving TNF-α, ILs, and other mediators. Although these inflammatory mediators play an integral role in the recovery of local tissue from trauma and infection, an uncontrolled systemic inflammatory response contributes to organ failure. Immunologically active cells and the coagulation cascade contribute to tissue ischemia and inflammation that may result in organ failure and CCI.[15]

Regulation of the systemic inflammatory response has been an active area of shock research for several decades. However, current efforts to regulate the inflammatory response have not been successful in improving outcomes after shock resuscitation.[18]

Pulmonary Response

The lungs are highly susceptible to systemic shock, often leading to ARDS, a severe form of pulmonary failure. This condition is driven by inflammatory mediators produced during shock.[19]

Renal Response

Sympathetic-induced renal vasoconstriction, along with angiotensin II and catecholamines, decreases renal blood flow and glomerular filtration rate (GFR), causing oliguria and prerenal azotemia. Prolonged ischemia can lead to acute tubular necrosis (ATN). Differentiating between oliguric renal failure and decreased renal perfusion can be achieved through urine sodium and osmolality analysis.

Hepatic Response

The liver plays a critical role in shock by releasing acute-phase reactants and managing toxic agents. Prolonged shock can cause hepatic necrosis and impaired synthesis of coagulation factors and proteins. Severe ischemia may deplete glycogen stores, though this is rare without preexisting conditions.

Genetic Regulation of the Response to Shock

Individuals vary considerably in their susceptibility to shock and in their ability to recover from its consequences. Unique host-specific responses have been identified as important determinants of the outcome of sepsis and septic shock. Genetic predispositions in an individual's immunoinflammatory response may dictate whether an infection is adequately or inadequately countered.[20] These differences in response may be partially explained by single-nucleotide polymorphisms (SNPs) in the genetic sequences for various inflammatory mediators. These subtle nucleotide variations may affect the transcription or translation of associated genes or the secretion or function of the corresponding proteins. These subtle but significant alterations in the genomic makeup of individuals may be responsible for the various organ responses seen in individual patients to shock.[21,22]

LOSS OF COMPENSATORY RESPONSES TO SHOCK

Prolonged shock causes arteriolar and precapillary sphincter relaxation, increasing capillary hydrostatic pressure, and leading to intravascular volume depletion. Cellular membrane function deteriorates, resulting in increased permeability and swelling due to cellular hypoxia and impaired Na+–K+ pump function.

Organ dysfunction progresses as endothelial injury leads to fluid leakage and reduced nutrient and gas diffusion, exacerbated by microcirculatory thrombosis. This condition underlies the late-stage organ failure seen in uncompensated shock.

COMPLICATIONS OF SHOCK

Ischemia–Reperfusion Injury

Inadequate microvasculature flow results in the activation of leukocytes and converts local endothelial cells to a

proinflammatory, prothrombotic phenotype. On reperfusion, the reintroduction of oxygen prompts these cells to generate
7 superoxide anion, hydroxyl radicals, and hydrogen peroxide, further injuring local tissue. Microvascular endothelial adherence, monolayer transmigration, and local oxidative burst by activated neutrophils, along with the profound loss of endothelial monolayer integrity (ie, microvascular capillary leak), contribute to massive interstitial edema after reperfusion. Although all tissues are sensitive to varying degrees, ischemia–reperfusion injury appears to be most detrimental to the pulmonary vasculature and the splanchnic circulations. Pulmonary interstitial edema and alveolar fluid accumulation are associated with the development of ARDS, whereas extensive visceral edema may contribute to the development of ACS and mesenteric ischemia.

Multiple Organ Dysfunction Syndrome and CCI

The development of MODS is complex but appears to depend significantly on changes in the splanchnic and pulmonary microcirculations during shock. These vascular beds appear to be major sites of the activation and subsequent immunoinflammatory mediator production. During shock that is primarily due to hypovolemia, homeostatic vasoconstrictive responses reduce splanchnic microcirculatory flow, leading to excessive and prolonged hypoperfusion of the gut. This results in extensive microvascular injury and subsequent activation of endothelium, neutrophils, and macrophages.[23]

Moreover, the disruption of the mucosal barrier permits the translocation of bacteria and bacterial toxins into the circulation, reaching the large tissue-fixed macrophage population in the liver. The extensive activation of Kupffer cells in the liver releases inflammatory mediators, which cause distant organ injury through the systemic activation of other immune cells.

Not only is there a proinflammatory innate phase, but there is also a concurrent anti-inflammatory adaptive phase designed to counter the locally generated hyperimmune response and prevent the systemic spread of proinflammatory mediators. If this concurrent anti-inflammatory response syndrome results in excessive immunosuppression, it may increase susceptibility to primary and secondary infections, further perpetuating organ failure. These variable inflammatory responses can lead to the development of MODS, and associated chronic dysfunction termed CCI.

Abdominal Compartment Syndrome

ACS is a highly morbid complication of reperfusion injury to the splanchnic viscera. This syndrome appears to be increasingly prominent due to aggressive resuscitation techniques that enable the salvage of profoundly hypotensive and hypovolemic patients. Splanchnic ischemia and reperfusion result in extensive visceral capillary leak and interstitial edema of the bowel. Excessive volume resuscitation during this phase leads to grossly edematous viscera within the closed space of the abdomen, which dramatically increases intra-abdominal pressure, compromises intra-abdominal organ function, increases renovascular resistance, limits diaphragmatic excursion, and may decrease CO and elevate intracranial pressure. The clinical hallmarks of ACS are a distended and tense abdomen, diminished tidal volume, increased plateau pressure on mechanical ventilation, pulmonary edema, decreased CO, oliguria, and elevated urinary bladder pressure. The presence of all or a major part of this syndrome should prompt consideration of an urgent operative laparotomy to decompress the abdomen and treat it by leaving the abdomen open.

Hypothermia

Hypothermia, defined as a core temperature below 35 °C, is common during severe shock due to impaired energy-dependent homeostatic processes. This reduction in oxygen delivery directly contributes to progressive hypothermia if uncorrected, resulting in a loss of ATP generation and heat production. Exposure to cold environments before hospital admission and after, can exacerbate hypothermia through conductive, convective, and evaporative heat loss, all of which should be minimized. Additionally, the administration of room-temperature intravenous fluids and cold-stored blood also contributes to hypothermia. Hypothermia increases fluid requirements and independently raises acute mortality rates.[24] As the core temperature decreases, the rate of oxygen consumption drops to approximately 50% of normal at 28 °C. Hypothermia also causes a leftward shift in the oxyhemoglobin dissociation curve, though this is partially compensated by acidosis. CNS effects progress from confusion and loss of manual dexterity to obtundation and coma as the core temperature falls from 35 °C to 26.5 °C. The heart rate decreases to approximately half of the baseline at 28 °C, with a concomitant reduction in CO. All cardiac electrical conduction intervals are prolonged, consistent with the changes in heart rate, and both atrioventricular dissociation and refractory ventricular fibrillation occur at 28 °C. Other potential physiologic effects include ileus and pancreatitis due to cold enzyme activation at temperatures below 35 °C.

Compensatory responses to hypothermia include increased excretion of catecholamines, resulting in doubling of the basal metabolic rate, and increased production of thyroid hormones, further raising the basal metabolic rate to five times baseline. Shivering can increase heat production but represents a significant energy expenditure and is inhibited during episodes of hypotension or hypoxemia.[25] Compensatory responses to hypothermia are lost at temperatures below 30 °C, and a state of complete poikilothermy is reached.

The primary treatment for hypothermia is to address the underlying cause of shock. However, in cases of severe hypothermia, shock reversal may need to be accompanied by passive and active rewarming. The core temperature should be obtained on admission of patients in shock. Patients whose core temperatures are 33 °C to 35 °C can be treated with passive rewarming, warm blankets, and hot packs. Patients with core temperatures lower than 33 °C require active rewarming. If the patient is unconscious, airway control should first be obtained. Due to severe hypothermia-induced vasoconstriction, noninvasive blood pressure measurements may be inaccurate, necessitating the placement of an arterial line for monitoring and blood–gas sampling. The inspired gas through the ventilator should be heated to 41 °C and fully saturated with water vapor to increase heat conductance in the lung. Intravenous fluids should also be warmed by using rapid infusion systems with countercurrent heating elements. For extreme hypothermia, continuous mechanical arteriovenous rewarming via cardiac bypass or extracorporeal membrane oxygenation can provide both circulatory support and rewarming. Recently developed microtechnology permits core rewarming by percutaneous placement of countercurrent warming coils directly in the inferior vena cava (IVC). Additional warming methods include lavage of heated saline through nasogastric and thoracostomy tubes, as well as peritoneal lavage, though these are effective.

Coagulopathy

Coagulopathy frequently complicates shock, particularly in patients who have received large volumes of crystalloid solution and blood for resuscitation. The issue, while not fully understood, is multifactorial, influenced by the presence of shock, the volume of fluid resuscitation, hypothermia, and preexisting diseases. Recent studies have further elucidated these complexities.[26]

Dilutional thrombocytopenia is a significant factor in coagulopathy, occurring after massive volume resuscitation. Bleeding times can be prolonged with platelet counts below 100,000 cells/mL, but counts of 50,000 cells/mL or higher are usually adequate for surgical hemostasis. Dilutional thrombocytopenia becomes more likely with infusions exceeding one blood volume, and each unit of platelets administered increases the count by 10,000 to 15,000 cells/mL. It is prudent to control surgically remediable hemorrhage before platelet transfusion to prevent the loss of the transfused platelets.

Dilution of other coagulation factors also contributes to coagulopathy. Factors V and VIII are particularly labile in banked blood, but levels of less than 10% of normal for factors VII, X, XI, XII, and XIII are associated with abnormalities in hemostasis, demonstrated by prolonged partial thromboplastin time and prothrombin time. Fresh–frozen plasma can provide all the soluble coagulation factors, and cryoprecipitate may be necessary as a concentrated source of factor VIII and fibrinogen if fresh–frozen plasma does not achieve adequate hemostasis.

Evidence supports the use of tranexamic acid (TXA) for patients with exsanguinating hemorrhage.[27] TXA prevents fibrinolysis, resulting in more rapid hemorrhage control. Its benefits are most evident in patients with severe hemorrhagic shock when administered within the first 3 hours. Though theoretically associated with thrombotic complications such as pulmonary embolism, myocardial infarction, and stroke, current data do not show this association.

Prothrombin complex concentrates (PCCs) and fibrinogen administration have shown promise in rapidly reversing anticoagulant effects, improving outcomes in trauma-induced coagulopathy (TIC). Rotational thromboelastometry (ROTEM) is increasingly used to assess and manage coagulopathy in trauma patients, offering detailed insights into coagulation status and guiding targeted treatment interventions.[28]

Finally, early aggressive use of fresh–frozen plasma following massive blood loss can minimize coagulopathy and hemorrhage. Studies have shown that a 1:1 ratio of packed red blood cells to fresh–frozen plasma is associated with reduced mortality in both civilian and military settings.[29] However, this practice may increase the risk of ARDS and organ dysfunction, highlighting the need for cautious generalization beyond massively injured patients.[30]

TREATMENT

Fluid Therapy

8 Providing fluid beyond the amount of blood loss improved survival in both clinical and experimental studies of hemorrhagic shock, leading to the widespread acceptance of aggressive fluid infusion. However, current research indicates that crystalloid overresuscitation significantly increases morbidity and mortality due to increased risk of ARDS, MODS, increased intracranial pressure, and ACS.[31] Because massive volumes of fluid are provided to patients with severe shock, it is unclear whether these complications are due to excessive fluid or underlying shock.

For adults, a minimum of two large-bore (14- to 16-gauge) intravenous catheters should be established. Isotonic fluid is then infused while blood is obtained for analysis, screening, and typing. Fluid can be infused at a rate up to 200 mL/min through a 14-gauge catheter and up to 220 mL/min through a 7-Fr catheter. A fluid challenge of 10 to 25 mL/kg is administered to the hypotensive patients, and the response is assessed. Patients with hypovolemia due to hemorrhage should undergo early blood and blood product resuscitation rather than crystalloid infusion, with early activation of a massive transfusion protocol. Persistent hypotension despite active blood product resuscitation should prompt early surgical intervention for control.

In patients with nonhemorrhagic shock, an initial crystalloid therapeutic challenge helps determine the extent of volume loss. If the blood pressure normalizes and stabilizes, the volume loss is relatively small, and isotonic fluid may suffice. If the increase in blood pressure is transient after fluid bolus, then hemorrhage or continued fluid losses should be considered. Persistent hypotension without evidence of hemorrhage requires a careful assessment of other shock etiologies, including septic, neurogenic, and cardiac with the potential need for vasopressor support.

Crystalloids

Balanced salt solutions are commonly used in resuscitation, significantly reducing the need for transfusions in mild-to-moderate hemorrhagic shock. Balanced salt solutions, such as Lactated Ringer and Plasma-Lyte, are isotonic and readily available. They rapidly replace the depleted interstitial fluid compartment and do not aggravate any preexisting electrolyte abnormalities. Normal saline is also effective for hypovolemic resuscitation, though the risk of hypernatremic, hyperchloremic metabolic acidosis with large volumes should be considered.

Colloids

Colloids theoretically increase colloid oncotic pressure and require smaller volumes for resuscitation compared to crystalloids. Common colloids for volume expansion in hypovolemia include albumin, dextran 70, dextran 40, and hydroxyethyl starch. Despite their unique properties, routine use of colloids over balanced salt solutions is not justified and may increase mortality risk, especially with hydroxyethyl starch.[32]

Albumin is used during resuscitation to increase colloid oncotic pressure and, hypothetically, to protect the lung from interstitial edema. However, it rapidly crosses pulmonary capillaries and is quickly cleared within the lymphatics, thus prolonging the resuscitation phase and delaying postresuscitation diuresis. It may also depress immunoglobulin levels and suppress albumin synthesis.

Dextran 40 (10%) is hyperoncotic and initially exerts a volume-expanding effect but is rapidly excreted, making it useful for peripheral vascular disease and hyperviscosity syndromes. Dextran 70 (6%), conversely, provides greater volume expansion lasting up to 48 hours but can decrease platelet adhesiveness and decreased factor VIII activity, with allergic reactions in up to 5% and anaphylaxis in 0.6% of cases.[33]

Hydroxyethyl starch, an amylopectin, expands volume for about 36 hours and has fewer side effects than dextran. Its newer version, pentastarch, has a shorter duration (2.5 hours) and even fewer side effects.

The debate between crystalloids and colloids in resuscitation continues. Both restore circulating volume, but crystallized decreased plasma oncotic pressure, leading to lung edema at lower pressures, while colloids can extravasate during pulmonary injury, promoting edema. A meta-analysis indicated higher mortality in colloid resuscitated patients due to pulmonary complications.[34] Therefore, colloids are not currently recommended over crystalloids for managing hypovolemic shock.

Resuscitative Strategy

7 Aggressive fluid resuscitation is clearly a lifesaving modality and a key strategy in the treatment of shock and prevention of secondary consequences. However, resuscitation is not a substitute for early hemorrhage control, and indiscriminate fluid loading causes problematic edema in the lungs, gut, brain, and other organs. It can also worsen the bleeding due to dislodgement of fresh clot, thrombocytopenia, coagulopathy, and hemodilution.

Permissive Hypotension

Elevation of systemic arterial pressure in patients with disruption of the arterial system or major solid organ injury, especially after penetrating trauma, may cause acceleration of hemorrhage, disrupt natural clotting mechanisms, and cause dilution of clotting factors. Current evidence supports the judicious use of fluid resuscitation until hemorrhage is controlled by surgery, angiography, or direct pressure for penetrating trauma.[35] Aggressive fluid resuscitation before hemorrhage control has been demonstrated to worsen outcomes by increasing blood loss. As a result, current guidelines recommend maintaining a systolic blood pressure between 80 to 90 mm Hg in these patients to limit further bleeding until definitive control of the hemorrhage is achieved.

Fluid resuscitation for patients with multisystem blunt trauma, especially with concomitant traumatic brain injury (TBI), presents a more complex decision process. In such cases, maintaining cerebral perfusion pressure is crucial to prevent secondary brain injury. Balancing the need to avoid hypotension, which can worsen TBI, with the risk of exacerbating hemorrhage requires careful monitoring and often a tailored approach based on the patient's condition.

The avoidance of both excessive fluid administration and prolonged hypoperfusion is best achieved in all patients by rapid surgical or angiographic intervention to control bleeding. Current protocols now emphasize the importance of early and aggressive hemorrhage control strategies, including the use of hemostatic agents and damage control surgery, to improve survival rates and outcomes in patients in shock due to hemorrhage.

Transfusion

Anemia can indicate blood loss or hematologic disease but rarely leads to tissue ischemia. Hemoglobin levels causing concern should be based on the adequacy of oxygen delivery mechanisms, such as arterial oxygen saturation and CO, specific clinical situations, and the organs most at risk, balanced against the risk of transfusion. Current evidence suggests that hemoglobin values above 7 g/dL are adequate for most patients, including the critically ill, although this has not been thoroughly explored in patients in shock, or with active bleeding.

Hemoglobin Thresholds and Clinical Evidence

For most patients, including the elderly with significant cardiac disease, a restrictive transfusion strategy (transfusion trigger of hemoglobin level of 7 g/dL) is typically sufficient.[36] In critically ill patients, a prospective randomized trial demonstrated a reduction in complications and improved survival with lower hemoglobin values, though this study excluded patients with hypovolemia, active bleeding, acute coronary syndrome, and sepsis.

Shock and Resuscitation

In patients with class I or II shock, balanced salt solutions alone can often be resuscitated without the need for blood. However, patients who lose more than 25% to 30% of total blood volume or have persistent inadequate end-organ perfusion require blood transfusions. The urgency of the situation determines the extent of blood cross-matching before transfusion. Fully typed and cross-matched blood carries the least risk of transfusion reactions but takes the longest to obtain. Other options include using type O or type-specific blood (**Table 7.4**).

Type O Blood

Type O blood, the universal donor, is available without a crossmatch and is relatively safe for all patients. Males can receive type O Rh-positive blood, while prepubescent females and females of childbearing age should receive type O Rh-negative blood to avoid sensitization complications in future pregnancies. More than four units of type O blood to a non–type-O blood patient can result in an admixture of blood type. A pretransfusion blood specimen should be sent to the blood bank upon patient admission, and type-specific blood should be transfused as soon as available

Type-Specific Blood

Type-specific blood is available from most blood banks within 5 to 10 minutes after receiving a blood specimen. Though not cross-matched, this blood can be administered safely, as demonstrated in both military and civilian experiences.[37]

Whole Blood

Recent studies highlight the benefits of early whole blood (WB) transfusions in injured patients, significantly improving survival rates at 24 hours and 30 days postinjury.[38] Despite these potential benefits, only a minority of trauma centers currently use WB. Early administration, ideally within minutes of injury, shows the most significant reduction in mortality. As a result, WB should be considered as part of the resuscitation of hemorrhagic shock, if available.

Autotransfusion

Autotransfusion involves collecting and reinfusing shed blood through a filter. This can range from simple systems to more elaborate systems, which deliver washed, packed red blood cells. Benefits include using warm, compatible blood with no delays or risk of transmitting blood-borne pathogens. However, autotransfused blood can lead to complications like disseminated intravascular coagulation and bacterial contamination from enteric-injured cavities. Despite its benefits, autotransfusion is underutilized, with no evidence suggesting it improves outcomes compared to homologous blood transfusions.[39]

Endpoints of Resuscitation

Endpoints of resuscitation can be categorized as either global or regional indicators of perfusion. Blood pressure and pulse are global measures and are relatively poor determinants of tissue oxygenation. They must be interpreted in the context of the patient's age and preexisting medical conditions. Tachycardia, part of SIRS, does not always resolve with increased preload. Arterial pressure is maintained by various compensatory mechanisms and is influenced by baseline pressures, age, and preexisting medical conditions.

Base deficit and serum lactate are also global indicators that help detect compensated shock. Acidosis from regional tissues may not appear in peripheral blood, as seen in patients with intestinal ischemia, where systemic acidosis is a late finding. Elevated base deficit and lactate can result from electrolyte abnormalities, accelerated glycolysis, or decreased liver clearance. They may also indicate resolved dysfunction from past hypoperfusion. A positive correction response indicates effective resuscitation, particularly for base deficit over lactate.[40]

Table 7.4. Comparison of Blood Availability

Blood	Typing	Antibody Screen	Cross-Match	Time
Type O	No	No	No	Immediate
Type Specific	Yes	No	No	<10 min
Type and Screen	Yes	Yes	Yes	20–30 min
Type and Cross-Match	Yes	Yes	Yes	45–60 min

Central venous oxygen saturation ($ScvO_2$) helps to assess the balance between oxygen delivery and consumption. It is measured from the superior vena cava (SVC) and reflects the amount of oxygen returning to the heart. During resuscitation, maintaining an adequate ScvO2 indicates that tissues are receiving adequate oxygen, which is crucial for preventing progressive organ dysfunction and improving outcomes in critically ill patients. It helps guide fluid therapy, inotropes, and other interventions to optimize hemodynamic status and oxygen delivery.[41]

Resuscitation adequacy can also be assessed by end-organ function and perfusion. Blood flow to vital organs (brain and heart) is preserved during shock, sacrificing flow to the skin, muscles, gut, and kidneys. Detecting ischemia in less vital organs can identify compensated shock despite normal global indicators.

Low urine output (<0.5 to 1.0 mL/kg/h) indicates inadequate end-organ perfusion, though it may initially be maintained by peripheral vasoconstriction and tachycardia-maintained CO. Gastric tonometry to measure intramucosal pH highlights uneven shock recovery by visceral organs. Persistent visceral hypoperfusion, shown by intramucosal acidosis despite normal hemodynamics, is linked to organ failure and poor outcomes. Measuring visceral hypoperfusion is challenging due to labor-intensive, unreliable devices not widely used.

Several biomarkers show promise, including procalcitonin for the early recognition of sepsis. However, in addition to being significantly elevated during sepsis, procalcitonin has recently been demonstrated, like lactate and base deficit, to be prognostic of outcomes from hypovolemia based on the rate of clearance.[42] Thus, this biomarker, along with potential others, may lead to early recognition and treatment of shock.

MONITORS

Central Venous Pressure

CVP is used to estimate venous return to the right heart and preload, which is crucial in shock management. Measured via a central venous catheter positioned at the cavoatrial junction, CVP helps guide fluid resuscitation. Despite limitations and debates about its efficacy, CVP goals of 8 to 12 mm Hg are incorporated in specific resuscitation protocols, such as sepsis, though recent studies question the survival benefits of such targets.[43] CVP is most useful at its extremes and when evaluated within the clinical context, such as in hypovolemic shock indicated by a CVP <5 mm Hg, or in cases of congestive heart failure where a CVP of 15 mm Hg needs further context for proper assessment. As such, CVP is one measure that can help to guide shock resuscitation when evaluated in the proper context.

Pulmonary Artery Catheter

The PAC was once a standard in shock treatment but is now questioned due to studies linking its use with increased mortality and potential data misinterpretation by clinicians. Nearly half of the physicians in a study struggled to determine wedge pressure or identify oxygen delivery determinants correctly. Improved outcomes have been observed in ICUs staffed by critical care specialists who frequently use PACs. However, complications such as endocarditis and pulmonary artery injury are associated with PACs, raising concerns about their overall benefit.

Minimally Invasive CO Monitors

Newer cardiac monitoring devices like LiDCO, PiCCO, and FlowTrac require arterial lines to measure CO and PPV. The LiDCO device combines pulse contour analysis with lithium dilution for SV measurement and continuous CO calculation. The PiCCO device uses pulse contour analysis and transpulmonary thermodilution but requires both central and arterial lines. The FlowTrac device relies on the linear relationship between pulse pressure and SV, offering good correlation with PAC without needing external calibration, except during severe radial artery vasoconstriction.

Arterial Wave Contour Analysis

Analysis of the arterial wave contour in mechanically ventilated patients helps predict fluid responsiveness. Positive-pressure ventilation increases intrathoracic pressure, decreasing venous return to the right heart, left ventricular preload, SV, and CO. This effect is more pronounced in hypovolemic patients, with a PPV greater than 12.5% indicating fluid responsiveness.[44] This method is dynamic and provides more information than static measures like CVP or PCWP.

Bedside Ultrasound and Echocardiography

Improved ultrasound technology has enhanced its use in emergency and critical care settings. Noninvasive, real-time, and reproducible, ultrasound provides valuable information on ventricular function and volume status. It can identify pericardial effusion and tamponade physiology. Ultrasound is also useful in assessing volume status and fluid responsiveness, with measurements of the SVC, IVC, and left ventricular stroke area (LVSA) guiding resuscitation. IVC measurement via bedside ultrasound is particularly useful in trauma and shock settings, with an IVC diameter of <1 cm indicating fluid responsiveness.

Future Monitoring Devices

Recent advancements in hemodynamic monitoring include both invasive and noninvasive technologies, enhancing accuracy and ease of use. Capillary refill time (CRT) is effective in assessing circulatory efficiency, especially in septic shock resuscitation, and continuous noninvasive arterial pressure technology (CNAP) offers dynamic parameters for better surgical and emergency care.

PHARMACEUTICAL SUPPORT

Therapeutic adjustments of preload and afterload form the basis of treatment strategies in all forms of shock. Optimal volume resuscitation should always precede measures to augment the contractile function of the heart. Inotropic augmentation of CO may, therefore, be required when restoration of venous preload fails to provide sufficient CO to satisfy tissue oxygen demands. The effect of inotropic agents depends on the specific adrenergic receptor affinity, chronotropic effects, and demands placed on myocardial oxygen consumption of the individual agents (**Table 7.5**). Vasodilators reduce demands on the myocardium and augment cardiac function via reduction in systemic vascular resistance (SVR) or afterload or by dilating the venous system and reducing cardiac preload. Afterload reduction may preserve SV in the face of a failing myocardium, whereas venodilation reduces pulmonary capillary wedge pressure and pressure-driven pulmonary edema. Agents that increase afterload may be needed when blood pressure falls below the autoregulatory range of the coronary, cerebral, and renal vascular beds.

Inotropes and Vasopressors

Dopamine

Dopamine is an endogenous amine, precursor to epinephrine, and functions as a neurotransmitter. Its effects vary by dose: low doses (<2 to 3 μg/kg/min) increase renal blood flow and urine output without preventing acute renal failure. Moderate doses (3 to 5 μg/kg/min) increase heart contractility and rate. High doses (>5 μg/kg/min) increase heart rate and blood pressure, and doses >10 μg/kg/min elevate blood pressure and peripheral resistance. Individual titration is required to achieve desired effects.

Dobutamine

Dobutamine, a synthetic catecholamine, targets β-adrenergic receptors. At 5 to 20 μg/kg/min, it enhances myocardial

Table 7.5. Pharmacodynamics of Inotropic/Vasoconstrictor Agents

		Sites of Action				Hemodynamic Response			
Drug	**Metabolism**	**Heart β_1**	**Heart β_2**	**Vessels α**	**Vessels β_2**	**Renal Perfusion**	**CO**	**SVR**	**BP**
Isoproterenol 1 mg/250 mL 1–2 µg/min initially	Renal	+++	+++	0	+++	+/–		–	+/–
Dobutamine 250 mg/250 mL 3 µg/kg/min initially	Hepatic	+++	0/+	0/+	0/+			–	0/+
Dopamine 200 mg/250 mL 2–5 µg/kg/min low dose 20–50 µg/kg/min high dose	Hepatic	+++	+	0	Low dose High dose		Low dose High dose	0/+	
Epinephrine 2 mg/250 mL 2 µg/min initially	Renal	+++	+++	+++	++	–		–	
Norepinephrine 4 mg/250 mL 4 µg/min initially	Renal	++	++	+++	0	–	+/–		
Phenylephrine	Renal	0	0	+++	0	–	–		

α (alpha), vasoconstrict peripheral arterioles; β_1 (beta-1), myocardial inotropy, chronotropy, enhance atrioventricular conduction; β_2 (beta-2), chronotropy, vasodilate mesenteric/skeletal bed, bronchodilation; dopaminergic, vasodilate mesenteric/renal bed.
BP, blood pressure; CO, cardiac output; SVR, systemic vascular resistance.

contractility and causes peripheral vasodilation, making it suitable for increasing CO without raising blood pressure. It's ideal for cardiogenic shock postmyocardial infarction or cardiac dysfunction requiring contractility support and peripheral resistance reduction.

Epinephrine

Epinephrine, released during stress, has significant cardiovascular effects. At 0.01 to 0.05 µg/kg/min, it predominantly stimulates β1-adrenergic receptors, increasing SV, heart rate, and contractility. Higher doses stimulate α-adrenergic receptors, increasing blood pressure and SVR but can cause renal and splanchnic vasoconstriction, dysrhythmias, and increased oxygen demand. It's a short-term option for impaired cardiac function not responsive to dobutamine.

Norepinephrine

Norepinephrine predominantly has α-constrictor effects with some β-stimulation, suitable for hypotensive patients unresponsive to dopamine. It increases afterload and renal perfusion, preserving CO. It's associated with increased urine output and creatinine clearance in septic patients. Adequate volume resuscitation is essential to avoid tissue damage from excessive vasoconstriction in hypovolemic patients.

Isoproterenol

Isoproterenol, a synthetic catecholamine, has potent β-adrenergic effects, increasing heart contractility, rate, and conduction, with significant chronotropic response and peripheral vasodilation, increasing CO and pulse pressure. It's indicated for significant bradyarrhythmias while preparing for electrical pacing.

Phenylephrine

Phenylephrine, a pure α-agonist, increases peripheral vascular resistance and arterial blood pressure without directly affecting the myocardium. It increases left ventricular work and oxygen demand, potentially reducing SV and CO. It is often used in neurogenic shock or for hypotensive patients who can't tolerate increased doses of other agents.

Vasopressin

Vasopressin acts on V_1 receptors to cause vasoconstriction and enhances vascular response to catecholamines. Effective in increasing SVR and mean arterial pressure in septic shock, it doesn't have inotropic properties but can cause splanchnic and coronary vasoconstriction, potentially decreasing CO and worsening acidosis. Early use at physiologic doses may reduce the need for other pressors.

Amrinone and Milrinone

Amrinone and milrinone, noncatecholamine inotropes, enhance cardiac contractility and output with minimal chronotropic effect by inhibiting phosphodiesterase and increasing cAMP. They reduce afterload, making them useful for cardiogenic shock or as dobutamine alternatives. Their long half-lives necessitate caution in hypotensive patients.

Vasodilators

Vasodilators are used to augment cardiac function through optimization of preload and afterload, both of which reduce demands on the myocardium. The failing ventricle responds to afterload reduction with significant increases in SV. The reason for this is that the compromised myocardium is working past the plateau and on the down slope of the Starling curve. As a result, afterload reduction with vasodilator agents may allow CO to increase, resulting in improved oxygen delivery.

Nitroprusside

Nitroprusside is a balanced but potent arterial and venous smooth muscle vasodilator. It causes a reduction in afterload that increases CO and has a less prominent venodilatory effect that reduces pulmonary venous pressure and preload. Hypotension may limit its use, particularly in the presence of contractility deficits or inadequate preload. Infusions (>3 μg/kg/min) continued for greater than 48 hours require monitoring of serum thiocyanate levels and arterial pH to detect complications of cyanide toxicity.

Nitroglycerin

Nitroglycerin is primarily a venous smooth muscle vasodilator, with less significant arterial vasodilation effects than nitroprusside. Thus, although nitroprusside predominantly decreases afterload, nitroglycerin predominantly increases venous capacitance. It is an effective treatment for acute myocardial ischemia because it reduces excessive preload and ventricular end-diastolic pressure, thereby diminishing myocardial oxygen demand.

Miscellaneous Therapeutics

Corticosteroids

In shock, ACTH resistance may diminish the normal cortisol response. As a result of this hypoadrenal response, the administration of physiologic concentrations of corticosteroids may be appropriate in selected patients. However, this should only be considered in patients who have achieved adequate intravascular volume but remain in shock despite high vasopressor administration. Therefore, the use of corticosteroids at only physiologic doses, with immediate tapering once hemodynamics has improved, should be used with caution.

Metabolites and Electrolytes

Severe shock is frequently associated with hypocalcemia, which, if causing cardiac dysfunction or electrical instability, should be treated rapidly. Calcium chloride quickly corrects calcium deficits, while calcium gluconate acts slower but has fewer tissue reaction risks. Without cardiac dysfunction, restoring plasma calcium during shock isn't necessary, as ischemia decreases cell membrane ATP and calcium pump function.

Reduced serum calcium in severe shock likely results from ionized calcium moving into cells. Increased cytosolic calcium releases lysosomal enzymes and activates phospholipases, protein kinases, and proteases, damaging membranes and cytoskeletons. Administering exogenous calcium may worsen this intracellular calcium influx, while effective resuscitation typically normalizes circulating calcium levels.

Electrolyte imbalances in shock, including potassium, magnesium, and calcium, must be closely monitored and corrected. In septic shock, balanced crystalloid solutions like Lactated Ringer or Plasma-Lyte are preferred over normal saline, as they better mimic plasma composition and improve outcomes.

Shock resuscitation protocols often focus on correcting metabolic acidosis with fluids and inotropes. An anion gap indicates lactic acidosis, whereas non–anion-gap acidosis with a worsening base deficit can occur from large volumes of normal saline. Correcting non–anion-gap acidosis with unnecessary fluids risks fluid overload.

Future Therapies

When initiating therapy for shock, clinicians often face uncertainty regarding whether the treatment is started early enough to allow for recovery or too late when irreversible cellular damage has occurred. Failure to respond to fluids, inotropes, and vasopressors with the restoration of normal oxygen consumption and aerobic metabolism likely indicates a defect in cellular and subcellular functions within critical organ systems. Recent advances reflect a deeper understanding of shock and are moving the field beyond the basics of fluid resuscitation and hemodynamic monitoring.

Efforts to control ischemia–reperfusion injury include controlled reperfusion with carbon monoxide or other compounds to reduce oxidative stress. Induced hypothermia may interrupt the generation of harmful byproducts of ischemia, allowing the restoration of circulation and repair of structural injuries in a less critically hypoxic environment. New biomarkers, such as procalcitonin, may facilitate early diagnosis and treatment of sepsis and shock. Innovative biosensors using near-infrared light may enable transcutaneous identification of blood flow limitations, allowing clinicians to target areas of regional hypoperfusion more accurately.[45]

Research is ongoing to find agents that optimize microvascular circulation by preventing endothelial activation. Such agents could enhance resuscitative efforts by ensuring that oxygen reaches cells as needed for normal respiration and nutrient supply. Further understanding of functional genomics could eventually allow clinicians to target transcriptional and translational events triggered by shock, potentially altering patient outcomes.

SCIENTIFIC PRINCIPLES

References

1. Cannon WB. Pharmacological injections and physiological inferences. *Science.* 1929;70(1821):500–501.
2. Blalock A, Mason MF. Blood and blood substitutes in the treatment and prevention of shock: with particular reference to their uses in warfare. *Ann Surg.* 1941;113(5):657–676.
3. Wiggers HC, Ingraham RC. Hemorrhagic shock: definition and criteria for its diagnosis. *J Clin Invest.* 1946;25(1):30–36.
4. Weil MH, Shubin H. Proposed reclassification of shock states with special reference to distributive defects. *Adv Exp Med Biol.* 1971;23(0):13–23.
5. Haider AA, Azim A, Rhee P, et al. Substituting systolic blood pressure with shock index in the National Trauma Triage Protocol. *J Trauma Acute Care Surg.* 2016;81(6):1136–1141.
6. Chaterjee K. The Swan-Ganz Catheter: past, present, and future: a viewpoint. *Circulation.* 2009;119(1):147–152.
7. Vitek V, Cowley RA. Blood lactate in the prognosis of various forms of shock. *Ann Surg.* 1971;173(2):308–313.
8. Davis JW, Shackford SR, Holbrook TL. Base deficit as a sensitive indicator of compensated shock and tissue oxygen utilization. *Surg Gynecol Obstet.* 1991;173(6):473–476.
9. Davis JW, Shackford SR, Mackersie RC, Hoyt DB. Base deficit as a guide to volume resuscitation. *J Trauma.* 1988;28(10):1464–1467.
10. Mira JC, Cuschieri J, Ozrazgat-Baslanti T, et al. The epidemiology of chronic critical illness after severe traumatic injury at two level-one trauma centers. *Crit Care Med.* 2017;45(12):1989–1996.
11. American College of Surgeons. *Advanced Trauma Life Support for Doctors: Student Course Manual.* 8th ed. American College of Surgeons; 2008.
12. Rahod KS, Sirker A, Baumbach A, Mathur A, Jones DA. Management of cardiogenic shock in patients with acute coronary syndromes. *Br J Hosp Med.* 2019;80(4):204–210.
13. Lee J, Levy MM. Treatment of patients with severe sepsis and septic shock: current evidence-based practices. *R I Med J.* 2019;102(10):18–21.
14. Kollef MH. Broad-spectrum antimicrobials and the treatment of serious bacterial infections: getting it right up front. *Clin Infect Dis.* 2008;47(suppl 1):S3–S13.
15. Brakenridge SC, Wang Z, Cox M, et al. Distinct immunologic endotypes are associated with clinical trajectory after severe blunt trauma and hemorrhagic shock. *J Trauma Acute Care Surg.* 2021;90(2):257–267.
16. Winfield RD, Delano MJ, Dixon DJ, et al. Differences in outcome between obese and nonobese patients following severe blunt trauma are not consistent with an early inflammatory genomic response. *Crit Care Med.* 2010;38(1):51–58.
17. Peters J, Mack GW, Lister G. The importance of the peripheral circulation in critical illnesses. *Intensive Care Med.* 2001;27(9):1446–1458.
18. Barie PS, Hydo LJ. Epidemiology of multiple organ dysfunction syndrome in critical surgical illness. *Surg Infect (Larchmt).* 2000;1(3):173–185; discussion 185–186.
19. Bhatia M, Moochhala S. Role of inflammatory mediators in the pathophysiology of acute respiratory distress syndrome. *J Pathol.* 2004;202(2):145–156.

20. Imahara SD, O'Keefe GE. Genetic determinants of the inflammatory response. *Curr Opin Crit Care.* 2004;10(5):318–324.
21. Shalhub S, Junker CE, Imahara SD, Mindrinos MN, Dissanaike S, O'Keefe GE. Variation in the TLR4 gene influences the risk of organ failure and shock posttrauma: a cohort study. *J Trauma.* 2009;66(1):115–122.
22. Xiao W, Mindrinos MN, Seok J, et al; Inflammation and Host Response to Injury Large-Scale Collaborative Research Program. A genomic storm in critically injured humans. *J Exp Med.* 2011;208(13):2581–2590.
23. Huber-Lang M, Lambris JD, Ward PA. Innate immune responses to trauma. *Nature Immunology.* 2018;19:327–341.
24. Gentilello LM. Advances in the management of hypothermia. *Surg Clin North Am.* 1995;75(2):243–256.
25. Stoner HB. Studies on the mechanism of shock. The impairment of thermoregulation by trauma. *Br J Exp Pathol.* 1969;50(2):125–138.
26. Gubler KD, Gentilello LM, Hassantash SA, Maier RV. The impact of hypothermia on dilutional coagulopathy. *J Trauma.* 1994;36(6):847–851.
27. Roberts I, Shakur H, Coats T, et al. The CRASH-2 trial: a randomized controlled trial and economic evaluation of the effects of tranexamic acid on death, vascular occlusive events and transfusion requirement in bleeding trauma patients. *Health Technol Assess.* 2013;17(10):1–79.
28. Drotarova M, Zolkova J, Belakova KM, et al. Basic Principles of Rotational Thromboelastometry (ROTEM®) and the role of ROTEM-guided fibrinogen replacement therapy in the management of coagulopathies. *Diagnostics (Basel).* 2023;13(20):3219.
29. Holcomb JB, Tilley BC, Baraniuk S, et al; PROPPR Study Group. Transfusion of plasma, platelets, and red blood cells in a 1:1:1 vs a 1:1:2 ratio and mortality in patients with severe trauma: the PROPPR randomized clinical trial. *JAMA.* 2015;313(5):471–482.
30. Robinson BRH, Cohen MJ, Holcomb JB, et al; PROPPR Study Group. Risk factors for the development of acute respiratory distress syndrome following hemorrhage. *Shock.* 2018;50(3):258–264.
31. Gonzalez EA, Moore FA. Resuscitation beyond the abdominal compartment syndrome. *Curr Opin Crit Care.* 2010;16(6):570–574.
32. Perner A, Haase N, Guttomsen AB, et al; 6S Trial Group:Scandinavian Critical Care Trials Group. Hydroxethyl starch 130/0.42 versus Ringer's acetate in severe sepsis. *N Engl J Med.* 2012;367(2):124–134.
33. London MJ, Ho JS, Triedman JK, et al. A randomized clinical trial of 10% pentastarch (low molecular weight hydroxyethyl starch) versus 5% albumin for plasma volume expansion after cardiac operations. *J Thorac Cardiovasc Surg.* 1989;97(5):785–797.
34. Finfer S, Bellomo R, Boyce N, French J, Myburgh J, Norton R; SAFE Study Investigators. A comparison of albumin and saline for fluid resuscitation in the intensive care unit. *N Engl J Med.* 2004;350(22):2247–2256.
35. Tran A, Yates J, Lau A, Lampron J, Matar M. Permissive hypotension versus conventional resuscitation strategies in adult trauma patients with hemorrhagic shock: a systematic review and meta-analysis of randomized controlled trials. *J Trauma Acute Care Surg.* 2018;84(5):802–808.
36. Hebert PC, Wells G, Blajchman MA, et al. A multicenter, randomized, controlled clinical trial of transfusion requirements in critical care. Transfusion requirements in critical care investigators, Canadian Critical Care Trials Group. *N Engl J Med.* 1999;340(6):409–417.
37. Gervin AS, Fischer RP. Resuscitation of trauma patients with type-specific uncrossmatched blood. *J Trauma.* 1984;24(4):327–331.
38. Torres CM, Zenzik KM, Saillant NN, et al. Timing to first whole blood transfusion and survival following severe hemorrhage in trauma patients. *JAMA Surg.* 2024;159(4):374–381.
39. Jurkovich GJ, Moore EE, Medina G. Autotransfusion in trauma. A pragmatic analysis. *Am J Surg.* 1984;148(6):782–785.
40. Davis JW, Dirks RC, Kaups KL, Tran P. Base deficit is superior to lactate in trauma. *Am J Surg.* 2018;215(4):682–685.
41. Dueck MH, Klimek M, Appenrodt S, Weigand C, Boerner U. Trends but not individual values of central venous oxygen saturation agree with mixed venous oxygen saturation during varying hemodynamic conditions. *Anesthesiology.* 2005;103(2):249–257.
42. Seligman R, Meisner M, Lisboa TC, et al. Decreases in procalcitonin and C-reactive protein are strong predictors of survival in ventilator-associated pneumonia. *Crit Care.* 2006;10(5):R125.
43. Boyd JH, Forbes J, Nakada T, Walley KR, Russell JA. Fluid resuscitation in septic shock: a positive fluid balance and elevated central venous pressure are associated with increased mortality. *Crit Care Med.* 2011;39:259–265.
44. Alvarado Sánchez JI, Caicedo Ruiz JD, Diaztagle Fernández JJ, Amaya Zuñiga WF, Ospina-Tascón GA, Cruz Martínez LE. Predictors of fluid responsiveness in critically ill patients mechanically ventilated at low tidal volumes: systematic review and meta-analysis. *Ann Intensive Care.* 2021;11(1):28.
45. Hopf HW. Molecular diagnostics of injury and repair responses in critical illness: what is the future of "monitoring" in the intensive care unit? *Crit Care Med.* 2003;31(suppl 8):S518–S523.

8

Critical Care

William C. Chiu and Samuel A. Tisherman

SCIENTIFIC PRINCIPLES

Key Points

1. In 1957, Peter Safar from the Baltimore City Hospital Department of Anesthesiology (later from the University of Pittsburgh School of Medicine), first reported on his new technique of mouth-to-mouth respiration using an artificial airway, leading to the development of cardiopulmonary resuscitation (CPR). In 1958, the first "intensive care unit" (ICU) was established at the Baltimore City Hospital, to provide optimal medical and nursing care to all critically ill patients.
2. A recent systematic review and practice management guideline evaluated the use of focused echocardiography (ECHO) and pulse waveform analysis in patients with shock. The results were variable regarding the benefits of either modality in predicting fluid responsiveness, reduction in organ failure or complications, or mortality. However, the recommendations were that, in appropriate subpopulations and with adequate training in the technology, ECHO and pulse waveform analysis protocols can be associated with favorable outcomes.
3. In the recent Berlin definition of acute respiratory distress syndrome (ARDS), the ARDS spectrum is classified by the PaO_2/FiO_2 (P/F) ratio as mild (201 to 300), moderate (101 to 200), or severe (≤100). Conventional ventilatory strategies incorporate a low-stretch philosophy. Evidence-based adjunctive strategies include prone positioning, airway pressure release ventilation (APRV), inhaled prostacyclins, and extracorporeal support.
4. Venous thromboembolism (VTE) is a significant problem in surgical ICU patients and chemical prophylaxis beneficially impacts outcome. A recent systematic review and meta-analysis showed that low–molecular-weight heparin (LMWH) is probably more effective than unfractionated heparin (UFH) in reducing incidence of deep vein thrombosis (DVT), and should be considered the primary pharmacologic agent for thromboprophylaxis. Since LMWH is primarily eliminated by the kidneys, LMWH should be avoided in those with renal dysfunction. Increasing the prophylactic dose of LMWH may be appropriate in morbidly obese patients. Laboratory monitoring of anti-Xa activity should be considered when using LMWH in patients with renal impairment or obesity.
5. A conservative transfusion trigger (<7 g/dL hemoglobin) may be appropriate in most surgical ICU patients, including those with gastrointestinal bleeding, neurotrauma, cardiac disease, and sepsis. A recent systematic review and meta-analysis showed that RBC transfusions at the threshold of hemoglobin <7 g/dL did not result in significant difference in short-term mortality when compared with transfusions administered at a more liberal threshold.
6. ICU patients should receive routine assessment and adequate support of their nutritional status to preserve lean body mass, maintain immune function, and avert metabolic complications. Enteral nutrition is strongly preferred over parenteral nutrition. The most recent recommendations for prophylaxis against stress-related gastrointestinal bleeding (SRGIB) suggest using either proton pump inhibitors or histamine-2 antagonists for patients with coagulopathy, shock, or chronic liver disease. Mechanical ventilation alone may not be a significant risk factor.
7. Acute kidney injury (AKI) is a common complication in the ICU and is associated with worse outcomes. Rapid restoration of normal hemodynamics and treatment of sepsis, as well as avoidance of nephrotoxic agents, are the best preventative measures. Both continuous and intermittent dialysis play an important role with severe AKI.
8. Successful management of sepsis requires rapid identification, appropriate cultures, early antibiotics, fluid resuscitation, and hemodynamic support with goals of normalizing perfusion. Catheter-associated infections are often preventable with proper maintenance and removal as soon as possible.
9. Delirium is common in critically ill patients and is associated with increased length of stay, increased postintensive care syndrome, and, possibly, mortality. The causes are multifactorial. Trying to maintain normal day/night cycles can help. There are no drugs that directly improve delirium. Drugs that can aggravate delirium, such as anticholinergics or benzodiazepines, should be avoided. Pharmacologic therapy is mainly useful for managing patients with hyperactive delirium with the main goal of preventing harm.

The history of intensive care dates back to the 1854 Crimean War with Florence Nightingale, the founder of professional nursing. Nightingale was known to have separated the most severely injured soldiers into close proximity to the nursing station to provide more intensive care. During the 1952 poliomyelitis epidemic in Denmark, Bjorn Ibsen advanced the concept of artificial respiration outside the operating room in a special department at the University of Copenhagen. The majority of severe polio patients treated with the standard iron lung negative-pressure respirator tanks were still dying.

The new strategy employed was that patients with paralysis and respiratory failure underwent tracheotomy and manual intermittent positive-pressure ventilation performed by medical students at bedside in 6-hour shifts.

1 In 1957, Peter Safar from the Baltimore City Hospital Department of Anesthesiology (later from the University of Pittsburgh School of Medicine), first reported on his new technique of mouth-to-mouth respiration using an artificial airway, leading to the development of cardiopulmonary resuscitation (CPR). In 1958, the first "intensive care unit" (ICU) was established at the Baltimore City Hospital, to provide optimal medical and nursing care to all critically ill patients. This ICU maintained early emphasis on airway, ventilation, and resuscitation. Also in 1958, cardiologists Max Harry Weil and Herbert Shubin created the Shock Ward at the Los Angeles County General Hospital of the University of Southern California. This unit had early emphasis on acute circulatory failure and hemodynamics, employing new continuous monitoring techniques and physiologic measurements to manage patients with life-threatening critical illness. This evolving concept of multidisciplinary patient care with medicine, anesthesiology, surgery, nursing, and various collaborators would come to be known as the modern-day ICU.

While patients admitted to the ICU make up a large proportion of hospital cost and resources, estimated to be roughly 1% of gross domestic product, both surgical and medical ICUs continue to find themselves understaffed. The supply of critical care practitioners is inadequate and the demand is extensive, largely from aging patients with complex comorbidities undergoing complicated procedures. There are approximately 3000 board-certified surgical intensivists with less than 200 completing training annually, most of whom do not practice critical care exclusively. In the United States, these surgical intensivists serve largely in surgical specialty units of academic medical centers that account for approximately 10% to 15% of the nearly 6500 ICUs with roughly 100,000 beds and 5 million admissions annually. The largest growing demographic in hospitals and ICUs is the group over 65 years of age, now accounting for over half of all admissions.[1]

HEMODYNAMIC MONITORING

Oxygen Transport

The transport of oxygen to the microcirculation and tissues is mediated by four general parameters: (1) arterial oxygen content (CaO_2), (2) rate of oxygen delivery (DO_2) to tissues, (3) rate of oxygen uptake from tissues, and (4) fraction of oxygen in blood that is extracted by tissues. DO_2, the rate at which oxygen is transported to the microcirculation, is the product of cardiac output (CO) and CaO_2 and is normally about 1000 mL/min. DO_2 falls in instances of cardiac failure, hypovolemia, and anemia, but less so due to poor oxygenation. Oxygen consumption (VO_2), the rate at which oxygen is removed from the blood by the microcirculation, is the product of CO and the arteriovenous O_2 difference and is normally 250 mL/min in an average adult. The oxygen extraction (OE) ratio or the ratio of VO_2 to DO_2 is normally about 25%. The myocardium has the body's highest extraction ratio at approximately 75%. VO_2 remains constant over a wide range of DO_2 by changes in OE. For example, in situations of decreased DO_2 such as hemorrhagic or cardiogenic shock, VO_2 can be maintained by increasing extraction ratio. This mechanism may be altered in critically ill patients who show marked increases in VO_2 under the influence of stress hormones and catecholamines.

To evaluate the balance between systemic DO_2 and VO_2, the oxygen saturation of hemoglobin in mixed venous blood can be assessed. Mixed venous blood is obtained from the pulmonary artery using a pulmonary artery catheter (PAC) and reflects the final destination of circulating blood from all tissue beds prior to reoxygenation in the lung. Mixed venous oxygen saturation (SvO_2) may be used as a measure of tissue oxygenation, and is expressed as $1 - VO_2/DO_2$, with normal values of 60% to 80% that can be continuously displayed with an oximetric PAC. Reductions in SvO_2 reflect a mismatch between DO_2 and VO_2, commonly from a reduction in DO_2 and/or an elevation in VO_2 (**Table 8.1**).

More recently, central venous blood obtained from a central venous catheter in the superior vena cava (SVC) has been a more practical source for measurement of venous saturation. The normal values of central venous oxygen saturation ($ScvO_2$) are 65% to 85%, slightly shifted up compared to SvO_2. While large studies have revealed discordant results demonstrating the utility of monitoring $ScvO_2$, for common practice we recommend that $ScvO_2$ may be used as a helpful adjunct, but not as the only endpoint of resuscitation.

Volume Assessment

Assessment of volume status and cardiac function in the critically ill patient continues to evolve. Traditional static measures of volume assessment using central venous catheters and PACs are being replaced in many settings by dynamic or functional measures such as pulse waveform analysis and focused

Table 8.1. Normal Hemodynamic Parameters

Parameter	Equation	Normal Range	Units
Oxygen delivery	$DO_2 = CO \times CaO_2 \times 10$	950–1150	mL/min
Arterial oxygen content	$CaO_2 = SaO_2 \times 0.0138 \times Hgb + 0.003 \times PaO_2$	17–20	mL/dL
Oxygen consumption	$VO_2 = CO \times (CaO_2 - CvO_2) \times 10$	200–250	mL/min
Oxygen extraction ratio	$OE = VO_2/DO_2 \times 100$	22–30	%
Mixed venous oxygen saturation	$SvO_2 = (1 - VO_2/DO_2) \times 100$	60–80	%
Cardiac output	$CO = HR \times SV/1000$	4–8	L/min
Stroke volume	$SV = CO/HR \times 1000$	60–100	mL/beat
Stroke volume variation	$SVV = (SV_{max} - SV_{min})/SV_{mean} \times 100$	10–15	%

DO_2, oxygen delivery; CO, cardiac output; CaO_2, arterial oxygen content; SaO_2, oxygen saturation; PaO_2, partial pressure of oxygen in arterial blood; VO_2, oxygen consumption; CvO_2, mixed venous oxygen content; OE, oxygen extraction; SvO_2, mixed venous oxygen saturation; HR, heart rate; SV, stroke volume; SVV, stroke volume variation.

echocardiogram (ECHO). Similarly, indirect measurement of cardiac function by PACs is being succeeded by pulse waveform analysis and systolic and diastolic evaluation of left and right regional function using ECHO.

2 A recent systematic review and practice management guideline evaluated the use of ECHO and pulse waveform analysis in patients with shock. The results were variable regarding the benefits of either modality in predicting fluid responsiveness, reduction in organ failure or complications, or mortality. However, the recommendations were that in appropriate subpopulations, and with adequate training in the technology, ECHO and pulse waveform analysis protocols can be associated with favorable outcomes.[2]

Fluid Responsiveness

The concept of volume status using static measures has evolved to "volume responsiveness" using dynamic or functional measures to assess whether a fluid bolus will improve stroke volume (SV) and cardiac performance of a critically ill patient. Static measures such as central venous pressure (CVP) and pulmonary artery occlusion pressure (PAOP) can give inferential data of cardiac filling pressures at a single time-point, which then extrapolates to cardiac preload (end-diastolic volume [EDV]) and volume status of the patient. However, these pressures can be altered depending on cardiopulmonary physiology, do not always correlate with Frank–Starling principles, and give no indication of whether the patient will respond to a fluid bolus.

Measurements of CVP and PAOP are made at end-expiration when the pleural pressure is closest to atmospheric pressure. Normal venous waveform components include the "a" wave (corresponding to right atrial contraction), the "c" wave (tricuspid valve closure and isovolumic right ventricular contraction), and the "v" wave (ventricular ejection driving venous filling of the atrium) (**Fig. 8.1**). Clinically, the high point of the "a" wave is the atrial pressure at maximum contraction, where atrial pressure is greater than ventricular diastolic pressure. Here, the right atrium is contracted and the tricuspid valve is open, which is synonymous with right ventricular end-diastolic pressure, making the ventricle, atrium, and vena cava interconnected.

The use of CVP to guide resuscitation has not been demonstrated to be beneficial in many large clinical series. A large meta-analysis revealed a very poor relationship between CVP and blood volume.[3] Additionally, several large recent trials of sepsis resuscitation demonstrated that resuscitation targeted to CVP endpoints did not improve outcome.[4,5]

PAC-based volume assessment employs the principle that a single column of fluid forms from the pulmonary artery to the left ventricle during diastole. For a given left ventricular end-diastolic pressure (LVEDP) and compliance, left ventricular end-diastolic volume (LVEDV) can be estimated. Based on the Frank–Starling principle, the force of ventricular contraction is proportional to muscle stretch and LVEDV. As PAOP estimates LVEDV for a given CO, preload may be determined. Numerous physiologic changes may alter the relationship between PAOP and LVEDV, including pulmonary vascular disease, pulmonary hypertension, acute respiratory distress syndrome (ARDS), increased intrathoracic pressure, valvular disease, and altered cardiac compliance. Finally, large clinical trials have failed to demonstrate a benefit to outcome for those resuscitated to a PAOP endpoint.

Dynamic and functional assessment of volume responsiveness include those on both the arterial and venous side of the heart. Normally, the inspiratory increase in pleural pressure during positive-pressure breathing reduces right ventricular preload and SV. Left ventricular SV reduction is maximal during expiration. These normal physiologic changes during the mechanically supported respiratory cycle are augmented with hypovolemia that is volume responsive.

Pulse waveform analysis from arterial catheter transduction is minimally invasive and uses a proprietary algorithm analysis of the arterial pressure waveform. The area under the curve corresponding to systole (ie, before the dicrotic notch) is used to calculate SV (**Fig. 8.2**). Computer calculation is made of the maximal and minimal amplitudes of the curve. In general, a stroke volume variation (SVV) of greater than 13% to 15% reflects volume responsiveness, whereas values below this threshold imply that the patient is beyond the upper inflection point of the Frank–Starling curve and will not benefit from further volume loading. There are instances where it is possible to misinterpret these values. For example, arrhythmias, high vasopressor burden, or lack of arterial compliance may alter blood flow and arterial wave morphology. However, clinical applications of SVV as a volume assessment tool have been promising.

ECHO can provide arterial and venous volume assessment with both static and dynamic values. Many static measures can be rendered functional by performing measurements before and after a passive leg raise, a maneuver that replicates volume loading. In spontaneously breathing patients, a breath results in an increase in SV and systolic pressure. Static values include measurement of the diameter of the inferior vena cava (IVC), the SVC, or the internal jugular vein

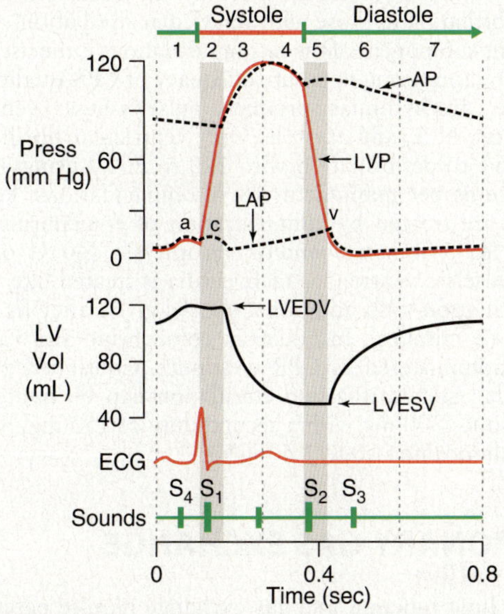

Figure 8.1. Normal venous waveform with ECG (a, c, and v waves).

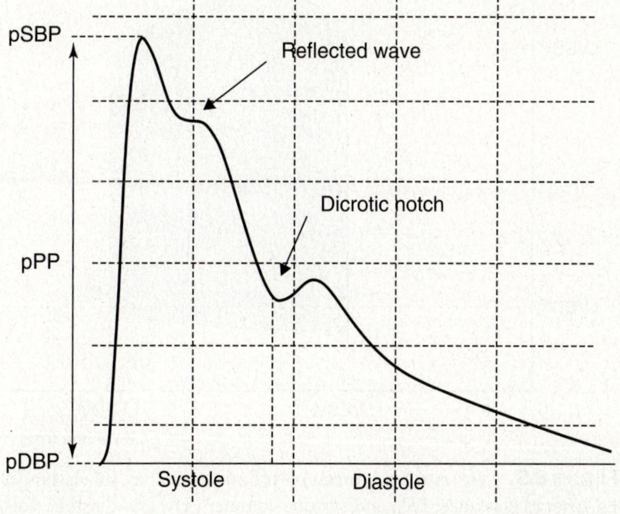

Figure 8.2. Arterial pressure waveform. Area under systole curve is used to calculate stroke volume. pSBP, peripheral systolic blood pressure; pPP, peripheral pulse pressure; pDBP, peripheral diastolic blood pressure.

SCIENTIFIC PRINCIPLES

(IJV) on the venous side or calculation of the velocity time integral (VTI) on the arterial side. Collapsibility of the IVC (or SVC/IJV) of at least 15% and as much as 50% during respiration predicts fluid responsiveness. Right heart failure may alter the size relationships of the central veins, thus providing an underestimate of fluid responsiveness using venous measurements.

In summary, ECHO, SVV, and passive leg raise are complementary tools to predict fluid responsiveness. Each technique has its own benefits and drawbacks, but in combination, depending upon local expertise, they can provide a multifaceted approach. Repeated measures during resuscitation can allow the provider to further fine tune fluid management.

Cardiac Function

Assessment of cardiac function is best understood by referring to the cardiac pressure–volume curve depicting the cardiac cycle (**Fig. 8.3**). Starting at the top right at "A," the aortic valve opens and blood is ejected into the outflow tract. At "B" systole ends as the aortic valve closes. A period of isovolumic relaxation occurs and ventricular pressure falls until the mitral valve opens at "C," the start of diastole. Diastole ends as the mitral valve closes at "D" and then there is a period of isovolumic contraction with both valves closed until the cycle repeats. Note that the distance across the box represents SV, the amount of blood ejected per heartbeat, and is determined by preload, afterload, and contractility. The product of SV and heart rate is CO. Ejection fraction (EF), a more valid estimate of cardiac function, is the proportion of preload or EDV ejected per beat or SV/EDV.

PACs determine CO by thermodilution. This technique measures temperature changes sensed by a thermistor at the distal end of the catheter after a cold saline injection through the proximal port. Based on the modified Stewart–Hamilton equation, which constructs a plot of temperature change against time, measurements of CO can be obtained. The thermodilution technique assumes that complete mixing of the blood occurs, that there is constant blood flow in the heart, and that there is no loss in concentration of the cold saline between the point of injection and the distal catheter tip. Pulse waveform analysis using an arterial catheter is now a less invasive method to measure SV and CO, with acceptable accuracy.

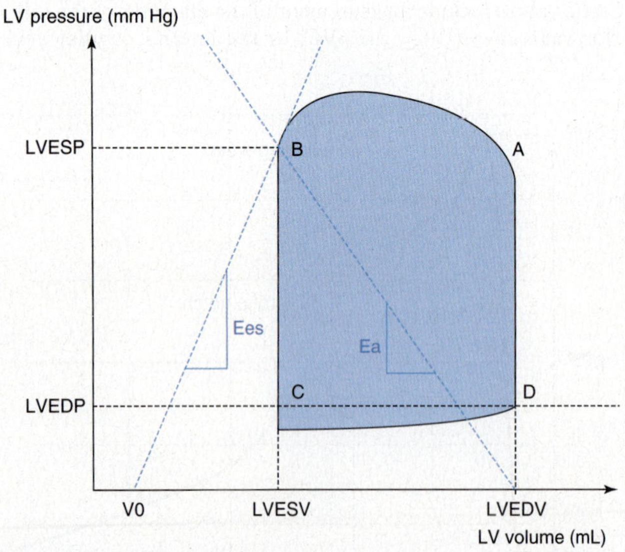

Figure 8.3. Left ventricular pressure–volume curve. Ees, LV elastance; Ea, arterial elastance; ESV, end-systolic volume; EDV, end-diastolic volume; ESP, end-systolic pressure; EDP, end-diastolic pressure; LV, left ventricle. *A* aortic valve opens; *B* aortic valve closes; *C* mitral valve opens; *D* mitral valve closes.

ECHO does not suffer from many of the shortcomings of CVP, PAC, or arterial line assessment of cardiac function, such as static measurement and requiring an invasive catheter. ECHO can provide information about heart function in a qualitative or quantitative fashion, can be used to assess left and right heart morphology and size, dynamics, can determine the difference in EF and SV, and can perform quantitative estimates of pulmonary artery and right ventricular pressure. ECHO can distinguish whether a shock state is due to impaired EF or contractility, or due to diminished volume status and SV, and can be readily repeated as frequently as needed based on the clinical situation.[6]

CARDIAC ARREST AND DYSRHYTHMIAS

Dysrhythmias are common in both cardiac and noncardiac surgical ICU patients. The most life-threatening dysrhythmias can be treated by following current American Heart Association Advanced Cardiac Life Support (ACLS) guidelines.[7] For patients who become pulseless in the ICU, rapid restoration of the circulation employing basic life support (BLS) is vital. The most important features of the current BLS guidelines include the recognition that CPR, when indicated, be delivered by pushing hard and fast with complete recoil at a rate of at least 100 compressions/min to a depth of 2 inches in adults. CPR providers should deliver no more than 2 minutes of chest compressions each (or five cycles of compressions) until a personnel switch is made. In adults, if two providers are present, the ratio of 30 compressions to 2 breaths is maintained until respirations can be controlled by intubation and controlled ventilation.

The rapid use of a defibrillator is key to improving postarrest survival. Cardiac arrest from a rhythm other than ventricular fibrillation, such as from bradycardia progressing to asystole or pulseless electrical activity (PEA), portends a poor prognosis, often as the result of acidosis or profound hypoxia. Another important feature of the current BLS and ACLS guidelines that may impact surgical ICU patients is the recognition of the need for postcardiac arrest care. This includes fluid resuscitation and administration of vasopressors and inotropes as needed. However, there may also be a need to interrogate via coronary angiography and treat for acute coronary syndrome if anticoagulation can be tolerated and for consideration of postarrest targeted temperature management (goal of 33 °C to 36 °C for 24 hours) to preserve neurologic function. Although targeted temperature management protocols were established to address out of hospital cardiac arrest with coma, there has been increasing use of the modality for hospitalized patients as well. Current guidelines also address new technology with biphasic electrical sources that deliver shocks for dysrhythmias with a pulse and defibrillation in those with ventricular fibrillation. Another important component of the recommendations is the use of end-tidal CO_2 monitoring to ensure adequacy of CPR quality.

Three dysrhythmias produce pulselessness: ventricular fibrillation, PEA, and asystole. Only ventricular fibrillation is responsive to defibrillation with 120 to 200 J using a biphasic device as per manufacturer's recommendations. PEA and asystole are treated by administration of epinephrine (1 mg every 3 to 5 minutes) and/or vasopressin (40 U one-time dose). Pulseless ventricular tachycardia is treated like ventricular fibrillation with additional shocks given after five cycles of CPR (2 minutes). In addition, epinephrine and vasopressin are administered as CPR continues. Continued pulseless ventricular tachycardia and fibrillation can be treated with amiodarone (300 mg with a second dose of 150 mg, if refractory) or lidocaine (1.0 to 1.5 mg/kg).

PULMONARY GAS EXCHANGE

Oxygenation

Normal lung function and gas exchange require patent alveoli and pulmonary capillaries. Once red blood cells become

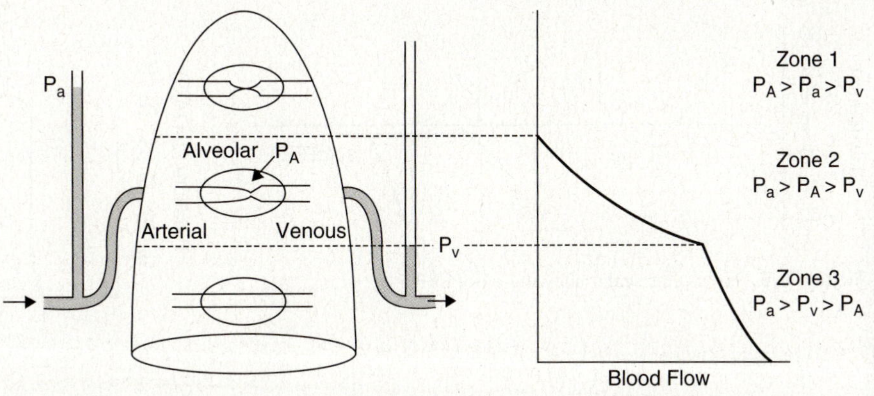

Figure 8.4. West lung zones. **Zone 1:** Not observed in healthy lung. Alveolar pressure exceeds pulmonary blood vessel pressure leading to alveolar dead space. **Zone 2:** Located approximately 3 cm above heart. Pulmonary vessel pressure exceeds alveolar pressure in a pulsatile fashion and allows pulmonary blood flow and alveolar distention. **Zone 3:** Majority of healthy lungs with continuous blood flow and oxygenation. P_A, alveolar pressure; P_a, arterial pressure; P_V, venous pressure.

saturated with oxygen, additional oxygen dissolves into the plasma and the measured partial pressure of oxygen (PO_2) is 100 mm Hg with an oxygen saturation (SaO_2) of 100%. Since a small portion of oxygenated blood is diverted away from the pulmonary circulation (via bronchial vessels), a normal PaO_2 is 90 mm Hg with 98% saturation. Insufficient blood oxygenation is termed hypoxemia. This is to be differentiated from hypoxia, which is abnormally low oxygen content in a tissue or organ. The alveolar to arterial (A-a) oxygen gradient is a common measure of oxygenation ("A" denotes alveolar and "a" denotes arterial oxygenation).

Perturbations causing hypoxia and hypoxemia may be the result of ventilation/perfusion (V/Q) mismatch, impaired diffusion, or shunt. Hypoventilation, a result of neuromuscular dysfunction and impaired diffusion (occurring with pulmonary edema or interstitial lung disease) can be treated by exogenous administration of oxygen. The A-a gradient is normal in hypoxemia due to pure hypoventilation and increased in V/Q mismatch. V/Q mismatch, the most frequent cause of hypoxemia in the ICU, occurs with decreased airflow to the alveoli in relation to the amount of pulmonary capillary blood flow. In the normal lung, there is V/Q mismatch because perfusion and ventilation are heterogeneous. Both ventilation and perfusion are greater in the bases than in the apices. However, the difference between apical and basilar ventilation is less than the difference between apical and basilar perfusion. Therefore, the V/Q ratio is higher in the apices than in the bases. In the diseased lung, V/Q mismatch increases because heterogeneity of both ventilation and perfusion worsen resulting in hypoxemia. Common causes of hypoxemia due to V/Q mismatch include obstructive lung diseases, pulmonary vascular diseases, and interstitial diseases. Shunting occurs when there is adequate ventilation of the alveoli but decreased pulmonary capillary blood flow. Hypoxia due to shunting with venous admixture as with severely depressed CO or anemia cannot be overcome by administration of oxygen (**Fig. 8.4**).

Ventilation

Ventilation refers to the exchange of air from the lungs and alveoli. The rate at which alveolar ventilation occurs determines the amount of carbon dioxide (CO_2) excreted. The respiratory quotient (RQ) is the ratio of CO_2 produced to O_2 consumed and is normally 0.8, and can be altered by the amount of dietary carbohydrates and fats. Chemoreceptors in the medulla are responsive to pH changes and when patients become acidemic, hyperventilation decreases $PaCO_2$ to maintain normal pH. End-tidal CO_2 may be lower than $PaCO_2$ whenever portions of the respiratory tract and lungs are ventilated but not perfused (dead space).

VENTILATOR MODES

One of the initial steps in evaluating a patient with respiratory failure is to confirm a patent and protected airway. The ICU team must determine if the patient has an acute issue causing the respiratory failure that can be treated without mechanical ventilation. Through the use of physical examination, bedside ultrasound and radiography, the ICU team may diagnose a pneumothorax or acute pulmonary edema that can be treated without intubation. If the patient has acute respiratory failure without an easily treatable process, intubation and mechanical ventilation may be safest. When setting up the mechanical ventilator there are several options and modalities from which to select.

Mechanical ventilation may improve oxygenation and ventilation by improving V/Q mismatch and decreasing the amount of shunt. Current recommendations are for low tidal volume (Vt) settings of 6 to 8 mL/kg for the prevention of barotrauma in surgical ICU patients.[8] Respiratory rate (RR) is typically set at 12 to 16 breaths/min. RR is altered to achieve an optimal $PaCO_2$ or end-tidal CO_2. Positive end-expiratory pressure (PEEP) is applied to prevent alveolar collapse (atelectotrauma) during expiration and is particularly important in low–lung-volume ventilation strategies. PEEP is typically started at 5 cm H_2O but can be titrated up to improve oxygenation. The initial setting for patients with respiratory failure is an FiO_2 of 1.0. After initial check of ABG or O_2 saturation, the FiO_2 is weaned down to maintain a minimal PaO_2 of ≥60 mm Hg and O_2 saturation of ≥90% with goals of FiO_2 ≤0.4 to prevent O_2 toxicity.

Pulmonary Mechanics

Pulmonary mechanics can be displayed graphically and include scalars and loops. Scalars are plots against time—either flow, pressure, or volume. Several loops are helpful clinically and include the pressure–volume and flow–volume loops. Each graphic can be important in demonstrating a physiologic abnormality. The flow–time scalar is helpful for identifying air trapping or auto-PEEP (**Fig. 8.5**). Auto-PEEP occurs when the next mechanical breath is delivered before expiration is complete. This can result in barotrauma or hemodynamic instability. Measures to decrease auto-PEEP include decreasing tidal volume, RR, inspiratory time, or increasing flow rate. The pressure–time scalar allows the practitioner to view and calculate compliance (**Fig. 8.6**). Elevations in peak airway pressure may occur as a result of bronchospasm, mucus plugging, a pneumothorax or kinked endotracheal tube, and a sudden decrease may represent an airway leak or disconnection. The volume–time scalar allows one to identify an airway leak as well (**Fig. 8.7**).

Conventional Modes

Ventilators often display all three scalars simultaneously. A spontaneously breathing patient is identified by the negative deflection in the pressure–time scalar at breath initiation (**Fig. 8.8**). Distinct ventilator modes have unique methods of cycling, triggering, and limitations of breaths. In volume-controlled ventilation, breaths are volume cycled, time triggered, and flow limited (**Fig. 8.9**). In pressure-controlled ventilation, breaths are time cycled, time triggered, and pressure limited. Note the distinct difference in the flow- and pressure–time scalars between volume- and pressure-controlled modes (**Fig. 8.10**).

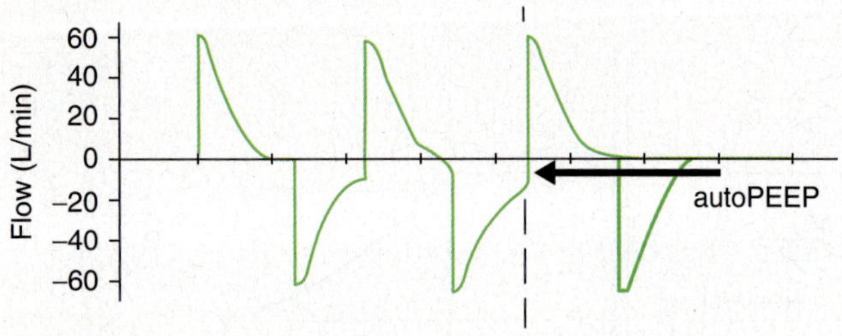

Figure 8.5. Flow–time scalar showing autoPEEP.

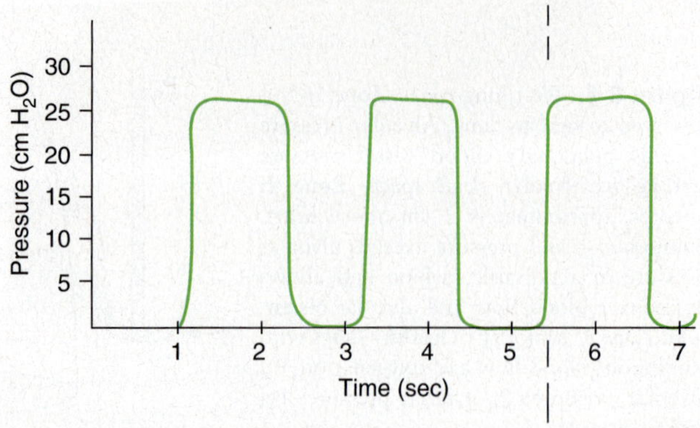

Figure 8.6. Pressure–time scalar.

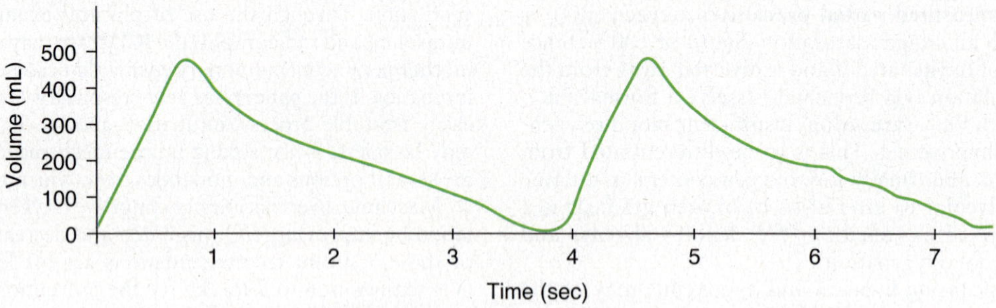

Figure 8.7. Volume–time scalar.

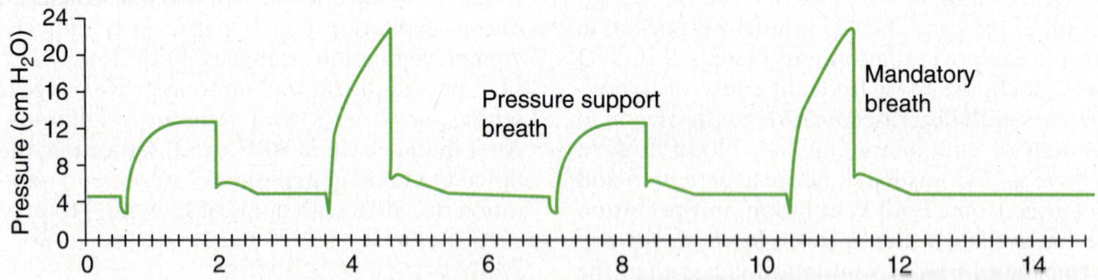

Figure 8.8. Pressure–time scalar with alternating ventilator-assisted breaths and spontaneous breaths.

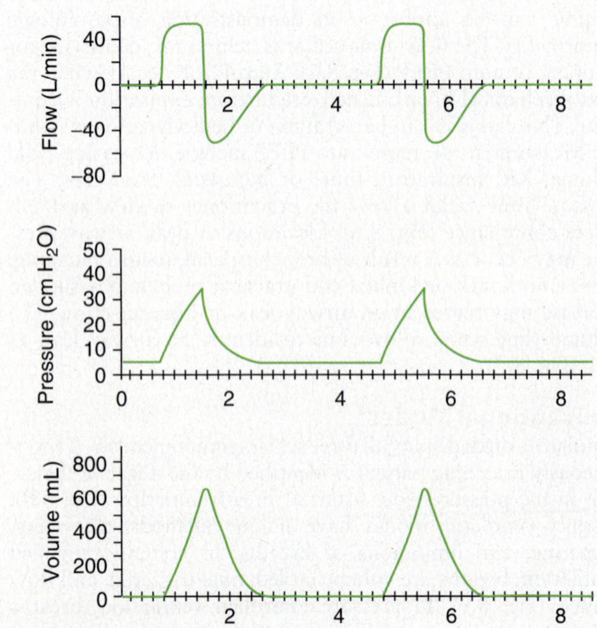

Figure 8.9. Controlled mandatory ventilation. Breaths are volume cycled, time triggered, and flow limited.

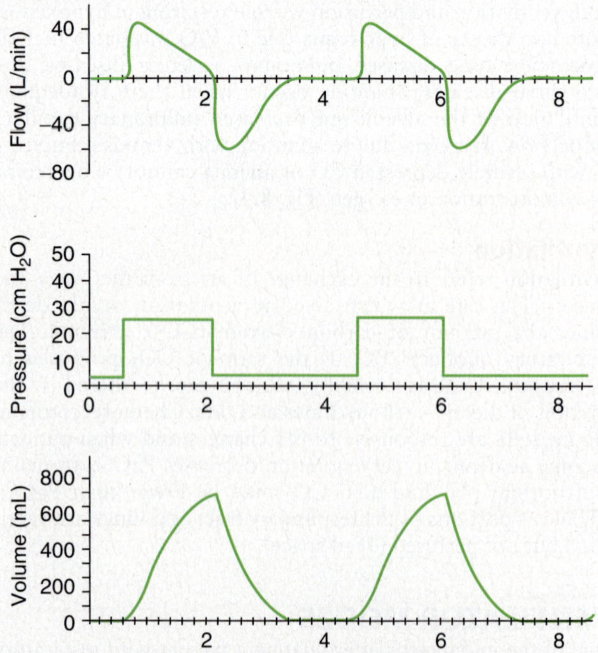

Figure 8.10. Pressure-controlled ventilation: Breaths are time cycled, time triggered, and pressure limited.

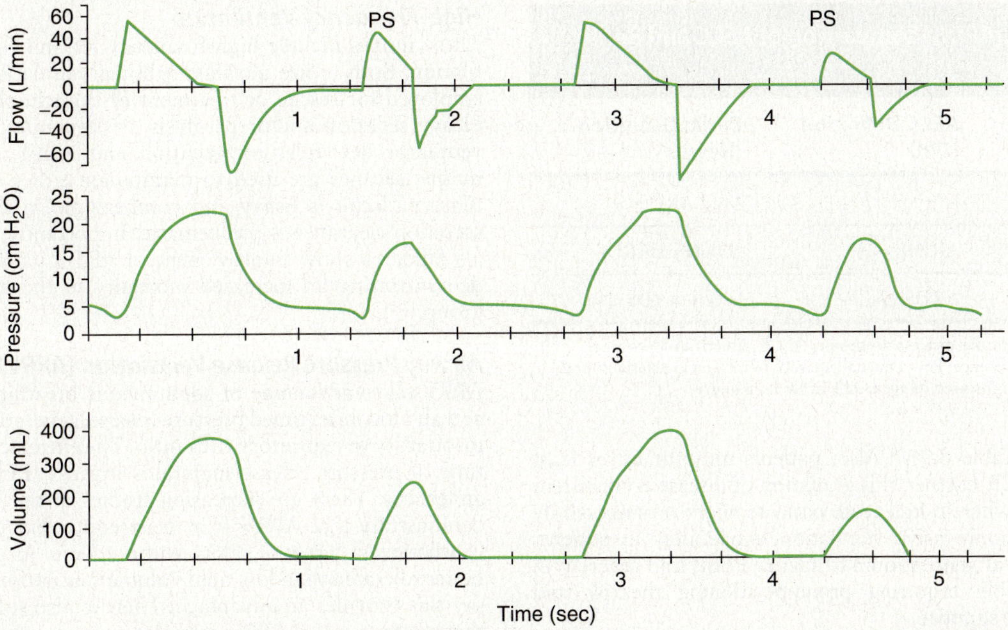

Figure 8.11. Pressure support (PS). Breaths are flow cycled, patient triggered, and pressure limited. Pressure support breaths are second and fourth breaths.

In pressure-support ventilation (PSV) mode, breaths are flow cycled, patient triggered, and pressure limited (**Fig. 8.11**). Pressure- and volume-controlled ventilation can be set in an assist control (AC) mode or synchronized intermittent mandatory ventilation (SIMV) mode (**Table 8.2**). With either mode, the patient receives a minimum number of breaths delivered per minute. In the AC mode, if the patient triggers additional breaths, the full pressure or volume is delivered, whereas these breaths are pressure-supported in the SIMV mode. Patients who are critically ill may require AC for full support, but these patients may be weaned to a PSV mode to prevent respiratory muscle atrophy.

A newer ventilator mode is proportional pressure support (PPS), a variation of the traditional PSV. In this mode, during spontaneous breathing, the pressure support is applied proportional to the inspiratory effort for each breath. This is in contrast to traditional PSV which gives a fixed pressure support regardless of effort. This variable pressure support can be set to either proportional to volume or flow. A recent systematic review and meta-analysis showed that proportional modes were associated with a reduction in asynchrony, weaning failure, and duration of mechanical ventilation.[9]

ACUTE RESPIRATORY FAILURE

Diagnosis

3 Past consensus definitions of ARDS and acute lung injury (ALI) categorized them by acute-onset hypoxemia, bilateral infiltrates on chest radiography, and absence of cardiac etiology. ALI and ARDS were differentiated by the degree of hypoxia, with ALI typified by a ratio of PaO_2/FiO_2 (P/F) ≤300 and ARDS with P/F ≤200. The newer Berlin definition makes an attempt at describing timing of ARDS relative to a known insult. Most importantly, ALI is now part of the ARDS spectrum that is classified as mild, moderate, or severe, if the PaO_2/FiO_2 ratio is between 200 and 300, between 100 and 200, and less than 100,

Table 8.2. Ventilator Modes Breath Types

Ventilator Mode	Mandatory Breaths	Spontaneous Breaths
Continuous Mandatory Ventilation	Yes	None
Volume Assist Control	Yes	Assisted to set volume
Pressure Assist Control	Yes	Assisted to set pressure
Volume SIMV	Yes	Fixed pressure supported
Pressure SIMV	Yes	Fixed pressure supported
Volume Support Ventilation	No	Fixed volume supported
Pressure Support Ventilation	No	Fixed pressure supported
Proportional Pressure Support	No	Variable pressure supported
Continuous Positive Airway Pressure	No	Unassisted
Airway Pressure Release Ventilation	No	Unassisted

SIMV, synchronized intermittent mandatory ventilation.

Table 8.3. ARDS: Comparison of AECC and Berlin Definitions

PaO_2/FiO_2 (P/F)	AECC Definition (Old)	Berlin Definition (New)
201–300	ALI	Mild ARDS
101–200	ARDS	Moderate ARDS
≤100	ARDS	Severe ARDS

ARDS, acute respiratory distress syndrome; AECC, American–European Consensus Conference; PaO_2, partial pressure of oxygen in arterial blood; FiO_2, fraction of inspired oxygen; ALI, acute lung injury.

respectively (**Table 8.3**).[10] Also, patients must be on at least 5 cm H_2O PEEP. Further, this gradation of disease is consistent with therapy, wherein less acute patients might be successfully treated with noninvasive ventilation, moderately ill patients with mechanical ventilation and higher PEEP, and severely ill patients possibly requiring prone-positioning therapy and extracorporeal support.

Ventilator Management

Standard Management

The standard of care of volume-controlled ventilation with low tidal volume was set forth as a result of an early study from the NIH ARDS Network. Patients ventilated at 6 mL/kg tidal volume had better outcome than those who received 12 mL/kg. Thus, the standard of care for ventilating ARDS patients became the use of low tidal volumes to diminish the incidence of ventilator-associated barotrauma.

Adjunctive Therapies

High PEEP

Ideally, to prevent atelectasis and avoid overdistension, PEEP is titrated to the safe window between the lower and upper inflection points of the pressure–volume curve (**Fig. 8.12**). The precise PEEP level to optimize outcome from ARDS has been the subject of several trials. The Assessment of Low Tidal Volume and Elevated End-Expiratory Pressure to Obviate Lung Injury (ALVEOLI) trial did not demonstrate a benefit to adding high PEEP to those ventilated with lower tidal volumes. Two other trials (LOVS and EXPRESS) reached similar conclusions. A systematic review and meta-analysis showed no statistically significant difference in hospital mortality overall but worse mortality in those with severe established ARDS treated with high PEEP.[11]

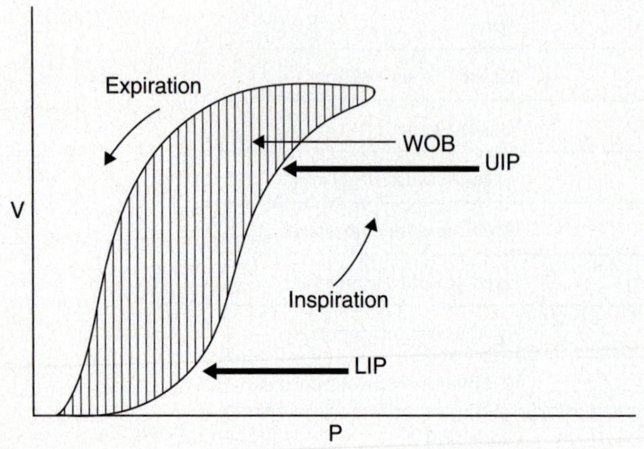

Figure 8.12. Pressure–volume curve with added PEEP. V, volume; P, pressure; LIP, lower inflection point; UIP, upper inflection point. Ideal PEEP is set between LIP and UIP.

High-Frequency Ventilation

These modes include high-frequency jet and oscillatory ventilation. Both utilize ultrafast subtidal ventilation and can be employed for rescue or treatment of bronchopleural fistulae. Heavy sedation and/or paralysis are generally required. The ventilator decouples oxygenation and ventilation such that unique settings are used to manipulate either one. The ventilatory circuit is heavy and cumbersome in this mode and secretion clearance is problematic. Importantly, two large trials failed to show improvement in ARDS patients, with one demonstrating an increased mortality in the high-frequency group.[12,13]

Airway Pressure Release Ventilation (APRV)

APRV takes advantage of spontaneous breathing with CPAP and an ultra-brief timed pressure release, generating a very high inspiratory to expiratory (I:E) ratio. The extremely short phase time of pressure release maintains intrinsic PEEP to prevent atelectasis. There are increasing studies in the literature that demonstrate that APRV is at least equivalent to low-stretch ventilation in terms of safety and outcome. As APRV may be better tolerated than low tidal volume ventilation, some would say this provides an advantage. There is also some suggestion that routine use of APRV may decrease the incidence of, and mortality from ARDS.

Inhaled Nitric Oxide and Prostacyclin

Inhaled nitric oxide (iNO) relaxes smooth muscle for selective vasodilation of the pulmonary vasculature without systemic effect. It improves oxygenation and lowers pulmonary artery pressures. Five of the early meta-analyses showed improved oxygenation without a mortality benefit, with three of them demonstrating increased renal failure. A more recent meta-analysis failed to show a mortality advantage for iNO use for ARDS.[14] Inhaled prostacyclins such as epoprostenol can also lower pulmonary artery pressures and improve oxygenation. A 2010 Cochrane review demonstrated no safety or outcome differences between iNO and epoprostenol. Although neither agent improves mortality, it seems reasonable to employ prostacyclin in ARDS patients with concomitant pulmonary hypertension.

Positional Therapy

Prone-positioning therapy can be used in conjunction with many other therapies previously described. It can be accomplished on a conventional ICU bed or one specially equipped to provide this therapy. Either way, extreme caution must be taken to avoid tube and line dislodgement and development of pressure-related skin complications. The ideal amount of time to keep a patient in the prone position is of debate. A recent large multicenter study in ICU patients demonstrated a significant improvement in mortality in ARDS patients treated with prone-positioning therapy. This multicenter, prospective, randomized, controlled trial was from the French Proning Severe ARDS Patients (PROSEVA) study investigators.[15] They concluded that in patients with ARDS and severe hypoxemia, early application of prolonged (16 hours) prone-positioning sessions significantly decreased mortality. Similarly, a systematic review and meta-analysis reinforced the mortality benefit of nearly 25% by prone positioning therapy for ARDS.[16]

Fluid Management

In ARDS, fluid management strategies should maintain the concept of providing sufficient circulating volume, but avoiding excessive extravascular lung water. A large trial conducted by the ARDSNet group Fluid and Catheter Treatment Trial (FACTT) demonstrated that ARDS patients have better outcome if managed with a conservative fluid strategy. These findings must be reconciled with extensive data supporting improved outcome in septic patients who received more robust fluid resuscitation.[17] Another controversial topic concerns the utility and timing of diuretics in ARDS patients. Diuretics may improve lung compliance, oxygenation, and possibly ventilator duration, but there is little evidence for a survival benefit.

Rescue Therapies

Extracorporeal Support

Extracorporeal membrane oxygenation (ECMO) was thought to provide a beneficial effect to those patients in the European Conventional Ventilation versus ECMO for Severe Adult Respiratory Failure (CESAR) trial. However, it was apparent on further analysis that patients with severe ARDS benefit most from transfer to a center that had ECMO capabilities, whether or not the therapy was actually used. Data from recent viral pneumonia epidemics are similarly confusing. Regardless of the effect on mortality, it is apparent that ECMO may be thought of as a rescue effort to improve oxygenation. Current technology involving smaller access catheters, more portable oxygenators, and venovenous deployment has made ECMO a viable rescue therapy for ARDS, with survival rates of around 65%.

Ventilator-Associated Events

Ventilator-associated pneumonia (VAP) is the most common life-threatening health care–associated infection. VAP is associated with increased ICU and hospital length of stay and costs, and may often be preventable. Nonetheless, it can be extraordinarily difficult to define, particularly in injured patients who may be febrile and have pulmonary infiltrates for reasons other than pneumonia. Further, if attempts are made to diagnose the entity predominantly by microbiologic criteria (using bronchoalveolar lavage to culture >10^4 organisms), then the incidence of VAP may be overstated. Thus, the CDC has worked with various critical care societies to define the surveillance definition of ventilator-associated events (VAE) which are publicly reportable and include probable and possible VAP, which are not reportable. Briefly, VAE require patients to have a baseline period of more than 2 calendar days on the ventilator followed by a sustained decrement in oxygenation. Note there are no longer radiographic criteria for VAE or VAP. An infection-related VAE requires a change in temperature or white blood cell count and the initiation of a new antibiotic that is continued for 4 days. The differentiation between possible and probable VAP involves positive cultures as previously prescribed.[18]

Liberation from Ventilation

It is now apparent that the need for ventilation can be approached in a more bimodal, on–off approach, rather than the concept of sequential "weaning" of ventilator support. Thus, current practice is to complete daily spontaneous breathing trials (SBTs) to assess patients' readiness for liberation from ventilation. Of course, SBTs should not be conducted in patients with hypoxia or hemodynamic instability. SBTs may be accomplished using CPAP with or without low PSV (<10 mm Hg), the latter to enable ventilatory monitoring of work of breathing and respiratory effort. If patients develop tachypnea, tachycardia, hypoxia, hypercapnia, and/or use accessory muscles during the SBT, they are not ready to be extubated. Typically, the parameter that predicts extubation success most accurately is the rapid shallow breathing index (RSBI) or the respiratory frequency divided by the tidal volume with a level of less than 105 most predictive of success.

Further, the requirement for airway support, as might be expected in those with burns, head injury, or anasarca must be considered separately from the requirement for ventilatory support. Checking for a cuff leak, although conceptually of benefit in identifying patients with airway edema, may not be an accurate metric of those with a stable airway. Trials in the medical literature suggest that a short course of steroids may benefit some to diminish airway edema; these have not been replicated in surgical patients. Finally, some patients, such as those with COPD, may benefit from extubation to noninvasive modes of ventilation such as bilevel positive airway pressure (BiPaP) or CPAP. Additionally, the use of high-flow nasal cannula oxygen, typically delivered at 40 L/min or greater may prevent reintubation.[19]

VENOUS THROMBOEMBOLISM PROPHYLAXIS

Venous thromboembolism (VTE) is a common cause of preventable morbidity and mortality in critical care patients. Many VTE complications occur following surgery and injury. Further, the risk of bleeding in the injured, immobile, and/or postoperative ICU patient may be heightened. Safe administration of a chemoprophylactic agent must also take into account drug metabolism that may be altered with renal insufficiency.

Incidence

The incidence of deep vein thrombosis (DVT) can vary from less than 10% (in mobile patients undergoing brief, minor surgery) to over 80% (in those with spinal cord injury or elderly hip fracture patients) in the absence of prophylaxis. Upper extremity DVT is more common than previously appreciated and may result in pulmonary embolism at a higher rate than thought in the past, thus affecting VTE rates. The incidence of fatal pulmonary embolism in surgical patients ranges from less than 1% in most undergoing elective general surgery to as high as 5% to 8% in those receiving operations for hip fractures.

Risk Factor Scoring

Surgical ICU patients are at increased risk of VTE via Virchow triad of stasis, vessel wall injury, and hypercoagulability. Acquired risk factors in surgical critical care patients are a consequence of surgery, trauma, immobilization, obesity, malignancy, advanced age, and invasive monitoring devices. The American College of Chest Physicians (ACCP) 2012 guidelines stratify surgical patients into four risk categories: very low, low, moderate, and high. The most widely used tool to assist in classification is the Caprini score (**Tables 8.4A and 8.4B**).[20]

Approaches to Prevention of VTE

Screening

One prevention strategy involves the early detection of subclinical venous thrombosis by regular screening tests. These tests include duplex ultrasonography scans and laboratory assays such as evaluation of D-dimer. As most ICU patients will fall into moderate and high-risk categories for VTE (in whom D-dimer assays are usually elevated), there is virtually no role for utilizing D-dimer results for diagnostic purposes. Further, the safety of early administration of chemoprophylactics is now being proven in even the highest-risk patients (eg, neurotrauma).

Mechanical Devices

Mechanical devices for thromboprophylaxis include graduated compression stockings and intermittent pneumatic compression devices. The use of mechanical devices alone, without chemical prophylaxis, is only considered for surgical ICU patients at the lowest risk for VTE, or for those patients with a contraindication to a chemoprophylaxis agent. Intermittent compression devices may afford additional protection from VTE in those in high-risk groups if used in concert with chemical agents.

Chemical

UFH and LMWH

4 Few studies have performed a direct comparison of these agents for VTE prophylaxis in surgical ICU patients. A study of injured patients completed by Geerts and published in 1996 demonstrated that use of low-molecular-weight heparin (LMWH)

Table 8.4A. Caprini Risk Assessment for Venous Thromboembolism (VTE) in Surgical Patients

1 Point	2 Points	3 Points	5 Points
41–60 y old	61–74 y old	>75 y old	Hip, pelvis, or leg fracture
BMI >25 kg/m^2	Arthroscopic surgery	PMH of VTE	Elective arthroplasty
Minor surgery	Major open surgery	FH of VTE	Stroke (<1 mo)
Swollen legs	Laparoscopic surgery	Factor V Leiden	Spinal cord injury (<1 mo)
Varicose veins	Malignancy	Prothrombin 20210 A	
Pregnancy/Postpartum	Bed rest >72 h	Lupus anticoagulant	
PMH of spontaneous abortion	Immobilizing cast	Anticardiolipin antibodies	
Oral contraceptives/hormone therapy	Central venous access	Elevated serum homocysteine	
Pneumonia (<1 mo)		HIT	
Sepsis (<1 mo)		Other thrombophilia	
Abnormal pulmonary function			
Acute MI			
CHF (<1 mo)			
PMH of inflammatory bowel disease			
Medicine patient on bed rest			

BMI, body mass index; PMH, past medical history; MI, myocardial infarction; CHF, congestive heart failure; FH, family history; HIT, heparin-induced thrombocytopenia.

resulted in a significantly lower incidence of VTE (31% vs 44%). This likely drove the 2009 ACCP recommendation that moderate- and high-risk ICU patients should preferentially receive LMWH for prophylaxis. However, in the interim, Dr. Geerts and colleagues performed a multicenter, RCT (PROTECT) that did not demonstrate a difference in the development of DVT or proximal DVT in those who received LMWH in the form of dalteparin compared to those administered twice-daily unfractionated heparin (UFH). There was no difference in bleeding rate, but a higher incidence of PE was noted in the UFH patients. This study, undoubtedly, drove the 2012 ACCP recommendation that UFH or LMWH can be used interchangeably. However, it is vital to mention that the authors excluded injured, orthopedic, and neurosurgical patients from this study. Geerts himself provides guidelines suggesting that ICU patients at high risk for VTE including injured and major surgery patients should receive LMWH preferentially (**Table 8.5**). UFH should be reserved for moderate-risk ICU patients. High-risk patients at risk for bleeding should receive mechanical prophylaxis until the risk for bleeding is abrogated, and then LMWH should be initiated. Literature suggests that this may be substantially earlier than we might have thought in the past. A recent systematic review and meta-analysis showed that LMWH is probably more effective than UFH in reducing incidence of DVT, and should be considered the primary pharmacologic agent for thromboprophylaxis.[21]

Since LMWH is primarily eliminated by the kidneys, LMWH should be avoided in those with renal dysfunction. Increasing the prophylactic dose of LMWH may be

Table 8.4B. Caprini VTE Percentage Risk Based on Score

Risk	Score	Estimated VTE Percentage Risk Without Prophylaxis
Very low	0	<0.5%
Low	1–2	1.5%
Moderate	3–4	3%
High	>5	6%

From Caprini JA. Risk assessment as a guide to thrombosis prophylaxis. *Curr Opin Pulm Med.* 2010;16:448–452, with permission.

Table 8.5. VTE Prophylaxis in the ICU

ICU Patient Population	Thromboprophylaxis
Moderate VTE risk	(LMWH [40 mg QD] or LDUH [5000 units TID]) + IPC
High VTE risk	LMWH (40 mg QD) + IPC
Trauma	LMWH (30 mg BID) + IPC
High bleeding risk	IPC until bleeding risk decreases
Renal impairment	LDUH (5000 units TID) + IPC
Morbid obesity	LMWH increased dose + anti-Xa monitoring

VTE, venous thromboembolism; ICU, intensive care unit; LMWH, low-molecular-weight heparin; QD, daily; LDUH, low-dose unfractionated heparin; TID, thrice daily; IPC, intermittent pneumatic compression; BID, twice daily; anti-Xa, antiactivated factor X.

appropriate in morbid obesity (body mass index ≥40 kg/m^2). Laboratory monitoring of anti-activated factor X (anti-Xa) activity should be considered when using LMWH in patients with renal impairment or obesity.

Factor Xa Inhibitors

Fondaparinux is a synthetic injectable indirect factor Xa inhibitor and has been studied in the orthopedic and general surgery populations. In both these populations, it may be more efficacious than LMWH without an increase in bleeding risk. How this extrapolates to the ICU population is unknown; however, it may be helpful in those with heparin-induced thrombocytopenia.

There is even less experience using oral direct factor Xa inhibitors (rivaroxaban and apixaban) and direct thrombin II inhibitors (dabigatran) in the ICU. These agents may be less than helpful because of a long half-life. Nonetheless, we should appreciate that all three agents had a lower rate of significant bleeding such as intracranial hemorrhage in outpatients who were being treated for atrial fibrillation. Rivaroxaban is metabolized renally and apixaban both hepatically and renally. Due to similar concerns of time and ability to reverse, the use of warfarin may be limited in the ICU.

TRANSFUSION

5 Transfusion of packed red blood cells to promote DO_2 is common in surgical ICU patients (**Table 8.6**). Nearly 85% of those who remain in the SICU after a week and over 40% overall will be transfused, many of whom are not actively bleeding. It was common practice a decade ago to prescribe a transfusion for ICU patients whose hemoglobin levels fell below 10 g/dL with at least two units being administered. However, packed red blood cell transfusion may not dramatically improve DO_2, particularly in situations where the oxygen dissociation curve has been shifted to the left, as with decreased 2,3-diphosphoglycerate concentrations (**Table 8.7**). In addition, in many patient populations, transfusion of packed red blood cells has been associated with increased infections and organ failure. The Transfusion Requirements in Critical Care (TRICC) trial published in 1999 provided data to question the universal practice of red blood cell transfusion. This multi-institutional trial of patients in Canadian ICUs was designed as a noninferiority trial comparing a restrictive transfusion strategy, aimed at maintaining a hemoglobin level 7 to 9 g/dL (transfusion trigger of 7 g/dL), to a liberal one, targeting a level of 10 to 12 g/dL. Hebert and colleagues demonstrated no difference in mortality between the groups. Although patients with significant cardiac history were excluded a priori, nearly 300 were studied, and there was no outcome difference in this group either.

Table 8.6. Indications for RBC Transfusion in the General Critically Ill Patient

- RBC transfusion is indicated for patients with evidence of hemorrhagic shock.
- RBC transfusion may be indicated for patients with evidence of acute hemorrhage and hemodynamic instability.
- A "restrictive" strategy (transfuse when Hb <7 g/dL) is as effective as a "liberal" strategy (transfuse when Hb <10 g/dL) in critically ill patients with hemodynamically stable anemia, except possibly in patients with acute myocardial ischemia.
- The use of only Hb level as a "trigger" for transfusion should be avoided.
- In the absence of acute hemorrhage, RBC transfusion should be given as single units.
- RBC transfusion should not be considered as an absolute method to improve tissue oxygen consumption.

Adapted from Napolitano LM, Kurek S, Luchette FA, et al. American College of Critical Care Medicine of the Society of Critical Care Medicine and the Eastern Association for the Surgery of Trauma Practice Management Workgroup. Clinical practice guideline: Red blood cell transfusion in adult trauma and critical care. *Crit Care Med.* 2009;37(12):3124–3157.

Table 8.7. Factors Altering the Oxygen Dissociation Curve

Left Shift	Right Shift
Decreased temperature	Increased temperature
Decreased 2,3-DPG	Increased 2,3-DPG
Increased pH	Decreased pH
High altitude, carbon monoxide	

Oxygen dissociation curve describes how our blood carries and releases oxygen. Right shift represents a decreased affinity for oxygen by hemoglobin favoring to the ability to release oxygen to tissues in need. Left shift represents increased affinity by hemoglobin for oxygen.
2,3-DPG, 2,3-diphosphoglycerate.

Despite widespread dissemination of this landmark article, transfusion practice did not rapidly change in many surgical ICUs, and there is still a minority viewpoint that older, cardiac, actively bleeding, neurosurgical, and septic patients should be excluded from restrictive transfusion practices. Subsequent studies have further questioned this dogma. A large propensity-matched study analyzed the effect of transfusion on ICU patients who were not actively bleeding. It revealed that nontransfused patients (including those with a significant cardiac history) had a lower hospital mortality and incidence of infection and acute kidney injury (AKI).[22] The RELIEVE trial was a multicenter randomized controlled trial of ventilated ICU patients over the age of 55, including one-third with ischemic cardiac disease. Those in the restrictive group received almost a quarter fewer transfusions and had over a 30% lower mortality rate.[23] A meta-analysis of the effect of blood transfusion during myocardial infarction noted that the therapy was associated with a relative risk of 2.91 for mortality and 2.04 for a subsequent MI with a number to treat of 8.[24] Further, a British propensity-matched study of cardiac surgery patients revealed odds ratios of 3.8 and 3.5, respectively, for infection and ischemia after transfusion and ratios of 6.69 and 1.32, respectively, for 30-day and 1-year mortality in transfused patients. Finally, a recent systematic review and meta-analysis showed that RBC transfusions at the threshold of hemoglobin <7 g/dL did not result in significant difference in short-term mortality when compared with transfusions administered at a more liberal threshold.[25]

This risk of transfusion in cardiac surgery patients is apparent even with administration of small-volume (ie, one or two units of packed red blood cells) transfusions.[26] A large, randomized controlled trial of cardiac surgery patients over the age of 18 undergoing a bypass or valve replacement revealed no change in 30-day all-cause mortality or morbidity utilizing a transfusion trigger of 8 g/dL versus 10 g/dL of hemoglobin. Further, a large single center study randomized those with severe acute upper gastrointestinal bleeding—almost 75% variceal—to a transfusion target of 7 g/dL versus 9 g/dL of hemoglobin. Nearly half of those in the restrictive group did not receive a transfusion. This study reinforced the findings of a previous observation study that a liberal transfusion target in active upper gastrointestinal bleeding doubled the risk of rebleeding and increased mortality by 28%, presumably by promoting "popping the clot."[27] In a randomized clinical trial of patients with traumatic brain injury, a hemoglobin target of

10 compared to 7 g/dL was associated with no improvement in neurologic outcome at 6 months but a higher incidence of adverse events including thromboembolism.[28]

METABOLISM AND NUTRITION

Critically ill patients are at significant risk for developing severe malnutrition because the stress response to critical illness, surgery, and/or trauma significantly increases metabolic demands. The result is worse outcomes, including inability to wean from mechanical ventilation, inability to heal wounds (surgical or hospital acquired pressure injuries), and increased risk of nosocomial infections.

Starvation in a noncritically ill person leads to rapid depletion of hepatic glycogen stores as the brain and cellular components of blood require glucose. Once glycogen stores are depleted, gluconeogenesis from protein breakdown and, later, fat oxidation is required. Adaptation to more prolonged starvation includes shifting neuronal metabolism to free fatty acids, ketones, and glycerol, as well as a decrease in overall metabolic demands. These adaptations are quite limited in critically ill patients. Stress hormones, including cortisol and catecholamines, further drive protein catabolism. The overall goals for nutritional support include preservation of lean body mass, wound healing, and immune function.

Severely ill patients may develop the persistent inflammation, immunosuppression, and catabolism syndrome (PICS), a combination of the systemic inflammatory response syndrome (SIRS) and the compensatory anti-inflammatory response syndrome (CARS). These patients remained chronically critically ill. There is currently no specific test for this syndrome nor any specific treatment. It seems logical, however, that providing sufficient nutritional and organ system support is the best approach.[29]

Metabolic Requirements and Assessment

6 Assessment of nutritional status and risk for severe malnutrition begins with a careful history and physical examination. Key information includes diet, recent weight loss, the severity of critical illness, and the nature of any surgical procedures or trauma. Various scoring systems for nutritional risk have been developed. One commonly used score is the NUTRIC score (**Table 8.8**), which takes into account age, illness severity using the Acute Physiologic and Chronic Health Evaluation (APACHE), Sequential Organ Failure Assessment (SOFA), comorbidities, days in the hospital prior to ICU admission, and interleukin-6 level (if available).[30]

Table 8.8. NUTRIC Score Table

Variable	Range	Points
Age (years)	<50	0
	50–<75	1
	≥75	2
APACHE II	<15	0
	15–<20	1
	20–28	2
	≥28	3
SOFA	<6	0
	6–<10	1
	≥10	2
Number of comorbidities	0–1	0
	≥2	1
Days from hospital to ICU admission	0–<1	0
	≥1	1
IL-6	0–<400	0
	≥400	1

APACHE, Acute Physiologic Assessment and Chronic Health Evaluation; SOFA, Sequential Organ Failure Assessment; ICU, intensive care unit; IL, interleukin.

Because of the severely catabolic state of critically ill patients, meeting protein requirements are critical. Though it's possible to measure nitrogen balance by comparing nitrogen input via nutritional support with output (urinary urea nitrogen) in 24 hours, this is cumbersome and does not clearly improve outcomes. Generally, providing 1.2 to 2.0 g/kg/d of protein is sufficient. [31] The highest requirements are for patients with major surgical procedures, multitrauma, and burns. Measurement of serum protein markers, such as prealbumin, transferrin, and retinol-binding protein, may demonstrate trends in nutritional status, but the utility is questionable, particularly since these proteins are acute phase reactants.

Meeting patients' caloric requirements is also important for improving outcomes. Hypocaloric feeding within the first several days of ICU admission does not seem to be helpful or harmful. Several equations, including Harris–Benedict and Mifflin St. Jeor, have been used to calculate resting energy expenditure (REE). These equations take height, weight, age, and gender into account.

Indirect calorimetry, by measuring VO_2 and carbon dioxide production (VCO_2) and calculating the respiratory quotient ($RQ = VCO_2/VO_2$), can be used, but the measurement is complicated. Like nitrogen balance, use of indirect calorimetry does not clearly impact outcomes.

In general, critically ill patients should receive 12 to 25 kcals/kg/d in the first 7 to 10 days of critical illness.[31] It is worth considering that hypothermia, coma, stable quadriplegia, barbiturates, sedatives, anesthesia, and muscle relaxants can decrease metabolic needs, while fever, sepsis, stress, shivering, and seizures can increase these needs.

How best to estimate energy requirements in obese patients is unclear. A high-protein, hypocaloric strategy is favored to reduce fat mass, improve insulin sensitivity, and preserve lean body mass. Obese patients should receive 2.0 to 2.5 g/kg ideal body weight per day of protein.

Nutritional Support

Macronutrients include carbohydrates, fat, and protein. Carbohydrates provide 3.4 kcal/g and have the highest RQ of 1.0. While a higher RQ from administration of a large amount of carbohydrates, compared to fats, may mildly increase the need for CO2 removal via the lungs, the bigger issue can be overfeeding as overfeeding leads to increased glycogenesis and lipogenesis, which have an RQ higher than 1. Thus, overfeeding may impact the ability to wean a patient from mechanical ventilation.

Fat provides 9.0 kcal/g with an RQ of 0.7. Free fatty acid deficiency can cause anemia, thrombocytopenia, respiratory distress, and rash, but this deficiency is easily prevented. Fatty acids exist in two varieties, omega-3 and omega-6. Omega-3 fatty acids are derived from linolenic acid, found in fatty fish such as salmon, and are less pathogenic than omega-6 fatty acids derived from linoleic acid. It has been difficult, however, to demonstrate a benefit of using formulas such as SMOFlipid® (soybean oil, medium chain triglycerides, olive oil, and fish oil) with monounsaturated and omega-3 fatty acids, designed to decrease the SIRS response to critical illness and trauma.

Protein delivers 4.0 kcal/g with an RQ of 0.8. Essential amino acids cannot be synthesized endogenously and must be provided in the diet.

Current nutritional formulas contain sufficient trace elements and vitamins to make deficiency of these micronutrients in ICU patients extremely rare. These formulas generally include vitamin K, which could impact anticoagulation using vitamin K antagonists.

Routes of Nutritional Support

Enteral nutrition is preferred over parenteral nutrition as it preserves the gut mucosa and is associated with fewer complications and costs. Standard formulas have a calorie density of 1 kcal/mL. More concentrated formulas may provide more nutrition with less fluid volume. For patients who have malabsorption with resultant diarrhea and/or fail to tolerate standard formulas, use of an elemental diet, which includes the basic building blocks of the energy substrates, for example, proteins as free amino acids, fats as medium chain triglycerides, and carbohydrates as oligosaccharides, may be beneficial. Formulas with high osmolarity may also cause diarrhea with tube feeds. Decreasing the osmolarity or adding bulking agents can help.

There are several complications related to enteral nutrition in the ICU. The most significant of which is aspiration. The risk for aspiration can be decreased by maintaining head-of-bed elevation at 30 to 45 degrees or greater. Though monitoring gastric residuals has been standard, the benefit of such monitoring has been questioned, at least in patients who have not undergone abdominal procedures. In general, there is no difference in aspiration risk between gastric versus postpyloric feedings. When patients don't tolerate gastric feedings, use of prokinetic agents or placement of a postpyloric feeding tube may help.

Placement of any feeding tube carries risk. Placement of transnasal feeding tubes can result in intrapulmonary or even transpulmonary placement. Having a dedicated team with a protocol for tube placement can minimize these risks. Surgically placed tubes in the stomach or jejunum can become dislodged, leading to intra-abdominal leak and peritonitis.

For patients who have an artificial airway in place and may need to undergo multiple operations that do not involve the airway or abdomen continuing tube feedings up to, and possibly during, the operation is safe.

When provision of adequate enteral nutrition is not possible, parenteral nutrition may be indicated.[31] Parenteral nutrition requires the insertion of a central line, adding risks for mechanical complications and infection. Some complications related to parenteral nutrition, such as cholestasis, can be decreased by the provision of at least a small amount of enteral feedings to maintain the trophic effects of gut hormones on the liver and to prevent biliary stasis.

Overall, there is no significant difference in clinical outcomes between the use of enteral or parenteral nutrition as the primary modality for nutritional support in the first week of illness. Supplementing enteral nutrition with parenteral nutrition does not provide benefit.

Timing of Nutritional Support

Nutritional support should be initiated within 24 to 48 hours of ICU admission following adequate resuscitation. Initiating enteral nutrition while the patient remains in shock can lead to bowel ischemia. On the other hand, patients who are relatively stable on low doses of vasoactive agents may tolerate feedings quite well. Having an open abdomen is not an absolute contraindication to enteral feedings, depending upon the status of the bowel. The use of prone positioning for the management of the ARDS is also not an absolute contraindication.

Enteral feeding does not need to immediately provide full nutritional support. Ideally, nutritional goals should be met within 5 to 7 days. If it is anticipated that the patient will not be able to tolerate enteral feedings for at least 7 days, early use of parenteral nutrition may be indicated. In patients with evidence of severe malnutrition at the time of admission, there may be benefit in earlier parenteral nutritional support.

Patients often don't actually receive the amount of enteral nutritional support that is ordered. Tube feedings get held for many reasons, including procedures, baths, and ventilator weaning trials. One approach to make up for this decrease in support has focused on volume-based feeding. If the patient falls behind, the nurse can increase the feeding rate for a period of time to make up for the difference. Another approach to achieving feeding goals quickly is to start with a semielemental feeding formula that is readily absorbed, combined with the volume-based feeding approach and liberal use of prokinetic medications.

Organ Specific Nutritional Support

A variety of formulas have been developed to potentially improve outcomes of specific organ dysfunction. Recognizing that a higher RQ is associated with increased CO_2 production, enteral formulas have been developed that are high in fat and low in carbohydrates. Use of such formulas has not improved weaning from mechanical ventilation or improved survival. Formulas with large quantities of antioxidants have also been tested in patients with the ALI without success.

Volume status, potassium load, and urea production may affect patients with AKI. Formulas that are low in potassium and nutrient dense can help. In general, minimizing protein intake to decrease urea production is counterproductive because these patients are very catabolic and need protein to support recovery.

For patients with hepatic dysfunction, aromatic amino acids can cross the blood–brain barrier and worsen encephalopathy. Formulas that are high in branched chain amino acids but low in aromatic amino acids do not seem to have benefit, however.

In patients with acute pancreatitis, enteral nutrition, if tolerated, may decrease length of stay, improve resolution of SIRS, and decrease infection rate. The concept of "resting" the pancreas has little benefit. The choice of post-Ligament of Treitz, postpyloric, or gastric feeding is dependent upon individual patient tolerance, not on an expected difference in outcome. Parenteral nutrition should be reserved for patients who clearly do not tolerate enteral feedings.

Immunonutrition

A number of additives to nutritional formulas could improve immune function and thereby decrease the risk for infection and, perhaps, mortality. Immune modulating formulas containing arginine, glutamine, nucleotides, and omega-3 fatty acids did seem to improve some aspects of immune function, but did not clearly improve outcomes. There may be marginal benefit for these formulas in patients who have undergone major surgery or trauma, but not in nonsurgical patients. Glutamine, which can be used as a substrate for gut metabolism to improve gut barrier function and thereby decrease translocation and infection, also lacks clear benefit.[31]

Stress-Related Gastrointestinal Bleeding

The pathophysiology of stress-related gastrointestinal bleeding (SRGIB) is thought due to be impaired mucosal protection, mostly related to blood flow, and not acid hypersecretion or *Helicobacter pylori* infection. Overt bleeding, that is, coffee ground upper intestinal aspirates or hemoccult positive stool, is not uncommon in the ICU. Clinically significant bleeding resulting in the need for a blood transfusion and/or hemodynamic instability has become much less common over the past 20 to 30 years, with or without pharmacologic prophylaxis most likely due to more aggressive resuscitation and early initiation of enteral nutrition. The strongest risk factors for SRGIB seem to be coagulopathy, shock, and chronic liver disease. Mechanical ventilation does not appear to be a significant, independent risk factor. It seems prudent that pharmacologic prophylaxis of SRGIB be limited to those with one of these significant risk factors. If pharmacologic prophylaxis is prescribed, proton pump inhibitors seem to be equivalent to histamine-2 receptor antagonists in terms of risk for gastrointestinal bleeding, mortality, prolonged length of stay, pneumonia, or *Clostridium difficile* colitis.[32]

ACUTE KIDNEY INJURY

AKI complicates at least 5% and as many as 30% of all surgical ICU admissions with a mortality of over 50%, though it

Table 8.9. Workup for Acute Kidney Injury

Diagnostic Study	Prerenal	Acute Tubular Necrosis
Urinalysis	Normal	Casts and epithelial cells
Serum BUN:creatinine	20:1	Normal
Urine osmolality	>500 mOsm/kg	<350–450 mOsm/kg
FENa	<1%	>2%

BUN, blood urea nitrogen; FENa, fractional excretion of sodium.

is not clear how much the AKI contributes to mortality or is more of a marker of illness severity.

Etiology

The causes of AKI are typically divided into prerenal, intrinsic renal, and postrenal. Prerenal causes relate to renal blood flow and may include hypovolemia, shock, and low CO. Heart failure can also impair renal function by significantly increasing the pressure in renal veins and, thereby, impeding renal blood flow. Sometimes, the renal dysfunction, as manifest by low urine output, is the first sign of an underlying problem, for example, heart failure or sepsis. Initially, the kidney is able to maintain perfusion by selectively dilating the afferent arteriole and vasoconstricting the efferent arteriole of the juxtaglomerular apparatus. As hypotension persists and the renin–angiotensin system is activated, systemic vasoconstriction occurs, and cortical perfusion decreases.

Renal parenchymal causes of AKI are the most common. Differentiating prerenal from renal AKI is not always obvious. Serum and urinary studies can help (**Table 8.9**).

The most common cause of intrinsic renal AKI is acute tubular necrosis (ATN), though other causes, such as acute interstitial nephritis can occur. ATN is often caused by ischemia (initially a prerenal cause) or nephrotoxic agents. Numerous medications may cause ATN. Common culprits include antimicrobials and chemotherapeutic agents.[33]

Iodinated contrast-induced nephropathy is uncommon and, in fact, it's existence has been debated. Age, preexisting kidney disease, diabetes, and vascular disease have been touted as risk factors. If iodinated contrast is clearly necessary, the best approach to prevention is administration of intravenous fluids before contrast administration. The use of *N*-acetyl cysteine, bicarbonate, or prophylactic dialysis before or after the contrast load are not beneficial. Though gadolinium does not seem to be as directly toxic to the kidneys as iodinated contrast, it may cause nephrogenic systemic fibrosis in patients with preexisting renal dysfunction. It, too, should be used with caution in patients with renal dysfunction. As a general rule, the benefits of obtaining accurate information with a contrasted study in critically ill patients outweigh the theoretical risks.

Large amounts of pigments, such as myoglobin or hemoglobin, can cause AKI. Hemoglobin pigment rarely causes ATN in surgical ICU patients, except perhaps after a severe transfusion reaction. Myoglobinuria as a consequence of rhabdomyolysis is far more common, particularly after severe trauma, compartment syndrome, electrical burns, seizures, or coma with prolonged immobilization. Myoglobinuria should be suspected in patients with dark urine and a positive urine dipstick without red cells on microscopy. Patients with a serum myoglobin level exceeding 10,000 ng/mL or a creatinine phosophokinase (CPK) greater than 20,000 IU/L are at risk for pigment nephropathy. Myoglobin is both a potent vasoconstrictor and a direct tubular toxin when converted to ferrihemate in an acid environment. However, alkalinization of the urine by administration of sodium bicarbonate does not prevent AKI. Volume administration and forced diuresis to achieve a urine output of 2 mL/kg/h, along with source control of rhabdomyolysis, are the most important interventions. There is also no evidence that early initiation of dialysis improves outcomes, even if it decreases myoglobin levels.[34]

The best approach to prevention of AKI is early resuscitation to restore renal blood flow, which should include appropriate volume expansion, vasopressors and inotropes, and avoidance of nephrotoxic agents.[35] There is little evidence that colloids are better than crystalloids. Hydroxyethyl starch preparations should be avoided, however, as they are nephrotoxic through tubular obstruction. There is no role for the use of low-dose dopamine or fenoldopam for protection against AKI or improvement of diuresis.

Postrenal AKI is caused by obstruction, usually from urinary retention, rarely from bilateral ureteral obstruction or unilateral ureteral obstruction in a patient with one functioning kidney. Evaluation begins with placement of a urinary catheter, if one is not already present and patent. Renal ultrasound or abdominal computed tomography can also help.

Severity

There has been interest in developing markers for early development of AKI with the thought that earlier detection could lead to earlier intervention and improved outcomes. Markers involved in cell-cycle arrest during the early phase of renal cell injury include insulin-like growth factor-binding protein 7 (IGFBP7) and tissue inhibitor of metalloproteinases 2 (TIMP-2). The NephroCheck® point of care device can measure these markers. Neutrophil gelatinase–associated lipocalin (NGAL) is also produced after ischemic or toxic insults to the kidney. So far, however, measurement of these markers has not led to improved outcomes in terms of need for renal replacement therapy (RRT) or mortality.

Several grading systems for AKI, based upon serum creatinine and urine output, have been used (**Table 8.10**). These include the Risk to Injury to Failure to Loss to End stage kidney disease (RIFLE) as defined by the Acute Dialysis Quality Initiative (ADQI), the Acute Kidney Injury Network (AKIN) criteria, and the Kidney Disease Improving Global Outcomes (KDIGO) work group criteria. None of these systems are better or worse than the others at predicting outcome from AKI.[36]

Treatment of Acute Kidney Injury

7 The most important issues in the management of patients with AKI are: (1) Minimizing any further injury to the kidney through adequate resuscitation and avoidance of nephrotoxic agents; (2) Adjusting the dosing regimens for medications that are excreted by the kidneys. Consultation with a critical care pharmacist can be invaluable; (3) Management of the physiologic effects of AKI, including electrolyte disturbances, acid–base disorders, and hypervolemia.[36] Hyperkalemia is the most immediately life-threatening electrolyte disturbance. The absolute level of potassium may not be as important as the presence of changes on electrocardiography, such as peaked T waves or prolonged QRS. Depending upon severity, medical management can include the administration of calcium to stabilize the myocardium, administration of insulin and glucose, bicarbonate, and/or an inhaled beta agonist to drive potassium intracellularly. Administration of sodium zirconium cyclosilicate or polystyrene sulfonates can bind potassium in the gastrointestinal tract and facilitate elimination. Ultimately, RRT may be needed.

RRT is often required for patients who develop severe AKI.[37] The urgent indications for RRT include severe, refractory acidosis (eg, pH <7.1 without respiratory acidosis),

Table 8.10. Acute Kidney Injury Severity Scores

Stage	RIFLE	AKIN	KDIGO	Urine Output
1	Risk = SCr ↑ ≥1.5 or GFR ↓ >25% × baseline	SCr ↑ ≥0.3 mg/dL or 1.5–2 × baseline	SCr ↑ ≥0.3 mg/dL or 1.5–1.9 × baseline	<0.5 mL/kg/h for 6–12 h
2	Injury = SCr ↑≥2 or GFR ↓>50% × baseline	SCr ↑ 2–3 × baseline	SCr ↑ 2.0–2.9 × baseline	<0.5 mL/kg/h for >12 h
3	Failure = SCr ↑≥3 or GFR ↓ >75% × baseline, or SCr >4 mg/dL with an acute ↑ >0.5 mg/dL	SCr ↑ >3 × baseline, or SCr ≥4.0 mg/dL with an acute ↑ >0.5 mg/dL, or on RRT	SCr ↑ ≥3 × baseline or SCr ≥4.0 mg/dL or initiation of RRT	<0.3 mL/kg/h for ≥24 h or anuria for ≥12 h
4	Loss = Complete loss of kidney function >4 wk			
5	ESRD >3 mo			

RIFLE, risk, injury, failure, loss, end-stage renal disease (ESRD); AKIN, Acute Kidney Injury Network; KDIGO, Kidney Disease Improving Global Outcomes; SCr, serum creatinine; GFR, glomerular filtration rate; RRT, renal replacement therapy.

electrolyte abnormalities (particularly hyperkalemia), intoxication with agents that can be dialyzed, hypervolemia, and uremia, as manifest by pericarditis or severe encephalopathy. The latter can be difficult to separate from other causes of altered mental status in the ICU. Platelet dysfunction is also associated with AKI, particularly in face of a BUN in excess of 100 mg/dL. The administration of desmopressin (DDAVP) or analogues help temporarily.

Timing of RRT has remained controversial. Though some studies have suggested benefit from early initiation, others have suggested that waiting for a clear indication as outlined above is reasonable.

Once a decision is made to initiate RRT, the next question is whether or not to utilize intermittent hemodialysis (IHD) or continuous RRT (CRRT). In general, the latter is preferred in patients with hemodynamic instability, but the benefit of this approach is unclear. Studies of using high flux CRRT or specialized adsorbers to remove cytokines or endotoxin have been disappointing.

LIVER DYSFUNCTION

Patients with liver dysfunction can present to the ICU with acute liver failure (ALF) or with complications of chronic liver disease such as variceal hemorrhage, encephalopathy, spontaneous bacterial peritonitis (SBP), and hepatorenal syndrome. In addition, liver disease, as a comorbid condition, can have a significant impact upon patients who present with other disease processes.

Variceal Bleeding

The management of a patient with potential variceal bleeding should proceed like that for any other patient with an upper GI bleed. If necessary, the patient may need to be intubated to prevent aspiration. At the same time, fluid resuscitation, including transfusion of packed red blood cells, should be initiated. To minimize the effect of acid on the varices and potentially treat concomitant peptic ulcer disease, high-dose proton pump inhibitor therapy should be started. Administration of octreotide, a synthetic analogue of somatostatin, can decrease portal pressure and decrease bleeding. Vasopressin also reduces portal pressure but may cause myocardial ischemia and is less specific than octreotide. Terlipressin, an analog of vasopressin, can be effective, but it is currently only approved for treatment of hepatorenal syndrome in the United States.

Definitive control of hemorrhage usually requires endoscopic intervention, with either banding or sclerotherapy. Complications include perforation, ulceration, and delayed stricture. In the face of massive, uncontrolled bleeding, balloon tamponade, using the Sengstaken–Blakemore or Minnesota tube, can temporarily control hemorrhage to allow time for adequate resuscitation. Complications of balloon tamponade include aspiration and esophageal ischemia or perforation. If other interventions fail, a portosystemic shunt, such as the transjugular intrahepatic portal systemic shunt (TIPS) or surgical shunt, can be performed to reduce the pressure in the varices.

Patients with variceal bleeding are also at risk for worsening encephalopathy or infection, particularly SBP. Prophylactic antibiotics are often administered.

The effects of liver disease on the clotting system are complex.[38] The liver synthesizes key coagulation factors, as well as anticoagulant proteins, such as protein C and protein S. Patients may have an elevated international normalized ratio (INR) but are actually hypercoagulable. Patients with liver disease are also often thrombocytopenic. Monitoring thromboelastography may be the best way to understand the patient's coagulation status and, thereby, titrate the use of blood component therapy.

Hepatic Encephalopathy

Hepatic encephalopathy is often precipitated by gastrointestinal hemorrhage or infection. The diagnosis may be difficult because of other causes of an altered mental status such as hypoglycemia, hypoxemia, uremia, and medications. Hepatic encephalopathy results from increased blood ammonia and aromatic amino acid levels from nitrogenous substances within the gut lumen resulting in increased stimulation of γ-aminobutyric acid (GABA) receptors. Ammonia levels, however, do not correlate well with the severity of encephalopathy. In addition to controlling precipitating factors, management includes pharmacologically reducing the production and/or absorption of ammonia from the gut. The mainstay of therapy is lactulose, which acts to acidify the colon, trapping nonabsorbable ammonium in the gut lumen and causing diarrhea, eliminating nitrogen from the body. Reduction of urease-producing gut flora with antibiotics, such as neomycin or rifaximin, may also help relieve severe encephalopathy.

Ascites and Spontaneous Bacterial Peritonitis

Severe ascites may result in respiratory distress and, rarely, the development of abdominal compartment syndrome. Paracentesis is a temporizing measure for refractory ascites. SBP can occur in any patient with ascites. Common clinical manifestations include fever, abdominal pain, and unexplained encephalopathy. Paracentesis is the appropriate diagnostic test for SBP. Finding greater than 250 neutrophils/mL suggests SBP, with or without a positive culture. Treatment is based on the organism sensitivity if the culture is positive, but empiric therapy with third-generation cephalosporins or fluoroquinolones is reasonable. The addition of 25% albumin infusions may decrease the risk for AKI and mortality.

Hepatorenal Syndrome

Portal hypertension can lead to splanchnic vasodilation and reduced renal blood flow leading to decreased effective circulatory volume and activation of the renin–angiotensin system leading to worsening renal function, the hepatorenal syndrome.[39] The diagnosis is made by identifying AKI in a patient with liver disease and demonstrating that the renal function does not improve with withholding diuretics and volume loading with albumin. Infection or bleeding can cause a rapid decline in renal function. Medical management focuses on improving renal blood flow with midodrine or norepinephrine (if in an ICU) as a vasoconstrictor and octreotide to inhibit vasodilation. Terlipressin can also be used effectively. Albumin administration may be helpful. Patients with severe hepatorenal syndrome may require RRT, but the most definitive therapy is liver transplantation.

Liver Failure

Liver transplantation is the most effective treatment for chronic liver failure. The prognostic model for end-stage liver disease (MELD) score predicts liver-related mortality based on a formula involving the serum creatinine, serum bilirubin, and INR. The MELD score is used to allocate donor livers to the most appropriate patient.

ALF in patients with previously normal liver function or previously compensated liver disease is defined by a rapid decline in liver synthetic function combined with encephalopathy not attributable to another cause.[40] Support for patients with ALF may include management of respiratory failure, hypotension, coagulopathy, gastrointestinal bleeding, renal failure, sepsis, and encephalopathy. As the primary cause of death in ALF is cerebral edema, aggressive management of elevated ICP, with or without invasive intracranial pressure monitoring, is employed. In rare circumstances, extracorporeal liver support systems, such as molecular adsorbent recirculating system, can bridge patients to recovery or transplantation.

ENDOCRINE ISSUES

Glucose Control

Hyperglycemia is common in critically ill patients due to elevated cortisol, growth hormone, and catecholamine levels, leading to increased hepatic gluconeogenesis, insulin resistance, and, ultimately, poor clinical outcomes. Complications of hyperglycemia include an increased risk of infection and worse outcomes in patients with acute neurologic disorders such as stroke or traumatic brain injury. Though intensive insulin therapy, maintaining glucose levels of 80 to 110 mg/dL, originally demonstrated benefit in medical or cardiac surgery patients, subsequent studies did not demonstrate the same benefit, perhaps because of an increased rate of hypoglycemia or the use of enteral, rather than parenteral, nutrition. There is also evidence that glucose variability, in addition to absolute values, is associated with worse outcomes. Current guidelines recommend maintaining blood glucose less than 180 mg/dL, ideally with a protocol that minimizes the risk of iatrogenic hypoglycemia.[41]

Adrenal Insufficiency

The presence or absence of adrenal insufficiency in critically ill patients has been controversial for years. Absolute adrenal insufficiency is extremely rare, but relative adrenal insufficiency, also known as critical illness–related corticosteroid insufficiency, manifested by hypotension and fever (and, rarely, with electrolyte abnormalities), is more common in ICU patients and may be associated with worse outcomes.[42]

Critically ill patients may have total levels of cortisol that are normal, but they may not respond appropriately to the stress of critical illness and lack the typical diurnal variation of cortisol seen in normal subjects. In the past, relative adrenal insufficiency was defined by a random cortisol level of less than 10 mcg/dL and/or failure to raise the level by more than 9 mcg/dL after stimulation by high-dose (250 mcg) adrenocorticotropin hormone. However, there is much debate as to what cortisol level is appropriate in septic shock, what constitutes an adequate response to ACTH stimulation, and what dose of ACTH should be used. Current consensus is that ACTH stimulation tests are not helpful for determining which patients may benefit from steroid administration. The current Surviving Sepsis Campaign (SSC) guidelines recommend adding hydrocortisone at a dose of 200 mg/d for patients with refractory shock despite adequate fluid resuscitation and vasopressors without doing any ACTH stimulation tests.[43]

Another controversial question regarding adrenal insufficiency is the potential effect of the induction agent etomidate, which is frequently used for intubation in the ICU because of its lack of significant hemodynamic effects. Etomidate is a reversible inhibitor of 11-beta-hydroxylase, and thus, may cause transient adrenal insufficiency. Studies have not definitively demonstrated worse outcome between patients intubated using etomidate versus other induction agents such as ketamine.

Critically ill patients who were on therapeutic steroids prior to their current illness are at risk for developing true adrenal insufficiency if the steroids are abruptly stopped or the relative dosing decreased. The stress dose of steroids currently recommended for refractory septic shock (200 mg hydrocortisone/d) may actually be less than the equivalent baseline dose of steroid the patient was receiving prior to admission.

Thyroid Abnormalities

New onset of clinically important thyroid abnormalities in ICU patients is extremely rare. Nonthyroidal illness, previously called euthyroid sick syndrome, seems to be more of a laboratory finding marked by high reverse T3 levels and total T3, normal or low free T4 and thyroid-stimulating hormone levels. The actual clinical significance is questionable. No treatment is required.

True hypothyroidism in the ICU is very rare. Consequently, there is little utility in testing thyroid function in chronically critically ill patients without a specific indication. Although the half-life of commonly administered thyroid medications is long, it is possible that critically ill patients with preexisting hypothyroidism could develop severe hypothyroidism without supplementation in the ICU. Patients with severe hypothyroidism develop hypothermia, bradycardia, and obtundation with low serum sodium and glucose levels. The treatment includes supportive care and administration of thyroxine and hydrocortisone.

Thyroid storm can occur in patients with Graves disease or toxic nodular goiters who become stressed by infection, pregnancy, trauma, or surgery. Supportive management includes monitoring hemodynamics and arrhythmias, cooling, and hydration. Beta adrenergic antagonists, for example, propranolol, can ameliorate many of the physiologic effects of thyroid storm. Propylthiouracil (PTU) or methimazole is administered to inhibit the release of T4. PTU also blocks the conversion of T4 to T3. Thereafter, iodine as saturated solution of potassium iodide (SSKI) or Lugol solution is given after PTU or methimazole have been administered to inhibit T4 release. Glucocorticoids are often administered as prophylaxis against concomitant relative adrenal insufficiency related to the hypermetabolic state of thyroid storm.

INFECTIOUS DISEASE ISSUES

Sepsis is the primary cause of death from infection, especially if not recognized and treated promptly. Sepsis-induced organ dysfunction may be occult; unrecognized infection should be considered as the cause of new-onset organ dysfunction. In addition, specific infections may result in local organ dysfunction, for example, acute respiratory failure from pneumonia.

The working definition of sepsis has evolved over the years. The most recent, Sepsis-3, definition states that sepsis is a life-threatening organ dysfunction caused by a dysregulated host response to infection.[44] In other words, it is the patient's immune response to the infection that leads to the organ failure. Operationally, a patient can be diagnosed with sepsis in the presence of a suspected infection and either an increase by at least 2 in the SOFA score or at least 2 of 3 quick SOFA criteria (RR of ≥22/min, altered mentation, systolic blood pressure ≤100 mm Hg). Septic shock is defined as a vasopressor requirement to maintain mean arterial pressure (MAP) of at least 65 mm Hg and serum lactate level >2 mmol/L in the absence of hypovolemia.

Sepsis Guidelines

8 The management of patients with sepsis and septic shock has continued to evolve over the years. The comprehensive SSC guidelines for management cover resuscitation, antibiotic coverage, and source control, as well as many aspects of organ-specific supportive care.[43] The initial resuscitation of the patient with sepsis focuses on rapid restoration of normal hemodynamics and normalization of lactate level, termed early goal directed therapy.

The SSC guideline for initial fluid resuscitation includes the administration of 30 mL/kg intravenous crystalloid in every patient who is hypotensive or has a lactate of at least 4 mmol/L. Additional fluids should be given as needed. There is no indication for the use of albumin unless the patient requires substantial crystalloids. Starches should not be administered. The goal MAP is 65 mm Hg. If this is not achieved with the initial fluid bolus, initiation of a vasopressor, for example, norepinephrine, is indicated. Second-line agents include vasopressin and epinephrine. Dobutamine or epinephrine may also help if myocardial dysfunction is identified. There is no indication for blood transfusion unless the patient's hemoglobin is <7 gm/dL. The response to these interventions should be reassessed by serial lactate levels, central venous oxygen saturation, echocardiography (ECHO), passive leg raising, and/or focused physical examination.

If hemodynamic stability is not restored with adequate fluid resuscitation and vasopressor therapy, intravenous hydrocortisone at a dose of 200 mg/d delivered by bolus dosing or continuous infusion should be considered. There is no indication for performing the ACTH stimulation test. The hydrocortisone can be stopped without a taper once the patient is off vasoactive agents or the patient has received 7 days of therapy.

Administration of antimicrobials should be initiated as soon as possible, with a goal of within 1 hour after recognition of sepsis or septic shock. Appropriate cultures should be obtained prior to starting antimicrobial therapy as long as doing so does not delay the start of antimicrobials. The initial empiric regimen should have activity against all likely pathogens. This regimen should be deescalated as soon as possible once cultures and sensitivities are known. The duration of antimicrobial therapy should generally be 7 to 10 days. Longer courses are appropriate in patients who have a slow clinical response, undrainable foci of infection, bacteremia with *S. aureus*, some fungal and viral infections, or immunologic deficiencies. Procalcitonin levels may be utilized to shorten the course of antimicrobials or discontinue antimicrobials when there is limited evidence of sepsis.

For patients with surgical infections that require drainage, debridement, device removal, or definitive control (eg, resection), a target of source control within 6 to 12 hours is sufficient in most cases. Adequate hemodynamic resuscitation is important prior to the administration of a general anesthetic.

Table 8.11. Sepsis Bundles

To Be Completed within 3 h	To Be Completed within 6 h
Measure lactate level	Apply vasopressors for hypotension after that does not respond to initial fluid resuscitation
Obtain blood cultures	Reassess volume status and tissue perfusion
Administer broad-spectrum antibiotics	Remeasure lactate if initial lactate elevated
Administer 30 mL/kg crystalloid for hypotension or lactate ≥4 mmol/L	

The SSC has encouraged the use of bundles of care (**Table 8.11**). Within the first 3 hours of sepsis recognition, one should measure a lactate level, obtain blood cultures prior to administration of antibiotics, administer broad-spectrum antibiotics (though now this should be within 1 hour), and administer 30 mL/kg crystalloid for hypotension or lactate ≥4 mmol/L in all patients, regardless of previous heart or renal failure. Within 6 hours, one should initiate vasopressors if hypotensive after a fluid bolus, reassess volume status and tissue perfusion, and reassess lactate level.

Hospital-Acquired Infections

CLABSI can be an important cause of morbidity, resource utilization, and even attributable mortality in ICU patients. The Center for Disease Control defines a CLABSI as a positive blood culture in a patient who has a central line in place within 2 calendar days of the culture and no identifiable secondary sources of bacteremia. Typically, the management includes appropriate antimicrobial therapy and removal of the line. If more clinical proof is needed because of the potential risks and challenges related to catheter removal, quantitative blood cultures or differential time to positivity can be compared between paired cultures drawn from the line and from a peripheral vein. Blood cultures drawn from an infected line should have a higher quantity of organisms that should also become positive more quickly than blood drawn peripherally.

Preventative measures, including use of an antimicrobial coated catheter (minocycline/rifampin or chlorhexidine/silver sulfadiazine), maximal sterile barrier precautions (handwashing, sterile gloves, large drape, sterile gown, mask, and cap) during insertion, use of a chlorhexidine-impregnated dressing, meticulous care of the insertion site, and rapid removal of catheters that are no longer needed, have significantly decreased the rate of CLABSI. The best site for line placement has been debated for years. Though it has been thought that subclavian has the least risk for infection, there may be reasons for choosing a separate site because of the risk for pneumothorax or venous stricture in a patient who may require long-term dialysis access. The internal jugular or femoral sites may be reasonable choices.

Catheter-associated urinary tract infections (CAUTI) are a common cause of bacteremia, leading to significant morbidity, but rarely mortality, in ICU patients. Maintenance of sterility during insertion and careful attention to care of the catheter following insertion are helpful. The most important strategy is assessing the need for the catheter on a daily basis and removing it when appropriate.

NEUROLOGIC ISSUES

Analgesia and Sedation

Surgical patients who require intensive care need appropriate levels of analgesia.[45] Pain management in the ICU can be challenging because patients may not be able to describe or quantify their pain. Numerical pain scales or visual analog scales are commonly used, but these require subjective input from the patient. Behavioral scales, which assess the patient's pain based upon behaviors, may be more objective. Narcotics are frequently prescribed, either enterally or intravenously. The minimum dose of narcotic to achieve an acceptable level of pain should be utilized. Dosing should balance analgesia with the potential for mental status changes, respiratory depression, hypotension, prolonged need for mechanical ventilation, and constipation. Nonnarcotic alternatives, such as acetaminophen, nonsteroidal anti-inflammatories, gabapentin, muscle relaxants, regional blocks, lidocaine patches, and environmental modifications, should be utilized as much as possible.

Sedation is often used for patients on mechanical ventilation.[45] As with analgesics, the minimum dose required to achieve the desired effect should be utilized. Short-acting agents, such as propofol or dexmedetomidine, are used as a continuous infusion. There are a number of sedation scales available. Regardless of which one is used, the goal is usually to have a calm, but responsive patient. Daily interruption or at least titration of the infusion is an important way to prevent over sedation. Deeper levels of sedation may be required in some circumstances, such as difficulty with ventilation requiring high airway pressures, intracranial hypertension, or an open abdomen.

Delirium

9 Delirium, defined as a state of altered or fluctuating mental status and inattention, plus disordered thinking or altered level of consciousness, is very common in critically ill patients. Delirium may be further classified as hypoactive (lethargic) or hyperactive (agitated).[45] Common causes for delirium include patient factors (eg, alcoholism, endocrine disorders), acute illness (eg, sepsis [sometimes occult], stroke, head trauma), complications of acute illnesses (eg, hypoxemia, hypoglycemia, hypovolemia, electrolyte abnormalities), and iatrogenic factors (eg, medications). Lack of sleep and loss of the usual day/night cycles contribute substantially to delirium. Trying to maintain normal day/night cycles by keeping the patient active during the day and turning off lights, minimizing disturbance at night, and assisting sleep with mild medication, such as melatonin, can help.

The workup for a patient with delirium should focus on ruling out reversible causes. Any focal findings should be evaluated with a CT of the head. Without focal findings, a CT scan is likely to be unrevealing, but may still be indicated. If the patient remains unarousable, an electroencephalogram should be considered for ruling out nonconvulsive status epilepticus before assuming the issue is hypoactive delirium.

Management is mostly supportive. There are no drugs that directly improve delirium. Pharmacologic therapy is mainly useful for managing patients with hyperactive delirium with the main goals of preventing harm, for example, from an unplanned extubation, and promoting sleep. Drugs that can aggravate the delirium, such as anticholinergics or benzodiazepines, should be avoided. Antipsychotics, such as haloperidol or droperidol, which can be administered intravenously, are helpful in the acute situation. For ongoing issues, the atypical antipsychotics, such as risperidone, olanzapine, and quetiapine, can be very effective. The risk of arrhythmias related to prolonged QTc with these agents seems to be small, but periodic monitoring of QTc is worthwhile. Dexmedetomidine infusion is also very effective in the acute situation, but its use may be limited by bradycardia, hypotension, or cost.

Delirium is associated with increased length of stay and, possibly, mortality. In addition, delirium can increase the risk for development of the postintensive care syndrome, which may include impairments of memory, concentration, and judgment. Posttraumatic stress disorder can also occur.

ORGANIZATIONAL STRUCTURE OF CRITICAL CARE

Though critical care can be provided anywhere, the ICU provides an environment that allows close monitoring and care by experienced physicians, nurses, respiratory therapists, pharmacists, and other ancillary staff. Current ICUs have the following common features: (1) a designated geographical space, (2) specialized monitoring and therapeutic capabilities, (3) resources to provide continuous care, and (4) appropriate staffing. ICU nurse to patient ratios vary from 1:3 to 2:1 depending on patient acuity and therapeutic needs that may be addressed with a scoring system such as the therapeutic intervention severity score (TISS). Dedicated pharmacists, dieticians, therapists (physical, occupational, and speech language), and advanced practice providers improve process of care compliance and patient outcomes. Diagnostic and therapeutic capabilities may include invasive and minimally invasive cardiac monitoring, basic and rescue modes of ventilation and adjuncts, extracorporeal circulatory support, dialysis, hepatic support, and neurologic monitoring.

There is controversy, particularly in adult surgical ICUs, as to how super specialized they should be (eg, trauma, visceral transplant, cardiac surgery, noncardiac thoracic surgery, neuro). Practically, this is an issue of institutional volume and expertise as there is little data to support superspecialization in surgical units. Some of these decisions are based around the use of specific technology, such as intra-aortic balloon pumps or ECMO in a cardiac surgery ICU or intracranial pressure monitoring in a neuro ICU.

Traditionally there are two types of ICU organizational structures: open and closed. In an open ICU, the patients are admitted under the supervision and care of the primary medical or surgical team, which is responsible for decision making, order entry, and communication with the staff and family. They have the option of consulting other services, perhaps including an intensivist service. This team also continues to care for patients in other areas of the hospital, providing continuity, but decreasing their focus on care of the most acutely ill and injured in the ICU.

Within a closed ICU, the patient's care is transferred to an intensivist whose only responsibility is to manage patients within the ICU. Of course, hybrid models exist. Some units have a mandatory intensivist consult. In some units, both the surgical team and the critical care team can write orders or share other responsibilities.

A multidisciplinary team led by an intensivist can function in either closed or open structures. A high-intensity staffing model (with an intensivist-led team or mandatory intensivist consultation) can improve adherence to national guidelines, shorten ICU stay, decrease costs, and improve outcomes.[46] A ratio of one intensivist to a maximum of 14 patients should be maintained to ensure timely completion of rounds, staff satisfaction, and provision of high-quality patient care, and education of trainees. Extending this model to 24/7 attending intensivist coverage does not seem to improve outcomes, at least in large academic medical centers. There may be a benefit of 24/7 coverage in units with a lower-intensity staffing model during the day. Good communication between members of the health care team and patients/families, processes for performance improvement, development of protocols, and institutional support are critical for good outcomes.[47]

The role of telemedicine in the ICU environment continues to evolve. Clinicians, including physicians and advanced practice providers, have developed the skills necessary to be able

Table 8.12. Organ Failure Scores

Multiple Organ Dysfunction Syndrome Score

Organ System	0	1	2	3	4
Respiratory (PO_2/FiO_2)	>300	226–300	151–225	76–150	<75
Renal (Serum creatinine) (μmol/L)	<100	101–200	201–350	351–500	>500
Hepatic (Serum bilirubin) (μmol/L)	≤20	21–60	61–120	121–240	>240
Cardiovascular (Pressure-adjusted heart rate) (HR × CVP/MAP)	≤10	10.1–15	15.1–20	20.1–30	>30
Hematologic (Platelet) (mL × 10^3)	>120	81–120	51–80	21–50	≤20
Neurologic (Glasgow Coma Scale)	15	13–14	10–12	7–9	≤6

Sequential Organ Failure Assessment Score

Organ System	0	1	2	3	4
Respiratory (PO_2/FiO_2)	>400	400–300	299–200	200–100 + mechanical ventilation	<100 + mechanical ventilation
Renal (Serum creatinine) (mg/dL)	<1.2	≥1.2–≤2	≥2–≤3.5	≥3.5–≤5	≥5 or Dialysis
Hepatic (Serum bilirubin) (mg/dL)	<1.2	≥1.2–≤2	≥2–≤6	≥6–≤12	≥12
Cardiovascular (MAP or vasopressor required)	≥70	<70	dopamine ≤5 μg/kg/min or dobutamine (any dose)	dopamine ≤5 μg/kg/min OR epinephrine ≤0.1 μg/kg/min norepinephrine ≤0.1 μg/kg/min	dopamine >15 μg/kg/min OR epinephrine >0.1 μg/kg/min norepinephrine >0.1 μg/kg/min
Hematologic (Platelet) (mL × 10^3)	>150	100–150	50–99	49–20	≤20
Neurologic (Glasgow Coma Scale)	15	13–14	10–12	6–9	<5

Denver

Organ System	0	1	2	3	4
Respiratory (PO_2/FiO_2) (mm Hg)	>250	250–175	175–100	<100	
Renal (Serum Creatinine) (mg/dL)	<1.6	≥1.6–≤2.1	≥2.11–≤4.2	>4.2	
Hepatic (Serum Bilirubin) (mg/dL)	<2	≥2–≤4	>4–≤8	>8	
Cardiovascular (inotrope required)	None	1 inotrope, small dose	1 inotrope, moderate dose, or >1 inotrope, small dose	1 inotrope, large dose, or >2 inotropes, moderate dose	

to closely monitor critically ill patients from a distance and work closely with the health care providers at the patient's bedside. The technology for compliance with the Health Insurance Portability and Accountability Act continues to improve. Also, the requirements for third-party pay or reimbursement have been defined. Use of telemedicine has been associated with improved patient safety, and decreased mortality, length of stay, and, possibly, malpractice claims in some systems. The responses from trainees working with the telemedicine intensivist have generally been positive.[48]

Evidence-Based Care

National and international organizations have developed numerous evidence-based guidelines for various aspects of ICU care. Good examples of comprehensive guidelines are those developed by the SSC, discussed above. Recommended bundles of care that accompany guidelines provide actionable items that can be addressed routinely during patient care. Such guidelines and bundles lend themselves to the development of multidisciplinary, multiprofessional, institutional protocols, and clinical practice guidelines. The electronic health record can often help with order sets or electronic prompts to improve compliance. The use of a daily-goals checklist in the ICU enables practitioners to ensure that important components of care, such as ventilator weaning and removal of central venous and/or urinary catheters, are addressed. Discussing the goals assures that all members of the critical care team understand the game plan.

The bundle of care developed by the ICU Liberation ABCDEF Initiative includes *A*ssess, prevent, and manage pain; *B*oth spontaneous awakening and breathing trials: Choice of analgesia and sedation; *D*elirium: assess, prevent, and manage; *E*arly mobility and exercise; and *F*amily engagement/empowerment. Implementation of this bundle is associated with decreased mortality, mechanical ventilation use, coma, delirium, need for restraints, and ICU readmissions, and improved post-ICU discharge disposition.[49]

Severity of Illness

Several ICU scoring systems have been developed to provide a framework to describe patients' severity of illness for the routine evaluation of ICU performance and quality improvement initiatives.[50] They have been designed more for evaluation of an ICU cohort and less for prognostication in an individual case. The most robust prognostication systems compare observed and risk-adjusted hospital mortality for critically ill patient groups derived from analysis of large data sets, based mainly on early physiologic derangements. Other systems have been developed to quantify organ dysfunction in a longitudinal fashion.

The most frequently used severity of illness scores in an adult ICU used to prognosticate hospital mortality are APACHE, the Mortality Probability Model (MPM), and the Simplified Acute Physiology Score (SAPS) with higher scores portending increased hospital mortality. Some versions of these systems can be calculated manually, while others require inputting data into a proprietary software program, which can be embedded in the electronic health record. The ideal scoring system should be valid, reliable, calibrated, discriminating, and simple. The future of ICU prognostication may well involve interpretation of "big data" that relies less on traditional data acquisition and storage and more on linear or logistic regression modeling. Artificial intelligence also has the potential to further improve our ability to prognosticate ICU outcomes and to predict which patients may deteriorate and require ICU admission.

Several organ failure scores for initial and/or serial assessments exist as well for use in clinical trials or quality assessment (**Table 8.12**). The SOFA and Marshall Multiple Organ Dysfunction Score consider variables in six categories (respiratory, cardiovascular, hematologic, central nervous system, renal, and hepatic). The Denver score excludes the hematologic and neurologic components.

References

1. Halpern NA, Pastores SM, Oropello JM, Kvetan V. Critical care medicine in the United States: addressing the intensivist shortage and image of the specialty. *Crit Care Med.* 2013;41(12):2754–2761.
2. Plurad DS, Chiu W, Raja AS, et al. Monitoring modalities and assessment of fluid status: a practice management guideline from the Eastern Association for the Surgery of Trauma. *J Trauma Acute Care Surg.* 2018;84(1):37–49.
3. Marik PE, Cavallazzi R. Does the central venous pressure predict fluid responsiveness? An updated meta-analysis and a plea for some common sense. *Crit Care Med.* 2013;41:1774–1781.
4. The ProCESS Investigators. A randomized trial of protocol-based care for early septic shock. *N Engl J Med.* 2014;370(18):1685–1693.
5. The ARISE Investigators and the ANZICS Clinical Trials Group. Goal-directed resuscitation for patients with early septic shock. *N Engl J Med.* 2014;371:1496–1506.
6. Levitov A, Frankel HL, Blaivas M, et al. Guidelines for the appropriate use of bedside general and cardiac ultrasonography in the evaluation of critically ill patients—Part II: cardiac ultrasonography. *Crit Care Med.* 2016;44:1206–1227.
7. Panchal AR, Berg KM, Hirsch KG, et al. 2019 American Heart Association focused update on advanced cardiovascular life support: use of advanced airways, vasopressors, and extracorporeal cardiopulmonary resuscitation during cardiac arrest. An update to the American Heart Association Guidelines for Cardiopulmonary Resuscitation and Emergency Cardiovascular Care. *Circulation.* 2019;140:e881–e894.
8. Futier E, Constantin JM, Paugam-Burtz C, et al; IMPROVE Study Group. A trial of intraoperative low-tidal-volume ventilation in abdominal surgery. *N Engl J Med.* 2013;369(5):428–437.
9. Kataoka J, Kuriyama A, Norisue Y, Fujitani S. Proportional modes versus pressure support ventilation: a systematic review and meta-analysis. *Ann Intensive Care.* 2018;8(1):123.
10. ARDS Definition Task Force; Ranieri VM, Rubenfeld GD, Thompson BT, et al. Acute respiratory distress syndrome: the Berlin Definition. *JAMA.* 2012;307:2526–2533.
11. Santa Cruz R, Rojas JI, Nervi R, Heredia R, Ciapponi A. High versus low positive end-expiratory pressure (PEEP) levels for mechanically ventilated adult patients with acute lung injury and acute respiratory distress syndrome. *Cochrane Database Syst Rev.* 2013;6:CD009098.
12. Young D, Lamb SE, Shah S, et al; OSCAR Study Group. High-frequency oscillation for acute respiratory distress syndrome. *N Engl J Med.* 2013;368(9):806–813.
13. Ferguson ND, Cook DJ, Guyatt GH, et al; OSCILLATE Trial Investigators; Canadian Critical Care Trials Group. High-frequency oscillation in early acute respiratory distress syndrome. *N Engl J Med.* 2013;368(9):795–805.
14. Adhikari NK, Dellinger RP, Lundin S, et al. Inhaled nitric oxide does not reduce mortality in patients with acute respiratory distress syndrome regardless of severity: systemic review and meta-analysis. *Crit Care Med.* 2014;42(2):404–412.
15. Guérin C, Reignier J, Richard JC, et al. PROSEVA study group. Prone positioning in severe acute respiratory distress syndrome. *N Engl J Med.* 2013;368:2159–2168.
16. Sud S, Freidrich JO, Adhikari NK, et al. Effect of prone positioning during mechanical ventilation on mortality among patients with acute respiratory distress syndrome: a systemic review and meta-analysis. *CMAJ.* 2014;186(10):E381–E390.
17. Lee SJ, Ramar K, Park JG, Gajic O, Li G, Kashyap R. Increased fluid administration in the first three hours of sepsis resuscitation is associated with reduced mortality: a retrospective cohort study. *Chest.* 2014;146:908–915.
18. Boyer AF, Schoenberg N, Babcock H, McMullen KM, Micek ST, Kollef MH. A prospective evaluation of ventilator-associated conditions and infection-related ventilator-associated conditions. *Chest.* 2014;147(1):68–81.
19. Zhao H, Wang H, Sun F, Lyu S, An Y. High-flow nasal cannula oxygen therapy is superior to conventional oxygen therapy but not to noninvasive mechanical ventilation on intubation rate: a systematic review and meta-analysis. *Crit Care.* 2017;21(1):184.
20. Caprini JA. Risk assessment as a guide to thrombosis prophylaxis. *Curr Opin Pulm Med.* 2010;16:448–452.
21. Fernando SM, Tran A, Cheng W, et al. VTE prophylaxis in critically ill adults: a systematic review and network meta-analysis. *Chest.* 2022;161(2):418–428.
22. Leal-Noval SR, Muñoz-Gómez M, Jiménez-Sánchez M, et al. Red cell transfusion in non-bleeding critically ill patients with moderate anemia: is there a benefit? *Int Care Med.* 2013;39:445–453.
23. Walsh TS, Boyd JA, Watson D, et al; RELIEVE Investigators. Restrictive versus liberal transfusion strategies for older

mechanically ventilated critically ill patients: a randomized pilot trial. *Crit Care Med.* 2013;41(10):2354–2363.

24. Chatterjee S, Wetterslev J, Sharma A, Lichstein E, Mukherjee D. Association of blood transfusion with increased mortality in myocardial infarction: a meta-analysis and diversity-adjusted study sequential analysis. *JAMA Intern Med.* 2013;173(2):132–139.
25. Yao RQ, Ren C, Zhang ZC, Zhu YB, Xia ZF, Yao YM. Is haemoglobin below 7.0 g/dL and optimal trigger for allogenic red blood cell transfusion in patients admitted to intensive care units? A meta-analysis and systematic review. *BMJ Open.* 2020;10(2):e030854.
26. Paone G, Likosky DS, Brewer R, et al; Membership of the Michigan Society of Thoracic and Cardiovascular Surgeons. Transfusion of 1 and 2 units of red blood cells is associated with increased morbidity and mortality. *Ann Thorac Surg.* 2014;97(1):87–93.
27. Villanueva C, Colomo A, Bosch A, et al. Transfusion strategies for acute upper gastrointestinal bleeding. *N Engl J Med.* 2013;368(1):11–21.
28. Robertson CS, Hannay HJ, Yamal JM, et al. Effect of erythropoietin and transfusion threshold on neurological recovery after traumatic brain injury: a randomized clinical trial. *JAMA.* 2014;312(1):36–47.
29. Efron PA, Brakenridge SC, Mohr AM, et al. The persistent inflammation, immunosuppression, and catabolism syndrome 10 years later. *J Trauma Acute Care Surg.* 2023;95:790–799.
30. Heyland DK, Dhaliwal R, Jiang X, Day AG. Identifying critically ill patients who benefit the most from nutrition therapy: the development and initial validation of a novel risk assessment tool. *Crit Care.* 2011;15(6):R268.
31. Compher C, Bingham AL, McCall M, et al. Guidelines for the provision of nutrition support therapy in the adult critically ill patient: the American Society for Parenteral and Enteral Nutrition. *J Parenter Enteral Nutr.* 2022;46:12–41.
32. MacLaren R, Dionne JC, Granholm A, et al. Executive Summary-Society of Critical Care Medicine guideline and American Society of Health-System Pharmacists for the prevention of stress-related gastrointestinal bleeding in critically ill adults. *Crit Care Med.* 2024;52:1295–1299.
33. Darmon M, Ostermann M, Cerda J, et al. Diagnostic work-up and specific causes of acute kidney injury. *Intensive Care Med.* 2017;43(6):829–840.
34. Kodadek L, Carmichael li SP, Seshadri A, et al. Rhabdomyolysis: an American Association for the surgery of trauma critical care Committee Clinical consensus document. *Trauma Surg Acute Care Open.* 2022;7:e000836.
35. Joannidis M, Druml W, Forni LG, et al. Prevention of acute kidney injury and protection of renal function in the intensive care unit: update 2017: expert opinion of the Working Group on Prevention, AKI section, European Society of Intensive Care Medicine. *Intensive Care Med.* 2017;43(6):730–749.
36. Patel PP, Egodage T. Failing kidneys: renal replacement therapies in the ICU. *Trauma Surg Acute Care Open.* 2024;9:e001381.
37. Bagshaw SM, Darmon M, Ostermann M, et al. Current state of the art for renal replacement therapy in critically ill patients with acute kidney injury. *Intensive Care Med.* 2017;43(6):841–854
38. Premkumar M, Sarin SK. Current concepts in coagulation profile in cirrhosis and acute-on-chronic liver failure. *Clinical Liver Disease.* 2020:16(4):158–167.
39. Badura K,Frak W, Hajdys J, et al. Hepatorenal syndrome-Novel insights into diagnostics and treatment. *Int J Mol Sci.* 2023;24:17469.
40. Nanchal R, Subramanian R, Karvellas CJ, et al. Guidelines for the management of adult acute and acute-on-chronic liver failure in the ICU: cardiovascular, endocrine, hematologic, pulmonary and renal considerations: executive summary. *Crit Care Med.* 2020;48(3):415–419.
41. Honarmand K, Sirimaturos M, Hirshberg EL, et al. Society of critical care medicine guidelines on glycemic control for critically ill children and adults 2024. *Crit Care Med.* 2024;52(4):e161–e181.
42. Annane D, Pastores SM, Rochwerg B, et al. Guidelines for the diagnosis and management of critical illness-related corticosteroid insufficiency (CIRCI) in critically ill patients (Part I): Society of Critical Care Medicine (SCCM) and European Society of Intensive Care Medicine (ESICM) 2017. *Crit Care Med.* 2017;45(12):2078–2088.
43. Evans L, Rhodes A, Alhazzani W, et al. Executive summary: surviving Sepsis Campaign: International guidelines for the management of sepsis and septic shock 2021. *Crit Care Med.* 2021;49:1974–1982.
44. Singer M, Deutschman CS, Seymour CW, et al. The third international consensus definitions for sepsis and septic shock (sepsis-3). *JAMA.* 2016;315(8):801–810.
45. Devlin JW, Skrobik Y, Gélinas C, et al. Executive summary: clinical practice guidelines for the prevention and management of pain, agitation/sedation, delirium, immobility, and sleep disruption in adult patients in the ICU. *Crit Care Med.* 2018;46(9):1532–1548.
46. Weled BJ, Adzhigirey LA, Hodgman TM, et al; Task Force on Models for Critical Care. Critical care delivery: the importance of process of care and ICU structure to improved outcomes: an update from the American College of Critical Care Medicine Task Force on Models of Critical Care. *Crit Care Med.* 2015;43(7):1520–1525.
47. Writing Group for the CHECKLIST-ICU Investigators and the Brazilian Research in Intensive Care Network (BRICNet); Cavalcanti AB, Bozza FA, Machado FR, et al. Effect of a quality improvement intervention with daily round checklists, goal setting, and clinician prompting on mortality of critically ill patients: a randomized clinical trial. *JAMA.* 2016;315(14):1480–1490.
48. Guinemer C, Boeker M, Fürstenau D, et al. Telemedicine in intensive care units: scoping review. *J Med Internet Res.* 2021;23(11):e32264
49. Pun BT, Balas MC, Barnes-Daly MA, et al. Caring for critically ill patients with the ABCDEF bundle: results of the ICU liberation collaborative in over 15,000 adults. *Crit Care Med.* 2019;47(1):3–14.
50. Kramer AA, Zimmerman JE, Knaus WA. Severity of illness and predictive models in Society of Critical Care Medicine's first 50 years: a tale of concord and conflict. *Crit Care Med.* 2021;49:728–740.

9

Fluids, Electrolytes, and Acid–Base Balance

Louis J. Magnotti and Bellal Joseph

Key Points

1 The human body is composed of two main fluid compartments: extracellular fluid (ECF) and intracellular fluid (ICF), separated by cellular membranes.

2 The ECF can be subdivided into interstitial fluid, plasma, transcellular fluid, and bone/connective tissue fluid. Blood is a composite compartment containing both ECF (plasma) and ICF (red cell volume).

3 Sodium and potassium are the dominant cations of the ECF and ICF, respectively.

4 Extracellular tonicity is under tight regulation by osmoreceptors found in the hypothalamus. As sodium accounts for the majority of ECF tonicity, these receptors function essentially as ECF monitors.

5 Effective circulating volume (ECV) is sensed by volume receptors (capacitance vessels, atria, hepatic, and central nervous system [CNS]) and pressure receptors (aortic arch, carotid, and intrarenal). These receptors influence sodium and water balance via regulatory systems such as renin–angiotensin, aldosterone, atrial natriuretic peptide (ANP), dopamine, and renal prostaglandins (PGs).

6 Water losses consist of both sensible (ie, measurable) losses via urine, stool, and sweat and insensible (ie, immeasurable) via evaporative loss from the skin, respiratory tract, or open abdomen.

7 The goals of fluid therapy, are to normalize body fluid compartment volumes and electrolyte concentrations, can be achieved with crystalloid (preferable) or colloid infusion by correcting deficits and/or matching ongoing and expected losses.

8 The major electrolytes (Na^+, K^+, Ca^{2+}, Mg^{2+}, Cl^-, HCO_3^-, and HPO_4^{2-}) should be monitored and replaced, when possible, with respect to the pathophysiology of various disease states.

9 Acid–base balance is carefully buffered within narrow limits. Acid–base disturbances are frequently mixed, involving combined respiratory and metabolic derangements.

In this chapter, the normal physiology of fluid and electrolyte homeostasis, inclusive of acid–base physiology, are reviewed, and will be the starting point for a discussion of fluid and electrolyte pathophysiology and the management of specific clinical situations. With a thorough understanding of disease- and injury-related alterations from normal fluid volume and electrolyte physiology, one can effectively care for all surgical and critically ill patients.

BODY FLUIDS

Total Body Water and Body Fluid Compartments

Total body water (TBW) is defined as the total amount of water contained within the body varies according to the percentage of body fat. The average TBW in adult men is 60% of total body weight and 55% in adult women. In infants, water makes up approximately 75% to 80% of body weight. This figure decreases to approximately 65% by 1 year of age and continues to decrease slowly throughout life, primarily related to decreases in lean body mass and increases in adipose tissue.[1]

1 TBW is distributed into the intracellular fluid (ICF) and extracellular fluid (ECF) compartments which are in dynamic equilibrium (**Table 9.1**). ICF makes up approximately two-thirds of the TBW, and the remaining one-third is composed of ECF.[1,2]

2 The ECF compartment is subdivided into the interstitial fluid, intravascular plasma volume, and transcellular fluids. The intravascular space accounts for 25% of the ECF and contains the plasma volume, which is approximately 8% of the TBW. The transcellular space is lined by epithelial cells such as gastrointestinal tract, renal tubular epithelium, pleural and peritoneal spaces and comprises part of the ECF.[2]

Composition of Body Fluids

3 Sodium and potassium are the dominant cations in the body. Sodium is restricted primarily to the ECF, while potassium is the dominant cation in the ICF[2] (**Table 9.2**).

An equilibrium exists between the ICF and ECF because of the high concentration of intracellular protein and nondiffusible phosphates. ECF cations are in electrochemical balance with chloride, bicarbonate, phosphate, and sulfate anions, with chloride being the major contributor to this balance. Anionic proteins contribute to ion balance in plasma but not in interstitial fluid, which is essentially an ultrafiltrate of plasma that normally contains little protein. As a result, the content of both cations and anions in interstitial fluid is slightly higher than in plasma (**Table 9.2**).

Osmotic Activity of Body Fluids

When two solutions are separated by a semipermeable membrane, water moves across the membrane to equalize the concentration of osmotically active particles to which the membrane is impermeable. The unit of measurement of osmotically active particles is the osmole (Osm) or milliosmole (mOsm) rather than the conventional units of solute concentration such as milliequivalents per liter (mEq/L). In solution, osmolarity (mOsm/L) and osmolality (mOsm/kg water) define the osmotic activity of particles.[3]

Cells are bounded by a semipermeable membrane. Adding free water to the fluid surrounding a cell causes water to move

Table 9.1. Body Fluid Compartments

	Total Body Weight
Total Body Water	60%
Intracellular Fluid	40%
Extracellular Fluid	20%
Intravascular fluid (Plasma)	5%
Interstitial fluid	12%
Transcellular fluid	3%

into the cell. On a larger scale, adding free water to the ECF of the body causes an immediate expansion of the extracellular space, followed by a redistribution of water into the intracellular compartment. Conversely, loss of free water from the extracellular space leads to a shift of water from the intracellular to the extracellular space.

Colloid Oncotic Pressure (Colloid Osmotic Pressure)

Plasma proteins are confined primarily to the intravascular space and contribute to the osmotic pressure developed between the plasma and the interstitial fluid. Normal plasma protein levels of 7 g/dL contribute approximately 0.8 mOsm/L.

Osmoregulation

Role of Osmoreceptors and Antidiuretic Hormone

4 Osmolality of body fluids remains fairly constant at approximately 285 to 295 mOsm/L as a result of tightly regulated water balance. Osmoreceptors (cells in the paraventricular and supraoptic nuclei of the hypothalamus) exert central control over the thirst mechanism and antidiuretic hormone (ADH) secretion from the posterior pituitary.[4] In the presence of excess free water, ECF osmolality approaches 280 mOsm/kg H_2O, thirst is inhibited, and ADH levels decline. Absence of ADH decreases the permeability of renal collecting tubules to water increasing its excretion. Urine osmolality (U_{osm}) can decline to 50 mOsm/kg H_2O. As excess free water is eliminated, P_{osm} rises.

Conversely, free water depletion increases P_{osm}. As P_{osm} approaches 295 mOsm/kg H_2O, thirst is stimulated and ADH levels increase. With rising ADH levels, the renal collecting tubules become maximally permeable to water. Both the permeability of the collecting ducts and the concentration of renal

Table 9.2. Electrolyte Concentrations of Extracellular and Intracellular Fluid Compartments

	Extracellular Fluid (mEq/L)		Intracellular Fluid (mEq/L)
	Plasma	Interstitial	
Cations			
Na^+	140	146	12
K^+	4	4	150
Ca^{2+}	5	3	10^{-7}
Mg^{2+}	2	1	7
Anions			
Cl^-	103	114	3
HCO_3^-	24	27	10
SO_4^{2-}	1	1	—
HPO_4^{3-}	2	2	116
Protein	16	5	40
Organic anions	5	5	—

medullary interstitium determine the final concentration of urine with maximal U_{osm} approaching 1200 mOsm/kg H_2O.[4] The net effect of these mechanisms is to promptly return high or low P_{osm} to normal.

Role of Angiotensin II and Baroreceptors

Angiotensin II and neural input from renal medullary baroreceptors also influence ADH secretion and thirst. Relatively small changes in pressure have little effect on ADH secretion, but large decreases in pressure can cause tremendous increases in ADH release.

FLUID BALANCE

Volume Control

5 Changes in circulating volume (10% to 20% blood volume loss), detected by both osmoreceptors and baroreceptors, can modify the osmoregulation of ADH and lead to nonosmotic stimulation of ADH release. Cardiac atrial baroreceptors control volume through sympathetic and parasympathetic neural mechanisms, whereas atrial natriuretic peptide (ANP) released by atrial myocytes in response to atrial wall distention may influence sodium-linked volume control by inhibition of renal sodium reabsorption.[6]

Osmoreceptors

Osmoreceptors can respond to changes in tonicity as small as a few percent. For example, these cells shrink in response to an increase in plasma tonicity triggering the release of ADH and/or the sensation of thirst.

Baroreceptors

Effective circulating volume (ECV), described as portion of the extracellular volume that perfuses the organs of the body, is regulated by baroreceptors. The ECV normally corresponds to the intravascular volume.

Changes in the ECV are sensed by volume receptors in the intrathoracic capacitance vessels and atria, pressure receptors of the aortic arch and carotid arteries, intrarenal baroreceptors, and hepatic and cerebrospinal volume receptors. These stretch receptors respond through a complex system of neural and hormonal actions to alter sodium and water balance in the kidneys.

Hormonal Mediators

Hormonal effects are mediated by the renin–angiotensin system, aldosterone, ANP, dopamine, and renal prostaglandins (PGs).

Renin–Angiotensin System

Renin is a proteolytic enzyme released from the juxtaglomerular cells of afferent arterioles in the kidney in response to changes in arterial pressure and sodium chloride delivery to the macula densa of the distal convoluted tubule, increases in β-adrenergic activity, and increases in cellular cyclic adenosine monophosphate (cAMP).

Renin cleaves angiotensinogen, produced by the liver, into angiotensin I, which in turn is cleaved to angiotensin II by angiotensin-converting enzyme (ACE), produced by pulmonary vascular endothelial cells. The multiplicity of actions of angiotensin II is depicted in **Figure 9.1**.

Aldosterone

Aldosterone, a mineralocorticoid produced in the *zona glomerulosa* of the adrenal cortex, enhances sodium reabsorption in the renal tubules by directly acting on distal tubule cells. By modifying gene expression, it stabilizes the epithelial Na+ channels in the open state and increases the number of these channels in the apical membrane.[4] This leads to increased Na+ influx and higher Na^+-K^+-ATPase activity. The net result is increased sodium reabsorption and the obligate loss of potassium via the renal outer medullary potassium (ROMK) channel. Although

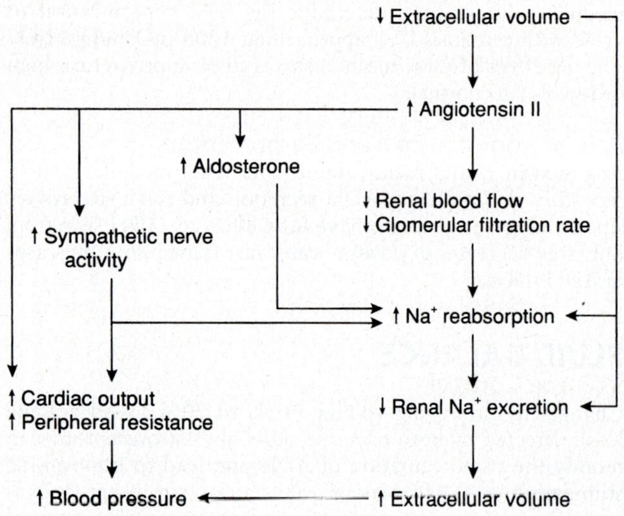

Figure 9.1. Effects of increased angiotensin II in response to decreased extracellular volume.

the primary regulator of aldosterone secretion is angiotensin II, increased potassium levels, adrenocorticotropic hormone, endothelins, and PGs also stimulate aldosterone release.

Atrial and Renal Natriuretic Peptides

ANP, released by atrial myocytes in response to atrial wall distention, exerts a direct inhibitory effect on renal sodium reabsorption.[6] Although pharmacologic doses of ANP can cause changes in both renal blood flow and glomerular filtration rate (GFR), physiologic levels do not appear to have any major effect on these parameters. Other active fragments of the ANP prohormone have been found to have natriuretic activity. The best described is urodilatin, also known as *renal natriuretic* peptide.

Renal Prostaglandins

PGs appear to play a role in volume control, although under normal physiologic conditions, this role may be minimal.

PGE_2 and PGI_2 are the main PGs produced in the kidney. PGE_2 increases sodium excretion without changing GFR, while PGI_2, a vasodilator, increases renal blood flow and GFR by reducing renal vascular resistance. PGI_2 production is stimulated by angiotensin, catecholamines, and sympathetic tone. Nonsteroidal anti-inflammatory drugs (NSAIDs), which inhibit cyclooxygenase, can cause renal failure in patients with renal dysfunction (eg, cirrhosis) by blocking the protective effects of renal PGs.

Endothelins

Endothelins, released by endothelial cells to act on adjacent smooth muscle cells, are peptide vasoconstrictors involved in volume and pressure regulation.

Endothelin increases ANP secretion, activates ACE, and inhibits renin release. At low concentrations, endothelin-1 causes natriuresis and diuresis.[7] Endothelin also modulates the biosynthesis of aldosterone, thereby inhibiting water reabsorption.

Nitric Oxide

Nitric oxide, produced in renal smooth muscle cells, mesangial cells, tubules, and endothelial cells, contributes to tubuloglomerular feedback, regulating sodium and chloride delivery and reabsorption in the renal tubules. Nitric oxide also regulates renin release by the juxtaglomerular apparatus and mediates the effects of angiotensin on tubular reabsorption.[8]

Normal Water Exchange

6 Water losses are both sensible (measurable) and insensible (unmeasurable). Measurable losses include urinary and intestinal. **Table 9.3** summarizes the normal sensible and insensible losses encountered in a 24-hour period. The volumes of these losses may vary considerably, especially in disease states. Under normal conditions, the minimal amount of water needed to excrete normal metabolic waste products is approximately 300 to 500 mL/d.

Table 9.3. Water Losses in a 60- to 80-kg Man

	Average Daily Volume (mL)	Minimal Daily Volume (mL)
Sensible losses		
Urinary	800–1500	300
Intestinal	0–250	0
Sweat	0	0
Insensible losses		
Lungs and skin	600–900	600–900

Adapted from Shires GT, Canizaro PC. Fluid and electrolyte management of the surgical patient. In: Sabiston DC, ed. *Textbook of Surgery.* WB Saunders; 1986:77, with permission.

The GI tract has a net secretory action down to the level of the jejunum. After that, the resorptive capacity of the remainder of the small and large bowel acts to keep further water loss to a minimum. Fecal water loss is usually trivial: ~150 mL/d. In disease conditions like bowel obstruction, severe diarrhea, and enterocutaneous fistulas, GI losses of water and electrolytes can be significant causing secondary pathophysiologic conditions.

Sweating and diaphoresis are active processes involving the secretion of a hypotonic mixture of electrolytes and water.

Evaporative skin losses are maximized with an increase in body surface area (especially infants and small children), patient temperature, and the relative humidity of the environment. Overall, normal insensible water losses average approximately 8 to 12 mL/kg/d. Insensible water loss increases 10% for each degree of body temperature above 37.2 °C (99 °F). Patients who are on ventilators or who breathe air that is 100% humidified have no respiratory losses and may gain free water.

Surgical patients are prone to fluid and electrolyte abnormalities. It is important to recognize that disease states, trauma, and stress-related abnormalities especially those caused by a surgical procedure alter many of the body's fundamental homeostatic mechanisms. It is therefore important to understand normal fluid and electrolyte balance to avoid additional iatrogenic perturbations of these mechanisms.

FLUID AND ELECTROLYTE THERAPY

Parenteral Solutions

Timely administration of fluid therapy and increasing the circulating blood volume are main treatments for traumatic patients presenting with shock.[9] The choice of IV fluids depends on their ability to increase ECV, and to impact osmolarity.[3] Moreover, it requires assessment of the patient's maintenance fluid needs, existing fluid deficits, and anticipated ongoing fluid losses.

Crystalloids

7 The most widely used parenteral solutions are composed of sodium and chloride, collectively referred to as *crystalloids* (based on the solid, room temperature form of the primary ingredient sodium chloride).[9] Crystalloids are inexpensive and highly effective for fluid maintenance and rapid volume replacement.[10] Commonly used crystalloid solutions in clinical practice and their compositions are found in **Table 9.4**.

Normal Saline

Isotonic saline (0.9% NaCl or *normal saline*) contains 154 mEq of both sodium and chloride. Although this solution can be

Table 9.4. Electrolyte Content of Commonly Used Intravenous Crystalloids

	Electrolyte (mEq/L)					
Solution	Na^+	K^+	Ca^{2+}	Mg^{2+}	Cl^-	…
Hypotonic						
0.45% NaCl	77	—	—	—	77	—
0.33% NaCl	56	—	—	—	56	—
0.2% NaCl	34	—	—	—	34	—
Isotonic						
0.9% NaCl	154	—	—	—	154	—
Lactated Ringer	130	4	4	—	109	28
Hypertonic						
3.0% NaCl	513	—	—	—	513	—
5.0% NaCl	855	—	—	—	855	—

useful in patients with hyponatremia or hypochloremia, the excess of both sodium and chloride can lead to acid–base disturbances including hyperchloremic metabolic acidosis.[9]

Lactated Ringer Solution

Lactated Ringer solution is a buffered solution composed of the conjugate-base lactate. The solution has a lower sodium (130 mEq/L) and chloride content and adds a small amount of potassium and calcium (4 mEq/L each). It is ideal for the replacement of acute fluid losses where serum electrolyte concentrations are initially normal. Extended use of lactated Ringer, however, can cause hyponatremia.

Sodium Bicarbonated Ringer Solution

Sodium bicarbonated Ringer solution is a new type of crystalloid solution containing electrolytes such as sodium, potassium, calcium, and magnesium. It is active in increasing circulating blood volume and improving metabolic acidosis. Moreover, it has been found effective in improving outcomes for patients with traumatic shock and multiple injuries by reducing complications, improving coagulation and lactic acid metabolism.[9]

Hypotonic Solutions

For preoperative maintenance fluid therapy, particularly when the patient is *nil per os (NPO)* or following correction of any fluid deficits, less concentrated saline solutions are preferred to replace ongoing fluid losses, such as those from a nasogastric tube. The choice of crystalloid should be based on calculated requirements. These fluids are hypoosmotic and hypotonic relative to plasma. Rapid infusion of such hypotonic solutions can theoretically cause red blood cell lysis. To prevent this, 5% dextrose (50 g of dextrose per liter) is often added to increase the solution's tonicity, and also to deliver sugar during the NPO period.

Hypertonic Saline

Hypertonic saline (HTS) solutions (3% NaCl, 5% NaCl, 7.5% and 23% NaCl) are used as resuscitation fluids and/or for sodium delivery. HTS appears to increase intravascular volume more rapidly than isotonic solutions.[11] This effect, in turn, may decrease the total resuscitation volume requirement. When HTS is used for resuscitation of patients with severe sepsis, it has been shown to improve oxygen transport, cardiac output, and pulmonary capillary wedge pressure.

The osmotic effect of HTS may benefit patients with acute traumatic brain injury.[12,13] By reducing the water content of the brain, HTS can help to control intracerebral pressure. In addition, HTS has well-documented immunomodulatory effects,[14] by reducing the systemic inflammatory response syndrome. However, with HTS, patients are at increased risk for hypernatremia, hyperchloremia, and subsequent metabolic acidosis.

Colloids

Colloids are composed of large molecules (eg, albumin) that have a greater tendency to stay within the intravascular space. Colloid solutions offer the potential benefits of promoting fluid retention in the intravascular space and reducing excess interstitial fluid (edema). Colloids are typically confined to the intravascular space resulting in transient plasma volume expansion. However, abnormal capillary membrane permeability (as occurs with sepsis and hemorrhagic shock) allows for the extravasation of colloids into the interstitial space, potentially worsening edema and tissue oxygenation. The CRISTAL trial (crystalloids vs colloids) found no overall difference in survival between the groups.[15,16]

Albumin

Albumin is the primary protein in plasma responsible for the oncotic pressure. Exogenous human albumin is derived from human plasma. It is available in a 5% (50 g/L) and a 25% solution (250 g/L) in isotonic saline. These solutions work by increasing plasma oncotic pressure, which can theoretically slow or reverse the movement of water into the interstitial space.

Hetastarch

Hydroxyethyl starches (HES) are synthetic colloids derived from hydrolyzed amylopectin. Because of its higher colloid osmotic pressure, HES is slightly more effective than 5% albumin as a colloid and has been used as a resuscitative solution with variable results.[17] Coagulopathy and bleeding complications have been widely reported.[18] The Surviving Sepsis Campaign recommends against HES administration in septic patients.[19]

Dextrans

Dextrans are glucose polymers. Their use involves risks of anaphylaxis, hyperglycemia, renal dysfunction and failure, coagulopathy, and increased thrombosis. The use of dextran solutions is no longer favored given a higher relative risk of mortality compared to HES.[20]

Gelatins

Gelatin solutions produced from bovine collagen are effective as plasma volume expanders. These are currently only available outside the United States and were used in similar clinical settings to HES, with similar clinical results. Adverse effects include renal impairment, allergic reactions, and anaphylaxis.

Artificial Oxygen Carriers

Non–red blood cell hemoglobin-based oxygen-carrying solutions (eg, PolyHeme, Northfield Laboratories, Inc.)[21] are made from polymerized human hemoglobin. PolyHeme was originally used in military trauma situations involving massive blood loss, particularly when fresh whole blood was not readily available. On May 9, 2009, Northfield Laboratories, Inc. shut down operations after it failed to secure a biologic license application for PolyHeme from the FDA.

Goals of Fluid and Electrolyte Therapy

Maintenance Fluid Therapy

Maintenance fluid volume requirements can be calculated based on body weight (**Table 9.5**). A 10-kg child requires 100 mL/kg/d or 1000 mL/d. A 70-kg man requires 1000 mL/d for the first 10 kg (100 mL/kg × 10 kg), plus 500 mL/d for the second 10 kg (50 mL/kg × 10 kg), plus 1000 mL/d for the last 50 kg (20 mL/kg × 50 kg), for a total daily water requirement of 2500 mL/d. In patients who may not tolerate hypervolemia (ie, cardiac disease, elderly patients), the requirement per kilogram over 20 kg is decreased to 15 mL/kg/d.

Maintenance Electrolyte Therapy

One to 2 mEq/kg/d of sodium is required, with any administered excess managed by urinary sodium excretion. Potassium requirements are approximately 0.5 to 1 mEq/kg/d. If

Table 9.5. Calculation of Maintenance Fluid Requirements

Body Weight	Fluid Requirements[a]	
For 0–10 kg	Give 100 mL/kg/d	A
For the next 10–20 kg	Give an additional 50 mL/kg/d	B
For weight >20 kg[b]	Give 20 mL/kg/d	C

[a]Maintenance fluid requirements = A + B + C.
[b]For elderly patients or patients with cardiac disease, this amount should be reduced to 15 mL/kg/d.

sodium is replaced at 2 mEq/kg/d and potassium is replaced at 1 mEq/kg/d, a 70-kg patient requires 2500 mL of water containing 140 mEq of sodium and 70 mEq of potassium. Each liter of parenteral solution would contain 56 mEq of sodium and 28 mEq of potassium. The solution that best fits this patient's daily maintenance requirements is 0.33% saline solution (56 mEq/L Na^+). Potassium chloride can be added to each liter of solution (20 to 30 mEq/L), with appropriate adjustments for the patient's electrolyte and renal functional status.

Additional Electrolyte Therapy

Short-term maintenance therapy typically does not require adding calcium, phosphate, or magnesium. However, in patients with acute and/or chronic disorders, significant volume shifts, or those requiring long-term parenteral fluid therapy, these electrolytes should be measured and corrected by the enteral route. If the enteral route is unavailable, electrolytes, along with trace elements, vitamins, and appropriate caloric sources, should be included in parenteral nutrition solutions. Adjustments must be made for disease states that alter electrolyte needs, such as potassium management in renal failure.

CORRECTION OF VOLUME ABNORMALITIES

Volume Deficits

Hypovolemia is common in surgical and trauma patients due to blood loss or fluid depletion. Large fluid volumes can be sequestered in extravascular spaces (third-space losses) because of inflammation, sepsis, or shock-related endothelial injury and increased permeability. Disorders causing third-space losses include bowel obstruction with bowel wall edema and fluid transudation into the bowel lumen, pancreatitis with retroperitoneal fluid extravasation, and extensive soft tissue injury in trauma. As the underlying condition resolves and microvascular permeability normalizes, these fluid losses decrease, and the sequestered fluid gradually returns to the intravascular space at variable rates.

Volume deficits can be acute or chronic. Chronic volume deficits may present with decreased skin turgor, sunken eyes, oliguria, weight loss, hypothermia, tachycardia, orthostatic hypotension, and a high blood urea nitrogen (BUN)/creatinine ratio (above 15:1). Acute volume losses typically present with an increased heart rate, eventually leading to hypotension and decreased urine output. Fluid resuscitation for hypovolemia is initiated with an isotonic solution such as normal saline, or lactated Ringer solution. In critically ill patients, urine flow is monitored with an indwelling Foley catheter, with a desired goal of at least 0.5 mL/kg/h.

Volume Excess

Volume excess can result from significant resuscitative fluid, blood product administration, or excessive parenteral volume administration. If fluid therapy is not adjusted as the patient's clinical status changes, volume overload may occur, presenting as weight gain, truncal and peripheral edema, and pulmonary congestion. Treatment for intravascular volume excess involves a combination of volume restriction and diuresis.

Table 9.6. Electrolyte Concentrations in Gastrointestinal Secretions

	Electrolyte (mEq/L)					
Secretion	Na^+	K^+	Cl^-	...	H^+	Rate (mL/d)
Salivary	50	20	40	30	—	100–1000
Gastric						
Basal	100	10	140	—	30	1000
Stimulated	30	10	140	—	100	4200
Bile	140	5	100	—	—	500–1000
Pancreatic	140	5	75	—	—	1000
Duodenum	140	5	80	—	—	100–2000
Ileum	140	5	70	—	—	100–2000
Colon	60	70	15	—	—	—

REPLACEMENT OF ONGOING FLUID LOSSES

Continuous monitoring and recording of fluid losses from stomas, fistulae, open body compartments (such as abdomen or chest), and all tubes (including nasogastric tubes) and drains are essential throughout the course of patient care. Once the net "ins and outs" have been calculated, any existing volume deficits should be corrected with fluid replacement therapy. The electrolyte content of these fluids can be estimated or measured and used to guide the choice of replacement fluid type (**Table 9.6**).

Intraoperative Fluid Therapy

Fluid losses during operative procedures arise from evaporative losses in open wounds, blood loss, and third-space sequestration into extravascular spaces. While blood loss can be quantified relatively easily, evaporative losses and shifts of intravascular fluid are difficult to measure but should be anticipated. Intraoperative replacement typically involves crystalloid solutions administered at rates of 500 to 1000 mL/h, approximately matching the hourly insensible loss rate during open celiotomy cases. The choice of intraoperative fluid is dependent on many factors. Buffered solutions like Ringer lactate are effective and safe alternatives to nonbuffered saline-based fluids, potentially mitigating postoperative hyperchloremic metabolic acidosis. Close monitoring of blood pressure, blood loss, urine output, and invasive monitoring techniques aids surgeons and anesthesiologists in managing fluid shifts and potential problems associated with intraoperative volume depletion.

Postoperative Fluid Therapy and Monitoring

Routine monitoring of intraoperative and postoperative fluid status consists of serial vital signs such as blood pressure and heart rate, measurements of outputs from all tubes, lines, and drains including urine output. The total fluid input (all drips, intravenous, and enteral) minus the output (losses) allows for daily and length-of-stay volume assessments. Daily weight should be recorded and compared to the patient's presurgical "dry" weight, if available. In the postsurgical patient, rapid fluctuations in weight are generally related to changes in TBW. In the absence of any extenuating circumstances (eg, renal dialysis, kidney transplantation), adequate fluid is usually given to maintain a urine output of greater than 0.5 mL/kg/h in adult patients.

Urine specific gravity serves as an indicator of both volume status and renal ability to concentrate or dilute urine. A urine specific gravity above 1.010 to 1.012 indicates concentrated urine compared to plasma, while a urine specific gravity less than 1.010 indicates the production of more dilute urine.

Renal failure in the postoperative period may be accompanied by low urine volume (oliguric renal failure, <0.5 mL/kg/h, or <500 mL/d). In addition, normal or high urine volumes (nonoliguric or high-output renal failure) may also indicate renal dysfunction. Fractional excretion of sodium (FeNa) compared to creatinine measurement helps distinguish renal dysfunction causes: FeNa <1% suggests prerenal states (eg, dehydration), while FeNa >2% indicates acute tubular necrosis.

$$FeNa = (Urine_{Na})(Serum_{Creat})/(Urine_{Creat})(Serum_{Na})$$

Central venous pressures (CVPs) have also been extensively used to gauge fluid status and responsiveness. Normal CVP may range from 5 to 12 mm Hg. Higher pressures usually indicate volume overload or cardiac failure, whereas pressures below this range indicate intravascular volume depletion. However, the use of CVP measurements alone has been shown to be highly variable in assessing intravascular volume and venous return.

Recent methods for assessing fluid status include the following: (1) Bedside echocardiography (eg, transthoracic) measures ventricular function; (2) Ultrasound measures vena caval diameter; (3) Peripheral arterial pulse-volume variability [stroke volume variation (SVV)] calculates stroke volume changes during ventilation, indicating fluid responsiveness reliably. The efficacy of these techniques may be altered in abnormal right and/or left ventricular compliance, increased intrathoracic pressure (via elevated levels of positive end expiratory pressure and intra-abdominal pressure), valvular heart disease (eg, mitral stenosis), and cardiac dysrhythmias (eg, atrial fibrillation). To solve any serious questions of volume status, the gold standard technique remains pulmonary artery catheterization in critically ill patients.

ELECTROLYTES

8 An electrolyte is defined as a substance that ionizes when dissolved in an appropriate solvent, most commonly water.

In order to maintain homeostasis, the human body has a complex yet stable distribution of electrolytes in different concentrations in the intracellular and extracellular environments (**Table 9.7**). In clinical practice, only measurements of serum values (extracellular space excluding the interstitial space) are performed and used to infer disruptions of homeostasis, which cause organ damage. For instance, with hyperkalemia, the serum concentration itself does not directly cause injury. It initiates depolarization leading to impairment of cardiac conduction resulting in an end pathway of ventricular fibrillation or asystole.

Given that serum derangements can only be discovered on lab evaluation or clinically, it is important to anticipate potentially life-threatening electrolyte abnormalities. This concept is especially important in surgical patients in whom the loss of electrolyte-rich GI fluids occurs and can cause predictable serum derangements.

Sodium

Where Sodium Goes, Water Follows

There is a distinct correlation between sodium and fluid status. This relationship can help establish both the etiology and treatment of various derangements. For example, with hyponatremia, it is clinically important to assess the patient's volume status as well as check laboratory studies, including serum sodium, serum osmolality, and urine electrolytes. Other values such as serum glucose, serum protein, and serum lipids may also help to differentiate hyponatremia from pseudohyponatremia.

Table 9.7. Electrolyte Concentrations in Plasma and Intracellular Fluid

	Normal Ranges	
Solute	**Plasma**	**Intracellular**
Na^+	136–145 (mEq/L)	10–15 (mEq/L)
K^+	3.5–5.0 (mEq/L)	120–150 (mEq/L)
Ca^{++}	8.4–10.2 mg/dL	0.1 µM
Mg^{++}	1.5–2.0 (mEq/L)	5–20 mmol/L
Cl^-	95–105 (mEq/L)	3–20 mmol/L
HCO_3	22–28 (mEq/L)	10–15 mmol/L
pH	7.37–7.43	7.0–7.2
Osmolarity	280–290 (**mOsm/kg**)	280–290 (**mOsm/kg**)

mEq/L, milliequivalents per liter; µM, micromoles; mmol = millimoles.

Pseudohyponatremia

Marked elevations in serum lipid or protein result in a reduction in the fraction of serum that is water/sodium and thus produce a "dilutional" hyponatremia. Examples include hyperlipidemia, hyperproteinemia (eg, multiple myeloma), hyperglycemia, and mannitol administration.

Hyponatremia

The most common pathophysiology is retention of water, which most often stems from oral intake or iatrogenic use of intravenous hypotonic fluids. The kidney has an enormous ability to dilute urine, however, in most surgical/trauma patients who experience hyponatremia, there is an inability to suppress ADH, as it is normally elevated during a stress response. In this case, the sodium rarely falls below 130 mEq/L because the hyponatremia itself, as well as volume expansion, decreases the effects of ADH on the renal collecting tubules.

In significant cases (ie, serum sodium <130 mEq/L), it is helpful to take a more systematic approach. This entails assessing serum and urine osmolality as well as urine sodium (**Algorithm 9.1**).

Clinical Manifestations

Hyponatremia affects multiple organ systems including the CNS, GI, and musculoskeletal. In acute hyponatremia, symptoms often manifest when serum sodium is less than 130 mEq/L; whereas in chronic hyponatremia, symptoms typically do not occur until serum sodium falls below 120 mEq/L.

Treatment

Treatment depends on the patient's volume status. Hypovolemic patients are treated by rehydration with isotonic saline, with caution not to correct serum sodium faster than 0.5 mEq/L/h and less than 10 mEq/L over 24 hours. If correction is faster than this rate, the patient may develop *central pontine myelinolysis* or "*locked in*" *syndrome*, which consists of quadriplegia, dysarthria, and dysphagia. To prevent this rare, yet highly morbid complication, the following calculation is recommended:

$$Na^+ \text{ required (in mEq)} = (\text{Desired } Na^+ - \text{Actual } Na^+) \times TBW$$

$$TBW = 0.6 \times \text{Weight (kg)}$$

Rapid correction with 3% or higher-concentration saline solutions should be avoided unless significant CNS symptoms

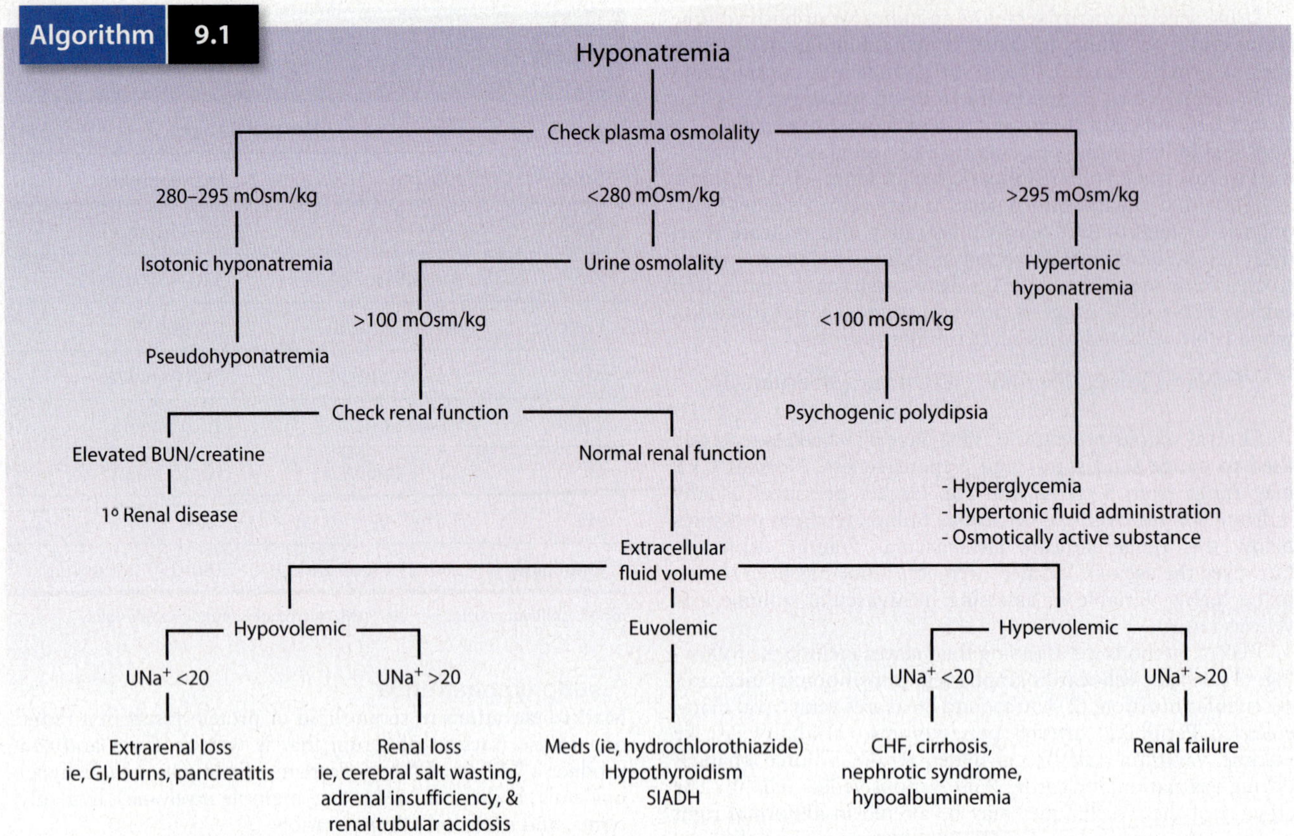

Algorithm 9.1. Hyponatremia.

such as coma or seizures are present and should be done using the equation above to prevent overcorrection. A reasonable initial dose in an emergent situation would be 100 mL of 3% saline given as a bolus; this can be repeated in 10-minute intervals with a definite need for follow-up laboratory evaluation to prevent overly rapid correction.

Cerebral Salt Wasting and Syndrome of Inappropriate Antidiuretic Hormone

Cerebral salt wasting (CSW) and syndrome of inappropriate antidiuretic hormone (SIADH) are both seen in the setting of CNS disease, which is especially pertinent in trauma patients. CSW is much rarer and typically occurs within the first 10 days following CNS insult/injury. The pathophysiology is likely related to impaired sodium reabsorption leading to volume depletion, followed by increased ADH release causing hyponatremia from water retention. Laboratory findings are nearly identical among CSW and SIADH. Both have elevated urine osmolality compared to serum. However, CSW is associated with ECF depletion (hypovolemic hyponatremia) and thus hypotension and/or elevated hematocrit, whereas SIADH patients are often net positive in fluid balance (euvolemic hyponatremia).

Treatment

Given the volume status (hypovolemia) associated with CSW the treatment is usually isotonic fluids which will suppress the release of ADH. On the contrary if isotonic fluid is given for SIADH it can worsen the hyponatremia. Other options to treat CSW include salt tablets and if needed fludrocortisone.

The initial treatment for SIADH is often fluid restriction of <800 mL/d. For more significant cases, the use of oral salt tablets or 3% HTS is recommended. Finally, vasopressin receptor antagonists such as conivaptan (IV) and tolvaptan (PO) can be used; however, these do carry risks such as hepatotoxicity and can rapidly overcorrect serum sodium levels if not monitored closely. Furthermore, they are fairly expensive in the United States and should only be used in select cases.

Hypernatremia

Although a less common problem in surgical patients, hypernatremia has a variety of etiologies which, like hyponatremia, can be categorized based on the patient's volume status (**Table 9.8**). The most common scenario is excessive free water loss associated with hypovolemia.

Clinical Manifestations

Symptoms of hypernatremia typically do not develop until serum sodium exceeds 160 mEq/L or serum osmolality is higher than 320 to 330 mOsm/kg. Acute hypernatremia can cause symptoms at lower levels than chronic hypernatremia. The majority of symptoms experienced are CNS related with early signs being irritability, restlessness, and spasms. Later symptoms include ataxia and seizures.

Table 9.8. Causes of Hypernatremia

Volume Status	Cause
Low	▪ Free water loss ▪ Insensible—skin, respiratory ▪ Gastrointestinal loss ▪ Excessive hyperosmotic peritoneal dialysis ▪ Renal: diuretics, diabetes insipidus, nonoliguric renal failure
Normal	Same as "Low" volume status but with improper correction
High	▪ Free water loss ▪ Increased mineralocorticoids—hyperaldosteronism, hypercortisolism ▪ Iatrogenic ▪ Excessive sodium administration

Treatment

The treatment of hypernatremia, like hyponatremia, should not occur too rapidly, otherwise complications can ensue. A rate >0.7 mEq/L/h is considered dangerous as it can lead to cerebral edema and brainstem herniation. The most judicious way to correct hypernatremia involves calculating the free water deficit to obtain a desired sodium level suing the following equation.

$$\text{Water requirement} = (\text{Desired change in Na}^+ \times \text{TBW})/\text{Desired Na}^+$$

$$\text{TBW} = 0.6 \times \text{Weight (kg)}$$

This equation fails to account for ongoing free water losses such as urinary or GI loss. Further calculations can be done to quantify urine losses if this is a major concern.

Potassium

Potassium is the most abundant intracellular cation with a normal intracellular concentration of 150 mEq/L as opposed to an extracellular level ranging from 3.5 to 5 mEq/L. This large gradient produces a strong membrane potential, especially in cardiac, skeletal, and smooth muscles. The overall potassium balance is determined by potassium intake and renal/extrarenal excretion. Renal excretion accounts for 90% of excreted potassium. Thus, renal failure leads to hyperkalemia. Humoral factors such as aldosterone, vasopressin, and β-agonists stimulate renal excretion of potassium. Intracellular shifting is another strong causative agent for extracellular potassium change. For instance, insulin and alkalosis both cause K^+ to shift intracellular, one for glycolysis, the other in exchange for H^+ as a buffer. Conversely, acidosis causes K^+ to shift extracellular in exchange for H^+, again to buffer serum pH.

Hyperkalemia

Renal insufficiency is the leading cause of hyperkalemia in surgical patients (**Table 9.9**).

Clinical Manifestations

Regardless of the etiology, the clinical manifestations are due to dysfunctional membrane depolarization, the most lethal scenario affecting cardiac membranes. On an electrocardiogram (EKG) this can be seen, in the mildest form, as peaked T waves, and, in a more severe state, flattened P waves, prolongation of the QRS, or deep S waves. The final pathway can yield ventricular fibrillation with or without cardiac arrest.

Table 9.9. Causes of Hyperkalemia

Major Causes of Hyperkalemia
Renal failure (leading cause)
Blood transfusions
Crush injury
Reperfusion injury
Tumor lysis syndrome
Burns
Succinylcholine
ACE inhibitors

Treatment

The initial medication of choice for hyperkalemia is intravenous calcium for membrane stabilization, which lasts approximately 30 to 60 minutes. Subsequent therapy can include insulin coadministered with dextrose, β_2-agonist, and sodium bicarbonate, which are designed to shift extracellular potassium into the intracellular space. Resin-binding agents such as Kayexalate can decrease potassium absorption and thus are more important in the management of chronic hyperkalemia. Loop diuretics can assist by promoting renal potassium excretion, but should only be used if the patient is not hypovolemic. A last resort in situations of complete renal failure or critical levels of potassium is hemodialysis. The treatment utilized not only depends upon the laboratory value, but more importantly the clinical scenario and EKG findings (**Algorithm 9.2**).

Hypokalemia

Hypokalemia is characterized by low serum potassium levels. Among major causes of hypokalemia are vomiting, diarrhea, and loop diuretics (**Table 9.10**).

Clinical Manifestations

The reference level of 3.5 mEq/L is often cited as the lowermost level of normal serum potassium. Below this level, minor disturbances including intestinal ileus, premature ventricular

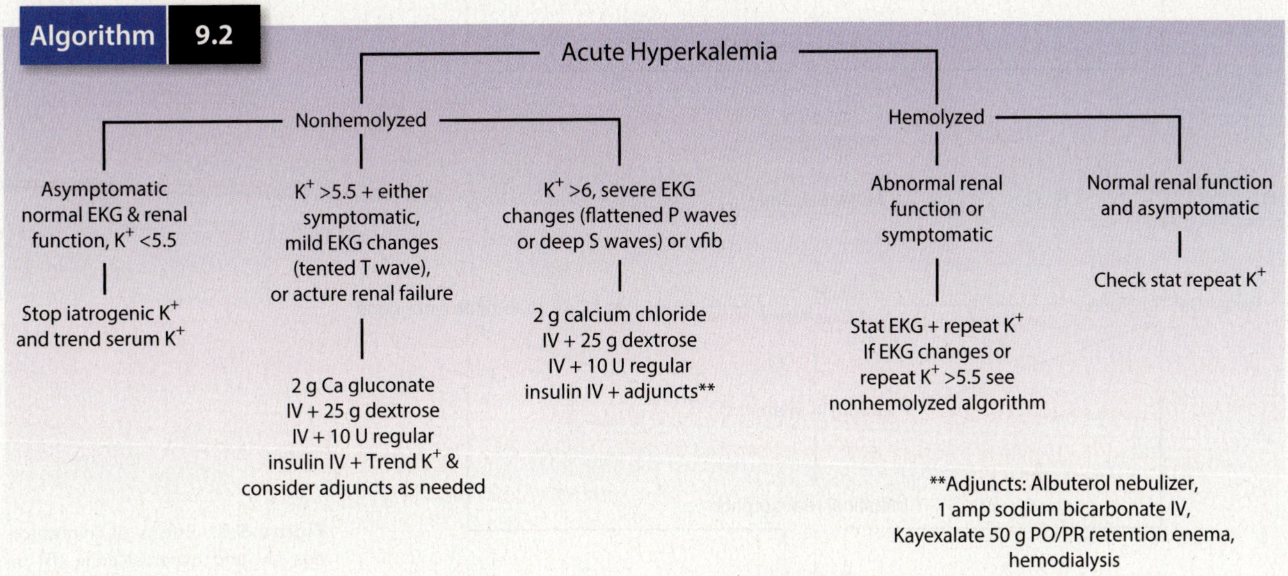

Algorithm 9.2. Acute hyperkalemia.

Table 9.10. Causes of Hypokalemia

Causes of Hypokalemia
Vomiting/diarrhea
Diuretics (ie, loop diuretic)
Catecholamines (endogenous or exogenous)
Renal tubular acidosis
Refeeding syndrome
Insulin
Hypomagnesemia
Acute alkalosis

complexes, and nonfatal arrhythmias can occur. Severe cardiac and muscle manifestations often do not occur until levels fall below 2.5 mEq/L. Findings at this dangerous level include significant muscle weakness and major EKG changes including prolonged QT, flattened T waves, ST depression, prominent U waves, and most dangerously, ventricular arrhythmias.

Treatment

Initial treatment consideration must include elucidation of possible etiologies. Without correction of the underlying cause, the hypokalemia itself may not be correctable. Examples of this include hypomagnesemia, acute alkalosis, hyperaldosteronism, and mucus secreting villous adenoma. The mainstay of initial treatment for hypokalemia is enteral or intravenous potassium replacement. If the patient is symptomatic, then the replacement or at least a portion of it should be given intravenously to achieve a more rapid effect. Limiting the rate of intravenous potassium infusion is necessary to prevent caustic injury to veins. Maximal recommended rates include 10 to 20 mEq/h via a peripheral IV or up to 40 mEq/h via central access.

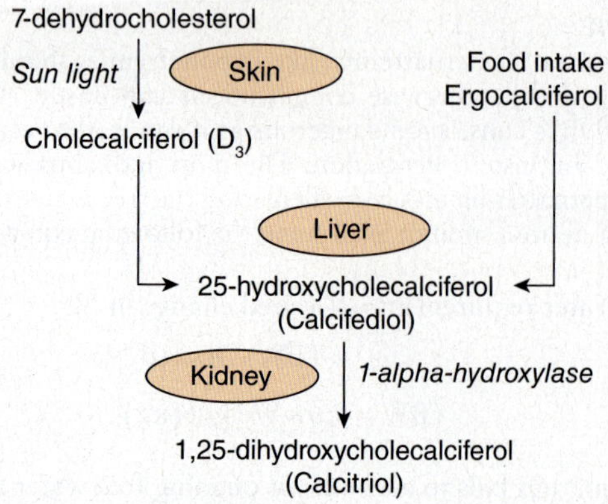

Figure 9.2. Vitamin D synthesis.

Calcium

Calcium (Ca^{2+}) is essential for human life and participates in numerous processes including cardiac membrane depolarization, muscle contraction, enzymatic reactions, coagulation, and formation of bone/teeth. Approximately 99% of total body calcium is located in bone. In plasma, calcium exists in three forms. Ionized calcium, which makes up approximately 45% of total calcium, is responsible for most of the physiologic actions of calcium in the body. Another 40% of plasma calcium is bound to albumin and nearly 15% to anions. Normal serum concentration of ionized calcium is approximately 4.5 mg/dL and this level is tightly regulated. Both pH and plasma protein level can affect the proportion of calcium in the ionized state. A change in albumin concentration of 1 g/dL changes protein-bound calcium by 0.8 mg/dL in the same direction. The fundamentals of the regulation of calcium homeostasis are depicted in **Figures 9.2** and **9.3**.

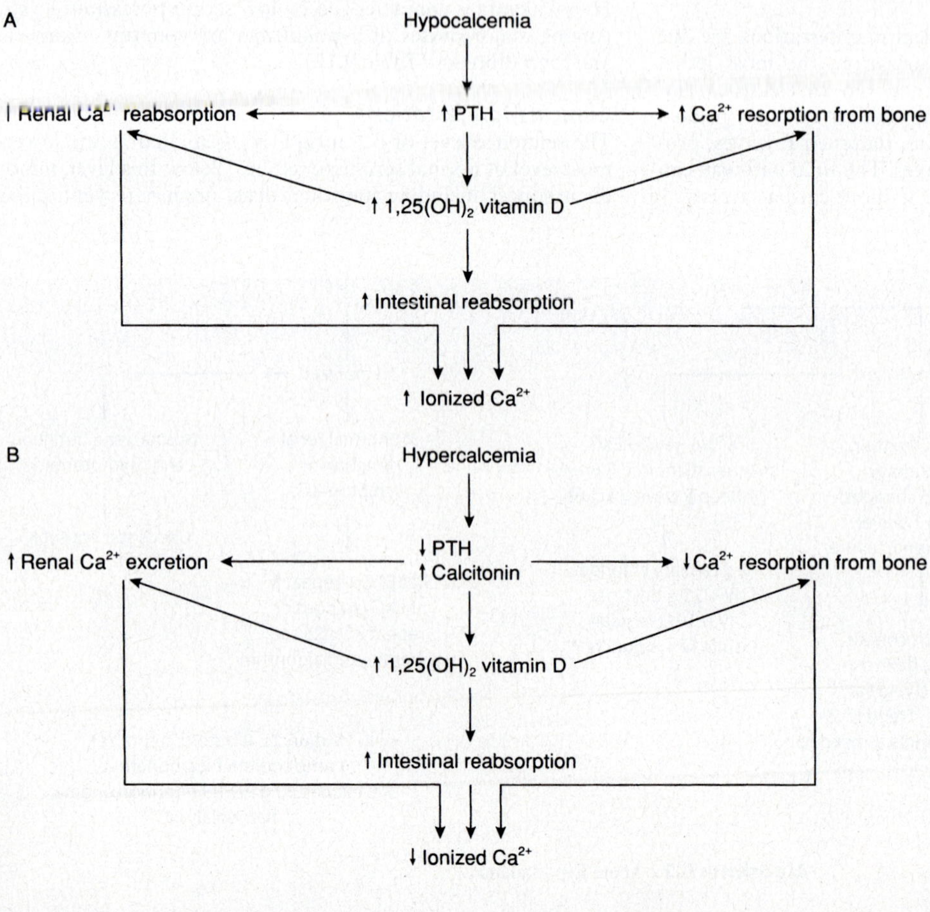

Figure 9.3. Effects of hypocalcemia (**A**) and hypercalcemia (**B**) on the mediators of calcium homeostasis.PTH, parathyroid hormone.

Table 9.11. Other Causes of Hypercalcemia

PTH mediated	▪ Lithium ▪ Familial hypocalciuric hypercalcemia (FHH)
Cancer	▪ PTHrp-mediated breast, lung, renal cancer ▪ Bone metastases ▪ Multiple myeloma
Calcitriol mediated	▪ End-stage renal disease ▪ Sarcoid/granulomatous ▪ Lymphoma (ectopic 1,25 vit D) ▪ Milk alkali syndrome ▪ Exogenous vitamin D
Other causes	▪ Vitamin A toxicity ▪ Thyrotoxicosis ▪ Paget disease ▪ Adrenal insufficiency ▪ Medications (ie, Thiazide)

Hypercalcemia

The most common causes of hypercalcemia are hyperparathyroidism and malignancy (**Table 9.11**).[22,23]

Primary hyperparathyroidism occurs when one or more parathyroid glands inappropriately produce increased amounts of parathyroid hormone (PTH). Parathyroid adenomas account for ~85% of cases followed by chief cell hyperplasia (15%) and cancer (less than 1%).

Secondary hyperparathyroidism arises from elevated PTH due to renal failure. This condition results from poor renal excretion of phosphate and decreased intestinal absorption of calcium secondary to impaired renal hydroxylation of vitamin D.

Tertiary hyperparathyroidism is parathyroid hyperplasia with autonomous PTH production. The most common scenario involves a patient who, after experiencing renal failure with secondary hyperplasia, undergoes a renal transplant but continues to have hypercalcemia (**Table 9.12**).

Clinical Manifestations

Regardless of cause, hypercalcemia has characteristic clinical manifestations classically taught as "stones, moans, and psychiatric overtones," meaning renal, abdominal/GI, and neuropsychiatric symptoms (**Table 9.13**). The earliest symptoms are usually neuromuscular and mild GI symptoms. Cardiac and renal complications typically occur later in the disease progression.

Table 9.13. Signs and Symptoms of Hypercalcemia

Constitutional symptoms	Weakness, fatigue, anorexia
CNS	Drowsiness, lethargy, altered mental status, stupor, coma
Cardiac	Short QT interval
Renal	Nephrolithiasis, nephrocalcinosis, nephrogenic diabetes insipidus, polyuria, renal failure
GI	Constipation, abdominal pain, acute pancreatitis
Ophthalmologic	Calcific-band keratopathy (calcium deposits in cornea)

Treatment

Serum calcium concentration >14 mg/dL requires prompt treatment. If combined with hyperphosphatemia, this situation is even more concerning due to the potential for metastatic calcification.

Initial treatment should include aggressive hydration with 0.9% normal saline with 20 mEq/L potassium with a goal urine output of greater than 200 mL/h. Once the patient is adequately hydrated a trial of furosemide can be performed provided a positive fluid balance is maintained, and potassium and magnesium are adequately replaced. Other adjuncts include calcitonin (especially for inhibition of bone resorption), bisphosphonates (especially to treat malignancy), and in patients with renal failure the use of low-calcium dialysate. Patients with hematologic malignancies and granulomatous disease can be considered for treatment with steroids. Finally, for those with hyperparathyroidism, parathyroidectomy of some form is clearly indicated, with operation type dependent upon the etiology (adenoma vs hyperplasia). In medically refractory secondary or tertiary hyperparathyroidism, total parathyroidectomy with parathyroid autotransplantation or subtotal parathyroidectomy should be considered.

Hypocalcemia

There are many causes of hypocalcemia (**Table 9.14**).

Postsurgical Hypocalcemia

Postsurgical hypocalcemia can occur following any neck operation, especially parathyroidectomy. In nonneck surgery, hypocalcemia can occur because of hypoalbuminemia; this does

Table 9.12. Differential Diagnosis of Hypercalcemia

Cause	Ca^{+}	Phosphate	PTH	24-h UCa
Primary PTH	Increased	Decreased	Elevated/normal	Elevated
Secondary PTH	Low or normal (can be high w/ prolonged disease)	High	Elevated	N/A
FHH	Increased	Normal	Elevated/normal	Decreased
PTHrp mediated	Increased	Decreased	Decreased	Elevated
Tertiary PTH	Increased	Decreased	Very elevated	Elevated

PTHrp, parathyroid hormone–related peptide; UCa, urine Ca^{+}.

SCIENTIFIC PRINCIPLES

Table 9.14. Causes of Hypocalcemia

Low PTH (hypoparathyroidism)	■ Postsurgical (thyroidectomy, parathyroidectomy, radical neck dissection, hungry bone syndrome) ■ Autoimmune ■ Infiltration of the parathyroid gland (granulomatous, iron overload, metastases) ■ Radiation-induced destruction of parathyroid glands ■ HIV infection
High PTH (secondary hyperparathyroidism in response to hypocalcemia)	■ Vitamin D deficiency ■ Pseudohypoparathyroidism ■ Hypomagnesemia ■ Renal disease ■ Loss of calcium in circulation (ie, hyperphosphatemia, tumor lysis, acute pancreatitis, osteoblastic metastases, acute respiratory alkalosis, sepsis)
Drugs	■ Bisphosphonate, calcitonin, phenytoin, foscarnet, calcium chelators

not affect ionized calcium levels. Other postsurgical causes of hypocalcemia include atrophy of the remaining parathyroid glands (ie, after removal of a large parathyroid adenoma), venous congestion, devascularization, or *hungry bone syndrome*. Transient hypoparathyroidism is seen in up to 20% of thyroid cancer surgery; this is permanent in 1% or less of cases.

Other surgery-related etiologies include pancreatitis, small bowel fistula, renal failure, massive blood transfusion, and severe hypomagnesemia. Pancreatitis-induced hypocalcemia occurs due to calcium precipitation in peripancreatic tissue. Small bowel fistula can lead to hypocalcemia by loss of calcium-rich effluent and vitamin D deficiency from malnutrition. Renal failure hypocalcemia is due to deficiency in 1,25-dihydroxyvitamin D and hyperphosphatemia. Massive transfusion hypocalcemia does not affect total calcium but decreases ionized calcium as a result of citrate binding to ionized calcium.

Clinical Manifestations

Symptoms typically do not occur until calcium levels are below 8 mg/dL. Symptoms are described as acute or chronic (**Table 9.15**).

Tetany, defined as repetitive discharges after a single stimulus, usually does not occur until serum total calcium is less than 7.0 mg/dL. The earliest symptoms of hypocalcemia are perioral and acral paresthesias. Motor symptoms such as *Trousseau sign* (induction of carpopedal spasm by inflation of sphygmomanometer above systolic pressure for 3 minutes) and *Chvostek sign* (tap facial nerve and ipsilateral facial muscles twitch) occur later. Of note, Chvostek sign is seen in up to 10% of normal patients. The last findings to occur are cardiac, in the form of ST segment prolongation.

Treatment

Asymptomatic hypocalcemia requires no treatment as it is most commonly attributed to hypoalbuminemia with normal ionized calcium. Symptomatic hypocalcemia is best treated with intravenous infusion of calcium gluconate or calcium chloride. Calcium chloride is faster acting as it does not require hepatic metabolism to dissociate into an active form, hence is usually

Table 9.15. Clinical Manifestations of Hypocalcemia

Acute	■ Neuromuscular ■ Paresthesia (initially perioral) ■ Seizures ■ Tetany (ie, Trousseau/Chvostek sign) ■ Pulmonary ■ Laryngospasm, bronchospasm ■ Cardiac ■ Prolonged QT, hypotension, heart failure, arrhythmias ■ Ocular ■ Papilledema
Chronic	■ Abnormal dentition ■ Extrapyramidal signs ■ Ectopic calcification ■ Subcapsular cataracts

the drug of choice if severely symptomatic. A study during the anhepatic stage of liver transplantation found equally rapid increase in calcium after administration of calcium chloride and gluconate. Calcium chloride carries a higher risk of venous irritation and tissue damage should extravasation occur; hence calcium gluconate should be the drug of choice except in emergent situations. In order to minimize caustic damage to veins, any form of calcium should be administered at a rate not to exceed 1.5 mEq/min. If prolonged calcium replacement is needed, it is recommended to check vitamin D levels and replace any deficiency with calcitriol, in addition to giving an oral form of calcium such as calcium carbonate, calcium citrate, or calcium lactate.

Magnesium

Half of the total body magnesium is confined to bone. Most of the remaining magnesium is intracellular, with less than 1% of total body magnesium found extracellular. Magnesium is primarily absorbed in the small intestine and is influenced by 1,25-dihydroxyvitamin D_3.

Hypermagnesemia

With the exception of renal failure, hypermagnesemia is rare (**Table 9.16**), as the kidneys have a strong ability to excrete large amounts of magnesium.

Clinical Manifestations

Symptoms of hypermagnesemia include loss of deep tendon reflexes at levels greater than 8 mg/dL. Once levels are greater than 12 mg/dL, paralysis can occur. Cardiac arrest can occur if levels exceed 18 mg/dL.

Table 9.16. Causes of Hyper- and Hypomagnesemia

Hypermagnesemia ■ Renal failure (leading cause) ■ Severe burns ■ Crush injury ■ Rhabdomyolysis
Hypomagnesemia ■ Chronic malnutrition ■ Diarrhea ■ Prolonged IV fluids without Mg^{+2} ■ Loop diuretics ■ Pancreatitis ■ Diabetic ketoacidosis

Treatment

The mainstay of treatment is intravenous calcium to antagonize the effect of magnesium, volume expansion or loop diuretic depending on volume status, correction of acid–base disturbances and if needed, hemodialysis.

Hypomagnesemia

Kidneys are also able to conserve magnesium quite well with about 40% reabsorption in the proximal tubule. Most instances of hypomagnesemia occur with chronic malnutrition (**Table 9.16**).

Clinical Manifestations

Magnesium functions as a cofactor for many neuromuscular functions, thus deficiency can lead to muscle fasciculation or tetany.

Treatment

The treatment depends on the severity. For instance, if serum magnesium level is less than 1 mEq/L or if the patient is hemodynamically unstable or is in a torsade de pointes arrhythmia, then immediate infusion of intravenous magnesium sulfate is indicated. The maximum recommended rate would be 150 mg/min excluding the above emergent situations where it can be given as IV push or over 5 minutes for torsade de pointes. If the patient has chronic or mild hypomagnesemia, oral doses of magnesium should be used, with options including magnesium oxide, magnesium chloride, and magnesium hydroxide (milk of magnesia) depending on side-effect profiles. It should be noted that doses greater than 80 mEq/d can become cathartic.

ACID–BASE

An acid is defined as a chemical that can donate a hydrogen ion (H^+), for example, HCl and H_2CO_3. A base is a chemical that can accept an H^+, for example, OH^- and HCO_3^-. Bases are commonly anions, but neutral substances can also function as bases (eg, ammonia and creatinine). Some chemicals do not fit the classic definition of an acid, although they retain acidic properties when dissociated in water. For example, when $CaCl_2$ is dissolved in water, the Ca^{2+} accepts OH^- to form $Ca(OH)_2$.[2]

The concentration of hydrogen ions [H^+] determines the acidity of a solution. The pH is the negative logarithm of [H^+] expressed in moles per liter (mol/L). The degree to which an acid dissociates determines its strength.

The *Henderson–Hasselbalch* equation describes pH as a measure of acidity in a biologic system.[2]

$$pH = pK_a + \log_{10}([A^-])/[HA])$$

$$pK_a = \text{Negative log of the acid dissociation constant}$$

$$A^- = \text{Conjugate base}$$

$$HA = \text{Acid–base pair}$$

Table 9.17. Major Buffer Systems of Human Body

Intracellular	Bicarbonate Organic phosphates Peptides
RBCs	Hemoglobin
Extracellular fluid	Bicarbonate

Buffer Systems

Buffers are chemicals in solution that tend to minimize changes in pH that would otherwise occur after the addition of an acid or alkali. For instance, if a strong base is added to a weak acid, the base is neutralized:

$$NaOH + H_2CO_3 \rightarrow NaHCO_3 + H_2O$$

The buffer pair carbonic acid/bicarbonate (H_2CO_3/HCO_3^-) is the primary buffer system of the body (**Table 9.17**). This buffer system is efficient because of the presence of large amounts of bicarbonate, the conversion of its acid H_2CO_3 to CO_2 that is rapidly excreted through the lungs, and an inexhaustible supply of CO_2 from metabolism.

Acid–Base Balance

To maintain a steady state, acid produced by the body during metabolism must equal net acid excreted by the kidneys. Acid or alkali produced by the cells is transported into the ECF via plasma membrane proteins, and eventually eliminated in the urine: acid as NH_4^+ and acid phosphates and alkali as HCO_3^- to maintain an acid–base balance.[2]

Acid–Base Disturbances

Acid–base disturbances are commonly seen in critically ill patients. Early identification and correction of these disturbances are of utmost importance in surgical intensive care unit (ICU) patients. Arterial blood gas (ABG) and serum chemistry profile are often used to identify these disorders. Serum bicarbonate (HCO_3^-) accurately predicts metabolic acidosis in surgical ICU patients[24] and can act as a substitute for arterial base deficit.

There are four primary acid–base disturbances, each of which is related to changes in either [HCO_3^-] or PCO_2. These are categorized as metabolic and/or respiratory (**Table 9.18**). In each of these disorders, compensatory changes occur to minimize changes in the relative ratio of [HCO_3^-] to PCO_2 and thereby blunt the effect of the primary disturbance on pH (**Table 9.19**).

Metabolic Acidosis

Anion Gap

The difference in the measured serum cations and anions yields the anion gap. The most common equation used in practice is as follows:

$$\text{Anion gap} = [Na^+] - ([Cl^-] + [HCO_3^-])$$

Table 9.18. HCO_3^- and PCO_2 Derangements in Primary and Secondary Acid–Base Disturbances

Disorder	pH	HCO_3^-	PCO_2	Compensatory Response
Metabolic acidosis	↓	↓	↓	Hyperventilation
Metabolic alkalosis	↑	↑	↑	Hypoventilation
Respiratory acidosis	↓	↑	↑	↑renal [HCO_3^-] reabsorption
Respiratory alkalosis	↑	↓	↓	↓renal [HCO_3^-] reabsorption

↑ and ↓ represent primary disturbance.

Table 9.19. Compensatory Mechanisms for Acid–Base Disorders

Disorder	Compensation	Time
Metabolic acidosis	PCO_2 = serum HCO_3^- + 15 PCO_2 = 1.5 × serum HCO_3^- + 8 ± 2	12–24 h
Metabolic alkalosis	0.7 mm Hg PCO_2 per 1 mEq/L HCO_3^-	12–24 h
Acute respiratory alkalosis	2 mEq/L HCO_3^- per 10 mm Hg PCO_2	<3 d
Chronic respiratory alkalosis	4–5 mEq/L HCO_3^- per 10 mm Hg PCO_2	3–5 d
Acute respiratory acidosis	1 mEq/L HCO_3^- per 10 mm Hg PCO_2	<3 d
Chronic respiratory acidosis	~4 mEq/L HCO_3^- per 10 mm Hg PCO_2	3–5 d

The normal value of serum anion gap is approximately 3 to 10.

Anion gap can be utilized to identify the etiology of a metabolic acidosis. The differentials for elevated and normal anion gap metabolic acidosis are given in **Table 9.20**.

Mechanisms of Metabolic Acidosis

Four mechanisms result in a decrease in extracellular bicarbonate concentration and metabolic acidosis:

1. Dilutional acidosis (Rapid infusion of an alkali-free solution [eg, normal saline], results in dilution of the bicarbonate concentration)
2. Diminished renal acid excretion (eg, renal failure or type I renal tubular acidosis [RTA][2])
3. Increased acid generation (eg, lactic acidosis, ketoacidosis, salicylate poisoning)
4. Decreased body bicarbonate content (eg, severe diarrhea, fistula, type II RTA)

Clinically significant metabolic acidosis in surgical patients is most commonly related to net loss of bicarbonate. One means of classification would be renal acidosis versus extrarenal acidosis. Renal acidosis is not as readily compensated because the kidney's ability to regulate acid base is compromised. Extrarenal acidosis can be further subdivided into increased acid production (eg, lactic acidosis in shock) or increase bicarbonate loss (eg, fistula).

Nonrenal Loss of Bicarbonate

Diarrhea, intestinal or pancreatic fistulas, and burns can cause metabolic acidosis secondary to loss of bicarbonate. Urinary diversion with segments of the GI tract (ureterosigmoidostomy and ureteroileostomy) can result in loss of bicarbonate with reabsorption of NH_4Cl from the urine. The potential for fistulas to result in metabolic acidosis depends on the concentration of bicarbonate in the fluid and the rate of external drainage. For instance, metabolic acidosis is less common with biliary fistulas than pancreatic fistulas.

Table 9.20. Differentials of Metabolic Acidosis

Elevated Anion Gap (MUDPILES)	Normal Anion Gap
Methanol	Hyperchloremia
Uremia (CKD)	Addison disease
Diabetic ketoacidosis	Renal tubular acidosis
Propylene glycol	Diarrhea
Iron tablets or isoniazid	Acetazolamide
Lactic acidosis	Spironolactone
Ethylene glycol	Saline infusion
Salicylates poisoning	

Ketoacidosis

Ketoacids are produced from the beta oxidation of fatty acids forming acetoacetate and β-hydroxybutyrate. During prolonged starvation, production of ketoacid increases modestly. In DKA, insulin deficiency leads to excessive ketoacid production. This results in osmotic diuresis, causing the kidneys to excrete more sodium, potassium, and water. Despite total body potassium depletion, serum potassium often remains high. The typical clinical presentation includes dehydration, polyuria, polydipsia, hyperglycemia, hyperventilation, and anion gap metabolic acidosis.

Lactic Acidosis

Lactic acid is a common cause of metabolic acidosis, and can be seen in patients with sepsis[25] and hemorrhagic shock. Its levels are predictive of outcomes in shock states. In the setting of hypoxia, the cellular dependence on anaerobic metabolic pathways increases lactic acid generation which correlates with oxygen debt, degree of hypoperfusion, and the severity of shock. Lactic acidosis is managed by optimizing tissue perfusion with volume resuscitation. Once perfusion is restored, the liver rapidly metabolizes lactic acid, normalizing serum pH.

Renal Acidosis

The most common renal-associated acidosis in surgical patients is due to acute or chronic renal failure. The kidneys play a crucial role in acid excretion, and a decrease in GFR impairs this function.

Type I RTA

The impaired ability of the kidney to excrete acid may be secondary to a decrease in the number of functioning nephrons termed as RTA. Type I (distal) RTA is most commonly caused by autoimmune diseases (eg, Sjögren syndrome or rheumatoid arthritis) and hypercalciuria in adults. Distal RTA leads to impaired distal acidification.

Type II RTA

Type II (proximal) RTA is caused by a reduction in proximal bicarbonate reabsorption—the most common cause in adults being monoclonal gammopathies or medications such as carbonic anhydrase inhibitors.

Clinical Features of Acute Metabolic Acidosis

The major cardiovascular effects of acute metabolic acidosis are peripheral arteriolar dilatation, decreased cardiac contractility, and central venous constriction. These can lead to cardiovascular collapse and pulmonary edema. In addition, metabolic acidosis can increase oxygen delivery by shifting the oxygen–hemoglobin dissociation curve to the right.

Renal Compensation

The kidney is extremely sensitive to changes in serum bicarbonate concentration and responds by increasing net acid excretion primarily in the form of ammonia. Maximal renal compensation requires 2 to 4 days. In addition, the maximal amount of ammonia excreted during acidosis depends on factors such as glutamine delivery, GFR, and the type of anion that accompanies the acid.

Respiratory Compensation

A decrease in blood pH causes an immediate stimulus to hyperventilate. Although effective in promptly raising blood pH, early ventilatory compensation is only partial. Full respiratory compensation can occur in 12 to 24 hours. The magnitude of the decrease in PCO_2 in response to a given degree of metabolic acidosis can be used to determine whether the metabolic acidosis is complicated by concomitant respiratory acidosis or respiratory alkalosis. There are multiple equations that can describe this relationship:

$$\text{Arterial } PCO_2 = \text{Serum } HCO_3^- + 15$$

$$\text{Arterial } PCO_2 = 1.5 \times \text{Serum } HCO_3^- + 8 \pm 2 \text{ (Winter equation)}$$

The PCO_2 can fall no lower than 8 to 12 mm Hg in response to a severe metabolic acidosis and this compensation can only be maintained for a limited period due to respiratory muscle fatigue.

Treatment of Acute Metabolic Acidosis

Volume resuscitation alone may correct metabolic acidosis. Correcting acidosis with exogenous bicarbonate without addressing tissue perfusion will be unsuccessful. In addition, bicarbonate administration can cause respiratory alkalosis and a left shift in the oxygen–hemoglobin dissociation curve, leading to tissue hypoxia.

Metabolic Alkalosis

Sustained metabolic alkalosis occurs only if extracellular bicarbonate concentration is increased and renal excretion of excess bicarbonate is inhibited. In surgical patients, loss of HCl is a frequent cause of metabolic alkalosis, most commonly due to vomiting or nasogastric suction in the presence of gastric outlet obstruction. External loss of gastric acid results in a net gain in bicarbonate, which causes alkalosis. Although the kidney can excrete excess bicarbonate, this must be accompanied by excretion of sodium. Renal excretion of sodium is limited in the presence of the volume depletion that occurs with external loss of gastric secretions. As volume depletion progresses, sodium is conserved in exchange for hydrogen, leading to acidic urine even in severe metabolic alkalosis, a phenomenon known as *paradoxical aciduria.*

Metabolic alkalosis can occur with the administration of either bicarbonate or its precursors, such as lactate, citrate, or calcium carbonate, or as a result of increased renal bicarbonate production. It can also occur in conditions like moderate potassium depletion, excess mineralocorticoids, and high PCO_2, when acid excretion exceeds acid production and the renal threshold for bicarbonate reabsorption increases.

Hypokalemia results in enhanced proximal tubular bicarbonate reabsorption and distal tubular acid excretion. When potassium leaves the cell, it is exchanged for either sodium or hydrogen to maintain electrical neutrality. Loss of potassium from the body then results in a net gain in bicarbonate in the ECF.

Volume contraction leads to a decrease in renal blood flow and GFR thus reducing the filtered load of bicarbonate. This, in addition to increased proximal tubular reabsorption, maintains high extracellular concentrations of bicarbonate. High PCO_2 causes an increase in renal threshold for bicarbonate secondary to decreased intracellular pH of the renal tubular cell. The net result is increased bicarbonate reabsorption.

Diuretics can cause or exacerbate metabolic alkalosis by both causing rapid contraction of intravascular volume and increasing renal excretion of acid. Chloride deficiency is another common factor that maintains an alkalotic state. In some instances of metabolic alkalosis, urinary excretion of chloride is markedly reduced. Reversal of metabolic alkalosis in these cases can be readily achieved by administration of chloride-containing solutions. Metabolic alkalosis can be categorically divided into chloride-responsive and chloride-resistant types.

Clinical Features

Clinical signs of metabolic alkalosis develop slowly. Acute manifestations include confusion, obtundation, stupor, and coma as well as tetany or neuromuscular irritability.

Respiratory Compensation

Respiratory compensation for metabolic alkalosis should raise the PCO_2 by 0.7 mm Hg for every 1 mEq/L elevation in serum HCO_3^-. Typically the arterial PCO_2 does not go above 55 mm Hg. Among the four major acid–base disorders, this compensatory mechanism is the least effective.

Treatment

Treatment for metabolic alkalosis focusses on the underlying cause. Generally, reversing potassium and volume depletion corrects the metabolic alkalosis. Persistent volume depletion impairs renal bicarbonate excretion, which should be managed with chloride-containing solutions. In patients without volume deficits, administration of acetazolamide (a carbonic anhydrase inhibitor) can enhance bicarbonate excretion.

In rare cases of severe alkalosis or renal insufficiency, acids like ammonium chloride or dilute hydrochloric acid may be used to titrate excess bicarbonate. Partial correction of the alkalosis is the initial goal and a specialist should be involved before instituting this care. In cases of severe renal failure, dialysis may be required to remove excess bicarbonate.

Respiratory Alkalosis

Respiratory alkalosis is defined as increased extracellular pH secondary to decreased PCO_2 with hyperventilation (**Table 9.18**). Hyperventilation and the ensuing fall in PCO_2 may be secondary to hypoxia, reflex stimulation from decreased pulmonary compliance, drugs, mechanical ventilation, or other causes.

Hypoxia stimulates ventilation via peripheral chemoreceptors in the carotid and aortic bodies, with arterial pO_2 being the main stimulus. Acute drops in pO_2 cause sustained hyperventilation only when PCO_2 falls below 60 mm Hg. Mild hypoxia induces hyperventilation, but increased cerebral pH suppresses this response unless hypoxia is severe. Chronic hypoxia leads to hyperventilation even with mildly decreased PCO_2 due to metabolic compensation lowering cerebral pH. The two most common causes of hypoxia resulting in respiratory alkalosis are pulmonary disease and exposure to high altitudes.

Clinical Features

Chronic respiratory alkalosis is typically asymptomatic due to effective compensatory mechanisms maintaining near-normal pH. Acute respiratory alkalosis may cause breathlessness, dizziness, nervousness, circumoral and extremity paresthesias, altered consciousness, and tetany. These symptoms arise from decreased cerebral blood flow due to low PCO_2 and reduced ionized calcium from increased blood pH.

Compensatory Mechanisms

Tissue buffering is the initial response to a decrease in PCO_2. Red blood cells provide one-third of this buffering. Cellular

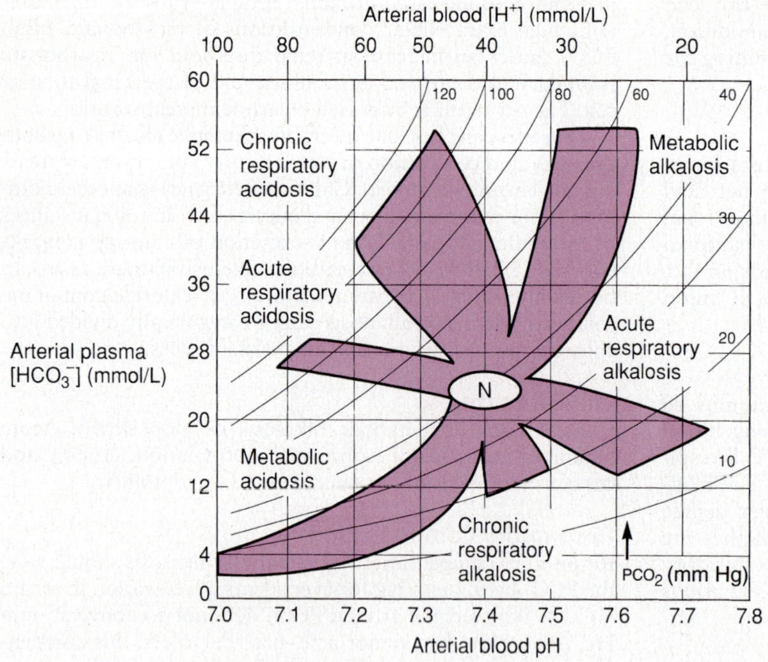

Figure 9.4. Acid–base nomogram.Shown are the 95% confidence limits of the normal respiratory and metabolic compensations for primary acid–base disturbances. (Reproduced with permission from Cogan MG, Rector FC Jr. Acid-base disturbances. In: Brenner BM, Rector FC Jr, eds. *The Kidney.* WB Saunders; 1986:473.)

liberation of H^+ consumes bicarbonate. Tissue buffering is relatively weak compared to renal compensation, achieved by decreasing net acid excretion, particularly ammonia. Chronic compensation is stronger and takes at least 3 days to develop, unlike acute compensation (**Table 9.19**).

Treatment

The underlying stimulus for the hyperventilation and the cause of hypoxemia should be determined and corrected. In acute symptomatic respiratory alkalosis, temporary relief can be achieved with rebreathing or breathing 5% CO_2. If caused by mechanical ventilation, reducing tidal volume or respiratory rate should resolve the alkalosis.

Respiratory Acidosis

Respiratory acidosis is defined by a decrease in extracellular pH arising from a primary increase in PCO_2, due to inadequate ventilation. Causes of hypoventilation include CNS depression, impaired pulmonary mechanics (respiratory muscles weakening), airway obstruction, chronic obstructive pulmonary disease (COPD) and opioids. In addition, inappropriate ventilator settings may result in respiratory acidosis in patients on mechanical ventilation.

Clinical Features

Clinical manifestations of respiratory acidosis vary depending on its chronicity and rate of development. Acute increases result in cerebral acidosis, presenting as drowsiness, restlessness, and tremor, and severe cases may progress to stupor or coma. Acidosis leads to cerebral vasodilation thereby increasing cerebral blood flow. This may result in increased intracranial blood pressure, headache, and papilledema. Systemic acidosis results in peripheral vasodilatation, depressed cardiac contractility, and reduced sensitivity to catecholamines.

Compensatory Mechanisms

Increased pCO_2 leads to elevated H_2CO_3, which dissociates into H^+ and HCO_3^-. Cellular exchange of Na^+ and K^+ for H^+ promotes this reaction, increasing extracellular bicarbonate. This tissue buffering is accomplished within minutes. Persistently elevated PCO_2 also stimulates increased renal acid excretion, primarily as the chloride salt of ammonia, generating more HCO_3^-. Full renal compensation takes over 3 to 5 days (**Table 9.19**).

Treatment

Treatment should be directed to the underlying cause of hypoventilation. Endotracheal intubation to achieve adequate ventilation is paramount to the treatment of acute respiratory acidosis of any cause.

In select cases of respiratory acidosis, namely patients with COPD, noninvasive positive pressure ventilation (ie, CPAP/BiPAP) has proven effective. However, patients must be able to protect their airway and have no major concern for aspiration (ie, not appropriate in the setting of a bowel obstruction). Furthermore, there must be close follow-up to ensure the acidosis is resolving.

The treatment of chronic, compensated respiratory acidosis may be complicated by the accompanying hypoxemia. In chronic hypercapnia, the central chemoreceptors may become insensitive, with hypoxemia driving respiration via peripheral chemoreceptors. In such patients, complete correction of the hypoxemia may further suppress respiration, worsening acidosis.

In addition, rapid normalization of PCO_2 should be avoided as cerebral bicarbonate equilibration lags systemic changes. Thus, even if PCO_2 is normal, cellular and cerebral metabolic alkalosis may develop.

Mixed Acid–Base Disorders

Combinations of two or more of the four primary acid–base disorders may occur and should be suspected when blood pH approaches normal despite abnormal PCO_2 and $[HCO_3^-]$, or when compensatory changes appear excessive or inadequate (**Fig. 9.4**).

References

1. Forbes GB. Body composition: overview. *J Nutr.* 1999;129(1S Suppl):270s–272s.
2. Seifter JL, Chang HY. Extracellular acid-base balance and ion transport between body fluid compartments. *Physiology (Bethesda).* 2017;32(5):367–379.
3. Vujovic P, Chirillo M, Silverthorn DU. Learning (by) osmosis: an approach to teaching osmolarity and tonicity. *Adv Physiol Educ.* 2018;42(4):626–635.
4. Stockand JD. New ideas about aldosterone signaling in epithelia. *Am J Physiol Renal Physiol.* 2002;282(4):F559–576.
5. Thompson CA, Tatro DL, Ludwig DA, Convertino VA. Baroreflex responses to acute changes in blood volume in humans. *Am J Physiol.* 1990;259(4 Pt 2):R792–798.

6. Rosati F, de Maat GE, Valente MAE, et al. Surgical clip closure of the left atrial appendage. *J Cardiovasc Electrophysiol*. 2021;32(10):2865–2872.
7. Benigni A, Buelli S, Kohan DE. Endothelin-targeted new treatments for proteinuric and inflammatory glomerular diseases: focus on the added value to anti-renin-angiotensin system inhibition. *Pediatr Nephrol*. 2021;36(4):763–775.
8. Carlström M, Wilcox CS, Arendshorst WJ. Renal autoregulation in health and disease. *Physiol Rev*. 2015;95(2):405–511.
9. Ma J, Han S, Liu X, Zhou Z. Sodium bicarbonated Ringer's solution effectively improves coagulation function and lactic acid metabolism in patients with severe multiple injuries and traumatic shock. *Am J Transl Res*. 2021;13(5):5043–5050.
10. Arabi YM, Belley-Cote E, Carsetti A, et al. European Society of Intensive Care Medicine clinical practice guideline on fluid therapy in adult critically ill patients. Part 1: the choice of resuscitation fluids. *Intensive Care Med*. 2024;50(6):813–831.
11. Joseph B, Aziz H, Snell M, et al. The physiological effects of hyperosmolar resuscitation: 5% vs 3% hypertonic saline. *Am J Surg*. 2014;208(5):697–702.
12. Joseph B, Haider A, Rhee P. Traumatic brain injury advancements. *Curr Opin Crit Care*. 2015;21(6):506–511.
13. Mangat HS, Chiu YL, Gerber LM, et al. Hypertonic saline reduces cumulative and daily intracranial pressure burdens after severe traumatic brain injury. *J Neurosurg*. 2015;122(1):202–210.
14. Junger WG, Rhind SG, Rizoli SB, et al. Resuscitation of traumatic hemorrhagic shock patients with hypertonic saline-without dextran-inhibits neutrophil and endothelial cell activation. *Shock*. 2012;38(4):341–350.
15. Hohertz B, Seupaul RA, Holmes TM. Are colloids better than crystalloids for fluid resuscitation in critically ill patients? *Ann Emerg Med*. 2015;65(4):443–444.
16. Annane D, Siami S, Jaber S, et al. Effects of fluid resuscitation with colloids vs crystalloids on mortality in critically ill patients presenting with hypovolemic shock: the CRISTAL randomized trial. *JAMA*. 2013;310(17):1809–1817.
17. Wiedermann CJ, Eisendle K. Comparison of hydroxyethyl starch regulatory summaries from the Food and Drug Administration and the European Medicines Agency. *J Pharm Policy Pract*. 2017;10:1–6.
18. Schramko AA, Suojaranta-Ylinen RT, Kuitunen AH, et al. Rapidly degradable hydroxyethyl starch solutions impair blood coagulation after cardiac surgery: a prospective randomized trial. *Anesth Analg*. 2009;108(1):30–36.
19. Rhodes A, Evans LE, Alhazzani W, et al. Surviving sepsis campaign: International Guidelines for Management of Sepsis and Septic Shock: 2016. *Crit Care Med*. 2017;45(3):486–552.
20. Perel P, Roberts I, Ker K. Colloids versus crystalloids for fluid resuscitation in critically ill patients. *Cochrane Database Syst Rev*. 2013;(2):Cd000567.
21. Bernard AC, Moore EE, Moore FA, et al. Postinjury resuscitation with human polymerized hemoglobin prolongs early survival: a post hoc analysis. *J Trauma*. 2011;70(5 Suppl):S34–37.
22. Cooper MS, Gittoes NJ. Diagnosis and management of hypocalcaemia. *BMJ*. 2008;336(7656):1298–1302.
23. Hannan FM, Thakker RV. Investigating hypocalcaemia. *BMJ*. 2013;346:f2213.
24. Martin MJ, FitzSullivan E, Salim A, et al. Use of serum bicarbonate measurement in place of arterial base deficit in the surgical intensive care unit. *Arch Surg*. 2005;140(8):745–751.
25. Dellinger RP, Levy MM, Schorr CA, Townsend SR. 50 years of sepsis investigation/enlightenment among adults—the long and winding road. *Crit Care Med*. 2021;49(10):1606–1625.

10

Burns: Medical, Surgical, Critical Care, and Reconstruction of the Burn Patient

Samuel P. Mandell, Chiaka O. V. Akarichi, Naveen F. Sangji, and Benjamin Levi

Key Points

1. Most chemical injuries should be treated with dilution of the chemical rather than neutralization.
2. Early excision and grafting within 72 hours of the injury remains a pillar of burn care.
3. Resuscitation is of crucial importance for burn patient outcome and physicians must be aware when to begin resuscitation (>20% total body surface area [TBSA]) and to monitor the patient response to avoid over resuscitation.
4. New technologies have a role to play in scar rehabilitation, improving quality and pain associated with these scars.

Burn injuries represent a major source of trauma, scarring, and debilitation throughout the world. Improved worker safety programs, building codes, fire prevention efforts, and fire detection systems have significantly decreased the prevalence of major burn injuries. Burn survival has also been impacted by improvements in surgical critical care in areas such as lung protective ventilation, blood glucose control, and antibiotic stewardship. Overall, survival after burn injuries today is high, leading to a need for improved reconstructive treatment options for burn survivors.

EPIDEMIOLOGY

According to the Centers for Disease Control and Prevention (CDC), approximately 404,000 people received emergency department treatment for burns in the United States in 2021.[1] Overall, more than 67% of reported cases had burn sizes <10% total body surface area (TBSA).[2] Men account for 67% and women account for 33% of reported injuries. Men make up the majority of burns in every age group except for those aged >80 years. Of those injured, 59% are Caucasian, 21% are African American, and 11% are Hispanic. The cause of these burn injuries vary with 41% from fire or flame burns, 35% from scald burns, 10% from contact burns, and 7% from electrical and chemical burns. Approximately 13% of these injuries are work related. The majority of all burn injuries happen at home. In 2020, there were 29,165 hospital admissions in the United States and 3790 deaths from fire and smoke inhalation.[3,4] Of the patients who died, 72% of the deaths resulted from home fires and an estimated 16% of deaths were due to highway vehicle fires.[3]

As in other trauma populations, children are affected to a greater degree. Children under 16 years of age comprise 26% of total burns, and adults 20 to 59 years make up 55% of burns. Older adults >60 years represent 15% of cases, but 37% of deaths from burns. Fire/flame is the most common etiology of injury for adults, whereas children under the age of 5 years typically suffer from scald burns caused by spilling of hot liquids. With improved surgical critical care and understanding of burn injury physiology, over 96% of burn patients survive.

Children

Scald burns caused by hot liquids are the most common cause of pediatric burns and occur most often in the home.[2,5,6] The number of burns decreases from age 9 until adolescence and increases again after the age of 15, presumably due to greater exposure to hazards, experimentation, risk-taking, and employment.[6] Intentional burns account for around 10% of all cases of child abuse.[7] Common etiologies of intentional burns include hot water, and contact with heated objects including cigarettes, irons, and heated kitchen utensils.

Adults

Flame burns are the most common cause of burns in adults. Cooking is the most common cause of home fires, accounting for 49% of all residential fires between 2016 and 2020.[8]

Older Adults

The burn-related mortality rate increases greatly for adults aged 60 years or older. The mortality rate for a burn >20% TBSA is 15% for adults 60 years and older.[2] Individuals over the age of 65 comprise 12% of all burn unit admissions. The average age of those admitted is 76 ± 7 years.[9] The most frequent cause of burns that led to death in elderly women is clothing ignition during cooking.[10] Elderly burn patients treated for scald burns had relatively small burns (<13% of TBSA) but high mortality rates (30%).[11–13] Overall, burns are the fourth leading cause of mortality among the elderly population. Those aged 80 years and older have an overall mortality rate of 20% from burn injury. The mortality rate for a burn >20% TBSA is >60% for those aged 80 or older.

Socioeconomic Status

Socioeconomic status (SES) factors such as low household income, crowded household living conditions, and unemployment increase the risk of burns. Children in the lowest SES groups requiring hospitalization for treatment in US burn centers are twice the proportion of all children in the general population.[4] Furthermore, the incidence of house fires was eight times greater in low-income families compared to high incomes.[14] The higher incidence of house fires has been attributed to the frequent absence of functioning smoke detectors.[14]

ETIOLOGY

A burn is an injury to the skin caused by thermal energy. There are numerous modalities, including fire or flame, scalds, contact, electrical conduction, and chemicals that can produce burns. Between 2008 and 2017, 41% of burns were produced by fire or flame, 33% by scald, 9% by contact, and 3% by electricity, and 3% by chemicals.[2]

The depth of the burn injury is proportional to the temperature and duration of exposure. Burn depth is also dependent on the body region due to differences in skin thickness and blood flow.

Flame Burns

Thermal injuries, caused by fire or flames, are the most common burn etiology reported over the past decade.[2] These injuries usually occur because of flammable liquids, motor vehicle crashes, cooking fires, or ignited clothing. Flame injuries are associated with the highest risk of death and complications compared to all other burn etiologies. When evaluating thermal injuries, it is important to consider the possibility of smoke inhalation as its presence significantly impacts the morbidity and mortality of patients with flame burns. Inhalation injury occurs in 17% of patients with flame burns. The presence of smoke inhalation in burn patients is associated with an overall mortality rate of 24%, compared to the mortality rate of 4% in those patients without smoke inhalation.

Scald Burns

Scald burns are most commonly caused by water in the community. Once the water temperature exceeds 156 °F, only 1 second is needed for a full-thickness burn injury. Hot water heaters are factory set at a low enough temperature (120 °F) to minimize scald injuries as a prevention measure.

Though water scalds do not always cause full-thickness injury due to the variation in temperature, grease burns very commonly cause a deep partial- or full-thickness burn. Grease is usually 400 °F and thus even minimal exposure will cause significant thermal injury. Tar and asphalt also exceed 400° to 500 °F making them a high burn injury risk for industrial workers. Water and grease injury sites should be cleansed with aqueous solutions. Tar, however, requires a petroleum-based solution to remove it from the burn wound.

Contact Injuries

Contact burns occur as the result of direct contact with hot surfaces and material, most frequently glass, metal, or plastic. There has also been an increase in the incidence of hot concrete burns in hot geographic areas of the country. The depth of the injury depends on the temperature of the material and the length of contact. Frequent sites of injury include the palms of the hands as people, especially toddlers, will often fall with outstretched hands. Other commonly seen contact injuries are due to hot metal devices such as space heaters, curling irons, motorcycle exhaust systems, and vaping devices.

Electrical

Electrical injury is the result of electrical current that flows through tissues. Most electrical injuries result from occupational exposure. The degree of the electrical injury is divided into two categories: high voltage and low voltage, which are arbitrarily set at greater than or equal to 1000 V (high voltage) and less than 1000 V (low voltage). At high voltages, no tissue in the human body will experience a safe level of electrical current. Tissue resistance in decreasing order includes bone, fat, tendon, skin, muscle, vessel, and nerve. Increasing resistance to electrical current generates heat. Bone heats to a high temperature resulting in increased temperatures to adjacent tissue. Tissue, especially muscle located between two bones, as in the wrist and the ankle, can undergo significant thermal damage leading to muscle swelling and compartment syndrome. This is common in high-voltage electrical injuries.

Electrical exposure can cause significant injuries to organ systems. Arrhythmias are common at the scene (any voltage) or in the hospital (high voltage ≥1000). The cardiac rhythm should be monitored continuously for at least 24 hours if cardiac injury is suspected at the scene or if a high-voltage injury has occurred. Ventricular fibrillation is the most common cause of death after an electrical injury. Advanced cardiac life support should be instituted immediately. Sinus tachycardia, sinus bradycardia and isolated premature atrial and ventricular complexes are the most common arrhythmias in electrical injuries presenting to the emergency department.[15] A normal cardiac rhythm on admission, means dysrhythmia is unlikely and thus 24-hour monitoring is not needed.[16] Myoglobinuria may result from direct damage to muscle tissue and patients should be monitored for the presence of compartment syndrome. Additionally, injury to solid organs, acute bowel perforation, and gallstones after myoglobinuria have been described. Intravenous fluid for high-voltage injuries should be given to maintain urine output of 75 to 100 cc/hr and 1 cc/kg/hr in pediatric patients.

When taking the patient to the operating room for debridement and grafting of electrical injuries, the surgeon should perform serial debridement and allow the tissue to completely declare. These injuries will often evolve with progressive muscle necrosis and early grafting (within the first week) often fails to fully close the burn wound.

1 Chemical Burns

Types of Chemical Burns

Alkali (pH >7.0) causes liquefaction necrosis and protein denaturation and is found in oven and drain-cleaning products, fertilizers, and industrial cleaners. Alkali injuries extend deeper into tissues following exposure and are especially disruptive to eyes. **Acids** (pH <7.0) cause damage to tissue via coagulation necrosis and protein precipitation. Acid burns tend to be self-limited secondary to pain as the patient will quickly react to the offending agent and the formation of a leathery eschar that may hinder deeper spread. **Organic compounds** (phenol and petroleum) cause damage due to fat-solvent action (cell membrane–solvent action) and systematic absorption with toxic effects on the liver and kidneys. These agents also can cause significant erythema in the surrounding areas that can be mistaken for cellulitis.

Special Types of Chemical Burns

Hydrofluoric acid is a potent and corrosive acid used for rust removal, glass etching, and to clean semiconductors. It is a weak acid but the fluoride ion is toxic as it leaches calcium from cells. Hydrofluoric acid causes severe pain and local necrosis and should be treated with copious water irrigation. The fluoride ion is neutralized with topical calcium gel (one ampule of calcium gluconate in 100-g lubricating jelly). If symptoms persist, intra-arterial calcium infusion (10-mL calcium gluconate diluted in 80 mL of saline, infused over 4 hours) and/or subeschar injection of dilute (10%) calcium gluconate solution should be administered. Fluoride ion binds free serum calcium and magnesium and inhibits the Na-K ATPase pump. Thus it is crucial to monitor the cardiac rhythm and serum calcium, magnesium, and potassium levels, replacing with IV calcium as needed.

Phenol (carbolic acid) is commonly used in disinfectants and chemical solvents; it is an acidic alcohol with poor water solubility. Phenol causes protein disruption and denaturation resulting in coagulation necrosis. Systemically, phenol can cause cardiac arrhythmias and liver toxicity. Thus, patients should have cardiac and liver function monitored. Additional adverse effects include renal injury and demyelination. Given phenol's anesthetic effect, pain is not a reliable indicator of injury. Treatment is copious water irrigation and cleansing with 30% polyethylene glycol or ethyl alcohol.

Tar is used in the paving and roofing industry and can be heated to 260 °C (~500 °F) prior to application. Tar causes thermal injury and then solidifies as it cools, often becoming enmeshed with hair and skin. Patients with tar injuries should be cooled with copious water irrigation to stop the burning process. Tar removers promote micelle formation to break the tar–skin bond. Sterile surfactant mixture (De-Solv-it® or Shur-Clens®) allows tar to be wiped away quickly. Wet dressings using polysorbate (Tween® 80) or Neomycin cream for 6 hours prior to tar removal can also be effective.

White phosphorus is used to manufacture military explosives, fireworks, and methamphetamine. Obvious particles should be brushed off. Skin should be irrigated with a 0.5% copper sulfate solution. Copper sulfate stains the particles black for identification. Copper sulfate will also prevent ignition when particles are submerged in water. After copper sulfate irrigation, the exposed area should be placed in a water bath and the white phosphorous debrided.

PHYSIOLOGY OF BURNS

Burn Shock

Most patients with large burn or inhalation injuries will meet criteria for systemic inflammatory response syndrome (SIRS). Burn shock does not equate to septic shock in the acute setting as true sepsis from a burn injury with subsequent infection usually does not occur until after the first 48 to 72 hours.

Burn shock is unique in the degree of vascular permeability coupled with increased hydrostatic pressure.[17] This increased permeability is thought to result from the release of histamine from mast cells in burned skin following burn injury.[18] Histamine interferes with the venous tight junctions and thereby allows efflux of fluid and proteins causing intravascular hypovolemia despite total-volume hypervolemia.

Platelet activation products such as eicosanoids and serotonin also act to increase pulmonary vascular resistance and amplification of the vasoconstrictive effects of norepinephrine and angiotensin II.[19] In addition to the increased vascular leak, platelet-activating factor in addition to clotting factor dysregulation creates a hypercoagulable state with bleeding that resembles disseminated intravascular coagulation. This coagulation disorder is further amplified if patients become hypothermic during their resuscitation.[20] Thus, patient temperature monitoring and maintenance is crucial during resuscitation.

Changes in cardiac output are also seen in burn patients acutely as patients often have an increase in heart rate and systemic vascular resistance but hypovolemia. Though not defined as "cardiogenic shock," cardiac function is altered due to inflammatory mediators.[21–23] With appropriate burn resuscitation, cardiac output should return to normal levels within 24 to 72 hours.

Metabolic Response to Burn Injury

A physiologic response unique to burn injury is the extent of hypermetabolism. This hypermetabolism is characterized by increased body temperature, glycolysis, gluconeogenesis, proteolysis, lipolysis, and prolonged substrate cycling.[24,25] The degree of the hypermetabolic response is proportional to the size of burn injury and appears to plateau at 70% TBSA. Overall, the basal level of glucose is elevated despite a high insulin state which can complicate outcomes and exacerbate muscle catabolism.

Lipolysis also occurs at a rate that is higher than normal due to abnormal substrate cycling. This results in an accumulation of triglycerides causing steatosis. Recent work to combat this peripheral lipolysis has had some success using propranolol.[26]

Proteolysis is increased in burn patients compared to nonburn patients. This is due to a combination of increased muscle breakdown and increased plasma protein production by the liver.

Catecholamines are also significantly elevated following a burn injury and are thought to play a role in the hypermetabolic response. Burn injuries also cause alterations in diurnal glucocorticoid levels leading to persistent hypercortisolemia.

There are three ways to influence hypermetabolism: nutrition, medication, and surgery as discussed in subsequent sections in the chapter.

Immunologic Response to Burn Injury

The immune system in burn patients demonstrates significant dysregulation that may explain their increased risk of infection. Serum levels of IgA, IgG, and IgM are decreased indicating decreased B-cell function. T-cell function or cell-mediated immunity is also impaired and that is why prolonged homograft and xenograft take is seen. Interleukin 2 (IL-2) production is also decreased whereas IL-10 is increased. Similar to other types of nonthermal trauma, burn patients also have elevated tumor necrosis factor alpha (TNF-a) and IL-6. With regard to the innate immune system, polymorphonuclear neutrophils have impaired chemotaxis as well as decreased oxygen consumption and impaired bactericidal capabilities.

2 BURN SEVERITY

TBSA is useful to guide fluid resuscitation administration and defines the overall prognosis. Only partial- and full-thickness burns are totaled to calculate TBSA.

There are several methods for determining TBSA. The "rule of the palm" states that the patient's palm size is approximately 1% of the patient's TBSA. Another useful guide is the "rule of 9's", in which the adult body is partitioned into several areas that each constitutes 9% of the TBSA (**Fig. 10.1**). In children and infants, the body surface area of the lower extremities constitutes a lower percentage while the head is higher. Other tools such as the Lund & Browder chart, software programs, or Apps are available that may provide more precise estimations. Adult patients who have burns of more than 20% TBSA commonly require resuscitation, whereas 15% TBSA is the threshold for the pediatric burn patient.

EMERGENCY CARE

The initial care of burn patients should follow the primary survey, ABCDE (airway, breathing, circulation, disability, exposure) principles of the American College of Surgeons Advanced Trauma Life Support (ATLS) and the American Burn Association Advanced Burn Life Support (ABLS). These programs have standardized emergency care and have improved patient outcomes. A complete history and physical examination should be performed with specific focus placed on the cause and timing of the injury, risk of smoke inhalation injury, concomitant injuries, and treatments including intravenous fluids received prior to patient arrival. The American Burn Association (ABA) has published criteria to follow regarding the transfer and consultation of a patient to a verified burn center that is listed in **Table 10.1**.[27]

Stop the Burning

Fire or flame will typically be extinguished in the field, however some causal agents can persist into the hospital setting. Health care providers should use personal protective equipment—always considering that the chemicals are still present. With few exceptions, chemical burns should be copiously irrigated with water. Water dilutes but does not neutralize the chemical and cools the injured area. Water irrigation is contraindicated or ineffective following exposure to elemental sodium, potassium, and lithium (precipitates an explosion). Dry chemicals should be brushed off, prior to irrigation. Phenol is water insoluble and should be wiped from the skin with polyethylene glycol–soaked sponges.

For thermal burns, cool wounds with cool, running tap water for 20 minutes. This can be effective up to 3 hours after injury. Care must be taken to avoid hypothermia (especially in larger burns). Do not use ice. Once the burning process has been stopped, cover the patient with warm, clean, dry linens to prevent hypothermia.

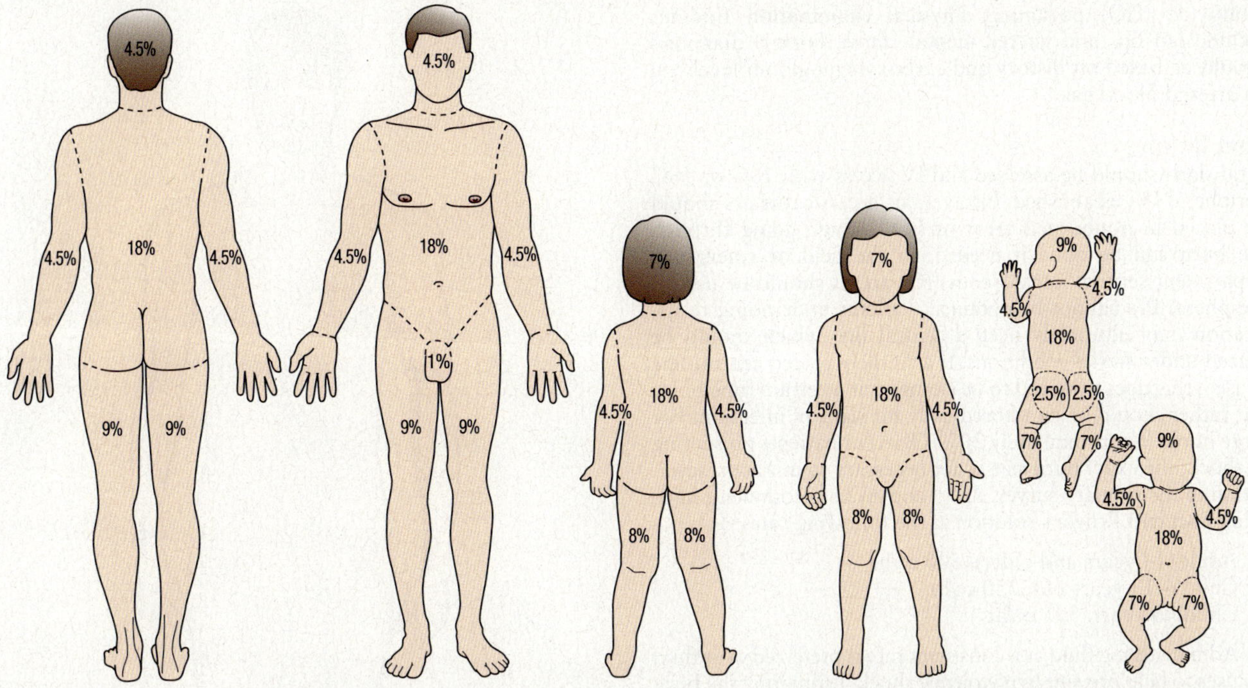

Figure 10.1. Rule of 9s used to estimate percent burns in adults and kids.

Primary Survey

Airway

Inhalation injuries occur in approximately 10% of all burn patients, but are present in 70% of those who die of their burn injury.[28] Risk for inhalation injury can be first assessed by the history. In general, patients burned outside (not in an enclosed space) rarely suffer inhalational injuries. Prolonged exposure to burning material or fumes in an enclosed space should raise suspicion of inhalation injury. Patients in respiratory distress should be immediately endotracheal intubated. Physical examination should note facial burns, changes in voice, shortness of breath, singed nasal vibrissae, carbonaceous sputum, and intraoral swelling. These physical exam findings may point to inhalation injury, but do not themselves mandate intubation in the absence of respiratory symptoms. If a patient is transferred with an endotracheal tube that the accepting physician feels is no longer needed, a spontaneous breathing trial should be performed followed by an assessment for a cuff leak before removing the endotracheal tube.

Breathing

During the primary survey, burn patients should be administered 100% oxygen if there is a concern for inhalation injury. Oxygenation in a burned patient may be altered by carbon

Table 10.1. American Burn Association Burn Guidelines for Burn Center Referral (Advice on Transfer and Consultation)

	Immediate Consultation with Consideration for Transfer	Consultation Recommendation
Thermal Burns	▪ Full-thickness burns ▪ Partial thickness ≥10% TBSA ▪ Any deep partial- or full-thickness burns involving the face, hands, genitalia, feet, perineum, or over any joints ▪ Patients with burns and other comorbidities ▪ Patients with concomitant traumatic injuries ▪ Poorly controlled pain	▪ Partial-thickness burns <10% TBSA ▪ All potentially deep burns of any size
Inhalation Injury	▪ All patients with suspected inhalation injury	▪ Patients with signs of potential inhalation such as facial flash burns, signed facial hairs, or smoke exposure
Pediatrics (≤14 years, or <30 kg)	▪ All pediatric burns may benefit from burn center referral due to pain, dressing change needs, rehabilitation, patient/caregiver needs, or nonaccidental trauma	
Chemical Injuries	▪ All chemical injuries	
Electrical Injuries	▪ All high voltage (≥1000 V) electrical injuries ▪ Lightning injury	▪ Low voltage (<1000 V) electrical injuries should receive consultation and consideration for follow-up in a burn center to screen for delayed symptom onset and vision problems

monoxide (CO) poisoning. Physical examination findings include red lips and altered mental status. Formal diagnosis should be based on history and carboxyhemoglobin levels on an arterial blood gas.

Circulation

Vital signs should be assessed and IV access with 16G or 18G peripheral IVs established. Intravenous access catheters should be placed in nonburned areas of skin though going through the burn can be done if needed. In the field or emergency department setting, intraosseous (IO) access should be used if peripheral IVs cannot be obtained. Patients undergoing resuscitation may ultimately need a central line which should be placed under sterile conditions. If a sterilely placed central line is used, this does not need to be changed at a certain time point but rather should be monitored daily for signs of infection. For large burns (>approximately 20% TBSA) or patients presenting in shock, the exact burn size is not necessary to initiate resuscitation in the primary survey. ABLS and ATLS recommend initiating Lactated Ringer's solution at the following rates:

- Adult (14 years and older): 500 cc/hr
- Child 6-13 years old: 250 cc/hr
- Child <6 years: 125 cc/hr

Administering fluid at a consistent rate is preferred over fluid boluses to help prevent hypovolemic shock. Estimating the burn size and calculating adjusted fluid rates tailored to the patient are done in the secondary survey as described below. However, patients in shock with hypotension may require boluses to manage their hypotension. Isolated burns rarely result in hemorrhage, however patients with other signs of trauma should be evaluated for hemorrhage according to ATLS principles.

Peripheral perfusion may be impaired by full-thickness burn injuries and edema formation. Pulses in all extremities, with particular attention to burned extremities, should be assessed. Nearly circumferential or circumferential full-thickness burns may cause compartment syndrome. The signs of compartment syndrome, including pain, pallor, and paresthesia, may not be reliable in a burned extremity, and a high index of suspicion is needed throughout resuscitation. Any sign of compartment syndrome such as loss of Doppler signals or reduced pulses warrants escharotomy. This is rarely necessary in the field or the emergency department as it takes time for tissue edema to occur. Escharotomies are typically performed at bedside using electrocautery. The burn eschar is released, down through the entire dermis, taking care not to unnecessarily divide the fat. Fasciotomies are rarely required in the absence of electrical injury.

In the case of circumferential, full-thickness burns to the chest, chest wall compliance can be reduced such that peak and/or plateau airway pressures rise and impair ventilation. Escharotomy is performed in an "H" pattern along the bilateral anterior axillary lines and horizontally across the chest or as a "checkerboard." Incision lines for escharotomies are illustrated in **Figure 10.2**.

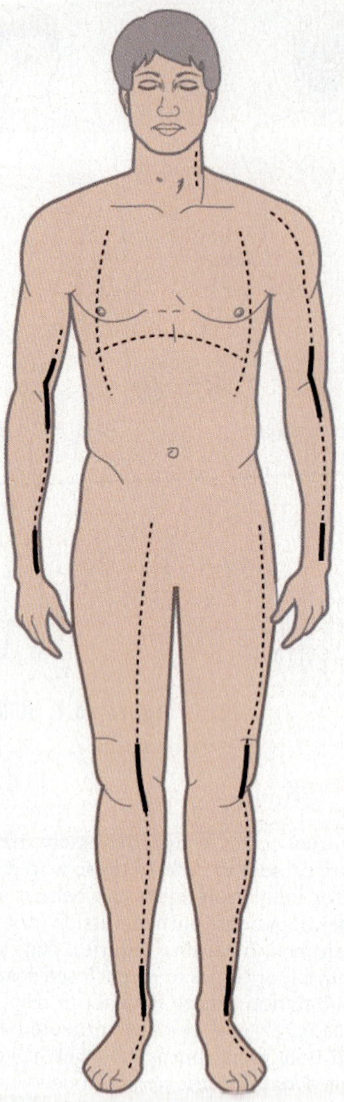

Figure 10.2. Incision lines for escharotomies. In general, incisions should be kept on the lateral aspect of extremities to avoid damage to neurovascular structures.

Disability

Evaluate and document the patient's neurologic status. Commonly, burn patients are alert and oriented on arrival. For those with altered mental status, hypoxia, CO, and hydrogen cyanide should be ruled out.

Carbon Monoxide

Symptoms of CO poisoning typically begin with headaches at levels around 10%, while CO in the blood becomes lethal at around 50% to 70%. The half-life of CO is normally 4 hours when breathing room air. Treatment with 100% oxygen (FiO_2 100%) reduces the half-life of CO to 30 to 90 minutes. Hyperbaric oxygen treatment can reduce the half-life of CO to 15 to 23 minutes. However, if the patient has additional burn injuries or is unstable, the patient should not be placed in a hyperbaric chamber. Also, the time needed to transfer patients to hyperbaric facilities and the subsequent difficulty of resuscitating a critically ill patient in a closed chamber make hyperbaric oxygen an impractical option.

Hydrogen Cyanide

Incomplete combustion can result in the gaseous form of cyanide. Cyanide binds to cytochrome C oxidase stopping cellular respiration. Tissue hypoxia is profound in such cases and results in elevated lactate levels as cells are dependent on anaerobic energy production. Symptoms of cyanide toxicity include unresponsiveness, respiratory failure, seizure, hypotension, and cyanosis. Treatment is empirical as tests for cyanide levels are time consuming and not widely available. The current recommended antidote is hydroxycobalamin (Cyanokit®). Hydroxycobalamin chelates cyanide, producing cyanocobalamin (vitamin B12) which is renally excreted. There are no large studies of its use but it appears safe and without major side effects. There is, however, a potential for renal injury with its use. We use Cyanokit® for patients according to the following pathway (**Algorithm 10.1**).

Exposure

Burn patients should be exposed with a care toward maintaining normothermia. Once burned clothing is removed, take care to keep the patient covered with clean, warmed blankets.

Algorithm 10.1

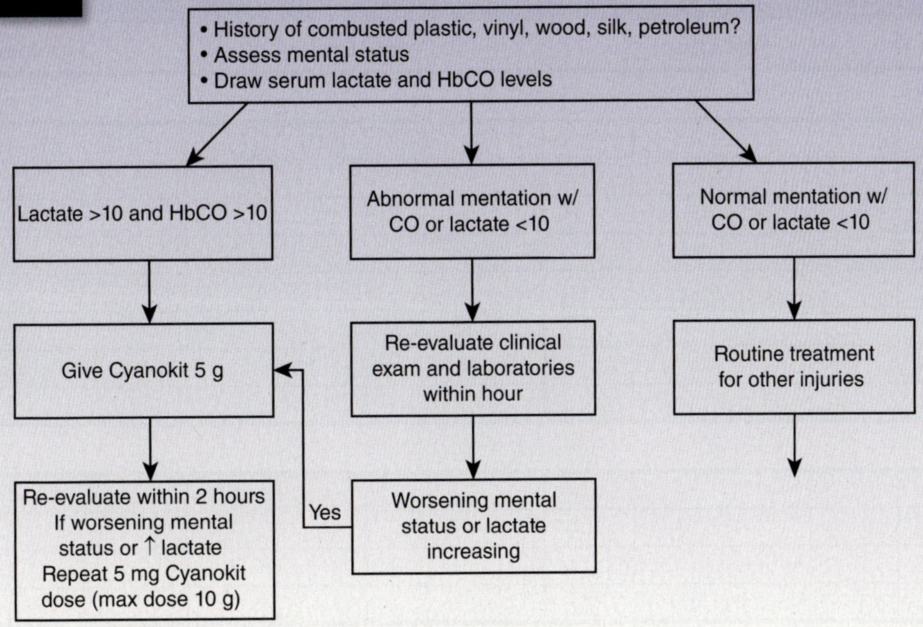

Algorithm 10.1. Cyanokit triage protocol.

One should be mindful to remove all items in contact with the patient, including contacts, jewelry, diapers, etc.

Secondary Survey

Following the primary survey, key aspects of the patient's medical history, including preburn weight and the circumstances of injury should be obtained. Burn size and depth should also be determined.

3 Fluid Resuscitation

The ABA Consensus Formula should be used to calculate the adjusted fluid rate. It is a starting point and not a prescription of the total fluid volume to be given during the first 24 hours. The consensus formula is based on **Table 10.2**.

$$\frac{\text{Age} \times \text{TBSA Burn} \times \text{Weight(kg)}}{16}$$

For example, a 70-kg 30-year-old patient with 20% TBSA flame burn would be started on an initial lactated Ringer's fluid rate of 500 mL/hr (14 years and older). His adjusted fluid rate would be calculated as 2 mL × 20 (%TBSA burn) × 70 (weight in kg) or 2800 mL over 24 hours, with an estimate of half given over the first 8 hours and the remaining half over the subsequent 16 hours. Lactated Ringer's crystalloid solution is recommended as the first-choice fluid to avoid metabolic acidosis when using large volumes of normal saline.[29] Currently the data do not support the use of hypertonic saline or dextran.[30,31] Studies, however, have suggested that albumin usage may play a role in reducing the rate of abdominal compartment syndrome when the patient requires substantially more fluid administration than estimated by the Parkland Formula (>1.5 times).[32–34] Additionally, D5LR is commonly used for maintenance fluids in children under 1 year of age to avoid hypoglycemia. After 24 hours, there are data to suggest that providing albumin reduces crystalloid volume.

The use of colloids may minimize the total volume of fluids administered during resuscitation, although whether or not this improves outcomes such as mortality and respiratory complications is debated.[30,32,34] Colloids should be considered for patients with extensive burns, or for those requiring fluid volumes in excess of those predicted by the Consensus Formula. Albumin is the colloid of choice, typically at 5% concentration. Albumin can be started at a rate of 0.3 to 0.5 cc/kg/%TBSA, and subsequently titrated alongside the crystalloid rate based on resuscitation endpoints.

During resuscitation, the patient's vital signs and urine output should be closely monitored, and laboratory studies should be drawn frequently, since proper fluid resuscitation should be guided by overall clinical response and the trend of vital

Table 10.2. Category of Burn

Category of Burn	Age and Weight	Adjusted Fluid Rates	Urine Output
Flame or Scald	Adults and older children (≥14 yrs old)	2 mL LR × kg × % TBSA	0.5 mL/kg/hr 30–50 mL/hr
	Children (<14 yrs old)	3 mL LR × kg × % TBSA	1 mL/kg/hr
	Infants and young children (≤30 kg)	3 mL LR × kg × % TBSA Plus a sugar-containing solution at maintenance rate	1 mL/kg/hr
Electrical Injury	All ages	4 mL LR × kg × % TBSA until urine clears	1–1.5 mL/kg/hr until urine clears

Table 10.3. Burn Resuscitation Flowsheet

	First 8 hrs				Next 16 hrs				Post Burn Day 2			
Time Since Injury												
pH												
Bicarb												
CO_2												
BD												
Lactate												
CVP												
U/O												
Central Venous Sat.												
PiCCO #s												
SVV												
SVRi												
ELWi												
GEDi												

signs as well as several laboratory values (**Table 10.3**). Intravenous fluid infusion rate should be increased or decreased based on the response of the patient on an hourly basis with fluid administration titrated to maintain urine output goals of 0.5 to 1 mL/kg/hr in adults and 1 to 1.5 mL/kg/hr in children. Computerized decision support is utilized in some burn centers to guide this resuscitation. Using such platforms reduces the total volume of fluid administered during resuscitation. Blood pressure and heart rate should also be monitored, however, burn patients are often tachycardic regardless of the degree of resuscitation. Close monitoring of the patient's laboratory parameters is necessary to determine the trend in organ perfusion (**Table 10.3**). Although none of these values alone provide a sensitive marker of the patient status. Trending these values during resuscitation can help direct resuscitation adjustments if the current fluid rate is causing a positive trend.

In the second 24 hours, all patients should receive crystalloid fluids that are sufficient to maintain urine output and parameters of perfusion including lactate, pulse pressure variation, and cardiac output. This will often be at a maintenance rate plus adjustment for losses of fluid into the burn wound. Enteral nutrition should be started within 24 hours. After 24 to 36 hours, fluids can be decreased by one-third as long as the patient continues to make adequate urine. Fluids may be decreased once again for hours 36 to 48. Colloid can be given after initial crystalloid resuscitation (5% albumin at 0.3 to 0.5 mL/kg per %TBSA over 24 hours).

Pediatric fluid resuscitation does have some differences with regard to fluid management. Due to the limited reserve in children under 20 kg, an additional glucose-based maintenance fluid is recommended based upon patient using D5-containing solutions. Additionally, pediatric fluid requirements may be as high as 6 mL/kg per TBSA and their urine output should be 1.0 to 1.5 mL/kg/hr.[35] Since burn resuscitation should be considered in the setting of a 15% TBSA in children, transfer to a burn center is recommended.

Difficult to Resuscitate Patients

If the fluid resuscitation required during the first 24 hours is 1.5 times greater than initially estimated or >6 mL/kg/hr, the physician should reassess the clinical picture. If estimates predict these high levels of fluid will be given, clinicians should consider changing the crystalloid to colloid. Additionally, continuous renal replacement therapy (CRRT) should be considered for cases where excessive fluid is estimated, and the patient has kidney injury.[36] Giving excessive crystalloid fluids and failure to use appropriate early resuscitation adjuncts is associated with worse outcomes. Physicians often will give additional fluid due to low urine output not realizing that the kidney, like other organs during burn shock often lag behind the clinical picture. Specific complications associated with excessive resuscitation include compartment syndrome of the extremities and the abdomen. Signs of abdominal compartment syndrome include abdominal distention, decreased urine output, and elevated ventilator pressures. Diagnosis can be made both by observing clinical signs as well as by assessment of bladder pressure transduced through a Foley catheter. Pressures over 20 mm Hg are considered abnormal and pressures greater than 25 mm Hg with evidence of organ failure indicate the urgent need for intervention. Strategies to intervene should begin with decreasing the rate of fluid administration. If the patient has full-thickness burns on the abdomen or torso, escharotomies should be performed. The bed should be reclined, and neuromuscular blockade can be given to relax the musculature. If elevated bladder pressures remain despite these maneuvers, a decompressive laparotomy may be required.

When patients are difficult to resuscitate, additional monitoring devices can be used including monitors of cardiac output and cardiac index. Examples include esophageal Doppler, bedside echo, and a formal transthoracic echo. Serial echo examinations after providing a fluid bolus allow monitoring of cardiac filling, IVC variation, and wall motion changes.[37,38]

CRITICAL CARE OF THE BURN PATIENT

Treatment for Inhalational Injury

If inhalation injury is suspected, the patient should undergo airway assessment and be placed on supplemental oxygen. Inhalation injury has three components that must be considered: (1) upper airway thermal injury which can cause swelling and obstruction, (2) CO poisoning, and (3) lower airway chemical injury from toxic agents found in smoke. The acute management of the airway is described above.

Lower airway injury is diagnosed by evidence of soot or mucosal irritation on bronchoscopy. Airway mucosal injury from chemical pneumonitis leads to increased secretions while compromising the patient's ability to clear those secretions. This leads to increased risk of mucus plugging. Airway mucosal sloughing can also result in bleeding and clot formation that further obstruct airways. The use of aerosolized heparin, albuterol, and Mucomyst (HAM) following smoke inhalation to promote airway clearance is advocated in some centers, however, larger studies are needed to validate these treatments.[37–41]

Early endotracheal intubation and mechanical ventilator support is important in patients with inhalation injury or in large TBSA burns expected to receive large-volume resuscitation. Ventilator management should follow ARDSnet protocol recommendations.[42,43] Recruitment maneuvers may be needed to improve oxygenation and/or ventilation. Permissive hypercapnia is preferred over large tidal volumes to avoid lung barotrauma. Limited studies have shown a potential role for high-frequency percussive ventilation in burn patients.[44]

Pulmonary infection in burn patients occurs in 30% to 50% of patients. Patients with three of the following five clinical criteria should be assessed for pneumonia with culture samples and placed on empiric antibiotic therapy: purulent sputum production, fever, elevated WBC, infiltrate on chest radiograph, and increasing supplemental oxygen requirements. If the patient has pneumonia and been in the hospital for over 48 hours, they should be treated for hospital-acquired pneumonia. Sputum or a bronchoalveolar lavage sample should be sent for aerobic, anaerobic, and quantitative cultures. Empiric antibiotics including coverage of Pseudomonas species and MRSA should be started until culture results become available.

Electrolyte Abnormalities and Acute Renal Failure

The immediate effects of burn injury on kidney function are secondary to hypovolemia and circulating inflammatory mediators. The diuresis phase occurs at 48 to 72 hours after "third-space" fluid is reabsorbed. Hyponatremia is often seen due to large-volume resuscitation with hypotonic IV fluids and will usually self-correct. Open burn wounds or the use of topical silver nitrate can also cause hyponatremia. Renal hypoperfusion exacerbates hyponatremia by decreasing glomerular filtration. Hypernatremia may also occur due to insensible and evaporative water losses. Hypophosphatemia can result from dilution or refeeding syndrome. Hypocalcemia can result from the use of silver nitrate.

Acute Kidney Injury

Risk factors include sepsis, large TBSA burns, organ failure, and antibiotic administration. Renal function is compromised by hypoperfusion, pharmacologic nephrotoxic insult, and sepsis which are all common following major burn injury. Physiologically there is a decrease in renal perfusion, glomerular filtration rate, and renal blood flow. Patients present with oliguria and decreased creatinine clearance. Early renal failure often results from hypovolemia-induced ischemic injury. However, over resuscitation can also compromise renal perfusion by causing abdominal compartment syndrome. Late renal failure occurs after fifth postburn day and is frequently caused by sepsis or nephrotoxic antibiotics. CRRT and pharmacologic treatments such as dopamine have not definitively been shown to improve outcomes. The initial care of acute renal failure patients should focus on reversing underlying causes and correcting any fluid and electrolyte imbalances.

Metabolic Response and Nutrition

Burn patients are catabolic and may be more so than in other critically ill populations leading to accelerated lean body mass wasting. Positive nitrogen balance is key to prevent skeletal muscle breakdown and highlights the importance of early nutritional support. The general composition of enteral feeding should include at least 60% calories from carbohydrates not exceeding 1600 kcal/day, 12% to 15% from lipids and essential fatty acids, and 20% to 25% from protein. Failure to meet large energy and protein requirements can impair wound healing and alter end-organ function. While adequate nutrition is crucial, overfeeding must be avoided. A randomized, double-blind, prospective study demonstrated that aggressive high-calorie feeding with enteral and parenteral nutrition was associated with increased mortality.[45] The daily caloric requirements can be calculated using the Curreri formula: [(25 kcal)(body weight (kg))] + [(40)(%TBSA burn)] 1 to 2 g/kg/day of protein for synthetic needs of the patient. In the ICU setting, however, indirect calorimetry is the gold standard and should be used to determine caloric needs in appropriate patients. Burn patients should receive lower percentage of calorie requirements from fat than other ICU patients. The liver in a burn patient has less VLDL causing hepatic triglyceride elevation. Increased fat leads to increased complications including fatty liver, infection, hyperlipidemia, hypoxia, and mortality. Decreased gastrointestinal absorption and increased urinary losses can also lead to deficiencies in vitamins C, E, and zinc, iron, and selenium.

Acute response to thermal injury is biphasic with the hypodynamic shock state at 24 to 72 hours and hyperdynamic catabolic state beginning on the fifth postburn day. Patients have supraphysiologic cardiac output, elevated body temperature, supranormal oxygen consumption, supranormal glucose consumption and altered glucose metabolism, increased CO_2 production and accelerated tissue catabolism. This response is thought to be caused by excessive release of catabolic hormones including catecholamines, glucagon, and cortisol. There is a shift from anabolic–catabolic homeostasis to hypercatabolic state requiring increased substrates for energy including skeletal muscle, which is broken down to maintain sufficient glucose and amino acids. The resting metabolic rate is directly related to the severity of burn injury. This hypermetabolism can be reduced by promptly treating sepsis as well as performing early excision and grafting of burn wounds. Recent studies have shown efficacy of a nonselective beta blocker such as propranolol which inhibits the effect of catecholamines and slows muscle catabolism. Propranolol in acute burns in the pediatric population improved net muscle synthesis and increased lean body mass.[46] Oxandrolone improves muscle synthetic activity, increases expression of muscle anabolic genes, and increases net muscle protein synthesis improving lean body mass composition and has been shown to reduce weight loss, improve donor-site wound healing and decreased hospital stay. Patients with burn injuries greater than 30% should receive oxandrolone for 1 year as the hypermetabolic state has been shown to persist following major burn injury. In the United States, Oxandrolone is no longer available for use. Other testosterone alternatives have been suggested, but are less well tolerated and do not have supporting data in the burn population.[47,48] Human growth hormone and insulin-like growth factor have also been investigated but results have been indeterminate.

Glucose Control

Glucose control in burn patients is similar to other critically ill populations. Currently, the literature does not support strict glucose control (<110 mg/dL) but moderate blood glucose control is recommended (<180 mg/dL) and may decrease infectious complications.[49]

WOUND MANAGEMENT

There are a variety of burn wound dressing materials. Patient factors such as burn wound depth, condition, location of the burn, and comfort during dressing changes dictate the choice utilized.[31] It is generally recommended to use a topical antimicrobial. For dry, deep wounds, topical ointments or soaks may help provide a moist healing environment. Silver sulfadiazine (SSD) is a silver-containing cream that has broad-spectrum coverage against both gram-negative and gram-positive bacteria. SSD is commonly used on the skin of both partial- and full-thickness burn injuries. Its use is contraindicated in patients with sulfa allergies and over wounds near the eyes.[50] A self-limited leukopenia may be seen during the initial days of SSD treatment, but its use can be continued as leukocyte counts recover quickly without intervention. Mafenide acetate cream (MA) is used over cartilaginous areas such as the nose or ear due to increased tissue penetration compared to other dressing materials. Both the cream and a 5% solution of MA are equally effective.[51] Recently, however, MA solution has been removed from the market and is no longer available. MA cream is useful for ear burns when there is risk of cartilage exposure. MA may cause increased pain in the burn wound. Bacitracin and petroleum-bismuth gauze are additional examples of antimicrobial type dressing regimens when an ointment is desired.

Silver nitrate can also be used by soaking dressings in a 0.5% to 1.0% concentration solution and applied three to four times a day. The use of silver nitrate in burn patients remains slightly controversial as nitrates are toxic to tissues and wound healing may be delayed by its use. The nitrates impair reepithelization and this effect partially offset the benefits of silver in these compounds.[52] Furthermore, it can cause leaching of cations causing hyponatremia. Dakin's solution can also be utilized for soaked dressings.

For partial-thickness wounds or when less frequent dressing changes are desirable, long-term antimicrobial impregnated dressings can be used. Silver impregnated dressings are one such option. These dressings consist of silver-impregnated sheets or foams that have antimicrobial properties and can be changed less frequently, reducing pain and cost.[53]

Following skin grafting, Donor sites can be the most painful area for the patient. Like other wounds, these wounds heal in a moist environment and though dry petroleum gauze can be used, this can be extremely painful. Long-term dressings, or long-term antimicrobial dressings that can be used to maintain wound moisture should be considered.

OPERATIVE INTERVENTIONS

Excision and Grafting

After initial stabilization of the patient, which generally takes 24 to 48 hours, surgical intervention should occur as soon as possible. Early excision of devitalized tissue reduces the local and systemic effects of mediators released from burned tissue, thus reducing the progressive pathophysiologic derangements.[54,55] It also removes dead skin which can serve as a nidus for wound infection. Tangential excision with a sharp blade on a guarded device removes necrotic tissue while preserving as much of the underlying viable tissue as possible. For large burn wounds, excision should begin within 2 to 4 days of the initial injury. If there are insufficient donor sites to autograft the entire burn wound, the excised burn should be covered temporarily with allograft or a skin substitute[56] (**Fig. 10.3**).

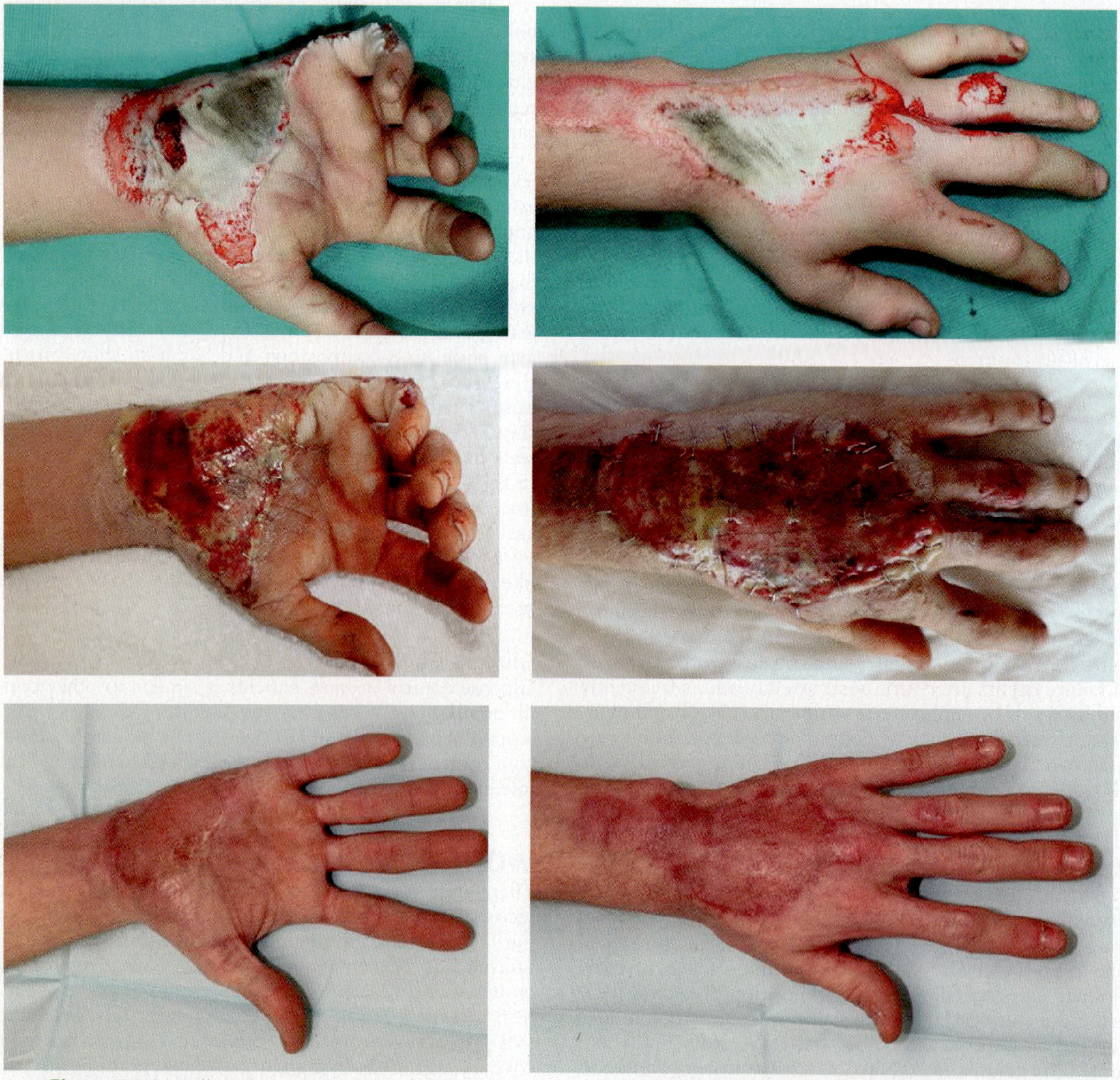

Figure 10.3. Full-thickness friction burn staged with Integra to allow for full declaration of the wound prior to grafting.

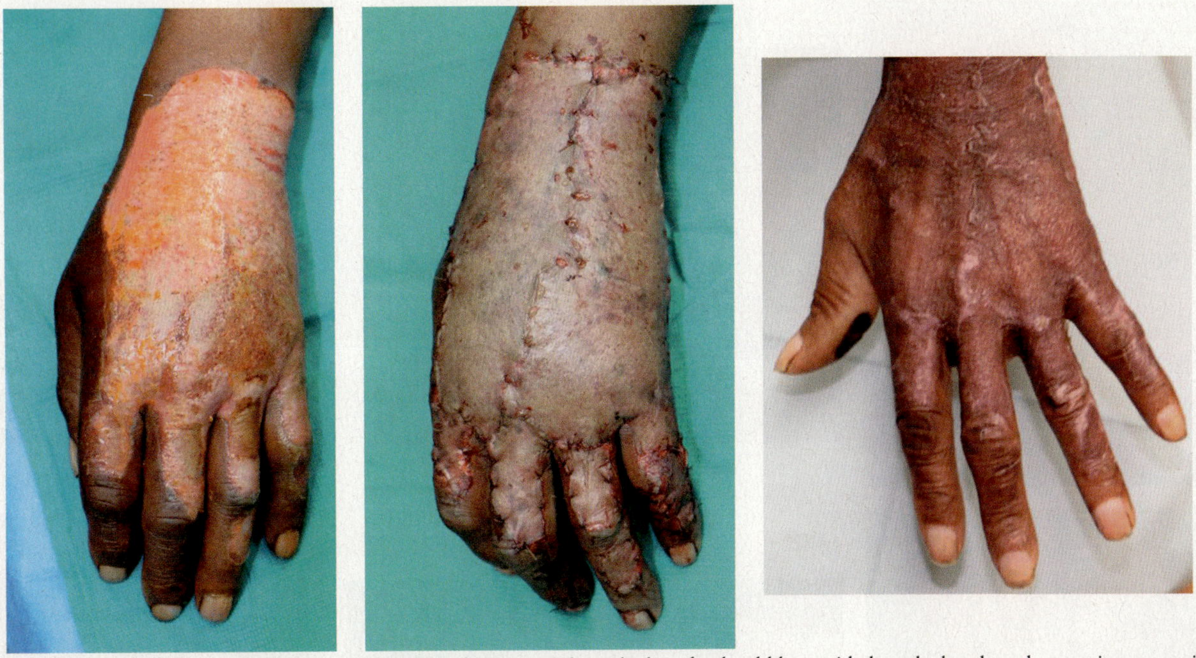

Figure 10.4. Sheet grafting of full-thickness hand burns. In general, meshed grafts should be avoided on the hands and across important joints to avoid scar contracture. (**Left**) Preop photo. (**Middle**) Intraop photo. (**Right**) 1-month postop photo.

Serial excisions and grafting is the backbone of burn care in those suffering from large TBSA burns. The use of allograft also allows the surgeon to assess the depth of the injury and the adequacy of their excision. If the allograft has good take, then it is likely that an autograft will also take.

After a decision regarding the use of allograft versus autograft has been made, attention is turned to the size and thickness of the skin graft. Commonly, split-thickness skin grafts (STSGs) composed of the epidermis and a thin layer of dermis are utilized to minimize donor-site morbidity and optimize graft take. Thin grafts are more likely to succeed than thick grafts as it is easier to adhere and for neovascularization to occur. However, there are certain areas where full-thickness skin grafts are preferred as they cause less secondary contracture and have better tone matching. Areas of function, such as the hands and feet, lose a remarkable amount of utility if afflicted by scar contracture and may benefit from full-thickness grafts.[57] If split-thickness skin is used on the feet and hands, the grafts should be harvested on the thick side and meshing should be avoided when possible (**Fig. 10.4**).

Similarly, aesthetically important areas, such as the face, are also more amenable to full-thickness skin grafting to optimize color tone match and minimize contracture over such areas.[58] The abdomen can offer a site for large full-thickness harvest using an abdominoplasty incision (**Fig. 10.5**).

Other areas include the inguinal crease, inner upper arm and the posterior auricular area. Areas above the level of the nipples tend to have better facial tone matching. Full-thickness grafts require closing the tissues primarily to avoid additional wounds. There is also more difficulty with successful healing of the graft given that a more robust blood supply within the wound bed is necessary. The split-thickness graft can be meshed to increase the surface area that may be covered. Meshing allows for fluid egress, which minimizes the risk of fluid accumulation beneath the graft, a common cause of skin graft failure. Meshing should not be performed, however, over cosmetically sensitive areas as the meshed pattern will be apparent even after complete healing. Both types of skin grafts benefit from bolstering once placed to minimize shear, improve contact, and allow for imbibition and inosculation. **Table 10.4** summarizes the key steps involved in a burn excision.

When burn injuries lead to large regions of exposed tendons, especially in the distal one-third of the upper and lower extremity, free tissue transfer should be considered (**Fig. 10.6**). It is necessary to ensure that all dead tissue is debrided prior to coverage with a free flap to mitigate infection and flap failure. Additionally, if the patient is elderly or has vascular insufficiency, a preoperative CT angiogram should be obtained.

Skin Substitutes

Allograft

In larger burn wounds, patients may not have an adequate surface area available for donor sites. In such cases, allograft can be used instead for initial coverage. This homograft will serve as a temporary coverage and its take will ensure that the initial excision was performed at the correct depth. Allografts will eventually be rejected as the body recognizes the newly engrafted skin as foreign material after 10 to 13 days. The process is initiated by the placement of the allografts, which is associated with an inflammatory process, leading to the activation of the innate immune response. Donor dendritic cells migrate from the graft to the recipient's secondary lymphoid organs where they present donor antigens and elicit an adaptive immune response. This response results in activated effector T cells from the donor leaving the secondary lymphoid organs and infiltrating the graft where they mediate the rejection of the allograft.[59]

Cultured Epidermal Autograft

If insufficient autograft donor sites exist even after temporary allograft, the surgeon may consider use of cultured epidermal autografts. Cultured epidermal autografts utilize the ability to grow keratinocytes in vitro to generate cohesive sheets of stratified epithelium, which maintains the characteristics of authentic epidermis.[60] Two 2 × 3 cm full-thickness skin biopsies must be obtained from a nonburned area, typically at the same time as the initial excision. After 3 to 4 weeks, the cultured epidermal autograft sheets are 8 to 10 cells thick.[61] These constructs require advanced planning as it takes at least 3 to 4 weeks to develop. Additionally, risks and benefits should be discussed with the family and patient as there is a high percentage of graft loss due to fragility. Case reports of squamous cell cancer developing from cultured epidermal autograft sites do exist.

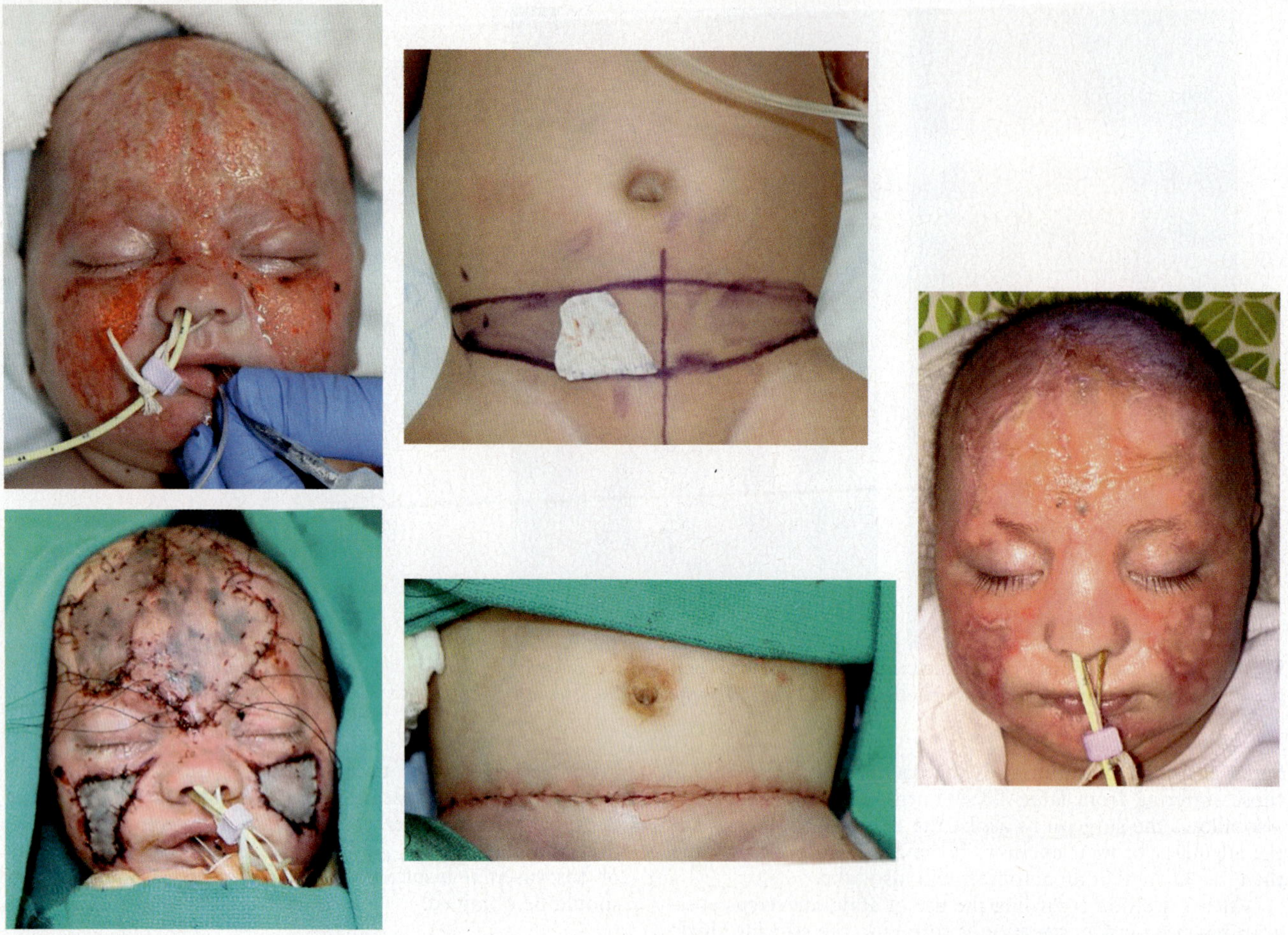

Figure 10.5. Use of full-thickness skin graft to prevent facial ectropion. Full-thickness graft harvested from the abdomen. (**Left column**) Intraop photos. (**Middle figures**) Intraop donor-site photos. (**Right column**) Postop 2-week photo.

Integra®

Integra® Bilayer Wound Matrix is an alternative for temporary coverage and creation of a neodermis in a wound after excision. Composed of bovine collagen and silicone film, this construct is designed to mimic the epidermis and dermis of the missing tissue.[62] Its structure allows for the growth of healthy granulation tissue into a wound bed to optimize the wound niche to promote greater and healthier take of the skin graft that will eventually be placed over the site of injury. This is especially important over areas of function, such as the hand, which has the potential for significant debilitation if scar or graft contracture occurs over the traumatized site. Integra® is also important for areas that do not have enough viable or vascularized tissue to support a skin graft. Integra®, however, often fails in burn patients due to infection Additionally, clinicians should examine the Integra frequently and remove any areas of silicone under which there is concern for infection.

ReCell® Spray-On Skin™

A newer technology known as the ReCell® Autologous Cell Harvesting Device (or ReCell® Spray-On Skin™) is a point-of-care preparation and application of a suspension of noncultured, disaggregated, autologous skin cells. A 1 cm^2 of donor-site skin can be used to treat up to 80 cm^2 of excised burn.[63] It is used with widely meshed STSG (eg, 6:1). Small trials have demonstrated noninferiority to STSG for small surface areas of mixed depth burn. However, the data are still lacking on effectiveness measures for this technology to be widely adopted.

Biodegradable Temporizing Matrix®

Biodegradable Temporizing Matrix® (BTM) is a biodegradable, synthetic dermal substitute composed of a polyurethane matrix and a nonbiodegradable, transparent sealing membrane. The 2-mm matrix permits infiltration of cellular material that once integrated forms a neodermis. The sealing membrane mimics normal skin function by preventing loss of moisture and serving as a barrier to infection.[64] BTM is indicated for use in the management of partial- and full-thickness burn wounds. Unlike biologic dermal substitutes (ie, Integra®), BTM is less prone to infection due to its synthetic composition. There is evidence that BTM may decrease scarring and contracture.[65–67] Once the burn wound is surgically excised to healthy, viable tissue, BTM is applied and secured with good apposition to the wound bed. After about 3 to 43 weeks, the matrix integrates into the wound forming a fully vascularized neodermis, The sealing membrane is delaminated and grafted with autograft for definitive wound closure.

Matriderm®

Matriderm® is a dermal substitute composed of a 1- to 2-mm bovine collagen-elastin matrix. It is indicated in the management of partial- and full-thickness burn wounds. Once the burn wound is surgically excised, Matriderm is applied to the healthy wound bed and definitive closure with an autograft is performed in one stage. Matriderm is meant to promote tissue growth and wound healing. The elastin component is responsible for improved wound healing and scar formation.[68]

Kerecis Graftguide®

Kerecis Graftguide® is a newer skin substitute. It is a freeze-dried, decellularized, intact fish skin graft (IFSG) sourced from North Atlantic cod (Gadus morhua). It is FDA approved for use in chronic wounds and partial-thickness burns. Animal studies have demonstrated noninferiority to allograft for temporary coverage of full-thickness burn wounds and human studies have shown promising data for its use as temporary

Table 10.4. Pre- and Intraoperative Steps for a Burn Excision and Grafting Procedure

1. Preoperatively, it is helpful to correct hematologic and metabolic derangements given potential for large amount of blood loss.
2. The preoperative time-out should include a discussion of expected blood loss, the blood products available, and the transfusion triggers for the case.
3. In any burn over 20%, a preoperative blood type and crossmatch should be performed and PRBCs should be available in the operating room, and given appropriately, to avoid intraoperative acute blood loss anemia.
4. Arterial lines as well as large-bore IVs and often a central line should be in place before beginning the operation.
5. Techniques to decrease intraoperative blood loss include:
   a. The use of tourniquets on the extremities
   b. Use of topical spray thrombin and epinephrine-soaked Telfa pads placed immediately after excision followed by wrapping with Kerlix gauze soaked in a 1:1,000,000 epinephrine in saline solution
   c. In regions where circumferential wrapping cannot be performed, this epinephrine solution can be used as an injectable solution to perform dermatoclysis with an 18G spinal needle on the end of a 60 cc syringe or injection device
   d. This epinephrine injection solution is also used as a preharvest tumescent solution for donor sites, helping to create a flat surface on which to run the dermatome as well as decrease postharvest blood loss
   e. If working on an extremity, a good strategy is to start proximally and perform the excision followed by inflation of the tourniquet. Subsequently, the distal excision can be performed under tourniquet control
6. After achieving a healthy and well-vascularized wound bed, proceed with allografting or autografting.
7. If autografting is carried out, grafts can be excised in thicknesses ranging from 0.010 to 0.018 in. We typically use 0.012 in for standard grafts.
   a. Thinner grafts lead to faster donor-site healing, hence are helpful if there is a need to reharvest donor sites, or if the patient has thin skin due to increased age or chronic immunosuppression.
   b. Thinner grafts increase the likelihood of skin graft take and decrease the risk of superficial epidermolysis of the graft, however, result in greater secondary contracture.
8. Grafts are meshed in 1:1 or 1:1.5 ratio to allow fluid egress.
9. Backgrafting: If backgrafting of the donor site is needed, the same area of graft harvested should be harvested next to the donor site then meshed 4:1 and placed over the entire donor site (**Fig. 10.4**).

coverage for full-thickness burns requiring staged grafting.[69–72] The main advantage of Kerecis over allograft is the 3-year shelf life of Kerecis, and unlike allograft, it does not require cryopreservation. It is placed on the wound bed for 1 week to encourage wound bed healing, at which time it is removed and replaced with an STSG.

PAIN MANAGEMENT

Burn injuries are among the most painful traumatic injuries sustained given their extensive nature. Thermal injury to the overlying epidermis leads to exposed nerve endings which are sensitive to stimulation. Thus, superficial partial-thickness burn injuries often cause the most pain to the patient. Deeper partial- and full-thickness injuries may not cause as much pain to palpation; however, these regions are still painful due to the inflammatory response. Given the multifactorial nature of burn pain, elimination of pain in burn patients is not possible. Outcomes are often improved if a dedicated physician with expertise in pain management is a part of the burn team. When establishing a pain regimen, the physician should focus on treating acute procedural, as well as background pain. A successful regimen often includes the use of short- to intermediate-acting narcotics to treat the acute procedural pain as well as a long-acting narcotic such as methadone for the background pain.[73] Some patients will also benefit from gabapentin (Neurontin) to alleviate neurologic pain. Balancing of narcotic dosing over time is essential to preserve their acute pain relief effect and to avoid situations in which tolerance renders all available agents and doses ineffective.

WOUND INFECTIONS

Burn wound sepsis is a severe sequelae of burn injuries caused by colonization of the damaged skin and soft tissues with infectious bacteria or fungi. The most common organisms are *Staphylococcus aureus, Streptococcus pneumoniae,* and *Pseudomonas aeruginosa.* Despite the morbidity of this complication, its incidence has decreased dramatically with the use of early excision and grafting and appropriate topical antibiotic therapy. General critical care infection protocols should be followed with burn wound excision if the patient does not yet have skin grafts placed. If adequate excision was performed and the patient already has skin grafts placed, then antibiotic soaks or cream dressing changes.

BURN RECONSTRUCTION

Optimizing Acute Treatment to Minimize the Need for Reconstruction

During the acute burn injury stages, emphasis should be placed on general coverage of burn wounds and large flaps and local tissue rearrangements should be delayed. However, if there is a high likelihood that the patient might need a flap or local tissue rearrangement in the future, the region of graft harvest should be carefully planned. For example, if a patient has a large neck burn or exposed lower extremity tendons or bone and an anterolateral thigh flap would help, then the thigh should be avoided as a donor site. Surgeons should consider the fact that a meshed skin graft will have an abnormal appearance once it heals and has an increased risk of hypertrophic scarring. Donor sites should be harvested from inconspicuous locations in case a hypertrophic scar results. Other examples requiring acute reconstructive surgery include eyelid contracture with exposure keratitis and cervical contractures causing airway issues. Once acute grafts and donor sites have healed patients and physicians should focus on maximizing normal scar healing. Normal wound healing requires a balance in the hydration of the wound and water-based moisturizers should be encouraged. Compression garments are also commonly used to decrease formation of hypertrophic scarring, though their efficacy is still debated.[74,75]

4 Hypertrophic Scarring

Thermal burn injures can cause tremendous morbidity, leaving the patient with cosmetic and functional impairments. Hypertrophic scarring is a major sequelae of burn injury with a prevalence of 32% to 72%. Several risk factors have been identified that contribute to its development including the localization of the burn injury, burn depth, time to heal, and skin color.[76,77] While the precise mechanism by which hypertrophic scarring occurs remains unclear, strong, and persistent expression of transforming growth factor beta (TGF-β), focal adhesion kinase-1 (FAK-1), and its receptors have been associated with postburn hypertrophic scarring. Furthermore, a critical step in the healing process that is altered is the transition from granulation tissue into normal scarring. During this remodeling process, wound epithelization and scar collagen is formed but accompanied by a gradual decrease in cellularity

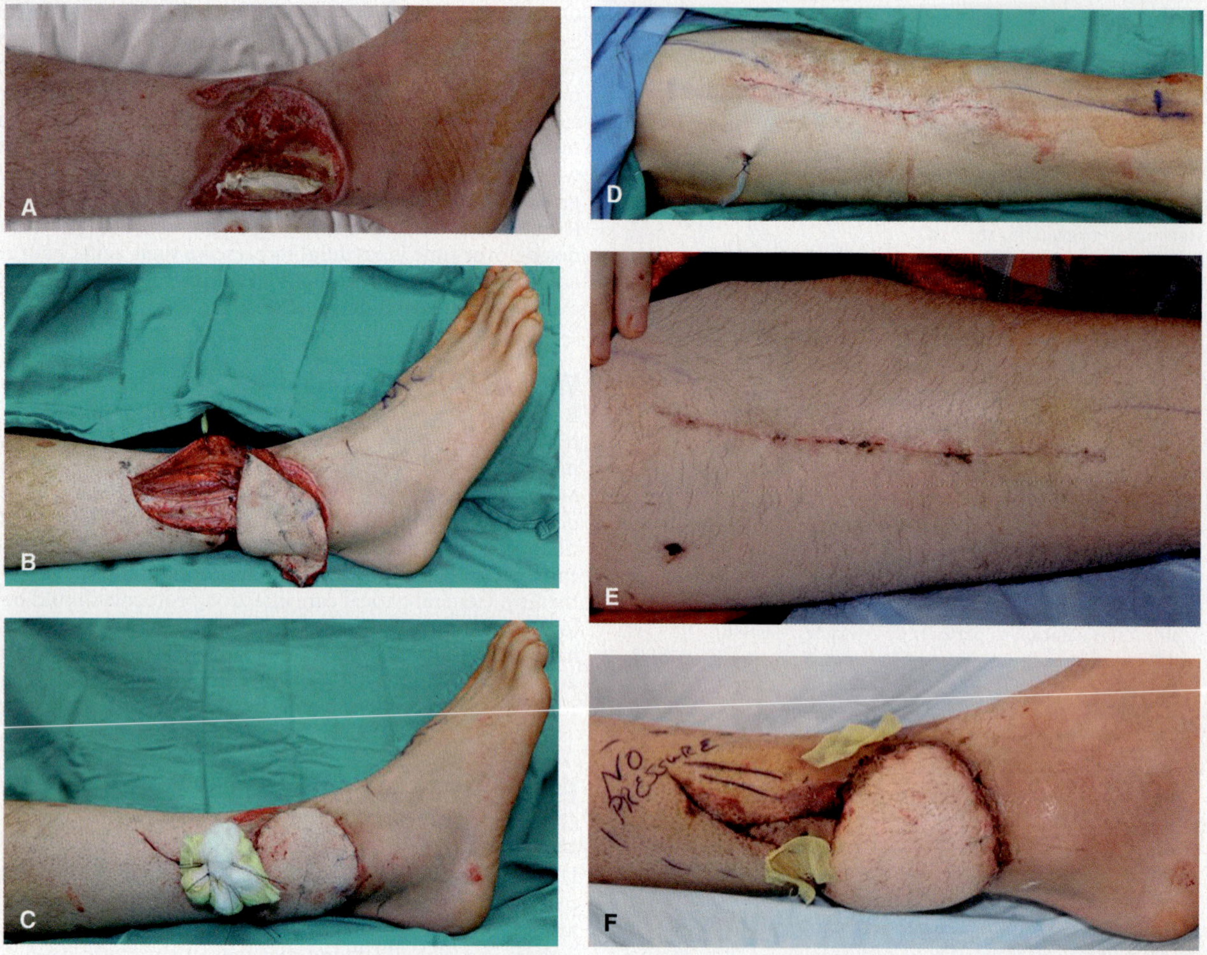

Figure 10.6. Use of free anterolateral thigh flap for reconstruction of lateral full-thickness ankle burn with exposed tendon. **A:** Wound bed. **B:** Free flap, intraoperative. **C:** Free flap, postoperative. **D:** Donor site. **E:** Healed donor site. **F:** Postoperative free flap appearance.

due to apoptosis. However, early immature hypertrophic scars caused by burns are hypercellular and during the process of remodeling and maturing, fibroblast density does not resemble that of normal healing.[78] More specifically, apoptosis of myofibroblasts occur 12 days after injury in normal wound healing, but in hypertrophic scar tissue, the maximum apoptosis occurs much later at 19 to 30 months.[79] These events result in a significantly higher percentage of myofibroblast and the hypertrophy of the scar tissue following severe burn injuries.

One of the key pathologic factors that must be addressed in any hypertrophic scar is tension. The concept of "scar rehabilitation" maintains the key idea to improve the environment of the scar without actually excising the scar. The most important step in rehabilitating the scar is to release the tension. Rather than excising the scar, the focus in on releasing the area of greatest tension. Despite not removing any tissue, a large defect is often created once the tension is released. This defect can then be treated by adding new tissue such as an FTSG or a thick STSG. Additional ways to relieve tension involve the use of tissue rearrangements such as a Z-plasty. A Z-plasty lengthens the scar at the expense of width, alleviating tension along the central access of the hypertrophic scar. In general Z-plasty rearrangements are made with 60-degree angles to maximize tissue gain without causing excess tension on the donor-site closure. Alternative V-Y advancements are useful if there is healthy tissue surrounding the scar and can be advanced into the area of the contracture release. Both Z-plasties and V-Y advancements relieve the tension on the scar. By relieving this tension, the scars can heal in a more normal environment and often will do so without the raised erythematous characteristics initially present. The physiology of the Z-plasty is thought to result from improved collagen remodeling after relief of tension.[80,81] Z-plasties can be used to flatten a hypertrophic scar or elevate a depressed scar as long as the lateral limbs extend into normal tissue. The classic design of a Z-plasty has a central segment with limbs oriented at 60 degrees (although can be 30 to 90 degrees) with all three lines of equal length (**Fig. 10.7**). Widening the angle of the limbs increases percent gain in length along the central limb. Multiple Z-plasties can be designed in series to improve contracture release in large hypertrophic scars.

Although less well studied, postburn pruritus is another significant problem affecting almost 100% of pediatric and 87% adult patients and may persist for many years, resulting in a scratching/inflammation cycle leading to hypertrophic scarring. Treatment options are limited for postburn pruritus, commonly involving antihistamines and moisturization of the skin with only incomplete resolution of symptoms and thus significant deterioration in the quality of life.[82]

Current treatment strategies for hypertrophic scars include surgical manipulation, intralesional corticosteroid injections, cryotherapy, and laser therapy. Surgical manipulation to remove the excess skin remains the traditional treatment for hypertrophic scar. Recent studies investigating the role of fat grafting into scars have shown promise to further improve function and appearance.[83] Patients who have undergone fat transfer reported satisfactory results 6 months after the procedure, indicating considerable improvement in the features of the skin, skin texture, and thickness. Histologic examination demonstrated new collagen deposition, neovascularization, and dermal hyperplasia in regions treated with fat grafting, which mimicked surrounding undamaged skin. Additionally, intralesional corticosteroids suppress the inflammatory

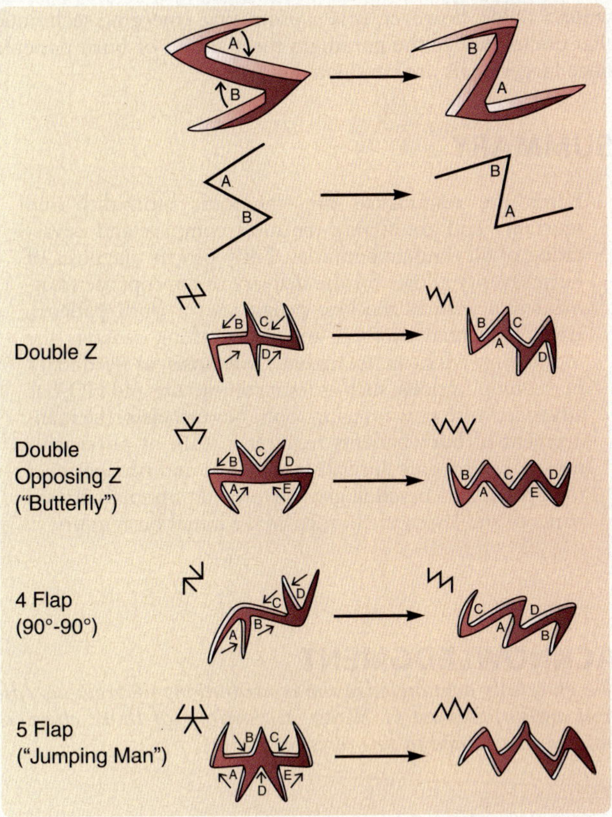

Figure 10.7. Z-plasty diagrams demonstrated tissue rearrangement used for hypertrophic burn scars.

process in wounds, diminish collagen synthesis, and enhance collagen degradation.[84] Conversely, cryotherapy induces vascular damage that leads to anoxia and ultimately tissue necrosis and has yielded marked improvement of hypertrophic scars.[85] However, its efficacy is limited to the management of small scars.

Lastly, since the introduction of laser treatment in the mid-1980s, additional lasers with different wavelengths have been employed. Encouraging results have been obtained with the 585-nm wavelength pulsed-dye laser (PDL), which has been recognized as an excellent therapeutic option for the treatment of younger hypertrophic scars.[86] PDL induces the dissociation of disulfide bonds in collagen fibers and leads to collagen fiber realignment, decreased fibroblast proliferation, and neocollagenesis. However, it is necessary for repeated treatments, generally between two and six treatments, for the optimal resolution. Shorter-pulse durations are generally more effective for scar improvement.[87] Unlike vascular malformations and hemangiomas, scars also tend to respond better to low or medium PDL fluences, about 4 to 7 J/cm^2, than to higher fluences.[88] Low, short-pulse duration PDL fluences induce local damage to the vascular endothelium followed by mural platelet thrombi, while high PDL fluences at longer-pulse durations tend to cause immediate intravascular coagulation with cessation of blood flow.[89] Side effects include erythema/purpura for 7 to 14 days, hyperpigmentation, and hypopigmentation. Though these lasers are effective in improving scar erythema, they do not have a substantial effect on the thickness or contour of hypertrophic scars. Controversy still exists about how much of this redness would subside if given adequate time compared to laser treatments.

Recently, studies have demonstrated the benefit of fractional photo thermolysis in the treatment of hypertrophic scarring. Though the exact mechanism is unknown, this concept uses a CO_2 laser (10,600 nm), an ablative laser that targets water in the underlying tissues. The laser creates columns of tissue destruction, which stimulates collagen production in adjacent uninjured columns of tissue. Only a portion of the epidermis and dermis is treated with columns of energy to create targeted areas of thermal damage (microthermal treatment zones, or MTZs). The untreated areas are a reservoir of collagen and promote tissue regrowth. Fractional lasers, as opposed to nonfractional lasers allow for greater penetration with decreased risk of scarring. This healing will take place outside of the acute inflammation period and thus allow for a more normal wound healing cascade than existed at the time of the initial excision and graft. The adjacent uninjured tissue allows for more rapid tissue regeneration from their follicles and sweat glands. Ablative lasers have a greater potential depth of treatment compared to nonablative lasers (4.0 mm compared to 1.8 mm). Ablative lasers appear to be more effective for thicker scars and those associated with restriction. Overall, this creates a smoother appearance and allows meshed grafts to appear less obvious. Patients have described less tightness as well as decreased pruritus and improved overall appearance.[90–94]

Tissue Expansion

As a reconstructive technique, tissue expansion is versatile, reliable, and repeatable, and can be applied to many regions of the body. A tissue expander (TE) is an artificial filling device that is used to grow and expand local tissue to reconstruct an adjacent soft tissue defect. A silicone elastomer reservoir is placed beneath the donor tissue and slowly filled over time with saline, causing the overlying soft tissue envelope to stretch with a net increase in surface area per unit volume. Advantages to TE is that it allows the surgeon to reconstruct "like with like" using donor and recipient tissues that share similarities in color, thickness, texture, and hair-bearing patterns. Larger soft tissue defects that would usually require a local flap for reconstruction can be closed primarily using expanded local tissue, limiting donor-site morbidity. A robust angiogenic response is achieved histologically within the expanded local tissue resembling an incisional delay phenomenon. Predictable amounts of donor tissue can be gained through the expansion process. Disadvantages of tissue expansion include the need for multiple operations (at least two for placement and removal of the expander) and outpatient visits. Definitive reconstruction is delayed secondary to the expansion process. Specific complications related to the presence of foreign material can be as high as 30% (eg, infection, exposure, or extrusion). This complication risk is even higher in the extremities and scalp.

Specific Anatomic Concerns

Neck contractures are the most common wound healing complication of burn injury. Functionally this can limit range of motion and oral competence. Surgical release of the scar contracture down to platysmal or subplatysmal layer followed by coverage with large FTSG or thick STSG followed by aggressive range of motion 5 days after having patient in neck brace is an option for correction. If the contraction is severe, a free tissue transfer may be required after neck release. Postoperatively, it is crucial to use compression garments for 6 to 18 months and neck bracing to maintain neck extension to reduce contracture recurrence.

Ectropion is a common complication after periorbital burns. This deformity is caused by inadequate tissue, therefore, to release the contracture the surgeon needs to insert tissue. If the ectropion is caused by an extrinsic contracture, scar release and provision of additional tissue are needed to prevent recurrence.

The axilla also represents a common area of contracture because it is difficult to maintain adequate positioning in the acute phase of burn wound healing. Anatomically, the axilla can be divided into the anterior axillary fold, midaxillary line, and posterior axillary line. The shoulder should be kept 90 to 120 degrees abduction and 15 to 20 degrees flexion

(60 to 80 degrees arm elevation). There are three grades of axillary contractures:

1A: Involves anterior axillary fold
1B: Involves posterior axillary fold
2: Involves both axillary folds
3: Involves both folds and axillary dome

Type 1 and 2 contractures can be treated with sequential release and thick STSGs or FTSGs. Type 3 contractures require local and distant flaps including parascapular and latissimus flaps. It is important to pay attention to where hair-bearing regions are transposed. Postoperative occupational therapy and splinting are necessary to prevent recurrence.

Heterotopic Ossification

Heterotopic ossification (HO) is the pathologic formation of bone in extraskeletal regions of soft tissue including muscle, joint spaces, and often encasing major nerves. This complication of burn injury causes significant pain, joint restriction, and contractures.[95] The incidence of HO is proportional to the severity of the injury with an increased incidence in severely burned patients. It may affect all areas of the body but is most frequently encountered in the elbow joint.[95,96] While the etiology of HO remains elusive, common risk factors that have been identified include upper extremity burns, large TBSA burns, young age, prolonged immobilization,[97] and a delay in time to wound closure.[98]

Early detection and diagnosis of heterotopic bone formation is critical in the clinical management of this complication, which oftentimes involves surgical resection. However, surgical intervention is associated with a high recurrence rate. Perioperative radiotherapy has been suggested as an adjunct to surgical resection and has been shown to reduce the recurrence rate to some extent.[99]

Pharmacologic interventions have been shown to have some efficacy in limiting the severity of HO. Bisphosphonates and NSAIDs have been used for prophylaxis and treatment of HO with some success.[100,101] While there is no consensus on choice or timing of therapy, it has been proposed that bisphosphonates should be prescribed as soon as elevated alkaline phosphatase is noted or imaging studies establish the presence of HO. Other studies have shown that NSAIDs limit the severity of HO when delivered as a preventative therapy.

Marjolin Ulcer

Similar to chronic wounds from other etiologies, chronic untreated burn scars can lead to malignant degeneration. Squamous cell carcinoma is the most common type of malignancy observed. However, these malignancies are rare in an era of early excision and grafting. Malignancy requires wide excision with at least a 2-cm margin as well as sentinel lymph node biopsy. If the sentinel node is observed to be positive, a compete lymph node excision should be performed.

EMERGING TECHNIQUES

A recent notable advance in burn care involves enzymatic debridement of partial- and full-thickness thermal burn wounds. NexoBrid® is a topical gel that contains proteolytic enzymes that have shown, in an initial trial, effective debridement of thermal burn wounds in patients with TBSA up to 33%, with shorter time for complete eschar removal compared to standard of care, that is, surgical debridement, and noninferiority wound closure at 1 year and scar appearance at 2 years.[102] The process is extremely painful and requires intensive monitoring of the patient during the application of the gel. The challenges include identifying the ideal patient population that would benefit from this debridement rather than surgical standard of care. It is currently recommended for use on up to 20% body surface area. NexoBrid has not been studied for chemical burns, electrical burns, or contaminated wound fields, however, it is a promising emerging technique that could change the paradigm for a subset of burn patients once larger trials are conducted.

SUMMARY

Burns are responsible for significant morbidity and mortality and are among the most complex and devastating of all traumatic injuries. Early proper diagnosis of burn severity allows for the delivery of appropriate treatment and ensures the best prognosis for burn patients. Early tangential excision and autografting remains the foundation of burn treatment. Diagnosis of secondary burn complications, such as joint contracture and HO, has advanced with new imaging tools. Nevertheless, the management of burn patients requires a team of physicians, nurses, critical care specialists, physical and occupational therapists, and psychologists to provide optimal care to patients and lessen the burden of the initial burn injury.

ACKNOWLEDGMENT

We gratefully acknowledge the contributions of previous edition author, Stewart C. Wang, as portions of those chapters have been retained in this revision.

References

1. Cairns C, Kang K. *National Hospital Ambulatory Medical Care Survey: 2020 Emergency Department Summary Tables*. National Center for Health Statistics (U.S.); 2022.
2. American Burn Association. National Burn Repository. Report of data from 2008–2017. 2017.
3. (AHRQ) AfHRaQ. AHRQ releases 2020 National Inpatient Sample (NIS) (September 2022) 2020 [cited 2024 September 19]. https://hcup-us.ahrq.gov/news/announcements/nis2020.jsp.
4. Association NFP. Fire loss in the United States Quincy, MA: National Fire Protection Association; 2023 https://www.nfpa.org/education-and-research/research/nfpa-research/fire-statistical-reports/fire-loss-in-the-united-states.
5. Shields BJ, Comstock RD, Fernandez SA, Xiang H, Smith GA. Healthcare resource utilization and epidemiology of pediatric burn-associated hospitalizations, United States, 2000. *J Burn Care Res*. 2007;28(6):811–826.
6. Conner KA, Williams LE, McKenzie LB, Shields BJ, Fernandez SA, Smith GA. Pediatric pedestrian injuries and associated hospital resource utilization in the United States, 2003. *J Trauma*. 2010;68(6):1406–1412.
7. Ballesteros M, Thigpen S, Faul M, Kresnow M-J, Middlebrooks J. *161 An evaluation of CDC's web-based injury statistics query and reporting system (WISQARS)*. Injury Monitoring; 2016/09: BMJ Publishing Group Ltd; 2016, p. A59.2-A.
8. Pressel DM. Evaluation of physical abuse in children. *Am Fam Physician*. 2000;61:3057–3064.
9. Davidge K, Fish J. Older adults and burns. *Geriatrics and Aging*. 2008;11:270–275.
10. Ryan CM, Thorpe W, Mullin P, et al. A persistent fire hazard for older adults: cooking-related clothing ignition. *J Am Geriatr Soc*. 1997;45(10):1283–1285.
11. Ryan CM, Schoenfeld DA, Thorpe WP, Sheridan RL, Cassem EH, Tompkins RG. Objective estimates of the probability of death from burn injuries. *N Engl J Med*. 1998;338(6):362–366.
12. Muller MJ, Pegg SP, Rule MR. Determinants of death following burn injury. *Br J Surg*. 2001;88(4):583–587.
13. Wibbenmeyer LA, Amelon MJ, Morgan LJ, et al. Predicting survival in an elderly burn patient population. *Burns*. 2001;27(6):583–590.
14. Istre GR, McCoy M, Carlin DK, McClain J. Residential fire related deaths and injuries among children: fireplay, smoke alarms, and prevention. *Inj Prev*. 2002;8(2):128–132.

15. Pilecky D, Vamos M, Bogyi P, et al. Risk of cardiac arrhythmias after electrical accident: a single-center study of 480 patients. *Clin Res Cardiol*. 2019;108(8):901–908.
16. Purdue GF, Hunt JL. Electrocardiographic monitoring after electrical injury: necessity or luxury. *J Trauma*. 1986;26(2):166–167.
17. Gibran NS, Heimbach DM. Mediators in thermal injury. *Semin Nephrol*. 1993;19(4):344–358.
18. Santos FX, Arroyo C, García I, et al. Role of mast cells in the pathogenesis of postburn inflammatory response: reactive oxygen species as mast cell stimulators. *Burns*. 2000;26(2):145–147.
19. Zhang X-J, Irtun Ø, Zheng Y, Wolfe RR. Methysergide reduces nonnutritive blood flow in normal and scalded skin. *Am J Physiol Endocrinol Metab*. 2000;278(3):E452–E61.
20. García-Avello A, Lorente JA, Cesar-Perez J, et al. Degree of hypercoagulability and hyperfibrinolysis is related to organ failure and prognosis after burn trauma. *Thromb Res*. 1998;89(2):59–64.
21. Maass DL, White J, Horton JW. IL-1beta and IL-6 act synergistically with TNF-alpha to alter cardiac contractile function after burn trauma. *Shock*. 2002;18(4):360–366.
22. Maass DL, Hybki DP, White J, Horton JW. The time course of cardiac NF-kappaB activation and TNF-alpha secretion by cardiac myocytes after burn injury: contribution to burn-related cardiac contractile dysfunction. *Shock*. 2002;17(4):293–299.
23. White DJ, Maass DL, Sanders B, Horton JW. Cardiomyocyte intracellular calcium and cardiac dysfunction after burn trauma. *Crit Care Med*. 2002;30(1):14–22.
24. Herndon DN, Tompkins RG. Support of the metabolic response to burn injury. *Lancet*. 2004;363(9424):1895–1902.
25. Fagan SP, Bilodeau M-L, Goverman J. Burn intensive care. *Surg Clin North Am*. 2014;94(4):765–779.
26. Morio B, Irtun O, Herndon DN, Wolfe RR. Propranolol decreases splanchnic triacylglycerol storage in burn patients receiving a high-carbohydrate diet. *Ann Surg*. 2002;236(2):218–225.
27. Guidelines for Burn Patient Referral: American Burn Association. https://ameriburn.org/wp-content/uploads/2024/04/one-page-guidelines-for-burn-patient-referral-1.pdf.
28. Bezuhly M, Fish JS. Acute burn care. *Plast Reconstr Surg*. 2012;130(2):349e–358e.
29. Chung KC. *Grabb and Smith's Plastic Surgery*. Lippincott Williams & Wilkins; 2007.
30. Cartotto R, Callum J. A review of the use of human albumin in burn patients. *J Burn Care Res*. 2012;33(6):702–717.
31. Melinyshyn A, Callum J, Jeschke MC, Cartotto R. Albumin supplementation for hypoalbuminemia following burns. *J Burn Care Res*. 2013;34(1):8–17.
32. Park SH, Hemmila MR, Wahl WL. Early albumin use improves mortality in difficult to resuscitate burn patients. *J Trauma Acute Care Surg*. 2012;73(5):1294–1297.
33. Greenhalgh DG. Burn resuscitation: the results of the ISBI/ABA survey. *Burns*. 2010;36(2):176–182.
34. Lawrence A, Faraklas I, Watkins H, et al. Colloid administration normalizes resuscitation ratio and ameliorates "Fluid Creep". *J Burn Care Res*. 2010;31(1):40–47.
35. Graves TA, Cioffi WG, McManus WF, Colonel, Mason AD, Pruitt BA. Fluid resuscitation of infants and children with massive thermal injury. *J Trauma*. 1988;28(12):1656–1659.
36. Chung KK, Juncos LA, Wolf SE, et al. Continuous renal replacement therapy improves survival in severely burned military casualties with acute kidney injury. *J Trauma*. 2008;64(2):S179–S87.
37. Stawicki SP, Hoff WS, Cipolla J, deQuevedo R. Use of non-invasive esophageal echo-Doppler system in the ICU: a practical experience. *J Trauma*. 2005;59(2):506–507.
38. Wang G-Y, Ma B, Tang H-T, et al. Esophageal echo-Doppler Monitoring in burn shock resuscitation: Are hemodynamic variables the critical standard guiding fluid therapy? *J Trauma*. 2008;65(6):1396–1401.
39. Kashefi NS, Nathan JI, Dissanaike S. Does a nebulized heparin/N-acetylcysteine protocol improve outcomes in adult smoke inhalation? *Plast Reconstr Surg Glob Open*. 2014;2(6):e165.
40. Miller AC, Rivero A, Ziad S, Smith DJ, Elamin EM. Influence of nebulized unfractionated heparin and N-acetylcysteine in acute lung injury after smoke inhalation injury. *J Burn Care Res*. 2009;30(2):249–256.
41. Palmieri TL, Enkhbaatar P, Bayliss R, et al. Continuous nebulized albuterol attenuates acute lung injury in an ovine model of combined burn and smoke inhalation. *Crit Care Med*. 2006;34(6):1719–1724.
42. Salman D, Finney SJ, Griffiths MJD. Strategies to reduce ventilator-associated lung injury (VALI). *Burns*. 2013;39(2):200–211.
43. Peck MD, Koppelman T. Low-tidal-volume ventilation as a strategy to reduce ventilator-associated injury in ALI and ARDS. *J Burn Care Res*. 2009;30(1):172–175.
44. Chung KK, Wolf SE, Renz EM, et al. High-frequency percussive ventilation and low tidal volume ventilation in burns: a randomized controlled trial. *Crit Care Med*. 2010;38(10):1970–1977.
45. Herndon DN, Barrow RE, Stein M, et al. Increased mortality with intravenous supplemental feeding in severely burned patients. *J Burn Care Rehabil*. 1989;10(4):309–313.
46. Herndon DN, Hart DW, Wolf SE, Chinkes DL, Wolfe RR. Reversal of catabolism by beta-blockade after severe burns. *N Engl J Med*. 2001;345(17):1223–1229.
47. Ferrando AA, Sheffield-Moore M, Wolf SE, Herndon DN, Wolfe RR. Testosterone administration in severe burns ameliorates muscle catabolism. *Crit Care Med*. 2001;29(10):1936–1942.
48. Gus EI, Shahrokhi S, Jeschke MG. Anabolic and anticatabolic agents used in burn care: What is known and what is yet to be learned. *Burns*. 2020;46(1):19–32.
49. Wahl WL, Arbabi S, Zalewski C, Wang SC, Hemmila MR. Intensive care unit core measures improve infectious complications in burn patients. *J Burn Care Res*. 2010;31(1):190–195.
50. Atiyeh BS, Costagliola M, Hayek SN, Dibo SA. Effect of silver on burn wound infection control and healing: Review of the literature. *Burns*. 2007;33(2):139–148.
51. Falcone PA, Harrison HN, Sowemimo GOA, Reading GP. Mafenide acetate concentrations and bacteriostasis in experimental burn wounds treated with a three–layered laminated mafenide–saline dressing. *Ann Plast Surg*. 1980;5(4):266–269.
52. Klasen HJ. A historical review of the use of silver in the treatment of burns. II. Renewed interest for silver. *Burns*. 2000;26(2):131–138.
53. Fong J, Wood F. Nanocrystalline silver dressings in wound management: a review. *Int J Nanomedicine*. 2006;1(4):441–449.
54. Engrav LH, Heimbach DM, Reus JL, Harnar TJ, Marvin JA. Early excision and grafting vs. nonoperative treatment of burns of indeterminant depth: a randomized prospective study. *J Trauma*. 1983;23(11):1001–1004.
55. Gray DT, Pine RW, Harnar TJ, Marvin JA, Engrav LH, Heimbach DM. Early surgical excision versus conventional therapy in patients with 20 to 40 percent burns. *Am J Surg*. 1982;144(1):76–80.
56. Steiner M, Walsh PC, Retik AB, Vaughan ED, Wein AJ. *Campbell's Urology*. 7th ed. W.B. Saunders Co.; 1998.
57. Sterling J, Gibran NS, Klein MB. Acute management of hand burns. *Hand Clinics*. 2009;25(4):453–459.
58. Klein MB, Moore ML, Costa B, Engrav LH. Primer on the management of face burns at the University of Washington. *J Burn Care Rehabil*. 2005;26(1):2–6.
59. Benichou G, Yamada Y, Yun S-H, Lin C, Fray M, Tocco G. Immune recognition and rejection of allogeneic skin grafts. *Immunotherapy*. 2011;3(6):757–770.
60. Ronfard V, Rives J-M, Neveux Y, Carsin H, Barrandon Y. Long-term regeneration of human epidermis on third degree burns transplanted with autologous cultured epithelium grown on a fibrin matrix. *Transplantation*. 2000;70(11):1588–1598.
61. Paddle-Ledinek JE, Cruickshank DG, Masterton JP. Skin replacement by cultured keratinocyte grafts: an Australian experience. *Burns*. 1997;23(3):204–211.
62. Brown DL, Adidharma W, Hespe GE. *Michigan Manual of Plastic Surgery*. Lippincott Williams & Wilkins; 2004.
63. Holmes JH, Molnar JA, Shupp JW, et al. Demonstration of the safety and effectiveness of the RECELL® System combined

with split-thickness meshed autografts for the reduction of donor skin to treat mixed-depth burn injuries. *Burns*. 2019;45(4): 772–782.

64. Greenwood JE, Schmitt BJ, Wagstaff MJD. Experience with a synthetic bilayer biodegradable temporising matrix in significant burn injury. *Burns Open*. 2018;2(1):17–34.
65. Greenwood JE, Dearman BL. Comparison of a sealed, polymer foam biodegradable temporizing matrix against Integra® Dermal regeneration template in a porcine wound model. *J Burn Care Res*. 2012;33(1):163–173.
66. Greenwood JE, Dearman BL. Split skin graft application over an integrating, biodegradable temporizing polymer matrix. *J Burn Care Res*. 2012;33(1):7–19.
67. Wagstaff MJD, Salna IM, Caplash Y, Greenwood JE. Biodegradable Temporising Matrix (BTM) for the reconstruction of defects following serial debridement for necrotising fasciitis: A case series. *Burns Open*. 2019;3(1):12–30.
68. Rnjak J, Wise SG, Mithieux SM, Weiss AS. Severe burn injuries and the role of elastin in the design of dermal substitutes. *Tissue Eng Part B Rev*. 2011;17(2):81–91.
69. Lee YJ, Han HJ, Shim HS. Treatment of hard-to-heal wounds in ischaemic lower extremities with a novel fish skin-derived matrix. *J Wound Care*. 2024;33(5):348–356.
70. Stone R 2nd, Saathoff EC, Larson DA, et al. Comparison of intact fish skin graft and allograft as temporary coverage for full-thickness burns: a non-inferiority study. *Biomedicines*. 2024;12(3):680.
71. Luze H, Nischwitz SP, Smolle C, Zrim R, Kamolz LP. The use of acellular fish skin grafts in burn wound management-a systematic review. *Medicina (Kaunas)*. 2022;58(7):912.
72. Staubach R, Glosse H, Loff S. The use of fish skin grafts in children as a new treatment of deep dermal burns-case series with follow-up after 2 years and measurement of elasticity as an objective scar evaluation. *J Clin Med*. 2024;13(8):2389.
73. Wiechman Askay S, Patterson DR, Sharar SR, Mason S, Faber B. Pain management in patients with burn injuries. *Int Rev Psychiatry*. 2009;21(6):522–530.
74. Tandara AA, Mustoe TA. The role of the epidermis in the control of scarring: evidence for mechanism of action for silicone gel. *J Plast Reconstr Aesthet Surg*. 2008;61(10):1219–1225.
75. Mustoe TA. Evolution of silicone therapy and mechanism of action in scar management. *Aesthetic Plast Surg*. 2007;32(1):82–92.
76. Saulis A. Silicone occlusive treatment of hypertrophic scar in the rabbit model. *Aesthetic Surg J*. 2002;22(2):147–153.
77. Gangemi EN, Gregori D, Berchialla P, et al. Epidemiology and risk factors for pathologic scarring after burn wounds. *Arch Facial Plast Surg*. 2008;10(2):93–102.
78. Nedelec B, Shankowsky H, Scott PG, Ghahary A, Tredget EE. Myofibroblasts and apoptosis in human hypertrophic scars: The effect of interferon-alpha2b. *Surgery*. 2001;130(5):798–808.
79. Armour A, Scott PG, Tredget EE. Cellular and molecular pathology of HTS: basis for treatment. *Wound Repair Regen*. 2007; 15(s1):S6–17.
80. Longacre JJ, Berry HK, Basom CR, Townsend SF. The effects of Z plasty on hypertrophic scars. *Scand J Plast Reconstr Surg*. 1976;10(2):113–128.
81. Davis JS. The relaxation of scar contractures by means of the Z-, or reversed Z-type incision: stressing the use of scar infiltrated tissues. *Ann Surg*. 1931;94(5):871–884.
82. Parnell LKS, Nedelec B, Rachelska G, LaSalle L. Assessment of pruritus characteristics and impact on burn survivors. *J Burn Care Res*. 2012;33(3):407–418.
83. Klinger M, Marazzi M, Vigo D, Torre M. Fat injection for cases of severe burn outcomes: a new perspective of scar remodeling and reduction. *Aesthetic Plast Surg*. 2008;32(3):465–469.
84. Reish RG, Eriksson E. Scar treatments: preclinical and clinical studies. *J Am Coll Surg*. 2008;206(4):719–730.
85. Zouboulis CC. Outcomes of cryosurgery in keloids and hypertrophic scars. *Arch Dermatol*. 1993;129(9):1146.
86. Alster TS, Handrick C. Laser treatment of hypertrophic scars, keloids, and striae. *Semin Cutan Med Surg*. 2000;19(4): 287–292.
87. Manuskiatti W, Wanitphakdeedecha R, Fitzpatrick RE. Effect of pulse width of a 595-nm flashlamp-pumped pulsed dye laser on the treatment response of keloidal and hypertrophic sternotomy scars. *Dermatol Surg*. 2007;33(2):152–161.
88. Manuskiatti W, Fitzpatrick RE, Goldman MP. Energy density and numbers of treatment affect response of keloidal and hypertrophic sternotomy scars to the 585-nm flashlamp-pumped pulsed-dye laser. *J Am Acad Dermatol*. 2001;45(4): 557–565.
89. Garden JM, Tan OT, Kerschmann R, et al. Effect of dye laser pulse duration on selective cutaneous vascular injury. *J Invest Dermatol*. 1986;87(5):653–657.
90. Manstein D, Herron GS, Sink RK, Tanner H, Anderson RR. Fractional photothermolysis: a new concept for cutaneous remodeling using microscopic patterns of thermal injury. *Lasers Surg Med*. 2004;34(5):426–438.
91. Patel SP, Nguyen HV, Mannschreck D, Redett RJ, Puttgen KB, Stewart FD. Fractional CO_2 laser treatment outcomes for pediatric hypertrophic burn scars. *J Burn Care Res*. 2019;40(4): 386–391.
92. Madni TD, Lu K, Nakonezny PA, et al. Treating hypertrophic burn scar with 2940-nm Er:YAG laser fractional ablation improves scar characteristics as measured by noninvasive technology. *J Burn Care Res*. 2019;40(4):416–21.
93. Hultman CS, Friedstat JS, Edkins RE, Cairns BA, Meyer AA. Laser resurfacing and remodeling of hypertrophic burn scars: the results of a large, prospective, before-after cohort study, with long-term follow-up. *Ann Surg*. 2014;260(3):519–529.
94. Zuccaro J, Muser I, Singh M, Yu J, Kelly C, Fish J. Laser therapy for pediatric burn scars: focusing on a combined treatment approach. *J Burn Care Res*. 2017;39(3):457–462.
95. Elledge ES, Smith AA, McManus WF, Pruitt BA. Heterotopic bone formation in burned patients. *J Trauma*. 1988;28(5): 684–687.
96. Esselman PC, Thombs BD, Magyar-Russell G, Fauerbach JA. Burn rehabilitation. *Am J Phys Med Rehabil*. 2006;85(4): 383–413.
97. Evans EB. Orthopaedic measures in the treatment of severe burns. *J Bone Joint Surg*. 1966;48(4):643–669.
98. Klein MB, Logsetty S, Costa B, et al. Extended time to wound closure is associated with increased risk of heterotopic ossification of the elbow. *J Burn Care Res*. 2007;28(3):447–450.
99. Maender C, Sahajpal D, Wright TW. Treatment of heterotopic ossification of the elbow following burn injury: Recommendations for surgical excision and perioperative prophylaxis using radiation therapy. *J Shoulder Elbow Surg*. 2010;19(8): 1269–1275.
100. Orzel JA, Rudd TG. Heterotopic bone formation: clinical, laboratory, and imaging correlation. *J Nucl Med*. 1985;26(2): 125–132.
101. Neal BC, Rodgers A, Clark T, et al. A systematic survey of 13 randomized trials of non-steroidal anti-inflammatory drugs for the prevention of heterotopic bone formation after major hip surgery. *Acta Orthop Scand*. 2000;71(2):122–128.
102. Shoham Y, Rosenberg L, Hickerson W, et al. Early enzymatic burn debridement: results of the DETECT multicenter randomized controlled trial. *J Burn Care Res*. 2024;45(2):297–307.

11

Anesthesiology and Pain Management

Paul Picton, Sachin Kheterpal, and Michael R. Mathis

SCIENTIFIC PRINCIPLES

Key Points

1 Anesthetics are generalized depressants of consciousness, pain, cardiopulmonary function, motor function, and recall.

2 To prevent movement and to facilitate the surgical exposure, neuromuscular blocking agents are generally used. Commonly used drugs are competitive inhibitors of the neurotransmitter acetylcholine at the neuromuscular junction. Residual neuromuscular blockade is a common and underappreciated phenomenon that impacts postoperative adverse events such as hypoxemia, pneumonia, reintubation, and prolonged recovery room stay. Sugammadex, a novel medication capable of reversing deep neuromuscular blockade, has permeated perioperative care for high-risk patients.

3 Opioids produce profound analgesia and respiratory depression. They have no amnesic properties, minimal direct myocardial depressive effects, and no muscle-relaxant properties.

4 Propofol is a lipid-soluble substituted isopropyl phenol that produces a rapid induction of anesthesia followed by awakening in 4 to 8 minutes after a single bolus. However, as the duration and dose of the maintenance infusion are increased, the time to return to consciousness is also significantly increased.

5 Although neuraxial techniques (spinal and epidural) may decrease pulmonary complications, they are contraindicated in patients with systemic infection, coagulopathy, receiving ongoing anticoagulation, or exhibiting severe flow-dependent cardiovascular diseases.

6 Peripheral nerve blockade (PNB) can be used in lieu of general anesthesia as a primary anesthetic for surgery, or in conjunction with general anesthesia to serve as a postoperative pain management technique. Use of long-acting local anesthetics or placement of an indwelling continuous catheter provides long-term (16 hours to several days) pain relief.

7 The concept of airway management should be focused on not just endotracheal intubation, but also mask ventilation. Until the airway can be secured via intubation, the patient must be supported through mask ventilation. The key elements of an airway examination are an assessment of obesity, mouth opening, neck flexion and extension, Mallampati oropharyngeal classification, presence of beard, and mandibular protrusion ability.

8 More than 8% of patients undergoing major noncardiac inpatient surgery will experience postoperative myocardial ischemia, elevating their risk of 30-day mortality. The optimal management of the patient at high risk of cardiac complications has evolved significantly, now focusing on optimizing the patient using guidelines consistent with long-term cardiac risk modification and interventions.

9 The three goals of the preoperative evaluation are (a) to develop an anesthetic plan that considers the patient's medical condition, the requirements of the surgical procedure, and the patient's preferences; (b) to ensure that the patient's chronic disease is under appropriate medical therapy before an elective procedure; and (c) to gain rapport with and the confidence of the patient, answer any questions, and allay fears.

10 A variety of outpatient medication classes require careful management in the perioperative period, including but not limited to (a) anticoagulants and antiplatelets, (b) cardiovascular medications (beta blockade, antihypertensives, antiarrhythmics, pulmonary hypertension therapy), (c) chronic pain and opioid use disorder medications (opioids, buprenorphine), (d) glycemic agents (insulin, oral hypoglycemics, and SGLT-2 inhibitors), (e) obesity medications (GLP-1 agonists), and (f) pulmonary medications (novel biologics, inhaled steroids, and beta agonists). Failure to adhere to relevant guidelines can increase clinical risk and delay time-sensitive procedures.

11 Enhanced recovery programs incorporating preoperative optimization, and standardized surgical and anesthesia protocols may improve patient outcomes and reduce costs. Goal-directed intraoperative fluid therapy has conflicting evidence basis and cannot be considered a standard of care at this time.

12 Postoperative acute pain management may require a multimodal approach that incorporates opioids, PNB, and nonopioid analgesics. Chronic pain patients may require preoperative optimization and care coordination led by an anesthesiologist.

INTRODUCTION

The goal of anesthesia is to enable the safe conduct of procedures with maintenance of physiologic homeostasis while optimizing procedural conditions. The state of general anesthesia is a combination of hypnosis, amnesia, analgesia, and muscle relaxation, achieved by the administration of single or multiple anesthetic agents via inhalational or intravenous routes. Anesthesia is typically achieved by using a balance of multiple pharmacologic agents, each targeted to produce a specific effect—hypnotic/sedatives, analgesics, and neuromuscular blocking agents. As

Table 11.1. Common Inhalation Agents: Minimum Alveolar Concentrations and Effects

Agent	Minimum Alveolar Concentration (%)	Strengths	Weaknesses
Nitrous oxide	105	Analgesia Rapid uptake and elimination Less cardiac or respiratory depression	Sympathetic stimulation Expansion of closed air spaces Interference with vitamin B_{12} metabolism Limitation of inspired oxygen fraction
Isoflurane	1.15	Good muscle relaxation Stable cardiac rate and rhythm Usability in neurosurgery	Airway irritant, may cause coughing
Desflurane	6	Rapid induction and emergence	Airway irritant, may cause coughing High vapor pressure (Boiling point 23.5 °C) requiring special pressurized vaporizer High cost
Sevoflurane	1.71	Rapid induction and emergence Less pungent, does not cause airway irritation	Moderate cost

the concentration of hypnotic/sedative and analgesic agents increases, cardiovascular and respiratory functions may be progressively blunted; titration is necessary to optimize surgical conditions while maintaining cardiovascular stability.

Despite serious potential complications, anesthesia is administered with a high degree of safety 30 to 40 million times a year in the United States. Good patient outcomes may be attributed to the efforts of thousands of surgeons and anesthesiologists who have advanced the art and science of their field. Although modern surgical techniques, regional or neuraxial blockade procedures, and systemic analgesics help to ameliorate perioperative pain, significant challenges remain; pain is not only unpleasant but can also provoke the stress response and is associated with significant adverse effects.

ANESTHETIC MEDICATIONS AND THEIR PHYSIOLOGIC EFFECTS

Inhalation Agents

1 Inhalational anesthetics produce dose-dependent depression of consciousness, pain, cardiopulmonary function, motor function, and recall. Comparative potency of inhalation agents is expressed as the minimum alveolar concentration (MAC), an empirically derived number defined as the expired percent concentration required to prevent movement on painful stimulation (incision) in half of experimental subjects. There is significant patient-to-patient variability independent of underlying comorbidities. Compounding this variability are the effects of age, weight, preexisting heart disease, liver disease, and coadministered medications. **Table 11.1** lists the commonly used inhalation agents, their MACs, and side effects. In general, all agents cause hypotension by myocardial depression and vasodilation. There is also a generalized depression of cerebral function and cerebral metabolic rate for oxygen, although cerebral blood flow may increase because of cerebrovascular dilatation and a loss of flow–metabolism coupling. Renal blood flow and glomerular filtration rate are reduced by 20% to 50%. The body's regulation of core body temperature is lost, resulting in a redistribution of heat from the core to the periphery; the cold environment of the operating room and open body cavities make anesthetized patients extremely vulnerable to hypothermia (core body temperature <36 °C).

Intravenous Sedatives/Hypnotics

Intravenous sedative/hypnotic medications can also be used, by intravenous infusion, in lieu of an inhalational anesthetic to achieve maintenance of anesthesia. Unlike inhalational agents, there is currently no methodology to measure the patient's expired or blood concentration of these agents. As a result, the infusion rate is titrated to effect by observing patient movement (if muscle relaxants are not used concurrently), hemodynamic responses to procedural stimuli, and more recently to commercially available processed electroencephalographic monitoring (EEG). The sedative/hypnotic intravenous agents do not possess clinically useful muscle-relaxant or analgesic properties and must be combined with other agents to deliver a "balanced" anesthetic. The most commonly used intravenous agent for maintenance of anesthesia is propofol, a lipid-soluble substituted isopropyl phenol that produces dose-dependent hypnosis and sedation through interactions with γ-aminobutyric acid (GABA), the primary inhibitory neurotransmitter of the central nervous system. Propofol infusions are the foundation of total intravenous anesthesia (TIVA), a specific general anesthetic technique that avoids the use of inhaled volatile agents or nitrous oxide and their associated side effects such as nausea and vomiting. Additional details regarding the use of propofol are discussed later. The highly specific α_2-receptor agonist, dexmedetomidine, may also be used as an intravenous sedative/hypnotic and also has analgesic effects and does not produce significant respiratory depression. In the perioperative setting, it is currently limited to use as an adjunct to propofol and inhalational anesthetics for general anesthesia or as a sole agent during procedural sedation.

Muscle Relaxants and Antagonism

2 To facilitate endotracheal intubation, surgical exposure, and minimize unintended patient movement, neuromuscular blocking agents are generally used. These drugs are competitive or noncompetitive inhibitors of the neurotransmitter acetylcholine at the neuromuscular junction. The only noncompetitive inhibitor used clinically is succinylcholine. This drug rapidly binds to the nicotinic receptors and produces depolarization at the neuromuscular junction, clinically manifesting as fine-muscle fasciculations occurring 30 to 60 seconds after injection. Succinylcholine cannot be reversed but has a short duration of action (<10 minutes) because it is quickly hydrolyzed in the plasma by cholinesterase. Because of rapid onset and short duration of action, succinylcholine is classically used to facilitate endotracheal intubation when it must be accomplished quickly, or when quickly regaining neuromuscular function is beneficial.

All other clinically useful muscle relaxants compete with endogenous acetylcholine at the neuromuscular junction, are termed *competitive inhibitors* and do not cause depolarization (nondepolarizing). The block produced is in direct proportion

Table 11.2. Common Neuromuscular Blocking Drugs and Reversal Agents

Muscle Relaxant	Intubating Dose (mg/kg)	Strengths	Weaknesses
Depolarizing			
Succinylcholine	1.0	Fastest onset (30–60 s) Short duration[a] (5–10 min)	Associated with malignant hyperthermia, dysrhythmias, bradycardia, and hyperkalemia, especially in patients with burns or neurologic injury
Nondepolarizing			
Cisatracurium	0.2	Spontaneous degradation, not affected by renal or liver disease	Moderate cost
Vecuronium	0.1	No cardiovascular effects	
Rocuronium	0.8	Fast onset, no cardiovascular effects	

[a]Duration is dramatically increased in patients with abnormal plasma pseudocholinesterase.

to the concentration of the agent relative to the concentration of acetylcholine. The common neuromuscular blocking drugs and their doses, durations, and side effects are listed in **Table 11.2**; common regimens of reversal agents are shown in **Table 11.3**.

Postoperative residual neuromuscular blockade is recognized as a common problem after routine administration of nondepolarizing muscle relaxants and may underlie many common postoperative care unit clinical issues such as delayed emergence, airway obstruction, and hypoxemia. Muscles in the body are not equally sensitive to muscle relaxants. The diaphragm is most resistant to neuromuscular blockade, whereas the neck and pharyngeal muscles that support the airway are most sensitive. It is therefore possible for an intubated patient to exhibit adequate spontaneous ventilation and produce a large negative inspiratory pressure and yet develop complete airway obstruction when extubated.

Competitive relaxants can be antagonized by two different classes of medications: (1) anticholinesterases (eg, neostigmine) that block acetylcholine metabolism to increase the concentration of acetylcholine relative to the neuromuscular blockade agent and (2) selective relaxant binding agents (eg, sugammadex) which can bind and sequester steroidal nondepolarizing neuromuscular blocking agents. When anticholinesterases are used, the neuromuscular blocking agent is still present and unbound, but motor function returns when acetylcholine concentration is high enough to overwhelm the blocking agent. Anticholinesterases hence exhibit a ceiling effect. There are systemic consequences to increasing the plasma concentration of acetylcholine. Acetylcholine is the predominant neurotransmitter in the preganglionic sympathetic and parasympathetic nervous systems and in the postganglionic parasympathetic nervous system. To counter the undesirable effects of systemic acetylcholine an anticholinergic drug (atropine or glycopyrrolate) must be given with the anticholinesterase.

Selective relaxant binding agents—currently comprised of only one FDA-approved drug, sugammadex—are now widely used for the reversal of neuromuscular blockade. Such compounds are able to rapidly reverse the effects of profound muscle relaxation (0/4 twitches) created by steroidal nondepolarizing muscle-relaxant agents rocuronium and vecuronium. These agents physically bind free muscle-relaxant molecules within a cyclodextrin ring structure and decrease the concentration of free muscle relaxant allowing acetylcholine to function normally at the neuromuscular junction. The cyclodextrin–muscle-relaxant combination is eliminated via the kidney. Sugammadex rapidly (<3 minutes) reverses profound muscle relaxation without cholinergic side effects offering considerable advantage over

Table 11.3. Drugs for Antagonizing Nondepolarizing Neuromuscular Blockade[a]

Dose	Time to Peak Effect (min)	Dose	Use with	Comments
Anticholinesterases				
Edrophonium	1–2	0.5–1.0 mg/kg	Atropine	Very fast onset, not commonly used
Neostigmine	3–15	0.04–0.07 mg/kg	Glycopyrrolate	Most commonly used
Pyridostigmine	10–12	0.2–0.3 mg/kg	—	Not used clinically for neuromuscular reversal
Selective Relaxant Binding Agents				
Sugammadex	2–3	2–16 mg/kg	—	Used for reversal of rocuronium and vecuronium

[a]For reliable results in reversing the effects of nondepolarizing muscle relaxants, administration of anticholinesterases is delayed until spontaneous recovery permits three to four twitch responses to a train-of-four stimulus. For patients with more profound blockade, larger amounts of anticholinesterases may be required, but doses of neostigmine higher than 0.14 mg/kg are unlikely to produce additional improvement.

CNS, central nervous system.

Adapted from Watling SM, Dasta JF. Prolonged paralysis in intensive care unit patients after the use of neuromuscular blocking agents: a review of the literature. *Crit Care Med.* 1994;22:884.

Table 11.4. Analgesics

	Potency	Sedation Dose	Duration	Infusion Dose
Opioids				
Morphine	1	0.02–0.1 mg/kg IV	2–7 h	—
Fentanyl	100	0.5–1 mcg/kg IV	30–60 min	—
Sufentanil	1000	Not recommended	—	—
Alfentanil	25	10–20 mg/kg IV	10–15 min	—
Remifentanil[a]	—	Not recommended	10 min	0.1–0.2 mg/kg/min
Other Analgesics and Anesthetics				
Propofol		0.1–0.5 mg/kg IV[b,c]		100–200 mcg/kg/min[b]
Ketamine		0.1–0.5 mg/kg IV[b] 1.0–2.0 mg/kg IM		1–2 mg/min (anesthetic dose) 500 mcg/kg (analgesic dose)
Dexmedetomidine		0.2–1.0 µg/kg/h		0.2–1.0 µg/kg/h

[a]Will produce apnea.
[b]May produce apnea.
[c]Produces pain on injection that can be reduced by treatment with 20 mg of lidocaine IV.
IM, intramuscular; IV, intravenous.

the traditional approach. Sugammadex cannot reverse neuromuscular blockade achieved with benzylisoquinolinium muscle relaxants (atracurium, cisatracurium) given incompatibility in chemical structures.

Opioids (Narcotics) and Other Intravenous Analgesics

Narcotics and synthetic analogs belong to the class of drugs called *opioids*. The most commonly used drugs in this family are morphine, fentanyl, and hydromorphone. Since the mid-1980s, a series of synthetic opioids have been developed with
3 fentanyl as the prototype. More recently developed synthetics (sufentanil, alfentanil, and remifentanil) are more potent and of varying duration (**Table 11.4**). Opioids produce profound analgesia and respiratory depression. They have no amnesic properties, minimal direct myocardial depressive effects, and no muscle-relaxant properties. Opioids can produce significant hemodynamic effects indirectly by releasing histamine or blunting the patient's sympathetic vascular tone. Because of the lack of direct myocardial depression and the absence of histamine release with the synthetic opioids, they are frequently used as the primary anesthetic in combination with an amnesic agent and a muscle relaxant in patients with significant myocardial dysfunction.

All opioids can be reversed with naloxone. The duration of action of naloxone can be shorter than that of the opioid, and patients must be observed carefully for renarcotization after they have been treated with naloxone. Naloxone treatment has been associated with acute pulmonary edema and myocardial ischemia and should not be used electively to reverse the effects of a narcotic.

Propofol

Propofol is a lipid-soluble substituted isopropyl phenol that
4 produces a rapid induction of anesthesia in 30 seconds followed by awakening in 4 to 8 minutes after a single bolus. Intravenous propofol can effectively produce total anesthesia (for less stimulating procedures), including amnesia, some analgesia, and some degree of muscle relaxation. As the duration and dose of the maintenance infusion are increased, the time to return to consciousness is also significantly increased. This context-sensitive half-life of propofol must be incorporated into expectations of a "quick wake-up." Propofol has direct antiemetic properties and is an excellent alternative to inhalational anesthetics in patients who have demonstrated a history of refractory postoperative nausea and vomiting. It has an important role in intensive care units (ICUs) when used as a continuous infusion sedative. Due to dose-dependent direct myocardial depression and peripheral vasodilation, propofol can produce significant hypotension when IV induction doses are administered. It also produces pain on injection in peripheral veins.

Ketamine

Ketamine is a phencyclidine derivative that produces anesthesia characterized by dissociation between the thalamus and limbic systems. Induction of anesthesia is achieved within 60 seconds after IV injection of 1 to 2 mg/kg or within 2 to 4 minutes of intramuscular (IM) injection of 5 to 10 mg/kg. Patients appear to be in a cataleptic state in which their eyes remain open with a slow nystagmic gaze. The drug produces intense amnesia and analgesia but has been associated with unpleasant visual and auditory hallucinations that can progress to delirium. The incidence of these problems can be significantly reduced if benzodiazepines are coadministered. At low doses (0.1 to 0.2 mg/kg IV or 2 mg/kg IM), patients continue to spontaneously ventilate. At higher doses, ketamine acts as a respiratory depressant and produces complete apnea. Ketamine also has direct and indirect sympathetic nervous system stimulatory effects, which can be useful in hypovolemic patients or in patients likely to encounter bronchospasm. These effects are diminished or absent in patients who are catecholamine depleted. The sympathetic stimulatory effect increases myocardial oxygen consumption and intracranial pressure. IM ketamine (1 to 2 mg/kg) is also very useful for sedating patients who have difficulty cooperating with preoperative IV line placement (eg, combative patients or those with intellectual disabilities). While observational research purported the value of intraoperative ketamine for improved acute and chronic pain outcomes, prospective clinical trials have not been able to support this practice pattern.

Amnesics and Anxiolytics

Benzodiazepines are the primary class of agents used as amnesics and anxiolytics. The prototype drug, diazepam, has been

Table 11.5. Anxiolytics and Amnesics (Benzodiazepines)

Name	Dose (mg)	Duration (h)	Strengths	Weaknesses
Midazolam (Versed)	0.5–2 IV	0.5	Water soluble Short duration Good for sedation for short procedures	Acute respiratory depression
Diazepam (Valium)	5–10 IV	1	Intermediate duration	Irritation on IV injection Phlebitis Acute respiratory depression after IV overdose
Lorazepam (Ativan)	2–4 IV	6–8	Long duration	—
Benzodiazepine Reversal				
Flumazenil (Romazicon)	0.2 IV (0.2 mg repeated every 2–10 min until reversal is achieved) Maximum dose 1 mg	45–90 min	—	May produce seizures, panic, arrhythmias

IV, intravenous.

mostly replaced by its water-soluble analog of shorter duration, midazolam. Lorazepam also belongs to this family of agents, but because it has a very long duration of action, it is not routinely used intraoperatively. Lorazepam has ICU applications (**Table 11.5**). Benzodiazepines have no analgesic properties but can be used in combination with the short-acting opioid fentanyl to produce conscious sedation for minor procedures. Benzodiazepines can produce apnea and have synergistic adverse effects with narcotics. As with all anesthetics, benzodiazepines used as IV agents for sedation should be given in small incremental doses to achieve the desired effect. A reversal agent is also available for benzodiazepines (flumazenil). The recommended dosages of these drugs and the reversal agents appear in **Table 11.5**.

Local Anesthetics

Local anesthetics temporarily block nerve conduction by binding to neuronal sodium channels. As the concentration of the local anesthetic increases around the nerve, autonomic transmission will be blocked first, followed by sensory transmission, and then motor nerve transmission. These drugs can be injected locally into tissue to produce a field block; around peripheral nerves to produce a specific dermatomal block; around nerve plexuses to produce a major conductive block; and into the subarachnoid or epidural space to produce extensive neuraxial blockade.

Adverse consequences associated with the use of local anesthetics fall into three categories: acute central nervous system toxicity due to excessive plasma concentration; hemodynamic and respiratory consequences due to excessive conduction block of the sympathetic or motor nerves; and allergic reactions. Whenever a local anesthetic is injected, there can be inadvertent intravascular injection or an overdose of the drug because of rapid uptake from the tissues. Overdose can produce seizures, as well as cardiovascular collapse from ensuing arrhythmias. Agents differ in duration of action (**Table 11.6**) which may be prolonged by the coadministration of epinephrine. Epinephrine works, for this purpose, by local vasoconstriction and hence delays the distribution of local anesthetic from tissues to the bloodstream; it is not recommended for any

Table 11.6. Local Anesthetics

	Maximum Single Dose (mg/kg)	Duration (h)	Comments
Amides			
Lidocaine	4.5	1[a]	Fast onset
Ropivacaine	3	4–12[a]	Less cardiac toxicity than bupivacaine
Bupivacaine	3	4–12[a]	Exaggerated cardiotoxicity with IV injection Slow onset Long duration
Esters[b]			
2-Chloroprocaine	12	0.5–1[a]	Fast onset Lowest toxicity, rapid metabolism
Tetracaine	3	0.5–1	Slow onset

[a]Addition of 100 μg of epinephrine (0.1 mL of 1:1000) lowers the toxicity and increases the duration of the local anesthetic.
[b]Metabolism to para-aminobenzoic acid may cause allergic reactions.
IV, intravenous.

SCIENTIFIC PRINCIPLES

anatomic site that may be subject to ischemia such as penis and digits.

Local anesthetics are chemically divided into two groups: esters and amides. Esters (2-chloroprocaine and tetracaine) produce metabolites that are related to *p*-aminobenzoic acid and have been associated with allergic reactions. Amides (eg, lidocaine and bupivacaine) are rarely associated with allergic reactions. If an allergic reaction does occur, it is most likely due to the preservative (methylparaben) used in multidose vials of lidocaine.

NEURAXIAL BLOCKADE

The two primary neuraxial techniques, a "single-shot" spinal and continuous epidural catheter, can be used for lower extremity and lower abdominal procedures. In the case of a "single-shot" spinal anesthetic—also known as a subarachnoid block—the intrathecal sac surrounding the cauda equina is located using a sterile, small-caliber needle (25 gauge typically). Once cerebrospinal fluid is observed in the hub of a needle, 1 to 3 mL of preservative-free local anesthetic (typically bupivacaine or lidocaine) is injected into the intrathecal space. The needle is then completely withdrawn. Blockade of sensory, motor, and sympathetic nerves occurs at the nerve roots. The spread of local anesthetic within the subarachnoid space is primarily determined by three factors: (a) the vertebral interspace accessed, (b) the density of the local anesthetic in relation to the density of cerebrospinal fluid (a concept known as *baricity*), and (c) the position of the patient during injection and immediately thereafter. In order to eliminate the risk of needle puncture of the spinal cord, subarachnoid blocks are only performed below L2–L3 in adults and L3–L4 in children. The local anesthetic solution may be combined with vasoconstrictors such as epinephrine or opioids such as fentanyl or morphine in order to increase the density or duration of the sensory blockade. Surgical anesthesia ranging from 1 to 2 hours can be achieved. Because of concerns regarding permanent nerve damage, intrathecal catheters are typically not used.[1]

In the case of epidural techniques, the nerve roots are blocked outside the thecal sac in a potential space between the ligamentum flavum and dura mater. This space is accessed sterilely using a 19-gauge introducer needle and a loss of resistance technique. Once the space is identified, a 21-gauge catheter is inserted into the space via the introducer needle and the needle is removed leaving the catheter in place and redosing is therefore possible. Dilute local anesthetics combined with vasoconstrictors or opioids are the mainstay of epidural therapy. Epidural neuraxial techniques can be used for surgical anesthesia, as an adjunct to general anesthesia, or for postoperative pain relief. Epidural catheters can be placed in the thoracic or lumbar regions because the intrathecal sac is not being accessed; associated dermatomal spread and analgesia are observed. Epidural techniques often fail to result in a dense sacral nerve root blockade making it a suboptimal choice for surgical anesthesia below the knee.

When local anesthetics are administered for a spinal or epidural block, they produce a progressive blockade of the sympathetic nervous system, which produces systemic vasodilation. Sympathetic nerves travel along the thoracolumbar region with the first four thoracic branches, including the cardiac sympathetic accelerators. A sympathetic blockade of this entire region produces a characteristic profound systemic vasodilatation and bradycardia. This condition is referred to as *total sympathectomy.* Affected patients are bradycardic, hypotensive, unconscious, and usually apneic. This disastrous situation is easily remedied if treated quickly with a vasopressor (phenylephrine or ephedrine) and atropine or small doses of epinephrine (increments of 10 μg for an adult). If not treated promptly, the situation proceeds to cardiac arrest. The required doses of epinephrine are higher than in a usual cardiac arrest because of the total sympathectomy. Because the level of sympathetic block is two to six dermatomal levels higher than the sensory block, it is often difficult to obtain a high spinal sensory level without approaching a total sympathectomy. For this reason, spinal or epidural techniques can present a prohibitively high risk in patients with severe flow-dependent cardio-
5 vascular disease.

PERIPHERAL NERVE BLOCKADE

Peripheral nerve blockade (PNB) has been used for surgical anesthesia of the extremities since the days of intravenous regional anesthesia described by Bier in 1908. Upper extremity, lower extremity, and visceral peripheral nerves are targets.
6 Much like neuraxial blockade, PNB can be used to achieve intraoperative surgical anesthesia, intraoperative analgesia as an adjunct to general anesthesia, or postoperative analgesia. Use of long-acting local anesthetics or placement of an indwelling continuous catheter provides long-term (16 hours to several days) pain relief. A PNB may be contraindicated if a neurologic examination performed at or near the surgical site in the early postoperative period is necessary.

Because of the limited distribution of sympathetic blockade, PNB has a much smaller hemodynamic effect than general or neuraxial anesthesia. In addition, if general or neuraxial anesthesia can be supplemented by a PNB, the residual unwanted side effects of these anesthetics can be limited. However, PNB is not without side effects; the impact of phrenic nerve motor blockade associated with specific upper extremity blocks (common with interscalene and rare with supraclavicular) may have significant consequences for patients with underlying pulmonary disease.

Most anesthesiologists employ real-time ultrasound guidance of needle under direct visualization for the placement of PNB. Despite direct visualization using ultrasound, PNB in adults is typically performed in the awake state to minimize the risk of intraneural injection, which may be detected via patient complaint of significant pain upon injection. PNB can be extremely difficult or contraindicated in patients with challenging body habitus, local superficial infection, significant coagulopathy, or implants near the area to be visualized or injected.

While PNB targets named major peripheral nerves resulting in both motor and sensory blockade sufficient for surgical anesthesia, field blocks target small cutaneous sensory nerve fibers, used more commonly to achieve moderate sensory blockade for postoperative analgesia alone. Procedures such as transversus abdominis plane (TAP), adductor canal, quadratus lumborum, intercostal nerve, and local infiltration enable postoperative analgesia.

SEDATION ANALGESIA FOR MINOR SURGICAL PROCEDURES

Sedation occurs on a continuum from minimal sedation (responds normally to verbal stimuli) to general anesthesia (unarousable). "Deep sedation" describes a drug-induced depression of consciousness from which a patient cannot easily be aroused but maintains the ability to respond purposefully to repeated or painful stimuli; since inadvertent progression to general anesthesia is a risk, providers are held to similar standards to those who provide anesthesia services by federal code. The term "monitored anesthesia care" (MAC) does not describe a level of sedation but is rather a specific anesthesia service in which an anesthesiologist participates. There are a variety of minor surgical procedures that can be accomplished safely and comfortably with anesthesia provided by infiltration of local anesthetics (most commonly 1% lidocaine or 0.25% bupivacaine) and minimal sedation/anxiolysis provided by IV agents. All IV benzodiazepines, narcotics, and other IV anesthetics produce apnea with substantial patient-to-patient variation;

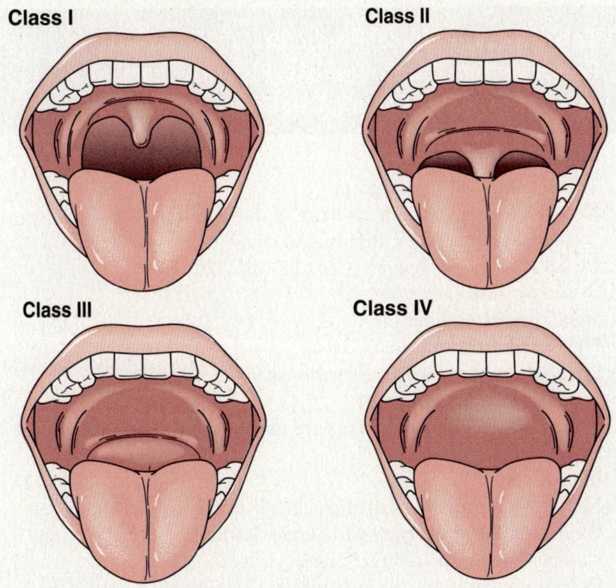

Figure 11.1. Classification of the patient's upper airway based on the size of the tongue and the pharyngeal structures visible on mouth opening.Class I, soft palate and anterior/posterior tonsillar pillars, and uvula visible; Class II, tonsillar pillars and part of uvula hidden by base of tongue; Class III, soft and hard palate visible; Class IV, soft palate not visible, only hard palate visible. (Redrawn from Stoelting RK, Miller RD. *Basics of Anesthesia*. 5th ed. Churchill Livingston; 2007:146.)

small incremental doses are recommended to achieve a safe sedated state. Inadequate infiltration of local anesthetic cannot be compensated by increased doses of IV sedatives. Because of the potentially serious consequences of an apneic episode, The Joint Commission has required that all patients receiving sedation for minor surgical or medical procedures undergo the following as a minimum standard[2]:

1. A preprocedure evaluation including an airway examination (**Fig. 11.1**)
2. Appropriate monitoring: pulse oximetry as a minimum
3. Documentation of the patient's vital signs and arterial saturation as well as the dose and timing of sedatives provided during the procedure
4. Documentation of a recovery period and a return to a safe recovered state

The preprocedure evaluation should include current medications, coexisting disease, and a brief physical examination including an evaluation of the airway. The most common drug used to provide sedation and anxiolysis is midazolam. This is a fast-onset, relatively short-acting benzodiazepine that can be easily titrated to produce a sedated yet cooperative arousable state. It is usually given to adults in incremental doses of 1 mg (0.01 mg/kg in children). Narcotics such as fentanyl even in small doses act synergistically with benzodiazepines to cause a more sedated state with a much higher incidence of apnea. To assess the effect of the drug, a validated sedation scale can be of value. The scale used at the University of Michigan is presented in **Table 11.7**.[3]

AIRWAY EVALUATION FOR THE NONANESTHESIOLOGIST

7 An essential skill for all clinicians is the assessment of a patient's airway to determine how difficult it may be to obtain control of the airway if a patient requires ventilatory support. The concept of airway management should be focused on not just endotracheal intubation, but also mask ventilation. Until the airway can be secured via intubation, the patient must be supported through mask ventilation.[4] Supraglottic airway devices (laryngeal mask airways) are of additional consideration, used for both intraoperative airway management as well as a rescue technique for failed mask ventilation or failed intubation. Limitations to supraglottic airway devices, however, include a relative lack of protection from aspiration, as well as a limited ability to provide adequate positive-pressure ventilation in patients prone to airway obstruction (eg, morbidly obese, sleep apnea). The key elements of an airway examination are an assessment of obesity, mouth opening, neck flexion and extension, Mallampati oropharyngeal classification, presence of beard, and mandibular protrusion ability (**Table 11.8**). The presence of abnormalities in three or more of the aforementioned elements increases the likelihood of a difficult mask ventilation and/or difficult intubation by more than eightfold.[5] Assessment of oropharyngeal classification is performed by having patients open their mouth and maximally protrude the tongue without phonation. This Mallampati oropharyngeal assessment can be classified depending on whether the uvula can be completely seen (class 1), only partly seen (class 2), or not seen, with the hard and soft palate visible (class 3), or only the hard palate visible (class 4) (**Fig. 11.1**).[6]

Table 11.7. Sedation Scale

Sedation Scale	Description
0	Awake and alert
1	Minimally sedated: tired/sleepy, appropriate response to verbal conversation and/or sound
2	Moderately sedated: somnolent/sleeping, easily aroused with light tactile stimulation or a simple verbal command
3	Deeply sedated: deep sleep, arousable only with significant repeated physical stimulation
4	Unarousable

Table 11.8. Standard Airway Examination for Nonanesthesiologists

Exam Element	Concerning Findings
Body mass index (kg/m^2)	Body mass index ≥31
Mouth opening	Interincisor or intergingival distance <3 cm
Mallampati classification	Class III or IV (see **Fig. 11.1**)
Mandibular protrusion	Inability to protrude lower incisors to meet or extend past upper incisors
Neck anatomy	Radiation changes, or thick obese neck
Cervical spine mobility	Limited extension or possibly unstable cervical spine
Beard	Presence of full beard

SCIENTIFIC PRINCIPLES

RISKS ASSOCIATED WITH ANESTHESIA

With the advent of newer agents and monitoring techniques, it is estimated that the mortality rate directly attributable to anesthesia has decreased from about 1 in 10,000 patients in the 1950s to as low as 1 in 200,000 or less for healthy patients today.[7] When patients are placed in a condition in which they cannot breathe, there is always the possibility of a technical or judgmental error resulting in hypoxia and brain damage or death. It has been estimated that between 50% and 75% of anesthetic-caused deaths are due to human error and are preventable.

Efforts to improve outcome can be approached at three levels: (a) reduction of the incidence of rare but catastrophic anesthetic-related problems, (b) improvement of the care and experience of every patient undergoing anesthesia and surgery, and (c) improvement of the preparation and management of patients with preexisting medical conditions that have higher morbidity and mortality rates. Historically, the most common problems associated with adverse outcomes were related to the airway and included inadequate ventilation, unrecognized esophageal intubation, unrecognized extubation, and unrecognized disconnection from the ventilator. The incidence of these problems has been significantly reduced by including capnometry and pulse oximetry in addition to other noninvasive monitors, although a cause-and-effect relation has been difficult to prove. Standardized anesthesia machine checklists, anesthesiology training, pain management programs, and improved understanding of preexisting comorbidities have also had positive impact.

Cardiovascular Diseases

Hypertension

Hypertension is the most common preexisting medical disease in patients presenting for surgery and is a major risk factor for renal, cerebrovascular, peripheral vascular, and coronary artery diseases, as well as congestive heart failure (CHF). It is particularly associated with lipid disorders, diabetes, and obesity. It is these associated comorbidities that are most likely to lead to morbidity and mortality in the perioperative period. Hypertensive patients should be treated medically to render them normotensive before elective surgery. In general, antihypertension medications should be continued throughout the perioperative period. However, patients treated with angiotensin receptor blockers (ARBs), such as valsartan, candesartan, losartan, or angiotensin-converting enzyme inhibitors (ACE-Is), such as lisinopril, captopril, or ramipril, who are exposed to general anesthesia, are at risk for developing profound, refractory intraoperative hypotension requiring terlipressin, vasopressin, or methylene blue treatment.[8–10] Many medical centers recommend withholding ACE-Is/ARBs the morning of surgery. Recent multicenter trials evaluating strategies of withholding versus continuing ACE-Is/ARBs on the day of surgery have confirmed a higher risk of clinically significant intraoperative hypotension, but no clear impact on short- and long-term end-organ injury (eg, acute kidney injury, myocardial ischemia).

The incidence of hypotension and myocardial ischemia intraoperatively is higher in untreated hypertensive patients than in adequately treated hypertensive patients if the preoperative diastolic pressure is 110 mm Hg or higher.[11] Inadequately treated hypertensive patients undergoing carotid endarterectomies have an increased incidence of neurologic deficits, and those with a history of prior myocardial infarctions have an increased incidence of reinfarction. Hypertensive patients can have exaggerated responses to painful stimuli and have a higher incidence of perioperative ischemia.

Coronary Artery Disease

Coronary artery disease or its risk factors are present in about 30% of patients who undergo major surgery. It is the leading cause of death in the United States and continues to be a major cause of postoperative morbidity and mortality.[12] The goal of the preoperative cardiac evaluation is to identify patients who are at increased risk of perioperative cardiac morbidity and ensure that their chronic conditions are optimized. Although perioperative cardiac events are the leading cause of death following anesthesia and surgery, it has been difficult to define patient characteristics that accurately predict a high risk of adverse outcome.[13] It has been even more difficult to modify that risk effectively.[14] Preoperative CHF is clearly a significant risk factor, as is recent myocardial infarction or unstable angina (**Table 11.9**). Diabetes mellitus (DM), atherosclerotic vascular disease, and hypertension also appear to confer risk, although less than with CHF or unstable angina. Perioperative risk in patients with valvular heart disease varies with the severity of the disease as represented by CHF, pulmonary hypertension, and dysrhythmias. Dysrhythmias are also a concern in the presence of coronary artery disease. The value of revascularization remains controversial as well. The ability to climb two flights of stairs without stopping or experiencing symptoms of angina or shortness of breath is considered a good practical test of cardiac reserve. Unfortunately, many patients with ischemic heart disease have concomitant pulmonary or musculoskeletal diseases that limit their activity. A history of myocardial infarction is important information. Large retrospective studies have found that the incidence of reinfarction is related to the time elapsed since the previous myocardial infarction.[15] The incidence of reinfarction appears to stabilize at about 6% (50-fold higher than patients without myocardial infarction) after 6 months. The highest rate of reinfarction occurs in the 0- to 3-month period. Mortality from reinfarction, for patients undergoing noncardiac surgery (**Table 11.10**), has been reported to be between 20% and 50% and usually occurs within the first 48 hours after surgery.

Table 11.9. Clinical Predictors of Increased Perioperative Cardiovascular Risk (Myocardial Infarction, Heart Failure, Death)

Major
Unstable coronary syndromes
Acute or recent MI[a] with evidence of important ischemic risk by clinical symptoms or noninvasive study
Unstable or severe[b] angina (Canadian class III or IV)[c]
Decompensated heart failure
Significant arrhythmias
High-grade atrioventricular block
Symptomatic ventricular arrhythmias in the presence of underlying heart disease
Supraventricular arrhythmias with uncontrolled ventricular rate
Severe valvular disease
Intermediate
Mild angina pectoris (Canadian class I or II)
Previous MI by history or pathologic Q waves
Compensated or prior heart failure
Diabetes mellitus (particularly insulin dependent)
Renal insufficiency
Minor
Advanced age
Abnormal ECG (left ventricular hypertrophy, left bundle-branch block, ST–T abnormalities)
Rhythm other than sinus (eg, atrial fibrillation)
Low functional capacity (eg, inability to climb one flight of stairs with a bag of groceries)
History of stroke
Uncontrolled systemic hypertension

[a]The American College of Cardiology National Database Library defines recent MI as >7 d but ≤1 mo (30 d); acute MI is within 7 d.
[b]May include "stable" angina in patients who are unusually sedentary.
[c]From Campeau L. Grading of angina pectoris. *Circulation.* 1976;54:522.
ECG, electrocardiogram; MI, myocardial infarction.

Table 11.10. Cardiac Risk Stratification for Noncardiac Surgical Procedures

High (reported cardiac risk often >5%)[a]
Emergent major operations, particularly in the elderly
Aortic and other major vascular surgery
Peripheral vascular surgery
Anticipated prolonged surgical procedures associated with large fluid shifts and/or blood loss
Intermediate (reported cardiac risk generally <5%)
Carotid endarterectomy
Head and neck surgery
Intraperitoneal and intrathoracic surgery
Orthopedic surgery
Prostate surgery
Low[b] (reported cardiac risk generally <1%)
Endoscopic procedures
Superficial procedures
Cataract surgery
Breast surgery

[a]Combined incidence of cardiac death and nonfatal myocardial infarction.
[b]Do not generally require further preoperative cardiac testing.

Perioperative cardiac adverse event risk reduction has undergone significant changes over the past decade. Despite[4]
8 these efforts, a large, international prospective study across 15,000 patients demonstrated that more than 8% of patients undergoing major inpatient surgery still experience postoperative myocardial ischemia.[16] These patients have significantly increased 30-day mortality, even though only 15% of perioperative ischemic episodes included typical cardiac symptoms. Previous retrospective studies demonstrating value of coronary revascularization spurred aggressive preoperative coronary artery disease identification and management. However, recent data have questioned the value of coronary revascularization among asymptomatic patients in not only the perioperative period but also in the general medical population.[17] Furthermore, large retrospective and prospective studies have demonstrated that perioperative beta blockade also bears significant risks that must be weighed against possible benefits.[18] As a result, the most recent ACC/AHA guidelines reserve the commencement of beta-blocker therapy for only high-risk patients that would warrant blockade independent of the surgical procedure and with sufficient time to titrate the medication dosing and assess tolerability.[17] Patients already on beta-blocker therapy should continue throughout the perioperative period.[17] Although prospective data establishing the value of instituting preoperative statin therapy are limited, there is general consensus that these medications should not be withdrawn.[19] A large randomized controlled trial evaluating the benefit of other promising agents—clonidine and aspirin—as perioperative optimization standards failed to demonstrate benefit.[20]

All patients in high-risk groups or with a history of ischemic heart disease must be evaluated and properly treated before elective surgery. All elective surgery should be delayed for 6 months after myocardial infarction. If this is not feasible, invasive monitoring should be considered in the perioperative period and intensive postoperative observation should continue for at least 48 hours. The intrusiveness of the surgical procedure also plays a part in the overall risk and need for preoperative workup of heart disease.[17]

Percutaneous Coronary Intervention with Stenting

An increasing number of patients present for surgery following percutaneous coronary interventions via stenting (with or without drug-eluting coating). In-stent thrombosis is a feared complication with profound morbidity and mortality. Given the known proinflammatory and prothrombotic physiologic state induced by acute illness, surgery, and anesthesia, coronary stents may be at elevated risk for thrombosis during the perioperative period. The risk of perioperative in-stent thrombosis is increased if noncardiac surgery is performed soon after percutaneous coronary intervention.[21,22] The appropriate duration to defer elective surgery after coronary stenting remains controversial, but recent ACC/AHA guidelines recommend 6 ("reasonable") to 12 ("ideal") months for drug-eluting stents and 30 days for bare-metal stents.[17] Data suggest that cessation of recommended antiplatelet therapy in the perioperative period may have significant coronary thrombotic risks without major reduction in bleeding.[21,22] The decision to stop antiplatelet therapy prior to recommended guidelines should be limited to specific procedures that demand a nearly bloodless surgical field or in procedures involving closed spaces incapable of tolerating minor bleeding (intracranial, minimally invasive spine surgery). The continuation of aspirin therapy throughout the perioperative period in patients with coronary artery stents should be the standard of care.[17]

Congestive Heart Failure

CHF has been described as the single most important factor predicting postoperative cardiac morbidity[23]; patients are less tolerant of the fluid shifts associated with surgery and the myocardial depression associated with the anesthetic. All elective procedures should be deferred until heart failure is medically optimized. If surgery cannot be deferred, aggressive management to enhance cardiac output is warranted. In contrast to isolated ischemic heart disease, CHF is more easily diagnosed by history, physical examination, and basic preoperative laboratory workup, electrocardiography (ECG), chest radiography, and echocardiography.

Pulmonary Disease

Recent data demonstrate that although cardiac complications have been the focus of surveillance and prevention, pulmonary and infectious complications may warrant similar attention. Pulmonary disease is classically divided into acute and chronic restrictive and obstructive disease. Restrictive disease is defined by processes that reduce lung volumes; obstructive disease is characterized by reduced flow rates. Obstructive diseases are present in patients with forced expiratory volume in 1 second (FEV_1)/forced vital capacity (FVC) ratios of less than 50%. Obstructive pulmonary disease can be either chronic or acute. Any reversible component of obstruction should be reversed before surgery. Patients should be maintained on bronchodilator and biologic medications. Reactive bronchospasm can complicate anesthetic induction and the emergence; severe bronchospasm is potentially life threatening. Administration of potent local (albuterol) and systemic (epinephrine) bronchodilators in a timely fashion is essential.

Regional or neuraxial techniques that allow airway manipulation to be avoided have particular advantage. However, for sensory and motor levels of T6 and above, patients lose significant accessory motor function that can decrease expiratory reserve volume and the ability to cough and clear secretions. Any intubated patient with severe respiratory disease should be extubated with caution only when they meet adequate extubation criteria relative to preoperative test data. Patients undergoing upper abdominal surgery are at particular risk. Because of the potential adverse effects of systemic narcotics on respiratory drive, the use of epidural narcotics and local anesthetics for postoperative pain control is very popular.

Cerebrovascular Disease

Following stroke there is local inflammation, cerebral autoregulation is impaired, and for a time, the brain is more susceptible to the inflammatory consequences of surgery and exquisitely sensitive to perturbations in blood pressure, cerebral blood flow, hemorrhage, and anemia. The risk of perioperative stroke and death is significantly increased if surgery is conducted during this phase and delaying elective surgery is therefore a critical strategy for the prevention of stroke. The American Heart Association and American Stroke Association released a consensus guideline in 2021 indicating that individuals should wait at least 6 months and possibly as long as 9 months after stroke to reduce the risk of recurrent stroke in the perioperative period.[24] These recommendations were based largely on data from a Danish Nationwide Registry including patients aged 20 years and older undergoing noncardiac surgery. The investigative team reported a 68-fold increase in perioperative stroke if surgery was performed less than 3 months following a stroke. The risk decreased markedly as the time interval between stroke and surgery increased and stabilized at approximately 9 months.[25]

Obesity

Obesity is defined as a body mass index (BMI) greater than or equal to 30 kg/m². The pathophysiologic changes associated with morbid obesity (BMI ≥40 kg/m²) affect the respiratory, cardiovascular, and gastrointestinal systems. Patients develop external restrictive lung disease that reduces functional residual capacity and is exacerbated by supine positioning. Increased airway pressures required to maintain adequate ventilation in obese patients predispose this patient group to barotrauma, furthering their risk of pulmonary complications. Obese patients frequently desaturate at night and have a high incidence of sleep apnea. Because of increased blood volume and frequent desaturations, obese patients can develop pulmonary hypertension and right-sided heart failure. Obese individuals have a high incidence of coronary artery disease. Because of size alone, they have increased cardiovascular demands with limited cardiac reserve and exercise tolerance. Obese patients have a high incidence of hiatal hernia and gastroesophageal reflux, increasing the risk for aspiration on induction and emergence from anesthesia. Venous access, positioning, and blood pressure measurement are often difficult.

The combined problems of aspiration risk, rapid desaturation caused by reduced functional residual capacity and increased oxygen demand, and technical difficulties associated with intubation due to anatomic fat deposits make intubation a high-risk procedure. Awake intubation can be useful or necessitated. Epidural analgesics for postoperative pain management may enable improved recovery for these patients.

Diabetes Mellitus

The incidence of DM is rising, particularly, type 2 DM. This systemic disorder affects the vascular, renal, nervous, and immune systems. Patients with DM should be evaluated for the presence of concomitant coronary artery disease, peripheral vascular occlusive disease, renal failure, and autonomic and peripheral neuropathy. Problems with cardiovascular instability, fluid balance, and aspiration due to gastroparesis should be expected. In addition, these patients are more prone to infection and have problems with temperature control. Hypoglycemia during anesthesia is a feared complication because of challenges in prompt diagnosis. Although there are compelling data associating perioperative hyperglycemia with adverse postoperative events, there are no randomized controlled trials demonstrating improved outcomes in noncardiac surgery with aggressive intraoperative hyperglycemia management.[26] Furthermore, complications from hypoglycemia are arguably greater than those from hyperglycemia and are more likely as insulin therapy becomes more aggressive during the perioperative period. As a result, modern intraoperative glucose control protocols with insulin infusions include frequent (every 60 minutes) glucose checks.

Renal Insufficiency and Failure

Because the kidneys play a vital role in metabolic, synthetic, and fluid homeostasis, renal failure is associated with many effects on the cardiovascular, pulmonary, hematologic, gastrointestinal, and immune systems. Preexisting renal insufficiency is a known risk factor for postoperative myocardial infarction and renal failure.[27] Optimizing fluid and metabolic status of a patient with end-stage renal disease is of vital importance. Elective surgery should be delayed until such optimization is performed.[28] In emergent situations, hemodialysis should be considered to avoid life-threatening electrolyte and fluid derangements. Nearly 15% of patients undergoing general surgery procedures experience postoperative acute kidney injury, as defined by a 0.3 mg/dL increase in serum creatinine within 7 postoperative days. Risk factors for postoperative acute kidney injury in patients undergoing general surgery are listed in **Table 11.11** and should be considered during the patient consent.

Table 11.11. Predictors of Postoperative Acute Kidney Injury after General Surgery Procedures

Age ≥56 y
Male sex
Emergency surgery
Intraperitoneal procedures
Preoperative renal insufficiency (serum creatinine >1.2 mg/dL)
Ascites
Active congestive heart failure
Diabetes mellitus requiring oral hypoglycemic or insulin therapy
Hypertension requiring chronic medication

From Kheterpal S, Tremper K, Heung M, et al. Development and validation of an acute kidney injury risk index for patients undergoing general surgery. *Anesthesiology.* 2009;110:505–515.

Obstructive Sleep Apnea

With increasing obesity prevalence, obstructive sleep apnea (OSA) is emerging as a major comorbidity that has impact on postoperative outcomes and costs. The physiologic changes in the upper airway, lungs, pulmonary circulation, heart, and brain are extensive and challenge immediate perioperative and postoperative management. These patients are prone to airway collapse at induction and emergence, hypoxemia, delayed emergence, respiratory depression, and cardiovascular collapse. Data demonstrate increased sensitivity to the effects of opiates[29] and a relationship between OSA treatment and a reduction in postoperative complications.[30] The standard protocol for all preoperative evaluations should be the use of a locally accepted OSA screening tool (STOP-BANG questionnaire, Perioperative Sleep Apnea Prediction Score) and ensuring postoperative access to continuous positive airway pressure therapy for patients currently prescribed such therapy as outpatients. Some undiagnosed or noncompliant patients may require initiation of therapy in the immediate postoperative period and the perioperative resources to fulfill clinical urgency are essential.

Risks Associated with Regional Techniques in Patients Being Treated with Anticoagulants

As the indications for anticoagulant therapy have increased, ranging from drug-eluting stents to atrial fibrillation and venous thromboembolism prophylaxis, the number of patients and types of anticoagulant therapy has continued to increase. In particular, low–molecular-weight heparin (LMWH) and oral direct factor Xa inhibitors are often part of a patient's pre- or postoperative therapy plan. The use of neuraxial or PNB in patients with preoperative anticoagulation requires careful planning and assessment of the risks and benefits of specific anesthetic techniques and withdrawal of anticoagulant therapy. LMWH raises specific concerns about epidural hematoma formation when neuraxial techniques are used. The American Society of Regional Anesthesia has published specific guidelines for central conduction block (spinal and epidural anesthesia) to try to minimize the incidence of this devastating complication.[31] In general, LMWH therapy requires coordination of neuraxial administration at least 12 hours after the last dose. Coumadin, clopidogrel, and ticlopidine should be held for at least 5, 7, and 10 days prior to neuraxial techniques, respectively. The absence of any reversal agents or reliable diagnostic testing for oral direct Xa inhibitors requires a conservative approach to withdrawal of therapy and limited data guide withholding these medications for at least 72 hours prior to neuraxial techniques.[31] Data regarding risks for PNB are even more scarce and local protocols should be established and followed.

PREOPERATIVE EVALUATION

9 The three goals of the preoperative evaluation are (a) to develop an anesthetic plan that considers the patient's medical condition, the requirements of the surgical procedure, and the patient's preferences; (b) to ensure that any chronic disease is under appropriate control; and (c) to establish rapport, answer questions and allay fears.

Optimization of a patient's medical conditions is best performed by the primary care physician, with medical specialty consultation, if necessary. The following questions must be answered when evaluating a patient undergoing an elective surgical procedure: What must be included in the preoperative evaluation? Who should be involved in this process? When and where are all the steps in this process to be conducted? How should all the information be coordinated so that it is available to the appropriate personnel at the appropriate time? If the procedure is deemed a surgical emergency, the anesthesiologist is responsible for assessing the patient quickly, developing the appropriate anesthetic plan, and proceeding to the operating room as soon as possible. During such scenario, the anesthesiologist is not obligated to seek medical consultation to evaluate chronic medical problems.

The following steps must be completed before moving the patient into the operating room:

1. A comorbidity-focused history and physical examination
2. Appropriate laboratory studies and medical consultations
3. An anesthesiologist's preoperative evaluation with assignment of an American Society of Anesthesiologists (ASA) physical status (PS)
4. Discussion with the patient of the options and risks
5. Development and communication of the anesthetic plan to the patient and surgeon
6. Acute optimization of any pertinent medical conditions

The history and physical examination have repeatedly been shown to be the most valuable parts of the preoperative assessment. The anesthesiologist must review previous anesthetic problems experienced by the patient or blood relatives, the patient's exercise tolerance, and additional details regarding general medical conditions. This evaluation not only determines the laboratory tests that may be required but also allows for the assignment of ASA PS (**Table 11.12**). The classification serves as a general measure of the patient's state of well-being, considering all problems the patient brings to the operating room, including systemic disturbances caused by the surgical illness. Although studies of anesthetic mortality show a correlation with the PS classification, this categorization does not describe the risk directly. The risk of any operation is determined not only by patient-related factors but also by procedure-specific ones. For patients with complex medical problems, it is frequently helpful to supplement the surgical history and physical examination with a recent assessment by the patient's primary physician in order to assess the patient's long-term health trajectory. There are no data demonstrating the value of routine preoperative medical consultation.

Table 11.12. Physical Status Classification of the American Society of Anesthesiologists

Physical Status Classification	Description
PS-1	A normal, healthy patient
PS-2	A patient with mild systemic disease that results in no functional limitation *Examples:* Hypertension, diabetes mellitus, chronic bronchitis, morbid obesity, extremes of age
PS-3	A patient with severe systemic disease that results in functional limitation *Examples:* Poorly controlled hypertension, diabetes mellitus with vascular complications, angina pectoris, prior myocardial infarction, pulmonary disease that limits activity
PS-4	A patient with severe systemic disease that is a constant threat to life *Examples:* Congestive heart failure, unstable angina pectoris, advanced pulmonary, renal, or hepatic dysfunction
PS-5	A moribund patient who is not expected to survive without the operation *Examples:* Ruptured abdominal aneurysm, pulmonary embolus, head injury with increased intracranial pressure
PS-6	A declared brain-dead patient whose organs are being removed for donor purposes
Emergency operation (E)	Any patient in whom an emergency operation is required *Example:* An otherwise healthy 30-year-old woman who requires dilation and curettage for moderate but persistent vaginal bleeding (PS-1E)

The value of preoperative laboratory studies has undergone substantial reevaluation since the mid-1980s. The current thinking is that a laboratory test should not be ordered unless a change in the surgical or anesthetic plan is anticipated. For procedures with significant anticipated blood loss, a type and cross match is ordered, and a preoperative hematocrit is also required. An ECG can be justified for men older than 50 years of age and women older than 60 years of age recorded within 1 year of planned surgery. All other tests should have an indication based on history and physical examination. A simple strategy to evaluate physical robustness is presented in **Table 11.13**. Electronic patient questionnaires have also been developed, allowing the appropriate laboratories to be selected based on the patient's response to questions.

Outpatient Medication Regimen Management

The patient's medication regimen must be reviewed to ensure that appropriate medications are continued or discontinued in the days and hours leading up to an elective procedure. A variety of outpatient medication classes require careful management in the perioperative period, including but not limited to (a) anticoagulants and antiplatelets; (b) cardiovascular medications (beta blockade, antihypertensives, antiarrhythmics, pulmonary hypertension therapy); (c) chronic pain and

Table 11.13. Simplified Strategy for Preoperative Testing

Estimated Energy Requirements for Various Activities

1 MET ↓ 4 METs	Can you take care of yourself? Eat, dress, or use the toilet? Walk indoors around the house? Walk a block or two on level ground at 2 to 3 mph or 3.2 to 4.8 km/h? Do light work around the house like dusting or washing dishes?	4 METs ↓>10 METs	Climb a flight of stairs or walk up a hill? Walk on level ground at 4 mph or 6.4 km/h? Run a short distance? Do heavy work around the house like scrubbing floors or lifting or moving heavy furniture? Participate in moderate recreational activities like golf, bowling, dancing, doubles tennis, or throwing a baseball or football? Participate in strenuous sports like swimming, singles tennis, football, basketball, or skiing?

MET, metabolic equivalent; mph, miles per hour.

opioid use disorder medications (opioids, buprenorphine); (d) glycemic agents (insulin, oral hypoglycemics, and SGLT-2 inhibitors); (e) obesity medications (GLP-1 agonists); and (f) pulmonary medications (novel biologics, inhaled steroids and beta agonists). Failure to adhere to relevant guidelines can increase clinical risk and delay time-sensitive procedures. 10 Guidelines continue to evolve.

Several important classes of medications should be continued as per the patient's normal regimen: aspirin for patients with coronary stents, chronic pain therapy (including opioids), opioid use disorder therapy, beta blockers, statins, and proton pump inhibitors. The decision regarding anticoagulant therapy is complex and must consider the indication for therapy, the likelihood and impact of surgical bleeding, and the risk of perioperative thrombosis. Insulin and oral hypoglycemic agents should be continued at a reduced dose.

Patients receiving chronic pain or opioid use disorder therapy with high doses (ie, more than 16 mg daily dosing) of buprenorphine (Subutex, Suboxone) can be challenging to manage in the postoperative period. Buprenorphine, a mixed opioid agonist/antagonist, tightly binds at the μ receptor and has a long and varied half-life (24 to 60 hours). Although prospective clinical trials are lacking, general consensus exists that continuation of buprenorphine therapy at low and moderate doses (≤16 mg daily dose) is safe, effective, and allows use of supplemental opioid therapy for perioperative acute pain management.[32] Patients undergoing scheduled elective surgery with high daily buprenorphine dosing may require tailored buprenorphine and acute pain therapies. A management protocol used at the University of Michigan is demonstrated in **Algorithm 11.1**.

The increasing prevalence of obesity, DM, renal disease, heart failure, and metabolic syndrome has resulted in many patients presenting for surgery with ongoing treatment with sodium-glucose cotransporter-2 inhibitors (SGLT-2), glucagon-like peptide-1 agonists (GLP-1), and gastric inhibitory polypeptide (GIP) agonists. SGLT-2 inhibitors (eg, canagliflozin, dapagliflozin, and empagliflozin) can cause difficulty to diagnose life-threatening euglycemic diabetic ketoacidosis in the perioperative period due to concomitant fasting and stress. Many protocols recommend discontinuing these agents at least 72 to 96 hours prior to scheduled surgery. GLP-1 agonists such as semaglutide (trade name Ozempic and Wegovy) and tirzepatide (trade name Mounjaro and Zepbound) delay gastric emptying and may increase the risk of regurgitation and pulmonary aspiration when traditional perioperative fasting guidelines are implemented. Data are rapidly evolving regarding

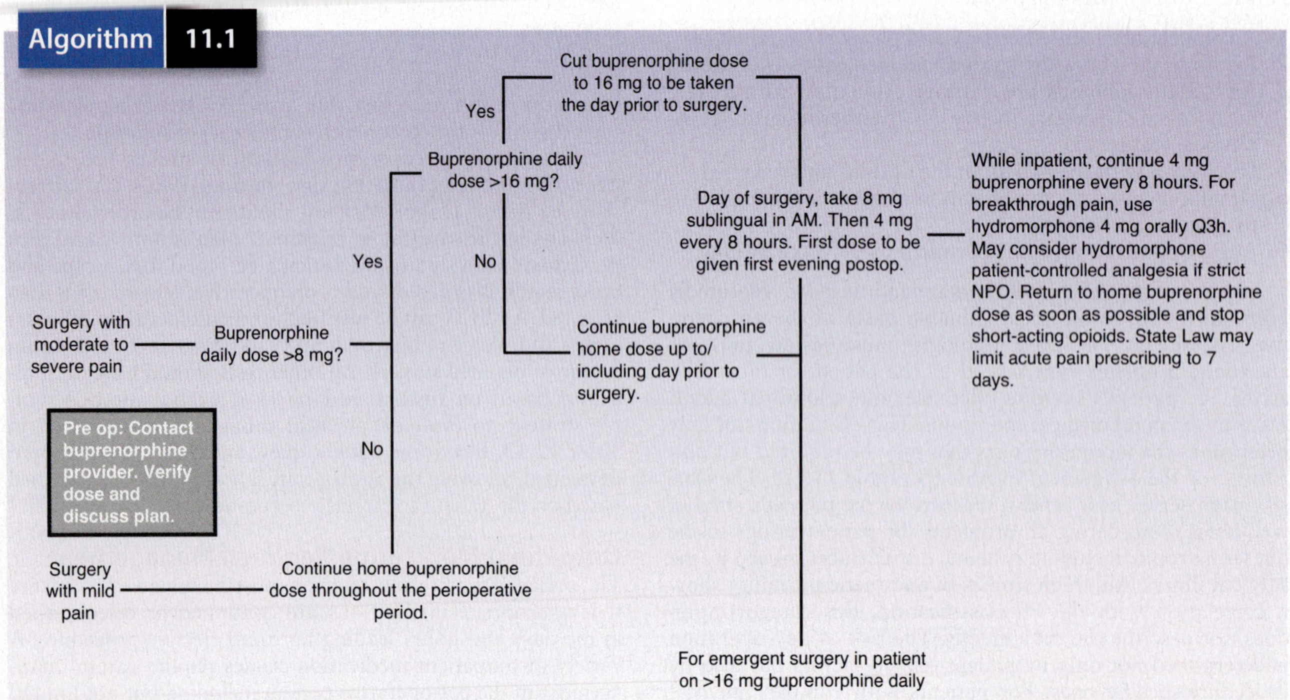

Algorithm 11.1. Algorithm for managing a patient on chronic buprenorphine therapy. APS, acute pain service; ICU, intensive care unit; PCA, patient-controlled anesthesia; NSAIDs, nonsteroidal anti-inflammatory drugs.

the optimal handling of these medications, but many centers currently incorporate one of several consensus guideline recommendations) discontinuing the medication for 7 to 14 days, altered fasting guidelines (eg, liquid diet for 24 hours), delaying elective surgery if in the dose escalation phase or symptomatic with nausea or vomited or medication continuation if the underlying conditions warrant it.

Airway Assessment

The potential of a difficult intubation is of fundamental concern and should be evaluated as previously discussed (**Fig. 11.1** and **Table 11.8**). While videolaryngoscopy has revolutionized the management of the difficult and routine airway,[33] awake fiberoptic intubation remains a crucial skill in patients with difficult mask ventilation, difficult laryngoscopy, and reduced oxygen reserves. The requirement of an awake fiberoptic technique takes planning and can cause delay without prior warning. A variety of advanced airway management techniques such as rigid videolaryngoscopy, flexible fiberoptic laryngoscopy, transnasal humidified rapid-insufflation ventilatory exchange (THRIVE) have replaced historical devices. Despite these advances, the risk of failed intubation or mask ventilation with hypoxemia and death or anoxic brain injury remains an important complication that affects modern surgical patients every day.

MONITORING THE SURGICAL PATIENT

The routine use of an array of electronic monitors to provide continuous surveillance of physiologic status is well established. Because the art and science of anesthesiology involves titrating pharmacologic agents to produce desired physiologic effects, there must be a measured parameter to which drug dosages are titrated. Depending on the severity of preexisting disease and the extent of the surgical procedure, invasive techniques can be used to provide comprehensive continuous data to guide the titration of fluid therapy and cardiovascular agents.

Monitors of Oxygenation

Pulse oximetry continuously, noninvasively, and inexpensively provides arterial hemoglobin saturation (SaO_2) and peripheral pulse by measuring light absorption in a manner similar to that of a laboratory cooximeter. Each hemoglobin species absorbs light in direct proportion to its concentration (Beer–Lambert law). The traditional pulse oximeter uses two wavelengths of light, one red and one infrared that shine through a tissue bed, usually a finger. Oxyhemoglobin absorbs light maximally in the infrared band and deoxyhemoglobin in the red band. Opposite the light sources is a photodiode that measures the transmitted light intensity. The device analyzes only the pulsatile component of absorption and assumes that anything that pulses within the tissue bed is arterial blood, hence the name *pulse oximeter*. The ratio of the pulsatile component of red light absorbed to the pulsatile component of the infrared light absorbed is measured and this ratio changes with SaO_2. The exact relation between this ratio and SaO_2 has been empirically determined from volunteer studies and is programmed into the electronics of the oximeter. If any artifacts occur in a pulsatile nature, they may be erroneously integrated into the equation, causing erroneous SaO_2 estimates.

Several things should be remembered when interpreting a pulse oximeter's output: (1) The device measures SaO_2 and not arterial oxygen tension (PaO_2); (2) The PaO_2 must drop below 80 mm Hg before any significant change in SaO_2 occurs; (3) As the PaO_2 drops below 60 mm Hg, the SaO_2 rapidly falls as the inflection point of the sigmoidal oxyhemoglobin dissociation curve is approached; and (4) The pulse oximeter measures saturation and not arterial content or oxygen delivery to tissues.

Pulse oximeters are generally not capable of detecting carboxyhemoglobin or methemoglobin unless they incorporate additional wavelengths of light. Such devices are not widely used clinically.

Ventilation Monitors

Capnography, or end-tidal CO_2 monitoring, is the visual display of the CO_2 concentration in the airway. To understand the utility of capnography, one must understand dead-space (DS) components and how they affect CO_2 removal from the body. DS is defined as the portion of the tidal volume (V_T) that does not participate in gas exchange.

$$V_T = DS + V_A$$

The alveolar volume (V_A) is the volume of the inspired gas that reaches well-perfused alveoli. The remainder of the V_T, which equals the DS, can be divided into three subcomponents: apparatus dead space (DS_{ap}), anatomic dead space (DS_{an}), and alveolar dead space (DS_{al}). At the end of inspiration, the respiratory apparatus (eg, endotracheal tube) is filled with inspired gas that should not contain CO_2. Similarly, all the anatomic airways (trachea, bronchi, and all conducting airways down to the alveoli) should be filled with inspired gas and should therefore contain no CO_2. In this model, there are two types of alveoli: those that are well perfused and those that are not perfused. The alveolar gas should completely equilibrate with the arterial blood and contain CO_2 at the same tension as the arterial blood; ideally, $PaCO_2$ should equal 40 mm Hg. As the patient expires, the CO_2 detected at the patient's mouth first reflects the DS_{ap} gas having no CO_2 followed by the DS_{an} gas, again with no CO_2, and finally the alveolar gases, containing both DS and well-perfused alveolar gas (ideally at 40 mm Hg). With inspiration, the CO_2 value again drops to 0 until another expiration, and a square wave appears again as the alveolar gas is detected at the mouth. With each breath, there should be a square wave, the height of which approaches the $PaCO_2$ value as the amount of the DS_{al} gas approaches 0.

The presence of a capnogram itself implies that there is metabolism (the production of CO_2), circulation (blood flow to the lungs), and ventilation (respiratory rate and an intact ventilator circuit). Providing this information on a breath-to-breath basis, the continuous capnogram is extremely useful in many critical situations and can be used as a surveillance monitor of both the respiratory circuit and the cardiovascular system. Any acute decrease in cardiac output will decrease blood flow to the lungs and increase the DS_{al}, causing an acute drop in end-tidal CO_2. The only acute catastrophic cardiopulmonary problem that will not be detected by the capnometer is arterial desaturation. Therefore, the combination of the capnometer and the pulse oximeter creates a dynamic beat-to-beat and breath-to-breath surveillance of metabolism, circulation, ventilation, and oxygenation.

Circulation Monitors

Hemodynamic stability can be monitored by a variety of methods, the most basic of which is systemic arterial blood pressure. Intermittent, noninvasive measurement of systemic blood pressure with an oscillometric blood pressure cuff is the standard in the operating room, and its accuracy equals that of clinical measurements by auscultation. Blood pressure cuffs can be cycled as quickly as once per minute, but when used for an extended duration, they should be cycled no more than once every 3 to 5 minutes. When tighter control or observation is required in patients with significant comorbidities or large swings in hemodynamics due to surgical circumstances, invasive arterial monitoring is recommended. Pressure measurements provided by invasive and noninvasive techniques, usually coincide closely. A continuous invasive arterial tracing can also be used to assess the adequacy of fluid resuscitation by following the systolic pressure variation (SPV) with positive-pressure ventilation. As positive-pressure ventilation impedes venous return within a closed thorax, decreases in systolic pressure associated with a respiratory pattern can be detected. In patients with sinus rhythm with stable cardiac contractility, the degree of SPV is inversely related to the intravascular volume status. The normal range of SPV is 5 to 10 mm Hg. A systolic pressure decrease of greater than 10 mm Hg during positive-pressure ventilation implies inadequate preload and the need for more aggressive fluid resuscitation.

In this context, central venous access may be reserved for patients and procedures with the potential for large, rapid-volume resuscitation requirements or expected need for potent vasoactive medication. Transesophageal echocardiography (TEE) is now commonly used to quickly assess systolic and diastolic function as well as valvular dysfunction. Increasing familiarity with the use of TEE by noncardiac anesthesiologists may result in the pulmonary artery catheter being reserved for very specific patients demonstrating the need for pulmonary artery pressure monitoring or frequent quantitative cardiac output trending.

Finally, a wave of noninvasive continuous cardiac output monitors has gained the attention of surgeons and anesthesiologists alike. These monitors, promising the realization of goal-directed therapy, use indirect means to assess the missing aspect of blood pressure–focused hemodynamic management—stroke volume. Thoracic electrical bioimpedance, pulse wave transit time, peripheral pulse contour analysis, volume clamp, and other methods of estimating stroke volume have been in existence for decades, but have seen a recent rise in interest as variation in intraoperative fluid management may impact surgical outcomes. However, conflicting studies in real-world critically ill patients have failed to establish an outcome benefit.[34] Despite the absence of compelling clinical data, many enhanced recovery protocols have begun including some type of noninvasive cardiac output monitoring to guide fluid therapy.[35]

Neuromuscular Blockade Monitors

The evaluation of depth of muscle relaxation is a subjective process based on empirical pharmacokinetics or visual inspection of a patient's peripheral nerve response to external electrical stimulation. During peripheral nerve stimulator monitoring, two electrode patches are placed on the patient's skin along the course of a peripheral nerve which innervates an observable muscle group. Commonly used monitoring locations include the ulnar nerve, ophthalmic branch of the facial nerve, or the posterior tibial nerve. Electrodes are connected to a hand-held device that delivers four short transcutaneous bursts of electricity, ranging from 10 to 100 mA every 0.5 seconds, hence the term "train-of-four monitoring." Due to competitive blocking of the neuromuscular junction nicotinic receptor, each successive stimulation results in a weaker response because sequentially fewer receptors are available for stimulation. The ratio between the strength of the fourth twitch and the first twitch is known as the train-of-four ratio. In a patient without any pharmacologic neuromuscular blockade (ie, normal neuromuscular transmission), the strength of the fourth muscle response (or "twitch") matches that of the first. Historically, a ratio of 0.7 was considered adequate muscular strength for extubation. However, more recent literature suggests that a ratio between 0.7 and 0.9 still exposes the patient to significant risks of atelectasis, hypoxemia, aspiration, pneumonia, and possibly reintubation.

In routine practice, a clinician visually inspects the response to each electrical stimulation and simply counts the number of twitches observed, and a subjective train-of-four count is typically reported (eg, 0/4, 1/4, 2/4, 3/4, 4/4). In the face of complete pharmacologic competitive inhibition of neuromuscular transmission, no muscular twitches are observed at all. At varying levels of neuromuscular blockade in between, the fourth, third, or second twitch may be absent. A patient with 3/4 or 4/4 twitches is capable of responding to cholinesterase inhibitors and returning to normal function. A patient with 0/4, 1/4, or 2/4 is unlikely to adequately respond to cholinesterase inhibitors and may require the administration of a high dose of a selective relaxant binding agent (eg, sugammadex).

The use of subjective train-of-four monitors is inferior to quantitative acceleromyography, a calibrated device used to accurately establish the "true" train-of-four ratio. Although clinically effective at eliminating the limitations of subjective train-of-four monitoring, its use remains limited because of the time necessary for set up, and an underappreciation of the frequency of residual neuromuscular blockade.

Processed EEG Monitors

When delivering a general anesthetic, one of the major imperatives is to achieve and maintain a loss of consciousness and prevention of intraoperative recall. Historically, this was achieved through careful observation of hemodynamic vital signs (heart rate, blood pressure), physical examination signs (movement in a patient without neuromuscular blockade), and delivery of inhalational or intravenous agents at doses consistent with a loss of consciousness. However, this indirect approach to assessing the neurologic impact of sedative/hypnotic agents has many limitations. As a result, patients may rarely experience "unintended intraoperative awareness under anesthesia"—a state characterized not only by consciousness but also by recall of intraoperative events. The lay press and public have increased their scrutiny of this perioperative event.

First, appropriate expectations and effective communication of the anesthetic are required. Literature has demonstrated that patients undergoing regional anesthesia are as likely to report unpleasant "awareness" as patients undergoing a general anesthetic.[36] This is despite the reality that loss of consciousness is only a goal of general anesthesia.

Second, several intraoperative processed EEG monitors have been developed in hopes of providing the anesthesiologist with additional objective data to guide their assessment and actions. The current generation of monitors generally uses real-time automated EEG analysis of gelled single-use electrodes placed on a patient's forehead. These monitors typically provide a raw EEG waveform display, a proprietary calculated "index" purporting to reflect "depth" of anesthesia, and several physiologic parameters related to EEG analysis such as suppression ratio (the percentage of the time the EEG reflex burst suppression), and EEG frequency measures. Data evaluating the value of these EEG-based monitors in improving any outcomes (eg, intraoperative awareness, postoperative delirium, morbidity/mortality, or quality of recovery) are conflicting. As a result, the ASA has not adopted awareness monitors as a standard of care and leaves the decision to use such monitoring technology for each provider, patient, and situation.[37] The largest, trials have failed to demonstrate a measurable reduction in awareness.[38]

COMMON PROBLEMS IN THE POSTOPERATIVE PERIOD

Postanesthesia care units (PACUs) are required in any setting where surgical procedures are conducted. The increased scope of surgery and the invasive technology used to monitor sicker patients have increased the service and training required to operate these facilities. In 2024, the ASA revised the Standards for Postanesthesia Care (**Table 11.14**).

The scoring systems used to assess the postoperative patient direct attention to the primary areas of concern. The postanesthesia recovery score is an attempt to evaluate postanesthesia patient status (**Table 11.15**).[39] This basic information should be incorporated in a record that provides clear documentation of postoperative events. Documentation should also include details of postoperative outpatient care, with a note indicating postoperative telephone contact made to elucidate problems. Problems should receive appropriate follow-up, and written postoperative discharge instructions should be provided for the patient.

Table 11.14. Standards for Postanesthesia Care

Standards		Criteria to Be Fulfilled
Standard I[a]	All patients who have received general, regional, or monitored anesthesia care shall receive appropriate postanesthesia management.	1. A PACU or an area that provides equivalent postanesthesia care shall be available to receive patients after anesthesia care. All patients who receive anesthesia care shall be admitted to the PACU or its equivalent *except* by specific order of the anesthesiologist responsible for the patient's care. 2. The medical aspects of care in the PACU shall be governed by policies and procedures that have been reviewed and approved by the department of anesthesiology. 3. The design, equipment, and staffing of the PACU shall meet requirements of the facility's accrediting and licensing bodies.
Standard II	A patient transported to the PACU shall be accompanied by a member of the anesthesia care team who is knowledgeable about the patient's condition. The patient shall be continually evaluated and treated during transport with monitoring and support appropriate to the patient's condition.	
Standard III	On arrival in the PACU, the patient shall be reevaluated and a verbal report provided to the responsible nurse by the member of the anesthesia care team who accompanies the patient.	1. The patient's status on arrival in the PACU shall be documented. 2. Information concerning the preoperative condition and the surgical/anesthetic course shall be transmitted to the receiving nurse. 3. The member of the anesthesia care team shall remain with the patient until the receiving nurse accepts responsibility for the nursing care of the patient.
Standard IV	The patient's condition shall be evaluated continually in the PACU.	1. The patient shall be observed and monitored by the methods appropriate to the patient's medical condition. Particular attention shall be given to monitoring oxygenation, ventilation, circulation, and temperature. During recovery from all anesthetics, a quantitative method of assessing oxygenation such as pulse oximetry shall be employed in the initial phase of recovery. This is not intended for application during the recovery of the obstetric patient in whom regional anesthesia was used for labor and vaginal delivery. 2. An accurate written report of the recovery period shall be maintained. Use of an appropriate scoring system is encouraged to assist with management and discharge readiness. 3. General medical supervision and coordination of patient care in the PACU should be the responsibility of an anesthesiologist. 4. There shall be a policy to ensure the availability in the facility of a physician capable of managing complications and providing cardiopulmonary resuscitation for patients in the PACU.
Standard V	A physician is responsible for discharging the patient from the PACU.	1. When discharge criteria are used, they must be approved by the department of anesthesiology and the medical staff. They may vary depending on whether the patient is discharged to a hospital room, to the ICU, to a short-stay unit, or home. 2. In the absence of the physician responsible for the discharge, the PACU nurse shall determine that the patient meets the discharge criteria. The name of the physician accepting responsibility for discharge shall be noted on the record.

[a]For nursing care issues, refer to Standards of Postanesthesia Nursing Practice, published by the American Society of Postanesthesia Nurses.
ICU, intensive care unit; PACU, postanesthesia care unit.
Based on American Society of Anesthesiologists (ASA)'s *Standards for Postanesthesia Care*. A copy of the full text can be obtained from ASA, 1061 American Lane, Schaumburg, IL 60173. https://www.asahq.org/standards-and-practice-parameters/standards-for-postanesthesia-care

Almost one-fourth of patients experience a complication within the PACU. Nausea, vomiting, and the need for airway support constitute 70% of these (**Fig. 11.2**).[40] The need to maintain airway support is by far the most common respiratory complication. The duration of the procedure, ASA classification, and type of procedure appear to be important determinants. Hypothermia is also noteworthy, slowing drug metabolism, delaying recovery, and is associated with prolonged postoperative PACU stay.

Among cardiovascular complications in the postoperative period, none is more important or more difficult to diagnose than myocardial ischemia. The association of perioperative myocardial ischemia with cardiac morbidity has been clearly documented. Diagnosis is complicated by the fact that only 10% to 30% of patients suffering from documented myocardial infarction have pain and that postoperative ECG T-wave changes are often nonspecific. Instead, one must seek secondary indications of ongoing ischemia such as hypotension, arrhythmias, elevated

Table 11.15. Postanesthesia Recovery Score

Parameter	Score[a]
Activity	
Voluntary movement of all limbs to command	2
Voluntary movement of two extremities to command	1
Unable to move	0
Respiration	
Breathes deeply and coughs	2
Dyspnea, hypoventilation	1
Apneic	0
Circulation	
Blood pressure equals 80% of preanesthetic level	2
Blood pressure equals 50–80% of preanesthetic level	1
Blood pressure equals <50% of preanesthetic level	0
Consciousness	
Fully awake	2
Arousable	1
Unresponsive	0
Color	
Pink	2
Pale, blotchy	1
Cyanotic	0

[a]Patients should score at least 7 before discharge from the postanesthesia care unit.

filling pressures, or postoperative oliguria. Arrhythmias are common and are significant primarily because of the association with myocardial ischemia or hypoxemia.

The most important neurocognitive outcomes following anesthesia and surgery include stroke and delirium. Perioperative stroke can be defined as any embolic, thrombotic, or hemorrhagic cerebral event with clinical manifestations of brain injury that persist for at least 24 hours and occur within 30 days of surgery. It is devastating, diagnosis is frequently delayed and is associated with high mortality and disability. Most perioperative strokes are ischemic and for patients undergoing noncardiac, nonneurologic surgery the reported incidence of between 0.1% and 1% which increases with the number of risk factors is generally accepted. Most risk factors are nonmodifiable but intraoperative hypotension and either low- or high–end-tidal carbon dioxide concentrations have been independently associated with stroke[41] representing modifiable and biologically plausible targets for further investigation. Delirium is acute disorder of attention and cognition and may serve as a marker of brain vulnerability. It is associated with significant decline in cognitive trajectory, prolonged impairment, and increased mortality[42] when encountered in the postoperative setting.

Nausea and vomiting are rarely unifactorial and cause considerable discomfort. Opioids and inhaled anesthetics are responsible for stimulating the emesis center in a significant cohort of patients. These patients may provide a clear history of opioid or inhaled anesthesia sensitivity and regimens may be tailored to limit exposure. In general, however, there is little evidence to favor one inhaled anesthetic over another, although propofol-based TIVA has consistently demonstrated lower rates of nausea and vomiting in prospective clinical trials. It is not unusual for an antiemetic agent to be included preoperatively or as part of the anesthetic technique, especially in patients with a positive history or those deemed to be at risk, such as menstruating young women undergoing laparoscopy. Standard usage includes phenothiazines, butyrophenones, $5HT_3$ antagonists, NK_1 antagonists, and steroids. A multimodal approach that avoids redosing of a given medication class is most beneficial.[43]

The most common cause of delayed emergence is the residual effects of anesthesia. The differential diagnosis is best approached by ruling out physiologic, pharmacologic, and neurologic cases, in this order (**Table 11.16**). There should be little confusion about the implication of muscle relaxants because physical indications of ventilatory distress, combined with

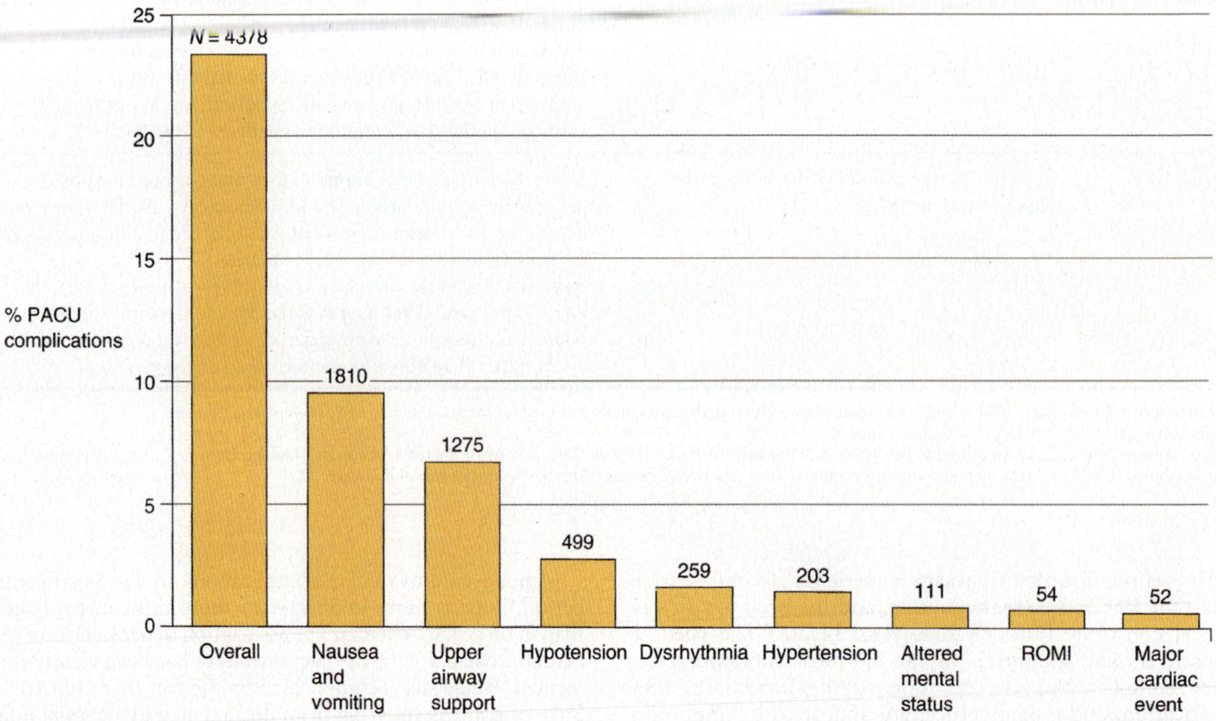

Figure 11.2. Major postanesthesia care unit complications by percentage of occurrence and number of patients experiencing each complication. Nausea and vomiting were the most frequently observed complications. ROMI, rule out myocardial infarction. (Reproduced with permission from Hines R, Barash PG, Watrous G, O'Connor T. Complications occurring in the postanesthesia care unit: a survey. *Anesth Analg*. 1992;74:505.)

Table 11.16. Differential Diagnosis of Delayed Emergence

Metabolic Abnormalities
Hypoxia
Hypercarbia
Hypoglycemia
Hypotension
Hypothermia
Hyponatremia
Drug Effects
Muscle relaxants
Opioids
Barbiturates
Benzodiazepines
Ketamine
Anticholinergics
Inhalational anesthetics
Neurologic Injury
Ischemia
Mass lesions
Seizure disorders

the readings of the blockade monitor are diagnostic. Where appropriate, opioids can be reversed using titrated doses of naloxone. Flumazenil can be used for reversal of benzodiazepines.

ENHANCED RECOVERY PROTOCOLS

11 With the increasing adoption of minimally invasive surgical techniques and a realization that postoperative complications may be impacted by intraoperative management, nearly every surgical subspecialty establish efforts toward enhanced recovery protocols. These comprehensive care management plans dictate the preoperative preparation, intraoperative management, surgical technique, and postoperative management. While a consistent decrease in length of stay, complications, and costs have been observed across the many trials assessed in many surgical specialties, there are very few consistent protocols. The process of collaboration and standardization may be the most important element.

ARTIFICIAL INTELLIGENCE AND ANESTHESIOLOGY

Artificial intelligence (AI)–based technologies continue to gain traction within the healthcare setting. Within anesthesiology, new opportunities have emerged related to preoperative risk stratification and outcome prediction, operating room resource allocation, and depth of anesthesia monitoring.[44] As limitations to computational processing power necessary for training machine learning algorithms on massive, complex datasets have been largely overcome, new opportunities keep emerging. However, major challenges remain in order for AI applications to be implemented within a perioperative setting, and have safe and sustained impact over time. These core challenges—which remain outside the scope of this text—include concerns regarding ethics and regulatory oversight, a paucity of prospective trials establishing clinical impact, and underlying data heterogeneity, quality, and shift.

POSTOPERATIVE ACUTE PAIN MANAGEMENT

Postoperative pain is an inevitable consequence of surgery. Its severity is site dependent, but the magnitude of the pain experienced by individual patients after similar surgical

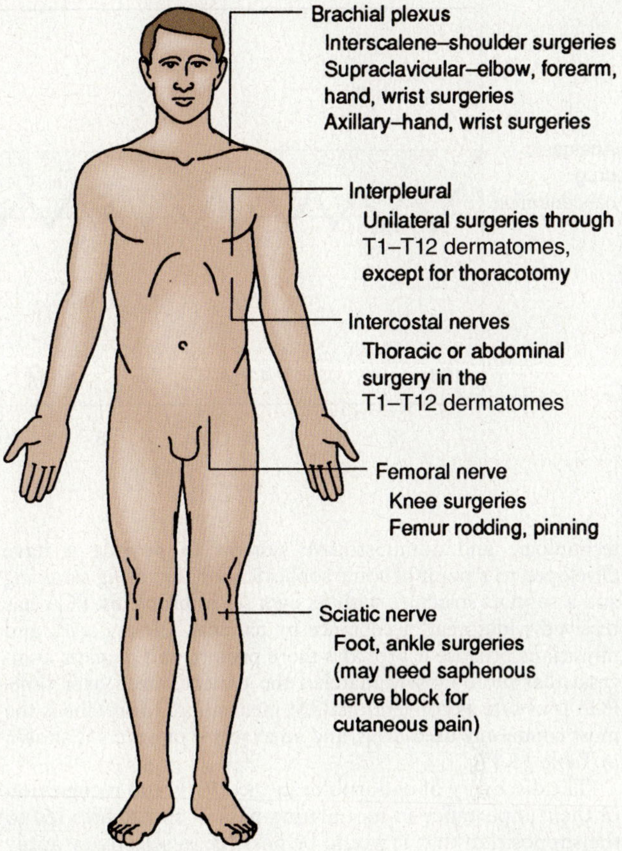

Figure 11.3. Surgical procedures in which peripheral nerve blockade can provide postoperative pain relief.

procedures is influenced by a multitude of factors. Variation in patient experience has been clearly demonstrated by several authors and is reflected in deficiencies in postoperative pain control.[45]

Superficial somatic pain is well localized and has a protective function. Superficial somatic pain is readily treated by common analgesic techniques. Deep somatic pain may not be well localized, may have some protective function, and is fairly responsive to a variety of analgesics. Visceral pain, served almost entirely by C fiber activity, is poorly localized, often referred to, and difficult to treat. In major operations, all modes can be activated. The use of nonsteroidal anti-inflammatory drugs with or without the injection of local anesthetics into the wound is very effective. If done preemptively at the time of surgery, this approach can significantly benefit the patient's postoperative experience. Examples of nerve blocks for various procedures are shown in **Figure 11.3**.

Including potent opioids in the treatment of deep pain, both somatic and visceral, has been routine. However, the responses to standard regimens have been notoriously unreliable, from inadequate pain relief to narcosis. It was not until the 1980s that variations in response were linked to variable serum concentrations of analgesic drugs. Interpatient variation in serum levels to any standard dose can be fivefold, and interpatient therapeutic concentrations can vary on a similar scale. When factored together, there is the potential for a 25-fold variation in patient response to a standard drug prescription. Each patient has an individual therapeutic window. The clinical implications are enormous.

In 1968, investigators demonstrated the virtue of small IV doses given on demand. As a result, the patient experienced greater pain relief, yet used the same or less total narcotic (**Fig. 11.4**). Patient-controlled analgesia (PCA) and the

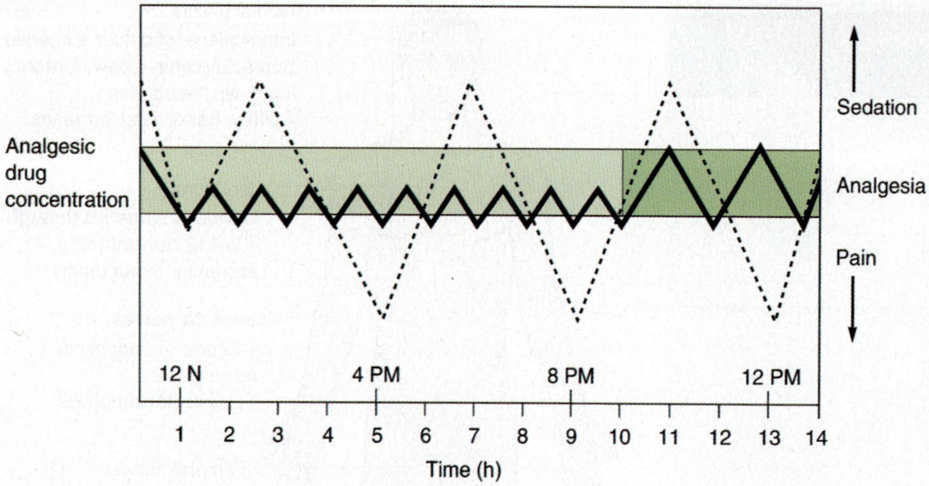

Figure 11.4. Theoretical relation among dosing interval, analgesic drug concentration, and clinical effects when comparing a patient-controlled analgesia system (*solid line*) to conventional intramuscular therapy (*dashed line*). (Reproduced with permission from White PF. Patient-controlled analgesia: a new approach to the management of postoperative pain. *Semin Anesth*. 1985;4:261.)

technologic and administrative systems to provide it have developed to a point of some sophistication, requiring servicing and a support structure with its own set of problems. PCA has received widespread acceptance by patients, nursing staff, and physicians because it provides more prompt and painless analgesia that more closely matches the patient's need over time. PCA is as safe as conventional IM medication. Morphine is the most commonly used drug, and an example of orders is shown in **Table 11.17**. 12

The discovery of endorphins in the 1970s and recognition of their importance in modulating pain at spinal sites led to the supposition that it would be possible to selectively apply opioids directly to receptors. This led to the development of epidural opiate analgesia, in which opioids are applied directly to the receptors at spinal sites. The goal of epidural analgesia is to obtain maximal analgesia while minimizing systemic side effects. For severe acute postoperative pain caused by major surgery, epidural analgesia has proved to be a superior modality for pain control. In high-risk cases, there is evidence that it has an overall beneficial effect on morbidity.

The effective use of this sophisticated modality requires education and the establishment of protocols with rigorous attention to detail. The potential for respiratory depression demands adherence to monitoring standards. Morphine and fentanyl, often in combination with a dilute local anesthetic solution, are most often prescribed (**Table 11.18**).

A comprehensive postoperative pain management service demands resources and must use the physical and pharmacologic modalities available while recognizing the significant subjective component of any individual's pain. The ability to recognize the impact of acute pain or an underlying chronic pain disorder requires experience and the active involvement of nursing staff and surgeons is essential.

Postoperative acute pain management may require a multimodal approach that incorporates opioids, PNB, and nonopioid analgesics. Chronic pain patients can be particularly difficult to manage and may require preoperative optimization and opiate tapering. These patients require very large doses of IV analgesics and need to be maintained orally. A typical way to evaluate an appropriate starting dose is to convert the preoperative opioid regimen to an IV morphine equivalent, and then add what would be required to treat the acute surgical pain. The use of nonopioid and nonpharmacologic treatments is essential in the management of acute postoperative pain in this patient population. PNB, aggressive use of acetaminophen nonsteroidal anti-inflammatory agents, and agents such as dexmedetomidine may be necessary to minimize the adverse effects associated with uncontrolled postoperative pain. The relationship between the administration of opiates during the intraoperative and immediate postoperative phase of care with the "opiate crisis" remains to be fully determined.

Table 11.17. Example of Orders for Patient-Controlled Analgesia (PCA)

1. Patient is to be initiated on PCA with standard monitoring protocol		
2. Drug selection	Morphine 5 mg/mL	Hydromorphone 1 mg/mL
3. Loading initial dose (start PRN for pain)	2–5 mg	0.2–0.5 mg
Maximum total loading dose	10 mg	1 mg
4. Pump setting PCA dose	1–2 mg	0.1–0.2 mg
Lockout interval	6–10 min	6–10 min
4-h limit	30–45 mg	4–5 mg

From University of Michigan Hospitals online order form Acute Pain Service, Patient Controlled Analgesia Standard Orders.

Table 11.18. Opioid Protocols in Epidural Opiate Analgesia

	Morphine[a]	Fentanyl[b]
Length of onset	Longer (30–60 min)	Shorter (15–30 min)
Duration	Longer (6–24 h for single bolus)	Shorter (1–2 h for single bolus)
Cephalad spread and side effects	More prone	Less prone
Indication	Favored for lumbar administration after abdominal surgery	Favored for thoracic administration after chest surgery
Dose	Typically 3–5 mg, q6–8 h	Typically 50–75 mg/h (±dilute bupivacaine)

[a]Hydrophilic: slow in, slow out.
[b]Lipophilic: fast in, fast out.

ACKNOWLEDGMENTS

We gratefully acknowledge the contributions of previous edition authors, Kevin K. Tremper and Timothy W. Rutter, as portions of those chapters have been retained in this revision.

References

1. Standl TG. Catheter tip position and baricity of the local anesthetic have an impact on maldistribution in microcatheter CSA. *Anesthesiology*. 1999;90(4):1227–1229.
2. *Comprehensive Accreditation Manual for Hospitals: CAMH 2025*. Joint Commission Resources 2025. ISBN 9781635854046.
3. Malviya S, Naughton N, Tremper K. *Sedation Analgesia for Diagnostic and Therapeutic Procedures*. Humana Press; 2003.
4. Apfelbaum JL, Hagberg CA, Connis RT, et al. 2022 American Society of Anesthesiologists Practice Guidelines for management of the difficult airway. *Anesthesiology*. 2022;136(1):31–81.
5. Kheterpal S, Han R, Tremper KK, et al. Incidence and predictors of difficult and impossible mask ventilation. *Anesthesiology*. 2006;105(5):885–891.
6. Mallampati SR, Gatt SP, Gugino LD, et al. A clinical sign to predict difficult tracheal intubation: a prospective study. *Can Anaesth Soc J*. 1985;32(4):429–434.
7. Lienhart A, Auroy Y, Péquignot F, et al. Survey of anesthesia-related mortality in France. *Anesthesiology*. 2006;105(6):1087–1097.
8. Sparicio D, Landoni G, Zangrillo A. Angiotensin-converting enzyme inhibitors predispose to hypotension refractory to norepinephrine but responsive to methylene blue. *J Thorac Cardiovasc Surg*. 2004;127(2):608.
9. Medel J, Boccara G, Van de Steen E, Bertrand M, Godet G, Coriat P. Terlipressin for treating intraoperative hypotension: can it unmask myocardial ischemia? *Anesth Analg*. 2001;93(1):53–55, TOC.
10. Talbot MP, Tremblay I, Denault AY, Bélisle S. Vasopressin for refractory hypotension during cardiopulmonary bypass. *J Thorac Cardiovasc Surg*. 2000;120(2):401–402.
11. Stoelting R. *Anesthesia and Co-Existing Disease*. 3rd ed. Churchill Livingstone; 1993.
12. Davenport DL, Ferraris VA, Hosokawa P, Henderson WG, Khuri SF, Mentzer RM Jr. Multivariable predictors of postoperative cardiac adverse events after general and vascular surgery: results from the patient safety in surgery study. *J Am Coll Surg*. 2007;204(6):1199–1210.
13. Mangano DT. Perioperative cardiac morbidity. *Anesthesiology*. 1990;72(1):153–184.
14. Fleisher LA, Poldermans D. Perioperative beta blockade: where do we go from here? *Lancet*. 2008;371(9627):1813–1814.
15. Rao TL, Jacobs KH, El-Etr AA. Reinfarction following anesthesia in patients with myocardial infarction. *Anesthesiology*. 1983;59(6):499–505.
16. Botto F, Alonso-Coello P, Chan MTV, et al. Myocardial injury after noncardiac surgery: a large, international, prospective cohort study establishing diagnostic criteria, characteristics, predictors, and 30-day outcomes. *Anesthesiology*. 2014;120(3):564–578.
17. Thompson A, Fleischmann KE, Smilowitz NR, et al. 2024 AHA/ACC/ACS/ASNC/HRS/SCA/SCCT/SCMR/SVM guideline for perioperative cardiovascular management for noncardiac surgery: a report of the American college of cardiology/American Heart Association Joint Committee on clinical practice guidelines. *Circulation*. 2024;150(19):e351–e442.
18. POISE Study Group, Devereaux PJ, Yang H, et al. Effects of extended-release metoprolol succinate in patients undergoing non-cardiac surgery (POISE trial): a randomised controlled trial. *Lancet*. 2008;371(9627):1839–1847.
19. Le Manach Y, Coriat P, Collard CD, Riedel B. Statin therapy within the perioperative period. *Anesthesiology*. 2008;108(6):1141–1146.
20. Devereaux PJ, Mrkobrada M, Sessler DI, et al. Aspirin in patients undergoing noncardiac surgery. *N Engl J Med*. 2014;370(16):1494–1503.
21. Rabbitts JA, Nuttall GA, Brown MJ, et al. Cardiac risk of noncardiac surgery after percutaneous coronary intervention with drug-eluting stents. *Anesthesiology*. 2008;109(4):596–604.
22. Nuttall GA, Brown MJ, Stombaugh JW, et al. Time and cardiac risk of surgery after bare-metal stent percutaneous coronary intervention. *Anesthesiology*. 2008;109(4):588–595.
23. Goldman L, Caldera DL, Nussbaum SR, et al. Multifactorial index of cardiac risk in noncardiac surgical procedures. *N Engl J Med*. 1977;297(16):845–850.
24. Benesch C, Glance LG, Derdeyn CP, et al. Perioperative neurological evaluation and management to lower the risk of acute stroke in patients undergoing noncardiac, nonneurological surgery: a scientific statement from the American Heart Association/American Stroke Association. *Circulation*. 2021;143(19):e923–e946.
25. Jørgensen ME, Torp-Pedersen C, Gislason GH, et al. Time elapsed after ischemic stroke and risk of adverse cardiovascular events and mortality following elective noncardiac surgery. *JAMA*. 2014;312(3):269–277.
26. Abdelmalak BB, Bonilla A, Mascha EJ, et al. Dexamethasone, light anaesthesia, and tight glucose control (DeLiT) randomized controlled trial. *Br J Anaesth*. 2013;111(2):209–221.
27. Kheterpal S, O'Reilly M, Englesbe MJ, et al. Preoperative and intraoperative predictors of cardiac adverse events after general, vascular, and urological surgery. *Anesthesiology*. 2009;110(1):58–66.
28. Fielding-Singh V, Vanneman MW, Grogan T, et al. Association between preoperative hemodialysis timing and postoperative mortality in patients with end-stage kidney disease. *JAMA*. 2022;328(18):1837–1848.
29. Brown KA, Laferrière A, Lakheeram I, Moss IR. Recurrent hypoxemia in children is associated with increased analgesic sensitivity to opiates. *Anesthesiology*. 2006;105(4):665–669.
30. Abdelsattar ZM, Hendren S, Wong SL, Campbell DA Jr, Ramachandran SK. The impact of untreated obstructive sleep apnea on cardiopulmonary complications in general and vascular surgery: a cohort study. *Sleep*. 2015;38(8):1205–1210.
31. Horlocker TT, Vandermeuelen E, Kopp SL, Gogarten W, Leffert LR, Benzon HT. Regional anesthesia in the patient receiving antithrombotic or thrombolytic therapy: American Society of Regional Anesthesia and Pain Medicine Evidence-Based Guidelines (fourth edition). *Reg Anesth Pain Med*. 2018;43(3):263–309.
32. Kohan L, Potru S, Barreveld AM, et al. Buprenorphine management in the perioperative period: educational review and recommendations from a multisociety expert panel. *Reg Anesth Pain Med*. 2021;46(10):840–859.
33. Ruetzler K, Bustamante S, Schmidt MT, et al. Video laryngoscopy vs direct laryngoscopy for endotracheal intubation in the operating room: a cluster randomized clinical trial. *JAMA*. 2024;331(15):1279–1286.
34. Minto G, Scott MJ, Miller TE. Monitoring needs and goal-directed fluid therapy within an enhanced recovery program. *Anesthesiol Clin*. 2015;33(1):35–49.
35. Wuethrich PY, Burkhard FC, Thalmann GN, Stueber F, Studer UE. Restrictive deferred hydration combined with preemptive norepinephrine infusion during radical cystectomy reduces postoperative complications and hospitalization time: a randomized clinical trial. *Anesthesiology*. 2014;120(2):365–377.
36. Avidan MS, Zhang L, Burnside BA, et al. Anesthesia awareness and the bispectral index. *N Engl J Med*. 2008;358(11):1097–1108.
37. Bonner S. *Admission and Discharge Criteria. Post Anesthesia Care*. Prentice Hall International; 1990.
38. Avidan MS, Jacobsohn E, Glick D, et al. Prevention of intraoperative awareness in a high-risk surgical population. *N Engl J Med*. 2011;365(7):591–600.
39. Hines R, Barash PG, Watrous G, O'Connor T. Complications occurring in the postanesthesia care unit. *Anesth Analg*. 1992;74(4):503–509.
40. Breslow MJ, Miller CF, Parker SD, Walman AT, Rogers MC. Changes in T-wave morphology following anesthesia and surgery. *Anesthesiology*. 1986;64(3):398–401.
41. Vlisides PE, Mentz G, Leis AM, et al. Carbon dioxide, blood pressure, and perioperative stroke: a retrospective case-control study. *Anesthesiology*. 2022;137(4):434–445.

42. Gottesman RF, Grega MA, Bailey MM, et al. Delirium after coronary artery bypass graft surgery and late mortality. *Ann Neurol*. 2010;67(3):338–344.
43. Charbit B, Funck-Brentano C. Droperidol-induced proarrhythmia: the beginning of an answer? *Anesthesiology*. 2007;107(4): 524–526.
44. Hashimoto DA, Witkowski E, Gao L, Meireles O, Rosman G. Artificial intelligence in anesthesiology: current techniques, clinical applications, and limitations. *Anesthesiology*. 2020;132(2): 379–394.
45. Melzack R, Wall PD. Pain mechanisms: a new theory. *Science*. 1965;150(3699):971–979.

12

The Pregnant Patient

Dalya M. Ferguson and Lillian S. Kao

Key Points

1. A medically necessary surgery should never be denied or delayed in a pregnant woman, as this is associated with adverse outcomes for both the mother and the fetus.
2. Understanding the relative increase in the size of the gravid uterus and the displacement of intra-abdominal and pelvic structures is a critical step in surgical planning, specifically with regard to incision location, laparoscopic port placement, and patient positioning in the operating room.
3. Maternal administration of antenatal corticosteroids is one of the most significant advances in the reduction of morbidity of prematurity.
4. There is no evidence that tocolytic therapy directly improves neonatal outcomes, except for the short-term prolongation of pregnancy to allow for administration of antenatal steroids.
5. Fetal heart rate (FHR) monitoring, the most commonly performed procedure during pregnancy, is associated with a substantial decrease in early neonatal morbidity, particularly in preterm fetuses.
6. In most cases, ultrasonography is the first-line diagnostic imaging modality in the pregnant surgical patient, but other or additional modalities should be utilized when necessary. Computed tomography (CT) is the imaging modality of choice in pregnant patients after major trauma.
7. Acute appendicitis is the most common nonobstetric cause of acute surgical abdomen during pregnancy, and delays in diagnosis and treatment can have serious consequences for both mother and fetus. Appendectomy is recommended over nonoperative management in pregnant patients.
8. Biliary tract disease is the most common cause of maternal hospitalization in the first year after delivery.
9. Pregnant patients with breast cancer should be managed by similar treatment strategies as nonpregnant patients, without delay of treatment, but with a few adjustments to account for potentially teratogenic interventions.
10. A multidisciplinary approach is essential for safely managing pregnant patients.

Nearly every general surgeon will encounter a pregnant patient with a surgical diagnosis. While many basic principles of care remain consistent, some critical differences must be noted. To provide appropriate pre-, intra-, and postoperative care, the general surgeon must possess a complete understanding of the unique physiology of the pregnant patient. Moreover, any surgeon managing a gravid patient must be aware of the effects
1 that diagnostic and therapeutic interventions might have on the fetus. However, tests or treatments that are medically necessary for the mother should never be denied or delayed due to concern about risk to the fetus. Failure to diagnose and treat a surgical condition in a timely fashion may result in serious harm to both the pregnant woman and the fetus. To ensure the safety of the mother and fetus, a multidisciplinary approach is essential for managing pregnant patients. This chapter will review the most common surgical diseases that present during pregnancy, along with current management recommendations.

ANATOMY OF THE CHANGING UTERUS

In a nonpregnant woman, the uterus resides within the pelvis,
2 weighs approximately 70 g, and has a cavity volume of 10 mL. By the end of the first trimester, the uterus expands out of the pelvis, and it reaches the level of the umbilicus by 20 weeks. The uterus eventually comes in contact with the anterior abdominal wall, displacing the bowel laterally and cranially, and it nearly reaches the liver by 36 weeks (**Fig. 12.1**).[1] Coupled with its ascent from the pelvis, the uterus usually rotates to the right due to the presence of the sigmoid colon and rectum in the left pelvis. By the completion of the first trimester, the size of the uterus typically precludes abdominal entry below the level of the umbilicus, thus altering port placement for minimally invasive surgery and incision location for open surgery. Furthermore, when the pregnant woman lies supine, the gravid uterus can compress the inferior vena cava, decrease cardiac preload, and potentially cause hypotension. As such, proper patient positioning during pregnancy (in the left lateral decubitus position) is essential to avoid aortocaval compression.

DEVELOPMENT OF THE FETUS

Accurate determination of gestational age is imperative to guide patient counseling and surgical and obstetric decision making. Before 20 weeks of gestation, ultrasonography provides a better estimate of fetal gestational age than the last menstrual period. Ultrasonographic estimation of fetal age is most accurate during the first trimester, when crown–rump length is within 5 days of the date of conception.[2] Major developmental stages and milestones are listed in **Table 12.1**.

Fetal Viability and Corticosteroid Administration

By the beginning of the third trimester, the fetus may survive if born prematurely, though the functional status of the respiratory system is crucial in determining viability.[3] Surfactant production, which begins by the 20th week of gestation, is necessary for reduction of surface tension at the alveolar–air interface and

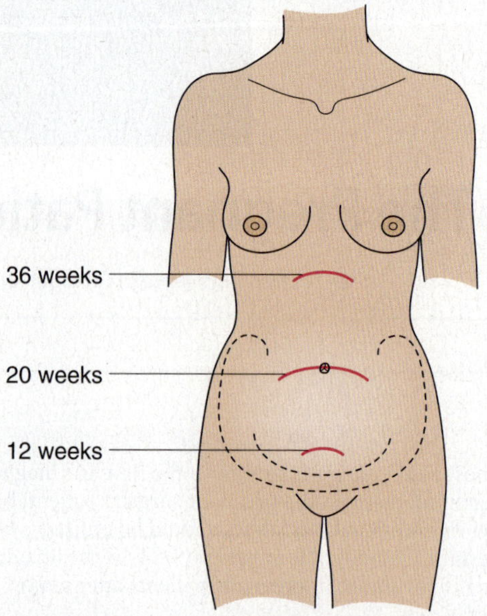

Figure 12.1. Enlarging uterus during gestation. At 12 weeks, the uterus rises out of the pelvis into the abdomen. At 20 weeks, the fundus is at the height of the umbilicus, and at 36 weeks, the uterus reaches the upper abdomen.

proper oxygen exchange. In general, surfactant is present in only small amounts before 24 weeks, but this can be augmented
3 by maternal administration of antenatal corticosteroids, one of the most significant advances in the reduction of morbidity of prematurity.[3] Corticosteroids not only increase surfactant secretion in the fetal lung, but also induce morphologic development of pulmonary epithelial cells and increase lung compliance. Corticosteroids also stimulate development of other organ systems, decreasing the incidence of necrotizing enterocolitis, intraventricular hemorrhage, periventricular leukomalacia, and death. The maximum developmental effects can be seen as early as 24 hours after maternal administration of dexamethasone or betamethasone, and administration at the first sign of premature onset of labor can improve survival, particularly in births between 22 and 25 weeks.[4] The decision to administer corticosteroids depends on accurate determination of gestational age and, therefore, this decision should always be made in conjunction with an obstetrician.

PREMATURE ONSET OF LABOR

Preterm birth is defined as birth prior to 37 weeks of gestation. The etiology of preterm labor is often multifactorial, but the onset of labor from fetal and uterine stress or trauma during surgical manipulation or intra-abdominal inflammatory processes is of principal concern to the surgeon.[5] The complex interactions between the inflammatory response, uterine and/or maternal trauma, and early initiation of labor may represent the body's attempt to expel the fetus from a hostile uterine environment.

Tocolysis

4 Tocolytic therapy can improve neonatal outcomes via short-term prolongation of pregnancy to allow for the administration of antenatal corticosteroids and/or transportation of the patient to a tertiary care facility and by providing fetal neuroprotection.[6] Tocolysis is indicated in women with preterm contractions with cervical change between the 24 and 34 weeks of gestation. The four most commonly utilized tocolytic agents are prostaglandin synthesis inhibitors, magnesium sulfate, beta$_2$-adrenergic agonists, and calcium channel blockers. Nifedipine is now considered the agent of choice by the World Health Organization (WHO), based on its safety profile, efficacy, and cost.[6] Because all tocolytic agents carry risks of maternal and fetal side effects, the decision to use tocolytics must be made only after the diagnosis of premature onset of labor is confirmed and determination that the benefits of prolonging gestation outweigh the risks of tocolysis. This decision should always be made in conjunction with an obstetrician.

MONITORING OF THE FETUS

The utility of perioperative fetal monitoring arises from the relationship between the degree of fetal acidemia and the presence and depth of decelerations and decreased or absent fetal heart rate (FHR) variability.[7,8] Established FHR patterns and variable cardiac responses to fetal and maternal stimuli reflect an intact, well-oxygenated central nervous system (CNS). Use of fetal monitoring to identify deviation from normal patterns, indicative of metabolic acidosis, has been associated with a substantial decrease in early neonatal morbidity, particularly
5 in preterm fetuses.[9] FHR monitoring may be performed externally or internally (**Fig. 12.2**). Tracings are printed on a continuous strip of paper, with the FHR plotted at the top of the graph and uterine activity at the bottom.

Fetal Heart Rate

A normal FHR ranges between 110 and 160 beats/min. Minute-to-minute variations away from a baseline FHR are known as accelerations or decelerations. Normal FHR tracings express continuous adjustment in the vagal tone through variability in the heart rate (**Fig. 12.3**).

Selected findings on FHR tracings, the underlying causes, and their clinical significance are outlined in **Table 12.2**. Intraoperative fetal compromise, indicated by an ominous heart rate tracing, must be treated by correcting maternal hypotension or increasing oxygen delivery with increased FiO_2, positional changes, aggressive fluid resuscitation, or blood transfusion. The inability to improve the intrauterine milieu can necessitate an emergent cesarean section to prevent fetal demise.[10]

Fetal Heart Rate Monitoring During Nonobstetric Surgery

The decision to use continuous FHR monitoring during nonobstetric surgery in pregnancy is controversial and should be based on gestational age and procedure type, site, and duration. For previable pregnancies (<23 weeks), documentation

Table 12.1. Human Developmental Stages and Associated Milestones

Stage	Time Frame	Important Milestones
Embryonic period	Conception through end of 8th week of gestation	Critical development of brain and central nervous system, heart, lungs, diaphragm, intestines, and abdominal wall Exposure to toxins, medications, or ionizing radiation can have catastrophic effects
Fetal period	9th week of gestation through birth	Further development of tissues and organs Surfactant production begins by 20th week of gestation

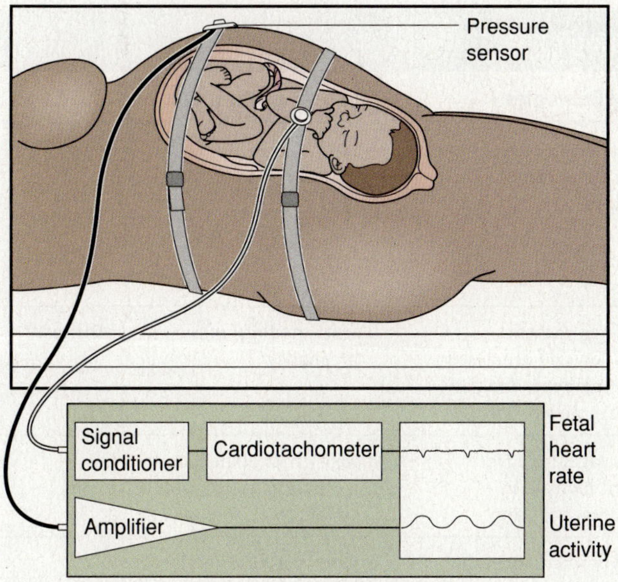

Figure 12.2. Intraoperative and postoperative fetal monitoring using noninvasive surface Doppler and pressure sensor to monitor uterine contractions. (Reproduced from Miller DA, Paul R. Antepartum–intrapartum monitoring. In: Scott JR, DiSaia PJ, Hammond CB, et al., eds. *Danforth's Obstetrics and Gynecology.* 8th ed. Lippincott Williams & Wilkins; 1999:243–255.)

of fetal heart activity by Doppler before and after the procedure suffices.[11] For viable gestations, there is mixed support for FHR monitoring, but at a minimum, simultaneous electronic FHR and contraction monitoring should be performed before and after the procedure to assess fetal well-being and the absence of contractions. If intraoperative electronic FHR monitoring is performed, then all the necessary provisions should be made to provide optimal safety for the mother and the fetus. These include availability of obstetric care providers, anesthesiologists, neonatologists, and nurses working as a team and ready to intervene during the surgical procedure for maternal or fetal indications. Informed operative consent should thus be obtained in anticipation of a possible emergency delivery.[12]

IMAGING THE PREGNANT PATIENT

The most commonly used imaging modalities during pregnancy include plain radiography, ultrasonography, magnetic resonance imaging (MRI), and computed tomography (CT). The first and latter modalities generate ionizing radiation. Anxiety about the risks of ionizing radiation on the part of health care providers and patients may influence the diagnostic approach in pregnant patients, potentially placing both the mother and the fetus in greater danger due to misdiagnosis. Although experimental data regarding the effects of ionizing radiation on the developing human fetus are impossible to obtain, data are available from animal experiments and retrospective studies in patients with inadvertent exposure, atomic bomb survivors in Hiroshima and Nagasaki, and victims of the atomic power plant disaster in Chernobyl.[13,14]

Ionizing Radiation

Fetal effects of ionizing radiation depend on the dose absorbed by tissue and the stage of development during exposure. Exposure is defined as the amount of ionic charge created by radiation when passing through a defined mass of air. It is a misconception to assume that the radiation dose a pregnant woman absorbs is the same as that absorbed by the fetus, as the latter is partially protected by a pregnant woman's soft tissues and uterus, both of which generally stop alpha and beta particles from penetration if they are not ingested, injected, or inhaled.[15,16] Radiographic evaluation of the abdomen and pelvis is most likely to expose the fetus to direct ionizing radiation, whereas examination of the extremities and chest leads to exposure from scatter radiation only (**Table 12.3**).[16] The potential deleterious consequences of radiation-induced ionization of vital cellular structures can be divided into four categories: (1) lethal effects, (2) teratogenic effect, (3) growth retardation, and (4) oncogenic potential. The occurrence of each effect depends upon gestational age at the time of exposure, dose absorbed by the fetus, and fetal cellular repair mechanisms. The first three categories of adverse pregnancy outcomes have a deterministic effect. A threshold, or no-adverse-effect level exists; after exceeding this threshold, a predictable relationship is observed between the absorbed dose and the severity of the effect. On the contrary, cancer appears to have a stochastic effect, in which the probability of an effect increases as radiation dose increases, but the severity of the effect is unpredictable, and no safe threshold exists.

Lethal Effects of Ionizing Radiation

The developing human is most sensitive to the lethal effects of ionizing radiation during the first 14 days after conception (3 to 4 weeks gestational age), during which the "all or none" principle applies: the radiation-exposed embryo either survives undamaged or succumbs. The lethal threshold increases throughout pregnancy, and at full term, the fetal risk equals the pregnant woman's risk.[17,18]

Teratogenic Effects of Ionizing Radiation

Teratogenic effects of radiation occur during early organogenesis, corresponding to weeks 2 to 4 in human development. CNS malformations, including microcephaly, retinal pigmentary changes, hydrocephalus, and optic nerve atrophy, are the only malformations that can be specifically linked to radiation exposure during organogenesis.[19]

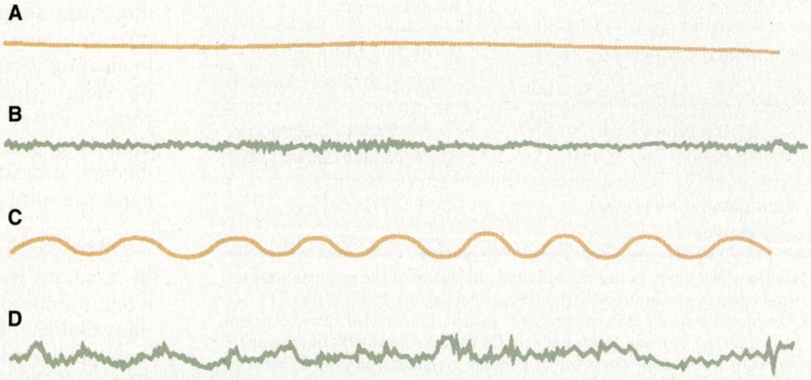

Figure 12.3. Fetal heart variability. **A:** Short-term and long-term variability both absent: abnormal. **B:** Short-term variability present, long-term variability absent: abnormal. **C:** Long-term variability present, short-term variability absent: abnormal. **D:** Both short- and long-term variability present: normal. (Reproduced from Miller DA, Paul R. Antepartum–intrapartum monitoring. In: Scott JR, DiSaia PJ, Hammond CB, et al., eds. *Danforth's Obstetrics and Gynecology.* 8th ed. Lippincott Williams & Wilkins; 1999:243–255.)

SCIENTIFIC PRINCIPLES

Table 12.2. Selected Findings on Fetal Heart Rate Monitoring

Term	Description	Potential Etiologies	Clinical Significance
FHR variability	Fluctuation in FHR (amplitude range) over time Variability may be absent, minimal (amplitude <5 BMP), moderate (6–25 BMP), or marked (>25 BMP).	Fetal sleep–wake cycle Maternal medications CNS acidosis	Absent or minimal FHR variability can indicate hypoxia or acidosis Moderate FHR variability effectively rules out fetal hypoxia and acidosis
Accelerations	Abrupt increase in FHR above baseline	Increased sympathetic stimulation and decreased parasympathetic stimulation with fetal movements	Normal findings in the second half of pregnancy
Early decelerations	Gradual decrease and return of the FHR that mirrors uterine contractions	Increased vagal tone from transient increase in intracranial pressure	Benign physiologic manifestation of a functioning autonomic nervous system
Variable decelerations	Abrupt decrease in FHR by at least 15 BPM with the change lasting at least 15 s but less than 2 min	Umbilical cord compression	Isolated variable decelerations have little clinical significance, but if persistent with inadequate recovery between contractions, fetal hypoxemia and acidosis can occur
Late decelerations	Gradual decrease and return of the FHR that lags behind uterine contractions	Uteroplacental insufficiency	Can indicate serious physiologic derangement, which can be due to maternal dehydration, anemia, hypoxia, hypotension, placental abruption, or uterine tachysystole

FHR, fetal heart rate; BPM, beats per minute; CNS, central nervous system.

Growth Retardation from Ionizing Radiation

Growth retardation results from radiation-induced cellular depletion. Although catch-up growth can occur if exposure happens early in gestation, permanent cell depletion and growth retardation occur with exposure during later fetal stages.[20] Reduced head circumference, height, and weight was observed in children within 1500 m of the Japanese atomic blasts while in utero, whereas those beyond 1500 m from the blast had normal growth.[21]

Table 12.3. Radiation Dosing to the Conceptus and Uterus From Selected Radiographic Examinations

Examination	Dose
Endoscopic retrograde cholangiopancreatography with no permanent films and shielding of abdomen	4 mrad
Routine chest radiograph	8–50 mrad
Routine mammography	<50 mrad
Abdomen (flat plate)	250–300 mrad
Computed tomography, chest	25–1000 mrad (uterus shielded and not exposed)
Computed tomography, upper abdomen	670–3000 mrad (uterus shielded and not exposed)
Computed tomography, abdomen	2000–3000 mrad

Data from Wagner L, Lester R, Saldana L. Exposure of the pregnant patient to diagnostic radiation. Medical Physics Publishing; 1997; Wyte CD. Diagnostic modalities in the pregnant patient. *Emerg Med Clin North Am.* 1994;12(1):9–43; and From Baillie J, Cairns SR, Cotton PB. Endoscopic management of choledocholithiasis during pregnancy. *Surgery Gynecol Obstet.* 1990;171(1):1–4.

Oncogenic Potential of Ionizing Radiation

Although the cause-and-effect relationship between in utero exposure to radiation and childhood cancer cannot be definitively established, even small exposures have been correlated with increased rates of childhood cancer.[22] Exposure to diagnostic levels of radiation likely increases the risk of future cancer; therefore, this risk must be weighed against the utility of the information provided by the study, and patients should be appropriately counseled.

Ultrasound

In general, ultrasonography is considered the first-line diagnostic imaging modality of the pregnant surgical patient because it is nonionizing, widely available, portable, and often provides adequate diagnostic performance. Ultrasonography has been used in obstetrics for more than 60 years without
6 reported fetal damage or harmful effects.[23] Ultrasonography is, however, a form of energy, producing effects on the tissues it penetrates. The two major mechanisms of potential effects are direct, resulting from the alternation of positive and negative pressures (mechanical or cavitation effects), or indirect, caused by heating of tissues secondary to transformation of the acoustic energy (thermal effects). Because of these theoretical concerns, several organizations have recommended that this diagnostic procedure be performed only when there is a valid medical indication and using the lowest possible ultrasonic exposure setting.[24]

Computed Tomography

In pregnant women, CT is indicated after major trauma and when nonionizing imaging modalities are inconclusive or unavailable.[25] Because of its sensitivity for detecting abdominal, pelvic, and retroperitoneal injuries, CT is the diagnostic test of choice in injured pregnant patients. Dose-reduction protocols (eg, abdominal and internal barium shielding) reduce the probability of adverse effects on the fetus without sacrificing image quality.[26]

Magnetic Resonance Imaging

Like ultrasonography, MRI does not generate ionizing radiation. Theoretical concerns include the effects of fluctuating electromagnetic fields and high sound intensity levels with potential damage to the fetal ear. Despite these concerns, present data have not documented any deleterious effects of MRI exposure on the developing conceptus.[27] Other known dangers of MRI exposure are not specific to pregnant women or fetuses: trauma from projection of metal, interference with implantable electronic devices, reposition of metallic implants, and burns from heating of conductive materials in implants.

APPENDICITIS IN THE PREGNANT PATIENT

Acute appendicitis is the most common nonobstetric cause of acute surgical abdomen during pregnancy.[28] Appendicitis is
7 confirmed in 65% to 75% of suspected cases, with an incidence of approximately 1:1500 births.[29] The incidence of appendicitis during pregnancy is similar to the rest of the population, however, appendiceal perforation rates are higher during pregnancy when compared with nonpregnant populations (4% to 57% vs 4% to 19%).[28] This difference may be attributable to delays in diagnosis, which allow for progression to perforation. However, it is possible that a number of cases of uncomplicated appendicitis get misdiagnosed as other infectious pathologies and are inadvertently but successfully treated with antibiotics. This would mean that the incidence of uncomplicated appendicitis during pregnancy has been underestimated, resulting in a falsely elevated proportion of perforated appendicitis. Regardless, perforated appendicitis presents a greater infectious risk in the pregnant patient than in the population as a whole. The gravid uterus interferes with omental migration, preventing the omentum from successfully walling off the inflammatory process. Additionally, Braxton Hicks contractions disrupt adhesion formation, and the general increase in vascularity of the abdomen with greater lymphatic drainage allows for rapid dissemination of infection.

Diagnosis

Anatomic and physiologic changes of the gravid state make diagnosis of appendicitis more difficult. Delays in diagnosis may be due to attributing abdominal pain to other etiologies (eg, pyelonephritis, false labor, or gastroenteritis), failure to pursue further investigation, and fear of surgically-induced premature labor. Delays are more common as pregnancy progresses; several studies have documented a correlation between a delay in diagnosis and gestational age.[30]

All of the classic signs and symptoms of appendicitis can be masked by pregnancy (**Table 12.4**). Anorexia, nausea, and vomiting occur in 58% to 77% of pregnant patients with appendicitis.[30] Although anorexia, nausea, and vomiting are common in the first trimester of pregnancy, their occurrence during the second or third trimesters, especially if associated with abdominal pain, should prompt a thorough investigation. In a large study of pregnant women with appendicitis, abdominal pain was present in all patients. Location of pain in the right lower quadrant, however, was common only early in gestation, and a portion of patients reported pain in the right upper quadrant. This change in symptomatology is easily understood if the anatomic changes of the appendix are taken into consideration. In the classic 1932 study, Baer and colleagues evaluated the migration of the appendix through the duration of pregnancy with barium enemas.[31] Beginning in the first trimester, the appendix and the cecum are gradually displaced by the uterus and start a caudal migration out of the pelvis into the upper abdomen. By the third trimester, the

Table 12.4. Variation in Signs and Symptoms of Appendicitis During Pregnancy

Signs and Symptoms	First Trimester (%)	Second Trimester (%)	Third Trimester (%)
Right lower quadrant pain	100	50	14
Right upper quadrant pain	0	17	57
Guarding (muscle spasm)	80	50	43
Nausea and vomiting	53	60	23
Tenderness on rectal examination	60	17	0
Perforation rate	20	49	70

Data from Weingold AB. Appendicitis in pregnancy. *Clin Obstet Gynecol.* 1983;26(4):801–809; Tamir IL, Bongard FS, Klein SR. Acute appendicitis in the pregnant patient. *Am J Surg.* 1990;160(6):571–575; and from Cunningham FG, McCubbin JH. Appendicitis complicating pregnancy. *Obstet Gynecol.* 1975;45:415–420.

appendiceal tip can abut the gallbladder (**Fig. 12.4**). The vague, referred epigastric pain due to early appendiceal obstruction is not changed by this anatomic consideration, but the location of the somatic pain is.

Laboratory investigations to assist in the diagnosis of appendicitis are also obscured by pregnancy. The physiologic leukocytosis of pregnancy, ranging from 5000 to 12,000 white blood cells (WBCs)/mL, overlaps that of appendicitis. In one series, only 25% of patients with proven appendicitis had WBC counts above 15,000, 50% had WBC counts ranging between 10,000 and 15,000, and 25% had less than 10,000 WBCs/mL.[32] Urinalysis, a useful adjunct in the workup of appendicitis, again presents a dilemma in pregnancy. Urinary tract infection and asymptomatic bacteriuria are common in pregnancy, as the enlarging uterus compresses the right ureter. Dilatation and stagnant flow in the right collecting system can contribute to bacterial overgrowth and infection. Pyuria without bacteria can also indicate involvement of the right ureter in the appendiceal inflammatory process. The presence of pyuria or bacteriuria does not rule out appendiceal inflammation, because the two conditions may coexist in 40% of pregnant patients.[30]

Imaging

Ultrasonography is the initial nonionizing imaging modality of choice in patients with suspected appendicitis. Findings suggesting appendicitis include visualization of a blind-ending tubular structure with a diameter greater than 6 mm, wall thickness greater than 3 mm, and lack of peristalsis (**Fig. 12.5**).[33] The utility of ultrasonography may be limited by patient body habitus, intraluminal air, and operator level of experience. Distortion of anatomic landmarks and displacement of the appendix make ultrasonography more challenging during pregnancy. Other structures, such as an inflamed salpinx, can also mimic appendicitis on ultrasonogram.[34] Chest radiography should be considered in the evaluation of patients with suspected appendicitis because right lower lobe pneumonia may manifest with lower abdominal pain.

CT is a highly reliable modality for the diagnosis of appendicitis. Appendiceal CT with rectally administered contrast can be performed within 10 to 20 minutes and does not require a waiting period for oral contrast to progress down through the cecum; it also exposes the patient to only one-third the radiation of a regular CT scan.[35] CT findings of appendicitis

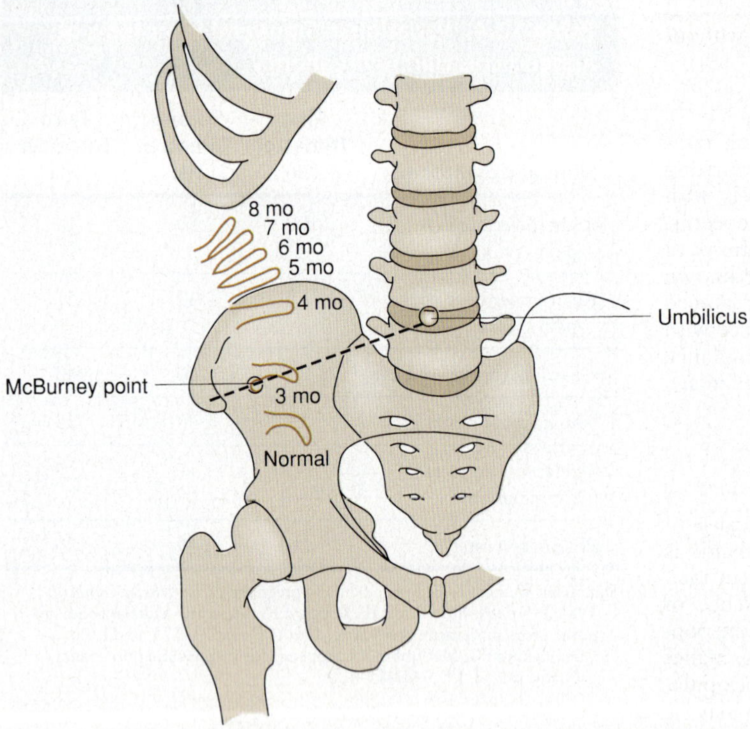

Figure 12.4. Changing location of the appendix throughout gestation.

in pregnant women are the same as in nonpregnant individuals, aside from the altered appendiceal position. Radiation exposure is 300 mrad with a limited helical CT scan, which is one-third the amount of a typical abdominopelvic CT scan.[36] Because in utero radiation exposure may increase the incidence of childhood cancer, CT should be selectively utilized in pregnant patients when the clinical history, physical examination, and imaging are indeterminate (**Fig. 12.6**).

MRI utilizes nonionizing radiation and, like CT, has the potential to image the whole abdomen. Again, imaging findings in appendicitis are unchanged from the general population. Additionally, a normal appendix on MRI has a high specificity (98% to 100%) and negative predictive value (94% to 100%) for excluding acute appendicitis.[37] Intravenous gadolinium contrast has no known adverse effects in humans but its use should be based on whether the potential benefits to the patient exceed theoretical risks to the fetus.[38]

Diagnostic Laparoscopy

When unable to satisfactorily rule out appendicitis by other means, laparoscopy may be used to evaluate the appendix, though this becomes more difficult during later gestation. Trocar position is shifted cranial to the gravid uterus and abdominal entry under direct visualization (the Hassan technique)

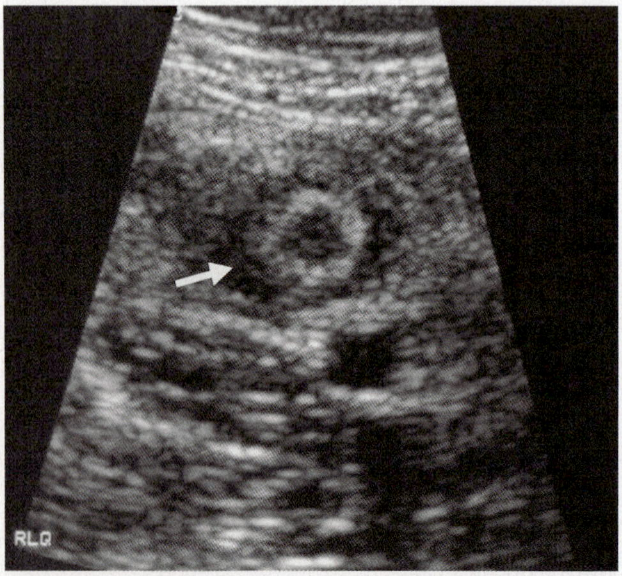

Figure 12.5. Ultrasonographic appearance of appendicitis. The appendix appears as a thick, noncompressible tubular structure with central hypoechogenicity. The walls are 5 mm thick, over the 3-mm limit for a normal appendix. (Courtesy of Dr. Beverly Coleman, Department of Radiology, Hospital of the University of Pennsylvania, Philadelphia, PA.)

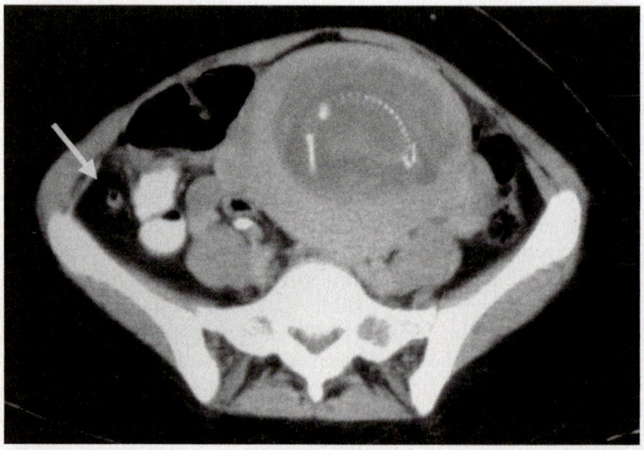

Figure 12.6. Computed tomographic (CT) scan of a woman in the 18th week of gestation presenting with a 12-hour history of right-sided abdominal pain. Abdominal examination on presentation revealed significant tenderness, and after a nondiagnostic ultrasonography, a laparotomy was considered for presumed appendicitis. A CT scan is obtained instead, revealing a normal, air-filled appendix with no sign of periappendiceal inflammation (*arrow*). The laparotomy was postponed, and 12 hours later, the patient aborted a septic fetus. An unnecessary laparotomy for an atypical presentation of chorioamnionitis was avoided by the judicious use of the CT scan. (Courtesy of Dr. David Weiss, Chestnut Hill Hospital, University of Pennsylvania Health System, Philadelphia, PA.)

Table 12.5. Guidelines for Laparoscopic Surgery During Pregnancy

1. Diagnostic laparoscopy is safe and effective when used selectively in the workup and treatment of acute abdominal processes in pregnancy.
2. Laparoscopic treatment of acute abdominal disease has the same indications in pregnant and nonpregnant patients.
3. Laparoscopy can be safely performed during any trimester of pregnancy.
4. Gravid patients should be placed in the left lateral decubitus position to minimize compression of the vena cava.
5. Initial abdominal access can be safely accomplished with an open (Hassan) technique, Veress needle, or optical trocar, if the location is adjusted according to fundal height and previous incisions.
6. CO_2 insufflation of 10–15 mm Hg can be safely used for laparoscopy in the pregnant patient.
7. Intraoperative CO_2 monitoring by capnography should be done during laparoscopy in the pregnant patient.
8. Intraoperative and postoperative pneumatic compression devices in early postoperative ambulation are recommended prophylaxes for deep venous thrombosis in the gravid patient.
9. Laparoscopic cholecystectomy is the treatment of choice in the pregnant patient with gallbladder disease, regardless of trimester.
10. Cholelithiasis during pregnancy may be managed with preoperative endoscopic retrograde cholangiopancreatography (ERCP) with sphincterotomy, followed by laparoscopic cholecystectomy, laparoscopic common bile duct exploration, or postoperative ERCP.
11. Laparoscopic appendectomy may be performed safely in pregnant patients with appendicitis.
12. Obstetric consultation can be obtained pre- and/or postoperatively on the basis of the severity of the patient's disease, gestational age, and availability of the consultant.

Adapted from the SAGES guidelines for the use of laparoscopy during pregnancy. *Surg Endosc.* 2017;31(10):3767–3782.

is thought to be the safest approach.[39] Maneuvers to enhance operative safety of laparoscopy in pregnancy have been outlined by the Society of American Gastrointestinal Endoscopic Surgeons (SAGES) (**Table 12.5**).[39]

Management

Antibiotics should be started at the time of diagnosis. The selected agent or agents should be broad spectrum and include Gram-negative and anaerobic coverage, with care taken to avoid teratogenic medications.

The surgical management of uncomplicated appendicitis in nonpregnant patients has shifted over recent years, as several high-quality randomized trials have demonstrated the safety of nonoperative management and treatment with antibiotics alone has gained popularity. However, it is critical to note that pregnant patients were excluded from all of these trials.[40,41] Additionally, observational evidence suggests significantly increased risk of harm to both the mother and fetus after failed nonoperative management of acute appendicitis.[42] As such, American and European Surgical Societies continue to recommend appendectomy as the treatment of choice for appendicitis during pregnancy.[43,44] The 2024 SAGES guideline for the use of laparoscopy during pregnancy conditionally recommends appendectomy for pregnant patients with acute appendicitis, regardless of trimester at the time of diagnosis.[43] This recommendation is based on very low-certainty evidence of reduced rates of sepsis, cesarean section and peritonitis, which are thought to outweigh slightly increased rates of pregnancy loss and preterm birth. Additionally, the American College of Obstetricians and Gynecologists (ACOG) clinical practice guideline on nonobstetric surgery during pregnancy affirms that medically necessary surgeries should never be withheld from pregnant patients due to concern over risk to the fetus.[45]

Laparoscopy is almost always used to treat appendicitis during the first two trimesters, with increased utilization of an open approach during the third trimester. Laparoscopic appendectomy is safe in all trimesters, with a complication rate similar to that for nonpregnant laparoscopy.[43] Abdominal entry may be riskier in a pregnant patient, but this can be mitigated by the use of an open Hassan technique and direct visualization of trocar insertion after careful consideration of fundal height.[39] In addition, limiting intra-abdominal pressures to less than 12 mm Hg and reducing operative time may reduce maternal hypercarbia and subsequent fetal acidosis. To date, the risks and benefits of robotic assistance for laparoscopic appendectomy during pregnancy have not been studied.

If an open approach is selected, a muscle-splitting incision is made over the *point of maximum tenderness* because the appendix typically lies beneath that point. This differs from the classic right lower quadrant paramedian incision, which usually necessitates medial retraction of the gravid uterus for exposure and thus increases the risk of precipitating premature labor. In addition, by tilting the patient 30 degrees to the left, the uterus is shifted away from the operative field and off the inferior vena cava. Because of the migration of the appendix, the classic incision over McBurney point in the late second and third trimesters is not optimal. If diffuse peritonitis is present, a midline incision is usually performed. Perforated appendicitis or pus in the abdominal cavity demands thorough peritoneal cleansing along with the appendectomy. A periappendiceal abscess, just as with nonpregnant patients, can be treated with percutaneous drainage, followed by an interval appendectomy 2 to 3 months later.

If exploration reveals a normal appendix, an appendectomy still should be performed; removal of the normal appendix adds little to morbidity while eliminating potential confusion if symptoms recur.[30] Unless there is perforation, antimicrobial therapy can be discontinued postoperatively, and the duration of therapy in perforated appendicitis should be the same as that in nonpregnant patients.

BILIARY TRACT DISEASE IN PREGNANCY

Acute cholecystitis is the second most common nonobstetric
8 indication for surgery in pregnant women.[28] Pregnancy and the postpartum period appear to predispose women to gallstone formation. This is attributed to hormonal changes during pregnancy that result in biliary stasis, prolonged intestinal transit, and increased cholesterol saturation of bile. Multiparity and obesity are two major independent risk factors for cholelithiasis in pregnancy. One study found that gallstones occurred in 7% of nulliparous women versus 19% of women with two or more pregnancies. This risk of gallstones appears to increase throughout gestation, with sludge or stones found in 5% of 3254 prospectively studied women in the first trimester, 8% in the second trimester, and 10% by 4 to 6 weeks after delivery.[46] However, among women with sludge or stones, only 1% developed symptoms attributable to the gallbladder during pregnancy.[28] Despite the increased incidence of cholelithiasis during pregnancy, the incidence of acute cholecystitis is unchanged. Data suggest that cholecystitis affects only 0.1% of pregnant women.[28] Most patients with symptomatic gallstones present with complaints of typical biliary colic, likely resulting from gallbladder contractions and increased pressure and luminal expansion, characteristically exacerbated by a fatty meal. Less frequently, the symptoms are those of one of the complications of gallstones: acute cholecystitis, cholangitis, or pancreatitis. Signs and symptoms are the same as those in nonpregnant patients, discussed elsewhere in this text.

Laboratory studies should be normal in patients with uncomplicated cholelithiasis. However, mild elevations in serum aminotransferases and amylase may occur after passage of small stones or sludge. It is important to note that serum alkaline phosphatase levels increase during pregnancy because of production of an alkaline phosphatase isozyme by the placenta. Significant elevations in aminotransferases, hyperamylasemia, or increased direct bilirubin may be signs of complicated gallbladder disease. The differential diagnosis includes appendicitis, pancreatitis, peptic ulcer disease, pyelonephritis, right-sided pneumonia, acute fatty liver of pregnancy, and preeclampsia.

Abdominal ultrasound is a reliable diagnostic tool for identifying gallstones, sludge, and acute or chronic cholecystitis, with a high sensitivity and specificity.[28] A diagnosis of acute cholecystitis is supported by the presence of sludge or stones, gallbladder distention, gallbladder wall thickening, and/or pericholecystic fluid on ultrasonography. Transabdominal ultrasonography is relatively insensitive for the detection of common bile duct stones, whereas endoscopic ultrasound is 9
highly accurate for that purpose. Magnetic resonance cholangiopancreatography (MRCP) may be used when extrahepatic ductal stones are suspected or in cases when ultrasound is nondiagnostic. Endoscopic retrograde cholangiopancreatography (ERCP), with its associated radiation exposure, can be performed safely in pregnant patients but should be limited to cases in which treatment of ductal stones is required.

Management of Symptomatic Cholelithiasis and Acute Cholecystitis

While there is little high-quality evidence to guide the management of symptomatic cholelithiasis and acute cholecystitis during pregnancy, the safety of laparoscopic surgery during pregnancy is well established. As in nonpregnant patients, the decision to proceed with cholecystectomy should be based on the patient's constellation and severity of symptoms and individual preferences, as well as the potential risks and benefits of the procedure.

The 2024 SAGES guideline for the use of laparoscopic surgery during pregnancy conditionally recommends laparoscopic cholecystectomy over nonoperative management for biliary disease during any trimester of pregnancy.[43] This recommendation is based on low certainty of evidence in acute cholecystitis and very low certainty of evidence in biliary colic. SAGES provides an additional conditional recommendation based on expert opinion (due to low quality of evidence) that nonoperative management or laparoscopic cholecystectomy may be considered for biliary colic during the third trimester.[43] The development of acute cholecystitis during pregnancy is associated with increased odds of adverse pregnancy outcomes, regardless of management approach; however, management with cholecystectomy is associated with lower odds of adverse 10
outcomes compared with nonoperative management.[47]

Cholecystectomy can be performed safely and effectively during all trimesters, though the second trimester is the optimal time for laparoscopic surgery. Organogenesis is complete, and the gravid uterus is not yet large enough to impinge on the operating field. Either an open or laparoscopic approach may be chosen, however, laparoscopic cholecystectomy is the preferred technique.[43] As with nonpregnant patients, laparoscopy is associated with shorter postoperative stay, earlier diet initiation, reduced pain, and a lower rate of incisional hernia.[39] As in laparoscopic appendectomy, the risks and benefits of robotic assistance for laparoscopic cholecystectomy during pregnancy have not been specifically studied.

Management of Choledocholithiasis

Indications for evaluation of the common bile duct are no different in the pregnant patient than in the population as a whole—namely, an elevated bilirubin, a dilated common bile duct, or gallstone pancreatitis. ERCP can be performed during pregnancy.[43] With proper lead shielding, judicious use of fluoroscopy time, and avoidance of permanent roentgenographic films, ERCP has been performed with no direct exposure of the fetus to radiation. Calculated scatter radiation on the order of 4 mrad during the whole examination presents the only risk from ionizing radiation.[28] Evaluation of the biliary tree, stone retrieval, and sphincterotomy can be performed under these conditions without maternal or fetal complications.[39] SAGES conditionally recommends ERCP over laparoscopic common bile duct exploration (LCBDE) for treatment of choledocholithiasis during pregnancy; this recommendation is based on expert opinion due to the scarcity of literature on LCBDE during pregnancy and the fact that LCBDE expertise is not widespread.[43]

BREAST CANCER IN THE PREGNANT PATIENT

Breast cancer diagnosed during pregnancy poses a complex clinical situation. In general, pregnant patients should be managed by similar treatment strategies as nonpregnant patients, with a few adjustments to account for potentially teratogenic interventions. The most critical component of managing breast cancer in the pregnant patient is timing, as treatment should not be delayed due to pregnancy. The management of breast cancer in pregnant patients is discussed in detail elsewhere within this text.

MANAGEMENT OF THE PREGNANT PATIENT WITH TRAUMA

The most important principle of managing the pregnant patient after major trauma is that any diagnostic test or treatment should be performed if that intervention is required to save the mother's life, even if that intervention is potentially dangerous for the fetus. This topic is covered in detail elsewhere within this text and, therefore, will not be addressed in detail here.

SUMMARY

Management of the pregnant patient poses unique challenges for the general surgeon. A thorough understanding of the unique anatomic and physiologic characteristics of mother and fetus is necessary. While the first priority of surgical management of the pregnant patient is ensuring the health and safety of the mother, a surgeon must constantly be aware of the effects that interventions may have on the fetus. We have reviewed the diagnostic and therapeutic management strategies for the most common surgical pathologies encountered during pregnancy. A multidisciplinary approach to the pregnant patient is ideal for ensuring the safety of the mother and the fetus.

ACKNOWLEDGMENTS

We gratefully acknowledge the contributions of previous edition authors, Eugene S. Kim and Michael J. Zobel, as portions of those chapters have been retained in this revision.

References

1. Spong CY. Maternal physiology. In: Cunningham FG, Leveno KJ, Bloom SL, et al., eds. *Williams Obstetrics*. 24th ed. McGraw-Hill Companies; 2014:46–77.
2. Verburg BO, Steegers EA, De Ridder M, et al. New charts for ultrasound dating of pregnancy and assessment of fetal growth: longitudinal data from a population-based cohort study. *Ultrasound Obstet Gynecol*. 2008;31(4):388–396.

3. Moore K, Persaud T. *The Developing Human*. 8th ed. WB Saunders; 2008.
4. Carlo WA, McDonald SA, Fanaroff AA, et al. Association of antenatal corticosteroids with mortality and neurodevelopmental outcomes among infants born at 22 to 25 weeks' gestation. *JAMA*. 2011;306(21):2348–2358.
5. Romero R, Avila C, Brekus CA, Morotti R. The role of systemic and intrauterine infection in preterm parturition. *Ann N Y Acad Sci*. 1991;622:355–375.
6. WHO recommendation on tocolytic therapy for improving preterm birth outcomes. World Health Organization; 2022. Licence: CC BY-NC-SA 3.0 IGO.
7. Hon EH. The fetal heart rate patterns preceding death in utero. *Am J Obstet Gynecol*. 1959;78(1):47–56.
8. Paul RH, Suidan AK, Yeh S, Schifrin BS, Hon EH. Clinical fetal monitoring. VII. The evaluation and significance of intrapartum baseline FHR variability. *Am J Obstet Gynecol*. 1975;123(2):206–210.
9. Chen HY, Chauhan SP, Ananth CV, et al. Electronic fetal heart rate monitoring and its relationship to neonatal and infant mortality in the United States. *Am J Obstet Gynecol*. 2011;204(6):491.e1–491.e10.
10. Miller DA, Paul R. Antepartum–intrapartum. In: Scott J, Disaia P, Hammond C, et al., eds. *Danforth's Obstetrics and Gynecology*. 8th ed. Lippincott Williams & Wilkins; 1999:243–255.
11. Kendrick JM, Neiger R. Intraoperative fetal monitoring during nonobstetric surgery. *J Perinatol*. 2000;20(4):276–277.
12. ACOG Committee on Obstetric Practice. ACOG Committee Opinion No. 474: nonobstetric surgery during pregnancy. *Obstet Gynecol*. 2011;117(2 Pt 1):420–421.
13. Otake M, Schull WJ. A review of forty-five years study of Hiroshima and Nagasaki atomic bomb survivors. Radiation cataract. *J Radiat Res*. 1991;32(Suppl):283–293.
14. Wertelecki W. Malformations in a chornobyl-impacted region. *Pediatrics*. 2010;125(4):e836–e843.
15. Groen RS, Bae JY, Lim KJ. Fear of the unknown: ionizing radiation exposure during pregnancy. *Am J Obstet Gynecol*. 2012;206(6):456–462.
16. Harrison JD, Stather JW. The assessment of doses and effects from intakes of radioactive particles. *J Anat*. 1996;189(Pt 3):521–530.
17. Wagner L, Lester R, Saldana L. *Exposure of the Pregnant Patient to Diagnostic Radiation*. Medical Physics Publishing; 1997.
18. Brent RL. Saving lives and changing family histories: appropriate counseling of pregnant women and men and women of reproductive age, concerning the risk of diagnostic radiation exposures during and before pregnancy. *Am J Obstet Gynecol*. 2009;200(1):4–24.
19. Donnelly EH, Smith JM, Farfan EB, et al. Prenatal radiation exposure: background material for counseling pregnant patients following exposure to radiation. *Disaster Med Public Health Prep*. 2011;5(1):62–68.
20. Brent RL. The effect of embryonic and fetal exposure to x-ray, microwaves, and ultrasound: counseling the pregnant and nonpregnant patient about these risks. *Semin Oncol*. 1989;16(5):347–368.
21. Wood JW, Keehn RJ, Kawamoto S, et al. The growth and development of children exposed in utero to the atomic bombs in Hiroshima and Nagasaki. *Am J Public Health Nations Health*. 1967;57(8):1374–1380.
22. Doll R, Wakeford R. Risk of childhood cancer from fetal irradiation. *Br J Radiol*. 1997;70:130–139.
23. American College of Obstetricians and Gynecologists. ACOG Practice Bulletin No. 101: ultrasonography in pregnancy. *Obstet Gynecol*. 2009;113(2 Pt 1):451–461.
24. American Institute of Ultrasound in Medicine. AIUM practice guideline for the performance of obstetric ultrasound examinations. *J Ultrasound Med*. 2013;32(6):1083–1101.
25. Shetty MK. Abdominal computed tomography during pregnancy: a review of indications and fetal radiation exposure issues. *Semin Ultrasound CT MR*. 2010;31(1):3–7.
26. Yousefzadeh DK, Ward MB, Reft C. Internal barium shielding to minimize fetal irradiation in spiral chest CT: a phantom simulation experiment. *Radiology*. 2006;239(3):751–758.
27. Ray JG, Vermeulen MJ, Bharatha A, Montanera WJ, Park AL. Association between MRI exposure during pregnancy and fetal and childhood outcomes. *JAMA*. 2016;316(9):952–961.
28. Gilo NB, Amini D, Landy HJ. Appendicitis and cholecystitis in pregnancy. *Clin Obstet Gynecol*. 2009;52(4):586–596.
29. Mazze RI, Kallen B. Appendectomy during pregnancy: a Swedish registry study of 778 cases. *Obstet Gynecol*. 1991;77(6):835–840.
30. Weingold AB. Appendicitis in pregnancy. *Clin Obstet Gynecol*. 1983;26(4):801–809.
31. Baer JL, Reis RA, Arens RA. Appendicitis in pregnancy. *JAMA*. 1932;98:1359–1364.
32. Babaknia A, Parsa H, Woodruff JD. Appendicitis during pregnancy. *Obstet Gynecol*. 1977;50(1):40–44.
33. Freeland M, King E, Safcsak K, et al. Diagnosis of appendicitis in pregnancy. *Am J Surg*. 2009;198(6):753–758.
34. Paulman AA, Huebner DM, Forrest TS. Sonography in the diagnosis of acute appendicitis. *Am Fam Physician*. 1991;44(2):465–468.
35. Rao PM, Rhea JT, Novelline RA, et al. Helical CT combined with contrast material administered only through the colon for imaging of suspected appendicitis. *AJR Am J Roentgenol*. 1997;169(5):1275–1280.
36. Ames Castro M, Shipp TD, Castro EE, et al. The use of helical computed tomography in pregnancy for the diagnosis of acute appendicitis. *Am J Obstet Gynecol*. 2001;184(5):954–957.
37. Long SS, Long C, Lai H, et al. Imaging strategies for right lower quadrant pain in pregnancy. *AJR Am J Roentgenol*. 2011;196(1):4–12.
38. Gilk T, Kanal E. Interrelating sentinel event alert #38 with the ACR guidance document on MR safe practices: 2013. An MRI accreditation safety review tool. *J Magn Reson*. 2013;37(3):531–543.
39. Pearl JP, Price RR, Tonkin AE, Richardson WS, Stefanidis D. SAGES guidelines for the use of laparoscopy during pregnancy. *Surg Endosc*. 2017;31(10):3767–3782.
40. CODA Collaborative; Flum DR, Davidson GH, et al. A randomized trial comparing antibiotics with appendectomy for appendicitis. *N Engl J Med*. 2020;383(20):1907–1919.
41. Salminen P, Sippola S, Haijanen J, et al. Antibiotics versus placebo in adults with CT-confirmed uncomplicated acute appendicitis (APPAC III): randomized double-blind superiority trial. *Br J Surg*. 2022;109(6):503–509.
42. Ashbrook M, Cheng V, Sandhu K, et al. Management of complicated appendicitis during pregnancy in the US. *JAMA Netw Open*. 2022;5(4):e227555.
43. Kumar SS, Collings AT, Wunker C, et al. SAGES guidelines for the use of laparoscopy during pregnancy. *Surg Endosc*. 2024;38(6):2947–2963.
44. Adamina M, Andreou A, Arezzo A, et al. EAES rapid guideline: systematic review, meta-analysis, GRADE assessment, and evidence-informed European recommendations on appendicitis in pregnancy. *Surg Endosc*. 2022;36(12):8699–8712.
45. ACOG Committee Opinion No. 775: Nonobstetric surgery during pregnancy. *Obstet Gynecol*. 2019;133(4):e285–e286.
46. Ko CW, Napolitano PG, Lee SP, et al. Physical activity, maternal metabolic measures, and the incidence of gallbladder sludge or stones during pregnancy: a randomized trial. *Am J Perinatol*. 2014;31(1):39–48.
47. Hantouli MN, Droullard DJ, Nash MG, et al. Operative vs nonoperative management of acute cholecystitis during the different trimesters of pregnancy. *JAMA Surg*. 2024;159(1):28–34.

13

Measuring the Quality of Surgical Care: Surgeons, Hospitals, Systems, and Neighborhoods

Andrew M. Ibrahim and Justin B. Dimick

Key Points

1. Quality measures fall into three categories: structure, process, and outcomes. Health care structure refers to fixed attributes of the system in which patients receive care. Process of care measures are the clinical details of care provided to patients. Outcome measures reflect the end result of care, from a clinical perspective or as judged by the patient.
2. Common widely adopted programs for national surgery quality improvement rely on sampling of cases that may misclassify more than half of high- or low-performing hospitals.
3. Choosing the right measure depends on whether the underlying goal is (a) quality improvement–raising the level of performance for all providers or (b) optimizing delivery–directing patients to providers and hospitals best aligned to their needs.
4. Choosing the right measure also relies on the characteristics of the procedure. For example, high-volume procedures with frequent complications (eg, colorectal surgery) are well suited for measuring outcomes. In contrast, less common operations with frequent complications (eg, Whipple) may be better evaluated with structure.
5. Measurement alone rarely results in quality improvement and should be coupled with meaningful plans for intervention targeting a specific goal.
6. To make comparisons fair, quality outcome measures often need to be risk adjusted using various techniques. In addition, when sample size is small, statistical techniques such as reliability adjustments also need to be applied.
7. Surgical quality can be measured at multiple levels including individual surgeon, hospital, and health system levels. In parallel, there is a growing recognition to understand the broader context of where patients live—before and after hospitalization for surgery—and how that may impact our common measures of surgical quality. Proposals for neighborhood and social risk adjustment are being considered as way to measure quality of surgical care delivered.

With growing recognition that the quality of surgical care varies widely, good measures of performance are in high demand. Patients and their families need accurate information to help them choose the safest hospitals for surgery.[1] Employers and payers need reliable measures for their value-based purchasing programs.[2] Motivated in part by these external pressures, clinical leaders need better measures to guide their quality improvement efforts.[3]

Despite a broadening array of measures, there remains considerable uncertainty about which measures are most useful. Current measures are remarkably heterogeneous, encompassing different elements of health care structure, process, and outcomes. With the proliferation of value-based purchasing, which requires a global assessment of quality that has significant implications on reimbursement, growing attention has been placed on evaluating the performance measures themselves.[4,5] Although each of these measurement approaches has strengths, each is also associated with conceptual, methodologic, and/or practical problems (**Table 13.1**).

This chapter provides an overview of existing quality indicators, followed by a review of the main strengths and limitations of each type of measure: structure, process, and outcomes. For common limitations, the chapter outlines established statistical techniques now applied routinely in measuring surgical quality. The chapter then closes with how these measurement tools are moving from evaluating surgeons and hospitals toward the performance across an entire health care system and the community context in which they deliver care.

TRADITIONAL QUALITY MEASURES

1 Quality measures fall into three categories: structure, process, and outcomes.

Structure

Health care structure refers to fixed attributes of the system in which patients receive care. Many structural measures describe hospital-level attributes, such as the resources or staff coordination and organization (eg, nurse-to-patient ratios, hospital teaching status). Other structural measures reflect attributes of individual physicians (eg, subspecialty board certification, procedure volume).

Strengths

Structural measures of quality have several attractive features. First, they are strongly related to patient outcomes. For example, many of our complex operations (eg, esophagectomy and pancreatic resection), operative mortality rates at high-volume hospitals are often 10% lower, in absolute terms, than low-volume centers. In some instances, structural measures such as procedure volume are more predictive of subsequent hospital performance than any known processes of care or even direct mortality measures.[6]

Table 13.1. Examples, Strengths, and Limitations of Different Approaches to Measuring Surgical Performance

	Examples	Strengths	Limitations
Structure	Hospital or surgeon volume Surgeon specialty training	Inexpensive and readily available Strong relationship to important outcomes	Not actionable for quality improvement Not good at discriminating individual provider performance
Process	Appropriate selection, timing, and duration of antibiotic prophylaxis Use of internal mammary artery for coronary artery bypass grafting	Actionable as targets for improvement Everybody can achieve 100% compliance	Most known processes relate to secondary outcomes High-leverage processes are unknown for most procedures
Outcome	Risk-adjusted mortality Risk-adjusted morbidity	Seen as the bottom line of patient care Buy in from providers	Sample sizes too small at individual hospitals

Perhaps the most important advantage of structural variables is the ease with which they can be assessed. Many can be determined using readily available sources, such as administrative billing data. Although some structural measures require surveying hospitals or providers, such data are much less expensive to collect than measures requiring detailed patient-level information.

Limitations

The use of structure for quality measure has two primary limitations. First, structure is not readily actionable for most hospitals. For example, a small hospital cannot readily make itself a high-volume center. In fact, many small, low-volume hospitals exist within a network with a high-volume hospital in their system.[7] Such a finding underscores the potential challenges of achieving higher volume within a network. Second, these measures are also limited in their ability to discriminate between the performance of individual providers. Capturing quality differences of an individual surgeon may take hundreds of operations before a quality concern is identified. As such, this measure tends to be used at the hospital level with volumes that are higher.

Process of Care

Process of care measures are the clinical details of care provided to patients. Although long the predominant quality indicators for medical care, their popularity in surgery ebbs and flows. Common process measures are often managed through checklists and have predominantly focused on the wrong-site surgery, prevention of surgical site infections, postoperative cardiac events, venous thromboembolism, and respiratory complications.

Strengths

Since processes of care reflect the care actually delivered by physicians, they have face validity and enjoy greater buy-in from providers. They are also directly actionable and provide good substrate for quality improvement activities. Moreover, process measures have a lower overhead burden because they do not require the additional risk adjustment that is needed for outcomes. For example, the appropriate prophylaxis against postoperative venous thromboembolism is a widely used process measure. Since virtually all patients undergoing open abdominal surgery should be offered some form of prophylaxis, there is little need to collect detailed clinical data for risk adjustment.

Limitations

The biggest limitation of process measures is the lack of correlation between processes of care and important outcomes. For example, adherence to the Joint Commission and CMS process measures for acute myocardial infarction explained only 6% of the observed variation in risk-adjusted mortality for acute myocardial infarction.[8] Similarly, in surgery, several studies have failed to identify improvement in surgical site infections related to adherence to SCIP measures.[9] Even adherence to a broad collection of process measures, such as those needed to become a bariatric center of excellence, fails to correlate with improved surgical outcomes.[10]

There are several reasons why existing process measures explain very little of the variation in important surgical outcomes. First, most process measures currently used in surgery relate to secondary outcomes. While none would dismiss the value of prophylactic antibiotics in reducing risks of superficial wound infection, this process is not related to the most important adverse events of major surgery, including death.

Second, process measures in surgery often relate to complications that are very rare. In fact, process measures are often used instead of outcome measures because the outcomes are too rare to detect meaningful differences in quality.

Outcomes

Outcome measures reflect the end result of care, from a clinical perspective or as judged by the patient. Although mortality is by far the most commonly used measure in surgery, other outcomes that could be used as quality indicators include complications, hospital readmission, and a variety of patient-centered measures of quality of life or satisfaction. For example, a recent evaluation of Medicare revealed that a significant drop in hospital readmissions among surgical patients after payment incentives were announced. While some readmissions after surgery may in fact be good and represent high-quality care, the significant drop suggests that there were also avoidable readmissions that were prevented.[11]

Strengths

There are at least two key advantages of outcome measures. First, outcome measures have obvious face validity, and thus, are likely to get the greatest "buy-in" from hospitals and surgeons. Surgeon enthusiasm for adopting objective measurement of quality and joining quality collaboratives centered on outcomes clearly underlines this point. Second, outcomes are also seen as valuable by payers. As such, many payers are willing to place incentives and resources around agreed-upon measures. For example, CMS recently announce a new TEAMS model that will, beginning 2026, place financial incentives around quality measures for major surgery.[12] This represents an opportunity for hospitals to be rewarded for improving outcomes seen as valid.

Limitations

Hospital- or surgeon-specific outcome measures are severely constrained by small sample sizes. For the large majority of surgical procedures, very few hospitals (or surgeons) have sufficient adverse events (numerators) and cases (denominators) for meaningful, procedure-specific measures of morbidity or mortality. As such, data either needs to be aggregated over multiple surgeons, multiple sites, or multiple years to generate enough statistical power to identify meaningful differences.

2 Another significant limitation of outcome assessment is the expense of data collection. Reporting outcomes requires the costly collection of detailed clinical data for risk adjustment. For example, it costs over $125,000 annually for a private sector hospital to participate in the ACS-NSQIP. Because of the expense of data collection, the ACS-NSQIP currently collects data on only a sample of patients undergoing surgery at each hospital. Although this sampling strategy decreases the cost of data collection, it creates new challenges. For example, a recent study of hospital quality found that such sampling strategies identify less than half of the hospitals with higher-than-expected postoperative mortality.[13]

CHOOSING THE RIGHT MEASURE

3 No quality measure is perfect. Clinical leaders, patient advo-
4 cates, payers, and policy makers will have to make decisions about when imperfect measures are good enough to act upon. A measure should be implemented only with the expectation that acting on it will result in net improvement in health quality. Thus, the direct benefits of implementing a particular measure cannot be outweighed by the indirect harms. Unfortunately, these benefits and harms are often difficult to measure and heavily influenced by the specific context and who—patients, payers, or providers—is doing the accounting. For this reason, there is no simple answer for where to "set the bar."

3 It is important to ensure a good match between the performance measure and the primary goal of measurement. The right measure depends on whether the underlying goal is (a) quality improvement–raising the performance of all providers or (b) selective referral–directing patients to higher-quality hospitals and/or providers. Although many pay-for-performance initiatives have both goals, one often predominates. For example, the ultimate objective of the CMS's pay-for-performance initiatives are improving quality at all hospitals (quality improvement).[12] Conversely, the Leapfrog Group's efforts, which sets minimum volume standards for high-risk operations, are primarily aimed at getting patients to hospitals likely to have the best outcomes (selective referral).[11]

5 For quality improvement purposes, a good performance measure must be actionable. Measurable improvements in the given process should translate to clinically meaningful improvements in patient outcomes. Although quality improvement activities are rarely "harmful," their major downsides relate to their opportunity cost. Initiatives hinged on bad measures divert resources (eg, time and focus of physicians and other staff) away from more productive activities.

With selective referral, a good measure will steer patients to better hospitals or physicians. As a basic litmus test, a measure based on prior performance should reliably identify providers likely to have superior performance now and in the future. At the same time, an ideal measure would not incentivize perverse behaviors (eg, surgeons doing unnecessary procedures to meet a specific volume standard) or negatively affect other domains of quality (eg, patient autonomy, access, and satisfaction).

Many believe that a good performance measure must discriminate performance at the individual level. From the provider perspective in particular, a "fair" measure must reliably reflect the performance of individual hospitals or physicians. Unfortunately, as described earlier, small caseloads (and sometimes case mix variation) conspire against this objective for most procedures. Patients, however, should value information that improves their odds of good outcomes on average. Many measures meet this latter interest while failing on the former (eg, hospital volume standards). There may be no simple solution to resolving the basic tension implied by performance measures that are unfair to providers yet informative for patients. However, it underscores the importance of being clear about both the primary purpose (quality improvement or selective referral) and whose interests are receiving top priority (provider or patient).

IMPROVING OUR ABILITY TO MEASURE

6 Over the last two decades significant progress has been made in the science of quality measurement for surgical outcomes addressing two major constraints: low volume and appropriate risk adjustment.

Low Volume

At noted multiple times throughout, one of the biggest limitations of surgical quality measurement is the statistical "noise" from the small sample sizes at most hospitals. This problem makes it difficult to isolate the quality signal from the background statistical noise. In other words, it is often hard to know whether hospitals or surgeons have poor performance because they provide low-quality care or because they were unlucky. For obvious reasons, labeling surgeons and hospitals correctly is extremely important.

Reliability adjustment directly addresses the problem of statistical noise secondary to low volume.[15] This technique, based on hierarchical modeling, quantifies and subtracts statistical noise from the measurement process. Essentially, it "shrinks" providers' performance back toward average unless they deviate to such an extreme that it is safe to assume they are truly different. A similar technique, taken from professional sports, uses cumulative probability-based metrics that weight outcomes based on volume and similar address statistical noise. Such techniques have been applied to surgical quality with similar discrimination as reliability adjustment.[16]

Risk Adjustment

Risk adjustment has become an increasing area of scrutiny. Understandably, when presented with poor outcomes, many surgeons and hospitals may respond that their patients or case-mix are higher risk. Traditional approaches to handling these differences in risk have included applying a logistic regression model that takes into account these measurable differences between groups. In addition, instrumental variables may be applied that may also account for "unmeasurable" differences between groups to help mimic true randomization.[17]

Additional strategies aiming to achieve better risk adjustment for surgical outcomes include the application of machine learning algorithms, propensity weighting, and balanced entropy. These techniques are still emerging, and their advantage over traditional risk adjustment has not yet been determined.

APPROACHES TO MEASURE AND IMPROVE SURGICAL CARE ACROSS HEALTH CARE SYSTEMS

While previous measures of surgical quality have focused on individual surgeons and hospitals (as discussed above), increasing attention is now being focused on health care systems. As a result of continual mergers and acquisitions, the majority of hospitals now belong to a larger system. The interest in measuring quality of surgical care at the systems level can be understood through **Figure 13.1**. The figure displays rates of failure to rescue (death after a complication) for surgical patients across 87 hospitals in 16 major health care systems.[18] Each dot in the same column is part of the same health care system. On the far left is a health care system with low complication rates that are consistent across their system. In contrast, on the far right, the complication rates vary widely within the same system.

There are multiple reasons why measuring quality at the health care system level has appeal. First, doing so reflects the day-to-day reality of health care leadership who now assume

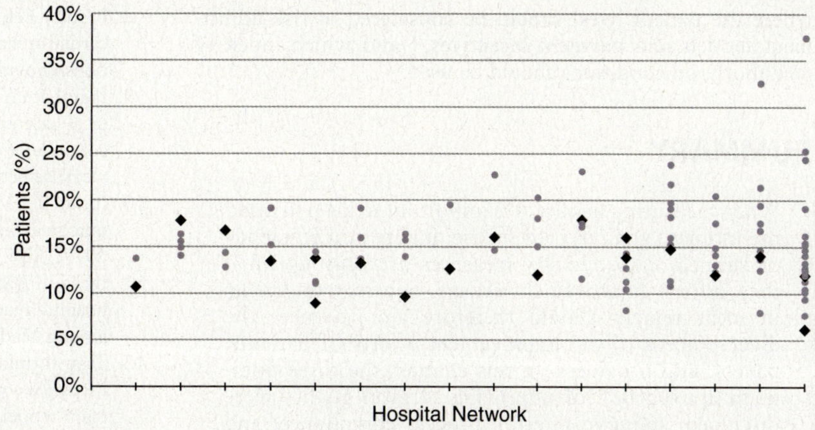

Figure 13.1. Variation in failure to rescue rates within and across hospital systems. Each dot is a hospital, and each column of dots is within the same health care system. (Modified from Sheetz KH, Claflin J, Dimick JB. Trends in the adoption of robotic surgery for common surgical procedures. *JAMA Netw Open*. 2020;3(1):e1918911.)

responsibility for care delivery across multiple sites. Second, payers and policy makers have increasingly explored and adopted systems-level metrics as a novel way to incentivize quality. Third, patients now increasingly recognize the trusted brand of a health care system and assume uniform quality across multiple sites of care. Taken together, systems-level metrics reflect an optimism that the parts together can function at a higher quality than when they were alone by taking advantage of shared resources and expertise.

As our expertise around hospital networks grows, we focus on three domains that build on previous quality measures and apply them toward measuring health care system (**Fig. 13.2**).

Centralize Complex Procedures

Multiple surgical procedures, particularly those that are high risk, have known volume–outcome relationships. With the creation of new hospital networks, it has become fertile ground for in-network regionalization. The percentage of patients undergoing high-risk procedures at a high-volume center could be an important systems metric. For example, a recent evaluation by Kalata and colleagues[7] demonstrated that 79% of patients undergoing high-risk surgery at a low-volume center had a high-volume hospital in the same network with a median travel distance of only 29 miles.

Decentralize Ambulatory Procedures

With accumulated assets of a newly formed network, surgical procedures can be provided at multiple sites. For common procedures that are low risk, these can be performed at multiple sites that have lower overhead and are located closer to patients. In doing so, health care systems can improve access for patients and also decrease the cost of the procedure. Measures to assess this level of systems delivery could include patient travel time and procedure expenses.

Delivery Coordination

As patients will likely move across multiple sites within a health care system, there will need to be ways to measure how well their care is coordinated. Possible measures may include patient wait times or redundant tests and imaging.

These collective strategies are increasingly becoming more common among hospital leaders as possible levers to improve surgical quality across their newly formed network.

EMERGING NEEDS TO UNDERSTAND AND MEASURE THE NEIGHBORHOODS OF OUR PATIENTS

7 Traditional hospital quality measurement and improvement for surgery has focused on what happens within the hospital. However, we are increasingly understanding that several factors outside of the hospitals, such as the patient's neighborhood environment, likely influence their outcomes after surgery. For example, Diaz and colleagues identified a 23% increase in risk-adjusted rates of mortality after common surgical operations based on the patient's neighborhood exposure to historic housing discrimination.[19] Similarly, Bonner and colleagues identified that the extent of neighborhood deprivation translates to a higher cost of $2654 for an episode of surgical care.[20] Such findings have led payers to consider whether or not these additional factors (eg, neighborhood conditions

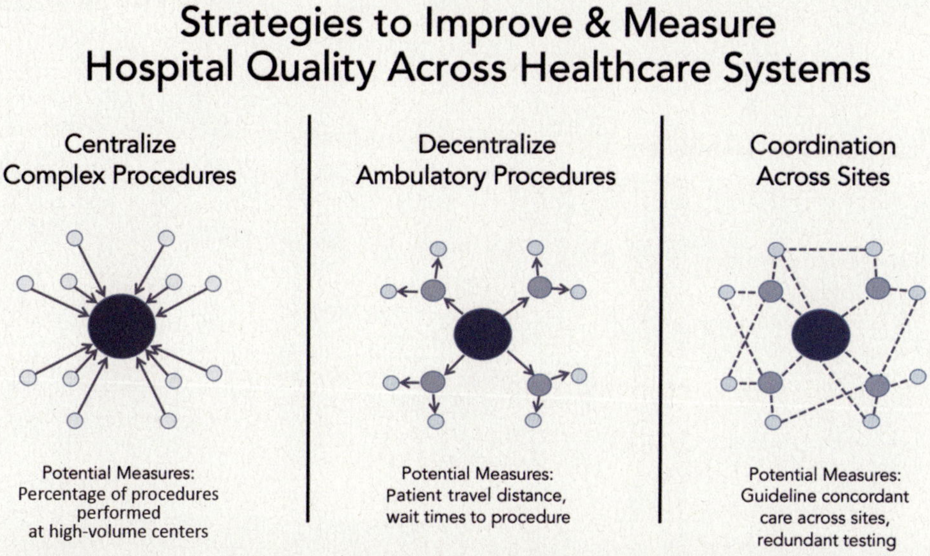

Figure 13.2. Measuring and improving systems delivery of surgical care.

SCIENTIFIC PRINCIPLES

where the patient lives) should be considered in risk-adjustment models and payment incentives,[21] and which index of neighborhood conditions should be used.[22]

SUMMARY

When measuring quality, it is important to keep in mind the ultimate goal: improving the quality and efficiency of surgical care. Quality measures are only useful if they inform improvement efforts. Future refinements in measurement should therefore aim to meet the diverse needs of the improvement efforts of patients, payers, and providers. In this chapter, the three dominant approaches for improving surgical quality were discussed: selective referral, process compliance, and outcome measurement. These three policy approaches roughly mirror the three types of quality measures (structure, process, and outcomes), providing real-world examples of how various stakeholders weigh the pros and cons of quality indicators and ultimately choose an assessment approach by matching the measure to the purpose.

References

1. Diaz A, Harbaugh C, Dimick JB, Kunnath N, Ibrahim AM. Variation in postoperative outcomes across federally designated hospital star ratings. *JAMA Surg*. 2024;159(8):918–926.
2. Joynt Maddox KE, Shashikumar SA, Ryan AM. Medicare's bundled payment models-progress and pitfalls. *JAMA*. 2022;327(18):1761–1762.
3. Liao JM, Wong SL, Chu D. Going beyond one size fits all in surgical bundled payments. *JAMA Surg*. 2020. Online ahead of print.
4. Bilimoria KY. Facilitating quality improvement: pushing the pendulum back toward process measures. *JAMA*. 2015;314(13):1333–1334.
5. Bilimoria KY, Barnard C. An Evolving hospital quality star rating system from CMS: aligning the stars. *JAMA*. 2021;325(21):2151–2152.
6. Ibrahim AM, Dimick JB. What Metrics Accurately Reflect Surgical Quality? *Annu Rev Med*. 2018;69:481–491.
7. Kalata S, Schaefer SL, Nuliyahu U, Ibrahim AM, Nathan H. Low-volume elective surgery and outcomes in Medicare beneficiaries treated at hospital networks. *JAMA Surg*. 2024;159(2):203–210.
8. Bradley EH, Herrin J, Elbel B, et al. Hospital quality for acute myocardial infarction: correlation among process measures and relationship with short-term mortality. *JAMA*. 2006;296(1):72–78.
9. Ingraham AM, Cohen ME, Bilimoria KY, et al. Association of surgical care improvement project infection-related process measure compliance with risk-adjusted outcomes: implications for quality measurement. *J Am Coll Surg*. 2010;211(6):705–714.
10. Ibrahim AM, Ghaferi AA, Thumma JR, Dimick JB. Variation in outcomes at bariatric surgery centers of excellence. *JAMA Surg*. 2017;152(7):629–636.
11. Ibrahim AM, Nathan H, Thumma JR, Dimick JB. Impact of the hospital readmission reduction program on surgical readmissions among Medicare beneficiaries. *Ann Surg*. 2017;266(4):617–624.
12. Transforming Episode Accountability Model (TEAM). CMS.gov. https://www.cms.gov/priorities/innovation/innovationmodels/team-model
13. Chen VW, Chidi AP, Rosen T, et al. Case sampling vs universal review for evaluating hospital postoperative mortality in US surgical quality improvement programs. *JAMA Surg*. 2023;158(12):1312–1319.
14. Urbach DR. Pledging to eliminate low-volume surgery. *N Engl J Med*. 2015;373(15):1388–1390.
15. Krell RW, Hozain A, Kao LS, Dimick JB. Reliability of risk-adjusted outcomes for profiling hospital surgical quality. *JAMA Surg*. 2014;149(5):467–74.
16. Jones DW, Simons JP, Osborne NH, Schermerhorn M, Dimick JB, Schanzer A. Earned outcomes correlate with reliability-adjusted surgical mortality after abdominal aortic aneurysm repair and predict future performance. *J Vasc Surg*. 2024;80(3):715–723 e1.
17. Sheetz KH, Ibrahim AM, Regenbogen SE, Dimick JB. Surgeon experience and Medicare expenditures for laparoscopic compared to open colectomy. *Ann Surg*. 2017;268(6):1036–1042.
18. Sheetz KH, Ibrahim AM, Nathan H, Dimick JB. Variation in surgical outcomes across networks of the highest-rated US hospitals. *JAMA Surg*. 2019;154(6):510–515.
19. Diaz A, O'Reggio R, Norman M, Thumma JR, Dimick JB, Ibrahim AM. Association of historic housing policy, modern day neighborhood deprivation and outcomes after inpatient hospitalization. *Ann Surg*. 2021;274(6):985–991.
20. Bonner SN, Kunnath N, Dimick JB, Ibrahim AM. Neighborhood deprivation and Medicare expenditures for common surgical procedures. *Am J Surg*. 2022;224(5):1274–1279.
21. Tran LD. Social risk adjustment in health care performance measures. *JAMA Netw Open*. 2020;3(6):e208020.
22. Rollings KA, Noppert GA, Griggs JJ, Ibrahim AM, Clarke PJ. Comparing deprivation vs vulnerability index performance using medicare beneficiary surgical outcomes. *JAMA Surg*. 2024;159(12):1404–1413.

Improving Surgical Quality

Kristan L. Staudenmayer

Key Points

1. Metrics are key to improvement, but it is important to understand the strengths and limitations of each metric used.
2. The foundation for quality metrics in health care was established by Donabedian in 1966 when he proposed using the framework of structure, process, and outcome to evaluate quality.
3. Improving the quality with which we conduct quality improvement efforts is increasingly seen as important.
4. High-reliability organizations have been associated with improved outcomes.
5. Payers and regulators continue moving toward value-based payment models to improve quality.

The landmark publication by the Institute of Medicine in 2000, "To Err is Human," raised the alarm bells on the state of quality in health care in the United States.[1] The report estimated that 44,000 to 98,000 lives were lost in hospitals every year as a result of medical errors, and that costs from medical errors were estimated to be as high as $29 billion. The last three decades have seen much work go into quality improvement. Despite some successes,[2,3] issues still remain, such as preventable mortality and morbidity, disparities in outcomes, and medical errors.[4] This suggests that we have not yet fully achieved solving for quality in health care.

Quality is crucial in surgery due to its inherently invasive nature and the technical precision it demands. Historically, surgeons have led quality efforts and been deeply aware of the importance and role of quality improvement. As we move forward, it is essential for surgeons to maintain their leadership in this area, which requires a strong grasp of the key elements of quality improvement.

QUALITY METRICS

Over the years, there has been a proliferation of quality metrics.[5] Complicating matters, different metrics do not always correlate. For example, it has been shown that publicly available commercial quality awards (such as U.S. News and World Report) do not always correlate with measures of quality with regard to
1 surgical procedures.[6] Given the complexity of quality metrics, it is important to understand the history and to have a framework for how they are constructed.

2 The foundation for quality metrics in health care was established by Donabedian in 1966 when he proposed using the framework of structure, process, and outcome to evaluate quality.[7] This construct continues to guide quality efforts today. For example, process metrics are endorsed by the National Quality Forum, structural metrics are used in surgical quality programs to verify and accredit centers of excellence, and outcome metrics are promoted by various organizations such as Medicare (**Table 14.1**).

Structural metrics consist of characteristics possessed by a hospital or a provider that are associated with desired outcomes. These metrics are attractive for quality improvement as they are relatively easy to measure. The limitation of structural metrics is that they can be too high level and may not be actionable. However, there are certain cases where they may be helpful. One example is with surgical volume in specific cases. The volume–outcome relationship was first recognized as early as 1979.[8] In 2002, Birkmeyer et al. confirmed the existence of a volume–outcome relationship for selected surgical procedures,[9] and others have validated these findings. However, the relationship does not hold true for all surgical procedures, and the relationship between volume and outcomes is not linear. For example, in abdominal aneurysm repairs, there are diminishing returns in outcomes as the number of surgeries increases. It has since been recognized that there are specific scenarios in which surgical volume or other structural metrics are ideal. For example, for surgical cases that are low in volume but high in risk, such as pancreatectomies.[10,11]

Another category of quality metrics consists of process measures. Process measures are similarly easy to measure but have the added benefit of helping to identify possible quality improvement solutions. While attractive in theory, process measures have also not proved successful. One example of a process measure is the now-retired Surgical Care Improvement Project (SCIP), a collaboration between the Centers for Disease Control (CDC) and the Centers for Medicare and Medicaid Services (CMS) intended to reduce surgical site infections. SCIP process measures included the timely delivery of appropriate antibiotics and other factors known to be associated with infection (eg, hyperglycemia, hypothermia). The program was found not to improve outcomes and so was retired in 2015.[12] The reason process measures may not work is that their simplicity may not be sufficient to capture the complexity of disease. The third type of quality improvement metrics consists of outcome metrics. Outcome metrics are attractive for quality improvement because they are simple to understand (eg, mortality, length of stay, infection) and are aligned with the concept of health shared by providers and patients. Despite this, outcome metrics present different implementation challenges. Most importantly, outcome metrics can be difficult to analyze because appropriate risk adjustment is necessary and because risk adjustment can be limited by the availability of important variables.

Despite these limitations, the importance of outcomes in patient care continues to drive the use of these metrics. Two newer outcome metrics include patient-reported outcome

Table 14.1. Process Metrics

	Process	Structure	Outcomes
Example	Checklists	Surgical volume	30-d mortality
Pros	Easy to measure Based on known process–outcome relationships	Easy to measure Based on known structure–outcome relationships	Directly measures outcomes that are desired
Cons	Policies that employ these metrics are not universally successful	Policies that employ these metrics are not universally successful Might not reflect factors amenable to change	Hard to measure and analyze No single measures for all patients, conditions, or procedures

measures (PROMs) and failure to rescue (FTR). PROMs are attractive as they are derived directly from patient values. The downside is that collecting PROMs can be expensive, and that there is no standardized methodology. A recent review of PROM implementation studies in surgery found variability in how PROMs were implemented (eg, pre- or postsurgery), a lack of method to identify "success," and lack of consistent reporting of costs.[13]

FTR is another newer metric. The FTR concept is that in the case where a patient has a complication after surgery, the team can "rescue" the patient from clinical deterioration and death. While the concept is simple, the calculation and implementation of the metric have been variable. Specifically, there is variability in the number and types of complications used, in the timing of postoperative outcome measurement, as well as in how the PROM implementation efforts' success is measured.[13] Despite these complications, FTR remains a popular metric. The Agency for Healthcare Research has FTR as a Quality Patient Safety Indicator, and it is publicly reported by the Centers for Medicare and Medicaid Services Hospital Compare program.

Over time, the measurement has expanded to frameworks that encompass a more comprehensive view of patient care. One of the most influential was created by the Institute of Medicine (IOM, now the National Academies of Medicine), and includes six domains: safety, effectiveness, patient-centeredness, timeliness, efficiency, and equity.[11] An advantage to these measures is that the public can relate to the measures. They can be derived from administrative health records. While relatable, calculating the scores is complex, and improvements based on them may be difficult to implement. Further, there is a question of validity for measures derived from administrative data versus clinical data.[15]

The Agency for Healthcare Research and Quality similarly has created a suite of measures they call "Quality Indicators (QIs)".[16] The QIs are standardized, evidence-based measures that can also be derived from administrative data. These include prevention quality indicators in inpatient settings, inpatient quality indicators, patient safety indicators, pediatric quality indicators, and prevention quality indicators in emergency department settings, and Consumer Assessment of Healthcare Providers and Systems. These metrics are subject to the same limitations as those created by the IOM.

One of the newer approaches to assessing quality takes a very different approach—the review of operative videos. There is some data on how such data can be put to use; however, it remains a relatively new approach.[17] In one review of video-based studies, a positive association between surgical quality and clinical outcomes was shown.[18] Analytic approaches continue to evolve, and artificial intelligence (AI) will likely play a role in analyzing videos.

QUALITY IMPROVEMENT PROCESSES

It is known that having data and metrics is not sufficient to ensure quality. The science of quality improvement processes is just as important, and it requires specific resources, skills, and expertise.[19]

Outcome Based

3 Quality improvement is where surgeons have historically led. Peer review has served as the cornerstone of these quality efforts, and how this is done has evolved over the years. For example, one advancement has been to formalize the peer review within surgical departments to ensure fair and transparent processes. Some frameworks for this focus primarily on the system, rather than the individual surgeon. These efforts are often coupled with other activities, such as the establishment of a Surgical Quality Council within a surgical department. The American College of Surgeons has recently published a guide that describes the role of such a council, as well as how such a structure fits into the broad array of surgical quality.[20]

Extending peer review further is the development of locoregional collaboratives, where surgeons compare outcomes and best practices across hospitals in a geographic region. The leading example for this is the Michigan Surgical Quality Collaborative (MSQC). The MSQC is a collaborative of over 2000 surgeons and 70 Michigan hospitals that share data and best practices. This collaborative has been shown to both reduce complications and save costs.[3]

At the national level, quality programs evaluate hospitals' quality by specialty. Examples of these networks include the American College of Surgeons National Surgical Quality Improvement Program (ACS NSQIP). Such programs allow participants to track their progress through the regular issuance of reports and to identify best practices by learning from others in the network.

Culture and Quality

More recently has been the recognition that organizational culture can have a strong influence on quality. This has been described as a "culture of safety." The concept did not originate within health care, but in other industries where it was recognized that there were organizations that consistently
4 minimized adverse events. These companies were deemed to be "high-reliability" organizations. High-reliability companies achieved success through commitment at every level toward promoting a culture of safety. Components of such a culture involve ones where communication is founded on mutual trust, where the importance of safety is recognized at all levels of the organization, and where there is confidence that measures undertaken to improve outcomes will be successful. This contrasts with a culture that seeks to place blame on individuals and/or groups for bad outcomes. These concepts are now being applied to the challenges with improving quality in health care. Health care organizations have made resources available for those interested in improving the culture of safety, including the Agency for Healthcare Research and Quality (AHRQ),[21] the Institute for Healthcare Improvement,[22] and The Joint Commission.[23]

QUALITY IMPROVEMENT POLICY AND REGULATION—THE MOVE TOWARD VALUE

Health care is one of the most heavily regulated industries with multiple layers of quality-ensuring policies and regulations. 5 These mechanisms range from physician level (board certification and licensing) to the hospital level (The Joint Commission, and quality-based reimbursement models). Many of these mechanisms are under continuous evolution and exist in various stages of maturity. Of these, the most notable in recent history has been the shift from fee-for-service (FFS) toward value-based reimbursement. Collectively, these are called value-based purchasing (VBP) models. The notion behind VBP is that incentives in a pure FFS payment structure encourage poor quality—incursion of a complication will result in more payments to a provider rather than less. Shifting the burden of risk onto the provider financially aligns the interests of payers and providers. These reimbursement strategies are being employed by both private and public payers, and the CMS plan to transition completely from FFS to VBP models.

An example of a VBP program is the CMS Hospital-Acquired Condition (HAC) Reduction Program. The program began to reduce payments to hospitals for a list of conditions that were deemed preventable in 2008. The success of the program is still largely argued. The reason for this is due to challenges inherent to the use of outcome metrics—appropriate risk adjustment and avoidance of bias. There is no universal agreement that the HAC methodology is sufficient to produce fair results and, therefore that it can accomplish its intended goals.

Another VBP model is the concept of an Accountable Care Organization (ACO). The ACO is a provider or a collaborative of providers who work together to ensure that the patients cared for by the entity remain healthy. This is achieved through aligning incentives via capitated payments for each covered life. If an ACO can keep patients out of the hospital or from receiving costly care, it receive a greater margin. While the alignment of incentives is an attractive mechanism to ensure high-performing providers are rewarded for delivering quality care, it is not clear that these arrangements work. Initial results from the 2014 CMS ACO implementation did not show financial savings. Furthermore, with regard to surgery and ACOs, surgery has not been prioritized as a target area for improvement. Surgical-specific VBP has largely been focused on specific procedures such as hip replacement surgery or coronary artery bypass surgery.

New VBP-based programs continue to be developed, and existing programs evolve. No dominant model has yet been determined. That said, it is reasonable to expect that the concept of reimbursement based on value rather than services rendered is one that will continue to drive quality improvement efforts from payers in the foreseeable future.

SUMMARY

There are opportunities to improve the quality of surgical care at every level, from the individual provider to policymakers. Surgeons have led in the quality improvement space, and there is a need for them to continue to do so. Peer review processes and benchmarking remain a cornerstone of these efforts. It is important that surgeons continue to strive to make these even more effective tools than they are today. Furthermore, policymakers and payers require guidance from those with experience caring for surgical patients and improving quality at home as they make the change to value-based strategies. The need for continued surgical quality leadership is clear.

References

1. Kohn LT, Corrigan J, Donaldson MS, Institute of Medicine (U.S.). *Committee on Quality of Health Care in America. To err is Human: Building a Safer Health System.* National Academy Press; 2000.
2. Montroy J, Breau RH, Cnossen S, et al. Change in Adverse events after enrollment in the National Surgical Quality Improvement Program: a systematic review and meta-analysis. *PLoS One.* 2016;11(1):e0146254.
3. Share DA, Campbell DA, Birkmeyer N, et al. How a regional collaborative of hospitals and physicians in Michigan cut costs and improved the quality of care. *Health Aff (Millwood).* 2011;30(4):636–645.
4. 2023 National Healthcare Quality and Disparities Report. December 2023. (AHRQ Pub. No. 23(24)-0091-EF).
5. Yu J, Massarweh NN. Surgical quality improvement: working toward value or a work in progress? *J Surg Res.* 2019;235:160–166.
6. Cobb AN, Erickson TR, Kothari AN, et al. Commercial quality "awards" are not a strong indicator of quality surgical care. *Surgery.* 2018;164(3):379–386.
7. Ayanian JZ, Markel H. Donabedian's lasting framework for health care quality. *N Engl J Med.* 2016;375(3):205–207.
8. Luft HS, Bunker JP, Enthoven AC. Should operations be regionalized? The empirical relation between surgical volume and mortality. 1979. *Clin Orthop Relat Res.* 2007;457:3–9.
9. Birkmeyer JD, Siewers AE, Finlayson EV, et al. Hospital volume and surgical mortality in the United States. *N Engl J Med.* 2002;346(15):1128–1137.
10. Ibrahim AM, Dimick JB. What metrics accurately reflect surgical quality? *Annu Rev Med.* 2018;69:481–491.
11. Sahni NR, Dalton M, Cutler DM, Birkmeyer JD, Chandra A. Surgeon specialization and operative mortality in United States: retrospective analysis. *BMJ.* 2016;354:i3571.
12. Hawn MT, Vick CC, Richman J, et al. Surgical site infection prevention: time to move beyond the surgical care improvement program. *Ann Surg.* 2011;254(3):494–499; discussion 499–501.
13. Sokas C, Hu F, Edelen M, Sisodia R, Pusic A, Cooper Z. A review of PROM implementation in surgical practice. *Ann Surg.* 2022;275(1):85–90.
14. Institute of Medicine (U.S.). Committee on Quality of Health Care in America. *Crossing the Quality Chasm: A New Health System for the 21st Century.* National Academy Press; 2001.
15. Maass C, Kuske S, Lessing C, Schrappe M. Are administrative data valid when measuring patient safety in hospitals? A comparison of data collection methods using a chart review and administrative data. *Int J Qual Health Care.* 2015;27(4):305–313.
16. Agency for Healthcare Quality and Research (AHRQ). (2025). AHRQ Quality Indicators; Measures. https://qualityindicators.ahrq.gov/measures/qi_resources
17. O'Mahoney PR, Yeo HL, Lange MM, Milsom JW. Driving surgical quality using operative video. *Surg Innov.* 2016;23(4):337–340.
18. Gruter AAJ, Van Lieshout AS, van Oostendorp SE, et al. Video-based tools for surgical quality assessment of technical skills in laparoscopic procedures: a systematic review. *Surg Endosc.* 2023;37(6):4279–4297.
19. Ko CY, Martin G, Dixon-Woods M. Three observations for improving efforts in surgical quality improvement. *JAMA Surg.* 2022;157(12):1073–1074.
20. Surgeons TACo. *Optimal Resources for Surgical Quality and Safety.* 2021.
21. Quality AfHRa. Patient Safety Resources by Setting. https://www.ahrq.gov/patient-safety/settings/index.html
22. Improvement IoH. Patient Safety Essentials Toolkit. https://www.ihi.org/resources/tools/patient-safety-essentials-toolkit
23. Commission TJ. Patient Safety Resources. https://www.jointcommission.org/resources/patient-safety/#0dfe29bba39f4993b-3000d2e481a67d4_719da3f0a3944b58847b141864a7f45a

15

Patient Safety

Ali B. Abbasi and Elizabeth C. Wick

Key Points

1 Safety events are usually rare occurrence, but when examined in aggregate, may reveal themes.

2 Most safety events occur because of poorly defined systems as opposed to an error on the part of an individual.

3 A "just culture" requires a system of institutional accountability that prioritizes improvement and learning over assigning blame.

4 Culture, communication, and teamwork are key contributors to patient safety in the perioperative setting.

5 Emerging technologies like artificial intelligence (AI) could enhance patient safety, but could also pose novel threats.

1 In 1999, the National Academy of Medicine (NAM, formerly called the Institute of Medicine) published *To Err is Human: Building a Safer Health System,* which highlighted the large number of Americans dying every year from medical errors and has been largely credited with catalyzing the modern patient safety movement.[1] Before *To Err is Human*, it was largely believed that errors in medicine resulted from "bad apples," but the report elucidated how mistakes in health care frequently result from poor system design. Many began to draw analogies to and learn from other high-stakes industries such as aviation, pointing out how broad system reform that prioritized safety had led to better outcomes in other fields. This shift in thinking launched sweeping efforts to improve the safety of the health care delivery system in the United States, prompting important changes in measurement of safety, event reporting, culture, training, regulation, and technology. While the distinction between patient safety and quality can be blurred at times, it is important to note that patient safety is considered only one aspect of high-quality care, which is defined as care that is not only safe but also effective, patient centered, timely, efficient, and equitable.[2]

Much progress has been made over the last two decades, and we have seen significant improvements in many measures of patient safety, especially in the inpatient setting.[3] Unfortunately, the COVID-19 pandemic appears to have reversed some of the trends, as rates of health care–acquired infections increased significantly during the first year of the pandemic.[4] These developments highlight that improving patient safety requires an ongoing commitment from health care organizations, especially in complex procedural areas like operating rooms. To be effective in helping to transform surgical culture and ensuring safe care for patients, it is critical that all surgeons have a working knowledge of patient safety as well as a general awareness of the principles of improvement.

ADVERSE EVENTS AND ERRORS

In health care, adverse patient outcomes can result from both underlying disease processes and medical care received. The latter are typically referred to as adverse events, or medical harm which is defined by the Institute for Healthcare Improvement as: "unintended physical injury resulting from or contributed to by medical care (including the absence of indicated medical treatment) that requires additional monitoring, treatment, or hospitaliza-
2 tion, or that results in death."[5] Adverse events can be further subdivided into those that are thought not to be preventable, resulting from appropriate medical care without any error, and those that are preventable, resulting from errors on the part of an individual, a poorly functioning system, or a combination of both. In health care, an error or mistake is defined as "an act of commission (doing something wrong) or omission (failing to do the right thing) that leads to an undesirable outcome or significant potential for such an outcome."[6] Not all errors or mistakes lead to adverse outcomes for patients, and one that does not may be referred to as a "near miss." Within the field of patient safety, the focus has shifted from measuring and reducing errors to measuring and reducing the totality of preventable adverse events or preventable harm. It is important to acknowledge that what is defined as preventable harm may continue to evolve over time. For example, central line–associated blood stream infections (CLABSIs) were once thought not to be preventable, and now it is well established that with proper techniques and protocols in place, CLABSI rates can be driven close to zero.[7]

While medical errors can occur across all health care settings, there are some forms of harm that are unique to the perioperative area (**Table 15.1**). Some of the errors that receive the most attention include patients undergoing surgery on the wrong limb, retention of foreign objects after the patient leaves the operating room, and mislabeling of critical specimens. As the science of safety has advanced, systems have been put in place to try to prevent these events such as marking of the planned surgical site and side prior to the patient going back to the operating room (wrong-site surgery), using radio frequency identification or digital counting to account for all surgical laparotomy pads (retained foreign objects), and implementing team debriefings (mislabeled surgical specimens). But, despite these interventions, events still occur. In this chapter, we provide a brief background on patient safety; summarize the role of culture, teamwork, communication, and technology in improving safety; and highlight the importance of working toward zero preventable harms in surgical patients.

MEASUREMENT CHALLENGES

Despite advances in the field of patient safety over the last two decades, measuring safety remains an ongoing challenge,

Table 15.1. Surgical "Never Events"[a]

Surgical "Never Events"[a]
1. Surgical or Invasive Procedure Events
1A. Surgery or other invasive procedure performed on the wrong site (updated) Applicable in: hospitals, outpatient/office-based surgery centers, ambulatory practice settings/office-based practices, long-term care/skilled nursing facilities
1B. Surgery or other invasive procedure performed on the wrong patient (updated) Applicable in: hospitals, outpatient/office-based surgery centers, ambulatory practice settings/office-based practices, long-term care/skilled nursing facilities
1C. Wrong surgical or other invasive procedure performed on a patient (updated) Applicable in: hospitals, outpatient/office-based surgery centers, ambulatory practice settings/office-based practices, long-term care/skilled nursing facilities
1D. Unintended retention of a foreign object in a patient after surgery or other invasive procedure (updated) Applicable in: hospitals, outpatient/office-based surgery centers, ambulatory practice settings/office-based practices, long-term care/skilled nursing facilities
1E. Intraoperative or immediately postoperative/postprocedure death in an ASA Class 1 patient (updated) Applicable in: hospitals, outpatient/office-based surgery centers, ambulatory practice settings/office-based practices

[a]Excerpt from the National Quality Forum Never Events.

and some have aptly stated that "what you see depends on how you look."[8] For example, many health care systems have established voluntary "incident-reporting systems," in which employees can share information about errors, mistakes, and near misses. However, these databases are subject to reporting bias: It can be hard to tell whether fluctuation in the rate of reported incidents reflects changes in the culture of reporting or true changes in safety.

Voluntary reports can also perpetuate harmful biases and inequities. For example, one study suggests that physicians who are female or identify as racial or ethnic minorities might be more likely to be reported for communication issues, while others have found that white patients are overrepresented among reports filed in incident-reporting systems.[9] To better understand and mitigate these disparities, it is important to capture demographics in safety event reports, to examine safety criteria and systems for bias, and to develop measures of health equity in patient safety.[10,11]

Using administrative data, the Agency for Healthcare Research and Quality (AHRQ) developed patient safety indicators (PSIs) as triggers to identify safety issues.[12] Over time and not without controversy, PSIs have been incorporated into public-reporting and pay-for-performance programs.[12,13] Beyond administrative data and incident reporting, organizations use a variety of other tools to measure safety and identify harm, including publicly reported quality measures, retrospective chart review, trigger tools, and even patient-reported concerns. Because each of these measurement techniques has unique strengths and limitations, it is essential to avoid overly emphasizing a single source, and relying on a variety of data to track patient safety.[14–16]

SYSTEMS THINKING

A key shift in patient safety since *To err is human*, has been the realization that adverse events often occur because of poorly designed or poorly functioning systems, rather than because of the actions of a single individual The adoption of "systems" thinking in health care—the idea that humans are human and as such will inevitably make mistakes and that systems need to be designed to be resilient, mitigating the possibility of error or identifying risk before harm results—has transformed the ability to realize safety. Systems thinking often involves redesigning systems using a combination of frontline provider input, human factors principles, systems engineering, and health information technology to significantly decrease the risk of adverse events and harm. This approach results in systems that anticipate human error by simplifying processes and building in the use of tools such as checklists and read backs to create redundancy wherever possible.[17] James Reason's "Swiss cheese model" is frequently referred to when discussing how a series of defects in a system can align to cause inadvertent harm, and is worth becoming familiar with.[18]

HIGH-RELIABILITY ORGANIZATIONS

Health care is considered a high-risk industry with a high error rate, but other high-risk industries, such as nuclear power and commercial aviation, have managed to achieve and maintain an impeccably low error rate.[18] Organizations in these industries are frequently referred to as high-reliability organizations (HROs). Beyond systems thinking, these organizations are thought to encourage a collective mindfulness that is shared by all individuals in these organizations and reflected in the organizational processes. This mindfulness is made up of five basic principles: Constant preoccupation with the potential for failure regardless of when the last adverse event occurred; Reluctance to simplify procedures or explanations; Sensitivity to the operational needs of the organization and situational awareness; Deference to expertise by organizational leaders; Resilience and rapid recovery in the face of failure.[19] While most health care organizations remain far from achieving the admirably low error rate of HROs in other industries, HROs can provide a pathway for instituting a culture of safety in health care.[20]

CREATING A JUST CULTURE

3 Culture is to an organization what personality is to an individual—a difficult-to-precisely define, yet unifying set of characteristics and attributes that provide meaning and direction.[21] Historically, the culture of surgery strongly valued professional autonomy, promoting individualism over cooperation, often to the detriment of patient care.[22] Surgeons have been hesitant to discuss errors as mistakes have been equated with incompetence. Such a "blame culture" disincentivizes transparency about threats to patient safety, which stifles organizational learning.

Recently, there has been recognition of the need for developing a "just culture" that fosters an environment of trust where individuals are willing to provide essential safety-related information.[23] In a just culture, individuals are empowered to speak up because they feel psychologically safe that they will not experience negative consequences for reporting unsafe practices and because they trust that safety reports will be dispositioned in a fair process that is focused on preventing recurrence and improving the safety of the organization.[24,25] However, a just culture does not relieve individuals and organizations from accountability, but rather provides a transparent framework for response. Instances of human error are met by adapting the environment to reduce the risk of recurrence, while providing support to the individuals involved. At-risk behaviors that involve violations of established procedures are met with creating incentives for positive behavioral change and coaching the individual in question. Remedial or punitive actions are reserved for acts that are reckless or grossly negligent.[23]

Achieving a just culture requires leadership commitment to these principles, and a willingness to empower and educate all individuals in the organization from the frontlines (learners, technicians, clerks, nurses, anesthesia providers, surgeons, sterile processing staff) to the leadership (perioperative executives, chief operating officers, clinical department leadership). It also requires implementing processes for accountability and implementing open channels of communication that are free from judgment across the institution.[26]

COMMUNICATION

Research in HROs such as commercial aviation has demonstrated a strong correlation between better communication and improved safety performance. Cockpit crew members' reluctance to question a captain's judgment was long ago identified as a root cause of aviation accidents. In health care, The Joint Commission identified communication breakdown as a contributing factor in over 60% of sentinel events reported to the Joint Commission on Accreditation of Healthcare Organizations in 2011.[27]

Good communication is especially important in the OR, one of the most complex work environments in health care. Unfortunately, the traditional surgical hierarchy can prevent OR personnel from communicating openly and expressing safety concerns. One perioperative field study showed a 30% rate of communication failure in the OR, with 36% of these breakdowns having a substantial impact on patient safety.[28] It is important to note that not only the content, but also the delivery matters for excellent communication in the operating room. A study found that exposure to rude or incivil communication reduced the performance of anesthesiology residents on all performance measures in a simulated OR.[29] On the other hand, improving communication has been associated with improved patient outcomes in ICUs, decreased nurse turnover in the OR, and improved job satisfaction.[30]

MEASURING CULTURE AND COMMUNICATION

Efforts to foster cultural change within an organization with regard to patient safety have been limited in the past by the inability to measure the impact of any given intervention. However, there is evidence that improvements in culture survey scores correlate with error reduction behaviors in aviation and with decreased rates of CLABSIs in health care.[7] The Safety Attitudes Questionnaire (SAQ) and the Survey on Patient Safety Culture (SOPS) are validated survey instruments that can be used to measure culture in a health care setting.[31]

These surveys have identified significant discrepancies in perceptions regarding the safety climate. In a survey of operating room personnel across 60 hospitals, the SAQ identified substantial differences in the perception of communication in the OR depending on one's role.[32] Physicians frequently rated the teamwork of others as good, while nurses at the same institutions perceived teamwork as poor. These discrepancies can be attributed to differences in the communication skills that are valued by surgeons and nurses. For example, nurses describe good collaboration as having their input respected, while physicians describe good collaboration as having nurses who can anticipate their needs and follow instructions. Empowering well-respected surgeons to promote principles of teamwork and communication can go a long way toward transforming attitudinal and behavioral changes in fellow physicians as well as other members of the surgical team.

Safety culture surveys can be used to measure culture and communication and provide benchmarks for departments or hospitals seeking to measure and improve their teamwork climate.[33] While The Joint Commission encourages all hospitals to measure baseline safety culture every 18 months to 2 years, these survey scores can also be used to evaluate the effectiveness of interventions by comparing survey scores after implementation to baseline values.

TOOLS FOR IMPROVING TEAMWORK AND COMMUNICATION

4 A hallmark of HROs is the frequent use of tools such as prompts, checks, standard operating protocols, and communication interventions such as team briefings and debriefings. These same interventions have been shown to improve patient safety in ORs and ICUs.[34,35] These tools help "engineer out" human error, particularly when it comes to errors of omission which are more likely to occur when there is information overload, multiple steps in a process, repetitions in steps, planned departures from routine processes, and when there are other interruptions and distractions present while the process is being executed.

Preoperative briefings or checklists are a safety intervention that is by now ubiquitous in the perioperative setting. Briefings allow personnel to discuss potential problems before they become a "near miss" or cause actual harm and ensure adherence to evidence-based measures such as the appropriate administration of preoperative antibiotics and deep vein thrombosis (DVT) prophylaxis. They have been associated with an improved safety culture, including increased awareness of wrong-site/wrong-procedure errors, early reporting of equipment problems, reduced operational costs, and fewer unexpected delays. In one study, 30.9% of OR personnel reported a delay before the institution of OR briefings, and only 23.3% reported delays after briefings were instituted.[36,37]

The World Health Organization (WHO) has developed a comprehensive perioperative checklist as a primary intervention of the "Safe Surgery Saves Lives" program—an effort to reduce surgical deaths across the globe.[38] The WHO checklist includes prompts to ensure that infection prevention measures are followed, potential airway complications are precluded (eg, anesthesia has necessary equipment and assistance for a patient with a difficult airway), and the groundwork for effective surgical teamwork is established (eg, proper introductions of all OR personnel). The initial WHO checklist study was associated with significant reduction in mortality worldwide, but follow-up studies evaluating the efficacy of the checklist in governmental programs have failed to reproduce the same impact on morbidity and mortality. It is now understood that the efficacy of checklists is largely dependent on the safety culture in which they are implemented.[37] Simply mandating use is unlikely to change the quality of care delivered, but comprehensive interventions to improve safety culture and implement checklists will likely result in meaningful improvement. Therefore, it is important to adapt checklists to the local environment (**Fig. 15.1**).

Provider handoffs are another high-risk aspect of patient care that could benefit from standardization. Standardized patient handoffs in eight intensive care units across two hospital systems improved providers' preparedness for their shifts, but were not associated with improvements in patient outcomes such as duration of mechanical ventilation or reintubations.[39] This highlights a challenge in studying the efficacy of safety interventions: because the majority of adverse events in critically ill patients are related to the nature of the disease, proving the impact of safety interventions like structured handoffs is challenging. Therefore, studies in patient safety may require

Surgical Safety Checklist

UCSF Health

1 Time out

- All tasks cease
- Introductions and roles

Surgeon/Proceduralist

- ☐ Patient name and MRN
- ☐ Procedure/site/side with consent form
- ☐ Implants
- ☐ EBL
- ☐ Allergies
- ☐ Systemic meds (ABX, DVT, etc.)
- ☐ Specimens planned
- ☐ Disposition postop

Anesthesia Providers

- ☐ Comorbidity concerns
- ☐ Lab results of concern

Circulating Nurse

- ☐ Surgical fire risk/prep solutions
- ☐ Blood products available
- ☐ Confirm implants available
- ☐ Confirm equipment available
- ☐ When feasible, write names on board

Scrub Person

- ☐ Instrument concerns
- ☐ Meds on field

Other Members

- ☐ Monitoring (Neuro, Fetal heart, etc.)
- ☐ Cell saver, perfusion, vendors

2 Final verification

Before procedure begins

All team members verbally agree

- ☐ Patient name
- ☐ Procedure
- ☐ Side/site marking visible
- ☐ Confirm ABX given
- ☐ Additional concerns

If no prep and drape then Time Out will serve as Final Time Out

3 Debrief

Before patient leaves the OR

Surgeon/Proceduralist

- ☐ Verify procedure
- ☐ Verify wound class
- ☐ EBL
- ☐ Confirm specimens with RN
- ☐ Confirm patient disposition

Anesthesia Providers

- ☐ Postop management concerns
- ☐ Key concerns for postop management (airway mgt, etc.)
- ☐ Significant labs/meds
- ☐ I's and O's

Circulating Nurse

- ☐ Confirm with Provider
  - Specimens (type and location)
  - Counts correct
- ☐ Verify with provider
  - Implants used
- ☐ Verify ID band on patient before leaving the OR/procedural room

Figure 15.1. University of California, San Francisco perioperative briefing and debriefing checklist. Courtesy of Ali Abbasi and Elizabeth C. Wick, UCSFHealth.

using surrogate markers such as measures of teamwork, communication, and safety culture as described above. Specialties that have incorporated structured handoffs, such as anesthesia, have made impressive strides in patient safety.

MACHINE LEARNING AND ARTIFICIAL INTELLIGENCE IN PATIENT SAFETY

5 Technology has the potential to significantly improve patient safety. For example, the use of bar-code technology reduced medication administration errors by 54%.[40] As novel technologies like machine learning (ML) and artificial intelligence (AI) are being developed, their role in patient safety is being considered. The vast majority of research relating to ML in patient safety has focused on predicting adverse events, such as the occurrence of venous thromboembolism or clinical decompensation.[41] However, many of these algorithms are developed in single-institution datasets, which limits their generalizability to other settings, and few have convincingly demonstrated that prediction algorithms can reduce the occurrence of adverse events. Recent developments in AI, including the development of large language models, could accelerate developments in this field, because these algorithms can ingest unstructured text, audio, and video data, which makes integration into clinical workflows easier. For example, computer vision can be used to identify whether critical steps of an operation have been completed before advancing to the next step.[42]

The rise of AI also presents novel threats to patient safety. Many algorithms have not been externally validated or tested in prospective studies.[41,43] An external validation of an algorithm to detect sepsis that is widely implemented in EHRs found that the algorithm identified only 7% of patients with sepsis who did not receive timely antibiotics, indicating limited utility of the algorithm beyond clinician judgment.[44] In addition, AI models are known to perpetuate biases present in training data, which could worsen health disparities. As AI models are becoming increasingly common, health systems must implement safeguards, including continuous assurance of algorithm performance, ensuring traceability of outcomes and tracking of metadata, and monitoring how providers interact with AI, using the principles of human-factors engineering that are common in other high-risk professions.[45]

INVESTIGATING A SAFETY EVENT

5 The approach to analyzing adverse events and mistakes has shifted from assigning blame to using frameworks that help elucidate contributing factors so that improvements can be put in place to make the system more resilient, thereby preventing similar harms or near misses from occurring in the future.

There are several tiers of investigation that can be deployed, depending on the severity of the event. While sentinel events such as wrong-site surgery always require a full event review and analysis, other events can be reviewed using different formats. For example, the UK national health service patient safety incident response framework identified several different approaches that can be taken, depending on the severity and type of incidents, including a complete incident investigation for a near miss for significant safety event, after action reviews to capture learning from a particular event, thematic reviews to identify patterns in data and identify issues, and swarm huddles that involve staff huddling to analyze the incident as soon as it occurs and prevent recurrence.[46] The idea behind these tiered approaches is to integrate safety reviews into everyday practice by providing a flexible set of tools that can be deployed.

In surgery, division and department morbidity and mortality conferences (M&Ms) have long provided a protected space in which clinicians from similar fields can openly discuss clinical decision making, including errors. However, M&Ms are not always the optimal forum for discussing cases in which broad systems issues beyond the purview of a particular division or department may have played a role. There are several best practices that can be employed to ensure M&Ms contribute to patient safety.[47] First, cases should be referred and presented using a standardized format, with a detailed and organized review of the event and contributing systemic factors. Second, the discussions should strive to follow the tenants of a "just culture" focused on learning over attributing blame. Finally, the M&M should be integrated with departmental quality improvement efforts and provide mechanisms to implement learnings as part of a broader system of safety and quality.

When so-called sentinel events or never events do occur, institutions should conduct detailed systematic reviews, with the engagement of hospital leadership. This process is required in many states and by The Joint Commission. Traditionally, this process has been referred to as a root cause analysis, although this term is falling out of favor, because the primary purpose of an event review is not to identify a single "root" cause, but rather to prevent recurrence by identifying and ameliorating the many systemic and human factors contributing to an event.[48] Investigations should utilize trained reviewers who investigate the event and interview participants in a timely fashion. The information collected should be protected from disclosure by organization policies, and emphasize the principles of a just culture, focusing on facts rather than faults.

ESTABLISHING A COMPREHENSIVE SAFETY PROGRAM

Historically, safety issues and concerns were managed in a fragmented manner within divisions and departments. However, there is now recognition that improving patient safety requires multidisciplinary action, consistent institutional investments, and leadership buy in. Nationwide Children's Hospital reported their progress in patient safety, which involved increasing the budget for patient safety from $690K in 2007 to $3.3M in 2012, and growing their safety team from 8 to 33 employees. Between 2010 and 2012, the institution experienced an 83.3% reduction in the rate of serious safety events and a 53% decline in preventable harm.[49]

Many larger organizations have now developed robust infrastructure dedicated to managing safety at an institutional level. These safety programs should be empowered to work across different layers of the institution using evidence-based approaches. For example, the comprehensive unit-based safety program (CUSP) is an effective approach for improving both safety culture and clinical outcomes.[50] Every clinical area that implements CUSP assembles a multidisciplinary team and follows five iterative steps: training on the science of safety, identifying patient safety hazards, partnering with senior executive, learning from defects and implement tools to improve teamwork, and improving communication. All teams include providers from relevant disciplines such as nurses, physicians, hospital infection control practitioners, technicians, advanced practice providers, resident physicians, and clerks. This approach has been successfully used to reduce colorectal SSIs from 27% to 18% in a university-based setting.[50]

SUMMARY

The fields of quality and safety have evolved tremendously in the past two decades. Much of the terminology is now commonplace, and many frontline providers are routinely engaged in efforts related to quality and safety. Yet, there remains tremendous opportunity to adopt learnings from HROs such as commercial aviation or nuclear power, by implementing systems thinking, a just culture, high-fidelity communications strategies, and safely deploying technology. As surgeons, we must be dedicated to acquiring competency in the areas described above so that we can serve as leaders in advancing patient safety in our hospitals and operating rooms.

References

1. Kohn LT, Corrigan JM, Donaldson MS. *To Err Is Human: Building a Safer Health System.* National Academies Press; 1999.
2. Medicine I. Committee on Quality of Health Care in America. *Crossing the Quality Chasm: A New Health System for the 21st Century*. National Academies Press US; 2001.
3. Eldridge N, Wang Y, Metersky M, et al. Trends in adverse event rates in hospitalized patients, 2010–2019. *JAMA.* 2022;328(2):173–183.
4. Weiner-Lastinger LM, Pattabiraman V, Konnor RY, et al. The impact of coronavirus disease 2019 (COVID-19) on healthcare-associated infections in 2020: a summary of data reported to the National Healthcare Safety Network. *Infect Control Hosp Epidemiol.* 2022;43(1):12–25.
5. Agency for Healthcare Research and Quality. Adverse Events, Near Misses and Errors [Internet]. 2020. https://psnet.ahrq.gov/primer/adverse-events-near-misses-and-errors
6. Agency for Healthcare Research and Quality. AHRQ Patient Safety Network Glossary [Internet]. 2020. https://psnet.ahrq.gov/glossary?glossary%5B0
7. Pronovost PJ, Goeschel CA, Colantuoni E. Sustaining reductions in catheter related bloodstream infections in Michigan intensive care units: observational study. *BMJ.* 2010;340:c309.
8. Shojania KG. The elephant of patient safety: what you see depends on how you look. *Jt Comm J Qual Patient Saf.* 2010;36(9):399–401.
9. Thomas AD, Pandit C, Krevat SA. Race differences in reported harmful patient safety events in healthcare system high reliability organizations. *J Patient Saf.* 2020;16(4):e235–e239.
10. Gandhi TK, Schulson LB, Thomas AD. Bringing the equity lens to patient safety event reporting. *Jt Comm J Qual Patient Saf.* 2024;50(1):87–89.
11. Chin MH. Advancing health equity in patient safety: a reckoning, challenge and opportunity. *BMJ Qual Saf.* 2020;bmjqs-2020-012599.
12. Kubasiak JC, Francescatti AB, Behal R. Patient safety indicators for judging hospital performance. *Am J Med Qual.* 2017;32(2):129–133.
13. Rajaram R, Barnard C, Bilimoria KY. Concerns about using the patient safety indicator-90 composite in pay-for-performance programs. *JAMA.* 2015;313(9):897–898.
14. Caplan RA, Posner KL, Cheney FW. Effect of outcome on physician judgments of appropriateness of care. *JAMA.* 1991;265(15):1957–1960.
15. Schildmeijer K, Nilsson L, Arestedt K. Assessment of adverse events in medical care: lack of consistency between experienced teams using the global trigger tool. *BMJ Qual Saf.* 2012;21(4):307–314.
16. Lilford R, Pronovost P. Using hospital mortality rates to judge hospital performance: a bad idea that just won't go away. *BMJ.* 2010;340:c2016.
17. Wachter RM, Gupta K. *Understanding Patient Safety.* 3rd ed. McGraw-Hill Education; 2018.
18. Reason JT. *Human Error*. Cambridge University Press; 1990.

19. Weick KE, Sutcliffe KM. *Managing the Unexpected [Internet]*. John Wiley & Sons, Ltd; 2015. https://onlinelibrary.wiley.com/doi/abs/10.1002/9781119175834.fmatter
20. Chassin MR, Loeb JM. The ongoing quality improvement journey: next stop, high reliability. *Health Aff (Millwood)*. 2011; 30(4):559–568.
21. Ruchlin HS, Dubbs NL, Callahan MA. The role of leadership in instilling a culture of safety: lessons from the literature. *J Healthc Manag*. 2004;49(1):58–59.
22. Amalberti R, Auroy Y, Berwick D. Five system barriers to achieving ultrasafe health care. *Ann Intern Med*. 2005;142(9): 756–764.
23. Reason J. *Managing the Risks of Organizational Accidents [Internet]*. Ashgate; 1997. https://books.google.com/books?id=ZnhRAAAAMAAJ
24. Boysen PG. Just culture: a foundation for balanced accountability and patient safety. *Ochsner J*. 2013;13(3):400–406.
25. Murray JS, Kelly S, Hanover C. Promoting psychological safety in healthcare organizations. *Mil Med*. 2022;187(7–8):808–810.
26. Murray JS, Lee J, Larson S, Range A, Scott D, Clifford J. Requirements for implementing a 'just culture' within healthcare organisations: an integrative review. *BMJ Open Qual*. 2023;12(2):e002237.
27. Joint Commission Standards [Internet]. 2010. https://www.jointcommission.org/en-us/standards
28. Lingard L, Espin S, Whyte S. Communication failures in the operating room: an observational classification of recurrent types and effects. *Qual Saf Health Care*. 2004;13(5):330–334.
29. Katz D, Blasius K, Isaak R, et al. Exposure to incivility hinders clinical performance in a simulated operative crisis. *BMJ Qual Saf*. 2019;28(9):750–757.
30. Sexton JB, Berenholtz SM, Goeschel CA. Assessing and improving safety climate in a large cohort of intensive care units. *Crit Care Med*. 2011;39(5):934–939.
31. Makary MA, Sexton JB, Freischlag JA. Patient safety in surgery. *Ann Surg*. 2006;243(5):632–635.
32. Fan CJ, Pawlik TM, Daniels T. Association of safety culture with surgical site infection outcomes. *J Am Coll Surg*. 2016;222(2): 122–128.
33. Makary MA, Holzmueller CG, Thompson D. Operating room briefings: working on the same page. *Jt Comm J Qual Patient Saf*. 2006;32(6):351–355.
34. Pronovost PJ, Berenholtz SM, Goeschel CA. Creating high reliability in health care organizations. *Health Serv Res*. 2006; 41(4 Pt 2):1599–1617.
35. Makary MA, Mukherjee A, Sexton JB. Operating room briefings and wrong-site surgery. *J Am Coll Surg*. 2007;204(2):236–243.
36. Nundy S, Mukherjee A, Sexton JB. Impact of preoperative briefings on operating room delays: a preliminary report. *Arch Surg*. 2008;143(11):1068–1072.
37. Hicks CW, Rosen M, Hobson DB. Improving safety and quality of care with enhanced teamwork through operating room briefings. *JAMA Surg*. 2014;149(8):863–868.
38. Patient Safety WA. WHO Surgical Safety Checklist and Implementation Manual [Internet]. https://www.who.int/teams/integrated-health-services/patient-safety/research/safe-surgery/tool-and-resources
39. Parent B, LaGrone LN, Albirair MT, et al. Effect of standardized handoff curriculum on improved clinician preparedness in the intensive care unit: a stepped-wedge cluster randomized clinical trial. *JAMA Surg*. 2018;153(5):464–470.
40. Paoletti RD, Suess TM, Lesko MG, et al. Using bar-code technology and medication observation methodology for safer medication administration. *Am J Health Syst Pharm*. 2007;64(5): 536–543.
41. Bates DW, Levine D, Syrowatka A, et al. The potential of artificial intelligence to improve patient safety: a scoping review. *NPJ Digit Med*. 2021;4(1):54.
42. Hashimoto DA, Rosman G, Witkowski ER, et al. Computer vision analysis of intraoperative video: automated recognition of operative steps in laparoscopic sleeve gastrectomy. *Ann Surg*. 2019;270(3):414–421.
43. Loftus TJ, Altieri MS, Balch JA, et al. Artificial intelligence-enabled decision support in surgery: state-of-the-art and future directions. *Ann Surg*. 2023;278(1):51–58.
44. Wong A, Otles E, Donnelly JP, et al. External validation of a widely implemented proprietary sepsis prediction model in hospitalized patients. *JAMA Intern Med*. 2021;181(8):1065–1070.
45. Ratwani RM, Bates DW, Classen DC. Patient safety and artificial intelligence in clinical care. *JAMA Health Forum*. 2024;5(2): e235514.
46. NHS England. Patient Safety Learning Response Toolkit [Internet]. [cited 2024 Aug 19]. https://www.england.nhs.uk/publication/patient-safety-learning-response-toolkit/#heading-2
47. JAMA Network. JAMA Surgery. Defining a High-Quality and Effective Morbidity and Mortality Conference: A Systematic Review. [cited 2024 Aug 19]. https://jamanetwork.com/journals/jamasurgery/article-abstract/2810740
48. Agency for Healthcare Research and Quality. System-Focused Event Investigation and Analysis Guide [Internet]. [cited 2024 Aug 19]. https://www.ahrq.gov/patient-safety/settings/hospital/candor/modules/guide4.html
49. Brilli RJ, McClead RE, Crandall WV, et al. A comprehensive patient safety program can significantly reduce preventable harm, associated costs, and hospital mortality. *J Pediatr*. 2013;163(6). 1638–1645.
50. Wick EC, Hobson DB, Bennett JL. Implementation of a surgical comprehensive unit-based safety program to reduce surgical site infections. *J Am Coll Surg*. 2012;215(2):193–200.

16

Artificial Intelligence in Surgery

Daniel A. Hashimoto and Anai Kothari

Key Points

1. AI is not objective like data, and the interpretation of models trained on that data can be biased.
2. Surgeons must be aware of AI's potential to introduce biases in clinical practice and the importance of critically evaluating AI-driven recommendations to ensure they do not perpetuate inequities in patient care.
3. Surgeons are encouraged to actively participate in AI development to ensure these technologies address practical clinical needs and challenges.
4. Surgeons should understand the fundamentals of AI algorithms, particularly machine learning (ML) models, as these are increasingly being explored to enhance surgical precision and predict patient outcomes.
5. Ethical and legal considerations, such as data privacy and algorithmic bias, are crucial in the integration of AI in surgical practice.
6. Surgeons should recognize the potential of generative AI models, such as large language models (LLMs), to assist in creating medical documentation, drafting surgical notes, and even generating synthetic data for research, while also being aware of the challenges these tools pose in maintaining accuracy and avoiding the propagation of errors.

Artificial intelligence (AI) has seemingly exploded into public consciousness over the last several years as advances in computing have offered the promise of automation and complex software functions previously confined to science fiction books and movies. Within surgery, AI has teased tools that enhance diagnostic accuracy, optimize treatment plans, and offer clinical decision support with the aim of improving patient outcomes. However, the translation of AI advances into clinical practice remains in its infancy.

AI has experienced several boom (often called "AI spring") and bust ("AI winter") cycles since its inception. These periods are characterized by high expectations followed by disappointment and reduced funding when these expectations are unmet. The concept of AI winters highlights the challenges faced in translating AI from theoretical models to practical applications, particularly in surgery. Thus, while recent advances in generative AI have brought new excitement, with capabilities such as generating realistic images, videos, and even entire conversations, it is crucial for surgeons to recognize the many additional considerations that must be carefully weighed.

This chapter offers an overview of methodologies and applications of AI in surgery, emphasizing its transformative potential while highlighting its dangers and obstacles to implementation. Key vocabulary terms essential for understanding AI are defined, followed by a discussion on the types, sources, and quality of data critical for AI applications. We describe various AI methods and examine their specific applications in predictive modeling, computer vision (CV), natural language processing (NLP), and generative AI. The chapter also addresses the challenges in adopting AI for clinical use, the importance of AI literacy among health care professionals, and ethical considerations to ensure equitable and unbiased implementation.

TERMINOLOGY

While there are different definitions of AI throughout the literature and the lay press, for this chapter, we define AI as the study of algorithms that enable machines to approximate intelligent human functions, such as problem solving, object or word recognition, inference of world states, and decision making. AI can be considered a broader parent field of study under which several subfields may fall. Machine learning (ML) refers to the study of algorithms and mathematical models that enable machines to learn and perform tasks, while deep learning is a specific technique within ML (**Fig. 16.1**).[1] We cover several strategies for ML and applications facilitated by AI techniques, including NLP and CV. It is important to recognize that ML is not necessary for NLP and CV; however, as described below, modern techniques tend to leverage ML advances to optimize such applications.

DATA

Fundamental to developing and applying AI in surgery is the multitude of data that provides the foundation for accurate, effective, and reliable AI-enabled systems. Since AI algorithms rely on training data to learn patterns and encode knowledge, the quality and quantity of this data directly impact the performance of the AI models.[2]

Sources of Data

1 Sources of data are quite varied and multimodal. Data can be structured, that is, organized in a standardized format to facilitate analysis, or unstructured. Structured data is commonly stored in tabular (ie, tables such as spreadsheets), relational (ie, databases where relationships are maintained across data points in a queryable manner [eg, structured query language [SQL]), or hierarchical (ie, tree-type structures such as extensible markup language [XML]) formats. Structured data includes elements drawn from electronic health records (EHRs), such as lab results, imaging studies, and structured clinical notes. These are often stored in relational databases, making them easier to query and analyze.

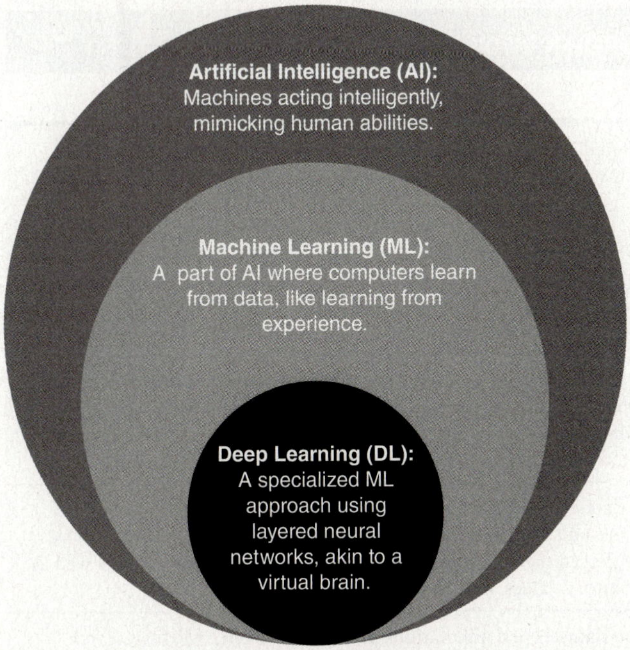

Figure 16.1. Relationship between AI, machine learning, and deep learning. (From Turner L, Hashimoto DA, Vasisht S, Schaye V. Demystifying AI: current state and future role in medical education assessment. *Acad Med.* 2024;99(4S Suppl 1):S42–S47. Figure 1.)

Unstructured data includes free-text clinical notes, surgical videos, radiology images, and pathology slides. These data types are often more challenging to process due to their lack of standardized structure and may require advanced AI techniques from NLP or CV to extract meaningful insights. Multimodal data combines data from different modalities, including both structured and unstructured data. These data types necessitate unique approaches for management and storage since they can exceed the capacity of traditional database systems and on-premise computing. Large-scale data management solutions, such as data lakes or nonrelational systems, are often required to manage the volume and complexity of multimodal health care data. This has led to shifts in handling data on local computers and networks to instead using the cloud (ie, remote computing resources that are accessed over the Internet).[3,4] These systems must be capable of integrating diverse data types while maintaining data integrity, security, and accessibility.

One helpful frame for considering sources of data in surgery is the phase of care (eg, preoperative, intraoperative, postoperative) from which the data is acquired. **Table 16.1** provides examples of potential data sources for each phase of care.

Data can be obtained from either proprietary or public sources. Proprietary data sources are held by individual institutions, companies, or consortia and are typically available only internally. As these datasets are often created to address the specific needs of an institution or project, they often contain more detailed and extensive information, including high-resolution imaging, longitudinal data, and specific annotations that are not available in public datasets. These datasets can be customized to meet the specific needs of the institution or the AI model being developed, allowing for more precise and targeted research. However, institutions may worry about data security and privacy in allowing outside access. Furthermore, access to proprietary data can give organizations a significant advantage in developing AI models that are more accurate and applicable to their specific patient populations.

Public datasets are more readily available to the research community and often curated by academic institutions, government agencies, or consortia. These datasets are crucial for advancing AI research as they provide a common ground for benchmarking algorithms, enabling reproducibility of results and fostering transparency in scientific inquiry. Examples of public datasets in surgery are found in **Table 16.2.** Unlike proprietary datasets, public datasets allow researchers to validate and replicate the findings of others, fostering a culture of transparency and scientific rigor. They can allow the effectiveness of AI models to be objectively compared across studies. From an equity perspective, open access to data enables a wide range of researchers, including those from institutions with limited resources, to participate in research.

Both proprietary and public datasets have limitations. Proprietary datasets are limited in accessibility and transparency, thus reducing the ability for other researchers to reproduce findings or leverage the data for additional insights. This, combined with potentially limited capture of clinical scenarios or patient populations, can limit the generalizability of the data. While public datasets are more amenable to transparency and reproducibility by outside investigators, the depth and variety of data within public datasets may be limited by the interests and missions of those creating and maintaining the publicly available data. Researchers should note that "*public*" does not necessarily mean the data are free. Depending on the license type under which datasets are released, researchers may be required to pay a licensing fee to facilitate dataset maintenance or sign data-use agreements.

There has been increasing interest in the FAIR (Findable, Accessible, Interoperable, and Reusable) principles of data sharing, a set of guidelines designed to improve the management and accessibility of data. The FAIR principles strive to produce data that can be (1) easily found by both humans and computers (findable); (2) accessed, downloaded, and retrieved using standard protocols (accessible); (3) integrated with other data and used with various tools and applications (interoperable); and (4) reused in future research and applications (reusable).[5]

Table 16.1. Potential Sources of Surgical Data Found in Each Phase of Care

Preoperative	Intraoperative	Postoperative
EHR data (eg, clinical notes, laboratory data)	EHR data	EHR data
Imaging (eg, axial imaging, ultrasound, nuclear studies)	Imaging (eg, fluoroscopy, ultrasound, axial imaging)	Imaging (eg, axial imaging, ultrasound, nuclear studies)
Wearable sensors	Wearable sensors (surgeon and patient)	Wearable sensors
Genomics, proteomics, metabolomics, etc.	Anesthesia monitors Instrument tracking data (eg, robotic kinematics)	Patient-reported outcome measures

Table 16.2. Examples of Publicly Available Datasets That Include Surgical Data

Database	Description
American College of Surgeons National Safety and Quality Improvement Program (ACS NSQIP) https://www.facs.org/quality-programs/data-and-registries/acs-nsqip/	A risk-adjusted database of surgical outcomes collected from participating hospitals. Data is drawn from patient charts rather than from claims data.
Medicare Claims Data https://data.cms.gov/	Collection of billing and health care utilization data from services provided to Medicare beneficiaries, encompassing inpatient, outpatient, and physician encounters.
Healthcare Cost and Utilization Project (HCUP) https://hcup-us.ahrq.gov/	A collection of nation- or state-wide data on health care utilization, access, charges, quality, and outcomes. HCUP includes the nationwide inpatient sample (NIS), the largest publicly available all-payer inpatient care database in the United States.
Medical Information Mart for Intensive Care-IV (MIMIC-IV) https://physionet.org/content/mimiciv/3.0/	Deidentified dataset of patients admitted to the emergency department or intensive care unit at Beth Israel Deaconess Medical Center in Boston, MA. It contains deidentified patient and provider data, chest x-ray data, as well as notes, laboratory values, and vital sign data.
Research Group CAMMA http://camma.u-strasbg.fr/datasets/	Surgical video datasets and annotations provided by the CAMMA research group of the University of Strasbourg. Includes videos of laparoscopic cholecystectomy and gastric bypass.

Quality of Data

The quality of data is critical for the development of effective
2 and reliable computational models in surgery. High-quality data ensures that algorithms can learn from accurate, complete, and representative datasets.[2] Key aspects of data quality include accuracy, representation, completeness, and consistency.

Accuracy refers to the correctness of data entries and measurements within a dataset. Accurate data precisely reflects the real-world phenomena it represents, whether that be patient demographics, imaging results, or surgical outcomes. Inaccurate data can lead to faulty models, as AI systems will learn from erroneous information, leading to predictions or classifications that do not reflect true clinical scenarios.

Representation, the extent to which the data reflects the diversity of the target patient population and clinical scenarios, is an important consideration when building and analyzing models. Representation includes demographic diversity (eg, age, gender, ethnicity) as well as variability in disease presentation and treatment approaches. A dataset that is not representative may result in models that perform well on certain subgroups of patients but poorly on others.

Completeness refers to the extent to which all necessary data is available and recorded without gaps or omissions. Incomplete data can introduce biases, as models may be trained on partial information that does not fully represent the clinical context. Thus, missing data can significantly impair model performance, leading to inaccurate predictions or the inability to recognize certain patterns.

Consistency refers to the standardization of data entry formats, units, and methods across different sources and time points. Consistent data ensures that similar information is recorded in a uniform manner, making it easier to integrate and analyze. Inconsistencies in data can lead to confusion and errors during analysis, as AI models might interpret similar data points differently due to variations in format or units. For example, variations in the recording of drug dosages can lead to incorrect dose–response relationships being learned by the model.

Each of these elements raises the potential to bias datasets and thus the outputs of models. However, there may be scenarios in which inconsistencies in data labels reflect the realities of the clinical environment. For example, multiple annotators labeling safe and unsafe areas of dissection in laparoscopic cholecystectomy can disagree on the exact delineation between a safe and unsafe plane, reflecting the preferences of different surgeons.[2,6] The same may hold for incomplete data as well, where complete data may never truly be available for clinical decision making. Therefore, the degree of representation, completeness, and consistency required for a given model may vary depending on the goals and needs of a given project. However, every effort should be made to maximize and optimize data quality for a given circumstance.

OVERVIEW OF METHODS

Classes of Learning

ML encompasses a variety of methods designed to enable machines to learn from data and make decisions or predictions. These methods are broadly categorized based on the nature of the learning process. The common classes of learning in ML for surgical applications include supervised, unsupervised, semisupervised, weakly supervised, and reinforcement learning (RL).

Supervised learning involves training a model on a labeled dataset, where the input data is paired with the correct output. The goal is for the model to learn the relationship between inputs and outputs so that it can predict the output for new, unseen data.[7] The primary tasks in supervised learning are classification (eg, identifying whether an image is of a gallbladder) and regression (eg, predicting length of stay based on features such as operative time and American Society of Anesthesiologists [ASA] classification).

Unsupervised learning deals with data that does not have labels (**Fig. 16.2**). The model attempts to learn the underlying structure or distribution in the data, often through clustering or association. In other words, the algorithm tries to find patterns or relationships without guidance on what the correct output should be. Common tasks include clustering (eg, grouping patients by comorbidities or other measures of similarity) and dimensionality reduction (eg, reducing the number of features in a dataset while preserving its essential information).

Semisupervised learning leverages elements from both supervised and unsupervised learning. It uses a small amount of labeled data along with a large amount of unlabeled data, using the labeled data to guide the learning process and make use of the unlabeled data to improve the model's performance.

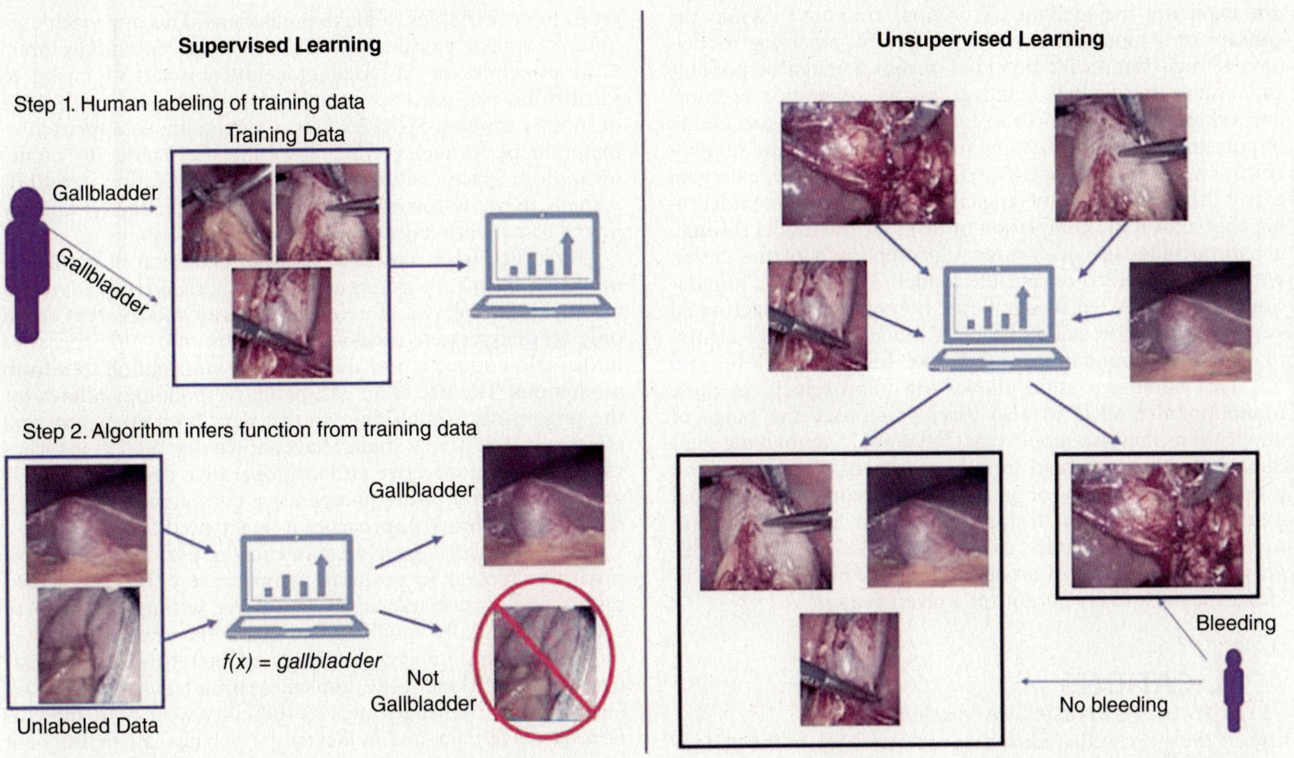

Figure 16.2. In supervised learning, human-labeled data are fed to a machine learning algorithm to teach the computer a function, such as recognizing a gallbladder in an image or detecting a complication in a large claims database. In unsupervised learning, unlabeled data are fed to a machine learning algorithm, which then attempts to find a hidden structure to the data, such as identifying bright red (eg, bleeding) as different from nonbleeding tissue. (From Hashimoto DA, Rosman G, Rus D, Meireles OR. Artificial Intelligence in surgery: promises and perils. *Ann Surg*. 2018;268(1):70–76. Figure 1.)

This approach is often used when obtaining labeled data is expensive or time consuming, but unlabeled data is plentiful. Weakly supervised learning refers to learning from data where the labels are noisy, imprecise, or incomplete. Thus, existing labels may provide supervision to the model that is noisy or otherwise not fully reliable. For CV applications, weakly supervised learning approaches have been utilized when labels are not as fine grained as needed (eg, only the presence of an instrument is labeled, but not its exact location). These approaches can have value in scenarios where acquiring precise and comprehensive labels is difficult or expensive.

RL involves training an "agent" (ie, a model) to make a sequence of decisions by rewarding it for correct actions and punishing it for incorrect ones. The learning process involves trial and error, where the agent continually improves its strategy based on the rewards it accumulates. Thus, the agent learns to maximize cumulative rewards over time by exploring different strategies. This is akin to operant conditioning, wherein biologic organisms learn a behavior by associating a reward or punishment (eg, a mouse pressing a lever to get a food reward). RL is the technique that was used to great success in training AI algorithms to consistently beat human players in complex games such as Go and chess. Surgically, RL has been used in research environments to train surgical robots to perform some autonomous tasks, such as tissue manipulation and suturing.[8,9]

Generative Artificial Intelligence

Advancements in generative artificial intelligence (GenAI) have led to a new era of technologic possibility and applications. What distinguishes GenAI from nongenerative AI is the ability to create new, original content, produce variable (and logical) outputs based on the same inputs, and adapt to new tasks without retraining.[10,11] OpenAI's release of ChatGPT in November 2022 marked a significant milestone in making GenAI accessible to the general public. While similar AI approaches had been attempted previously without widespread success, ChatGPT's user-friendly interface allowed for ease of interaction with the underlying foundation model (a very large-scale, pretrained AI model), catalyzing rapid adoption and exploration.[12]

The success of ChatGPT and similar large language models (LLMs) has led to the "GPT era" in AI development. These models, though primarily designed for text generation and understanding, have demonstrated versatility in tackling complex tasks across numerous domains. In the context of surgery, LLMs show promise in areas such as preoperative planning, medical literature analysis, patient education, and real-time decision support.[13,14] However, it is crucial to note that the effective application of these technologies in surgical settings requires consideration of ethical implications, data privacy, and the need for rigorous validation in clinical environments.

As the field progresses, there is an emergence of both proprietary and open-source GenAI models from many organizations. This also includes model frameworks that allow more than text generation, such as image generation (eg, DALL-E, Midjourney, Stable Diffusion), audio generation (eg, Jukebox, MusicLM), and video generation (eg, Imagen Video). Generative models in these domains offer additional opportunities for surgeons to consider in the application of AI. For example, these models could generate detailed visualizations of surgical procedures for training purposes or patient education. Additionally, they could generate customized models of patient-specific anatomy to augment surgical planning, create educational audio or video, or other adjuncts to enhance surgical training.

A crucial element "under the hood" to all GenAI systems is the foundation models upon which they are built. A foundation model is characterized by training on a broad dataset, enabling adaptation to perform downstream tasks that were not explicitly included in its original training.[15] While the concept of a foundation model is not new, emerging models have shown significant potential across a range of possible capabilities that include language, vision, robotics, reasoning, and others. With advances in foundation models also comes important cautions that center around emergence and homogenization. One of the unexpected, and unexplained, emergent capabilities of foundation language models is in-context learning that allows the completion of tasks by the model through a natural language description ("prompting") of the action without the need to retrain the model. Additionally, foundation models have led to significant homogenization across AI systems, with most state-of-the-art models now built on top of a few key foundation models like BERT, RoBERTa, and T5. This homogenization allows any improvement in these foundational models to also quickly improve the range of applications they are supporting ("leverage"), amplifying their impact. However, it also introduces the risk of widespread propagation of biases or problems inherent in the original models across various AI applications.[16] It is also important to note that GenAI models do not encode knowledge. As with many AI models, GenAI models encode for probability, calculating the most likely output for a given prompt.

APPLICATIONS

Perioperative Predictive Models

One of the most well-studied uses of AI and ML in the perioperative setting is the prediction of the risk of postoperative complications. An early example of this was the development of the American College of Surgeons National Safety and Quality Improvement (NSQIP) risk calculator. In its original form, data obtained through a national surgical outcomes registry was used to train a logistic regression model to provide risk estimates for a total of 21 postoperative outcomes. Importantly, the model inputs and outputs were made easily accessible through a web-based application, allowing for widespread use.[17] Surgeons, patients, families, and other health providers had the ability to use a risk model to understand the anticipated impact an operation would have on the postoperative patient course.

Fundamentally, the surgical risk calculator positions a mathematical model in real-world clinical scenarios to help consider what might happen after surgery, what risk looks like compared to an average patient, and the decision to proceed with surgery in some cases. Predictive models for perioperative risk stratification have evolved significantly since the original surgical risk calculator. This includes the adoption of more advanced analytic techniques to improve the performance and applicability of personalized risk prediction. Specific examples of this include POTTER (Predictive OpTimal Trees in Emergency Surgery Risk), SURPAS (Surgical Risk Preoperative Assessment System), and MySurgeryRisk, each of which demonstrates the evolution of predictive models for postoperative risk prediction.[18–20]

POTTER utilizes an AI methodology known as optimal classification trees, allowing for better handling of complex, nonlinear interactions between variables. This approach has resulted in superior performance in predicting postoperative mortality and morbidity compared to earlier models. POTTER has demonstrated high accuracy across various complications, including septic shock and respiratory failure. Moreover, its availability as an interactive smartphone application enhances its accessibility, enabling real-time decision making at the bedside. The performance gains seen with POTTER emphasize the potential of using AI-based tools over conventional methods, especially when rigorously assessed and made available through user-friendly platforms.

Another advancement in surgical risk prediction is seen in the development of SURPAS, which uses a more streamlined set of input variables to make predictions. This approach may initially appear paradoxical to some of the commonly practiced principles in AI-based modeling. Instead of trying to identify unseen patterns in a large feature space with 100s of input variables, SURPAS uses a parsimonious approach to maintain performance while lowering the barrier to implementation. Specifically, this facilitates its integration into EHR systems to allow for real-time risk assessment that is directly linked to patient records and clinical workflows.

MySurgeryRisk represents another evolution in predictive modeling by incorporating data from both preoperative and intraoperative phases of care. Unlike prior models that relied only on preoperative variables, the inclusion of intraoperative information added a new dimension of information to inform predictions. The use of an ML-based methodology allows for the processing of multidimensional data both efficiently and effectively. Additional studies have shown that models incorporating both preoperative and intraoperative data significantly outperform those using preoperative data alone, highlighting the role of AI-based approaches to make predictions.

Several societies now recommend the use of preoperative predictive models to promote preoperative optimization and resource allocation, especially in elective settings where these can be potentially modified based on the estimated risk.[21] However, despite a growing body of literature demonstrating validity of these tools, implementation has been slow and inconsistent. Challenges such as difficulty with EHR integration, access to data, and model trustworthiness all are ongoing barriers to wider adoption.

Computer Vision

CV is the field of study that enables machines to interpret and analyze visual data such as images and videos. AI techniques have been applied to CV, but it is important to note that CV has not and does not require modern AI techniques.[22] While CV has most frequently been applied to radiology, pathology, and dermatology, CV has been applied to surgical applications, including analysis of surgical video,[23] assessment of technical skills,[24] and evaluation of surgical wounds.[25]

Automated analysis of operative video to estimate workflow, analyze procedural steps, and identify key anatomic structures has been an emphasis of surgical applications of CV. While such methods feel relatively new, some of the earliest work in this area dates to 2006.[26] Advances have since included the demonstration of automated segmentation of procedural steps in various minimally invasive surgical cases, including general, bariatric, endoscopic, and oncologic surgery. Furthermore, deep learning methods have been leveraged to identify critical anatomic structures[23] and safe versus unsafe areas of dissection[6] (including in real time), demonstrating the feasibility of using AI tools to guide surgeons (**Fig. 16.3**). Deep learning methods in CV have also enabled automated assessment of surgical techniques—both in comparison to examples from other surgeons[27] and in relation to patient outcomes.[28]

OBSTACLES

Culture of Data

For surgical applications of AI to advance, researchers and developers must be able to access large, diverse datasets on
3 which to train AI models. As discussed earlier in the chapter, tradeoffs between public and proprietary datasets can limit the scope and function of AI models. Sharing of data across institutions is often limited, though collaborations such as the Observational Medical Outcomes Partnership (OMOP) and Common Data Model (CDM)[29] are establishing standards to facilitate at least interoperability of datasets. Additionally, while some types of health care data are captured in a structured manner during routine clinical care (eg, laboratory work, vital signs), much of the clinical encounter is captured in

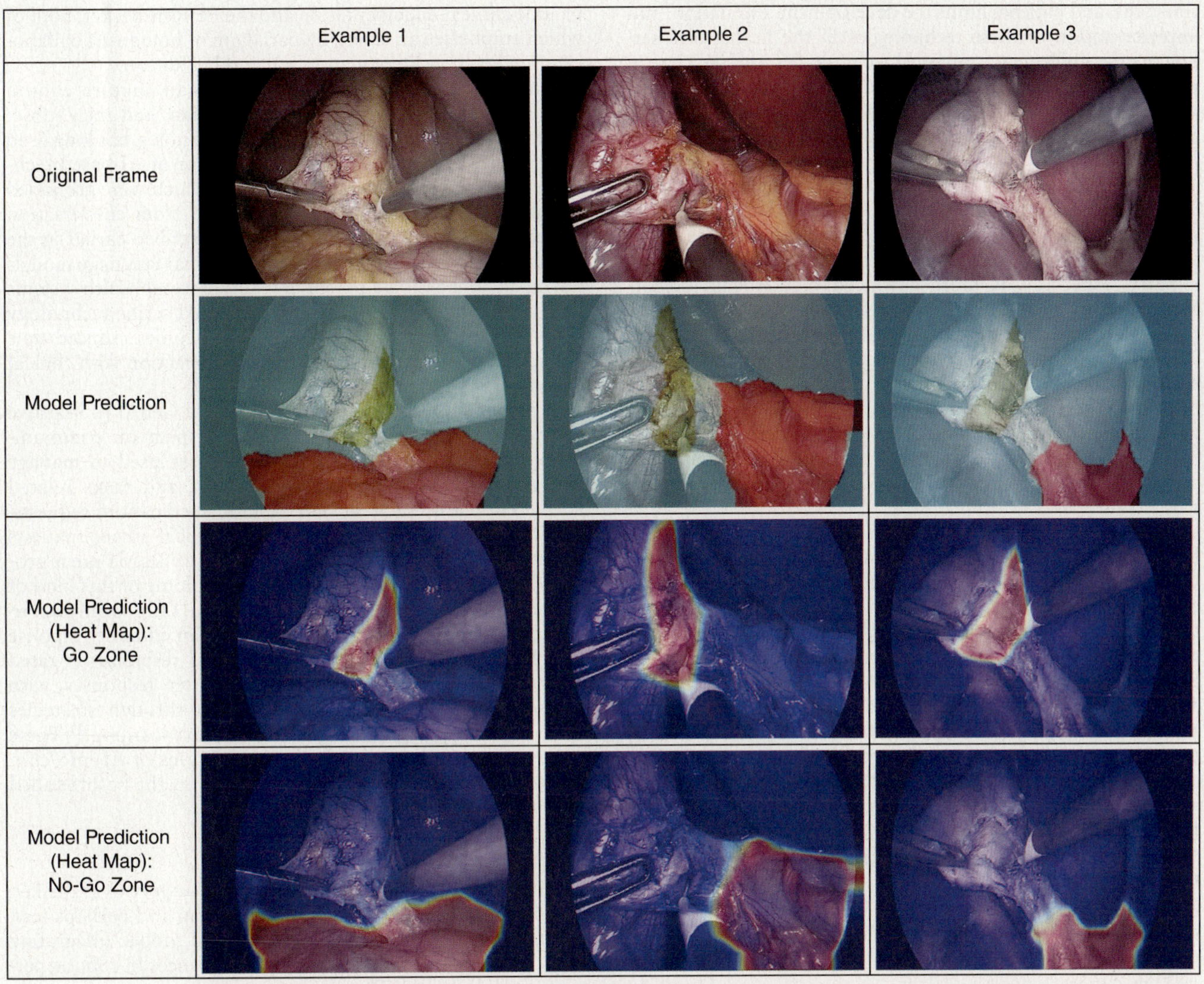

Figure 16.3. Deep learning models used to generate safe (Go) and unsafe (No-Go) zones of dissection in laparoscopic cholecytectomy to facilitate review of cholecystectomy videos and potentially offer real-time intraoperative guidance to surgeons. (From Madani A, Namazi B, Altieri MS, et al. Artificial intelligence for intraoperative guidance: using semantic segmentation to identify surgical anatomy during laparoscopic cholecystectomy. *Ann Surg*. 2022;276(2):363–369. Figure 3.)

an unstructured manner (eg, clinician notes, radiology images) or not recorded and stored at all (eg, operative video). Mazer et al. found that a minority of surgeons record and store video of their operations. While the reasons for not doing so are varied, they include ambiguity around hospital policies on video recording, the lack of infrastructure to store the data in a secure, accessible manner, and the lack of perceived benefit of capturing and storing video data.[30]

Standards for data interoperability across devices have been proposed and implemented (eg, HL7, DICOM); however, some forms of operative data (eg, robotic systems, electrosurgical energy units) are proprietary and inaccessible to surgeons or researchers without specific agreements with the companies that manufacture the devices.

Policymakers, hospital leaders, clinicians, and patients will likely need to consider changes to the regulation of health care data to maximize the protection of patient privacy while optimizing the use of data to develop tools that can improve the efficacy and efficiency of patient care. AI techniques such as federated learning (ie, an ML approach where models are trained collaboratively across multiple devices or servers using local data without sharing that data centrally) offer methods to achieve privacy-preserving AI. However, the culture of capturing, storing, and sharing surgical data must evolve to leverage these powerful techniques for ultimate translation to the bedside.

AI Knowledge and Literacy

The proliferation of AI technologies in health care has sparked
4 a vibrant and interdisciplinary research domain.[31] However, incorporating these technologies into practice has been limited, with only a few achieving widespread clinical use.[32,33] One factor contributing to this limited adoption is the variable trust and acceptance of AI technologies among health care professionals and patients.[34,35] This lack of trust may also result from knowledge deficits about AI, given its complex and rapidly evolving nature. Thus, AI knowledge and literacy (the understanding of the concepts fundamental to AI technologies) are of growing importance.[36] In health care, the need for AI literacy is particularly pressing. Clinicians require AI literacy to effectively utilize AI tools in clinical practice and contribute to the development of new tools. For patients, AI literacy may enhance their understanding of digital health literacy, with potential implications for health equity, safety, and access to care.[37]

Most clinicians lack formal training in data science, ML, or AI despite recognizing such training as a key competency for future physicians.[38] Prior studies indicate that while most of the public acknowledges the existence of AI technologies, they do not possess a deep understanding of the concepts fundamental to developing these technologies.[39] This "digital divide" between the developers of AI technologies and its users, clinicians, and patients limits the development, evaluation, and implementation of these technologies in the health care setting. As the implementation of AI technologies into the clinical workflow increases, it will be critical for surgeons and surgical trainees to improve their understanding of these concepts to facilitate patient care and optimize clinical workflows.[7]

Trustworthiness

Significant and rapid progress in AI has led to substantial interest in actually adopting these tools into routine clinical care. Despite this enthusiasm, understandable skepticism remains, especially as more advanced models gain performance improvement through increasing complexity. This often means that model weights, input features, feature importance, and other important aspects needed for interpretability are no longer available. This is often referred to as the black box problem, where the end user receives a model output without having a clear understanding of how it was derived. In sensitive industries such as health care, this comes with immediate apprehension since many proposed AI applications impact patients directly.

To assess trustworthiness of an AI model, surgeons can focus their AI literacy on the evaluation of AI models, including models' performance and usability. AI trustworthiness can be addressed by rigorous review and measurement of model outputs, even when the underpinnings of the model may not be immediately transparent. Several frameworks to guide the implementation of AI systems have recently been proposed.[33,40,41] Some commonalities across these include assessment of the model validity (both internal and external), generalizability and safety, and adoption (both technical and user centered). For example, model validity can be assessed using standard metrics such as discrimination and calibration, augmented by tools that include decision curves or usability measures. Generalizability and safety can be assessed through systematic review of bias, data drift, and privacy. Finally, adoption can be evaluated by understanding the fit with existing workflows and domain alignment.[42,43]

REGULATORY CONSIDERATIONS

Regulation of AI varies depending on the country in which an application is meant to be used. As of 2024, the European
5 Union has enacted the AI Act as a legal framework for developing and using AI in Europe. This framework puts into place rules defining high–risk-use cases, prohibited-use cases, the obligations of developers and distributors of AI systems, and other guidance.[44] In the United States, an executive order on AI was signed in 2023 to outline guidance on the safe, secure, and trustworthy use and development of AI. While the specific implementation of the executive order is unclear as of this writing, the order defines terminology regarding development, testing, privacy, and security. It offers key areas of consideration that developers and distributors of AI technologies should follow.[45] Furthermore, the US Food and Drug Administration (FDA) has classified AI and ML tools as software as a medical device (SaMD). It has established a digital health advisory committee to support regulating digital tools, including AI. While there have been hundreds of FDA-approved AI/ML devices and tools,[46] the regulatory environment around AI tools continues to evolve as new AI capabilities are unlocked and officials' understanding of these tools' promise and risk improves.

EMERGING AREAS

GenAI to Improve Surgical Workflows

6 Early-use cases of GenAI in surgical workflows center on improving clinical efficiency and addressing common pain points faced by practitioners on a day-to-day basis. These include clinical documentation and the EHR in-basket, both of which emphasize an emerging paradigm of human-AI collaboration when considering adoption and health care.

The concept of ambient technologies to capture clinical conversations between patient and clinician, and then subsequently transfer these into finalized clinical notes, has long been described. Realization of this potential use of AI-based technology was limited by language models, which were grounded in rule-based NLP, making the transition from conversation to text inaccurate and ineffective.[47] As described earlier in the chapter, substantial advances in foundational language models now make this vision a potential reality. Several health systems have now implemented at scale ambient AI scribe technology with high satisfaction from users. This includes reduced time on clinical documentation and higher satisfaction with clinical encounters.[48]

Another successful and emerging use of GenAI to improve clinical efficiency is to reduce the time spent on communications through EHR in-baskets which are used to manage and organize incoming messages, alerts, and tasks related to patient care, such as lab results, medication requests, appointment scheduling, and patient medical advice requests (PMARs). PMARs are a specific area where LLMs are a proposed solution to help address the high volume of this kind of request. Similar to ambient AI scribing, the LLM would act to collaborate with the surgeon by drafting an editable response to a PMAR. The quality of LLM-drafted responses is rated similarly to those created by human-written responses, with potential to improve the LLM's output through strategies such as prompt engineering and in-context learning.[49] These successes set the stage for future integrations of AI into clinical settings where language-based tasks might be offloaded to these tools.

Robotics

Given the rapid rise of AI applications in surgery over the last decade, there has been increasing attention, and perhaps fear, of a near future with autonomous surgical robots. Integrating AI techniques into robotics has led to advances in robotic perception and control. This has been quite pronounced in daily life with the increasing visibility of advanced driving assist capabilities and even some autonomous vehicles. A classification system of surgical autonomy that parallels that of autonomous vehicles has been proposed (**Fig. 16.4**).

Semiautonomous suturing robots have been reported in the literature.[9] However, they still require human setup of a bowel anastomosis in a specific configuration and for an enterotomy to be performed by a human surgeon. Furthermore, the time required to complete the anastomosis is beyond what is clinically feasible. While such reported semiautonomous robots are not quite ready for clinical use today, new generations of surgical robots that can change surgical care are likely to arise as advances in robotics grow in parallel with advances in AI techniques.

However, it is important to consider the example of autonomous vehicles as a cautionary tale in overestimating the speed at which autonomous surgical robots may develop. While the attention on autonomous vehicles over the last decade may make it seem like these cars have been developed over the last few years, some of the earliest autonomous vehicles were exhibited in the 1980s.[50] Forty years later, there are still not fully autonomous (ie, level V) vehicles on the road. Thus, while the combination of visual features and kinematics (ie, the precise positions and motions) of robotic instrument arms offers the promise of augmented understanding of an operation and improvement of its execution, significant advances are still required to achieve truly autonomous surgery. It is instead more conceivable that surgical robots may facilitate specific tasks during an operation, similar to how surgical staplers now facilitate bowel anastomoses.

Human Driver Monitors Environment			System Monitors Environment		
0 No Automation	1 Driver Assistance	2 Partial Automation	3 Conditional Automation	4 High Automation	5 Full Automation
Solely reliant on human control and guidance.	Human control; systems to assist navigation or speed.	Automated assistance Eg, cruise control, lane keeping.	Automated navigation and monitoring, human backup	Fully automated, human backup only in limited circumstances.	Fully automated "smart vehicle" capable of operating in any circumstance.

Human vs. Robot Surgeons					
0 No Automation	1 Some Assistance	2 Partial Automation	3 Conditional Automation	4 High Automation	5 Full Automation
Traditional surgery: Human surgeon performs all tasks.	Eg, Intraoperative image guidance; human still physically performs all surgery.	Eg, ROBODOC hip arthroplasty robot: reduced level of human input required but range of procedures.	Eg, Cyberknife, automated preoperative planning and radiosurgery (but not technically "surgery").	Eg, Robot capable of performing most, if not all parts of a complex procedure. Negligible human input required.	Eg, Robot for deep space exploration? Fully autonomous, versatile; no human assistance needed.

Figure 16.4. Comparison of the five levels of autonomy between vehicles (**top**) and robots (**bottom**). (From Panesar S, Cagle Y, Chander D, Morey J, Fernandez-Miranda J, Kliot M. Artificial intelligence and the future of surgical robotics. *Ann Surg.* 2019;270(2):223–226. Figure 1.)

SUMMARY

Integrating AI into surgical practice represents a potential paradigm shift to significantly enhance patient outcomes and surgical efficiency. As AI continues to evolve, surgeons should stay informed about these tools' underlying technologies, ethical considerations, and practical applications. By participating in the development and implementation of AI, surgeons can ensure that these innovations are aligned with clinical needs and improve patient care. The future of surgery will increasingly rely on a synergistic relationship between human expertise and AI-driven insights, making it imperative for the surgical community to embrace this technologic advancement while maintaining a critical eye on its limitations and both its positive and negative implications.

ACKNOWLEDGMENTS

Artificial intelligence tools, including custom-trained instances of chatGPT (Version 4o, OpenAI, San Francisco, CA), ChatLLM Teams (Abacus.AI, San Francisco, CA), and Grammarly (Grammarly, San Francisco, CA), were utilized to optimize word choice, organization, spelling, and grammar. The authors thank Vivek Singh for his assistance in collating and summarizing reference materials and for his expertise in the health care AI literacy portions of the chapter.

References

1. Hashimoto DA, Rosman G, Meireles OR. *Artificial Intelligence in Surgery: Understanding the Role of AI in Surgical Practice.* McGraw Hill Professional; 2021.
2. Jogan M, Kurada S, Vasisht S, Singh V, Hashimoto DA. Quality over quantity? The role of data quality and uncertainty for AI in surgery. *GSE JASE.* 2024;3:1–9.
3. Gupta NS, Kumar P. Perspective of artificial intelligence in healthcare data management: a journey towards precision medicine. *Comput Biol Med.* 2023;162:107051.
4. Agapito G, Cannataro M. An overview on the challenges and limitations using Cloud Computing in healthcare corporations. *Big Data Cogn Comput.* 2023;7:68.
5. Wilkinson MD, Dumontier M, Aalbersberg IJ, et al. The FAIR Guiding Principles for scientific data management and stewardship. *Scientific Data.* 2016;3:1–9.
6. Madani A, Namazi B, Altieri MS, et al. Artificial intelligence for intraoperative guidance: using semantic segmentation to identify surgical anatomy during laparoscopic cholecystectomy. *Ann Surg.* 2022;276:363–369.
7. Hashimoto DA, Rosman G, Rus D, Meireles OR. Artificial intelligence in surgery: promises and perils. *Ann Surg.* 2018;268:70–76.
8. Nguyen ND, Nguyen T, Nahavandi S, Bhatti A, Guest G. Manipulating Soft Tissues by Deep Reinforcement Learning for Autonomous Robotic Surgery. *2019 IEEE International Systems Conference (SysCon).* Orlando, FL, USA. 2019; pp. 1–7. https://ieeexplore.ieee.org/abstract/document/8836924?casa_token=Jf-3NFsaREwkAAAAA:rU0UT83dXeFp_kBL0UOnw2wSw2FB8x1gUkL8_quRNWuF4DA2zRI6gSHAfKho_JXNk0mRolBr0cI
9. Shademan A, Decker RS, Opfermann JD, Leonard S, Krieger A, Kim PC. Supervised autonomous robotic soft tissue surgery. *Sci Transl Med.* 2016;8:337ra64.
10. Cao Y. A comprehensive survey of AI-generated content (AIGC): a history of generative AI from GAN to ChatGPT. *arXiv [cs.AI].* 2023.
11. Epstein Z, Hertzmann A; Investigators of Human Creativity, et al. Art and the science of generative AI. *Science.* 2023;380:1110–1111.
12. Stokel-Walker C, Van Noorden R. What ChatGPT and generative AI mean for science. *Nature.* 2023;614:214–216.
13. Rengers TA, Thiels CA, Salehinejad H. Academic surgery in the era of large language models: a review: a review. *JAMA Surg.* 2024;159:445–450.
14. Haltaufderheide J, Ranisch R. The ethics of ChatGPT in medicine and healthcare: a systematic review on Large Language Models (LLMs). *NPJ Digit Med.* 2024;7:183.
15. Moor M, Banerjee O, Abad ZSH, et al. Foundation models for generalist medical artificial intelligence. *Nature.* 2023;616:259–265.
16. Bommasani R, Hudson DA, Adeli E, et al. On the opportunities and risks of foundation models. *arXiv [cs.LG].* 2021.
17. Bilimoria KY, Liu Y, Paruch JL, et al. Development and evaluation of the universal ACS NSQIP surgical risk calculator: a decision aid and informed consent tool for patients and surgeons. *J Am Coll Surg.* 2013;217:833–42.e1–3.
18. Bertsimas D, Dunn J, Velmahos GC, Kaafarani HMA. Surgical risk is not linear: derivation and validation of a novel, user-friendly, and machine-learning-based Predictive OpTimal Trees in Emergency Surgery Risk (POTTER) calculator: derivation and

SCIENTIFIC PRINCIPLES

validation of a novel, user-friendly, and machine-learning-based predictive OpTimal trees in emergency surgery risk (POTTER) calculator. *Ann Surg*. 2018;268:574–583.
19. Meguid RA, Bronsert MR, Juarez-Colunga E, Hammermeister KE, Henderson WG. Surgical risk preoperative assessment system (SURPAS): I. parsimonious, clinically meaningful groups of postoperative complications by factor analysis. *Ann Surg*. 2016;263:1042–1048.
20. Bihorac A, Ozrazgat-Baslanti T, Ebadi A, et al. MySurgeryRisk: development and validation of a machine-learning risk algorithm for major complications and death after surgery. *Ann Surg*. 2019;269:652–662.
21. Vernooij JEM, Koning NJ, Geurts JW, et al. Performance and usability of pre-operative prediction models for 30-day peri-operative mortality risk: a systematic review. *Anaesthesia*. 2023;78:607–619.
22. Forsyth DA, Ponce J. *Computer Vision: A Modern Approach: International Edition*. Pearson Higher Ed; 2015.
23. Mascagni P, Alapatt D, Sestini L, et al. Computer vision in surgery: from potential to clinical value. *NPJ Digit Med*. 2022;5(1):163.
24. Cui Z, Ma R, Yang CH, et al. Capturing relationships between suturing sub-skills to improve automatic suturing assessment. *NPJ Digit Med*. 2024;7:1–10.
25. Reifs D, Casanova-Lozano L, Reig-Bolaño R, Grau-Carrion S. Clinical validation of computer vision and artificial intelligence algorithms for wound measurement and tissue classification in wound care. *IMU*. 2023;37:101185.
26. Ahmadi SA, Sielhorst T, Stauder R, Horn M, Feussner H, Navab N. Recovery of surgical workflow without explicit models. *Med Image Comput Comput Assist Interv*. 2006;9:420–428.
27. Igaki T, Kitaguchi D, Matsuzaki H, et al. Automatic surgical skill assessment system based on concordance of standardized surgical field development using artificial intelligence. *JAMA Surg*. 2023;158:e231131.
28. Ma R, Ramaswamy A, Xu J, et al. Surgical gestures as a method to quantify surgical performance and predict patient outcomes. *NPJ Digit Med*. 2022;5:1–8.
29. Hallinan CM, Ward R, Hart GK, et al. Seamless EMR data access: integrated governance, digital health and the OMOP-CDM. *BMJ Health Care Inform*. 2024;31(1):e100953.
30. Mazer L, Varban O, Montgomery JR, Awad MM, Schulman A. Video is better: why aren't we using it? A mixed-methods study of the barriers to routine procedural video recording and case review. *Surg Endosc*. 2021;36:1090–1097.
31. Secinaro S, Calandra D, Secinaro A, Muthurangu V, Biancone P. The role of artificial intelligence in healthcare: a structured literature review. *BMC Med Inform Decis Mak*. 2021;21:125.
32. Yin J, Ngiam KY, Teo HH. Role of artificial intelligence applications in real-life clinical practice: systematic review. *J Med Internet Res*. 2021;23:e25759.
33. Aristidou A, Jena R, Topol EJ. Bridging the chasm between AI and clinical implementation. *Lancet*. 2022;399:620.
34. Quinn TP, Senadeera M, Jacobs S, Coghlan S, Le V. Trust and medical AI: the challenges we face and the expertise needed to overcome them. *J Am Med Inform Assoc*. 2021;28:890–894.
35. Richardson JP, Smith C, Curtis S, et al. Patient apprehensions about the use of artificial intelligence in healthcare. *NPJ Digit Med*. 2021;4:140.
36. Ng DTK, Leung JKL, Chu SKW, Qiao MS. Conceptualizing AI literacy: an exploratory review. *AIED*. 2021;2:100041.
37. van Kessel R, Wong BLH, Clemens T, Brand H. Digital health literacy as a super determinant of health: more than simply the sum of its parts. *Internet Interv*. 2022;27:100500.
38. Charow R, Jeyakumar T, Younus S, et al. Artificial Intelligence Education Programs for Health Care Professionals: scoping review. *JMIR Med Educ*. 2021;7:e31043.
39. Cadario R, Longoni C, Morewedge CK. Understanding, explaining, and utilizing medical artificial intelligence. *Nat Hum Behav*. 2021;5:1636–1642.
40. Gama F, Tyskbo D, Nygren J, Barlow J, Reed J, Svedberg P. Implementation frameworks for artificial intelligence translation into health care practice: scoping review. *J Med Internet Res*. 2022;24:e32215.
41. Reddy S. Generative AI in healthcare: an implementation science informed translational path on application, integration and governance. *Implement Sci*. 2024;19:27.
42. Binuya MAE, Engelhardt EG, Schats W, Schmidt MK, Steyerberg EW. Methodological guidance for the evaluation and updating of clinical prediction models: a systematic review. *BMC Med Res Methodol*. 2022;22(1):316.
43. Riley RD, Archer L, Snell KIE, et al. Evaluation of clinical prediction models (part 2): how to undertake an external validation study. *BMJ*. 2024;384:e074820.
44. European Commission. Act AI. *Shaping Europe's digital future*. https://digital-strategy.ec.europa.eu/en/policies/regulatory-framework-ai
45. House TW. Executive Order on the Safe, Secure, and Trustworthy Development and Use of Artificial Intelligence. The White House. https://www.federalregister.gov/documents/2023/11/01/2023-24283/safe-secure-and-trustworthy-development-and-use-of-artificial-intelligence
46. Devices C, Intelligence RHA and Learning M (AI/ML)-Enabled Medical Devices. *U.S. Food and Drug Administration*. https://www.fda.gov/medical-devices/software-medical-device-samd/artificial-intelligence-enabled-medical-devices 2024.
47. Quiroz JC, Laranjo L, Kocaballi AB, Berkovsky S, Rezazadegan D, Coiera E. Challenges of developing a digital scribe to reduce clinical documentation burden. *NPJ Digit Med*. 2019;2:114.
48. Hassan H, Zipursky AR, Rabbani N, et al. Ambient artificial intelligence scribes to alleviate the burden of clinical documentation. *NEJM Catalyst*. 2024;5. Online ahead of print.
49. Yan S, Knapp W, Leong A, et al. Prompt engineering on leveraging large language models in generating response to InBasket messages. *J Am Med Inform Assoc*. 2024;31(10):2263–2270.
50. Kanade T, Thorpe C, Whittaker W. Autonomous land vehicle project at CMU. *Proceedings of the DOE/CESAR Workshop on Planning and Sensing for Autonomous Navigation. Oak Ridge National Laboratory, UCLA*, Los Angeles, 1985;71–80.

17

Global Surgery

Jennifer L. Rickard and Sherry M. Wren

SCIENTIFIC PRINCIPLES

Key Points

1 Global surgery is the multidisciplinary field focused on the goal to provide equitable and improved surgical care across international health systems.
2 Surgery is a cross-cutting discipline, impacting multiple disease processes, which translates to a significant burden of disease.
3 Multiple determinants of health impact surgical care, further exacerbating health care disparities.
4 Systems of care are essential to overall population health and surgical outcomes.
5 Opportunities and solutions exist and need to be contextually appropriate, bidirectional, and ethical.

Global surgery is a multidisciplinary field within health care that focuses on improving and providing surgical services to underserved populations worldwide. This chapter will explore the challenges and opportunities in delivering surgical care in resource-limited settings, including discussions on infrastructure, capacity building, ethical considerations, and innovative solutions to improve surgical outcomes on a global scale.

DEFINITIONS

Health disparities exist everywhere, including in high-resource settings (such as the United States). The phrase "global is local" is often employed to highlight that you don't need to travel to find these disparities—often, they are in our backyard.

Global health and global surgery have many different definitions.[1] Global surgery refers to all underserved populations that face inequitable or inadequate surgical care delivery,
1 chronically or acutely. Broadly defined, global surgery is an area of research, study, practice, and advocacy that seeks to improve health outcomes and achieve health equity for all who need surgical, obstetric, and anesthesia care.[2] Using this definition, global surgery can be broadly characterized and classified into the field of health care disparities.

In 2015, The Lancet Commission on Global Surgery proposed six metrics to evaluate a nation's surgical capacity to care for the population.[3] These measures have since been refined and further characterized in the Utstein consensus.[4] These metrics are designed to assess health care at a population level, with less guidance on individual, patient, or local targets. Briefly, these measures are:

- Number (rate) of surgeries performed
- Perioperative mortality rate
- Surgery/Anesthesia/Obstetrics provider density per 100,00 population
- Percentage of the population that can access surgical care within 2 hours
- Protection against catastrophic health expenditure

Built into all of these definitions is the understanding that provision of surgical care requires infrastructure including shelter, supplies, equipment, perioperative care, medications, blood, diagnostics, and trained health care providers that provide anesthesia and a wide range of surgical procedures for adult, obstetrical, and pediatric patients.

HISTORY AND EVOLUTION OF GLOBAL SURGERY

The history of global surgery traces back to health care providers from high-income areas (Global North) providing care in less-resourced regions, primarily in the Global South. This assistance has been viewed through the spectrum of humanitarian efforts to colonialism. The terminology describing the national and/or health care resources of a country or region has also evolved: Initially, First World versus Third World, developed versus underdeveloped, high- versus low-resource, high-income versus low- and middle-income, and most recently, Global North versus Global South. Each term can be considered biased, and none accurately reflects the whole picture.

Missionary doctors, most often with religious affiliation, would travel and work for years in under-resourced locations, providing medical care. These physicians and surgeons were dedicated to improving the lives of their communities and filled the significant void due to inadequate numbers of trained health care providers. Even today, missionary doctors provide significant care in many lower-resourced areas. Advances in air travel facilitated the development of short-term surgical missions where visiting doctors would provide surgical care in time-limited engagements.[5] One of the first was Amref Health Africa, officially founded in 1957 by British surgeons to deliver mobile health services and provide mission hospitals with surgical support. Soon, numerous organizations in multiple specialties were developed, and many are still working today. However, there was a growing recognition that these programs often left gaps in coverage, potentially displaced local surgeons when free services were being provided, and often did not address skills and knowledge transfer to local physicians and surgeons.[5,6] Next, a new focus developed on capacity-building programs where institutions or organizations partner to build up and strengthen the training of local health care workers within their home country, especially in the nations with significant deficits in surgical workforce.

The goal is to achieve a self-sustaining education and training system where there are enough sites and faculty to provide sufficient surgical workforce for the needs of the population. There are many challenges that partnerships can address: supplementation of faculty, codevelopment of training sites, faculty development, advanced skills training, and system development for diseases (eg, injury, cancer). One challenge difficult

Table 17.1. Common Models of Global Surgery

Domain	Type of Model	Characteristics (defining)
Clinical care	Short-term surgical mission/camp	Short-term mission where surgeons from high-income countries travel for 1–2 wks and provide clinical care Surgical camps where surgeons in low- or middle-income countries work in remote areas within their home country
	Missionary	Works with a faith-based organization to provide medical care
	Domestic	US-based programs working in less-resourced settings ▪ Indian health services ▪ Rural surgery ▪ OB/Gyn as part of primary care ▪ Public Health Service/Corps ▪ Urban programs (Operation Access)
	Humanitarian (Informal)	Organizations that provides care, material, and logistic assistance to people in need
	Formal humanitarian actors	Médecins Sans Frontiérs, International Committee of the Red Cross, Emergency: organizations that are formal humanitarian actors in conflict settings and function under legal framework governing Law of Armed Conflict
	Disaster relief	Organizations that specifically respond acutely to disasters (often natural disasters)
Education and capacity building	Short courses	Courses provided over a short duration (often <1 wk) to teach a specific skill or topic
	Simulation and tele-education	Education provided through simulation or teleconferencing techniques
	Degree-granting programs	Degree granting program developed in home country Degree obtained in another country
Research	Research partnerships	Research partnerships between high-income and low- and middle-income country partners to enhance research in low- and middle-income country ▪ Best practice—follow guidelines to ensure equitability especially in regard to authorship
	Quality improvement programs	Specific field of research aimed to monitor and ensure quality of care provided ▪ Not necessarily involving publication
Advocacy		Organizations to promote and advocate for global health/surgery principles at national and international levels

to address is "brain drain," namely the retention of trained workforce. Internal "brain drain" occurs in many countries as evidenced by the rural–urban divide and difficulty keeping rural surgical access for patients. There are now multiple US states sponsoring medical school tuition or other incentives with the recipients' commitment to remain in a rural practice. Low- and middle-income countries (LMICs) have similar rural challenges and in addition emigration of surgical workforce to other countries due complex issues including: financial, professional and academic growth, conflict or political issues, and poor health systems management.

Over time, global surgery has evolved into a recognized field with specialized training programs, fellowships, and career pathways. Practitioners in global surgery often concentrate on specific areas such as clinical care, education, research, or a blend of these domains (**Table 17.1**). Advocacy and leadership are vital components of the field. Challenges persist in establishing it as a sustainable career option, particularly regarding time commitments and funding limitations.

EPIDEMIOLOGY OF SURGICAL BURDEN OF DISEASE

The Lancet Commission on Global Surgery estimated that 5 billion people lack access to safe, timely, and affordable surgical care.[3] Though widely quoted, this number characterized access and an economic qualifier, not actual surgical needs based on the disease burden or aversion of mortality.[7]

There are significant challenges and limitations when estimating the burden of disease requiring a surgical procedure. 2 Most data collection on disease burden focuses on specific disease entities. However, surgery is a cross-cutting discipline across many disease categories. Another challenge is the lack of data in low-resource settings, and current data is often extrapolated based on minimal reported data. Based on modeling using 2010 world data with a global population of 6.9 billion, it was estimated that a minimum of 321.5 million surgical procedures would be required to address the disease burden.[8] The unmet rates of surgical procedures varied by geographic region, from approximately 4,000 procedures/100K population in Central Latin America to 6,500/100K in Western Sub-Saharan Africa. In addition, specific surgical needs varied across different categories of diseases, with the low end of the range of 131K procedures for Nutritional Deficiencies to the high end of 45.8 million procedures for unintentional injuries.

Noncommunicable Disease (NCD)

Advancements in treating infectious diseases have led to higher survival rates into adulthood and increased life expectancy. This demographic shift has resulted in a higher prevalence of noncommunicable diseases (NCDs. NCDs now account for 74% of deaths ages 30 to 69, 85% of which occur in LMICs.[9] They are caused in ranked order by cardiovascular disease, cancer, respiratory disease, and diabetes. Access to surgery is crucial in diagnosing, treating, and palliating NCDs.

Injury

Injuries and violence account for an estimated 10% of all years lived with disability and 8% of global mortality.[10] Approximately 2 million die from road traffic crashes (RTCs) per year, and they are the leading cause of death for people aged 5 to 29 years.[11] LMICs have a disproportionate mortality burden, with 92% of the world's RTC fatalities occurring in LMICs. Trauma and injury disproportionally impact young and healthy individuals in their prime work years as well as their families. The estimated cost of RTCs to most countries is 3% of their gross domestic product.[7]

Communicable Disease

Infectious disease has long been a primary driver of global health. The characterization of surgical needs for infection has yet to be fully quantitated. A wide range of communicable diseases exist, such as bone and soft tissue infections, gastrointestinal diseases from parasites or pathogens, and rheumatic heart disease.[12] The emergence of drug-resistant pathogens and limited antibiotic options in many countries further complicate the treatment of these conditions.

Maternal/Child Health

Maternal and neonatal disorders account for 2 million deaths worldwide, with 30 countries accounting for 80% of maternal deaths.[13] Obstructed labor, postpartum hemorrhage, and hypertensive emergency are critical drivers of maternal mortality. Cesarean sections are the most common surgery performed globally, and access to timely and quality surgical care can affect outcomes for both the mother and the infant. Globally, 25% of the population is <15 years old, and a significant number of them require procedures for infections, congenital abnormalities, neoplasms, injury, and reconstruction.[14]

DETERMINANTS OF HEALTH

The conditions in the environments where people live, learn, and work can affect various health outcomes and disease risks. 3 Social determinants of health are associated with longevity in different countries.[15] The combination of multiple factors can further compound this impact on health. These determinants often worsen gaps in disparities, as it is often the lowest-resourced populations who are most vulnerable.

Socioeconomic Factors

Sex

In many places around the world, females have less access or referral to health care interventions. This has been characterized in multiple high-income nations even with procedures with strict guideline algorithms, such as myocardial infarction.[16] Possible factors are unconscious bias of providers, patient autonomy or agency to seek/receive care, women's needs not being prioritized within the family structure, and less financial means to seek care. They are often tasked with caring for the children, home, and animals, which does not allow them the flexibility to seek medical attention. Once reaching the health care system, women may not be granted the autonomy to make their own medical decisions. Afghanistan is a complex nation where women's access to health care and, concomitantly, their children's health has flip-flopped in the very recent past with significant detriment to the female population.[17]

Culture/Religion/Ethnicity/Race

Culture and religion play an important role in how we access and manage our health care. Certain individuals or groups may be granted less agency or autonomy to make their own decisions. Beliefs or perceptions about health care are often influenced by our culture and religion (eg, Jehovah's Witness and blood products). Even in the United States, surgical outcomes vary for different ethnic groups.[18] Many nations have nonmajority populations whose health access and metrics may differ from those of the dominant population. Surgical care can be impacted in cultures that prevent male practitioners from caring for female patients due to the significant gender imbalance among surgeons in most countries, leaving females with diminished care options.

Education and Literacy

Education and literacy can have significant effects on health. In general, with better education comes greater wealth, knowledge, and awareness of how to care for one's health. It also provides greater access to health care. Being literate means that you have access to written communication that can be shared about your health. It also offers better empowerment in managing and coordinating your health care. A recent meta-analysis demonstrated each additional year of education showed a dose–response relationship with all-cause adult mortality.[19] Globally, there are gender and regional differences in educational attainment, which have downstream health impacts.[20]

Occupation and Downstream Risk for Surgical Procedures

Many jobs are associated with higher rates of injury or exposure to carcinogens, including construction, agriculture, fishing, and manufacturing.[21] This is true for both high-income and LMICs, but the burden of disease and disability is much more significant in LMICs, where occupational health protections are less well-developed or enforced. Globally, there are millions of people trafficked for bonded or slave labor, as well as child laborers, in hazardous conditions that lead to high rates of injury and disability.[22]

Poverty and Ability to Pay for Care

Poverty also has profound effects on health outcomes. There are multiple classifications of poverty, including absolute versus relative poverty and current versus cumulative poverty. Poverty has a profound impact on mortality risks, with cumulative (more than 10 years of uninterrupted poverty) having the most significant association with mortality.[23] Poverty factors into surgical care in the many countries where universal health care is absent. This may play a role in the perception that surgery was "too expensive" and not cost-effective in lower-resourced areas. However, multiple studies have demonstrated the cost-effectiveness of surgery, especially compared to treatment for other diseases.[24]

Whether something is cost-effective or not, cost considerations play a critical role in decisions about obtaining health care. It is not simply the cost of health care, but who can and will bear the burden—patient/family versus hospital versus insurance versus government. National advocacy for health cost coverage is essential because economic analyses demonstrate that investment in surgical care is effective since the burden of surgical conditions disproportionally affects the working-age population and children and, thus, the country's economic output.[25] Increased investment in health care, particularly surgical care, improves the health of these people and, therefore, leads to economic growth.

Unfortunately, even in the United States, health care costs increasingly cause patients and/or families to declare bankruptcy.[26] Catastrophic health expenditure is defined as health expenditures exceeding 40% of household income net of subsistence needs, and impoverishing health expenditure refers to out-of-pocket health expenditures that push a family further into poverty.[3] To date, there is limited data on these metrics and there are challenges with their data capture. They do not capture whether a family has had to sell off assets. Nor do they capture other financial impacts, such as the decision not to send children to school (to balance finances). Universal health insurance has been promoted to offset the economic impact of unanticipated health care costs. The availability of health insurance varies widely around the globe, with many different models ranging from government-sponsored to private health insurance programs. Some countries have poor or limited options for health insurance. Other countries have broad health insurance coverage. Life expectancy is higher in countries with publicly funded health care compared with countries without publicly funded health care.[15]

Physical Environment

Access to Water

Access to clean, safe water is a significant factor in health and disease. Myriad diseases are transmitted through unclean water and cause diseases in the population, some requiring surgery (eg, typhoid intestinal perforation). Hospitals are also dependent on ready access to and supply of water, especially for the operating room to have the capacity to clean and sterilize instruments and perform hand hygiene. Reports of hospitals' access to water in LMICs vary, with many in some regions lacking consistent access to this vital resource.[27]

Access to Food and Nutrition

Malnutrition is a serious global issue that disproportionally affects the poor, women, and children. Climate, conflict, and famine are reversing years of improvement in international nutrition. Children suffer from stunting of their growth, which has lifelong implications on their cognitive and physical abilities. Malnutrition is a known cause of poor surgical outcomes, with many prehabilitation programs existing in high-income countries to try and optimize patients before surgery.[28]

Transportation

Access to transportation can significantly impact health and access to surgery. A 2020 report on global access to health care reported that even if everyone had access to motorized transportation, only 8.9% (646 million people) of the global population would reach a health care facility within 1 hour. If access was defined as being able to walk to the facility within 1 hour, only 43.3% (3.16 billion) could get there in the hour.[29] Transportation costs can also be a significant barrier for patients to seek care.

Natural Disasters

Not only do natural disasters cause direct physical injury, but they can also disrupt the health care infrastructure, thereby further worsening the insult. Earthquakes, in particular, generate large numbers of injured patients compared with other natural disasters such as tsunamis, floods, and wildfires.[30] The Haiti earthquake in 2010 caused direct injury to 220,000 individuals, and an additional 5,899 died from a cholera outbreak.[31] Additional loss was experienced with the destruction of the health care infrastructure, which frustrated recovery efforts. With the worsening climate change, more natural disasters are predicted, and greater adverse health outcomes can be expected.

Conflict or War

Conflict and war directly contribute to the burden of disease through injury, untreated disease, destruction of the health care infrastructure, and loss of health care providers. A relevant example is the Syrian conflict (2011–2021), which included 595 attacks on 350 health facilities; in some regions, 59% of civilians were significantly impacted, with 24% reporting inability to receive medical treatment due to direct attacks on centers and for the country an estimated loss of 70% of the health care workforce who died or left the country.[32] Conflict numbers and duration are increasing with devastating consequences on populations.

Delays in Care

In health care, time can matter. The landmark Three Delays Model first described how delays in care affected expectant mothers and subsequently was applied to other medical and surgical conditions.[23] The model outlines a delay in deciding to seek care (First Delay), a delay in reaching the health facility (Second Delay), and a delay in receiving appropriate treatment at the facility (Third Delay). The First Delay is linked to family and community factors: care affordability, and past experiences with the health system. The Second Delay involves challenges in accessibility: such as distance, availability, and cost of transportation. The Third Delay relates to the quality of service at the facility: which may be inadequate due to lack of supplies and equipment, unwelcoming environment (including disrespectful care), and poorly trained staff.[33]

HEALTH CARE SYSTEMS

Most modern health care is comprised of systems, oftentimes
4 in a tiered approach. These are not simple systems, but systems within systems. These systems promote efficient, timely, cost-effective care. Each tiered health care system is unique, but there are common themes.

One example of this tiered system is the organization of trauma care in the United States, with lower-tiered trauma facilities prepared to manage the most basic traumas but higher facilities expected to manage the more complex cases. This organization helps direct trauma patients to the appropriate level of care. Similarly, around the globe, many public systems are organized in a tiered system with increasing complexity, ranging from health centers to districts, then provincial and referral hospitals. Health centers are often staffed with nurses and health care workers, whereas referral hospitals will have a wide cadre of health care professionals, including physicians, specialists, and subspecialists. Increasingly, in both higher- and lower-resourced countries, regionalization of more complex care is being focused in regional centers to achieve economies of scale for imaging equipment, medical/surgical expertise, drugs, trained staff, and specialists. A successful example is cancer care systems that demonstrated increased access, better care and survival metrics, and more controllable costs.[34]

Health care systems and their design are critical to the health of the population and access to surgical care, as reflected in the global surgery indicators–the percentage of the population that has access to a facility with a surgeon within 2 hours, as well as the economic stress paying for care, has on a patient. National or regional systems are complex and include other elements such as prehospital care and transportation to the health center. Ambulances do not exist everywhere due to many factors such as cost, lack of roads, and relevance (island nations). In many countries, community members, police officers, and transportation drivers have been trained as first responders with demonstrable benefits.[35–37]

Systems are also reliant on material resource availability and maintenance of existing equipment. Supply chains are being affected by a myriad of stressors, such as a lack of raw materials and transportation disruption due to conflict, climate change, worker shortages, and natural disasters. The procurement process for medical supplies, drugs, and equipment is very complex, and supply flow disruptions can negatively impact patient care, with a disproportionate effect on lower-resourced settings.

Finally, medical equipment maintenance is another area where disparities exist across nations and systems. Lower-resourced nations often have minimal to no trained biomedical engineers to perform basic equipment maintenance and repair. In addition, hospitals in low-resource settings are working with old and outdated, donated medical equipment, often not appropriate for their setting or in good working order. This is increasingly being recognized by the biomedical engineering community and organizations with programs, training, and support to try to facilitate and improve access to trained personnel in more settings.[38,39]

OPPORTUNITIES AND SOLUTIONS

There are key concepts and principles that must be under-
5 stood and followed when participating in global surgery. First and foremost, global surgeons must follow basic principles of medical ethics. Ethics focuses on the principles of autonomy, beneficence, nonmaleficence, and justice. *Primum non nocere*, which translates to "First, do no harm," is a medical adage that captures general principles of medical care regardless of location. Surgeons should provide the same standard of care irrespective of location and maintain the same scope of practice, unless there are truly no other options, and then carefully examine whether their intervention can be justified. There are far too many tales of health care providers working outside their usual scope of practice, with unfortunate results. Medical tourism to get operative experience that a trainee or surgeon would not be allowed to do at home also needs to be closely examined as to whose interests are being served.

Each setting has its own unique strengths and limitations, including the infrastructure, workforce, capacity, resources, and information management system. It is important to understand the mission and values of the program or group that you are partnering with. Preparation is key. Read about the country, region, ongoing sociopolitical issues, religion, and culture before working on the ground. Look to see if there is National, Surgical, Obstetric, and Anesthetic Plans (NSOAPs) for the country. The NSOAPs framework aims to strengthen surgical systems through focused attention to infrastructure, service delivery, workforce, information management, financing, and governance.[40] These plans help delineate gaps in health care services, define opportunities for engagement, and help prioritize activities. With this in mind, global partners can better coordinate efforts with other implementing partners. To date, the largest barrier to implementation of NSOAPs remains financial and innovative solutions are needed to overcome this barrier.[41]

Cultural competency builds on the recognition of differences in perceptions across cultures. Cultural competence is a set of skills for efficient communication with those from other cultures through understanding social rules, norms, and rituals that are not one's own.[42] This includes understanding local health practices and developing skills which are relevant to the local context. One method to address cultural competency is to develop a predeparture training which can include education on the history of the region, social determinants of health, and ethics.[42]

Within this dynamic it is important to respect the local health care system and the impact on that system. The presence of a visiting surgeon can actually result in a negative economic impact for the local system.[42] Visiting surgeons can displace or compete with local surgeons, especially when they are offering free services, depriving the local surgeons of workload. Visiting surgeons may also disrupt the local supply chain development through importation of medical equipment and materials.

For optimal efficacy, engage with local partners. This should be a respectful, bilateral, and equitable partnership that considers the needs and strengths of all partners. Unfortunately, there are many instances of inequitable partnerships. A common example in research partnerships is the unequal representation of LMIC authors on peer-reviewed publications. In a bibliometric analysis of scientific studies published in LMICs, over one-quarter of all publications did not list a local author and most have no first or corresponding author from the LMIC.[43]

At the end of the day, what is the measure of success? One true measure of success would be the complete elimination of health care disparities and the need for a field of "global" surgery. As we slowly but consistently break down the disparities in care, the need for a separate field of study will slowly disappear. Successful global surgeons should work themselves out of a job and successful global surgery partnerships will either end or transition to new goals. Programs and partnerships should grow and develop over time so that facilities in low-resource settings are less dependent on high-resource partners. Perhaps the partnerships will remain, but the aim and focus of those partnerships should grow and evolve over time.

SUMMARY

Global surgery represents a field of health care disparities focused on addressing inadequate or inequitable surgical care delivery. The field has grown and evolved over the past decades with increased focus on metrics and ensuring equity among partners.

ACKNOWLEDGMENTS

We gratefully acknowledge the contributions of previous edition author(s), Tiffany E. Chao and Jahnavi K. Srinivasan, as portions of those chapters have been retained in this revision.

References

1. Dare AJ, Grimes CE, Gillies R, et al. Global surgery: defining an emerging global health field. *Lancet*. 2014;384(9961):2245–2247.
2. Bath M, Bashford T, Fitzgerald JE. What is 'global surgery'? Defining the multidisciplinary interface between surgery, anaesthesia and public health. *BMJ Glob Health*. 2019;4(5):e001808.
3. Meara JG, Greenberg SL. The Lancet Commission on Global Surgery Global surgery 2030: Evidence and solutions for achieving health, welfare and economic development. *Surgery*. 2015;157(5): 834–835.
4. Davies JI, Gelb AW, Gore-Booth J, et al. Global surgery, obstetric, and anaesthesia indicator definitions and reporting: An Utstein consensus report. *PLoS Med*. 2021;18(8):e1003749.
5. Nthumba PM. "Blitz surgery": redefining surgical needs, training, and practice in sub-Saharan Africa. *World J Surg*. 2010;34(3):433–437.
6. Ginwalla R, Rickard J. Surgical missions: the view from the other side. *JAMA Surg*. 2015;150(4):289–290.
7. Gupta S, Groen RS, Kyamanywa P, et al. Surgical care needs of low-resource populations: an estimate of the prevalence of surgically treatable conditions and avoidable deaths in 48 countries. *Lancet*. 2015;385 Suppl 2:S1.
8. Rose J, Weiser TG, Hider P, Wilson L, Gruen RL, Bickler SW. Estimated need for surgery worldwide based on prevalence of diseases: a modelling strategy for the WHO Global Health Estimate. *Lancet Glob Health*. 2015;3 Suppl 2(Suppl 2):S13–S20.
9. WHO. Noncommunicable diseases: Mortality: World Health Organization; 2024. Available from: https://www.who.int/data/gho/data/themes/topics/topic-details/GHO/ncd-mortality
10. WHO. Injuries and violence: World Health Organization; 2024. Available from: https://www.who.int/news-room/fact-sheets/detail/injuries-and-violence
11. WHO. Road traffic injuries: World Health Organization; 2023. Available from: https://www.who.int/news-room/fact-sheets/detail/road-traffic-injuries
12. Rickard J, Beilman G, Forrester J, et al. Surgical infections in low- and middle-income countries: A global assessment of the burden and management needs. *Surg Infect (Larchmt)*. 2020;21(6):478–494.
13. IHME. Maternal health: Institute for Health Metrics and Evaluation; Available from: https://www.healthdata.org/research-analysis/health-risks-issues/maternal-health
14. Investigators A-P. Outcomes after surgery for children in Africa (ASOS-Paeds): a 14-day prospective observational cohort study. *Lancet*. 2024;403(10435):1482–1492.
15. Galvani-Townsend S, Martinez I, Pandey A. Is life expectancy higher in countries and territories with publicly funded health care? Global analysis of health care access and the social determinants of health. *J Glob Health*. 2022;12:04091.
16. Cenko E, Yoon J, Bergami M, et al. Coronary revascularization and sex differences in cardiovascular mortality after myocardial infarction in 12 high and middle-income European countries. *Eur Heart J Qual Care Clin Outcomes*. 2024:qcae035.
17. Glass N, Jalalzai R, Spiegel P, Rubenstein L. The crisis of maternal and child health in Afghanistan. *Confl Health*. 2023;17(1):28.
18. Haider AH, Scott VK, Rehman KA, et al. Racial disparities in surgical care and outcomes in the United States: a comprehensive review of patient, provider, and systemic factors. *J Am Coll Surg*. 2013;216(3):482–492.e12.
19. Collaborators I-C. Effects of education on adult mortality: a global systematic review and meta-analysis. *Lancet Public Health*. 2024;9(3):e155–e165.
20. Local Burden of Disease Educational Attainment Collaborators. Mapping disparities in education across low- and middle-income countries. *Nature*. 2020;577(7789):235–238.
21. Mock CN, Smith KR, Kobusingye O, et al. Injury prevention and environmental health. *The International Bank for Reconstruction and Development, 3rd ed*. The World Bank; 2017.
22. Zimmerman C, Hargreaves S, Lau K, Kiss L, Chia-Yin Lin R, Pocock N. Addressing labour exploitation in the global workforce. *Lancet*. 2024;403(10438):1748.
23. Brady D, Kohler U, Zheng H. Novel estimates of mortality associated with poverty in the US. *JAMA Intern Med*. 2023;183(6):618–619.

24. Chao TE, Sharma K, Mandigo M, et al. Cost-effectiveness of surgery and its policy implications for global health: a systematic review and analysis. *Lancet Glob Health*. 2014;2(6):e334–e345.
25. Jumbam DT, Reddy CL, Makasa E, et al. Investing in surgery: a value proposition for African leaders. *Lancet*. 2020;396(10243):7–9.
26. Himmelstein DU, Lawless RM, Thorne D, Foohey P, Woolhandler S. Medical bankruptcy: still common despite the affordable care act. *Am J Public Health*. 2019;109(3):431–433.
27. Chawla SS, Gupta S, Onchiri FM, Habermann EB, Kushner AL, Stewart BT. Water availability at hospitals in low- and middle-income countries: implications for improving access to safe surgical care. *J Surg Res*. 2016;205(1):169–178.
28. Williams DGA, Molinger J, Wischmeyer PE. The malnourished surgery patient: a silent epidemic in perioperative outcomes? *Curr Opin Anaesthesiol*. 2019;32(3):405–411.
29. Weiss DJ, Nelson A, Vargas-Ruiz CA, et al. Global maps of travel time to healthcare facilities. *Nat Med*. 2020;26(12):1835–1838.
30. Bartholdson S, von Schreeb J. Natural disasters and injuries: what does a surgeon need to know? *Curr Trauma Rep*. 2018;4(2):103–108.
31. DEC. 2010 Haiti Earthquake Facts And Figures: Disaster Emergency Committee; 2024. https://www.dec.org.uk/article/2010-haiti-earthquake-facts-and-figures
32. IRC. A Decade of Destruction: Attacks on health care in Syria: International Rescue Committee; 2021. https://www.rescue.org/sites/default/files/document/5648/adecadeofdestructionattacksonhealthcareinsyria.pdf
33. Actis Danna V, Bedwell C, Wakasiaka S, Lavender T. Utility of the three-delays model and its potential for supporting a solution-based approach to accessing intrapartum care in low- and middle-income countries. A qualitative evidence synthesis. *Glob Health Action*. 2020;13(1):1819052.
34. Prager GW, Braga S, Bystricky B, et al. Global cancer control: responding to the growing burden, rising costs and inequalities in access. *ESMO Open*. 2018;3(2):e000285.
35. Husum H, Gilbert M, Wisborg T, Van Heng Y, Murad M. Rural prehospital trauma systems improve trauma outcome in low-income countries: a prospective study from North Iraq and Cambodia. *J Trauma*. 2003;54(6):1188–1196.
36. Slingers M, De Vos S, Sun JH. Ten years of the community-based emergency first aid responder (EFAR) system in the Western Cape of South Africa: What has happened, what has changed, and what has been learned. *Afr J Emerg Med*. 2022;12(4):299–306.
37. Jayaraman S, Mabweijano JR, Lipnick MS, et al. Current patterns of prehospital trauma care in Kampala, Uganda and the feasibility of a lay-first-responder training program. *World J Surg*. 2009;33(12):2512–2521.
38. Inagaki D, Nakahara S, Chung UI, Shimaoka M, Shoji K. Need for improvements in medical device management in low- and middle-income countries: Applying Learnings from Japan's Experience. *JMA J*. 2023;6(2):188–191.
39. De Maria C, Díaz Lantada A, Jämsä T, Pecchia L, Ahluwalia A. Biomedical engineering in low- and middle-income settings: analysis of current state, challenges and best practices. *Health Technol (Berl)*. 2022;12(3):643–653.
40. Truché P, Shoman H, Reddy CL, et al. Globalization of national surgical, obstetric and anesthesia plans: the critical link between health policy and action in global surgery. *Global Health*. 2020;16(1):1.
41. Reddy CL, Peters AW, Jumbam DT, et al. Innovative financing to fund surgical systems and expand surgical care in low-income and middle-income countries. *BMJ Glob Health*. 2020;5(6):e002375.
42. Yang G, Bekele A, Krishnaswami S, et al. Cultural competency and ethical behavior for collaboration in limited-resource settings: Guidelines from the Society of University Surgeons Academic Global Surgery Committee and the Association for Academic Global Surgery. *Surgery*. 2024;176(1):108–114.
43. Ghani M, Hurrell R, Verceles AC, McCurdy MT, Papali A. Geographic, subject, and authorship trends among LMIC-based scientific publications in high-impact global health and general medicine journals: A 30-month bibliometric analysis. *J Epidemiol Glob Health*. 2021;11(1):92–97.

Section A:
TRAUMA

18

Trauma and Trauma Care: General Considerations

John W. Scott and Hasan B. Alam

Key Points

1 Injuries are the leading cause of death in young Americans, and account for 1 out of every 10 deaths in the world.
2 The three most common mechanisms of injury-related deaths are firearms, motor vehicle collisions, and falls.
3 Establishment of trauma systems that use evidence-based triage and treatment protocols saves lives.
4 The vast majority of trauma-related deaths are within the first few hours (<6 hours) after sustaining injuries.
5 Bleeding is the number one cause of preventable deaths.
6 Advance Trauma Life Support (ATLS) provides a systematic approach for rapid assessment and treatment of injured patients.
7 Massive transfusion protocols and hemostatic resuscitations are key components of strategies to prevent trauma-induced coagulopathy.
8 The two treatment priorities for bleeding patients are early hemorrhage control and prevention of trauma-induced coagulopathy.
9 Throughout time military conflicts have rapidly advanced trauma care in many domains, and these developments continue to inform and improve the care of injured patients in the civilian trauma settings.
10 As inpatient survival after major injury continues to improve, more emphasis is being placed on understanding and improving long-term outcomes among survivors of nonfatal injury.

EPIDEMIOLOGY OF INJURIES IN THE UNITED STATES

Injuries and violence affect everyone, regardless of age, sex, race, or economic status. Injuries are the number one cause of death for children in America, they are the number one cause of death and disability among working-age adults, and the incidence of injury-related deaths among older adults is
1 increasing at an alarming rate year after year.[1,2] According to the Centers for Disease Control and Prevention (CDC), National Center for Injury Prevention and Control, injuries account for nearly 200,000 deaths per year, excluding drug overdoses.[1] On the global scale, injuries account for over 10% of the entire global burden of disease.[2] Each year, almost 100 million people are injured and nearly 5 million people die from injuries—more deaths than HIV/AIDS, malaria, and tuberculosis, combined.[2]

Figure 18.1 shows the top 10 causes of death in different age groups in the United States, whereas **Figure 18.2** shows the top
2 10 causes of injury-related deaths.[1] Excluding drug overdoses/poisoning, the top three mechanisms of injury-related deaths in the United States are firearms, motor vehicle collisions (MVCs), and falls—*each* of which account for approximately 44,500 to 48,000 deaths annually (**Table 18.1**).[1] This heterogeneous group of injury mechanisms have a dynamic relationship with societal and demographic changes over time (**Fig. 18.3**).

For example, better roads, safer cars, more frequent use of seatbelts, and a reduction in drunk driving over the last few decades led to a marked decrease in the MVC fatality rate from the 1970s through the mid-2010s despite a marked increase in the number of cars on the roads and overall miles driven (**Fig. 18.4**). However, from 2019 to 2021, annual motor vehicle traffic fatalities rose 19% from roughly 36,000 to over 43,000, and the deaths per 100 million vehicles for 2020 to 2023 is nearly 20% higher than the nadir of 1.08 in 2013.[3] Conversely, falls—which are more common in older adults—are rapidly becoming a major health care issue due to the increasing age of the population.[4] In the United States today, 1 in 6 Americans is aged 65 or older, which by 2050 will increase to 1 in 4.5.[5] The fall-related death rates have been climbing since the early 1990s (**Fig. 18.5**) and are expected to increase even more dramatically over the next few decades (see Chapter 29: Geriatric Trauma for more information).

10 Leading Causes of Death, United States
2022, Both sexes, All ages, All races

	<1	1–4	5–9	10–14	15–24	25–34	35–44	45–54	55–64	65+	All Ages
1	Congenital Anomalies 3,970	Unintentional Injury 1,288	Unintentional Injury 726	Unintentional Injury 926	Unintentional Injury 14,669	Unintentional Injury 33,058	Unintentional Injury 36,972	Malignant Neoplasms 33,363	Malignant Neoplasms 1,05,133	Heart Disease 5,67,365	Heart Disease 7,02,880
2	Short Gestation 2,884	Congenital Anomalies 441	Malignant Neoplasms 393	Suicide 493	Homicide 6,262	Suicide 8,663	Heart Disease 12,258	Heart Disease 32,298	Heart Disease 85,733	Malignant Neoplasms 4,52,490	Malignant Neoplasms 6,08,371
3	Sids 1,529	Homicide 343	Congenital Anomalies 241	Malignant Neoplasms 442	Suicide 6,040	Homicide 6,712	Malignant Neoplasms 11,177	Unintentional Injury 31,394	Unintentional Injury 34,017	Covid-19 1,46,320	Unintentional Injury 2,27,039
4	Unintentional Injury 1,354	Malignant Neoplasms 266	Homicide 180	Homicide 366	Malignant Neoplasms 1,421	Heart Disease 3,789	Suicide 8,185	Covid-19 9,678	Covid-19 24,252	Cerebrovascular 1,42,513	Covid-19 1,86,552
5	Maternal Pregnancy Comp. 1,215	Influenza & Pneumonia 129	Influenza & Pneumonia 77	Congenital Anomalies 205	Heart Disease 848	Malignant Neoplasms 3,641	Liver Disease 5,501	Liver Disease 9,401	Diabetes Mellitus 17,410	Chronic Low. Respiratory Disease 1,25,803	Cerebrovascular 1,65,393
6	Placenta Cord Membranes 649	Heart Disease 103	Heart Disease 73	Heart Disease 145	Covid-19 447	Liver Disease 1,786	Homicide 4,765	Suicide 7,781	Chronic Low. Respiratory Disease 17,138	Alzheimer's Disease 1,18,525	Chronic Low. Respiratory Disease 1,47,382
7	Bacterial Sepsis 636	Covid-19 101	Covid-19 62	Covid-19 69	Congenital Anomalies 412	Covid-19 1,640	Covid-19 3,841	Diabetes Mellitus 7,364	Liver Disease 16,484	Unintentional Injury 72,616	Alzheimer's Disease 1,20,122
8	Respiratory Distress 456	Perinatal Period 62	Chronic Low. Respiratory Disease 48	Chronic Low. Respiratory Disease 58	Diabetes Mellitus 324	Diabetes Mellitus 1,188	Diabetes Mellitus 2,879	Cerebrovascular 5,563	Cerebrovascular 14,173	Diabetes Mellitus 71,985	Diabetes Mellitus 1,01,209
9	Intrauterine Hypoxia 362	Septicemia 60	Cerebrovascular 45	Cerebrovascular 55	Chronic Low. Respiratory Disease 197	Cerebrovascular 599	Cerebrovascular 2,150	Chronic Low. Respiratory Disease 2,987	Suicide 7,864	Nephritis 47,086	Nephritis 57,937
10	Circulatory System Disease 356	Cerebrovascular 49	Septicemia 33	Influenza & Pneumonia 54	Influenza & Pneumonia 168	Complicated Pregnancy 591	Nephritis 1,029	Homicide 2,740	Nephritis 6,668	Parkinson's Disease 38,931	Liver Disease 54,803

Data Source: National Vital Statistics System, National Center for Health Statistics, CDC.
Adapted from: National Center for Injury Prevention and Control, CDC using WISQARS™

Figure 18.1. Ten leading causes of death by age group in the United States (2022). (Data Source: National Vital Statistics System, National Center for Health Statistics, CDC. Adapted from National Center for Injury Prevention and Control, CDC using WISQARS™. Accessed December 31, 2024. https://wisqars.cdc.gov/lcd/)

10 Leading Causes of Injury Deaths by Age Group United States
Highlighting Falls, Motor Vehicles, and Firearms
2022, Both sexes, All ages, All races

	<1	1–4	5–9	10–14	15–24	25–34	35–44	45–54	55–64	65+	All Ages
1	Unintentional Suffocation 1,146	Unintentional Drowning 461	Unintentional Mv Traffic [illegible]	Unintentional Mv Traffic [illegible]	Unintentional Mv Traffic [illegible]	Unintentional Poisoning [illegible]	Unintentional Poisoning [illegible]	Unintentional Poisoning 21,364	Unintentional Poisoning 19,334	Unintentional Fall 40,919	Unintentional Poisoning 102,958
2	Homicide Unspecified 111	Unintentional Mv Traffic 315	Unintentional Drowning 123	Homicide Firearm 300	Unintentional Poisoning 6,205	Unintentional Mv Traffic 8,249	Unintentional Mv Traffic 6,918	Unintentional Mv Traffic 5,889	Unintentional Mv Traffic 6,331	Unintentional Mv Traffic 9,104	Unintentional Fall 46,630
3	Unintentional Mv Traffic 77	Unintentional Suffocation 124	Unintentional Hot Object Or Substance 103	Suicide Suffocation 256	Homicide Firearm 5,814	Homicide Firearm 5,836	Homicide Firearm 3,861	Suicide Firearm 3,838	Suicide Firearm 4,412	Suicide Firearm 7,367	Unintentional Mv Traffi c 44,534
4	Undetermined Suffocation 62	Unintentional Hot Object Or Substance 89	Homicide Firearm 95	Suicide Firearm 175	Suicide Firearm 3,246	Suicide Firearm 4,230	Suicide Firearm 3,759	Suicide Suffocation 2,092	Unintentional Fall 3,247	Unintentional Poisoning 6,780	Suicide Firearm 27,032
5	Homicide Other Spec., Classifiable 55	Homicide Unspecified 88	Unintentional Suffocation 38	Unintentional Drowning 107	Suicide Suffocation 1694	Suicide Suffocation 2,830	Suicide Suffocation 2,716	Homicide Firearm 1,947	Suicide Suffocation 1,571	Unintentional Suffocation 4,264	Homicide Firearm 19,651
6	Unintentional Drowning 39	Homicide Firearm 77	Homicide Unspecified 29	Unintentional Poisoning 88	Suicide Poisoning 569	Suicide Poisoning 807	Suicide Poisoning 963	Suicide Poisoning 1,204	Suicide Poisoning 1,237	Unintentional Unspecified 4,096	Suicide Suffocation 12,247
7	Unintentional Poisoning 28	Unintentional Poisoning 75	Unintentional Other Land Transport 28	Unintentional Other Land Transport 63	Unintentional Drowning 488	Undetermined Poisoning 671	Undetermined Poisoning 810	Unintentional Fall 1,200	Homicide Firearm 1,080	Adverse Effects 2,466	Unintentional Suffocation 7,416
8	Undetermined Poisoning 26	Undetermined Poisoning 66	Unintentional Firearm 15**	Unintentional Fire/Flame 56	Homicide Cut/ Pierce 234	Unintentional Drowning 547	Unintentional Fall 682	Undetermined Poisoning 706	Unintentional Suffocation 896	Unintentional Hot Object Or Substance 1,742	Suicide Poisoning 6,150
9	Homicide Poisoning 23	Homicide Other Spec., Classifiable 55	Adverse Effects 13**	Suicide Poisoning 42	Suicide Fall 202	Homicide Cut/ Pierce 430	Unintentional Drowning 549	Unintentional Drowning 483	Unintentional Hot Object Or Substance 703	Unintentional Natural/ Environment 1,592	Unintentional Unspecified 5,273
10	Unintentional Natural/Environment 22	Unintentional Pedestrian, Other 52	Homicide Other Spec., Nec 13**	Unintentional Suffocation 37	Undetermined Poisoning 186	Unintentional Fall 383	Homicide Cut/ Pierce 363	Unintentional Suffocation 391	Adverse Effects 653	Suicide Poisoning 1,328	Unintentional Drowning 4,509

Data Source: National Vital Statistics System, National Center for Health Statistics, CDC.
Adapted from: National Center for Injury Prevention and Control, CDC using WISQARS™
Note: ** indicates unstable value (<20 deaths); Note also that the CDC includes poisoning with injuries, though they do not meet the clinical definition of injury as accepted by the trauma community.

Figure 18.2. Ten leading causes of injury deaths by age group in the United States (2022), highlighting unintentional causes. Note: **indicates unstable value (<20 deaths); Also, the CDC includes poisoning with injuries, though they do not meet the clinical definition of injury as accepted by the trauma community. (Data Source: National Vital Statistics System, National Center for Health Statistics, CDC. Adapted from National Center for Injury Prevention and Control, CDC using WISQARS™. Accessed December 31, 2024. https://wisqars.cdc.gov/lcd/)

Table 18.1. Crude Death Rates by Mechanisms, All Ages (United States, 2022)[a,b]

Mechanisms	Number of Deaths	Crude Death Rate (Per 100,000 Population)
All Injury Mechanisms[b]	**195,057**	**58.5**
Firearm	48,204	14.5
Fall	47,984	14.4
Motor vehicle, traffic	44,534	13.4
Suffocation	20,197	6.1
Drowning and water transport	5384	1.6
Fire/Flame, Hot object/ Substance	4096	1.2
Natural/Environmental	3140	0.9
Cut/Pierce	3011	0.9
Transport, other land	1590	0.5
Struck by/against	1184	0.4
Pedestrian, other	955	0.3
Machinery	645	0.2
Transport, other	480	0.1
Pedal cyclist, other	432	0.1
Other/Unspecified	13,221	4.0

[a]Data obtained from the National Vital Statistics System, National Center for Health Statistics, CDC. Adapted from National Center for Injury Prevention and Control, CDC using WISQARS.™ Accessed December 31, 2024. https://wisqars.cdc.gov/lcd/

[b]Excludes deaths due to poisoning.

Firearm deaths also demonstrate the complex interplay of injury and society. The overall firearm death rate, including both homicide and suicide, decreased significantly from the mid-1970s through the mid-2000s (**Fig. 18.3**), mirroring the national trends in overall violent crimes. However, over the past decade, firearm-related deaths are steadily increasing. Gun suicide rates have been increasing since 2006, and gun homicide rates have been increasing since 2014 (**Fig. 18.6**).[1] Both of these trends are mostly concentrated among males. In 2022, there were over 48,200 firearm-related deaths in the United States, 56% of which were suicides.[1] The crude and age-adjusted firearm-related death rates in 2022 were the highest recorded rates in the last 20 years, up to 45% from 2009.[1] Over the past few years, there has been an increasing awareness that reducing firearms-related deaths will require a public health approach, as advocated for by the multiple Medical Summits on Firearm Injury Prevention led by the American College of Surgeons' Committee on Trauma (ACS-COT)[6] (see Chapter 21: Injury Prevention and Gun Violence for more information).

Although striking, the mortality data do not tell the entire story. In 2022, there were nearly 22 million injured patients treated and released from US emergency departments, and there were approximately 3.9 million nonfatal hospitalizations for injuries.[1] The overwhelming majority of these patients survive, but they may face lifelong mental, physical, social, and financial challenges. At the population level, the resultant economic toll on our society is staggering. In 2022, the medical costs and work loss costs associated with nonfatal injuries amounted to nearly $450 billion.[1] According to the CDC's value of statistical life calculations, the costs of fatal injuries were $3.0 trillion in 2022 alone.[1] At the patient level, patient's injuries may greatly impair a patient's functional status and limit their ability to return to school, work, or preinjury activity level, which can result in significant financial hardship for many patients.[7] As such, there has been increased attention on understanding and optimizing long-term outcomes after injury by addressing postinjury functional limitation, mental health needs, and health-related social needs.[8]

BIOMECHANICS OF INJURY TO GUIDE CLINICAL MANAGEMENT

At the most basic level injuries are caused by energy transfer that results in deformation and damage of bodily tissues. In general, mechanisms of injury are categorized as blunt (eg, falls and MVCs), penetrating (eg, stab and gunshot wounds), or thermal (eg, flame burns and electrocution). Blunt trauma causes damage either through crush or shear forces, whereas penetrating trauma causes injury to the tissues that are in the path of the foreign body. Different types of energy transfer will result in different classically described patterns of injury. Understanding this link between the mechanism of energy transfer and their associated patterns of injury will greatly aid the initial patient evaluation and subsequent management priorities in the prehospital setting, the trauma bay, the operating room, and the ICU.

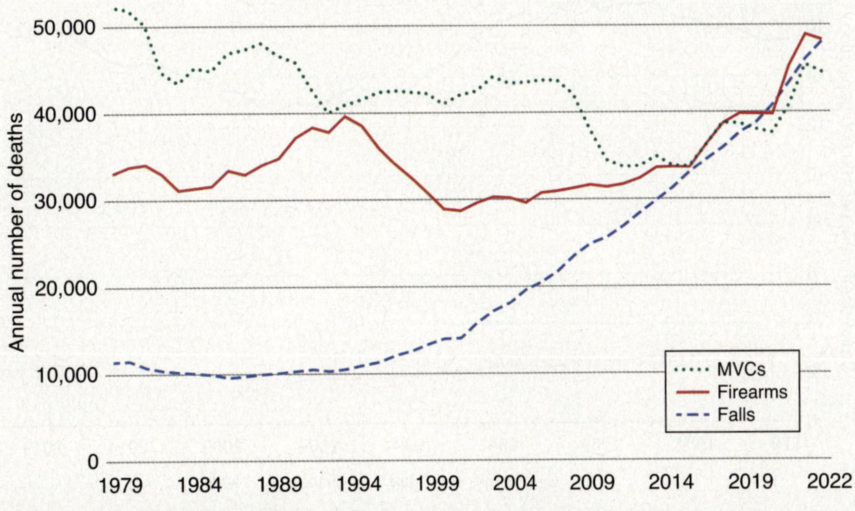

Figure 18.3. Top three causes of injury-related mortality over time in the United States. (From CDC WISCARS. *Fatal Injury Data.* Accessed December 31, 2024. https://wisqars.cdc.gov/create-tables/)

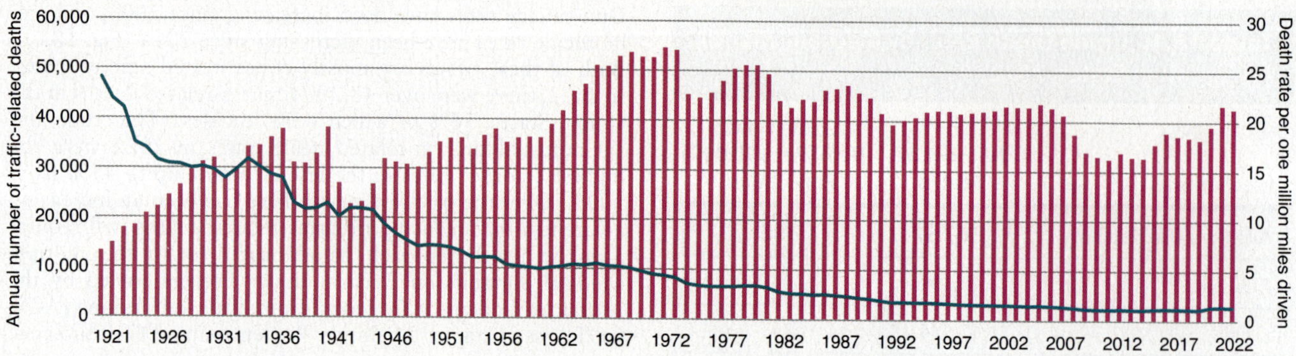

Figure 18.4. Motor vehicle-related fatalities over time in the United States. (From National Highway Traffic Safety Administration. *Summary of Motor Vehicle Traffic Crashes*. Accessed December 31, 2024. https://crashstats.nhtsa.dot.gov/Api/Public/Publication/813643)

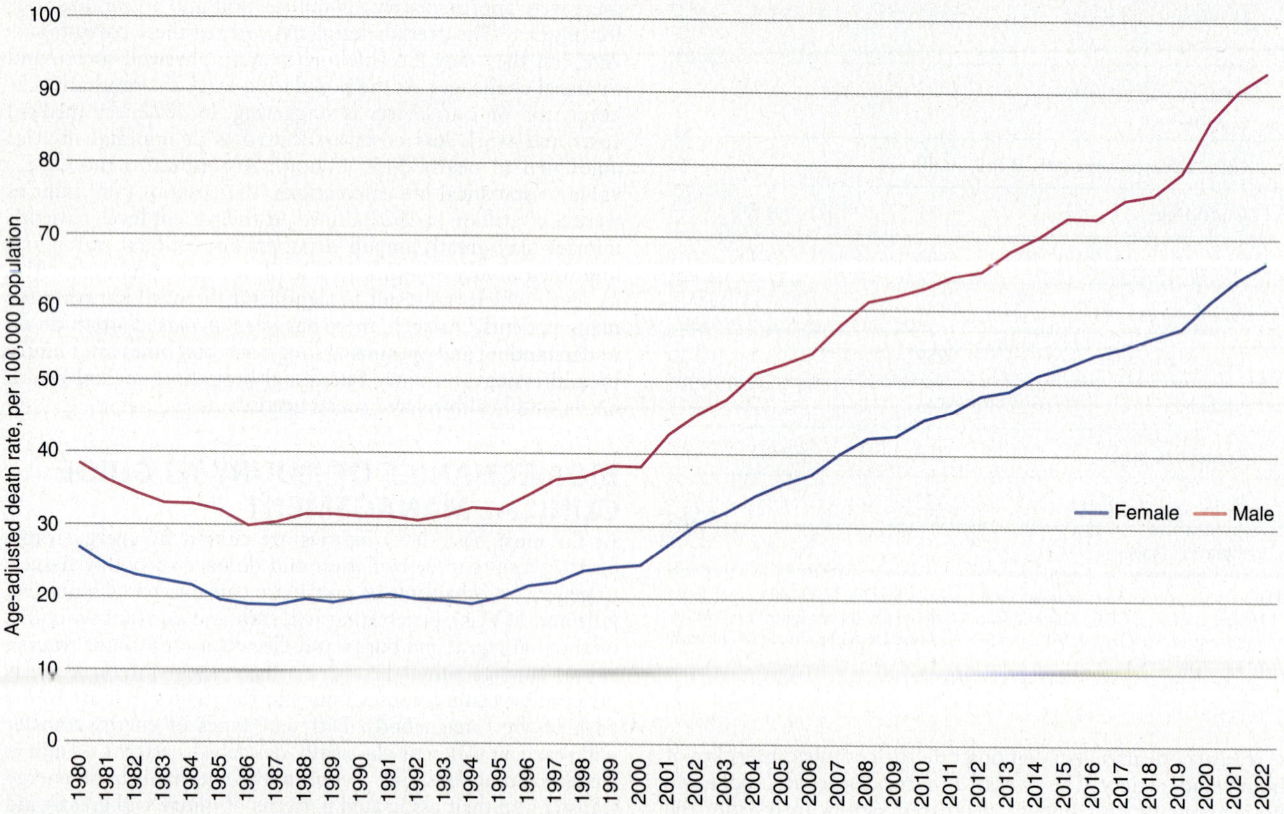

Figure 18.5. Age-adjusted death rates from unintentional falls for ages 65 years and older, by sex. (From CDC WISCARS. *Fatal Injury Data*. December 31, 2024. https://wisqars.cdc.gov/create-tables/)

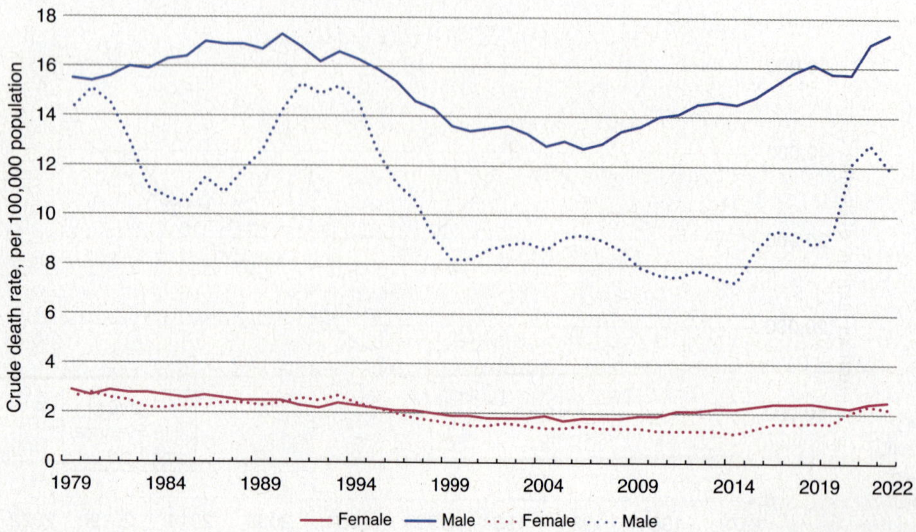

Figure 18.6. Gun-related crude death rates for ages 15 years and older, by sex. *Solid lines* represent gun suicide rates and *dotted lines* represent gun homicide rates. Gun-related death rates fell dramatically from a peak in the early 1990s through the mid-2000s. Since 2013, however, gun-related death rates are now increasing dramatically over the last 5 years. (From CDC WISCARS. *Fatal Injury Data*. December 31, 2024. https://wisqars.cdc.gov/create-tables/)

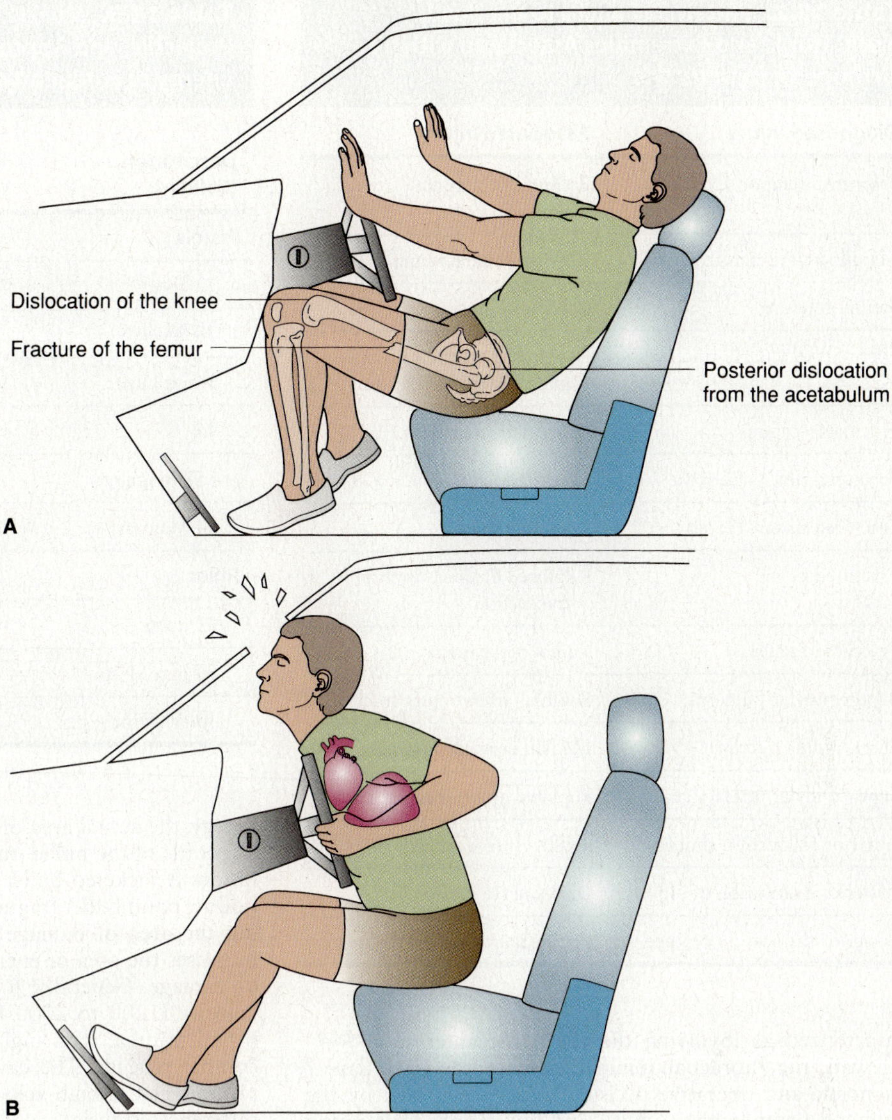

Figure 18.7. A, B: Frontal deceleration impact.

Blunt Injuries

Blunt trauma is best understood by applying the rules of kinetic energy transfer: KE = (M × V)/2, where KE is kinetic energy, M is mass of the object, and V is velocity. Thus, a head-on collision between two large sport utility vehicles (~6000 lb each) traveling at 65 mph can generate enormous amounts of forces. Various safety mechanisms in the modern vehicles direct this energy transfer away from the occupants of the vehicle, it is impossible to fully appreciate the forces and vectors involved in the collision. Relatedly, MVCs can involve frontal impact, rear impact, lateral impact, rollover crashes, rotational forces, and ejection from the vehicle all have implications for some classically described injury patterns (**Fig. 18.7**).

Additional factors from the scene of the crash, such as ejection from the vehicle or the death of another occupant, act as surrogates for the severity of impact or the complexity of the forces involved and can inform risk stratification for underlying injuries. Because the force vectors from blunt trauma are nearly impossible to known in the trauma bay, the clinician also must specifically look for clinical evidence of energy transfer. For example, a "seat belt sign" across the abdomen must raise suspicion for energy transfer across the bowel, mesentery, pancreas, and lumbar spine. Similarly, wedge fracture of L1 vertebra in this setting mandates ruling out a pancreatic injury as the pancreatic body drapes across the anterior aspect of L1. In fact, orthopedic injuries should always be considered markers of kinetic energy transfer and make the clinicians proactively look for injuries to adjacent organs, nerves, vessels, and tendons (**Table 18.2**).

Penetrating Injuries

Penetrating injuries can be categorized as either low energy (eg, stab or slash wounds with a knife or sharp surface) or high–high (eg, gunshot wounds). Low-energy lacerations are usually straightforward as the structures in the depth of the wound can be examined and injuries to critical organs ruled out by careful visual inspection. Conversely, low-energy puncture wounds (eg, stabs wounds from a knife or ice pick) often present a greater challenge when it comes to ruling out occult injury to deeper structures. For example, a stab wound to the neck can cause injuries to the airway, esophagus, blood vessels, thyroid gland, or intrathoracic organs. In the absence of obvious vascular or aerodigestive tract injury, a complete workup may include a computerized tomography (CT) scan to evaluate the blood vessels in the neck, laryngoscopy and bronchoscopy to evaluate for a missed airway injury, and both a video esophagoscopy and a confirmatory esophagram to rule out an occult esophageal injury (see Chapter 22: Neck Injuries for more information). Another example is stab wounds to the trunk, in which the appropriate evaluation and treatment is based on the underlying structures at risk for injury. Truncal stab wounds may be

Table 18.2. Patterns of Injury to the Head, Neck, Trunk, and Extremities Associated with Orthopedic Injuries

Diagnosed Injury	Associated Injury
Fracture—temporal, parietal bone	Epidural hematoma
Maxillofacial fracture	Cervical spine fracture
Sternal fracture	Cardiac contusion
First and second rib fracture	Descending thoracic aorta, intra-abdominal bleeding
Fractured scapula	Pulmonary contusion
Fractured ribs 8–12, right	Lacerated liver
Fractured ribs 8–12, left	Lacerated spleen
Fractured pelvis	Ruptured bladder, urethral transection
Fractured humerus	Radial nerve injury
Supracondylar humerus	Brachial artery injury fracture
Distal radius fracture	Median nerve compression
Supracondylar femur fracture	Popliteal artery thrombosis
Anterior dislocation shoulder	Axillary nerve injury
Posterior dislocation of hip	Sciatic nerve injury
Posterior dislocation of knee	Popliteal artery thrombosis

Table 18.3. Muzzle Velocity, Kinetic Weight of Projectile, and Approximate Maximum Kinetic Energy of Frequently Used Firearms

Description (Caliber)	Projectile Weight (g)	Muzzle Velocity (ft/s)	Kinetic Energy (ft/lb)
Pistols			
22 Short	29	1000	72
38 Special	158	870	263
9-mm Luger	125	1150	440
45	250	860	410
357 Magnum	158	1430	695
44 Magnum	240	1470	1150
Rifles			
22 Long	40	1150	150
56-mm M-16	55	3200	1248
30–30 Winchester	170	2200	1830

characterized as involving the chest, the anterior abdominal wall, the thoracoabdominal area, or the back/flank.[9] Diagnostic and operative decision making is driven by the likelihood of underlying injury, and low-energy penetrating wounds to each of these body regions merits ruling out of different types of injuries via different diagnostic modalities.[9] Hemodynamically normal patients with stab wounds to the chest often require placement of a chest tube and close evaluation of both initial and ongoing chest tube output. For patients with stab wounds to the anterior abdominal wall who are not hypotensive, the decision to operate is based on evidence of intraperitoneal penetration. In patients with stab wounds to the thoracoabdominal region (ie, from the nipples to the costal margin) the surgeon must rule out injuries in the chest, to the diaphragm, and in the upper abdomen; and thus may require a chest tube and a diagnostic laparoscopy. Flank stab wounds may involve retroperitoneal structures that will not elicit peritonitis on exam and thus often require evaluation with a CT scan enhanced with intravenous, oral, and rectal contrast. In all four scenarios, a hypotensive patient is assumed to have uncontrolled hemorrhage and should thus be immediately taken to the operating room for emergency exploration and prompt hemorrhage control.

High-velocity penetrating injuries, such as bullet wounds, differ from stab wounds not only in the fact that the bullets impart significant kinetic energy depending upon their velocity and weight (**Table 18.3**) but can also cause "cavitation" effect. Cavitation occurs as tissues impacted by the bullet recoil and transmit the kinetic energy outward, creating a cavity due to the rapid acceleration and deceleration. This can injure organs/tissues that are adjacent to the bullet track, even if not hit directly by the projectile. In addition to the kinetic energy, the actual area of injury is influenced by factors such as profile of the bullet, tumble (spin and yaw), and fragmentation. A jacketed bullet does not deform much, whereas a hollow point bullet fragments, spreads, and deforms (increasing the area of damage). Similarly, tumbling of the bullet increases the area of energy exchange and much larger zone of damage. Generally, low-velocity (<1200 ft/s) or medium velocity (1200 to 2000 ft/s) firearms are more common in urban trauma, with high-velocity wounds seen typically in combat settings. The cavitation effect is significantly more pronounced in high-velocity injuries, and the kinetic energy differences translate into a much larger area of destruction, more devitalized tissues, and contamination (cavitation can pull in debris, clothes, etc, into the wound). Injuries to multiple organs and structures, even in different body cavities, are possible with bullet wounds. For example, a bullet injury to the anterior wall of the stomach can easily pass through the posterior wall, through the pancreas, duodenum, vena cava, and the kidney, depending upon the trajectory. While trying to determine the trajectory, it is important to *not* assume that the subject was in a "normal" anatomical position (standing straight front facing with arms by his side) when shot. Typically, victims assume a variety of odd positions in an effort to avoid getting hit. In addition, bullets do not necessarily travel in a linear track and can bend and bounce off in atypical directions. Thus, gunshot wound to the chest can easily result in injuries not only in the chest (ipsilateral or contralateral), but also in the abdomen, pelvis, or the neck, depending upon the course of the projectile. It is also wrong to notice two holes and assume that they represent a through-and-through gunshot wound. It is equally likely to be two separate gunshot wounds with both bullets still inside the body. As a general rule, the number of gunshot wounds and the number of retained bullets should add up to an even number; otherwise, you are missing either a hole or a bullet. Even in critically ill patients, quick x-rays of the chest/abdomen/pelvis, as a "bullet survey" can be very helpful before rushing to the operating room. This information can be critically important in planning the surgical approach, and in deciding which body cavity to tackle in what sequence.[10]

THE TRIMODAL MODEL OF INJURY-RELATED MORTALITY: IMMEDIATE, EARLY, AND LATE DEATHS

Though life-threatening injuries result from a variety of mechanism, deaths tend to occur in a well-described temporal pattern and due to only a few underlying causes. The classical trimodal distribution of trauma deaths was first described by Trunkey[11] in 1983, based upon the patterns of posttraumatic deaths in several counties of Northern California. In that report, nearly half of the deaths occurred within minutes after injury due to disruption of major blood vessels, devastating central nervous system (CNS) injuries or combination. A smaller second peak, lasting a few hours, followed that first major peak in mortality (~30% of the deaths) where depending upon the mechanism of trauma, ongoing hemorrhage and CNS injuries played an almost equal role. The third peak was noted days to weeks after injury due to infections, multiple organ failure, and various late complications. An understanding of these patterns of death has led to significant advances in the arenas of injury prevention, trauma systems development, early hemorrhage control, balanced resuscitation, avoidance of trauma-induced coagulopathy (TIC), and improvements in surgical critical care.

Immediate Deaths

"Immediate deaths" that occur within first few seconds to minutes after injury will only be avoided by altering the nature and severity of the energy transfer to the body, or by prevention of the injury altogether. As mentioned above, improved roads, safer car design, increased seat belt use, and enforcement of speeding and drunk driving laws result in thousands of avertable deaths each year. For MVCs that do occur, these same factors may reduce the energy transfer to the body and covert what would have been an instantly fatal injury into a survivable injury that can be attended to by modern trauma care. Based on a multi-institutional review of preventable trauma deaths by the Western Trauma Association,[12] 60% of preventable prehospital deaths were due to hemorrhage and 30% were due to neurotrauma. As more patients survive the first few moments of injury and as prehospital transfer to definitive care improves, opportunities to reduce preventable deaths exist in the prehospital setting, the trauma bay, the operating room, and early intensive care.

Early Deaths

"Early deaths," those occurring within the first 1 to 24 hours after injury, are overwhelming due to exsanguination and trau-
3 matic brain injury (TBI).[11-13] Of these two conditions,[4] bleeding is clearly more treatable, which makes it the number one cause of *preventable* deaths. If patients can survive these first few hours, modern data show that even among massively bleeding patients (without head injuries), mortality beyond the first 24 hours is only ~10%.[14] Though there is still a great deal of work to do in reducing preventable mortality among this patient population, tremendous advances in survival have been made among patients at risk of "early death" due to massive hemorrhage primarily due to reducing early exsanguination from hemorrhage and reducing TIC. Key advances in trauma systems have led to shortened time to definitive hemorrhage control through the development of robust protocols that guide prehospital care and time in the trauma bay. Similarly, multiple advances involving "hemostatic resuscitation" in the prehospital and early hospital phase as well as implementation of inhospital massive transfusion protocols (MTP)
4 have led to a reduced incidence of TIC and improved survival. These two management principles are explored in more depth in the subsequent section on clinical priorities.

Once in the operating room, early deaths are avoided by continued prioritization of hemorrhage control and avoidance of TIC. Though an in-depth description of operative decision making in trauma are outside of the scope of this introductory chapter, the basic principles of the trauma laparotomy include: prepping and draping from chin to knees and from table to table, rapid entry into the abdominal cavity, early control of bleeding, temporary control of contamination, exploration of the entire intra-abdominal cavity, and finally either definitive repair of injured structures or a damage control operation with temporary abdominal closure. "Damage control" surgery refers to an abbreviated operation focused on hemorrhage control and temporary control of contamination followed by temporary closure, resuscitation in the intensive care unit (ICU), and a return to the operating room for definitive management within 24 to 48 hours.[15,16] This serves to reduce the likelihood of entering the deadly "bloody vicious cycle" of uncontrolled acidosis, coagulopathy, and hypothermia[17] that will develop when the severely injured patient who undergoes a prolonged operation. Although opinions are evolving, and there is a potential for overuse, traditionally held indications for a damage control operation are found in **Table 18.4**.

Table 18.4. List of Proposed Indications for Damage Control, Including Range of Values Reported in Various Articles

1. Core temperature <35 °C (34–35 °C)
2. pH <7.20 (7.10–7.30)
3. Base deficit >14
4. Systolic blood pressure persistently <80 mm Hg (70–90 mm Hg)
5. Blood transfusion >10 units packed red blood cells
6. Estimated blood loss >4 L
7. Operating room fluid replacement >10 L
8. Associated life-threatening injuries in second anatomical location
9. Vascular injuries in inaccessible locations
10. Inability to close the abdomen due to visceral edema
11. Clinical evidence of coagulopathy (nonsurgical bleeding)

Late Deaths

Finally, some of the most obvious gains in injury-related mortality reduction have occurred among the so-called "late deaths" occurring weeks to months after injury. In more contemporary studies, the initial spike in early deaths remain, but beyond 24 hours deaths slowly taper off with no discernable late peak.[13] Unlike the classic trimodal distribution, the late peak has markedly diminished, most likely due to significant improvements in surgical intensive care. Mortality rates for many of the reasons for late death are rapidly dropping with wider adoption of best care practices for managing critical care illnesses.[13,18,19] For example, due to more judicious resus-
5 citation practices severe respiratory failure after trauma has become a fairly rare occurrence. Advances in critical care have helped to "flatten" the third peak in two ways: through a lower incidence of late complications and an increased ability to "rescue" patients even if they develop the complications. More information regarding Postinjury Management can be found in Chapter 31: Postinjury Management.

CLINICAL PRIORITIES FOR INITIAL MANAGEMENT OF INJURED PATIENTS

Broadly speaking, the trauma patients can be divided into three categories: patients with (a) rapidly fatal injuries, (b) potentially fatal injuries, and (c) all others. A key component of effective prehospital triage is to properly place the injured into these categories based on the available data (mechanism of injury, age of the patient, comorbid diseases, physiologic status, and injury patters), and then make a rapid decision about what type of facility is the most appropriate for the patient. The ACS-COT

National Guideline for the Field Triage of Injured Patients

RED CRITERIA
High Risk for Serious Injury

Injury Patterns	Mental Status & Vital Signs
• Penetrating injuries to head, neck, torso, and proximal extremities • Skull deformity, suspected skull fracture • Suspected spinal injury with new motor or sensory loss • Chest wall instability, deformity, or suspected flail chest • Suspected pelvic fracture • Suspected fracture of two or more proximal long bones • Crushed, degloved, mangled, or pulseless extremity • Amputation proximal to wrist or ankle • Active bleeding requiring a tourniquet or wound packing with continuous pressure	**All Patients** • Unable to follow commands (motor GCS < 6) • RR < 10 or > 29 breaths/min • Respiratory distress or need for respiratory support • Room-air pulse oximetry < 90% **Age 0-9 years** • SBP < 70 mm Hg + (2 x age in years) **Age 10-64 years** • SBP < 90 mm Hg or • HR > SBP **Age ≥65 years** • SBP < 110 mm Hg or • HR > SBP

Patients meeting any one of the above RED criteria should be transported to the highest-level trauma center available within the geographic constraints of the regional trauma system

YELLOW CRITERIA
Moderate Risk for Serious Injury

Mechanism of Injury	EMS Judgment
• High-Risk Auto Crash – Partial or complete ejection – Significant intrusion (including roof) • >12 inches occupant site OR • >18 inches any site OR • Need for extrication for entrapped patient – Death in passenger compartment – Child (age 0-9 years) unrestrained or in unsecured child safety seat – Vehicle telemetry data consistent with severe injury • Rider separated from transport vehicle with significant impact (eg, motorcycle, ATV, horse, etc.) • Pedestrian/bicycle rider thrown, run over, or with significant impact • Fall from height > 10 feet (all ages)	**Consider risk factors, including:** • Low-level falls in young children (age ≤5 years) or older adults (age ≥65 years) with significant head impact • Anticoagulant use • Suspicion of child abuse • Special, high-resource healthcare needs • Pregnancy > 20 weeks • Burns in conjunction with trauma • Children should be triaged preferentially to pediatric capable centers **If concerned, take to a trauma center**

Patients meeting any one of the YELLOW CRITERIA WHO DO NOT MEET RED CRITERIA should be preferentially transported to a trauma center, as available within the geographic constraints of the regional trauma system (need not be the highest-level trauma center)

Figure 18.8. 2021 National Guidelines for the Field Triage of Injured Patients. From Newgard CD, Fischer PE, Gestring M, et al; the Writing Group for the 2021 National Expert Panel on Field Triage. National guideline for the field triage of injured patients: recommendations of the National Expert Panel on Field Triage, 2021. *J Trauma Acute Care Surg*. 2022;93(2):e49–e60. https://www.facs.org/media/2zdltley/field-triage-handout-vfinal-review.pdf

has developed detailed criteria for designating hospitals into different levels depending upon the resource availability, from the highest (level I) to the lowest (level IV).[20] The ACS-COT also provides recommendations on transfer criteria to ensure that patients with critical injuries, complex resource needs, or conditions exceeding the capabilities of a Level III center are promptly transferred to Level I or II centers when necessary.[20] In addition, the ACS-COT has worked with the CDC to develop a guideline for the prehospital triage of the injured patients to ensure that injured patients get to the right facility based on initial field triage (**Fig. 18.8**).[21] As a result of improved prehospital and trauma systems, we know that appropriate and timely triage to the right
6 facility saves lives. Results from the landmark National Study on the Costs and Outcomes of Trauma were published in the *New England Journal of Medicine (NEJM)* in 2006 and demonstrated that treatment at a level 1 trauma center, compared to treatment at a nontrauma center, was associated with a 20% lower odds of death—with even larger benefits among those with more severe injuries.[22] Please see Chapter 19: Prehospital and New Advances in Resuscitation for a detailed discussion on prehospital care and advances in early resuscitation strategies for injured patients, including the use of prehospital plasma, the use of whole blood, and the appropriate application of permissive hypotension[23] until hemorrhage control is achieved.

Advance Trauma Life Support

While appropriate interventions begin in the prehospital setting, the trauma bay is the point of entry to the hospital system for severely injured patients. A systematic approach is needed to ensure rapid assessment for and treatment of life-threatening injuries, identification of all non–life-threatening injuries, and determination of the appropriate disposition from the trauma bay. These priorities are the basis of the Advance Trauma Life Support (ATLS) program that is utilized in every trauma center in the United States and in thousands of trauma centers around the world.[24] ATLS was developed by the ACS-COT and was first introduced in 1980, and is now taught in 60 countries across the world. The ATLS program provides participants with a safe, reliable method for immediate management of the injured patient and the basic knowledge necessary to:

1. Assess the patient's condition rapidly and accurately
2. Resuscitate and stabilize the patient according to priority
3. Determine if the patient's needs exceed a facility's capacity
4. Arrange appropriately for the patient's interhospital transfer (who, what, when, and how)
5. Assure that optimum care is provided and that the level of care does not deteriorate at any point during the evaluation, resuscitation, or transfer process.

The basic concepts of ATLS include a primary survey focusing on the ABCDE (airway, breathing, circulation, disability, and exposure) to identify and address the life-threatening issues, followed by a secondary survey to identify all the injuries. The specific treatments of various injuries have been addressed in the different chapters that follow. However, the key points to emphasize are that the two main killers during the early hospital period ("golden hour") are the same as the prehospital setting—*bleeding and TBI*. As treatments for TBI remain mostly supportive, bleeding remains the number one cause of *preventable* deaths during the first 6 hours following trauma.

Immediate Hemorrhage Control

In a bleeding patient, the priorities are to identify and control the source of bleeding as quickly as possible.[25] Sometimes the bleeding source is obvious and can be controlled by direct compression (eg, stab wound to the femoral artery in the groin), tourniquets (eg, mangled extremity), or sutures (eg, scalp laceration), but often it is inside a body cavity—and is thus categorized as noncompressible hemorrhage which will require additional interventions beyond manual compression or tourniquets. Localization of the hemorrhage source is relatively easy for penetrating trauma that is limited to a specific body region, but is notoriously difficult in the blunt polytrauma patients. In these patients, it helps to remember that a person can only lose significant volumes of blood in five locations: (1) pleural space, (2) intra-abdominal, (3) pelvis/retroperitoneal space, (4) soft tissues at the site of long bone fractures/sheer injuries, and (5) externally. With a quick examination and a chest x-ray, three of these possibilities can be easily ruled out, and the choice typically comes down to deciding between the abdomen and the pelvis/extraperitoneal space as the site of intervention. Focused assessment with sonography for trauma (FAST) can also be helpful in determining the source of hemorrhage. If it shows free fluid in the abdomen in a hypotensive patient, then emergent laparotomy for hemorrhage control is justified. While the reported false negative rate in the literature has been reported to be as low as 2%,[26] others have reported a significant false negative rate even in experienced hands. Although diagnostic peritoneal lavage has largely been abandoned, a bedside percutaneous diagnostic peritoneal aspiration (DPA) can be very helpful in these patients. If a high-quality FAST is negative and the pelvic x-ray shows a significant pelvic fracture, then the possibility of a pelvic bleeding source is significant, and a pelvic binder should be applied promptly (or pelvis wrapped tightly with a sheet) for appropriate fracture patterns (eg, suitable for open-book fracture but potentially harmful for severe lateral compression). Depending on institutional protocols, such patients may benefit from immediate pelvic angioembolization from the trauma bay, or after preperitoneal packing in the operating room.

Hemostatic Resuscitation and Massive Transfusion Protocols

In addition to hemorrhage control, it is imperative to prevent or mitigate the risks of TIC in patients that are actively bleeding.[27] Normal coagulation homeostasis depends on a delicate balance between clot formation and breakdown. Normally, trauma tilts the balance in favor of clot formation at the site of injuries to stop the bleeding. However, major injuries, excessive blood loss, prolonged tissue hypoperfusion, and TBI with disruption of the blood–brain barrier have all been shown to upset the normal coagulation homeostasis, resulting in TIC.[27] This can manifest as abnormal clot formation and/or excessive or rapid clot breakdown (fibrinolysis). Unless treated promptly, this coagulopathy leads to further bleeding, which sets up a vicious cycle resulting in the "lethal triad" of coagulopathy, acidosis, and hypothermia that is associated with an extremely high mortality.[17] In TIC, depletion coagulopathy results in abnormalities of traditional coagulation parameters (international normalized ratio, partial thromboplastin time) and predicts mortality, whereas fibrinolytic coagulopathy predicts infection, end-organ failure, and mortality, without a detectable difference in international normalized ratio or partial thromboplastin time.[27]

7

Damage Control Resuscitation (DCR) or Hemostatic resuscitation has recently emerged as a potential solution for the prevention and reversal of TIC.[28,29] This approach advocates early hemorrhage control, permissive hypotension (until control of hemorrhage),[23] avoidance of crystalloids, and a balanced resuscitation with either whole blood or precise ratios of blood components (such as packed red blood cells [RBCs], fresh frozen plasma, and platelets). A massive transfusion is usually defined as either receiving 10 units of RBCs in the first 24 hours after admission or 4 units of RBCs in the first hour (or until death).[27] An MTP is a standardized, evidence-based system that rapidly provides blood products (using either whole blood or balanced ratios of RBCs, plasma, and platelets) to patients with life-threatening hemorrhage. Despite some debate about precise ratios of blood products and/or the best way to integrate the use of whole blood, there is general agreement that implementation of an MTP with balanced blood product ratios has been shown to reduce early and overall mortality, decrease intraoperative and postoperative blood product use, and limit crystalloid administration.[30] These benefits are particularly pronounced in patients with blunt trauma. The 2015 Pragmatic, Randomized Optimal Platelet and Plasma Ratios (PROPPR) trial enrolled 680 patients with severe trauma and major bleeding to test two different blood component ratios.[14] In this study, early administration of plasma, platelets, and RBCs in a 1:1:1 ratio compared with a 1:1:2 ratio did not result in significant differences in mortality at 24 hours or at 30 days. However, more patients in the 1:1:1 group achieved hemostasis and fewer experienced death due to exsanguination by 24 hours.[14] It must be emphasized, however, that high-ratio protocols have not been shown to improve survival in patients who do not require massive transfusion. More recent data have explored the use of whole blood as a part of MTPs. A 2023 retrospective analysis of data from the ACS Trauma Quality Improvement Program database used propensity score matching and hierarchical mixed-effects multivariable logistic regression to evaluate whether the use of whole blood as an adjunct to component therapy—MTP, compared with MTP alone, was associated with improved survival among patients presenting with severe hemorrhage.[31] This retrospective analysis found a lower risk of death at 24 hours (hazard ratio, 0.63; 95% CI, 0.41–0.96; $P = .03$) and 30 days (HR, 0.53; 95% CI, 0.31–0.93; $P = .02$). Though retrospective studies have significant risk of bias that may be unaccounted for, the Trauma Resuscitation with Group O Whole Blood Or Products (TROOP) trial is currently underway which is a pragmatic, multicenter, phase III randomized clinical trial evaluating the effectiveness and safety of whole blood versus component therapy in trauma patients requiring massive transfusion. Please see Chapter 19: Prehospital and New Advances in Resuscitation for further discussion regarding the use of low-titer whole blood as a part of trauma resuscitation.

We also know that development of a clot is just the initial part of the process, and rapid breakdown of the clot may be equally detrimental. It has been shown that development of fibrinolysis is a highly lethal event in severely injured patients, and treatment with blood products alone is incapable of reversing this process.[27] In a bleeding patient, initiating DCR is a great idea, but the patient's eventual survival depends on the ability (or inability) to obtain rapid and reliable hemorrhage control. It should therefore be emphasized, that hemostatic resuscitation via MTP is an adjunct to early hemorrhage control and not a substitute. In addition, prevention and active reversal of hypothermia (eg, use of fluid warmers, body warming devices) and correction of acidosis and hypocalcemia are critically important while resuscitation protocols are carried out.

LESSONS LEARNED FROM THE BATTLEFIELD

Every major war has catalyzed rapid advances in trauma care. As the medical systems grapple with the challenges of taking

Table 18.5. Lethality of War Wounds among US Soldiers

	No. Wounded or Killed in Action[a]	No. Killed in Action[a]	Lethality of War Wounds (%)
Revolutionary War, 1775–1783	10,623	4435	42
War of 1812, 1812–1815	6765	2260	33
Mexican War, 1846–1848	5885	1733	29
Civil War (Union Force), 1861–1865	422,295	140,414	33
Spanish–American War, 1898	2047	385	19
World War I, 1917–1918	257,404	53,402	21
World War II, 1941–1945	963,403	291,557	30
Korean War, 1950–1953	137,025	33,741	25
Vietnam War, 1961–1973	200,727	47,424	24
Persian Gulf War, 1990–1991	614	147	24
Operation Enduring Freedom, 2001–2014	21,994	1845	8
Operation Iraqi Freedom, 2003–2010	35,475	3482	10
Three conflicts since 2010, 2010–2015[b]	1529	138	9

[a]For recent conflicts these numbers are taken from the publicly available DCAS data and include total hostile wounded in action and total hospital deaths.

[b]Summation of data from Operation New Dawn (2010–2011), Operation Inherent Resolve (2014–2015), and Operation Freedom's Sentinel Resolve (2015).

From Gawande A. Casualties of war—Military care for the wounded from Iraq and Afghanistan. *N Engl J Med.* 2004;351:2471–2475. US Defense Casualty Analysis System (DCAS). Accessed January 1, 2025. https://dcas.dmdc.osd.mil/dcas/

care of massive numbers of injured people (military and civilian), often in very austere settings, they quickly evolve, adapt, and improvise. Wars also prompt significant financial investment by the governments in research and development, and attract some of the best minds to the field. Many of the things (various operative interventions, drugs, fluids, dressings, rapid transport systems, trauma teams, in-field care, and many more) that are taken for granted today in the civilian trauma centers can be traced back to the wars of the past. Interestingly, as war medicine improves and evolves to take care of worse injuries, the war industry responds by developing more lethal weaponry. Thus, the percentage of injured that die in the battlefield (Killed in action or KIA rate) has remained relatively static during the 20th century, hovering around 25% (**Table 18.5**). However, for more recent conflicts, the KIA rate has dropped down to 10%
8 for the first time in modern warfare. This dramatic drop is clearly multifactorial in etiology, and reflects the focus on prevention strategies with widespread use of superior protective body armor, and deployment of better-designed[7] military vehicles. In addition, the current ongoing conflicts have fundamentally altered how we take care of the injured, which has informed landmark clinical trials and national initiatives that have saved lives and improved functional outcomes.[32–37] A brief list of the key advancements can be found in **Table 18.6**.

FUTURE DIRECTIONS

The future of trauma care will require novel advances spanning basic science, health care delivery systems, and cross-disciplinary patient-centered care. Even with development of robust trauma systems, improvements in early hemorrhage control, a focus on balanced resuscitation, institution of MTP, and adoption of standardized best practices in modern surgical critical care, estimated one-in-five trauma deaths are still preventable.[38] Many of these individuals have underlying injuries that are potentially survivable, but they die before getting definitive care. In addition, while resuscitation restores tissue perfusion, by the time the injured gets to the hospital nothing can be done to reverse the seemingly irreversible shock. In the not-too-distant future, early trauma resuscitation may be very different from what we currently practice due to advances in our understanding of the cellular response to injury. Promising, ongoing work suggests that one day we may see advances such as: the development of specific prosurvival drugs that can be given in the prehospital setting to keep the injured alive long enough to get evacuated to higher levels of care; ability to temporarily "suspend" life using hypothermia or hibernation strategies for patients that have potentially survivable injuries, but need more time for surgery or transfer; individualized therapy with administration of specific pharmacologic agents based upon the individual's cellular disturbances; and monitoring of response to therapy that goes beyond measurement of physiology, and looks at the reversal of cellular disturbances.

At the other end of the spectrum, there is significant work underway at health systems level to better understand which deaths are potentially preventable and how the current organization of trauma delivery systems can be further optimized. In the 2016 report by the National Academies of Science, Engineering, and Medicine (NASEM),[38] "A National Trauma Care System: Integrating Military and Civilian Trauma Systems to Achieve Zero Preventable Deaths," the ACS-COT joined a broad coalition of trauma stakeholders including the National Highway Traffic Safety Administration (NHTSA), the US Department of Defense, NASEM, and the National Institutes of Health to develop a national trauma action plan. The action plan identified existing gaps in our current trauma care systems including regional variation in EMS care, mismatch of level 1 and 2 trauma center location and population

Table 18.6. Translating Lessons from Military Experience to Civilian Trauma Care

Domain of Trauma Care	Lessons from Military Experience	Translation to Civilian Trauma Care
Prevention	– Improvements in body armor and armored transportation have resulted in changing injury patterns and decreased case-fatality rates.[a,b] – Kevlar helmets have made otherwise lethal injuries now survivable, such that mild TBI was the most common injury from the Iraq war.[a] – Mortality from direct chest trauma has fallen to 10%, with the most common injury being pulmonary contusion as opposed to lethal injury to vital organs in the chest.[b]	– The Multi-Disciplinary Multi-Institutional Mortality Investigation in the Civilian Prehospital Environment (MIMIC) study is funded by the US Department of Defense and will help create reliable measures for prehospital time and distance to definitive care and also help determine which injured civilians who die before reaching the hospital had a potentially preventable cause of death.[36]
Management of extremity hemorrhage	– Advanced hemostatic bandages were quickly developed, rigorously tested, and expeditiously deployed by the military.[c–e] – Military experience demonstrated that survival rates improved markedly for casualties that had injuries suitable for tourniquets.[f]	– These same hemostatic dressings are now used widely for intracavitary hemorrhage control in the operating room.[f] – Both advanced hemostatic dressings and windlass tourniquets are used widely by EMS first responders for temporary control of compressible or extremity hemorrhage. Increased tourniquet use in the civilian population has been associated with a survival benefit in patients with extremity vascular injuries.[g] – The ACS-COT's "Stop the Bleed" Course has trained over 1 million civilian first responders in the application of direct pressure, the use of advanced hemostatic dressings, and windlass tourniquets for compressible hemorrhage. Bleeding control kits are increasingly available in public places such as airports, stadiums, schools; akin to automatic external defibrillators.[33]
Management of junctional and truncal hemorrhage, including resuscitative endovascular balloon occlusion of the aorta (REBOA)	– Junctional injuries to the very proximal extremities are not amenable to windlass tourniquets, but the Combat Ready Clamp and the SAM Junctional Tourniquet have been developed and tested in the military setting.[h] – Military and civilian collaboration has led to the development and refinement of the resuscitative endovascular balloon occlusion of the aorta (REBOA) device.[i] – Military guidelines suggest a role for REBOA in the prehospital setting when used by advanced combat medical personnel with specialized training in an effort to reduce death from noncompressible hemorrhage.[j,k] – DARPA-funded research led to development of novel injectable foam to temporize pelvic hemorrhage.[l]	– Junctional tourniquet devices are now used for temporary hemorrhage control by prehospital EMS personnel and at trauma centers around the US.[m] – REBOA is now used in many trauma centers in the United States. While there have been multiple observational studies demonstrating promising results,[n,o] the most recent data to date suggest that further work is needed to properly define when and in which patient population REBOA offers benefit.[p–r] – The Reducing Exsanguination Via In-Vivo Expandable Foam (REVIVE) Trial is still recruiting patients at civilian trauma centers in the United States.[r]
Damage control resuscitation and the prevention and treatment of trauma-Induced coagulopathy	– Many DoD agencies, such as the Office of Naval Research (ONR), the US Army Medical Research and Material Command (MRMC), and Defense Advanced Research Projects Agency (DARPA), just to name a few, have been long-standing sponsors of resuscitation research. – In the late 1990s and early 2000s, experts from three national consensus conferences agreed that aggressive resuscitation is deleterious, an "ideal" fluid is yet not available, and that low-volume resuscitation (hypertonic, colloid, or combination) is the most logical choice for the military needs – Tactical Combat Casualty Care (TCC) guidelines emphasize hypotensive resuscitation, avoidance of crystalloids, early blood product use, high ratios of plasma and platelets to red cells, and administration of TXA when appropriate. – The Military Application of Tranexamic Acid in Trauma Emergency Resuscitation (MATTERs II) took place in a Role 3 Combat Surgical Hospital in southern Afghanistan and showed that the addition of cryoprecipitate independently added to the benefits of TXA in the seriously injured in the battlefield.[34] However, this study also showed higher rates of VTE among soldiers receiving TXA.	– DOD-funded Prospective, Observational, Multicenter, Major Trauma Transfusion (PROMMTT) study was performed at 10 US level 1 trauma centers and showed that higher ratios of plasma and platelets early in resuscitation was associated with lower mortality.[35] – As a follow-up to the MATTERs trial, the Clinical Randomization of an Antifibrinolytic in Significant Hemorrhage (CRASH-2) trial took place in 40 countries and again showed that all-cause mortality and death due to hemorrhage were both lower in TXA-treated patients, compared with placebo.[36] – Massive Transfusion Protocols (MTPs) have been shown to save lives among bleeding patients[24] and are now standard of care at civilian trauma centers and these are based on military data and DOD-funded research that prioritize avoidance of crystalloids, use of TXA in appropriate patients, and 1:1:1 ratio of RBCs, plasma, and platelets.[14,35] – The US Army Medical Research and Materiel Command funded the recent PAMPer trial which demonstrated a survival benefit from prehospital administration of plasma in hypotensive blunt trauma patients requiring air medical transport.[37]

(*continued*)

Table 18.6. Translating Lessons from Military Experience to Civilian Trauma Care (*Continued*)

Domain of Trauma Care	Lessons from Military Experience	Translation to Civilian Trauma Care
Rapid-evacuation and long-distance transport	– In 2009, the US military mandated that the prehospital helicopter transport of critically injured combat casualties should be ≤60 min. Median transport time was cut in half and follow-up data showed significant reductions in total casualty rate and case fatality rate, resulting in hundreds of lives saved.[r] – Operation Iraqi Freedom and Operation Enduring Freedom provided new insight regarding the rapid movement of critically injured casualties within hours of wounding. Review of the Critical Care Air Transport Team and Joint Theater Trauma Registry databases shows that for severely injured (mean ISS 23.7) that were evacuated to Landstuhl Regional Medical Center in Germany, the en route mortality rate was less than 0.02%.[u]	– The lessons learned regarding the safety, and the survival benefit, of long-distance transport for severely injured patients have important applications to civilians injured in rural areas; where they may be far from the nearest level 1 trauma center
Rehabilitation	– Lower-extremity injuries account for 60% of all injuries to the US troops in Iraq and Afghanistan, which are mostly due to explosive devices. But unlike previous wars, temporary vascular shunts have been used more widely, and early vascular reconstruction has being performed more frequently with excellent outcomes.[v,w] – Modern development and implementation of comprehensive rehabilitation strategies, and cutting edge technology in prosthetic limbs to treat the injured service members with complex lower-extremity trauma from combat has resulted in some of the best functional outcomes in the history of warfare.[x]	– Care of complex extremity care in civilian trauma systems has learned a great deal from the more recent military experience with regard to both initial injury management and the needs of longer-term functional recovery[y]

Note: For additional reading, please see the articles referenced in this table: From a. Eskridge et al. Injury, 2012. b. Keneally and Szpisjak. *J Trauma Acute Care Surg*, 2013. c. Pusateri et al. *J Trauma*, 2006. d. Sims et al. *J Spec Oper Med*, 2016. e. Bennett et al. *J Spec Oper Med*, 2014. f. Tompeck et al. *J Trauma Acute Care Surg*, 2020. g. Teixeira et al. *J Am Coll Surg*, 2018. h. Kragh et al. *J Spec Oper Med*, 2013. i. Rasmussen and Eliason. *J Trauma Acute Care Surg*, 2017. j. Glaser et al. *J Trauma Acute Care Surg*, 2019. k. REBOA Hemorrhagic Shock. Joint Trauma Systems Clinical Practice Guideline, 2017. l. Duggan et al. *J Trauma Acute Care Surg*, 2013. m. Smith et al. *J Trauma Acute Care Surg*, 2019. n. DuBose et al. *J Trauma Acute Care Surg*, 2016. o. Brenner et al. *J Am Coll Surg*, 2018. p. Davidson et al. *J Trauma Acute Care Surg*, 2018. q. Joseph et al. *JAMA Surg*, 2019. r. Brenner et al. *Trauma Surg Acute Care Open*, 2018. s. NCT02880163. NIH ClinicalTrials.gov, 2024. t. Kotwal et al. *JAMA Surg*, 2016. u. Ingalls et al. *JAMA Surg*, 2014. v. Gifford et al. *J Vasc Surg*, 2009. w. Casey et al. *J Vasc Surg*, 2015. x. Hoyt et al. *Curr Trauma Rep*, 2015. y. Blair et al. *J Ortho Trauma*, 2016.

distribution, and inadequate funding for research to improve care of the injured patient. The NASEM report highlighted the need to develop a national trauma research plan, share innovation between the military and civilian sectors, engage the public through programs such a Stop the Bleed campaign, and empower trauma survivors and their families to be key advocates for advancing trauma care.

10 Finally, as the inpatient mortality rate for US adult trauma patients has fallen to less than 5%, there is an increasing appreciation for the importance of optimizing long-term outcomes after injury. Trauma survivors follow highly variable recovery trajectories as they navigate postinjury risks such as reduced in functional status, new mental health challenges, and lower health-related quality of life. These recovery trajectories are further influenced by patient's varying levels of social support, health-related social needs, and financial risk protection.[7,8,39] Work led by the ACS-COT, the National Trauma Research Action Plan (NTRAP),[40] and other researchers has been leading the way to identify knowledge gaps in need of rigorous inquiry, interventions in need of implementation, and cross-disciplinary innovation as they continue to support efforts that "ensure optimal patient outcomes across the continuum of care."[20]

References

1. Centers for Disease Control and Prevention (CDC). Web-based Injury Statistics Query and Reporting System (WISQARS). Accessed December 31, 2024. https://wisqars.cdc.gov
2. Norton R, Kobusingye O. Injuries. *N Engl J Med*. 2013;368(18):1723–1730.
3. National Center for Statistics and Analysis. Early estimate of motor vehicle traffic fatalities for the first 9 months (January-September) of 2024 (Crash Stats Brief Statistical Summary. Report No. DOT HS 813 670). National Highway Traffic Safety Administration. 2024. Accessed January 1, 2025. https://crashstats.nhtsa.dot.gov/Api/Public/ViewPublication/813670
4. Centers for Disease Control and Prevention (CDC). Trends in nonfatal falls and fall-related injuries among adults aged ≥65 years—United States, 2012–2018. *MMWR Morb Mortal Wkly Rep*. 2020;69(27):833–837. Accessed January 1, 2025. https://www.cdc.gov/mmwr/volumes/69/wr/pdfs/mm6927a5-H.pdf
5. Population Reference Bureau. Aging in the United States: Fact Sheet. Published 2022. Accessed January 1, 2025. https://www.prb.org/resources/fact-sheet-aging-in-the-united-states
6. Bulger EM, Kuhls DA, Campbell BT, et al. Proceedings from the medical summit on firearm injury prevention: a public health approach to reduce death and disability in the US. *J Am Coll Surg*. 2019;229(4):415–430.
7. Scott JW, Knowlton LM, Murphy P, Neiman PU, Martin RS, Staudenmayer K; AAST Health Economics Committee. Financial toxicity after trauma and acute care surgery: From understanding to action. *J Trauma Acute Care Surg*. 2023;95(5):800–805.
8. Sakran JV, Ezzeddine H, Schwab CW, et al; Patient reported outcome consortium. Proceedings from the consensus conference on trauma patient-reported outcome measures. *J Am Coll Surg*. 2020;230(5):819–835.

9. Martin MJ, Brown CVR, Shatz DV, et al. Evaluation and management of abdominal stab wounds: A Western Trauma Association critical decisions algorithm. *J Trauma Acute Care Surg.* 2018;85(5):1007–1015.
10. Martin MJ, Brown CVR, Shatz DV, et al. Evaluation and management of abdominal gunshot wounds: A Western Trauma Association critical decisions algorithm. *J Trauma Acute Care Surg.* 2019;87(5):1220–1227.
11. Trunkey DD. Trauma. Accidental and intentional injuries account for more years of life lost in the U.S. than cancer and heart disease. Among the prescribed remedies are improved preventive efforts, speedier surgery and further research. *Sci Am.* 1983;249:28–35.
12. Callcut RA, Kornblith LZ, Conroy AS, et al; Western Trauma Association Multicenter Study Group. The why and how our trauma patients die: A prospective Multicenter Western Trauma Association study. *J Trauma Acute Care Surg.* 2019;86(5):864–870.
13. Bardes JM, Inaba K, Schellenberg M, et al. The contemporary timing of trauma deaths. *J Trauma Acute Care Surg.* 2018;84(6):893–899.
14. Holcomb JB, Tilley BC, Baraniuk S, et al; PROPPR Study Group. Transfusion of plasma, platelets, and red blood cells in a 1:1:1 vs a 1:1:2 ratio and mortality in patients with severe trauma: the PROPPR randomized clinical trial. *JAMA.* 2015;313(5):471–482.
15. Rotondo MF, Schwab CW, McGonigal MD, et al. Damage control: An approach for improved survival in exsanguinating penetrating abdominal injury. *J Trauma.* 1993;35(3):375–382.
16. Roberts DJ, Bobrovitz N, Zygun DA, et al. Indications for use of damage control surgery in civilian trauma patients: A content analysis and expert appropriateness rating study. *Ann Surg.* 2016;263(5):1018–1027.
17. Kashuk JL, Moore EE, Millikan JS, Moore JB. Major abdominal vascular trauma—a unified approach. *J Trauma.* 1982;22:672–679.
18. Cuschieri J, Johnson JL, Sperry J, et al; Inflammation and Host Response to Injury, Large Scale Collaborative Research Program. Benchmarking outcomes in the critically injured trauma patient and the effect of implementing standard operating procedures. *Ann Surg.* 2012;255:993–999.
19. van Breugel JMM, Niemeyer MJS, Houwert RM, Groenwold RHH, Leenen LPH, van Wessem KJP. Global changes in mortality rates in polytrauma patients admitted to the ICU-a systematic review. *World J Emerg Surg.* 2020;15(1):55.
20. Resources for the Optimal Care of the Injured Patient 7th Edition (2022 Standards). American College of Surgeons, Committee on Trauma. https://www.facs.org/quality-programs/trauma/quality/verification-review-and-consultation-program/standards/. Last accessed December 3, 2025.
21. Newgard CD, Fisher PE, Gestring M, et al.; Writing Group for the 2021 National Expert Panel on Field Triage. National guideline for the field triage of injured patients: Recommendations of the National Expert Panel on Field Triage, 2021. *J Trauma Acute Care Surg.* 2022;93(2):e49–e60.
22. MacKenzie EJ, Rivara FP, Jurkovich GJ, et al. A national evaluation of the effect of trauma-center care on mortality. *N Engl J Med.* 2006;354(4):366–378.
23. Bickell WH, Wall MJ Jr, Pepe PE, et al. Immediate versus delayed fluid resuscitation for hypotensive patients with penetrating torso injuries. *N Engl J Med.* 1994;331:1105–1109.
24. American College of Surgeons Committee on Trauma. *ATLS® Student Course Manual.* 10th ed. American College of Surgeons; 2018.
25. Chang R, Kerby JD, Kalkwarf KJ, et al; PROPPR Study Group. Earlier time to hemostasis is associated with decreased mortality and rate of complications: Results from the Pragmatic Randomized Optimal Platelet and Plasma Ratio trial. *J Trauma Acute Care Surg.* 2019;87(2):342–349.
26. Schwed AC, Wagenaar A, Reppert AE, et al. Trust the FAST: Confirmation that the FAST examination is highly specific for intra-abdominal hemorrhage in over 1,200 patients with pelvic fractures. *J Trauma Acute Care Surg.* 2021;90(1):137–142.
27. Moore EE, Moore HB, Kornblith LZ, et al. Trauma-induced coagulopathy. *Nat Rev Dis Primers.* 2021;7(1):30.
28. Cannon JW, Khan MA, Raja AS, et al. Damage control resuscitation in patients with severe traumatic hemorrhage: A practice management guideline from the Eastern Association for the Surgery of Trauma. *J Trauma Acute Care Surg.* 2017;82(3):605–617.
29. LaGrone LN, Stein D, Cribari C, et al. American Association for the Surgery of Trauma/American College of Surgeons Committee on Trauma: Clinical protocol for damage-control resuscitation for the adult trauma patient. *J Trauma Acute Care Surg.* 2024;96(3):510–520.
30. Consunji R, Elseed A, El-Menyar A, et al. The effect of massive transfusion protocol implementation on the survival of trauma patients: a systematic review and meta-analysis. *Blood Transfus.* 2020;18(6):434–445.
31. Torres CM, Kent A, Scantling D, Joseph B, Haut ER, Sakran JV. Association of whole blood with survival among patients presenting with severe hemorrhage in US and Canadian Adult Civilian Trauma Centers. *JAMA Surg.* 2023;158(5):532–540.
32. Medrano NW, Villarreal CL, Price MA, et al. Multi-Institutional Multidisciplinary Injury Mortality Investigation in the Civilian Pre-Hospital Environment (MIMIC): a methodology for reliably measuring prehospital time and distance to definitive care. *Trauma Surg Acute Care Open.* 2019;4(1):e000309.
33. Goolsby C, Jacobs L, Hunt RC, et al. Stop the Bleed Education Consortium: Education program content and delivery recommendations. *J Trauma Acute Care Surg.* 2018;84(1):205–210.
34. Morrison JJ, Ross JD, Dubose JJ, Jansen JO, Midwinter MJ, Rasmussen TE. Association of cryoprecipitate and tranexamic acid with improved survival following wartime injury: findings from the MATTERs II Study. *JAMA Surg.* 2013;148:218–225.
35. Holcomb JB, del Junco DJ, Fox EE, et al; PROMMTT Study Group. The prospective, observational, multicenter, major trauma transfusion (PROMMTT) study: comparative effectiveness of a time-varying treatment with competing risks. *JAMA Surg.* 2013;148(2):127–136.
36. CRASH-2 trial collaborators; Shakur H, Roberts I, Bautista R, et al. Effects of tranexamic acid on death, vascular occlusive events, and blood transfusion in trauma patients with significant hemorrhage (CRASH-2): a randomized, placebo-controlled trial. *Lancet.* 2010;376:23–32.
37. Sperry JL, Guyette FX, Brown JB, et al; PAMPer Study Group. Prehospital plasma during air medical transport in trauma patients at risk for hemorrhagic shock. *N Eng J Med.* 2018;379(4):315–326.
38. National Academies of Sciences, Engineering, and Medicine. *A National Trauma Care System: Integrating Military and Civilian Trauma Systems to Achieve Zero Preventable Deaths After Injury.* The National Academies Press; 2016. Accessed January 5, 2024. https://www.nap.edu/catalog/23511/a-national-trauma-care-system-integrating-military-and-civilian-trauma
39. Salim A, Stein DM, Zarzaur BL, Livingston DH. Measuring long-term outcomes after injury: current issues and future directions. *Trauma Surg Acute Care Open.* 2023;8(1):e001068.
40. Herrera-Escobar JP, Castillo-Angeles MA, Das S, et al; National Trauma Research Action Plan (NTRAP) Investigators Group. Long-term patient-reported outcome and patient-reported outcome measures after injury: the National Trauma Research Action Plan (NTRAP) scoping review protocol. *Trauma Surg Acute Care Open.* 2020;5(1):e000512.

19

Prehospital and New Advances in Resuscitation

Jason L. Sperry and Kristina J. Nicholson

Key Points

1. Triage is an active process with the goal of transporting the patient to the most appropriate trauma center in the shortest time, while avoiding over- or undertriage.
2. Prehospital assessment should follow ABCDE (Airway, Breathing, Circulation, Disability, and Environment); providers should perform only necessary critical interventions while avoiding delays in transfer to definitive care.
3. Direct pressure and hemostatic dressings can be used for control of hemorrhage; however, large-volume extremity hemorrhage may need to be addressed with placement of a tourniquet.
4. Prehospital fluid resuscitation follows damage-control principles of permissive hypotension and whole blood or balanced blood products if available, while minimizing crystalloid.
5. Prehospital use of resuscitative endovascular balloon occlusion of aorta (REBOA) is not recommended at this time.

Trauma continues to be the leading cause of death for 1- to 44-year-olds, and has risen to the overall third leading cause of death for all age groups.[1] The care of the injured patient is a tightly integrated exercise combining the expertise of the prehospital care team and the trauma team once they arrive at the hospital. The likelihood of patient survival is vastly increased by timely transport and proper interventions on arrival at definitive care centers. The care of the injured patient begins immediately following injury. This may be rendered initially by nearby civilian bystanders or a variety of trained first responders. The main goal of a prehospital system is expedient assessment and care for the injured patient, with rapid transportation to the most appropriate hospital for definitive care. At times the most appropriate hospital may be the closest, and at others, it may be more distant but with resources needed for a specific patient. Most commonly, a phone call placed to a 911 dispatcher activates the emergency medical system (EMS) and quickly allocates resources to the location where help is needed.

PREHOSPITAL CARE

Personnel

Prehospital personnel are comprised of civilians, emergency medical technicians (EMTs), paramedics, firefighters, police, nurses, and, less commonly, physicians. The Hartford Consensus III placed nonmedical civilians on the forefront of hemorrhage control as a ready force of immediate responders; prompted by this call to action, more than three million civilians to date have received basic training in bleeding control principles to provide immediate care until first responders arrive.[2] There are multiple levels of EMTs whose capabilities vary slightly by system. In general, the EMT-B or basic level has training capable of providing basic life support (BLS). BLS maneuvers include triage and transport, external hemorrhage control, administration of supplementary oxygen, spine immobilization, cardiopulmonary resuscitation, and application of an automated external defibrillator (AED). Prehospital advanced life support (ALS) may be provided by paramedics and was first employed as a "mobile intensive care unit" in 1967.[3] Paramedics require additional training—upward of 1200 hours—and may administer ALS techniques. In addition to the maneuvers administered by BLS personnel, an ALS unit can typically provide cardiac drugs, pain control, blood pressure management, glucose control, needle decompression of tension pneumothoraces, and anticonvulsant medication. There is debate as to whether ALS is superior to BLS in the prehospital setting for injured patients. A recent meta-analysis demonstrated no survival or neurologic advantage for patients receiving ALS services in controlled trials, and in fact demonstrated longer scene time and higher mortality in observational studies.[4] However, there may be some benefit to the presence of ALS providers for injured patients who require advanced life-saving maneuvers in the prehospital environment, even at the expense of prolonged scene time, especially as advanced technologies such as video laryngoscopy become more widely available.[5] In certain US cities, a physician medical director of EMS is available at all times to advise ground crews and dispatch centers. There may be selected physician response to calls for quality control, education, and approval of drug administration outside of set protocols. While physician presence may increase in survival in patients with acute myocardial infarction and respiratory distress, it also increases transport time, which is not beneficial for most trauma patients.[6]

Triage

1 Triage takes into account multiple factors with the goal of transporting the patient to the most appropriate trauma center in the shortest amount of time. The Centers for Disease Control and Prevention publish guidelines helping to facilitate proper triage of injured patients, which were most recently updated in 2011 and use physiologic and anatomic data, as well as the mechanisms of the injury to guide the triage of the patient.[7] While the goal of these guidelines is to prevent both under- and overtriage of the acutely injured patient, data suggest that undertriage of severely injured patients is significant,

particularly among the elderly.[8] This leads to prolonged time to definitive care for injuries, multiple transfers to identify the correct level of care, and overall worse outcomes for the patient while creating a greater burden on systems resources. The development and validation of quick prehospital triage models, especially for geriatric patients, is an area of ongoing investigation.

Triage of multiple simultaneously injured patients creates a challenging scenario. A multicasualty event is defined by a hospital being able to manage the number of casualties with local resources. The majority of level 1 trauma centers are able to take care of a small multicasualty event without significant strain on their work environment. A mass casualty event exists when the numbers, severity, and diversity of injuries overwhelm the local medical resources. Mass casualty events require coordination at the state and national level, and extensive practice implementing triage criteria.

Scoop and Run versus Stay and Play

Traditionally, two paradigms that dictate the amount and type of care that patients receive in the prehospital setting are the "Scoop and Run" and the "Stay and Play." The premise of the Scoop and Run technique is rapid transport of the injured patient to a facility that can provide definitive care, while Stay and Play advocates that the early control of life-threatening injuries may improve patient survival.[9] Which strategy is best likely depends on multiple factors for a given situation, including injury complex, skill set of first responders, and proximity to definitive care. In an urban setting with readily accessible trauma facilities, it makes sense to extract the patient and get them to the closest center, performing limited, life-saving interventions during transport. In a rural environment, where access to a hospital may be delayed by prolonged ground transport time or wait for helicopter transport arrival, it may be necessary to provide initial care on site for unstable injuries.

SCENE ASSESSMENT AND MANAGEMENT

Airway

Once on scene, it is paramount for the prehospital provider to assess the patient's airway quickly. Evaluating the patient's Glasgow Coma Scale (GCS), chest rise, and extent and nature of injuries provide vital insight into whether or not the patient
2 will be able to maintain their airway. Supplemental maneuvers such as suctioning, chin lift/jaw thrust, placement of oropharyngeal airways, and use of bag–mask devices can temporarily restore oxygenation in the acutely injured patient (**Table 19.1**). These maneuvers will usually maintain airway patency for the patient during their transport to definitive care; for those who are unable to do so, advanced airway maneuvers are key to securing a patent airway. Tracheal intubation provides a definitive airway with a cuffed endotracheal tube that will facilitate oxygenation, ventilation, and prevent aspiration. The skills required to successfully intubate are difficult to achieve and even more difficult to maintain, as this is a low-frequency event often performed under challenging conditions.

Table 19.1. Prehospital Assessments and Interventions

A	Chin lift/jaw thrust, oropharyngeal airway, nasopharyngeal airway
B	Laryngeal mask airways (LMA), King tube, surgical airway, needle decompression, chest tube, capnography
C	Tourniquet, needle decompression, permissive hypotension, early blood products
D	C-spine immobilization, backboard placement, splinting of extremity fractures
E	Clothing removal, exposure of wounds, warming devices

Field Intubation

The majority of studies regarding prehospital intubation suggest that prehospital intubation does not improve survival and prolongs time to definitive care.[10] A meta-analysis evaluating emergency intubation for the acutely ill did not show a benefit for trauma patients in the urban environment.[11] Moreover, a pediatric cohort from a conflict region showed increased mortality with prehospital intubation after controlling for other factors associated with death.[12] One study that did show a mortality benefit was a retrospective review of blunt trauma patients with severe head injury, who had a statistically significant decrease in mortality when intubated in the field compared to those who were not.[13] While the majority of situations in the prehospital setting do not require intubation, there are certain scenarios in which it may be prudent to secure an airway. For instance, patients who have evidence of extensive facial trauma with airway compromise and those patients who are apneic due to suspected cervical injury may be appropriate to be intubated in the prehospital setting. In most cases, however, the reflexive intubation to "protect" the airway in patients who are breathing and maintaining reasonable oxygen saturation (pulse oximetry) should be avoided, and further randomized studies are required to truly answer the question of who and when to intubate in the prehospital setting.

Alternate Airways

Due to the unclear benefit and challenge of mastering endotracheal intubation techniques in the prehospital setting, laryngeal mask airways (LMA) have been suggested as an alternative when a definitive airway is desired. A multivariable regression analysis of a retrospective data set from a level 1 trauma center showed similar outcomes in patients managed with LMA in the prehospital setting.[14] Prospective data on the utility of prehospital LMA in trauma patients is forthcoming.

While video-assisted airway insertion devices are commonly utilized in the hospital setting for "difficult" airways and increasingly for standard airways as well, data regarding their use in the prehospital setting is limited and primarily in European physician-staffed air units, therefore not generalizable to the US model of prehospital care. A randomized controlled trial of direct laryngoscopy versus video laryngoscopy in a prehospital cohort failed to show a difference in intubation success rate, tracheal intubation times, number of attempts, or difficulty. Notably, the number of technical problems with the equipment was increased in the video group.[15] As technology advances, the use of video-assisted airway devices may allow for more successful prehospital intubation, though whether this will translate to a survival benefit is unknown at this time.

A surgical cricothyroidotomy (CRIC) can provide an emergency airway in the hands of skilled practitioners. This maneuver requires much training and is utilized infrequently, mainly by personnel in austere environments or after failed orotracheal intubation efforts. A review of the physician-staffed Netherlands Hospital EMS database reported a 94% success rate, which was consistent with prior studies.[16] In spite of this high success rate, however, only 33% of patients arrived alive at the hospital, and only 11% survived till discharge. A retrospective review of the Department of Defense Trauma Registry reported that CRIC was an infrequent event in combat settings that did not confer a survival advantage over the less technically challenging supraglottic airway in a comparable cohort.[17]

Breathing

Assessment of the patient's breathing occurs concurrently with airway assessment. Evaluation for symmetric chest rise, obvious signs of chest trauma, and presence of bilateral breath sounds give the first responder an idea of the patient's status. The presence of a tension pneumothorax is a life-threatening event that may lead to obstructive shock, hemodynamic collapse, and potentially death. Signs of tension pneumothorax may include tracheal deviation, neck vein distention, and cyanosis. Prompt decompression of the thoracic cavity with a needle is necessary to reverse the tension effect. While the traditional landmark has been the midclavicular line, cadaver and computerized tomography evaluations have demonstrated more consistent evacuation of air using the anterior axillary, especially in females.[18] Further management with tube thoracostomy will be addressed once the patient arrives at their receiving facility. Large sucking chest wounds that permit the rapid equilibration of pleural and atmospheric pressure can be rapidly fatal. These wounds prevent the lung from expanding and preclude alveolar ventilation. These large wounds cause hemodynamic collapse rapidly unless an airway is obtained that allows for positive-pressure ventilation. The very rare smaller open sucking chest wounds are amenable to a three-sided dressing that allows for gas to exit from the chest wall defect but prevents gas from entering the chest wall. These can be fashioned in a field expedient manner and function as a temporizing action until definitive therapy with a chest tube can be achieved.

Mismanagement of ventilation in the intubated patient, specifically those with traumatic brain injury (TBI), can result in inadvertent harm. Intentional hyperventilation in the prehospital setting had been previously advocated and is unfortunately, still occasionally practiced. Current recommendations from the Brain Trauma Foundation target $PaCO_2$ between 35 and 45 mm Hg, as overventilation causes acute vasospasm and an overall decrease in the cerebral blood flow in patients with a severe TBI.[19] Additionally, hypoxemia (arterial hemoglobin saturation <90%) should be avoided. The resulting cerebral ischemia is one mechanism for secondary brain injury and increased mortality in patients with severe TBI.[20,21] Unintentional hyperventilation can be an issue as bag–valve device volumes can exceed 1200 mL. The Brain Trauma Foundation guidelines advocate for both continuous capnography and continuous pulse oximetry to facilitate optimal ventilation of the brain-injured patient.[19]

Circulation

Prehospital Control of Hemorrhage

3 Evaluation of circulatory status begins with initial evaluation of mental status and inspection for obvious signs of active hemorrhage. Direct pressure and hemostatic dressings can be used for control of hemorrhage, even by a layperson with minimal training[1]; however, large-volume extremity hemorrhage may need to be addressed with placement of a tourniquet.

Tourniquets

Tourniquet use for injury has documentation as far back as 6 BC in Hindu texts for the treatment of a snakebite.[22] Recent experience in combat environments supports the extension of this historically military practice to the provision of civilian trauma care. In the Vietnam War, surgeons recognized that of the casualties killed in the war, 2590 lives could have been saved with better prehospital hemorrhage control.[23] Analysis of the casualties of Operation Gothic Serpent, the 1993 battle fought between US forces and the militias in Somalia, showed 7% of fatalities resulted from penetrating extremity trauma and that hemorrhage control in the form of tourniquet use should be more widely adopted.[22] The recent conflict in Iraq and Afghanistan provided the strongest data supporting the use of prehospital tourniquets. A prospective study of casualties over a 7-month period in 2006 at a combat hospital in Baghdad showed tourniquet application with the absence of shock was strongly associated with survival, no amputations resulted solely from tourniquet use, and only four nerve palsies at the level of the tourniquet occurred, all of which resolved.[23]

Studies have detailed successful civilian application of this concept. A multicenter retrospective review of all patients sustaining peripheral vascular injuries admitted to 11 level I trauma centers compared tourniquet and nontourniquet groups. Mortality was 5.2% in the nontourniquet group compared with 3.9% in the tourniquet group, with adjusted odds ratio of survival = 5.86 in tourniquet group. Delayed amputation rates were not significantly different between the two groups.[24] A systematic review in 2018 included eight trauma centers (n = 718) and one national database (n = 2048) study reporting prehospital tourniquet use. The aggregate data reported >90% effectiveness of tourniquet, 6% mortality rate, 5.4% amputation rate, 4% extremity compartment syndrome, 3.7% peripheral nerve dysfunction, and 4% wound infection.[25] The overall mortality and limb amputation rate was less than that seen in similar cohorts of military patients. Additional quality research in civilian trauma patients is required to support whether tourniquet use leads to increased survival and limb salvage. In addition to their use in adult combat and civilian trauma, CAT tourniquets have been shown to be effective in preschool and school-age children and are recommended by the Pediatric Trauma Society in the prehospital setting and during the resuscitation of children suffering from exsanguinating hemorrhage from severe extremity trauma.[26,27]

Control of Junctional Hemorrhage

A final, more fatal, type of hemorrhage is junctional hemorrhage, defined as bleeding from the pelvis, groin, perineum, axilla, and neck. These wounds are seen extensively in the current era of combat as the use of improvised explosive devices (IEDs) has increased. Holcomb et al. reviewed preventable causes of death in US Special Forces Soldiers in 2007 and found that junctional or noncompressible trauma was implicated in 47% of deaths.[28] The junctional tourniquet has shown in healthy volunteers to occlude blood flow to the lower extremity, and requires effectiveness and implementation data prior to widespread utilization in prehospital trauma protocols.[29]

Resuscitation

Once the circulatory status of the patient has been addressed and sites of rapid compressible exsanguination identified and treated, the decision is made for intravenous access and possible use of intravenous fluid. Placement of peripheral intravenous or intraosseous access should be performed only if it does not delay the transport of the patient. In patients without evidence of ongoing hemorrhage or in prehospital settings where blood and blood products are not available, numerous choices of fluid are available. However, most fluid options are actually poor choices for resuscitation of injured patients. Normal saline (0.9% sodium chloride) has an average pH of 5.5, with a sodium and chloride concentration of 154 mEq/L. Normal saline is often preferred as a universal solution for prehospital settings as it is "compatible with blood," contains no potassium, and is cheap to carry; with a low overall cost and extended shelf life. Lactated Ringer solution (LR), initially developed to support organs in the lab (because of calcium content) and later championed for treating cholera, has only a slightly better physiologic profile. LR gives the clinician a better average pH of 6.5, with lower sodium (130 mEq/L) and chloride content (109). The optimal fluid, however, is plasmalyte/normosol which has an average pH of 7.4 and an electrolyte content that more closely resembles a normal metabolic profile. In addition to its superior profile, Plasmalyte is compatible with all blood products and has been shown in a randomized trial to result in improved acid–base status and less hyperchloremia at 24 hours postinjury.[30]

[1] *See https://www.stopthebleed.org/ for additional information.*

Prehospital Transfusion Protocols

Resuscitation practice is rapidly evolving based on the imperative that the prehospital setting is the ideal place to begin early resuscitation with blood products. Hemorrhage is the leading cause of preventable death in trauma, responsible for one-third to one-half of prehospital casualties. Trauma-induced coagulopathy is common in severely injured trauma patients and contributes to morbidity and mortality. Severely injured patients are now receiving blood and blood-product transfusion in the prehospital setting to facilitate early hemostatic resuscitation and prevention of coagulopathy complications.

Early studies focused on transfusion of packed red blood cells (RBCs) versus standard practice (crystalloid); the evidence overwhelmingly supports transfusion of RBCs for patients in hemorrhagic shock. Shackelford et al. described a cohort of military combat casualties with traumatic amputation or hemorrhagic shock. In comparing those who received blood-product transfusion prehospital (RBCs, plasma, or both) to those who received delayed or no transfusion, patients who received early product transfusion had decreased 24-hour (adjusted HR = 0.26) and 30-day (adjusted HR = 0.39) mortality.[31] Brown et al. conducted a retrospective, case-controlled analysis of patients who received prehospital RBCs (n = 240) against those who did not (n = 480).[32] Those receiving prehospital transfusion had an increased likelihood of 24-hour survival, lower odds of shock, and lower overall 24-hour blood products transfusion. A subsequent study from these investigators evaluated over 2000 blunt trauma patients presenting to care within 2 hours of injury, comparing those who received RBCs in the prehospital setting (n = 3.5%) to those who did not.[33] Those who received prehospital RBCs had a 95% reduction in the odds of 24-hour mortality, 64% reduction in 30-day mortality, and an 88% reduction in the incidence of trauma-induced coagulopathy. In a multicenter study of over 1400 injured patients with evidence of shock, patients receiving prehospital RBCs had increased 24-hour and 30-day survival, as well as less coagulopathy on arrival in those patients receiving prehospital RBC transfusions.[32] Subsequently, the Houston group published their aeromedical experience comparing patients who received prehospital plasma and RBC (n = 137) versus those who received crystalloid (n = 1540). Those who received products had improved acid–base status on hospital admission, decreased use of blood products over 24 hours, and reduced 6-hour mortality in the sickest cohort.[34] In another prehospital study comparing four different resuscitation groups (crystalloid only; PRBC; plasma; and PRBC + plasma), the group receiving plasma and PRBC had the greatest risk-adjusted 30-day mortality benefit.[35]

4 Further interest in prehospital plasma administration resulted in two concurrent trials: PAMPER and COMBAT. Sperry et al. enrolled 501 patients in a multicenter cluster-randomized trial comparing the administration of thawed plasma with standard-care resuscitation during air medical transport. Mortality at 30 days was significantly lower in the plasma group than in the standard-care group, as was median prothrombin time on arrival to the trauma center.[36] In the COMBAT trial, 125 eligible patients in the as-treated analysis dataset were compared, 65 receiving plasma and 60 receiving crystalloid. There was no difference in 28-day mortality, the lack of benefit posited to be due to short transport times and rapid presentation to high-volume, high-quality care centers[37]; a posthoc analysis of these combined datasets did show a significant mortality benefit when transport times were greater than 20 minutes.[38] Further research is focusing on the use of freeze-dried plasma (FDP) to increase the shelf-life in systems and locations, where maintaining a supply of fresh frozen plasma is not practical. Early studies indicate that the use of FDP in military combat settings at the point of injury and in prehospital civilian trauma systems is feasible and acceptable.[39–41]

There has also been a renewed interest in cold-stored platelets (CSPs, 1 °C to 6 °C), as they perform better on in vitro coagulation testing than room-temperature platelets.[42] Importantly, cold storage also extends acceptable storage time, theoretically facilitating maintenance of a supply of platelets for prehospital transfusion.[43] Attempts have been made to evaluate the feasibility of maintaining a dual supply of platelets, as CSP have a shorter half-life following transfusion as compared to room-temperature platelets, which are preferred for prophylactic transfusion. A modeling study using data from a Canadian Blood Services regional center predicted increased platelet wastage with a dual supply of platelets.[44] It is unclear, however, if this would be true across other blood-product supply chains, and further study is necessary to elucidate whether this prediction is generalizable and whether it is justifiable for the hemostatic benefit in the bleeding patient.

Current transfusion practice emphasizes a balanced transfusion strategy with high ratios of plasma and platelets to packed RBCs that attempts to mimic or "reconstitute" whole blood composition. The foundation for this practice comes from the landmark PROPPR trial, which included patients who received blood transfusion prehospital and showed that more patients resuscitated in the 1:1:1 group versus the 1:1:2 group achieved hemostasis, and fewer experienced death due to exsanguination by 24 hours.[45] In the last decade, in keeping with the desire to transfuse in 1:1:1 ratios, the pendulum has swung back toward utilizing whole blood as opposed to reassembling it from its component part. Transfusion of cold-stored low-titer group O whole blood (LTOWB) as the first resuscitative fluid is now the standard of care in over 70 civilian trauma centers and prehospital settings in the United States.[43] Despite theoretical concerns about hemolysis, studies in both adult and pediatric trauma patients demonstrate an excellent safety profile and no increased risk of hemolysis among the non–group O recipients compared to the group O recipients of WB who are not susceptible to hemolysis following LTOWB transfusion.[46,47] Advantages to whole blood include higher hematocrit, greater platelet and factor concentrations, and less saline and additive solution compared to an equivalent volume of "reconstituted" whole blood (**Table 19.2**). Further, LTOWB is a single product that can be transfused more efficiently than multiple component products, as evidenced by the significantly faster time to transfusion of at least one unit of RBCs, plasma, and platelets among pediatric trauma patients who received LTOWB versus conventional components (median = 15 minutes vs 303 minutes, respectively).[46] In a single-center comparison of LTOWB versus component therapy in adult trauma patients, LTOWB was associated with a 53% reduction in post-ED blood-product transfusion and twofold increase in likelihood of 28-day survival compared to component therapy after controlling for

Table 19.2. Components of Whole Blood versus Reconstituted Component Products

	Whole Blood	Components
	1 unit whole blood	1 unit red blood cells 1 unit plasma 1 pack platelets 1 unit cryoprecipitate
Product volume (mL)	570	675
Hematocrit (%)	38–50	29
Platelet count	150,000–400,000	88,000
Factor activity (%)	100	65
Fibrinogen (mg)	1000	750

age, injury severity, and prehospital physiology.[48] These findings were recapitulated in another prospective cohort study of over 1300 patients, and two additional cohort studies with a total of over 4000 patients also show a survival benefit with whole blood resuscitation of trauma patients.[49–51] Those receiving fewer transfusions are therefore exposed to fewer donors overall, decreasing risk. Further study is required to determine if whole blood transfusion will improve other outcomes.

Permissive Hypotension

The concept of permissive hypotension involves keeping the blood pressure low enough to avoid exsanguination while maintaining perfusion of end organs.[52] It is an integral part of damage-control resuscitation protocols dating back to World War I. The work of Walter Cannon and John Fraser while serving with the Harvard Medical Unit in France involved the observation that artificial elevations in blood pressure may dislodge the clot that is preventing further hemorrhage, and the patient will lose sorely needed blood.[53] In 1994, Bickell et al. presented a randomized controlled trial showing delayed fluid resuscitation in adults with penetrating torso injuries led to greater survival and overall shorter hospital length of stay.[54] These results have been repeated in subsequent studies showing no benefit to targeting physiologic or supernormal blood pressures in either blunt or penetrating trauma. A multicenter study randomized hypotensive blunt trauma patients to receive small boluses of fluid (250 mL) if they had no radial pulse or a systolic blood pressure lower than 70 mm Hg, or to receive a 2-L fluid bolus and additional fluid needed to maintain a systolic of 110 mm Hg or greater.[55] The permissive hypotension group received 1 L less of fluid and had less deaths (5% vs 15%) at 24 hours after admission; and among patients with blunt abdominal trauma 24-hour mortality was 3% versus 18%, all statistically significant. There was, however, no difference in mortality among patients with penetrating trauma. These data suggest that controlled resuscitation in the prehospital setting may offer an early survival advantage to the blunt trauma patient.

This strategy of permissive hypotension is not applicable to patients with severe TBI, in light of well-described evidence on secondary brain injury and poor outcomes due to even a single episode of prehospital hypotension. Further confusion is generated for prehospital providers as recommendations for permissive hypotension in trauma literature on damage-control resuscitation directly contradict the Advanced Trauma Life Support guidelines that advocate for early administration of 2-L crystalloid bolus for those patients manifesting signs of shock.[56] Additional studies are necessary to clarify this issue and at which level fluid administration may be paused; however, the general paradigm prehospital trauma providers should follow includes minimizing intravenous fluids, tolerating systolic blood pressures in the 90 mm Hg range, and not resuscitating to supernormal values with crystalloids. Importantly, children do not tolerate hypotension. They have the physiologic reserve to maintain normotension to the verge of circulatory collapse; hypotension therefore is a sign that a child is in extremis and should be treated with expedient fluid resuscitation, not observation.

CONTROVERSIES

Resuscitative Endovascular Balloon Occlusion of Aorta

5 REBOA is achieved with a balloon placed via the femoral artery to occlude the aorta and prevent life-threatening hemorrhage. While the technology is relatively new, the concept was described in the journal Surgery in 1954.[57] While initially popularized as a substitute for resuscitative thoracotomy, it is probably best suited for temporizing pelvic hemorrhage (before the patient has lost pulses) as a bridge to embolization in interventional radiology, or as an adjunct in the operating room.[58] High-volume centers who utilize REBOA in a protocolized fashion report feasibility, faster time to aortic occlusion, fewer early deaths, and improved overall survival as compared with resuscitative thoracotomy (37.5% vs 9.7%).[59,60] However, the 2023 UK-REBOA randomized clinical trial, which is the only randomized controlled trial to examine the use of REBOA, was halted early due to demonstrated harm, with an odds ratio of 1.58 for all-cause mortality at 90 days, likely due to delay in achieving definitive hemorrhage control.[61] While the majority of US trauma centers do not perform REBOA placement, and those that do perform only a few each year (median = 6), it is feasible that continued training in endovascular skills may lead to greater implementation of this skill.[62]

Safety concerns with REBOA include the following: (1) prolonged aortic occlusion may lead to spinal cord ischemia; (2) ischemia reperfusion injury can lead to acute kidney injury and multisystem organ failure; (3) femoral access complications (dissection, hematoma, pseudoaneurysm, etc.) may result in limb loss or need for complex vascular repair/reconstruction; (4) balloon rupture or overinflation can result in rupture or thrombosis of aorta or iliac vessels; (5) Prolonged attempts to complete the procedure, in particular in obtaining vascular access, can delay definitive hemorrhage control.[63] Measures to reduce the risks and maximize success of REBOA include adequate training and preparedness of a skilled multidisciplinary team, having the resources for urgent operative or catheter-based hemostasis following REBOA placement as soon as possible, using a smaller-diameter sheath devices (<8 Fr), limiting aortic occlusion time, and attentive assessment of lower extremity perfusion.[62]

There have been case reports of REBOA placement by physicians in prehospital settings outside of the United States. However, prehospital placement of REBOA is not recommended in the United States at this time due to lack of clear "safe" duration of aortic occlusion, difficulty defining reliable and appropriate patient selection criteria, lack of safety data in prehospital settings, and potential to delay transport to definitive care.

LTOWB Rh-Positive Transfusion in Children and Women of Childbearing Potential

Concerns regarding the transfusion of Rh(D)-positive whole blood to Rh(D)-negative children and women of childbearing potential (WCP) are sometimes raised as a barrier to the transfusion of whole blood to these populations in emergencies. The risk in this scenario is that a woman who is Rh(D) negative will be exposed to Rh(D)-positive RBCs in the transfusion of whole blood and could become alloimmunized to Rh antigen. If she goes on to carry a Rh(D)-positive fetus, maternal anti-D antibodies would cross the placenta, and bind and destroy fetal RBCs. This hemolytic disease of fetus and newborn (HDFN), if untreated, may cause death or significant developmental neurologic morbidity in the child.

One strategy to avoid this would be transfusion of group O Rh(D)-negative whole blood, which is the practice in some pediatric protocols currently. However, this is an incredibly rare product and is not available in quantities sufficient to support all whole blood programs. In light of this, women should be transfused LTOWB when indicated, as it is ethically questionable to withhold a superior lifesaving treatment in an emergency from a woman who may or may not bear children in the future. Further, the risk of demise of a future fetus as a result of receiving Rh(D)-positive whole blood is 0.3% in adult women, and even lower in children due to decreased alloimmunization rates after exposure to Rh antigen.[64] This number is small compared to the lifesaving benefits of early blood-product administration in a bleeding emergency. Additionally, with current practices for timely diagnosis and treatment, severe HDFN is much less common than in the past.

SUMMARY

Prehospital trauma care is a constantly evolving field. Advance in trauma care from recent military conflicts are being rapidly implemented in the civilian prehospital setting. Uncertainty remains regarding how to best care for the most critically injured trauma patients in the prehospital setting. Further research and developments are necessary to continue to optimize the distribution of care between the prehospital and in-hospital settings.

ACKNOWLEDGMENT

We gratefully acknowledge the contributions of previous edition author, Christine M. Leeper, as portions of those chapters have been retained in this revision.

References

1. Heron M. *National Vital Statistics Reports*. Vol 68. 6th ed.; 2017.
2. Jacobs LM Jr; Joint Committee to Create a National Policy to Enhance Survivability from Intentional Mass-Casualty and Active Shooter Events. The Hartford Consensus III: implementation of bleeding control: if you see something do something. *Bull Am Coll Surg*. 2015;100(1Suppl):40–46.
3. Beuran M, Paun S, Gaspar B, et al. Prehospital trauma care: a clinical review. *Chirurgia (Bucur)*. 2012;107:564–570.
4. Kondo Y, Fukuda T, Uchimido R, et al. Advanced life support vs. basic life support for patients with trauma in prehospital settings: a systematic review and meta-analysis. *Front Med (Lausanne)*. 2021;8:660367.
5. Chen X, Gestring ML, Rosengart MR, et al. Speed is not everything: identifying patients who may benefit from helicopter transport despite faster ground transport. *J Trauma Acute Care Surg*. 2018;84:549–557.
6. Haas B, Nathens AB. Pro/con debate: is the scoop and run approach the best approach to trauma services organization? *Crit Care*. 2008;12(5):224.
7. Sasser SM, Hunt RC, Faul M, et al; Centers for Disease Control and Prevention. Guidelines for field triage of injured patients: recommendations of the National Expert Panel on Field Triage, 2011. *MMWR Recomm Rep*. 2012;61(RR-1):1–20.
8. Newgard CD, Uribe-Leitz T, Haider AH. Undertriage remains a vexing problem for even the most highly developed trauma systems: the need for innovations in field triage. *JAMA Surg*. 2018;153(4):328.
9. Gausche M, Lewis RJ, Stratton SJ, et al. Effect of out-of-hospital pediatric endotracheal intubation on survival and neurological outcome: a controlled clinical trial. *JAMA*. 2000;283(6):783–790.
10. Nolan B, Haas B, Tien H, Saskin R, Nathens A. Causes of delay during interfacility transports of injured patients transported by air ambulance. *Prehosp Emerg Care*. 2020;24(5):625–633.
11. Lecky F, Bryden D, Little R, Tong N, Moulton C. Emergency intubation for acutely ill and injured patients. *Cochrane Database Syst Rev*. 2008;2008(2):CD001429.
12. Schauer SG, Naylor JF, Hill GJ, Arana AA, Roper JL, April MD. Association of prehospital intubation with decreased survival among pediatric trauma patients in Iraq and Afghanistan. *Am J Emerg Med*. 2018;36(4):657–659.
13. Winchell RJ, Hoyt DB. Endotracheal intubation in the field improves survival in patients with severe head injury. *Arch Surg*. 1997;132(6):592–597.
14. Kempema J, Trust MD, Ali S, et al. Prehospital endotracheal intubation vs extraglottic airway device in blunt trauma. *Am J Emerg Med*. 2015;33(8):1080–1083.
15. Kreutziger J, Hornung S, Harrer C, et al. Comparing the McGrath Mac Video Laryngoscope and Direct Laryngoscopy for prehospital emergency intubation in air rescue patients: a multicenter, randomized, controlled trial. *Crit Care Med*. 2019;47(10):1362–1370.
16. Schober P, Biesheuvel T, de Leeuw MA, Loer SA, Schwarte LA. Prehospital cricothyrotomies in a helicopter emergency medical service: analysis of 19,382 dispatches. *BMC Emerg Med*. 2019;19(1):12.
17. Schauer SG, Naylor JF, Chow AL, et al. Survival of casualties undergoing prehospital supraglottic airway placement versus cricothyrotomy. *J Spec Oper Med*. 2019;19(2):91–94.
18. Inaba K, Branco BC, Eckstein M, et al. Optimal positioning for emergent needle thoracostomy: a cadaver-based study. *J Trauma*. 2011;71(5):1099–1103.
19. Lulla A, Lumba-Brown A, Totten AM, et al. Prehospital guidelines for the management of traumatic brain injury–3rd edition. *Prehosp Emerg Care*. 2023;27(5):507–538.
20. Warner KJ, Cuschieri J, Copass MK, Jurkovich GJ, Bulger EM. Emergency department ventilation effects outcome in severe traumatic brain injury. *J Trauma*. 2008;64(2):341–347.
21. Davis DP, Hoyt DB, Ochs M, et al. The effect of paramedic rapid sequence intubation on outcome in patients with severe traumatic brain injury. *J Trauma*. 2003;54(3):444–453.
22. Mabry RL, Holcomb JB, Baker AM, et al. United States army rangers in Somalia: an analysis of combat casualties on an urban battlefield. *J Trauma*. 2000;49(3):515–528.
23. Kragh JF Jr, Walters TJ, Baer DG, et al. Survival with emergency tourniquet use to stop bleeding in major limb trauma. *Ann Surg*. 2009;249(1):1–7.
24. Teixeira PGR, Brown CVR, Emigh B, et al. Civilian prehospital tourniquet use is associated with improved survival in patients with peripheral vascular injury. *J Am Coll Surg*. 2018;226(5):769–776.e1.
25. Kauvar DS, Dubick MA, Walters TJ, Kragh JF Jr. Systematic review of prehospital tourniquet use in civilian limb trauma. *J Trauma Acute Care Surg*. 2018;84(5):819–825.
26. Kelly JR, Levy MJ, Reyes J, Anders J. Effectiveness of the combat application tourniquet for arterial occlusion in young children. *J Trauma Acute Care Surg*. 2020;88(5):644–647.
27. Cunningham A, Auerbach M, Cicero M, Jafri M. Tourniquet usage in prehospital care and resuscitation of pediatric trauma patients-Pediatric Trauma Society position statement. *J Trauma Acute Care Surg*. 2018;85(4):665–667.
28. Holcomb JB, McMullin NR, Pearse L, et al. Causes of death in U.S. special operations forces in the global war on terrorism: 2001-2004. *Ann Surg*. 2007;245(6):986–991.
29. Lyon M, Johnson D, Gordon R. Use of a novel abdominal aortic and junctional tourniquet to reduce or eliminate flow in the brachial and popliteal arteries in human subjects. *Prehosp Emerg Care*. 2015;19(3):405–408.
30. Young JB, Utter GH, Schermer CR, et al. Saline versus plasma-lyte A in initial resuscitation of trauma patients: a randomized trial. *Ann Surg*. 2014;259(2):255–262.
31. Shackelford SA, Del Junco DJ, Powell-Dunford N, et al. Association of prehospital blood product transfusion during medical evacuation of combat casualties in Afghanistan with acute and 30-day survival. *JAMA*. 2017;318(16):1581–1591.
32. Brown JB, Sperry JL, Fombona A, Billiar TR, Peitzman AB, Guyette FX. Pre-trauma center red blood cell transfusion is associated with improved early outcomes in air medical trauma patients. *J Am Coll Surg*. 2015;220(5):797–808.
33. Brown JB, Cohen MJ, Minei JP, et al. Pretrauma center red blood cell transfusion is associated with reduced mortality and coagulopathy in severely injured patients with blunt trauma. *Ann Surg*. 2015;261(5):997–1005.
34. Holcomb JB, Donathan DP, Cotton BA, et al. Prehospital transfusion of plasma and red blood cells in trauma patients. *Prehosp Emerg Care*. 2015;19(1):1–9.
35. Guyette FX, Sperry JL, Peitzman AB, et al. Prehospital blood product and crystalloid resuscitation in the severely injured patient: a secondary analysis of the prehospital air medical plasma trial. *Ann Surg*. 2021;273(2):358–364.
36. Sperry JL, Guyette FX, Brown JB, et al. Prehospital plasma during air medical transport in trauma patients at risk for hemorrhagic shock. *N Engl J Med*. 2018;379(4):315–326.

37. Moore HB, Moore EE, Chapman MP, et al. Plasma-first resuscitation to treat haemorrhagic shock during emergency ground transportation in an urban area: a randomised trial. *Lancet.* 2018;392(10144):283–291.
38. Pusateri AE, Moore EE, Moore HB, et al. Association of prehospital plasma transfusion with survival in trauma patients with hemorrhagic shock when transport times are longer than 20 minutes: a post hoc analysis of the PAMPer and COMBAT clinical trials. *JAMA Surg.* 2020;155(2):e195085.
39. Shlaifer A, Siman-Tov M, Radomislensky I, et al. Prehospital administration of freeze-dried plasma, is it the solution for trauma casualties? *J Trauma Acute Care Surg.* 2017;83(4):675–682.
40. Sunde GA, Vikenes B, Strandenes G, et al. Freeze dried plasma and fresh red blood cells for civilian prehospital hemorrhagic shock resuscitation. *J Trauma Acute Care Surg.* 2015;78:S26–S30.
41. Oakeshott JE, Griggs JE, Wareham GM, Lyon RM; Kent Surrey Sussex Air Ambulance Trust. Feasibility of prehospital freeze-dried plasma administration in a UK Helicopter Emergency Medical Service. *Eur J Emerg Med.* 2019;26(5):373–378.
42. Pidcoke HF, McFaul SJ, Ramasubramanian AK, et al. Primary hemostatic capacity of whole blood: a comprehensive analysis of pathogen reduction and refrigeration effects over time. *Transfusion.* 2013;53(1):137S–149S.
43. Zhu CS, Pokorny DM, Eastridge BJ, et al. Give the trauma patient what they bleed, when and where they need it: establishing a comprehensive regional system of resuscitation based on patient need utilizing cold-stored, low-titer O+ whole blood. *Transfusion.* 2019;59(S2):1429–1438.
44. Blake JT, Krok E, Pavenski K, Pambrun C, Petraszko T. The operational impact of introducing cold stored platelets. *Transfusion.* 2023;63(12):2248–2255.
45. Holcomb JB, Tilley BC, Baraniuk S, et al. Transfusion of plasma, platelets, and red blood cells in a 1:1:1 vs a 1:1:2 ratio and mortality in patients with severe trauma: the PROPPR randomized clinical trial. *JAMA.* 2015;313(5):471–482.
46. Leeper CM, Yazer MH, Cladis FP, Saladino R, Triulzi DJ, Gaines BA. Use of uncross matched cold-stored whole blood in injured children with hemorrhagic shock. *JAMA Pediatr.* 2018;172(5):491–492.
47. Harrold IM, Seheult JN, Alarcon LH, et al. Hemolytic markers following the transfusion of uncrossmatched, cold-stored, low-titer, group O+ whole blood in civilian trauma patients. *Transfusion.* 2020;60(S3):S24–S30.
48. Williams J, Merutka N, Meyer D, et al. Safety profile and impact of low-titer group O whole blood for emergency use in trauma. *J Trauma Acute Care Surg.* 2020;88(1):87–93.
49. Brill JB, Tang B, Hatton G, et al. Impact of incorporating whole blood into hemorrhagic shock resuscitation: analysis of 1,377 consecutive trauma patients receiving emergency-release uncrossmatched blood products. *J Am Coll Surg.* 2022;234(4):408–418.
50. Torres CM, Kent A, Scantling D, Joseph B, Haut ER, Sakran JV. Association of whole blood with survival among patients presenting with severe hemorrhage in US and Canadian Adult Civilian Trauma Centers. *JAMA Surg.* 2023;158(5):532–540.
51. Hazelton JP, Ssentongo AE, Oh JS, et al. Use of cold-stored whole blood is associated with improved mortality in hemostatic resuscitation of major bleeding: a multicenter study. *Ann Surg.* 2022;276(4):579–588.
52. Geeraedts LMG Jr, Kaasjager HAH, van Vugt AB, Frölke JPM. Exsanguination in trauma: a review of diagnostics and treatment options. *Injury.* 2009;40(1):11–20.
53. Beuran M, Negoi I, Păun S, Runcanu A, Gaspar B. [History of trauma care]. *Chirurgia (Bucur).* 2011;106(5):573–580.
54. Bickell WH, Wall MJ Jr, Pepe PE, et al. Immediate versus delayed fluid resuscitation for hypotensive patients with penetrating torso injuries. *N Engl J Med.* 1994;331(17):1105–1109.
55. Schreiber MA, Meier EN, Tisherman SA, et al. A controlled resuscitation strategy is feasible and safe in hypotensive trauma patients: results of a prospective randomized pilot trial. *J Trauma Acute Care Surg.* 2015;78:687–695.
56. Holcomb JB, Jenkins D, Rhee P, et al. Damage control resuscitation: directly addressing the early coagulopathy of trauma. *J Trauma.* 2007;62(2):307–310.
57. Hughes CW. Use of an intra-aortic balloon catheter tamponade for controlling intra-abdominal hemorrhage in man. *Surgery.* 1954;36(1):65–68.
58. Vella MA, Dumas RP, DuBose J, et al. Intraoperative REBOA: an analysis of the American Association for the Surgery of Trauma AORTA registry. *Trauma Surg Acute Care Open.* 2019;4(1):e000340.
59. Moore LJ, Brenner M, Kozar RA, et al. Implementation of resuscitative endovascular balloon occlusion of the aorta as an alternative to resuscitative thoracotomy for noncompressible truncal hemorrhage. *J Trauma Acute Care Surg.* 2015;79(4):523–530.
60. Romagnoli A, Teeter W, Pasley J, et al. Time to aortic occlusion: it's all about access. *J Trauma Acute Care Surg.* 2017;83(6):1161–1164.
61. Jansen JO, Hudson J, Cochran C, et al. Emergency department resuscitative endovascular balloon occlusion of the aorta in trauma patients with exsanguinating hemorrhage: the UK-REBOA randomized clinical trial. *JAMA.* 2023;330(19):1862–1871.
62. Bulger EM, Perina DG, Qasim Z, et al. Clinical use of resuscitative endovascular balloon occlusion of the aorta (REBOA) in civilian trauma systems in the USA, 2019: a joint statement from the American College of Surgeons Committee on Trauma, the American College of Emergency Physicians, the National Association of Emergency Medical Services Physicians and the National Association of Emergency Medical Technicians. *Trauma Surg Acute Care Open.* 2019;4(1):e000376.
63. Joseph B, Zeeshan M, Sakran JV, et al. Nationwide analysis of resuscitative endovascular balloon occlusion of the aorta in civilian trauma. *JAMA Surg.* 2019;154(6):500–508.
64. Yazer MH, Delaney M, Doughty H, et al. It is time to reconsider the risks of transfusing RhD negative females of childbearing potential with RhD positive red blood cells in bleeding emergencies. *Transfusion.* 2019;59(12):3794–3799.

20

Head Injuries

Jacob R. Joseph, Venkatakrishna Rajajee, and Krishnan Raghavendran

TRAUMA

Key Points

1 Traumatic brain injury (TBI) accounts for a significant mortality and morbidity worldwide.

2 Factors that worsen primary brain insult such as hypoxia and hypotension should be aggressively treated.

3 A noncontrast computed tomography (CT) is the preferred imaging modality in any trauma patient with suspected TBI.

4 Management goals for treatment of severe TBI include appropriate resuscitation with priority for maintenance of airway, breathing, and circulation.

5 We recommend the use of invasive intracranial pressure (ICP) monitoring in all patients with severe TBI.

6 A tiered approach for the management of elevated ICP is recommended.

7 Prompt surgical intervention should be performed in patients with large mass lesions and refractory medical management of elevated ICP.

1 Craniocerebral injuries account for the majority of deaths and disability following trauma across the world. In the current chapter, we will discuss the epidemiology, clinical assessment, treatment paradigms, and prognostic elements associated with head injuries and in particular traumatic brain injury (TBI).

DEFINITION AND CLASSIFICATION

TBI is a heterogeneous disease and has been variably defined. It can vary from physiologic disturbances in the brain to significant macroscopic anatomic alterations that lead to loss of brain function, death, and disability. A unified definition of TBI across the spectrum of injury was adopted in 2010 by the International Interagency Initiative toward common data elements for research in TBI and psychological health.[1] TBI was defined as an alteration in brain function, or other evidence of brain pathology, caused by an external force. This definition emphasizes "brain" rather than "head" injury and allows for imaging or laboratory evidence of injury. The clinician must use judgment in determining the potential confounding effect of intoxication, drug abuse, or medical illness on the patient's clinical condition. This definition also recognizes that evidence of brain injury may be delayed, rather than present at the time of the event.

TBI is also categorized by the nature of the traumatic mechanism (eg, blunt vs. penetrating injuries, blast injury) that impacts the type and severity of the pathologic insult. Finally, the importance of extracranial injuries in a multisystem trauma cannot be overemphasized. These injuries are present in about 35% of trauma patients.[2] Systemic hypotension, frequently caused by blood loss, and hypoxia have been identified as important causes of secondary brain injury.

Clinical Scoring System

Severity of injury is best characterized by a scoring system that is simple, easy to use, and reproducible. The Glasgow Coma Scale (GCS) is the most commonly used TBI scoring system worldwide. It includes three separate components: eye opening, motor score, and a verbal score (**Table 20.1**). A GCS of 13 to 15 is considered mild injury, 9 to 12 is considered moderate injury, and 8 or less is considered severe TBI. Advantages of the GCS include simplicity, reproducibility, and prognostic value.

Table 20.1. Glasgow Coma Scale

Response	Score
Eye Opening	
No eye opening	1
To pain	2
To speech	3
Spontaneously	4
Best Verbal Response	
None	1
Incomprehensible sounds	2
Inappropriate words	3
Patient confused	4
Patient oriented	5
Best Motor Response	
None	1
Extensor response to painful stimulus	2
Flexion to painful stimulus	3
Withdraws from pain	4
Localizes to pain stimulus	5
Obeys commands	6

Table 20.2. Marshall Classification for Radiologic Assessment of TBI

Diffuse Injury I (no visible pathology) ■ No visible intracranial pathology
Diffuse Injury II ■ Midline shift of 0–5 mm ■ Basal cisterns remain visible ■ No high- or mixed-density lesions >25 cm³
Diffuse Injury III (swelling) ■ Midline shift of 0–5 mm ■ Basal cisterns compressed or completely effaced ■ No high- or mixed-density lesions >25 cm³
Diffuse Injury IV (shift) ■ Midline shift >5 mm ■ No high- or mixed-density lesions >25 cm³
Evacuated Mass Lesion V ■ Any lesion evacuated surgically
Nonevacuated Mass Lesion VI ■ High- or mixed-density lesions >25 cm³ ■ Not surgically evacuated

Used with permission of Mary Ann/Liebert, Inc. Publishers, from Marshall LF, Marshall SB, Klauber MR, et al. The diagnosis of head injury requires a classification based on computed axial tomography. *J Neurotrauma.* 1992;9 Suppl 1: S287–S292; permission conveyed through Copyright Clearance Center, Inc.

Table 20.3. Rotterdam Scale for Radiologic Assessment of TBI

Basal Cisterns ■ 0: normal ■ 1: compressed ■ 2: absent
Midline Shift ■ 0: no shift or ≤5 mm ■ 1: shift >5 mm
Epidural Mass Lesion ■ 0: present ■ 1: absent
Intraventricular Blood or Traumatic SAH ■ 0: absent ■ 1: present

From Maas AI, Hukkelhoven CW, Marshall LF, et al. Prediction of outcome in traumatic brain injury with computed tomographic characteristics: a comparison between the computed tomographic classification and combinations of computed tomographic predictors. *Neurosurgery.* 2005;57(6):1173–1182.

The GCS is therefore recognized as the single most important assessment for an injured patient with suspected TBI. While it is considered a single score, the separate components are important to assess and document. A patient with a GCS of 8 is better described as E2V3M3. The primary reason is that the motor score has been recognized as the single most important portion of the score in terms of severity and prognosis, particularly with severe TBI. The presence of an endotracheal tube obviates the verbal score, which by tradition is scored as a "1" followed by the letter "T" in intubated patients. A limitation of the GCS includes the potential confounding effect of sedation, neuromuscular blockade, and intoxication with drugs and alcohol, particularly in patients with a low GCS.[3] The eye-opening and verbal responses appear to be more helpful for the characterization of mild TBI. The GCS has also been applied to describe conscious states other than TBI and has found broad application for serial neurologic assessments in the ICU.

Neuroimaging Scales

A detailed discussion of the radiologic tools for diagnosis is described under the radiologic assessment section. Computed tomography (CT) scan remains the cornerstone for early diagnosis of intracranial pathology in patients with TBI. The Marshall scale uses CT findings to classify injuries in six different categories based on the compression of basal cisterns, presence of high or mixed-density lesions with volume >25 mL, and midline shift >5 mm (**Table 20.2**).[4] Multiple studies have shown an increase in mortality with higher Marshall grades. The Marshall grade does not consider the presence of traumatic subarachnoid hemorrhage (SAH), type of lesion (epidural/subdural/parenchymal), or the extent of compression of basal cisterns.

The Rotterdam scale is a more recent CT-based classification developed to overcome the limitations of the Marshall scale (**Table 20.3**). It includes the presence of SAH or intraventricular hemorrhage (IVH), presence or absence of an epidural lesion, and severity of compression of cisterns (compression vs complete effacement). Though the Rotterdam scale has shown promising early results,[5] broader validation is required.

EPIDEMIOLOGY

The Global Burden of Disease (GBD) study reported 27.16 million new cases of TBI worldwide in 2019.[6] In the United States, the Centers for Disease Control and Prevention (CDC) reported 586 TBI-related hospitalizations in 2020 and 190 TBI-related deaths in 2021.[7] Although TBI has traditionally been a disease of the young, its epidemiology is shifting toward an elderly population due to falls and the wider use of anticoagulation. Worldwide, falls were the leading cause of TBI in the GBD 2019 study,[6] followed by pedestrian road injuries, motor vehicle road injuries, and conflict and terrorism. The proportion of TBI caused by motor vehicle road injuries is lower in higher-income countries, likely a result of enforcement of traffic regulations. In the United States, people over the age of 75 years have the highest rate of hospitalization and death related to TBI, accounting for 32% of all TBI-related hospitalizations and 28% of TBI-related deaths.[7] Men are twice as likely to be hospitalized and three times as likely to die as women following TBI.[7] In addition to falls, intentional injuries (homicide and suicide) rose as a cause of TBI-related deaths in the United States between 2007 and 2017, surpassing motor vehicle injuries.[8] This shift was driven in part by a 32% increase in firearm-related suicides among non-Hispanic White patients. Risk factors for TBI include lower socioeconomic status, the use of alcohol and drugs, and the presence of neurologic and neuropsychiatric disorders.[9] In adolescents, sports-related injuries account for a substantial proportion of TBI.[10]

It is estimated that between 70% and 90% of hospital admissions for TBI fall into the category of mild TBI (GCS 13 to 15). The definition of mild TBI has evolved over time. A recent World Health Organization (WHO) Task Force included confusion and disorientation in the diagnostic criteria, instead of altered mental status. Additional criteria include the presence of focal signs, seizure, and an intracranial lesion that does not require any surgical intervention. The WHO definition allows for the GCS to be estimated at later time points, beyond 30 minutes. Overall, mild TBI continues to be a problem with varying diagnostic elements and definitions. An emerging body of evidence suggests that neuropsychological evaluation and targeted interventions may promote recovery from mild TBI.[11]

PATHOPHYSIOLOGY OF TBI

The pathophysiology of brain injury includes primary and secondary injuries. Primary brain injury occurs at the time of impact and primarily involves disruption of the brain parenchyma and blood vessels. Secondary injury occurs as a result of hypotension, hypoxemia, intracranial pressure (ICP) elevation, and biochemical factors that worsen the primary structural damage. The management of TBI is focused on mitigation of secondary insults to improve long-term outcomes. The identification, prevention, and treatment of secondary injury is therefore the mainstay of TBI care in the ICU.

Primary Brain Injury

The International Interagency Initiative toward common data elements for research in TBI has identified six categories of external force that may result in TBI[1]:

- The head being struck by an object
- The head striking an object
- Acceleration/deceleration of the brain without direct external impact
- A foreign body penetrating the brain
- The force from a blast/explosion
- Other forces yet to be defined

Movement of the brain within the skull will result in impact with the inner table. "Coup" injuries occur adjacent to the site of impact, while "contrecoup" injuries occur as a result of the impact on the opposite side of the brain against the skull. As an example, direct frontal impact has the potential to produce frontal lobe injuries whereas a contrecoup injury may occur in the occipital lobe. Rapid acceleration and deceleration injuries are typically sustained in a high-speed motor vehicular accident or fall from a height. Penetrating bullet wounds with cavitation effects on the brain parenchyma are particularly devastating. Bullet wounds that are bihemispheric are associated with significant mortality and early herniation. Injury from explosions primarily occurs because of blast waves.[12] These waves have the potential to cause devastating injury, while the presence of a helmet does not adequately protect the brain from acoustic injuries. Through these varied mechanisms, external energy transfer results in serious injuries to brain parenchyma, vascular injury, and disruption of the blood–brain barrier. Diffuse axonal injury (DAI) is a specific form of injury from rotational forces inside the cranium causing disruption of white matter.[13] Magnetic resonance imaging (MRI) is more sensitive than CT for the detection of DAI.[14] Rotational and torsion injuries, particularly in the brain stem, may result in profound neurologic dysfunction.

Traumatic intracranial hemorrhages are another form of primary brain injury. These may include cerebral contusions and extra-axial hematomas. Subdural or epidural hemorrhage can result in direct mass effect on the brain, while traumatic SAH can be indicative of damaged parenchyma.

Secondary Brain Injury

Secondary brain insults, which may otherwise be well tolerated can exacerbate neuronal injury in cells made vulnerable by the initial TBI. The cellular processes involved with secondary injury to the brain are complex and include mitochondrial dysfunction, neuronal apoptosis, and secondary ischemic
2 insults. Remediable causes of secondary injury[15] include hypotension and hypoxemia which decrease substrate delivery of oxygen and glucose to injured brain; fever and seizures which may further increase metabolic demand; increased ICP resulting in ischemic injury; and hyperglycemia causing immune modulation.[16]

Hypotension

Systemic hypotension has long been recognized as a potential source of secondary brain injury and predictor of poor long-term outcome following TBI. In a meta-analysis, hypotension (systolic blood pressure [BP] <90 mm Hg) was present in 30% of patients,[17] and was an independent predictors of poor outcome (odds ratio, OR 2.67). In a more recent study, a mean arterial pressure (MAP) of less than 65 mm Hg at presentation was associated with a fourfold increase in mortality.[18] A single episode of hypotension predicts adverse outcomes following severe TBI. Episodes of hypotension can be particularly devastating in patients with severe TBI and elevated ICP, as a result of a fall in cerebral perfusion pressure (CPP), discussed in the next section. Appropriate resuscitation, with maintenance of MAP over 65 mm Hg is therefore critical following TBI.

Hypoxemia

Neurons are particularly sensitive to hypoxemia. In a meta-analysis, a PaO_2 <60 mm Hg was present in about 50% of TBI patients and was an independent predictor of poor outcome (OR 2.14).[17] Multisystem trauma patients are prone to hypoxemia from aspiration-induced lung injury, lung contusions, and rib fractures with associated atelectasis. Additionally, therapeutic measures such as crystalloid resuscitation and blood product transfusion (particularly administration of fresh frozen plasma [FFP]) have all been linked to respiratory failure and ARDS. Patients with severe TBI are typically unable to protect their airway and require endotracheal intubation. Oxygen saturation <90% is an independent risk factor for mortality.[19]

Intracranial Hypertension and Cerebral Autoregulation

The Monroe–Kellie doctrine states that total volume remains constant within the skull, which is rigid and nonexpansile. The contents of the cranial cavity include the brain, the vasculature, and the CSF. Therefore, expansion of injured brain tissue volume occurs at the cost of reduction in other components, which typically involve compression of the venous reservoir and the CSF. However, once a threshold of displacement of the venous system and CSF is reached, the ICP begins to increase.

The CPP is the difference between MAP and the ICP. Precapillary arterioles have the regulatory ability to undergo vasoconstriction and dilatation. This response is mainly controlled by MAP. Through autoregulation, the cerebral vasculature maintains an adequate cerebral blood flow (CBF) across a wide range (50 to 150 mm Hg) of MAP (**Fig. 20.1**). There appears to be a direct correlation between the degree of brain injury and loss of autoregulation. Cerebral autoregulation is disrupted in approximately one-third of patients with severe TBI.[20,21] In these patients, a rise in MAP can lead to elevated ICP due to increased CBF and blood volume, while a decrease in MAP may result in hypoperfusion and ischemia. A goal CPP of 60 to 70 mm Hg is recommended for all patients with moderate and severe TBI. However, ICP elevation should be treated first to achieve CPP goals, prior to the institution of vasopressors to elevate the MAP.

Severely elevated ICP may lead to cerebral herniation. Herniation occurs across compartments with incomplete barriers. Global ICP elevation leads to downward movement of the cerebral neuraxis, with axial (transtentorial) herniation. Progressive brainstem compression will result in loss of consciousness, respiratory arrest, and death. Hemispheric lesions, particularly with involvement of the temporal lobe, may result in herniation of the uncus and compression of the midbrain. Predominantly unilateral hemispheric injury can result in herniation of the cingulate gyrus under the cerebral falx. Tonsillar herniation involves displacement of a part of the cerebellum through the foramen magnum. Cerebral herniation may result in ischemic injury through compromise of the CPP, as well as direct arterial compression. Transtentorial herniation may result in infarction through direct compression of the bilateral posterior cerebral arteries, while cingulate herniation may result in compression of the anterior cerebral arteries.

Hyperglycemia and Hypoglycemia

Intensive insulin therapy targeting a blood glucose of 80 to 110 mg/dL is no longer routinely used, as the benefits of tight

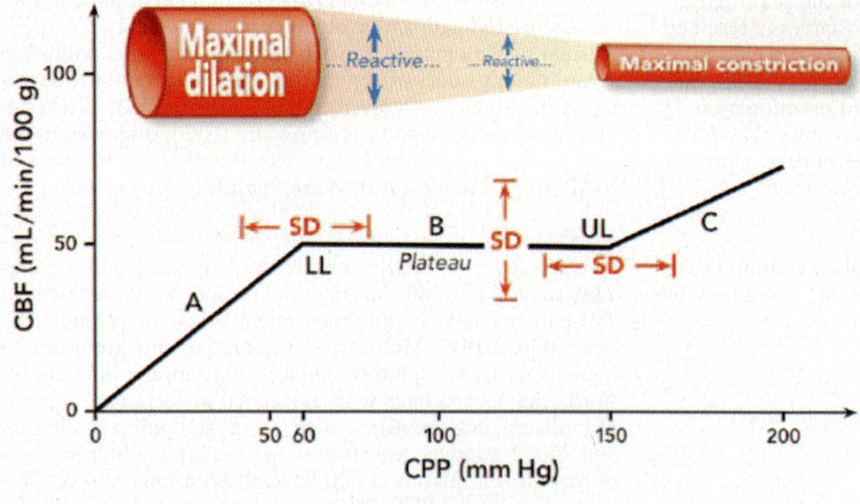

Figure 20.1. Cerebral autoregulation depicted in a graph with cerebral blood flow (CBF) in y-axis and cerebral perfusion pressure (CPP) in x-axis. Typically, the autoregulation is maintained at CPP of 50 to 150 mm Hg. Cerebral vascular reactivity is additionally illustrated. (Adapted from Meng L, Gelb AW. Regulation of cerebral autoregulation by carbon dioxide. *Anesthesiology.* 2015;122:196–205.)

glycemic control are offset by a higher incidence of hypoglycemia. Hypoglycemia can be particularly ominous in comatose TBI patients as the symptoms may not be easily recognized. Both hyper- and hypoglycemia are associated with worsened outcomes in severe TBI.[22,23] Hyperglycemia may lead to aggravation of secondary brain injury through mechanisms such as free-radical generation and alteration of the blood–brain barrier.

Coagulopathy

It is estimated that coagulopathy is present in about one-third of patients with severe TBI. The presence of coagulopathy, either from the primary neurologic injury or from blood loss and multivisceral trauma, is associated with worsening of neurologic outcomes and death.[24,25] Patients with TBI on anticoagulant or antiplatelet therapy are at high risk for expansion of intracranial hemorrhage.

Other factors with the potential to worsen brain injury include the use of hypotonic intravenous fluid that worsens cerebral edema, and elevated intrathoracic or intra-abdominal pressure that compromises cerebral venous return. Fever and seizure activity that increases cerebral metabolic demand may compromise the adequacy of cerebral oxygen delivery.

Molecular and Cellular Mechanisms in TBI

The complexity of the brain and the heterogeneous nature of TBI make it harder to characterize the precise biochemical and cellular changes following brain injury. Neuroinflammation and neurodegeneration may contribute significantly to neurologic disability following TBI. While the acute traumatic event involves tissue and vascular disruption, TBI is characterized by abundant activation of glial cells, generation of inflammatory cytokines, and neutrophil recruitment. The microglia are the primary resident immune cells in the brain. Additional changes that have been documented in the acute phase include alteration of calcium channels and sensors, apoptotic cell death, and generation of reactive oxygen species, further increasing injury and inflammation. Disruption of the blood–brain barrier leads to protein deposition in the extravascular space, a process that can continue for prolonged periods of time. Persistent and chronic changes associated with microglial inflammation and posttraumatic neurodegeneration contribute to long-term disability. Modulation of these molecular and cellular pathways has yet to translate into meaningful clinical therapeutic interventions.

CLINICAL ASSESSMENT

Assessment of a TBI patient in the emergency department should follow the guidelines and principles of advanced trauma life support (ATLS). Evaluation and management are therefore focused on airway, breathing, and circulation, prior to disability.

The identification and treatment of associated injuries in a multisystem trauma patient cannot be overemphasized. Injuries that cause hypotension and hypoxia in patients with TBI have to be emergently addressed and additional secondary brain insults mitigated.

RADIOLOGIC ASSESSMENT

A noncontrast CT is the preferred imaging modality in any trauma patient with suspected TBI. This test should be completed as soon as possible in accordance with ATLS protocols. Noncontrast CT will detect skull fractures, intracranial hematomas, and presence of cerebral edema. In addition to a GCS of ≤14, a complete list of indications for CT and other radiologic imaging in patients with mild TBI is outlined in **Table 20.4**.

A follow-up CT scan should be performed immediately in patients who suffer clinical deterioration. Repeat imaging in 6 hours should also be considered in patients with an intracranial hematoma with a propensity to expand, including patients on anticoagulation or antiplatelet therapy. Additional CT scans may also be indicated in patients with a GCS <9,[26] particularly in patients where an awake examination cannot be safely performed. Evolution of CT findings is common and can change the treatment strategy in a significant proportion of patients. In the absence of clinical deterioration, contrast extravasation within the brain parenchyma may predict a higher risk of

Table 20.4. Indications for Obtaining CT Scan in Mild TBI

High Risk for Neurosurgical Intervention
GCS less than 15 at 2 h after injury
Suspected open or depressed skull fracture
Any sign of basilar skull fracture (raccoon eyes, CSF otorrhea or rhinorrhea, hemotympanum)
Vomiting (more than 2 episodes)
Age more than 65 y
Use of anticoagulants
Moderate Risk of Brain Injury on CT
Loss of consciousness (LOC) for more than 5 min
Amnesia before impact (more than 30 min)
Dangerous mechanism (pedestrian vs. motor vehicle, fall more than 3 ft or 5 stairs)

From Steill IG, Wells GA, Vandemheen K, et al. Canadian CT head rule for minor head injury. *Lancet.* 2001;357(9266):1391–1396.

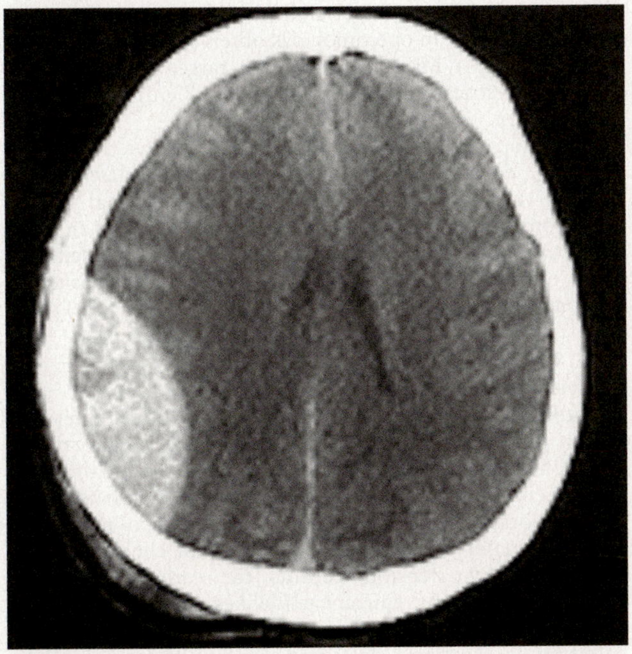

Figure 20.2. CT showing acute posttraumatic epidural hematoma.

hemorrhage progression.[27] In patients with normal neurologic exam, and no additional risk factors for progression of the brain lesion, there is no reason to obtain a "routine" repeat CT scan. Recently developed Brain Injury Guideline (BIG) can be a useful tool to identify patients who require repeat CT scans and/or neurosurgical consultation.[28]

Findings on CT imaging that raise concern for neurologic deterioration and cerebral herniation include cisternal compression and a midline shift of >5 mm. Widespread sulcal effacement may also indicate the presence of diffuse cerebral edema, and possible ICP elevation. Epidural hematomas are typically in the temporoparietal region and do not cross suture lines. They are lenticular in shape, with mixed or high density depending on the time of presentation (**Fig. 20.2**). Subdural hematomas (SDHs) are crescentic lesions that cross suture lines over the cerebral convexity,

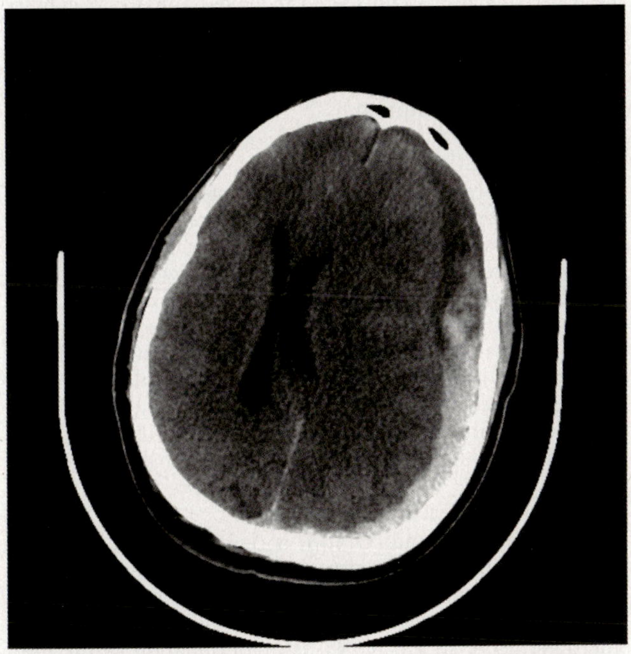

Figure 20.3. CT showing acute left subdural hematoma with severe midline shift.

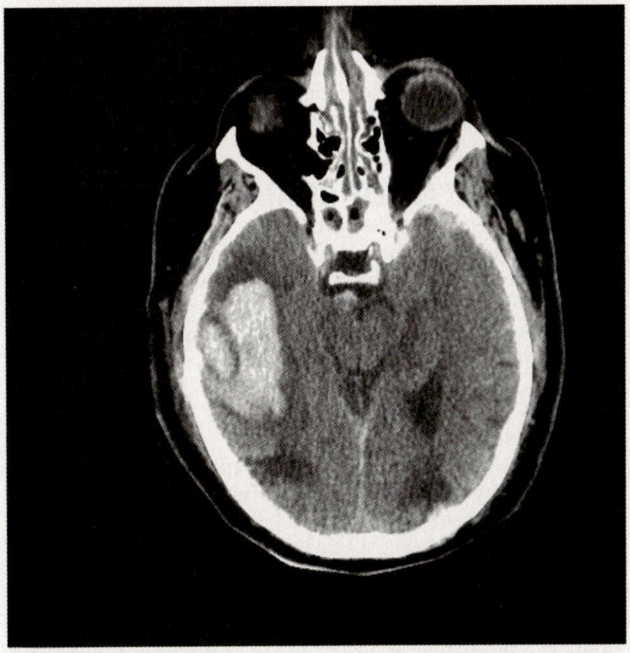

Figure 20.4. CT showing large right temporal contusion.

and typically occur as a result of disruption of the bridging cortical veins (**Fig. 20.3**). Underlying brain injury, with cerebral edema, seizures, and elevated ICP, is more likely to be present in association with subdural than epidural hematomas. The underlying brain injury, rather than the hematoma itself, is the primary determinant of long-term neurologic outcome. Intraparenchymal hematomas are common following trauma and present as high- or mixed-density lesions on CT (**Fig. 20.4**). Their distribution is related to the site of impact on the skull. Intraparenchymal hematomas, also referred to as cerebral contusions, frequently expand ("blossom") in the hours following presentation, necessitating close neurologic observation and repeat imaging.

SAH appears as a thin layer of blood on the surface of the parenchyma (**Fig. 20.5**). The distribution of blood may help differentiate traumatic from aneurysmal SAH.

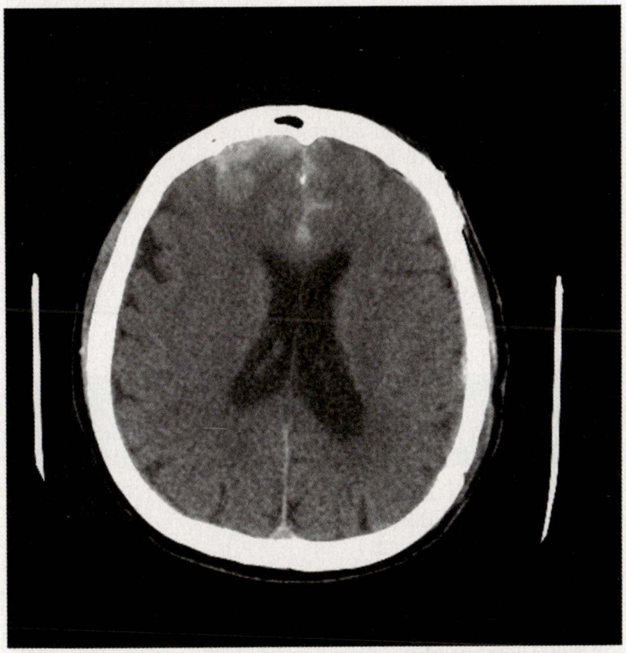

Figure 20.5. CT showing acute bifrontal traumatic subarachnoid hemorrhage.

TRAUMA

3 Other radiologic tools such as MRI and diffusion tensor imaging[29] may be helpful in specific circumstances but are not used routinely in the acute management of TBI. Nuclear medicine cisternography is sometimes indicated to identify and localize CSF leaks following TBI.

MANAGEMENT OF BRAIN INJURIES

Broad Goals of Management

The key principles of management of a trauma patient remain the same, regardless of the specifics of injury. A major goal is to avoid the development of the "lethal triad" of hypothermia, acidosis, and coagulopathy. Additional goals include adequate oxygen delivery, prioritization of injuries, reducing ongoing blood loss, and treatment of hypotension.

Initial Resuscitation

Following stabilization of airway, breathing, and circulation, a clinical assessment with GCS and assessment of the pupillary light response (PLR) needs to be performed. Quantitative pupillometry may detect subtle impairment of the PLR, which often precedes life-threatening ICP elevation and cerebral herniation.[30,31] In addition, manual determination of pupillary nonreactivity may be inaccurate, particularly with small pupils. Pupillary dilation or loss of the PLR without significant changes either in the level of consciousness or other indicators of worsening brain injury should raise the possibility of local ocular injury or oculomotor dysfunction.

4 Endotracheal intubation should be performed for all patients with a GCS <9.[32,33] Other indications for emergent intubation include inability to protect the airway (often in the context of intoxication with drugs or alcohol) and hypoxemic respiratory failure, with inability to maintain SpO_2 >90% despite the use of supplemental oxygen. Patients with TBI and signs of clinical herniation or impending herniation should also undergo emergent endotracheal intubation. Signs of cerebral herniation include pupillary asymmetry, rapid worsening in level of consciousness, decorticate or decerebrate posturing, and the Cushing reflex of hypertension with bradycardia.[34]

The initial resuscitation fluid of choice in patients with TBI is an isotonic crystalloid solution such as normal saline. The SMART ICU clinical trial demonstrated a reduction in mortality overall with the use of balanced IV fluid such as lactate Ringer or Plasmalyte A for resuscitation in critically ill patients, compared to normal saline.[35] However, no benefit was seen with the use of balanced fluids in the subgroup of patients with TBI. Electrolyte imbalances are common in patients with TBI and should be regularly assessed and corrected.

Trauma patients with active bleeding should preferentially receive transfusion of blood products rather than crystalloid. A 1:1:1 ratio of packed red blood cells (pRBCs), FFP, and platelets, or transfusion of whole blood, is preferred.[36,37] Most trauma centers follow the principles outlined in damage control resuscitation (**Table 20.5**). The appropriate threshold for blood transfusion in TBI patients without active bleeding is unclear. In the HEMOTION clinical trial, no statistically significant difference in outcomes was observed between patients managed with a liberal (hemoglobin target >10g/dL) compared to a restrictive (hemoglobin target >7 g/dL) transfusion strategy.[38]

Table 20.5. Principles of Damage Control or Hemostatic Resuscitation

Damage Control or Hemostatic Resuscitation
- Prioritize hemorrhage control
- Permissive hypotension
- Avoid crystalloids
- Early component therapy (protocol driven)
- Adjuncts:
  - Correct hypothermia, acidosis, hypocalcemia
  - Antifibrinolytics

Coagulopathy in patients who require massive transfusion should be identified and characterized with viscoelastic assays such as thromboelastography (TEG) or rotational thromboelastometry (ROTEM) where available, rather than standard coagulation assays.[39] Of note, the value of resuscitation based on viscoelastic assays has not yet been established in randomized clinical trials.

Neuromonitoring

ICP Monitoring

5 Elevated ICP is a predictor of subsequent neurologic deterioration in patients with severe TBI.[40] The primary rationale for ICP monitoring is therefore, to detect potentially life threatening, but clinically occult, intracranial hypertension before clinical deterioration, cerebral herniation, and death, or permanent neurologic injury occurs. Early detection of clinically occult intracranial hypertension permits the early initiation of ICP-targeted therapy. Current guidelines recommend the use of invasive ICP monitoring in all patients with severe TBI, based on observational data that suggest reduction in short-term mortality with the use of ICP-targeted management.[41]

6 An external ventricular drain (EVD) connected to a transducer is considered the gold standard, and a cost-effective method of ICP monitoring. Additionally, an EVD can be used to treat elevated ICP with appropriate drainage of CSF. The presence of midline shift and compressed ventricles (slit ventricles) may increase the technical difficulty of EVD placement. Intraparenchymal monitor placement is technically easier to
7 perform, with a lower risk of hemorrhage and infection.[42] An ICP goal ≤22 mm Hg is recommended as values above this level are associated with increased mortality and unfavorable neurologic outcomes.[41]

While the use of ICP monitoring has been considered the standard of care during management of severe TBI, a randomized clinical trial (BEST TRIP) demonstrated equivalent long-term neurologic outcomes with the use of invasive ICP measurement compared to serial clinical and radiologic assessment.[43] The study was conducted in a limited-resource environment, with multiple differences in treatments used between the trial arms and is considered to have limited applicability to clinical settings in high-income nations where invasive ICP monitoring is routinely used. Observational studies[44,45] have demonstrated a reduction in in-hospital mortality with the use of invasive ICP monitoring.

Pressure Reactivity Index

Cerebral autoregulation is an important mechanism to preserve tissue perfusion in patients with severe TBI and increased ICP. The pressure reactivity index (PRx), which is the continuously monitored correlation coefficient between mean MAP and ICP, may be used to quantify cerebral autoregulation. A direct correlation of ICP with MAP (PRx value = 1) suggests a complete loss of autoregulation, while a negative correlation or PRx of zero suggests preservation of autoregulation. A PRx <0.05 predicted favorable outcome in one study.[46] Measurement of pressure reactivity may also help identify the optimal CPP in individual patients.[47]

Noninvasive ICP Monitoring

Optic nerve ultrasound (ONUS) is one of the best-evaluated noninvasive tools for the detection of intracranial hypertension and is already in clinical use in several emergency departments and in settings where ICP monitoring is unavailable.[48–51] The optic nerve sheath (ONS) is a continuation of the dura and contains the subarachnoid space. An increase in ICP is transmitted through the subarachnoid space and results in distension of the retrobulbar ONS.[48–51] The optic nerve sheath diameter (ONSD) can be measured posterior to the globe using point-of-care ultrasound, and a threshold ONSD used to identify the presence of elevated ICP. Several studies have reported high accuracy of ONSD for the detection of elevated ICP.[48–51] However, the ONSD threshold to identify elevated ICP has varied greatly between studies.[52] The use of ONUS to assess ICP is considered investigational and cannot be recommended for routine use. Transcranial Doppler has also been evaluated for noninvasive ICP assessment, with mixed results.[53,54]

Role of Cerebral Oximetry and Microdialysis

Tissue oximetry has been investigated as a marker of tissue perfusion in many different vascular beds. Notable examples include sublingual, gastric, and cutaneous circulations. Measurement of brain tissue oxygen tension ($PbtO_2$) by placement of an oxygen electrode into the white matter helps assess the adequacy of cerebral oxygen delivery. While $PbtO_2$ values >20 mm Hg are considered normal, persistent levels below 10 to 15 mm Hg are associated with worsened outcome.[33] A phase-2 randomized clinical trial (BOOST-2) concluded that ICP and brain tissue oxygenation monitoring with the use of specific protocols reduced brain tissue hypoxia compared to the use of ICP monitoring alone.[55] A more definitive phase 3 trial (BOOST-3) is underway.

Cerebral microdialysis uses an intraparenchymal probe to measure solute concentration in the brain. The products of anaerobic (lactate) and aerobic oxidative phosphorylation (glucose, pyruvate, etc.) are measured, and the lactate: pyruvate ratio used as a surrogate of cellular distress.[56,57] The use of cerebral microdialysis to improve outcomes following TBI has not been validated in clinical trials.

Medical Management of ICP Elevation

Basic principles of medical management of elevated ICP include elevation of the head of bed, with the head in the neutral position to avoid compression of the jugular veins and compromise of venous return. Intra-abdominal hypertension should be recognized and managed appropriately, to maximize cerebral venous return.

Sedation and Analgesia

Effective analgesia is a critical first step in the management of intubated mechanically ventilated TBI patients. The empiric use of an opioid infusion is typically necessary, since comatose patients with severe TBI are unable to report the presence or severity of pain. Fentanyl is often the analgesic of choice because of a short half-life and better hemodynamic profile compared with morphine and hydromorphone. Effective sedation lowers the ICP by lowering metabolic demand, thereby decreasing CBF and volume.[57] Propofol is the preferred agent for sedation in view of its very short half-life, which facilitates rapid neurologic assessment on discontinuation, and efficacy in decreasing ICP through a reduction in metabolic demand.[58] Bradycardia and hypotension are common with propofol, necessitating a vasopressor infusion to maintain the CPP. For patients with severe TBI with appropriate control of ICP, a Richmond Agitation–Sedation Scale (RASS) target of 0 to −2, representing light sedation, is preferred.[57] Deep sedation, with a RASS goal of −4 to −5, may be required when ICP is difficult to control. The routine use of neuromuscular blocking agents for the control of ICP is not recommended because of side effects such as critical illness polymyopathy and neuropathy.

Cerebrospinal Fluid Drainage

Drainage of CSF in patients with an EVD is often the first intervention for lowering ICP. Guidelines recommend continuous over intermittent CSF drainage for better control of ICP.[33] However, caution is necessary to avoid excessive drainage, which may lead to ventricular collapse and occlusion of the catheter, particularly with slit ventricles.

Osmotic Therapy

Hyperosmolar agents decrease cerebral edema through diffusion of water along an osmolar gradient from brain into the vascular space. Hyperosmolar therapy is typically a first- or second-line therapy in ICP management in conjunction with sedation, analgesia, and CSF drainage. The most common agents used are hypertonic saline and mannitol. Hypertonic saline is available in a wide variety of concentrations, ranging from 1.8% to 23.4% NaCl, and is effective for the control of elevated ICP.[59,60] While bolus doses of 23.4% NaCl are frequently used for acute life-threatening ICP elevation, 3% NaCl is typically used as a continuous infusion in the ICU, titrated to an initial sodium goal of approximately 145 to 155 mEq/L to maintain control of ICP. Although hypertonic saline can be used for limited periods of time through peripheral venous access, central venous delivery is preferred because of concern for tissue injury from extravasation. Mannitol is also effective for ICP control, the dose is 0.25 to 1 g/kg administered every 4 to 6 hours as necessary for elevation in ICP. Mannitol is, in addition, a free-radical scavenger. Hypertonic saline is preferred over mannitol, particularly when there is concern for active bleeding, since mannitol may cause hypovolemia and hypotension.[59] Meta-analyses also suggest superior ICP control with hypertonic saline compared to mannitol.[61] Side effects of hypertonic saline include circulatory overload, pulmonary edema, hyperchloremia, and nonanion gap metabolic acidosis.

Seizure Prophylaxis

Seizure prophylaxis is recommended for all patients with severe TBI. The incidence of seizures following TBI ranges from approximately 15% to 30%[62] in the first 2 weeks following injury. The use of antiseizure prophylaxis decreases the incidence of early seizures, but does not improve long-term outcomes or decrease the incidence of long-term epilepsy.[63] In the early period following TBI, seizures may worsen secondary brain injury by increasing cerebral metabolic demand, CBF, and ICP. Up to a quarter of all patients with TBI may suffer nonconvulsive seizure activity, identified on continuous EEG monitoring.[62,64] While phenytoin was previously the preferred agent for prophylaxis, levetiracetam at a dose of 1 g twice daily is now widely used for antiseizure prophylaxis instead, because of concerns with worsened long-term cognitive and functional outcomes with the use of phenytoin in other disease states. In a small randomized clinical trial, levetiracetam and phenytoin achieved equivalent seizure prevention, but the use of levetiracetam was associated with improved 6-month functional outcome.[65]

Role of Tranexamic Acid

Over the last decade, there has been increased attention to the role of pathologic fibrinolysis following trauma in ongoing bleeding, coagulopathy, and increased mortality. Tranexamic acid (TXA) has been validated in clinical trials to decrease mortality in the setting of traumatic hemorrhage. The CRASH-3 trial was a large international multicenter clinical trial that evaluated the administration of TXA within 3 hours of TBI. The use of TXA reduced the risk of head injury–related death with moderate (RR 0.78 [95% CI 0.64–0.95]) but not severe (0.99 [95% CI 0.91–1.07]) head injury.[66] TXA should therefore be administered to patients with moderate TBI within 3 hours of injury, as a 1-g IV infusion over 10 to 15 minutes followed by a gram administered every 8 hours for the first 24 hours in these patients.

Early Enteral Nutrition

Early enteral nutrition either through a nasogastric tube or postpyloric silastic tube is recommended for all patients with TBI. Although earlier studies suggested a reduction in pneumonia and mortality with early enteral nutrition,[67] a subsequent randomized clinical trial did not confirm these benefits.[68]

Others

Trauma including TBI is identified as a unique high-risk factor for the development of thromboembolism. We typically initiate early thromboprophylaxis with enoxaparin 40 mg daily after follow-up CT imaging confirms stability in the extent of intracranial hemorrhage.[69]

Fever increases cerebral metabolism, CBF, and ICP.[70] Therefore, fever control is required, with the use of antipyretics, as well as external and intravascular cooling devices. Patients with severe TBI also commonly exhibit signs of paroxysmal sympathetic hyperactivity (PSH), a sign of central autonomic dysfunction. As the name suggests, PSH is episodic, and presents as paroxysms of hypertension, tachycardia, rigidity, posturing, fever, and diaphoresis. First-line management of PSH includes abortive therapy with benzodiazepines and opioids, as well as treatment to decrease the frequency, intensity, and duration of episodes. Commonly used agents include nonselective beta blockers such as propranolol, and alpha-2 agonists such as clonidine. Dopamine agonists such as bromocriptine and antiseizure medications such as gabapentin are also widely used. Symptomatic treatment includes management of fever with antipyretic agents such as acetaminophen, and treatment for rigidity with muscle relaxants such as baclofen.

Therapeutic Intensity Level and Management Parameters to Control ICP

The therapeutic intensity level (TIL) is a standardized tool to assess the intensity of ICP-targeted treatments following TBI.[2] The basic scale is outlined in **Table 20.6**. Subsequent study has validated the TIL scoring system of ICP management in the ICU at 4- and 24-hour time points.

Management of Impending Cerebral Herniation

Patients admitted with severe TBI should undergo serial neurologic assessments at least every 2 hours in the initial period following admission. Neurologic signs of herniation include sudden worsening in the GCS, new-onset fixed and dilated pupils, decorticate or decerebrate posturing, and hypertension with bradycardia. Treatment measures for cerebral herniation are listed in **Table 20.7**. These interventions include endotracheal intubation, brief hyperventilation,[71] and high-dose osmotherapy.[72,73] Typical doses include 23.4% NaCl at 30 to 60 mL over 10 minutes, and mannitol 1 g/kg. Urgent repeat CT imaging is typically required to evaluate the need for surgical intervention.

Table 20.6. Basic Scale for Therapeutic Intensity Level (TIL)

TIL 0—No Specific ICP-DIRECTED THERAPY
TIL 1—Basic ICU Care ▪ Sedation for ventilator/endotracheal tube tolerance ▪ Volume/vasopressors for non-CNS cause (eg, sepsis, myocardial injury) ▪ Head-up positioning (ventilator bundle) ▪ Normocapnia ($PaCO_2$ ≥40 mm Hg)
TIL 2—Mild ▪ Higher levels of sedation ▪ Vasopressors/volume for CPP support ▪ Low-dose osmotic therapy ▪ Mild hypocapnia ($PaCO_2$ 4.6–5.3 kPa; 35–40 mm Hg) ▪ CSF drainage <120 mL/d (<5 mL/h)
TIL 3—Moderate ▪ Higher doses of osmotic therapy ▪ Moderate hypocapnia ($PaCO_2$ 4.0–4.5 kPa; 30–35 mm Hg) ▪ Mild hypothermia (>35 °C) ▪ CSF drainage ≥120 mL/d (>5 mL/h)
TIL 4—Extreme ▪ Profound hypocapnia ($PaCO_2$ <4.0 kPa; <30 mm Hg) ▪ Hypothermia <35 °C ▪ Metabolic suppression for control of ICP ▪ Surgery for refractory ICP (decompression, lobectomy)

Table 20.7. Immediate Management of Impending Cerebral Herniation

Endotracheal intubation, if not already performed
Elevation of the head of bed (HOB) to 30–45 with the head in neutral position to promote venous drainage
Brief hyperventilation to a pCO_2 of approximately 30 mm Hg[73]
Osmotherapy with either mannitol 1–1.5 g/kg[75] or 23.4% hypertonic saline 30–60 mL over 10 min[76]
Higher mean arterial pressure (MAP), to approximately 80–100 mm Hg, to maintain an adequate cerebral perfusion pressure (CPP) with fluids ± vasopressors
Definitive surgical interventions when indicated

SURGICAL APPROACH

Skull Fracture

Skull fractures are variable in both their presentation and management. Closed linear convexity skull fractures without significant displacement can typically be managed conservatively without any specific restrictions or precautions. Conversely, open fractures with significant depression causing mass effect upon the brain parenchyma typically require washout and elevation of bony fragments. Skull base fractures require special care and evaluation. Clinically, skull base fractures may present with CSF rhinorrhea or otorrhea, raccoon eyes (bruising around the orbit), or Battle sign (bruising behind the ears). On imaging, fluid within the mastoid air cells or sphenoid sinus should raise concern for a skull base fracture. Pneumocephalus can also help identify fractures. Due to their proximity to the intracranial circulation, skull base fractures pose a risk for cerebrovascular injury such as dissection or pseudoaneurysm formation (Fig. 20.6). Fracture lines that are in close approximation to structures such as the carotid canal warrant further imaging with CT angiography. Skull base fractures also pose a risk for CSF leak, particularly with fractures in the frontal sinus, cribriform plate, or ethmoid/sphenoid sinuses. Surgical repair may be indicated in these cases. Surgical treatment entails cranialization of the frontal sinus (removal of the posterior wall of the frontal sinus), stripping of the mucosa in the sinus, and pericranial flap placement along the anterior skull base. Abdominal fat may be harvested to pack the sinuses. In certain cases, endoscopic endonasal approaches may be appropriate rather than open craniotomy.

Epidural Hematoma

Epidural hematomas are typically thought to arise from laceration of intracranial arteries by skull fractures, causing arterial bleeding between the dura and skull. In many cases, a skull fracture in the pterion results in laceration of the middle meningeal artery (MMA). Smaller epidural hematomas, particularly in other locations, can be due to dural lacerations and skull fractures. Hematomas that cross the midline may involve injury to the dural venous sinuses. Given the high pressure and high flow through the arteries such as the MMA, epidural hematomas can rapidly expand, leading to sudden coma and death. Classically, a "lucid interval" is described, where a patient is initially neurologically intact, with subsequent rapid deterioration. Emergent surgical decompression is warranted for evacuation. A temporal craniotomy is usually sufficient to evacuate the hematoma and coagulate the torn MMA. If performed prior to a herniation syndrome, patient outcomes can be excellent.[74]

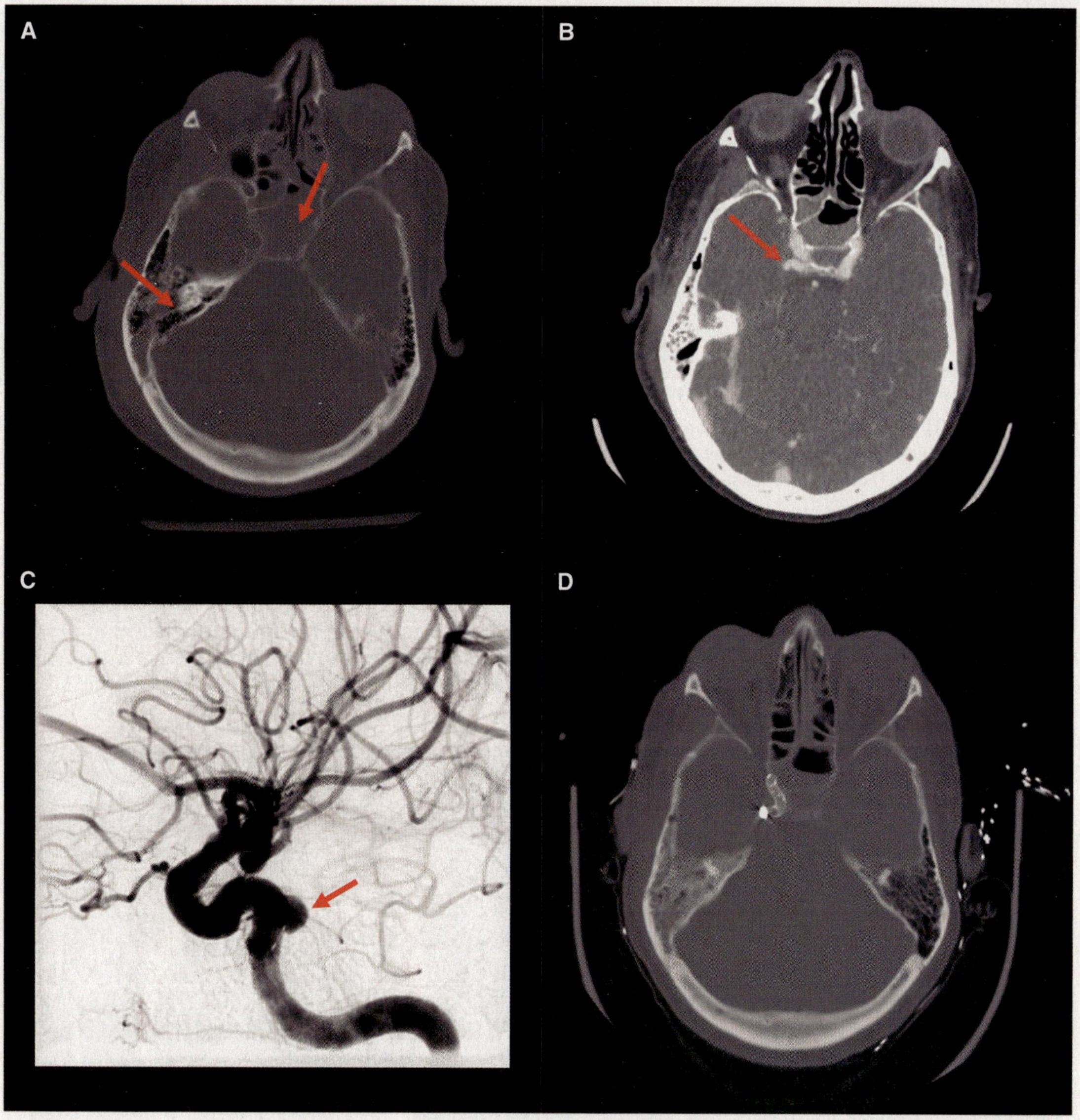

Figure 20.6. **A:** Initial CT showing fluid in the right mastoid air cells and sphenoid sinus (*red arrows*), raising suspicion for skull base fracture. **B:** CT angiography and (**C**) digital subtraction angiography showing a pseudoaneurysm (*red arrows*) of the right cavernous internal carotid artery. **D:** Stent-coil embolization of the pseudoaneurysm.

Subdural Hematoma

SDHs can present acutely after severe trauma or in a subacute fashion from minor trauma or even in the absence of a history of trauma. In acute severe TBI, an SDH causing significant midline shift (>5 mm) and neurologic deficits may warrant an emergent surgical evacuation. In certain circumstances, ICP monitoring may be pursued in lieu of immediate surgery. Surgery for acute SDH typically involves a large unilateral craniotomy in order to adequately evacuate the gelatinous clot. Burr hole drainage is typically not successful in treatment of acute SDH. In many circumstances with elevated ICP, a craniectomy is pursued in order to ensure that the brain is sufficiently decompressed. A randomized clinical trial to evaluate the use of craniectomy and craniotomy in patients with SDH showed similar outcomes in disability and quality-of-life outcomes.[75] As opposed to acute SDH, chronic or subacute SDH is a disorder of the elderly. As SDHs age, they tend to liquefy. Chronic or subacute SDH causing neurologic symptoms may therefore be evacuated through burr holes or a small craniotomy (**Fig. 20.7**).

Parenchymal Contusions

Parenchymal contusions pose a difficult dilemma for management. They tend to occur in the basal frontal lobes or in the temporal lobes. Contusions typically “blossom” or enlarge over the course of several days. Therefore, contusions rarely require emergent surgery at initial presentation. However, due to their enlargement, coupled with a significant edematous reaction of the surrounding parenchyma, patients tend to deteriorate 2 to 7 days post trauma. Close neurologic monitoring should be carried out during this time, and ICP monitoring may be warranted. Patients with temporal contusions are at particular risk for developing uncal herniation even in the absence of ICP elevations. Conversely, patients with bifrontal contusions may develop global ICP elevations. Decompressive craniectomy (DC) is warranted if medical management is unsuccessful. For bifrontal contusions, a bifrontal craniectomy is typically performed. In the case of temporal contusions, a unilateral craniectomy is performed.

Diffuse Axonal Injury

Diffuse axonal injury (DAI) occurs due to shearing forces from blunt trauma affecting axons throughout the brain. DAI can be difficult to identify on CT but is readily seen on MRI. DAI can also occur concurrently with other traumatic intracranial pathology. DAI is typically a nonsurgical entity and is managed medically with ICP monitoring.

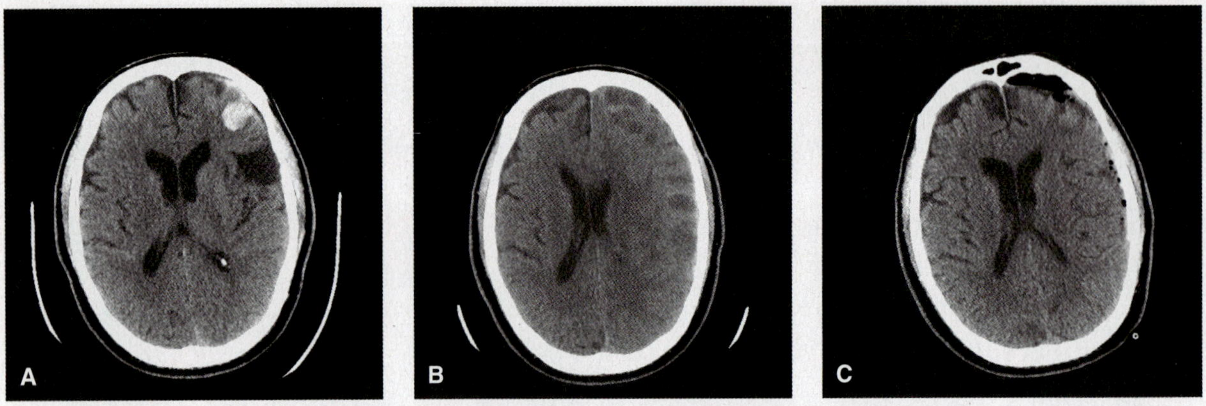

Figure 20.7. **A:** Initial CT showing a left frontal contusion with associated small subarachnoid and subdural hemorrhage. **B:** Follow-up CT at 2 months showing resolution of the contusion, but development of a large loculated subdural hemorrhage causing significant mass effect and midline shift. **C:** Postoperative CT showing evacuation of the hemorrhage with resolution of mass effect.

Penetrating Injuries to the Brain

Gunshot wounds (GSWs) comprise the vast majority of penetrating brain injuries. Most patients with GSWs to the head either die in the field or do not survive initial resuscitation. Physical examination and CT should be used to evaluate the path of the bullet. Bihemispheric injury, and particularly bithalamic injury, portends an extremely grim prognosis. However, if a patient is able to be stabilized hemodynamically and has evidence of brain function, emergent surgical treatment is necessary. Due to the cavitation injury by the bullet, patients develop rapid malignant cerebral edema (**Fig. 20.8**). Therefore, surgery should involve a large DC. Due to the

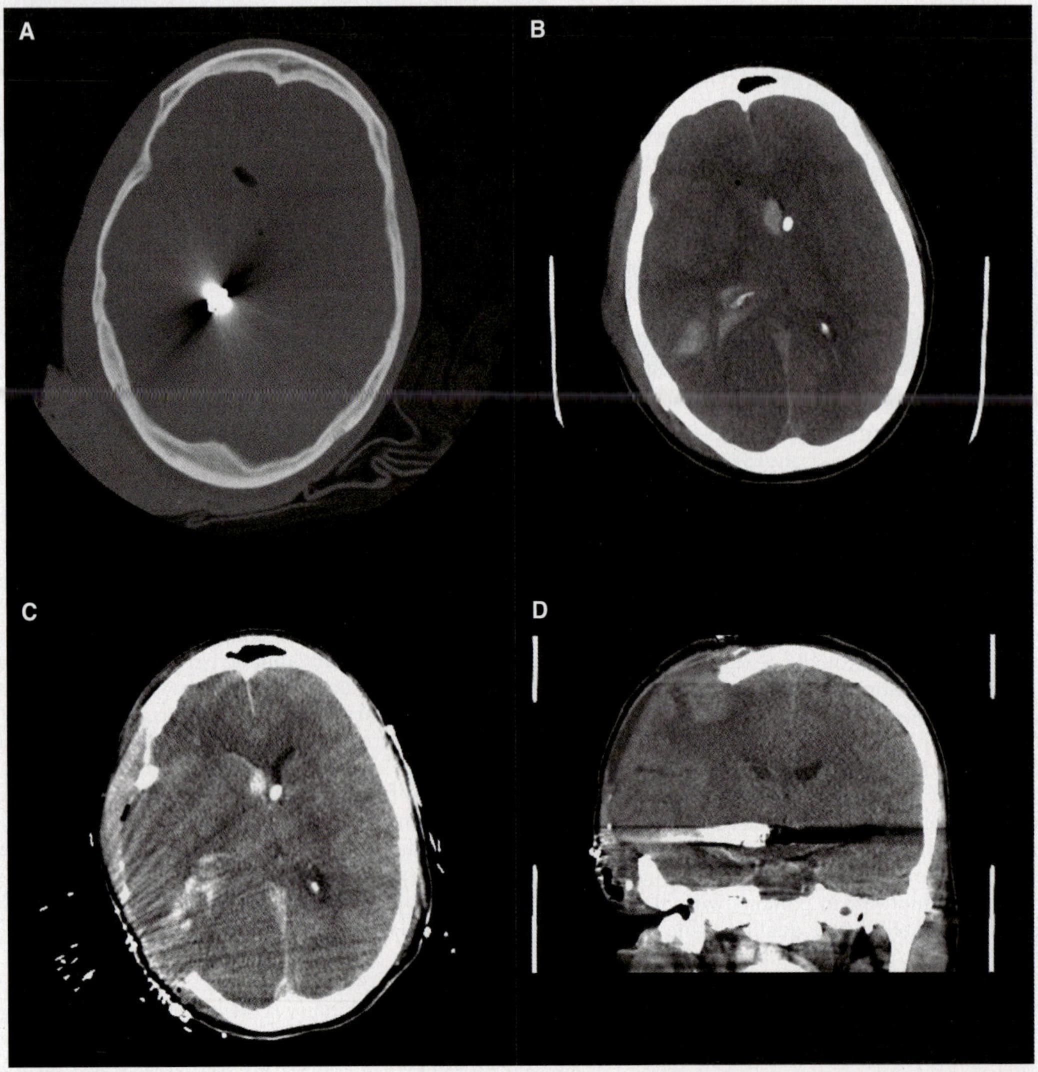

Figure 20.8. **A:** Initial CT showing intracranial bullet fragment. **B:** Development of progressive hemorrhage and mass effect. Ventriculostomy catheter can be seen on the left side. **C, D:** After right decompressive craniectomy, mass effect is relieved and brain parenchyma can be seen herniating through the craniectomy defect.

significant risk of direct blood vessel injury, voluminous blood loss is typical and intraoperative death is a major concern. During decompression, any concomitant hematomas should be evacuated. Similarly, devitalized scalp should be resected, and any air sinuses encountered should be exenterated. Bone and bullet fragments that are deep in the parenchyma should not be retrieved due to the risk of causing further injury.

Non–gunshot-penetrating trauma usually involves low-velocity objects such as knives, arrows, nails, etc. In these cases, preoperative CT angiography is helpful to identify if there is an injury to a major blood vessel. If the object is still embedded when the patient presents, it should not be removed until in surgery. In these cases, a craniectomy is typically necessary with careful extraction of the embedded object. If the object is not embedded, the patient may be managed similar to a closed head injury.

Role of Decompressive Craniectomy

DC continues to be a mainstay in the surgical treatment of severe TBI. The rationale for DC is that it is a rapid, reliable, and sustainable intervention to decrease ICP. It may be performed either immediately at the time of severe TBI (primary DC), or in a delayed fashion if nonsurgical methods for ICP control have failed (secondary DC). Clinical trials and observational studies have established DC as a life-saving intervention following TBI, with a significant proportion of survivors achieving good long-term functional outcome.

There have been two major randomized trials evaluating secondary DC. The DECRA trial was first published in 2011.[76] In this study, 155 patients were randomized to bifrontal craniectomy versus standard of care nonsurgical treatments. The inclusion criteria were patients within 72 hours of injury with diffuse severe TBI who had intracranial hypertension. This was defined as ICP >20 mm Hg for over 15 minutes within a 1-hour time period, despite standard of care medical interventions. Surgical treatment was standardized to be a bifrontal craniectomy. Outcomes were measured with the GOS-E at 6-month follow-up. The results of the trial found that while DC led to improved ICP control, no improvement in mortality was observed, with higher rates of severe disability and vegetative state in the craniectomy arm. DECRA was limited by significant flaws. Patients in the craniectomy arm were more likely to have bilateral nonreactive pupils at the time of enrollment. Only diffuse TBI was included and patients who required hematoma evaluation were excluded. The threshold to perform a large craniectomy was lower than typical for clinical practice. Finally, a large bifrontotemporoparietal craniectomy was used in all patients, which may have been more extensive than required to achieve ICP control in several patients.

RESCUEicp was published in 2016.[77] In this trial, 408 patients were again randomized to DC or standard nonsurgical management. Differing from DECRA, the investigators included any severe TBI with an abnormal CT. ICP for inclusion was >25 mm Hg for 1 to 12 hours despite nonsurgical methods. In addition, patients who underwent craniotomy for mass lesion earlier in their course remained eligible. The surgical approach for decompression was tailored to the nature of injury. Primary outcome was GOS-E at 6 months, while secondary outcomes were assessed at 12 months. The results showed that DC again led to a large improvement in survival. An increase in rates of severe disability and vegetative state were again observed in the craniectomy arm, likely among patients who would otherwise have died with medical management alone. However, at 12 months, surgical patients showed an increased rate of living independently when compared to the medical group. RESCUEicp benefitted from being a more "real-world" situation but was significantly limited by crossover (37.2% of the medical group eventually had a craniectomy), which may have diluted the benefit seen from DC.

Table 20.8. Factors that Determine Prognosis in Patients with TBI

GCS at Presentation (Motor Score—Most Important Prognosticator)
CT—High-grade subarachnoid hemorrhage, cisternal effacement, midline shift
Pupillary function
Age—Older age associated with poor prognosis
Presence of factors that cause secondary brain injury—Hypotension, hypoxemia, and fever
Elevated intracranial pressure (ICP) and reduced cerebral perfusion pressure (CPP)
Associated coagulopathy
Diffuse axonal injury and brain stem injury

PROGNOSIS

Outcome from severe head injury is dependent on a range of factors (**Table 20.8**). No single factor is reliable for the prediction of outcome following TBI, and multimodal evaluation is always necessary.

Clinical prediction models that incorporate known predictors of death and poor long-term functional outcome have been developed. The CRASH prediction model, which incorporates age, country, GCS, pupillary reactivity, the presence of extracranial injury, and CT findings to predict 2-week mortality and 6-month functional outcome, was developed using data from a large international multicenter clinical trial of glucocorticoids in TBI.[74] The IMPACT model, derived from 8509 patients, uses age, GCS, pupillary reactivity, the occurrence of hypoxemia and hypotension, the Marshall CT grade, presence of traumatic SAH, presence of epidural hematoma, and glucose and hemoglobin levels to predict 6-month mortality and functional outcome.[78] These models are best applied to large cohorts, however, and should not be used to guide management decisions in individual patients. Both models have been shown to overestimate poor outcomes in the current era of neurotrauma management.

Mortality following severe TBI is about 30% to 40%, while long-term disability is expected in approximately half of all severe TBI patients. Conversely, half or more will regain independence in activities of daily living.[79] Recovery following severe TBI typically occurs over many months, and may continue beyond 1 year.[80] Approximately 10% to 25% of severe TBI patients will be discharged in a vegetative (unresponsive wakeful) state, the majority of whom will eventually recover responsiveness to the outside environment but remain severely disabled.[81] Psychosocial factors may play an important role in the long-term prognosis of TBI patients.[82] Since patients with severe TBI may recover very slowly,[83] recent guidelines recommend waiting 2 weeks or longer before attempting prognostication.[84] Patients with severely impaired consciousness at 2 to 4 weeks also frequently recover to good long-term outcomes.

References

1. Menon DK, Schwab K, Wright DW, Maas AI, Demographics and Clinical Assessment Working Group of the International and Interagency Initiative toward Common Data Elements for Research on Traumatic Brain Injury and Psychological Health. Position statement: definition of traumatic brain injury. *Arch Phys Med Rehabil.* 2010;91(11):1637–1640.
2. Maas AI, Harrison-Felix CL, Menon D, et al. Standardizing data collection in traumatic brain injury. *J Neurotrauma.* 2011;28(2):177–187.
3. Balestreri M, Czosnyka M, Chatfield DA, et al. Predictive value of Glasgow Coma Scale after brain trauma: change in trend over the past ten years. *J Neurol Neurosurg Psychiatry.* 2004;75(1):161–162.

4. Marshall LF, Chesnut RM. Head injury and shock. *J Neurosurg.* 1993;79(4):637.
5. Maas AI, Hukkelhoven CW, Marshall LF, Steyerberg EW. Prediction of outcome in traumatic brain injury with computed tomographic characteristics: a comparison between the computed tomographic classification and combinations of computed tomographic predictors. *Neurosurgery.* 2005;57(6):1173–1182; discussion 1173–1182.
6. Guan B, Anderson DB, Chen L, Feng S, Zhou H. Global, regional and national burden of traumatic brain injury and spinal cord injury, 1990-2019: a systematic analysis for the Global Burden of Disease Study 2019. *BMJ Open.* 2023;13(10):e075049.
7. CDC. https://www.cdc.gov/traumatic-brain-injury/data-research/index.html.
8. Daugherty J, Waltzman D, Sarmiento K, Xu L. Traumatic brain injury-related deaths by race/ethnicity, sex, intent, and mechanism of injury–United States, 2000–2017. *MMWR Morb Mortal Wkly Rep.* 2019;68(46):1050–1056.
9. Liao CC, Chiu WT, Yeh CC, Chang HC, Chen TL. Risk and outcomes for traumatic brain injury in patients with mental disorders. *J Neurol Neurosurg Psychiatry.* 2012;83(12):1186–1192.
10. Ilie G, Boak A, Adlaf EM, Asbridge M, Cusimano MD. Prevalence and correlates of traumatic brain injuries among adolescents. *JAMA.* 2013;309(24):2550–2552.
11. Prince C, Bruhns ME. Evaluation and treatment of mild traumatic brain injury: the role of neuropsychology. *Brain Sci.* 2017;7(8):105.
12. Bukowski J, Nowadly CD, Schauer SG, Koyfman A, Long B. High risk and low prevalence diseases: blast injuries. *Am J Emerg Med.* 2023;70:46–56.
13. Moen KG, Brezova V, Skandsen T, Haberg AK, Folvik M, Vik A. Traumatic axonal injury: the prognostic value of lesion load in corpus callosum, brain stem, and thalamus in different magnetic resonance imaging sequences. *J Neurotrauma.* 2014;31(17):1486–1496.
14. Moen KG, Skandsen T, Folvik M, et al. A longitudinal MRI study of traumatic axonal injury in patients with moderate and severe traumatic brain injury. *J Neurol Neurosurg Psychiatry.* 2012;83(12):1193–1200.
15. Centers for Disease Control and Prevention. *Surveillance Report of Traumatic Brain Injury-related Emergency Department Visits, Hospitalizations, and Deaths-United States, 2014.* U.S. Department of Health and Human Services; 2019.
16. Chesnut RM, Marshall LF, Klauber MR, et al. The role of secondary brain injury in determining outcome from severe head injury. *J Trauma.* 1993;34(2):216–222.
17. McHugh GS, Engel DC, Butcher I, et al. Prognostic value of secondary insults in traumatic brain injury: results from the IMPACT study. *J Neurotrauma.* 2007;24(2):287–293.
18. Fuller G, Hasler RM, Mealing N, et al. The association between admission systolic blood pressure and mortality in significant traumatic brain injury: a multi-centre cohort study. *Injury.* 2014;45(3):612–617.
19. Silverston P. Pulse oximetry at the roadside: a study of pulse oximetry in immediate care. *BMJ.* 1989;298(6675):711–713.
20. Bouma GJ, Muizelaar JP, Bandoh K, Marmarou A. Blood pressure and intracranial pressure-volume dynamics in severe head injury: relationship with cerebral blood flow. *J Neurosurg.* 1992;77(1):15–19.
21. Muizelaar JP, Ward JD, Marmarou A, Newlon PG, Wachi A. Cerebral blood flow and metabolism in severely head-injured children. Part 2: autoregulation. *J Neurosurg.* 1989;71(1):72–76.
22. Oddo M, Schmidt JM, Carrera E, et al. Impact of tight glycemic control on cerebral glucose metabolism after severe brain injury: a microdialysis study. *Crit Care Med.* 2008;36(12):3233–3238.
23. Rovlias A, Kotsou S. The influence of hyperglycemia on neurological outcome in patients with severe head injury. *Neurosurgery.* 2000;46(2):335–342; discussion 342–343.
24. Allard CB, Scarpelini S, Rhind SG, et al. Abnormal coagulation tests are associated with progression of traumatic intracranial hemorrhage. *J Trauma.* 2009;67(5):959–967.
25. Harhangi BS, Kompanje EJ, Leebeek FW, Maas AI. Coagulation disorders after traumatic brain injury. *Acta Neurochir (Wien).* 2008;150(2):165–175; discussion 175.
26. Brown CV, Zada G, Salim A, et al. Indications for routine repeat head computed tomography (CT) stratified by severity of traumatic brain injury. *J Trauma.* 2007;62(6):1339–1344; discussion 1344–1245.
27. Huang AP, Lee CW, Hsieh HJ, et al. Early parenchymal contrast extravasation predicts subsequent hemorrhage progression, clinical deterioration, and need for surgery in patients with traumatic cerebral contusion. *J Trauma.* 2011;71(6):1593–1599.
28. Joseph B, Obaid O, Dultz L, et al. Validating the brain injury guidelines: results of an American Association for the surgery of trauma prospective multi-institutional trial. *J Trauma Acute Care Surg.* 2022;93(2):157–165.
29. Edlow BL, Giacino JT, Hirschberg RE, Gerrard J, Wu O, Hochberg LR. Unexpected recovery of function after severe traumatic brain injury: the limits of early neuroimaging-based outcome prediction. *Neurocrit Care.* 2013;19(3):364–375.
30. Chen JW, Vakil-Gilani K, Williamson KL, Cecil S. Infrared pupillometry, the Neurological Pupil index and unilateral pupillary dilation after traumatic brain injury: implications for treatment paradigms. *Springerplus.* 2014;3:548.
31. Khan MN, Shallwani II, Khan MU, Shamim MS. Noninvasive monitoring intracranial pressure—A review of available modalities. *Surg Neurol Int.* 2017;8:51.
32. Bernard SA, Nguyen V, Cameron P, et al. Prehospital rapid sequence intubation improves functional outcome for patients with severe traumatic brain injury: a randomized controlled trial. *Ann Surg.* 2010;252(6):959–965.
33. Brain Trauma Foundation; American Association of Neurological Surgeons; Congress of Neurological Surgeons; et al. Guidelines for the management of severe traumatic brain injury. VI. Indications for intracranial pressure monitoring. *J Neurotrauma.* 2007;24 Suppl 1:S37–44.
34. Bullock MR, Chesnut R, Ghajar J, et al. Surgical management of acute epidural hematomas. *Neurosurgery.* 2006;58(3):S7–15; discussion Si–iv.
35. Semler MW, Self WH, Wanderer JP, et al. Balanced crystalloids versus saline in critically ill adults. *N Engl J Med.* 2018;378(9):829–839.
36. Holcomb JB, Tilley BC, Baraniuk S, et al. Transfusion of plasma, platelets, and red blood cells in a 1:1:1 vs a 1:1:2 ratio and mortality in patients with severe trauma: the PROPPR randomized clinical trial. *JAMA.* 2015;313(5):471–482.
37. Novak DJ, Bai Y, Cooke RK, et al. Making thawed universal donor plasma available rapidly for massively bleeding trauma patients: experience from the Pragmatic, Randomized Optimal Platelets and Plasma Ratios (PROPPR) trial. *Transfusion.* 2015;55(6):1331–1339.
38. Turgeon AF, Fergusson DA, Clayton L, et al. Liberal or restrictive transfusion strategy in patients with traumatic brain injury. *N Engl J Med.* 2024;391(8):722–735.
39. Gonzalez E, Moore EE, Moore HB, et al. Goal-directed hemostatic resuscitation of trauma-induced coagulopathy: a pragmatic randomized clinical trial comparing a viscoelastic assay to conventional coagulation assays. *Ann Surg.* 2016;263(6):1051–1059.
40. Juul N, Morris GF, Marshall SB, Marshall LF. Intracranial hypertension and cerebral perfusion pressure: influence on neurological deterioration and outcome in severe head injury. The Executive Committee of the International Selfotel Trial. *J Neurosurg.* 2000;92(1):1–6.
41. Carney N, Totten AM, O'Reilly C, et al. Guidelines for the management of severe traumatic brain injury, Fourth Edition. *Neurosurgery.* 2017;80(1):6–15.
42. Maas AI, Stocchetti N, Bullock R. Moderate and severe traumatic brain injury in adults. *Lancet Neurol.* 2008;7(8):728–741.
43. Chesnut RM, Temkin N, Carney N, et al. A trial of intracranial-pressure monitoring in traumatic brain injury. *N Engl J Med.* 2012;367(26):2471–2481.
44. Agrawal D, Raghavendran K, Schaubel DE, Mishra MC, Rajajee V. A propensity score analysis of the impact of invasive intracranial pressure monitoring on outcomes after severe traumatic brain injury. *J Neurotrauma.* 2016;33:853–858.
45. Farahvar A, Gerber LM, Chiu YL, Carney N, Hartl R, Ghajar J. Increased mortality in patients with severe traumatic brain injury

treated without intracranial pressure monitoring. *J Neurosurg.* 2012;117(4):729–734.
46. Sorrentino E, Diedler J, Kasprowicz M, et al. Critical thresholds for cerebrovascular reactivity after traumatic brain injury. *Neurocrit Care.* 2012;16(2):258–266.
47. Needham E, McFadyen C, Newcombe V, Synnot AJ, Czosnyka M, Menon D. Cerebral perfusion pressure targets individualized to pressure-reactivity index in moderate to severe traumatic brain injury: a systematic review. *J Neurotrauma.* 2017;34(5):963–970.
48. Hansen HC, Lagreze W, Krueger O, Helmke K. Dependence of the optic nerve sheath diameter on acutely applied subarachnoidal pressure—an experimental ultrasound study. *Acta Ophthalmol.* 2011;89(6):e528–532.
49. Kimberly HH, Shah S, Marill K, Noble V. Correlation of optic nerve sheath diameter with direct measurement of intracranial pressure. *Acad Emerg Med.* 2008;15(2):201–204.
50. Masquere P, Bonneville F, Geeraerts T. Optic nerve sheath diameter on initial brain CT, raised intracranial pressure and mortality after severe TBI: an interesting link needing confirmation. *Crit Care.* 2013;17(3):151.
51. Moretti R, Pizzi B. Optic nerve ultrasound for detection of intracranial hypertension in intracranial hemorrhage patients: confirmation of previous findings in a different patient population. *J Neurosurg Anesthesiol.* 2009;21(1):16–20.
52. Agrawal D, Raghavendran K, Zhao L, Rajajee V. A prospective study of optic nerve ultrasound for the detection of elevated intracranial pressure in severe traumatic brain injury. *Crit Care Med.* 2020;48(12):e1278–e1285.
53. Cardim D, Robba C, Bohdanowicz M, et al. Non-invasive monitoring of intracranial pressure using transcranial Doppler ultrasonography: is it possible? *Neurocrit Care.* 2016;25(3):473–491.
54. Rasulo FA, Bertuetti R, Robba C, et al. The accuracy of transcranial Doppler in excluding intracranial hypertension following acute brain injury: a multicenter prospective pilot study. *Crit Care.* 2017;21(1):44.
55. Okonkwo DO, Shutter LA, Moore C, et al. brain oxygen optimization in severe traumatic brain injury phase-II: a phase II randomized trial. *Crit Care Med.* 2017;45(11):1907–1914.
56. de Lima Oliveira M, Kairalla AC, Fonoff ET, Martinez RC, Teixeira MJ, Bor-Seng-Shu E. Cerebral microdialysis in traumatic brain injury and subarachnoid hemorrhage: state of the art. *Neurocrit Care.* 2014;21(1):152–162.
57. Rajajee V, Riggs B, Seder DB. Emergency neurological life support: airway, ventilation, and sedation. *Neurocrit Care.* 2017;27(Suppl 1): 4–28.
58. Kelly DF, Goodale DB, Williams J, et al. Propofol in the treatment of moderate and severe head injury: a randomized, prospective double-blinded pilot trial. *J Neurosurg.* 1999;90(6):1042–1052.
59. Boone MD, Oren-Grinberg A, Robinson TM, Chen CC, Kasper EM. Mannitol or hypertonic saline in the setting of traumatic brain injury: what have we learned? *Surg Neurol Int.* 2015;6:177.
60. Sakellaridis N, Pavlou E, Karatzas S, et al. Comparison of mannitol and hypertonic saline in the treatment of severe brain injuries. *J Neurosurg.* 2011;114(2):545–548.
61. Burgess S, Abu-Laban RB, Slavik RS, Vu EN, Zed PJ. A systematic review of randomized controlled trials comparing hypertonic sodium solutions and mannitol for traumatic brain injury: implications for emergency department management. *Ann Pharmacother.* 2016;50(4):291–300.
62. Vespa PM, Nuwer MR, Nenov V, et al. Increased incidence and impact of nonconvulsive and convulsive seizures after traumatic brain injury as detected by continuous electroencephalographic monitoring. *J Neurosurg.* 1999;91(5):750–760.
63. Temkin NR, Dikmen SS, Wilensky AJ, Keihm J, Chabal S, Winn HR. A randomized, double-blind study of phenytoin for the prevention of post-traumatic seizures. *N Engl J Med.* 1990;323(8): 497–502.
64. Zimmermann LL, Diaz-Arrastia R, Vespa PM. Seizures and the role of anticonvulsants after traumatic brain injury. *Neurosurg Clin N Am.* 2016;27(4):499–508.
65. Szaflarski JP, Sangha KS, Lindsell CJ, Shutter LA. Prospective, randomized, single-blinded comparative trial of intravenous levetiracetam versus phenytoin for seizure prophylaxis. *Neurocrit Care.* 2010;12(2):165–172.
66. CRASH-3 trial collaborators. Effects of tranexamic acid on death, disability, vascular occlusive events and other morbidities in patients with acute traumatic brain injury (CRASH-3): a randomised, placebo-controlled trial. *Lancet.* 2019;394(10210):1713–1723.
67. Hartl R, Gerber LM, Ni Q, Ghajar J. Effect of early nutrition on deaths due to severe traumatic brain injury. *J Neurosurg.* 2008;109(1):50–56.
68. Chourdakis M, Kraus MM, Tzellos T, et al. Effect of early compared with delayed enteral nutrition on endocrine function in patients with traumatic brain injury: an open-labeled randomized trial. *JPEN J Parenter Enteral Nutr.* 2012;36(1):108–116.
69. Margolick J, Dandurand C, Duncan K, et al. A systematic review of the risks and benefits of venous thromboembolism prophylaxis in traumatic brain injury. *Can J Neurol Sci.* 2018;45(4):432–444.
70. Andrews PJ, Sleeman DH, Statham PF, et al. Predicting recovery in patients suffering from traumatic brain injury by using admission variables and physiological data: a comparison between decision tree analysis and logistic regression. *J Neurosurg.* 2002;97(2): 326–336.
71. Cadena R, Shoykhet M, Ratcliff JJ. Emergency neurological life support: intracranial hypertension and herniation. *Neurocrit Care.* 2017;27(Suppl 1):82–88.
72. Koenig MA, Bryan M, Lewin JL III, Mirski MA, Geocadin RG, Stevens RD. Reversal of transtentorial herniation with hypertonic saline. *Neurology.* 2008;70(13):1023–1029.
73. Qureshi AI, Geocadin RG, Suarez JI, Ulatowski JA. Long-term outcome after medical reversal of transtentorial herniation in patients with supratentorial mass lesions. *Crit Care Med.* 2000;28(5): 1556–1564.
74. Collaborators MCT, Perel P, Arango M, et al. Predicting outcome after traumatic brain injury: practical prognostic models based on large cohort of international patients. *BMJ.* 2008;336(7641): 425–429.
75. Hutchinson PJ, Adams H, Mohan M, et al. Decompressive craniectomy versus craniotomy for acute subdural hematoma. *N Engl J Med.* 2023;388(24):2219–2229.
76. Cooper DJ, Rosenfeld JV, Murray L, et al. Decompressive craniectomy in diffuse traumatic brain injury. *N Engl J Med.* 2011; 364(16):1493–1502.
77. Hutchinson PJ, Kolias AG, Timofeev IS, et al. Trial of decompressive craniectomy for traumatic intracranial hypertension. *N Engl J Med.* 2016;375(12):1119–1130.
78. Steyerberg EW, Mushkudiani N, Perel P, et al. Predicting outcome after traumatic brain injury: development and international validation of prognostic scores based on admission characteristics. *PLoS Med.* 2008;5(8):e165; discussion e165.
79. Jiang JY, Gao GY, Li WP, Yu MK, Zhu C. Early indicators of prognosis in 846 cases of severe traumatic brain injury. *J Neurotrauma.* 2002;19(7):869–874.
80. Andelic N, Hammergren N, Bautz-Holter E, Sveen U, Brunborg C, Roe C. Functional outcome and health-related quality of life 10 years after moderate-to-severe traumatic brain injury. *Acta Neurol Scand.* 2009;120(1):16–23.
81. Levin HS, Saydjari C, Eisenberg HM, et al. Vegetative state after closed-head injury. A Traumatic Coma Data Bank Report. *Arch Neurol.* 1991;48(6):580–585.
82. Seagly KS, O'Neil RL, Hanks RA. Pre-injury psychosocial and demographic predictors of long-term functional outcomes post-TBI. *Brain Inj.* 2018;32(1):78–83.
83. McCrea MA, Giacino JT, Barber J, et al. Functional outcomes over the first year after moderate to severe traumatic brain injury in the prospective, longitudinal TRACK-TBI Study. *JAMA Neurol.* 2021;78(8):982–992.
84. Muehlschlegel S, Rajajee V, Wartenberg KE, et al. Guidelines for neuroprognostication in critically ill adults with moderate-severe traumatic brain injury. *Neurocrit Care.* 2024;40(2):448–476.

21

Injury and Violence Prevention: A Public Health Approach

Joseph V. Sakran and Nicole Lunardi

Key Points

1. Injuries are preventable, and we should therefore avoid using the term "accident."
2. Violence is a public health problem.
3. Injury prevention requires multidisciplinary teams, including education, healthcare, criminal justice, legislature, communications/media, business, and community organizations.
4. Injury and violence prevention takes place on a continuum: before the injury occurs (primary prevention) or after the injury occurs by minimizing the mortality, likelihood of reoccurrence (secondary prevention), and reducing long term morbidity (tertiary prevention).
5. Healthcare systems must engage the community in addressing the social determinants of health and disease, which contribute to structural violence in underserved communities.
6. Our medical organizations must commit to working together in order to provide constructive actions that reduce injury and death in communities across America.
7. Surgeons have a critical role in social movements, and advocating for evidence-based solutions.

HISTORY OF INJURY PREVENTION

1 The field of injury prevention began with occupational hazards in the first half of the 20th century. Injuries, at the time, were considered true accidents: random, unavoidable, or, even, acts of God. Thus, the notion of systematically preventing "accidents" was novel. In 1913, the National Safety Council was created and distributed industrial hazard information. Simultaneously, thought leaders were studying national trends and circumstances of workplace "accidents." Julian Harvey put forth the first framework of "accident control" in 1923, which became known as the "three Es": education, engineering, and enforcement. Despite these advancements, many workplace injuries were still considered unavoidable accidents.[1,2]

Starting in the mid-20th century, the paradigm shifted toward evidence-based injury prevention. Federal agencies teamed up with local health departments to educate the public and implement prevention programs. Epidemiologists applied the principles used to describe disease to injuries: host demographics, causal agents, environments, seasonal/cyclical trends, distributions, and epidemic episodes.[3–5] In 1966, the National Academy of Sciences landmark paper, "Accidental Death and Disability: The Neglected Disease of Modern Society," identified the need for improved care of the injured patient.[6] By 1972, William Haddon Jr, the director of the National Highway Safety Bureau, proposed a framework to describe the interaction between causal factors regarding the host, agent, and environment before, during and after the injury. The Haddon Matrix allowed for strategic prevention efforts. He is credited as the father of modern injury epidemiology.[7]

In the same period, basic scientists were describing the mechanisms by which energy transfer (kinetic, electric, chemical, etc.) caused tissue damage for the first time.[8] These discoveries resulted in the development of safer products, like padded dashboards, air bags, and seat belts in cars. Product safety along with the development of the first regional trauma systems worked to decrease the severity of injuries, and to increase survival.[8]

By the late 20th century, a robust group of stakeholders, including basic scientists, engineers, epidemiologists, healthcare workers, local, state and national health agencies, and nonprofit organizations were building a coalition to establish the science of injury prevention. Representing a true shift in understanding, the word "accident" was replaced with the word "injury" in International Statistical Classification (ICD) codes in 1979.[1,2] The trauma community has worked to shift daily terminology to reflect the firmly grounded principle that injuries are preventable, that is, avoiding the use of "motor vehicle accident" and shifting to "motor vehicle crash."

Advancements in the field were contemporaneous with the emergence of injury as a leading cause of death in the United States. In fact, injury has been in the top 15 causes of death of all Americans since 1965 (https://www.cdc.gov/injury/wisqars/LeadingCauses_images.html).[9] In 1985, the Department of Transportation along with the National Academy of Sciences and Institute of Medicine drew attention to injury being responsible for more life years lost than cancer and heart disease, but having the smallest funding allocation with no central agency in "Injury in America."[10] That very year, the Centers for Disease Control and Prevention (CDC) Injury Control Pilot Program was created. It oversaw and funded multidisciplinary research centers and demonstration projects. The pilot program was found to be efficacious in a 1988 review. By 1990, the Injury Control Act was signed reauthorizing the CDC-based program.[2]

2 Over the course of the century, the field of injury prevention was created with the overarching goal to reduce the morbidity, mortality, and economic burden of injury. The field is, by definition, multidisciplinary, drawing on the expertise from basic scientists, engineers, epidemiologists, health systems and administrators, healthcare workers, educators, the private sector, and numerous others.

EPIDEMIOLOGY OF INJURY: DEFINING THE PROBLEM

The CDC's National Center for Injury Prevention and Control (NCIPC) collects and stores national injury data on the web-based Injury Statistics Query and Reporting System (WISQARS: cdc.gov/injury/wisqars/index.html).[9] Made available for the first time in 2000, WISQARS includes the 2001–2022 data on fatal and nonfatal injury, leading causes of death and injury, violent deaths (homicides and suicides), years of potential life lost, and cost of injury. This data is compiled from sources, including the National Vistal Statistics System, National Electronic Injury Surveillance System—All Injury Program, the Pacific Institute for Research and Evaluation, and the National Violent Death Reporting System (NVDRS: cdc.gov/violenceprevention/datasources/nvdrs/index.html).[11]

In 2002, the NVDRS started collecting homicide and suicide data from six states and has grown to include all 50 states, Puerto Rico, and Washington DC by 2018. The NVDRS is unique in that it collects data from law enforcement, medical examiners, and death certificates regarding the violent incident (geography, weapon used), characteristics of the victim (mental and physical health problems, toxicology reports, substance abuse, financial problems), and the relationship between victim and suspect (nature of relationship, relationship problems, and intimate partner violence [IPV]).

Injury data can be studied from many different perspectives, with the two most common being by intent and mechanism. Intent, as captured by the ICD codes, falls into the following major categories: unintentional, suicide/self-harm, homicide/assault, and legal intervention. There is a small percentage of cases each year for which the intent is not determined (1.8% in 2022). Mechanism describes the way by which the injury occurred. Common mechanisms of injury include transportation (motor vehicle collision, pedestrian, cyclist), penetrating injury (firearm, cut/pierce), blunt injury (stuck, fall), drowning, suffocation, burns, and poisonings (drug, nondrug). For the purposes of a complete discussion, trends regarding both intent and mechanism will be explored.

Unintentional Injury

Unintentional injury has consistently been among the leading causes of death for Americans regardless of age, race/ethnicity, and sex, claiming 227,039 lives in 2022 alone. It was single leading cause of death for all Americans aged 1 to 44 between 2001 and 2022. The most common mechanisms of these deaths varied based on age: drowning (ages 1 to 4), motor vehicle crashes (ages 5 to 24), and poisonings (ages 24 to 44). For every single fatality, there were 108 nonfatal unintended injuries in 2022.

From 2001 to 2022, 12,805 fatal and 419,517 nonfatal unintended injuries involved a firearm. While the age-adjusted rates of unintended firearm fatalities have been steadily

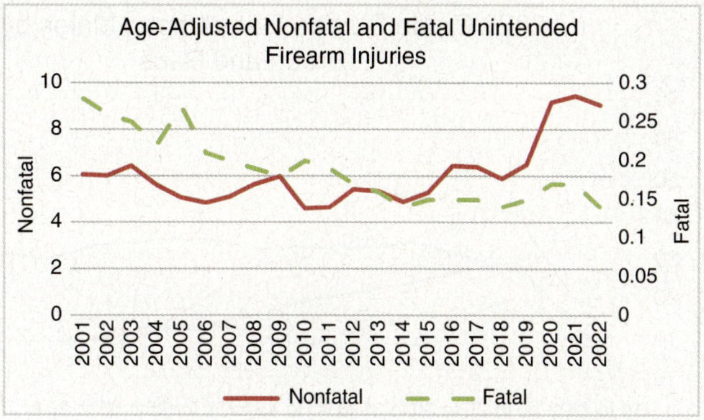

Figure 21.1. Age-adjusted fatal and nonfatal unintended firearm injuries per 100,000 persons. (Data sourced from WISQARS Data from National Center for Injury Prevention and Control. WISQARS [Web-based Injury Statistics Query and Reporting System], Injury Center, Centers for Disease Control and Prevention: Injury Prevention & Control Data and Statistic [WISQARS]. https://www.cdc.gov/injury/wisqars/index.html. Published March 30, 2020.)

decreasing (0.28 in 2001 to 0.14 deaths/100,000 population 2022), the trend in nonfatal firearm injuries has been increasing (**Fig. 21.1**).[9]

Suicide and Self-Harm

Overall, suicide is the 11th leading cause of death for all Americans with 49,476 deaths in 2022. Greater than half of all suicide deaths are committed with a firearm. Suicide rates are higher in men than women. Age-adjusted suicide rates with a firearm are higher than non-firearm among men, whereas the opposite is true among women (**Fig. 21.2**).

Among American men, older White and younger American Indian men have higher suicide rates than Blacks or Asians (**Fig. 21.3**).[9] This racial and age disparity has been well documented.[12,13] Between 2001 and 2022, for every single suicide there were 11 self-harm injuries. These nonfatal injuries are more common among women (**Fig. 21.4**) and are most likely to involve poisoning or cutting. There are so few failed suicide attempts involving a firearm that the absolute number is not reported. Surviving a suicide attempt with a firearm is very unlikely given the high lethality of the weapon.[9]

Homicide and Assault

While the prevalence of homicides has varied overtime in the United States, they are consistently less common than unintentional injury and suicides. It has been well documented that the homicide rate increased during the COVID pandemic, but has since begun to decrease.[14,15] There is also data to suggest that while the absolute number of homicides may fluctuate, the intensity of violence of each act is increasing.[16]

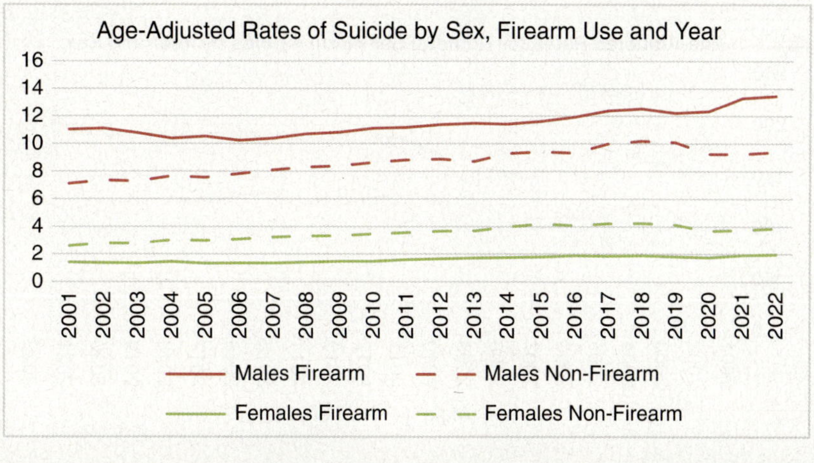

Figure 21.2. Age-adjusted rates of suicide per 100,000 people by sex, firearm use, and year. (Data sourced from WISQARS Data from National Center for Injury Prevention and Control. WISQARS [Web-based Injury Statistics Query and Reporting System], Injury Center, Centers for Disease Control and Prevention: Injury Prevention & Control Data and Statistic [WISQARS]. https://www.cdc.gov/injury/wisqars/index.html. Published March 30, 2020.)

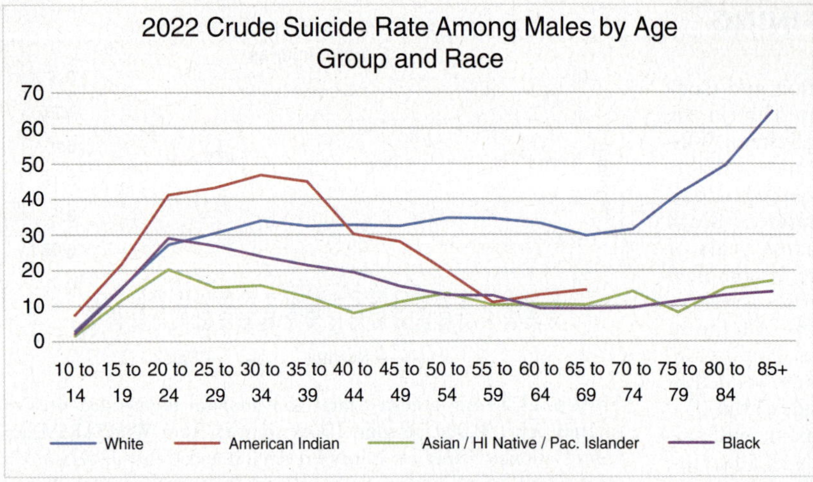

Figure 21.3. Crude death rate by age group and race among 2018 male suicides. (Data sourced from WISQARS Data from National Center for Injury Prevention and Control. WISQARS [Web-based Injury Statistics Query and Reporting System], Injury Center, Centers for Disease Control and Prevention: Injury Prevention & Control Data and Statistic [WISQARS]. https://www.cdc.gov/injury/wisqars/index.html. Published March 30, 2020.)

In 2022, there were 24,849 homicides. The majority of deaths were among males 15 to 44 years of age (**Fig. 21.5**). Racial and ethnic minorities' risk of death from homicide is significantly higher than non-Hispanic Whites. Young, Black males (aged 15 to 34), in particular, have the highest homicide rate (**Fig. 21.6A,B**). In fact, it is the leading cause of death in this population. Of all homicides between 2001 and 2022, 71% used a firearm. In 2022, there were 60 nonfatal assaults for every homicide death. Approximately 4% of nonfatal assaults involve a firearm.[9]

These acts of fatal and nonfatal violence occur daily between strangers, community members, partners, and families. Experiencing or, even, witnessing violence, in all of its forms, increases the risk of being a future victim or perpetrator of violence. Thus, to truly understand the pervasiveness of the problem is to understand the different permutations of interpersonal violence.

Mass Shootings

Mass shootings, as they are discussed here, include four or more shooting victims. Between 2006 and 2023 there were 475 mass shooting incidents in 47 states and Washington DC. The majority (65%) occurred in residences and 35% occurred in public places. Ninety-one percent of these shootings were committed by a single male shooter. Over 2523 people were killed in this time frame, with thousands more injured. Approximately 60% of the victims are known to the shooter. Mass shootings have been more deadly and occurring more frequently, bringing the topic of gun violence into the public eye. It is important to acknowledge that while they grip the nation's attention, mass shootings account for <1% of gun deaths each year.[17]

Legal Intervention

Deaths or injury attributed to legal intervention are acts inflicted by on-duty law enforcement agents. Within the WISQARS database, there is no indication of legal circumstances of these events. In 2022, there were 817 fatalities and 74,150 nonfatal injuries.[9] There is data to suggest, however, that these incidents are vastly unreported, particularly if the injured individual is lower socioeconomic class or a minority.[18] The overwhelming majority of these deaths were among males (94%) younger than 39 years old (58%). Eighty percent of deaths involved a firearm. Age-adjusted death rates were highest among American Indians (0.84) and Blacks (0.46) followed by Whites (0.23) and Asians (0.07). This disparity is consistent with studies that have shown officers are more likely to shoot a Black individual holding weapons faster and more often when compared to White individuals in the same circumstance.[18,19]

Intimate Partner Violence

IPV encompasses physical, sexual, emotional, and psychological violence between current or past spouses. In fact, 47% of women and 44% of men have experienced some form of IPV in their lifetime. The majority of individuals experienced IPV for the first time before the age of 25. Thirty-three percent of women and 25% of men have experienced severe physical violence from a partner.[20] One in four homicides in 2021 involved intimate partners. Half of all female homicide victims are killed by their spouse.[9] It is estimated that the medical, legal, and lost productivity of IPV cost $3.6 trillion annually.[21]

Child Abuse

Child abuse is defined as physical, sexual, emotional abuse or neglect of a minor by a caregiver. In 2022, there were over 550,000 victims of child abuse or neglect with a national victimization rate of 7.7 per 1000 children. Survivors are at increased risk of future injury and violence. While rare, 1990 children were killed as result of abuse in 2022.[22]

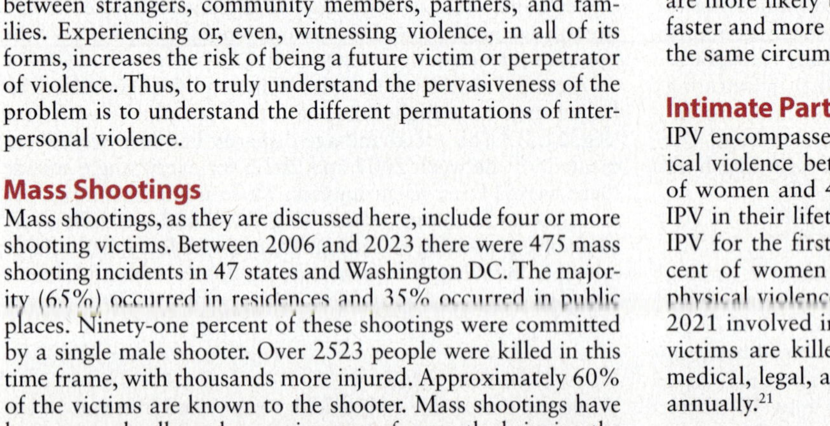

Figure 21.4. Age-adjusted rates for nonfatal self-harm injuries per 100,000 people by year and sex. (Data sourced from WISQARS Data from National Center for Injury Prevention and Control. WISQARS [Web-based Injury Statistics Query and Reporting System], Injury Center, Centers for Disease Control and Prevention: Injury Prevention & Control Data and Statistic [WISQARS]. https://www.cdc.gov/injury/wisqars/index.html. Published March 30, 2020.)

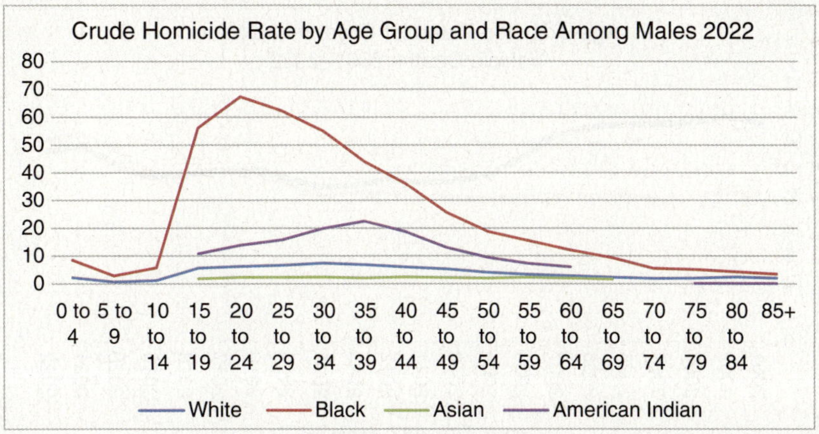

Figure 21.5. Crude homicide rate by age group and sex in 2022. (Data sourced from WISQARS Data from National Center for Injury Prevention and Control. WISQARS [Web-based Injury Statistics Query and Reporting System], Injury Center, Centers for Disease Control and Prevention: Injury Prevention & Control Data and Statistic [WISQARS]. https://www.cdc.gov/injury/wisqars/index.html. Accessed August 28, 2024.)

Firearms

The public health burden of injuries has been well documented since the mid-20th century. Prevention initiatives have aimed to reduce the morbidity and mortality attributed to common vectors like motor vehicles, since the 1930s, and firearms, since the 1980s. Over the last 15 years, the age-adjusted death rates for firearm injury first equalized and have now surpassed that of motor vehicles (**Fig. 21.7**). As such, it is an unprecedented time in the history of the field of injury prevention.

Firearms play an intricate role in injury mortality in that they are a highly lethal, common vector within unintentional, suicide, homicide, and legal intervention injuries.[23] Firearms are among the top five mechanisms of injury deaths. In 2022, 48,204 deaths were caused by a firearm. The majority, 56%, were suicides. Forty-one percent were homicides, 1% legal intervention, 1% unintentional, and 1% undetermined. There was over 1,100,000 years of productive life lost. Nonfatal and fatal firearm injuries resulted in $521.4 billion dollars in medical costs, lost wages, and quality-of-life loss cost in 2022.[9]

LANDMARK INJURY PREVENTION INITIATIVES

Workplace, motor vehicle, and childhood injuries have been the subject of injury prevention initiatives since the inception of the field. As such, these three areas are heavily represented in the field's landmark achievements.

The Occupational Health and Safety Act created the CDC's National Institute for Occupational Safety and Health in 1970 (NIOSH; https://www.cdc.gov/niosh/).[24] NIOSH aims to keep America's workforce safe through research, partnership, and program implementation covering topics like needlestick injury. The OSHA blood-borne pathogen standards (1992) along with NIOSH recommendations (1999) aimed to reduce the nearly 800,000 needlestick injuries each year. Interventions targeted safer sharps and sharp container design, universal precautions, worker education, free hepatitis B vaccinations, and postexposure evaluation and treatment.[25–32] These efforts have proven to be effective, with a decrease in total needlesticks to less than 400,000 by 2015.

Nation-wide motor vehicle and road safety policies, programs, and behaviors have developed over the last century. Starting in the 1920s there was a call for national, uniform, enforced road safety laws, including speed limits, seat belts, child car seats, and maximum blood alcohol limits.[2,33–41] As a mechanism to ensure national adoption of these policies, a stipulation was made that any state that failed to pass these laws would not receive federal highway funding.[33] Widespread behavior change came about with both law enforcement (i.e., sobriety checkpoints) and public education campaigns (Mothers Against Drunk Driving, "Click it or ticket"). Seatbelt use, for example, increased from 11% in 1981 to 91% in 2019. Nearly 15,000 lives were saved by seat belt use in 2017 alone.[33,37,42] States have varying degrees of graduated drivers' license for new, young adult drivers.[43,44] Furthermore, over this time frame, cars have become safer.[35] Despite the 10-fold increase in number of miles driven per year in America between 1920 and 1990, the death rate per mile traveled has decreased by 90%.[33,45]

In addition to the widespread success in car seat use, there have been several other initiatives to mitigate childhood injuries in all settings.[46] The Child Safety Network of the Health Resources and Services Administration spearheads national and state wide efforts on diverse topics like poison control, sports safety, child abuse, and fall prevention (https://www.childrenssafetynetwork.org/).[47] Window guards, stair gates, bike helmets, energy-absorbing playground surfacing, and

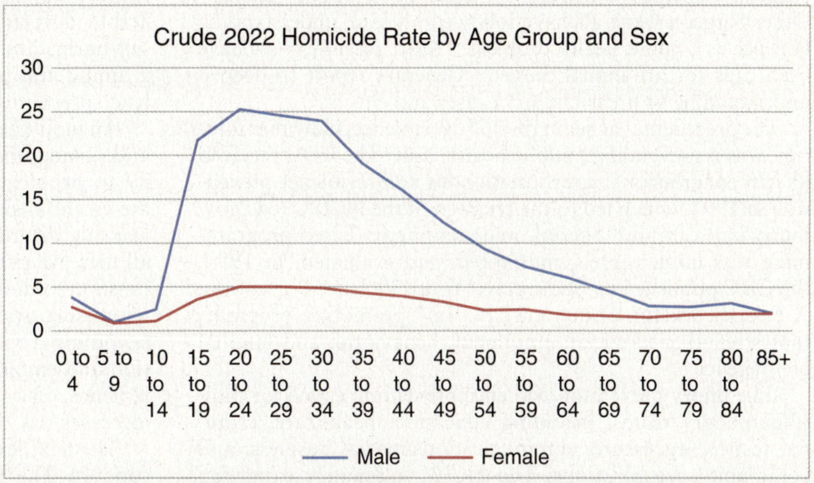

Figure 21.6. Crude homicide rate by age group and race among males in 2022. (Data sourced from WISQARS Data from National Center for Injury Prevention and Control. WISQARS [Web-based Injury Statistics Query and Reporting System], Injury Center, Centers for Disease Control and Prevention: Injury Prevention & Control Data and Statistic [WISQARS]. https://www.cdc.gov/injury/wisqars/index.html. Accessed August 28, 2024.)

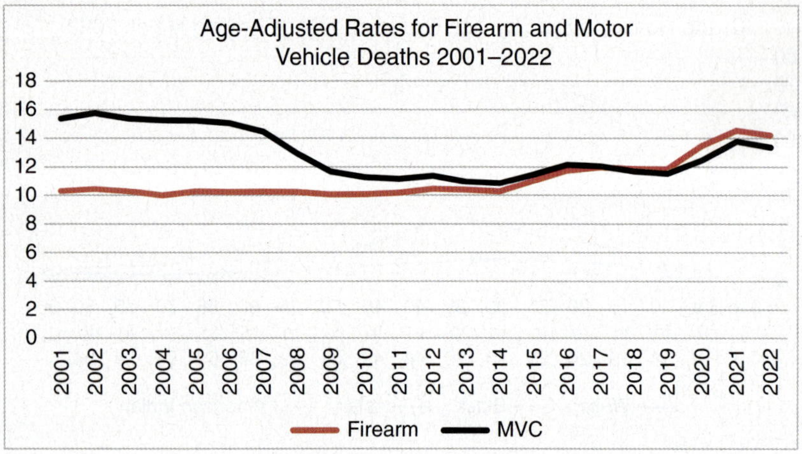

Figure 21.7. Age-adjusted rates for firearm and motor vehicle deaths 2001–2022. (Data sourced from WISQARS Data from National Center for Injury Prevention and Control. WISQARS [Web-based Injury Statistics Query and Reporting System], Injury Center, Centers for Disease Control and Prevention: Injury Prevention & Control Data and Statistic [WISQARS]. https://www.cdc.gov/injury/wisqars/index.html. Accessed August 28, 2024.)

child supervision improvements have all been shown to successfully reduce falls.[48–56] One specific program example includes the "Children Can't Fly" campaign in New York City. This 1974 initiative required window guards in homes with children less than 10 years old. The result was a 96% decrease in falls from windows.[57] While workplace, motor-vehicle, and childhood injury prevention has developed over the last century, violent injury prevention came into the purview of the field much more recently.

Violence as Public Health Problem

3 Violence was considered purely a criminal justice issue until 1968. It was then that President Lyndon B. Johnson appointed the National Commission on the Causes and Prevention of Violence with the goal of identifying the social underpinnings of violent acts.[58] Thereafter, data was collected and analyzed regarding the morbidity, mortality, and healthcare cost of violent injuries. The Healthy People 1979 report was the first instance in which injury and violent behavior was described as a public health priority.[59] Subsequently, the 1980 Promoting Health/Preventing Disease Report outlined specific objectives for child abuse, homicides, suicides, privately owned guns, and data collection.[60] Violent injury has been identified as a priority in all subsequent Healthy People Reports (https://www.healthypeople.gov/).[61] The CDC then created the Violence Epidemiology Branch in 1983 and the Extramural Research Program for injury and violence in 1986. An infrastructure to treat violence as a public health issue was thereby created.

Two milestones occurred in 1985. The first was the Secretary's Task Force on Black and Minority Health Report which outlined the heavy contribution of violent firearm injury to health disparities among Blacks.[62] This disparity persists to this day. Second, Surgeon General C. Everett Koop convened the first Surgeon General's Workshop on Violence in Public Health.[63] Other Surgeon Generals have followed his lead, understanding violence as a public health problem.[64] More recently, there have been calls for an annual Surgeon General's report to deepen understanding of firearm injury causes and effects.[65]

The precedent was set in the 1980s: violence, like other injuries, was a preventable, public health issue. The CDC received its first congressional appropriation for youth violence prevention in 1992, which led to the creation of the NCIPC (cdc.gov/injury/index.html).[66] School- and community-based programming was implemented, monitored, and evaluated. In 1993, the CDC published its findings in "Youth Violence Prevention: A Framework for Community Action" promoting programs that strengthened social, emotional, behavioral, and familial competencies.[67]

Like injury prevention, violence prevention called for multidisciplinary teams, including education, healthcare, criminal justice, legislature, communications/media, business, and community organizations. The NCIPC ultimately expanded its prevention efforts beyond youth violence to include IPV, sexual violence, child maltreatment, elder maltreatment, and suicide.[2] By 2001, public health violence prevention initiatives were proven to be both efficacious and cost effective in the "Youth Violence: A Report of the Surgeon General."[68]

Federally funded injury and violence prevention research in the 1990s included gun violence. Initial studies identified having a firearm in the home was an independent risk factor of homicide. Unfortunately, firearms have not been a bipartisan topic. Controversy ensued. Through the National Rifle Association's strong lobby and, ultimately, the Representative Jay Dickey's 1996 Omnibus Appropriations Act, the CDC was banned from conducting research that may ultimately promote gun control. In 2012, this ban was extended to the US Department of Health and Human Services.[69] Attempts were made to repeal the ban of firearms research in both 2015 and 2017. Both failed. Firearm possession by private citizens remains a controversial, partisan topic of debate in the public arena.[70] However, recent data would suggest a majority of Americans actually agree on particular gun restrictions.[71] The goal of this chapter is to refocus the conversation on the health and well-being of the patients encountered in the trauma bay—in preventing injury, increasing survival, and improving long-term outcomes for the individual, communities, and the nation.

THE SOCIAL ECOLOGIC MODEL

4 The social ecologic model is used as a framework for the dynamic risk and protective factors of gun violence on various levels, including individual, interpersonal, community, and society (**Fig. 21.8**). This framework is vital in identifying opportunities to reduce risk, bolster protective factors, and identify stakeholders. The preponderance of factors is unifying across different types of violence (child abuse, IPV, suicide/self-harm, and assault/homicide).[72] Therefore, relevant programing and policy should be recognized as generalized violence prevention.

An individual's personal characteristics, health, experiences, and demographics affect the likelihood of violence. The ability to problem-solve, manage anger, and control impulsivity are essential skills in conflict resolution. A personal history of learning disorders, mental health issues, and substance abuse all increase risk. Prior adverse childhood experiences, chronic or severe emotional distress, attitudes toward violence, and witnessing or experiencing violence increase the likelihood of becoming a victim or perpetrating violence. Level of education and employment have also been shown to correlate with violence. Easy access to unlocked and unprotected firearms increases risk of suicide and homicide.[68,71–77]

The next level, interpersonal relationships, hinges on social support. The presence or absence of stable, positive social

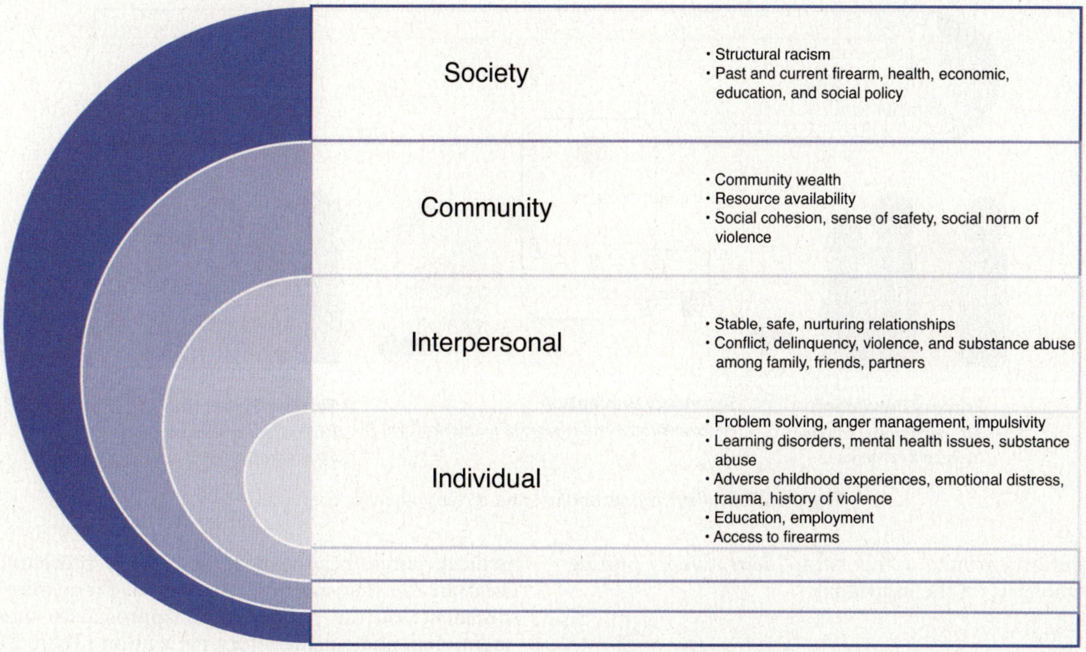

Figure 21.8. Social ecologic model for violence.

connections among family, friends, and partners can contribute as a risk or protective factor. Unstable, conflict-ridden relationships along with the presence of delinquent, violent (toward self or others), and substance abuse behaviors among family, friends, and partners can negatively impact the individual. Nurturing, safe, stable relationships, however, have the ability to positively influence outcomes even in the setting of other individual, community, or societal risk factors.[68,72,74,75]

Neighborhoods, schools, workplaces, and places of worship are part of the community level of the social ecologic model. It is where an individual lives, learns, works, prays, and plays. Community wealth is measured directly by unemployment and poverty levels and indirectly by the residential instability, crowded housing, concentration of liquor stores, and availability of green space and fresh food. Pertinent resource availability includes readily accessible health services (mental health, primary care, trauma centers, and substance abuse programs) and a trusting relationship with law enforcement. The sense of social cohesion and community safety at this level are important factors. Crime levels and the social norm of violence and substance abuse contribute to the sense of safety. Community-level poverty, lack of resources, and low sense of safety and social cohesion all increase the risk of violence. The violence that results acts as a positive feedback mechanism in that violence lowers property values, drives out resources, and propagates low sense of safety.[77–82]

Society-level factors can be at city, state, and national level. This includes past as well as current firearm, health, economic, education, and social policy that tickle down to lower social ecologic levels. It has been well documented that individual, interpersonal, and community risk factors for violence are not evenly distributed. In fact, this was discussed on the national level as early as President Johnson's National Commission on the Causes and Prevention of Violence.[58] They identified violence as a reflection of a myriad of social problems, including, but not limited to, racial segregation, low income, low levels of education, low home ownership, physical deterioration, and broken homes. The range of extreme concentration of risk factors to extreme concentration of protective factors exists to this day. The dichotomy begs the question: are there forces on a societal level that concentrate risk versus protective factors?

The discussion necessitates careful consideration of structural violence, or the unequal power and opportunity driving social determinants of health.[83,84] The long-standing history of race-based inequity, therefore, is at the root of health disparities. This goes far beyond interpersonal acts of racism, to the institutional level discriminatory policies and practices based on race. As this has occurred across sectors including housing, education, employment, healthcare, and criminal justice, these discriminatory systems reinforce one another to result in the phenomenon of structural racism.[85–87] The role institutional and structural racism play in the outcome of firearm injury can be illustrated with the example of housing.

When communities were still legally segregated by race, they were economically diverse. In the early 1930s, the Federal Housing Administration initiated a mortgage lending process called Redlining, by which the housing market prices were determined based on race, ethnicity, and religion. After neighborhoods were legally desegregated in the 1960s, only wealthy minorities could afford to move into nicer communities. This combination resulted in the concentration of poverty among the disenfranchised minority still evident today.[88] Multiple studies have shown that racially segregated, low-income communities have higher rates of firearm injury.[89–94] Even further, restrictive firearm policies may be less effective at decreasing injury in these communities.[95]

Despite the 1960 Civil Rights Act, many laws have systematically targeted poverty-stricken minority populations. The War on Drugs provides just one example. With the crack cocaine epidemic, national rhetoric created a discriminatory stereotype of "crack babies," "crack whores," "gangbangers," and "welfare queens." From 1980 to 2010, crack cocaine sentencing laws were 100 times those for powder cocaine. Even with the Fair Sentencing Act of 2010, the sentencing is still 18 times greater. Laws such as these have contributed to incarceration rates of Blacks being 3 to 10 times higher than non-Hispanic Whites. Mass incarceration has destabilized minority families and communities and further reduced education, employment, and housing opportunities. Similar examples could be discussed within education, policing, and health sectors.[85,96]

This is not to suggest impoverished White communities and wealthy minority communities do not have varying degrees of risk and protective factors. Rather, it is to bring attention to the societal-level forces which have systematically concentrated risk factors among minorities over time. Without knowing the societal forces at play, it is all too easy to oversimplify

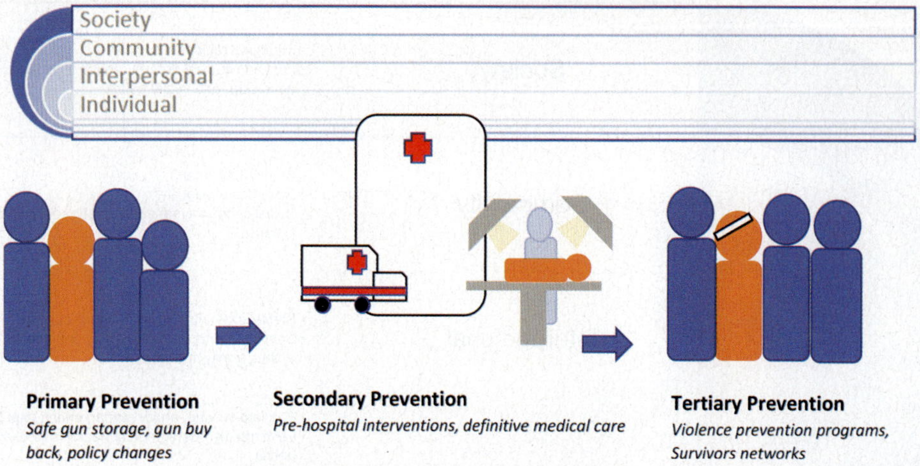

Figure 21.9. Primary, secondary, and tertiary violence prevention.

prevention efforts around a "bootstrap" narrative by putting the entire emphasis on the individual.

THE SURGEON'S ROLE IN FIREARM-RELATED INJURY AND VIOLENCE PREVENTION

The scope of the firearm-related injury and violence prevention is vast. It encompasses injury and violence in multiple forms (unintentional, suicide, interpersonal, intimate partner, child abuse) with pertinent risk factors throughout the life span across all ecologic levels (individual, interpersonal, community, and society). Thus, there are nearly endless opportunities for preventative programming and policy.[97]

5 Firearm-related injury and violence prevention takes place on a continuum: before the injury occurs (primary prevention) or after the injury occurs by minimizing the mortality, likelihood of reoccurrence (secondary prevention), and reducing long-term morbidity (tertiary prevention). The social ecologic risk and protective factors span the timeline of an injury (**Fig. 21.9**). Prevention initiatives, including programs and policies, should involve an array of stakeholders, including gun owners, vulnerable communities, law enforcement, educators, health professionals, public health professionals, and lawmakers.[98] Prior to discussing specific opportunities for surgeon involvement in prevention, it is important to review the standpoint of the surgical community on gun violence.[99–101]

There have been a variety of Association statements, including the American Association for the Surgery of Trauma, Eastern Association for the Surgery of Trauma, and the American College of Surgeons Committee on Trauma (ACS-COT).[102–104] The ACS-COT published a Consensus on firearm-related injury based on member survey (93% response rate) and meetings with surgeon leaders in town halls and professional organization meetings. While the community had varying personal opinions on gun ownership, there was agreement on the need to address the preventable morbidity and mortality of firearm injury. The majority supported healthcare worker rights, education, and training to counsel patients on safe firearm ownership (90%), federal funding for gun violence research, and the development of a research agenda (92%), universal background checks (86%), severe penalties for individuals who illegally supply guns to others (92%), and trauma center involvement in addressing the root causes of firearm injury.[105,106] The ACS-COT also created the Firearm Strategy Team (FAST), a group of firearm-owning surgeons as they offer a truly unique perspective on safe gun ownership and the prevention of injury.[71,107,108]

6 In September of 2022, the ACS hosted the second Medical Summit on Firearm Injury Prevention, joining together 46 medical, public health, legal, and injury prevention associations. In the first meeting of its kind, there were consensus statements on the public health approach to unintentional, intentional, and suicide injury prevention (**Table 21.1**). In the second meeting a new coalition was formed, the Healthcare Coalition for Firearm Injury Prevention with the directives to educate and engage healthcare professionals, advocate for effective policy, and engage in community-centered violence prevention.[99,104]

Thus, the surgical community, along with the general medical community, has reached a consensus that firearm injury and violence is a cause of preventable morbidity and mortality. It is within the surgeon's scope practice for their patients, hospitals, and communities to address the root causes of violence and make gun ownership safer. The following are specific
7 mechanisms to do so.

Primary Prevention

Primary prevention initiatives target the upstream causes of gun injury and violence to prevent incidents in the first place.

Access to a firearm is an independent risk factor for homicide and suicide.[109–111] Physicians and their representative professional associations, including internists, pediatricians and surgeons, have agreed physicians should screen and counsel patients on firearm safety.[112–117] However, the available data suggests few attending physicians and even fewer residents are discussing the topic despite the majority of patients being receptive to the conversation.[118–120] Studies regarding firearm safety counseling in outpatient and hospital settings have demonstrated an increase in the safe storage of firearms decreased firearm access among suicidal teens, and reduction in firearm injury recurrence. Supplying safety devices to patients increases sustained safe storage of firearms.[118,121–125]

In outpatient and inpatient settings, surgeons can and should be systematically screening and counseling patients on safe firearm storage much like the way we counsel on smoking cessation or weight loss. Various tools can be found to guide this conversation include courses by the American Medical Association, Massachusetts Medical Society, the University of Michigan and Scrubs Addressing the Firearm Epidemic. The ACS-COT has a Gun Safety Brochure available in English and Spanish.[126–130]

The surgeon should illicit access to firearm, safe storage, and intent to harm. Easy access to firearms is particularly risky in households with children and/or individuals with cognitive impairment, dementia, substance use disorder, mental illness, and history of violence. Nearly 5 million American children live in a home where a gun is not safely stored.[131] The patient should be asked to share their opinions regarding firearm storage. Other adults in the home may have similar or conflicting opinions. Patients should be educated that guns should

Table 21.1. Medical Summit on Firearm Injury Prevention Consensus Statements

February 2019 Medical Summit on Firearm Injury prevention Consensus Statements
Firearm injury is a public health crisis.
A comprehensive public health and medical approach is required to reduce death and disability from firearm injury.
Research is needed to better understand the root causes of violence, identify people at risk, and determine the most effective strategies for firearm injury prevention.
Federal and philanthropic research funding must be provided to match the burden of disease.
Engaging firearm owners and populations at risk is critical in developing programs and policies for firearm injury prevention.
Healthcare providers should be encouraged to counsel patients and firearm safety and safe storage. Educational and research efforts are needed to support culturally competent messaging.
Screening for the risk of depression, suicide, intimate partner violence, and interpersonal violence should be conducted across all healthcare settings and in certain high-risk populations (such as those with dementia). Comprehensive resources and interventions are needed to support patients and families identified as high risk for firearm injury and who have access to a firearm.
Hospitals and healthcare systems must genuinely engage the community in addressing the social determinants of health of disease, which contribute to structural violence in underserved communities.
Our professional organizations commit to working together and continuing to meet to ensure these statements lead to constructive actions that improve the health and well-being of our fellow Americans.

From Bulger EM, Kuhls DA, Campbell BT, et al. Proceedings from the Medical Summit on Firearm Injury Prevention: A public health approach to reduce death and disability in the US. *J Am Coll Surg*. 2019;229(4):415–430.e12.

TRAUMA

be stored locked, unloaded, separate from ammunition away from any individuals at risk for unsafe use or harm to self or others. If the patient has access to a gun, the physician to assess suicidal or homicidal intention. Any expressed intent to harm should result in the patient being committed for emergent psychiatric evaluation.[132] In some states, there are Extreme Risk Protection Orders which allows healthcare professionals, family, or law enforcement to file petitions for temporary removal of a firearm from the home.[133] Patients can and should also be made aware of any local gun buy-back programs for unwanted firearms.[134]

Surgeons can be advocates for local, state, and federal policy changes to prevent firearm injury without infringing upon the rights of firearm owners. Data-driven legislation may affect gun licensing, sales and use, firearm and ammunition availability, and research funding.[104] The number of state firearm laws varies widely (<10 to >100).[135] Studies have demonstrated cities and states with stricter firearm laws are correlated with fewer associated mortalities.[136–142] A state's homicide rates are not only associated with their own laws, but also the laws of surrounding states.[143] Restrictive laws include comprehensive background checks, which may identify a history of protective/restraining orders, domestic violence charges, fugitive status, psychiatric disorders, and misdemeanor crimes in addition to state or federal crime convictions. These features have been associated with overall decreased homicide, including intimate partner homicide, and suicide rates.[144–151] Importantly, studies have identified these laws only have an effect when properly enforced.[152,153] Restrictive legislation, however, is not uniformly beneficial. In particular, these laws were not correlated with lower homicide rate among Blacks.[95,154,155] Given the historical and contemporary structural violence and racism to this population, beneficial legislation may need to target the etiology.

In addition to tighter regulation on who can purchase a firearm, legislation also dictates the type of firearms and ammunition available to the public. High-capacity magazines, gun caliber, semiautomatic weapons, and bump stocks are all features that increase a firearm's lethality, or its capacity to render more severe injuries in a shorter time frame.[156–158] In 2004, the federal ban on assault weapons expired. Seven states have since passed new assault weapon bans. Such laws are vital given that the rate and severity of firearm injuries has been increasing.[159] While there is data to support the merit of stricter firearm legislation, there is a paucity of funding allocated for firearm injury research. This dates back to the Dickey Amendment in 1996, which dried up federal funding for gun violence prevention research. Therefore, legislation to increase and maintain the federal appropriation for firearm injury research is imperative.[160]

Surgeons are poised to leverage clinical experience to advocate for data-driven legislation regarding gun licensing, firearm and ammunition regulation, and research funding.[104,161–164] The ACS advocates on behalf of and alongside surgeons and their patients. In 2019, this included legislation which would increase in the appropriation for firearm injury prevention research. For the first time in more than 20 years, Congress appropriated federal dollars for gun violence research. Federal agencies received $25 million from Congress to study gun violence in a government spending deal reached by House and Senate negotiators. The deal included $12.5 million each for the CDC and National Institutes of Health to study gun violence and ways to prevent it.[161,165] The College and the Healthcare Coalition for Firearm Injury Prevention and the American College of Surgeon are major resources for advocacy resources ad activities.[104] Partnering with nonprofit and grassroots organizations, including the Brady Campaign, Gifford's, Mom's Demand Action, is another practical mechanism to identify advocacy opportunities on the local, state, and federal levels.[161]

Social media campaigns have also proven to be an effective mechanism to educate the public and inform policy. In the fall of 2018, front-line trauma workers joined together to share collective experiences treating firearm injury patients using the #ThisIsOurLane. This campaign was in response to the National Rifle Association's tweet suggesting physicians should "stay in their lane," suggesting a lack of expertise in firearm policy. The public and many policy makers were galvanized as a result of the campaign.[161] While advocacy work may seem overwhelming to some, there are many practical ways for a surgeon to share their professional opinion with the public, local organizations, and policy makers. In 2018, 67 pieces of gun reform legislation were passed.[166] Hopefully, this trend will continue with the support of the surgical community.

Secondary and Tertiary Prevention

Secondary and tertiary prevention initiatives aim to decrease the mortality and morbidity after an injury occurs. Survival after a firearm injury depends on location and severity of the injury as well as expedient and effective prehospital stabilization and definitive hospital care.

Unfortunately, not all regional trauma systems provide the same care resulting in a wide range of geographic-based survival rates. In the 2016 National Academies of Science Engineering and Medicine report entitled "A National Trauma Care System" the argument is made up to 20% of the annual trauma deaths may have been preventable. This landmark paper calls for a national trauma system in which the military and civilian trauma experience is shared to improve quality of care and patient outcomes.[167] These two sectors have relied on one another for high-quality preclinical and clinical research on countless topics including nonoperative versus nonoperative management, prehospital and hospital resuscitation, and mass casualty care.[168–175] This proposed system would provide infrastructure to a longstanding relationship between the military and civilian traumatologists with the goal of having zero preventable deaths due to trauma.[167]

Uncontrolled hemorrhage was found to be a major cause of preventable deaths in the military. To address this problem, the Tactical Combat Casualty Care training was developed. It taught soldiers immediate life-saving maneuvers like applying a tourniquet and combat gauze and relieving an obstructed airway. This program proved to be efficacious.[176,177] These skills translate to civilian traumatic injury.[178] In the aftermath of the Sandy Hook Elementary School shooting in 2013, a wide variety of stakeholders joined to develop the Hartford Consensus. They identified bystanders to injury as the true "first care responders" who, with the proper skill set, can control hemorrhage while waiting for first responders to arrive (EMS, police-fire). In 2015, the White House National Security Council's Office of Medical Preparedness Policy announced the Stop the Bleed campaign which would aim to target the same skill set as the Hartford Consensus based on the military's successful program (https://www.dhs.gov/stopthebleed). In 2016, the initiatives joined to train nonmedical first responders (police and fire) and, ultimately, the public.[179–182] These trainings taught the same skills and made tourniquets available in public settings. Participants reported increased ability and willingness to apply this skills should the need arise.[183]

Survivors of firearm injury face a long mental and physical recovery.[184] There are hospital-based and national trauma survivors networks to assist patients in the aftermath of injury.[185] Victims of violent injury are at increased risk of future victimization or perpetration of violence. These negative effects are felt not only by the victim, but also the community where the violence occurred.[186–188] For these reasons, community- and hospital-based prevention programs intervene after an injury as a teachable moment to address modifiable risk factors. This is a similar principle used in cardiac rehabilitation programs used to change diet and exercise following a myocardial infarction.

While these violence prevention programs are diverse in activities and scope, there are several unifying principles. Employees are typically from the community, who will be deemed credible and relatable to the patients. They are charged with the task of building and maintaining a relationship as mentors and case managers. The program assists the patient overcome barriers to meet basic needs and achieve goals. This is not an easy task, as it requires navigating the systems that have all too often already failed the individual including healthcare (mental, physical, and substance abuse) employment, education, housing, and legal aid. The patient continues to work with the program after discharge with the ultimate goal of reducing risk and increasing protective factors for future injury.[189]

The Wraparound Program based out of University of California, San Francisco and Violence Intervention Program at University of Maryland are among the well-established and well-studied hospital-based programs.[189,190] Across 22 randomized control trials of 14 different programs, there was an increase in service utilization, change in attitude regarding violence, decrease in violent behavior, and decreased repeat injury. There was a cost–benefit among the intervention arms from reduced hospital readmissions and legal costs of conviction and incarceration.[189,191–198] As the evidence as grown, several states have increased funding availability for these programs including California, New Jersey, and Virginia.[189]

The Health Alliance for Violence Interventions, formerly called the National Network of Violence Prevention Programs aims to provide infrastructure to the hospital-, community- and health department-based programs across the country HAVI has partnered with ACS-COT and the American Foundation for Firearm Injury Reduction. They provide technical assistance, conduct research, and issue best practice guidelines. While guidelines and evidence have been produced based on program experience, this infrastructure will allow for rigorous evaluation across institutions and program models.[199–201]

SUMMARY

The victims of gun injuries reflect the diversity of circumstances in which guns are used. This should come as no surprise to the surgical community. It is the older adult suicide attempt, the hunting injury, the child unintentionally wounded after finding and playing with a gun, the teenager shot during an altercation, the battered spouse, and the store patrons present during a mass shooting—all of whom are rolled into the trauma bay with devastating injuries. Despite the heavily charged political debate about firearms in the United States, decreasing firearm-related deaths and disability should be approached as a multidisciplinary public health priority with an emphasis on minimizing death and suffering through broadly based prevention efforts. Surgeons may find opportunities to support firearm prevention initiatives in and out of the hospital, locally and nationally.

References

1. Loimer H, Guarnieri M. Accidents and acts of God: a history of the terms. *Am J Public Health*. 1996;86(1):101–107.
2. Sleet DA, Baldwin G, Marr A, et al. History of Injury and Violence as public health problems and emergence of the National Center for Injury Prevention and Control at CDC. *J Safety Res*. 2012;43(4):233–247.
3. Godfrey ES. Role of the health department in the prevention of accidents. *Am J Public Health Nations Health*. 1937;27(2):152–155.
4. Gordon JE. The epidemiology of accidents. *Am J Public Health Nations Health*. 1949;39(4):504–515.
5. American Public Health Association. *Accident Prevention: The Role of the Physician and Public Health Workers*. McGraw Hill; 1961.
6. National Research Council. *Accidental Death and Disability: the Neglected Disease of Modern Society*. National Academies Press (US); 1966.
7. Haddon W Jr. A logical framework for categorizing highway safety phenomena and activity. *J Trauma*. 1972;12(3):193–207.
8. Guarnieri M. Landmarks in the history of safety. *J Safety Research*. 1992;23(3):151–158.
9. National Center for Injury Prevention and Control. WISQARS (Web-based Injury Statistics Query and Reporting System)|Injury Center|Centers for Disease Control and Prevention: Injury

Prevention & Control Data and Statistic (WISQARS). https://www.cdc.gov/injury/wisqars/index.html. Published March 30, 2020. Accessed June 15, 2024.
10. National Research Council. *Injury in America: A Continuing Health Care Problem*. National Academies Press; 1985.
11. National Violent Death Reporting System|NVDRS|Violence Prevention|Injury Center| Centers for Disease Control and Prevention. https://www.cdc.gov/violenceprevention/datasources/nvdrs/index.html. Published November 07, 2019. Accessed June 18, 2020.
12. Cook A, Osler T, Hosmer D, et al. Gunshot wounds resulting in hospitalization in the United States: 2004–2013. *Injury.* 2017;48(3):621–627.
13. Fowler KA, Dahlberg LL, Haileyesus T, et al. Firearm injuries in the United States. *Prev Med.* 2015;79:5–14.
14. Major Cities Chiefs Police Association. Violent Crime Reports. https://majorcitieschiefs.com/resources/. Published August 8, 2024. Accessed September 15, 2024.
15. Houry DE, Simon TR, Crosby AE. Firearm homicide and suicide during the COVID-19 pandemic: implications for clinicians and health care systems. *JAMA.* 2022;327(19):1867–1868.
16. Sakran JV, Lunardi N, Mehta A, et al. Increasing injury intensity among 6500 violent deaths in the state of Maryland. *J Am Coll Surg.* 2024;238(4):710–717.
17. Washing Post Staff. There have been 22 mass killings with guns in 2024. *The Washington Post.* https://www.washingtonpost.com/nation/interactive/mass-shootings/. Updated September 4, 2024. Accessed August 15, 2024.
18. Feldman JM, Gruskin S, Coull BA, Krieger N. Quantifying underreporting of law-enforcement-related deaths in United States vital statistics and news-media-based data sources: A capture- recapture analysis. *PLoS Med.* 2017;14(10):e1002399.
19. Mooney AC, McConville S, Rappaport AJ, Hsia RY. Association of legal intervention injuries with race and ethnicity among patients treated in emergency departments in California. *JAMA Netw Open.* 2018;1(5):e182150.
20. Leemis RW, Friar N, Khatiwada S, et al. *National Intimate Partner and Sexual Violence Survey: 2016/2017 Report on Intimate Partner Violence*. Center for Disease Control and Prevention; 2022.
21. Peterson C, Kearns MC, McIntosh WL, Estefan LF, Nicolaidis C, McCollister KE, Florence C. Lifetime economic burden of intimate partner violence among US adults. *Am J Prev Med.* 2018;55(4):433–444.
22. U.S. Department of Health & Human Services, Administration for Children and Families, Administration on Children, Youth and Families, Children's Bureau. Child Maltreatment 2022. 2024. https://www.acf.hhs.gov/cb/data-research/child-maltreatment
23. Webster DW, Cerdá M, Wintemute GJ, Cook PJ. Epidemiologic evidence to guide the understanding and prevention of gun violence. *Epidemiol Rev.* 2016;38(1):1–4.
24. CDC—The National Institute for Occupational Safety and Health (NIOSH). Centers for Disease Control and Prevention. https://www.cdc.gov/NIOSH/. Published May 25, 2018. Accessed July 15, 2020.
25. National Institute for Occupational Safety and Health. *ALERT: Preventing Needlestick Injuries in Health Care Settings*. NIOSH Publications Dissemination; 1999.
26. Occupational Safety and Health Administration (OSHA) United States Department of Labor. OSHA Directives 2-2.44D—Enforcement procedures for the occupational exposure to bloodborne pathogens. https://www.osha.gov/enforcement/directives/cpl-2-244d/. Published November 5, 1999. Accessed July 15, 2020.
27. Cardo DM, Culver DH, Ciesielski CA, et al. A case-control study of HIV seroconversion in health care workers after percutaneous exposure. Centers for Disease Control and Prevention Needlestick Surveillance Group. *N Engl J Med.* 1997;337(21):1485–1490.
28. Jagger J, Hunt EH, Brand-Elnaggar J, Pearson RD. Rates of needle-stick injury caused by various devices in a university hospital. *N Engl J Med.* 1988;319(5):284–288.
29. Gartner K. Impact of a needleless intravenous system in a university hospital. *Am J Infect Control.* 1992;20(2):75–79.
30. Lawrence LW, Delclos GL, Felknor SA, et al. The effectiveness of a needleless intravenous connection system: an assessment by injury rate and user satisfaction. *Infect Control Hosp Epidemiol.* 1997;18(3):175–182.
31. Yassi A, McGill ML, Khokhar JB. Efficacy and cost-effectiveness of a needleless intravenous access system. *Am J Infect Control.* 1995;23(2):57–64.
32. Sharps Safety for Healthcare Settings. Centers for Disease Control and Prevention. https://www.cdc.gov/sharpssafety/. Published February 11, 2015. Accessed July 18, 2020.
33. Gielen AC, Green LW. The impact of policy, environmental, and educational interventions: a synthesis of the evidence from two public health success stories. *Health Educ Behav.* 2015;42(1 Suppl):20S–34S.
34. Bergen G, Pitan A, Qu S, et al. Publicized sobriety checkpoint programs: a community guide systematic review. *Am J Prev Med.* 2014;46(5):529–539.
35. Institute of Medicine (US) Committee on Injury Prevention and Control, Bonnie RJ, Fulco CE, Liverman CT, eds. *Reducing the Burden of Injury: Advancing Prevention and Treatment.* National Academies Press (US); 1999.
36. Centers for Disease Control and Prevention. Ten great public health achievements—United States, 1900–1999. *MMWR Morb Mortal Wkly Rep.* 1999;48(12):241–243. https://www.cdc.gov/mmwr/preview/mmwrhtml/00056796.htm. Published April 2, 1999. Accessed July 15, 2020.
37. Nichols JL. Changing public behavior for better health: is education enough? *Am J Prev Med.* 1994;10(3 Suppl):19–22.
38. Rivara FP, Thompson DC, Beahler C, MacKenzie EJ. Systematic reviews of strategies to prevent motor vehicle injuries. *Am J Prev Med.* 1999;16(1 Suppl):1–5.
39. Waller PF. Public health's contribution to motor vehicle injury prevention. *Am J Prev Med.* 2001;21(4 Suppl):3–4.
40. Zwerling C, Jones MP. Evaluation of the effectiveness of low blood alcohol concentration laws for younger drivers. *Am J Prev Med.* 1999;16(1 Suppl):76–80.
41. Tung GJ, Vernick JS, Stuart EA, Webster DW, Gielen AC. Federal actions to incentivise state adoption of 0.08 g/dL blood alcohol concentration laws. *Inj Prev.* 2017;23(5):309–313.
42. Seat Belts. National Highway Traffic Safety Administration. United Stated Department of Transportation. https://www.nhtsa.gov/risky-driving/seat-belts. Published January 15, 2020. Accessed July 15, 2020.
43. Chen LH, Baker SP, Li G. Graduated driver licensing programs and fatal crashes of 16-year-old drivers: a national evaluation. *Pediatrics.* 2006;118(1):56–62.
44. Shope JT, Molnar LJ, Elliott MR, Waller PF. Graduated driver licensing in Michigan: early impact on motor vehicle crashes among 16-year-old drivers. *JAMA.* 2001;286(13):1593–1598.
45. Nader R. Unsafe at any speed: the designed-in dangers of the American automobile. 1965. *Am J Public Health.* 2011;101(2):254–256.
46. Eriksen MP, Gielen AC. The application of health education principles to automobile child restraint programs. *Health Educ Q.* 1983;10(1):30–55.
47. Children's Safety Network. Health resources and services administration. https://www.childrenssafetynetwork.org/. Published June 19, 2020. Accessed July 15, 2020.
48. Pressley JC, Barlow B. Child and adolescent injury as a result of falls from buildings and structures. *Inj Prev.* 2005;11(5):267–273.
49. Gielen AC, McDonald EM, Wilson ME, et al. Effects of improved access to safety counseling, products, and home visits on parents' safety practices: results of a randomized trial. *Arch Pediatr Adolesc Med.* 2002;156(1):33–40.
50. Kendrick D, Illingworth R, Woods A, et al. Promoting child safety in primary care: a cluster randomised controlled trial to reduce baby walker use. *Br J Gen Pract.* 2005;55(517):582–588.
51. Phelan KJ, Khoury J, Xu Y, Liddy S, Hornung R, Lanphear BP. A randomized controlled trial of home injury hazard

reduction: the HOME injury study. *Arch Pediatr Adolesc Med.* 2011;165(4):339–345.

52. Hubbard S, Cooper N, Kendrick D, et al. Network meta-analysis to evaluate the effectiveness of interventions to prevent falls in children under age 5 years. *Inj Prev.* 2015;21(2):98–108.
53. Owen R, Kendrick D, Mulvaney C, Coleman T, Royal S. Non-legislative interventions for the promotion of cycle helmet wearing by children. *Cochrane Database Syst Rev.* 2011;(11):CD003985.
54. Sibert JR, Mott A, Rolfe K, et al. Preventing injuries in public playgrounds through partnership between health services and local authority: community intervention study. *BMJ.* 1999; 318(7198):1595.
55. Chalmers DJ, Marshall SW, Langley JD, et al. Height and surfacing as risk factors for injury in falls from playground equipment: a case-control study. *Inj Prev.* 1996;2(2):98–104.
56. Schnitzer PG, Dowd MD, Kruse RL, Morrongiello BA. Supervision and risk of unintentional injury in young children. *Inj Prev.* 2015;21(e1): e63–e70.
57. Barlow B, Niemirska M, Gandhi RP, Leblanc W. Ten years of experience with falls from a height in children. *J Pediatr Surg.* 1983;18(4):509–511.
58. National Commission on the Causes and Prevention of Violence. *To Establish Justice, to Insure Domestic Tranquility: Final Report of the National Commission on the Causes and Prevention of Violence.* U.S. Government Printing Office; 1969.
59. Department of Health and Human Services. *Healthy People: the Surgeon General's Report on Health Promotion and Disease Prevention.* U.S. Government Printing Office; 1979.
60. Department of Health and Human Services. *Promoting Health, Preventing Disease; Objectives for the Nation.* U.S. Government Printing Office; 1980.
61. Healthy People Office of Disease Prevention and Health Promotion. https://www.healthypeople.gov/. Accessed June 15, 2020.
62. Department of Health and Human Services. *Report if the Secretary's Task Force on Black and Minority Health.* National Center for Environmental Health and Injury Control Division of Injury Control, Office of the Assistant Director for Minority Health; 1985.
63. Department of Health and Human Services, Department of Justice. *Surgeon General's Workshop on Violence in Public Health Report.* Health Resources and Services Administration; 1985.
64. Carmona R. Life on both sides of the gun: a surgeon general's call to action. *CurrTrauma Rep.* 2020;6(1):1–4.
65. Maa J, Darzi A. Firearm injuries and violence prevention—the potential power of a surgeon general's report. *N Engl J Med.* 2018;379(5):408–410.
66. National Center for Injury Prevention and Control |Injury Center|Centers for Disease Control and Prevention. https://www.cdc.gov/injury/index.html. Published May 11, 2020. Accessed June 18, 2020.
67. Fenley MA. *The Prevention of Youth Violence: a Framework for Community Action.* Centers for Disease Control and Prevention, National Center for Injury Prevention and Control, Office of the Assistant Director for Minority Health; 1993.
68. Office of the Surgeon General, National Center for Injury Prevention and Control, National Institute of Mental Health, Center for Mental Health Services. *Youth Violence: a Report of the Surgeon General.* Department of Health and Human Services, U.S. Public Health Service; 2001.
69. Kellermann AL, Rivara FP. Silencing the science on gun research. *JAMA.* 2013;309(6):549–550.
70. Strong BM, Sangji NF, Barrera K. Gun violence and firearm policy in the U.S.: A brief history and the current status. *Bull Am Coll Surg.* 2018;103(7):26–33.
71. Barry CL, Webster DW, Stone E, Crifasi CK, Vernick JS, McGinty EE. Public support for gun violence prevention policies among gun owners and non-gun owners in 2017. *Am J Public Health.* 2018;108(7):878–881.
72. Wilkins, N, Tsao, B, Hertz, M, et al. *Connecting the Dots: An Overview of the Links Among Multiple Forms of Violence.* National Center for Injury Prevention and Control, Centers for Disease Control and Prevention: Prevention Institute; 2014.
73. Lubell KM, Vetter JB. Suicide and youth violence prevention: the promise of an integrated approach. *Aggress Violent Behav.* 2006;11(2):167–175.
74. American Psychological Association. *Gun violence: Prediction, Prevention, and Policy.* American Psychological Association; 2013. http://www.apa.org/pubs/info/reports/gun-violence-report.pdf
75. David-Ferdon C, Vivolo-Kantor AM, Dahlberg LL, et al. *A Comprehensive Technical Package for the Prevention of Youth Violence and Associated Risk Behaviors.* National Center for Injury Prevention and Control, Centers for Disease Control and Prevention; 2016.
76. Milam AJ, Furr-Holden CD, Leaf P, Webster D. Managing conflicts in urban communities: youth attitudes regarding gun violence. *J Interpers Violence.* 2018;33(24):3815–3828.
77. McGinty EE, Webster DW. The roles of alcohol and drugs in firearm violence. *JAMA Intern Med.* 2017;177(3):324–325.
78. Franklin FA, Laveist TA, Webster DW, et al. Alcohol outlets and violent crime in Washington DC. *West J Emerg Med.* 2010;11(3): 283–290.
79. Rohrer JE, Arif AA, Pierce JR Jr, Blackburn C. Unsafe neighborhoods, social group activity, and self-rated health. *J Public Health Manag Pract.* 2004;10(2):124–129.
80. Widener MJ, Metcalf SS, Bar-Yam Y. Dynamic urban food environments a temporal analysis of access to healthy foods. *Am J Prev Med.* 2011;41(4):439–441.
81. Molnar BE, Gortmaker SL, Bull FC, Buka SL. Unsafe to play? Neighborhood disorder and lack of safety predict reduced physical activity among urban children and adolescents. *Am J Health Promot.* 2004;18(5):378–386.
82. McNeely CA, Nonnemaker JM, Blum RW. Promoting school connectedness: evidence from the National Longitudinal Study of Adolescent Health. *J Sch Health.* 2002;72(4):138–146.
83. Galtung J. Violence, peace, and peace research. *J Peace Res.* 1969;6(3):167–191.
84. Farmer PE, Nizeye B, Stulac S, Keshavjee S. Structural violence and clinical medicine. *PLoS Med.* 2006;3(10):e449.
85. Bailey ZD, Krieger N, Agénor M, Graves J, Linos N, Bassett MT. Structural racism and health inequities in the USA: evidence and interventions. *The Lancet.* 2017;389(10077):1453–1463.
86. Boeck MA, Strong B, Campbell A. Disparities in firearm injury: consequences of structural violence. *Curr Trauma Rep.* 2020;6(1):10–22.
87. Bonne S, Dicker RA. Hospital-based violence intervention programs to address social determinants of health and violence. *Curr Trauma Rep.* 2020;6(1):23–28.
88. Pietila A. *Not in My Neighborhood: How Bigotry Shaped a Great American City.* Ivan R Dee, Inc; 2012.
89. Knopov A, Rothman EF, Cronin SW, et al. The role of racial residential segregation in black-white disparities in firearm homicide at the state level in the United States, 1991–2015. *J Natl Med Assoc.* 2019;111(1):62–75.
90. Rowhani-Rahbar A, Quistberg DA, Morgan ER, Hajat A, Rivara FP. Income inequality and firearm homicide in the US: a county-level cohort study. *Inj Prev.* 2019;25(Suppl 1):i25–i30.
91. Kalesan B, Vyliparambil MA, Bogue E, et al. Race and ethnicity, neighborhood poverty and pediatric firearm hospitalizations in the United States. *Ann Epidemiol.* 2016;26(1):1–6.e62.
92. Carter PM, Cook LJ, Macy ML, et al. Pediatric Emergency Care Applied Research Network (PECARN). Individual and neighborhood characteristics of children seeking Emergency Department care for firearm injuries within the PECARN Network. *Acad Emerg Med.* 2017;24(7):803–813.
93. Krieger N, Feldman JM, Waterman PD, Chen JT, Coull BA, Hemenway D. Local residential segregation matters: stronger association of census tract compared to conventional city-level measures with fatal and non-fatal assaults (total and firearm related), using the Index of Concentration at the Extremes (ICE) for Racial, Economic, and Racialized Economic Segregation, Massachusetts (US), 1995–2010. *J Urban Health.* 2017;94(2):244–258.

94. Beardslee J, Docherty M, Mulvey E, Pardini D. The direct and indirect associations between childhood socioeconomic disadvantage and adolescent gun violence. *J Clin Child Adolesc Psychol.* 2021;50(3):326–336.
95. Resnick S, Smith RN, Beard JH, et al. Firearm deaths in America: can we learn from 462,000 lives lost? *Ann Surg.* 2017;266(3):432–440.
96. Alexander M. *The New Jim Crow: Mass Incarceration in the Age of Colorblindness.* New Press; 2012.
97. Hemenway D, Miller M. Public health approach to the prevention of gun violence. *N Engl J Med.* 2013;368(21):2033–2035.
98. Barber C, Frank E, Demicco R. Reducing suicides through partnerships between health professionals and gun owner groups beyond Docs vs Glocks. *JAMA Intern Med.* 2017;177(1):5–6.
99. Bulger EM, Kuhls DA, Campbell BT, et al. Proceedings from the Medical Summit on Firearm Injury Prevention: A public health approach to reduce death and disability in the US. *J Am Coll Surg.* 2019;229(4):415–430.e12.
100. American Association for the Surgery of Trauma (AAST) Board of Managers. AAST statement on firearm injury. *Trauma Surg Acute Care Open.* 2018;3(1):e000204.
101. Stewart RM, Kuhls DA. Firearm injury prevention: A consensus approach to reducing preventable deaths. *J Trauma Acute Care Surg.* 2016;80(6):850–852.
102. Streib E, Blake D, Christmas AB, et al. American Association for the Surgery of Trauma statement on firearm injuries. *J Trauma Acute Care Surg.* 2016;80(6):849.
103. Eastern Association for the Surgery of Trauma Firearm Injury Prevention Statement. *J Trauma Acute Care Surg.* 2019;86(1):168–170.
104. Sakran JV, Bornstein SS, Dicker R, et al. Proceedings from the Second Medical Summit on Firearm Injury Prevention, 2022: creating a sustainable healthcare coalition to advance a multidisciplinary public health approach. *J Am Coll Surg.* 2023;236(6):1242–1260.
105. Kuhls DA, Campbell BT, Burke PA, et al. Survey of American College of Surgeons Committee on trauma members on firearm injury: Consensus and opportunities. *J Trauma Acute Care Surg.* 2017;82(5):877–886.
106. Puls MW, Kuhls DA, Campbell BT, et al. Survey of the American College of Surgeons Board of governors on firearm injury prevention: consensus and opportunities. *Bull Am Coll Surg.* 2017;102(10):30–36.
107. Stewart RM, Kuhls DA, Rotondo MF, Bulger EM. Freedom with Responsibility: A consensus strategy for preventing injury, death, and disability from firearm violence. *J Am Coll Surg.* 2018;227(2):281–283.
108. Talley CL, Campbell BT, Jenkins DH, et al. Recommendations from the American College of Surgeons Committee on Trauma's Firearm Strategy Team (FAST) Workgroup: Chicago Consensus I. *J Am Coll Surg.* 2019;228(2):198–206.
109. Anglemyer A, Horvath T, Rutherford G. The accessibility of firearms and risk for suicide and homicide victimization among household members: a systematic review and meta-analysis. *Ann Intern Med.* 2014;160(2):101–110.
110. Siegel M, Rothman EF. Firearm ownership and suicide rates among US Men and Women, 1981–2013. *Am J Public Health.* 2016;106(7):1316–1322.
111. van Aalst JA, Shotts SD, Vitsky JL, et al. Long-term follow-up of unsuccessful violent suicide attempts: risk factors for subsequent attempts. *J Trauma.* 1992;33(3):457–464.
112. McLean RM, Harris P, Cullen J, et al. Firearm-related injury and death in the United States: a call to action from the nation's leading physician and public health professional organizations. *Ann Intern Med.* 2019;171(8):573–577.
113. Butkus R, Weissman A. Internists' attitudes toward prevention of firearm injury. *Ann Intern Med.* 2014;160(12):821–827.
114. Cassel CK, Nelson EA, Smith TW, Schwab CW, Barlow B, Gary NE. Internists' and surgeons' attitudes toward guns and firearm injury prevention. *Ann Intern Med.* 1998;128(3):224–230.
115. Dowd MD, Sege RD; Council on Injury, Violence, and Poison Prevention Executive Committee, American Academy of Pediatrics. Firearm-related injuries affecting the pediatric population. *Pediatrics.* 2012;130(5):e1416–e1423.
116. Campbell BT, Thaker S, Fallat ME, et al. A multicenter evaluation of a firearm safety intervention in the pediatric outpatient setting. *J Pediatr Surg.* 2020;55(1):140–145.
117. Frattaroli S, Webster DW, Wintemute GJ. Implementing a public health approach to gun violence prevention: the importance of physician engagement. *Ann Intern Med.* 2013;158(9):697–698.
118. Wintemute GJ, Betz ME, Ranney ML. Yes, you can: physicians, patients, and firearms. *Ann Intern Med.* 2016;165(3):205–213.
119. Wallace LN. Concealed ownership: Americans' perceived comfort sharing gun ownership status with others. *Sociological Spectrum.* 2017;37(5):267–281.
120. Betz ME, Azrael D, Barber C, Miller M. Public opinion regarding whether speaking with patients about firearms is appropriate: results of a national survey. *Ann Intern Med.* 2016;165(8):543–550.
121. Violano P, Bonne S, Duncan T, et al. Prevention of firearm injuries with gun safety devices and safe storage: An Eastern Association for the Surgery of Trauma Systematic Review. *J Trauma Acute Care Surg.* 2018;84(6):1003–1011.
122. Rowhani-Rahbar A, Simonetti JA, Rivara FP. Effectiveness of interventions to promote safe firearm storage. *Epidemiol Rev.* 2016;38(1):111–124.
123. Albright TL, Burge SK. Improving firearm storage habits: impact of brief office counseling by family physicians. *J Am Board Fam Pract.* 2003;16(1):40–46.
124. Vernick JS, O'Brien M, Hepburn LM, Johnson SB, Webster DW, Hargarten SW. Unintentional and undetermined firearm related deaths: a preventable death analysis for three safety devices. *Inj Prev.* 2003;9(4):307–311.
125. Crifasi CK, Doucette ML, McGinty EE, Webster DW, Barry CL. Storage practices of US gun owners in 2016. *Am J Public Health.* 2018;108(4):532–537.
126. O'Reilly KB. Talking firearms in the exam room: 3 cases where it matters. American Medical Association. https://www.amaassn.org/delivering-care/public-health/talking-firearms-exam-room-3-cases-where-it-matters. Published December 20, 2018. Accessed June 18, 2020.
127. Talking to Patients About Gun Safety. Massachusetts Medical Society: Talking to Patients About Gun Safety. https://www.massmed.org/Continuing-Education-and-Events/Online-CME/Courses/Patient-Conversations-About-Firearms/Talking-to-Patients--About-Gun-Safety/. Accessed June 18, 2020.
128. Naughton M, Rajput S, Hashikawa A, et al. Pilot of an asynchronous web-based video curriculum to improve firearm safety counseling by pediatric residents. *Acad Pediatr.* 2020;20(4):565–568.
129. SAFE's Mission. SAFE: Scrubs Addressing the Firearm Epidemic. https://www.standsafe.org/projects. Accessed July 18, 2020.
130. Gun Safety and Your Health: A Proactive Guide to Protect You and Those Around You. American College of Surgeons Committee on Trauma Firearm Injury Prevention Activities. https://www.facs.org/quality-programs/trauma/advocacy/ipc/firearm-injury. Accessed June 18, 2020.
131. Azrael D, Cohen J, Salhi C, Miller M. Firearm storage in gun-owning households with children: results of a 2015 National Survey. *J Urban Health.* 2018;95(3):295–304.
132. Butkus R, Doherty R, Bornstein SS, et al. Reducing firearm injuries and deaths in the United States: A position paper from the American College of Physicians. *Ann Intern Med.* 2018;169(10):704–707.
133. Gondi S, Pomerantz AG, Sacks CA. Extreme risk protection orders: an opportunity to improve gun violence prevention training. *Acad Med.* 2019;94(11):1649–1653.
134. Hazeltine MD, Green J, Cleary MA, et al. A review of gun buybacks. *CurrTrauma Rep.* 2019;5(4):174–177.
135. Siegel M, Pahn M, Xuan Z, et al. Firearm-related laws in all 50 US states, 1991–2016. *Am J Public Health.* 2017;107(7):1122–1129.

136. Jehan F, Pandit V, O'Keeffe T, et al. The burden of firearm violence in the United States: stricter laws result in safer states. *J Inj Violence Res.* 2018;10(1):11–16.
137. Safavi A, Rhee P, Pandit V, et al. Children are safer in states with strict firearm laws: a National Inpatient Sample study. *J Trauma Acute Care Surg.* 2014;76(1):146–151.
138. Fleegler EW, Lee LK, Monuteaux MC, Hemenway D, Mannix R. Firearm legislation and firearm-related fatalities in the United States. *JAMA Intern Med.* 2013;173(9):732–740.
139. Madhavan S, Taylor JS, Chandler JM, Staudenmayer KL, Chao SD. Firearm legislation stringency and firearm-related fatalities among children in the US. *J Am Coll Surg.* 2019;229(2): 150–157.
140. Crandall M, Eastman A, Violano P, et al. Prevention of firearm-related injuries with restrictive licensing and concealed carry laws: An Eastern Association for the Surgery of Trauma systematic review. *J Trauma Acute Care Surg.* 2016;81(5): 952–960.
141. Zeoli AM, Webster DW. Firearm policies that work. *JAMA.* 2019;321(10):937–938.
142. Crifasi CK, Merrill-Francis M, Webster DW, Wintemute GJ, Vernick JS. Changes in the legal environment and enforcement of firearm transfer laws in Pennsylvania and Maryland. *Inj Prev.* 2019;25(Suppl 1):i2–i4.
143. Olson EJ, Hoofnagle M, Kaufman EJ, Schwab CW, Reilly PM, Seamon MJ. American firearm homicides: the impact of your neighbors. *J Trauma Acute Care Surg.* 2019;86(5):797–802.
144. Sen B, Panjamapirom A. State background checks for gun purchase and firearm deaths: an exploratory study. *Prev Med.* 2012;55(4):346–350.
145. Sumner SA, Layde PM, Guse CE. Firearm death rates and association with level of firearm purchase background check. *Am J Prev Med.* 2008;35(1):1–6.
146. Vigdor ER, Mercy JA. Do laws restricting access to firearms by domestic violence offenders prevent intimate partner homicide? *Eval Rev.* 2006;30(3):313–346.
147. Kalesan B, Mobily ME, Keiser O, Fagan JA, Galea S. Firearm legislation and firearm mortality in the USA: a cross-sectional, state-level study. *Lancet.* 2016;387(10030):1847–1855.
148. Castillo-Carniglia A, Webster DW, Wintemute GJ. Effect on background checks of newly-enacted comprehensive background check policies in Oregon and Washington: a synthetic control approach. *Inj Epidemiol.* 2019;6:15.
149. Vittes KA, Webster DW, Frattaroli S, Claire BE, Wintemute GJ. Removing guns from batterers: findings from a pilot survey of domestic violence restraining order recipients in California. *Violence Against Women.* 2013;19(5):602–616.
150. Webster DW, Wintemute GJ. Effects of policies designed to keep firearms from high-risk individuals. *Annu Rev Public Health.* 2015;36:21–37.
151. McGinty EE, Webster DW, Barry CL. Gun policy and serious mental illness: priorities for future research and policy. *Psychiatr Serv.* 2014;65(1):50–58.
152. Castillo-Carniglia A, Kagawa RMC, Webster DW, Vernick JS, Cerdá M, Wintemute GJ. Comprehensive background check policy and firearm background checks in three US states. *Inj Prev.* 2018;24(6):431–436.
153. Castillo-Carniglia A, Kagawa RMC, Cerdá M, et al. California's comprehensive background check and misdemeanor violence prohibition policies and firearm mortality. *Ann Epidemiol.* 2019;30:50–56.
154. Crifasi CK, Merrill-Francis M, McCourt A, Vernick JS, Wintemute GJ, Webster DW. Association between Firearm Laws and Homicide in Urban Counties. *J Urban Health.* 2018;95(3): 383–390.
155. Vernick JS, Webster DW. Policies to prevent firearm trafficking. *Inj Prev.* 2007;13(2):78–79.
156. de Jager E, Goralnick E, McCarty JC, Hashmi ZG, Jarman MP, Haider AH. Lethality of civilian active shooter incidents with and without semiautomatic rifles in the United States. *JAMA.* 2018;320(10):1034–1035.
157. Braga AA, Cook PJ. The Association of Firearm Caliber with likelihood of death from gunshot injury in criminal assaults. *JAMA Netw Open.* 2018;1(3):e180833.
158. Fackler ML, Malinowski JA, Hoxie SW, Jason A. Wounding effects of the AK-47 rifle used by Patrick Purdy in the Stockton, California, schoolyard shooting of January 17, 1989. *Am J Forensic Med Pathol.* 1990;11(3):185–189.
159. Joseph B, Bible L, Hanna K. Developing data-driven solutions to firearm violence. *Curr Trauma Rep.* 2020;6(1):44–50.
160. He K, Sakran JV. Elimination of the moratorium on gun research is not enough: the need for the CDC to set a budgetary agenda. *JAMA Surg.* 2019;154(3):195–196.
161. Sakran JV, Maa J, Masiakos PT. Turning experience into action: this is our lane. *Curr Trauma Rep.* 2020;6(1):5–9.
162. Rubin R. Physicians are steering the conversation about gun violence. *JAMA.* 2019;321(2):133–135.
163. Galea S. Physicians' voices on gun violence and other important-public health issues. *JAMA.* 2019;321(2):141–142.
164. Masiakos PT, Griggs C. The quiet room. *N Engl J Med.* 2017; 377(25):2411–2412.
165. American College of Surgeons. American College of Surgeons Leadership & Advocacy Summit Participants Discuss Health Policy Priorities with Legislators. https://giffords.org/lawcenter/trendwatch/gun-law-trendwatch-december-14-2018/.
166. Anderman A. Gun Law Trend Watch 2018 Year-End Review. Giffords Law Center to Prevent Gun Violence. https://lawcenter.giffords.org/wp-content/uploads/2018/12/Giffords-Law-Center-Year-End-Trendwatch-2018_Digital-Spreads.pdf. Published December 14, 2018. Accessed July 18, 2020.
167. National Academies of Sciences, Engineering, and Medicine. A National Trauma Care System: Integrating military and civilian trauma systems to achieve zero preventable deaths after injury. *Mil Med.* 2017;182(5):1563–1565.
168. Welch CE. War wounds of the abdomen. *N Engl J Med.* 1947; 237(6):187–194.
169. Shaftan GW. Indications for operation in abdominal trauma. *Am J Surg.* 1960;99:657–664.
170. Propper BW, Rasmussen TE, Davidson SB, et al. Surgical response to multiple casualty incidents following single explosive events. *Ann Surg.* 2009;250(2):311–315.
171. Eastridge BJ, Mabry RL, Seguin P, et al. Death on the battlefield (2001-2011): implications for the future of combat casualty care. *J Trauma Acute Care Surg.* 2012;73(6 Suppl 5):S431–S437.
172. Borgman MA, Spinella PC, Perkins JG, et al. The ratio of blood products transfused affects mortality in patients receiving massive transfusions at a combat support hospital. *J Trauma.* 2007;63(4):805–813.
173. Gonzalez E, Moore EE, Moore HB, et al. Goal-directed hemostatic resuscitation of trauma-induced coagulopathy: a pragmatic randomized clinical trial comparing a viscoelastic assay to conventional coagulation assays. *Ann Surg.* 2016;263(6): 1051–1059.
174. Sperry JL, Guyette FX, Brown JB, et al. Prehospital Plasma during air medical transport in trauma patients at risk for hemorrhagic shock. *N Engl J Med.* 2018;379(4):315–326.
175. Cooper G, Laskowski-Jones L. Development of trauma care systems. *Prehospital Emergency Care.* 2006;10:328–331.
176. Kragh JF Jr, Walters TJ, Baer DG, et al. Practical use of emergency tourniquets to stop bleeding in major limb trauma. *J Trauma.* 2008;64(2 Suppl):S38–S50.
177. Kotwal RS, Montgomery HR, Kotwal BM, et al. Eliminating preventable death on the battlefield. *Arch Surg.* 2011;146(12): 1350–1358.
178. Rasmussen TE, Baer DG, Goolsby C. The giving back: Battlefield lesson to national preparedness. *J Trauma Acute Care Surg.* 2016;80(1):166–167.
179. Jacobs LM, Warshaw AL, Burns KJ. Empowering the public to improve survival in mass casualty events. *Ann Surg.* 2016; 263(5):860–861.
180. Callaway D, Bobko J, Smith ER, et al. Building community resilience to dynamic mass casualty incidents: A multiagency white

paper in support of the first care provider. *J Trauma Acute Care Surg.* 2016;80(4):665–669.
181. Department of Homeland Security. Stop the Bleed. https://www.dhs.gov/stopthebleed. Published July 14, 2020. Accessed July 18, 2020.
182. Knudson MM, Velmahos G, Cooper ZR. Response to mass casualty events: from the battlefield to the Stop the Bleed campaign. *Trauma Surg Acute Care Open.* 2016;1(1):e000023.
183. Jacobs LM, Burns KJ, Langer G, Kiewiet de Jonge C. The hartford consensus: A national survey of the public regarding bleeding control. *J Am Coll Surg.* 2016;222(5):948–955.
184. Joseph B, Hanna K, Callcut RA, Coleman JJ, Sakran JV, Neumayer LA. The hidden burden of mental health outcomes following firearm-related injuries. *Ann Surg.* 2019;270(4):593–601.
185. American Trauma Society. Trauma Survivors Network—Survive Connect Rebuild. https://www.traumasurvivorsnetwork.org/pages/home. Accessed June 18, 2020.
186. Corbin TJ, Purtle J, Rich LJ, et al. The prevalence of trauma and childhood adversity in an urban, hospital-based violence intervention program. *J Health Care Poor Underserved.* 2013;24(3):1021–1030.
187. Reese C, Pederson T, Avila S, et al. Screening for traumatic stress among survivors of urban trauma. *J Trauma Acute Care Surg.* 2012;73(2):462–468.
188. Gillikin C, Habib L, Evces M, Bradley B, Ressler KJ, Sanders J. Trauma exposure and PTSD symptoms associate with violence in inner city civilians. *J Psychiatr Res.* 2016;83:1–7.
189. Smith R, Evans A, Adams C, Cocanour C, Dicker R. Passing the torch: evaluating exportability of a violence intervention program. *Am J Surg.* 2013;206(2):223–228.
190. Cooper C, Eslinger DM, Stolley PD. Hospital-based violence intervention programs work. *J Trauma.* 2006;61(3):534–540.
191. James TL, Bibi S, Langlois BK, Dugan E, Mitchell PM. Boston violence intervention advocacy program: A qualitative study of client experiences and perceived effect. *Acad Emerg Med.* 2014;21(7):742–751.
192. Juillard C, Cooperman L, Allen I, et al. A decade of hospital-based violence intervention: benefits and shortcomings. *J Trauma Acute Care Surg.* 2016;81(6):1156–1161.
193. Juillard C, Smith R, Anaya N, Garcia A, Kahn JG, Dicker RA. Saving lives and saving money: hospital-based violence intervention is cost-effective. *J Trauma Acute Care Surg.* 2015;78(2):252–258.
194. Loveland-Jones C, Ferrer L, Charles S, et al. A prospective randomized study of the efficacy of "Turning Point," an inpatient violence intervention program. *J Trauma Acute Care Surg.* 2016 81(5):834–842.
195. Purtle J, Dicker R, Cooper C, et al. Hospital-based violence intervention programs save lives and money. *J Trauma Acute Care Surg.* 2013;75(2):331–333.
196. Whitehill JM, Webster DW, Frattaroli S, Parker EM. Interrupting violence: how the CeaseFire Program prevents imminent gun violence through conflict mediation. *J Urban Health.* 2014;91(1):84–95.
197. Whitehill JM, Webster DW, Vernick JS. Street conflict mediation to prevent youth violence: conflict characteristics and outcomes. *Inj Prev.* 2013;19(3):204–209.
198. Webster DW, Whitehill JM, Vernick JS, Curriero FC. Effects of Baltimore's safe streets program on gun violence: a replication of Chicago's CeaseFire Program. *J Urban Health.* 2013;90(1):27–40.
199. Dicker RA, Gaines BA, Bonne S, et al. Violence intervention programs: a primer for developing a comprehensive program for trauma centers. *Bull Am Coll Surg.* 2017;102(10):20–29.
200. Karraker N, Cunningham RA, Becker M, et al. Violence is preventable: a best practices guide for launching and sustaining hospital-based program to break the cycle of violence. Youth ALIVE! https://www.ojp.gov/library/publications/violence-preventable-best-practices-guide-launching-sustaining-hospital-based.
201. The Health Alliance for Violence Intervention. https://www.thehavi.org/. Accessed June 18, 2020.

22

Neck Injuries

Mira H. Ghneim, Brandon R. Bruns, and Thomas M. Scalea

Key Points

1 A comprehensive understanding of the neck anatomy is necessary for optimal management of injuries in this region.

2 Obtaining a secure airway is vital for management of all major injuries, especially those in the neck.

3 Gentle digital pressure or balloon tamponade may control life-threatening hemorrhage from vascular injuries in the neck while definitive measures are arranged.

4 A rapid assessment of the neurologic exam must be performed and carefully documented, as this provides insight into the degree of vascular injury.

5 Though classic teaching mandated exploration of all zone II injuries with penetration of the platysma, modern trauma care allows some discretion.

6 Endovascular techniques may be used as either temporizing bridge to surgical repair or for definitive treatment of penetrating vascular injuries.

7 A high index of suspicion and recognition of injury patterns are necessary to diagnose blunt cerebrovascular injury (BCVI).

8 BCVI is often present in patients who do not manifest traditional screening criteria, and recognition is important as untreated injuries may lead to strokes.

While traumatic neck injuries constitute only 5% to 10% of all trauma cases,[1] the anatomic complexity of the neck and the diverse injury mechanisms make diagnosing and treating these
1 injuries particularly challenging. Many vital structures, including the aerodigestive tract, major vasculature, and the spinal cord, are situated within the neck and reside in close proximity to one another. This often results in multiple injuries affecting a variety of structures within a relatively small area. Neck injuries are caused by both blunt and penetrating trauma. Penetrating trauma results from gunshot injuries, stab injuries, or penetrating blunt objects. While stab wounds occur at a higher rate than gunshot wounds,[2,3] 35% of gunshot wounds and 20% of stab wounds result in significant injuries.[4] Blunt trauma to the neck often occurs from direct blows or hyperextension of the neck in the setting of motor vehicle collisions (MVCs), falls, assault, and various hanging mechanisms. Given the unique challenges posed by the intricate anatomy and the varied mechanisms of injury, understanding the nuances of neck trauma is essential.

FUNCTIONAL ANATOMY

The exterior anatomic barriers of the neck include the lower border of the mandible anteriorly, to the nuchal line of the occipital bone posteriorly. Inferiorly, the clavicles serve as the anterior border, with a line drawn toward the seventh cervical vertebral spinous process encompassing the posterior border.

Triangles are classically used to divide the neck into zones; however, they are only rarely used to classify and plan treatment in trauma patients. The posterior triangles are bordered by the sternocleidomastoid muscles anteriorly, the trapezius muscles posteriorly, and the clavicles inferiorly. The sternocleidomastoid muscles, the midline, and the angles of the mandible border the anterior triangles bilaterally.

In 1969, Monson and colleagues[5] arbitrarily divided the neck into three anatomic zones: zone I consisted of the area below the sternal notch, zone II was the area between the clavicles and the mandibles, and zone III was described as the upper cervical region and consisted of the area above the mandibles. Roon and Christensen[6] introduced a more modern version of the neck zones in 1979 and defined zone II as the area between the cricoid and the angle of the mandible, zone I as the area below the cricoid cartilage, and zone III remained the area above the mandibular angle. Zone I contains aortic arch, brachiocephalic and subclavian vessels, the lung apices, esophagus, trachea, thoracic duct, and thyroid gland. Zone II contains the carotid sheath (common and internal carotid, internal jugular vein, vagus nerve, cranial nerves 9–12), vertebral arteries, esophagus, trachea, pharynx, and the recurrent laryngeal nerve. Zone III contains the distal carotid and vertebral arteries, distal jugular vein, and salivary and parotid glands. Overall, Zone II is the most injured zone, followed by Zone III, then Zone I. In 16% of patients, more than one zone is involved (**Fig. 22.1**).[7]

INITIAL MANAGEMENT

Basic trauma management of patients with injury to the neck should proceed as outlined in the American College of Sur-
2 geons course, Advanced Trauma Life Support (ATLS). Initial priority is given to securing the airway. Early control of the airway with intubation is considered in every patient with a neck injury. Even in seemingly stable nonbleeding patients, a cough may dislodge a thrombus, producing sudden hemorrhage. An airway that had previously been straightforward to control is now much more complicated and may require advanced techniques.

Obvious injury to the neck, presenting with hard signs of vascular injury (pulsatile hemorrhage, expanding pulsatile hematoma, thrill, bruit), should lead the provider to obtain definitive endotracheal access as the first step in the resuscitation. Similarly, air bubbling through the wound, subcutaneous emphysema, hoarseness, or an obviously transected trachea should guide the treatment team toward immediate and definitive airway control.

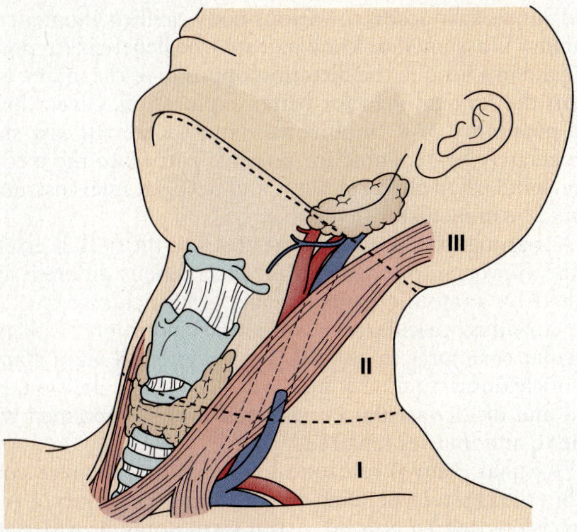

Figure 22.1. Zones of the neck.

If orotracheal intubation cannot be accomplished (rapidly expanding hematoma, destructive laryngeal trauma, patient habitus, excessive debris within the oropharynx), an emergent surgical airway should be expeditiously obtained. Cricothyroidotomy and emergency tracheostomy remain the safest and most reliable methods of emergent surgical control of the airway. Some investigators have shown promising results with percutaneous tracheostomy performed in the emergency setting, though this should only be contemplated by experienced clinicians.[8] If tracheal transection is visualized in the wound, intubation of the distal tracheal segment with an endotracheal tube, or any available airway device, can be lifesaving.

Though obtaining a safe and definitive airway is the priority in all injured patients with airway compromise, blunt trauma patients are at high risk for cervical spine injury. Maintaining the head and neck in neutral position, with the help of a competent assistant trained in such maneuvers, accomplishes cervical stabilization during intubation attempts. The same caution is not needed in patients with penetrating trauma, as patients presenting alive and neurologically intact are highly unlikely to have unstable cervical spine fractures.[9,10]

After securing an adequate airway, the next priorities are breathing and circulation. In evaluating the chest, the clinician must remain aware that penetrating injury to zone I can violate the cupula of the lung and result in pneumothorax or hemothorax, which may require evacuation. Circulatory issues focus on intravenous access with resuscitation and assessment of the blood pressure, but it also entails control of any obvi-
3 ously bleeding focus. Pulsatile bleeding emanating from a neck wound is best managed with gentle digital compression. Occasionally, a urinary catheter or a Fogarty catheter can be delicately placed into a bleeding neck wound with gradual inflation of the balloon in an attempt to tamponade hemorrhage. Insert the catheter until it no longer goes easily; inflate the balloon slowly until the bleeding stops.

Physical examination is the most reliable diagnostic tool. In
4 fact, a rapid assessment of the neurologic exam of the patient must be performed and carefully documented, as this can give insight into the nature of a neck injury as a dense hemiplegia may be the result of carotid arterial injury and subsequent ischemic stroke. It is imperative to recognize the patient with a lateralizing neurologic defect early, as revascularization may result in hemorrhagic conversion of a cerebral infarction.

After the primary survey and adjunctive radiographic procedures (chest radiograph, abdominal sonography), a thorough secondary survey should be performed, with focus on the structures of the neck. A hematoma across the base of the neck caused by an automobile seatbelt may portend a blunt cerebrovascular injury (BCVI). Extensive subcutaneous emphysema in the tissues of the neck usually represents air tracking up from a pneumothorax but can represent an injury to the airway. Injury to the esophagus is possible, but subcutaneous air is rarely the only symptom of esophageal injury. Similarly, an audible bruit or palpable thrill may indicate major vascular injury that requires prompt attention.

PENETRATING NECK TRAUMA

Mandatory Versus Selective Exploration

Few would argue that penetrating wounds to the neck with hard signs of injury (pulsatile hemorrhage, expanding hematoma, shock, massive hemoptysis and hematemesis, air bubbling from the wound, massive subcutaneous emphysema) mandate immediate surgical exploration. However, in the absence of these hard signs of injury, a selective approach with clinical examination and diagnostic workup should be undertaken. This includes computed tomography (CT), CT angiography (CTA), laryngoscopy, flexible esophagoscopy, flexible bronchoscopy, and gastrografin swallow/esophagography. In asymptomatic patients with platysma penetration, management options include observation with serial physical examination every 6 to 8 hours for up to 36 hour or further evaluation by CT/CTA and discharge if no injuries are identified.[11]

5 Traditional surgical teaching calls for neck exploration in patients with penetrating zone II neck injuries that violate the platysma muscle.[6] Those supporting the concept of mandatory surgical exploration cite the low incidence of significant morbidity with surgical exploration, despite the high likelihood of negative exploration.[10,12] Proponents of operation also point to the lack of physical examination findings in patients that did proceed to have positive findings.[12] In contrast to mandatory exploration, many investigators advocate a more selective approach to operative therapy, suggesting surgery only in symptomatic patients. Authors supportive of the more limited approach cite a low morbidity and mortality associated with observation of zone II injuries and high likelihood of negative exploration.[2]

The Utility of Computed Tomography as a Diagnostic Adjunct

In recent years, CT has become the imaging modality of choice to evaluate neck injuries. CT is extremely attractive as it provides a three-dimensional evaluation of the neck and is rapidly available. In patients with injury patterns that put the upper mediastinal structures at risk as well, CT can simultaneously evaluate both areas for injury.

CT may be very effective at excluding injuries in certain cases. For example, a patient with a gunshot wound to the neck has a clearly demonstrated CT trajectory that avoids all vital structures. In this case, close observation without additional studies is appropriate. Other patients, such as those with significant amounts of subcutaneous air or a trajectory that is close to vital structures, may need additional diagnostic testing (angiography, endoscopy).

In 2002, Gonzalez et al. prospectively evaluated patients with penetrating injury to zone II of the neck who did not have an indication for emergent surgical exploration.[13] Patients then underwent dynamic CT imaging and had a barium esophagram, followed by mandatory surgical exploration of the neck. Investigators noted a total of four esophageal injuries. Two of the four were seen on surgical exploration only and were not identified on either CT scan or esophagram; however, both injuries missed on imaging were less than 0.5 cm and were the result of stab wounds. The authors speculated that the injuries may have healed spontaneously. The most commonly missed injury by CT scan was jugular venous injury, which likely needed no therapy.[13]

In a large prospective study involving Los Angeles County, the University of Southern California Medical Center, and the R Adams Cowley Shock Trauma Center at the University of

Maryland, all asymptomatic patients presenting with a penetrating neck injury and no signs of injury were safely observed, and investigators reported zero missed injuries. In the same series, patients with soft signs of injury (venous oozing, nonexpanding or nonpulsatile hematomas, minor hemoptysis, dysphonia, dysphagia, and subcutaneous emphysema), underwent multidetector CTA. Investigators achieved 100% sensitivity and 97.5% specificity in detecting all clinically significant injuries.[14]

The Utility of Digital Subtraction Angiography (DSA) as a Diagnostic Adjunct

DSA provides high-resolution, dynamic imaging and historically was the gold standard for detection and characterization of both blunt and penetrating cerebrovascular injury (PCVI). However, DSA is more labor intensive, time intensive, and less widely available than CTA. Additionally, CTA has a documented specificity of 100%, positive predictive value of 100%, and negative predictive value of 98% compared to DSA.[15] As a result, the role of DSA has largely moved from its use as a screening tool to a vehicle for endovascular intervention. However, it is important to note that arteriovenous fistulas (AVF) and carotid-cavernous fistulas (CCF) are often missed by CTA. Additionally, CTA interpretation is challenging in the setting of artifacts from metallic fragments or excessive air in the surrounding neck tissue. In these cases, DSA continues to play an important role in diagnosis and management of penetrating neck injuries.[16]

General Considerations for Management

While diagnostic exploration may make sense for some zone II injuries, diagnostic preoperative evaluation certainly makes sense for injuries in zone I and zone III. Penetrating injury in zone I puts vascular structures, trachea, and esophagus at risk. Physical examination can be misleading, and different incisions may be needed depending on which structures are injured and the level at which they are injured. Thus, in stable patients, additional imaging is indicated. This includes endoscopy, contrast studies, or both to investigate the possibility of an esophageal injury, bronchoscopy for tracheal injuries, and CTA for vascular injuries.

Unfortunately, in unstable patients with a zone I trajectory, localization of the injury may not be possible preoperatively. In such a case, the clinician should make an estimate as to which structures are most likely to be injured. The initial incision should be tailored to quickly expose that area. If exposure is inadequate or a different structure has been injured, the incision should be lengthened, or a second incision should be made. This process continues until the injury is controlled or the patient dies.

Aerodigestive injuries are not an issue in zone III; however, the difficulty in surgical management of vascular injuries in zone III makes preoperative imaging very attractive. In the past, angiography was used as the sole diagnostic test in stable patients. If patients are unstable, clinicians must weigh the difficulty of diagnostic exploration against the time it would take to use alternative hemostatic methods. In some cases, if catheter hemostasis is immediately available, temporary control with finger pressure or a balloon, as a bridge to rapid diagnostic angiography and catheter hemostasis, may actually be quicker than direct operative exploration. In most areas of the world, this approach is only appropriate in a few highly advanced centers. In most centers, while difficult, direct surgical exploration is the wisest course in the unstable patient.

Incision Selection

As many general surgeons do not routinely operate in the neck, early consideration of potential injuries is important. Immediate availability of vascular instruments, advanced airway devices, endoscopic towers, and scopes is important.

The patient is positioned supine, with a full surgical prep from the chin to the knees. Utilizing a widely prepped surgical field allows easy access to various body cavities. If unilaterality of injury is assumed or known, it may be beneficial to position the patient's head in the direction opposite to the injury, which opens the surgical field for better exploration. Given the very real possibility of a "multizone" injury, a sternal saw should immediately be available for possible entry into the mediastinum. Similarly, a chest retractor and deep vascular instruments should be immediately available.

A thorough knowledge of the zones of the neck is essential, as the approach to injury within each zone is different and is limited by anatomic barriers. This is particularly true when one considers vascular exposure, as exploration of all major vascular structures in zone II is accomplished via a standard sternocleidomastoid neck incision. Via a single incision, proximal and distal vascular control can both be obtained within zone II, and injuries repaired.

Proximal control for zone I injuries may require control within the chest. Depending on the location of injury, a variety of incisions can be utilized. A full sternotomy provides access to the mediastinal great vessels and the proximal left subclavian artery, along with the origin of the left common carotid artery. A partial sternotomy allows control of the innominate artery through a smaller incision. A periclavicular incision provides access to the bilateral subclavian arteries. In short, full exposure is achieved through a variety of incisions. After proximal control, subsequent distal control is obtained in zone II.

Proximal control for zone III injuries can be achieved in zone II without much difficulty; however, distal control may be difficult as the mandible and skull base prevent wide exposure. Several methods, such as mandibular subluxation or osteotomy, have been described to control the carotid artery at the base of the skull.[17] A muscle-splitting incision can also help give access to the carotid artery and the base of the skull.[18]

The inferior and lateral extensions of zone I are often contested and debated. While this is not well described, our practice is to classify lateral and inferior (superior mediastinal) injuries by zone I principles. Because proximal control involves a thoracic incision, we believe zone I extends to the junction of the subclavian and axillary arteries laterally and inferiorly to the mediastinal great vessels.

Injury to the posterior neck is inherently different than injury to the anterior neck. It makes sense that tracheal and esophageal injuries would be less common with posterior injury, as they are protected by the spine. Injuries to the spine should be more common in this anatomical region.

Often, more than one zone can be injured by a single trajectory, such as an injury through both zone II and zone I. Management of these "multizone" injuries is guided by the standard principles used for the more challenging zone, usually zone I or zone III.

BLUNT NECK TRAUMA

Blunt injuries most commonly result from MVCs but may occur with strangulation, assault, and sports injuries. These often result in laryngotracheal, cervical spine, spinal cord, and cerebrovascular (carotid and vertebral artery) injuries. Clinical presentation of blunt neck injuries includes neck bruising/swelling, hoarseness, dysphonia, tracheal deviation, hemoptysis, subcutaneous air, expanding hematoma, cervical spine tenderness, and neurologic deficits. The primary modality for diagnosis blunt neck injuries is a CTA.

MANAGEMENT OF SPECIFIC INJURIES

Penetrating Cerebrovascular Injury

Clinical Presentation and Classification System

The presenting symptoms of penetrating vascular injury in the neck are dependent on the vessel injured and its location. Arterial injuries, specifically the carotid arteries, may present with pulsatile arterial hemorrhage emanating from the wound, a palpable thrill, an audible bruit, or a rapidly expanding hematoma. Cerebral ischemia secondary to carotid artery injury can lead to stroke and long-term neurologic sequelae, or even death. In some series, patients who present in hemorrhagic shock have a mortality of 41% but have 50% mortality when presenting with stroke.[19] Patients presenting with any neurologic deficit, short of coma, should undergo carotid arterial repair with revascularization if technically feasible, as results are improved with revascularization. In patients presenting with a Glasgow Coma Scale (GCS) <8, a poor outcome is likely regardless of the therapy selected.[20,21] Venous injuries tend to have a more insidious presentation and may be clinically undetectable. Penetrating vertebral artery injury is rarer, given the relatively protected position of the artery within the osseous spinal canal. A vascular injury is often identified in 20% of patients presenting with penetration neck trauma. The common carotid artery is the most frequently injured vessel.[22]

Unlike BCVI, PCVI lacks a widely accepted classification system. Instead, clinicians often extrapolate treatment options for PCVI from the Biffl criteria, originally developed for BCVI.[23] However, it's crucial to recognize that in PCVI, higher-grade injuries such as those involving vessel dissection, pseudoaneurysm (PSA), or occlusion, often signify vessel transection by virtue of mechanism of injury. This distinction is vital when devising a management strategy, as transected vessels in PCVI can lead to different clinical outcomes and may necessitate a more aggressive or tailored therapeutic approach than BCVI.

Operative Repair

Often, diagnosis of carotid injury occurs intraoperatively, as there is no time for preoperative imaging. Carotid artery injuries are managed using standard principles of vascular repair. Exploration of the neck is through a generous sternocleidomastoid incision. Control of the proximal carotid artery is obtained at the base of zone II. If possible, it is wise to control the artery distally, before entering the hematoma. Unfortunately, distal control is often not possible. As the neck is a compact region, during dissection to control the distal carotid artery, the contained hematoma often ruptures. Digital control should then be utilized to prevent exsanguinating hemorrhage while the distal dissection is performed. Once the distal carotid artery (whether it is the internal carotid artery or distal common artery) is controlled, digital pressure is released, and careful dissection is performed.

Injuries to the common carotid artery can be primarily repaired, particularly if the injury is caused by a stab wound and has clean edges. More complex injuries, as those from gunshot wounds, usually require resection of the injured segment. Even after resection of a segment of the carotid artery, primary anastomosis may be possible. Full mobilization of the common carotid artery will often give additional length and allow for a tension-free anastomosis. For injuries located more distally, ligating the external carotid artery will give additional mobility to the common carotid artery. If primary anastomosis or repair is not feasible, a bypass graft using either saphenous vein or PTFE is equally acceptable. PTFE should be avoided in the event of contamination or concomitant tracheal or esophageal injury.

Internal carotid artery injury represents a distinct subset of carotid artery injuries. Unlike common carotid artery injury, the initial neurologic presentation is not a good predictor of final neurologic presentation. Injuries to the internal carotid artery have 20% mortality, and the majority of these deaths are secondary to cerebral ischemia.[24] Interventional techniques, including embolization, may be effective in some injuries, thus obviating the need for exploration.[25]

Control of the internal carotid artery proceeds along the same principles as with common carotid artery injuries, though distal control may be even more problematic. During the dissection, one must take care not to injure the hypoglossal nerve, which passes across the distal internal carotid artery. The surgeon should ascertain adequacy of back bleeding from

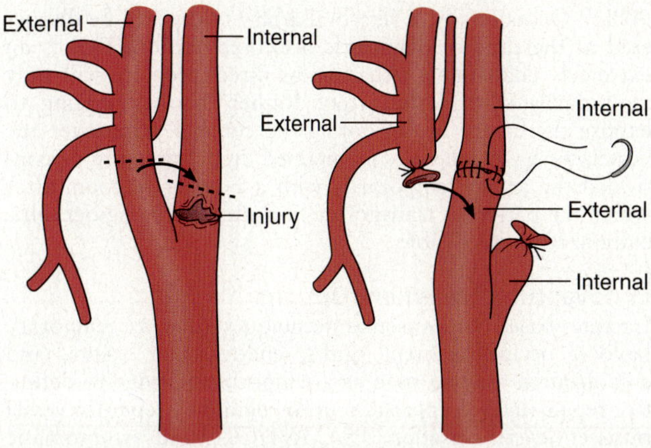

Figure 22.2. A proximal internal carotid artery injury managed with resection and transposition of the external carotid artery to obtain inflow to the native internal carotid artery.

the distal internal carotid artery. Pulsatile back bleeding confirms patency of the circle of Willis. In patients with poor back bleeding, use of a shunt should be considered. We routinely use full-dose IV heparin unless there is a contraindication.

The internal carotid artery is repaired using the same principles as mentioned for the common carotid artery, though several scenarios require special mention. If there is injury to the proximal internal carotid artery and the distal vessel is thrombosed, dissection should be carried out as distal as possible. If the vessel is thrombosed as far as is surgically accessible, the surgeon should avoid the temptation to do catheter thrombectomy as this is virtually never complete and once revascularized, the patient has significant risks of embolic stroke. In addition, one should avoid ligating the thrombosed internal carotid artery at the base. If one forcefully ligates the internal carotid artery, there is high likelihood that distal clot will be dislodged, causing a stroke of clinical significance.

Occasionally, one will encounter an injury in the very proximal internal carotid artery. Once the vessels are controlled, consideration should be given to using the external carotid artery as the conduit if primary repair is not feasible. The damaged internal carotid artery can be dissected down to the level of the bifurcation (**Fig. 22.2**). The external carotid is ligated at the level of the first branch and the external carotid artery rotated over to use as the conduit. A single vascular suture line then connects the external to the internal carotid artery.

For the most part, the external carotid artery is expendable. If an external carotid artery injury is diagnosed at the time of surgical exploration, it can simply be ligated. Those that are diagnosed preoperatively, with images, are often amenable to catheter-based hemostatic techniques.[26] If there is a distal injury to a branch of an external carotid artery, such as the facial or lingual arteries, particularly if caused by penetrating facial trauma, catheter-based hemostasis is by far the most attractive option. Proximal ligation of the external carotid artery will decrease inflow, but the robust collateral circulation from the contralateral external carotid may be sufficient to cause continued hemorrhage. Angiographic options are then essentially nil, as the ligated external carotid prevents an angiographic solution.

Secondary to the posterior anatomic location and protection provided by the cervical spine, penetrating vertebral artery injuries are less likely. Additionally, injuries to the vertebral arteries are less likely to cause neurologic sequelae than those to the carotids.[19] Operative exposure of the vertebral artery is quite difficult secondary to its protected location in the posterior neck. If necessary, it is best approached via an anterior approach with proximal ligation of vertebral artery.[20]

Combined carotid and vertebral artery penetrating injuries are very morbid, with mortality rates of approximately

50%.[21] Occasionally, a vertebral artery injury will be discovered at the time of diagnostic neck exploration. This is an extremely challenging situation, as direct pressure will only temporarily control the artery. Rather than attempting to expose the artery by unroofing the cervical spine over the vessel, we have generally maintained digital pressure or controlled the artery temporarily with a Fogarty balloon, after which the patient is transported to a site where angiographic embolization is possible.

Endovascular Treatment Options

Catheter-based endovascular techniques such as temporary balloon occlusion, stent grafts, endovascular stents, and embolization may be used as a temporizing bridge to definitive repair (hybrid approach) or for definitive repair in vessel transection/extravasation, PSA, AVF/CCF, and symptomatic dissections. Preservation of an arterial patency is the main goal of treatment. Vessel sacrifice is sometimes indicated, however, as a last resort.[27] These techniques are particularly useful in Zones I and III, which are difficult to access with an open surgical approach. Angiography with endovascular intervention should be considered in the following hemodynamically appropriate patient with one of the following injury types: (1) distal internal carotid artery injury, (2) AVF or CCF, (3) injury to branches of the external carotid artery with associated ongoing facial or intraoral hemorrhage, (4) small intimal defects or PSAs in surgically inaccessible locations or high-risk patients, and (5) vertebral artery injuries (**Fig. 22.3**).

Multiple studies in the literature have reported on the endovascular treatment of penetrating traumatic injuries to the carotid and vertebral arteries.[7,27,28] A recent 1-year prospective study involving Ukrainian soldiers (n = 30) with penetrating
6 vertebral artery injuries showed that endovascular interventions (n = 14) were performed based on anatomical location and severity of the injury, severity of concomitant injuries, and the presence of collateral circulation.[29] In this study, endovascular procedures were performed in all patients with V3 segment injuries, 46.7% of those with V2 segment injuries, and 27.3% with V1 segment injuries. Additionally, the frequency of endovascular interventions increased with the severity of the injury (grade I [0%], grade 2 [3%], grade III [10%], and grade [IV]). Endovascular interventions included embolization, stent placement with and without thrombectomy, and placement of microvascular plugs. Dual antiplatelet therapy was initiated in patients who underwent stent graft placement and had no contraindications to therapy.[29]

Laryngeal and Tracheal Injuries

The clinical presentation of laryngotracheal injuries includes hemoptysis, hoarseness, dysphonia, subcutaneous emphysema, and air bubbling from an open wound. Management focuses on rapid airway control, either via endotracheal intubation or via a surgical airway. In the rare instance of tracheal transection in the neck with two visible lumens, the distal lumen should be intubated with any available airway device. Concomitant esophageal injury is a source of major morbidity; therefore, the esophagus should be evaluated with early endoscopy or operative exploration.[30]

Blunt laryngotracheal trauma is uncommon[31] and low-grade injuries can be clinically occult. Thus, these injuries require a high index of suspicion. The most typical mechanism of injury involves an anterior-to-posterior vector of force that drives the thyroid cartilage into the rigid cervical spine. Such forces can be the result of a motor vehicle collision with compression of the neck against the steering wheel or dashboard of the automobile. The most common symptoms include hoarseness, dyspnea, and dysphagia.[31,32] Careful attention must be paid to the airway as laryngotracheal separation can be catastrophic. Definitive

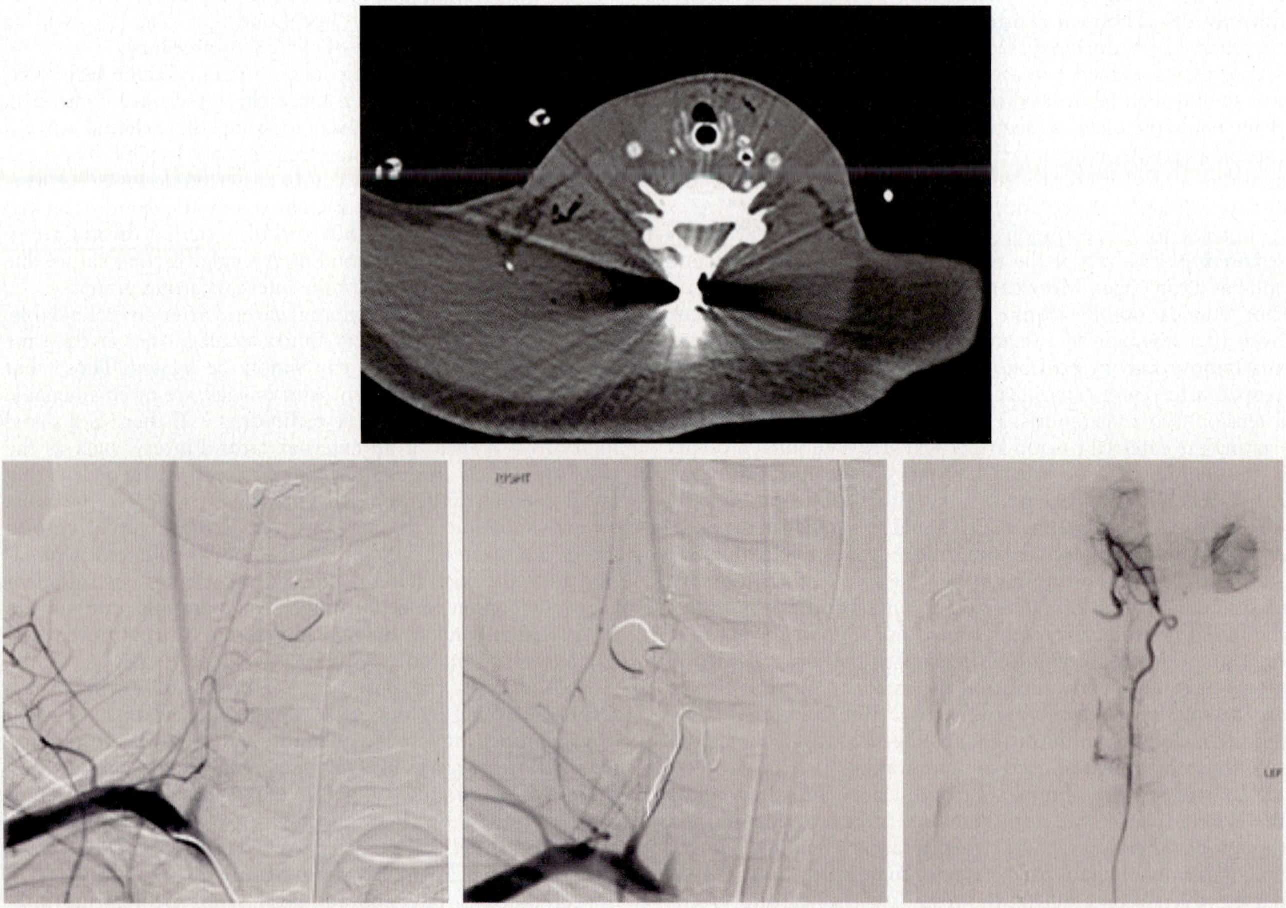

Figure 22.3. Vertebral artery occlusion with subsequent angioembolization in a patient with an intact Circle of Willis.

diagnosis is made with a combination of CT scanning and endoscopy. Definitive airway management is best obtained with tracheostomy if endotracheal intubation is not prudent.[33]

Cervical tracheal injuries, particularly if they are isolated, are best approached via a collar incision performed approximately two fingerbreadths above the sternal notch. If other injuries are present and/or if full exploration is needed, the trachea can be exposed and repaired using a sternocleidomastoid incision. If a collar incision is used, subplatysmal flaps are created and the strap muscles are then divided in the midline. The thyroid isthmus can be retracted cephalad, and the entire cervical trachea is then clearly visualized. If the location of the tracheal injury in the neck is clearly in zone II, surgical exploration confirms the diagnosis and allows for prompt therapy.

Occasionally, tracheal injuries are located closer to the thoracic inlet. In these cases, preoperative bronchoscopy is vital in order to plan the best operative course. If the injury is located in the upper mediastinum, several options exist. The patient can be explored via a collar incision, and the anterior trachea identified. The trachea can be mobilized using digital dissection into the upper mediastinum. The trachea can then be grasped with a tracheal hook and retracted up into the neck. It is possible to mobilize the trachea for approximately three rings, thus allowing the surgeon to repair these injuries with a relatively small incision. Injuries that are located in the more distal mediastinum are best approached with a right-sided posterolateral thoracotomy.

Occasionally, tracheal injuries will be located at a level above the endotracheal balloon. When performing diagnostic bronchoscopy, the endotracheal tube must be withdrawn (with the cuff deflated) over the bronchoscope, up to the level of the vocal cords. This allows complete visualization of the proximal trachea. Not pulling back the endotracheal tube risks missing proximal tracheal injuries.

Injuries to the posterior membranous trachea are relatively difficult to approach. In patients with blunt trauma, small injuries may be observed; however, if repair is thought to be prudent, the best way to approach this is through the anterior trachea. The anterior trachea is opened transversely at the level of the injury, and the posterior injury is then visualized and repaired. The anterior trachea is closed primarily. Intraoperative bronchoscopy can help locate the level of the injury.

The blood supply to the trachea enters posterolaterally on both sides; therefore, circumferential mobilization of the trachea risks causing ischemia, which may manifest either as tracheal necrosis, dehiscence of a repair, or postoperative tracheal stenosis. In addition, the recurrent laryngeal nerve runs in the tracheoesophageal groove, and care must be taken to avoid damage to it during mobilization or tracheal repair. Postoperatively, patients undergoing tracheal repair should be extubated as soon as possible. It is often tempting to think that the tracheal repair is protected with longer-term tracheal intubation, but the chances of complications are less if the patient is extubated at the end of the operative procedure. One should avoid a tracheostomy in a patient with tracheal repair, because stenosis at the level of tracheostomy and the level of tracheal repair can make future reconstruction exceedingly difficult.

In the event that the injury extends into the thoracic inlet, a partial sternal split (**Fig. 22.4**) or full sternotomy can be performed for better visualization. Tracheal injuries are preferentially repaired primarily with single-layer absorbable suture, though resection of up to 2 to 4 cm with primary anastomosis is technically feasible. Suture lines should be buttressed with autologous, well-vascularized tissue, such as strap muscle.

Esophagus

Early diagnosis of esophageal injury is imperative, as missed injury and/or a delay in diagnosis can lead to disastrous consequences. In a review of 109 penetrating esophageal injuries, the mortality rate was 2% with immediate operation. Mortality increased to 44% with delayed diagnosis and operation. In this same series, mortality increased to 100% for patients with a delayed diagnosis and no operative procedure.[34]

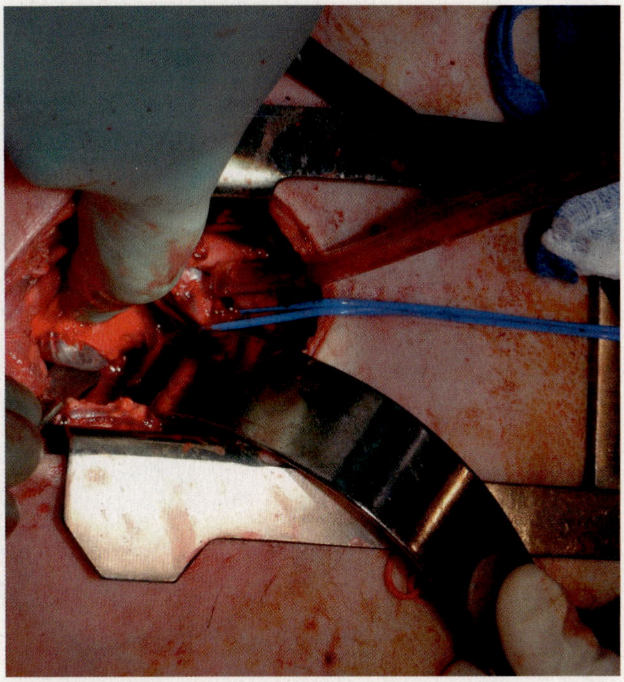

Figure 22.4. Partial sternal split for evaluation of tracheal injury. The endotracheal tube balloon is visualized within the lumen of the injured trachea.

As the course of the esophagus is relatively superficial within the neck, diagnosis can occasionally be made on physical examination findings alone. Food particles or salivary secretions within the wound are highly suggestive of esophageal injury. Additional physical examination findings may include esophageal or oropharyngeal bleeding, subcutaneous emphysema, and neck hematoma. Plain film radiographic findings may include air within the subcutaneous tissues and pneumomediastinum.[35] In a review of 77 patients with noniatrogenic esophageal injury, 58% occurred in the cervical esophagus, with physical examination findings present in only 26% of the cohort.[36]

Given the pervasive nature of CT scanning in the trauma patient, investigators have evaluated the utility of this imaging modality for esophageal injury. A study from the Aga Khan University Hospital showed 53% sensitivity for CT scanning in diagnosing esophageal injuries.[37] The gold standard for diagnosis of most esophageal injuries remains a combination of esophagoscopy and contrast-enhanced esophagography. When these two imaging modalities are used in combination, an accuracy of almost 100% is achieved.[38] The sensitivity of esophagography alone varies from 50% to 90%, while the sensitivity of endoscopy alone varies from 29% to 100%.[39]

As with the trachea, the location of the esophageal injury defines the approach for repair. Those injuries that are clearly in zone II can easily be approached via a sternocleidomastoid incision. Those in the chest are best approached via a posterolateral right thoracotomy. As with the trachea, localization of the injury, particularly those at the junction between the neck and chest, is the easiest way to ensure optimal exposure. Intraoperative endoscopy can be very helpful in positively identifying the location of an injury and helping to direct therapy.

Small, nondestructive injuries in the hypopharyngeal region can occasionally be managed nonoperatively with antibiotics, upright positioning, limited oral intake, and close clinical observation.[40] The vast majority of cervical esophageal injuries are best managed operatively. Cervical esophageal injuries are most easily approached via a left anterior sternocleidomastoid incision (**Fig. 22.5**). If a collar incision has been initiated, it can be extended to the left, along the anterior border of

TRAUMA

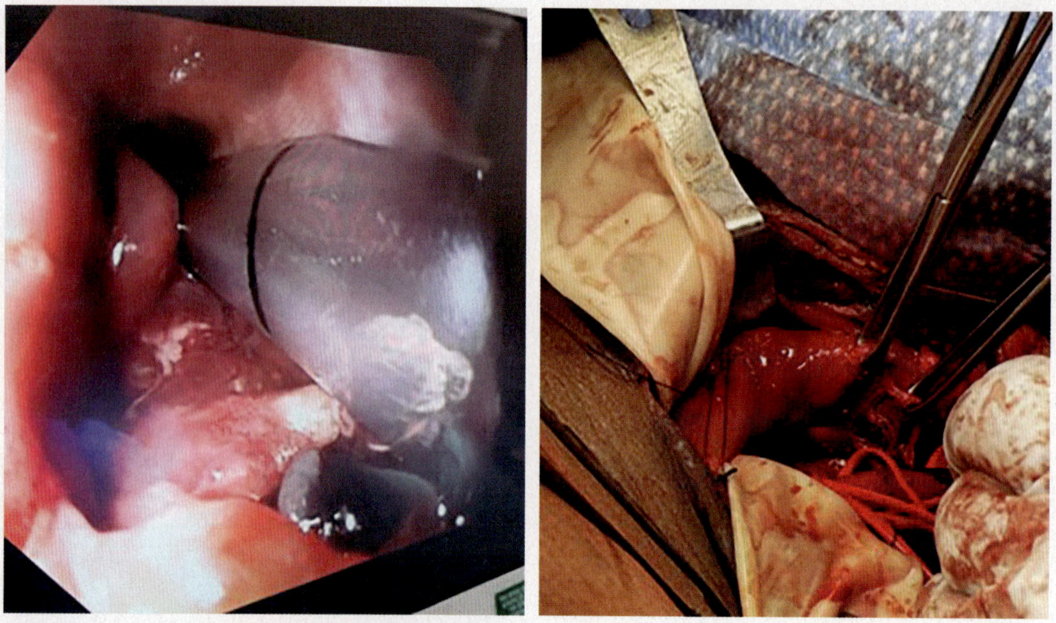

Figure 22.5. Esophageal injury identified on endoscopy and managed operatively.

the sternocleidomastoid muscle to facilitate better exposure. Preoperative placement of a nasogastric tube may assist with identification of the esophagus in the neck, as the hard nasogastric tube can be palpated within the lumen. After lateral retraction of the sternocleidomastoid muscle, the dissection progresses medially until the esophagus is encountered. Care must be taken to avoid injury to the recurrent laryngeal nerve in the tracheoesophageal groove.

Circumferential dissection of the esophagus and placement of large rubber drain around the organ can facilitate retraction and mobilization. As the blood supply of the esophagus runs vertically within the muscle, the esophagus can be circumferentially mobilized without risk of ischemia. Thus, injuries located in the superior mediastinum can be mobilized into the neck and repaired. After repair, liberal drainage of the injured area is highly recommended in an effort to avoid salivary fistula and deep neck infection.[35,40] Delays in diagnosis of more than 12 hours are associated with poor outcomes, and in these cases, proximal diversion and wide drainage may be the safest option.

Primary repair of the injury is the goal in most circumstances. During repair, the entirety of the mucosal injury must be visualized, as it may extend beyond the field of view under the longitudinal outer muscle of the esophagus. Debridement of all devitalized tissue is required. Repairs are typically performed in two layers with absorbable sutures, though single-layer repair is possible.[35,41] Similar to tracheal repair, a well-vascularized muscle is highly recommended to buttress the repair. Given the likelihood that the patient will be on a restricted oral diet, placement of a small-bore enteral tube, distal to the repair, should be considered intraoperatively. Imaging repairs at 7 to 10 days with a contrast-enhanced swallow study is recommended prior to removal of drains.

BCVI

Mechanism of Injury, Symptoms, and Incidence of BCVI

Blunt injuries to the carotid and vertebral arteries are the result of a direct blow to the vessel itself or an extreme flexion, extension, or lateral rotational injury. BCVI of the carotid artery 7 typically occurs at the base of the skull, while vertebral artery injuries occur along the segment located within the cervical spine transverse foramina. Given that BCVI affects cerebral blood flow, leading to ischemia, a symptomatic lesion presents as a stroke. The severity of the symptoms is also dependent on the absence or presence of collateral circulation and/or any underlying cerebrovascular disease.[42] BCVI is reported to occur in 1% to 3% of blunt trauma patients and the incidence of stroke is approximately 25%, with a mortality rate of up to 13%, if left untreated.[23,43–46]

The Role of CTA

Historically, DSA was considered the gold standard for diagnosing BCVI. However, due to the limitations of DSA and the need for CT imaging in patients with concomitant injuries, CTA emerged as a more attractive alternative for diagnosis. In a study of 146 patients at risk for BCVI, investigators imaged all patients with 16-slice CTA and four-vessel cerebral angiography. They noted a sensitivity of 97.7% and a specificity of 100% with the utilization of CTA for the diagnosis of BCVI.[47] Authors in Memphis examined 684 patients and found the sensitivity of CTA to be 51% with a specificity of 97%.[48] Despite the disparate findings, survey results illustrate that 90% of trauma surgeons utilize CTA as their preferred diagnostic modality for BCVI.[49] Whole-body multidetector-row CT scan is now employed more often in trauma centers. This scan offers the advantage of more rapid imaging, utilizing a single dose of contrast for the entire body. Sliker et al. demonstrated the accuracy equivalence of the whole-body multidetector scan to the 16-slice CTA in identifying BCVI, allowing for early identification and treatment of BCVI.[42,50]

Screening Criteria

The work of Biffl and colleagues in 1999[23,46] highlighted the importance of screening for BCVI when certain anatomic injuries or injury patterns were observed (**Table 22.1**). Subsequently, organizational guidelines have been disseminated by the Eastern Association for the Surgery of Trauma (EAST) based on review of the literature with the aim of guiding screening practices for BCVI (**Table 22.2**).[25] Investigators have shown that up to 30% of patients diagnosed with BCVI may have no radiographic or clinical risk factor that would guide the clinician to screen for these injuries.[51] Recent data has also identified an association between BCVI and nontraditional risk factors such as serious chest injury.[47] Thus, a high index of suspicion must be maintained in order to effectively diagnose and treat BCVI. Given the seeming inability of screening guidelines to accurately identify patients at risk for BCVI, some centers have gone to blanket screening.[51] All polytrauma patients with a blunt mechanism of injury undergo CT scan of the cervical spine with contrast, timed to image the carotid and

Table 22.1. Signs and Symptoms of Blunt Cerebrovascular Injury

Hemorrhage of potential arterial origin
Expanding cervical hematoma
Cervical bruit in a patient <50 y old after trauma
Unexplained lateralizing neurologic deficits, transient ischemic attack, amaurosis fugax, or Horner syndrome after trauma
Cranial neurologic deficits incongruous with brain CT findings
Evidence of cerebral infarction on CT scan

From Biffl WL, Moore EE, Elliott JP, Brega KE, Burch JM. Blunt cerebrovascular injuries. *Curr Probl Surg.* 1999;36(7):505–599.

vertebral arteries in conjunction with a chest and abdominal CT scan, obviating the need for a second contrast study. While data on this blanket screening is limited, it does enable the identification of injuries early in the course of workup and identifies injuries in patients that would otherwise not be screened secondary to lack of criteria.[51] Patients with identified injuries generally receive a formal CT angiogram as their follow-up study.

Injury Grading Scale and Associated Stroke Rate by Injury Grade

The Denver injury grading scale was developed to provide an accurate description of the injury, define the stroke risk, and provide guidance regarding the appropriate therapy per vessel injured and grade of injury[42] (**Table 22.3**). The overall stroke rates of untreated BCVI in asymptomatic patients are 25% versus <8% for those who receive therapy. Stroke rates increase with increasing injury of carotid but not vertebral artery injuries.[52,53]

Treatment

Antithrombotic Therapy

Medical treatment for BCVI is centered on antiplatelet therapy and systemic anticoagulation to decrease the risk of stroke. A Western Trauma Association study of 492 patients with BCVI-related stroke found that the median time to stroke was 48 hours from admission. Additionally, the peak incidence of stroke occurs between 13 to 24 hours postinjury and then declines out to day 5.[42,54] Early recognition and initiation of treatment have been shown to decrease the rate of cerebral
8 ischemia.[24,55] If stroke can be avoided with prompt initiation of therapy, functional outcomes after BCVI are good;[48] however, many patients with BCVI have multisystem trauma and are thus deemed not suitable for antiplatelet therapy or systemic anticoagulation. In a 2009 study, almost one-third of patients with BCVI were identified as not candidates for therapy, with an overall stroke rate of 12% and stroke-related mortality of 50%.[43] Experience with BCVI and stroke has led our institution to a fairly aggressive stance on treating BCVI judged to be severe, even in the face of concomitant injuries (including traumatic brain injury in certain circumstances).

Table 22.2. Screening Criteria for Blunt Cerebrovascular Injury

Injury Mechanism
Severe cervical hyperextension/rotation or hyperflexion
Displaced midface or complex mandibular fracture
Closed-head injury inconsistent with diffuse axonal injury
Near hanging result in anoxic brain injury
Physical Exam Signs
Seat belt abrasion or other soft tissue injury of the neck resulting in swelling or altered mental status
Fracture in proximity to internal carotid or vertebral artery
Basilar skull fracture involving the carotid canal
Cervical vertebral body fracture

From Bromberg WJ, Collier BC, Diebel LN, et al. Blunt cerebrovascular injury practice management guidelines: the Eastern Association for the Surgery of Trauma. *J Trauma.* 2010;68(2):471–477.

Table 22.3. Stroke Rate Associated With Carotid and Vertebral BCVI Classified by Grade of Injury

		Stroke Rate	
Injury	Grade of Injury	Carotid	Vertebral
I	Irregularity of the vessel wall or a dissection/intramural hematoma with <25% luminal stenosis	8	6
II	Intraluminal thrombosis, raised intimal flap, dissection, intramural hematoma >25% luminal stenosis	14	38
III	Pseudoaneurysm	26	27
IV	Vessel occlusion	50	28
V	Vessel Transection	100	100

From Cothern CC, Moore EE. Blunt cerebrovascular injuries. *Clinics.* 2005;60(6):498–496

It is tempting to assign treatment for BCVI to a relatively lower priority. Patients with BCVI often have concomitant injuries such as intra-abdominal solid visceral injury or traumatic brain injury. The traditional approach has been to simply decide that these patients are not candidates for anticoagulation and defer therapy. While this may be acceptable with low-grade injuries, given the relatively high rate of stroke with higher-grade injuries, this may not be wise. Recent data suggest that in Grade IV carotid injuries (complete occlusion), recanalization and subsequent stroke are extremely common.[26] This would seem to suggest that the presence of higher-grade injuries mandates therapy. For instance, in a patient with splenic injury and carotid artery injury, one should consider whether splenectomy followed by anticoagulation is wiser than nonoperative management and withholding treatment for the BCVI.

It is important to acknowledge that the optimal treatment regimen, including the choice of antiplatelet and anticoagulant therapy, as well as the duration of treatment and long-term surveillance imaging, remains controversial due to the availability of mainly retrospective and prospective observational data, with no randomized controlled trials. The experience at our institution has been to manage grade I injuries with low-dose aspirin, grade II injuries with full-dose aspirin, grade III and IV injuries with aspirin and Plavix. Patients are reimaged at 1, 3, and 12 months. At 3 months, if the lesion is resolved the therapy is discontinued. Stable or worsening injuries are managed in conjunction with the trauma endovascular service.

Open and Endovascular Interventions

Open surgical intervention is rare in BCVI, and the injuries are often inaccessible. Additionally, the indications for endovascular interventions in the setting of traumatic carotid and vertebral artery injuries are not well defined. This can be attributed to the fact that while some groups report a good safety profile for endovascular stenting, the risks (stent occlusion) may outweigh the benefits, leading to a decrease in stent usage over time. Additionally, the stroke rate is found to be similar regardless of treatment (medical vs. endovascular), suggesting that anticoagulation alone is sufficient for most BCVI.[56] At our institutions, stents are placed in the setting of flow-limiting stenosis, AVF, and PSAs. Endovascular embolization of grade IV/V injuries to control hemorrhage and prevent distal embolization if the artery recanalizes (**Fig. 22.3**).

SUMMARY

Management of injuries to the neck requires a thorough understanding of three-dimensional anatomy and an appreciation for the severity of injuries possible in this region. A relatively small anatomic region, the neck contains many structures vital to meaningful survival. Attention to airway is of the utmost importance because without a secure airway, the remainder of workup is meaningless. In the presence of vascular injury, all management options must be rapidly reviewed, and the most easily obtained and efficacious maneuver should be chosen. As nonoperative management of many traumatic injuries continues to expand, it is the obligation of the surgeon to remember basic surgical principles and apply them in an expeditious and safe manner as the situation mandates.

References

1. Nowicki JL, Stew B, Ooi E. Penetrating neck injuries: a guide to evaluation and management. *Ann R Coll Surg Engl*. 2018; 100(1):6–11.
2. Nason RW, Assuras GN, Gray PR, Lipschitz J, Burns CM. Penetrating neck injuries: analysis of experience from a Canadian trauma centre. *Can J Surg J Can Chir*. 2001;44(2):122–126.
3. Bishara RA, Pasch AR, Douglas DD, Schuler JJ, Lim LT, Flanigan DP. The necessity of mandatory exploration of penetrating zone II neck injuries. *Surgery*. 1986;100(4):655–660.
4. Vassiliu P, Baker J, Henderson S, Alo K, Velmahos G, Demetriades D. Aerodigestive injuries of the neck. *Am Surg*. 2001;67(1):75–79.
5. Monson DO, Saletta JD, Freeark RJ. Carotid vertebral trauma. *J Trauma*. 1969;9(12):987–999.
6. Roon AJ, Christensen N. Evaluation and treatment of penetrating cervical injuries. *J Trauma*. 1979;19(6):391–397.
7. Demetriades D, Salim A, Brown C, Martin M, Rhee P. Neck injuries. *Curr Probl Surg*. 2007;44(1):13–85.
8. Davidson SB, Blostein PA, Walsh J, Maltz SB, VandenBerg SL. Percutaneous tracheostomy: a new approach to the emergency airway. *J Trauma Acute Care Surg*. 2012;73(2 Suppl 1):S83–88.
9. Medzon R, Rothenhaus T, Bono CM, Grindlinger G, Rathlev NK. Stability of cervical spine fractures after gunshot wounds to the head and neck. *Spine*. 2005;30(20):2274–2279.
10. Ramasamy A, Midwinter M, Mahoney P, Clasper J. Learning the lessons from conflict: pre-hospital cervical spine stabilisation following ballistic neck trauma. *Injury*. 2009;40(12):1342–1345.
11. Moore E, Feliciano D, Mattox K. Neck and larynx. In: *Trauma*. 9th ed. McGraw-Hill Medical; 2020.
12. Saletta JD, Lowe RJ, Lim LT, Thornton J, Delk S, Moss GS. Penetrating trauma of the neck. *J Trauma*. 1976;16(7):579–587.
13. Gonzalez RP, Falimirski M, Holevar MR, Turk B. Penetrating zone II neck injury: does dynamic computed tomographic scan contribute to the diagnostic sensitivity of physical examination for surgically significant injury? A prospective blinded study. *J Trauma*. 2003;54(1):61–64; discussion 64–65.
14. Inaba K, Branco BC, Menaker J, et al. Evaluation of multidetector computed tomography for penetrating neck injury: a prospective multicenter study. *J Trauma Acute Care Surg*. 2012;72(3):576–583; discussion 583–584; quiz 803–804.
15. Lauzier DC, Chatterjee AR, Kansagra AP. Neurointerventional management of cerebrovascular trauma. *J Neurointerventional Surg*. 2022;14(7):718–722.
16. Zampakis P, Panagiotopoulos V, Kalogeropoulou C, et al. Computed tomography angiography scoring systems and the role of skull defects in the confirmation of brain death. *Sci Rep*. 2021; 11(1):15081.
17. Simonian GT, Pappas PJ, Padberg FT, et al. Mandibular subluxation for distal internal carotid exposure: technical considerations. *J Vasc Surg*. 1999;30(6):1116–1120.
18. Shaha A, Phillips T, Scalea T, et al. Exposure of the internal carotid artery near the skull base: the posterolateral anatomic approach. *J Vasc Surg*. 1988;8(5):618–622.
19. Ramadan F, Rutledge R, Oller D, Howell P, Baker C, Keagy B. Carotid artery trauma: a review of contemporary trauma center experiences. *J Vasc Surg*. 1995;21(1):46–55; discussion 55–56.
20. Feliciano DV. Management of penetrating injuries to carotid artery. *World J Surg*. 2001;25(8):1028–1035.
21. Liekweg WG, Greenfield LJ. Management of penetrating carotid arterial injury. *Ann Surg*. 1978;188(5):587–592.
22. DiBartolomeo AD, Williams B, Weaver FA, et al. Risk factors for stroke in penetrating cerebrovascular injuries. *J Vasc Surg*. 2024;80(4):1064–1070.
23. Biffl WL, Moore EE, Elliott JP, Brega KE, Burch JM. Blunt cerebrovascular injuries. *Curr Probl Surg*. 1999;36(7):505–599.
24. Eastman AL, Muraliraj V, Sperry JL, Minei JP. CTA-based screening reduces time to diagnosis and stroke rate in blunt cervical vascular injury. *J Trauma*. 2009;67(3):551–556; discussion 555–556.
25. Bromberg WJ, Collier BC, Diebel LN, et al. Blunt cerebrovascular injury practice management guidelines: the Eastern Association for the Surgery of Trauma. *J Trauma*. 2010;68(2):471–477.
26. Lauerman MH, Feeney T, Sliker CW, et al. Lethal now or lethal later: the natural history of Grade 4 blunt cerebrovascular injury. *J Trauma Acute Care Surg*. 2015;78(6):1071–1074; discussion 1074–1075.
27. Herrera DA, Vargas SA, Dublin AB. Endovascular treatment of penetrating traumatic injuries of the extracranial carotid artery. *J Vasc Interv Radiol JVIR*. 2011;22(1):28–33.
28. Vellimana AK, Lavie J, Chatterjee AR. Endovascular considerations in traumatic injury of the carotid and vertebral arteries. *Semin Interv Radiol*. 2021;38(1):53–63.
29. Sirko A, Cherednychenko Y, Dowlati E, Perepelytsia V, Armonda RA. Incidence and management of traumatic vertebral artery injuries: wartime experience in Ukraine. *J Neurosurg*. 2024;141(2):445–454.
30. Grewal H, Rao PM, Mukerji S, Ivatury RR. Management of penetrating laryngotracheal injuries. *Head Neck*. 1995;17(6):494–502.
31. Sofferman RA. Management of laryngotracheal trauma. *Am J Surg*. 1981;141(4):412–417.
32. Myers EM, Iko BO. The management of acute laryngeal trauma. *J Trauma*. 1987;27(4):448–452.
33. Fuhrman GM, Stieg FH, Buerk CA. Blunt laryngeal trauma: classification and management protocol. *J Trauma*. 1990;30(1):87–92.
34. Sankaran S, Walt AJ. Penetrating wounds of the neck: principles and some controversies. *Surg Clin North Am*. 1977;57(1):139–150.
35. Glatterer MS, Toon RS, Ellestad C, et al. Management of blunt and penetrating external esophageal trauma. *J Trauma*. 1985;25(8): 784–792.
36. Defore WW, Mattox KL, Hansen HA, Garcia-Rinaldi R, Beall AC, DeBakey ME. Surgical management of penetrating injuries of the esophagus. *Am J Surg*. 1977;134(6):734–738.
37. Kazi M, Junaid M, Khan MJ, Ali NS, Masoom A. Utility of clinical examination and CT scan in assessment of penetrating neck trauma. *J Coll Physicians Surg Pak*. 2013;23(4):308–309.
38. Weigelt JA, Thal ER, Snyder WH, Fry RE, Meier DE, Kilman WJ. Diagnosis of penetrating cervical esophageal injuries. *Am J Surg*. 1987;154(6):619–622.
39. Carducci B, Lowe RA, Dalsey W. Penetrating neck trauma: consensus and controversies. *Ann Emerg Med*. 1986;15(2):208–215.
40. Stanley RB, Armstrong WB, Fetterman BL, Shindo ML. Management of external penetrating injuries into the hypopharyngeal-cervical esophageal funnel. *J Trauma*. 1997;42(4):675–679.

41. Winter RP, Weigelt JA. Cervical esophageal trauma. Incidence and cause of esophageal fistulas. *Arch Surg*. 1990;125(7):849–851; discussion 851–852.
42. Asensio JA, Meredith JW. Blunt cerebrovascular injuries. In: *Current Therapy of Trauma and Surgical Critical Care*. 3rd ed. Elsevier; 2024.
43. Stein DM, Boswell S, Sliker CW, Lui FY, Scalea TM. Blunt cerebrovascular injuries: does treatment always matter? *J Trauma*. 2009;66(1):132–143; discussion 143–144.
44. Miller PR, Chang MC, Hoth JJ, Holmes JH, Meredith JW. Colonic resection in the setting of damage control laparotomy: is delayed anastomosis safe? *Am Surg*. 2007;73(6):606–609; discussion 609–610.
45. Cothren CC, Moore EE, Biffl WL, et al. Anticoagulation is the gold standard therapy for blunt carotid injuries to reduce stroke rate. *Arch Surg*. 2004;139(5):540–545; discussion 545–546.
46. Biffl WL, Moore EE, Offner PJ, Brega KE, Franciose RJ, Burch JM. Blunt carotid arterial injuries: implications of a new grading scale. *J Trauma*. 1999;47(5):845–853.
47. Eastman AL, Chason DP, Perez CL, McAnulty AL, Minei JP. Computed tomographic angiography for the diagnosis of blunt cervical vascular injury: is it ready for primetime? *J Trauma*. 2006;60(5):925–929; discussion 929.
48. DiCocco JM, Emmett KP, Fabian TC, Zarzaur BL, Williams JS, Croce MA. Blunt cerebrovascular injury screening with 32-channel multidetector computed tomography: more slices still don't cut it. *Ann Surg*. 2011;253(3):444–450.
49. Harrigan MR, Weinberg JA, Peaks YS, et al. Management of blunt extracranial traumatic cerebrovascular injury: a multidisciplinary survey of current practice. *World J Emerg Surg*. 2011;6:11.
50. Sliker CW. Blunt cerebrovascular injuries: imaging with multidetector CT angiography. *Radiographics*. 2008;28(6):1689–1708.
51. Bruns BR, Tesoriero R, Kufera J, et al. Blunt cerebrovascular injury screening guidelines: what are we willing to miss? *J Trauma Acute Care Surg*. 2014;76(3):691–695.
52. Murphy PB, Severance S, Holler E, Menard L, Savage S, Zarzaur BL. Treatment of asymptomatic blunt cerebrovascular injury (BCVI): a systematic review. *Trauma Surg Acute Care Open*. 2021;6(1):e000668.
53. Cothren CC, Moore EE. Blunt cerebrovascular injuries. *Clinics*. 2005;60(6):489–496.
54. Burlew CC, Sumislawski JJ, Behnfield CD, et al. Time to stroke: a Western Trauma Association multicenter study of blunt cerebrovascular injuries. *J Trauma Acute Care Surg*. 2018;85(5):858–866.
55. Fabian TC, Patton JH, Croce MA, Minard G, Kudsk KA, Pritchard FE. Blunt carotid injury. Importance of early diagnosis and anticoagulant therapy. *Ann Surg*. 1996;223(5):513–522.
56. Shahan CP, Sharpe JP, Stickley SM, et al. The changing role of endovascular stenting for blunt cerebrovascular injuries. *J Trauma Acute Care Surg*. 2018;84(2):308–311.

23

Thoracic Trauma

Jacqueline J. Blank and Marc de Moya

Key Points

1 The mortality associated with penetrating thoracic trauma is higher than blunt trauma.

2 The most common blunt thoracic injury is rib fracture and the most effective pain relief is thoracic epidural analgesia. Data regarding rib fracture stabilization is mixed.

3 Small simple pneumothoraces do not necessitate drainage, but if drainage is needed for larger pneumothoraces, it can be accomplished effectively with a small caliber catheter (eg, 8- to 14-Fr pigtail catheter).

4 Small caliber chest tubes (14 to 28 Fr) are effective at draining hemothoraces. Those with 28-Fr chest tubes should undergo thoracic irrigation at time of tube insertion. If there is a significant retained hemothorax after tube thoracostomy, early operative evacuation with video-assisted thoracoscopy should be employed.

5 Operative repair of blunt aortic injuries, particularly low grade, may be delayed and treated medically in the face of severe associated injuries.

Thoracic trauma is a common occurrence with an incidence of approximately 25% of all traumas.[1] The most common blunt thoracic injury is rib fracture; mortality and morbidity increase as the number of rib fractures increases. Mortality is most pronounced in the elderly with a 19%[1] increase in mortality with
1 each additional rib fracture.[2] The majority of deaths from thoracic trauma are due to a penetrating mechanism. Regardless of the mechanism or associated injuries, one should always proceed with a systematic approach to the trauma patient, using the Advanced Trauma Life Support (ATLS) protocols.[3]

INITIAL IMAGING

The initial imaging in the trauma bay for suspected chest trauma is the screening chest x-ray (CXR) and the extended focused assessment with sonography for trauma (eFAST) examination. The screening CXR can help identify additional injuries such as bony fractures, mediastinal hematoma, pneumothorax, hemothorax, lung contusions, elevated diaphragm, and large diaphragmatic rupture. It can also confirm position of breathing tubes, gastric decompression tubes, and central lines.[4] If the spine is cleared, particularly in the case of penetrating trauma, then an upright AP film may be obtained, which increases sensitivity for diagnosing hemothoraces and pneumothoraces (**Fig. 23.1**).

The FAST exam has become a standard adjunct in the trauma bay. The standard FAST examination views include the right upper quadrant, left upper quadrant, pelvic view, and the pericardium. Hemopericardium is typically the result of penetrating trauma to the heart but may also be due to blunt rupture of the heart.[5] Rozycki et al.[6] used the FAST examination to evaluate for pericardial fluid in 1540 patients with truncal injuries, with 100% sensitivity and 99.3% specificity. The extended FAST exam, or eFAST, includes the evaluation of lung and pleural spaces to detect pneumothoraces or hemothoraces.[7] Sonographic findings of pneumothorax include absence of lung sliding, presence of A-lines, loss of comet tails, and the presence of a lung point sign.[8]

In stable patients, computed tomographic (CT) scans are often employed in thoracic trauma after the secondary survey and provide additional information as they are highly sensitive for hemothoraces, pneumothoraces, rib and spine fractures, vascular injuries, and lung contusions or lacerations. CT scans are typically performed with intravenous contrast to better visualize vascular injuries and lung parenchyma. It is advantageous to administer contrast contralateral to the suspected injury, if possible, to avoid obscuring the pathology. CT scans, in contrast to eFAST and CXR, are both sensitive and specific for a wide array of traumatic thoracic injuries that may be missed on simple US or x-ray examinations and should be considered in the stable patient when there is a high suspicion of thoracic injury.[7]

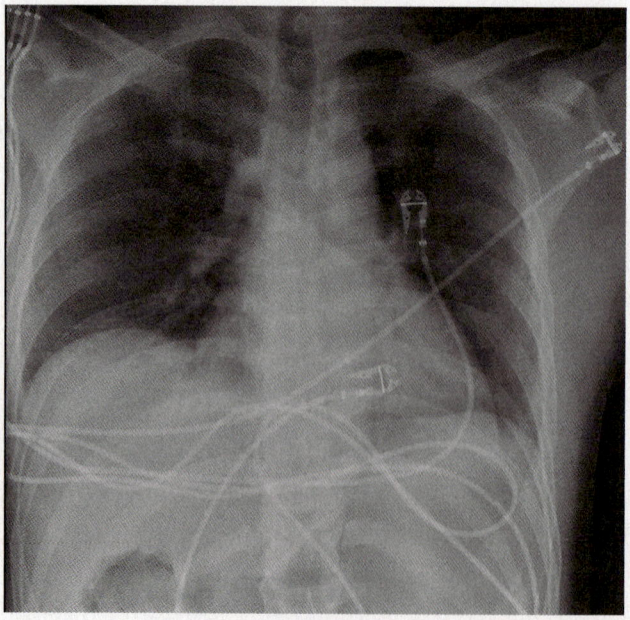

Figure 23.1. Supine AP CXR in the trauma bay.

COMMON INJURIES

Rib Fractures

The most common injury in thoracic trauma is the rib fracture, occurring in approximately 10% of all trauma patients. These most commonly occur after blunt trauma to the thorax, though gunshot wounds to the chest may also cause rib fractures. The spectrum of injury patterns ranges from a single nondisplaced rib fracture to large flail segments with severe displacement. Injury patterns are related to age and degree of flexibility of ribs. The younger population has innately more flexible ribs and therefore requires a higher force to create fractures. This higher force also translates to a higher degree of underlying lung injury, most notably pulmonary contusions. The older population with more brittle ribs requires less force to fracture the ribs and therefore may not have severe associated injuries. The diagnosis is usually made by initial physical examination, which may elicit tenderness, crepitus, and instability. While CXR only visualizes 30% of rib fractures, CT scan is extremely sensitive for diagnosing rib fractures, and also allows for quantification of any associated hemothorax, pneumothorax, or contusion.

Flail chest is defined as three or more consecutive ribs broken in two or more places. These segments may exhibit a "mechanical" flail which is the paradoxical movement of the flail segment in relation to the surrounding chest wall. As the patient inspires and expands the chest to produce a negative intrathoracic pressure, the flail segment is pulled inward (**Fig. 23.2A**). The opposite occurs during expiration and the flail segment bulges outward (**Fig. 23.2B**). A flail segment may be identified radiographically but may not be clinically evident; however, the converse may not be true. That is, one cannot have clinical flail chest without a radiographic flail segment. The respiratory compromise that occurs in the face of a flail segment is multifactorial: (1) underlying lung contusion, (2) pain with respirations, and (3) mechanical disadvantage. Pain control and contusion have a larger impact on clinical outcomes when compared to the mechanical disadvantage.

TRAUMA

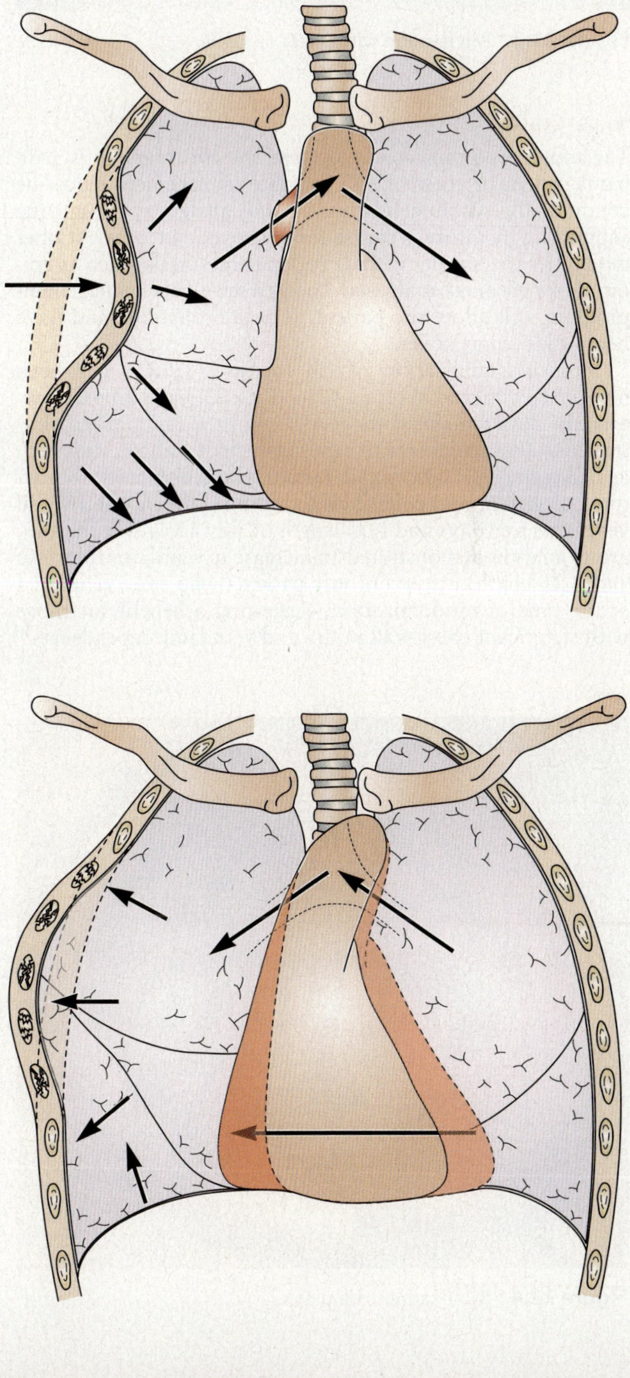

Figure 23.2. Pathophysiology of flail chest. **A:** Inspiratory phase: Chest wall collapses inward, causing air to move out of the bronchus of the involved lung into the trachea and bronchus of the uninvolved lung, causing a shift of mediastinum to the uninvolved side. **B:** Expiratory phase: Chest wall balloons outward so that air is expelled from the lung on the uninvolved side and enters the lung on the involved side with an associated shift of mediastinum to the involved side.

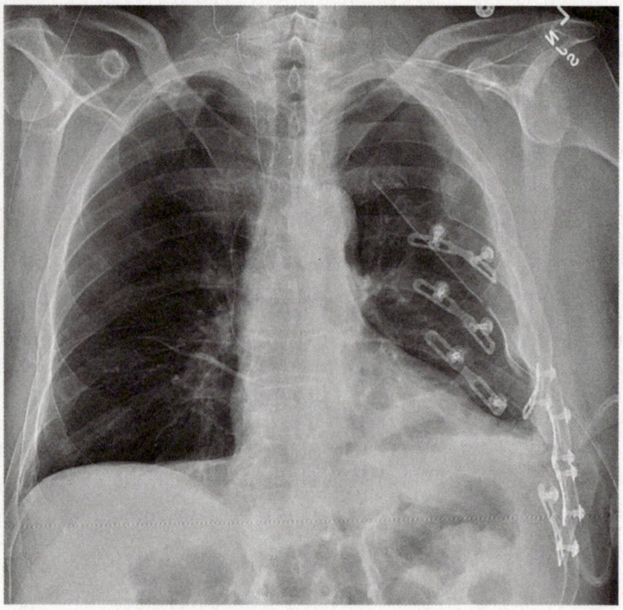

Figure 23.3. Rib fixation with plates on CXR.

Treatment

2 The most important aspect of care for rib fractures is pain management. A recent EAST practice management guideline conditionally recommends multimodal analgesia, though the supporting literature is sparse for improved outcomes.[9] Other modalities to consider include regional anesthesia, such as epidural or neuraxial analgesia. An aggressive pain management program will allow the patient to be more mobile and have better pulmonary toilet.

Surgical stabilization of rib fractures (SSRF) has been increasingly utilized in recent years (**Figs. 23.3** and **23.4**). However, the data remains controversial. In their randomized controlled trial of patients with significant chest wall injuries, such as flail segments, chest wall deformities, and displaced rib fractures, Dehghan and colleagues found no difference in overall ventilator free days and ICU length of stay. However, the subgroup analysis demonstrated an increase in ventilator free days and ICU length of stay in those patients who were ventilated at the time of randomization, suggesting a benefit for those with significant chest wall injury and ventilator dependence.[10]

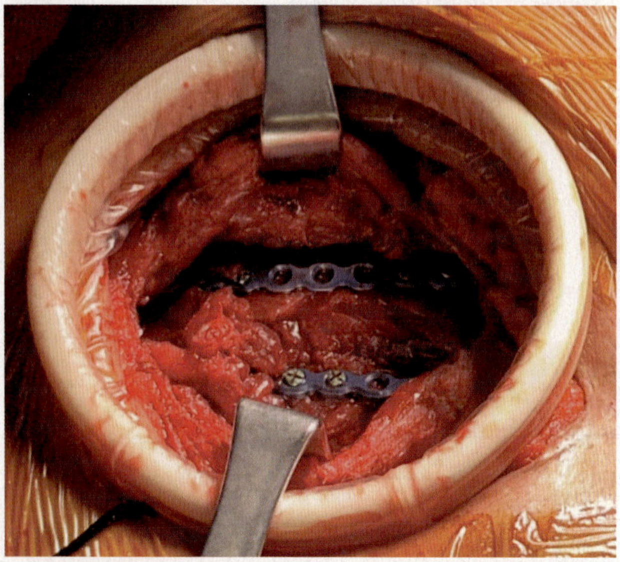

Figure 23.4. Rib fixation with plates.

Contradicting data still exists regarding nonintubated patients with flail chest: a large RCT of patients with radiographic flail chest failed to demonstrate improvement in pain scores and quality of life for up to 6 months after injury.[11] On the other hand, a multicenter prospective trial demonstrated improvement in pain scores at 2 weeks postoperatively when patients underwent SSRF within 72 hours of injury.[12] SSRF data has also been mixed regarding elderly patients and those with preexisting pulmonary comorbidities.[13] As new rib-plating systems, and adjuncts such as cryoablation of intercostal nerves become available, SSRF will likely continue to be an active area of research. It is the authors' position that the decision to undergo SSRF is patient specific and should be undertaken with thorough discussion between the surgeon and the patient, with careful consideration to the radiographic, clinical, and lifestyle factors for each individual patient.

Pneumothorax

Pneumothoraces can be classified into three subtypes: occult, simple, and tension. The diagnosis of pneumothorax can be made with physical examination, CXR, or eFAST. The standard of care in the trauma bay is upright or supine AP CXR, pending spinal clearance. Although radiographs are less sensitive than ultrasound for small pneumothoraces, they are used to screen for other associated injuries as described above. The pathophysiology of pneumothorax is the accumulation of air in the pleural space secondary to underlying pulmonary parenchymal injury or entrapment of atmospheric air from penetrating injury.

Occult pneumothoraces, which are detected on CT scan but not CXR, are detected in 15% to 20% of blunt thoracic trauma patients (**Fig. 23.5A,B**). Subcutaneous emphysema on screening CXR should alert the clinician to possible pneumothorax (**Fig. 23.6**). A simple pneumothorax is one that is seen on either CT scan or CXR but is not associated with hemodynamic compromise. A pneumothorax with concurrent hemodynamic compromise must be considered a tension pneumothorax until proven otherwise. A tension pneumothorax is a pneumothorax that has progressed to the point of pressurizing the pleural space, resulting in shifting of the mediastinum and compromising the venous return to the heart. Compression of the great vessels leads to an acute decrease in cardiac output and shock. Signs and symptoms of a tension pneumothorax include shortness of breath, dyspnea, tachypnea, hypotension, distended neck veins, and tracheal deviation away from the site of injury. If any of these signs are present, immediate decompression is necessary. Even temporary decompression, converting a tension pneumothorax into a simple pneumothorax, is warranted in an emergent situation. This is most easily done with a needle decompression or finger thoracostomy.

Treatment of Pneumothorax

If the patient is hemodynamically unstable and a tension pneumothorax is suspected, needle decompression or finger thoracostomy may be considered. For needle decompression, a large gauge angiocatheter of at least 5 cm length is inserted into the pleural space at the 5th intercostal space in the midaxillary line. There is cadaveric data that suggest that the 5th intercostal space in the midaxillary line has the shortest distance from the skin to the pleural cavity and therefore, may be superior to the anterior position, which is in the 2nd intercostal space along the midclavicular line, and is thus advocated in the ATLS guidelines.[14] Needle decompression is not without its risks; namely iatrogenic pneumothorax due to lung injury caused by the needle itself.[15] It should therefore only be undertaken in cases with high suspicion of tension pneumothorax in the face of not having a tube thoracostomy immediately available.

Finger thoracostomy achieves the same pleural depressurization as needle decompression. The procedure for finger thoracostomy is identical to the first steps of a traditional tube

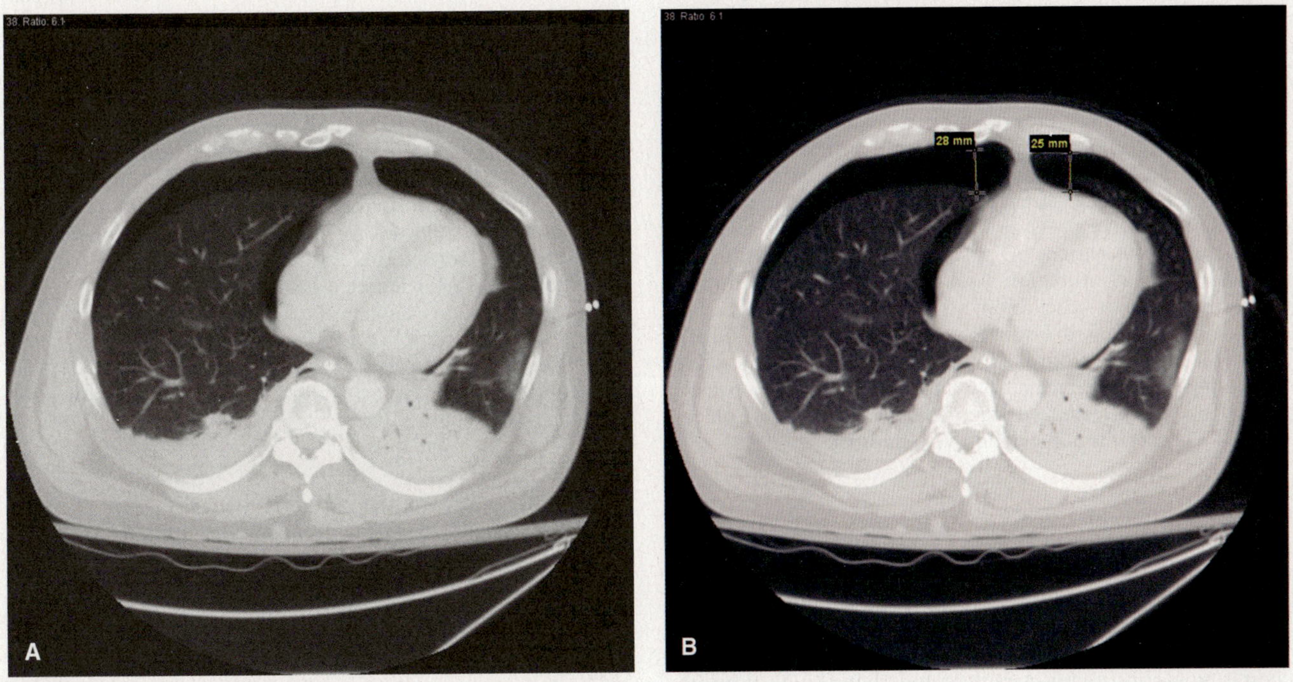

Figure 23.5. **A:** Occult pneumothorax seen on CT scan. **B:** Measurement of largest air pocket in a line drawn perpendicular to the chest wall.

thoracostomy. An incision is made in the 4th or 5th intercostal space in the midaxillary line and carried down sharply above the rib to incise the intercostal muscles and parietal pleura. The pleural space can then be entered with a finger or clamp to provide pleural decompression.

If one has access to a chest tube quickly, there is no need to perform a needle decompression or finger thoracostomy. A tube thoracostomy placed in the zone of safety, outlined by the pectoralis major lateral border, the nipple line in men, or two fingerbreadths above the inframammary fold in women, and the anterior border of the latissimus dorsi may be performed expeditiously (**Fig. 23.7**). If the tube is placed too far caudal, it can inadvertently enter the abdominal cavity. The inferior border of the axillary hair-line along the midaxillary line is another topographical landmark that can be used to identify a safe area. A 28-Fr chest tube suffices and larger tubes are unnecessary and only serve to increase the pain associated with the
3 procedure with no added benefit.[3] If there is no appreciable hemothorax and the major component is a pneumothorax, an even smaller tube may be used.[16] In those patients with a pure pneumothorax, an 8.3- to 14-Fr pigtail catheter is acceptable and may be superior, given the significantly less pain and discomfort of the tube as described in a randomized clinical trial.[17]

Drainage of all traumatic pneumothoraces via chest tube or pigtail catheter is no longer mandatory, even for patients on positive-pressure ventilation. For those with small pneumothoraces, defined as <35 mm distance between the visceral pleura and parietal pleura in a line perpendicular to the chest wall (radial line) of the largest air pocket on axial imaging. In a series of 146 patients with pneumothoraces, 90% of pneumothoraces that were 35 mm or less on chest CT scan were successfully observed. Therefore, if the patient is stable, we recommend repeating the CXR in 4 to 6 hours, and only treating the pneumothorax if it has significantly increased in

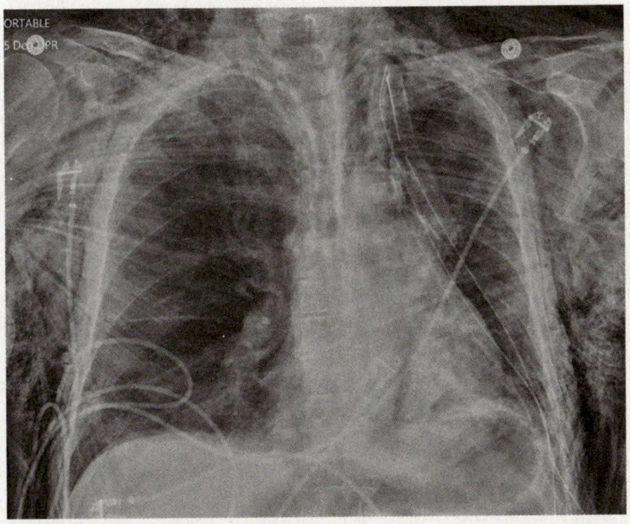

Figure 23.6. Subcutaneous emphysema.

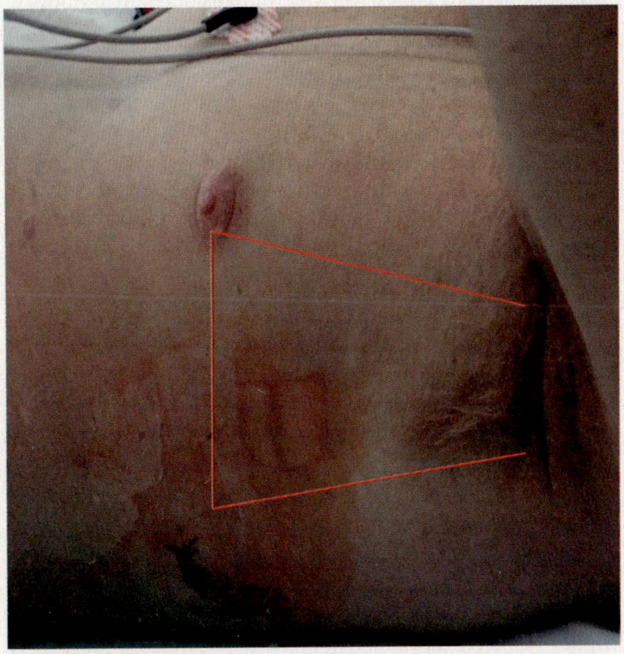

Figure 23.7. Zone of safety.

size or if the patient becomes symptomatic. A more objective guideline for placement of chest tubes using volumetric measurements has been shown to decrease the number of unnecessary chest tubes.[18]

In the rare circumstance of an open pneumothorax, where there is a loss of a portion of the chest wall, the normal negative pressure of the pleural space is lost. Due to the intrinsic elastic nature of the lung parenchyma it will collapse. One must establish a negative pressure in the pleural space to expand lung or place the patient on positive-pressure ventilation via oral endotracheal intubation. As a temporary measure during transport or early resuscitation, a partially occluding dressing can be applied. This dressing is sealed on three sides, which allows air to escape from the fourth side of the dressing while preventing atmospheric air from entering the pleural space.[19] Formal operative closure of the chest wall defect and placement of a chest tube is the definitive treatment.

Pulmonary Contusion

The transmission of energy across the chest wall can result in pulmonary contusion. Lung contusion is the extravasation of blood into the interstitial space of the lung parenchyma impairing gas exchange from alveoli to the pulmonary capillary bed. One may observe a significant decrease in the PaO_2:FiO_2 ratio with severe pulmonary contusions. Hypoxia in flail chest is most consistently a result of underlying lung contusion rather than a function of the disruption chest wall mechanics. Diagnosis of pulmonary contusion is typically made with CT scan, as it is more sensitive and specific than CXR.

Treatment

The treatment for lung contusion is primarily supportive care to include minimizing intravenous crystalloid fluid administration, early mobilization, and aggressive pulmonary hygiene. For hypoxia due to contusion, treatment includes the application of positive end-expiratory pressure. Intubations did not necessarily occur on the first day but often on the second day as the contusion "blooms" with surrounding interstitial edema. Fluid overload should be avoided, with the goal of judicious use of intravenous fluids while still maintaining adequate tissue perfusion. Diuretics may be helpful in this setting.[20]

Hemothorax

The causes of hemothorax are varied. Initial imaging to detect a hemothorax is the screening trauma bay CXR. The eFAST examination has a high sensitivity for detecting a hemothorax.

Treatment

The urgency of the treatment of a hemothorax is dictated by the physiologic state of the patient with rapid control of hemorrhage being the first priority. ATLS guidelines dictate that hemothoraces associated with hemodynamic instability or those that drain >1500 cc immediately or >200 cc/h for >4 hours after placement of a chest tube should be taken expeditiously to the operating room for hemorrhage control. Contemporary data suggest that there is no difference in the ability of the 28-Fr versus the 36-Fr chest tube to effectively drain a hemothorax. Ample high-quality data have demonstrated
4 equivalent efficacy of 14-Fr pigtail catheters and larger bore chest tubes in hemothorax drainage.[21–23] In general, patients with a hemothorax greater than approximately 300 cc require drainage when estimated using the Mergo volumetric formula on CT scan.[24]

Retained Hemothorax

Hemothoraces that persist despite drainage, or retained hemothoraces, may occur in 30% of patients.[25] Consequences of retained hemothorax include increased risk of empyema, entrapped lung parenchyma, and fibrothorax. Kugler and colleagues reported thoracic irrigation at the time of chest tube placed decreased the rate of retained hemothorax requiring secondary intervention.[26] This data has been expanded to a multicenter study of nearly 500 patients. Thoracic irrigation at the time of chest tube placement decreased need for secondary intervention, namely a VATS or additional chest tube, in 44% of patients.[27] For retained hemothoraces, there are two therapeutic options: (1) early video-assisted thoracostomy for evacuation or (2) tissue plasminogen activator (TPA) with or without DNase administered via the chest tube. The key is that early intervention allows for clot evacuation and prevention of fibrothorax formation. A meta-analysis of 476 patients undergoing VATS for retained hemothorax demonstrated that earlier intervention (days 1 to 3) was superior.[28] There are no trials comparing VATS to TPA, however, EAST guidelines recommend VATS for evacuation of retained hemothorax in all appropriate operative candidates, reserving TPA for poor operative candidates only.[29]

Aortic Injury

Penetrating injury to the aorta is typically fatal as most patients exsanguinate in the prehospital setting. A CT of the chest should be considered in bluntly injured patients with a high-risk mechanism, or with the following features on CXR: widened mediastinum >8 cm, loss of aortic knob, loss of aortopulmonary window, depression of left mainstem bronchus >110 degrees, deviation of nasogastric tube, apical cap, or tracheal deviation. CT scan with intravenous contrast has become the standard of care for diagnosis and classification of aortic injuries. Blunt aortic injuries most commonly occur at points of aortic fixation. These locations in decreasing order of occurrence include: (1) ligamentum arteriosum, just distal to the left subclavian artery, (2) diaphragmatic hiatus, (3) root of the aorta, and (4) left mainstem bronchus. The current classification of aortic injuries divides the extent of injury into four grades: (I) intimal tear, (II) intramural hematoma, (III) pseudoaneurysm, and (IV) periaortic rupture (**Fig. 23.8A,B**). Identification of blunt thoracic aortic injury has increased with advances in CT imaging, and the rate of intervention, particularly endovascular management, has risen since the FDA approval of thoracic stent grafts.[30]

Treatment

Treatment of blunt aortic injury is dictated by grade of injury. The Society for Vascular Surgery consensus guidelines for management of blunt aortic injury recommends medical management of grade I injuries.[31] Medical management consists of aggressive heart rate and blood pressure control. The recommended goal HR is <80 beats/min and goal systolic blood pressure is <120 mm Hg. This control is achieved with the administration of short-acting beta blocker (ie, esmolol) with additional agents such as nicardipine or nitroprusside as needed. Repeat CT angiogram to evaluate for progression of the injury is recommended, though the time interval to repeat imaging is variable. The management of grade II aortic injuries is evolving. Traditionally, it was recommended that these injuries undergo repair either via thoracic endovascular aortic repair (TEVAR) or an open approach, however, there is a trend toward treating these lesions with medical management alone.[32]

The EAST and SVS practice management guideline for blunt aortic injuries agree that Grade III and IV injuries should undergo timely endovascular repair.[33] When compared to open repair, incidence of paraplegia and mortality is lower in the endovascular treatment group,[34] which has resulted in its adoption as the contemporary standard of care (**Fig. 23.9**). Timing of repair is dictated by both grade of injury and the presence of other life-threatening injuries. For traumatic aortic pseudoaneurysms (grade III injuries), these do not need to be
5 repaired immediately if impulse control can be achieved. Delayed repair has been shown to be safe and actually has a lower overall mortality rate.[35] Grade IV injuries are repaired emergently in most situations.

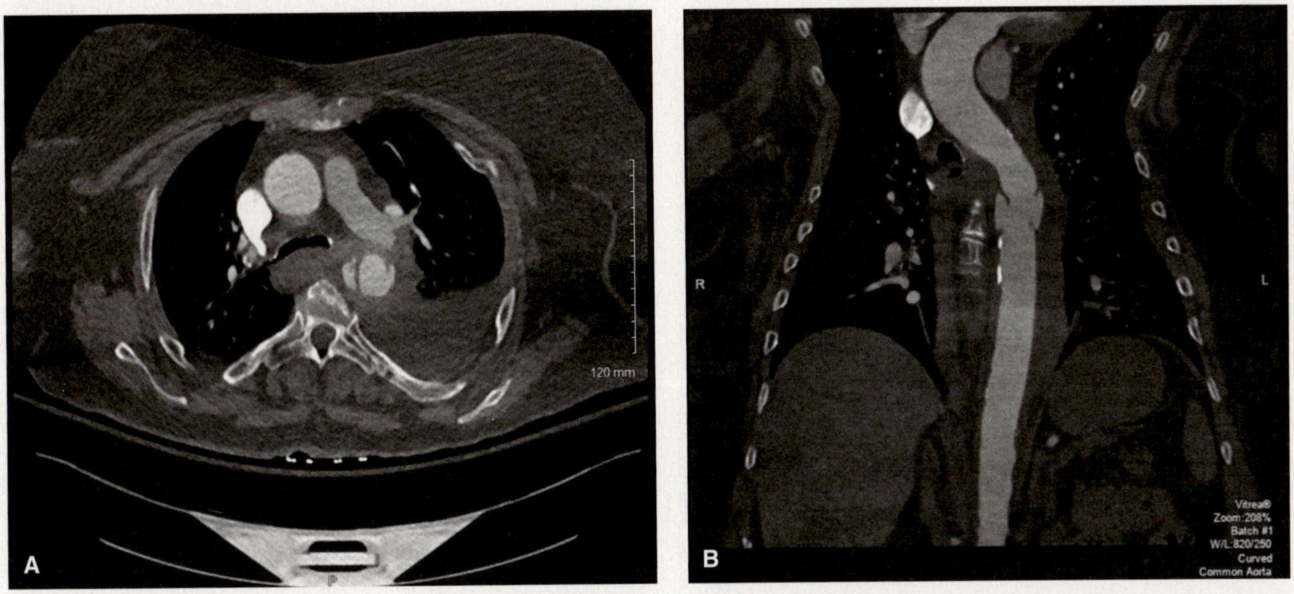

Figure 23.8. **A:** Axial view of type IV blunt aortic injury. **B:** Coronal view of type IV blunt aortic injury.

Diaphragmatic Injuries

Injuries to the diaphragm may be the result of either penetrating or blunt trauma. In a 2015 review, there were 3873 diaphragmatic injuries among the sample size of 833,309 trauma patients giving an incidence of 0.46%.[36] The average size of a diaphragmatic injury is approximately 2 cm for penetrating mechanisms and is 8 cm for blunt mechanisms. For the small injuries seen in penetrating trauma, one must maintain a high index of suspicion for diaphragmatic injury based on the trajectory of the knife or bullet. EAST guidelines recommend laparoscopy over CT scan for the diagnosis of left-sided diaphragm injuries.[37]

Treatment

Once the diagnosis is made, repair of left-sided diaphragm injuries should occur; injuries to the right hemidiaphragm may be safely observed in stable patients with no evidence of peritonitis or biliary fistula.[37] In the case of the penetrating trauma patient who is undergoing a diagnostic laparoscopy, the repair can be done laparoscopically. For those with an acute rupture following blunt trauma, the repair is usually performed via laparotomy to evaluate the abdominal organs for injury. For chronic hernia defects, strong consideration is made for repairing from the chest via a thoracotomy or via video-assisted thoracoscopy, as these are often associated with intrathoracic adhesions.

Diaphragmatic injuries should be repaired with nonabsorbable sutures in an interrupted horizontal mattress fashion; irrigation of the chest and tube thoracostomy may also be necessary. When primary suture repair is not possible due to tissue loss, a synthetic or biologic mesh may be used. Alternatively, the diaphragm may be sewn to a more cephalad rib, transposing it to a slightly higher position to achieve closure of the hemithorax.

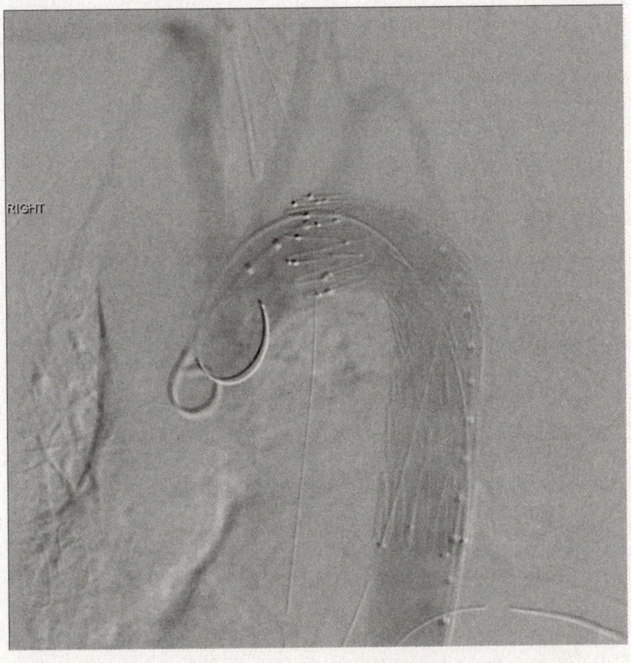

Figure 23.9. Aortic stent graft for blunt rupture.

Cardiac Injuries

Cardiac injury can occur with either penetrating or blunt mechanisms. The most common chamber affected with penetrating injury is the right ventricle since it has the largest anterior surface area; the thin-walled right atrium is the most commonly ruptured chamber in blunt mechanisms. The diagnosis of hemopericardium is usually made via the pericardial view of the FAST examination which is 95% sensitive and specific for pericardial fluid.[5] The presence of hypotension and hemopericardium defines cardiac tamponade and should be treated emergently.

Treatment

For an awake trauma patient with pericardial fluid, emergent transport to the operating room for median sternotomy is preferred. There is no role for pericardiocentesis in the acute trauma scenario, given the difficulties in evacuating clot from the pericardium, though this may be attempted by nonsurgeons to temporize a patient for transport to a trauma center. A pericardial window is typically a diagnostic test restricted to those patients who have confounding medical issues or to rule out cardiac injury in patients with a concerning trajectory with an equivocal pericardial fluid on the FAST exam. Typically, a positive pericardial FAST mandates surgical exploration via a sternotomy or thoracotomy, without any need for a pericardial window. If the patient has lost vital signs in the trauma bay or is rapidly deteriorating with loss of consciousness, then a resuscitative thoracotomy is indicated.[38] This allows rapid opening of the pericardium to relieve tamponade and temporize underlying cardiac injuries.

With impending cardiac tamponade due to hemopericardium, it is important to note that the decrease in preload with induction of anesthesia and positive-pressure ventilation may cause the patient to lose vital signs. The patient should be prepped and draped from the chin to the thighs prior to the induction of anesthesia and should be volume loaded to counteract periinduction drop in cardiac preload, and an acute afterload increase due to positive-pressure ventilation.

Once in the chest, the pericardium is opened and the cardiac injury identified. The injury can usually be controlled with digital pressure or other adjuncts such as a skin stapler, a Foley catheter, with special care not to rip the thin right ventricle with the balloon, or two stay sutures on either side of the injury that are crossed to close the wound. Formal repair with 3-0 Prolene on a larger needle (ie, MH) is then performed with or without pledgets in an interrupted fashion. If the injury is juxtaposed to a coronary vessel, one should perform a horizontal mattress and pass the needle deep to the coronary artery to avoid occluding the artery. If the proximal two-thirds of a coronary vessel are injured, it should be bypassed or repaired. Injuries to the distal third of a coronary vessel can be ligated, which is usually tolerated well. Intra- or postoperative echocardiography should be performed to evaluate for valve or septal injury, both of which are indications for cardiopulmonary bypass and expert consultation with a cardiac surgeon.

Blunt Cardiac Injury

There is a spectrum of blunt cardiac injuries. Injuries may cause mild dysrhythmias or lead to wall rupture (**Fig. 23.10**) and death. The most common sign of blunt cardiac injury is dysrhythmia, particularly sinus tachycardia. Any patient who undergoes a rapid deceleration mechanism is at risk for blunt cardiac injury. These patients are screened with a 12-lead ECG and troponin I; if both are normal, then blunt cardiac injury is ruled out and the patient does not require observation.[39] There is ongoing debate on the utility, timing, and sensitivity of obtaining cardiac enzymes. If an EKG demonstrates a new arrhythmia or conduction abnormality, or troponin elevation is present, then the patient requires admission for cardiac monitoring. If ST segment changes occur, a cardiac catheterization is necessary to rule out coronary dissection; echocardiography should be used to evaluate for valvular or other structural damage.

Tracheobronchial Injury

Tracheobronchial tree injury can occur from either blunt or penetrating mechanisms and usually presents with voice changes, pneumothorax, subcutaneous emphysema, pneumomediastinum, and air leak after chest tube placement. The majority of penetrating injuries to the tracheobronchial tree occur in the cervical trachea, while blunt injuries are typically in proximity to the carina, likely due to deceleration mechanisms and relative tethering of the carina.[40]

Treatment

Treatment must focus on maintaining a secure airway and secondarily, treating the injury. If necessary, an endotracheal tube may be advanced past the site of injury to allow for adequate oxygenation, ventilation, and attention to repair.[40] In rare cases, there may be the need for selective lung ventilation with a bronchoscopically placed bronchial blocker or may even require extracorporeal membrane oxygenation (ECMO) to temporize and allow for surgical repair. The majority of intrathoracic injuries are to the right mainstem bronchus and therefore, a right posterolateral thoracotomy is the best surgical approach as this also grants access to the carina. Left thoracotomy is reserved for injuries to the left bronchus. Once surgically exposed, the bronchus or trachea can usually be primarily repaired using a 3-0 absorbable suture. The repair can be buttressed with intercostal muscle or pleural flaps. Care should be taken not to devascularize the tracheal repair with excessive circumferential dissection. Ideally, these patients should be taken off positive-pressure ventilation as soon as possible, even immediately postoperatively.

Thoracic Esophageal Injury

Esophageal injuries are almost exclusively secondary to penetrating trauma as blunt rupture of the esophagus is exceedingly rare.[41] If the trajectory of the penetrating injury crosses the midline, the mediastinal structures must be evaluated. Hemodynamically unstable patients with penetrating torso trauma should be promptly operated upon for hemorrhage control and evaluation of injury. If the patient is stable, one may perform diagnostic studies to evaluate the esophagus. Secondary signs of esophageal injury may be present including pneumomediastinum, pleural effusion, or mediastinal hematoma. The spectrum of esophageal injuries ranges from a contusion or partial thickness laceration (grade I) to segmental loss or devascularization >2 cm (grade V).[42] An AAST multicenter retrospective review reported a 19% overall mortality rate for patients with esophageal injury with increasing mortality directly related to AAST grade of injury.[43]

The initial imaging study is a CT scan of the chest with IV contrast to better delineate the track of the missile (**Fig. 23.11A**). The most commonly utilized diagnostic modality is flexible endoscopy, which has been shown to have high sensitivity and specificity.[44] Otherwise, diagnostic imaging with water-soluble contrast followed by a barium-contrast study is warranted. The water-soluble contrast is used first in case there is a large leak (**Fig. 23.11B**). If no obvious leak is identified, then the water-soluble contrast study should be followed up with a barium study to increase the sensitivity for a

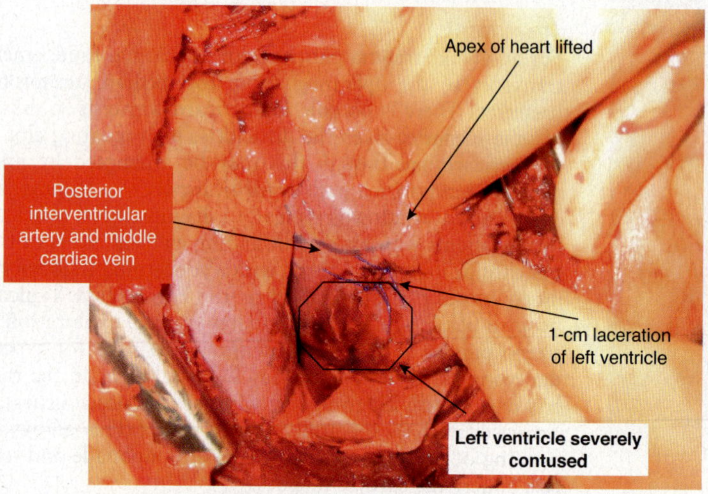

Figure 23.10. Blunt cardiac rupture/contusion.

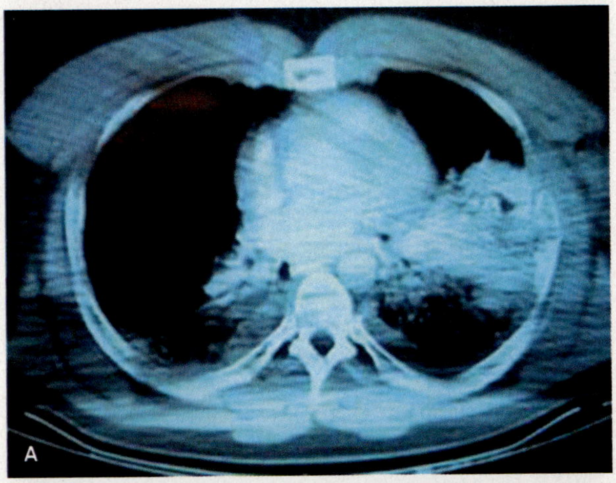

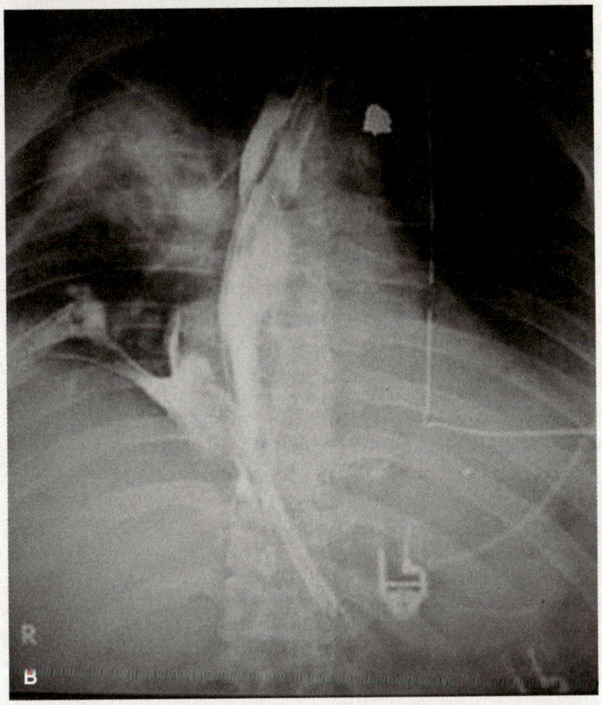

Figure 23.11. **A:** Tract of bullet coursing to posterior mediastinum. **B:** Contrast leaking from an injury to the esophagus.

small leak.[45] A CT esophagram may also be used if a patient is unable to participate in esophagography.[45]

Distal thoracic esophageal injuries are repaired via a left thoracotomy and the proximal two-thirds repaired via a right thoracotomy. Once the esophageal injury is identified, it should be debrided and repaired in two layers: absorbable suture should be used on mucosa, and the muscular layer may be repaired with permanent suture. The repair should be buttressed with either a pedicled intercostal muscle flap or a pleural patch. Some have used a tongue of omentum for distal esophageal repairs. Feeding access, either with a nasogastric tube or a gastrostomy tube, may be necessary to ensure adequate nutrition and enteral access in the perioperative period.[46]

RESUSCITATIVE THORACOTOMY

Resuscitative thoracotomy is an emergent procedure done primarily to control lethal hemorrhage. It provides exposure for control of vascular injuries, relieve cardiac tamponade, repair cardiac injury, perform internal cardiac massage, gain control of the pulmonary hilum, and cross-clamp the aorta to gain proximal control of intra-abdominal hemorrhage (**Fig. 23.12**). Mortality rates are high: up to 93% of patients injured in a blunt mechanism and 79% of patients injured in a penetrating mechanism succumb to their injuries.[47] Given the low likelihood of survival, EAST guidelines recommend resuscitative thoracotomy for patients with penetrating thoracic injuries without pulses but with signs of life.[1] A conditional recommendation for resuscitative thoracotomy is made for patients without pulses or signs of life with a thoracic injury, patients without pulses with extrathoracic penetrating injuries, and patients who present pulseless but with signs of life after blunt injury. For patients without pulses nor signs of life after blunt injury, a resuscitative thoracotomy is not recommended.[48]

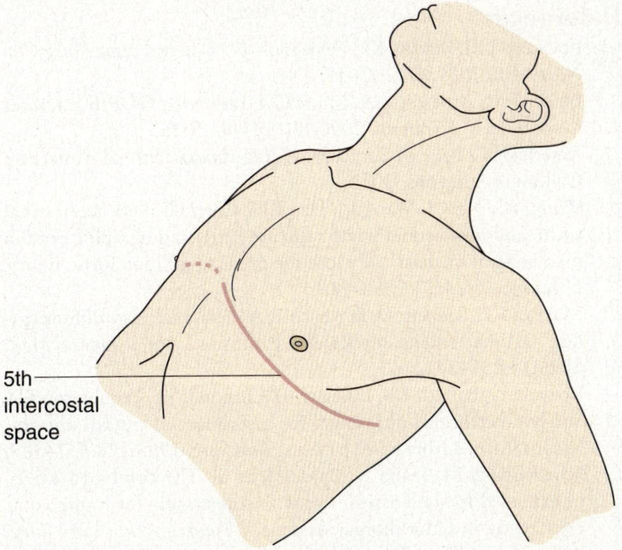

Figure 23.12. Left anterolateral thoracotomy incision.

A resuscitative thoracotomy gives fast access to a variety of intrathoracic structures. Of paramount importance is identification and quick control of injuries. First, the source of arrest must be addressed, which in most cases requires quick control of the bleeding site. In cases of cardiac injuries, pericardium must be opened to assess the heart. Second, descending thoracic aortic can be temporarily clamped to maintain perfusion to the brain and the heart, and to decrease bleeding if the source is downstream. After these steps are taken, the thoracic cavity must be evaluated quickly for other sources of bleeding, such as to the intercostal arteries, lungs, and pulmonary vessels. If needed, open cardiac massage can be performed. The patients that survive the resuscitative thoracotomy and regain perfusing cardiac rhythm should be rapidly taken to the operating room for definitive repair of injuries.

SUMMARY

Thoracic injuries are a common entity with rib fractures being the most common injury. A careful and systematic approach to the trauma patient is key to uncovering significant thoracic injuries. Life-threatening injuries, that is, massive truncal hemorrhage, tension pneumothorax, or cardiac tamponade must be identified quickly within the trauma bay and treated without delay.

ACKNOWLEDGMENT

We gratefully acknowledge the contributions of previous edition author, Jill Streams, as portions of those chapters have been retained in this revision.

References

1. LoCicero J III, Mattox KL. Epidemiology of chest trauma. *Surg Clin North Am.* 1989;69(1):15–19.
2. Bulger EM, Arneson MA, Mock CN, Jurkovich GJ. Rib fractures in the elderly. *J Trauma.* 2000;48(6):1040–1046.
3. American College of Surgeons. *ATLS Manual.* 9th ed. American College of Surgeons; 2012.
4. Wong YC, Ng CJ, Wang LJ, Hsu KH, Chen CJ. Left mediastinal width and mediastinal width ratio are better radiographic criteria than general mediastinal width for predicting blunt aortic injury. *J Trauma.* 2004;57(1):88–94.
5. Maenza RL, Seaberg D, D'Amico F. A meta-analysis of blunt cardiac trauma: ending myocardial confusion. *Am J Emerg Med.* 1996;14:237–241.
6. Rozycki G, Ballard RB, Feliciano DV, Schmidt JA, Pennington SD. Surgeon-performed ultrasound for assessment of truncal injuries: lessons learned from 1540 patients. *Ann Surg.* 1998;228:557–567.
7. Schellenberg M, Inaba K, Bardes J, et al. The combined utility of extended focused assessment with sonography for trauma and chest x-ray in blunt thoracic trauma. *J Trauma Acute Care Surg.* 2018;85(1):113–117.
8. Kirkpatrick AW, Sirois M, Laupland KB, et al. Hand-held thoracic sonography for detecting post-traumatic pneumothoraces: the Extended Focused Assessment with Sonography for Trauma (EFAST). *J Trauma.* 2004;57(2):288–295.
9. Galvagno SM Jr, Smith CE, Varon AJ, et al. Pain management for blunt thoracic trauma: a joint practice management guideline from the Eastern Association for the Surgery of Trauma and Trauma Anesthesiology Society. *J Trauma Acute Care Surg.* 2016;81(5): 936–951.
10. Dehghan N, Nauth A, Schemitsch E, et al; Canadian Orthopaedic Trauma Society and the Unstable Chest Wall RCT Study Investigators. Operative vs nonoperative treatment of acute unstable chest wall injuries: a randomized clinical trial. *JAMA Surg.* 2022;157(11):983–990.
11. Meyer DE, Harvin JA, Vincent L, et al. Randomized controlled trial of surgical rib fixation to nonoperative management in severe chest wall injury. *Ann Surg.* 2023;278(3):357–365.
12. Pieracci FM, Leasia K, Bauman Z, et al. A multicenter, prospective, controlled clinical trial of surgical stabilization of rib fractures in patients with severe, nonflail fracture patterns (Chest Wall Injury Society NONFLAIL). *J Trauma Acute Care Surg.* 2020;88(2):249–257.
13. Pieracci FM, Leasia K, Hernandez MC, et al. Surgical stabilization of rib fractures in octogenarians and beyond-what are the outcomes? *J Trauma Acute Care Surg.* 2021;90(6):1014–1021.
14. Inaba K, Branco BC, Eckstein M, et al. Optimal positioning for emergent needle thoracostomy: a cadaver-based study. *J Trauma.* 2011;71(5):1099–1103.
15. Travis HJ, Andry GV, Rutner CC, et al. Prehospital needle decompression of suspected tension pneumothorax: outcomes and consequences. *Am Surg.* 2024;90:2124–2126.
16. Inaba K, Lustenberger T, Recinos G, et al. Does size matter? A prospective analysis of 28-32 versus 36-40 French chest tube size in trauma. *J Trauma Acute Care Surg.* 2012;72(2):422–427.
17. Kulvatunyou N, Erickson L, Vijayasekaran A, et al. Randomized clinical trial of pigtail catheter versus chest tube in injured patients with uncomplicated traumatic pneumothorax. *Br J Surg.* 2014;101:17–22.
18. Al Tannir AH, Biesboer EA, Tentis M, et al. Implementation of the 300-mL rule for the management of traumatic hemothorax. *J Am Coll Surg.* 2024;239(5):422–429.
19. Kong VY, Liu M, Sartorius B, Clarke DL. Open pneumothorax: the spectrum and outcome of management based on Advanced Trauma Life Support recommendations. *Eur J Trauma Emerg Surg.* 2015;41(4):401–404.
20. Simon B, Ebert J, Bokhari F, et al. Management of pulmonary contusion and flail chest: an Eastern Association for the Surgery of Trauma practice management guideline. *J Trauma Acute Care Surg.* 2012;73(5 Suppl 4):S351–361.
21. Bauman ZM, Kulvatunyou N, Joseph B, et al. Randomized clinical trial of 14-French (14F) pigtail catheters versus 28-32F chest tubes in the management of patients with traumatic hemothorax and hemopneumothorax. *World J Surg.* 2021;45(3):880–886.
22. Beeton G, Ngatuvai M, Breeding T, et al. Outcomes of pigtail catheter placement versus chest tube placement in adult thoracic trauma patients: a systematic review and meta-analysis. *Am Surg.* 2023;89(6):2743–2754.
23. Kulvatunyou N, Bauman ZM, Zein Edine SB, et al. The small (14 Fr) percutaneous catheter (P-CAT) versus large (28-32 Fr) open chest tube for traumatic hemothorax: a multicenter randomized clinical trial. *J Trauma Acute Care Surg.* 2021;91(5):809–813.
24. Mergo PJ, Helmberger T, Didovic J, Cernigliaro J, Ros PR, Staab EV. New formula for quantification of pleural effusions from computed tomography. *J Thorac Imaging.* 1999;14:122–125.
25. DuBose J, Inaba K, Demetriades D, et al. Management of post-traumatic retained hemothorax: a prospective, observational, multicenter AAST study. *J Trauma Acute Care Surg.* 2012;72(1):11–22.
26. Kugler NW, Carver TW, Milia D, Paul JS. Thoracic irrigation prevents retained hemothorax: a prospective propensity scored analysis. *J Trauma Acute Care Surg.* 2017;83(6):1136–1141.
27. Carver TW, Berndtson AE, McNickle AG, et al. Thoracic irrigation for prevention of secondary intervention after thoracostomy tube drainage for hemothorax: a Western Trauma Association multicenter study. *J Trauma Acute Care Surg.* 2024;97:724–730.
28. Ziapour B, Mostafidi E, Sadeghi-Bazargani H, Kabir A, Okereke I. Timing to perform VATS for traumatic-retained hemothorax (a systematic review and meta-analysis). *Eur J Trauma Emerg Surg.* 2020;46(2):337–346.
29. Patel NJ, Dultz L, Ladhani HA, et al. Management of simple and retained hemothorax: a practice management guideline from the Eastern Association for the Surgery of Trauma. *Am J Surg.* 2021;221(5):873–884.
30. Scalea TM, Feliciano DV, DuBose JJ, Ottochian M, O'Connor JV, Morrison JJ. Blunt thoracic aortic injury: endovascular repair is now the standard. *J Am Coll Surg.* 2019;228(4):605–610.
31. Lee WA, Matsumura JS, Mitchell RS, et al. Endovascular repair of traumatic thoracic aortic injury: clinical practice guidelines of the Society for Vascular Surgery. *J Vasc Surg.* 2011;53(1):187–192.
32. Sandhu HK, Leonard SD, Perlick A, et al. Determinants and outcomes of nonoperative management for blunt traumatic aortic injuries. *J Vasc Surg.* 2018;67(2):389–398.
33. Fox N, Schwartz D, Salazar JH, et al. Evaluation and management of blunt traumatic aortic injury: a practice management guideline from the Eastern Association for the Surgery of Trauma. *J Trauma Acute Care Surg.* 2015;78(2):136–146.
34. Moainie SL, Neschis DG, Gammie JS, et al. Endovascular stenting for traumatic aortic injury: an emerging new standard of care. *Ann Thorac Surg.* 2008;85(5):1625–1629.
35. Marcaccio CL, Dumas RP, Huang Y, Yang W, Wang GJ, Holena DN. Delayed endovascular aortic repair is associated with reduced in-hospital mortality in patients with blunt thoracic aortic injury. *J Vasc Surg.* 2018;68(1):64–73.
36. Uhlich R, Kerby JD, Bosarge P, Hu P. Diagnosis of diaphragm injuries using modern 256-slice CT scanners: too early to abandon operative exploration. *Trauma Surg Acute Care Open.* 2018; 3(1):e000251.
37. McDonald AA, Robinson BRH, Alarcon L, et al. Evaluation and management of traumatic diaphragmatic injuries: a Practice Management Guideline from the Eastern Association for the Surgery of Trauma. *J Trauma Acute Care Surg.* 2018;85(1):198–207.
38. Karmy-Jones R, Nathens A, Jurkovich GJ, et al. Urgent and emergent thoracotomy for penetrating chest trauma. *J Trauma.* 2004;56(3):664–668; discussion 668–669.
39. Clancy K, Velopulos C, Bilaniuk JW, et al. Screening for blunt cardiac injury: an Eastern Association for the Surgery of Trauma practice management guideline. *J Trauma Acute Care Surg.* 2012; 73(5 Suppl 4):S301–S306.
40. Dennis BM, Bellister SA, Guillamondegui OD. Thoracic trauma. *Surg Clin North Am.* 2017;97(5):1047–1064.
41. Xu AA, Breeze JL, Paulus JK, Bugaev N. Epidemiology of traumatic esophageal injury: an analysis of the National Trauma Data Bank. *Am Surg.* 2019;85(4):342–349.

42. Moore EE, Jurkovich GJ, Knudson MM, et al. Organ injury scaling. VI: extrahepatic biliary, esophagus, stomach, vulva, vagina, uterus (nonpregnant), uterus (pregnant), fallopian tube, and ovary. *J Trauma*. 1995;39(6):1069–1070.
43. Asensio JA, Chahwan S, Forno W, et al. American Association for the Surgery of Trauma. Penetrating esophageal injuries: a multicenter study of the American Association for the Surgery of Trauma. *J Trauma*. 2001;50(2):289–296.
44. Arantes V, Campolina C, Valerio SH, et al. Flexible esophagoscopy as a diagnostic tool for traumatic esophageal injuries. *J Trauma*. 2009;66(6):1677–1682.
45. Biffl WL, Moore EE, Feliciano DV, et al. Western Trauma Association Critical Decisions in Trauma: diagnosis and management of esophageal injuries. *J Trauma Acute Care Surg*. 2015;79(6):1089–1095.
46. Chirica M, Kelly MD, Siboni S, et al. Esophageal emergencies: WSES guidelines. *World J Emerg Surg*. 2019;14:26.
47. Liu A, Nguyen J, Ehrlich H, et al. Emergency resuscitative thoracotomy for civilian thoracic trauma in the field and emergency department settings: a systematic review and meta-analysis. *J Surg Res*. 2022;273:44–55.
48. Seamon MJ, Haut ER, Van Arendonk K, et al. An evidence-based approach to patient selection for emergency department thoracotomy: a practice management guideline from the Eastern Association for the Surgery of Trauma. *J Trauma Acute Care Surg*. 2015;79(1):159–173.

24

Abdominal Trauma

Kazuhide Matsushima, Anaar E. Siletz, and Kenji Inaba

Key Points

1. There is a fundamental difference in the diagnostic approach to patients who present with penetrating versus blunt abdominal trauma. A combination of clinical examination and focused imaging, running concurrent to active resuscitation, will be required for the accurate diagnosis and timely treatment of injuries.
2. After blunt abdominal trauma, patients with peritonitis or hemodynamic instability with a positive Focused Assessment with Sonography for Trauma (FAST) require immediate laparotomy. For those not requiring immediate exploration, computed tomography (CT) is a high-yield diagnostic modality for intra-abdominal organ injuries.
3. Penetrating abdominal trauma patients who present with hemodynamic instability, peritonitis, or those who cannot be evaluated, should be taken to the operating room immediately. In hemodynamically stable and evaluable patients without peritonitis or evisceration, selective nonoperative management can be considered when appropriate resources are available.
4. Damage-control laparotomy, which consists of rapid control of bleeding and contamination followed by temporary abdominal closure, should be considered for any patient with, (1) severe physiologic derangements, (2) a significant injury burden for which definitive repair may be detrimental, or (3) an injury profile beyond the scope of the surgeon's skillset or facility resources.
5. Angioembolization is an important adjunct in the management of abdominal trauma and may be of particular benefit in patients with ongoing bleeding from complex solid organ injuries or pelvic fractures.

For patients who have sustained blunt multisystem trauma or penetrating trauma including stab wounds (SW), gunshot wounds (GSW), and shotgun wounds, the abdominal cavity is at risk of potentially life-threatening injuries. Unlike injuries to the extremities or neck, where bleeding often occurs externally, significant bleeding and enteric spillage into the abdominal cavity can occur before the patient exhibits obvious symptoms and physiologic changes. Therefore, a systematic approach with the rapid diagnosis and treatment of these injuries is essential. This chapter will provide a pragmatic approach, focusing on the initial resuscitation, diagnosis, and treatment in patients with clinically relevant injuries to the abdominal organs.

BLUNT TRAUMA: INITIAL EVALUATION AND DIAGNOSTICS

Resuscitation

In contrast to extremity hemorrhage, which can be controlled with direct pressure, packing, or tourniquet placement, there are currently no validated prehospital methods for direct or indirect control of abdominal hemorrhage. In the appropriate clinical setting with trained personnel, resuscitative endovascular balloon occlusion of the aorta (REBOA) could theoretically be performed in the prehospital setting.[1] However, rapid transport to definitive care at a trauma center remains the primary-scene goal for any patient at risk of abdominal injury. The general principles of resuscitation that apply to all trauma patients as outlined elsewhere in this textbook should be followed. In patients with suspected abdominal trauma, intravenous or if not possible, intraosseous access should be rapidly obtained in the upper limbs or torso. Access in the lower limbs including femoral central venous catheters may not allow adequate resuscitation if there are injuries to the iliac veins or inferior vena cava (IVC), as transfused blood products and medications may extravasate rather than circulate systemically. Once the diagnosis of an intra-abdominal injury requiring operative repair has been made, immediate transfer to the operating room should take precedence over continued resuscitative efforts which can be continued concurrent to definitive hemorrhage control.

Diagnostics

The diagnostic approach to the patient in the resuscitation area can be categorized based on the presenting hemodynamic status: cardiac arrest, unstable, or stable.

Cardiac Arrest Patient

In blunt trauma, patient outcomes following resuscitative thoracotomy are exceedingly poor, especially if the source of hemorrhage is in the abdomen. However, survival to discharge and organ donation have been reported.[2] Along with airway control and gaining venous access for resuscitation with blood products and medication administration, resuscitative left anterolateral thoracotomy and concurrent evaluation of the right chest with tube or finger thoracostomy are the immediate priorities. If a resuscitative thoracotomy is performed and return of spontaneous circulation is achieved, the patient should be taken immediately to the operating room for exploratory laparotomy, if there is any evidence of an intra-abdominal injury. It is important to note that the performance of abdominal FAST in the setting of cardiac arrest has been documented to be poor.[3]

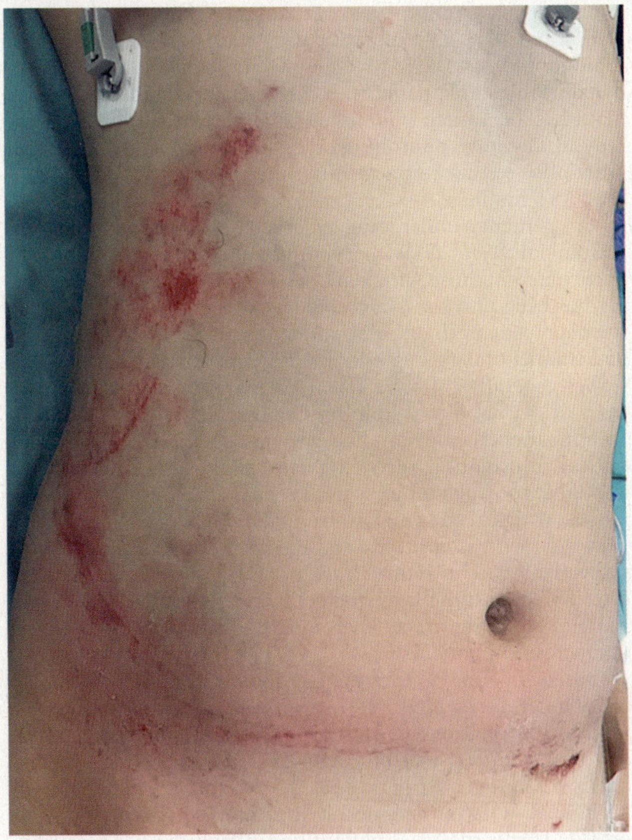

Figure 24.1. Abdominal seatbelt sign.

Hemodynamically Unstable Patient

In hemodynamically unstable patients, aggressive, balanced resuscitation with blood products should be initiated immediately. An abdominal FAST should be performed simultaneously to evaluate for intra-abdominal hemorrhage. If abdominal free fluid is visualized on the FAST, the patient should immediately be taken to the operating room for an emergency laparotomy. Even if the FAST is negative, given the suboptimal sensitivity and negative predictive value of FAST, a diagnostic peritoneal aspirate (DPA) looking for gross blood should be considered to confirm the result.[4] In the setting of persistent hypotension, with a negative FAST and negative DPA, alternative sources for the hemorrhage should be sought.

Hemodynamically Stable Patient

A diagnostic workup in stable patients begins with an external examination for any evidence of significant soft tissue injuries. A seatbelt sign, for example, has been associated with an eightfold increase in the incidence of intra-abdominal injuries, impacting both the solid organs and hollow viscera[5] (**Fig. 24.1**). While the presence of a seatbelt sign is not sufficient to warrant mandatory laparotomy, a very low threshold for obtaining an abdominal computed tomography (CT) should be maintained, and the patient should undergo a period of observation or diagnostic laparoscopy based on their clinical and radiographic findings.[6]

1 If the patient already has peritonitis on their initial examination, immediate laparotomy should be performed. This is a high-yield indication for emergency operation in the setting of trauma. In patients without peritonitis, the initial imaging modality is FAST to look for intra-abdominal free fluid. The presence of free fluid should trigger further imaging work-up with an abdominal CT. CT should be also considered in stable patients with clinical evidence of significant force to the abdomen or significant abdominal tenderness on examination. Additionally, high-energy injury mechanisms or a history of direct, focused energy transfer to the abdomen should be worked up with an abdominal CT.

Based on the CT results, patients can be categorized into two groups: those with normal versus abnormal CT findings. If the CT demonstrates no abnormalities including abdominal free fluid or other nonspecific findings such as mesenteric stranding, the likelihood of a clinically significant injury is extremely low.[7,8] For patients with intra-abdominal injuries seen on CT, the nature of the injuries will determine management. Any hollow viscus injury or intraperitoneal bladder injury will require operative repair. For solid organ injuries, the indications for operative management will depend on the hemodynamic status, the extent of injury, and other associated injuries. This will be further elucidated in the organ-specific sections below. Patients with hollow viscus injuries may have subtle CT findings such as mesenteric fat stranding, free fluid in the absence of solid organ injury, and bowel wall thickening. These patients should be monitored clinically for collateral evidence of hollow viscus injuries such as leukocytosis, tachycardia, fever, and worsening abdominal examination.

PENETRATING TRAUMA: INITIAL EVALUATION AND DIAGNOSTICS

General Approach to Penetrating Abdominal Injury

Due largely to the experience of World Wars I and II, characterized by high rates of destructive injuries, penetrating abdominal trauma was historically treated with mandatory surgical exploration. Starting in the 1960s with SWs, followed by GSWs, this paradigm began to shift toward selective nonoperative management. Patient selection criteria for operative versus nonoperative management based on clinical assessment and radiologic evidence have been developed and validated in multiple studies.[9] Due to the morbidity associated with nontherapeutic operations, contemporary evidence now supports a nonoperative approach to the management of penetrating abdominal trauma in select circumstances. A Western Trauma Association multicenter study including 359 patients with anterior abdominal SW found that 64% of patients did not require laparotomy.[10] The need for laparotomy is even lower after SWs to the back with only 15% of patients noted to have clinically significant injury.[11] Patients with abdominal GSW are more likely to require operative exploration, but the presence of a GSW to the abdomen alone does not mandate laparotomy. In an analysis of 1856 patients with abdominal GSWs, had a policy of mandatory laparotomy been employed, 47% of patients would have undergone an unnecessary laparotomy.[12] Similar to SW, posterior and transpelvic injuries are less likely than anterior injuries to require exploration.[13,14]

2 The balance between prompt surgical management of traumatic injury and avoiding unnecessary surgery remains a central diagnostic and management challenge in penetrating abdominal trauma. In patients who present with hemodynamic instability, peritonitis, or are unevaluable, immediate operation is mandated. In the remaining patients, the practice of universal exploration would result in a high rate of nontherapeutic laparotomy which is associated with a high incidence of postoperative morbidity.[15] This not only impacts patient outcome and quality of life, but also trauma resource utilization as nontherapeutic laparotomy is associated with increased hospital length of stay and health care costs.

Indications and Contraindications for Selective Nonoperative Management

Peritonitis and hemodynamic instability in the setting of penetrating abdominal trauma remain absolute indications for emergency laparotomy. Although soft tissue injury from a SW or GSW can cause local abdominal tenderness, diffuse peritonitis after penetrating abdominal trauma is associated with a 97% chance of finding an intra-abdominal injury at laparotomy.[16] As the detection of peritonitis on exam is so critical, unevaluable patients including those with concomitant head or spinal cord injury or those undergoing urgent nonabdominal operations are not candidates for selective nonoperative management. Abdominal exploration can be considered in patients with omental or visceral evisceration after penetrating abdominal trauma as significant intra-abdominal injury is present in 46% to 85% of patients with omental evisceration, and even higher rates with visceral evisceration.[17] Peritoneal penetration alone after penetrating trauma is not an absolute indication for operative exploration. For this reason, invasive evaluation including diagnostic laparoscopy or local-wound exploration for the sole purpose of determining peritoneal violation should not be considered.

Diagnostics

Radiologic imaging is a key component of the diagnostic workup in patients who have sustained penetrating abdominal trauma, especially those undergoing a trial of selective nonoperative management. In hemodynamically stable, evaluable patients without peritonitis, a detailed evaluation of the external wounds and retained fragments using plain radiographs is imperative to plot missile trajectories. External wounds do not always correspond to internal injury and, especially in the setting of multiple missiles, trajectory may be misleading from external wounds alone. Management of the patient may change significantly based on the internal trajectory. For example, paired lateral abdominal wall bullet wounds may represent a superficial tangential trajectory or two separate destructive transabdominal trajectories with retained missiles.

The primary use of the FAST in penetrating trauma is to evaluate for pericardial fluid. A positive pericardial FAST can occur after penetrating abdominal trauma and mandates immediate median sternotomy given the high specificity for cardiac injury.[18] For the abdominal windows, while the FAST is highly specific for intra-abdominal free fluid, the sensitivity is poor.[18] In hemodynamically unstable patients who could potentially have multiple cavitary sources of ongoing bleeding, FAST can still be helpful, particularly with positive results, as a rapid tool for operative planning. On the other hand, in hemodynamically stable patients, it rarely impacts clinical decision making. The patient will either undergo exploratory laparotomy if they have peritonitis or are unevaluable, or they meet criteria for selective nonoperative management, irrespective of the FAST findings.

For patients undergoing emergent exploration following abdominal SW or GSW, CT should not be routinely obtained, particularly in those with hemodynamic instability. In contrast, CT has been universally accepted as an integral component of the diagnostic evaluation of patients with penetrating abdominal trauma undergoing selective nonoperative management.[19] GSWs generally follow a linear path and have an associated tract of air bubbles visible on CT that allows for trajectory identification. Understanding the missile trajectory provides critical information regarding potentially injured structures and those to which injury is unlikely. CT imaging after abdominal GSW has been shown to be highly reliable for injury identification, with a sensitivity and specificity of 90.5% and 96%, respectively.[19] The injury tract on CT is often more subtle after SW due to the lower velocity and smaller volume of air bubbles along the tract. Therefore, CT is not always a useful adjunct in SW patients.[20]

Based on the CT findings, patients with penetrating trauma can be divided into four groups. (1) Patients with no peritoneal violation. In this group, it is unlikely that operative intervention will be required. The patient may be discharged after a short period of observation. (2) Patients with peritoneal violation but no obvious intra-abdominal injuries on CT. This is the ideal patient population for selective nonoperative management with close clinical monitoring. (3) Patients with peritoneal violation and CT findings concerning for vascular or hollow viscus injuries. These patients require laparotomy. Findings concerning for injury include bowel wall irregularity, mural defect, abnormal wall enhancement, mesenteric hematoma, and free air or fluid[21] (**Fig. 24.2**). (4) Patients with peritoneal violation and solid organ injuries. In the absence of hollow viscus injuries, solid organ injuries alone would not mandate laparotomy.[22] If the patient remains

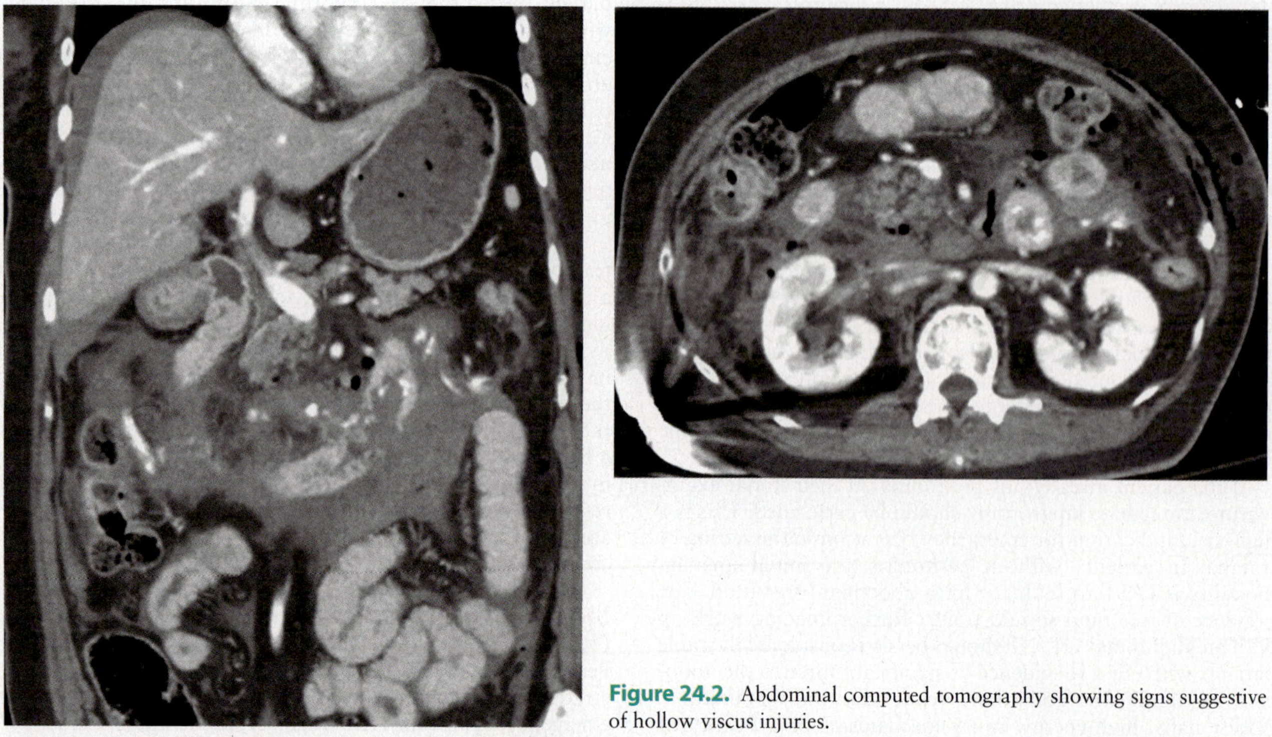

Figure 24.2. Abdominal computed tomography showing signs suggestive of hollow viscus injuries.

hemodynamically stable, nonoperative management can be attempted in this group. Adjunctive use of angioembolization may be considered for CT findings suggestive of vascular injuries (eg, contrast extravasation, pseudoaneurysm, arteriovenous fistula).

In patients undergoing nonoperative management, clinical observation becomes an important next step. This is the most time-consuming and resource-intensive aspect of nonoperative management, and one of the primary reasons it is not always feasible at institutions with limited resources. This observation should be performed ideally by the same group of providers, who can carefully examine for changes in abdominal tenderness, collateral signs of occult injury such as tachycardia or fever, and laboratory abnormalities such as anemia or leukocytosis. During the observation period, it is expected that a certain percentage of patients initially selected for nonoperative management will require operative interventions based on changes in clinical examination and/or laboratory results. Patients should not receive any opioid analgesics or antibiotics that may mask the symptoms and signs of ongoing hemorrhage or occult hollow viscus injuries. Strict adherence to an established protocol is necessary to ensure early identification of patients who fail nonoperative management and require operative intervention. The duration of observation should meet a minimum standard. After abdominal GSWs, a review of 270 patients found that all injuries requiring laparotomy became apparent within 24 hours of observation.[23,24] Similar results have been described for abdominal SWs with injuries requiring laparotomy detected within 24 hours of observation.[25]

Penetrating left-sided thoracoabdominal injuries, bounded by the nipple line, scapular tip, and costal margin, present a unique challenge due to the risk of occult diaphragmatic injury. Diaphragmatic injuries following penetrating trauma are notoriously difficult to identify on CT and are often asymptomatic during the early postinjury period. Because the size of injury will likely increase over time, the patient will be at risk of visceral herniation and strangulation. The incidence of complications related to diaphragm injuries are lower after right-sided injuries due to buttressing of the injury by the liver. The incidence of diaphragmatic injury after penetrating left-sided thoracoabdominal injury is reported to be as high as 42%.[26] For that reason, patients treated nonoperatively for left-sided thoracoabdominal injury should undergo evaluation for diaphragm injuries during the same admission. If the patient develops peritonitis during their clinical observation, which in general should be for 24 hours, the diaphragm can be examined at laparotomy. If the patient passes the trial of nonoperative management and other associated intra-abdominal injuries have been excluded, diagnostic laparoscopy should be offered to evaluate the left-sided diaphragm.[27]

3 THE TRAUMA LAPAROTOMY

For all emergent trauma laparotomies, the patient should be placed in the supine position with arms abducted. Even with a concomitant thoracic injury, this is the preferred starting position. Rarely, for patients with a penetrating injury with a transpelvic trajectory, where endoscopic evaluation of rectal injury can be required, lithotomy position may be required. Similarly, in the blunt trauma patient where there is external perineal injury associated with pelvic fractures, the patients should be positioned accordingly for proper exposure of the perineum. At a minimum, the torso, neck, and upper half of the lower extremities should always be prepared into the field for maximum flexibility. With any concurrent limb injuries, the entire extremity should be prepared. If there is any concern for a urethral or bladder injury, the Foley catheter should be prepared into the field to allow manipulation by the surgeon. Forced air warming on the lower half of the extremities, and other warming adjuncts should be utilized to prevent hypothermia. All preoperative patient preparation including venous and arterial access, preoperative antibiotics, and confirmation of patient identification should be a team effort with full participation by the surgical team.

The trauma laparotomy incision typically extends from the xiphoid process to the symphysis pubis. For the patient in extremis, all layers are made with a scalpel to gain access to the abdomen as quickly as possible. For all other patients, electrocautery can be utilized to minimize bleeding. This extensile midline incision can be extended across the right or left inguinal ligament for distal iliac and femoral vascular injuries. Superiorly, a subcostal extension (L- or J-shaped extension) can be added to improve access to the liver on the right, especially with retrohepatic venous injuries, or to the left for gastroesophageal (GE) junction injuries. The incision can be extended into a sternotomy for concurrent thoracic cavity injuries or to facilitate intrapericardial suprahepatic vena cava control for high-grade liver injuries not amenable to packing. If the patient has a preexisting right thoracotomy, this can be joined to the laparotomy with incision of the diaphragm to afford the same view of the liver, retrohepatic venous structures, and intrapericardial vena cava.

On entry to the abdomen, the falciform should be taken down so as to minimize traction damage to the liver. The next step is to survey the abdominal contents, including the retroperitoneum, to identify and temporize any major sources of bleeding. Traditionally, routine four quadrant packing was advocated. This maneuver is not always helpful in penetrating trauma or blunt trauma with preoperative CT identifying injured areas.[28] In order to prevent iatrogenic damage, it is preferable to remove large amounts of central clotted blood, followed by selected packing of any areas with active bleeding. A rapid examination of the retroperitoneum should also be performed. Injuries that are not immediately life threatening, such as hollow viscus injuries, may be encountered during this initial rapid survey. However, assessing for and temporizing life-threatening bleeding should proceed in a systematic fashion first, prior to focusing on repair of other injuries. A plan for surgical hemorrhagic control is then made. This includes notifying the circulator of any necessary additional equipment and close communication with the anesthesia team to optimize the resuscitation needs of the patient. Early consideration of damage-control maneuvers, addressed later in the chapter, should be considered. The need for adjunctive services such as angioembolization by the interventional radiology team should be considered and initiated early to allow lead time for preparation. Once active hemorrhage has been temporized, a careful and complete survey of all the abdominal contents should be performed. In the exsanguinating patient who is undergoing a damage-control procedure, this may not be possible, but in the stable patient, this is critical. The potential for a missed injury can be mitigated by always conducting a comprehensive, systematic approach to evaluating the abdominal contents. We recommend that the entire abdomen be reviewed in the same manner for every case, regardless of the mechanism. There are specific areas that warrant extra care during the examination. For blunt injuries without preoperative imaging, duodenal injuries may present with only a subtle hematoma in the retroperitoneum. If you see a hematoma in this area, a right medial visceral rotation should be performed. If the injury mechanism is penetrating, the actual visible injury can be subtle. For shotgun wounds or in GSW where the projectile fragments after hitting bone, this can be especially problematic, leading to missed injuries. Hollow viscus injuries, especially on the mesenteric surface, may only be visible as a small bloodstain or hematoma in the overlying fat. These need to be inspected carefully. The posterior surface of the stomach is also a common area for missed injuries. Even in the absence of an anterior gastric injury, the undersurface of the stomach should be inspected carefully.

While exceedingly uncommon with blunt injuries, ureteral injuries due to GSW and SW can be difficult to diagnose.

Therefore, in the event of any penetrating trauma trajectory in the region of the ureters, care should be taken to inspect the at-risk segment of the ureter without devascularizing the structure. Likewise, whereas blunt bladder injuries are often large and located near the dome, penetrating intraperitoneal bladder injuries can be small and asymptomatic. Most small extraperitoneal injuries can be managed nonoperatively with urinary catheter drainage. However, large injuries, especially those with an intact connection to the skin, can be problematic. In order to rule this out, if there is an intraperitoneal component of bladder injury, this should be extended as needed to visualize the interior of the bladder prior to repair. If not, we recommend retrograde filling of the bladder with methylene blue in sterile water to look for any visible extravasation while the bladder is distended. If an injury is identified, the bladder should be mobilized as needed for full evaluation and repair of these injuries. Genitourinary trauma is discussed in detail elsewhere in this book.

For retroperitoneal hematomas, the abdomen is traditionally divided into three zones. Zone I is the central portion of the retroperitoneum, extending from the aortic hiatus of the diaphragm to the sacral promontory craniocaudally and between the psoas muscles laterally. Zone I contains the aorta, IVC, and their major branches. Zone II includes the lateral retroperitoneum which contains the kidneys. Finally, zone III is the pelvis, which encompasses the sacral venous plexus and iliac vessels. The approach to the retroperitoneum differs according to the mechanism. All zones undergo exploration after penetrating trauma because of the high likelihood of vascular injury requiring surgical repair. This differs from blunt injuries where traditionally only zone I hematomas are explored routinely, while in zones II and III, hematomas are only explored if they are large, expanding or pulsatile. Bleeding in the retrohepatic retroperitoneum carries unique risks and intraoperative considerations; this area is sometimes referred to as zone IV. The retrohepatic retroperitoneum contains the retrohepatic IVC and major hepatic veins. This area is difficult to expose and attempts to do so may release tamponade of venous injuries, resulting in catastrophic bleeding. As such, if a retrohepatic hematoma can be controlled with packing, it should not be explored for either blunt or penetrating injuries.

DAMAGE-CONTROL LAPAROTOMY

In contemporary trauma management, the concept of damage control has become common, and has been credited with saving more lives than many of the other surgical techniques developed over the last two decades.[29] Abdominal damage-control techniques are a critical component of the overarching concept of damage-control resuscitation, which includes early empiric balanced blood component therapy or whole-blood transfusion and minimizing crystalloid usage. Abdominal damage-control surgery includes three key components: (1) temporary rapid control of bleeding and contamination with early termination of the operation, (2) perioperative resuscitation with correction of coagulopathy, hypothermia,
4 and acidosis, and (3) delayed definitive repair of injuries.

In this era of trauma surgery, while the concepts of damage control permeate all operative interventions regardless of the patient physiology or injury burden, damage control should be explicitly considered in the following situations: (a) severe physiologic compromise with coagulopathy, hypothermia, or acidosis, (b) significant overall injury burden which will result in physiologic compromise if attempts are made to definitively complete all repairs at the index operation, and (c) resource limitations, which include austere environments such as a rural or combat setting, or situations where there is inadequate human resources required to complete the definitive operation. Early initiation of damage control, even prior to physiologic decompensation, may be associated

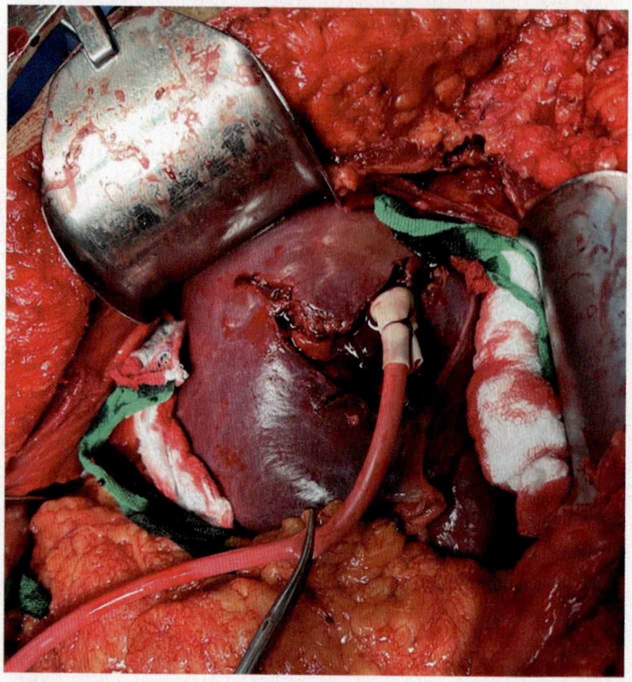

Figure 24.3. Hemorrhage control of liver injuries with a tamponade balloon.

with improved survival. Therefore, patients with a large injury burden at risk of becoming physiologically depleted should also be considered as candidates for damage-control surgery. The exact timing of damage control should be determined by the complexity of the injuries, the physiologic condition of the patient, the available resources, and the experience of the surgical team.

Hemorrhage control is the primary concern and can usually be achieved by mechanical compression or packing. If however, this is not effective, for example with major vascular injuries, surgical control with ligation or shunting may be necessary. For deep tracts, for example in the liver, balloon tamponade can be very effective (**Fig. 24.3**). Angioembolization may be a useful adjunct for abdominal damage control. Angioembolization should be considered early and performed immediately following the operation, or in conjunction with surgery if a hybrid operating room is available.[30]

Control of intestinal spillage is also an integral part of damage control. Stapled resection of injured segments of the bowel, without reestablishing intestinal continuity, should be considered for unstable patients. Definitive reconstruction can then be performed at a later stage when the patient is stabilized. However, this temporary iatrogenic complete bowel obstruction may also promote bacterial and toxin translocation, especially in patients requiring vasopressors. Also, performing an anastomosis at a later stage when the bowel is distended and the bowel wall is edematous, can be technically challenging. Decision to defer anastomosis is a tradeoff, and therefore, reconstruction of the bowel should be performed at the index operation whenever possible. Exceptions to this include patients with severe physiologic depletion in whom the benefit of expeditious termination of the operation outweighs the risks of complete bowel obstruction (leaving the bowel in discontinuity).[31]

A temporary closure of the abdomen should always be utilized following damage-control surgery. The abdominal fascia or skin should never be closed because of the high risk of intra-abdominal hypertension and abdominal compartment syndrome.[32] There are several methods for temporary closure, but all should preserve the fascia and abdominal wall domain, facilitate effective removal of intraperitoneal fluid, protect

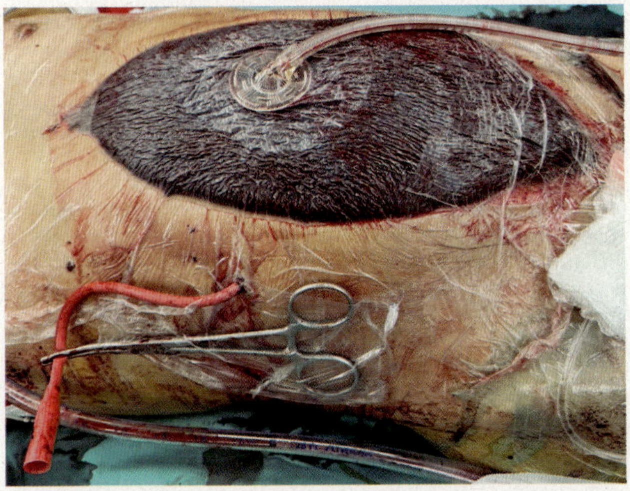

Figure 24.4. Temporary abdominal closure with negative wound pressure therapy.

the hollow viscus and reduce the risk of enteroatmospheric fistula (**Fig. 24.4**). Both commercially available and surgeon-constructed temporary closure devices can be utilized, depending on the local practice and resources.

After undergoing the initial index laparotomy and temporary abdominal closure, the next step is continued resuscitation in the ICU setting. There is no mandatory time set for the ICU phase of care, and as soon as physiologic status has normalized, the patient should return to the OR for definitive repair of all injuries. Even prior to normalization of the patient's physiology, if significant bleeding is noted, the patient should return to the operating room for reexploration. Even with a temporary abdominal wall closure in place, it is important that bladder pressures are monitored in the ICU after damage-control laparotomy as intra-abdominal hypertension and abdominal compartment syndrome can occur.

DIAPHRAGM

Anatomy

The diaphragm consists of a central aponeurotic portion which fuses with the pericardium and a peripheral muscular portion which is attached to the lower sternum, the lower six ribs, and the lumbar spine. Because the diaphragm rises to the level of the nipples at the 4th to 5th intercostal space during exhalation, penetrating injuries of the lower chest have the potential to cause diaphragmatic injury.

Epidemiology

For patients who have sustained blunt trauma, three different mechanisms can cause injury to the diaphragm: a sudden increase in intra-abdominal pressure causing bursting of the diaphragm; fractured ribs perforating the diaphragm; and deceleration injuries causing detachment of the diaphragm from the ribs. A diaphragmatic injury is found in approximately 7% of all laparotomies following blunt trauma, and in about 7.5% of autopsy studies. There is laterality to the injury with the left hemidiaphragm being injured in approximately 70% of cases and the right in 30%, a difference presumably due to the bolstering effect of the liver. Blunt injuries, create larger diaphragmatic defects than penetrating (**Fig. 24.5**) usually in the 7 to 10 cm range as compared with 2 to 3 cm for penetrating trauma (**Fig. 24.6**). A right diaphragmatic rupture indicates more severe force application, and as a result, in almost all cases, there are associated intra-abdominal injuries.

Diagnostics

Isolated diaphragmatic injuries can be challenging to diagnose as they may be completely asymptomatic or present with minor, nonspecific signs. Classic physical findings such as shortness of breath or bowel sounds in the chest are rare and indicate acute herniation of abdominal contents. The natural history of unrecognized diaphragmatic injuries is unknown, and although some small injuries may heal, this is not universal. For right hemidiaphragm injuries, the presence of the liver generally protects against herniation of abdominal viscera through smaller diaphragmatic injuries. However, on the left side, unrepaired diaphragm injuries commonly result in a diaphragmatic hernia. Diaphragmatic hernias may present within hours, days, or years after the injury.

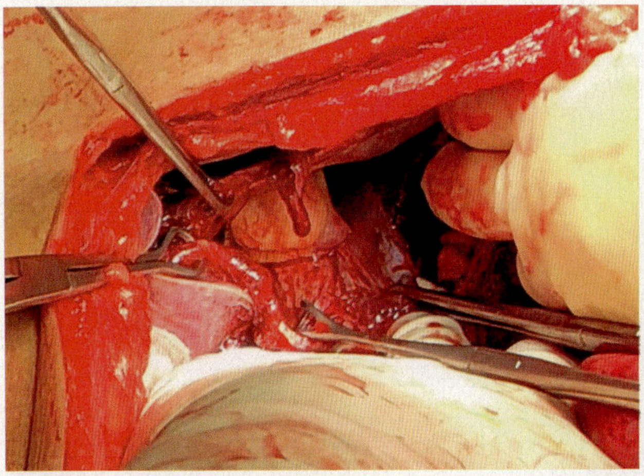

Figure 24.5. Blunt diaphragmatic injury.

Imaging can be useful in the diagnosis of blunt diaphragmatic injuries. Classic plain radiologic findings suspicious of diaphragmatic injury include an elevated diaphragm, an irregular diaphragmatic contour, and nonvisualization of the diaphragm. While rare, a nasogastric tube may also be seen in the thoracic cavity. Once herniation of the stomach, small, or large bowel has occurred, chest x-ray (**Fig. 24.7**) and CT (**Fig. 24.8**) have higher sensitivity. Although injuries are not always detected on CT, this modality is the highest yield study to evaluate for diaphragmatic injury as it allows concurrent evaluation of any associated intra-abdominal injuries. Diagnostic imaging is less helpful in the evaluation of penetrating diaphragmatic injuries due to the typically small size of such injuries. Chest x-ray has a very limited role in diagnosis. The sensitivity of CT for penetrating diaphragmatic injuries is also reported to be only around 65%.[33] As a result, for patients with penetrating injuries to the right thoracoabdominal region that do not undergo laparotomy, after a period of observation to ensure there is no missed hollow viscus injury, we recommend a diagnostic laparoscopy to evaluate the diaphragm for injuries.

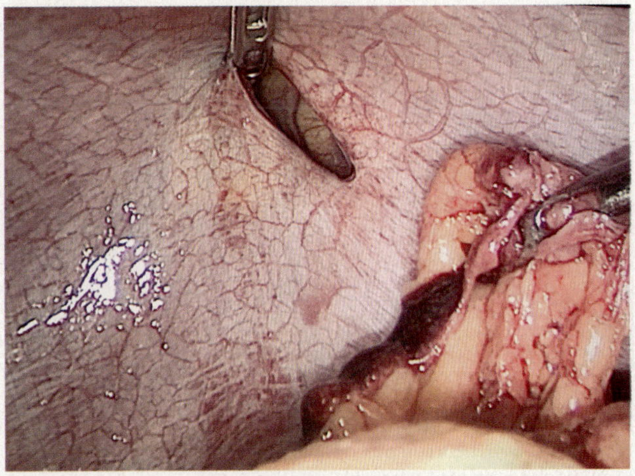

Figure 24.6. Penetrating diaphragmatic injury.

TRAUMA

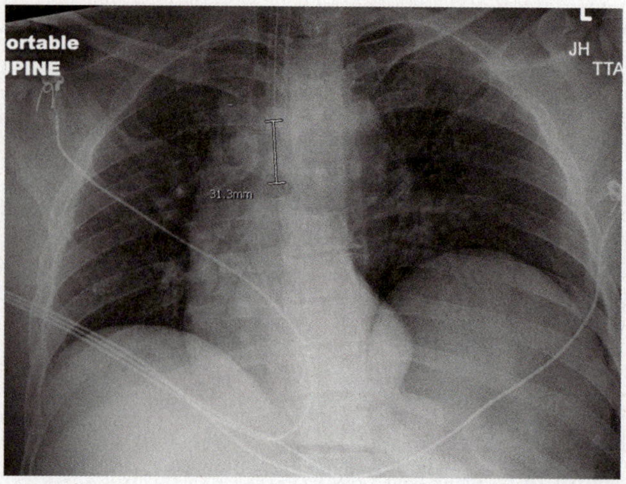

Figure 24.7. Chest plain radiograph showing elevation of the left diaphragm.

Treatment

All diaphragm injuries should ultimately have the herniated abdominal contents reduced and the defects repaired. In the acute setting, diaphragmatic injuries should be approached through a laparotomy to facilitate evaluation of the remaining intra-abdominal organs for injuries. The repair can be performed with interrupted or running nonabsorbable sutures. If there is contamination of the pleural cavity due to associated hollow viscus injuries such as the stomach, extending the diaphragmatic injury to wash out the thoracic cavity may be warranted. Tube thoracostomy should be considered in most cases. If the diaphragm has been avulsed from the chest wall, careful reconstruction of the diaphragmatic architecture utilizing nonabsorbable sutures is required. In some cases where there is significant tissue loss, apposition of the remaining diaphragm to the chest wall, a few rib spaces higher than the original insertion may be required to create a tension-free repair. It is extremely rare to require synthetic prosthetic reconstruction, but this remains a viable option for large areas of tissue loss. In patients with delayed presentation of diaphragmatic hernia, access and repair of the hernia can be performed through either the chest or the abdomen, often in a minimally invasive fashion.

LIVER AND BILIARY TRACT

Anatomy

The anatomical division of the liver into the classic Couinaud segments has no practical application in trauma. This is because the resection of nonviable liver tissue does not need to follow anatomical boundaries. However, an understanding of the blood supply is important. The vascular outflow of the liver consists of the three major hepatic veins (right, middle, and left), along with numerous short hepatic veins, all draining into the retrohepatic IVC. Only the proximal 1 to 2 cm of the major hepatic veins are extrahepatic. In approximately 70% of individuals, the middle hepatic vein joins the left hepatic vein near the IVC. The retrohepatic IVC is approximately 8 to 10 cm long and in most patients, is partially covered by the liver parenchyma. In approximately 7% of individuals the IVC is completely embedded in the liver. The vascular inflow of the liver consists of the portal vein and hepatic artery. The portal vein provides approximately 70% of hepatic blood flow and 50% of hepatic oxygenation. It divides into right and left branches at the level of the liver hilum. The common hepatic artery originates from the celiac artery. In most individuals, it branches into the left and right hepatic arteries at the hilum of the liver. In 10% to 15% of patients, the right hepatic artery originates from the superior mesenteric artery, and travels in the hepatoduodenal ligament to reach the liver along with the other structures of the portal triad. In 5% to 10% of patients, the left hepatic artery originates from the left gastric artery, and travels in the lesser omentum to reach the hilum of the liver. The porta hepatis contains the common hepatic artery to the left, and the common bile duct to the right. The portal vein lies posteriorly and between the common bile duct and the common hepatic artery. The left hepatic duct, the left hepatic artery, and the left portal vein enter the undersurface of the liver near the falciform ligament.

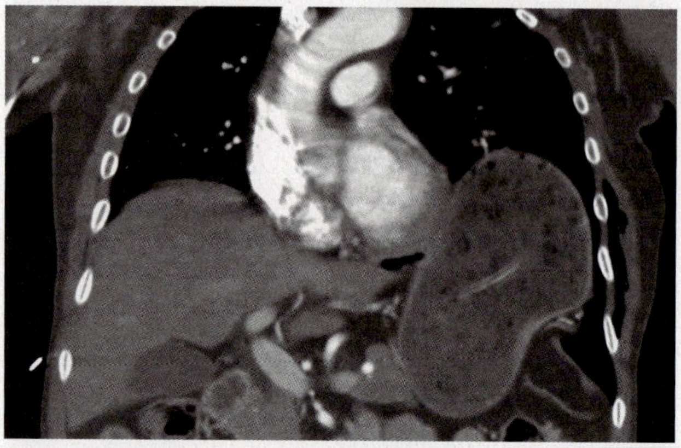

Figure 24.8. Chest computed tomography showing diaphragmatic rupture with herniated stomach.

Epidemiology

The liver is one of the most commonly injured intra-abdominal organs following both penetrating and blunt trauma. Gunshot and close-range shotgun blasts can cause massive tissue destruction and are associated with high mortality. The American Association for the Surgery of Trauma Organ Injury Scale (AAST-OIS) grading system (**Table 24.1**) ranges from a

Table 24.1. OIS-AAST Grading Scale for the Liver

Grade[a]	Type	Injury Description
I	Hematoma	Subcapsular, <10% surface area
	Laceration	Capsular tear, <1 cm parenchymal depth
II	Hematoma	Subcapsular, 10–50% surface area; intraparenchymal, <10 cm in diameter
	Laceration	1–3 cm parenchymal depth, <10 cm in length
III	Hematoma	Subcapsular, >50% surface area or expanding; ruptured subcapsular or parenchymal hematoma; intraparenchymal hematoma, >10 cm or expanding
	Laceration	>3 cm parenchymal depth
IV	Laceration	Parenchymal disruption involving 25–75% of hepatic lobe or 1–3 Couinaud segments within a single lobe
V	Laceration	Parenchymal disruption involving >75% of hepatic lobe or >3 Couinaud segments within a single lobe
	Vascular	Juxtahepatic venous injuries; ie, retrohepatic vena cava/central major hepatic veins
VI	Vascular	Hepatic avulsion

[a]Advance one grade for multiple injuries, up to grade III.
From Moore EE, Cogbill TG, Jurkovich GJ, et al. Organ injury scaling: spleen and liver (1994 revision). *J Trauma.* 1995;38:323–324.

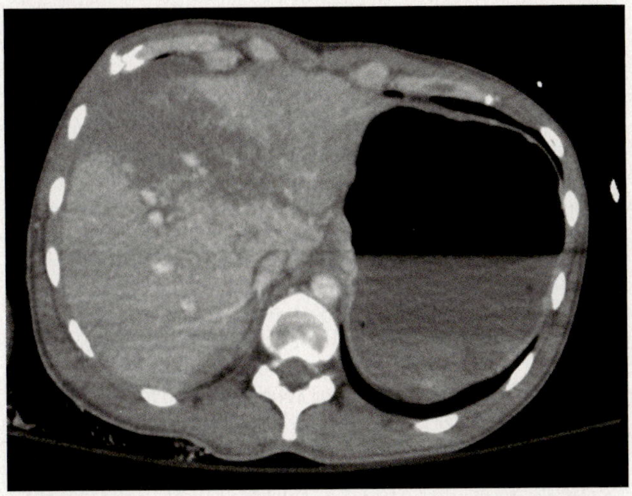

Figure 24.9. Abdominal computed tomography showing high-grade liver injury from blunt trauma.

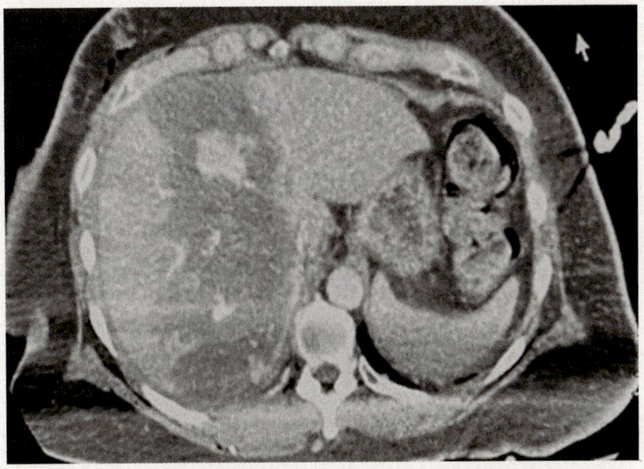

Figure 24.11. Computed tomography showing high-grade liver injury from abdominal gunshot wounds with active contrast extravasation.

mild grade I injury to a grade V injury which involves >75% of parenchymal disruption or juxtrahepatic venous injuries. In the modern era of selective nonoperative management of solid organ injuries, the organ injury grading system was updated in 2018 to include radiologic criteria of vascular injury as a component of risk stratification for failure of nonoperative management.[34]

Diagnostics

An abdominal FAST will detect free intraperitoneal bleeding, but it does not provide any information about the source of this bleeding. In hemodynamically stable patients, an abdominal CT with intravenous contrast is the highest-yield imaging modality. CT provides accurate information about the architecture of the injury, the amount of intraperitoneal blood, the presence of active bleeding, pseudoaneurysms or arteriovenous fistulas, and the presence of associated injuries. CT is a valuable tool in the selection of patients for operation, angiographic embolization, or observation (**Fig. 24.9**).

Treatment

Selective nonoperative management of blunt liver trauma has become the standard of care for both blunt and penetrating injuries. Patients undergoing nonoperative management should be selected based on clinical examination, CT findings, and associated intra-abdominal injuries. Hemodynamic stability and the absence of peritonitis are absolute requirements for nonoperative management. The success rate of nonoperative management for blunt hepatic trauma, including those with high-grade injuries, is high. In a multicenter study of 393 patients with grade IV or V blunt liver injuries, a trial of nonoperative management was attempted in 66.7% with a 91.3% success rate.[35] For these high-grade injuries, especially with evidence of contrast extravasation, angiointervention has been shown to be an independent predictor of survival and should be used liberally (**Fig. 24.10**).[36] Most failures of nonoperative management occur within the first 24 hours of admission. There is some evidence that patients with high injury severity score (ISS), severe grade IV or V liver injuries, multiple transfusions, major associated injuries, and associated chronic conditions such as cirrhosis, are at an increased risk for failure of nonoperative management. While angiographic embolization increases the success rate of nonoperative management of high-grade injuries as well as hospital survival, the risk of liver-related complications requiring percutaneous drainage following angioembolization is significantly increased.[36,37] Similarly, selective nonoperative management of liver injury has been more frequently used in penetrating trauma (**Fig. 24.11**).[22,38] For both blunt and penetrating injuries being managed nonoperatively, close monitoring in the ICU and frequent serial clinical examinations are critical

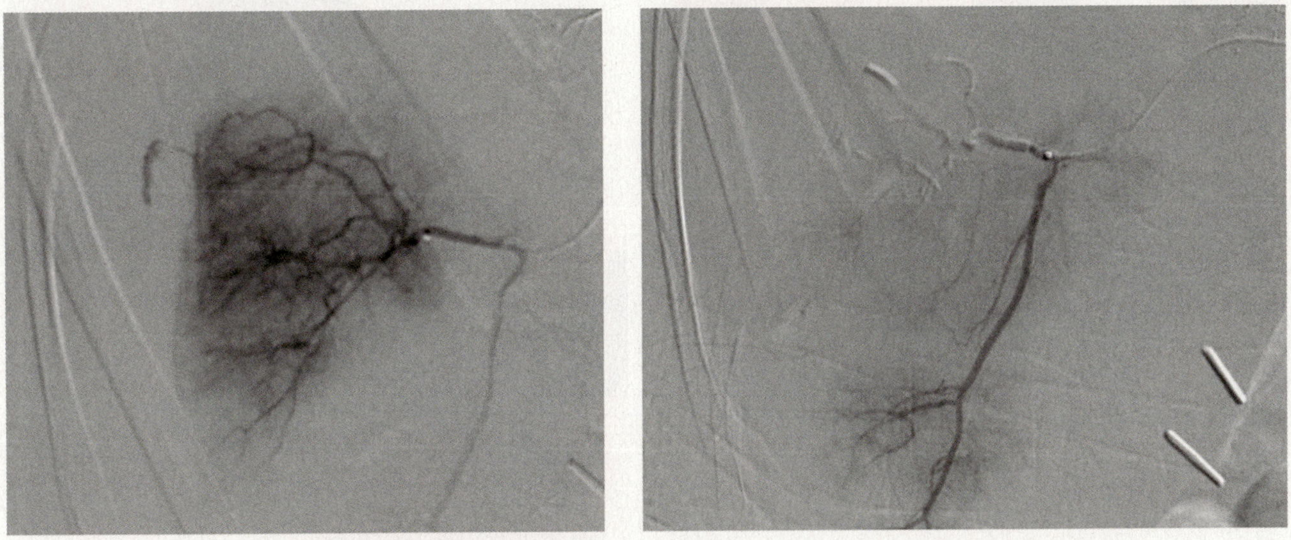

Figure 24.10. Selective angioembolization performed for liver injury with active contrast extravasation.

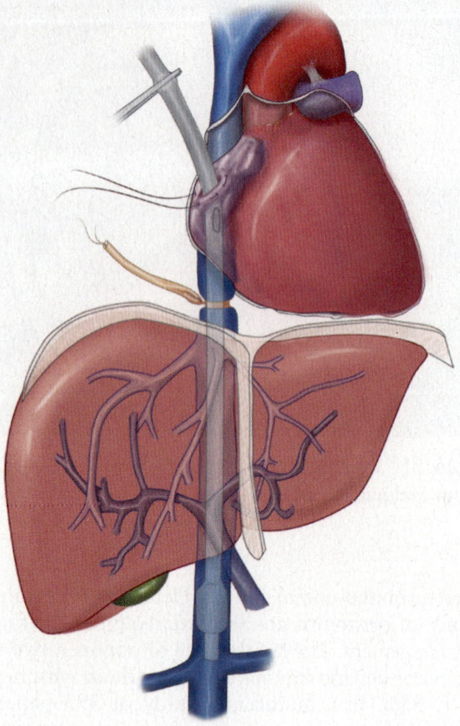

Figure 24.12. Schematic demonstrating an atriocaval shunt.

to avoid any delay in identifying patients with failed nonoperative management.

For the surgical management of liver injuries, adequate exposure is critical. The initial incision should be a midline laparotomy. For improved access to the posterolateral part of the liver, a right transverse or subcostal incision may be added. In rare occasions, a median sternotomy may be required to obtain access to the intrapericardial IVC for total vascular isolation of the liver or exposure of the heart for placement of an atriocaval shunt (**Fig. 24.12**). Alternatively, as discussed earlier in the chapter, if the patient has a right thoracotomy, often seen for a right thoracic GSW that enters the chest, traverses the diaphragm and injures the retrohepatic venous structures, the thoracotomy and laparotomy can be joined with incision of the diaphragm for unimpeded access to the posterior liver and suprahepatic segment of the IVC.

In approximately 80% to 85% of patients, the liver injury can be managed using relatively simple surgical techniques, such as application of local hemostatic agents, electrocoagulation, or suture repair. Bleeding from deep liver lacerations can be controlled by clipping or suture ligation of any major vessels, followed by deep figure-of-eight sutures using a large blunt liver needle. Omental packing of large liver defects can be useful in providing tamponade, especially at the take back operation if packing was utilized at the index operation. Significant bleeding from deep bullet or knife tracts in the liver may require a tractotomy for peripheral wounds or temporary balloon catheter tamponade for central wounds (**Fig. 24.13**).

High-grade liver injuries from blunt trauma or high-velocity GSWs are often associated with extensive parenchymal damage and not amendable to simple maneuvers. The liberal use of perihepatic packing and other damage-control techniques is critical in the management of these complex liver
5 injuries. In general, packing is highly effective and major hepatic resections are rarely indicated in the acute setting. Angioembolization following perihepatic packing may be considered early postoperatively, or intraoperatively if a hybrid operating room is available (**Fig. 24.14**). Soon after correction of coagulopathy and other physiologic abnormalities in the ICU, the patient should return to the OR for removal of perihepatic packing and reassessment of the liver injuries for findings suggestive of persistent hemorrhage or ischemic changes of the liver parenchyma.

Contained retrohepatic hematomas from blunt or penetrating injury should not be explored due to the risk of uncontrollable hemorrhage. If the hematoma is not contained and perihepatic packing fails to control the hemorrhage, or bleeding worsens with anterior retraction of the liver, injuries to the hepatic veins or retrohepatic IVC should be suspected. As exploration and repair or ligation of the bleeding vessels is usually required in these cases, total vascular isolation of the liver may need to be considered to control bleeding prior to exposing the injury. This procedure consists of first occluding inflow through the supraceliac abdominal aorta, followed by occlusion of the supra- and infrahepatic IVC, and the hepatic artery by occluding the hepatoduodenal ligament (Pringle maneuver). Control of the suprahepatic IVC below the diaphragm can be extremely challenging, as this segment of the

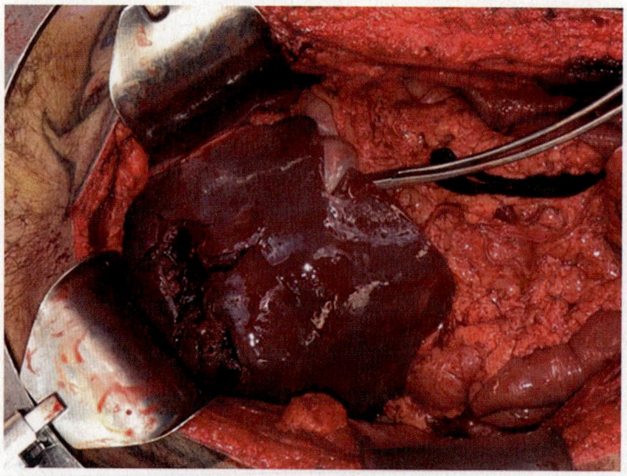

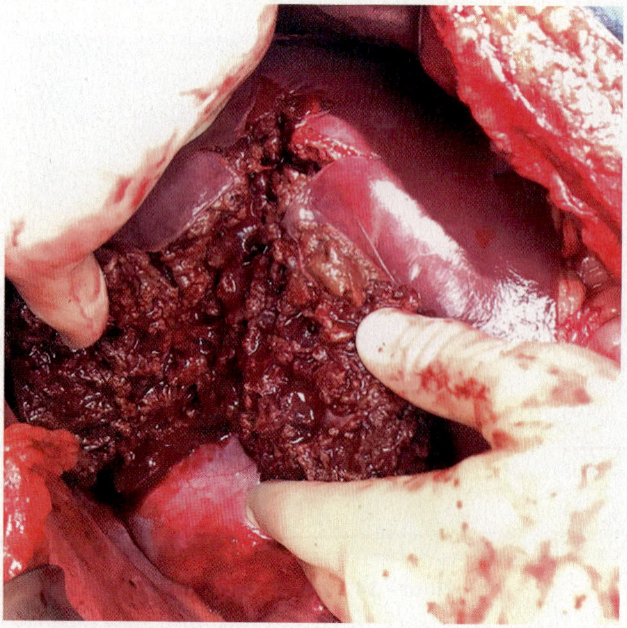

Figure 24.13. Tractotomy for complex liver injuries.

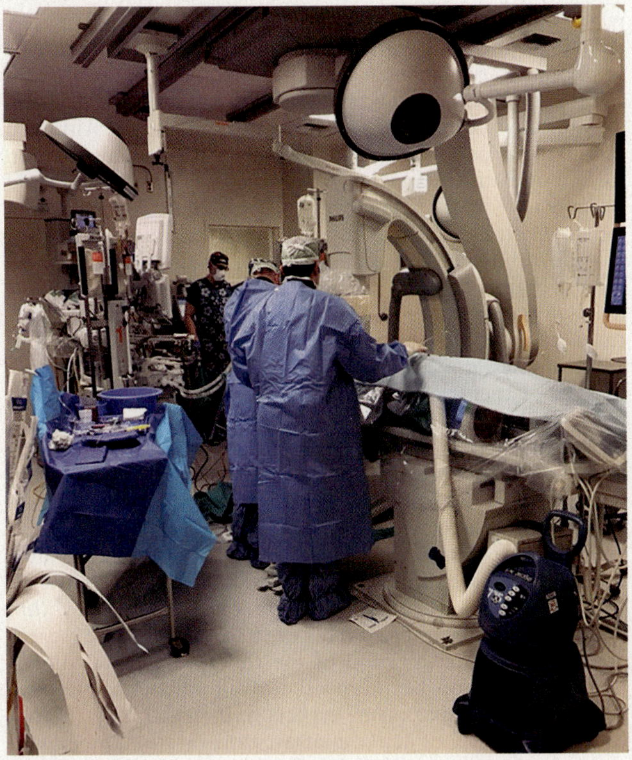

Figure 24.14. Hybrid operating room used in trauma.

IVC is usually the primary source of bleeding necessitating the procedure. Alternatively, the uninjured intrapericardial segment of the IVC can be accessed through a median sternotomy. Addition of a subcostal incision improves exposure of the liver and the retrohepatic veins. As described earlier, an alternative to the subcostal incision is a median sternotomy or, if the patient already has a right anterolateral thoracotomy, the diaphragm may be divided to further expose the IVC. Division of the falciform and coronary ligaments allows inferior-medial rotation of the liver and direct visualization of the retrohepatic IVC and the right hepatic vein.

The use of an atriocaval shunt is an invasive and complicated procedure that should be considered only in cases with complex retrohepatic venous injuries which cannot be controlled with other operative approaches. The procedure involves extension of the laparotomy incision into a median sternotomy and opening of the pericardium. A tape tourniquet is then applied around the IVC inside the pericardium. A purse-string suture is placed in the right atrial appendage and a size 8 endotracheal tube with a side hole cut at approximately 8 to 10 cm from the clamped proximal end, is then inserted through the purse-string and advanced to the infrahepatic segment of the IVC. The balloon of the endotracheal tube is then inflated just above the renal veins and the tape tourniquet around the intrapericardial IVC is tightened. Alternatively, a 36-Fr chest tube, with fenestrations cut into the proximal segment of the tube to allow blood flow from the IVC into the right atrium may be used. Nevertheless, the reported results on the use of atriocaval shunts are generally poor, and it should be considered only if all other techniques have failed. Other techniques which have been described in the management of retrohepatic venous injuries include intravascular balloons inserted through the femoral vein, extracorporeal membrane oxygenation (ECMO), and liver transplantation.[39]

Postoperative Complications

The incidence of postoperative liver-related complications after high-grade liver injuries has been reported to be as high as 50%.[40] These complications may occur days, or even months, after the initial injury. Complications include hemorrhage, pseudoaneurysm formation, arteriovenous fistula, biloma, biliary fistula, liver necrosis leading to abscess, hemobilia, and intrahepatic biliary strictures. Approximately 35% of patients with significant liver-related postoperative complications diagnosed on CT are asymptomatic. The majority of these complications can be managed nonoperatively, but often require percutaneous, endovascular, or endoscopic interventions.

Extrahepatic Biliary Tract Injury

Trauma to the extrahepatic biliary tree is rare and is usually due to a penetrating mechanism. Bile duct injuries are usually diagnosed during laparotomy, although some cases may present late, even days after injury. The diagnosis may be confirmed with a hepatobiliary iminodiacetic acid (HIDA) scan, magnetic resonance cholangiopancreatography (MRCP), or endoscopic retrograde cholangiopancreatography (ERCP). The management of injuries to the biliary tree is determined by the location and extent of the biliary injury, the time of diagnosis, and the presence of associated intra-abdominal injuries. Injuries to the gallbladder are treated by cholecystectomy. Complete duct transections are best managed with a Roux-en-Y biliary-enteric anastomosis because primary repair is associated with a high stricture rate.

Incomplete injuries to the extrahepatic ductal system involving less than 50% of the duct circumference can be managed with primary repair. Placement of a T-tube can be considered to prevent future stricture. Transactions involving more than 50% of the circumference of the duct, especially with questionable tissue viability, should be treated in the same manner as a complete transection, described above. All repairs of the biliary tract should be drained externally with closed suction drains.

In the damage-control setting, the transected duct may be ligated, or an external catheter may be placed into the proximal duct and exteriorized through the skin. Definitive repair can be performed after physiologic stabilization of the patient or once subspecialty care becomes available.

SPLEEN

Anatomy

Anatomically, the spleen is tethered in place by four ligaments which include the splenogastric ligament medially, the splenocolic ligament inferiorly, and both the splenophrenic and splenorenal ligaments posterolaterally. The splenogastric ligament is the only ligament containing vascular structures which consist of five to seven short gastric vessels, which originate from the distal splenic artery. The tail of the pancreas is in close proximity to the splenic hilum and is at risk of injury during splenectomy or hilar clamping. The splenic artery courses along the superior border of the pancreas, and divides into upper and lower pole arteries. The splenic vein is located posterior and inferior to the splenic artery, receives the inferior mesenteric vein and joins the superior mesenteric vein to form the portal vein.

Epidemiology

The spleen is a commonly injured intra-abdominal organ following blunt and penetrating trauma. The severity of splenic injury is graded by the AAST-OIS (**Table 24.2**). Generally, grades I and II are considered low-grade injuries and grades III to V are high-grade injuries.

Diagnostics

The clinical presentation of a splenic injury depends on the volume of blood loss and the presence of associated injuries. Many low-grade splenic injuries may be asymptomatic or cause only minor local tenderness. Classically, those with large splenic hematomas may experience pain in the left upper quadrant, radiating to the left shoulder (Kehr sign), especially when

TRAUMA

Table 24.2. OIS-AAST Grading Scale for the Spleen

Grade[a]	Type	Injury Description
I	Hematoma	Subcapsular, <10% surface area
	Laceration	Capsular tear, <1 cm parenchymal depth
II	Hematoma	Subcapsular, 10–50% surface area, <5 cm in diameter
	Laceration	1–3 cm parenchymal depth not involving a trabecular vessel
III	Hematoma	Subcapsular, >50% surface area or expanding; ruptured subcapsular or parenchymal hematoma; intraparenchymal hematoma, ≥5 cm or expanding
	Laceration	>3 cm parenchymal depth or involving trabecular vessels
IV	Laceration	Laceration involving segmental or hilar vessels producing major devascularization (>25% of the spleen)
V	Laceration	Shattered spleen
	Vascular	Hilar vascular injury with devascularized spleen

[a]Advance one grade for multiple injuries, up to grade III.
From Moore EE, Cogbill TG, Jurkovich GJ, et al. Organ injury scaling: spleen and liver (1994 revision). *J Trauma*. 1995;38:323–324.

placed in the Trendelenburg position. Although chest x-ray is not diagnostic, the presence of fractures of the left lower ribs or an elevated left hemidiaphragm can be associated with an underlying splenic injury. A FAST exam may show free fluid around the spleen. An abdominal CT with intravenous contrast is the highest-yield imaging modality for characterizing the architecture of the spleen injury (**Fig. 24.15**). It provides accurate information about the grade of injury, the amount of intraperitoneal bleeding, evidence of active bleeding, and associated injuries.

Treatment

The vast majority, upward of 80% of blunt splenic injuries in adults and 90% to 95% in children can be safely managed nonoperatively. This is different from penetrating injuries,

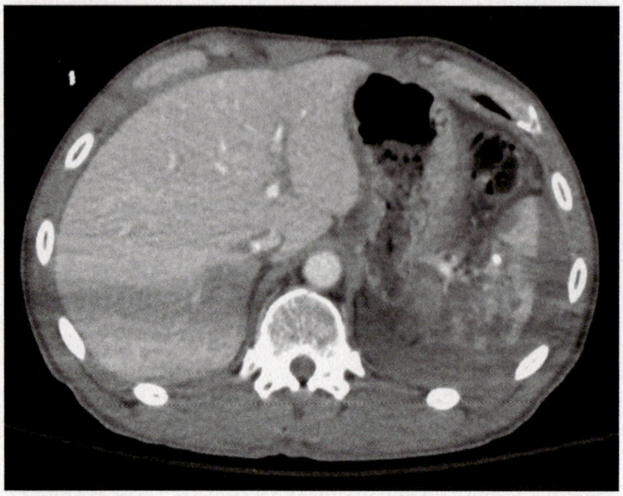

Figure 24.15. Abdominal computed tomography showing high-grade splenic injury.

where only 10% are successfully managed nonoperatively.[41,42] Similar to other solid organ injuries, the selection of patients for nonoperative management should be based on clinical examination and CT findings. The patient should be hemodynamically stable and have no signs of peritonitis. Although associated head trauma is not an absolute contraindication for nonoperative management, it should lower the threshold for operative intervention, because brain injury related coagulopathy increases the risk of splenic bleeding, and hypotensive episodes from the splenic injuries can be detrimental to the injured brain.

Low-grade (grades I and II) splenic injuries are more likely to be successfully managed nonoperatively, but most high-grade injuries (grades III to V) can be managed nonoperatively as well.[43] Patients with high-grade splenic injuries undergoing nonoperative management should be observed in the ICU. Development of hemodynamic instability, peritonitis, or the need for blood transfusion should trigger operative exploration. Nonoperative management failures occur within the first few days in most cases, although for those with subcapsular hematomas or pseudoaneurysms, delayed hemorrhage may occur days to weeks after the injury. Therefore, a follow-up CT should be considered for high-grade splenic injuries within 2 to 3 days of admission to rule out the development of a pseudoaneurysm or progression of the subcapsular hematoma.[44] Angioembolization has been used as an adjunct to selective nonoperative management, especially in high-grade injuries with CT evidence of active contrast extravasation, pseudoaneurysm, or arteriovenous fistula.[43]

The operative management of splenic injuries starts with the assessment of the location and severity of the injury to determine whether the spleen is salvageable. To accomplish a full surgical exposure, the spleen is rotated inferomedially, and several laparotomy pads are placed under the left diaphragm, behind the spleen. Excessive traction on the stomach or the splenic flexure of the colon may cause an avulsion injury to the splenic capsule, resulting in bleeding. Active bleeding from the spleen can temporarily be controlled with digital compression of the hilum or direct digital compression of the injured splenic parenchyma. A vascular clamp can also be placed across the hilum, taking care not to injure the tail of the pancreas. The critical move for a quick and safe splenectomy is adequate mobilization of the spleen. This is achieved by dividing the splenophrenic, splenorenal, and splenocolic ligaments to allow medial rotation of the spleen. The next step is division and ligation of the vascular gastrosplenic ligament far enough from the stomach in order to avoid injury or ischemic necrosis of the gastric wall. Finally, the splenic artery and vein should be divided close to the splenic hilum to avoid injury to the tail of the pancreas. Although this stepwise approach for mobilization of the spleen is applicable to most patients, the order of steps in a splenectomy should be individualized based on the anatomy and injury pattern. In cases with severe bleeding, clamping and division of the vessels at the splenic hilum may be the initial step once the spleen is adequately exposed. Division of ligamentous attachments of the spleen can then proceed after hemorrhage is controlled.

Preservation of the spleen should be considered in low-grade injuries if the patient is hemodynamically stable with a low overall injury burden.[45] For minor lacerations to the splenic capsule, hemostasis can be achieved with electrocautery and local hemostatic agents. Splenic lacerations may be repaired primarily with figure-of-eight or horizontal mattress sutures. If the splenic parenchyma is so fragile that the sutures tear through tissue, pledgets may be used to buttress the repair (**Fig. 24.16**). An absorbable splenic mesh can also be used as an adjunct to facilitate splenorrhaphy, especially in those with multiple stellate parenchymal injuries. However, extensive efforts to save the spleen are difficult to justify, as splenectomy is well tolerated, and a repaired spleen still exposes the patient to the risk of delayed rupture/bleeding.

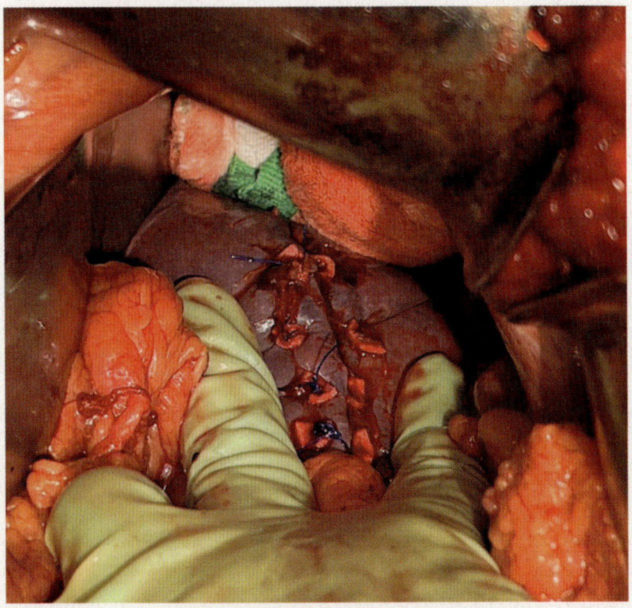

Figure 24.16. Splenorrhaphy with pledget sutures.

Postoperative Complications

Early complications following splenectomy include recurrent bleeding, pancreatic complications (pancreatitis, pseudocyst, and pancreatic fistula), gastric complications (gastroparesis, perforation/necrosis of the greater curvature), subdiaphragmatic abscess, splenic vein thrombosis, splenic arteriovenous fistula, left lower lobe atelectasis, or pleural effusion. Complications after splenic-preserving surgery include intrasplenic hematoma or abscess, splenic infarcts, and pseudoaneurysms or arteriovenous fistulas. Common hematologic changes following total splenectomy include leukocytosis and thrombocytosis. The leukocytosis is usually moderate and may last several weeks. More severe leukocytosis may indicate an infectious complication, especially in the presence of fever or tachycardia. Thrombocytosis is usually moderate and may last for a few weeks.

Infectious complications may occur in the early or late postsplenectomy period. There is evidence that splenectomy is associated with an increased risk of early postsplenectomy infections. A recent prospective observational, multicenter study of 269 patients with blunt splenic injury surviving at least 72 hours, demonstrated that patients who underwent splenectomy had a significantly higher incidence of early infectious complications compared to those with splenic preservation.[46] Overwhelming postsplenectomy infection (OPSI) is a rare but life-threatening complication, especially in children. The reported mortality ranges from 10% to 80%. Encapsulated organisms, such as *H. influenza*, *S. pneumonia*, and *N. meningococcus*, are the most common pathogens. Although the majority of infections occur within the first 3 to 4 years, OPSI may occur at any time after splenectomy. While it remains controversial, the timing of postsplenectomy vaccination may be optimal around 14 days after splenectomy.[47]

PANCREAS

Anatomy

The pancreas is a retroperitoneal organ with its head directly located over the IVC and its neck, and uncinate process located in close proximity to the superior mesenteric vessels and the proximal portal vein. The body extends over the suprarenal aorta and the left renal vessels. The splenic artery runs along the superior border of the pancreas. As described for the spleen section of this chapter, the splenic vein courses inferior to the splenic artery and joins the superior mesenteric vein at a right angle to form the portal vein behind the neck of the pancreas. The inferior mesenteric vein drains into the splenic vein behind the body of the pancreas (**Figs. 24.17** and **24.18**).

The major pancreatic duct of Wirsung travels down the entire length of the pancreas and drains into the ampulla of Vater, approximately 8 cm downstream from the pylorus. The accessory duct of Santorini branches off the superior aspect of the major duct, at the level of the neck of the pancreas. This drains into the duodenum, approximately 2 to 3 cm proximal to the ampulla of Vater. The pancreatic head and the proximal duodenum receive their blood supply from the anterior and posterior pancreaticoduodenal arcades. Because these arcades lie on the surface of the pancreas, close to the duodenal loop, separating these organs can result in ischemic damage to the duodenum.

Epidemiology

Injury to the pancreas is relatively uncommon and occurs in approximately 0.2% of blunt trauma and 1% of penetrating trauma patients. Overall, about 60% of patients with blunt trauma and about 90% with penetrating trauma will have

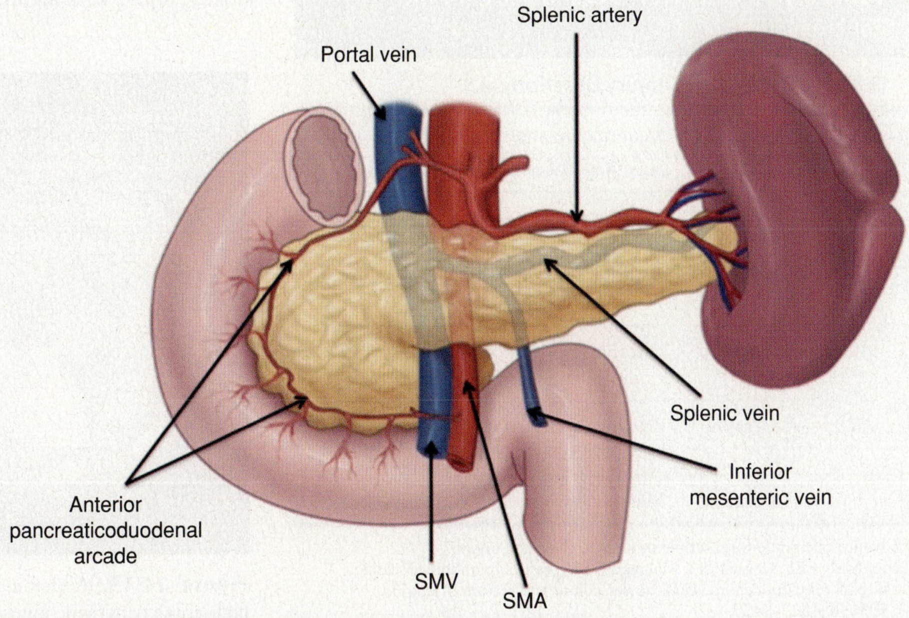

Figure 24.17. Pancreatic anatomy demonstrating relationship to vascular structures and spleen.

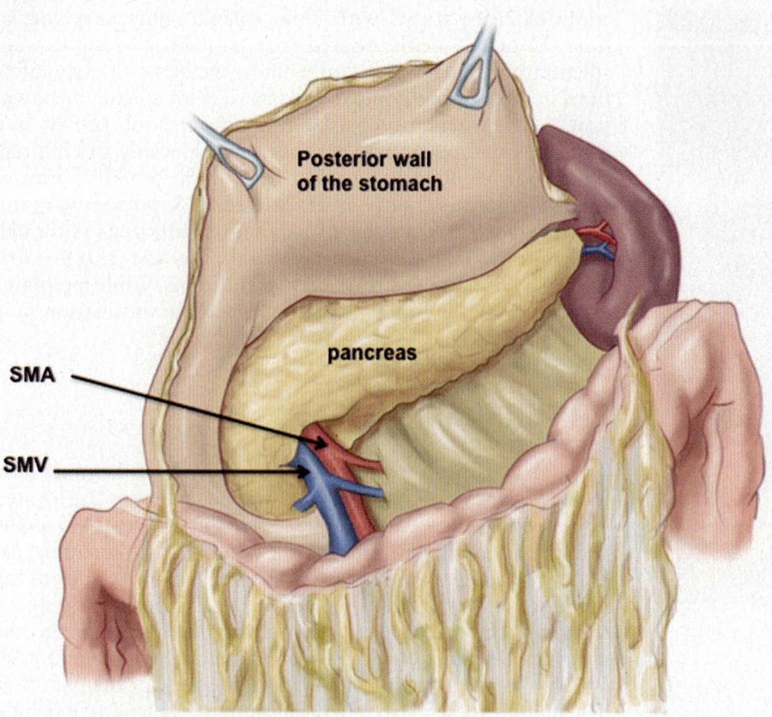

Figure 24.18. Pancreatic anatomy demonstrating relationship to stomach.

associated intra-abdominal injuries. The most common associated injury is the spleen in blunt trauma. Associated intra-abdominal vascular injuries to structures such as the IVC or superior mesenteric vein are common in penetrating trauma and are found in more than 75% of penetrating injuries to the head of the pancreas. A concomitant major vascular injury increases the likelihood of a poor outcome. The most widely used grading system (**Table 24.3**) is the AAST-OIS. The classification is based on CT and operative findings.

Diagnostics

The diagnosis of penetrating pancreatic injury is usually made intraoperatively. Preoperatively, in blunt trauma, especially for isolated injuries, the diagnosis may be challenging as the injury can be occult. Clinical signs may take hours or even days to manifest. Serial serum amylase and lipase levels may be useful as a screening test for pancreatic trauma, but isolated values have poor sensitivity and specificity. Contrast-enhanced CT (**Fig. 24.19**) is the investigation of choice in patients with suspected pancreatic trauma, although in the AAST multicenter study, the sensitivity and specificity to detect pancreatic injuries on 64-slice multidetector CT are 47.2% and 52.4%, respectively.[46] Its accuracy increases with time from injury and in cases with an equivocal initial test, a repeat CT 6 to 8 hours after the initial investigation should be considered. MRCP or ERCP can be considered in selected cases with pancreatic trauma to establish the integrity of the main pancreatic duct.

Treatment

The management of pancreatic trauma is dictated by the mechanism of injury and the presence of main pancreatic duct injury. Penetrating pancreatic injuries usually require operative management. However, most patients with isolated blunt pancreatic injury with an intact main pancreatic duct can safely be

Table 24.3. OIS-AAST Grading Scale for the Pancreas

Grade[a]	Type	Injury Description
I	Hematoma	Minor contusion without duct injury
	Laceration	Superficial laceration without duct injury
II	Hematoma	Major contusion without duct injury or tissue loss
	Laceration	Major laceration without duct injury or tissue loss
III	Laceration	Distal transection or parenchymal injury with duct injury
IV	Laceration	Proximal transection or parenchymal injury involving ampulla
V	Laceration	Massive disruption of pancreatic head

[a]Advance one grade for multiple injuries to the same organ.
From Moore EE, Cogbill TH, Malangoni MA, et al. Organ injury scaling, II: pancreas, duodenum, small bowel, colon, and rectum. *J Trauma*. 1990;30:1427–1429.

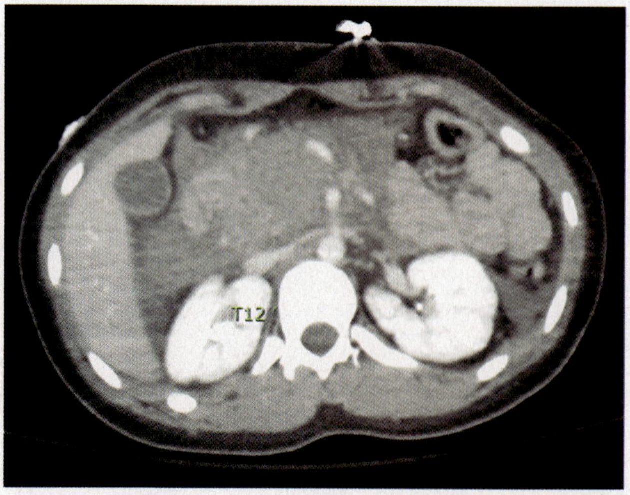

Figure 24.19. Abdominal computed tomography suggestive of high-grade pancreatic injuries.

managed nonoperatively. Known complications related to the nonoperative management of pancreatic injury include pancreatic pseudocyst and pancreatitis.

For patients undergoing operative management, the pancreas can be exposed through the lesser sac. This allows access to the anterior, superior, and inferior surfaces of the body and tail of the pancreas. The posterior aspect of the pancreas can be mobilized by incising the peritoneum over the inferior border of the pancreas and retracting upward. Further exposure of the distal pancreas can be achieved by mobilizing and rotating the spleen and tail of the pancreas medially. The pancreatic head and uncinate processes can be exposed with the Kocher maneuver.

As a general rule, all peripancreatic hematomas, even stable ones, should be explored to examine for any underlying main pancreatic duct injuries.[48] However, small stable hematomas localized specifically to the head of the pancreas may be left undisturbed, because the duct in this area is deep in the parenchyma. These injuries should be drained externally with closed drains and postoperatively the integrity of the duct can be evaluated using MRCP or ERCP and potentially treated with endoscopic pancreatic duct stent placement. Low-grade injuries without obvious ductal disruption should be treated with the debridement of nonviable tissue, hemostasis, and wide external drainage. For severe parenchymal injuries with known or suspected ductal disruption, the optimal surgical procedure will depend on the patient condition and the location of the pancreatic injury (head and neck vs. body and tail). Severe pancreatic injuries involving the body and tail of the pancreas are best treated by distal pancreatectomy, with or without splenic preservation (**Fig. 24.20**). In contrast, there are several surgical options for destructive injuries to the head of the pancreas, often with concurrent duodenal injury. If isolated, and the duodenum is intact, drainage is an option. If however, there is a destructive duodenal injury that is unable to be reconstructed, an en bloc resection is recommended. If the patient's hemodynamic status requires damage-control surgery or the procedure is beyond the skill set of the operating surgeon, temporary hemorrhage control and external drainage followed by delayed pancreatic resection and biliopancreatic reconstruction may be considered. If, however, a pancreaticoduodenectomy is to be performed, even for hemodynamically stable patients with an experienced surgeon, a two-stage procedure is often recommended. The initial operation includes hemorrhage control and, in appropriate cases, arterial shunting and/or ligation of concomitant venous injuries. Similarly, the common bile duct stump can be ligated or drained externally (**Fig. 24.21**). The definitive reconstruction should be scheduled soon after adequate resuscitation in the ICU, ideally within 24 to 48 hours after the index operation. The reconstruction, which includes pancreaticojejunostomy, hepaticojejunostomy, and gastroenterostomy, is similar to that in elective cases and can be performed in concert with hepatobiliary surgeons when appropriate.

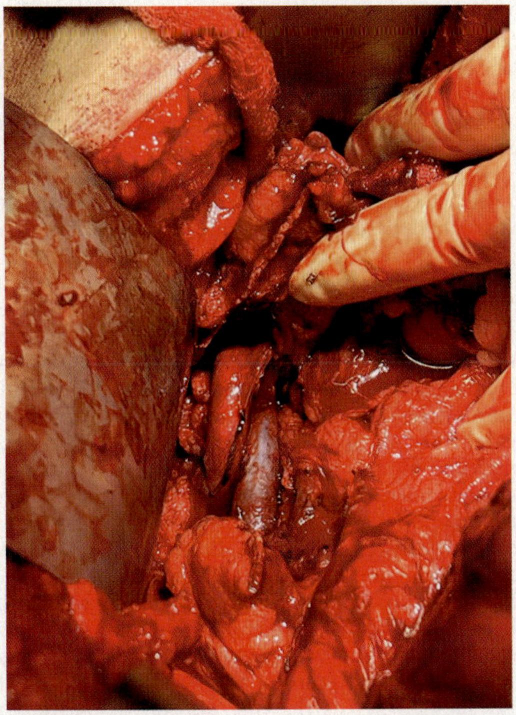

Figure 24.20. Spleen-preserving distal pancreatectomy.

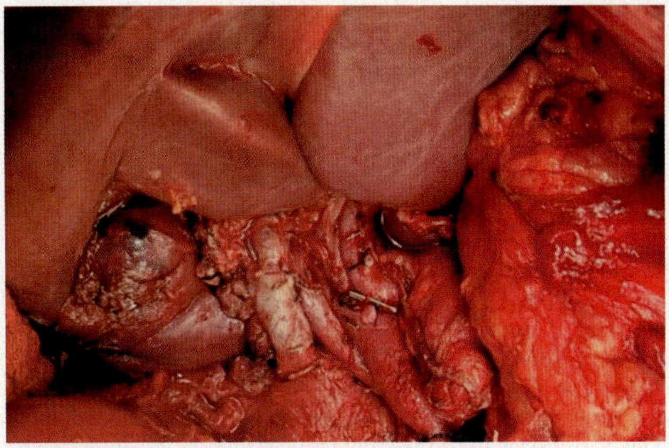

Figure 24.21. Surgical clip applied on the common bile duct stump following pancreaticoduodenectomy.

Postoperative Complications

Pancreas-related local complications occur in about 25% of patients with pancreatic injuries and include pancreatic fistulas, pseudocysts, pancreatitis, and perihepatic infection. Most of these complications can successfully be managed nonoperatively or with percutaneous drainage and endoscopic stenting of the main pancreatic duct. Endocrine pancreatic insufficiency may occur after major pancreatic resections, particularly proximal resections.[49] The risk of exocrine pancreatic insufficiency after partial pancreatic resection is very low.

STOMACH

Anatomy

The stomach is a hollow viscus organ located in the left upper quadrant of the abdomen with the GE junction, fundus, and often a significant portion of the body lying above the costal margin. The stomach has a robust blood supply including the left and right gastric arteries, the right and left gastroepiploic arteries, and the short gastric arteries. This level of vascularity can result in significant bleeding after injury but also provides redundancy, making devascularization and necrosis of the stomach relatively rare even with significant injury.

Diagnostics

Gastric injury usually results from either significant blunt force trauma or after penetrating trauma to the left upper abdomen or lower chest. The presence of blood upon placement of a nasogastric tube is concerning for gastric injury. Most patients with full-thickness gastric injury after trauma will present with spillage of gastric contents and peritonitis resulting in direct transfer to the operating room. Blunt injury to the stomach can cause local contusion with gastric wall hematoma or hollow viscus rupture, similar to bladder rupture, with a large full-thickness defect. After blunt or penetrating trauma, in the absence of peritonitis or hemodynamic instability, additional diagnostic workup with CT imaging is appropriate. CT findings concerning gastric injury include intra-abdominal free air or fluid, localized wall thickening, or enhancement and discontinuity of the gastric wall.

Treatment

Gastric resection is generally well tolerated due to the redundancy of tissue and a rich blood supply of the stomach. In the setting of penetrating injury, if a single injury is identified on the anterior wall of the stomach, the operating surgeon must assume that there is another injury corresponding to the entry or exit site. A single gastric injury is rare; therefore, even a linear laceration should not be mistaken for a tangential wound. The anterior stomach is fully inspected from the GE junction to pylorus. The left lobe of the liver may need to be mobilized for better visualization of the proximal third of the stomach. The posterior wall of the stomach is evaluated by entering the lesser sac below the gastroepiploic vessels. The posterior gastric wall must be fully evaluated and visualized all the way up to the GE junction to avoid missing an injury. Blood or fluid upon entry into the lesser sac should prompt the surgeon to look for gastric and/or pancreatic injury. Care must be taken when inspecting the GE junction and greater curvature as excess tension on the gastric fundus may result in iatrogenic tearing of the splenic capsule.

Low-grade injuries including contusions and intramural hematoma should be evaluated and evacuated as appropriate. After hematoma evacuation and hemostasis is achieved, the injured area may be reinforced with seromuscular sutures. Full-thickness injuries can be repaired in one or two layers. In gunshot injuries, it is important to debride the devitalized tissue at the edge of the injury prior to primary repair. Injuries to the greater curvature or larger injuries to the body can be controlled with wedge resection using a stapler. Care must be taken, however, to avoid narrowing the GE junction or pylorus. Injuries involving the pylorus may be managed with a pyloroplasty to prevent severe stenosis. Destructive injuries or those involving the GE junction or pylorus may require a proximal or distal gastrectomy with reconstruction. In rare cases, a total gastrectomy with esophagojejunostomy is required. Proximal gastric injuries or those at the GE junction may present technical challenges for surgeons not accustomed to operating in this area. If the surgeon's skillset does not allow for a single-stage definitive reconstruction, a staged procedure should be considered. During the initial operation, the distal esophagus or proximal stomach may be stapled off and internally drained with a nasogastric tube thus controlling the injury in a damage-control manner. The second operation includes a delayed gastrointestinal reconstruction performed under optimal conditions with all of the requisite expertise present.

DUODENUM AND SMALL BOWEL

Anatomy

The duodenum is the first portion of the small intestine and forms a C-loop around the head of the pancreas. The duodenum is divided into four parts, an anatomic distinction that is important in operative management. The first portion is intraperitoneal and directly associated with the portal structures and gastroduodenal artery. The second and third portions are retroperitoneal and curve around the head of the pancreas. As discussed above, the common bile and pancreatic ducts drain into the ampulla in the second portion of the duodenum. The fourth portion of the duodenum ascends to the ligament of Treitz to join the jejunum. The jejunum and ileum, comprising most of the length of the bowel, extend on the relatively mobile small bowel mesentery from the upper abdomen just to the left of the midline to the right lower quadrant and the ileocecal junction. The vascular supply to the bowel from the jejunum through the transverse colon is the superior mesenteric artery. Drainage is from the superior mesenteric vein.

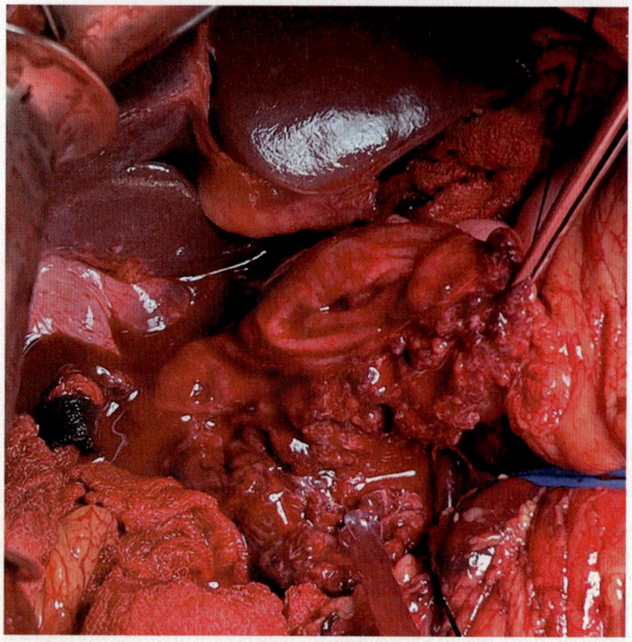

Figure 24.22. Transected second portion of the duodenum following abdominal gunshot wounds.

Epidemiology

Injury to the duodenum is relatively uncommon, occurring in less than 5% of all trauma patients, but when it does happen, it is associated with high morbidity and mortality. The majority of duodenal trauma is secondary to penetrating injury (**Fig. 24.22**) and is often identified during operative exploration. Patients with duodenal trauma frequently have additional intra-abdominal injury, most commonly of the liver, pancreas, and small bowel. Overall, small bowel injury occurs in less than 1% of blunt trauma and in less than 17% of penetrating trauma.[50] The proximal jejunum and distal ileum are the most common sites of blunt small bowel injury due to the relatively fixed position of the mesentery in these locations.[51]

Treatment

Duodenal hematomas secondary to blunt trauma can be managed nonoperatively with nasogastric tube decompression and parenteral nutrition. All duodenal hematomas encountered intraoperatively require exploration to evaluate for underlying perforation.

Mobilization of the duodenum is achieved with the Kocher maneuver. This maneuver allows full exposure of the second and third portions of the duodenum, evaluation of the posterior wall, and access to the underlying vascular structures to evaluate for any injuries. Although various complex procedures were historically described for the surgical management of duodenal injuries, most duodenal injuries can be repaired primarily in one or two layers with a transverse closure to avoid luminal narrowing.[52] The injury can be buttressed with omentum or the serosal surface of a segment of small bowel. Segmental resection is rarely indicated but is an option, with primary, end-to-end anastomosis. Segmental resection is not recommended for the second portion of the duodenum because the ampulla is located on the medical aspect. There is also a risk of ischemia due to disrupting the blood supply of the duodenum as it is mobilized away from the pancreas. For destructive, complex injuries that can be reconstructed, pyloric exclusion with gastrojejunostomy may be utilized to protect the repair, however, routine exclusion should not be used for all duodenal injuries. For exclusion of the pylorus, external stapling across the first portion of the duodenum with a TA stapler and internal cerclage with sutures are both

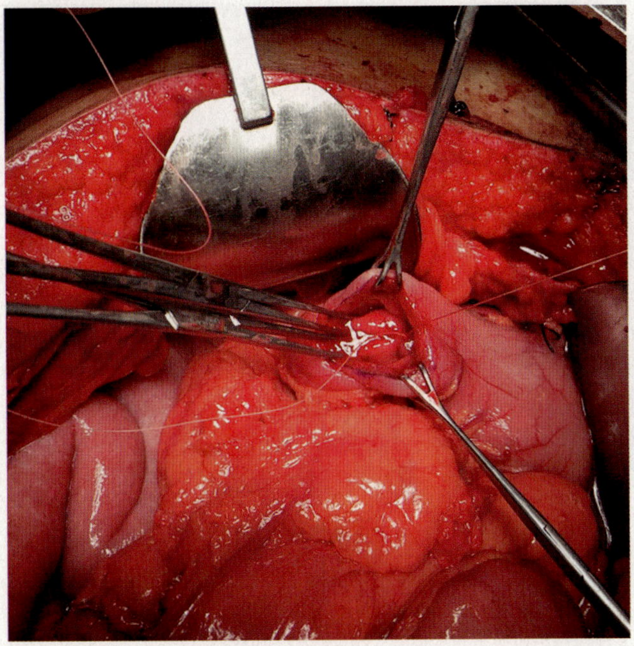

Figure 24.23. Surgical exclusion of the pylorus by sutures.

well-accepted techniques (**Fig. 24.23**). Other surgical options include jejunal serosal patch and duodenojejunostomy. In unstable patients, damage-control techniques may be applied followed by delayed reconstruction. The traumatic pancreaticoduodenectomy is rarely indicated and carries a high mortality. Therefore, it should be considered only in patients with complex destructive injuries to the pancreaticoduodenal complex where reconstruction of the duodenum is not possible, as discussed earlier in the chapter. One of the major complications after duodenal injury operation is fistula formation, occurring in 4% to 33% of patients. These cases can often be managed with percutaneous drainage.

For the remainder of the small bowel distal to the ligament of Treitz, from jejunum to ileum, injuries can nearly always be managed with either primary repair or resection and anastomosis. The principles of repair and anastomosis are similar to those described for colon injuries below.

COLON

Epidemiology

Colon injuries occur in approximately 30% of abdominal GSW and 20% of SW undergoing laparotomy. In blunt trauma, approximately 10% of patients undergoing laparotomy have a colon injury. Many blunt colonic injuries are superficial; with only 3% of patients undergoing laparotomy having a full-thickness perforation. The presence of an external seatbelt sign is associated with an increased risk of colon injury.

Diagnostics

The definitive diagnosis of colon injury is almost always made intraoperatively. The preoperative diagnosis of colon injury following blunt trauma is difficult, especially in unevaluable patients. If a CT is obtained, collateral findings of mesenteric stranding, bowel wall thickening, or unexplained fluid may be seen, increasing the level of suspicion for a hollow viscus perforation. Free extraluminal air is rare. Intraoperatively, all colonic hematomas should be explored to rule out any underlying colon injury, taking care not to devascularize the colon wall. Particular care should be taken for penetrating injuries, especially due to stab or shotgun wounds, where the injury can be subtle and hidden within pericolonic or mesenteric fat. The severity of colon injury can be graded by the AAST-OIS

Table 24.4. OIS-AAST Grading Scale for the Colon

Grade[a]	Type	Injury Description
I	Hematoma	Contusion or hematoma without devascularization
	Laceration	Partial thickness, no perforation
II	Laceration	Laceration <50% of circumference
III	Laceration	Laceration ≥50% of circumference without transection
IV	Laceration	Transection of the colon
V	Laceration	Transection of the colon with segmental tissue loss
	Vascular	Devascularized segment

[a]Advance one grade for multiple injuries to the same organ.
From Moore EE, Cogbill TH, Malangoni MA, et al. Organ injury scaling, II: pancreas, duodenum, small bowel, colon, and rectum. *J Trauma.* 1990;30:1427–1429.

colon injury scale (**Table 24.4**), which is based on the operative findings. A practical classification used by many surgeons divides injuries into two severity groups: nondestructive injuries involving less than 50% of the bowel wall; and destructive injuries involving more than 50% of the bowel wall or involving devascularization.

Treatment

The management of colon injuries has undergone major changes over the last two decades. For nondestructive injuries, a primary repair of the injury can be performed irrespective of traditional risk factors such as the site of colon injury, associated injuries, or physiologic status. In contrast, the surgical management of destructive colon injuries, defined as those with >50% of the bowel wall circumference or with devascularization, remains controversial. Destructive colon injuries were traditionally managed with routine diversion because of the perceived high risk for anastomotic leak and intra-abdominal sepsis. A prospective multicenter observational study published in 2001 examined clinical outcomes associated with colonic diversion versus primary anastomosis in patients with penetrating colon injuries.[53] The overall colon-related mortality was 1.3% and all deaths occurred in the diversion group. The incidence of anastomotic leaks was 6.6%. Multivariate analysis identified severe fecal contamination, ≥4 units of blood transfusions within the first 24 hours, and single-agent prophylactic antibiotics as independent risk factors for abdominal complications, whereas the surgical management of colonic injuries (ie, anastomosis vs. diversion) did not impact outcomes. For both blunt and penetrating destructive injuries, if the patient meets criteria for a damage-control procedure, contamination control with stapling of the colon should be performed expeditiously. Primary anastomosis may be considered during the index operation when appropriate.[54]

Postoperative Complications

Abdominal complications after colon injuries are relatively common, and approximately 20% of patients develop abdominal sepsis. Colonic leaks with associated abdominal sepsis after repair or resection of colonic injuries have been examined in detail. In a review of 35 prospective and retrospective studies including 2964 primary repairs, the rate of colonic leaks was 2.2%.[55] For patients undergoing resection and anastomosis, the leak rate was 5.5%. Anastomotic leaks occur more commonly with a colon–colon anastomosis when compared to an ileocolic anastomosis. The majority of colonic leaks

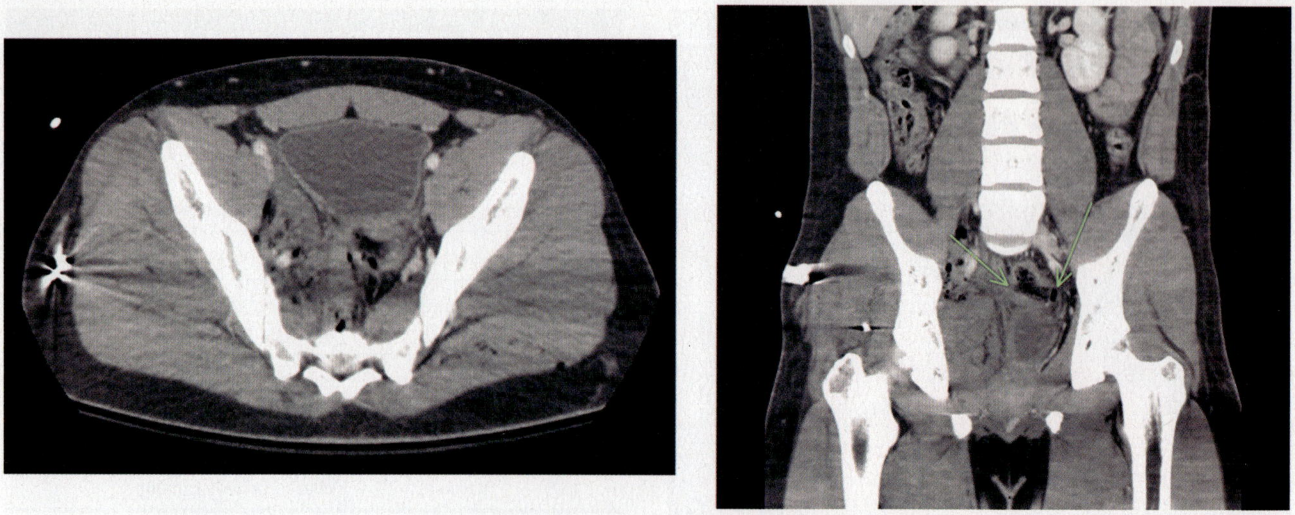

Figure 24.24. Pelvic computed tomography suggestive of rectal injury following transpelvic gunshot wounds.

can be managed nonoperatively with percutaneous drainage. CT should be obtained to evaluate for any intra-abdominal fluid collections amenable to percutaneous drainage. Surgical exploration of the abdomen is only required when the patient fails percutaneous drainage or develops evidence of generalized peritonitis.

RECTUM

Anatomy

The rectum begins where the tenia coli coalesce as the terminal part of the colon. This segment of the GI tract is approximately 12 to 15 cm long and is considered both an intra- and extraperitoneal organ. Anteriorly, the upper two-thirds and laterally, the upper one-third are intraperitoneal, with the lower third being completely extraperitoneal. The blood supply is derived from the superior rectal artery branching from the inferior mesenteric artery; the middle rectal artery branching from the internal iliac artery; and the inferior rectal artery branching from the internal pudendal artery.

Epidemiology

Most rectal injuries result from a penetrating mechanism, usually secondary to a GSW although injuries caused by anally inserted foreign body or endoscopic procedures are also seen. Because of its protected location within the pelvis, rectal injury is only seen in approximately 5% to 10% of blunt trauma patients and is often associated with a pelvic fracture.

Diagnostics

The clinical presentation of rectal injuries that are intraperitoneal does not differ from that of colon injuries. For extraperitoneal injuries, the clinical symptomatology can be masked by containment of the perforation in the retroperitoneal tissues. In most cases, rather than physical examination, the diagnosis of rectal injuries is made during the operative exploration or a combination of proctoscopy and abdominopelvic CT.[56]

Treatment

Most blunt rectal injuries occur in the intraperitoneal rectum, and the same surgical principles apply as for other colonic injuries. On the other hand, both intraperitoneal and extraperitoneal injuries can be seen in penetrating trauma patients. Patients with penetrating injury with peritonitis, hemodynamic instability, or those that are unexaminable, should be taken directly to the operating room. Patients with known or suspected rectal injuries may be placed in the lithotomy position to facilitate perineal examination or proctoscopy, although hemorrhage control in the abdomen and pelvis should always be prioritized. In patients with abdominal or transpelvic GSW, who meet the criteria for a trial of nonoperative management, the highest-yield initial examination is abdominopelvic CT (**Fig. 24.24**). If the CT findings suggest intra-abdominal injuries, including rectal injuries above the level of the peritoneal reflection, the patient should be taken to the operating room for laparotomy. For intraperitoneal rectal injuries, the management principles are the same as those that apply to colon injuries. Most injuries can be repaired primarily without the need for fecal diversion.

For patients with CT findings suggestive of rectal injuries below the peritoneal reflection, proctoscopy should be performed for evaluation of rectal injuries. In such cases, the abdomen should also be prepared for additional abdominal procedures as indicated. The classic surgical dogma in extraperitoneal rectal injuries includes Debridement, Diversion, presacral Drainage, and Distal rectal washout ("Four Ds"), although this is no longer the mainstay of surgical management. For distal extraperitoneal injuries that are accessible through a transanal approach, a primary repair can be performed without fecal diversion. For more proximal injuries inaccessible in this manner, fecal diversion is usually performed without repairing the injury or presacral drainage. However, the absolute need for colostomy has never been demonstrated.[57]

ACKNOWLEDGMENTS

We gratefully acknowledge the contributions of previous edition authors, Elizabeth R. Benjamin and Demetrios Demetriades, as portions of those chapters have been retained in this revision.

References

1. Henry R, Matsushima K, Henry RN, et al. Who would have benefited from the prehospital use of Resuscitative Endovascular Balloon Occlusion of the Aorta (REBOA)? An autopsy study. *J Am Coll Surg.* 2019;229(4):383–388.
2. Rhee PM, Acosta J, Bridgeman A, Wang D, Jordan M, Rich N. Survival after emergency department thoracotomy: review of published data from the past 25 years. *J Am Coll Surg.* 2000;190(3):288–298.
3. Ghafil C, Matsushima K, Guzman R, et al. Performance of focused assessment with sonography for trauma following resuscitative thoracotomy for traumatic cardiac arrest. *World J Surg.* 2022;46(1):91–97.
4. Liasidis PK, Garapati H, Ghafil C, et al. Diagnostic peritoneal aspiration revisited: its diagnostic accuracy for the detection of intraabdominal hemorrhage. *Am Surg.* 2021;87(10):1551–1555.

5. Velmahos GC, Tatevossian R, Demetriades D. The "seat belt mark" sign: a call for increased vigilance among physicians treating victims of motor vehicle accidents. *Am Surg.* 1999;65(2):181–185.
6. Santos J, Delaplain PT, Tay-Lasso E, et al. Development and validation of a novel hollow viscus injury prediction score for abdominal seatbelt sign: a pacific coast surgical association multicenter study. *J Am Coll Surg.* 2023;237(6):826–833.
7. Delaplain PT, Tay-Lasso E, Biffl WL, et al. Excluding hollow viscus injury for abdominal seat belt sign using computed tomography. *JAMA Surg.* 2022;157(9):771–778.
8. Benjamin ER, Siboni S, Haltmeier T, Lofthus A, Inaba K, Demetriades D. Negative finding from computed tomography of the abdomen after blunt trauma. *JAMA Surg.* 2015;150(12):1194–1195.
9. Inaba K, Demetriades D. The nonoperative management of penetrating abdominal trauma. *Adv Surg.* 2007;41:51–62.
10. Biffl WL, Kaups KL, Pham TN, et al. Validating the Western Trauma Association algorithm for managing patients with anterior abdominal stab wounds: a Western Trauma Association multicenter trial. *J Trauma.* 2011;71(6):1494–1502.
11. Demetriades D, Rabinowitz B, Sofianos C, et al. The management of penetrating injuries of the back. A prospective study of 230 patients. *Ann Surg.* 1988;207(1):72–74.
12. Velmahos GC, Demetriades D, Toutouzas KG, et al. Selective nonoperative management in 1,856 patients with abdominal gunshot wounds: should routine laparotomy still be the standard of care? *Ann Surg.* 2001;234(3):395–402; discussion 402–403.
13. Velmahos GC, Demetriades D, Foianini E, et al. A selective approach to the management of gunshot wounds to the back. *Am J Surg.* 1997;174(3):342–346.
14. Velmahos GC, Demetriades D, Cornwell EE III. Transpelvic gunshot wounds: routine laparotomy or selective management? *World J Surg.* 1998;22(10):1034–1038.
15. Schnüriger B, Lam L, Inaba K, Kobayashi L, Barbarino R, Demetriades D. Negative laparotomy in trauma: are we getting better? *Am Surg.* 2012;78(11):1219–1223.
16. Brown CV, Velmahos GC, Neville AL, et al. Hemodynamically "stable" patients with peritonitis after penetrating abdominal trauma: identifying those who are bleeding. *Arch Surg.* 2005;140(8):767–772.
17. Arikan S, Kocakusak A, Yucel AF, Adas G. A prospective comparison of the selective observation and routine exploration methods for penetrating abdominal stab wounds with organ or omentum evisceration. *J Trauma.* 2005;58(3):526–532.
18. Matsushima K, Khor D, Berona K, et al. Double jeopardy in penetrating trauma: get FAST, get it right. *World J Surg.* 2018;42(1):99–106.
19. Velmahos GC, Constantinou C, Tillou A, et al. Abdominal computed tomographic scan for patients with gunshot wounds to the abdomen selected for nonoperative management. *J Trauma.* 2005;59(5):1155–1160; discussion 1160–1161.
20. Inaba K, Okoye OT, Rosenheck R, et al. Prospective evaluation of the role of computed tomography in the assessment of abdominal stab wounds. *JAMA Surg.* 2013;148(9):810–816.
21. Lian T, Ashbrook M, Myers L, et al. Diagnostic accuracy of computed tomography findings for hollow viscus injuries following thoracoabdominal gunshot wounds. *J Trauma Acute Care Surg.* 2023;94(1):156–161.
22. Demetriades D, Hadjizacharia P, Constantinou C, et al. Selective nonoperative management of penetrating abdominal solid organ injuries. *Ann Surg.* 2006;244(4):620–628.
23. Inaba K, Branco BC, Moe D, et al. Prospective evaluation of selective nonoperative management of torso gunshot wounds: when is it safe to discharge? *J Trauma Acute Care Surg.* 2012;72(4):884–891.
24. Inaba K, Barmparas G, Foster A, et al. Selective nonoperative management of torso gunshot wounds: when is it safe to discharge? *J Trauma.* 2010;68(6):1301–1304.
25. Owattanapanich N, Cremonini C, Schellenberg MA, et al. Prospective evaluation of the selective nonoperative management of abdominal stab wounds: when is it safe to discharge? *J Trauma Acute Care Surg.* 2022;93(5):639–643.
26. Murray JA, Demetriades D, Cornwell EE III, et al. Penetrating left thoracoabdominal trauma: the incidence and clinical presentation of diaphragm injuries. *J Trauma.* 1997;43(4):624–626.
27. Murray JA, Demetriades D, Asensio JA, et al. Occult injuries to the diaphragm: prospective evaluation of laparoscopy in penetrating injuries to the left lower chest. *J Am Coll Surg.* 1998;187(6):626–630.
28. Jakob DA, Liasidis P, Schellenberg M, et al. Intra-abdominal hemorrhage control: the need for routine four-quadrant packing explored. *World J Surg.* 2021;45(4):1014–1020.
29. Rotondo MF, Schwab CW, McGonigal MD, et al. 'Damage control': an approach for improved survival in exsanguinating penetrating abdominal injury. *J Trauma.* 1993;35(3):375–382; discussion 382–383.
30. Matsushima K, Hogen R, Piccinini A, et al. Adjunctive use of hepatic angioembolization following hemorrhage control laparotomy. *J Trauma Acute Care Surg.* 2020;88(5):636–643.
31. Talving P, Chouliaras K, Eastman A, et al. Discontinuity of the bowel following damage control operation revisited: a multi-institutional study. *World J Surg.* 2017;41(1):146–151.
32. Raeburn CD, Moore EE, Biffl WL, et al. The abdominal compartment syndrome is a morbid complication of postinjury damage control surgery. *Am J Surg.* 2001;182(6):542–546.
33. Cremonini C, Lewis MR, Jakob D, et al. Diagnosing penetrating diaphragmatic injuries: CT scan is valuable but not reliable. *Injury.* 2022;53(1):116–121.
34. Kozar RA, Crandeall M, Shanmuganathan K, et al. Organ injury scaling 2018 update: spleen, liver, and kidney. *J Trauma Acute Care Surg.* 2018;85(6):1119–1122.
35. van der Wilden GM, Velmahos GC, Emhoff T, et al. Successful nonoperative management of the most severe blunt liver injuries: a multicenter study of the research consortium of new England centers for trauma. *Arch Surg.* 2012;147(5):423–428.
36. Sivrikoz E, Teixeira PG, Resnick S, Inaba K, Talving P, Demetriades D. Angiointervention: an independent predictor of survival in high-grade blunt liver injuries. *Am J Surg.* 2015;209(4):742–746.
37. Samuels JM, Carmichael H, Kovar A, Urban S, Vega S, Velopulos C, McIntyre RC Jr. Reevaluation of hepatic angioembolization for trauma in stable patients: weighing the risk. *J Am Coll Surg.* 2020;231(1):123–131.
38. Schellenberg M, Benjamin E, Piccinini A, et al. Gunshot wounds to the liver: no longer a mandatory operation. *J Trauma Acute Care Surg.* 2019;87(2):350–355.
39. Plackett TP, Barmparas G, Inaba K, Demetriades D. Transplantation for severe hepatic trauma. *J Trauma.* 2011;71(6):1880–1884.
40. Demetriades D, Karaiskakis M, Alo K, Velmahos G, Murray J, Asensio J. Role of postoperative computed tomography in patients with severe liver injury. *Br J Surg.* 2003;90(11):1398–1400.
41. Peitzman AB, Heil B, Rivera L, et al. Blunt splenic injury in adults: multi-institutional study of the Eastern Association for the Surgery of Trauma. *J Trauma.* 2000;49(2):177–187; discussion 187–189.
42. Berg RJ, Inaba K, Okoye O, et al. The contemporary management of penetrating splenic injury. *Injury.* 2014;45(9):1394–1400.
43. Aoki M, Onogawa A, Matsumoto S, Matsushima K. Recent trends in the management of isolated high-grade splenic injuries: a nationwide analysis. *J Trauma Acute Care Surg.* 2023;94(2):220–225.
44. Schellenberg M, Owattanapanich N, Emigh B, et al. Pseudoaneurysms after high-grade blunt solid organ injury and the utility of delayed computed tomography angiography. *Eur J Trauma Emerg Surg.* 2023;49(3):1315–1320.
45. Tang-Tan A, Chien CY, Park S, et al. Clinical factors and outcomes of spleen-conserving surgery versus total splenectomy in splenic injuries: a nationwide database study. *Am J Surg.* 2024;233:142–147.
46. Demetriades D, Scalea TM, Degiannis E, et al. Blunt splenic trauma: splenectomy increases early infectious complications: a prospective multicenter study. *J Trauma Acute Care Surg.* 2012;72(1):229–234.
47. Shatz DV, Romero-Steiner S, Elie CM, Holder PF, Carlone GM. Antibody responses in postsplenectomy trauma patients receiving

the 23-valent pneumococcal polysaccharide vaccine at 14 versus 28 days postoperatively. *J Trauma.* 2002;53(6):1037–1042.

48. Schellenberg M, Inaba K, Bardes JM, et al. Detection of traumatic pancreatic duct disruption in the modern era. *Am J Surg.* 2018;216(2):299–303.
49. Mansfield N, Inaba K, Berg R, et al. Early pancreatic dysfunction after resection in trauma: an 18-year report from a Level I trauma center. *J Trauma Acute Care Surg.* 2017;82(3):528–533.
50. Bonomi AM, Granieri S, Gupta S, et al. Traumatic hollow viscus and mesenteric injury: role of CT and potential diagnostic-therapeutic algorithm. *Updates Surg.* 2021;73(2):703–710.
51. Iaselli F, Mazzei MA, Firetto C, et al. Bowel and mesenteric injuries from blunt abdominal trauma: a review. *Radiol Med.* 2015;120(1):21–32.
52. Aiolfi A, Matsushima K, Chang G, et al. Surgical trends in the management of duodenal injury. *J Gastrointest Surg.* 2019;23(2):264–269.
53. Demetriades D, Murray JA, Chan L, et al. Penetrating colon injuries requiring resection: diversion or primary anastomosis? An AAST prospective multicenter study. *J Trauma.* 2001;50(5):765–775.
54. Mitchao DP, Lewis MR, Strickland M, Benjamin ER, Wong MD, Demetriades D. Destructive colon injuries requiring resection: is colostomy ever indicated? *J Trauma Acute Care Surg.* 2022;92(6):1039–1046.
55. Curran TJ, Borzotta AP. Complications of primary repair of colon injury: literature review of 2,964 cases. *Am J Surg.* 1999;177(1):42–47.
56. Trust MD, Veith J, Brown CVR, et al; AAST Contemporary Management of Rectal Injuries Study Group. Traumatic rectal injuries: is the combination of computed tomography and rigid proctoscopy sufficient? *J Trauma Acute Care Surg.* 2018;85(6):1033–1037.
57. Brown CVR, Teixeira PG, Furay E, et al; AAST Contemporary Management of Rectal Injuries Study Group. Contemporary management of rectal injuries at Level I trauma centers: the results of an American Association for the Surgery of Trauma multi-institutional study. *J Trauma Acute Care Surg.* 2018;84(2):225–233.

Genitourinary Trauma

Farris Serio, Bradley A. Rittenhouse, and Martin A. Schreiber

Key Points

1 Hematuria is the most sensitive indicator of genitourinary trauma, but the absence of hematuria is insufficient to rule out a genitourinary injury.

2 CT scan with IV contrast is the primary modality for evaluating genitourinary injuries. It must include a delayed phase to evaluate the renal collecting system and ureter and a cystogram to evaluate the bladder if indicated.

3 Renal injuries in hemodynamically stable patients can most often be treated nonoperatively.

4 Genitourinary injuries can result in multiple complications including abscess, sepsis, urine leak, stricture of urethra or ureter, hypertension, and renal insufficiency.

5 Intraperitoneal bladder injuries require repair, while many extraperitoneal bladder injuries can be managed nonoperatively with Foley catheter drainage.

6 Urethral injuries are most commonly associated with pelvic fractures and are evaluated with a retrograde urethrogram.

Trauma produces a large burden on health care both in the United States and throughout the world. As of 2022, unintentional injuries were the leading cause of death for people 1 to 44 years of age.[1–3] The genitourinary system is infrequently injured in isolation. Of these organs, the kidney is the most frequently injured, with renal injuries seen in 5% of all trauma patients, 10% of all patients with abdominal trauma, and accounting for up to 24% of all solid organ injuries.[2–5] Multiple organizations have guidelines for the evaluation and management of injuries to the genitourinary system including the American Urological Association, European Association of Urology, and the Société Internationale d'Urologie. These recommendations as well as recent updates are reviewed to provide an efficient organized method to evaluate genitourinary injuries in the trauma patient.

KIDNEY

Injuries to the kidneys are commonly the result of blunt trauma, including motor vehicle collisions and falls.[6,7] The kidneys are somewhat protected, being located within the rib cage in the retroperitoneum and surrounded by perinephric fat and Gerota's fascia. Nearby structures that are susceptible to concurrent injury include the liver, adrenal gland, duodenum, and colon on the right and the spleen, adrenal gland, and colon on the left. Within the kidney, the collecting system begins with the renal pelvis which then becomes the ureter as it leaves the kidney at the ureteropelvic junction (UPJ). Injuries to the renal parenchyma or the collecting system result from external impact or from impact against the nearby ribs. Rapid deceleration can also induce shearing forces at fixed points near the renal pelvis and vasculature, resulting in avulsion injuries.

Evaluation

1 The evaluation for renal injury includes a focused history and physical exam. Findings suspicious for renal trauma include a history of hematuria, blunt or penetrating injury to the flank, lower rib fractures, flank hematoma/ecchymosis, and injuries to nearby organs such as the liver or spleen. Both macroscopic and microscopic hematuria can be seen and a urine dipstick is
2 appropriate in the initial evaluation for genitourinary trauma, but it is neither sensitive nor specific enough to stratify injury severity.[2,8] As with any trauma patient, ensuring hemodynamic stability is paramount before proceeding to additional diagnostic testing. In hemodynamically stable patients with concern for renal injury, **Algorithm 25.1** provides an algorithm for evaluation.[5,9,10]

The primary method for evaluation of renal injuries is the CT scan. The ideal protocol to evaluate for renal injuries is a three-phase contrast CT scan with an arterial phase to evaluate for active extravasation, a venous or nephrographic phase to evaluate the renal parenchyma, and a 5-minute delayed phase to evaluate the urinary collecting system. Addition of a 5- to 10-minute delayed phase CT to the initial trauma contrast-enhanced CT protocol is sufficient to detect injuries to the kidneys and the collecting system.[5,9] CT imaging is the primary modality for grading the severity of injury. The American Association for the Surgery of Trauma (AAST) organ injury scale (OIS) is the most commonly used grading system, and the 2018 guidelines combine imaging, operative, and autopsy findings (**Table 25.1**).[11,12] If CT is unavailable, a single-shot intravenous pyelogram may be used intraoperatively to verify the presence of a contralateral kidney. Ultrasound is generally not recommended as initial evaluation (E-FAST excluded) of the genitourinary system, but contrast-enhanced ultrasound and Doppler imaging may play a role in the minimally injured pregnant and pediatric populations.[3] MRI offers no benefit over CT, has increased logistical challenges, and is not recommended.[5,9]

Treatment

3 AAST grading provides a basis for treatment decisions. In blunt injury, nonoperative management is the preferred treatment of mild (Grade I and II), moderate (Grade III), and most severe (Grade IV–V) injuries. Even grade III to V injuries can be successfully managed without operative intervention in
4 80% of blunt injuries without increased hospital stay or complication.[3,10,13] Angiography and embolization is indicated in hemodynamically normal patients and most transient

Algorithm 25.1

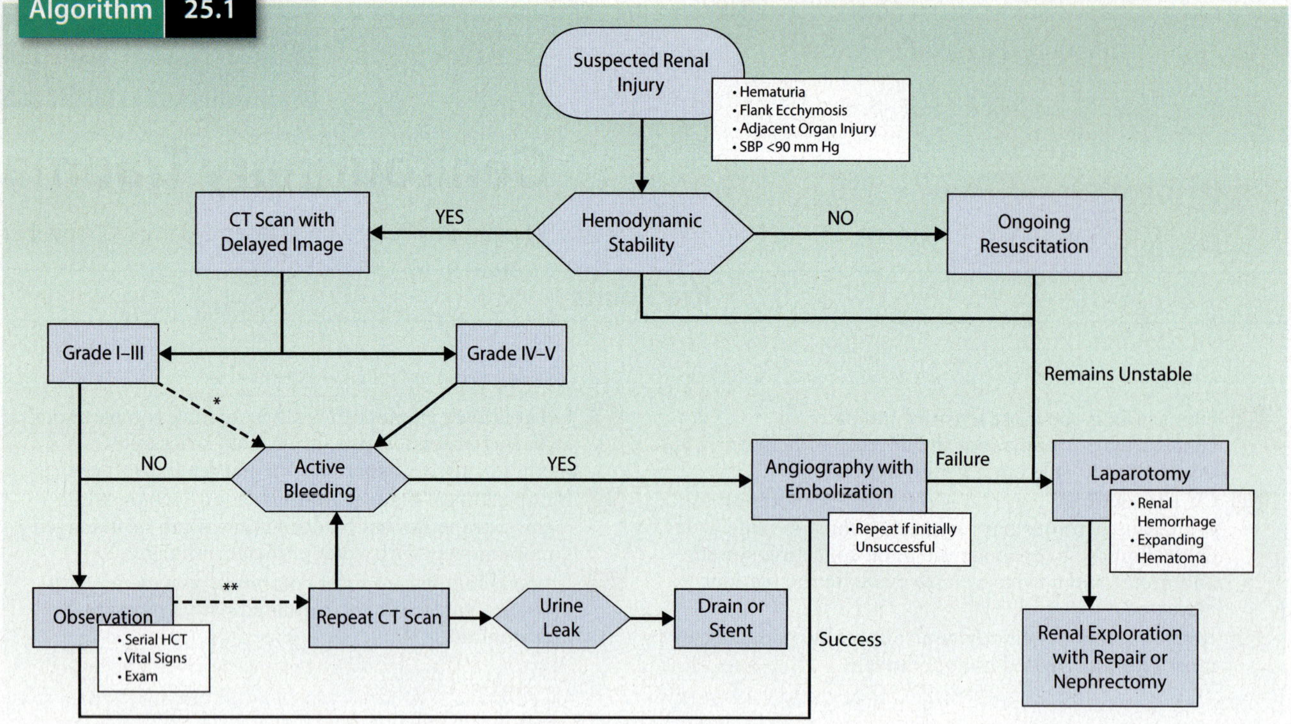

Algorithm 25.1. Evaluation of renal trauma. *Grade III with active extravasation is frequently self-limited. **Grade IV–V should have routine repeat CT scan at 48 hours. Grade I–III routine repeat CT is not recommended, but should be performed selectively.

Table 25.1. AAST Grading of Injuries to Urologic Structures

Injured Structure	AAST Grade	Description of Injury
Kidney	I	▪ Subcapsular hematoma/contusion without laceration
	II	▪ Laceration <1 cm in depth without collecting system involvement
		▪ Perinephric hematoma within Gerota fascia
	III	▪ Laceration >1 cm in depth without collecting system involvement
		▪ Active bleeding or vascular injury within Gerota fascia
	IV	▪ Urine extravasation from laceration
		▪ Laceration of renal pelvis or ureteropelvic disruption
		▪ Injury to segmental artery or vein/segmental infarct
		▪ Active bleeding outside Gerota fascia
	V	▪ Shattered kidney
		▪ Avulsion or devascularization at renal hilum
Ureter	I	▪ Contusion or hematoma without devascularization
	II	▪ Laceration with <50% transection
	III	▪ Laceration with >50% transection
	IV	▪ Complete transection with <2 cm of devascularization
	V	▪ Avulsion/Laceration with >2 cm of devascularization
Bladder	I	▪ Contusion, intramural hematoma
		▪ Partial thickness laceration
	II	▪ Extraperitoneal bladder wall laceration <2 cm
	III	▪ Extraperitoneal laceration >2 cm
		▪ Intraperitoneal laceration <2 cm
	IV	▪ Intraperitoneal laceration <2 cm
	V	▪ Laceration of involving bladder neck or ureteral orifice
Urethra	I	▪ Contusion with blood at urethral meatus, retrograde urethrography (RUG) normal
	II	▪ Stretch with elongation of urethra without extravasation
	III	▪ Partial disruption with contrast extravasation at injury site and within bladder
	IV	▪ Complete disruption with contrast extravasation at injury site and none progressing to bladder <2 cm of urethral separation
	V	▪ Complete disruption >2 cm
		▪ Extension of disruption into the prostate or vagina

If injuries are bilateral, increase one grade up to III (in table refers to kidney and ureter).
If there are multiple injuries in one organ, use the highest grade (in table refer to kidney, ureter, bladder and urethra).

responders with arterial contrast extravasation, pseudoaneurysm, arteriovenous fistula, and non–self-limiting gross hematuria.[3,14] Operative management in blunt injury is reserved for hemodynamically unstable patients and some transient responders who don't improve with resuscitation. In these patients, nephrectomy is required in 0.4% to 4.5% in grade III, 15% to 24% in grade IV, and 57% to 62% in grade V injuries.[3,15–18] (**Fig. 25.1**).

AAST grade is similarly used in penetrating trauma, but penetrating injuries result in operative management more frequently. In stable patients, 88% of injuries posterior to

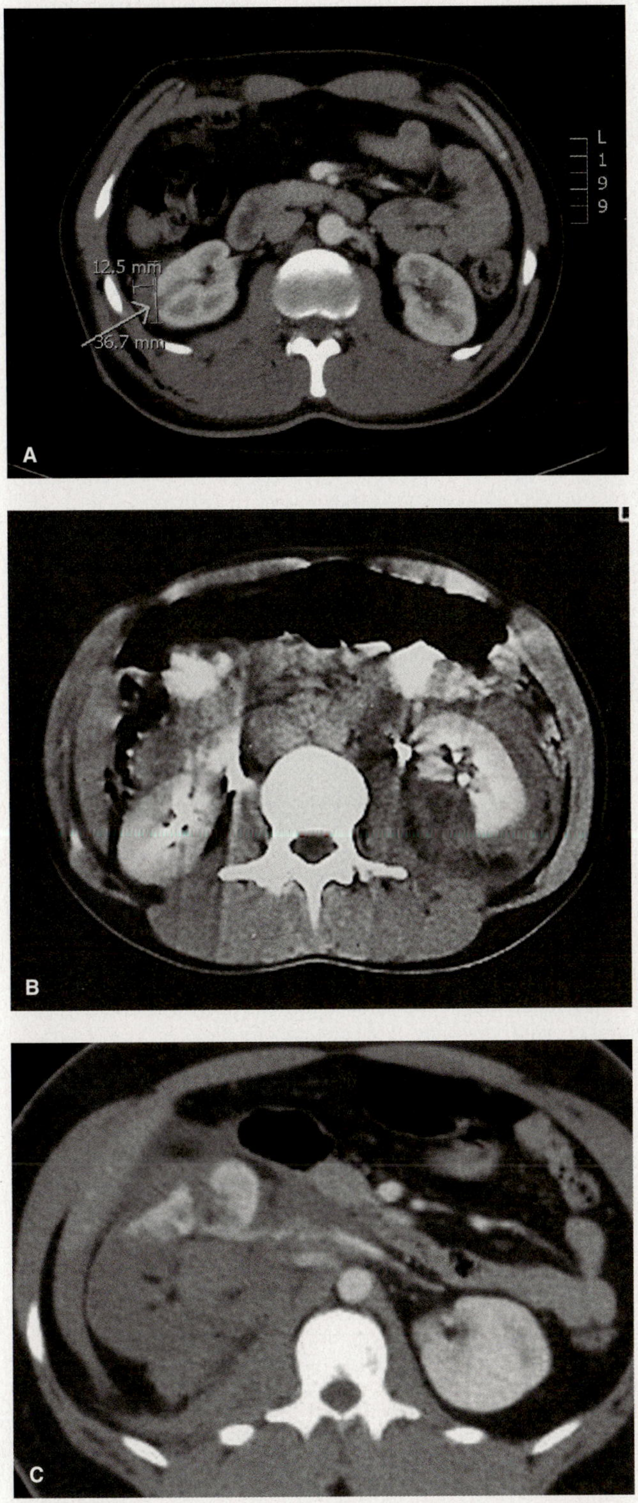

Figure 25.1. CT scan of renal injuries. **A:** Grade I. **B:** Grade III. **C:** Grade V.

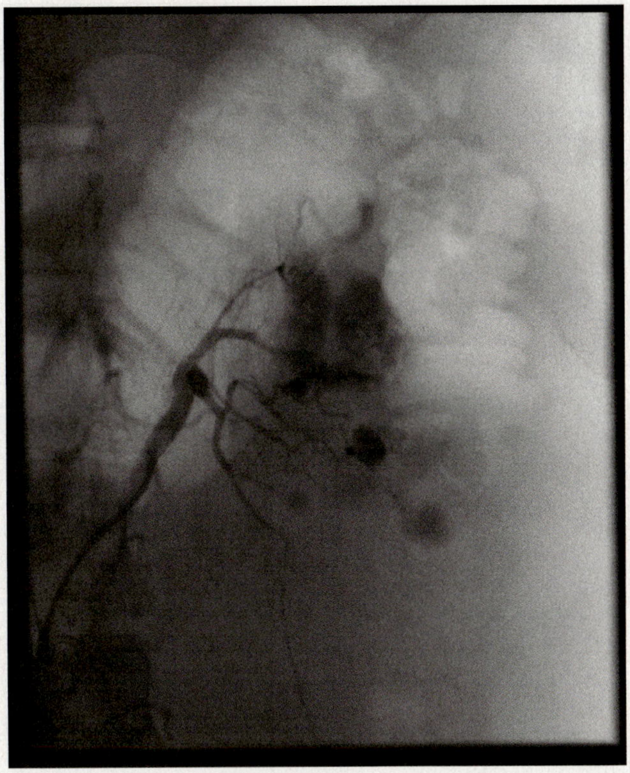

Figure 25.2. Angiogram of grade V renal injury.

the axillary line may be managed nonoperatively.[3] This is successful more commonly in low-velocity injuries such as stab wounds, whereas in high-velocity injuries like gunshot wounds, closer to 40% are amenable to nonoperative management.[3,19,20] (**Fig. 25.2**).

Should operative exploration be required, exposure of the kidney and upper urinary tract is accomplished through an upper midline incision as outlined in **Table 25.2.** Early complications (<1 month) and late complications (>1 month) are also outlined in **Table 25.2.** Hypertension from renal trauma is a rare complication but is initially treated medically with ACE inhibitors. Additional options for treatment include interventions to drain perinephric hematomas or even nephrectomy if hypertension cannot be controlled.[4,21]

URETER

3 Ureteral trauma is rare due to the small size and relative mobility of the ureter. Injury to the ureter accounts for only 1% to 2.5% of urinary tract trauma. Penetrating injuries frequently occur due to gunshot wounds and blast injuries with most blunt injuries associated with pelvic fractures.[22–24] The collecting system begins with the renal pelvis which then becomes the ureter as it leaves the kidney at the UPJ. The ureter remains in the retroperitoneum, traversing along the psoas muscle then crosses over the common iliac vessels to enter the pelvis. In women, the ureter runs below the uterine artery. Blood supply to the ureter is segmental with supply to the upper third from the renal artery, middle third from the gonadal and iliac arteries, and distal third from the internal iliac artery and uterine artery in women.

Evaluation

4 Evaluation for ureteral trauma should be performed in high-energy blunt trauma or in penetrating abdominal trauma that involves the retroperitoneum. Hematuria is a poor predictor of ureteral injury.[3,25,26] The diagnosis of penetrating ureteral injuries is most often made at laparotomy and should be suspected when nearby structures are damaged including the

Table 25.2. Key Technical Steps, Pearls and Pitfalls: Repair of the Kidney, Ureters, and Bladder

KIDNEY	
Key Technical Steps	1. Access via upper midline incision 2. Vascular control: a. Centrally by incising the peritoneum medial to inferior mesenteric vein[27] b. Rapidly by medial visceral rotation[28] 3. Nonviable tissue debrided 4. Repair of kidney or collecting system vs nephrectomy 5. Place retroperitoneal drain
Pearls	■ Stability of the patient dictates vascular control options: stable patient may allow for mesenteric dissection but in an unstable patient, medializing the kidney via right or left visceral rotation to obtain control is much faster ■ Attempt to preserve renal capsule when debriding to allow for closure ■ Use absorbable suture for repair to avoid stone disease ■ Vascular injuries often require nephrectomy ■ Left renal vein may be ligated if necessary, drainage will occur via gonadal and lumbar vein collaterals
Pitfalls	■ Early complications (<1 mo) include abscess, urinary leak, and urinary fistula ■ Urine leak can be diagnosed if high drain output has creatinine level greater than serum ■ Late complications (>1 mo) include hydronephrosis, pseudoaneurysm, calculus, or hypertension ■ Hypertension can be caused by perirenal hematoma (Page kidney), renal artery thrombosis or stenosis (Goldblatt kidney)[21] ■ Hypertension is often managed medically but may require drainage of hematoma or even nephrectomy[4,21]
URETER	
Key Technical Steps	1. Access via midline laparotomy with mobilization of viscera to expose retroperitoneum 2. If hemodynamically normal, ureters can be repaired at the index operation, with type of repair dictated by location of injury and amount of tissue destruction.[5,9] 3. **Figures 25.3** and **25.4** demonstrate anatomic considerations and operative techniques 4. Unstable patients require urinary diversion: a. proximal control via either nephrostomy or percutaneous ureterostomy tube b. Retroperitoneal drainage at the site of injury c. Bladder drainage distally
Pearls	■ Any repairs should be performed using absorbable suture and aim to be watertight, with mucosal apposition over a ureteral stent, minimizing tension on the anastomosis.
Pitfalls	■ Delayed presentations should not undergo immediate repair. Instead, urinary diversion should be performed ■ After 3–6 mo, repair can be attempted to maximize chances of success ■ Complications include urine leak, stricture, obstruction, and infection
BLADDER	
Key Technical Steps	1. Exposure can be extraperitoneal or intraperitoneal depending on location and extent of associated injuries 2. Repair of bladder lacerations is performed in 2 layers with absorbable suture and should be water tight 3. Postoperative Foley catheter drainage (rather than suprapubic catheter) is typically adequate and can be removed in 7–10 d after repeat cystogram.[4,5,9,29]
Pearls	■ To fully explore bladder injuries, the bladder wall, ureteral orifices, and bladder neck can be accessed via an anterior cystotomy or the injury itself. It is critical to avoid narrowing of the ureteral orifices. ■ Closed suction drainage of the peritoneum or extraperitoneal perivesical space **allows** for detection of urine leaks. Drain creatinine greater than serum suggests urine leak.[4,5,9,29]
Pitfalls	■ Intraperitoneal rupture requires repair; undrained urine can lead to infection, peritonitis, sepsis, and death.[4]
URETHRA	
Key Technical Steps	1. Operative vs nonoperative management is determined by location, concomitant injuries, and grade of injury to the urethra.[4,25–27] 2. Endoscopic realignment is performed by placing a guidewire across the defect using a flexible/rigid cystoscope then advancing a catheter over this.[4]
Pearls	■ Suprapubic catheterization is a good solution in urgent situations. ■ Placement of a urethral catheter can be attempted in many cases and has a low risk of causing additional damage.[4]
Pitfalls	■ Risks of stricture, impotence, or incontinence can be reduced with endoscopic realignment ■ Immediate urethroplasty is associated with higher rates of impotence, incontinence, and stricture ■ Suprapubic catheterization may be difficult when distortions occur due to pelvic fracture or hematoma.[4,30–32]

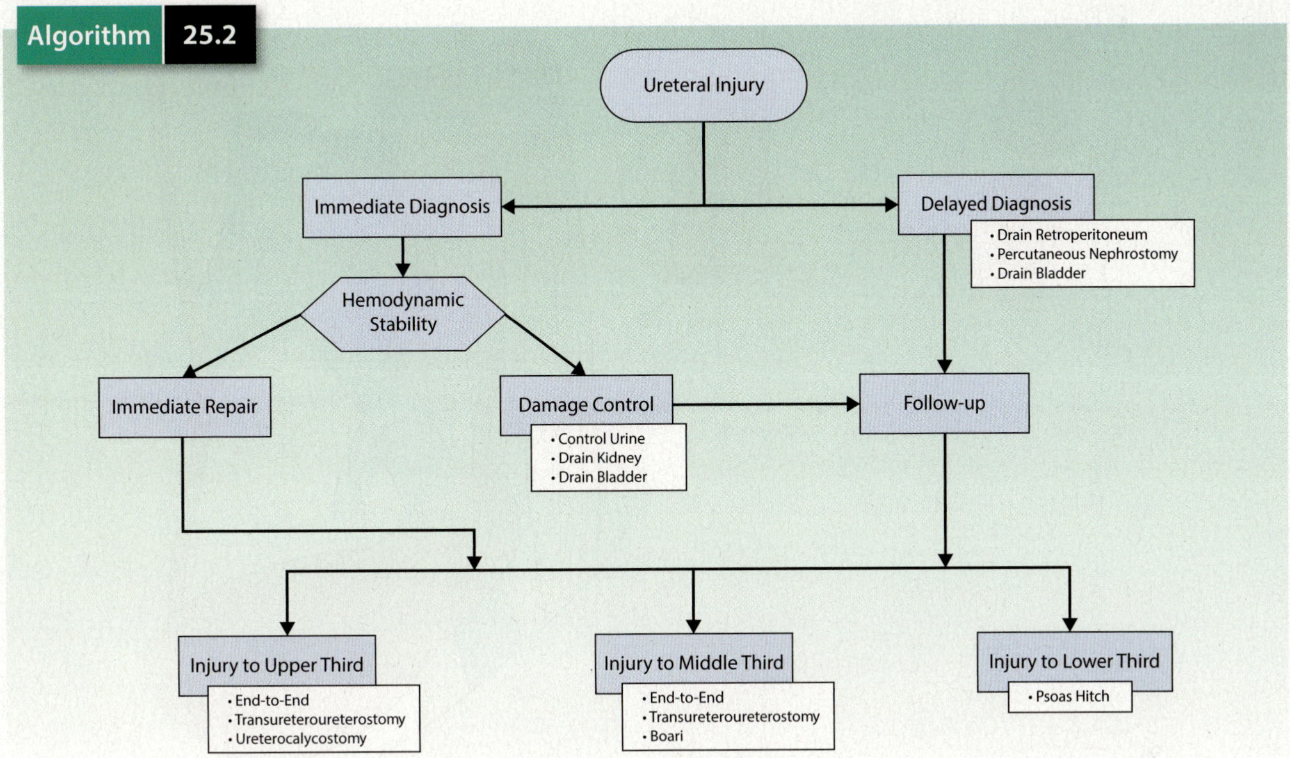

Algorithm 25.2. Evaluation of ureteral injury.

psoas muscle, kidney, bladder, and colon. In stable patients, contrast-enhanced CT scan with delayed imaging is the evaluation of choice. In addition to extravasated contrast on the delayed images, unilateral ureteral dilation, urinoma, or ascites may be indications of injury. Exploration is recommended if laparotomy is required for other injuries. Retrograde urography may be performed if the diagnosis is unclear.[5,7,9] Delayed presentation with fever, flank pain, tenderness atelectasis, urinoma, hematoma, or oliguria is evaluated in a similar manner with contrast-enhanced CT scan (**Algorithm 25.2**).

Treatment

The management of ureteral trauma is operative repair in most instances. Grading is based upon the AAST system (**Table 25.1**). Patients with ureteral injuries often require laparotomy for other associated injuries. During this exploration, the ureter should be examined for injury and viability while avoiding its devascularization. Operative treatment is described in **Table 25.2** along with complications related to injury and repair. **Figure 25.3** demonstrates anatomic considerations for type of repair and **Figure 25.4** describes the techniques utilized. Patients who have sustained a high-grade ureteral injury should have repeat imaging with ultrasound, radionucleotide scan, or CT urography to evaluate for stricture or urinoma.

BLADDER

Bladder injuries most commonly occur as a result of blunt trauma.[33] Pelvic fracture is associated with 60% to 90% of these injuries, and other abdominal organ injuries occur 55% to 68% of the time. Conversely, less than 10% of pelvic fractures have associated urogenital injuries.[9,29,34] Bladder injuries are characterized as either extraperitoneal or intraperitoneal. Extraperitoneal injuries are almost always associated with pelvic fractures, whereby distortion of the pelvic ring causes shearing on the bladder at its fascial attachments or the bladder is lacerated by a bony shard.[3] The highest risk for bladder injuries occurs with pelvic ring fractures with >1 cm of displacement.[5,35,36]

Evaluation

Evaluation for bladder injury must involve a high degree of suspicion when pelvic fractures or injury to other pelvic organs are present. Gross hematuria occurs in greater than 90% of

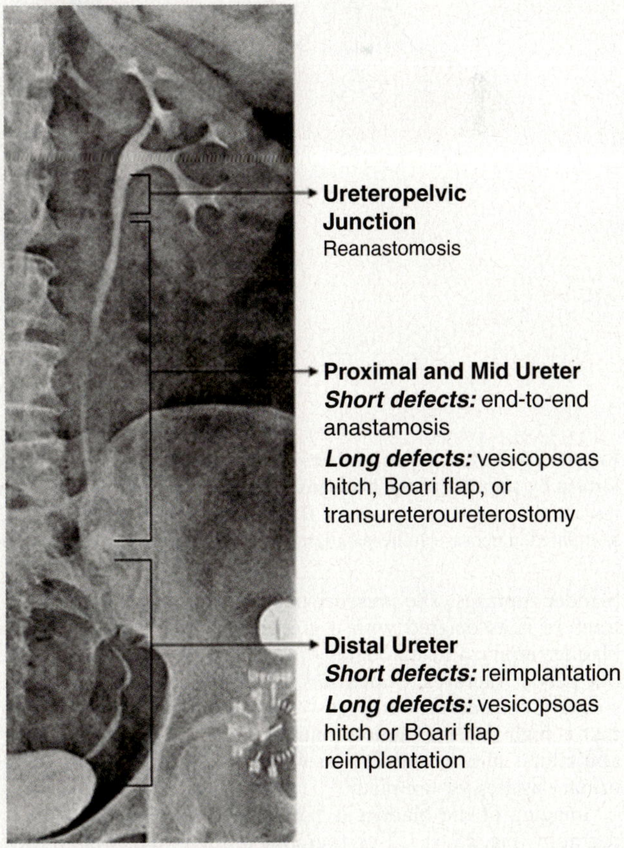

Figure 25.3. Locations of ureteral injury.

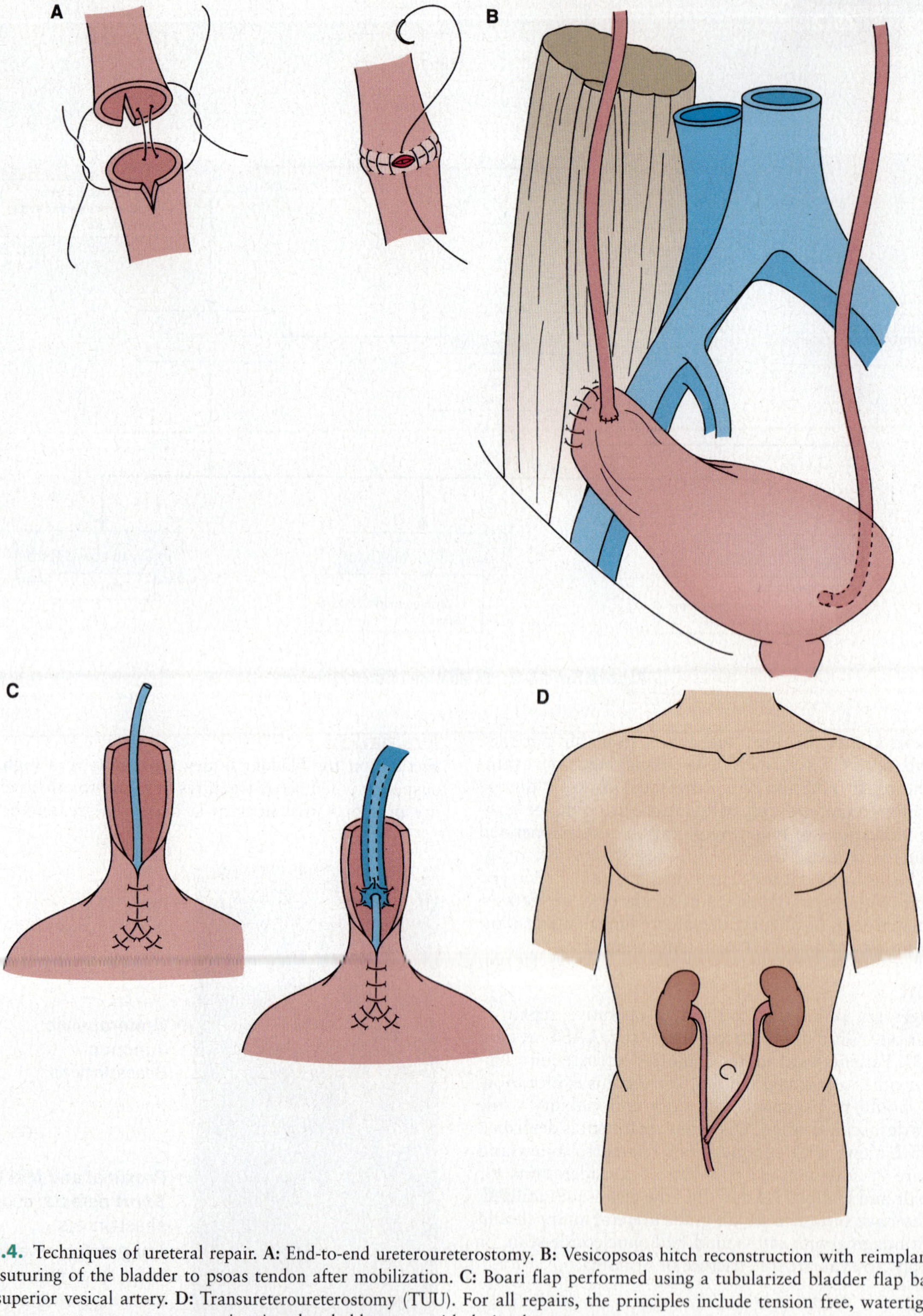

Figure 25.4. Techniques of ureteral repair. **A:** End-to-end ureteroureterostomy. **B:** Vesicopsoas hitch reconstruction with reimplantation performed by suturing of the bladder to psoas tendon after mobilization. **C:** Boari flap performed using a tubularized bladder flap based on the ipsilateral superior vesical artery. **D:** Transureteroureterostomy (TUU). For all repairs, the principles include tension free, watertight, stented, spatulated, mucosa-to-mucosa anastomosis using absorbable suture with drain placement.

bladder ruptures. The presence of gross hematuria with pelvic fracture is associated with a greater than 30% incidence of bladder injury and mandates evaluation.[5,37] In patients without pelvic fractures, evaluation for bladder injury should be strongly considered with gross hematuria and a mechanism that is high risk for bladder injury such as high-impact lower abdominal injury, inability to void, imaging consistent with urinary ascites, or uremia.[4,5,9]

Imaging of the bladder is performed with retrograde cystography (**Fig. 25.5**). CT cystography or high-quality plain film cystography are acceptable choices however, CT cystography may be better at identifying bony fragments in the bladder as well as bladder neck injuries.[5,9,38,39] CT cystography involves instilling 300 to 350 mL of contrast into the bladder through a Foley catheter prior to CT of the pelvis. Simply clamping the Foley catheter during the standard trauma CT scan is inadequate to rule out bladder rupture.[39] Intraperitoneal injuries are identified by visualizing free flow of contrast material into the abdomen where it outlines bowel loops and intraperitoneal organs. Extraperitoneal bladder injuries produce more localized extravasation of contrast that is often described as flame shaped.

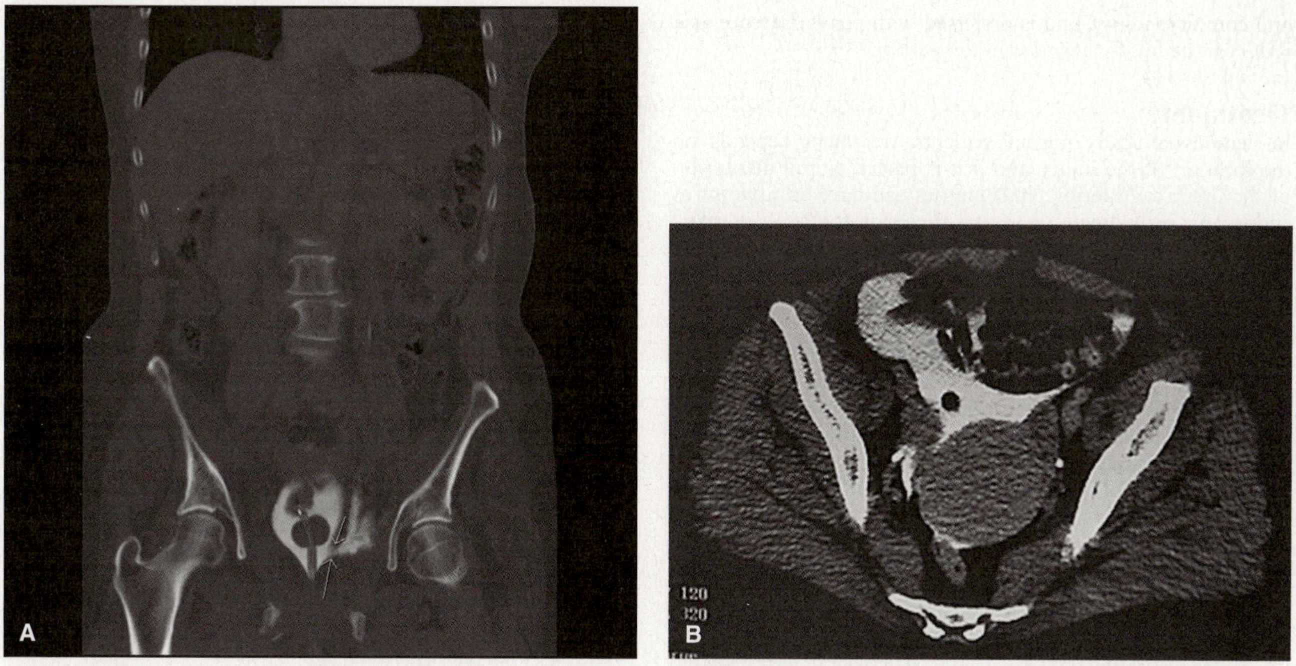

Figure 25.5. CT cystogram with bladder injury. **A:** Extraperitoneal bladder rupture. **B:** Intraperitoneal bladder rupture.

Treatment

5 Management of bladder injuries depends on the location of rupture (extraperitoneal or intraperitoneal) and associated injuries. Nonoperative management is common for uncomplicated extraperitoneal bladder rupture and involves Foley catheter drainage for 2 to 3 weeks to allow healing. This observation period is typically followed by repeat cystogram to ensure healing. Complicated extraperitoneal bladder rupture which includes the presence of pelvic fracture requiring operative repair, boney shards within the bladder, concomitant rectal or vaginal injuries, or injuries to the bladder neck or ureters should be repaired surgically.[4,5,37]

Intraperitoneal bladder injuries must be explored and repaired. The size of these injuries and risk of peritonitis preclude nonoperative treatment.[4,5,9,29] Operative management is described in **Table 25.2.**

URETHRA

6 Urethral injuries are most commonly the result of blunt trauma and much more common in males than females. The male urethra can be divided into anterior and posterior portions and injuries are classified as either partial or full disruptions. Injuries to the anterior portion can result from a straddle mechanism or perineal kicks causing compression against the pubic symphysis. Posterior injuries are associated with pelvic fractures.[4,5,9,34]

Evaluation

Blood at the urethral meatus and injuries to the perineum warrant evaluation for urethral injury. Other signs that suggest urethral injury include inability to void with a distended bladder, pain, hematuria, or difficulty/inability to pass a urethral catheter. A rectal examination should be performed to rule out concomitant rectal injury. A "high-riding prostate," meaning the prostate is not palpated on rectal exam, may be identified, although this is unreliable.[4,5,9,34] If there is concern for a urethral injury, a retrograde urethrogram should be performed prior to the placement of a urethral catheter. Retrograde urethrography (RUG) is performed by instilling 20 to 30 mL of contrast into the urethra through a Foley catheter placed at the tip of the meatus. An x-ray is then taken at a 30-degree oblique angle while infusing contrast. Any contrast extravasation from the urethra is indicative of an injury (**Fig. 25.6**).[5,35,37] Flexible cystourethroscopy is helpful to differentiate between partial

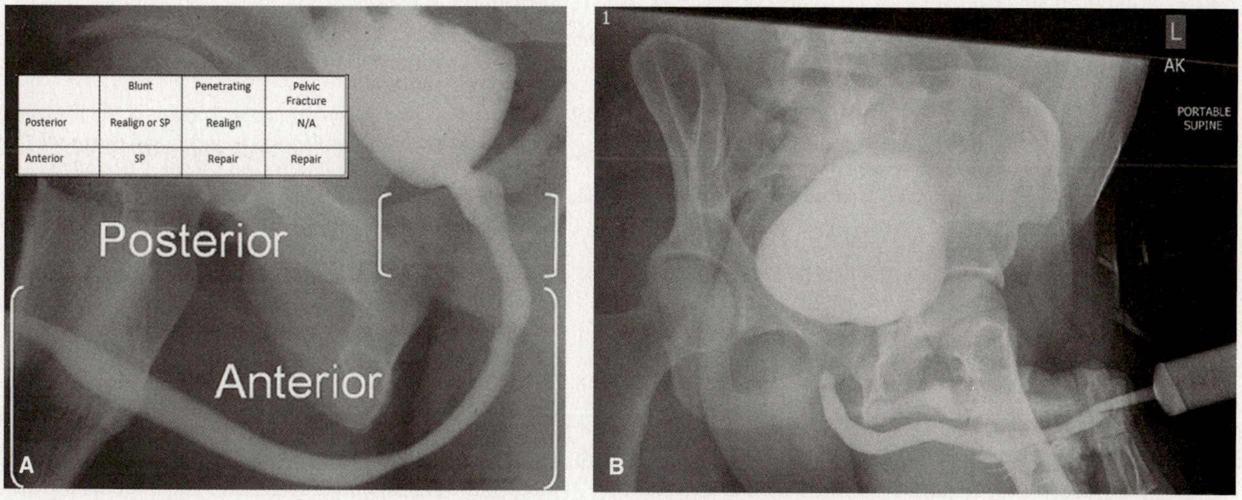

Figure 25.6. Retrograde urethrogram. **A:** Normal. **B:** Partial injury. (Demonstrated by contrast in corpus cavernosum and incompletely opacified posterior urethra.)

and complete injury, and is preferred with penile fracture as a RUG can be falsely negative in this setting.[9,30,31,37]

Treatment

In hemodynamically normal patients, treatment depends on the location of the injury and if it is partial or full disruption of the urethra. Anterior blunt injuries can have an attempt at endoscopic realignment or urinary diversion for 2 to 3 weeks.[4] Penetrating injuries or those associated with penile fracture may require early exploration and repair. Early realignment may decrease the risk of stricture from nearly 80% to 45% without increased risk of incontinence (5%) or erectile dysfunction (20%).[9,30–32] If realignment is not possible, urethral injuries are repaired in a delayed fashion when swelling and hematomas have decreased. In cases of urethral injury that involve high-energy destructive mechanisms or additional injuries, suprapubic drainage with delayed reconstruction may be appropriate.[4,5,9]

References

1. Injury Prevention and Control: Ten leading causes of death, United States [Internet]. [cited 2024 August 20]. https://www.cdc.gov/injury/wisqars/LeadingCauses.html
2. European Association of Urology. EAU Guidelines on Urological Trauma 2018 [Internet]. 2018 [cited 2024 August 20]. https://cdn.dal.ca/content/dam/dalhousie/pdf/faculty/medicine/departments/department-sites/urology/ClinicalClerkshipBook/EAU-Guidelines-on-Urological-Trauma-2018-large-text.pdf
3. Coccolini F, Moore EE, Kluger Y, et al. Kidney and uro-trauma: WSES-AAST guidelines. *World J of Emerg Surg.* 2019;14:54.
4. Bryk DJ, Zhao LC. Guideline of guidelines: a review of urological trauma guidelines. *BJU Int.* 2016;117(2):226–234.
5. Morey AF, Brandes S, Dugi DD 3rd, et al. Urotrauma: AUA guideline. *J Urol.* 2014;192(2):327–335.
6. McAninch JW. Genitourinary trauma. *World J Urol.* 1999;17(2):65.
7. Serafetinides E, Kitrey ND, Djakovic N, et al. Review of the current management of upper urinary tract injuries by the EAU Trauma Guidelines Panel. *Eur Urol.* 2015;67(5):930–936.
8. Chandhoke PS, McAninch JW. Detection and significance of microscopic hematuria in patients with blunt renal trauma. *J Urol.* 1988;140(1):16–18.
9. Kitrey ND, Djakovic N, Hallscheidt P, et al. European Association of Urology Guidelines: Urological Trauma [Internet]. [cited 2019 October 5]. https://uroweb.org/guideline/urological-trauma/# 1_4
10. Brown CVR, Alam HB, Brasel K, et al. Western Trauma Association critical decisions in trauma: Management of renal trauma. *J Trauma Acute Care Surg.* 2018;85(5):1021–1025.
11. Kozar RA, Crandall M, Shanmuganathan K, et al; AAST Patient Assessment Committee. Organ injury scaling 2018 update: spleen, liver, and kidney. *J Trauma Acute Care Surg.* 2018;85(6): 1119–1122.
12. Bjurlin MA, Jeng EI, Goble SM, Doherty JC, Merlotti GJ. Comparison of nonoperative management with renorrhaphy and nephrectomy in penetrating renal injuries. *J Trauma.* 2011;71(3): 554–558.
13. Keihani S, Xu Y, Presson AP, et al; Genito-Urinary Trauma Study Group. Contemporary management of high-grade renal trauma: Results from the American Association for the Surgery of Trauma Genitourinary Trauma study. *J Trauma Acute Care Surg.* 2018;84(3):418–425.
14. Hampson LA, Radadia KD, Odisho AY, McAninch JW, Breyer BN. Conservative management of high-grade renal trauma does not lead to prolonged hospital stay. *Urology.* 2018;115:92–95.
15. McClung CD, Hotaling JM, Wang J, Wessells H, Voelzke BB. Contemporary trends in the immediate surgical management of renal trauma using a national database. *J Trauma Acute Care Surg.* 2013; 75(4):602–606.
16. van der Wilden GM, Velmahos GC, Joseph DK, et al. Successful nonoperative management of the most severe blunt renal injuries: a multicenter study of the research consortium of New England Centers for Trauma. *JAMA Surg.* 2013;148(10):924–931.
17. Wright JL, Nathens AB, Rivara FP, Wessells H. Renal and extrarenal predictors of nephrectomy from the National Trauma Data Bank. *J Urol.* 2006;175(3 Pt 1):970–975; discussion 975.
18. Carroll PR, Klosterman P, McAninch JW. Early vascular control for renal trauma: A critical review. *J Urol.* 1989;141(4):826–829.
19. El Hechi MW, Nederpelt C, Kongkaewpaisan N, et al. Contemporary management of penetrating renal trauma—A national analysis. *Injury.* 2020;51(1):32–38.
20. Nuss GR, Morey AF, Jenkins AC, et al. Radiographic predictors of need for angiographic embolization after traumatic renal injury. *J Trauma.* 2009;67(3):578–582; discussion 582.
21. Pereira BMT, Ogilvie MP, Gomez-Rodriguez JC, et al. A review of ureteral injuries after external trauma. *Scand J Trauma Resusc Emerg Med.* 2010;18:6.
22. McGeady JB, Breyer BN. Current epidemiology of genitourinary trauma. *Urol Clin North Am.* 2013;40(3):323–334.
23. Siram SM, Gerald SZ, Greene WR, et al. Ureteral trauma: patterns and mechanisms of injury of an uncommon condition. *Am J Surg.* 2010;199(4):566–570.
24. Medina D, Lavery R, Ross SE, Livingston DH. Ureteral trauma: preoperative studies neither predict injury nor prevent missed injuries. *J Am Coll Surg.* 1998;186(6):641–644.
25. Elliott SP, McAninch JW. Ureteral injuries from external violence: the 25-year experience at San Francisco General Hospital. *J Urol.* 2003;170(4 Pt 1):1213–1216.
26. Brandes S, Coburn M, Armenakas N, McAninch J. Diagnosis and management of ureteric injury: an evidence-based analysis. *BJU Int.* 2004;94(3):277–289.
27. Gonzalez RP, Falimirski M, Holevar MR, Evankovich C. Surgical management of renal trauma: Is vascular control necessary? *J Trauma.* 1999;47(6):1039–1042; discussion 1042–1044.
28. Dopson SJ, Jayakumar S, Velez JCQ. Page kidney as a rare cause of hypertension: Case report and review of the literature. *Am J Kidney Dis.* 2009;54(2):334–339.
29. Johnsen NV, Dmochowski RR, Young JB, Guillamondegui OD. Epidemiology of blunt lower urinary tract trauma with and without pelvic fracture. *Urology.* 2017;102:234–239.
30. Barros R, Silva M, Antonucci V, Schulze L, Koifman L, Favorito LA. Primary urethral reconstruction results in penile fracture. *Ann R Coll Surg Engl.* 2018;100(1):21–25.
31. Elshout PJ, Veskimae E, MacLennan S, et al. Outcomes of early endoscopic realignment versus suprapubic cystostomy and delayed urethroplasty for pelvic fracture-related posterior urethral injuries: A systematic review. *Eur Urol Focus.* 2017;3(6):545–553.
32. Barrett K, Braga LH, Farrokhyar F, Davies TO. Primary realignment vs suprapubic cystostomy for the management of pelvic fracture-associated urethral injuries: a systematic review and meta-analysis. *Urology.* 2014;83(4):924–929.
33. Barnard J, Overholt T, Hajiran A, et al. Traumatic bladder ruptures: A ten-year review at a level 1 trauma center. *Adv Urol.* 2019;2019:2614586.
34. Figler BD, Hoffler CE, Reisman W, et al. Multi-disciplinary update on pelvic fracture associated bladder and urethral injuries. *Injury.* 2012;43(8):1242–1249.
35. Phillips B, Holzmer S, Turco L, et al. Trauma to the bladder and ureter: a review of diagnosis, management, and prognosis. *Eur J Trauma Emerg Surg.* 2017;43(6):763–773.
36. Lumen N, Kuehhas FE, Djakovic N, et al. Review of the current management of lower urinary tract injuries by the EAU Trauma Guidelines Panel. *Eur Urol.* 2015;67(5):925–929.
37. Quagliano PV, Delair SM, Malhotra AK. Diagnosis of blunt bladder injury: A prospective comparative study of computed tomography cystography and conventional retrograde cystography. *J Trauma.* 2006;61(2):410–421; discussion 421–422.
38. Wirth GJ, Peter R, Poletti P-A, Iselin CE. Advances in the management of blunt traumatic bladder rupture: Experience with 36 cases. *BJU Int.* 2010;106(9):1344–1349.
39. Kamdar C, Mooppan UMM, Kim H, Gulmi FA. Penile fracture: preoperative evaluation and surgical technique for optimal patient outcome. *BJU Int.* 2008;102(11):1640–1644; discussion 1644.

Vascular Trauma

Kendal M. Endicott, Shahab Toursavadkohi, and Todd E. Rasmussen

Key Points

1. Vascular injury is the leading cause of mortality and morbidity in both civilian and military trauma.
2. Mechanisms of vascular injury are broadly categorized as either blunt or penetrating.
3. Patient examination is the most important step in evaluation of a suspected vascular injury.
4. Hard signs of vascular injury suggest near or complete disruption of the vessel in question and include pulsatile bleeding, expanding hematoma, palpable thrill, audible bruit, or evidence of acute ischemia distal to the injury site.
5. Contrast-enhanced computed tomography angiography (CTA) is the most widely used diagnostic imaging modality to identify and localize arterial and venous injuries in patients with suspected vascular injury in the emergency setting.
6. In the trauma patient, hemorrhage leads to both the overall metabolic consequences of shock and end-organ ischemia specific to the injured vessel.
7. Basic tenants of the operative management of vascular trauma include hemorrhage control, restoration of blood flow, and prevention of further reperfusion injury.
8. While open surgical therapy remains the gold standard for treatment for traumatic injuries, endovascular management presents an alternative option particularly with injury to the arch vessels and thoracic aorta.

BACKGROUND

1 Vascular disruption and hemorrhage is the leading cause of mortality and morbidity in both civilian and military trauma.[1–3] Arterial and venous injuries often occur concomitantly due to their anatomic proximity and are frequently associated with injury to other vital structures. Optimal management of traumatic vascular injury requires an understanding of the epidemiology and anatomic distribution of vascular injury patterns, consideration of mechanism, and attention to key tenants of diagnosis and management. The objective of this chapter is to familiarize the reader with current knowledge pertaining to the topic of vascular trauma including the circumstances in which vascular injury occurs and different approaches to diagnosis. Additionally, this chapter will provide guidance to the management of different patterns of vascular injury including extremity, cervical, and torso traumatic injury.

EPIDEMIOLOGY AND MECHANISMS OF VASCULAR TRAUMA

The epidemiology of vascular trauma can be broadly categorized into contextual circumstances (military and civilian), mechanism of injury (blunt and penetrating), and anatomical location of injury (extremity, cervical, and torso).

Wartime Vascular Injury

Contemporary data confirm that exsanguination is the major cause of death in wounded service personnel. The prevalence of wartime vascular trauma has increased markedly over the past century (**Fig. 26.1**).[1–3] Estimates from allied surgeons in World War I (WWI) suggest overall vascular trauma rates of 0.4% to 1.3%.[4] DeBakey characterized the vascular injury burden in World War II (WWII) and the Korean and Vietnam wars at 0.96% and 2% to 3%, respectively.[4–6]

Coalition militaries engaged in recent combat operations in Afghanistan and Iraq have reported rates of vascular trauma higher than the previously mentioned military campaigns.[2,7–9] In a study reporting the US military experience, White and colleagues analyzed vascular cases entered into the US Joint Theater Trauma Registry (JTTR) from 2002 to 2009 (**Fig. 26.2**).[2] Defining the denominator as battle-related injuries sufficiently severe to prevent return to duty in the combat theater, the specific incidence of vascular injury (defined as the *total incidence injury*) was found to be 12% (1570 of 13,076 cases). The incidence of injuries requiring an operation (defined as the *operative incidence*) was found to be 9% (1212 of 13,076 cases). Injuries were most common in the extremities (79%) followed by those in the torso (12%) and cervical regions (8%).

Overall, the authors concluded that the rate of vascular injury in these modern wars was five times that previously reported from Vietnam and Korea (**Figs. 26.1** and **26.2**). An update of that data from the final years of war in Afghanistan from 2009 to 2015 estimated 17.6% of injuries to involve the vasculature, with most involving the extremities (45%). That study also cited an increase in endovascular methods of vascular injury management.[10] In a contemporary study examining management and outcomes particular to 597 wartime lower extremity injuries, explosive versus firearm injuries were more likely to involve the tibial vasculature and associated with lower rates of limb salvage. Since the mortality associated with immediate limb salvage attempts was low, authors recommended delayed amputation with aggressive attempts at vascular repair and limb salvage.[11]

Civilian Population Vascular Trauma

The impact of vascular trauma in the civilian setting is less well characterized than wartime vascular injury. According to data from the National Center for Injury Prevention and

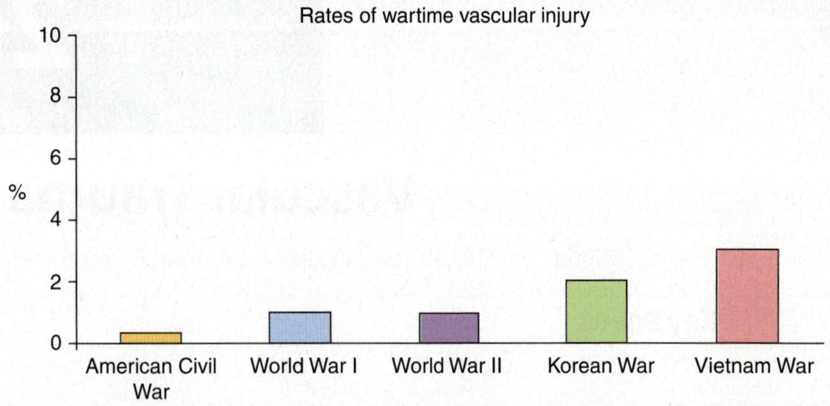

Figure 26.1. The rate of vascular injury reported from the wars of the previous two centuries. (From White JM, Stannard A, Burkhardt GE, et al. The epidemiology of vascular injury in the wars in Iraq and Afghanistan. *Ann Surg*. 2011; 253(6):1184–1189.)

Control, in 2011 in the United States, injuries accounted for 51.3% of all deaths among persons 1 to 44 years of age, which is more deaths than those caused by noncommunicable and infectious diseases combined.[12] Fatalities stemmed mainly from motor vehicle accidents (32%), gunshot wounds (22%), and falls (9%). Vascular injuries represented 1% to 2% of total trauma patients but accounted for more than 20% of all trauma-related deaths and had the highest utilization of resources among the trauma population.[3]

In 2010, Barmparas and colleagues characterized vascular injury in 22,089 patients drawn from a population of more than 1.8 million in the National Trauma Data Bank (NTDB).[13] Acknowledging the reporting bias that accompanies analysis of such retrospective data, it was determined that the incidence of vascular injury (2002 to 2006) was 1.6%. Four-fifths of the injured were male, and the average age was 34 years. Half of the patients (51%) sustained a penetrating mechanism. Just under a quarter of patients presented in hemorrhagic shock and over half had an Injury Severity Score of more than 15. Abdominal and chest injuries accounted for more than 25% and 24% of the injury burden, respectively, with arm and leg injuries contributing 26% and 18%, respectively. Mortality among those with vascular trauma was 23%, and vessels associated with the highest rates of amputation were the axillary (upper limb amputation rate of 6%) and popliteal arteries (lower limb amputation rate of 15%).[13]

In other reports of vascular trauma from civilian centers in New York and El Paso, the rates of injury, in the context of all presenting to each trauma center, were 2.3% and 3.4%, respectively.[14,15] These reports confirm the "at-risk demographic" to be young and male, and demonstrate that mortality in those with vascular trauma is twice that of patients without this injury pattern. Not surprisingly, penetrating mechanisms are overrepresented in patients with vascular injury. A single-center study of vascular trauma from Houston in 1988 demonstrated that the wounding pattern in civilian circumstances does not follow that seen in wartime, even where ballistic penetrating injury is common.[3] Torso and neck injuries accounted for two-thirds of all injuries, while lower extremity injuries (including the groin) comprised only 20%.

Mechanism of Vascular Trauma

2 Vascular injuries are broadly categorized by mechanism as either blunt or penetrating. Either mechanism can disrupt the normal integrity of the blood vessel wall (intima, media, and adventitia) with varying degrees of integrity. Blunt vascular trauma is produced by local tissue compression or acceleration–deceleration resulting in disruptive shear forces. Motor vehicle crashes are the main cause of blunt vascular trauma in the civilian setting, and these patients usually have injuries to other areas of the body including extremity fractures or dislocation, brain injury, and injury to structures in the abdomen or thorax including aortic disruption. Blunt mechanism is also recognized as a source of vascular disruption with specific extremity fractures or dislocation patterns (e.g., posterior knee dislocation, tibial plateau fracture, and supracondylar fracture of humerus) (**Fig. 26.3**).

Penetrating mechanisms typically result in direct injury of the vessel causing either laceration or contusion of the wall as well as separation or destruction of soft tissues surrounding the vessel. Penetrating vascular injury may result from simple, low-velocity sharp objects (i.e., knife or glass), irregular fragments from explosives, and uniform munitions fired from a weapon. For ballistic injuries, damage to the vessel and surrounding soft tissues often results from a concussive shockwave that is conducted through the tissues as the object moves through the body dissipating energy. Unlike blunt injuries, which more commonly affect torso vascular structures, penetrating injuries more commonly affect the extremity vasculature.

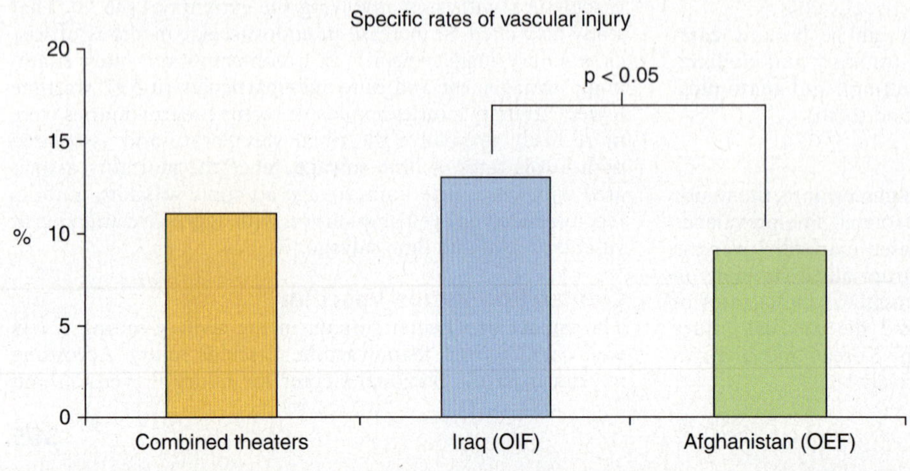

Figure 26.2. The rate of vascular injury reported during the wars in Afghanistan and Iraq.This specific rate refers to the 1,570 US service personnel identified within the Department of Defence Joint Theater Trauma Registry (JTTR) as having sustained vascular injury during the wars (between 2002 and 2009). Note that the overall rate of 12% is severalfold higher than the rate of vascular injury reported in previous wars. (From White JM, Stannard A, Burkhardt GE, et al. The epidemiology of vascular injury in the wars in Iraq and Afghanistan. *Ann Surg*. 2011;253(6):1184–1189.)

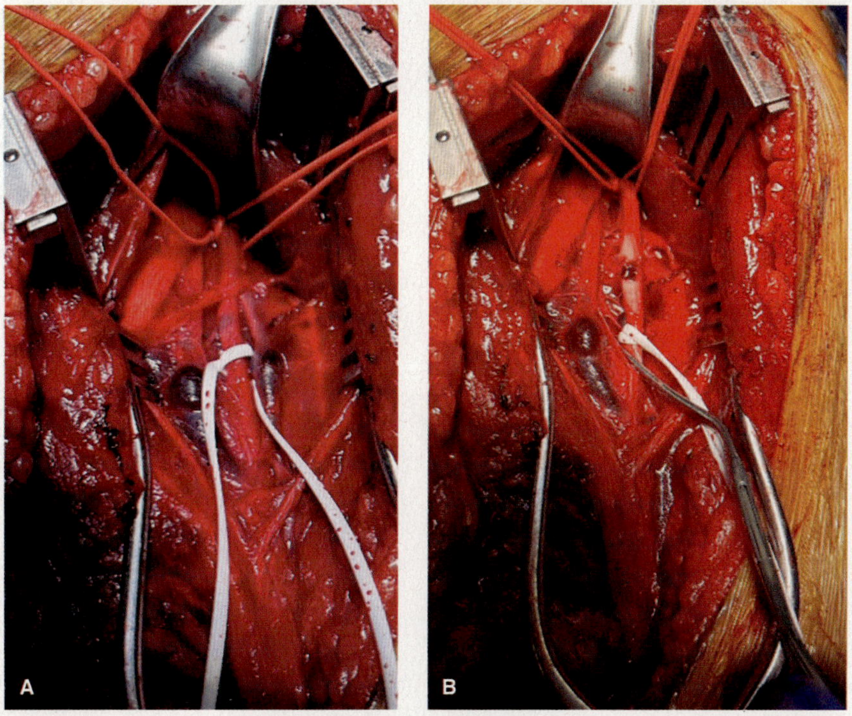

Figure 26.3. (**A**) Posterior approach to the popliteal artery in the setting of a knee dislocation with distal malperfusion. Exploration demonstrated a focal, blunt injury to the popliteal artery. (**B**) Upon arteriotomy, focal intimal disruption vas visualized. The injury was repaired with a short segment interposition saphenous vein graft.

DIAGNOSIS OF VASCULAR INJURY

Physical Examination

3 Patient examination is the most important step in evaluation of a suspected vascular injury. The physical examination should include complete exposure of the patient, identification of all wounds, and palpation of all extremities to assess for fracture or dislocation. The extremity vascular examination should also include assessment of distal perfusion by examination of the general appearance of the extremity and identification of pulses. Similarly, the neck and cervical region should be examined for signs of penetrating wounds, the presence of carotid pulses, and bruising or hematoma.[16,17]

4 Vascular trauma physical examination findings can be divided into hard versus soft signs of injury. Hard signs of vascular injury suggest near or complete disruption of the vessel in question and include pulsatile bleeding, expanding hematoma, palpable thrill, audible bruit, or evidence of acute ischemia distal to the injury site. Depending on the degree of extremity ischemia, a patient may exhibit one or more of the classic six "P's" including pulselessness, pain, pallor, paresthesia, paralysis, and poikilothermia. Soft signs of vascular injury suggest partial disruption of the vessel in proximity and include trauma in proximity to a named vessel (i.e., certain fracture or dislocation patterns) (**Figs. 26.4** and **26.5**), diminished pulse distal to the site of injury, nonexpanding hematoma or severe bruising, and a peripheral neurologic deficit. Although torso vascular injury is more difficult to diagnose with physical examination alone, it should be suspected in

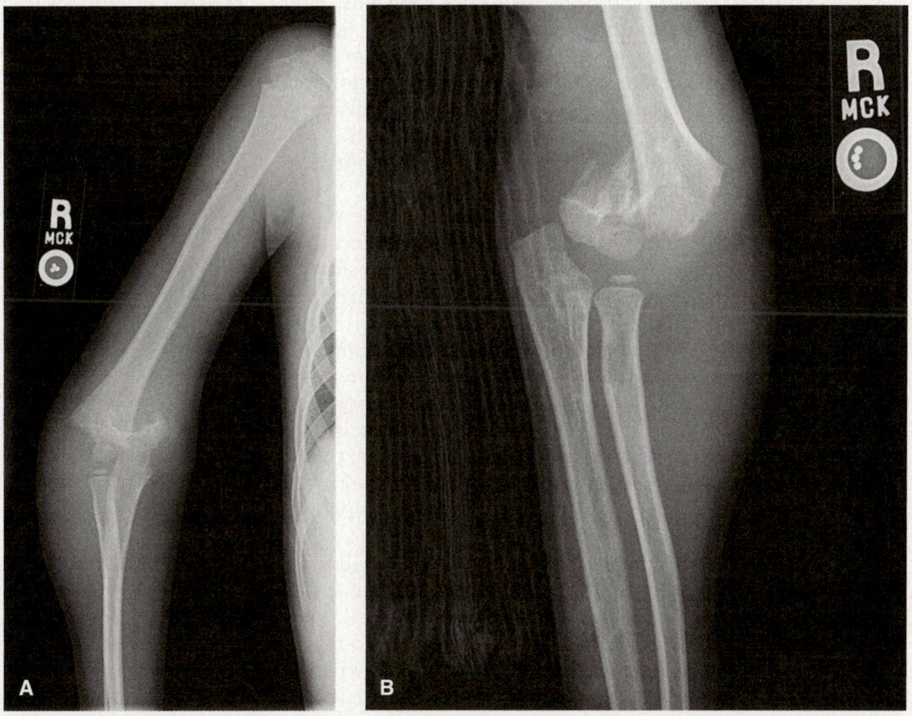

Figure 26.4. **A, B:** Radiographic images of a Gartland type III fracture of the right supracondylar humerus which is commonly associated with brachial artery injury.

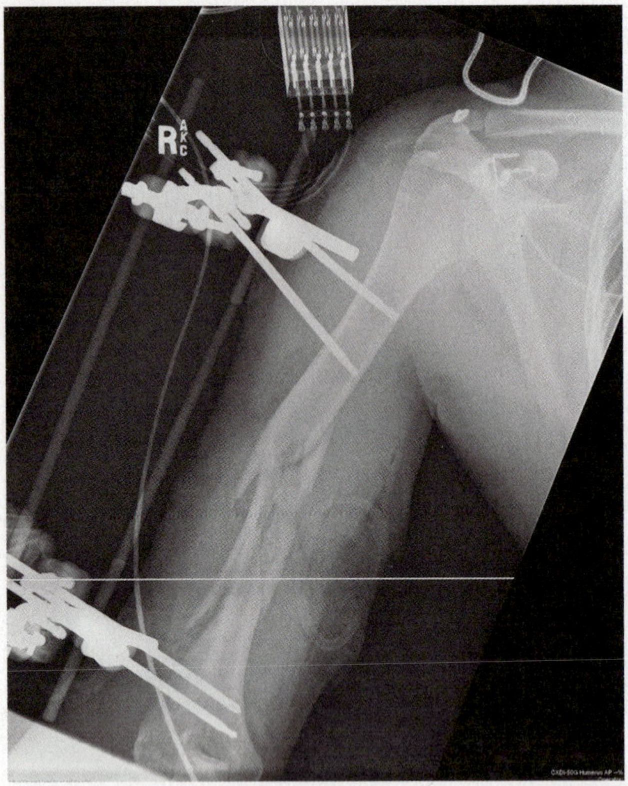

Figure 26.5. Radiograph of right upper extremity demonstrating an open humerus fracture.The brachial artery was found to be severed by the fracture.

patients with asymmetric arm pulses or pressures and those presenting in shock with evidence of fluid in the peritoneum or thoracic cavity.

Adjuncts to the Physical Examination

A plain chest radiograph is frequently performed during the initial evaluation of the trauma bay and is a useful adjunct in the diagnosis of blunt aortic injury. Classic signs of this injury pattern include a widened mediastinum (greater than 8 to 10 cm), an apical cap, loss of the characteristic aortic nob, downward displacement of the left mainstem bronchus, and hemothorax. Although multiple rib fractures are not a sign of aortic injury itself, it is a marker of severe blunt injury with significant shear and should raise one's index of suspicion for injury to the thoracic aorta. In addition, a persistent discrepancy of blood pressure cuff measurements from both arms greater than 20 mm Hg suggests a proximal vascular injury to the subclavian or axillary arteries.

Continuous-wave Doppler is another adjunct to the physical examination of patients in whom there is a concern for vascular injury. Doppler signals in the distal extremity should be recorded as present or absent and, if present, graded as strong and bi- or triphasic or weak and monophasic.[17,18] In the lower extremity, signals should be assessed in the dorsalis pedis and posterior tibial arteries, while in the upper extremity, signals should be examined over the radial, ulnar, and brachial arteries. While describing the quality of Doppler signals can be somewhat subjective, identifying the presence of extremity perfusion by noting the presence of an arterial signal is an important step that is typically less subjective than palpation for a pulse with one's finger.

The addition of a manual blood pressure cuff to continuous-wave Doppler allows one to calculate an ankle branchial index (ABI) or injured extremity index (IEI). The normal ABI or IEI is 0.9 or greater, although caution should be used in interpreting the ratio in patients who are hypotensive, in severe pain, or hypothermic.[17–19] Peripheral vasoconstriction is a normal response to significant trauma and shock and may result in a transiently decreased ABI or IEI in the absence of an injured axial vessel. In this context, assessment of the Doppler occlusion pressures and measurement of ratios should be viewed as dynamic and repeated after resuscitation, administration of pain control, and rewarming.

Ultrasound is another noninvasive modality that can be used in the evaluation of patients with vascular trauma. Brightness or B-mode ultrasound is ubiquitous in most emergency departments and critical care settings and allows one to make basic assessments that provide insight into the presence and severity of some patterns of vascular injury.[16,17] The focused assessment with sonography for trauma (FAST) examination of the abdomen is based on B-mode ultrasound and is commonly used to determine the presence or absence of fluid in the peritoneum following severe injury. Although not specific for vascular injury, fluid seen on a positive FAST examination in a hypotensive trauma patient should be assumed to be blood. In these cases, the source of bleeding may be a solid organ injury (liver, kidney, or spleen) or a larger named vessel.

Computed Tomography for Vascular Trauma

5 Contrast-enhanced computed tomography angiography (CTA) is the most widely used diagnostic imaging modality to identify and localize arterial and venous injuries in patients with suspected vascular injury in the emergency setting.[20] CTA has a high degree of sensitivity in identifying dissection, occlusion, and active extravasation of blood into a contained space (i.e., pseudoaneurysm) or into an open space or cavity (**Fig. 26.6**). CTA is particularly useful in the assessment of anatomic regions where physical examination of the vasculature is limited. Growing experience with CTA in the assessment of the peripheral vasculature and several clinical reports now demonstrate this modality's sensitivity and specificity in the diagnosis of extremity vascular injury.[21] Extremity CTA is particularly appealing for the polytrauma patient who has soft signs of vascular injury as it can be performed with imaging of other body regions (i.e., head, neck, abdomen, and pelvis).[21]

Contrast Angiography

CTA has largely replaced the need for diagnostic contrast angiography in the trauma setting. Exception to this statement is the unstable patient who does not undergo imaging prior to operative exploration. In this circumstance, on-table angiogram can be performed in the operating room while other injuries are addressed with ongoing resuscitation.[22] Angiogram can demonstrate active extravasation of contrast if bleeding from an injured vessel is brisk and ongoing. Extravasation may not however be visualized if the bleeding is slow or under tamponade. Bleeding may also be missed if a contrast bolus is too small, mistimed, or injected into a different vessel not in direct continuity with the injury. Angiographic interruption of vessel continuity usually indicates disruption or thrombosis. With sufficient contrast and time delay, distal reconstitution of flow beyond the injured segment from collateral vessels can typically be demonstrated. Imaging of distal arterial beds can be compromised by hypoperfusion and vasoconstriction, typical manifestations of shock. Vasospasm with tapering of arteries (sometimes to occlusion) and slow flow can be prominent in young patients who have a greater degree of vasomotor reactivity.[20–22] Endovascular therapies such as embolization and placement of covered stents or stent grafts can be placed immediately following injury diagnosis when appropriate.

MANAGEMENT OF THE PATIENT WITH VASCULAR TRAUMA

Trauma Patient Pathophysiology

6 In the trauma patient, hemorrhage leads to both the overall metabolic consequences of shock and end-organ ischemia of

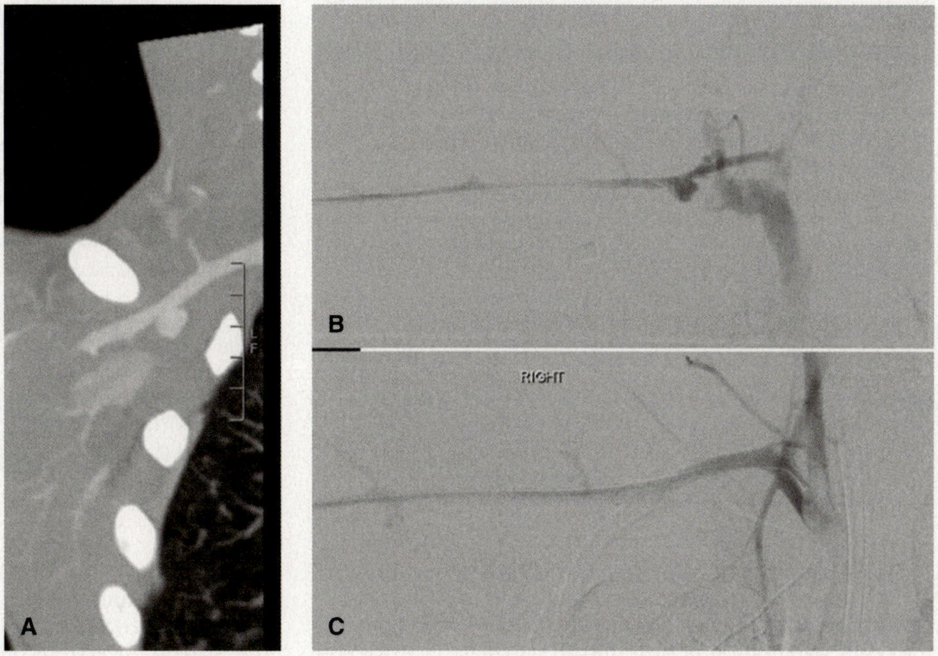

Figure 26.6. A: CT angiogram demonstrating a traumatic right proximal axillary artery injury as a result of ballistic injury. B: Angiogram demonstrating a small pseudoaneurysm and large arteriovenous (AV) connection with immediate filling of the right axillary vein. C: A 7 × 50 mm covered stent was placed across the injury with resolution of both the pseudoaneurysm and AV fistula.

the specific injured vessel. Ischemia of both types results in anoxic cell death. Resuscitation is directed toward minimizing ischemia and the "lethal triad" of acidosis, hypothermia, and coagulopathy. Hypoperfusion or ischemia leads to acidosis which causes platelet morphology changes and dysfunction and declining coagulation factor activity leading to decreased thrombin generation and the degradation of fibrinogen. Hypothermia likewise causes platelet dysfunction, less coagulation factor activity, and the induction of fibrinolysis. Both of these pathways lead to coagulopathy and endothelial damage. Unbalanced massive blood transfusions can also lead to tissue injury, hypoperfused vascular beds, hemodilution, and depletion or dilution of clotting factors and platelets, all of which can contribute to a coagulopathic state.

Reperfusion injury following revascularization can precipitate additional metabolic insults in the trauma patient. Reperfusion of ischemic tissues releases reactive oxygen species and activates multiple proinflammatory processes including lipid peroxidation. This activation causes injury to the microvasculature which increases cell permeability and edema. An increase in interstitial pressure in turn leads to more stasis in microvasculature and therefore worsened ischemia. Ensuing cell lysis, also called rhabdomyolysis, leads to hyperkalemia, metabolic acidosis, and eventually myoglobin-induced renal failure.

Resuscitation of the Trauma Patient

Recent literature has shifted from the tradition airway, breathing, circulation (ABC) approach in trauma resuscitation to a perfusion first strategy.[23] CAB approaches have demonstrated improved outcomes, much of which is thought to stem from the avoidance of postintubation hypotension and decreased venous return associated with positive pressure ventilation. As such, recent trauma protocols at high volume centers have prioritized hemorrhage control over airway management with guidelines focused on delayed intubation in eligible patients.[24,25] Similarly, the Stop the Bleed campaign has empowered first responders with the tools to effectively halt bleeding in the field. This approach has created a critical frontline defense in hemorrhage control.[23]

Resuscitation of the trauma patient should begin immediately following initial assessment of injuries. Venous access with large-bore catheters in peripheral veins of uninjured extremities is preferred over central access in the emergent setting. Venous cutdowns are sometimes necessary. Radial or femoral arterial lines are also often placed for hemodynamic monitoring.[26] Damage control resuscitation, a term coined in 2005, involves permissive hypotension with a goal of a palpable radial pulse in patients without head injury.[27] Massive transfusion of packed red blood cells, plasma, and platelets should be conducted in a 1:1:1 ratio.[28–30]

General Intraoperative Considerations and Pearls

7 The principles of "damage control" guide the surgical management of vascular trauma. Basic tenants include hemorrhage control, restoration of blood flow, and prevention of further reperfusion injury.

1. Prep widely, considering all possible sites of injury given the mechanism of disability. In particular, consider the need for autogenous venous conduit, namely saphenous vein. With chest or abdominal injuries, prep down to bilateral knees. With leg injuries, prep circumferentially and include the chest and abdomen. With neck or upper extremity wounds, include the shoulders and chest.
2. Patients should receive preoperative antibiotics based on local guidelines.
3. Longitudinal incisions parallel to neurovascular bundles should be used for the wide exposure and best control. This may necessitate and "S"-shaped incision over joint spaces.
4. Proximal and distal control for any vascular injury is critical. This may be obtained with a digit, vessel loop, vascular clamps, or a Foley or Fogarty balloon. Consider remote proximal control when hematomas or open blast wounds impede visualization. Shunts should also be considered to decrease ischemic time when orthopedic stabilization or other lifesaving procedures must occur first. Nonbleeding wounds should not be disturbed including removal of debris or foreign objects until surgical control is obtained.
5. Temporary application of a lower extremity tourniquet may be helpful with complex wounds prior to obtaining surgical proximal control. An inappropriately applied tourniquet inflated to venous pressure can however increase exsanguinating hemorrhage. As systemic blood

Table 26.1. Exposures in Vascular Trauma Surgery

Vessel Injured	Exposure/Maneuver
Right subclavian artery Ascending aorta Innominate artery	Median sternotomy
Left subclavian artery Descending thoracic aorta	Left thoracotomy
Paravisceral, infrarenal aorta Left renal artery Left iliac artery	Left colon mobilization
Inferior vena cava Right renal artery Right iliac artery	Right colon mobilization, extended Kocher maneuver (duodenal mobilization)

Table 26.2. Options for Treatment of Vascular Injuries

Type of Repair	Description of Injury
Primary repair	<25% vessel compromise
Patch angioplasty	<50% vessel compromise
End-to-end anastomosis	<2 cm defect, ends mobilized, spatulated (smaller vessels)
Interposition graft	>2 cm defect, reversed vein graft, or synthetic conduit
Extra-anatomic bypass	Extensive defect, multiple level injury, contamination

pressure increases with resuscitation, tourniquet pressure may need to be increased to remain effective.

6. Injury may require orthopedic fracture reduction and limb stabilization prior to formal vascular, nerve, or soft tissue repair. Relining of the bony structures will often improve vessel spasm, and vascular examination should be repeated following any orthopedic intervention.
7. Use of systemic heparin is individualized and contingent upon multiple factors including preoperative blood loss, hemodynamic stability, the presence of brain injury, and the overall physiologic status of the patient with regard to acidosis, hypothermia, and coagulopathy. Local administration of heparin and papaverine can be used in the wound and flushed directly into the vessel during repair. In general, systemic heparin can be obviated in young patients with healthy vessels and adequate revascularization.
8. Choice of surgical incision is dictated by the injury pattern and anatomic exposure needed for proximal control and subsequent revascularization (**Table 26.1**). Aggressive debridement of devitalized tissue may be necessary for adequate visualization and postoperative healing.
9. Inflow and outflow must be assessed before beginning an anastomosis. Thrombectomy of both the inflow and outflow vessels with a Fogarty embolectomy catheter may be required.
10. Decision to perform immediate vascular reconstruction versus shunt placement with delayed reconstruction should consider the overall physiologic status of the patient. Arterial reconstruction should be prioritized over venous reconstruction in most cases.
11. Decision for direct repair with and without patching, primary anastomosis, or interposition grafting should consider factors outlined in **Table 26.2**.
12. Appropriate conduit is obtained, if applicable. Reversed greater saphenous vein of the uninvolved leg is the ideal conduit although synthetic grafts can be used if needed.
13. Repair is performed with nonabsorbable, monofilament running suture.
14. Adjuvant hemostatic agents can be parenteral (tranexamic acid for hyperfibrinolysis) or topical (**Table 26.3**).
15. Following completion of repair, perfusion should be assessed in the operating room with Doppler and arteriogram when indicated.
16. Soft tissue coverage over vascular repairs is necessary to prevent contamination, vessel desiccation, and anastomotic disruption. If large tissue defects are present, vacuum-assisted dressings are useful for tissue approximation and temporary closure.
17. Reperfusion injury and compartment syndrome must be considered and fasciotomies performed as clinically indicated.

Table 26.3. Topical Hemostatic Agents

	Indications	Agent Potency/Mechanism	Uses	Examples
Level I (mechanical hemostat)	Min or mild bleeding, localized	Contact activation ± platelet aggregation	Capillary, arteriolar ooze	Gelfoam, porcine gelatin, bovine collagen, surgical, nu-knit, Arista
Level II (Thrombin)	Min or mild bleeding diffuse	Converts fibrinogen to fibrin-activated platelet aggregation Contact activation + fibrinogen converted to fibrin	Capillary, ooze Capillary, arteriolar ooze, spurting	Bovine thrombin, recombinant thrombin Collagen or gelatin + thrombin; Floseal, Surgiflo
Level III (fibrin sealant, combination hemostat)	Mild bleeding diffuse; moderate bleeding	Fibrin sealant, replicates final stage of clotting cascade Synthetic sealant, covalently and mechanically bond Other	Capillary, arteriolar ooze High-pressure sealing	Thrombin + fibrinogen ± fibrinolysis inhibitor; Tisseel, EvicelPEG polymer; CoSealBioGlue

Adapted from Shander A, Kaplan LJ, Harris MT, et al. Topical hemostatic therapy in surgery: Bridging the knowledge and practice gap. *J Am Coll Surg*. 2014;219(3): 570–579.e4.

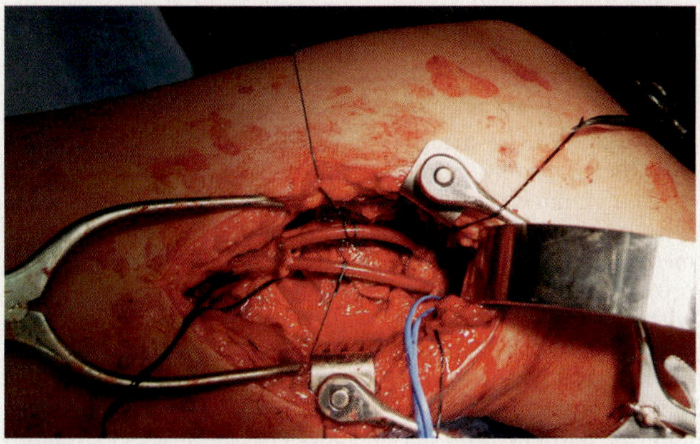

Figure 26.7. Operative photograph showing temporary vascular shunt placement as a damage control maneuver in the proximal popliteal artery and vein of the left lower extremity. The shunts were secured with silk suture ties, and both were patent with Doppler flow several hours following the injury.

MANAGEMENT OF SPECIFIC INJURY PATTERNS—EXTREMITY

Extremity trauma requiring operative intervention is often readily identifiable from physical examination alone. Exceptions to this statement include more proximal vessel injury entering the chest or pelvis including the subclavian and femoral arteries. For all extremity trauma, the goals of management include hemorrhage control, revascularization of an ischemic extremity, and limb stabilization to minimize future disability.[31] Injuries with hard signs of vascular injury should be taken immediately to the operating room for open or endovascular exploration without further imaging workup. Decision to perform immediate reconstruction versus temporary shunt placement should be dictated by the overall physiologic status of the patient (**Figs. 26.7** and **26.8**). "Soft signs" of vascular injury suggest less devastating injury allowing time for further workup, imaging, and potential nonoperative management.[32,33]

The classic teaching in time to revascularization in the ischemic limb is 6 hours. Recent translational literature has suggested that critical ischemic injury begins immediately, and early restoration of perfusion (within 3 hours) significantly reduces ischemic injury.[34–36] Further data from porcine models suggest a dose response of increasing ischemic times on loss of functional recovery. These animal model findings are supported by the literature which demonstrates that limb salvage following lower extremity arterial injuries decline rapidly after just 3 hours.[11] The physiologic consequences of hemorrhagic shock further exacerbate ischemia by compromising collateral circulation, increasing perfusion compromise of the injured extremity. A recent review of military injuries from 2003 to 2013 of 129 limbs demonstrated a 10% reduction in the probability of limb salvage for every delay to revascularization. As such, many groups advocate the use of early shunting to decrease ischemic times.[37] Polcz et al. showed a threefold reduction in amputation rates with early shunting in civilians compared to matched controls without shunt use.[38]

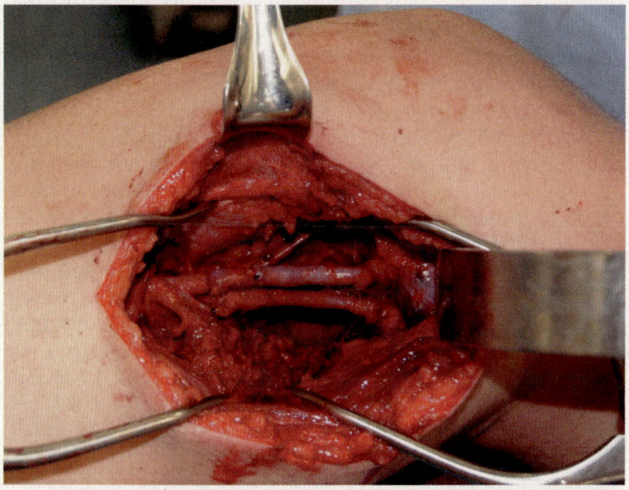

Figure 26.8. Operative photograph showing an interposition vein graft repair of the left proximal popliteal artery and vein. The interposition greater saphenous vein grafts were harvested from the right (contralateral) leg and performed following removal of the temporary vascular shunts.

An additional critical issue in all extremity trauma management is evaluation for compartment syndrome. Elevated fascial compartment pressures can be due to reperfusion, hematoma, swelling from crush injury, or major fractures. Compartment syndrome should be suspected in cases of delayed revascularization, crush injuries, combined arterial and venous injuries, vessel ligation, and tense muscle compartments on examination. The classic physical examination finding in the awake patient concerning for compartment syndrome is calf pain with passive motion and paresthesia in the 2nd dorsal web space. Compartment pressures can be measured as an adjunctive aid in diagnosis with pressures greater than 30 mm Hg considered abnormal, however, normal pressures in a patient in whom compartment syndrome is clinically suspected should not discourage compartment release. Low threshold for fasciotomy should be adopted as risk of limb loss is high if a compartment syndrome goes undiagnosed or if the treatment is delayed.

Postoperatively, patient should be started on low-dose aspirin once hemodynamics permit. Deep vein thrombosis (DVT) prophylaxis is also an essential component of treatment in the polytrauma patient to prevent thromboembolic complications. Elevation of the injured extremity will reduce swelling. Twenty-four hours of antibiotics is adequate following isolated vascular repairs.

Upper Extremity

The axillary artery is defined proximally by the lateral margin of the first rib and distally by the lateral edge of the teres major muscle. The artery is protected proximally within the shoulder from penetrating injury but susceptible to forceful blunt trauma due to its fixation. Proximal exposure may require infra- and supraclavicular incisions to gain control with potential sternotomy if more proximal intrathoracic control of the subclavian artery is needed. In centers with endovascular capabilities, proximal balloon occlusion should be considered as this may be more expeditious. The mid- and distal axillary artery can be approached through a traditional infraclavicular incision. Complications with more distal exposure are due to increasing branches and associated nerve supply in the shoulder and arm. An endovascular approach to repair with stent grafts may be particularly advantageous in subclavian and axillary injuries.[39,40] It is also worth noting that upper extremities tolerate more prolonged ischemia time than lower extremities due to the dense arterial collateral network originating off the subclavian and axillary arteries.

The axillary artery becomes the brachial artery after passing the lower margin of the teres major. The brachial artery runs in the anterior compartment of the arm with the median nerve. The basilic and brachial veins accompany and often crossover the artery in the upper arm. The brachial artery is most often injured during penetrating trauma, but injury should be considered with any humeral fracture, especially posterior or lateral fractures. The brachial artery's main proximal branch, the profunda brachii, can provide significant perfusion to the distal upper extremity if it remains intact.

The radial artery is a terminal branch of the brachial just distal to the elbow and travels in the anterior compartment to become the deep palmar arch. The ulnar artery is the larger terminal branch of the brachial artery and runs to the wrist to form the superficial palmar arch and joins the deep arch. If temporary control of bleeding is needed, a blood pressure cuff can be used as a tourniquet. Evaluation should include a neurovascular examination with addition of the Allen test to determine patency of the palmar arch. Single-vessel injury with no ischemic changes can be ligated if the palmar arch is intact. If both forearm arteries are injured, repair of the usually dominant ulnar is preferred with either mobilization and primary end-to-end repair or interposition vein graft.

Lower Extremity

Femoral artery trauma constitutes 20% of all traumatic arterial injuries. Supracondylar femur and tibial plateau fractures are associated with distal superficial femoral artery and popliteal artery injuries. In the case of exsanguinating hemorrhage, an assistant's digit may be prepped into the field until more formal proximal control can be obtained. Options include tourniquet, temporary balloon catheter, or exposure of the distal external iliac artery in the preperitoneal space with compression against the iliac fossa for femoral triangle injuries. Incision should be longitudinal just below the inguinal ligament. Primary repair or interposition grafting is the mainstay of therapy as acute ligation of the femoral artery leads to 50% amputation rate.[40] Although vein conduit is always preferred, prosthetic graft can be used when necessary in larger vessels with good muscle coverage.[41] Prosthetic grafts have also been described as a bridge to definitive therapy in the setting of severely injured patients in wartime injuries.[42]

Popliteal trauma is classically due to posterior knee dislocation. Historically, amputation rates were 20% for both penetrating and blunt popliteal injuries.[43] Failure to repair a popliteal occlusion results in amputation rates as high as 60%. Incision should be medial, employing the use of a bump under a slightly flexed leg (**Figs. 26.7** and **26.8**). Repair can be performed primarily following debridement to healthy tissue or with an interposition graft. Primary repair should be attempted only with defects less than 1 cm which can be repaired without tension. In select cases of isolated popliteal injuries, a posterior approach may provide direct exposure leading to more expeditious revascularization with shorter interposition grafts.

A single terminal vessel including the anterior and posterior tibial artery and peroneal artery can be ligated in the lower extremity in a patient with no signs of ischemia and no preexisting peripheral vascular disease. When all three arteries are damaged, repair of the anterior or posterior tibial artery via lateral and medial calf incisions, respectively, should be performed. Injury to all three tibial vessels typically equates to high rates of limb loss.

MANAGEMENT OF SPECIFIC INJURY PATTERNS—CERVICAL

The location of penetrating trauma in the neck is classically divided into three zones to identify which structures are at risk for injury. Zone I is from the thoracic inlet to the cricoid cartilage, zone II is between the cricoid cartilage and the angle of the mandible, and zone III is above the angle of the mandible to the base of the skull. The carotid and vertebral arteries are at risk in all three zones.[44] In addition to the carotid artery, injury to the jugular veins and branches, nerves (vagus, hypoglossal), trachea, and esophagus must also be considered with wounding in the neck. Hard signs of vascular injury include expanding hematoma, bruit, and hemiparesis.

Zone II of the neck is the most injured region in penetrating neck injuries with vascular injuries in up to 20% of cases. Prior to widespread CTA use, zone II neck injuries mandated operative exploration if the injury violated the platysma. This mantra led to a high negative exploration rate which has now been negated by CT imaging. Currently, CTA of the neck through the aortic arch is utilized in stable patients to rule out injury. Multiple studies have demonstrated a 90% sensitivity and near 100% specificity rate for vascular injuries requiring treatment.[45–47] Of note, significant ballistic fragments in the neck may obscure arterial segments. In these cases, conventional angiography should be considered.

Zone I injuries with hard signs of vascular injury should raise suspicion for injury to the great vessels and may require median sternotomy or a high anterolateral thoracotomy for proximal control. Endovascular attempts at proximal control with balloon occlusion can be attempted, however, should not delay definitive operative control.

Injuries in zone II of the neck with hard signs of injury mandate neck exploration via a cervical incision along the anterior border of the sternocleidomastoid muscle. Occasionally a collar incision may be utilized if both sides of the neck require exploration. Exposure with proximal and distal control of the carotid artery should be performed expeditiously. The internal carotid artery should always be repaired as there is a high reported mortality with ligation (up to 45%).[48] Stab wounds can often be repaired primarily or with a patch as dictated by the degree of vessel disruption, while ballistic injuries typically require segmental resection with an interposition graft. Greater saphenous vein should be used as conduit whenever possible. Heparinization with or without shunting is employed during these repairs unless major contraindications exist in the multi-injured trauma patient. The external carotid artery can be ligated without significant consequence. The internal jugular vein can be ligated in an emergent setting but if possible, should be repaired, especially if injury is bilateral.

Zone III injuries are more difficult to expose using an open approach and can require subluxation of the mandible or mandibulotomy. Endovascular or hybrid strategies can be lifesaving in high injuries inaccessible to open repair.[49]

Vertebral artery injuries are less common and more difficult to expose operatively compared to carotid artery injuries. Vertebral artery injuries are most often associated with cervical spine transverse process fractures, subluxations, or penetrating injuries to the back of the neck. Open exposure is similar to that for the common carotid artery, however, more lateral. After the sternocleidomastoid and anterior scalene muscles are mobilized, the vertebral artery can be isolated and ligated. In this procedure, care must be taken to avoid injury to the phrenic nerve and thoracic duct. Proximal and distal control of a more distal vertebral artery injury may require endovascular techniques as with a zone III carotid injury. In a recent review of the contemporary management of combat-related vertebral artery injuries, injuries included occlusion, pseudoaneurysms, dissection, and arteriovenous fistula. Injury was most commonly in the V2 segment, and treatment included coils and covered stents.[50]

Blunt cerebrovascular injury (BCVI) includes both carotid and vertebral injuries. While BCVI represents less than 1% of admissions for blunt trauma, these injuries can lead to mortality rates from 23% to 28% with 48% to 58% of survivors having permanent severe neurologic deficits.[51] Given the high morbidity of unrecognized BCVI in the asymptomatic patient, many screening protocols recommend screening CTA in trauma patients presenting with petrous bone fractures, diffuse axonal injury, Glasgow Coma Scale score less than 8, complex C1 to C2 cervical fractures, and Le Fort II or III facial fractures.[52] Treatment is dictated by the severity of the injury as defined by Biffl's grading score (**Table 26.4**, **Fig. 26.9**).[53] While no prospective data exist to define optimal treatment regiments, low-grade injuries should be treated with antithrombotic agents such as aspirin or heparin. Grade III injuries rarely resolve with observation and medical therapy alone, therefore surgical therapy should be considered. Patients presenting with severe deficits generally do not improve with revascularization.[52]

Table 26.4. Grading of Blunt Cerebrovascular Injury

Injury Grade	CT Characteristics
Grade 1	Intimal irregularity with <25% narrowing
Grade 2	Dissection or intramural hematoma with >25% narrowing
Grade 3	Pseudoaneurysm
Grade 4	Occlusion
Grade 5	Transection with extravasation

MANAGEMENT OF SPECIFIC INJURY PATTERNS—TORSO

Control of bleeding from vascular disruption within the torso is not readily amenable to control with direct pressure and is therefore referred to as noncompressible torso hemorrhage (NCTH). Civilian studies demonstrate that NCTH accounts for 60% to 70% of mortality following otherwise survivable injuries clearly emphasize the lethality of this injury pattern. Hemorrhage is also a significant problem in the wartime setting, accounting for up to 60% of deaths in potentially survivable injury scenario. The distinction between compressible extremity hemorrhage and NCTH is notable. There has been a demonstrable reduction in mortality from extremity injury with a better understanding of its epidemiology and the need to rapidly control hemorrhage with tourniquets and topical hemostatic agents. To date, there has been no such reduction in mortality in the setting of NCTH.[54]

The initial management of torso hemorrhage is dictated by a patient's hemodynamic stability and the site of injury. A proportion of patients with NCTH and penetrating trauma present with circulatory collapse with profound hypotensive or cardiac arrest. Management of patients presenting in such a fashion has been extensively studied, and the current civilian standard of care is a resuscitative thoracotomy (RT) which permits the following maneuvers:

- Release of cardiac tamponade
- Management of thoracic bleeding
- Control of massive air leaks
- Internal cardiac massage
- Thoracic aortic occlusion

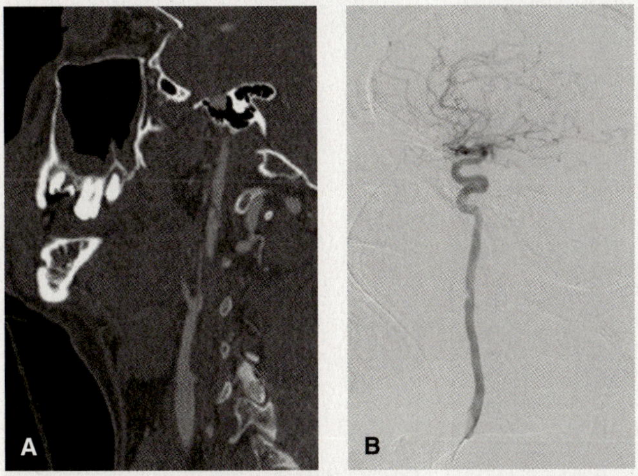

Figure 26.9. **A:** CT angiogram demonstrating a grade 3 blunt cerebrovascular injury to the left internal carotid artery with small pseudoaneurysm. **B:** Corresponding cerebral angiogram of the internal carotid artery.

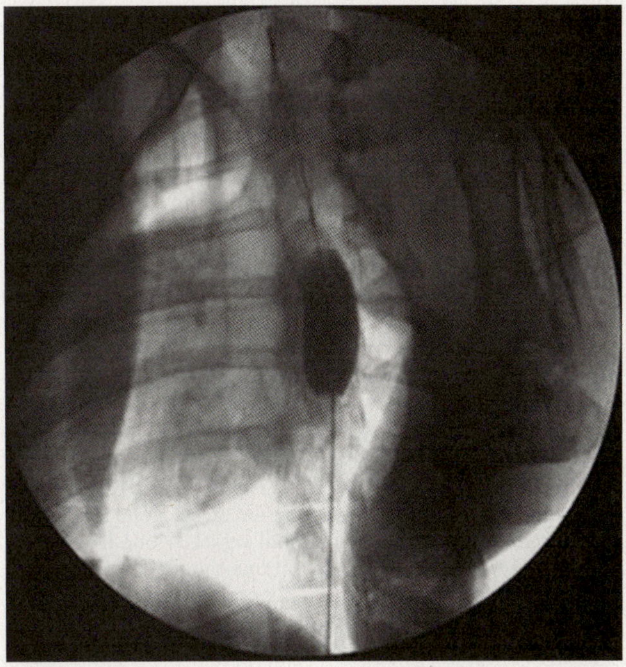

Figure 26.10. Fluoroscopic image of a compliant balloon inflated in the descending thoracic aorta (resuscitative endovascular balloon occlusion of the aorta or REBOA). This endovascular maneuver was accomplished through a percutaneous sheath in the right femoral artery and can be accomplished in certain scenarios in lieu of resuscitative thoracotomy with aortic clamping. (From Scott DJ, Eliason JL, Villamaria C, et al. A novel fluoroscopy-free, resuscitative endovascular aortic balloon occlusion system in a model of hemorrhagic shock. *J Trauma Acute Care Surg.* 2013;75(1):122–128.)

RT provides rapid access to the thoracic cavity via an anterolateral thoracotomy through the 4th interspace with the patient in the supine position. This approach allows extension of this incision across the sternum called a "clam-shell incision" permitting access to both the mediastinum and contralateral thoracic cavity if needed.

Aortic control permits time for transfusion and enhances cerebral and myocardial perfusion until definitive operative repair can occur. Published neurologically intact survival rates following RT range from 3.9% to 11.7%[55] with penetrating thoracic injury. Patients presenting pulseless with blunt injury demonstrated neurologically intact survival rates from 0.7% to 2.4%. Given the dismal outcomes with RT in the setting of blunt trauma, many centers do not perform RT in the absence of penetrating injury.

The use of resuscitative endovascular balloon occlusion of the aorta (REBOA) has been introduced and studied as an adjunct for temporary hemorrhage control with NCTH (**Fig. 26.10**).[56–58] This technique for hemorrhage control has been used in trauma as early as the Korean War.[59] While increased data have led to more widespread use of REBOA in tertiary care trauma centers across the world,[60–62] the role of REBOA in the control of exsanguinating torso hemorrhage both in the prehospital and emergency room setting remains controversial.[58]

Thoracic Cavity

Patients with vascular trauma to the aortic arch and its major branch vessels often present in shock requiring immediate surgical intervention in the form of tube thoracostomy, RT, or median sternotomy. Aortic arch injuries are associated with multiple other vascular injuries including vena cava, innominate vein, and pulmonary artery injuries. Median sternotomy provides the widest and most versatile exposure for the arch vessels with the exception of the proximal left subclavian artery. This vessel injury is best approached via a left anterior lateral thoracotomy in the 3rd rib space given its origin in the posterior mediastinal. Sternotomy followed by division of the innominate vein allows the pericardium to be opened for release of cardiac tamponade as well as evaluation and repair of a cardiac injury. Exposure of aortic branches more distally can be facilitated by extending the sternotomy incision proximally as a supraclavicular incision with division of the sternocleidomastoid muscle. The descending aorta and pulmonary hilum can be approached most rapidly via a left anterolateral thoracotomy or if patient stability permits, a left posterolateral thoracotomy.

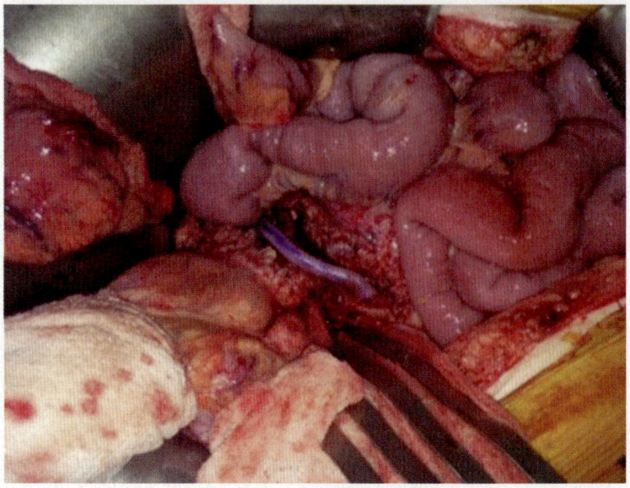

Figure 26.11. End-to-end interposition graft repair of midsuperior mesenteric artery injury with great saphenous vein.

Abdomen and Retroperitoneum

Abdominal vascular trauma is conventionally divided into the intraperitoneal and retroperitoneal area. The retroperitoneum can further be divided into four zones. Zone I is centrally located and contains the aorta and major branches as well as the inferior vena cava (IVC). This zone is further divided into the supramesocolic and inframesocolic areas. Zone II (left and right) contains the kidneys and renal vessels. Zone III includes the pelvic retroperitoneal and contains the iliac vessels. Zone IV includes the perihepatic area containing the retrohepatic IVC and hepatic vines.

The abdomen should be opened through a midline incision from the xiphoid process to the pubic symphysis to permit access to all four quadrants. Initial packing remains the best method of initial hemostasis, allowing time for resuscitation. Packs are then removed in a stepwise fashion allowing for more directed hemostasis. In penetrating trauma, all retroperitoneum hematomas should be explored with the exception of zone IV retrohepatic hematoma. In blunt trauma, only zone I hematomas should be opened unless expanding. Hematomas at the root of the mesentery in the presence of ischemic bowel should be explored to rule out injury to the superior mesenteric artery.

In zone I injuries, proximal control should be obtained of the supraceliac aorta by cross-clamping at the diaphragm. In cases where a retroperitoneal hematoma extends to the aortic hiatus, proximal control may be best approached with surgical control of the thoracic aorta or placement of a REBOA. Supramesocolic bleeding involving the origin of major aortic branch vessels should be exposed via a left medial visceral rotation (the Mattox maneuver) by mobilizing the left colon, spleen, tail of the pancreas, stomach fundus, and left kidney medially. If supramesocolic IVC bleeding is suspected, bleeding can be identified with a right visceral rotation (the Cattell–Braasch maneuver) by mobilization of the right colon, hepatic flexure, and Kocher mobilization of the duodenum and pancreatic head. Inframesocolic bleeding can be exposed with cephalad retraction of the transverse colon and displacement of the small bowel to the right of the abdomen.

Zone II injuries require partial medial visceral rotation on the affected side. Nephrectomy may be required. If there

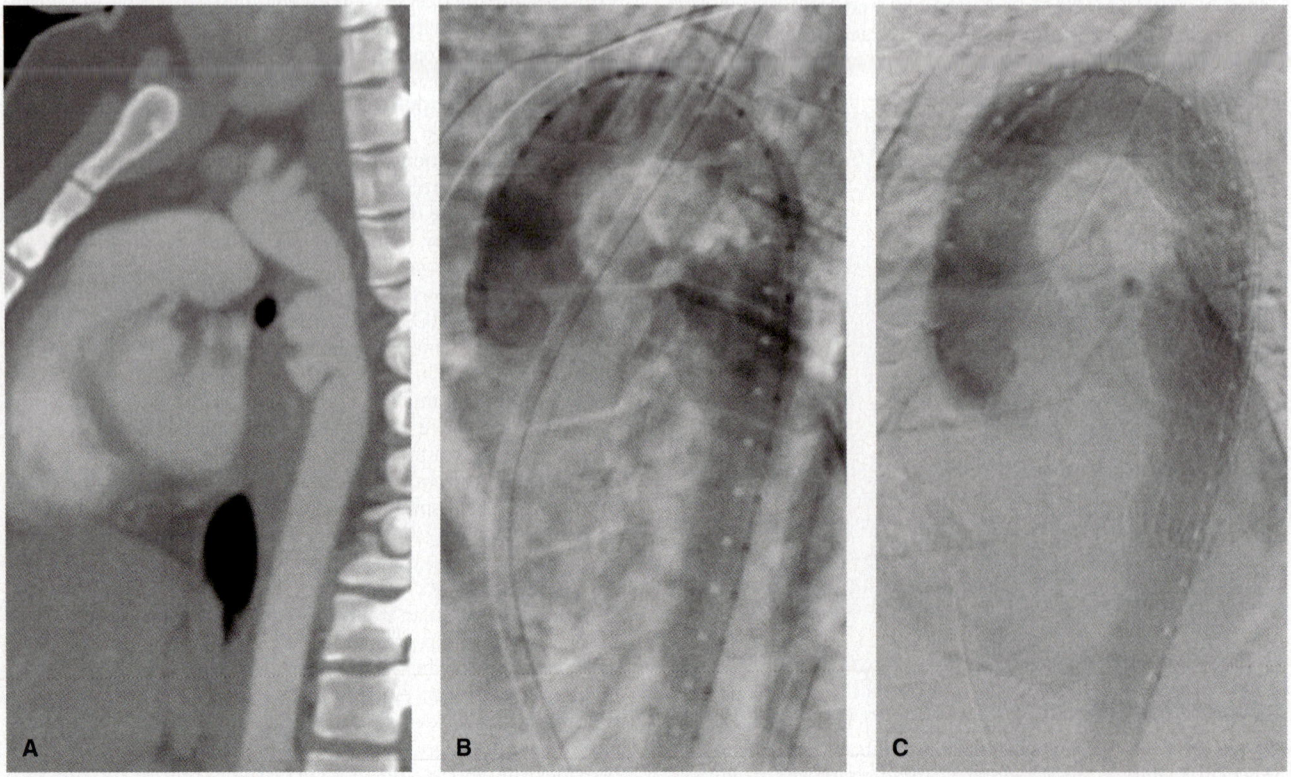

Figure 26.12. **A:** CT Angiogram depicting a grade 4 thoracic aortic injury. **B, C:** Angiograms demonstrating active extravasation with subsequent stent graft repair.

Table 26.5. Grading of Blunt Thoracic Aortic Injury

Injury Grade	CT Characteristics
Grade 1	Intimal tear
Grade 2	Intramural hematoma
Grade 3	Pseudoaneurysm
Grade 4	Free rupture

is concern for injury or violation of the collecting system, drains should be left in the perinephric retroperitoneal space. Zone III injuries should only be explored if large vessel injury is suspected. Dissection of the paracolic peritoneum and medial rotation of the right or left colon may be necessary, as well as mobilization of the terminal aorta. Operative management of zone IV is fraught with difficulty and high mortality. In the absence of exsanguinating hemorrhage, these contained venous injuries should be managed with packing alone.

In general, reconstruction of any major vessel should utilize autogenous vein (typically greater saphenous vein) especially in the presence of intestinal spillage (**Fig. 26.11**). In the setting of damage control laparotomy for patients with severe physiologic derangements, temporary shunting with later definitive repair may be appropriate. Small venous injuries should be ligated; however, large venous injuries should be repaired whenever possible. Because large veins often do not tolerate clamps in the setting of trauma and hematoma, direct pressure should be applied with sponge-sticks or smaller Kittner dissector sponges to allow for visualization.

ENDOVASCULAR MANAGEMENT OF TRAUMATIC VASCULAR INJURIES

8 While open surgical therapy remains the gold standard for treatment for traumatic injuries, endovascular management presents an alternative option particularly with injury to the arch vessels and thoracic aorta. The injury pattern in which endovascular therapy has revolutionized treatment algorithms is blunt thoracic aortic injury (BTAI). In those 20% of patients who arrive to the hospital alive following BTAI, endovascular treatment has essentially replaced open aortic repair as the gold standard of treatment due to improved outcomes (**Fig. 26.12**).[63,64] The BTAI grading system can be used to determine which patients are candidates for medical therapy alone versus repair (**Table 26.5**).[65] Studies have also demonstrated that in the absence of free rupture, delayed repair if preferred.[63]

SUMMARY

Vascular trauma remains a leading cause of mortality and morbidity following civilian and military injuries despite improvement in damage control protocols and an improved understanding of resuscitation principles. While the operative management of vascular trauma has changed with the growth of endovascular approaches to hemorrhage control, the principles of proximal and distal control remain paramount. Regardless of experience and training level, the foundational principles provided in this chapter will guide one's attempts to improve management of one of the most challenging and devastating injury patterns in trauma.

References

1. Eastridge BJ, Mabry RL, Seguin P, et al. Death on the battlefield (2001-2011): Implications for the future of combat casualty care. *J Trauma Acute Care Surg.* 2012;73(6 Suppl 5):S431–S437.
2. White JM, Stannard A, Burkhardt GE, Eastridge BJ, Blackbourne LH, Rasmussen TE. The epidemiology of vascular injury in the wars in Iraq and Afghanistan. *Ann Surg.* 2011;253(6):1184–1189.
3. Mattox KL, Feliciano DV, Burch J, Beall AC Jr, Jordan GL Jr, De Bakey ME. Five thousand seven hundred sixty cardiovascular injuries in 4459 patients. Epidemiologic evolution 1958 to 1987. *Ann Surg.* 1989;209(6):698–705; discussion 706–707.
4. Debakey ME, Simeone FA. Battle injuries of the arteries in World War II: An analysis of 2471 cases. *Ann Surg.* 1946;123(4):534–579.
5. Hughes CW. The primary repair of wounds of major arteries; an analysis of experience in Korea in 1953. *Ann Surg.* 1955;141(3): 297–303.
6. Rich NM, Baugh JH, Hughes CW. Acute arterial injuries in Vietnam: 1,000 cases. *J Trauma.* 1970;10(5):359–369.
7. Stannard A, Brown K, Benson C, Clasper J, Midwinter M, Tai NR. Outcome after vascular trauma in a deployed military trauma system. *Br J Surg.* 2011;98(2):228–234.
8. Clouse WD, Rasmussen TE, Peck MA, et al. In-theater management of vascular injury: 2 years of the Balad Vascular Registry. *J Am Coll Surg.* 2007;204(4):625–632.
9. Fox CJ, Gillespie DL, O'Donnell SD, et al. Contemporary management of wartime vascular trauma. *J Vasc Surg.* 2005;41(4): 638–644.
10. Patel JA, White JM, White PW, Rich NM, Rasmussen TE. A contemporary, 7-year analysis of vascular injury from the war in Afghanistan. *J Vasc Surg.* 2018;68(6):1872–1879.
11. Sharrock AE, Tai N, Perkins Z, et al. Management and outcome of 597 wartime penetrating lower extremity arterial injuries from an international military cohort. *J Vasc Surg.* 2019;70(1):224–232.
12. Norton R, Kobusingye O. Injuries. *N Engl J Med.* 2013;368: 1723–1730.
13. Barmparas G, Inaba K, Talving P, et al. Pediatric vs adult vascular trauma: A National Trauma Databank review. *J Pediatr Surg.* 2010;45(7):1404–1412.
14. Loh SA, Rockman CB, Chung C, et al. Existing trauma and critical care scoring systems underestimate mortality among vascular trauma patients. *J Vasc Surg.* 2011;53(2):359–366.
15. Galindo RM, Workman CR. Vascular trauma at a military level II trauma center (1). *Curr Surg.* 2000;57(6):615–618.
16. Sise MJ. Diagnosis of vascular injury. In: Rasmussen TE, Tai NRM, eds. *Vascular Trauma.* 3rd ed. Elsevier Inc; 2016:35–43.
17. Fox N, Rajani RR, Bokhari F, et al. Evaluation and management of penetrating lower extremity arterial trauma: An Eastern Association for the Surgery of Trauma practice management guideline. *J Trauma Acute Care Surg.* 2012;73(5 suppl 4):S315–S320.
18. Frykberg ER, Dennis JW, Bishop K, Laneve L, Alexander RH. The reliability of physical examination in the evaluation of penetrating extremity trauma for vascular injury: Results at one year. *J Trauma.* 1991;31(4):502–511.
19. Frykberg ER. Advances in the diagnosis and treatment of extremity vascular trauma. *Surg Clin North Am.* 1995;75(2):207–223.
20. Dawson DL. Imaging for the evaluation and treatment of vascular trauma. In: Rasmussen TE, Tai NRM, eds. *Vascular Trauma.* 3rd ed. Elsevier Inc; 2016:44–55.
21. Miller-Thomas MM, West OC, Cohen AM. Diagnosing traumatic arterial injury in the extremities with CT angiography: Pearls and pitfalls. *Radiographics.* 2005;25(suppl 1):S133–S142.
22. Holcomb JB, Fox EE, Scalea TM, et al; Catheter-Based Hemorrhage Control Study Group. Current opinion on catheter-based hemorrhage control in trauma patients. *J Trauma Acute Care Surg.* 2014;76(3):888–893.
23. Ferrada P, Ferrada R, Jacobs L, et al. Prioritizing circulation to improve outcomes for patients with exsanguinating injury: A literature review and techniques to help clinicians achieve bleeding control. *J Am Coll Surg.* 2024;238(1):129–136.
24. Ferrada P, Callcut RA, Skarupa DJ. Circulation first – the time has come to question the sequencing of care in the ABCs of trauma;

TRAUMA

an American Association for the Surgery of Trauma multicenter trial. *World J Emerg Surg*. 2018;13:8.

25. Ferrada P, García A, Duchesne J, et al. Comparing outcomes in patients with exsanguinating injuries: an Eastern Association for the Surgery of Trauma (EAST), multicenter, international trial evaluating prioritization of circulation over intubation (CAB over ABC). *World J Emerg Surg*. 2024;19(1):15.
26. Dua A, Desai SS, John B, et al., eds. *Clinical Review of Vascular Trauma*. Springer Berlin Heidelberg; 2014.
27. Dutton RP. Resuscitative strategies to maintain homeostasis during damage control surgery. *Br J Surg*. 2012;99(Suppl 1):21–28.
28. Hess JR, Holcomb JB, Hoyt DB. Damage control resuscitation: The need for specific blood products to treat the coagulopathy of trauma. *Transfusion*. 2006;46(5):685–686.
29. Holcomb JB, del Junco DJ, Fox EE, et al; PROMMTT Study Group. The prospective, observational, multicenter, major trauma transfusion (PROMMTT) study: Comparative effectiveness of a time-varying treatment with competing risks. *JAMA Surg*. 2013;148(2): 127–136.
30. Holcomb JB, Tilley BC, Baraniuk S, et al; PROPPR Study Group. Transfusion of plasma, platelets, and red blood cells in a 1:1:1 vs a 1:1:2 ratio and mortality in patients with severe trauma: The PROPPR randomized clinical trial. *JAMA*. 2015;313(5):471–482.
31. Shander A, Kaplan LJ, Harris MT, et al. Topical hemostatic therapy in surgery: Bridging the knowledge and practice gap. *J Am Coll Surg*. 2014;219(3):570–579.e4.
32. Dua A, Patel B, Desai SS, et al. Comparison of military and civilian popliteal artery trauma outcomes. *J Vasc Surg*. 2014;59(6): 1628–1632.
33. Gill H, Jenkins W, Edu S, Bekker W, Nicol AJ, Navsaria PH. Civilian penetrating axillary artery injuries. *World J Surg*. 2011; 35(5):962–966.
34. Alarhayem AQ, Cohn S, Cantu-Nunez O, Eastridge BJ, Rasmussen TE. The impact of time to repair on outcomes in patients with lower extremity arterial injuries. *J Vasc Surg*. 2019;69:1519–1523.
35. Burkhardt GE, Gifford SM, Propper B, et al. The impact of ischemic intervals on neuromuscular recovery in a porcine survival model of vascular injury. *J Vasc Surg*. 2011;53:165–173.
36. Hancock HM, Stannard A, Burkhardt GE, et al. Hemorrhagic shock worsens neuromuscular recovery in a porcine model of hind limb vascular injury and ischemia-reperfusion. *J Vasc Surg*. 2011;53:1052–1062.
37. Perkins ZB, Kersey AJ, White JM, et al. Impact of Ischemia duration on lower limb salvage in combat casualties. *Ann Surg*. 2022;276(3):532–538.
38. Polcz JE, White JM, Ronaldi AE, et al. Temporary intravascular shunt use improves early limb salvage after extremity vascular injury. *J Vasc Surg*. 2021;73(4):1304–1313.
39. Branco BC, Boutrous ML, DuBose JJ, et al. Outcome comparison between open and endovascular management of axillo-subclavian arterial injuries. *J Vasc Surg*. 2016;63(3):702–709.
40. Moore WS. *Vascular and Endovascular Surgery: A Comprehensive Review*. 7th ed. Saunders Elsevier; 2006.
41. Vertrees A, Fox CJ, Quan RW, et al. The use of prosthetic grafts in complex military vascular trauma: A limb salvage strategy for patients with severely limited autologous conduit. *J Trauma*. 2009;66(4):980–983.
42. Watson JDB, Houston R 4th, Morrison JJ, Gifford SM, Rasmussen TE. A retrospective cohort comparison of expanded polytetrafluorethylene to autologous vein for vascular reconstruction in modern combat casualty care. *Ann Vasc Surg*. 2015;29(4):822–829.
43. Wagner WH, Calkins ER, Weaver FA, Goodwin JA, Myles RA, Yellin AE. Blunt popliteal artery trauma: One hundred consecutive injuries. *J Vasc Surg*. 1988;7(5):736–743.
44. Núñez DB Jr, Torres-León M, Múnera F. Vascular injuries of the neck and thoracic inlet: Helical CT-angiographic correlation. *Radiographics*. 2004;24(4):1087–1098.
45. Múnera F, Soto JA, Nunez D. Penetrating injuries of the neck and the increasing role of CTA. *Emerg Radiol*. 2004;10(6):303–309.
46. Múnera F, Soto JA, Palacio D, Velez SM, Medina E. Diagnosis of arterial injuries caused by penetrating trauma to the neck: Comparison of helical CT angiography and conventional angiography. *Radiology*. 2000;216(2):356–362.
47. Inaba K, Múnera F, McKenney M, et al. Prospective evaluation of screening multislice helical computed tomographic angiography in the initial evaluation of penetrating neck injuries. *J Trauma*. 2006;61(1):144–149.
48. du Toit DF, van Schalkwyk GD, Wadee SA, Warren BL. Neurologic outcome after penetrating extracranial arterial trauma. *J Vasc Surg*. 2003;38(2):257–262.
49. Cohen JE, Ben-Hur T, Rajz G, Umansky F, Gomori JM. Endovascular stent-assisted angioplasty in the management of traumatic internal carotid artery dissections. *Stroke*. 2005;36(4):e45–e47.
50. Greer LT, Kuehn RB, Gillespie DL, et al. Contemporary management of combat-related vertebral artery injuries. *J Trauma Acute Care Surg*. 2013;74(3):818–824.
51. Biffl WL, Moore EE, Ryu RK, et al. The unrecognized epidemic of blunt carotid arterial injuries: Early diagnosis improves neurologic outcome. *Ann Surg*. 1998;228(4):462–470.
52. Bromberg WJ, Collier BC, Diebel LN, et al. Blunt cerebrovascular injury practice management guidelines: The Eastern Association for the Surgery of Trauma. *J Trauma*. 2010;68(2):471–477.
53. Biffl WL, Moore EE, Offner PJ, Brega KE, Franciose RJ, Burch JM. Blunt carotid arterial injuries: Implications of a new grading scale. *J Trauma*. 1999;47(5):845–853.
54. Kotwal RS, Montgomery HR, Kotwal BM, et al. Eliminating preventable death on the battlefield. *Arch Surg*. 2011;146(12): 1350–1358.
55. Seamon MJ, Haut ER, Van Arendonk KV, et al. An evidence-based approach to patient selection for emergency department thoracotomy: A practice management guideline from the Eastern Association for the Surgery of Trauma. *J Trauma Acute Care Surg*. 2015; 79(1):159–173.
56. Stannard A, Eliason JL, Rasmussen TE. Resuscitative endovascular balloon occlusion of the aorta (REBOA) as an adjunct for hemorrhagic shock. *J Trauma*. 2011;71(6):1869–1872.
57. Sadeghi M, Nilsson KF, Larzon T, et al. The use of aortic balloon occlusion in traumatic shock: First report from the ABO trauma registry. *Eur J Trauma Emerg Surg*. 2018;44(4):491–501.
58. Biffl WL, Fox CJ, Moore EE. The role of REBOA in the control of exsanguinating torso hemorrhage. *Trauma Acute Care Surg* 2015;78(5):1054–1058.
59. Hughes CW. Use of an intra-aortic balloon catheter tamponade for controlling intra-abdominal hemorrhage in man. *Surgery*. 1954;36(1):65–68.
60. Brenner ML, Moore LJ, DuBose JJ, et al. A clinical series of resuscitative endovascular balloon occlusion of the aorta for hemorrhage control and resuscitation. *J Trauma Acute Care Surg*. 2013;75(3): 506–511.
61. Moore LJ, Brenner M, Kozar RA, et al. Implementation of resuscitative endovascular balloon occlusion of the aorta as an alternative to resuscitative thoracotomy for noncompressible truncal hemorrhage. *J Trauma Acute Care Surg*. 2015;79(4):523–530.
62. DuBose JJ, Scalea TM, Brenner M, et al; AAST AORTA Study Group. The AAST prospective Aortic Occlusion for Resuscitation in Trauma and Acute Care Surgery (AORTA) registry: Data on contemporary utilization and outcomes of aortic occlusion and resuscitative balloon occlusion of the aorta (REBOA). *J Trauma Acute Care Surg*. 2016;81(3):409–419.
63. Fox N, Schwartz D, Salazar JH, et al. Evaluation and management of blunt traumatic aortic injury: A practice management guideline from the Eastern Association for the Surgery of Trauma. *J Trauma Acute Care Surg*. 2014;78(1):136–146.
64. Scalea TM, Feliciano DV, DuBose JJ, et al. Blunt thoracic aortic injury: Endovascular repair is now the standard. *J Am Coll Surg*. 2019;228(4):605–610.
65. Demetriades D. Blunt thoracic aortic injuries: Crossing the rubicon. *J Am Coll Surg*. 2012;214(3):247–259.

Orthopedic Trauma

Raymond Malcolm Smith

Key Points

1. Orthopedic trauma surgery is an essential part of the trauma team and system.
2. Establishing bony stability significantly reduces local bleeding.
3. Major pelvic fractures occur in recognizable patterns that predict other injuries.
4. Obtaining bony stability can significantly reduce pelvic bleeding and is an essential part of their initial care.
5. Early stabilization of major fractures in polytrauma patients facilitates general patient care and saves lives.
6. Early radical management of open fractures with adequate debridement by wound excision, bony stabilization, and early healthy soft tissue cover significantly reduces the risk of infection and decreases morbidity.
7. Establishing reliable bony stability is the key for local soft tissue healing.
8. The principles of accurate reduction, stable fixation, preservation of a healthy soft tissue envelope, and early rehabilitation with joint and patient mobility are the keys to general fracture management.

AIMS AND PRIORITIES IN ORTHOPEDIC TRAUMA CARE

While the management of musculoskeletal problems caused by injury has always accounted for a significant part of orthopedic practice, over recent years the subspecialty of orthopedic traumatology has progressively developed and is now a fully established subspecialty with its specialist society (the Orthopedic Trauma Association in the United States and many similar organizations around the world) and recognized fellowship training programs. Today orthopedic traumatologists are an essential member of any trauma system managing all the aspects of major skeletal reconstruction after injury and contributing to the overall management of these patients. This ranges from the management of routine fractures to the more complex problems presented by very severe localized high-energy injury and combination multisystem polytrauma. In critical multisystem injury, life-saving issues dominate and it is very important to correctly manage the orthopedic injuries which can easily be underestimated. Their management has a critical role in ensuring patient survival and ensuring practical overall clinical management. In severe local injury, life is also at risk but useful limb salvage needs orthopedic management often combined with plastic surgery to manage severe soft tissue injury. Patients with less severe fractures still have major problems, the orthopedic care should limit the medium- and long-term disability caused by fractures and severe peripheral soft tissue injuries. This overview is illustrated in **Table 27.1**.

Table 27.1. Why We Operate on Fractures: Priorities in Trauma Care

Orthopedic surgery to save a life
Orthopedic surgery to save a limb
Orthopedic surgery to limit disability

1 THE OVERALL ROLE OF THE ORTHOPEDIC TRAUMATOLOGIST IN THE TRAUMA CENTRE

Organization of trauma centers in the United States in governed by the Committee on Trauma of the American College of Surgery. Orthopedic surgeons are closely involved in this and represented on the relevant committees. The ACS requires specific standards of trauma care organized in different levels of hospitals, with Level 1 representing the highest level of care concentrated at one committed specialist site. The ACS trauma Quality Improvement Program (TQIP) details the specific requirements for each specialty, in orthopedics it defines the need for trauma fellowship trained orthopedic surgeons staffing high-level centers and being involved in their management committees.[1,2] Specific standards are defined for the management of open fractures, damage control orthopedic (DCO) surgery in polytrauma, management of the mangled extremity, compartment syndrome, pelvic fractures associated with hemorrhage, geriatric hip fractures, pediatric supracondylar humeral fracture, and rehabilitation in the multisystem trauma patient. Similar recommendations exist in other developed countries[3] and it is essential that these are understood and are continued to be developed and improved.

ORTHOPEDIC TRAUMA SURGERY TO SAVE LIFE

In patients with severe multisystem trauma, musculoskeletal injuries are commonly a major part of the trauma burden and a threat to life. This threat comes from hemorrhage (from individual or multiple injury sites), the general effect of multiple major skeletal injuries and specific injuries such as vascular injury and compartment syndrome or later complications such as infection, immobility, and thromboembolic disease.[4]

Hemorrhage

The most immediate and absolute need for surgery in trauma is the control of bleeding; this critically involves the

orthopedic traumatologist in two scenarios, massive bleeding from multiple high-energy fractures or severe localized bleeding associated with a specific major injury, most typically from the pelvis. Bleeding from multiple fractures is common and
2 often underestimated. In general, early transfusion protocols and early fracture management control the situation. Bleeding from fractures will be invariably slow and usually stops spontaneously when the fracture is reduced, stabilized, and the compartment tension restored. However, it is very easy to underestimate the collective blood loss from multiple injuries and get too far behind in resuscitation, a situation that can then become uncontrollable. Aggressive transfusion protocols with appropriate attention to replace volume and clotting factors with early use of blood with plasma and platelets are essential in parallel with the provision of skeletal stabilization for early hemorrhage control.[5] This may involve wound debridement and hemostasis in the complex open injury or early long-bone stabilization in multiple closed fractures. Occasionally, temporary external fixation may be required to provide rapid control of skeletal instability when the more extensive surgery required for definitive stabilization would be inappropriate.

The Bleeding Pelvis

Put simply, patients with major pelvic ring injuries can bleed to death. Often presenting after a high-energy injury, the signs of major hemorrhage from the pelvis may be obvious with massive local swelling and clear instability. At presentation, a primary plain pelvic x-ray remains the best way to quickly understand the fracture. It will allow immediate assessment of the fracture pattern, energy involved, degree of displacement and leads to an estimate of the risk of local bleeding and presence of local or distal associated injuries.[6–10] Today many patients have a binder applied in the field for transport. This is a very effective way to initially control pelvic volume and tamponade bleeding but may reduce the deformity and also lead to the initial x-ray, underestimating the degree of injury.

Understanding the pelvic fracture is essential, Young and Burgess[6,7] (**Fig. 27.1**) presented a classification system based on the implied direction of the initial force and defined injuries essentially as anterior–posterior compression (APC), lateral compression (LC), and vertical shear (VS) injuries. This allows an assessment of the direction of the force applied, the resultant instability, and can predict mortality, transfusion requirements,
3 and associated injuries. In general, injuries that make the pelvic ring bigger bleed locally while ones that make it smaller can bleed but are more commonly markers of the injury mechanism and remote injuries, specifically, the associated ipsilateral chest and abdominal injury. The Tile[11,12] (**Fig. 27.1**) system considers the injury with regard to the resultant instability and has now been adopted by the AO Foundation (AO) and Orthopedic Trauma Association (OTA). An "A"-type fracture has a stable pelvic ring and essentially includes more minor avulsion fractures and mechanically stable pelvic ring injuries (includes APC I and LC I). "B"-type injuries are rotationally unstable but vertically stable with an intact posterior soft tissue hinge providing some stability (corresponding to APC II or LC II/III injuries), while "C"-type injuries are both rotationally and vertically unstable, implying that the posterior hinge is torn (corresponding to APC III and VS injuries). The latter carry the highest risk of bleeding and death.

From a surgical management perspective, A-type injuries are unlikely to be a source of major bleeding while B type and, specifically, C types are increasingly life threatening. After initial assessment, primary radiology, and consideration of the response to initial resuscitation, pelvic fractures can then be considered by the mechanical stability resulting from the injury and the resultant hemodynamic response (**Table 27.2**).

The role of the orthopedic surgeon is to assess the injury with regard to the local and associated problems and to provide pelvic mechanical stability when required. A hemodynamically stable patient with a stable pelvic ring injury does not require major active orthopedic management, although it should be noted that rarely even the most apparently simple injury can cause local bleeding and transfusion may be required.[13] The hemodynamically stable patient with a mechanically unstable pelvic ring injury needs early but not emergent surgery to restore mechanical stability to the pelvis

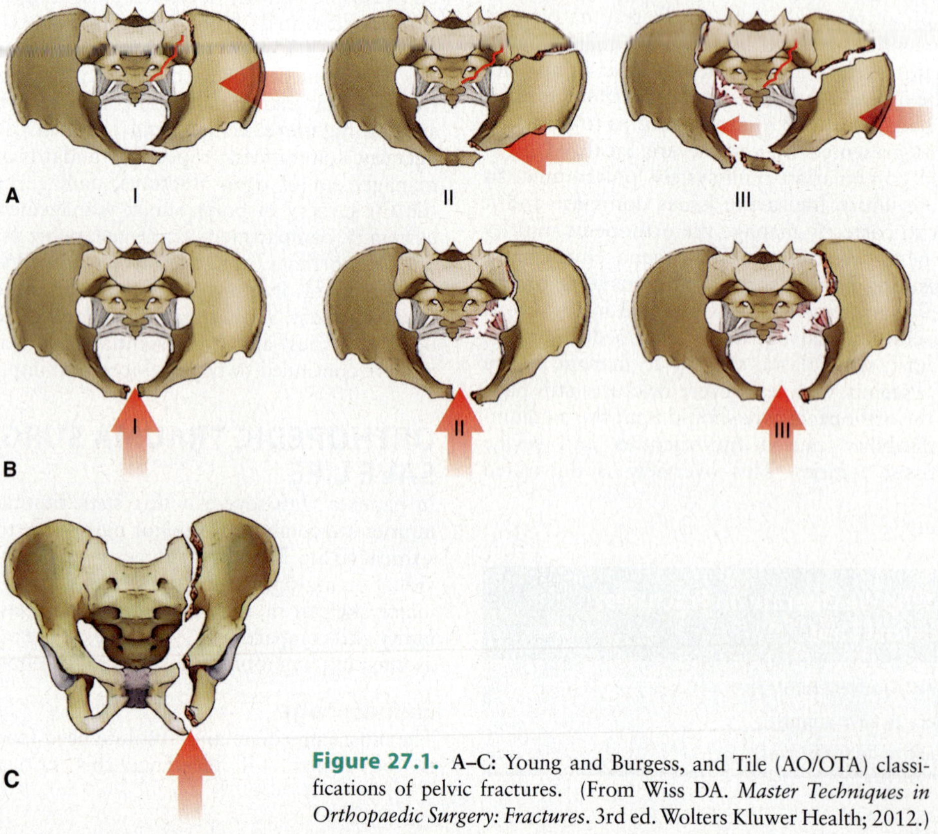

Figure 27.1. A–C: Young and Burgess, and Tile (AO/OTA) classifications of pelvic fractures. (From Wiss DA. *Master Techniques in Orthopaedic Surgery: Fractures*. 3rd ed. Wolters Kluwer Health; 2012.)

Table 27.2. Principles of Management of Major Pelvic Ring Injuries

	Mechanically Stable Pelvis	Mechanically Unstable Pelvis
Hemodynamically stable	Nonoperative	Early, planned operative stabilization of pelvic ring
Hemodynamically unstable	Likely extrapelvic cause Angiography/embolization	Emergent provision of mechanical stability ± Packing/angio

for pain relief, normal daily care, and mobilization. Hemodynamically unstable patients need emergent care to restore their physiologic stability. If the pelvis is mechanically stable, orthopedic intervention has little to offer, either there is an extrapelvic cause for the bleeding or hemostasis should be obtained by provision of appropriate clotting factors and platelets, packing or angiographically, *in extreme cases REBOA has been used.*

The patient in hemorrhagic shock with a major unstable pelvic ring is a very different problem.[13,14] Early coordinated multidisciplinary care in the right hospital is essential, with appropriate resuscitation within an established massive transfusion protocol. It is well established that the site of hemorrhage in most bleeding major pelvic fractures is from the fractured bone surfaces and extensive soft tissue injury, and
4 rarely from major named arteries. Fortunately, the majority of pelvic bleeding will slow or stop when skeletal stability is achieved. However, rapid stabilization of the pelvic ring is a major expert intervention at best and is rarely easily achievable in the acute bleeding situation. Initial reduction, stability, and some local tamponade is provided by a pelvic binder. In critical cases, it should not be removed without an available alternative method to provide stability. Internally rotating the hips, slightly flexing the knees, and binding the legs at the thigh should also be used if possible and provides additional effective control. The provision of early pelvic fixation or a primary angiographic approach to bleeding control depends on local expertise and protocol. Recently, a move to emergent operative provision of skeletal stability and packing of bleeding from the pelvis has entered common practice.[5,15] The major bleeding pelvic injury is considered similar to a bleeding liver and where general hemorrhage control is achieved with packing for local pressure. For the severe pelvic injury, a systematic protocol of bleeding control and transfusion that emphasizes the importance of not getting out of control or reacting too late, "The Denver Protocol"[5,15] begins with a patient with shock, a pelvic ring injury, and a failure to respond to 2 L of crystalloid resuscitation and 2 units of blood transfusion (Algorithm 27.1). The essential principle is an early trigger to aggressive surgical management for hemorrhage control with preperitoneal packing and rapid blood and factor replacement before the patient becomes grossly coagulopathic. From the orthopedic point of view, restoring skeletal stability is a critical part of this process and close cooperation with the general traumatologist is essential. *While an early response to hemorrhage is essential to gain control of the situation, many pelvic fractures do require transfusion in the first few hours without the bleeding becoming uncontrollable. Accordingly, the trigger of a 2-unit transfusion in this protocol has been challenged and no difference found with a trigger of 4 units.*[16] *Clearly, responding rapidly in a critical situation is essential and requires a co-operative multi specialist approach.*

Pelvic Packing

The procedure of packing a pelvis for hemorrhage is well within the capabilities of most surgeons but some form of pelvic bony stability has to be achieved first to give a solid base to pack into. In the emergency situation, this commonly means the application of an anterior external fixation frame although if possible, internal fixation has many advantages. Occasionally, emergency provision of posterior stability with emergent percutaneous sacroiliac fixation or application of a "C clamp" can be dramatically effective in restoring stability and markedly

Algorithm 27.1

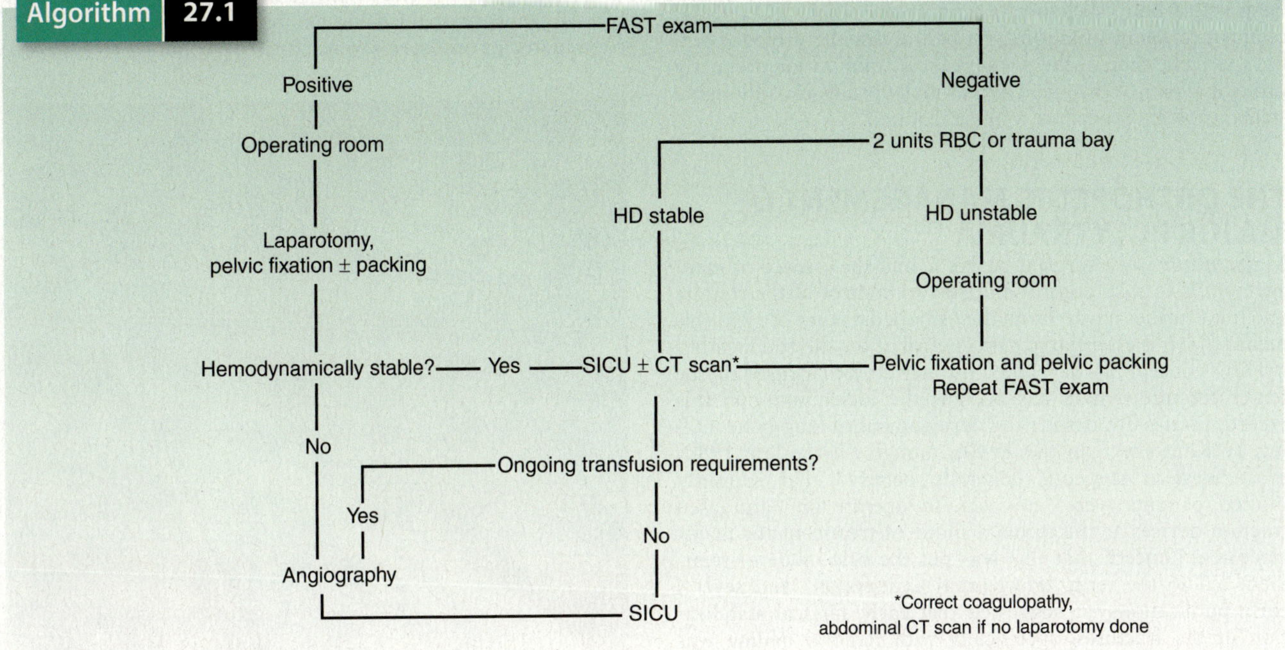

Algorithm 27.1. The Denver Protocol for management of major pelvic fractures. (Used with permission of the British Editorial Society of Bone and Joint Surgery. Mauffrey C, Cuellar DO III, Pieracci F, et al. Strategies for the management of haemorrhage following pelvic fractures and associated trauma-induced coagulopathy. *Bone Joint J*. 2014;96(9):1143–1154. Permission conveyed through Copyright Clearance Center, Inc.)

slowing bleeding. Preperitoneal packing is done through a small anterior incision just above the pubis. After separating the rectus muscles (which may be avulsed from the pubis), the cavity created by the trauma is entered, the hematoma evacuated and rapid mechanical stability obtained (often temporarily, applying a bone-reduction clamp across the pubis). The bleeding cavity, already produced by the trauma, is then packed with as many packs as required. These should be placed as far back into the true pelvis as possible. The hematoma cavity created by the injury will be obvious and it is not required or desirable to extend the dissection outside this area but it is essential to get the packs right to the back of the cavity. Assuming hemostasis is achieved, the packs are left in, often for 48 hours and under an open but sealed abdomen before they are changed or simply removed depending on the physiologic response.

COMPLICATED PELVIC INJURIES—OPEN FRACTURES OR ASSOCIATED VISCERAL INJURY

The initial assessment of any patient with a pelvic fracture must also include an inspection of the perineum with rectal and vaginal examination to check for complex open injuries or associated urologic injuries. Open pelvic fractures and those associated with local visceral damage carry significant mortality and need specific treatment based on the wound or specific injury sustained.[17,18] The degree of contamination and size of the zone of injury in the pelvis massively worsens the situation such that it may prove fatal. Aggressive decontamination and protection of this extensive zone of injury from further contamination by diversion of the fecal stream may be essential.

Complex urologic injuries are commonly seen with specific patterns of pelvic fracture. A significant APC injury is commonly associated with an extraperitoneal bladder rupture of the anterior bladder wall directly in line with the plane of injury. LC injuries may be associated with urethral tears as the inferior ramus cuts the male membranous urethra as it is forced across the midline by the injury. In all cases, the presence of hematuria or blood at the meatus is the pathognomonic sign of injury and necessitates appropriate investigation and joint management with the urologic service. Again, from the orthopedic point of view, no soft tissue reconstruction can work without an underlying stable bony skeleton to support the repair and prevent reinjury. In many situations, the best access the urologist will have is at the time of the primary bony stabilization and early urologic repair or diversion avoids many problems, although a staged urologic procedure may be required.

THE ORTHOPEDIC MANAGEMENT OF MAJOR POLYTRAUMA

5 Major trauma is a surgical problem, and the essence of management is to take control and stay in control of the trauma and limit further harm. From the orthopedic point of view, this means that it is essential to gain control of the skeletal instability. This concept has developed through studies focused on the femur fracture, which has become the index injury in this regard. Essentially, despite the development of long-bone nailing by Küntscher[19] in the 1940s, though till the late 1980s most Western surgeons generally believed that seriously injured patients were "too sick to operate on" and used traction devices as the primary mode of treatment for major fractures. Concern that this was not the best mode of treatment led to the term "Horizontal Crucifixion" and several early publications[19–21] suggested that early surgical stabilization of the fractures, specifically with femoral nailing was valuable. Johnson[22] confirmed this effect and showed that it appeared to be greater the more severely the patient was injured. In 1989, Bone[23] published his landmark paper, a prospective randomized trial of early against late femoral nailing after severe injury. Essentially, he showed that there was a major advantage in early nailing and the pendulum now swung from nonoperative care to enthusiastic universal early skeletal stabilization after polytrauma. The patient was considered "too sick not to operate on" and a management philosophy now termed "Early Total Care" developed. This practice was soon questioned, specifically in Germany where the orthopedic trauma surgeon is closely involved with intensive care and inevitably observed the combined effect of other injures. Pape et al.[24] again considering the femur, looked specifically at the effect of early and late femoral nailing in severe polytrauma and showed a deleterious effect of an associated chest injury in association with femur fractures treated by early reamed nailing. While statistically the effect seemed more related to the chest injury than the nailing, this alerted the profession to the combination effect of these injuries and stimulated an outpouring of research looking at the general and immunologic effects of orthopedic procedures and specifically of reaming the femur.[25–40] Eventually, an understanding of the general effects of polytrauma and bony injury has become more widely accepted and a concept of the appropriate surgery (DCO) for the most severely injured patients developed.

Damage Control Surgery in Orthopedics

Damage control in orthopedics means taking control of the musculoskeletal elements of the injury without creating an increased trauma load due to increased surgical bleeding or a lengthy surgery associated with definitive care of complex fractures (**Fig. 27.2**). The priorities are hemorrhage control, wound management, tissue revascularization (including compartment decompression), and general restoration of major skeletal stability, usually by the rapid application of temporary external fixation. The basic physiologic parameters are then normalized in a critical care environment unit and definitive stabilization is delayed until the peritraumatic immunologic storm has settled.[29,30,32,33] The most critical element is the speed and accuracy of the initial surgery as the critical injured patient cannot tolerate a long orthopedic procedure. However, the principle of establishing early skeletal stability remains; this is the major and lasting lesson from Johnson and Bone[22,23] and is not disputed. The issue is not if, but how this is obtained. Today's question is how do we identify which patients are too sick for definitive fixation? Long orthopedic procedures and protracted bleeding must be avoided and nailing the femur in a sick, under resuscitated patient seems to be particularly poorly tolerated. A

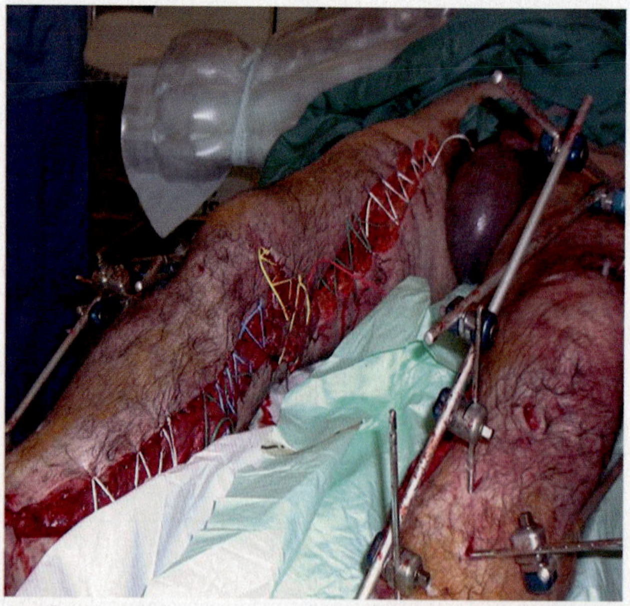

Figure 27.2. Early damage control of extensive limb injuries with external fixation.

Table 27.3. Essential Priorities in Orthopedic Damage Control

Principle	Example
Surgical hemorrhage control	Direct control, pelvic packing, long-bone stabilization
Cavity decompression	Compartment syndrome
Debridement/ decontamination	Major open wounds/fractures
Revascularization	Repair vascular injury to revascularize the limb if patient is well enough, if not amputate
Fracture stabilization	Usually rapid external fixation of major long-bone injury/pelvis
Critical care	Ongoing resuscitation, rewarming, and factor replacement prior to delayed secondary surgery
Delay reconstructive surgery	Conversion of external fixation to nails, definitive joint reconstruction

variety of parameters have been investigated to understand this,[29] despite early enthusiasm, interleukin-6[28] has proved mainly to be a research tool and today a spectrum of parameters considering the patient's general condition are commonly used.[34] This essentially means close communication and protocol agreement with the anesthetic/general trauma team to decide what extent of surgery should be done. Basic parameters to be considered include the hemoglobin/hematocrit, ventilation parameters, platelet count and coagulation studies, patient temperature, and a measure of acidosis, usually the lactate level. The latter is now the primary decision-making parameter used by many orthopedic surgeons. Currently, Vallier et al.[34] have suggested a lactate level of 4 mmol/L is a safe cutoff above which it is not safe to continue surgical reconstruction and only
6 DCO can proceed (**Table 27.3**). If DCO has been performed to obtain temporary skeletal stability, it is accepted that the definitive reconstruction should be delayed until the patient is well enough, usually at least 5 days.

Special Polytrauma Situations—Head Injury

There are specific scenarios that change priorities, the most obvious being the associated head injury. When the brain is at risk, the primary aim of care is to maintain cerebral oxygenation and cerebral perfusion pressure (CPP). Orthopedic procedures, especially those that would lead to bleeding, swings in blood pressure and thus episodes of reduced CPP should be avoided. However, this does not eliminate the benefit of the stable skeleton in general critical care such that DCO and appropriate bony stabilization at the right time are strongly indicated.[41,42]

Special Polytrauma Situations—Chest Injury and Femur Fractures

The effect of the chest injury is discussed above. It was emphasized by Pape and Tscherne and innumerable papers that followed.[24] While multiple studies have shown the advantages of early skeletal stabilization, there is no doubt that the lungs are vulnerable to further insults after injury, and that the acute lung injury can be worsened by fat embolization especially during instrumentation of the femoral canal. While improvements in reamer design reduce canal pressurization and smaller nails have been advocated, delaying definitive nailing for 5 days after initial external fixation in the most critical patient is probably the standard of care. The patient with bilateral femur fractures is at a significantly increased risk and some surgeons avoid bilateral femoral nailing at the same time even in healthy patients.[43–46]

Table 27.4. Open Fracture Surgical Principles

Debridement to healthy margins and profuse lavage/decontamination
Bony stabilization
Early, healthy soft tissue cover

SPECIFIC ORTHOPEDIC SCENARIOS

Major Wounds

The ongoing effect of major wounds can be critical. In the first instance, debridement of necrotic tissue from the trauma is essential and is commonly inadequately done at the initial surgery. Wounds will never stabilize until adequately excised and when associated with fractures, will not heal until bony stability has been established. The management of open fractures is described below; in polytrauma cases the principles remain the same but the ability to obtain early definitive care and specifically complex closure techniques may be compromised by the patient's general situation.

ORTHOPEDIC TRAUMA SURGERY TO SAVE LIMBS

Open Fracture Principles

Open fractures can range from simple to destructive injuries but in all, the important feature is that the fracture hematoma communicates with the outside environment and the fracture is contaminated. As such, the specific management revolves around preventing this contamination converting to established infection. General emergency measures include the provision of tetanus cover, early broad-spectrum antibiotics, early splintage, and wound dressing and are followed by early surgical management. The latter is designed to reduce the degree of contamination, to remove necrotic or threatened tissue likely to become infected, and to protect the limb by making it unlikely to develop further infection due to the unstable fracture and critical open wound (**Tables 27.4** and **27.5**).

The debridement of an open fracture is one of the most difficult surgical procedures; it should not be relegated to inexperienced staff and, if possible, not attempted out of normal hours unless the limb is very seriously threatened. The whole zone of injury must be assessed and all dead and dying tissue removed, only nerve and vessel must be preserved and poor muscle specifically removed. It may more appropriately be termed wound excision. Any free bone or fragments attached by flimsy soft tissue should also be removed and the resulting defect dealt with accordingly, although only rarely is a significant defect produced. Wound extensions need to be placed with specific

Table 27.5. Open Fracture Classification (after Gustilo and Anderson[47])

Grade I	Small low-energy wound <1 cm, no high-energy features
Grade II	Small low-energy laceration over fracture 1–10 cm, no high-energy features
Grade IIIa	High-energy open fracture (degloving, periosteal stripping, bone comminution) with adequate soft tissue cover
Grade IIIb	High-energy open fracture with inadequate soft tissue cover
Grade IIIc	Any open fracture with a vascular injury requiring repair for viability

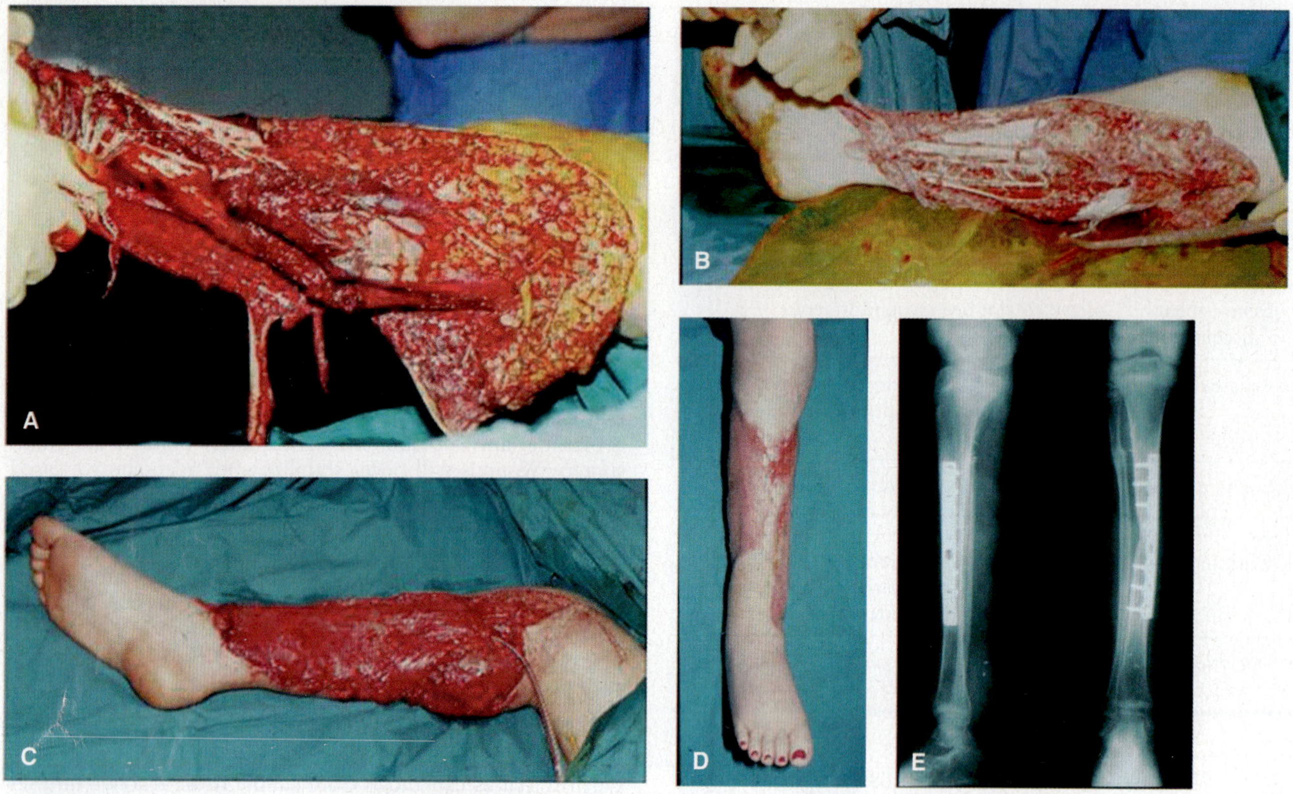

Figure 27.3. A–E: Management sequence of a major open fracture. This is a III-C injury in a 12-year-old treated by immediate "fix and flap" incorporating the anastomosis for the latissimus dorsi free flap into the vascular repair. The subsequent course shows good soft tissue and bony healing.

consideration for the later closure and must not make the soft tissue reconstruction more complex. An adequate appropriate debridement must be performed the first time. Repeated debridements "to make sure" are usually because there was an inadequate initial operation. This tends to lead to recruitment of additional necrotic tissue requiring debridement that can be avoided if the first debridement is adequate and soft tissue cover established quickly. The associated delay with repeated procedures massively increases the infection rate.

7 Establishing early bone stability is essential, this reduces the chance of late infection and facilitates the subsequent soft tissue reconstruction. In truth, the ability to perform an adequate debridement and the best bony reconstruction depends directly on the orthopedic surgeons' confidence in the subsequent soft tissue closure and thus the working relationship with the plastic surgery team. While soft tissue reconstruction is often delayed for practical reasons, there is excellent evidence that the earlier a healthy closure is obtained the better. This is true to the extent that the best data in the most complex (IIIb) injuries are with immediate flap cover after an adequate initial debridement and definitive bony reconstruction as one primary procedure (**Fig. 27.3**). While current TQIP recommendations require coverage within 7 days, UK (BOAST) recommendations ask for soft tissue coverage within 48 hours of definitive fixation and seems to be reflected in a much improved infection rate. Outside the most advanced orthoplastic reconstruction units few units can achieve such early cover. But as suggested by BOAST, definitive debridement, fracture stabilization, and appropriate soft tissue assessment at the primary procedure followed by definitive soft tissue cover at the second visit to the OR (at about 48 hours) after the patient has been appropriately counseled is probably the best achievable standard. Cooperative care with the plastic surgical service from the start is essential.[48–54]

VASCULAR INJURIES

An acutely ischemic limb with a fracture or dislocation is a major surgical emergency. At presentation, all fractures must have the distal circulation assessed and documented; if the blood supply is affected, the fracture or dislocation must be rapidly reduced. Fortunately, this commonly results in restoration of circulation and normal fracture care can continue. If not an emergent, combined vascular–orthopedic procedure is required. Sometimes a temporary shunt will be used to obtain distal flow while a bony reconstruction is performed. Bony stability at the correct length must be obtained before definitive vascular reconstruction, both to allow the vascular repair to be at the correct level and tension, and to protect it from disruption. Any subsequent reconstruction must be done with provision for awareness and care of the vascular repair and should include fasciotomy to prevent reperfusion compartment syndrome.

COMPARTMENT SYNDROME

A compartment syndrome is a major surgical emergency as the muscle is acutely ischemic due to an increased compartment pressure reducing tissue perfusion to below a critical level. Accordingly, the classical presentation is pain out of proportion to the injury due to the muscle ischemia. The compartment may be obviously hard with loss of muscle function and distal neurologic symptoms due to pressure on the nerves passing through the compartment. Loss of arterial flow through the compartment is exceedingly rare and not useful diagnostically, the presence of a distal pulse does not contribute to the diagnosis of compartment syndrome. While the diagnosis is often clinical and straightforward, a formal measurement of the perfusion pressure of the compartment (similar to CPP in head injuries) has been popularized by McQueen.[55] Assessing the anterior compartment of the lower leg after tibial fractures with constant compartment pressure monitoring, they showed that if the compartment pressure remained at least 30 mm Hg below the diastolic blood pressure (known as the D*p* >30), the consequences of compartment syndrome (muscle necrosis and contractures) did not occur. Accordingly, today the definitive test for compartment syndrome is a direct measurement of the compartment pressure and comparison to the diastolic pressure. This is particularly seen in situations when the patient is not able to respond appropriately to pain. These include, during anesthesia, particularly under regional anesthesia; patients sedated on intensive care; patients where any strong analgesia is being used; or if the patient is poorly responsive after a medication overdose.[56] The diagnosis must not be missed, as immediate fasciotomy is needed to restore muscle perfusion.

Unfortunately, "compartment syndromes" can present late when muscle necrosis is established. Commonly this "acute dead muscle syndrome" is commonly seen in the "Found Down Syndrome". In this presentation, there is usually established muscle necrosis associated with a missed crush syndrome commonly associated with the unconscious patient after drug abuse or intoxication. This is not acute compartment syndrome. There will be rhabdomyolysis, a high creatinine kinase level, myoglobinuria, and even frank renal failure if several compartments are involved. If muscle necrosis is the driving factor and established at presentation, and certainly if diagnosed after 12 to 24 hours, fasciotomy is not indicated as it will only expose the necrotic compartment to infection. Unless additional progressive vascular or neurologic compromise develops decompression is not helpful. Occasionally, radical muscle debridement is the only way to reduce the myoglobin level and reduce the renal damage but that commonly means amputation. While this is a very difficult management dilemma unless these specific situations are present decompression will be harmful. The tight limb should be simply observed intensive medical management, possibly even dialysis continued and the subsequent distal contracture more safely dealt with later by specific muscle or tendon releases.[57]

INDICATIONS FOR AMPUTATION/ FAILURE OF RECONSTRUCTION

The indications for amputation can be remembered as the three "D's" referring to a limb that is "Dead," "Dangerous," or a "Damn" nuisance. In the early trauma situation, this may be clearly obvious and early amputation may be lifesaving while the latter refers to later reconstructive scenarios. While limb salvage is always the aim, the injury may be too severe and should not be attempted if it puts life at risk. This requires experienced decision making at the acute stage and, when possible, agreement between staff surgeons. In an isolated injury situation, the decision essentially depends on the degree and site of necrotic tissue and the functional potential of the limb after reconstruction. This can be a most difficult decision and should be made by a surgeon experienced in reconstructive options and their functional outcome. In many situations, an amputee will function as well as, if not better than a poor reconstruction especially if several muscle compartments have been lost. This is clearly a decision for experienced staff and should involve the patient as much as possible. The application of a temporary external fixator to the critically injured limb with a view to appropriate discussion prior to initiating further treatment has much to recommend it.

ORTHOPEDIC TRAUMA SURGERY TO LIMIT DISABILITY—MANAGEMENT OF FRACTURES

The management of fractures has been a core medical discipline for millennia and has developed from primitive bone setting, through the guild of army barber surgeons to the modern-day orthopedic traumatologist. In general orthopedic practice today, almost half of the work is the care of injury and in most modern trauma centers 80% to 90% of the surgical care of the injured falls to the orthopedic service.

Fortunately, fractures have an intrinsic tendency to heal, and bone is one of only two tissues to heal by reforming its own tissue and not with a scar. There are four essential phases in fracture management: assessment, position, healing, and rehabilitation. The first mandates a full limb assessment with documentation of the relevant clinical signs. This must include assessment and documentation of the neurovascular state of the distal limb. X-rays need to be taken of the whole bone involved and centered on the fracture. For example, an x-ray of the humerus which includes the shoulder is inadequate to assess a specific shoulder injury and separate views of the relevant part must be obtained. These views must include an AP and appropriate lateral specifically of the appropriate part. In many situations, the injury anatomy is still not adequately defined by these views and specific additional x-ray views or a computed tomography (CT) scan will be required to fully understand the injury and for surgical planning. Fracture management then centers on obtaining and holding the position of the fracture through healing. Essentially, mid-diaphyseal fractures need to be held in a position to maintain overall length, alignment, and rotation but do not need an anatomical reduction of individual fragments. In modern practice, this is usually achieved by intramedullary nailing which also provides the relative stability needed at the fracture site and facilitates healing with callus (**Fig. 27.4**). As a contrast, articular fractures usually need a direct open approach to ensure accurate reduction of the joint surface and stabilization with absolute stability. The recovery of joint function is directly related to the quality of the reduction, the provision of stable fixation and health local soft tissues to allow early motion. In this situation, the bone at the joint would be expected to heal by primary bone union without callus (**Fig. 27.5**).

Essentially, the method chosen to hold the position of the fracture will be more or less stable depending on how firmly it holds the bone. A traditional cast on the tibia will provide only relative stability and should lead to a high rate of healing with callus. There can be a very good functional recovery if an adequate position is maintained and cast complications are avoided, but it essentially provides a less reliable hold than an implant directly applied to the bone. Accordingly, the patient undergoing nonoperative management in cast has to be followed closely, often with weekly x-rays for up to a month or until the position is deemed stable. The cast then stays until bone healing is considered adequate to maintain the position faced with functional loads and the cast can be removed. A stable, painless fracture on clinical examination suggests adequate healing to stay out of cast which should be confirmed by good bone healing on x-ray.

Nonoperative fracture management is a highly skilled art that has been practiced for years but in the developed world is used today only for stable relatively undisplaced fractures. This includes undisplaced articular fractures, low-energy nonarticular fractures, and many fractures in children who have a large capacity for remodeling during and after bone healing and obtain bony healing in about half the time of adults with excellent function results (**Table 27.6**).

The phase of bone healing from fracture to a stable skeleton progresses from an inflammatory reaction through fibrous tissue and cartilage formation before immature bone and finally mature remodeling. A number of biologic stimulatory molecules and specific mechanical features then drive the normal healing response. Overall, there is a progressive stiffening of the fracture environment until bone can form when the local strain is at or below 2%.[58,59] This may be produced by the gradual tissue stiffening provided by the natural healing process or by an orthopedic implant that creates a local strain environment in conjunction with the specific fracture anatomy and intrinsic fracture stability. Normal healing with splintage or with devices that produce relative stability (some fracture motion under physiologic loads) lead to the progressive stiffening effect described briefly above and healing by callus when the strain reduces to a level where bone can form. If an implant confers absolute stability, usually through direct compression of the fracture surfaces, the strain is less than 2% from the

TRAUMA

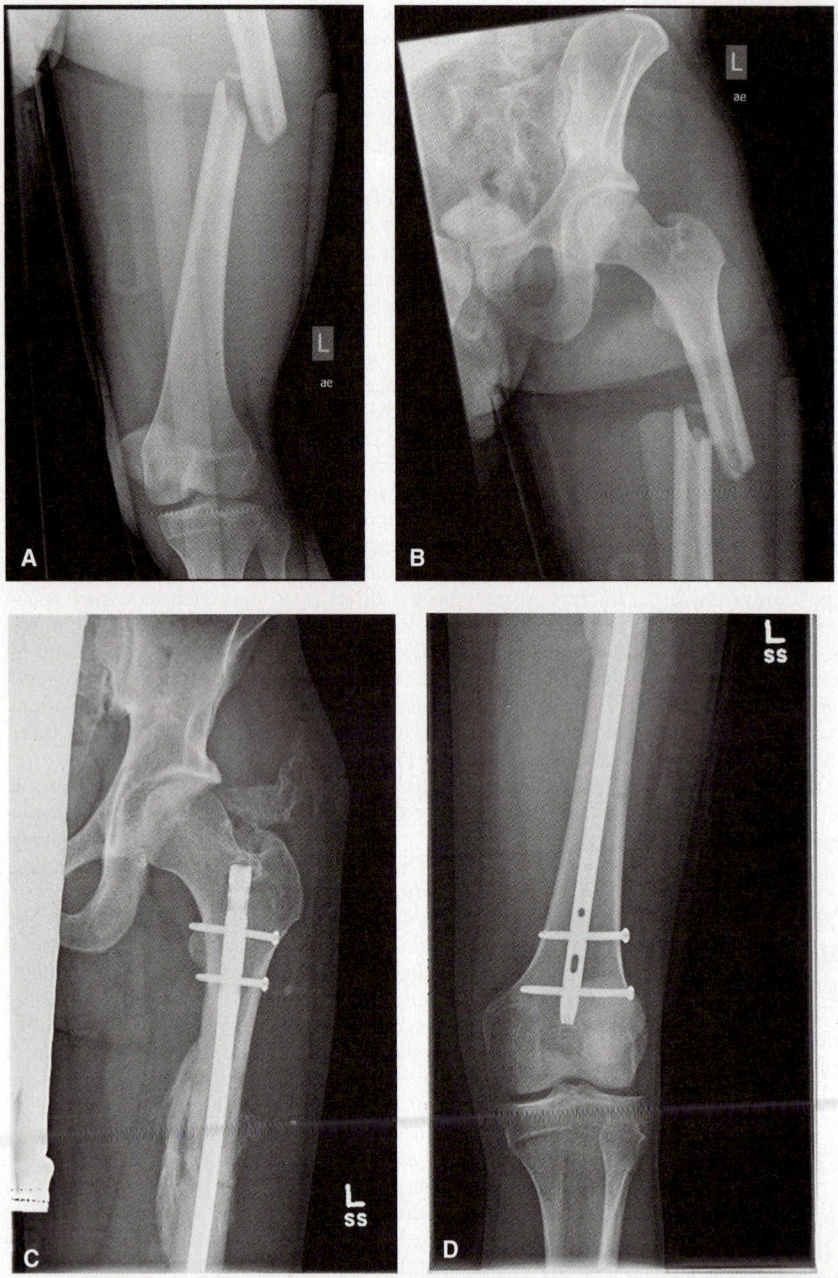

Figure 27.4. Assessment and surgical management of a diaphyseal fracture of the femur. **A, B:** Anteroposterior x-rays of a diaphyseal femur fracture. **C, D:** Reamed fully locked intramedullary nailing of a diaphyseal femur fracture showing progressive healing.

start and the bone heals by a modified remodeling process termed "primary bone healing," callus does not form. In planning a bony reconstruction, the surgeon specifically decides what degree of stability is required to treat a specific fracture
8 and the appropriate implant to do this. This follows basic AO[60,61] principles which are the key to fracture surgery. Essentially, diaphyseal fractures need treatment with relative stability and indirect reduction techniques to maximize the local healing process. In contrast, articular fractures usually require a direct reduction for perfect anatomy and subsequent fixation with absolute stability (no deformation occurs under physiologic load) to facilitate joint recovery.

The rehabilitation process should be considered as soon as the soft tissues are stable enough to allow dependency and joint motion. This confers the major advantages of mobility to the limb and whole patient. With articular fractures, the cartilage is only nourished by diffusion from joint fluid which is effectively pumped into the hyaline cartilage as a secondary effect of motion. Accordingly, fracture fixation must be stable enough to allow early range of motion (ROM) exercises as tolerated but weight bearing is usually limited to protect the reconstruction from early displacement.

Complex Articular Fractures

Major joint injuries are significant threat to joint function.[62–64] The aim of care involves articular reconstruction with perfect joint anatomy and stable fixation with absolute stability. Surgical reconstruction often requires detailed preoperative assessment with a CT scan and application of specific implants often designed for the specific joint and side involved. The basic principles used for surgical reconstruction of these injuries were developed over 50 years ago by the AO and have only seen minor modifications since. However, modern implants and particularly the development of locking plates have improved the capability of our implants to hold fractures securely and specifically allow fractures to be held in position with less extensile exposures. Occasionally, the primary injury (even if closed) is associated with significant degloving of the local soft tissues, manifest by major fracture blisters and precludes an early open surgical approach.[65] Surgical management then takes the form of temporary bridging external fixation, applied outside the zone of injury which confers some stability and allows the soft tissues to settle prior to conversion to an internal fixation often after 1 to

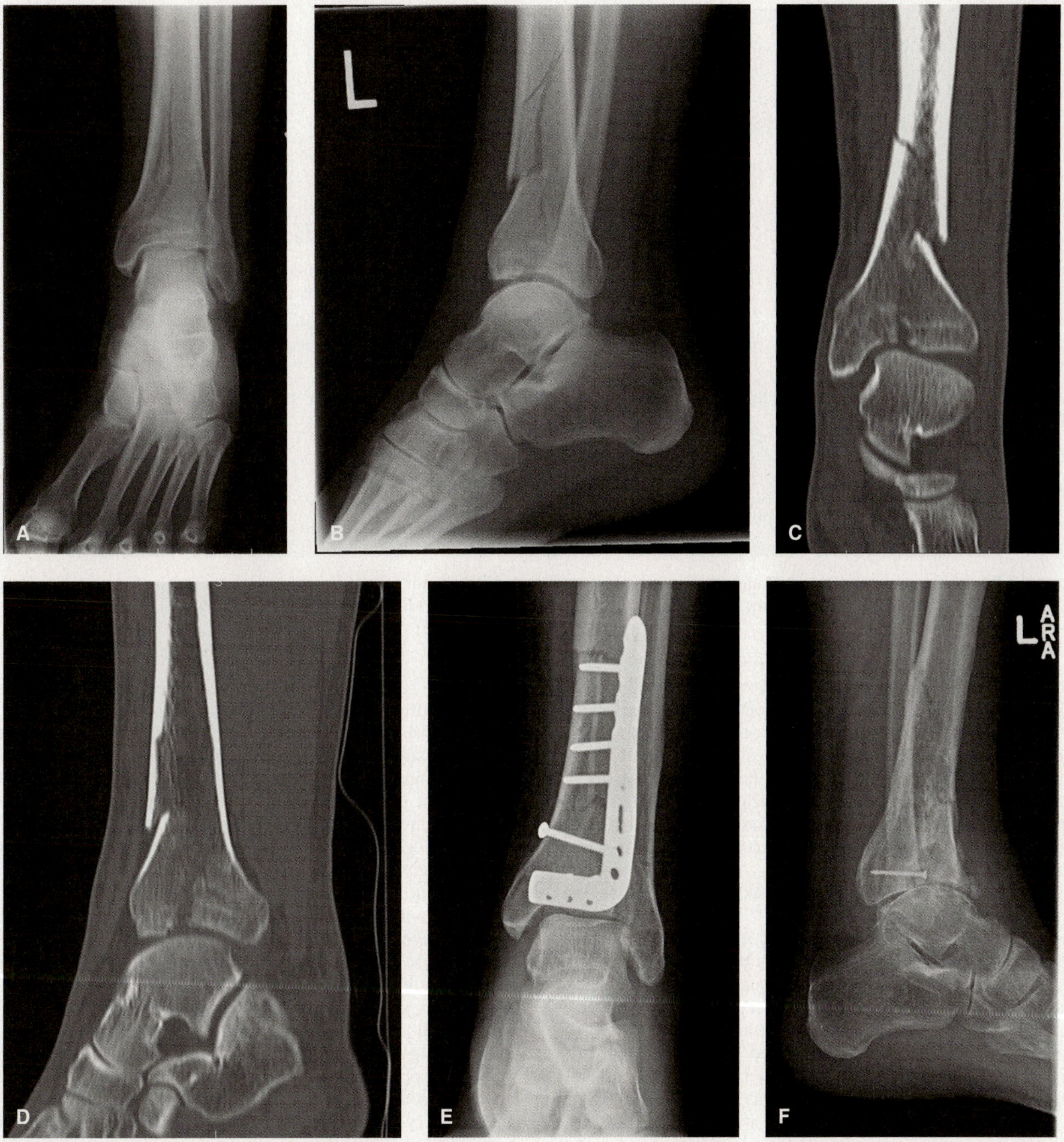

Figure 27.5. Assessment and surgical management of a complex articular fracture of the distal tibia (pilon).Despite virtually anatomic reduction, it progresses to degenerative arthritis in the medium term. **A, B:** AP and lateral x-rays of an intra-articular fracture of the distal articular surface of the tibia. **C, D:** CAT scans show the marked damage and displacement at the joint surface, underappreciated by initial x-rays. **E:** Open reduction and internal fixation to restore the joint surface for function and joint longevity. **F:** After healing and removal of the majority of the hardwear, there is significant degenerative arthritis of the joint that may need joint arthrodesis.

2 weeks. However, in most fractures, excellent results can be obtained by much earlier surgery which is much easier than a delayed reconstruction.[65,66]

Table 27.6. Bone Healing Timeframes

Guideline Fracture Healing Times (in Cast)	Upper Limb (wks)	Lower Limb (wks)
Children	3	6+
Adults	6	12

SPECIAL FRACTURE GROUPS—PROXIMAL FEMUR

Like many injuries, fractures of the proximal femur have a bimodal distribution with rarer high-energy injuries in the young and extremely common bone fragility fractures in the elderly. As a public health issue, osteoporosis and its related fractures are at epidemic proportions and specifically covered by TQIP reccomendations.[67] The general medical care of the elderly dominates the clinical picture where the mortality is of the order of 15% to 20% in the 3 months after fracture, and the injured frail elderly produce a major load on hospital and rehabilitation services. In addition, specific attention to long-term bone health is essential. The orthopedic issues of

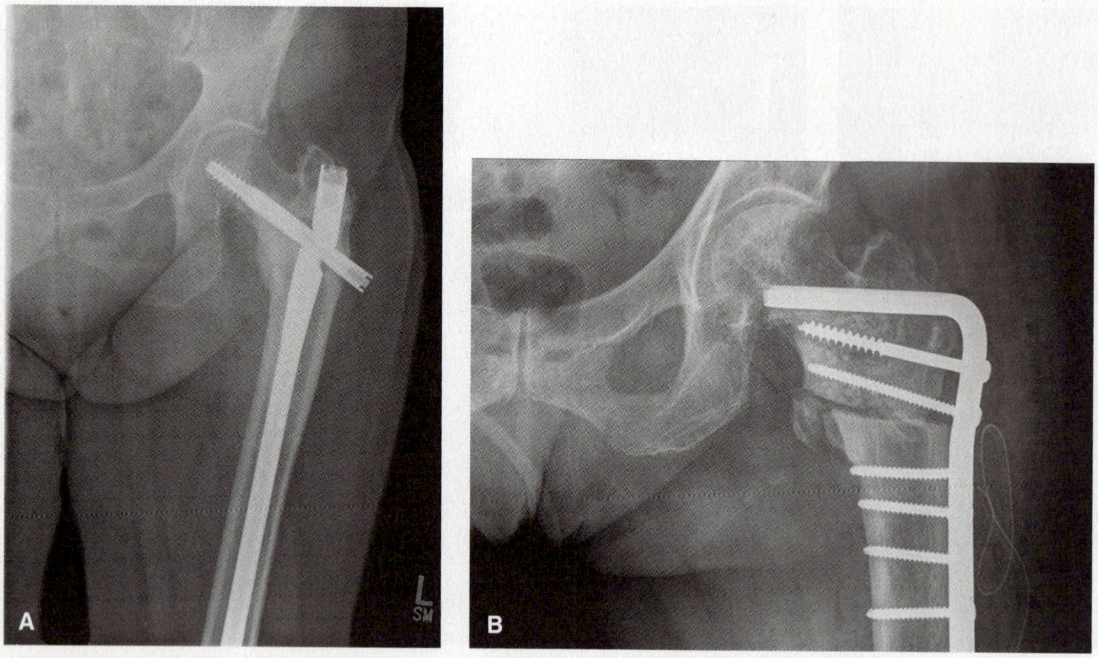

Figure 27.6. Assessment and surgical management of a proximal femoral malunion after implant failure. **A:** Proximal femoral malunion (collapsed into varus) with a broken implant in place. **B:** Correction of the malunion with a valgus osteotomy held with a blade plate.

proximal femoral fracture take two forms and produce specifically different problems and solutions. The fractures essentially occur inside (intracapsular) or outside the hip capsule (extracapsular). Intracapsular fractures carry a risk of avascular necrosis (AVN) of the femoral head depending on the displacement of the fracture, while intratrochanteric fractures are mechanically unstable due to the anatomy and offset of the proximal femur creating marked mechanical instability with a tendency to collapse into varus.

Intracapsular fractures (femoral neck) are classically classified by Garden.[68] Garden grade 1 and 2 injuries are essentially undisplaced and carry a low risk of AVN, they are usually treated by fixation unless the patient's bone quality is considered too poor for fixation. In that situation and in displaced fractures (Garden grades 3 and 4), a replacement of the femoral head with hemiarthroplasty or total hip replacement in a biologically younger patient is required.[69,70]

Extracapsular fractures (trochanteric) are mechanically unstable. They will collapse into varus without fixation and have a tendency to settle and shorten with healing due to the intrinsic bone weakness and pull of local muscles. Accordingly, fixation devices need the ability to mechanically control the angle of the femoral neck and accommodate some shortening without protrusion of the device into the hip. The instability is associated with the degree and position of any comminution which also indicates which device is appropriate to use. Essentially, a sliding hip screw device can be used for any trochanteric fracture unless the lateral wall is incompetent (reverse obliquity injuries or their equivalent) or where there is subtrochanteric extension. In these cases, an intramedullary nail with a retrograde locking device is specifically indicated, although many surgeons use these nails for most fractures. When using a sliding hip screw for a trochanteric fracture, it is essential to get the tip of the screw close to the articular surface.[71,72]

COMPLICATIONS

Infection Nonunion and Malunion

Specific healing problems may require later specialist care.[73] Infection is unfortunately common after complex fracture care, especially if the initial injury was open. Failure of healing (nonunion) is not usually diagnosed before 6 months and commonly suggested by persistence of pain on loading and failure of progression of bone healing on x-ray. Malunion is assessed with regard to the specific deformity and may require corrective surgery for limb alignment, joint function, or longevity. Commonly, infection and failure of bone healing occur together. In principle, infection after fracture creates a similar situation to osteomyelitis with acute and chronic clinical pictures. In general, the management of infection involves the same principles as the management of open fractures with debridement and lavage, skeletal stability and healthy soft tissue cover; with the addition of long-term antibiotics guided by perioperative cultures and under the supervision of an infectious disease specialist. Again, adequate debridement of the poor often dead infected bone, the provision of bony stability and healthy soft tissue cover is the key to management.

Surgical management of the acute infection before fracture healing involves urgent washout of the wound, biopsy, cultures, appropriate antibiotics, and healthy wound management, often necessitating delayed primary closure after a secondary washout. While unstable fixation should be removed and stability restored, stable fixation should be maintained even if superficially contaminated until adequate fracture union. An implant can then be safely removed and usually any residual infection eradicated. Chronic infection with a united fracture needs similar treatment but if the fracture is stable, the key here is removal of a contaminated implant and debridement of dead bone to remove the source of infection. Local washout and healthy soft tissue closure then proceeds as above. However, in the chronic situation, affected tissues are stiff and nonpliable such that bone and soft tissue debridement may produce a dead space, soft tissue defect, or skeletal instability with a bony defect, each of which may require specific management.[74,75] Unfortunately, while possible, limb salvage often carries significant morbidity with additional personal and social consequences and is often not be the best option for the patient.

Malunions cause considerable disability and can be very rewarding to correct (**Fig. 27.6**). Each needs to be fully assessed for the specifics of the deformity and consideration to a variety of methods of correction given. There are champions of a variety of acute correction methods with an osteotomy and fixation or gradual correction usually with a ring-fixation device.

Orthopedic Injury/Disaster Triage

Given the predominance of orthopedic injuries in the injured patient and the frequency of multiple patient events, surgeons are often faced with prioritizing the care of a number of injuries in one complex patient or of a number of patients at the same time. In common day practice, a major motor vehicle crash with several victims can stress a system and require appropriate prioritization. In major international disasters, these situations can be extreme. In these situations, simple reliable rules are needed to guide staff through the process especially when there are multiple problems to consider and the situation is critical. ATLS dealt with this superbly with the A, B, C, alphabetic system for the primary survey. While this remains an excellent system for initial patient evaluation and can guide some immediate surgical decisions, it does not help the surgeon who will have to make critical priority decisions beyond this. From the orthopedic traumatology point of view, the variety of injuries often cover the whole spectrum of clinical need and produce complex decision-making situations. The easiest way for the supervising surgeon to plan the care of an individual is to stand back and work along simple priority guidelines, asking "what is needed here to save the life," "what is needed to save a limb," and "what is disability limiting." Considering each injury in turn then allows a logical plan to be made to prioritize the care required. In multiple patient scenarios, the process is the same but modified by the number of patients involved and the medical resources available. With adequate resources, each patient's problems are dealt with individually as needed and no consideration to major disaster triage is required. If resources are available although stressed, patients with life-threatening problems are dealt with first prioritized by their individual acuity while others with important but initially stable issues can be managed later. In the massive disaster situation, priorities change, resources are overwhelmed, and first priority is given to the group of patients who will gain the most while not tying up or exhausting scarce resources. This is extremely difficult to do as the critical patient who would often be dealt with first if more resources were available is not prioritized as their care would swamp the resources available and not allow simpler care to many others.[57] Going into situations (such as the immediate medical relief after the 2010 Haiti earthquake or conflict situations) without preplanning or the experience to deal with difficult decisions like this is not advisable.

References

1. Rotondo MF, Cribari C, Smith RS. Resources for optimal care of the injured patient. American College of Surgeons Committee on Trauma; 2014.
2. https://www.facs.org/quality-programs/trauma/quality/best-practices-guidelines/
3. BOA Standards for Trauma and Orthopaedics (BOASts) www.boa.ac.uk/standards-guidance/boasts.html
4. Bucholz RW, Heckman JD, Court-Brown CM, eds. *Rockwood and Green's Fractures in Adults*. 6th ed. Lippincott Williams & Wilkins; 2006.
5. Mauffrey C, Cuellar DO 3rd, Pieracci F, et al. Strategies for the management of haemorrhage following pelvic fractures and associated trauma-induced coagulopathy. *Bone Joint J*. 2014;96B:1143–1154.
6. Burgess AR, Eastridge BJ, Young JW, et al. Pelvic ring disruptions: Effective classification systems and treatment protocols. *J Trauma*. 1990;30:848–856.
7. Dalal SA, Burgess AR, Siegel JH, et al. Pelvic fracture in multiple trauma: Classification by mechanism is key to pattern of organ injury, resuscitative requirements, and outcome. *J Trauma*. 1989;29(7):981–1000.
8. Poole GV, Ward EF, Muakkassa FF, Hsu HS, Griswold JA, Rhodes RS. Pelvic fracture from major blunt trauma. Outcome is determined by associated injuries. *Ann Surg*. 1991;213(6):532–538.
9. Demetriades D, Karaiskakis M, Toutouzas K, Alo K, Velmahos G, Chan L. Pelvic fractures: Epidemiology and predictors of associated abdominal injuries and outcomes. *J Am Coll Surg*. 2002;195(1):1–10.
10. Starr AJ, Griffin DR, Reinert CM, et al. Pelvic ring disruptions: Prediction of associated injuries, transfusion requirement, pelvic arteriography, complications, and mortality. *J Orthop Trauma*. 2002;16(8):553–561.
11. Tile M, Pennal GF. Pelvic disruption: Principles of Management. *Clin Orthop Relat Res*. 1980;151:56–64.
12. Tile M. Classification of fractures of the pelvis and acetabulum. In: Tile M, ed. *Fractures of the Pelvis and Acetabulum*. 2nd ed. Williams & Wilkins; 1995:66–101.
13. Bramos A, Velmahos GC, Butt UM, Fikry K, Smith RM, Chang Y. Predictors of bleeding from stable pelvic fractures. *Arch Surg*. 2011;146(4):407–411.
14. Gruen GS, Leit ME, Gruen RJ, Peitzman AB. The acute management of hemodynamically unstable multiple trauma patients with pelvic ring fractures. *J Trauma*. 1994;36(5):706–711.
15. Biffl WL, Smith WR, Moore EE, et al. Evolution of a multidisciplinary clinical pathway for the management of unstable patients with pelvic fractures. *Ann Surg*. 2001;233(6):843–850.
16. Pesante BD, Moore EE, Pieracci FM, Kim YJ, Mauffrey C, Parry JA. Increasing the threshold to perform preperitoneal pelvic packing decreases morbidity without affecting mortality. *J Orthop Trauma*. 2024;38(8):426–430.
17. Rothenberger DA, Fischer RP, Strate RG, Velasco R, Perry JF Jr. The mortality associated with pelvic fractures. *Surgery*. 1978;84(3):356–361.
18. Rothenberger D, Velasco R, Strate R, Fischer RP, Perry JF Jr. Open pelvic fracture: A lethal injury. *J Trauma*. 1978;18(3):184–187.
19. Küntscher G. The intramedullary nailing of fractures. *Clin Orthop Relat Res*. 1968;60:5–12.
20. Riska EB, von Bonsdorff H, Hakkinen S, Jaroma H, Kiviluoto O, Paavilainen T. Primary operative fixation of long bone fractures in patients with multiple injuries. *J Trauma*. 1977;17(2):111–121.
21. Goris RJ, Gimbrère JS, van Niekerk JL, Schoots FJ, Booy LH. Early osteosynthesis and prophylactic mechanical ventilation in the multitrauma patient. *J Trauma*. 1982;22:895–903.
22. Johnson KD, Cadambi A, Seibert GB. Incidence of adult respiratory distress syndrome in patients with multiple musculoskeletal injuries: Effect of early operative stabilization of fractures. *J Trauma*. 1985;25:375–384.
23. Bone LB, Johnson KD, Weigelt J, Scheinberg R. Early versus delayed stabilization of femoral fractures. A prospective randomized study. *J Bone Joint Surg Am*. 1989;71(3):336–340.
24. Pape HC, Auf'm'Kolk M, Paffrath T, Regel G, Sturm JA, Tscherne H. Primary intramedullary femur fixation in multiple trauma patients with associated lung contusion—a cause of posttraumatic ARDS? *J Trauma*. 1993;34(4):540–547.
25. Bosse MJ, MacKenzie EJ, Riemer BL, et al. Adult respiratory distress syndrome, pneumonia, and mortality following thoracic injury and a femoral fracture treated either with intramedullary nailing with reaming or with a plate. A comparative study. *J Bone Joint Surg Am*. 1997;79(6):799–809.
26. Pape HC, Hildebrand F, Pertschy S, et al. Changes in the management of femoral shaft fractures in polytrauma patients: From early total care to damage control orthopedic surgery. *J Trauma*. 2002;53(3):452–461.
27. Giannoudis PV, Smith RM, Banks RE, Windsor AC, Dickson RA, Guillou PJ. Stimulation of inflammatory markers after blunt trauma. *Br J Surg*. 1998;85:986–990.
28. Giannoudis PV, Smith RM, Bellamy MC, Morrison JF, Dickson RA, Guillou PJ. Stimulation of the inflammatory system by reamed and unreamed nailing of femoral fractures. An analysis of the second hit. *J Bone Joint Surg Br*. 1999;81(2):356–361.
29. Pape HC, Grimme K, Van Griensven M, et al. Impact of intramedullary instrumentation versus damage control for femoral

fractures on immunoinflammatory parameters: Prospective randomized analysis by the EPOFF Study Group. *J Trauma.* 2003; 55(1):7–13.
30. Harwood PJ, Giannoudis PV, Van Griensven M, Krettek C, Pape HC. Alterations in the systemic inflammatory response after early total care and damage control procedures for femoral shaft fracture in severely injured patients. *J Trauma.* 2005;58(3): 446–452.
31. Giannoudis PV, Pape HC, Cohen AP, Krettek C, Smith RM. Review: systemic effects of femoral nailing: From Küntscher to the immune reactivity era. *Clin Orthop Relat Res.* 2002;(404): 378–386.
32. Pape HC, Rixen D, Morley J, et al.; EPOFF Study Group. Impact of the method of initial stabilization for femoral shaft fractures in patients with multiple injuries at risk for complications (borderline patients). *Ann Surg.* 2007;246(3):491–499.
33. Nahm NJ, Vallier HA. Timing of definitive treatment of femoral shaft fractures in patients with multiple injuries: A systematic review of randomized and nonrandomized trials. *J Trauma Acute Care Surg.* 2012;73(5):1046–1063.
34. Vallier HA, Wang X, Moore TA, Wilber JH, Como JJ. Timing of orthopaedic surgery in multiple trauma patients: Development of a protocol for early appropriate care. *J Orthop Trauma.* 2013;27(10):543–551.
35. Vallier HA, Cureton BA, Ekstein C, Oldenburg FP, Wilber JH. Early definitive stabilization of unstable pelvis and acetabulum fractures reduces morbidity. *J Trauma.* 2010;69(3):677–684.
36. Nahm NJ, Como JJ, Wilber JH, Vallier HA. Early appropriate care: Definitive stabilization of femoral fractures within 24 hours of injury is safe in most patients with multiple injuries. *J Trauma.* 2011;71(1):175–185.
37. Vallier HA, Super DM, Moore TA, Wilber JH. Do patients with multiple system injury benefit from early fixation of unstable axial fractures? The effects of timing of surgery on initial hospital course. *J Orthop Trauma.* 2013;27(7):405–412.
38. O'Toole RV, O'Brien M, Scalea TM, Habashi N, Pollak AN, Turen CH. Resuscitation before stabilization of femoral fractures limits acute respiratory distress syndrome in patients with multiple traumatic injuries despite low use of damage control orthopedics. *J Trauma.* 2009;67(5):1013–1021.
39. Canadian Orthopaedic Trauma Society. Reamed versus unreamed intramedullary nailing of the femur: Comparison of the rate of ARDS in multiple injured patients. *J Orthop Trauma.* 2006;20(6): 384–387.
40. Weninger P, Figl M, Spitaler R, Mauritz W, Hertz H. Early unreamed intramedullary nailing of femoral fractures is safe in patients with severe thoracic trauma. *J Trauma.* 2007;62(3):692–696.
41. Brundage SI, McGhan R, Jurkovich GJ, Mack CD, Maier RV. Timing of femur fracture fixation: Effect on outcome in patients with thoracic and head injuries. *J Trauma.* 2002;52(2): 299–307.
42. Giannoudis PV, Veysi VT, Pape HC, Krettek C, Smith MR. When should we operate on major fractures in patients with severe head injuries? *Am J Surg.* 2002;183(3):261–267.
43. Giannoudis PV, Abbott C, Stone M, Bellamy MC, Smith RM. Fatal systemic inflammatory response syndrome following early bilateral femoral nailing. *Intensive Care Med.* 1998;24: 641–642.
44. Copeland CE, Mitchell KA, Brumback RJ, Gens DR, Burgess AR. Mortality in patients with bilateral femoral fractures. *J Orthop Trauma.* 1998;12(5):315–319.
45. Nork SE, Agel J, Russell GV, Mills WJ, Holt S, Routt ML Jr. Mortality after reamed intramedullary nailing of bilateral femur fractures. *Clin Orthop Relat Res.* 2003;(415):272–278.
46. Kobbe P, Micansky F, Lichte P, et al. Increased morbidity and mortality after bilateral femoral shaft fractures: Myth or reality in the era of damage control? *Injury.* 2013;44(2):221–225.
47. Gustilo RB, Anderson JT. Prevention of infection in the treatment of one thousand and twenty-five open fractures of long bones: retrospective and prospective analyses. *J Bone Joint Surg Am.* 1976;58(4):453–458.
48. Blachut PA, Meek RN, O'Brien PJ. External fixation and delayed intramedullary nailing of open fractures of the tibial shaft. A sequential protocol. *J Bone Joint Surg Am.* 1990;72(5): 729–735.
49. Gopal S, Majumder S, Batchelor AG, Knight SL, De Boer P, Smith RM. Fix and Flap: The radical orthopaedic and plastic treatment of severe open fractures of the tibia. *J Bone Joint Surg Br.* 2000;82: 959–966.
50. Gopal S, Giannoudis PV, Murray A, Matthews SJ, Smith RM. The functional outcome of severe, open tibial fractures managed with early fixation and flap coverage. *J Bone Joint Surg Br.* 2004;86(6):861–867.
51. Wood T, Sameem M, Avram R, Bhandari M, Petrisor B. A systematic review of early versus delayed wound closure in patients with open fractures requiring flap coverage. *J Trauma Acute Care Surg.* 2012;72(4):1078–1085.
52. Hull PD, Johnson SC, Stephen DJ, Kreder HJ, Jenkinson RJ. Delayed debridement of severe open fractures is associated with a higher rate of deep infection. *Bone Joint J.* 2014;96:379–384.
53. Lack WD, Karunaker MA, Angerame MR, et al. Type III open tibia fractures: Immediate antibiotic prophylaxis minimizes infection. *J Orthop Trauma.* 2015;29(1):1–6.
54. Pincus D, Byrne JP, Nathens AB, et al. Delay in flap coverage past 7 days increases complications for open tibia fractures: A cohort study of 140 North American trauma centers. *J Orthop Trauma.* 2019;33(4):161–168.
55. McQueen MM, Court-Brown CM. Compartment monitoring in tibial fractures: The pressure threshold for decompression. *J Bone Joint Surg Br.* 1996;78:99–104.
56. Harrington P, Bunola J, Jennings AJ, Bush DJ, Smith RM. Acute compartment syndrome masked by intravenous morphine from a patient-controlled analgesia pump. *Injury.* 2000;31:387–389.
57. Smith RM, Dyer GS, Antonangeli K, et al. Disaster triage after the Haitian earthquake. *Injury.* 2012;43(11):1811–1815.
58. Perren SM. Physical and biological aspects of fracture healing with special reference to internal fixation. *Clin Orthop Relat Res.* 1979;138:175–196.
59. Perren SM. Evolution of the internal fixation of long bone fractures. The scientific basis of biological internal fixation: Choosing a new balance between stability and biology. *J Bone Joint Surg Br.* 2002;84(8):1093–1110.
60. Mueller ME, Allgower M, Schneider R, et al. *Manual of Osteosynthesis.* Springer Verlag; 1970.
61. Helfet DL, Haas NP, Schatzker J, Matter P, Moser R, Hanson B. AO philosophy and principles of fracture management—its evolution and evaluation. *J Bone Joint Surg Am.* 2003;85(6): 1156–1160.
62. Schatzker J, McBroom R, Bruce D. The tibial plateau fracture. The Toronto experience 1968–1975. *Clin Orthop Relat Res.* 1979;(138):94–104.
63. Matta JM. Fractures of the acetabulum: Accuracy of reduction and clinical results in patients managed operatively within three weeks after the injury. *J Bone Joint Surg Am.* 1996;78: 1632–1645.
64. Moed BR, Yu PH, Gruson KI. Functional outcomes of acetabular fractures. *J Bone Joint Surg Am.* 2003;85(10):1879–1883.
65. Sirkin M, Sanders R, DiPasquale T, Herscovici D Jr. A staged protocol for soft tissue management in the treatment of complex pilon fractures. *J Orthop Trauma.* 1999;13(2):78–84.
66. White TO, Guy P, Cooke CJ, et al. The results of early primary open reduction and internal fixation for treatment of OTA 43.C-type tibial pilon fractures: A cohort study. *J Orthop Trauma.* 2010;24(12):757–763.
67. Donaldson LJ, Cook A, Thomson RG. Incidence of fractures in a geographically defined population. *J Epidemiol Community Health.* 1990;44(3):241–245.
68. Garden RS. Low-angle fixation in fractures of the femoral neck. *J Bone Joint Surg Br.* 1961;43:647–663.
69. Parker MJ, Gurusamy K. Arthroplasties (with and without bone cement) for proximal femoral fractures in adults. *Cochrane Database Syst Rev.* 2006;(3):CD001706.

70. Bhandari M, Devereaux PJ, Swiontkowski MF, et al. Internal fixation compared with arthroplasty for displaced fractures of the femoral neck: A meta-analysis. *J Bone Joint Surg Am.* 2003; 85:1673–1681.
71. Queally JM, Harris E, Handoll HH, Parker MJ. Intramedullary nails for extracapsular hip fractures in adults. *Cochrane Database Syst Rev.* 2014;(9):CD004961.
72. Baumgaertner MR, Curtin SL, Lindskog DM, Keggi JM. The value of the tip-apex distance in predicting failure of fixation of peritrochanteric fractures of the hip. *J Bone Joint Surg Am.* 1995;77(7):1058–1064.
73. Schatzker J. Intraarticular malunions and nonunions. *Orthop Clin North Am.* 1990;21(4):743–757.
74. Masquelet AC, Begue T. The concept of induced membrane for reconstruction of long bone defects. *Orthop Clin North Am.* 2010;41(1):27–37.
75. García-Cimbrelo E, Martí-González JC. Circular external fixation in tibial nonunions. *Clin Orthop Relat Res.* 2004;(419):65–70.

28

Pediatric Trauma

Meera Kotagal, Marissa Ray, and Peter T. Masiakos

Key Points

1 **Epidemiology:** Pediatric trauma remains a significant public health problem. Traumatic injuries are the top cause of mortality for children and adolescents in the United States and account for more than 50% of deaths in children younger than 18 years. Management strategies should include emergency medical care as well as injury prevention and systems of trauma care to meet the needs for pediatric patients.

2 **ABCs:** The primary survey should focus on the identification of acute life-threatening injuries. Attention to the airway, breathing, and circulation (ABCs) supersedes all other interventions in the initial resuscitation phase. Centers that care for children should have pediatric resuscitation equipment, such as appropriately sized endotracheal tubes, laryngoscopes, catheters, passive warming lamps, and the Broselow Pediatric Emergency Tape which aides in estimating the weight of the child and facilitates safe, weight-based resuscitation.

3 **Child physical abuse:** Abuse may be difficult to recognize, and a high index of suspicion is needed when evaluating children with injuries. The Pediatric Trauma Society and Western Trauma Association published an evaluation and management algorithm in 2020 as unrecognized cases of abuse can represent with serious or even fatal injuries.

4 **Injury prevention:** As policy makers struggle to allocate limited resources to improve population health, injury prevention programs will play a particularly important role. Regulatory efforts specifically aimed at primary and secondary injury prevention, can reduce health care costs, thereby freeing resources for other concerns.

OVERVIEW AND EPIDEMIOLOGY

Injury has a significant impact on the lives of children and families in the United States and around the world. Traumatic injuries remain the leading killer of children and adolescents in the United States. Injury, both unintentional and nonaccidental, accounts for more than 50% of deaths in children younger than 18 years.[1] The pediatric mortality rate from trauma in the United States is double that of other developed countries, and for every pediatric death there are more than 2,000 emergency department visits.[2] In the United States alone, more than 50,000 children are permanently disabled after trauma, most commonly as the result of traumatic brain injury (TBI).[2] These disabilities account for $14 billion in lifetime medical spend-
1 ing and $66 billion in future wages lost.[3] Therefore, pediatric trauma is a significant public health problem, and management strategies should target not only emergency medical care but also injury prevention and systems of trauma care to meet the needs for pediatric patients.[3]

Although there is a rise in the incidence of penetrating trauma, which now accounts for up to 10% to 20% of trauma activations, the vast majority of pediatric injuries result from blunt trauma with associated closed head injuries that require nonoperative management.

TRAUMA SYSTEMS

The concept of a trauma system was shaped by the publication of a US government report in 1966 "Accidental Death and Disability: the Neglected Disease of Modern Society"[4] and has led to improvements in infrastructure, processes of emergency response, communication, and outcome measurements and quality indicators of responding hospital centers. The Committee on Trauma first categorized Trauma Center designations in 1976.[2] The first Pediatric trauma centers were organized in the 1970s to 1980s; however, even today in the United States, there are too few designated pediatric trauma centers to care for all pediatric trauma patients. The vast majority of pediatric patients are cared for at adult trauma centers[5,6]; as such, the exchange of ideas between adult and pediatric trauma centers and the development of integrated regional trauma systems remain critically important for our care of injured children.[2,7]

Inclusive trauma systems are comprised of facilities within a region according to a tiered-triage system. Each participating facility receives a level designation, and this is used to appropriately triage and refer patients as necessary. Along with these regionalization efforts, advances in pediatric transport have also improved how we care for injured children. Inclusive systems have been shown to improve outcomes because more timely and appropriate transfers can occur. It has become increasingly important to develop and study various "performance indicators" of the quality of care that is delivered to injured pediatric patients. For example, rate of successful splenic salvage is a commonly cited quality indicator in pediatric trauma, and there are reports that children cared for at an adult trauma center have a fivefold higher risk of splenectomy than those at pediatric trauma center.[6–9] Beyond benchmarking mortality rates, which is a rare outcome, other measurable quality indicators include availability of a pediatric intensive care unit with in-house intensivists, radiation exposure from imaging, early neurosurgical intervention for severe head injury, early fixation of femur fractures, operative rates for solid organ injuries, and participation in registry databases to monitor performance over time, such as the Trauma

Quality Improvement Program set up by the American College of Surgeons-Committee on Trauma.[10,11] It is unclear whether superior care is offered to injured children in a dedicated pediatric hospital, compared to an adult hospital; however, it has been demonstrated that pediatric trauma certification and expertise in care of trauma patients are both important factors in optimal care.[12–17]

INITIAL ASSESSMENT, RESUSCITATION, AND STABILIZATION

The evaluation and treatment of traumatic injuries of infants and children requires specific knowledge of pediatric physiology and the physiologic response to injury. Generally, the trauma resuscitation of children follows similar rules that have been described for adults by advanced trauma life support standards. However, there are several special considerations in the initial assessment and subsequent care for children and specific paradigms regarding ancillary studies that are different from those in adults.

As in adults, the primary survey should focus on the identification of acute life-threatening injuries. Attention to the airway, breathing, and circulation (ABCs) is critical in the 2 initial resuscitation phase (**Table 28.1**). All centers that care for children should have sequestered resuscitation equipment designed for children, such as endotracheal tubes (ETTs), laryngoscopes, catheters, and passive warming lamps. Room temperature should be kept warm to limit insensible heat losses in small children. The Broselow Pediatric Emergency Tape aids in estimating the weight of the child by measuring his or her length. A color-coded bar on the tape measures the length of the child and indicates the appropriate equipment sizes and medication doses to perform emergency resuscitation on the child. Designated resuscitation equipment is contained in corresponding, color-coded equipment pouches or drawers (**Fig. 28.1**).

Vital Signs

Pediatric vital signs vary by age (**Table 28.2**). Children are able to maintain normal blood pressures until late hemorrhagic shock (>30% blood loss), and, therefore, subtle changes in heart rate and respiratory rate must be noted. As a general rule, the lower limit of acceptable systolic blood pressure = (age × 2) + 70 mm Hg. For newborns, acceptable systolic blood pressure is 60 mm Hg or greater. Initial fluid resuscitation is indicated when there are signs of hypovolemic shock.

Table 28.1. Pediatric Resuscitation ABCs

Airway "A"
▪ Cardiac arrest most often of respiratory etiology
▪ Use jaw thrust technique and in-line cervical stabilization
▪ Key anatomic differences: larger tongue, more narrow and anterior glottis, and shorter trachea
▪ Miller blade may be easier than the curved Mac blade because the epiglottis is floppy
▪ Size of ETT can be estimated by the size of pinkie finger or Broselow Pediatric Emergency Resuscitation Tape
▪ Consider using an uncuffed ETT in a child less than 8 y or 60 lb
▪ With acute airway obstruction, needle cricothyroidotomy with a 14-g catheter is preferential to open cricothyroidotomy
Breathing "B"
▪ Assess for potential life-threatening thoracic injuries: pneumothorax (open chest wound or tension pneumothorax), hemothorax, flail chest/pulmonary contusions, and rib fractures
▪ Mediastinum of a child is very compliant and can lead to rapid decline from a tension pneumothorax
▪ Children are diaphragmatic breathers; ensure stomach is decompressed with nasogastric tube or orogastric tube in infants, who are obligate nose breathers
Circulation "C"
▪ Hemorrhage is the most common etiology of circulatory compromise in trauma
▪ Also consider obstructive etiologies (cardiac tamponade and tension pneumothorax) and distributive etiologies (neurogenic shock)
▪ Assessment of volume status and shock is difficult because children have impressive physiologic reserve
▪ Tachycardia, tachypnea, altered level of consciousness, and poor peripheral perfusion (mottled cool extremities, weak thready pulses, narrowed pulse pressure, delayed capillary refill) are early but subtle signs of blood loss
▪ Peripheral intravenous (IV) lines are ideal, but when they cannot be obtained, intraosseous lines are quick, reliable, and allow high-volume infusion of any fluid
▪ Definitive IV access can be obtained with a central line
▪ Initial fluid resuscitation is indicated when there are signs of hypovolemic shock. Initial bolus consists of 20 mL/kg of warmed normal saline or lactated Ringer solution
▪ After two initial boluses, all subsequent volume resuscitation should be performed with blood products (10 mL/kg = "1 unit") (**Table 28.3**)
▪ Massive transfusion protocols may be initiated if indicated
▪ Once resuscitated, maintenance fluid requirements (**Table 28.3**) can be estimated using the "4-2-1" rule and isotonic fluids should be administered for all children greater than 28 d
Disability "D"
▪ Perform a brief neurologic assessment
▪ Head injury accounts for the highest degree of morbidity and mortality in children
▪ Secondary insults include ischemia, hypoxia, hypotension, hyperthermia, hypercapnia, acidosis, and increased intracranial pressure (ICP)
▪ The Glasgow Coma Scale (GCS) is modified in young children who are preverbal to measure neurologic function and prognosis. The motor response scale tends to provide the most reliable assessment of function in a preverbal or intubated child (**Table 28.4**)
Exposure ("E")
▪ Allows for a complete head-to-toe physical examination
▪ Children have a larger body surface area ratio and, therefore, lose heat and water quickly and can become hypothermic
▪ Use warm fluids, forced-air warmers (eg, Bair Hugger), warming lights, and warm ambient room temperature to prevent heat loss

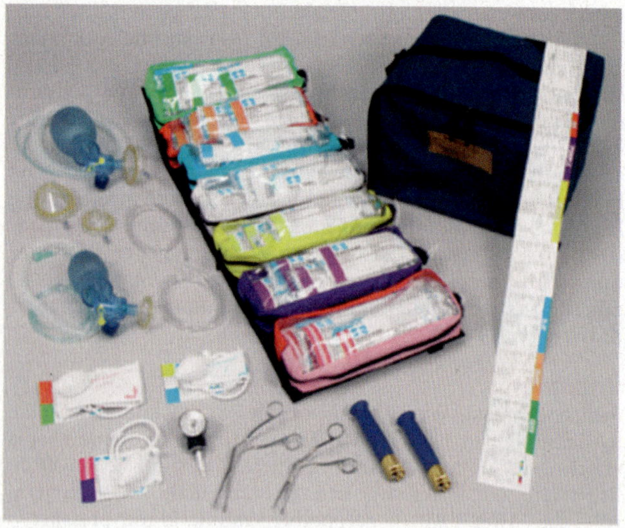

Figure 28.1. Broselow pediatric emergency resuscitation tape.

Fluid Resuscitation

Initial bolus consists of 20 mL/kg of warmed normal saline or lactated Ringer solution. This may be repeated if there is no response or only a transient response, but subsequent volume resuscitation should be performed with blood products (10 mL/kg = "1 unit") (**Table 28.3**). Crystalloid resuscitation should be <40 mL/kg to avoid dilutional coagulopathy and development of ascites/edema.[18] If there is no time for cross-matched, type-specific blood, "O-negative" blood is indicated. Massive transfusion protocols may be initiated at this time if indicated and should include hemostatic resuscitation with packed red blood cells, fresh frozen plasma, and platelets, targeting high plasma-to-red blood cell and platelet-to-red blood cell ratios.[19] In the most recent advanced trauma life support protocols, this has become known as "damage control resuscitation,"[20] espousing permissive hypotension, minimizing crystalloid resuscitation, and promoting early blood product administration for the treatment of the lethal triad (acidosis, coagulopathy, and hypothermia) of severe uncontrolled hemorrhage. There is, however, no evidence-based support for permissive hypotension strategies in pediatric trauma patients. In patients requiring massive transfusion, diagnostic assays such as thromboelastography (TEG) and rotation thromboelastometry (ROTEM) are used to assess whole blood clotting and guide product-based resuscitation with demonstrated decreases in mortality.[21,22] Sources of bleeding can be thought of in terms of body compartments: including the chest, peritoneal cavity, retroperitoneum/pelvis, femur fracture/thigh compartment, and external injury (especially the scalp). In an infant, prior to suture closure of the skull, intracranial hemorrhage may produce hemodynamic instability. Once resuscitated, maintenance fluid requirements (**Table 28.3**) can be estimated using the "4-2-1" rule and isotonic fluids should be administered for all children >28 days (**Fig. 28.2**).[23]

Table 28.3. Fluid Management in Children

Resuscitation Fluids (NS or LR)	
If hypotension or signs of shock	Bolus 20 mL/kg. Repeat if transient or no response and then switch to blood transfusions (10 mL/kg)
Daily Maintenance Fluid Requirements (D5 1/2NS or D10 1/2NS)	
Weight <10 kg	100 mL/kg/d
Weight 11–20 kg	1000 mL + 50 mL/kg/d (for every kg over 10)
Weight >20 kg	1500 mL + 20 mL/kg/d (for every kg over 20)

SECONDARY SURVEY AND ADJUNCT DIAGNOSTIC MODALITIES

Only after the primary assessment is complete, and ABCs are secured, do we move on to the full secondary survey. In reality, with a team approach to management of the pediatric trauma patient, much of the supportive care happens concurrently with the primary and secondary surveys, including placement of intravenous (IV) lines, drawing laboratories, applying monitors and oxygen, and obtaining ancillary diagnostic tests. Adjunct diagnostic modalities and imaging may be used to provide additional information in the evaluation of a pediatric trauma patient. Although diagnostic peritoneal aspiration has been traditionally used to evaluate intra-abdominal injuries in the unstable patient, it has no role in the pediatric population where solid organ injuries are unlikely to require surgery. Focused assessment with sonography in trauma (FAST) examination has significant advantages over more invasive diagnostic maneuvers: the FAST examination can be performed quickly and exposes the patient to no potential harm from delay or ionizing radiation. However, children with intra-abdominal injuries are more frequently managed nonoperatively, and thus the need for rapid decision making regarding operative management is less common. Children also have a relatively higher incidence of solid organ injury without free fluid, and consequently, a negative FAST examination may not obviate the need for an abdominal computed tomography (CT) when there is a clinical suspicion of significant injury.

Table 28.2. Pediatric Vital Signs

	Pulse (Beats/Min)	Systolic Blood Pressure (mm Hg)	Respiration (Breaths/Min)
Newborn (<1 mo)	95–145	60–90	30–60
Infant (1 mo to 1 y)	125–170	75–100	30–60
Toddler (1–2 y)	100–160	80–110	24–40
Preschool (3–4 y)	70–110	80–110	22–34
School age (4–12 y)	70–110	85–120	18–30
Adolescent (>12 y)	55–100	95–120	12–16

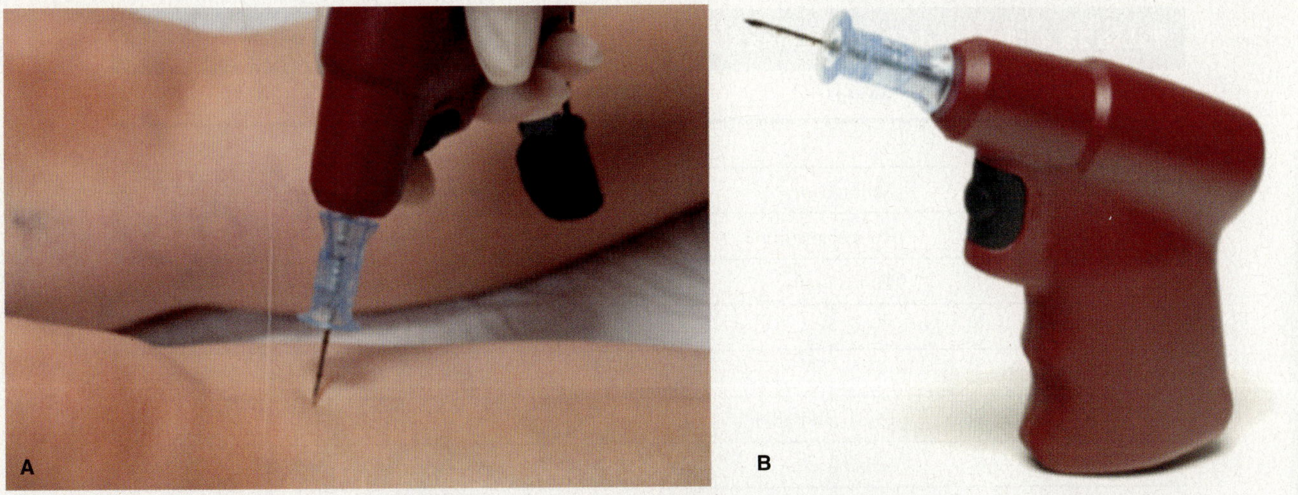

Figure 28.2. **A:** Intraosseous line placement. **B:** EZ-IO drive.

The FAST examination should not be relied on as a standalone screening tool in the pediatric population.[24,25] To date, the largest prospective trial of FAST in stable pediatric trauma patients showed no evidence of benefit, leading the authors to conclude that their findings do not support the routine use of FAST among hemodynamically normal children treated in an ED following blunt trauma.[26] In practice, only 13% of pediatric trauma patients with a suspicion for intra-abdominal injuries undergo FAST examination.[27] Sensitivity in pediatric patients ranges from 50% to 92%, with a rigorous meta-analysis suggesting the sensitivity to be around 66%.[24,25,28,29] Specificity is also very low, and in a hemodynamically normal patient, a positive FAST examination should be followed up with an urgent CT. Bedside FAST may have utility in hemodynamically unstable patients to rapidly identify or rule out intraperitoneal hemorrhage when patients cannot undergo CT, but decision making should include other features such as patient physiology, mechanism, clinical suspicion, and responsiveness to initial resuscitation measures.[25] As its use in children increases, it is likely that FAST will become more reliable, with greater sensitivity and specificity. Findings from chest radiography, anteroposterior pelvis radiography, and the FAST examination, along with the primary and secondary surveys, guide decisions regarding further radiographic examination, including CT or plain radiography.

In addition to a full physical examination, a brief history is essential and is often provided by emergency medical services (EMS) personnel or the parents. An "AMPLE" history helps the provider focus on essential information such as Allergies, Medications, Past medical history, Last meal, and Events surrounding the traumatic incident. Blunt trauma is the most common mechanism after which children present for evaluation. Children are more prone to multisystem trauma due to their small body size and more compliant body (less protective bones, muscle, and torso fat). Blunt trauma can result in injury patterns that resemble penetrating injuries, without significant external signs of trauma. Careful attention to a bruise on the abdominal wall resulting from a bicycle handlebar should lead to a more thorough investigation of the abdomen. A lap belt mark across the abdomen may raise concerns of lumbar spine fracture (Chance fracture), with an associated risk of small bowel injury. Therefore, a thorough history, mechanism of injury, and focused examination of the entire child is mandated so that signs of forceful impact can be elucidated.

MANAGEMENT OF SPECIFIC INJURIES

Traumatic Brain Injury

TBI is the leading cause of death and disability in children,[30–32] and is an important determinant of outcome. Child physical abuse (CPA) is the most common cause of head injury in children younger than 2 years, and blunt head trauma from motor vehicle crashes (MVCs), falls, or bicycle/pedestrian crashes are responsible for most injuries in children older than 2 years. Injury prevention strategies are necessary for improving outcomes of the primary TBI. However, reduction of secondary injury patterns is critical in children, who have impressive physiologic reserve and potential for rehabilitation after brain injury. The focus must be on preserving cerebral oxygenation and perfusion, and mitigation of toxic exposures to minimize secondary brain injury. This includes treating or preventing hypotension, hypo/hyperoxia, hyper/hypocarbia with generation of ischemia reperfusion free-radicals, hyperthermia, seizures, and intracranial hypertension. The Glasgow Coma Scale (GCS) (and modified GCS for infants) is a universal tool that can be used for rapid assessment of neurologic function and is based on verbal response, motor function, and eye opening. Moderate TBI is considered GCS score of 9 to 12 or 13 and severe TBI includes GCS score of ≤8, the definition of a coma (**Table 28.4**).

Mild Traumatic Brain Injury

Children with minor head trauma can present the greatest challenge to emergency department personnel. Eastern Association for the Surgery of Trauma (EAST) guidelines define mild traumatic brain injury (MTBI) to be interchangeable with the term "Concussion," involving a blunt force mechanism with alteration in brain function (ie, GCS score of 13 to 15) but by definition must have a normal head CT if performed.[33] CT scans provide the most accurate and expeditious means of diagnosis but expose many pediatric patients to unnecessary radiation. Evidence-based clinical decision tools have helped identify the population of children who benefit most from radiologic evaluation. The TBI study group for PECARN (Pediatric Emergency Care Applied Research Network) has developed tools for assessment of children after blunt head injury.[33–38] The "PECARN Rules"[35] (**Algorithm 28.1**) identify children at very low risk (<0.05%) of having clinically important TBI requiring intervention. These patients can avoid CT and be discharged safely with appropriate instructions. Children with MTBI (GCS score of 14 to 15) who underwent CT can be safely discharged home without further neurologic monitoring, if their head CT scan is normal.[33,36] Even those with an isolated skull fracture can be discharged home from the emergency department with strict discharge instructions and return precautions.[37–40] At this point, routine structural or functional imaging modalities such as magnetic resonance imaging, functional magnetic resonance imaging, or positron emission tomography for diagnosis or prognosis of MTBI are not supported.[33]

Table 28.4. Modified Glasgow Coma Scale in Children

	Infant	Child
Eye Opening		
4	Spontaneous	Spontaneous
3	To verbal stimuli	To verbal stimuli
2	To pain only	To pain only
1	None	None
Verbal Response		
5	Coos and babbles	Oriented, appropriate
4	Irritable cries	Confused
3	Cries to pain	Inappropriate words
2	Moans to pain	Incomprehensible sounds
1	None	None
Motor Response[a]		
6	Moves spontaneously and purposefully	Obeys commands
5	Withdraws to touch	Localizes painful stimuli
4	Withdraws in response to pain	Withdraws in response to pain
3	Abnormal flexion posture to pain	Flexion in response to pain
2	Abnormal extension posture to pain	Extension in response the pain
1	None	None

[a]If patient is intubated, unconscious, or preverbal, the most important part of this scale is motor response and should be closely evaluated.

Prognosis and outcome in MTBI, especially as it relates to "return to learn or return to play" after concussion, is still hotly debated. Standardized tools, such as the Immediate Postconcussion Assessment and Cognitive Testing Battery (ImPACT), exist to aid clinicians in functional assessment of patients with MTBI.[41] The well-known NCAA Concussion Study from 2003 found that high-level athletes were more likely to sustain repeat concussions, which were associated with a longer recovery time,[42] and it has been increasingly recognized that repeat concussions can have permanent and sometimes devastating effects. In 2010, the American Academy of Pediatrics officially endorsed the International Conference on Concussion in Sport recommendations for a graduated "Return to Play" protocol.[43,44] The CDC HEADS UP guidelines also incorporate these recommendations[45] and provide resources for schools, coaches, and primary care providers on returning to school and sports after a concussion. Data are lacking in the efficacy of these guidelines and their role in preventing recurrent concussions.[46] Patients may also suffer from lingering symptoms of headache, dizziness, fatigue, sleep disturbance, irritability, anxiety or depression, and impaired memory and concentration, commonly referred to as "postconcussive syndrome," a poorly understood entity.[33]

Moderate to Severe TBI

More serious head injury needs to be evaluated and treated expeditiously. The goal of initial assessment and resuscitation in a severely brain-injured patient is to minimize or prevent secondary brain injury. Attention to ABCs is critical, with maintenance of normotension and normoxia. Prehospital management should include supplemental oxygen, with equal or worse outcomes with endotracheal intubation compared to bag-mask ventilation, likely due to higher rates of procedural failure.[47] Supraglottic airways are often used in adults but are less commonly employed in the pediatric population. Children with severe TBI benefit from treatment in a pediatric trauma center over adult trauma center, especially in very young children.[48,49] Management of severe TBI in the pediatric intensive care unit is largely focused on management of elevated intracranial pressure (ICP) and maintenance of cerebral perfusion pressure.[50] The first guidelines for acute medical management of severe TBI in infants, children, and adolescents were published in 2003 then revised in 2012 and most recently updated in 2019.[51–54] These guidelines, composed mostly of class II or III evidence, incorporate clinical evidence and expert panel opinion. From these guidelines, an algorithm for the management of acute intracranial hypertension was developed (**Algorithm 28.2**), which has served as a template for clinical protocols for patient care and research. The 2012 and 2019 guidelines updated and expanded recommendations in the domains of management (**Table 28.5**), thresholds (**Table 28.6**), and treatments (**Table 28.7**). Of note, these guidelines incorporate evidence with two separate primary outcomes: improvement of overall outcomes and ICP control, which may at times seem contradictory. For example, moderate hypothermia (30 °C to 33 °C) is not recommended over normothermia to improve overall outcomes including mortality (Cool Kids trial)[55]; however, moderate hypothermia has been shown to improve ICP control.[56,57] Overall, there is still a paucity of high-quality, level I evidence to make specific treatment plans for children with severe TBI, but this allows for a wide variety of clinical approaches that are considered within the guidelines of pediatric care.

Spine Trauma

Cervical spine injuries (CSIs) in blunt trauma pediatric patients occur in less than 2% of seriously injured children.

Algorithm 28.1

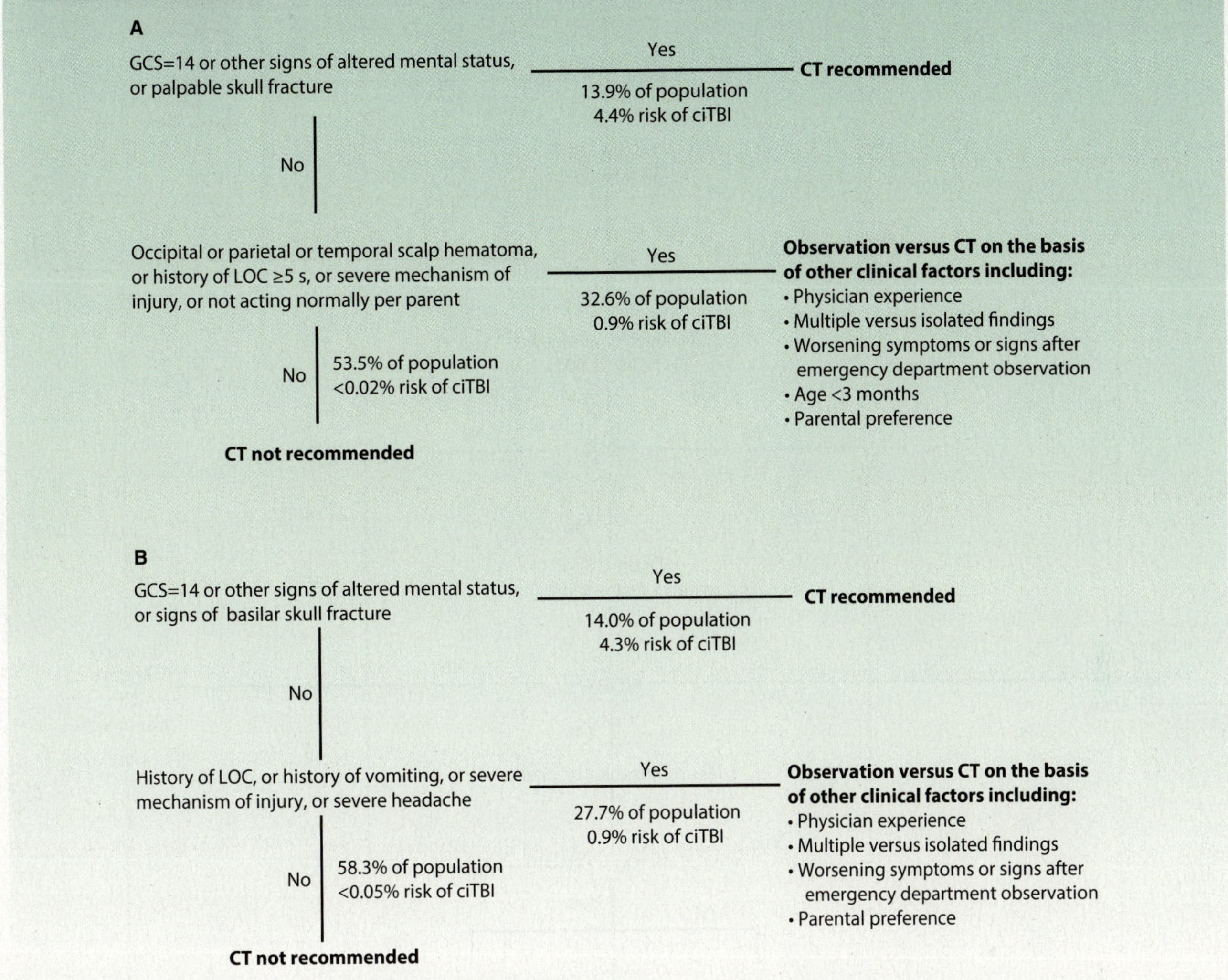

Algorithm 28.1. PECARN rules to identify children at very low risk of clinically important TBI. CT algorithm for children younger than 2 years (**A**) and for those aged 2 years and older (**B**) with GCS scores of 14 to 15 after head trauma. ciTBI, clinically important traumatic brain injury; GCS, Glasgow Coma Scale; LOC, loss of consciousness. (From Kuppermann N, Holmes JF, Dayan PS, et al. Identification of children at very low risk of clinically-important brain injuries after head trauma: a prospective cohort study. *Lancet*. 2009;374[9696]:1160–1170.)

Despite this low incidence, many clinicians obtain radiographs to exclude CSI. The added benefit of routine imaging in the pediatric trauma evaluation is debatable. In recent years, concerns have been raised about the liberal use of plain films, CT scans, and magnetic resonance images in children with reference to imaging-related short- and long-term morbidity, resource consumption, and cost. The increased risk of fatal and nonfatal cancers associated with CT-related radiation has gained attention both by physicians and consumers. Both the US Food and Drug Administration (FDA) Center for Devices and Radiological Health and the National Cancer Institute have published guidelines designed to limit unnecessary imaging in children, and initiatives such as the Choosing Wisely campaign have contributed to eliminating unnecessary imaging from everyday practice. Although proponents of liberal imaging argue that a single missed CSI may cost more than multiple diagnostic tests, the use of non–evidence-based tests may inspire suboptimal practice with an undefined risk–benefit ratio.

Two seminal studies (NEXUS and Canadian Cervical Spine Rules [CCR])[58,59] have examined whether clinical criteria (neurologic deficit, cervical spine tenderness, intoxication, decreased mental status, and distracting injuries) can rule out CSI in adults without the need of imaging. These criteria have been applied to pediatric patients in a manuscript by Viccellio and colleagues, who found that nearly 20% of ordered imaging could have been avoided.[60] The American College of Radiology published updated guidelines for obtaining imaging based on current evidence and a panel of expert pediatric specialists.[61] The PECARN, NEXUS, and Pieretti–Vanmarcke criteria for imaging in accidental spine trauma are summarized in **Table 28.8**.[62–64] For children younger than 16 years with suspected thoracolumbar spine trauma, plan radiographs are usually appropriate as the initial imaging. There was a lack of high-level evidence and no consensus among the panel regarding the use of CT or MRI as initial imaging modality for suspected cervical, thoracic, or lumbar spine injuries.[53]

Mechanism and Location of Injury

MVC remains the most common mechanism of CSI for the youngest age group with falls the most common mechanism for ages 2 to 9 years old.[65]

Conventional wisdom has taught that the position of a CSI in children was related to age, with the predominance of upper C-spine injuries seen in infants and toddlers and lower C-spine injuries seen in adolescents. However, National Trauma Data

Algorithm 28.2A

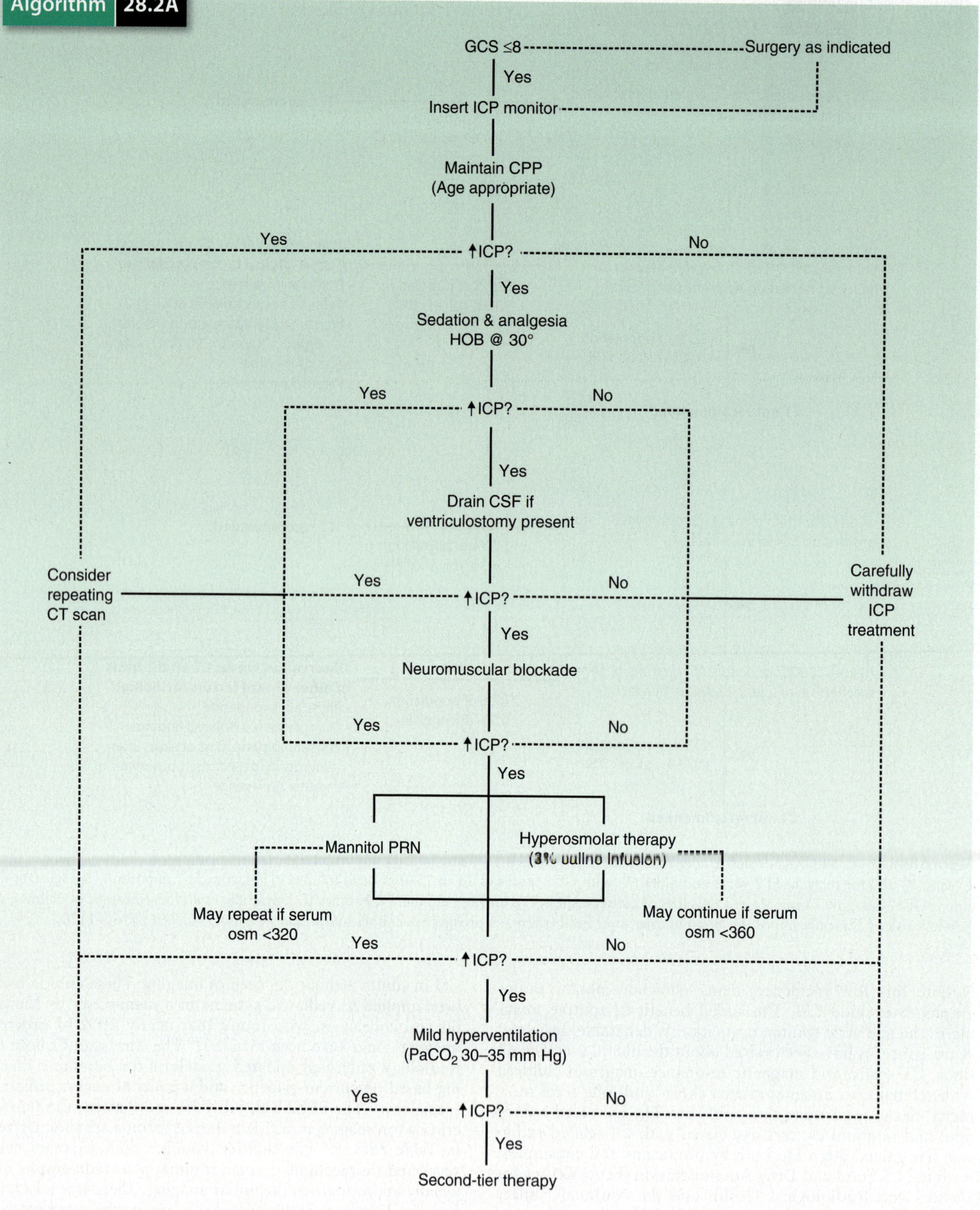

Algorithm 28.2A. Algorithm generated by the Brain Trauma Foundation Committee for the third edition of the *Guidelines for the Medical Management of Severe Traumatic Brain Injury in Infants, Children, and Adolescents* for first-tier therapies (A) and second-tier therapies (B).

Bank data show that the number of fractures to the upper C-spine and lower C-spine was nearly equal (53% and 47%, respectively) in young patients (age <8).[66] Despite the low incidence of CSI, until the cervical spine is cleared, it should be immobilized, ideally with an age/size appropriate hard collar. Such collars should be stocked in all trauma centers that care for pediatric patients.

Spinal Cord Injury without Radiographic Abnormality

Spinal cord injury without radiographic abnormality was first defined in a series of children with signs of acute traumatic spinal cord injury in the absence of bony findings on cervical spine radiographs, flexion–extension films, or CT scans.[67] The authors noted that these patients had neurologic deficits or a

Algorithm 28.2B

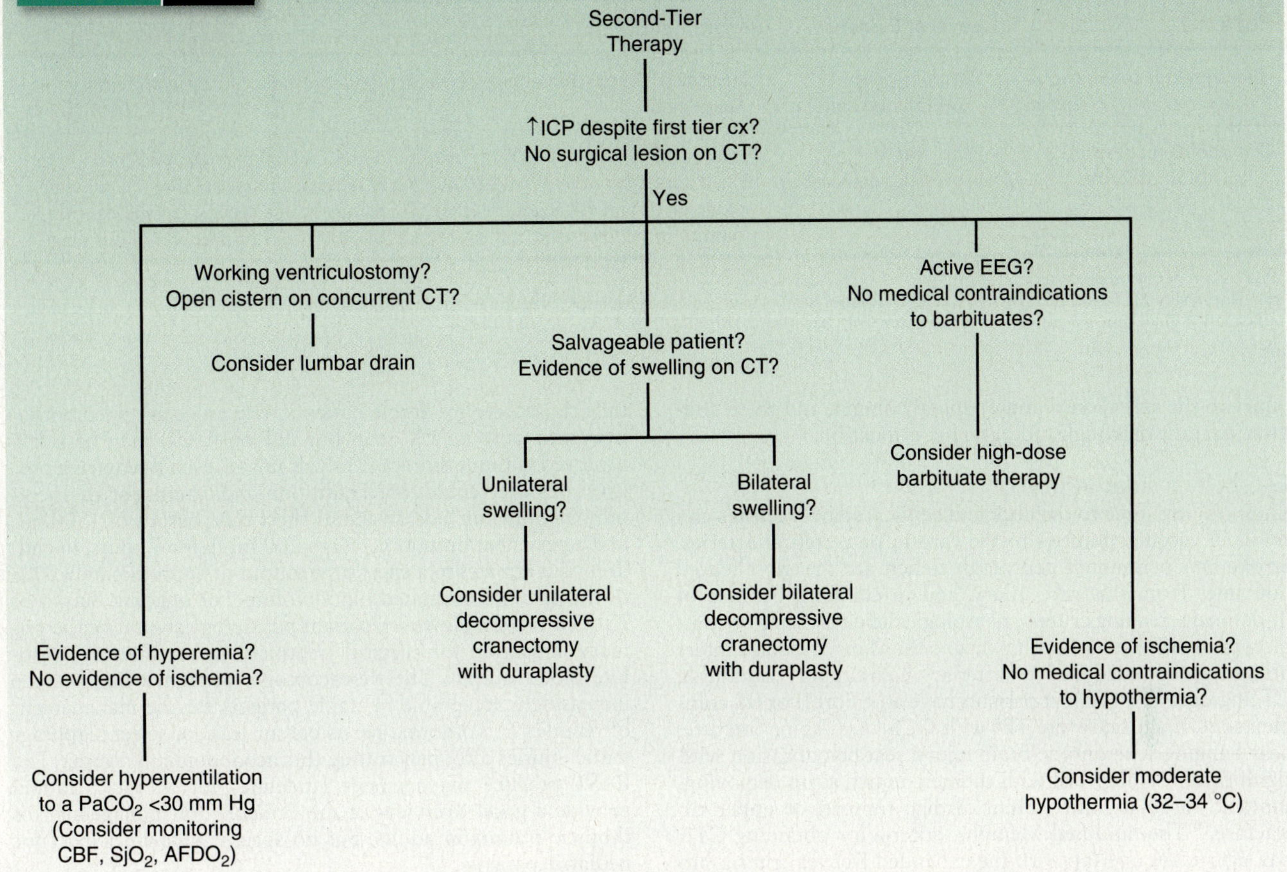

Algorithm 28.2B. (*Continued*) CBF, cerebral blood flow, EEG, electroencephalogram, ICP, intracranial pressure, PRx, pressure reactivity index, TCD, transcranial Doppler untrasonography. (From Kochanek PM, Tasker RC, Bell MJ, et al. Management of pediatric severe traumatic brain injury: 2019 consensus and guidelines-based algorithm for first and second tier therapies. *Pediatr Crit Care Med*. 2019;20(3):269–279.)

history of transient paresthesia, numbness, or paralysis, and a delay of symptoms occurred in approximately half of the patients.

In recent years, as efforts to limit ionizing radiation exposure in children have increased, magnetic resonance imaging has become a mainstay in the workup of children with presumed CSI or neurologic deficits on physical examination. As a result, more children have been found to have demonstrable injury to the spinal cord or soft tissue components of the spinal column vertebral body growth plates.[68,69] As a result of this advent of new neuroimaging paradigms, the diagnosis of spinal cord injury without radiographic abnormality has become questionable. Although the trend has been to limit radiography in children (with good reason), it is important to remember that young patients with blunt trauma who have a history of any transient neurologic symptom may have a significant

Table 28.5. Summary of Evidence Generated from 2019 Pediatric TBI Guidelines: Monitoring

Topic	Level of Evidence	Recommendation
Intracranial pressure monitoring	III (to improve overall outcomes)	"Use of ICP monitoring is suggested"
Advanced neuromonitoring	III (to improve overall outcomes)	"If $PbrO_2$ monitoring is used, k maintaining a level >10 mm Hg is suggested"
Neuroimaging	III (to improve overall outcomes)	"Excluding the possibility of elevated ICP on the basis of a normal initial (0–6 h after injury) CT examination of the brain is not suggested in comatose pediatric patients" "Routinely obtaining a repeat CT scan >24 h after the admission and initial follow-up is not suggested for decisions about neurosurgical intervention, unless there is either evidence of neurologic deterioration or increasing ICP"

ICP, intracranial pressure.
From Kochanek PM, Tasker RC, Carney N, et al. Guidelines for the management of pediatric severe traumatic brain injury, third edition: update of the brain trauma foundation guidelines, executive summary. *Pediatr Crit Care Med*. 2019;20(3):280–289. *Neurosurgery*, 84(6):1169–1178. https://doi.org/10.1093/neuros/nyz051.

Table 28.6. Summary of Evidence Generated from the 2019 Pediatric TBI Guidelines: Thresholds

Topic	Level of Evidence	Recommendation
Threshold for treatment of intracranial hypertension	III (to improve overall outcomes)	"Treatment of intracranial pressure targeting a threshold of <20 mm Hg is suggested"
Thresholds for cerebral perfusion pressure	III (to improve overall outcomes)	"Treatment to maintain CPP at a minimum of 40 mm Hg is suggested" "A CPP target between 40 and 50 mm Hg is suggested to ensure that the minimum value of 40 mm Hg is not breached. There may be age-specific thresholds with infants at the lower end and adolescents at or above the upper end of this range"

CPP, cerebral perfusion pressure.
From Kochanek PM, Tasker RC, Carney N, et al. Guidelines for the management of pediatric severe traumatic brain injury, third edition: update of the brain trauma foundation guidelines, executive summary. *Pediatr Crit Care Med*. 2019;20(3):280–289.

injury to the spinal cord and/or spinal column, and these children warrant thorough radiographic evaluation.

Cerebrovascular Injury

Blunt trauma force to the neck and cervical spine fractures can result in vascular injuries to the carotid or vertebral arteries. Stroke and permanent neurologic deficit are the most feared outcomes from this rare injury, and in children, because of ill-defined screening criteria, neurologic deficit is the most common presenting symptom for diagnosis. Many trauma centers utilize the expanded Denver criteria, which supports obtaining CT angiography (CTA) if patients have a Le Fort II or III, complex skull fracture, severe TBI with GCS <6, C-spine fracture, near hanging with anoxic brain injury, seat belt abrasion with significant swelling, TBI with thoracic injury, scalp degloving, thoracic vascular injury, blunt cardiac rupture, or upper rib fracture.[70] The modified Memphis criteria for obtaining CTA has significant overlap with the expanded Denver criteria but includes Horner syndrome and neurologic exam findings not otherwise explained by imaging.[71] In patients with imaging-confirmed BCVI, antithrombotic treatment should commence as soon as safe and continue for at least 3 months with follow-up imaging. A recent meta-analysis of pediatric blunt cerebrovascular injury recommended screening high-risk pediatric patients with CTA of the neck and treatment with anticoagulation in patients with confirmed injuries.[72]

Thoracic Trauma

The primary survey is designed to identify acute life-threatening thoracic injuries that require immediate intervention (**Table 28.9**).[73] Once bilateral breath sounds and adequate ventilation and oxygenation are confirmed, chest x-ray (CXR) is an urgent part of any pediatric trauma evaluation and can identify most other acute thoracic injuries. FAST examination can evaluate for pericardial fluid and in experienced hands can identify pneumothorax or pleural effusion.

Blunt Thoracic Injury

Blunt trauma, most commonly from MVCs, is the most common mechanism for thoracic trauma in pediatric patients. Children have a more flexible, cartilaginous rib cage, and, therefore, serious intrathoracic injuries can occur in the absence of obvious external trauma or rib fractures. Children also have a more mobile mediastinum, predisposing them to tension pneumothorax with subsequent cardiopulmonary collapse from impaired venous return.

Pulmonary contusions are one of the most common thoracic injuries after blunt trauma. The diagnosis is made on CXR in which infiltrates are identified that do not follow anatomic boundaries. Parenchymal edema peaks at 24 to 36 hours postinjury, as the contusion "blossoms" on CXR, and requires admission for monitoring, oxygen therapy, or intubation and respiratory support if needed. Any evidence of hemothorax or pneumothorax seen on CXR should be managed initially with tube thoracostomy. Stable patients with an occult pneumothorax (seen only on CT scan but not on CXR) may be safely observed without thoracostomy drainage, even if requiring positive pressure ventilation. Traditional indications for thoracotomy in adults include an initial chest tube output of 1500 mL and a persistent output of 150 to 200 mL/h for 4 hours. In children, this equates to a chest tube output of approximately 20% of the patient's estimated blood volume, or ongoing output of 2 to 3 mL/kg/h. However, patient physiology should be the primary indication for surgical treatment rather than the absolute blood output. The thoracoscopic approach has become increasingly acceptable in stable patients for the management of retained hemothorax, persistent air leak, or select diaphragmatic injuries after penetrating thoracoabdominal trauma. The EAST practice management guidelines for thoracic trauma provide a good overview of the evidence for management of thoracic trauma in adults, but no specific guidelines exist for pediatric patients.[74]

Penetrating Thoracic Injury

Only around 10% to 20% of thoracic trauma in the pediatric population is from penetrating injury, most often from firearms, with high levels of morbidity and mortality.[75] Emergency bedside thoracotomy is indicated for patients who present pulseless to the emergency department with signs of life and penetrating thoracic trauma. Pediatric patients have worse outcomes after ED thoracotomy, which is thought to be attributed to disproportionately higher incidence of blunt trauma rather than penetrating trauma as the cause of thoracic injury in children.[76] An analysis of the National Trauma Data Bank found that no pediatric patients survived ED thoracotomy after blunt trauma, and there is no role for emergency thoracotomy for patients without signs of life after blunt trauma.[77,78]

Cardiac and Aortic Injury

Other serious thoracic injuries are very rare in children but include blunt aortic injury and blunt cardiac injury. CXR is a useful initial test as there is limited value in chest CT when a patient has a normal CXR.[79] Widened mediastinum on CXR from a physiologic thymic shadow is quite commonly seen in young children. However, with the appropriate mechanism, including blunt thoracic trauma with a significant deceleration mechanism, and abnormal contour of mediastinum, CT chest should be obtained to identify intrathoracic vascular injuries.[79,80] Treatment, as in adults, relies on strict antihypertensive therapy and operative repair, including an endovascular approach in children big enough to accommodate a stent (although this has not been standardized in pediatric patients). Blunt cardiac injury (most commonly myocardial contusion) can also be challenging to diagnose but occurs most commonly after motor vehicle collision or pedestrian trauma. Abnormalities on EKG are the main findings in myocardial contusion. Traditional risk factors such as sternal fracture or

Table 28.7. Summary of Evidence Generated from the 2019 Pediatric TBI Guidelines: Treatments

Topic	Level of Evidence	Recommendation
Hyperosmolar therapy	II (for ICP control)	"Bolus hypertonic saline (3%) is recommended in patients with intracranial hypertension. Recommended effective doses for acute use range between 2 and 5 mL/kg over 10–20 min."
	III (for ICP control)	"Continuous infusion of hypertonic saline is suggested in patients with intracranial hypertension, the minimum dose needed to maintain intracranial pressure <20 mm Hg is suggested" "Bolus of 23.4% hypertonic saline is suggested for refractory ICP, suggested dose is 0.5 mL/kg with a maximum of 30 mL"
Analgesics, sedatives, and neuromuscular blockade	III (for ICP control)	"With use of multiple ICP-related therapies, as well as appropriate use of analgesia and sedation in routine ICU care, avoiding bolus administration of midazolam and/or fentanyl during ICP crises is suggested due to risks of cerebral hypoperfusion"
Cerebrospinal fluid drainage	III (for ICP control)	"Cerebrospinal fluid drainage through an external ventricular drain is suggested to manage increased ICP"
Seizure prophylaxis	III (for seizure prevention)	"Prophylactic treatment is suggested to reduce the incidence of early (within 7 d) PTS" "insufficient evidence to recommend levetiracetam over phenytoin based on either efficacy in preventing early PTS or toxicity"
Ventilation therapies	III (to improve overall outcomes)	"Prophylactic severe hyperventilation to a $PaCO_2$<30 mm Hg in the initial 48 h after injury is not suggested" "If hyperventilation is used in the management of refractory intracranial hypertension, advanced neuromonitoring for evaluation of cerebral ischemia is suggested"
Temperature control/ hypothermia	II (to improve overall outcomes)	"Prophylactic moderate (32 °C–33 °C) hypothermia is not recommended over normothermia to improve overall outcomes"
	III (for ICP control)	"Moderate (32 °C–33 °C) hypothermia is suggested for ICP control"
Barbiturates	III (for ICP control)	"High-dose barbiturate therapy is suggested in hemodynamically stable patients with refractory intracranial hypertension despite maximal medical and surgical management"
Decompressive craniectomy	III (for ICP control)	"Decompressive craniectomy is suggested to treat neurologic deterioration, herniation, or intracranial hypertension refractory to medical management"
Nutrition	II (to improve overall outcomes)	"Use of an immune-modulating diet is not recommended"
	III (to improve overall outcomes)	"Initiation of early enteral nutritional support (within 72 h from injury) is suggested to decrease mortality and improve outcomes"
Corticosteroids	III (to improve overall outcomes)	"The use of corticosteroids is not suggested to improve outcome or reduce ICP"

ICP, intracranial pressure, PTS, posttraumatic seizures.
From Kochanek PM, Tasker RC, Carney N, et al. Guidelines for the management of pediatric severe traumatic brain injury, third edition: update of the brain trauma foundation guidelines, executive summary. *Pediatr Crit Care Med*. 2019;20(3):280–289.

upper rib fractures do not appear to correlate with blunt cardiac injury. The EAST guidelines, although designed for adult patients, recommend an EKG and troponin I if blunt cardiac injury is suspected.[81] If both studies are normal, this effectively rules it out. If either is abnormal, the child should be admitted to a monitored bed.

Traumatic Asphyxia

Traumatic asphyxia occurs in children because of their flexible thoracic wall in the setting of direct blunt compression, most often after a motor vehicle collision or crush injury. At the time of injury, if the glottis is closed and the thoracoabdominal muscles are tensed, the increased intrathoracic pressure is transmitted through the central venous system (inferior and superior vena cava) to the brain and solid organs. Typical signs of traumatic asphyxia include subconjunctival hemorrhage and petechiae of the chest, shoulders, and head, with subsequent bronze discoloration of the skin. Supportive care in a monitored setting is the standard of care for these children, watching for signs of airway edema.

Abdominal Trauma

Blunt mechanism of injury is the most common cause of abdominal trauma in children. Assessment of abdominal trauma in pediatric patients can be challenging. Vomiting, abdominal tenderness, and seat belt signs are signs and symptoms that

Table 28.8. American College of Radiology Appropriateness Criteria

Name of Rule	Study Age Group	Criteria
PECARN	0 to <16 y	High risk for cervical spine injury (do imaging) if one or more of the following are present: 1. Altered mental status 2. Focal neurologic findings 3. Neck pain 4. Torticollis 5. Substantial torso injury 6. Conditions predisposing to cervical spine injury 7. Diving 8. High-risk motor vehicle crash
NEXUS	2–100 y	Low risk for cervical spine injury (no imaging) if patients have all of the following: 1. Absence of tenderness at the posterior midline of the C-spine 2. Absence of a focal neurologic deficit 3. Normal level of alertness 4. No evidence of intoxication 5. Absence of clinically apparent pain that might distract the patient from the pain of a C-spine injury
Pieretti–Vanmarcke	≤3 y	Low risk: Weighted score 0 to 1 points (negative predictive value 99.83%) High Risk: Weighted score ≥2 to 8 points GCS < 14 (3 points) GCS_{EYE} = 1 (2 points) Motor vehicle crash (2 points) Age 25–36 mo (1 point)

GCS, Glasgow Coma Scale.
From Expert Panel on Pediatric Imaging; Kadom N, Palasis S, Pruthi S, et al. ACR appropriateness criteria® suspected spine trauma-child. *J Am Coll Radiol.* 2019;16(5S):S286–S299.

increase the likelihood of abdominal injuries. CT scan with IV contrast is the best assessment tool for abdominal trauma and despite concerns for radiation exposure, is an important diagnostic tool if indicated. PECARN has similarly developed rules and algorithms to identify a low-risk patient who can safely avoid abdominal CT.[82–84] If an examinable child (GCS score of >13) had no evidence of abdominal or chest wall trauma (including seat belt sign), no abdominal pain, tenderness or vomiting, and normal bilateral breath sounds, the rule had a 99.9% negative predictive value for intra-abdominal injuries requiring intervention[82,84] and was more sensitive than clinical suspicion.[83] Another widely used clinical prediction tool designed by Streck et al. found that patients without abdominal pain, normal abdominal exam, normal CXR, low AST, and normal pancreatic enzymes are at extremely low risk for intra-abdominal injury and can forgo CT scan.[85] After a normal abdominal CT scan, most patients can safely be discharged if otherwise stable (sensitivity 97.8%). However, most missed injuries were hollow viscous injuries, which are difficult to identify on CT and should be suspected in patients with seat belt sign, free fluid on CT, or leukocytosis.[86]

Penetrating abdominal trauma is much less common in children than in adults but should be managed similarly. Laparotomy is indicated in the hemodynamically unstable

Table 28.9. Acute Life-Threatening Thoracic Injuries

Injury	Diagnosis	Management
Airway obstruction	Apnea or stridor, maxillofacial trauma.	Definitive tracheal intubation (oro- or nasotracheal) or cricothyroidotomy
Flail chest	Paradoxical chest wall motion.	Positive pressure ventilation
Tension pneumothorax (PTX)	Respiratory distress, tracheal deviation, hypotension, distended neck veins, absent unilateral breath sounds, **hyperresonance to percussion**	Needle decompression (2nd interspace, midclavicular line), followed by placement of chest tube (4th interspace, anterior axillary line)
Open pneumothorax	Open wound into chest → **"sucking chest wound"**	Sterile gauze (secure on three sides) and placement of chest tube
Hemothorax	Absent breath sounds, **dullness to percussion**, hypotension	Chest tube placement. Massive hemothorax necessitates thoracotomy
Cardiac tamponade	Distended neck veins, muffled heart sounds, hypotension (**Beck triad**), pulsus paradoxus	Pericardiocentesis (or emergency thoracotomy if pulseless)

patient, in patients with evisceration, or those with peritonitis on physical exam. Patients with abdominal stab wounds without the aforementioned findings may be watched with serial examinations to avoid the morbidity associated with negative laparotomy.[87] Laparoscopy can also be considered for hemodynamically normal patients with penetrating injury to determine whether it has violated the peritoneum and further exploration of intra-abdominal contents is needed.

Damage control laparotomy is an established operative approach for hemodynamically unstable trauma patient in hemorrhagic shock and is utilized in approximately 5% of all laparotomies for trauma in both adults and children.[88] The goal of this approach is to avoid the onset of the lethal triad: hypothermia, coagulopathy, and acidosis. The procedure is abbreviated and focused on maintaining the priorities of hemorrhage control, followed by control of contamination and temporary abdominal closure, with plans to return for definitive repairs after resuscitation and warming in the ICU, usually 24 to 48 hours later. The decision for damage control should be made early in the operative course to minimize exposure time in the operating room and avoid irreversible shock and its sequelae. Although well described and widely adopted within the adult trauma population, data are less available in the pediatric population but theoretically of even greater importance as children have small circulating blood volumes and are more prone to hypothermia.[88]

Solid Organ Injuries

Most solid organ injuries (spleen, liver, and kidney) are managed nonoperatively after blunt trauma.[89] Most of these injuries are identified or evaluated by CT and can be graded according to American Association for the Surgery of Trauma (AAST) grading system for prognostic value.[90] APSA guidelines recommend admission to an ICU if patient has abdominal vital signs after initial resuscitation and should be treated with bedrest, labs every 6 hours, and NPO until vital signs normalize. Indications for laparotomy include ongoing hemodynamic instability with hematocrit drop and blood transfusion requiring greater than 20 mL/kg of product or evidence of hollow viscous injury. If admitted to the floor, patients should have no activity or diet restrictions with minimization of blood draws during observation. Discharge is based on clinical condition rather than injury grade and patients may be safely discharged if they have normal vital signs, no abdominal pain, and can tolerate a diet. Postdischarge activity should be restricted to injury grade plus 2 weeks and patients who continue to remain asymptomatic do not need follow-up imaging.[91,92] The American College of Surgeons' pediatric trauma consortium (ATOMAC) developed a practice management algorithm for solid organ injury, which is now used at many pediatric trauma centers throughout the United States (**Algorithm 28.3**).[93] Similar to APSA guidelines, this algorithm also supports management on the basis of hemodynamic status rather than injury grade.

Angioembolization in Solid Organ Injury

While used more often in adults, angioembolization performed by interventional radiologists has been shown to be safe and effective in pediatric patients with radiographic findings that demonstrate ongoing bleeding from a solid organ injury.[94] APSA guidelines support the use of interventional radiology for embolization in ongoing bleeding to improve organ salvage and maximize nonoperative interventions.[95,96]

Hollow Viscous Injury

Hollow viscous injuries occur after blunt abdominal trauma, such as bicycle handlebar injuries or lap belt injuries (often associated with Chance vertebral fracture). Diagnosis can be challenging with current radiographic techniques. Findings on CT might include free fluid in the absence of solid organ injuries, free intraperitoneal air, or extravasation of oral contrast. In the setting of abdominal wall ecchymosis (seat belt sign), leukocytosis, or abdominal tenderness, patients should be closely monitored with serial abdominal examinations and blood count. Evidence for evolving peritonitis, fever, leukocytosis, or systemic inflammatory response syndrome physiology should prompt surgical exploration, either laparoscopic or by laparotomy. Intramural duodenal hematomas are managed conservatively without surgical intervention but may take several weeks to resolve, requiring nasogastric tube (NG) drainage and total parenteral nutrition (TPN) in the interim. Delayed stricture after partial thickness luminal injury or mesenteric injury can present days to weeks after an injury, with symptoms of partial or complete small bowel obstruction.

Pancreatic and Biliary Injury

Pancreatic injury classification by AAST injury grade divides patients into those without ductal injury (grades 1 to 2) and those with duct disruption (grades 3 to 5). Lipase is useful to screen for pancreatic injury but may be normal immediately after trauma; by 3 hours after trauma, they are universally elevated (100% sensitivity), although with low specificity.[97] Abdominal CT scan and/or MRCP can determine the integrity of the duct.[98] Endoscopic retrograde cholangiopancreatography (ERCP) may be a useful adjunct as it can both diagnose ductal injury and manage late complications such as stricture or fistula.[99] The Pediatric Trauma Society proposed a nonoperative pathway for high-grade pancreatic injuries that begins with obtaining baseline lipase and initiation of oral diet once pain improves with repeat ultrasound/labs if pain persists for a week.[100] Following nonoperative management, patients commonly develop organized fluid collections that may or may not require drainage procedures.[101,102] Higher-grade pancreatic injuries with duct disruption typically require operative intervention, with evidence suggesting improved outcomes, reduced need for drainage procedures, and decreased length of stay with operative intervention (most commonly a distal pancreatectomy) in these patients.[103–105]

Biliary injury is rare in children, representing <0.1% of all trauma patients, and includes intrahepatic and extrahepatic ductal injuries, biloma, and gallbladder injury. Literature is sparse but many injuries can be managed nonoperatively with ERCP with biliary stent placement and percutaneous peritoneal drainage. These patients are at risk for delayed stricture and require close follow-up. Hepaticojejunostomy remains the definitive repair for extrahepatic biliary tract transections.[106]

Anorectal Injuries

Anorectal injuries are uncommon in children and usually occur after penetrating mechanism. Isolated anal trauma can be repaired primarily, including sphincter repair. Extraperitoneal rectal injuries should be repaired primarily, if possible, and often require fecal diversion and/or presacral drainage. Intraperitoneal rectal injuries can be managed similarly to colon injuries, with or without fecal diversion. Associated genitourinary injuries should be sought with examination under anesthesia.[107,108]

Pelvic Fracture and Extremity Trauma

Fractures represent one of the most common injuries in pediatric trauma patients. Children have more malleable bones, more absorptive cartilage, and a higher potential for bone remodeling and healing than adults. Anatomic differences in radiology of pediatric bones can make recognition of injuries challenging. Injury to the growth plates can result in premature fusion and asymmetric limb growth. Greenstick fractures occur when the bone bends before it breaks. Options for stabilization include casting, splinting, traction, internal fixation, or external fixation. Open fractures occur when fracture fragments communicate with the environment and should be treated with irrigation and debridement of exposed bone, surgical fixation, and systemic antibiotic coverage of gram-positive organisms as soon as possible after injury (ideally within 60 minutes). A thorough neurovascular examination is essential. Although

Algorithm 28.3

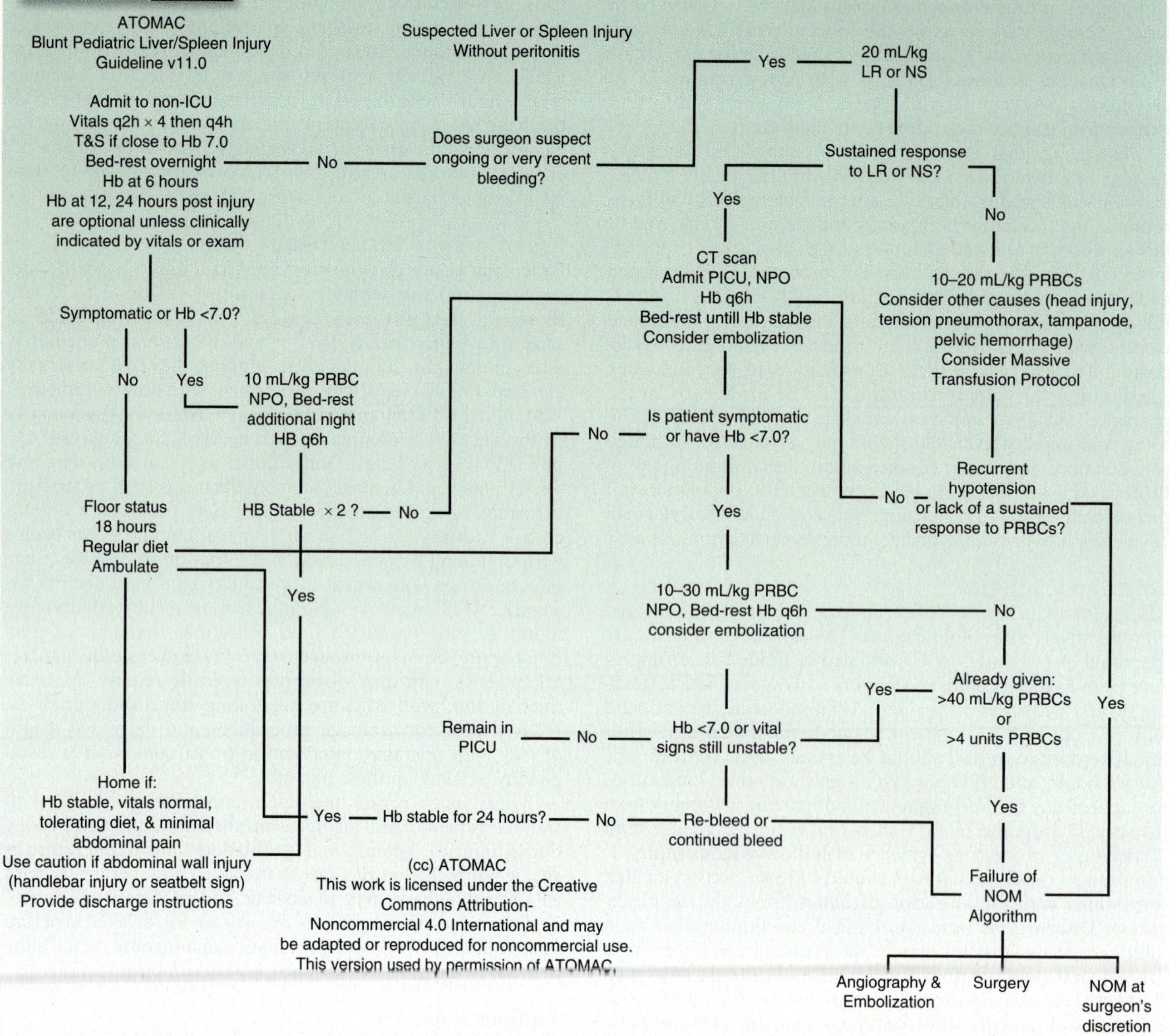

Algorithm 28.3. ATOMAC guidelines for management of pediatric solid organ injury. Hb, hemoglobin; ICU, intensive care unit; LR, lactated Ringer's; NOM, nonoperative management; NPO, non per os; NS, normal saline; PICU, pediatric intensive care unit; PRBC, packed red blood cell; q6h, every 6 hours. (From Notrica DM, Eubanks JW III, Tuggle DW, et al. Nonoperative management of blunt liver and spleen injury in children: evaluation of the ATOMAC guideline using GRADE. *J Trauma Acute Care Surg*. 2015;79[4]:683–693, with permission.)

vascular injury requiring repair is rare, children are more prone to vascular spasm, resulting in asymmetric pulse examination and transient ischemic symptoms.[109]

Pelvic fractures are a source of morbidity and mortality in pediatric patients and occur most commonly after high-mechanism blunt trauma such as MVC or pedestrians struck. Pelvic fractures are usually present in the setting of multiple injuries including TBI, abdominal injuries, and genitourinary trauma. The Young–Burgess Classification system for pelvic fractures is most commonly used in adults and categorizes injuries into lateral compression, anterior–posterior compression, and vertical shear injuries to the pelvic ring. Pediatric classifications exist but are not standard. The pediatric pelvis is more elastic, allowing for significant displacement before fracture. Pelvic hematoma and ongoing hemorrhage requiring angiographic intervention or preperitoneal packing occurs less commonly in children than in adults, but should be a major consideration in the hemodynamically unstable child. The 2011 EAST guidelines for the treatment of hemorrhage in pelvic fracture are limited to adult data, but many principles can be extrapolated to the pediatric population.[110] These guidelines recommend the use of early external stabilization, particularly with a size-appropriate pelvic orthotic device, to stabilize fractures, reduce pelvic volume, and theoretically limit blood loss. The hemodynamically unstable pediatric patient with a pelvic fracture represents a diagnostic challenge—does one proceed to the operating room for abdominal exploration or to the angiography suite for embolization? FAST examination does not have the sensitivity to rule out abdominal hemorrhage. If stable enough, a CT scan of the abdomen and pelvis is preferable to help identify the injuries and determine treatment course. Despite classification systems, fracture patterns on anteroposterior pelvic plain film do not predict bleeding or need for angiographic embolization. Angiographic embolization should be considered in hemodynamically unstable patients after other sources of hemorrhage have been ruled out. In the adult literature, arterial contrast extravasation on CT scan warrants empiric embolization, even in a stable patient, but these data are unclear in the pediatric population. Similarly, preperitoneal packing is a newer technique for the control of pelvic hemorrhage, and its use can be considered alongside pelvic embolization.[110] Treatment of pelvic fractures in children is usually nonoperative with non–weight-bearing, Spica casts, or traction. In some cases, external fixation or open reduction internal fixation (ORIF) is necessary. Fractures involving the acetabulum are complex, especially when the triradiate cartilage complex is involved, as premature fusion can result in long-term problems with leg-length discrepancy and acetabular failure.

Venous Thromboembolism

The incidence of venous thromboembolism in pediatric trauma patients is very low, ranging from 0.02% to 0.3%.[111] Practice guidelines from the Trauma EAST and Pediatric Trauma Societies proposed the following guidelines for the use of chemical prophylaxis in the pediatric trauma population. In children hospitalized after trauma who are at low risk of bleeding, pharmacologic prophylaxis should be considered in children older than 15 years and in younger postpubertal children with an injury severity score greater than 25. Routine pharmacologic prophylaxis in prepubertal children, even with ISS greater than 25 is not currently recommended. Mechanical prophylaxis should be considered either alone or as an adjunct to pharmacologic prophylaxis in children older than 15 years and in younger postpubertal children with ISS greater than 25.[112] It is worth noting that these guidelines were developed from a thorough summary of the limited literature regarding VTE prophylaxis in children hospitalized after trauma, and many centers are lowering age of consideration for pharmacologic VTE prophylaxis to 12 years old.[113] As such, prophylaxis and detection of venous thromboemobolism in the pediatric trauma population continues to be an area of ongoing study.

Child Physical Abuse

3 CPA is a leading cause of trauma in children, with 650,000 confirmed cases of physical abuse annually in the United States, accounting for 1500 deaths per year, mostly in children younger than 4 years. CPA may be difficult to recognize and a high index of suspicion is needed when evaluating children with injuries. The Western Trauma Association and Pediatric Trauma Society created a clinical decisions algorithm in 2020 to guide evaluation and management.[114] Features of the history that should increase suspicion include unexplained significant injury, denial of trauma, changes in the story or differences in the story by different witnesses, explanation that is inconsistent with the pattern, age, or severity of injury or with the child's developmental capabilities, and delay in seeking medical care. Findings on examination that may suggest abuse include any injury in a preambulatory infant, multiple organ system injuries or multiple injuries at different stages of healing, patterned injuries, injuries to unusual locations (mnemonic "TEN-4" = injury to torso, ears, or neck in a child younger than 4 years), or other evidence of neglect (failure to thrive, dental caries, poor hygiene). Burns with sharply demarcated edges, bite marks, cigarette burns, and other markers of being hit with an object are high-risk injuries. Certain fracture patterns should raise concern for abuse including fractures in nonambulatory patients, multiple fractures, rib fractures, infants and toddlers with midshaft femur or humerus fractures, and other unusual fractures such as scapular and metaphyseal fractures. Skeletal survey is recommended in children younger than 2 years who have suspicion for abuse.[115,116] If there is a reasonable suspicion that a child has been abused, a report to child protective services for further investigation is mandated by law.

4 INJURY PREVENTION

In 1968, the National Traffic and Motor Vehicle Safety Act established the National Highway Traffic Safety Administration, which has influenced the improvement of road infrastructure, automobile, and driver and passenger safety, resulting in precipitous drops in roadway fatalities.

There are many examples where comprehensive state and federal laws have resulted in statistical drops in injuries and deaths.[117–119] In the following section, we provide several examples where federal mandates and state laws have been implicated in the reduction of pediatric injuries. In many cases, surgeon advocates were integral in the legislative process.

Smoke Detectors and Carbon Monoxide Detectors

Smoke detectors have been legislated into building codes in all 50 states. As a result, the early warnings of a fire are thought to have prevented thousands of deaths. More than 10,000 Americans are poisoned by carbon monoxide and more than 500 people in the United States die annually from carbon monoxide poisoning. As of August 2015, 30 states have enacted statutes regarding carbon monoxide detectors, and another 11 have promulgated regulations on CO detectors. Several states now require CO detectors in hotels and schools.

Drunken Driving Laws

Alcohol is known to play a role in many MVCs. Drivers younger than 21 years are more likely than older drivers to be involved in fatal crashes, and alcohol use adds to the risk of fatal crashes. This group has been the target of several interventions to reduce alcohol-impaired driving, including "zero tolerance" blood alcohol concentration standards for drivers under the legal drinking age with mandatory license revocation after a first offense.[120]

Junior Driver Laws/Safe Driving Laws

The increased risk of car crashes associated with texting and cell phone use has been well documented—among adults and teens alike. But for teens, who are immersed in a world of smart phones and texting, these types of laws send a powerful message that driving demands their undivided attention. Although not exclusive to children or adolescents, "safe driving laws" ban text messaging for all drivers, prohibit junior drivers from using cell phones, and institute new license renewal procedures for mature drivers, among other provisions. Graduated driver licensing programs that require new drivers to progress through stages allowing them increased driving privileges as they gain experience have, in some form, been enacted in all 50 states. Many states have also incorporated parental education and curfews to these laws and have seen up to a 40% decrease in the number of injuries and fatalities as novice drivers have become engaged in this process.[121,122]

Child Passenger Restraints

Seat belt use around the country has steadily increased. There is mounting evidence that seat belt use and airbag implementation have been the greatest cause for decreased road fatalities per miles driven, which is at an all-time low according to National Highway Traffic Safety Administration statistics. Furthermore, there is evidence that educating pediatricians improves the use of car seats for children. Although the rate of use of car seats for newborns and infants is approximately 75%, their use in toddlers is estimated at only 29%, and more than half of car seats for children are not used correctly. In the child older than 4 years or 40 lb, there is ample evidence that booster seats should be used rather than adult-type restraints. Many states now have legislation aimed at this population.

All-Terrain Vehicle Laws

In the United States, all-terrain vehicle crashes account for a rising number of injuries and deaths in all age. Approximately 30% of the injured/dead are children. In 1988, in response to this trend, the Consumer Product Safety Commission and the all-terrain vehicle industry agreed upon a set of standards designed to limit injury. This included regulations that restricted operators younger than 16 years halted the sale of three-wheeled vehicles and included a mandatory educational safety training module and improved safety warnings. However, in 1998, 10 years after they were established, these consent decrees expired and since that time, the rate of injuries has risen steeply. Several states have recently enacted restrictions on ridership and in Massachusetts, where these restrictions have included an age cutoff, the number of injuries have fallen dramatically (unpublished data).

Finally, as policy makers struggle to allocate limited resources to improve population health, injury prevention programs will play a particularly important role. The rationale is straightforward: regulatory efforts specifically aimed at injury primary and secondary prevention, if well designed, can be very successful at health care cost reduction, thereby freeing resources for other concerns.

GUN VIOLENCE PREVENTION

Between 2009 and 2018, mass shootings took center stage in the nation's consciousness. A total of 194 mass shootings resulted in the death or serious injury of nearly 2000 Americans, and one in four of them were children or adolescents.[123] However, these numbers represent a small fraction of the yearly death toll (nearly 40,000) from modern American gun violence—now an undeniable health epidemic for children and adults living in the United States. In 2020, firearm-related injuries surpassed MVCs as the leading cause of death for children and adolescents in the United States.[124] Without understanding their implications of the psyche of our children, active shooter drills have become a routine part of school preparedness and emergency planning in over 95% of our nations' schools.[125] While we are constantly reminded about mass shootings, deaths from suicide and homicide contribute far more American lives to this toll and their determinants are poorly understood. Furthermore, nonfatal injuries, estimated to be greater than 150,000 per year, also strain our health care systems and impose a cost that has been shown to exceed the budget of the US department of Education.[126] Recognizing the important perspective that surgeons and health care providers bring to the public debate over gun control policy, organized medicine has developed working groups and published statements with the goal of influencing the nation's policy makers. In November 2018, the American College of Surgeons Committee on Trauma (ACS COT) released its initial set of recommendations to develop an effective and durable strategy for reducing firearm injury, death, and disability in the United States through their Injury Prevention and Control Committee as well as a Medical Summit on Firearm Injury Prevention.[127] In 2020, the federal budget included $25 million dedicated to the Centers for Disease Control and the National Institutes of Health for gun violence research, the first time federal funding has been dedicated to this cause since the Dickey Amendment was passed in 1996. Organizations such as Everytown for Gun Safety, Sandy Hook Promise, and March for our Lives and campaigns such as Asking Saves Kids (ASK) have formed to address and combat this growing public health crisis.

ACKNOWLEDGMENTS

We gratefully acknowledge the contributions of previous edition authors, Cornelia L. Griggs and Danielle B. Cameron, as portions of those chapters have been retained in this revision.

References

1. Osterman MJ, Kochanek KD, MacDorman MF, Strobino DM, Guyer B. Annual summary of vital statistics: 2012–2013. *Pediatrics.* 2015;135(6):1115–1125.
2. Wesson DE. Pediatric trauma centers: coming of age. *Tex Heart Inst J.* 2012;39(6):871–873.
3. American Academy of Pediatrics Section on Orthopaedics; American Academy of Pediatrics Committee on Pediatric Emergency Medicine; American Academy of Pediatrics Section on Critical Care; American Academy of Pediatrics Section on Surgery; American Academy of Pediatrics Section on Transport Medicine; American Academy of Pediatrics Committee on Pediatric Emergency Medicine; Pediatric Orthopaedic Society of North America, Krug SE, Tuggle DW. Management of pediatric trauma. *Pediatrics.* 2008;121(4):849–854.
4. Committee on Trauma and Committee on Shock, Division of Medical Sciences, National Academy of Sciences, Nation Research Council. *Accidental Death and Disability: The Neglected Disease of Modern Society.* The National Academies Press; 1966.
5. Segui-Gomez M, Chang DC, Paidas CN, Jurkovich GJ, Mackenzie EJ, Rivara FP. Pediatric trauma care: an overview of pediatric trauma systems and their practices in 18 US states. *J Pediatr Surg.* 2003;38(8):1162–1169.
6. Simpson AJ, Rivara FP, Pham TN. Quality care in pediatric trauma. *Int J Crit Illn Inj Sci.* 2012;2(3):149–155.
7. Kelly ML, Banerjee A, Nowak M, Steinmetz M, Claridge JA. Decreased mortality in traumatic brain injury following regionalization across hospital systems. *J Trauma Acute Care Surg.* 2015;78(4):715–720.
8. Bowman SM, Zimmerman FJ, Christakis DA, Sharar SR, Martin DP. Hospital characteristics associated with the management of pediatric splenic injuries. *JAMA.* 2005;294(20):2611–2617.
9. Hamlat CA, Arbabi S, Koepsell TD, Maier RV, Jurkovich GJ, Rivara FP. National variation in outcomes and costs for splenic injury and the impact of trauma systems: a population-based cohort study. *Ann Surg.* 2012;255(1):165–170.
10. http://www.emscnrc.org/emsc-resources/toolboxes/emergency-department-pediatric-performance-measures-toolbox. Accessed June 27, 2016.
11. http://www.emscnrc.org/~/media/emsc/files/pdf/emsc_resources/hospitalbased_performance_measures/trauma.ashx?la=en. Accessed June 27, 2016.
12. Lorch SA, Myers S, Carr B. The regionalization of pediatric health care. *Pediatrics.* 2010;126:1182–1190.
13. MacKenzie EJ, Rivara FP, Jurkovich GJ, et al. A national evaluation of the effect of trauma-center care on mortality. *N Engl J Med.* 2006;354:366–378.
14. Densmore JC, Lim HJ, Oldham KT, Guice KS. Outcomes and delivery of care in pediatric injury. *J Pediatr Surg.* 2006;41: 92–98; discussion 92–98.
15. Amini R, Lavoie A, Moore L, Sirois MJ, Emond M. Pediatric trauma mortality by type of designated hospital in a mature inclusive trauma system. *J Emerg Trauma Shock.* 2011;4: 12–19.
16. Hulka F, Mullins RJ, Mann NC, et al. Influence of a statewide trauma system on pediatric hospitalization and outcome. *J Trauma.* 1997;42:514–519.
17. Pracht EE, Langland-Orban B, Tepas JJ III, Celso BG, Flint L. Analysis of trends in the Florida Trauma System (1991–2003): changes in mortality after establishment of new centers. *Surgery.* 2006;140: 34–43.
18. Hussmann B, Lefering R, Kauther MD, Ruchholtz S, Moldzio P, Lendemans S; TraumaRegister DGU®. Influence of prehospital volume replacement on outcome in polytraumatized children. *Crit Care.* 2012;16(5):R201.
19. Camazine MN, Hemmila MR, Leonard JC, et al. Massive transfusion policies at trauma centers participating in the American College of Surgeons Trauma Quality Improvement Program. *J Trauma Acute Care Surg.* 2015;78(6 suppl 1):S48–S53.
20. Hughes NT, Burd RS, Teach SJ. Damage control resuscitation: permissive hypotension and massive transfusion protocols. *Pediatr Emerg Care.* 2014;30(9):651–666; quiz 657–658.
21. Phillips R, Moore H, Bensard D, et al. It is time for TEG in pediatric trauma: unveiling meaningful alterations in children who undergo massive transfusion. *Pediatr Surg Int.* 2021;37(11): 1613–1620.
22. Deng Q, Hao F, Wang Y, Guo C. Rotation thromboelastometry (ROTEM) enables improved outcomes in the pediatric trauma population. *J Int Med Res.* 2018;46(12):5195–5204.

23. Feld LG, Neuspiel DR, Foster BA. Clinical practice guideline: maintenance intravenous fluids in children. *Pediatrics.* 2018;142(6): e20183083.
24. Murphy R, Ghosh A. Towards evidence based emergency medicine: best BETs from the Manchester Royal Infirmary. The accuracy of abdominal ultrasound in paediatric trauma. *Emerg Med J.* 2001;18(3):208–209.
25. Scaife ER, Rollins MD, Barnhart DC, et al. The role of focused abdominal sonography for trauma (FAST) in pediatric trauma evaluation. *J Pediatr Surg.* 2013;48(6):1377–1383.
26. Holmes JF, Kelley KM, Wootton-Gorges SL, et al. Effect of abdominal ultrasound on clinical care, outcomes, and resource use among children with blunt torso trauma: a randomized clinical trial. *JAMA.* 2017;317(22):2290–2296.
27. Menaker J, Blumberg S, Wisner DH, et al. Intra-abdominal Injury Study Group of the Pediatric Emergency Care Applied Research Network (PECARN). Use of the focused assessment with sonography for trauma (FAST) examination and its impact on abdominal computed tomography use in hemodynamically stable children with blunt torso trauma. *J Trauma Acute Care Surg.* 2014;77(3): 427–432.
28. Ben-Ishay O, Daoud M, Peled Z, Brauner E, Bahouth H, Kluger Y. Focused abdominal sonography for trauma in the clinical evaluation of children with blunt abdominal trauma. *World J Emerg Surg.* 2015;10:27.
29. Holmes JF, Gladman A, Chang CH. Performance of abdominal ultrasonography in pediatric blunt trauma patients: a meta-analysis. *J Pediatr Surg.* 2007;42(9):1588–1594.
30. National Center for Injury Prevention and Control. *Traumatic Brain Injury in the United States: Assessing Outcomes in Children.* Centers for Disease Control and Prevention; 2006.
31. http://www.cdc.gov/TraumaticBrainInjury/. Accessed November 2, 2015.
32. Daley BJ, Lee S, Raju R, et al. Emedicine. Considerations in pediatric trauma. Accessed September 9, 2015. http://emedicine.medscape.com/article/435031-overview#al
33. Barbosa RR, Jawa R, Watters JM, et al. Eastern Association for the Surgery of Trauma. Evaluation and management of mild traumatic brain injury: an Eastern Association for the Surgery of Trauma practice management guideline. *J Trauma Acute Care Surg.* 2012; 73(5 suppl 4):S307–S314.
34. Kuppermann N, Holmes JF, Dayan PS, et al. Pediatric Emergency Care Applied Research Network (PECARN). Identification of children at very low risk of clinically-important brain injuries after head trauma: a prospective cohort study. *Lancet.* 2009;374(9696):1160–1170.
35. Lee LK, Monroe D, Bachman MC, et al. Traumatic Brain Injury (TBI) Working Group of Pediatric Emergency Care Applied Research Network (PECARN). Isolated loss of consciousness in children with minor blunt head trauma. *JAMA Pediatr.* 2014;168(9):837–843.
36. Holmes JF, Borgialli DA, Nadel FM, et al. TBI Study Group for the Pediatric Emergency Care Applied Research Network. Do children with blunt head trauma and normal cranial computed tomography scan results require hospitalization for neurologic observation. *Ann Emerg Med.* 2011;58(4):315–322.
37. Powell EC, Atabaki SM, Wootton-Gorges S, et al. Isolated linear skull fractures in children with blunt head trauma. *Pediatrics.* 2015;135(4):e851–e857.
38. Dayan PS, Holmes JF, Hoyle J Jr, et al. Pediatric Emergency Care Applied Research Network (PECARN). Headache in traumatic brain injuries from blunt head trauma. *Pediatrics.* 2015;135(3):504–512.
39. Metzger RR, Smith J, Wells M, et al. Impact of newly adopted guidelines for management of children with isolated skull fracture. *J Pediatr Surg.* 2014;49(12):1856–1860.
40. Blackwood BP, Bean JF, Sadecki-Lund C, Helenowski IB, Kabre R, Hunter CJ. Observation for isolated traumatic skull fractures in the pediatric population: unnecessary and costly. *J Pediatr Surg.* 2016;51(4):654–658.
41. Schatz P, Pardini JE, Lovell MR, Collins MW, Podell K. Sensitivity and specificity of the ImPACT Test Battery for concussion in athletes. *Arch Clin Neuropsychol.* 2006;21(1):91–99.
42. McCrea M, Guskiewicz KM, Marshall SW, et al. Acute effects and recovery time following concussion in collegiate football players: the NCAA Concussion Study. *JAMA.* 2003;290(19):2556–2563.
43. Halstead ME, Walter KD; Council on Sports Medicine and Fitness. American Academy of Pediatrics. Clinical report-sports-related concussion in children and adolescents. *Pediatrics.* 2010;126(3): 597–615.
44. https://www.cdc.gov/heads-up/guidelines/returning-to-sports.html. Accessed September 12, 2024.
45. Patricios JS, Schneider KJ, Dvorak J, et al. Consensus statement on concussion in sport: the 6th International Conference on Concussion in Sport–Amsterdam, October 2022. *Br J Sports Med.* 2023;57(11):695–711.
46. Cancelliere C, Hincapié CA, Keightley M, et al. Systematic review of prognosis and return to play after sport concussion: results of the International Collaboration on Mild Traumatic Brain Injury Prognosis. *Arch Phys Med Rehabil.* 2014;95(3 suppl): S210–S229.
47. Weihing VK, Crowe EH, Wang HE, Ugalde IT. Prehospital airway management in the pediatric patient: a systematic review. *Acad Emerg Med.* 2022;29(6):765–771.
48. Johnson DL, Krishnamurthy S. Send severely head-injured children to a pediatric trauma center. *Pediatr Neurosurg.* 1996;25(6): 309–314.
49. Khalil M, Alawwa G, Pinto F, O'Neill PA. Pediatric mortality at pediatric versus adult trauma centers. *J Emerg Trauma Shock.* 2021;14(3):128–135.
50. Dawes AJ, Sacks GD, Cryer HG, et al. Los Angeles County Trauma Consortium. Intracranial pressure monitoring and inpatient mortality in severe traumatic brain injury: a propensity score-matched analysis. *J Trauma Acute Care Surg.* 2015;78(3): 492–501; discussion 501–502.
51. Adelson PD, Bratton SL, Carney NA, et al. American Association for Surgery of Trauma; Child Neurology Society; International Society for Pediatric Neurosurgery; International Trauma Anesthesia and Critical Care Society; Society of Critical Care Medicine; World Federation of Pediatric Intensive and Critical Care Societies. Guidelines for the acute medical management of severe traumatic brain injury in infants, children, and adolescents. Chapter 5. Indications for intracranial pressure monitoring in pediatric patients with severe traumatic brain injury. *Pediatr Crit Care Med.* 2003;4(suppl 3):S19–S24.
52. Bell MJ, Kochanek PM. Pediatric traumatic brain injury in 2012: the year with new guidelines and common data elements. *Crit Care Clin.* 2013;29(2):223–238.
53. Kochanek PM, Carney N, Adelson PD, et al. Guidelines for the acute medical management of severe traumatic brain injury in infants, children and adolescents: second edition. *Pediatr Crit Care Med.* 2012;13(suppl 1):S1–S82.
54. Kochanek PM, Tasker RC, Bell MJ, et al. Management of pediatric severe traumatic brain injury: 2019 consensus and guidelines-based algorithm for first and second tier therapies. *Pediatr Crit Care Med.* 2019;20(3):269–279.
55. Adelson PD, Wisniewski SR, Beca J, et al. Paediatric Traumatic Brain Injury Consortium. Comparison of hypothermia and normothermia after severe traumatic brain injury in children (Cool Kids): a phase 3, randomised controlled trial. *Lancet Neurol.* 2013;12(6): 546–553.
56. Li H, Lu G, Shi W, Zheng S. Protective effect of moderate hypothermia on severe traumatic brain injury in children. *J Neurotrauma.* 2009;26:1905–1909
57. Hutchison JS, Ward RE, Lacroix J, et al. Hypothermia Pediatric Head Injury Trial Investigators and the Canadian Critical Care Trials Group. Hypothermia therapy after traumatic brain injury in children. *N Engl J Med.* 2008;358(23):2447–2456.
58. Hoffman JR, Wolfson AB, Todd K, Mower WR. Selective cervical spine radiography in blunt trauma: methodology of the National Emergency X-Radiography Utilization Study (NEXUS). *Ann Emerg Med.* 1998;32(4):461–469.
59. Steill IG, Wells GA, Vandemheen KL, et al. The Canadian C-Spine rule for radiography in alert and stable trauma patients. *JAMA.* 2001;286(15):1841–1848.

60. Viccellio P, Simon H, Pressman BD, Shah MN, Mower WR, Hoffman JR; NEXUS Group. A prospective multicenter study of cervical spine injury in children. *Pediatrics.* 2001;108(2):E20.
61. Expert Panel on Pediatric Imaging; Kadom N, Palasis S, Pruthi S, et al. ACR appropriateness criteria® suspected spine trauma-child. *J Am Coll Radiol.* 2019;16(5S):S286–S299.
62. Leonard JC, Kuppermann N, Olsen C, et al. Pediatric Emergency Care Applied Research Network. Factors associated with cervical spine injury in children after blunt trauma. *Ann Emerg Med.* 2011;58(2):145–155.
63. Hoffman JR, Mower WR, Wolfson AB, Todd KH, Zucker MI. Validity of a set of clinical criteria to rule out injury to the cervical spine in patients with blunt trauma. *N Engl J Med.* 2000; 343(2):94–99.
64. Pieretti-Vanmarcke R, Velmahos GC, Nance ML, et al. Clinical clearance of the cervical spine in blunt trauma patients younger than 3 years: a multi-center study of the American Association for the Surgery of Trauma. *J Trauma.* 2009;67(3):543–549; discussion 549–550.
65. Leonard JR, Jaffe DM, Kuppermann N, Olsen CS, Leonard JC; Pediatric Emergency Care Applied Research Network (PECARN) Cervical Spine Study Group. Cervical spine injury patterns in children. *Pediatrics.* 2014;133(5):e1179–e1188.
66. Polk-Williams A, Carr BG, Blinman TA, Masiakos PT, Wiebe DJ, Nance ML. Cervical spine injury in young children: a National Trauma Data Bank review. *J Pediatr Surg.* 2008;43(9):1718–1721.
67. Pang D, Wilberger JE Jr. Spinal cord injury without radiographic abnormalities in children. *J Neurosurg.* 1982;57(1):114–129.
68. Pang D. Spinal cord injury without radiographic abnormality in children, 2 decades later. *Neurosurgery.* 2004;55(6):1325–1342; discussion 1342–1343.
69. Yucesoy K, Yuksel KZ. SCIWORA in MRI era. *Clin Neurol Neurosurg.* 2008;110:429–433.
70. Burlew CC, Biffl WL, Moore EE, Barnett CC, Johnson JL, Bensard DD. Blunt cerebrovascular injuries: redefining screening criteria in the era of non-invasive diagnosis. *J Trauma Acute Care Surg.* 2012;72(2):330–335.
71. Circelli A, Ciapetti M, Spina R, et al. Diagnosis of carotid and vertebral artery injury in major trauma with head injury. *Crit Care.* 2010;14(Suppl 1):P297.
72. Malhotra A, Wu X, Kalra VB, Goodman TR, Schindler J, Forman HP. Screening for pediatric blunt cerebrovascular injury: review of literature and a cost-effectiveness analysis. *J Pediatr Surg.* 2015;50(10):1751–1757.
73. Sharma MS, Kupferschmid J. Pediatric thoracic trauma. Updated September 15, 2013. Accessed September 13, 2024. http://emedicine.medscape.com/article/905863-overview#a1
74. Mowery NT, Gunter OL, Collier BR, et al. Practice management guidelines for management of hemothorax and occult pneumothorax. *J Trauma.* 2011;70(2):510–518.
75. Nance ML, Sing RF, Reilly PM, Templeton JM Jr, Schwab CW. Thoracic gunshot wounds in children under 17 years of age. *J Pediatr Surg.* 1996;31(7):931–935.
76. Moore HB, Moore EE, Bensard DD. Pediatric emergency department thoracotomy: a 40-year review. *J Pediatr Surg.* 2016;51(2): 315–318
77. Flynn-O'Brien KT, Stewart BT, Fallat ME, et al. Mortality after emergency department thoracotomy for pediatric blunt trauma: analysis of the National Trauma Data Bank 2007–2012. *J Pediatr Surg.* 2016;51(1):163–167.
78. Seamon MJ, Haut ER, Van Arendonk K, et al. An evidence-based approach to patient selection for emergency department thoracotomy: a practice management guideline from the Eastern Association for the Surgery of Trauma. *J Trauma Acute Care Surg.* 2015;79(1):159–173.
79. Golden J, Isani M, Bowling J, et al. Limiting chest computed tomography in the evaluation of pediatric thoracic trauma. *J Trauma Acute Care Surg.* 2016;81(2):271–277.
80. Fox N, Schwartz D, Salazar JH, et al. Evaluation and management of blunt traumatic aortic injury: a practice management guideline from the Eastern Association for the Surgery of Trauma. *J Trauma Acute Care Surg.* 2015;78(1):136–146.
81. Clancy K, Velopulos C, Bilaniuk JW, et al. Eastern Association for the Surgery of Trauma. Screening for blunt cardiac injury: an Eastern Association for the Surgery of Trauma practice management guideline. *J Trauma Acute Care Surg.* 2012;73(5 suppl 4):S301–S306.
82. Holmes JF, Lillis K, Monroe D, et al. Pediatric Emergency Care Applied Research Network (PECARN). Identifying children at very low risk of clinically important blunt abdominal injuries. *Ann Emerg Med.* 2013;62(2):107–116.e2.
83. Mahajan P, Kuppermann N, Tunik M, et al. Intra-abdominal Injury Study Group of the Pediatric Emergency Care Applied Research Network (PECARN). Comparison of clinician suspicion versus a clinical prediction rule in identifying children at risk for intra-abdominal injuries after blunt torso trauma. *Acad Emerg Med.* 2015;22(9):1034–1041.
84. Adelgais KM, Kuppermann N, Kooistra J, et al. Intra-Abdominal Injury Study Group of the Pediatric Emergency Care Applied Research Network (PECARN). Accuracy of the abdominal examination for identifying children with blunt intra-abdominal injuries. *J Pediatr.* 2014;165(6):1230–1235.e5.
85. Streck CJ, Vogel AM, Zhang J, et al. Pediatric Surgery Research Collaborative. Identifying children at very low risk for blunt intra-abdominal injury in whom CT of the abdomen can be avoided safely. *J Am Coll Surg.* 2017;224(4):449–458.e3.
86. Kerrey BT, Rogers AJ, Lee LK, et al. Pediatric Emergency Care Applied Research Network. A multicenter study of the risk of intra-abdominal injury in children after normal abdominal computed tomography scan results in the emergency department. *Ann Emerg Med.* 2013;62(4):319–326.
87. Ertekin C, Yanar H, Taviloglu K, Güloglu R, Alimoglu O. Unnecessary laparotomy by using physical examination and different diagnostic modalities for penetrating abdominal stab wounds. *Emerg Med J.* 2005;22(11):790–-794.
88. Lamb CM, MacGoey P, Navarro AP, Brooks AJ. Damage control surgery in the era of damage control resuscitation. *Br J Anaesth.* 2014;113(2):242–249.
89. Stassen NA, Bhullar I, Cheng JD, et al. Eastern Association for the Surgery of Trauma. Selective nonoperative management of blunt splenic injury: an Eastern Association for the Surgery of Trauma practice management guideline. *J Trauma Acute Care Surg.* 2012; 73(5):S294–S300.
90. *Injury Scoring Scales: A Resource for Trauma Care Professionals.* Accessed November 8, 2015. http://www.aast.org/library/traumatools/InjuryScoringScales.aspx
91. Williams RF, Grewal H, Jamshidi R, et al. Updated APSA guidelines for the management of blunt liver and spleen injuries. *J Pediatr Surg.* 2023;58(8):1411–1418.
92. Wisner DH, Kuppermann N, Cooper A, et al. Management of children with solid organ injuries after blunt torso trauma. *J Trauma Acute Care Surg.* 2015;79(2):206–214; quiz 332.
93. Notrica DM, Eubanks JW III, Tuggle DW, et al. Nonoperative management of blunt liver and spleen injury in children: evaluation of the ATOMAC guideline using GRADE. *J Trauma Acute Care Surg.* 2015;79(4):683–693.
94. Kiankhooy A, Sartorelli KH, Vane DW, Bhave AD. Angiographic embolization is safe and effective therapy for blunt abdominal solid organ injury in children. *J Trauma.* 2010;68(3):526–531.
95. Gates RL, Price M, Cameron DB, et al. Non-operative management of solid organ injuries in children: an American Pediatric Surgical Association Outcomes and Evidence Based Practice Committee systematic review. *J Pediatr Surg.* 2019;54(8):1519–1526.
96. Naiditch JA, Notrica DM, Sayrs LW, et al. The use and timing of angioembolization in pediatric blunt liver and spleen injury. *J Trauma Acute Care Surg.* 2024;96(6):915–920.
97. East Guidelines for the Diagnosis and Management of Pancreatic Trauma. Eastern association for the surgery of trauma practice management guidelines. Accessed November 8, 2015. https://www.east.org/education/practice-management-guidelines/pancreatic-trauma-diagnosis-and-management-of
98. Adamson WT, Hebra A, Thomas PB, Wagstaff P, Tagge EP, Othersen HB. Serum amylase and lipase alone are not cost-effective screening methods for pediatric pancreatic trauma. *J Pediatr Surg.* 2003;38(3):354–357; discussion 354–357.

99. Rosenfeld EH, Vogel A, Russell RT, et al. Comparison of diagnostic imaging modalities for the evaluation of pancreatic duct injury in children: a multi-institutional analysis from the Pancreatic Trauma Study Group. *Pediatr Surg Int.* 2018;34(9):961–966.
100. Rosenfeld EH, Vogel AM, Klinkner DB, et al. Pancreatic Trauma Study Group. The utility of ERCP in pediatric pancreatic trauma. *J Pediatr Surg.* 2017:S0022-3468(17)30660-7.
101. Naik-Mathuria BJ, Rosenfeld EH, Gosain A, et al; the Pancreatic Trauma Study Group (PTSG) Collaborators. Proposed clinical pathway for nonoperative management of high-grade pediatric pancreatic injuries based on a multicenter analysis: a pediatric trauma society collaborative. *J Trauma Acute Care Surg.* 2017;83(4):589–596.
102. Bhakta D, de Latour R, Khanna L. Management of pancreatic fluid collections. *Transl Gastroenterol Hepatol.* 2022;7:17.
103. Wales PW, Shuckett B, Kim PC. Long-term outcome after nonoperative management of complete traumatic pancreatic transection in children. *J Pediatr Surg.* 2001;36(5):823–827.
104. Mattix KD, Tataria M, Holmes J, et al. Pediatric pancreatic trauma: predictors of nonoperative management failure and associated outcomes. *J Pediatr Surg.* 2007;42(2):340–344.
105. Iqbal CW, St. Peter SD, Tsao K, et al. Pancreatic Trauma in Children (PATCH) Study Group. Operative vs nonoperative management for blunt pancreatic transection in children: multi-institutional outcomes. *J Am Coll Surg.* 2014;218(2):157–162.
106. Wood JH, Partrick DA, Bruny JL, Sauaia A, Moulton SL. Operative vs nonoperative management of blunt pancreatic trauma in children. *J Pediatr Surg.* 2010;45(2):401–406.
107. Soukup ES, Russell KW, Metzger R, Scaife ER, Barnhart DC, Rollins MD. Treatment and outcome of traumatic biliary injuries in children. *J Pediatr Surg.* 2014;49(2):345–348.
108. Russell KW, Soukup ES, Metzger RR, et al. Fecal continence following complex anorectal trauma in children. *J Pediatr Surg.* 2014;49(2):349–352.
109. Samuk I, Steiner Z, Feigin E, Baazov A, Dlugy E, Freud E. Anorectal injuries in children: a 20-year experience in two centers. *Pediatr Surg Int.* 2015;31(9):815–819.
110. Mommsen P, Zeckey C, Hildebrand F, et al. Traumatic extremity arterial injury in children: epidemiology, diagnostics, treatment and prognostic value of Mangled Extremity Severity Score. *J Orthop Surg Res.* 2010;5:25.
111. Cullinane DC, Schiller HJ, Zielinski MD, et al. Eastern Association for the Surgery of Trauma practice guidelines for hemorrhage in pelvic fracture—update and systematic review. *J Trauma.* 2011;71(6):1850–1868.
112. Thompson AJ, McSwain SD, Webb SA, Stroud MA, Streck CJ. Venous thromboembolism prophylaxis in the pediatric trauma population. *J Pediatr Surg.* 2013;48(6):1413–1421.
113. Mahajerin A, Petty JK, Hanson SJ, et al. Prophylaxis against venous thromboembolism in pediatric trauma: a practice management guideline from the Eastern Association for the Surgery of Trauma and the Pediatric Trauma Society. *J Trauma Acute Care Surg.* 2017;82(3):627–636.
114. Christian CW; Committee on Child Abuse and Neglect, American Academy of Pediatrics. The evaluation of suspected child physical abuse. *Pediatrics.* 2015;135(5):e1337–e1354.
115. Rosen NG, Escobar MA Jr, Brown CV, et al. Child physical abuse trauma evaluation and management: a Western Trauma Association and Pediatric Trauma Society critical decisions algorithm. *J Trauma Acute Care Surg.* 2021;90(4):641–651.
116. Wood JN, Fakeye O, Feudtner C, Mondestin V, Localio R, Rubin DM. Development of guidelines for skeletal survey in young children with fractures. *Pediatrics.* 2014;134(1):45–53.
117. Mendelson KG, Fallat ME. Pediatric injuries: prevention to resolution. *Surg Clin North Am.* 2007;87(1):207–228, viii.
118. Brussoni M, Towner E, Hayes M. Evidence into practice: combining the art and science of injury prevention. *Inj Prev.* 2006(6);12: 373–377.
119. Tepas JJ III. The national pediatric trauma registry: a legacy of commitment to control of childhood injury. *Semin Pediatr Surg.* 2004;13(2):126–132.
120. Brehaut JC, Miller A, Raina P, McGrail KM. Childhood behavior disorders and injuries among children and youth: a population based study. *Pediatrics.* 2003;111(2):262–269.
121. Kaafarani HMA, Lee J, Cropano C, et al. The impact and sustainability of the graduated driver licensing program in preventing motor vehicle crashes in Massachusetts. *J Trauma Acute Care Surg.* 2015;78(2):265–270; discussion 270–271.
122. Rajaratnam SMW, Landrigan CP, Wang W, Kaprielian R, Moore RT, Czeisler CA. Teen crashes declined after Massachusetts raised penalties for graduated licensing law restricting night driving. *Health Aff (Millwood).* 2015;34(6):963–970.
123. https://everytownresearch.org/massshootingsreports/mass-shootings-in-america-2009-2019. Accessed February 3, 2020.
124. Goldstick JE, Cunningham RM, Carter PM. Current causes of death in children and adolescents in the United States. *N Engl J Med.* 2022;386(20):1955–1956.
125. Sacks CA, Masiakos PT. Confronting moral obligations in an active shooter incident: a reminder to focus on prevention. *J Law Med Ethics.* 2020;48(2):352–353.
126. Lee J, Quraishi SA, Bhatnagar S, Zafonte RD, Masiakos PT. The economic cost of firearm-related injuries in the United States from 2006 to 2010. *Surgery.* 2014;155(5):894–898.
127. https://www.facs.org/quality-programs/trauma/advocacy-and-injury-prevention/firearm-injury-prevention-activities/. Accessed September 13, 2024.

29

Geriatric Trauma

Tatiana C. P. Cardenas, Marc D. Trust, and Carlos V. R. Brown

Key Points

1 The physiology of aging affects nearly every organ system, including cardiovascular, pulmonary, renal, and gastrointestinal. Altered physiology may also be associated with comorbid conditions in the elderly patient, including hypertension, cardiac disease, chronic obstructive pulmonary disease (COPD), chronic renal insufficiency, and altered drug metabolism.

2 The American Geriatrics Society has published the Beers Criteria for potentially inappropriate medication use in older adults that can be used to refine inpatient medication management for elderly trauma patients.

3 Falls are far and away the most common mechanism of injury in elderly trauma patients, causing almost 75% of injuries in elderly patients; nearly one in three adults over 65 years old will experience ground-level falls each year.

4 An underreported but important mechanism of injury in elderly trauma patients is elderly abuse.

5 Imaging with head CT in elderly trauma patients should be used liberally.

6 Severely injured older patients may not display standard signs of hemodynamic instability.

7 Due to the broad range of age-related factors that can contribute to injury and adversely affect recovery in geriatric patients, injured individuals should receive a comprehensive geriatric assessment during their hospital stay.

8 Frailty is a syndrome of decreased physiologic reserve distinct from the normal aging process and other comorbidities. Frailty is associated with higher mortality and complications, and worse functional outcomes after trauma, and is more predictive than age or injury severity of hospital complications, in-hospital mortality, or discharge to an institution.

9 Goals of care, advanced directives and surrogate decision makers should be discussed and clarified as early as possible in the hospital course.

The elderly population in the United States is steadily growing, and according to the U.S. Census Bureau, the number of Americans >65 years old is expected to reach over 82 million by the year 2030.[1]

Trauma and acute care surgeons will be increasingly responsible for caring for this complex population of patients. Even prior to injury, the elderly patient brings unique challenges, including altered physiology, numerous comorbid conditions, and preinjury medications. The epidemiology and triage complexities of elderly trauma patients make it challenging to ensure these patients are transported to the appropriate receiving facility. Elderly patients are most often injured by a blunt mechanism and are particularly at risk for falls from standing. In addition, they sustain unique injuries that may escape diagnosis during the initial evaluation. Trauma centers may need to alter activation criteria for elderly trauma patients in order to avoid the pitfall of undertriage that is associated with poor outcomes in this population. Though the initial trauma evaluation for elderly patients is similar to younger adults, the trauma surgeon must understand the nuances associated with caring for the injured elderly patient. The elderly trauma patient more frequently has issues that relate to end-of-life care in the postinjury period.

PHYSIOLOGY, COMORBIDITY, AND PREINJURY MEDICATIONS

1 Elderly individuals present with a vast array of body systems affected by the deranged physiology associated with aging. The physiology of aging affects nearly every organ system, including cardiovascular, pulmonary, renal, and gastrointestinal. Altered physiology may also be associated with comorbid conditions in the elderly patient, including hypertension, cardiac disease, chronic obstructive pulmonary disease (COPD), chronic renal insufficiency, and altered drug metabolism.

Cardiovascular

The cardiovascular system is most commonly affected by the physiology of aging and has a significant impact on care of the injured elderly patient. Alterations to physiology of the vascular system in the aging adult are primarily the result of changes in the large arteries, including elongation, dilatation, and arterial wall thickening as a result of changes in the intima and media.[2] Changes in both small and large arteries lead to decreased compliance, stiffness, and hypertension or other cardiovascular diseases in elderly adults. The aging process will affect cardiac physiology, including reduced systolic and diastolic functions of the right ventricle as well as left ventricular hypertrophy with associated impaired contractility and relaxation. Resting cardiac output and ejection fraction are preserved.[2] While there are significant changes in cardiac and vascular physiology in elderly patients at baseline, the lack of cardiovascular response to stress may be the most important component of altered cardiovascular physiology in elderly patients, especially in the setting of hemorrhagic shock. The diminished response to alpha-adrenergic stimulation can limit vasoconstriction, while lack of response to beta-adrenergic stimulation limits the ability to mount a tachycardic response.[2] Elderly individuals are also at increased risk of developing atrial fibrillation, ischemic heart disease, and congestive heart failure.

Table 29.1. Changes in Cardiovascular and Pulmonary Physiology and Commonly Encountered Comorbidities in the Elderly

System Involved	Physiologic Changes	Common Comorbidity
Cardiovascular	Elongation, dilatation, and wall thickening of large arteries Decreased arterial compliance and stiffness Reduced systolic and diastolic function of right ventricle Left ventricular hypertrophy Lack of cardiovascular response	Hypertension Ischemic heart disease Atrial fibrillation Congestive heart failure
Pulmonary	Kyphosis Decreased intervertebral height Decreased muscular strength Loss of elasticity and recoil Emphysematous changes Dysfunction of mucociliary system Alterations in lung volumes, gas exchange, and respiratory drive Diminished physiologic response to hypoxia and hypercapnia	Chronic obstructive pulmonary disease (COPD) Asthma Obstructive sleep apnea

Pulmonary

The aging process also brings significant baseline anatomic and physiologic changes to the pulmonary system. The chest wall of the elderly individual changes over time with decreasing strength of intercostal muscles and diaphragm. A decrease in height of intervertebral spaces and the development of kyphosis are associated with decline in FEV1/FVC ratio.[3] Chest wall stiffness resulting from calcification of costal cartilage and joints leads to decreased chest wall compliance.[3] After trauma, these anatomic changes place elderly patients at risk for earlier or more rapid respiratory failure as well as difficulty in liberation from the ventilator.[3] In addition to alterations in the chest wall, there are several changes in the pulmonary parenchyma of elderly individuals. These changes lead to increased compliance due to loss of elasticity and elastic recoil, emphysematous changes, and dysfunction of the mucociliary system. While anatomic changes are important, the altered pulmonary physiology of aging may lead to significant clinical implications when caring for the injured elderly patient. The elderly individual will have changes to pulmonary physiology, including alterations in lung volumes, gas exchange, and respiratory drive.[3] Lung volumes in elderly patients will have increased residual volume and functional residual capacity but decreased vital capacity and FEV1.[3] Alterations of pulmonary gas exchange in elderly patients include increased ventilation–perfusion mismatch as well as decreased diffusion across the alveolar–arterial membrane, both associated with a decrease in baseline PaO_2.[3] Some of the most common pulmonary comorbidities in the elderly trauma patients include COPD, asthma, and obstructive sleep apnea. **Table 29.1** displays changes in cardiovascular and pulmonary physiology as well as common comorbidities encountered in the elderly trauma patient.

Renal and Gastrointestinal

Aging causes deterioration in renal function over time due to alterations in renal vasculature, microanatomy, as well as changes in renal physiology. Over time, glomerular tissue is replaced with fibrous tissue, causing 30% to 50% loss of cortical glomeruli by 70 years of age.[4] The aging kidneys also have a diminished capacity to preserve their own function as a result of renovascular dysautonomy.[4] These changes put elderly patients at increased risk for development of acute kidney injury after trauma. Avoiding nephrotoxic agents, intravenous contrast, hyperglycemia, and hypovolemia can help prevent acute kidney injury in elderly trauma patients. Gastrointestinal derangements in the elderly patient may include dysphagia, gastroesophageal reflux, gastroparesis, and diarrhea or constipation. In addition, many elderly trauma patients will present in a state of malnutrition established long before the time of injury. It is important to screen elderly trauma patients for nutritional status and begin enteral nutrition early in the postinjury course.

Elderly trauma patients present with a wide array of altered physiology and comorbid conditions. These preexisting medical conditions are usually treated in the outpatient setting by primary care providers, and the mainstay of treatment is often a long list of medications. These preinjury medications can have a profound effect on the management and outcomes of elderly trauma patients. In addition, elderly individuals have an altered ability to metabolize the medications they encounter prior to injury as well as during their hospitalization.

Medications

Elderly trauma patients may be taking a variety of medications that may affect initial presentation, evaluation, and treatment, and eventually outcomes. As hypertension is the most common comorbidity, elderly trauma patients will often be taking preinjury antihypertensive medications. Diuretics will cause patients to present in a hypovolemic state prior to injury or hemorrhage. Preinjury beta blockers will blunt the tachycardic response and may confound the initial presentation.[5] The most significant preinjury medications in elderly trauma patients are anticoagulants and antiplatelet agents. Elderly patients may be on anticoagulants or antiplatelet agents for a variety of conditions, including atrial fibrillation, ischemic cardiac disease, valvular heart disease, cerebrovascular accidents, or thromboembolic disease. The most common outpatient anticoagulant is coumadin (vitamin K antagonist). Its use is associated with many food and drug interactions and the need for frequent monitoring. Over the last decade, the pharmaceutical industry has developed and brought several novel oral anticoagulants to the market, and their use is rapidly increasing. These newer anticoagulants include the direct thrombin inhibitor, dabigatran, as well as the Xa inhibitors, rivaroxaban, apixaban, and edoxaban. The most common antiplatelet agents include aspirin (cyclooxygenase inhibitor) and clopidogrel (ADP inhibitor). Newer antiplatelet agents include newer ADP inhibitors, prasugrel and ticagrelor.

Reversal of anticoagulants and antiplatelet agents in elderly trauma patients can be a challenging and complex clinical scenario. The clinician must balance the reversal to eliminate hemorrhage and thromboembolic complications associated with reversing anticoagulation or antiplatelet agents. Coumadin may be reversed with prothrombin complex concentrate (PCC) or plasma, if PCC is not available.[6] In recent years, there has been more evidence regarding the reversal of direct thrombin inhibitors and Xa inhibitors.[7,8] Dabigatran may be reversed with idarucizumab (Praxbind), a 2015 FDA-approved antidote that binds to dabigatran with 350 times affinity than

Table 29.2. Common Preinjury Anticoagulants in the Elderly

Mechanism of Action	Drugs	Reversal Strategies
Vitamin K antagonist	Warfarin	FFP or PCC
Direct thrombin inhibitor	Dabigatran	Idarucizumab (Praxbind) Consider intragastric charcoal Hemodialysis Consider PCC (although data is inconsistent)
Xa inhibitors	Rivaroxaban Apixaban Edoxaban	Andexanet alfa Consider intragastric charcoal Consider PCC
Antiplatelet agents	Aspirin Aspirin dipyridamole Clopidogrel Prasugrel Ticagrelor	DDAVP Platelet transfusion

dabigatran to thrombin.[7] Treatment resulted in complete reversal of the anticoagulant effects of dabigatran, with over 98% of patients reaching a median reversal of 100%.[7] Thrombotic complications occurred in 4.8% of patients at 30 days.[7] Intragastric-activated charcoal may be administered if drug has been taken within 2 hours of presentation, or hemodialysis may be considered. PCC may be considered for the reversal of dabigatran however, the data and consensus guidelines are inconsistent.[6] Plasma is unlikely to have any therapeutic effect on reversing dabigatran. Andexanet alfa is an option for the reversal of Xa inhibitors. Recent data on the use of Andexanet alfa in patients taking Xa inhibitors with intracerebral hemorrhage showed better control of hematoma expansion compared to usual care but was associated with thrombotic events, including ischemic stroke. The risk of thrombotic events seemed to be highest in patients with a history of myocardial infarction or stroke.[8] Other reversal strategies for Xa inhibitors include activated charcoal (if ingested within 2 hours) or PCC. Finally, a new drug called ciraparantag is under investigation by the FDA. It was designed as a universal reversal agent for novel oral anticoagulants, unfractionated heparin, and low–molecular-weight heparin activity. Antiplatelet agents may be reversed with either DDAVP or platelet transfusion, but the indications for either therapy have not been elucidated. A new monoclonal antibody targeted at ticagrelor reversal, named bentracimab, is also under investigation. **Table 29.2** displays common preinjury anticoagulants and antiplatelet agents in the elderly trauma patient.

Once hospitalized, particular attention must be paid to medications ordered for the elderly trauma patient. Elderly patients have changes in pharmacokinetics and pharmacodynamics, including alterations in absorption, bioavailability,
2 distribution, metabolism, and elimination. The American Geriatrics Society has published the 2023 updated Beers Criteria for potentially inappropriate medication use in older adults that can be used to refine inpatient medication management for elderly trauma patients.[9] Of particular importance to the management of the elderly trauma patients is the plan for pain control. Pain medications may have significant side effects in elderly patients, including delirium, nausea, vomiting, constipation, renal dysfunction, and gastrointestinal bleeding. A multimodal approach with the lowest effective dose for pain control should be used for elderly trauma patients.

MECHANISM AND INJURIES

Mechanisms of injury for elderly trauma patients are most often a result of blunt trauma with falls, motor vehicle crashes,
3 and pedestrian struck by auto being the most frequent. Falls are far and away the most common mechanism in elderly trauma patients, causing almost 75% of injuries.[5] Nearly one in three adults over 65 years old will experience ground-level falls each year.[4] There are a variety of reasons that elderly individuals are at risk for falls, including weakness, deconditioning from chronic illness, vision loss, gait and balance disturbances, slowed reaction time, and cognitive impairments.[5] The American Geriatrics Society has developed clinical practice guidelines (**Table 29.3**) for the prevention of falls in older adults.[10]

Elderly Abuse

4 An underreported but extremely important mechanism of injury in elderly trauma patients is abuse. Elderly abuse is committed by an individual who has a relationship with and is responsible for the well-being of an elderly individual. Abuse can be further classified as physical abuse, verbal or psychological abuse, sexual abuse, financial abuse, and neglect.[11] Perpetrators of elderly abuse may include family members or caregivers, either in the home or at an assisted-living facility. Abuse of the elderly is associated with depression, cognitive impairment, loss of functional capacity, and increased morbidity and mortality.[11] Several risk factors and warning signs for elderly abuse have been identified and are listed in **Table 29.4**.[12] If elderly trauma patients appear to be at risk for or display warning signs of possible abuse, they may be assessed using a variety of available screening tools[12] including the American Medical Association (AMA) screening tool, the Conflict Tactics Scale (CTS), the Brief Abuse Screen for the Elderly (BASE), the Elder Assessment Instrument (EAI), or the Comprehensive Geriatric Assessment (CGA). Some recommended strategies for intervention in suspected cases of elder abuse are outlined in **Table 29.5**.[11]

Traumatic Brain Injury

Traumatic brain injury (TBI) is a significant cause of morbidity and mortality in elderly trauma patients.[13] People aged 75 years and older account for about 32% of TBI-related hospitalizations and 28% of TBI-related deaths.[14] The most common mechanism causing TBI in elderly patients is falls,
5 followed by motor vehicle collisions. Falls account for 55% of all TBIs in patients 65 to 74 years old and 85% of TBIs in patients >85 years old.[13] Imaging with head CT in elderly trauma patients should be used liberally for several reasons: (1) elderly patients have progressive brain atrophy leading to stretching of bridging veins and increased risk of subdural hemorrhage after trauma, (2) clinical tools such as the Canadian CT Head Rule exclude elderly patients,[15] and (3) neurologic examination may be unreliable in elderly trauma patients. The catastrophic combination of TBI and preinjury anticoagulation should prompt the rapid reversal of anticoagulation.[6]

Fractures

Elderly patients have decreased cortical bone mass, increasing their risk for fractures at lower levels of kinetic energy. Consequently, older patients have an increased risk of rib, spinal, pelvic, and extremity fractures after falls and other low-impact mechanisms than younger patients.

Rib fractures are a significant cause of morbidity and mortality among older patients. Retrospective studies show that in-hospital mortality for patients >65 years is double that of younger patients.[16] The risk of mortality and pneumonia

Table 29.3. AGS/BGS Clinical Practice Guideline: Prevention of Falls in Older Persons

Summary of Recommendations

Screening and Assessment

1. All older individuals should be asked whether they have fallen (in the past year).
2. An older person who reports a fall should be asked about the frequency and circumstances of the fall(s).
3. Older individuals should be asked if they experience difficulties with walking or balance.
4. Older persons who present for medical attention because of a fall, report recurrent falls in the past year, or report difficulties in walking or balance (with or without activity curtailment) should have a multifactorial fall risk assessment.
5. Older persons presenting with a single fall should be evaluated for gait and balance.
6. Older persons who have fallen should have an assessment of gait and balance using one of the available evaluations.
7. Older persons who cannot perform or perform poorly on a standardized gait and balance test should be given a multifactorial fall risk assessment.
8. Older persons who have difficulty or demonstrate unsteadiness during the evaluation of gait and balance require a multifactorial fall risk assessment.
9. Older persons reporting only a single fall and reporting or demonstrating no difficulty or unsteadiness during the evaluation of gait and balance do not require a fall risk assessment.
10. The multifactorial fall risk assessment should be performed by a clinician (or clinicians) with appropriate skills and training.
11. The multifactorial fall risk assessment should include the following:

Focused History

a. History of falls: detailed description of the circumstances of the fall(s), frequency, symptoms at time of fall, injuries, and other consequences
b. Medication review: all prescribed and over-the-counter medications with dosages
c. History of relevant risk factors: acute or chronic medical problems (eg, osteoporosis, urinary incontinence, cardiovascular disease)

Physical Examinations

a. Detailed assessment of gait, balance, and mobility levels and lower extremity joint function
b. Neurologic function: cognitive evaluation, lower extremity peripheral nerves, proprioception, reflexes, and tests of cortical, extrapyramidal, and cerebellar function
c. Muscle strength (lower extremities)
d. Cardiovascular status: heart rate and rhythm, postural pulse, blood pressure, and, if appropriate, heart rate and blood pressure responses to carotid sinus stimulation
e. Assessment of visual acuity
f. Examination of the feet and footwear

Functional Assessment

a. Assessment of activities of daily living (ADLs) skills including use of adaptive equipment and mobility aids, as appropriate
b. Assessment of the individual's perceived functional ability and fear related to falling (assessment of current activity levels with attention to the extent to which concerns about falling are protective [ie, appropriate given abilities] or contributing to deconditioning and/or compromised quality of life [ie, individual is curtailing involvement in activities he or she is safely able to perform due to fear of falling])

Environmental Assessment

a. Environmental assessment including home safety

increases with increasing number of ribs fractured, and patients with more than three fractures have worse outcomes.[16] Up to a third of older patients with rib fractures develop pneumonia, and rib fractures are associated with longer mechanical ventilation days and ICU length of stay.[16]

Osteoporosis, prior fracture, and functional impairment are all risk factors for pelvic fracture. Over 85% of pelvic fractures are caused by falls, and morbidity and mortality after pelvic fractures are significant.[17] Many patients after pelvic fracture require a cane or a walker, over 80% are institutionalized, and 12% to 25% will die within a year of injury.[17] Most do not regain prior functional abilities, and patients after pelvic fracture are five times more likely to live in an institution a year after injury. Pelvic fracture in older patients often leads to decline in mental health, social isolation, and overall health. Up to half of patients with pelvic fractures experience pain for many months after injury.[18]

Spinal trauma is increasingly common in elderly patients. The risk of cervical fracture after falls increases with age due to higher rates of cervical stenosis and degenerative disk disease.[5] An estimated 5% to 10% will sustain spinal injury and permanent neurologic deficit after cervical fracture, and 1-year mortality is estimated to be 20% to 30%.[19]

TRIAGE CRITERIA FOR OLDER PATIENTS

Trauma center care reduces mortality for older trauma patients, and the benefit of treatment at trauma centers for older patients increases with age. However, triage of older
6 patients can be quite challenging. Even severely injured older patients may not display standard signs of hemodynamic instability. Using standard adult trauma triage criteria for older adults leads to delays in recognition of injury severity and undertriage.[20] For these reasons, trauma activation protocols must have criteria specific for older adults. A recent systematic review of prehospital trauma triage criteria showed age cut-offs anywhere from 55 to 70 years of age, with ≥65 most frequently reported.[21] The National Trauma Triage Protocol suggests that a systolic blood pressure of ≤110 mm Hg should trigger transport to a trauma center, to decrease the incidence of undertriage.[22] Shock index (SI) can also be incorporated into triage criteria. In a retrospective study using the National Trauma Data Bank, Pandit et al. showed that SI (HR/SBP) ≥1 was associated with higher rates of blood transfusions, exploratory laparotomy, in-hospital complications, and in-hospital mortality. Based on these findings, the authors recommend that patients with an SI ≥1 should be transferred to level I trauma centers.[23] The Eastern Association for Trauma

Table 29.4. Risk Factors and Warning Signs for Elderly Abuse

History
Advanced age (>80 y)
Disability in self-care
Dementia
Depression
History of hip fracture
History of stroke
Social isolation
Poor socioeconomic status
External family stressors
Unfavorable caretaker characteristics (mental illness, substance abuse, history of violent or antisocial behavior, depression, or financial dependency on the victim)
Institutional staffing shortages
Inappropriate or excessive medications; failure to get needed medications; lack of appropriate monitoring of medications and their effects
Substance abuse
Physical/Mental Status Examination
Indicators of sexual abuse: pain, bruises, lacerations, bleeding in anal–genital areas; bruised breasts or abdomen; signs of venereal diseases
Lacerations (including large skin tears, abrasions, burns, and bruises) without adequate explanation, especially on the trunk or other unusual locations
Suspicious fractures in sites other than those seen in osteoporotic fractures, that is, wrist, hip, or vertebral body
Malnutrition
Focal findings on neurologic examination
Signs of dehydration
Pressure ulcers
Dementia, psychiatric disorders, lack of mental capacity

Table 29.5. Strategies for Intervention by Physicians in Suspected Cases of Elder Abuse

Suspected Type of Abuse	Intervention Strategies
Neglect	Optimize assistance, including home care Address burden and stress on the caregiver Educate caregiver that care being provided may be aberrant Identify alternative potential caregivers Arrange for social work assistance to ensure benefits and services are optimized Consider nursing home placement Consider adult day care and other respite programs
Verbal abuse	Refer victim for psychiatric or social work assistance Recognize and treat depression and other mental health issues Address burden and stress on the caregiver Educate caregiver that care being provided may be aberrant Identify alternative potential caregivers Address substance abuse
Financial exploitation	Stop the loss of resources as soon as possible Consider power of attorney, daily money management, or guardianship Alert banks and financial institutions to victim's vulnerability Consider referral to local law enforcement, district attorney, or both
Physical/sexual abuse	Evaluate, treat, and document physical and sexual violence Refer case to local law enforcement and district attorney Consider filing an order of protection with assistance of law enforcement Consider referral to a shelter for victims of elder abuse Emphasize the need for a safety plan

(EAST) geriatric triage guidelines suggest that older patients should be transferred to a level I center if they have a base deficit of −6 or greater, or one body system AIS is >3.[24]

Despite evidence supporting higher triage, multiple studies show that older patients are routinely undertriaged. Data from the Washington State database showed that the likelihood of being transferred to a trauma center decreased above age 45.[25] Compared to younger patients in the cohort, patients 81 years and older were only 11% as likely to be transported to a level I trauma center from the scene, and only 24% as likely to be transferred from a lower level center to a level I center. The relationship between trauma center admission and longer-term outcome is controversial.

EVALUATION AND MANAGEMENT

Trauma Evaluation

Initial evaluation of all geriatric trauma patients, regardless of mechanism of injury, should follow advanced trauma life support (ATLS) principles. As described previously, older patients are much more likely to have medical comorbidities and extensive lists of medications. These comorbidities, along with the changes in physiology described previously, should be taken into consideration in the assessment of hemodynamic stability. With this in mind, a thorough medical and medication history should be reviewed with patients or their surrogates, with specific focus on beta blockers, ACE inhibitors, anticoagulant, and antiplatelet medications. Standard laboratory evaluation should include complete blood counts, comprehensive metabolic panel, coagulation studies such as prothrombin time with international normalized ratio and partial thromboplastin time, lactate, and cardiac enzymes. Initial imaging should include a chest and pelvis x-ray and focused assessment for sonography and trauma (FAST) exam for all mechanisms, as even low-energy mechanisms can produce significant injury in this population. CT imaging should also be used liberally.[26]

Comprehensive Geriatric Assessment

7 Due to the broad range of age-related factors that can contribute to injury and adversely affect recovery in geriatric patients, patients should receive a CGA during their hospital stay. This is a multidimensional and multidisciplinary evaluation including functional ability, physical health, cognition and mental health, and medication review. A previously published meta-analysis of 22 randomized trials showed that hospitalized elders who receive a CGA are less likely to die in hospital, have higher rates of discharge to home, and improved long-term functional outcomes.[27] Functional status is evaluated with a review of activities of daily living (ADLs) (eating, dressing, bathing, transfers, toileting, continence) and instrumental ADLs (housework, bills, meal preparation, medication management, using the telephone).[28] Physical and occupational therapists can assess gait, balance, home safety, and ability to carry out ADL. Medications that can exacerbate or cause

injuries should be reviewed. Patients should also receive a nutritional assessment. Social workers can assess social supports, caregiver needs, and financial assets and identify resources for the patient and family after hospital discharge. In cases where it is impractical to thoroughly evaluate each condition during hospitalization, patients should be referred for outpatient follow-up at discharge.

Assessing Frailty

8 Frailty is a syndrome of decreased physiologic reserve, includes physical, cognitive, social, and psychological components that can worsen over time, and is distinct from the normal aging process and other comorbidities.[29] It is associated with higher mortality and complications, worse functional outcomes after trauma, and is more predictive than age or injury severity as a predictor of hospital complications, in-hospital mortality, or discharge to an institution.[30] Components of the frailty syndrome include shrinkage, weakness, exhaustion, low physical activity, and slowness. Presence of three or more of these indicates frailty.[31]

While frailty can be assessed using a number of different instruments, the Trauma Specific Frailty Index and the Rockwood Frailty Score were recently shown to be better predictors of poor outcomes compared to other commonly used instruments.[32] Sarcopenia can also be used as a surrogate for frailty, and can easily be measured using psoas CT diameter. The Vulnerable Elders-13 Survey (VES-13), an assessment of functional status, has also been validated as a screening tool to predict discharge to a nursing facility and surgical complication or death in trauma patients 65 years or older.[33]

Patient Management

Data published over the last decade have shown that geriatric trauma patients benefit from care at trauma centers and management by multidisciplinary teams. Various studies have shown that trauma centers with higher volumes and proportions of geriatric trauma patients have lower mortality, fewer complications, and lower rates of failure to rescue.[34,35] This suggests that the greater experience of these centers leads to improved outcomes. Furthermore, there is a great deal of interest in the value of geriatricians to the care of trauma patients. Data also show that routine geriatric consultation leads to lower mortality rates, lower rates of delirium, fewer discharges to facilities among patients admitted from home, and better long-term functional recovery.[36–38]

Some centers have reported success in developing clinical pathways for geriatric trauma patients. Previously, Mangram et al.[39] described their experience with a dedicated geriatric service and hospital unit, known as the G-60 service, which is a multidisciplinary service aimed at providing comprehensive care. As compared to historical controls, patients on the G-60 service had significantly shorter ED length of stay, time to OR, hospital length of stay, and ICU length of stay. Although mortality was unchanged, there were also significantly lower rates of medical complications. Furthermore, when applied to patients based on frailty rather than age, the use of this multidisciplinary approach was shown to decrease delirium and readmission.[40] The evidence supporting multidisciplinary care of geriatric trauma patients is strong, and organizations such as the American Association for the Surgery of Trauma and American College of Surgeons Committee on Trauma advocate for their implementation at centers caring for these patients.

OUTCOMES

Mortality Outcomes

As compared to younger patients, in-hospital mortalities for older patients are 4.4% versus 1.6% for low severity injuries and 5.9% versus 1.4% for moderate severity injuries. Furthermore, in patients over the age 85 and older, mortality has been reported as high as 60%.[41] Moreover, mortality among older trauma patients increases with the number of comorbidities; patients with minor injuries and comorbidities are at increased risk of death compared to age-matched counterparts without comorbidities.[42] It is important for clinicians to recognize that significant numbers of geriatric trauma patients die shortly after hospital discharge, and 30-day postdischarge mortality rates have been shown to be double in-hospital mortality.[43] Other than the impact of age and comorbidities on mortality, in-hospital complications such as respiratory failure and delirium are associated with increased mortality and diminished quality of life postdischarge. Medications, including analgesics and their effect on delirium, are well understood. It is imperative to use nonnarcotic options for pain control as first-line treatment in the geriatric patient. Regional anesthesia has long been advocated to minimize narcotic use, and was recently shown to decrease the risk of delirium in geriatric patients with rib fractures.[44]

Functional Outcomes

A significant portion of patients experience long-term functional decline after injury. In a prospective study of patients older than 65 years of age, Kelley-Quon et al.[45] showed that most patients had lost one ADL at 12 months. More recent data from this group show that a geriatric consultation during the index hospitalization is associated with less long-term functional decline.[38] Quality of life in older patients is significantly impaired. Among patients 1 year after hip fracture, 90% have reduced mobility, 69% have pain, and 33% who were independent live in a nursing home. As compared to patients without TBI, a cohort of patients >50 years old had poorer cognitive and psychosocial function a year postinjury.

TRAUMA

PALLIATIVE AND END-OF-LIFE CARE IN THE GERIATRIC TRAUMA PATIENT

Palliative care is an approach to medical care aimed at relieving suffering and improving quality of life for patients with serious illness and for their families. Palliative care is appropriate in the management of a broad range of injured patients who die or suffer from acute and chronic pain, functional disability, or life-limiting conditions such as severe frailty and underlying organ failure.[46] Clinical domains of palliative care encompass symptom management. Spiritual, religious, psychosocial, and bereavement support can be delivered alongside aggressive life-prolonging care and should not be limited to only those patients near the end of life.[47] Thus, palliative care can be provided to patients who are expected to recover from injury. Palliative care should not be confused with hospice care, which is an administrative benefit provided to patients with terminal illness and typically provided to patients expected to survive less than 6 months.

End-of-Life Care

9 Advanced directives, including living wills and proxy forms, are intended to guide medical decisions in the event a patient loses capacity to make decisions. Unfortunately, many patients, even those with terminal illness, do not have advanced directives or the advanced directives are too specific or too broad to be useful. Therefore, it is critically important that clinicians make every effort to engage patients and their families in conversations about resuscitation status, the overall goals of care, and expectations for recovery early in the hospital course. Patients may forego heroic measures and prolonged life-sustaining treatments if all possible outcomes are not acceptable to them. Furthermore, lack of decision-making capacity, whether it be from preexisting comorbidities, sequelae of injuries, or delirium, often complicates this discussion with the patient. It is advisable for clinicians to identify health care proxies as early in the hospital course as possible, should this be the case. Palliative care services, which focus on improving quality of life in seriously ill patients, are an integral part of critically ill geriatric trauma patients.

Physicians play an important role in providing a comfortable death experience for patients and families. In death, patients want to minimize discomfort, to avoid a prolonged dying process, to achieve a sense of control, and to have time to strengthen relationships with loved ones.[48] Survivors and surrogates suffer high rates of depression, posttraumatic stress disorder, and complicated grief after a loved one dies in the ICU.[49] Better outcomes for survivors are achieved when they feel that they have been well informed and have had appropriate responsibility in decision making.[50] It is important for physicians to provide emotional support for surrogates who are often conflicted and distressed.

References

1. Projected Population by Age Group and Sex for the United States, Main Series: 2022–2100. U.S. Census Bureau, Population Division. 2023.
2. Martin RS, Farrah JP, Chang MC. Effect of aging on cardiac function plus monitoring and support. *Surg Clin North Am.* 2015; 95:23–35.
3. Tran D, Rajwani K, Berlin DA. Pulmonary effects of aging. *Curr Opin Anaesthesiol.* 2018;31(1):19–23.
4. Brooks SE, Peetz AB. Evidence-based care of geriatric trauma patients. *Surg Clin North Am.* 2017;97(5):1157–1174.
5. Bonne S, Schuerer DJ. Trauma in the older adult. Epidemiology and evolving geriatric trauma principles. *Clin Geriatr Med.* 2013;29:137–150.
6. Frontera JA, Lewin JJ III, Rabinstein AA, et al. Guideline for reversal of antithrombotics in intracranial hemorrhage: executive summary. A statement for healthcare professionals from the Neurocritical Care Society and the Society of Critical Care Medicine. *Crit Care Med.* 2016;44(12):2251–2257.
7. Rose DK, Bar B. Direct oral anticoagulant agents: pharmacologic profile, indications, coagulation monitoring, and reversal agents. *J Stroke Cerebrovasc Dis.* 2018;27(8):2049–2058.
8. Connolly SJ, Sharma M, Cohen AT, et al. ANNEXA-I investigators. Andexanet for factor Xa inhibitor-associated acute intracerebral hemorrhage. *N Engl J Med.* 2024;390(19):1745–1755.
9. 2023 American Geriatrics Society Beers Criteria® Update Expert Panel. American Geriatrics Society 2023 updated AGS Beers Criteria® for potentially inappropriate medication use in older adults. *J Am Geriatr Soc.* 2023;71(7):2052–2081.
10. Kenny RAM, Rubenstein LZ, Tinetti ME, et al. Panel on Prevention of Falls in Older Persons, American Geriatrics Society and British Geriatrics Society. Summary of the Updated American Geriatrics Society/British Geriatrics Society clinical practice guideline for prevention of falls in older persons. *J Am Geriatr Soc.* 2011;59(1): 148–157.
11. Lachs MS, Pillemer KA. Elder abuse. *N Engl J Med.* 2015;373(20): 1947–1956.
12. Halphen JM, Dyer CB. Elder mistreatment: abuse, neglect, and financial exploitation. In: Schmader KE, Sokol HN, eds. *UpToDate.* Wolters Kluwer; 2014.
13. Gardner RC, Dams-O'Connor K, Morrissey MR, Manley GT. Geriatric traumatic brain injury: epidemiology, outcomes, knowledge gaps and future directions. *J Neurotrauma.* 2018;35(7): 889–906.
14. Centers for Disease Control and Prevention. National Center for Health Statistics: Mortality Data on CDC WONDER. Accessed June, 2024. https://wonder.cdc.gov/mcd.html
15. Stiell IG, Wells GA, Vandemheen K, et al. The Canadian CT Head Rule for patients with minor head injury. *Lancet.* 2001;357: 1391–1396.
16. Witt CE, Bulger EM. Comprehensive approach to the management of the patient with multiple rib fractures: a review and introduction of a bundled rib fracture management protocol. *Trauma Surg Acute Care Open.* 2017;2(1):e000064.
17. Moreland BL, Legha JK, Thomas KE, et al. Hip fracture-related emergency department visits, hospitalizations and deaths by mechanism of injury among adults aged 65 and older, United States 2019. *J Aging Health.* 2023;35(5–6):345–355.
18. Herrick C, Steger-May K, Sinacore DR, Brown M, Schechtman KB, Binder EF. Persistent pain in frail older adults after hip fracture repair. *J Am Geriatr Soc.* 2004;52(12):2062–2068.
19. Harris MB, Reichmann WM, Bono CM. Mortality in elderly patients after cervical spine fractures. *J Bone Joint Surg Am.* 2010; 92(3):567–574.
20. Benoit E, Stephen AH, Monaghan SF, Lueckel SN, Adams CA Jr. Geriatric trauma. *R I Med J (2013).* 2019;102(8):19–22.
21. Boulton AJ, Peel D, Rahman U, Cole E. Evaluation of elderly specific pre-hospital trauma triage criteria: a systematic review. *Scand J Trauma Resusc Emerg Med.* 2021;29:127.
22. Brown JB, Gestring ML, Forsythe RM, et al. Systolic blood pressure criteria in the National Trauma Triage Protocol for geriatric trauma: 110 is the new 90. *J Trauma Acute Care Surg.* 2015;78(2):352–359.
23. Pandit V, Rhee P, Hashmi A, et al. Shock index predicts mortality in geriatric trauma patients: an analysis of the National Trauma Data Bank. *J Trauma Acute Care Surg.* 2014;76(4):1111–1115.
24. Jacobs DG, Plaisier BR, Barie PS, et al. Practice management guidelines for geriatric trauma: the EAST Practice Management Guidelines Work Group. *J Trauma Acute Care Surg.* 2003;54(2): 391–416.
25. Gage AM, Traven N, Rivara FP, et al. Compliance with Centers for Disease Control and Prevention field triage guidelines in an established trauma system. *J Am Coll Surg.* 2012;215(1):148–154; discussion 154–156.
26. American College of Surgeons. *Best Practice Guidelines: Geriatric Trauma Management I.* 2023. Accessed June 30, 2024. https://www.facs.org/media/ubyj2ubl/best-practices-guidelines-geriatric-trauma.pdf
27. Ellis G, Whitehead MA, Robinson D, Langhorne P, Robinson D. Comprehensive geriatric assessment for older adults admitted to hospital: meta-analysis of randomised controlled trials. *BMJ.* 2011;343:d6553.
28. Katz S, Ford A, Moskowitz RW, Jackson BA, Jaffe MW. Studies of illness in the aged. The index of ADL: a standardized measure of biological and psychosocial function. *JAMA.* 1963;185:914–919.
29. Cubitt M, Downie E, Shakerian R, et al. Timing and methods of frailty assessments in geriatric trauma patients: a systematic review. *Injury.* 2019;50(11):1795–1808.
30. Pandit V, Joseph B, Rhee PM, et al. Frailty is superior to age in predicting outcomes in geriatric trauma patients: a prospective analysis. *J Am Coll Surg.* 2013;217(3 Suppl):S59.
31. Fried LP, Tangen CM, Walston J, et al. Cardiovascular Health Study Collaborative Research Group. Frailty in older adults: evidence for a phenotype. *J Gerontol A Biolo Sci Med Sci.* 2001; 56(3):M146–M157.
32. Hamidi M, Haddadin Z, Zeeshan M, et al. Prospective evaluation and comparison of the predictive ability of different frailty scores to predict outcomes in geriatric trauma patients. *J Trauma Acute Care Surg.* 2019;87(5):1172–1180.
33. Min L, Ubhayakar N, Saliba D, et al. The vulnerable elders survey-13 predicts hospital complications and mortality in older adults with traumatic injury: a pilot study. *J Am Geriatr Soc.* 2011; 59(8):1471–1476.
34. Matsushima K, Schaefer EW, Won EJ, et al. Positive and negative volume-outcome relationships in the geriatric trauma population. *JAMA Surg.* 2014;149(4):319–326.
35. Olufajo OA, Metcalfe D, Rios-Diaz A, et al. Does hospital experience rather than volume improve outcomes in geriatric trauma patients? *J Am Coll Surg.* 2016;223(1):32–40.e1.
36. Grigoryan KV, Javedan H, Rudolph JL. Ortho-geriatric care models and outcomes in hip fracture patients: a systematic review and meta-analysis. *J Orthop Trauma.* 2014;28(3):e49–e55.
37. Lenartowicz M, Parkovnick M, McFarlan A, et al. An evaluation of a proactive geriatric trauma consultation service. *Ann Surg.* 2012;256(6):1098–1101.
38. Tillou A, Kelley-Quon L, Burruss S, et al. Long-term postinjury functional recovery: outcomes of geriatric consultation. *JAMA Surg.* 2014;149(1):83–89.
39. Mangram AJ, Mitchell CD, Shifflette VK, et al. Geriatric trauma service: a one-year experience. *J Trauma Acute Care Surg.* 2012; 72(1):119–122.
40. Bryant EA, Tulebaev S, Castillo-Angeles M, et al. Frailty identification and care pathway: an interdisciplinary approach to care for older trauma patients. *J Am Coll Surg.* 2019;228(6):852–859.e1.

41. de Vries R, Reininga IHF, de Graaf MW, et al. Older polytrauma: mortality and complications. *Injury.* 2019;50(8):1440–1447.
42. McGwin G Jr, MacLennan PA, Fife JB, et al. Preexisting conditions and mortality in older trauma patients. *J Trauma.* 2004;56(6): 1291–1296.
43. Clark DE, DeLorenzo MA, Lucas FL, et al. Initial presentation of older injured patients to high-volume hospitals is not associated with lower 30-day mortality in Medicare data. *Crit Care Med.* 2007;35(8):1829–1836.
44. O'Connell KM, Quistberg DA, Tessler R, et al. Decreased risk of delirium with use of regional analgesia in geriatric trauma patients with multiple rib fractures. *Ann Surg.* 2018;268(3): 534–540.
45. Kelley-Quon L, Min L, Morley E, et al. Functional status after injury: a longitudinal study of geriatric trauma. *Am Surg.* 2010; 76(10):1055–1058.
46. Grossman MD, Miller D, Scaff DW, et al. When is an elder old? Effect of preexisting conditions on mortality in geriatric trauma. *J Trauma.* 2002;52(2):242–246.
47. American College of Surgeons Task Force on Surgical Palliative Care. *Statement of Principles of Palliative Care.* 2005. Accessed June, 2024. https://www.facs.org/about-acs/statements/principles-of-palliative-care
48. Steinhauser KE, Clipp EC, McNeilly M, et al. In search of a good death: observations of patients, families, and providers. *Ann Intern Med.* 2000;132(10):825–832.
49. Siegel MD, Hayes E, Vanderwerker LC, et al. Psychiatric illness in the next of kin of patients who die in the intensive care unit. *Crit Care Med.* 2008;36(6):1722–1728.
50. Gries CJ, Engelberg RA, Kross EK, et al. Predictors of symptoms of posttraumatic stress and depression in family members after patient death in the ICU. *Chest.* 2010;137(2):280–287.

30

Trauma in Pregnancy

Felix Y. Lui and Kimberly A. Davis

Key Points

1. The management of the pregnant patient presents challenges that can impact outcomes for both the mother and child.
2. Treatment priorities remain the same as for the nongravid patient but plans should be tailored for the anatomic and physiologic changes in the gravid trauma patient based on stage of pregnancy.
3. Relative hypervolemia of pregnancy may mask physiologic changes associated with massive hemorrhage.
4. Compression of the inferior vena cava (IVC) and hypotension can result from supine positioning. Left-sided decubitus positioning with a wedge is recommended.
5. A Kleihauer–Betke (KB) test should be performed in all pregnant trauma patients >12 weeks of gestation and prophylactic anti-D immune globulin given within 72 hours for high-risk patients.
6. The increased risk for deep venous thrombosis (DVT) should be mitigated with low–molecular-weight heparin prophylaxis.
7. Angiography and angioembolization may be useful in life-threatening hemorrhage, recognizing the risks of increased radiation exposure.
8. Intimate partner violence (IPV) and substance abuse are increased in pregnancy and should be screened for.

Trauma is the leading cause of nonobstetric death in women of child-bearing age, with homicide leading all obstetric causes (hypertensive, disorders, hemorrhage, and sepsis) in the United States.[1] Pregnant patients present a unique scenario in that treatment is required for two (or more) patients simultane-
1 ously.[2] The management of pregnant women who suffer trauma is complicated by altered physiology, anatomic distortions, and additional diagnostic considerations. These complexities are associated with increased mortality as compared to nonpregnant women.[2] More than 1 in 20 pregnancies are complicated by trauma of varying degree which leads to increased rates of preterm labor, placental abruption, and fetal demise.[3] Evaluation of pregnant women after trauma can be challenging but should follow the same priorities as for nonpregnant patients. Recognition of the predictable changes of anatomy and physiology as gestation progresses, pregnancy-related conditions, and specific challenges in critical care and operative management are critical to management of these patients. Early consultation with an obstetrical provider should be strongly considered.

Pregnancy is a well-known risk factor for intimate partner violence (IPV) but is underrecognized by health care providers and leads to increased risk of adverse outcomes including preterm birth and NICU admission.[4] The primary focus of resuscitation should be to stabilize the mother. While fetal survival and outcome must be considered, preterm and emergency deliveries are associated with poorer outcomes for infants.

EPIDEMIOLOGY

Women seek medical attention following trauma in 5% to 7% pregnancies but few require hospitalization.[5] More than 40% of maternal deaths in the United States are due to trauma. Fetal death is reported in nearly half of pregnancies when the mother has life-threatening injuries, but even minor trauma can be associated with fetal loss. In fact, the majority of fetal loss occurs after minor injuries due to their much higher incidence.[6] Most traumas occur in the third trimester. Motor vehicle collisions are the most common mechanism of injury, followed by falls and interpersonal violence. Motor vehicle collisions are a leading cause of fetal death due to their frequency (207 cases per 100,000 pregnancies).[7,8] IPV occurs in up to 30% of pregnant women, with a fetal mortality of 5%. While it is more common earlier in pregnancies, violence is prevalent throughout gestation and increases immediately after delivery.[9,10] Almost 10% of trauma in pregnant patients is intentional.[11]

MECHANISMS OF INJURY

Phases of fetal maturation and uterine size during pregnancy correlate with injury patterns. Before 12 weeks of gestation, the uterus remains thick walled and within the bony pelvis. As the uterus enlarges, it becomes increasingly thin walled and emerges from the protection conferred by the bony pelvis. By week 20, the uterus reaches the level of the umbilicus and by week 34, the costal margin. Additionally, the relative volume of amniotic fluid decreases further limiting the cushion for the fetus to blunt trauma.

Falls during pregnancy are common and underreported. When surveyed, 27% of pregnant women reported a fall during their pregnancy.[12] Expected changes in pregnancy (ie, increased weight, increased joint laxity, and hypermobility) predispose women to falls. Fortunately, most falls result in only minor trauma to the mother, but a risk to the fetus.

Trauma after motor vehicle collisions, the most common mechanism of significant trauma for pregnant women can be mitigated with the use of restraint devices resulting in improved outcomes and decreased fetal mortality.[13] With increasing gestational age, the fetus is at higher risk for direct blunt force. Trauma to the fetus can results in skull fracture and/or intracranial hemorrhage. Placental abruption, separation of the placenta from the uterus, is the most common direct cause of fetal demise after trauma. Uterine rupture, while rare, is exceptionally lethal with rare fetal survival and maternal mortality of 10%. Maternal pelvic fractures, a high-energy marker, should raise concern for retroperitoneal hemorrhage of the mother and direct injury to the fetal head especially late in pregnancy.

Penetrating trauma in pregnant woman has a high fetal mortality rate, ranging from 40% to 80%, depending on mechanism, gestational age, and location. Gunshot wounds (GSWs) result in represent 73% of penetration abdominal wounds in pregnancy.[11] Fetal injury is identified in 70% these cases. All abdominal GSWs should be explored but stab wounds may be managed nonoperatively in the stable patient if there is no fascial violation.[14]

EVALUATION OF THE PREGNANT TRAUMA PATIENT

2 The American College of Surgeons' Advanced Trauma Life Support guidelines apply for both pregnant and nonpregnant trauma patient.[15] Evaluation begins with a primary survey, according the ABCDE approach pausing to correct immediately life-threatening problems as identified. The secondary survey, a complete head-to-toe assessment, follows in order to identify other associated injuries. Prioritizing resuscitation of the mother leads to improved outcomes for the fetus. A detailed obstetric history including gestational age, prenatal care, complications, and names of obstetrical providers can be invaluable information.

The goals of fetal assessment are to evaluate for fetal injury or death, uteroplacental integrity, and signs of maternal fetal hemorrhage (MFH). Key to the assessment is knowing gestational age and sonography. For viable pregnancies (≥23 weeks) at least 4 hours of electronic fetal heart rate (FHR) and uterine activity monitoring is recommended to start as soon as feasible. Heart tones can be heard as early as 10 weeks and should be confirmed but previable fetal monitoring is not indicated.[16] As fetal distress often precedes maternal signs, FHR monitoring can help guide resuscitation. Fetal tachycardia (FHR >160) and bradycardia (FHR <120) are signs of fetal distress and should prompt additional resuscitation for the mother (see **Table 30.1**).

Table 30.1. Physiologic Changes in Pregnancy

Cardiovascular	Increased heart rate (10–15 bpm) Increased plasma volume Decreased systemic vascular resistance Decreased blood pressure (first and second trimesters)
Pulmonary	Elevated diaphragm Increased tidal volume Increased minute ventilation Increased oxygen consumption Decreased functional residual capacity Decreased PCO_2 (30 mm Hg)
Gastrointestinal	Decreased lower esophageal sphincter competency Decreased gastric motility Increased transaminase levels Impaired gallbladder contractions
Genitourinary	Increased glomerular filtration rate Increased renal plasma flow Decreased blood urea nitrogen levels Decreased creatinine levels Hydronephrosis/hydroureter
Hematologic	Relative anemia but increased overall RBC volume Increased WBC counts (9.8–15 k) Increased clotting factors VII, VIII, IX, X, XII (hypercoagulability) Increased fibrinogen Decreased fibrinolytic activity (hypercoagulability)

Airway

Pregnant women have increased oxygen consumption (30% to 60%) and have a decreased functional expiratory reserve volume and functional residual capacity. The space occupied by a gravid uterus limits diaphragmatic excursion into the abdomen diminishing respiratory reserve and potentially leading to precipitous hypoxia of mother and fetus.

Normal weight gain during pregnancy increases BMI and Mallampati scores making airway management more challenging with higher morbidity and more failed intubations.[17] Hormone-related fluid retention leads to generalized edema, including in the tongue, oropharynx, and trachea, further complicating laryngoscopy and intubation. These difficulties lead to much higher rate of failed intubation during pregnancy.[18] The physiologic changes of pregnancy should be accounted for while avoiding hypoxia and hypotension.[15] Pregnant women should be considered high risk for aspiration due to decreased esophageal sphincter tone and upward compression of the stomach.

Pulmonary System

Supplemental oxygen should be provided to pregnant women during the primary survey. Chronic hyperventilation and a 30% to 40% increase in minute ventilation during pregnancy is compensatory for a decrease total lung capacity and functional residual capacity due to anatomical changes. Chronic respiratory alkalosis, a side effect of hyperventilation, sets up a gradient for diffusion of fetal CO_2 to the maternal circulation. Overaggressive correction of maternal alkalosis can impact the fetus negatively.[19] Hypocapnia ($PaCO_2$ of <30 mm Hg) is normal in pregnancy and a "normal" CO_2 (~40 mm Hg) may be a sign of impending hypercarbic respiratory failure.

Mechanical ventilation is poorly studied in pregnant patients and there is no consensus on optimal mode for support. However, as a general principle, hypercapnea should be avoided and oxygenation should be optimized.

If chest tubes are required for pneumothorax or hemothorax, they should be placed in the 3rd or 4th interspaces to avoid inadvertent injury to the hemidiaphragm and intra-abdominal structures.

Cardiovascular System

3 Relative hypervolemia of pregnancy can blunt typical signs of shock after hemorrhage. As much as 35% of maternal blood volume can be lost prior to signs and symptoms of shock. The pulse rate is 10 to 15 beats/min faster until delivery and circulating blood volume increases steadily during pregnancy to 150% or more at term. Early and robust volume resuscitation is recommended to maintain maternal circulation as maternal hypovolemia will lead to fetal compromise. During resuscitation, the patient should be placed in a slight left decubitus
4 position with a wedge to tilt her >15 to 30 degrees or manually displacing the uterus to her left to alleviate the inferior vena cava (IVC) compression improve venous return. Spinal precautions should be maintained. If CPR is needed, this position decreases effectiveness of chest compressions. Standard advanced cardiac life support (ACLS) voltage should be used for defibrillation of shockable rhythms for pregnant patients.

Resuscitation should be balanced emphasizing early use of blood and blood products for suspected life-threatening hemorrhage.[20,21] Resolution of fetal distress signs may lag up to 30 minutes after maternal stabilization.[22] When deemed appropriate for transfusion, O-negative blood products should be used until type specific or cross-matched blood is available. Vasopressors should be avoided and reserved only for fluid-refractory shock because uteroplacental perfusion is highly sensitive to their use resulting in decreased fetal perfusion.[16,23] If needed, phenylephrine is the pressor of choice given its high efficacy and ease of titration in pregnant patients. Norepinephrine and epinephrine can be considered, especially in those without a viable pregnancy.[24,25] The use of tranexamic acid is safe and its use should be considered early in the bleeding patient.[26]

Hematologic System

There is a disproportionate increase in plasma volume relative to the approximately 15% increase in red blood cell (RBC) mass initially yielding a functional physiologic anemia as early 10 weeks. RBC production augments as pregnancy progresses and hematocrits are near normal by term. A hematocrit of 32 is considered normal until the third trimester. White blood cell counts (WBCs) are also elevated ranging from 9,800 to 15,000/mm³.[4]

Maternal and fetal circulations are normally separate but as little as 0.001 mL of fetal blood crossing into the maternal system can trigger sensitization in a Rh-negative mother. Up to a third of pregnant trauma patients have some degree of MFH.[16] Therefore, anti-D immune globulin (RhoGAM™) should be
5 given within 72 hours to all Rh-negative mothers with confirmed or suspected MFH.[5] Kleihauer–Betke (KB) testing is advocated for all Rh-negative mothers with >12 weeks of gestation; its utility in Rh-positive women is less clear.[27,28]

Pregnancy is a hypercoagulable state and increases the risk of venous thromboembolic events (VTEs) fivefold.[29] The phenomenon is attributed to an increase in coagulation factor production, decreased fibrinolysis, and venous stasis from aortic and IVC compression. The hypercoagulability of trauma
6 compounds this risk. The heightened risk warrants prophylactic treatment with low–molecular-weight heparin, or unfractionated heparin in patients with decreased creatinine clearance, as well as pneumatic compression devices, in conjunction with early ambulation.[29,30] Warfarin, a known teratogen, should be avoided.[31] Direct-acting oral anticoagulants (DOACs) are not recommended in pregnancy.[32,33]

FETAL EVALUATION AND MONITORING

After maternal evaluation and resuscitation, evaluation of the fetus should be performed, including an obstetrical history and examination, including estimation of uterine size and fundal height. A vaginal examination should be performed cautiously, looking for bleeding, a nonspecific sign of many unfavorable obstetrical conditions including premature cervical dilation, early labor, abruption placentae, and placenta previa. Cervical dilatation, bleeding, strong contractions, or bulging of the perineum can signal impending delivery. Early involvement of obstetrics and neonatology is advised (see **Table 30.2**).

Table 30.2. Obstetrical Examination Points

Fundal height
Evaluation for vaginal bleeding
Rupture of membranes
Bulging perineum
Contractions
Fetal heart rate and rhythm
Amniotic fluid pooling
Gestational tissue
Perineal lacerations
Cervical dilation and effacement
Bleeding
Fetal presentation
Fetal engagement

DIAGNOSTIC IMAGING

During pregnancy, radiation exposure should be avoided or minimized whenever possible. Low levels of exposure, less than 5 rad of radiation at any gestational age, is deemed safe and has not been associated with fetal anomalies or fetal demise. The risk is highest in weeks 5 to 10 during organogenesis.[16] Radiation exposure to the fetus can be reduced with proper shielding during plain films (**Table 30.3**). Indicated radiologic examinations should proceed without delay for concerns over fetal radiation exposure to protect the life of the mother. Patients and families should be reassured by the health care team that the radiation exposure from a single diagnostic test is not sufficient to cause harmful effects to the fetus.[34]

Focused abdominal sonography for trauma (FAST) is a useful imaging modality to guide initial resuscitation and is safe for both mother and fetus. It has a reported sensitivity of 61% to 83% and a specificity of 94% to 100% in detecting intraperitoneal free fluid consistent with hemoperitoneum.[34] Pregnant women with direct blunt force to the uterus can have massive hemorrhage from engorged uterine vessels. FAST has excellent negative predictive value in detecting pericardial, pleural, and peritoneal free fluid in the hemodynamically unstable mother.[3] Fetal ultrasound is recommended to evaluate for gestational age, cardiac activity, and movement. Ultrasound is particularly useful in the evaluation of intrauterine contents, but can miss 50% to 80% of placental abruptions.[35]

Computed tomography (CT) scans are a staple in trauma evaluations because of their high sensitivity for identifying injuries. Providers should utilize dose-reduction strategies when possible and minimize unnecessary and/or repeated imaging.[36–40] Head and neck CT scans can be performed with minimal radiation exposure to the fetus. Radiation levels from chest, abdomen, and pelvis CT scans vary but newer scanning techniques and algorithms can reduce radiation dosing by 25% without significantly degrading image quality and thus diagnostic accuracy.[41–45]

Magnetic resonance imaging (MRI) poses minimal risk to the fetus but it has very limited role in initial evaluation of trauma patients. It's use is largely restricted to the evaluation of the spine, spinal cord, and neurologic injuries in a delayed fashion. The utility of this modality is limited due to availability, scheduling, length of the examination, and inconvenience

Table 30.3. Estimated Fetal Radiation Doses from Common Imaging Studies

Diagnostic Test	Fetal Dose (rad)
Chest x-ray	<0.01
Abdominal x-ray	0.1–0.3
Pelvis x-ray	0.04–0.24
Extremity x-ray	<0.01
CT head	<0.05
CT chest	0.1–0.45
CT abdomen	0.24–2.6
CT pelvis	0.73–4.6

Adapted from Williams PM, Fletcher S. Health effects of prenatal radiation exposure. *Am Fam Physician.* 2010;82(5):488–493.
From Brown MA, Sirlin CB, Farahmand N, et al. Screening sonography in pregnant patients with blunt abdominal trauma. *J Ultrasound Med.* 2005;24(2):175–181; quiz 183–184.

relative to imaging techniques. MRI should only be performed in hemodynamically normal patients without ongoing resuscitative efforts.

7 Angiography and endovascular treatments are increasingly a part of trauma care to control life-threatening hemorrhage. Radiation dosage increases with duration fluoroscopic examination and generally range from 2 to 10 rad/min. Embolization of nonuterine pelvic vessels is feasible and potentially lifesaving in pelvic fractures. However, embolization of the gravid uterus is not recommended (see **Table 30.3**).[46]

The American College of Obstetricians and Gynecologists position on diagnostic imaging for pregnant women states, "With few exceptions, radiation exposure through radiography, CT scan, or nuclear medicine imaging techniques is at a dose much lower than the exposure associated with fetal harm. If these techniques are necessary in addition to ultrasonography or MRI or are more readily available for the diagnosis in question, they should not be withheld from a pregnant patient."[37,47]

Pelvic Fractures

Of all fractures in pregnancy, pelvic fractures have the worst outcomes. They are associated intrauterine fetal demise (IUFD) up to 40% of the time.[48] Hemorrhage from engorged pelvic veins and the hyperdynamic circulation of pregnancy can combine to produce maternal shock leading to fetal death. Angiography and embolization can be helpful to control maternal hemorrhage.

The direct and high-energy blunt force associated with pelvic fractures is also transmitted to the uterus, placenta, and fetus. This can result in abruption or direct injury to the fetus, especially traumatic brain injuries. If the pregnancy continues, a pelvic ring fractures does not contraindicate vaginal delivery, but there is a higher cesarean section rate from multiple factors.[49–52]

Abruptio Placentae

Abruption, the separation of the placenta from the uterus, is the most frequent etiology of late maternal hemorrhage and the primary cause of intrauterine fetal death following trauma. Severe trauma is associated with a six-fold increase in incidence of abruption, but it can also occur with even minor trauma.[53] Both direct impact and rapid deceleration confer shear forces on the interface of an unyielding placenta against a comparatively pliable uterus resulting in separation, maternal bleeding, and compromised perfusion to the fetus. Fetal mortality may be as high as 70%. More severe cases, more than 50% disruption by surface area, are considered highly lethal and may lead to preterm labor. Smaller insults, less than 30% disruption, may not even show signs of fetal distress.

Abruption can lead to life-threatening intrauterine bleeds. Even at lower volumes of blood loss, mothers may develop disseminated intravascular coagulation (DIC) and hemodynamic collapse.[3] Delayed presentation of abruptio placentae has been reported but fortunately, the majority presents within the first 6 hours after trauma and nearly all in the first 24. Monitoring of pregnant women with blunt injury to the abdomen is widely accepted as standard. The signs and symptoms, abdominal or back pain with vaginal bleeding, are unfortunately nonspecific. All vaginal bleeding after trauma must be evaluated with at least a sonogram.[3] Ultimately, diagnosis of abruption is clinical and treatment decisions are based on laboratory data and fetal evaluation. Severe placental abruption is potentially fatal for the fetus; expedient cesarean delivery may result in higher fetal survival (see **Table 30.4**).[28,54]

Table 30.4. Evaluation of Abruption

Maternal Risk Factors	Signs	Symptoms
Previous abruption	Vaginal bleeding	Abdominal pain
Diabetes mellitus/HTN	Intense uterine contractions	Back pain
Advanced maternal age		
Multiparity		
Tobacco use		
Cocaine or methamphetamine use		
Prior cesarean delivery		

Uterine Rupture

Traumatic uterine rupture, which accounts for 17.5% of MVC-related perinatal deaths, is uncommon, but is seen more commonly in women with uterine scarring from cesarean sections or other causes.[55,56] Maternal mortality risk is up to 10% and fetal survival is negligible.[6,12] Like pelvic fractures, and placental abruption, uterine ruptures result from direct high-energy blunt force and resulting in a constellation of injuries. Patients may present with abdominal pain as the only symptom of uterine rupture. Excellent outcomes in subsequent pregnancies can be achieved in those with prior uterine rupture who undergo uterine repair.[57]

Amniotic Fluid Embolism

Amniotic fluid embolism is exceptionally rare but may accompany uterine rupture and is thought to be caused by the maternal proinflammatory reaction to exposure of fetal tissue in her circulation. It manifests suddenly as respiratory distress and hemodynamic collapse. It has 20% to 60% mortality.[58] Diagnosis is rooted in clinical suspicion. Chest imaging may show evidence of pulmonary vascular congestion or bilateral scattered infiltrates like ARDS. DIC may also develop in 30% of these women. There are no proven interventions available, only supportive management of affected systems.[59]

Eclampsia

Preeclampsia is new-onset gestational hypertension with evidence of significant end-organ dysfunction. In the context of trauma, preeclampsia is important because it is relatively common (5% of pregnancies), and it can progress to eclampsia, with the new onset of seizures. Development of seizures is infrequent, occurring in about 0.05% to 0.2% of pregnancies. When diagnosed or suspected treatment with intravenous magnesium sulfate is recommended and emergency cesarean delivery should be considered (see **Table 30.5**).

Disseminated Intravascular Coagulation

DIC is a dysregulation of the clotting cascade triggered by many pathologic conditions in pregnancy, some of which can arise from trauma. Normal pregnant women are prone to clot due to

Table 30.5. Eclampsia

Risk Factors	Signs
Advanced maternal age (>35 y)	Hypertension (most reliable)
Obesity	Edema
Diabetes mellitus	Proteinuria
Prior or family history of preeclampsia	Hyperactive reflexes

TRAUMA

Table 30.6. Indications for Emergency Cesarean

Maternal shock
Massive exsanguination
Unstable thoracolumbar spinal injuries
High risk of fetal demise
Facilitation of maternal treatment

the marked elevation of their coagulation factors. The departure from the normal state predisposes their hematologic system to DIC when activated by trauma. Major trauma, especially those with hypoperfusion, abruption, uterine rupture, eclampsia, HELLP (hemolysis, elevated liver enzymes, low platelet count), and amniotic fluid embolism, can lead to DIC. Treatment consists of blood component therapy and supportive care.[53,60–62]

EMERGENCY CESAREAN SECTION

Cesarean section should be deferred in favor of vaginal delivery when it is feasible. Labor can continue in appropriate patients; even the onset of labor precedes completion of the trauma evaluation and treatment of identified injuries. This is true even if treatment includes laparotomy or other operative intervention (**Table 30.6**).

Perimortem cesarean section should be considered for fetuses greater than 20 to 22 weeks of gestation depending on local availability of neonatology. This decision can be difficult but must be made expediently as the best fetal outcomes are correlated with time from arrest to delivery. There is also evidence that 60% of mothers have improved circulation after perimortem cesarean sections. Current recommendations advocate for perimortem cesarean section for the viable fetus within 4 minutes of maternal cardiac arrest without return of spontaneous circulation or malignant arrhythmia.[63–65] Early involvement of the obstetrics team facilitates the decision to perform an emergent cesarean section and ensures the timeliest delivery of the child should one be necessary.

SOCIAL CONSIDERATIONS

Intimate partner violence (IPV) during pregnancy is underrecognized and endangers both the mother and child. It is reported in 10% to 30% of pregnancies and women from any age group, religion, ethnic background, income level, educational attain-
8 ment, and sexual orientation are victims of IPV. Universal screening of pregnant patients for IPV is strongly recommended. Women with multiple episodes of trauma, suspicious patterns of injury, or injuries inconsistent with the reported history are concerning indicators. Screening during trauma evaluation may not be possible. Effective brief screening tools are available that can be used at a (slightly) delayed fashion. It is important that screening be performed confidentially in order to obtain accurate information. Identifying the signs and providing options for safety with referrals to social work and local resources, best ensures the safety of both mother and fetus.[66–68]

Substance abuse issues also occur in the pregnant patient. In some urban facilities 50% to 80% of women were screened positive for illicit drugs.[69] Traumas affecting pregnant women were alcohol or drug related 12.9% and 19.6% respectively according to National Trauma Data Bank.[44,69]

TEAM APPROACH TO TRAUMA IN THE PREGNANT PATIENT

Collaborative care delivery with input from prehospital providers, the Emergency Medicine, Nursing, Obstetrics, Critical Care, Neonatology, and Surgery optimizes management of the pregnant trauma patient. Early notification obstetrics (even prior to arrival of the patient) may provide the critical time that can be invaluable for both mother and fetus in extremis.

SUMMARY

Fetal survival is best achieved by appropriate resuscitation and care of the mother. Recognition of the unique issues and potential complications associated with trauma in pregnancy ensure the best possible outcome for both mother and fetus. Optimal treatment requires special attention to the evolving anatomical and physiologic changes of gestation. Evaluation and management should be tailored to the stage of pregnancy and requires a multidisciplinary team approach.

ACKNOWLEDGMENT

We gratefully acknowledge the contributions of previous edition author, Dirk C. Johnson, as portions of those chapters have been retained in this revision.

References

1. Wallace M, Gillispie-Bell V, Cruz K, Davis K, Vilda D. Homicide during pregnancy and the postpartum period in the United States, 2018–2019. *Obstet Gynecol.* 2021;138(5):762–769.
2. Deshpande NA, Kucirka LM, Smith RN, Oxford CM. Pregnant trauma victims experience nearly 2-fold higher mortality compared to their nonpregnant counterparts. *Am J Obstet Gynecol.* 2017;217(5):590.e1–590.e9.
3. Kirkpatrick AW, Ball CG, D'Amours SK, Zygun D. Acute resuscitation of the unstable adult trauma patient: bedside diagnosis and therapy. *Can J Surg.* 2008;51(1):57–69.
4. Hill CC, Pickinpaugh J. Trauma and surgical emergencies in the obstetric patient. *Surg Clin North Am.* 2008;88(2):421–440, viii.
5. Schiff MA, Holt VL. Pregnancy outcomes following hospitalization for motor vehicle crashes in Washington State from 1989 to 2001. *Am J Epidemiol.* 2005;161(6):503–510.
6. Mead JS, Pollack CC, Paris AE, Emeny RT, Puleo RA, St Ivany AR. Obstetric outcomes among women with a history of intimate partner violence in the United States. *Obstet Gynecol.* 2023; 142(1):80–89.
7. Peckham CH, King RW. A study of intercurrent conditions observed during pregnancy. *Am J Obstet Gynecol.* 1963;87:609–624.
8. Kuczkowski KM. Trauma during pregnancy: a situation pregnant with danger. *Acta Anaesthesiol Belg.* 2005;56(1):13–18.
9. Drost TF, Rosemurgy AS, Sherman HF, Scott LM, Williams JK. Major trauma in pregnant women: maternal/fetal outcome. *J Trauma.* 1990;30(5):574–578.
10. Lavin JP, Polsky SS. Abdominal trauma during pregnancy. *Clin Perinatol.* 1983;10(2):423–438.
11. Mattox KL, Goetzl L. Trauma in pregnancy. *Crit Care Med.* 2005;33(10 Suppl):S385–S389.
12. Crosby WM. Traumatic injuries during pregnancy. *Clin Obstet Gynecol.* 1983;26(4):902–912.
13. Weiss HB. Pregnancy-associated injury hospitalizations in Pennsylvania, 1995. *Ann Emerg Med.* 1999;34(5):626–636.
14. Weiss HB, Songer TJ, Fabio A. Fetal deaths related to maternal injury. *JAMA.* 2001;286(15):1863–1868.
15. Weiss HB, Lawrence BA, Miller TR. Pregnancy-associated assault hospitalizations. *Obstet Gynecol.* 2002;100(4):773–780.
16. Poole GV, Martin JN Jr, Perry KG Jr, Griswold JA, Lambert CJ, Rhodes RS. Trauma in pregnancy: the role of interpersonal violence. *Am J Obstet Gynecol.* 1996;174(6):1873–1877; discussion 1877–1878.
17. Rogers FB, Rozycki GS, Osler TM, et al. A multi-institutional study of factors associated with fetal death in injured pregnant patients. *Arch Surg.* 1999;134(11):1274–1277.
18. Petrone P, Talving P, Browder T, et al. Abdominal injuries in pregnancy: a 155-month study at two level 1 trauma centers. *Injury.* 2011;42(1):47–49.
19. Dunning K, LeMasters G, Bhattacharya A. A major public health issue: the high incidence of falls during pregnancy. *Matern Child Health J.* 2010;14(5):720–725.

20. Klinich KD, Flannagan CAC, Rupp JD, Sochor M, Schneider LW, Pearlman MD. Fetal outcome in motor-vehicle crashes: effects of crash characteristics and maternal restraint. *Am J Obstet Gynecol.* 2008;198(4):450.e1–450.e9.
21. Franger AL, Buchsbaum HJ, Peaceman AM. Abdominal gunshot wounds in pregnancy. *Am J Obstet Gynecol.* 1989;160(5 Pt 1): 1124–1128.
22. Iliya FA, Hajj SN, Buchsbaum HJ. Gunshot wounds of the pregnant uterus: report of two cases. *J Trauma.* 1980;20(1):90–92.
23. Pearlman MD, Tintinallli JE, Lorenz RP. A prospective controlled study of outcome after trauma during pregnancy. *Am J Obstet Gynecol.* 1990;162(6):1502–1507; discussion 1507–1510.
24. Brooks D, Oxford C. The pregnant surgical patient. In: Souba WW, Fink MP, Jurkovich GJ, eds. *ACS Surgery: Principles & Practice.* BC Decker; 2007.
25. Ngan Kee WD, Khaw KS. Vasopressors in obstetrics: what should we be using? *Curr Opin Anaesthesiol.* 2006;19(3):238–243.
26. American College of Surgeons (ACS). Trauma in pregnancy and intimate partner violence. In: The Committee on Trauma, ed. *Advanced Trauma Life Support: Student Course Manual.* American College of Surgeons; 2018:226–229.
27. Jain V, Chari R, Maslovitz S, et al. Guidelines for the management of a pregnant trauma patient. *J Obstet Gynaecol Can.* 2015;37(6):553–574.
28. Muench MV, Baschat AA, Reddy UM, et al. Kleihauer–Betke testing is important in all cases of maternal trauma. *J Trauma.* 2004;57(5):1094–1098.
29. Pilkington S, Carli F, Dakin MJ, et al. Increase in Mallampati score during pregnancy. *Br J Anaesth.* 1995;74(6):638–642.
30. Russell R. The difficult airway: risk assessment, prophylaxis, and treatment. In: Chestnut DH, Wong CA, Tsen LC, et al., eds. *Chestnut's Obstetric Anesthesia: Principles and Practice.* Elsevier; 2019:671–691.
31. Gabbe SG, Niebyl J, Galan H, et al. *Obstetrics: Normal and Problem Pregnancies.* 6th ed. Elsevier/Saunders; 2012.
32. Hytten FE, Leitch I. *The Physiology of Human Pregnancy.* 2nd ed. Blackwell Scientific Publications Ltd; 1971.
33. Xue X, Liu L, Rao Z. Management of postpartum hemorrhagic shock and disseminated intravascular coagulation with damage control resuscitation. *Am J Emerg Med.* 2013;31(8):1291.e1–1291.e2.
34. Cotton BA, Au BK, Nunez TC, Gunter OL, Robertson AM, Young PP. Predefined massive transfusion protocols are associated with a reduction in organ failure and postinjury complications. *J Trauma.* 2009;66(1):41–48; discussion 48–49.
35. Oxford CM, Ludmir J. Trauma in pregnancy. *Clin Obstet Gynecol.* 2009;52(4):611–629.
36. Dildy GA, Saade G, Phelan J, Hankins G, Clark SL, Belfort sMA. *Critical Care Obstetrics.* 4th ed. Blackwell Pub; 2004:xii, 691.
37. ACOG Committee on Obstetric Practice. ACOG Committee Opinion. Number 299, September 2004 (replaces No. 158, September 1995). Guidelines for diagnostic imaging during pregnancy. *Obstet Gynecol.* 2004;104(3):647–651.
38. Richards JR, Ormsby EL, Romo MV, Gillen MA, McGahan JP. Blunt abdominal injury in the pregnant patient: detection with US. *Radiology.* 2004;233(2):463–470.
39. Goodwin H, Holmes JF, Wisner DH. Abdominal ultrasound examination in pregnant blunt trauma patients. *J Trauma.* 2001;50(4):689–693; discussion 694.
40. Brown MA, Sirlin CB, Farahmand N, Hoyt DB, Casola G. Screening sonography in pregnant patients with blunt abdominal trauma. *J Ultrasound Med.* 2005;24(2):175–181; quiz 183–184.
41. Sadro C, Bernstein MP, Kanal KM. Imaging of trauma: part 2, Abdominal trauma and pregnancy—a radiologist's guide to doing what is best for the mother and baby. *AJR Am J Roentgenol.* 2012;199(6):1207–1219.
42. McCollough CH, Primak AN, Braun N, Kofler J, Yu L, Christner J. Strategies for reducing radiation dose in CT. *Radiol Clin North Am.* 2009;47(1):27–40.
43. Higashigaito K, Becker AS, Sprengel K, Simmen HP, Wanner G, Alkadhi H. Automatic radiation dose monitoring for CT of trauma patients with different protocols: feasibility and accuracy. *Clin Radiol.* 2016;71(9):905–911.
44. Barraco RD, Chiu WC, Clancy TV, et al; EAST Practice Management Guidelines Work Group Practice management guidelines for the diagnosis and management of injury in the pregnant patient: the EAST Practice Management Guidelines Work Group. *J Trauma.* 2010;69(1):211–214.
45. Williams PM, Fletcher S. Health effects of prenatal radiation exposure. *Am Fam Physician.* 2010;82(5):488–493.
46. American College of Obstetricians and Gynecologists' Committee on Obstetric Practice. Committee Opinion No. 656: guidelines for diagnostic imaging during pregnancy and lactation. *Obstet Gynecol.* 2016;127(2):e75–e80.
47. Liggett MR, Amro A, Son M, Schwulst S. Management of the pregnant trauma patient: a systematic literature review. *J Surg Res.* 2023;285:187–196.
48. El Kady D, Gilbert WM, Xing G, Smith LH. Association of maternal fractures with adverse perinatal outcomes. *Am J Obstet Gynecol.* 2006;195(3):711–716.
49. Weinlein JC, Mashru RP, Perez EA, Johnson SE. Lateral compression-I pelvic ring injury: not benign to the developing fetus. *J Orthop Trauma.* 2018;32(2):100–103.
50. Amorosa LF, Amorosa JH, Wellman DS, Lorich DG, Helfet DL. Management of pelvic injuries in pregnancy. *Orthop Clin North Am.* 2013;44(3):301–315, viii.
51. Crosby W. Trauma in the pregnant patient. *Conn Med.* 1986; 50(4):251–258.
52. Cheng HT, Wang YC, Lo HC, et al. Trauma during pregnancy: a population-based analysis of maternal outcome. *World J Surg.* 2012;36(12):2767–2775.
53. Bates SM, Middeldorp S, Rodger M, James AH, Greer I. Guidance for the treatment and prevention of obstetric-associated venous thromboembolism. *J Thromb Thrombolysis.* 2016;41(1): 92–128.
54. Higgins SD, Garite TJ. Late abruptio placenta in trauma patients: implications for monitoring. *Obstet Gynecol.* 1984;63(3 Suppl): 10S–12S.
55. Schrinsky DC, Benson RC. Rupture of the pregnant uterus: a review. *Obstet Gynecol Surv.* 1978;33(4):217–232.
56. Weintraub AY, Leron E, Mazor M. The pathophysiology of trauma in pregnancy: a review. *J Matern Fetal Neonatal Med.* 2006;19(10):601–605.
57. Fox NS, Gerber RS, Mourad M, et al. Pregnancy outcomes in patients with prior uterine rupture or dehiscence. *Obstet Gynecol.* 2014;123(4):785–789.
58. Balinger KJ, Lam MTC, Hon HH, Stawicki SP, Anasti JN. Amniotic fluid embolism: despite progress, challenges remain. *Curr Opin Obstet Gynecol.* 2015;27(6):398–405.
59. Judich A, Kuriansky J, Engelberg I, Haik J, Shabtai M, Czerniak A. Amniotic fluid embolism following blunt abdominal trauma in pregnancy. *Injury.* 1998;29(6):475–477.
60. Pomp ER, Lenselink AM, Rosendaal FR, Doggen CJ. Pregnancy, the postpartum period and prothrombotic defects: risk of venous thrombosis in the MEGA study. *J Thromb Haemost.* 2008;6(4):632–637.
61. Ley EJ, Brown CVR, Moore EE, et al. Updated guidelines to reduce venous thromboembolism in trauma patients: a Western Trauma Association critical decisions algorithm. *J Trauma Acute Care Surg.* 2020;89(5):971–981.
62. Beyer-Westendorf J. DOACS in women: pros and cons. *Thromb Res.* 2019;181(Suppl 1):S19–S22.
63. Vanden Hoek TL, Morrison LJ, Shuster M, et al. Part 12: cardiac arrest in special situations: 2010 American Heart Association Guidelines for cardiopulmonary resuscitation and emergency cardiovascular care. *Circulation.* 2010;122(18 Suppl 3): S829–S861.
64. American College of Obstetricians and Gynecologists. ACOG Practice Bulletin No. 100: critical care in pregnancy. *Obstet Gynecol.* 2009;113(2 Pt 1):443–450.
65. Chu J, Johnston TA, Geoghegan J; The Royal College of Obstetricians and Gynaecologists (RCOG). Maternal Collapse in Pregnancy

and the Puerperium (Green-top Guideline No. 56). 2011. [Cited September 27, 2019]. https://www.rcog.org.uk/en/guidelines-research-services/guidelines/gtg56/#:~:text=56)-,Maternal%20Collapse%20in%20Pregnancy%20and%20the%20Puerperium%20(Green%2Dtop%20Guideline,56)&text=This%20guideline%20covers%20the%20different,the%20management%20of%20maternal%20 collapse.&text = Delineate%20the%20initial%20and%20continuing% 20management%20of%20maternal%20collapse

66. Dyer I, Barclay DL. Accidental trauma complicating pregnancy and delivery. *Am J Obstet Gynecol*. 1962;83:907–929.
67. McFarlane J, Parker B, Soeken K, Bullock L. Assessing for abuse during pregnancy. Severity and frequency of injuries and associated entry into prenatal care. *JAMA*. 1992;267(23):3176–3178.
68. Krimm J, Heinzer MM. Domestic violence screening in the emergency department of an urban hospital. *J Natl Med Assoc*. 2002;94(6):484–491.
69. Patteson SK, Snider CC, Meyer DS, et al. The consequences of high-risk behaviors: trauma during pregnancy. *J Trauma*. 2007;62(4):1015–1020.

Postinjury Management

Audrey C. Pendleton and Paula Ferrada

Key Points

1 Coagulopathy is common in trauma and is multifactorial, with dilution and consumption being contributing factors. Empiric replacement of coagulation factors is an important aspect of early resuscitation.

2 Damage control resuscitation (DCR) involves limited use of crystalloid fluids, and early, more liberal use of blood products in a balanced ratio to restore volume and maintain organ perfusion.

3 Multiple metrics should be used to determine adequate endpoints of resuscitation since vital signs alone can be falsely reassuring.

4 Abdominal compartment syndrome, characterized by increased intra-abdominal pressures and a tense, distended abdomen, causes oliguria, multiorgan failure, decreased venous return and impaired cardiac output, and emergent decompressive laparotomy is required in severe cases.

5 Traumatic brain injury (TBI) is a major cause of mortality and morbidity in trauma patients. Care of these patients must be focused on preventing secondary brain injury.

6 Early nutritional support is important in trauma patients and enteral nutrition is preferred over parenteral nutrition when possible.

7 Trauma patients can be a source of organ donation. Therefore, resuscitation should be continued even after brain death or irreversible neurologic devastation is determined and until the necessary conversations can be held with the families.

8 Chest trauma and rib fractures are a major cause of mortality and morbidity in trauma patients, especially in the geriatric population. Early, aggressive pain control and pulmonary toilet are essential in preventing pneumonia and respiratory failure. Surgical rib fixation is sometimes indicated to restore chest wall mechanics and improve breathing.

9 Blunt cardiac injury (BCI) can often be managed with supportive measures. A high index of suspicion must be maintained for more serious cardiac injury as this can be fatal without surgical intervention.

Trauma is now the leading cause of death for ages 46 and below in the United States.[1] Hemorrhagic shock is the most common cause of mortality during the first 6 hours following trauma and 16% to 80% of those deaths may be preventable.[2] Postinjury management predominantly focuses on two goals: early control of bleeding and resuscitation.

ACUTE TRAUMATIC COAGULOPATHY

1 Coagulopathy will worsen posttraumatic hemorrhage and is associated with increased mortality and worse outcomes. Interestingly, up to 25% of trauma patients are already coagulopathic upon arrival to the hospital.[3,4] Current data suggest that coagulopathy develops in the early posttraumatic period even before resuscitation begins and is now referred to as acute traumatic coagulopathy.[4–6] Diffuse endothelial damage, activation of the protein C pathway, and massive catecholamine release are some of the proposed mechanisms for acute traumatic coagulopathy.[7] Acute traumatic coagulopathy is exacerbated by hypothermia, acidosis, and dilution of clotting factors. Hypothermia in trauma patients results from a multitude of factors that include radiant heat losses to the environment, failure of shivering response during anesthesia, intraoperative heat loss from exposed peritoneal surfaces, and tissue hypoxia during hemorrhagic shock with decreased metabolism. Another major cause of hypothermia is the use of relatively cool room temperature resuscitation fluids or cold refrigerated blood products that were not warmed before infusion.[8–10] These cumulative factors produce qualitative and quantitative defects in platelet function and decrease coagulation factor activity.[11–13]

In addition to reducing coagulation factor activity, dilutional coagulopathy from large-volume crystalloid resuscitation and acidosis from prolonged tissue hypoxia perpetuates the bloody vicious cycle.[14,15] The combined presence of three factors, hypothermia, acidosis, and coagulopathy, is known as the "lethal triad." Modern trauma resuscitation is defined as damage control resuscitation (DCR) and aimed at reducing the iatrogenic development of this "lethal triad."

DETECTION OF TRAUMATIC COAGULOPATHY

The early identification of acute traumatic coagulopathy remains a challenge. Conventional coagulation assays like PT, aPTT, and INR are insensitive and unreliable in trauma patients, as they do not provide an accurate assessment of the in vivo state of coagulation. Moreover, these assays are performed at physiologic pH and temperature; because of this, they are unable to account for the effects of hypothermia and acidosis on coagulation.[7] Acute traumatic coagulopathy involves changes in both coagulation and fibrinolytic pathways, and detection requires a more dynamic view of all components of the coagulation cascade, which is provided by viscoelastic tests, that is, thromboelastography and rotational thromboelastometry. These assays rely on changes in

Table 31.1. Components of Damage Control Resuscitation

Permissive hypotension
Early definitive hemorrhage control
Reduced crystalloid use
Use of hypertonic saline
Early correction of coagulopathy with drugs (Factor Vila, PCC, TXA)
Increased use of blood products in 1:1:1 ratios

PCC, prothrombin complex concentrate; TXA, tranexamic acid.

clot strength to detect coagulation defects and provide an in vivo picture of the coagulation and fibrinolytic processes. These tests also assess the interaction between coagulation factors and platelets and can detect functional changes in platelet function even with normal platelet counts. They can be performed with much more rapidity and have been shown to detect coagulation abnormalities with higher sensitivity as compared to conventional coagulation assays.[16–18]

Viscoelastic tests have also shown to be more accurate in predicting blood product requirements and massive transfusion and can therefore guide blood transfusion in trauma patients.[19,20] Despite these advantages, viscoelastic tests come with inherent disadvantages such as cost and the need for greater expertise in performance and interpretation.

DAMAGE CONTROL RESUSCITATION

2 The primary objective of resuscitation following hemorrhage is to restore effective circulating volume to allow adequate tissue perfusion and oxygenation. Historically, the standard of practice had been to aggressively resuscitate patients with high volumes of crystalloids to restore volume and blood pressure. In recent years, there has been a paradigm shift away from the large-volume resuscitation, and specifically away from large volumes of crystalloid. Current strategies combine the principles of permissive hypotension, liberal use of blood products instead of isotonic fluids, the use of hypertonic saline to pull water back into the vascular system, and early correction of coagulopathy with blood products as well as drugs (**Table 31.1**).

Permissive hypotension aims at restoring systolic blood pressure to 90 mm Hg so that adequate tissue perfusion can be maintained while not exacerbating blood loss, before definitive hemorrhage control is achieved. Large-volume resuscitation with crystalloids before definitive hemostasis can raise blood pressure which can "pop off" the clot and worsen hemorrhage.[21] A target mean arterial pressure (MAP) of around 60 mm Hg is thought to maintain adequate tissue perfusion without the potential for increased blood loss.[22–25] A brief period of hypotension with a MAP around 60 mm Hg can be safely maintained for short periods of time without risk of irreversible damage or an increase in mortality.[26] Permissive hypotension has been shown to reduce the risk of death and development of coagulopathy.[3,27] However, in patients with hemorrhagic shock and concurrent traumatic brain injury (TBI), the safety of permissive hypotension has not been demonstrated and thus it is not yet recommended.[28] It is important to note that permissive hypotension is intended for young, otherwise healthy patients with penetrating trauma in hemorrhagic shock. It should not be applied to patients with blunt trauma or in elderly patients, especially since the latter are more likely to have comorbidities such as cardiac and carotid disease where hypotension may lead to catastrophic results. Furthermore, hypotension in TBI may worsen outcomes and should thus be avoided in that patient population. Up to 5% of civilian trauma patients require massive transfusion, defined as the need for more than 10 units of red blood cells in 24 hours. These patients are at greatest risk for developing dilutional coagulopathy from large volumes of resuscitation even if packed red cell transfusion is used early in the resuscitation phase.

DCR utilizes massive transfusion protocols and early use of red cells, fresh frozen plasma (FFP), and platelets in a 1:1:1 ratio in an attempt to reconstitute whole blood. The use of blood products early in the course of resuscitation is not only an attempt to combat the coagulopathy in trauma patients requiring massive transfusion but to also minimize the use of crystalloids and colloids.[29–31] The use of predefined massive transfusion protocols has shown improved survivals and decrease in adverse outcomes.[32,33] This approach requires the ability to predict the need for massive transfusion in trauma patients at the time of arrival which is often difficult even for experienced surgeons. Multiple scoring systems have been developed to help define the cohort requiring massive transfusion.[34,35]

The appropriate ratios of packed red cells, FFP, and platelets in exsanguinating trauma patients have been debated. The concept of a 1:1:1 ratio stems from military data that show improved survival with the use of fresh whole blood. Since civilian trauma centers do not have fresh whole blood available, component therapy is an attempt to reconstitute whole blood by giving red cells, FFP, and platelets in a nearly physiologic ratio. Most studies have shown improved mortality with the use of high plasma and pRBC ratios with even greater survival in those with early (6 to 12 hours) use of high ratios.[5,8,36–41] The use of a 1:1 ratio for pRBC and platelets has also shown improved survival.[38] Despite the survival advantage with the use of a 1:1:1 ratio for transfusion, the potentially lethal complications of blood transfusion need to be kept in mind. The PROPPR trial was a multicenter prospective randomized study in hemorrhagic trauma patients that demonstrated an early survival benefit when the patients were resuscitated with a 1:1:1 ratio compared to a 2:1:1 ratio but the 28-day mortality was not statistically significantly different. FFP is an essential component of MTP but it is logistically challenging to use because it needs to be stored at −18 °C and needs about 30 minutes lead time before use. These requirements can make it difficult to use in a hemorrhaging patient. In patients who require immediate MTP, prethawed FFP, which can be stored for 5 days, can be used immediately.[42]

Hypertonic saline has many potential advantages in that it can resuscitate with low volume by pulling water into the vascular space and thus avoids excess water during resuscitation. This concept has advantages especially in the military field environment. Hypertonic saline is also thought to be an immune modulator that potentially decreases inflammation associated with resuscitation injury.[43] However, a multicenter prospective trial in trauma patients with hemorrhagic shock was halted before completion as the outcome was similar between the groups. Overall there was no survival disadvantage in the hypertonic saline arm of the study except in a small subset of patients who did not require blood transfusion. This subset of patients had higher mortality if given hypertonic saline in the field. There was also a subset that required ICU treatment that showed higher survival and decreased multiple organ failure when hypertonic saline was given.[44] Since 7.5% hypertonic saline is not commercially available, an alternative is to use 5% hypertonic saline. Those who use 5% hypertonic saline administer it as a one-time bolus in the initial phase of resuscitation. This approach may be beneficial in patients with TBI. The safety of using 5% hypertonic saline has been shown in two studies.[45,46]

A caveat of using hypertonic saline is that it causes hyperchloremic acidosis, but clinical significance has not yet been demonstrated. Because of the capability of increasing intravascular volume, the ideal time and place for hypertonic saline use may be in the field, especially in the military setting.[47] Hyperfibrinolysis associated with traumatic coagulopathy may decrease levels of fibrinogen. High plasma:pRBC ratios adequately replenish the fibrinogen pool required for adequate hemostasis and thus the use of cryoprecipitate rich in fibrinogen as an adjunct to DCR is rational.[8] The use of cryoprecipitate has additional advantages as it provides particles that act as a low-volume colloid resuscitation and draw water into the vascular system, and is an adjunct in resuscitation. Tranexamic acid is an antifibrinolytic agent found to be safe and effective in reducing the risk of bleeding if used within 3 hours of injury.[48] The military Tactical Combat Casualty Care Committee has recommended its use in the military setting.

Several other novel strategies have also been used as an adjunct in DCR including the use of activated recombinant factor VII (rFVIIa). rFVIIa activates factor Xa at the site of tissue injury by complexing with tissue factor on the surface of platelets. Use of rFVIIa in the initial studies appeared to reduce blood loss and mortality in trauma patients; but subsequent larger randomized trials failed to confirm these benefits.[49] Prothrombin complex concentrate (PCC) is another cost-effective option that reverses coagulopathy in traumatic injury; however, it is not appropriate for every trauma patient and is mostly used as a second-line therapy as part of a massive transfusion protocol. While each component of resuscitation is important, it is the combination of these methods that is essential. Specifically, avoiding hypothermia and acidosis, early temporizing measures and expeditious definitive control of hemorrhage with surgical or angiographic methods, use of the correct ratios of blood products and adjunctive pharmacologic agents, such as tranexamic acid and use of viscoelastic assays all compose the hemorrhage control bundle, which has been associated with decreased mortality from hemorrhage and overall improved outcome.

The discussion of DCR should also include damage control laparotomy (DCL). The principle of the DCL is to explore the patient, control hemorrhage, contain contamination, and temporize the damage but to refrain from definitive repairs that may subject the patient to a prolonged operation before they are properly resuscitated, which would exacerbate the lethal triad and increase chance of death. In these cases, the abdomen remains open and the patient is brought to the ICU for continued resuscitation. One hallmark study suggested that DCL is of benefit in trauma patients with numerous major visceral injuries that also have vascular injury; this study also showed that DCL in patients without major injuries was associated with worse outcome. While the use of DCL is necessary in certain circumstances, there can be significant morbidity associated with them. Specific complications include abdominal abscesses, gastrointestinal fistulas, as well as complex ventral hernias and loss of domain. Furthermore, the prolonged ICU course and multiple trips to the operating room that occur in the patient with an open abdomen contribute to the associated morbidity.

A more recent study evaluated the variability in practice of DCL. There is no strict practice management guideline for its use, but the standard general criteria are major abdominal vascular injury, coagulopathy, acidosis, and hypothermia. Outside of these criteria, its use is left to the discretion of the surgeon. This study examined the variability of DCL in level 1 trauma centers by evaluating patients from the PROPPR Trial who underwent immediate laparotomy and categorized them to having either DCL or definitive surgical management (DSM). The study found that there is significant variability among centers in the use of DCL but that there was no difference in mortality. DCL was associated with higher rates of sepsis and VAP. This study suggests that reducing the use of DCL might lessen the morbidity burden while not affecting the mortality. Definitive laparotomy may have survival benefit with decrease in morbidities known to accompany DCL, such as open abdomens and enterocutaneous fistulas. Because of the decreased number of surgeries and morbidities, the cost benefits were significant.

ENDPOINTS OF RESUSCITATION

3 The ultimate goal of resuscitation is to ensure adequate oxygen delivery to tissues. Prolonged tissue hypoxia is associated with multiorgan dysfunction syndrome, risk of infection, and increased mortality. Advanced trauma life support (ATLS) guidelines define the correction of vital signs like blood pressure and heart rate as markers of adequate resuscitation. However, up to 86% of severely injured patients with normalized vital signs have ongoing occult ischemia that is associated with adverse outcomes. While normalization of vital signs may describe the current perfusion status, they do not assess oxygen debt, defined as ongoing oxygen deficits that have accumulated during the period of shock. Oxygen debt is known to be associated with increased mortality. Arterial lactate and base deficit may serve as indicators for severity of shock and may help to stratify patients. Trends in serum lactate levels indicate adequacy of resuscitation.

Invasive monitoring with central venous pressure (CVP) and pulmonary artery catheter (PAC) has been extensively used to guide resuscitation. CVP and pulmonary capillary wedge pressure monitoring provide information regarding the intravascular volume, but concurrent factors like mechanical ventilation and changes in ventricular compliance from myocardial dysfunction limit their efficacy in accurately guiding resuscitation. Moreover, PAC use in critically ill trauma patients has not been shown to improve outcomes. $ScVO_2$ and SVO_2 measure central venous oxygen saturation from the upper body and mixed venous oxygen saturation from both the upper and lower body, respectively. Inadequate oxygen supply from ongoing shock or increased oxygen demand leads to an increased tissue extraction of oxygen, which is reflected as a decrease in the values of $ScVO_2$ and SVO_2. SVO_2 of less than 65%, even in the presence of normal vital signs, indicates blood loss and need for transfusion to optimize oxygen supply and demand. Therefore, $ScVO_2$ and SVO_2 provide a real-time picture of tissue perfusion and are able to detect very subtle changes in oxygen delivery. The ideal marker for resuscitation may be to determine blood volume, but there is currently no simple way to determine ideal circulating blood volume.

ABDOMINAL COMPARTMENT SYNDROME

4 Abdominal compartment syndrome is an undesired consequence of elevated intra-abdominal pressure and a cause of morbidity and mortality. The incidence of abdominal compartment syndrome is decreasing with recent evolution in resuscitation strategy, suggesting a possible iatrogenic etiology. Intra-abdominal hypertension is defined as a pressure of greater than or equal to 12 mm Hg. Intra-abdominal hypertension is graded based on increasing intra-abdominal pressure (**Table 31.2**). Abdominal compartment syndrome is defined as

Table 31.2. Grades of Intra-Abdominal Hypertension

Grade	Intra-Abdominal Pressure (mm Hg)
I	12–15
II	16–20
III	21–25
IV	>25

TRAUMA

a sustained intra-abdominal pressure greater than 20 mm Hg (with or without an abdominal perfusion pressure of less than 60 mm Hg) with new organ dysfunction or failure. Experimental data indicate that hepatic arterial, portal venous, and hepatic microcirculatory blood flow are markedly reduced when intra-abdominal pressure is increased.

Typically, abdominal compartment syndrome is observed after severe abdominal trauma with intra-abdominal hemorrhage, severe liver and kidney injuries, and in both operatively and nonoperatively managed settings (primary abdominal compartment syndrome). Excessive large-volume resuscitation, even in the absence of any direct abdominal trauma, can also lead to abdominal compartment syndrome (secondary abdominal compartment syndrome). Recurrent or tertiary abdominal compartment syndrome refers to a condition following a previously treated primary or secondary abdominal compartment syndrome. Risk factors for development of abdominal compartment syndrome include diminished abdominal wall compliance, increased intraluminal and intra-abdominal content, crystalloid resuscitation/leak, and other risk factors such as age, shock, high BMI, coagulopathy, and mechanical ventilation.

Abdominal compartment syndrome can even occasionally occur in patients with an open abdomen. The diagnosis often begins with findings of a tense and distended abdomen in the presence of high end-inspiratory airway pressures and other signs of organ dysfunction (ie, oliguria, rising serum creatinine). Additional clinical signs consistent with abdominal compartment syndrome are a reduced cardiac output, elevated systemic vascular resistance, and elevated pulmonary capillary wedge pressure with simultaneous low or normal calculated estimates of end-diastolic volume. The standard for monitoring intra-abdominal pressure is bladder pressure measurement via intravesical technique. Bladder pressure is measured in end expiration with the patient supine, by distending the bladder with 25 mL of sterile saline. Surgical decompression of the abdomen is an option for established abdominal compartment syndrome with associated organ dysfunction and persistent shock with no absolute thresholds for urine output and airway pressure. Protocols on fluid resuscitation are recommended to avoid a sustained increase in intra-abdominal pressure.

In addition to decompressive laparotomy for abdominal compartment syndrome, numerous medical and minimally invasive therapies have been proposed such as sedation and analgesia for anxiety relief and brief trials of neuromuscular blockade as temporizing measures. Body positioning and colonic/nasogastric decompression are also suggested noninvasive treatment options. Patients with abdominal compartment syndrome may have ascites and drainage of fluid with various catheters can be tried before performing decompressive laparotomy as a less invasive alternative. A common factor among all cases of abdominal compartment syndrome seems to be the use of aggressive crystalloid resuscitation causing resuscitation injury. Use of excessive crystalloid resuscitation is discouraged in DCR and studies show decreased rates of abdominal compartment syndrome in association with decreased rates of crystalloid resuscitation. Attempts to achieve "supranormal" endpoints (cardiac index of >4 L/min/m^2 or oxygen delivery index of >600 mL/min/m^2), while theoretically desirable, have not been shown to be effective as this often requires excessive resuscitation volumes that contribute to abdominal compartment syndrome.

As resuscitation has changed with DCR, the incidence of abdominal compartment syndrome has been decreasing. In the trauma setting, abdominal compartment syndrome has been disappearing rapidly but in the general surgery setting, it is more common. Sepsis as a source of inflammation can create abdominal compartment syndrome even when resuscitation injury is minimized. Source control of the bacterial contamination is the best treatment for abdominal compartment syndrome. End-organ failure with microcirculatory disruption and endothelial leak is another source of the syndrome.

TRAUMATIC BRAIN INJURY

TBI remains one of the leading causes of injury-related deaths. Initial management of TBI includes hyperosmolar resuscitation, intracerebral pressure (ICP) monitoring, and prevention of hypoxia and hypotension.

Secondary Brain Injury

5 Injury prevention and better safety are the mainstays for primary brain injury. After the initial insult, the main goal is to prevent or minimize secondary brain injury. Secondary brain injury can be influenced by a cascade of inflammatory responses, occurring as a consequence of the primary injury. Secondary brain injury is also exacerbated by potentially preventable factors such as hypotension, hyperthermia, seizure activity, hyperglycemia, hyperventilation, hyponatremia, and hypoxemia. Hypotension at any point (even brief time periods) is associated with a doubling of mortality in patients with severe TBI. Although hyperventilation temporarily reduces intracranial pressure and may help to prevent herniation, evidence suggests that excessive hyperventilation may be harmful for patients with TBI. Therefore, brief hyperventilation is only recommended in order to reduce ICP temporarily until surgical decompression can be performed.

Imaging in TBI

Computed tomography (CT) scanning remains an essential tool in the initial evaluation and postinjury management of TBI. Patients with mild and moderate TBI who are examinable and not on any anticoagulant medications can be monitored by clinical examination without the need for routine serial CT scans of the head. With technologic improvements made to the CT scanners around the world, the incidence of TBI has been increasing. Small insignificant intracranial radiologic findings are the main reason for the increase in the diagnosis of TBI. With increased awareness of mild TBI and with the increased attention to mild TBI with posttraumatic stress disorder, CT scans of the head are being ordered more often and routinely. In trauma, the single most common reason for obtaining a CT scan of the head has been loss of consciousness. Thus increased screening for TBI and improved technology identifying small clinically insignificant intracranial injuries has resulted in the increase of incidence of TBI.

TBI is a clinical diagnosis and not just a radiographic diagnosis. There are patients with TBI with normal CT scans of the head who have cognitive deficits as well as posttraumatic stress disorder and there are many with radiographic TBI that do not have clinical deficits. Therefore, significant deterioration in neurologic examination should be considered in the decision for whether repeat head CT scan or consultation of a neurosurgeon is needed. CT scans and neurosurgical consultations are valuable resources with costs to the health care system as well as to the patient. The use of routine repeat head CT and neurosurgical consultations should be restricted to patients on prehospital antiplatelet and anticoagulants, and those with depressed skull fractures. A Brain Injury Guideline has been developed which helps guide when the resources should be used (**Table 31.3**). Progression of lesions on repeat head CT scan promptly identifies patients who require more invasive neurosurgical interventions and medical therapies. Routine repeat head CT is still recommended for those patients with Glasgow Coma Scale (GCS) less than 8 and for those who do not have a reliable clinical examination such as patients that are under general anesthesia or patients that are in the ICU under sedation.

Coagulopathy in TBI

A decreased platelet count (less than 100,000/μL) and/or impaired platelet function after TBI is associated with progression of intracranial hemorrhage, need for neurosurgical intervention, and mortality. Admission INR greater than 1.5 also predicts progression of intracranial hemorrhage. The

Table 31.3. Brain Injury Guideline

Variables	BIG 1[a]	BIG 2
Neurologic Examination	Normal	Normal/abnormal
Intoxication	Yes/no	Yes/no
CAMP	No	Yes/no
Skull fracture	No/simple, nondisplaced	Other
SDH	<4 mm	>4 mm
EDH	<4 mm	>4 mm
IPH/Contusion	One location and <4 mm	Other
SAH	Trace/pinpoint	Other
Therapeutic Plan		
Neurosurgical Consult	No	Yes
RHCT	No	Yes
ICU Admission	No	Yes

[a]Patients should meet all criteria for BIG 1.
Intoxication, alcohol/drugs; CAMP, Coumadin, aspirin, Motrin, Plavix; SDH, subdural hematoma; EDH, epidural hematoma; IPH, intraparenchymal hemorrhage; SAH, subarachnoid hemorrhage; IVH, intraventricular hemorrhage; RHCT, repeat head CT; NSC, neurosurgical consult.

treatment of coagulopathy after TBI is multipronged due to the complexity of the problem. Therapeutic strategies should focus on the treatment of the primary cause and controlling the progression of intracranial bleeding. FFP, platelets, recombinant factor VII, and PCC can be used in various combinations to improve outcomes.

Antiplatelet and Anticoagulation Therapy in TBI

Antiplatelet medications, anticoagulants, and nonsteroidal antiinflammatory drugs are among the most frequently encountered medications in TBI patients, especially the elderly. Existing evidence shows an increased risk of progression of intracranial bleeding in patients on high-dose aspirin and clopidogrel, whereas low-dose aspirin and ibuprofen do not cause progression on CT or neurologic examination. A platelet count of less than 135,000/μL in patients on antiplatelet therapy is predictive of both radiographic and clinical worsening. Reversal of the effect of anticoagulants and antiplatelets is suggested to improve the outcomes. Use of newer oral anticoagulants like direct thrombin inhibitors and factor Xa inhibitors is increasing. Despite their safety advantage over Coumadin, concerns for progression of intracranial bleed, and adverse outcomes exist in TBI patients. There are limited reversal agents for the newer oral anticoagulants. Andexanet Alfa is used to reverse Apixaban and Rivaroxaban, but is very expensive and not widely available yet. Oral charcoal administration, hemodialysis, PCC, and rFVIIa have shown some efficacy in the reversal of these agents.

Seizure Prophylaxis after TBI

Posttraumatic seizures increase the cerebral metabolic rate, ICP, and may cause secondary brain injury. Seizures after TBI are associated with worse outcome. It is not known if poor outcomes are due to underlying injury which is associated with posttraumatic seizures or if posttraumatic seizures exacerbate injury. Studies have shown that prophylactic therapy with phenytoin during the first 7 days after injury is effective in reducing the number of early posttraumatic seizures. Long-term use of prophylactic anticonvulsants has not been shown to be of benefit. Anticonvulsant prophylaxis is not indicated for late-onset posttraumatic seizures (after 7 days). Because phenytoin is cumbersome to use, as it requires frequent drug-level monitoring and can lead to neurodepressive side effects, the use of levetiracetam has become common. However, recent studies have shown that the seizure rate after TBI is very low and the use of levetiracetam has not equated to reduced seizures.

Penetrating Brain Injury

Gunshot wounds to the brain are the most lethal of all firearm injuries. Aggressive postinjury resuscitation is associated with significant improvement in both survival and organ donor eligibility. Early aggressive management includes blood products, hyperosmolar therapy, vasopressors, and/or PCC. Early aggressive T4 (levothyroxine) therapy and correction of coagulopathy increases the organ donation rate in nonsurvivable patients.

NUTRITIONAL AND METABOLIC SUPPORT

Nutritional support after injury imparts significant acute and long-term effects on outcomes. Understanding of the nutritional and metabolic derangements following injury has increased exponentially over the past few decades. This has resulted in a more focused and goal-oriented approach toward nutritional support. Once patients are stabilized and recovered from shock, attention should be directed to metabolic and nutritional support. The route of administration and timing of initiation of nutritional support have been issues of contro-
6 versy. Current evidence supports the use of enteral nutrition in all trauma patients as soon as possible. There are certain situations where enteral nutrition is not a feasible option; in such patients, total parenteral nutrition is an alternative. Even in cases where enteral nutrition cannot be administered due to frequent or impending operative intervention or intolerance of enteral feeding, total parenteral nutrition should be used as a bridging measure. The literature on nutritional support in critically injured trauma patients consistently reports higher septic morbidity in patients on total parenteral nutrition. Current guidelines on the nutritional support provide a level 1 recommendation on the advantages of enteral nutrition over nutritional support via the parenteral route. Recent recommendations aim for early enteral nutrition. The definition of early varies in the literature, ranging from a few hours after injury up to hours. Although the benefits are yet to be established, safety of early (within 24 hours of injury) enteral feeding is well documented. In patients with severe burns, it is recommended to initiate enteral feeding within 18 hours of injury. Early feeding in this group of patients reduces the risk of gastroparesis. In the case of severe TBI, enteral feeding is safe and should be administered early.

Nasogastric and nasojejunal routes are the preferred modes of initial nutritional access. If long-term nutritional support is required, the planning of feeding access should be based on individual patient circumstances. In patients undergoing laparotomy, insertion of a surgical feeding tube either in the stomach or small intestine is a feasible option. For patients in need of long-term nutritional support and not requiring surgical intervention the preferred route is via endoscopically guided percutaneous feeding tube. The percutaneous endoscopic route is increasingly popular, but the literature is not well established on its safety and complications. While choosing one route over the other, special consideration should be given to individual patient factors as there is no single feeding access that stands out among the others for safety and efficacy.

The goal of nutritional support during postinjury phase is twofold, first to provide enough calories to meet basal energy expenditure and second to complement the special micronutrient requirements of ongoing inflammation. Basal energy expenditure during postinjury phase ranges from 30 to 35 kcal/kg/d. Basal energy expenditure is higher in TBI patients and lower in spinal cord injury patients. The estimation of basal energy expenditure in critically ill patients remains challenging and current calculators frequently overestimate caloric requirements. A high-caloric dietary supplementation is associated with hyperglycemia, hypercapnia, and higher in-hospital complications. While underfeeding is also a concern in critically ill patients, a more balanced approach is permissive underfeeding. Permissive underfeeding focuses more on maintaining nitrogen balance than meeting caloric requirements alone. Diets containing higher protein content and lower caloric value than target serve such a purpose. Permissive underfeeding results in better glycemic control, rapid recovery, and overall better in-hospital patient outcomes.

In the setting of trauma and critical illness, the ongoing catabolic response demands special micronutrients and dietary considerations along with standard protein and caloric replacement. Nonessential amino acids such as arginine and glutamine become conditionally essential. Addition of these amino acids along with omega-3 fatty acids to standard dietary formulas has been shown to improve outcomes and immune function. Enhanced diets containing higher protein content, and including a combination of arginine, glutamine, omega-3 fatty acids, minerals (zinc, copper, etc.), nucleic acids, and vitamins have shown to improve overall immune function. The assessment of nutritional requirement in critically ill patients is primarily done by the indirect calorimetry method. The standard measure of nutritional requirement uses a metabolic cart, but this is expensive and cumbersome. An alternative approach uses predictive equations but these are imprecise and often over- or underestimate the nutritional requirement. In recent years, several handheld indirect calorimeters have been marketed. They provide ease of use as they are portable and relatively accurate. To assess the adequacy of nutritional supplementation, anthropometric measurements and biochemical data can be utilized. While there is no single measure which accurately predicts adequacy of nutritional support, prealbumin levels provide a reliable estimate compared to albumin, transferrin, and retinol-binding protein.

ORGAN DONATION

Trauma donors are the major contributor in the organ donation pool. There remains great potential to enhance the conversion rate in this group of trauma donors. Over the past decade significant changes occurred in resuscitation protocols in general and specifically in potential organ donors. These changes in resuscitation have resulted in better organ donation in this group of potential donors. Wide spread acceptance of DCR has led to better end-organ preservation, which not only improves outcomes in surviving patients but can improve
7 overall organ donation rates in brain-dead patients. The guidelines defining organ donor management recommend continuation of this aggressive resuscitative support even after declaration of brain death. A feasible goal for resuscitating any potential donors is to follow a rule of 100s, that is, maintaining a systolic blood pressure of >100 mm Hg, heart rate of 100 mL/hr, and PaO_2 > 100 mm Hg. Along with hemodynamic resuscitation, focus should also be given to pulmonary edema, coagulopathy, and hypothermia. Coagulopathy and hypothermia are not only associated with adverse outcomes in trauma patients but also render them ineligible for organ donation.

The focus of resuscitative efforts after declaration of brain death shifts from cerebral preservation to organ preservation. The shift in resuscitation focus is a continuum of ongoing resuscitation. Donors should be managed in a critical care setting and attention should be directed toward moderation of post brain death physiologic changes. Along with ongoing resuscitation, initiation of a T4 protocol should ensue. T4 protocol or hormone replacement therapy takes into account the disruption of hypothalamic–pituitary axis. The essential components of the T4 protocol include methylprednisolone, triiodothyronine (T3)/levothyroxine (T4), arginine, vasopressin, and insulin. The goal of this resuscitative cocktail is to prevent potential cardiac arrhythmias, diabetes insipidus, hypotension, and metabolic acidosis. Early initiation of hormonal therapy has shown improved organ donation rates and should be considered in all brain-dead potential organ donors.

Organ donation is a legitimate outcome in trauma patients. As aggressive resuscitation protocols for trauma patients closely align with donor management goals, the spectrum of care in potential organ donors can easily be extended to address organ preservation. Trauma patients presenting with previously fatal neurologic injuries provide an excellent cohort where aggressive resuscitation can not only improve survival rates but also the organ donation rates. The care of a potential organ donor is a multidisciplinary task. Involvement of organ procurement networks and social services can improve the communication between the treatment team, procurement agency, and the donor's relatives. Bridging this gap is of utmost importance as family decline still remains a major cause of the loss of potential donors.

Rib Fractures

Traumatic rib fractures are most often caused by blunt force
8 trauma to the chest. The mainstay of management is to control the pain and prevent the pulmonary sequelae, such as pneumonia and respiratory failure, which increases mortality. Rib fractures are associated with significant morbidity and mortality and therefore early recognition and aggressive proactive pain control are essential to good outcomes. Rib fractures occur in approximately 10% of trauma patients and are often markers for significant concomitant internal injuries, such as pulmonary contusion, pneumo- or hemothorax, diaphragm injury, or blunt cardiac injury (BCI). There are numerous associated pulmonary complications, most notably pneumonia, retained hemothorax, aspiration, and ARDS. The number of rib fractures correlates to the mortality and associated complications, which has been demonstrated in several studies. One study that looked at patients in the National Trauma Data Bank (NTDB) over 7 years found that one rib fracture was associated with a 5.8% mortality and the chance of death increased with each rib fractured, culminating in a mortality rate of 34.4% in patients with eight or more rib fractures. Furthermore, increased number of rib fractures was associated with more complications, specifically ARDS, pneumonia, pneumothorax, empyema, and ICU and hospital length of stay. Flail chest is defined both radiographically and clinically. On imaging, it is multiple consecutive rib fractures (>4) unilaterally with fractures in two or more locations in a single rib. Clinically, it is when a segment of the chest wall moves paradoxically within the respiratory cycle. This type of injury has a greater impact on respiratory function and is associated with increased complications.

A particularly vulnerable patient population is the elderly who experience the most significant morbidity and mortality secondary to rib fractures. Patients over the age of 65 with rib fractures have twice the rate of mortality than younger patients with similar injury patterns. Furthermore, for each rib fractured, there is an increase in mortality of 19.4%. The overall mortality in elderly patients with rib fractures has been shown to 20.1% while the mortality rate in this population without rib fractures has been reported at 7.6%. Given the higher risk of death and complications in this patient population, trauma centers often admit elderly patients with rib fractures to the ICU. One study compared two groups of elderly patients once there was a change in protocol regarding admission criteria for patients with rib fractures. Patients over the age of 65 with blunt thoracic trauma and three or more rib fractures were automatically admitted to the ICU regardless of other injuries or respiratory status. The two groups had comparable ISS. They compared outcomes of the patients from before and after the change in admission ICU admission criteria and found that patients in the latter group had shorter lengths of stay, lower mortality rates, lower rates of unplanned ICU admission, and few complications. The improved outcomes were attributed to the more concentrated nursing care that could provide aggressive pulmonary hygiene, the comprehensive care provided by the multidisciplinary teams and the continuous monitoring that allows for earlier recognition of clinical deterioration.

The cornerstone of management of blunt thoracic trauma with rib fractures is aggressive pain control and pulmonary hygiene so that patients can breathe effectively and mobilize, which helps reduce the risk of pulmonary complications and death. Multimodal pain therapy has become the standard of care and involves a combination of medications including opiates, NSAIDs, acetaminophen, and sometimes ketamine. A common strategy is to use standing doses of acetaminophen and NSAIDs with on-demand opiates via an oral or intravenous route. Each drug class has advantages and disadvantages. NSAIDs are readily available, do not dampen respiratory drive, and have no addictive potential but carry the risk of peptic ulceration and some clinicians are hesitant to use them when there is a concern for bleeding. Opiates are also readily available but depress respiratory function and are addictive. Lidocaine and ketamine infusions are also reasonable options but should be managed with the help of pain specialists. Early consultation of an acute pain service has been shown to be beneficial to patients and outcomes. Regional anesthesia is another mode of therapy that has demonstrated benefits in rib fracture management and includes intercostal blocks, paravertebral catheters, and epidural catheters. Paravertebral catheters are most beneficial in unilateral rib fractures as opposed to bilateral fractures. Studies have reported decreased delirium with the use of regional anesthesia in the management of multiple rib fractures, which is especially important in the elderly population.

Surgical fixation involves open reduction and internal fixation of the fractures. There is no clear consensus on which patients benefit the most from rib fixation or the optimal timing of the procedure and there is much debate among trauma surgeons. However, some common accepted indications include flail chest, symptoms with displaced segments, refractory pain or persistent respiratory failure, and fixation in conjunction with a thoracotomy for another reason. Several randomized studies have been conducted and have demonstrated decreased rates of pneumonia and fewer days on the ventilator. On meta-analysis, there was no significant difference in mortality but there was a lower rate of pneumonia. The randomized studies have been small and of lower quality so larger multicenter studies are still needed. A single-institution prospective study compared nonoperative and surgical fixation for specific indications (flail chest, >3 displaced fractures, >30% volume loss, and failure of medical therapy) and found that the operative group had a reduced likelihood of respiratory failure and tracheostomy. A different study performed in two trauma centers in Canada demonstrated contradictory results and showed significantly improved outcomes in the nonoperative group in terms of rates of pneumonia, ventilator days, and length of stay in the ICU and in the hospital overall. Given the variable data on the role of surgery in rib fractures and the lack of consensus, each patient should be evaluated individually with regard to the risks and benefits of the procedure. Regarding the technical aspects of the procedures, preoperative imaging with CT scan and 3D reconstruction of the chest wall is important in operative planning. The procedure is usually performed through a thoracotomy incision and there are various plating systems available. The goal of the procedure is to stabilize the ribcage while restoring mechanical function to the chest wall. Careful attention should be paid not to overly restrict the chest wall with excessive fixation so that the breathing mechanics are impaired.

Blunt Cardiac Injury

9 BCI refers to the trauma to the myocardium secondary to blunt trauma. There is a wide range of clinical manifestations, from asymptomatic and clinically silent to life threatening. Due to this spectrum in severity, there is a range in management from monitoring to open heart surgery, however, the majority of cases are managed with telemetry and supportive care.

Severe cardiac injuries often result in instant death. Up to 25% of deaths from trauma were found to have cardiac or aortic injuries. The most common cause is motor vehicle collisions, motorcycle collisions, falls, and crush injuries. Most patients with BCI who survive to the hospital have relatively minor cardiac injury. Therefore, there should be a high index of suspicion whenever there is significant blunt force trauma to the chest. Specifically, if there is a sternal fracture, hemopneumothorax, esophageal injury, or multiple rib fractures and pulmonary contusion, since many patients present insidiously and delay in diagnosis increases morbidity and mortality. In a retrospective study that examined NTDB blunt trauma patients over 8 years found that a 0.3% incidence of BCI with hemopneumothorax being the strongest independent risk factor for BCI, followed by sternal fracture and esophageal injury.

There are various types of BCI, including myocardial injury, which involves a laceration of the walls of the heart or papillary muscles, myocardial contusion, for which there is no clear consensus for diagnostic criteria but is generally thought to be bruising of the heart, pericardial laceration, septal injuries, and valvular injuries. The most common chamber injured is the right ventricle due to its anterior location. Myocardial injury carries a high mortality rate, especially when the pericardium is intact because of tamponade.

There is a spectrum of clinical presentations, including chest pain and bruising, arrhythmias, hypotension, and flash pulmonary edema from valvular injury and dysfunction. In addition to ATLS, when evaluating for BCI, the initial workup should include an EKG and a troponin. The negative predictive value of a normal EKG and negative troponin is approximately 100%, so if both are normal then no further evaluation or monitoring for BCI is necessary. If these tests are abnormal then the patient should be admitted to a telemetry unit, and if there are arrhythmias or any hemodynamic instability, then an echocardiogram should be obtained to evaluate for any wall motion abnormalities, effusion, and valvular issues. Elevated troponin has been associated with higher mortality rates in BCI in retrospective analysis. Hypotension may occur and bleeding should be ruled out as is the case in all trauma patients. Once bleeding has been addressed and ruled out, hypotension secondary to cardiac dysfunction in patients with BCI should be managed with vasopressor support in a monitored setting. Most BCI can be managed nonoperatively, however, if there is valvular, pericardial, or myocardial disruption, rupture or laceration, then surgery is required, often emergently.

References

1. Rhee P, Joseph B, Pandit V, et al. Increasing trauma deaths in the United States. *Ann Surg*. 2014;260(1):13–21.
2. Spinella PC, Holcomb JB. Resuscitation and transfusion principles for traumatic hemorrhagic shock. *Blood Rev*. 2009;23(6):231–240.

TRAUMA

3. Maegele M, Lefering R, Yucel N, et al. Early coagulopathy in multiple injury: an analysis from the German Trauma Registry on 8724 patients. *Injury*. 2007;38(3):298–304.
4. MacLeod JB, Lynn M, McKenney MG, et al. Early coagulopathy predicts mortality in trauma. *J Trauma*. 2003;55(1):39–44.
5. Maegele M, Lefering R, Paffrath T, et al. Red-blood-cell to plasma ratios transfused during massive transfusion are associated with mortality in severe multiple injury: a retrospective analysis from the Trauma Registry of the Deutsche Gesellschaft für Unfallchirurgie. *Vox Sang*. 2008;95(2):112–119.
6. Brohi K, Singh J, Heron M, Coats T. Acute traumatic coagulopathy. *J Trauma*. 2014;20(4):638–645.
7. Palmer L, Martin L. Traumatic coagulopathy—part 1: pathophysiology and diagnosis. *J Vet Emerg Crit Care (San Antonio)*. 2014;24(1):63–74.
8. Duchesne JC, Hunt JP, Wahl G, et al. Review of current blood transfusions strategies in a mature level I trauma center: were we wrong for the last 60 years. *J Trauma*. 2008;65(2):272–276; discussion 276–278.
9. Burch JM, Denton JR, Noble RD. Physiologic rationale for abbreviated laparotomy. *Surg Clin North Am*. 1997;77(4):779–782.
10. Kirkpatrick AW, Chun R, Brown R, Simons RK. Hypothermia and the trauma patient. *Can J Surg*. 1999;42(5):333–343.
11. Rohrer MJ, Natale AM. Effect of hypothermia on the coagulation cascade. *Crit Care Med*. 1992;20(10):1402–1405.
12. Valeri CR, Feingold H, Cassidy G, Ragno G, Khuri S, Altschule MD. Hypothermia-induced reversible platelet dysfunction. *Ann Surg*. 1987;205(2):175–181.
13. Vella MA, Jenner C, Betteridge DJ, Jowett NI. Hypothermia-induced thrombocytopenia. *J Royal Soc Med*. 1988;81(4):228–229.
14. Meng ZH, Wolberg AS, Monroe DM III, Hoffman M. The effect of temperature and pH on the activity of factor VIIa: implications for the efficacy of high-dose factor VIIa in hypothermic and acidotic patients. *J Trauma*. 2003;55(5):886–891.
15. Dirkmann D, Hanke AA, Gorlinger K, Peters J. Hypothermia and acidosis synergistically impair coagulation in human whole blood. *Anesth Analg*. 2008;106(6):1627–1632.
16. Doran CM, Woolley T, Midwinter MJ. Feasibility of using rotational thromboelastometry to assess coagulation status of combat casualties in a deployed setting. *J Trauma*. 2010;69(Suppl 1):S40–S48.
17. Levrat A, Gros A, Rugeri L, et al. Evaluation of rotation thrombelastography for the diagnosis of hyperfibrinolysis in trauma patients. *Br J Anaesth*. 2008;100(6):792–797.
18. Martini WZ, Cortez DS, Dubick MA, Park MS, Holcomb JB. Thrombelastography is better than PT, aPTT, and activated clotting time in detecting clinically relevant clotting abnormalities after hypothermia, hemorrhagic shock and resuscitation in pigs. *J Trauma*. 2008;65(3):535–543.
19. Cotton BA, Faz G, Hatch QM, et al. Rapid thrombelastography delivers real-time results that predict transfusion within 1 hour of admission. *J Trauma*. 2011;71(2):407–414; discussion 414–417.
20. Plotkin AJ, Wade CE, Jenkins DH, et al. A reduction in clot formation rate and strength assessed by thrombelastography is indicative of transfusion requirements in patients with penetrating injuries. *J Trauma*. 2008;64(2 Suppl):S64–S68.
21. Alam HB. An update on fluid resuscitation. *Scand J Surg*. 2006;95(3):136–145.
22. Kentner R, Safar P, Prueckner S, et al. Titrated hypertonic/hyperoncotic solution for hypotensive fluid resuscitation during uncontrolled hemorrhagic shock in rats. *Resuscitation*. 2005;65(1):87–95.
23. Sondeen JL, Coppes VG, Holcomb JB. Blood pressure at which rebleeding occurs after resuscitation in swine with aortic injury. *J Trauma*. 2003;54(5 Suppl):S110–S117.
24. Alam HB, Koustova E, Rhee P. Combat casualty care research: from bench to the battlefield. *World J Surg*. 2005:29(Suppl 1):S7–S11.
25. Alam HB, Rhee P. New developments in fluid resuscitation. *Surg Clin North Am*. 2007;87(1):55–72.
26. Palmer L, Martin L. Traumatic coagulopathy—part 2: resuscitative strategies. *J Vet Emerg Crit Care (San Antonio)*. 2014;24(1):75–92.
27. Mapstone J, Roberts I, Evans P. Fluid resuscitation strategies: a systematic review of animal trials. *J Trauma*. 2003;55(3):571–589.
28. Chesnut RM, Marshall LF, Klauber MR, et al. The role of secondary brain injury in determining outcome from severe head injury. *J Trauma*. 1993;34(2):216–222.
29. Alam HB, Stanton K, Koustova E, Burris D, Rich N, Rhee P. Effect of different resuscitation strategies on neutrophil activation in a swine model of hemorrhagic shock. *Resuscitation*. 2004;60(1):91–99.
30. Rhee P, Koustova E, Alam HB. Searching for the optimal resuscitation method: recommendations for the initial fluid resuscitation of combat casualties. *J Trauma*. 2003;54(5):S52–S62.
31. Koustova E, Stanton K, Gushchin V, Alam HB, Stegalkina S, Rhee PM. Effects of lactated Ringer's solutions on human leukocytes. *J Trauma*. 2002;52(5):872–878.
32. Cotton BA, Au BK, Nunez TC, Gunter OL, Robertson AM, Young PP. Predefined massive transfusion protocols are associated with a reduction in organ failure and postinjury complications. *J Trauma*. 2009;66(1):41–48; discussion 48–49.
33. Cotton BA, Gunter OL, Isbell J, et al. Damage control hematology: the impact of a trauma exsanguination protocol on survival and blood product utilization. *J Trauma*. 2008;64(5):1177–1182; discussion 1182–1183.
34. Yucel N, Lefering R, Maegele M, et al. Trauma associated severe hemorrhage (TASH)-score: probability of mass transfusion as surrogate for life threatening hemorrhage after multiple trauma. *J Trauma*. 2006;60(6):1228–1236.
35. Nunez TC, Voskresensky IV, Dossett LA, Shinall R, Dutton WD. Early prediction of massive transfusion in trauma: simple as ABC (assessment of blood consumption). *J Trauma*. 2009;66(2):346–352.
36. Borgman MA, Spinella PC, Perkins JG, et al. The ratio of blood products transfused affects mortality in patients receiving massive transfusions at a combat support hospital. *J Trauma*. 2007;63(4):805–813.
37. Gunter OL Jr, Au BK, Isbell JM, Mowery NT, Young PP, Cotton BA. Optimizing outcomes in damage control resuscitation: identifying blood product ratios associated with improved survival. *J Trauma*. 2008;65(3):527–534.
38. Holcomb JB, Wade CE, Michalek JE, et al. Increased plasma and platelet to red blood cell ratios improves outcome in massively transfused civilian trauma patients. *Ann Surg*. 2008;248(3):447–458.
39. Snyder CW, Weinberg JA, McGwin G Jr, et al. The relationship of blood product ratio to mortality: survival benefit or survival bias? *J Trauma*. 2009;66(2):358–362; discussion 362–364.
40. Sperry JL, Ochoa JB, Gunn SR, et al. An FFP:PRBC transfusion ratio ≥1:1.5 is associated with a lower risk of mortality after massive transfusion. *J Trauma*. 2008;65(5):986–993.
41. Teixeira PG, Inaba K, Shulman I, et al. Impact of plasma transfusion in massively transfused trauma patients. *J Trauma*. 2009;66(5):693–697.
42. Yan PY, Holcomb J, Schreiber MA. Novel concepts for damage control resuscitation in trauma. *Curr Opin Crit Care*. 2017;23(6):498–502.
43. Junger WG, Coimbra R, Liu FC, et al. Hypertonic saline resuscitation: a tool to modulate immune function in trauma patients? *Shock*. 1997;8(4):235–241.
44. Bulger EM, May S, Kerby JD, et al. Out-of-hospital hypertonic resuscitation after traumatic hypovolemic shock: a randomized, placebo controlled trial. *Ann Surg*. 2011;253(3):431–441.
45. DuBose JJ, Kobayashi L, Lozornio A, et al. Clinical experience using 5% hypertonic saline as a safe alternative fluid for use in trauma. *J Trauma*. 2010;68(5):1172–1177.
46. Joseph B, Aziz H, Snell M, et al. The physiologic effects of hyperosmolar resuscitation: 5% vs. 3% hypertonic saline. *Am J Surg*. 2014;208(5):697–702.

47. Rhee P. Noncolligative properties of intravenous fluids. *Curr Opin Crit Care*. 2010;16(4):317–322.
48. Williams-Johnson JA, McDonald AH, Strachan GG, Williams EW. Effects of tranexamic acid on death, vascular occlusive events, and blood transfusion in trauma patients with significant haemorrhage (CRASH-2) a randomised, placebo-controlled trial. *West Indian Med J*. 2010;59(6):612–624.
49. Perkins JG, Schreiber MA, Wade CE, Holcomb JB. Early versus late recombinant factor VIIa in combat trauma patients requiring massive transfusion. *J Trauma*. 2007;62(5):1095–1099.

32

The Outdoors—Venomous Bites and Stings and Environmental Exposure

Joshua Person, John Patrick Walker, and Gregory J. Jurkovich

Key Points

1. Of the 3700 species of snakes worldwide, only 200 are significantly venomous, with approximately 6 deaths per year in the United States caused by snakebite. In contrast, there are over 150,000 species of Hymenoptera in the world that cause approximately 40 deaths per year, mostly as a result of severe anaphylactic reactions.
2. Snakebite morbidity depends on the type of snake and the degree of envenomation. Venoms consist of numerous polypeptides that can disrupt endothelial cells and blood flow, produce neuromuscular blockade, or generate a coagulopathy via procoagulants. Some snakes (particularly Elapids [represented by the coral snakes in North America]) also have direct neurotoxins and cardiotoxins.
3. Snakebite produces immediate pain, edema, and erythema at the site. Spread of the swelling greater than 10 cm/hr indicates severe envenomation. Initial incision and suction and the use of a proximal tourniquet are contraindicated. Use of purified ovine antivenin is effective for serious Crotalidae envenomation and has replaced equine antivenin with its associated risk of serum sickness. Because of the presumed safety of the newer antivenom, overuse is more likely.
4. Spider bites produce toxicity by local tissue necrosis (brown recluse and hobo spiders) and painful muscle contractions (black widow spider). Death may be caused by stinging Hymenoptera, including bees (particularly aggressive Africanized bees), fire ants, and scorpions. The death is usually secondary to anaphylaxis, but occasionally massive envenomation occurs—especially with Africanized honeybees. The estimated lethal dose is approximately 20 stings/kg in most mammals.
5. The initial response to hypothermia is an intensive sympathetic type reaction with tremulousness, profound vasoconstriction, marked increase in oxygen consumption, and accelerated heart rate and minute ventilation. As core temperature falls to between 33° and 30 °C this response is lost and deeper core hypothermia rapidly develops.
6. Hypothermia risk is high in the severely injured patient as a result of exposure, loss of normal protective metabolism (ie, shivering), rapid massive infusion of cold fluids/blood, and open thoracic and abdominal cavities.
7. Hypothermia increases risk of mortality at every level of traumatic injury. There is no improvement in outcome when hypothermia is applied to the severe TBI; trauma patients rapidly rewarmed require less resuscitation volume and have improved survival.
8. Treating hypothermia begins by preventing further heat loss and allowing endogenous rewarming. Active rewarming has many adjuncts, including warm blankets, heating pads and lights, and immersion in warm water or internally by core rewarming. Internal core rewarming is more effective and includes heated intravenous fluids; heated body cavity lavage; heated moist inhaled air; extracorporeal circulatory rewarming (ECMO or CPB) or closed circuit intravascular countercurrent heat-exchange devices.
9. Frostbite involves ice crystal formation and unpredictable loss of tissue. Early definitive rewarming (avoiding refreezing) by submersion in 40° to 42 °C water is preferable with subsequent meticulous care, awaiting demarcation, and avoidance of early debridement to optimize outcomes and tissue salvage.
10. Early thrombolytic therapy might be beneficial in select frostbite patients.

BITES AND STINGS

Snakebites

The legends and lore of snakes are spread across history; with serpents mentioned in 42 Bible verses, implicated in the death of Cleopatra, and the medical field—the snake is essential to the rod of Aesculapius and the Caduceus. Few emergencies have been surrounded with as many types of attempted but ineffective treatments (eg, electrical shock and TASER®, tourniquets with ice emersion, crosscut of the bite with suction of the wound) and little scientific fact as a snakebite. We will address the management of snakebites and related envenomation with scientific evidence.

Snake Epidemiology

The World Health Organization (WHO) estimates 5.4 million people worldwide are bitten by snakes each year, with 1.8 to 2.7 million cases of envenomation. This organization also estimates between 81,000 and 138,000 deaths a year and three times as many amputations and permanent disabilities. High-quality snake antivenoms are considered essential medicines by the WHO. In the United States, the Centers for Disease Control (CDC) estimates there are 7000 to 8000 bites per year with 5 to 6 deaths. Most of the deaths are secondary to rattlesnake envenomation, with only two fatalities from copperhead

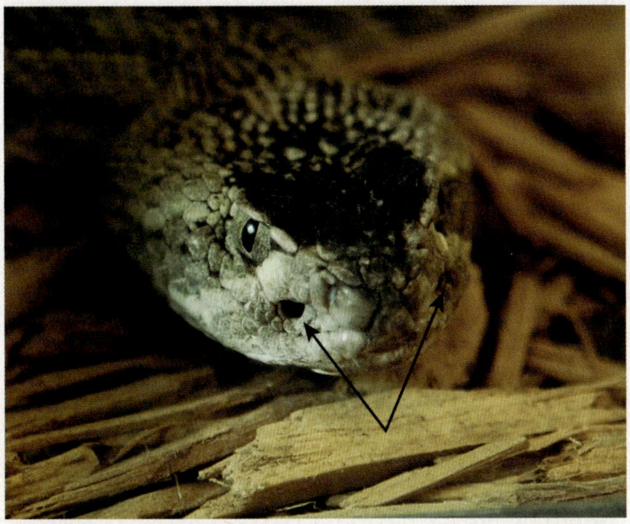

Figure 32.1. Depiction of nasal pits that are located between the nose and the eye. These are excellent sensory organs that can differentiate a temperature differential of 0.003 °C. (Photo courtesy of Ronny Stewart, MD.)

Table 32.1. Crotalus Species

US Rattlesnakes—Genus Crotalus:
Timber rattlesnake (Canebrake)—*Crotalus horridus*
Eastern diamondback—*Crotalus adamanteus*
Western diamondback—*Crotalus atrox*
Prairie rattlesnake—*Crotalus viridis*
Mojave rattlesnake—*Crotalus scutulatus*
Rock rattlesnake—*Crotalus lepidus*
Black-tailed rattlesnake—*Crotalus molossus*
Red diamond rattlesnake—*Crotalus ruber*
Speckled rattlesnake—*Crotalus mitchellii*
Sidewinder rattlesnake—*Crotalus cerastes*
Tiger rattlesnake—*Crotalus tigris*
Twin-spotted rattlesnake—*Crotalus pricei*
Ridge-nosed rattlesnake—*Crotalus willardi*
Western rattlesnake—*Crotalus oreganus*

1 snakebite in the past 5 years. More than 3700 species of snakes exist in the world of which approximately 200 are deadly. They range in size from 10 cm to greater than 9 m. Nonvenomous snakes predominate on all continents except for Australia.

There are four families of poisonous snakes worldwide: Colubridae, Elapidae (which now include the Hydrophiliinae—the sea snakes), Viperidae, and Atractaspididae. The boomslang and the bird snake represent the Colubridae—found mostly in Africa. The Elapids are found throughout the world and include snakes such as mambas, kraits, adders, and cobras. The only Elapids in North America are the coral snakes. The Viperids have long hinged fangs. They include the pit vipers that, like the nonvenomous Boidae family (boas and pythons), have infrared sensors in a nasal pit that is located between the nose and the eye (**Fig. 32.1**). These are excellent sensory organs that can differentiate a temperature differential of 0.003 °C.

All venomous snakes in North America except for the coral snakes are in this Viperidae family. The phylogeny of poisonous snakes in North America are therefore of the phylum Chordata, class Reptilia, order Squamata, suborder Serpentes, and of the Crotalidae (subfamily Crotalinae) or Elapidae family. Venomous snakes are distributed throughout the United States with at least one species in every state except for Hawaii, Alaska, and Maine. Water moccasins are found primarily in the southeastern United States. Copperheads are found from Massachusetts westerly to Illinois and to the south from Florida to Texas. Rattlesnakes are found coast to coast. The genus Crotalus—the true rattlesnakes—are found only in the Americas.

Snakes are easily identifiable reptiles, marked anatomically by the large number (greater than 120) of precloacal vertebral bodies. They also have a reduced (almost absent) left lung, a single ventricle (no ventricular septum), and no muscles in the ciliary body of the eye. Despite the absence of a ventricular septum, oxygenated and deoxygenated blood channels separately though the heart. All snakes are strictly carnivores. The size of the snake dictates the size of the prey.

In the management of snakebite one of the most important steps is identification of the species of the offending serpent. In the United States, this is less important than in other countries, as almost all venomous bites are from the genera Crotalus and Sistrurus (eg, rattlesnakes and pigmy rattlers) and the genera Agkistrodon (eg, copperheads and water moccasins). All of these are treated in a similar fashion, with the same antivenom. The only exception is envenomation by the Coral snakes (an Elapid). Note that manufacture of antivenom for coral snakes was discontinued in the United States (however available in other countries), although a few vials may still exist, likely of decreased potency.

In North America, there are two genera of rattlesnakes: Crotalus (**Table 32.1**)—the true rattlesnakes and Sistrurus (**Table 32.2**)—the pigmy rattlers. There are 14 species of Crotalus in North America. The remainder of the pit vipers fall into the members of the Agkistrodon genus—moccasins and copperheads (**Table 32.3**).

The largest species of rattlesnake in North America is the eastern diamondback (*Crotalus adamanteus*), which is slightly larger than its cousin the western diamondback (*Crotalus atrox*). These pit vipers (ie, genus Crotalus, Sistrurus, and Agkistrodon) are morphologically distinguished by elliptical pupils and a triangular head (**Fig. 32.2**) and retractable fangs. The fangs are tubular, injecting venom similar to a hypodermic needle. This is in contradistinction to the Elapids in which the fangs are fixed and grooved, wicking the venom into the victim. Venomous snakes have a single row of caudal plates distal to the anal plate, whereas nonvenomous snakes have a double row of caudal plates.

Table 32.2. Sistrurus Species

Genus Sistrurus (Ground Rattlers/Swamp Rattlers):
Massasauga—*Sistrurus catenatus* Eastern—*Subsp. catenatus* Western—*Subsp. tergeminus* Desert—*Subsp. edwardsii*
Western pigmy rattlesnake—*Sistrurus miliarius streckeri*
Carolina pigmy rattlesnake—*Sistrurus miliarius miliarius*
Dusky pigmy rattlesnake—*Sistrurus miliarius barbouri*

Table 32.3. Agkistrodon Species

US Copperheads and Moccasins:
Northern copperhead—*Agkistrodon contortrix mokasen*
Osage copperhead—*Agkistrodon contortrix phaeogaster*
Southern copperhead—*Agkistrodon contortrix contortrix*
Broad-banded copperhead—*Agkistrodon contortrix laticinctus*
Trans-Pecos copperhead—*Agkistrodon contortrix pictigaster*
Eastern cottonmouth—*Agkistrodon piscivorus piscivorus*
Florida cottonmouth—*Agkistrodon piscivorus conanti*
Western cottonmouth—Agkistrodon piscivorus leucostoma

There are thirty-two species of rattlesnakes in the Americas, ranging from southern Alberta to central Argentina. Rattlesnakes are only found in the Americas. All true rattlesnakes have a rattle (except for an endangered species in Mexico—the Santa Catalina rattlesnake, which has only a vestigial rattle). The rattle is a series of interlocking segments. A new segment is added with each shedding of the skin. Venom is produced in Duvernoy glands on the dorsal sides of the head (corresponding to parotid glands) enhancing the triangular appearance. During envenomation the venom is forced through the fangs by the palatine muscles. If a fang is broken off, it will be replaced by the next in a row of "proto fangs." Any clothing may limit the amount and depth of envenomation. The purpose of the venom is to immobilize or kill the prey and begin digestion.

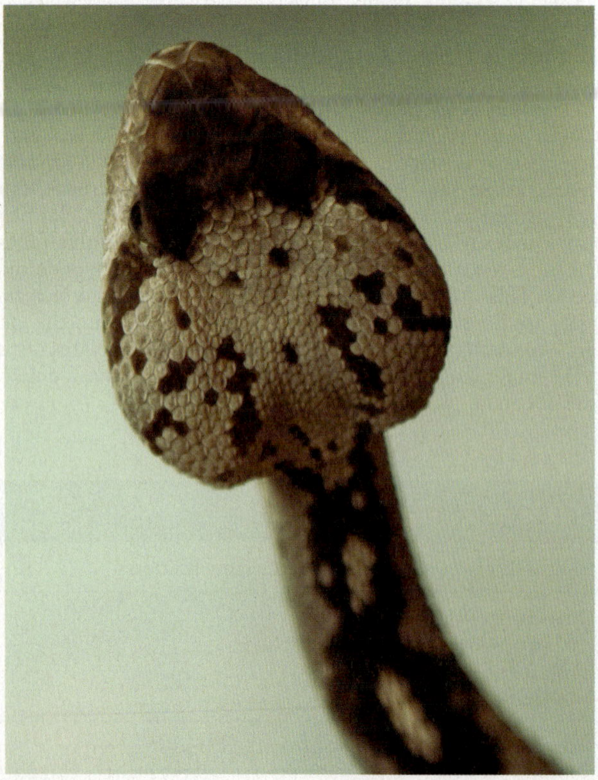

Figure 32.2. Pit vipers (ie, genus Crotalus, Sistrurus, and Agkistrodon) are morphologically distinguished by elliptical pupils and a triangular head. (Photo courtesy of Ronny Stewart, MD.)

Table 32.4. Composition of Venom

Main Enzymes of Snake Venom:
Dehydrogenase lactate
L-Amino acid oxidase
Catalase
Alanine amino transferase
Phospholipase A_2
Lysophospholipase
Acetylcholinesterase
5′-Nucleotidase
Phosphodiesterase
Deoxyribonuclease
Ribonuclease 1
Adenosine triphosphatase
Hyaluronidase
NAD-Nucleotidase
Factor-X activator
α-Fibrinogenase
Prothrombin activator
Collagenase
Elastase

Snake Venom Composition and Consequences

Pit viper venoms are complex with up to 30 different proteins and enzymes identified. Over 90% of the dry weight of venom is proteinaceous in nature. Although it is common to classify the venoms as neurotoxic or digestive in nature, all snakes have varying compositions of venoms. The Crotalids will have a higher percentage of digestive/enzymatic type proteins than the Elapids, which will contain a higher percentage
2 of neurotoxins. Common enzymes are phospholipases, metalloproteases, collagenase, and hyaluronidase (**Table 32.4**). These peptides and polypeptides act by damaging vascular endothelium and other cellular membranes. Compliment is activated, fibrin is degraded, and platelets are activated. The increased permeability of the membranes leads to peripheral and pulmonary edema, hemorrhage, and hypotension. L-amino acid oxidase splits fibrinogen contributing to the induction of disseminated intravascular coagulation (DIC). The Elapids contain a higher percentage of proteins that block acetylcholine receptor sites. This can lead to dysphagia, slurred speech, seizures, coma, and death. Despite the very high toxicity of coral snake venom, only one fatality has been recorded in the United States in the past 50 years.

Snakebite Management

By far the most critical step in management of snakebite is identification of the offending species. Most snakebites are nonvenomous and require no treatment. Most bites, such as those of copperheads and pigmy rattlers, are almost always self-limiting and require little more than observation. Others such as the Diamondback Rattlesnake (**Fig. 32.3**) and Mojave rattlers can require intense medical management, occasional

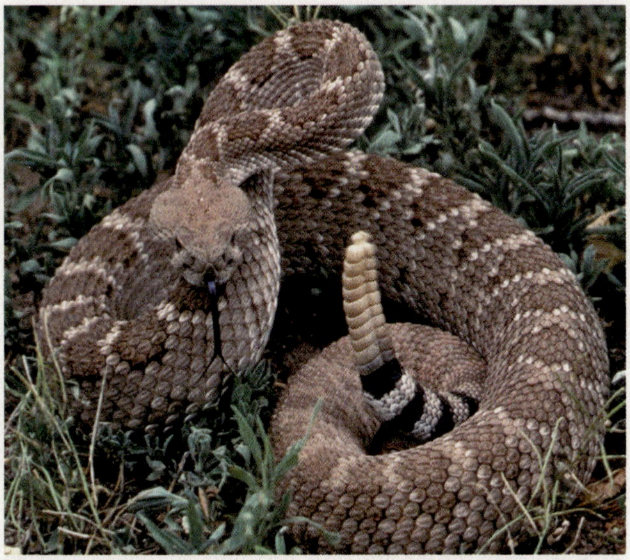

Figure 32.3. Diamondback Rattlesnake—geographically distributed located in the southwestern United States and Mexico. (Photo courtesy of Ronny Stewart, MD.)

surgical intervention, and even rarely cause death. Identification of the species by the patient is notoriously invalid; however, a detailed description of the offending snake should be taken. In the United States and Canada, the only snake where color is useful in identification is the coral snake—"red and yellow kill a fellow, red and black venom lack" (**Fig. 32.4**). Note that this saying is true only in North America, as there are venomous coral snakes in Central and South America that have red bands touching black bands. Other clues, such as geography and topography (proximity to water), can also at least help with identification of the genus. All snakebites should, at least initially, be considered an event with potential morbidity and possible mortality. As snakes are cold-blooded animals, snakebites generally occur in the warm months, with an increase in incidence in the spring and fall. Most snakebites occur in young men, *with up to 60% of bites occurring in victims that were deliberately provoking the snakes.*

Field Treatment of Snakebites

The initial treatment of snakebite begins with first aid. Although identification of the snake is important, one should not risk a second bite to try to catch the snake. Do not delay treatment while looking for the offending reptile and do not assume that a stationary snake is dead. Do not try to handle a dead snake directly, as a reflexive bite can occur. Remove any jewelry or tight clothing from the affected extremity. Initial first aid on the scene should involve immobilization and splinting in a functional position. There are no data to confirm this will limit the spread of venom, but it will be more comfortable. The application of ice or heat seems to have little effect on results. Limit exertion, particularly extended ambulation in lower extremity bites. The application of pressure bandages—specifically a constrictor band—is species specific. In countries where systemic neurotoxicity is more likely than necrosis (ie, an Elapid bite in Australia) a pressure bandage or constrictor band should be considered and placed between the wound and the heart at approximately 55 mm Hg. This has been demonstrated to reduce systemic toxicity in an animal model.[1] However, in the United States, where the envenomation is most likely to be from a Crotalid, the application of a constrictor band is likely to result in concentration of the venom in the extremity with increased necrosis and local enzymatic injury. The patient should be promptly brought to appropriate medical care, if possible, a center with experience in management of snakebite. It is probable that if there is no pain or erythema by the time that the patient arrives in the emergency department, no envenomation has occurred.

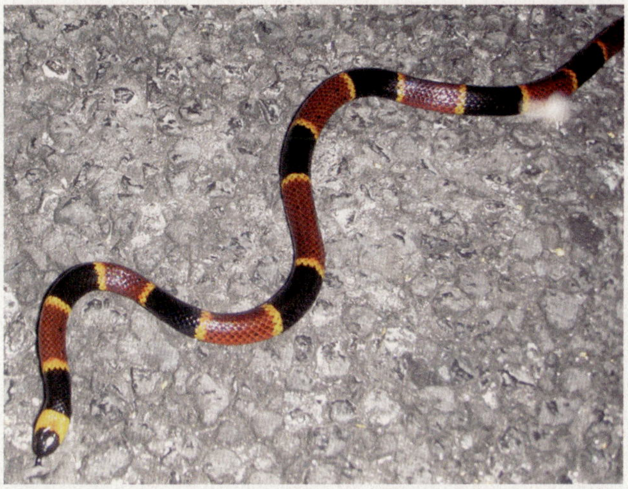

Figure 32.4. In North America, the only snake where color is useful in identification is the coral snake.

When evaluating the snakebite victim, it is important to document both local and systemic signs and symptoms. Vital signs should be recorded and repeated at intervals guided by the clinical response. Pain, edema, and erythema at the site are common. Secondary symptoms include muscle twitching, perioral paresthesia, and a metallic taste in the mouth. The wound should be cleansed, and the location of the puncture sites documented. The distance between the two fang marks is related to the size of the snake. In countries where a rapid venom identification kit is available to swab the wound and guide antivenom therapy (eg, Australia and Papau New Guinea) do not wash the wound. In other areas, gentle cleansing is acceptable.

Avoidable Treatments for Snakebites

Several historical treatments should specifically be avoided. Do not massage the wound and particularly—*do not incise the wound.* Incision and suction, previously advocated for decades, has not been recommended since 1980. A surgical incision in the field by a nonsurgeon can possibly involve vessels, tendons, and nerves and increase morbidity, and only a small amount of venom can be extracted with suction. Several animal studies have proven electrical shock therapy (such as a Taser) to be ineffective in snakebite.

Hospital Evaluation and Treatment of Snakebites

3 Once in the emergency department, initial focus should be on evaluation of the airway, breathing, and circulation. Intravenous access should be obtained. In the event of a bite to the head, neck, or face early intubation should be considered to protect the airway. Laboratory evaluation should include a CBC with platelet count, PT, PTT, CPK, fibrinogen level, BUN, creatinine, and urinalysis. Viscoelastic assays such as TEG or ROTEM can also be used to monitor coagulopathy. Marking the area of ecchymosis can help the clinician follow the progression of the envenomation (**Fig. 32.5**). Swelling in the affected digit or limb

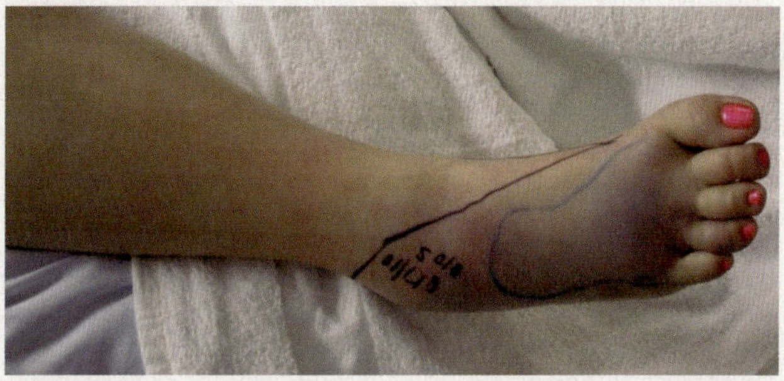

Figure 32.5. Progression of envenomation being monitored using serial skin marking.

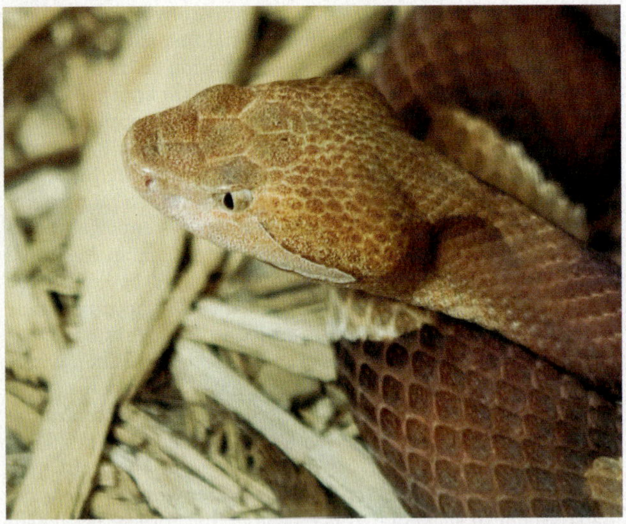

Figure 32.6. Copperhead, from the *Agkistrodon* genus, bites account for many of the treated snakebites in the United States.

should be measured (circumference), compared to the unaffected side, and followed closely with serial measurements. The amount of local tissue destruction is an accurate marker of the degree of envenomation. The presence of additional symptoms such as nausea/vomiting, diarrhea, headache, arthralgias should raise suspicion for envenomation.

Crotalid venom primarily causes local tissue destruction and hematologic toxicity, although other organ systems can be involved. Up to 30% of Crotalid envenomation will show an abnormality in the coagulation profile, most commonly hypofibrinogenemia with elevated prothrombin time and thrombocytopenia. Clinical bleeding is exceedingly rare. In Lavonas' (2004) review of 400 copperhead (**Fig. 32.6**) bites from the Carolinas, no hypotension, no respiratory failure, and no deaths occurred.[2] Eight patients did have laboratory abnormalities, but none developed bleeding complications. However, in a severe envenomation by one of the larger rattlesnakes, diffuse capillary leakage can lead to pulmonary edema, hypotension, and shock. A consumptive coagulopathy may rapidly develop. In the rare patient that develops clinical bleeding, such as hemoptysis, intracranial hemorrhage, or gastrointestinal bleeding, correction of the coagulopathy should be undertaken with appropriate blood products. Antivenom should be given in these patients as initial therapy. Do not routinely treat thrombocytopenia or severe coagulopathy in the absence of bleeding. Delayed coagulopathy can recur up to 2 weeks later.

Such patients may bleed spontaneously from any site. Acute renal failure may result from nephrotoxins as well as myoglobinuria. An electrocardiogram, or at least continuous cardiac monitoring, should be considered. Tetanus toxoid should be administered. If there appears to be no evidence of envenomation, the patient may be observed in the emergency department for several hours and discharged home. Although several series have noted that observation alone is an appropriate treatment of Agkistrodon (copperhead and moccasin) bites,[3,4] extrapolation of this data to rattlesnakes could be misleading. In the rattlesnake bite victim with a moderate or severe envenomation, early use of antivenom is appropriate, and should be strongly considered (see section that follows). In locals such as Australia where there is a preponderance of Elapid envenomations the observation time should be extended, as local skin changes may be minimal. With evidence of envenomation, general recommendations are for admission to a monitored bed in the hospital for observation and possible intervention for at least 24 hours.

Although there are a number of snakebite severity indices (grading systems) published, a modification of the simple system proposed by Dart in 1996 is probably the most useful.[5] A grade 1 envenomation is limited to the immediate bite site; a grade 2 envenomation extends proximately to less than a full extremity and may have non–life-threatening symptoms such as nausea, vomiting, mild tachycardia, and mild hypotension. A grade 3 envenomation involves more than an extremity and includes systemic signs such as severe hypotension/tachycardia or blood dyscrasias or clinically significant clotting abnormalities. Although enzyme-linked immunosorbent assays (ELISAs) have been developed that can directly measure serum venom antigens as well as identify the offending snake, clinical applicability of these types of tests are limited.

Steroids have no benefit in humans although these are often used by veterinarians. Steroids do have a role in treating the infrequent acute allergic as well as delayed-onset serum sickness that may occur after the use of sheep-derived antivenom, as noted below. The prophylactic use of antibiotics has been evaluated by several studies and does not seem to reduce infection rates.[6] Infection after snakebite is surprisingly uncommon and while patients are often given an antibiotic, there is no good clinical evidence for their use. Although many patients will have erythema, edema, and tissue necrosis and will appear infected, these are usually sterile; culture-proven infection occurring after snakebite should be treated appropriately. Culture of organisms in the mouth of the rattlesnake includes Pseudomonas, Enterobacteriaceae, Staphylococcus, and Clostridia. If the species is a coral snake or a nonindigenous Elapid, the administration of cholinergic agonists should occur at the first sign of symptoms. Calcium infusion may reduce the onset of seizures.

Antivenom Administration for Crotalid Envenomation

Certainly, the most controversial decision point in management of snakebite is the administration of antivenom. Although hundreds of antivenoms are available worldwide for various species, for all practical purposes in North America, the envenomation is limited to Crotalids. Snakebite by coral snakes is uncommon in North America, and while the venom is exceedingly toxic, the treatment is only supportive, as antivenom is no longer available in the United States for coral snake bites. *Cranial advancement of the area of ecchymosis at a rate greater than 10 cm per hour is generally considered an indication for initiation of antivenom therapy.*

Prior to 2000, the primary antivenom available in the United States for the bite of a Crotalid was a hyperimmune serum produced by envenomation of horses. Its use was associated with a high incidence of side effects: anaphylaxis, hypersensitivity, and delayed serum sickness. In 2000, CroFab® (Crotalidae Polyvalent Immune Fab [Ovine]) was introduced, obviating the use of now unavailable horse serum products. This is now complimented by another purified product—Anavip®. CroFab is composed of small Fab fragment antibodies, while Anavip is made from larger V-shaped F(ab')2 fragments. Anavip® has a much longer half-life. This may result in a lower incidence of late coagulopathy. Note that the Crotalidae Immune F(ab')2 antivenom is of Equine origin and may be problematic in those patients with horse allergies. A detailed review of antivenom therapy for pit vipers is provided by Weinstein.[7]

CroFab is truly an elegant drug. It is produced by immunizing sheep with the venom from the western diamondback rattlesnake (*C. atrox*), the eastern diamondback rattlesnake (*C. adamanteus*), the Mojave rattlesnake (*Crotalus scutulatus*) or the cottonmouth water moccasin (Agkistrodon). The monovalent immunoglobulin from the sheep is prepared by fractionation of the immunoglobulin from the serum, digesting it with papain, and then utilizing ion exchange and affinity chromatography to separate the Fab fragments specific to each species. The Fc portion of IgG is generally thought to be responsible for high rates of hypersensitivity and serum sickness seen with the horse serum product developed by Wyeth in 1954, and hence this ovine (sheep) version is generally

Table 32.5. Components of Antivenom—CroFab®

Antibodies LD50 Neutralizing Units
Crotalus atrox (Western diamondback) 1350
Crotalus adamanteus (Eastern diamondback) 800
Crotalus scutulatus (Mojave rattler) 5210
Agkistrodon piscivorus (Cottonmouth water moccasin) 460

considered safer. The four different monospecific antivenins are then mixed (**Table 32.5**). In a murine model there is good antigenic crossover in treating other North American Crotalid envenomations.

Utilizing CroFab to treat Crotalid envenomation is somewhat controversial, primarily because of the cost/benefit ratio. The cost of this drug is a significant factor with wholesale prices up to $3200 per vial in 2023. Certainly, any patient with life-threatening symptoms should immediately be given 4 to 6 vials of the antivenom.[8] Treatment is not based on the body mass of the patient—as the antivenom neutralizes the poison that is injected—this will vary with each envenomation. The lyophilized powder is reconstituted with 18 mL of normal saline, followed by dilution in 250 mL. Each dose is given over 1 hour. It is thought that venom is rapidly tissue bound, therefore the earlier the antivenom can be given, the more likely a favorable response. The packaging information states that treatment should begin within 6 hours of the bite.

If one can ascertain that the snake is one of the less virulent types (Agkistrodon or Sistrurus species), the patient can usually be treated without the use of antivenom. However, in the patient with a deteriorating clinical condition, antivenom treatment should always be given. Repeated dosing should be given until clinical stability is achieved, although this is highly unlikely after 30 to 40 vials. The patient should be monitored for recurrence of symptoms and retreated if necessary. CroFab has an estimated half-life of 12 to 23 hours.

CroFab has been used extensively in children as young as 14 months, although there are beginning to be reports of overuse of CroFab in both children and adults. A special consideration is in the use of antivenom in the pregnant patients. Certainly, coagulopathy could be lethal to the mother and fetus, but there have been limited reports of use of CroFab in pregnancy. Reports of fetal loss of up to 20% are noted in the worldwide literature with snakebites of a variety of species. This seems to be improved with the use of antivenom.[9] Certainly, the risk/benefit ratio must be carefully weighed, but the general recommendation is to treat pregnant women with CroFab when indicated.

Consequences of Antivenom Administration for Snakebites

Immediate adverse drug reactions to CroFab will occur in 6% to 8% of patients. This may be related to the rate of infusion, although at least one study from Sri Lanka showed no difference in severe hypersensitivity reactions when the antivenom was over 20 minutes versus IV infusion of 2 hours. Although anaphylaxis would occur in up to 50% of patients treated with the older equine antivenin, it is a lesser occurrence with CroFab—but still up to 14% of patients. It should be treated aggressively when occurring: The antivenin infusion should be stopped and a combination of antihistamines (diphenhydramine), epinephrine, and steroids administered, depending on the severity of the response to anaphylaxis. The airway should be assessed and secured if necessary. Appropriate volume resuscitation should be instituted. Steroid dosing ranges from a single 125-mg intravenous bolus of methylprednisolone to short-course prednisone pulse dosing (60 mg daily for 5 days).

Table 32.6. Components of Antivenom—ANAVIP

Antibodies LD50 Neutralizing Units
Bothrops asper (Terciopelo or fer-de-lance) 780
Crotalus simus (formerly Crotalus durissus—Central American Rattlesnake) 790
Crotalus adamanteus (Eastern Diamondback Rattlesnake) 244
Crotalus atrox (Western Diamondback Rattlesnake) 147
Crotalus scutulatus (Mohave Rattlesnake) 185
Agkistrodon contortrix (Copperhead) 28
Agkistrodon piscivorus (Water Moccasin) 61

Serum sickness will occur in 13% to 16% of patients treated with ovine antivenom (CroFab), certainly less common than with the older Wyeth equine antivenom.

Serum sickness is a type III hypersensitivity reaction in which soluble antigen–antibody complexes are deposited diffusely in the presence of antigen excess. Symptoms such as urticaria, itching, nephritis, and arthralgia can occur for weeks after the infusion. The treatment for serum sickness is a pulse of corticosteroids tapered over 7 to 14 days. There is no question that the purified ovine antivenin (CroFab), and now ANAVIP (Crotalidae immune $F(ab')_2$ [equine]), are much safer than the older horse product.[10] It may be that ANAVIP (**Table 32.6**) may be a better choice for several reasons: less expensive, longer half-life, it can be stored at room temperature, and it can be reconstituted more rapidly. Each CroFab vial costs about $3198, with 4 to 12 vials usually given, with ANAVIP costing $1220 with a starting dose of 10 vials. While CroFab has a half-life of about 15 hours, ANAVIP has a half-life of about 133 hours—therefore theoretically lessening the need for redosing. However, a recent publication indicates that, in patients bitten by rattlesnakes, more ANAVIP was utilized and more redosing was required.[11]

The decreased toxicity of modern antivenom has led to some indiscriminate and increasing usage in emergency departments across the country, as there is at least one report of effective use of antivenom after significant delay. Thus is the conundrum—there are certainly snakebites that initially appear innocuous that later become life-threatening. This has led physicians in the emergency room to overtreat large numbers of patients who do not require therapy, and why it is so important that every attempt be made to identify the offending species. In a recent study, up to 84% of pit viper envenomations were treated with antivenom.[12] The reason for the high usage may be medicolegal, as it is certainly not to reduce mortality, but in some cases, it may reduce morbidity. It should be recognized that the vast majority of snakebite victims will recover uneventfully with only supportive treatment. Each patient must be individually clinically evaluated and antivenom use limited to those in whom the potential benefits outweigh the risk of side effects.

The Role of Surgery in Snakebites

The use of surgery in the management of snakebite has a limited role. Although historically snakebite has been treated with various surgical procedures, it should be in an unusual patient that more than simple debridement is needed. Crosscut and aspiration of the puncture sites was utilized for decades, but this is no longer recommended. Several studies have shown the limitations of this practice. In dogs, up to one-half of the venom can be removed, but only if incision and suction are begun within 3 minutes. However, in human studies only about 11% of the venom may be removed. It is rapidly

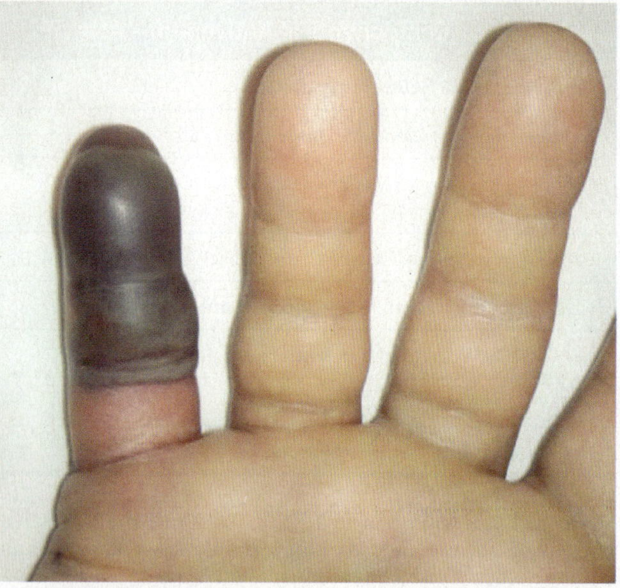

Figure 32.7. Snakebite resulting in local cytolytic response with hemolytic bulla.

bound to tissues and is difficult to be removed by suction. Both partial and radical surgical excision of the involved bite area has likewise been attempted with no proven benefit. A not uncommon finding is a local cytolytic response (**Fig. 32.7**) that produces a hemolytic bulla and requires debridement (**Figs. 32.8 and 32.9**).

Actual tissue loss occurs in 7.8% of rattlesnake bites and 3.8% of Copperhead bites. These injuries can be expected to heal by secondary intention with a satisfactory cosmetic response (**Fig. 32.10**).

Another use of antivenom is in the patient with impending compartment syndrome. The great majority of snakebites deposit venom in the subcutaneous tissues, not subfascial. It can sometimes be difficult to differentiate a swollen painful extremity from a true compartment syndrome. A recent review of the North American snake bite registry found 22 cases of suspected extremity compartment syndrome in 1604 reported envenomations by North American native crotalids over a 9-year period from 2013 to 2021. This represents an incidence of approximately 1% of crotalid envenomations. When in doubt, compartment pressures should be measured. With rising pressures (greater than 30 to 40 mm), antivenom therapy should be initiated (or repeated). With failure of response to adequate dosing of antivenom, appropriate surgical fasciotomy can save an extremity. Prophylactic fasciotomy has no role in

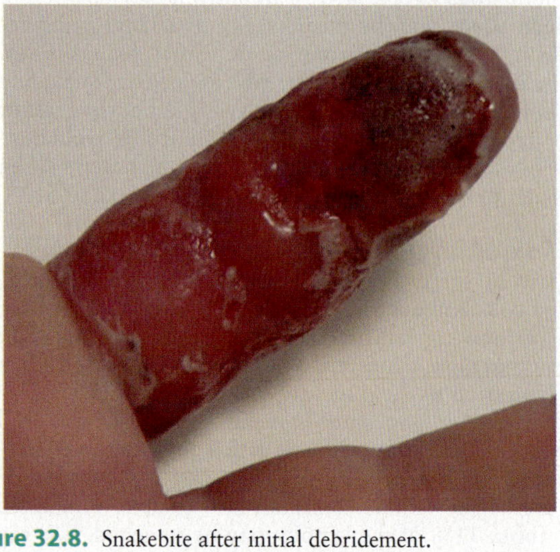

Figure 32.8. Snakebite after initial debridement.

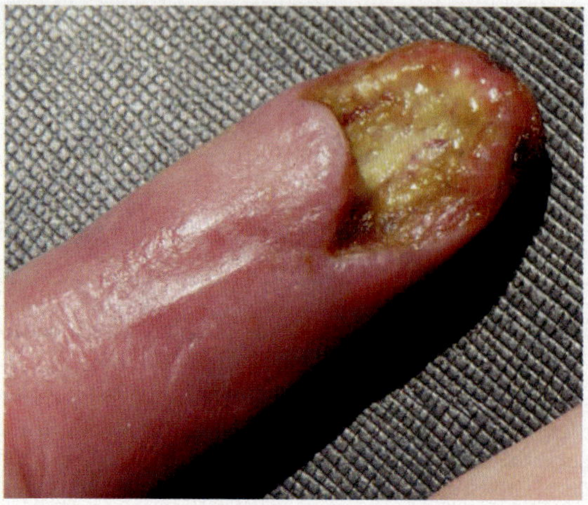

Figure 32.9. After second debridement.

treatment. Stewart et al. at the University of Texas Health Science Center in San Antonio have an extensive experience with rattlesnake bites.[13] They have randomized animals to receive an intracompartmental injection of venom from the western diamondback rattlesnake. The animals received fasciotomy with debridement alone, antivenom alone, or antivenom with fasciotomy and debridement. Antivenom therapy prevented muscle loss and improved survival. Surgery alone did not. It was noted that muscle that had been debrided would have survived if treated with antivenom alone. Fasciotomy may increase the severity of local tissue loss. When fasciotomy is required because of rising compartment pressures that do not respond to antivenom, consideration for postoperative negative pressure wound therapy should be given.

Elapid Snake Epidemiology, Envenomation, and Treatment

As noted, there are only three species of Elapids in the United States—the Eastern coral snake, the Texas coral snake, and the Arizona coral snake. The eastern coral snake (*Micrurus fulvius*) is found in the southeastern United States up to Kentucky and North Carolina. The Texas coral snake (*Micrurus tener*) is found west of the Mississippi across Arkansas, through Louisiana into eastern Texas. The eastern and Texas coral snakes inhabit forests and shrubbery. The Arizona coral snake (Micruroides *euryxanthus*) is found in the desert climates of the southwestern United States into Mexico. Coral snakes are more active at night and hide under ground cover. Their

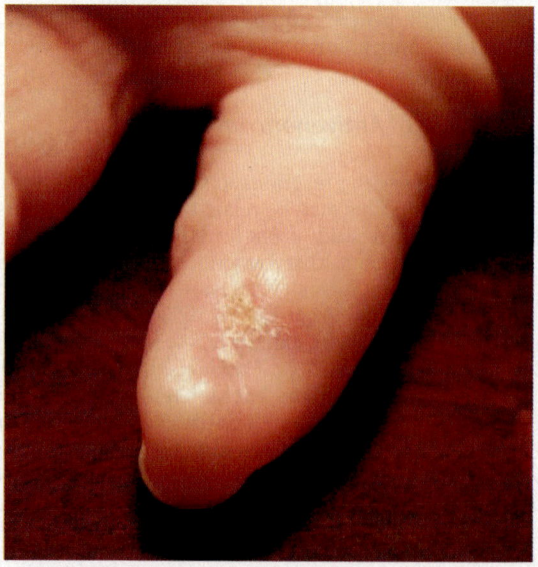

Figure 32.10. Healed snakebite.

behavior is elusive, and they will generally try to flee when disturbed.

This family of snakes has a common feature—bilateral upper maxillary fangs that are fixed into position and angled down and back. The fangs are grooved for instillation of the venom, which is predominately a neurotoxin. The snakes are oviparous (lay eggs) and have round pupils. Their head is flat, with a smooth tapered tail and of course no rattles. They have characteristic coloration which is mimicked by several other nonvenomous species (such as the king snake and the scarlet king snake) in an evolutionary phenomenon referred to as Batesian mimicry. Although the North American coral snakes are relatively small (less than 5 ft), some Elapids from other continents are very large; the Black mamba is 14 to 15 ft, and the king cobra can be up to 18 ft and weigh 25 lb. Although nonnative elapids bites have a substantial risk for death, only one known death from a coral snake has occurred in the United States since 1967 (Bonita Springs Florida, 2006).

The bite of an Elapid is likely to produce much less tissue injury than the bite of a Crotalid. There may be minimal pain. Envenomation may result in immediate neurotoxicity (within 15 to 30 minutes in the case of the mamba or Australian brown snake) or be delayed (2 to 5 hours with coral snakes). There is no longer any antivenom available for North American coral snakes, but local zoos and other countries may be able to provide antivenom for more exotic Elapidae. First aid should involve a compression bandage over the wound. The poison generally spreads by lymphatics; therefore, field compression to occlude lymph flow at the site of envenomation can slow toxicity. Symptoms will be related to the neurotoxicity—confusion, muscle spasm, nausea, vomiting, and dizziness. Blurred vision and difficulty with speech will occur. Finally, respiratory paralysis of the diaphragm occurs with resultant death. Cardiovascular and pulmonary support is essential to salvage patients that progress to this state.

It should be noted that venom of an Elapid is incredibly toxic. Micrurus venoms contain a complex mixture of proteins which include presynaptic phospholipase A_2 neurotoxin and postsynaptic alpha neurotoxin. The treatment should include neostigmine in the regimen. Deaths are usually from respiratory failure. The Taipan and Belcher Sea snakes have an LD50 in mice of as little as 0.025 mg/kg of venom. Any suspected Elapid bite should be managed with the possibility of rapid demise of the patient. If the bite is of a nonnative Elapid, antivenom (if it can be found) should be administered promptly at the first sign of clinical demise. Death rates for untreated nonnative Elapids vary from 20% to 30% for cobras to nearly 100% for the mambas. Antivenom for exotic snakebites may be obtained from the local zoo or through their national organization—the Association of Zoos and Aquariums (www.aza.org/antivenom-index) or through the American Association of Poison Control Centers at 1-800-222-1222 or visit www.poisonhelp.org. In the absence of coral snake antivenom, care remains supportive.

Venomous Lizards

There are two venomous lizards in North America: the Gila monster (*Heloderma suspectum*) and the Mexican beaded lizard (*Heloderma horridum*). Both species have heavy bodies with large heads. The Gila monster is found in the southwestern United States, ranging primarily in Arizona, extending into southeastern California, southwestern Utah and New Mexico, and into northern Mexico. There are two subspecies: the banded Gila monster (**Fig. 32.11**) that is found in the northern portion of the habitat and the reticulated that exists in the southern portion of the range. It is the largest lizard in the United States with a length of up to 56 cm. The Gila monster has generated substantial lore in the southwestern United States, because of its characteristic appearance and apparent fetid breath. It lives below ground and spends most of its life in or near its burrow. It is primarily seen in the spring, in the

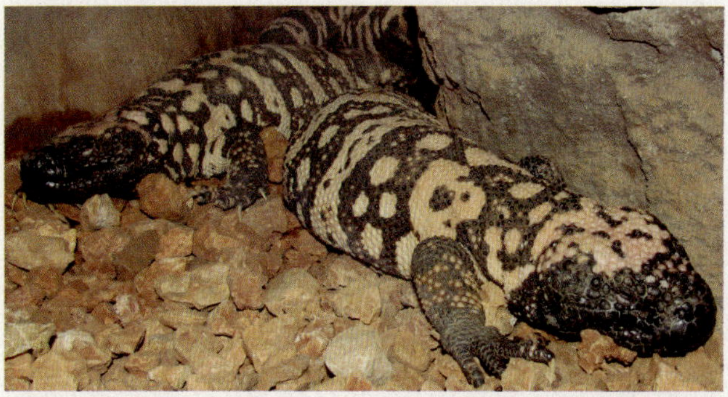

Figure 32.11. The venomous lizard, the banded Gila monster, *Heloderma suspectum*, which is found in the southwestern United States.

morning hours during breeding season. It has powerful jaws, and the bite is characterized by the tendency to hang on with the animal difficult to dislodge. The Poison Control Center reported 105 Gila to human bite-related calls from 2000 to 2011; 40% were seen in a hospital, 16% admitted, about 1/3 to an ICU. There were no deaths.[14]

The Gila lizard has eight labial glands on either side of the lower jaw. The venom is secreted into the floor of the Gila monster mouth where it is wicked into the victim via grooved lower canine teeth. Envenomation is limited and deaths are virtually unknown. The morbidity is usually secondary to local effects from the toxins present: serotonin, phospholipase A, amine oxidases, hyaluronidase, and proteases. These produce pain at the site that usually resolves in less than 24 hours. Hypotension, coagulopathy, and myocardial infarction have been reported. Nausea and vomiting can occur. Malaise may persist for several days. Recent study has shown a similarity between the venom of Gila monsters and Monitor lizards (Varanid species). This shows neurotoxins blocking channels of sodium and calcium ion transport as a mode of paralysis. The patient should be admitted for observation and a low threshold for surgical exploration/ debridement is given because the teeth often shed into the bite and can serve as a nidus for infection. The Mexican beaded lizard is found from Sonora to Guatemala and is represented by four subspecies. They are larger than the North American Gila monster; with a maximum size of up to 91 cm. They have similar venom as the Gila monster and bites should be managed in a supportive fashion. There is no antivenom available for Gila monster bites.

Insect Bites and Stings

4 Although the bite of a venomous snake will certainly draw more attention in the emergency department, in fact insects kill many more Americans (greater than 100 deaths per year) than snakes (about 5 deaths per year). Although most of these deaths are from anaphylactic reactions, some are from overwhelming envenomation, particularly from those of the Africanized honeybee (the "killer" bee).[15] Most of the treatment recommendations below are from expert opinion; few randomized trials have been performed.

Spiders

There are six genera of spiders in the United States that can produce painful bites, tissue necrosis, and rarely death. These fall into three groups—the brown recluse (**Fig. 32.12**), the black widow (**Fig. 32.13**), and the hobo spiders. Spider bites are notoriously difficult to diagnose—as the insects are often not seen, the bites are often painless and numerous dermatosis mimic spider bites.

Brown Recluse

There are 13 species of Loxosceles, of which 5 have been known to produce tissue necrosis. Probably the species producing the most pathology is the brown recluse (*Loxosceles*

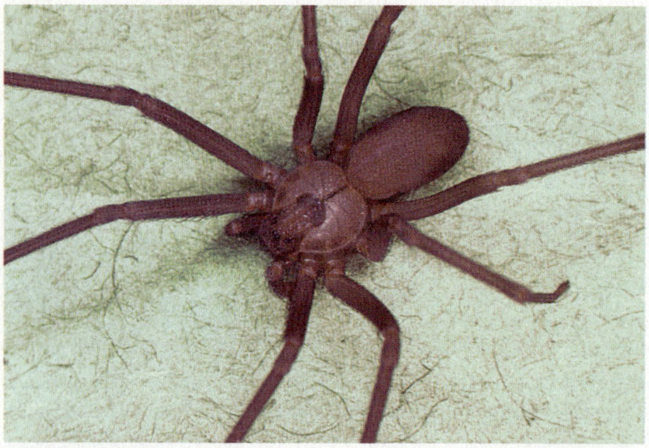

Figure 32.12. The brown recluse, *Loxosceles reclusa*, spider, nicknamed the fiddleback spider, brown fiddler, or violin spider. Its characteristic dark line coming from its head, looks like a violin, with the neck of the violin pointing to the rear of the spider.

reclusa). Envenomation by the hobo spiders (*Tegenaria agrestis*) produces a similar wound. The brown recluse is generally found in the southern states. Hobo spiders are found in the Pacific Northwest.[16] Bites from these two species generally are initially painless and the victim may not recall being bitten. Pain and erythema develop over the next 6 hours. The venom can produce a painful, necrotic, slow-healing wound over the next 48 to 72 hours. Two to 7 days after the bite, an eschar develops with surrounding soft tissue induration. The eschar can conceal an underlying tissue necrosis that can persist for months. The presence of adenopathy generally indicates another etiology for the necrosis.

Treatment is highly variable depending on the severity: eschars can require extensive debridement leading to skin grafting and even amputation, or they can be left alone and allowed to heal spontaneously, often with a residual shallow crater from loss of fat and soft tissue. The venom is both hemolytic and cytotoxic. The enzyme that is thought to produce the "desmonecrotic arachnidosis" is sphingomyelinase D. The venom also contains hyaluronidase, lipase, arachidonic acid, and prostaglandins. Systemic symptoms occur in less than 10% of victims, more commonly in children. Rarely hemolysis, hemodynamic instability, and death have occurred.[17] Initial treatment should include analgesia, wound care, and tetanus prophylaxis. Antibiotics should be reserved for infection/cellulitis. Early debridement should be withheld. Consideration for oral dapsone therapy should be given. Dapsone is thought to work as an inhibitor of polymorphonuclear leukocyte chemotaxis. It has significant side effects and can produce hemolysis in G6PD-deficient patients. Its use is somewhat controversial. It has been shown to reduce the size of the skin lesion and lessen the amount of surgical debridement, but these are no prospective studies. A controlled study in guinea pigs of dapsone, electroshock therapy, and no treatment showed some improvement with dapsone, but none with the electrical therapy. Hyperbaric oxygen has been studied in rabbits and pigs and has failed to demonstrate significant improvement. A trial of hyperbaric oxygen, dapsone, and cyproheptadine in rabbits failed to show any improvement. Systemic steroids have not been shown to help. Initial surgical excision of the lesion has no clear benefit. Others have reported a favorable response with high-dose diphenhydramine, calling it a "uniquely conservative," but this has not been replicated. The same can be said for topical application with diethyl azelate (DEA), a plasma membrane fluidizer. Delayed excision of the area of necrosis with skin grafting can be necessary. Recurrent necrosis in the same site can return even years later.

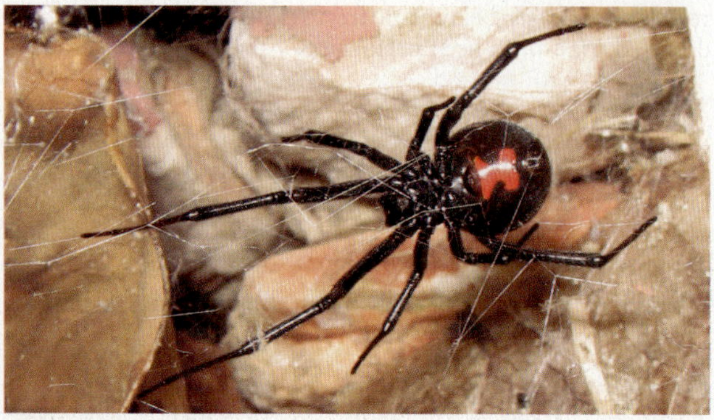

Figure 32.13. The black widow spider, with its characteristic red hourglass on the underside of the abdomen.

Black Widow Spiders

There are 31 species of the genus Latrodectus, the Black Widow spider, of which 4 are found in North America. These are marked by a prominent red hourglass figure on the ventral aspect of the thorax. Although both the male and the female possess venom, only the bite of the female can penetrate human skin. The female is four times the size of the male. The female of the species is known for eating the male after mating, which may or may not occur. The bite may produce only minimal local symptoms, with only a small area of redness, or a "target" appearance, or more dramatic erythema, induration, and purpura (**Fig. 32.14**). The venom contains α-latrotoxin, which is neurotoxic. This can produce chest and abdominal pain, and the patient's presentation may be confused as an acute surgical abdomen. Marked cramping and abdominal rigidity may be present. Fasciculations of facial muscles with periorbital edema, lacrimation, and blepharospasm may occur produce *Latrodectus facies*. Hyperreflexia, paresthesia, cutaneous hyperesthesia, and nausea may also occur. Symptoms may occur within an hour and resolve over several days. A recent review of 59 cases from a single center in China reported that all patients were anxious, irritable, restless, and had difficulty breathing, with 71% having painful muscle spasm, sometimes called "lactrodectism."[18] The muscle spasm should initially be treated with benzodiazepines. Antivenom is available and should be considered in the very young, and in other age groups is simply to augment relief from pain, which usually last 3 to 7 days, but sometimes for several weeks. The dose is 1 ampule given in 50 mL of saline, and the response can be quite dramatic and immediate. The antivenom is equine and hypersensitivity testing should be done prior to giving the antivenom. A 1-mL test dose of horse serum is included with the antivenom for topical conjunctival testing. Calcium gluconate was often given in the past but is no longer recommended. Mortality is exceedingly rare.

Hymenoptera

More than 150,000 species of Hymenoptera exist. This includes the winged Hymenoptera—the Apidae family (honeybees and bumble bees), and the Vespidae family (yellow jackets, yellow hornets, white faced hornets, and paper wasps) and the wingless Hymenoptera—the Formicidae family (fire ants, harvester ants, bulldog ants, and jack jumper ants). The venom injected by these insects is at least as toxic as that of the rattlesnake, but the volume is much less. The venom is primarily a hemolysin and neurotoxin. Anaphylaxis is a common clinical problem produced by the envenomation. The incidence of systemic allergic reactions after a sting is currently estimated to be between 0.15% to 0.8% in children, and up to 8.9% in adults.[19] The anaphylaxis is modulated by preformed IgE that activates mast cells leading to massive histamine release. This leads to laryngeal edema, pulmonary edema, and cardiovascular collapse. This must be treated aggressively with intravenous diphenhydramine, epinephrine and fluid resuscitation, as well as with management of the airway and supplemental oxygen. Most stings are mild, however, resulting in only dermal reactions—pain,

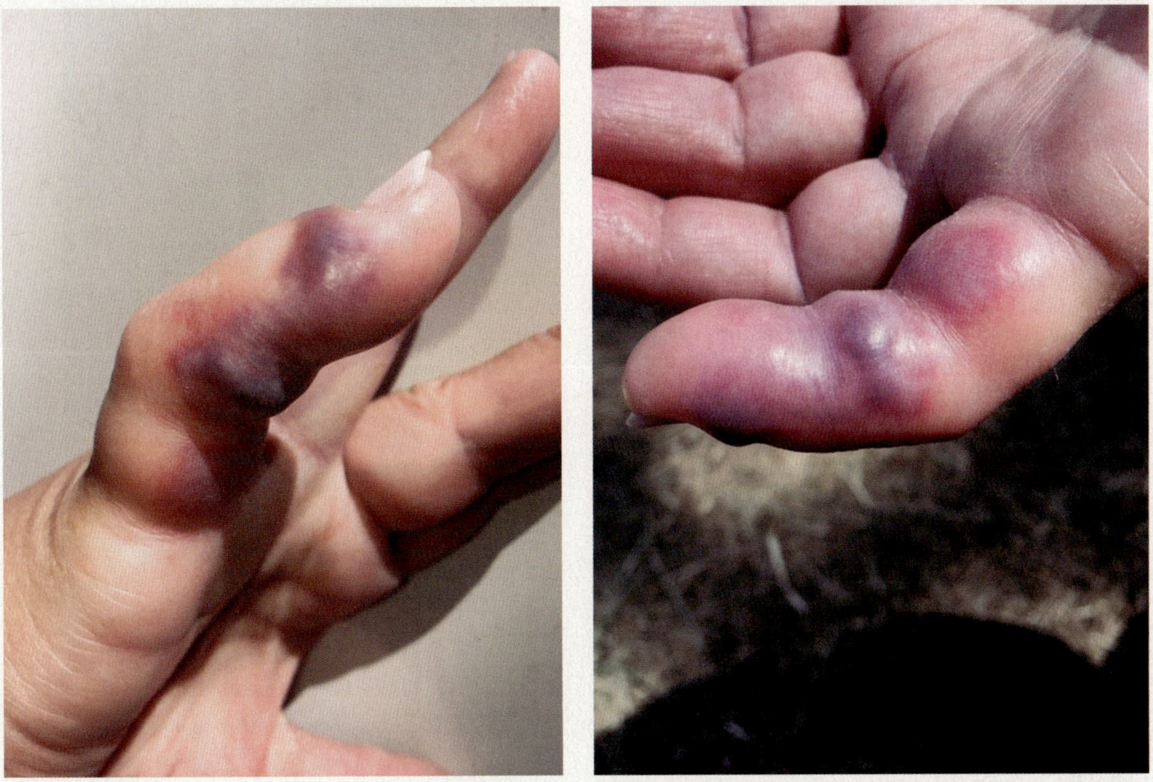

A B

Figure 32.14. Erythema, induration, and purpura associated with a black widow bite.

erythema, and edema. The stinger should be removed, and ice applied to the site. Bees, and some yellow jackets have a barbed stinger that once inserted injects the venom from a sac that is torn from the insect. This takes a few seconds and if the stinger can be "flicked" off in the first few seconds—the amount of venom may be limited. Application of meat tenderizer might be of some benefit. Patients with a history of insect sting anaphylaxis should be given a prescription for an epinephrine pen and be considered for venom immunotherapy. This is almost 100% successful in desensitization but can take up to 3 years.

Killer Bees

Africanized honeybees (killer bees) are hybrids of the African honeybee and the European honeybee, the one commonly found in the United States. The Africanized honeybee was originally brought from Tanzania to Brazil in 1957, with the hope of better honey production. The bees have spread up through Central America, Mexico, and into southwestern United States. They are continuing to advance at about 100 miles/yr, with some evidence of slowing in more recent years. Africanized honeybees are morphologically indistinguishable from the European honeybee, so DNA (usually mitochondrial DNA) analysis is necessary to differentiate the subspecies. They are termed "killer bees" because of increased aggressive traits. They show greater defensiveness of the hive, they have a larger "alarm" area, and they deploy in greater numbers and will pursue perceived threats over much greater distances. Although their venom is of the same potency as the European bees, the number of stings received will usually be much greater. With more than 50 stings, nausea, vomiting, shock, hemolysis, rhabdomyolysis, coagulopathy, coma, and death may occur. Usually most patients will just complain of pain but delayed toxic reactions—6 to 48 hours—may also occur. It is recommended that any patient presenting with more than 50 stings be hospitalized and observed. Laboratory evaluation with coagulation studies, platelet count, and liver function studies should be obtained.

Fire Ants

Fire ants, *Solenopsis invicta*, are wingless members of the Hymenoptera order. They were brought to the United States from South America around 1918 and have spread throughout the southern United States (**Fig. 32.15**). The imported red

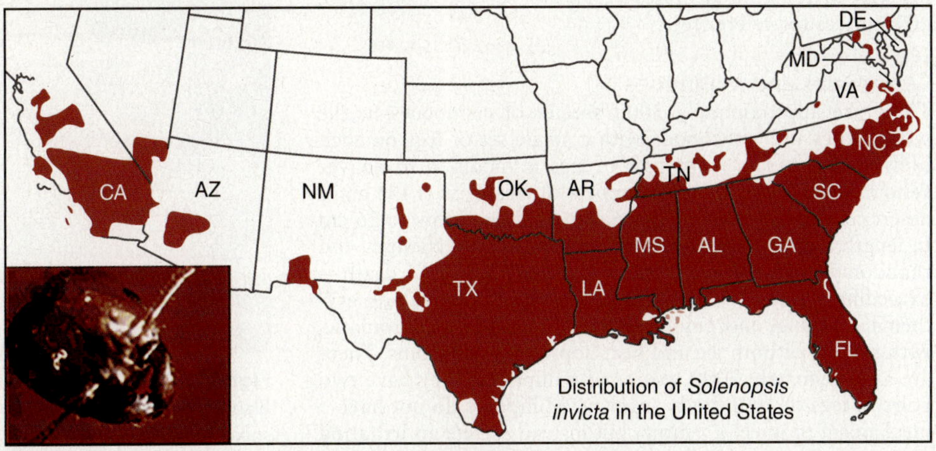

Figure 32.15. Fire ant, *Solenopsis Invicta*, distribution around the southern United States (used with permission from University of California, Berkely, UC Museum of Paleontology https://evolution.berkeley.edu/fire-ants-invade-and-evolve/fire-ants-in-the-u-s-a/)

fire ants appear to have been introduced on a ship through Mobile, Alabama. Shipments of infested nursery stock and other agricultural products, natural mating flights, and floating on flood waters and lack of natural enemies have contributed to their spread. There are now five times more ants per acre in the United States than in their native South America. Two species of imported fire ant now infect large areas of the Gulf Coast states. Fire ants aggressively attack any perceived danger to themselves or their mound. Each ant can produce multiple stings. The venom is a dialkylpiperidine that induces the release of histamine from increased mast cell reactivity. The fire ant sting produces a sterile pustule, which does not usually require antibiotic therapy. Infectious complications can occur at the site may be more common in diabetic or immunocompromised patients. More than 80 fatalities have been reported from fire ant anaphylaxis, notably in Australia and southern United States. The treatment is the same as with bee/wasp sting anaphylaxis. Fire ant venom shares at least four antigenic proteins with bees and wasps.

Scorpions

More than 1500 species of scorpions can be found worldwide. Only about 20 or 25 are considered dangerous. They are in the class Arachnida, close relatives of ticks, mites, and spiders. Scorpions prefer dry habitats but may be found throughout the southern United States. Scorpions are nocturnal, hiding during the day and becoming active at night. The scorpion's body has a 5-segmented tail that can be arched over the back and becomes slenderer toward the end. On the end of the tail is the bulb-like poison gland/stinger. Between the last pair of legs are comb-like structures called the pectines—sensory organs used to sense surface textures and detect prey. The venom toxicity varies greatly depending on the species, season, and age of the scorpion. Stings from dangerous species may cause paralysis, severe convulsions, cardiac irregularities, breathing difficulties, and death. In the United States most scorpion bites are not life-threatening and only result in local effects. In parts of Brazil, Mexico, North Africa, and Israel, however, the sting may be lethal. In Brazil the mortality rate is as high as 12% for adults and 60% in children. In India, of 34 children admitted to a hospital for a scorpion sting, 14 had hypertension, 9 had acute pulmonary edema, 5 had a myocardial infarction, and 1 died. Antivenins are typically available in areas where dangerous species are found, either from a local zoo or state or university agricultural extension departments. Only one species in the North America is particularly venomous—the Arizona bark scorpion (*Centruroides exilicauda*) (**Fig. 32.16**). The Bark Scorpion is relatively diminutive, reaching only an inch and a half at maturity. The sting produces a dramatic neuromotor syndrome and respiratory insufficiency. It has produced several deaths in the United States and hundreds in Mexico. Anascorp (an immune F(ab)2 equine antivenom) is now available for patients with systemic symptoms.[20] It (like CroFab) is very expensive (about $12,000 per vial in the United States—or $100 per vial in Mexico; 2013 prices for reference).

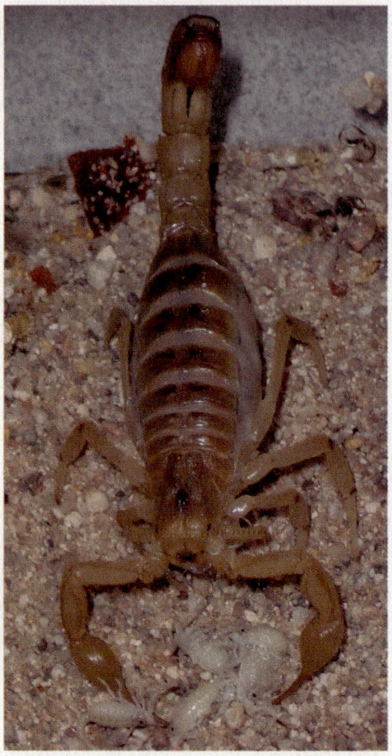

Figure 32.16. The venomous Arizona bark scorpion (*Centruroides exilicauda*).

Centipedes and Millipedes

There are approximately 3000 species of centipedes in the world. They are arthropods with a single set of legs on each body segment. The front pair of legs is modified to deliver venom. One of the largest members of this class is the giant desert centipede (*Scolopendra gigantea*). It can grow to 26 cm in length. Significant morbidity, including ECG changes and rhabdomyolysis, can occur from centipede bites, but death is exceedingly rare. The most common symptoms include erythema, swelling, and pain. Treatment is largely symptomatic, with reports of both ice and heat improving symptoms. There are approximately 7000 species of millipedes. They have two pairs of legs on each body segment. Millipedes do not have a mechanism to inject a venom, but instead secrete an irritating liquid from pores covering their body. This can produce a superficial burn that is self-limiting. Only symptomatic therapy is indicated.

Asp Caterpillars

The asp is a venomous caterpillar found in the southern United States. It is the larval stage of the Southern Flannel Moth (*Megalopyge opercularis*) (**Fig. 32.17**). It has the appearance of soft furry ball, encouraging the unwary to touch it (also referred to as the Puss moth, given its cat-like appearance). The long hairs of the asp conceal shorter spikes that discharge venom. Typically, an intense throbbing and pain occurs almost immediately. Erythematous spots occur at the site of envenomation (erucism). Symptoms include headache, nausea, vomiting, and the development of lymphadenopathy. Chest pain occurs occasionally. Rarely shock and respiratory distress have been reported. Death is exceedingly rare and is almost

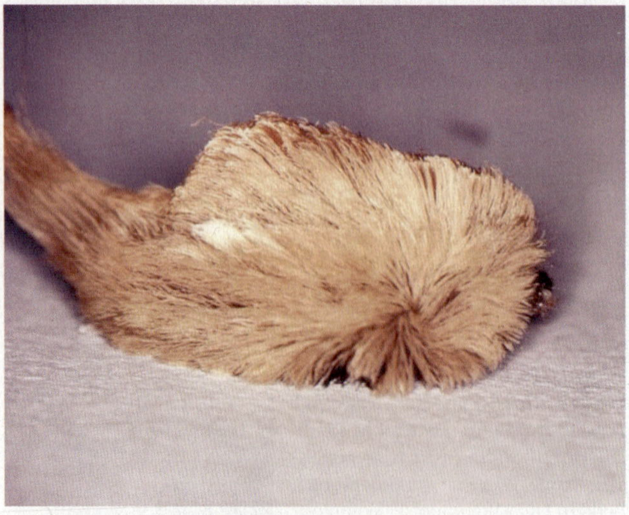

Figure 32.17. The long hairs of the asp caterpillar, aka Southern Flannel Moth and Puss moth (Megalopyge opercularis), conceal shorter spikes that discharge venom.

certainly because of a hypersensitivity reaction. A similar caterpillar found in South America—Lonomia—has a death rate of 1.7%. The initial treatment should be to apply adhesive tape and pull it off to remove the spines. Ice packs, NSAIDs, acetaminophen, and antihistamines may provide symptomatic relief. Intravenous calcium and steroids have been suggested as a treatment regimen.

ENVIRONMENTAL EXPOSURE

Hypothermia

Humans, like all mammals, will always attempt to maintain a constant body temperature despite changes in environmental temperature. Normal human body temperature is thought physiologically vary between 36.1 °C and 37.2 °C . It also varies by body location: 37 °C sublingually, 38 °C in the rectum, 32 °C at the skin, and 38.5 °C deep in the liver; we tolerate poorly even minor deviations from these norms. Although humans have a remarkable capacity to dissipate heat by evaporating body water, our tropical evolutionary heritage has provided us with far less ability to cope with cold conditions. As a result, hypothermia can occur in a variety of clinical settings and from several causes (**Table 32.7**).

Hypothermia is defined in humans as a core temperature below 35 °C. Hypothermia is usually classified by temperature zones: mild (32° to 35 °C); moderate (28° to 32 °C); or severe (<28 °C). *Primary* accidental (verses intentional) hypothermia is defined as a decrease in core temperature that occurs because of overwhelming environmental cold stress, such as recreational misadventures that lead to cold-water immersion or prolonged environmental exposure. *Secondary* accidental hypothermia is triggered by, or at least associated with, underlying disease. Secondary accidental hypothermia occurs in patients with impaired thermoregulation, decreased heat production, or increased heat loss. These patients become cold despite only mild cold stress. The most significant risk factors are advanced age, mental impairment, and substance abuse (alcohol, primarily), although hypothyroidism, hypoadrenalism, trauma, and hypoglycemia are other risk factors. Chronic hypothermia develops in patients with impaired heat generation (ie, the elderly and infirm) who live in unheated apartments, are under continual cold stress, and after a time are found to have a chronically low temperature as if they have autoregulated to a new, lower-set core temperature.

Table 32.7. Risk Factors for Hypothermia

Prehospital phase
Severity of injury
Head injury
Spinal cord injury
Shock
Extremes of age
Wet clothing
General anesthesia and prehospital intubation
Suspected medical conditions
Thyroid disease, adrenal disease, diabetes, cardiac dysfunction, hepatic disease, malnutrition, autonomic nervous system dysfunction
Hospital phase
Exposure
Cold intravenous fluids and blood products
Burns
General anesthesia
Epidural and spinal anesthesia
Observation phase
Size of surgery
General anesthesia >3 h
Intravenous crystalloids, blood products
SAPS II scores

SAPS II, Simplified Acute Physiology II Score.
From Perlman R, Callum J, Laflamme C, et al. A recommended early goal-directed management guideline for the prevention of hypothermia-related transfusion, morbidity, and mortality in severely injured trauma patients. *Crit Care*. 2016;20(1):107.

It is estimated that each year about 1500 patients in the United States have hypothermia listed on their death certificate, although the exact incidence and associated morbidity and mortality remain poorly characterized. The 2015–2017 death rate from accidental hypothermia per 100,000 in the United States is depicted in **Figure 32.18.** This figure emphasis

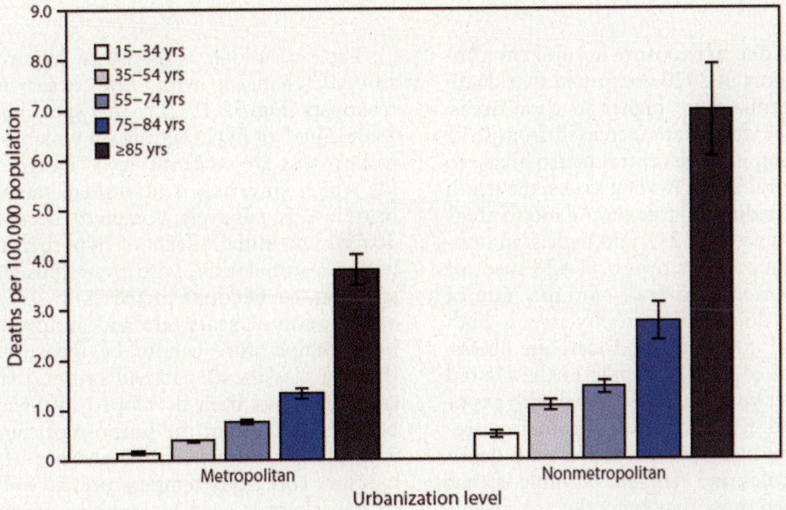

Figure 32.18. Death rates* attributed to excessive cold or hypothermia† among persons aged ≥15 years, by urbanization level§ and age. (From *QuickStats:* Death rates attributed to excessive cold or hypothermia among persons aged ≥15 years, by urbanization level and age group — National Vital Statistics System, 2015–2017. *MMWR Morb Mortal Wkly Rep*. 2019;68:187.)* Crude rate of deaths per 100,000 population; 95% confidence intervals indicated by error bars. †Deaths attributed to excessive cold or hypothermia were identified using the *International Classification of Diseases, Tenth Revision* underlying cause of death code X31 (Exposure to excessive natural cold) or multiple cause-of-death code T68 (Hypothermia). §Urbanization level is based on the Office of Management and Budget's February 2013 delineation of metropolitan statistical areas (MSA), in which each MSA must have at least one urbanized area of ≥50,000 inhabitants. Areas with <50,000 inhabitants are grouped into the nonmetropolitan category.

TRAUMA

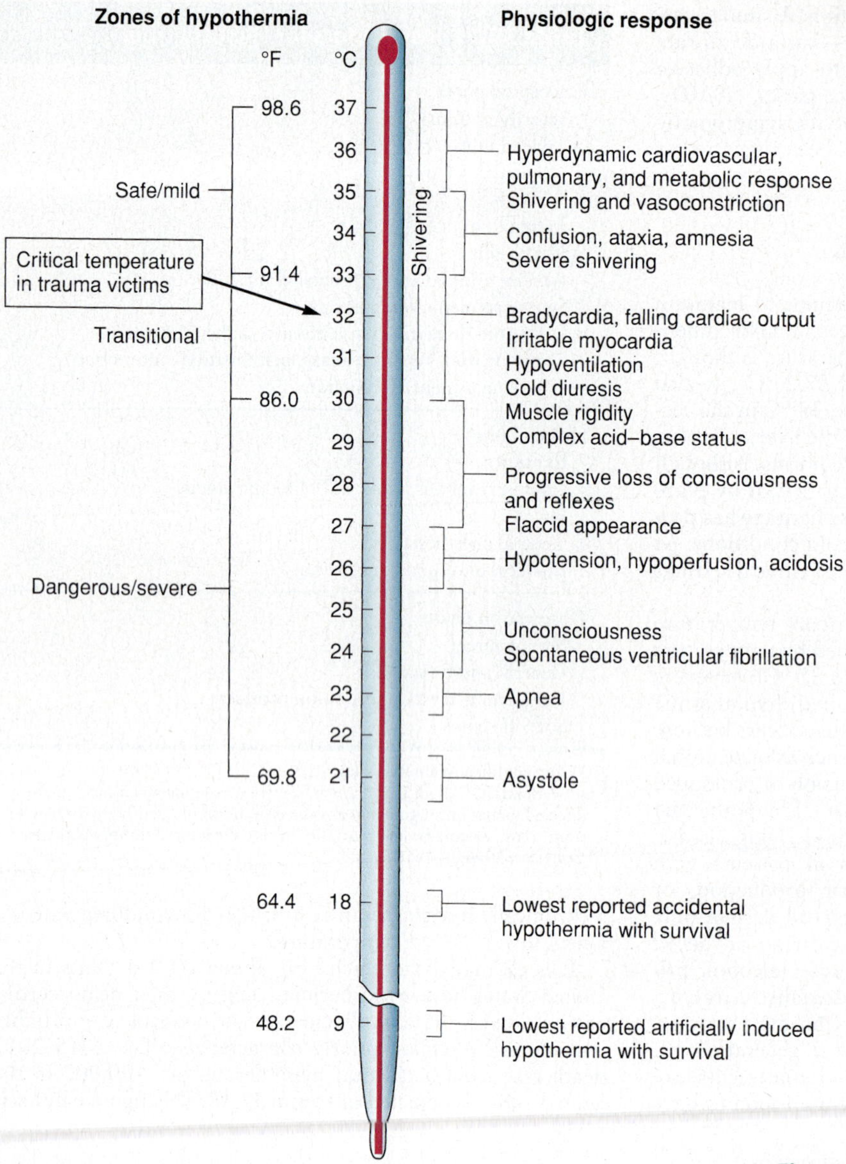

Figure 32.19. Physiologic responses to hypothermia.

the problem of hypothermia due to exposure in rural environments. An updated CDC report in 2020 confirmed that death rates attributed to hypothermia were higher in rural areas, such that among females, the death rate increased from 0.11 per 100,000 for those residing in large central metro areas, to 0.40 for those in noncore, rural areas. Among males, the death rates were lowest for those residing in large central metro areas (0.29) and large fringe metro areas (0.24), and highest in noncore, rural areas (0.93). A multicenter review of 428 cases of accidental hypothermia reported an overall mortality rate of 17%, although other reports document mortality rates as high as 80%, primarily a result of infection and underlying illness. From 1999 to 2011, a total of 16,911 deaths in the United States, an average of 1301 per year, were associated with exposure to excessive natural cold. Most reported hypothermia-related deaths (67%) occurred in males, but the overall death rate is the same for both males and females. Notable is that deaths occur in all states, even those that generally are considered to have warm climates. Hypothermia-related deaths are reported by states with characteristically milder climates that experience rapid temperature changes and by western states that have high elevations and experience considerable changes from daytime to nighttime temperatures. In the United States, the greatest overall death rates caused by hypothermia are Alaska, New Mexico, Wyoming, and Montana.

The physiologic response to hypothermia is one of transitional changes, with few exact temperature-dependent responses (**Fig. 32.19**). Broadly speaking, the transition from a "safe zone" of hypothermia (in which physiologic adaptations to heat loss are working) to a "danger zone" of hypothermia (in which shivering is abolished, metabolism decreases, and heat loss is passively accepted) occurs between 33 °C and 30 °C. The initial effects of hypothermia mimic intense sympathetic stimulation, with tremulousness, profound vasoconstriction, tremendous increases in oxygen consumption, and acceleration of heart rate and minute ventilation. When core body temperature cannot be measured, a four-stage hypothermia classification based on vital signs and level of consciousness has been developed by Swiss clinicians. It should be emphasized that the purpose of the Swiss clinical grading is to direct treatment in the absence of the ability to actually measure core body temperature, as well as to predict the risk of hypothermic cardiac arrest, so it should have its primary purpose in the austere or field care environment.

5 The most current modification of the Swiss System for hypothermia and risk of cardiac arrest is shown in **Figure 32.20**. In this latest revision shivering is not used as a stage-defining sign, although its presence usually means that the core temperature is >30 °C, a temperature at which hypothermic cardiac arrest is unlikely. The estimated risk of cardiac arrest is based

	Stage 1	Stage 2	Stage 3	Stage 4
Clinical findings*	"Alert" from AVPU	"Verbal" from AVPU	"Painful" or "Unconscious" from AVPU AND Vital signs present	"Unconscious" from AVPU AND No detectable Vital signs
Risk of cardiac arrest[Δ]	Low	Moderate	High	Hypothermic cardiac arrest

Figure 32.20. Swiss Staging System for hypothermia.

on accidental hypothermia being the only cause of clinical findings. If other conditions impair consciousness, such as asphyxia, intoxication, high-altitude cerebral edema, or trauma, the Revised Swiss System may falsely predict a higher risk of cardiac arrest. Be cautious with patients who remain "alert" or "verbal" but show signs of hemodynamic or respiratory instability (eg, bradycardia, bradypnea, hypotension); they may be at a transitional stage with a higher risk of cardiac arrest.

The cardiovascular response to hypothermia begins with tachycardia, but followed by progressive bradycardia, which starts at approximately 34 °C and results in a 50% heart rate decrease at 28 °C. Cardiac output initially increases with the tachycardia, and then progressively decreases, with a concomitant fall in blood pressure. The conduction system is particularly sensitive to hypothermia: the PR interval, then the QRS complex, and finally the QT interval become progressively prolonged. As temperature falls below 30 °C, atrial fibrillation, bradycardia, and ventricular dysrhythmia become common, with asystole occurring at temperatures below 25 °C.

Perhaps the most challenging management of an accidental hypothermia patient is the one with temperatures between 28 °C and 32 °C (Swiss stage 2), as these patients are prone to develop poorly perfusing arrhythmias, yet they often can be rewarmed with active external and environmental rewarming if such arrhythmias do not occur. Hence gentle manipulation of such patients is required. Because palpating pulses or measuring blood pressure in cold, stiff, hypothermic patients is difficult, the presence of an organized cardiac electrical rhythm should be taken as a sign of life that contraindicates cardiopulmonary resuscitation chest compressions, despite the absence of a palpable pulse. Such a rhythm may provide diminished but sufficient circulation in patients with severely reduced metabolism, and it is likely that vigorous chest compressions will convert this perfusing rhythm to fibrillation. Rewarming should occur with close monitoring of rhythm, pulse, and blood pressure. If cardiac arrest occurs (Swiss stage 3 or 4), cardiopulmonary bypass (CPB) or extracorporeal membrane oxygenation (ECMO) for perfusion and rewarming is indicated.[21]

Among patients with what is likely Swiss stage 4, those treated with CPB or ECMO have a reported survival rate without neurologic impairment of 47% to 63%, compared to 37% for similar patients treated without active core rewarming and oxygenation techniques. One report noted excellent long-term functional outcomes in 15 of 32 young patients successfully rewarmed with CPB. All patients were intubated and ventilated and had received ongoing cardiac massage during transportation, and all 15 survivors had documented circulatory arrest (ventricular fibrillation [VF] or asystole) and fixed, dilated pupils. The mean interval from discovery of the patient to rewarming with cardiopulmonary bypass was 141 ± 50 minutes; the mean temperature was 21.8 °C ± 2.5 °C. A report from Finland documents a 61% (14 of 23) survival to hospital discharge for adults undergoing cardiopulmonary bypass after a mean of 70 minutes of cardiopulmonary resuscitation following hypothermic arrest primarily from cold-water immersion or exposure. A recent review of 18 studies in the literature and 286 hypothermic patients in cardiac arrest who underwent extracorporeal support documented a 37% survival rate, with 84% good neurologic outcome.[22] Finally, the lowest recorded temperature from which a person has been successfully resuscitated following accidental or secondary hypothermia is 13.7 °C.

Respiratory drive is increased during the early stages of hypothermia, but below 33 °C progressive respiratory depression occurs, resulting in a decrease in minute ventilation. This decrease is not usually a significant problem until temperatures below 29 °C is reached. Occasionally, hypothermia results in the production of a large amount of mucus (cold bronchorrhea). This development predisposes to atelectasis and aspiration as ciliary action and the cough reflex are also depressed. Noncardiogenic pulmonary edema is also occasionally reported, especially in elderly patients and especially after prolonged periods of hypothermia.

The effect of core hypothermia on arterial blood gas interpretation warrants a comment. Arterial blood gas samples are typically warmed to 37 °C before measurement. A nomogram of Severinghaus mathematical corrections is then used to estimate the blood gas values at the patient's actual body temperature. With each 1 °C temperature drop, the P_{CO_2} decreases by 4.4% and the P_{O_2} decreases by 7.2%. Gas solubility increases with decreasing fluid temperature, hence the decrease in partial pressure is related to the increased solubility of gases in cold fluids and is not a result of a change in carbon dioxide content, oxygen content, or serum bicarbonate level. Clinicians often assume that the "normal" P_{CO_2} and P_{O_2} at 37 °C are the values that should be attained at all temperatures. However, if normothermic endpoints for P_{CO_2} were attained in a hypothermic patient, they would have increased total-body CO_2 stores, which would manifest by a rising P_{CO_2} and a falling pH during rewarming. Likewise, attempts at increasing a P_{O_2} that reflects normal oxygen content at a lower temperature are also inappropriate. A far simpler strategy is to assess the blood gases at 37 °C without temperature correction. Values that are normal and acceptable when reported at 37 °C (without temperature correction) correspond to normal values and contents when "corrected" for hypothermic temperatures.

Temperature correction of blood gases for pH management is also unnecessary. The pH of water rises with cooling, causing the pH of blood to rise by 0.015 pH units/°C, without a change in bicarbonate content. Treating a patient with a temperature of 30 °C with a pH of 7.40 instead of 7.47 fails to maintain the normal pH offset above the neutral point of water (relative alkalinity) and results in an acidotic cellular and chemical environment that has a multiplicity of effects on enzyme systems. Because blood with a pH of 7.40 assessed at 37 °C is reported as having a pH of 7.47 when temperature corrected to 32 °C, the simplest strategy when confronted with a patient with a temperature of 32 °C is to assess the blood gas at 37 °C only and to use the 37 °C uncorrected pH value for management.[23]

The neurologic response to hypothermia is heralded by progressive loss of lucidity and deep tendon reflexes and, eventually, by flaccid muscular tone. Patients are often amnestic below 32 °C, and between 31 °C and 27 °C they usually lose consciousness. Pupillary dilatation and loss of cerebral autoregulation occur at temperatures below 26 °C, and electroencephalography becomes silent at 19° to 20 °C. These findings, combined with an unobtainable pulse and apparent rigor mortis, may cause the patient to appear dead. It is important to remember that patients have been revived from core temperatures as low as 13.7 °C and hence the saying "No one is dead until warm and dead."[24] An exception to this admonition includes the patient who has sustained an anoxic event while still normothermic and has a serum potassium level greater than 10 mmol/L, although the Bernese criteria for trauma and hypothermia have picked a level of 12 mmol/L as being nonsalvageable.[25,26]

The role of hypothermia in brain death determination remains controversial. Brain death is a medically and legally accepted mechanism of death in the United States and worldwide. Yet significant variability in individual institutional policies regarding the determination of brain death occurs.[27] A 2020 report recommended and suggested that determination of the clinical criteria for brain death should include a minimum core temperature of 36 °C.[28]

In classic surgical physiology research, Moyer and Debakey showed that with hypothermia, reduction in blood pressure and cardiac output decreases glomerular filtration rate, but urinary output is maintained because of impairment in renal tubular Na^+ reabsorption (the so-called "cold diuresis"). Vasoconstriction also results in an initial increase in central blood volume that prompts a diuresis. Ileus, bowel wall edema, depressed hepatic drug detoxification, punctate gastric erosions (Wischnevsky ulcers), hyperamylasemia, and, rarely, hemorrhagic pancreatitis are hallmarks of the intestinal response to hypothermia. Hypothermia inhibits insulin release and insulin uptake at receptor sites, making hyperglycemia a relatively common finding, especially at temperatures below 30 °C. Exogenous insulin administration is unwarranted because it may result in rebound hypoglycemia during rewarming. Serum electrolyte changes are unpredictable, but serum potassium is often slightly increased in hypothermic patients because of renal tubular dysfunction, acidosis, and the breakdown of liver glycogen. Hypothermia also appears to affect endothelial cell adhesion molecule function, which may partially explain increased infectious complications in hypothermic patients. One study demonstrated a drop of 1.9 °C core hypothermia triples the incidence of surgical wound infection following colon resection and increases the duration of hospitalization by 20%, leading to the now standard perioperative checklist monitoring of body temperature during surgery.

Body temperature also has a significant effect on oxygen uptake. Oxygen consumption (VO_2) initially increases dramatically with any fall in body temperature. When involuntary muscle contractions in the form of shivering occur, oxygen consumption increases by three- to fivefold. This process is inefficient because shivering produces heat near the surface of the body, causing most of the heat to be lost to the environment, with less than 45% being retained by the patient. As core temperatures fall to between 33 °C and 30 °C, shivering is abolished, and the patient will rapidly sink to ambient temperature.

The thermoregulatory drive is such a powerful one that it takes precedence over many other homeostatic functions. The resultant increase in oxygen utilization may result in anaerobic metabolism, acidosis, and significant cardiopulmonary stress. One study noted a 35% increase in oxygen consumption and a 65% increase in CO_2 production in postoperative patients after resolution of anesthesia, when the thermostatic drive reappeared. In another study, a core temperature decrease of as little as 0.3 °C in postoperative patients was associated with a 7% increase in VO_2, and temperature reductions between 0.3 °C and 1.2 °C were associated with a 92% increase in VO_2, with proportional increases in minute ventilation. Shivering can be abolished with low doses of meperidine (Demerol®). Ondansetron (Zofran®, Zuplenz®) will reduce postoperative shivering, but it is unknown if it is effective in primary hypothermia.[29]

6 Hypothermia in Trauma Patients

Mild hypothermia is very common after traumatic injury. The thermoneutral environment for humans is a humid and warm 28 °C (82.5 °F) like a tropical island. When ambient temperature falls below the thermoneutral temperature (ie, the temperature at which no thermogenesis or heat dissipation is necessary), an increase in heat production is required to maintain a normal body temperature. Combustion is the only source of endogenous heat production, and this process requires an increase in oxygen utilization. After shock or injury, however, oxygen supplies are often limited and further heat loss occurs owing to cold emergency department and operating room environments, cold fluid resuscitation, and open thoracic and abdominal cavities. Anesthetic and neuromuscular blocking agents that prevent the heat-producing shivering response further aggravate this. Thus, the occurrence of hypothermia in surgical or critically injured patients is most often a form of secondary accidental hypothermia.[30]

One study found that 57% of trauma patients admitted to a level 1 trauma center were hypothermic at some time and that temperature loss was most significant in the emergency department. Another study reported that the average initial temperature for 94 intubated major trauma victims was 35 °C, with no seasonal variation. Of patients in this study, 66% were hypothermic on admission; 43% were mildly hypothermic (34° to 36 °C), and 23% had temperatures below 34 °C. Likewise, Jurkovich and Luterman reported that 42% of 71 adult trauma victims with an injury severity score (ISS) of 25 or higher had core temperatures below 34 °C and in 13% the core temperature fell below 32 °C.[31] Importantly, there were no survivors when core body temperature was below 32 °C. Inaba reported that of 118 patients requiring emergent surgery following traumatic injury, hypothermia (<35 °C) was present in nearly 30% of patients upon presentation to the operating room, and that a continued decrease in core tem-
7 perature was associated with increased mortality. This mortality rose to 50% if temperature fell below 32 °C. Both mortality rate and the incidence of hypothermia increase with higher ISS, massive fluid resuscitation, and the presence of shock, but controlling for these variables still demonstrates that the mortality rate of the hypothermic trauma patient is greater than that of the warm trauma patient. Although the mortality rate for moderate (28° to 32°C) degrees of primary accidental hypothermia is approximately 20%, moderate levels of hypothermia in trauma and critically ill patients are associated with a much higher mortality rate. Rutherford et al. reported that 9.4% of surgical intensive care unit patients had a core body temperature less than 35 °C; the mortality rate of the hypothermic trauma patients was 53%.* In fact, compared with other patient populations, the mortality rate associated with hypothermia in the trauma victim is so high that the definition of mild, moderate, and severe hypothermia in the trauma patient warrants special classification (**Table 32.8**). These

Table 32.8. Classification of Hypothermia

Classification	Conventional	Trauma Patient
Mild hypothermia	35–32 °C (95.0–89.6 °F)	36–34 °C (96.8–93.2 °F)
Moderate hypothermia	32–28 °C (89.6–82.4 °F)	34–32 °C (93.2–89.6 °F)
Severe hypothermia	28–20 °C (82.4–68.0°F)	32 °C (89.6 °F)
Profound hypothermia	20–14 °C (68.0–57.2 °F)	

From Perlman R, Callum J, Laflamme C, et al. A recommended early goal-directed management guideline for the prevention of hypothermia-related transfusion, morbidity, and mortality in severely injured trauma patients. *Crit Care*. 2016;20(1):107.

data have resulted in the standard incorporation of aggressive techniques to prevent the occurrence of hypothermia in trauma patient beginning with field transport with warm blankets and heated IV fluids to routine use of body and fluid rewarmers in emergency departments and operating rooms. Hypothermia is simply not acceptable in any trauma patient, and if it occurs, should prompt a quality-of-care review.

Hypothermia appears to occur primarily in victims of relatively severe trauma. Little and Stoner, while reporting on a heterogeneous group of 82 trauma patients, observed that hypothermia occurred only in those patients with an ISS greater than 12. Hypothermia did not occur in less severely injured patients, and shivering, which should be expected, was noted in only one of the hypothermic patients. Mild degrees of injury have, in fact, been associated with small elevations in core body temperature, particularly when the shivering response mechanism has not been abated.[32] The recognition that hypothermia can be prevented has resulted in substantial changes in the management of the acute injured patient. As a result, the "lethal triad" of coagulopathy, acidosis, and hypothermia is much less frequently observed.[33]

The detrimental effect of hypothermia in the human trauma victim is contrasted by a large body of experimental evidence in animals suggesting that hypothermia has a protective role in shock. This extensive body of literature is reviewed elsewhere, but in general, animals subjected to combined hypothermia and shock (hemorrhage, burn, and blunt trauma) usually survive longer than similarly injured but actively warmed animals. Blalock and Mason (1941) were among the first in modern times to recognize the ability of hypothermia to prolong survival times after shock, but they emphasized that the overall survival rate was unchanged, an observation reaffirmed in 2003.* However, increases in both survival times and survival rates have been shown in a number of animal models of induced hypothermia after hemorrhagic shock. The protective effects of hypothermia in preventing ischemia–reperfusion injury have been described in a number of models, including muscle, intestine, and rabbit ear.[34] These observations have prompted some to suggest that there is a role for iatrogenic-induced hypothermia in severe trauma patients, with the goal being a reduction of oxygen consumption in the setting of limited oxygen delivery (hypovolemic shock) to allow surgeons time to repair injured structures and then rewarm and resuscitate the patients.[35]

Evidence further supporting the harmful effect of hypothermia in the trauma patient is provided by a prospective, randomized trial of rapid rewarming versus conventional rewarming of 57 multiple-trauma patients.[36] In this study, trauma patients who were rapidly rewarmed with continuous arteriovenous rewarming (CAVR) from less than 34.5 °C to greater than 36 °C required less resuscitation fluid volume and had a lower early mortality rate than those rewarmed more slowly. Failure to rewarm in either group was uniformly fatal. The survival rate at 3 days after injury was 82% in the rapid rewarm group versus 62% in conventionally managed patients. Approximately 50% of the patients in both groups had a severe head injury, defined as a head abbreviated ISS of 3 or greater. In this well-controlled study, maintenance of hypothermia not only failed to confer an advantage but also was detrimental to early survival.[37]

The systems most affected by hypothermia in victims of injury are those involved in clotting. Focused attention on the coagulation mechanisms in trauma patients over the past decade has exposed the lack of a comprehensive understanding of the complex relationship between injury, inflammation, and coagulopathy. Temperature is yet another variable in this complexity. Reports of coagulation abnormalities in patients with apparently normal clotting factor levels surfaced shortly after the introduction of hypothermic cardioplegia for cardiac surgery. Although hemodilution with volume expanders deficient in clotting factors and platelets is a cause of nonsurgical bleeding, cold platelets are known to undergo morphologic changes that affect adherence, including loss of shape, cytoplasmic swelling, and dissolution of cytoplasmic microtubules necessary for normal motility. Platelet activation is also associated with activation of cell membrane phospholipases that hydrolyze phospholipids to arachidonic acid, a precursor to prostaglandin endoperoxides and thromboxane A_2, a potent vasoconstrictor necessary for normal platelet aggregation. Valeri et al. induced systemic hypothermia to 32 °C in baboons but kept one forearm warm using heating lamps and a warming blanket.* Simultaneous bleeding time measurements in the warm and cold arm were 2.4 and 5.8 minutes, respectively. This effect, which was reversible with rewarming, appeared to be mediated by cold-induced slowing of the enzymatic reaction rate of thromboxane synthetase, which resulted in decreased production of thromboxane A_2. Bleeding observed at mildly reduced temperatures (33° to 37°C) results primarily from a platelet adhesion defect and not reduced enzyme activity or platelet activation; however, at temperatures below 33 °C, both reduced platelet function and enzyme activity likely contribute to the coagulopathy, perhaps helping to explain why 32 °C is such a critical temperature in the coagulopathic injured patient.

As with blood gases, clinical tests of coagulation are temperature standardized to 37 °C. Fibrometers contain a thermal block that heats the plasma and reagents to 37 °C before initiating the assay. Thus, tests of coagulation reflect clotting factor deficiencies but are corrected for any potential effect of hypothermia on clotting factor function. A detailed study of the kinetic effects of hypothermia on clotting factor function has been undertaken by Reed et al. He performed clotting tests (PT, PTT, and thrombin time) on reference human plasma–containing normal clotting factor levels at temperatures ranging from 25° to 37°C. The results showed a significant slowing of all coagulation tests at temperatures below 35 °C that was proportional to the degree of hypothermia. The prolongation of clot formation occurred at clinically relevant levels of hypothermia and was equivalent to that seen in normothermic patients with significant clotting factor depletion. For example, assays conducted at 35 °C, 33 °C, and 31 °C prolonged the PTT to the same extent as would occur in a euthermic patient with reductions in factor IX levels to 66%, 32%, and 7% of normal, respectively.

Clotting factor supplementation is not the answer to a hypothermia-induced coagulopathy; rewarming is. However, in many seriously injured patients, clotting factor depletion exists in conjunction with hypothermia. A potentiating effect of hypothermia on coagulation dysfunction occurs in plasma of patients with deficient clotting factor levels, although there does not appear to be synergy between the two conditions. Hypothermic, coagulopathic trauma patients still benefit from coagulation profile testing. If prolongation of PT and PTT is evident in plasma warmed to 37 °C, clotting factor replacement is indicated. If PT and PTT are near normal, rewarming alone reverses the clinically apparent coagulopathy.

8 Treatment of Primary or Accidental Hypothermia

Treatment of accidental hypothermia remains highly variable. A study from Amsterdam reported that over an 8-year period (2000 to 2008) a total of 84 patients with accidental hypothermia were treated with 14 different rewarming techniques, with an overall mortality of 28.6%. There are several excellent publications from European societies and authors on a step wise, algorithmic approach to resuscitation the primary or accidental or exposure hypothermic patients. Perhaps it is the long-standing history of mountaineering or the presence of Emergency Physicians in the field that is responsible. **Algorithm 32.1** is an example of this approach, based on the European Resuscitation Council that has addressed the management of cardiac arrest in a number of special circumstances, including hypothermia.

*The resource(s) mentioned are readily available online for further review.

Algorithm 32.1

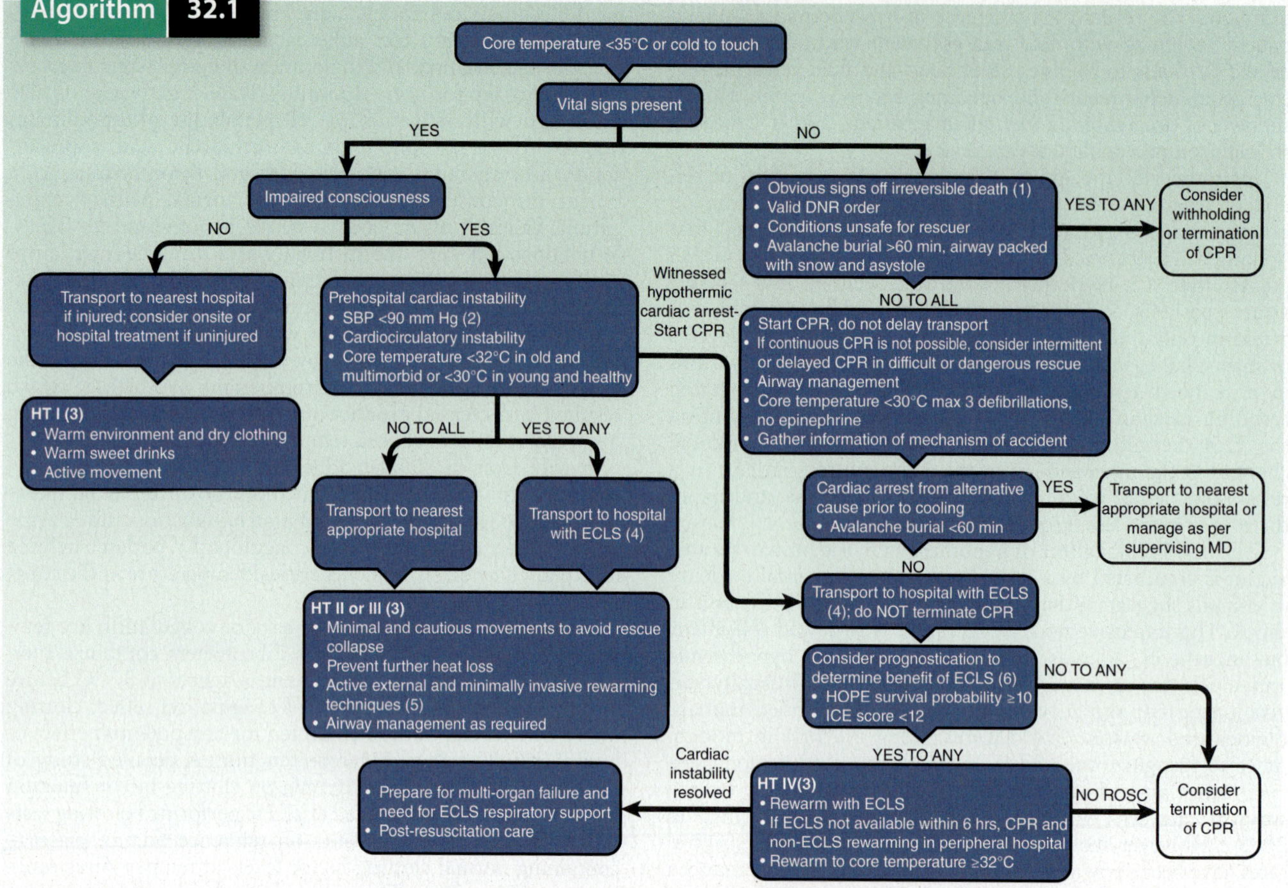

Algorithm 32.1. Management of hypothermia from the European Resuscitation Council. AVPU, alert, verbal, painful (ie, responds to pain), unconscious; GCS: Glasgow Coma Scale. * In the Revised Swiss System, "alert" corresponds to a GCS score of 15, "verbal" corresponds to a GCS score of 9 to 14 and includes confused patients, and "painful" and "unconscious" correspond to a GCS score <9. ¶ No respiration, no palpable carotid or femoral pulse, no measurable blood pressure. Check for signs of life (pulse and, especially, respiration) for up to 1 minute. Δ The transition of colors between stages represents the overlap of patients within groups. From Lott C, Truhlar A, Alfonzo A, et al. European Resuscitation Council Guidelines 2021: Cardiac arrest in special circumstances. *Resuscitation*. 2021;161:152–219.

The key points to this treatment (shown in **Algorithm 32.1**) are the following:

- Check for the presence of vital signs for up to 1 minute to account for bradycardia and depressed ventilation.
- Accurate assessment of core temperature needs low temperature thermometers.
- Prehospital insulation to prevent further heat loss.
- Prompt transfer to a hospital with core rewarming capabilities and extracorporeal life support capabilities in severe cases.
- Prehospital cardiac instability is defined as systolic BP <90 mm Hg or core temperature <32 °C in a patient with vital signs of life.
- Hypothermic cardiac arrest patients should receive continuous CPR during transfer. Chest compression and ventilation rate should not be different to CPR in normothermic patients.
- If VF persists after three shocks, delay further attempts until the core temperature is >30 °C.
- Withhold adrenaline if the core temperature is <30 °C and increase administration intervals for adrenaline to 6 to 10 minutes if the core temperature is >30 °C.
- If prolonged transport is required or the terrain is difficult, use of a mechanical CPR device is recommended.
- In hypothermic arrested patients <28 °C delayed CPR may be used when CPR on site is too dangerous or not feasible, intermittent CPR can be used when continuous CPR is not possible.

Rewarming techniques are usually classified as passive external rewarming, active external rewarming, or active core rewarming. Passive external rewarming simply implies allowing spontaneous rewarming to occur with the patient removed from a hypothermic environment and is usually used only for the mildly hypothermic patient. Active external rewarming techniques include surrounding the patient with warm blankets or heating pads, infrared heating lights, and immersion in warm water. Active core rewarming includes heated intravenous fluids, as well as heated peritoneal or thoracic lavage; heated gastric, bladder, or colonic lavage; heated and water-saturated inhaled air; and extracorporeal circulatory rewarming. Blood rewarming is currently limited to a maximum temperature of 42 °C by the American Association of Blood Banks, but rewarming to 49 °C with inline microwave blood rewarmers has been reported as safe, as has intravenous fluid rewarming to 65 °C.

The advantages and disadvantages of each technique are regularly debated, particularly regarding the role of external versus core rewarming. It is clear, however, that the rate of heat transfer to the hypothermic patient is greatest using active core rewarming, particularly extracorporeal circulation rewarming.

The technique of rewarming the hypothermic victim by extracorporeal circulation has been described by numerous authors, initially based on small personal experiences and using cardiopulmonary bypass techniques of open-heart surgery. This technique has appeal in cases of primary accidental hypothermia, in which maintenance of circulation, correction of hypoxia, and replenishment of intravascular volume may play a role as large as correcting the temperature change itself. The need for systemic anticoagulation has, however, generally limited the usefulness of full cardiopulmonary bypass rewarming in the trauma patient. More recently the use of ECMO for core hypothermia rewarming has been the subject of numerous publications as more centers become more experienced with this tool.[38] A technique of extracorporeal active core rewarming that makes use of the patient's own blood pressure to drive an extracorporeal circuit through an efficient, but small countercurrent heat-exchange device was developed, with demonstrated efficacy via improved survival,[36] but is no longer in commercial production.

The use of body cavity lavage with warm solutions is a simple, less invasive method of accomplishing active core rewarming; however, rewarming rates with body cavity lavage vary greatly based on initial core temperature, dialysate temperature, infusion rate, and dwell time. Several studies support the notion that active core rewarming by peritoneal lavage is preferable to active external rewarming. Moss examined three techniques of rewarming hypothermic and cardiac-arrested dogs, concluding that both peritoneal lavage (55 °C dialysate) and partial extracorporeal circulation were faster than active external rewarming with a heating blanket. A frequently stated disadvantage of external rewarming is that the peripheral tissues are rewarmed in advance of the still cool "core," resulting in peripheral vasodilation leading to shock. In the presence of inadequate volume resuscitation, this rewarming method may result in vascular collapse ("rewarming shock") and a subsequent fall in central temperature ("afterdrop") as the cold peripheral blood returns to the core. Whether this process is the mechanism of the core afterdrop is debatable because continued cooling of a patient's core temperature during the initial states of rewarming has been noted to occur in animal models even during complete circulatory arrest. Volume contraction caused by vasoconstriction, cold diuresis, and cellular swelling coupled with inadequate fluid resuscitation may be a more appropriate explanation for circulatory collapse during rewarming.

The thermodynamic principles of heat transfer to the hypothermic patient are reviewed in greater detail elsewhere,[39] but a sense of rewarming rates and quantity of heat transferred by various techniques is instructional. Ventilating a patient with a core temperature of 32 °C with water-saturated air at 41 °C results in a maximum heat transfer rate of 9 kcal/hr. For comparison, basal metabolic heat generation produces approximately 70 kcal/hr, and shivering produces up to 250 kcal/hr. Given the specific heat of the body (0.083 kcal/kg/°C), 58 kcal is required to raise the temperature of a 70-kg patient by 1 °C. Thus, more than 6 hours would be required to warm a 32 °C patient using 41 °C humidified inspired air.

Heat transfer rates using body cavity lavage can be similarly calculated based on the specific heat of water (1 kcal/kg/°C). If 1 L of 44 °C water infused into a body cavity dwells long enough to exit at 40 °C, 4 kcal of heat will have been transferred to the patient. Thus, over 14 L of fluid is needed to increase core temperature by 1 °C. However, warming becomes less efficient as the patient rewarms because a longer dwell time is required to reduce the temperature of the infusate to 40 °C.

Warming by cardiopulmonary bypass or ECMO or CAVR is the most efficient method of core heating. With flow rates of 15 to 30 L/hr, it is possible to deliver 120 to 240 kcal/hr. if the reinfused blood is heated to 40 °C, a rate of heat transfer over 10 times that of the other methods. In any case, the urgency with which rewarming must be accomplished depends on how adversely the hypothermia is affecting the patient. Except for extracorporeal circulatory methods, most rewarming techniques serve primarily to prevent loss of endogenously generated heat and are ineffective in circumstances in which rapid rewarming is indicated. Early and direct attention to preventing heat loss is therefore essential in surgical patients. With more widespread adoption of ECMO capabilities for treating severe lung disease, centers are starting to report on the use of this modality as a rewarming technique. The combination of injury and hypothermia represents a particular challenge. Swiss physicians with experience in treating injured and hypothermia avalanche victims have developed the Bernese Hypothermia Algorithm, a detailed approach to rewarming techniques and injury care priorities in this population.

Cold Injury and Frostbite

Frostbite is a cold injury limited to digits, extremities, or exposed surfaces that is the result of direct tissue freezing. Chilblain (aka pernio) and trench foot are the result of more chronic exposure to an environment just above freezing. Both types of cold injury have been a major cause of morbidity during war experiences. They resulted in more than 7 million lost soldier fighting days by Allied forces in World War II and were reportedly the most common major injury sustained by British soldiers in the Falklands expedition. Upton Sinclair's novel *The Jungle* used the cold exposure of Chicago's meatpacking industry in the early 20th century to depict the pain of frostbite and chilblains and deplored the working conditions and exploitation of immigrants.

The terms *chilblain* and *pernio* describe a form of local cold injury characterized by pruritic, red-purple papules, macules, plaques, or nodules on the skin. Chilblains can result in a specific form of a dermopathy secondary to cold-induced skin vasculitis. The lesions are often associated with edema or blistering and are caused by a chronic vasculitis of the dermis; this entity does not appear to be related to hereditary protein C or S deficiency. This pathologic process is provoked by repeated exposure to cold, but not freezing, temperatures. This injury typically occurs on the face, the anterior surface of the tibia, or the dorsum of the hands and feet, areas poorly protected or chronically exposed to the environment. With continued exposure, ulcerative or hemorrhagic lesions may appear and progress to scarring, fibrosis, and atrophy. Treatment consists of sheltering the patient, elevating the affected part, and allowing gradual rewarming at room temperature. Rubbing and massage are contraindicated because they can cause further damage and secondary infection. Chronic treatment strategies are similar to frostbite injury treatment, with similar limited success (see section that follows).

Trench foot or cold immersion foot (or hand) describes a nonfreezing injury of the hands or feet, typically in sailors, fishermen, or soldiers, that is caused by chronic exposure to wet conditions and temperatures just above freezing. It appears to involve an alternating arterial vasospasm and vasodilatation, with the affected tissue first cold and anesthetic and then hyperemic after 24 to 48 hours of exposure. With the hyperemia comes an intense, painful burning and dysesthesia; tissue damage is characterized by edema, blistering, redness, ecchymosis, and ulceration. Complications of local infection or cellulitis, lymphangitis, and gangrene may occur. A post hyperemic phase occurs 2 to 6 weeks later and is characterized by tissue cyanosis with increased sensitivity to cold. Treatment is best started during or before the reactive hyperemia state and consists of immediate removal of the extremity from the cold, wet environment with exposure of the feet (or hands) to warm, dry air. Elevation to minimize edema, protection of pressure spots, and local and systemic measures to combat infection are indicated. Massage, soaking of the feet, or rapid rewarming is not indicated. Demyelination of nerves, muscle atrophy, fallen arches, and osteoporosis may all present long-term complications, and a tendency toward marked vasospasm during subsequent exposure to cold develops in some patients.

Frostnip is the mildest form of cold injury. It is characterized by initial pain and pallor, with subsequent numbness of the affected body part. Skiers and other winter outdoor enthusiasts are most likely to experience this cold injury to the nose, ears, or tips of digits. The injury is reversible and warming of

Table 32.9. Grading Frostbite Severity

Frostbite Injuries of the Extremities	Grade 1	Grade 2	Grade 3	Grade 4
Extent of initial lesion at day 0 after rapid rewarming	Absence of initial lesion	Initial lesion on distal phalanx	Initial lesion on intermediary (and) proximal phalanx	Initial lesion on carpal/tarsal
Bone scanning at day 2	Useless	Hypofixation of radiotracer uptake area	Absence of radiotracer uptake area on the digit	Absence of radiotracer uptake area on the carpal/tarsal
Blisters at day 2	Absence of blisters	Clear blisters	Hemorrhagic blisters on the digit	Hemorrhagic blisters over carpal/tarsal
Prognosis at day 2	No amputation	Tissue amputation	Bone amputation of digit	Bone amputation of the limb
				± Systemic involvement
				± sepsis
	No sequelae	Fingernail sequelae	Functional sequelae	Functional sequelae

the cold tissue results in return of sensation and function with no tissue loss. Frostbite is a more severe and common form of cold injury that can result in debilitating long-term irreversible morbidity. Frostbite damage is caused by direct ice crystal formation at the cellular level with cellular dehydration and microvascular occlusion. Indirect cellular injury, also referred to as progressive dermal ischemia is a progressive microvascular insult. Following thawing, microvascular thrombosis, endothelial damage, intravascular sludging and reperfusion injury all occur, resulting in continued cell injury and death. Current treatment modalities have focused on minimizing the indirect cellular or reperfusion injury as discussed in the section that follows.

Frostbite is traditionally classified into four grades of injury severity (**Table 32.9**).

The affected body part nearly always initially appears hard, cold, white, and anesthetic, regardless of the depth of injury. Because the appearance of the lesion changes frequently during the course of treatment and because the initial treatment regimen (see **Algorithm 32.2**) is applicable for all degrees of insult, some authorities suggest discarding this classification as a prognostic impossibility and simply classifying frostbite as either superficial or deep.[40]

Weather conditions, altitude, degree of protective clothing, duration of exposure, and degree of tissue wetness are all contributing external factors to the development of frostbite injury. Because sensory nerve activity is abolished at 7° to 9 °C, the disappearance of pain is an early warning sign of cold injury. Acclimation to cold may be protective, whereas a previous history of frostbite probably predisposes to another cold tissue injury. Smoking and a history of arterial disease also are contributing factors. In urban environments, more than 50% of frostbite injuries are alcohol-related and in one report, 16% of these patients also had a significant underlying psychiatric illness.

As noted, frostbite injury has two components—the initial freeze injury and a reperfusion injury that occurs during rewarming. The initial response to tissue cooling is vasoconstriction and arteriovenous shunting, intermittently relieved (every 5 to 7 minutes) by vasodilation, the so-called "hunting response." With prolonged exposure, this response fails, and the temperature of the freezing tissue approximates ambient temperature until −2 °C. At this point, extracellular ice crystals form, and as these crystals enlarge, the osmotic pressure of the interstitium increases resulting in movement of intracellular water out of cells and into the interstitium. Cells begin to shrink and become hyperosmolar, disrupting cellular enzyme function. If freezing is rapid (>10 °C/min), intracellular ice crystal formation will occur, resulting in immediate cell death. In addition, endothelial cell disruption and red cell sludging associated with freezing result in cessation of circulation. During rewarming, red cell, platelet, and leukocyte aggregation occurs and results in patchy thrombosis of the microcirculation.[41] These accumulated blood elements are thought to release, among other products, the toxic oxygen free radicals and the arachidonic acid metabolites PGF_{2a} and thromboxane A_2, which further aggravate vasoconstriction and platelet and leukocyte aggregation. However, the exact mechanism of tissue destruction and death after freeze injury remains poorly defined.

Treatment of Cold Injury

Prehospital or field care of the victim of cold injury should focus on removing the patient from the hostile environment and protecting the injured body part from further damage. Rubbing or exercising the affected tissue does not augment blood flow and risks further cold injury or mechanical trauma. Because repeated bouts of freezing and thawing worsen the injury, it is preferable for the patient with frostbite of the hands or feet immediately to seek definitive shelter and care rather than rewarm the tissue in the field and risk refreezing. Although the initial symptoms may be mild and overlooked by the patient, severe pain, burning, edema, and even necrosis and gangrene may appear with rewarming. With severe injury the range of motion progressively decreases, and edema becomes prominent. The injury may progress to numbness and, eventually, to loss of all sensation in the affected tissue.

The emergency room treatment of a frostbite victim should first focus on the basic ABCs (airway, breathing, and circulation) of trauma resuscitation and then systemic hypothermia should be identified and corrected. Most patients are dehydrated, and resuscitation with warm fluids is an important part of early management. Fractures are often accompanied by frostbite in mountaineers, and although manipulation may be required to treat vascular compromise, open reduction is hazardous, and application of traction should be delayed until after postthawing edema has been assessed.

9 Rapid rewarming is the goal. Gradual, spontaneous rewarming is inadequate, particularly for deeper injuries, and rubbing the injured part in ice or snow often delays warming and results in marked tissue loss. Rapid rewarming should be achieved by immersing the tissue in a large water bath of

Algorithm 32.2

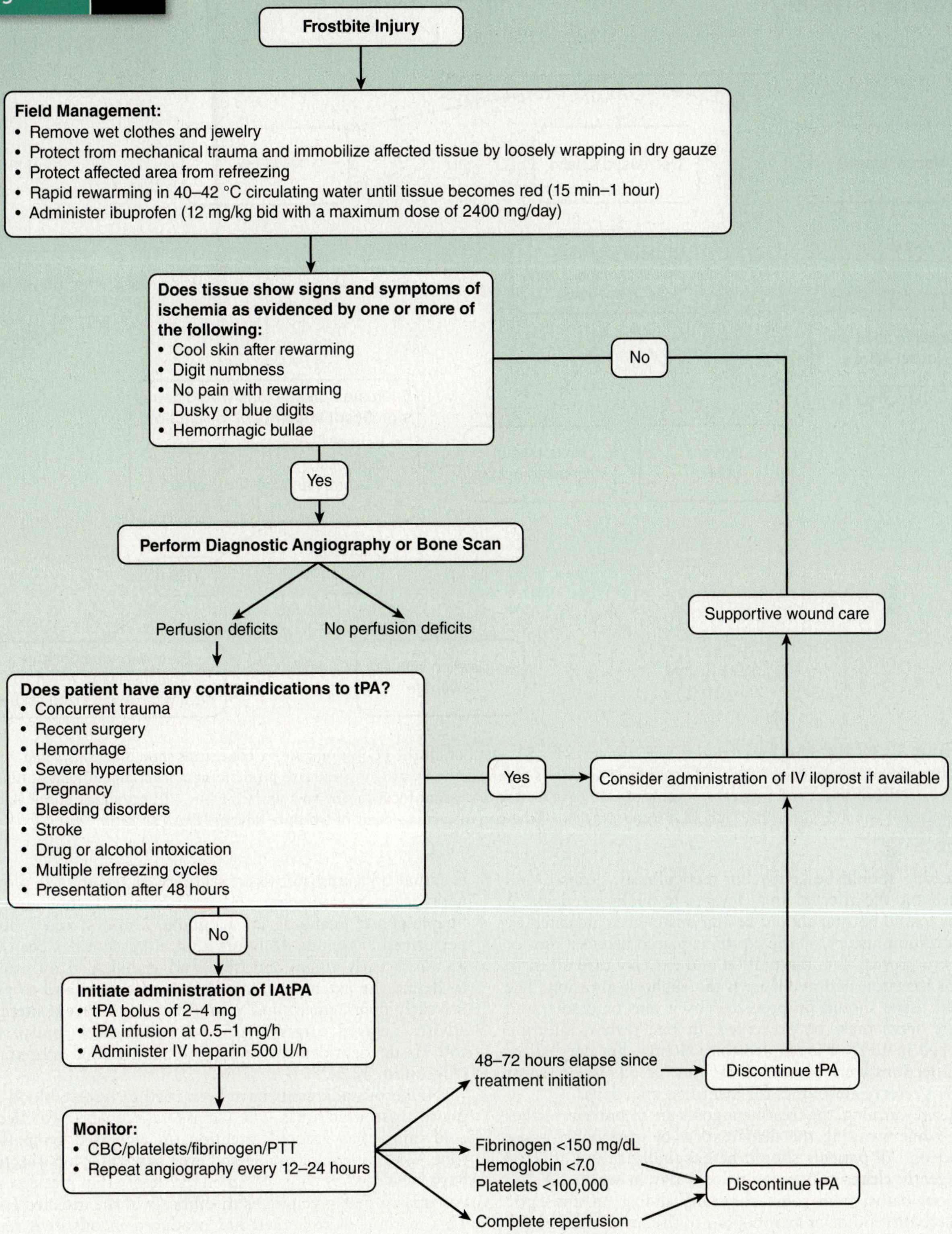

Algorithm 32.2. Frostbite management algorithm. Key management of frostbite injury begins with proper field management, and rapid rewarming. Following rewarming, identification of tissue ischemia with diagnostic angiography or bone scans is often necessary. If tPA is administered, patients require monitoring of CBC/platelets/fibrinogen and PTT to avoid hemorrhagic events. CBC, complete blood count; PTT, partial thromboplasmin time. From Zaramo TZ, Green JK, Janis JE. Practical review of the current management of frostbite injuries. *Plast Reconstr Surg Glob Open*. 2022;10(10):e4618.

40° to 42 °C (104° to 108 °F). The water should feel warm, but not hot, to the normal hand. The bath should be large enough to prevent rapid loss of heat, and the water temperature should be maintained. Dry heat is not advocated because it is difficult to regulate, and the result of using excessive heat is often disastrous. The rewarming process should take approximately 30 to 45 minutes for digits, with the affected area appearing flushed when rewarming is complete and good circulation has been reestablished. Narcotics can be required because the rewarming process can be quite painful.

Algorithm 32.3

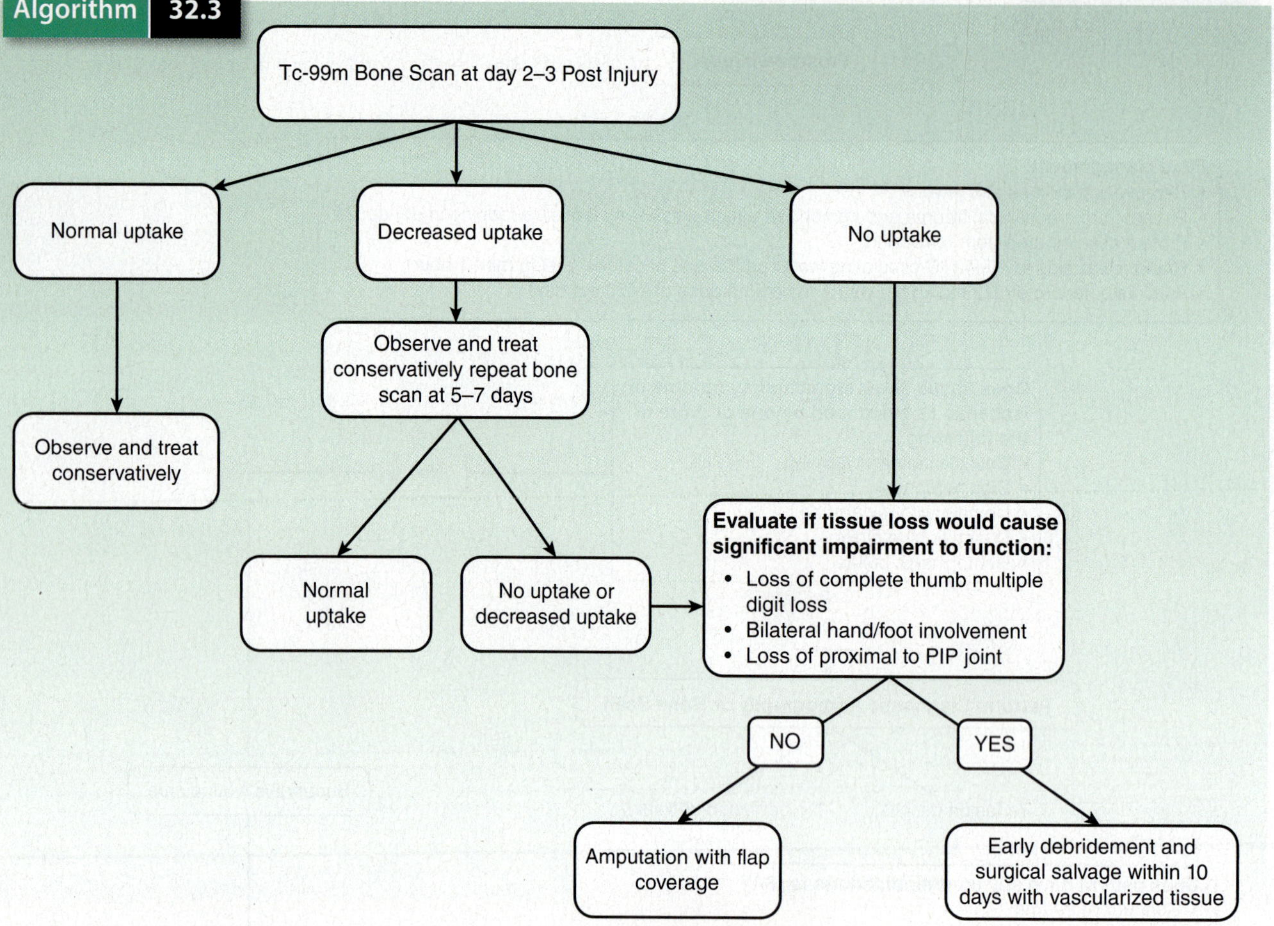

Algorithm 32.3. Algorithm for surgical salvage. Patients with decreased or absent Tc-99m uptake on bone scans should be considered for surgical salvage by assessing affected area and quantifying tissue loss. Injuries that are prognosticated to promote significant impairment of function requires early debridement and surgical salvage within 10 days (before dry eschar forms) using vascularized tissue. PIP, proximal interphalangeal joint. From Zaramo TZ, Green JK, Janis JE. Practical review of the current management of frostbite injuries. *Plast Reconstr Surg Glob Open.* 2022;10(10):e4618.

The skin should be gently but meticulously cleansed and air-dried and the affected area elevated to minimize edema. A tetanus toxoid booster should be administered as indicated by immunization history. Sterile cotton is placed between toes or fingers to prevent skin maceration and extreme care taken to prevent infection and avoid even the slightest abrasion. The affected tissue should be protected by a tent or cradle, and pressure spots must be prevented. In one review, infection developed in 13% of urban frostbite victims, but one-half of these infections were present at the time of admission. Most clinicians reserve antibiotics for identified infections.

After rewarming, the treatment goals are to prevent further injury while awaiting the demarcation of irreversible tissue destruction. All patients should be hospitalized, and affected tissue gently cleansed once or twice a day in warm (38 °C) whirlpool baths, with some clinicians adding an antiseptic such as chlorhexidine or an iodophor to the bath. Based on the findings of arachidonic acid metabolites in the blisters of frostbite victims, some authors advocate the use of topical aloe vera (thromboxane inhibitor) and systemic ibuprofen or aspirin.
10 Uninfected blebs should be left intact because they provide a sterile biologic dressing for 7 to 10 days and protect underlying epithelialization. After resolution of edema, digits should be exercised during the whirlpool bath and physical therapy begun. Tobacco, nicotine, and other vasoconstrictive agents must be withheld. Weight bearing is prohibited until complete resolution of edema.

The use of technetium-99m methylene diphosphonate bone scanning has shown some promise in the early detection of eventual bone and soft tissue viability, as has the use of magnetic resonance imaging and arteriogram. Technetium-99m "triple-phase" scanning (at 1 minute, 2 hours, and 7 hours) performed beginning 48 hours after admission has been used to assess early tissue perfusion and viability, in an attempt to define the extent of fatally damaged tissues and to allow for early debridement and wound closure. Current literature advises delayed surgery (~2 to 4 weeks after injury) with soft tissue debridement and bone scan-guided amputation (**Algorithm 32.3**).[40]

Numerous adjuvants have been tried to restore blood supply to frostbitten areas. The intense vasoconstrictive effect of cold injury has focused attention on increased sympathetic tone. Sympathetic blockade and even surgical sympathectomy have been used by some based on the theory that it releases the vasospasm that precipitates thrombosis in the affected tissue. This method of treatment has produced inconsistent results and is difficult to evaluate clinically, with no prospective, randomized trials available. Although sympathectomy appears to mollify the pain and hyperhidrosis and vasospasm of cold injuries, it may increase vascular shunting and adversely affect healing. In one series of patients from cold injuries in Alaska, a more proximal demarcation of injury in sympathectomized limbs was noted than in non-sympathectomized ones, despite apparently equal bilateral injury.

Experience with intra-arterial vasodilatory reserpine, tolazoline, and papaverine have also been unrewarding. In a controlled clinical study, immediate (mean 3 hours) ipsilateral intra-arterial reserpine infusion coupled with early (mean 3 days) ipsilateral operative sympathectomy failed to alter the natural history of acute frostbite injury compared with the contralateral limb. Low–molecular-weight dextran has been shown to alleviate post thawing circulatory obstruction as late as 2 hours after thawing and markedly reduced tissue loss in rabbit feet, but similar results in humans has not been demonstrated. Heparin, thrombolytic agents, and hyperbaric oxygen have also failed to demonstrate any substantial treatment benefit, but hyperbaric enthusiasts continue to tout its role. None of these adjuncts is considered routine care.

Intra-arterial infusion of tissue plasminogen activator (tPA) has shown to be of benefit. In a nonrandomized study of a small number (n = 7) of patients who received intra-arterial tPA, the burn team at the University of Utah demonstrated that tPA infusion improved tissue perfusion and reduced amputations (10% vs 41%) when administered within 24 hours of injury (6 of the 7), as compared with 25 patients managed in a more traditional fashion. Since this 2007 report, isolated case reports have also suggested that this therapy is effective. During tPA administration, serial angiography should be serially performed to determine improvement in perfusion and discontinued if no improvement is noted after 48–72 hours. IV heparin should be co-administered with IAtPA to prevent the propagation of thrombosis.[40]

In 2024 the FDA formally approved the use of iloprost (Aurlumyn®) to treat frostbite.[42] The primary data source for this approval was a study from 2011. Iloprostis is a synthetic analog of prostacyclin PG12. It works by binding with equal affinity to human prostacyclin (Prostanoid IP) and prostaglandin EP1 receptors and acts as a vasodilator, relaxing the muscles in artery walls. This intravenous agent is touted to increase blood flow, relieves high blood pressure, and inhibit platelet aggregation. The effectiveness of iloprost was determined by an open-label, randomized controlled trial that involved 47 patients, mean age 33 years, 94% were men. Of those studied, 70% had frostbite involving the feet, 62% had frostbite involving the hands, and 32% had frostbite involving both feet and hands. Those assigned to the groups that received iloprost IV for 6 hours daily for up to 8 days were reported to have a significantly lower presence of bone scintigraphy anomaly (a marker that is expected to predict the risk of amputation) than those assigned to received buflomedil (Loftyl®) a vasoactive drug usually used to treat claudication but not FDA approved.

What is termed the "Helsinki frostbite protocol" involves the use of intra-arterial fibrinolytics (tPA) and/or intravenous vasodilator iloprost. Candidates for this therapy should have minimal risk of bleeding from other injuries, have the tPA administered (intra-arterial or intravenously) within 24 hours of frostbite, with no episodes of rewarming or refreezing between injury and treatment, and have clear evidence of full-thickness tissue involvement, as well as abnormal perfusion on either angiogram or pyrophosphate scanning. In one study, 20 patients with frostbite were diagnosed between 2013 and 2016.[43] Nine patients underwent fibrinolytic treatment with tPA and/or iloprost. The overall digital salvage rate was 74.8%. However, as of January 2020 the American Burn Association guidelines state that the data are insufficient to support routine treatment of all patients with frostbite with thrombolytics,[44] but do state that patients with cyanosis persisting proximal to the distal phalanx (grade 3 or 4 frostbite injury) and demonstrated loss of perfusion at or proximal to the middle phalanx immediately after rewarming can be treated with thrombolytic therapy in accordance with local hospital protocols. The guidelines also support the concept that time to treatment is an important quality metric in the treatment of frostbite. The work from Hennepin County Burn Center supports the notion that "time is tissue" similar to that of the treatment of ischemic stroke or myocardial infarction. Nice summaries of the body of work on the history and treatment of frostbite injuries, and the paucity of data on effective treatment, were recently compiled.[40,45]

The difficulty in determining the depth of tissue destruction in cold injury has led to a conservative approach to the care of frostbite injuries.[46] For digit frostbite, the Hennepin score may provide a useful way to track progress and compare experimental therapies. As a general rule, amputation and surgical debridement are delayed for 2 to 3 months unless infection with sepsis intervenes, hence the adage: "frostbite in January, amputate in June." The natural history of a full-thickness frostbite injury is the gradual demarcation of the injured area with dry gangrene or mummification clearly delineating nonviable tissue. Often the permanent tissue loss is much less than originally suspected. In an Alaskan series, only 10.5% of patients required amputation, usually involving only phalanges or portions of phalanges. The need for emergency surgery is unusual, but vigilance should be maintained during the rewarming phase for the development of a compartment syndrome requiring fasciotomy. Open amputations are indicated in patients with persistent infection and sepsis that is refractory to debridement and antibiotics. Mills convincingly demonstrated that of all the factors in the treatment of frostbite that may influence outcome, premature surgical intervention by any means, in any amount, was by far the greatest contributor to poor results.

Frostbitten tissues seldom recover completely. Some degree of cold insensitivity invariably remains. Hyperhidrosis (in up to 72% of patients), neuropathy, decreased nail and hair growth, and a persistent Raynaud phenomenon in the affected part are frequent sequelae to cold injury.[47] The affected tissue remains at risk for reinjury and should be carefully protected during any cold exposure. Treatment with antiadrenergic agents (prazosin hydrochloride, 1 to 2 mg/day) or calcium channel blockers (nifedipine, 30 to 60 mg/day) and careful protection from further exposure is often helpful. However, few therapies afford significant relief to the chronic symptoms after tissue freeze injury, although β- and α-adrenergic blocking agents, calcium channel blockers, topical and systemic steroids, and a host of home remedies have been tried with occasional individual success.

SUMMARY

Of the 3700 species of snakes worldwide, only 200 are significantly venomous, with approximately 6 deaths per year in the United States caused by snakebite. In contrast, there are over 150,000 species of Hymenoptera (a large order of insects, comprising the sawflies, wasps, bees, and ants) in the world that cause approximately 40 deaths per year, mostly because of severe anaphylactic reactions.

Snakebite morbidity depends on the type of snake and the degree of envenomation. Venoms consist of numerous polypeptides that can disrupt endothelial cells and blood flow, produce neuromuscular blockade, or generate a coagulopathy via procoagulants. Some snakes (particularly Elapids, as represented by the coral snakes in North America) also have direct neurotoxins and cardiotoxins. Snakebite produces immediate pain, edema, and erythema at the site. Spread of the swelling greater than 10 cm/hr indicates severe envenomation. Initial incision and suction and the use of a proximal tourniquet are contraindicated. Use of purified ovine antivenin is effective for serious Crotalidae envenomation and has replaced equine antivenin given its associated risk of serum sickness. Because of the presumed safety of the newer antivenom, overuse is more likely.

Spider bites produce toxicity by local tissue necrosis (brown recluse and hobo spiders) and painful muscle contractions (black widow spider). Death may be caused by stinging Hymenoptera, including bees (particularly aggressive Africanized bees), fire ants, and scorpions. The death is usually secondary to anaphylaxis, but occasionally massive envenomation occurs—especially with Africanized honeybees. The estimated lethal dose is approximately 20 stings/kg in most mammals.

Hypothermia risk is high in the severely injured patient because of exposure, loss of normal protective metabolism (ie, shivering), rapid massive infusion of cold fluids/ blood, and open thoracic and abdominal cavities. The initial response to hypothermia is an intensive sympathetic type of reaction with tremulousness, profound vasoconstriction, marked increase in oxygen consumption, and accelerated heart rate and minute ventilation. As core temperature falls to between 33 °C and 30 °C this response is lost, and deeper core hypothermia rapidly develops. Hypothermia increases risk of mortality at every level of traumatic injury. There is no improvement in outcome when hypothermia is applied to the severe TBI; trauma patients rapidly rewarmed require less resuscitation volume and have improved survival.

Treating hypothermia begins by preventing further heat loss and allowing endogenous rewarming. Active rewarming has many adjuncts, including warm blankets, heating pads and lights, and immersion in warm water or internally by core rewarming. Internal core rewarming is more effective and includes heated intravenous fluids; heated body cavity lavage; heated moist inhaled air; extracorporeal circulatory rewarming (ECMO or CPB) or closed circuit intravascular countercurrent heat-exchange devices. Frostbite involves ice crystal formation and unpredictable loss of tissue. Early definitive rewarming (avoiding refreezing) by submersion in 40° to 42 °C water is preferable with subsequent meticulous care, awaiting demarcation, and avoidance of early debridement to optimize outcomes and tissue salvage. Early thrombolytic and/or prostaglandin vasodilator therapy might be beneficial in select frostbite patients.

References

1. Meggs WJ, Courtney C, O'Rourke D, Brewer KL. Pilot studies of pressure-immobilization bandages for rattlesnake envenomations. *Clin Toxicol (Phila)*. 2010;48(1):61–63.
2. Lavonas EJ, Gerardo CJ, O'Malley G, et al. Initial experience with Crotalidae polyvalent immune Fab (ovine) antivenom in the treatment of copperhead snakebite. *Ann Emerg Med*. 2004;43(2): 200–206.
3. Walker JP, Morrison RL. Current management of copperhead snakebite. *J Am Coll Surg*. 2011;212(4):470–474; discussion 474–475.
4. Whitley RE. Conservative treatment of copperhead snakebites without antivenin. *J Trauma*. 1996;41(2):219–221.
5. Dart RC, Hurlbut KM, Garcia R, Boren J. Validation of a severity score for the assessment of crotalid snakebite. *Ann Emerg Med*. 1996;27(3):321–326.
6. LoVecchio F, Klemens J, Welch S, Rodriguez R. Antibiotics after rattlesnake envenomation. *J Emerg Med*. 2002;23(4):327–328.
7. Weinstein SA. The pharmacotherapy for pit viper envenoming in the United States: a brief retrospective on roots, recurrence, and risk. *Clin Toxicol (Phila)*. 2015;53(1):1–4.
8. Lavonas EJ, Ruha AM, Banner W, et al; Rocky Mountain Poison and Drug Center, Denver Health and Hospital Authority. Unified treatment algorithm for the management of crotaline snakebite in the United States: results of an evidence-informed consensus workshop. *BMC Emerg Med*. 2011;11:2.
9. Langley RL. Snakebite during pregnancy: a literature review. *Wilderness Environ Med*. 2010;21(1):54–60.
10. Corneille MG, Larson S, Stewart RM, et al. A large single-center experience with treatment of patients with crotalid envenomations: outcomes with and evolution of antivenin therapy. *Am J Surg*. 2006;192(6):848–852.
11. Brandehoff N, Dalton A, Daugherty C, Dart RC, Monte AA; ToxIC Snakebite Study Group. Total CroFab and Anavip antivenom vial administration in US rattlesnake envenomations: 2019–2021. *J Med Toxicol*. 2023;19(3):248–254.
12. Ruha AM, Kleinschmidt KC, Greene S, et al. The epidemiology, clinical course, and management of snakebites in the North American Snakebite Registry. *J Med Toxicol*. 2017;13(4):309–320.
13. Stewart RM, Page CP, Schwesinger WH, McCarter R, Martinez J, Aust JB. Antivenin and fasciotomy/debridement in the treatment of the severe rattlesnake bite. *Am J Surg*. 1989;158(6):543–547.
14. French R, Brooks D, Ruha AM, et al. Gila monster (Heloderma suspectum) envenomation: descriptive analysis of calls to United States Poison Centers with focus on Arizona cases. *Clin Toxicol (Phila)*. 2015;53(1):60–70.
15. Rahimian R, Shirazi FM, Schmidt JO, Klotz SA. Honeybee stings in the era of killer bees: anaphylaxis and toxic envenomation. *Am J Med*. 2020;133(5):621–626.
16. Swanson DL, Vetter RS. Bites of brown recluse spiders and suspected necrotic arachnidism. *N Engl J Med*. 2005;352(7): 700–707.
17. Sams HH, Dunnick CA, Smith ML, King LE Jr. Necrotic arachnidism. *J Am Acad Dermatol*. 2001;44(4):561–573; quiz 573–576.
18. Zhou HJ, Xu K, Zheng PY, Gu W. Clinical characteristics of patients with black widow spider bites: a report of 59 patients and single-center experience. *World J Emerg Med*. 2021;12(4): 317–320.
19. Pesek RD, Lockey RF. Management of insect sting hypersensitivity: an update. *Allergy Asthma Immunol Res*. 2013;5(3):129–137.
20. Boyer L, Degan J, Ruha AM, Mallie J, Mangin E, Alagón A. Safety of intravenous equine F(ab')2: insights following clinical trials involving 1534 recipients of scorpion antivenom. *Toxicon*. 2013;76:386–393.
21. Walpoth BH, Walpoth-Aslan BN, Mattle HP, et al. Outcome of survivors of accidental deep hypothermia and circulatory arrest treated with extracorporeal blood warming. *N Engl J Med*. 1997;337(21):1500–1505.
22. Pasquier M, Paal P, Blancher M, Darocha T. Higher survival chances of hypothermic vs. normothermic cardiac arrest patients with ECLS re-warming. *Resuscitation*. 2019;134:161–162.
23. Brix DM, Tvingsholm SA, Hansen MB, et al. Release of transcriptional repression via ErbB2-induced, SUMO-directed phosphorylation of myeloid zinc finger-1 serine 27 activates lysosome redistribution and invasion. *Oncogene*. 2019;38(17):3170–3184.
24. Iyer A, Rajkuman V, Sadasivan S, Bruce J, Gilfillan I. No one is dead until warm and dead. *J Thorac Cardiovasc Surg*. 2007;134: 1042–1043.
25. Brown DJ, Brugger H, Boyd J, Paal P. Accidental hypothermia. *N Engl J Med*. 2012;367(20):1930–1938.
26. Deslarzes T, Rousson V, Yersin B, Durrer B, Pasquier M. An evaluation of the Swiss staging model for hypothermia using case reports from the literature. *Scand J Trauma Resusc Emerg Med*. 2016;24:16.
27. Greer DM, Kirschen MP, Lewis A, et al. Pediatric and adult brain death/death by neurologic criteria consensus guideline. *Neurology*. 2023;101(24):1112–1132.
28. Greer DM, Shemie SD, Lewis A, et al. Determination of brain death/death by neurologic criteria: the world brain death project. *JAMA*. 2020;324(11):1078–1097.
29. Zheng G, Zhang J, Liu J, Chen C, Zhang L, Cao F. A meta-analysis of randomized controlled trials: efficiency and safety of ondansetron in preventing post-anesthesia shivering during cesarean section. *Arch Gynecol Obstet*. 2023;307(1):223–231.
30. Paal P, Brugger H, Strapazzon G. Accidental hypothermia. *Handb Clin Neurol*. 2018;157:547–563.
31. Little R, Stoner H. Body temperature after accidental injury. *Br J Surg*. 1981;68:221–224.
32. Jurkovich GJ. *Hypothermia in the Trauma Patient, in Advances in Trauma*. Maull KI, ed. Yearbook; 1989:111–140.
33. Perlman R, Callum J, Laflamme C, et al. A recommended early goal-directed management guideline for the prevention of

hypothermia-related transfusion, morbidity, and mortality in severely injured trauma patients. *Crit Care.* 2016;20(1):107.

34. Jurkovich GJ, Pitt RM, Curreri PW, Granger DN. Hypothermia prevents increased capillary permeability following ischemia-reperfusion injury. *J Surg Res.* 1988;44(5):514–521.
35. Tisherman SA. Salvage techniques in traumatic cardiac arrest: thoracotomy, extracorporeal life support, and therapeutic hypothermia. *Curr Opin Crit Care.* 2013;19(6):594–598.
36. Gentilello LM, Jurkovich GJ, Stark MS, et al. Is hypothermia in the victim of major trauma protective or harmful? A randomized, prospective study. *Ann Surg.* 1997;226(4):439–447; discussion 447–449.
37. Granfeldt A, Holmberg MJ, Nolan JP, Soar J, Andersen LW; International Liaison Committee on Resuscitation (ILCOR) Advanced Life Support Task Force. Targeted temperature management in adult cardiac arrest: systematic review and meta-analysis. *Resuscitation.* 2021;167:160–172.
38. Darocha T, Jarosz A, Ziętkiewicz M, et al. ECMO in treating patients in critical, life-threatening medical condition brought on by severe hypothermia-criterion standard. *Ann Emerg Med.* 2016;67(4):558–559.
39. Gentilello L, Jurkovich G, Moujaes S. Hypothermia and injury: thermodynamic principles of prevention and treatment. In: Levine B, ed. *Perspectives in Surgery*. Quality Medical Publishers; 1991.
40. Zaramo TZ, Green JK, Janis JE. Practical review of the current management of frostbite injuries. *Plast Reconstr Surg Glob Open.* 2022;10(10):e4618.
41. Mileski WJ, Raymond JF, Winn RK, Harlan JM, Rice CL. Inhibition of leukocyte adherence and aggregation for treatment of severe cold injury in rabbits. *J Appl Physiol. (1985).* 1993;74(3):1432–1436.
42. Harris E. FDA approves iloprost as first drug to treat severe frostbite. *JAMA.* 2024;331(11):907.
43. Lindford A, Valtonen J, Hult M, et al. The evolution of the Helsinki frostbite management protocol. *Burns.* 2017;43(7):1455–1463.
44. Hickey S, Whitson A, Jones L, et al. Guidelines for thrombolytic therapy for frostbite. *J Burn Care Res.* 2020;41(1):176–183.
45. Sheridan RL, Goverman JM, Walker TG. Diagnosis and treatment of frostbite. *N Engl J Med.* 2022;386(23):2213–2220.
46. Petrone P, Kuncir EJ, Asensio JA. Surgical management and strategies in the treatment of hypothermia and cold injury. *Emerg Med Clin North Am.* 2003;21(4):1165–1178.
47. Heil KM, Oakley EH, Wood AM. British Military freezing cold injuries: a 13-year review. *J R Army Med Corps.* 2016;162(6):413–418.

33

Section B: TRANSPLANTATION

Clinical Transplant Immunology

Seth A. Waits and Kyle H. Sheetz

Key Points

1 Understanding clinical transplant immunology is predicated on understanding mechanisms of innate and adaptive immunity, as well as T- and B-cell signal pathways.

2 T cells are responsible for regulatory and effector mechanisms in the immune response. T-cell effector activity is coordinated by regulatory cells driven by three signals of antigen presentation.

3 Acute rejection has a clinical phenotype and may involve cellular infiltration of the allograft as well as antibody-mediated mechanisms. Chronic rejection, or chronic transplant dysfunction, is driven by immune and nonimmune mechanisms and results in progressive graft fibrosis that is heretofore irreversible.

4 Clinical immunosuppression involves induction and maintenance therapies.

5 Induction therapies are used to prevent early acute rejection of allografts, and are generally aimed at reducing T-cell signaling. Commonly used drugs are lymphocyte depletion agents, IL-2 receptor antibodies, and agents to block costimulatory signals.

6 Maintenance immunosuppression consists of calcineurin inhibitors, mTOR inhibitors, antimetabolite agents, and steroids. All agents have a clinically significant side-effect profile.

7 Major side effects of chronic immunosuppression include calcineurin inhibitor–related nephrotoxicity, major and minor infections, and cancer.

Solid organ transplantation has evolved rapidly over the past 65 years. Advances in surgical technique and biologic science have saved the lives of thousands of patients. The bedrock of success in clinical transplantation is the result of growth in transplant immunology. The discovery era of the immune response to alloantigens and identification of molecular targets for immunosuppressive agents have solidified clinical transplantation as the treatment of choice for patients with organ failure.

1 Understanding transplant immunology requires an in-depth understanding of the molecular mechanisms that lead to acute and chronic rejection. Transplant rejection is the clinical phenotype of organ injury brought on by the recipient immune system's recognition of allogeneity. The aim of this chapter is to review the scientific principles behind the use of modern immunosuppressive agents, the interplay between cell types involved in the alloimmune response, and an in-depth discussion of modern therapeutics. Additionally, the complications of immunosuppressive therapy and evolving therapies will be discussed.

SCIENTIFIC BASIS FOR MODERN CLINICAL IMMUNOSUPPRESSION

The Immune Response to a Solid Organ Transplant

As the field of transplant immunology has matured, it is clear that the interaction of a host's immune system with foreign antigen is central to understanding the pathways that modulate organ-directed effector responses. T- and B-cell activation and regulatory pathways are primary targets for conventional immunosuppressive regimens. Immunosuppressive regimens have been developed to impact isolated pathways in T-cell activation by recipient antigen-presenting cells (APCs). Increasingly more specific suppressive pharmacotherapies have become targeted and less toxic to the host immune system.

The development of mature T cells begins with nascent thymocytes. Thymocytes contain T-cell receptors (TCRs) arranged and rearranged in a random, individual-specific manner. These TCR-containing thymocytes are challenged by "self" antigen and undergo programmed cell death if they express "high affinity" and activate. In contrast, these immature cells are programmed not to proliferate if they express "too low" an affinity. Thymocytes with an intermediate affinity are fostered to survive and differentiate into specific CD4- and CD8-expressing cells which interact with self-restricted major histocompatibility complexes (MHCs) on APCs, such as dendritic cells, in the peripheral blood.

The foundation of the adaptive immune response lies in the presentation of antigen to T cells, which takes place via macrophages, B cells, and dendritic cells. Dendritic cells present antigen via their MHC class I or II molecules to $CD8^+$ T cells and $CD4^+$ T cells, respectively. The most common scenario occurs when a T cell interacts with an APC–MHC complex—presenting "self" antigen. In normal (nonautoimmune) circumstances, this is usually a very weak bond, and the T cell removes itself from the interaction and begins to recirculate. In the context of infection or transplantation, the APC–MHC complex presents a foreign peptide which the T cells recognize as "nonself" and begin the cascade of activation as well as clonal expansion.

2 T cells are activated by a process that requires three sequential signals. The "three-signal" process of T-cell activation begins with **signal 1** as the TCR interacts with the MHC–foreign peptide complex presented by an APC. T cells become maximally activated only after a threshold number of TCRs have been occupied. Multiple costimulatory–supporting molecules on the periphery of both the APC and T cells travel to the immunologic synapse and begin to interact with each other, comprising **signal 2**. The engagement of TCR by MHC–peptide complexes in combination with the interaction of costimulatory, accessory, and adhesion molecules results in a cascade of

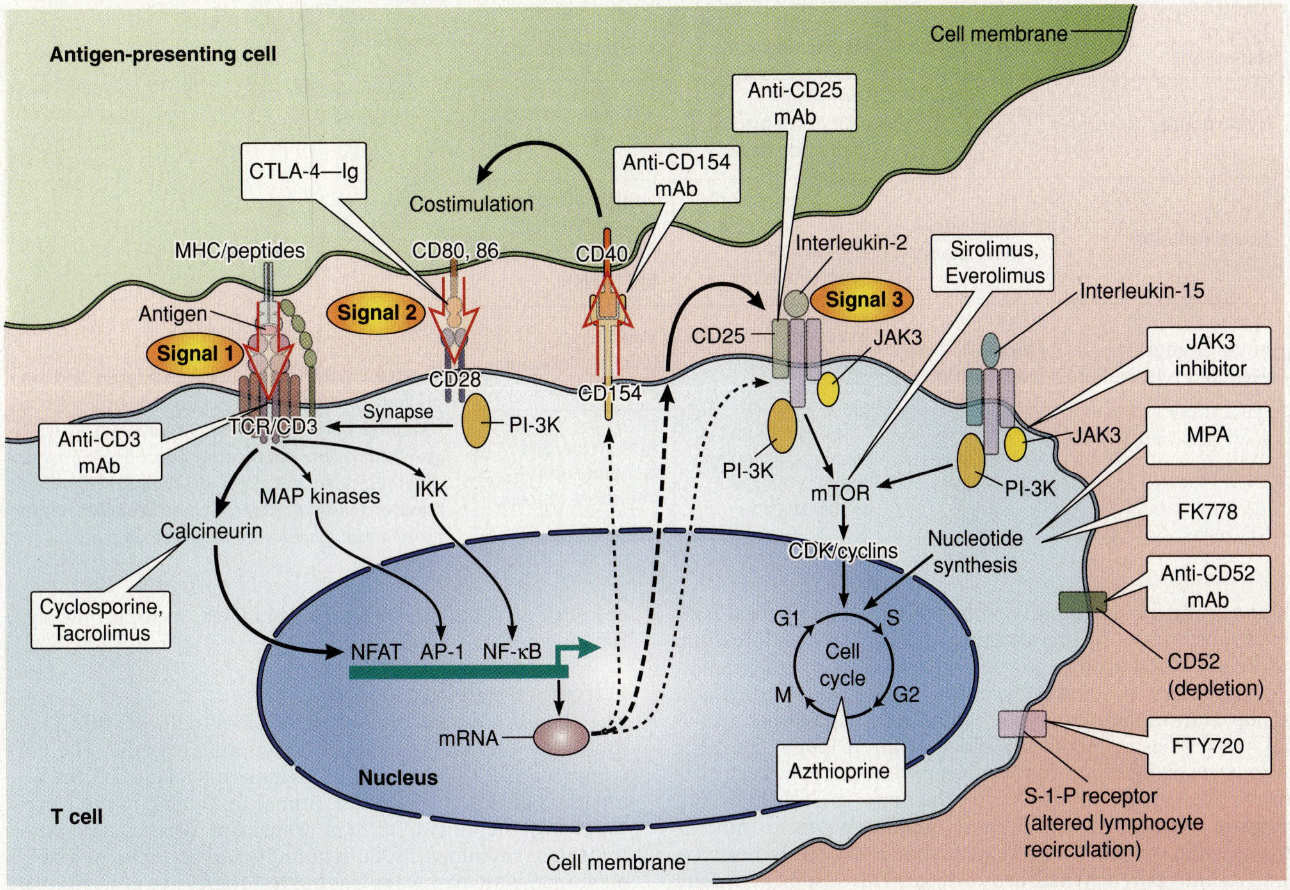

Figure 33.1. The signal hypothesis of T-cell activation and molecular targets of modern clinical immunosuppression. T-cell activation requires three signals to initiate an effector response: antigen presentation of nonself MHC, costimulatory signal, and regulation of cytokine signaling at the cell surface. These three signals are thus targets for therapeutic drugs used in modern clinical immunosuppression in both induction and maintenance phases, as well as in the treatment of rejection. The figure demonstrates the site of action of these agents.

signaling pathways. This includes activation of NF-κB and translocation of the nuclear factor of activation and transcription (NFAT) to the nucleus of the T cell, which translates and transcribes proteins such as interleukin-2 (IL-2). IL-2, formerly known as T-cell growth factor, then contributes to the clonal expansion of other T-cell populations, allowing for cellular expansion to fight against the inciting foreign antigen. IL-2 also engages with CD25 on the T cell itself, thereby activating a doublet complex known as the mammalian target of rapamycin, or mTOR. Signaling through mTOR constitutes **signal 3** of activation, which affects cell cycling and cytokine production, cellular proliferation, and T-cell differentiation into an effector cell against the grafted organ. This pathway initiates the slower, more sophisticated, adaptive immune response (**Fig. 33.1**).

Immediately following implantation and reperfusion of an organ allograft, markers of inflammation are upregulated, which attract effector T cells. These inflammatory mediators also allow for a more efficient uptake of antigen by dendritic cells. Organ-derived dendritic cells are released to the host's secondary lymphoid tissue. Termed "passenger leukocytes," these dendritic cells are primed to present antigen to naive host T cells. These activated CD4$^+$ T cells specialize into subsets of helper T cells, each identified by a distinct signature of cytokines. Interferon-γ (IFN)–secreting TH1 cells are central to various cell-mediated rejection responses, including acute and chronic or delayed-type hypersensitivity responses. TH2 cells support B-cell production of antibody and secrete cytokines with a suppressive capacity, such as IL-4 and IL-10.

Memory T-cell subsets react in a more rapid manner to the graft and incite an accelerated rejection response. Seminal studies investigating memory responses to allografts proved that antigen-experienced memory T-cell subsets can cause graft destruction in the absence of secondary lymphoid tissue. Clinically, these "memory" T cells are generated throughout the life span of a potential recipient due to various infections that the patient may have experienced. Memory T-cell subsets that have been generated by these infections may then react against an organ at the time of transplant if the antigenic response from the organ mimics that of the previous infectious episodes. It is now established that these memory T cells are spared by conventional induction immunosuppression, allowing their graft alloreactivity to induce acute rejection responses. Thus, circulating memory responses remain a roadblock to immunologic tolerance.

REJECTION IN SOLID ORGAN TRANSPLANTATION

Immunologic rejection can occur minutes to years after an organ transplant. The early phases of rejection, termed **hyperacute rejection**, can occur on the operating room table to 24 hours after surgery and are mediated by the humoral immune system. **Acute rejection** is a cell-mediated phenomenon that often manifests days to months after transplant. **Chronic rejection** occurs in the months to years after transplant and continues to be one of the leading causes of graft loss in the long term. Acute and chronic antibody-mediated rejection (AMR) is a separate phenomenon that may occur days to years after transplant and remains an important barrier to successful engraftment of organs.

Hyperacute Rejection

Hyperacute rejection is rare in modern clinical transplantation. Hyperacute rejection is generally attributed to ABO

Type of Rejection	Time of Onset	Mechanism	Morphology
Hyperacute	Minutes to few hours	Preformed antibodies bind to graft endothelium	Vessel thrombosis; Ischemic necrosis
Acute Cellular	Days to weeks, months to years	T cells injure graft by direct cytotoxicity and type IV hypersensitivity	Interstitial infiltrates of lymphocytes; Focal necrosis of graft tissue
Acute Humoral (Rejection Vasculitis)	Days to weeks, months to years	Antidonor antibodies against graft antigens	Vasculitis; Intimal thickening; Thrombosis
Chronic	Months to years (Irreversible)	T-cell cytokines stimulate vascular smooth muscle proliferation	Arteriosclerosis; Ischemic atrophy; Interstitial fibrosis

Figure 33.2. Time course, mechanism, and morphology of transplant rejection. Allograft rejection responses have many different phenotypes, which also lead to different therapies. This figure provides a summary of the types of clinically significant rejection episodes, the root cause behind them, and histopathologic features identified on biopsy.

blood group incompatibility or the presence of preformed anti-HLA antibodies. In the allograft, the capillary endothelium expresses blood group antigens which may join with circulating antibodies to A and B glycoproteins. For example, a blood group B transplant candidate would have circulating anti-A IgG antibodies in blood. If a blood group A kidney allograft were transplanted into that recipient without any other treatment, these antibodies react with the donor endothelium and activate complement and humoral immunity effector mechanisms, which would lead to endothelial injury, thrombosis, as well as intraparenchymal hemorrhage. This response usually happens within minutes after reperfusion of the allograft and requires removal of the allograft to prevent a systemic inflammatory response, which may lead to multiorgan failure. Prevention of this type of rejection is central to the practice of clinical transplantation, and mandates confirmation of donor and recipient compatibility via ABO blood group verification and cross-matching prior to implantation of the allograft (**Fig. 33.2**).

Acute Rejection

3 Induction protocols in combination with immunosuppressive therapy successfully prevent the acute rejection episodes. In the case of renal transplantation, induction therapies in combination with maintenance therapies have fostered a significant improvement in 1-year outcomes. Less than 10% of organs experience clinically significant acute cellular rejection (ACR) episodes leading to graft loss at 1 year. ACR is an adaptive response characterized by T-cell interactions with donor antigens, either presented directly by the donor APC or indirectly by the recipient professional-presenting cells. Once clonal expansion occurs, "effector" T cells then infiltrate the graft and mediate various methods of organ injury.

The gold standard in pathologic categorization of renal transplant rejection is the Banff classification model. The Banff classification originated at a consensus conference in 1991 aimed at ranking the levels of rejection seen on kidney transplant biopsies based on degree of structural damage, such as tubulitis, arteritis, and cellular infiltrate. In renal transplantation, the diagnosis of ACR occurs with tissue confirmation after ruling out other causes for declining graft function. Treatment of ACR is usually dictated by the Banff classification. For example, borderline rejection characterized by Banff class IA or IB is often treated with pulse corticosteroids and increases in maintenance immunosuppression whereas, more severe ACR (Banff 2 to 4) is more often treated with multiple doses of thymoglobulin. Today, ACR is often the result of inadequate immunosuppression due to noncompliance/adherence or early immunosuppression withdrawal/underdosing. Repeated episodes of acute rejection are associated with chronic dysfunction and early graft failure.

Chronic Rejection

The clinical sequelae of chronic rejection (chronic transplant dysfunction or CTD) are varied and organ specific. The unifying factor of CTD among all organs transplanted is the histopathologic effect of arterial intimal thickening in the vessels supplying the organ, termed transplant arteriosclerosis or transplant vasculopathy. Both immune and nonimmune stimuli may upregulate pathways leading to progressive graft fibrosis. Immune-dependent mechanisms, including HLA mismatching, inadequate immunosuppression, and episodes of acute rejection, promote the development of CTD and eventual graft failure. Additionally, immune-independent mechanisms, such as prolonged ischemia time and usage of brain-dead donor organs, as well as recipient factors such as native hypertension may also play a role in the onset of CTD.

Clinically, the manifestations of CTD depend on the type of organ allograft. Recipients of renal allografts with CTD often manifest with proteinuria, decreases in glomerular filtration rate (GFR), increases in plasma creatinine, and arterial hypertension. Patients who have undergone liver transplantation may present with abnormal liver function tests or an increase in serum bilirubin secondary to the so-called *vanishing bile duct syndrome*. Bronchiolitis obliterans, detected by computed tomography and altered pulmonary function tests, indicate the onset of CTD in lung transplant recipients. Patients receiving cardiac allografts may present with a range of symptoms from arrhythmias to fatal myocardial infarction.

Antibody-Mediated Rejection

AMR can occur in both the acute and chronic phases of transplantation. AMR starts with production of donor-specific antibody (DSA) directed to the endothelial lining of organ allografts. DSA–endothelial cell interactions lead to complement activation as well as innate responses, resulting in allograft injury. In the chronic setting, persistent DSA leads to microthrombotic events and late graft failure. Diagnostically, along with serum titers of circulating DSA, tissue biopsy reveals deposition of complement split products, including C4d, and inflammation of capillaries and renal tubules.[1] AMR has also been diagnosed using newer endothelial, cell-specific biomarkers of capillaritis. Liver allografts have shown susceptibility to AMR and DSA in recent studies.

The treatment of acute AMR is based on removal of inciting antibodies. Although there are no high-quality evidence-based treatments for acute AMR, strategies include plasmapheresis, immunoadsorption, use of B-cell toxic antibodies such as rituximab, newer proteasome inhibitors such as bortezomib, and even splenectomy. In patients with drug-resistant AMR, small trials have suggested that monoclonal antibodies to complement C5 (eculizumab) have been used with encouraging results.

IMMUNOLOGIC PHARMACOTHERAPY IN SOLID ORGAN TRANSPLANTATION

Induction

Human immunity depends on innate and adaptive responses to foreign antigens. The innate response is rapid and nonspecific when foreign antigen is encountered, while the adaptive response develops over time and is focused on recall of foreign
4 antigen. While the innate immune system sets the scene for the adaptive response, it is the specificity of antigens that allows for the activation and proliferation of effector cells to rid the system of the pathogenic insult.[2] Current therapies in clinical immunosuppression target global T-cell activation and proliferation. Induction immunosuppression is used perioperatively as a prophylactic treatment to attenuate acute rejection.

CELL SURFACE RECEPTOR BLOCKADE

To interrupt the signal 3 T-cell activation pathway, various pharmacotherapies have targeted signal 2, or costimulation. This effectively targets the clonal proliferation of effector
5 T cells. Costimulation pathways have been targeted by monoclonal antibodies as well as recombinant fusion proteins.

IL-2 Receptor Blockade

Basiliximab is a chimeric mouse/human IgG1 monoclonal antibody to the α-chain of CD25 (IL-2 receptor), which has proven to reduce acute rejection rates in adult and pediatric renal and pancreas transplant recipients. In clinical trials with 6-month follow-up, basiliximab had a significant impact on acute rejection rates with no increase in infectious complications. Basiliximab can be used as induction therapy for kidney transplant recipients or in liver transplant recipients to spare the nephrotoxic effects of tacrolimus. Recent studies have cast doubt on the renal protective effects of basiliximab induction and CNI reduction, however, long-term follow-up remains to be provided.

LEUKOCYTE DEPLETION

In order to achieve tolerance to an organ transplant, it may be necessary to maximize the potential of engraftment by depleting the alloreactive effector T cells (and B cells in some therapeutic regimens), which mediate a rejection response. Depleting the recipient of leukocytes creates a window of opportunity for an allograft to "settle in" without attack by effector immunocytes.[3] The recipient's transient immunodeficiency is dictated by the strength and duration of depletion. Many investigators have identified the value of monoclonal or polyclonal antibodies designed to bind to peripheral alloreactive lymphocytes. The short-term depletion of leukocytes using antithymocyte globulin, anti-CD3, anti-CD2, anti-CD4, and anti-CD8 has proven successful in terms of long-term graft survival in animal models.

Polyclonal leukocyte–depleting antibodies, such as thymoglobulin (rabbit antithymocyte globulin [rATG]), are useful as induction agents and are mainstays of induction therapy in renal transplant recipients. Upon binding various T-cell epitopes, rATG lyses leukocytes using complement-dependent pathways and opsonization, leading to mononuclear cell phagocytosis of T cells. rATG also binds to surface receptors on dendritic cells, which impair antigen presentation. Polyclonal antithymocyte globulin is wrought with serious side effects, including a predisposition to posttransplant lymphoproliferative disorder and the cytokine release syndrome.

MAINTENANCE IMMUNOSUPPRESSION

Calcineurin Inhibitors

6 One of the greatest medical discoveries of the 20th century was the identification of the CNIs with their effects on T-cell signaling. This class of agents has potent biologic activity and minimal myelosuppressive effects, which were a significant limitation in early clinical transplantation. CNIs, as a class, disrupt regulatory T-cell signaling and lead to a downregulation of IL-2 production, which eventually decreases the activity of cytotoxic T cells. Antigen presentation at the TCR leads to an increase in cytoplasmic calcium levels through a protein kinase and G-protein reaction within regulatory T cells. This calcium binds to calmodulin, a regulatory subunit of the phosphatase calcineurin, prevalent in immunocompetent lymphocytes and nerve cells. Calcineurin is responsible for cleaving the phosphate bound to NFAT (nuclear factor of activated T cells), which in its activated form traverses the T-cell nuclear membrane and promotes transcription of IL-2. Inhibition of calcineurin occurs through the activation of immunophilins, such as cyclophilin and FK-binding protein, which are endogenous cytosolic peptides. The cyclosporine–cyclophilin complex and its counterpart, the FK506-FKBP12 complex, prevent dephosphorylation of NFAT, which in turn leads to reduced IL-2 production and diminished T-cell signal transduction to effector lymphocytes.[4]

Cyclosporine A was the first of these drugs identified, initially found in a soil sample from the fungus *Tolypocladium inflatum*. The clinical efficacy of cyclosporine A was demonstrated in human kidney transplantation, opening the gates to a new era for clinical organ transplantation. Cyclosporine remained the mainstay of clinical immunosuppression for several years and was used across organ types by thousands of patients. In 1984, FK506 (tacrolimus) was identified as another CNI with a similar mechanism of action. FK506 is a macrolide immunosuppressant that was approved by the U.S. Food and Drug Administration for use in liver transplantation. Tacrolimus has become the mainstay of maintenance immunosuppression in solid organ transplant programs due to a gentler side-effect profile and potency of immunosuppression, and is used in virtually all solid organ types.

CNIs have a variety of side effects that present challenges in the clinical management of transplant recipients. The most significant long-term effects include chronic nephrotoxicity that may precipitate end-stage renal disease, as well as new-onset diabetes mellitus after transplantation. Registry analyses suggest that 7% to 21% of nonrenal transplant recipients are at risk for renal failure, and patients treated with CNIs are at significantly increased risk of requiring dialysis treatment in the months and years after transplant.[5] As implied by the name, calcineurin is also present in nerve tissue as well as lymphocytes. Drug activity in nerve tissue leads to several clinical effects including tremors, seizures, and posterior reversible encephalopathy syndrome. Additional side effects include hyperkalemia, hypercholesterolemia, and gastrointestinal dysfunction, including diarrhea. Cyclosporine has also been associated with gingival hyperplasia which is seen less frequently with tacrolimus. Consultation with a transplant pharmacist is integral to the successful management of the posttransplant patient to prevent toxicity and achieve therapeutic immunosuppression goals.

Steroids

7 Steroids have been a bedrock of immunosuppressive therapy since the beginning of clinical transplantation. Glucocorticoids are steroids that arise from the zona fasciculata in the adrenal gland. These molecules have a plethora of effects in humans, and their receptors are omnipresent across human cell types. In lymphocytes, glucocorticoids act on cytosolic receptors that, in turn, lead to a variety of intracellular signals that are responsible for gene transcription, and decrease the expression of several cytokines, including IL-2. Glucocorticoids also reduce the number and function of both T cells and B cells.

Steroid therapy is used in a variety of clinical treatments, including maintenance immunosuppression and in high doses as a rescue therapy in patients presenting with acute rejection. There are several side effects to chronic corticosteroid use, which have prompted transplant clinicians and researchers to develop protocols that reduce the need for chronic steroid use. Common side effects include glucose intolerance, weight gain, skin and tissue frailty, osteopenia and osteoporosis, muscle breakdown, neuropsychiatric dysfunction, glaucoma and cataracts, secondary hypercortisolemia, and other effects. Many transplant programs are shifting toward steroid avoidance in maintenance immunosuppression in low-risk patients.[6]

mTOR Inhibitors

Like CNIs, mTOR inhibitors lead to decreased IL-2 proliferation. The first discovered mTOR inhibitor was sirolimus. Sirolimus (rapamycin) is a bacterial macrolide derived from *Streptomyces hygroscopicus*, found initially in a soil sample from Easter Island (Rapa Nui). Sirolimus binds to FK-binding protein 12, as does tacrolimus. The site of action of the sirolimus–FKBP12 complex is known as the mammalian target of rapamycin, or mTOR. Despite having structural similarity to tacrolimus, sirolimus has limited activity on calcineurin when bound to FKBP12. The complex disrupts signal transduction of the IL-2 receptor and decreases nuclear transcription of molecules active in lymphocyte homing. Sirolimus also has significant antiproliferative properties and inhibits cell cycle activity in lymphocytes and fibroblasts.

Sirolimus has been adopted in a variety of clinical protocols. Sirolimus is currently used primarily in place of CNIs, most commonly in patients who are weeks to months out from the transplant operation. Sirolimus has less nephrotoxicity than CNIs, but has been associated with a higher risk of acute rejection in some studies. In liver transplantation, conversion from tacrolimus to sirolimus in patients with reduced kidney function was associated with more acute rejection episodes but did not have a tangible benefit in terms of kidney function in a randomized controlled trial. Some have advocated for lower-dose CNIs as maintenance therapy in patients with impaired renal function compared to sirolimus monotherapy, and studies have demonstrated the potential of low-dose CNIs in conjunction with sirolimus for maintenance immunosuppression. Importantly, there is an FDA black box warning against using sirolimus in conjunction with higher-dose CNIs due to higher risk of mortality and graft loss in liver transplantation, as well as an increased risk of hepatic artery thrombosis within the first month after transplant. Everolimus is another mTOR inhibitor approved for use in kidney and liver transplantation with a similar mechanism of action via FKBP12 binding and mTORC1 inhibition. In a multicenter prospective clinical trial, patients with reduced-dose tacrolimus and everolimus had improved GFR at 2 years posttransplant compared to patients on standard tacrolimus-based regimens, without any higher risk of biopsy-proved acute rejection or major side effects.

Sirolimus has been associated with impaired wound healing after transplant, including anastomotic dehiscence in lung transplantation, surgical site infections, and fascial union problems. Surgeons confronted with transplant patients who are on mTOR inhibitors should consult with transplant professionals prior to operative intervention, if possible, in order to guide alterations in immunosuppressive therapy to minimize complications. Several other complications have been noted in patients on mTOR inhibitors. Pulmonary toxicity manifested as pneumonitis has been identified, and caution should be taken in administering the drug to patients with preexisting lung disease. In low- to moderate-risk renal transplant recipients, conversion from tacrolimus to mTOR inhibitors was associated with a higher risk of acute rejection, higher rates of proteinuria, hypercholesterolemia, and anemia.

Antimetabolite Drugs

Antimetabolite drugs in solid organ transplantation comprise a class of agents aimed at suppressing lymphocyte proliferation by reducing the rate of de novo purine synthesis, which prevents effective nucleotide synthesis and DNA transcription. Typically, these drugs are used in combination with CNIs and steroids. One of the first antimetabolite drugs applied in clinical transplantation was azathioprine. While it is effective in reducing T- and B-cell propagation, azathioprine is also a potent suppressive agent of bone marrow, increases the risk of anemia, and is associated with pancreatitis. A newer antimetabolite, mycophenolic acid (MPA), has emerged as a mainstay in solid organ transplantation. MPA was identified in a *Penicillium* fungal species and is hepatically metabolized. MPA has less myelosuppressive activity than azathioprine, but side effects are common.

Myelosuppression and leukopenia are common side effects of this class of agents. Mycophenolate is also associated with a significant risk of gastrointestinal dysfunction, including diarrhea, nausea, and vomiting. Azathioprine has been recognized as a group 1 carcinogen by the National Toxicology Program in the United States, related to length of use and dosage. Mycophenolate should be avoided in pregnancy or in transplant recipients trying to conceive due to the risk of miscarriage and congenital malformations.

Infections after Transplant

Posttransplant infections are directly related to the level of immunosuppression in the host. In the early period after transplant, when levels of immunosuppression are high and proximal to the use of T-cell–depleting induction agents, the risk of opportunistic infection is highest, and management is focused on antimicrobial prophylaxis. Further from transplant, less immunosuppression is typically required, and prophylaxis is not necessary. However, the prevalence and incidence of infectious diseases in solid organ transplant recipients mandate close monitoring of clinical signs and symptoms, and appropriate diagnostic testing when a clinical suspicion arises of a bacterial, viral, parasitic, or fungal infection. Infections after transplant may consist of donor-derived infections transmitted with the organ, recipient-derived infections due to colonization or other pretransplant exposure, nosocomial infections acquired in the healthcare setting, and community-acquired infections. **Figure 33.3** demonstrates the peak incidence of common opportunistic infections as a function of time after transplant. When faced with a transplant patient with a high clinical suspicion of an infection, transplant providers and infectious disease specialists use this information, clinical history, affected organs and systems, and a battery of cause-oriented diagnostic tests to establish the diagnosis and treatment strategy (see **Fig. 33.3**).

Donor-Derived Infections

Deceased organ donors may be exposed to community-acquired infections prior to death, infectious risk related to lifestyle exposures (ie, intravenous drug abuse), as well as nosocomial infections acquired during hospital care. Several infectious transmissions have occurred as a result of donor transmission, including human immunodeficiency virus (HIV), West Nile virus, rabies, Chagas disease, and lymphocytic choriomeningitis virus. Careful attention must be paid to the circumstances surrounding the donor's death as well as reported signs and symptoms such as fever and altered mental status. Prior to organ recovery, organ donors are routinely serologically screened for several infectious pathogens, including HIV, hepatitis, cytomegalovirus (CMV), EBV, and syphilis. Routine blood, urine, and sputum cultures may be used in premortem care. Serologic testing consists of antibody testing, which is not 100% sensitive, but the recent inclusion of nucleic acid testing in many centers may help mitigate risk in organ acceptance and aid patient counseling. In the case of CMV, hepatitis, and EBV serologic testing, serologic matching between donors and recipients drives the perception of posttransplant infectious risk and guides antimicrobial prophylaxis decisions and selection of immunosuppression.

Time from Transplant

<1 month	1–6 months	>6 months
Surgical infections – wound complications, anastomotic/deep space infections Nosocomial infections, *Clostridium difficile* colitis Donor-derived infections: Nosocomial exposures, HSV, LCMV, rabies, West Nile virus, HIV, *Trypanosoma cruzi* Recipient-derived infection (colonization): MRSA, VRE, Candida, Aspergillus, Pseudomonas	With PCP and antiviral (CMV, HBV) prophylaxis: BK polyomavirus infection, *C. Difficile* colitis HCV infection Influenza, adenovirus *Cryptococcus neoformans* infection *Mycobacterium* species infection Anastomotic complications Late donor-derived infections (viral reactivation)	Community-acquired pneumonia, urinary tract infection Infection with Aspergillus, endemic fungal species (*Coccidioidomycosis, Histoplasma,* etc.), molds, Mucormycosis *Nocardia, Rhodococcus* species Late viral infections: CMV HSV encephalitis HBV, HCV SARS, West Nile virus infection JC polyomavirus (PML) EBV-related PTLD (EBV mismatch patients)

Figure 33.3. Timeline of common infections after transplantation. Immunosuppression predisposes transplant recipients to infection by deterring host defenses. In this context, bacterial, viral, and fungal infections may arise, which have distinct peaks of onset. Treatment of these infections usually involves withdrawal or reduction of immunosuppression in most cases, particularly when infections are life threatening or are causing significant morbidity. (Adapted from Fishman JA. Infection in solid-organ transplant recipients. *N Eng J Med.* 2007;357[25]:2601–2614.)

Recipient-Derived Infections

The incidence of posttransplant infections that arises from pretransplant exposure to the recipient is increasingly recognized. Transplanting patients with active infections should be undertaken with extreme caution due to the risk of dissemination of disease with early immunosuppression. Nosocomial pathogens may colonize the recipient prior to transplant, when healthcare utilization may be high due to organ failure, or may infect patients at any point after transplant. Pathogens may acquire antibiotic resistance, which may make treatment difficult, such as in cases with vancomycin-resistant *Enterococcus*, methicillin-resistant *Staphylococcus*, azole-resistant *Candida*, as well as in *Clostridium difficile* colitis, several gram-negative enteric pathogens, and fungi. Recipient exposure via travel or residence in geographically endemic areas can also be a risk for infection (fungal infections such as histoplasmosis, aspergillosis, coccidioidomycosis, atypical bacterial infections such as *Mycobacterium tuberculosis*, parasitic infections caused by *Strongyloides* or *Trypanosoma cruzi*), as well as reactivation of dormant viruses (hepatitis, CMV, or varicella-zoster virus). Exposures to relatively benign pathogens may result in major infections after transplant. Respiratory viruses may further weaken natural tissue defenses in the bronchopulmonary tree and lead to superinfection with other pathogens. Fungal infections derived from the soil, such as *Nocardia* or *Aspergillus* may arise in this fashion and require changes in immunosuppression to prevent exacerbation of infection. Common posttransplant infections are listed in **Figure 33.4.**

Pathogen	Site of Disease	Disease Manifestations	Prophylaxis	Treatment
Cytomegalovirus (CMV)	CNS, respiratory, GI tract, bone marrow	Fever, neutropenia, pneumonitis, diarrhea, mucosal ulceration, chorioretinitis, meningoencephalitis, graft dysfunction	Low-risk patients: Acyclovir High-risk patients: Valganciclovir	Valganciclovir Ganciclovir CMV-immunoglobulin Minimization of immunosuppression
Epstein–Barr Virus (EBV)	Bone marrow, spleen, CNS	B-cell–derived post transplant lymphoproliferative disease (PTLD)	Antiviral prophylaxis such as acyclovir or valganciclovir	Minimization of immunosuppression Chemotherapy Radiation therapy (CNS) Anti-CD20 antibody therapies
BK Virus	Kidney	Renal Dysfunction	None	Minimization of immunosuppression Experimental antiviral therapies (cidofovir)
Pneumocystis	Respiratory	Pneumonia/pneumonitis	Trimethoprim/ sulfamethoxazole Pentamidine Dapsone	

Figure 33.4. Common infections after transplantation, prophylaxis, and treatment strategies. After transplant, while predisposed to multiple infections related to immunosuppression, certain infections are particularly common and virulent. Clinical decisions regarding prophylaxis against these pathogens and how this affects immunosuppression are key decision points in managing the posttransplant patient.

Cancer

Chronic immunosuppressive therapy weakens host defenses against neoplastic processes. There is well-established evidence that solid organ transplant recipients of every type have an increased risk of malignancy, both related to immunosuppression and oncogenic viral infections. The most common cancers incurred by solid organ transplant recipients are skin cancers, followed by posttransplant lymphoproliferative disease. In this context, posttransplant patients are strongly recommended to have yearly skin examinations by a dermatologist. Screening for malignancy in chronically immunosuppressed patients follows general screening guidelines. Treatment of cancers is driven by site and extent of disease, but in all cases includes reduction in the amount of immunosuppression.

ACKNOWLEDGMENTS

We gratefully acknowledge the contributions of previous edition authors, Amit K. Mathur and Satish N. Nadig, as portions of those chapters have been retained in this revision.

References

1. Djamali A, Kaufman DB, Ellis TM, Zhong W, Matas A, Samaniego M. Diagnosis and management of antibody-mediated rejection: current status and novel approaches. *Am J Transplant.* 2014;14(2): 255–271.
2. Kirk AD. Induction immunosuppression. *Transplantation.* 2006; 82(5):593–602.
3. Penninga L, Wettergren A, Wilson CH, Chan AW, Steinbrüchel DA, Gluud C. Antibody induction versus corticosteroid induction for liver transplant recipients. *Cochrane Database Syst Rev.* 2014;(5): CD010252.
4. Warty V, Diven W, Cadoff E, Todo S, Starzl T, Sanghvi A. FK506: a novel immunosuppressive agent. Characteristics of binding and uptake by human lymphocytes. *Transplantation.* 1988;46(3): 453–455.
5. Ojo AO, Held PJ, Port FK, et al. Chronic renal failure after transplantation of a nonrenal organ. *N Eng J Med.* 2003;349(10):931–940.
6. Pascual J, Zamora J, Galeano C, et al. Steroid avoidance or withdrawal for kidney transplant recipients. *Cochrane Database Syst Rev.* 2009;(1):CD005632.

Organ Retrieval and Preservation

Mary T. Killackey and Kiara A. Tulla

Key Points

1 Despite advances in survival and expanded indications for transplant, the gap between organ availability and organ supply persists.

2 Efforts to expand organ donation are critical to save lives. Organ donation must be done within a regulated system that is deeply rooted in ethical standards of care.

3 A balance must be maintained between using every viable donor organ and ensuring each patient a chance of successful posttransplant outcome.

4 Organ retrieval requires coordination of a multidisciplinary team including surgeons, anesthesiologists, nurses, and organ perfusion technicians. Careful retrieval and perfusion techniques are necessary for a successful outcome.

5 Organ retrieval and storage result in significant alterations in the homeostasis of the organ. The degree of organ preservation injury contributes to organ dysfunction. Current trials aim to rehabilitate injured or otherwise discarded organs.

1 Organ transplantation has become the standard of care for end-organ failure, and often it is the only lifesaving therapy available. The gap between organ availability and organ supply has continued to be at a deficit to the expanding waitlist patient population. From 2012 to 2022, more solid transplants have been performed than ever before in the United States with an increase of greater than 50% for heart, lung, kidney, and liver transplants.[1] The total number of transplants has been increasing, surpassing 41,000 in 2022, due in large part to the increase in opioid-related deaths and the support of living donation year after year.[1] Yet the disparity continues as a new patient is added to the waitlist every 10 minutes and on average, 22 patients die each day waiting for transplant (**Fig. 34.1A,B**).[2]

ORGAN DONATION (FIG. 34.2)

Living Donation

Considering high waitlist mortality and long wait times, early transplant for patients with end-organ failure has significant benefits. For example, patients who receive a kidney transplant prior to initiating dialysis (a preemptive transplant) have a lower rate of allograft failure and mortality and a higher quality of life compared to patients who receive a transplant after beginning dialysis (**Table 34.1**).[3] Five-year graft survival after living-donor kidney transplant (LDKT) compared with deceased-donor kidney transplants (DDKT) was 90.0% versus 81.4% for recipients aged 18 to 34 years and 80.8% versus 67.8% for recipients aged 65 years or older, respectively.[1]

In the United States, 23% of liver and kidney transplants utilize living-donor organs. In certain parts of the world, living donation predominates due to multiple ethnic, social, cultural, and religious factors, as well as weak regional networks and infrastructure, resulting in low rates of deceased donation. Living donation has been in a steady decline since 2004, however, with recent intentional efforts to increase living donation, the annual volume of living donors has increased and reached a new peak in 2019 (**Table 34.2**).[1]

In paired kidney exchange programs, donor–recipient pairs that were previously determined to be incompatible can swap donors with another pair if appropriately matched by blood type, HLA type, and antibody sensitization (**Fig. 34.3**). Living donors must be excellent surgical candidates with minimal

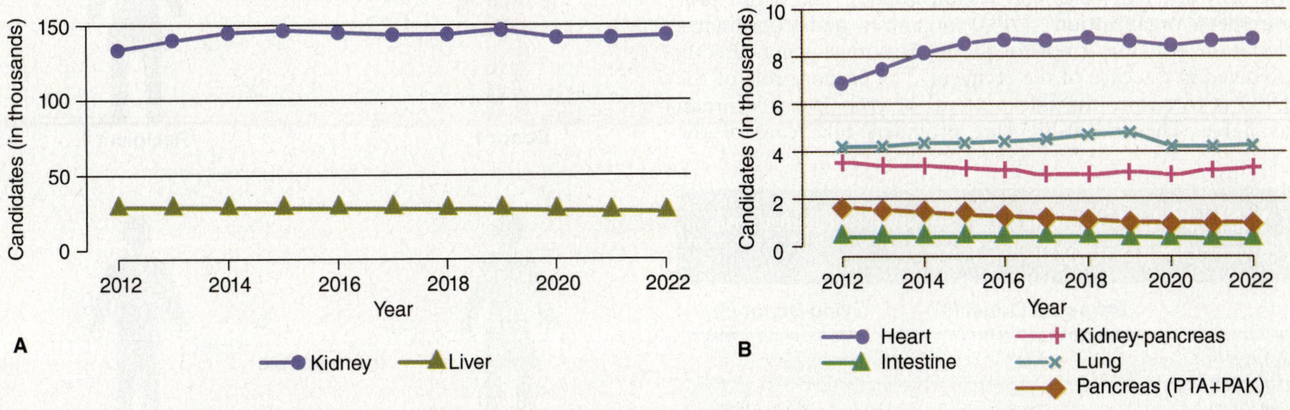

Figure 34.1. Active candidates on the UNOS waitlist as of 12/31/2022 by organ.[1] (Data from UNOS.)

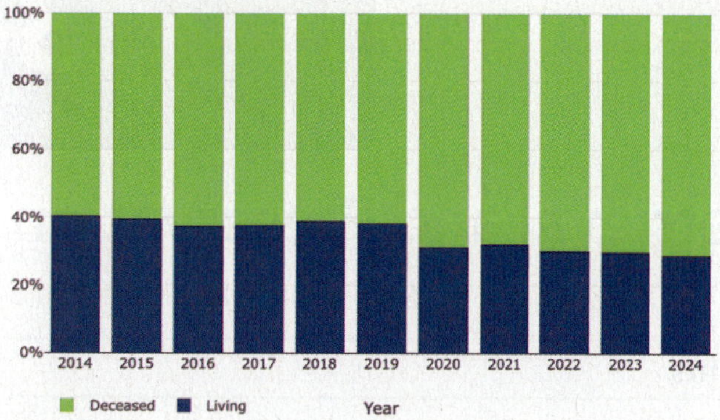

Figure 34.2. National Donors by Type[1] (Data from OPTN Metrics. Accessed September 2024. https://insights.unos.org/OPTN-metrics/)

medical comorbidities and a stable psychosocial assessment. Regulations are in place to ensure the donors have not been coerced.

Deceased Donation

In 2022, in the United States, the majority (>80%) of organs used for transplantation were from deceased donation. There was a 7.5% increase in the number of donors from 2012, with a similar increase in organs utilized from those donors. The COVID-19 pandemic did change the landscape of transplantation, donation, and offer acceptance. The number of patients listed for kidney transplant has decreased, but the number of new candidates that are listing each month is returning to the pre-COVID numbers. Organ discard didn't dramatically increase. There is a notable increase in donation after circulatory death (DCD), rising to 32.1% of deceased donors, but the rate is lagging from international peers, where DCD rates are rising due to change in donation policies and the utilization of normothermic regional perfusion (NRP).[1,4]

Declaration of Death

In the United States, a patient is considered dead when they have irreversible cessation of brain function (brain death) or irreversible cessation of circulatory and respiratory functions (DCD). The definition of brain death is established locally by hospitals using rules that conform to the *Harvard Criteria* and comply with the Uniform Determination of Death Act (UDDA).[5] Donation increased in 2010, when the American Academy of Neurology updated its established guidelines for determination of death (**Table 34.3**).[6] Donors who are declared brain dead are supported to allow for the organs to maintain perfusion before and during the procurement process.

In deceased donation cases, the division of labor amongst the stakeholders in the transplant and donation process is ascribed different roles and responsibilities. The organ procurement organization (OPO) organizes and coordinates donation, which is a not-for-profit entity that is not directly involved in the care of the recipient. The primary role of the OPO is to ensure the safe retrieval of every possible organ available. The end-of-life care providers take care of the patient and declare they to then allow the transplant or recovery team to participate in the recovery of the organs for donation (**Fig. 34.4**).

If a donor is not determined to be brain dead, but has sustained irreversible neurologic injury, these patients can become donors when they lose cardiopulmonary function to allow declaration of death. Following family wishes, ventilatory and circulatory support are withdrawn. The patient is declared dead by the end-of-life caring physician upon cessation of circulation. Each hospital establishes policies and procedures for retrieval of DCD donor organs, and it is critical that members of the transplant teams are not involved in the process of declaration of death. After declaration, 2 to 5 minutes must elapse prior to the organ recovery surgery. If the patient does not reach criteria for death within 120 minutes, most organ recovery efforts are stopped, and the patient is able to pass with continued end-of-life care. The maximal time that is used for each organ varies due to ischemic injury and organ recovery metrics. Kidneys can still have reasonable functional recovery with a functional warm ischemia time (time from a donor withdrawal to cold perfusion flushing) as high as 120 minutes long, while organs like the liver, can only tolerate shorter times (20 to 30 minutes) due to the long-term ischemic consequences. Traditionally, the transplant team rapidly recovers the organs (**Fig. 34.5**).

Advances in Donation after Circulatory Death: Advent of Normothermic Regional Perfusion (NRP)

DCD organs, due to the additional hypoxia during organ recovery, have decreased graft survival; however, standardized techniques have allowed for improvements in organ and patient outcomes.[7] To increase organ availability, an international push opened the idea of recirculating blood in the

Table 34.1. Five-Year Graft Survival of Kidney and Liver Transplant by Donor Type

	Deceased Donor (%)	Living Donor (%)
Liver	71.9	77.3
Kidney	74.4	85.6

From OPTN National Data Report: Survival Rates for Transplant Performed 2008–2015. Accessed January 20, 2020. https://optn.transplant.hrsa.gov/data/view-data-reports/national-data/

Table 34.2. Efforts to Increase Living Donation in the Last Decade

- Improved public education from transplant centers
- Utilization of social media to connect potential pairs
- Transplant center participation in local and/or national paired exchange programs
- Development of protocols for immunologically high-risk transplants

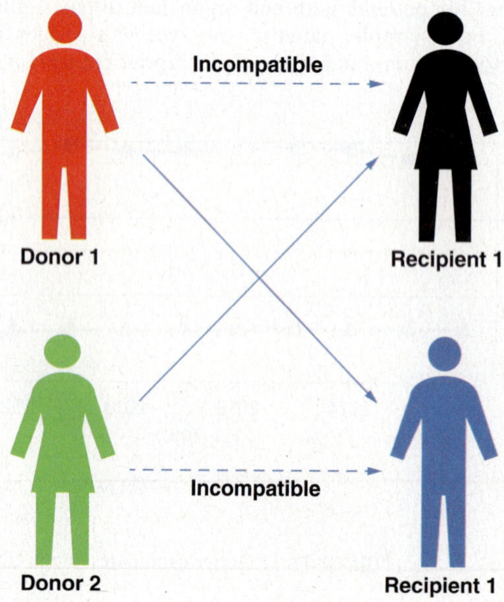

Figure 34.3. Schematic for paired exchange kidney transplant.

Table 34.3. Criteria for Brain Death

- All reversible causes of coma excluded
  - Hypothermia
  - Shock
  - Severe electrolyte abnormality
  - Pharmacologic sedation or paralysis
- Loss of all function of the entire brain, including brain stem[a]
  - No response to noxious stimuli
  - No pupillary light reflex
  - No corneal reflex
  - No oculocephalic reflex
  - No gag reflex
  - No spontaneous respirations
- Preferred confirmatory diagnostic tests (one must be completed)
  - Cerebral angiogram (gold standard)
  - EEG
  - Nuclear medicine perfusion scan

[a]In the United States, one neurologic examination is sufficient in most states.
Data from Wijdicks E, Varelas P, Gronseth G, Greer DM; American Academy of Neurology. Evidence-based guideline update: determining brain death in adults. *Neurology.* 2010;74(23):1911–1918.

donor body after declaration of death in DCD recoveries to allow for reduction in the effects of reperfusion injury and ischemia coined as NRP. NRP occurs immediately after the 2 to 5 minutes after the declaration of death in a DCD organ retrieval case. The arterial and venous cannulas for extracorporeal recirculation of blood centrally or peripherally are started after the ligation of the cerebral vasculature or the occlusion of the supraceliac aorta (**Fig. 34.6**) to restore oxygenated, pulsatile warm blood to the donor organs available for recovery.

In 1989, a porcine DCD model with NRP demonstrated improved liver and kidney graft viability when compared to traditional rapid recovery DCD.[8] During the period of functional warm ischemia, ATP declines progressively; during NRP, cellular energy increases due to partial restoration of ATP content, therefore, an ischemic conditioning effect can be observed.[9] NRP with DCD donors[4] are progressively showing improved graft and patient survival outcomes.[10]

However, the ethical question of whether DCD recovery with NRP violates the UDDR spurred a desire to edit the law. Two arguments support how the practice is in line with the ethical rule:[11] (1) organ procurement does not cause or interrupt the trajectory to death, (2) death is the loss of the organism's capacity to function as an integrated whole (the interrelated system consisting of the brain, heart, and lungs), with the brain at its core. By not restoring flow to the brain, the integral being is not restored.[11] However, the dilemma lies in how NRP allows for restarting circulation, causing what was just declared to be the irreversible cessation of circulatory and respiratory function to be reversed. Because of the concerns by experts regarding the UDDA's shortcomings, efforts by the Uniform Law Commission (ULC) in 2021 created a committee to edit the law; however, the efforts were paused in September of 2023 as the feasibility of enacting change was questioned.

Consent for Donation

Permission for organ donation is obtained from the patient's next of kin prior to organ donation. Organized efforts over the past several decades have resulted in more than 60% of the U.S. adult population registered as an organ, eye, or tissue donor, often associated with driving licensure.[12] A signed and witnessed organ donor card is sufficient indication of the decedent's wishes to allow organ donation. Despite this declaration, the family's consent is routinely obtained even when a valid organ donor card is present. In conjunction with the OPO, many hospitals have trained specialists who approach families to consent to donation. Explanation of the organ donation process by a trained and empathetic party not directly involved in the care of the deceased patient yields the highest consent rates.

Organ Allocation

2 Considering the desperate need for lifesaving organs, regulations are necessary to ensure fair and equitable distribution across populations. In 2018, a lawsuit was filed arguing the current system of distribution violated federal law. The United Network for Organ Sharing (UNOS) was ordered to remove artificial geographic boundaries from the organ allocation policy in 2019.[13]

Organ allocation schemes have transitioned to acuity circles (AC) distribution policies rather than regional systems started in February 2020 for liver donors. Using concentric circles capturing candidates from a specific geographic distance from the donor hospital can improve equity in organ distribution. Data supports that waitlist mortality has neither been improved nor worsened since its implementation. With time, the hope is that this model will provide more equity nationally.[14]

ORGAN SELECTION

3 Organ quality is closely linked to recipient outcomes. A careful balance must be maintained between using every viable organ and ensuring the best possible outcome for each recipient.

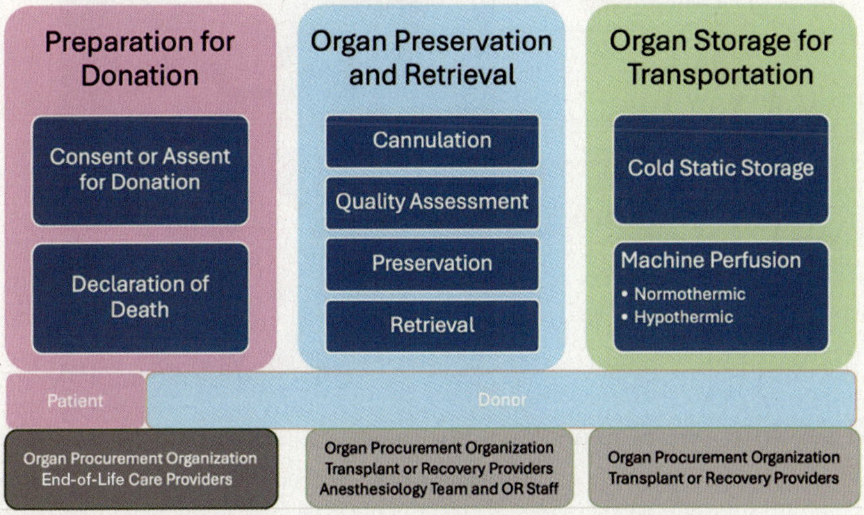

Figure 34.4. Stages of organ donations.

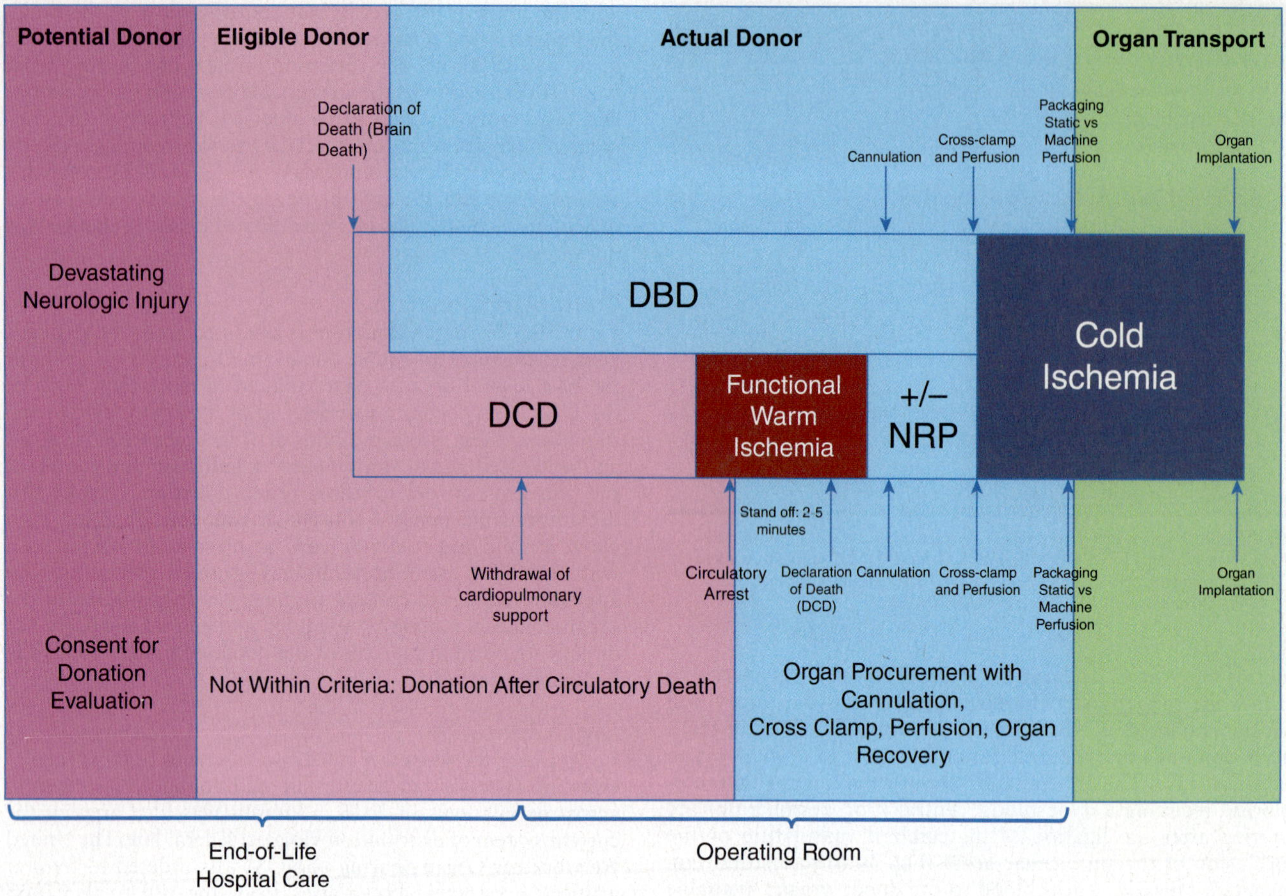

Figure 34.5. Brain dead versus donation after circulatory death timelines.

Donor History of Cancer

Potential organ donors should be free of cancer as transmission to the organ recipient may result in early death related to cancer progression in the setting systemic immunosuppression. For most major cancers associated with systemic progression, organ donors should be disease free for 5 years. Some donor cancers have been shown to have minimal risk of transmission to the recipient. These include nonmelanoma skin cancers without nodal involvement, small renal cell and prostate cancers, and many intracranial malignancies that have not recently had surgical intervention. Donors with a history of melanoma, leukemia, lymphoma, or small-cell carcinoma are excluded from donation. Criteria and guidelines for suitability for donation among cancer survivors are well detailed in the literature.[12]

Donor History of Infectious Disease

All donors are screened for transmissible disease, and the recipients must be tested prior to and after transplant (**Tables 34.4 and 34.5**).[15] Risk criteria and donor behavior questions have

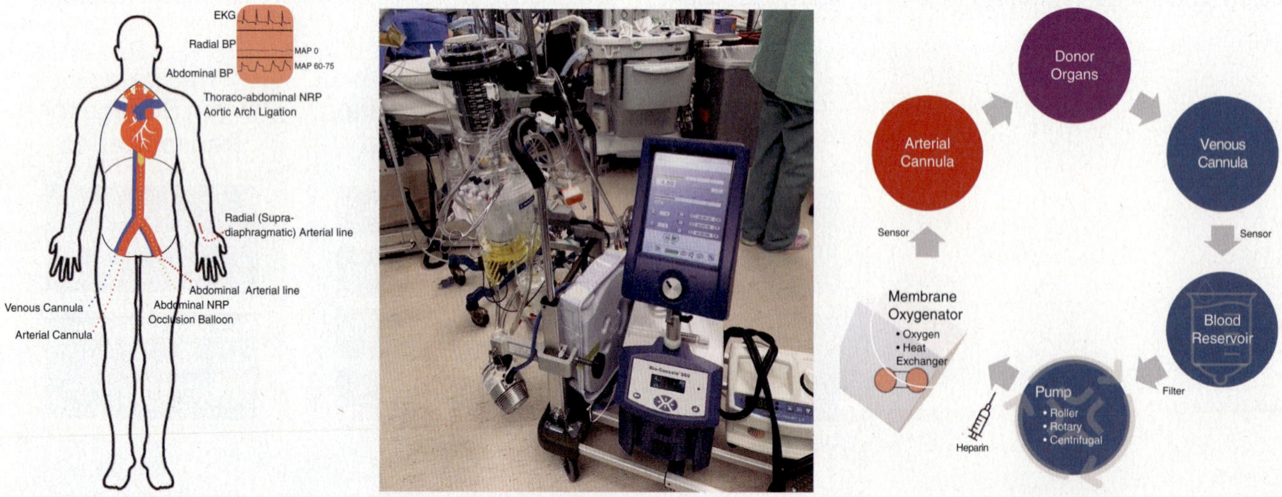

A: Depiction of Peripheral Cannulation B: Picture of compact portable circuit C: Depiction of circuit components

Figure 34.6. Normothermic regional perfusion (NRP).

Table 34.4. Conditions That Are Transmitted by Donor to Recipients

- Infections
  - Syndromes
    - Unknown infection of central nervous system (encephalitis, meningitis)
    - Multisystem organ failure due to overwhelming sepsis
  - Bacterial infections
    - Bacterial meningitis
    - Bacteremia
    - Pneumonia
    - Syphilis
    - Tuberculosis
  - Fungal infections
    - Endemic mycoses: blastomycosis, histoplasmosis, coccidioidomycosis
    - Cryptococcal infection
    - Fungal sepsis (eg, *Candidemia*)
  - Parasitic infections
    - *Trypanosoma cruzi*
    - *Leishmania*
    - *Naegleria fowleri*
    - Strongyloides
    - Toxoplasmosis
  - Viral infections
    - Active hepatitis A, B, or C
    - Herpes simplex encephalitis or documented viremia
    - Human immunodeficiency virus/AIDS
    - HTLV-I
    - History of JC virus infection (progressive multifocal leukoencephalopathy)
    - West Nile virus infection
    - Cryptococcal infection of any site
    - Rabies
    - SARS, MERS-CoV, influenza
  - Prion disease, including Creutzfeldt–Jakob disease
- Malignancies
  - Melanoma, Merkel cell, and Kaposi sarcoma
  - Hodgkin disease and non-Hodgkin lymphoma
  - Multiple myeloma
  - Leukemia
  - Aplastic anemia agranulocytosis
    - Any historic malignancies
- Others: Inborn errors of metabolism, drug or food allergies

Data summarized from Theodoropoulos N, Ison MG. Donor-derived infections: incidence, prevention, and management. *Transpl Infect.* 2016:113–127.

Table 34.5. Updated U.S. Public Health Service Guideline 2020 for Assessing Solid Organ Donors and Monitoring Transplant Recipients for Infectious Diseases (HIV, Hepatitis B and C)

Risk Assessment of Living and Deceased Donors—Risk criteria (during the 30 days before organ procurement):

1. Sex (ie, any method of sexual contact, including vaginal, anal, and oral) with a person known or suspected to have HIV, HBV, or HCV infection
2. Man who has had sex with another man
3. Sex in exchange for money or drugs
4. Sex with a person who had sex in exchange for money or drugs
5. Drug injection for nonmedical reasons
6. Sex with a person who injected drugs for nonmedical reasons
7. Incarceration (confinement in jail, prison, or juvenile correction facility) for ≥72 consecutive hours
8. Child breastfed by a mother with HIV infection
9. Child born to a mother with HIV, HBV, or HCV infection
10. Unknown medical or social history

Living and deceased solid organ donor testing AND Recipient Testing:

- HIV: NAT and anti-HIV (antigen/antibody combination [4th generation]) immunoassay (HIV-1/2 ab and HIV-1 p24 antigen)
- HBV: NAT, anti-HBc, HBsAg, anti-HBs
- HCV: NAT and anti-HCV

Timing of Testing:

- Deceased donor: collected within 96 hours before organ procurement with results of available at the time of organ procurement.
- Living Donor: as close to surgery as possible with a maximum of 28 days of transplant
- Pre-Transplant Recipient: Prior to transplant during hospital admission
- Post-Transplant Recipient: 4–6 weeks post-transplant

anti-HBc, antibodies to hepatitis B virus core antigen; anti-HCV, antibodies to hepatitis C virus; anti-HIV-1/2, antibodies to HIV-1/2; HbsAg, hepatitis B surface antigen; HBV, hepatitis B virus; HCV, hepatitis C virus; HIV, human immunodeficiency virus; IRD, increased risk donor; OPO, organ procurement organization; NAT, nucleic acid testing.

This is a summary of the guidelines modifications for risk criteria that were published in Jones JM, Kracalik I, Levi ME, et al. Assessing solid organ donors and monitoring transplant recipients for human immunodeficiency virus, hepatitis B virus, and hepatitis C virus infection – U.S. Public Health Service Guideline, 2020. *MMWR Recomm Rep.* 2020;69(4):1–16.

been modified based on data from infectious transmissions and clearer guidance was delineated in the 2020 update.[16] Any risk criteria information is discussed with recipients during the informed consent process, and contextualized as the risk of donor transmission to recipients is incredibly low and transplantation is lifesaving.[17]

Treated systemic bacteremia is acceptable in most cases, while donors who have had recent fungemia or untreatable viral illnesses are passed in many cases. The transplant center needs to follow donor culture data and make sure that the recipient is appropriately treated.

Donors with active hepatitis B virus (HBV) (surface antigen positive) are excluded from transplant; however, those with a previous history of hepatitis B infection (core antibody positive) can be used in recipients who have been immunized against HBV. Depending on the organ and the recipient serology, they may antiviral therapy.

With the development of highly effective antiviral regimens over the last decade, and current literature supporting the utilization of HCV viral-positive donors in patients who are HCV naïve, most transplant programs accept these organs for transplant. Detailed informed consent is essential, and access to the antiviral therapy with the intent to treat for cure is paramount.[18]

The HOPE Act, which was passed in 2015 allows HIV-positive donors to be used for donation to HIV positive recipients as part of IRB-approved research protocols. This legislation allowed the transplantation of these organs and recipients exclusively at specific transplant hospital defined by the NIH and approved by the Organ Procurement Transplant Network (OPTN).[19]

Rare and highly infections pathogens should be discussed with a transplant infectious disease expert prior to accepting any questionable organ offer. Understanding donor and recipient cytomegalovirus (CMV), Epstein–Barr virus (EBV), herpes virus (HSV), and more are just a few infections that affect prophylaxis for prevention of reactivation or worsening infections posttransplant.

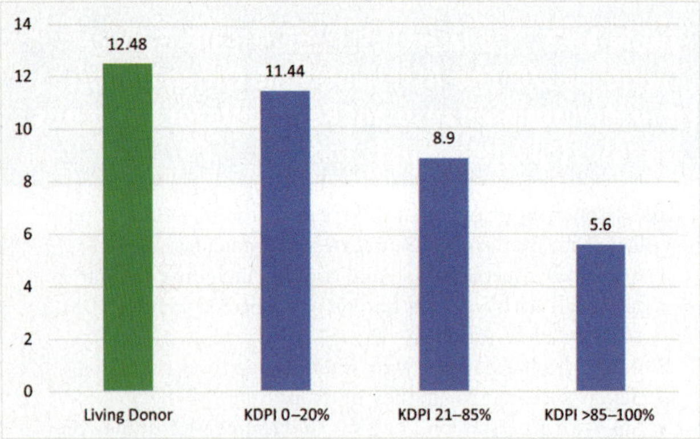

Figure 34.7. Estimated graft half-lives (years) by KDPI as compared to living-donor transplant.

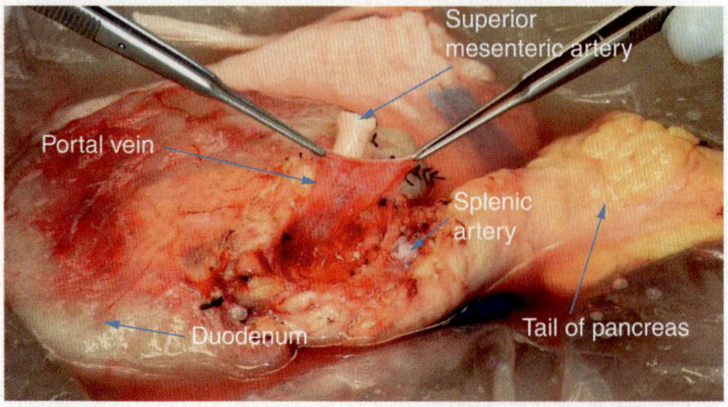

Figure 34.8. Pancreas allograft following procurement, with ample length of portal vein, superior mesenteric artery, and splenic artery.

Organ-Specific Issues

All donors are subject to a global assessment, including age, medical history, social history, and cause of death. Each organ has specific considerations:

Kidney

In 2014, the kidney allocation system (KAS) was significantly revised and included a continuous metric known as the Kidney Donor Profile Index (KDPI) to better capture kidney quality. This number combines a variety of donor factors to estimate the likelihood of graft failure after deceased donor transplant (**Fig. 34.7**) This included an expected posttransplant survival (EPTS, defined by age, time on dialysis, diabetes status, and prior organ transplants) into the matching criteria, and increased the prioritization of patients who were highly sensitized. Priority was given to patients listed based on time with end-organ failure rather than time of listing.[20]

Informed consent is required to be listed for high KDPI organs and both renal biopsies (read by renal pathologist, >16% glomerular sclerosis is associated with graft failure), assessing for glomerular fibrosis, and organ preservation pumping, assessing for circulatory resistance, can aid in graft selection. Kidneys may be preserved for up to 36 hours, preferably within 24 hours.

Liver

Up-to-date donor liver function and graft size are essential considerations for liver transplant success. A liver biopsy is frequently available from donors with risk factors for liver disease. Greater than 30% macrosteatosis with or without parenchymal fibrosis (septate) may preclude use for transplantation. More than a grade 2 liver laceration generally precludes transplantation. Greater than 10% diffuse necrosis and severe macroangiopathy are also avoided. Efforts should be made to keep the CIT to less than 12 hours, preferably within 4 to 6 hours.

Pancreas

Selection of pancreas allografts must be done with care since recipient complications are common and can be fatal. Donors ideally should be less than 40 years old and be free of major comorbidities. On inspection, the pancreas should be soft without significant fat infiltration or parenchymal edema. Donor iliac vessels used for the vascular conduit should be free of atherosclerotic disease. Pancreatic branches from the splenic and superior mesenteric arteries must be intact (**Fig. 34.8**) with care to identify the drainage of the inferior pancreaticoduodenal artery (IPDA) for adequate collateral circulation to the head of the pancreas. Injury to pancreatic parenchyma precludes use of the organ. Efforts should be made to keep the cold ischemia time (CIT) to less than 12 hours.

Heart

Heart allografts area assessed via an echocardiogram as significant structural cardiac disease or abnormal cardiac function precludes donation. Donors with risk factors for cardiac disease undergo cardiac catheterization to rule out significant coronary artery disease. The relationship between the donor and recipient body size should be considered. Prior to retrieval, the procuring surgeon should examine the beating heart for size and function before the recipient surgeon begins the heart transplant operation. Efforts should be made to keep the CIT to less than 4 hours.

Lungs

Initial assessment of lung donors must determine if there is a history of smoking or pulmonary disease and must consider the events surrounding death (ie, aspiration or accident with chest injury). Predonation workup includes chest x-rays, arterial blood gases, CT scan, and a bronchoscopy with airway cultures. Lung contusions or pneumonia may preclude transplantation. Donors are ventilated on 100% oxygen to assure high blood oxygen levels. The relationship between the donor and recipient body size is considered. At the time of retrieval, the donor surgeon performs a repeat bronchoscopy and a median sternotomy to physically inspect the lungs for damage, infection, underlying lung disease, or masses. Efforts should be made to keep the CIT to less than 6 hours.

THE ORGAN RETRIEVAL OPERATION

4 The organ retrieval operation requires coordination of a multidisciplinary team including surgeons, anesthesiologists, nurses, and organ perfusion technicians. By convention, transplant centers send their own teams to procure the heart, liver, lungs, and pancreas, however, with the COVID pandemic and use of normothermic and machine perfusion, the use of local recovery teams or recovery surgeons has increased in adoption and utility. The kidneys are procured by one of the abdominal teams and are shipped to the appropriate transplant center. In most cases, retrieval teams travel to the hospital where the donor is admitted; both air and ground transportation are usually required. With more regularity, the donors are transported to a centralized retrieval facility or hospital. This has been shown to reduce costs, travel time, and CITs.[21] The recipient liver, lung, and heart operations usually begin before organs return to the transplant center; thus, continuous communication and coordination are needed between transplant centers and the recovery teams.

Upon arrival in the donor operating room, the transplant surgeon must check the appropriate documentation. This includes identification of the donor, consent for donation, and the donor's medical chart. The surgery team should discuss hemodynamic and anticoagulation management with the anesthesia team. The donor is placed supine with the arms

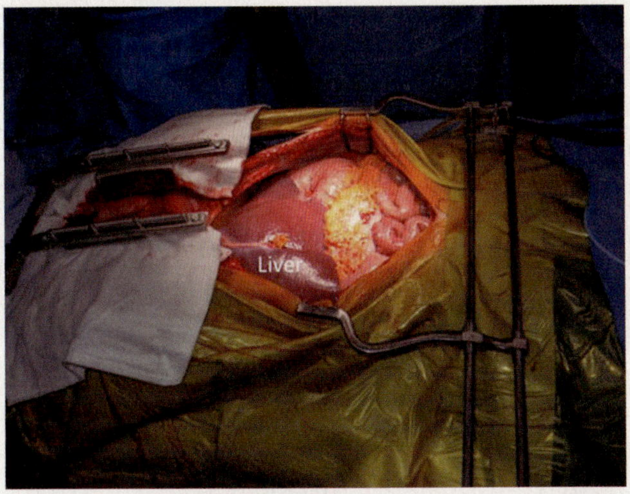

Figure 34.9. Procurement incision/exposure allowing for inspection of thoracic and abdominal cavities.

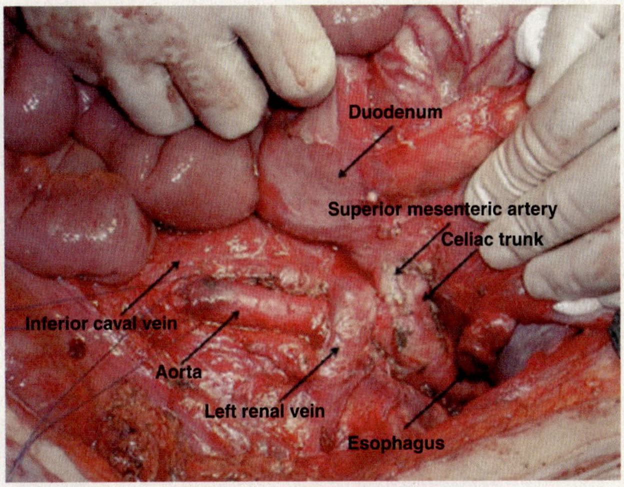

Figure 34.11. Exposure of retroperitoneum following Kocher and Cattell maneuvers.

tucked to facilitate multiple teams working on the donor simultaneously. Prior to incision, it is common to observe a moment of silence to honor the donor and the magnitude of the act of giving. An incision is made from the sternal notch to the symphysis pubis; the abdomen and sternum are opened, and the cavities inspected for gross pathologic disease that would contraindicate donation (**Fig. 34.9**). The key organ-specific steps are detailed below. Of note, the steps are described below as they are done in the brain-dead donor for ease of understanding, during DCD and NRP recoveries, all the same steps are completed as well, but the order and timing of the steps vary.

Heart and Lung Retrieval

A bronchoscopy is done to examine anatomy, remove secretions, and rule out pneumonia. The sternum is opened, and a chest retractor is placed. The thymus gland is dissected, and the innominate vein is identified. The pericardium is incised, and stay sutures are placed. The aorta is mobilized, freeing it from the main pulmonary artery and the right pulmonary artery. The superior and inferior vena cava (IVC) are mobilized. The chest and abdominal teams must agree on where to transect the IVC.

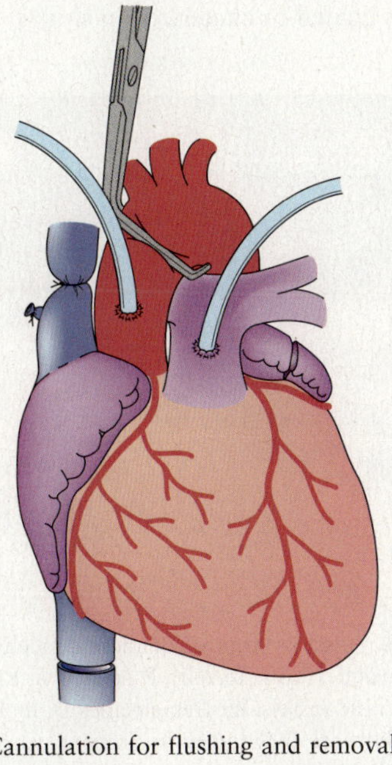

Figure 34.10. Cannulation for flushing and removal of heart then lungs.

When all teams are ready, systemic heparin is administered and the organs are preserved and removed (**Fig. 34.10** and **Table 34.4**).

Liver Retrieval

Prior to coordinated cold storage perfusion, the right colon and small bowel are mobilized to expose the entirety of the retroperitoneum, including the IVC and aorta. The inferior mesenteric vein (IMV) is identified and cannulated for eventual portal perfusion. The superior mesenteric artery is identified and may be encircled at the root of the mesentery close to the aorta (**Fig. 34.11**). The gallbladder is opened, and the bile is removed. The left lateral segment of the liver is mobilized, and the gastrohepatic ligament is inspected for a replaced or accessory left hepatic artery. If an artery is noted, the surgeon must carefully dissect all the branches from the proximal left gastric artery, staying close to the lesser curvature of the stomach. The porta hepatis is palpated to assess the location of the arteries. If present, a replaced right hepatic artery is noted to the right and posterior to the common bile duct (**Fig. 34.12**).

The aorta is dissected at its bifurcation to facilitate proximal and distal control (**Fig. 34.10**). The surgeon should assure that there are no renal arteries from the distal aorta or iliac arteries. If there are, the cannulation should occur distal to these arteries to make sure they are flushed. The supraceliac aorta is exposed by retracting the caudate lobe and the left lateral segment of the liver to the right, grasping the crux of the diaphragm, and dividing it with electrocautery. Sufficient exposure of the supraceliac aorta is needed for occlusive clamping (**Fig. 34.13**). When all teams are ready and heparin is administered, the aorta is clamped, and ice is placed into both cavities (**Fig. 34.14**). The abdominal surgeon works simultaneously with the thoracic surgeon (**Table 34.5**).

Arterial anatomy has many variations, and failure to identify the variation may jeopardize the transplant operation (**Fig. 34.9**). On occasion, dissection of the replaced right hepatic artery can jeopardize the pancreas allograft, but usually both teams can agree to an acceptable dissection plane. The reconstruction of the replaced right hepatic artery can be done in many ways; most common anastomotic variations include superior mesenteric artery (SMA), gastroduodenal artery (GDA), or splenic artery with the celiac artery as inflow.

Kidney Retrieval

Kidney retrieval is the final step in the procurement operation. It is important to identify the SMA to avoid injury to the renal arteries during recovery of both kidneys.

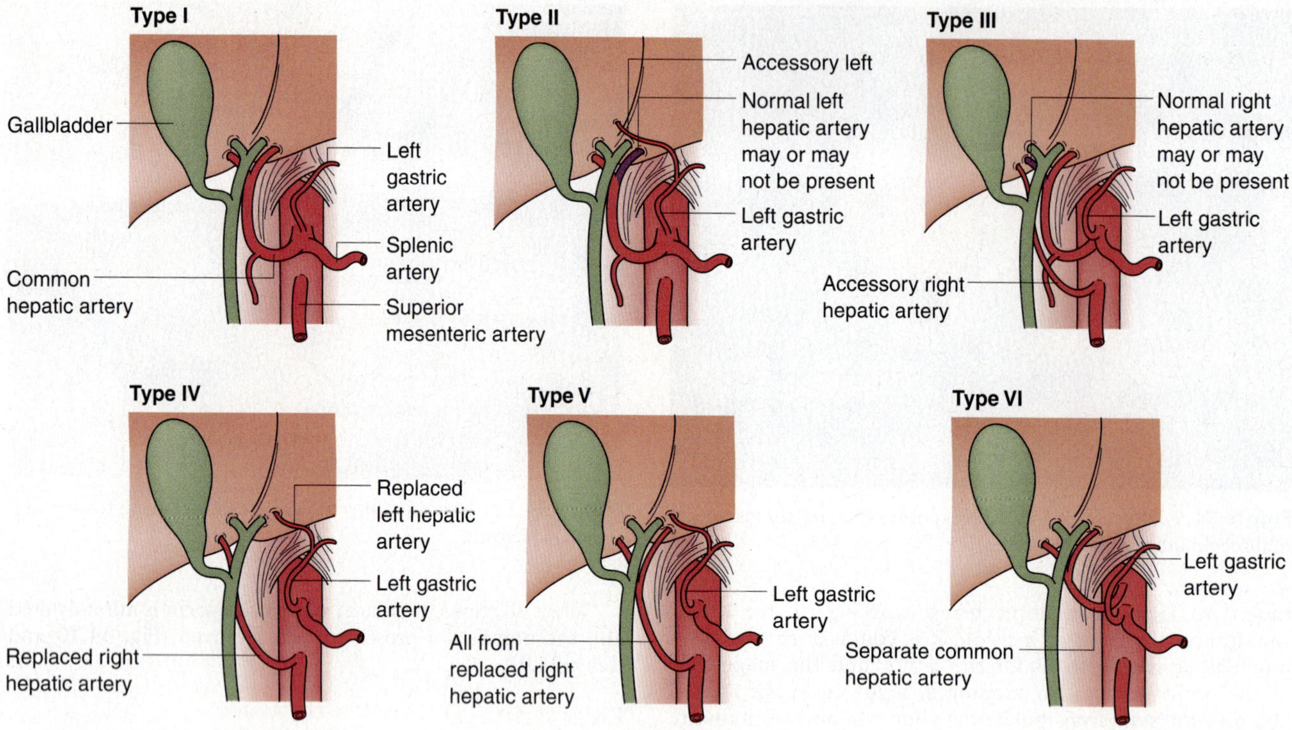

Figure 34.12. Variations in hepatic arterial anatomy. Lack of identification of this anatomy may jeopardize the transplant operation.

Prior to perfusion, the kidneys are mobilized posteriorly to facilitate packing with ice at the time of the cold perfusion. After flushing, the ureters are divided bilaterally in the pelvis and mobilized upward toward the kidney. The periureteral tissue should be left intact to maintain sufficient blood supply to the ureter. The IVC and the aorta are divided at the iliac bifurcation, and the two vasculatures, along with the ureters, are retracted superiorly, and the tissue posterior to the vessels is incised. The left renal vein is divided at the level of the IVC, leaving the entire IVC with the right kidney to allow for extension of the short right renal vein utilizing the cava. If the donors are <35 kg or the kidneys smaller than 8 cm in size, the kidneys can be explanted together along with a piece of bladder to allow for en bloc implantation, at the discretion of the recipient surgeon. The kidneys are placed in cold storage or on a perfusion pump.

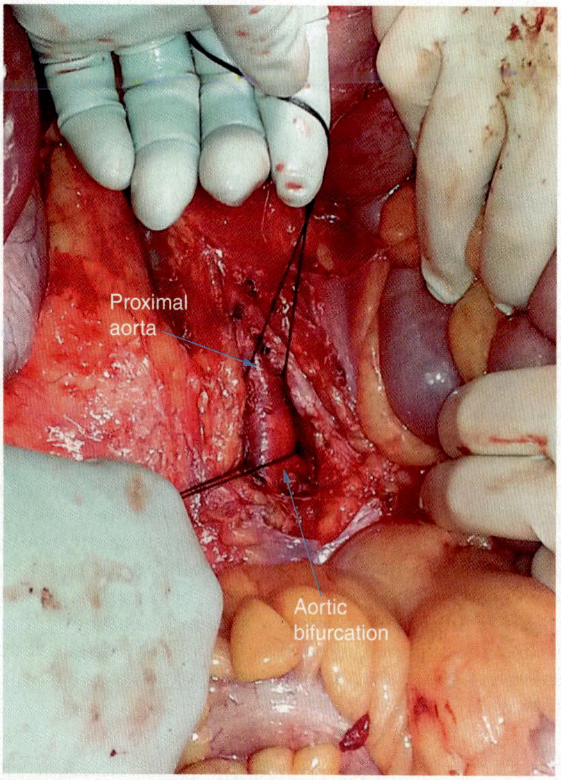

Figure 34.13. Exposure of the distal abdominal aorta in preparation for aortic cannulation.

Pancreas Retrieval

All the steps necessary for the liver retrieval up to the point of perfusion are completed. The pancreas must be mobilized out of the retroperitoneum with care. This can be done in the cold following perfusion, but mobilization prior to this allows for a careful examination of the organ as well as ensuring that the vasculature is ligated or cauterized in situ.

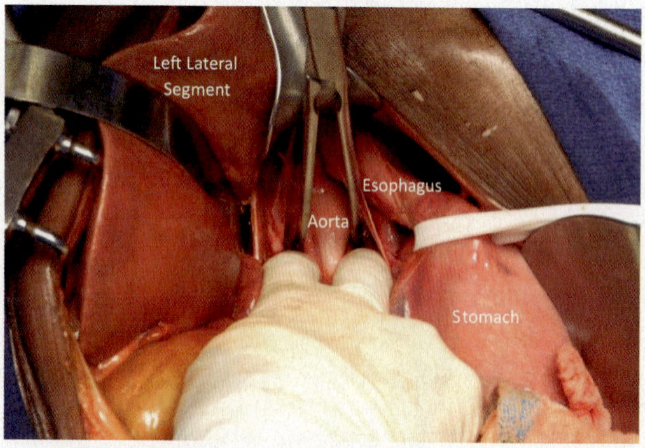

Figure 34.14. Vascular control of the supraceliac aorta in preparation for perfusion. (From Teixeira P, Magee G, Rowe V. Abdominal aorta and splachnic vessels. In: Demetriades D, Inaba K, Velmahos G, eds. *Atlas of Surgical Techniques in Trauma*. Cambridge University Press; 2020:268–285.)

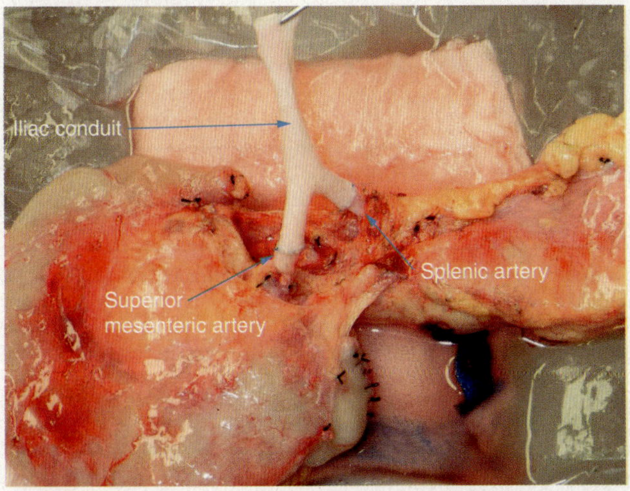

Figure 34.15. Donor superior mesenteric artery and splenic artery with arterial conduit created from the donor iliac artery.

The short gastric vessels are divided to widely expose the pancreas. The gland is assessed for fatty infiltration or firmness, both of which may preclude transplantation. The retroperitoneal tissue inferior to the pancreas and behind the spleen is incised. The spleen is retracted both anteriorly and medially. The tissue behind the spleen and pancreas is divided until the aorta is reached. The duodenum is divided distal to the pylorus. A vessel loop is placed around the splenic artery, and cold perfusion is initiated.

After perfusion, the pancreas can be removed in situ or en bloc with the liver. The proximal jejunum is divided as it exits the retroperitoneum. It is critical that the root of the mesentery is securely divided with a vascular stapler. Division of the portal vein (at the level of the coronary vein), the SMA, and splenic artery should be done in communication with the liver surgeon (**Fig. 34.9**). Identification of the IPDA is essential when a replaced right hepatic artery is anatomically present to ensure adequate arterial blood supply to the head of the pancreas. The iliac artery is retrieved for creation of the Y graft for the transplant operation. The iliac vein is retrieved in case an extension graft is needed for the portal vein (**Fig. 34.15**).

METHODS FOR ORGAN OPTIMIZATION AND PRESERVATION

5 Organ retrieval and storage result in significant alterations in the homeostasis of the organ. The degree of organ preservation injury contributes to the degree to which normal organ function is delayed or prevented following transplantation. Organ preservation injury is largely mediated by ischemia and hypothermia. The duration when the organ is in cold storage is termed "cold ischemic time." Minimizing this time, as well as careful organ preservation, is critical for successful outcomes (**Table 34.6**).

Cold ischemia and subsequent warm reperfusion cause much of the cellular organ damage. As a result, novel strategies for warm perfusion of organs are being used. These techniques involve perfusion with blood or a bloodlike analog with or without oxygenation.[22] Trials of ex vivo liver perfusion machines appear to enhance preservation of donor organs, extending viability and potentially evaluating function in organs previously considered too marginal for transplant.[23] These perfusion techniques offer great promise of optimized organ function and are expanding donor organs via data collection and rehabilitation. The issues are the accessibility due to the personnel, expertise, and cost needed for the machines to be utilized (**Tables 34.7** and **34.8**). These modalities are also allowing for organs to have extended cold ischemic time, with minimal consequence due to the conditioning that is occurring with machine and/or normothermic perfusion techniques.

Machine-cold perfusion is commonly done in renal transplantation and, in some regions, is the standard of care for renal preservation (**Tables 34.9** and **34.10**). Some of the injury during cold ischemia and reperfusion is related to the accumulation of metabolites; perfusion may mitigate these effects by washing out deleterious metabolites and by maintaining patency of the microvasculature of the organ with pressure and pulsitlity (**Fig. 34.16**).[24]

Several strategies have been developed to mitigate the effects of ischemia on organs obtained following DCD retrieval procedures. These include the infusion of antifibrinolytics into the donor organ at the time of transplant.[25] Early reports suggest these strategies result in fewer postliver transplant biliary complications. Similarly, NRP with concurrent DCD retrievals, depending on the length of time, allows both the thoracic and abdominal organs to be oxygenated and perfused. This

Table 34.6. Steps for Flushing and Removal of Heart Then Lungs

- The aortic root is cannulated with a standard needle-tipped cannula.
- A purse-string suture is placed on the distal main pulmonary artery through which an "L"-shaped cannula is placed in the pulmonary artery. Prostaglandin is administered into the pulmonary artery.
- The superior vena cava is ligated; the inferior vena cava is incised at the level agreed upon by the liver surgeon.
- An incision is made to vent the heart and the aortic cross clamp is placed distal to the coronary perfusion cannula.
- The heart and lung cold perfusion is started and the organs are surrounded by ice.
- After the flush, the left atrium is divided, leaving an oval cuff of atrial tissue for the pulmonary veins on each lung.
- The pulmonary artery is divided, taking care not to damage the left main pulmonary artery. The aorta is divided just distal to the aortic arch and the heart is removed.
- The lateral and posterior borders of the pericardium are divided.
- The innominate vein is divided and the anterior trachea is identified and encircled as high in the chest as possible.
- The lungs are inflated and the main bronchus and left main bronchus are stapled. The trachea is divided proximal to the stale line and the inflated lungs are removed.

Table 34.7. Steps for Flushing and Removal of Abdominal Organs

- The aorta is cannulated, the supraceliac aorta is clamped, and the abdominal organs are flushed with cold preservation solution.
- The liver is surrounded with ice and flushed with approximately 5 L of preservation solution in the aortic cannula and 2 L in the portal cannula.
- After the flush, the diaphragm is divided with a cuff around the suprahepatic inferior vena cava.
- The infrahepatic inferior vena cava is divided just above the renal veins.
- The bile duct and portal vein are divided.
- The aorta is divided between the SMA and the renal arteries.
- The liver is removed, and the portal vein is flushed on the back table if not done in situ and placed in cold storage.

Table 34.8. Key Concepts in Organ Preservation

Prevent thrombosis	▪ Anticoagulation of donor ▪ Rapid and complete organ flush
Maintain organ structural integrity	▪ Maintenance of cell membrane lipid bilayer ▪ Cold storage results in conformational changes of cell membrane resulting in cell swelling ▪ Hypertonic preservation solutions mitigate some of these effects
Maintain ionic composition	▪ Preservation solution electrolyte composition is similar to intercellular composition of Na^+ and K^+ ▪ H^+ accumulated as a result of anaerobic glycolysis ▪ Preservation solution buffers H^+ effects
Maintain cellular energy	▪ Hypothermia reduces metabolism 12-fold ▪ Hypothermia affects the activity of mitochondrial enzymes ▪ Mitochondrial dysfunction results in changes in cellular energy
Reperfusion injury—oxygen-free radicals	▪ The majority of organ injury happens at reperfusion and not during cold ischemia ▪ The sudden availability of O_2 results in the production of reactive oxygen intermediates (O^{2-} and OH^-) ▪ Free radicals cause cellular injury, largely through lipid peroxidation ▪ Glutathione protects against peroxidation and is useful in preservation solutions
Reperfusion injury—cytokines	▪ Tissue injury results in the release of cytokines ▪ Tumor necrosis factor, interferon gamma, interleukin-1, and interleukin-8 are released at reperfusion ▪ Cytokine exposure results in the upregulation of adhesion molecules, resulting in platelet plugging and leukocyte adherence to the endothelium

Table 34.9. Comparing Organ Storage Options

	Static Cold Storage	Hypothermic Machine Perfusion	Normothermic Machine Perfusion
Cost	Inexpensive	Moderate expense	Expensive
Resources	Minimal	Moderate	Extensive
Personnel	None	Single operator	Team
Device Malfunction	Low risk of organ loss	Low risk	High risk
Intervention	None	Limited capacity	Extensive capacity
Operation and organ evaluation	Simple/minimal	Moderate complexity and capibility	Extensive complexity and capability
Perfusate	Crystalloid	Crystalloid or erythorcyte based	Erythrocyte based
Temperature	0–4 °C	4–10 °C	34–39 °C

Table 34.10. Commercially Available Machine Perfusion Devices

	Hypothermic Machine Perfusion	Normothermic Machine Perfusion
Kidney	LifePort Kidney Transporter RM3 Kidney Perfusion System Kidney Assist	Kidney Assist
Liver	LifePort Liver Transporter Liver Assist	OrganOx Metra TransMedics Organ Care System Liver Assist
Lung	Lung Assist	TransMedics Organ Care System XVIVO XPS Lung Assist
Heart	LifeCradle by Organ Transport System	TransMedics Organ Care System

From Tatum R, O'Malley TJ, Bodzin AS, Tchantchaleishvili V. Machine perfusion of donor organs for transplantation. *Artif Organs*. 2021;45:682–695.

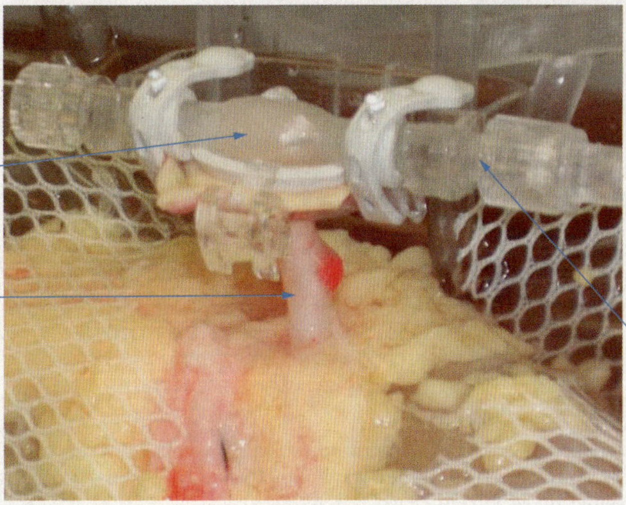

Figure 34.16. Renal machine-cold perfusion circuit with renal artery cannula.

strategy allows for restoring organ function and rehabilitating organs to make them as optimal to low-risk, younger brain-dead organ recoveries.

References

1. From OPTN/SRTR 2022 Annual Data Report: Preface. *Am J Transplant*. 2024;24(2S1):S1–S556.
2. Weiner SG, Malek SK, Price CN. The opioid crisis and its consequences. *Transplantation*. 2017;101(4):678–681.
3. Abramowicz D, Hazzan M, Maggiore U, et al. Does pre-emptive transplantation versus post start of dialysis transplantation with a kidney from a living donor improve outcomes after transplantation? A systematic literature review and position statement by the Descartes Working Group and ERBP. *Nephrol Dial Transplant*. 2016;31(5):691–697.
4. Lomero M, Gardiner D, Coll E, et al. Donation after circulatory death today: an updated overview of the European landscape. *Transpl Int*. 2020;33(1):76–88.
5. Guidelines for the determination of death. Report of the medical consultants on the diagnosis of death to the President's Commission for the Study of Ethical Problems in Medicine and Biomedical and Behavioral Research. *JAMA*. 1981;246(19):2184–2186.
6. Wijdicks EF, Varelas PN, Gronseth GS, Greer DM. Evidence-based guideline update: determining brain death in adults: report of the Quality Standards Subcommittee of the American Academy of Neurology. *Neurology*. 2010;74(23):1911–1918.
7. Morrissey PE, Monaco AP. Donation after circulatory death: current practices, ongoing challenges, and potential improvements. *Transplantation*. 2014;97(3):258–264.
8. Rojas-Pena A, Reoma JL, Krause E, et al. Extracorporeal support: improves donor renal graft function after cardiac death. *Am J Transplant*. 2010;10(6):1365–1374.
9. Arias-Diaz J, Alvarez J, Gomez M, et al. Changes in adenine nucleotides and lipid hydroperoxides during normothermic cardiopulmonary bypass in a porcine model of type II non-heart-beating donor. *Transplant Proc*. 1997;29(8):3486–3487.
10. De Carlis R, Di Sandro S, Lauterio A, et al. Liver grafts from donors after circulatory death on regional perfusion with extended warm ischemia compared with donors after brain death. *Liver Transpl*. 2018;24(11):1523–1535.
11. Nielsen Busch EJ, Mjaaland MT. Does controlled donation after circulatory death violate the dead donor rule? *Am J Bioeth*. 2023;23(2):4–11.
12. Nalesnik MA, Woodle ES, Dimaio JM, et al. Donor-transmitted malignancies in organ transplantation: assessment of clinical risk. *Am J Transplant*. 2011;11(6):1140–1147.
13. Snyder JJ, Salkowski N, Wey A, Pyke J, Israni AK, Kasiske BL. Organ distribution without geographic boundaries: a possible framework for organ allocation. *Am J Transplant*. 2018;18(11):2635–2640.
14. Giorgakis E, Ivanics T, Wallace D, et al. Acuity circles allocation policy impact on waitlist mortality and donation after circulatory death liver transplantation: a nationwide retrospective analysis. *Health Sci Rep*. 2023;6(2):e1066.
15. Theodoropoulos N, Ison MG. Donor-derived infections: incidence, prevention, and management. *Transpl Infect*. 2016:113–127.
16. Jones JM, Kracalik I, Levi ME, et al. Assessing solid organ donors and monitoring transplant recipients for human immunodeficiency virus, hepatitis B virus, and hepatitis C virus infection – U.S. Public Health Service Guideline, 2020. *MMWR Recomm Rep*. 2020;69(4):1–16.
17. Croome KP, Lee DD, Pungpapong S, Keaveny AP, Taner CB. What are the outcomes of declining a public health service increased risk liver donor for patients on the liver transplant waiting list? *Liver Transpl*. 2018;24(4):497–504.
18. Werbel WA, Durand CM. Pro: use of hepatitis C virus-positive donors should be considered standard of care. *Clin Liver Dis (Hoboken)*. 2018;12(4):100–104.
19. Durand CM, Zhang W, Brown DM, et al. A prospective multicenter pilot study of HIV-positive deceased donor to HIV-positive recipient kidney transplantation: HOPE in action. *Am J Transplant*. 2021;21(5):1754–1764.
20. Samoylova ML, Shaw BI, Irish W, et al. Decreased graft loss following implementation of the kidney allocation score (KAS). *Am J Surg*. 2020;220(5):1278–1283.
21. Doyle MB, Vachharajani N, Wellen JR, et al. A novel organ donor facility: a decade of experience with liver donors. *Am J Transplant*. 2014;14(3):615–620.
22. Tatum R, O'Malley TJ, Bodzin AS, Tchantchaleishvili V. Machine perfusion of donor organs for transplantation. *Artif Organs*. 2021;45(7):682–695.
23. Chapman WC, Barbas AS, D'Alessandro AM, et al. Normothermic machine perfusion of donor livers for transplantation in the United States: a randomized controlled trial. *Ann Surg*. 2023;278(5):e912–e921.
24. Moers C, Smits JM, Maathuis MH, et al. Machine perfusion or cold storage in deceased-donor kidney transplantation. *N Engl J Med*. 2009;360(1):7–19.
25. Jayant K, Reccia I, Virdis F, Shapiro AMJ. Systematic review and meta-analysis on the impact of thrombolytic therapy in liver transplantation following donation after circulatory death. *J Clin Med*. 2018;7(11):425.

35

Kidney Transplantation

Jayme E. Locke and Peter G. Stock

Key Points

1 The presence of antidonor HLA antibodies is a relative contraindication to kidney transplantation and is screened by a "virtual cross-match" with increased frequency.

2 Methods to expand living kidney donation include kidney paired exchange and incompatible kidney transplantation.

3 Methods to expand the deceased-donor pool of kidneys include the use of donation after cardiac death donors, high kidney donor profile index (KDPI) kidneys, hepatitis C+ kidneys, and HIV+ kidneys.

4 The etiology of kidney disease resulting in end-stage failure, and the necessity for transplantation is led by glomerulonephritis, diabetes, and hypertension.

5 As a result of the increasing wait times across the United States, the presence of a cardiovascular system that will tolerate a major operation is the biggest barrier to successful transplantation.

6 The kidney transplant is heterotopically placed in the extraperitoneal iliac fossa.

7 Surgical complications of kidney transplantation include vascular, urologic, lymphocele, and wound problems.

8 Hyperacute rejection is humorally mediated by preformed anti-HLA antibodies. Hyperacute rejection occurs within minutes to hours following reperfusion of the kidney.

9 Acute cell-mediated rejection most typically occurs between 1 week and 3 months following transplantation.

10 Chronic rejection leads to loss of graft function over the course of months to several years.

Kidney transplantation has evolved to become the preferred therapeutic modality for patients with end-stage kidney failure. Improved patient survival and quality of life as compared with dialysis have been established, with cost-effectiveness achieved after a minimum of 18 months of allograft function. The importance of minimizing time on dialysis, compounded by the exponential growth of patients on the wait list, has led to several strategies to increase the number of deceased- and living-donor organs in an effort to decrease waiting time and mortality on the wait list. These new strategies have been the focus of clinical research in kidney transplantation and will be discussed in this chapter. Other important topics that will be reviewed include immunologic considerations specific to kidney transplantation; preoperative assessment of kidney allograft recipients; the standard surgical approach in kidney transplantation and advances in minimally invasive technology for the donor; current strategies in immunosuppression; management of the technical and immunosuppressive complications; new kidney allocation policies affecting wait list management; and future trends.

IMMUNOLOGY OF KIDNEY TRANSPLANTATION

The immunologic response to allografted tissue is well defined and under the influence of both T- and B-cell–derived reactions. The cells and cytokines responsible for rejection vary with time posttransplant (hyperacute, acute, and chronic rejection) and have a differential response to currently available immunosuppressive agents.

The HLA system is made up of well-defined antigens present on most cell types that are genetically determined for each patient and are termed the *major histocompatibility complex*. These genes reside on chromosome 6 and are distributed in a Mendelian fashion to offspring. The HLA system includes several loci, but the most commonly characterized are the HLA-A, HLA-B, and HLA-D regions. Given that each human has two alleles for each locus, there are six potential HLA antigens of clinical significance. These are characterized using tissue-typing techniques and can be used to determine the degree of matching between a donor and potential recipient, that is, one- to six-antigen match. Improved graft survival is seen when the degree of matching reaches the six-antigen level.

Class I antigens include the HLA antigens A, B, and C, whereas class II antigens include the DP and DR loci. Class I antigens act as targets for cytotoxic T lymphocytes, and class II antigens are important for antigen presentation. Class II antigens are also responsible for triggering lymphocyte proliferation in the mixed lymphocyte culture system.

1 Before a kidney transplant is undertaken, histocompatibility of the donor and recipient is determined. HLA matching is not a prerequisite for proceeding with transplantation. However, the presence of recipient antibodies directed against the donor HLA usually precludes transplantation. Standard pretransplant workup consists of several assays that will help to determine future compatibility with a potential donor. First, donors and recipients undergo tissue typing, which involves characterization of their respective HLA type. Secondly, recipient serum is tested against a panel of antigens that contains the known HLA types to identify anti-HLA antibodies. The sensitivity for detecting anti-HLA antibodies continues to improve, and newer technology uses single antigen beads with next generation sequencing to detect antibodies against a specific HLA

antigen. The amount of reactivity that a potential recipient has against a panel of HLA antigens is indicative of the degree of sensitization. Based on the number of anti-HLA antibodies detected, a calculated percent reactive antibody (cPRA) can be estimated. A cPRA of 70% would suggest that the potential recipient would have anti-HLA antibodies against 70% of the potential donor pool. Sensitization to HLA antigens occurs as a result of previous exposure to foreign HLA antigen, either from pregnancy, previous blood transfusion, or a previous organ transplant. A patient who is highly sensitized is more difficult to transplant because of the greater likelihood of having antibodies to a potential donor.

The last critical test performed prior to transplantation is commonly known as the *final cross-match*. This final cross-match can be performed in several ways. Recipient serum samples collected at different times are mixed with donor lymphocytes in a culture system. This assay will detect preformed cytotoxic antibodies that would result in a hyperacute rejection if the transplantation were performed (see Rejection, later). A more sensitive method of detecting these antibodies uses a fluorescent-activated cell scanner cross-match and is commonly used when evaluating potential recipients who are highly sensitized or receiving second transplants. Many transplant centers have adopted "virtual cross-matching" based on the detection 2
of anti-HLA antibodies present in a given recipient. The most sensitive technology will be used to detect the presence of anti-HLA antibodies in a given recipient. Based on these antibodies, each recipient will have a list of unacceptable donor antigens. Compatibility with each donor will be determined in the absence of the serum-based final cross-match by eliminating a potential donor based on the presence of unacceptable antigens. This strategy facilitates an expedited transplant and minimization of cold ischemia times, as it avoids the additional time and expense associated with the serum-based final cross-match. The use of the virtual cross-matching is particularly beneficial for determining potentially compatible kidneys allocated to highly sensitized recipients, a scenario occurring with increasing frequency as a result of the kidney allocation system (KAS) algorithm initiated in December 2014.[1]

In general, kidney transplantation is done between ABO-compatible donor and recipients using the same guidelines as for blood transfusion. However, several groups have reported successful kidney transplantation across ABO blood group barriers, using aggressive pretransplant immunosuppression, plasmapheresis to decrease anti-ABO titers, and in some cases splenectomy.[2,3] This strategy has been implemented in the United States as a result of the marked increases in the waiting times for blood group O and B recipients.[4] However, ABO-incompatible transplants in the United States have not enjoyed the same success as in Japan, where ABO-incompatible living-related donor transplants are the only option for transplantation. Based on the better results observed in ABO-compatible transplants in the United States, most centers have opted to participate in the paired exchange program (see below) rather than proceed with ABO-incompatible transplants. The exception to this is transplantation of blood type A2 and A2B–deceased-donor allografts to blood type B recipients, provided the anti-A titers are acceptably low. In this circumstance, outcomes are comparable to ABO-compatible transplants, and this exception has become part of the United Network for Organ Sharing (UNOS) allocation system in order to decrease the length of waiting times for blood type B recipients.[5]

THE DONOR POOL: LIVING DONORS, DECEASED DONORS, AND DONATION AFTER CARDIAC DEATH

There is marked improvement in graft survival for both living and deceased donors when a transplant can be completed before the initiation of dialysis.[6] The significantly better outcomes achieved with preemptive transplantation and 3
minimizations of dialysis times have given rise to several strategies to increase the number of available kidneys.

Living Donors

The first long-term success in kidney transplantation over 70 years ago involved a live-donor transplant between twin brothers. Introduction of laparoscopic and robotic donor nephrectomy has further revolutionized the field. Despite initial concerns about the safety and efficacy of these techniques for the donor procedure, morbidity and mortality rates remain low and comparable with those of the open technique.[7–9]

The evaluation of a potential living kidney donor includes a comprehensive medical, surgical, and psychosocial evaluation. Diabetes, hypertension, and cardiovascular disease generally rule out a potential donor.[10] Testing of a potential donor also involves anatomic definition of the two kidneys and is typically done with either a computed tomography angiogram or MR angiogram, both of which avoid the arterial needlestick and catheters associated with a conventional angiogram. The results of these studies are used to detect any anatomic abnormalities that would exclude a donor and to decide which kidney will be removed. In general, the left kidney is favored for transplant because it has a longer renal vein.

Several strategies are currently being considered to increase the frequency of living donation. Potential donors with well-controlled hypertension on a single antihypertensive agent are being considered, although this remains controversial. Multiple national exchange systems have been developed that match living donors who were incompatible with their intended recipient (either because of ABO incompatibility or a positive cross-match test) with other recipients with incompatible living donors and in some cases compatible pairs choose to participate. Such exchange systems have been successful, with one in five living-donor kidney transplants in 2021 the result of such exchanges.[11] Extending this to a single national system has the potential to permit many more successful exchanges and further expand the living-donor pool.[12] In addition, for those pairs unable to identify a compatible transplant via paired exchange, an important strategy currently being implemented in the United States, as well as internationally, involves the use of desensitization protocols to facilitate transplantation across a known positive anti-HLA cross-match. These protocols may involve pretransplant infusion of gamma globulin in the recipient to bind circulating antibody, plasmapheresis of the recipient to remove circulating antibody, and/or the use of agents, such as rituximab and imlifidase, to decrease antibody production.[13,14] Finally, a hybrid approach for the highly sensitized recipient with a cross-match–incompatible donor could involve finding a kidney that is "less incompatible" through an exchange program, and then converting the positive cross-match to a compatible cross-match with desensitization techniques.

Deceased Donors

Procurement of kidneys from brain-dead deceased donors has increased over the last decade, but continues to be outpaced by the number of patients in need of a lifesaving kidney transplant. Although most deceased donors are brain-dead, there has been an increased use of kidneys from donors who do not meet the strict definitions of brain death but have cardiopulmonary support withdrawn because of a severe brain injury or high spinal cord injury, with little hope of living without the use of ongoing mechanical ventilation and/or the possibility of existing in a persistent vegetative state. Organs are recovered after withdrawal of support, once the heart stops beating, hence the terminology of *donors by cardiac death* or *DCD donors*. Usually, support is withdrawn in a controlled setting so that the time of warm ischemia and poor organ perfusion can be minimized. Minimizing the time from cessation of the heart to perfusion of organs with preservation fluid requires an experienced procurement team, and the successful use of these organs is dependent on rapid procurement. Kidneys procured from DCD donors are proving to be an important source of donor kidneys, and studies have demonstrated comparable graft success between kidneys procured from DCD donors and brain-dead donors, although the incidence of initial delayed graft function is higher in DCD kidneys. The percentage of DCD donors in the United States has progressively increased over the last decade and presently represents about 30% of deceased donors.[15]

Placement of deceased-donor kidneys is guided by a series of complex allocation rules established by the UNOS. Donor kidneys are now assigned a kidney donor profile index (KDPI) score, which is used to define donor organ longevity, with a lower score corresponding to better-predicted survival of the kidney (better-quality kidney). The new allocation system attempts to match the predicted longevity of the deceased-donor organ, quantified by the KDPI, with the estimated posttransplant survival (EPTS) of the recipient. The top 20% of kidneys (KDPI scores less than 20%) will be transplanted to recipients with the longest EPTS. In the new allocation scheme, the highest KDPI kidneys (KDPI >85%) will be allocated to recipients who have consented to receive an expanded criteria donor (ECD). Highly sensitized patients will receive a significant number of allocation points, so if, in the rare event that a compatible kidney becomes available, that kidney will be allocated to the compatible highly sensitized recipient. Highly sensitized recipients with cPRAs of 99% or 100% will get access to the regional and national lists, respectively, to increase the chances of finding a compatible kidney. Finally, waiting times will be backdated to the time of the initiation of dialysis, although patients can still be listed when the glomerular filtration rate drops below 20 mL/min.[16]

Further Strategies for Increasing the Number of Donor Kidneys

Many of the unique approaches for increasing the number of potential living donors, including kidney paired exchange and incompatible transplantation, have been previously discussed in the chapter. Additional strategies include programs aimed at separating the advocacy role from the recipient and including programs such as the Johns Hopkins Champion Program and the University of Alabama at Birmingham Living Donor Navigator Program. Both programs have demonstrated early success, but widespread adoption of such programs remains limited.[17,18]

Further strategies have recently been implemented to expand the number of kidneys procured from deceased donors. In addition to the use of kidneys from DCD donors described earlier, transplant centers have considered using kidneys from donors that are less than optimal (KDPI ≥85%), previously designated as ECDs. These kidneys clearly had a shorter survival compared to younger, healthier donors, and therefore, potential recipients are required to give consent to receive these kidneys before transplant. The advantage to certain patient groups who were predicted to do poorly on dialysis (ie, older patients or patients with diabetes) was an increased overall patient survival if they received a timely transplant rather than wait a prolonged time on the list. As mentioned above, the new allocation system also affords the opportunity for blood group–incompatible kidney transplantation in select scenarios, specifically blood group A, subtype A2 donors into blood group B recipients, with the overall goal to increase access to transplantation for ethnic minorities, which have a disproportionate number of blood group B donors. Most recently, in the era of direct-acting antiviral therapy with 99% sustained viral response, kidneys from hepatitis C donors are being offered to select hepatitis C–naive recipients with excellent results.[19] Finally, an additional source of potential deceased-donor kidneys is now available to HIV+ candidates. With the passage of the HIV Organ Policy Equity Act, HIV+ individuals may donate their organs upon their death. HIV+ to HIV+ kidney transplantation, which is still performed under research protocols in the United States, has met with good success and excellent long-term outcomes abroad.[20]

THE TRANSPLANT PROCEDURE

Recipient Preoperative Assessment

4 The etiologies of kidney disease resulting in end-stage failure and the necessity for transplantation are led by glomerulonephritis, diabetes, and hypertension (**Table 35.1**).[15] Because of the high incidence of cardiovascular disease associated with many of these conditions, most notably diabetes, a careful

Table 35.1. Etiology of Renal Disease as Indications for Renal Transplantation, Ranked in Order of Prevalence

Diabetes mellitus (types I and II)
Hypertension
Polycystic kidney disease
IgA nephropathy
Chronic glomerulonephritis
Focal sclerosis
Systemic lupus
Membranous glomerulonephritis
Pyelonephritis
Focal segmental glomerulosclerosis
Congenital obstructive uropathy
Nephritis
Alport syndrome
Hypoplasia, dysplasia
Wegener granulomatosis
Postinfectious glomerulonephritis
Obstructive uropathy
Hemolytic uremia
Membranoproliferative glomerulonephritis
Goodpasture syndrome
Membranous nephropathy
Analgesic nephropathy
Prune belly syndrome
Medullary cystic disease
Henoch–Schönlein purpura
Nephronophthisis
Scleroderma
Sickle cell anemia
Amyloidosis
Oxalosis

Adapted from Cecka JM. The OPTN/UNOS renal transplant registry. In: Cecka JM, Terasaki PI, eds. *Clinical Transplants 2003*. UCLA Immunogenetics Center; 2004:1–12, with permission.

assessment of the cardiovascular status of the potential recipi-
5 ent is critical. As a result of the increasing wait times across the United States, the presence of a cardiovascular system that will tolerate kidney transplantation is the biggest barrier. For patients at risk, this assessment should include, at a minimum, an echocardiogram and an exercise or pharmacologic stress test as a screen for reversible ischemia requiring cardiac catheterization. Controversy remains with regard to the accuracy of noninvasive studies in terms of identifying significant disease of the coronary arteries, particularly in diabetic patients. Nonetheless, for most centers, this remains the standard screening strategy, and updated studies should be obtained within 1 year of the transplant procedure. If either coronary artery bypass or stenting has taken place in preparation for kidney transplantation, follow-up angiograms and/or stress tests should be repeated within 1 to 2 years of the actual transplant. If stenting of the coronary arteries is required, patients with drug-eluting stents will commonly require clopidogrel (Plavix) for an extended period of time. Although controversial, many centers will proceed with transplantation while recipients are on Plavix, after a waiting period of 6 months following the stenting procedure.

Although the evaluation of potential recipients is focused on the assessment of cardiovascular status, further studies must exclude malignancies and infections that would contraindicate transplantation and immunosuppression. Potential kidney recipients who are infected with hepatitis C should be evaluated by a hepatologist to determine the risks of immunosuppression causing progression to end-stage liver disease. Potential kidney recipients with evidence of advanced liver disease should be evaluated for a combined liver and kidney transplant. For patients with less advanced liver disease, consideration could be given to treatment with newer antiviral drugs before proceeding with kidney transplantation to provide the opportunity for viral clearance.[21] Kidney transplantation was previously contraindicated in people with HIV infection secondary to concerns of exacerbating an already immunologically compromised state. Recent advances in antiretroviral therapy and the ability to provide effective prophylaxis against opportunistic infections have prompted several centers to perform transplantation in people with end-stage kidney disease and HIV infection. Early results suggest that progression of HIV to AIDS has not been seen following transplantation and immunosuppression, with allograft success rates comparable to those in non–HIV-positive recipients.[22] Potential patients with a previous history of tuberculosis or conversion to purified protein derivative positivity should be evaluated for active disease.

Colonoscopy, mammography, and Pap smear should be performed as dictated by age-specific standard guidelines. For most malignancies, a disease-free interval of 5 years is recommended before kidney transplantation. Controversy exists about pretransplant waiting times for certain malignancies, such as early-stage breast cancer or prostate cancer, and some centers will not require any pretransplant waiting.[23] Similarly, pretransplant wait times are probably not necessary for nonmelanoma skin cancers and early-stage renal cancers.[24] For patients with congenital abnormalities as the cause of kidney failure, a complete workup of the genitourinary systems is necessary, including urodynamics and voiding cystourethrograms. These studies are particularly important in children with end-stage disease resulting from posterior urethral valves, to ensure that the bladder will serve as an adequate conduit for the kidney transplant. For patients with severe reflux disease and chronic pyelonephritis, native nephroureterectomy may be required to prevent posttransplant infection secondary to chronic reflux into the native ureters. For patients with inadequate bladder capacity and function, pretransplant-reconstructive procedures such as ileal augmentation or ileal conduits may be required.

For patients with suspected clotting disorders based on a previous history of thromboembolic events (frequent clotting problems with dialysis access) or diseases associated with an increased frequency of clotting disorders (ie, lupus), a hematologic workup is necessary to determine the necessity for anticoagulation at the time of the transplant. The length of time for anticoagulation is dependent on the severity of the clotting disorder and a history of a previous thrombotic event. This workup should include a determination of serum levels of protein C, protein S, anticardiolipin antibody, factor V Leiden, antithrombin III levels, and the G20210 A prothrombin gene mutation.

Living-Donor Nephrectomy: Open and Minimally Invasive

A living kidney donor operation is a unique surgical procedure for two reasons. First, the donor has no medical reason to be in the operating room, and the process is driven only by his or her willingness to help another person with the gift of donation. Second, the removed tissue must be in perfect condition because it will be reimplanted into the recipient. These two features, therefore, necessitate that the donor operation is done safely and well. The original donor operation was done through a generous flank incision, allowing for good exposure and careful dissection of the renal vessels. Unfortunately, this flank approach generally left a large incision, with its accompanying morbidity, pain, and sometimes adverse cosmetic result. The development of minimally invasive techniques to remove kidneys has revolutionized the field. With the explosive growth and dissemination of this procedure, it has now become the standard for donor nephrectomy.

The procedure is most commonly done through a transperitoneal approach, although some surgeons prefer to remain retroperitoneal. Once the operative space is expanded with carbon dioxide gas and the scope is inserted, most commonly two to three additional ports are placed to allow for the passage of instruments to dissect the kidney (**Fig. 35.1**). Some centers also favor the use of a gastight "hand port," which allows placement of the surgeon's hand in the operative space to assist in exposure and to have available if sudden bleeding is encountered. Once the kidney vessels are transected and the vessel stumps are controlled by laparoscopic staples, the kidney can be removed through a 2- to 3-in incision, which can be placed in a position that leaves minimal scarring and avoids cutting muscle tissue. Most commonly, this is via a Pfannenstiel incision, and recently, the use of natural orifice approaches has been described. Additionally, some centers have adopted the use of a robotic technique. Donors who undergo minimally invasive procedures typically have reduced pain medicine requirements, have a slightly shorter hospital stay, and are able to return to their usual activities sooner.[7–9]

The safety of minimally invasive donor nephrectomy has been established, in addition to the demonstration that kidneys recovered through a laparoscopic approach function as well as kidneys removed in an open operation. There has been an increased interest in live donation, coincident with the introduction of the laparoscopic procedure, suggesting that this procedure has removed some of the disincentives of the donation process.

Recipient Operative Procedure

6 The kidney transplant is heterotopically placed in the extraperitoneal iliac fossa. Attention to detail is imperative to optimize immediate graft function and avoid technical complications resulting in loss of the kidney transplant.

The operation is initiated by exposure of the iliac fossa through a curvilinear incision and can be done on either the right or left side. The incision extends from 1 cm above the symphysis pubis to approximately 2 cm medial to the anterior iliac spine (**Fig. 35.2**). The fascia is divided along the lateral border of the rectus sheath, and the contents of the peritoneal cavity are reflected cephalad and medially, exposing the iliac vessels in the retroperitoneum. Lymphatics overlying the iliac vessels are ligated and divided to prevent the development of

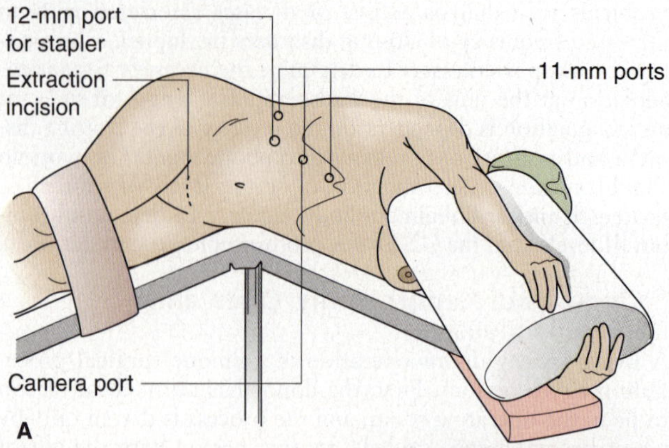

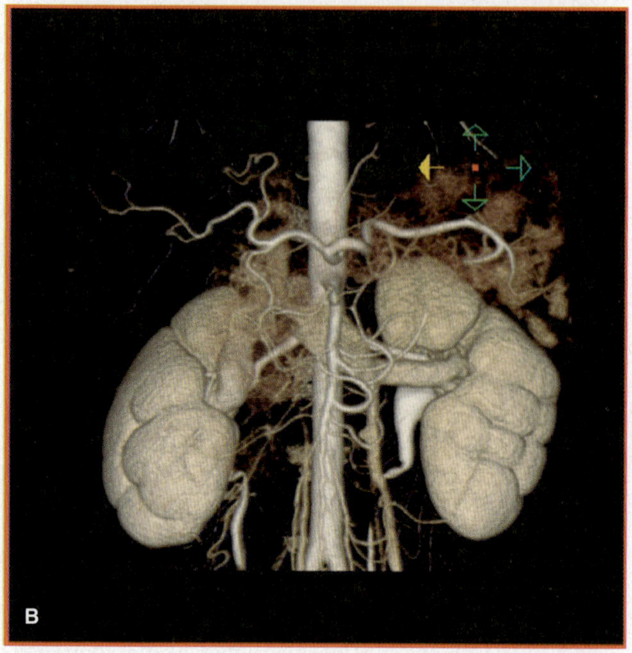

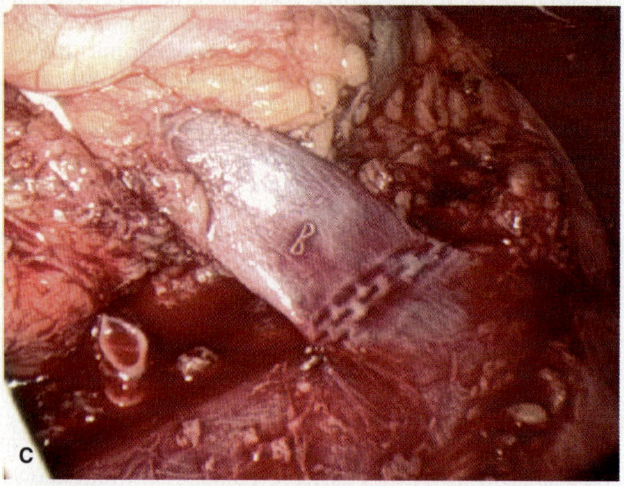

Figure 35.1. **A:** The laparoscopic donor procedure is performed with the donor in a lateral position, typically using three to four ports, with extraction of the kidney through a 6- to 8-cm incision. **B:** Preoperative computed tomography angiogram revealing the arterial and venous anatomy. **C:** Intraoperative photograph of laparoscopic view of right kidney just prior to transection of the renal vein. The artery has already been divided.

lymphoceles. In males, the spermatic cord is secured with a vessel loop and can be retracted away from the operative field. In females, the round ligament is suture ligated and divided. The inferior epigastric artery and vein are typically divided to prevent potential compression of the transplanted ureter. Placement of a mechanical retractor should avoid compression of the iliac artery and vein as well as the femoral nerve to prevent neuropraxias.

The living- or deceased-donor kidney is inspected for the presence of multiple vessels, duplication of the urinary collecting system, and parenchymal abnormalities. The artery and vein are dissected from surrounding structures to provide the necessary length for transplantation. In the case of multiple arteries, a decision must be made as to whether to perform ex vivo reconstruction to achieve a single implantable conduit versus implanting the vessels separately. This decision is in part dependent on the quality of the recipient vessels and an assessment as to whether the anastomosis of multiple vessels directly into the recipient would require an unacceptable period of warm ischemia to the kidney. In general, in an adult, the anastomosis of the renal artery and vein is performed in an end-to-side fashion to the external iliac vessels, although occasionally the presence of atherosclerotic disease requires transplantation to the common iliac vessels. In children who

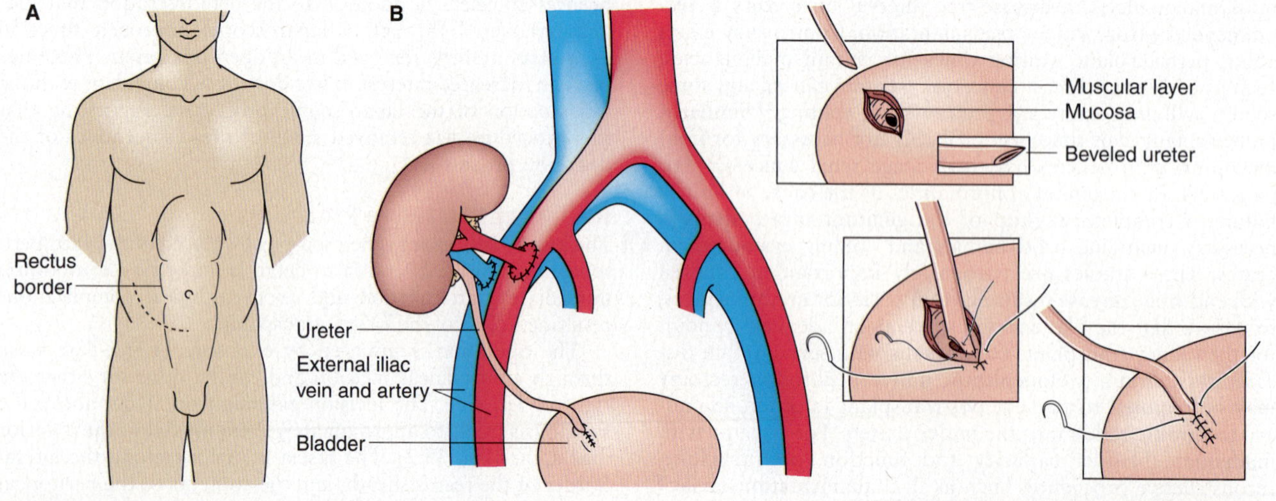

Figure 35.2. **A:** Curvilinear iliac fossa incision used for the kidney-transplant recipient procedure. **B:** Vascular anastomoses completed between the recipient external iliac artery and vein and donor renal artery and vein. *Insets:* ureteral anastomosis performed using the external ureteroneocystostomy technique.

weigh less than 20 kg, or for third transplants in adults, an intraperitoneal approach is used, and the vascular anastomoses are frequently performed to the aorta and inferior vena cava. For kidneys from deceased donors, a Carrel patch of aorta is used to prevent stenosis and to provide a common patch for multiple arteries. Warm ischemia time should be minimized to prevent delayed graft function. Ensuring adequate intravascular volume and stable hemodynamics at the time of reperfusion is extremely important to achieve optimal function of the transplant.

The reimplantation of the ureter is most frequently performed through an extravesicular technique. Following positioning of the revascularized kidney in the iliac fossa and assurance of hemostasis, the ureter is shortened to permit a tension-free anastomosis with adequate blood supply to the distal ureter. In men, the ureter is placed under the spermatic cord to prevent ureteral obstruction. The bladder is distended to identify a suitable area for ureteral implantation on the dome of the bladder, and a cystotomy is made at this site. An anastomosis between the mucosa of the bladder and transplanted ureter is constructed using an absorbable suture to prevent stone formation. A second layer of the bladder musculature is closed over the distal portion of the ureter to prevent reflux during micturition.

There are alternative techniques to reimplant the ureter, including the Politano–Leadbetter transvesical ureteroneocystostomy. This technique involves tunneling the ureter through the bladder wall from the inside of the bladder. This technique is still preferred by some surgeons who believe the long-term prevention of reflux is superior with the transvesicular approach. However, this technique requires a second cystotomy, and posttransplant hematuria is more common than with the extravesicular technique. A third technique for ureteral implantation in recipients with normal native ureters is ureteroureterostomy over a double-J stent. In general, this technique is reserved as a salvage procedure for reimplantation of transplanted ureters with distal strictures secondary to ischemia. It can also be used as a primary technique if there are questions regarding the blood supply to the distal ureter at the time of transplant. This technique is preferred if the donor ureter was damaged or inadvertently stripped of its blood supply at the time of procurement, but is dependent on the availability of normal native ureters to serve as an adequate conduit. The routine placement of a double-J stent is center dependent, with some centers reserving placement of the stent for challenging extravesicular anastomosis to poor-quality bladders.

The surgical procedure has changed little over the last 70 years, with the exception of recent reports of robotic implantation of the kidney. The purported advantage is smaller incisions, which appear to have an advantage in obese patients, avoiding some of the frequent wound complications. Widespread adaptation of this technique has not occurred.[25,26]

COMPLICATIONS

Early Graft Dysfunction

Most kidneys begin to function immediately after implantation, especially in the case of a living donor. When the initial function results in only a slow drop in serum creatinine, the diagnosis of slow graft function is made. When dialysis is needed in the first week because of poor function, the diagnosis of delayed graft function is made. Delayed graft function typically occurs in 15% to 30% of deceased-donor transplants. The diagnosis of slow graft function or delayed graft function is important to establish because other problems, such as rejection, vascular occlusion, or ureteral obstruction, can also result in low urine output and need for dialysis. These other causes must be eliminated before the diagnosis of slow graft function or delayed graft function can be made.

In the immediate postoperative period, careful attention to fluid status is critical. In cases of immediate graft function, fluid orders should include replacement for urine output as well as a maintenance fluid rate. This approach ensures that the patient does not become volume-depleted and compromise perfusion to the new kidney. In cases of delayed graft function, fluid should be restricted and dialysis instituted when electrolyte imbalance or fluid overload are evident.

A decrease in urine output in the early postoperative period requires immediate diagnostic and therapeutic intervention. A stepwise algorithm to assist in diagnosing the etiology of oliguria is shown in **Figure 35.3**. Once mechanical obstruction of the indwelling Foley catheter has been excluded by irrigation, the volume status of the patient should be assessed. Fluid replacement to restore intravascular volume should be initiated in the volume-depleted patient.

Radiologic evaluation using various imaging techniques is required if urine output remains low in the face of adequate volume status. Ultrasonography is most helpful to diagnose ureteral obstruction caused by technical complications at the anastomosis or fluid collections that may be obstructing the ureter by extrinsic compression. With the addition of duplex and color Doppler imaging, blood flow to the kidney can be evaluated, and technical problems with the vessels can be assessed. Nuclear medicine techniques are also valuable for assessing renal function. Technetium-99m diethylenetriamine pentaacetic acid (DTPA) and iodine-131 iodohippurate (Hippuran) are the two major radionuclides used in the evaluation of kidney allograft function. DTPA renal scans evaluate the vascular flow pattern of the kidney as well as the gross anatomy of the ureter and bladder. Scans are performed over 30 minutes, with uptake of contrast within 6 seconds indicating adequate flow to the graft. Peak activity in the parenchyma should be reached within 2 minutes, followed by a gradual decline in radioactivity in the renal parenchyma and an increase in radioactivity in the urinary collecting system and bladder. Iodine-131 iodohippurate scans are more sensitive in evaluating kidney function. Peak activity is also reached in 2 to 4 minutes, with gradual decline over the next 30 minutes. In rejection, acute tubular necrosis and drug toxicity, poor uptake, and poor excretion are the typical findings with a nuclear medicine scan.

If these imaging techniques do not provide an explanation for poor urine output, the diagnosis of delayed graft function is made. Immunosuppression can then be adjusted to minimize or avoid the calcineurin inhibitors, which can prolong the recovery from delayed graft function, and also to initiate antibody therapy to protect the kidney from rejection. The combination of delayed graft function and early rejection is clearly associated with worse outcome in the long term, and an early biopsy of the kidney that is functioning poorly is helpful to diagnose rejection and guide therapy.

Technical Complications

7 Most surgical complications are experienced in the immediate postoperative period. The two main types of complications can be classified as vascular and urologic.

Renal artery thrombosis is a rare complication occurring in about 1% of transplants. The risk of this complication is higher with size mismatch of donor renal artery and recipient internal iliac artery when an end-to-end anastomosis is performed, in kidneys with multiple renal arteries, in kidneys traumatized because of rough handling, and in the presence of an unidentified renal artery intimal flap. Sudden loss of urinary output, not the result of an obstructed Foley catheter or inadequate vascular volume, should necessitate a workup with duplex Doppler ultrasound. Loss of signal is indicative of no flow to the kidney. Alternatively, a nuclear medicine renal scan is informative, with lack of isotope uptake by the kidney indicating no blood flow. Prompt return to the operating room for correction of a technical problem is imperative, but often the diagnosis is not made quickly enough to salvage the kidney.

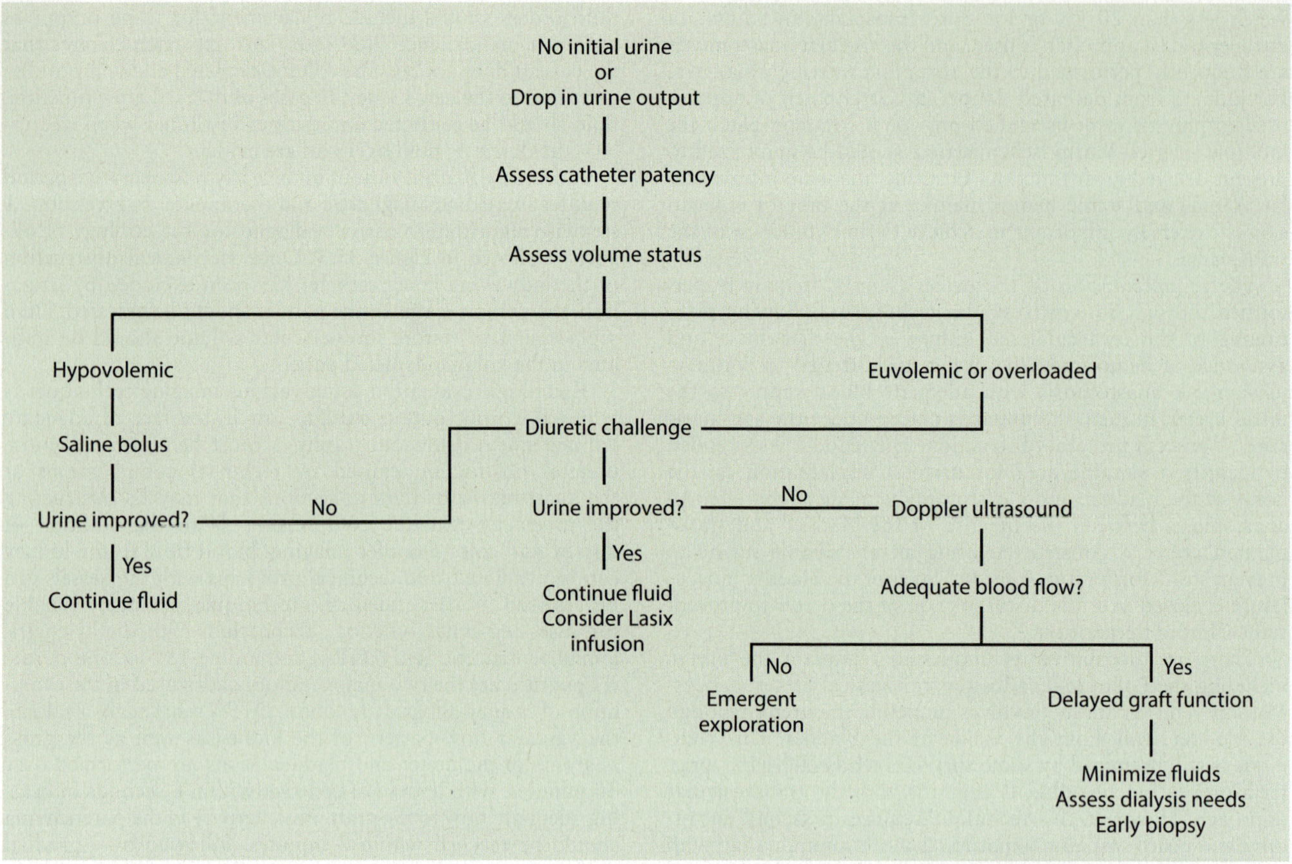

Figure 35.3. Stepwise approach to the management of decreased low urine output posttransplant.

Renal artery stenosis occurs in up to 15% of transplanted kidneys. Difficult-to-control hypertension should suggest the possibility of stenosis. Diagnosis with renal duplex ultrasound followed by arteriography to better define the anatomy and degree of stenosis, should be done before operative repair or angioplasty. Initial success rates for both methods are similar (75% to 80%), but the restenosis rate following angioplasty is not well defined. Anastomotic strictures respond less well to angioplasty and probably should be repaired by operative intervention.

Aneurysms that occur in the renal artery are either pseudoaneurysms at the anastomotic site or mycotic aneurysms secondary to bacterial or fungal infection. A rapidly expanding, tender pulsatile mass in the region of the kidney suggests a mycotic aneurysm. Arteriography is confirmatory for diagnosis. Treatment consists of appropriate antibiotics and removal of the transplanted kidney.

Venous complications are less frequent, with thrombosis occurring in 1% to 4% of transplants. Causative factors include intimal damage during retrieval, kinking at the iliac vein anastomosis, or pressure secondary to a lymphocele, urinoma, or hematoma. Occasionally, severe rejection can result in venous occlusion. Heparin infusion for incomplete occlusion and transplant nephrectomy for complete occlusion are the indicated therapies. Occasionally, graft salvage is possible if the diagnosis is made before progression of clot into the kidney itself. The classic sign of new-onset hematuria may be an early hint of a renal vein problem and should lead to an ultrasound.

Urologic complications include ureteral obstruction, urinary fistula, or bladder leak. These complications all present with decreased urine output and a rise in serum creatinine. With a urine leak, pain in the region of the transplant may be severe. Mechanical obstruction of the Foley catheter must first be eliminated. Ureteral obstruction occurs in 1% to 9% of transplants, and diagnosis can be made with ultrasonography demonstrating hydronephrosis. A leak is usually diagnosed with a nuclear medicine renal scan. Further definition of a leak or stricture can be obtained via an antegrade pyelogram (**Fig. 35.4**). Early obstruction of the transplant ureter at the site of the bladder anastomosis may respond to internal stenting. Late strictures usually require reoperation, and urine and blood polymerase chain reaction for the polyoma virus should be done in that circumstance, because polyoma viral infection can lead to ureteral stricture. The surgical correction of a ureteral stricture may require reimplantation of the ureter into the bladder, the creation of a Boari flap, or the use of the recipient's native ureter for a ureteroureterostomy (**Fig. 35.5**).

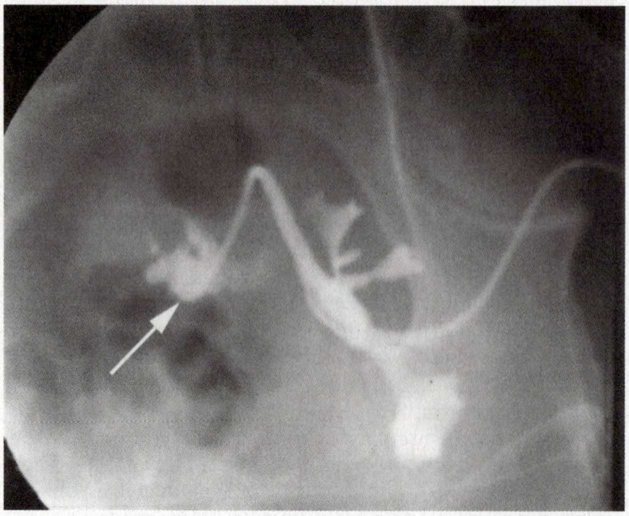

Figure 35.4. Percutaneous nephrostogram revealing a urine leak (*arrow*) from the ureterovesical anastomosis.

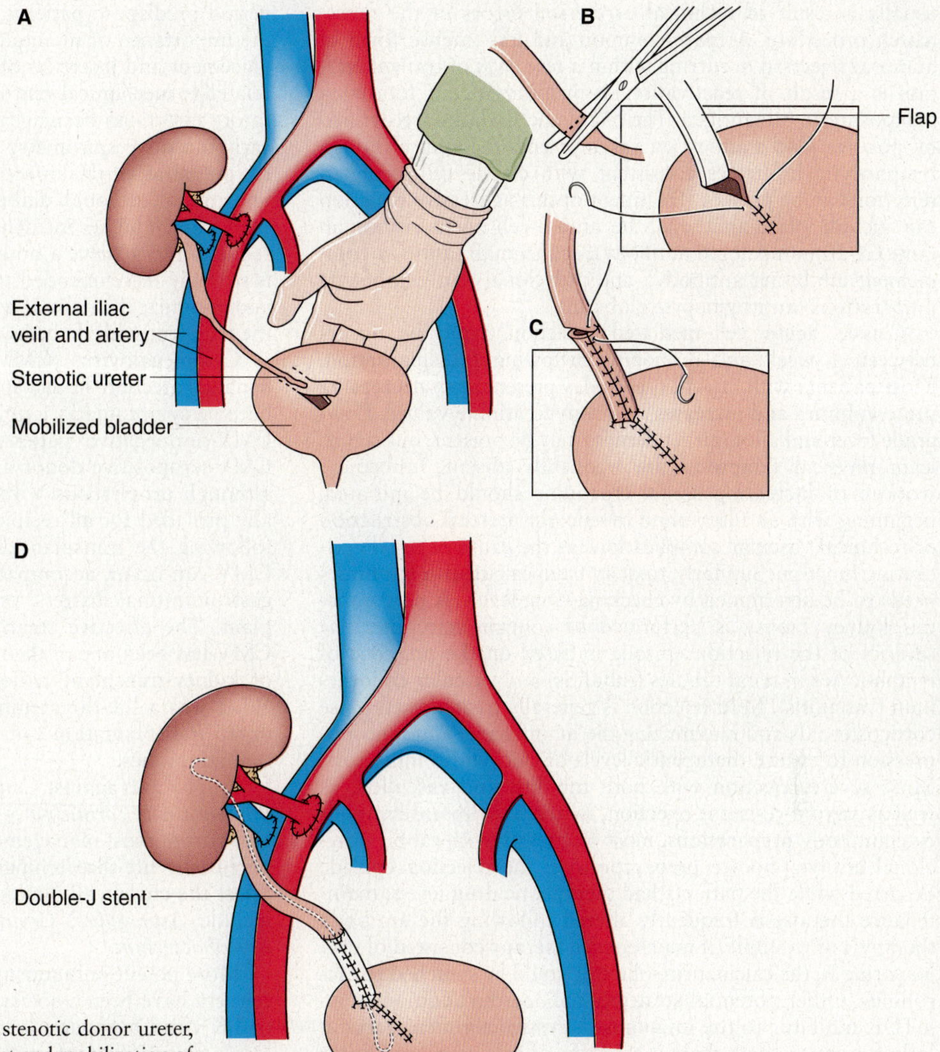

Figure 35.5. **A:** Reconstruction of a stenotic donor ureter, showing resection of the stenotic segment and mobilization of the bladder. **B–D:** A Boari flap is constructed from a tabularized segment of bladder wall and anastomosed end-to-end to the proximal donor ureter.

TRANSPLANTATION

IMMUNOSUPPRESSION, REJECTION, AND IMMUNOSUPPRESSIVE COMPLICATIONS

Immunosuppression

Major advances in the ability to block immune-mediated destruction of the kidney have taken place in the past few years, resulting in a significant decrease in the incidence of acute rejection and improvement in long-term allograft survival rates. This advance is the result of numerous agents that have been added during the past decade to the immunosuppressive armamentarium of prednisone, azathioprine, and cyclosporine A. These agents include tacrolimus, mycophenolate mofetil, sirolimus, and everolimus (mTOR inhibitors), anti–interleukin-2 receptor blockers, antithymocyte globulin (a polyclonal anti–T-cell agent), rituximab (an anti-CD20 monoclonal agent), and most recently, costimulatory blockade with CTLA4-Ig. The addition of various newer drugs targeting different pathways in the alloimmune cascade has permitted the development of regimens that are less dependent on the calcineurin inhibitors or prednisone.[27]

Newer strategies in the immunosuppressive pipeline are targeted to block costimulatory pathways—signaling pathways that activate T cells and T-cell proliferation—and trafficking and recruitment of immune cells. The most promising biologic agents targeted to block the costimulatory pathways include a second-generation CTLA4Ig (LEA29Y), a humanized anti-CD11a (anti-LFA1), and a humanized anti-B7.1/B7.2. Promising agents designed to block T-cell activation and proliferation are the inhibitors of the Janus protein tyrosine kinase (JAK3) and the leflunomide analog FK778. Finally, drugs to block the trafficking and recruitment of immune cells are antagonists against the chemokine receptors CCR1, CXCR3, and CCR5. The chemokine antagonists have been effective in experimental transplantation and will likely be transitioned to clinical trials in the near future.[28]

Rejection

8 Hyperacute rejection is extremely rare and is humorally mediated by preformed anti-HLA antibodies. Hyperacute rejection occurs within minutes to hours following reperfusion of the kidney, whereas classic cell-mediated rejection typically does not occur until 1 to 2 weeks after the transplant. In hyperacute rejection, the anti-HLA antigens bind to the vascular endothelium of the kidney transplant, resulting in activation of the complement cascade and rapid graft thrombosis. The kidney appears blue-black with poor tissue turgor despite adequate blood flow. The characteristic histologic appearance includes the triad of polymorphonuclear leukocytes in the glomerular capillary loops, fibrin deposition, and platelet thrombi. The kidney cannot be salvaged, and a transplant nephrectomy is necessary. The presence of anti-HLA antibodies should be detected in the pretransplant cross-match, and with the sensitivity of current immunologic assays, hyperacute rejection is

usually a result of technical or clerical errors in the crossmatch procedure. A more common and less intense form of humoral rejection occurring within a few days of transplantation is a result of reactivation of memory B cells following reexposure to alloantigen. The histologic findings are defined by positive C4d staining on vascular endothelium, although lymphocytic infiltrates consistent with classic cell-mediated rejection can be present. Treatment of this aggressive rejection can include plasmapheresis, the anti–B-cell agent rituximab (anti-CD20 monoclonal antibody), eculizumab (anti-C5 complement inhibiting antibody), and polyclonal antilymphocyte preparations (antithymocyte globulin).

9 Classic acute cell–mediated rejection typically occurs between 1 week and 3 months following transplantation. Most patients with rejection episodes present with decreasing urine volumes and increases in serum creatinine values. Low-grade fever and allograft tenderness may be present, but significant physical symptoms are frequently absent. Immediate workup of increasing serum creatinine should be initiated, beginning with an ultrasound to rule out ureteral obstruction or technical vascular complications as the cause of the deteriorating function. Similarly, toxicity from calcineurin inhibitors needs to be determined by checking drug levels. A percutaneous kidney biopsy is performed to confirm rejection. The severity of the rejection episode is based on the presence of lymphocytes in renal tubules (tubulitis) and vascular endothelium (vasculitis). Mild rejection is generally treated with pulse corticosteroids and maximizing the maintenance immunosuppression to ensure therapeutic levels of calcineurin inhibitors. More severe rejection with both tubulitis and vasculitis, as well as steroid-resistant rejection, is treated with antilymphocyte antibody preparations, most frequently with rabbit polyclonal antilymphocyte preparations. If the rejection episode occurred while the patients had therapeutic drug levels, maintenance therapy is frequently altered following the antibody therapy. For example, if maintenance therapy consisted of cyclosporine A, the calcineurin inhibitor could be switched to tacrolimus. Other potential strategies include the addition of an mTOR inhibitor to the immunosuppressive regimen, particularly for cases where there is evidence of calcineurin inhibitor toxicity on biopsy.

Each rejection episode takes a toll on long-term function of the kidney transplant. Even well-controlled acute rejection episodes initiate a cascade of events leading to interstitial fibrosis and proliferative changes affecting the vascular endothelium.
10 These histologic and progressive degenerative changes are classified as chronic rejection or chronic allograft nephropathy. These changes lead to loss of graft function over the course of months to several years. Current strategies minimizing calcineurin inhibitor nephrotoxicity are being used to prolong function in kidneys with these chronic changes and involve the addition of TOR inhibitors to replace the calcineurin inhibitors. It remains unclear whether the marked decrease in acute rejection episodes, from greater than 50% to less than 20% observed in recent years, will translate to better long-term function of transplants. Nonetheless, it is evident that immunosuppression strategies minimizing prednisone and calcineurin inhibitors are providing safer and more effective immunosuppression for kidney-transplant recipients while decreasing long-term toxicities associated with immunosuppression.[29]

Immunosuppressive Complications

It would be naive to assume that the intensification of immunosuppressive regimens resulting in decreased acute and chronic rejection rates can be accomplished without sequelae. Infections and malignancy remain significant complications associated with long-term immunosuppression and are the driving force for drug-minimization strategies. Early infections during the perioperative period are commonly iatrogenic and involve bladder infections or intravenous catheter use. Higher doses of immunosuppressive drugs used in the early postoperative period predispose patients to these infections and emphasize the importance of maintaining sterility during Foley catheter placement and insertion of intravenous catheters. Pneumonia related to mechanical ventilation and poor postoperative inspiratory effort can occur in the early postoperative period, and early incentive spirometry should be encouraged to decrease the potential for this infection. Wound infections are relatively uncommon, although diabetes and obesity are both associated with a much higher incidence of wound complications. Weight reduction to achieve a body mass index of less than 40 kg/m^2 is strongly recommended to facilitate the operative procedure and minimize the risks of wound complications, particularly in the recipient with diabetes mellitus.

Cytomegalovirus (CMV), a herpesvirus, remains a problematic infection in the immunosuppressed patient and can become symptomatic 1 to 2 months following the transplant. CMV-seronegative patients who receive a kidney from a CMV-seropositive donor are at the highest risk for infection, although prophylaxis with acyclovir or ganciclovir is generally provided for all recipients for a period of 3 to 6 months following the transplant. Despite prophylaxis, activation of CMV can occur, accompanied by fever, malaise, pneumonia, gastrointestinal distress, or dysfunction of the kidney transplant. The effective treatment of blood- or tissue-invasive CMV has been one of the major advances in the management of kidney-transplant patients within the past two decades. What was a life-threatening disease in the early era of solid organ transplantation can today be effectively managed with oral antibiotics.

Prophylaxis against *Candida albicans* with fluconazole and *Pneumocystis carinii* with trimethoprim–sulfamethoxazole is also part of most management strategies posttransplant. Other potentially life-threatening opportunistic organisms that can affect the chronically immunosuppressed transplant recipient include *Aspergillus, Cryptococcus, Listeria, Nocardia,* and *Mycobacterium.*

More potent immunosuppression regimens used in the current era have been associated with the emergence of polyoma or BK virus, a previously rare infection that may cause graft loss in up to 5% of infected patients. Reduction in immunosuppression is necessary to prevent progression of viral tubulitis. There has been some experience with the use of leflunomide, ironically an immunosuppressive agent, but with an active metabolite, A77 1726, that has substantial antiviral activity in vitro and in animals. Another potential medication, cidofovir, is a nucleotide analog that inhibits viral DNA polymerase but, unfortunately, is also nephrotoxic, and its in vivo efficacy has not been proved. Probably the best method to prevent graft loss due to polyoma is the use of monitoring of urine and serum levels of BK virus, with lowering of immunosuppression when early evidence of polyoma is detected.

Patients with a previous history of active tuberculosis or conversion to purified protein derivative positivity should receive appropriate prophylaxis for 6 months to 1 year following the transplant procedure.

More potent immunosuppression regimens will also have an impact on the development of neoplasms following transplantation.[30] Skin cancers are the most common malignancy following transplantation, with more than 90% being squamous or basal cell cancers. The incidence of skin cancers is staggering, with 50% or more of white recipients ultimately developing lesions. The immunosuppressed patient also has a higher incidence of nodal spread, and educating the patient about the importance of avoiding direct sun exposure is essential. Other malignancies that have a particularly high incidence in transplant recipients include non-Hodgkin lymphomas and carcinomas of the anogenital areas. The etiology of anogenital carcinoma is related to the presence of human papillomavirus. Although there have been no prospective trials to date, there is some evidence that TOR inhibitors are advantageous in the setting of malignancies as the preferred immunosuppressive agent based on their antiproliferative qualities. Conversion to mTOR inhibitors and minimization of calcineurin inhibitors is a strategy that has been used with increasing frequency in the scenario of malignancies following transplantation.

Posttransplant lymphoproliferative disease is the second most common form of malignancy in transplant recipients and is associated with Epstein–Barr virus. These lymphoproliferative syndromes present as a spectrum of pathology, extending from polyclonal lymphoproliferation to monoclonal B-cell lymphomas. Polyclonal disease has been managed by decreasing or withdrawing immunosuppression, whereas progression to monoclonal lymphomas has required chemotherapy. CD20-positive lymphomas have been successfully managed with rituximab, an anti-CD20 antibody, with no significant side effects.

CURRENT RESULTS AND FUTURE TRENDS

Over the past three decades, progressive improvement has been made in patient and graft survival, independent of donor source. Overall graft survival, as well as the half-life of the graft, improved incrementally for live-donor transplants, standard deceased-donor transplants, and even deceased-donor transplants using suboptimal or ECDs.[12] This change is related to improved organ preservation, perfected operative technique, and most importantly, improved immunosuppressive agents. Current 1-year graft survival rates for living- and deceased-donor transplants are 97.5% and 93.2%, respectively.[31] These remarkable 1-year results continue to be overshadowed by the specter of late graft loss due to chronic rejection. This problem remains unsolved in kidney transplantation, and future improvement in long-term survival will be achieved only when the mechanisms of this process are understood.

The ongoing critical shortage of organs will continue to stimulate creative means of increasing living- and deceased-donor pools, as well as the development of alternative organ sources such as xenografts. Expansion in the number and types of immunosuppressive agents has resulted in marked decreases in the incidence of acute rejection, which it is hoped will translate to prolongation in the long-term function of kidney transplants. Newer strategies in immunosuppressive regimens that minimize nephrotoxic cyclosporine and tacrolimus by adding nonnephrotoxic agents will also benefit the long-term function of transplanted kidneys. The effect of ischemia-reperfusion injury on both early and late graft function, as well as its impact on the development of chronic rejection and transplant glomerulopathy, is an area of active research, and potential therapeutic interventions to minimize this injury are being evaluated. The induction of tolerance to foreign antigen remains the "holy grail" of transplantation. A paucity of tolerizing regimens has been applied clinically, although the use of donor bone marrow or stem cells will likely have a future role in achieving the elusive goal of transplantation tolerance.

References

1. Roll GR, Webber AB, Gae DH, et al. A virtual crossmatch based strategy facilitates sharing of deceased donor kidneys for highly sensitized recipients. *Transplantation.* 2020;104(6):1239–1245.
2. Kakuta Y, Okumi M, Unagami K, et al. Outcomes, complications, and economic impact of ABO-incompatible living kidney transplantation: a single-center Japanese cohort study. *Clin Transplant.* 2019;33(6):e13591.
3. Maenosono R, Unagami K, Kakuta Y, et al. Association between response to rituximab and antibody-mediated rejection in ABO-incompatible living kidney transplantation. *Int J Urol.* 2019; 26(12):1114–1120.
4. Mustian MN, Cannon RM, MacLennan PA, et al. Landscape of ABO-incompatible live donor kidney transplantation in the US. *J Am Coll Surg.* 2018;226(4):615–621.
5. Martins PN, Mustian MN, MacLennan PA, et al. Impact of the new kidney allocation system A2/A2B → B policy on access to transplantation among minorities. *Am J Transplant.* 2018;18(8):1947–1953.
6. Haller MC, Kainz A, Baer H, Oberbauer R. Dialysis vintage and outcomes after kidney transplantation: a retrospective cohort study. *Clin J Am Soc Nephrol.* 2017;12(1):122–130.
7. Ahearn AJ, Posselt AM, Kang SM, Roberts JP, Freise CE. Experience with laparoscopic donor nephrectomy among more than 1000 cases: low complication rates, despite more challenging cases. *Arch Surg.* 2011;146(7):859–864.
8. Nogueira JM, Jacobs SC, Haririan A, et al. A single center comparison of long-term outcomes of renal allografts procured laparoscopically versus historic controls procured by the open approach. *Transpl Int.* 2008;21(9):908–914.
9. Creta M, Calogero A, Sagnelli C, et al. Donor and recipient outcomes following robotic-assisted laparoscopic living donor nephrectomy: a systematic review. *Biomed Res Int.* 2019;2019: 1729138.
10. Sawinski D, Locke JE. Evaluation of kidney donors: core curriculum 2018. *Am J Kidney Dis.* 2018;71(5):737–747.
11. Garg N, Thiessen C, Reese PP, et al. Temporal trends in kidney paired donation in the United States: 2006–2021 UNOS/OPTN database analysis. *Am J Transplant.* 2024;24(1):46–56.
12. Aull MJ, Kapur S. Kidney paired donation and its potential impact on transplantation. *Surg Clin North Am.* 2013;93(6):1407–1421.
13. Orandi BJ, Luo X, Massie AB, et al. Survival benefit with kidney transplants from HLA-incompatible live donors. *N Engl J Med.* 2016;374(10):940–950.
14. Kumar V, Locke JE. New perspectives on desensitization in the current era – an overview. *Front Immunol.* 2021;12:696467.
15. 2022 Organ Transplants Again Set Annual Records; Organ Donation From Deceased Donors Continues 12-Year Record-Setting Trend. OPTN. Accessed August 20, 2024. hrsa.gov
16. Stewart DE, Kucheryavaya AY, Klassen DK, Turgeon NA, Formica RN, Aeder MI. Changes in deceased donor kidney transplantation one year after KAS implementation. *Am J Transplant.* 2016;16(6):1834–1847.
17. Garonzik-Wang JM, Berger JC, Ros RL, et al. Live donor champion: finding live kidney donors by separating the advocate from the patient. *Transplantation.* 2012;93(11):1147–1150.
18. Locke JE, Reed RD, Kumar V, et al. Enhanced advocacy and health systems training through patient navigation increases access to living-donor kidney transplantation. *Transplantation.* 2020;104(1):122–129.
19. Reese PP, Abt PL, Blumberg EA, et al. Twelve-month outcomes after transplantation of hepatitis C-infected kidneys into uninfected recipients: a single-group trial. *Ann Intern Med.* 2018;169(5): 273–281.
20. Selhorst P, Combrinck CE, Manning K, et al. Longer-term outcomes of HIV-positive-to-HIV-positive renal transplantation. *N Engl J Med.* 2019;381(14):1387–1389.
21. Shelton BA, Sawsinski D, Linas BP, et al. Population level outcomes and cost-effectiveness of hepatitis C treatment pre- vs. postkidney transplantation. *Am J Transplant.* 2018;18(10):2483–2495.
22. Locke JE, Mehta S, Reed RD, et al. A national study of outcomes among HIV-infected kidney transplant recipients. *J Am Soc Nephrol.* 2015;26(9):2222–2229.
23. Al-Adra DP, Hammel L, Roberts J, et al. Pretransplant solid organ malignancy and organ transplant candidacy: a consensus expert opinion statement. *Am J Transplant.* 2021;21(2):460–474.
24. Al-Adra DP, Hammel L, Roberts J, et al. Preexisting melanoma and hematological malignancies, prognosis, and timing to solid organ transplantation: a consensus expert opinion statement. *Am J Transplant.* 2021;21(2):475–483.
25. Tzvetanov I, Giulianotti PC, Bejarano-Pineda L, et al. Robotic-assisted kidney transplantation. *Surg Clin North Am.* 2013;93: 1309–1323.

26. Broering DC, Raptis DA, Malago M, Clavien P; MIOT Collaborative. Revolutionizing organ transplantation with robotic surgery. *Ann Surg*. 2024;280(5):706–712.
27. Sawinski D, Trofe-Clark J, Leas B, et al. Calcineurin inhibitor minimization, conversion, withdrawal, and avoidance strategies in renal transplantation: a systematic review and meta-analysis. *Am J Transplant*. 2016;16(7):2117–2138.
28. Abramowicz D, Oberbauer R, Heeman U, et al. Recent advances in kidney transplantation from the Descartes advisory board. *Neprhol Dial Transplant*. 2018;33(10):1699–1707.
29. Vincenti F, Rostaing L, Grinyo J, et al. Belatacept and long-term outcomes in kidney transplantation. *N Engl J Med*. 2016;374(4):333–343.
30. Engles EA, Pfeiffer RM, Fraumeni JF Jr, et al. Spectrum of cancer risk among US solid organ transplant recipients. *JAMA*. 2011;306(17):1891–1901.
31. U.S. Department of Health & Human Services. HRSA. Organ Procurement and Transplantation Network. *National Data*. Accessed August 20, 2024. https://optn.transplant.hrsa.gov/data/view-data-reports/national-data.

Hepatic Transplantation

Benjamin Samstein and Christopher J. Sonnenday

Key Points

1. Liver transplantation remains the only definitive therapy for patients with end-stage liver disease (ESLD).
2. The three primary indications for liver transplantation in the United States are alcohol-related liver disease (ALD), metabolic-associated steatotic liver disease (MASLD), and hepatocellular carcinoma (HCC).
3. Transplantation for early-stage HCC is associated with low recurrence rates and excellent survival, driving interest in expanding criteria for liver transplantation to patients with more extensive but localized tumor burdens.
4. The multidisciplinary evaluation of a patient for liver transplantation involves thorough scrutiny of medical, surgical, and psychosocial domains to ensure the benefits of transplant are realized.
5. Recipient, donor, and technical factors dictate the likelihood of major posttransplant complications, which tend to occur in a predictable continuum.

1 Over the past 50 years, liver transplantation has evolved from an experimental procedure to the definitive treatment for patients with end-stage liver disease (ESLD), specific metabolic diseases, and select hepatic malignancies. Dr. Thomas Starzl reported the first three cases of orthotopic liver transplantation in 1963, for a child with biliary atresia, a man with alcohol-related cirrhosis and hepatocellular carcinoma (HCC), and a man with hilar cholangiocarcinoma.[1] None of these patients survived more than 22 days after the operation, but the foundations for the donor and recipient operations were established. Each of those diagnoses remains an indication for liver transplantation today, and the survival of liver transplant recipients has improved dramatically. Current 1-year patient survival rates following liver transplantation are 90% to 97%, with median life expectancy for recipients of more than 15 years posttransplant.[2]

As is true of all solid organ transplantation, advances in immunosuppression strategies have had an equivalent or greater impact on outcome than advances in surgical technique. Following the discouraging initial experience in liver transplantation in the 1960s in the United States and the United Kingdom, a relative moratorium on liver transplantation was established by Dr. Starzl and his contemporaries. Very few liver transplants occurred worldwide until the 1980s, following the development of the calcineurin-inhibitor cyclosporine by Sir Roy Calne in 1979.[3] This discovery transformed the field, and cyclosporine quickly became the primary maintenance immunosuppression drug for all solid organ transplant recipients. Over the ensuing decade, liver transplantation rapidly expanded such that more than 2,000 cases were performed in the United States in 1989. In 1991, liver transplantation of adults with decompensated cirrhosis was approved for Medicare Coverage by the Centers for Medicare and Medicaid Services.[4]

A fundamental challenge in solid organ transplantation is to ensure that supply of donor organs increases to meet increasing demand. In recent years, more than 12,000 candidates await liver transplantation in the United States and annual transplant volume has exceeded 10,000.[2] The disparity in supply of donor livers and the lack of an alternative life-sustaining therapy for ESLD translate to approximately 2,000 deaths on the waiting list annually. Many of the recent innovations in liver transplantation over the last 20 years have focused on expanding the number of available donors for liver transplantation, including use of elderly deceased donors, use of grafts with significant steatosis, use of organs from donors with risk of transmission of donor disease (eg, donors with hepatitis B, hepatitis C, HIV, or malignancy), novel preservation techniques, use of livers from donation after circulatory death (DCD) donors, and living-donor liver transplantation (LDLT).

INDICATIONS FOR LIVER TRANSPLANTATION

2 One of the most noticeable changes in liver transplantation over the past three decades has been the significant change in the patients undergoing transplantation—recipients are older, have more comorbidities, and have different primary diagnoses as their indication for liver transplantation. For more than two decades, decompensated cirrhosis related to chronic hepatitis C infection was leading indication for liver transplantation in the United States. The development of direct-acting antiviral agents that can effectively eradicate hepatitis C viremia in greater than 95% of treated patients has led to a rapid fall in the number of patients with hepatitis C–related cirrhosis referred for liver transplantation.[5] This change, accompanied by the substantial rise in number of patients with metabolic-associated steatotic liver disease (MASLD), alcohol-related cirrhosis, and hepatic malignancy referred for liver transplantation, has significantly changed the recipient population (**Fig. 36.1**). Patients with alcohol-related liver disease (ALD), MASLD, and HCC account for ~60% of patients currently transplanted in the United States, with the remainder accounted for with the diagnoses in **Table 36.1**. Biliary atresia is the most common indication for liver transplantation in infants and children. The cholestatic liver diseases (primary sclerosing cholangitis, primary biliary cirrhosis, Alagille syndrome) and autoimmune hepatitis tend to occur in younger adults and occasionally adolescents, requiring transplant.

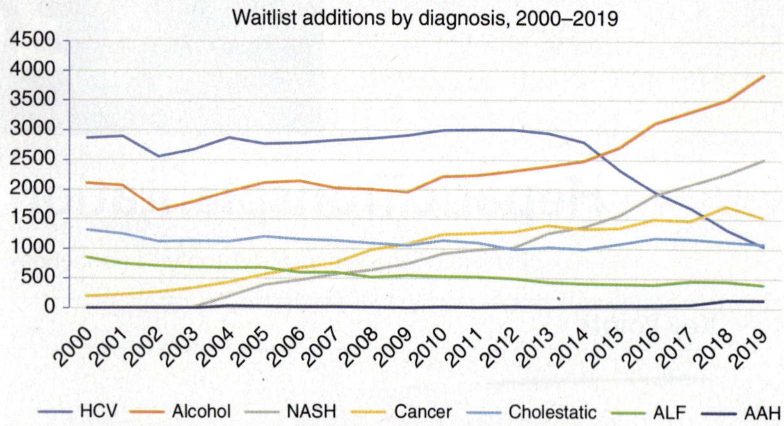

Figure 36.1. Liver transplant waitlist additions by diagnosis, United States, 2000–2019. ALF, acute liver failure; AAH, acute alcoholic hepatitis. (Based upon Organ Procurement and Transplant Network data as of June 30, 2020. https://optn.transplant.hrsa.gov/)

Metabolic-Associated Steatotic Liver Disease

The epidemic of obesity, metabolic syndrome, and associated MASLD has changed the epidemiology of liver disease in the United States and other developed nations. Projections are that ESLD secondary to MASLD will continue to rise as a primary indication for liver transplantation, advancing a patient population with other substantial comorbidities toward transplant.[6] The increasing incidence of hepatic steatosis has also begun to affect the health of the deceased-donor organ pool, with steatotic-donor livers recognized as higher-risk organs with a higher risk of early allograft dysfunction. The obesity and comorbid disease associated with MASLD recipients have raised concern that posttransplant outcomes will be inferior in this patient group, but published studies to date do not appear to validate that concern.[7] Clearly though, MASLD can recur in the transplanted liver, and programs to engage patients in improving their overall health and nutrition posttransplant will be critical to achieving durable outcomes in this patient population.

Table 36.1. Indications for Liver Transplantation by Diagnosis

Diagnosis	Examples
Metabolic-associated steatotic liver disease	
Alcohol-related liver disease	
Hepatic malignancy	Hepatocellular carcinoma Cholangiocarcinoma Metastatic neuroendocrine tumor Hepatoblastoma Metastatic colon cancer
Viral hepatitis	Hepatitis B Hepatitis C
Cholestatic liver disease	Primary sclerosing cholangitis Primary biliary cirrhosis Biliary atresia Alagille syndrome
Autoimmune hepatitis	
Budd–Chiari syndrome	
Fulminant hepatic failure	
Metabolic liver disease	Amyloidosis Ornithine transcarbamylase (OTC) deficiency Maple syrup urine disease Crigler–Najjar syndrome Tyrosinemia Cystic fibrosis Wilson disease Alpha-1 antitrypsin deficiency Hemochromatosis

Alcohol-Related Liver Disease

ALD remains a primary indication for liver transplantation, and recent data suggest a substantial rise in the incidence of alcohol-use disorder and associated transplant referrals in the United States, a trend that was accelerated during the COVID-19 pandemic.[8] Furthermore, the utilization of liver transplantation for select patients with acute alcoholic hepatitis without cirrhosis is a growing indication for liver transplantation.[9,10] Traditional arbitrary policies about length of sobriety necessary to be considered a liver transplant candidate have been replaced with more comprehensive evaluations for ALD patients, as evidence demonstrates that select patients without concomitant untreated mental illness and possessing adequate social support can be transplanted with limited sobriety with outcomes similar to other diagnosis groups. In general, the ALD patient population is younger and otherwise healthier than other liver transplant candidates, but poses substantial psychosocial challenges in evaluation and posttransplant management for centers.[11]

Of note, ALD and MASLD together account for the primary risk factor for approximately 50% of HCC cases in the United States,[12] and epidemiologic evidence exists that obesity and type 2 diabetes mellitus increase the risk of HCC among ALD patients. There are, however, distinctions between the presentation of patients with HCC in the setting of ALD versus MASLD. ALD patients most often develop HCC in the setting of cirrhosis (~80% of cases), have a higher incidence of vascular invasion, and appear to have worse overall survival than patients with MASLD-related HCC. As many as 50% of HCC cases in MASLD patients may not yet have cirrhosis at the time of diagnosis and appear to more often present with a large solitary HCC as opposed to multifocal disease. MASLD-related HCC also may more often be well-differentiated tumors, and less prone to AFP production, which poses additional challenges to screening protocols.[13]

3 Transplant for Malignancy

The indications for transplant for patients with hepatobiliary malignancies have expanded (**Fig. 36.2**), and new challenges in recipient selection, immunosuppression management, and cancer surveillance have therefore emerged. Liver transplantation has been established as definitive therapy for select patients with HCC, for the rare neoplasm hepatic epithelioid hemangioendothelioma, for pediatric patients with unresectable hepatoblastoma, and for a select population of patients with hilar cholangiocarcinoma and metastatic neuroendocrine tumor. In addition, emerging data have documented the

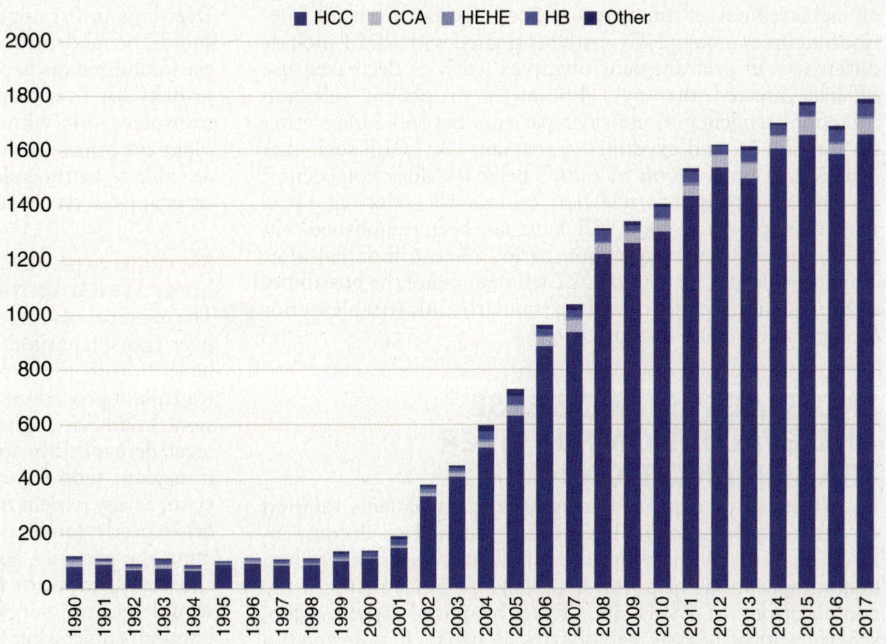

Figure 36.2. Liver transplants performed for malignancy, United States, 2000–2017. HCC, hepatocellular carcinoma; CCA, cholangiocarcinoma; HEHE, hepatic epithelioid hemangioendothelioma; HB, hepatoblastoma. (Based upon Organ Procurement and Transplant Network data as of January 15, 2018. https://optn.transplant.hrsa.gov/)

benefit of liver transplantation in highly select candidates with intrahepatic cholangiocarcinoma and metastatic colorectal cancer.[14,15]

Early series reporting transplantation of HCC patients documented excessively high recurrence rates (75%+) with expedited cancer-related mortality.[16] It was not until Mazzaferro's seminal series of patients with early-stage HCC undergoing successful liver transplantation that the primacy of patient selection and tumor burden was established.[17] The Milan criteria established in that study—cirrhotic patients with T2 tumors (**Table 36.2**), who do not have a resection option either due to tumor burden or severity of liver disease—remain the benchmark for predicting low recurrence risk. Numerous efforts have been made to expand eligibility criteria beyond Milan criteria, although none have been universally accepted. Alternative criteria may be evaluated on the balance between expanding eligibility for transplant to additional patients with HCC, with the increased risk of recurrent disease. Consensus in the transplant community has generally established 60% 5-year overall posttransplant survival as the lowest acceptable survival to balance the utility of transplant for HCC with other diagnoses. Though select experiences have documented similar outcomes among patients with HCC beyond Milan criteria, there has not yet been consensus in the United States to change Organ Procurement and Transplantation Network (OPTN) policy to extend selection criteria for HCC candidates.

Table 36.2. OPTN Modified TNM Staging for Hepatocellular Carcinoma

T stage	T1	Solitary tumor <2 cm
	T2	Solitary tumor 2–5 cm; 2–3 nodules all less than 3 cm
	T3	Solitary tumor >5 cm; 2–3 nodules with at least one >3 cm
	T4a	Four or more tumors
	T4b	T2, T3, or T4b tumor with gross vascular involvement
N stage	N1	Regional lymph node involvement
M stage	M1	Any extrahepatic metastatic disease beyond regional nodes

While extension of HCC eligibility criteria at the time of transplant has not been endorsed broadly in the United States, liver-directed therapy to downstage patients diagnosed beyond Milan criteria, such that they meet OPTN T2 criteria at the time of transplant, has been increasingly utilized.[18] Despite this increasing experience and expert opinion supporting the use of downstaging to expand access to transplantation, there is no consensus about the most effective modality for liver-directed therapy.[19,20] A systematic review of published series of downstaging suggested that up to 60% of candidates will be successfully downstaged to within Milan criteria, but no clear advantage was demonstrated according to liver-directed therapy modality (transarterial chemoembolization versus transarterial radioembolization).[21] A critical element of downstaging is the utilization of standard criteria for measuring response to therapy by imaging. The modified RECIST (mRECIST) criteria were created by expert consensus convened by the American Association for the Study of Liver Diseases (AASLD) and remain the gold standard for evaluating response to therapy on contrast-enhanced CT or MRI.[22] The extent of residual viable tumor, rather than measurement of treatment cavity or previous tumor size, is utilized to determine the amount of residual disease. Patients should be monitored for intrahepatic and extrahepatic progression every 3 months until transplant. Allocation policy for deceased-donor liver transplant must balance the survival benefit of transplantation for HCC patients against the need of patients with noncancer diagnoses. Furthermore, evidence exists that "expedited" transplant of HCC patients may lead to inferior outcomes, as patients with HCC with shorter waiting times for transplant have higher recurrence rates relative to HCC patients with longer wait times.[23] Current OPTN allocation policy delays assignment of HCC exception points for 6 months (with restaging imaging and serum alfa-fetoprotein (AFP) required every 3 months). After 6 months listing with their natural MELD score, patients with T2 HCC are granted an exception score near the median MELD at transplant. The delay in granting the HCC exception for 6 months allows for observation of tumor biology and dropout of patients who progressed beyond T2 criteria.

Since waiting time may help select the most appropriate patients for transplantation for HCC, the use of LDLT for HCC recipients poses interesting challenges. While among patients with non-HCC diagnoses, LDLT offers equivalent or superior survival outcomes to deceased-donor liver transplantation,[24] LDLT for HCC patients appears to be associated with an increased risk of tumor recurrence.[25] Explanations for inferior outcomes among HCC patients treated with LDLT include differences in pretransplant therapies (such as decreased use of liver-directed therapy), differences in patient selection (potential tendency to consider patients beyond Milan criteria for LDLT), and expedited transplant via LDLT such that a period of observation of tumor behavior does not occur.[26] The most appropriate selection criteria for selecting HCC patients appropriate for LDLT have not been established, but utilization of some observation period (3 to 6 months) after diagnosis of HCC prior to LDLT may eliminate the possibility of transplanting patients with particularly unfavorable tumor biology and increased recurrence risk.

END-STAGE LIVER DISEASE AND EVALUATION FOR LIVER TRANSPLANTATION

Regardless of their primary diagnosis, most patients referred for liver transplantation have ESLD, defined as decompensated cirrhosis with symptoms of hepatic synthetic failure and complications of portal hypertension. Since many of the complications of ESLD are driven by portal hypertension, replacement of healthy hepatocytes alone (such as through a cellular-based therapy, or heterotopic or auxiliary transplant) would not cure portal hypertension. Orthotopic liver transplantation addresses not only the synthetic failure but also serves to correct portal hypertension by replacing the fibrotic liver that serves as a high-resistance circuit to portal blood flow with a healthy, low-resistance liver. Patients without significant synthetic failure but with significant complications of portal hypertension (refractory ascites or recurrent variceal hemorrhage) might be treated effectively with procedures to address portal hypertension, such as a transjugular intrahepatic portosystemic shunt (TIPS) procedure or a surgical therapy for portal hypertension (splenorenal or mesocaval shunt).

While laboratory measures of hepatic function exist, and the Model of End-Stage Liver Disease (MELD) score serves as a helpful predictor of mortality of ESLD,[27] patients referred for liver transplantation should have clinical symptoms that justify transplantation. The most common symptoms include jaundice, fatigue, loss of muscle mass and cachexia, and hepatic encephalopathy. Complications of portal hypertension include ascites, hepatic hydrothorax, variceal hemorrhage, and splenomegaly with thrombocytopenia. The development of hepatorenal syndrome, associated with a particularly poor prognosis in ESLD, should also prompt consideration of liver transplantation.[28] The clinical trajectory of patients with chronic liver disease can be variable and difficult to predict, and may depend on whether the cause of liver injury can be treated or removed, such as antiviral therapy for chronic hepatitis or alcohol cessation in ALD. Medical therapies to manage symptoms of decompensated cirrhosis have improved substantially over the past decades, but ultimately, no definitive therapies for ESLD exist other than liver transplantation.

Acute Liver Injury and Fulminant Hepatic Failure

Currently, less than 5% of liver transplants in the United States are performed for fulminant hepatic failure, a profound syndrome that may be precipitated by diverse etiologies. Common causes of acute liver injury among liver transplant candidates include acetaminophen toxicity, autoimmune hepatitis, drug-induced injury, viral disease, hepatic ischemia, Wilson disease, and idiopathic causes.[29] Fortunately, many patients with acute liver injury will recover with supportive care, but patients who develop fulminant hepatic failure may be considered for urgent liver transplantation. Patients present with jaundice and hepatic encephalopathy and develop multisystem organ failure. Importantly, the urgency of liver transplantation is driven by the development of cerebral edema and brain injury, including herniation that occurs in patients with fulminant hepatic failure. Decisions to list appropriate patients for liver transplantation should be made in under 24 hours, and patients meeting criteria for fulminant hepatic failure are granted special expedited priority for liver transplantation (Status 1a) with the goal of transplantation within 48 to 72 hours of presentation. Transplant outcomes in the select patients with this diagnosis who are able to be transplanted rapidly are similar to other diagnosis groups in recent studies.[30]

Medical and Surgical Evaluation for Liver Transplantation

4 The medical and surgical evaluation of patients referred for liver transplantation is focused on identifying patients whose benefit from the procedure outweighs the risks of the liver transplant procedure and the need for chronic immunosuppression. In addition, given the lack of sufficient donor organs to meet demand, transplant centers must choose candidates for transplant who have a high likelihood of posttransplant survival, as any patient transplanted competes to some degree with other needy candidates. The evaluation therefore, must determine the presence and impact of medical comorbidities, psychosocial fitness for transplant, and any technical factors that would increase surgical risk. In addition, given the need for immunosuppression posttransplant, the evaluation must identify risk factors for conditions that could be exacerbated with chronic immunosuppression (eg, chronic infections and extrahepatic malignancy). While the specific risk–benefit analysis for any individual patient is subject to transplant center practices, guidelines exist to guide standard evaluation processes.[31]

As the success of liver transplantation has increased, medical conditions previously thought to be contraindications to transplant have diminished. Broadly speaking, conditions with limited life expectancy, and/or those that compromise short-term transplant outcomes, are still considered relative contraindications to transplant. MELD score predicts mortality risk among patients with ESLD, but certain patient populations have conditions where MELD does not reflect their mortality risk (ie, hepatopulmonary syndrome, portopulmonary syndrome, hepatic malignancy, metabolic disease). Both deceased-donor liver transplantation and, when available, LDLT may provide a survival benefit for lower MELD patients with significant clinical decompensation refractory to medical management.[32]

Challenging elements of the liver transplant evaluation in current practice focus on the evaluation of older candidates with obesity and medical comorbidities, particularly cardiac disease. Obese patients have been shown to have increased perioperative complications and diminished long-term outcomes following liver transplantation in older studies.[33] However, traditional measures of obesity, such as BMI, may be difficult to interpret in liver transplant candidates with ascites and anasarca, and more recent studies suggest similar outcomes in selected obese patients relative to nonobese recipients.[34] Obesity and metabolic syndrome are common among liver transplant candidates, particularly those with MASLD-related cirrhosis, which has markedly increased the demand for transplant among obese candidates.

Pretransplant cardiac evaluation focuses primarily on identifying risk factors that would compromise perioperative outcomes. The hemodynamic changes experienced during the liver transplant period, associated with the challenges of total hepatectomy, the systemic vasodilation of cirrhosis, and the circulatory collapse that can be associated with reperfusion injury and early graft dysfunction, require that liver transplant candidates have acceptable cardiac function. All liver transplant candidates should undergo noninvasive cardiac testing, typically with echocardiography and a test for inducible ischemia (dobutamine echocardiography or nuclear medicine perfusion scan). Patients with concern for ischemia should be evaluated with coronary angiography if otherwise appropriate transplant candidates and considered for revascularization when treatable lesions are identified.[35] In addition, the cardiac evaluation should scrutinize valvular dysfunction, ventricular dysfunction, and evidence of pulmonary hypertension, all of which would require further evaluation to determine appropriateness for transplant.

Waitlist Management and Organ Allocation

Once the decision has been made to list a patient for transplant, the patient's priority for transplant is established by the OPTN policy. Current liver transplant allocation in the United States is based upon the MELD 3.0 score, an adaptation of the MELD-based allocation first adopted in 2002.[36] MELD-based allocation is predicated on the ability of MELD to predict waitlist mortality, and the addition of MELD 3.0 recognizes the impact of hyponatremia, hypoalbuminemia, and gender on outcomes of patients with ESLD. MELD 3.0 is a relatively sensitive indicator of changes in clinical condition, allowing the sickest patients to rise to the top of the waiting list. Current liver transplant allocation distributes livers according to proximity circles determined by distance of the candidate transplant center from the donor hospital, allowing broader sharing of livers to limit geographic variation in transplant access.

As the MELD system does not represent the waitlist mortality or dropout rate for all patients, a system of MELD exception scores has been created to assign additional points to patients who meet established criteria for specific diagnoses. Patients being transplanted for HCC represent the largest group of MELD exception candidates, though other standard criteria exist for other diagnoses (hepatopulmonary syndrome, portopulmonary syndrome, polycystic liver disease, other hepatic malignancies, etc.). OPTN policy dictates that exception applications are reviewed by a national review board, with standardized appeal policies when necessary. The system aims to assign appropriate waitlist priority to patients awaiting transplant. OPTN policy prioritizes children, who are allocated livers from young donors preferentially before adults. This policy attempts to overcome the disadvantage children on the waitlist may face due to size mismatch between pediatric candidates and available donor organs. Pediatric waitlist mortality remains low in the current system, although the smallest infants continue to face challenges in identifying appropriate donors.[37]

SURGICAL PROCEDURE: LIVER TRANSPLANTATION

Donor Selection, Procurement, and Preservation

The ideal deceased donor is less than age 50, previously healthy, without liver injury or disease, hemodynamically stable, without risk factors for blood-borne infections, and has been declared brain dead prior to recovery of organs.[38] The graft itself should be without steatosis. Though many factors act in synergy to affect recipient outcomes, donor age has repeatedly proven to be the most important donor factor in predicting allograft failure and posttransplant death.[39] The proportion of available deceased donors that meet this exclusive definition is decreasing (likely 40% or less of current donors in the United States), and current allocation of acuity circles directs these donors to the highest priority candidates.[40] Increased demand has led to consideration of expanded criteria donors, including elderly donors (age >70), donors with evidence of resolving liver injury, and donor livers with steatosis. Such donor livers can be used with acceptable outcomes, particularly when chosen for transplant in lower MELD patients with less severe portal hypertension.

The significant increase in deceased-donor liver transplantation in recent years has been facilitated by a marked increase in the use of DCD donor livers. These donors do not fulfill the strict criteria for brain death but have suffered an irreversible neurologic injury or other medical condition from which meaningful recovery is deemed exceedingly unlikely. Once the decision for possible donation from next of kin has been confirmed, the donor is brought to the operating room (or nearby location) for withdrawal of life-sustaining therapies. Prior to extubation high-dose intravenous heparin is administered, and life-sustaining care is withdrawn by the team caring for the potential donor. Rapid procurement is then performed to facilitate organ recovery. Selection of DCD donor livers appropriate for transplantation is largely based on donor functional warm ischemic time, defined as the time when the donor demonstrates agonal perfusion (defined variably, but with SBP <80 mm Hg and/or oxygen saturation <80% being a common definition) until donor cross-clamp, interpreted in the context of other donor risk factors such as age and steatosis. Historically, DCD donor livers have carried a higher risk of graft loss and the development of ischemic cholangiopathy from biliary ischemia. However, improved donor selection and innovation in preservation technology have facilitated the safe use of DCD donor livers with outcomes largely equivalent to brain-dead allografts.

The donor procurement operation has the goals of evaluation for donor conditions that could compromise recipient outcome (eg, occult donor infection or malignancy), assessment of organ quality, and safe and efficient organ retrieval. In the case of brain-dead donor procurement, steps include exploration through an incision from sternal notch to pubis, assessment of liver quality including a liver biopsy when indicated (concern for steatosis, fibrosis, or focal lesion), placement of aortic cannulae for perfusion, supraceliac aortic cross-clamp, rapid cooling with cold perfusate and sterile ice instillation into the body cavity, exsanguination of the donor with cessation of cardiac activity, followed by methodical removal of the organs without injury. The donor liver is further assessed for vascular disease or anomalies that may complicate implantation. In the case of DCD donor procurement, the steps above are accelerated with the goal of cannulation, cross-clamp, and flush within 5 to 10 minutes of declaration of death to limit further injury from donor functional warm ischemic time. An alternative emerging technique, normothermic regional perfusion, for DCD procurement is to instead rapidly cannulate and initiate extracorporeal circulation after declaration of death to reinitiate perfusion to the potential donor organs.[41]

Historic practice has included cold perfusion with fortified preservation solutions, and cold storage of the liver at 4 °C. Cold ischemic time beyond 6 to 8 hours was associated with compromised recipient outcomes using cold storage. Clinical trials performed in the past decade have demonstrated the benefits of machine perfusion of organs using normothermic oxygenated devices using packed red blood cells as the perfusate, or hypothermic oxygenated perfusion using preservation solution.[42–44] In clinical practice, use of these devices has allowed expansion of organ utilization in more expanded criteria donors, mitigated the pressure of cold ischemic time, allowing greater travel of organs, and mitigation of some of the reperfusion injury associated with expanded criteria donor organs, especially DCD donor livers. In addition, these devices allow the potential for more refined selection of donor livers based upon functional metrics while on machine perfusion systems.

Anesthetic Management

An anesthesiologist with experience in liver transplantation is essential to the transplant team. Proper anesthetic management and effective communication between the surgery and anesthesiology teams are critical to optimize care during the procedure. For adult patients, cardiac monitoring is often performed either by pulmonary artery catheterization or intraoperative transesophageal echocardiography. An arterial catheter is placed for blood pressure monitoring. Adequate vascular access, often including central venous catheters, is required for the administration of blood products and the potential for rapid resuscitation in the case of massive blood loss. A device for rapid infusion and the ability to warm blood products or intravenous fluids is required. Low central venous pressures maintained during the hepatectomy phase of the procedure help avoid excess bleeding.

Intraoperative Management of Coagulopathy

Liver transplantation has the potential for massive blood loss for several reasons. Liver transplant candidates with cirrhosis often have synthetic deficiencies in circulating coagulation factors as well as severe portal hypertension associated with thrombocytopenia and extensive venous collaterals. Intraoperative coagulopathy may be worsened during the anhepatic phase of the procedure and immediately after reperfusion when hepatic function may be impaired. Finally, liver transplantation involves extensive dissection of major vascular structures, including the inferior vena cava, portal vein, and hepatic artery, all with an inherent risk for bleeding. Intraoperatively, coagulation is best assessed by functional assays such as thromboelastography (TEG) and rotational thromboelastometry (ROTEM).[45] Use of these point-of-care tests may reduce transfusion requirements.[46] Normal coagulation is also helped by maintaining normal pH, calcium levels, and normothermia. Following reperfusion of the donor liver, a fibrinolytic state may be encountered. This is related to the global reduction of all coagulation factors and simultaneous generation of tissue plasminogen activator.[47] As long as graft function is not significantly impaired, fibrinolysis gradually resolves.

Surgical Technique

Transplantation of the liver is among the most technically demanding surgical procedures. The donor liver must be prepared on the back table for implantation (**Fig. 36.3A**). Bench preparation includes meticulous ligation of tributaries from the vena cava (adrenal vein, phrenic vein, and lumbar branches) is performed. The artery is freed from surrounding tissues from the aortic patch to the gastroduodenal artery. Dissection more distally along the proper hepatic artery is avoided to prevent unnecessary injury. The portal vein is circumferentially dissected free, with small branches ligated. Tissues surrounding the common bile duct are left intact to avoid injury to the blood supply. Assessment for vascular anomalies, specifically hepatic artery variants that may require reconstruction, is performed.

The most used recipient incision is a unilateral or bilateral subcostal incision with a midline extension to the xiphoid process (**Fig. 36.3B**). After dividing the fascia, any ascites is evacuated. The ligamentum teres hepatis is divided between clamps and ligated because a large recannulized umbilical vein is often present in patients with severe portal hypertension. After dividing the falciform ligament, a mechanical retractor is used to retract the bilateral costal margins anteriorly and superiorly for exposure of the upper abdomen. The abdominal cavity and liver are then inspected for any abnormalities, including unsuspected malignancy. Following this, liver transplantation occurs in three stages: recipient hepatectomy, anhepatic phase, and postrevascularization.

Recipient Hepatectomy

During the recipient hepatectomy phase, the liver is mobilized from its ligamentous attachments, and the porta hepatis is skeletonized. Attention is first directed to dissecting and skeletonizing the structures of the portal triad. The peritoneum overlying the portal triad is divided with electrocautery. The right and left hepatic arteries are dissected free, ligated, and divided, leaving adequate length to provide options for the arterial anastomosis. The proper hepatic artery is also dissected free to the level of the gastroduodenal artery allowing enough length for clamping during the anastomosis. A replaced or accessory right hepatic artery typically arises as a branch of the proximal superior mesenteric artery and travels in a posterior position to the common bile duct and lateral to the portal vein. When the replaced right hepatic artery is relatively large and the proper hepatic artery is diminutive in size, the replaced right hepatic artery can be left long and used for arterial inflow for the donor liver. A replaced or accessory left hepatic artery is rarely adequate for arterial inflow and is securely ligated.

Conceptually, the common bile duct and common hepatic duct should be dissected free with as much length as possible and without injuring the blood supply to the bile duct. Leaving the recipient bile duct as long as possible allows the length of the donor bile duct, which may have a tenuous blood supply, to be shorter and still avoid tension at the time of anastomosis.

Once the bile duct and the hepatic artery are freed from surrounding tissues, the portal vein can be easily approached from its anterior, medial, and lateral aspects. In general, the portal vein is freed circumferentially from the edge of the

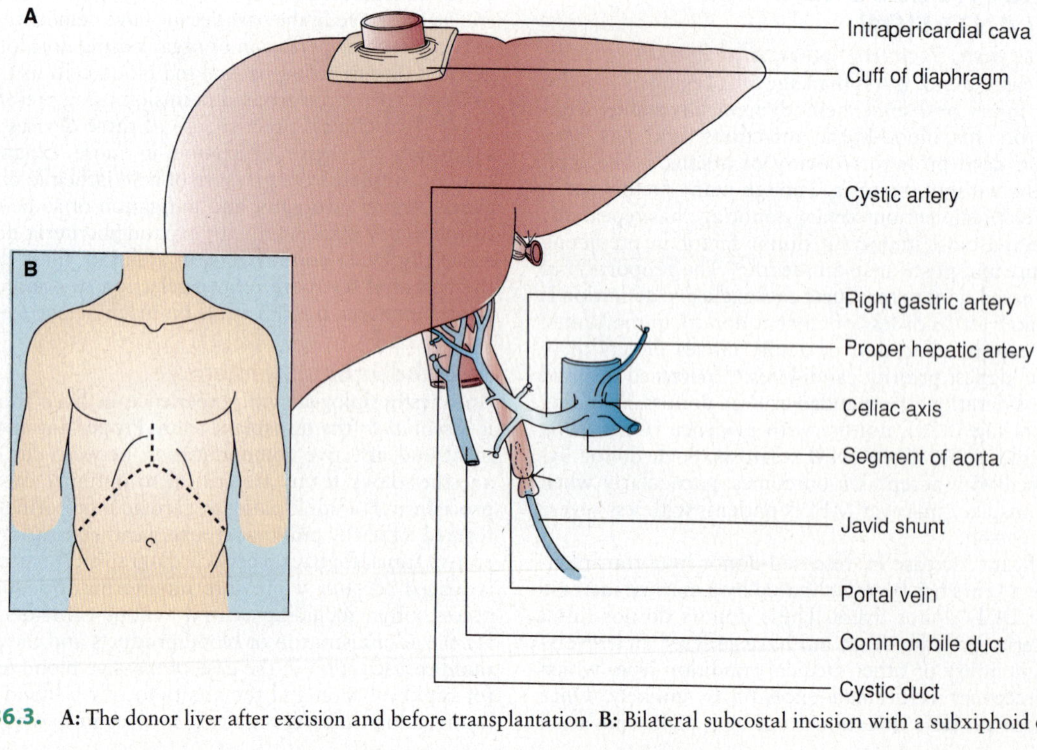

Figure 36.3. **A:** The donor liver after excision and before transplantation. **B:** Bilateral subcostal incision with a subxiphoid extension.

duodenum up to its bifurcation into the right and left portal veins. Most patients with severe portal hypertension will not develop hypotension, small bowel edema, or ischemia if the portal vein is clamped and divided because of the presence of portal venous collaterals. However, patients without portal hypertension, such as those undergoing liver transplantation for fulminant hepatic failure, metabolic deficiency, or those who have had a TIPS, may develop small bowel edema or hypotension when the portal vein is clamped. Small bowel edema can lead to limited exposure in the right upper quadrant, making implantation of the liver difficult. In these situations, the portal vein should be left in continuity for as long as possible, particularly when the use of venovenous bypass or a temporary portocaval shunt is not intended.

For those patients with portal vein thrombosis, portal venous flow can be restored in most cases. A mature portal vein thrombosis may require an eversion endovenectomy. If this maneuver is unsuccessful, the junction of the splenic vein and superior mesenteric vein may be patent. Dissection of the portal vein behind the pancreatic neck to this junction can then be performed to allow for a patent anastomosis. Dissection to the confluence of the splenic and superior mesenteric veins is sometimes necessary in pediatric recipients because of the small caliber of the portal vein within the porta hepatis. In rare cases, all of these maneuvers may be unsuccessful and a venous bypass graft from the superior mesenteric vein may be necessary (**Fig. 36.4**). If the superior mesenteric vein is also occluded, the inferior vena cava or left renal vein can be used for portal inflow, procedures termed cavoportal or renoportal transposition (**Fig. 36.5**) which may be successful in addressing both hepatic inflow and alleviation of portal hypertension when significant portosystemic shunts exist.

During mobilization of the liver, the left and right triangular and coronary ligaments are divided using electrocautery. The bare area of the liver is dissected along a plane just superficial to the capsule of the liver. If a bicaval venous anastomosis technique is used, the vena cava can be circumferentially mobilized near the diaphragm above the hepatic veins as well as in an infrahepatic position. However, if a piggyback or cavocavostomy (side-to-side caval anastomosis) technique is intended, the dissection of the dorsal aspect of the vena cava is unnecessary and risks bleeding from collateral or lumbar venous branches in this area. If caval preservation is being performed, the liver is then dissected off of the anterior aspect of the inferior vena cava. Small venous branches from the inferior vena cava to the caudate lobe are ligated and divided. Larger branches, such as an inferior hepatic vein, are clamped, divided, and oversewn. Division of the portal vein facilitates exposure for this dissection, but is not required. The liver may be gradually retracted and dissected from either the right or left aspects until the right, middle, and left hepatic veins are reached. The hepatocaval ligament along the right lateral aspect of the vena cava is ligated and divided.

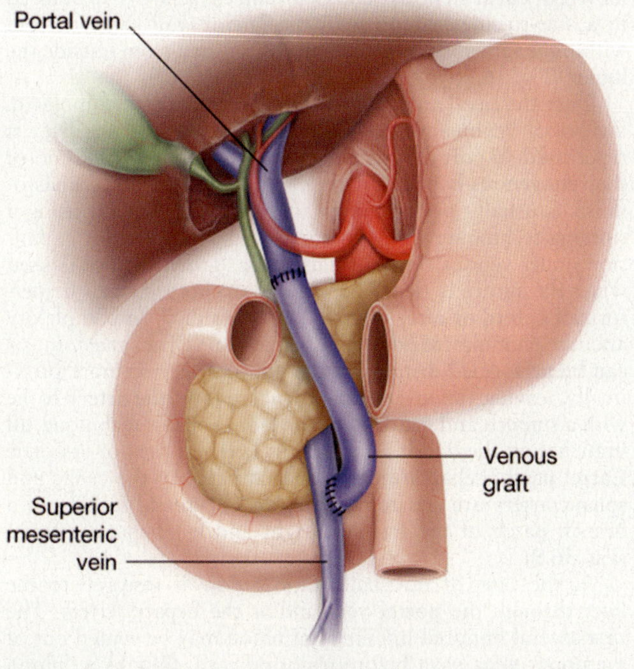

Figure 36.4. Mesoportal venous jump graft in the setting of portal vein thrombosis. The venous conduit is sewn to the superior mesenteric vein and tunneled retrogastric to anastomosis end to end to the donor portal vein.

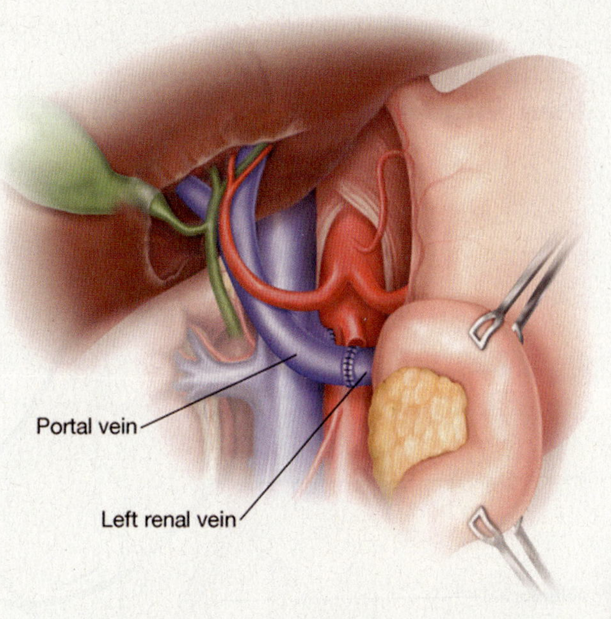

Figure 36.5. Renoportal anastomosis in the setting of portal vein thrombosis. The duodenum and pancreatic head have been mobilized to expose the left renal vein, which is divided at its drainage to the IVC and anastomosed end to end to the donor portal vein.

Anhepatic Phase and Implantation of the Donor Liver

At this point, the liver has been completely mobilized except for its attachments of the hepatic veins to the inferior vena cava and in some cases, the portal vein. Most patients will tolerate clamping of both the portal vein and the inferior vena cava without difficulty. At this point, communication with the anesthesiologist is essential and the vena cava should be test clamped before division to make sure that adequate cardiac filling and blood pressure can be maintained. If the patient becomes hypotensive during test clamping, the clamps should be removed, and additional volume or vasopressor support can be administered. Occasionally, patients will require venovenous bypass, but its use is no longer routine at most centers.

If necessary, venovenous bypass can be accomplished by drainage from both the portal vein and inferior vena cava simultaneously, or a single cannula in either the portal vein or the inferior vena cava may be used (**Fig. 36.6**). There are several accepted methods of placing cannulas for venovenous bypass. Cannulas may be placed percutaneously in the internal jugular vein and femoral vein prior to beginning the procedure. These cannulas are advanced into the superior and inferior vena cava, respectively. Alternatively, one or both of the bypass cannulas may be placed by cutdown on the axillary and/or the femoral vein. Inferior vena caval and mesenteric blood is returned to the superior vena cava by a centrifugal pump. The cannulas, tubing, and centrifugal pump head are heparin bonded to reduce the chance of thrombus formation

TRANSPLANTATION

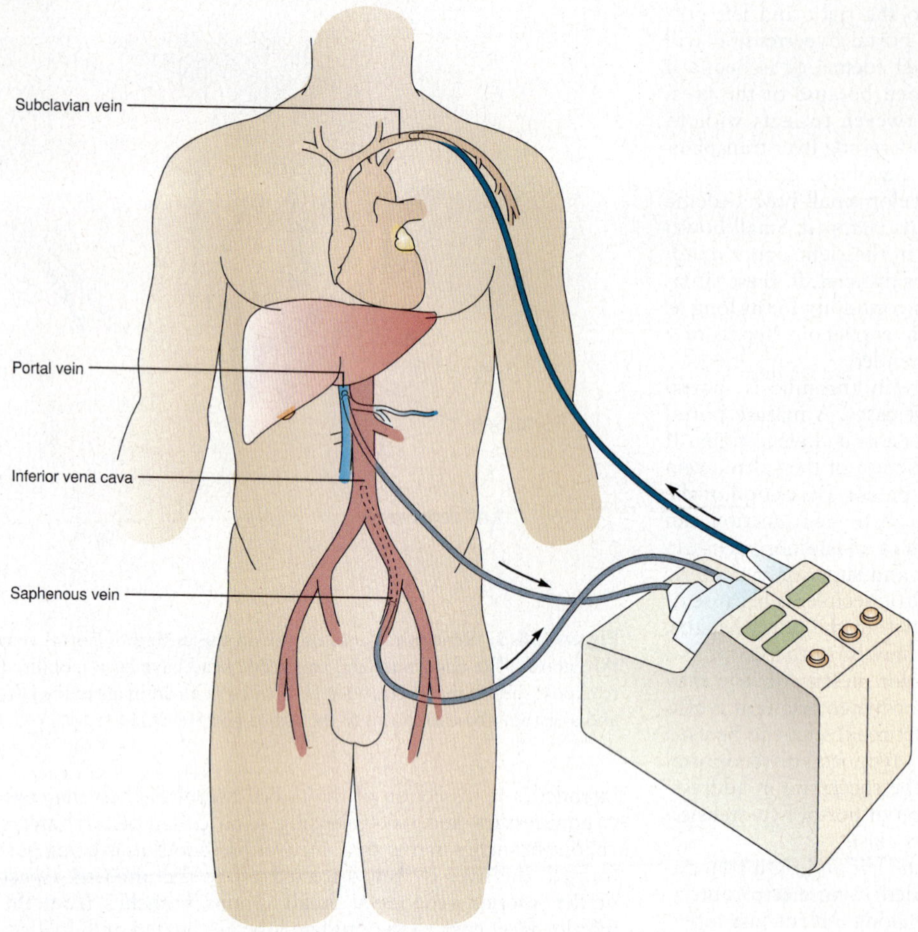

Figure 36.6. Setup for venovenous bypass during hepatic transplantation. Cannulas are placed into the portal vein and inferior vena cava (through the greater saphenous vein). A centrifugal pump is used to deliver bypassed blood to the central circulation by means of a cannula passed into the axillary vein.

and subsequent embolism. Flow rates of 1 to 2 L/min are typical. Once venovenous bypass has been established or the decision to forego bypass has been made, the recipient hepatectomy is completed. If still intact, the portal vein is divided as high in the hilum as possible, and the hepatic veins are divided. Three methods are commonly used for orthotopic liver transplantation: the bicaval technique, the piggyback technique, cavocavostomy (side-to-side caval technique).

For the **bicaval** technique, the recipient liver is excised en bloc with the retrohepatic inferior vena cava after caval clamps have been placed in a suprahepatic and infrahepatic position. The hepatic veins are divided within the substance of the native liver to allow the creation of a large suprahepatic cuff compromising the left, middle, and right hepatic veins. This technique has the disadvantages of: (a) occluding inferior vena cava flow, resulting in renal congestion and decreased cardiac filling with associated hypotension, (b) requiring two vena caval anastomoses prolonging the warm ischemic time, (c) may require increased mobilization of the recipient vena cava possibly leading to bleeding. However, dissection of the caudate lobe off the vena cava is not necessary in this technique, making the recipient hepatectomy phase often faster.

For the **piggyback** technique, a clamp is placed transversely, partially occluding the vena cava at the level of the hepatic veins. The vena cava is left in continuity, and the hepatic veins are divided within the substance of the native liver, allowing the creation of a common patch of the right, middle, and left hepatic veins for a wide anastomosis. While the intention is to only partially occlude the vena cava, allowing venous return to the heart, often a clamp placed for the piggyback technique either occludes or nearly occludes the inferior vena cava. This technique does have the advantage of only requiring a single vena caval anastomosis, helping to limit warm ischemic time (**Fig. 36.7**).

For the **cavocavostomy** technique, the native hepatic veins are stapled or oversewn (**Fig. 36.8**). Advantages of the cavocavostomy anastomosis include: (a) minimal time that the vena cava is clamped, (b) the vena caval clamp is placed longitudinally only occluding the anterior third of the vena cava leading to minimal or no changes in the recipient's hemodynamics, (c) a broad anastomosis is performed limiting the likelihood of caval stenosis. The two vena cavae are then sutured in a side-to-side fashion with the lateral wall sutured from within the lumen and the medial wall sutured from outside the lumen (**Fig. 36.8**).

Once the caval anastomosis or anastomoses are completed, the portal venous anastomosis is completed, and the liver is reperfused. If portal bypass has been used, the portal limb of the venovenous bypass circuit is removed. The portal anastomosis is usually performed in an end-to-end fashion using a running technique. To avoid narrowing and allow for expansion under venous flow, a small air or "growth" knot is used when the suture is tied. The arterial anastomosis can be performed before or after reperfusion, depending on complexity and the cumulative warm ischemic time. The anastomosis can be performed distally on the donor artery or more proximally, leaving the artery long, which allows the artery to lie with a smooth and gentle curve or loop. For this technique, all branches on the donor artery are ligated and the donor aortic Carrel patch, celiac artery, or branch patch of the celiac and splenic artery are anastomosed in an end-to-end fashion to a branch patch of the recipient right and left hepatic arteries (**Fig. 36.9**).

At the time of revascularization, flow is restored to the liver through the portal vein and/or the hepatic artery. The first several hundred milliliters of blood may be vented out of the donor vena cava before restoring caval flow as a "blood flush" to eliminate cold perfusate and other cellular metabolites. Close coordination between the surgeon and anesthesiologist is necessary during this phase, as hypotension and bradycardia are routinely encountered and cardiac arrest may

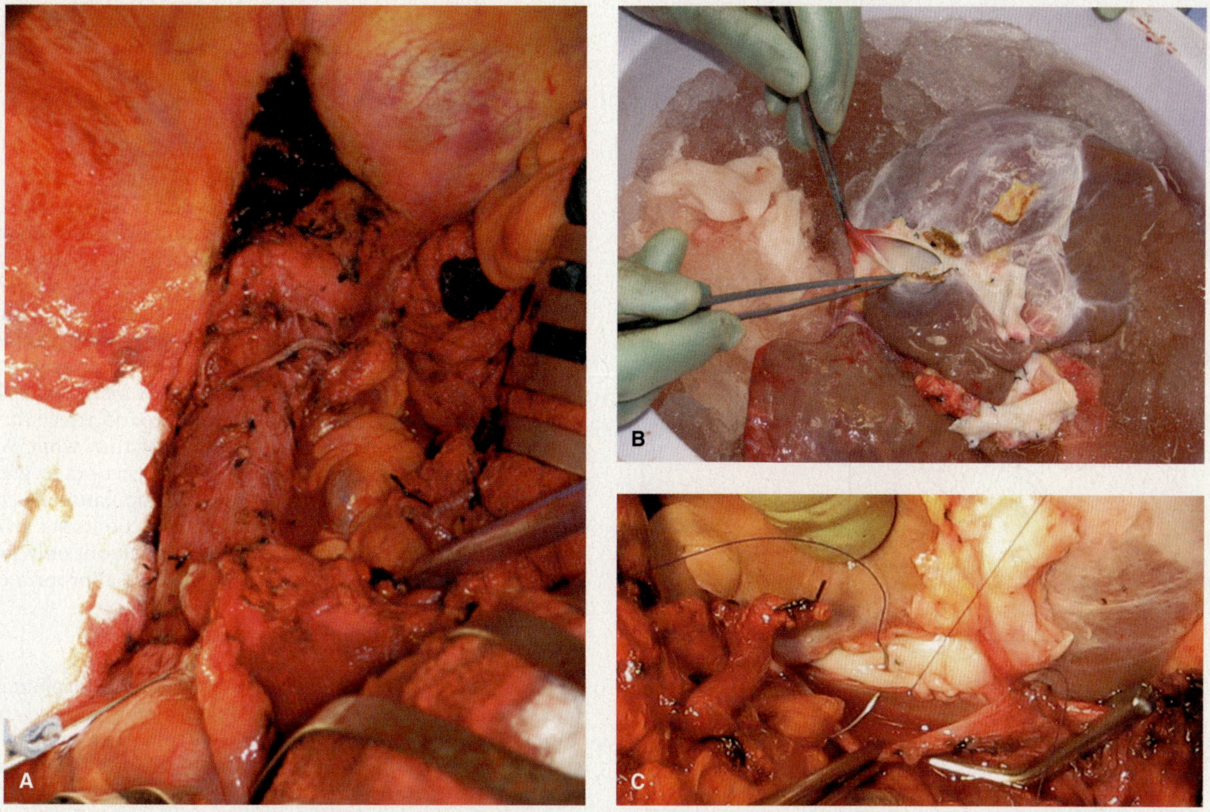

Figure 36.7. Cavocavostomy. **A:** The recipient right and junction of the middle and left hepatic veins are stapled and the inferior vena cava is left in continuity. **B:** The supra- and infrahepatic vena cavae are stapled and a venotomy is made longitudinally on the posterior aspect of the donor liver. **C:** A side-to-side caval anastomosis is performed with a running suture.

rarely occur. If venovenous bypass has been used during the anhepatic phase, it can be discontinued.

Postrevascularization Phase

Following revascularization, the liver should assume a normal color and consistency within several minutes. If the liver remains pale or is overly soft, problems with portal inflow should be considered. Alternatively, if the liver becomes edematous and overly firm, outflow obstruction should be excluded. Bile production should be seen while in the operating room and is among the first evidence of liver function. Inspection for surgical bleeding should be performed and entails examination of the vascular anastomoses as well as a search for branches of the major vessels that may not have been ligated. If bleeding continues after all surgical bleeding has been resolved, attention should be directed toward correction of coagulopathy as described above. Adequate time should be allowed after reperfusion for correction of coagulopathy and hemodynamic stabilization before the biliary anastomosis and fascial closure are considered.

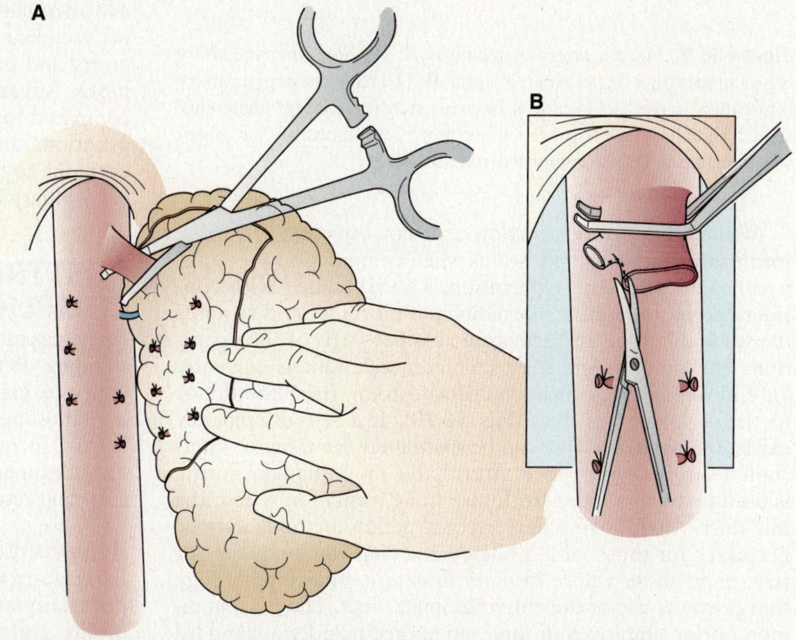

Figure 36.8. Piggyback technique. **A:** Recipient liver is dissected off native inferior vena cava by dividing veins draining directly into the inferior vena cava up to the level of the hepatic veins. **B:** Clamp placed on recipient hepatic veins in preparation for excision of the recipient's native liver and performance of a piggyback anastomosis.

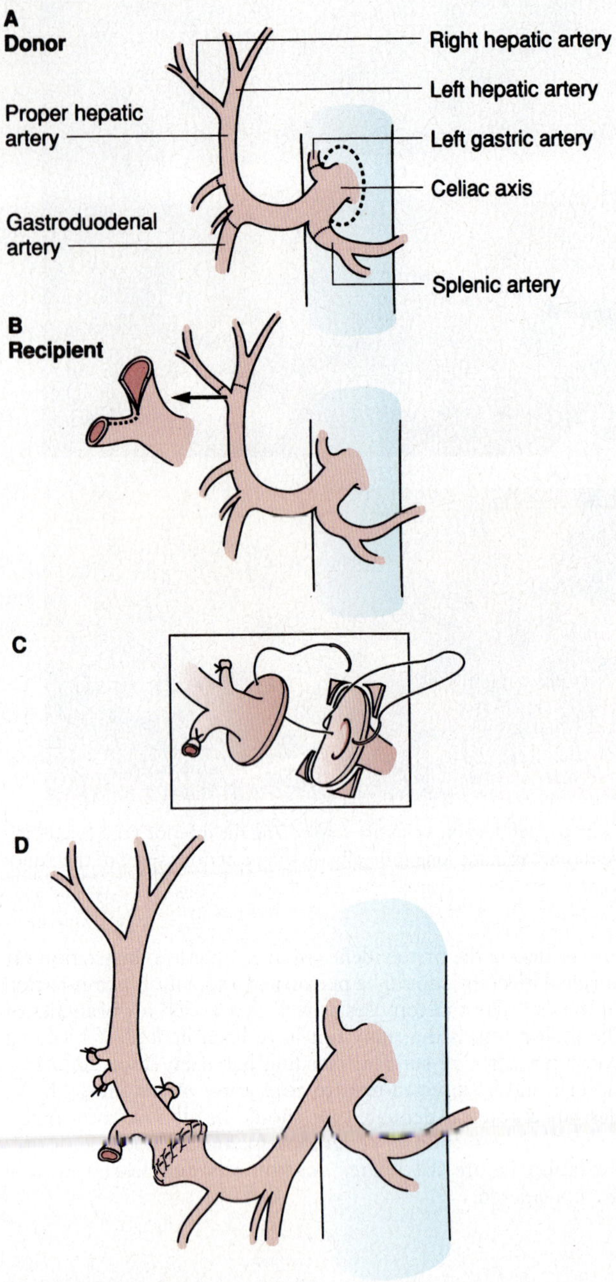

Figure 36.9. Hepatic artery anastomosis. **A:** The donor hepatic artery is procured with a Carrel patch of aorta. **B:** The recipient hepatic artery bifurcation is used to fashion a branch patch for a larger anastomosis. **C:** The anastomosis is carried out using continuous monofilament suture material. **D:** The completed anastomosis.

While biliary reconstruction does not carry the same risk for intraoperative complications when compared to the recipient hepatectomy and reperfusion, it is associated with considerable postoperative morbidity and mortality and requires the same diligence and attention as other steps of the operation. The simplest and most common technique is currently an end-to-end choledochocholedochostomy from the donor to the recipient bile duct (**Fig. 36.10**). If a size discrepancy exists, the narrower duct can be spatulated. Running or interrupted sutures can be used. Absorbable monofilament suture is used to avoid a nidus for future stone formation within the bile duct. Alternative biliary reconstruction methods may be necessary for those with a bile duct of inadequate quality or size, or in those whose primary disease is biliary pathology that prevents use of the native recipient duct. The most common option employed in these situations includes a standard Roux-en-Y choledochojejunostomy, though choledochoduodenostomy may be considered. Placement of drains may be considered to manage ascites or monitor for biliary leak. Abdominal wall and skin closure are then performed in the standard fashion.

Technique for Partial Liver Transplantation

Use of partial allografts may increase donor organs available for transplant, and techniques for split and living-donor grafts based on Couinaud segmental anatomy (**Fig. 36.11**) have been developed. Split liver transplantation allows two segmental allografts to be transplanted into separate recipients, either a child and an adult, or two adults.[48] Split liver transplantation may provide equivalent patient outcomes to whole graft transplantation but has been associated with an increased risk of early technical complications, including hepatic artery thrombosis and biliary complications. Because of this, while widespread adoption of allocation policies to encourage greater utilization of split liver grafts in the adult population has been suggested, split liver transplantation only accounts for a small proportion of transplants performed. In addition, only grafts from "ideal" deceased donors are considered appropriate for this form of transplantation.

Living-Donor Liver Transplantation

Experiences with deceased donor split liver transplantation and ongoing shortages of deceased donor allografts led to the adoption of the techniques utilized in split liver transplantation for LDLT. While LDLT now accounts for approximately 5% of all liver transplants performed in the United States, it is the predominant pathway to liver transplantation in many countries without robust deceased-donor organ donation. Although initially used in the pediatric recipients, adult LDLT has become more frequent.

In many respects, transplantation of a graft from a living donor is like transplantation of a whole liver from a deceased donor. However, the recipient vena cava must be left intact. A direct hepatic vein to vena caval anastomosis is used. Establishing adequate outflow of hepatic venous blood is necessary to help prevent congestion of the anterior segment of the right lobe. Therefore, any veins draining not draining into the right hepatic vein greater than 3 to 5 mm in diameter should be reconstructed either by direct anastomosis to the vena cava or using an interposition graft (**Fig. 36.12**). In addition, the length of the portal vein, hepatic artery, and bile duct on the donor graft is considerably shorter than that available from a deceased donor. Therefore, during the recipient hepatectomy, considerable care should be given to preserving the length of the recipient bile duct as well as the right and/or left hepatic artery and portal vein, which are intended for future anastomosis. Advantages of LDLT include lower recipient mortality compared to waiting for a deceased donor, less medical complications, and optimization of timing of transplant.[35,49] However, due to the technical complexity, there is a higher risk of early biliary and vascular complications.

POSTTRANSPLANT CARE AND COMPLICATIONS

5 Management of the postliver transplant patient requires understanding of the continuum of care from acute perioperative issues to long-term health maintenance and management of immunosuppression. While transplant patients may be challenging to manage, they develop complications across a predictable timeline, and the best clinicians anticipate complications such that rescue may occur (**Table 36.3**).

Recipient Factors

Early posttransplant complications occur in the first 90 days posttransplant and are most threatening to the survival of the graft and patient. Three elements dictate the early

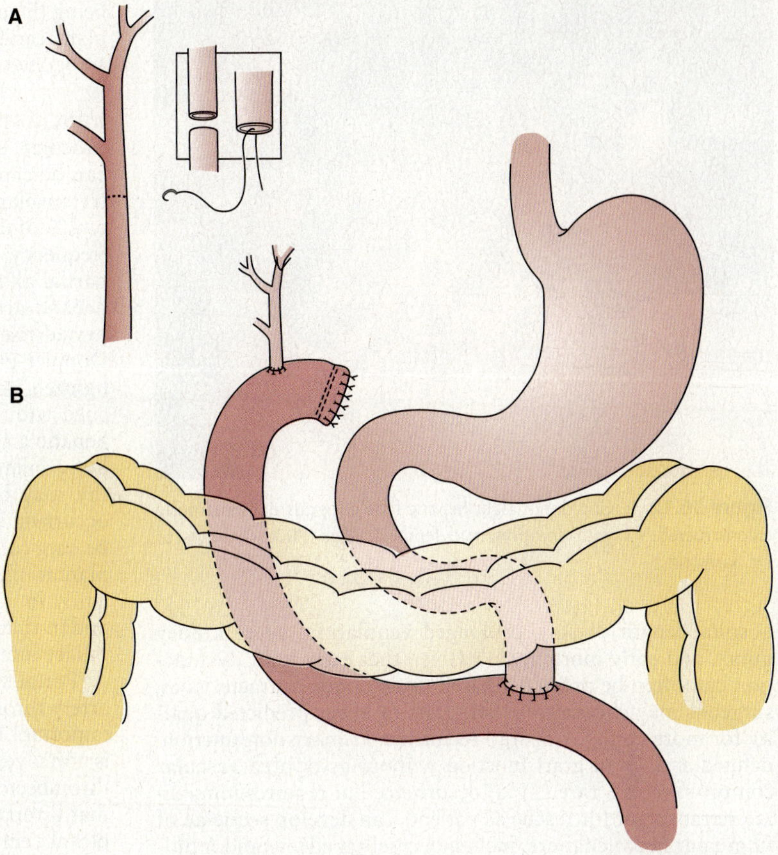

Figure 36.10. Biliary anastomosis. A: In most cases, a choledochocholedochostomy is performed, possibly over an internal stent. B: Patients with a diseased or unsuitable common bile duct may require biliary reconstruction with a Roux-en-Y choledochojejunostomy.

posttransplant course: recipient health and comorbidity at time of transplant, donor organ quality, and technical details of the transplant operation. Comprehensive care of the recipient requires detailed knowledge of all three to guide perioperative care. Given the current MELD 3.0 based allocation system, recipients may often have significant renal dysfunction and hyponatremia at the time of transplant. These factors, coupled with an aging recipient population with a higher comorbidity, explain the high incidence of posttransplant renal dysfunction, with acute kidney injury occurring in up to 50% of recipients and up to 15% of patients requiring some duration of renal replacement therapy following transplant.[50] Other aspects of recipient clinical status at the time of transplant, beyond renal dysfunction, such as frailty, obesity, and malnutrition, can increase recipient vulnerability to posttransplant complications, particularly sepsis. Clinical pathways to promote early extubation, mobilization, and optimization of nutrition act to mitigate these recipient challenges in the early posttransplant period.

Donor Factors

Donor quality has long been associated with risk of perioperative complications and early graft loss.[51] With increasing demand, transplant centers have increasingly used more marginal grafts (older donors, more steatosis, DCD donors) at risk of early allograft dysfunction. Donor livers of lesser quality, and particularly DCD donor livers, are associated with more robust reperfusion injury and associated downstream consequences for the recipient, including but not limited to coagulopathy and need for more transfusions, prolonged ICU and

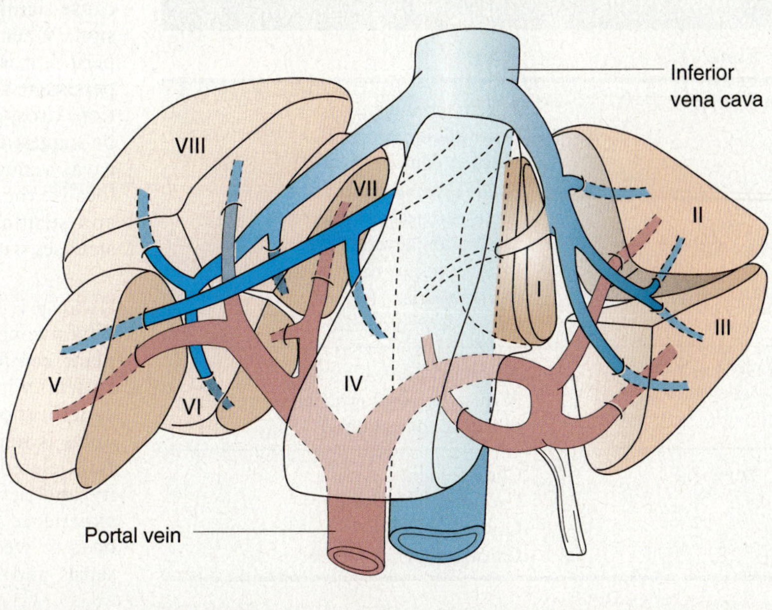

Figure 36.11. Segmental anatomy of the liver based on Couinaud nomenclature.

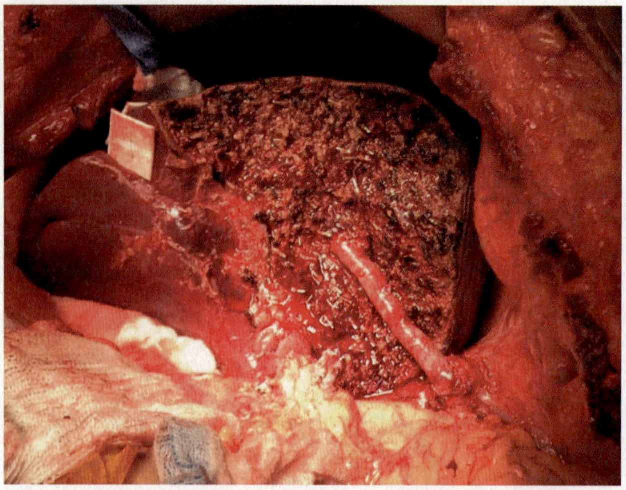

Figure 36.12. Living donor right hepatic lobe allograft demonstrating reconstructed V5 with cryopreserved femoral vein. (Photo belongs to Dr. Samstein.)

hospital length of stay, prolonged ventilation, acute kidney injury, and early mortality.[52,53] Given that early graft dysfunction can often be predicted based upon donor characteristics, surgeons may choose to avoid grafts of lower predicted quality for more complex or frail recipients. Primary nonfunction, defined as lack of graft function without associated vascular compromise, is a rare (≤1%) occurrence but requires immediate retransplant for rescue as patients can develop sequelae of fulminant hepatic failure, including cerebral edema and multisystem organ failure.

Technical Factors

In addition to recipient health and donor quality, the difficulty of the transplant operation has a significant impact on the initial perioperative course. Risk factors for increased perioperative risk include retransplantation, previous abdominal surgery, and portal vein thrombosis. In addition, patients in specific diagnosis groups may pose greater technical challenges, including candidates with Budd–Chiari syndrome, polycystic liver disease, and acute alcoholic hepatitis. Technical factors that complicate vascular inflow or outflow to the transplant liver are especially challenging, with portal vein thrombosis being the most common vascular challenge among liver transplant candidates, occurring in up to 15% of candidates and associated with increased risk of graft loss and patient death.[54]

Table 36.3. Continuum of Postliver Transplant Complications

Time	Event
0–90 d	Primary nonfunction Acute kidney injury Vascular complications Biliary complications Sepsis; surgical site infections Medication adverse reactions Perioperative cardiac events Acute rejection Donor-derived disease
90 d to 1 y	Acute rejection Atypical/opportunistic infections Biliary complications
Beyond 1 y	Chronic kidney disease Cardiovascular disease Cancer Chronic allograft failure

Vascular Complications

Vascular complications in the early posttransplant period can be catastrophic and may lead to the need for immediate retransplantation. Hepatic artery thrombosis, occurring in 1% to 2% of deceased donor whole grafts, may occur at increased frequency in higher-risk grafts, including DCD donor livers, partial allografts, and pediatric donor livers. The diagnosis of hepatic artery thrombosis may be associated with an unexpected rise in serum transaminase levels and is diagnosed by Doppler ultrasonography and/or CT angiography. When recognized immediately, hepatic artery thrombosis may be rescued with surgical revision and thrombectomy, but given the hepatic artery's preferential blood supply to the biliary epithelium, biliary complications, including ischemic cholangiopathy, may be predictable sequelae. Hepatic artery thrombosis occurring in the first 1 to 2 weeks posttransplant that cannot be surgically corrected is an indication for immediate retransplantation. Hepatic artery thrombosis may occur more indolently in a delayed fashion, weeks to months posttransplant, and in that setting, the consequences to graft function and the biliary integrity may be less severe.

Portal vein thrombosis occurs less commonly than hepatic artery thrombosis in the acute posttransplant setting. The most important risk factor for posttransplant portal vein thrombosis is portal vein thrombosis in the transplant candidate. Inadequate thrombectomy, and/or inadequate flow due to robust collaterals that divert mesenteric venous return away from the transplant portal vein, may predispose recipients to portal vein thrombosis and persistent or recurrent portal hypertension. Portal vein thrombosis that occurs in the immediate posttransplant period should prompt operative exploration and revision to ensure there is not a technical error in construction of the anastomosis. Management of posttransplant portal vein thrombosis that occurs more indolently requires understanding of mesenteric venous anatomy, such that a venous-phase CT or more formal mesenteric angiography with venous runoff is needed. Ligation or embolization of collateral venous channels may be necessary to ensure adequate flow to keep the transplant portal vein patent following thrombectomy or thrombolysis.

Hepatic venous outflow stenosis is a rare complication that can be complicated to diagnose and treat. When outflow stenosis presents in the immediate posttransplant period, or even in the primary operation, graft congestion and dysfunction can develop immediately. Surgical revision of the outflow may be necessary, which is a high-risk and difficult procedure that can cause significant graft injury during a time of vascular exclusion. When outflow stenosis develops in the posttransplant period, it is typically characterized by a clinical syndrome of persistent ascites, lower extremity edema, and renal dysfunction. Cross-sectional imaging studies and ultrasonography can be suggestive but not definitive for outflow stenosis, so direct caval venography with manometry is needed to make and localize the diagnosis of outflow stenosis. Balloon angioplasty and stenting can fortunately address most subacute venous stenoses without the need for operative revision.

Biliary Complications

Biliary complications are among the most common posttransplant complications, affecting 15% to 30% of recipients.[55] Patients with partial allografts are at the highest risk for biliary complications, particularly when reconstruction of segmental ducts is required. Biliary complications are likely multifactorial, related to technical factors, duct size, donor liver quality, and ischemia. Approximately 4% to 12% of patients will experience biliary leaks, which typically present in the first days to weeks posttransplant. Biliary leaks can present with sepsis and peritonitis and should be suspected in any early

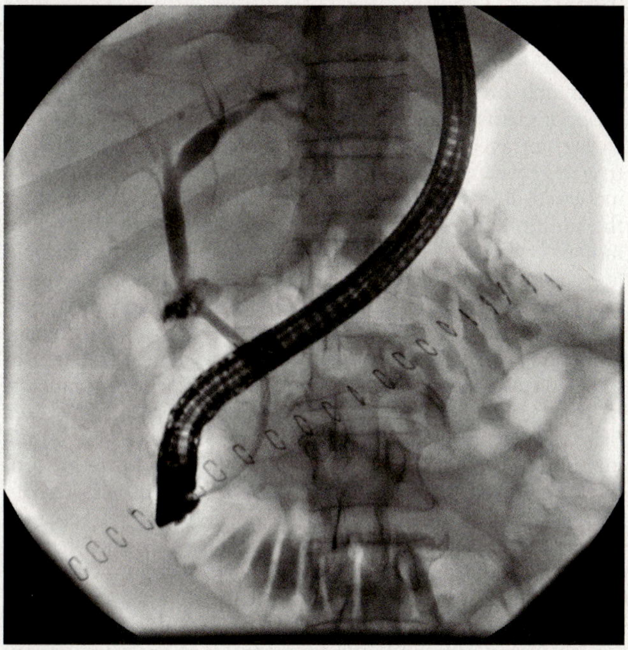

Figure 36.13. Endoscopic retrograde cholangiogram demonstrating a biliary anastomotic leak. (Photo belongs to Dr. Sonnenday.)

posttransplant patient who develops infectious symptoms, ileus, or other evidence of clinical decline. In the absence of a direct evidence of bile from a surgical drain or peritoneal aspirate, direct cholangiography via endoscopic retrograde cholangiopancreatography (ERCP) or percutaneous cholangiography is needed for diagnosis (**Fig. 36.13**). Management of biliary leaks should be catered to the clinical context and patient condition. Early leaks, particularly when associated with evidence of intra-abdominal sepsis, should prompt consideration of reoperation, washout, and surgical revision. Less acute leaks in stable patients can be managed with drainage of bilomas or ascites and endoscopic stenting. Percutaneous transhepatic cholangiography and placement of an external biliary drain may be necessary with a biliary-enteric anastomosis.

Biliary stricture occurs in 10% to 20% of liver transplant recipients and may present months or even years posttransplant. Recipients with a previous leak are at risk for stricture development, as well as patients who receive DCD donor livers and patients with hepatic artery complications.[56] The majority of biliary strictures are anastomotic and can be dealt with effectively with endoscopic or percutaneous dilatation and stenting. Use of self-expanding fully covered metal stents has further expanded nonoperative management options with fewer endoscopic procedures.[57] Surgical revision should be reserved for patients who fail endoscopic management.

Cellular Rejection

Typical acute rejection in liver transplant recipients is cell mediated and manifests most commonly in the first 2 postoperative months, occurring in up to 25% of patients in the first year posttransplant. In modern practice, rejection is a far less common cause of graft loss than are primary nonfunction or vascular complications. Still, the effectiveness of therapy requires early diagnosis and treatment of acute rejection, which is, in turn, the result of careful monitoring by frequent laboratory testing and compliance by the patient. Treatment of acute rejection with enhanced immunosuppressive therapy is highly effective, and an episode of rejection typically does not affect long-term graft survival. This is very different from renal transplantation, where an episode of rejection may markedly decrease long-term graft survival. The diagnosis of cellular-mediated rejection is made primarily on a histologic basis, as the patient is completely asymptomatic. Laboratory evaluation of peripheral blood may demonstrate leukocytosis and occasionally eosinophilia. Biochemical changes associated with rejection include elevated and rising levels of serum transaminases and alkaline phosphatase. A prolonged serum prothrombin time and an abnormal serum bilirubin also suggest the possibility of rejection, but frequently these parameters are normal if rejection is detected early. Any of these findings without an obvious vascular or biliary cause should prompt a biopsy.

The diagnosis of cellular-mediated rejection rests on the finding of a triad of portal lymphocytosis, endothelialitis (subendothelial deposits of mononuclear cells), and bile duct infiltration and damage (**Fig. 36.14**). Various classification schemes have been devised to grade the severity of the rejection based on the degree of cellular involvement or injury. Cell characterization studies have documented that the cells in the portal triads are primarily T cells, with fewer macrophages and neutrophils. Bile duct epithelial cells appear to be a prime target of immune attack, and they are known to express large amounts of class II HLA antigen.

TRANSPLANTATION

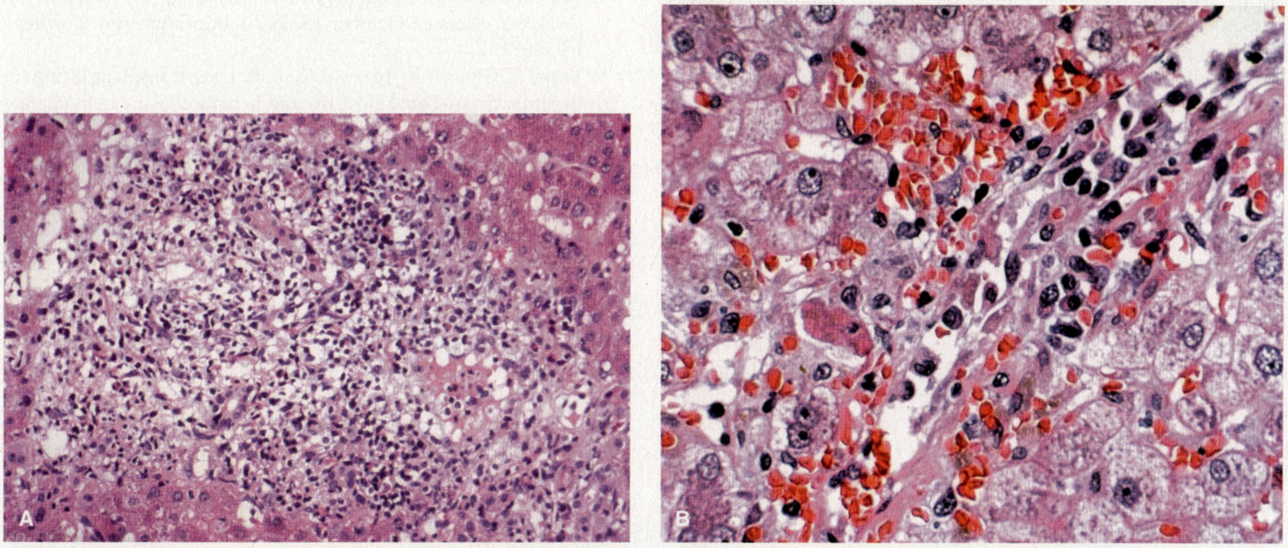

Figure 36.14. Acute rejection of a liver transplant. **A:** A portal tract is expanded by a polymorphous inflammatory infiltrate consisting of large and small lymphocytes, plasma cells, macrophages, and neutrophils. The bile ducts (*arrows*) are damaged and inflamed. **B:** A central vein from the same biopsy exhibits endothelialitis, characterized by swollen endothelial cells and infiltrating lymphocytes. Reprinted from Thung SN, Gerber MA. Histopathology of liver transplantation. In: Fabry TL, Klion FM, eds. *Guide to Liver Transplantation*. Igaku-Shoin Medical Publishers; 1988.

Antibody-Mediated Rejection

The liver is relatively resistant to injury from recipient antibodies, regardless of whether they are present at the time of transplant or develop later. This is very different compared to recipients of other solid organ transplants who experience rapid graft destruction, termed hyperacute rejection, due to complement-fixing antibodies directed against the donor organ, particularly the endothelium. Hepatic graft injury from preexisting antibodies directed at donor ABO antigens does occur, but in a much less pronounced fashion than in other organ transplants. The overall results of ABO-incompatible liver transplants are somewhat inferior to those of ABO-compatible transplantations, but only by about a 10% to 20% decrease in 1-year graft survival rates compared to ABO-compatible grafts. Because preformed antibodies do not seem to be clinically important, most transplantation programs do not perform prospective crossmatch between recipient serum and donor cells before liver transplantation, and determination of recipient and donor HLA type is no longer considered mandatory. The clinical impact of antibody-mediated injury in liver transplantation is still being deciphered, with evidence to suggest cumulative injury may compromise allograft function.[58,59]

Chronic Rejection

Chronic rejection is characterized by ongoing and often subacute immune injury, with impact on small bile ducts. Clinically, the pattern is one of gradual elevation of alkaline phosphatase and bilirubin, in the absence of obstruction of the large bile ducts. Histologically, small bile ducts are obliterated or completely absent, with a less pronounced cellular infiltrate than is seen with acute rejection. This finding has been termed vanishing bile duct syndrome, when bile ducts are absent in 15 of 20 portal triads examined. The loss of small bile ducts is partly the result of lymphocyte-directed attack on biliary epithelium. Relative to other cells in the liver, biliary epithelium tends to express more class I antigen. Thus, biliary epithelial cells are vulnerable targets for host attack because of their antigenicity. Loss of bile ducts may also occur indirectly as the result of ischemia secondary to immune-mediated obliteration of small to medium arteries. While the biliary injury and ductopenia may not improve significantly histologically, patients may stabilize clinically with increased tacrolimus-based immunosuppression.[60]

Immunosuppression Management

Multiple immunosuppressive protocols achieve acceptable suppression of allograft rejection for liver transplant recipients. Induction with antithymocyte globulin or other induction agents is no longer considered to be mandatory, but is used at some centers. Similarly, prednisone therapy, once considered a mainstay of a successful immunosuppressive protocol, is often tapered off rapidly (within 7 to 28 days). Treatment with a calcineurin inhibitor is still considered to be imperative for most liver transplant recipients. These agents are associated with significant long-term morbidity, particularly the development of chronic renal failure, and therefore, target serum trough levels are progressively lowered as the transplant becomes more remote. Antiproliferative agents, most commonly mycophenolate mofetil, are added to calcineurin inhibitors for maintenance therapy in most protocols. Because immunosuppression predisposes to infection, prophylactic anti-infective drugs are usually administered. Trimethoprim–sulfamethoxazole, dapsone, or pentamidine is recommended to prevent *Pneumocystis carinii* infection. Oral mycostatin or fluconazole therapy is used to prevent fungal infections, particularly esophageal *Candida albicans*. Either ganciclovir or valganciclovir is prescribed for patients who are at risk for CMV infection, which includes any patient exposed to CMV in the past and any patient transplanted with organs from a donor who has been exposed to CMV. The duration of prophylactic anti-infective therapy has not been rigorously defined by evidence-based trials and is therefore dependent on each center's experience with the prevalence of these infections in its patient population.

Several options are available for treatment of acute rejection, depending on the clinical circumstances. Traditionally, high doses of methylprednisolone are administered (usually 500 mg to 1 g) intravenously daily for 3 days. This treatment is effective in reversing most acute rejection episodes. Alternatively, increased doses of oral prednisone, a calcineurin inhibitor, or the addition of an antimetabolite drug, such as mycophenolate mofetil, will also reverse most episodes of rejection, particularly if the rejection is mild. Rejection that is resistant to these maneuvers or severe is treated with antilymphocyte therapy, typically a polyclonal antilymphocyte therapy such as thymoglobulin. These treatments are typically administered daily for 3 to 7 days. These agents are highly effective, and it is unusual to lose an allograft secondary to acute rejection. However, these treatments are associated with profound and long-lasting immunosuppression, and it is usually advisable to restart prophylactic anti-infective therapies when they are administered.

Liver transplantation remains the definitive therapy for patients with ESLD, select metabolic diseases, and hepatic malignancies. Despite an aging patient population with more comorbid disease, short and long-term outcomes after transplantation continue to improve. Graft loss due to immunologic causes is rare, and long-term threats to graft and patient survival include chronic kidney disease, cardiovascular disease, and malignancy, all of which are associated with exposure to chronic immunosuppression. Given the success of liver transplantation as a durable therapy for ESLD, the primary challenge in the field remains expanding donor organ availability to allow expansion of this life-saving therapy to more patients with chronic liver disease.

References

1. Starzl TE, Marchioro TL, Vonkaulla KN, Hermann G, Brittain RS, Waddell WR. Homotransplantation of the liver in humans. *Surg Gynecol Obstet.* 1963;117:659–676.
2. Organ Procurement and Transplantation Network (OPTN) and Scientific Registry of Transplant Recipients (SRTR). *OPTN/SRTR 2022 Annual Data Report.* U.S. Department of Health and Human Services, Health Resources and Services Administration; 2024. Accessed September 5, 2024. http://srtr.transplant.hrsa.gov/annual_reports/Default.aspx
3. Calne RY, Rolles K, White DJ, et al. Cyclosporin A initially as the only immunosuppressant in 34 recipients of cadaveric organs: 32 kidneys, 2 pancreases, and 2 livers. *Lancet.* 1979;2:1033–1036.
4. Federal Register: 56 Fed. Reg. 14837 (April 12, 1991). Library of Congress. Accessed October 13, 2020. https://www.loc.gov/item/fr056071/
5. Vaziri A, Gimson A, Agarwal K, et al. Liver transplant listing for hepatitis C-associated cirrhosis and hepatocellular carcinoma has fallen in the United Kingdom since the introduction of direct-acting antiviral therapy. *J Viral Hepat.* 2019;26:231–235.
6. Wong RJ, Aguilar M, Cheung R, et al. Nonalcoholic steatohepatitis is the second leading etiology of liver disease among adults awaiting liver transplantation in the US. *Gastroenterology.* 2015;148:547–555.
7. Yong JN, Lim WH, Ng CH, et al. Outcomes of nonalcoholic steatohepatitis after liver transplantation: an updated meta-analysis and systematic review. *Clin Gastroenterol Hepatol.* 2023;21(1):45–54.
8. Anderson MS, Valbuena VSM, Brown CS, et al. Association of COVID-19 with new waiting list registrations and liver transplantation for alcoholic hepatitis in the United States. *JAMA Netw Open.* 2021;4(10):e2131132.
9. Lee BP, Mehta N, Platt L, et al. Outcomes of early liver transplantation for patients with severe alcoholic hepatitis. *Gastroenterology.* 2018;155:422–430.
10. Cotter TG, Sandıkçı B, Paul S, et al. Liver transplantation for alcoholic hepatitis in the United States: excellent outcomes with profound temporal and geographic variation in frequency. *Am J TransPlant.* 2021;21(3):1039–1055.

11. Giard JM, Dodge JL, Terrault NA. Superior wait-list outcomes in patients with alcohol-associated liver disease compared with other indications for liver transplantation. *Liver Transpl.* 2019;25: 1310–1320.
12. Welzel TM, Graubard BI, Quraishi S, et al. Population-attributable fractions of risk factors for hepatocellular carcinoma in the US. *Am J Gastroenterol.* 2013;108:1314–1321.
13. Llovet JM, Willoughby CE, Singal AG, et al. Nonalcoholic steatohepatitis-related hepatocellular carcinoma: pathogenesis and treatment. *Nat Rev Gastroenterol Hepatol.* 2023;20:487–503.
14. Hernandez-Alejandro R, Ruffolo LI, et al. Recipient and donor outcomes after living-donor liver transplant for unresectable colorectal liver metastases. *JAMA Surg.* 2022;157(6):524–530.
15. Sapisochin G, Javle M, Lerut J, et al. Liver transplantation for cholangiocarcinoma and mixed hepatocellular cholangiocarcinoma: working group report from the ILTS Transplant Oncology Consensus Conference. *Transplantation.* 2020;104(6):1125–1130.
16. Iwatsuki S, Gordon RD, Shaw BW, et al. Role of liver transplantation in cancer therapy. *Ann Surg.* 1985;202:401–407.
17. Mazzaferro V, Regalia E, Doci R, et al. Liver transplantation for the treatment of small hepatocellular carcinomas in patients with cirrhosis. *New Engl J Med.* 1996;334:693–700.
18. Tabrizian P, Holzner ML, Mehta N, et al. Ten-year outcomes of liver transplant and downstaging for hepatocellular carcinoma. *JAMA Surg.* 2022;157(9):779–788.
19. Heimbach JK, Kulik LM, Finn RS, et al. AASLD guidelines for the treatment of hepatocellular carcinoma. *Hepatology.* 2018; 67(1):358–380.
20. Clavien PA, Lesurtel M, Bossuyt PM, et al. Recommendations for liver transplantation for hepatocellular carcinoma: an international consensus conference report. *Lancet Oncol.* 2012;13:e11–e22.
21. Parikh ND, Waljee AK, Singal AG. Downstaging hepatocellular carcinoma: a systematic review and pooled analysis. *Liver Transpl.* 2015;21:1142–1152.
22. Lencioni R, Llovet JM. Modified RECIST (mRECIST) assessment for hepatocellular carcinoma. *Semin Liver Dis.* 2010;30:52–60.
23. Halazun KJ, Patzer RE, Rana AA, et al. Standing the test of time: outcomes of a decade of prioritizing patients with hepatocellular carcinoma, results of the UNOS natural geographic experiment. *Hepatology.* 2014;60:1957–1962.
24. Olthoff KM, Abecassis MM, Emond JC, et al. Outcomes of adult living donor liver transplantation: comparison of the Adult-to-adult Living Donor Liver Transplantation Cohort Study and the national experience. *Liver Transpl.* 2011;17:789–797.
25. Fisher RA, Kulik LM, Freise CE, et al. Hepatocellular carcinoma recurrence and death following living and deceased donor liver transplantation. *Am J Transplant.* 2007;7:1601–1608.
26. Kulik LM, Fisher RA, Rodrigo DR, et al. Outcomes of living and deceased donor liver transplant recipients with hepatocellular carcinoma: results of the A2ALL cohort. *Am J Transplant.* 2012;12:2997–3007.
27. Kamath PS, Wiesner RH, Malinchoc M, et al. A model to predict survival in patients with end-stage liver disease. *Hepatology.* 2001;33:464–470.
28. Modi RM, Patel N, Metwally SN, et al. Outcomes of liver transplantation in patients with hepatorenal syndrome. *World J Hepatology.* 2016;8:999–1011.
29. Koch DG, Speiser JL, Durkalski V, et al. The natural history of severe acute liver injury. *Am J Gastroenterol.* 2017;112:1389–1396.
30. Karvellas CJ, Leventhal TM, Rakela JL, et al. Outcomes of patients with acute liver failure listed for liver transplantation: a multicenter prospective cohort analysis. *Liver Transpl.* 2023;29(3):318–330.
31. Martin P, DiMartini A, Feng S, et al. Evaluation for liver transplantation in adults: 2013 practice guideline by the American Association for the Study of Liver Diseases and the American Society of Transplantation. *Hepatology.* 2014;59(3):1144–1165.
32. Jackson WE, Malamon JS, Kaplan B, et al. Survival benefit of living-donor liver transplant. *JAMA Surg.* 2022;157(10):926–932.
33. Nair S, Verma S, Thuluvath PJ. Obesity and its effect on survival in patients undergoing orthotopic liver transplantation in the US. *Hepatology.* 2002;35:105–109.
34. Leonard J, Heimbach JK, Malinchoc M, et al. The impact of obesity on long-term outcomes in liver transplant recipients-results of the NIDDK liver transplant database. *Am J Transplant.* 2008;8:667–672.
35. Azarbal B, Poommipanit P, Arbit B, et al. Feasibility and safety of percutaneous coronary intervention in patients with end-stage liver disease referred for liver transplantation. *Liver Transpl.* 2011;17:809–813.
36. Kim WR, Mannalithara A, Heimbach JK, et al. MELD 3.0: the model for end-stage liver disease updated for the modern era. *Gastroenterology.* 2021;161(6):1887–1895.
37. Hsu EK, Shaffer ML, Gao L, et al. Analysis of liver offers to pediatric candidates on the transplant wait list. *Gastroenterology.* 2017;153:988–995.
38. Routh D, Naidu S, Sharma S, et al. Changing pattern of donor selection criteria in deceased donor liver transplant: a review of literature. *J Clin Exp Hepatol.* 2013;3(4):337–346.
39. Lué A, Solanas E, Baptista P, et al. How important is donor age in liver transplantation? *World J Gastroenterol.* 2016;22(21): 4966–4976.
40. Kwong AJ, Ebel NH, Kim WR, et al. OPTN/SRTR 2020 annual data report: liver. *Am J TransPlant.* 2022;22 Suppl 2:204–309.
41. Brubaker AL, Sellers MT, Abt PL, et al. US liver transplant outcomes after normothermic regional perfusion vs standard super rapid recovery. *JAMA Surg.* 2024;159(6):677–685.
42. Chapman WC, Barbas AS, D'Alessandro AM, et al. Normothermic machine perfusion of donor livers for transplantation in the United States: a randomized controlled trial. *Ann Surg.* 2023;278(5):e912–e921.
43. Markmann JF, Abouljoud MS, Ghobrial RM, et al. Impact of portable normothermic blood-based machine perfusion on outcomes of liver transplant: the OCS Liver PROTECT Randomized Clinical Trial. *JAMA Surg.* 2022;157(3):189–198.
44. Panayotova GG, Lunsford KE, Quillin RC III, et al. Portable hypothermic oxygenated machine perfusion for organ preservation in liver transplantation: a randomized, open-label, clinical trial. *Hepatology.* 2024;79(5):1033–1047.
45. Abeysundara L, Mallett SV, Clevenger B. Point-of-care testing in liver disease and liver surgery. *Semin Thromb Hemost.* 2017; 43:407–415.
46. Leon-Justel A, Noval-Padillo JA, Alvarez-Rios AI, et al. Point-of-care haemostasis monitoring during liver transplantation reduces transfusion requirements and improves patient outcome. *Clin Chim Acta.* 2015;446:277–283.
47. Clevenger B, Mallett SV. Transfusion and coagulation management in liver transplantation. *World J Gastroenterol.* 2014;20: 6146–6158.
48. Emond JC, Whitington PF, Thistlethwaite JR, et al. Transplantation of two patients with one liver. Analysis of a preliminary experience with "split-liver" grafting. *Ann Surg.* 1990;212:14–22.
49. Samstein B, Smith AR, Freise CE, et al. Complications and their resolution in recipients of deceased and living donor liver transplants: findings from the A2ALL Cohort Study. *Am J Transplant.* 2016;16:594–602.
50. Durand F, Francoz C, Asrani SK, et al. Acute kidney injury after liver transplantation. *Transplantation.* 2018;102:1636–1649.
51. Feng S, Goodrich NP, Bragg-Gresham JL, et al. Characteristics associated with liver graft failure: the concept of a donor risk index. *Am J Transplant.* 2006;6:783–790.
52. Olthoff KM, Kulik L, Samstein B, et al. Validation of a current definition of early allograft dysfunction in liver transplant recipients and analysis of risk factors. *Liver Transpl.* 2010;16:943–949.
53. Agopian VG, Harlander-Locke MP, Markovic D, et al. Evaluation of early allograft function using the liver graft assessment following Transplantation Risk Score Model. *JAMA Surg.* 2018;153:436–444.
54. Conzen KD, Pomfret EA. Liver transplant in patients with portal vein thrombosis: medical and surgical requirements. *Liver Transpl.* 2017;23:S59–S63.
55. Axelrod DA, Lentine KL, Xiao H, et al. National assessment of early biliary complications following liver transplantation: incidence and outcomes. *Liver Transpl.* 2014;20:446–456.

56. Foley DP, Fernandez LA, Leverson G, et al. Biliary complications after liver transplantation from donation after cardiac death donors: an analysis of risk factors and long-term outcomes from a single center. *Ann Surg*. 2011;253:817–825.
57. Coté GA, Slivka A, Tarnasky P, et al. Effect of covered metallic stents compared with plastic stents on benign biliary stricture resolution: a randomized clinical trial. *JAMA*. 2016;315:1250–1257.
58. O'Leary JG, Shiller SM, Bellamy C, et al. Acute liver allograft antibody-mediated rejection: an inter-institutional study of significant histopathological features. *Liver Transpl*. 2014;20:1244–1255.
59. O'Leary JG, Demetris AJ, Friedman LS, et al. The role of donor-specific HLA alloantibodies in liver transplantation. *Am J Transplant*. 2014;14:779–787.
60. Blakolmer K, Jain A, Ruppert K, et al. Chronic liver allograft rejection in a population treated primarily with tacrolimus as baseline immunosuppression: long-term follow-up and evaluation of features for histopathological staging. *Transplantation*. 2000;69:2330–2336.

37

Cardiac Transplantation

Benjamin Bryner

Key Points

1. Heart transplantation is the gold standard of therapy for end-stage heart failure; however, its availability is limited by a paucity of suitable donors and its long-term success in recipients is limited by perioperative infections, cellular rejection, malignancies, and allograft vasculopathy.
2. Left ventricular assist devices (LVADs) are an effective means of circulatory support and can serve as a bridge to transplant or a destination therapy themselves, but complications include driveline infection, pump thrombosis, strokes, allosensitization, and gastrointestinal bleeding.
3. Temporary mechanical support (MCS) is emerging as the most common therapy to allow heart transplantation as technology has advanced for longer-term univentricular and biventricular support.
4. Advances in donor heart preservation and ex situ perfusion have allowed for expansion of the donor pool by allowing heart donation after cardiac death (DCD) and long-distance transplantation while preserving posttransplant survival.

1 HISTORICAL PERSPECTIVE

The original technique developed in the Stanford laboratories by Lower and Shumway in the 1960s confirmed that a denervated donor heart could support circulation in a recipient (**Fig. 37.1**).[1] Christiaan Barnard gained worldwide recognition by applying this innovative technique in performing the first human heart transplant in Cape Town on December 3, 1967.[2] Adrian Kantrowitz performed the first pediatric heart transplant in New York and laid the foundation for brain death criteria later codified at Harvard.[3] The development of a technique to perform transvenous endomyocardial biopsies for immunologic surveillance was another breakthrough at Stanford. This innovation allowed for characterization of acute cellular rejection and earlier detection of rejection. One of the most influential advances was the development of cyclosporine led by the Stanford group and Roy Calne at Cambridge University in the early 1980s. Other immune suppression therapies, better control of infections, and mechanical circulatory support (MCS) have led to dramatic improvements in outcomes for recipients.[4]

INDICATIONS AND ASSESSMENT FOR HEART TRANSPLANTATION

Over 5 million Americans suffer from heart failure and more than 250,000 die annually. Heart transplantation represents a last-line therapy after advanced medical therapy for heart failure, and early recognition of patients who will benefit can be challenging.[5] Heart transplantation is the treatment of choice for selected patients with advanced heart failure who have extraordinary limitations in terms of their overall physical well-being and limited life expectancy, approaching less than 2 years. Patients with advanced heart failure and coronary disease should be evaluated for benefit from conventional interventions (angioplasty or coronary bypass) often including myocardial viability testing.[6]

Cardiopulmonary exercise testing is the most reliable and objective criterion, to determine the extent of advanced heart failure and the likely morbidity and mortality associated with

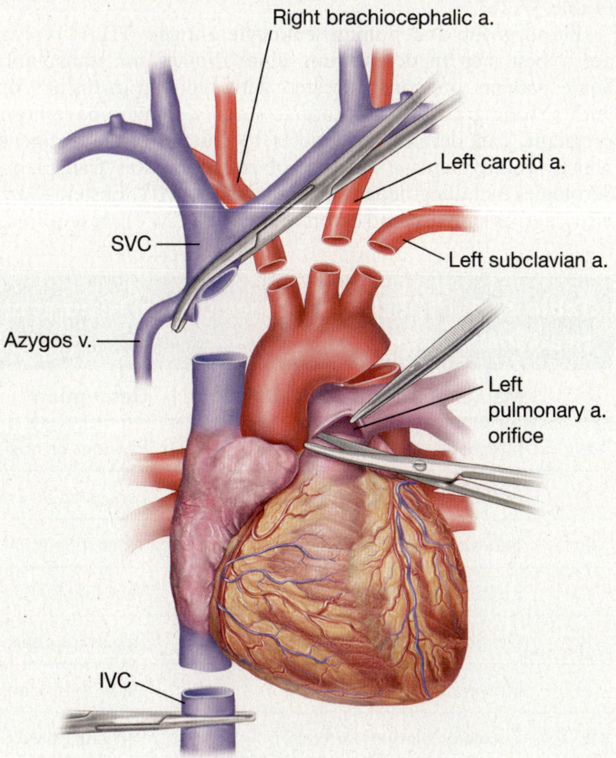

Figure 37.1. The explanted donor heart. (Redrawn from Camp PC, Heart transplantation: donor operation for heart and lung transplantation. *Oper Tech Thorac Cardiovasc Surg.* 2010;15(2):125–137.)

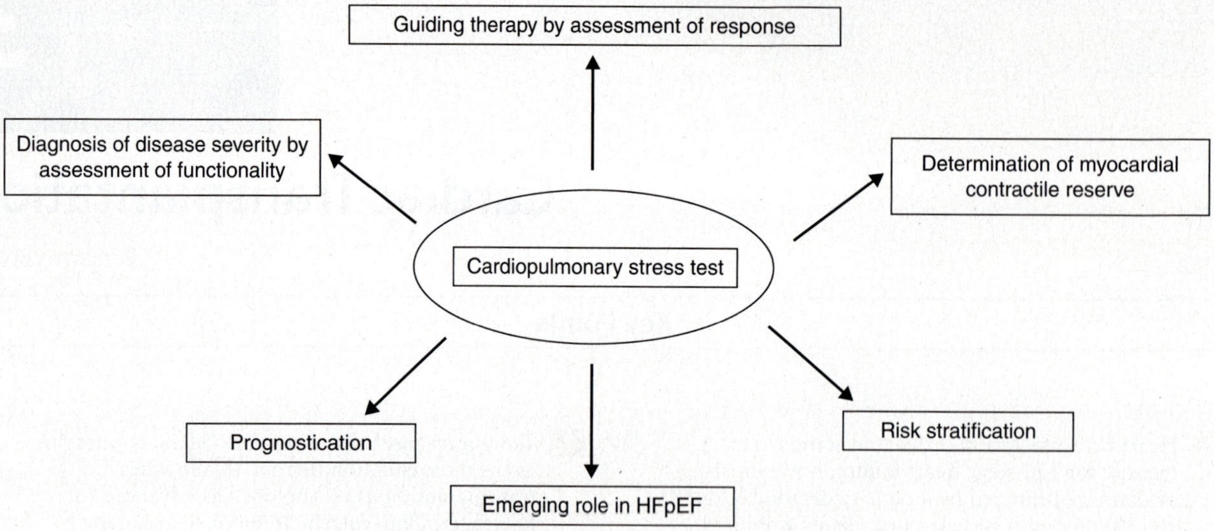

Figure 37.2. Uses of cardiopulmonary stress tests in heart failure.

class for heart failure (**Fig. 37.2**).[7] The measurement of peak oxygen consumption (VO_2) has been shown to correlate with functional capacity and mortality.

A detailed clinical assessment complements the above quantitative criteria. Repeated hospitalizations for heart failure therapy, progressive increases in heart failure medications, and especially the need for inotropes, should prompt evaluation for transplant and direct symptomatic management (**Table 37.1**).

The International Society for Heart and Lung Transplant (ISHLT) most recently issued consensus listing criteria for heart transplantation in 2024.[8] Selection criteria for heart transplantation have been well defined and should be evaluated by a multidisciplinary team of healthcare professionals (**Table 37.2**).[9]

2 Blood group and human leukocyte antigen (HLA) typing are a first step in determining compatibility for transplant. Some patients previously treated with blood transfusions or with a homograft in prior cardiac surgery, or who have been pregnant, can develop antibodies to foreign tissue antigens which would increase the risk of rejection after transplant. Serologies including hepatitis B, hepatitis C, HIV, Epstein–Barr virus, herpes simplex, and cytomegalovirus (CMV) are required, as are assessments of other organ function (creatinine, platelet count, hepatic enzymes, hemoglobin A1c). Computed tomography (CT) of the chest is performed to assess for anatomic abnormalities that would complicate transplant, such as patients with congenital heart disease who may have persistent left SVC, aortic arch abnormalities dextrocardia, etc., which affect the operative strategy. Patients who have had prior cardiac surgery must undergo CT to assess the location of prior bypass grafts, mechanical support devices, etc. These results should be discussed in multidisciplinary conferences and further testing may be required (**Table 37.3**).

PRETRANSPLANT MANAGEMENT

The last 20 years have seen significant advancements in medical therapy for heart failure. The use of beta-adrenergic blockers, angiotensin receptor-neprilysin inhibitors (angiotensin-converting enzyme [ACE] inhibitors and angiotensin receptor blockers [ARBs]), mineralocorticoid receptor antagonists, and sodium-glucose co-transporter 2 (SGLT2) inhibitors comprise the "four pillars" of guideline-directed pharmacologic therapy for advanced heart failure.[10]

Table 37.1. "I NEED HELP" Mnemonic for Features of Advanced Heart Failure that Should Prompt Workup for Heart Transplantation

	Marker of Advanced Heart Failure	Description
I	Inotropes	Previous or ongoing requirement for dobutamine, milrinone, dopamine, or levosimendan
N	NYHA class/natriuretic peptides	Persisting NYHA class III or IV and/or persistently high BNP or NT-pro-BNP
E	End-organ dysfunction	Worsening renal or liver dysfunction in the setting of heart failure
E	Ejection fraction	Very low LVEF <20%
D	Defibrillator shocks	Recurrent appropriate defibrillator shocks
H	Hospitalizations	More than 1 hospitalization with HF in the last 12 mo
E	Edema/escalating diuretics	Persisting fluid overload and/or increasing diuretic requirement
L	Low blood pressure	Consistently low blood pressure with systolic <90–100 mm Hg
P	Prognostic medication	Inability to up-titrate (or need to decrease/cease) GDMP

BNP, B-type natriuretic peptide; HF, heart failure; LVEF, left ventricular ejection fraction; NT-Pro-BNP, N-terminal pro–b-type natriuretic peptide; NYHA, New York Heart Association.
Adapted from Baumwol J. "I Need Help"—A mnemonic to aid timely referral in advanced heart failure. *J Heart Lung Transplant*. 2017;36(5):593–594.

Table 37.2. Indications and Contraindications for Heart Transplantation

Indications for Heart Transplantation
Cardiogenic shock requiring inotropes or mechanical circulatory support
New York Heart Association (NYHA) class IV heart failure symptoms refractory to optimal medical therapy
Intractable angina without percutaneous or surgical therapeutic options
Intractable unstable arrhythmias refractory to ablation and medical therapy
Cardiac allograft vasculopathy (severe)
Restrictive cardiomyopathy, severe hypertrophic cardiomyopathy, and congenital heart disease refractory to or not amenable to medical or surgical therapy
Above conditions treated with durable left ventricular assist device and now amenable to transplantation
Contraindications for Heart Transplantation
Severe pulmonary hypertension
Advanced age (70 yr is a relative contraindication)
Life expectancy <2 yr from other comorbidities
Malignancy <5 yr ago (<2 in nonmelanoma skin cancers or carefully selected low-grade tumors)
Cerebrovascular disease impairing cognitive function
Frailty/debility precluding functional recovery from transplant surgery
Severe peripheral vascular disease
Lack of adequate support network
Psychosocial obstacles to follow-up and adherence to medical and procedural regimens
Severe obesity (body mass index >35)
Uncontrolled diabetes
Active infection
Other end-stage organ failure (unless multiorgan transplant is a viable option)
Anatomic features (postoperative or congenital) posing excessive risk for sternal re-entry, transplantation, or recovery

Implantable cardioverter defibrillators (ICDs) and cardiac resynchronization therapy (CRT) devices (biventricular pacemakers) have been shown to improve mortality in patients with advanced heart failure.[11]

The majority of patients with advanced heart failure have secondary end-organ dysfunction, potentially including renal failure, liver congestion, evolution of secondary pulmonary hypertension. While these conditions improve with better cardiac output after transplant, in the immediate posttransplant period, pulmonary hypertension in particular can cause right ventricular failure in particular. Right heart catheterization data is essential in assessing this, and medications including nitroprusside, nesiritide, dobutamine, and inhaled nitric oxide can assess for the responsiveness of the pulmonary vascular bed and therefore its reversibility with better heart function. Other parameters on right heart catheterization help guide medical therapy and diuretic management. A number of prognostic heart failure scores have been developed, including the Seattle Heart Failure Model and the Heart Failure Survival Score in advanced heart failure populations.[12]

3 DONOR HEART AVAILABILITY AND ALLOCATION

In 2018, the United States updated the adult heart allocation system to better stratify the most medically urgent heart transplant candidates, reflect the increased use of temporary mechanical circulatory support, and address geographic disparities in access to donors among heart transplant candidates (**Table 37.4**). Recipients are ranked on a match list to individual organ offers by UNOS status, distance from the donor, and wait time. Ongoing efforts to reform the allocation system may eventually yield a numerical heart allocation score similar to the Lung Allocation Score (LAS) and the Model for End-stage Liver Disease (MELD) scores used in lung and liver allocation.

Table 37.3. Components of Assessment for Heart Transplantation Candidacy

Domain of Assessment	Elements
Cardiac	Coronary angiogram Echocardiogram
Functional	Cardiopulmonary exercise test
Other end-organ function	Creatinine Pulmonary function tests Lower extremity Doppler, carotid ultrasound, abdominal ultrasound as needed
Pulmonary vascular resistance	Right heart catheterization
Infectious	Hepatitis B and C; human immunodeficiency virus; Ebstein–Barr virus; herpes simplex virus; cytomegalovirus serologies Vaccination history
Psychosocial	Treatment adherence and health behaviors, mental health history, substance use history, cognitive status, social support
Anatomic	Computed tomography (CT) of the chest
Nutrition	Hemoglobin A1c Body mass index and overall nutritional assessment

2 DURABLE MECHANICAL CIRCULATORY SUPPORT

Durable MCS began in the 1990s with the first generation of left ventricular assist devices (LVADs). Two general treatment paradigms were developed and tracked: VAD as a bridge to transplant (BTT) and as lifelong destination therapy (DT). As VAD technology has improved these categories have blurred substantially as some patients may improve, or may not initially be a candidate for transplant but become one later. The initial generation of devices relied on pneumatically driven pulsatile flow. Advancements in technology led to axial-flow pumps and then to centrifugal pumps in the current generation of LVADs. The only currently commercially available pump, the HeartMate 3 (Abbott, Abbott Park, IL), drains blood from the apex of the left ventricle via magnetically levitated rotor with blades spinning perpendicularly to the outflow port, which leads to the aorta (**Fig. 37.3**). The device is more resistant to thrombus than prior generations of pumps: In the key trial establishing the superiority of Heartmate 3 over its predecessor, 1.6% of patients with a HeartMate 3 needed the pump replaced within 2 years, compared to about 12.2% of those with a HeartMate II.[13] That study also showed that 77.9% of recipients of a HeartMate 3 survived to 2 years after implant without requiring a pump replacement, as compared to 56.4% after HeartMate II implant.

Table 37.4. Summary of US Adult Heart Allocation Statuses (2018 Changes)

OPTN Heart Allocation Status	Qualifying Criteria (Simplified)
1	Venoarterial extracorporeal membrane oxygenation (VA-ECMO); nondischargeable nonendovascular biventricular support device; mechanical circulatory support (MCS) with unstable arrhythmia
2	Nondischargeable left ventricular assist device (LVAD); total artificial heart/ durable biventricular support device; percutaneous MCS device (axial flow pump or intra-aortic balloon pump); ventricular tachycardia/arrhythmia
3	Multiple inotropes with hemodynamic monitoring; temporary or durable MCS with one of several defined complications
4	Dischargeable LVAD; inotropes; congenital heart disease
5	Multiorgan transplants
6	All other active candidates
7	Temporarily inactive candidates

Through documentation and reporting in clinical databases like the Society of Thoracic Surgeons' INTERMACS and the ISHLT Registry, LVADs have demonstrated effective performance profiles, improved systemic perfusion, and enhanced outcomes.[14] Complications of LVADs are still common: driveline infections, cannula or graft obstruction, gastrointestinal bleeding, and electrical faults can occur.[15] Predisposing factors include shear stresses in blood flow, cannula malposition, disturbances in von Willebrand factor levels (deficiency), and heparin-induced thrombocytopenia.

3 TEMPORARY MECHANICAL CIRCULATORY SUPPORT

While LVADs are designed to serve as BTT or as destination therapy, a growing number of temporary devices are designed for a bridge to recovery, to transplant, or to durable LVAD.[16] The oldest of these, the intra-aortic balloon pump (IABP), is the simplest and commonest. A 25- to 50-cc balloon is inserted peripherally over a wire and rests in the descending aorta. The console rapidly drives helium gas into the balloon in diastole and deflates it immediately before systole. This increases the pressure within the aortic root as well as the diastolic perfusion-time index, thereby increasing coronary blood flow. When the IABP deflates immediately prior to systole, the reduction in left ventricular (LV) afterload reduces myocardial oxygen demand.

The micro axial-flow pumps (mAFP) devices function on the Archimedes' screw principle: When positioned across the aortic valve, rotation of an in-line impeller displaces blood from the LV into the aorta.[10] This augments cardiac output and unloads the LV directly. The commercially available axial pump is Impella (Abiomed, Danvers, MA). The Impella CP model is inserted percutaneously, using the femoral artery, or via surgical cutdown on the axillary artery. The Impella 5.5 is inserted through the axillary artery, or directly through the ascending aorta, via a 10-mm graft. Impella 5.5 offers up to 5.5 L/min of output, and incremental technologic improvements have made this device more resistant to blood trauma and hemolysis than earlier iterations allowing longer support.

Venoarterial (VA) extracorporeal membrane oxygenation (ECMO) is used as short-term support in cases of refractory cardiogenic shock or cardiac arrest to provide circulatory and respiratory support. A VA-ECMO circuit consists of a venous

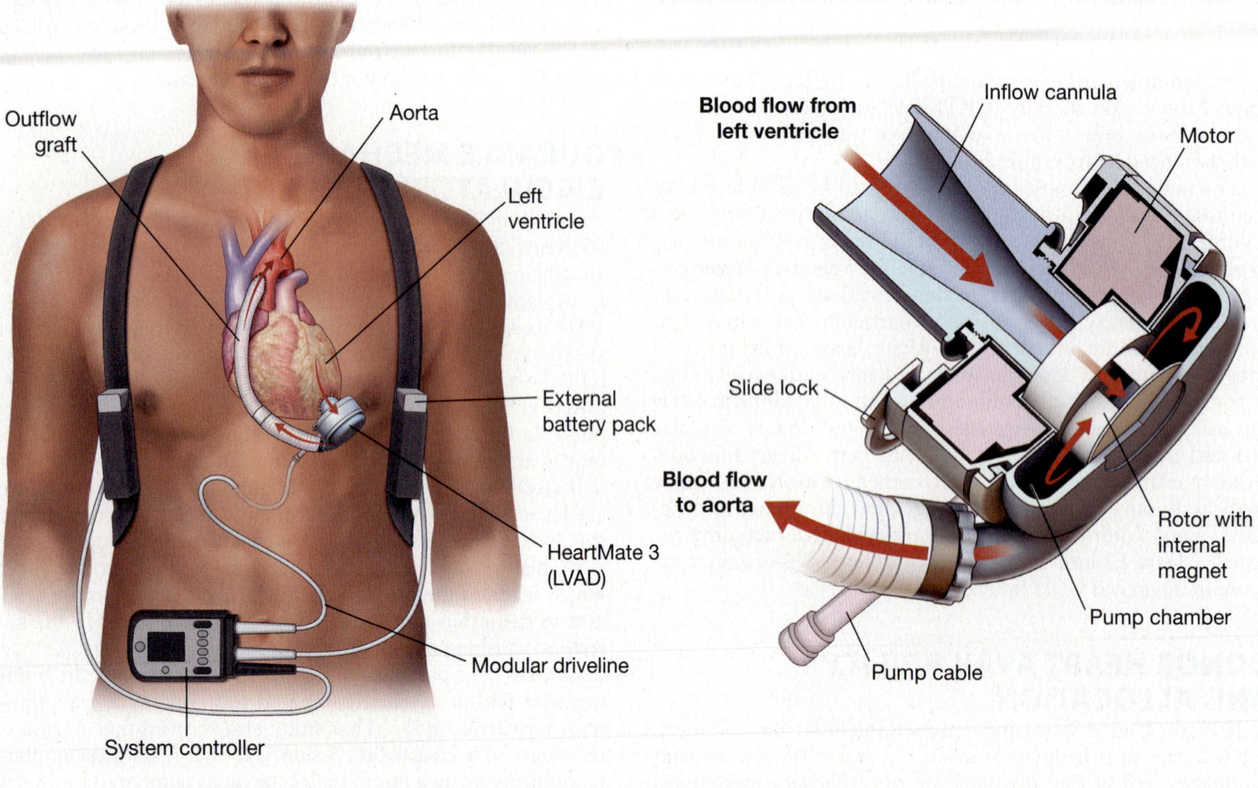

Figure 37.3. The HeartMate 3 left ventricular assist device (LVAD) system and cross-sectional schematic.

Table 37.5. Forms of Temporary Left-Sided Mechanical Circulatory Support

Form of Mechanical Support	Intra-aortic Balloon Pump	Impella CP or Impella 5.5	TandemHeart Cannula	Venoarterial ECMO
Mechanism	Helium balloon inflation and deflation	Microaxial flow pump across aortic valve	Centrifugal pump; transseptal puncture for percutaneous drainage from left atrium	Centrifugal pump; venous drainage and arterial reinfusion
Access site	Femoral or axillary artery	Femoral or axillary artery	Femoral vein	Femoral vein and artery; axillary vein and artery, or central
Size	7–8 Fr	13–21 Fr	12–19 Fr	14–19 Fr arterial; 19–25 Fr venous
Advantages	Speed of insertion, small caliber	Direct left ventricular unloading	Direct left atrial unloading	Speed of insertion; high level of support; lung support
Disadvantages	Incremental increase in cardiac output, requires stable rhythm	Not usable with intracardiac thrombus or mechanical aortic valve	Requires transseptal access, still requires arterial access	Retrograde blood flow; increases afterload; high rate of vascular complications

ECMO, extracorporeal membrane oxygenation.
Adapted from Truesdell AG, Davies R, Eltelbany M, Megaly M, Rosner C, Cilia LA. Mechanical circulatory support for complex high-risk percutaneous coronary intervention. *US Cardiol.* 2023;17:e03.

drainage cannula, membrane gas exchanger (oxygenator) and arterial reinfusion cannula. It is useful in reversible causes of cardiogenic shock such as postoperative myocardial stunning and myocarditis. Its advantage lies in its rapid deployability and ability to deliver high flow, but complication rates are high from arterial access, bleeding, and LV afterload increase exacerbating LV dysfunction. It is less commonly used for bridge directly to transplant, but also used as a bridge to a mAFP or durable LVAD.

A modified form of ECMO in which centrally placed cannulas drain the left atrium and reinfuse into the aorta, or drain the right atrium and reinfuse into the pulmonary artery, are termed paracorporeal VADs, and can be tunneled through the chest wall and allow patient mobilization during the wait for transplantation. A special cannula designed for femoral venous insertion and transseptal placement in the left atrium for drainage (TandemHeart) provides similar benefits with peripheral insertion (**Table 37.5**).

Finally, percutaneous right ventricular support is available via dual-lumen ECMO cannulas which are positioned similarly to a pulmonary artery catheter, and drain blood from the right atrium and reinfuse it past the pulmonic valve. An alternative form of the Impella mAFP designed for RV support (Impella RP Flex) is positioned similarly and drains blood from the right atrium and propels it forward into the pulmonary artery (**Table 37.6**).

DONOR SELECTION AND MANAGEMENT

Choosing to accept or decline an offered donor heart is a complex decision. Particular attention should be paid to the age of the donor, function and quality of the donor heart, donor–recipient compatibility (gender, height, and body mass index), ischemic time, and preformed antibodies. Despite the scarcity of organs, over the past 30 years, the median donor age in the United States has remained between 25 and 30 years of age whereas in Europe the median age is around 45.[17]

Gender discordance has been recognized as a posttransplant risk particularly when female hearts are transplanted to male recipients. Donor height, weight, body surface area, predicted heart mass, and body mass index have all been associated with posttransplant outcomes.[18] In heart transplantation, even more so than other organs, a major factor in outcomes is the ischemic time between the donor cross-clamp and reperfusion in the recipient. Historically, cold storage has limited the acceptable ischemic time to 4 hours. Longer ischemic times were associated with worse survival, more rejection episodes, and higher rates of allograft vasculopathy.[19]

Table 37.6. Forms of Temporary Right-Sided Mechanical Circulatory Support

Form of Mechanical Support	Impella RP Flex (Abiomed)	Protek Duo Cannula (LivaNova) or Spectrum Medical Dual-lumen Cannula
Mechanism	Microaxial flow pump across tricuspid and pulmonic valves	With centrifugal pump for right atrial drainage and pulmonary arterial reinfusion
Access site	Femoral or internal jugular vein	Internal jugular or subclavian vein
Size	22 Fr	27–31 Fr
Advantages	Smaller cannula, allows patient mobility	Can also use oxygenator for venovenous ECMO; allows patient mobility
Disadvantages	No oxygenator support; hemolysis	Larger cannula in patient's neck

ECMO, extracorporeal membrane oxygenation.

Assessing the quality and function of the donor heart is crucial. The first step is considering the donor's cause of death. Most suitable heart donors have died of an anoxic brain injury, stroke, or trauma: A mechanism of death attributable to the heart like an arrhythmia, myocardial infarction, or traumatic injury would preclude most uses. Often donors' cause of death is unclear, in which case a higher level of scrutiny to rule out cardiac causes is warranted. Scrutiny of the electrocardiogram at admission and serially as well as serial troponin values can help exclude coronary pathology. Donors may undergo cardiac catheterization with coronary angiogram to exclude coronary disease as a cause of death. In donors with hypertensive stroke as the cause of death (or more generally with hypertension), careful evaluation must be made to ensure that the left ventricle is not overly hypertrophied (ideal LV interventricular septum is <1.3 cm), as hypertrophy can cause restrictive dysfunction of the allograft and poor myocardial preservation during organ recovery.

An essential part of the evaluation of the potential donor is an echocardiogram, which demonstrates the ejection fraction, anatomic and physiologic abnormalities, ventricular hypertrophy, right heart function, the exclusion of masses or vegetation, and regional wall abnormalities. While vasopressor requirement does not necessarily affect heart function, the number of and the dosage of inotropic support can serve as an important prognostic measure for the posttransplant primary graft dysfunction (PGD) and should be considered while interpreting the echocardiogram.

In patients with risk factors for coronary arterial disease (age >40, smoking, hypertension, diabetes mellitus, regional wall motion abnormality on echocardiogram), a left heart catheterization can provide information of coronary anatomy as well as LV function and LV end-diastolic pressure. A right heart catheterization can be an adjunct test in patients where heart function (especially of the RV) is in question.

DONOR HEART RECOVERY PROCEDURE

Once a donor heart has been accepted, the goals of recovery are to minimize ischemic time, ensure no technical injury to important structures, and to ensure optimal myocardial protection during the procurement and transportation.[20] Due to the high sensitivity of the heart to ischemic time, the heart recipient operation is often underway during the remote recovery operation, so constant communication on findings and timing is essential.

In donor heart recovery, a sternotomy is performed and the heart is inspected for functional status, size, and the presence of congenital abnormalities.[21] Less dissection of structures is necessary than for abdominal organ transplant: The superior vena cava is dissected off the right pulmonary artery and the aorta and pulmonary artery are separated (**Fig. 37.4**). After the systemic administration of heparin, a cardioplegia line is placed in the aorta. Once all teams are ready, the superior vena cava is clamped, the inferior vena cava is cut just above the diaphragm, and the left atrium is vented through its appendage or wall. The aorta is then clamped and the preservation solution is flushed into the aortic root and down the coronaries. The surgeon must constantly check for correct pressurization of the root, distention of the LV, and adequate venting of the heart, while applying ice for topical cooling. The goals are to avoid distention of the heart, ensure adequate cooling, and preserve appropriate cuffs for safe anastomosis to the recipient, specifically:

- the ascending aorta to the level of the great vessels,
- the pulmonary artery at the pulmonary bifurcation a safe distance from the pulmonary valve,
- as much length on the SVC as possible (typically to the confluence of the internal jugular and brachiocephalic vein),
- a safe distance on the IVC away from the coronary sinus without compromising the suprahepatic cava for the liver team, and

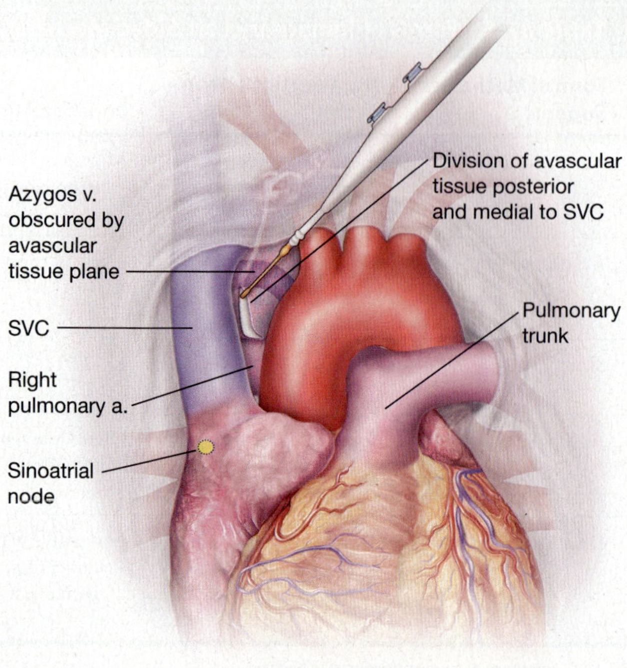

Figure 37.4. Preparation of the donor heart for recovery. (Redrawn from Camp PC, Heart transplantation: donor operation for heart and lung transplantation. *Oper Tech Thorac Cardiovasc Surg*. 2010;15(2): 125–137.)

- most importantly, enough of a left atrial cuff that allows safe course for the left circumflex artery and the coronary sinus while preserving the confluence of the pulmonary venous drainage for the lung team (see **Fig. 37.7**).

4 DONOR HEART PRESERVATION

Recent efforts have been made to overcome the limitations of simple storage in a bag of cold preservation solution inside a cooler. The Paragonix SherpaPak is a passive cooler but features cooling packs that do not drop below freezing, avoiding damage to the heart from overcooling and keeping the heart between 4 °C and 8 °C.[12] The Organ Care System (OCS; Transmedics, Andover, Massachusetts) involves perfusion of the donor heart with augmented blood obtained from the donor at 34 degrees.[22] Perfusate is pumped through the aorta, through the coronaries, and drained from the right side of the heart via the pulmonary artery, allowing for measurement of arterial and venous blood gases. The heart is paced, allowing qualitative, unloaded assessment of the donor heart on the device. This greatly extends the ischemic tolerance, allowing for long-distance transport. Other investigational devices such as the XVIVO Heart Box use cold coronary perfusion of banked blood at low flows, which does not allow for assessment of myocardial function but avoids a second period of cooling for the donor heart (**Fig. 37.5**).[23]

DONATION AFTER CIRCULATORY DETERMINATION OF DEATH (DCD)

Some potential donors, despite being neurologically devastated, do not meet criteria for brain death and can only donate organs after controlled withdrawal of life-sustaining therapy and being declared dead because their circulation has stopped. This pathway, donation after circulatory determination of death (DCD), was used in the first heart transplant. However, this approach poses unique challenges to heart donation. The inability to directly assess the function of a heart that has stopped beating before the organ recovery procedure has historically precluded the use of hearts from these donors, while

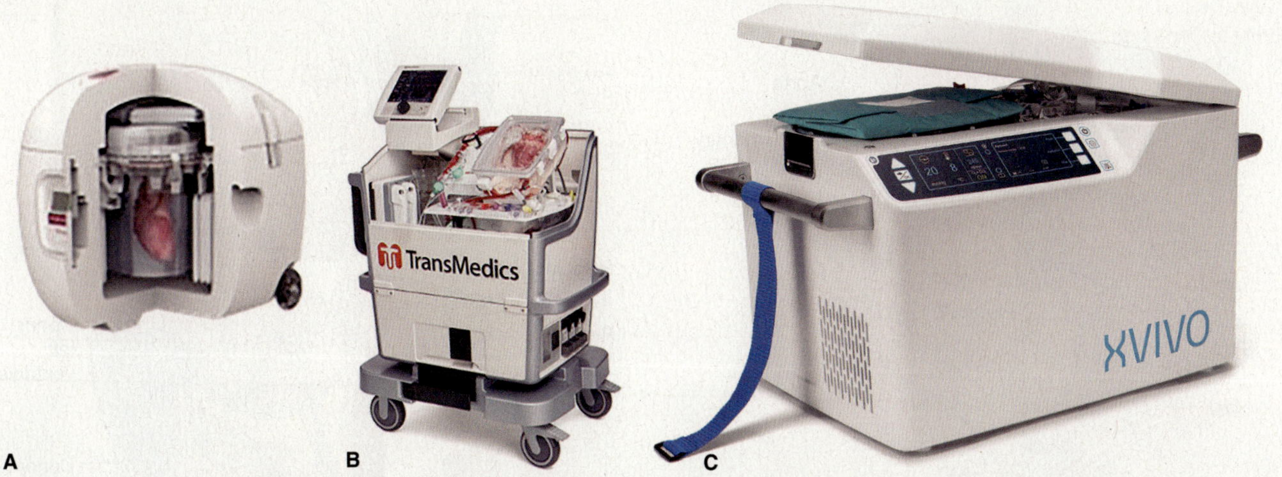

Figure 37.5. Novel methods of preservation and transportation for donor hearts. **A:** Sherpapak. (Image courtesy of Paragonix Technologies, Inc. All rights reserved.) **B:** Organ Care System. (Copyright © 2026, TransMedics, Inc. All rights reserved.) **C:** XVIVO Heart Box. (XVIVO Heart Assist Transport™ is a trademark of XVIVO Perfusion AB. The picture is published with permission from XVIVO Perfusion AB, 2026. All rights reserved.)

lung and liver recovery has long been accepted.[24,25] The first of two strategies for heart recovery in the setting of DCD is direct procurement and perfusion (DPP), or *ex vivo* machine perfusion.[26] In this approach, after the donor's care is withdrawn, circulation stops, and death is declared, an expedited median sternotomy is done. The heart is exposed and blood is drained from the right atrium for use in perfusate. A cardioplegia needle is inserted and the aorta is cross-clamped. The already-arrested heart is cooled and then quickly removed and prepared for perfusion on a device like OCS which allows for assessment of the heart before implant.

The second approach to DCD heart recovery is termed Thoraco-abdominal Normothermic Regional Perfusion (TA-NRP).[27] Similarly to DPP, the donor's family authorizes donation, the withdrawal of life-sustaining therapy, and the administration of heparin in connection with DCD. Once the donor progresses to circulatory arrest and death is declared, a median sternotomy is done rapidly. The next step is clamping and/or ligation of the arch vessels so the donor's brain is not reperfused.[28] Next the flaccid aorta and distended right atrium are cannulated. The cannulas are connected to a perfusion circuit (analogous to an ECMO circuit) and perfusion of the thoracic and abdominal organs is done. The reperfused heart is then slowly weaned from the perfusion circuit and assessed for suitability. When all teams are ready, the heart is arrested with cardioplegia and removed and packed in ice, similar to a DBD recovery. Advantages of this approach are greater flexibility in repurposing perfusion equipment (no devices are FDA approved specifically for NRP), potentially beneficial effects of having the heart reperfused in the donor, and better support for abdominal procurement. No trials have directly compared NRP and DPP, and long-term outcomes comparing the two are not yet available (**Fig. 37.6**).[29]

RECIPIENT PREPARATION AND TRANSPLANTATION

Patients taking warfarin or who have other coagulopathy should have their effects reversed. Induction of anesthesia is followed by vascular access for rapid volume infusion, pulmonary artery catheter for hemodynamic monitoring, transesophageal echocardiogram, and arterial line monitoring.

Explant of the native heart is performed with the major principle of not taking on undue risks while minimizing warm ischemic time.[30] Once the donor heart is confirmed to be suitable, the recipient operation can begin. Bicaval cannulation is required and done via the SVC as well as the IVC (or percutaneously via the femoral vein). Central ascending aortic cannulation is preferred unless difficult sternal entry vascular abnormalities prompt use of the axillary. Once the donor heart is relatively close to the recipient center, the heart is isolated by caval snares and the aortic cross-clamp without cardioplegia.

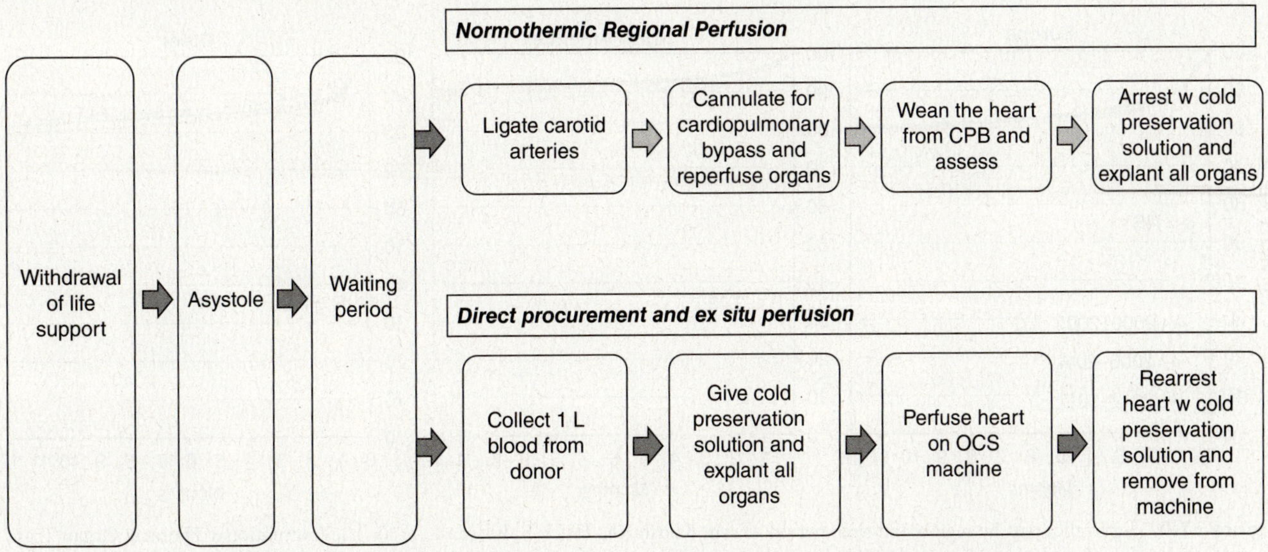

Figure 37.6. Two pathways to heart donation after circulatory declaration of death (DCD).

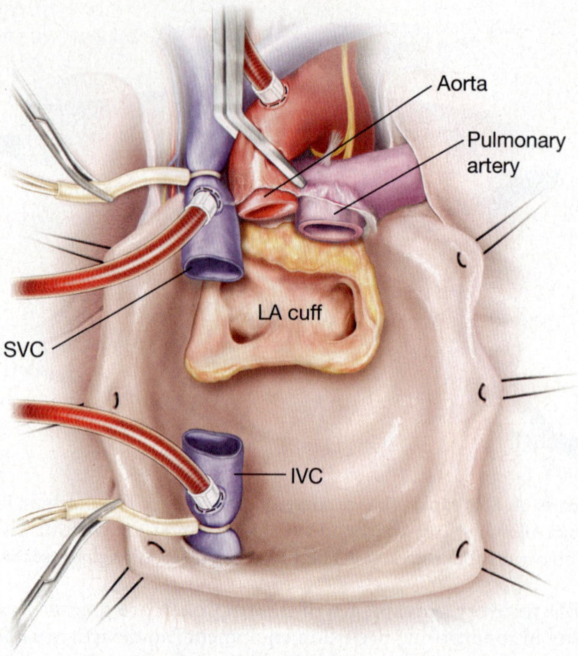

Figure 37.7. Recipient cardiectomy is done to leave adequate cuffs for anastomosis. (Redrawn from John R, Liao K, Orthotopic heart transplantation. *Oper Tech Thorac Cardiovasc Surg*. 2010;15(2):138–146.)

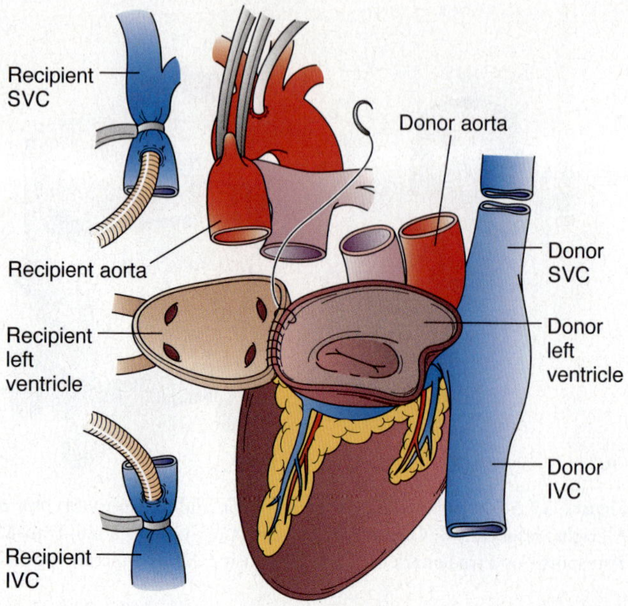

Figure 37.8. Bicaval implantation technique starting with left atrial anastomosis followed by inferior/superior vena cava anastomosis, pulmonary artery and aortic anastomosis. (Image credit Timothy Phelps.)

The heart is then removed while carefully preserving enough tissue to construct cuffs for anastomosis (**Fig. 37.7**).

The most common implant technique today is the bicaval approach, in which the SVC and IVC are separately anastomosed to the same structures in the donor. Remaining tissue is trimmed away from the SVC, IVC, left atrium, pulmonary artery, and aorta. Once the heart arrives and safety checks are performed, careful assessment and backtable preparation of the heart is done. A patent foramen ovale should be closed if found, and preparation of the donor vascular cuffs is done.

The donor heart is implanted by performing the left atrial anastomosis first, since it is posterior (**Fig. 37.8**). All four pulmonary veins are visualized as the heart is lowered into the chest. The remaining order of anastomosis varies, but once the aortic anastomosis is done the clamp can be removed to minimize the ischemic time. When time allows, it is still easier to perform at least portions of the pulmonary artery and IVC anastomoses with the clamp on, which also allows for venting through the open front wall of the anastomosis. Care must be taken during the SVC anastomosis to avoid narrowing the anastomosis, as it can lead to SVC syndrome, or difficulty with access for percutaneous jugular endomyocardial biopsies to detect graft rejection. Once all anastomoses are complete, the heart is de-aired and slowly weaned off cardiopulmonary bypass. Atrial and ventricular pacing is done to minimize distention. Inhaled pulmonary vasodilators including nitric oxide, inotropes, and vasopressor agents are used to facilitate weaning from bypass.

OUTCOMES

Survival

Outcomes following heart transplantation have improved significantly since the first technically successful heart transplant in 1967. The first decade of heart transplantation saw dismal postoperative outcomes with about 60% of patients surviving to 1 year posttransplant. The current 1-year survival now exceeds 90% (**Fig. 37.9**). The many improvements in heart transplantation have included better recipient selection and optimization, improved methods of assessment of donors, safer myocardial preservation, more options for

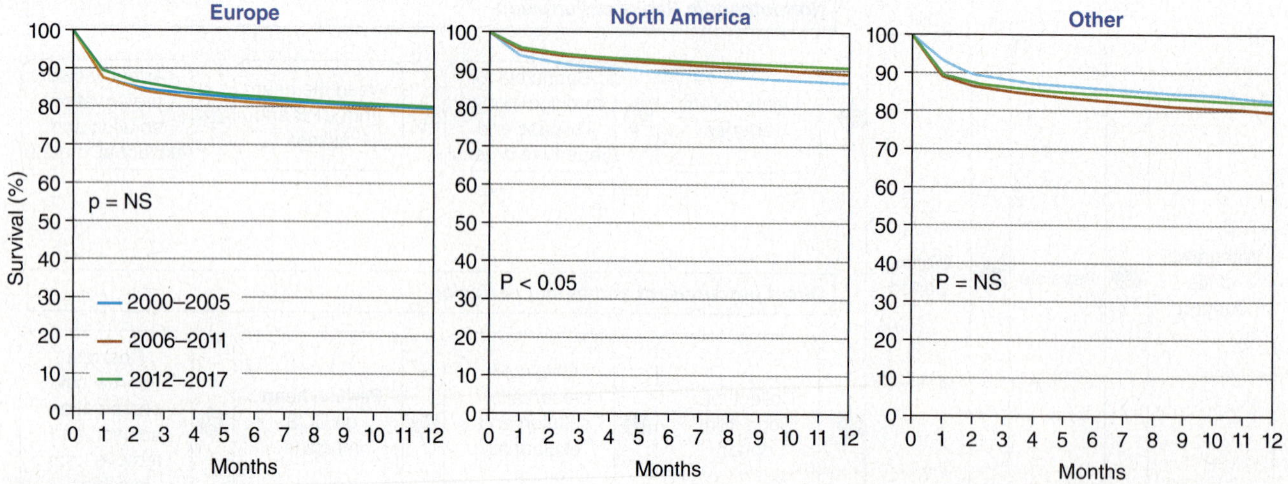

Figure 37.9. Survival curves by region and time period. (From Khush KK, Hsich E, Potena L, et al. The International Thoracic Organ Transplant Registry of the International Society for Heart and Lung Transplantation: thirty-eighth adult heart transplantation report—2021; Focus on recipient characteristics. *J Heart Lung Transplant*. 2021;40(10):1035–1049.)

Table 37.7. ISHLT Standardized Cardiac Biopsy Grading: Acute Cellular Rejection

2004		1990	
Grade 0 R	No rejection	Grade 0	No rejection
Grade 1 R, mild	Interstitial and/or perivascular infiltrate with up to one focus of myocyte damage	Grade 1, mild A—Focal B—Diffuse	 Focal perivascular and/or interstitial infiltrate without myocyte damage Diffuse infiltrate without myocyte damage
Grade 2 R, moderate	Two or more foci of infiltrate with associated myocyte damage	Grade 2 moderate (focal) Grade 3, moderate A—Focal B—Diffuse	One focus of infiltrate with associated myocyte damage Multifocal infiltrate with myocyte damage Diffuse infiltrate with myocyte damage
Grade 3 R, severe	Diffuse infiltrate with multifocal myocyte damage ± edema, ± hemorrhage ± vasculitis	Grade 4, severe	Diffuse, polymorphous infiltrate with extensive myocyte damage ± edema, ± hemorrhage + vasculitis

immunosuppression, defined methods of graft surveillance, and refined techniques in suppressing rejection episodes with patient-specific immunomodulation. The improvements in survival by era can clearly be seen with the current median survival after heart transplant exceeding 12 years (**Fig. 37.9**).[31]

The effects of the 2018 donor heart allocation changes are still being examined: Higher rates of transplant from ECMO and temporary MCS, and lower rates of transplant after LVAD, with slightly lower overall survival, have been noted.[32]

In many regards, the quality of life and functional capacity that is restored after heart transplantation is as important as the time of survival posttransplantation. The improvement in quality of life allows patients to resume full activity, return to work, and have a higher perception of themselves with improved self-esteem. These metrics are adversely affected by the presence of and severity of rejection episodes, highlighting the importance of reduction and management of complications.

Complications

The most immediate and morbid complication following heart transplantation is PGD. PGD after heart transplantation manifests as failure to wean from cardiopulmonary bypass after reperfusion of the heart, or cardiogenic shock within 24 hours of reperfusion of the heart. A consensus statement defines PGD-left ventricle and PGD-right ventricle and graded as mild, moderate, or severe.[33] It was estimated that the incidence of PGD was approximately 7% with an accompanying 30-day mortality of 30% and a 1-year mortality of nearly 35%. Treatment modalities typically involve mechanical circulatory support, most commonly IABP or conversion of the bypass cannulas to ECMO, to allow time for recovery.

Immune Suppression and Rejection

Most immunosuppressive regimens for heart transplant consist of a two- or three-drug regimen, including a calcineurin inhibitor (typically tacrolimus), an antimetabolite agent (typically mycophenolate mofetil), and tapering doses of glucocorticoids over the first year.[4]

Current regimens use IL-2 receptor antagonists for induction therapy and these drugs are now used in 30% of patients undergoing heart transplantation. The currently available agent, basiliximab (Simulect), is a monoclonal antibody that selectively binds to the IL-2 receptor of T lymphocytes, inhibiting T-lymphocyte proliferation.

Rejection of a heart allograft can be divided into early (<3-month posttransplant) and late (>3-month posttransplant) time periods and can be categorized by the mechanism of rejection—cellular, antibody mediated, or mixed rejection.

ISHLT developed a biopsy grading system to ensure a more consistent grading across centers for cardiac allograft rejection.[34] The differences between this system and the previous definitions from 1990 are highlighted in **Table 37.7**. Antibody-mediated rejection (AMR) has also been defined based on pathologic diagnosis (**Table 37.8**).

Table 37.8. The 2013 ISHLT Working Formulation for Pathologic Diagnosis of Cardiac Antibody-Mediated Rejection

Grade	Definition	Substrates
pAMR 0	Negative for pathologic AMR	Histologic and immunopathologic studies are both negative.
pAMR 1 (H+)	Histopathologic AMR alone	Histologic findings are present and immunopathologic findings are negative.
pAMR 1 (I+)	Immunopathologic AMR alone	Histologic findings are negative and immunopathologic findings are positive (CD68+ and/or C4D+).
pAMR 2	Pathologic AMR	Histologic and immunopathologic findings are both present.
pAMR 3	Severe pathologic AMR	Interstitial hemorrhage, capillary fragmentation, mixed inflammatory infiltrates, endothelial cell pyknosis, and/or karyorrhexis, and marked edema and immunopathologic findings are present. These cases may be associated with profound hemodynamic dysfunction and poor clinical outcomes.

AMR, antibody-mediated rejection.
Reprinted from Berry GJ, Angelini J, Burk MM, et al. The ISHLT working formulation for pathologic diagnosis of antibody-mediated rejection in heart transplantation: evolution and current status (2005–2011). *J Heart Lung Transplant.* 2011;30(6):601–611.

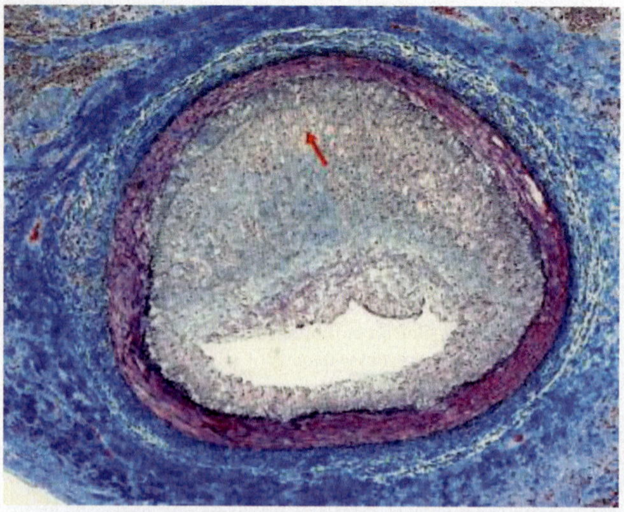

Figure 37.10. Trichrome elastic stain of a coronary artery demonstrating progressive arterial occlusion with lipid-laden foam cell macrophages (*arrow*) in a patient with cardiac allograft vasculopathy (CAV). (Used with permission from Zimmer R, Lee M. Transplant coronary artery disease. *JACC Cardiovasc Interv.* 2010;3(4):367–377.)

All three types of rejection—cellular, AMR, and mixed—are associated with increased risk of mortality and loss of graft function. Roughly 25% of all patients will have an episode of acute rejection in the first year.[35] In a more chronic form of rejection, cardiac allograft vasculopathy (CAV) can develop in a process of coronary endothelial inflammation, injury, fibrosis, and dysfunction after chronic rejection (**Fig. 37.10**).[36] Unlike acute rejection, which has surveillance diagnosis by endomyocardial biopsies, CAV is usually evaluated by invasive coronary angiography. By 5 years posttransplant, a third of heart transplant recipients develop CAV, which is the most common cause of death among recipients in the long term.

Technical issues with transplantation usually arise in the immediate postoperative period: Anastomotic narrowing, damage to coronary arteries or the coronary sinus, infections, bleeding or inappropriate patient–donor size matching. Complications can also arise from chronic immunosuppression which can include infectious complications such as viral, bacterial, or fungal infections. Particular attention should be paid to recipients who are CMV negative who receive donor CMV-positive organs. CMV prophylactic therapy during the early postoperative course is routinely employed when immunosuppression is greatest during the first 6 months posttransplant. Another complication from immunosuppression can be the development of malignancies such as skin cancer, posttransplant lymphoproliferative disease, and visceral cancers.[37] Lastly, patients on chronic immunosuppression can develop diabetes mellitus, hypertension, and renal failure.

4 FUTURE DIRECTIONS

The annual number of heart transplants in the United States has continued to rise within the last 5 years with improvements in expansion of the donor pool. These incremental improvements are multifactorial and stem from meticulous patient selection, donor selection, operative technique, posttransplant immunosuppression, protocol-driven surveillance biopsies to detect early, nonclinical rejection and maintenance of long-term healthcare needs.

Immunosuppression in its present state is far from perfect and causes infectious, autoimmune, and oncologic complications. Reliance on serial, surveillance endomyocardial biopsies to assess for rejection, as well as yearly cardiac angiography for accelerated chronic rejection leading to atherosclerotic coronary disease, is being augmented by noninvasive methods such as AlloMap testing that test genetic expression to detect early rejection.[38] In addition, better understanding of the differences between AMR and acute cellular rejection will enable targeted treatment options based upon the specific type of rejection in the future.

There has already been an increased awareness of the utilization of nontraditional donors. With novel medications to treat and cure hepatitis C, hearts from hepatitis-C–positive

Table 37.9. Key Steps, Pearls, and Pitfalls in Heart Transplantation

	Donor Heart Procurement	Recipient Cardiectomy	Heart Transplantation
Key Steps	▪ Functional assessment ▪ Anatomic assessment (left SVC, calcified coronaries, etc.) ▪ SVC mobilization ▪ Aorta and pulmonary artery mobilization	▪ Bicaval and central aortic cannulation ▪ Remove the heart ▪ Preserve aortic, pulmonary artery, left atrial, superior vena cava and inferior vena cava cuffs	▪ Backtable prep of donor heart ▪ Left atrial anastomosis ▪ Surgeon's preference for remaining anastomosis (aorta, PA, SVC, IVC) ▪ Remove clamp, pace, de-air ▪ Wean slowly from cardiopulmonary bypass
Pearls	▪ Constant communication with the recipient surgeon about the donor heart, timing of recovery, and unexpected findings is essential.	▪ Balance safety and readiness for the donor heart with minimization of excess time on bypass	▪ Keep the PA relatively short to avoid kinking and the aorta relatively long to facilitate inspection for bleeding ▪ Biventricular pacing at high rate may help keep end-diastolic volume low
Pitfalls	▪ Distention of the donor heart (from excessively high perfusion pressure, inadequate venting of the pulmonary drainage, or unrecognized aortic insufficiency) ▪ Damage to the circumflex artery or coronary sinus during left atrial dissection	▪ Injury on redo sternotomy to the RV, innominate vein, or VAD outflow graft ▪ Injury to the IVC or pulmonary veins after prior sternotomy	▪ Purse-stringing anastomoses, especially the SVC ▪ Weaning too quickly from cardiopulmonary bypass ▪ Failing to recognize early signs of PGD or to respond quickly with MCS

IVC, inferior vena cava; MCS, mechanical circulatory support; PA, pulmonary artery; PGD, primary graft dysfunction; RV, right ventricle; SVC, superior vena cava.

donors are being transplanted with good results.[39] Heart donation after cardiac death (DCD) has led to a significant expansion in the donor pool and a more general reconsideration of what makes a suitable donor.

SUMMARY

Over the past 60 years, heart transplantation has changed from a daring endeavor with dismal early outcomes to the gold standard for patients suffering from end-stage heart failure. This remarkable transformation came from decades of innovation, perseverance, and commitment by thousands of dedicated heart failure physicians and surgeons, immunologists and scientists, organ recovery technicians and professionals, researchers, nurses and coordinators, regulatory and administrative policy experts, and infectious disease experts. There have been over 70,000 heart transplants in the UNOS registry at this time, with 1-year survival surpassing 90%. Careful attention to recipient and donor selection, advanced methods of heart preservation, meticulous surgical technique (**Table 37.9**), surveillance, and individualized detection and treatment of rejection will push the field into even greater heights in the future.

ACKNOWLEDGMENTS

We gratefully acknowledge the contributions of previous edition authors, Ahmet Kilic and Robert S. D. Higgins, as portions of those chapters have been retained in this revision.

References

1. McRae D. *Every Second Counts: The Race to Transplant the First Human Heart*. G.P. Putnam's Sons; 2006.
2. Barnard CN. The operation: a human cardiac transplant: an interim report of a successful operation performed at Groote Schuur Hospital, Cape Town. *S Afr Med J*. 2017;107(12):1271–1274.
3. Hines GL, Gooding R. Ethical issues in early cardiac transplantation. *Cardiol Rev*. 2022;30(2):57–58.
4. Velleca A, Shullo MA, Dhital K, et al. The International Society for Heart and Lung Transplantation (ISHLT) guidelines for the care of heart transplant recipients. *J Heart Lung Transplant*. 2023;42(5):e1–e141.
5. Baumwol J. "I Need Help"-A mnemonic to aid timely referral in advanced heart failure. *J Heart Lung Transplant*. 2017;36(5):593–594.
6. Bakaeen FG, Gaudino M, Whitman G, et al. 2021: The American Association for Thoracic Surgery Expert Consensus Document: coronary artery bypass grafting in patients with ischemic cardiomyopathy and heart failure. *J Thorac Cardiovasc Surg*. 2021;162(3):829–850.e1.
7. Malhotra R, Bakken K, D'Elia E, Lewis GD. Cardiopulmonary exercise testing in heart failure. *JACC Heart Fail*. 2016;4(8):607–616.
8. Peled Y, Ducharme A, Kittleson M, et al. International Society for Heart and Lung Transplantation Guidelines for the evaluation and care of cardiac transplant candidates—2024. *J Heart Lung Transplant*. 2024;43(10):1529–1628.e54.
9. Dew MA, DiMartini AF, Dobbels F, et al. The 2018 ISHLT/APM/AST/ICCAC/STSW recommendations for the psychosocial evaluation of adult cardiothoracic transplant candidates and candidates for long-term mechanical circulatory support. *J Heart Lung Transplant*. 2018;37(7):803–823.
10. Malgie J, Clephas PRD, Brunner-La Rocca HP, de Boer RA, Brugts JJ. Guideline-directed medical therapy for HFrEF: sequencing strategies and barriers for life-saving drug therapy. *Heart Fail Rev*. 2023;28(5):1221–1234.
11. Heidenreich PA, Bozkurt B, Aguilar D, et al. 2022 AHA/ACC/HFSA guideline for the management of heart failure: a report of the American College of Cardiology/American Heart Association Joint Committee on Clinical Practice Guidelines. *Circulation*. 2022;145(18):e895–e1032.
12. Silvestry S, Leacche M, Meyer DM, et al. Outcomes in heart transplant recipients by bridge to transplant strategy when using the SherpaPak Cardiac Transport System. *ASAIO J*. 2024;70(5):388–395.
13. Mehra MR, Uriel N, Naka Y, et al. A fully magnetically levitated left ventricular assist device—Final report. *N Engl J Med*. 2019;380(17):1618–1627.
14. Yuzefpolskaya M, Schroeder SE, Houston BA, et al. The Society of Thoracic Surgeons INTERMACS 2022 annual report: focus on the 2018 heart transplant allocation system. *Ann Thorac Surg*. 2023;115(2):311–327.
15. Weber MP, Stulak J, Maltais S, Pagani FD, Cowger J, Tchantchaleishvili V. Quality of life metrics in LVAD patients after hemocompatibility-related adverse events. *Artif Organs*. 2022;46(8):1616–1625.
16. Saeed D, Feldman D, Banayosy AE, et al. The 2023 International Society for Heart and Lung Transplantation guidelines for mechanical circulatory support: a 10-year update. *J Heart Lung Transplant*. 2023;42(7):e1–e222.
17. Khush KK, Zuckermann A, Cherikh WS, et al. The International Thoracic Organ Transplant Registry of the International Society for Heart and Lung Transplantation: 37th Adult Heart Transplantation Report—2020; Focus on deceased donor characteristics. *J Heart Lung Transplant*. 2020;39(10):1003–1015.
18. Kransdorf EP, Kittleson MM, Benck LR, et al. Predicted heart mass is the optimal metric for size match in heart transplantation. *J Heart Lung Transplant*. 2019;38(2):156–165.
19. Jernryd V, Stehlik J, Metzsch C, et al. Donor age and ischemic time in heart transplantation: implications for organ preservation. *J Heart Lung Transplant*. 2025;44(3):364–375.
20. Copeland H, Hayanga JWA, Neyrinck A, et al. Donor heart and lung procurement: a consensus statement. *J Heart Lung Transplant*. 2020;39(6):501–517.
21. Camp PC. Heart transplantation: donor operation for heart and lung transplantation. *Oper Tech Thorac Cardiovasc Surg*. 2010;15(2):125–137.
22. Ardehali A, Esmailian F, Deng M, et al. Ex-vivo perfusion of donor hearts for human heart transplantation (PROCEED II): a prospective, open-label, multicentre, randomised non-inferiority trial. *Lancet*. 2015;385(9987):2577–2584.
23. Rega F, Lebreton G, Para M, et al. Hypothermic oxygenated perfusion of the donor heart in heart transplantation: the short-term outcome from a randomised, controlled, open-label, multicentre clinical trial. *Lancet North Am Ed*. 2024;404(10453):670–682.
24. Page A, Messer S, Large SR. Heart transplantation from donation after circulatory determined death. *Ann Cardiothorac Surg*. 2018;7(1):75–81.
25. Truby LK, Casalinova S, Patel CB, et al. Donation after circulatory death in heart transplantation: history, outcomes, clinical challenges, and opportunities to expand the donor pool. *J Card Fail*. 2022;28(9):1456–1463.
26. Connellan M, Dhital K. Donor heart procurement from the donation after circulatory death pathway. *Oper Tech Thorac Cardiovasc Surg*. 2017;22(1):58–67.
27. Hoffman JRH, McMaster WG, Rali AS, et al. Early US experience with cardiac donation after circulatory death (DCD) using normothermic regional perfusion. *J Heart Lung Transplant*. 2021;40(11):1408–1418.
28. Hoffman JRH, Hartwig MG, Cain MT, et al. Consensus Statement: technical standards for thoracoabdominal normothermic regional perfusion. *Ann Thorac Surg*. 2024;118(4):778–791.
29. Kearns MJ, Brann A, White R, et al. (229) A single center comparison of DCD heart transplantation using two procurement strategies: direct procurement and perfusion versus normothermic regional perfusion. *J Heart Lung Transplant*. 2023;42(4):S112–S113.

30. John R, Liao K. Orthotopic heart transplantation. *Oper Tech Thorac Cardiovasc Surg*. 2010;15(2):138–146.
31. Khush KK, Hsich E, Potena L, et al. The International Thoracic Organ Transplant Registry of the International Society for Heart and Lung Transplantation: thirty-eighth adult heart transplantation report—2021; focus on recipient characteristics. *J Heart Lung Transplant*. 2021;40(10):1035–1049.
32. Maitra NS, Dugger SJ, Balachandran IC, Civitello AB, Khazanie P, Rogers JG. Impact of the 2018 UNOS heart transplant policy changes on patient outcomes. *Heart Fail*. 2023;11(5): 491–503.
33. Kobashigawa J, Zuckermann A, Macdonald P, et al. Report from a consensus conference on primary graft dysfunction after cardiac transplantation. *J Heart Lung Transplant*. 2014;33(4): 327–340.
34. Berry GJ, Angelini A, Burke MM, et al. The ISHLT working formulation for pathologic diagnosis of antibody-mediated rejection in heart transplantation: evolution and current status (2005–2011). *J Heart Lung Transplant*. 2011;30(6):601–611.
35. Gemelli M, Doulamis IP, Tzani A, et al. Rejection requiring treatment within the first year following heart transplantation: the UNOS insight. *J Pers Med*. 2023;14(1):52.
36. Spartalis M, Spartalis E, Siasos G. Cardiac allograft vasculopathy after heart transplantation: pathophysiology, detection approaches, prevention, and treatment management. *Trends Cardiovasc Med*. 2022;32(6):333–338.
37. Mudigonda P, Berardi C, Chetram V, Barac A, Cheng R. Implications of cancer prior to and after heart transplantation. *Heart*. 2021;108(6):414–421.
38. Goldberg JF, Truby LK, Agbor-Enoh S, et al. Selection and interpretation of molecular diagnostics in heart transplantation. *Circulation*. 2023;148(8):679–694.
39. Kilic A, Hickey G, Mathier M, et al. Outcomes of adult heart transplantation using hepatitis C–positive donors. *J Am Heart Assoc*. 2020;9(2):e014495.
40. Truesdell AG, Davies R, Eltelbany M, Megaly M, Rosner C, Cilia LA. Mechanical circulatory support for complex high-risk percutaneous coronary intervention. *US Cardiol*. 2023;17:e03.

38

Lung Transplantation

Alfred J. Casillan and Errol L. Bush

Key Points

1 Annual numbers of lung transplants in the United States have been increasing and in 2022, 2,743 lung transplants were performed in the United States.

2 Each transplant center's multidisciplinary candidate selection committee carefully considers candidates' individual underlying disease severity, medical comorbidities, psychosocial factors, and surgical risk.

3 Idiopathic pulmonary fibrosis (IPF) is the most common indication for lung transplantation in the United States, and in 2022, restrictive lung diseases represented nearly 60% of all lung transplants performed in the United States.

4 The donor recovery lung evaluation is as important to the success of the lung transplant as the implantation.

5 Eighty percent of recipients received a bilateral-lung transplant. Double-lung transplantation now involves a bilateral, sequential technique that can be performed via a median sternotomy, bilateral thoracosternotomy (clamshell) incision, bilateral anterior thoracotomies without sternal division, or bilateral muscle-sparing axillary thoracotomies.

6 Most transplant centers attempt to limit organ ischemic time to less than 6 total hours, but many centers have experience comfortably extending cold ischemic time with careful donor selection, organ preservation, and utilization of ex vivo lung perfusion (EVLP) to evaluate extended criteria donors.

7 Primary graft dysfunction (PGD), an acute lung injury syndrome characterized by inexplicable diffuse allograft infiltrates and hypoxemia defined as a PaO_2/FiO_2 ratio (P/F) <300, occurs within the first 72 hours following transplantation and results in significant morbidity and mortality.

8 Donor availability remains a limiting factor to successful and timely transplantation, which has led to innovative utilization of techniques that increase donor utilization, such as use of EVLP, donation after cardiac death donors, and hepatitis C virus–infected organs.

EARLY YEARS OF LUNG TRANSPLANTATION

In 1963, James Hardy from the University of Mississippi reported the first human lung transplant in a patient with end-stage emphysema, an obstructive left mainstem carcinoma, and chronic renal disease.[1] While the surgery was regarded as a success, the recipient died from renal failure after 18 days, but reportedly still had a functioning lung allograft. Over the next 20 years, less than 40 attempted lung or heart–lung transplants were performed, with all but one dying in less than a month from bronchial dehiscence.[2] In 1983, improved surgical technique, better recipient selection, and the emergence of cyclosporine enabled the University of Toronto group to perform the first lung transplant with long-term success,[3] in which the recipient survived for 7 years.[2]

CURRENT STATUS OF LUNG TRANSPLANTS IN THE UNITED STATES

1 In 2022, 2,743 lung transplants were performed in the United States.[4] Eighty percent of candidates received a bilateral-lung transplant, and 97.1% of candidates received a primary lung transplant.[4] In 2022, 3,161 recipients were added to the waitlist, continuing a trend of donor shortage and resulting in 10.7% of recipients dying or becoming too sick for transplant while listed.[4] Although lung transplantation still has the worst survival outcome among solid organ transplants, progressive improvements in survival have been realized: 87.8% of recipients survived to 1 year and 59.6% to 5 years.[4]

INDICATIONS

Prior to 2005, lung allocation priority for lung transplantation was based upon wait times, geography, and blood type, which resulted in significantly prolonged wait times and high waitlist mortality. The Lung Allocation Score (LAS) was implemented in 2005 as a weighted combination of the predicted risk of death on the waiting list and the predicted likelihood of survival during the first year after transplantation.[5] In March 2023, the LAS was replaced by the Composite Allocation Score (CAS), which uses a continuous distribution approach to more efficiently consider all patient factors in the allocation process. Four disease diagnosis groups are considered in the CAS: obstructive lung disease (group A); pulmonary vascular disease (group B); cystic fibrosis (CF) and immunodeficiency disorders (group C); and restrictive lung disease (group D) (**Table 38.1**).

2 Each transplant center's multidisciplinary candidate selection committee carefully considers candidates' individual underlying disease severity, medical comorbidities, psychosocial factors, and surgical risk. In 1998, the International Society for Heart and Lung Transplantation (ISHLT) produced a multiorganizational consensus document, entitled "International Guidelines for the Selection of Lung Transplant Candidates."[6] The document has undergone updates, most recently in 2021,[7] and is generally considered by lung transplant programs in their selection criteria (**Table 38.2**). The statement recommends that, in general, lung transplantation should be considered for adults with end-stage lung disease who have:

1. High (>50%) risk of death from lung disease within 2 years if lung transplantation is not performed.

Table 38.1. Pulmonary Disease Diagnosis Groups

Group A: Obstructive	Group B: Pulmonary Vascular	Group C: Cystic Fibrosis and Immunodeficiency	Group D: Restrictive
Allergic bronchopulmonary aspergillosis Alpha-1 antitrypsin deficiency Bronchiectasis Bronchopulmonary dysplasia Chronic obstructive pulmonary disease/emphysema Ehlers–Danlos syndrome Granulomatous lung disease Inhalation burns/trauma Kartagener syndrome Lymphangioleiomyomatosis Obstructive lung disease Primary ciliary dyskinesia Sarcoidosis with mean pulmonary artery pressure of 30 mm Hg or less Tuberous sclerosis Wegener granuloma—bronchiectasis	Congenital malformation CREST—pulmonary hypertension Eisenmenger syndrome Portopulmonary hypertension Primary pulmonary hypertension/pulmonary arterial hypertension Pulmonary capillary hemangiomatosis Pulmonary telangiectasia—pulmonary hypertension Pulmonary thromboembolic disease Pulmonary vascular disease Pulmonary veno-occlusive disease Pulmonic stenosis Right hypoplastic lung Scleroderma—pulmonary hypertension Secondary pulmonary hypertension Thromboembolic pulmonary hypertension	Common variable immune deficiency Cystic fibrosis Fibrocavitary lung disease Hypogammaglobulinemia Schwachman–Diamond syndrome	ABCA3 transporter mutation Alveolar proteinosis Amyloidosis Acute respiratory distress syndrome or pneumonia Bronchioloalveolar carcinoma (BAC) Carcinoid tumorlets Chronic pneumonitis of infancy Constrictive bronchiolitis CREST—restrictive Eosinophilic granuloma Fibrosing mediastinitis Graft-versus-host disease (GVHD) Hermansky–Pudlak syndrome Hypersensitivity pneumonitis Idiopathic interstitial pneumonia Idiopathic pulmonary hemosiderosis Lung retransplant or graft failure Lupus mixed connective tissue disease Obliterative bronchiolitis: nonretransplant Occupational lung disease Paraneoplastic pemphigus–associated Castleman disease Polymyositis Pulmonary fibrosis: other Pulmonary hyalinizing granuloma Pulmonary lymphangiectasia (PL) Pulmonary telangiectasia—restrictive Rheumatoid disease Sarcoidosis with mean pulmonary artery pressure higher than 30 mm Hg Scleroderma—restrictive Secondary pulmonary fibrosis Silicosis Sjogren syndrome Surfactant protein B or C mutation Teratoma Wegener granuloma—restrictive

Adapted from the U.S. Organ Procurement and Transplantation Network Policy 10.1.F.i (Effective February 27, 2020).

2. High (>80%) likelihood of surviving at least 90 days after lung transplantation.
3. High (>80%) likelihood of 5-year posttransplant survival from a general medical perspective provided that there is adequate graft function.

Table 38.3 lists disease-specific listing considerations for the most common disease diagnoses undergoing lung transplantation.

Table 38.2. ISHLT General Recommendations for Consideration for Lung Transplantation[8]

High (>50%) risk of death from lung disease within 2 y if lung transplantation is not performed
High (>80%) likelihood of surviving at least 90 d after lung transplantation
High (>80%) likelihood of 5-y posttransplant survival from a general medical perspective, provided that there is adequate graft function

Idiopathic Pulmonary Fibrosis

3 Idiopathic pulmonary fibrosis (IPF) is a progressive fibrosing interstitial lung disease with less than 5 years expected survival following diagnosis, although the prognosis is better at younger ages.[8] IPF is the most common subtype of interstitial lung disease and is the most common indication for lung transplantation in the United States.[9] In 2022, restrictive lung diseases represented 59.1% of all lung transplants performed in the United States.[4]

Chronic Obstructive Pulmonary Disease

COPD is the second most common indication for lung transplantation. It is the most common disease indication in the obstructive diagnosis group, which represented 27.3% of all lung transplants in the United States.[4] Recipients with COPD share the best 1-year survival with those recipients with CF, but a lower 10-year survival compared to all diagnoses except IPF.[10]

Cystic Fibrosis

CF is the third most common indication for lung transplantation, but the proportion of patients transplanted for CF

Table 38.3. Disease-Specific Considerations for Listing for Lung Transplantation[8]

Interstitial Lung Disease—Early Referral Following Radiologic or Histologic Diagnosis, Regardless of Lung Function
Decline in FVC ≥10% during 6 mo of follow-up (Note: A 5% decline is associated with a poorer prognosis and may warrant listing.)
Decline in DLCO ≥15% during 6 mo of follow-up
Desaturation to <88% or distance <250 m on 6-min walk test or 450 m decline in 6-min walk distance over a 6-mo period
Pulmonary hypertension on right heart catheterization or 2-dimensional echocardiography
Hospitalization because of respiratory decline, pneumothorax, or acute exacerbation
Chronic Obstructive Pulmonary Disease (COPD)
BODE index ≥7
FEV_1 <15–20% predicted
Three or more severe exacerbations during the preceding year
One severe exacerbation with acute hypercapnic respiratory failure
Moderate to severe pulmonary hypertension
Cystic Fibrosis—Early Referral When FEV_1 Has Fallen to 30% or a Patient with a Rapidly Falling FEV_1 Despite Optimal Therapy (Particularly in a Female Patient) or Increasing Frequency of Life-Threatening Lung Disease Complications
Chronic hypoxic or hypercapnic respiratory failure
Long-term noninvasive ventilation therapy
Pulmonary hypertension
Frequent hospitalization
Rapid lung function decline
World Health Organization Functional Class IV
Pulmonary Hypertension
NYHA functional class III or IV despite a trial of at least 3 mo of combination therapy including prostanoids
Cardiac index of <2 L/min/m²
Mean right atrial pressure of 415 mm Hg
6-min walk test of <350 m
Development of significant hemoptysis, pericardial effusion, or signs of progressive right heart failure

Table 38.4. Contraindications to Lung Transplant

Absolute Contraindications
Recent history of malignancy
Multiorgan dysfunction unless combined multiorgan transplant considered correctable
Uncorrected atherosclerotic disease
Acute medical instability, including, but not limited to, acute sepsis, myocardial infarction, and liver failure
Uncorrectable bleeding diathesis
Chronic infection with highly virulent and/or resistant microbes that are poorly controlled pretransplant
Evidence of active *Mycobacterium tuberculosis* infection
Significant chest wall or spinal deformity expected to cause severe restriction after transplantation
Class II or III obesity (body mass index [BMI] ≥35.0 kg/m²)
Current or history of nonadherence to medical therapy
Psychosocial barriers to posttransplant care adherence
Severely limited functional status with poor rehabilitation potential
Substance abuse or dependence
Relative Contraindications
Age >65 y in association with low physiologic reserve and/or other relative contraindications
Class I obesity (BMI 30.0–34.9 kg/m²), particularly truncal (central) obesity
Progressive or severe malnutrition
Severe, symptomatic osteoporosis
Extensive prior chest surgery with lung resection
Mechanical ventilation and/or extracorporeal life support (ECLS)
Colonization or infection with highly resistant or highly virulent bacteria, fungi, and certain strains of mycobacteria
For patients infected with hepatitis B and/or C, a lung transplant can be considered in patients without signs of cirrhosis or portal hypertension
For patients infected with human immunodeficiency virus (HIV), a lung transplant can be considered in compliant patients with controlled disease with undetectable HIV RNA
Infection with *Burkholderia cenocepacia*, *Burkholderia gladioli*, and multidrug-resistant *Mycobacterium abscessus*
Prior chest surgery or pleurodesis (surgical or chemical)
Patients requiring a mechanical (ventilator or circulatory) bridge to transplant

Adapted from ISHLT Consensus Statement.[8]

continues to slowly fall, now representing 13% of adult lung transplants worldwide[10] and only 2.8% in the United States.[4] Recipients with CF share the best 1-year survival with those who have COPD and have the highest overall survival, with some recipients living up to 20 years following their transplant.[10] Colonization of the airway with multi- or pan-resistant organisms is common in CF, and some transplant programs consider colonization with pan-resistant strains of *Pseudomonas aeruginosa* or *Burkholderia* species as contraindications to transplantation because of the poorer demonstrated posttransplant outcomes. A comprehensive review by Morrell et al. found that lung transplant patients with pan-resistant *Pseudomonas* have poorer outcomes than sensitive patients with CF, but comparable outcomes to overall UNOS registrants, and only patients infected with *Burkholderia gladioli* and specific nonepidemeic *Burkholderia cenocepacia* strains demonstrate excess mortality in the first 6 months after transplant.[11]

Pulmonary Hypertension

Pulmonary vascular diseases represented 10.8% of the US transplants in 2022.[4] Natural history registry data reported a 3-year median survival of 75%,[12] which has improved with optimal medical therapies.[13] Because of the relative success and good response to medical therapies, timing for referral to transplant is variable among centers, as optimization of therapies may significantly delay the need for transplant. However, clinical deterioration can occur rapidly and not allow time for a full evaluation, so earlier referral for evaluation is recommended. Recipients with IPAH have the lowest 1-year survival, but their 10-year conditional 1-year median survival approaches the best of all recipients at 12 years.[10]

CONTRAINDICATIONS

Table 38.4 lists absolute consensus and relative contraindications to lung transplantation.[7] The list represents common patient comorbidities and balances the benefits of transplantation, organ stewardship, and the expected recipient and allograft survival. An individualized candidate evaluation should carefully consider a candidate's underlying disease severity, medical comorbidities, psychosocial factors, and risk of perioperative morbidity and mortality based on the program's relevant experience and expertise. Ultimately, candidate selection is decided by the transplant program's selection committee. A patient may be considered a suitable or unsuitable candidate at any particular center and, hence, is free to be evaluated and/or listed at more than one program, if desired. Moreover, a patient who is not a candidate at a particular

Table 38.5. Sequential Steps in Donor Lung Recovery

1	Review donor blood group, history, and imaging
2	Perform bronchoscopy
3	Perform median sternotomy
4	Intraoperative inspection of lungs and thoracic cavity
5	Lung recruitment maneuvers and assessment of lung function and suitability for transplantation
6	Dissection of great vessels as needed
7	Systemic donor heparinization
8	Cannulation of main PA
9	Prostaglandin E1 (500 mg) injected into main pulmonary
10	Division of systemic venous return to decompress right heart
11	Aortic cross-clamp
12	Left atrial division to decompress left heart
13	Initiation of cold lung preservation flush
14	Topical cooling of ventilated lungs
15	Cardiectomy
16	Retrograde lung flush
17	Recovery of lung

center due to a relative contraindication should be referred to another center that has pertinent expertise.

OPERATIVE PROCEDURES

Donor Recovery Operation

4 The donor recovery lung evaluation, which is summarized in **Table 38.5**, is as important to the success of the lung transplant as the implantation. Before accepting the organ, the recovery surgeon should review the donor's ABO blood group, history, and imaging. Additionally, a bronchoscopy and manual inspection of the lung(s) is performed to ensure the donor lungs' usability or a lack of problematic anatomy.

A median sternotomy is performed, often concomitant with a laparotomy by the abdominal team. The sternal retractor's crossbar is placed cephalad to minimize interference with the abdominal operation. If there is no urgency for cardiac evaluation, the pericardium should be left closed during the lung evaluation to decrease hemodynamic instability with excessive lung manipulation. The bilateral pleura are opened widely with care to avoid damage to the lung parenchyma. Visual and manual inspection then ensues of the pleural cavity and lungs for nodules, masses, consolidation, atelectasis, and/or infarction. Compliance is checked by temporarily disconnecting the ventilator, which should result in an immediate collapse of the lungs. If necessary, positive pressure lung recruitment maneuvers are performed, with peak pressures restricted to 20 to 30 cm H_2O to minimize the risk of barotrauma. If an intraoperative systemic arterial blood gas (ABG) is satisfactory (usually a PaO_2/FiO_2 >300 on PEEP 5 cmH_2O with normal CO_2 levels), then proceeding with the intended lung recovery and transplant is appropriate. However, if the ABG is not satisfactory or there is a clinical concern about the function or suitability of the lung, individual pulmonary vein gases may be sampled to further evaluate the lobar contributions to total pulmonary function.

If no contraindications arise during the organ evaluation, the pericardium is opened, and exposure is optimized using stay sutures. The SVC is encircled caudal to the azygos vein, while care is taken to separate the right PA from the posterior SVC and ascending aorta. The paratracheal tissue is accessed between the SVC and the ascending aorta with gentle retraction of both vessels. The trachea is then manually exposed circumferentially. The authors prefer to wait on circumferential exposure of the trachea until after cross-clamping in order to minimize bleeding risk and/or airway injury.

Once all teams have completed their dissection, the donor is heparinized as per protocol, usually with 250 to 300 units/kg. A purse-string suture is placed in the main PA near its midpoint, and a perfusion cannula is inserted and secured. To achieve equal distribution of preservation solution, the cannula is preferably oriented in a retrograde fashion toward a competent pulmonary valve. Prostaglandin E1 (500 μg) is injected directly into the main PA less than 1 minute prior to intended cross-clamping, since systemic vasodilation and potential hemodynamic compromise may ensue. Next, the SVC is ligated and the IVC divided at an appropriate level to facilitate intended heart and/or liver transplant. The aorta is cross-clamped. The left atrial appendage is amputated prior to starting the pulmonary flush in order to allow left heart decompression. Three to 4 liters of cold Perfadex flush is initiated, and the chest is cooled with iced saline. Care must be taken to avoid thermal injury from direct ice contact with the organ. Ventilation is continued throughout the duration of the flush to facilitate even distribution of perfusate. At completion of the flush, ventilation may be temporarily ceased until just prior to lung extraction. The heart is then extracted by sharply mobilizing the IVC to the level of the right inferior pulmonary vein. While lifting the heart, an incision is made in the left atrium at the midpoint between the left and right inferior pulmonary veins. The atriotomy can be retracted with a suction device to allow visualization, and scissors are used to extend the opening superiorly while visualizing the venous orifices. The remaining left atrium is then divided. The great vessels are divided by cutting the SVC distal to the ligature, the ascending aorta proximal to the head vessels, and the main PA at the level of cannulation.

With the heart now removed, a Foley or self-inflating retrograde perfusion catheter is utilized to provide 500 mL of Perfadex flush into each vein orifice until the effluent from the PA is clear of residual blood and clots. The en bloc lungs can then be removed by dividing the bilateral inferior pulmonary ligaments and herniating the left lung toward the right chest to visualize and develop an anterior paraesophageal plane. Division of the mediastinal pleura just anterior to the esophagus completely into the right chest during gentle upward retraction of the lungs protects the lung and its vasculature, while avoiding enteric contamination with esophageal injury or division. At this point, the trachea remains as only remaining connection. The endotracheal tube is withdrawn into the proximal trachea, a gentle Valsalva maneuver is performed until atelectasis is resolved, and then the Valsalva is released just before the proximal trachea is divided with a linear stapler distal to the endotracheal tube. To minimize air leak, two staple firings are usually placed on the extracted trachea. If the lungs will be split for two different recipients, the proximal left main bronchus is divided with a liner stapler to maintain inflation before dividing the left atrium and PA at the midline. The lungs are then bagged in a cold preservation solution and transported to the recipient center.

Recipient Preparation

Before anesthetic induction, patients have epidural catheters placed to aid in perioperative pain management and facilitate

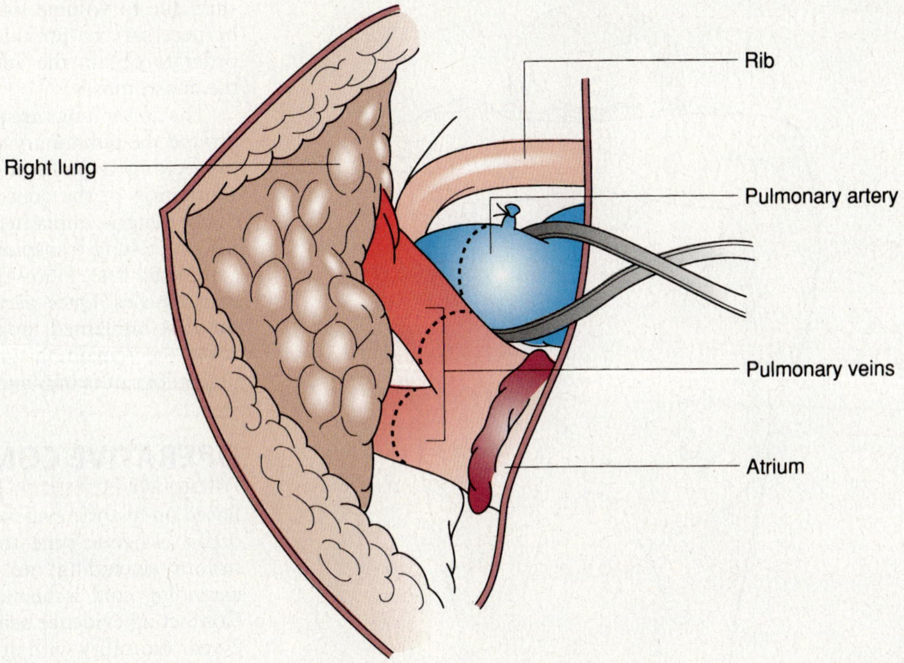

Figure 38.1. Mobilization of the hilum of the right lung. The pulmonary artery is encircled, and the first branch is ligated and divided. The superior and inferior pulmonary veins have been exposed. Both the artery and veins are taken as close to the lung as possible. The bronchus is divided at the level of the takeoff of the upper lobe to minimize ischemia of the airway.

faster extubation and ambulatory rehabilitation. If cardiopulmonary bypass (CPB) is needed intraoperatively, use of ECMO is preferred, since it usually limits the heparinization requirement to less than 5,000 total units. Double-lumen endotracheal intubation with an appropriately sized tube is performed, but the tubes must be large enough to allow vigorous suctioning of purulent secretions through an adult fiberoptic bronchoscope. Two internal jugular central venous lines are routinely placed for both volume and medication administration. A Foley catheter with a bladder temperature monitor, radial and femoral arterial lines, and a transesophageal echocardiography probe are also placed. With these adjuncts, we have not needed a Swan–Ganz catheter for perioperative management and have therefore avoided the inherent risks associated with it during pneumonectomy or with fresh anastomoses. The patient is then placed either into a supine position with all extremities padded, shoulders medially rotated and arms tucked at sides for bilateral-lung transplants or into the lateral recumbent position for single-lung transplants. A heating blanket may be utilized.

Single-Lung Transplantation

In the recipient operation, a standard fifth intercostal space posterolateral thoracotomy is preferred. The groin should always be included in the sterile field, so that CPB can be performed by femoral cannulation, if necessary. The hilar dissection (**Fig. 38.1**, shown with stapler) differs from that of a pneumonectomy in that the main pulmonary artery and veins should be divided within the pulmonary hilum at the level of the lung parenchyma, thereby leaving as much of a vascular stump as possible to facilitate anastomotic reconstruction. The pericardium is opened around the left atrial cuff, allowing the left atrium to be clamped proximal to the branch point of the superior and inferior veins. On the right, the veins are elongated by developing Sondergaard groove. To provide exposure of the bronchus, the artery and vein stumps are gently retracted using 2-0 silk sutures through the staple lines. Care should be taken to preserve the peribronchial lymphatic and areolar tissue in order to maintain the vascular supply of the mainstem bronchus just proximal to the origin of the upper lobe bronchus. However, care should be taken to clip any divided bronchial or lymphatic vessels during the dissection. In addition, injury to the phrenic nerve must be avoided, especially in the setting of pleural adhesions from previous surgery, severe emphysema, or pulmonary fibrosis. Diaphragmatic dysfunction from phrenic injury can adversely affect posttransplant functional recovery.

The donor lung is prepared by dissecting the left atrial cuff and the proximal pulmonary artery from the surrounding tissues. Retrograde perfusion with cold Perfadex is administered to the superior and inferior pulmonary veins while the lung is still inflated. The bronchial cuff is prepared by transecting the mainstem bronchus approximately two cartilaginous rings from the orifice of the upper lobe bronchus to maximize retrograde blood flow to the bronchial anastomosis.

Implantation of the donor lung progresses in a posterior-to-anterior fashion, with the anastomosis between the donor and recipient bronchus being performed first. An end-to-end anastomosis is performed with a running 4-0 polydioxanone suture at the cartilaginomembranous junction, continuing along the membranous airway, before reapproximation of the cartilaginous airway. Care to not purse string the anastomosis is accomplished when the assistant maintains equal tension along the suture until completion. Absorbable sutures are used instead of polypropylene to reduce the risk of suture granuloma formation.

The venous and arterial anastomoses are then performed sequentially using running 4-0 and 6-0 nonabsorbable polypropylene sutures, respectively. The recipient's two pulmonary vein stumps are prepared by unifocalization into a single left atrial cuff in order to reduce the risk of pulmonary venous obstruction. In constructing the pulmonary arterial anastomosis, the donor PA must be trimmed to the appropriate length to avoid kinking of the low-pressure vessel. Once the vascular anastomoses are completed, the lungs are gently ventilated as the vessels are deaired with the patient in the Trendelenburg position and with the left atrial clamp followed by the PA clamp being removed prior to tying the anastomotic sutures. A 500-mg dose of methylprednisolone is usually given prior to reperfusion to minimize an expected systemic inflammatory response. In our institution, inhaled nitric oxide is routinely initiated prior to lung reperfusion to minimize the risk and complications of primary graft dysfunction (PGD).[14] Progressive reperfusion to the allograft is manually controlled. Anterior and posterior chest tubes are placed, and the chest is then closed in standard fashion.

Bilateral-Lung Transplantation

5 The technique of double-lung transplantation has evolved considerably since the late 1980s from an en bloc technique

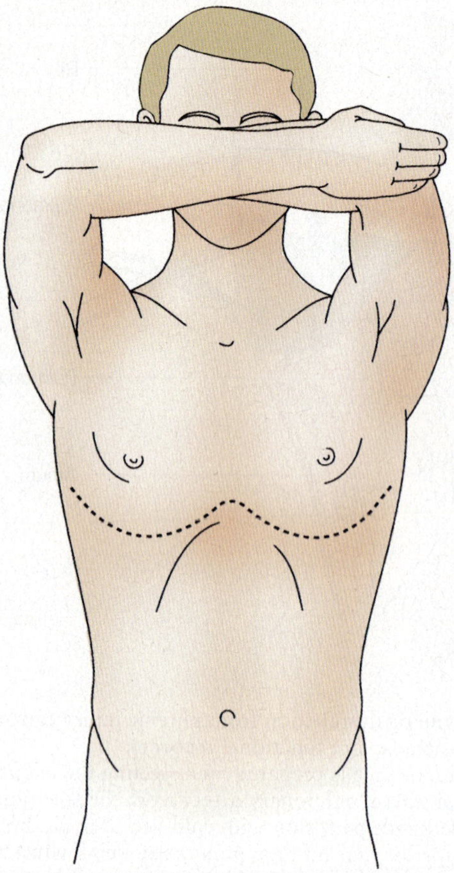

Figure 38.2. Patient positioning for a bilateral, sequential lung transplant. Bilateral anterior thoracotomies are made in the fourth intercostal space with a transverse sternotomy when needed for exposure (clamshell incision).

to a bilateral, sequential technique.[15,16] With the patient in the supine position, this operation can be performed through a median sternotomy, bilateral thoracosternotomy (clamshell) incision (Fig. 38.2, shown with arms tucked at sides), bilateral anterior thoracotomies without sternal division, or bilateral muscle-sparing axillary thoracotomies. The bilateral thoracosternotomy incision is our preference for bilateral-lung transplants, as it provides the widest exposure, facilitates dissection and mobilization of the hilar structures, and permits cannulation of the right atrium and ascending aorta when CPB is necessary. This exposure is particularly important in recipients with diffuse dense pleural adhesions, as is often seen in patients with chronic infections (ie, bronchiectasis or CF), previous pleurodesis, or severe apical adhesions following lung volume reduction in emphysema patients.

Although both lungs are replaced, the operation can often be performed without CPB unless the recipient has significant pulmonary hypertension or severely limited gas exchange. By replacing the lung that has the least function first, as determined by the quantitative ventilation perfusion scan or intraoperative pulmonary arterial test clamping, oxygenation and ventilation can be maintained by the contralateral native lung. If the patient is unable to tolerate single-lung ventilation due to inadequate gas exchange or worsening right ventricular dysfunction occurs with near- or suprasystemic pulmonary hypertension, then CPB is initiated. If recipient hemodynamics are significantly impaired during retraction and exposure of the left atrial anastomosis during left lung recipient pneumonectomy or allograft implantation, CPB should be utilized to facilitate the operation. In patients with severe mediastinal shift due to volume loss from pulmonary fibrosis, CPB may be necessary to provide sufficient cardiac decompression in order to obtain the adequate exposure needed to construct the anastomoses.

The donor lungs are prepared by leaving a cuff of left atrium around the pulmonary veins on each side. The recipient pneumonectomy is performed one side at a time, with single-lung ventilation of the contralateral lung being maintained. Each donor lung is implanted using the same technique described for single-lung transplantation. The bronchial anastomosis is completed first, followed by the atrial and pulmonary arterial anastomoses. Once perfusion and ventilation are restored to the first implanted lung, this lung then supports the patient while the remaining native lung is removed and the second lung allograft is implanted.

OPERATIVE CONSIDERATIONS

Allograft Ischemic Time

6 Based on historic evidence, most transplant centers try to limit organ ischemic time to <6 hours. However, multiple institutions (including our own) have experience comfortably extending cold ischemic times with careful donor selection. Conflicting evidence using older registry data found increased 2-year mortality with donor age >50 years and ischemic times of 7 hours or more,[17] yet another analysis demonstrated that prolonged ischemic time was not an independent predictor of mortality.[18] In the current era of widening donor shortages and improved organ preservation techniques, 10% of recipients were reported to have ischemic times >8 hours, and ischemic times up to 12 hours were demonstrated to not be associated with primary graft failure nor survival.[19]

Single- versus Bilateral-Lung Transplant

Although bilateral-lung transplants constitute 80% of cases, there remains a persistent debate over whether single or bilateral-lung transplantation is the best strategy. While many institutions prefer bilateral-lung transplants for recipients without technical and comorbid contraindications to bilateral transplantation, single-lung transplants are suggested to be a better utilization strategy given the limited number of available allografts. A comprehensive review of literature during the LAS era concluded that the level of evidence supporting either conclusion is conflicted, limited, and varied by disease and patient factors. In the absence of a randomized trial, which will likely never be performed, the decision regarding a single- versus double-lung transplant should be made on a case-by-case basis.[20]

Intraoperative Cardiopulmonary Support

Traditionally, recipients who demonstrate inadequate pulmonary reserve during single-lung ventilation or inadequate cardiovascular reserve during implantation are placed onto intraoperative CPB or venoarterial extracorporeal membrane oxygenation (ECMO). Intraoperative ECMO is currently favored over CPB, since the absence of a venous reservoir and less circuit components necessitate less heparinization. Additionally, compared to intraoperative CPB, ECMO is associated with lower incidences of bleeding, prolonged mechanical ventilation, PGD, and in-hospital mortality.[21–25] Some programs selectively use intraoperative ECMO only when cardiopulmonary support is necessary, while other programs advocate routine intraoperative ECMO for all lung transplant procedures.[26] Comparisons of the selective versus routine use of intraoperative ECMO during lung transplantation are an ongoing focus of research.

Special Patient Populations

Some patient-specific factors may complicate or alter the course of the operation or predispose them toward postoperative complications. Patients with severe pulmonary hypertension and right ventricular failure are at risk for hemodynamic collapse with induction of general anesthesia, and the surgical team and perfusionist should be readily available for emergent institution of CPB or ECMO, if needed. In cases of near- or suprasystemic PA pressures, preinduction institution of ECMO should be considered. In patients with severe peripheral vascular disease, Raynaud disease, or digital ischemia, the radial arterial line may either be deferred or kept in place for a minimal period of time.

Surgical Complications

Primary Graft Dysfunction

7 PGD is an acute lung injury syndrome occurring within the first 72 hours following lung transplantation and is characterized by inexplicable diffuse allograft infiltrates and hypoxemia, defined as a PaO_2/FiO_2 ratio (P/F) <300 (**Table 38.6**).[27] PGD is also characterized by low pulmonary compliance, interstitial/alveolar edema, pulmonary infiltrates on chest radiographs, increased pulmonary vascular resistance, intrapulmonary shunt, and acute alveolar injury, as revealed by diffuse alveolar damage (DAD) on pathology.[28] Recipients who suffer from severe PGD have a significantly increased short- and long-term mortality.[29,30] The risk of developing PGD is thought to result from complex immunomechanistic interactions and the conduct of the donor and recipient operations.

Table 38.6. Grading of Primary Graft Dysfunction Severity

Grade	PaO_2/FiO_2	Radiographic Infiltrate Consistent with Pulmonary Edema
0	>300	Absent
1	>300	Present
2	200–300	Present
3	<200	Present

Table 38.7. Summary of Multicenter Clinical Trials Investigating Utilization of Ex Vivo Lung Perfusion Prior to Lung Transplant

Trial, Start Year	Donor Type	Protocol/ Device	Study Design	Number of Subjects	Number of Centers	Primary Endpoint	Donor Inclusion Criteria	Key Findings
NOVEL, 2011	Extended criteria	Toronto/ XPS	Nonrandomized	110 EVLP, 116 control	17	Absence of PGD grade 3 within first 72 h, 1-y survival	PaO_2/FiO_2 ≤300 mm Hg OR one or more of the following: (1) multiple blood transfusions; (2) pulmonary edema detected via chest x-ray, bronchoscopy, or palpation of lungs; (3) donation after circulatory death donors; (4) investigator evaluation of donor lung as "unsuitable" for standard criteria for lung transplant.	Conversion rate of 50.9%; PGD3 within 72 h (EVLP 8.9% vs control 9.5%, P = .12); 1-y survival (EVLP 93.2% vs control 96.5%, P = .84)
INSPIRE, 2011	Standard criteria	OCS/OCS Lung	Randomized	151 EVLP, 169 control	21	Absence of PGD grade 3 within first 72 h, 30-d survival	Age <65 y with PaO_2/FiO_2 >300 mg and no active pulmonary disease	PGD3 within 72 h (EVLP 17.7% vs 29.7% control, P = .015); 30-d survival (EVLP 95.7% vs control 100%, P = .009)
DEVELOP-UK, 2012	Extended criteria	Lund/ Vivoline LS1	Nonrandomized	18 EVLP, 184 control	5	1-y survival	Depended on assessment by individual centers	Conversion rate of 34%; 1-y survival (EVLP 67% vs control 80%)
EXPAND, 2014	Extended criteria	OCS/OCS Lung	Single-arm	79 EVLP	8	Absence of PGD grade 3 within first 72 h, with an objective of 65%	One or more of the following: (1) $PaO_2:FiO_2$ ratio ≤300 mm Hg; (2) expected ischemic time >6 h; (3) age ≥55 y; (4) donors after circulatory death	Conversion rate of 87%; PGD3 within 72 h found in 44%; 99% 30-d survival

XPS, XVIVO Perfusion System (From XVIVO Perfusion AB, Göteborg, Sweden); PGD, primary graft dysfunction; EVLP, ex vivo lung perfusion; OCS, Organ Care System Lung (From TransMedics, Andover, MA, USA).

Airway Complications

The lung has a dual blood supply from both the pulmonary and bronchial arteries. Conventional lung transplantation techniques interrupt and do not revascularize the bronchial artery supply, so postlung transplant airway complications remain a concern. Airway complication rates have ranged from 2% to 18% in larger contemporary studies.[31]

In 1970, Haglin et al. performed the first lung transplant with bronchial artery revascularization (BAR) as a method to 8
restore bronchial artery circulation.[32] The technique is infrequently used due to its added complexity, operative time, and uncertain benefit. The largest report on BAR involved 65 patients, of whom 47 underwent double-lung transplantation with the left mammary artery used as BAR conduit; excellent success and long-term survival were demonstrated.[33]

STRATEGIES FOR EXPANDING THE DONOR ORGAN POOL

Ex Vivo Lung Perfusion

Donor lungs are utilized in only approximately 20% of multiorgan donors, thereby making lungs the lowest utilized donor organ.[34] Ex vivo lung perfusion (EVLP) has been proposed as a technique to assess marginal donor lungs prior to transplantation. Since the original EVLP description for the evaluation of lungs from a DCD donor,[35] three basic EVLP techniques have been reported,[36] but the underlying premise of these techniques is the same. The donor lungs are normothermically perfused and ventilated on an ex vivo platform that facilitates assessment of physiologic parameters and reconditioning of the lungs, if necessary.

While the use of EVLP may be more readily accepted for marginal or nonutilized lungs, the benefit of using EVLP for standard lungs may raise questions. Slama et al. demonstrated that EVLP can safely be used in standard donor lungs, with comparable perioperative outcomes to using standard donor lung preservation techniques, with the added potential to exclude lungs with functional impairment and safely extend total preservation time.[37]

In order to evaluate the safety and efficacy of EVLP, several major multicenter prospective clinical trials have been completed, including the NOVEL trial (United States; XVIVO), the INSPIRE and EXPAND trials (Europe and the United States; Transmedics), and the DEVELOP trial (United Kingdom; Vivoline). A summary of these trials is provided in **Table 38.7**.[38]

While all of these aforementioned options include the use of significant resources and staff from the recipient hospital to recover, resuscitate, monitor, and evaluate organs during EVLP, Lung Bioengineering (Silver Spring, MD) is currently investigating the ability of a centralized facility to evaluate marginal donor lungs utilizing the Toronto EVLP system, usually for targeted recipients, in the EVP-DEV-301 trial (NCT02234128).

Hepatitis C Virus–Infected Organs (HCV)

Prior to 2016, only five HCV+ donor lung transplants had been performed. In 2017, however, an increased willingness by patients and programs to perform HCV+ transplants resulted from earlier success in abdominal transplant organs and the advent of more effective second-generation direct-acting antivirals (DAAs) that demonstrate an over 90% sustained HCV cure rate.[39] In 2019, DONATE trial, an open-label phase IV trial involving 36 recipients who received lungs from hepatitis C viremic donors, showed that a 4-week DAA regimen prevented the establishment of HCV infection.[40] These findings have resulted in the progressive adoption of HCV protocols at many institutions. Use of HCV-viremic donors in HCV-seronegative recipients has resulted in noninferior 3-year outcomes compared to HCV-seronegative donors.[41] Furthermore, use of HCV donors is associated with lower waitlist mortalities.[42]

SUMMARY

The field of lung transplantation, which is a time-tested treatment for end-stage respiratory disease, continues to evolve. While lung transplant outcomes continue to lag behind other solid organ transplants, improvements in technique, perioperative care, and allocation adjustments continue to advance survival and volume benchmarks. Donor availability remains a limiting factor to successful and timely transplantation, which has led to innovative techniques that increase donor utilization. However, PGD is still a concern with the use of underutilized donor populations, and several clinical trials are investigating the effect that these strategies will have on the incidence or severity of PGD.

References

1. Hardy JD, Webb WR, Dalton ML Jr, Walker GR Jr. Lung homotransplantation in man. *JAMA*. 1963;186:1065–1074.
2. Venuta F, Van Raemdonck D. History of lung transplantation. *J Thorac Dis*. 2017;9(12):5458–5471.
3. Toronto Lung Transplant Group. Unilateral lung transplantation for pulmonary fibrosis. *N Engl J Med*. 1986;314(18):1140–1145.
4. Valapour M, Lehr CJ, Schladt DP, et al. OPTN/SRTR 2022 annual data report: lung. *Am J Transplant*. 2024;24(Suppl s1):394–356.
5. Kosztowski M, Zhou S, Bush E, Higgins RS, Segev DL, Gentry SE. Geographic disparities in lung transplant rates. *Am J Transplant*. 2019;19(5):1491–1497.
6. International guidelines for the selection of lung transplant candidates. The American Society for Transplant Physicians (ASTP)/American Thoracic Society (ATS)/European Respiratory Society (ERS)/International Society for Heart and Lung Transplantation (ISHLT). *Am J Respir Crit Care Med*. 1998;158(1):335–339.
7. Leard LE, Holm AM, Valapour M, et al. Consensus document for the selection of lung transplant candidates: an update from the International Society for Heart and Lung Transplantation. *J Heart Lung Transplant*. 2021;40(11):1349–1379.
8. Raghu G, Chen SY, Yeh WS, et al. Idiopathic pulmonary fibrosis in US Medicare beneficiaries aged 65 years and older: incidence, prevalence, and survival, 2001–11. *Lancet Respir Med*. 2014; 2(7):566–572.
9. McShane PJ, Garrity ER Jr. Impact of the lung allocation score. *Semin Respir Crit Care Med*. 2013;34(3):275–280.
10. Chambers DC, Cherikh WS, Harhay MO, et al. International Society for Heart and Lung Transplantation. The International Thoracic Organ Transplant Registry of the International Society for Heart and Lung Transplantation: thirty-sixth adult lung and heart-lung transplantation Report—2019; Focus theme: donor and recipient size match. *J Heart Lung Transplant*. 2019;38(10):1042–1055.
11. Morrell MR, Pilewski JM. Lung transplantation for cystic fibrosis. *Clin Chest Med*. 2016;37(1):127–138.
12. D'Alonzo GE, Barst RJ, Ayres SM, et al. Survival in patients with primary pulmonary hypertension. Results from a national prospective registry. *Ann Intern Med*. 1991;115(5):343–349.
13. Benza RL, Miller DP, Barst RJ, Badesch DB, Frost AE, McGoon MD. An evaluation of long-term survival from time of diagnosis in pulmonary arterial hypertension from the REVEAL Registry. *Chest*. 2012;142(2):448–456.
14. Bhatraju P, Crawford J, Hall M, Lang JD Jr. Inhaled nitric oxide: current clinical concepts. *Nitric Oxide*. 2015;50:114–128.
15. Pasque MK, Cooper JD, Kaiser LR, Haydock DA, Triantafillou A, Trulock EP. Improved technique for bilateral lung transplantation: rationale and initial clinical experience. *Ann Thorac Surg*. 1990;49(5):785–791.
16. Lau CL, Patterson GA. Technical considerations in lung transplantation. *Chest Surg Clin N Am*. 2003;13(3):463–483.

17. Meyer DM, Bennett LE, Novick RJ, Hosenpud JD. Effect of donor age and ischemic time on intermediate survival and morbidity after lung transplantation. *Chest.* 2000;118(5):1255–1262.
18. Hennessy SA, Hranjec T, Emaminia A, et al. Geographic distance between donor and recipient does not influence outcomes after lung transplantation. *Ann Thorac Surg.* 2011;92(5):1847–1853.
19. Grimm JC, Valero V III, Kilic A, et al. Association between prolonged graft ischemia and primary graft failure or survival following lung transplantation. *JAMA Surg.* 2015;150(6):547–553.
20. Subramanian MP, Meyers BF. Bilateral versus single lung transplantation: are two lungs better than one? *J Thorac Dis.* 2018; 10(7):4588–4601.
21. Ius F, Kuehn C, Tudorache I, et al. Lung transplantation on cardiopulmonary support: venoarterial extracorporeal membrane oxygenation outperformed cardiopulmonary bypass. *J Thorac Cardiovasc Surg.* 2012;144(6):1510–1516.
22. Bermudez CA, Shiose A, Esper SA, et al. Outcomes of intraoperative venoarterial extracorporeal membrane oxygenation versus cardiopulmonary bypass during lung transplantation. *Ann Thorac Surg.* 2014;98(6):1936–1942; discussion 1942–1943.
23. Biscotti M, Yang J, Sonett J, Bacchetta M. Comparison of extracorporeal membrane oxygenation versus cardiopulmonary bypass for lung transplantation. *J Thorac Cardiovasc Surg.* 2014; 148(5):2410–2415.
24. Hoechter DJ, Dossow VV, Winter H, et al. The Munich Lung Transplant Group: intraoperative extracorporeal circulation in lung transplantation. *Thorac Cardiovasc Surg.* 2015;63(8):706–714.
25. Machuca TN, Collaud S, Mercier O, et al. Outcomes of intraoperative extracorporeal membrane oxygenation versus cardiopulmonary bypass for lung transplantation. *J Thorac Cardiovasc Surg.* 2015;149(4):1152–1157.
26. Hoetzenecker K, Benazzo A, Stork T, et al. Vienna Lung Transplant Group. Bilateral lung transplantation on intraoperative extracorporeal membrane oxygenator: an observational study. *J Thorac Cardiovasc Surg.* 2019;160(1):320–327.e1.
27. Christie JD, Carby M, Bag R, Corris P, Hertz M, Weill D. ISHLT Working Group on Primary Lung Graft Dysfunction. Report of the ISHLT Working Group on primary lung graft dysfunction part II: definition. A consensus statement of the International Society for Heart and Lung Transplantation. *J Heart Lung Transplant.* 2005;24(10):1454–1459.
28. Christie JD, Raemdonck DV, de Perrot M, et al. ISHLT Working Group on Primary Lung Graft Dysfunction. Report of the ISHLT Working Group on primary lung graft dysfunction part I: Introduction and methods. *J Heart Lung Transplant.* 2005;24(10): 1451–1453.
29. Kreisel D, Krupnick AS, Puri V, et al. Short- and long-term outcomes of 1000 adult lung transplant recipients at a single center. *J Thorac Cardiovasc Surg.* 2011;141(1):215–222.
30. Diamond JM, Lee JC, Kawut SM, et al. Lung Transplant Outcomes Group. Clinical risk factors for primary graft dysfunction after lung transplantation. *Am J Respir Crit Care Med.* 2013;187(5): 527–534.
31. Crespo MM, McCarthy DP, Hopkins PM, et al. ISHLT Consensus Statement on adult and pediatric airway complications after lung transplantation: definitions, grading system, and therapeutics. *J Heart Lung Transplant.* 2018;37(5):548–563.
32. Haglin JJ, Ruiz E, Baker RC, Anderson WR. Histologic studies of human lung allotransplantation [Chapter]. In: Wildevuur CRH, ed. *Morphology in Lung Transplantation: Symposium, Held at the 7th Congress of the European Society for Experimental Surgery, Amsterdam, April 1972.* Karger Medical and Scientific Publishers; 1973.
33. Pettersson G, Nørgaard MA, Arendrup H, et al. Direct bronchial artery revascularization and en bloc double lung transplantation–surgical techniques and early outcome. *J Heart Lung Transplant.* 1997;16(3):320–333.
34. Israni AK, Zaun D, Hadley N, et al. OPTN/SRTR 2018 annual data report: deceased organ donation. *Am J Transplant.* 2020;20(Suppl s1):509–541.
35. Steen S, Sjöberg T, Pierre L, Liao Q, Eriksson L, Algotsson L. Transplantation of lungs from a non-heart-beating donor. *Lancet.* 2001;357(9259):825–829.
36. Reeb J, Cypel M. Ex vivo lung perfusion. *Clin Transplant.* 2016;30(3):183–194.
37. Slama A, Schillab L, Barta M, et al. Standard donor lung procurement with normothermic ex vivo lung perfusion: a prospective randomized clinical trial. *J Heart Lung Transplant.* 2017;36(7): 744–753.
38. Zhou AL, Larson EL, Ruck JM, Ha JS, Casillan AJ, Bush EL. Current status and future potential of ex vivo lung perfusion in clinical lung transplantation. *Artif Organs.* 2023;47(11): 1700–1709.
39. Wang JH, Gustafson SK, Skeans MA, et al. OPTN/SRTR 2018 annual data report: hepatitis C. *Am J Transplant.* 2020;20(Suppl s1):542–568.
40. Woolley AE, Singh SK, Goldberg HJ, et al. DONATE HCV Trial Team. Heart and lung transplants from HCV-infected donors to uninfected recipients. *N Engl J Med.* 2019;380(170029): 1606–1617.
41. Ruck JM, Zeiser LB, Zhou Al, et al. Trends in use and three-year outcomes of hepatitis C virus-viremic donor lung transplants for hepatitis C virus-seronegative recipients. *J Thorac Cardiovasc Surg.* 2023;165(4):1587–1595.
42. Ruck JM, Bowring MG, Durand CM, et al. To decline or not to decline: consequences of decision-making regarding lung offers from donors with hepatitis C. *J Thorac Cardiovasc Surg.* 2024; 167(6):1967–1976.

39

Pancreas and Islet Transplantation

Ty B. Dunn and Emre Arpali

Key Points

1. The Diabetes Control and Complications Trial (DCCT) demonstrated that tight control of blood glucose and minimization of hemoglobin A1C delays the progression of secondary complications of diabetes.
2. Recipients with functioning pancreas transplants have normal glycemic control without the need for exogenous insulin, and pancreas transplantation has a beneficial impact on diabetic complications.
3. Pancreas allograft survival rates are >90% at 1 year.
4. The vast majority of pancreas transplants are performed in patients with end-stage kidney disease (ESKD), either concomitant with or following a kidney transplant.
5. In general, eligibility criteria for pancreas transplantation are more stringent than for kidney transplantation alone.
6. Pancreas transplant outcome is dependent on the careful selection of donors, pancreas recovery technique, and backbench preparation.
7. Immunosuppression for pancreas transplantation is similar to that for kidney transplantation, while the incidence of rejection is slightly higher for pancreas than for kidney.
8. Pancreas after kidney transplant improves patient survival and kidney graft survival.
9. Insulin independence after islet transplant is less frequent and less durable than whole-pancreas transplants, but continues to improve.

Diabetes mellitus is a spectrum of impaired glucose regulation that ranges from gestational glucose intolerance to severe hyperglycemia and ketoacidosis. Diabetes affects approximately 34 million people, or 10.5% of the US population. The incidence of diabetes in those under age 19 continues to increase. The prevalence of diabetes is highest among American Indians/Alaska Natives (14.5%), people of Hispanic origin (12.5%), and non-Hispanic Blacks (11.7%).

While both hyperglycemic episodes from poorly controlled diabetes and hypoglycemic events from insulin may be life threatening, the major morbidity of diabetes stems from chronic microvascular injury resulting in the long-term manifestations of this chronic disease, particularly in loss of function (blindness, neuropathy, renal failure) and accelerated atherosclerosis.

PATHOPHYSIOLOGY

The classic pathophysiology of diabetes is that of insulin secretory failure in type 1 diabetes and peripheral insulin resistance in patients with type 2 diabetes. Type 3c diabetes can occur when the gland is damaged by another disease, such as cystic fibrosis, hemochromatosis, or chronic pancreatitis, or surgical resection, and hence, both endocrine and exocrine compartments can be affected and precipitate insulin dependence and a need for pancreatic enzyme replacement therapy. The etiology, epidemiology, and pathogenesis of diabetes are complex and outlined below.

Type 1 diabetes is classically described as an autoimmune disorder manifested by destruction of β-cells, with proinsulin being the most likely primary target. Although there are rare monogenic, immune-mediated forms of type 1 diabetes, the common form is thought to be determined by multiple genetic and environmental factors. The concordance for type 1 diabetes in monozygotic twins is less than 100%, and although type 1 diabetes aggregates in some families, it does not segregate with any clear mode of inheritance. While the mean age of type 1 diabetes onset is in the early teenage years, the disease may present as early as the first year of life and afflicts approximately one in every 400 to 500 children and adolescents. The disease classically presents in a lean patient with polyuria, polydipsia, and polyphagia. It may present at the time of a concurrent illness. While there may be a brief "honeymoon" period after presentation, where insulin is not required, exogenous insulin is always required due to the complete destruction of β-cell mass.

Susceptibility to type 1 diabetes is multigenic. Genes within the human leukocyte antigen (HLA) region, especially those that encode antigen-presenting molecules, confer the greatest part of the genetic risk of type 1 diabetes. The likelihood that these many genes may individually only have weak effects may explain the heterogeneity of inheritance of type 1 diabetes. This genetic susceptibility background is thought to interact with environmental triggers that lead to autoimmunity and insulitis, the characteristic pathologic lesion of type 1 diabetes.

The incidence of type 1 diabetes has been progressively increasing during the past several decades, particularly among children younger than 5 years. In children at genetic risk, diabetes-related autoantibodies appear, followed by the evolution of metabolic abnormalities and the eventual clinical appearance of the disease. If individuals identified by genetic markers subsequently undergo seroconversion and develop two or more diabetes-related autoantibodies, their risk of progression to type 1 diabetes is 75% over 10 years and appears to be almost certain over 20 years.[1] A recent study of patients with diabetes-related autoantibodies who were treated with teplizumab, a monoclonal antibody that reduces the actions of CD8+ T lymphocytes on targets such as β-cells, showed significant reductions in annualized rates of type 1 diabetes and an increase in the median time to diagnosis of type 1 diabetes.[2]

In type 2 diabetes, while β-cell hypersecretion initially may exist, ultimately, loss of β-cell mass ensues. β-cell apoptosis is mediated by glucotoxicity from insulin resistance, and is exacerbated by fatty acids, lipoproteins, leptins, and cytokines, all of which are elevated in type 2 diabetes and obesity. Because of peripheral insulin resistance, many patients require insulin in amounts that exceed one unit per kilogram, far greater than typically required by type 1 diabetics.

The observation that type 1 and type 2 diabetes frequently occur in the same family has raised the possibility that they are opposite ends of the same disease spectrum, and ample evidence suggests the two are more similar than initially believed. Families with mixed diabetes histories tend to have an intermediate diabetes phenotype: insulin resistance in type 1 and lower body mass index (BMI) and C-peptide concentrations in type 2 patients. β-Cell destruction is common to both types, and obesity and insulin resistance have both been shown to be risk factors for childhood type 1 as well as type 2 diabetes. The "accelerator hypothesis" of diabetes proposes three determinants of disease in all types of diabetes: the intrinsic rate of β-cell apoptosis, insulin resistance, and autoimmunity (which would apply only to a subset). Genetic studies suggest there may be a common predisposition. However, the cytokines, signal transduction pathways, and other soluble mediators of apoptosis are quite different between the insulitis of type 1 diabetes and the lipotoxic or glucotoxic processes of type 2 diabetes, and thus, at minimum, represent distinct mechanisms of β-cell destruction.

SECONDARY COMPLICATIONS OF DIABETES

Diabetes mellitus is responsible for tens of thousands of deaths each year in the United States. The high incidence of cardiovascular complications in diabetics is primarily responsible for the twofold increase in the risk of death in diabetics compared with those without diabetes. Clinical complications of diabetes include end-stage kidney disease (ESKD), retinopathy, peripheral vascular disease, coronary artery disease, and neuropathy. Diabetic nephropathy is responsible for nearly 40% of all cases of ESKD; diabetes is also the leading cause of blindness and amputations in the United States. The total direct estimated costs of diagnosed diabetes in the United States increased from $188 billion in 2012 to $306.6 billion in 2022, underscoring the unrelenting financial burden of this chronic disease.[3]

Improvements in diabetes care have reduced the long-term impact to some extent. Rates of all five major diabetes complications (acute myocardial infarction, hyperglycemic crisis, stroke, amputations, and ESKD) have declined since 1990, with the smallest decline in ESKD. However, when expressed as rates for the overall population, in which a change in prevalence also affects complication rates, there was a decline in rates of acute myocardial infarction and death from hyperglycemic crisis, but not in rates of amputation, stroke, or ESKD. Thus, while rates of diabetes-related complications have declined substantially in the past two decades, a large burden of disease persists because diabetes is the driver of multiple long-term conditions and impacts health resource utilization and quality and quantity of life.[4]

While diabetic complications have a multifactorial etiology, they are ultimately secondary to structural alterations in nerves, blood vessels, and connective tissue. Excess glucose is converted to sorbitol by aldose reductase, leading to the reduction of cellular content of myoinositol, abnormal phosphoinositide metabolism, and reduction in Na^+-K^+-ATPase activity. The accumulation of advanced glycosylation end products (AGEs), due to abnormal nonenzymatic glycosylation of proteins, and extensive crosslinking of these proteins, is pathogenic. Ligation of endothelial cell receptors by AGEs results in the release of proinflammatory cytokines and activation of the coagulation cascade. Microangiopathy is characterized by thickening of capillary basement membranes, which increases with the duration of disease, and altered capillary permeability.

1 The Diabetes Control and Complications Trial (DCCT) demonstrated that tight control of blood glucose prevents and delays the progression of secondary complications of diabetes This study, in which patients with type 1 diabetes were randomized to conventional treatment with one or two doses of daily insulin versus intensive treatment with three or more injections per day, demonstrated a dramatic reduction in the risk of progression of retinopathy, microalbuminuria, albuminuria, peripheral neuropathy, and cardiovascular disease in the subjects randomized to intensive treatment. A follow-up study reported a long-term decreased risk of cardiovascular disease.[5] Unfortunately, the major side effect of intensive treatment was a threefold increase in the risk of severe hypoglycemic episodes; approximately 10% of patients in the intensive insulin therapy cohort experienced five or more episodes of seizure or coma during the study period. Even in the absence of overt brain injury, multiple episodes of severe hypoglycemia have been associated with cerebral perfusion abnormalities and poor neuropsychiatric performance. If hypoglycemia becomes more frequent and autonomic neuropathy worsens, patients may develop impaired awareness of hypoglycemia, where the typical symptoms of tremor and anxiety do not occur. Such patients are at risk for accidental trauma, seizure, neurologic injury, or death when unable to detect the onset of severe hypoglycemia and initiate treatment and/or obtain aid from another person.

More contemporary cohorts examined the impact of type 1 diabetes on life expectancy and found a loss of 11.1 and 12.9 years of life for men and women respectively, and while there was a reduction in fatal outcomes over time, the incidence of cardiovascular disease remained substantial and linked to excess mortality.[6,7]

The management of diabetes is focused upon maintaining blood glucose as close to normal range as possible while attempting to minimize significant hypoglycemic episodes. Although the frequency and extent of hyperglycemia are important in the assessment of glucose management, long-term glycemic control is best assessed by evaluation of blood levels of HbA1c, which measures the extent of glycosylation of hemoglobin. Although the incidence of diabetes is increasing, the overall treatment efficacy has improved through the use of newer insulin formulations, the increasing utilization of subcutaneous insulin pumps and continuous glucose monitors have provided improved safety and simplified the diabetic patient's self-care. Fully automated artificial-pancreas systems have been developed that link glucose sensors with insulin pumps through computerized control algorithms, which automate insulin delivery in response to real-time sensor data. Recent studies in both inpatient and outpatient populations have shown that such systems can improve glucose control and reduce the risk of nocturnal hypoglycemia in children, adolescents, and adults.[8,9]

Nevertheless, many diabetics still have difficulty maintaining tight glucose control without hypoglycemic complications. Even for those patients fortunate enough to have access to state-of-the-art technology, there is still the potential for technology failure and death. Most type 1 diabetics, even if on optimal insulin therapy, are unable to maintain HbA1c levels in the normal range, and are at risk for developing progressive diabetic complications.[10]

PANCREAS TRANSPLANTATION

Overview

2 Pancreas transplantation, while not technically a cure, represents an important therapeutic insulin-replacement option

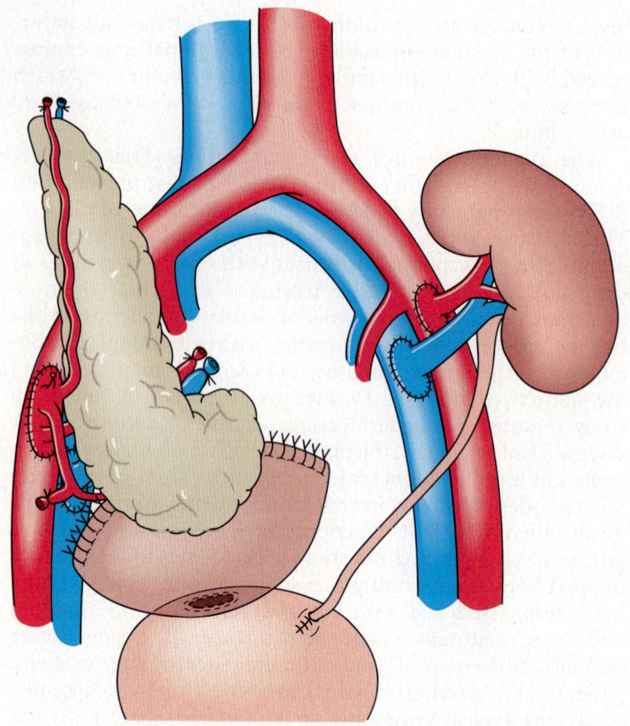

Figure 39.1. Simultaneous pancreas kidney transplantation performed with drainage of the pancreatic exocrine secretions into the urinary bladder (bladder drainage). This technique had been predominant until the last couple decades. Note that a portion of the duodenum is left attached to the pancreas. Despite its heterotopic location, the transplanted pancreas responds to gastrointestinal hormones with a marked increase in secretion of pancreatic juice that has very high bicarbonate content. Also note that the portal vein drains into the iliac vein (ie, systemic venous drainage).

for selected insulin-dependent diabetics. Initial experience with pancreas transplantation, from the first pancreas transplant performed by Kelly and Lillehei in 1966, was marked by low success rates and high mortality.[11] In 1980, the 1-year graft survival rate for pancreas transplantation was only 21%, and there was tremendous skepticism about the utility of the
3 procedure. Iterative advances in surgical technique and immunosuppression dramatically improved graft survival rates to more than 90% at 1 year. The introduction of bladder drainage of the donor pancreas by Sollinger in 1985 used a button of donor duodenum, and was subsequently modified by Nghiem and Corry in 1986 to anastomose a segment of duodenum to the urinary bladder. This modification dramatically improved the technical results of pancreas transplantation *and* provided an easy way to monitor the allograft for rejection, which can be signaled by decreasing urinary amylase levels (**Fig. 39.1**).[12] In the 1990s, the introduction of tacrolimus and valganciclovir further improved graft and patient survival, and decreased the risk of graft loss from occult rejection, which was especially problematic for isolated pancreas transplantation (pancreas after kidney transplantation [PAK] and pancreas transplantation alone [PTA]) compared to simultaneous pancreas–kidney (SPK) transplantation. Because rejection rates are now lower than the morbidity of bladder drainage, most pancreas transplants now utilize an enteric exocrine drainage technique.

Patient Selection

Pancreas transplantation is performed mostly in patients with type 1 diabetes, predominantly in those with ESKD. The recognition of now excellent outcomes of pancreas transplantation, in combination with allocation policy changes, has resulted in an increase in the use of pancreas transplantation for highly selected candidates classified as having type 2 diabetes, which now represents 22.4% of transplants and 23.2% of waitlisted candidates. A small percentage (3%) of pancreas transplant recipients do not have type 1 or type 2 diabetes but have diabetes from other causes. Some pancreas transplants (<1%) are performed as part of a multivisceral transplant that includes liver and small intestine in patients who do not have diabetes; in these transplants, the pancreas is included in the graft to facilitate the technical conduct of the operation and to reduce complications.[13]

4 Most individuals evaluated for pancreas transplantation have chronic kidney disease. These patients may present prior to the onset of dialysis, while currently receiving dialysis, or following kidney transplantation. Potential transplant options include simultaneous deceased-donor SPK, living-donor kidney transplantation followed by PAK, simultaneous pancreas with living donor kidney transplant, or deceased-donor kidney transplant followed by PAK. Of these options, the former two are by far the most common. Segmental pancreas transplantation from a living donor was performed first in 1979, and activity increased through the 1990s as the procedure was associated with improved immunologic outcomes compared to deceased-donor pancreas transplantation.[14] With the introduction of more effective immunosuppression and organ allocation policies, this procedure then waned until a single case was done in 2008 and finally in 2013 (OPTN data accessed Aug 8, 2024). Few US centers have retained the skillset to perform this operation, although it is still performed in Japan and South Korea due to an extreme shortage of deceased-donor pancreata.

Simultaneous Kidney–Pancreas Transplantation

SPK from a deceased donor is by far the most commonly performed pancreas transplant option, with the number exceeding all other types of pancreas transplants combined. An SPK transplant has the advantage of requiring only one operation for both transplants. Since alloreactivity against the transplanted pancreas is often concordant with activity against the kidney, pancreas rejection may be heralded by signs of kidney rejection. Consequently, SPK pancreas outcomes have been historically superior to those of solitary pancreas transplants.

Pancreas after Kidney Transplantation

If a living kidney donor is available, candidates have the option of receiving a living-donor transplant, followed by a deceased-donor pancreas transplant. This approach has the disadvantage of requiring two separate operations, but the recipient enjoys the benefit of a living-donor kidney transplant that, in many circumstances, occurs sooner than would an SPK from a deceased donor. Since the primary survival benefit of the kidney–pancreas transplant mostly comes from the restoration of renal function, this is a significant advantage. However, since a PAK is essentially a solitary pancreas transplant—immunologically distinct from the kidney transplant and alloreactivity is more difficult to detect and treat, and thus long-term pancreas graft survival is decreased compared to SPK.

Simultaneous Living-Donor Kidney–Deceased-Donor Pancreas Transplantation

SPLK is another option previously performed at a few centers, but now is done rarely.[15] Candidates with identified living donors are listed for deceased-donor pancreas transplantation. When a deceased-donor pancreas becomes available, the living kidney donor transplant is performed at the same time as the pancreas transplant. This approach has the advantages of a single operation and a single course of induction therapy. It does require that the potential living donor be available to donate at any time, a requirement that is unappealing to many donors. Because the waiting time for a solitary pancreas has become longer than for SPK, and because kidney donors may donate via a paired exchange program at a time most convenient to them and their intended recipient, the SPLK option is now very infrequently performed.

Pancreas transplant candidates with kidney failure may be counseled in a variety of ways depending on their estimated time until needing renal replacement therapy and the availability of a living kidney donor. How individuals are counseled depends on factors particular to the potential living donor and recipient, and on the recipient's blood type and associated expected waiting time for SPK and PAK transplantation, which vary greatly by geographic region. Since the mortality benefit of SPK or PAK is derived primarily from the kidney transplant, priority is generally given to achieving a kidney transplantation expeditiously. If the individual's estimated waiting time for SPK is longer than a year, living-donor kidney transplantation is typically advised. Because the date of listing is the beginning of solitary pancreas waiting time, it is advantageous for candidates medically eligible for pancreas transplant to be listed for SPK even if a living-donor kidney transplant is planned, as this practice will result in a more competitive waiting time for subsequent PAK.

Even when SPK wait times are very short, it is important to consider the option of living kidney donation through a paired exchange program, especially for younger adults. This would result in a voucher credit to facilitate an opportunity for a preemptive future living-donor kidney retransplant, since younger patients may require kidney retransplantation later in their lifetime when they may no longer have an available living donor and when returning to dialysis has increased mortality. This enables the candidate to have the benefits of an initial SPK (one operation with longer pancreas allograft survival) and is an important consideration since both late PAK and SPK retransplantation are rare.

Pancreas-Alone Transplantation

A small number of type 1 diabetics are evaluated for PTA. These individuals are generally extremely labile diabetics who have progressive complications but do not have nephropathy. In these individuals, the risk/benefit equation is quite different from that for uremic diabetics evaluated for SPK. For nonuremic diabetics evaluated for PTA, the risk of immunosuppression in addition to the surgical procedure must be weighed against the potential benefits from transplantation. The risk of nephrotoxicity due to calcineurin inhibitor (CNI)–based immunosuppression is commonly cited as justification to not perform PTA, with an estimated 10-year risk of ESKD of at least 20%, depending on the pretransplant estimated glomerular filtration rate.[16] PTA for type 1 diabetes results in a significant survival benefit is controversial and must be contextualized to the individual candidate's near-term risk of diabetes-related mortality, cadence of progression of diabetic comorbidities, and quality of life. The most common indication for PTA is impaired awareness of hypoglycemia with difficult-to-control diabetes.

Evaluation and Screening

5 In general, eligibility criteria for pancreas transplantation are more stringent than for kidney transplantation alone. Candidates should have excellent functional status in anticipation of the more extensive surgery and more frequent complications. Age is not tightly related to outcome, but patients over the age of 60 are carefully scrutinized.[17] A detailed history of the patient's diabetes and treatment is obtained, including current glycemic control, hypoglycemic events, secondary complications, insulin requirements, and overall quality of life. Obesity in and of itself is not a contraindication, but BMI >30 is associated with an increased risk of technical failure due to surgical complications. Selection practices vary widely—for some centers, pancreas transplantation is reserved for type 1 diabetics with significant complications and poor glycemic control who have failed alternative treatments, while for others, the presence of insulin-dependent diabetes and a full understanding of the risks and benefits are sufficient, with patient preferences playing a significant role. Because of the need for the new burden of immunosuppression in the absence of kidney disease, PTA criteria are often more stringent than for SPK or PAK.

All candidates should undergo noninvasive cardiac stress testing. Potential candidates with reversible myocardial defects undergo coronary angiography, and some centers perform angiography on all candidates. The decision to perform pretransplantation coronary revascularization must be made with consideration of both peritransplant mortality and long-term survival. Although survival outcomes are diminished in recipients with coronary artery disease, a history of coronary revascularization is not necessarily a contraindication. Individuals with significant myocardium at risk who are without revascularization options are typically excluded.

In addition to a thorough physical examination, screening for significant arteriosclerosis may include noninvasive flow studies and/or abdominal and pelvic computerized tomography (CT). Candidates should be screened for hemodynamically significant carotid occlusive disease. Although distal peripheral vascular occlusive disease is characteristic of long-standing diabetes, aortoiliac disease and femoral popliteal vascular disease may also be present. Femoral popliteal disease is generally not a contraindication to transplantation unless there are clinical signs of arterial insufficiency, such as severe claudication or nonhealing ulcers. The presence of iliac disease is more problematic, as it can compromise inflow to the transplanted organ or preclude pancreas transplantation even in the absence of flow abnormalities, such as when there are limited or absent surgical targets for transplant. In these situations, a kidney-alone transplant may still be feasible.

As with other types of organ transplantation, the evaluation is tailored to the individual's medical history and differs among centers. Common themes are screening for malignancy in accordance with established guidelines for the general population. Individuals with a prior history of treated cancer and who are judged to be at low risk for recurrence are usually candidates following an appropriate disease-free interval. This interval is decreasing as greater experience with transplantation in individuals with a history of cancer has accumulated, and as oncology treatment options have expanded in recent years. Screening for chronic viral infections such as hepatitis B, hepatitis C, and human immunodeficiency virus (HIV) is commonly performed, as is the serostatus of other viral exposures that serve to guide pre- and posttransplant prophylaxis or treatment. As with liver and kidney transplantation, early experience with pancreas transplantation in carefully selected individuals with HIV infection has been encouraging.[18] Social work and/or psychiatric evaluation is performed to assess for the presence of uncontrolled psychiatric issues or inadequate social support that may impact the recipient's ability to safely navigate the necessary posttransplant management.

The Waiting List and Recipients

The number of patients on the waiting list for pancreas transplant has gradually decreased from over 3,500 in 2007 to approximately 3,037 in 2024 (OPTN data accessed August 8, 2024). In contrast to historical data, the majority of waitlisted patients are non-White (56%), a phenomenon which occurred after policy changes relaxed restrictions around type 2 candidates, which improved access to SPK transplant for insulin-dependent Black, Asian, and Hispanic candidates with renal failure. The age distribution of the pancreas waitlist has shifted upward. While the majority (51% in 2024) are ages 35 to 49, the percentage who are older (ages 50 to 64) and younger (18 to 34) are increasing slightly. The annual death rate on the pancreas waiting list was 4.7 per 100 patient years in 2022, which is stable in the post-COVID era when death on the waitlist peaked at 6.2 per 100 patient years.[13]

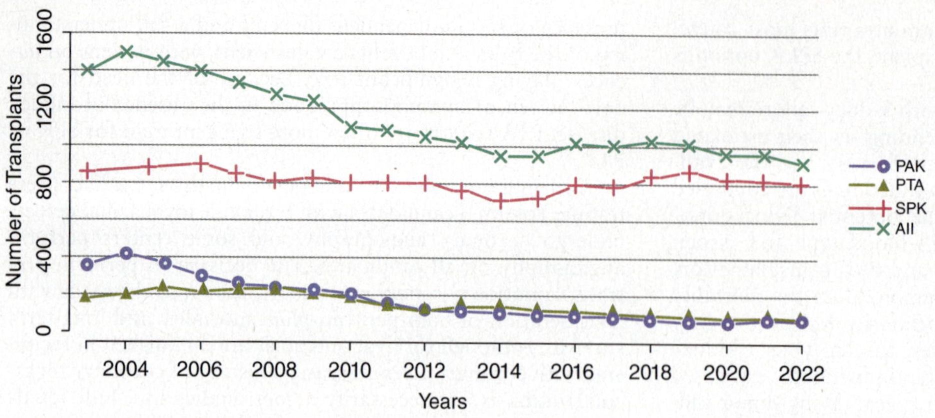

Figure 39.2. The number of pancreas transplants in total and by transplant type (simultaneous pancreas–kidney [SPK], pancreas after kidney transplantation [PAK], and pancreas transplantation alone [PTA]) performed in the United States between 2003 and 2022. (Adapted from the 2013 and 2022 OPTN/SRTR Annual Report: Pancreas.)[13,19]

The overall number of pancreas transplants performed in the United States has continued to decline. There were 914 pancreas transplants performed in 2023, compared with a peak of 1,484 in 2004. The decrease has mostly been due to decreases in PAK and PTA (**Fig. 39.2**).[13,19] Median times to transplant have increased over the past 3 years and now average 1 to 2 years but vary widely by region, with isolated pancreas wait times being longer than for SPK. The age and race distribution of recipients generally parallels that of the waiting list.

Deceased-Donor Pancreas Allocation

As with other organs, pancreata are allocated according to nationally determined policies. The pancreas waitlist includes candidates who need any type of pancreas (or islet) transplant. If the pancreas candidate also requires a kidney, then a kidney from the same donor is allocated to the SPK candidate, independent of the candidate's place on the kidney waiting list. Beginning in 2021, the distribution of pancreata was based on a 250 nautical mile circle from the donor hospital in order to eliminate inequities based on smaller geographic boundaries. Within the circle, up to 2 proximity points are assigned, and outside the circle, up to 4 proximity points are assigned to maximize placement efficiency. Pancreas allocation is mostly prioritized by a combination of candidate waiting time and proximity to the donor hospital, with some additional priority assigned to candidates who have zero mismatches with a donor or who are highly sensitized.

Pancreas allocation is complicated by the fact that the pancreas donor selection criteria for islet transplant and whole-organ transplant overlap, leading to competition among certain types of organs. In determining whether a given pancreas will be allocated to a solid organ or islet transplant candidate, donor age and BMI are considered. Few islet transplants are currently performed as they can only be done under a biologic license agreement and are categorized as a research procedure in the pancreata. Donors under age 50 and with BMI <30 are allocated first for whole-organ pancreas transplant. If there is no candidate for whole pancreas, the pancreas is then allocated for islets. For donors older than age 50 *or* with BMI >30, whose pancreata are rarely used for whole-organ transplant, the organ is first offered locally then nationally for pancreas or kidney–pancreas transplant for 0 mismatched or cPRA >80% candidates, then if unplaced and also no local accepting pancreas or kidney–pancreas candidates, the pancreas is then offered for islets locally then nationally.[20]

In general, pancreata are significantly underutilized compared to other solid organs, and donor selection criteria are more rigorous. There is significant geographic variation in pancreas use, which correlates with activity by local transplant centers. Restrictions on cold ischemia time for whole-pancreas transplantation and particularly for islet transplantation make the placement of pancreata challenging when distances are longer between the donor and recipient center.

Donor Evaluation

6 The selection of appropriate pancreas donors is perhaps the most important determinant of successful pancreas transplantation. Many complications early after pancreas transplantation are thought to be secondary to processes related to ischemia and reperfusion injury, rather than the technical conduct of the recipient operation. While the ideal donor is young, nonalcoholic, nonobese, and hemodynamically fairly stable, very few donors meet this description, and the surgeon frequently needs to consider pancreata from imperfect donors. Donor selection criteria vary among surgeons and transplant centers, and depend significantly on surgeon and programmatic experience, waiting time, and access to next offer. Primary criteria are the age of the donor, donor BMI, donor cause of death, and the gross appearance of the organ at the time of recovery. Additional information that may influence organ acceptance rates includes aspects of the medical and social history, donor hemodynamics, laboratory values, anticipated preservation time, and (less frequently) HLA matching. As with donor selection for other organs, the decision-making process often involves consideration of multiple factors in aggregate.

The importance of donor age on patient and graft survival outcomes has been confirmed by multiple studies of risks for early technical as well as later graft loss, but the mechanism by which age affects outcomes is not firmly established. The survival benefit of pancreas transplantation is blunted with the use of older donors as well as in older recipients.[21,22] As such, the maximum age threshold is significantly lower than for heart, liver, and kidney transplantation.

Donor BMI has been found to be a determinant of early graft failure by single-center and transplant registry analyses. Very few pancreata from donors with BMI greater than 30 are used for pancreas transplantation, and are more likely to be recovered for islet transplant. More recent registry data suggest that carefully selected donors with BMI up to 35 can successfully be used as pancreas donors.[23]

The mechanism of death in combination with other donor characteristics greatly influences donor selection. Pancreata from donors with stroke as a cause of death have reduced graft survival. Although experience from donors after cardiac death (DCD) remains relatively limited (<5% of all pancreas transplants), outcomes have been good with careful donor selection. Laboratory values, including serum lipase, play a relatively minor role in donor selection. Insulin administration during donor management is not considered a contraindication to pancreas donation since, in the presence of a normal HbA1c, donor hyperglycemia reflects the administration of dextrose-containing solutions, corticosteroids for cerebral edema, and high-dose catecholamines for blood pressure support rather than latent pancreatic endocrine insufficiency. Abnormal HbA1c has been utilized as a relative contraindication, but recent single-center data suggest that levels up to 6.2 mg/dL are not associated with adverse graft outcomes.[24] Donor ischemic insults that result in

Table 39.1. Summary of Pancreas Donor Risk Index

Donor Characteristics	Reference Donor (DRI = 1.00)	Change Factor Value to	DRI
Gender	Male	Female	0.87
Age	28	45	1.56
Black race	No	Yes	1.27
Asian race	No	Yes	1.17
BMI	24	30	1.17
Height (cm)	173	190	0.9
Cause of death: CVA/stroke	No	Yes	1.23
Cause of death: CVA/stroke in PAK	No	Yes	0.93
Pancreas preservation time (hours)	12	20	1.13
DCD	No	Yes	1.39
SCr >2.5	No	Yes	1.22

Equation: pDRI = exp(−0.13792 × I[Female Donor]) – 0.034455 × I[Donor Age <20] × [Donor Age – 20] + 0.026149 × [Donor Age – 28] + 0.19490 × I[Donor Creatinine > 2.5] + 0.23951 × I[Donor Black Race] + 0.15711 × I[Donor Asian Race] – 0.000986347 × [Donor BMI – 24] + 0.033274 × I[Donor BMI > 25] × [Donor BMI – 25] – 0.006073879 × (Donor Height – 173) + 0.21018 × I[Donor COD CVA] – 0.28137 × I[Donor COD CVA for PAK txp] + 0.014678 × [Preservation Time – 12] + 0.33172 × I[DCD].[25]

ongoing dysfunction of other organs are an important consideration for assessing the risk of significant ischemia/reperfusion injury to the pancreas allograft.

As with other organ transplants, careful review of the donor's social history, medical history, and diagnostic testing is required to assess the risk of transmission of donor-derived infection or cancer, relative to the benefit of the transplant.

Intraoperative evaluation of the donor organ is said to be the most important determinant of pancreas donor selection. Significant fatty infiltration of the pancreas, mass, direct trauma, or fibrosis/atrophy are contraindications to transplantation. Severe pancreatic edema is also an adverse finding, although it may be correctable with donor management. A prior splenectomy is not a contraindication, provided that the tail can be dissected atraumatically.

Factors not intrinsic to the donor may also influence the decision for donor acceptance. The higher risk of graft failure associated with solitary pancreas transplants leads some centers to have more stringent selection criteria for PTA and PAK. While cold ischemia is a risk factor for graft survival, pancreata from highly selected donors can be transplanted with cold ischemic times approaching 24 hours with good outcomes. Attention to HLA matching varies by center; several analyses suggest that matching does not have a very significant impact on graft outcome.

As for deceased-donor livers and kidneys, a Pancreas Donor Risk Index (PDRI) has been described in an attempt to provide an assessment of certain donor characteristics that are associated with the risk of pancreas graft failure (**Table 39.1**).[25] With the elimination of race-based calculations in 2023, the emerging use of normothermic preservation for DCD, and the change in the definition of graft failure, it remains to be seen how the PDRI might be recalibrated in the future in order to remain a useful tool for donor selection.

Procurement Technique

The importance of the donor pancreas procurement technique cannot be overstated. It is thought by many pancreas transplant surgeons to be more critical to the success of the transplant than the recipient procedure. Because the pancreas is susceptible to traumatic injury, it must be carefully dissected and manipulated to avoid injury to the pancreatic parenchyma. Typically, the pancreas is recovered along with the liver and kidneys via a midline incision, which extends from the sternal notch to the pubic symphysis. After a Cattell–Braasch maneuver exposes the retroperitoneum, the aorta and inferior mesenteric vein (IMV) are prepared for future cannulation and clamping. The pancreas is visualized by dividing the gastrocolic omentum and entering the lesser sac. This dissection continues with division of the short gastric vessels and the avascular gastrosplenic ligament. The mobilization of the pancreas may be performed either prior to or following the aortic perfusion procedure described below. An antibiotic and/or a betadine-containing solution is frequently instilled into the duodenum through a nasogastric tube for decontamination. The pancreas is dissected from the pancreatic bed using the spleen as a handle, affording minimal manipulation of the parenchyma. The duodenum is divided at the pylorus using a stapler. The proximal jejunum is transected distal to the ligament of Treitz. Division of the middle colic vessels permits exposure of the proximal small bowel mesentery, which is divided distal to the pancreas, typically with a stapler.

Perfusion of the abdominal organs is generally achieved by cannulating the distal aorta and clamping the supraceliac aorta. This is typically achieved with approximately 3 to 5 L of University of Wisconsin (UW) or histidine–tryptophan–ketoglutarate (HTK) solution while the abdominal organs are packed in saline slush. The portal system of the liver is perfused on the back table with 1 to 2 L preservation solution, or via the IMV in situ, but this approach is less common due to risk of causing pancreatic edema. Overperfusion may result in pancreatic edema and an increased risk of complications. Many centers prefer UW preservation for pancreas procurements since HTK use is associated with decreased graft survival.[26]

The pancreas can be removed either en bloc with the liver and kidneys, en bloc with the liver, or separately, following removal of the liver. Whatever the technique, the portal triad is dissected out in cooperation with the liver recovery team.

Table 39.2. Pancreas Procurement for Transplantation: Key Technical Steps, Pearls, and Potential Pitfalls

Key Technical Steps

1. Midline laparotomy and full exploration. Mobilize the right colon and perform generous Kocher maneuver. Assess for variant hepatic artery anatomy
2. Open the lesser sac and assess the pancreas for fat, texture, and edema. Mobilize the left colon away from the pancreas, and release the spleen
3. Identify the origins of the superior mesenteric artery, splenic artery, and gastroduodenal artery
4. Lavage the duodenum with amphotericin B or ½ strength betadine irrigation. Ligate and divide the bile duct, and incise and irrigate the gallbladder with saline
5. Place aortic and IMV cannulae
6. Cross-clamp and flush donor viscera with preservation solution, venting into the chest
7. Divide (and tag) the splenic artery, ligate the GDA, and divide the portal vein
8. Use a blue load GIA stapler to divide the proximal duodenum, proximal jejunum, and the colonic and small bowel mesentery
9. Using the spleen as a handle, excise the pancreas
10. Procure the donor Y graft (common, external, and internal iliac artery) and iliac vein segment

Pearls

- Communicate pancreas assessment to the recipient team upon visualization
- Minimize manipulation of the gland
- Keep the pancreas cold while awaiting removal of other organs

Potential Pitfalls

- Violating the pancreas capsule
- Overflushing or venous outflow obstruction of preservation fluid
- Stapling the mesentery too close to the uncinate process
- Y graft surgical injury, shortening, or donor disease

The portal vein is shared by dividing it at the level of the coronary vein. Only in the rarest of circumstances should there be any difficulty using both the liver and the pancreas from the same donor, even in the presence of hepatic arterial anomalies. In the case of a replaced right hepatic artery, the superior mesenteric artery (SMA) can be divided just peripheral to the replaced right hepatic artery, leaving a very short SMA with the pancreas. Alternatively, if a replaced right hepatic artery is large enough to be safely reconstructed without a cuff of SMA, it can be transected as it exits superiorly from behind the head of the pancreas. This is also true in the rare case where a completely replaced hepatic artery emerges from the superior aspect of the head of the pancreas; usually, the artery in this case is long enough and large enough to be used for liver transplant without a celiac axis or aortic cuff. The bile duct is ligated on the pancreas side, as is the gastroduodenal artery (GDA) (only in the cold), and divided on the liver side. Dissection then proceeds along the superior aspect of the pancreas along the proper hepatic artery. The splenic artery, which provides the arterial blood supply to the body and tail of the pancreas, is divided a few millimeters from its origin to allow for adequate length on the pancreas while allowing the stump to be oversewn without compromising flow to the liver. The key steps, pearls, and pitfalls are outlined below (**Table 39.2**). Once the pancreas is removed or split from the liver, the pancreas is packed in preservation solution; a Y-graft consisting of the entire donor common iliac artery and its two main branches, the internal and external iliac arteries, and a segment of donor iliac vein are packaged and transported with the pancreas for use in back-table reconstruction.

Back-Table Preparation of the Pancreas

The pancreas is placed in ice-cold preservation solution and should remain cold at all times. The spleen is removed by dividing all vessels near the spleen, either by ligature or stapling, taking care to avoid injury to the tail of the pancreas. Peripancreatic fat should be trimmed. The bile duct, GDA, and IMV are resecured. The pylorus is resected, and the duodenal staple line is oversewn with silk or polypropylene sutures. The distal duodenum is mobilized to the uncinate process. It can be transected on the back-table or after reperfusion, and the staple line oversewn with silk or polypropylene. The mesenteric staple line is oversewn with polypropylene suture. The portal vein is mobilized by freeing the surrounding adventitial tissue to the confluence of the splenic vein and superior mesenteric vein (SMV) to allow an adequate length of portal vein for anastomosis. Some surgeons routinely add an end-to-end venous extension graft of donor iliac vein to lengthen the portal vein, but this is usually not necessary. A ganglionectomy is performed to secure all cut lymphatics and to enhance future hemostasis. The dual arterial circulation of the pancreas allograft is then reconstructed using the donor iliac artery Y-graft by anastomosing the internal iliac artery to the splenic artery and the external iliac artery to the SMA (**Fig. 39.3**). In the absence of a Y-graft, the splenic artery may be implanted in end-to-side fashion to the SMA or an interposition graft can be created.

Recipient Operation

Pancreas transplantation is typically performed through a midline incision, although a lower quadrant incision similar

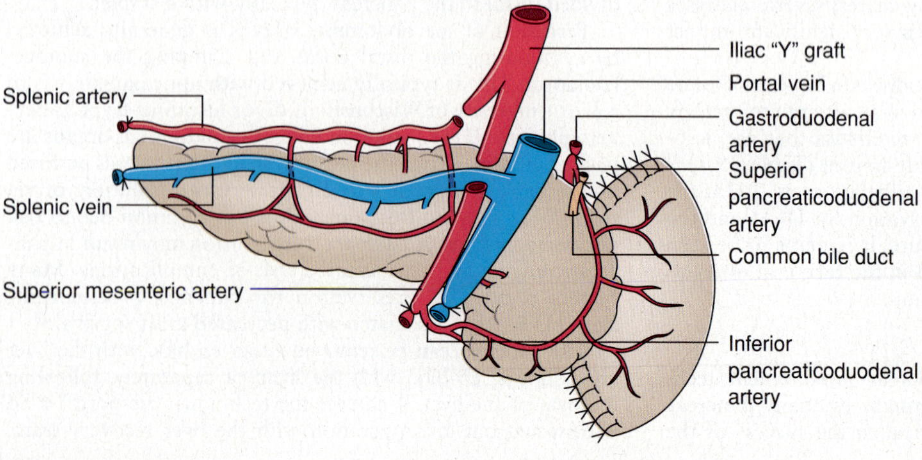

Figure 39.3. Back-table preparation of the pancreas. During back-table preparation, donor splenectomy is performed, the duodenal cuffs are prepared, and the mesenteric vessels are secured. The dual blood supply of the pancreas is unified using a Y graft of donor iliac artery; the donor external iliac artery is anastomosed to the donor superior mesenteric artery and the donor internal iliac artery to the donor splenic artery. The donor common iliac artery is used for anastomosis to the recipient iliac artery.

to a kidney transplant incision may be used. The recipient should receive broad-spectrum antibiotics preoperatively. The pancreas transplant is placed preferably on the right side to facilitate systemic venous drainage, and can be oriented either head up or head down. After dissection of the targeted recipient artery and vein, the donor portal vein is anastomosed in an end-to-side fashion to the systemic vein. The distal inferior vena cava (IVC), common iliac vein, or external iliac vein may be used; the recipient vein segment should be mobile enough for the portal vein to reach without tension after reperfusion. The common iliac artery component of the donor Y-graft is then anastomosed in end-to-side fashion to either the recipient external iliac artery or common iliac artery; the distal aorta can also serve as the site of anastomosis. A pancreas placed on the left side in the recipient may be placed either medial or lateral to the sigmoid colon. Multiple variations have been described.

Venous drainage typically utilizes the systemic circulation (IVC or iliac vein) but can also be directed into the recipient portal circulation via the SMV. Since 50% of insulin is removed with the first pass through the liver and hyperinsulinemia has been associated with dyslipidemia and accelerated atherosclerosis, the technique of portal venous drainage for pancreas transplantation was developed as a more physiologic approach compared to systemic drainage (**Fig. 39.4**).[27] However, despite more than 30 years of experience with the

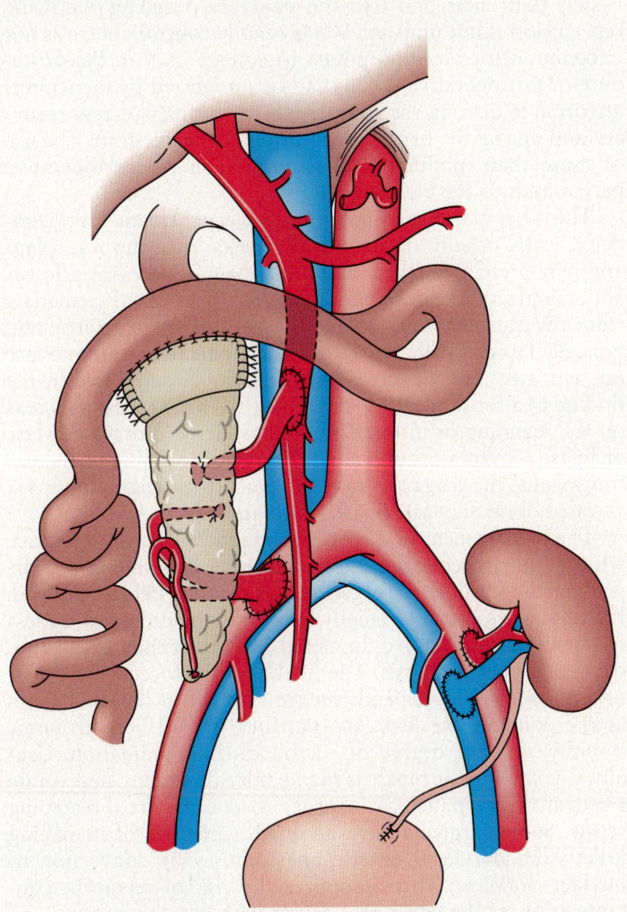

Figure 39.4. Simultaneous pancreas kidney transplantation performed with enteric drainage of the pancreatic exocrine secretions into the proximal jejunum (enteric drainage). This technique has been adopted by most US transplant centers for simultaneous pancreas–kidney transplants. For solitary pancreas transplantation, some centers still utilize bladder drainage to allow monitoring of the urinary amylase. Note that the donor portal vein drains into the recipient superior mesenteric vein (portal venous drainage), but most centers utilize the IVC or iliac vein (systemic venous drainage), depending on if the gland is placed in the head-up or head-down configuration.

technique, no difference in cardiac morbidity or mortality has been observed, and graft and patient survival are essentially equivalent with systemically drained pancreas transplants.

For portal venous drainage, the SMV is dissected out just below the transverse mesocolon. The right common iliac artery is typically prepared. An end-to-side anastomosis of the donor portal vein to the recipient SMV is performed with the pancreas in the head-up position. The Y-graft of the donor is then passed through a hole created in the small bowel mesentery and anastomosed to the recipient common iliac artery.

Although the type of venous drainage selected typically depends on the preferences of individual surgeons or transplant centers, the decision to perform portal or systemic drainage may also depend upon the anatomy of an individual patient. Patients with multiple previous abdominal operations, a thickened mesentery, may be more suited for systemic venous drainage. Alternatively, patients who have had multiple transplants or have limited venous targets may be better candidates for portal venous drainage.

The majority of centers now manage the exocrine secretions via enteric drainage, but some centers still use bladder drainage, mostly for solitary pancreas transplants or unique situations. The major advantage of bladder drainage is the ability to monitor urinary amylase—a decrease in which may be the earliest sign of rejection. This can be helpful in solitary pancreas transplants, but is perhaps less important for SPK transplants, where rejection rates are lower and signs of donor alloreactivity can also be monitored by serum creatinine. Improved immunosuppression and an increased utilization of pancreas biopsies to diagnose rejection have led to a decreased reliance on urinary amylase for graft monitoring, which contributed to a decrease in utilization of the bladder drained technique. This change in clinical practice was also due to recognition of the longer-term significant morbidity that can be associated with bladder-drained pancreas transplants; about 25% of recipients required enteric conversion due to complications such as acute kidney injury from dehydration, bicarbonate wasting contributing to metabolic acidosis, recurrent urinary tract infections, hematuria, and chemical urethritis and cystitis.

Enteric drainage is achieved by creating a side-to-side or end-to-side anastomosis of donor duodenum to recipient small bowel. This is most commonly done by using a loop of proximal jejunum, but a Roux-en-Y configuration may be created if needed. For bladder drainage, a side-to-side anastomosis between the donor duodenum and the bladder is performed. Enteric drainage is always used for pancreas transplants with portal venous drainage or those with systemic venous drainage in the head-up configuration because the orientation of the gland precludes anastomosis of the graft duodenum to the bladder.

During a SPK transplant, the kidney allograft is traditionally placed in the left iliac fossa, although ipsilateral placement of both organs on the right iliac system may simplify the operation when the vasculature is suitable and when the pancreas is in the head-up configuration. The intraperitoneal location of the kidney increases the potential for medial torsion of the kidney on its vascular pedicle compared with kidney-alone transplants placed in a retroperitoneal location. To mitigate this risk, some surgeons create a retroperitoneal flap or "pocket," or pexy remnant perinephric fat to the lateral abdominal wall.

Following revascularization of the pancreas, attention is paid to bleeding from the pancreas, which can be significant. This is controlled with ties, clips, or suture ligatures. Since thrombosis is a common complication of pancreas transplantation, anticoagulation in the perioperative period may be employed, particularly for solitary pancreas transplantation or in patients with known hypercoagulable states. Thrombosis is less frequent in SPK transplantation, where uremic platelet dysfunction is protective. The preferred anticoagulation regimen ranges from intraoperative administration of heparin prior to clamping the recipient vessels, followed by postoperative aspirin or other antiplatelet agents, to more aggressive regimens such as low-dose heparin infusion and oral anticoagulation with warfarin or apixaban. Whatever the approach, patients should be closely monitored for bleeding since postoperative hemorrhage (along with concern for thrombosis) is the most common cause for reoperation (up to 10%).[28]

Following revascularization, serum glucose levels are obtained hourly. It is common for the blood glucose to decline significantly following revascularization, and it is not uncommon for it to fall to normal levels soon after the patient's arrival in the recovery room. At some point, maintenance intravenous fluids should be converted to a dextrose-containing solution in order to prevent hypoglycemia. Pancreas transplant recipients with enteric drainage require only maintenance fluid calculated to support obligatory third-space losses. SPK recipients require additional fluid replacements similar to what would be administered following kidney-alone transplantation. Individuals who receive bladder-drained pancreas transplants require replacement of bicarbonate and pancreatic exocrine volume loss, which can be quite profound.

Immunosuppression

7 Immunosuppression for pancreas transplantation is fairly similar to that for kidney transplantation. The immunogenicity of a pancreas transplant is considered to be greater than the majority of solid-organ transplants because of the extensive lymphoid component of the gland.

The use of induction therapy to inhibit lymphocyte function is common. Several large randomized multicenter trials utilizing either T-cell–depleting antibody induction (OKT3, ATGAM, and thymoglobulin) or interleukin-2 (IL-2) receptor antibody inhibition (daclizumab and basiliximab) showed a reduction in the incidence of acute rejection but failed to demonstrate a significant effect on patient or graft survival. These findings were also replicated by analyses done with registry data by the International Pancreas Transplant Registry. Despite the modest impact on overall outcomes, 86.3% of pancreas transplant recipients received T-cell–depleting therapy and 3.7% used IL-2 receptor antibody for induction in 2022.[13]

Due to the difficulty in diagnosing rejection compared to other solid-organ transplants, the choice of maintenance immunosuppression is center specific, with most centers using triple therapy, which includes a CNI, an antiproliferative agent, and steroids. Steroid-free regimens have decreased in frequency over the last decade, but were used by 22.8% of programs.[13] Steroid-free maintenance immunosuppression regimens are used in concert with T-cell–depleting induction therapy such as antithymocyte globulin or alemtuzumab. Solumedrol is utilized only for premedication for these agents and is typically given only over the first several days posttransplant. These regimens typically target slightly higher tacrolimus trough level goals and are used in combination with mycophenolic acid or sirolimus. Steroid minimization protocols, as in kidney transplantation, aim to avoid the significant short- and long-term side effects associated with corticosteroids. Several groups have reported excellent 10-year patient and graft outcomes utilizing steroid minimization protocols.[29,30]

Complications

Thrombosis of the pancreas transplant is the most common cause of graft loss in the early postoperative period, occurring in 5% to 10% of transplants. Why pancreas transplants are more prone to thrombosis than other solid-organ transplants is uncertain, but the most likely mechanism is that ischemia reperfusion injury of the pancreas is characterized by the release of cytokines, edema, and activation of pancreatic enzymes which leads to decreased microvascular blood flow and a procoagulant state in an organ that receives only about 1% of the total cardiac output. Diabetic patients have impaired fibrinolysis and are, therefore, relatively hypercoagulable at baseline. The decreased blood flow through the portal vein after transplant, due to the lack of outflow from the spleen and small bowel as compared to the native state, may be contributory. Thrombosis is slightly more common in solitary pancreas transplantation than in SPK, probably due to the absence of uremic platelet dysfunction present in SPK recipients. The risk of thrombosis has been associated with donor factors such as older patient age, renal dysfunction, cold ischemic time, BMI, DCD status, and cerebrovascular cause of death.[31]

Pancreas transplant thrombosis is usually heralded by a sudden rise in postoperative baseline blood glucose. Confirmation of the diagnosis is usually obtained with duplex ultrasound. Although anecdotal reports have described successful surgical and angiographic thrombectomy or thrombolysis in restoring flow to the pancreas, the usual treatment is removal of the infarcted pancreas. In contrast, asymptomatic thrombosis, whether partial or even complete, has been successfully managed with anticoagulation, especially if late in onset. Because of the high risk of thrombosis, some form of anticoagulation is frequently employed after pancreas transplantation. It is likely due to these efforts and improvements in donor selection and immunosuppression that the thrombosis rate for all types of pancreas transplants is at an all-time low.

Bleeding is another frequent cause for reoperation in the early postoperative period. Because of the large number of vessels that enter and exit the pancreas, bleeding following reperfusion is not unusual. While readily controllable, it is not uncommon for bleeding points to emerge later in the procedure or postoperatively. This can be minimized by meticulous attention to ligating vascular structures during pancreas recovery and during the bench preparation of the allograft. The use of more than minimal anticoagulation in the perioperative period adds to the bleeding risk.

The other major early complication is pancreatic leak. Duodenal leaks usually occur 1 to 2 weeks after the transplant and may present as fever, abdominal pain, leukocytosis, lower abdominal tenderness, or persistent ileus. Leak can also emanate from any capsular violation and present earlier after transplant, typically less clinically impactful, as the pancreatic enzymes are not activated. The diagnosis of a leak may be supported by the finding of a focal fluid collection near the head of the pancreas on CT scanning or ultrasound, and/or elevated drain amylase or lipase >3 times serum values. For bladder-drained pancreas transplants, the diagnosis may be made by cystography or via elevated drain amylase, lipase, or creatinine.

The management of a suspected duodenal leak is operative with the aim of achieving control of enteric contamination. The peritoneum should be lavaged and all necrotic debris removed. If a leak is present, it is usually located at the proximal (or less frequently distal) stapled duodenal cuff rather than at the duodenoenteric anastomosis. The likelihood of success for repair of a duodenal leak depends on the viability of the duodenum at the point of the leak, the patient's overall hemodynamic stability, and the degree of surrounding inflammation. Usually, one attempt at repair is made, but failure may necessitate removal of the pancreas in order to control life-threatening sepsis. Some surgeons have adopted a practice of managing leaks from duodenal enteric anastomoses by conversion to bladder drainage. This minimizes the risk of recurrent contamination of the peritoneal cavity with enteric contents and allows for Foley catheter decompression of the duodenum, but is not possible when the graft is oriented head-up. Drainage of infection without primary repair of the duodenal leak has been successfully employed in situations where inflammation is so profound that the leak could not be primarily repaired, typically via diversion of the enteric stream by creation of a Roux-Y in combination with wide drainage. The morbidity associated with duodenal fistulas dictates that the aforementioned options be employed only when definitive repair is not possible and the patient is clinically well-compensated.

Peripancreatic abscess can also occur in the absence of a frank duodenal leak. Patients with abscess and without systemic sepsis can be treated with early surgical washout or percutaneous CT-guided drainage, depending on abscess location and time posttransplant.

In contrast to renal transplantation, the complications of pancreas transplantation can be severe and life threatening if not properly managed. Even in the most experienced centers, occasional patients may require extended hospitalization. This is a consequence of both the tenuous medical status of long-standing diabetics and the potential for substantial morbidity from complications of pancreas transplantation. Nevertheless, the risk of death from perioperative complications is low (0.5% in the first month after transplant). Given the limited gain in short-term survival benefit of pancreas transplantation, particularly compared with kidney transplantation, patients should be counseled frankly about the potential magnitude of these complications so that they have a realistic expectation of outcomes. Even with honest discussion and informed consent, most individuals will elect pancreas transplantation, and a surprising number will pursue a repeat pancreas transplant even with a history of complications from a prior pancreas transplant, which speaks to the improved quality of life experienced through freedom from intensive insulin therapy.

Diagnosis and Treatment of Rejection

The timely and accurate diagnosis of pancreas transplant rejection is one of the most important and challenging aspects of posttransplant management. The incidence of pancreas rejection was <12% in the first year for all pancreas transplant types performed in 2022. The incidence of rejection is highest in recipients not receiving lymphocyte-depleting induction and in PTA. Pancreas rejection is associated with inferior graft survival. Therefore, the implications of delayed or missed treatment for rejection can be profound.

There is no single laboratory abnormality capable of diagnosing rejection. Amylase and lipase serum levels may be elevated for a number of reasons, and so can arouse suspicion for rejection, but are not specific. Hyperglycemia is also nonspecific. If hyperglycemia is due to rejection, it occurs late in the process and reflects significant pancreatic endocrine injury and a dismal prognosis. While imaging modalities, including ultrasound, may identify abnormalities in the parenchyma or perfusion, they too are neither sensitive nor specific.[32] Hence, the diagnosis of rejection is best made with histologic examination of a pancreatic biopsy specimen once other causes of dysfunction are ruled out. SPK transplant recipients benefit from monitoring of the kidney transplant by serum creatinine, as there is some degree of concordance rate for rejection between kidney and pancreas grafts. However, isolated pancreas rejection clearly occurs, and neither a normal creatinine nor a normal kidney biopsy can rule out pancreas rejection in recipients of SPK or PAK. Improvements in the outcome of solitary pancreas transplants are attributable to improvements in immunosuppression, and to more timely and accurate diagnosis and treatment of pancreas rejection.

The technique of pancreas transplant biopsy has evolved over the years. In the era of bladder-drained pancreas transplants, cystoscopic biopsy of both the pancreas and transplant duodenum was common. As more enteric-drained pancreas transplants have been performed, a greater experience with percutaneous biopsy was developed, using either ultrasound or CT-guided techniques. Laparoscopic-assisted or open pancreas biopsy may be utilized for patients whose pancreas transplant is not accessible to percutaneous approaches. Endoscopic biopsy has been described, and a proximal jejunal or duodenal anastomosis can facilitate the utilization of this method. The indications for pancreatic biopsy include hyperlipasemia, hyperamylasemia, hyperglycemia, or unexplained pain in the vicinity of the pancreas transplant. The differential diagnosis includes pancreatitis, cytomegalovirus (CMV) infection, and toxicity from CNIs and, in the early postoperative period, peripancreatic infection. The histologic grading system developed at the University of Maryland for determining rejection grade in pancreas biopsies has been updated by the Banff 2022 Pancreas Work Group.[33] Indeterminate or mild rejection may be treated with increases in CNI target trough levels and/or pulse corticosteroids. Steroid-resistant or higher-grade rejection is generally treated with antilymphocyte depleting antibody therapy.

As long-term survival of pancreas transplants becomes more commonplace, chronic rejection is now an important problem. As with kidney transplantation, newer agents have improved short-term survival by preventing acute rejection, but this has not translated to an increase in long-term graft survival. Chronic rejection is histologically characterized as expansion of fibrous septa within the pancreatic parenchyma. This may progress to lobular atrophy or loss of both acini and β-cells. Although there are parallels to chronic allograft nephropathy, whether chronic CNI toxicity contributes to chronic pancreas rejection is unknown.

Recurrent Autoimmune Diabetes

Selective β-cell destruction in pancreas transplants due to recurrent autoimmune diabetes may manifest in a pattern similar to the insulitis seen in type 1 diabetes. This pattern is histologically distinct from cellular rejection. Although recurrent autoimmune diabetes has been documented in both immunosuppressed pancreas transplant recipients and nonimmunosuppressed living-donor recipients from identical twin siblings, well-documented case series have been infrequent. A variety of associations have been suggested with autoantibodies to glutamic acid decarboxylase and islet cells, but patterns of autoantibody expression have not proven reliable enough to establish their etiologic relevance or prognostic value.

Posttransplant Viral Infections

The higher level of immunosuppression given to pancreas transplant recipients compared with kidney transplant recipients, particularly with respect to lymphocyte-depleting induction therapy, places pancreas transplant recipients at risk for conditions known to be influenced by overall immunosuppressive exposure. While rates of CMV infection are generally higher than for kidney recipients, especially when the donor is known to carry the virus, the use of oral valganciclovir has reduced the incidence of significant CMV-associated disease. The incidence of CMV disease may also be lower in those recipients receiving steroid-free immunosuppression. Data are mixed with respect to the incidence of polyomavirus infection (BK) nephropathy. As with kidney-alone recipients, SPK recipients with BK nephropathy have inferior kidney graft survival. Posttransplant lymphoproliferative disorder, often associated with Epstein–Barr virus (EBV) infection, has a 1-year incidence of approximately 1%, which is similar to that seen after kidney-alone transplantation, but has been reported as high as 6.4% in EBV naïve PTA recipients at 5 years posttransplant, likely reflecting their higher risk of rejection and immunosuppression exposure.

Outcomes

8 Registry analyses have demonstrated a significant survival benefit of SPK transplantation compared with dialysis or any type of kidney alone transplantation in a candidate with diabetes, underscoring the long-term benefit of correcting diabetes. Whether an isolated pancreas transplantation positively impacts patient survival has historically been controversial.[34,35] Fridell et al.[36] in 2019 reported the long-term survival advantage conferred by PAK to be similar to SPK, and that PAK transplantation increases the kidney allograft survival when applied to either deceased- or living-donor kidney-alone transplants. A matched cohort analysis was done comparing patients waitlisted for PTA and not transplanted with PTA

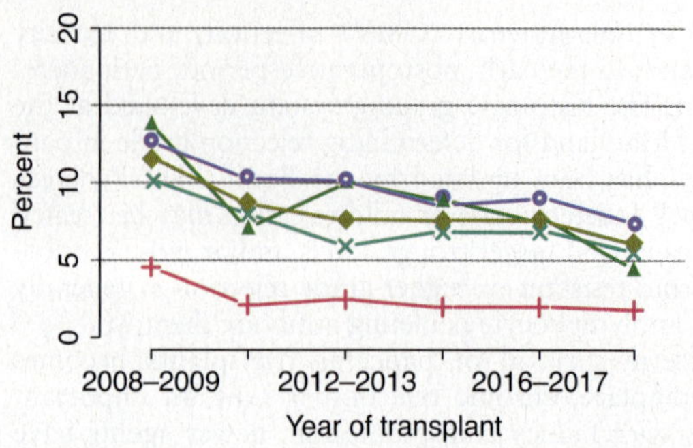

Figure 39.5. Graft failure within the first 90 days posttransplant among adult pancreas transplant recipients by transplant type and year. (Adapted from the 2021 OPTN/SRTR Annual Data Report: pancreas)[38]

recipients, which showed the median patient survival to be 7.8 versus 11.8 years.[37] In summary, patient survival at 1 year following pancreas transplantation is high, at 96.3%, 97.5%, and 98.7% for SPK, PAK, and PTA, respectively and at 10 years posttransplant, patient survival is 76.3%, 77.9%, and 82.4% for SPK, PAK, and PTA, respectively.[13]

Since return to insulin can occur due to modifiable pancreas dysfunction or insulin resistance, and there was previously no defined threshold of C-peptide level or insulin use, center reporting of graft failure had been variable for events other than pancreatectomy, relisting, or death. In 2018, the OPTN updated the definition of pancreas graft failure to the use of ≥0.5 units/kg/d of insulin for 90 consecutive days (and eliminated the "partial function" reporting category) with the aim of making reporting more consistent. Registry data from 2020 was the first year that graft failure data was reported using the new definition. Pancreas 1-year graft survival rates decreased across all pancreas transplant types in the first 2 years of data collection (2019 and 2020): from 92.8% to 89.5% for SPK, 93.2% to 85.4% for PAK, and 89.7% to 84.4% for PTA, perhaps influenced by the stringency in the definition change or an effect of the COVID-19 pandemic.[38] The number of HLA mismatches has not been shown to impact pancreas or kidney graft survival in SPK. Technical causes of graft loss (defined as graft failure in the first 90 days) continue to decline over time and in 2022 was low at 6.1%, 5.3%, and 8.8% for SPK, PAK, and PTA, respectively (**Fig. 39.5**).[13] A relationship between low center volume and increased risk of graft failure has been reported.[39,40]

The impact of the change in graft failure definition on longer-term data will not be available for many years, but it has previously been shown that recipient risk factors for decreased pancreas allograft survival include African American race, retransplantation, and high allosensitization. It is important to recognize the improvement in pancreas graft survival rates over time; for SPK 1-year graft survival rates of 85% were reported for SPK transplants done between 2000 and 2004, in contrast to the >90% pancreas graft survival currently reported in the modern era.

For PAK, the 1-year reported pancreas graft survival improved from 78% to 93.2% for transplants performed in 2005 versus 2019.[38] Longer-term graft survival also has improved, with 5-year graft survival reported in 2011 at 53% in contrast to the most recent *10-year* graft survival for PAK of 63.2%.[36]

Likewise, PTA graft survival has improved over time, with 1- and 5-year pancreas graft survival in the United States improved from 76% and 52.2% (transplant cohort 2000 to 2009) compared to 80% and 58.8% for the cohort transplanted from 2010 to 2020.[41] Important differences between the cohorts included improved donor selection with statistically lower CIT and graft failure rates due to graft pancreatitis, vascular thrombosis, and chronic rejection, signifying further maturation of the surgical and medical management of this population.

Effect of Pancreas Transplantation on Secondary Complications of Diabetes Mellitus

The favorable impact of pancreas transplantation on the course of secondary complications of diabetes is clear. This could be predicted from the results of the DCCT, in that pancreas transplantation leads to a complete normalization of blood glucose and glycosylated hemoglobin levels that are superior to even those achievable by intensive insulin therapy.

For example, while type 1 diabetic recipients of kidney-alone transplants develop typical findings of diabetic nephropathy in the allograft, successful SPK transplantation prevents recurrent diabetic nephropathy. The microvascular structural abnormalities in native diabetic nephropathy have demonstrated reversal 10 years following successful isolated pancreas transplantation.[42,43] These reports demonstrate that pancreas transplantation has a significant impact on diabetic nephropathy.

Effects on diabetic neuropathy have also been documented using nerve conduction studies, which are significantly improved following pancreas transplantation.[44] Furthermore, clinical progression of diabetic neuropathy is significantly diminished compared to nontransplanted controls. It has also been shown that pancreas transplantation can impact autonomic neuropathy, with clinical improvement in epinephrine responses to hypoglycemia. Despite commonly described clinical improvements in neuropathy, additional research is needed in this area.

While the DCCT demonstrated a relationship between glycemic exposure and retinopathy, the effect of pancreas transplantation on retinopathy is only modest. Early acceleration of retinopathy, a phenomenon that has been noted with other methods of improving glycemic control, can occur in the first 6 to 12 months following transplant. While stabilization of moderate retinopathy has been demonstrated, long-term graft function (>3 years) is required. Many pancreas transplant candidates have advanced retinopathy, and improvement has not been demonstrated in these individuals.

Pancreas transplantation also appears to have a modest impact on cardiovascular disease parameters. Despite the DCCT trial findings, assessment of the clinical impact of pancreas transplantation on the progression of cardiovascular disease lacks a definitive large-scale study. Positive effects on lipid profiles, hypertension, carotid intimal thickness, and left ventricular ejection fraction have been demonstrated. A positive impact on peripheral vascular occlusive disease has been reported.[45]

Regardless of the magnitude of objectively demonstrable benefits of pancreas transplantation, the freedom from insulin and the avoidance of hyper- and hypoglycemia offered by a functioning pancreas transplant is a primary motivator for many candidates. The fervor with which some patients pursue pancreas transplantation, especially retransplantation, is an indication of the significant benefit on quality of life for these individuals.[46]

ISLET TRANSPLANTATION

Overview

The notion that insulin-producing β-cells could be physically separated from the pancreas and transplanted for the treatment of diabetes has long been recognized. Islet transplantation, as a cellular transplant, has significant potential advantages over whole-organ pancreas transplant due to the minimally invasive nature of the procedure as well as the avoidance of complications of the exocrine pancreas. In addition, the potential ability to preserve islets opens up possibilities with regard to distribution, allocation, and transportation of the islet cell mass. Recipients of successful islet transplants can have glucose metabolism and insulin secretion profiles that are close to normal and maintain metabolic control in a manner equivalent to whole-pancreas transplantation. Although effects on long-term mortality and progression of diabetic complications are unproven, these benefits are also anticipated. From a long-range perspective, technologic advances in islet isolation and autotransplantation following pancreatic resection have paved the way for optimization of allotransplantation (and vice versa), and the development of human islet allotransplantation has informed some of the procedural, technical, and regulatory groundwork for the eventual establishment of stem-cell–derived β-cell transplantation.

History

The development of islet allotransplantation was historically limited by poor graft survival. The first human islet allograft in a type 1 diabetic was performed in 1974 by the University of Minnesota. The first islet autograft for the treatment of chronic pancreatitis was performed at Minnesota in 1977.[47] Despite intense research in islet transplantation over the next nearly three decades, clinical islet allotransplantation was met with minimal success; of the 270 recipients transplanted through 1999, only 6 had achieved insulin independence for greater than 2 years. The dramatic improvement in islet transplant outcome reported by the Edmonton Group in 2000 stimulated an increase in islet transplant activity.[48] Several important refinements in islet isolation and immunosuppression were credited for the improvement, including careful attention to pancreas recovery, minimization of cold ischemia time of the pancreas prior to islet isolation, avoidance of xenoproteins in the isolation process, and avoidance of steroids in the immunosuppressive regimen. The use of sequential infusions to achieve insulin independence has been critical to success for many centers. Subsequently, the enthusiasm that accompanied this success was tempered by (1) the inability for many new centers to replicate the success of more established centers, (2) the disappointing long-term function of the allografts, and (3) the costs associated with islet transplants, which are still not reimbursed by third-party payers and Medicare in the United States, despite abundant evidence of good outcomes in a phase 3 clinical trial.[49] As a result, the volume of islet transplants and the number of centers performing transplants under research protocols contracted over the next decade, and are currently at a steady state of almost nonexistent case volume due to persistent classification as an experimental treatment. The requirement for (and cost of) a biologic license by the US Food and Drug Administration to allow islet transplantation is a significant barrier to adoption of this treatment modality in the United States.[50]

Islet Isolation

The separation of the islets from the other tissues of the pancreas (exocrine cells, lymphatics, and vascular structures) is the most important determinant of successful islet transplantation and is accomplished by a combination of enzymatic digestion of the pancreas by mechanical distension and parenchymal disruption. Following digestion, the separation of islets from non-islet tissue is performed via density gradient centrifugation. After suspension in culture media, islets are counted and assessed for sterility, purity, viability, and functional capacity. Many elements of the process, such as collagenase batch or type, gradient preparation, the use of culture and culture conditions, and additives to prevent islet loss, introduce inherent variability in the process. Stringent product release criteria ensure the quality and suitability of the isolated islets for transplantation. The percentage of islet isolations that result in a transplantable preparation varies widely among centers, between 25% and 70%, and depends on the center's expertise and donor selection practices. One of the limitations of islet isolation is the difficulty in getting a large number of high-quality islets to meet release criteria for transplant, and consistent success in islet isolation is a combination of science, art, and experience.

Patient Selection

Candidate selection for islet transplantation is slightly different from whole-organ pancreas transplantation. Islet transplantation is currently limited to adult type 1 diabetics with progressive diabetic complications who have failed intensive insulin therapy (unlike pancreas transplantation, which is available for patients with non–type 1 diabetes etiologies). Because islet transplantation in the United States is extremely limited in availability, the procedure is generally offered only to ideal candidates with minimal extraneous medical conditions. Nonuremic candidates should be free of renal insufficiency, due to concerns about aggravation of nephropathy by CNIs. Since efficacy of the islet transplant appears to be related to the number of islets transplanted per kilogram of recipient body weight, only lean type 1 candidates are typically selected.

Donor Selection/Recovery/Preservation

Donor selection for islet isolation differs from that for whole-pancreas transplantation in several respects. While the ideal donor for islet isolation is also young and healthy, donors greater than age 50, donors on vasopressors, and obese donors are all suitable for islet isolation. Since the ideal pancreas is easily distensible and digestible, fatty pancreata are felt to be especially suitable, whereas fibrotic pancreata are not.

The pancreas is recovered in a manner similar to whole-pancreas transplantation. However, less attention to preservation of vascular structures is required. Surface cooling following flushing of preservation solution and the avoidance of pancreatic injury is paramount. Use of the two-layer technique of pancreas preservation, using a standard preservation solution (UW solution or HTK) and oxygenated perfluorocarbon solution, has resulted in increased islet yields and permits cold ischemia time up to 18 hours.

Transplant Techniques

The preferred site for islet transplantation is into the portal circulation (**Fig. 39.6**). This can be performed by a mini-laparotomy with infusion of the islets into a peripheral mesenteric vein, but most centers utilize percutaneous transhepatic cannulation of the portal venous system under ultrasound or fluoroscopic guidance using a small gauge (4-French) catheter, which avoids both a surgical incision and general anesthesia. Either approach employs catheter-based infusion of islets into the portal vein. The islets lodge in the hepatic sinusoids and experience passive oxygenation and subacute engraftment through microvascularization. Portal vein pressure is monitored intermittently throughout the procedure. Following the infusion of islets, hemostasis is achieved using a combination of coils and gelfoam. Recipients receive systemic heparinization as well as heparin in the islet preparation. In the perioperative period, patients receive systemic heparinization for prophylaxis against portal vein thrombosis, a now rare but serious complication.

Perioperative Care

Although islet transplantation is in theory an outpatient procedure, it is not uncommon for recipients to receive a few days of inpatient care to be monitored for bleeding. A liver ultrasound is frequently done to assess portal venous flow and to check for hematoma. Intensive glycemic control with insulin in the immediate posttransplant period "rests" the islets and has been shown to enhance medium and long-term islet function.

Immunosuppression

Immunosuppressive regimens for islet transplantation have evolved over time and now commonly employ antilymphocyte antibody therapy for induction, minimize CNIs, and avoid steroid maintenance.[51]

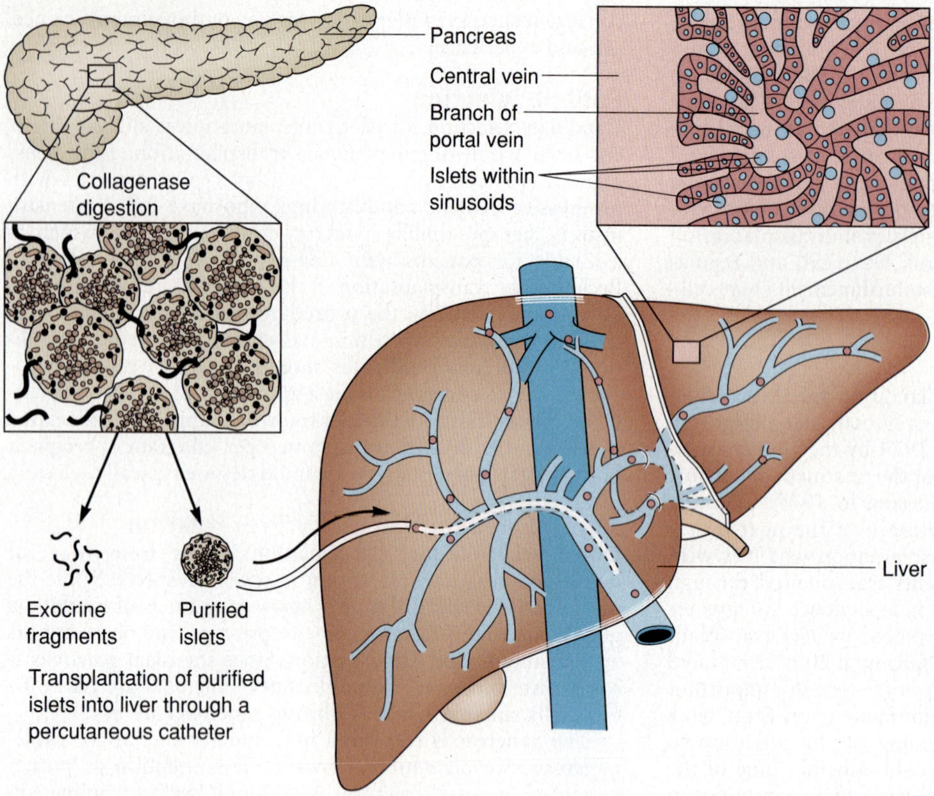

Figure 39.6. Islet transplantation. The pancreas is recovered as a whole organ from the donor. The islets are isolated from the pancreas and are purified and infused into a cannula placed in a branch of the recipient's portal vein.

Metabolic Control

9 Islet recipients show significant improvement in metabolic function and glycemic reserve. Although hormonal counterregulation to hypoglycemia is diminished, actual hypoglycemic events are rare. Islet recipients also demonstrate a reduction in behaviors adopted in avoiding hypoglycemia and an attenuation of concerns about hypoglycemic episodes. However, islet recipients have significantly diminished β-cell reserve and an inability to monitor for rejection compared to recipients of whole-pancreas transplants, which may account for their reduced long-term allograft survival. The Edmonton group recently reported the largest single-center cohort of long-term outcomes of islet allotransplantation, with insulin independence rates of 61% and 32% at 1 and 5 years, respectively, but remarkably, 20% were insulin independent at 10 years and 11% at 20 years follow-up.[52] Insulin independence is approximately 10% lower in islet-after-kidney recipients. In addition to insulin independence, a very important outcome metric for recipients of islet transplantation is freedom from severe hypoglycemic episodes, which has been shown to occur in over 95% of recipients at 5 years posttransplant when donor and recipient factors are ideal.[53]

Complications

Morbidity from islet transplantation is much less than for whole-pancreas transplantation. The most common serious complication is bleeding (1% to 5%), with other complications mostly attributed to immunosuppression. Most cases of bleeding can be managed nonoperatively with adjustments in anticoagulation, however, laparotomy is occasionally required. Transient elevations of portal venous pressure during islet infusion and elevations of liver function tests following infusion are common and usually well tolerated. Renal insufficiency is an uncommon but longer-term serious consequence. CMV infection is rare. Mortality from procedural complications is virtually nil.

Sensitization and the development of posttransplant donor-specific antibody (DSA), which was originally thought not to occur following allogenic islet transplantation, are now recognized as a significant risk. Recent experience has shown that most recipients have increases in DSA or autoantibody (de novo expression or titer increase) after islet transplantation. Recipients who develop an increase in posttransplant antibody have similar initial performance but significantly lower graft survival compared to patients who do not experience an increase. Patients with complete graft loss who discontinue immunosuppression had significantly higher levels of anti-HLA antibodies than those with functioning grafts still on immunosuppression, which may decrease access to whole-organ transplantation. Ways to minimize sensitization in these recipients include minimizing the number of islet donors used per recipient, and avoiding repeating HLA mismatches in subsequent islet infusions.

Results

The short-term results of islet transplantation at high-volume centers continue to approach those of whole-pancreas transplantation, but the long-term rates of insulin independence are lower than observed in whole-pancreas transplants. Recently reported outcomes from a multicenter French study reported 5-year insulin independence rates of 46% for recipients of islet transplantation compared to 73% in PTA (**Fig. 39.7**).[54]

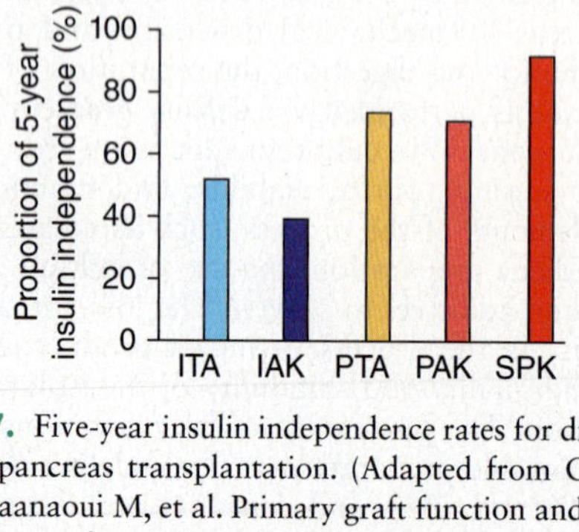

Figure 39.7. Five-year insulin independence rates for different types of islet and pancreas transplantation. (Adapted from Chetboun M, Masset C, Maanaoui M, et al. Primary graft function and 5 year insulin independence after pancreas and islet transplantation for type 1 diabetes: a retrospective parallel cohort study. *Transpl Int.* 2023;36:11950.)[54]

One of the major shortcomings of islet transplantation compared with whole-pancreas transplantation is the potential inability to reverse diabetes with the islets from one pancreas. This is due to extensive early β-cell loss from recipient inflammatory responses to the transplanted islets, as well as inefficient engraftment. Most recipients in the modern era have required two or more islet infusions to achieve insulin independence, but some centers have successfully employed single-donor islet transplantation by utilizing careful donor and recipient selection—usually by transplanting islets from pancreata from large donors into small recipients. Long-term outcome appears to be related to β-cell mass and the avoidance of diabetogenic immunosuppression regimens, and the inability to histologically diagnose and treat islet rejection, since the islets are scattered about the liver parenchyma. Most outcome measures focus on insulin independence as the most stringent definition of graft failure; however, an important benefit of islet transplantation is protection from severe hypoglycemic episodes; this occurs even in the absence of complete insulin independence and contributes to the challenge in describing the functional outcomes and defining success of the procedure.[55] The ability of islet transplantation to favorably compare to whole-pancreas transplantation will depend on minimization of donor pancreas utilization and durability (improved medium- and long-term outcomes) balanced with total cost of the transplant episode.

Alternative Methods

The emergence of pancreatic stem cells as a potential renewable source of insulin-producing cells to treat diabetes has shifted interest and funding somewhat away from islet allotransplantation. β-cells can be isolated from mature islets but can also be derived from either mature or embryonic stem cells, as the biology of β-cell development and differentiation has been well established.[56] These engineered β-cells produce insulin and exhibit glucose responsiveness in vitro. They also reverse diabetes in animal models and in early results of clinical trials. Despite this promise, technical hurdles with scalability and the requirement for systemic immunosuppression remain as potential limitations in this approach.

Islets can be encapsulated in materials designed to be permeable enough to permit the passage of insulin and glucose, but to isolate the islet from the immune system. Pilot clinical trials in humans with encapsulated islets transplanted into the peritoneal cavity without immunosuppression have been reported, which confirms the safety of the procedure and the demonstration of graft function, if not insulin independence. No allo- or autoantibody has been detected in this small number of recipients. Encapsulated human islets can also be shipped safely for long distances after encapsulation and culture without compromising viability and function. The major barriers to graft function and longevity so far have been the tendency of the capsules to cluster and fibrose, which so far has limited their efficacy.

Artificial delivery systems that contain β-cells or islets have been developed that can be implanted either in the abdomen or subcutaneous tissue. These artificial pancreata have semipermeable barriers that allow diffusion and neovascularization but afford immunoprotection and have the advantage of being reloadable and less prone to fibrosis. Other devices are vascularized, which are more complex to implant and can be complicated by thrombosis, but provide better oxygenation and fast exchange of nutrients. They also better maintain concentration gradients by preventing the local buildup of molecules, which is a potential limitation of nonvascularized systems.

Cotransplanting mesenchymal stem cells with islets has been shown to have a beneficial effect on engraftment and islet function by downregulating deleterious cytokine responses, providing multiple growth factors, and their proangiogenic and immunomodulatory effects.[57]

THE FUTURE OF PANCREAS AND ISLET TRANSPLANTATION

Many challenges remain in developing ideal insulin-replacement therapies for insulin-dependent diabetics. The current allocation system is designed to maximize whole-pancreas transplantation and ensures the most efficient use of donor pancreata. Pluripotent mesenchymal stem cell therapy may eventually supersede the supply and outcomes of alloislet transplantation. Importantly, the ability to tailor an "off the shelf" islet product to reduce the number of human pancreata used for transplant, regulatory relief, and the minimization of systemic immunosuppression are key hurdles to the mainstream application of islet transplantation.

ACKNOWLEDGMENT

We gratefully acknowledge the contributions of the previous edition author, Randall S. Sung, as portions of those chapters have been retained in this revision.

TRANSPLANTATION

References

1. Ziegler AG, Rewers M, Simell O, et al. Seroconversion to multiple islet autoantibodies and risk of progression to diabetes in children. *JAMA*. 2013;309(23):2473–2479.
2. Herold KC, Bundy BN, Long SA, et al. An anti-CD3 antibody, teplizumab, in relatives at risk for type 1 diabetes. *N Engl J Med*. 2019;381(7):603–613.
3. Parker ED, Lin J, Mahoney T, et al. Economic costs of diabetes in the U.S. in 2022. *Diabetes Care*. 2024;47(1):26–43.
4. Gregg EW, Pratt A, Owens A, et al. The burden of diabetes-associated multiple long-term conditions on years of life spent and lost. *Nat Med*. 2024;30(10):2830–2837.
5. Nathan DM, Cleary PA, Backlund JY, et al; Diabetes Control and Complications Trial/Epidemiology of Diabetes Interventions and Complications (DCCT/EDIC) Study Research Group. Intensive diabetes treatment and cardiovascular disease in patients with type 1 diabetes. *N Engl J Med*. 2005;353(25):2643–2653.
6. Livingstone SJ, Levin D, Looker HC, et al; Scottish Diabetes Research Network epidemiology group; Scottish Renal Registry. Estimated life expectancy in a Scottish cohort with type 1 diabetes, 2008–2010. *JAMA*. 2015;313(1):37–44.
7. Rawshani A, Rawshani A, Franzen S, et al. Mortality and cardiovascular disease in type 1 and type 2 diabetes. *N Engl J Med*. 2017;376(15):1407–1418.
8. Brown SA, Kovatchev BP, Raghinaru D, et al; iDCL Trial Research Group. Six-month randomized, multicenter trial of closed-loop control in type 1 diabetes. *N Engl J Med*. 2019;381(18):1707–1717.
9. Pelkey MN, Boyle ME, Long A, Castro JC, Cook CB, Thompson B. Hybrid closed-loop insulin pump technology can be safely used in the inpatient setting. *Endocr Pract*. 2023;29(1):24–28.
10. McCune K, Owen-Simon N, Dube GK, Ratner LE. The best insulin delivery is a human pancreas. *Clin Transplant*. 2023;37(4):e14920.
11. Kelly WD, Lillehei RC, Merkel FK, Idezuki Y, Goetz FC. Allotransplantation of the pancreas and duodenum along with the kidney in diabetic nephropathy. *Surgery*. 1967;61(6):827–837.
12. Nghiem DD, Corry RJ. Technique of simultaneous renal pancreatoduodenal transplantation with urinary drainage of pancreatic secretion. *Am J Surg*. 1987;153(4):405–406.
13. Kandaswamy R, Stock PG, Miller JM, et al. OPTN/SRTR 2022 annual data report: pancreas. *Am J Transplant*. 2024;24(2S1):S119–S175.
14. Gruessner RS, Sutherland DER, ed. *Transplantation of the Pancreas*. Springer; 2004.
15. Farney AC, Cho E, Schweitzer EJ, et al. Simultaneous cadaver pancreas living-donor kidney transplantation: a new approach for the type 1 diabetic uremic patient. *Ann Surg*. 2000;232(5):696–703.
16. Kim SJ, Smail N, Paraskevas S, Schiff J, Cantarovich M. Kidney function before pancreas transplant alone predicts subsequent

risk of end-stage renal disease. *Transplantation.* 2014;97(6):675–680.
17. Shah AP, Mangus RS, Powelson JA, et al. Impact of recipient age on whole organ pancreas transplantation. *Clin Transplant.* 2013;27(1):E49–E55.
18. Roll GR, Posselt AM, Freise J, et al. Long-term follow-up of beta cell replacement therapy in 10 HIV-infected patients with renal failure secondary to type 1 diabetes mellitus. *Am J Transplant.* 2020;20(8):2091–2100.
19. Kandaswamy R, Skeans MA, Gustafson SK, et al. OPTN/SRTR 2013 annual data report: pancreas. *Am J Transplant.* 2015;15 Suppl 2:1–20.
20. Organ Procurement and Transplantation Network (OPTN). Policy 11: Allocation of Pancreas, Kidney-Pancreas, and Islets. Accessed October 27, 2024. https://optn.transplant.hrsa.gov/media/eavh5bf3/optn_policies.pdf
21. Kayler LK, Wen X, Zachariah M, Casey M, Schold J, Magliocca J. Outcomes and survival analysis of old-to-old simultaneous pancreas and kidney transplantation. *Transpl Int.* 2013;26(10):963–972.
22. Mittal S, Smilevska R, Franklin R, et al. An analysis of the association between older recipient age and outcomes after whole-organ pancreas transplantation – a single-centre, retrospective study. *Transpl Int.* 2020;33(5):529–535.
23. Alhamad T, Malone AF, Lentine KL, et al. Selected mildly obese donors can be used safely in simultaneous pancreas and kidney transplantation. *Transplantation.* 2017;101(6):1159–1166.
24. Arpali E, Scalea JR, Redfield RR III, et al. The importance and utility of hemoglobin A1c levels in the assessment of donor pancreas allografts. *Transplantation.* 2017;101(10):2508–2519.
25. Axelrod DA, Sung RS, Meyer KH, Wolfe RA, Kaufman DB. Systematic evaluation of pancreas allograft quality, outcomes and geographic variation in utilization. *Am J Transplant.* 2010; 10(4):837–845.
26. Stewart ZA, Cameron AM, Singer AL, Dagher NN, Montgomery RA, Segev DL. Histidine-tryptophan-ketoglutarate (HTK) is associated with reduced graft survival in pancreas transplantation. *Am J Transplant.* 2009;9(1):217–221.
27. Rosenlof LK, Earnhardt RC, Pruett TL, et al. Pancreas transplantation. An initial experience with systemic and portal drainage of pancreatic allografts. *Ann Surg.* 1992;215(6):586–595; discussion 596–597.
28. Kopp WH, van Leeuwen CAT, Lam HD, et al. Retrospective study on detection, treatment, and clinical outcome of graft thrombosis following pancreas transplantation. *Transpl Int.* 2019;32(4):410–417.
29. Cerise A, Shaker T, LeNguyen P, et al. Recipient and graft outcomes in simultaneous kidney and pancreas transplantation with steroid avoidance in the United States. *Transplantation.* 2023;107(2): 521–528.
30. Pierce DR, Gruessner A, Campara M, et al. Impact of early corticosteroid withdrawal on simultaneous pancreas-kidney transplant long-term outcomes: single center experience and comparison to the International Pancreas Transplant Registry. *Clin Transplant.* 2023;37(10):e15063.
31. Finger EB, Radosevich DM, Dunn TB, et al. A composite risk model for predicting technical failure in pancreas transplantation. *Am J Transplant.* 2013;13(7):1840–1849.
32. Kersting S, Ludwig S, Ehehalt F, Volk A, Bunk A. Contrast-enhanced ultrasonography in pancreas transplantation. *Transplantation.* 2013;95(1):209–214.
33. Drachenberg CB, Buettner-Herold M, Aguiar PV, et al. Banff 2022 pancreas transplantation multidisciplinary report: refinement of guidelines for T cell-mediated rejection, antibody-mediated rejection and islet pathology. Assessment of duodenal cuff biopsies and noninvasive diagnostic methods. *Am J Transplant.* 2024; 24(3):362–379.
34. Venstrom JM, McBride MA, Rother KI, Hirshberg B, Orchard TJ, Harlan DM. Survival after pancreas transplantation in patients with diabetes and preserved kidney function. *JAMA.* 2003;290(21): 2817–2823.
35. Gruessner RW, Sutherland DE, Gruessner AC. Survival after pancreas transplantation. *JAMA.* 2005;293(6):675; author reply 675–676.
36. Fridell JA, Niederhaus S, Curry M, Urban R, Fox A, Odorico J. The survival advantage of pancreas after kidney transplant. *Am J Transplant.* 2019;19(3):823–830.
37. Rana A, Gruessner A, Gruessner R. The unequivocal survival benefit of pancreas transplant alone with long-term follow-Up. *Transplantation.* 2014;98:691.
38. Kandaswamy R, Stock PG, Miller JM, et al. OPTN/SRTR 2021 annual data report: pancreas. *Am J Transplant.* 2023;23(2 Suppl 1):S121–S177.
39. Alhamad T, Malone AF, Brennan DC, et al. Transplant center volume and the risk of pancreas allograft failure. *Transplantation.* 2017;101(11):2757–2764.
40. Kopp W, van Meel M, Putter H, et al. Center volume is associated with outcome after pancreas transplantation within the Eurotransplant Region. *Transplantation.* 2017;101(6):1247–1253.
41. Moein M, Papa S, Bahreini A, Saidi R. Pancreas transplant alone in the USA, where do we stand? *World J Surg.* 2023;47(9):2250–2258.
42. Fioretto P, Steffes MW, Sutherland DE, Goetz FC, Mauer M. Reversal of lesions of diabetic nephropathy after pancreas transplantation. *N Engl J Med.* 1998;339(2):69–75.
43. Khairoun M, de Koning EJ, van den Berg BM, et al. Microvascular damage in type 1 diabetic patients is reversed in the first year after simultaneous pancreas-kidney transplantation. *Am J Transplant.* 2013;13(5):1272–1281.
44. Navarro X, Sutherland DE, Kennedy WR. Long-term effects of pancreatic transplantation on diabetic neuropathy. *Ann Neurol.* 1997;42(5):727–736.
45. Knight RJ, Ye Y, Graviss EA, et al. The impact of kidney/pancreas transplantation on peripheral arterial disease. *Clin Transplant.* 2024;38(7):e15413.
46. Scalea JR, Pettinato L, Fiscella B, et al. Successful pancreas transplantation alone is associated with excellent self-identified health score and glucose control: a retrospective study from a high-volume center in the United States. *Clin Transplant.* 2018;32(2): 10.1111/ctr.13177.
47. Sutherland DE, Matas AJ, Goetz FC, Najarian JS. Transplantation of dispersed pancreatic islet tissue in humans: autografts and allografts. *Diabetes.* 1980;29 Suppl 1:31–44.
48. Shapiro AM, Lakey JR, Ryan EA, et al. Islet transplantation in seven patients with type 1 diabetes mellitus using a glucocorticoid-free immunosuppressive regimen. *N Engl J Med.* 2000;343(4): 230–238.
49. Hering BJ, Clarke WR, Bridges ND, et al; Clinical Islet Transplantation Consortium. Phase 3 trial of transplantation of human islets in type 1 diabetes complicated by severe hypoglycemia. *Diabetes Care.* 2016;39(7):1230–1240.
50. Witkowski P, Odorico J, Pyda J, et al; On Behalf Of The Islets For Us Collaborative. Arguments against the requirement of a biological license application for human pancreatic islets: the position statement of the islets for US Collaborative Presented during the FDA Advisory Committee Meeting. *J Clin Med.* 2021;10(13): 2878.
51. Collaborative Islet Transplant Registry 11th Allograft Report. The Emmes Corporation, CITR Coordinating Center. Accessed August 8, 2024. https://www.citregistry.org/system/files/11th_CITR_Network_Report_Allograft_2022_0.pdf
52. Marfil-Garza BA, Imes S, Verhoeff K, et al. Pancreatic islet transplantation in type 1 diabetes: 20-year experience from a single-centre cohort in Canada. *Lancet Diabetes Endocrinol.* 2022;10(7): 519–532.
53. Hering BJ, Ballou CM, Bellin MD, et al. Factors associated with favourable 5 year outcomes in islet transplant alone recipients with type 1 diabetes complicated by severe hypoglycaemia in the Collaborative Islet Transplant Registry. *Diabetologia.* 2023;66(1): 163–173.
54. Chetboun M, Masset C, Maanaoui M, et al. Primary graft function and 5 year insulin independence after pancreas and islet

transplantation for type 1 diabetes: a retrospective parallel cohort study. *Transpl Int*. 2023;36:11950.

55. Rickels MR, Stock PG, de Koning EJP, et al. Defining outcomes for beta-cell replacement therapy in the treatment of diabetes: a consensus report on the Igls criteria from the IPITA/EPITA opinion leaders workshop. *Transplantation*. 2018;102(9):1479–1486.
56. Helman A, Melton DA. A stem cell approach to cure type 1 diabetes. *Cold Spring Harb Perspect Biol*. 2021;13(1):a035741.
57. Sionov RV, Ahdut-HaCohen R. A supportive role of mesenchymal stem cells on insulin-producing Langerhans islets with a specific emphasis on the secretome. *Biomedicines*. 2023;11(9): 2558.

Head and Neck

Kelly Michele Malloy

Key Points

1 Patients with new-onset hoarseness of 2 weeks or greater duration should be evaluated via flexible fiberoptic laryngoscopy.

2 Airway obstruction is a potential concern in many head and neck conditions, be they infectious or neoplastic. Assessment of the airway with nasopharyngolaryngoscopy (NPL) is crucial to safe management of these patients and should be considered early in the evaluation of patients with stridor or other signs of airway compromise.

3 A cystic neck mass in an adult represents a cervical metastasis until proven otherwise; this should be worked up with imaging and fine-needle aspiration (FNA) biopsy and should not be incised and drained.

4 Thoughtful, functional reconstruction of the oral cavity and pharynx is equally important as sound oncologic resection in head and neck surgery.

The head and neck comprises one of the most functionally sensitive anatomic regions of the human body. Disorders of hearing, sight, speech, swallowing, smell, and taste are some of the most frustrating and life altering. There is a great breadth and depth of disease that impacts the head and neck, from infectious abscesses and congenital cysts to cancer. This chapter provides a high-level review of the presentation, assessment, and management of more common head and neck disorders, as well as a template for consultation and collaboration with multidisciplinary specialists when needed.

PATIENT EVALUATION

History

A thorough patient history is critical to accurate diagnosis of head and neck disease. Symptoms such as mass/swelling, pain, drainage, and changes in breathing, swallowing, or speech need to be further explored with questions about timing of onset, pace of progression, and relationship to any constitutional symptoms like weight loss and fevers. Social history is particularly meaningful in head and neck patients. Habitual tobacco and alcohol use increases the risk of head and neck malignancy, with increasing pack years augmenting risk in dose-dependent fashion.[1] Sexual history has become important as increasing number of oral sexual partners is associated with an increased risk of human papilloma virus (HPV)–related oropharyngeal cancer (OPC).[2]

Examination

A complete head and neck examination includes systematic inspection of the head and neck, including each mucosal subsite (**Table 40.1**) via otoscopy, anterior rhinoscopy, and often flexible fiberoptic nasopharyngolaryngoscopy (NPL). Dentures should be removed prior to inspection and bimanual palpation of the oral cavity and oropharynx. Gross craniofacial and/or neck deformity, skin lesions, previous scars, and any radiation sequelae should be noted. Complete cranial nerve examination is critical as even subtle changes in function can
1 guide diagnosis. The head and neck examination also relies on auditory cues: hoarseness, garbled voice, stridor, stertor, and hyper- or hyponasality are all important features of head and neck disease.

Indirect mirror laryngoscopy to visualize the larynx and hypopharynx requires practice, skill, and specialized office equipment to perform well; moreover, patients with active gag reflexes or with larger tongues may be difficult to examine adequately via mirror examination. NPL examination provides improved visualization of the nasal cavity, nasopharynx, larynx and pharynx, including assessment of airway patency, dynamic function of the vocal folds, and sensation of the pharynx; NPL also affords the ability to record images and video when coupled with appropriate equipment, critical to assessing treatment response in cases of malignancy and for enhanced medical record keeping. **Figure 40.1** demonstrates the view of the larynx provided by office NPL.

The neck should be inspected and palpated carefully with particular attention to both salivary glands and cervical lymph nodes. Location of adenopathy or neck mass should be described by level, from I to VI as described by Robbins et al. (**Fig. 40.2**)[3]; tenderness and mobility should also be described. Lymph nodes tend to be mobile in all directions early in disease, but fixation to deep tissues or invasion of overlying skin indicates more advanced disease. A lateral neck mass that is mobile in the anteroposterior dimension, but not superior–inferiorly raises suspicion of paraganglioma or schwannoma. A pulsatile mass suggests a vascular pathology and should not be biopsied without imaging. The larynx and trachea should be palpated to determine any disruption to the normal architecture, tenderness, or deviation due to neck or thyroid masses. The thyroid gland is also palpated as part of every head and neck examination, the specifics of which are addressed in a separate chapter.

Cranial neuropathies deserve special attention, and the clinician must be vigilant for subtle neurologic signs of underlying disease. Hyposmia may be a sign of sinonasal pathology, either due to nasal obstruction or to direct involvement of the olfactory nerve. Extraocular movement abnormalities are presenting symptoms of orbital or skull base pathology.

Table 40.1. Anatomic Subsites of the Head and Neck

Subsite	Anatomy
Anterior skull base	Nasal cavity Paranasal sinuses Orbit
Oral cavity	Anterior 2/3 tongue/floor of mouth Lip/buccal mucosa/teeth/gingiva/retromolar trigone Hard palate
Pharynx	Nasopharynx Oropharynx (soft palate, palatine tonsils, posterior 1/3 tongue/lingual tonsils, posterior pharyngeal wall above the hyoid to level of palate) Hypopharynx (piriform sinuses, postcricoid space, posterior pharyngeal wall below the level of the hyoid)
Larynx	Supraglottis Glottis Subglottis
Salivary	Parotid Submandibular gland Sublingual gland Minor salivary glands
Lateral skull base	Parapharyngeal space Infratemporal fossa Temporal bone

Facial numbness or progressive facial pain raises concern for trigeminal nerve involvement by malignancy. Facial weakness in the setting of a parotid mass suggests malignancy. Bell palsy and trigeminal neuralgia are diagnoses of exclusion and underlying malignancy must first be considered during workup of these cranial neuropathies. Ipsilateral vocal fold paresis or impaired palatal elevation suggests involvement of

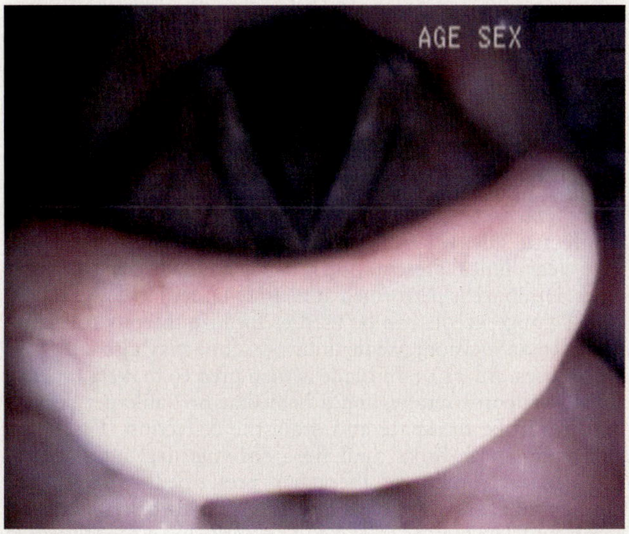

Figure 40.1. Office NPL demonstrates a normal larynx with glottis open.

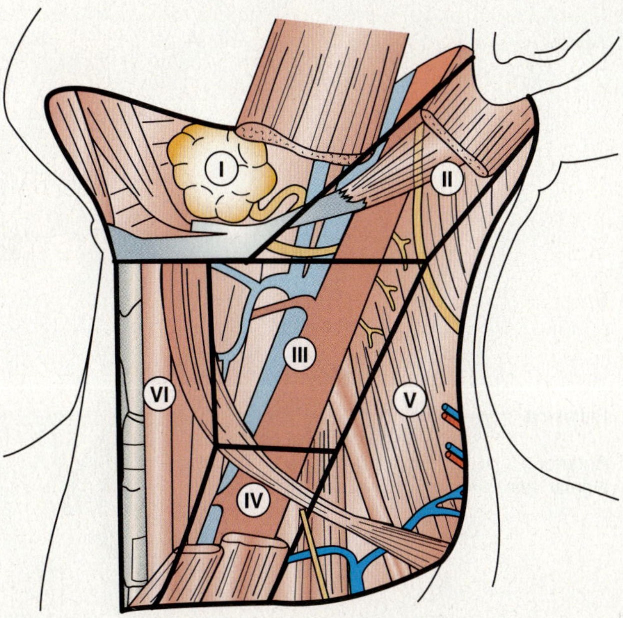

Figure 40.2. The anatomic levels of the cervical lymph nodes.

the vagus nerve by neoplasm. Shoulder weakness in the setting of cervical lymphadenopathy indicates spinal accessory nerve invasion by tumor and would prompt preoperative discussion of radical neck dissection over nerve- and muscle-sparing techniques. Tongue weakness/deviation raises concern for hypoglossal nerve involvement by primary tumor or by level I/II neck disease. Horner syndrome in the context of head and neck malignancy prompts suspicion for sympathetic chain invasion by deep cervical lymphatics.

Workup

In the setting of an accessible tumor (eg, oral tongue, tonsil), biopsy may be performed in the office under local anesthesia. For more distal tumors or in the presence of severe pain, trismus, or brisk gag, operative direct laryngoscopy is warranted. Fine-needle aspiration (FNA) biopsy of neck or salivary masses is recommended in the majority of cases and is enhanced by the use of office-based ultrasound guidance. Obtaining imaging prior to needle biopsy is reasonable in any circumstance when vascular pathology or proximity of pathology to vascular structures is of concern. CT with contrast is the preferred imaging modality for most head and neck pathologies. MRI is useful to evaluate for perineural spread of tumor and for orbital and dural assessment. When malignancy is diagnosed, metastatic workup with PET/CT or chest CT should be performed. National guidelines are available that provide detailed recommendations regarding workup that are more specific than the scope of the chapter; working with head and neck surgical oncology consultants promptly is recommended to avoid unnecessary delays in care.

Airway Concerns

2 The presence of head and neck disease may impact the patient's airway on presentation, but it may also complicate safe airway management during planned surgery. A number of patient factors have been described in the anesthesia literature as predictors of difficult direct laryngoscopy, including sternomental distance, thyromental distance, Mallampati score, and mouth opening; recent review of these bedside techniques reveals high degree of variability and low sensitivity in general.[4] Imaging may assist with assessment and NPL examination by an expert practitioner is critical to evaluate airway patency. A large laryngeal or oropharyngeal mass may lead to failure of mask ventilation and difficulty passing an orotracheal tube; lesions prone to bleeding may cause similar problems. Trismus

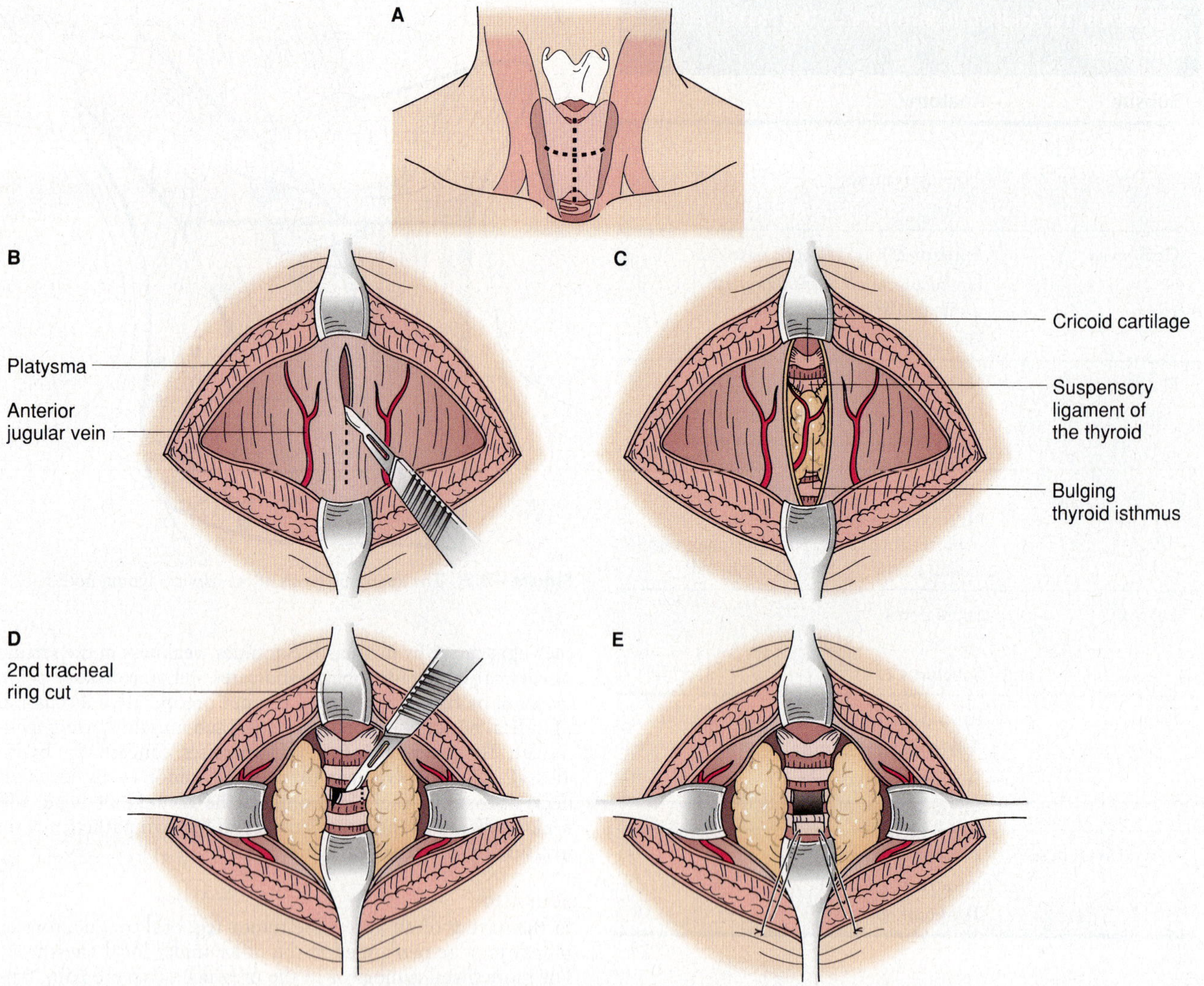

Figure 40.3. Tracheostomy. **A:** The incision for an elective tracheostomy is typically placed on a horizontal axis, approximately two-finger breadths above the sternal notch. A vertical incision allows for less bleeding when the procedure must be performed emergently. **B:** The strap muscles are separated in the midline. **C:** The thyroid isthmus is then encountered and may require division with cautery and/or inferior retraction. **D:** The trachea is entered horizontally, preferably between rings 2 and 3. **E:** An inferiorly based flap (ie, Bjork flap) is developed in the tracheal wall and sutured to the skin or subcutaneous tissues. This allows for easy access to the trachea while the tract is maturing.

secondary to advanced tumor or radiation fibrosis may also impede orotracheal intubation. Extrinsic compression or deviation of the airway by thyroid or neck nodal mass is another situation where head and neck surgeons can assist in airway assessment and management. A prospective study of intubation in patients with head and neck pathology found that a diagnosis of cancer, particularly of the supraglottis or glottis, as well as history of radiation, predicted difficult airway.[5] Surgeon and anesthesiologist thus must communicate clearly about the airway plan prior to induction.

Awake fiberoptic intubation (AFOI) may be safely performed in many such cases with the patient spontaneously breathing, using topical anesthesia and mild sedation to intubate via the nasotracheal or orotracheal route. A tracheotomy kit should always be available for emergent cricothyrotomy or tracheotomy should AFOI prove impossible or the airway becomes further compromised. In cases where NPL examination indicates imminent airway collapse, planned awake tracheotomy is the safest option. Early consultation with otolaryngology—head and neck surgery—is strongly encouraged in difficult airway cases. **Figure 40.3** demonstrates the steps of a tracheotomy.

INFECTIOUS AND INFLAMMATORY DISEASE OF THE HEAD AND NECK

Neck Abscesses

Peritonsillar abscess (PTA) is a complication of untreated or undertreated bacterial pharyngitis. Trismus is a hallmark of PTA, alongside symptoms of dysphagia, odynophagia, and a muffled "hot potato" voice. Physical examination reveals soft palate and tonsillar bulging with uvula deviation toward the unaffected side. CT neck is typically unnecessary in patients with clear clinical presentation but may have a role in equivocal cases. Drainage is performed at bedside under local anesthesia. An 18-gauge needle can be used to localize the pus collection and plan an incision; needle drainage alone may also suffice in some cases. An 11 or 15 blade is then used to make a cruciate incision superolaterally, and a hemostat or Yankauer suction used to probe the space and drain the collection (**Fig. 40.4**). Antibiotics with broad oral flora coverage (eg, amoxicillin–clavulanate) should be thereafter prescribed and adjusted once cultures are available. Patients with a history of multiple/recurrent PTAs may be considered for subsequent tonsillectomy.

Patients with epiglottitis may present similarly to PTA with odynophagia, muffled voice, and drooling; trismus, however,

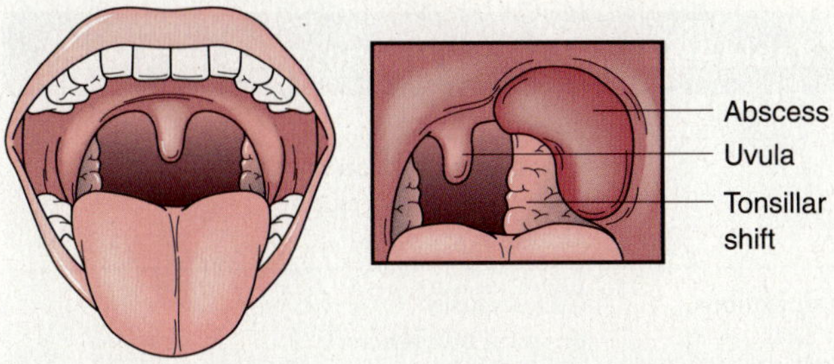

Figure 40.4. Schematic representation of a peritonsillar abscess. Purulence develops between the tonsillar capsule and the superior pharyngeal constrictor muscle. As a result, the palate bulges and the tonsil are deviated medially. Inflammation in the region of the pterygoid muscles results in pain and trismus which may be significant.

is usually absent. Epiglottitis patients have impending airway compromise and must be managed promptly. Lateral neck plain films demonstrate a classic "thumbprint sign" of an edematous epiglottis. NPL examination can be used to confirm the diagnosis, but early securing of the airway in the operating room via AFOI or awake tracheotomy is paramount.

Odontogenic and pharyngeal infections can progress to deep neck space infections, particularly in diabetic patients. Early evaluation of the patient's airway is critical as airway compromise may evolve rapidly. Elective intubation should be considered, and tracheotomy may be necessary in the setting of airway edema. Of particular concern are infections involving the floor of mouth, or Ludwig angina, which cause airway compromise via posterior displacement of the base of tongue. Infections in other neck spaces, including retropharyngeal, parapharyngeal, and prevertebral spaces, may spread quickly and cause rapid decompensation via mediastinitis. **Figure 40.5** lists the relevant deep neck spaces and paths of spread.

Incision and drainage with copious irrigation and placement of dependent drains is the treatment of choice for deep neck space infection. Surgical re-exploration is occasionally needed. Culture-guided antibiotics and control of blood glucose levels are also indicated. If odontogenic in origin, the source tooth should also be addressed. Sheikh et al.'s work reveals the paucity of high-level evidence around optimal management of neck abscesses in adults, however, drainage and antibiotics remain the mainstay of safe treatment of these patients.[6]

Complications of Rhinosinusitis

Acute rhinosinusitis may be viral or bacterial and presents with fever, facial pressure, pain, nasal obstruction, and

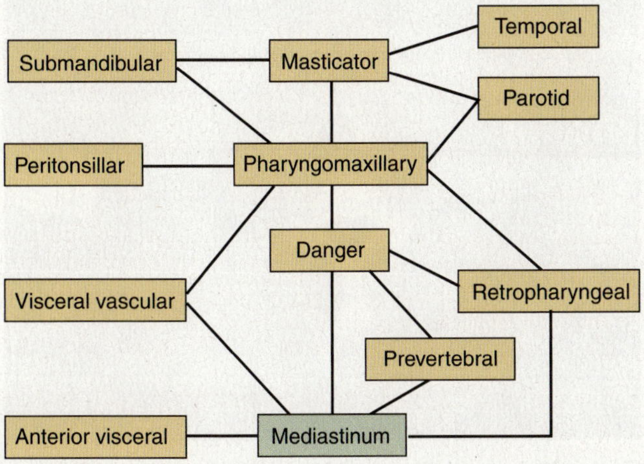

Figure 40.5. The deep spaces of the neck are distinct but interconnected compartments. Infections in any one of these may spread to involve other potential spaces and critical structures contained therein.

Table 40.2. Complications of Sinusitis

Local
Mucocele
Pott puffy tumor
Osteomyelitis
Orbital
Preseptal cellulitis
Orbital (postseptal) cellulitis
Subperiosteal abscess
Orbital abscess
Cavernous sinus thrombosis
Intracranial
Meningitis
Epidural abscess
Subdural abscess
Intracerebral abscess
Cavernous sinus thrombosis
Superior sagittal sinus thrombosis

From Epstein VA, Kern RC. Invasive fungal sinusitis and complications of sinusitis. *Otolaryngol Clin North Am.* 2008;39(3):497–524; with permission.

purulent or discolored nasal discharge. The American Academy of Otolaryngology-Head and Neck Surgery Clinical Practice Guideline for adult sinusitis notes that the vast majority of upper respiratory tract infections (URIs) are viral, and that bacterial rhinosinusitis should be suspected when symptoms persist after 10 days or worsen after a period of initial improvement.[7] Surgery is not indicated for patients with acute sinusitis unless orbital or intracranial complications occur. Complicated acute bacterial rhinosinusitis (**Table 40.2**) should be suspected when visual, mental status, or neurologic changes are present. Proptosis, chemosis, and periorbital edema may signify orbital abscess (**Fig. 40.6**). Contrast-enhanced CT and MRI are warranted in most cases.

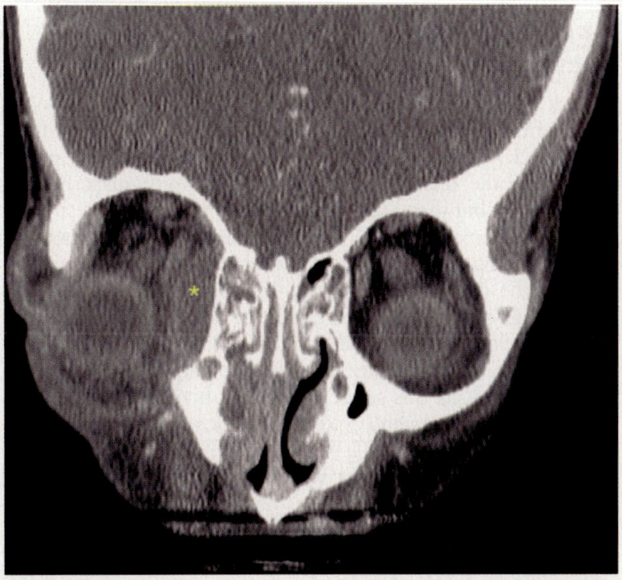

Figure 40.6. Coronal CT sinuses with contrast demonstrates a right-sided periorbital abscess (*asterisk*) arising in a child with acute bacterial ethmoid sinusitis. Urgent ophthalmologic consultation was obtained, which revealed increased intraocular pressure. The child was taken for endoscopic ethmoidectomy and orbital decompression.

Prompt consultation with otolaryngology, ophthalmology, and/or neurosurgery is imperative.

Rapid-onset, severe rhinosinusitis in the immunocompromised (neutropenic, HIV, poorly controlled diabetic or transplanted patients) prompts concern for acute invasive fungal sinusitis. Rapidly progressive and fatal if untreated, the organisms most commonly associated are from the genera *Aspergillus, Rhizopus, Mucor, Rhizomucor,* and *Absidia.*[8] Nasal endoscopy demonstrates pale or black necrotic mucosa of the turbinates or septum. Frozen section biopsy is performed as immediate diagnosis is imperative. The patient should be emergently and aggressively debrided to bleeding tissue in the operating room, tissue sent for cultures, and antifungal therapy initiated in consultation with Infectious Disease specialists. Reversal of the underlying immunocompromised state (ie, aggressive control of hyperglycemia) improves prognosis as well.

Sialadenitis

Patients who are debilitated, dehydrated, or have decreased salivary flow due to medications or xerostomia are predisposed to salivary gland infections. Sialadenitis is a clinical diagnosis, based on tense, tender swelling of the affected gland, fevers, and presence of purulence from Warthin or Stensen duct. Viral sialadenitis (mumps, HIV) tends to be bilateral. Bacterial sialadenitis is most often caused by *Staphylococcus aureus,* although a variety of anaerobes and other oral pathogens may be cultured.[9]

Patients with uncomplicated sialadenitis should be treated with hydration, sialogogues, gland massage, and broad-spectrum antibiotics if bacterial pathogens are suspected. Worsening of symptoms after initiation of therapy should prompt consideration of abscess development, and imaging with ultrasound or contrast-enhanced CT should be performed. Recurrent or chronic salivary infections should prompt suspicion for structural or inflammatory disorders. Structural disease includes salivary stones or strictures, while connective tissue disorders, such as Sjögren syndrome, rheumatoid arthritis, and sarcoidosis may present with or develop sialadenitis. When sialadenitis recurs, CT imaging should be undertaken to evaluate for stones or underlying duct-obstructing tumor. Abscess drainage must be thoughtful of the course of the facial nerve, with carefully placed incisions and dissection parallel to its branches.

NECK MASSES: CYSTIC NECK INFECTION OR MALIGNANCY?

3 A neck mass, solid or cystic, should be presumed malignant until definitive expert evaluation proves otherwise. Congenital cystic neck masses and infectious/inflammatory adenopathy remain on the differential diagnosis for adult neck masses (**Table 40.3**), but they are rare, and the first thought must be of neoplastic etiologies. HPV-related oropharyngeal squamous cell carcinoma (SCC) frequently presents with a cystic neck mass as the only symptom (**Fig. 40.7**); central necrosis with hemorrhage or superinfection can cause pain and rapid growth, thus mimicking an infected congenital mass or suppurative node. Incision and drainage must be avoided in cases of possible malignancy, as this seeds the neck soft tissues with tumor and may limit treatment options and efficacy. Prompt imaging with contrast-enhanced CT, FNA biopsy, and referral to a head and neck surgical oncologist will avoid delays in cancer diagnosis and treatment. If FNA does not yield sufficient material for diagnosis, repeat image-guided FNA or core biopsy in collaboration with a head and neck surgeon is preferrable over open excision. A complete head and neck exam, including possible operative direct laryngoscopy with biopsy should also be entertained to identify possible primary tumor sites.[10]

Algorithm 40.1 is a suggested approach to the adult with a lateral neck mass.

Table 40.3. Differential Diagnosis of a Neck Mass

Congenital	Branchial cleft cyst Vascular malformation Thyroglossal duct cyst Dermoid
Infectious	Tuberculosis Atypical mycobacteria Cat scratch disease Mononucleosis Odontogenic Sialadenitis
Inflammatory	Sarcoidosis Sialadenosis
Trauma	Hematoma Laryngocele
Neoplasm	Epithelial (SCC, melanoma, adenocarcinoma) Salivary Neurogenic (schwannoma, paraganglioma) Sarcoma Lipoma Lymphoproliferative

SALIVARY NEOPLASMS

Salivary tumors include a diverse array of benign and malignant pathologies (**Table 40.4**). The parotid is the most commonly affected gland and ~80% of parotid tumors are benign. Pleomorphic adenoma, or benign mixed tumor, is the most common benign tumor. Warthin tumor, or papillary cystadenoma lymphomatosum, another common pathology noted predominantly in male smokers, may be bilateral and tends to locate in the tail of the parotid gland.[11,12] These and other benign salivary tumors present as a painless firm mass of the affected gland, though those arising in the deep lobe of the gland or in the parapharyngeal space, may grow quite large before they are noted clinically. While Warthin tumor is often observed, surgical resection of pleomorphic adenoma via parotidectomy is recommended due the low but real rate of malignant transformation.

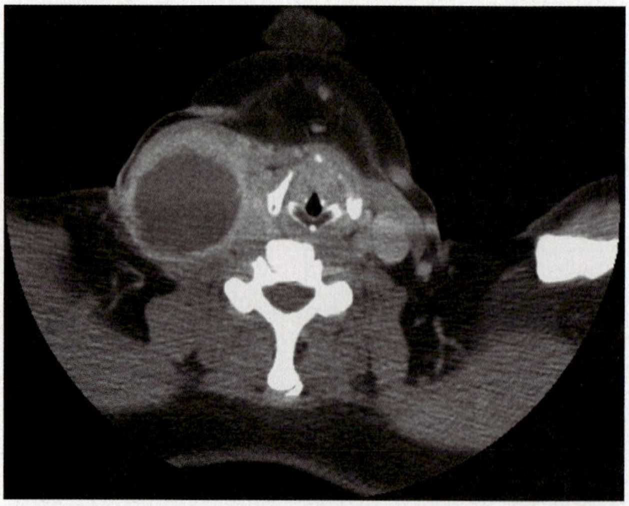

Figure 40.7. Axial CT neck with contrast shows a large cystic mass involving the right level III/IV neck. Image-guided FNA confirmed HPV-positive squamous cell carcinoma.

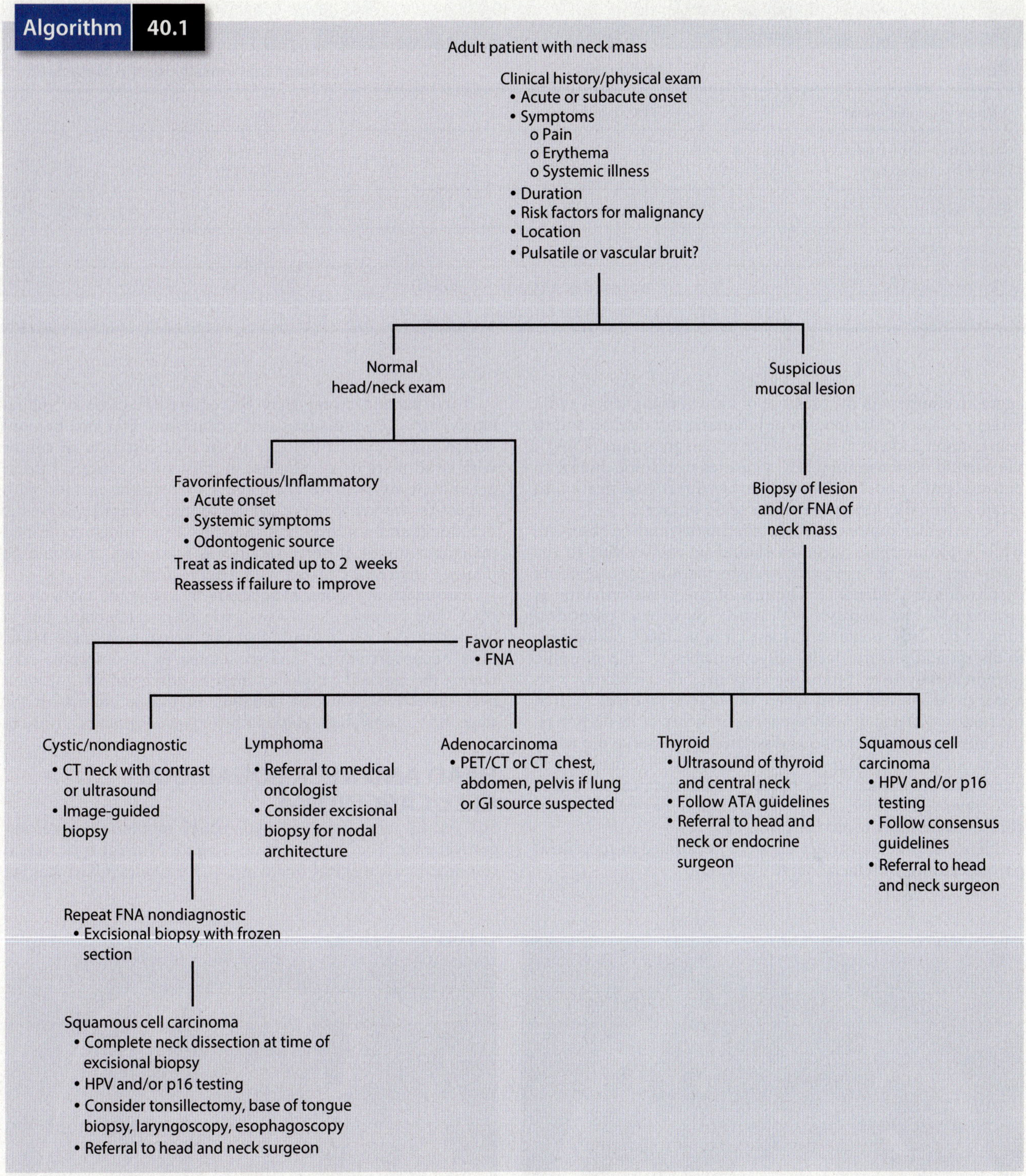

Algorithm 40.1. Workup of a neck mass in an adult patient.

Figure 40.8A,B demonstrates MRI characteristics of a pleomorphic adenoma on MRI.

A salivary mass that presents with pain, rapid growth, or facial nerve weakness must prompt immediate suspicion for malignancy. There is an inverse relationship between size of the gland and rate of malignancy: ~20% of parotid tumors harbor malignancy, 50% for the submandibular gland, and as high as 86% for the sublingual gland. Mucoepidermoid carcinoma (MEC) is the most common malignant salivary tumor, followed by adenoid cystic carcinoma (ACC) and adenocarcinoma.[11] The American Joint Committee on Cancer (AJCC) Cancer Staging Manual provides T-staging for salivary cancer.[13]

FNA biopsy should be considered prior to surgery alongside imaging (contrast-enhanced CT or MRI). The surgeon should be aware that historically the specificity of FNA for neoplasia and malignancy is high, however the sensitivity is lower.[14] A new cytopathology system, The Milan system for Reporting Salivary Gland Cytopathology (MSRSGC) was published in 2018 to better address the risk of malignancy (ROM) in various salivary cytopathologic entities. Retrospective application of the system indicates accuracy in ROM prediction with potential improvements in surgeons' ability to recommend and plan surgery as wider adoption of the MSRSGC rolls out.[15,16] That said, proper workup can direct the surgeon toward more

Table 40.4. Salivary Tumors

Benign	Malignant	Malignant Nonsalivary and Metastatic
Pleomorphic adenoma	Mucoepidermoid carcinoma	Lymphoma
Warthin tumor (papillary cystadenoma lymphomatosum)	Adenoid cystic carcinoma	Squamous cell carcinoma
Basal cell adenoma	Adenocarcinoma	Melanoma
Oncocytoma	Acinic cell carcinoma	
Hemangioma	Carcinoma ex pleomorphic adenoma Salivary ductal carcinoma	

aggressive surgery in the presence of known malignancy, avoid surgery in cases of lymphoma or inflammatory disease, and to help counsel patients in the presence of benign tumors. FNA of the parotid demonstrating SCC indicates metastatic disease to parotid lymph nodes and would further direct investigation to locate a primary skin cancer of the scalp or face.

Some benign tumors, like Warthin tumors, may be observed, while a pleomorphic adenoma should be excised due to the long-term risk of malignant transformation to carcinoma ex pleomorphic adenoma. The risk of this transformation is around 6%, and increases with time.[19] Superficial parotidectomy is typically adequate in these circumstances, taking care to dissect and preserve facial nerve branches.[17–19] Pleomorphic adenomas may have "tumor pseudopodia," thus resection with a margin of normal gland where possible is favored.[20] Often the tumor is sitting directly on nerve branches at its deep margin, however, and meticulous dissection to preserve the nerve and avoid tumor spillage is critical. Tumor spillage may lead to multifocal recurrence in the operative bed. Surgical salvage is recommended in these cases,[18] but radiation may provide local control in multiply recurrent cases.

Figure 40.9 demonstrates the steps performed in superficial parotidectomy with facial nerve dissection.

Total parotidectomy may be required in cases of malignancy, however, a diagnosis of malignancy may not be confirmed until final pathology; an en bloc resection of tumor with good margins is adequate in most small cancers.[19] Total parotidectomy is more challenging to perform en bloc with respect to the facial nerve, which should always preserved if functional and not grossly invaded by a pathology-confirmed malignant tumor. If nerve sacrifice is warranted, it should be immediately reconstructed with a nerve graft.

Parotidectomy alone is adequate in low-grade malignancy (ACC and polymorphous low-grade adenocarcinoma), but in high-grade cancers (salivary duct carcinoma, high-grade MEC, most adenocarcinomas, and carcinoma ex pleomorphic adenoma), the regional lymphatics must be addressed via ipsilateral neck dissection. Adjuvant radiation should be considered for stage III/IV disease, high-grade pathology, and perineural invasion.

HEAD AND NECK SQUAMOUS CELL CARCINOMA

SCC is the most common malignancy of the upper aerodigestive tract. The AJCC Cancer Staging Manual is a critical resource in all surgical oncology, and provides TNM staging

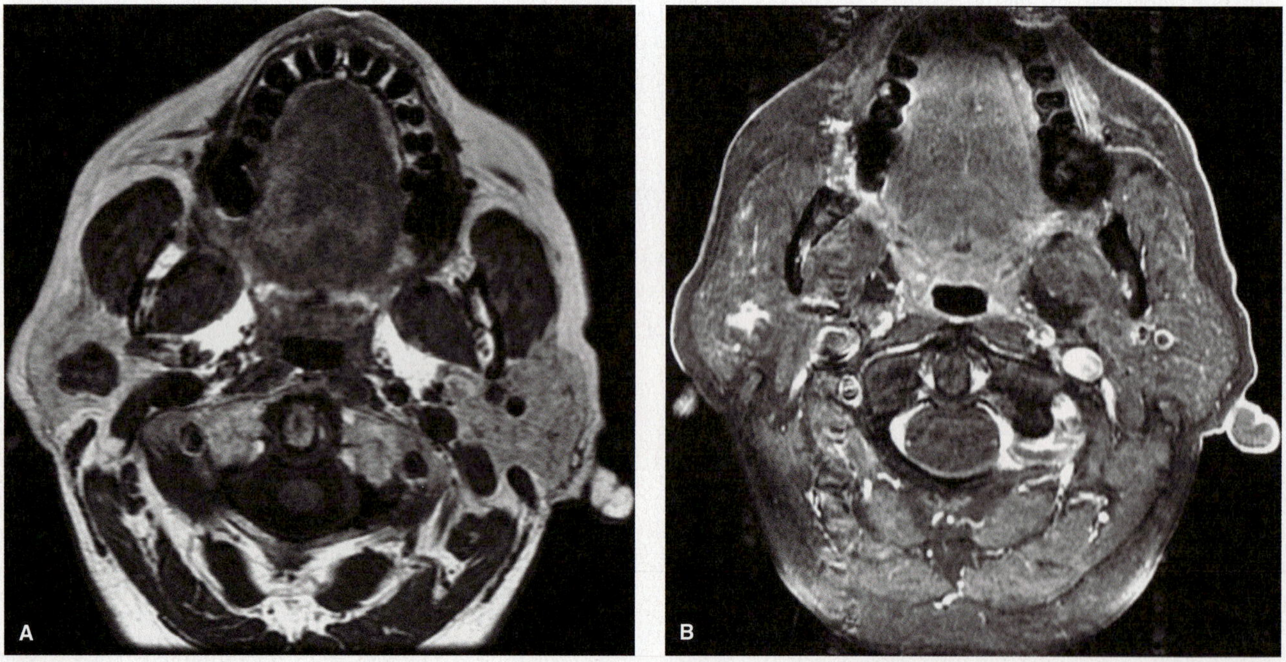

Figure 40.8. Precontrast (**A**) and postcontrast (**B**) T1 MRI demonstrate a lobulated, heterogeneous mass within the right parotid gland just posterior to the retromandibular vein, consistent with a pleomorphic adenoma.

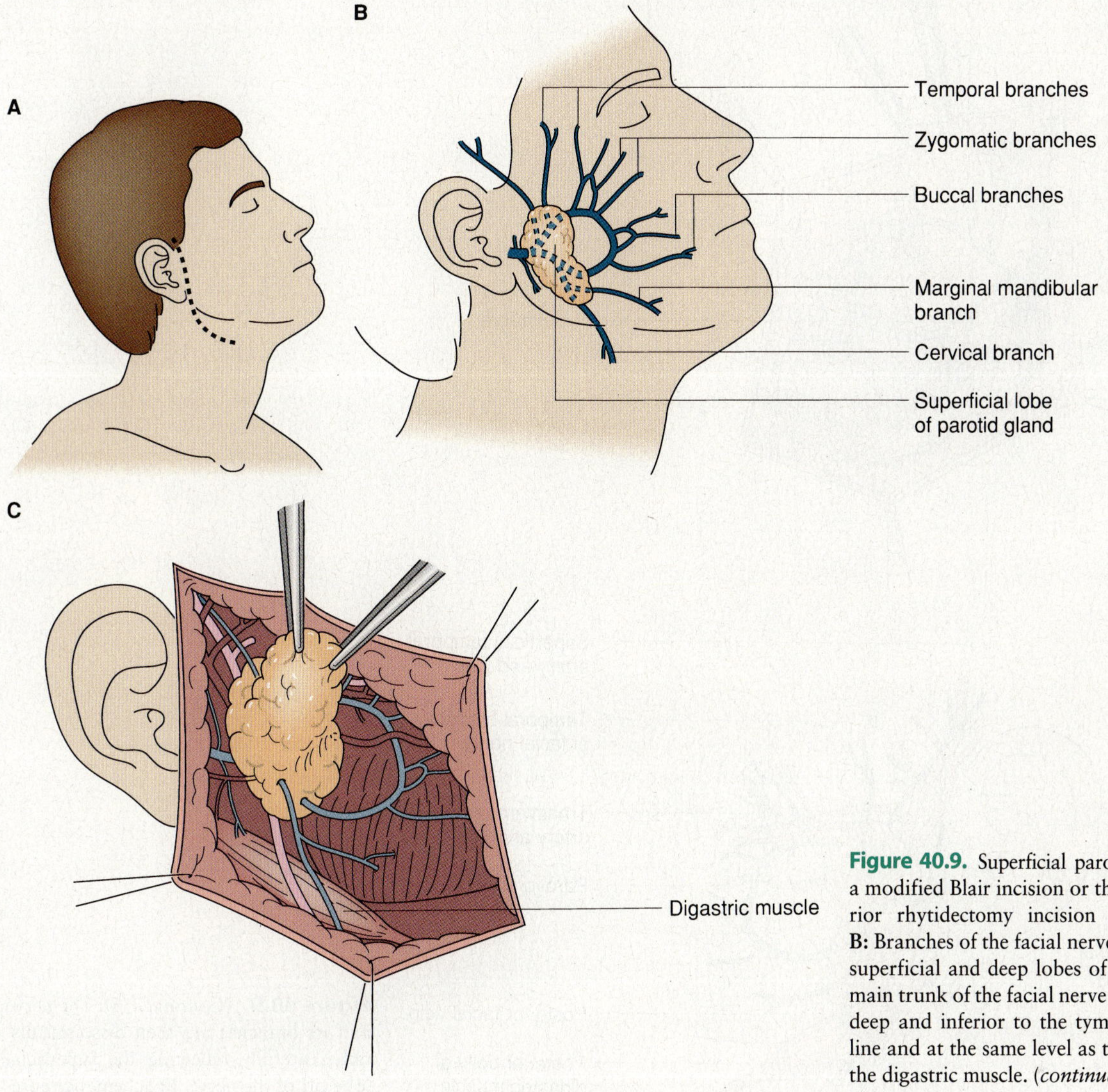

Figure 40.9. Superficial parotidectomy. **A:** Either a modified Blair incision or the cosmetically superior rhytidectomy incision may be employed. **B:** Branches of the facial nerve course between the superficial and deep lobes of the parotid. **C:** The main trunk of the facial nerve is located 3 to 4 mm deep and inferior to the tympanomastoid suture line and at the same level as the posterior belly of the digastric muscle. (*continued*)

for head and neck SCC, as well as updated nodal staging that accounts for the prognostic differences of nodal disease in HPV-positive versus HPV-negative SCC.[13] Generally speaking, patients with AJCC stage I/II tumors are often considered for single-modality treatment, either primary surgery or primary radiation in most cases. Patients with stage III/IV require multimodality treatment, often including systemic therapy; as such, most patients will benefit from evaluation and treatment in a multidisciplinary head and neck cancer program.

Oral Cavity

Cancers of the oral cavity should be considered for primary surgery to optimize oncologic outcomes and to avoid complications of definitive radiation or chemoradiation (ie, osteoradionecrosis of the mandible) whenever possible. Given the sensitive functional nature of the structures of the oral cavity, thoughtful reconstruction is as important as oncologically sound resection of malignancy for these patients to achieve quality survivorship. Microvascular free tissue reconstruction is a mainstay of oral cavity malignancy surgery as it restores structure and function of the oral cavity to maintain speech and swallowing.

4

Lip carcinomas pose both functional and cosmetic concerns. Lower lip cancer is more common than upper lip cancer and is most often caused by sun exposure; it has a very low incidence of occult cervical metastases (<15%) thus the bilateral necks may be observed in cT1–2 N0 disease as noted in consensus guidelines. The upper lip has unilateral nodal drainage but a higher incidence of occult nodal involvement compared to cancers of the lower lip. Reconstruction of the lip ranges from primary closure (after wedge resection of the primary) to local advancement or rotational flaps to free flap reconstruction for larger and more complex lip defects.[21]

Depth of invasion (DOI) in oral tongue and floor of mouth cancer is important for prognosis, so much so that the AJCC 8th edition added DOI to the staging system.[13] Thin tumors (<2 mm) have less regional lymphatic metastatic potential compared to thick tumors (>8 to 9 mm). Many head and neck surgeons recommend elective neck dissection for patients with T1 tumors and DOI >4 mm; sentinel node many be considered in experienced hands for tumors 2 to 4 mm DOI.[22,23] T1–T2 tongue tumors may be resected and closed primarily or with a skin or acellular dermis graft; larger defects and those involving the floor of the mouth require microvascular reconstruction to restore the tongue mound and facilitate recovery of articulation and swallowing. Similarly, small floor of mouth resections may be closed primarily or skin grafted, but free tissue is needed for larger defects, particularly when simultaneous neck dissection is performed.

SCC of the retromolar trigone and buccal mucosa/buccal space often demonstrates early involvement of the muscles of mastication. Pterygoid or masseter invasion causes trismus and pain and may make preoperative examination a challenge for both patient and surgeon. Marginal mandibulectomy

D

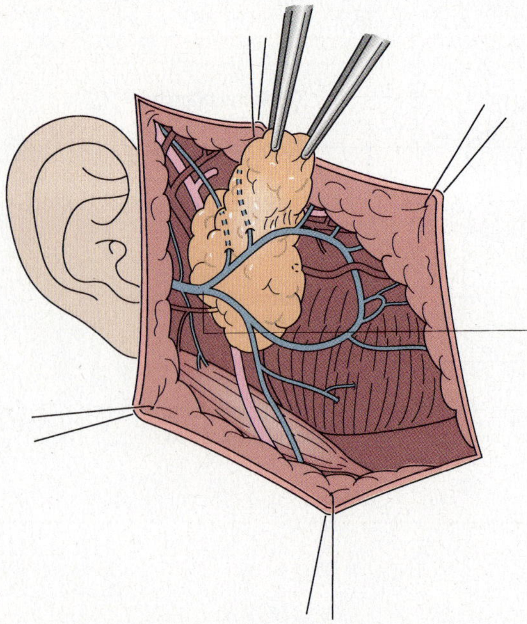

E

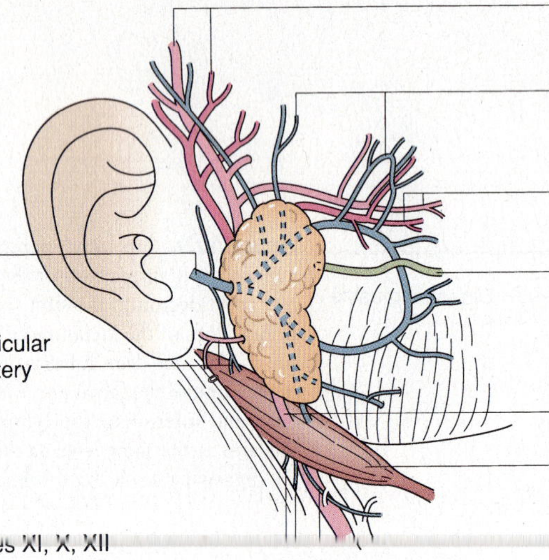

Figure 40.9. *(Continued)* **D:** The nerve and its branches are then dissected distally, carefully reflecting the superficial lobe off of the nerve. **E:** Schematic representation of the relationship between the parotid and surrounding structures.

is necessary when a retromolar trigone tumor is attached to mandibular periosteum. Composite resection of a segment of mandible should be performed when tumor invades bone. Osteocutaneous free tissue reconstruction is the gold standard for segmental defects. While an unreconstructed lateral mandible defect, or "mandibular swing," causes malocclusion and cosmetic asymmetry, failure to reconstitute the anterior mandibular arch leads to swallowing and airway compromise; loss of the anterior mandibular arch causes the lip and chin to migrate posteriorly and inferiorly into the neck, releases the tongue posteriorly, and thus adversely impacts oral competence, deglutition, speech, and airway. Tempting as it may be to place a titanium reconstruction plate across a segmental defect of the mandible, this should be avoided due to inevitable delayed hardware extrusion that occurs with mere plating and soft tissue coverage alone. This reinforces the need to refer complex oral cavity cancer patients to a center where microvascular free tissue reconstructive surgery of the head and neck is available.

Nasopharynx

Nasopharyngeal carcinoma (NPC) is endemic to certain parts of Asia, particularly southern China. The most important causal factor is Epstein–Barr virus (EBV).[24–26] The World Health Organization classifies NPC into three types: keratinizing SCC (I), nonkeratinizing SCC (II), and undifferentiated carcinoma (III). Endemic NPC is 95% type III, which is associated with the best prognosis, and types I and II are more common in nonendemic areas.[27]

NPC most commonly presents with bulky cervical adenopathy. Primary tumors do not typically cause symptoms until quite advanced. Unilateral otitis media in an adult should prompt a scope examination of the nasopharynx as this may be due to Eustachian tube obstruction by tumor. More advanced tumors may present with nasal obstruction or changes in speech due to palatal involvement. Cranial neuropathies are a hallmark of skull base invasion. Interestingly, large-volume lymphadenopathy alone is less prognostic in NPC than in other head and neck malignancies; it is the involvement of the supraclavicular nodes that portends a worse prognosis. This is reflected in a separate nodal staging paradigm for NPC.[13]

Endoscopic biopsy of the nasopharynx or FNA of lymph nodes confirms NPC; staining for EBV is also performed and is key to making the diagnosis from a neck node. Imaging should include contrast-enhanced CT and MRI to evaluate the skull base and infratemporal fossa. PET/CT is also obtained for complete staging and planning of radiation fields. The primary treatment for NPC is chemoradiation which has been shown to be superior to radiation alone in advanced disease.[28,29] Surgery is reserved for recurrent/persistent localized disease in select cases; small tumors may be amenable to an endoscopic approach but may require an open transfacial approach with maxillary disarticulation for adequate exposure and protection of the carotid artery.[30–32]

Oropharynx

The overall incidence of head and neck SCC in the United States has decreased in concert with the decrease in tobacco abuse in recent decades; a notable exception to this trend is in cancers of the oropharynx. OPC incidence has risen over the past two decades due to the increase in HPV transmission and chronic infection. HPV, particularly subtypes 16 and 18, appears to be responsible for approximately 80% of OPC.[33] Interestingly, HPV-associated OPC is associated with a more favorable prognosis compared to the tobacco-related "classic" HPV-negative cancers of the head and neck, even in advanced local and regional disease states.[34,35] This difference in prognosis led to changes in the AJCC staging system that account for the differences between HPV-positive and HPV-negative tumors. These include the findings that nodal metastases are less impactful on survival for HPV-positive OPC patients, and extranodal extension of tumor does not appear to impart the same poor prognosis as in HPV-negative SCC disease.[13]

T1 and T2 tumors of the palatine tonsils are typically amenable to transoral resection, but radiation and chemoradiation have been used since the 1990s to treat less accessible (ie, lingual tonsil) and larger tumors due to equivalent effectiveness and decreased morbidity and mortality compared to open surgical approaches (ie, mandibulotomy/transmandibular approach, transcervical and transpharyngeal approaches).[36] Both the increasing prevalence of HPV-positive OPC patients with favorable prognoses and the advent of transoral, minimally invasive surgical approaches to the oropharynx, have led to increased interest in primary surgery to avoid the long-term sequelae of chemotherapy and even radiation in these younger patients. Transoral laser microsurgery (TLM) and transoral robotic surgery (TORS) have emerged in the past 15 years as viable treatments for T1–T3 OPC with acceptable oncologic and functional outcomes.[37–40]

Hypopharynx

The hypopharynx is the area between the oropharynx and cervical esophagus. Cancers of the hypopharynx usually present in advanced stages as symptoms are delayed until the tumor is large enough to impede swallowing or invade the larynx. Patients report gradually increasing dysphagia, hoarseness, neck mass, and referred otalgia via Jacobson and Arnold nerves (branches of cranial nerves IX and X, respectively).

Hypopharyngeal SCC has the poorest prognosis of the head and neck subsites, with an overall survival of only 30% to 35% in early-stage cancer,[41] and a rate of distant metastases of up to 60%.[42] Surgical resection usually requires total laryngectomy with partial or complete pharyngectomy due to the intimate proximity of the piriform sinuses/postcricoid mucosa and the larynx; as such primary chemoradiation approaches predominate initial treatment algorithms. Small tumors of the posterior pharyngeal wall may be amenable to resection via transoral laser or robotic techniques.[43,44] Due to the rich lymphatics of the hypopharynx, bilateral neck treatment is required for regional control. Recurrent hypopharyngeal SCC following chemoradiation typically requires salvage total laryngopharyngectomy; free tissue reconstruction is critical to reconstitute the pharynx, either with a tubed fasciocutaneous free flap or an enteric flap such as the gastro-omental free tissue transplant.

Larynx

The glottic larynx, composed primarily by the true vocal folds, is the most common site of origin of laryngeal SCC, followed by the supraglottis (tip of the epiglottis to the laryngeal ventricle), and subglottis (just below the true vocal folds to the inferior border of the cricoid cartilage). The glottis consists of nonkeratinizing stratified squamous epithelium overlying a complex lamina propria over the thyroarytenoid ligament and muscle. Early glottic tumors have a low rate of metastasis to regional lymphatics due to the investing fibroelastic structure of the conus elasticus and quadrangular membrane. By way of contrast, supraglottic and subglottic are known for their risk of bilateral nodal metastasis even in early disease.

Early (T1–T2) glottis cancers may be managed with single-modality treatment—either radiation or endolaryngeal surgery—with long-term control rates of approximately 90% for T1 and 75% for T2 tumors. Surgical treatment is performed via transoral resection, often using CO_2 laser, or via open partial laryngectomy techniques. Surgery has no statistically significant difference in local control, overall or disease-free survival compared to narrow-field radiation, although laryngeal preservation rates appear to be higher in surgical patients based on retrospective studies.[45–47] Early supraglottic carcinoma has a high incidence of occult nodal metastasis and for both surgical and radiation based treatments of the supraglottis, bilateral levels II to IV neck nodes must be addressed alongside the primary tumor.

Advanced laryngeal cancer (T3–T4, N positive) requires multimodality treatment. This may be primary surgery followed by radiation or concurrent chemoradiation. The landmark "VA Larynx Trial" demonstrated equivalent survival between surgery followed by radiation versus induction chemotherapy followed by radiation, with 64% laryngeal preservation in the nonsurgical arm.[48] The RTOG 91–11 trial demonstrated the superiority of concurrent chemoradiation compared to radiation alone or after induction chemotherapy for laryngectomy-free survival and local control.[49] However, the 10-year follow-up to this study did not demonstrate an advantage of concurrent chemoradiation versus induction chemotherapy and radiation in overall survival, local control, or overall laryngeal preservation.[50]

Surgical treatment for advanced-stage laryngeal cancer is typically total laryngectomy with bilateral neck dissections. Speech is restored via esophageal speech training, tracheoesophageal puncture with prosthesis, or electrolarynx. These patients are permanent neck breathers and education for patients and caregivers on the implications of a separated airway and digestive tract is critical to ongoing safety. Open partial laryngectomy, including supraglottic or supracricoid partial laryngectomy, may be used in selected cases based on tumor anatomy but has long-term impact on swallowing and airway protection that requires both surgical and speech language pathology expertise to manage.

NECK DISSECTION

Given the risk of nodal metastasis in SCC of the head and neck, decision making regarding treatment of the neck is critical. In most cases, the cervical lymph nodes are treated via the same modality as the primary tumor. In the example of oral cavity cancer, neck dissection is performed alongside primary tumor extirpation and reconstruction. In the same vein, the radiation oncologist contours their treatment fields to incorporate draining lymphatic basins in oropharyngeal or laryngeal cancers selected for definitive radiation. Elective neck dissection or elective neck radiation is performed in the N0 neck when the risk of occult nodal metastasis is greater than 15%.

First described by George Crile in 1906, the radical neck dissection includes comprehensive removal of cervical lymphatics with sacrifice of the sternocleidomastoid (SCM) muscle, internal jugular vein (IJV), and spinal accessory nerve. The modified radical neck dissection removes levels I to V nodes with preservation of one or more of the aforementioned three structures.[3] By the 1950s, head and neck surgeons migrated to the concept of selective oncologic lymphadenectomy, based on tumor subsite drainage patterns, with decreased morbidity.[51]

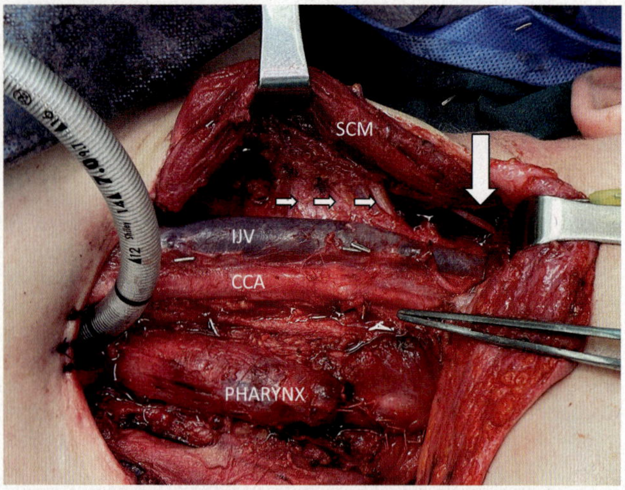

Figure 40.10. Intraoperative photograph demonstrating the right neck after performance of a selective, levels II to IV neck dissection. Selective neck dissection is generally a low-morbidity procedure. Vital structures such as the internal jugular vein (IJV), common carotid artery (CCA), and spinal accessory nerve (*large arrow*) are carefully preserved. Also preserved and noted here are the sternocleidomastoid muscle (SCM), and cervical sensory rootlets (*small arrows*). The forceps is highlighting the external carotid artery. This patient also underwent laryngectomy for laryngeal cancer; the endotracheal tube is positioned in the permanent tracheostomy and the pharyngeal reconstruction is noted superior to the stoma (PHARYNX).

Table 40.5. Complications of Head and Neck Surgeries

Tonsillectomy/Adenoidectomy
Hemorrhage
Velopharyngeal insufficiency
Lingual neuropraxia
Endoscopic Sinus Surgery
Intranasal adhesions
Hyposmia
Epistaxis
Orbital injury/hematoma
Cerebrospinal fluid leak
Internal carotid artery injury
Parotidectomy
Great auricular nerve injury
Hematoma/seroma
Frey syndrome (gustatory facial sweating)
Facial nerve injury
Submandibular Gland Removal
Hematoma/seroma
Marginal mandibular nerve injury
Lingual nerve injury
Neck Dissection
Spinal accessory nerve injury
Marginal mandibular nerve injury
Hypoglossal nerve injury
Great vessel injury
Chyle leak
Total Laryngectomy
Pharyngocutaneous fistula
Parathyroid injury with hypocalcemia
Hypoglossal nerve injury
Esophageal stricture

Known as selective neck dissection, careful but comprehensive removal of the at-risk nodal basins with preservation of normal structures is now the standard of care.[52] "Node plucking" or random sampling of neck nodes is inappropriate and should be avoided.

Head and neck patterns of lymphatic drainage are well described by Lindberg and Shah, and these studies allow for thoughtful subsite-based surgical planning.[53,54] As a general rule, oral cavity cancers require dissection of levels I to III, and possibly IV depending on nodal burden, while dissection of levels II to IV is performed for cancers of the oropharynx, larynx, and hypopharynx (Fig. 40.10). Level V is rarely involved except in NPC and some advanced skin cancers. Sentinel lymph node biopsy may be considered in early T-stage, clinically N0 oral cavity cancer, but does require technical expertise, and one should be prepared to complete the neck dissection at the time of biopsy[55]; this technique is under investigation in OPC as well.

The boundaries of the "lateral neck dissection," encompassing levels II to IV, extend from the posterior belly of the digastric muscle's insertion on the mastoid where it meets with the SCM superiorly to the plane of the clavicle inferiorly, and from the posterior edge of the SCM to the strap muscles anteriorly. The depth of the dissection is defined by the cervical sensory rootlets in level III and the deep layer of deep cervical fascia that invests the deep musculature in level II (levator scapulae) and level IV (anterior and middle scalenes). Care should be taken to preserve the deep layer of deep cervical fascia in order to protect the phrenic nerve and brachial plexus. As the dissection completes inferiorly in level IV, attention must be paid to controlling the lymphatics as they course toward the thoracic duct on the left and the lymphatic duct on the right. When level IB is dissected, the marginal mandibular nerve must be identified and preserved to allow for safe resection of the submandibular gland and perifacial nodes. Level V neck dissection requires identification of the spinal accessory nerve just above Erb point, followed by meticulous dissection to its entry into the trapezius. The nodes are then removed from the trapezius superiorly, the posterior edge of the SCM anteriorly and the clavicle inferiorly, all while preserving the accessory nerve.

COMPLICATIONS OF HEAD AND NECK SURGERY

Table 40.5 lists both common and rare complications of various head and neck procedures. Knowledge of these potential adverse outcomes, avoidance thereof, and disclosure of risk to patients during informed consent is crucial.

References

1. Sankaranarayanan R, Masuyer E, Swaminathan R, Ferlay J, Whelan S. Head and neck cancer: a global perspective on epidemiology and prognosis. *Anticancer Res.* 1998;18(6B):4779–4786.
2. D'Souza G, Kreimer AR, Viscidi R, et al. Case-control study of human papillomavirus and oropharyngeal cancer. *N Engl J Med.* 2007;356(19):1944–1956.
3. Robbins KT, Shaha AR, Medina JE, et al. Consensus statement on the classification and terminology of neck dissection. *Arch Otolaryngol Head Neck Surg.* 2008;134(5):536–538.
4. Roth D, Pace NL, Lee A, et al. Airway physical examination tests for detection of difficult airway management in apparently normal adult patients. *Cochrane Database Syst Rev.* 2018;5(5):CD008874.
5. Iseli TA, Iseli CE, Golden JB, et al. Outcomes of intubation in difficult airways due to head and neck pathology. *Ear Nose Throat J.* 2012;91(3):E1–E5.

6. Sheikh Z, Yu B, Heywood E, Quraishi N, Quraishi S. The assessment and management of deep neck space infections in adults: a systematic review and qualitative evidence synthesis. *Clin Otolaryngol*. 2023;48(4):540–562.
7. Rosenfeld RM, Piccirillo JF, Chandrasekhar SS, Walsh SA, Corrigan MD. Clinical practice guideline (update): adult sinusitis. *Otolaryngol Head Neck Surg*. 2015;152(2 Suppl):S1–S39.
8. Duggal P, Wise SK. Chapter 8: invasive fungal rhinosinusitis. *Am J Rhinol Allergy*. 2013;27(Suppl 1):S28–S30.
9. Fattahi TT, Lyu PE, Van Sickels JE. Management of acute suppurative parotitis. *J Oral Maxillofac Surg*. 2002;60(4):446–448.
10. Pynnonen MA, Gillespie MB, Roman B, et al. Clinical practice guideline: evaluation of the neck mass in adults. *Otolaryngol Head Neck Surg*. 2017;157(2_suppl):S1–S30.
11. Spiro RH. Salivary neoplasms: overview of a 35-year experience with 2,807 patients. *Head Neck Surg*. 1986;8(3):177–184.
12. Eveson JW, Cawson RA. Salivary gland tumours. A review of 2410 cases with particular reference to histological types, site, age and sex distribution. *J Pathol*. 1985;146(1):51–58.
13. Amin MB, Edge SB, Greene FL, et al., eds. *AJCC Cancer Staging Manual*. 8th ed. Springer; 2017.
14. Schmidt RL, Hall BJ, Wilson AR, Layfield LJ. A systematic review and meta-analysis of the diagnostic accuracy of fine-needle aspiration cytology for parotid gland lesions. *Am J Clin Pathol*. 2011;136(1):45–59.
15. Jalaly JB, Farahani SJ, Baloch ZW. The Milan system for reporting salivary gland cytopathology: a comprehensive review of the literature. *Diagn Cytopathol*. 2020;48(10):880–889.
16. Valstar MH, Andreasen S, Bhairosing PA, McGurk M. Natural history of recurrent pleomorphic adenoma: implications on management. *Head Neck*. 2020;42:2058–2066.
17. Mantsopoulos K, Koch M, Klintworth N, Zenk J, Iro H. Evolution and changing trends in surgery for benign parotid tumors. *Laryngoscope*. 2015;125(1):122–127.
18. Albergotti WG, Nguyen SA, Zenk J, Gillespie MB. Extracapsular dissection for benign parotid tumors: a meta-analysis. *Laryngoscope*. 2012;122(9):1954–1960.
19. Walvekar RR, Andrade Filho PA, Seethala RR, et al. Clinicopathologic features as stronger prognostic factors than histology or grade in risk stratification of primary parotid malignancies. *Head Neck*. 2011;33(2):225–231.
20. Zbären P, Stauffer E. Pleomorphic adenoma of the parotid gland: histopathologic analysis of the capsular characteristics of 218 tumors. *Head Neck*. 2007;29(8):751–757.
21. Papel ID, Frodel JL, Richard Holt G, et al. Lip reconstruction. In: DeFatta RJ, Williams EF III, eds. *Facial Plastic and Reconstructive Surgery*. 3rd ed. Thieme; 2009.
22. Huang SH, Hwang D, Lockwood G, Goldstein DP, O'Sullivan B. Predictive value of tumor thickness for cervical lymph-node involvement in squamous cell carcinoma of the oral cavity: a meta-analysis of reported studies. *Cancer*. 2009;115(7):1489–1497.
23. D'Cruz AK, Vaish R, Kapre N, et al. Elective versus therapeutic neck dissection in node-negative oral cancer. *N Engl J Med*. 2015;373(6):521–529.
24. de-Thé G. Epstein-Barr virus behavior in different populations and implications for control of Epstein-Barr virus-associated tumors. *Cancer Res*. 1976;36(2 pt 2):692–695.
25. Tsao SW, Tsang CM, To KF, Lo KW. The role of Epstein-Barr virus in epithelial malignancies. *J Pathol*. 2015;235(2):323–333.
26. Chang ET, Adami HO. The enigmatic epidemiology of nasopharyngeal carcinoma. *Cancer Epidemiol Biomarkers Prev*. 2006;15(10):1765–1777.
27. Badoual C. Update from the 5th edition of the World Health Organization Classification of head and neck tumors: oropharynx and nasopharynx. *Head Neck Pathol*. 2022;16(1):19–30.
28. Al-Sarraf M, LeBlanc M, Giri PG, et al. Chemoradiotherapy versus radiotherapy in patients with advanced nasopharyngeal cancer: phase III randomized Intergroup study 0099. *J Clin Oncol*. 1998;16(4):1310–1317.
29. Lee AWM, Tung SY, Chua DTT, et al. Randomized trial of radiotherapy plus concurrent-adjuvant chemotherapy vs radiotherapy alone for regionally advanced nasopharyngeal carcinoma. *J Natl Cancer Inst*. 2010;102(15):1188–1198.
30. Chan JYW. Surgical management of recurrent nasopharyngeal carcinoma. *Oral Oncol*. 2014;50(10):913–917.
31. Al-Sheibani S, Zanaion AM, Carrau RL, et al. Endoscopic endonasal transpterygoid nasopharyngectomy. *Laryngoscope*. 2011;121(10):2081–2089.
32. Tsang RK, To VS, Ho AC, Ho WK, Chan JY, Wei WI. Early results of robotic assisted nasopharyngectomy for recurrent nasopharyngeal carcinoma. *Head Neck*. 2015;37(6):788–793.
33. Chaturvedi AK, Engels EA, Pfeiffer RM, et al. Human papillomavirus and rising oropharyngeal cancer incidence in the United States. *J Clin Oncol*. 2011;29(32):4294–4301.
34. Ang KK, Harris J, Wheeler R, et al. Human papillomavirus and survival of patients with oropharyngeal cancer. *N Eng J Med*. 2010;363(1):24–35.
35. Posner MR, Lorch JH, Goloubeva O, et al. Survival and human papillomavirus in oropharynx cancer in TAX 324: a subset analysis from an international phase III trial. *Ann Oncol*. 2011;22(5): 1071–1077.
36. Parsons JT, Mendenhall WM, Stringer SP, et al. Squamous cell carcinoma of the oropharynx: surgery, radiation therapy, or both. *Cancer*. 2002;94(11):2967–2980.
37. Grant DG, Hinni ML, Salassa JR, Perry WC, Hayden RE, Casler JD. Oropharyngeal cancer: a case for single modality treatment with transoral laser microsurgery. *Arch Otolaryngol Head Neck Surg*. 2009;135(12):1225–1230.
38. Leonhardt FD, Quon H, Abrahao M, O'Malley BW Jr, Weinstein GS. Transoral robotic surgery for oropharyngeal carcinoma and its impact on patient-reported quality of life and function. *Head Neck*. 2012;34(2):146–154.
39. Shaw RJ, Holsinger FC, Paleri V, Evans M, Tudur-Smith C, Ferris RL. Surgical trials in head & neck oncology: renaissance and revolution? *Head Neck*. 2015;37(7):927–930.
40. Nichols AC, Theurer J, Prisman E, et al. Radiotherapy versus transoral robotic surgery and neck dissection for oropharyngeal squamous cell carcinoma (ORATOR): an open-label, phase 2, randomised trial. *Lancet Oncol*. 2019;20(10):1349–1359.
41. Lefebvre JL, Chevalier D, Luboinski B, Kirkpatrick A, Collette L, Sahmoud T. Larynx preservation in pyriform sinus cancer: preliminary results of a European Organization for Research and Treatment of Cancer phase III trial. EORTC Head and Neck Cancer Cooperative Group. *J Natl Cancer Inst*. 1996;88(13):890–899.
42. Kotwall C, Sako K, Razack MS, Rao U, Bakamjian V, Shedd DP. Metastatic patterns in squamous cell cancer of the head and neck. *Am J Surg*. 1987;154(4):439–442.
43. Park YM, Kim WS, De Virgilio A, Lee SY, Seol JH, Kim SH. Transoral robotic surgery for hypopharyngeal squamous cell carcinoma: 3-year oncologic and functional analysis. *Oral Oncol*. 2012;48(6):560–566.
44. Karatzanis AD, Psychogios G, Waldfahrer F, et al. T1 and T2 hypopharyngeal cancer treatment with laser microsurgery. *J Surg Oncol*. 2010;102(1):27–33.
45. Higgins KM, Shah MD, Ogaick MJ, Enepekides D. Treatment of early-stage glottic cancer: meta-analysis comparison of laser excision versus radiotherapy. *J Otolaryngol Head Neck Surg*. 2009;38(6):603–612.
46. Hartl DM, Ferlito A, Brasnu DF, et al. Evidence-based review of treatment options for patients with glottic cancer. *Head Neck*. 2011;33(11):1638–1648.
47. Caicedo-Granados E, Beswick DM, Christopoulos A, et al. Oncologic and functional outcomes of partial laryngeal surgery for intermediate-stage laryngeal cancer. *Otolaryngol Head Neck Surg*. 2013;148(2):235–242.
48. Department of Veterans Affairs Laryngeal Cancer Study Group; Wolf GT, Fisher SG, et al. Induction chemotherapy plus radiation compared with surgery plus radiation in patients with advanced laryngeal cancer. *N Eng J Med*. 1991;324(24):1685–1690.
49. Forastiere AA, Goepfert H, Maor M, et al. Concurrent chemotherapy and radiotherapy for organ preservation in advanced laryngeal cancer. *N Eng J Med*. 2003;349(22):2091–2098.

50. Forastiere AA, Zhang Q, Weber RS, et al. Long-term results of RTOG 91-11: a comparison of three nonsurgical treatment strategies to preserve the larynx in patients with locally advanced larynx cancer. *J Clin Oncol*. 2013;31(7):845–852.
51. Harrison BL, Sessions BR, Kies MS. *Head and Neck Cancer: A Multidisciplinary Approach*. 4th ed. Wolters Kluwer/Lippincott-Raven; 2014.
52. Byers RM. Modified neck dissection. A study of 967 cases from 1970 to 1980. *Am J Surg*. 1985;150(4):414–421.
53. Lindberg R. Distribution of cervical lymph node metastases from squamous cell carcinoma of the upper respiratory and digestive tracts. *Cancer*. 1972;29(6):1446–1449.
54. Shah JP. Patterns of cervical lymph node metastasis from squamous carcinomas of the upper aerodigestive tract. *Am J Surg*. 1990;160(4):405–409.
55. Schilling C, Stoeckli SJ, Haerle SK, et al. Sentinel European Node Trial (SENT): 3-year results of sentinel node biopsy in oral cancer. *Eur J Cancer*. 2015;51(18):2777–2784.

Section D:
ESOPHAGUS

41

Esophageal Anatomy and Physiology and Gastroesophageal Reflux Disease

Micaela M. Esquivel and Mary T. Hawn

Key Points

1 Esophageal anatomy: the cervical, thoracic, and abdominal esophagus each have distinct physiologic and pathologic differences.
2 The three layers of the esophageal wall: mucosa, submucosa, and muscularis propria. There is no serosa of the esophagus.
3 During a swallow, the lower esophageal sphincter (LES) relaxes at the initiation of the swallow and remains open until the peristaltic waves passes down through the body and through the LES.
4 The LES retains its competence as a barrier to prevent gastric reflux by three factors: length, resting pressure, and position.
5 Diagnostic modalities of the esophagus include endoscopy, fluoroscopy, manometry, ambulatory pH monitoring, and impedance planimetry.
6 Ambulatory pH monitoring remains the gold standard for confirming gastroesophageal reflux.
7 Endoluminal functional lumen imaging probe (EndoFlip) is an impedance planimetry system used to evaluate real-time pressure, diameter, and distensibility/compliance of the esophagus and gastrointestinal sphincters.
8 Barrett esophagus is defined as having the presence of both endoscopic mucosal changes and microscopic findings of cardiac mucosa with goblet cells or intestinal metaplasia.
9 Preoperative functional assessment of the esophagus and LES are pivotal to determining which type of antireflux operation is most appropriate.
10 Surgical treatment options for gastroesophageal reflux disease (GERD) include complete and partial fundoplication and magnetic sphincter augmentation. Concurrent hiatal hernia repair must be performed when present.
11 Endoscopic approaches for treating GERD include the Stretta procedure, transoral incisionless fundoplication (TIF 2.0), and evolving procedures such as anti-reflux mucosectomy (ARMS).

ESOPHAGEAL ANATOMY AND FUNCTION

1 The esophagus is an approximately 25- to 30-cm muscular tube that connects the pharynx to the stomach. It starts at cricopharyngeus, or upper esophageal sphincter (EUS), and travels from the superior mediastinum to the inferior mediastinum, ending at the lower esophageal sphincter (LES) as it enters to stomach (**Fig. 41.1**). The esophagus has specific anatomical relationships to critical structures and organs within the mediastinum and requires a detailed knowledge of these relationships to not only work-up esophageal pathology, but to also manage and expose the esophagus intraoperatively. The cervical, thoracic, and abdominal esophagus each have distinct physiologic and pathologic differences.

Cervical Esophagus

The cervical esophagus begins just below the cricopharyngeus muscle and is an apparent continuation of the inferior constrictor muscle of the pharynx. The cervical esophagus is the first 3 to 5 cm of the esophagus. A Zenker diverticulum occurs in the cervical esophagus at a natural area of weakening at Killian triangle. This is the space between the posterior left and right inferior constrictor muscles and immediately above the cricopharyngeus muscle (**Fig. 41.2**). The carotid sheaths lie laterally, and the recurrent laryngeal nerves lie in the grooves between the trachea and esophagus, important landmarks for thyroid and parathyroid

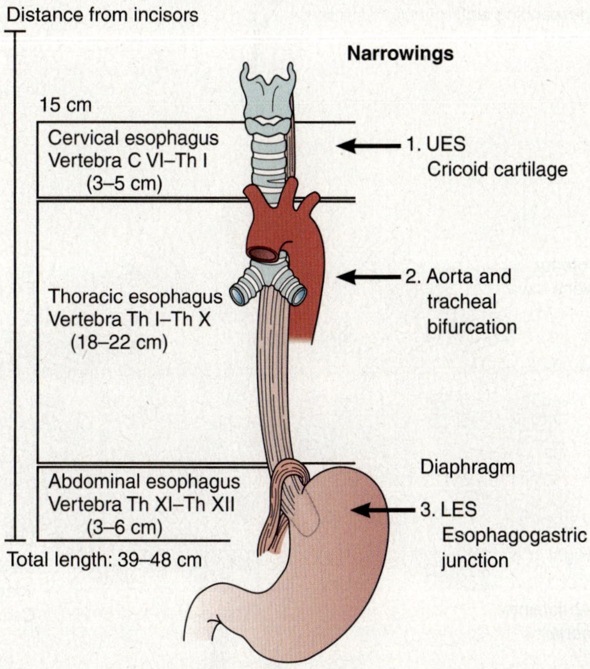

Figure 41.1. Anatomy of the esophagus.

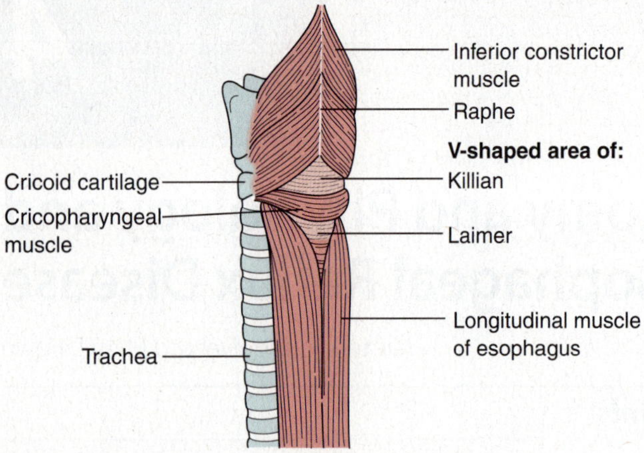

Figure 41.2. Posterior view of cervical esophagus.

operations. The cervical esophagus is more frequently approached surgically from the left due to the more variable course of the right recurrent laryngeal nerve. The trachea and larynx are immediately anterior to the cervical esophagus, while posteriorly is the prevertebral space, with the cervical esophagus immediately anterior to the vertebral bodies. The cervical esophagus passes from the retropharyngeal space superiorly to the posterior mediastinum inferiorly, allowing mediastinitis from oropharyngeal infections. When evaluating x-ray or CT imaging, the cervical esophagus is located from C6 to the lower border of T1.

Thoracic Esophagus

The thoracic esophagus begins at the thoracic inlet and is approximately 18 to 20 cm long (**Fig. 41.1**). In the upper thorax, the esophagus is immediately posterior to the trachea, and just above the level of the tracheal bifurcation, the esophagus lies to the right of the aortic arch and descending aorta. It then courses to the left as it passes behind the tracheal bifurcation and left main bronchus. The esophagus remains on the left in the lower thorax as it passes through the diaphragmatic hiatus. The thoracic esophagus can be constricted as it passes behind the aortic arch and left mainstem bronchus. The thoracic duct and azygos vein are both closely related to the esophagus and require particular consideration during esophagectomy (Chapter 42: Esophageal Tumors and Injury).

Abdominal Esophagus

The abdominal esophagus starts at the diaphragmatic hiatus, is approximately 3 to 6 cm in length, and consists of the abdominal portion of the LES. The phrenoesophageal membrane surrounds this section of the esophagus circumferentially and courses to approximately 1 to 2 cm above the level of the hiatus at its upper leaf. Its lower leaf merges with the serosa of the stomach, and in this area, there is a notable fat pad, marking the location of the gastroesophageal junction (GEJ) (**Fig. 41.3**).

The LES is a high-pressure zone about 3 to 4 cm in length at the distal esophagus. The LES has no visible macroscopic appearance changes on the inner mucosal lining or the outer surface of the esophagus. The left and right crura form the esophageal hiatus, and together they form a "sling" of diaphragmatic skeletal muscle around the esophagus.

These muscles originate from tendinous bands attached to the anterolateral surface of the first lumbar vertebra (**Fig. 41.4**). The median arcuate ligament, a tendinous arch, lies immediately anterior to the aorta, and attaches to the crura posterior to the esophagus.

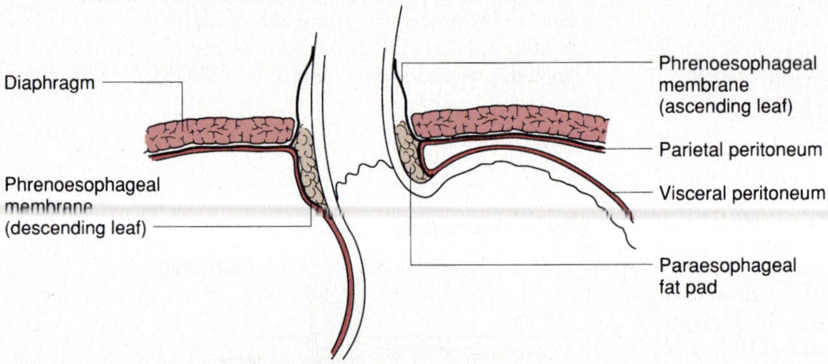

Figure 41.3. Anatomy of the esophageal hiatus and relationship to the phrenoesophageal membrane.

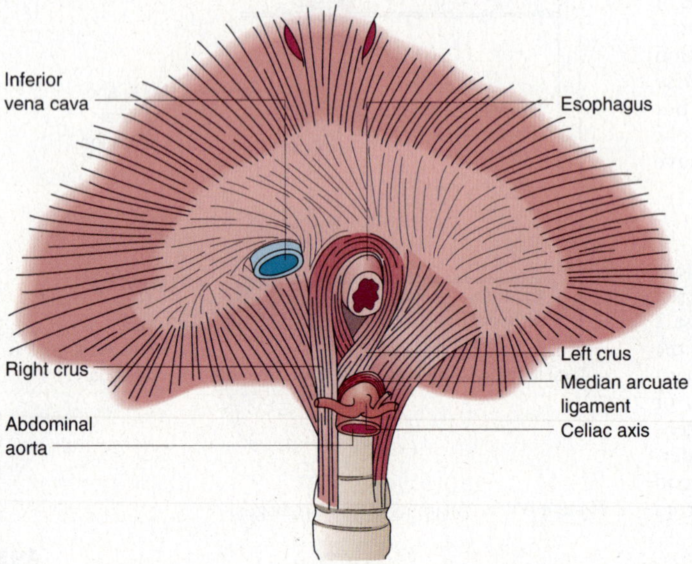

Figure 41.4. Inferior view of diaphragm and anatomy of the esophageal hiatus.

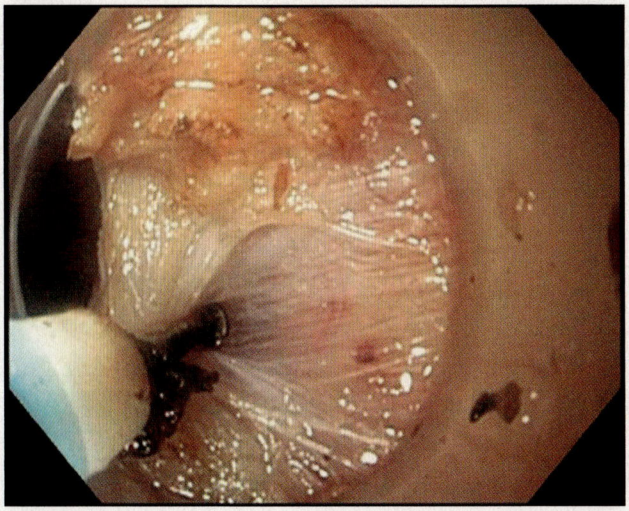

Figure 41.5. Endoscopic view of esophageal muscle layers during a peroral endoscopic myotomy (POEM) for achalasia. The endoscopic knife is lifting and cutting the circumferential circular muscle fibers, leaving the longitudinal muscle fibers intact.

Structure of the Esophageal Wall and Mucosa

2 The mucosa, submucosa, and muscularis propria are the three principal layers of the esophageal wall. In contrast to the rest of the gastrointestinal tract, there is no outer serosal layer, making the mucosa the strength layer of the esophagus. The mucosal layer is composed of nonkeratinized stratified squamous epithelium. The muscularis mucosa is located immediately below the basement membrane and above the submucosa. Tumors that penetrate this layer and into the submucosa carry a higher likelihood of lymph node metastases. The submucosa contains an extensive lymphatic plexus throughout the esophagus, with collecting branches that penetrate the muscularis propria to connect with the thoracic duct and regional lymph nodes. This lymphatic web is the reason esophageal cancers can spread longitudinally and produce skip metastases.

Intramucosal tumors have a <5% rate of regional lymph node metastases, compared to a 20% to 50% rate for submucosal tumors.[1] Additionally, the mucous glands of the esophagus are also located in the submucosal layer and drain into the esophageal lumen. The muscularis propria has an outer longitudinal muscle layer and a thicker inner circular muscle layer, composed of striated muscle in the uppermost portion that transitions to smooth muscle near the junction of the upper and middle third of the esophagus. Both the muscle layers have a spiraling orientation, with the longitudinal rotating nearly 90 degrees as it courses down to the stomach (**Fig. 41.5**). This organization of the two muscle layers allows for the esophageal waves of peristalsis.

Blood Supply, Lymphatics, and Innervation

The cervical, thoracic, and abdominal portions of the esophagus each have a specific blood supply (**Fig. 41.6**):

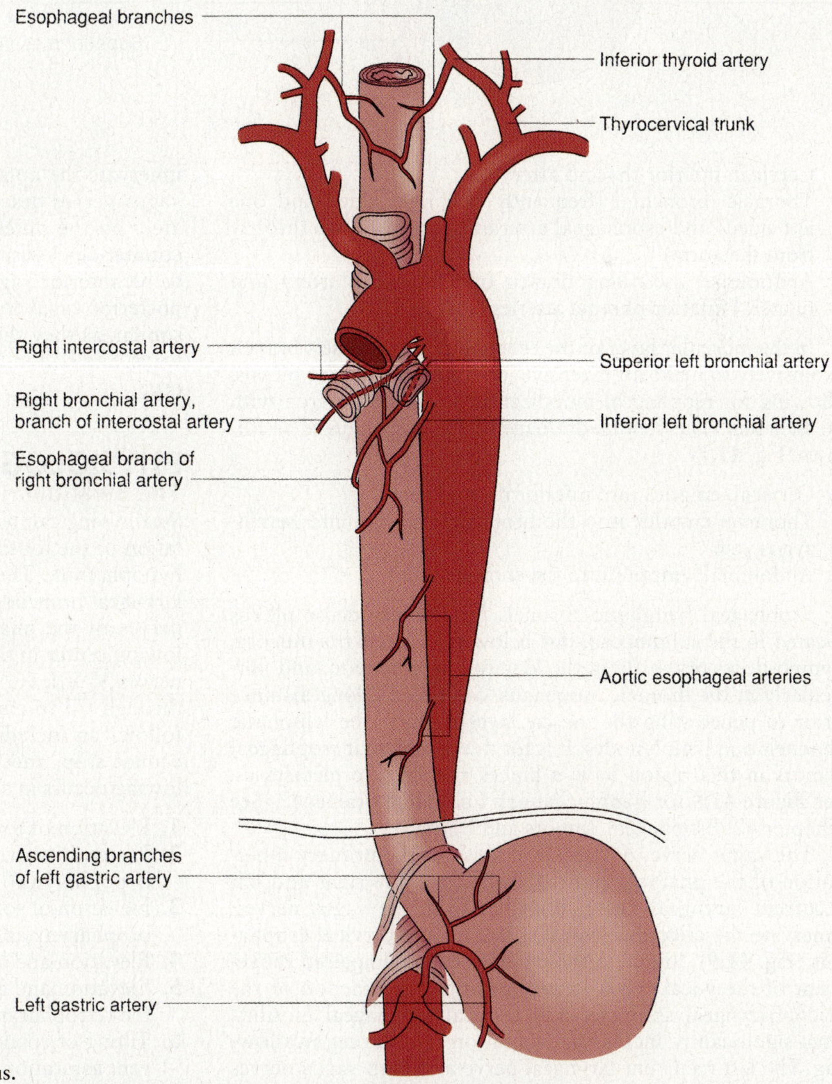

Figure 41.6. Arterial anatomy of the esophagus.

ESOPHAGUS

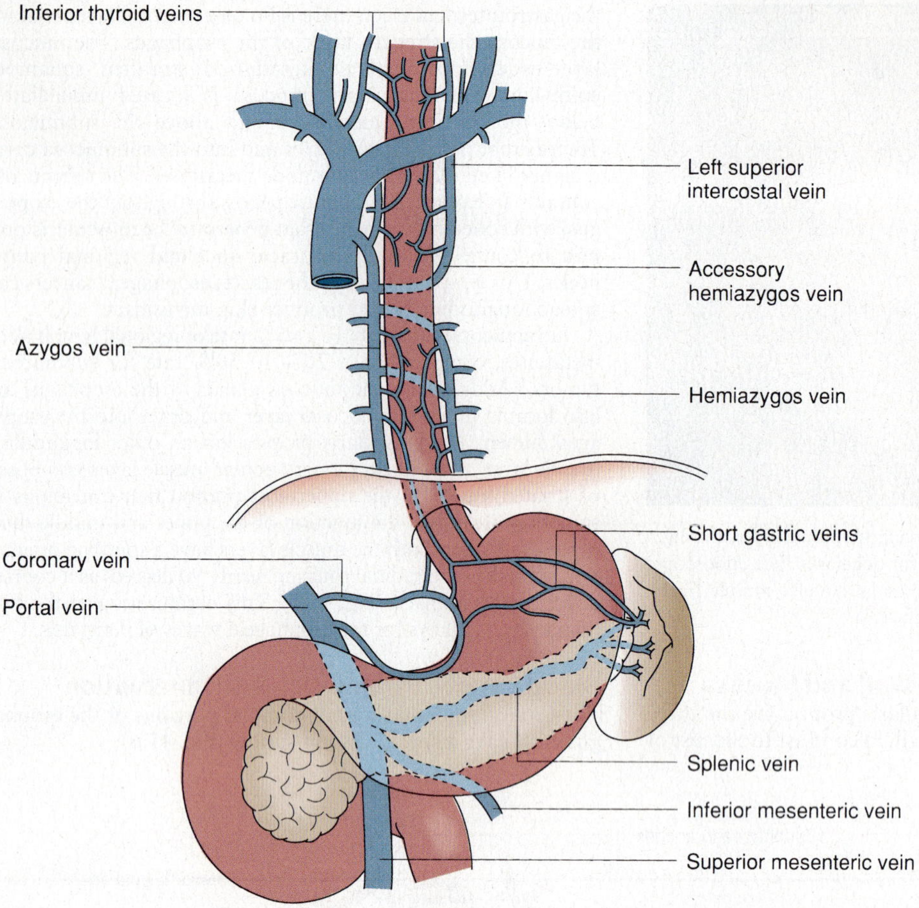

Figure 41.7. Venous anatomy of the esophagus.

- Cervical: inferior thyroid artery
- Thoracic: bronchial (frequently two right sided and one left sided) and esophageal arteries (frequently two directly from the aorta)
- Abdominal: ascending branch of left gastric artery and bilateral inferior phrenic arteries

In the muscular layer of the esophagus, these vessels branch extensively to make an extensive longitudinal vascular plexus, allowing for esophageal mobilization to the aortic arch with no ischemia. The venous drainage of the esophagus is as follows (**Fig. 41.7**):

- Cervical: empties into inferior thyroid vein
- Thoracic: empties into the bronchial, azygos, and hemiazygos vein
- Abdominal: empties into the coronary vein

Esophageal lymphatic channels form a very dense plexus located in the submucosa, just below the muscularis mucosa. Lymph flows primarily in the longitudinal direction, and particularly in the thoracic esophagus, can travel a long distance prior to penetrating the muscle layer to enter the lymphatic channels and lymph nodes. It is for this reason that esophageal tumors in this region have a higher rate of skip metastases. See **Figure 41.8** for lymph channels and nodal drainage.[2] (See Chapter 42: Esophageal Tumors and Injury.)

The vagus nerve, or cranial nerve X, is the primary innervation of the pharynx and the esophagus. The right and left recurrent laryngeal nerve, branches from the vagus nerves, innervate the cricopharyngeal sphincter and cervical esophagus (**Fig. 41.9**). Injury to these nerves causes impaired movement of the vocal cords as well as impaired function of the cricopharyngeal sphincter and cervical esophageal motility, thus significantly increasing aspiration risk during swallowing. The left recurrent laryngeal nerve and both vagus nerves innervate the upper thoracic esophagus. As the right and left vagus nerves descend into the mediastinum they lie immediately on the outer surface of the esophagus and rotate in a counter-clockwise fashion. Thus, the left vagus nerve rotates to be anterior vagal trunk, while the right rotates to become posterior vagal trunk. Esophageal and cardiac symptoms are similar, as they share the same afferent visceral sensory pathways, and end in the first four segments of the thoracic spinal cord.

PHYSIOLOGY

The Swallowing Mechanism

Swallowing can be intentional or reflexive secondary to stimulation of the tonsillar pillars or the posterolateral walls of the hypopharynx. The glossopharyngeal nerves and the superior laryngeal branches of the vagal nerves are the afferent sensory nerves of the pharynx. Once these are simulated, the swallowing center in the medulla then triggers neurons via cranial nerves V, VII, X, XI, and XII and the motor neurons of C1 through C3 to complete a swallow. This swallowing impulse follows an incredibly coordinated pattern that, once started, cannot stop, and lasts for approximately 0.5 seconds. Swallowing occurs in six distinct steps (**Fig. 41.10**):

1. Elevation of tongue
2. Posterior movement of tongue (propels food bolus into hypopharynx)
3. Elevation of soft palate (this closes the passage between the oropharynx and nasopharynx)
4. Elevation and anterior movement of hyoid
5. Elevation and anterior movement of larynx (thus enlarging the retropharyngeal space)
6. Tilting of epiglottis (thus closing the laryngeal inlet to prevent aspiration)

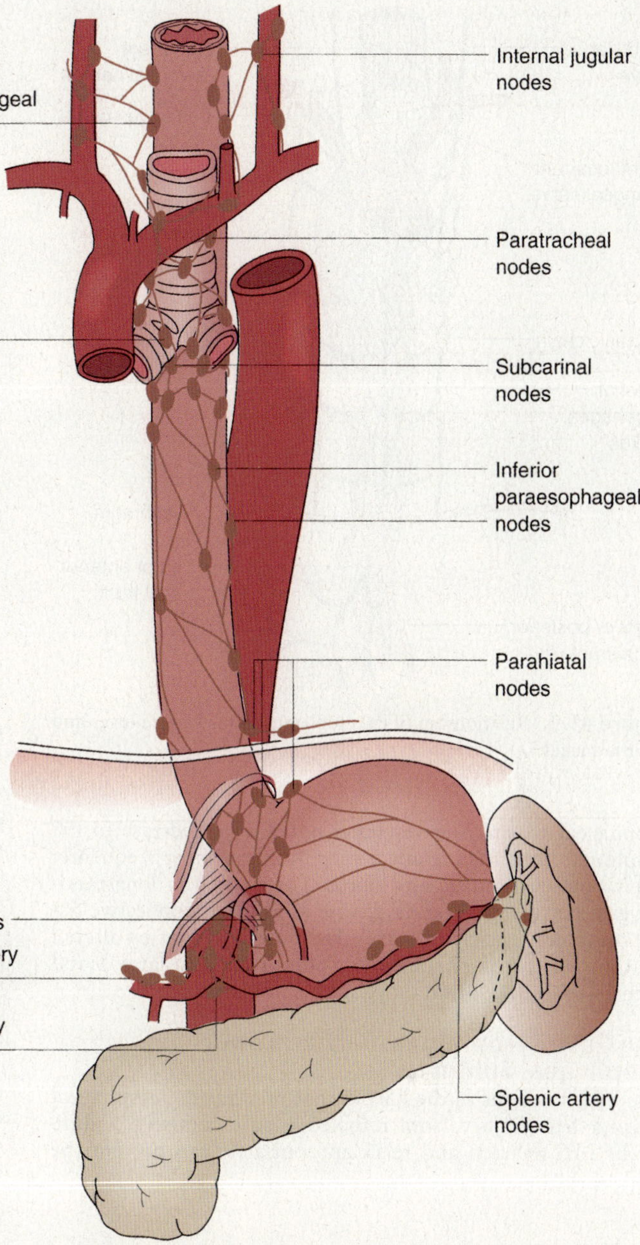

Figure 41.8. Lymphatic anatomy of the esophagus.

Pressure gradients initiated in the hypopharynx helps propel the movement of food from the hypopharynx into the esophagus as the cricopharyngeus, or EUS, relaxes.

The timing of relaxation of the UES and compliance of the cervical esophagus is pivotal to accepting the bolus. Deviations from this function may result in pharyngeal dysphagia. The elevation of the larynx (Step 5 in the previous section), pulls the hyoid bone by attached muscles and pulls the EUS open at the same time the EUS muscle is relaxing. The relaxation of the EUS is a neurologically mediated reflex that results in decreased tone of the cricopharyngeal muscle. The EUS then closes within half a second after the swallow is initiated, and the postrelaxation pressure is nearly two times the resting pressure (of 30 mm Hg). This high closing pressure of the EUS prevents reflux back into the pharynx. This postrelaxation contraction then flows down the esophagus to form a peristaltic wave (**Fig. 41.11**). At the conclusion of a swallow, the EUS returns to its baseline resting pressure.

3 When a swallow is initiated, the longitudinal muscles of the esophagus contract, or shorten, to then enlarge the lumen of the esophagus to better accept a bolus. The circular smooth muscle contraction is responsible for the peristaltic wave. The peristaltic waves produce an occlusive pressure of 30 to 120 mm Hg. The rise and fall of these contracts can engage one point in the esophagus for 3 to 5 seconds, as the wave rising peaks by 1 second, maintains peak pressure for 0.5 seconds, and subsides in about 1.5 seconds. After the initiation of a swallow, the peak of the primary peristaltic contraction waves down the esophagus 2 to 4 cm per second, and will reach the distal esophagus about 9 seconds later. The LES will relax at the start of the peristaltic wave and will remain open and relaxed until the wave passes through the LES. Similar to the UES, there is then a distinct postrelaxation contraction of the LES. This esophageal wave will be reproduced with a consecutive swallow 20 seconds after the first, though if a swallow occurs sooner, the esophagus will be functionally unresponsive (deglutitive inhibition).[3]

These peristaltic contractions must have sufficient amplitude or pressure to effectively occlude the esophageal lumen and be organized to successfully propel a bolus distal toward the stomach. There are three primary categories that cause impaired peristalsis. The first is a result of a neural abnormality resulting in defective organization of the peristaltic wave, resulting in a primary motility disorder, such a diffuse

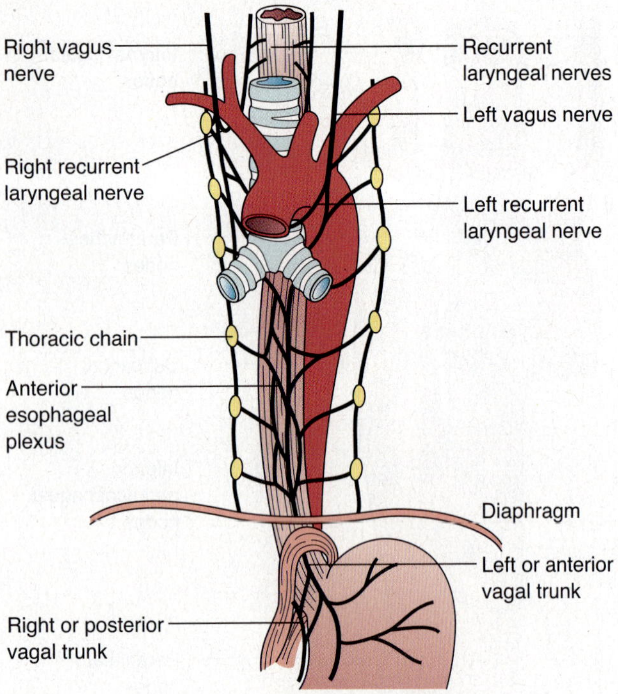

Figure 41.9. Relationship of the esophagus to the vagus nerves and their branches.

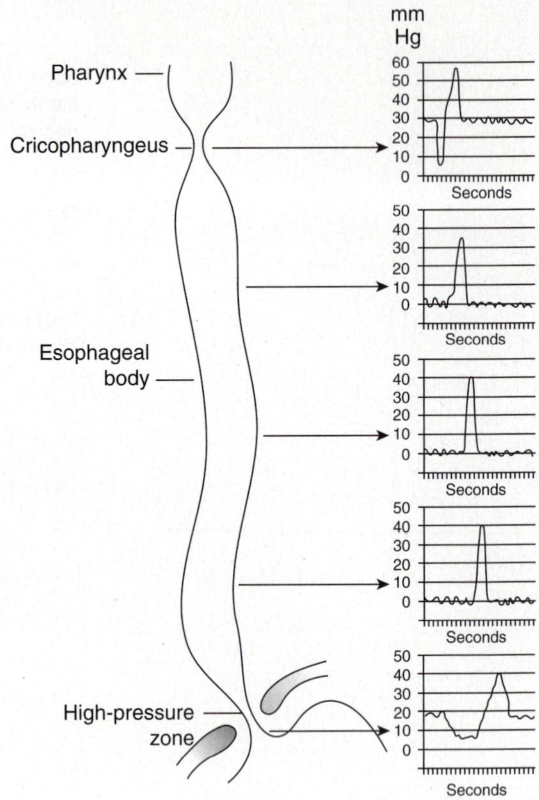

Figure 41.11. Overview of esophageal body peristalsis. (From Waters PF, DeMeester TR. Foregut motor disorders and their surgical management. *Med Clin North Am.* 1981;65[6]:1235–1268, with permission.)

esophageal spasm. The second is noted by a decrease in the amplitude with maintenance of peristalsis, most frequently due to muscle damage and fibrosis, often seen in longstanding gastroesophageal reflux disease (GERD) or connective tissue disorders (eg, scleroderma). The third is caused by altered anatomy of the esophagus, most often seen with large hiatal hernias, where the distal esophagus is not anchored.

The Gastroesophageal Barrier: Lower Esophageal Sphincter

The LES functions as the barrier that prevents the esophageal mucosa from injury from refluxed gastric contents. Failure of the LES to open and relax appropriately can prevent the esophagus from effectively pushing a bolus into the stomach, and if severe, can cause dysphagia. Failure of the LES to close effectively can lead to GERD, or increased exposure of the esophageal squamous epithelium to acidic gastric contents. Though the LES has no anatomical landmarks endoscopically, on manometry, it can be localized due to an area of pressure over baseline. At baseline, it is a "high-pressure zone" except during swallowing to allow a bolus to pass, or during belching to allow gas to be released. In early GERD, this is often due to a transient loss of the barrier, while in advanced GERD, it is frequently a permanent loss of LES barrier.[4]

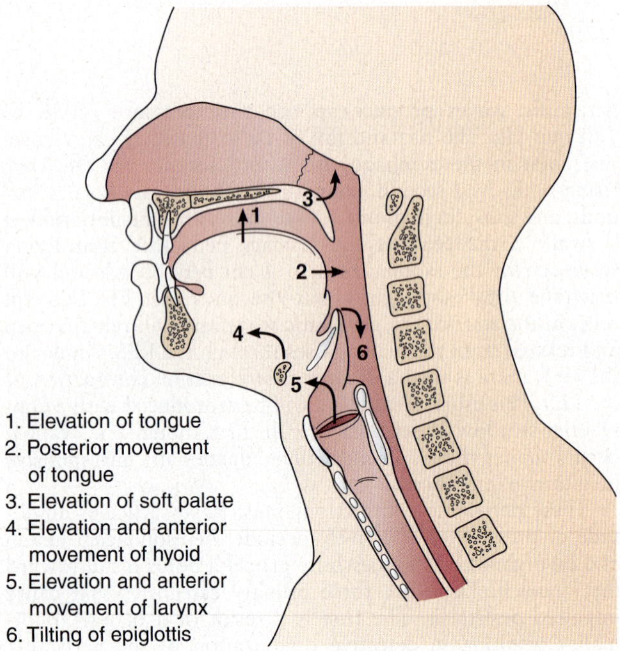

Figure 41.10. Overview of the act of swallowing.

There are three primary characteristics of the LES to allow it to maintain its function, even with high intragastric and intra-abdominal pressures. These LES characteristics include:

1. Length
2. Pressure
4 3. Position

The LES length and pressure work closely together to maintain LES effectiveness. The shorter the LES length, the higher the LES pressure must be to maintain competence. Additionally, the impact of a normal LES pressure can be negated by a short LES length and the impact of a normal LES length can be negated by a low LES pressure (**Fig. 41.12**).

The LES shortens due to gastric filling, as the terminal esophageal length is reduced by the expanding fundus—the greater the gastric volume, the shorter the LES length (**Fig. 41.13**). Overeating causes excessive gastric distension, which in turn critically shortens the LES to the point of impairing its ability to close. The LES pressure then abruptly drops and reflux occurs (**Fig. 41.14**). Additionally, if the LES is already permanently shortened, even normal-sized meals can cause postprandial reflux. The abnormal anatomy of the cardia, such as a sliding hiatal hernia, also impacts the ease in which the LES is shortened due to gastric distension. Less gastric distension is required to open the LES barrier in patients with a hiatal

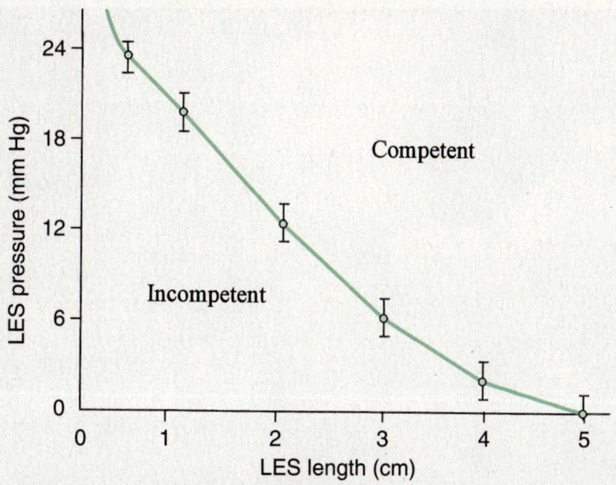

Figure 41.12. Relationship of the length and pressure of the lower esophageal sphincter in maintaining competence of the gastroesophageal barrier.

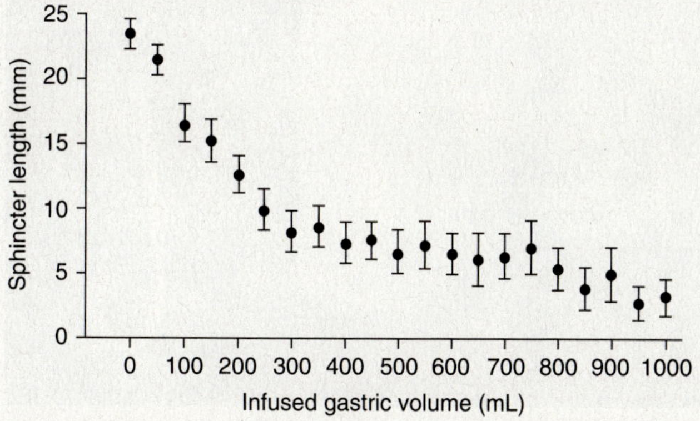

Figure 41.13. Effect of increasing gastric volume on the shortening of the lower esophageal sphincter length. As the stomach expands, the gastric body takes up the inferior aspect of the sphincter, causing its length to shorten. (Used with permission of Mason RJ, Lund RJ, DeMeester TR, et al. Nissen fundoplication prevents shortening of the sphincter during gastric distention. *Arch Surg.* 1997;132(7):719–724; discussion 724–726. Permission conveyed through Copyright Clearance Center, Inc.)

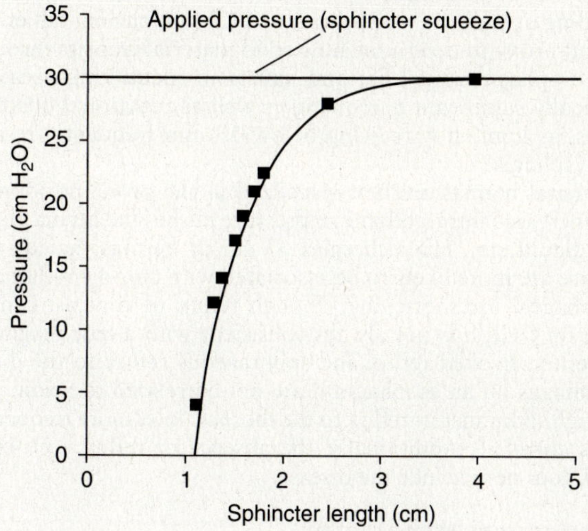

Figure 41.14. Representation of the loss of competence of the lower esophageal sphincter with shortening of its length. As a critical length is reached, there is a precipitous drop in sphincter pressure reflecting loss of competence. (From Pettersson GB, Bombeck CT, Nyhus LM. The lower esophageal sphincter: mechanisms of opening and closure. *Surgery*. 1980;88[2]:307–314, with permission.)

hernia. The funnel or dome shape of a hiatal hernia changes the wall tension and allows the barrier to be pulled open more easily, accounting for the frequent association of hiatal hernia with GERD. The position of the LES is also pivotal to its function. A segment of the LES is intra-abdominal and exposed to higher intra-abdominal pressures. If these pressures were only applied to the stomach, the barrier of the LES would be easily overcome (and therefore, reflux would occur) if the intra-abdominal LES were not also experiencing those same pressures. A minimum of 1 cm of abdominal LES is critical to its proper function.[5]

When LES length, pressure, and position are not adequate, this will lead to an incompetent LES. In these cases, even when fasting, continued reflux can occur, leading to chronic esophageal injury.

EVALUATION OF ESOPHAGEAL FUNCTION

5 Thorough assessment of esophageal anatomy and function is imperative to both medical and surgical management of esophageal disease. There are four core diagnostic tests commonly utilized, these include: upper endoscopy, barium esophagram, ambulatory pH monitoring, and high-resolution esophageal manometry. We also recommend esophageal impedance planimetry (endoluminal functional lumen imaging probe or Endoflip) for assessment of esophageal distensibility/compliance and function.

Upper Endoscopy

An esophagogastroduodenoscopy (EGD) is indicated in every patient being evaluated for GERD, and is a critical physical examination of the foregut. A thorough visual evaluation of the entire foregut is necessary with particular attention to the location and appearance of the squamocolumnar junction. This junction is noted by the transition of the lighter squamous epithelium and the darker rose (or velvet)-colored columnar epithelium. Narrow band imaging (NBI) is particularly helpful in distinguishing these two cellular types. If erosive esophagitis is encountered, application of the Los Angeles classification system should be applied (**Table 41.1**).[6]

If columnar metaplasia is observed during endoscopy, this raises a concern for Barrett esophagus, and the area must be biopsied (four-quadrant every 1 to 2 cm of columnar metaplasia). The cardia and GEJ should be visualized for abnormalities by retroflexion, as this will also assess the competency of the gastroesophageal barrier. The Hill grading system is

CLASSIFICATION

Table 41.1. Modified Los Angeles Classification of Esophagitis

Grade	Lesion
A	One (or more) mucosal break of longer than 5 mm that does not extend between the tops of two mucosal folds
B	One (or more) mucosal break more than 5 mm long that does not extend between the tops of two mucosal folds
C	One (or more) mucosal break that is continuous between the tops of two or more mucosal folds but that involves <75% of the circumference
D	One (or more) mucosal break that involves at least 75% of the esophageal circumference

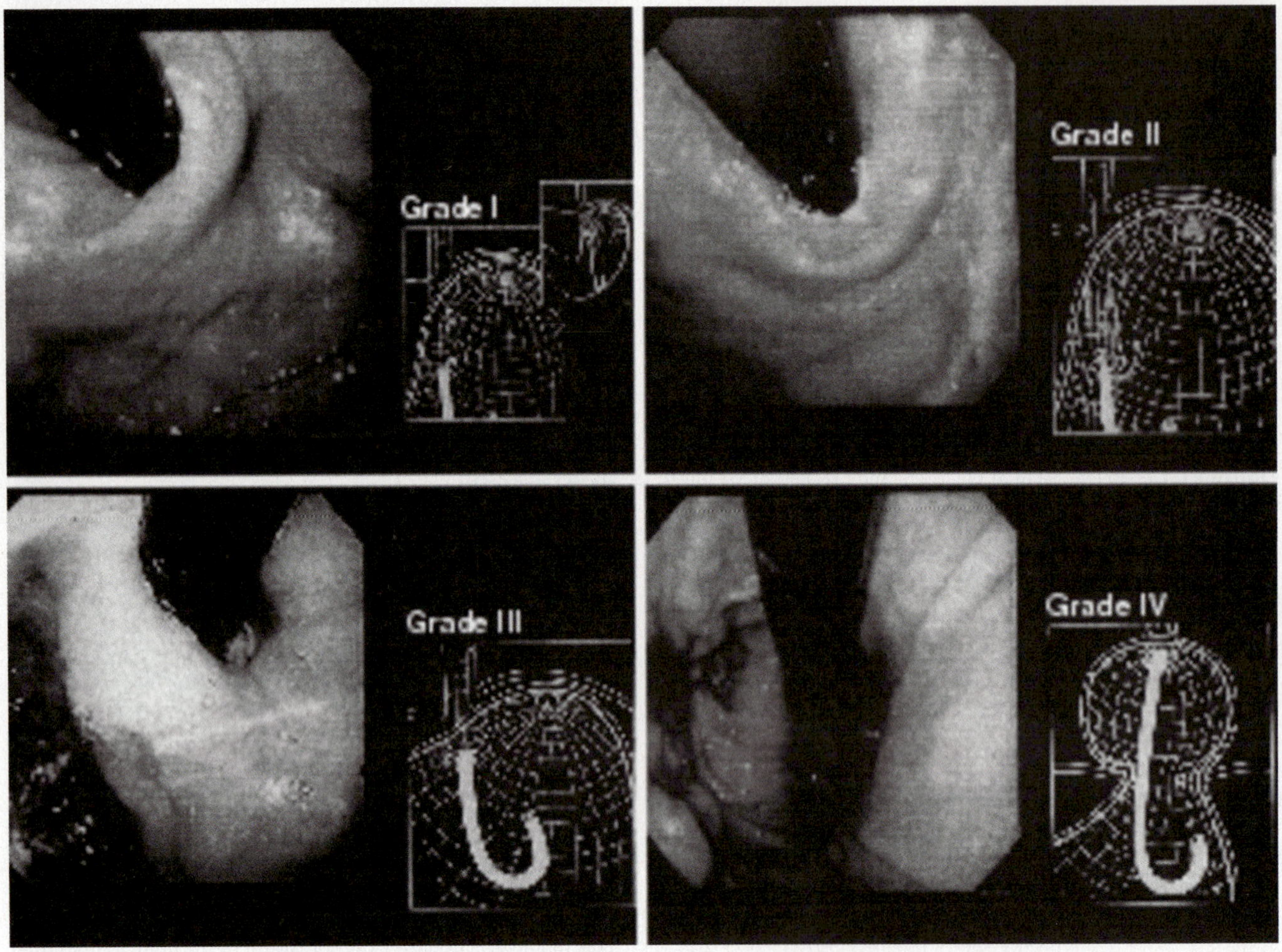

Figure 41.15. Endoscopic grading of the gastroesophageal junction during the retroflex view. (From Oberg S, Peters JH, DeMeester TR, et al. Endoscopic grading of the gastroesophageal valve in patients with symptoms of gastroesophageal reflux disease [GERD]. *Surg Endosc.* 1999;13(12):1184–1188, with permission.)

commonly used to categorize the appearance and competence of the gastroesophageal barrier (**Fig. 41.15**). The grading is I to IV, a higher grade with worsening architecture and thus higher likelihood of acid exposure through the GEJ.[7]

A hiatal hernia is seen when there is a separation of the GEJ from the crura, and by definition, is present when a minimum of 2 cm of rugal folds are above the pinch of the diaphragmatic crura. GERD is frequently associated with a notable sliding hiatal hernia. It is important to assess for presence of gastritis or Cameron ulcers within the hiatal hernia. During the removal of the endoscope, it is important to again slowly examine the esophagus. The larynx and vocal cords should also be visualized to assess inflammation and movement, as chronic acid reflux can injure these structures.

Radiologic Evaluation

A barium esophagram is a critical diagnostic test to assess the anatomy and function of the esophagus and upper stomach. Historically, the barium esophagram has been used as the "road map" of the esophagus as it can provide real-time visualization of bolus transport, esophageal motility, size of hiatal hernia, and structural abnormalities. The first part of the esophagram includes an assessment of the UES and pharynx in the upright position, to evaluate the coordination of pharyngeal transit. Bolus transit on esophagram complements information from esophageal manometry and clearance can be assessed with both liquids and solids (tablet), and is done in the upright and supine positions. A primary peristaltic wave strips the bolus through the esophagus and into the stomach during a normal swallow and adequate contractility is shown by full lumen approximation. Disorders of esophageal motility result in a segmented appearance of barium within the esophagus. This can be due to disorganized peristalsis or simultaneous esophageal contraction, resulting in a beading or corkscrew appearance. A 13-mm barium tablet is a useful proxy to determine how solid material transits through the esophagus and LES, and assists in identifying areas of clinically significant narrowing as well as functional obstructions, as luminal narrowing below 13 mm frequently results in dysphagia.

Hiatal hernias are best visualized in the prone position as the increased intra-abdominal pressure pushes the hernia above the diaphragm. Hiatal hernias >5 cm or hernias that do not reduce are more likely to be associated with chronic reflux and esophageal foreshortening. Though reflux of contrast can be seen on UGI, it is not always consistent with a true diagnosis of reflux. Evoked reflux and spontaneous reflux to the distal esophagus on an esophagram are not correlated to acidic pH, though spontaneous reflux to the thoracic inlet more frequently does correlate. Additionally, the absence of reflux seen on a UGI does not exclude the disease.

Esophageal Manometry

High-resolution manometry (HRM) provides a detailed assessment of esophageal contractility, coordination, and sphincter function. The most common HRM system utilizes 36 circumferential sensors spaced at 1-cm intervals, with each transducer able to detect pressure over a length of 25 mm in 12 radially dispersed sectors (**Fig. 41.16**).

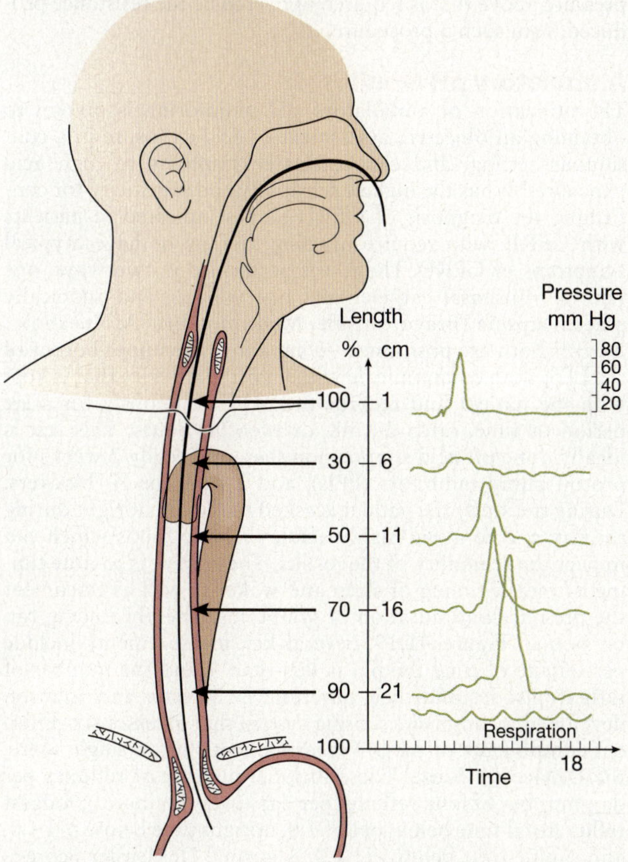

Figure 41.16. Illustration of the position of a five-channel esophageal motility catheter during the esophageal body portion of the study.

The pressures at each sector are averaged, providing a large amount of data that is then converted via a topographic plotting algorithm to a Clouse plot, or esophageal pressure topography (**Fig. 41.17**). HRM is generally performed by passing a lubricated catheter through the nasopharynx, into the esophagus and stomach, though endoscopic guidance is recommended in large paraesophageal hernias and achalasia

Table 41.2. Normal and Abnormal Lower Esophageal Sphincter Measurements on HRM

	Normal	Abnormal
Overall Length	**2.7–4.8 cm**	<2 cm
Pressure	13–43 mm Hg	<6 mm Hg

to confirm no coiling within the esophagus. The patient then completes 10 swallows (supine with head elevated), with at least 30 seconds between swallows (to prevent deglutitive inhibition) and quiet breathing between for better assessment of baseline resting pressures of UES and LES. The full HRM assessment includes contraction amplitude, waveform, esophageal body coordination, UES function, structural characteristics of the LES, and LES relaxation.[8]

HRM is indicated in symptoms of dysphagia, odynophagia, regurgitation, and heartburn. HRM plays a critical role in confirming and differentiating primary esophageal motility disorders including diffuse esophageal spasm, nutcracker esophagus, achalasia, and a hypertensive LES. Systemic diseases (including scleroderma, polymyositis, and dermatomyositis) as well as long-standing GERD can result in ineffective esophageal motility (IEM). HRM can identify a noncompetent LES and determine its location for placement of an ambulatory pH monitor.

Lower Esophageal Sphincter

Utilizing the HRM technique, expected LES measurements compared to noncompetent LES measurements are shown in **Table 41.2**.

Generally, the LES pressure drops to the baseline gastric pressure immediately after a swallow is initiated and will remain open and relaxed until the peristaltic wave reaches the stomach. After the passage of the bolus, the postrelaxation contraction of the LES is observed to ensure LES closure and prevention of reflux. The LES relaxation is assessed by the integrated relaxation pressure (IRP), which is a 4-second time period between initiation of swallow and when peristalsis reaches the LES. An IRP over 15 mm Hg is elevated and can result in resistance of flow through the LES.

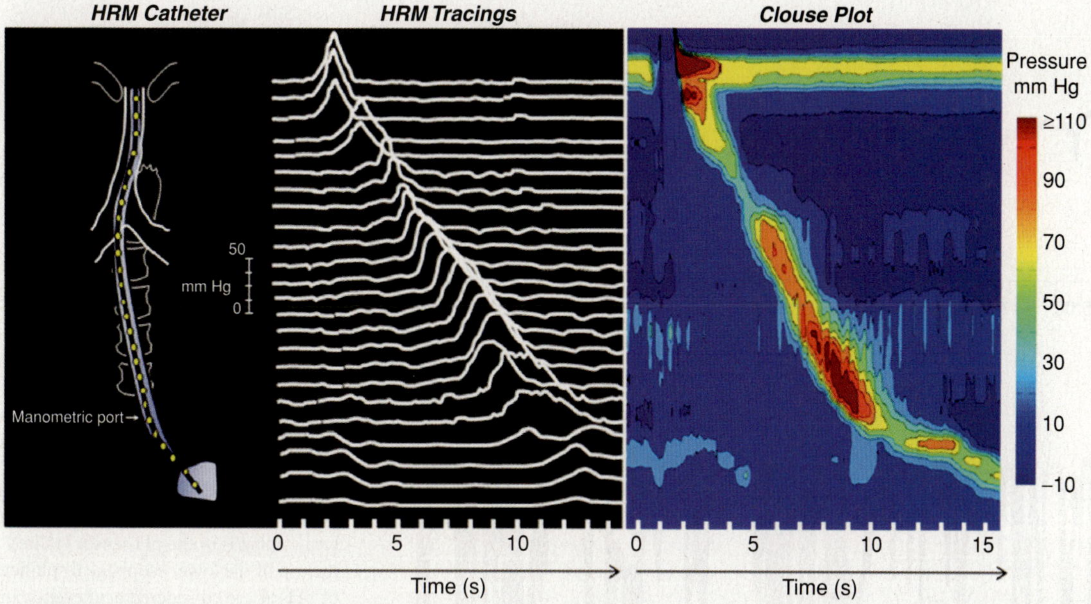

Figure 41.17. High-resolution manometry with line tracings and converted pressure topography or Clouse plot view. (From Pandalfino JE, Roman S. High-resolution manometry: an atlas of esophageal motility disorders and findings of GERD using esophageal pressure topography. *Thor Surg Clin.* 2011;21[4]:465–475, with permission.)

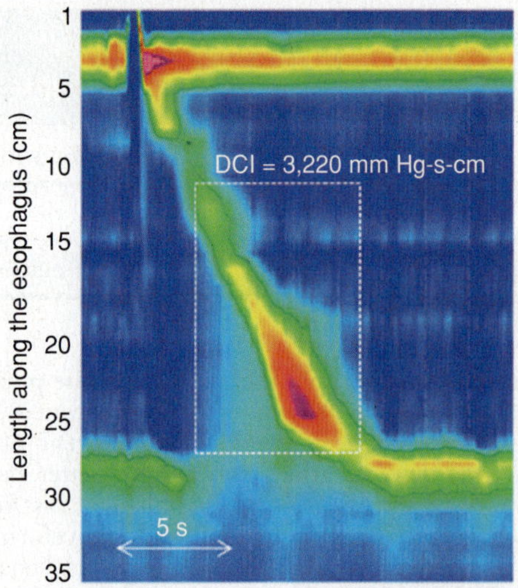

Figure 41.18. High-resolution esophageal manometry during a swallow. The initiation of swallowing is reflected by transient relaxation of the UES, followed by a peristaltic pressure wave progressing down the esophageal body. Note the LES relaxes at the initiation of swallowing. A characteristic peristaltic break is observed in the upper third of the esophageal body at the transition zone between the striated and smooth muscle. (From Pandalfino JE, Roman S. High-resolution manometry: an atlas of esophageal motility disorders and findings of GERD using esophageal pressure topography. *Thor Surg Clin.* 2011;21[4]:465–475, with permission.)

Esophageal Body Motility

HRM assesses esophageal body motility by quantifying contraction amplitude, duration, velocity, slope, and even morphology (type of peak of amplitude). Pathologic gaps in peristalsis occur if there are >2 cm long breaks in isobaric contour along the esophagus or any break at the LES. The distal contractile integral (DCI) provides a global assessment of esophageal contractile function and is calculated by: amplitude (mm Hg) duration (sec) × length (cm). Normal values for DCI range between 500 and 4,300 mm Hg·s·cm (**Fig. 41.18**). Current clinical practice recommends a DCI >500 to prevent postoperative dysphagia after an antireflux procedure, as a pressure above that is required to overcome the resistance produced from such a procedure.

Ambulatory pH Monitoring

6 The utilization of ambulatory pH monitoring is pivotal to obtaining an objective assessment of acid exposure in a continuous setting, and can correlate symptoms to high acid exposure.[9] It has the highest sensitivity and specificity for confirming the diagnosis of GERD and is indicated in patients with GERD who require ongoing therapy or have atypical symptoms of GERD. The test is performed in two ways, one with a transnasal catheter and one with an endoscopically placed capsule (Bravo capsule, Medtronic Inc., Minneapolis, MN).[10] Both are positioned ~6 cm above the upper border of the LES. Both communicate with a portable device that is kept with the patient and records the pH continuously for a set period of time, often 24, 48, or even 96 hours. This test is ideally done off acid suppression therapy; ideally 2 weeks for proton pump inhibitors (PPIs), and 2 days for H_2 blockers. During the study the patient is asked to remain upright during the day and to avoid highly acidic or basic foods which can impact the reliability of the results. The patient is to note timing of meals, timing of sleep and wake, as well as document the presence and duration of symptoms. The pH tracing can be seen in **Figure 41.19**. Several key measurements include percentage of time the pH is less than 4 and the number of reflux episodes and their duration. DeMeester and Johnson developed a composite scoring system that assesses six different components of the pH measurements into a single score, the DeMeester Score. These include: number of refluxes per day, number of long refluxes per day (over 5 minutes), longest reflux, total time below pH of 4.0, upright time below pH 4.0, and supine time below pH 4.0. A normal DeMeester Score is <14.7, and the normal total time spent in reflux is <4%.[9,10] The ambulatory pH study is the most reliable way to quantitatively measure the degree and pattern and of esophageal acid exposure, which can have an impact on the decision to operate for GERD.

Multichannel Impedance Testing

Multichannel intraluminal impedance (MII) uses a catheter with multiple pressure and impedance sensors separated by 1 to 2 cm, which evaluates the direction and effectiveness of bolus transit in addition to esophageal pressure abnormalities.

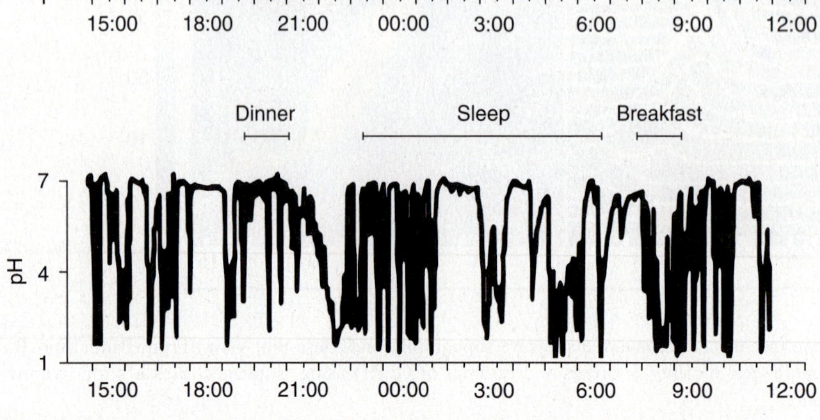

Figure 41.19. Dual-probe 24-hour pH tracing of patient. The top tracing is of the pH sensor located below the upper esophageal sphincter and the bottom tracing is of the pH sensor located 5 cm above the top of the lower esophageal sphincter. Episodes of pH <4 are considered acid events. In this example, the patient has abnormal acid exposure in the distal esophagus with several reflux events extending into the proximal esophagus.

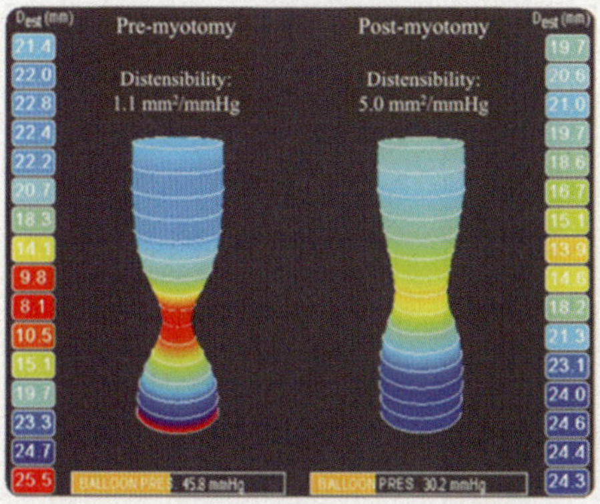

Figure 41.20. Visual representation of changes in the lower esophageal sphincter before and after myotomy for achalasia using EndoFlip with a 40-mL volume fill.

It also permits the detection of both acid and nonacid gastroesophageal reflux when combined with pH testing and can be done both on and off PPIs. This method is preferred for the assessment of patients with atypical symptoms and those with incomplete or no response to acid-suppressive therapy. MII-HRM classifies swallows as "complete bolus transit," "incomplete bolus transit" (no bolus exit identified at any one of the distal impedance-measuring sites), and "esophageal transit abnormality" (30% of liquid swallows or 40% of viscous swallows with incomplete bolus transit). MII-pH can establish the association of the patient's symptoms with reflux episodes by providing the symptom index (SI; 50% indicates symptomatic reflux on PPI therapy) and the symptom association probability (SAP; 95% is considered indicative of a good temporal association between the patient's symptoms and reflux).

Impedance Planimetry

7 Endoflip is an impedance planimetry system used to evaluate real-time pressure, diameter, and distensibility of the esophagus and gastrointestinal sphincters.[11,12] The balloon catheter can be passed transorally with endoscopic guidance or through the endoscope. There is an 8-cm long and a 16-cm balloon catheter, both of which can be used to assess the GEJ and LES, as well as the pylorus when indicated. The 16 cm is better suited for assessment of the esophagus proximal to the LES. The balloon is filled with 30 cc, 40 cc, 50 cc, 60 cc, or 70 cc, and the metrics documented (note, the 8-cm balloon should only be filled to 50 cc). There are several primary metrics and these include the maximum diameter (mm) of the narrowest luminal area, the cross-sectional area (mm^2), balloon pressure (mm Hg), the distensibility index (mm^2/mm Hg), and esophageal contractile pattern categories (repetitive antegrade contractions, repetitive retrograde contractions, absent contractile response, or disordered/diminished contractile response). Endoflip can be easily completed with upper endoscopy to immediately assess the competence of the LES, in workup for dysphagia, esophageal motility disorders such as achalasia, or symptoms of GERD. Endoflip allows an improved functional assessment of the LES, with detailed diameter assessment of the GEJ and of notable clinical importance, its distensibility, or ability to open at varying pressures (**Fig. 41.20**).

CONCLUSIONS

The anatomy and physiology of the esophagus is unique and requires a detailed understanding to ensure safe workup and management. A deep appreciation of the anatomic relationships to other critical structures is pivotal to safe operations on the esophagus. The anatomic and functional studies outlined guide clinical decision making and surgeons should closely consider their use and interpretation.

GASTROESOPHAGEAL REFLUX DISEASE

Definition and Epidemiology

The most widely used definition for GERD is "a condition which develops when the reflux of stomach contents causes troublesome symptoms and/or complications."[13] It is difficult to accurately estimate the prevalence of GERD due to heterogeneity in the design of published studies, but approximately 20% of people in the United States experience GERD symptoms at least weekly. Worldwide, GERD is most prevalent in South Asia and Southeast Europe (>25%) and lowest in Southeast Asia, Canada, and France (<10%).[14] However, it is still responsible for 110,000 hospital admissions annually in the United States.

The increasing prevalence of obesity, which is a significant risk factor for GERD, may be driving the increasing prevalence of GERD. Jacobson et al. have shown that compared to normal-weight women, underweight women (BMI <20) were one-third less likely and overweight women (BMI 25 to 27.4) two times more likely to have frequent GERD symptoms. Obese women (BMI >30) had a nearly three times higher risk of frequent GERD symptoms.[15] Recent meta-analyses confirm this association between increasing BMI and the presence of GERD.[14] High-resolution motility studies have shown a significant correlation with BMI and both increased intragastric pressure and abnormal gastroesophageal pressure gradients, providing a physiologic explanation for the BMI–GERD association. Specifically, central obesity has been shown to be especially associated with erosive esophagitis (OR 1.87), Barrett esophagus (OR 1.98), and esophageal adenocarcinoma (OR 2.51).[16]

There are two main categories of GERD: nonerosive disease (NERD) and erosive disease (ERD). Up to 70% of patients have NERD, but over time, patients may progress from NERD to erosive esophagitis and from ERD to Barrett esophagus. Risk factors for progression of disease included family history of GERD, baseline esophagitis or remaining unhealed after initial treatment, alcohol intake, and regular use of PPIs.[17]

Clinical Presentation

The most common symptoms in patients with GERD are heartburn, regurgitation, and dysphagia. Dysphagia may be an indication of more serious underlying pathology, including esophageal carcinoma, and should prompt an upper endoscopy. Heartburn is typically characterized as a substernal "burning" discomfort often radiating from the epigastrium to sternal notch. Occasionally, patients will refer to it as chest or epigastric pain or indigestion. Typically, heartburn occurs postprandially and is exacerbated by acidic foods, chocolate, coffee, and alcohol. It is commonly relieved by antacids, histamine-2 blockers, or PPIs. Importantly, the severity of symptoms is not necessarily related to the severity of the underlying disease as characterized by endoscopic findings (**Fig. 41.21**).

Regurgitation is the spontaneous return of gastric contents proximal to the GE junction, without necessarily reaching as high as the pharynx or mouth. It is typically worse at night in the recumbent position or when bending over or lying down after a meal. Patients commonly compensate by not eating late at night or by sleeping partially upright with several pillows or in a chair. This symptom is less often improved with antacid treatment. Dysphagia is generally described as the sensation of food being temporarily "stuck" in the esophagus. Dysphagia that is limited to solid food with normal passage of liquids is suggestive of a mechanical problem, such as a hiatal hernia, benign esophageal stricture, or tumor. Dysphagia with both solids and liquids is more typical of a functional or motor disorder, such as achalasia. Patients usually slowly adjust their eating habits as dysphagia progresses without realizing it, and dietary history including questions regarding the consistency of consumed food is an important component of patient assessment.

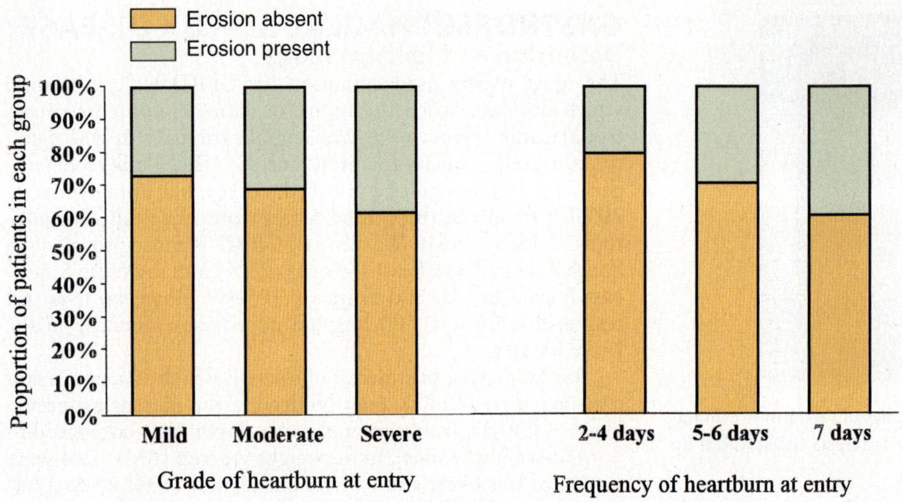

Figure 41.21. Prevalence of erosive esophagitis in 994 patients with varying severity and frequency of reflux symptoms. (Reproduced with permission from Venables TL, Newland RD, Patel AC, et al. Omeprazole 10 mg once daily, omeprazole 20 mg once daily, or ranitidine 150 mg twice daily, evaluated as initial therapy for the relief of symptoms of gastro-oesophageal reflux disease in general practice. *Scand J Gastroenterol.* 1997;32[10]:965–973.)

Some patients with GERD often also manifest extraesophageal symptoms, such as cough, asthma, hoarseness, and noncardiac chest pain. Atypical symptoms are the primary complaint in 20% to 25% of patients with GERD and are secondarily present in association with heartburn and regurgitation in many more. It is considerably more difficult to prove a cause-and-effect relationship between atypical symptoms and GE reflux than it is to do so for the typical symptoms, and the etiology of these symptoms is often multifactorial. Antireflux surgery can provide symptom relief in these patients, but careful testing to document GERD is critical, particularly in those with little or no response to medical therapy.

The symptoms above are not specific to GERD, and the differential diagnosis includes achalasia, diffuse spasm, esophageal carcinoma, pyloric stenosis, cholelithiasis, gastritis, gastric or duodenal ulcer, and coronary artery disease. This underlines the importance of objective diagnosis before the decision is made for surgical treatment.

Physiology of the Antireflux Barrier

The common feature of both physiologic or pathologic gastroesophageal reflux is the loss of the normal gastroesophageal high-pressure zone and the resistance it imposes to the flow of gastric juice from an environment of higher pressure (the stomach), to an environment of lower pressure (the esophagus). This barrier, composed of both anatomic (flap valve and diaphragm) and physiologic (LES) components, acts to prevent reflux. The key determinants of the barrier include:

1. The frequency of swallow- and nonswallow-induced transient relaxations of the LES
2. The structural integrity of the LES
3. Anatomic alterations of the diaphragmatic crura and gastroesophageal flap valve represented by the angle of His

The presence or absence of pathologic esophageal acid exposure (ie, abnormal pH studies) is not only influenced by the degree of barrier loss but also by esophageal and gastric functional characteristics, including esophageal clearance, intra-abdominal pressure, and gastric emptying abnormalities.

Structural Integrity of the Lower Esophageal Sphincter

The pressure, overall length, and the length exposed to the positive pressure environment of the abdomen are the three characteristics of the LES that maintain its resistance or barrier function to intragastric and intra-abdominal pressure increases. The resistance of the LES is a function of its pressure and the length over which this pressure is exerted. The shorter the overall length of the high-pressure zone, the higher the pressure must be to maintain sufficient resistance to remain competent (**Fig. 41.12**). If the overall length of the sphincter is abnormally short, then with minimal gastric distention there will be insufficient sphincter length for the existing pressure to maintain sphincter competency, and reflux will occur even in the presence of "normal" resting sphincter pressure.[5]

The third characteristic of the LES is its position, specifically the length of the high-pressure zone that is exposed to positive intra-abdominal pressure. If the abdominal length is inadequate, the sphincter cannot respond to an increase in applied intra-abdominal pressure by collapsing, and reflux is more likely. This usually occurs as a result of a hiatal hernia and is the most common cause of a permanently defective sphincter.

If the LES has an abnormally low pressure, a short overall length, or minimal exposure to the abdominal pressure environment in the fasting state, then uninhibited reflux of gastric contents into the esophagus occurs. Such a *permanently defective sphincter* is identified by having one or more of the following:

- high-pressure zone with an average pressure of less than 6 mm Hg
- average overall length of 2 cm or less
- an average length exposed to the positive pressure environment of the abdomen of 1 cm or less

A permanently defective sphincter is commonly associated with esophageal mucosal injury, difficulty to control symptoms with medical therapy, and esophageal dysmotility.

Anatomic Alterations

Hiatal Hernia

Hiatal hernia is a common abnormality in patients with GERD, and it has been demonstrated that the diaphragmatic crura are important in preventing reflux during periods of loss of LES pressure, and that the physiologic flap valve created by the angle of His is a contributing barrier to gastroesophageal reflux.[7] The presence of a normal acute angle of His versus the abnormal dome architecture of a sliding hiatus hernia influences the ease with which the sphincter is pulled open. A higher intragastric pressure is needed to open the sphincter in patients with an intact angle of His when compared to patients with a hiatal hernia (**Fig. 41.22**).

The presence of a hiatal hernia also leads to impaired esophageal clearance due to loss of anchorage of the esophagus in the abdomen. Kahrilas et al. have shown that complete esophageal emptying was achieved in 86% of swallows in control subjects without a hiatal hernia, 66% in patients with a sliding hiatal hernia, and only 32% of patients with a nonreducing hiatal hernia.[18] Thus, there is overwhelming evidence that hiatal hernia does indeed play a significant role in the pathophysiology of GERD.

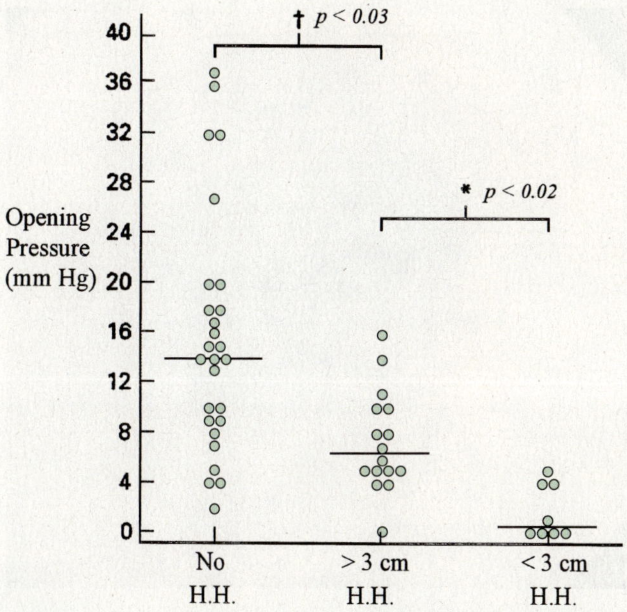

Figure 41.22. The intragastric pressure at which the lower esophagus endoscopically opened in response to gastric distention by air during endoscopy. Note that the dome architecture of a hiatus hernia (HH) influences the ease with which the sphincter can be pulled open by gastric distention. (Reproduced with permission from Ismail T, Bancewicz J, Barlow J. Yield pressure, anatomy of the cardia and gastro-oesophageal reflux. *Br J Surg.* 1995;82[7]:943–947.)

Gastric Distension

When the stomach is distended from overeating, aerophagia, or delayed gastric emptying, the vectors produced by gastric wall tension pull on the GE junction with a force that varies according to the geometry of the cardia. Thus, when increased intragastric pressure occurs in the presence of a hiatal hernia, the force is applied more directly. This pulls on the terminal esophagus, reducing the length of the sphincter until a critical length of 1 to 2 cm occurs, when the pressure drops precipitously, and reflux occurs. This results in postprandial reflux, which is a common complaint in the initial stages of GERD. After gastric venting, the length of the high-pressure zone is restored, and competence returns until the next episode of distention. This sequence results in the common complaints of repetitive belching and bloating in patients with GERD. The patients' repetitive swallowing is an effort to neutralize the refluxed acid, but then contributes to repeat gastric distension.

Repeated exposure of the squamous epithelium of the distal esophagus to gastric juice causes inflammation, columnarization, and carditis. In early disease, the esophagitis is mild and commonly limited to the very distal esophagus. The patient compensates by increased swallowing, allowing saliva to bathe the injured mucosa and alleviate the discomfort induced by exposure to gastric acid. Increased swallowing results in aerophagia, bloating, and repetitive belching. The distention induced by aerophagia leads to further exposure and repetitive injury to the terminal squamous epithelium and the development of cardiac-type mucosa (carditis). The process can lead to a fibrotic mucosal ring at the squamocolumnar junction (Schatzki ring). Extension of the inflammatory process into the muscularis propria causes a progressive loss in the length and pressure of the distal esophageal high-pressure zone associated with an increased esophageal exposure to gastric juice and the symptoms of heartburn and regurgitation. The loss of the barrier eventually results in the permanent loss of LES resistance and the extension of the disease into the esophagus with progression to severe esophagitis. Intestinalization of the cardiac-type mucosa can occur at any time during this process, setting the stage for malignant degeneration.

Implications

Implications of recognizing anatomic alterations as components of GE barrier:

1. Transient LES relaxation is likely a consequence of sphincter shortening by gastric distention and is the underlying mechanism for belching and physiologic reflux. It does not play a major role in patients with symptomatic gastroesophageal reflux, particularly those with ERD, Barrett esophagus, or those referred for surgery.
2. Efforts to augment the gastroesophageal barrier, either pharmacologically or endoscopically, will commonly fail when a hiatal hernia is present.
3. Patients with abnormal esophageal acid exposure in the presence of normal LES characteristics and no hiatal hernia have an uncommon reason for reflux and these patients require additional evaluation since gastric or esophageal clearance failure may be present and may impair the outcome of a fundoplication.
4. Both reduction of a hiatal hernia and augmentation of the LES are necessary to maximally restore gastroesophageal barrier competence.
5. Although acid control without regard to barrier incompetence will improve heartburn and heal esophageal ERD, it results in increasing numbers of patients with pulmonary manifestations of GERD.

Complications of Gastroesophageal Reflux Disease

The complications of gastroesophageal reflux result from the damage caused by the reflux of gastric juice onto the esophageal mucosa or laryngeal or respiratory epithelium (**Fig. 41.23**). Complications can be conceptually divided into (a) mucosal complications such as esophagitis and stricture; (b) extraesophageal

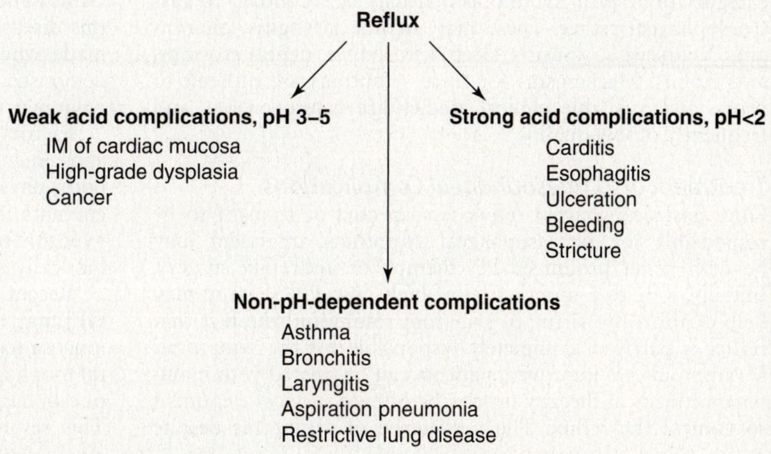

Figure 41.23. Schematic representation of the types of complications of gastroesophageal reflux disease.

ESOPHAGUS

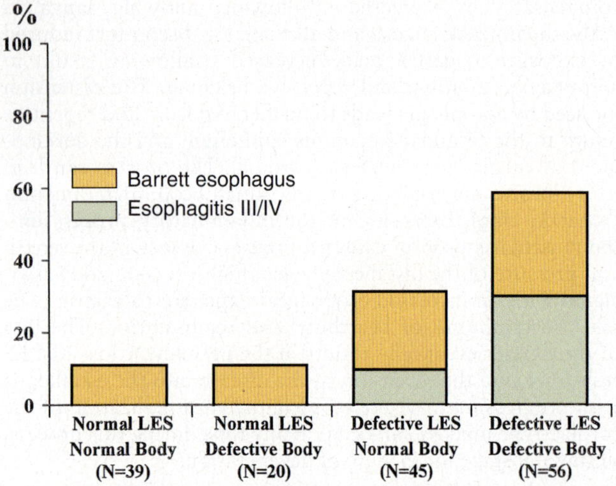

Figure 41.24. Prevalence of esophageal mucosal injury related to the presence of a defective lower esophageal sphincter, esophageal body motility, or both.

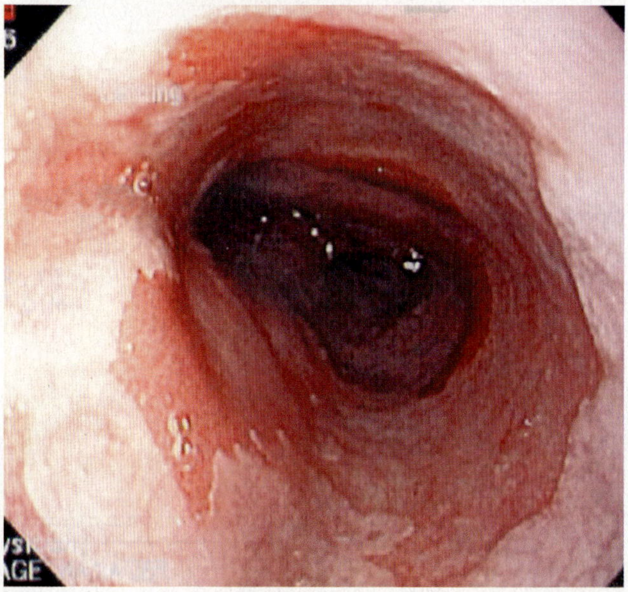

Figure 41.25. Endoscopic appearance of Barrett esophagus. Note the pink metaplastic mucosa as opposed to the normal whitish squamous lining of the esophagus.

or respiratory complications such as chronic cough, asthma, and pulmonary fibrosis; and (c) metaplastic (Barrett esophagus) and neoplastic (adenocarcinoma). The prevalence and severity of complications are related to the degree of loss of the gastroesophageal barrier, defects in esophageal clearance, and the content of refluxed gastric juice (**Fig. 41.24**).

Mucosal Complications

The potential injurious components that reflux into the esophagus include gastric secretions, such as acid and pepsin; biliary and pancreatic secretions that regurgitate from the duodenum into the stomach, and toxic compounds generated in the mouth, esophagus, and stomach by the action of bacteria on dietary substances. This exposure can cause esophagitis in the acute setting, and progress to Barrett esophagus with chronic exposure.

Respiratory Complications

Reflux has been implicated as causative of asthma and idiopathic pulmonary fibrosis (IPF), with 35% to 50% of asthmatics shown to have abnormal esophageal pH, esophagitis, and a hiatal hernia. Others have shown that the prevalence of reflux symptoms exceeded 50% in patients with asthma and CF. In addition, patients with COPD and gastroesophageal reflux are twice as likely to have significant COPD exacerbations than their nonreflux counterparts, and reflux symptoms correlate with airway obstruction in COPD patients.[19]

Laryngopharyngeal Reflux

The term *laryngopharyngeal reflux (LPR)* is used for a broad category of atypical symptoms that may be secondary to gastroesophageal reflux. These may include laryngitis, pharyngitis, hoarseness, sinusitis, sleep disturbance, dental erosions, and globus. Mechanisms for these symptoms are difficult to prove and available clinical studies are heterogeneous and frequently of low quality.[20]

Treatment of Extraesophageal Complications

Once gastroesophageal reflux is suspected or thought to be responsible for extraesophageal symptoms, treatment may be with either prolonged PPI therapy or antireflux surgery. Initially, a 3- to 6-month trial of high-dose PPI therapy may help confirm (by virtue of symptom resolution) the fact that reflux is partly or completely responsible for the symptoms. If symptoms are improved, patients can be treated with maintenance medical therapy or may be offered surgical treatment to control the reflux. The persistence of symptoms despite PPI treatment, however, does not necessarily rule out reflux as being a potential contributor. In patients with laryngopharyngeal reflux whose symptoms that are not relieved by acid suppression, small case series suggest that neuromodulating agents (tricyclic antidepressants, gabapentin, pregabalin) can provide some benefit.[21]

Based on reported observations, relief of RSs can be anticipated for 25% to 50% of patients with reflux-induced asthma treated with antisecretory medications. Fewer than 15% of asthmatics with symptom relief, however, have been shown to have objective improvements in their pulmonary function. Antireflux surgery has better outcomes, improving RSs in nearly 90% of children and 70% of adults with asthma and reflux disease.[22] Improvements in pulmonary function were demonstrated in around one-third of these patients. It is important to note that patients with nonreflux-induced esophageal dysmotility have inferior outcomes after antireflux surgery.

The lung transplantation literature shows that there is a benefit of antireflux surgery in improving both symptoms and pulmonary function tests in patients with bronchiolitis obliterans in pre- and post-lung transplant patients, with acceptable morbidity outcomes.[23]

Pathophysiology of Barrett Metaplasia and Complications

8 Barrett esophagus occurs in 7% to 10% of patients with GERD and represents the end stage of the natural history of this disease (**Fig. 41.25**).[24] Diagnosis of Barrett esophagus is made when any length of endoscopically visible tissue that demonstrates intestinal metaplasia on histology (**Fig. 41.26**) or columnar replacement of the esophagus of 3 cm or more.

Factors predisposing to the development of Barrett esophagus include early-onset GERD, abnormal LES, esophageal body physiology, and mixed reflux of gastric and duodenal contents into the esophagus.[24] In fact, increased esophageal exposure to duodenal juice in patients with GERD is most dramatically related to Barrett esophagus.[25]

Recent studies suggest that the metaplastic process at the GEJ may begin by conversion of distal esophageal squamous mucosa to cardiac-type epithelium due to exposure of the distal esophagus to excess acid and gastric contents via prolapse of esophageal squamous mucosa into the gastric environment. This results in inflammatory changes at the GEJ and/or a

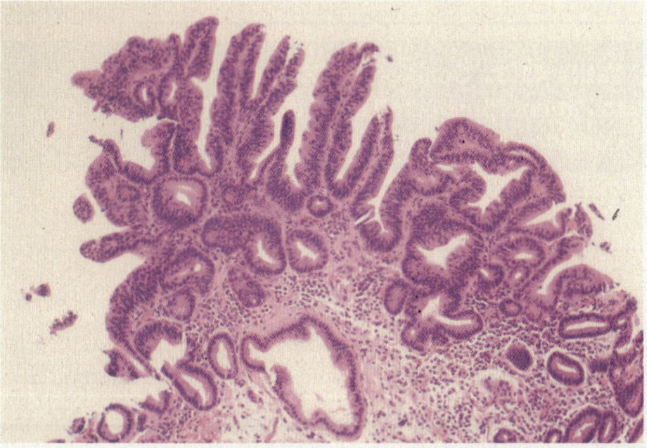

Figure 41.26. Histologic appearance of Barrett esophagus. To the left of the photograph, columnar mucosa with abundant goblet cells is seen. This is intestinal metaplasia, which is the histologic hallmark of Barrett esophagus. To the right of the photomicrograph, cardiac epithelium is present.

metaplastic process, both of which may result in the loss of muscle function and a mechanically defective sphincter, allowing free reflux with progressively higher degrees of mucosal injury.

Treatment

The goals of treatment in this patient population are the relief of symptoms, healing of esophageal mucosal injury, and the prevention of disease progression. Antireflux surgery should be considered when patient factors suggest severe disease or predict the need for long-term medical management, both of which are almost always true in patients with Barrett esophagus. PPI therapy is an acceptable treatment option in patients with Barrett esophagus. Once initiated, however, most patients with Barrett esophagus will require lifelong treatment. Complete control of reflux with PPI therapy can be difficult, and 40% to 80% of patients continue to experience abnormal esophageal acid exposure despite PPI administration.[24] An important consideration is that patients with Barrett esophagus generally have severe GERD, with its associated sequelae such as large hiatal hernia, stricture, shortened esophagus, and poor motility. Compared to mild and nonerosive reflux disease, severe ERD and Barrett esophagus are associated with significantly greater loss of the mechanical antireflux barrier because of associated hiatal hernias and a hypotensive LES. Antireflux surgery likely results in more reproducible and reliable elimination of reflux of both acid and duodenal content than medical treatment. Studies focusing on the symptomatic outcome following antireflux surgery in patients with Barrett esophagus document excellent results in 79% to 92% of patients at up to 12 months following surgery. Objective outcome studies suggest that histologic regression of Barrett metaplasia is seen in 22% to 41% of surgical patients post fundoplication, though as many as 25% of them will have persistent pathologic esophageal acid exposure confirmed by 24-hour pH studies.[26]

In addition to symptomatic and physiologic improvement in reflux after surgery, there is evidence that mediators of esophageal inflammation implicated in carcinogenesis are decreased as well, these include cyclooxygenase-2 (COX-2) and interleukin 8.[27]

Dysplasia in Barrett Esophagus

The prevalence of dysplasia at diagnosis in patients presenting with Barrett esophagus ranges from 15% to 25%, and approximately 5% of patients will develop dysplasia each year. Barrett metaplasia is currently classified into four broad categories:

1. No dysplasia
2. Indefinite for dysplasia
3. Low-grade dysplasia
4. High-grade dysplasia (HGD)

The overall annual risk of progression to esophageal adenocarcinoma among patients with Barrett esophagus is 0.29%, and the risk of progression is significantly higher in patients with low-grade dysplasia than in those without it at baseline.[28] Therefore, Barrett esophagus complicated by dysplasia should undergo aggressive therapy. Patients whose biopsies are interpreted as indefinite for dysplasia should be treated with a medical regimen consisting of 60 to 80 mg of PPI therapy for 3 months and rebiopsied. The presence of severe inflammation makes the microscopic interpretation of dysplasia difficult, and the purpose of acid suppression therapy is to resolve inflammation that may complicate the interpretation of the biopsy specimen. Persistent indefinite or low-grade dysplasia should be a relative indication for a Nissen fundoplication given the evidence that in most patients, low-grade dysplasia reverts to nondysplastic intestinal metaplasia after a fundoplication. Radiofrequency ablation or cryotherapy are acceptable alternative treatments to reduce the risk of progression to cancer in these patients.

Approximately 50% of patients thought to have only HGD will harbor a focus of invasive carcinoma somewhere in the columnar mucosa. Any patient with dysplasia, particularly HGD, requires careful endoscopic evaluation with high-definition white-light endoscopy to look for any nodules or lesions. If no lesion is present then ablation therapy should be performed to reduce the risk of progression to cancer in patients with HGD. If a lesion is present, endoscopic mucosal resection should be performed to determine if it is malignant and allow assessment of the depth of invasion and tumor characteristics. Endoscopic resection is preferred over esophagectomy for BE patients with intramucosal esophageal adenocarcinoma (T1a) given a significantly better safety profile, 96% complete response rate, and similar rates of recurrence. The remaining Barrett epithelium should be ablated after all visible lesions are resected. Risk factors for failure of endoscopic therapy include ultra–long segment (>8-cm) Barrett, poorly controlled reflux disease, and high-grade tumor differentiation. Metachronous lesions and local recurrences are treated following the same algorithm.[29] Treatment of more advanced esophageal cancers is discussed in Chapter 42: Esophageal Tumors and Injury.

Treatment of Gastroesophageal Reflux Disease

Medical Treatment

GERD is one of the most prevalent conditions encountered in general medical practice. As a result, medications for control of GERD comprise one of the largest pharmaceutical markets in the United States and abroad. Omeprazole is the seventh most commonly prescribed medication, and there are over 100 million PPI prescriptions given annually, accounting for over $10 billion in expenditures.[30] GERD is such a common condition that most patients with mild symptoms self-medicate with over-the-counter H_2-receptor antagonists (H_2RAs) and PPIs. When first seen with symptoms of heartburn or regurgitation without obvious complications, patients can reasonably be placed on 8 to 12 weeks of acid suppression therapy before further investigations are carried out. This is done in addition to counseling on dietary and lifestyle modification with avoidance of acidic foods, alcohol, tobacco, and weight loss for those with a BMI >25. In many situations, symptoms will successfully resolve. Patients should be advised to elevate the head of the bed; avoid tight clothing; eat small, frequent meals; avoid eating their nighttime meal shortly before retiring; lose weight; and avoid alcohol, coffee, chocolate, and peppermints, which may aggravate the symptoms.

Patients with persistent symptoms should be given PPIs, such as omeprazole, which result in up to 80% to 90%

reduction in gastric acidity and up to 95% reduction in esophageal acid exposure. H_2RAs are less effective in decreasing esophageal acid exposure (80%). PPI doses of 40 mg/d will usually heal mild esophagitis, though healing occurs in only three-fourths of patients with severe esophagitis. It is important to realize that in patients who reflux a combination of gastric and duodenal juice, inadequate acid suppression therapy may give symptomatic improvement while still allowing mixed reflux and persistent mucosal damage in an asymptomatic patient. Unfortunately, within 6 months of discontinuation of any form of medical therapy for GERD, 80% of patients have a recurrence of symptoms.

Despite their effectiveness, periods of acid breakthrough occur in 75% to 80% of patients taking PPIs, primarily at nighttime. Ranitidine 300 mg at bedtime appears superior to omeprazole 20 mg at bedtime in preventing acid breakthrough, likely due to the abolition of histamine-mediated acid secretion in the fasting state.

While PPIs are very well tolerated in the short term, there is increasing evidence suggesting potential adverse consequences to their long-term use. Increased relative risk of bone fractures due to calcium malabsorption, pneumonia, chronic kidney disease, dementia, myocardial infarction, renal disease, GI malignancies, B_{12} deficiency, hypomagnesemia, *Clostridium difficile* infection, and interactions with antiplatelet medications have all been reported. Most of the evidence is weak and obtained from observational studies. However, special attention should be given to elderly patients with significant comorbidities, those on many other medications, and patients with known osteoporosis when considering maintenance PPI therapy.[31]

Potassium-Competitive Acid Blockers (PCABs) are now available in the United States, and have demonstrated compelling outcomes in managing refractory reflux esophagitis. In meta-analyses, they have been more effective than PPIs in GERD management, and in particular for erosive esophagitis.[32]

Failure of acid suppression to control symptoms or immediate return of symptoms after stopping treatment suggests that either the diagnosis is incorrect or the patient has relatively severe disease. Endoscopic examination at this stage of the patient's evaluation provides the opportunity for assessing the severity of mucosal damage and the presence of Barrett esophagus. Both of these findings on initial endoscopy should prompt pH testing and manometry to assess the LES and the function of the esophageal body. These studies identify features that predict a poor response to medical therapy, frequent relapses, and the development of complications of GERD. Patients who have these risk factors should be given the option of surgery as a primary therapy.

Antireflux Surgery

Indications

Antireflux surgery is indicated for the treatment of objectively documented, relatively severe GERD. Candidates for surgery include patients with erosive esophagitis, stricture, Barrett esophagus, hiatal hernia as well as those who are dependent on PPIs for symptom relief.[33] Patients with atypical symptoms who have a good response to intensive medical treatment are also candidates. The option of antireflux surgery should be given to all patients who have demonstrated the need for long-term medical therapy, particularly if escalating doses of PPIs are needed to control symptoms. Antireflux surgery may be the preferred option in patients younger than 50 years, those who are noncompliant with their drug regimen, those for whom medications are a financial burden, and those who favor a single intervention over long-term drug treatment. It may be the treatment of choice in patients who are at high risk of progression despite medical therapy, such as those with nocturnal reflux on pH study, a structurally deficient LES, mixed reflux of gastric and duodenal juice, and mucosal injury at presentation.

DIAGNOSIS

Table 41.3. Goals of the Diagnostic Approach to Patients Suspected of Having GERD and Being Considered for Antireflux Surgery

Establish that GERD is the underlying cause of the patient's symptoms.
Estimate the risk of progressive disease.
Determine the presence or absence of esophageal shortening.
Evaluate esophageal body function and, occasionally, gastric emptying function.

GERD, gastroesophageal reflux disease.

Preoperative Evaluation

9 The preoperative evaluation of GERD is imperative to determining a diagnosis and establishing an optimal treatment plan for each individual patient. **Table 41.3** outlines four important goals in the diagnosis of suspected GERD and those being considered for antireflux surgery. Please refer to the prior section in this chapter for details on preoperative studies, the below will be a summary.

The preoperative work up includes endoscopic assessment to include grading of esophagitis if present (**Table 41.1**) and documentation of the Hill grade; ambulatory pH monitoring (24 hour, combined impedance-pH, or wireless Bravo capsule); radiographic evaluation with esophagram (**Fig. 41.27** and **Table 41.5**); and esophageal manometry (**Fig. 41.17**) with EndoFlip if available (**Fig. 41.20**).

Patient selection is critically important, and the studies outlined in the prior section of this chapter increase the degree of certainty of a diagnosis of GERD. In addition, three specific factors have been identified as predictive of a positive outcome

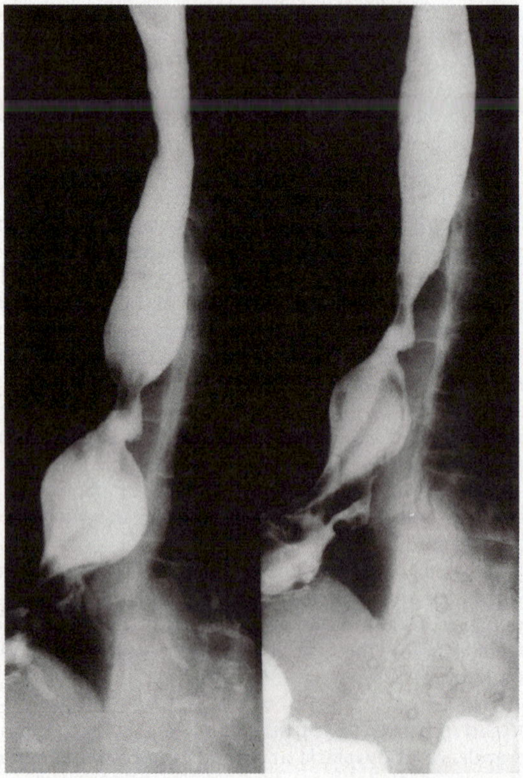

Figure 41.27. Barium-filled esophagogastric segment in a patient with a short esophagus. Note that the gastroesophageal junction is well above the hiatus.

Table 41.4. Predictors of Outcome after Laparoscopic Fundoplication: Stepwise Logistic Regression Results of 199 Patients

Predictor	Status	Adjusted Odds Ratio (95% Confidence Intervals)	Wald *P*-Value
Composite Acid score	Increased	5.4 (1.9–15.3)	<.001
	Normal	—	—
Symptom	Typical	5.1 (1.9–13.7)	<.001
	Atypical	—	—
Response to Medical Therapy	Complete/partial	3.3 (1.3–8.7)	.02
	Minor/none	—	—

Odds ratios and corresponding *P* values are adjusted for age and for all other factors in the model.
From Campos GM, Peters JH, DeMeester TR, et al. Multivariate analysis of the factors predicting outcome after laparoscopic Nissen fundoplication. *J Gastrointest Surg*. 1999;3(3):292–300.

after antireflux surgery. These factors include: abnormal score on esophageal pH monitoring, present of typical symptoms of GERD (heartburn or regurgitation), and symptomatic improvement in response to acid suppression therapy (**Table 41.4**).

Partial versus Complete Fundoplication

10 The decision between partial and complete fundoplication requires considerable judgment for specific patient factors. Though randomized studies have demonstrated overall equivalence in heartburn, regurgitation, and GERD control between Nissen and Toupet fundoplication. With longer-term evaluations showing equally low dysphagia prevalence at long-term follow up (10 to 15 years), as compared to the first 12 months after surgery.[34–36] Metanalysis also showed increased dysphagia, bloating, and inability to belch after Nissen fundoplication, but this also improved over time at longer-term follow up.[37] Additionally, with the use of intraoperative EndoFlip assessment, surgeons can now tailor or adjust their fundoplication in real time based on distensibility findings.[12,38] It is critical that surgeons complete a thorough review of the work-up and a deep understanding of the patient's symptoms and ensure surgeon–patient shared decision making when determining the optimal surgical approach.[39]

Laparoscopic Nissen Fundoplication

Table 41.6 lists the most critical steps in the performance of laparoscopic fundoplication and concurrent hiatal hernia repair as necessary.

Port Placement. For a laparoscopic repair, five ports are used. The camera is placed superiorly and to the left of the umbilicus, roughly one-third of the distance to the xiphoid process, to optimize the visualization of the hiatus. The liver is retracted with flexible retractor placed through a 5-mm

Table 41.5. University of Southern California Protocol for Video Esophagram Studies

Patient Position	Purpose	Technique
Prone RAO	Esophageal body function	Five separate 10-mL swallows, 15 s between each, follow bolus on videotape Video swallow over thoracic inlet and another over distal third of esophagus without panning
	Esophageal diameter	Rapid swallow of several gulps to distend esophagus maximally
	Gastric function	Video-record activity of stomach and duodenum for 30 s in prone position
Supine	Relationship of GE junction to hiatus	Two or three individual swallows focused on distal esophagus and GE junction
Erect	Cricopharyngeal function	Lateral and anteroposterior views of oropharynx and upper esophagus
	Mucosal injury	Spot of collapsed esophagus for mucosal detail
	Reducibility of hernia	Video images of one or two swallows focused on distal esophagus and GE junction
	Gas distention of distal esophagus	
Erect	Solid bolus transport	Record video images of passage of two contrast-coated hamburger boluses from oropharynx to stomach

GE, gastroesophageal; RAO, right anterior oblique.

Table 41.6. Elements of Laparoscopic Fundoplication

1. Crural dissection with identification and preservation of both vagus nerves
2. Circumferential dissection of the esophagus and mobilization of the gastric fundus
3. Crural closure
4. Creation of a short, loose fundoplication around the distal esophagus

incision in the right subcostal region along the anterior axillary line. A retraction port is placed slightly above the level of the umbilicus, in the left anterior axillary line. The surgeon's right-hand 11-mm port is placed 1 to 2 cm below the costal margin, approximately at the lateral rectus border to allow triangulation between the camera and the two working instruments. The surgeon's left-hand 5-mm port is placed last, after the left lateral segment of the liver has been retracted, to visualize the best trajectory under the falciform ligament toward the hiatus (**Fig. 41.28**).

Crural Dissection. In patients without a large hiatal or paraesophageal hernia dissection begins with division of the gastrohepatic omentum and identification of the right crus of the diaphragm. Care is taken to preserve the hepatic branch of the anterior vagus nerve. Alternatively, when a larger paraesophageal hernia is present, the hernia contents are reduced as much as possible first, and sac excision is started at the 2 o'clock position at the hiatus to avoid injuring the left gastric vessels that are routinely up in the chest on the right side of the hiatus.

A replaced left hepatic artery arising from the left gastric artery is present in up to 25% of patients; it should be identified and can typically be clipped and divided, but a pulse in the hepatoduodenal ligament should be confirmed first. The peritoneum overlying the anterior aspect of the right crus is incised and the plane between the esophagus and right crus developed (**Fig. 41.29**).

The dissection is then continued anteriorly, and the esophagus and anterior vagus nerve are swept downward away from the phrenoesophageal ligament. The anterior crural tissues are divided and the left crus identified. The anterior vagus nerve often "hugs" the left crus and can be injured in this portion of the dissection if not carefully searched for and protected. The left crus is dissected as completely as possible, including taking

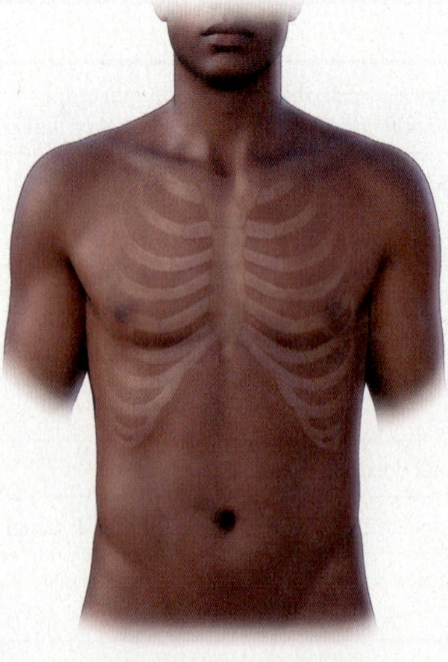

Figure 41.28. Laparoscopic port placement for hiatal hernia repair and fundoplication. SL, surgeon left; SR, surgeon right; C, camera; A, assist port; Liver, liver retractor.

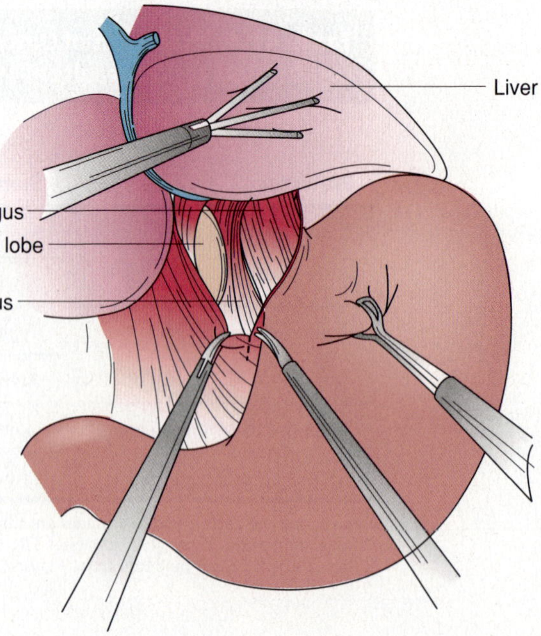

Figure 41.29. Illustration of the initial dissection of the esophageal hiatus. The right crus is identified and dissected toward its posterior confluence with the left crus.

down the angle of His and the attachments of the fundus to the left diaphragm (**Fig. 41.30**). The short gastric vessels are divided along with the posterior pancreatic vessels to completely mobilize the gastric fundus. A window behind the GE junction is then created, and a Penrose drain passed around the distal esophagus for retraction.

Esophageal Mobilization and Crural Closure. The esophagus is mobilized circumferentially into the posterior mediastinum centimeters to provide at least 3 cm of intra-abdominal esophageal length. Both the anterior and posterior vagus nerve should be identified and protected. The right and left pleural reflection often come into view and should be avoided, although if a pleural opening is created, it is well tolerated, provided the hole is made large enough to prevent a ball valve tension pneumothorax from developing. Following mobilization and an assessment of intra-abdominal esophageal length,

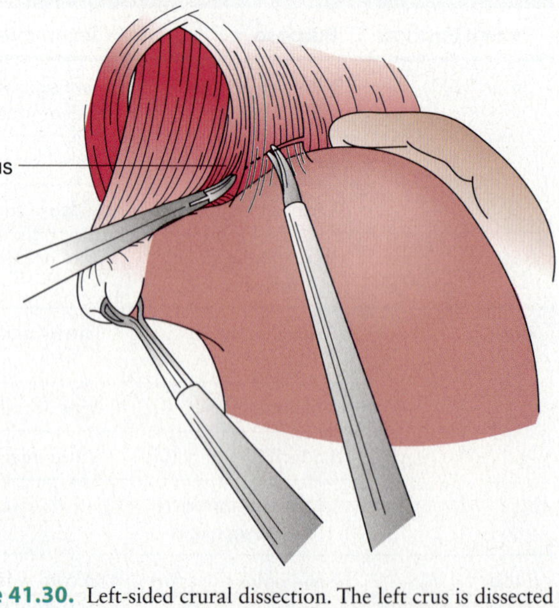

Figure 41.30. Left-sided crural dissection. The left crus is dissected as completely as possible, and the attachments of the fundus of the stomach to the diaphragm are taken down.

the hiatus is closed. The esophagus is retracted anteriorly and to the left, and the crura is approximated with interrupted 0 Ethibond sutures, starting just above the aortic decussation and working anteriorly. The authors prefer using pledgets to reinforce the repair. Care must be taken to identify the anterior surface of the aorta during this step in order to avoid inadvertent injury to it while suturing the left crus. If the crura cannot be approximated despite maximal mobilization, a right-sided relaxing incision in the diaphragm is recommended to allow the crura to be closed without tension. The defect created in the diaphragm is then repaired with permanent mesh to avoid herniation of abdominal contents into the thorax. The authors prefer a Gore-Tex patch for this purpose and reinforce the primary crural closure with an absorbable or biologic mesh. When the right-sided relaxing incision is inadequate (with a very large hernia or in reoperations), a left diaphragm relaxing incision may be necessary. Synthetic mesh bridging the crura should be avoided because it leads to the highest risk of mesh erosion. There are some studies showing that reinforcement of a primary crural closure with biologic or resorbable mesh may help prevent early hiatal hernia recurrence, but this advantage disappears with long-term follow-up, and may increase the complexity of a reoperation if one is necessary in the future.

Creation of the Fundoplication. A 2-cm in length, loose Nissen fundoplication is created after ensuring that there is no twisting of the wrap. The mid-posterior fundus is grasped and passed left to right behind the esophagus to ensure that the posterior fundus is used for the posterior aspect of the fundoplication. One should gently bring the posterior fundus behind the esophagus to the right side with an upward, rightward, and clockwise twisting motion. The anterior wall of the fundus is then folded over the esophagus to meet the posterior at about the 12 o'clock position, and confirmation is necessary to ensure the fundus is not twisted or spiraled around the esophagus.

The posterior and anterior fundic lips should be maneuvered (as in a "shoe shine") to allow the fundus to envelop the esophagus without twisting or tension. The esophagus should comfortably lie in the untwisted fundus prior to suturing. Adequate size of the posterior opening must be ensured to avoid any compression of the posterior fundus, and there must be sufficient mobilization of the posterior fundus to avoid undue

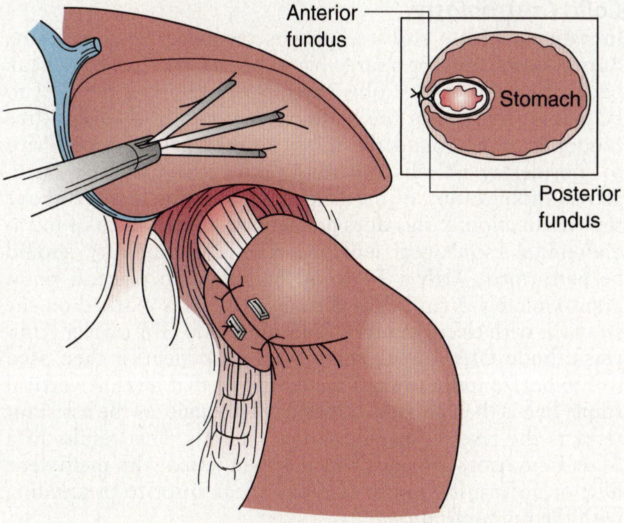

Figure 41.31. Fixation of the fundoplication. The fundoplication is sutured in place with interrupted 0 Ethibond sutures, and a 54- to 60-Fr bougie is in place to ensure the wrap is floppy and not too tight.

tension on the fundoplication. A 54-60-Fr bougie is passed to properly size the fundoplication prior to suturing, and the "lips" of the fundoplication sutured utilizing two to three 0 Ethibond sutures (**Fig. 41.31**). The authors prefer to incorporate the muscular wall of the esophagus with the sutures to facilitate a more secure fundoplication. The most common error is an attempt to grasp the anterior portion of the stomach to construct the right lip of the fundoplication rather than the posterior fundus.

Transthoracic Hiatal Hernia Repair and Fundoplication

The indications for performing an antireflux procedure by a transthoracic approach are given in **Table 41.7**, though these are solely considerations and a transabdominal is favored whenever possible, even with several of the indications and with recurrent hiatal hernias. A failed transabdominal attempt at a repair is also an indication for consideration of a transthoracic approach.

INDICATIONS/CONTRAINDICATIONS

Table 41.7. Indications for Performing an Antireflux Procedure by a Transthoracic Approach

Indication	Explanation
Previous hiatal hernia repair	In this situation, a peripheral circumferential incision in the diaphragm is made to provide simultaneous exposure of the upper abdomen. This allows safe dissection of the previous repair from both the abdominal and thoracic sides of the diaphragm.
Concomitant procedure	Concomitant esophageal myotomy for achalasia or diffuse spasm.
Short esophagus	This is usually associated with a stricture or Barrett esophagus. In this situation, the thoracic approach is preferred to allow maximum mobilization of the esophagus, the performance of a Collis gastroplasty, or, if necessary, placement of the repair without tension below the diaphragm.
Sliding hiatal hernia that does not reduce below the diaphragm during a roentgenographic barium study in the upright position	This can indicate esophageal shortening and, again, a thoracic approach is preferred for maximum mobilization of the esophagus and, if necessary, the performance of a Collis gastroplasty.
Associated pulmonary pathology	The nature of the pulmonary pathology can be evaluated, and the proper pulmonary surgery, in addition to the antireflux repair, can be performed.
Obesity	The abdominal repair is difficult because of poor exposure, whereas the thoracic approach gives better exposure and allows a more precise repair.

Collis Gastroplasty

In patients with a short esophagus secondary to a stricture, Barrett esophagus, or a large hiatal hernia, the esophagus can be lengthened with a Collis gastroplasty to allow the GEJ to be below the level of the hiatus and to ensure a tension-free fundoplication around the newly formed gastric tube. Prior to considering a Collis, one must perform an extensive mediastinal mobilization of the esophagus as far as feasible above the GE junction. If this does not achieve at least 2 cm of intra-abdominal esophageal length, a Collis gastroplasty should be performed. With a 54 to 60 Fr bougie in place, a point approximately 3 cm below the angle of His is marked on the stomach with electrocautery. A 45-mm Endo GIA stapler (Universal Endo GIA, USSC, Stamford, Connecticut) is then used to fire horizontally toward the bougie at that level. A vertical staple line is then created alongside the bougie, as the assistant retracts the resected gastric wedge laterally. This results in a 3- to 4-cm neoesophagus, which is then tested with methylene blue or air insufflation to rule out a leak prior to proceeding with thc fundoplication.[40]

Outcomes following Antireflux Surgery

Symptomatic and Objective Outcomes after Antireflux Surgery. Multiple studies of long-term outcomes following laparoscopic fundoplication document its ability to relieve typical reflux symptoms (heartburn, regurgitation, and dysphagia) in more than 90% of patients at follow-up intervals averaging 2 to 3 years and 80% to 90% of patients 5 years or more following surgery.[34,36,37] Of note, atypical reflux symptoms (cough, asthma, laryngitis) after surgery are relieved in only two-thirds of patients.

When compared to patients on PPIs, laparoscopic fundoplication leads to a better GERD-specific quality of life, fewer heartburn symptoms, but a higher risk of adverse events. The treatment failure rates are significantly lower after antireflux surgery in follow-up of 5 to 12 years,[41] with 5% to 18% requiring revision surgery. The most common reason for reoperation is dysphagia, which occurs in 2% to 16% of the patients. Rates of recurrent hiatal herniation are largely dependent on the size of the underlying hiatal hernia. While the need for reoperation after fundoplication for GERD is only approximately 5% over a patient's lifetime, it can be as high as 42% after repair of a giant paraesophageal hernia.[42]

When assessing some of the unpleasant side effects of antireflux surgery, such as hyperflatulence and inability to belch or vomit, these symptoms are significantly more common than in patients on medical therapy. Nevertheless, studies have shown an improvement in quality of life following antireflux surgery, outperforming medical therapy on some parameters.

Looking at objective physiologic outcomes, patients after antireflux surgery experience significantly greater reductions in ambulatory esophageal acid exposure when compared to the medical treatment cohort in long-term follow-up.[43] Laparoscopic fundoplication also results in a significant increase in LES pressure and length, generally restoring these values to normal. Based on these data, objective evidence of reflux should be obtained prior to restarting acid suppression medications in patients with symptoms after a fundoplication.

Complications of Antireflux Surgery. Laparoscopic Nissen fundoplication has been extensively studied and its complications are well documented. Postoperative complications occur in approximately 8% of patients, with the rate of conversion to an open procedure of about 4%. The most common perioperative complication is early wrap herniation (1.3%), defined as occurring within 48 hours of surgery.[44]

Both pneumothorax and pneumomediastinum have been reported secondary to the breach of either pleural membrane. Accumulated carbon dioxide usually dissipates following release of pneumoperitoneum by a combination of positive pressure ventilation and absorption, and creating a large pleural defect prevents tension pneumothorax. Intraoperative complications are rare, and include trocar injury, gastric or esophageal perforation, hemorrhage, retractor trauma to the liver, splenic injury, and vascular injury to the aberrant left hepatic vein or inferior vena cava. Generally, immediate recognition and repair of injury is the key to avoiding a major complication. Major vascular injury mandates immediate conversion to an open procedure to achieve hemostasis. Mortality rate has been reported at 0.08%.

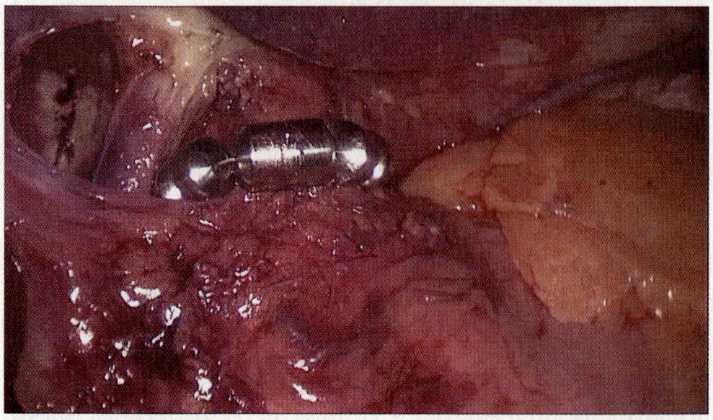

Figure 41.32. Magnetic sphincter augmentation device (LINX) placed around the gastroesophageal junction.

Roux-en-Y Gastric Bypass. Bariatric surgery is the procedure of choice in patients with refractory GERD and a BMI ≥35. Fundoplication alone in this patient population poses a significant risk of failure or hernia recurrence without significant weight loss. Of the available bariatric procedures, Roux-en-Y gastric bypass (discussed in detail Chapter 44: Management of Obesity) has been demonstrated to be the most effective at treating GERD, while sleeve gastrectomy carries the potential to exacerbate GERD symptoms and is contraindicated in patients with known esophagitis.

Magnetic Sphincter Augmentation. The LINX Reflux Management System (Torax Medical, Shoreview, MN) is a ring of titanium magnetic beads that is placed around the GEJ laparoscopically to mimic and augment the function of the LES (**Fig. 41.32**). The ring increases the natural resistance of the LES to opening but expands to allow food passage with swallowing and peristalsis. Concurrent hiatal hernia repair is performed during LINX placement, although patients with large hernias (>3 cm) and/or Barrett esophagus have traditionally been excluded from this procedure. Other exclusion criteria include those with allergies to titanium, stainless steel, nickel, or iron. Caution should be taken in those who need ongoing MRI screening, although the newest version of the device is compatible with 1.5-Tesla MRI.

Single-arm studies have shown that 80% to 90% of patients stop PPI use at up to 5 years after LINX placement, with a normalization of esophageal pH in 70%.[45] Importantly, all patients retain the ability to belch and vomit. Ganz et al.'s pivotal trial showed that dysphagia is present in about 68% of the patients in the first several months postoperatively, but decreases to 4% by 3 years. Five percent of patients required endoscopic balloon dilation or removal of the device for severe dysphasia. Subsequent studies have also demonstrated that device erosion occurs in about 1.2% of the patients.[45] Nonrandomized controlled trials have shown comparable outcomes of the LINX to Nissen fundoplication with lower rates of gas bloat and greater ability to belch and vomit in the LINX patients, with comparable safety, rates of PPI suspension, and postoperative GERD-HRQL scores. Long-term data on hernia recurrence in patients with magnetic sphincter augmentation and concurrent large hiatal or paraesophageal hernia repair is missing. However, short-term results show a

10% endoscopic recurrence rate reported at 12 months. Less than a third of these patients were symptomatic and required operative intervention.[46]

Endoscopic Management of GERD

11 Medical therapy for GERD and antireflux surgery both have inherent drawbacks. Major limitations of acid suppressive medications include the inability to prevent regurgitation of weakly acidic or nonacidic refluxate and the need for chronic, continual therapy, not to mention the cost, inconvenience, potential side effects, and need for ongoing dietary and lifestyle modifications. In addition, current therapy does not address the main pathophysiologic contributor to the presence of GERD, the mechanically defective LES. Fundoplications, while intended to permanently restore the LES, suffer from the potential for perioperative complications, a high initial cost, the risks inherent to general anesthesia, as well as possible short- and long-term side effects. For all these reasons, there is an interest in developing endoscopic means of restoring LES competence. The two main endoscopic approaches for treating GERD include the Stretta procedure and transoral incisionless fundoplication (TIF 2.0).

Radiofrequency Ablation. Stretta (Curon Medical, Sunnyvale, CA) involves the application of controlled radiofrequency energy (RFA) to the LES region using a four-channel RF generator and catheter system that is introduced endoscopically. Multiple lesions are created in the region 2 cm above and below the z-line, and thermocouples at each needle tip ensure that the lesion temperatures stay below 100 °C to minimize collateral tissue damage. Appropriate candidates for this procedure include patients who have relatively normal esophageal peristalsis and adequate relaxation of the LES, nonerosive reflux, or mild esophagitis (LA grade A or B), and are refractory to or wish to discontinue long-term medical therapy. Those with large hiatal hernias, significant dysphagia or esophageal aperistalsis, or advanced esophagitis are not good candidates for Stretta.

This procedure has been shown to reduce the rate of postprandial transient LES relaxations and esophageal acid exposure. Stretta also decreases the compliance of the GEJ and causes a reduction in esophageal acid sensitivity, leading to a decrease in GERD symptoms. RCTs and cohort studies show a significant reduction in PPI use at up to 10 years of follow-up.[47]

Nonrandomized studies comparing RFA to fundoplication show that 51% to 58% of the Stretta patients are able to discontinue PPI use at 5 years of follow-up, compared to 91% to 97% of the patients after a Nissen. Although there was a significant improvement in symptoms after RFA, up to 59% of those patients subsequently required antireflux surgery. The complication rate is very low at <1%, with small erosions and mucosal lacerations being the most common adverse events.[47]

Transoral Incisionless Fundoplication (TIF 2.0). TIF is performed using the EsophyX Z+ device (EndoGastric Solutions, Redmond, WA), which creates full-thickness plications with polypropylene H-shaped fasteners to reconstruct a valve that is 200 to 300 degrees in circumference and 3 cm in length,[48] mimicking a partial fundoplication. TIF 2.0 has been shown to reduce GEJ distensibility and increase resting LES pressures, thereby decreasing the number of transient LES relaxation episodes. It is appropriate for patients with a dysfunctional LES without a significant hiatal hernia (Hill grade I or II). Several RCTs comparing TIF 2.0 to PPI therapy showed that the procedure is superior to medical treatment in eliminating regurgitation and extraesophageal symptoms, and allowed 66% to 72% of patients to stay off PPIs for at least 5 years. The reported complication rate is 2% to 2.5%, and most commonly consists of gastrointestinal perforation, bleeding, and pneumothorax.[49]

ACKNOWLEDGMENT

We gratefully acknowledge the contributions of previous edition author, Yulia Zak, as portions of those chapters have been retained in this revision.

References

1. Nigro JJ, Hagen JA, DeMeester TR, et al. Prevalence and location of nodal metastases in distal esophageal adenocarcinoma confined to the wall: implications for therapy. *J Thorac Cardiovasc Surg.* 1999;117(1):16–23; discussion 23–25.
2. Liebermann-Meffert DM. Human foregut anatomy, adjacent structures, and their relation to surgical approaches. In: Yeo CJ, Matthews JB, eds. *Shackelford's Surgery of the Alimentary Tract.* 7th ed. Elsevier; 2013:9–31.
3. Pouderoux P, Lin S, Kahrilas PJ. Timing, propagation, coordination, and effect of esophageal shortening during peristalsis. *Gastroenterology.* 1997;112(4):1147–1154.
4. DeMeester TR, Peters JH, Bremner CG, Chandrasoma P. Biology of gastroesophageal reflux disease: pathophysiology relating to medical and surgical treatment. *Annu Rev Med.* 1999;50:469–506.
5. Kahrilas PJ, Shi G, Manka M, Joehl RJ. Increased frequency of transient lower esophageal sphincter relaxation induced by gastric distention in reflux patients with hiatal hernia. *Gastroenterology.* 2000;118(4):688–695.
6. Genta RM, Spechler SJ, Kielhorn AF. The Los Angeles and Savary-Miller systems for grading esophagitis: utilization and correlation with histology. *Dis Esophagus.* 2011;24(1):10–17.
7. Hill LD, Kozarek RA, Kraemer SJ, et al. The gastroesophageal flap valve: in vitro and in vivo observations. *Gastrointest Endosc.* 1996;44(5):541–547.
8. Ayazi S, Hagen JA, Zehetner J, et al. The value of high-resolution manometry in the assessment of the resting characteristics of the lower esophageal sphincter. *J Gastrointest Surg.* 2009;13(12):2113–2120.
9. Jamieson JR, Stein HJ, DeMeester TR, et al. Ambulatory 24-h esophageal pH monitoring: normal values, optimal thresholds, specificity, sensitivity, and reproducibility. *Am J Gastroenterol.* 1992;87(9):1102–1111.
10. Ayazi S, Lipham JC, Portale G, et al. Bravo catheter-free pH monitoring: normal values, concordance, optimal diagnostic thresholds, and accuracy. *Clin Gastroenterol Hepatol.* 2009;7(1):60–67.
11. Su B, Novak S, Callahan ZM, et al. Using impedance planimetry (EndoFLIP™) in the operating room to assess gastroesophageal junction distensibility and predict patient outcomes following fundoplication. *Surg Endosc.* 2020;34(4):1761–1768.
12. Su B, Dunst C, Gould J, et al. Experience-based expert consensus on the intra-operative usage of the Endoflip impedance planimetry system. *Surg Endosc.* 2021;35(6):2731–2742.
13. Vakil N, van Zanten SV, Kahrilas P, Dent J, Jones R; Global Consensus Group. The Montreal definition and classification of gastroesophageal reflux disease; a global evidence-based consensus. *Am J Gastroenterol.* 2006;101(8):1900–1920; quiz 1943.
14. Eusebi LH, Ratnakumaran R, Yuan Y, Solaymani-Dodaran M, Bazzoli F, Ford AC. Global prevalence of, and risk factors for, gastro-oesophageal reflux symptoms: a meta-analysis. *Gut.* 2018;67(3):430–440.
15. Jacobson BC, Somers SC, Fuchs CS, Kelly CP, Camargo CA Jr. Body-mass index and symptoms of gastroesophageal reflux in women. *N Eng J Med.* 2006;354(22):2340–2348.
16. Singh S, Sharma AN, Murad MH, et al. Central adiposity is associated with increased risk of esophageal inflammation, metaplasia, and adenocarcinoma: a systematic review and meta-analysis. *Clin Gastroenterol Hepatol.* 2013;11(11):1399–1412.e7.
17. Malfertheiner P, Nocon M, Vieth M, et al. Evolution of gastro-oesophageal reflux disease over 5 years under routine medical care—the ProGERD study. *Aliment Pharmacol Ther.* 2012;35(1):154–164.
18. Kahrilas PJ, Wu S, Lin S, Pouderoux P. Attenuation of esophageal shortening during peristalsis with hiatus hernia. *Gastroenterology.* 1995;109(6):1818–1825.

19. Sontag SJ. The spectrum of pulmonary symptoms due to gastroesophageal reflux. *Thorac Surg Clin.* 2005;15(3):353–368.
20. Durazzo M, Lupi G, Cicerchia F, et al. Extra-esophageal presentation of gastroesophageal reflux disease: 2020 update. *J Clin Med.* 2020;9(8):2559.
21. Norris BK, Schweinfurth JM. Management of recurrent laryngeal sensory neuropathic symptoms. *Ann Otol Rhinol Laryngol.* 2010;119(3):188–191.
22. Sontag SJ, O'Connell S, Khandelwal S, et al. Asthmatics with gastroesophageal reflux: long term results of a randomized trial of medical and surgical antireflux therapies. *Am J Gastroenterol.* 2003;98(5):987–999.
23. Davidson JR, Franklin D, Kumar S, et al. Fundoplication to preserve allograft function after lung transplant: systematic review and meta-analysis. *J Thorac Cardiovasc Surg.* 2020;160(3):858–866.
24. Peters JH, Hagen JA, DeMeester SR. Barrett's esophagus. *J Gastrointest Surg.* 2004;8:1–17.
25. Kauer WKH, Stein HJ. Bile reflux in the constellation of gastroesophageal reflux disease. *Thorac Surg Clin.* 2005;15(3):335–340.
26. Knight BC, Devitt PG, Watson DI, Smith LT, Jamieson GG, Thompson Sk. Long-term efficacy of laparoscopic antireflux surgery on regression of Barrett's esophagus using BRAVO wireless pH monitoring: a prospective clinical cohort study. *Ann Surg.* 2017;266(6):1000–1005.
27. Vallböhmer D, DeMeester SR, Oh DS, et al. Antireflux surgery normalizes cyclooxygenase-2 expression in squamous epithelium of the distal esophagus. *Am J Gastroenterol.* 2006;101(7):1458–1466.
28. Hvid-Jensen F, Pedersen L, Drewes AM, Sørensen HT, Funch-Jensen P. Incidence of adenocarcinoma among patients with Barrett's esophagus. *N Engl J Med.* 2011;365(15):1375–1383.
29. Sharma P, Shaheen NJ, Katzka D, Bergman JJGHM. AGA clinical practice update on endoscopic treatment of Barrett's esophagus with dysplasia and/or early cancer: expert review. *Gastroenterology.* 2020;158(3):760–769.
30. Gawron AJ, Feinglass J, Pandolfino JE, Tan BK, Bove MJ, Shintani-Smith S. Brand name and generic proton pump inhibitor prescriptions in the United States: insights from the national ambulatory medical care survey (2006–2010). *Gastroenterol Res Pract.* 2015;2015:689531.
31. Freedberg DE, Kim LS, Yang YX. The risks and benefits of long-term use of proton pump inhibitors: expert review and best practice advice from the American gastroenterological association. *Gastroenterology.* 2017;152(4):706–715.
32. Agago DE, Hanif N, Ajay Kumar et al. Comparison of potassium-competitive acid blockers and proton pump inhibitors in patients with gastroesophageal reflux disease: a systematic review and meta-analysis of randomized controlled trials. *Cureus.* 2024;16(7):e65141.
33. Pauwels A, Boecxstaens V, Andrews C, et al. How to select patients for antireflux surgery? The ICARUS guidelines (international consensus regarding preoperative examinations and clinical characteristics assessment to select adult patients for antireflux surgery). *Gut.* 2019;68:1928–1941.
34. Håkanson BS, Lundell L, Bylund A, Thorell A. Comparison of laparoscopic 270° posterior partial fundoplication vs total fundoplication for the treatment of gastroesophageal reflux disease: a randomized clinical trial. *JAMA Surg.* 2019;154(6):479–486.
35. Mardani J, Lundell L, Engström C. Total or posterior partial fundoplication in the treatment of GERD: results of a randomized trial after 2 decades of follow-up. *Ann Surg.* 2011;253(5):875–878.
36. Analatos A, Kakanson B, Ansorge C, Lindblad M, Lundell L, Thorell A. Clinical outcomes of laparoscopic total vs 270 partial fundoplication in chronic gastroesophageal reflux disease. *JAMA Surg.* 2022;157(6):473–480.
37. Du X, Hu Z, Yan C, Zhang C, Wang Z, Wu J. A meta-analysis of long follow-up outcomes of laparoscopic Nissen (total) versus Toupet (270°) fundoplication for gastro-esophageal reflux disease based on randomized controlled trials in adults. *BMC Gastroenterol.* 2016;16:88.
38. Wu H, Attaar M, Wong H, et al. Impedance planimetry (Endoflip) and ideal distensibility ranges for optimal outcomes after Nissen and Toupet fundoplication. *J Am Coll Surg.* 2022;235(3):420–429.
39. Slater B, Dirks R, McKinley S, et al. SAGES guidelines for the surgical treatment of gastroesophageal reflux (GERD). *Surg Endosc.* 2021;35:4903–4917.
40. Terry ML, Vernon A, Hunter JG. Stapled-wedge Collis gastroplasty for the shortened esophagus. *Am J Surg.* 2004;188(2):195–199.
41. Lundell L, Miettinen P, Myrvold HE, et al. Nordic GERD Study Group. Comparison of outcomes twelve years after antireflux surgery or omeprazole maintenance therapy for reflux esophagitis. *Clin Gastroenterol Hepatol.* 2009;7(12):1292–1298; quiz 1260.
42. Hashemi M, Peters JH, DeMeester TR, et al. Laparoscopic repair of large type III hiatal hernia: objective follow-up reveals high recurrence rate. *J Am Coll Surg.* 2000;190(5):553–560; discussion 560–561.
43. Hatlebakk JG, Zerbib F, Bruley des Varannes S, et al. Gastroesophageal acid reflux control 5 years after antireflux surgery, compared with long-term esomeprazole therapy. *Clin Gastroenterol Hepatol.* 2016;14(5):678–685.e3.
44. Carlson MA, Frantzides CT. Complications and results of primary minimally invasive antireflux procedures: a review of 10,735 reported cases. *J Am Coll Surg.* 2001;193(4):428–439.
45. Ganz RA, Peters JH, Horgan S, et al. Esophageal sphincter device for gastroesophageal reflux disease. *N Engl J Med.* 2013;368(8):719–727.
46. Ayazi S, Chowdhury N, Zaidi AH, et al. Magnetic sphincter augmentation (MSA) in patients with hiatal hernia: clinical outcome and patterns of recurrence. *Surg Endosc.* 2020;34(4):1835–1846.
47. Noar M, Squires P, Noar E, Lee M. Long-term maintenance effect of radiofrequency energy delivery for refractory GERD: a decade later. *Surg Endosc.* 2014;28(8):2323–2333.
48. Chang KJ, Bell R. Transoral incisionless fundoplication. *Gastrointest Endosc Clin N Am.* 2020;30(2):267–289.
49. Trad KS, Barnes WE, Prevou ER, et al. The TEMPO trial at 5 years: transoral fundoplication (TIF 2.0) is safe, durable, and cost-effective. *Surg Innov.* 2018;25(2):149–157.

42

Esophageal Tumors and Injury

Natalie S. Lui, Mark F. Berry, and Leah M. Backhus

Key Points

1. The incidence of esophageal adenocarcinoma is increasing, but squamous cell carcinoma is the most common cancer histology worldwide.
2. The American Joint Committee on Cancer (AJCC) esophageal cancer staging system separates the clinical, pathologic, and postneoadjuvant stage groups and has different staging systems for squamous cell and adenocarcinoma.
3. Resection remains essential to cure of esophageal cancer for most patients who do not have metastatic disease. The mortality of esophagectomy has improved over time, particularly in high-volume centers. Minimally invasive techniques are increasingly used, but the procedure remains complex with relatively high morbidity.
4. Esophagectomy without induction therapy is often recommended for superficial tumors that involve the submucosa (T1bN0M0) so that lymph nodes can be removed for diagnostic and therapeutic purposes, but less invasive endoscopic therapies are options in specific situations.
5. Whether to give neoadjuvant therapy before esophagectomy for T2N0M0 esophageal cancer is controversial.
6. Both neoadjuvant chemotherapy and neoadjuvant chemoradiation improve overall survival and disease-free survival over primary surgery in patients with locoregional disease.
7. Esophagectomy is rarely indicated for patients with metastatic esophageal cancer, but palliative procedures can improve comfort, possibly restore swallowing ability, and provide nutritional support.
8. Choice of esophagectomy (three incision, transhiatal, Ivor Lewis, or thoracoabdominal; open or minimally invasive) depends on the tumor location, patient characteristics, and surgeon experience.
9. Leiomyomas are the most common benign esophageal neoplasm and can often be resected by endoscopic submucosal dissection (ESD) or surgical enucleation.

MALIGNANT ESOPHAGEAL NEOPLASMS

Epidemiology and Histology

Esophageal cancer is the most common indication for esophagectomy. Although relatively uncommon in that it represents only 1.1% of all new cancer cases, the number of cases of esophageal cancer in the United States has risen from less than 14,000 new cases annually in the 2000s, to almost 17,000 new cases in 2012, and now to an estimate of 22,070 in the year 2025.[1–3] Adenocarcinoma and squamous cell carcinoma
1 are by far the most common esophageal cancer histologies, and squamous cell carcinoma is much more common worldwide. The epidemiology in the United States has evolved such that adenocarcinoma is more common than squamous cell carcinoma, with the incidence of adenocarcinoma rising and the incidence of squamous cell carcinoma falling in recent years.[2]

Esophageal cancer in the United States is most frequently diagnosed among people aged 65 to 74; adenocarcinoma more common in Caucasian patients, and squamous cell carcinoma more common in Black and Asian/Pacific Islander patients.[2] Tobacco use and a history of mediastinal radiation are risk factors for both tumor types.[3] Other risk factors for adenocarcinoma include male sex, gastroesophageal reflux disease (GERD), obesity, and Barrett esophagus.[3] Barrett esophagus with high-grade dysplasia is considered a premalignant condition, as 13% to 50% are found to harbor intramucosal carcinoma or invasive carcinoma at the time of biopsy or resection.[3] Additional risk factors for squamous cell carcinoma are conditions that cause chronic esophageal irritation and inflammation, such as alcohol abuse, achalasia, esophageal diverticuli, and frequent consumption of extremely hot beverages.[3] Approximately three-quarters of all adenocarcinomas are found in the distal esophagus, whereas squamous cell carcinomas are more evenly distributed throughout the distal two-thirds.[3]

Clinical Presentation and Diagnostic Evaluation

The Society of Thoracic Surgeons has published guidelines on the diagnosis and staging of patients with esophageal cancer.[4] The workup often starts because patients present with symptoms of dysphagia and weight loss, with less common symptoms being heartburn, odynophagia, shortness of breath, chronic cough, hoarseness, and hematemesis.[3] The physical examination is usually unremarkable.[3]

Upper gastrointestinal (GI) tract contrast studies and upper endoscopy with biopsy are commonly the initial diagnostic tests. An upper GI contrast study typically shows a stricture or ulceration when malignancy is present. Upper GI endoscopy typically shows a friable, ulcerated mass, and allows identification of tumor location and length and biopsy for pathologic examination. In addition to identifying the cancer and providing tissue for histologic confirmation, the endoscopy should also report detailed information on the location of the tumor as well as the presence of other areas of Barrett esophagus, which are particularly important for the selection of surgical approach. For distal tumors that involve the gastroesophageal junction, the extent of gastric involvement should be carefully evaluated. Tumors with epicenters in the lower esophagus that extend to the junction (Siewert Type I) and tumors of the true gastric cardia with epicenter within 1 cm above and 2 cm below the junction (Siewert Type II) should be treated as esophageal cancers. Tumors with epicenter between 2 cm and 5 cm from junction but infiltrate the junction from superior extension (Siewert Type III) should be treated as gastric cancers, though surgical approach will likely involve some degree of distal esophageal resection to obtain negative margins and complete resection.[5]

After a histologic cancer diagnosis has been obtained, subsequent studies are performed to determine clinical stage as accurately as possible before treatment is initiated to optimize esophageal cancer outcomes. Accurate staging and appropriate treatment can avoid both inadequate and unnecessary treatment to balance the potential benefits of improving prognosis with risks of treatment-related morbidity. A computed tomographic (CT) scan of the chest, abdomen, and pelvis with oral and intravenous contrast should be obtained when esophageal cancer is detected. This study is useful in evaluating for distant metastatic disease, such as in the liver or lungs, though CTs are not generally useful for detecting nodal disease or identifying or determining the extent of early-stage cancers localized to the superficial aspect of the esophageal wall.[4] Positron emission tomography (PET) scans improve staging and will detect previously unsuspected metastatic disease in up to 15% to 20% of patients.[6] They should be considered in place of CT scans or as an additional study when the CT scan does not show metastatic disease.[4] Further studies that evaluate T and N status would not typically impact treatment and therefore are generally unnecessary if distant disease is identified and subsequently confirmed by biopsy.

If CT and PET do not demonstrate distant disease, subsequent evaluation determines the extent of locoregional disease. Endoscopic ultrasound (EUS) is often the next test.[3] EUS provides more accurate evaluation of the depth of tumor invasion (T stage) and the extent of lymph node involvement (N stage) than both PET and CT.[3] However, the specific information obtained from EUS alone does not often change the clinical management of patients with esophageal cancer. For patients with significant symptoms from bulky tumors, the local extent of the tumor is almost certainly at least T3 with a high chance of local lymph node involvement. In these cases, EUS is likely only to confirm the clinical suspicion or to be unable to provide a complete evaluation due to luminal narrowing by the tumor, and therefore not changing the planned management. Conversely, EUS is generally less accurate for early-stage lesions such as T1 or T2 compared to more advanced tumors.[7] The accuracy of T staging can also be improved via endoscopic resection, which can be therapeutic in some cases as discussed below.[4] Finally, most incidences of understaging from EUS are due to missing nodal disease, and the specificity and the sensitivity for identifying lymph node disease are better when EUS is combined with fine-needle aspiration (FNA) compared to EUS alone.[8]

Additional studies prior to treatment may be indicated in certain circumstances. Bronchoscopy should be considered for tumors in the upper and middle esophagus to rule out airway invasion, which would preclude an eventual attempt at surgical resection. Airway evaluation is ideally done prior to starting any therapy in cases where there is a high suspicion due to imaging or clinical symptoms such as cough or pneumonia that could be due to an esophageal–airway fistula, as distinguishing between treatment changes and definite tumor invasion can be difficult after patients have been treated with chemotherapy and radiation. In addition, distant metastases are unfortunately missed even with completion of the staging evaluation described above. Small liver or lung metastases can be missed by both PET and CT scans, and patients can also have undetected pleural or peritoneal disease.[3,4] Staging via minimally invasive surgical techniques of thoracoscopy and laparoscopy improves the accuracy of the above noninvasive testing.[9] Use of these invasive techniques is relatively uncommon but should be considered in select patients, such as those who may be considered to have a high risk of treatment-related complications. Staging laparoscopy may particularly have a role for patients with signet cell adenocarcinomas of the distal esophagus or gastroesophageal junction that extend into the stomach at least 2 cm beyond the junction with at least T2 disease.[10]

Staging

Esophageal cancer staging is defined by the American Joint Committee on Cancer (AJCC) Staging System that establishes tumor–node–metastasis (TNM) subclassifications based on the depth of invasion of the primary tumor (T), involvement of regional lymph nodes in the adventitia or periesophageal tissue from the upper esophageal sphincter to the celiac artery (N), and presence of metastatic disease (M). The most recent 8th edition used the Worldwide Esophageal Cancer Collaboration database to expand on the 7th edition and provide distinctive and homogeneous stage groups with monotonically decreasing survival (Fig. 42.1).[11] Figure 42.2 and Tables 42.1 and 42.2 show the specific 8th edition TNM definitions. Grade is important for pathologic staging of early-stage cancers. Location is important to subgroup pT3N0M0 squamous cell carcinoma. The definition of the gastroesophageal junction was also revised in the new edition, such that cancers involving it with epicenters no

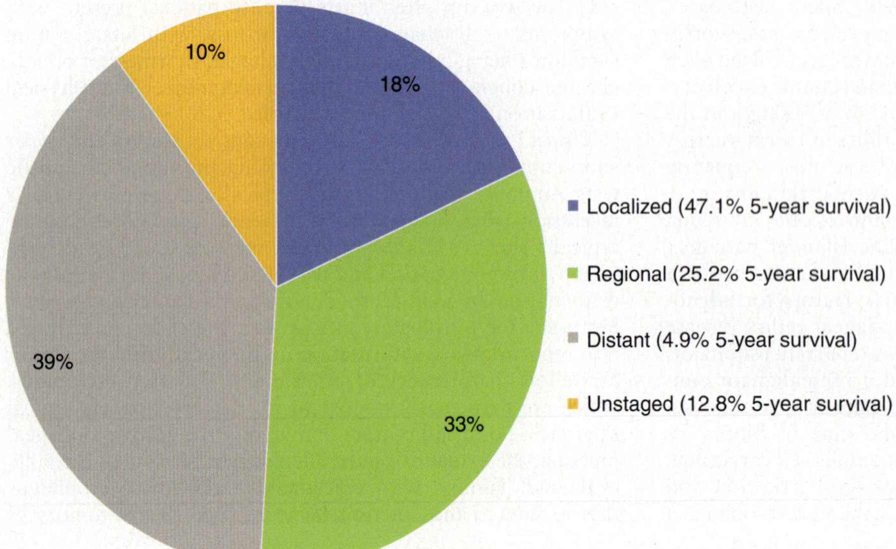

Figure 42.1. Distribution and survival of esophageal cancer by stage. (Adapted from Howlader N, Noone AM, Krapcho M, et al., eds. In: *SEER Cancer Statistics Review, 1975–2017, National Cancer Institute.* https://seer.cancer.gov/csr/1975_2017/, based on November 2019 SEER data submission, posted to the SEER web site, April 2020.)

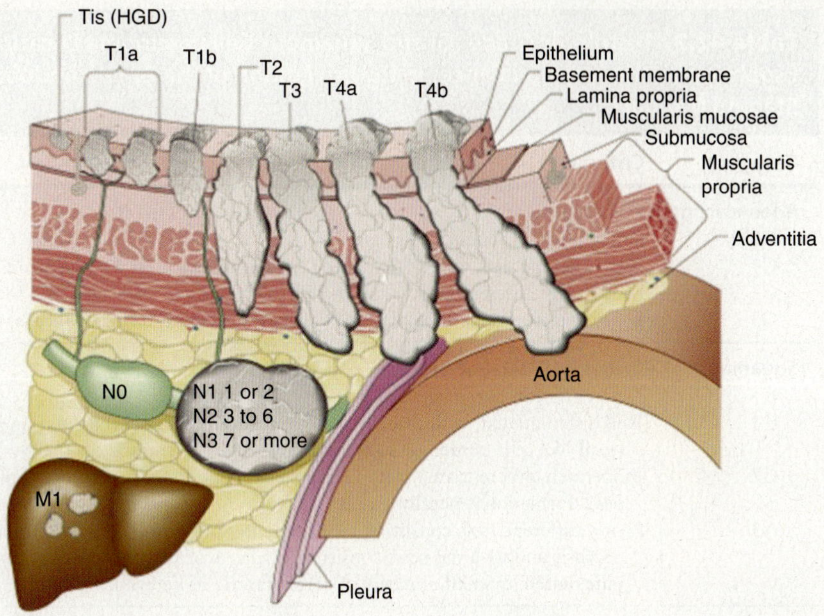

Figure 42.2. TNM categories. T is categorized as Tis: high-grade dysplasia (HGD). T1 is cancer that invades the lamina propria, muscularis mucosae, or submucosa and is subcategorized into T1a (cancer that invades the lamina propria or muscularis mucosae) and T1b (cancer that invades the submucosa); T2 is cancer that invades the muscularis propria; T3 is cancer that invades the adventitia; T4 is cancer that invades the local structures and is subcategorized as T4a (cancer that invades adjacent structures such as the pleura, pericardium, azygos vein, diaphragm, or peritoneum) and T4b (cancer that invades the major adjacent structures, such as the aorta, vertebral body, or trachea). N is categorized as N0 (no regional lymph node metastasis), N1 (regional lymph node metastases involving one to two nodes), N2 (regional lymph node metastases involving three to six nodes), and N3 (regional lymph node metastases involving seven or more nodes). M is categorized as M0 (no distant metastasis) and M1 (distant metastasis). (Reproduced from Rice TW, Ishwaran H, Ferguson MK, Blackstone EH, Goldstraw P. Cancer of the esophagus and esophagogastric junction: an eighth edition staging primer. *J Thoracic Oncol.* 2017;12(1):36–42.)

more than 2 cm into the gastric cardia are staged as esophageal cancers, and those with more than 2-cm involvement of the gastric cardia are staged as stomach cancers.

A major change from the 7th edition is that the 8th edition has separate classifications for clinical (cTNM), pathologic (pTNM), and postneoadjuvant (ypTNM) stage groups

Table 42.1. T, N, and M Categories for Esophagus and Esophagogastric Junction Cancer in the 8th Edition of the American Joint Committee on Cancer (AJCC) Cancer Staging Manual

Category	Criteria
T Category	
TX	Tumor cannot be assessed
T0	No evidence of primary tumor
Tis	High-grade dysplasia (malignant cells confined by the basement membrane)
T1a	Invasion into the lamina propria or muscularis mucosae
T1b	Invasion into the submucosa
T2	Invasion into muscularis propria
T3	Invasion into adventitia
T4a	Invades resectable adjacent structures (pleura, pericardium, azygos vein, diaphragm, or peritoneum)
T4b	Invades unresectable adjacent structures (aorta, vertebral body, or trachea)
N Category	
NX	Regional lymph nodes cannot be assessed
N0	No regional lymph node metastases
N1	1–2 positive regional lymph nodes
N2	3–6 positive regional lymph nodes
N3	7 or more positive regional lymph nodes
M Category	
M0	No distant metastases
M1	Distant metastases

Adapted from Rice TW, Ishwaran H, Ferguson MK, Blackstone EH, Goldstraw P. Cancer of the esophagus and esophagogastric junction: an eighth edition staging primer. *J Thoracic Oncol.* 2017;12(1):36–42.

2 (**Tables 42.3 to 42.5**). Clinical and pathologic groups were separated based on survival profiles. A separate postneoadjuvant pathologic stage group was added to account for pathologic information that may not have been available after induction therapy and different survival profiles across groups.[11]

Treatment

Consensus guidelines provide recommendations for the treatment of esophageal cancer. Treatment options include local mucosal resection or ablation therapies, esophagectomy, chemotherapy, and radiation therapy, with immunotherapy most recently being shown to improve outcomes in specific circumstances. Recommended treatment is primarily dictated by stage, tumor location, and patients' medical fitness for receiving a potential therapeutic modality. Data from randomized trials are increasingly available to help guide the treatment of esophageal cancer, but a spectrum of treatment regimens are often options for several clinical situations. Multidisciplinary evaluation by surgery, medical oncology, and radiation oncology should be considered for all patients before a treatment strategy is initiated. Treatment that does not follow guidelines should probably only be used in the context of clinical trials. In addition, all treatment strategies should include careful nutritional assessment and counseling, as well as smoking cessation advice if indicated. In some situations, placement of a pretreatment feeding tube can be integral in allowing a patient to adequately start and maintain therapy.

The stage groupings described above are very useful for both providing prognosis and guiding treatment. However, patients can be categorized more simply when considering treatment. The approach is initially dictated by whether the patients have been determined to have early-stage superficial cancers, cancers that are locally advanced with locoregional
3 disease but no distant metastases, and cancers with distant disease. The general treatment guidelines for each of these categories are discussed in the following sections.

Superficial Cancers

Patients with T1-2N0 esophageal cancer typically are recommended to undergo resection without induction therapy as noted in consensus guidelines. The prognosis for patients treated for intra- and submucosal (T1) esophageal cancers is significantly better than the prognosis for all other patients found to have esophageal cancer, even those also found in other relatively early-stage diseases.[12] These early-stage

Table 42.2. Histologic Grade (G) and Squamous Cell Carcinoma Location (L) Categories for Esophagus and Esophagogastric Junction Cancer in the 8th Edition of the American Joint Committee on Cancer (AJCC) Cancer Staging Manual

Category	Criteria
Adenocarcinoma G category	
GX	Differentiation cannot be assessed
G1	Well differentiated, with >95% of the tumor composed of well-formed glands
G2	Moderately differentiated, with 50–95% of the tumor showing gland formation
G3	Poorly differentiated, with tumors composed of nests and sheets of cells, with <50% of the tumor showing gland formation
Squamous Cell Carcinoma G category	
GX	Differentiation cannot be assessed
G1	Well differentiated, with prominent keratinization with pearl formation and a minor component of nonkeratinizing basal-like cells, tumor cells arranged in sheets, and mitotic counts low
G2	Moderately differentiated, with variable histologic features ranging from parakeratotic to poorly keratinizing lesions and pearl formation generally absent
G3	Poorly differentiated, consisting predominantly of basal-like cells forming large and small nests with frequent central necrosis and with the nests consisting of sheets or pavement-like arrangements of tumor cells that are occasionally punctuated by small numbers of parakeratotic or keratinizing cells
Squamous Cell Carcinoma L Category	
LX	Location unknown
Upper	Cervical esophagus to lower border of the azygos vein
Middle	Lower border of the azygos vein to lower border of the inferior pulmonary vein
Lower	Lower border of the inferior pulmonary vein to the stomach, including the esophagogastric junction

Adapted from Rice TW, Ishwaran H, Ferguson MK, Blackstone EH, Goldstraw P. Cancer of the esophagus and esophagogastric junction: an eighth edition staging primer. *J Thoracic Oncol.* 2017;12(1):36–42.

cancers are generally either found incidentally during endoscopies done for other reasons or during endoscopies done for Barrett monitoring.

Esophagectomy is effective oncologically for these superficial cancers but is associated with considerable morbidity and mortality despite improvements over time and the development of minimally invasive techniques.[13,14] Although recent data from high-volume centers have shown low mortality rates of 1% to 3.5%, studies involving population-based databases or multicenter trials have shown esophageal resection to have perioperative mortality rates as high as 8.8% to 14%.[14,15] Local treatments with modalities such as endoscopic mucosal resection (EMR), endoscopic submucosal dissection (ESD), radiofrequency ablation, cryotherapy, and photodynamic therapy can provide effective cancer treatment for superficial cancers with much less treatment-related morbidity.[16–18] These local treatments are good treatment options for patients with superficial tumors that involve only the mucosa (T1a), particularly when tumors are well or moderately differentiated without lymphovascular invasion. Pathologic examination should confirm complete resection with negative circumferential and deep/vertical margins. Endoscopic surveillance should be planned posttreatment, every 3 to 6 months for the first 2 years and then annually.

Local mucosal therapies were previously considered not appropriate for superficial tumors that involve the submucosa (T1b) due to potential for occult lymph node involvement, previously estimated to occur in as many as 50% of patients.[19]

Table 42.3. AJCC 8th Edition Clinical Stage Groupings

Adenocarcinoma				Squamous Cell Carcinoma			
c Stage	T	N	M	c Stage	T	N	M
0	is	0	0	0	is	0	0
I	1	0	0	I	1	0–1	0
IIA	1	1	0	II	2	0–1	0
IIB	2	0	0		3	0	0
III	2	1	0	III	1–2	2	0
	3–4a	0–1	0		3	1–2	0
IVA	1–4a	2–3	0	IVA	1–3	3	0
	4b	Any	0		4a–b	Any	0
IVB	Any	Any	1	IVB	Any	Any	1

Adapted from Rice TW, Ishwaran H, Ferguson MK, Blackstone EH, Goldstraw P. Cancer of the esophagus and esophagogastric junction: an eighth edition staging primer. *J Thoracic Oncol.* 2017;12(1):36–42.

Table 42.4. AJCC 8th Edition Pathologic Stage Groupings

Adenocarcinoma					Squamous Cell Carcinoma					
p Stage	T	N	M	Grade	p Stage	T	N	M	Grade	Location
0	is	0	0	Any	0	is	0	0	Any	Any
IA	1a	0	0	1	IA	1a	0	0	1	Any
IB	1a–b	0	0	2	IB	1a	0	0	2–3	Any
						1b	0	0	Any	Any
						2	0	0	1	Any
IC	1a–b	0	0	3						
	2	0	0	1–2						
IIA	2	0	0	3	IIA	2	0	0	2–3	Any
						3	0	0	1	Any
						3	0	0	2–3	Lower
IIB	1a–b	1	0	Any	IIB	1a–b	1	0	Any	Any
	3	0	0	Any		3	0	0	2–3	Upper or middle
IIIA	1a–b	2	0	Any	IIIA	1a–b	2	0	Any	Any
	2	1	0	Any		2	1	0	Any	Any
IIIB	2	2	0	Any	IIIB	2	2	0	Any	Any
	3	1–2	0	Any		3	1–2	0	Any	Any
	4a	0–1	0	Any		4a	0–1	0	Any	Any
IVA	1–3	3	0	Any	IVA	1–3	3	0	Any	Any
	4a	2–3	0	Any		4a	2–3	0	Any	Any
	4b	Any	0	Any		4b	Any	0	Any	Any
IVB	Any	Any	1	Any	IVB	Any	Any	1	Any	Any

Adapted from Rice TW, Ishwaran H, Ferguson MK, Blackstone EH, Goldstraw P. Cancer of the esophagus and esophagogastric junction: an eighth edition staging primer. *J Thoracic Oncol.* 2017;12(1):36–42.

Esophagectomy without induction therapy was therefore recommended for superficial tumors that involve the submucosa
4 (T1b) so that the lymph nodes can be removed for both diagnostic and therapeutic purpose. Patients undergoing esophagectomy without induction therapy should have at least 15 lymph nodes removed during surgery for adequate nodal staging.[20] However, endoscopic resection alone can be considered for pT1b tumors that are not poorly differentiated or have lymphovascular invasion when negative margins are achieved.[21] Shared decision making with patients is necessary to weigh a small risk of residual lymph node disease that is undetected and untreated versus the operative risks and lifestyle implications of surgery.

Table 42.5. AJCC 8th Edition Postneoadjuvant Pathologic Stage Groupings for Both Adenocarcinoma and Squamous Cell Carcinoma

yp Stage	T	N	M
I	0–2	0	0
II	3	0	0
IIIA	0–2	1	0
IIIB	0–2	2	0
	3	1–2	0
	4a	0	0
IVA	0–3	3	0
	4a	1–3	0
	4b	Any	0
IVB	Any	Any	1

Adapted from Rice TW, Ishwaran H, Ferguson MK, Blackstone EH, Goldstraw P. Cancer of the esophagus and esophagogastric junction: an eighth edition staging primer. *J Thoracic Oncol.* 2017;12(1):36–42.

The optimal management of esophageal cancer clinically
5 staged as T2N0M0 is somewhat more controversial. Clinical staging modalities for this subset are somewhat unreliable, with significant percentages of patients being both under and over staged.[22] Perhaps because clinical staging inaccuracies lead to a relatively high incidence of patients actually having nodal disease present at the time of surgical resection, induction therapy use is often used in this setting.[22] However, data that proves a survival benefit to induction therapy over surgery alone is still lacking, and patients who truly do not have nodal involvement may not benefit or need neoadjuvant therapy.[23] Consistent with the uncertainty of optimal treatment, consensus guidelines for medically fit patients allow a wide spectrum of treatment possibilities that include definitive chemoradiation and esophagectomy with or without induction or adjuvant therapy. One clinical approach to patients with cT2N0 disease is proceeding with primary esophagectomy when the tumor was incidentally found on endoscopy or during workup for very mild symptoms and using induction therapy in cases where patients had symptoms more consistent with a bulky or locally advanced tumor. In addition, an endoscopic resection of a small tumor can also be performed for more accurate T staging to direct therapy.

Locoregional or Locally Advanced Disease

Approximately 33% of esophageal cancer patients have regional disease at the time of diagnosis, with a 5-year survival of only 10% to 30%.[2] Surgery is considered integral to achieving cure in patients with esophageal cancer, as one study showed the 5-year survival rates for patients with stages I through III esophageal cancer treated with and without surgery to be 28% and 10%, respectively.[24] Definitive chemoradiation is generally reserved for those patients who refuse surgery or are not surgical candidates as noted in consensus guidelines. Areas of esophageal cancer in which definitive chemoradiation is recommended in place of surgical resection are squamous cell carcinoma of the cervical esophagus and patients with T4b (unresectable) tumors.[25] Some data suggest that definitive chemoradiation could be adequate for some patients with squamous cell carcinoma in other esophageal locations if a complete clinical response is obtained, but surgery has been considered integral to potential cure for adenocarcinoma in which pathologic complete response rates are generally less common.[26] However, active surveillance when a clinical complete response was obtained after neoadjuvant chemoradiation was demonstrated by the Surgery As Needed for Oesophageal cancer (SANO) trial to not be inferior to surgery in a cohort that included patients with adenocarcinoma, so avoiding surgery can be reasonable in select patients who are carefully counseled on the risks and benefits of both strategies.[27]

The treatment for locally advanced esophageal cancer that does not have distant metastases and is potentially resectable (T3-4aN0, T1-4aN1M0) is highly variable in practice.[28] The poor survival rate after esophagectomy alone for patients with locally advanced but not metastatic disease led to many studies of multimodality therapy in efforts to improve outcomes. Although not all trials demonstrated a benefit to induction therapy, induction chemoradiation followed by surgical resection has recently generally been considered the optimal 6 treatment for patients with T3-4a tumors or nodal disease[29] based on the Dutch Chemoradiotherapy for Oesophageal Cancer followed by Surgery Study (CROSS) randomized trial that demonstrated a survival benefit to induction chemoradiation followed by surgery compared to surgery alone (47% vs. 33% 5-year survival after an 84-month median follow-up) for esophageal or gastroesophageal junction cancer.[30,31] Patients who undergo surgery after chemoradiation and do not have a complete pathologic response in the resected specimen will also benefit from adjuvant immunotherapy.[32]

Although induction therapy is currently used in most patients with locally advanced disease,[33] the optimal induction regimen is still not completely clear. The benefit of induction chemoradiation on long-term follow-up of the CROSS trial patients was less pronounced for adenocarcinoma patients compared to squamous cell carcinoma patients.[34] Induction chemotherapy without radiation has also been shown to be beneficial for distal esophageal and gastroesophageal junction adenocarcinomas and is used by some high-volume centers.[35] Although combined chemoradiation has the theoretical advantage over chemotherapy alone of providing local benefit in addition to systemic control as well as possibly facilitating resectability, a definitive survival benefit has not been demonstrated.[36] The FLOT chemotherapy regimen (docetaxel, oxaliplatin, leucovorin, and fluorouracil) has survival advantages over previous standard chemotherapy regimens for gastric and gastroesophageal junction adenocarcinomas. Recently presented data from the ESOPEC multicenter prospective randomized trial comparing neoadjuvant CROSS chemoradiation versus perioperative FLOT chemotherapy actually showed that perioperative FLOT improved survival in resectable esophageal adenocarcinoma compared to neoadjuvant CROSS.[37] However, the specific choice of induction regimen should be based on specific patient characteristics, such as symptoms that may be better palliated if radiation is included, as well as the likelihood that a patient can tolerate both surgery and all doses of the somewhat more toxic FLOT regimen.

Metastatic or Unresectable Disease

Approximately 40% to 50% of patients have evidence of distant metastatic disease at the time of diagnosis.[2,3] Palliative therapy is recommended for these patients, and can include chemotherapy, clinical trial enrollment if available, or best supportive care. Best supportive care is often the most appropriate treatment option. Patients' performance status should determine whether chemotherapy is added to best supportive care. Specific symptoms that often need palliation include dysphagia, pain, and nausea. Oncologists generally avoid feeding tubes in patients with stage IV cancer, but feeding tubes may be reasonable options in some select patients with limited metastatic disease. Radiation or endoscopic management techniques, such as dilation and stenting, can be used to palliate dysphagia or cases of bleeding from esophageal tumors. Palliative esophagectomy for patients with metastatic disease may 7 have a role in very few cases and should be considered very selectively, given the morbidity of surgery and the poor prognosis with or without surgery.

Prognosis

Survival of esophageal cancer has improved from <5% at 5 years in 1975 to approximately 21.6% currently.[2,38,39] There are multiple factors responsible for this improvement, including a change in the stage distribution and more diagnoses of early-stage cancers secondary to the recognition of the importance and need for surveillance of Barrett esophagus, development of low-risk but highly effective endoscopic therapies for early-stage superficial cancers, improvements in the knowledge of the importance of multimodality for locally advanced cancers, and improvement in the outcomes associated with esophagectomy in general. As expected, survival correlates with the stage at presentation. Patients with localized disease have a 5-year survival of 48.1%, while patients with regional disease and distant disease have 5-year survival rates of 28.1% and 5.3%, respectively.[2] Specific survival is obviously impacted by not only stage, but therapy as discussed above. Survival curves after esophagectomy for various specific stage presentations are shown in **Figure 42.3**.[40]

ESOPHAGECTOMY

Surgery is recommended as possible treatment for most cases of esophageal cancer that do not have invasion of unresectable structures or distant metastatic disease. Several studies have provided evidence that complete surgical resection provides the best chance for cure for these patients.[24] However, surgery for locoregional esophageal cancer has been utilized in less than half of potentially resectable cases, perhaps because esophagectomy is historically associated with significant morbidity and mortality and disappointing long-term results.[24] Mortality following esophagectomy has decreased over time, but still exceeds that of most surgical procedures, and long-term survival generally remains poor. Consequently, minimizing perioperative morbidity in any manner possible is critically important, such that primary nonsurgical treatment is reserved for those who refuse surgery, have unresectable cancers, or are not thought to be surgical candidates for other reasons.

Techniques of Esophagectomy

Resection of the esophagus for malignancy is a technically complex procedure. The esophagus traverses three body regions (neck, chest, and abdomen), and the anatomy of the esophagus in the posterior mediastinum is such that its accessibility is very different at various positions in the chest. In addition, an appropriate conduit must be prepared in order to reestablish GI continuity, and this conduit must be placed in a location such that its blood supply will remain viable.

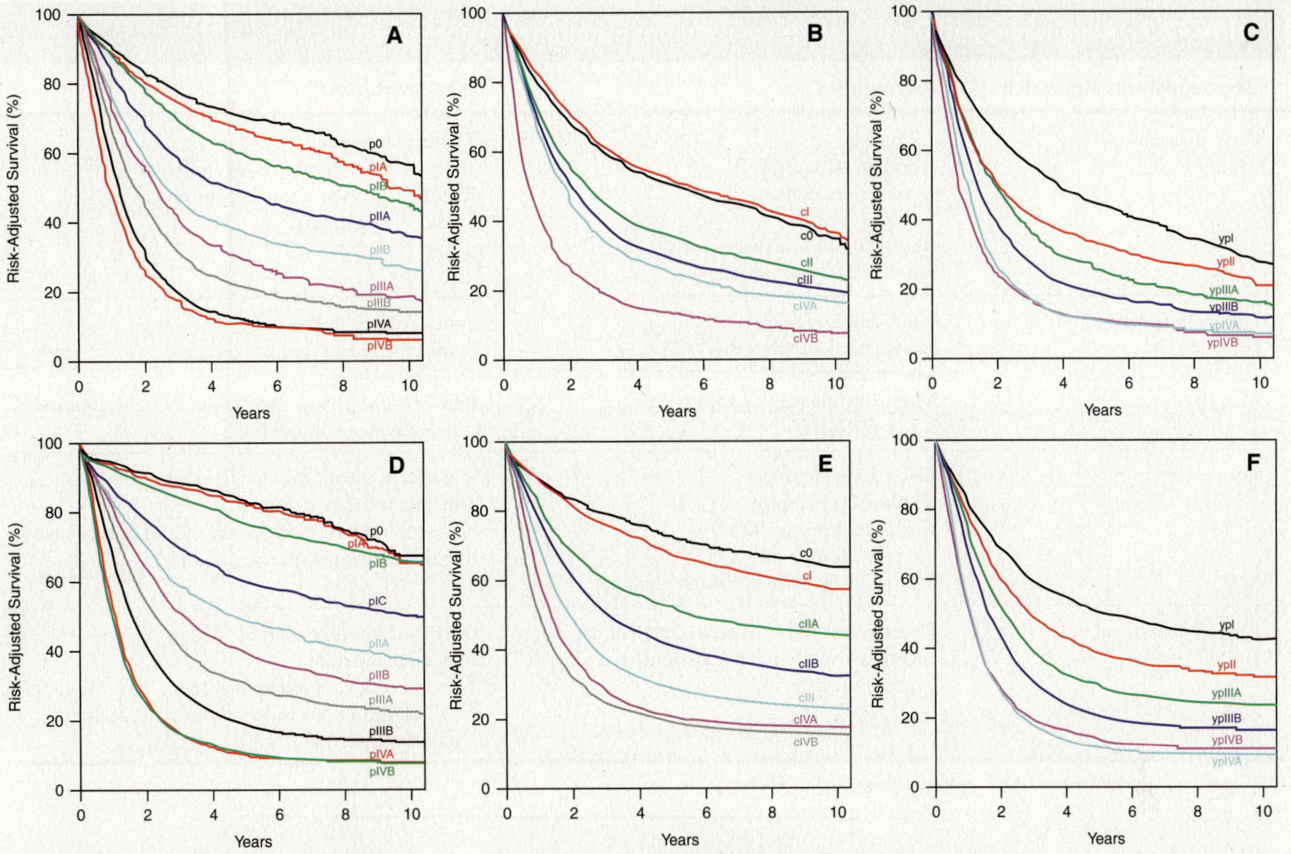

Figure 42.3. Risk-adjusted survival for squamous cell carcinoma (**A**) pathologic, (**B**) clinical, and (**C**) postneo adjuvant stage groups, as well as adenocarcinoma (**D**) pathologic, (**E**) clinical, and (**F**) postneoadjuvant stage groups. (Reproduced from Rice TW, Gress DM, Patil DT, Hofstetter WL, Kelsen DP, Blackstone EH. Cancer of the esophagus and esophagogastric junction-Major changes in the American Joint Committee on Cancer eighth edition Cancer Staging Manual. *CA Cancer J Clin.* 2017;67(4):304–317.)

Esophageal resection generally requires access to at least two body cavities, and often requires at least two incisions as well as patient repositioning and lung isolation with single-lung ventilation. Structures at risk of intraoperative injury include the spleen, trachea, and mainstem bronchi as well as major vascular structures in the chest such as the aorta.

Esophageal resection can be performed via several different techniques, with the most appropriate technique for any specific individual patient being dependent on both patient and surgeon factors. The most common surgical techniques used for esophagectomy are listed in **Table 42.6.** Minimally invasive techniques with either laparoscopy and/or thoracoscopy have been reported for all approaches except the left thoracoabdominal approach.

Specifics for each surgical technique are described below, with advantages and disadvantages listed in **Table 42.7.** The approach chosen for a patient depends on personal surgical experience and preference, institutional tradition, and patient
8 characteristics. Relevant factors include stage of disease, associated lesions such as Barrett esophagus or achalasia, other medical comorbidities, pulmonary function, and previous surgical history. In general, proximal and distal margins of at least 5 cm are desired; thus, the location of the tumor is a critical factor in determining surgical approach.[41] Also, the importance of the total number of lymph nodes involved and removed during surgery is increasingly recognized, so transthoracic approaches may be preferred over others that do not provide as optimal access to the relevant nodes.[42,43] Interestingly, an individual surgeon's skills are probably more critically important than variations in surgical approach in optimizing the long-term survival after esophagectomy for esophageal cancer.[44]

For all approaches, patients undergo preoperative upper endoscopy to confirm tumor location prior to resection to ensure the planned approach is appropriate. Patients with

Table 42.6. General Operating Room Set-Up for Different Esophagectomy Approaches

Procedure	Position	Order of Operation	Anastomosis	One-Lung Ventilation
Three-incision	(1) Left lateral (2) Supine	(1) Right thoracic (2) Abdominal with left cervical	Left cervical	Yes
Transhiatal	Supine	Abdominal with left cervical	Left cervical	No
Ivor Lewis	(1) Supine (2) Left lateral	1) Abdominal 2) Right thoracic	Right chest	Yes
Left thoracoabdominal	Supine with chest bumped 45 degrees	Left thoracoabdominal	Left chest	Yes

Table 42.7. Advantages and Disadvantages of Different Esophageal Approaches

Esophagectomy Approach	Advantages	Disadvantages
Three-incision	All tumors Good nodal access Maximal margins ↓ risk of GERD Access to thoracic duct No thoracic anastomosis	Thoracic incision ↑ risk of pulmonary complications Requires intraoperative repositioning ↑ risk of RLN injury
Transhiatal	No thoracic incision No thoracic anastomosis Maximal margins Minimally invasive approach possible ↓ risk of GERD	Poor access to nodes Blunt thoracic dissection ↑ risk of RLN injury Risk of hemorrhage, dysrhythmia, tracheal injury, hemodynamic instability
Ivor Lewis	Good access to nodes ↓ risk of RLN injury Access to thoracic duct No cervical incision Minimally invasive approach possible	Thoracic anastomosis Thoracic incision Not good for tumors in proximal third of esophagus Requires intraoperative positioning
Thoracoabdominal	Easier access to hiatal area of patient has extensive abdominal adhesions secondary to previous surgeries	Only for tumors beyond 30–35 cm Very large incision ↑ rate of residual positive margins ↑ risk of GERD due to low thoracic location of anastomosis

RLN, recurrent laryngeal nerve; GERD, gastroesophageal reflux disease.

tumors in the midesophagus or more proximal esophagus should have bronchoscopy to evaluate for airway involvement. Most surgeons place an orogastric or nasogastric (NG) tube prior to the start of the procedure to assist in esophageal mobilization. These tubes are manipulated during the procedure as requested and guided by the surgical team. Jejunostomy feeding tubes are routinely placed in many patients because there may be a delay in the return of normal eating during the postoperative period. However, feeding tubes themselves are associated with complications and some surgeons selectively place feeding tubes.[45]

Surgeons overwhelmingly choose to use the stomach as the final conduit and most of these patients have good or excellent functional results.[46] Patients generally express good satisfaction with their life after esophageal replacement with a gastric conduit, but postesophagectomy patients do fare worse in some physical and social functioning factors compared to the general population.[47] Patients who have had prior gastric surgery or another chronic condition, such as diabetic gastroparesis may require a colon or jejunal interposition to reestablish GI continuity.[48]

The optimal location for the esophageal anastomosis after resection (cervical vs. intrathoracic) is controversial, although the majority (almost 60%) in the past were placed in the cervical region.[46] The advantages of a cervical anastomosis include better access for a wider primary esophageal resection, avoidance of potentially morbid thoracotomy incisions, and less severe postoperative symptoms of reflux due to less residual esophageal mucosa.[49] Conversely, advantages of an intrathoracic anastomosis include a lower incidence of anastomotic leaks and injuries to the recurrent laryngeal nerves as well as a lower risk of postoperative stricture formation.[49] In the current era, mortality associated with cervical and intrathoracic leaks is similar, although intrathoracic leaks are more likely to require surgical intervention.[49]

Three-Incision Esophagectomy (McKeown)

The three-incision esophagectomy or McKeown approach combines left cervical, right thoracic, and abdominal incisions (**Fig. 42.4A**). This approach is especially useful for tumors of the mid and upper esophagus and for tumors when a long Barrett segment is present. The patient is initially positioned in the left lateral decubitus position for a right thoracotomy or thoracoscopy and one-lung ventilation is required for the thoracic portion of the case. The esophagus is mobilized from the thoracic inlet to the esophageal hiatus, and a lymph node dissection is performed. The azygos vein is routinely ligated in this approach, and recurrent laryngeal nerve injury can occur during this portion of the procedure. The thoracic incisions are closed after placement of a chest tube and the patient is repositioned in the supine position with a roll placed under the scapula to extend the neck. The head is turned to the right to maximally expose the left neck. An upper midline laparotomy or laparoscopy is then performed, and the gastric conduit is mobilized and created. Surgeons selectively place jejunostomy feeding tubes and perform pyloroplasty to enhance gastric emptying.

A left cervical incision is then made, and the cervical esophagus is dissected free in the neck. The recurrent laryngeal nerve is at risk of injury during this dissection. The NG tube is withdrawn to a specific depth under direct supervision of the surgeon, and the cervical esophagus is divided. A suture or a rubber drain is fastened to the distal end of the divided esophagus and the distal esophagus is withdrawn through the esophageal hiatus into the abdominal incision. The prepared gastric conduit is then pulled back through the hiatus and up into the neck with care to avoid torsion. The cervical anastomosis is then performed, and the NG tube is guided through the anastomosis under direct supervision by the surgical team.

Transhiatal Esophagectomy

The transhiatal esophagectomy combines abdominal and left cervical incisions (**Fig. 42.4B**). This approach is probably ideal for patients with Barrett and high-grade dysplasia, where lymph node dissection is not as critical for staging purposes. The abdominal portion of this procedure is performed as described above for the three-incision technique. The hiatus is dilated, and the surgeon's hand is inserted into the mediastinum to bluntly dissect the esophagus free from other intrathoracic

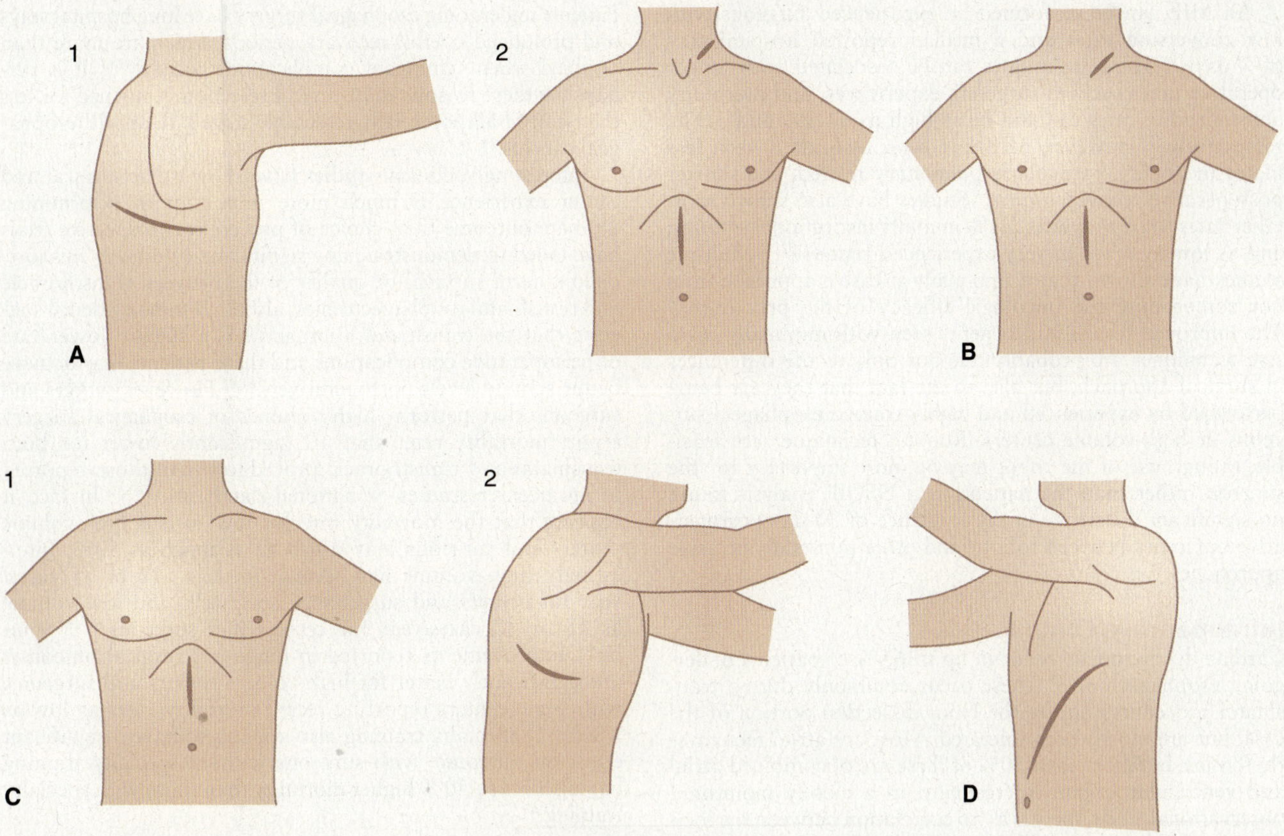

Figure 42.4. Incisions used for (A) three-incision or McKeown, (B) transhiatal, (C) Ivor Lewis, and (D) left thoracoabdominal esophagectomies.

structures. A left cervical incision is then made, and the esophagus is dissected in a similar manner from the neck into the chest but with special care to avoid injury to the recurrent laryngeal nerve. After complete esophageal mobilization, the esophagus is divided, and the anastomosis is performed in the neck as described above for the three-incision technique.

Excellent surgical outcomes for this technique have been reported by high-volume surgeons.[15] However, the use of this technique has decreased in the United States. An esophagectomy analysis of the American College of Surgeons-National Surgical Quality Improvement Project of the years 2005 to 2011 showed 52.5% of patients had a transhiatal approach, but a subsequent study that included the years 2005 to 2014 found that only 41.7% had the transhiatal approach.[50,51] The decrease in the utilization of this technique was probably influenced by both the recognition of the importance of lymph node resection to prognosis as well as the increasing use of minimally invasive techniques that also provides the transhiatal advantage of avoiding the morbidity of a thoracotomy.[52]

Ivor Lewis Esophagectomy

The Ivor Lewis esophagectomy resembles the modified McKeown approach, but involves only two incisions: right thoracic and upper abdominal (**Fig. 42.4C**). Although it also requires one-lung ventilation, the Ivor Lewis begins with the patient in the supine position for laparotomy or laparoscopy for preparation of the gastric conduit. The gastric tube is then advanced into the chest as far as possible and the abdomen is closed. The patient is then repositioned in the left lateral decubitus position for right thoracotomy or thoracoscopy. In the chest, the esophagus is mobilized and divided. The gastric conduit is pulled further into the chest and the anastomosis is performed. The thoracotomy or thoracoscopy incisions are closed after placement of a chest tube.

Left Thoracoabdominal Esophagectomy

The left thoracoabdominal approach (**Fig. 42.4D**) can be performed with acceptable morbidity and mortality but is generally only considered for patients with tumors limited to the distal esophagus, and even in those cases is associated with high rates of residual disease.[53] This approach necessitates one-lung ventilation, and the patient is positioned in the right lateral decubitus position but with the abdomen rolled back approximately 45 degrees. A thoracoabdominal incision is made along the 7th intercostal interspace across the costal margin, and the diaphragm is taken down circumferentially from the chest wall (**Fig. 42.4D**). Esophageal and gastric mobilization and resection are performed as described for the Ivor Lewis technique, but with reconstruction of the diaphragm prior to closure. This approach is not often utilized due to the limited amount of esophageal resection that can be achieved, and also the postoperative pain and morbidity associated with this approach. However, a thoracoabdominal option may be optimal for patients who have previous abdominal surgeries that could make a midline abdominal approach more difficult.

Minimally Invasive Esophagectomy

Minimally invasive techniques to achieve esophagectomy have been utilized for decades and are becoming increasingly more common. Essentially, the chest and the abdominal components of the different esophagectomy approaches described above can all be done using minimally invasive techniques via laparoscopic, thoracoscopic, and robotic approaches. Considering the multiple approaches that can be used to achieve an esophagectomy, specifically defining a minimally invasive esophagectomy (MIE), is not surprisingly problematic. One proposed MIE definition is "an operation that removes part or all of the esophagus, does not retract, lift, spread or remove any part of the chest or abdominal wall and the surgeon's and assistant's vision of the operative field is via a monitor, the patient's tissue is manipulated only by instruments that are controlled by the operating surgeon or team, except for during the neck portion if used."[54] Procedures that are done with not all but at least one component minimally invasively are generally considered to be "hybrid" procedures.[54]

An MIE can be performed by experienced surgeons with low conversion rates and a median reported hospital stay of 7 days.[52] These techniques can be associated with longer operative times early in surgeon's experiences, and morbidity and mortality rates can still be as high as 61.5% and 3.3%, respectively.[55] However, MIE has been associated with less major morbidity, particularly pulmonary related, and shorter postoperative recovery times.[56] Studies have also shown mortality rates to be as low as 2.1% in multi-institutional settings, and as low as 0.9% in very experienced centers.[52,57] Multiple studies have shown that a minimally invasive approach does not compromise the oncologic efficacy of the procedure.[56] The improved results and benefits seen with minimally invasive techniques are probably due not only to the differences in surgical approach, but also to the fact that they are being performed by experienced and highly trained esophageal surgeons at high-volume centers. Robotic techniques are feasible, though use of the robot may be more important for the surgeon rather than the patient, as a NSQIP analysis found no significant difference in the incidence of 30-day postoperative outcomes between robotic and other minimally invasive approaches.[58]

Intraoperative Complications

Cardiac dysrhythmias occur in up to 65% of patients undergoing esophagectomy.[59] These occur commonly during transhiatal procedures during the blunt dissection portion of the case, but are mostly well tolerated. Most are atrial tachydysrhythmias, but more than 50% of these are of combined atrial and ventricular origin. Interestingly, in a closely monitored observational study, there was no correlation between the incidence of dysrhythmias and that of hypotension, but there was a strong correlation between hypotension and the duration of manipulation.[59]

Other serious intraoperative events that can occur are hemorrhage and airway injury. While massive bleeding is rare, it may require rapid conversion from a minimally invasive to an open technique, or even an emergent change in patient position to facilitate surgical exposure of the involved vessel. In general, if severe bleeding occurs in the mid or upper esophagus, it may require conversion to a right thoracotomy for approach to the azygos vein; and if from the lower third of the esophagus, a left thoracotomy may be required to access a bleeding esophageal branch from the aorta. Fortunately, such vascular injuries occur in less than 2% of transhiatal esophagectomy cases.[60] Similarly, airway injury is rare, <1%.[60] These injuries are mostly limited to the distal membranous trachea or proximal bronchi and may be detected by the smell of inhaled anesthetic in the field or a feeling of airflow by the surgeon with each ventilator-delivered breath. Injuries are rarely large enough to be detected by loss of ventilator volume. If an airway injury is detected, deflation of the endotracheal tube cuff and advancement of the tube past the injury with manual guidance by the surgeon should be performed. An airway injury can be amenable to primary repair, though an intercostal muscle flap to buttress the repair is advisable. If the patient remains stable when an airway injury occurs, completing the procedure as planned should be accomplished. In any case of airway injury, though, extubating the patient immediately postoperatively is critically important to minimize pressure on or manipulation of the repair.

Immediate and Long-term Outcomes Following Esophagectomy

Even with advances in surgical technique, anesthetic, and critical care, esophagectomy continues to be a source of significant morbidity and mortality in both the immediate perioperative period and for long-term survivors. Perioperative mortality rates have historically been reported as 8.8% to 14% but was still 3.4% in a recent Society of Thoracic Surgeons General Thoracic Surgery Database; major morbidity is still 33%.[13–15,49,61] Patients undergoing esophageal surgery have long hospital stays and prolonged overall recovery periods, which are more than doubled when significant complications occur.[13,49,61] It is perhaps for these reasons that surgical resection is pursued for less than half of all potentially resectable stage I, II, and III esophageal cancers.[24]

Interestingly, clinical studies have shown that surgical and center experience is much more important in determining ultimate outcome than choice of procedure. Prospective trials have failed to demonstrate any significant differences in short- or long-term survival or quality of life between transthoracic and transhiatal esophagectomies, although some evidence suggests that the transhiatal approach has a slightly lower rate of perioperative complications and these patients may achieve better activity levels postoperatively.[61,62] However, centers and surgeons that perform high volumes of esophageal surgery report mortality rates that are significantly lower for both transhiatal and transthoracic procedures than those reported in multicenter studies or national databases.[15,63,64] In fact, it appears that the mortality rate for low- versus high-volume centers and surgeons may differ by as much as 50%. Interestingly, high volume has been defined as >12 or >5 cases/year for centers and surgeons, respectively, and low volume as <5 or <2 cases/year for centers and surgeons.[65–67] Similarly, improvements reported in long-term surgical outcomes are significantly better for high-volume centers and surgeons, with some centers reporting recent mortality rates as low as 1%.[13,15,68] Specialty training also appears to have a significant effect on outcome, with surgeons without specialty training having 37% to 50% higher mortality than those with specialty training.[65]

Morbidity Following Esophagectomy

A summary of complications following esophagectomy is listed in **Table 42.8.** Risk factors for major morbidity are pulmonary disease, older age, congestive heart failure, malnutrition, decreased functional status, and use of tobacco.[61,69] Preoperative predictors of mortality based on multivariable analysis include higher Charlson score (a measure of comorbid conditions), older age, renal dysfunction, diabetes, alcohol

Table 42.8. Perioperative Morbidity and Mortality After Esophagogastrectomy

Complication	Incidence
Technical	
Anastomotic stricture	16–48%
Anastomotic leak	6–14%
Conduit necrosis	0.5–2%
Vocal cord palsy	2–14%
Wound infection	5.3–12%
Fascial dehiscence	2–5%
Delayed gastric emptying	1.8–3.7%
Chylothorax	0.8–9%
Pulmonary (total)	28.5–29.7%
Pneumonia	8–26%
Reintubation	6–17%
Respiratory failure	1.8–16%
Aspiration	7%
Atelectasis requiring bronchoscopy	4.5%
Miscellaneous	
Deep venous thrombosis	0.9–2%
Myocardial infarction	0.7–1.2%
Pulmonary embolism	0.7–1.7%
Atrial fibrillation	14–17.5%
Renal failure	0.9–3.4%

abuse, decreased functional status, intraoperative transfusion, and ascites.[14,69] Tumor location and histology are also important, with squamous cell carcinomas and upper third esophageal tumors being associated with worse outcomes.[61] As noted above, undergoing surgery at a center where less than 12 esophagectomies are performed per year is also a risk factor for postoperative mortality.[14] Neoadjuvant therapy has been variably identified as a predictor of significant morbidity and mortality in the postoperative period.[69]

Considering the overall poor prognosis for esophageal cancer patients, the impact of surgical complications on survival and quality of life cannot be overstated.[62] However, surgical technique and perioperative care have implications beyond immediate perioperative survival. Improved long-term survival and quality of life are often directly related to avoidance of postoperative complications.[70] Measures that have been successful in reducing perioperative morbidity include aggressive preoperative conditioning, minimizing intensive care unit stays, aggressive pain management, early ambulation, involvement of a dedicated intensivist in the perioperative care team, and an overall multidisciplinary, multimodal approach to management.[15]

Anastomotic and Conduit Complications

Anastomotic leaks occur in 6% to 14% following esophagectomy and traditionally were associated with extremely high mortality. However, with improvements in surgical technique and critical care, mortality rates as low as 3.3% have been achieved.[61] Clinical features commonly associated with leaks include fever, leukocytosis, pleural effusion, and sepsis, although small leaks are often identified in asymptomatic patients.[71] Many leaks (57%) can be managed nonoperatively although operative alternatives include stent placement, primary anastomotic repair, anastomotic tissue reinforcement such as with a muscle flap, and esophageal diversion.[71] Necrosis of the gastric conduit is generally uncommon but is associated with high mortality and requires immediate intervention with resection of the compromised tissue and diversion.[72] High-volume centers have reported leak rates as low as 5%, though recent reports from the Society of Thoracic Surgeons showed leak rates even in recent years to be 12.9%.[52,61]

Anastomotic strictures are somewhat common after esophagectomy. Although generally not life threatening, strictures can cause significant patient discomfort and can put patients at risk for aspiration if they have dysphagia or regurgitation secondary to the stricture. The rate of stricture occurrence has been reported to be as high as almost 50%, though a recent population-based analysis found an incidence of 16.7%, with 6.6% of patients requiring three or more dilations as therapy.[73]

Respiratory Complications

Respiratory complications are the most common cause of death following esophagectomy.[49] Respiratory issues are typically due to poor clearance of secretions or postoperative aspiration. Factors that can increase the risk of aspiration or pulmonary complications include postoperative recurrent laryngeal nerve dysfunction, conduit emptying issues, and swallowing dysfunction. Risk of pneumonia appears to be highest in those approaches that involve a thoracotomy incision. Reducing pulmonary complications with the use of epidural analgesia and aggressive use of bronchoscopy for clearance of pulmonary secretions appears to reduce perioperative mortality. Other strategies include careful assessment of swallowing abnormalities and risk of aspiration by cineradiography or fiberoptic endoscopy before initiating oral intake.[49,63]

Issues with emptying of the conduit can also predispose patients to both short- and long-term pulmonary complications. Patients are at risk of aspirating contents from a full or dilated intrathoracic stomach, particularly when lying down after meals or when sleeping. A very important step to prevent this situation is to only pull the amount of stomach into the chest necessary to achieve a tension-free anastomosis and avoid having excessive redundant stomach in the chest. Performing a pyloric drainage procedure to enhance gastric drainage is also advocated by many surgeons, to avoid the risk of delayed gastric emptying that could occur from a functional gastric outlet obstruction secondary to resection of the vagus nerves during the esophagectomy.[15,52] However, a significant number of surgeons prefer very selective use of a pyloroplasty to avoid the risk of biliary reflux and dumping symptoms, as emptying issues can be somewhat easily managed with medications or endoscopic procedures such as balloon dilation, Botox injection, or a gastric per-oral endoscopic myotomy (POEM). The evidence supporting either strategy is variable. Early studies showed fewer issues with emptying when a gastric drainage procedure was performed, but more recent studies have not consistently shown a benefit.[74]

Recurrent laryngeal nerve injury manifesting as early postoperative hoarseness is a risk of esophagectomy, given the course of the recurrent laryngeal nerves in the trachea–esophageal groove. Such injuries occur in 4% to 11.2% who have a cervical anastomosis, and in 1% to 4.8% of patients who have an intrathoracic anastomosis.[15,52,75] Hoarseness is often transient and can resolve in 2 to 12 weeks if the injury was only a nerve palsy. Patients with persistent vocal cord paralysis require cord medialization procedures, as long-term persistent hoarseness is associated with debilitated performance status, as well as swallowing and pulmonary dysfunction.[76] Patients with evidence of aspiration should undergo early cord medialization, as this has been shown to decrease the incidence of pneumonia and need for bronchoscopy.[76]

BENIGN ESOPHAGEAL NEOPLASMS

There are several types of benign esophageal neoplasms that are rare and often asymptomatic (**Table 42.9**). They are important to distinguish from esophageal malignancy so they are managed appropriately. Some can be managed conservatively, while others should be removed (endoscopic or

Table 42.9. Classification of Benign Esophageal Neoplasms by Cell Type

Epithelial
Squamous cell papilloma
Fibrovascular polyp
Adenoma
Inflammatory pseudotumor
Inflammatory polyp
Nonepithelial
Leiomyoma
Schwannoma
Lymphangioma
Fibroma
Neurofibroma
Hemangioma
Rhabdomyoma
Lipoma
Hamartoma
Heterotopic
Granular cell tumor
Chondroma
Osteochondroma
Giant cell tumor
Eosinophilic granuloma

Adapted from Choong CK, Meyers BF. Benign esophageal tumors: Introduction, incidence, classification, and clinical features. *Semin Thoracic Cardiovasc Surg.* 2003;15(1):3–8.

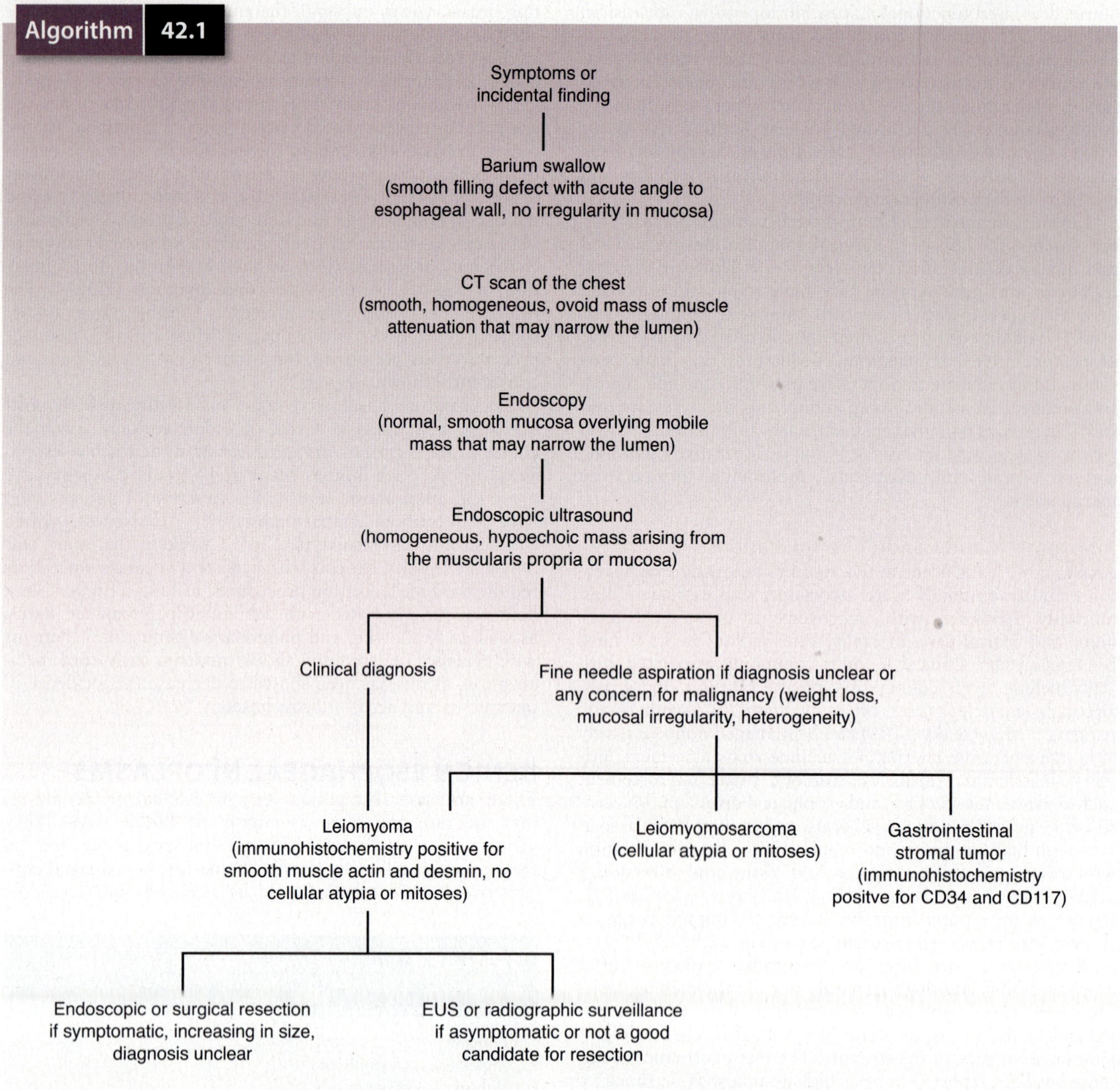

Algorithm 42.1. Evaluation and management of esophageal leiomyoma.

surgically) for definitive diagnosis, local symptoms, or rare malignant potential. Generally, if the tumor is subepithelial and resection is indicated, then surgical enucleation or ESD is performed. If the tumor is large or at a difficult location, such as the gastroesophageal junction, then a larger resection, such as esophagectomy may be required. It is important to coordinate care with an experienced thoracic surgeon and interventional gastroenterologist. The most common benign esophageal neoplasms are discussed here, but all of them should be considered during formulation of a differential diagnosis.

Leiomyoma

Leiomyomas comprise about two-thirds of the benign neoplasms of the esophagus.[77] The incidence of leiomyoma of the
9 esophagus reported in autopsy ranges from 0.005% to 5.1%. They arise from smooth muscle and thus are usually found in the middle and lower esophagus. Approximately 80% of leiomyoma originate from the muscularis propria and are located intramurally, but they have also been found arising from the muscularis mucosa and protruding into the esophageal lumen.[77] They are usually single lesions, but multiple lesions have been reported. They are generally slow-growing tumors and may not change for many years.

Patients have been diagnosed at all ages, with most at 20 to 69 years, and the incidence in men is almost twice that in women.[77] Most patients are asymptomatic, and slow onset of dysphagia and chest discomfort are the most common symptoms.[77] Rapid onset of symptoms and weight loss are concerning for malignancy.

Evaluation of a patient suspected of having a leiomyoma should begin with a barium swallow, CT scan of the chest, endoscopy, and EUS (**Algorithm 42.1**). Barium swallow demonstrates a smooth, rounded filling defect with an acute angle at the junction with the esophageal wall, indicating that the mucosa is not involved (**Fig. 42.5**). CT scan of the chest shows a smooth, ovoid mass of muscle attenuation that may narrow the lumen (**Fig. 42.6**). It is not always necessary but can confirm the differential diagnosis and rule out any other chest pathology. Endoscopy shows normal, smooth mucosa overlying a mobile mass that may narrow the lumen without obstruction (**Fig. 42.7**). Endoscopic biopsy is usually unsuccessful because of the subepithelial location. Any mucosal abnormality, such as

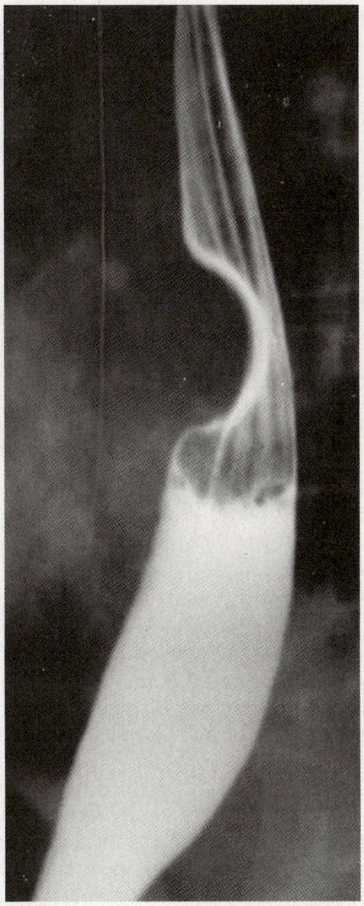

Figure 42.5. Esophagram of a leiomyoma. The acute angle at its junction with the esophageal wall is typical, indicating that the mucosa is not involved. (Reproduced with permission from Orringer MB. Tumors of the esophagus. In: Sabiston DC Jr, ed. *Textbook of Surgery.* 13th ed. AWB Saunders; 1986:736.)

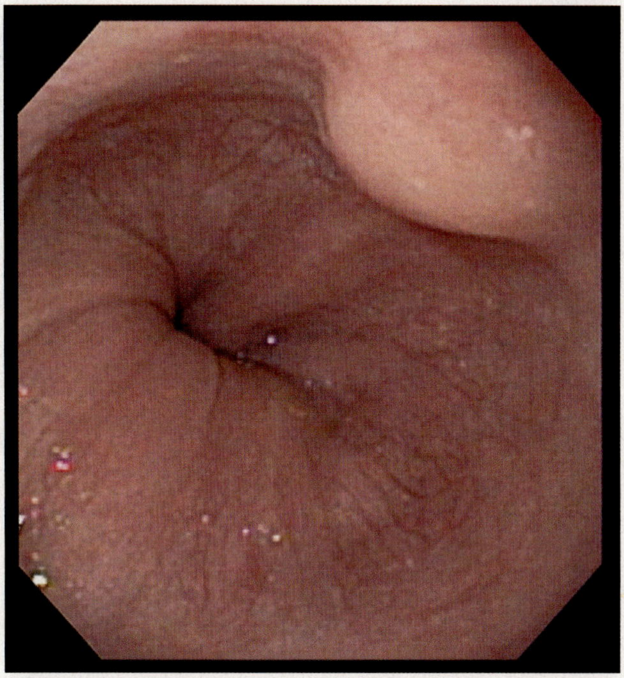

Figure 42.7. Endoscopic appearance of an esophageal leiomyoma in the distal esophagus just proximal to the gastroesophageal junction. The mucosa is smooth and normal overlying the mass, indicating that it is not involved. (Courtesy of Michael L. Kochman, MD, Hospital of the University of Pennsylvania, Philadelphia, PA.)

ulceration, is concerning for malignancy such as esophageal carcinoma or leiomyosarcoma.

EUS can confirm the layer of origin, and FNA can be used to obtain tissue for diagnosis and distinguish leiomyomas from the much rarer malignant gastrointestinal stromal tumor (GIST) and leiomyosarcomas. Leiomyomas are positive for smooth muscle actin and desmin, whereas GISTs are positive for CD117 and CD34. Leiomyosarcomas have significant cellular atypia. FNA should not be performed routinely if a clinical diagnosis can be made, since scarring may increase the risk of mucosal perforation during resection. If resection is not necessarily planned or there are any features concerning for malignancy, FNA should be performed.

Indications for resection are symptoms, increase in size, wish for a definitive diagnosis, and any concern for malignancy such as mucosal ulceration or heterogeneity. Small, asymptomatic leiomyomas may be monitored since they grow slowly

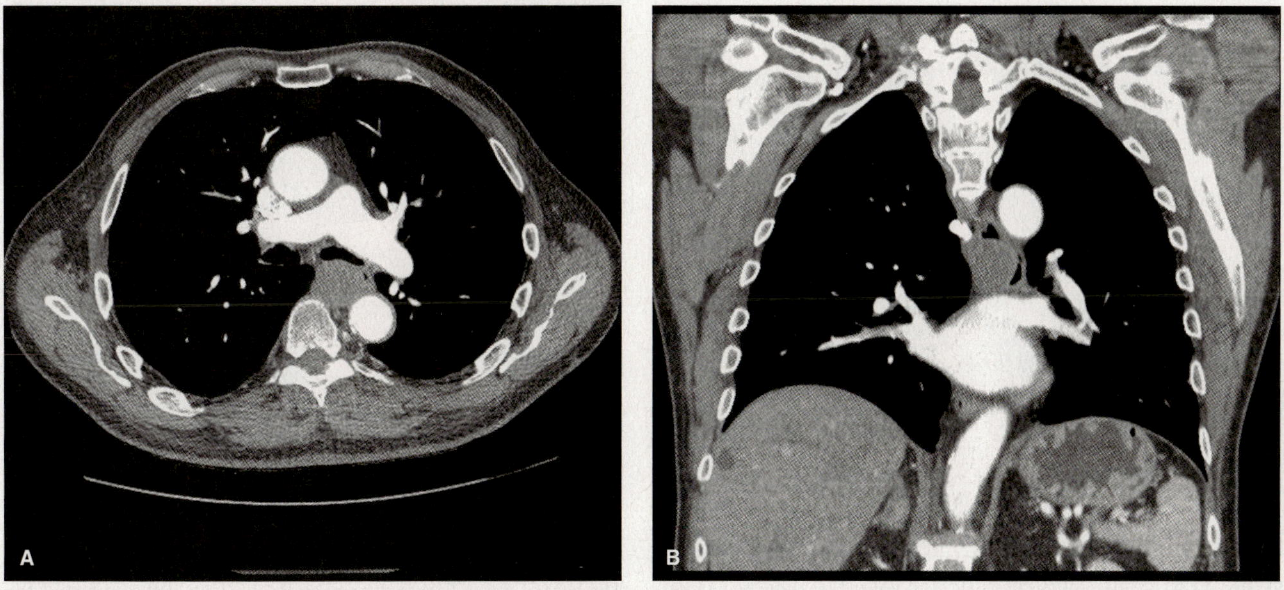

Figure 42.6. Axial (A) and coronal (B) computed tomography images of a midesophageal leiomyoma that was causing dysphagia. The smooth, ovoid mass of muscle attenuation partially occludes the esophagus. (Courtesy of Natalie S. Lui, MD, Division of Thoracic Surgery, Stanford University, Stanford, CA.)

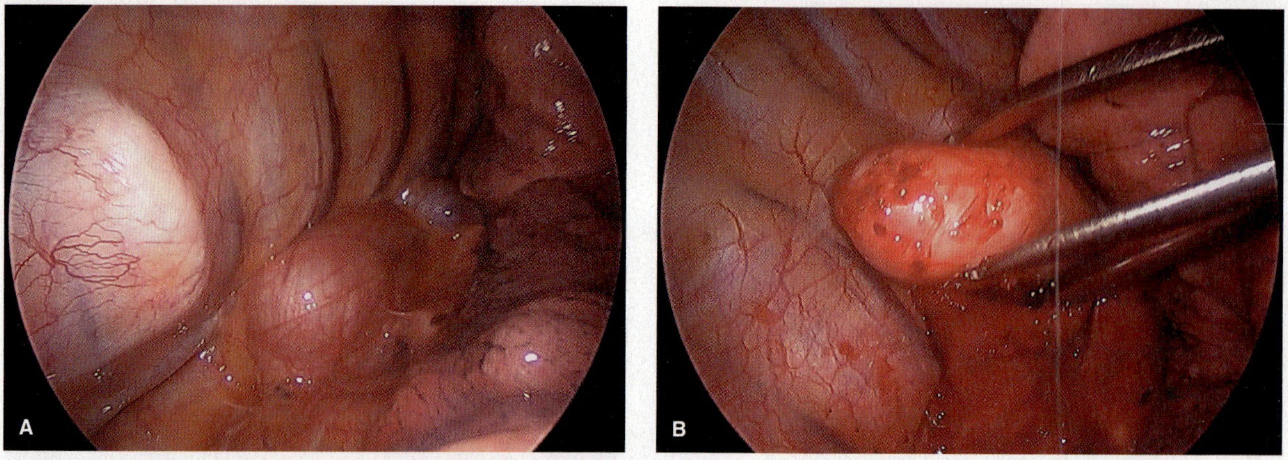

Figure 42.8. Intraoperative photos of a mid-esophageal leiomyoma before (**A**) and after (**B**) the pleura was opened via a right thoracoscopic approach. (Courtesy of Natalie S. Lui, MD, Division of Thoracic Surgery, Stanford University, Stanford, CA.)

and malignant transformation to leiomyosarcoma is rare.[77] ESD can be used for small tumors. Surgical resection is generally performed by enucleation, most commonly through the right chest (**Fig. 42.8**), but sometimes through the left chest for distal esophageal or abdomen for gastroesophageal junction tumors.[77] Minimally invasive approaches are increasingly used. The tumor is separated from the underlying mucosa, which must be repaired if injured, and the muscle layer is closed over the mucosa. Large tumors greater than about 8 cm and annular tumors may require esophagectomy. Most patients are free of symptoms after surgery and recurrence is rare.[77]

Fibrovascular Polyp

Fibrovascular polyps are rare benign neoplasms of the esophagus. They are extremely rare, described only in case reports and small case series. Recent studies have shown that many of these tumors may actually be liposarcomas, confirmed by review of morphology and MDM2 immunohistochemistry and fluorescence in situ hybridization.[78] They are intraluminal tumors that arise from a stalk near the cricopharyngeus muscle and range from small polyps to large tumors encompassing the entire esophagus (**Fig. 42.9**). They are thought to grow from excessive mucosal folds in the cervical esophagus that elongate with peristalsis.

Patients are most commonly diagnosed at 50 to 70 years of age, and the incidence is higher in men. They are usually symptomatic and most present with dysphagia. Odynophagia, regurgitation, neck pain, weight loss, and respiratory symptoms have also been reported.[79] Some patients describe coughing or vomiting the tumor out of their mouths, holding the tumor outside the mouth or between the teeth, and swallowing the tumor back into the esophagus.[79] Tumors can also cause airway obstruction leading to life-threatening presentations. On endoscopy, it may be difficult to identify the stalk, and the polyp may even be missed if it is mistaken for esophageal mucosa. CT scans reveal sausage-shaped tumors of fat or soft tissue density.

Resection is indicated to avoid symptoms, including airway obstruction, and has been described via endoscopic or surgical approaches, most commonly left cervical esophagotomy. For very large tumors, a combined approach may be required, with stalk division by endoscopy or left cervical esophagotomy and removal of the tumor by right thoracotomy or gastrotomy (**Fig. 42.10**). Control of the stalk is important since it contains feeding vessels.[79] Recurrence has been reported, so surveillance endoscopy has been recommended.

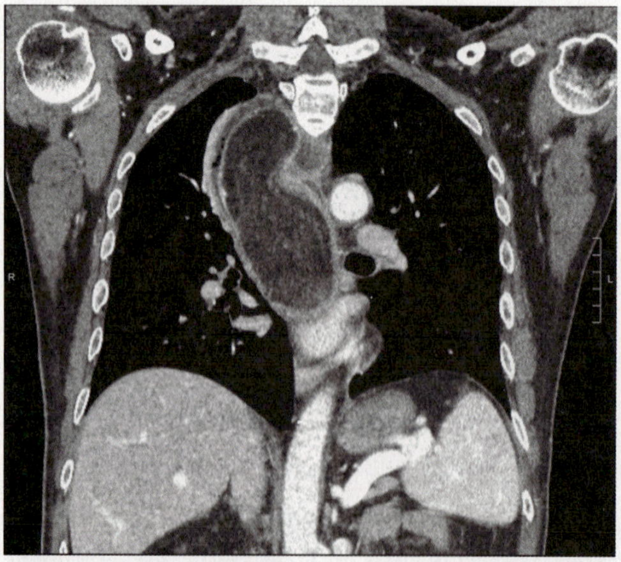

Figure 42.9. Computed tomography scan of the chest showing a large fibrovascular polyp that extended from the cervical to lower thoracic esophagus. (Courtesy of Joseph B. Shrager, MD and C. Jeffrey Yang, MD, Division of Thoracic Surgery, Stanford University, Stanford, CA.)

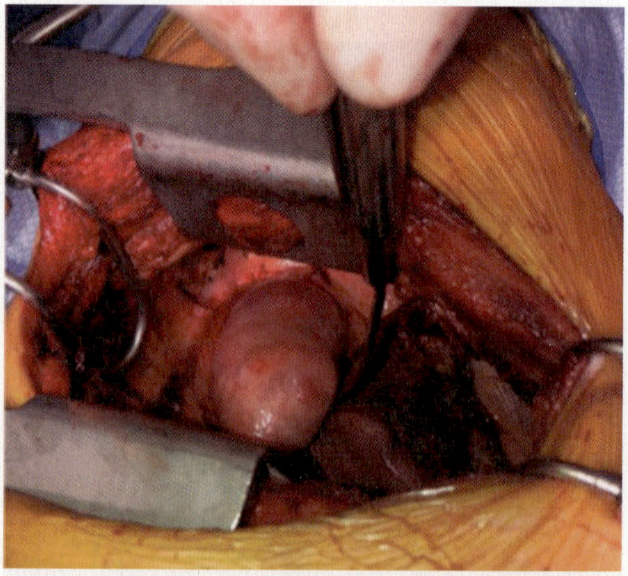

Figure 42.10. Intraoperative photos of a large fibrovascular polyp. The base of the stalk was divided endoscopically, and seen here is the tumor being removed through an esophagostomy via right thoracotomy. (Courtesy of Joseph B. Shrager, MD and C. Jeffrey Yang, MD, Division of Thoracic Surgery, Stanford University, Stanford, CA.)

Schwannoma

Schwannomas are neurogenic tumors that comprise less than 2% of benign neoplasms of the esophagus, described by case reports only.[80] They are thought to arise from the neural plexus within the esophageal wall and do not involve a distinct nerve, as compared to schwannomas that arise from the vagus nerve and grow into the esophagus.[80] They can present at all ages and are much more common in women. The most common symptom is dysphagia, but they can also cause compressive symptoms. They are most commonly located in the upper thoracic esophagus.

They can be difficult to distinguish preoperatively from the more common leiomyomas. CT scan of the chest reveals a homogeneous mass with smooth borders that may compress nearby structures such as the trachea.[80] Endoscopy shows smooth, normal mucosa overlying the mass. Of note, schwannomas have been found to be FDG-avid on PET scan.[80] EUS-FNA may be able to yield a preoperative diagnosis.

Resection is indicated if tumors are symptomatic, greater than about 3 cm, increasing in size, or concerning for malignancy. Endoscopic resection in small tumors and surgical enucleation are most common, while large tumors requiring esophagectomy have been reported.[80] Several case reports describe mucosal injury during enucleation, which was repaired. Pathologic examination shows palisading spindle cells that are positive for S-100 protein and neuron-specific enolase, but negative for smooth muscle actin or desmin (leiomyoma), or CD34 or CD117 (GIST). A few cases of malignant schwannoma have been reported, including one with lymph node involvement. Prognosis is good after resection.

Lymphangioma

Lymphangiomas are extremely rare benign neoplasms of the esophagus and are described only in case reports. They arise from dilated lymphatic vessels within the esophageal wall, most commonly in the lower esophagus. They most commonly present at 50 to 70 years of age, and they are more common in men. Patients present with dysphagia or chest or epigastric discomfort.[81]

Endoscopy shows a pale, translucent subepithelial tumor. Endoscopic biopsy is often unrevealing and should not be performed if tumor could possibly be an esophageal varix. CT and MRI of the chest show that the tumor has fluid density. Most tumors are smaller than 2 cm, but very large tumors have been reported. Resection is indicated if the tumor is symptomatic, large, increasing in size, or when the diagnosis is unclear. Resection has been described by EMR, ESD, surgery, and even laser treatment.[81] Recurrence after complete resection and malignant transformation have not been reported.

ESOPHAGEAL INJURY

Esophageal Perforation

Epidemiology

Esophageal perforations are a major source of morbidity (10% to 60%) and mortality (4% to 50%); accurate diagnosis and early treatment are essential to the successful management of these complicated and often significantly ill patients.

The causes of esophageal perforation are listed in **Table 42.10**. Generally speaking, the incidence of iatrogenic perforation (59%) far exceeds the second most common cause, that being spontaneous perforations (15%).[82] Other less common injuries include foreign-body ingestion (12%) and trauma (9%). Ingestion of foreign bodies or caustic materials most commonly causes perforations in the anatomic areas of narrowing: cricopharyngeus, level of aortic arch, and the level of left mainstem bronchus (**Fig. 42.11**). Also included in the area at risk is the lower esophageal sphincter zone. External penetrating trauma can occur at any level, but is seen more commonly in the cervical esophagus as the mediastinal portion is posterior and protected by the thorax. The morbidity and mortality of penetrating esophageal trauma are usually related to associated injuries, including major vascular and airway structures. Blunt traumatic perforation of the esophagus is exceedingly rare.

The incidence of perforation has risen in the modern era due to the rise in use of advanced endoscopic interventions, including EMR, ESD, and POEM for treatment of achalasia. A recent report examining the treatment trends for early-stage esophageal cancer identified utilization of endoscopic therapy increased from 42.7% to 50.6% with a reciprocal decrease in esophagectomy from 21.7% to 12.8% from 2010 to 2014.[83]

Table 42.10. Causes of Esophageal Perforation

Instrumental
Endoscopy
Dilation
Intubation
Sclerotherapy
Laser therapy
Noninstrumental
Barogenic trauma
Postemetic (Boerhaave syndrome)
Blunt chest or abdominal trauma
Other (eg, labor, convulsions, defecation)
Penetrating neck, chest, or abdominal trauma
Operative trauma
Esophageal reconstruction (anastomotic disruption)
Vagotomy, pulmonary resection, hiatal hernia repair, esophagomyotomy
Corrosive injuries (acid or alkali ingestion)
Erosion by adjacent infection
Swallowed foreign body

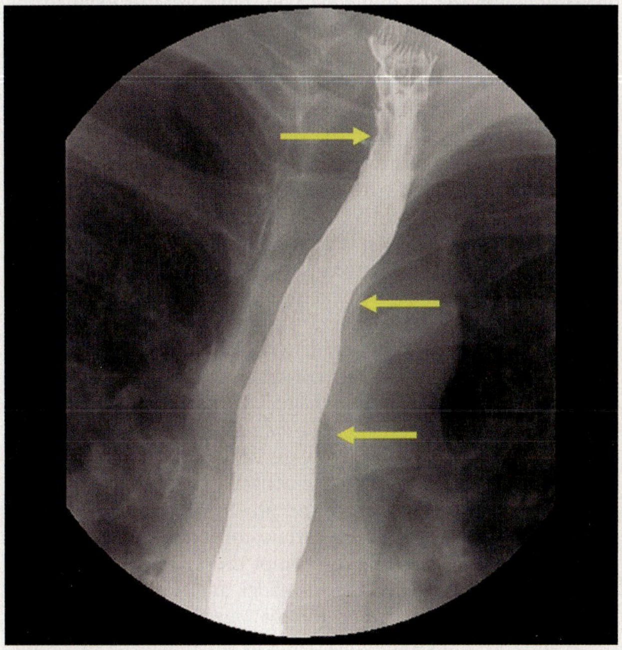

Figure 42.11. Barium esophagram showing the constrictions caused by the cricopharyngeal muscle, aortic arch, and left mainstem bronchus (*arrows*). Indentations of the esophagus made by external structures are important anatomic landmarks and are often sites of perforation due to instrumentation.

The incidence of esophageal perforation following EMR and ESD is estimated at 1.9% to 5.8%[83,84] and 2.8% to 6% following POEM.[85]

Spontaneous perforation results from a sudden increase in intraesophageal pressure. The most commonly reported is Boerhaave syndrome: spontaneous perforation of the distal esophagus following extensive ingestion of food or alcohol. This leads to violent emesis resulting in a distal esophageal perforation, frequently into the left chest. Perforation can also be associated with hyperemesis, childbirth, seizure, or prolonged coughing.

Clinical Features

The presenting features of esophageal perforation depend on the location of the injury and the time interval from injury to presentation. Underlying comorbidities may also have an influence on the presentation dictated by the patient's physiologic reserve. Patients with cervical perforation present with dysphagia, neck pain, dysphonia, and subcutaneous neck emphysema. Often, cervical perforations present earlier than distal perforations, given the intolerability of discomfort of neck symptoms. Intrathoracic perforations may present with a spectrum of clinical features ranging from simple persistent substernal chest pain to symptoms of frank mediastinitis and sepsis. Mediastinitis is characterized by chest pain, tachycardia, tachypnea, fever, and leukocytosis. Perforations of the intra-abdominal esophagus may present as an acute abdomen with diffuse abdominal pain in addition to the above. More significant perforations and longer intervals to presentation contribute to the features of systemic sepsis, shock, and rapid deterioration.

Diagnosis

The diagnosis of esophageal perforation begins with the clinician and their index of suspicion. Any patient who presents with pain following an endoscopic intervention needs to be carefully evaluated for perforation. The initial workup involves careful history and physical examination, laboratory studies including leukocyte count, and chemistry panel for acidosis. Chest x-ray is a good screening test for other diagnoses in the differential. Contrast esophagography remains the gold standard for diagnosis as the study will diagnose and localize the site of the perforation. This study also gives important information about coexisting pathology of the esophagus and the degree of extravasation and its trajectory. Water-soluble contrast (eg, Gastrografin) is the initial agent utilized, followed by thin barium to enhance the sensitivity of the study. Water-soluble agents demonstrate 50% of cervical perforations and 80% of intrathoracic perforations.[86] Thin barium will identify 60% of cervical and 90% of intrathoracic perforations.[87] If there is a chance of aspiration or high concern of tracheoesophageal fistula, thin barium should be used from the outset because the hyperosmolar water-soluble contrast agents may cause rapid pulmonary edema and respiratory compromise. Note that barium would interfere with any subsequent CT scan.

CT scan is very useful in the diagnostic evaluation of the patient with concern for esophageal perforation. Often a CT scan is the first test obtained following a chest x-ray as it affords the clinician the ability to narrow the differential diagnosis especially in the absence of available contrast esophagography. CT may be useful for identifying the site of perforation and any associated mediastinal or pleural fluid collections. It is very common for a CT scan finding to prompt thoracic surgical consultation or facility transfer as it provides additional information routinely utilized in forming the management plan. Although CT scan is very useful, its accuracy in the diagnosis of esophageal perforation is estimated at 38.7% thus it is still limited as a confirmatory test even when performed with the administration of properly timed oral contrast.[88] It should be emphasized that barium-swallow study is the procedure of choice for optimal diagnostic accuracy unless there is a significant risk of

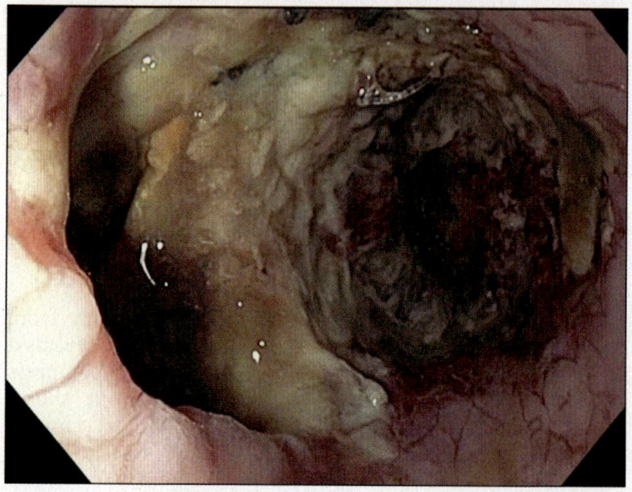

Figure 42.12. Endoscopy showing acute esophageal perforation at time of delayed presentation. (Courtesy of Joo Ha Hwang, MD, Division of Gastroenterology and Hepatology, Stanford University, Stanford, CA.)

aspiration. The barium esophagram is regarded as a real-time image, whereas the contrast delivery of the CT scan does not provide the same functional and anatomic details of the site and tracking of the leak; thus, we prefer both when possible.

Although flexible esophagoscopy raises the concern of worsening the clinical condition of the patient due to contamination of the mediastinum, use of insufflation, and aspiration, it should be utilized liberally in the diagnostic evaluation of the esophagus and in the planning of treatment options. Endoscopy also has a distinct advantage in potentially serving as a means of primary treatment intervention in a significant number of cases. The scope is utilized to directly visualize the area of perforation and identify any potential associated pathology. We routinely perform flexible endoscopy as the initial step in the operating room when considering all options for patient management (**Fig. 42.12**).

Management

Some investigators suggest aggressive operative intervention (eg, surgical exploration and repair or gastric conduit takedown with diversion), while others recommend nonoperative management with stenting, jejunostomy feeds, perianastomotic drainage, and broad-spectrum antibiotics. The decision is influenced by the location and size of the leak, the timing and degree of periesophageal soiling and extravasation, coexisting pathology of the esophagus, and the patient's overall clinical condition. The goal of treatment is to stabilize the patient, stop ongoing soilage, control infection, and maintain esophageal continuity if possible. Additional consideration should be given to the need for long-term enteral access predicted by the severity of the injury and condition. **Algorithm 42.2** provides general guidelines for the management of patients with esophageal perforations. Several well-established factors determine treatment strategy and prognosis: (1) time interval between injury and presentation, (2) location of the perforation along the esophagus, (3) severity and size of the perforation, (4) presence of signs of systemic sepsis, (5) presence of underlying esophageal pathology, and (6) experience of the care team.

Two potentially modifiable risk factors for poor outcomes are hospital volume and time to presentation. For patients presenting with spontaneous esophageal rupture (Boerhaave syndrome), diagnosis is often either missed or delayed, leading to a mortality rate approaching 60% if time to definitive treatment exceeds 48 hours. This is in stark contrast to the overall mortality in cases managed within 24 hours of presentation, which is associated with a 20% mortality.[89] Some have sought to address both delays in care and low-volume centers

Algorithm 42.2

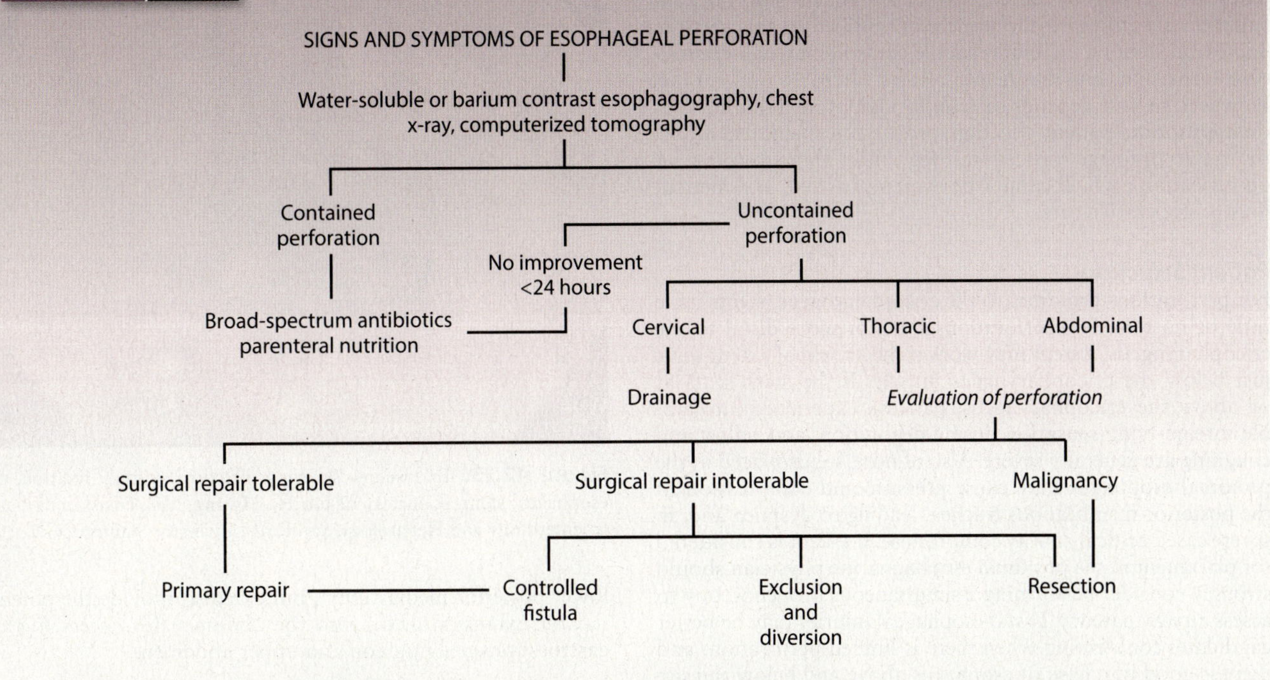

Algorithm 42.2. Evaluation and management of esophageal perforation.

by developing a regional esophageal emergency referral program emphasizing multidisciplinary care at high-volume institutions with early reports of favorable outcomes.[90] Still others report success in using the Perforation Severity Score (PSS) in an attempt to better triage patients.[91] The PSS is a clinical score based on preexisting esophageal pathology and clinical findings at the time of presentation (**Table 42.11**). Patients are risk stratified into low-, intermediate-, and high-risk groups according to increasing morbidity and mortality outcomes. The main benefit of such a score is its ability to identify patients at high risk for failure of nonoperative therapy, thereby lowering the threshold for operative intervention.

Table 42.11. Perforation Severity Scoring (PSS) Criteria

Clinical Criterion	Weighted Score
Age >75 y	1
Tachycardia	1
Leukocytosis	1
Pleural effusion	1
Fever >38.5 °C	2
Noncontained leak	2
Respiratory compromise	2
Presentation >24 h from injury	2
Hypotension	3
Malignancy	3

Adapted from Schweigert M, Sousa HS, Solymosi N, et al. Spotlight on esophageal perforation: a multinational study using the Pittsburgh esophageal perforation severity scoring system. *J Thorac Cardiovasc Surg*. 2016;151(4):1002–1009.

Nonoperative Treatment

For properly selected patients with esophageal perforation, nonoperative management may be appropriate. In fact, in more than 50% of patients presenting with known or suspected esophageal perforation, initial management is nonoperative,[88] with a success rate close to 60%.[91] Recently, the rates of nonoperative management have seen a significant increase from 48.6% between 2001 and 2003 to 54.9% between 2010 and 2012. Iatrogenic and traumatic perforations are more likely to be treated nonoperatively (68%), potentially due to the more immediate suspicion and presentation at the time of the procedure that resulted in the injury. By contrast, spontaneous perforations are more likely to be managed operatively, most likely due to their relatively delayed presentation.[92]

Current guidelines for patients who can be managed nonoperatively include those with no transmural perforation and those with a contained transmural perforation. Underlying esophageal pathology, such as malignancy or signs of systemic illness, must also be ruled out. The nonoperative approach begins with the administration of broad-spectrum antimicrobials, the suspension of oral intake, and vigilant clinical monitoring. Initial broad-spectrum antimicrobial therapy is directed to cover common gram-negative bacteria, anaerobic bacteria, and fungi. We generally use a beta-lactam agent in combination with fluconazole, which is usually sufficient. We adjust therapy to culture findings. Duration of therapy is patient dependent, but it is typically continued for 10 to 14 days after resolution.

The patient is followed clinically and reimaged as needed, generally within 48 to 72 hours with a CT scan and esophagram if clinically indicated. If the patient improves during that time and testing is favorable, the diet may be advanced to clear liquids, with the patient eventually being discharged on oral antibiotics and full liquids until reevaluation with imaging in the outpatient setting in 2 weeks. Any signs of sepsis, such as fever, tachycardia, or leukocytosis, suggest failure of this approach, and further intervention should be expeditiously considered.

Esophageal Stents

Endoscopic placement of endoluminal stents for esophageal perforations has increased dramatically to the point that they have become one of the main tools in the management of select cases.[93] Highly selected patients with perforations are candidates for stenting in the context of a thoracic surgical consultation according to the principles outlined in this section. Successful stenting facilitates source control, may reduce stricture formation, and frequently allows for early oral intake. However, success depends on a uniform approach that focuses on appropriate patient selection, proper placement technique, thorough drainage procedures (eg, tube thoracostomy or decortication), which cannot be overemphasized, and meticulous postoperative care.

Patient Selection

For perforations proximal to the cricopharyngeus, stents have little or no role. For perforations 2 cm or more distal to the cricopharyngeus, a stent may work if the proximal extent seats just below the cricopharyngeus muscle. If the stent seats at or above the cricopharyngeus, patients experience intolerable foreign-body sensation during deglutition, and reflux and coughing are generally severe. Also of note, stents placed in the proximal esophagus may cause pressure and compression of the posterior membranous trachea, leading to dyspnea and, in severe cases, critical airway compromise. If a stent is considered for placement in the proximal esophagus, the physician should strongly consider performing a simultaneous bronchoscopy to assess airway patency. Distal esophageal injuries may be better candidates for stenting when there is limited perforation, and there is good purchase of esophagus above and below the site of the perforation. This might include perforations associated with malignancy and in benign diseases such as iatrogenic perforation, Boerhaave syndrome, and select cases of achalasia. Patients with perforations from near-obstructing cancers can be ideal candidates for stents as the stent will purchase well against the tumor, leading to sealing of the perforation and relief of any coexisting blockage above or below the level of perforation. In addition, operating on perforated cancers can be a significant clinical challenge, as this may represent their initial diagnosis at the time of perforation without the benefit of clinical staging. Perforation may also occur during treatment for esophageal cancer with chemotherapy or radiation. In either event, the patient may have contamination from tumor spillage, thus making stenting our procedure of choice in the setting of malignancy.

We emphasize aggressive source control, and operative drainage of any extraluminal contamination. Stent placement without drainage in the setting of mediastinal soilage is a risky approach, and if it is done, one may question whether the perforation was small enough to need intervention. If larger, we would typically perform a VATS or thoracotomy to debride any soilage. If patients deteriorate clinically following any treatment, consideration of the presence of undrained sepsis should always be considered. At times, a patient might require several interventions to control the local and regional sepsis. In general, the presence of mediastinal air without fluid collection represents the highly select group for which antibiotics only, without additional source control measures as an adjunct to stent therapy, can be considered. The presence of mediastinal fluid collection or abscess most often requires formal operative drainage. The operative approach to drainage will vary by anatomical location. Cervical esophageal injuries with fluid collections in the neck and superior mediastinum can be approached through lower vertical neck incision with blunt mediastinal dissection, irrigation, open packing, and, if deemed appropriate, drain placement. Often, the use of a mediastinoscope can facilitate drainage of fluid collections extending down into the superior mediastinum without the need for formal chest exploration. Collections within the middle mediastinum are best approached via right thoracoscopy or thoracotomy with wide pleural incision, drainage, irrigation, and large-bore chest tube placement. Left thoracoscopy or thoracotomy is best reserved for isolated collections in the lower posterior mediastinum, but can also provide the potential for extension down into the abdomen for access to the gastroesophageal junction and upper abdomen.

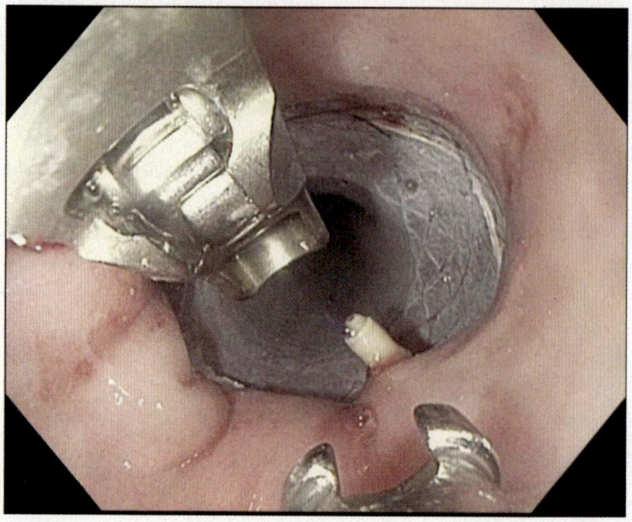

Figure 42.13. Endoscopy showing proximal suture fixation of esophageal stent. (Courtesy of Joo Ha Hwang, MD, Division of Gastroenterology and Hepatology, Stanford University, Stanford, CA.)

Stent Placement

Numerous stents are available for use. Longer stents (15 cm) that are fully covered work better to cover defects than uncovered stents. Newer covered stents which are uncovered at the proximal and distal end offer an advantage over fully covered stents to minimize migration. The procedure can be performed either in the endoscopy suite or the operating room. We prefer the latter with general anesthesia so that the stent can be placed immediately following diagnostic endoscopy followed by surgical exploration for mediastinal and pleural drainage in one setting. Fluoroscopy is useful to aid in optimal stent positioning using radiopaque skin markers. Additionally, fluoroscopy is useful if intraoperative esophagram is required for a small leak that is difficult to localize endoscopically. Ideal stent placement will depend on the location and size of the perforation. The goal is to cover at least 3 to 4 cm above and below the site of leak or perforation with a minimum distance from cricopharyngeus muscle (upper esophageal sphincter) of 1 to 2 cm. In the case of distal esophageal perforation centering the stent at the site of injury may result in crossing the GE junction which is associated with higher risk of stent migration. In this case, we suggest using a longer stent oriented such that the distal end is lodged against the greater curvature of the stomach which acts as an additional fixation point to minimize migration with peristalsis. Proximal stent fixation using endoscopic sutures or clips is also useful to reduce the risk of stent migration (**Fig. 42.13**). Following placement, intraoperative evaluation of stent position and proper sealing is confirmed with a final endoscopy. It is easier to "pull" a stent back more proximally than to "push" it more distally thus we recommend erring on the side of more distal placement and repositioning, if needed to be done via pulling technique.

Poststent Management

Enteral feeding access should be ensured as soon as possible, preferably at the time of endoscopic and operative interventions. This can be accomplished with laparoscopic or open jejunostomy, percutaneous gastrostomy (PEG), or nasoenteric tube in order of decreasing invasiveness. Anticipation of good stent placement with limited time estimate for enteral access can be managed with nasoenteric tube only, which can be placed at the conclusion of the endoscopy. PEG may be ideal for those not requiring laparotomy for other reasons and can also be placed at the time of endoscopy, but before stent placement. PEG placement after stent placement has the potential to displace the stent. Daily chest radiograph is performed to monitor stable stent location for several days following placement. We obtain chest radiography immediately after the procedure and daily thereafter to monitor for migration. Ongoing sepsis is generally due to poor source control and/or nonsealing of the perforation. Reintervention is tailored to the situation but might require aggressive surgical intervention and stent removal and/or replacement.

Outcomes

Outcomes for stent therapy for esophageal perforation have a reported success rate of 77% to 84%.[94] Stent migration is the leading complication following stent. It occurs in 30% to 55% of cases of stent placement and proximal fixation with sutures or clips is associated with a reduction in stent migration and need for replacement.[95] Once stent migration is confirmed radiographically, replacement is required unless the leak has resolved. This is typically not an emergency but should be addressed in a timely fashion. We generally repeat endoscopy at 3-week intervals and remove the stent each time. If a small leak persists, a new stent is placed so that the distal end of the stent is slightly proximal or distal to that of the previous stent to allow the area of inflamed mucosa to heal. Resumption of oral intake depends on the clinical scenario. A speech pathologist evaluates every patient before an esophagram. Only patients who are safe to swallow undergo an esophagram. Oral intake is then resumed and represents a major advantage of stent placement, which allows for the possibility of oral nutrition while the perforation is healing.

Esophageal stenting is also a useful tool in the setting of failed primary repair or anastomotic leak, with a high success rate. Secondary interventions following stent placement for patients with perforation are estimated at 33.7%. Major complications include sepsis (28.1%), pneumonia (17.1%), and multiorgan failure (11.6%). Overall mortality is 15.1%.[96] According to the latest systematic review, the overall technical and clinical success rates of esophageal stenting for esophageal perforation are 91% and 81%, respectively, with mortality of 13% likely reflective of diligent patient selection.[97]

Endoscopic Clipping

Advanced endoscopic interventions in the form of clipping or suturing are gaining in popularity with promising early results (**Fig. 42.14**). Endoscopic clipping can be performed either using a through-the-scope (TTS) method or an over-the-scope (OTSC) system. The OTSC system is a clipping method for mechanical compression of tissues in the GI tract first designed for the management of bleeding, perforation, and fistula. Similar to other interventions for perforation, endoscopic clipping is a viable option only when performed early after the injury. After 24 hours postinjury, tissue integrity becomes a major limitation hindering successful primary repair, and the rate of failure of endoscopic therapy increases significantly.[98] TTS clips are best for defects 10 mm or less in greatest dimension while bigger (<20 mm) lesions can be treated successfully with the OTSC method. Larger defects are best considered for stent placement or surgical repair. In either endoscopic treatment, a significant source of failure is overlooking the need for drainage and treatment for associated mediastinitis as a source of sepsis. Thus, concomitant surgical or nonsurgical drainage of the mediastinum is imperative to accompany the endoscopic intervention as outlined for stenting.

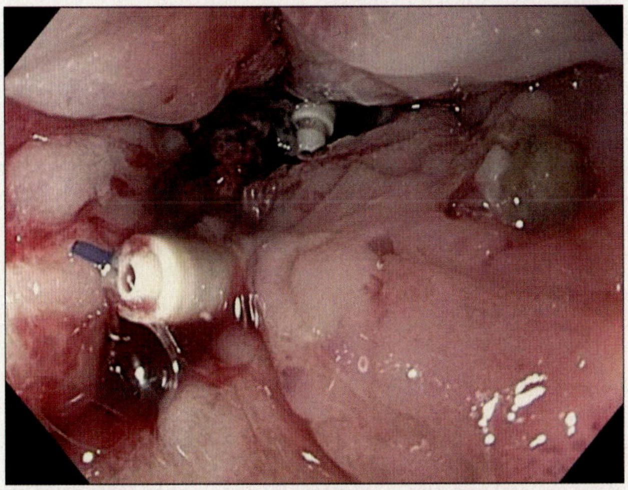

Figure 42.14. Endoscopy showing primary suture repair of esophageal perforation. (Courtesy of Joo Ha Hwang, MD, Division of Gastroenterology and Hepatology, Stanford University, Stanford, CA.)

Vacuum-Assisted Closure Therapy

Endoluminal vacuum-assisted closure (EVAC) therapy is a novel treatment modality for managing esophageal perforations. EVAC therapy facilitates tissue healing by overcoming physiologic negative pressure in the thorax, reducing mediastinal contamination and enabling tension-free approximation of tissue. The procedure can be performed in the endoscopy suite or the operating room under general anesthesia. The endosponge is created using a modified NG tube connected to a tailored wound vac sponge that is trimmed to size per endoscopic examination. The endosponge is then exteriorized for connection to the wound VAC suction system with continuous negative pressure at 175 mm Hg, on high intensity.[99] There are small series reporting success using EVAC therapy as primary treatment for esophageal perforations and leaks.[94] Successful closure is reported to range between 88% and 100% closed after a mean duration of 27 days requiring an average of six endosponge changes every 4.8 days. An additional advantage of EVAC therapy is the potential to treat patients outside of the 24-hour early presentation window with facilitated drainage of any mediastinal abscess cavity.

Surgical Repair

The operative management of esophageal perforation is dictated by the location of the injury, extent of injury, and underlying pathology. Operative approaches include drainage alone, primary reinforced repair, esophagectomy with immediate or delayed reconstruction, and esophageal exclusion. Among operative interventions, there has been a notable increase in the rates of primary surgical repair from 43% to 51% while diversion has decreased from 13% to 7% in the past 15 years.[100]

Perforations of the upper third of the esophagus to the level of the carina should be approached via a left neck incision (**Fig. 42.15**). Traditionally, it is not necessary to find or close the perforation when approached this way, as the injury will seal during the process of healing. In order for this to be successful, however, wide and complete drainage must be accomplished. Preoperative CT scan will aid in ensuring that the important areas of contamination are addressed surgically. In the operating room, we liberally use on-table flexible endoscopy to evaluate the defect and the location of the defect. If the defect is identified and it is small, we advocate for an attempt at primary closure. The neck incision is loosely reapproximated with staples over a passive drain without suction. Typically, a contrast esophagram is obtained 5 to 7 days postoperatively, the patient's diet is advanced, and the drain is removed. If there is continued leak, the patient is left nil per os (NPO) or on clear liquids and restudied in 1 week. There should be no distal obstruction on the contrast study, and if there is a stricture that prevents normal contrast flow, we advocate for dilation to aid in eventual closure of the esophageal fistula. As long as there is no underlying pathology or distal obstruction, most cervical injuries will heal spontaneously with adequate drainage.

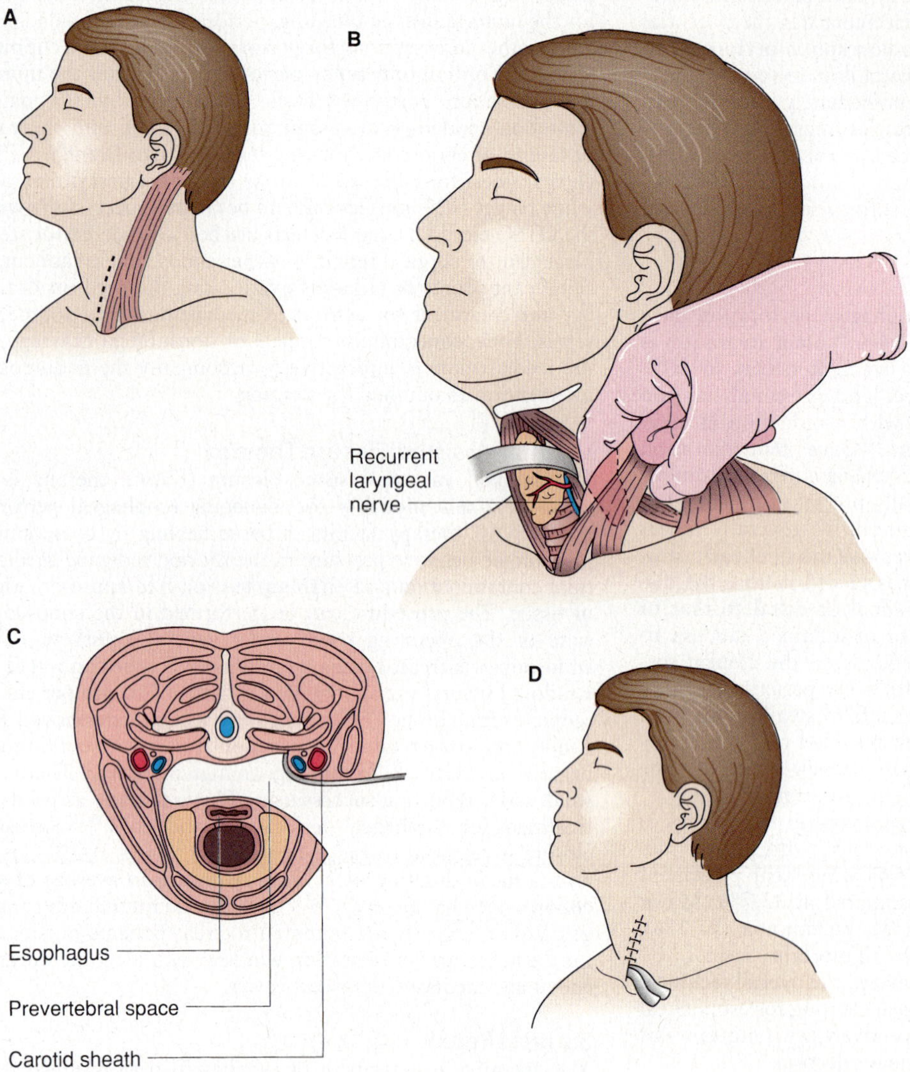

Figure 42.15. Approach for drainage of a cervical esophageal perforation. **A:** Skin incision parallel to the anterior border of the left sternocleidomastoid muscle, extending from the level of the cricoid cartilage to the sternal notch. **B:** With the sternocleidomastoid muscle and carotid sheath retracted laterally and the trachea and thyroid gland retracted medially, blunt dissection is performed along the prevertebral fascia in the superior mediastinum. Injury to the recurrent laryngeal nerve in the tracheoesophageal groove must be avoided. **C:** Schematic drawing of the prevertebral space drained by this cervical approach. **D:** Penrose drains placed into the superior mediastinum are brought out through the neck wound to allow establishment of an esophagocutaneous fistula, which usually heals spontaneously.

Perforations of the middle third of the esophagus are best approached via a right fifth interspace posterolateral thoracotomy. We routinely start thoracoscopically, but typically these patients are very ill thus, one should have a low threshold for conversion to thoracotomy. At the time of entry into the chest, an intercostal muscle flap is routinely taken. The mediastinal pleura is opened widely, and all pleural collections are drained, the lung is decorticated, and the site of perforation is identified. Necrotic tissue at the site of the perforation is debrided and the esophagus is mobilized. A vertical myotomy is performed to expose the mucosa and determine the full extent of the tear (**Fig. 42.16**). The mucosa is repaired with simple interrupted or running absorbable suture. The muscular layer is reapproximated with interrupted fine silk suture. On-table endoscopy is performed to ensure the leak is repaired. The intercostal muscle is then loosely secured as an onlay patch. Large chest tubes are placed and a malleable Blake drain is left in the area of the repair and placed to bulb suction. Nutritional access can be addressed at the index operation if the clinical condition of the patient is favorable. If not, this can be accomplished at a later date. On postoperative day 7, a contrast study is obtained, and if there is no leak, the diet is advanced. Persistent leaks are treated with continuation of the surgical drains and, potentially, placing additional drains via interventional radiology if there are any undrained collections. Esophageal stenting may be used to exclude any persistent leak as outlined above. If there are signs of clinical sepsis despite the above, esophageal exclusion may be required with cervical esophagostomy and establishment of

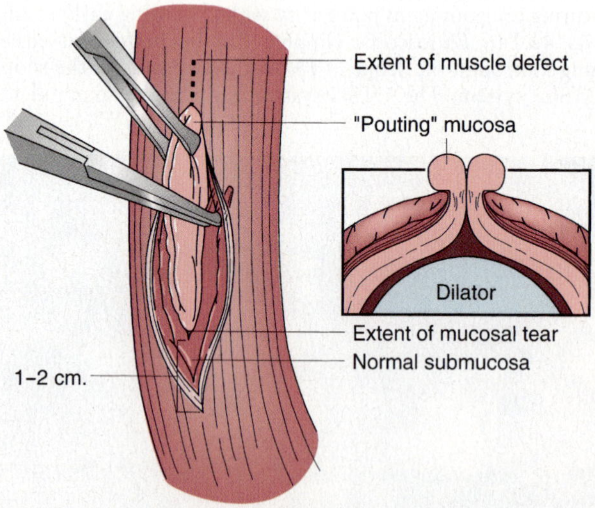

Figure 42.16. Primary repair of esophageal perforation. The edematous mucosa pouting through the muscular defect (*inset*) is grasped with Allis clamps and elevated. A 1-cm vertical esophagomyotomy is made at either end of the muscular defect to expose the entire limits of the mucosal tear. This is facilitated by using a right-angle clamp to direct muscularis away from underlying submucosa around the entire circumference of the tear. The result of this mobilization is exposure of a circumferential rim of normal submucosa that can then be closed.

long-term enteral access via jejunostomy or gastrostomy. Esophageal resection can be performed at the time of diversion or delayed depending on the clinical conditions. Patients can be considered for delayed reconstruction 6 to 12 months following perforation, most commonly approached as a gastric pull-up, colonic interposition, or jejunal flap placed in the substernal position. Perforations of the distal third of the esophagus can be approached via a left seventh intercostal space thoracotomy using the same principles for repair and drainage.

Operative treatment in the presence of underlying pathology deserves special attention and can be quite challenging. If there is distal obstruction, this must be dealt with. Strictures can be dilated or stented and often support the healing of a proximal perforation. Patients with achalasia who are perforated during pneumatic dilation are especially challenging. Many are candidates for nonoperative intervention as they have small perforations that are asymptomatic and the patients are clinically nontoxic. This is acceptable provided the distal obstruction has been relieved. For those who fail nonoperative management or are not candidates, operative management should be tailored to the individual and their pathology. In patients with preserved motility, the perforation should be repaired primarily and a vertical myotomy should be performed 180 degrees opposite the injury as in routine myotomy for achalasia patients. These patients, and those for whom esophageal motility status is unknown, should have a partial fundoplication performed. For stable patients with advanced achalasia, esophagectomy should be considered. For unstable patients, esophageal exclusion should be performed. Unstable patients with advanced pathology such as cancer should undergo esophageal stenting if appropriate or exclusion. This includes stapled esophageal diversion with resection of the diseased segment of the esophagus via a right transthoracic approach. A linear stapler is deployed on the esophagus proximally and at the gastroesophageal junction. The esophagus is resected. An end cervical esophagostomy is created saving as much esophageal length as possible. Pleural drainage is accomplished. Subsequently the patient undergoes placement of gastrostomy (± jejunostomy tube) with repair of the diaphragmatic defect from the abdominal side via laparoscopy or laparotomy. The components of operation may be staged based on the severity of patient illness. If the patient survives and is a candidate for reestablishment of continuity, this can be investigated later once they have recovered. Additionally, consideration should be given to end-of-life discussions depending on the extent of the cancer.

Surgical Resection

Fortunately, esophagectomy is necessary in only a small percentage of patients following perforation. It may be indicated following failed primary repair or as primary treatment with or without immediate reconstruction. The presence of preexisting benign or malignant stricture or large perforation (>5 cm) is associated with increased risk for need for an urgent esophagectomy.[101] When clinically indicated, emergent esophagectomy represents a safe treatment option with observational studies demonstrating mortality rates comparable between operative and nonoperative management (31% vs. 20%).[102]

Caustic Injury

Epidemiology

Caustic burns of the esophagus result from ingestion of substances with pH <2 or pH >12 (**Table 42.12**). In children, these ingestions are usually accidental, while in adults, they are most often associated with suicide attempts. Liquid alkaline agents (eg, household cleaner) are more likely to be swallowed and subsequently cause more injury. Although mortality from caustic ingestion is low, the morbidity associated with caustic ingestion is significant. Acute morbidities include perforation and necrosis. Late morbidities are more prevalent and include stricture formation and cancer.

The extent of injury to the esophagus caused by ingested caustic material is dependent on the volume and nature of

Table 42.12. Commonly Ingested Acids and Alkalines

Commonly Ingested Acids	Commonly Ingested Alkalines
Industrial cleaning solutions	Household cleaning products
Swimming pool cleaning solutions	Personal hygiene products
Battery fluids	Bleach (ammonia hydroxide)
Antirust compounds	

the ingestion. Injuries resulting from ingestion of liquids are much more severe than those caused by ingestion of solids. The patient usually spits particulate matter out and, thus, it rarely moves beyond the oropharynx. Liquid caustic agents contribute to pathology down the length of the esophagus. Strong acid and alkali ingestions comprise the majority of caustic ingestions.

Injury from alkaline ingestion tends to be more severe than acid ingestion, resulting in significantly higher rates of morbidity and mortality and higher incidence of associated stomach injuries. Alkaline burns are characterized by liquefactive necrosis, leading to far greater penetration at the level of the oropharynx however liquid alkali results in more distal esophageal and gastric injury. Frequently there is penetration of all layers of the esophagus causing substantial secondary edema. Commensurate with this, the potential for perforation and circumferential scar formation is greatest with an alkaline ingestion. In contrast to acid ingestion, alkali substances are typically odorless and tasteless, which enhances the potential for deeper injury.

Acids cause more severe damage to the stomach but similar damage to the esophagus when compared to alkalis. The burns from acid ingestion cause coagulative necrosis and a superficial eschar that protects the deeper layers of the esophagus from damage. Fortunately, acids tend to taste bitter and cause immediate pain, limiting the volume ingested prior to it reaching the esophagus and stomach. When acids are ingested in liquid form, they move quickly, typically spare the oropharynx, and produce skip injuries to the esophagus. Acids in liquid form cause gastric and duodenal injury more frequently than esophageal injury.

Clinical Presentation

The initial clinical presentation comprises oropharyngeal pain; irritability; and, in severe cases, excessive salivation, dysphagia, and airway compromise. Ingestion of particulate caustic substances results in signs of contact readily visible in the oropharynx. Hoarseness and stridor are signs of serious airway injury that mandate intubation. Retrosternal pain, neck crepitus, and sudden onset of epigastric pain imply full-thickness esophageal damage. Many patients present without symptoms and a significant proportion have injuries that will require intervention. Thus, a 24-hour period of observation is reasonable, even for asymptomatic patients, especially if there is any question about the circumstances of the ingestion or extent of injury.

As with any acute situation, management should begin with the standard assessment of the ABCs (airway, breathing, and circulation) (**Algorithm 42.3**). As with most foreign-body ingestions, the most common sites for pathology within the esophagus are its three areas of narrowing: the cricopharyngeus, the level of the aortic arch, and the gastroesophageal junction (**Fig. 42.11**). A stable patient may undergo imaging via posteroanterior and lateral upright chest and abdominal radiographs to evaluate for pleural effusion or free air. CT of the chest and abdomen can provide important anatomical definition of injury. Patients with no visible symptoms or only lip swelling or redness can be observed in the hospital or a short-stay unit for 24 hours to ensure they can tolerate oral

Algorithm 42.3

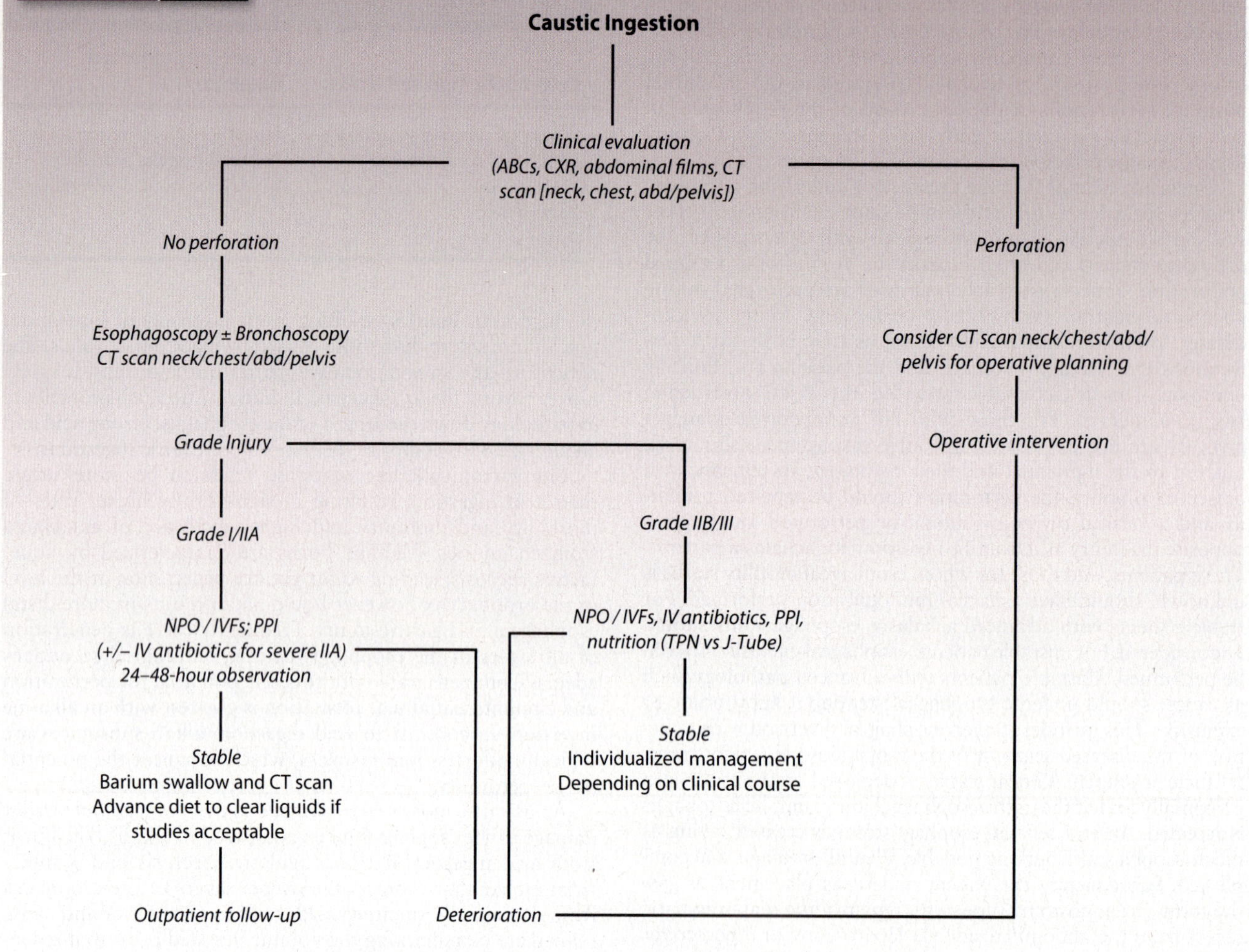

Algorithm 42.3. Evaluation and management of acute caustic ingestion.

feedings. This is typically for pediatric patients. Patients with oral lesions should undergo esophagoscopy and bronchoscopy. The bedside insertion of an NG or orogastric tube is discouraged when the extent and depth of injury have not been fully evaluated.

After radiographic imaging, esophagoscopy should be the next course of investigation to characterize the location and extent of injury. This should be performed within the first 24 hours as the risk of procedural complication increases with time. In a large retrospective study of 21,682 patients following caustic ingestion, patients undergoing endoscopy delayed greater than 48 hours after injury experienced a threefold increased risk for poor clinical outcome.[103] Others advocate for assessment with repeat endoscopy on postinjury day 5 reporting that delayed examination is a better predictor of esophageal and gastric cicatrization than day 1 exam alone, which significantly overestimates the grade of injury.[104] The indications for esophagoscopy include stridor, vomiting, drooling, and intentional ingestion. Caution should be used when moving beyond the first sign of pathology below the cricopharyngeus. If there are respiratory symptoms, laryngoscopy and bronchoscopy should be performed. The latter of which should direct the procedure to be done in the operating room. When injury is identified, the standard grading of the esophageal burn should be reported (**Table 42.13**).

Management

The initial clinical presentation comprises oropharyngeal pain, irritability and, in severe cases, excessive salivation, dysphagia, and airway compromise. Hoarseness and stridor are signs of serious airway injury that mandate intubation. Retrosternal pain, neck crepitus, and sudden onset of epigastric pain imply full-thickness esophageal damage. Many patients present without symptoms but have injuries that will require intervention. Thus, even asymptomatic patients should be observed closely for the first 24 hours. Acute management of caustic ingestion should be dictated by the endoscopic grading of the esophagus and the clinical status of the patient (**Algorithm 42.3**).

Patients with grade I injuries have superficial burns causing edema and hyperemia. These patients can be observed, a

CLASSIFICATION

Table 42.13. Endoscopic Grading of Acute Caustic Injury to the Esophagus

Injury	Endoscopic	Depth of Grade Appearance Injury
I	Superficial hyperemia	Mucosal
IIA	Sloughing mucosa, superficial ulceration	Patch partial thickness
IIB	Deep ulceration	Circumferential
III	Eschar, necrosis	Full thickness

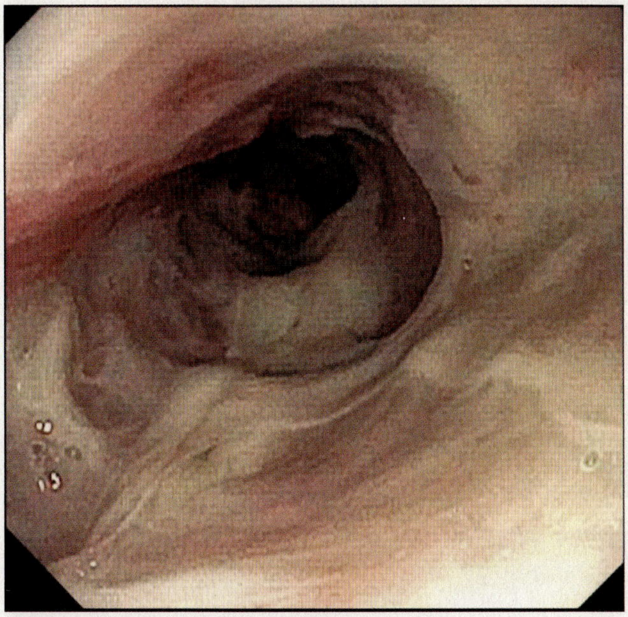

Figure 42.17. Endoscopy showing acute caustic ingestion. (Courtesy of Joo Ha Hwang, MD, Division of Gastroenterology and Hepatology, Stanford University, Stanford, CA.)

normal diet can be advanced, and the patient ultimately can be followed in an outpatient clinic. Superficial grade I injuries cause mucosal sloughing and should heal without a stricture. Grade II injuries penetrate into the muscular layer of the esophagus and can result in either patchy (IIA) or circumferential (IIB) injury. Ulcerations (superficial and deep) and pseudomembranes are found during endoscopy (**Fig. 42.17**). Once circumferential injury is identified, the risk of stricture formation increases dramatically. Generally, patients should be kept NPO until pain free. Enteral feedings can likely be introduced within 48 hours.

Grade III injuries are full-thickness injuries, and mediastinitis or peritonitis occurs within 48 hours. Grade III findings are characterized by gray mucosal slough, thrombosed submucosal vessels, and black eschar. All grade III burns and >75% of circumferential grade IIB burns cause esophageal stricture and, as expected, are associated with a higher incidence of infection.

Patients with grade IIB or grade III esophageal burns without evidence of perforation should be placed in a monitored setting, kept NPO, and given IV fluids and IV antibiotics (penicillin derivative or clindamycin). Patients should also be maintained on proton pump inhibitors to reduce acid exposure of the esophagus, as this may decrease the stricture incidence. Steroid administration is controversial, does not prevent stricture formation, and may mask findings in the serial abdominal examination. If corticosteroids (2 to 2.5 mg/kg/d) are used, they should be instituted within the first 24 hours of ingestion and for 3 weeks thereafter. Early introduction of parenteral nutrition is essential for all patients with esophageal perforation and for patients with poor gastric motility. Depending on the extent of injury, the patient may require mechanical ventilation. Esophagram (or CT scan with oral contrast) may be used as an adjunct evaluation. If free contrast extravasation into the mediastinum is visualized, drainage of the mediastinum into the pleural space is indicated. Further, esophageal resection may be required with findings of necrosis. On occasion, a contained mediastinal leak, which returns contrast material back into the esophagus, may be observed without the need for immediate drainage. Pneumoperitoneum is an absolute indication for laparotomy and resection of all dead tissues. Laparoscopic evaluation may be useful to evaluate the abdomen if there is isolated mediastinal pathology.

Surgical Resection

One of the challenges associated with esophagectomy for caustic ingestion is availability of the stomach as a possible replacement conduit. In the case of associated gastric necrosis, the stomach may itself be injured, thereby limiting its use as a conduit, or it may be completely necrotic, requiring concomitant gastrectomy. Initial resection can be performed as outlined above with or without immediate reconstruction. Delayed esophagectomy being done for sepsis or refractory stricture may be best performed in a staged fashion with esophagectomy and esophagostomy followed by substernal interposition graft of either colon or jejunum. Patients with extensive full-thickness esophageal and gastric necrosis should undergo total esophagogastrectomy with cervical esophagostomy and feeding jejunostomy. Of course, any operative intervention should include assessment of other organs involved and complete drainage/resection of necrotic tissue. Options for esophageal replacement have been outlined above.

Complications

Strictures of varying degrees occur in almost all patients following significant caustic ingestion and, thus, careful follow-up is recommended. The esophagus and stomach should be evaluated via barium swallow 3 weeks, 3 months, and 6 months after the ingestion to rule out stricture formation or gastric outlet obstruction. Esophagogastroduodenoscopy (EGD) is typically performed 3 weeks after the ingestion for full evaluation. Early endoscopy is warranted during the phase of cicatrix formation, and dilation is repeated at varying intervals. Risk factors for development of postingestion stricture include initial symptoms such as dysphagia or hematemesis, and grade IIa or higher esophagitis identified on initial endoscopy.[105]

Historically, management of esophageal strictures that develop as a result of caustic burns has been done with serial bougienage. This can be accomplished with an open gastrostomy and insertion of a string through the gastrostomy that exits transnasally. Four weeks after the burn, serial dilations using progressive antegrade bougienage from the oropharynx or retrograde stringing bougienage through the gastrostomy is effective (**Fig. 42.18**). Optimal caliber bougienage is 48 to 50 for adults and 34 to 36 for children. More commonly, serial dilatations are performed with endoscopy. Concomitant cricopharyngeal stricture, long stricture length, requiring frequent dilatation, and stricture refractory to greater than 11-mm dilatation are factors associated with failed dilatation.[106]

Esophageal stenting is another approach for second-degree esophageal burns, which can be done less frequently than dilatation. A removable, fully covered stent is placed endoscopically shortly after injury and left in place for 3 weeks. It can then be removed. Recent reports have suggested that this is an appropriate intervention to prevent stricture formation in some patients. Injection of the stricture with triamcinolone (30 mg/mL) may also be effective, especially in those strictures that are focal. Esophageal replacement is usually considered if a stricture fails to resolve after 1 year of dilations, stricture injections, and antacid therapy. Malignant degeneration is possible at the area of the stricture, and esophageal cancer occurs at a 1,000-fold greater frequency in individuals with a caustic injury to the esophagus than in the general population.

Esophageal Fistulas

The increasing use of endovascular and advanced interventional cardiology procedures has been associated with uncommon complications of fistulization between the esophagus, pericardium, aorta, or cardiac chambers. There were an estimated 120,000 cases of cryoablation done for atrial fibrillation worldwide since 2011.[107] Fortunately, despite increased use of cardiac ablation procedures, esophagopericardial fistulas are uncommon and are typically related to upper GI malignancy or as complications of esophageal injury, such as caustic ingestion, or prior surgery. Their rarity makes them a

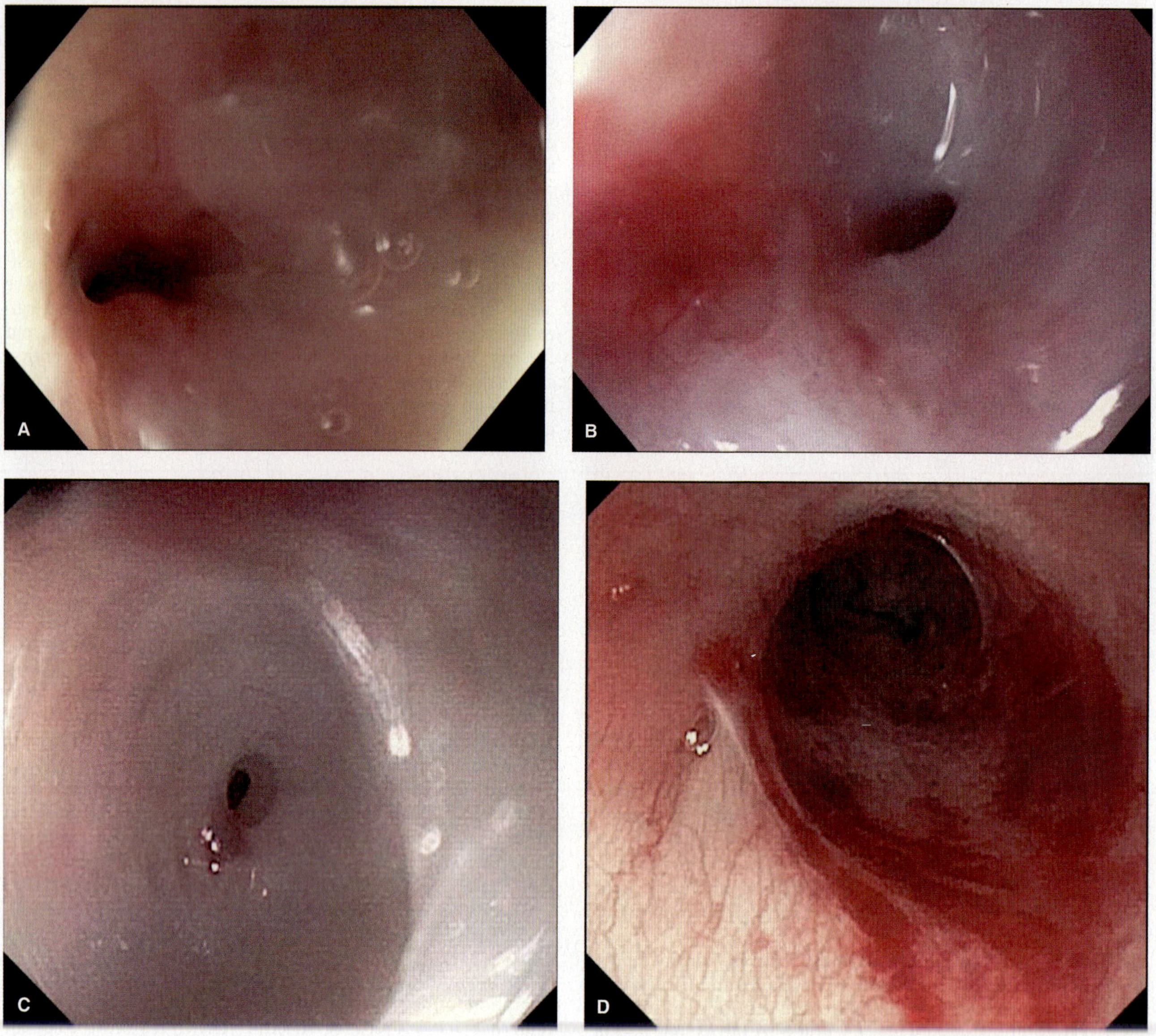

Figure 42.18. Endoscopy showing a stricture at the upper esophageal sphincter after caustic ingestion at baseline (**A**), 3 months after injury (**B**), 6 months after injury (**C**), and after balloon dilation (**D**). (Courtesy of Joo Ha Hwang, MD, Division of Gastroenterology and Hepatology, Stanford University, Stanford, CA.)

diagnostic challenge to clinicians. They are also a known complication of esophageal stents. The radial forces within esophageal stents, combined with motion from esophageal peristalsis, respirations, and cardiac pulsatility, can contribute to fistula formation if the stent is left in place for a prolonged period of time.[108]

Most patients will have a delayed presentation of weeks to months after initial insult or index procedure. A systematic review identified a median of 21 days between cardiac ablation and presentation, but patients may present as long as 60 days postprocedure. Most common presenting symptoms are fever (73%), neurologic (72%), GI (41%), and cardiac (40%) symptoms.[109] Cardiac tamponade may be present and its severity will depend on the size of the defect and rapidity with which air and/or fluid has accumulated within the pericardial space. Severe clinical symptoms only occur once the pressure in the pericardium exceeds a threshold and most patients do not require pericardial drainage. Plain radiographs may demonstrate pneumopericardium and echocardiography may show tamponade physiology if a large pericardial effusion is present. CT scan can be useful in diagnosing and localizing the site of the fistula. It is important to note that when atrioesophageal fistula is suspected, instrumentation of the esophagus with endoscopy or transesophageal echocardiography is contraindicated, as insufflation of the esophagus can result in the formation of air emboli causing devastating neurologic injury and death. If either are to be performed, they should be done at the time of surgical repair, and despite limiting the endoscopic examination, insufflation should not be used. Staged repairs may be the most appropriate way to deal with this highly morbid condition. In the case of aortoesophageal fistula, this may consist of a combined endovascular approach as a temporary measure to stabilize the patient followed by a definitive surgical repair or resection. In the case of atrioesophageal fistula repair, our approach has been via staged open intra-atrial repair for vascular control followed by thoracotomy and repair of the esophageal defect with muscle flap as detailed above. The condition carries a high mortality estimated at 55%. Mortality is significantly less for patients undergoing surgical repair (33%) compared with those undergoing endoscopic treatment (65%) or conservative management (97%).[109]

Esophageal Foreign Body

Foreign-body ingestion and food bolus impaction are common occurrences, with over 100,000 new cases occurring in the United States annually. Pediatric foreign-body ingestion is typically accidental and most frequently involves coins, followed by toy parts, batteries, bones, and food.[110] Typically, esophageal foreign bodies tend to pass through the GI tract spontaneously. However, roughly 10% to 20% of cases may require nonoperative intervention, and <1% require surgery.[111] A large percentage of objects that do not pass spontaneously remain in the cervical esophagus. Complete obstruction can lead to inability to tolerate secretions, airway compromise, and death. Pediatric patients are the most common population affected, while in adults, edentulous patients are at greatest risk.

Plain radiographs may be a sufficient diagnostic study if the object is known to be radio-opaque in order to determine location and number of foreign bodies. UGI or barium-swallow studies are not recommended because of the risk of aspiration and the presence of contrast that may potentially obscure visualization during any subsequent endoscopic examination.[112] Management in the setting of an asymptomatic patient usually consists of simple observation. Others have advocated for the use of glucagon and other effervescent agents as adjuncts to nonoperative treatment. Glucagon is known to decrease lower esophageal sphincter tone by causing smooth muscle relaxation, thus making it one of the most widely accepted agents for esophageal foreign-body impaction. This is despite the fact that the literature supporting its use is controversial and of poor quality.[113]

Following observation, endoscopy is the gold standard first-line treatment and is much more likely to lead to resolution of symptoms than medical therapy alone (98% vs. 28%).[114] Timing of endoscopy is indicated by the risk of esophageal wall damage or aspiration, as well as the clinical status of the patient. Urgent intervention using endoscopy may be required in patients with severe distress, unable to swallow their own secretions, or with foreign bodies that are batteries or have sharp edges. Patients who do not fit these criteria and have no evidence of severe obstruction can be handled less urgently. Retrieval is the goal when dealing with foreign bodies that are not subject to spontaneous passing. General anesthesia is recommended during the entirety of this procedure. Flexible endoscopy is the preferred method for most foreign bodies. A rigid endoscope is useful in the retrieval of foreign bodies lodged in the proximal esophagus at the level of the cricopharyngeus muscle. Rigid esophagoscopy is a rarer procedure and one should be familiar with the technique. The object should be reoriented with a grasper and removed safely. When using the flexible esophagoscope, we have found the overtube to be a very useful tool for removal of foreign bodies such that the esophagus is not injured proximally upon extrication of the object. Esophagotomy may be required when the lodged foreign bodies are large, have sharp edges, are embedded in the mucosa, or exceed the diameter of the rigid endoscope in all orientations. Following removal of the foreign body, completion esophagoscopy and contrast esophagoscopy should be performed to rule out injury. If there is a perforation, it should be managed according to the algorithm in **Algorithm 42.2**.

Perforation from esophageal foreign body is also rare, with an estimated incidence of 4%.[115] In an analysis of over 1,200 patients presenting with foreign-body impaction, independent risk factors for complications were age ≥60, duration of impaction longer than 1 day, impaction in the esophagus, and sharp foreign body (eg, chicken or fish bones). Duration of impaction longer than 1 day was associated with 2.5-fold increase in the risk of complications and increased risk of failure of endoscopic retrieval.[116] Sharp foreign-body ingestion is associated with worse outcomes than other object types; however, some have advocated for conservative management with good results.

Finally, the prevalence of concomitant motility disorders among patients presenting with esophageal foreign-body impaction cannot be overlooked. Its incidence is estimated at 10%,[115] thus, follow-up for these patients should include additional studies to examine for any underlying esophageal pathology, including motility testing.

ACKNOWLEDGMENT

We gratefully acknowledge the contributions of previous edition author, Yulia Zak, as portions of those chapters have been retained in this revision.

References

1. Siegel RL, Kratzer TB, Msph ANG, Sung H, Dvm AJ. Cancer statistics, 2025. 2025.
2. SEER Explorer: An interactive website for SEER cancer statistics [Internet]. Surveillance Research Program, National Cancer Institute; 2025. [cited 2025 Jul 16]. Available from: https://seer.cancer.gov/statistics-network/explorer/
3. Berry MF. Esophageal cancer: staging system and guidelines for staging and treatment. *J Thorac Dis*. 2014;6 Suppl 3(Suppl 3): S289–S297.
4. Varghese TK, Hofstetter WL, Rizk NP, et al. The society of thoracic surgeons guidelines on the diagnosis and staging of patients with esophageal cancer. *Ann Thorac Surg*. 2013;96(1): 346–356.
5. Rüdiger Siewert J, Feith M, Werner M, Stein HJ. Adenocarcinoma of the esophagogastric junction: results of surgical therapy based on anatomical/topographic classification in 1,002 consecutive patients. *Ann Surg*. 2000;232(3):353–361.
6. Luketich JD, Schauer PR, Meltzer CC, et al. Role of positron emission tomography in staging esophageal cancer. *Ann Thorac Surg*. 1997;64(3):765–769.
7. Rice TW, Mason DP, Murthy SC, et al. T2N0M0 esophageal cancer. *J Thorac Cardiovasc Surg*. 2007;133(2):317–324.
8. Vazquez-Sequeiros E, Wiersema MJ, Clain JE, et al. Impact of lymph node staging on therapy of esophageal carcinoma. *Gastroenterology*. 2003;125(6):1626–1635.
9. Krasna MJ, Reed CE, Nedzwiecki D, et al. CALGB 9380: a prospective trial of the feasibility of thoracoscopy/laparoscopy in staging esophageal cancer. *Ann Thorac Surg*. 2001;71(4):1073–1079.
10. de Graaf GW, Ayantunde AA, Parsons SL, Duffy JP, Welch NT. The role of staging laparoscopy in oesophagogastric cancers. *Eur J Surg Oncol*. 2007;33(8):988–992.
11. Rice TW, Ishwaran H, Ferguson MK, Blackstone EH, Goldstraw P. Cancer of the esophagus and esophagogastric junction: an eighth edition staging primer. *J Thorac Oncol*. 2017;12(1): 36–42.
12. Rice TW, Rusch VW, Ishwaran H, Blackstone EH; Worldwide Esophageal Cancer Collaboration. Cancer of the esophagus and esophagogastric junction: data-driven staging for the seventh edition of the American Joint Committee on Cancer/International Union Against Cancer Staging Manuals. *Cancer*. 2010;116(16): 3763–3773.
13. Dimick JB, Wainess RM, Upchurch GR, Iannettoni MD, Orringer MB. National trends in outcomes for esophageal resection. *Ann Thorac Surg*. 2005;79(1):212–216; discussion 217–218.
14. Ra J, Paulson EC, Kucharczuk J, et al. Postoperative mortality after esophagectomy for cancer: development of a preoperative risk prediction model. *Ann Surg Oncol*. 2008;15(6):1577–1584.
15. Orringer MB, Marshall B, Chang AC, Lee J, Pickens A, Lau CL. Two thousand transhiatal esophagectomies: changing trends, lessons learned. *Ann Surg*. 2007;246(3):363–372; discussion 372–374.
16. Worrell S, DeMeester SR. Endoscopic resection and ablation for early-stage esophageal cancer. *Thorac Surg Clin*. 2016;26(2): 173–176.
17. Sibille A, Lambert R, Souquet JC, Sabben G, Descos F. Long-term survival after photodynamic therapy for esophageal cancer. *Gastroenterology*. 1995;108(2):337–344.
18. Berry MF, Zeyer-Brunner J, Castleberry AW, et al. Treatment modalities for T1N0 esophageal cancers: a comparative analysis of local therapy versus surgical resection. *J Thorac Oncol*. 2013; 8(6):796–802.

19. Rice TW, Zuccaro G, Adelstein DJ, Rybicki LA, Blackstone EH, Goldblum JR. Esophageal carcinoma: depth of tumor invasion is predictive of regional lymph node status. *Ann Thorac Surg.* 1998;65(3):787–792.
20. Rizk NP, Ishwaran H, Rice TW, et al. Optimum lymphadenectomy for esophageal cancer. *Ann Surg.* 2010;251(1):46–50.
21. Fan X, Wang J, Xia L, et al. Efficacy of endoscopic therapy for T1b esophageal cancer and construction of prognosis prediction model: a retrospective cohort study. *Int J Surg Lond Engl.* 2023;109(6):1708–1719.
22. Crabtree TD, Kosinski AS, Puri V, et al. Evaluation of the reliability of clinical staging of T2 N0 esophageal cancer: a review of the Society of Thoracic Surgeons database. *Ann Thorac Surg.* 2013;96(2):382–390.
23. Speicher PJ, Ganapathi AM, Englum BR, et al. Induction therapy does not improve survival for clinical stage T2N0 esophageal cancer. *J Thorac Oncol.* 2014;9(8):1195–1201.
24. Paulson EC, Ra J, Armstrong K, Wirtalla C, Spitz F, Kelz RR. Underuse of esophagectomy as treatment for resectable esophageal cancer. *Arch Surg.* 2008;143(12):1198–1203; discussion 1203.
25. Uno T, Isobe K, Kawakami H, et al. Concurrent chemoradiation for patients with squamous cell carcinoma of the cervical esophagus. *Dis Esophagus.* 2007;20(1):12–18.
26. Swisher SG, Moughan J, Komaki RU, et al. Final results of NRG Oncology RTOG 0246: an organ-preserving selective resection strategy in esophageal cancer patients treated with definitive chemoradiation. *J Thorac Oncol.* 2017;12(2):368–374.
27. Van Der Wilk BJ, Eyck BM, Wijnhoven BPL, et al. LBA75 Neoadjuvant chemoradiotherapy followed by surgery versus active surveillance for oesophageal cancer (SANO-trial): a phase-III stepped-wedge cluster randomised trial. *Ann Oncol.* 2023;34:S1317.
28. Smith GL, Smith BD, Buchholz TA, et al. Patterns of care and locoregional treatment outcomes in older esophageal cancer patients: the SEER-Medicare Cohort. *Int J Radiat Oncol Biol Phys.* 2009;74(2):482–489.
29. Sjoquist KM, Burmeister BH, Smithers BM, et al. Survival after neoadjuvant chemotherapy or chemoradiotherapy for resectable oesophageal carcinoma: an updated meta-analysis. *Lancet Oncol.* 2011;12(7):681–692.
30. van Hagen P, Hulshof MCCM, van Lanschot JJB, et al. Preoperative chemoradiotherapy for esophageal or junctional cancer. *N Engl J Med.* 2012;366(22):2074–2084.
31. Shapiro J, van Lanschot JJB, Hulshof MCCM, et al. Neoadjuvant chemoradiotherapy plus surgery versus surgery alone for oesophageal or junctional cancer (CROSS): long-term results of a randomised controlled trial. *Lancet Oncol.* 2015;16(9):1090–1098.
32. Kelly RJ, Ajani JA, Kuzdzal J, et al. Adjuvant nivolumab in resected esophageal or gastroesophageal junction cancer. *N Engl J Med.* 2021;384(13):1191–1203.
33. Speicher PJ, Wang X, Englum BR, et al. Induction chemoradiation therapy prior to esophagectomy is associated with superior long-term survival for esophageal cancer. *Dis Esophagus.* 2015;28(8):788–796.
34. Eyck BM, van Lanschot JJB, Hulshof MCCM, et al. Ten-year outcome of neoadjuvant chemoradiotherapy plus surgery for esophageal cancer: the randomized controlled CROSS trial. *J Clin Oncol.* 2021;39(18):1995–2004.
35. Cunningham D, Allum WH, Stenning SP, et al. Perioperative chemotherapy versus surgery alone for resectable gastroesophageal cancer. *N Engl J Med.* 2006;355(1):11–20.
36. Liou DZ, Backhus LM, Lui NS, Shrager JB, Berry MF. Induction therapy for locally advanced distal esophageal adenocarcinoma: is radiation always necessary? *J Thorac Cardiovasc Surg.* 2018;155(6):2697–2707.
37. Hoeppner J, Brunner T, Lordick F, et al. Prospective randomized multicenter phase III trial comparing perioperative chemotherapy (FLOT protocol) to neoadjuvant chemoradiation (CROSS protocol) in patients with adenocarcinoma of the esophagus (ESOPEC trial). *J Clin Oncol.* 2024;42(17_suppl):LBA1–LBA1.
38. Siegel RL, Miller KD, Jemal A. Cancer statistics, 2020. *CA Cancer J Clin.* 2020;70(1):7–30.
39. Dubecz A, Gall I, Solymosi N, et al. Temporal trends in long-term survival and cure rates in esophageal cancer: a SEER database analysis. *J Thorac Oncol.* 2012;7(2):443–447.
40. Rice TW, Gress DM, Patil DT, Hofstetter WL, Kelsen DP, Blackstone EH. Cancer of the esophagus and esophagogastric junction-Major changes in the American Joint Committee on Cancer eighth edition cancer staging manual. *CA Cancer J Clin.* 2017;67(4):304–317.
41. Barbour AP, Rizk NP, Gonen M, et al. Adenocarcinoma of the gastroesophageal junction: influence of esophageal resection margin and operative approach on outcome. *Ann Surg.* 2007;246(1):1–8.
42. Peyre CG, Hagen JA, DeMeester SR, et al. The number of lymph nodes removed predicts survival in esophageal cancer: an international study on the impact of extent of surgical resection. *Ann Surg.* 2008;248(4):549–556.
43. Wolff CS, Castillo SF, Larson DR, et al. Ivor Lewis approach is superior to transhiatal approach in retrieval of lymph nodes at esophagectomy. *Dis Esophagus.* 2008;21(4):328–333.
44. Markar SR, Lagergren J. Surgical and surgeon-related factors related to long-term survival in esophageal cancer: a review. *Ann Surg Oncol.* 2020;27(3):718–723.
45. Kidane B, Kaaki S, Hirpara DH, et al. Emergency department use is high after esophagectomy and feeding tube problems are the biggest culprit. *J Thorac Cardiovasc Surg.* 2018;156(6):2340–2348.
46. Enestvedt CK, Perry KA, Kim C, et al. Trends in the management of esophageal carcinoma based on provider volume: treatment practices of 618 esophageal surgeons. *Dis Esophagus.* 2010;23(2):136–144.
47. Akkerman RDL, Haverkamp L, van Rossum PSN, van Hillegersberg R, Ruurda JP. Long-term quality of life after oesophagectomy with gastric conduit interposition for cancer. *Eur J Cancer.* 2015;51(12):1538–1545.
48. Luan A, Hunter CL, Crowe CS, Lee GK. Comparison of outcomes of total esophageal reconstruction with supercharged jejunal flap, colonic interposition, and gastric pull-up. *Ann Plast Surg.* 2018;80(5S Suppl 5):S274–S278.
49. Atkins BZ, Shah AS, Hutcheson KA, et al. Reducing hospital morbidity and mortality following esophagectomy. *Ann Thorac Surg.* 2004;78(4):1170–1176; discussion 1170–1176.
50. Papenfuss WA, Kukar M, Attwood K, et al. Transhiatal versus transthoracic esophagectomy for esophageal cancer: a 2005–2011 NSQIP comparison of modern multicenter results. *J Surg Oncol.* 2014;110(3):298–301.
51. Schlottmann F, Strassle PD, Patti MG. Transhiatal vs. Transthoracic esophagectomy: a NSQIP analysis of postoperative outcomes and risk factors for morbidity. *J Gastrointest Surg.* 2017;21(11):1757–1763.
52. Luketich JD, Pennathur A, Awais O, et al. Outcomes after minimally invasive esophagectomy: review of over 1000 patients. *Ann Surg.* 2012;256(1):95–103.
53. Forshaw MJ, Gossage JA, Ockrim J, Atkinson SW, Mason RC. Left thoracoabdominal esophagogastrectomy: still a valid operation for carcinoma of the distal esophagus and esophagogastric junction. *Dis Esophagus.* 2006;19(5):340–345.
54. Cerfolio RJ, Laliberte AS, Blackmon S, et al. Minimally invasive esophagectomy: a consensus statement. *Ann Thorac Surg.* 2020;110(4):1417–1426.
55. Sihag S, Kosinski AS, Gaissert HA, Wright CD, Schipper PH. Minimally invasive versus open esophagectomy for esophageal cancer: a comparison of early surgical outcomes from The Society of Thoracic Surgeons National Database. *Ann Thorac Surg.* 2016;101(4):1281–1288; discussion 1288–1289.
56. Straatman J, van der Wielen N, Cuesta MA, et al. Minimally invasive versus open esophageal resection: three-year follow-up of the previously reported randomized controlled trial: the TIME trial. *Ann Surg.* 2017;266(2):232–236.
57. Luketich JD, Pennathur A, Franchetti Y, et al. Minimally invasive esophagectomy: results of a prospective phase II multicenter

trial-the eastern cooperative oncology group (E2202) study. *Ann Surg*. 2015;261(4):702–707.

58. Harbison GJ, Vossler JD, Yim NH, Murayama KM. Outcomes of robotic versus non-robotic minimally-invasive esophagectomy for esophageal cancer: an American College of Surgeons NSQIP database analysis. *Am J Surg*. 2019;218(6):1223–1228.
59. Malhotra SK, Kaur RP, Gupta NM, Grover A, Ramprabu K, Nakra D. Incidence and types of arrhythmias after mediastinal manipulation during transhiatal esophagectomy. *Ann Thorac Surg*. 2006;82(1):298–302.
60. Parekh K, Iannettoni MD. Complications of esophageal resection and reconstruction. *Semin Thorac Cardiovasc Surg*. 2007;19(1): 79–88.
61. Raymond DP, Seder CW, Wright CD, et al. Predictors of major morbidity or mortality after resection for esophageal cancer: a Society of Thoracic Surgeons General Thoracic Surgery Database Risk Adjustment Model. *Ann Thorac Surg*. 2016;102(1):207–214.
62. de Boer AGEM, van Lanschot JJB, van Sandick JW, et al. Quality of life after transhiatal compared with extended transthoracic resection for adenocarcinoma of the esophagus. *J Clin Oncol*. 2004;22(20):4202–4208.
63. Berry MF, Atkins BZ, Tong BC, Harpole DH, D'Amico TA, Onaitis MW. A comprehensive evaluation for aspiration after esophagectomy reduces the incidence of postoperative pneumonia. *J Thorac Cardiovasc Surg*. 2010;140(6):1266–1271.
64. Griffin SM, Shaw IH, Dresner SM. Early complications after Ivor Lewis subtotal esophagectomy with two-field lymphadenectomy: risk factors and management. *J Am Coll Surg*. 2002;194(3):285–297.
65. Dimick JB, Goodney PP, Orringer MB, Birkmeyer JD. Specialty training and mortality after esophageal cancer resection. *Ann Thorac Surg*. 2005;80(1):282–286.
66. Birkmeyer JD, Siewers AE, Finlayson EVA, et al. Hospital volume and surgical mortality in the United States. *N Engl J Med*. 2002;346(15):1128–1137.
67. Birkmeyer JD, Stukel TA, Siewers AE, Goodney PP, Wennberg DE, Lucas FL. Surgeon volume and operative mortality in the United States. *N Engl J Med*. 2003;349(22):2117–2127.
68. Liu JF, Wang QZ, Ping YM, Zhang YD. Complications after esophagectomy for cancer: 53-year experience with 20,796 patients. *World J Surg*. 2008;32(3):395–400.
69. Bailey SH, Bull DA, Harpole DH, et al. Outcomes after esophagectomy: a ten-year prospective cohort. *Ann Thorac Surg*. 2003;75(1):217–222; discussion 222.
70. Ando N, Ozawa S, Kitagawa Y, Shinozawa Y, Kitajima M. Improvement in the results of surgical treatment of advanced squamous esophageal carcinoma during 15 consecutive years. *Ann Surg*. 2000;232(2):225–232.
71. Crestanello JA, Deschamps C, Cassivi SD, et al. Selective management of intrathoracic anastomotic leak after esophagectomy. *J Thorac Cardiovasc Surg*. 2005;129(2):254–260.
72. Athanasiou A, Hennessy M, Spartalis E, Tan BHL, Griffiths EA. Conduit necrosis following esophagectomy: an up-to-date literature review. *World J Gastrointest Surg*. 2019;11(3): 155–168.
73. Helminen O, Kytö V, Kauppila JH, Gunn J, Lagergren J, Sihvo E. Population-based study of anastomotic stricture rates after minimally invasive and open oesophagectomy for cancer. *BJS Open*. 2019;3(5):634–640.
74. Gaur P, Swanson SJ. Gastric emptying procedure after esophagectomy. In: Ferguson MK, ed. *Difficult Decisions in Surgery: An Evidence-Based Approach*. Vol. 1. Springer London; 2014:365–375. http://link.springer.com/10.1007/978-1-4471-6404-3_29
75. Rindani R, Martin CJ, Cox MR. Transhiatal versus Ivor-Lewis oesophagectomy: is there a difference? *Aust N Z J Surg*. 1999;69(3): 187–194.
76. Bhattacharyya N, Batirel H, Swanson SJ. Improved outcomes with early vocal fold medialization for vocal fold paralysis after thoracic surgery. *Auris Nasus Larynx*. 2003;30(1):71–75.
77. Lee LS, Singhal S, Brinster CJ, et al. Current management of esophageal leiomyoma. *J Am Coll Surg*. 2004;198(1):136–146.
78. Graham RP, Yasir S, Fritchie KJ, Reid MD, Greipp PT, Folpe AL. Polypoid fibroadipose tumors of the esophagus: "giant fibrovascular polyp" or liposarcoma? A clinicopathological and molecular cytogenetic study of 13 cases. *Mod Pathol*. 2018;31(2):337–342.
79. Levine MS, Buck JL, Pantongrag-Brown L, Buetow PC, Hallman JR, Sobin LH. Fibrovascular polyps of the esophagus: clinical, radiographic, and pathologic findings in 16 patients. *AJR Am J Roentgenol*. 1996;166(4):781–787.
80. Morales-Maza J, Pastor-Sifuentes FU, Sánchez-Morales GE, et al. Clinical characteristics and surgical treatment of schwannomas of the esophagus and stomach: a case series and systematic review. *World J Gastrointest Oncol*. 2019;11(9):750–760.
81. Arashiro M, Satoh K, Osawa H, et al. Endoscopic submucosal dissection of esophageal lymphangioma: a case report with a review of the literature. *Clin J Gastroenterol*. 2010;3(3):140–143.
82. Brinster CJ, Singhal S, Lee L, Marshall MB, Kaiser LR, Kucharczuk JC. Evolving options in the management of esophageal perforation. *Ann Thorac Surg*. 2004;77(4):1475–1483.
83. Semenkovich TR, Hudson JL, Subramanian M, et al. Trends in treatment of T1N0 esophageal cancer. *Ann Surg*. 2019;270(3): 434–443.
84. Weiman DS, Walker WA, Brosnan KM, Pate JW, Fabian TC. Noniatrogenic esophageal trauma. *Ann Thorac Surg*. 1995;59(4): 845–859; discussion 849–850.
85. Crespin OM, Liu LWC, Parmar A, et al. Safety and efficacy of POEM for treatment of achalasia: a systematic review of the literature. *Surg Endosc*. 2017;31(5):2187–2201.
86. Foley MJ, Ghahremani GG, Rogers LF. Reappraisal of contrast media used to detect upper gastrointestinal perforations: comparison of ionic water-soluble media with barium sulfate. *Radiology*. 1982;144(2):231–237.
87. Gollub MJ, Bains MS. Barium sulfate: a new (old) contrast agent for diagnosis of postoperative esophageal leaks. *Radiology*. 1997;202(2):360–362.
88. Sdralis EIK, Petousis S, Rashid F, Lorenzi B, Charalabopoulos A. Epidemiology, diagnosis, and management of esophageal perforations: systematic review. *Dis Esophagus*. 2017;30(8):1–6.
89. Connelly CL, Lamb PJ, Paterson-Brown S. Outcomes following Boerhaave's syndrome. *Ann R Coll Surg Engl*. 2013;95(8): 557–560.
90. Ceppa DP, Rosati CM, Chabtini L, et al. Development of a multidisciplinary program to expedite care of esophageal emergencies. *Ann Thorac Surg*. 2017;104(3):1054–1061.
91. Schweigert M, Sousa HS, Solymosi N, et al. Spotlight on esophageal perforation: a multinational study using the Pittsburgh esophageal perforation severity scoring system. *J Thorac Cardiovasc Surg*. 2016;151(4):1002–1009.
92. Sudarshan M, Elharram M, Spicer J, Mulder D, Ferri LE. Management of esophageal perforation in the endoscopic era: is operative repair still relevant? *Surgery*. 2016;160(4):1104–1110.
93. Freeman RK, Van Woerkom JM, Ascioti AJ. Esophageal stent placement for the treatment of iatrogenic intrathoracic esophageal perforation. *Ann Thorac Surg*. 2007;83(6):2003–2007; discussion 2007–2008.
94. Still S, Mencio M, Ontiveros E, Burdick J, Leeds SG. Primary and rescue endoluminal vacuum therapy in the management of esophageal perforations and leaks. *Ann Thorac Cardiovasc Surg*. 2018;24(4):173–179.
95. Wright A, Chang A, Bedi AO, et al. Endoscopic suture fixation is associated with reduced migration of esophageal fully covered self-expandable metal stents (FCSEMS). *Surg Endosc*. 2017 Sep;31(9):3489–3494.
96. Ali JT, Rice RD, David EA, et al. Perforated esophageal intervention focus (PERF) study: a multi-center examination of contemporary treatment. *Dis Esophagus*. 2017;30(11):1–8.
97. Dasari BVM, Neely D, Kennedy A, et al. The role of esophageal stents in the management of esophageal anastomotic leaks and benign esophageal perforations. *Ann Surg*. 2014;259(5):852–860.
98. Lázár G, Paszt A, Mán E. Role of endoscopic clipping in the treatment of oesophageal perforations. *World J Gastrointest Endosc*. 2016;8(1):13–22.

99. Mencio MA, Ontiveros E, Burdick JS, Leeds SG. Use of a novel technique to manage gastrointestinal leaks with endoluminal negative pressure: a single institution experience. *Surg Endosc.* 2018;32(7):3349–3356.
100. Wong LY, Leipzig M, Liou DZ, et al. Surgical management of esophageal perforation: examining trends in a multi-institutional cohort. *J Gastrointest Surg.* 2023;27(9):1757–1765.
101. Afifi RO, Mushtaq HH, Sandhu HK, Khalil K, Safi HJ, Estrera AL. Successful multistaged surgical management of secondary aortoesophageal fistula with graft infection. *Ann Thorac Surg.* 2016;101(6):e203–e205.
102. Abu-Daff S, Shamji F, Ivanovic J, et al. Esophagectomy in esophageal perforations: an analysis. *Dis Esophagus.* 2016;29(1):34–40.
103. Abbas A, Brar TS, Zori A, Estores DS. Role of early endoscopic evaluation in decreasing morbidity, mortality, and cost after caustic ingestion: a retrospective nationwide database analysis. *Dis Esophagus.* 2017;30(6):1–11.
104. Kochhar R, Ashat M, Reddy YR, et al. Relook endoscopy predicts the development of esophageal and antropyloric stenosis better than immediate endoscopy in patients with caustic ingestion. *Endoscopy.* 2017;49(7):643–650.
105. Le Naoures P, Hamy A, Lerolle N, Métivier E, Lermite E, Venara A. Risk factors for symptomatic esophageal stricture after caustic ingestion-a retrospective cohort study. *Dis Esophagus.* 2017;30(6):1–6.
106. Tharavej C, Pungpapong SU, Chanswangphuvana P. Outcome of dilatation and predictors of failed dilatation in patients with acid-induced corrosive esophageal strictures. *Surg Endosc.* 2018;32(2):900–907.
107. D'Silva A, Wright M. Advances in imaging for atrial fibrillation ablation. *Radiol Res Pract.* 2011;2011:714864.
108. Farkas ZC, Pal S, Jolly GP, Lim MMD, Malik A, Malekan R. Esophagopericardial fistula and pneumopericardium from caustic ingestion and esophageal stent. *Ann Thorac Surg.* 2019;107(3):e207–e208.
109. Han HC, Ha FJ, Sanders P, et al. Atrioesophageal fistula: clinical presentation, procedural characteristics, diagnostic investigations, and treatment outcomes. *Circ Arrhythm Electrophysiol.* 2017;10(11):e005579.
110. Berdan EA, Sato TT. Pediatric airway and esophageal foreign bodies. *Surg Clin North Am.* 2017;97(1):85–91.
111. Eisen GM, Baron TH, Dominitz JA, et al. Guideline for the management of ingested foreign bodies. *Gastrointest Endosc.* 2002;55(7):802–806.
112. Birk M, Bauerfeind P, Deprez PH, et al. Removal of foreign bodies in the upper gastrointestinal tract in adults: European Society of Gastrointestinal Endoscopy (ESGE) Clinical Guideline. *Endoscopy.* 2016;48(5):489–496.
113. Bodkin RP, Weant KA, Baker Justice S, Spencer MT, Acquisto NM. Effectiveness of glucagon in relieving esophageal foreign body impaction: a multicenter study. *Am J Emerg Med.* 2016;34(6):1049–1052.
114. Lin AY, Tillman BN, Thatcher AL, Graves CR, Prince ME. Comparison of outcomes in medical therapy vs surgical intervention of esophageal foreign bodies. *Otolaryngol–Head Neck Surg.* 2018;159(4):656–661.
115. Zamary KR, Davis JW, Ament EE, Dirks RC, Garry JE. This too shall pass: a study of ingested sharp foreign bodies. *J Trauma Acute Care Surg.* 2017;82(1):150–155.
116. Geng C, Li X, Luo R, Cai L, Lei X, Wang C. Endoscopic management of foreign bodies in the upper gastrointestinal tract: a retrospective study of 1294 cases. *Scand J Gastroenterol.* 2017;52(11):1286–1291.

Gastric Anatomy and Physiology

Trevor D. Crafts and Michael B. Ujiki

Key Points

1 The stomach is an extremely well-vascularized organ, supplied by a number of major arteries and protected by a large number of extramural and intramural collaterals.

2 Oxyntic glands occupy the fundus and body of the stomach and contain the oxyntic or parietal cells, which are the sites of acid production. Oxyntic glands also contain chief cells, the site of gastric pepsinogen synthesis.

3 Ghrelin and gastrin production are localized to the body and antrum, respectively.

4 The most important stimulant of gastrin release is a meal. Postprandial luminal pH also strongly affects gastrin secretion.

5 The basolateral membrane of the parietal cell contains specific receptors for histamine, gastrin, and acetylcholine, the three major stimulants of acid production.

6 Pepsins are a heterogeneous group of proteolytic enzymes that are secreted by the gastric chief cells.

7 The gastric mucosa is the site of production of intrinsic factor, which is necessary for the absorption of cobalamin from the ileal mucosa. Total gastrectomy is regularly followed by cobalamin malabsorption, as is resection of the proximal stomach or atrophic gastritis that involves the oxyntic mucosa.

8 Gastric motility is stimulated by slow wave myoelectric activity of the smooth muscle. There is differential emptying of liquids and solids from the stomach.

GROSS ANATOMY

Embryonic Development

The stomach and duodenum are derived from the embryonic foregut. During the fifth week of gestation, the future stomach is marked as a dilation in the caudal portion of the foregut. At this time, the primitive stomach is invested with both ventral and dorsal mesenteries. The embryonic ventral mesentery is represented in postnatal life by the falciform ligament and by the gastrohepatic and hepatoduodenal mesenteries that form the lesser omentum. The primitive dorsal mesentery ultimately forms three structures: the gastrocolic ligament, the gastrosplenic ligament, and the gastrophrenic ligament. It also contains the celiac artery, the major blood supply to the foregut structures.

Morphogenesis and gastric specification are driven by signaling pathways that include WNT, bone morphogenic protein (BMP), fibroblast growth factor (FGF), and retinoic acid.[1] During the sixth and seventh weeks of gestation, the typical morphology of the stomach is established. Accelerated growth of the left gastric wall, relative to the right, establishes the greater and lesser curvatures. This unequal growth also rotates the stomach and causes the left vagal nerve trunk to assume its anterior position, whereas the right vagal trunk is located posteriorly. The growth of structures cephalad to the stomach causes the organ to descend. During the sixth week, the primitive stomach lies between the T10 and T12 vertebral segments. In adult life, the stomach is most commonly located between the T10 and the L3 vertebral segments.

Structural Anatomy

The stomach can be divided into anatomic regions based on external landmarks (**Fig. 43.1**). Although these divisions are commonly referred to in surgical texts and are useful in discussing gastric resections, they do not necessarily reflect physiologic functionality. The gastric cardia is the region of the stomach just distal to the gastroesophageal junction. The acute angle formed by the esophagus and the cardia is termed the "angle of His."[2] The fundus is the portion of the stomach above and to the left of the gastroesophageal junction. The corpus constitutes the region between the fundus and the antrum. The acute angle between the lesser curve and antrum is the "incisura angularis." The margin between the corpus and antrum is not distinct externally but can be defined arbitrarily by a line from the incisura on the lesser curvature to a point one-fourth the distance from the pylorus to the esophagus along the greater curvature. The gastric antrum is bounded distally by the pylorus, which can be appreciated by palpation as a thickened ring of smooth muscle.

The stomach is mobile and is fixed at only two points, proximally by the gastroesophageal junction and distally by the retroperitoneal duodenum. Anteriorly, the stomach is in contact with the left hemidiaphragm, the left lobe and the anterior segment of the right lobe of the liver, and the anterior parietal surface of the abdominal wall. The posterior surface of the stomach is related to the left diaphragm; the left kidney and left adrenal gland; the neck, tail, and body of the pancreas; the aorta and celiac trunk; and the periaortic nerve plexuses. The greater curvature of the stomach is near the transverse colon and the transverse colonic mesentery. The concavity of the spleen contacts the left lateral portion of the stomach.

Arteriovenous Anatomy

1 The stomach is an extremely well-vascularized organ, supplied by a number of major arteries and protected by a large number of extramural and intramural collaterals.[3] Gastric viability can be preserved after ligation of all but one primary artery, an advantage that can be exploited during gastric reconstructive procedures. Also, the rich network of anastomosing vessels means that gastric hemorrhage cannot be controlled by the extramural ligation of gastric arteries. Most gastric blood flow is ordinarily derived from the celiac trunk (**Fig. 43.2**). The

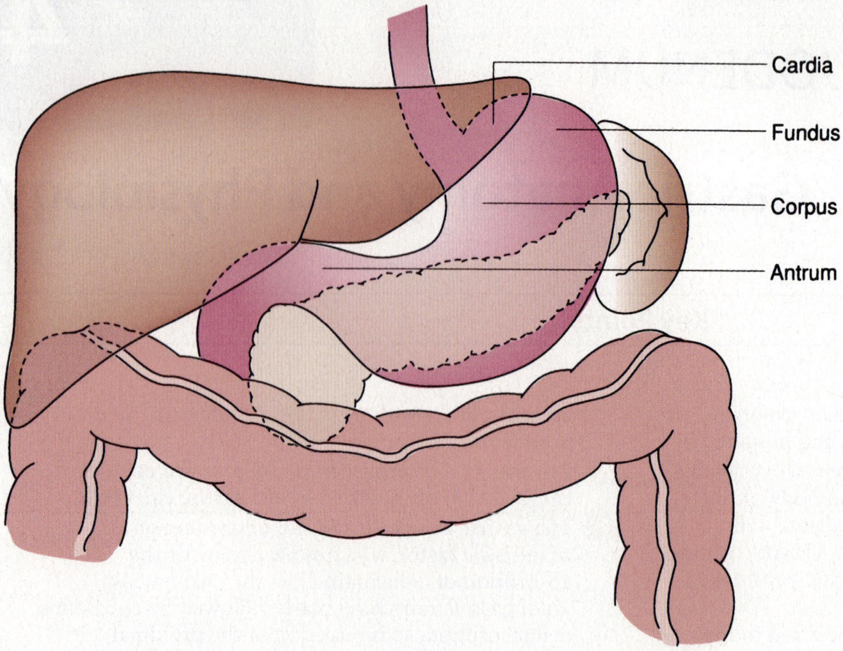

Figure 43.1. Topographic relations of the stomach.

lesser curvature is supplied by the left gastric artery, which is the first major branch of the celiac trunk, and by the right gastric artery, which is derived from the hepatic artery. Branches of the left gastric artery also supply the lowermost portion of the esophagus. The greater curvature is supplied by the short gastric and left gastroepiploic arteries, which are branches of the splenic artery, and by the right gastroepiploic artery, a branch of the gastroduodenal artery. In instances of celiac trunk occlusion, gastric blood flow is usually maintained from the superior mesenteric artery collaterally by way of the pancreaticoduodenal arcade. In general, venous effluent from the stomach parallels the arterial supply, noting that drainage is into the portal system. The venous equivalent of the left gastric artery is the coronary vein. At the distal border of the pylorus, the characteristic prepyloric veins course along the anterior and posterior surfaces (anterior termed the "vein of Mayo") before draining into the right gastric vein.[2]

Lymphatic Drainage

As a first approximation, the lymphatic drainage of the stomach parallels gastric arterial supply (**Fig. 43.3**). Lymph from the proximal portion of the stomach along the lesser curvature first drains into superior gastric lymph nodes surrounding the left gastric artery. The distal portion of the lesser curvature drains through suprapyloric nodes. The proximal portion of the greater curvature is supplied by lymphatic vessels that traverse pancreaticosplenic nodes, whereas the antral portion of the greater curvature drains into the subpyloric and omental nodal groups. Secondary drainage from each of these systems eventually traverses nodes at the base of the celiac axis. These

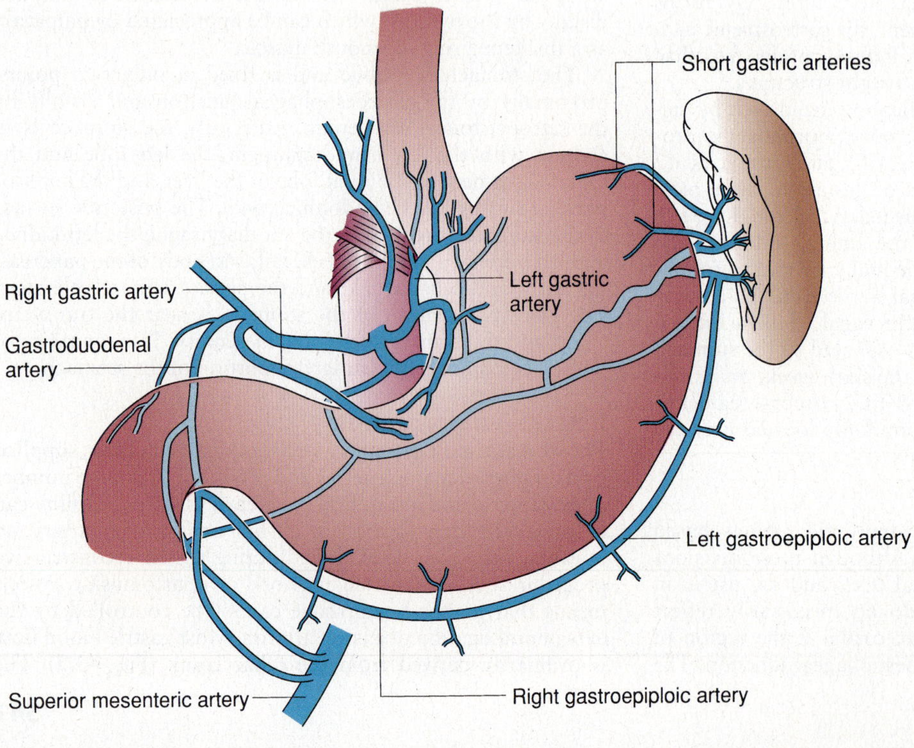

Figure 43.2. Arterial blood supply of the stomach.

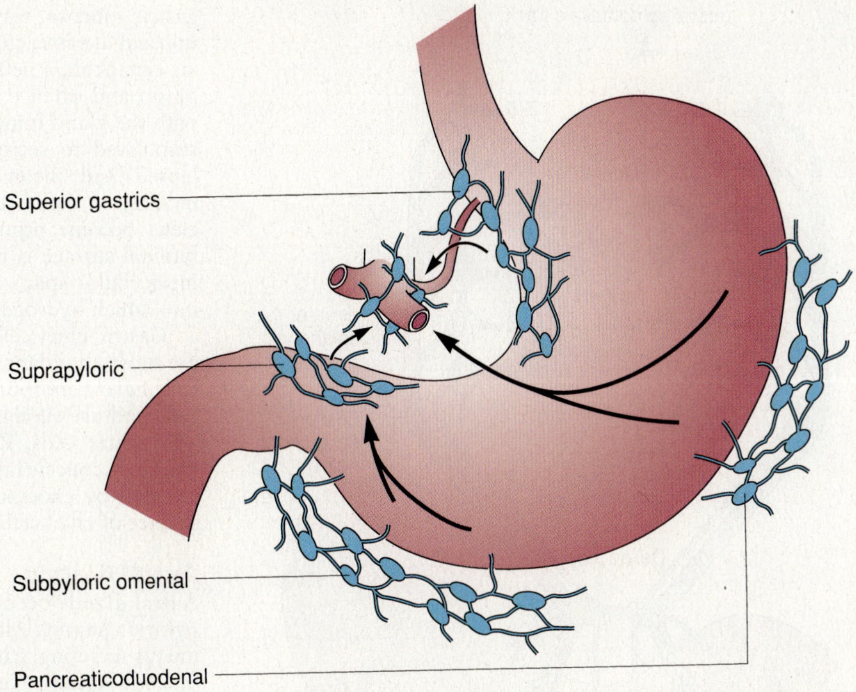

Figure 43.3. Lymphatic drainage of the stomach.

discrete anatomic groupings are misleading. The lymphatic drainage of the human stomach, like its blood supply, exhibits extensive intramural ramifications and a number of extramural communications. As a consequence, disease processes that involve the gastric lymphatics often spread intramurally beyond the region of origin and to nodal groups at a distance from the primary lymphatic zone.

Innervation

The left and right vagal nerves descend parallel to the esophagus within the thorax before forming a periesophageal plexus between the tracheal bifurcation and the diaphragm. From this plexus, two vagal trunks coalesce before passing through the esophageal hiatus of the diaphragm (**Fig. 43.4**). The left vagal trunk is usually closely applied to the anterior surface of the esophagus, whereas the posterior vagal trunk is often midway between the esophagus and the aorta. The anterior vagus supplies a hepatic division, which passes to the right in the lesser omentum before innervating the liver and biliary tract. The remainder of the anterior vagal fibers parallels the lesser curvature of the stomach, branching to the anterior gastric wall. The posterior vagus nerve branches into the celiac division, which passes to the celiac plexus, and a posterior gastric division, which innervates the posterior gastric wall.

Approximately 90% of the fibers in the vagal trunks are afferent, transmitting information from the gastrointestinal tract to the central nervous system (CNS). Parasympathetic afferent fibers are not responsible for the sensation of gastric pain. Only 10% of vagal nerve fibers are motor or secretory efferents. Parasympathetic efferent fibers travel from the dorsal nucleus of the medulla without synapse to contact postsynaptic neurons in the gastric wall in the myenteric and submucous plexuses. Secondary neurons directly innervate gastric smooth muscle or epithelial cells.

Gastric sympathetic innervation is derived from spinal segments T5 through T10. Sympathetic fibers leave the

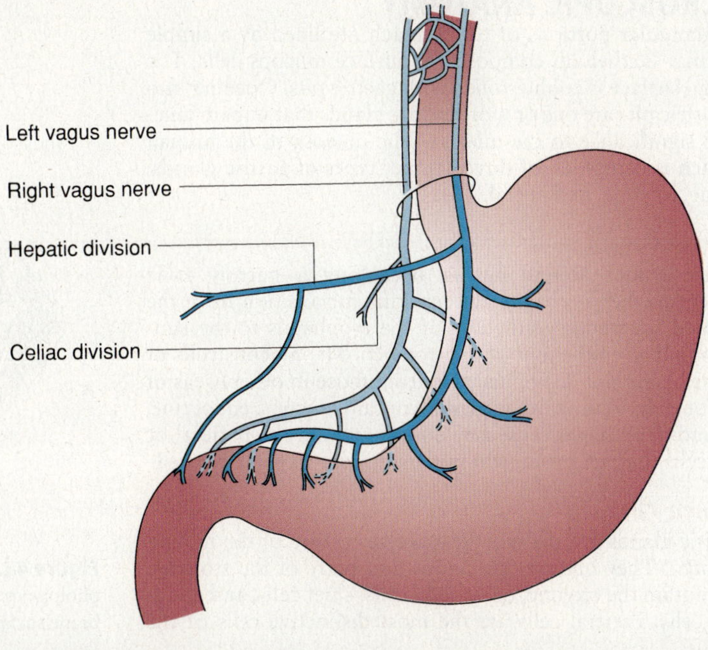

Figure 43.4. Vagal innervation of the stomach.

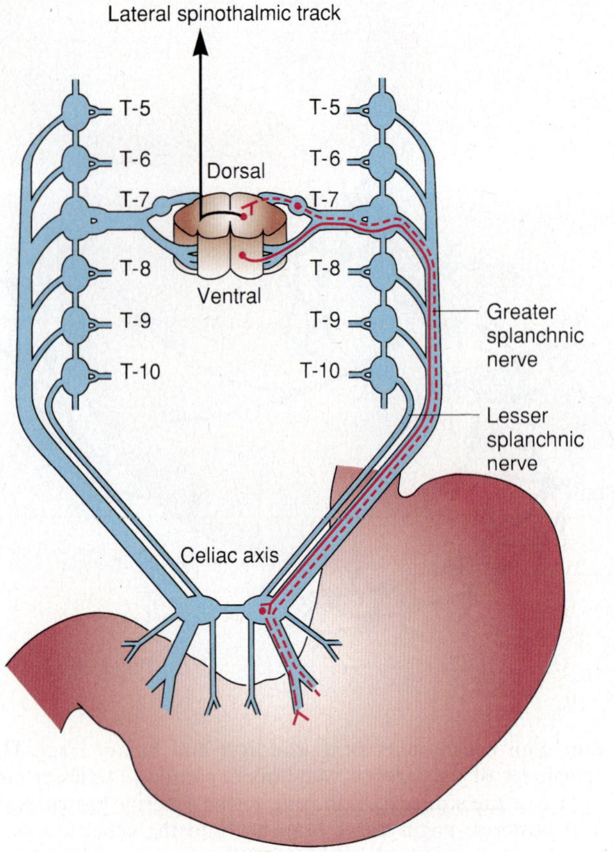

Figure 43.5. Derivation of gastric sympathetic innervation.

corresponding spinal nerve roots by way of gray rami communicantes and enter a series of bilateral prevertebral ganglia (**Fig. 43.5**). From these ganglia, presynaptic fibers pass through the greater splanchnic nerves to the celiac plexus, where they synapse with secondary sympathetic neurons. Postsynaptic sympathetic nerve fibers enter the stomach in association with blood vessels. Afferent sympathetic fibers pass without synapse from the stomach to dorsal spinal roots. Pain of gastroduodenal origin is sensed through afferent fibers of sympathetic origin.

MICROSCOPIC ANATOMY

The glandular portions of the stomach are lined by a simple columnar epithelium composed of surface mucous cells. The luminal surface is cobblestoned with gastric pits. Opening into the gastric pits are one or more gastric glands that impart functional significance to the mucosa. The mucosa of the human stomach is composed of three distinct types of gastric glands: cardiac, oxyntic, and antral.

Cardiac Glands

Cardiac glands secrete mucus, occupying a narrow zone adjacent to the esophagus and marking a transition from the stratified squamous epithelium of the esophagus to the simple columnar epithelium of the stomach. The mucous cells of the cardia are not distinguishable from those in other areas of the stomach. While cardiac glands contain mucous, endocrine, and undifferentiated cells, they do not contain the parietal or chief cells that are prominent in the adjacent oxyntic mucosa.

Oxyntic Glands

2 Oxyntic glands are the most distinctive feature of the human stomach.[4] They occupy the fundus and body of the stomach and contain the oxyntic, or *parietal* cells, chief cells, and endocrine cells. Parietal cells are the most distinctive cells of the gastric mucosa, responsible for acid secretion. They have an unusual ultrastructural specialization in the form of intracellular canaliculi, a network of clefts extending to the basal cytoplasm and often encircling the nucleus, which is continuous with the gland lumen (**Fig. 43.6**). In parietal cells that are not stimulated to secrete acid, the secretory canaliculi are collapsed and inconspicuous. On stimulation, a severalfold increase in canalicular surface area occurs, the intracellular clefts become prominent, and the communication with the luminal surface is readily identified. These changes create an intracellular space in communication with the gastric lumen into which hydrogen ions are secreted at high concentration.

Gastric chief cells synthesize and secrete pepsinogen. They are most abundant in the basal region of oxyntic glands. The cells have a morphology typical of protein-secreting exocrine cells and are similar in ultrastructural appearance to pancreatic acinar cells. Zymogen granules containing pepsinogen are most concentrated in the apical cytoplasm. Pepsinogen is released by exocytosis from secretory granules at the apical surface of chief cells.

Antral Glands

Antral glands occupy the mucosa of the distal stomach and pyloric channel. Although most cells in the antral glands are mucus secreting, gastrin cells are the distinctive feature of this mucosa. Gastrin cells (G-cells) are pyramid shaped, with a narrow area of luminal contact apically and a broad surface

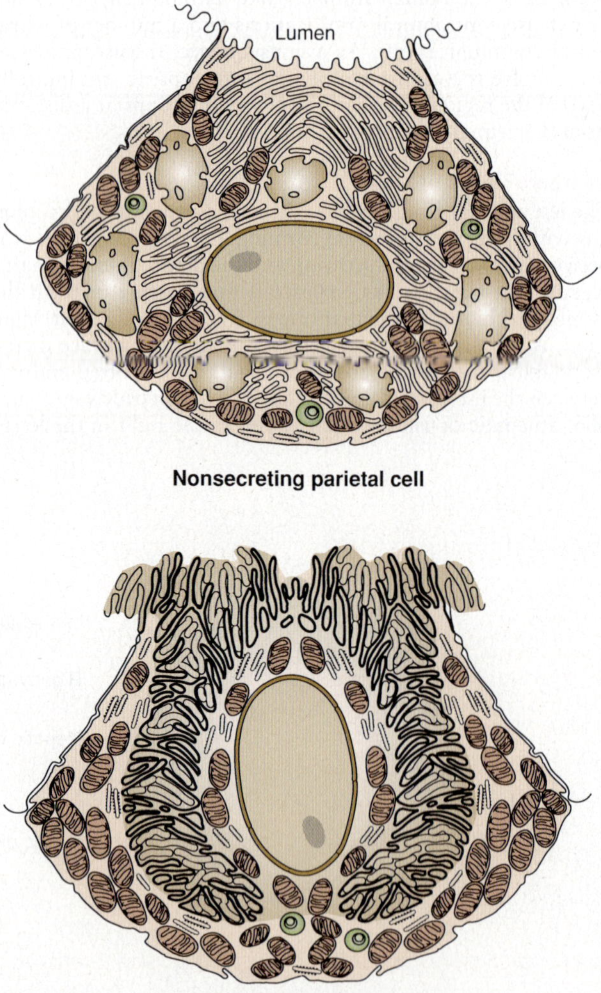

Figure 43.6. Resting and stimulated parietal cell, emphasizing morphologic transformation with increase in secretory canalicular membrane surface area that occurs with acid secretion.

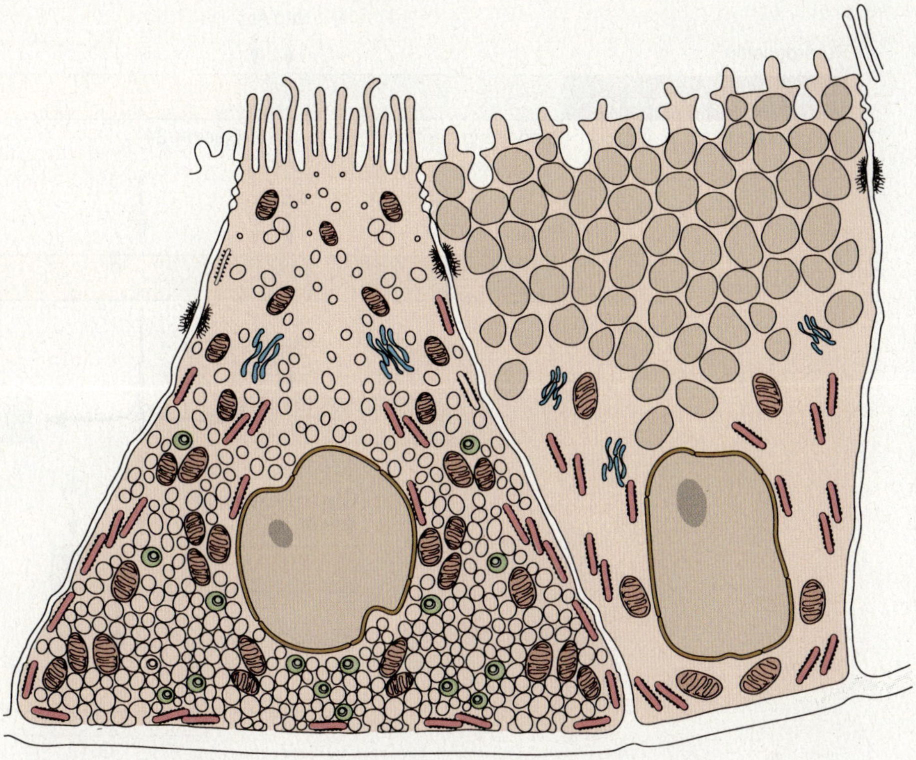

Figure 43.7. Contrasting morphology of antral gastrin cell (**left**) with basally oriented secretory granules, and gastric mucous cell (**right**) with apical mucous granules.

overlying the lamina propria basally (**Fig. 43.7**). Embryologic differentiation of gastrin cells is thought to be driven by transcription factors such as *Pdx1* and *Nkx6.3*.[5] Gastrin cells are identified immunocytochemically by the presence of the peptide. Gastrin is released by exocytotic fusion of the secretory granule with the plasma membrane. In contrast to luminal secretion from chief cells, emptying of gastrin-containing granules occurs at the basal membrane rather than at the apical region of the cell. Gastrin thus enters the circulation via submucosal capillaries in close apposition to the lamina propria.

GASTRIC PEPTIDES

The stomach contains a number of biologically active peptides in nerves and mucosal endocrine cells, including gastrin, somatostatin, ghrelin, gastrin-releasing peptide, vasoactive intestinal polypeptide (VIP), substance P, glucagon, calcitonin gene–related peptide, chromogranin A, and serotonin.

Gastrin

The synthesis, secretion, and action of gastrin have been extensively studied, and many aspects of the biology of gastrin appear to be shared by other gastrointestinal peptide hormones.[3] The human gastrin gene contains three exons, with the major
3 active product encoded by a single one of these. In adults, the gastrin gene is expressed primarily in mucosa cells of the gastric antrum, with lower levels of expression in the duodenum, pituitary, and testis.

The preprogastrin peptide contains the sequence of gastrin within its 101 amino acid sequence (**Fig. 43.8**). Preprogastrin consists of a signal peptide of 21 amino acids, an intervening peptide of 37 amino acids, the 34-residue region of the gastrin molecule, and a carboxyl-terminal extension of 9 amino acids. Gastrin is derived from its preprohormone by the sequential enzymatic cleavage of the signal peptide, the intervening peptide, and the carboxyl-terminal extension.

The signal peptide region of preprogastrin consists of a series of hydrophobic amino acids that direct the nascent peptide into the endoplasmic reticulum as it is translated from messenger RNA. In the rough endoplasmic reticulum, the signal peptide is removed. The remaining peptide is termed *progastrin*. Progastrin is further processed as it traverses the endoplasmic reticulum to mature secretory vesicles. There, it undergoes stepwise enzymatic cleavage, becoming glycine-extended gastrin, then gastrin 34 (G_{34}) after amidation of a carboxyl-terminal phenylalanine. Gastrin, like most gastrointestinal peptide hormones, requires terminal amidation for biologic activity. G_{34} is the predominate molecular form of gastrin in the duodenum. Gastrin 17 (G_{17}), the most abundant form of gastrin in the human antrum, is formed by further processing that removes the first 17 amino acids at the amino terminus of G_{34}.

4 The most important stimulant of gastrin release is a meal.[6] Small peptide fragments and amino acids that result from intragastric proteolysis are the most important food components that stimulate gastrin release, namely tryptophan and phenylalanine. Ingested fat and glucose do not cause gastrin release. Gastric distention by a meal activates cholinergic neurons and also stimulates gastrin release. As the meal empties and distention diminishes, VIP-containing neurons are activated, which stimulate somatostatin secretion and thus attenuate gastrin secretion.

Postprandial luminal pH also strongly affects gastrin secretion. Gastrin release is inhibited when acidification of an ingested meal causes the intraluminal pH to fall below 3.0. Conversely, maintaining intragastric pH above 3.0 potentiates gastrin secretion after ingestion of protein or amino acids.[4] Pernicious anemia and atrophic gastritis, which produce chronic achlorhydria, are associated with fasting hypergastrinemia and an exaggerated gastrin meal response. Release of mucosal somatostatin occurs with gastric acidification, and this peptide has been implicated in the inhibition of gastrin release that occurs when luminal pH falls.

The vagus nerve appears to both stimulate and inhibit gastrin release. In humans, vagally mediated stimulation of gastrin release can be demonstrated by sham feeding, insulin-induced hypoglycemia, and administration of the vagal stimulant γ-aminobutyric acid.[5] In contrast to these stimulatory vagal effects, hypergastrinemia, observed after vagotomy, suggests that inhibitory vagal effects on gastrin release may also exist.

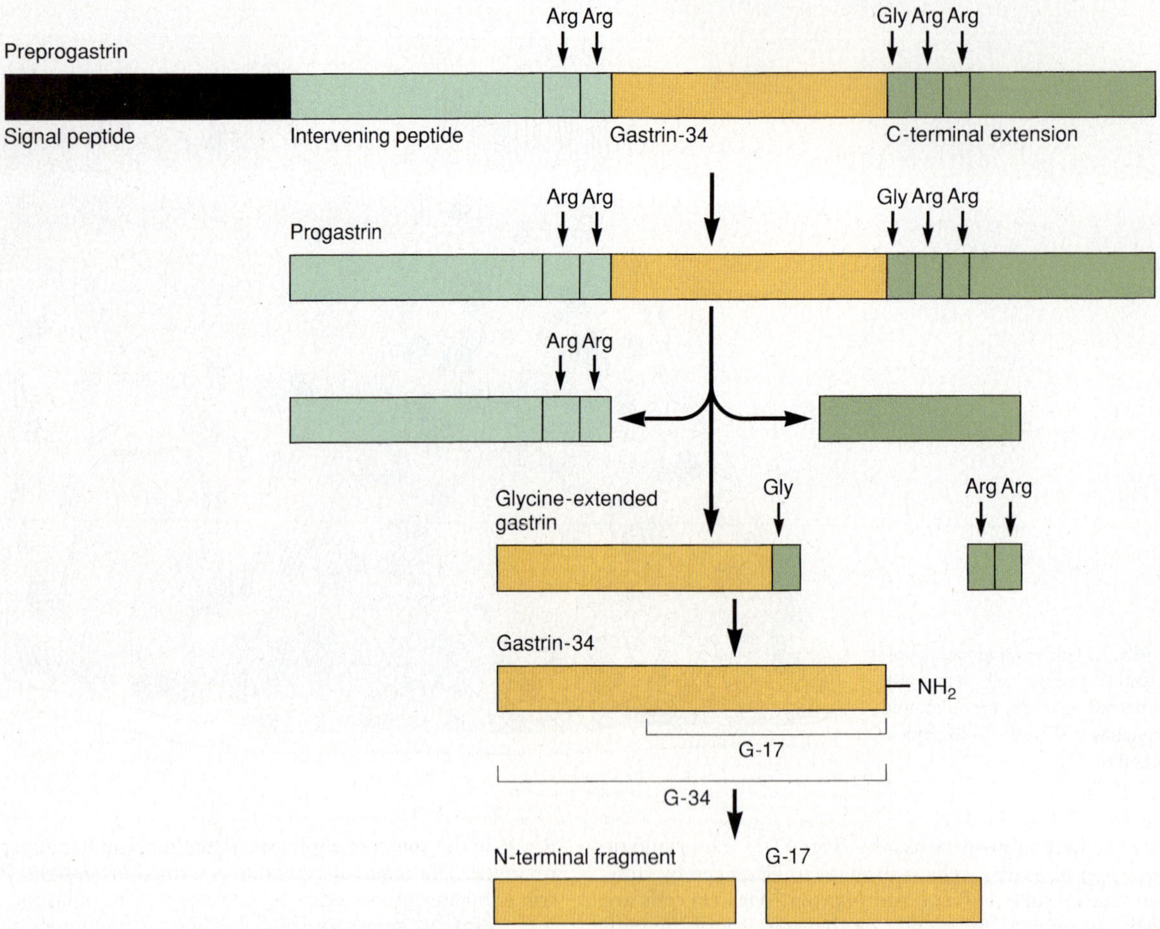

Figure 43.8. Sequential processing of preprogastrin molecule.

Cholinergic neurons stimulate gastrin secretion directly by actions on gastrin cells.

Chronic gastric infection with *Helicobacter pylori* causes increased acid secretion by altering gastrin release.[7,8] *H. pylori* has been observed to upregulate proinflammatory cytokines. Several inflammatory mediators have been demonstrated to stimulate gastrin release from isolated gastrin cells. The putative gastrin secretagogues include IL-1, IL-8, TNF-α, interferon-γ, and leukotrienes C4 and D4. The same factors that affect gastrin release also influence gastrin mRNA expression. Food ingestion increases gastrin mRNA abundance, whereas fasting and somatostatin decrease gastrin mRNA production. Chronic achlorhydria, as seen in pernicious anemia, increases gastrin mRNA production.

In addition to stimulating acid secretion from gastric parietal cells (detailed later in this chapter), gastrin has important physiologic actions in the control of gastrointestinal mucosal growth. The acid-secreting oxyntic mucosa is particularly sensitive to the trophic actions of gastrin, but the mucous membranes of the duodenum, colon, and pancreatic parenchyma are also affected. Stimulation of mucosal growth by gastrin is enhanced by the presence of solid food in the diet. Prolonged stimulation by high levels of gastrin, as seen in the Zollinger–Ellison syndrome, is associated with hypertrophy of the gastric mucosa. Smaller increases in circulating gastrin, such as those that follow vagotomy, do not cause mucosal hypertrophy.

Somatostatin

Somatostatin, like gastrin, is integral in gastric physiology. Somatostatin was first isolated from hypothalamic tissues and was named for its ability to inhibit the release of growth hormone. The peptide was subsequently localized in neurons in central and peripheral nervous systems, and in endocrine cells of the pancreas, stomach, and intestine. The wide tissue distribution of somatostatin suggested important regulatory functions, a concept validated by many investigations.[9] In the stomach, the highest concentration of somatostatin cells (D cells) is in the cardia and fundus.[10]

The human somatostatin gene is located on chromosome 3 and encodes for a precursor of 116 amino acids (**Fig. 43.9**). Gastric somatostatin release responds to luminal, hormonal, and neural signals. Luminal acidification is associated with increased somatostatin release, whereas somatostatin release decreases when luminal pH is increased. A number of peptides have been demonstrated experimentally to release somatostatin from the stomach, including gastrin, cholecystokinin (CCK), and secretin. β-Adrenergic agonists have also been shown to release somatostatin. In contrast, electrical stimulation of vagal nerves inhibits somatostatin release, as does the cholinergic agonist methacholine.

The most important gastric function of somatostatin is regulation of acid secretion and gastrin release. Circulating somatostatin appears to be important in modulating gastric acid secretion; locally released somatostatin functions to regulate gastrin release. In each instance, somatostatin serves an inhibitory function, decreasing acid secretion and diminishing the release of gastrin. Increases in circulating somatostatin are followed by decreased gastric acid secretion. Fittingly, infusion of exogenous somatostatin in doses similar to postprandial levels has also been shown to inhibit acid secretion. In humans, concentrations of somatostatin capable of inhibiting acid secretion can do so without altering serum gastrin levels, indicating a direct action on the acid-secreting fundic mucosa.

Somatostatin is believed to influence gastrin secretion through a locally active intramucosal mechanism. Local actions of somatostatin are supported by ultrastructural studies of

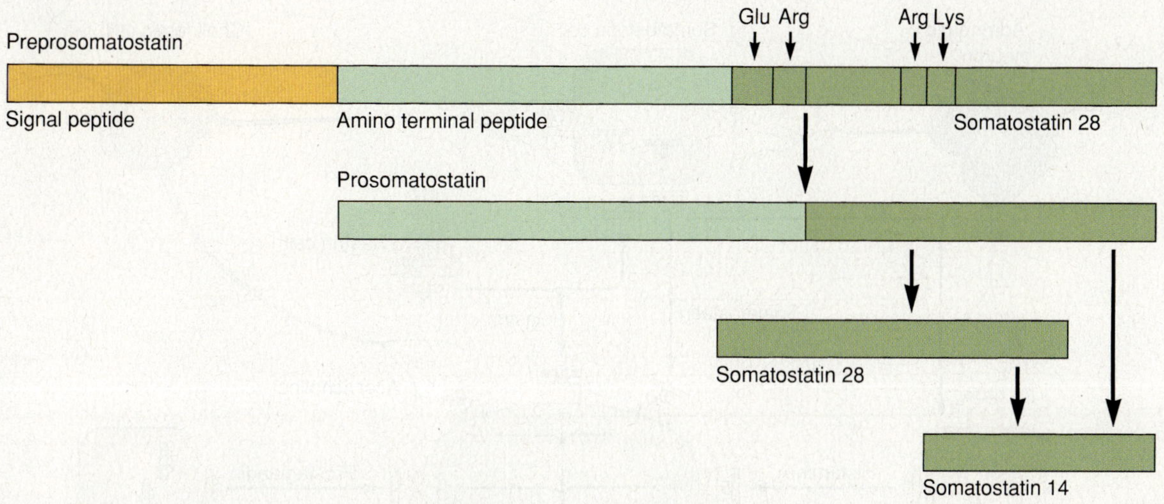

Figure 43.9. Derivation of somatostatin 14 from preprosomatostatin precursor.

antral somatostatin cells, which demonstrate long cytoplasmic processes that make intimate cell-to-cell contact with antral gastrin cells. The presence of somatostatin at these sites of cellular contact implies that somatostatin cells influence the function of gastrin cells through local release of the peptide. Increases in somatostatin release are often associated with decreased gastrin secretion. A family of five somatostatin receptors has been cloned. Inhibition of gastrin-stimulated gastric acid secretion is mediated by somatostatin receptor subtype 2.[11]

Ghrelin

Ghrelin is a gut hormone that is commonly known for being orexigenic or an appetite stimulant.[12] Additionally, it has numerous metabolic and endocrine functions.[10] Opposite of gastrin, ghrelin production characteristically takes place from enteroendocrine cells in the body of the stomach and is largely absent in the antrum.[12] The gene *GHRL* codes for a precursor peptide, preproghrelin, which is processed into biologically active products. This process takes place in the endoplasmic reticulum and is mediated by the availability of medium-chain fatty acids. Ghrelin then generates its effects by binding growth hormone secretagogue receptors of the hypothalamus. Ghrelin levels are decreased after consumption of food and increased in times of starvation. Ghrelin levels are inversely proportional to body mass index, with lower levels in patients with obesity.

Due to their implication in appetite and metabolism, there has been much recent attention given to ghrelin and the related adipokine, leptin. The role of these hormones in the pathophysiology and treatment of obesity continues to be elucidated. Surgical procedures that remove part of the body of the stomach, such as a sleeve gastrectomy, cause decreased levels of ghrelin. The reduction exceeds that seen in gastric bypass, suggesting a more complex role of ghrelin in the metabolic modulation of weight loss, beyond merely an anatomic restriction.[13]

GASTRIC ACID SECRETION

Cellular Events

An appreciation of the mechanisms that control gastric acid formation is essential to a discussion of gastric disease.[7] An understanding of the cellular basis of acid secretion by the gastric parietal cell also provides a foundation for discussing the
5 pharmacologic suppression of acid secretion. The basolateral membrane of the parietal cell contains specific receptors for histamine, gastrin, and acetylcholine, the three major stimulants of acid production.[14] Each stimulant reaches the parietal cell by a different route. Histamine is released from subepithelial enterochromaffin-like (ECL) cells and diffuses to the mucosa, acetylcholine is released in close proximity to the parietal cells from cholinergic nerve terminals, and gastrin is delivered by the systemic circulation to the fundic mucosa from its source in the antrum and proximal duodenum (**Fig. 43.10**).

Acetylcholine and related cholinergic agonists activate parietal cells after binding to muscarinic receptors. The stimulatory effects of acetylcholine and its congeners can be abolished by atropine. The action of acetylcholine is mediated by muscarinic receptor subtype 3 (M_3).

Although histamine, acetylcholine, and gastrin occupy separate receptors on the parietal cell, each secretagogue ultimately acts by means of a specialized ion transport system called the *parietal cell proton pump*. This membrane-bound protein is located in the secretory canaliculus of the parietal cell; the peptide has not been identified in other gastric cells or in significant amounts in other organs. The proton pump is an H^+-K^+-adenosine triphosphatase (ATPase) that electroneutrally exchanges cytosolic H^+ for luminal K^+. Hydrogen ions are concentrated 2.5-million-fold within the secretory canaliculus, and the hydrolysis of ATP is the energy source for transport against the steep electrochemical gradient generated. For each H^+ ion transported to the luminal surface of the canalicular membrane, one K^+ ion is transported to the cytosolic surface (**Fig. 43.11**).

Activation of the H^+-K^+-ATPase significantly increases intracellular OH^- generation, with potential cellular toxicity. Carbonic anhydrase, which is associated with the canalicular membrane, converts OH^- to HCO_3^-. The HCO_3^- produced is disposed of by exchange for Cl^- at the basolateral membrane. Intracellular Cl^-, thus acquired, supplies the necessary Cl^- on a one-to-one basis for each H^+ secreted. The transcellular exchange of H^+ for HCO_3^- ensures that the voluminous secretion of hydrochloride at the luminal surface of the gastric mucosa is matched by an equivalent delivery of base to submucosal capillaries. Parietal cell ionic transport pathways are shown in **Figure 43.12**.

The function of the proton pump is highly regulated. In the unstimulated state, the enzyme is sequestered in cytoplasmic structures termed *tubulovesicles* that are not connected to the gastric lumen. Tubulovesicle membranes in this state have a low permeability to KCl. Stimulation of acid secretion causes tubulovesicles to fuse with apical secretory membranes and increases membrane permeability to KCl. In this way, the fusion of the tubulovesicle membrane exposes the H^+-K^+ pump to the gastric lumen and simultaneously provides the K^+ substrate necessary for acid secretion.

Parietal cells also contain membrane receptors that inhibit acid secretion. Specific receptors for somatostatin have been identified using isolated gastric cells. Activation of isolated parietal cells by histamine, pentagastrin, or the cholinergic

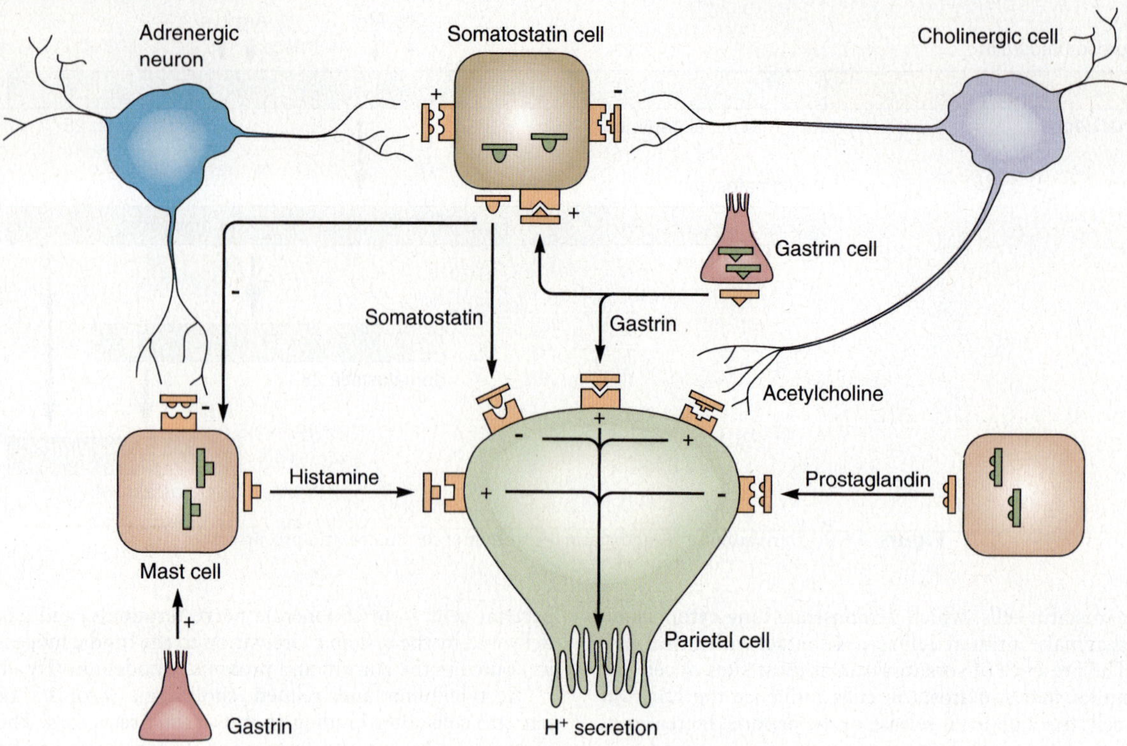

Figure 43.10. Interactions of cell types that affect parietal cell acid secretion.

agonist carbachol can be blocked by somatostatin 28. Gastric parietal cells also contain receptors for prostaglandins, notably prostaglandin E_2 and its derivatives. Prostaglandin E_2 is a potent inhibitor of histamine-stimulated parietal cell activation.

These considerations of the cellular basis of acid production demonstrate how parietal cell function can be altered pharmacologically. Gastric acid production can be blocked by receptor antagonists for each of the three primary stimulants—gastrin, acetylcholine, and histamine. Direct inhibition of acid production can be effected by derivatives of somatostatin or prostaglandin E_2. All forms of stimulated acid production can be blocked by agents that act as inhibitors of the parietal cell proton pump, such as traditional proton pump inhibitors (PPI's) and newer potassium-competitive acid blockers (PCABs).[15] The pharmacologic agents acting at each of the aforementioned points are detailed further in subsequent chapters.

Regulation of Acid Secretion

Given the multiple receptors on parietal cells, it is not surprising that a great deal of secretagogue interdependence, both stimulatory and inhibitory, exists in humans. Parietal cell activation and the resultant acid secretion is greater in response to a combination of agonists than it is in response to the total effect of agents used singly. This increase in responsiveness is defined as *potentiation*. Thus, histamine strongly potentiates the acid-secretory response to pentagastrin or to carbachol in humans. Conversely, blockade of receptors to one stimulant also decreases responsiveness to the other agonists. For example, blocking histamine receptors with agents such as cimetidine decreases responsiveness to pentagastrin, even though gastrin receptors are not directly affected. These inhibitory interactions are exploited therapeutically in the treatment of acid–peptic diseases.

Humans normally secrete 2 to 5 mEq/h of hydrochloride in the fasting state, constituting basal acid secretion. Both vagal tone and ambient histamine secretion are presumed to be important in determining the rate of basal acid secretion.

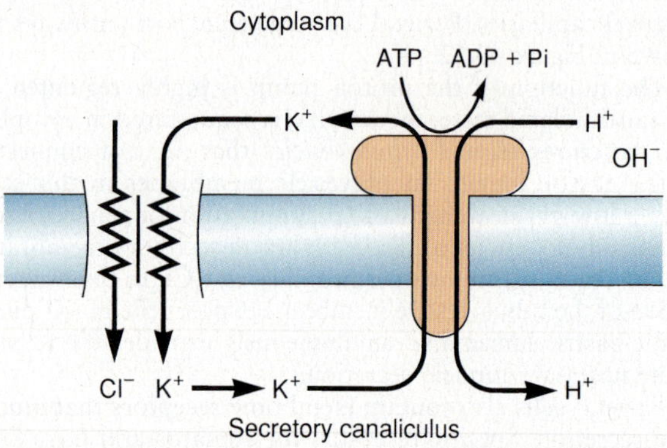

Figure 43.11. Gastric H+-K+-adenosine triphosphatase (ATPase). ADP, adenosine diphosphate; ATP, adenosine triphosphate; Pi, phosphate ion.

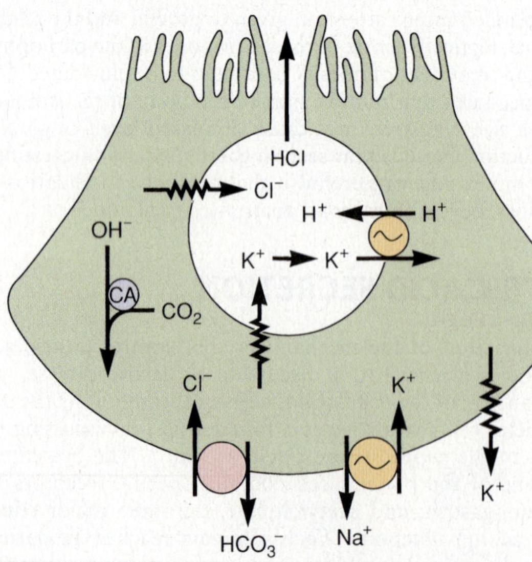

Figure 43.12. Ionic fluxes associated with acid secretion by the parietal cell.

In humans, truncal vagotomy decreases basal secretion by approximately 85%. Similarly, H_2-receptor antagonists also inhibit basal acid secretion by approximately 80%. Gastrin does not have an important role in determining basal acid secretion in normal people.

Stimulated acid secretion begins with the thought, sight, or smell of food. This *cephalic phase* of gastric acid secretion is mediated by the vagus nerve. Vagal discharge directs a cholinergic mechanism, and the cephalic phase of acid secretion can be inhibited by administering atropine. The cephalic component of acid secretion can be measured in normal people and is approximately 10 mEq/h. The cephalic phase approximates 40% of the maximal acid-secretory response to gastrin infusion.

The *gastric phase* of acid secretion begins when food enters the stomach. The presence of partially hydrolyzed food constituents, gastric distention, and the buffering capacity of food all stimulate acid secretion. In normal humans, acid-secretory rates after a mixed meal average 15 to 25 mEq/h, approximately 75% of the maximal response achieved with infusion of exogenous gastrin or histamine. The meal response is less than the maximal response to exogenous stimulants because food also causes the release of somatostatin and initiates other inhibitory responses. In humans, 90% of meal-stimulated acid secretion is mediated by gastrin release.[16]

In humans, the most important and clearly established gastric inhibitory influence is the suppression of gastrin release when the antral mucosa is exposed to acid. When luminal pH falls to 2.0, gastrin release stops. Antral acidification also suppresses the gastrin response to an ingested meal. Somatostatin acting locally in the gastric mucosa as a paracrine agent may mediate this important inhibitory response. Release of gastric somatostatin is reciprocally linked to that of gastrin; acidification of the antrum causes increases in somatostatin release and decreases in gastrin secretion. Antral distention also inhibits stimulated acid secretion.

The entry of digestive products into the intestine begins *intestinal phase* inhibition of gastric acid secretion. Acidification of the duodenal bulb inhibits acid secretion.

PEPSIN

6 Pepsins are a heterogeneous group of proteolytic enzymes that are secreted by gastric chief cells.[8] Pepsin is derived under acidic conditions from pepsinogen by the autocatalytic loss of a variable aminoterminal sequence. This conversion occurs slowly at pH values of 5.0 to 6.0 and occurs rapidly when luminal pH approaches 2.0. Pepsin catalyzes the hydrolysis of a wide variety of peptide bonds that contain acidic residues, with a pH optimum for hydrolysis between 1.5 and 2.5. Once activated, pepsin is sensitive to ambient pH values; it is irreversibly denatured at pH 7.0 or greater.

The most important stimulus for pepsinogen secretion is cholinergic stimulation. Acetylcholine and its derivatives stimulate pepsinogen secretion by a mechanism that can be antagonized by atropine, indicating a muscarinic receptor. Endogenous cholinergic stimulation through the vagal nerve results in the formation of a gastric secretion that is rich in pepsin. The oxyntic mucosa contains somatostatin cells near chief cells. Pepsinogen secretion in response to a variety of stimuli has been demonstrated to be inhibited by somatostatin.

The major physiologic function of pepsin is to initiate protein digestion. Pepsin is highly active against collagen and may be important in the digestion of animal protein. Intragastric protein hydrolysis by pepsin is incomplete, and relatively large peptides enter the intestine, although amino acids and small peptide fragments are released. These products of partial hydrolysis are important signals for gastrin and CCK release, which in turn regulate digestive processes. In this way, pepsin also contributes to the overall coordination of the digestive process.

INTRINSIC FACTOR

7 The gastric mucosa is the site of production of intrinsic factor, which is necessary for the absorption of cobalamin from the ileal mucosa.[9] The parietal cell is the site of intrinsic factor synthesis and storage in humans. Intrinsic factor secretion, like acid secretion, is stimulated by histamine, acetylcholine, and gastrin. Unlike acid production, intrinsic factor secretion peaks rapidly after stimulation and then returns to baseline. The amount of intrinsic factor secreted usually greatly exceeds the amount needed to bind and absorb available dietary cobalamin. However, cobalamin malabsorption can occur after stomach resection or when atrophic gastritis involves the oxyntic mucosa.

GASTRIC BLOOD FLOW

Because the gastric mucosa is metabolically highly active, control of mucosal blood flow is of great physiologic importance. In addition, studies have implicated perfusion abnormalities in the development of mucosal lesions during periods of stress. Mucosal blood flow is regulated by neural, hormonal, and locally active influences.

Postganglionic sympathetic nerve fibers innervate small mucosal arteries. Mucosal capillaries do not receive adrenergic innervation. Electrical stimulation of sympathetic nerves supplying the stomach is followed by decreased total gastric blood flow, decreased flow in celiac and gastroepiploic vessels, and diminished blood flow to the mucosa. Studies in animals demonstrate that vasoconstriction of the gastric vascular bed is mediated by α-adrenergic receptors and that vasodilation is mediated by β-adrenergic receptors.

Stimulation of the vagus nerve is followed by a prompt increase in blood flow, suggesting a dilatory effect of parasympathetic nerves. The effects of vagal stimulation on mucosal blood flow are complicated by accompanying increases in acid secretion. Almost all stimuli that increase acid production also increase blood flow secondarily.

A number of gastrointestinal peptide hormones affect gastric blood flow, mostly because of their ability to increase or decrease acid secretion. Thus, gastrin, because it is a potent stimulant of acid secretion, also increases mucosal blood flow. CCK appears to have direct vasodilatory effects on the gastric vasculature. Vasopressin has been well demonstrated to have direct vasoconstrictor activity. Nitric oxide modulates basal gastric vascular tone and controls gastric vasodilation and hyperemia, although the molecule has no direct stimulatory role in acid production.

Prostaglandins are important mucosally produced compounds that have clear effects on the gastric vasculature. Prostaglandins of the E class have been shown in animals and humans to increase gastric blood flow at doses that decrease acid secretion. Indomethacin, in doses sufficient to inhibit prostaglandin formation, decreases the diameter of submucosal blood vessels and reduces basal blood flow. Complete inhibition of cyclooxygenase activity causes an approximate 50% reduction in resting blood flow. These studies suggest that endogenous, locally produced prostaglandins are crucial to maintaining basal gastric blood flow in humans and probably act in concert with endogenous nitric oxide.

GASTRIC MOTILITY

Gastric Smooth Muscle

Consideration of gastric motility requires that the stomach be viewed in functional terms as two different regions, the proximal one-third and the distal two-thirds. These areas are distinct in terms of smooth muscle anatomy, electrical activity, and contractile function but do not correspond to traditional anatomic divisions.

In the proximal stomach, three layers of gastric smooth muscle can be distinguished: an outer longitudinal layer, a middle circular layer, and an inner oblique layer. In the distal two-thirds of the stomach, the longitudinal layer is most clearly defined, and the inner oblique layer is usually not distinct. The gastric smooth muscle ends at the pylorus.

The smooth muscle of the proximal stomach is electrically stable, whereas the smooth muscle of the distal stomach demonstrates spontaneous, repeated electrical discharges. Gastric smooth muscle exhibits myoelectric activity that is based on a highly regular pattern called the *slow wave*.[17] Pacemaker activity is mediated by networks of interstitial cells of Cajal (ICC) and platelet-derived growth factor alpha (PDGFRα^+) cells.[18] In the stomach, slow waves occur with a frequency of three cycles per minute. Slow waves do not, by themselves, lead to gastric contractions, but they do set the maximum rate of contractions at three per minute. Gastric contractions occur when action potentials are phase locked with the crest of the slow wave.[17]

Extracellular electrical recording from the serosal surface of the stomach also demonstrates the intrinsic electrical activity of the distal stomach in the form of pacesetter potentials. Pacesetter potentials reflect partial depolarization of the gastric smooth muscle cell and are recorded during relatively long periods (2 or 3 seconds). Pacesetters originate along the greater curvature at a point in the proximal third of the stomach. Pacesetter potentials, discharging at a rate of three times per minute in humans, drive cells located distally. Spread of the pacesetter potentials is faster along the greater curvature, so that a ring of electrical activity reaches the pylorus simultaneously along both curvatures. The pacesetter potentials do not result in smooth muscle contraction unless an additional depolarization is superimposed in the form of an action potential. When action potentials occur, a ring of smooth muscle contraction moves peristaltically along the distal stomach toward the pylorus.

The smooth muscle activity of the proximal stomach is fundamentally different from that of the distal stomach. There are no pacesetters or action potentials in the proximal stomach. As a result, peristalsis does not occur. Proximal gastric contraction is tonic and prolonged, and increases in luminal pressure are often sustained for several minutes.

Coordination of Contraction

Important vagally mediated reflexes influence intragastric pressure, presumably by affecting contractile activity of smooth muscle in the proximal stomach. The most important reflex is termed *receptive relaxation* and occurs with ingestion of a meal. Increasing gastric volumes are accommodated with little increase in intragastric pressure by relaxation of the proximal stomach. This receptive relaxation allows the proximal stomach to act as a storage site for ingested food in the immediate postprandial period. Afferent impulses, presumed to originate from stretch receptors in the gastric wall, are carried along vagal fibers; efferent vagal discharges are inhibitory. Receptive gastric accommodation is lost after either truncal or proximal gastric vagotomy. After the meal has been ingested, proximal contractile activity increases; alterations in proximal gastric tone cause the compressive movement of gastric content from the fundus to the antrum.

Food that enters the antrum from the proximal stomach is propelled peristaltically toward the pylorus. A number of observations indicate that the pylorus closes 2 or 3 seconds before the arrival of the antral contraction ring. This coordinate closing of the pylorus allows a small bolus of liquid and suspended food particles to pass while retropulsing the main mass of gastric contents back into the proximal antrum. The churning action that results mixes ingested food particles, gastric acid, and pepsin, and contributes to the grinding function of the stomach.

A consistent finding in humans ingesting a mixed solid–liquid meal is that liquids empty more quickly than solids. Characteristically, solid food empties only after a lag period, whereas liquid emptying begins almost immediately. A traditional interpretation of these observations has been that the proximal stomach is the dominant force in determining how quickly a liquid meal empties by the gastroduodenal pressure gradient generated by proximal gastric contractions. The distal gastric segment has been postulated to control solid emptying through its grinding and peristaltic actions.

This concept of the two-component stomach is useful in considering observations in patients who have undergone gastric operative procedures. After proximal gastric vagotomy, patients exhibit accelerated emptying of liquids but have normal solid emptying. Because of loss of receptive relaxation, the denervation of the proximal stomach is presumed to increase intragastric pressure and accelerate liquid emptying while leaving the distal gastric segment unaffected. Conversely, vagal denervation of the antrum interrupts gastric emptying of solids to a greater degree than liquids. Although this model of gastric emptying oversimplifies the many mechanisms (gastric, pyloric, and intestinal) that work in concert to control gastric emptying, it provides a useful framework for considering the effects of gastric surgical procedures.

Gastric motility is also regulated by numerous gut hormones. Prokinetic hormones include ghrelin and motilin. Those that inhibit gastric emptying include CCK, leptin, glucagon-like peptide 1, and peptide YY.[19] The action of pharmaceutical agents at these target receptors, either as intended or incidental, is likely to remain a burgeoning topic of study.

ACKNOWLEDGMENT

We gratefully acknowledge the contributions of previous edition author, Michael W. Mulholland, as portions of those chapters have been retained in this revision.

References

1. McCracken KW, Catá EM, Crawford CM, et al. Modelling human development and disease in pluripotent stem-cell-derived gastric organoids. *Nature*. 2014;516(7531):400–404.
2. Standring S. *Gray's Anatomy: The Anatomical Basis of Clinical Practice. Gray's Anatomy Series*. 41th ed. Elsevier Limited; 2016.
3. von Rosenvinge EC, Raufman JP. Gastrointestinal peptides and regulation of gastric acid secretion. *Curr Opin Endocrinol Diabetes Obes*. 2010;17(1):40–43.
4. Schubert M, Peura DA. Control of gastric acid secretion in health and disease. *Gastroenterology*. 2008;134(7):1842–1860.
5. Choi MY, Romer AI, Wang Y, et al. Requirement of the tissue-restricted homeodomain transcription factor Nkx6.3 in differentiation of gastrin-producing G cells in the stomach antrum. *Mol Cell Biol*. 2008;28(10):3208–3218.
6. Schubert ML. Gastric secretion. *Curr Opin Gastroenterol*. 2008;24(6):659–664.
7. Debas HT, Carvajal SH. Vagal regulation of acid secretion and gastrin release. *Yale J Biol Med*. 1994;67(3–4):145–151.
8. Cover TL. Role of *Helicobacter pylori* CagL in modulating gastrin expression. *Gut*. 2012;61(7):965–966.
9. Corleto VD. Somatostatin and the gastrointestinal tract. *Curr Opin Endocrinol Diabetes Obes*. 2010;17(1):63–68.
10. Choi E, Roland JT, Barlow BJ, et al. Cell lineage distribution atlas of the human stomach reveals heterogeneous gland populations in the gastric antrum. *Gut*. 2014;63(11):1711–1720.
11. Theodoropoulou M, Stalla GK. Somatostatin receptors: from signaling to clinical practice. *Front Neuroendocrinol*. 2013;34(3):228–252.
12. Cui H, López M, Rahmouni K. The cellular and molecular bases of leptin and ghrelin resistance in obesity. *Nat Rev Endocrinol*. 2017;13(6):338–351.
13. Alamuddin N, Vetter ML, Ahima RS, et al. Changes in fasting and prandial gut and adiposity hormones following vertical sleeve

gastrectomy or Roux-en-Y-Gastric bypass: an 18-month prospective study. *Obes Surg*. 2017;27(6):1563–1572.

14. Urushidani T, Forte JG. Signal transduction and activation of acid secretion in the parietal cell. *J Membr Biol*. 1997;159(2):99–111.
15. Jenkins H, Sakurai Y, Nishimura A, et al. Randomised clinical trial: safety, tolerability, pharmacokinetics and pharmacodynamics of repeated doses of TAK-438 (vonoprazan), a novel potassium-competitive acid blocker, in healthy male subjects. *Aliment Pharmacol Ther*. 2015;41(7):636–648.
16. Waldum HL, Brenna E, Kleveland PM, Sandvik AK. Gastrin—physiological and pathophysiological role: clinical consequences. *Dig Dis*. 1995;13(1):25–38.
17. Quigley EM. Gastric and small intestinal motility in health and disease. *Gastroenterol Clin North Am*. 1996;25(1):113–145.
18. Sanders KM, Ward SM, Koh SD. Interstitial cells: regulators of smooth muscle function. *Physiol Rev*. 2014;94(3):859–907.
19. Goyal RK, Guo Y, Mashimo H. Advances in the physiology of gastric emptying. *Neurogastroenterol Motil*. 2019;31(4):e13546.

44

Management of Obesity

Dana A. Telem and Robert W. O'Rourke

Key Points

1 Obesity is a chronic disease and is defined and categorized using body mass index (BMI, weight [kg]/height [m]^2) based on World Health Organization (WHO) definitions.

2 The severity of obesity directly correlates with the risk of multiple metabolic diseases and long-term mortality.

3 Lifestyle interventions as treatment for obesity, including diet, exercise, and psychological therapy, are of limited efficacy; evolving strategies directed toward environmental manipulation demonstrate potential.

4 Current pharmacotherapy for obesity includes a wide range of agents that act via multiple mechanisms and hold significant promise.

5 Bariatric surgery is safe and highly efficacious in treating obesity and metabolic disease, and includes a wide range of procedures that have evolved over the decades.

6 Current dominant bariatric surgery operations include gastric bypass and sleeve gastrectomy; however the duodenal switch is increasing in prevalence.

7 Classic mechanisms of action of bariatric surgery include restriction of caloric intake and malabsorption of ingested calories, but evolving data suggest that other mechanisms predominate, including but not limited to alterations in gut and satiety hormone homeostasis, bile acid metabolism, and enteroenteric and enterocentral nervous systemic communications.

DIAGNOSIS AND EPIDEMIOLOGY

Obesity and Metabolic Disease

Excess adipose tissue is the defining feature of obesity, and metabolic disease arises in adipose tissue. Metabolic disease is diverse, involving every organ system. The correlation between obesity and metabolic disease, while strong, is not perfect—some patients develop metabolic disease at low body weight, while others who are very obese are protected. Visceral adiposity imparts greater risk than subcutaneous adiposity, and heterogeneity of visceral and subcutaneous adiposities partly explains the imperfect correlation between obesity and metabolic disease. Lean patients also develop metabolic disease, albeit less frequently than the obese, demonstrating that non-adipose tissue–based mechanisms contribute to metabolic disease as well. It is beyond the scope of this chapter to discuss the wide spectrum of specific treatment strategies for individual metabolic diseases. Rather, we will discuss the treatment of obesity itself, the goal of which is reduction in adipose tissue mass, because despite the variable relationship between body weight and metabolic dysfunction, in the vast majority of patients, regardless of initial weight, weight loss has beneficial effects on virtually all metabolic diseases. Treatment options for obesity may be broadly divided into medical and surgical approaches.

Diagnosis

1 Body mass index (BMI, weight [kg]/height [m]^2) is the primary metric used to define obesity. Originally devised in the 19th century by the Belgian polymath Adolphe Quetelet as a general measure of human body habitus, BMI was co-opted in the 1940s by the insurance industry and used to stratify humans into high- and low-risk subpopulations based on actuarial data for the purpose of setting life insurance rates. The medical community subsequently used BMI to estimate risk of morbidity and mortality. Much debate exists regarding the appropriate BMI cutoff points for optimal health, with various health and professional organizations setting different values. World Health Organization (WHO) definitions, set in 1995 and agreed upon by the US Centers for Disease Control (CDC), are most commonly utilized and define overweight as BMI >25 and <30 and obesity as BMI ≥30, and categorize obesity into classes 1 (BMI 30 to 34.9), 2 (BMI 35 to 39.9), and 3 (BMI ≥40).[1]

BMI correlates with long-term mortality and metabolic dis-
2 ease in a J-shaped curve, the nadir of which is debated, but may be as low as 20 or as high as 25.[2] BMI in the obese range (≥30) is clearly associated with an increased risk for long-term mortality and multiple metabolic diseases relative to BMI <30. For individuals with BMI of 40 to 50, this risk translates into a 10-year decrease in life expectancy. In contrast to obesity, data demonstrating a correlation between overweight BMI and health risk are conflicting. Analyses are complicated by numerous confounding variables, including but not limited to sex, age, ethnicity, smoking, cancer, and diabetes. In addition, the choice of control/referent group alters outcomes; for example, the correlations between overweight BMI and clinical outcomes weaken significantly and may be masked when referent groups span a larger BMI range (eg, 18 to 25) relative to comparison with referent groups spanning a narrow BMI range (eg, 21 to 23). Despite these conflicting data, the preponderance of evidence suggests that BMI in the overweight range is associated with an increased risk of long-term mortality, albeit lower than the risk associated with BMI in the obese range.[3] Furthermore, mortality aside, compelling data demonstrate that overweight BMI is associated with an increased risk of cardiovascular disease, diabetes, and other metabolic diseases, and is associated with an increased risk of future progression to frank obesity with its attendant risks. Taken together, these observations suggest that being overweight should be considered a serious health risk and a predecessor to obesity.

These complex data demonstrate that BMI is not a perfect measure of adiposity. Indeed, muscular athletes may have BMI within the obese range despite low body fat levels and an absence of metabolic disease, while elderly people with a paucity of muscle mass may have low BMI despite increased adiposity and metabolic disease. Ethnic differences further confound the predictive power of BMI, as certain ethnicities, for example, Asians develop metabolic disease at lower BMI, prompting the WHO in 2004 to propose BMI cutoffs of 23 and 27.5 for overweight and obesity, respectively, in Asians. In certain subpopulations, including patients with heart failure, renal failure, and other chronic diseases, overweight and obesity are associated with decreased mortality, a phenomenon termed the "obesity paradox."[4]

Given the limitations of BMI, governing medical bodies recommend using other measures in addition to BMI to assess a person's health. Waist circumference and waist–hip ratio are easily measured and in many studies correlate more accurately with metabolic disease than BMI, reflecting the disproportionate effect of visceral adiposity on metabolic disease.[5] Water displacement, dual-energy x-ray absorptiometry scanning, double-labeled isotope water measurement, bioelectrical impedance analysis, and quantitative magnetic resonance imaging may provide more accurate measures of adiposity and better predict metabolic disease. More recently, a novel CT imaging approach, analytic morphomics, has been used to quantify adipose tissue and risk stratify various patient populations as well as determine adequate drug therapy dosing.[6] However, such methods have not gained widespread acceptance due to cost and complexity. Despite its limitations, BMI remains the most commonly used metric for obesity; however this is rapidly changing with a preference toward waist-to-hip ratio.

Epidemiology, Disease Burden

Human obesity has existed for millennia, as evidenced by prehistoric figurines of obese humans (eg, Venus of Willendorf) and periodic concerns regarding past obesity "epidemics" over the past two centuries. Nonetheless, the worldwide prevalence of overweight and obesity has increased dramatically over the past 50 years. BMI, like many clinical characteristics, spans a bell curve. Three large US epidemiologic datasets, the National Health and Nutrition Examination Survey (NHANES), the National Health Interview Survey (NHIS), and the Behavioral Risk Factor Surveillance System (BRFSS), demonstrate similar trends, with a rightward shift of the BMI bell curve over the past three decades, mean BMI increasing from 25.5 in the 1970s to 28.5 in 2005, and the prevalence of obesity more than doubling in the same interval.[7] The CDC reports that as of 2017 to 2018, 42% of US adults were obese and 18.5% of US children between 2 and 19 were obese.[8] To put this in context, the prevalence of obesity in adults increased 30.5% from 1999 to 2000. Sex, ethnic, and regional differences complicate obesity epidemiology. The rate of increase is higher in women compared to men, and while rates of increase are similar across ethnicities, mean BMI is highest in Blacks, followed by Hispanics, then Caucasians. Data regarding the association between obesity and socioeconomic status are conflicting; evidence suggests an inverse correlation between low socioeconomic status and obesity in low- and middle-income countries but a positive correlation in industrialized countries. Obesity prevalence is increased in rural compared to urban environments in the United States, although this relationship is inverted in developing countries.[8]

The disease burden associated with obesity is substantial. Multiple confounders complicate quantification of risk, not the least of which is variability in the degree of obesity itself, with increasing BMI being associated with increasing risk of mortality and disease in a dose-dependent but nonlinear fashion. Obesity is associated with decreased lifespan. Data from the Framingham Heart Study demonstrate a loss of 3 and 6 years of life for overweight and obese men, respectively,[9] while NHANES data demonstrate a loss of 13 years of life for severely obese men (BMI >45).[10] Overweight and obesity are associated with an increased risk of multiple diseases, among which type II diabetes is particularly important. The association between obesity and diabetes is robust; relative risks for diabetes range from 2 to 15 for BMI in the overweight range and 20 to 90 for BMI in the obese range. The CDC estimates that in the United States in 2018, the prevalence of type II diabetes was 13% among all adults and 27% among those over 65 years of age. Furthermore, 35% of all US adults, and 47% of US adults over 65 years of age have elevated fasting blood glucose or HbA1c consistent with prediabetes. If current trends persist, the prevalence of diabetes in the United States in 2050 will exceed 30%, and worldwide trends parallel these US data.[8]

Obesity is associated with an increased risk of multiple diseases, including atherosclerosis, hypertension, hyperlipidemia, hepatic steatosis and steatohepatitis, sleep apnea, osteoarthritis, gallbladder disease, endocrine disorders, autoimmune disease, allergy and atopy, multiple types of cancer, infertility, and depression. Metabolic disease encompasses all of physiology. Risk ratios for overweight and obesity-related diseases vary substantially depending on BMI, ranging from 2 to 5 for class I obesity, with dramatic dose-dependent increases in risk with increasing BMI. For example, the prevalence of hepatic steatosis in the general population is generally estimated to be approximately 30%, increases progressively with increasing BMI, and exceeds 90% in obese patients with BMI >40. In the NHANES population, the prevalence of sleep apnea was 3% in nonobese men and 12% in obese men (BMI >30),[11] but in a separate study of patients with severe obesity (BMI >40), prevalence exceeded 70%.[12] This disease burden is associated with significant economic costs. While accurate quantification of obesity-related healthcare costs is challenging and complicated by regional variability in payer systems and patient demographics, the estimated costs directly attributable to overweight and obesity in the United States exceed 100 billion dollars annually and constitute 5% to 10% of total US healthcare spending.[13]

MEDICAL MANAGEMENT

Treatment Strategies

The medical management of obesity falls into two primary categories: lifestyle intervention and pharmacotherapy. Both strategies, with rare exceptions, achieve similar results, with modest weight loss and high recidivism. Nonetheless, both strategies hold significant untapped promise, with advances expected in the coming decades, particularly in the areas of environmental engineering and pharmacotherapy.

Lifestyle Interventions

3 Lifestyle interventions for obesity include any or all of three basic components: diet modification, exercise, and psychological therapy. Interventions may be unsupervised or administered under the supervision of clinicians, dieticians, or commercial weight loss plans, and may be individualized or administered in group programs.

Diet modification is the mainstay of lifestyle intervention. Diet strategies vary with respect to macronutrient composition, daily caloric intake, and food and caloric measurement methods, and include low-carbohydrate diets, low-fat diets, meal replacement strategies, Mediterranean diets, very low-calorie diets, and multiple commercial diet plans. No clear evidence demonstrates advantages of any specific diet plan over others. Specifically, macronutrient composition does not impact weight loss when caloric intake is controlled—total calories, rather than the macronutrient composition of those calories, is the variable that determines weight loss. In contrast to weight loss, conflicting evidence exists regarding the role of macronutrient composition in improvement of metabolic disease, with some evidence suggesting that low-carbohydrate diets (which include low-glycemic index–high-fiber diets and very low–carbohydrate diets), when compared to low-fat diets, may be associated with greater improvements in insulin resistance and triglyceride levels, and higher resting energy expenditure. These studies must be interpreted with caution as follow-up is relatively short, and low-carbohydrate diets may be associated with adverse changes in low-density lipoprotein levels.[14] Low-carbohydrate diets also appear to provide better compliance than other diet strategies over short-term follow-up of less than 6 months, but compliance differences vanish at follow-up exceeding 1 year.

Physical activity is a central component of lifestyle intervention for obesity. Exercise alone achieves only modest weight loss, but exercise and diet potentiate each other. Importantly, exercise reduces obesity-related mortality and cardiovascular disease risk independent of weight loss. Data regarding the optimal type, duration, frequency, and intensity of exercise are conflicting, and specific evidence-based guidelines remain elusive. High intensity exercise may be more effective for weight loss, but many obese patients are unable to engage in even moderate intensity exercise due to comorbid diseases such as osteoarthritis. Increased daily activities such as walking and stair use nonetheless may provide modest weight loss and cardiovascular health benefits.

Of the wide range of psychological techniques used to treat obesity, cognitive-behavioral therapy is most common. Cognitive-behavioral therapy achieves modest weight loss in the obese of approximately 2 to 3 kg at 1-year follow-up, with increased weight loss when combined with diet and/or exercise. Increased frequency of psychological intervention and group therapy compared with individual therapy is associated with greater weight loss.[15]

Intensive lifestyle interventions are supervised multicomponent plans that involve a combination of diet, exercise, and behavioral modification, with periodic monitoring by coaches and dieticians, and individual or group psychological counseling. Two NIH-sponsored randomized controlled trials suggest that intensive lifestyle interventions provide more durable results than standard lifestyle interventions, although long-term outcomes of metabolic disease are conflicting. The Diabetes Prevention Program randomized 3,234 overweight or obese insulin-resistant patients (mean BMI 34) to one of three experimental arms: intensive lifestyle interventions, metformin treatment, or placebo treatment.[16] After a mean follow-up of 2.8 years, average weight loss in the intensive lifestyle interventions group was 5.6 kg compared with 2.1 kg and 0.1 kg for the metformin and placebo groups, respectively; at 10 years, an average weight loss of 2 kg was maintained in both intensive lifestyle interventions and metformin arms relative to the placebo arm. The cumulative risk of incident diabetes was 34% lower in the intensive lifestyle interventions arm and 18% lower in the metformin arm relative to the placebo arm. The NIH-sponsored Look AHEAD (Action for Health in Diabetes) study randomized 5,145 overweight or obese diabetic patients to a 4-year intensive lifestyle intervention involving diet and exercise modification with regular on-site visits and counseling, or standard primary care provider–supervised diabetes and weight loss education. After 8 years, mean weight loss was 4.7% and 2.1% in the intensive lifestyle intervention and standard care arms, respectively.[17] Nonetheless, the study was halted after 11 years after no difference in cardiovascular events was observed. These studies demonstrate that while modest, weight loss may be maintained over long periods with intensive lifestyle interventions, although the effects on metabolic disease are equivocal. Of importance, in Look AHEAD, a subset of patients in each arm (27% and 17% in intensive lifestyle intervention and standard care arms, respectively), maintained a loss of >10% of total starting weight, suggesting that subpopulations of patients are more responsive than others to lifestyle interventions, and that identification of predictors of responsiveness would permit better allocation of care.

Assessing the overall efficacy of lifestyle interventions for obesity is challenging, as results vary depending on the subgroup studied, follow-up is variable and often short, and program and outcome reporting methods are widely disparate. The resultant complex body of literature limits our current understanding of the efficacy of such interventions. Nonetheless, a preponderance of data suggests that results of lifestyle interventions for obesity are modest, with mean weight loss between 2% and 10% of total body weight over follow-up periods from 6 to 48 months. Unsupervised individual efforts underperform more intensive, multicomponent, supervised, group interventions. Compliance is a critical issue; individual diet programs are associated with attrition that may exceed 90% over a year or more while attrition for intensive supervised efforts is less. Weight regain after program discontinuation is common, and long-term adherence to lifestyle changes is low. Despite these limitations, modest weight loss, or exercise in the absence of weight loss, appears to have measurable, if modest, beneficial effects on metabolic disease, with a subset of patients being responsive to such interventions. As such, lifestyle interventions should be a component of the treatment of all obese patients, but only rarely achieve dramatic and durable results.

Pharmacotherapy

4 The history of pharmacotherapy for obesity is replete with drugs that have been introduced with much enthusiasm and variable efficacy but subsequently withdrawn due to unacceptable and, in many cases, life-threatening side effects that became apparent only after widespread use. Sheep thyroid extract was used in the late 19th century, while in the early 20th century, workers in the dye industry exposed to 2,4-dinitrophenol were observed to lose weight, leading to its use as a weight loss drug in the 1930s. Amphetamines were popular weight loss drugs in the 1950s to 1960s. All these agents were abandoned due to prohibitive side effects. The modest efficacy of weight loss drugs is testament to the multiple redundant physiologic systems that act to defend adipose tissue stores in the face of interventions designed to reduce those stores. The frequent adverse effects of weight loss drugs speak to the interface between body weight regulation and multiple fundamental physiologic processes, manipulation of which entails substantial risk.

Previously, the largest class of weight loss drugs targeted monoamine signaling mediators (norepinephrine, serotonin, dopamine, histamine) involved in CNS/hypothalamic control of satiety and hunger. Many of these agents regulate multiple pathways and demonstrate overlapping activities. Sympathomimetic agents that primarily potentiate norepinephrine release include phentermine, introduced in 1959 and still in use today, and phenylpropanolamine, used as a decongestant and also as a weight loss drug since the 1970s, but withdrawn from the market in 2000 after being associated with an increased risk of stroke. Drugs that primarily potentiate serotonin activity include fenfluramine, introduced in 1973 and withdrawn from the market in 1997, sibutramine (Meridia), a serotonin, norepinephrine, and dopamine reuptake inhibitor with primary effects on serotonin and norepinephrine, introduced in 1997 but withdrawn in 2010 after being linked to increased risks of myocardial infarction and stroke, and lorcaserin (Belviq), a selective serotonin 2C agonist approved by the Food and Drug Administration (FDA) in 2012, but withdrawn from the market in 2020 after being linked to a possible increased risk of cancer. Drugs that target dopamine signaling are currently being studied in clinical trials (eg, bupropion, tesofensine). Targeting multiple monoamine signaling pathways provides synergy. The combination drug fenfluramine/phentermine ("Fen-phen"), introduced in 1992, demonstrated increased efficacy over either agent alone, but was withdrawn from the market in 1997 after widespread use revealed serious morbidity attributable to fenfluramine, including pulmonary hypertension and cardiac valvular disease. In 2013, the FDA approved a combination drug of phentermine and topiramate, an antiepileptic with multiple CNS activities (Qsymia). A combination formulation of bupropion and naltrexone, an opioid antagonist that stimulates pro-opiomelanocortin neurons, is currently being studied in research trials.

Gut peptides have diverse metabolic functions including regulating satiety and hunger within the hypothalamic feeding center, and include glucagon-like peptide 1 (GLP-1), cholecystokinin, ghrelin, oxyntomodulin, pancreatic polypeptide, and amylin. Drugs based on these mediators show promise. Many gut peptides have short biologic half-lives and research has focused on long-acting analogs or mediators that target degradation pathways. GLP-1, secreted by ileal L cells in response to a meal, induces satiety and potentiates insulin secretion and peripheral insulin sensitivity. Long-acting GLP-1 analogs, including liraglutide (Victoza) and exenatide (Byetta), are FDA approved for treatment of type 2 diabetes and have proven beneficial in the treatment of obesity.[18] Ghrelin is an orexigenic hormone secreted by gastric fundus mucosal cells, and ghrelin antagonists, agonists of ghrelin degradation pathways, and antighrelin vaccines are in development. Amylin, released by pancreatic beta cells, induces satiety via CNS-based mechanisms and also potentiates peripheral insulin resistance; pramlintide (Symlin), a human amylin agonist, is approved for treatment of diabetes and induces modest weight loss. Orlistat (Xenical), approved by FDA in 1999, is a pancreatic lipase inhibitor that blocks intestinal absorption of fat, and the only drug to date that functions by reducing absorption of ingested calories. Side effects of orlistat include diarrhea, steatorrhea, and increased risks of kidney stones and pancreatitis. Second-generation lipase inhibitors are in development.

Agents designed to manipulate neuropeptide signaling within the hypothalamus, while not yet approved for use in humans, are important targets, and include drugs directed toward leptin, melanocortin-4 receptor (MC4R), neuropeptide Y, and melanin-concentrating hormone. While leptin resistance has confounded development of leptin as a therapeutic agent, recent data from animal models suggest that concomitant treatment of endoplasmic reticulum stress may abrogate leptin resistance,[19] while separate research demonstrates that amylin agonists also restore leptin sensitivity.[20] These lines of research have reinvigorated interest in leptin therapy. Mutations in the MC4R gene, a central hypothalamic satiety mediator, are implicated in up to 5% of cases of common human obesity, and MC4R agonists are currently in development. Other central-acting agents are directed toward endocannabinoid signaling: rimonabant (Acomplia), a selective endocannabinoid antagonist, was denied FDA approval in 2008 despite promising weight loss results in clinical trials due to an association with depression and suicide, but interest in manipulation of endocannabinoid signaling persists.

Manipulation of thermogenesis and metabolic rate remains an active field of research. Thyroid hormone achieves weight loss by increasing metabolic rate, but is associated with cardiac toxicity and has detrimental effects on glucose homeostasis. Despite these failures, research persists. Many agents discussed above that regulate food intake, most notably the sympathomimetics, also increase metabolic rate, and it is unclear to what extent these effects contribute to weight loss. Agents that regulate steroid metabolism, fatty acid oxidation, and other aspects of adipose tissue and skeletal muscle metabolism are under study. Dietary constituents also regulate thermogenesis, including methylxanthines (eg, caffeine), polyphenols (eg, resveratrol, quercetin), capsaicinoids (found in chili peppers and mustards), and medium-chain fatty acids, all of which represent potential therapeutic agents.

Overall efficacy of current obesity pharmacotherapy is the era of GLP1 agonists is promising. GLP-1 receptor agonists have shown significant promise in promoting weight loss and improving obesity-related comorbidities. Medications such as semaglutide and liraglutide have demonstrated an average weight loss of 10% to 15% in clinical trials, with some patients experiencing even greater reductions. This weight loss contributes to the resolution or improvement of comorbid conditions like hypertension, dyslipidemia, and obstructive sleep apnea. In the STEP trials, for example, semaglutide was associated with marked improvements in metabolic parameters, including reductions in blood pressure, triglycerides, and inflammatory markers.[21,22] These benefits highlight GLP-1 receptor agonists as a valuable therapeutic tool for both weight management and the reduction of obesity-related health risks.[23]

A complete summary of obesity pharmacotherapy is beyond the scope of this chapter, which has by necessity omitted important areas of research, including drugs that target steroid metabolism, lipid metabolism, adipocyte differentiation and proliferation, and efforts to shift white adipose tissue toward a brown adipose tissue phenotype (the "browning" of adipose tissue). This discussion has focused on agents designed to treat obesity directly with the goal of weight loss, but an important parallel class of drugs target metabolic disease independent of or in conjunction with weight loss. The activities of weight loss drugs are complex and overlapping, with many agents regulating body weight and metabolism via multiple mechanisms. Multiple redundancies in the regulation of energy homeostasis suggest that drug combinations will enhance efficacy. As an understanding of these mechanisms increases, safe and effective pharmacotherapy for obesity and metabolic disease will emerge.

SURGICAL MANAGEMENT

Bariatric Surgery—Beginnings

5 In contrast to lifestyle interventions and pharmacotherapy, surgical management of obesity is highly efficacious. Modern bariatric surgery (Gr. *baros,* heavy, burden) is the result of over half a century of evolution in surgical technique that has its genesis in the 1940s to 1950s with experiments in animals and isolated operations in humans that employed small intestinal resection and jejunocolic and ileocolic bypasses of various anatomic configurations. These operations involved substantial morbidity and did not achieve widespread acceptance, but set the stage for development of the *jejunoileal bypass,* the first bariatric operation to be widely applied in humans. Jejunoileal bypass involved division of the jejunum 14 in distal to the ligament of Treitz and creation of a jejunoileostomy 4 in proximal to the ileocecal valve, and was thus referred to as a "14–4 bypass." In 1969, Payne and DeWind[24] published the first report describing long-term clinical outcomes in a large group of patients who underwent jejunoileal bypass in the 1950 to 1960s, describing dramatic weight loss ("A total of 10,373 pounds have been lost by the [80] patients") along with improvements in insulin resistance, hypercholesterolemia, and hepatic steatosis. Jejunoileal bypass was widely used throughout the 1960s and early 1970s.

Despite its efficacy, as experience accumulated, it became clear that jejunoileal bypass was associated with significant morbidity. Diarrhea, steatorrhea, dehydration, electrolyte imbalances, and micro- and macronutrient deficiencies resulted from the highly malabsorptive nature of the operation. Patients also suffered a host of complications not obviously linked to malabsorption, including liver disease, nephropathy, arthropathy, neuropathy, and myopathy. While the cause of these latter complications was not completely clear, an immune response directed toward bacterial overgrowth in the blind intestinal limb was implicated. Overall morbidity afflicted as many as 70% of patients and led to abandonment of jejunoileal bypass by the late 1970s. Nonetheless, up to 30% of patients achieved good results, and the clinician may still encounter rare remaining patients. Indications for reversal or conversion to modern bariatric operations are not well established and must be considered on an individual basis, but include progressive liver or kidney disease not attributable to other causes. Some clinicians advocate reversal and conversion to a modern bariatric operation in all patients who are good operative candidates, regardless of the presence or absence of complications.

Gastric Bypass

With the decline of jejunoileal bypass, surgeons began searching for alternatives. In the 1960s, Edward Mason at the University of Iowa experimented with operations based on observations that patients who underwent gastric resections for ulcer disease had difficulty maintaining their weight. Mason's efforts led to the development of the *gastric bypass,* for which he earned the title "father of bariatric surgery." Mason's original gastric bypass consisted of a pouch gastroplasty with a loop gastrojejunostomy reconstruction. Gastric bypass subsequently evolved through a number of iterations, all with important clinical implications. Large horizontal fundal-based pouches were replaced with smaller vertical lesser curve–based pouches, which improve gastric emptying. Undivided gastric pouches were associated with high rates of staple-line dehiscence and gastro-gastric fistula, and were replaced with divided gastric bypass, expedited by the development of cutting staplers. Roux-en-Y reconstruction, compared to loop reconstruction, reduces tension on the gastrojejunal anastomosis and prevents bile reflux gastritis, but may be associated with higher rates of anastomotic ulcer disease. Retrocolic Roux limbs may improve pouch emptying and generate less tension on the gastrojejunostomy, but at the price of higher rates of mesocolic internal hernias. Banding of the gastrojejunal anastomosis may increase weight loss, but also increases risks of stenosis, obstruction, and erosion. Variations persist, including retrocolic Roux limbs, loop reconstructions ("minigastric bypass"), and prosthetic-banded gastric pouches. The modern gastric bypass practiced by the majority of surgeons today consists of a divided, unbanded, lesser curve-based pouch gastroplasty of 15 to 30 cc with an antecolic Roux-en-Y gastrojejunal reconstruction with a 100- to 150-cm Roux/alimentary limb and a 50- to 100-cm afferent/biliopancreatic limb (**Fig. 44.1**). The modern gastric bypass is a robust operation because within limits, subtle variations in technique, including pouch size and morphology and intestinal limb length and position, do not greatly affect efficacy or morbidity. Gastric bypass remains, as of this writing, the dominant bariatric operation worldwide and the gold standard against which all other operations are measured.

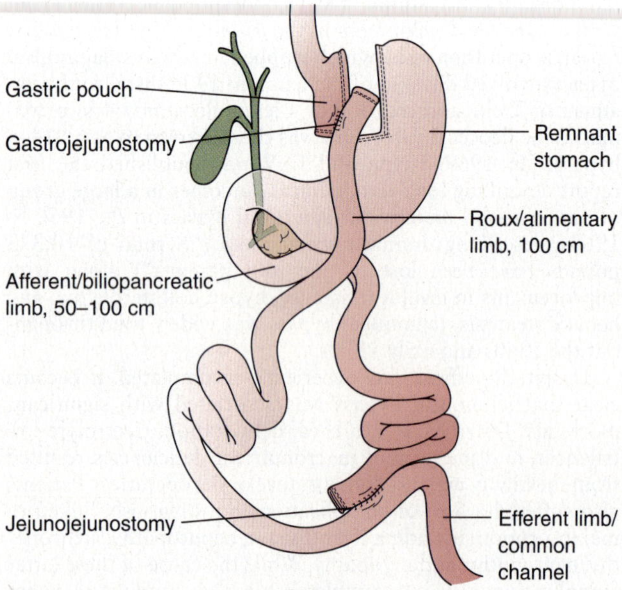

Figure 44.1. Anatomy of modern Roux-en-Y gastric bypass. Modern gastric bypass consists of a divided pouch gastroplasty with Roux-en-Y jejunojejunal reconstruction. The Roux limb is most commonly placed in the antecolic position. Intestinal limbs are termed with either standard Roux (Roux, afferent, efferent) or bariatric (alimentary, biliopancreatic, common channel) nomenclature as shown.

Malabsorption Revisited

Despite the failure of jejunoileal bypass, interest in operations that relied on small intestine bypass persisted. *Biliopancreatic diversion (BPD)* consists of an antrectomy with a gastrojejunostomy and distal Roux-en-Y jejunoileostomy. The *duodenal switch modification of the BPD* involves a sleeve gastrectomy, division of the duodenum distal to the pylorus, and a duodenojejunostomy and distal Roux-en-Y jejunoileostomy, thus maintaining the pylorus in the alimentary stream (**Fig. 44.2**). BPD/duodenal switch differs from jejunoileal bypass in two important regards. First, maintenance of forward flow of biliopancreatic effluent in the bypassed afferent limb prevents stasis and bacterial overgrowth. Second, common channel length was increased to 100 cm, reducing malabsorptive complications. BPD/duodenal switch provides weight loss and metabolic disease remission equivalent to, and in many series, greater than gastric bypass. Morbidity and mortality for BPD/duodenal switch span a wide range, with centers with significant expertise reporting low rates similar to gastric bypass. Nonetheless, when the literature as a whole is considered, BPD/duodenal switch is associated with higher morbidity and mortality than gastric bypass. Perioperative mortality reported by meta-analyses is at least twofold higher than gastric bypass, possibly due to a higher risk of anastomotic dehiscence, as laparoscopic creation of the duodenojejunal anastomosis associated with the duodenal switch modification is technically challenging.[25] Late malabsorptive complications, which may require surgical revision, while much improved over jejunoileal bypass, range from 2% to 20%. Unlike gastric bypass, in which small changes in pouch size or limb length do not substantially alter clinical outcome, outcomes of BPD/duodenal switch are relatively sensitive to differences in efferent limb length, small changes in which may make the difference between poor weight loss and malabsorptive complications. Predicting the correct efferent limb length for an individual patient is challenging. Most surgeons advocate a fixed length of 100 cm, while others advocate an ad hoc limb length proportional to total small intestine length. While advocated by select surgeons and associated with good outcomes in centers with significant experience, BPD/duodenal switch is nonetheless waning in use, currently comprising less than 2% of bariatric operations. Recently, the single anastomosis duodenal switch has emerged as an effective bariatric procedure for treating severe obesity and associated comorbidities. Technically simpler than the duodenal switch, it combines a sleeve gastrectomy with a single loop bypass of the small intestine, resulting in significant malabsorption and restriction. Clinical outcomes have shown impressive long-term weight loss, with patients often achieving a 75% to 85% excess weight loss. Studies have highlighted its benefits in achieving durable weight loss and metabolic improvements, though nutritional deficiencies remain a concern, requiring careful follow-up.[26]

Pure Restriction

In Mason's era, morbidity from gastric bypass was not trivial. In an effort to design a simpler and safer operation, Mason experimented with gastroplasties that precluded the need for small intestinal reconstruction. Like gastric bypass, these operations evolved through a number of iterations, eventually leading to the modern *vertical banded gastroplasty,* which involves creation of a partitioned upper stomach pouch with a prosthetic band restricting pouch outlet diameter. Vertical banded gastroplasty achieved widespread acceptance and peaked in the 1970s to 1980s. Vertical banded gastroplasty weight loss is substantially less and late weight regain substantially greater

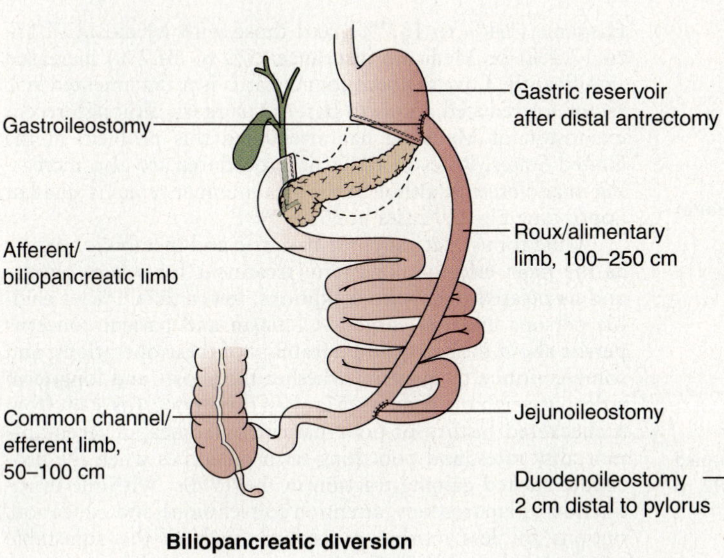

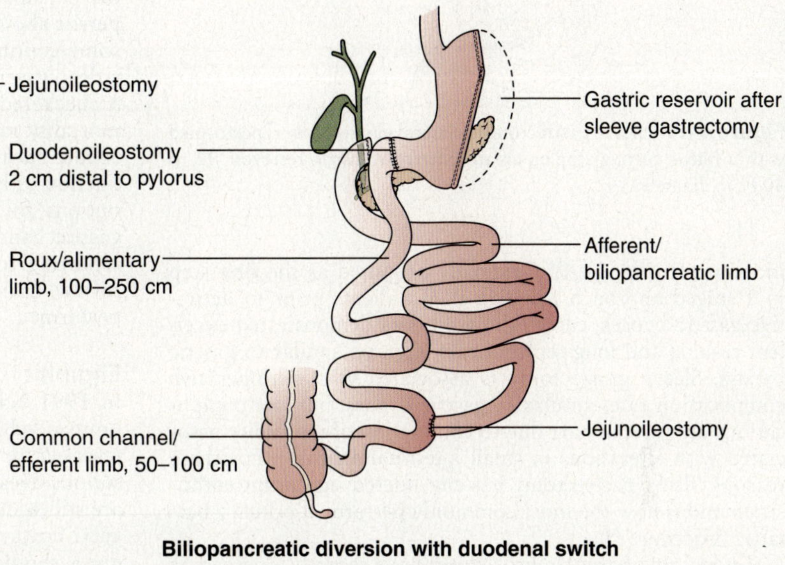

Figure 44.2. Biliopancreatic diversion (BPD). BPD involves a distal antrectomy with a Roux-en-Y jejunoileal reconstruction; BPD+DS involves a sleeve gastrectomy with a Roux-en-Y duodenoileal reconstruction, with the duodenoileostomy created 2 cm distal to the pylorus, thus preserving the pyloric emptying mechanism. Note that, unlike JIBP, the afferent/biliopancreatic jejunoileal limb is in continuity with biliopancreatic effluent, reducing limb stasis.

compared to gastric bypass, however, and vertical banded gastroplasty has therefore been relegated to a minority operation that is rapidly being eliminated from use.

Study of prosthetic bands applied to the upper stomach to limit food intake began in the late 1970s using devices made from Prolene, Marlex, and other materials. These devices were nonadjustable and plagued with complications related to erosion, migration, stenosis, and obstruction. Efforts persisted, eventually culminating in the modern *adjustable gastric band*, a silicone device that was FDA approved in the United States in 2001 (**Fig. 44.3**). A primary advantage of gastric band is its technical simplicity and low rates of major morbidity and mortality. Unlike gastric bypass, which continues to be associated with low but finite rates of anastomotic dehiscence and mortality, gastric band is associated with 5 to 10 lower rates of life-threatening complications and mortality. Much enthusiasm accompanied the introduction of gastric band in the late 1990s, but over the past decade, enthusiasm has waned for two reasons. First, therapeutic efficacy of gastric band in the majority of patients is substantially less than gastric bypass. Second, as years passed, late complication rates have increased. These complications, including band slippage, erosion, esophageal dilation, and development of gastroesophageal reflux disease (GERD), are usually not life threatening, but range between 10% and 50% and often lead to band removal.[27] Despite these problems, gastric band efficacy, while not as high as gastric bypass, is acceptable. Gastric band remains the bariatric operation with the lowest major morbidity and mortality rates, an appealing quality for risk-averse patients. Gastric band does not require Roux-en-Y reconstruction, an advantage in patients with complex abdominal surgical histories. However, given the known late-term complications and availability of sleeve gastrectomy, gastric bands have fallen out of favor and as of 2018 comprise only 1.1% of bariatric operations.[28]

Sleeve gastrectomy was introduced initially as a component of the duodenal switch modification of BPD, but did not gain significant attention as a stand-alone bariatric operation until the early 2000s. Sleeve gastrectomy involves a lateral gastrectomy, leaving a narrow "sleeve" of stomach 32 to 40 Fr

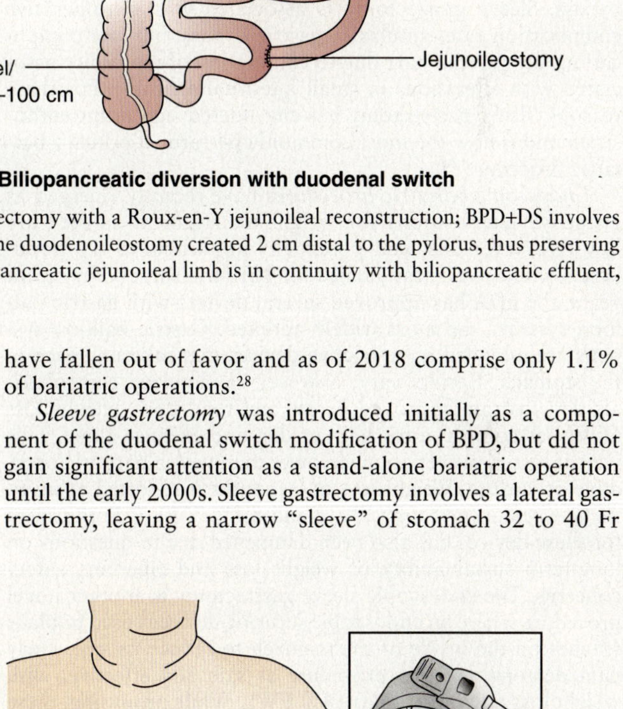

Figure 44.3. Gastric band. A silicone adjustable band is positioned around the upper stomach, creating a gastric pouch. A port attached to the band via silicone tubing is placed in the subcutaneous tissue in the abdominal wall, permitting percutaneous access and adjustment of band diameter.

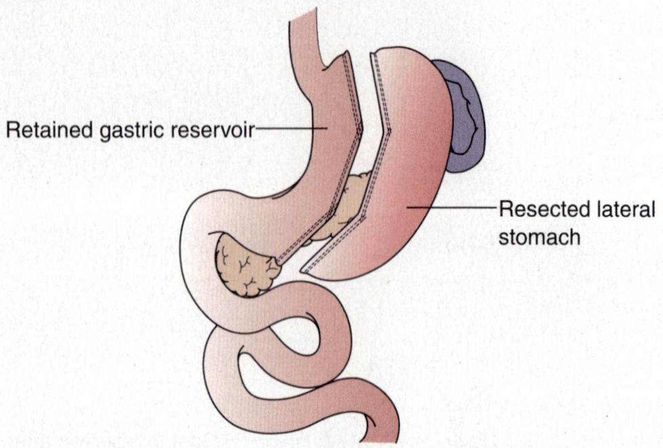

Figure 44.4. Sleeve gastrectomy. A lateral gastrectomy is performed with a linear cutting stapler, creating narrow gastric reservoir 32 to 40 Fr in diameter.

in diameter (**Fig. 44.4**). Originally proposed as the first step in a staged approach for high BMI patients prior to definitive gastric bypass, early follow-up data demonstrated excellent results, and long-term efficacy appears similar to gastric bypass. Sleeve gastrectomy is associated with perioperative complication rates similar to gastric bypass, but late complications are rare, in part due to elimination of morbidity associated with alterations in small intestinal anatomy. For these reasons, sleeve gastrectomy has engendered significant enthusiasm and is now the most commonly performed primary bariatric procedure.[28]

Endoscopic bariatric procedures have recently emerged as attractive interventions for weight management as they are low risk, reversible, and potentially applicable to the population who are not candidates for bariatric surgery. In recent years, the FDA has approved several devices with gastric balloon systems, the most widely adopted. Gastric balloon systems are intended as restrictive devices that take up space in the stomach. Results vary; however, randomized control trials demonstrate improved excess and total body weight loss (TWL) as compared to sham or diet and exercise alone. This weight loss, however, is much lower than with a bariatric operative procedure. Weight loss at 9 months is reported at up to 26% *excess weight lost* (EWL) and 8.8% TWL.[29] Enthusiasm for these devices has also been dampened due to questions on long-term sustainability of weight loss and emerging safety concerns. The endoscopic sleeve gastrectomy is another novel procedure where an endoscopic suturing device is used to place stitches on the inside of the stomach to reduce its size. Early data demonstrate this procedure as safe and effective, with weight loss outcomes up to 18% EWL. While promising, these procedures should be used in select patients and should not be used in lieu of bariatric surgical procedures where indicated.[30]

Epidemiology of Modern Bariatric Surgery

As of 2022, approximately 280,000 bariatric procedures were performed per year in the United States. Currently, sleeve gastrectomy accounts for the vast majority of primary bariatric procedures at 60%. Gastric bypass accounts for 18% of all procedures and the gastric band and duodenal switch each account for less than 3%. Revisions of bariatric procedures either for complication or weight recidivism have dramatically increased in recent time. In the last 3 years, approximately 14% all bariatric procedures were revisions.[28] The characteristics of the patient population undergoing bariatric surgery have also changed over the past two decades. Nationally representative data show that the mean age increased from 38.9 years in 1993 to 44.4 years in 2016 ($P < .001$).[3] Additionally, the proportion of male patients (15.3% to 20.4%), patients who self-identified as Black (11.6% to 17.7%) or Hispanic (1.4% to 13.7%), and those with Medicaid (8.1% to 17.2%) or Medicare insurance (5% to 14.2%) increased significantly. Low socioeconomic status is a documented risk factor for reduced access to bariatric surgery, although recent expansion of Medicaid has attenuated this problem in the United States. Rates of bariatric procedures are also increasing in adolescents, although the total number remains small at approximately 220 cases in 2016.[28,31–33]

While robust data support bariatric and metabolic surgery as the most effective long-term treatment for severe obesity and associated metabolic conditions, fewer than 1% of eligible persons undergo surgery. Clinician and patient concerns persist about the safety and durability of these operations, and some continue to question whether the short- and long-term risks outweigh the benefits. Many of these concerns stem from a checkered history of poor patient outcomes, unacceptable mortality rates, and poor long-term outcomes when the procedure started gaining traction in the 1990s. With the introduction of laparoscopy, attention to technique and education, options for less morbid procedures such as the adjustable gastric band, and accreditation programs requiring outcome reporting to a national registry and multidisciplinary team review, bariatric surgery is now among the safest operations performed.

Eligibility

In 1991 National Institutes of Health (NIH) guidelines recommended that the surgical treatment for obesity should be reserved for persons with a BMI ≥40 kg/m^2 or ≥35 kg/m^2 with serious obesity-related comorbid condition.[28] These guidelines are still widely used by insurers to determine eligibility for surgery; however, there is growing evidence that bariatric procedures should also be considered for patients with lower BMI (30.0 to 34.9 kg/m^2) and type II diabetes if hyperglycemia is inadequately controlled despite optimal medical treatment.[34] Recent guidelines also recommend the need for separate cutoff limits for Asian populations, and recommend consideration of surgery for BMI ≥35 kg/m^2 regardless of the existence of comorbidities, and BMI ≥35 kg/m^2 with the existence of a comorbid condition.[35] All persons who meet the BMI threshold should be further evaluated with a thorough history and physical to mitigate and optimize comorbid conditions, nutritional and psychological evaluation. Patients may be contraindicated for bariatric surgery if they have severe heart failure, unstable coronary artery disease, end-stage lung disease, active or recent history of cancer, cirrhosis with portal hypertension, uncontrolled drug or alcohol dependency, unstable psychiatric disorders, Crohn disease, severely impaired intellectual capacity, or if they are pregnant or planning to become pregnant within the next 1 to 2 years.[36]

Efficacy

Bariatric surgery achieves dramatic results. Weight loss was commonly reported as a percentage of EWL, defined as the difference between presurgical weight and ideal weight, with ideal weight calculated for BMI = 25 for height. Of note, there has been a recent effort to standardize weight loss reporting as percent TWL, total pounds lost divided but initial weight, to align with the medical literature, as TWL is less dependent than EWL on initial BMI.[37] Weight loss typically peaks 1 to 2 years after surgery and may approach 70% to 90% EWL, followed by partial weight regain at 3 to 10 years after surgery, leading to a plateau at 50% to 70% EWL at long-term follow-up.[37–67] The mechanisms underlying this weight loss pattern are unknown but may involve development of adaptive eating patterns that increase caloric intake over time. For gastric band, weight loss is typically slower and more gradual, with a plateau after 2 to 3 years. These varying patterns of weight loss complicate comparison of results of different operations and analysis of published data due to variable length of follow-up among studies. Analysis is further complicated

Table 44.1. Bariatric Surgery Long-Term Weight Loss Responses. Short-Term Comparative Outcomes at 2 Years

	RYGB	SG	BPD/DS
Weight Loss			
% EBWL	61.4–79.8 (21,22,32, 34,115)	60.8–77.8 (32,34,115)	65.1–69.4 (21,25)
% EBMIL	74.7–84.8 (3,19–22,33)	72.1–74.7 (11,33)	76.1–85.0 (16,21,25)
% TBWL	21.0–37.4 (19–22)	23.4–34.1 (23,24)	33.8–36.7 (21,25)
Comorbidities			
Diabetes remission; %	66.7–75.0 (21,69,70)	35.0–41.0 (70,71)	95.0–100 (21,69)
Hypertension remission; %	53.0–65.4 (75)	54.0–72.0 (36,37)	49.3–76.0 (37,76)
Dyslipidemia remission; %	52.0–57.0 (75,77)	60.0–65.2 (36,82)	70.0–92.1 (76,77)
GERD remission; %	61.0 (77)	77.4 (36)	48.0 (77)
OSA remission; %	29.0–100.0 (19,28,33, 35–39)	56.2–100.0 (19,28,33, 35–39)	80.0–100.0 (19,28,33, 35–39)

RYGB, Roux-en-Y gastric bypass; SG, sleeve gastrectomy; BPD/DS, biliopancreatic diversion with/without duodenal switch; % EBWL, percent excess body weight loss; % EBMIL, percent excess body mass index loss; % TBWL, percent total body weight loss; GERD, gastroesophageal reflux disease; OSA, obstructive sleep apnea.

by significant attrition of patients over long-term follow-up in most studies. Despite these challenges, meta-analyses, controlled trials, and uncontrolled case series provide estimates of the efficacy of bariatric operations (**Table 44.1**). Weight loss is highest for BPD/duodenal switch, ranging from 55% to 75% EWL, followed by gastric bypass and sleeve gastrectomy (50% to 70% EWL) and gastric band (40% to 60% EWL).[37–39]

Rates of improvement and remission of metabolic diseases parallel weight loss, with gastric bypass, sleeve gastrectomy, and BPD/duodenal switch associated with higher remission rates than gastric band. Diabetes, steatosis, sleep apnea, hypertension, and hyperlipidemia improvement/remission rates range from 60% to over 90% (**Table 44.1**). Weight loss is durable, lasting decades in most patients, and accompanied by marked reductions in long-term incident diabetes, cardiovascular disease, and cancer, increased quality of life, reduced long-term healthcare costs, and a 25% to 40% reduction in long-term mortality. Currently, 12 randomized controlled trials have been published and demonstrate that bariatric surgery is substantially more efficacious than medical therapy for weight loss and diabetes, and multiple medical societies, including the American Diabetes Association, the International Diabetes Federation, and the American Heart Association, endorse bariatric surgery as treatment for metabolic disease.[37–67]

Despite its efficacy, results of bariatric surgery are variable, with a substantial minority of patients achieving significantly better than average weight loss and disease response rates, while a similar minority experience suboptimal results. Anywhere from 10% to 30% of patients achieve <50% EWL, which may be due to insufficient initial weight loss or weight regain after a period of adequate weight loss. Mechanisms underlying insufficient weight loss are poorly defined, and identification of accurate predictors of response to surgery is an important area of research.[44] While suboptimal results are often attributed to lack of patient compliance with postoperative diet and exercise, these arguments ring false, echoing similar arguments that attribute obesity itself to a lack of "willpower." Instead, compelling evidence implicates genetic and epigenetic mechanisms. Like obesity itself, responses to bariatric surgery are highly heritable. Ethnicity is a predictor of outcome, with Caucasians and Hispanics experiencing greater weight loss than Blacks and Asians. Multiple single-nucleotide polymorphisms have been linked to surgical outcome. Future research will identify clinical and genetic predictors of response and permit optimization of allocation of surgical resources (**Table 44.2**).[37–67]

STOMACH AND DUODENUM

Perioperative Mortality and Morbidity

Morbidity and mortality associated with bariatric surgery have
6 decreased over the past two decades as surgeons experience increased and techniques evolved. Currently, gastric bypass and sleeve gastrectomy are associated with mortality risks similar to hip replacement. Perioperative mortality is highest for BPD/duodenal switch, followed by gastric bypass and sleeve gastrectomy, then gastric band (**Table 44.3**).[68–77] Life-threatening perioperative morbidity associated with gastric bypass and sleeve gastrectomy consists primarily of anastomotic dehiscence, staple-line leaks, hemorrhage, thromboembolic events, and cardiac events. Life-threatening perioperative morbidity associated with gastric band is rare and consists primarily of gastric perforation, thromboembolic events, and cardiac events.

The most dire perioperative complication of gastric bypass is anastomotic dehiscence of the gastrojejunostomy which usually occurs within 2 weeks of surgery. Incidences in most series range from 0.1% to 4%, although recent data suggest that anastomotic dehiscence rates are decreasing and high-volume centers report rates in the range of 0.1% to 0.2%. Signs and symptoms are similar to those of anastomotic dehiscence after any intestinal operation, but may be less apparent in the obese. Persistent tachycardia and abdominal pain are important but nonspecific sentinel signs. Upper GI radiographs may be of diagnostic utility but lack sensitivity. Abdominal CT scan, even within a few days of surgery, may be useful, as the lack of a fluid collection near the gastrojejunostomy has a high negative predictive value for leak, while contrast extravasation has a high positive predictive value. Nonetheless, data are conflicting regarding the sensitivity and specificity of radiologic studies for diagnosing anastomotic dehiscence, and laparoscopic reexploration should be employed aggressively in suspected cases. Operative management consists of washout, wide drainage, judicious attempt at repair, and consideration of distal enteral access, usually with a gastrostomy tube in the remnant stomach, although a jejunostomy tube in the distal Roux limb or biliary limb is an option if access to the remnant stomach is difficult. Anastomotic dehiscence can be managed laparoscopically in some cases, reducing the high risk of ventral hernia associated with laparotomy. Most will heal if sepsis is controlled. Endoscopic management of anastomotic dehiscence with suture, over-the-scope clipping systems, and endoscopic esophageal stent placement may also be employed for appropriate patients by advanced endoscopists with the appropriate skill set and training.

Staple-line leaks are an equally dire event after sleeve gastrectomy, occurring anywhere from 1 to 2 weeks to many months after surgery. Leaks may occur at any point along the staple line, but when involving the thicker tissue of the antrum may be less prone to heal, and interval conversion to gastric bypass with resection of the involved portion of gastric sleeve may be necessary. Depending on the acuity and location of the leak and the clinical status of the patient, a

Table 44.2. Bariatric Surgery Long-Term Comorbidity Responses. Mid- and Long-Term Comparative Outcomes at 3 to 10 Years

	RYGB			SG			BPD/DS		
	Mid Term	Long Term		Mid Term	Long Term		Mid Term	Long Term	
	3 y	5 y	10 y	3 y	5 y	10 y	3 y	5 y	10 y
Weight Loss									
% EBWL	61.7–83.0 (13,22,32,34,115)	66.6–74.8 (13,22,32)	57.1–69.0 (13,22)	61.1–68.5 (32,34,115)	60.3–65.1 (32,121)	52.5 (29)	83.0 (15)	63.8–79.3 (25,122,123)	67.9–73.4 (25,31)
% EBMIL	64.1–78.2 (19,3,4,33,13,22)	46.1–79.8 (4,13,17,19,22,26)	52.5–71.3 (13,19,22)	70.9–82.4 (27,33)	59.0–74.8 (28,121)	62.5[a] (27)	—	71.1–74.9 (17,25,26)	66.2–78.9 (25,30,31)
% TBWL	29.4–35.3 (13,19,22)	25.6–34.4 (13,17,19,22,26)	27.7–29.6 (13,19,22)	28.2–34.6 (24,27)	23.6–25.1 (24,28)	21.0[a]–26.3 (27,29)	45.2 (15)	31.1–40.7 (17,25,26)	33.4–39.0 (25,30,31)
Comorbidities									
Diabetes remission; %	77.0–90.0 (33,34,69)	37.0–66.7 (69,70)	42.6–54.7 (19,73)	60.0–91.2 (33,34,72)	26.0–80.0 (28,70–72)	—	90.0–93.1 (37,69)	63.0–91.7 (69)	91.3 (74)
Hypertension remission; %	52.0–71.2 (33,34,68)	42.0–57.0 (75,79)	20.4 (19)	65.2–80.0 (33,34,36,72)	52.9–54.5 (28,72)	—	68.0–85.8 (77,78)	70.6–88.4 (78,80)	80.9–91.4 (78,81)
Dyslipidemia remission; %	26.3–90.0 (34,77)	51.4–53.0 (39,75)	—	57.4–75.0 (34,36,72)	25.0–52.2 (28,72)	—	72.0–79.1 (77,80)	61.9 (83)	50.9–95.0 (74,81)
GERD remission; %	64.7–100 (33,34,77,86)	—	25.5 (19)	61.0–100 (33,34,36)	30.8–95.7 (38)	—	48.6 (77)	—	—
OSA remission%	74.0–85.0 (19,28,33,35–39)	50.0–93.5 (19,28,33,35–39)	54.7 (19,28,33,35–39)	23.0–100.0 (19,28,33,35–39)	33.0–88.9 (19,28,33,35–39)	—	74.0 (19,28,33,35–39)	—	—

RYGB, Roux-en-Y gastric bypass; SG, sleeve gastrectomy; BPD/DS, biliopancreatic diversion with/without duodenal switch; % EBWL, percent excess body weight loss; % EBMIL, percent excess body mass index loss; % TBWL, percent total body weight loss; GERD, gastroesophageal reflux disease; OSA, obstructive sleep apnea.

[a]Outcomes at 11+ years.

Table 44.3. Bariatric Surgery Perioperative Mortality and Morbidity. Early and Late Comparative Complications[78–84]

	RYGB	SG	BPD/DS
Early <30 d			
VTE; %	0.1–1.1 (10,11,79,117,118)	0.0–1.7 (10,11,37,117,118)	0.2–3.4 (10,15,15,37,117,124)
Leak; %	0.2–6.5 (10,11,16,19,79,114–117,125,126)	0.1–2.8 (10,11,24,37,114,117,121,127,128)	0.0–8.4 (10,15,16,37,116,117,124,129)
Bleeding; %	0.8–2.0 (10,11,19,114,115,117)	0.5–5.7 (10,11,24,37,114,115,117,121,128)	0.4–3.4 (10,15,37,117,123,124)
SBO/Sleeve Stenosis; %	0.1–5.3 (21,79,114,116,117)	0.1–3.5 (24,114,128,130)	0.5–7.7 (15,116,117,124,131)
Death; %	0.0–0.8 (16,114–116,132)	0.0–0.02 (24,114,115,121)	0.6–4.1 (16,74,116,129,133)
PNA; %	0.4 (11,16)	0.4–0.6 (11,121)	0.4–0.9 (15,16,123)
SSI; %	0.0–5.2 (11,16,19,79,114,115,117)	0.0–2.0 (11,114,115,117,121)	0.6–5.1 (15,16,117,123,124)
Readmission; %	0.4–1.9 (11,114)	1.6–4.5 (11,114,128)	2.8–6.7 (74,124)
Reoperation; %	1.0–3.9 (11,16,114,117)	1.2–5.6 (11,24,114,117)	0.6–3.5 (15,16,74,117,124)
Late >30 d; %			
Readmission; %	3.3–29.0 (114,120,126)	1.0–32.0 (114,120)	8.0–17.2 (74,126)
Reoperation; %	1.3–4.8 (11,16,19,114)	0.5–10.2 (11,114)	1.1–13.0 (16,74)

RYGB, Roux-en-Y gastric bypass; SG, sleeve gastrectomy; BPD/DS, biliopancreatic diversion with/without duodenal switch; VTE, venous thromboembolism; SBO, small bowel obstruction; PNA, pneumonia; SSI, surgical site infection.

wide variety of options may be used to manage sleeve leaks. Options range from nasogastric tube feeding and antibiotics with or without external drainage, to endoscopic interventions such as those mentioned above as well as internal drainage with a pigtail catheter, to operative intervention with wide drainage and potential conversion to RYGB. For chronic leaks that have matured and contain a fibrous septum, endoscopic septotomy has demonstrated reasonable success for definitive treatment. Proper stapler selection and use during primary operation with avoidance of overly narrow sleeves (current consensus recommends 32- to 40-Fr diameter) may reduce the risk of sleeve gastrectomy staple-line leaks, which currently occur with an incidence of approximately 1% to 3%. Gastric band is only rarely associated with perioperative septic complications, most often in the form of gastric perforation, which occurs in 0% to 0.5% of cases. Perforation, if not recognized, may be life threatening and is a primary cause of rare perioperative mortality and major morbidity after gastric band.

Perioperative hemorrhage after gastric bypass occurs with an incidence of 1% to 4%, often originating from staple lines, and may be intraperitoneal or intraluminal. Intraluminal bleeding presents with melena and is often self-limited, requiring only transfusion and observation. Infrequently, endoscopic or operative intervention may be necessary. Hemorrhage after sleeve gastrectomy ranges from 1% to 4%, is usually intraperitoneal from the gastric staple line, and may require operative intervention, although observation in the hemodynamically stable patient is a reasonable initial course. Early small bowel obstruction and thromboembolic, pulmonary, and cardiac events comprise the majority of the remainder of acute postoperative complications after bariatric surgery. Pathophysiology is not substantially different than after nonbariatric GI operations, although the obese may be at higher risk, reinforcing the importance of preoperative evaluation and preparation.

Late Morbidity

Late morbidity after bariatric surgery is similar to that associated with complex nonbariatric GI operations, may occur months or years later, and often presents with abdominal pain. Gallbladder disease and small bowel obstruction from adhesions and ventral/trocar hernias may occur after all bariatric operations. Other complications are operation specific. While definitions vary, overall late morbidity rates for gastric bypass range from 5% to 10%. Many late complications of gastric bypass result from Roux-en-Y anatomy. Internal hernias occur in 0.5% to 9% of patients, and are categorized as mesenteric (common to all Roux-en-Y reconstructions, in which bowel passes through the mesenteric split in the Roux limb), mesocolic (specific to retrocolic reconstructions, in which bowel passes through the mesocolic defect created for the Roux limb), and Petersen (more often associated with antecolic than retrocolic reconstructions, in which bowel passes under the Roux limb and its mesentery) (**Fig. 44.5**).[68] Closure of internal hernia defects at primary operation is straightforward and recommended, and recent meta-analyses suggest that this practice

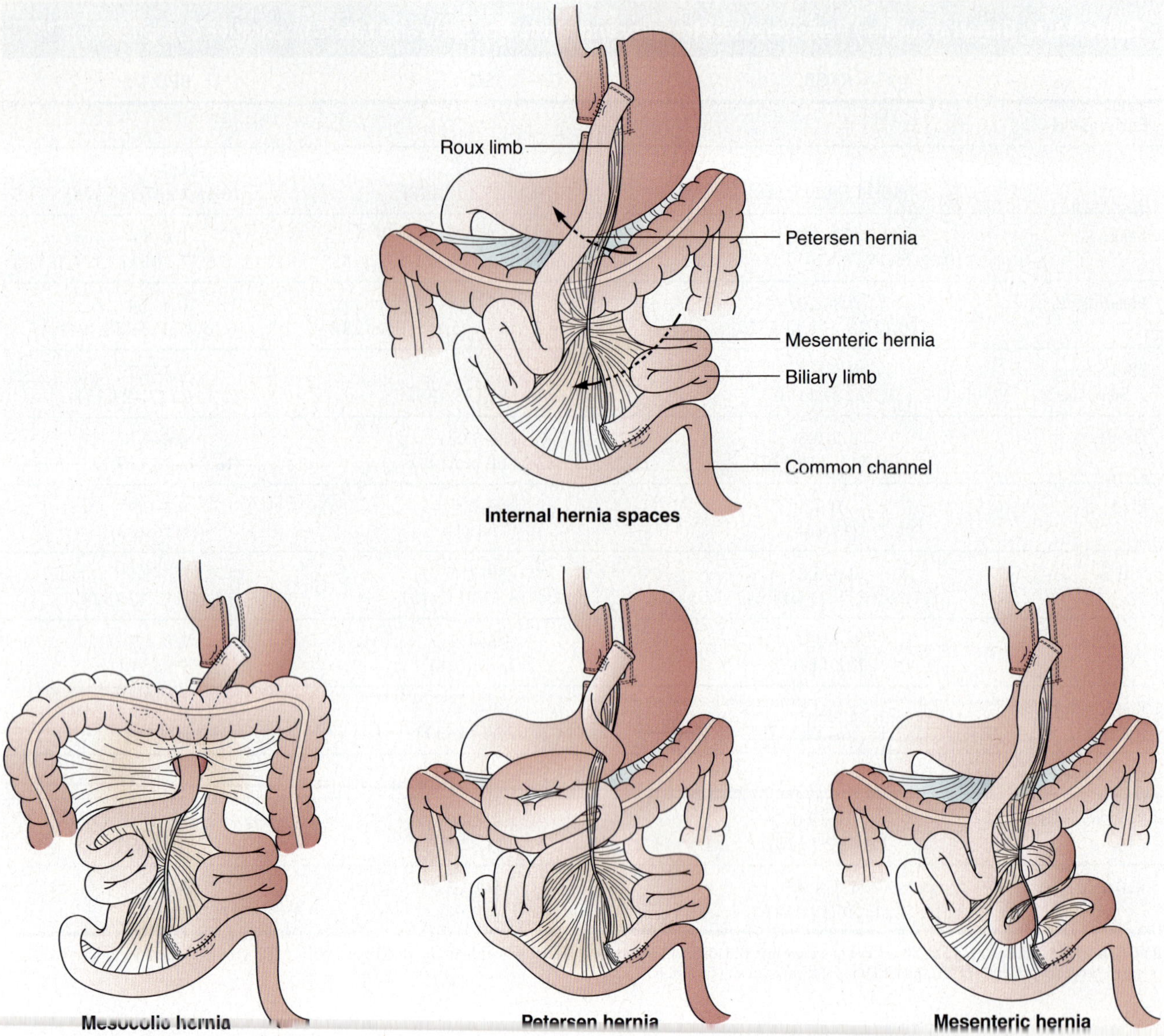

Figure 44.5. Internal hernias. Internal hernias may occur after any Roux-en-Y reconstruction, and include mesenteric, Petersen, and mesocolic hernias. Weight loss after gastric bypass and loss of adipose tissue in the intestinal mesentery may predispose to internal herniation.

likely reduces internal hernia rates, but does not obviate the future risk of hernia.[68] Patients often present years after surgery with a history of severe episodic abdominal pain. Diagnosis may be challenging, as obstipation may be absent and imaging normal even in the face of incarceration, especially if the biliopancreatic limb, which is out of continuity with the alimentary stream, is involved. A low threshold for operative exploration must be maintained in any patient with unrelenting abdominal pain after gastric bypass. Operative reduction and closure of internal hernia defects can usually be performed via a laparoscopic approach.

Gastrojejunal anastomotic ulcer occurs in 0.5% to 25% of patients after gastric bypass, with the majority of series reporting incidences between 2% and 8%. Tobacco or NSAID use increases risk, but ulcers may occur in the absence of these risk factors. Diagnosis by upper endoscopy is usually straightforward. Upper GI radiography is advisable to rule out an associated gastrogastric fistula, especially if an ulcer is recalcitrant to medical treatment or is associated with weight regain. Most ulcers heal with high-dose antacid therapy, and once healed, most surgeons recommend maintenance antacid therapy for life, although data supporting this practice are sparse. Rarely, ulcers recalcitrant to medical therapy require resection with anastomotic revision or reversal of the gastric bypass. Large pouches are a risk factor for ulcers due to retention of parietal cells in the distal gastric pouch that do not participate in negative inhibition of gastrin secretion, thus rationalizing pouch resection and anastomosis revision as a treatment strategy. Gastrogastric fistula occurs with an incidence of 0% to 2% and may be associated with ulcers. Gastrogastric fistula incidence has decreased substantially since the advent of divided gastric bypass. Gastrogastric fistula often results from incomplete division of the gastric pouch from the gastric remnant at primary operation. Stenosis of the gastrojejunostomy typically presents with intolerance of solid foods and vomiting within 1 to 3 months of surgery with a wide range of reported incidences from <1% to >20%, but most commonly 3% to 7%. Stenosis is usually easily treated with endoscopic dilation, although rare cases may require anastomotic revision. Retrograde intussusception at the jejunojejunostomy is a rare cause of abdominal pain after gastric bypass with a reported incidence of 0.1%. Pathogenesis is likely related to motility disorders resulting from disruption of enteroenteric nerves and divorce of the small intestine from duodenal pacemaker plexi with subsequent development of aberrant ectopic pacemakers in the involved intestinal limbs. Diagnosis may be challenging and imaging unreliable. Treatment consists of either plication/pexy of involved limbs or resection and revision of the

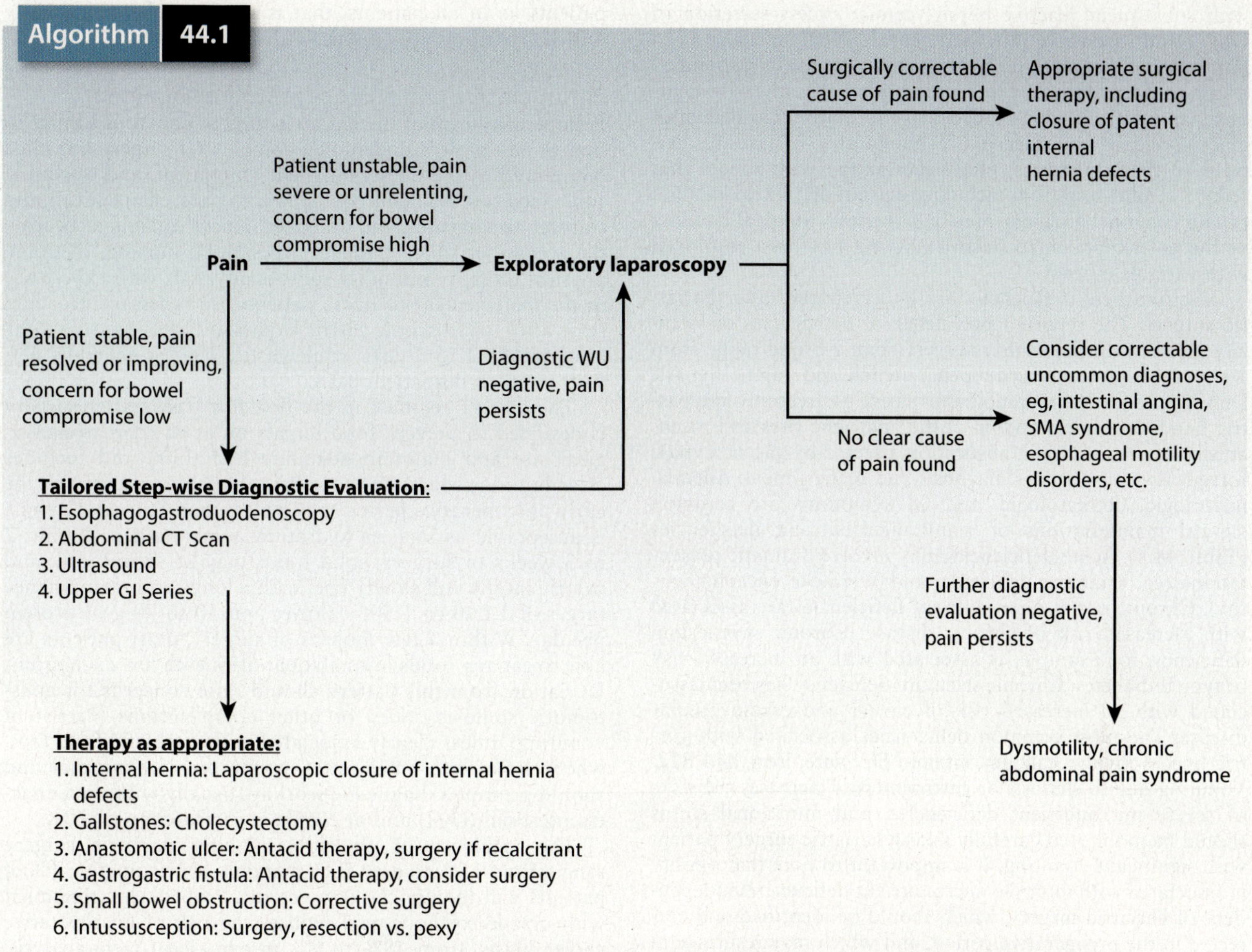

Algorithm 44.1. Algorithm for management of abdominal pain months or years after Roux-en-Y reconstruction.

jejunojejunostomy, with the latter approach associated with lower rates of recurrence.

The clinical presentation and differential diagnosis of abdominal pain after gastric bypass is diverse and diagnostic imaging may be unreliable. The clinician is not infrequently faced with a gastric bypass patient who presents with persistent pain in the absence of a clear cause after thorough diagnostic evaluation. Exploratory laparoscopy in such patients provides a diagnosis in up to 90% of cases. Even in the absence of intraoperative findings other than patent internal hernia defects without incarceration, closure of defects provides relief in the majority of patients. Less commonly, in the absence of a clear cause, pain is presumed to result from atypical motility disorders associated with Roux-en-Y anatomy and may be difficult to treat (**Algorithm 44.1**).

Rates of reoperation following bariatric surgery range from 5% to 22.1%, with higher rates of reoperation for the gastric bypass as compared to sleeve gastrectomy. However, two small randomized control trials reported no significant difference in 5-year rates of reoperations between the two operations. Specifically, the SLEEVEPASS trial reported an 8.3% reoperation rate following sleeve gastrectomy and a 15.1% rate of reoperation for gastric bypass.[77] Data from the SM-BOSS trial mirrored these finding with rates of reoperation at 15.8% for sleeve gastrectomy versus 22.1% for gastric bypass.[85] Later complications of sleeve gastrectomy include stricture, stenosis, or GERD. GERD is a more frequent complication for patients who undergo sleeve gastrectomy. While many patients respond to therapy with antacid medication, conversion to a gastric bypass may be required for those with refractory symptoms. As such, gastric bypass is often the procedure choice for patients with both severe obesity and GERD due to the reduction of acid in a small gastric pouch and a long Roux limb. There is increasing clinical concern that sleeve gastrectomy may worsen GERD or increase risk for development of Barrett esophagus. Studies are mixed in their findings of symptoms or complications of GERD after a sleeve gastrectomy.

Late complications after gastric band are common, afflicting 10% to 50% of patients, may occur years after primary operation, and include band slippage, band erosion, and development of GERD and esophageal motility disorders. Treatment often requires band explant, with late explant rates of 30% to 50% in some series.

Bariatric operations alter absorption of macro- and micronutrients. Protein and lipid malabsorption, steatorrhea, and protein wasting are rare after modern gastric bypass and virtually absent with gastric band and sleeve gastrectomy, but afflict anywhere from 2% to 20% of patients after BPD/duodenal switch.[86,87] The elimination of the pyloric emptying mechanism in gastric bypass is associated with dumping and hypoglycemic syndromes, the underlying mechanisms of which are not well understood. Early dumping occurs within 10 to 30 minutes of a meal, and is thought to result from intraluminal fluid shifts and acute intravascular volume depletion secondary to rapid emptying of hyperosmolar gastric contents into the small intestine. Early dumping is associated with tachycardia and diaphoresis. Aberrations in gut hormone secretion, including elevated secretion of vasoactive intestinal polypeptide, enteroglucagon, pancreatic polypeptide, and GLP-1, have been associated with a predisposition to early dumping. Late dumping occurs hours after a meal and is thought to be due to hypersecretion of insulin with subsequent reactive hypoglycemia; excess secretion of GLP-1 and vasoactive intestinal peptide (VIP) have also been implicated. Dumping and hypoglycemia typically respond to a low-carbohydrate diet and preprandial therapy with acarbose, an intestinal alpha glucosidase inhibitor that decreases glucose release from ingested carbohydrates. In cases recalcitrant to these measures, pharmacotherapy with agents that reduce insulin secretion, including octreotide, diazoxide, and calcium channel blockers, may be of benefit. Surgical banding of the gastric pouch to delay emptying has been employed with variable efficacy.

Micronutrient deficiencies are underreported after bariatric surgery. The reported prevalence of deficiencies of virtually all micronutrients after surgery span a broad range from 10% to >80% for BPD/duodenal switch and gastric bypass. Deficiencies are less common after sleeve gastrectomy and gastric band. An understanding of the anatomic sites and mechanisms of micronutrient absorption affected by gastric bypass foregut diversion guides diagnosis and management. Anemia, neurologic, dermatologic, and GI symptoms are common clinical manifestations of many micronutrient deficiencies (**Table 44.4**). Acute deficiencies may involve dramatic presentations (eg, thiamine deficiency and Wernicke encephalopathy). Chronic occult micronutrient deficiencies are associated with increased risk of chronic disease. Chronic magnesium deficiency, for example, is associated with an increased risk of type II diabetes. Chronic selenium deficiency has been associated with an increased risk of cancer and cardiovascular disease. The most common deficiencies associated with gastric bypass involve calcium, vitamin D, folate, iron, and B12. Vomiting due to stenosis or gastroenteritis increases the risks of severe micronutrient deficiencies, and nutritional status should be monitored carefully in any bariatric surgery patient with significant vomiting. It is important to note that obesity is associated with multiple micronutrient deficiencies independent of bariatric surgery, which should be identified and corrected in the preoperative period, and which may resurface in the postoperative period.

Operative Considerations

A thorough discussion of the technical aspects of bariatric surgery is beyond the scope of this chapter, but a few important issues warrant mention. Obesity is a risk factor for deep vein thrombosis (DVT), and aggressive DVT prophylaxis should be employed. Optimal prophylaxis agents and regimens have not been determined, but unfractionated or low–molecular-weight heparin during operation and continued through the hospitalization period is typical. Subtherapeutic dosing of these agents is common in the obese, and the American College of Chest Physicians recommends weight-based dosing.

Hand-sewn, linear stapler, and circular stapler techniques are used to create the gastrojejunostomy in gastric bypass. No single technique demonstrates a clear advantage, although stenosis rates may be higher with the circular stapler technique. Absorbable suture should be used for all anastomoses, as nonabsorbable suture is a nidus for ulcer formation. Routine intraoperative testing of the gastrojejunal anastomosis with EGD-air insufflation or methylene blue instillation may be associated with reduced anastomotic dehiscence rates and is advisable. The use of drains at the gastrojejunal anastomosis is practiced selectively, and no clear data demonstrate that routine drain placement aids in early detection or reduces morbidity of anastomotic dehiscence. Routine closure of internal hernia defects during gastric bypass is controversial, as data do not clearly demonstrate that this practice reduces late hernia incidence. Nonetheless, closure is straightforward, entails low morbidity, and is therefore recommended. Risk–benefit analyses do not support prophylactic cholecystectomy during laparoscopic bariatric surgery in the absence of cholelithiasis or in the presence of asymptomatic cholelithiasis. It is therefore reasonable to manage cholelithiasis in bariatric surgery patients as in all patients, that is, perform cholecystectomy only if symptoms are present.

Perioperative and Postoperative Management

Perioperative care of the bariatric surgery patient is similar to that of any patient undergoing complex GI surgery but must be tailored to the obese. Inpatient, outpatient, and operating room facilities should be equipped with beds, chairs, lifting and transfer apparatuses, and other equipment capable of bearing the weight of obese patients. Anesthesia, nursing, dietitian, physical therapy, and other subspecialty staff with experience in the management of obese patients are necessary. Hospital stays after laparoscopic gastric bypass and sleeve gastrectomy are typically 1 to 3 days, while gastric band is generally performed on an outpatient basis.

The dietary regimen in the first few weeks after surgery is designed to prevent food impaction at an edematous surgical site and maintain adequate hydration, and includes clear liquids progressing to soft foods. Caloric intake in the early postoperative period may be less than 500 cal/d, which is acceptable as long as hydration is maintained. Within 2 to 3 weeks of surgery, solid foods may be introduced, and caloric intake will slowly rise, with a long-term maintenance target of 1,200 to 1,500 calories and 50 to 70 g of protein per day. Within a few months of surgery, most patients are able to eat any foods in small quantities with few exceptions. Deviation from this pattern should raise concerns for anastomotic stenosis, ulcer, or other complications. Persistent vomiting, unless clearly associated with a specific food that, when eliminated, ameliorates symptoms, is abnormal and should prompt a diagnostic workup, usually with upper gastrointestinal (UGI) and/or esophagogastroscopy (EGD).

The incidence of cholelithiasis after bariatric surgery ranges from 15% to over 70%, but only approximately 7% of patients will require cholecystectomy. Prophylactic treatment with ursodeoxycholic acid reduces the risk of postoperative cholelithiasis, from 28% to 9% in one recent meta-analysis. Such therapy entails little morbidity, and a 6-month postoperative treatment regimen is common practice. Data are equivocal, however, regarding whether this practice reduces cholecystectomy rates or is cost effective.[88]

The variability in surveillance practices makes accurate estimation of the incidence of postoperative nutritional deficiencies challenging, and a wide range of supplementation practices exist. Interpretation of the data is made more difficult because obese patients are at high risk for preexisting micronutrient deficiencies independent of surgery. Vitamin D and zinc deficiencies, for example, afflict over 50% and 30% of obese patients, respectively. Abnormal serum levels of micronutrients after surgery are common, ranging from 10% to >80% depending on the micronutrient, operation, and patient population studied; clinically symptomatic deficiencies are less common. Consensus guidelines from the American Association of Clinical Endocrinologists, the Obesity Society, and the American Society for Metabolic and Bariatric Surgeons (ASMBS) recommend that gastric bypass patients undergo annual surveillance of 25-hydroxyvitamin D, calcium, iron, and B12 levels, along with a complete blood count, electrolyte and lipid panels, and liver function tests and periodic bone scans, and receive lifelong daily multivitamin (including folate), calcium citrate, vitamin D, and vitamin B12 supplementation, with iron supplementation in menstruating women.[89] Sleeve gastrectomy patients likely have a lower risk of nutritional deficiencies, but similar regimens are recommended. Gastric band patients receive a daily multivitamin, calcium, and vitamin D supplementation.

Clinical follow-up after bariatric surgery should be lifelong. Primary care providers play a critical role in preoperative and postoperative care. Endocrinology expertise may be required, especially in the early postoperative period when diabetes may resolve rapidly. A medical bariatrician subspecialty is evolving to care for this expanding patient population.

Table 44.4. Select Micronutrient Deficiencies Associated with Bariatric Surgery

Micronutrient	Signs, Symptoms of Deficiency	Site of Absorption	Mechanism of Absorption, Other Issues
B9 (folate)	Macrocytic megaloblastic anemia, leukopenia, thrombocytopenia, glossitis, elevated homocysteine levels, neural tube defects in pregnancy	Duodenum, jejunum, ileum	Water soluble, conserved via enterohepatic circulation; B12 required for folate activation, B12 deficiency can cause folate deficiency; multivitamin generally sufficient for supplementation after surgery
B1 (thiamine)	Wernicke encephalopathy (ophthalmoplegia, nystagmus, ataxia, dementia), Korsakoff psychosis, beri-beri, peripheral neuropathy	Jejunum, ileum	Water soluble, depletion may occur with 2–3 wks; rapid weight loss, vomiting increase risk of deficiency; symptoms of acute deficiency may mimic stroke
B6 (pyridoxine)	Seborrheic dermatitis, atrophic glossitis, conjunctivitis, neuropathy	Jejunum, ileum	Water soluble, passive absorption
B12 (cobalamin)	Macrocytic anemia, leukopenia, thrombocytopenia, glossitis, irreversible neuropathies	Ileum	Binds salivary R-proteins which prevent acid hydrolysis, then binds intrinsic factor secreted by parietal cells in gastric antrum; intrinsic factor-B12 complex absorbed in ileum; found in foods of animal origin—be alert for deficiency in vegetarians
C	Scurvy: malaise, myalgias, petechiae, mucosal bleeding, edema; iron deficiency	Jejunum	Symptomatic deficiency rare after bariatric surgery; potentiates iron absorption, should be used in iron deficient patients
D	Fatigue, myalgia, arthralgia, osteopenia	Jejunum, ileum	Fat soluble; deficiency common in obesity independent of surgery in up to 50% of patients
A	Xerophthalmia, night blindness, keratitis	Duodenum, jejunum, ileum	Fat soluble; deficiency associated with malabsorptive procedures
E	Ataxia, paresthesias, myopathy, arthropathy, anemia, retinopathy, immune dysfunction	Jejunum, ileum	Fat soluble; deficiency associated with malabsorptive procedures
K	Coagulopathy	Jejunum, ileum	Fat soluble; deficiency associated with malabsorptive procedures
Calcium	Tetany (Trousseau, Chvostek signs), paresthesias, QT prolongation, cardiac arrhythmias, petechiae, purpura, osteopenia	Duodenum, jejunum	Symptoms of acute deficiency rare; chronic deficiency common, manifests as osteopenia, related to vitamin D deficiency
Copper	Ataxia, anemia, demyelinating neuropathy, paresthesias; chronic deficiency associated with osteoporosis, cardiovascular disease, cancer	Stomach, duodenum	Involved in antioxidant metabolism
Iron	Microcytic anemia, fatigue, cold intolerance, atrophic glossitis, angular stomatitis	Duodenum	Conversion from ferric to ferrous form requires acid hydrolysis; supplements interfere with calcium absorption, should be taken at different times
Magnesium	Alopecia, muscle cramps, hypocalcemia, hypokalemia, hypoparathyroidism, chronic deficiency linked to increased risk of diabetes, cardiovascular disease	Duodenum	Deficiency common in obesity independent of surgery in up to 35% of patients
Selenium	Acute deficiency rare; chronic deficiency linked to increased risk of cancer, diabetes, long-term mortality	Duodenum	Involved in antioxidant metabolism; excess selenium is toxic
Zinc	Alopecia, dermatitis	Duodenum	Deficiency common in obesity independent of surgery in up to 50% of obese patients

Dominant anatomic sites of absorption are listed, but many micronutrients are absorbed throughout the GI tract. In cases of micronutrients absorbed via active transport mechanisms, passive absorption also occurs in lesser amounts, and supplementation with suprapharmacologic doses overcomes bypassed active uptake mechanisms via passive absorption (eg, B12).

Physiologic Mechanisms Underlying Bariatric Surgery Efficacy

7 Restriction of caloric intake and nutrient malabsorption are the classic presumed mechanisms of bariatric operations. These mechanisms are important, but their relationship to outcome is complex and nonlinear. For example, data are conflicting regarding the correlation between gastric bypass pouch size and weight loss. In general, pouch volumes <50 cc are associated with good results, with little evidence that smaller pouches achieve greater weight loss, while efficacy may decrease substantially as pouch sizes increase beyond 50 cc. Similar observations apply to sleeve gastrectomy: a recent MBSAQIP study of 189,477 sleeve gastrectomies demonstrated that bougie size ≥40 Fr was associated with greater weight loss relative to smaller bougies.[90] Similarly, common channel length teeters on a less well-defined threshold, above which weight loss is poor and below which malnutrition results. Other features of restriction are counterintuitive: more rapid gastric pouch emptying on oral contrast studies is associated with greater weight loss after gastric bypass, while sleeve gastrectomy is associated with increased gastric emptying rates compared to native anatomy. These observations suggest a complex relationship between weight regulation, metabolism, and gut anatomy and motility.

Complex mechanisms in addition to restriction and malabsorption contribute to weight loss and improved metabolism after surgery, with qualitatively different responses than those associated with diet-induced weight loss. Satiety is increased, hunger decreased, and metabolic rate increased after bariatric surgery, the opposite of responses observed with diet-induced weight loss. Bariatric surgery somehow "sidesteps" the normal compensatory responses that act to defend body weight with nonsurgical weight loss. The mechanisms underlying these counterintuitive responses are not well established. Among putative mechanisms are changes in gut hormone secretion secondary to altered intestinal anatomy. Decades ago, it was observed that an oral glucose load elicits a greater insulin response than an intravenous glucose load, leading to postulation of the existence of *incretins,* gut hormones secreted in response to a meal that regulate systemic glucose metabolism. Subsequent research led to the discovery of GIP and GLP-1, incretins secreted by duodenal K cells and ileal L cells, respectively, in response to nutrient delivery to the small intestine. Incretins have diverse effects on glucose homeostasis, potentiating central insulin secretion and peripheral insulin sensitivity. Alterations in incretin hormone secretion secondary to gut anatomic derangements were invoked to explain the observation that diabetes often improved within days of gastric bypass, well before substantial weight loss.

The *foregut and hindgut hypotheses* have been proposed to explain this phenomenon: bypass of the alimentary stream from the stomach, duodenum, and proximal jejunum (the foregut hypothesis), and increased caloric delivery to the distal jejunum and ileum (the hindgut hypothesis) alter secretion of gut hormones with improvement in glucose homeostasis. While data are less compelling for GIP and other putative foregut hormones, evidence supports the hindgut hypothesis, including data demonstrating increased serum GLP-1 levels after gastric bypass. While debate persists regarding the magnitude of these effects on diabetes remission after gastric bypass, an understanding of incretin physiology has led to the development of GLP-1 agonists as pharmacologic therapy for diabetes independent of bariatric surgery.

Gut anatomic derangements mediate additional metabolic changes. Gastric bypass and sleeve gastrectomy are associated with alterations in serum levels of the orexigenic hormone ghrelin, which is secreted by gastric fundus enteroendocrine cells, and peptide YY and oxyntomodulin, gut hormones secreted by L cells in parallel with GLP-1 in response to a meal that induce satiety and inhibit gut motility and are central mediators of the "ileal brake" mechanism. These changes may contribute to satiety and altered food responses after bariatric surgery. Gastric bypass and sleeve gastrectomy alter bile acid metabolism, increasing serum levels of conjugated bile acids with beneficial effects on glucose and lipid metabolism. Bariatric surgery disrupts vagal and enteroenteric innervations of the gut with downstream effects on CNS satiety responses. Finally, bariatric surgery is associated with alterations in gut microbiota that contribute to weight loss and resolution of metabolic disease, with data demonstrating that fecal transplant from mice that have undergone bariatric surgery transfers a lean, insulin-sensitive phenotype to obese, nonoperated mice. The precise mechanisms by which these diverse effects contribute to weight loss and metabolic disease remission remain unclear but are areas of active research.

Mechanisms other than restriction and malabsorption underlie the systemic effects of bariatric surgery. An emerging field of *metabolic surgery* is exploring operations designed to mimic the metabolic effects of gastric bypass (eg, ileal transposition, foregut exclusion, biliary diversion) in animals and lean diabetic humans with promising results. Also in development are endoscopic and laparoscopic gastric plications, intragastric balloon placement, vagal nerve blockade, gastric simulators, and impermeable intraluminal duodenal and jejunal stents designed to prevent caloric absorption. Bariatric surgery in the 21st century will evolve to include a broad array of procedures applied to a diverse patient population as these efforts mature.

References

1. Henderson RM. The bigger the healthier: are the limits of BMI risk changing over time? *Econ Hum Biol.* 2005;3(3):339–366.
2. Chen SE, Florax RJGM. Zoning for health: the obesity epidemic and opportunities for local policy intervention. *J Nutr.* 2010; 140(6):1181–1184.
3. Berrington de Gonzalez A, Hartge P, Cerhan JR, et al. Body-mass index and mortality among 1.46 million white adults. *N Engl J Med.* 2010;363(23):2211–2219.
4. Oreopoulos A, Padwal R, Kalantar-Zadeh K, Fonarow GC, Norris CM, McAlister FA. Body mass index and mortality in heart failure: a meta-analysis. *Am Heart J.* 2008;156(1):13–22.
5. Ashwell M, Gunn P, Gibson S. Waist-to-height ratio is a better screening tool than waist circumference and BMI for adult cardiometabolic risk factors: systematic review and meta-analysis. *Obes Rev.* 2012;13(3):275–286.
6. Englesbe MJ, Lee JS, He K, et al. Analytic morphomics, core muscle size, and surgical outcomes. *Ann Surg.* 2012;256(2):255–261.
7. Lewis CE, McTigue KM, Burke LE, et al. Mortality, health outcomes, and body mass index in the overweight range: a science advisory from the American Heart Association. *Circulation.* 2009;119(25): 3263–3271.
8. Centers for Disease Control and Prevention. Content source: Division of Nutrition, Physical Activity, and Obesity, National Center for Chronic Disease Prevention and Health Promotion; 2020. https://www.cdc.gov/obesity/data/adult.html
9. Peeters A, Barendregt JJ, Willekens F, Mackenbach JP, Al Mamun A, Bonneux L; Netherlands Epidemiology and Demography Compression of Morbidity Research Group. Obesity in adulthood and its consequences for life expectancy: a life-table analysis. *Ann Intern Med.* 2003;138(1):24–32.
10. Fontaine KR, Redden DT, Wang C, Westfall AO, Allison DB. Years of life lost due to obesity. *JAMA.* 2003;289(2):187–193.
11. Li C, Ford ES, Zhao G, Croft JB, Balluz LS, Mokdad AH. Prevalence of self-reported clinically diagnosed sleep apnea according to obesity status in men and women: National Health and Nutrition Examination Survey, 2005–2006. *Prev Med.* 2010;51(1):18–23.
12. Lopez PP, Stefan B, Schulman CI, Byers PM. Prevalence of sleep apnea in morbidly obese patients who presented for weight loss surgery evaluation: more evidence for routine screening for obstructive sleep apnea before weight loss surgery. *Am Surg.* 2008;74(9):834–838.
13. Trogdon JG, Finkelstein EA, Hylands T, Dellea PS, Kamal-Bahl SJ. Indirect costs of obesity: a review of the current literature. *Obes Rev.* 2008;9(5):489–500.

14. Samaha FF, Iqbal N, Seshadri P, et al. A low-carbohydrate as compared with a low-fat diet in severe obesity. *N Engl J Med.* 2003;348(21):2074–2081.
15. Alamout MM, Rahmanian M, Aghamohammadi V, Mohammadi E, Nasiri K. Effectiveness of mindfulness based cognitive therapy on weight loss, improvement of hypertension and attentional bias to eating cues in overweight people. *Int J Nurs Sci.* 2019;7(1):35–40.
16. Knowler WC, Barrett-Connor E, Fowler SE, et al; Diabetes Prevention Program Research Group. Reduction in the incidence of type 2 diabetes with lifestyle intervention or metformin. *N Engl J Med.* 2002;346(6):393–403.
17. Look AHEAD Research Group. Eight-year weight losses with an intensive lifestyle intervention: the look AHEAD study. *Obesity (Silver Spring).* 2014;22(1):5–13.
18. Cho YM, Wideman RD, Kieffer TJ. Clinical application of glucagon-like peptide 1 receptor agonists for the treatment of type 2 diabetes mellitus. *Endocrinol Metab (Seoul).* 2013;28(4):262–274.
19. Ozcan L, Ergin AS, Lu A, et al. Endoplasmic reticulum stress plays a central role in development of leptin resistance. *Cell Metab.* 2009;9(1):35–51.
20. Trevaskis JL, Coffey T, Cole R, et al. Amylin-mediated restoration of leptin responsiveness in diet-induced obesity: magnitude and mechanisms. *Endocrinology.* 2008;149(11):5679–5687.
21. Wilding JPH, Batterham RL, Calanna S, et al. *Once-Weekly Semaglutide in Adults with Overweight or Obesity.* New England Journal of Medicine; 2021.
22. Smith SR, Weissman NJ, Anderson CM, et al. Behavioral Modification and Lorcaserin for Overweight and Obesity Management (BLOOM) Study Group. Multicenter, placebo-controlled trial of lorcaserin for weight management. *N Engl J Med.* 2010;363(3):245–256.
23. Marso SP, Daniels GH, Brown-Frandsen K, et al. *Liraglutide and Cardiovascular Outcomes in Type 2 Diabetes.* New England Journal of Medicine; 2016.
24. Payne JH, DeWind LT. Surgical treatment of obesity. *Am J Surg.* 1969;118(2):141–147.
25. Sudan R, Jacobs DO. Biliopancreatic diversion with duodenal switch. *Surg Clin North Am.* 2011;91(6):1281–1293, ix.
26. Sakran N, et al. Single-anastomosis duodenal switch: short- and long-term outcomes. *Obes Surg.* 2020.
27. Ibrahim AM, Thumma JR, Dimick JB. Reoperation and Medicare expenditures after laparoscopic gastric band surgery. *JAMA Surg.* 2017;152(9):835–842.
28. American Society for Metabolic and Bariatric Surgery. Estimate of Bariatric Surgery Numbers, 2011–2018. Accessed August 1, 2019. https://asmbs.org/resources/estimate-of-bariatric-surgery-numbers
29. Telem DA, Ghaferi A. Gastric balloons for weight loss in 2020. *JAMA.* 2020;324(21):2206–2207.
30. Mohan BP, Asokkumar R, Khan SR, et al. Outcomes of endoscopic sleeve gastroplasty; how does it compare to laparoscopic sleeve gastrectomy? A systematic review and meta-analysis. *Endosc Int Open.* 2020;8(4):E558–E565.
31. Campos GM, Khoraki J, Browning MG, Pessoa BM, Mazzini GS, Wolfe L. Changes in utilization of bariatric surgery in the United States from 1993 to 2016. *Ann Surg.* 2020;271(2):201–209.
32. Gould KM, Zeymo A, Chan KS, et al. Bariatric surgery among vulnerable populations: the effect of the Affordable Care Act's Medicaid expansion. *Surgery.* 2019;166(5):820–828.
33. Kyler KE, Bettenhausen JL, Hall M, Fraser JD, Sweeney B. Trends in volume and utilization outcomes in adolescent metabolic and bariatric surgery at Children's Hospitals. *J Adolesc Health.* 2019;65(3):331–336.
34. NIH Conference. Gastrointestinal surgery for severe obesity. Consensus Development Conference Panel. *Ann Intern Med.* 1991;115(12):956–961.
35. Stegenga H, Haines A, Jones K, Jones K, Wilding J; Guideline Development Group. Identification, assessment, and management of overweight and obesity: summary of updated NICE guidance. *BMJ.* 2014;349:g6608.
36. Society of American Gastrointestinal and Endoscopic Surgeons. Guidelines for Clinical Application of Laparoscopic Bariatric Surgery. Accessed August 12, 2020. https://www.sages.org/publications/guidelines/guidelines-for-clinical-application-of-laparoscopic-bariatric-surgery/
37. van de Laar A. Bariatric Outcomes Longitudinal Database (BOLD) suggests excess weight loss and excess BMI loss to be inappropriate outcome measures, demonstrating better alternatives. *Obes Surg.* 2012;22(12):1843–1847.
38. Schauer PR, Kashyap SR, Wolski K, et al. Bariatric surgery versus intensive medical therapy in obese patients with diabetes. *N Engl J Med.* 2012;366(17):1567–1576.
39. Schauer PR, Bhatt DL, Kirwan JP, et al; STAMPEDE Investigators. Bariatric surgery versus intensive medical therapy for diabetes—3-year outcomes. *N Engl J Med.* 2014;370(21):2002–2013.
40. Schauer PR, Bhatt DL, Kirwan JP, et al; STAMPEDE Investigators. Bariatric surgery versus intensive medical therapy for diabetes—5-year outcomes. *N Engl J Med.* 2017;376(7):641–651.
41. Biertho L, Simon-Hould F, Marceau S, Lebel S, Lescelleur O, Biron S. Current outcomes of laparoscopic duodenal switch. *Ann Surg Innov Res.* 2016;10:1.
42. Nelson DW, Blair KS, Martin MJ. Analysis of obesity-related outcomes and bariatric failure rates with the duodenal switch vs gastric bypass for morbid obesity. *Arch Surg.* 2012;147(9):847–854.
43. Risstad H, Søvik TT, Engström M, et al. Five-year outcomes after laparoscopic gastric bypass and laparoscopic duodenal switch in patients with body mass index of 50 to 60: a randomized clinical trial. *JAMA Surg.* 2015;150(4):352–361.
44. Varban OA, Cassidy RB, Bonham A, et al. Factors associated with achieving a body mass index of less than 30 after bariatric surgery. *JAMA Surg.* 2017;152(11):1058–1064.
45. Mehaffey JH, LaPar DJ, Clement KC, et al. 10-Year outcomes after Roux-en-Y gastric bypass. *Ann Surg.* 2016;264(1):121–126.
46. Ikramuddin S, Billington CJ, Lee WJ, et al. Roux-en-Y gastric bypass for diabetes (the Diabetes Surgery Study): 2-year outcomes of a 5-year, randomised, controlled trial. *Lancet Diabetes Endocrinol.* 2015;3(6):413–422.
47. Mingrone G, Panunzi S, De Gaetano A, et al. Bariatric surgery versus conventional medical therapy for type 2 diabetes. *N Engl J Med.* 2012;366(17):1577–1585.
48. Higa K, Ho T, Tercero F, Yunus T, Boone KB. Laparoscopic Roux-en-Y gastric bypass: 10-year follow-up. *Surg Obes Relat Dis.* 2011;7(4):516–525.
49. Maghrabi AH, Wolski K, Abood B, et al. Two-year outcomes on bone density and fracture incidence in patients with T2DM randomized to bariatric surgery versus intensive medical therapy: Bone Density in Diabetes After Bariatric Surgery. *Obesity (Silver Spring).* 2015;23(12):2344–2348.
50. Seki Y, Kasama K, Hashimoto K. Long-term outcome of laparoscopic sleeve gastrectomy in morbidly obese Japanese patients. *Obes Surg.* 2016;26(1):138–145.
51. Sethi M, Chau E, Youn A, Jiang Y, Fielding G, Ren-Fielding C. Long-term outcomes after biliopancreatic diversion with and without duodenal switch: 2-, 5-, and 10-year data. *Surg Obes Relat Dis.* 2016;12(9):1697–1705.
52. Mingrone G, Panunzi S, De Gaetano A, et al. Bariatric-metabolic surgery versus conventional medical treatment in obese patients with type 2 diabetes: 5-year follow-up of an open-label, single-centre, randomised controlled trial. *Lancet.* 2015;386(9997):964–973.
53. Arman GA, Himpens J, Dhaenens J, Ballet T, Vilallonga R, Leman G. Long-term (11+years) outcomes in weight, patient satisfaction, comorbidities, and gastroesophageal reflux treatment after laparoscopic sleeve gastrectomy. *Surg Obes Relat Dis.* 2016;12(10):1778–1786.
54. Gadiot RPM, Biter LU, van Mil S, Zengerink HF, Apers J, Mannaerts GH. Long-term results of laparoscopic sleeve gastrectomy for morbid obesity: 5 to 8-year results. *Obes Surg.* 2017;27(1):59–63.
55. Felsenreich DM, Langer FB, Kefurt R, et al. Weight loss, weight regain, and conversions to Roux-en-Y gastric bypass: 10-year results of laparoscopic sleeve gastrectomy. *Surg Obes Relat Dis.* 2016;12(9):1655–1662.
56. Aasprang A, Andersen JR, Våge V, Kolotkin R, Natvig GK. Ten-year changes in health-related quality of life after

biliopancreatic diversion with duodenal switch. *Surg Obes Relat Dis*. 2016;12(8):1594–1600.

57. Topart P, Becouarn G, Delarue J. Weight loss and nutritional outcomes 10 years after biliopancreatic diversion with duodenal switch. *Obes Surg*. 2017;27(7):1645–1650.
58. Ignat M, Vix M, Imad I, et al. Randomized trial of Roux-en-Y gastric bypass versus sleeve gastrectomy in achieving excess weight loss. *Br J Surg*. 2017;104(3):248–256.
59. Peterli R, Wölnerhanssen BK, Vetter D, et al. Laparoscopic sleeve gastrectomy versus Roux-Y-Gastric bypass for morbid obesity—3-year outcomes of the prospective randomized Swiss multicenter bypass or sleeve study (SM-BOSS). *Ann Surg*. 2017;265(3):466–473.
60. Kehagias I, Karamanakos SN, Argentou M, Kalfarentzos F. Randomized clinical trial of laparoscopic Roux-en-Y Gastric bypass versus laparoscopic sleeve gastrectomy for the management of patients with BMI <50kg/m^2. *Obes Surg*. 2011;21(11):1650–1656.
61. Sarkhosh K, Switzer NJ, El-Hadi M, Birch DW, Shi X, Karmali S. The impact of bariatric surgery on obstructive sleep apnea: a systematic review. *Obes Surg*. 2013;23(3):414–423.
62. Albanopoulos K, Tsamis D, Natoudi M, Alevizos L, Zografos G, Leandros E. The impact of laparoscopic sleeve gastrectomy on weight loss and obesity-associated comorbidities: the results of 3 years of follow-up. *Surg Endosc*. 2016;30(2):699–705.
63. Biertho L, Lebel S, Marceau S, et al. Laparoscopic sleeve gastrectomy: with or without duodenal switch? A consecutive series of 800 cases. *Dig Surg*. 2014;31(1):48–54.
64. Chuffart E, Sodji M, Dalmay F, Iannelli A, Mathonnet M. Long-term results after sleeve gastrectomy for gastroesophageal reflux disease: a single-center French study. *Obes Surg*. 2017;27(11):2890–2897.
65. Sundbom M, Hedberg J, Marsk R, et al; Scandinavian Obesity Surgery Registry Study Group. Substantial decrease in comorbidity 5 years after gastric bypass: a population-based study from the Scandinavian obesity surgery registry. *Ann Surg*. 2017;265(6):1166–1171.
66. Buchwald H, Oien DM. Metabolic/bariatric surgery worldwide 2011. *Obes Surg*. 2013;23(4):427–436.
67. Sjöström L, Narbro K, Sjöström CD, et al.; Swedish Obese Subjects Study. Effects of bariatric surgery on mortality in Swedish obese subjects. *N Engl J Med*. 2007;357(8):741–752.
68. O'Rourke RW. Management strategies for internal hernia after gastric bypass. *J Gastrointest Surg*. 2011;15(6):1049–1054.
69. Chang SH, Stoll CRT, Song J, Varela JE, Eagon CJ, Colditz GA. The effectiveness and risks of bariatric surgery: an updated systematic review and meta-analysis, 2003–2012. *JAMA Surg*. 2014;149(3):275–287.
70. Lynch J, Belgaumkar A. Bariatric surgery is effective and safe in patients over 55: a systematic review and meta-analysis. *Obes Surg*. 2012;22(9):1507–1516.
71. Trastulli S, Desiderio J, Guarino S, et al. Laparoscopic sleeve gastrectomy compared with other bariatric surgical procedures: a systematic review of randomized trials. *Surg Obes Relat Dis*. 2013;9(5):816–829.
72. Banka G, Woodard G, Hernandez-Boussard T, Morton JM. Laparoscopic vs. open gastric bypass surgery: differences in patient demographics, safety, and outcomes. *Arch Surg*. 2012;147(6):550–556.
73. Finks JF, Kole KL, Yenumula PR, et al; Michigan Bariatric Surgery Collaborative, from the Center for Healthcare Outcomes and Policy. Predicting risk for serious complications with bariatric surgery: results from the Michigan Bariatric Surgery Collaborative. *Ann Surg*. 2011;254(4):633–640.
74. Carlin AM, Zeni TM, English WJ, et al. Michigan Bariatric Surgery Collaborative. The comparative effectiveness of sleeve gastrectomy, gastric bypass, and adjustable gastric banding procedures for the treatment of morbid obesity. *Ann Surg*. 2013;257(5):791–797.
75. Courcoulas AP, Christian NJ, Belle SH, et al; Longitudinal Assessment of Bariatric Surgery (LABS) Consortium. Weight change and health outcomes at 3 years after bariatric surgery among individuals with severe obesity. *JAMA*. 2013;310(22):2416–2425.
76. Flum DR, Belle SH, King WC, et al; Longitudinal Assessment of Bariatric Surgery (LABS) Consortium. Perioperative safety in the longitudinal assessment of bariatric surgery. *N Engl J Med*. 2009;361(5):445–454.
77. Salminen P, Helmiö M, Ovaska J, et al. Effect of laparoscopic sleeve gastrectomy vs laparoscopic Roux-en-Y gastric bypass on weight loss at 5 years among patients with morbid obesity: the SLEEVEPASS randomized clinical trial. *JAMA*. 2018;319(3):241–254.
78. Maggard-Gibbons M, Maglione M, Livhits M, et al. Bariatric surgery for weight loss and glycemic control in nonmorbidly obese adults with diabetes: a systematic review. *JAMA*. 2013;309(21):2250–2261.
79. Buchwald H, Avidor Y, Braunwald E, et al. Bariatric surgery: a systematic review and meta-analysis. *JAMA*. 2004;292(14):1724–1737.
80. Maggard MA, Shugarman LR, Suttorp M, et al. Meta-analysis: surgical treatment of obesity. *Ann Intern Med*. 2005;142(7):547–559.
81. O'Brien PE, McPhail T, Chaston TB, Dixon JB. Systematic review of medium-term weight loss after bariatric operations. *Obes Surg*. 2006;16(8):1032–1040.
82. Garb J, Welch G, Zagarins S, Kuhn J, Romanelli J. Bariatric surgery for the treatment of morbid obesity: a meta-analysis of weight loss outcomes for laparoscopic adjustable gastric banding and laparoscopic gastric bypass. *Obes Surg*. 2009;19(10):1447–1455.
83. Padwal R, Klarenbach S, Wiebe N, et al. Bariatric surgery: a systematic review of the clinical and economic evidence. *J Gen Intern Med*. 2011;26(10):1183–1194.
84. Genco A, Soricelli E, Casella G, et al. Gastroesophageal reflux disease and Barrett's esophagus after laparoscopic sleeve gastrectomy: a possible, underestimated long-term complication. *Surg Obes Relat Dis*. 2017;13(4):568–574.
85. Peterli R, Wolnerhanssen BK, Peters T, et al. Effect of laparoscopic sleeve gastrectomy vs laparoscopic Roux-en-Y gastric bypass on weight loss in patients with morbid obesity: the SM-BOSS randomized clinical trial. *JAMA*. 2018;319(3):255–265.
86. Mechanick JI, Apovian C, Brethauer S, et al. Clinical practice guidelines for the perioperative nutrition, metabolic, and nonsurgical support of patients undergoing bariatric surgery—2019 update: cosponsored by AACE/ACE, TOS, ASMBS, OMA, ASA. *Endocr Pract*. 2019;25(12):1346–1359.
87. Parrott J, Frank L, Rabena R, Craggs-Dino L, Isom KA, Greiman L. American Society for metabolic and bariatric surgery integrated Health Nutritional Guidelines for the surgical weight loss patient 2016 update: micronutrients. *Surg Obes Relat Dis*. 2017;13(5):727–741.
88. Warschkow R, Tarantino I, Ukegjini K, et al. Concomitant cholecystectomy during laparoscopic Roux-en-Y gastric bypass in obese patients is not justified: a meta-analysis. *Obes Surg*. 2013;23(3):397–407.
89. Telem DA, Gould J, Pesta C, et al. American Society for metabolic and bariatric surgery: care pathway for laparoscopic sleeve gastrectomy. *Surg Obes Relat Dis*. 2017;13(5):742–749.
90. Berger ER, Clements RH, Morton JM, et al. The impact of different surgical techniques on outcomes in laparoscopic sleeve gastrectomies: the first report from the metabolic and bariatric surgery accreditation and quality improvement program (MBSAQIP). *Ann Surg*. 2016;264(3):464–473.

Gastric Neoplasms

Donnele Daley and Sandra L. Wong

Key Points

1 While the incidence and mortality of gastric cancer have decreased substantially over the past several decades, it is still a leading cause of cancer-related mortality in many parts of the world.

2 *Helicobacter pylori* infection is the predominant risk factor for gastric carcinogenesis, and *H. pylori* eradication is responsible for a marked decline in intestinal-type gastric cancers.

3 The symptoms produced by gastric cancer are nonspecific and can mimic those associated with a number of nonneoplastic gastroduodenal diseases, especially benign gastric ulcer.

4 The extent of gastric resection is determined by the need to obtain a resection margin free of microscopic disease, and examination of a minimum of 16 nodes is suggested for adequate staging.

5 Multimodality treatment, including neoadjuvant therapy, should be the standard of care for treating locally advanced resectable gastric cancer.

Gastric cancer remains a relatively common and frequently lethal malignancy, noting that it is the fifth most commonly diagnosed cancer in the world.[1] The disease is often not recognized until it is at an advanced stage. Gastric cancer usually cannot be treated with resection alone, and surgical cure rates have remained disappointingly low. Multidisciplinary approaches must be considered the standard of care for these difficult neoplasms, noting some modest improvements in outcomes are finally being observed. Technical innovations and basic/translational scientific investigations must continue to be applied to this disease.

ADENOCARCINOMA

Epidemiology

1 The incidence of gastric cancer has declined dramatically in the United States over the past century, noting that it still constitutes a major global health problem in low- and middle-income countries. There is truly wide geographic variation in incidence, with a 15- to 20-fold difference between the high- and low-incidence regions. The rates are particularly high in Japan, Korea, and China, where gastric cancer is commonly diagnosed and a leading cause of cancer-related mortality. Globally, there were 968,784 cases and over 660,175 deaths in 2022.[1] In comparison, gastric cancer is an uncommonly diagnosed cancer in the United States, with an estimated 26,890 cases and an estimated 10,880 deaths in 2024.[2] Of note, Asian Americans appear to have a much higher incidence (15 cases per 100,000) compared to non-Hispanic Whites (6 per 100,000), and Korean Americans and Japanese Americans (40 per 100,000 and 30 per 100,000, respectively) face a particularly high risk of disease.[3]

Worldwide geographic variability in the incidence of gastric cancer is shown in **Figure 45.1**. The highest incidence occurs in Eastern Asia, but Central and Eastern Europe and South America also have high incidence of gastric cancer. The lowest incidence of gastric cancer is seen in Africa and North America. Factors including diet and associated issues of oral hygiene and food conservation have been linked to incidence, and variation in the gut microbiome, which is closely linked with both diet and environment, is being increasingly explored as a causal determinant.

Specifically, the intestinal histologic subtype of gastric adenocarcinoma appears to account for most of the geographical variation seen with this disease and is strongly related to environmental exposures. The strongest known risk factor for intestinal-type gastric cancer (with well-differentiated tumor cells) is infection with *Helicobacter pylori.* Approximately 75% of gastric cancer cases are, in fact, attributable to *H. pylori* infection, making this organism one of the dominant infectious cause of cancer in the world. It is associated with a sixfold increased risk of (noncardia) gastric cancer and eradication of *H. pylori* is a major factor in the marked declines of intestinal-type cancers of the distal stomach in the United States and much of the developed world.[4]

The anatomic distribution of gastric cancers also varies widely. Unfortunately, the incidence of diffuse type gastric cancer, characterized by undifferentiated tumor cells arranged in scattered formation in fibrous stoma, of the proximal stomach is rising. While distal tumors still predominate in developing countries, proximal cancers appear to occur more commonly in relatively younger, White, and male patients.

Premalignant Lesions

The risk for development of gastric cancer is greater in stomachs that harbor polyps. This risk is related most closely to polyp histologic type, size, and number. Variations in these three factors account for the wide range in reported risk associated with gastric polyps. In terms of malignant potential, gastric polyps can be divided into two broad categories—hyperplastic polyps and adenomatous polyps. Although not premalignant, hyperplastic polyps are discussed here because they are common, occurring in up to 1% of the general population and accounting for 75% of all gastric polyps. The hyperplastic polyp contains an overgrowth of histologically normal-appearing gastric epithelium. Atypia is rare, and hyperplastic gastric polyps have little to no neoplastic potential.

Hyperplastic polyps are generally asymptomatic. When hyperplastic polyps are discovered, endoscopic removal for

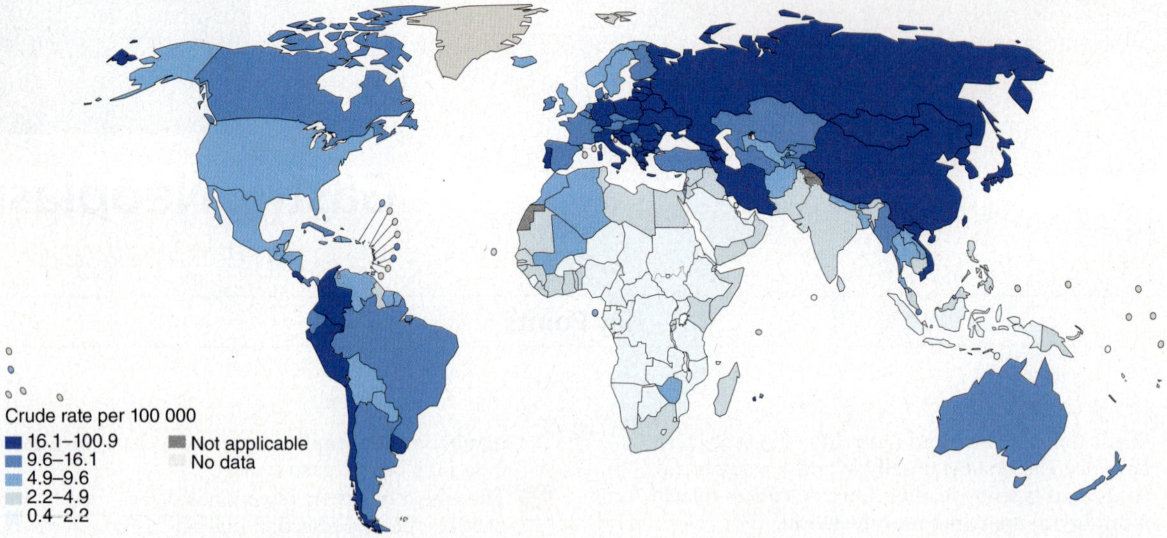

Figure 45.1. Worldwide geographic variability in gastric cancer incidence for both sexes. (Reprinted from GLOBOCAN 2022 v1.1 Cancer Incidence and Mortality Worldwide: Cancer TODAY/IARC [Internet] France: International Agency for Research on Cancer, 2024.)

histologic examination is indicated and such removal results in sufficient treatment. Subsequent surveillance is not necessary, given the lack of neoplastic potential in these polyps. Adenomatous polyps also tend to be asymptomatic, but in contrast to hyperplastic polyps, adenomatous polyps carry a distinct risk for the development of malignancy. Mucosal atypia is frequent, and mitotic figures are more commonly seen than in hyperplastic polyps. Dysplasia and carcinoma in situ have developed in adenomatous polyps observed over time. In fact, the risk for the development of carcinoma has been estimated at 10% to 20% and is greatest for polyps more than 2 cm in diameter. The presence of multiple adenomatous polyps increases the risk of cancer.

Endoscopic removal is indicated for pedunculated lesions and is sufficient if the polyp is completely removed and shows no evidence of invasive cancer on histologic examination. Operative excision is recommended for sessile lesions larger than 2 cm, for polyps with biopsy-proved invasive carcinoma, and for polyps complicated by pain or bleeding. Because the presence of gastric adenomatous polyp is a marker of increased risk for the development of cancer in the remaining gastric mucosa, repeat endoscopic surveillance is indicated. Enrollment in a surveillance program is indicated in order to rule out recurrence at the site of previous excision, evaluate for new or missed polyps or an early carcinoma, and confirm eradication of *H. pylori,* if applicable.

Gastritis

The incidence of atrophic gastritis and gastric cancer increases with age. Chronic gastritis is frequently associated with intestinal metaplasia and mucosal dysplasia, and these histologic features are often observed in mucosa adjacent to gastric cancer. Gastritis is frequently progressive and quite severe in the gastric mucosa of patients with cancer. Gastric malignancy seems to be increased in patients with chronic gastritis associated with pernicious anemia, although the risk appears to have been overstated in the past. Nevertheless, this disease, which is characterized by fundic mucosal atrophy, loss of parietal and chief cells, hypochlorhydria, and hypergastrinemia, is present in 3% of people older than 60 years. For people in whom pernicious anemia has been active for more than 5 years, the risk of gastric cancer is twice that of age-matched control subjects and there is increased risk for gastric neuroendocrine tumors as well.

Helicobacter Pylori

2 As outlined above, infection with *H. pylori* has been unequivocally associated with chronic inflammatory conditions in the stomach, and this association has stimulated interest in the role of chronic infection by this organism in gastric carcinogenesis. Childhood acquisition of *H. pylori* infection is frequent in areas of high gastric cancer incidence, and high rates of infection have been identified in patients with premalignant lesions and invasive cancer. Infection with *H. pylori* is associated with an increased risk of adenocarcinoma of both the body and the antrum of the stomach.[5] In contrast, *H. pylori* infection is not a risk factor for proximal cancers of the cardia or gastroesophageal junction, which are associated with mucosal abnormalities of Barrett esophagus and which seem to follow the metaplasia to dysplasia to carcinoma pattern of development.

The mechanism of carcinogenesis related to *H. pylori* infection is incompletely understood but is thought to be related to the chronic inflammation caused by the organism. Only ~1% of patients chronically infected with *H. pylori* will develop the gastric cancer phenotype, which consists of corpus-predominant gastritis, multifocal atrophic gastritis, high gastrin levels, hypo/achlorhydria, and low pepsinogen I/II ratio. The majority of subjects infected with *H. pylori* will develop the simple gastritis phenotype which is not associated with any significant clinical outcome, or the duodenal ulcer phenotype (10% to 15% of infected subjects), which consists of antral-predominant gastritis and high gastrin and acid secretion and actually provides protection from developing gastric cancer.[6] Of note, there is variable distribution of these three phenotypes geographically, with particular prevalence of the gastric cancer phenotype in certain parts of Asia where gastric cancer is common. While eradication of *H. pylori* is globally associated with decreased incidence of gastric cancer, it may not prevent the development of gastric cancer once premalignant lesions have already developed.[7]

Previous Gastric Surgery

A number of historical reports have suggested that gastric cancer is more likely to develop in people who have undergone previous partial gastrectomy, with patients who have undergone a gastrojejunal (Billroth II) anastomosis at apparently higher risk for carcinogenesis than those reconstructed with a gastroduodenal anastomosis (Billroth I). The so-called *gastric remnant cancer* is a true clinical entity, although the risk for development of this gastric neoplasm appears to have been overestimated. Several large, prospective studies with long-term follow-up indicate that the relative risk is not increased for up to 15 years after gastric resection, likely due to surgical removal of mucosa at risk for development of gastric cancer, followed by modest increases in cancer risk (three times the control value) observed only after 25 years.[8] The cellular mechanisms that contribute to the development of neoplasia in the remnant stomach are unknown. Decreased luminal pH, bacterial overgrowth with increased production of *N*-nitroso carcinogens, and reflux of bile acids into the stomach have been postulated to promote cancer development but remains unproved. Vagotomy, when performed in conjunction with (legacy) gastric surgery for benign disease, does not appear to promote cancer development. A population-based study from Sweden of 7,198 patients who had previously undergone vagotomy and then followed for up to 18 years did not seem to have increased risk of gastric cancer.[8]

A recent study explored genetic alterations in gastric remnant cancer and found that the microsatellite instability-high (MSI-H) phenotype was much more common (43%) in gastric remnant cancers than in sporadic gastric cancers (6%), and that this incidence was much higher in patients who had undergone a Billroth II anastomosis (67%) as compared to those who had undergone a Billroth I anastomosis (11%). The MSI-H phenotype in these tumors was associated with inactivation of the DNA mismatch repair genes hMLH1 and hMSH2, though the significance of this relationship is not yet clear.[9] Reported 5-year survival ranges from only 7% to 33% for gastric remnant cancers, but this poor prognosis is most likely due to the fact that these cancers are usually diagnosed at an advanced stage when treatment options are limited.

Hereditary Syndromes

Approximately 5% to 10% of gastric cancer may have a familial component, and 3% to 5% are associated with known inherited cancer syndromes. Hereditary diffuse gastric cancer (HDGC) is an autosomal dominant syndrome that is believed to confer a lifetime risk for the development of gastric cancer by age 80 years of 70% for men and 56% for women.[10] However, recent reports evaluating families with pathogenic variants observed that only 37% of these families met the clinical criteria for HDGC genetic testing, and the estimated penetrance of gastric cancer may be as low as 42% in males and 33% in females.[11] The average age at diagnosis is 37 years, and these cancers tend to be of the diffuse histologic type. Germline mutations in CDH1, a tumor suppressor gene that encodes the cell-to-cell adhesion protein E-cadherin, are found in most patients with HDGC. Mutations in α-Catenin (CTNNA1), another adhesion junction protein, account for a small minority of cases.[12] Carriers of pathogenic variants of CDH1 mutations commonly have foci of preinvasive signet ring cells throughout the gastric mucosa, suggesting the diagnosis of HDGC. Pathogenic CDH1 carriers, with a family history of diffuse gastric cancer, should be offered prophylactic total gastrectomy, with or without lymph node dissection at a young age (between 20 and 30 years of age).[12] Patients with pathogenic mutations without a family history of HDGC may be considered for prophylactic gastrectomy, and should undergo annual gastric endoscopic surveillance. If positive biopsies are obtained during surveillance, they should be recommended to undergo a total gastrectomy.[12] Prophylactic total gastrectomy should include confirmation of squamous esophageal mucosa along the proximal margin and duodenal mucosa along the distal margin to confirm removal of all gastric tissue. The clinical criteria for genetic testing are listed in **Table 45.1** as adapted from the 2020 Hereditary Diffuse Gastric Cancer Clinical Practice Guidelines.[12] CDH1 testing is recommended when one or more of these guidelines are met in the setting of confirmed cancer diagnoses. If CDH1 testing is found to be negative in individuals meeting these criteria, then CTNNA1 testing should also be carried out.

Other familial cancer syndromes associated with an increased risk of gastric cancer include Lynch syndrome (hereditary nonpolyposis colorectal cancer), juvenile polyposis syndrome, familial adenomatous polyposis (FAP), and Peutz–Jeghers syndrome. Given the autosomal dominant nature of these syndromes, screening upper endoscopy may be considered in these patients, often starting at a young age. Findings of polyps could lead to recommendations for surveillance upper endoscopy in patients with these syndromes, though no formal guidelines exist. In FAP, with germline mutations in the adenomatous polyposis coli (APC) gene on chromosome 5q21, the majority of polyps are benign (nonadenomatous). In individuals with FAP, 10% of gastric polyps are adenomatous in nature and could lead to gastric cancer, noting a 1% to 2% lifetime risk.[13]

Table 45.1. Criteria for Hereditary Diffuse Gastric Cancer Genetic Testing

Family Criteria (First- or Second-Degree Relatives):

- ≥2 cases of gastric cancer (with at least 1 diffuse gastric cancer) in the family at any age
- ≥1 case of lobular breast cancer at age <70 y, and ≥1 case of diffuse gastric cancer at any age, in different family members
- ≥2 cases of lobular breast cancer at age <50 y in the family

Individual Criteria:

- Diffuse gastric cancer at age <50 y
- Diffuse gastric cancer at any age of Māori ethnicity
- Diffuse gastric cancer at any age in persons with a personal or family history of cleft lip/palate (first-degree relative)
- History of diffuse gastric cancer and lobular breast cancer both diagnosed at <70 y of age
- Bilateral lobular breast cancer diagnosed at age <70 y
- Gastric in situ signet ring cells or pagetoid spread of signet ring cells in persons of age <50 y

Clinical Features

3 The symptoms produced by gastric cancer are nonspecific and can closely mimic those associated with a number of nonneoplastic gastroduodenal diseases, especially dyspepsia or benign gastric ulceration. In early gastric cancers, epigastric pain is present in over 70% of patients. Pain may be relieved, at least temporarily, by antacids or gastric antisecretory drugs. Anorexia, nausea, and weight loss are present in less than 50% of patients with early gastric cancers but become increasingly common with disease progression. Dysphagia is present in 20% of patients with proximal gastric lesions. Overt gastrointestinal hemorrhage (5%) and perforation (1%) are uncommon.

In most patients with early gastric cancers, physical examination is typically unremarkable. Stool tests positive for occult blood in one-third. There are no laboratory tests specific for gastric neoplasms. Abnormal physical findings usually reflect advanced disease (**Table 45.2**). Cachexia, abdominal mass, hepatomegaly, and supraclavicular adenopathy usually indicate advanced or metastatic disease.

DIAGNOSIS

Table 45.2. Common Symptoms and Physical Findings in Gastric Cancer

Symptoms	Physical Findings
Weight loss	Guaiac-positive stool
Pain	Cachexia
Nausea and vomiting	Abdominal mass or fullness
Anorexia	Abdominal tenderness
Dysphagia	Hepatomegaly
Melena	

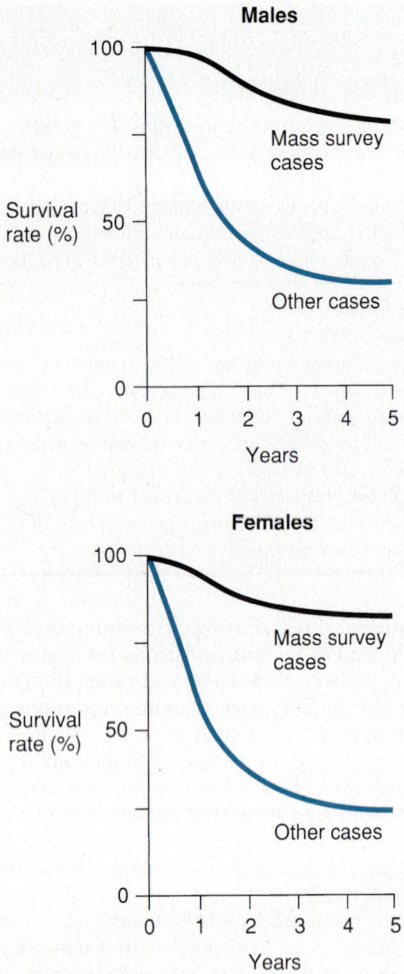

Figure 45.2. Early cancer survival rate in Japan. (From Kunisaki C, Ishino J, Nakajima S, et al. Outcomes of mass screening for gastric carcinoma. *Ann Surg Oncol*. 2006;13(2):221–228.)

Diagnosis and Staging

Fiberoptic endoscopy is the most definitive diagnostic method when gastric neoplasm is suspected. In the initial stages, gastric cancers can appear polypoid, as flat, plaque-like lesions, or as shallow ulcers. Advanced lesions are typically ulcerated. The ulcer border can have an irregular, beaded appearance because of infiltrating cancer cells, and the base is frequently necrotic and shaggy. The ulcer can appear to arise from an underlying mass. Although each of these features suggests a malignant ulcer, differentiation of benign from malignant gastric ulcers can be made definitively only with gastric biopsy. Multiple biopsies of any gastric ulcer should be performed, increasing sensitivity to 98% as compared to 70% for single biopsy. False-negative results occur in approximately 10% of patients, usually as the result of inadequate sampling, sampling error, or due to the absence of a mucosal abnormality as can occur with linitis plastica; false-positive results in this setting are rare.

Diagnostic accuracy can be further enhanced by the addition of endoscopic ultrasound (EUS) with fine-needle aspiration biopsy for infiltrative tumors involving the wall of the stomach without obvious mucosal abnormalities. EUS has added benefit of being able to provide staging information on the depth of tumor invasion when done by experienced endoscopists.

Annual mass screening programs have been instituted in some countries (eg, Japan, Venezuela, Chile) where there is a high incidence of gastric cancer. However, whether such programs significantly reduce gastric cancer mortality is unclear. In Japan, compliance with screening has been associated with a 50% decrease in gastric cancer mortality, but most of this

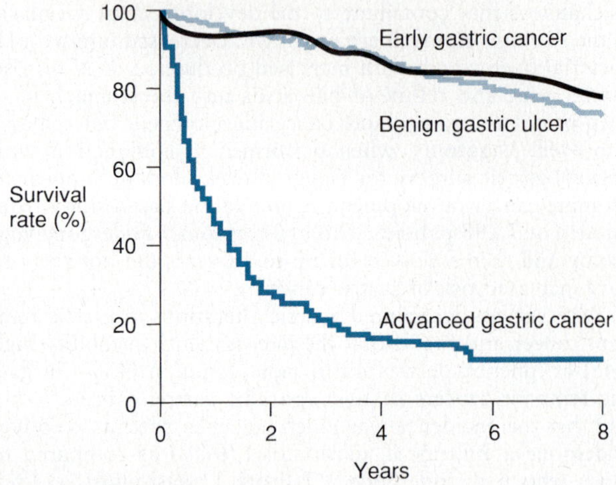

Figure 45.3. Early cancer survival rate in Europe. (From Moreaux J, Bougaran J. Early gastric cancer. A 25-year surgical experience. *Ann Surg*. 1993;217(4):344–355.)

benefit may actually be attributable to confounding factors such as good general health at baseline. Cancers detected in screened patients do tend to be earlier cancers with fewer nodal metastases,[14] and patients with resected gastric cancer diagnosed by screening in Japan have better survival than those diagnosed after development of symptoms (**Fig. 45.2**). However, a survival difference between screened and unscreened gastric cancer patients persists even after accounting for stage,[15] suggesting that patient selection confounds the effect of screening on mortality. The Japanese findings that early detection and identification of early gastric cancer can improve survival has been confirmed by European investigations, in which patients with early gastric cancers have been shown to have survival rates equivalent to those of patients with benign gastric ulcer (**Fig. 45.3**). Mass screening programs have been found to be cost effective in high-incidence countries such as South Korea,[16] but they are unlikely to be cost effective in lower-incidence countries such as the United States.

Barium-contrast radiographs have, in the past, been the standard method for diagnosing gastric neoplasm. Single-contrast examinations have a diagnostic accuracy of 80%. This diagnostic yield increases to approximately 90% when double-contrast (air and barium) techniques are used. Typical findings include ulceration, the presence of a gastric mass, loss of mucosal detail, and distortion of the gastric silhouette (**Fig. 45.4**). However, contrast radiography has been largely supplanted by endoscopy (with or without EUS) in contemporary practice because of the ability to obtain biopsy material concurrently by the latter technique.

Computed tomography (CT) can provide information about both the primary tumor and visceral metastatic disease. Because it is noninvasive and widely available, it is often the first staging modality that is employed in a patient diagnosed with gastric cancer. Patients who are found to have metastatic disease can be spared further, potentially invasive staging studies. When performed with intraluminal and intravenous contrast, CT can demonstrate infiltration of the gastric wall by tumor, gastric ulceration, and the presence of hepatic metastases (**Figs. 45.5 and 45.6**). While depth of invasion and serosal involvement can be assessed, CT is generally not as accurate as EUS for assessment of depth of tumor (T category).

EUS is a useful method of preoperative evaluation for local staging and diagnosis. As noted above, EUS can assess subepithelial lesions that may be confused with gastric cancer and guide biopsy of submucosal tumors within the wall of the stomach. Investigation of submucosal masses, infiltrative gastric disorders, and enlarged gastric epithelial folds, as well as differentiation of gastric lymphoma from gastric

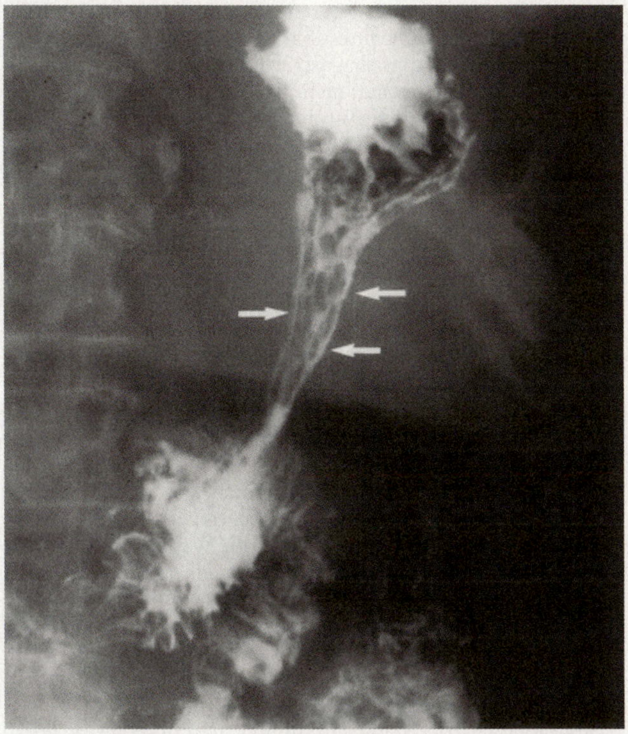

Figure 45.4. Barium-contrast radiograph demonstrating extensive involvement of the gastric body by infiltrating adenocarcinoma (linitis plastica). The gastric silhouette is narrowed (*arrows*), and the stomach is nondistensible.

adenocarcinoma, are all aided by EUS. This technique has the ability to assess the depth and pattern of gastric wall penetration by the tumor, as well as relationship to adjacent structures and has good correlation with intraoperative assessment and histologic findings. Perigastric lymph nodes involved with tumor are also reliably identified by EUS, though limitations with the transducer make visualization of more distant lymph nodes difficult. Nevertheless, EUS provides an accurate assessment of local stage of disease (TN status), with an accuracy of 46% to 88% for staging depth of tumor invasion and 30% to 90% for nodal involvement.[17]

EUS serves as a useful adjunct to cross-sectional imaging and can help guide selection of patients for further staging studies

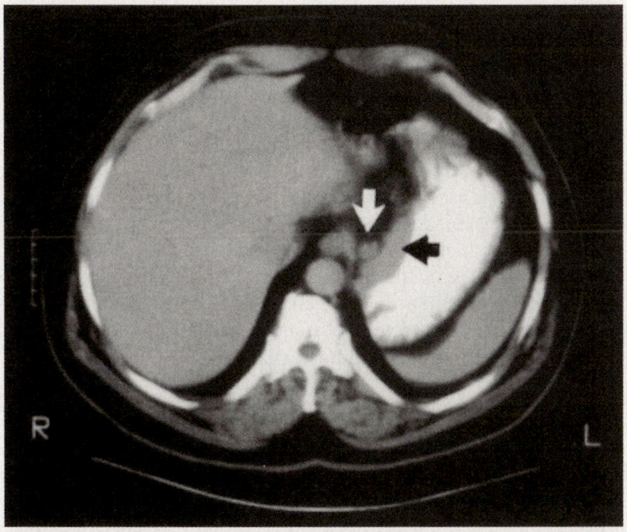

Figure 45.5. Computed tomography scan demonstrating mass along lesser curvature of the stomach (*black arrow*) and associated lymph node enlargement (*white arrow*).

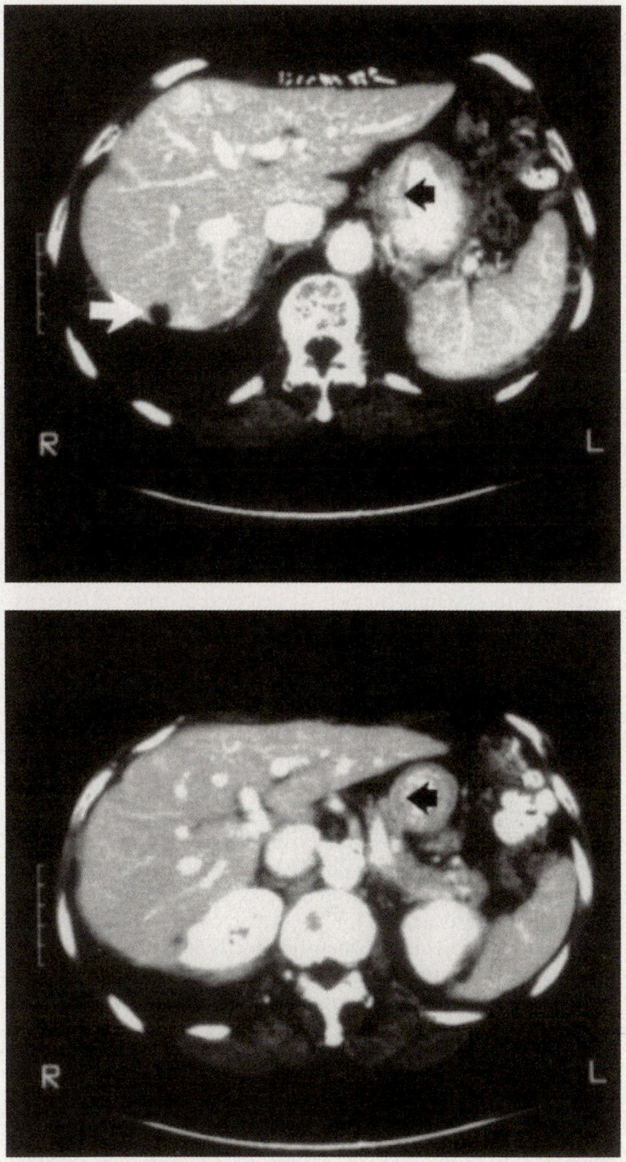

Figure 45.6. Computed tomography scans of the upper abdomen showing extensive thickening of the gastric wall (*black arrows*) caused by infiltrating adenocarcinoma and associated hepatic metastasis (*white arrow*).

or multimodality therapy. Evaluation of nodal disease by CT is very limited and CT is not reliable for detection of small peritoneal metastases, which may be missed in 30% of cases. Interestingly, the addition of 18-fluorodeoxyglucose (FDG) positive emission tomography (PET) has been found to be less accurate than cross-sectional imaging and EUS for assessing locoregional involvement, but more sensitive for detecting distant metastases in patients with gastric cancer. A meta-analysis comparing PET, ultrasound, CT, and magnetic resonance imaging (MRI) found that PET scan was the most sensitive imaging modality for detecting hepatic metastases.[18] A separate study found that tumors which demonstrated metabolic response to neoadjuvant chemotherapy on PET correlated highly with histopathologic response and improved patient survival.[19] Therefore, current recommendations regarding the use of PET for staging gastric cancer are for selective use for patients with locally advanced tumors where the metastatic potential is high and for cases in which neoadjuvant therapy is being considered.[18]

EUS is generally not useful for detecting metastatic disease, but it may help identify patients at risk for radiographically occult metastatic disease (eg, peritoneal metastases) for staging laparoscopy. However, even with adequate endoscopic

STOMACH AND DUODENUM

evaluation and cross-sectional imaging, occult metastases may be missed in 16% to 37% of patients. As such, staging laparoscopy is recommended for patients with potentially resectable gastric cancer.[20]

Staging Laparoscopy

The peritoneal lining, omentum, and liver capsule are common sites for gastric cancer metastasis that are difficult to evaluate preoperatively by CT scanning. In prospective studies, diagnostic laparoscopy has been superior to preoperative CT or percutaneous ultrasound in detection of peritoneal, hepatic, or lymphatic metastasis. Accurate identification of patients with metastatic disease is important in order to spare them futile, ultimately noncurative surgical procedures. Laparoscopy, that includes peritoneal lavage and acquisition of fluid for cytologic examination, will detect metastatic disease that precludes curative resection in up to 37% of patients[20] The highest yield for detection of occult metastatic disease is in those with T3 or T4 disease, and nodal involvement, noting low yield in cases that are T1 or T2, and N0.

Even in cases with planned upfront resection, staging laparoscopy should be performed prior to gastrectomy. Most patients with systemic metastasis detected at time of laparoscopy can be treated without the need for palliative surgical resection. Laparoscopy affords excellent visualization of the peritoneum, especially if care is taken to examine parietal and visceral surfaces, including the diaphragm, liver, spleen, bowel, and omentum. In addition to detection of grossly evident intra-abdominal metastatic disease, patients with findings of microscopic metastatic disease are at high risk for early recurrence and death after attempted curative resection.[21] Based on such a finding, patients with positive cytology in peritoneal washings are considered to have M1 disease. Approximately one-fourth of patients subjected to staging laparoscopy prior to planned curative resection of gastric cancer will have positive peritoneal cytology; one-third of these patients will not have had grossly apparent metastatic disease. The peritoneum also remains the most common organ of recurrence after R0 resection. Patients who clear their initially positive peritoneal cytology after systemic chemotherapy have an improved prognosis.[22] These considerations have led to recent work examining the role of heated intraperitoneal chemotherapy (HIPEC) with or without cytoreductive surgery for patients with evidence of carcinomatosis. Early results suggest that survival can be improved for comparable patients without peritoneal disease. However, long-term survival or cure remains highly unlikely in presence of peritoneal disease.[23]

Patients with locally advanced (T3–T4 or node-positive) tumors who are being considered for neoadjuvant therapy should undergo diagnostic laparoscopy with peritoneal washings prior to initiation of chemotherapy. In this situation, the finding of positive peritoneal cytology should prompt adoption of a noncurative paradigm of treatment in most cases. If carcinomatosis is limited or cytology positive only, patients may be eligible for ongoing trials of neoadjuvant HIPEC (with or without cytoreduction) with chance to treat the carcinomatosis and proceed with curative-intent gastrectomy.

Relative to laparotomy, the shorter hospitalization and reduced operative trauma following laparoscopy may both hasten recovery and facilitate earlier initiation of systemic chemotherapy. Despite strong evidence supporting benefits of accurate staging, laparoscopy is underused in the management of gastric cancer, noting that less than 10% of potentially eligible patients[24] undergo staging laparoscopy prior to planned gastrectomy or neoadjuvant treatment.

Pathology

Gastric adenocarcinoma occurs in two distinct histologic subtypes—intestinal and diffuse. These subtypes are characterized by differing pathologic and clinical features and by differing patterns of metastatic spread.

In the intestinal form of gastric cancer, the malignant cells tend to form glands. The intestinal form of malignancy is more frequently associated with gastric mucosal atrophy, chronic atrophic gastritis, intestinal metaplasia, and dysplasia. Gastric cancer with the intestinal histologic subtype is more common in populations at high risk (eg, Japan), and it occurs with increased frequency in men and older patients. Clinical studies suggest that this subtype more frequently demonstrates blood-borne metastases.

The diffuse form of gastric adenocarcinoma does not demonstrate gland formation and tends to infiltrate tissues as a sheet of loosely adherent cells. Lymphatic invasion is common. Intraperitoneal metastases are frequent. The diffuse form of gastric adenocarcinoma tends to occur in younger patients, in women, and in populations with a relatively low incidence of gastric cancer (eg, the United States). The prognosis is poorer for patients with the diffuse histologic subtype.

Additionally, signet ring cell carcinoma (SRC) is being investigated as a unique form of adenocarcinoma. SRC tumors contain scattered malignant cells containing intracytoplasmic mucin, and this prognostic importance in both Western and Eastern studies remains less than clear. A recent analysis that compared over 1,600 patients with SRC with well-to-moderately differentiated adenocarcinoma found that SRC has mixed prognosis, having better survival for early gastric cancer (ie, T1) but worse prognosis in advanced disease compared to well-to-moderately differentiated adenocarcinoma.[25]

Sporadic gastric adenocarcinomas demonstrate a number of chromosomal and genetic abnormalities. Cytometric analysis reveals that gastric tumors with a large fraction of aneuploid cells (with a greater-than-normal amount of nuclear DNA) tend to be more highly infiltrative and have a poorer prognosis. Amplifications of both the HER-2/*neu* and K-*ras* proto-oncogenes have been consistently detected in gastric adenocarcinomas, and in a small percentage of tumors, a lack of expression of the tumor suppressor gene *MKK4* is robustly associated with poor survival.

In the United States, the incidence of proximal gastric cancers has been increasing markedly over past few decades, while tumors of body and distal stomach are relatively stable.[26] Proximal cancers are more likely to occur in young White men and distal cancers are more likely to occur in Asian, African American, and Hispanic patients within the United States. In 10% of cases, the stomach is diffusely involved at the time of diagnosis based on historical data. Prognosis is poorer for tumors arising from the proximal stomach and for those with diffuse involvement of the organ relative to distal tumors. As such, these patients are much more likely to need neoadjuvant and adjuvant therapy.

The current staging system for gastric cancer is described in the 8th edition American Joint Committee on Cancer (AJCC).[27] The staging system accurately discriminates prognosis based on pathologic factors for tumors located 5 cm distal to the esophagogastric junction (EGJ) and below or arising within 5 cm of, but not crossing, the EGJ (Fig. 45.7). The AJCC recommends that cancers arising within 5 cm of the EGJ that cross into the EGJ or esophagus be staged and treated as esophageal cancers. A consideration of staging data illustrates the high frequency with which lymph node metastases are present at the time of diagnosis in the United States, and the severe impact lymphatic involvement has on survival. Even early gastric cancers (tumors restricted to the mucosa and submucosa) have a 15% prevalence of nodal metastasis.

Curative-Intent Treatment

Surgical resection is the only potentially curative therapy for gastric cancer, but an advanced stage of disease at the time of diagnosis precludes curative resection for most patients. Since the mid-1990s, the surgical treatment of gastric cancer has continued to evolve, with minimally invasive approaches increasingly pursued for early cancers and increasingly radical operations advocated by some for advanced tumors. The

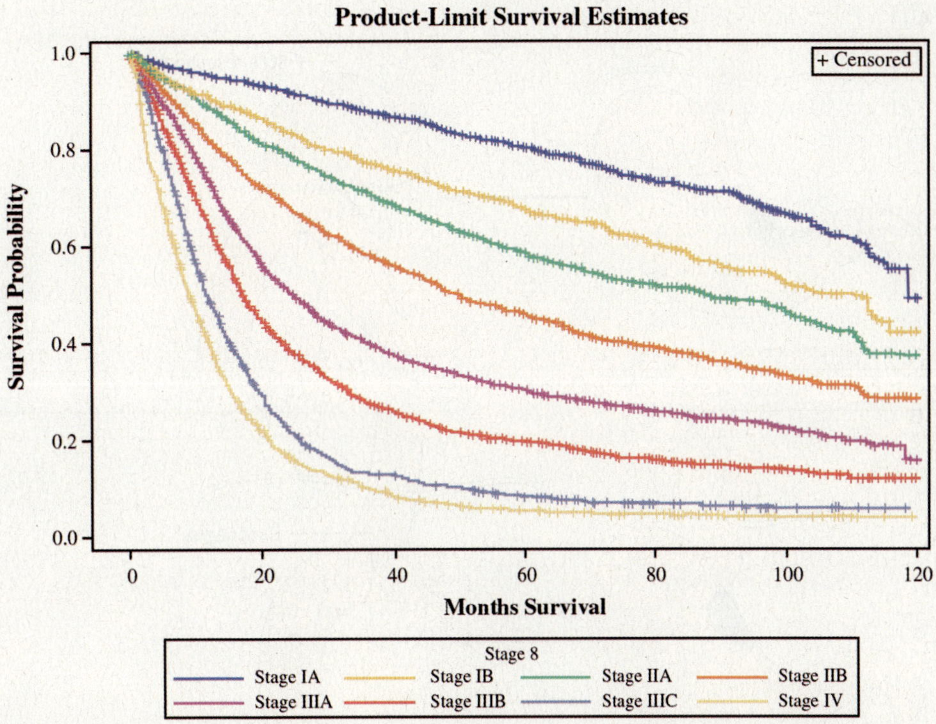

Figure 45.7. Gastric cancer 5-year survival by AJCC 8th edition pTNM stage groupings, based on data from the National Cancer Database. (From In H, Solsky I, Palis B, Langdon-Embry M, Ajani J, Sano T. Validation of the 8th edition of the AJCC TNM staging system for gastric cancer using the National Cancer Database. *Ann Surg Oncol.* 2017;24:3683–3691.)

Japanese Gastric Cancer Association defines early gastric cancer as tumor in which invasion is restricted to the mucosa or submucosa, noting that the presence or absence of lymph node metastasis is not considered in this classification. While the presence of lymphatic metastasis cannot be correctly judged by endoscopic findings, it is critically important in prognosis. For tumors confined to the mucosa, lymphatic metastasis is present in 1% to 3% of cases; with submucosal involvement, the rate of nodal positivity increases to 14% to 20%.[28]

Endoscopic Resection

Endoscopic approaches to the treatment of gastric cancer continue to evolve and advance. Endoscopic mucosal resection (EMR) and endoscopic submucosal dissection (ESD) may be considered as alternatives to surgical resection for very early-stage gastric cancer, especially by those with extensive experience with the techniques. For intestinal-type mucosal tumors less than 2 cm in size, without ulceration, or evidence of lymphovascular invasion, EMR may be performed with achievement of an R0 resection. EMR is performed by using a snare, with or without an electrosurgical current, to resect a mucosal lesion. With this approach, postoperative bleeding or perforation has been reported in up to 5%, and in up to 17% histologic examination revealed submucosal invasion that required further operative treatment. A Japanese series of 131 patients reported disease-free survival of 99% at 10 years[29] and others have demonstrated long-term results comparable to gastrectomy in terms of recurrence and mortality.[30] ESD is an emerging technique that may allow larger tumors (>3 cm) to be endoscopically resected. ESD is performed by injecting fluid into the submucosa to elevate the lesion, incising the mucosa around the lesion, then dissecting the lesion from the deeper submucosal layers. The main advantage of ESD is it allows for en bloc removal of tumors and lower rates of positive margins. However, even in experienced hands at high volume centers, there are higher associated rates of bleeding and perforation and there may not be any benefit over EMR for lesions less than 5 cm in size. Attention to surveillance endoscopy following EMR or ESD is mandatory. While the advantages of utilizing endoscopic resection for treating early cancers include avoiding the morbidity associated with surgical gastrectomy, endoscopic resection comes with its own disadvantages. Primarily, patients forgo lymph node staging with endoscopic resection since lymphadenectomy is not completed. The absence of lymphadenectomy is accompanied with the risk of pathologic understaging and the omission of adjuvant therapy that would otherwise be administered in pathologic lymph node positive disease. To minimize these risks, endoscopic resection is only recommended in patients with tumors limited to the mucosa (T1a) and with well/moderately differentiated histology, since these lesions have been shown to have a risk of lymph node metastasis less than 5%.[28]

Surgical Resection

4 The fundamental principle of surgical resection of gastric cancer is complete extirpation of the primary tumor. The extent of gastric resection is determined primarily by the need to obtain a resection margin free of microscopic disease (R0 resection) and requires formal, anatomic gastrectomy. Microscopic involvement of the resection margin by tumor cells (R1 resection) is associated with poor prognosis. Patients with positive surgical margins are at high risk for development of recurrent disease, and histologically positive margins are strongly correlated with the development of anastomotic recurrence. In the setting of ≥5 positive nodes, however, margin positivity itself does not impact survival, because these patients are at higher risk for systemic recurrence. In contrast to other gastrointestinal malignancies such as colon cancer, gastric cancer frequently demonstrates extensive intramural spread, especially the diffuse type. The propensity for intramural spread is related, in part, to the extensive anastomosing capillary and lymphatic network in the wall of the stomach. As such, wedge or segmental resections are inadequate and should not be performed. Based on retrospective studies as well as prospective data from the Italian Gastrointestinal Tumor Study Group, when performing a subtotal gastrectomy, a 3- to 6-cm (commonly cited as 5-cm) margin of resection is adequate and necessary to minimize anastomotic recurrence.[31]

For lesions in the distal two-thirds (middle or distal third) of the stomach, subtotal gastrectomy is usually sufficient for complete removal of the primary tumor.[32] In contrast, lesions in the upper third of the stomach generally require total gastrectomy (or esophagogastrectomy) to assure adequate resection (**Fig. 45.8**).[32] For tumors involving the cardia without

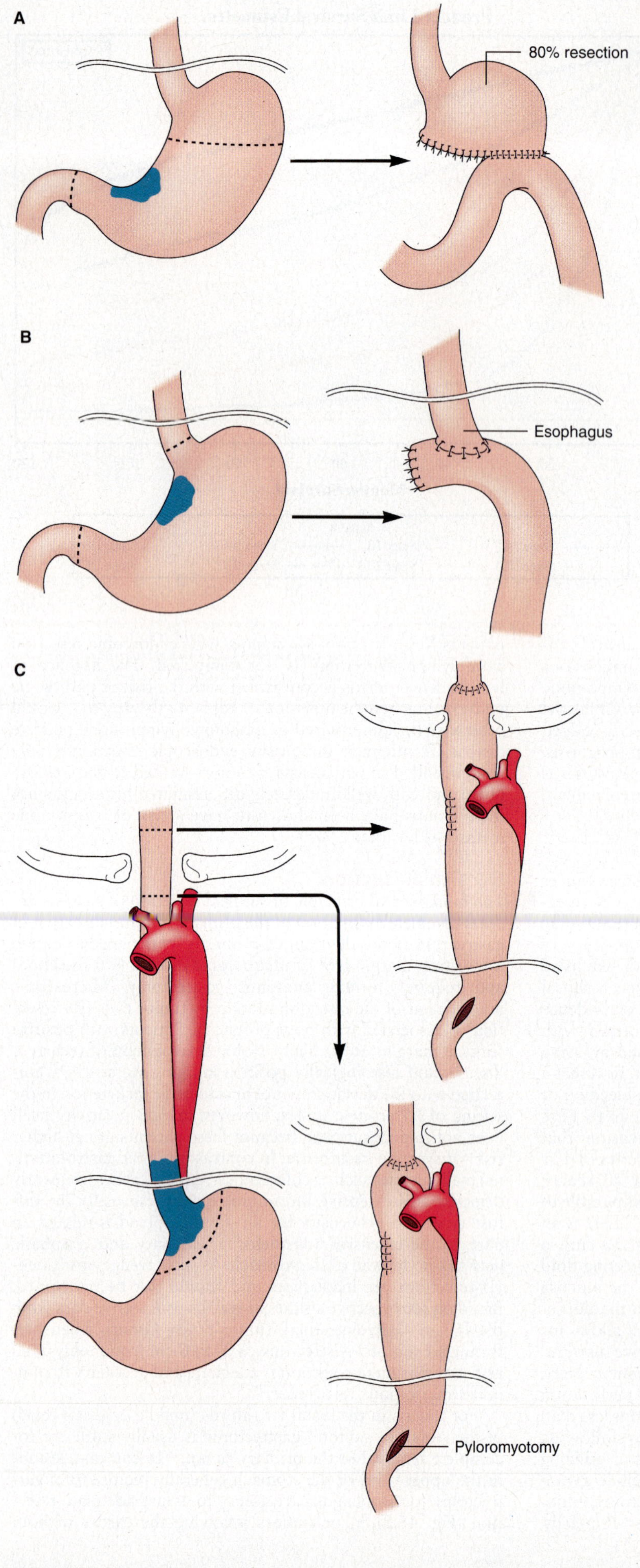

Figure 45.8. Surgical options for resection of gastric neoplasms. **A:** Subtotal gastrectomy with gastrojejunal reconstruction. **B:** Total gastrectomy with esophagojejunostomy. **C:** Esophagogastrectomy with anastomosis in cervical or thoracic position.

involvement of the gastroesophageal junction, some have advocated proximal gastrectomy as an alternative to total gastrectomy with esophagojejunostomy with the goal of preserving a gastric reservoir. This procedure does not compromise oncologic outcomes, but there is a significantly higher incidence of severe reflux esophagitis with proximal gastrectomy, and is generally not recommended even with jejunal interposition or fundoplication. The distal stomach is typically divided at the level of the duodenal bulb, beyond the pylorus. Local invasion into the duodenum on the distal margin can occur, though pancreaticoduodenectomy is rarely needed to assure clearance of disease. Frozen section evaluation of resection margins may be obtained prior to proceeding with reconstruction in order to improve the probability that radical (R0) resection is achieved, especially if gross margins are deemed closer than 3 cm. However, the decision to reresect in the setting of a positive frozen section margin is controversial and must take operative risk as well as tumor biology into account. Reresection has only been associated with improved survival in early-stage gastric cancer.[33] It is plausible that positive frozen section margins may be a surrogate for aggressive disease.

During the course of a radical resection, ligation of the right gastric and right gastroepiploic artery is standard. Ligation of the left gastric artery is a required part of a total gastrectomy, and is done selectively for partial gastrectomy. While the omentum is commonly removed en bloc as part of a radical gastrectomy, complete removal of the omental bursa (the peritoneum overlying the pancreas and anterior transverse mesocolon) is not indicated.[20] For some T4 tumors, a multivisceral resection is indicated if required to achieve complete removal of the tumor in the course of a curative-intent resection. Data evaluating the additional morbidity and mortality associated with multivisceral resection is variable and may be dependent on the organs removed, with higher risks associated with pancreatectomy than with splenectomy or colectomy.

Radical gastric operations can be performed with acceptable morbidity and low mortality rates in the older age groups at greatest risk for gastric cancer. In modern series, mortality rates for total gastrectomy range from 3% to 6%.[34] There is some evidence that outcomes are superior at higher-volume centers.[35] In the postacute setting, nutritional support in the immediate postoperative period is an important adjunctive measure as patients resume oral intake, and many surgeons place a jejunal feeding tube at the time of total gastrectomy to ensure that optimal enteral nutrition can be delivered in the postoperative period. Surgical reconstructions that interpose a small intestinal reservoir between the esophagus and the jejunum have been advocated after total gastrectomy, but a clear nutritional benefit has not been demonstrated. Postoperative complications, including malnutrition, adversely impact long-term survival in patients with gastric cancer due to a generalized failure to thrive or perhaps due, at least in part, to lower rates of adjuvant therapy.

Because gastric cancer metastasizes so frequently to lymph nodes, radical extirpation of draining lymph nodes has both diagnostic/staging and therapeutic implications. The value of routine-extended lymphadenectomy beyond the perigastric lymph nodes in the treatment of gastric adenocarcinoma, however, is controversial. The first favorable experience was reported from Japan, and extent of resection in the original Japanese system is shown in **Table 45.3**; the current nomenclature used to define extent of lymphadenectomy is shown in **Table 45.4** and **Figure 45.9**. Only retrospective studies of extended perigastric lymphadenectomy have been reported from Japan, and those reports suggested an improvement of approximately 10%, stage for stage, for patients with advanced disease treated with D2 or D3 operations. The benefits of extended lymphadenectomy have not been confirmed in non-Japanese centers, and several randomized trials in Western centers have failed to show a survival benefit for extended lymphadenectomy when the entire patient population was analyzed.[15] Long-term follow-up results from the Dutch trial of D1 versus D2 lymphadenectomy have shown a lower gastric cancer–related death rate in the D2 group (37% vs. 48%) and lower rates of local and regional recurrence.[36] The significance of this finding and implications for extended lymphadenopathy are unclear, given the absence of an overall survival benefit as well as intervening improvements in adjuvant therapy over the 15-year follow-up period. Additionally, in previous decades, the upstaging that results from positive lymph nodes found in extended lymphadenectomy could lead to the addition of adjuvant therapy, potentially conferring survival/recurrence-free benefit. However, in the current era where perioperative chemotherapy has become the standard for all patients with resectable disease, the therapeutic value of extended lymphadenectomy has been further questioned.

Data from a National Japanese Registry indicate a contemporary mortality of less than 1% associated with extended lymphadenectomy, and low mortality risks have been reported from multi-institutional trials conducted in Italy and Germany.[15,36–38] Investigations from the United States, Britain, and the Netherlands have been less optimistic, indicating increased short-term morbidity and in-hospital mortality.

MANAGEMENT

Table 45.3. Lymphadenectomy in the Original System of the Japanese Research Society for Gastric Cancer

Level	Description
R1	Resection of stomach, omentum, and perigastric lymph nodes
R2	Resection of stomach, omentum, and en bloc removal of the superior leaf of the transverse mesocolon, the pancreatic capsule, and lymph nodes along the branches of the celiac artery and in the infraduodenal and supraduodenal areas
R3	Resection of the above structures plus lymph nodes along the aorta and esophagus, along with the spleen and the tail of the pancreas, and skeletonization of vessels in the porta hepatis

MANAGEMENT

Table 45.4. Current Nomenclature Used to Describe the Extent of Lymphadenectomy Performed in Conjunction with Gastrectomy

Level	Description
D0	Any lymph node removal that is less than D1
D1	Resection of greater and lesser omenta, including the perigastric nodes along the right and left cardia, nodes along the lesser and greater curvatures, suprapyloric nodes along the right gastric artery, and infrapyloric nodes
D2	D1 dissection plus nodes along the left gastric artery, common hepatic artery, celiac trunk, splenic hilum, and splenic artery
D3	D2 dissection plus nodes in the hepatoduodenal ligament, retropancreatic nodes, and nodes at the root of the mesentery, the para-aortic lymph nodes
D4	D3 dissection plus paracolic and para-aortic nodes

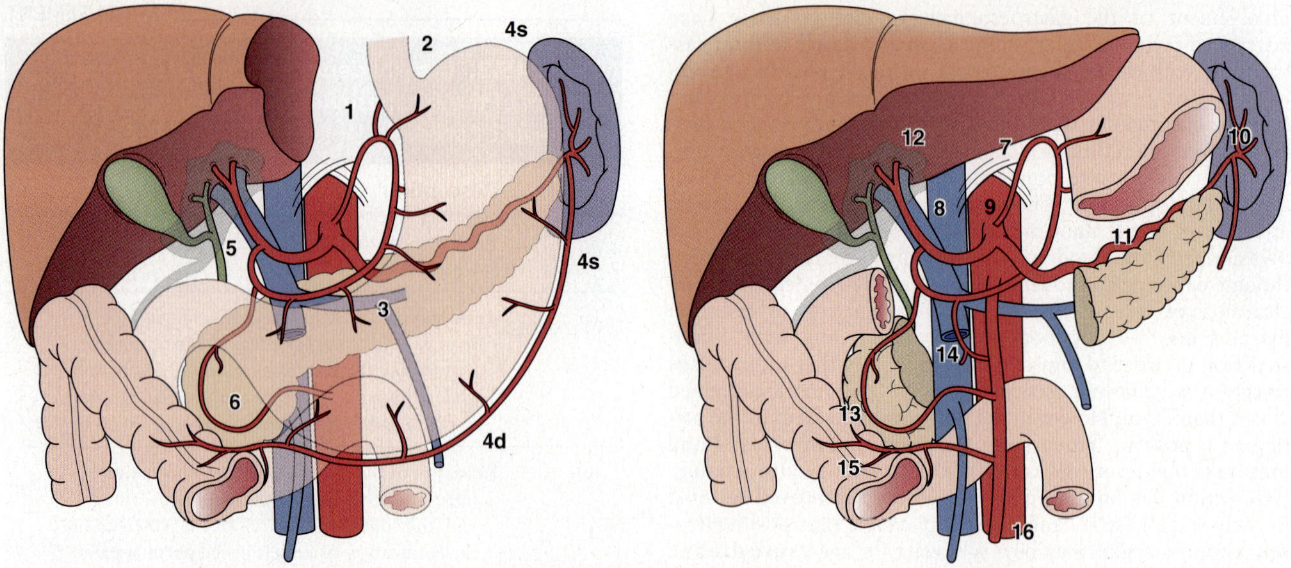

N1 Lymph nodes (perigastric)
1 Right cardiac nodes
2 Left cardiac nodes
3 Nodes along the lesser curvature
4d Lymph nodes along the short gastric and the left gastroepiploic vessels
4s Lymph nodes along the right gastroepiploic vessels
5 Suprapyloric nodes
6 Infrapyloric nodes

N2 Lymph nodes (celiac axis branches)
7 Nodes along root left gastric artery
8 Nodes along common hepatic artery
9 Nodes around celiac axis
10 Nodes at splenic hilum
11 Nodes along splenic artery

N3 Lymph nodes
12 Nodes at the hepatoduodenal ligament
13 Retropancreatic (periduodenal) nodes
14 Nodes at the root of the mesentery

N4 Lymph nodes
15 Nodes along the middle colic vein
16 Para-aortic nodes

Figure 45.9. Lymph node locations and groupings. D1 dissection: removal of N1 nodes. D2 dissection: removal of N1 and N2 nodes. D3 dissection: removal of N1, N2, and N3 nodes. D4 dissection: removal of N1–N4 nodes.

Histologically positive lymph nodes are frequently present in the splenic hilum and along the splenic artery, and routine splenectomy has been practiced in some centers. Splenectomy in this setting has not been demonstrated to improve outcome for similarly staged patients. Associated splenectomy or pancreatosplenectomy is only beneficial when there is direct extension or bulky adenopathy at the splenic hilum.

Recommendations for a minimum number of regional lymph nodes retrieved and examined with lymphadenectomy serve as a proxy for adequacy of resection. Emphasis on the total number of nodes removed rather than the location of the nodes (eg, D1 lymphadenectomy) continues to be debated. While the AJCC staging system does not strictly specify a minimum number of nodes, N3b disease is defined by metastases in 16 nodes. As such, current recommendations for gastric cancer staging suggest that a minimum of 16 nodes need to be retrieved and evaluated.[20,27,39]

The approach to resection can be via traditional open surgery or via a minimally invasive approach, either laparoscopic or using robotic surgical techniques. The main use of minimally invasive gastrectomy includes, but is not necessarily limited to, early and distal tumors. Resection of more advanced cancers or total gastrectomy have been reported for treatment of known gastric malignancy, but must take surgeon training and experience into account. Multiple studies from Japan, Korea, and Italy have demonstrated that distal, subtotal, or total gastrectomy with lymphadenectomy is feasible with acceptable morbidity and mortality. A meta-analysis of four small single-institution randomized trials from Asia demonstrated lower nodal harvests with a laparoscopic approach for early gastric cancer. Complication rates were lower in the laparoscopic group but did not translate into differences in time to oral intake or length of stay.[40] However, a single-institution Western randomized trial of laparoscopic versus open subtotal gastrectomy for distal gastric cancer (both early and locally advanced) did report equivalent lymph node retrieval (33.4 ± 7.4 in the open group vs. 30 ± 14.9 in the laparoscopic group), as well as similar rates of perioperative morbidity and mortality. Their 5-year overall and disease-free survival were also similar for both groups: 55.7% and 54.8% for the laparoscopic group versus 58.9% and 57.3% for the open group, respectively.[41] More recently, results of the Korean Laparoendoscopy Gastrointestinal Surgery Study (KLASS), a multicenter randomized trial focused on distal gastrectomy for early gastric cancer demonstrated improved perioperative morbidity and no differences in oncologic outcomes have been shown with short follow-up.[42] Early results from the Chinese Laparoscopic Gastrointestinal Surgery Study (CLASS) Group randomized clinical trial comparing the safety of laparoscopic versus open total gastrectomy with lymphadenectomy for patients with clinical stage I gastric cancer showed that overall morbidity and mortality rates were not significantly different between the groups.[43]

Neoadjuvant and Adjuvant Therapies

5 Given the largely disappointing outcomes of locoregional or locally advanced gastric cancer in Western countries, significant interest has focused on the use of multimodality therapy. Several neoadjuvant and adjuvant approaches have been explored. Although there is no consensus on the optimal approach, it is clear that all patients with locally advanced disease should be considered for multimodality therapy. Several landmark trials highlight a primary role for both adjuvant and neoadjuvant chemotherapy. Despite the limitations of these studies, which are beyond the scope of the present discussion, improved survival observed across trials makes it clear that a multimodality approach is superior to surgery alone for those patients with locally advanced gastric cancer. The addition of radiation to surgery has also been associated with improved local control

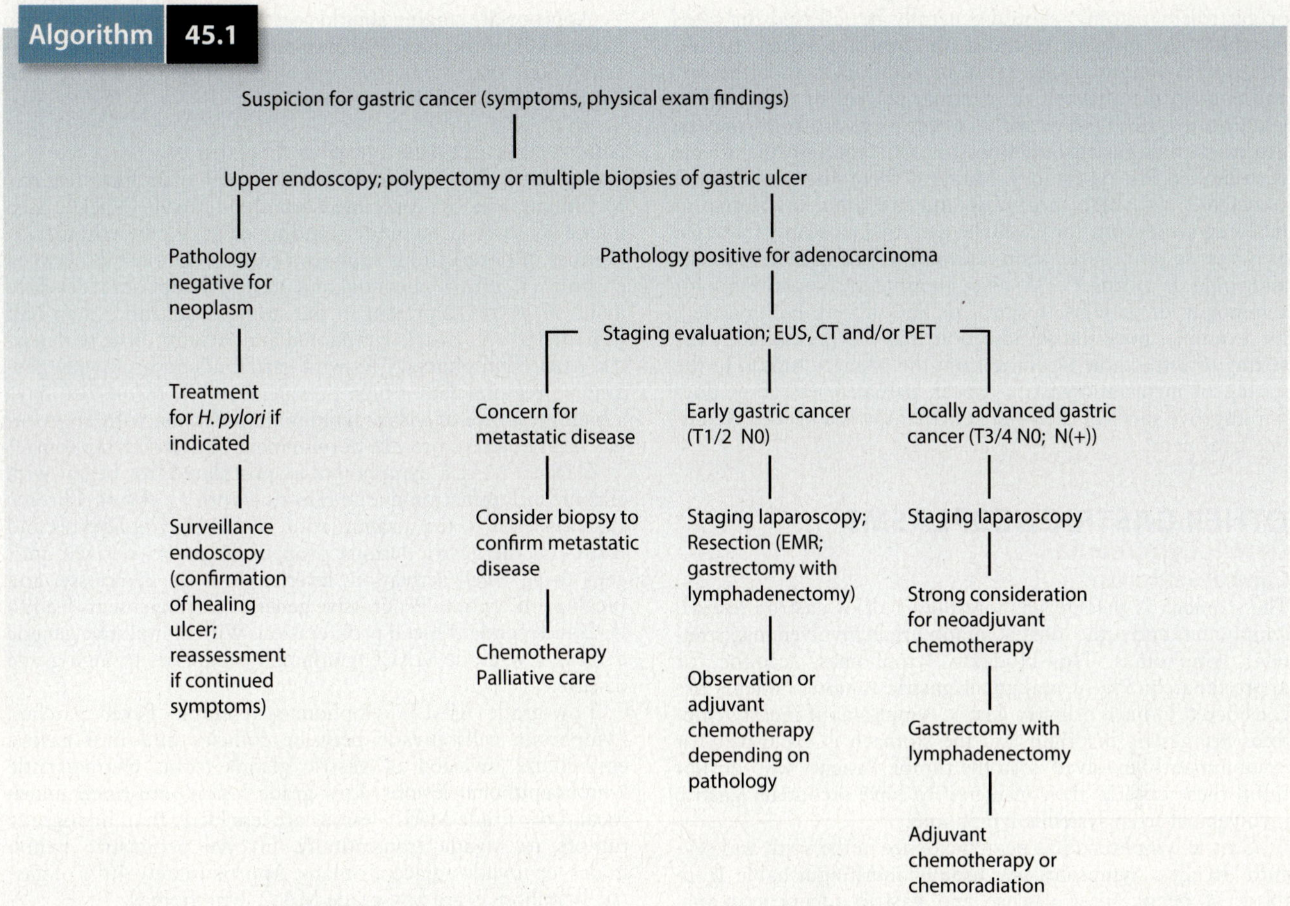

Algorithm 45.1. Diagnosis and management of gastric cancer.

and survival. A randomized phase III trial (CRITICS) comparing perioperative chemotherapy with preoperative chemotherapy followed by postoperative chemoradiation found no improvement in overall survival with the addition of postoperative radiation.[32] However, numerous ongoing studies are investigating the relative benefits of various chemotherapeutic regimens as well as the incremental benefit of chemoradiotherapy (with radiation in both the preoperative and postoperative settings) versus chemotherapy alone. This includes CRITICS II, which compares three preoperative strategies: chemotherapy, chemoradiation (concurrent), and sequential chemotherapy and chemoradiation treatments.

A neoadjuvant, or perioperative, approach is preferred for resectable disease. A randomized controlled phase II/III trial led to standard recommendations for fluorouracil, leucovorin, oxaliplatin, and docetaxel (FLOT) for patients with T2 or greater disease and/or node-positive disease if performance status is good.[44] Other regimens may be considered if performance status is more concerning, since a regimen of fluorouracil and oxaliplatin (FOLFOX) is better tolerated and has a lower chemotherapy-related toxicity profile. There are newer considerations for a total neoadjuvant therapy approach, meaning that all systemic therapy is administered in advance of the operation. In these cases, additional chemotherapy in the postoperative setting is only administered if microscopic disease or unexpectedly advanced nodal disease is found at time of gastrectomy. Some have advocated for the total neoadjuvant approach in order to mitigate against the adverse impact postoperative complications, and subsequent delays in adjuvant treatment may have on long-term survival[45] as it appears that rates of completion of multimodality treatment are much higher when given in the preoperative setting.

Targeted therapies, which are currently approved for use in recurrent, advanced, or metastatic disease, are also being actively investigated for use in the neoadjuvant setting. Treatment with trastuzumab is based on HER-2 status, with phase III trial evidence supporting first-line use in metastatic gastric cancer.[22] Treatment with neoadjuvant nivolumab and ipilimumab in patients with microsatellite instability-high/mismatch repair deficient (MSI-H/dMMR) disease in a phase II trial resulted in a 58.6% complete pathologic response.[46] A pooled analysis of perioperative chemotherapy trials evaluating patients with MSI-H/dMMR resectable gastric cancer highlighted that chemotherapy may lead to worse outcomes in these patients.[47,48] As a result, many centers now proceed with upfront surgery or perioperative immunotherapy in patients with MSI-H/dMMR resectable gastric cancer. Testing for MSI-H/dMMR is now recommended for all newly diagnosed patients, and HER-2 expression, and PD-L1 status are recommended in the setting of metastatic disease.

As preoperative strategies continue to evolve, patients with locally advanced resectable gastric cancer are optimally treated in a center where a collaborative multidisciplinary treatment approach can be devised and executed (**Algorithm 45.1**). Not only is discussion at a team meeting or tumor board important for decision making and treatment planning, but it also helps with careful coordination across the continuum of cancer care.

Palliative Surgical Treatment

When preoperative evaluation demonstrates disseminated disease, palliation of symptoms becomes a primary consideration. Palliation does not usually require surgical intervention. Obstruction and bleeding can be managed nonoperatively with endoscopic techniques, including intraluminal stents, or radiotherapy in selected patients. Dysphagia and bleeding caused by proximal lesions can also be alleviated endoscopically (laser therapy or stenting) in the majority of patients. Surgical palliation of obstructive symptoms (via formal resection or gastrojejunostomy) should generally be reserved for cases in which less invasive methods are contraindicated, technically infeasible, or unsuccessful. In addition to radiotherapy and endoscopic ablation or stenting, placement of a feeding jejunostomy tube with or without venting gastrostomy may be used to palliate gastric outlet obstruction, especially in patients with limited life expectancy. Many of these interventions are associated with high morbidity and are often ineffective at relieving symptoms; for example, gastrojejunostomy intended as a bypass procedure, often does not afford gastric drainage and could delay onset of systemic treatments. Nonetheless, for a minority of patients, surgical palliation may be indicated; for example, noncurative resection may be necessary in the setting of intractable bleeding from the primary tumor. In the setting of metastatic gastric cancer, palliative resection does not improve survival, and systemic therapy is considered first-line treatment.

OTHER GASTRIC NEOPLASMS

Gastric Lymphoma

Clinical Features

The stomach is the site of more than half of gastrointestinal lymphomas and is the most common organ involved in extranodal lymphomas. Non-Hodgkin lymphomas account for approximately 5% of malignant gastric tumors. Patients are considered to have primary gastric lymphoma if initial symptoms are gastric in origin and the stomach is exclusively or predominantly involved with the tumor. Patients who do not fulfill these criteria are considered to have secondary gastric involvement from systemic lymphoma.

Gastric lymphoma has peak incidence in the sixth and seventh decades. Symptoms are usually indistinguishable from those of peptic ulcer disease and gastric adenocarcinoma. Epigastric pain, weight loss, anorexia, nausea, and vomiting are common. Systemic B symptoms, such as fever and night sweats, occur in a minority of patients but may be suggestive of the diagnosis. Although gross bleeding is uncommon, occult hemorrhage and anemia are observed in more than half of patients. Patients rarely have spontaneous perforation.

Diagnosis

Radiologic findings are similar to those for adenocarcinoma (gastric thickening and lymphadenopathy). Endoscopic examination is the diagnostic method of choice. The endoscopic appearance of lesions may be ulcerated, polypoid, or infiltrative, and this morphology may be further characterized by EUS. Gastric lymphoma is most commonly localized to the middle or distal stomach and unusually involves the proximal stomach, in contrast to gastric adenocarcinoma. Endoscopic biopsy, combined with endoscopic brush cytology and EUS, provides positive diagnosis in 90% of cases. Submucosal growth without ulceration of the overlying mucosa can occasionally render endoscopic biopsy nondiagnostic. EUS-guided biopsy is useful in this circumstance.

Appropriate staging should search for evidence of systemic disease. CT of the chest and abdomen (to detect lymphadenopathy), bone marrow biopsy, and biopsy of enlarged peripheral lymph nodes are all appropriate.

Mucosa-Associated Lymphoid Tissue

The concept that low-grade gastric lymphomas have features resembling mucosa-associated lymphoid tissue (MALT) is a major advance in the understanding of gastric lymphomas. A number of observations support a causal relationship between chronic *H. pylori* infection and gastric lymphoma development. *H. pylori* is present in the stomachs of more than half of patients with gastric lymphoma and 90% of those with gastric MALT lymphoma.[49] As with gastric adenocarcinoma, geographic regions with a high prevalence of *H. pylori* also have a high incidence of gastric lymphoma. Infection with *H. pylori* has been noted to precede development of gastric lymphoma.

Gastric MALT lymphoma is postulated to begin with chronic inflammation due to infection with *H. pylori.* Chronic gastritis leads to the accumulation of CD4+ lymphocytes and B cells in the gastric lamina propria. *H. pylori*–derived antigens drive T-cell activation, interleukin-2 (IL-2) release, and B-cell proliferation. Progressive genetic rearrangements lead to IL-2–independent B-cell proliferation. With cumulative genetic defects, low-grade MALT lymphoma progresses to high-grade disease.

Low-grade MALT lymphomas resemble Peyer patches. Lymphoma cells invade between follicles and into gastric epithelium; invasion of gastric glands forms characteristic lymphoepithelial lesions. Low-grade lesions are often multifocal. Low-grade MALT lesions are less likely than high-grade tumors to invade transmurally, involve perigastric lymph nodes, or invade adjacent organs. Approximately 40% of gastric lymphomas are low-grade MALT lymphomas.

The concept that low-grade lymphoma depends on continued *H. pylori* antigenic stimulation supports eradication of *H. pylori* with antibiotics as first-line antineoplastic therapy. Complete regression of low-grade gastric MALT lymphomas with antibiotic treatment has been reported in 70% to 100% of cases. The median time to complete response is 5 months. Most patients with partial responses were also subsequently determined to have foci of high-grade lymphoma. Radiation and chemotherapy have been proposed as salvage for antibiotic treatment failures or for the minority of patients with *H. pylori*–negative gastric MALT lymphoma.

Non-MALT Lymphomas

Most non-MALT gastric lymphomas are diffuse large B-cell lymphomas (DLBCLs), including those that were previously called "high-grade MALT lymphomas." DLBCLs typically exhibit more aggressive behavior and worse prognosis than MALT lymphomas. Other histologies, such as mantle cell, follicular, and peripheral T-cell lymphomas, can also be seen. Survival for gastric lymphoma is closely linked to stage at diagnosis (**Fig. 45.10**).

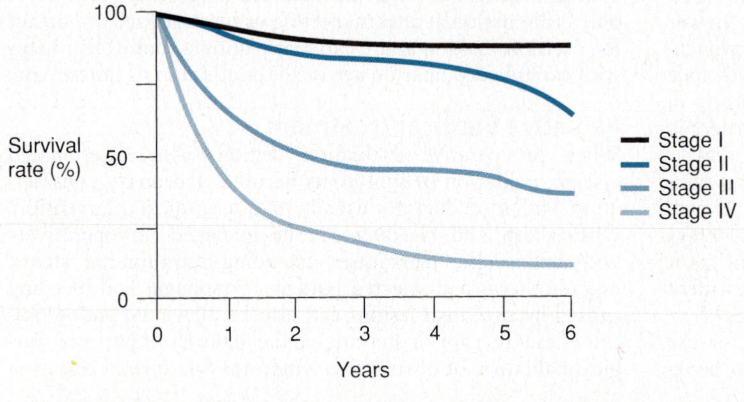

Figure 45.10. Survival with gastric lymphoma, by stage.

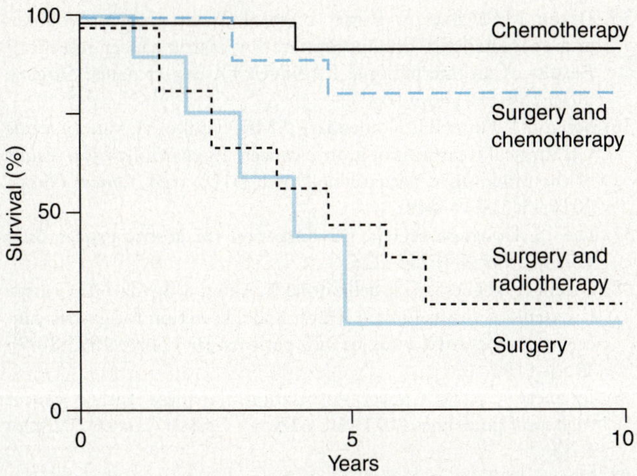

Figure 45.11. Relapse-free survival by treatment assignment for primary gastric diffuse large B-cell lymphoma.

In the past, a multimodality treatment program was used in most centers for primary gastric lymphomas, with gastrectomy as the first step in the therapeutic strategy. Even without prospective data to support gastrectomy, several advantages of this approach had been cited: (a) more accurate histologic evaluation was possible; (b) in cases with localized tumor, the procedure could be curative; and (c) gastrectomy eliminated the risk of life-threatening hemorrhage or perforation which may occur with the treatment of tumors involving the full thickness of the gastric wall However, the role of gastrectomy for both staging and treatment of gastric lymphoma has diminished significantly, based in part on results of a randomized trial demonstrating superior outcomes with CHOP (cyclophosphamide, doxorubicin, vincristine, and prednisone) chemotherapy compared with surgery, surgery plus radiotherapy, or surgery with CHOP (**Fig. 45.11**).[50] It has also been recognized that the incidence of perforation during chemotherapy is only 5%. Most patients are currently treated with chemotherapy (commonly CHOP with rituximab) with or without radiotherapy. Surgical intervention is generally reserved for complications such as obstruction, bleeding, or perforation.

Gastric Carcinoids

Neuroendocrine, or carcinoid, tumors of the stomach were previously considered to be very rare tumors, but more recent studies report that as many as 10% to 30% of all carcinoids occur in the stomach, and they account for at least 1% of all gastric neoplasms. Most patients with small gastric carcinoids are asymptomatic, and these tumors are most commonly diagnosed incidentally. Occasionally, however, larger tumors can present with abdominal pain, bleeding, or symptoms related to the secretion of bioactive substances (serotonin, histamine, or tachykinins) which can be produced by the tumor. When viewed endoscopically at an early stage, carcinoids are reddish-pink to yellow submucosal nodules in the proximal stomach. Endoscopic biopsy is usually diagnostic if sampling can be directed deep enough to sample submucosal tumor cells.

Classically, three types of gastric carcinoids have been described. Type 1 is the most common (65%) and is associated with chronic atrophic gastritis and pernicious anemia. These tumors tend to be small (<1 cm) and multiple, and exhibit indolent behavior and rarely metastasize. They can typically be followed and removed endoscopically, but surgery may be necessary for larger or very numerous tumors. Type 2 tumors comprise approximately 2% of gastric carcinoids and occur in patients with Zollinger–Ellison syndrome (gastrinomas), often in the setting of multiple endocrine neoplasia type 1 (MEN-1). Like type 1 tumors, they are often small, multiple, and indolent, and they can be treated endoscopically for the most part. Both type 1 and type 2 gastric carcinoid tumors are associated with hypergastrinemia. Type 1 and 2 gastric carcinoids arise from enterochromaffin-like (ECL) cells, which mediate the secretion of histamine and, in turn, stimulate parietal cells to secrete acid. Hypergastrinemia (due to chronic atrophic gastritis in type 1 and gastrinoma in type 2) is thought to cause ECL cell hyperplasia and lead to the development of gastric carcinoids over time.

Type 3 lesions account for 13% of gastric carcinoids. Type 3 gastric carcinoids tend to be larger, solitary lesions. They are associated with normal gastrin levels and behave much more aggressively than other gastric carcinoid tumors. Metastases are common, and these tumors can cause an atypical carcinoid syndrome. Type 3 carcinoids are best dealt with by resection and lymphadenectomy, the extent of which depends on the size of the tumor. Approximately 20% of gastric carcinoids have been associated with proton pump inhibitor use. These are not associated with atrophic gastritis, are seen in patients on long-term proton pump inhibitors (PPIs), and are generally indolent.[51]

ACKNOWLEDGMENT

We gratefully acknowledge the contributions of previous edition author, Andrew P. Loehrer, as portions of those chapters have been retained in this revision.

References

1. World Health Organization. International Agency for Research on Cancer. GLOBOCAN 2022: Stomach Cancer Fact Sheet. https://gco.iarc.who.int/media/globocan/factsheets/cancers/7-stomach-fact-sheet.pdf
2. American Cancer Society. *Cancer Facts & Figures 2024*. American Cancer Society; 2024.
3. Huang RJ, Koh H, Hwang JH; Summit Leaders. A summary of the 2020 Gastric Cancer summit at Stanford University. *Gastroenterology.* 2020;159(4):1221–1226.
4. Sitarz R, Skierucha M, Mielko J, Offerhaus GJA, Maciejewski R, Polkowski WJ. Gastric cancer: epidemiology, prevention, classification, and treatment. *Cancer Manag Res.* 2018;10:239–248.
5. Uemura N, Okamoto S, Yamamoto S, et al. Helicobacter pylori infection and the development of gastric cancer. *N Engl J Med.* 2001;345(11):784–789.
6. Amieva MR, El-Omar EM. Host-bacterial interactions in Helicobacter pylori infection. *Gastroenterology.* 2008;134(1):306–323.
7. Wong BCY, Lam SK, Wong WM, et al; China Gastric Cancer Study Group. Helicobacter pylori eradication to prevent gastric cancer in a high-risk region of China: a randomized controlled trial. *JAMA.* 2004;291(2):187–194.
8. Lundegårdh G, Ekbom A, McLaughlin JK, Nyrén O. Gastric cancer risk after vagotomy. *Gut.* 1994;35(7):946–949.
9. Aya M, Yashiro M, Nishioka N, Onoda N, Hirakawa K. Carcinogenesis in the remnant stomach following distal gastrectomy with Billroth II reconstruction is associated with high-level microsatellite instability. *Anticancer Res.* 2006;26(2B):1403–1411.
10. Hansford S, Kaurah P, Li-Chang H, et al. Hereditary diffuse gastric cancer syndrome CDH1 mutations and beyond. *JAMA Oncol.* 2015;1(1):23–32.
11. Roberts M, Ranola J, Marshall M, et al. Comparison of CDH1 penetrance estimates in clinically ascertained families vs families ascertained for multiple gastric cancers. *JAMA Oncol.* 2019;5(9): 1325–1331.
12. Blair VR, McLeod M, Carneiro F et al. Hereditary diffuse gastric cancer: updated clinical practice guidelines. *Lancet Oncology.* 2020; 21(8):e386–e297.
13. Anaya DA, Chang GJ, Rodriguez-Bigas MA. Extracolonic manifestations of hereditary colorectal cancer syndromes. *Clin Colon Rectal Surg.* 2008;21(4):263–272.
14. Kunisaki C, Ishino J, Nakajima S, et al. Outcomes of mass screening for gastric carcinoma. *Ann Surg Oncol.* 2006;13(2):221–228.
15. Siewert JR, Böttcher K, Stein HJ, Roder JD. Relevant prognostic factors in gastric cancer: ten-year results of the German Gastric Cancer Study. *Ann Surg.* 1998;228(4):449–461.

16. Sun D, Mülder D, Li Y, et al. The effect of nationwide organized cancer screening programs on gastric cancer mortality: a synthetic control study. *Gastroenterology*. 2024;166(3):503–514.
17. Spolverato G, Ejaz A, Kim Y, et al. Use of endoscopic ultrasound in the preoperative staging of gastric cancer: a multi-institutional study of the US gastric cancer collaborative. *J Am Coll Surg*. 2015;220(1):48–56.
18. Kinkel K, Lu Y, Both M, Warren RS, Thoeni RF. Detection of hepatic metastases from cancers of the gastrointestinal tract by using noninvasive imaging methods (US,CT, MR imaging, PET): a meta-analysis. *Radiology*. 2002;224(3):748–756.
19. Ott K, Herrmann K, Lordick F, et al. Early metabolic response evaluation by fluorine-18 fluorodeoxyglucose positron emission tomography allows in vivo testing of chemosensitivity in gastric cancer: long-term results of a prospective study. *Clin Cancer Res*. 2008;14(7):2012–2018.
20. American College of Surgeons and the Alliance for Clinical Trials in Oncology. Gastrectomy. In: *Operative Standards for Cancer Surgery*. Vol 2. Wolters Kluwer; 2019:67–178.
21. Mezhir JJ, Shah MA, Jacks LM, Brennan MF, Coit DG, Strong VE. Positive peritoneal cytology in patients with gastric cancer: natural history and outcome of 291 patients. *Ann Surg Oncol*. 2010;17(12):3173–3180.
22. Bang YJ, Van Cutsem E, Feyereislova A, et al; ToGA Trial Investigators. Trastuzumab in combination with chemotherapy versus chemotherapy alone for treatment of HER2-positive advanced gastric or gastro-oesophageal junction cancer (ToGA): a phase 3, open-label, randomised controlled trial. *Lancet*. 2010;376(9742):687–697.
23. Mazanedo I, Pereira F, Caro CR, et al. Cytoreductive surgery and hyperthermic intraperitoneal chemotherapy (HIPEC) for gastric cancer with peritoneal carcinomatosis: multicenter study of Spanish Group of Peritoneal Oncologic Surgery (GECOP). *Ann Surg Oncol*. 2019;26(8):2615–2621.
24. Zhao B, Blair SL, Katz MHG, Lowy AM, Kelly KJ. Adherence with operative standards in the treatment of gastric cancer in the United States. *Gastric Cancer*. 2020;23(3):550–560.
25. Chon HJ, Hyung WJ, Kim C, et al. Differential prognostic implications of gastric signet ring cell carcinoma: stage adjusted analysis from a single high-volume center in Asia. *Ann Surg*. 2017;265(5):946–953.
26. Honda M, Wong SL, Healy MA, et al. Long-term trends in primary sites of gastric adenocarcinoma in Japan and the United States. *J Cancer*. 2017;8(11):1935–1942.
27. American Joint Committee on Cancer. *AJCC Cancer Staging Manual*. 8th ed. Springer; 2017.
28. Kunisaki C, Shimada H, Takahashi M, et al. Prognostic factors in early gastric cancer. *Hepatogastroenterology*. 2001;48(37):294–298.
29. Uedo N, Iishi H, Tatsuta M, et al. Long-term outcomes after endoscopic mucosal resection for early gastric cancer. *Gastric Cancer*. 2006;9(2):88–92.
30. Choi KS, Jung HY, Choi KD, et al. EMR versus gastrectomy for intramucosal gastric cancer: comparison of long-term outcomes. *Gastrointest Endosc*. 2011;73(5):942–948.
31. Bozzetti F, Marubini E, Bonfanti G, Miceli R, Piano C, Gennari L. Subtotal versus total gastrectomy for gastric cancer: five-year survival rates in a multicenter randomized Italian trail. Italian Gastrointestinal Tumor Study Group. *Ann Surg*. 1999;230(2):170–178.
32. Cats A, Jansen EPM, van Grieken NCT, et al. Chemotherapy versus chemoradiotherapy after surgery and preoperative chemotherapy for resectable gastric cancer (CRITICS): an international, open-label, randomized phase 3 trial. *Lancet Oncol*. 2018;19(5):616–628.
33. Squires MH III, Kooby DA, Pawlik TM, et al. Utility of the proximal margin frozen section for resection of gastric adenocarcinoma: a 7-institutional study of the US Gastric Cancer Collaborative. *Ann Surg Oncol*. 2014;21(13):4202–4210.
34. Mamidanna R, Ni Z, Anderson O, et al. Surgeon volume and cancer esophagectomy, gastrectomy, and pancreatectomy: a population-based study in England. *Ann Surg*. 2016;263(4):727–732.
35. Dixon M, Mahar A, Paszat L, et al. What provider volumes and characteristics are appropriate for gastric cancer resection? Results of an international RAND/UCLA expert panel. *Surgery*. 2013;154(5):1100–1109.
36. Songun I, Putter H, Kranenbarg EMK, Sasako M, van de Velde CJ. Surgical treatment of gastric cancer: 15-year follow-up results of the randomised nationwide Dutch D1D2 trial. *Lancet Oncol*. 2010;11(5):439–449.
37. Lee JS, Douglass HO Jr. D2 dissection for gastric cancer. *Surg Oncol*. 1997;6(4):215–225.
38. Pacelli F, Doglietto GB, Bellantone R, Alfieri S, Sgadari A, Crucitti F. Extensive versus limited lymph node dissection for gastric cancer: a comparative study of 320 patients. *Br J Surg*. 1993;80(9):1153–1156.
39. Japanese Gastric Cancer Association. Japanese gastric cancer treatment guidelines 2021 (6th edition). *Gastric Cancer*. 2023;26:1–25
40. Ohtani H, Tamamori Y, Noguchi K, et al. A meta-analysis of randomized controlled trials that compared laparoscopy-assisted and open distal gastrectomy for early gastric cancer. *J Gastrointest Surg*. 2010;14(6):958–964.
41. Huscher CGS, Mingoli A, Sgarzini G, et al. Laparoscopic versus open subtotal gastrectomy for distal gastric cancer: five-year results of a randomized prospective trial. *Ann Surg*. 2005;241(2):232–237.
42. Kim W, Kim HH, Han SU, et al; Korean Laparo-endoscopic Gastrointestinal Surgery Study (KLASS) Group. Decreased morbidity of laparoscopic distal gastrectomy compared with open distal gastrectomy for stage I gastric cancer: short-term outcomes from a multi-center randomized controlled trial (KLASS-01). *Ann Surg*. 2016;263(1):28–35.
43. Liu F, Huang C, Xu Z, et al; Chinese Laparoscopic Gastrointestinal Surgery Study (CLASS) Group. Morbidity and mortality of laparoscopic vs open total gastrectomy for clinical stage I gastric cancer: the CLASS02 Multicenter Randomized Clinical Trial. *JAMA Oncol*. 2020;6(10):1590–1597.
44. Al-Batran SE, Homann N, Pauligk C, et al. Perioperative chemotherapy with fluorouracil plus leucovorin, oxaliplatin, and docetaxel versus fluorouracil or capecitabine plus cisplatin and epirubicin for locally advanced, resectable gastric or gastro-oesophageal junction adenocarcinoma (FLOT4): a randomised, phase 2/3 trial. *Lancet*. 2019;393(10184):1948–1957.
45. Li SS, Udelman BV, Parikh A, et al. Impact of postoperative complication and completion of multimodality therapy on survival in patients undergoing gastrectomy for advanced gastric cancer. *J Am Coll Surg*. 2020;230(6):912–924.
46. André T, Tougeron D, Piessen G, et al. Neoadjuvant nivolumab plus ipilimumab and adjuvant nivolumab in localized deficient mismatch repair/microsatellite instability-high gastric or esophagogastric junction adenocarcinoma: the GERCOR NEONIPIGA phase II study. *J Clin Oncol*. 2023;41(2):255–265.
47. Pietrantonio F, Miceli R, Raimondi A, et al. Individual patient data meta-analysis of the value of microsatellite instability as a biomarker in gastric cancer. *J Clin Oncol*. 2019;37(35):3392–3400.
48. Smyth EC, Wotherspoon A, Peckitt C, et al. Mismatch repair deficiency, microsatellite instability, and survival: an exploratory analysis of the Medical Research Council Adjuvant Gastric Infusional Chemotherapy (MAGIC) trial. *JAMA Oncol*. 2017;3(9):1197–1203.
49. Parsonnet J, Hansen S, Rodriguez L, et al. Helicobacter pylori infection and gastric lymphoma. *N Engl J Med*. 1994;330(18):1267–1271.
50. Avilés A, Nambo MJ, Neri N, et al. The role of surgery in primary gastric lymphoma: results of a controlled clinical trial. *Ann Surg*. 2004;240(1):44–50.
51. Rais R, Trikalinos N, Liu J, Chatterjee D. Enterochromaffin-like cell hyperplasia-associated gastric neuroendocrine tumors may arise in the setting of proton pump inhibitor use. *Arch Pathol Lab Med*. 2022;146(3):366–371.

Clinical Diagnosis and Management of Intestinal Obstruction, Ileus, and Pseudo-Obstruction of the Colon (Ogilvie Syndrome)

Allison R. Wilcox, Alexandra Briggs, and David I. Soybel

Key Points

1. In simple obstruction, the intestinal lumen is partially or completely occluded without imminent complications such as compromise of intestinal blood flow and ischemia with strangulation and necrosis.
2. Four key symptoms variably associated with acute mechanical bowel obstruction include abdominal pain, vomiting, distention, and obstipation.
3. Abdominal pain out of proportion to physical findings should raise concern about rapidly evolving closed-loop obstruction or ischemia and the need for urgent resuscitation and operation.
4. CT (computerized tomography) is the primary imaging modality to detect and identify the likely site and source of obstruction.
5. Intravenous hydration, nasogastric decompression, and restoration of electrolyte balance are cornerstones in the management of intestinal obstruction and preparing for surgery, if indicated.
6. For small bowel obstructions (SBOs) without indications for urgent operative intervention, the use of water-soluble contrast may be both diagnostic and therapeutic.
7. Peritoneal adhesions are the most common cause of obstruction of the small intestine.
8. Open and laparoscopic approaches are used in the treatment of unresolved SBO. Open operation is preferred in patients who are not stable, in surgically complex conditions (malignancy, radiation enteritis, multiple prior laparotomies) or when the abdomen will not permit safe insufflation. Laparoscopic approaches are safe in experienced hands.
9. Ileus denotes paralysis of the motility of the gastrointestinal tract and/or poor coordination of motility in different regions of the gastrointestinal tract, leading to a functional obstruction which must be differentiated from mechanical obstruction.
10. Postoperative ileus (POI) can be differentiated from SBO with the use of contrast CT and enteroclysis imaging techniques. POI is often self-limiting; less frequent interventions are required for prolonged POI, if proper precautions have been taken during surgery.
11. Pseudo-obstruction of the colon, also known as Ogilvie syndrome, is treated primarily via attention to underlying neurologic or metabolic disturbances, with medication management and decompressive colonoscopy as useful adjuncts. Colonic ischemia and perforation are the main complications that lead to surgical intervention.

The purpose of this chapter is to provide an overview of the etiologies, natural history, diagnosis, and management of: (1) mechanical obstruction of the small intestine; (2) ileus of the small intestine; and (3) neurogenic obstruction of the large intestine (Ogilvie syndrome). These conditions are linked by overlaps in underlying pathophysiology, differential diagnosis, approaches to resuscitation, and decisions about indications and timing of operation. The clinical approach to these conditions has evolved significantly in recent decades, giving improved imaging modalities, increased use of nonoperative management pathways, and the utilization of laparoscopy in patients requiring operative intervention.

The first portion of this chapter will focus on *mechanical obstruction* of the intestine, where luminal contents cannot pass through the intestine because the lumen is blocked. The second portion of this chapter will discuss *neurogenic* or *functional* causes of obstruction, in which luminal contents are prevented from passing because of disturbances in gut motility that prevent coordinated peristalsis from one region of the gut to the next. This latter form of obstruction is referred to as paralytic ileus in the small intestine and pseudo-obstruction of the large intestine.

MECHANICAL OBSTRUCTION OF THE INTESTINE

Terminology and Classification

1 Mechanical obstruction can be either complete, meaning that the lumen is totally occluded, or incomplete, meaning that the lumen is narrowed but permitting distal passage of some fluid and air. Incomplete obstructions are also commonly referred to as partial obstructions. As summarized in **Table 46A.1**, causes of obstruction can include intraluminal objects such as foreign bodies or gallstones, intramural obstructions such as tumors or intussusceptions, and extrinsic or extraluminal lesions, most commonly adhesions[1] and hernias—both abdominal wall as well as internal hernias. Another term often used in obstruction is *strangulation*, in which blood flow to the obstructed segment is compromised and tissue necrosis and gangrene are imminent. Strangulation usually implies that the

Table 46A.1. Classification of Adult Mechanical Intestinal Obstructions

Extrinsic	Intraluminal	Intramural
Adhesions	Foreign bodies	Congenital (rare in adult)
Congenital: Ladd or Meckel bands	Barium inspissation (colon)	Atresia, stricture, or stenosis
Postoperative	Bezoar	Web
Postinflammatory (after pelvic inflammatory disease)		Intestinal duplication
		Meckel diverticulum
Hernias	Inspissated feces	Inflammatory Process
Abdominal wall	Gallstone ileus	Crohn disease
Internal	Meconium (cystic fibrosis)	Diverticulitis
Groin		Stricture from ischemia
Volvulus		Radiation enteritis or stricture
External mass effect		Medication induced (NSAIDs, KCl tablets)
Abscess		
Annular pancreas	Parasites	Neoplasms
Pancreatic pseudocyst	Enterolith	Primary intestinal or colon (malignant or benign)
Carcinomatosis	Intussusception	
Endometriosis		Secondary (metastasis or carcinomatosis)
Pregnancy	Polypoid and exophytic lesions	Trauma (eg, intramural hematoma)

obstruction is complete, but some forms of partial obstruction can also be complicated by strangulation. Strangulation is also a concern for an incarcerated hernia as the hernia neck can impinge the blood flow to the incarcerated segment of bowel. Obstruction is "simple" when it is not complicated by strangulation (**Fig. 46A.1**).

An important concept and term in the classification of obstructions is the idea of a closed-loop obstruction (**Fig. 46A.2**). This occurs when inflow to the loop of bowel and outflow from the loop are both blocked, permitting gas and secretions to accumulate in a loop of intestine without a means of decompression, proximally or distally. Examples of closed-loop obstructions are torsion of a loop of small intestine around an adhesive band, incarceration of the bowel in a hernia, or volvulus.

Incarceration most commonly refers to obstructions caused by a herniated segment of intestine. If the hernia can be reduced, the obstruction may resolve. Incarceration refers to a nonreducible herniated segment of bowel and typically needs surgical reduction.

Mechanical causes of obstruction are contrasted with *neurogenic* or *functional* causes, in which luminal contents are prevented from passing because of disturbances in gut motility that prevent coordinated peristalsis from one region of the gut to the next. This latter form of obstruction is commonly referred to as *ileus* in the small intestine and *pseudo-obstruction* in the large intestine.

Clinical Presentation and Diagnosis of Small Bowel Obstruction

Initial History and Evaluation[2]

2 Four key symptoms associated with acute mechanical obstruction of the small intestine include abdominal pain, vomiting, distention, and obstipation. These symptoms and their associated physical signs can present in different combinations depending on the site of obstruction (**Table 46A.2**) and the type of obstruction, with or without complications (**Table 46A.3**).

A pertinent history should establish the quality of pain (colic/intermittent vs. steady), as well as the timeline of the appearance of symptoms, including last emesis as well as flatus/stool.
3 Uncomplicated obstructions typically present with intermittent, crampy pain localized to the midline and is often partially or completely relieved by NG decompression. Steady pain raises more concern for a complicated obstruction. A particularly worrisome combination of symptoms and signs occurs when abdominal pain has come on acutely and is worsening rapidly in severity, but not associated with physical findings (such as fever or localized tenderness) or laboratory abnormalities such as high leukocyte counts in the blood. Such a syndrome is known as "pain out of proportion to physical findings" and may represent a surgical emergency such as closed-loop obstruction (**Fig. 46A.2**) before strangulation has appeared (**Table 46A.2** and **Table 46A.3**). General symptoms that may reflect underlying malignancy as the cause should also be evaluated, including fatigue, deconditioning, anorexia, and weight loss. It is important to ask about prior abdominal surgeries and any prior bowel obstructions, along with personal and family history of malignancy.

A thorough abdominal exam is essential in the evaluation of patients presenting with possible bowel obstruction. Attention should be paid to prior incisions, and the exam should include evaluation for external evidence of ventral, incisional, or inguinal hernias. The location and severity of abdominal tenderness are important both for initial triage as well as for establishing a baseline exam in patients who will be managed medically with the inclusion of serial exams.

Basic laboratory evaluations with a basic metabolic panel, complete blood count, and lactate can aid in evaluating the extent of resuscitation for patients with electrolyte disturbances or volume depletion related to poor oral intake and emesis. Significant laboratory abnormalities may also raise the level of suspicion for more severe obstruction and possible bowel ischemia.

Systemic signs of illness and end organ dysfunction such as fever, tachycardia, hypotension, and oliguria also raise concern for severe illness and possible bowel ischemia and should prompt immediate resuscitation and, taken together with history and exam findings, consideration of urgent operative management.

Differential Diagnosis

Other abdominal conditions can usually be distinguished from small bowel obstruction (SBO), by clinical history, examination, basic laboratory data, and confirmation with imaging. The differential diagnosis includes appendicitis, diverticulitis, perforated peptic ulcer, cholecystitis, and choledocholithiasis. Obstruction of the colon is usually accompanied by varying levels of pain with massive abdominal distention and obstipation. It should also be emphasized that the presence of another abdominal process does not exclude the complication of SBO.

Imaging Modalities in Bowel Obstruction[3,4]

The role of initial imaging is to confirm the diagnosis of bowel obstruction while excluding other diagnoses, to locate the site of obstruction, and to gain insight into the etiology of the obstruction.

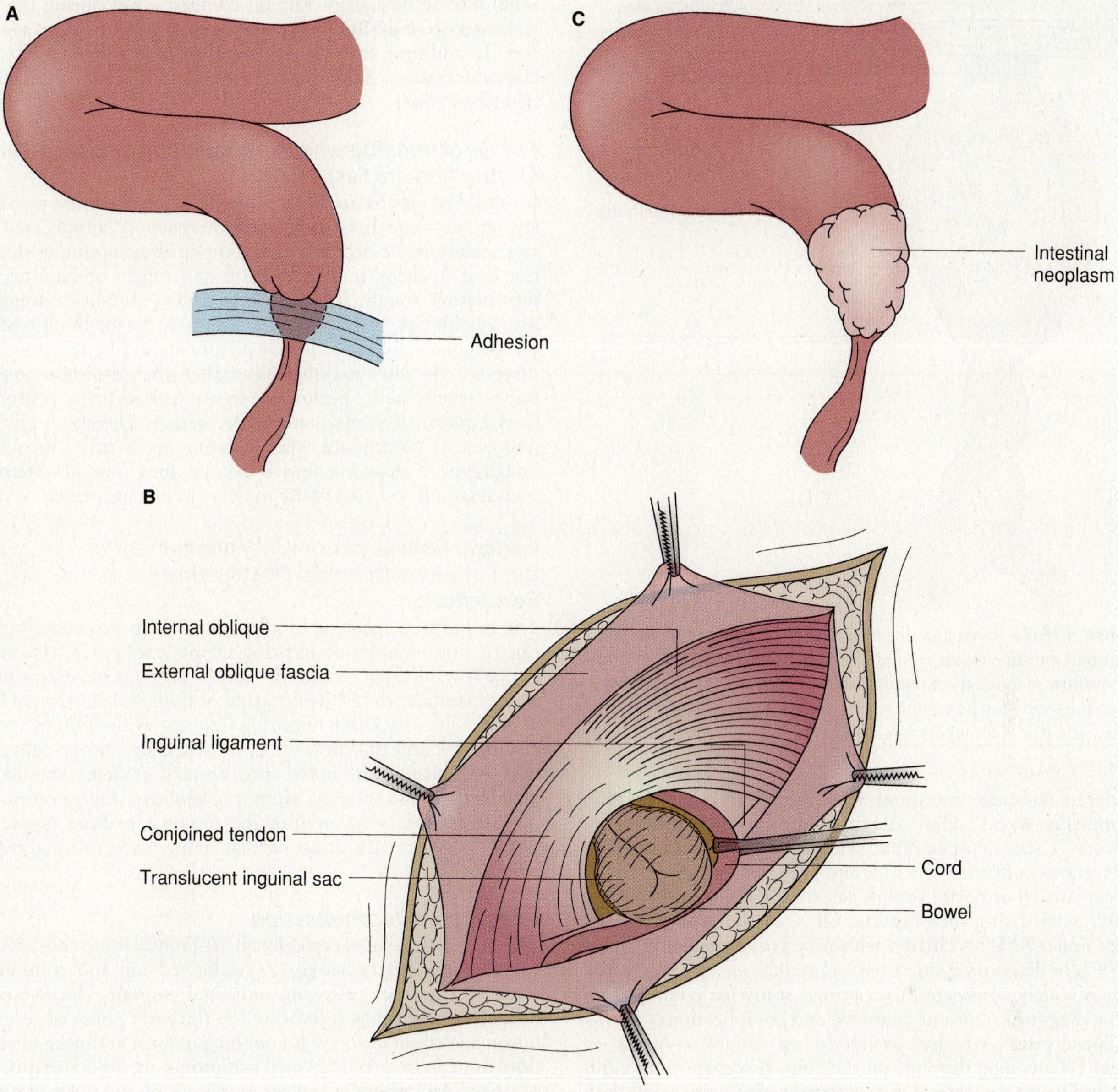

Figure 46A.1. Schematic illustration of different forms of simple mechanical obstruction. Simple obstruction is most often due to adhesion, (**A**), groin hernia, (**B**), or neoplasm, (**C**). The hernia can act as a tourniquet, causing a closed-loop obstruction and strangulation.

Plain Radiographs

When the clinical symptoms and signs make a simple obstruction likely, plain abdominal radiography can be diagnostic in 67% to 80% of patients. A plain, supine abdominal radiograph provides evidence of dilated loops of small bowel (>3 cm) proximally, and clearance of fluid and air distal to the point of obstruction (**Fig. 46A.3**). In the upright and lateral decubitus position, films classically reveal multiple air–fluid levels located at different levels on the upright film (**Fig. 46A.4**) or lateral decubitus film. Free air in the peritoneal cavity, reflecting perforation of a viscus, is best diagnosed on upright or lateral views, and is easily missed on the supine view. These considerations underscore the importance of obtaining all three views but also their limitations. One limitation, even with all three views, is that they are not consistently accurate in localizing the site of obstruction. In addition, the absence of air–fluid levels does not necessarily obviate the diagnosis of obstruction, especially in the initial presentation of a closed-loop obstruction, where air may be absent and yet loops of bowel may be overdistended by fluid in the lumen. Moreover, plain films do not provide adjunctive information about associated inflammation or free fluid. Lastly, in the postoperative patient, radiography may fail to distinguish ileus from an early obstruction, and the former condition may contribute to the development of the latter. Despite these limitations, it is important to be conversant with the role that plain films can play in the diagnosis and management of SBO, especially, in circumstances where other imaging modalities may not be easily accessed.

Computerized Tomography

4 The resolution and anatomic clarity afforded by computerized tomography (CT) provide several benefits, including improved localization of the obstructed segment and the points of transition, characterization of the completeness of obstruction, detection of ischemia and strangulation, and identification of the etiology of obstruction, and exclusion or confirmation of other diagnoses.

If the offending lesion is malignant, secondary information about local characteristics and stage can also be obtained. The anatomic information obtained, particularly if other diagnoses such as hernia are present, is equally valuable. Attributes of impending ischemia include mesenteric edema, vascular engorgement, high-density fluid in the peritoneal cavity, and

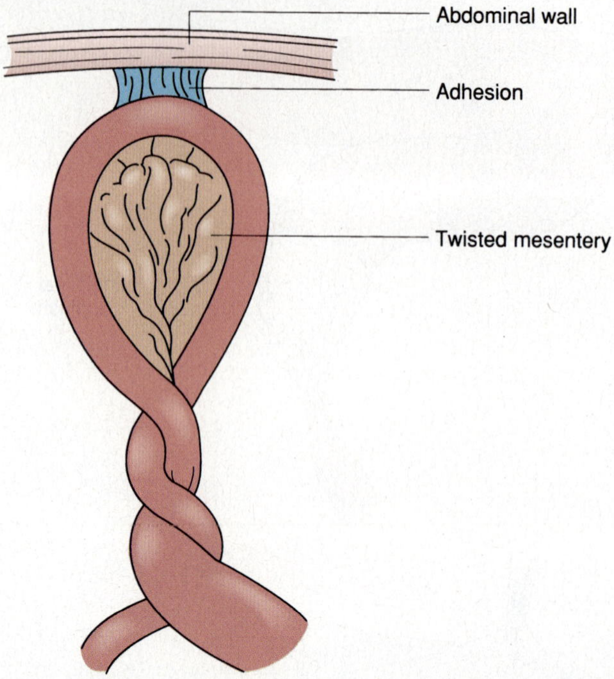

Figure 46A.2. Schematic illustration of a closed-loop obstruction. The small intestine twists around its mesentery, compromising inflow and outflow of luminal contents from the loop. Also, the vascular supply to the loop may be compromised due to the twisting of the mesentery. The risk of strangulation is high.

moderate-to-severe intestinal wall thickening (greater than 2 mm) (**Fig. 46A.5**). High attenuation of bowel wall on unenhanced CT scans, low or reduced attenuation of bowel wall on intravenous contrast CT scans, and presence of intramural air (pneumatosis) or portal venous gas are CT findings suggestive of ischemia. Using such criteria, CT scan has a >90% sensitivity and >90% specificity, with a negative predictive value of 99% in diagnosing intestinal strangulation. As a result, CT scan is widely considered the optimal study for confirmation of the diagnosis, relevant anatomy, and complications.

The decision whether or not to use enteric contrast on initial CT imaging depends on the clinical scenario and clinician judgment. In general, it is recommended to proceed with CT scan of the abdomen and pelvis with IV contrast alone, so long as the patient does not have contraindications such renal disease or allergy. Enteral contrast given during the initial workup of a SBO may place the patient at risk for aspiration. In addition, the lack of enteral contrast allows for better characterization of the small bowel wall and signs of ischemia, described above.

Pitfalls of Imaging when Strangulation or Closed-Loop Obstruction are Suspected

It should be emphasized that when the clinical picture provides strong suspicion for closed-loop obstruction complicated by strangulation, the decision for obtaining imaging studies should not lead to delay in resuscitation and timely operation. The information sought from imaging studies should be weighed against the risk of such delays. The message of the literature on imaging is that the clinical picture should be the principal driver of decision making, especially when multiple clinical signs (severe pain, peritoneal signs, leukocytosis, profound dehydration) of strangulation are present. Therefore, clinical judgment is paramount when determining whether to obtain imaging prior to proceeding to the operating room if obtaining such imaging will contribute to delay in management.

General Considerations in Management of the Patient with Bowel Obstruction

Resuscitation

5 The initial management of all patients with suspected bowel obstruction includes designating the patient "NPO" (Latin *nil per os* for "nothing by mouth") and starting intravenous infusion of isotonic fluids. Restoration of fluid and electrolyte balance is a priority, often requiring frequent evaluation of serum electrolytes and pH. In acute cases when significant dehydration is detected, an indwelling urinary catheter should be placed to monitor urine output. Hemodynamic monitoring may be necessary to monitor the response to fluid resuscitation in patients with severe cardiac, pulmonary, or renal insufficiency.

Nasogastric Decompression

The nasogastric tube, typically an 18-French sump tube, serves to prevent distal passage of swallowed air and minimizes the discomfort of refluxing intestinal content. Placement of decompressive tubes is indicated in the early phase of resuscitation and observation, with ongoing nausea, vomiting, distention, but can be avoided when symptoms are mild and quickly resolved. An important caveat in the use of any form of nasogastric decompression is the risk of aspiration during placement of the tube, which may incite gag and vomiting reflexes.[5]

Table 46A.2. Symptoms and Signs of Bowel Obstruction

Symptom/Sign	Prox. Small Bowel (Open Loop)	Dist. Small Bowel (Open Loop)	Small Bowel (Closed Loop)	Colon/Rectum
Pain	Intermittent, intense, colicky, often relieved by vomiting	Intermittent to constant	Progressive, intermittent to constant; rapidly worsens	Continuous
Vomiting	Large volumes, bilious, and frequent	Low volume and frequency, progressively feculent with time	May be prominent (reflex)	Intermittent, not prominent; when present, feculent
Tenderness	Epigastric or periumbilical; quite mild, unless strangulation is present	Diffuse and progressive	Diffuse, progressive	Diffuse
Distention	Absent	Moderate to marked	Often absent	Marked
Obstipation	May not be present	Present	May not be present	Present

Adapted from Schuffler MD, Sinanan MN. Intestinal obstruction and pseudo-obstruction. In: Sleisenger MH, Fordtran JS, eds. *Gastrointestinal Disease*. 5th ed. W. B. Saunders Co.; 1993:898–916.

Table 46A.3. Diagnosis and Decisions in Bowel Obstruction in Three Hypothetical Patients

	Patient I Early Closed-Loop Obstruction	Patient II Intestinal Obstruction with Strangulation	Patient III Open-Loop Obstruction of the Distal Small Intestine or Cecum
History/Symptoms	Crampy periumbilical pain rapidly evolving from colic to constant pain, with 2–3 episodes of emesis (sometimes dry emesis)	Diffuse, crampy abdominal pain over 24–48 h with many episodes of vomiting. Evolves to constant pain. Bowel movements or flatus not uncommon early in the illness, but not late	Progressive abdominal distention over previous 2 wks. Mild discomfort. No vomiting. Few bowel movements and little flatus
Physical Findings/ Signs	No distention, minimal flatus. Minimal disturbance in vital signs. Often with minimal or no tenderness. Peritoneal findings absent	Temperature >100 °F, heart rate >100/min, dehydrated. Mild distention; local tenderness often present with focal peritoneal signs. Strangulated segment may be palpable in thin individuals	Distention prominent, mild tenderness, often with minimal localizing tenderness and no peritoneal findings
Lab	No leukocytosis, pH, or electrolyte disturbances	WBC 16K. Serum Na^+ low, K^+ low, Cl^- low, pH alkalotic	WBC normal, serum electrolytes mildly decreased
X-Ray	Nonspecific gas pattern on plain film	Multiple dilated loops and air–fluid levels. No gas in colon	Multiple dilated small bowel loops and air–fluid levels. Some gas and stool in proximal colon
Differential Dx	Broad: includes appendicitis, closed-loop SBO, pancreatitis, nonsurgical conditions	Narrow: Complete SBO likely, strangulation cannot be excluded	Narrow: distal small bowel or proximal colon obstruction likely, possibly incomplete
Initial Rx	Admit with q3–4 h reevaluation by clinical examination, WBC. Repeat films q8–12 h. NG tube if vomiting persists. IVFs	Admit for rapid resuscitation with IVFs, IV antibiotics. Urinary catheter and NG intubation indicated	Admit for IVFs, NG intubation. Hypaque enema followed by barium to evaluate colon. CT if malignancy suspected
Indications for Surgery	If pain worsens, local tenderness or peritoneal signs evolve, WBC rises, urine output falls	Already present. Patient should be scheduled and brought to O.R. after adequate resuscitation (dramatic improvement with resuscitation may permit observation for 4 h)	Surgery performed when evaluation is complete or if clinical course deteriorates during evaluation

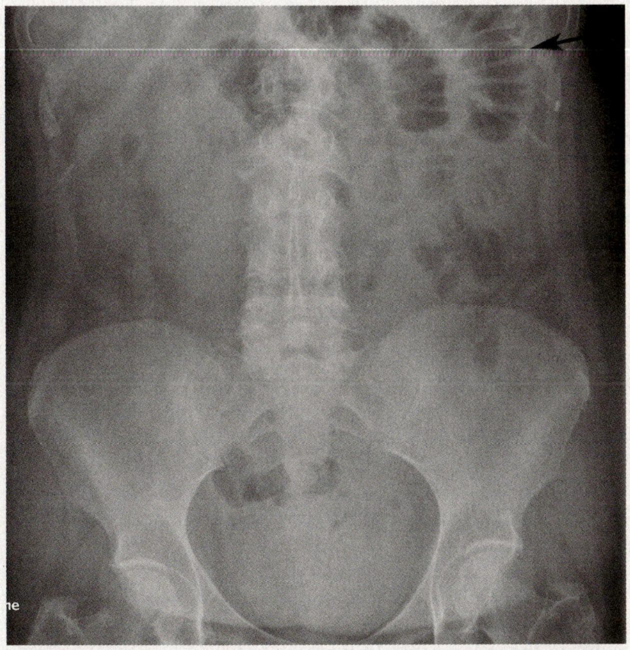

Figure 46A.3. Plain supine abdominal film of a patient with small intestinal obstruction. Note the multiple dilated loops of small intestine (*black arrow*) in the left upper quadrant, characterized by complete markings of the plicae. Also note absence of air in colon and rectum.

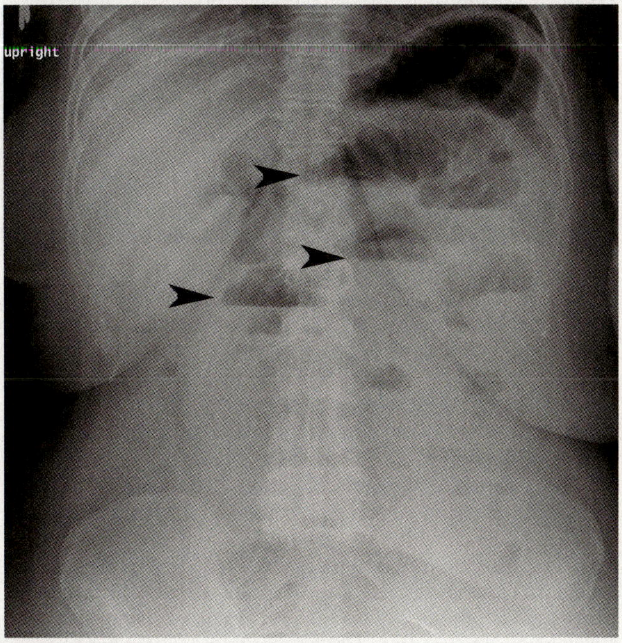

Figure 46A.4. Plain upright abdominal film of a patient with small intestinal obstruction. Note the air–fluid levels in the stomach and multiple dilated loops of small intestine (*arrowheads*), and absence of air in the colon or rectum.

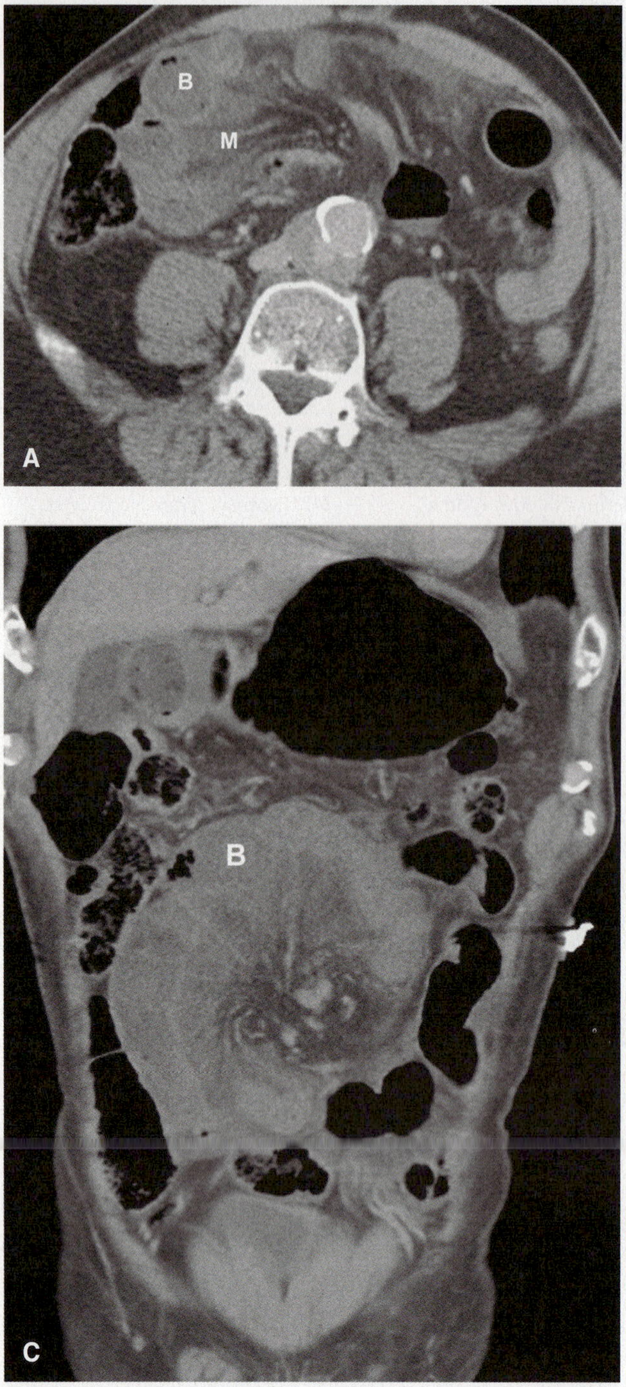

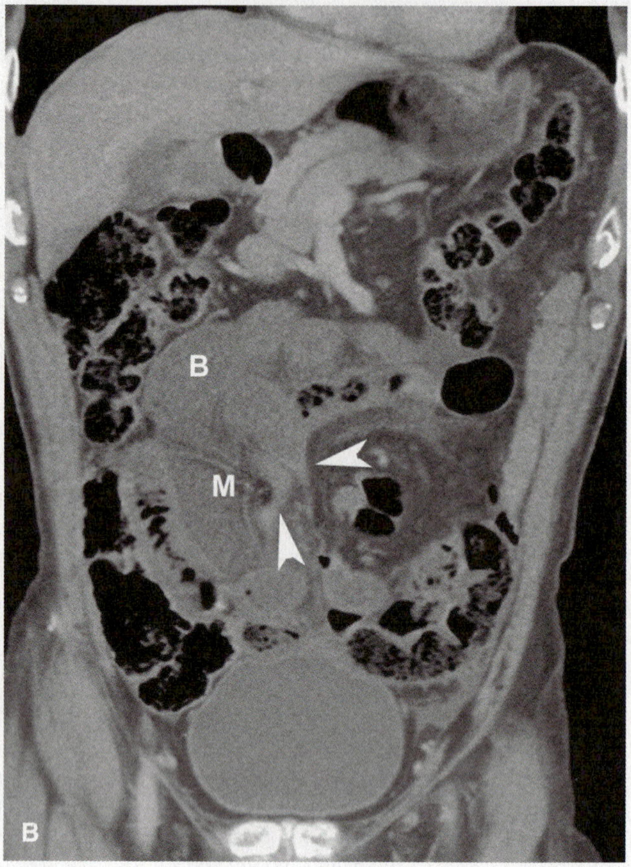

Figure 46A.5. Axial (Panel **A**), and coronal (Panel **B**), images of a closed-loop obstruction with strangulated small bowel secondary to a volvulus from an adhesive band. Distended fluid-filled loops of small bowel (**B**) in a radial distribution converging toward the point of torsion (*white arrowheads*). There is edema within the mesentery (M). Shown in Panel **C** is a coronal view of vascular engorgement and mesenteric edema in a closed-loop obstruction.

In turn, if a patient requires operative intervention to relieve their obstruction, nasogastric decompression is recommended prior to induction to reduce risk of aspiration.

Role of Contrast Studies in Management

6 When adhesive SBOs without ischemia or perforation are diagnosed based on clinical exam, history, and imaging findings, nonoperative management is first line, including nasogastric decompression and maintenance of fluid and electrolyte balance. Increasingly, a water-soluble contrast challenge is used as an adjunct to these traditional tenets of medical management. Though variations exist, a standard approach is to allow for a period of nasogastric decompression (at least 2 hours). Following this, 100 mL of Gastrografin, a hyperosmolar water-soluble contrast agent, is mixed with 50 mL of water and is instilled via the nasogastric tube. A plain abdominal x-ray is obtained 8 hours after contrast administration, and repeated every 8 hours for up to 24 hours. The appearance or absence of contrast within 8 hours after administration has greater than 90% sensitivity and specificity in predicting need for operative intervention.[6]

A water-soluble contrast challenge is diagnostic and also, theoretically, therapeutic. Due to its hyperosmolar nature, Gastrografin administration facilitates mobilization of fluid into the bowel lumen, which may decrease edema of the intestinal wall and increases the pressure gradient across obstructive site. It is thought that these fluid and pressure shifts can contribute to resolution in cases of incomplete obstruction. Utilization of the protocol has been found to decrease rates of surgery and hospital length of stay. In common clinical practice, Gastrografin challenge is typically considered a failure when contrast is not in the colon after 24 hours.

Of note, in the past and sometimes in the present, barium has been utilized as an enteral contrast agent. Although it does not stimulate motility as do water-soluble contrast agents, the use of barium provides the clearest images, in both small

Algorithm 46A.1

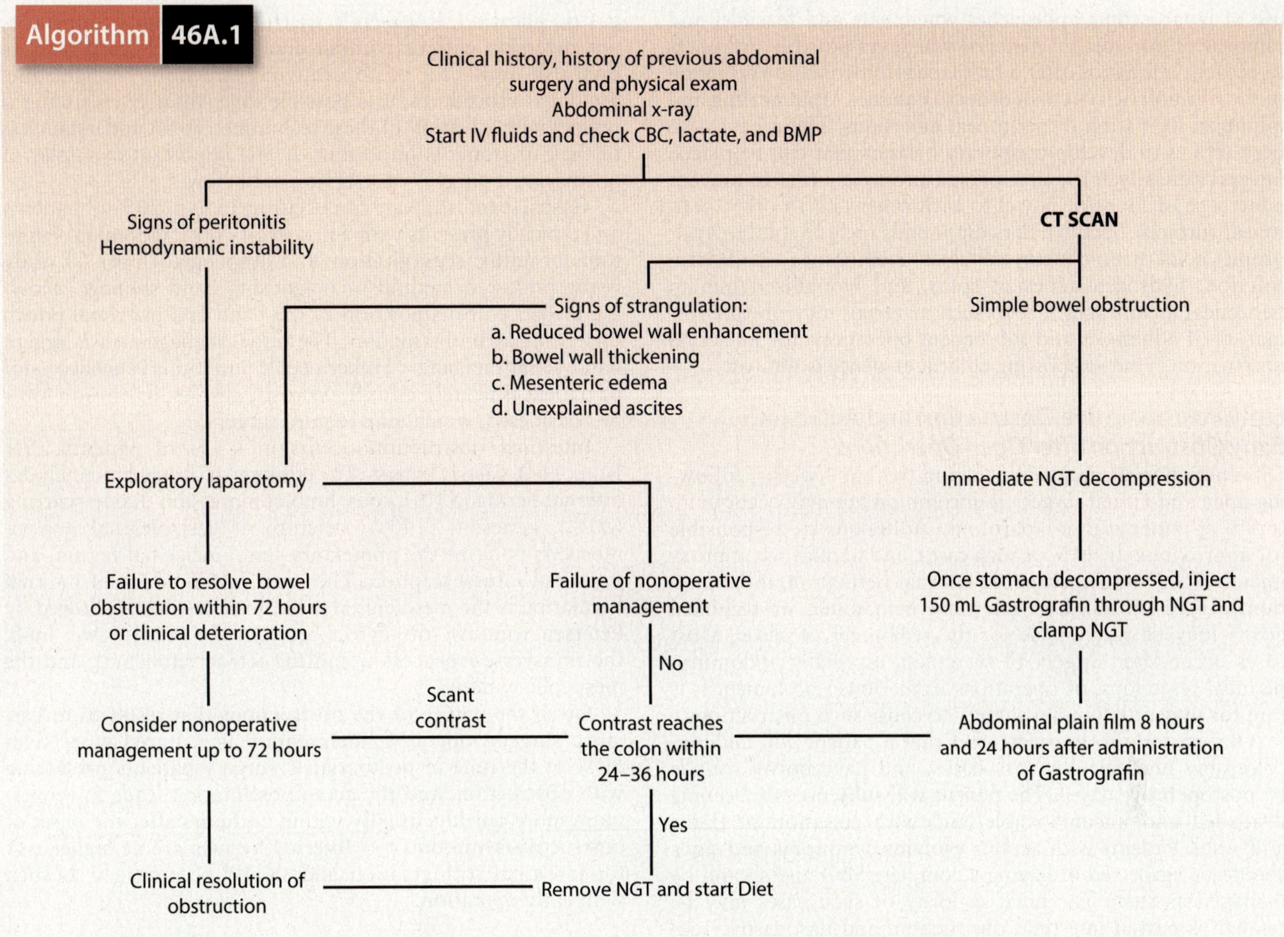

Algorithm 46A.1. Approach to recognition and management of early postlaparotomy obstruction of the small intestine.

bowel studies where the contrast is given from above and colon/rectum studies in which the contrast is given by enema. If barium leaks into the peritoneum, however, it elicits intense peritonitis. If there is any possibility of bowel perforation or gangrene, barium should not be used, and it is not traditionally used as an agent for contrast challenges in SBO. Failure of contrast to enter the colon by 24 hours, along with persistent symptoms and signs of obstruction, implies failure of nonoperative management.[7]

Indications and Timing of Operation

The decision to perform abdominal exploration to relieve intestinal obstruction should be made expeditiously, but not in the absence of critical information or before adequate resuscitation (**Algorithm 46A.1**). It should be emphasized that in patients with signs/symptoms concerning for bowel ischemia or necrosis, the safest course is to proceed to operation without undue delay. In patients without frank indications for operative intervention, medical management with resuscitation, restoration of electrolyte balance, serial examinations, Gastrografin challenge, and nasogastric suction when nausea, vomiting, and pain are prominent, as outlined above.

With management enhanced by administration of water-soluble contrast, there are circumstances in which uncomplicated obstruction may safely be observed unless and until clinical follow-up indicates failure of resolution. Similarly, patients with obstruction but without a history of prior operation, the so-called "virgin abdomen" may safely be observed to resolution. It is also important to recognize the circumstances under which scheduling for surgery may not be urgent but should not be unduly delayed. Such circumstances would include obstruction due to nonreducible hernia (internal or external) or malignancy amenable to curative resection. A decision for close observation, rather than early operation, may also be influenced by resources, expertise, and ancillary services that are available.[8] In all clinical scenarios, once the decision is made to proceed to the operating room for management of SBO, early administration of broad-spectrum antibiotics covering gram-negative aerobes and anaerobes is recommended, in order to reduce the incidence of postoperative infections and other adverse outcomes.[9]

Specific Types of Bowel Obstruction

Chronic Adhesions

7 Peritoneal adhesions account for more than half of SBO cases. Adhesions form secondary to peritoneal injury and inflammation, most commonly following surgical intervention, but also after nonoperative inflammatory insults, including endometriosis and radiation therapy.[7] Lower abdominal procedures, such as appendectomy, hysterectomy, colectomy, and abdominoperineal resection, are common precursor operations to adhesive obstruction. Adhesions may form after any abdominal procedure, however, including cholecystectomy, gastrectomy, and abdominal vascular procedures. In long-term follow-up, about 5% of patients undergoing laparotomy will develop adhesive obstruction; of these, 10% to 30% will suffer from additional episodes. Over 80% episodes of SBO due to adhesions may resolve nonoperatively.[10,11] An index episode and three recurrences indicate a likelihood of over 80% that there will be more recurrences.[12]

Current strategies to prevent adhesions at a first, or subsequent laparotomy, include first and foremost, minimizing tissue manipulation and injury to the peritoneal surfaces, meticulous attention to hemostasis and surgical technique, use of laparoscopic approaches where safe and feasible, and removal of any foreign material whenever possible. Adjuncts to prevent adhesions after a first laparotomy include targeting of the fibrinolytic system in order to enhance rapid healing and minimize formation of peritoneal adhesions. There have also been efforts to develop temporary barriers that can be placed intraperitoneally at the time of laparotomy in order to prevent adherence of loops of bowel to each other and to other peritoneal surfaces. Such barrier compounds include soluble hyaluronic acid–carboxymethylcellulose membranes, icodextrin solution, hydrogen adhesion spray, and lyophilized human peritoneal membranes. Use of such materials may obviate formation of adhesions and subsequent operations for intestinal obstruction,[13] but supporting clinical evidence is limited.

Early Postoperative Obstruction and Adhesions

Early Obstruction after Open Operations

Obstruction in the immediate period (within 4 weeks) following open abdominal surgery is uncommon but may occur in up to 1% of patients after laparotomy. Adhesions are responsible for approximately 90% of such cases, and hernias for approximately 7%.[14] Intussusception, internal herniation, inflammation, abscess, intramural intestinal hematoma, or technical errors may be responsible for the remainder of cases. Most cases occur after surgery of the colon, especially abdominoperineal resections, or operations in the lower abdomen. It is rare for upper abdominal surgery to cause such obstructions.

One scenario to be aware of is that a patient will undergo colectomy uneventfully, pass flatus, and have bowel sounds by postoperative day 3. The patient will subsequently become distended and uncomfortable, and with cessation of flatus and stool. Patients with acutely evolving symptoms and signs should be suspected of having a complete SBO and should be managed as such. The great majority of such cases may be treated as partial intestinal obstruction; and nasogastric suction and intravenous fluids will help resolve symptoms within a few days (**Algorithm 46A.1**). When the clinical course does not demand earlier intervention, a nonoperative approach may be tried for 10 to 14 days and will resolve the obstruction in over 75% of such cases. In one report,[15] patients who experienced early postoperative obstruction from adhesions were at higher risk of subsequent adhesive SBO than those who had not had an early event (26.5% vs. 7.5% at 5 years, $P < .001$).

Early Obstruction After Laparoscopic Procedures

Although less common than for open abdominal operations,[16] early obstructions can occur following laparoscopic procedures, and typically have different causes than postlaparotomy. Surgeons should maintain a high index of suspicion for port site hernia in patients with early SBO following laparoscopic surgery. Thick, vascular adhesions are formed in the early postoperative period when there is localized inflammation induced by injury, ischemia, or spillage of irritants such as gastric acid, intestinal succus, or infected bile or blood. Such adhesions are more likely to occur when procedures involve viscera of the lower abdomen (appendicitis, diverticulitis) or where there are extensively dissected surfaces, surgically stapled surfaces, or prosthetics placed intraperitoneally during hernia repair. Internal herniation is a risk when windows are opened in mesentery during laparoscopic procedures, such as in bariatric procedures or intestinal/colon resections. Based on these considerations, it should not be assumed that ileus is the most likely cause of early postoperative symptoms of abdominal pain, distension, or nausea and vomiting. When such symptoms appear after laparoscopic procedures, it is recommended that imaging be obtained and close clinical follow-up be practiced if expectant management is elected.

Bowel Obstruction after a Bariatric Procedure

There are numerous operative strategies for the management of obesity, including gastric banding, sleeve gastrectomy, gastric plication, Roux-en-Y gastric bypass, and biliopancreatic diversion with or without duodenal switch, each with its own risk profile for postoperative obstruction. Though some are dated procedures, it is possible that you may encounter a patient with a history of these techniques, so an understanding of their anatomy is important. A few important examples of postbariatric surgery obstruction are below.

Gastric band slippage can occur in 15% to 20% of patients and typically presents with a history of upper abdominal symptoms of reflux, regurgitation, and dysphagia. Upper GI study is the preferred method of diagnosing band slippage, showing evidence of malposition of the band and proximal pouch dilatation with obstruction. The initial management is urgent band deflation using a Huber needle and if this is unsuccessful or patient is acutely unwell, necrosis, abscess, or erosion must be considered, which may require surgery.

Intestinal obstruction occurs in 4.4% of patients after Roux-en-Y gastric bypass. The etiology of obstruction includes internal hernia (53%), roux limb compression due to scarring (20%), adhesion (14%), stricture at gastrojejunal anastomosis, kinking of the alimentary limb, incisional hernia, and intestinal intussusception. The most common site of internal herniation is the mesojejunal mesenteric window, followed by Petersen window (the defect between the small bowel limb, the transverse mesocolon, and the retroperitoneum), and the mesocolic window.

Given the nature of the obstructions that result from bariatric surgery, operative intervention is required more than 50% of the time in postbariatric surgery patients presenting with obstruction, and the acute presentation leads to reoperation more quickly, usually within 24 hours after the onset of obstructive symptoms.[17,18] Internal hernias are at higher risk for intestinal strangulation and should be managed as such with early operation.

Hernia

In high-income countries, hernias comprise the second most common group (after adhesions) of lesions causing obstruction of the small intestine. External hernias such as inguinal (**Fig. 46A.6**) or femoral hernias may present with the symptoms of obstruction. Femoral hernias are particularly prone to incarceration and bowel necrosis due to the small size of the hernia inlet. Other defects that may cause obstruction include umbilical, incisional, parastomal, and lumbar hernias. An attentive physical exam will frequently raise suspicion or provide explicit diagnosis of these external hernias as the source of obstruction. Imaging is usually required for hernia in unusual or occult locations such as the diaphragm, obturator foramen, or other pelvic foramina. Imaging is essential for suspected internal hernias such as those in the paraduodenal space, the foramen of Winslow (posterior to the porta hepatis), or within a mesentery. Occasionally, lumbar hernia may be a cause of intestinal obstruction.

When a hernia has been identified as the cause of the obstruction, particularly when there is incarceration, the patient is quickly resuscitated and taken to the operating room. The hernia is reduced and the viability of the bowel is assessed. If viable, the bowel is left alone; if not, it is resected. The hernia defect is then repaired.

One important consideration is the Richter hernia (**Fig. 46A.7**). In this variant, only a portion of the wall of the bowel is incarcerated and thus, incarceration and strangulation may not be associated with complete obstruction in this setting.

Use of Mesh in Repair of Obstruction-Associated Hernia

Inguinal Hernia. Historically, it was recommended to perform open tissue repair in the setting of obstructed inguinal hernia, saving mesh for recurrences should they occur. However, even in cases where bowel resection is necessary, prosthetic mesh repair is commonly utilized at the time of index operation and is well supported by recent literature. Laparoscopy,

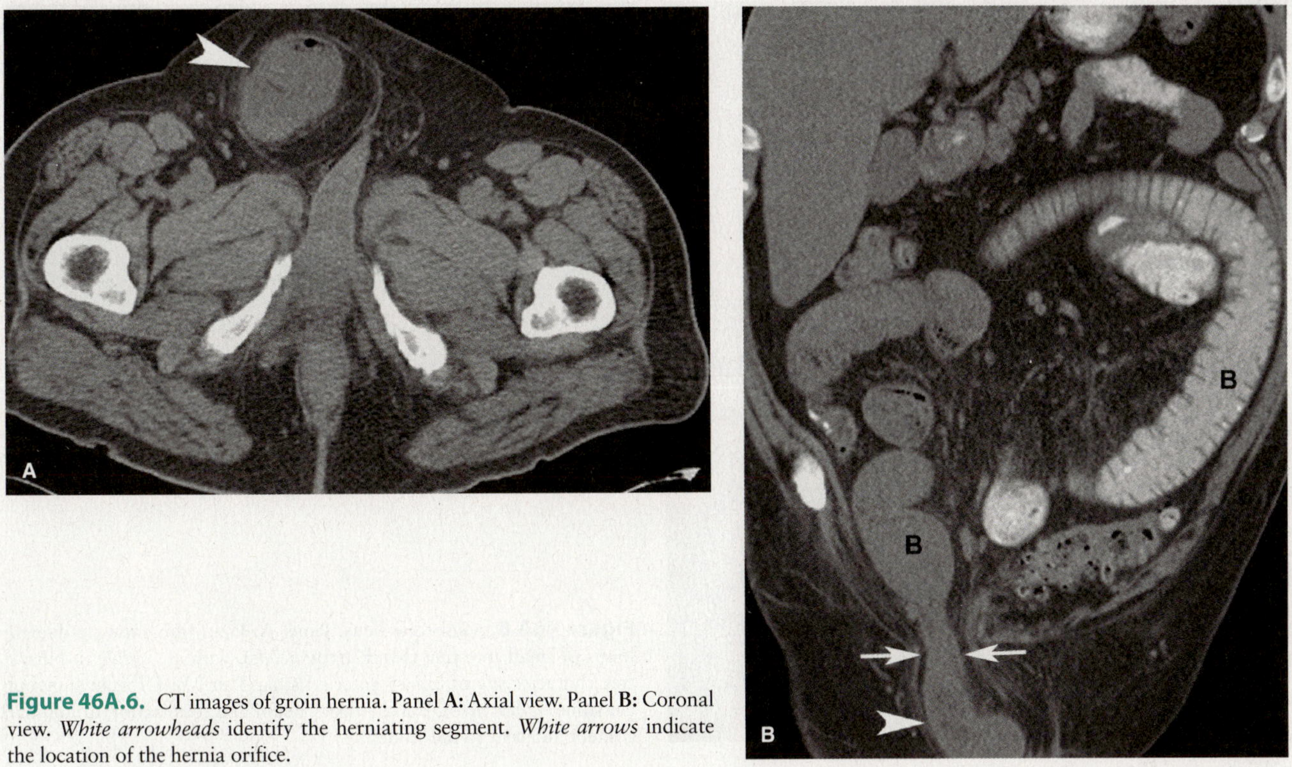

Figure 46A.6. CT images of groin hernia. Panel **A:** Axial view. Panel **B:** Coronal view. *White arrowheads* identify the herniating segment. *White arrows* indicate the location of the hernia orifice.

or laparotomy if necessary, is useful to assist in reduction and assess viability of bowel as needed. The laparoscopic approach to a nonreducible hernia, with reduction and placement of mesh, has been reported with acceptable results if bowel is viable with no evidence of perforation. In cases where there is significant contamination or when bowel required resection, a two-stage approach may be utilized, with repair delayed until healing after reduction, washout, and resection. Alternatively, in such cases, an anterior approach with open tissue repair may be utilized, recognizing the higher likelihood of recurrence. Clinical evidence favoring any specific approach is limited.[19,20]

Ventral Hernia. It remains uncertain whether repair of a ventral hernia can safely include use of permanent prosthetic mesh if it is the cause of an intestinal obstruction. Recent studies suggest that obstruction without ischemia or gangrene poses no special risk for postoperative wound occurrence or mesh infection. Complication rates have been found to increase if contamination occurs during hernia repair, due to perforation, enterotomy, or intestinal resection, leading to increased risks of postoperative wound infection, fistula, reoperation, and mortality. At the same time, recent studies have shown that such contamination need not lead to complication rates that are higher, even when permanent synthetic meshes are used. Even in contaminated fields, including the setting of bowel resection, stoma reversal or creation, and enterotomy, comparable rates of surgical site infection have been reported when repair is performed with biologic or synthetic mesh; in addition to which, significantly reduced rates of early hernia recurrence and cost at 2 years are reported for patients managed with synthetic mesh.[21] These considerations suggest that decisions are best individualized when a ventral hernia is present at the time of operation for, or is the cause of, an episode of acute intestinal obstruction.

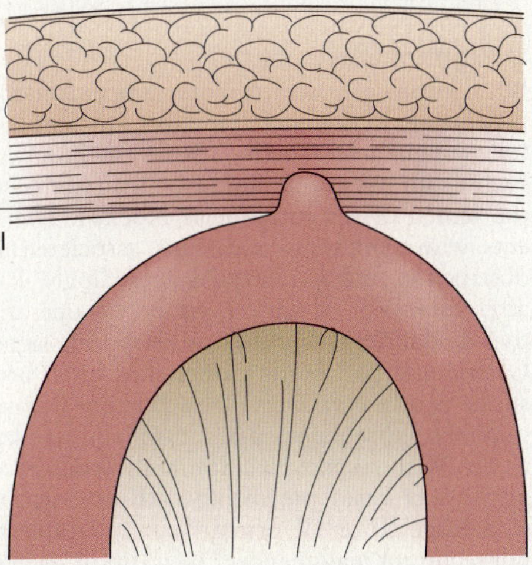

Figure 46A.7. Schematic diagram showing Richter hernia, in which the antimesenteric border (but not the whole wall) of the intestine is incarcerated.

Preoperative Reduction of Hernia to Relieve Obstruction (Taxis)

Reduction of acute inguinal and ventral hernias is often successful. This should only be attempted when there is no concern for strangulation of incarcerated contents (ie, no overlying skin changes, no hemodynamic instability or significant physiologic derangements).[22] In general, taxis should be followed by operative repair, though successful reduction is beneficial in that it often eliminates need to proceed to the operating room in an emergent fashion, facilitating safer operative intervention and optimal operative approach and timing.

Gallstone Ileus

A rare cause of obstruction, accounting for no more than 0.1% of cases, is gallstone ileus.[23] As a result of intense inflammation surrounding a gallstone, a fistula may develop between the biliary tree and the small or large intestine. Most fistulae develop between the gallbladder fundus and duodenum. If the stone is greater than 2.5 cm in diameter, it can lodge in the narrowest portion of the terminal ileum, which is just proximal to the ileocecal valve. Less common sites of impaction include the sigmoid colon and the duodenum (Bouveret syndrome). Typically, the patient is elderly and female, and presents with intermittent symptoms over several days, as the stone tumbles distally

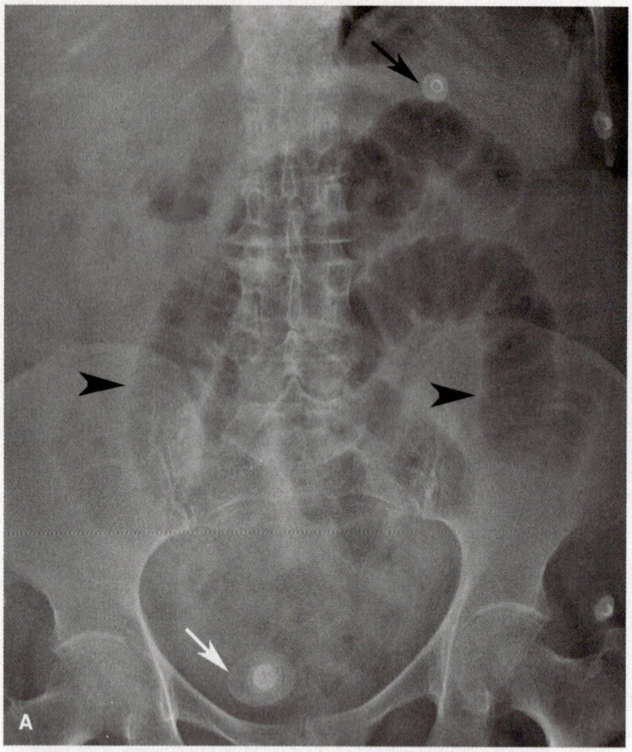

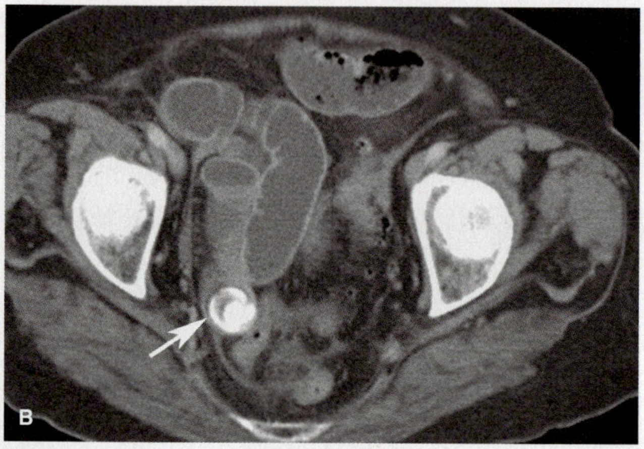

Figure 46A.8. Gallstone ileus. Panel **A:** Plain film showing dilated loops of small intestine (*black arrowheads*), with air visible in biliary tree characteristic of biliary enteric fistula. Panel **B:** CT scan showing gallstone (*white arrow*) in the distal ileum and fecalization of luminal content adjacent to the stone.

toward the ileum. Classic radiographic findings include those of intestinal obstruction, a stone lying outside the right upper quadrant, and air in the biliary tree (**Fig. 46A.8**). Treatment includes removal of the stone (via a proximal enterotomy), with resection of the obstructed segment only if there is evidence of tissue necrosis. The risk of a recurrent gallstone ileus is about 5% to 10%. Such recurrences usually occur within 30 days of the initial episode and are usually due to stones in the small intestine that were missed at the original operation.

Concurrent disconnection of the fistula and cholecystectomy is associated with higher morbidity; it should be considered only cautiously and performed very selectively.[24] A careful search of the entire intestine should be performed to exclude the possibility of additional large stones, which can occur in up to 25% of patients. For patients with Bouveret syndrome, particularly those with high operative risk, an endoscopic approach may be considered, as lithotripsy can often successfully relieve the obstruction.[25] It should be noted, however, that up to 15% of these patients may go on to require laparotomy due to the development of a more distal obstruction due to migration of a stone fragment.

Intussusception

About 5% of intussusceptions occur in adults. An intussusception occurs when one segment of bowel telescopes into an adjacent segment, resulting in obstruction and ischemic injury to the intussuscepting segment (**Fig. 46A.9**) and the obstruction may become complete, particularly if tissue inflammation and necrosis occur. Of adult cases, 90% are associated with pathologic processes. Tumors, benign or malignant, act as the lead point of intussusception in more than 65% of adult cases. It should also be noted that as CT scans have become more widely used, transient intussusceptions without evidence of bowel obstruction are not infrequently identified and do not typically require intervention. However, given the possibility occult and potential malignant lesions such as gastrointestinal stromal tumor or carcinoid, expectant management should probably not be initiated without additional studies such as enteroscopy or capsule endoscopy.[26–28]

Four types of intussusception are recognized: enteric, ileocolic (**Fig. 46A.9**), ileocecal, and colonic. In the ileocolic form, the ileum telescopes into the colon past a fixed ileocecal valve, and the valve itself may be the lead point of the intussusception. Radiographic features of intussusception are not specific. In adult patients, the mainstays of diagnosis are contrast studies or CT scans. Because of the high incidence of tumors, surgery has generally been recommended. Reduction by hydrostatic pressure, which is the standard of care in pediatric cases, is not usually attempted in adults. Clear indications for operation include long length and wide diameter of the intussusception, presence of a lead point, or evidence of bowel obstruction.

Crohn Disease

In this disease, obstruction occurs under two different sets of circumstances. When the disease has flared acutely, the lumen may be narrowed by a pharmacologically reversible inflammatory process. Alternatively, obstruction may occur in the setting of a chronic stricture. Management details and indications for surgery in Crohn disease are discussed elsewhere in this book.

Malignant Obstruction

Both intrinsic bowel tumors and extrinsic compression by peritoneal or nonbowel tumors are pathologies responsible for malignant obstruction. Most commonly, a primary lesion, such as an adenocarcinoma or lymphoma, will enlarge until the lumen of the intestine is blocked. The lesion then presents with symptoms and signs associated with the level of obstruction and is managed accordingly. Patients presenting after treatment of cancer, either via operative or nonoperative modalities, may also present with signs of obstruction. Gastric and pancreatic carcinomas often present with or are subsequently complicated by peritoneal carcinomatosis, and thus, the subsequent obstruction is most likely due to malignancy. With respect to colon and rectal carcinomas, as many as 50% of cases presenting with obstruction after resection of a Stage III or IV, primarily may be due to adhesions and not recurrent malignancy.[29] In addition, even if the obstruction is due to now unresectable disease, significant palliation may be obtained through bypass or enterostomy in up to 75% of patients (**Fig. 46A.10**). However, the underlying diagnosis of

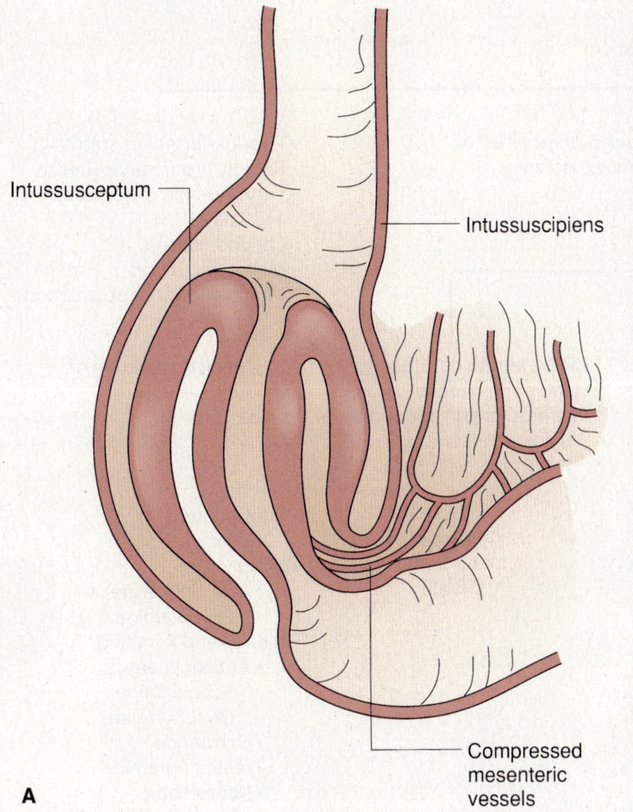

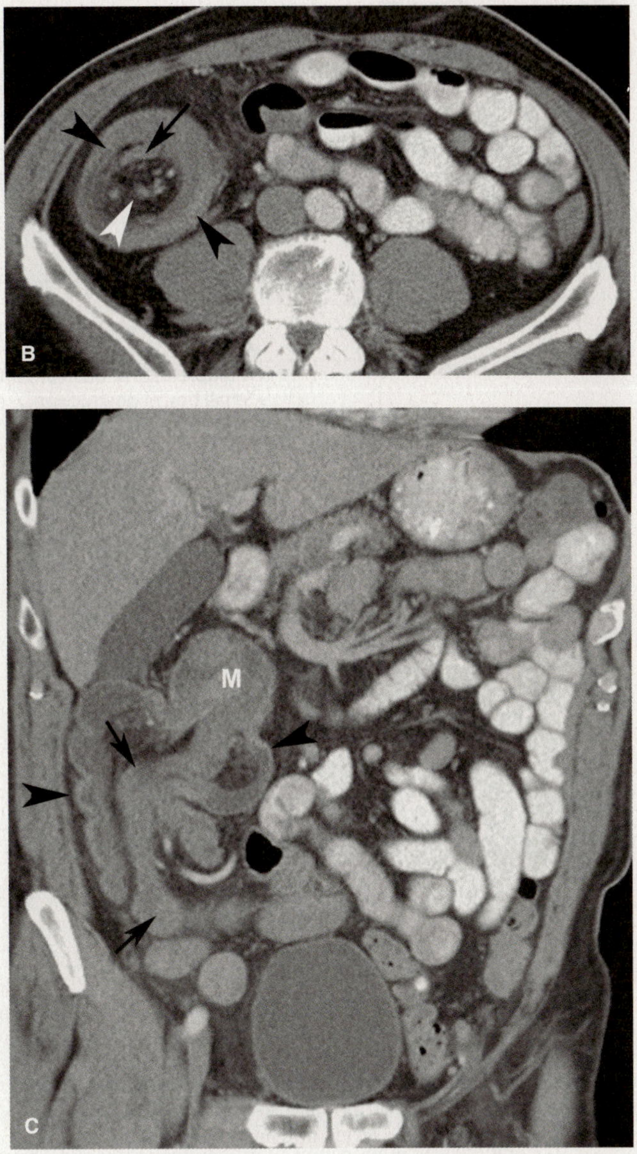

Figure 46A.9. Anatomy and CT views of intussusception. Panel A: The intussusceptum is the segment of bowel that invaginates into the intussuscipiens. Axial view, Panel B, *white arrowhead* shows the lumen, *thin arrow* shows the intussusceptum, and *thick black arrowheads* show the intussuscipiens. Coronal view, Panel C, M indicates the mesentery of the intussusceptum, while *black arrows* indicate the intussuscipiens. The *black arrowhead* indicates the edematous wall of the intussuscipiens.

cancer in this patient population mandates careful attention be paid to patient selection prior to any surgical intervention and risk factors for poor outcome (**Table 46A.4**).

Patients with advanced malignant obstruction in the absence of a solitary or correctable obstructing lesion are generally managed without surgery, with efforts aimed at supportive and palliative care. Patients are managed without a nasogastric tube, if possible. They are encouraged to eat as soon as obstructive symptoms resolve using a low-fiber diet. Antiemetics and opioids via continuous subcutaneous infusions are used to manage nausea, vomiting, and colic, respectively. Octreotide, a somatostatin analog, may be helpful in palliation

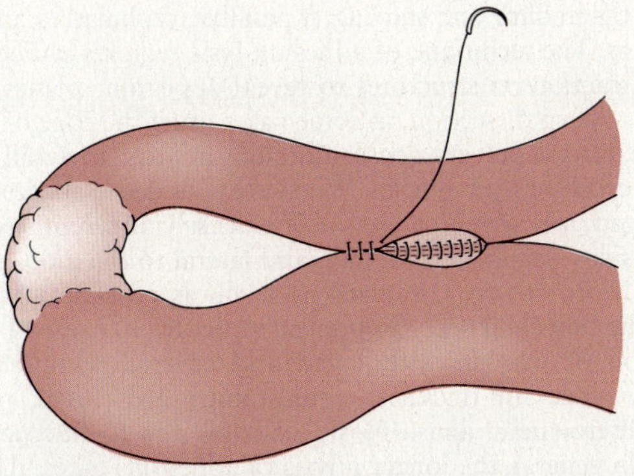

Figure 46A.10. Significant palliation can be achieved in a patient with obstructing, but unresectable malignancy. Enteroenterostomy is performed to bypass the obstructing segment.

Table 46A.4. Management of Malignant Obstructions: Risk Factors for Unfavorable Outcome

Advanced age (biologic/physiologic)
Poor performance status
Advanced stage of primary malignancy (previous treatments, availability of anticancer options, life expectancy)
Malnutrition/cachexia
Comorbidities
Absence of psychosocial support
Ascites (>100 cc associated with poor outcome)
Single vs. multiple sites of obstruction
Carcinomatosis (believed to respond poorly to surgical intervention)

Algorithm 46A.2

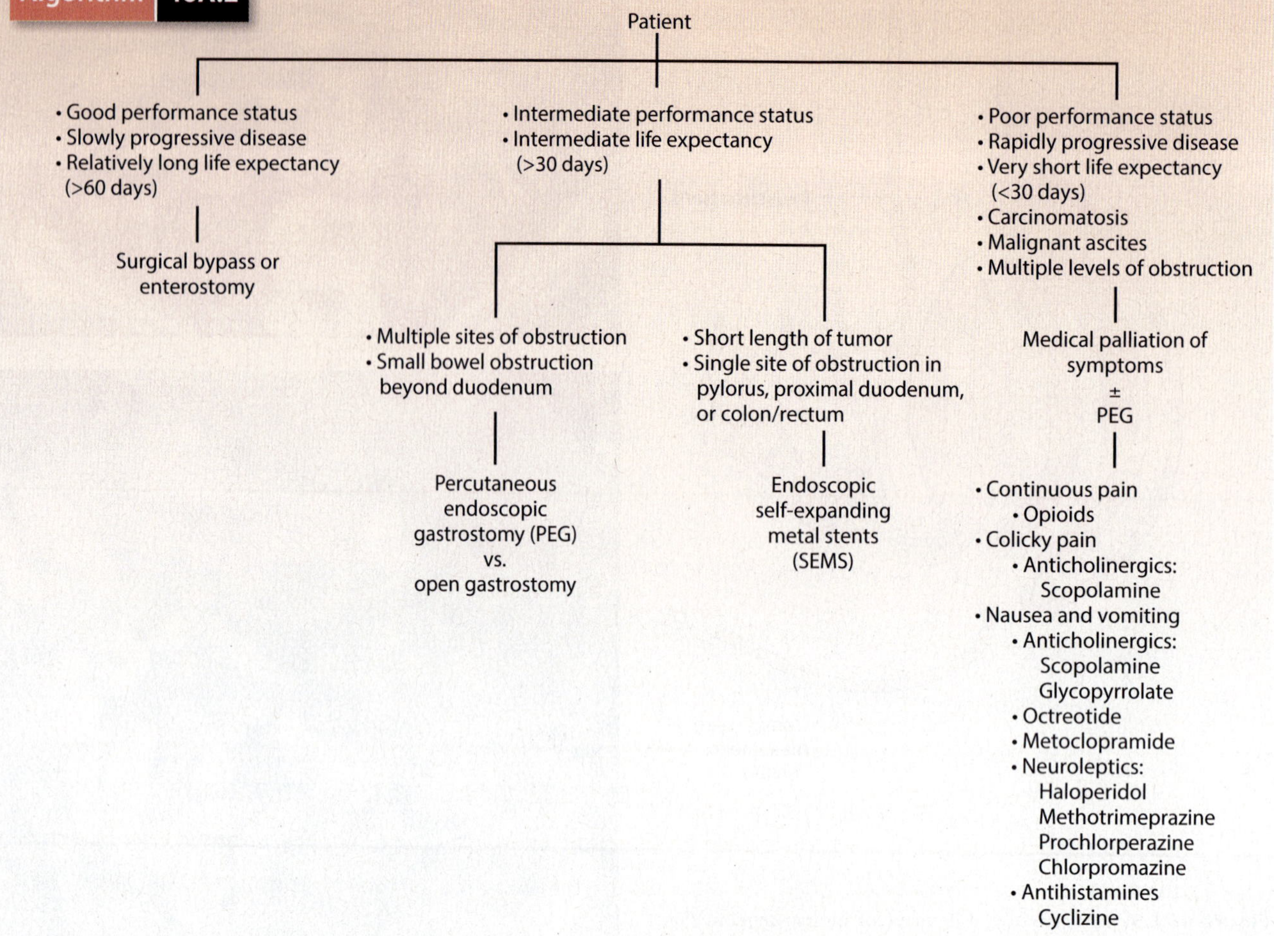

Algorithm 46A.2. Algorithm for management of malignant obstruction.

of refractory malignant intestinal obstruction by improving intestinal mucosal absorption, improving motility, reducing gastrointestinal hormone levels and intestinal secretions, and having a direct antineoplastic effect on the obstructing tumor.[30] This may allow true palliative care outside a hospital setting, saving patients the pain, discomfort, and complications of hospitalization and unproductive surgery. In patients presenting with gastroduodenal and colorectal obstructing lesions who are not candidates for surgical bypass or enterostomy, endoscopic management options include percutaneous endoscopic gastrostomy tube (PEG) placement, self-expanding metallic stent (SEMS) placement, and evolving forms of endoscopically assisted bypass in anatomically favorable circumstances.[31] These options have been associated with symptomatic relief in greater than 75% of patients (**Algorithm 46A.2**).

Radiation Enteritis

Radiation injury can elicit an underlying vasculitis and fibrosis that lead to chronic, recurring, low-grade partial obstruction of the small intestine or stricturing and bleeding in the colon and rectum. Operation is indicated for incapacitating symptoms and obstruction not resolved by conservative management. Recurrence of the original tumor as a cause of obstruction should be considered and excluded. A critical feature is preoperative malnutrition and diarrhea that is often associated with radiation enteritis, due to both malabsorption and maldigestion, leading to deficiencies in fat-soluble vitamins and interruption of the enterohepatic circulation. Surgical approaches include resection, when structuring disease is localized to distal segments and the intestinal loops are not too densely adherent to each other or other structures, such as major blood vessels. When resection is not feasible, it may be feasible and prudent to perform a bypass of the obstructing segment, as shown for a focal malignant obstruction in **Figure 46A.10**.

Open and Laparoscopic Operations in the Management of Small Bowel Obstruction

General Principles of Open Laparotomy and Lysis of Adhesions

8 Currently, open laparotomy is the preferred method for managing SBO complicated by strangulation or perforation, or in the setting of complex abdominal conditions such as malignancy, inflammatory bowel disease, or hernia. It is also generally the safest approach for operative management when multiple operations have been performed previously. An incision is made, usually in the midline and starting, if possible, cephalad to any prior incisions. The technique of adhesion lysis requires patience and gentle traction on structures to reveal opportune planes of dissection. Sharp dissection, in some cases using the edge of a fresh scalpel, is used on very dense adhesions in order to avoid unnecessary crush or tear injuries. When areas of dense adherence are visualized, it is wise to tease the less densely adherent structures on all sides—cephalad, caudad, and lateral to the most difficult areas. Moist sponges are used as much as possible when handling the bowel, in order to prevent desiccation. Areas of serosal abrasion or tear are imbricated and covered with uninjured serosa, while full-thickness enterotomies are closed, resected with enteroenteral anastomosis, or converted to enteroenterostomy. In general, the longer a lysis of adhesions takes, the more physiologic disturbance and the slower the recovery. Exploration of the peritoneal cavity for obstruction requires unhurried but steady progress, conscious of the clock but not driven by it.

Table 46A.5. Clinical Risk Factors for Prolonged Ileus after Abdominal Operations

Neurogenic	Metabolic	Pharmacologic	Infectious
Spinal cord lesions or injury	Hypokalemia Uremia	Anticholinergics Opiates	Systemic sepsis Pneumonia
Retroperitoneal process hematoma, tumor	Ca^{++}, Mg^{++} imbalance	Autonomic blockers	Peritonitis
Ureteral colic	Hypothyroidism Diabetic coma or ketoacidosis	Antihistamines Psychotropics Phenothiazines Haloperidol Tricyclic antidepressants Clonidine Vincristine	Herpes Zoster Tetanus Bacterial overgrowth (blind-loop)

General Principles of Laparoscopically Assisted Lysis of Adhesions

Over the past two decades, technical advances have permitted laparoscopy to enter the mainstream of surgical management for intestinal obstruction. According to a systematic review and meta-analysis, laparoscopic adhesiolysis was associated with reduced overall complication rate, with no significant difference in the occurrence of intraoperative injury to bowel and overall mortality. The benefits of laparoscopic management include faster recovery of bowel function, shorter hospital stay, less postoperative pain, reduced recovery time, and earlier return to full activity, and fewer postoperative complications, including a decreased incidence of wound infection and pneumonia. Additionally, laparoscopy is associated with decreased incidence, extent, and severity of intra-abdominal adhesions compared with open surgery. Thus, laparoscopic management of bowel obstruction may result in a decreased lifetime risk for recurrent bowel obstruction. Studies directly comparing laparoscopic to open surgical management of adhesive SBO highlight the benefits of the laparoscopic approach as indicated by statistically significant decreases in complication rates, time to return of bowel function, length of hospital stay, and even overall cost.[32,33]

The predictive factors for a successful laparoscopic adhesiolysis are fewer than two previous laparotomies, nonmedian previous laparotomy, appendectomy as prior surgery, unique band adhesion as the mechanism of SBO, early laparoscopic management (within 24 hours of the onset of symptoms), no signs of peritonitis on physical examination, and experience of the surgeon.[34] Reasons for conversion from laparoscopic to open operation include the overall burden of dense adhesions, inadvertent enterotomy, and inability to determine the underlying cause of obstruction.[35]

ILEUS AND PSEUDO-OBSTRUCTION

Ileus

Etiologic Factors

9 Ileus is distinct from obstruction, but has related features that will be discussed here, as the two processes may present with similarities but are managed in different ways. An *ileus* or "*eileos*" (ancient Greek root meaning "a twisting") reflects a loss of forward peristalsis and coordination of the motility of the different regions of the gastrointestinal tract, causing a functional, not mechanical obstruction. Clinically, passage of flatus and bowel movements have been used to signal the return of bowel function and coordination of peristalsis. Ileus is most commonly seen in the postoperative setting, especially after operations of the abdomen. Some impairment of intestinal function is considered normal after manipulation of the intestine, is usually self-limited, and easily tolerated. The overall duration of ileus is determined in part by the time required to restore electrical and motor activity in all regions of the alimentary tract viscera: stomach, small intestines, colon, and rectum. Duration of ileus is also dependent on the return of coordination of motor activity between these regions. Ileus is also a known consequence of systemic metabolic disturbances such as sepsis or ketoacidosis, activation of reflexes after injury to the central nervous system, direct contact of bowel with inflammation and infection (peritonitis). It is also observed in conditions or complications of surgery that cause irritation, infection, or bleeding in the retroperitoneum.

As summarized in the **Chapter 46B**: Small Intestine: Normal Anatomy, Physiology, and Pathophysiology of Obstruction and Ileus Syndromes, a diverse array of circulating peptides, inflammatory cytokines, neural pathways, and pharmacologic agents are implicated in the etiology and persistence of ileus. Clinically consequential medications include opioids and anti-serotoninergic/cholinergic medications such as clonazepam. A variety of clinical circumstances and laboratory tests may also increase suspicion for prolonged ileus and lessen concern for mechanical obstruction and associated complications. In addition to opiates, diverse medications have been associated with slow recovery of intestinal motor function (**Table 46A.5**). Isolated metabolic disturbances such as ketoacidosis, hypomagnesemia, hypercalcemia, hypokalemia can prolong ileus. Ileus can be caused and perpetuated by systemic inflammatory responses to sepsis, abscess, pneumonia, pancreatitis, and major burns. In addition, there is some clinical and experimental evidence to suggest that when there are preexisting micronutrient abnormalities that lead to systemic inflammation, recovery of intestinal motor function may be delayed. These considerations mandate careful attention to concurrent medical and surgical conditions, medications, diet, and psychosocial circumstances, physical examination, and laboratory studies for expeditious diagnosis and management of ileus.

Diagnosis

Clinically, it is important to distinguish between normal POI, pathologic, or the so-called paralytic ileus, and early postoperative mechanical obstruction. POI is self-limited, usually lasting 2 to 4 days, predominantly a reflection of colon dysmotility. Paralytic ileus lasts longer and reflects impaired coordination of electrical impulses and motor responses throughout the gastrointestinal tract. Symptoms and signs of normal POI include mild nausea and perhaps vomiting with mild distention and sparse but not absent bowel sounds. Plain Films (**Fig. 46A.11**) demonstrate distended loops of small and often large intestine, with air present in all segments of the gastrointestinal tract. Of note, it is difficult to use time alone as a criteria for defining a prolonged ileus, which depends as much on the clinical circumstances.[36]

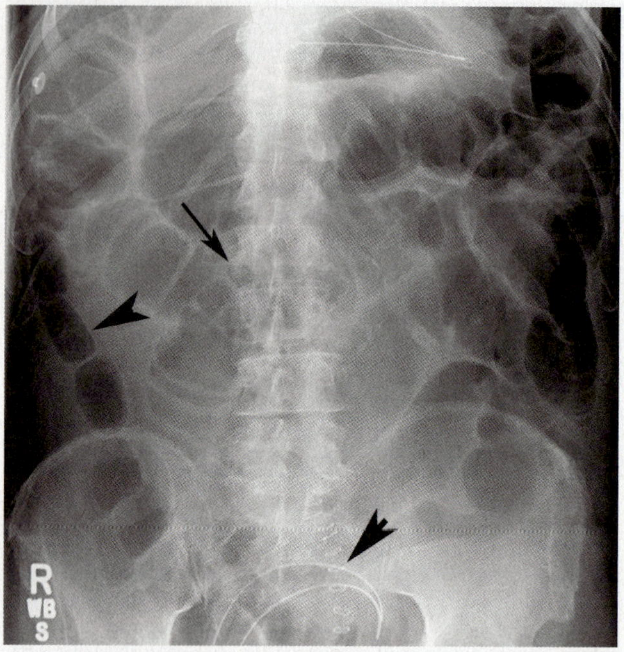

Figure 46A.11. Plain upright abdominal radiograph of a patient with ileus. Air–fluid levels are present in the small intestine (*thin black arrow*). Air is also seen in the ascending colon (*black arrowhead*) and the distal colon (*arrowhead* with short stem). These findings are characteristic of, but not specific for, ileus.

A prolonged postoperative ileus (PPOI) is manifest in protracted signs or symptoms of abdominal distention, bloating, diffuse and persistent and constant abdominal discomfort, nausea, vomiting, and inability to pass flatus or tolerate an oral diet. In contrast, mechanical obstruction is characterized by intense colicky pain, feculent emesis, or rapidly progressing pain or distention is more suggestive of SBO than PPOI. Differentiation of ileus from obstruction is often difficult without objective confirmation through imaging and systematic, serial clinical observations.

When the patient's POI has extended beyond the expected period, the patient may begin to experience some discomfort and distention, as swallowed air fills loops that do not have effective peristalsis. The differential diagnosis now includes the possibility of mechanical obstruction from early postoperative
10 adhesions. To differentiate early postoperative obstruction from ileus, contrast studies or CT scans are helpful. The latter may be useful if other abdominal pathology such as an abscess could be contributing to the clinical picture. If the diagnosis is uncertain after CT, upper GI contrast studies (enteroclysis) with water-soluble radio-opaque contrast material (eg, Gastrografin) are especially helpful in distinguishing ileus from partial SBO (which more closely mimics ileus than complete SBO) and in identifying the severity of partial obstruction. Recent developments suggest that point-of-care ultrasound may be useful in early recognition of gastric distention and luminal content as a hallmark of impending ileus.[37]

Management

The principal goal in managing a normal POI is to prevent uncomfortable distention, vomiting, and aspiration, as well as to attend to electrolyte disturbances and nutritional support in prolonged cases. A secondary goal is to limit its duration. Passage of flatus is used, in reliable patients, as the index indicating coordination of all segments of the gastrointestinal tract and resolution of ileus. Nasogastric suction is used selectively, mainly to relieve the discomfort associated with nausea and distention. In individual cases, use of nasogastric suction may be extended when, in the surgeon's judgment, the ileus is likely to be prolonged because of intraoperative findings such as peritonitis or because of extensive manipulation of the bowel due to widespread adhesions. Serial and standardized examinations will usually reveal that ileus is resolving as evidenced by passage of flatus. Until the patient's bowel functions are clearly restored, close attention to fluid and electrolyte balance is important, and alternate forms of nutrition should be considered. Of note, routine use of nasogastric suction after laparotomy provides no clear benefit, is uncomfortable, and may lead to more frequent pulmonary complications.[38]

In recent years, considerable attention has been given to identifying and systematically addressing the multiple and potentially interacting risk factors for prolongation of POI (**Table 46A.6**). Interventions include preventing perioperative fluid overload, electrolyte disturbance, and transient acute kidney injury. Early mobilization and walking are encouraged as activity stimulates bowel function, reduces the risk of pulmonary complications, and possibly improves cognition. Adjuncts such as gum chewing or use of hard candy theoretically stimulate vagal function and have been studied extensively, without strong evidence for or against their routine use. Use of epidural catheters and regional nerve blocks, when appropriate, has been shown to accelerate return of bowel function after laparotomy, not only by decreasing pain and use of opioid medications but also potentially by interfering with motility-inhibiting influences of the sympathetic nervous system. Early feeding also stimulates secretions, coordinated propulsive activity, and likely improves immune function, thereby reducing the risk of postoperative infection and metabolic disturbance.

Based on experimental studies, pharmacologic interventions have been proposed to shorten recovery of gastrointestinal motility and coordination between different regions of the gastrointestinal tract. Thus, opioid antagonists, somatostatin analogs, sympatholytic agents, injection of local anesthetics into mesenteric nerve roots, or nonsteroidal anti-inflammatory agents, such as ketorolac, all appear to promote faster recovery to normal myoelectric activity and intestinal transit times. Over the years, prokinetic agents that target vagal or other components of the enteric neuroendocrine system and including metoclopramide, erythromycin, and cisapride (currently not permitted for use in the United States), have also been studied but without clear, demonstrable benefit in accelerating resolution of POI and shortening hospital lengths of stay.[39] Laxatives have no proven benefit for earlier resolution of POI. Anecdotally, anorectal stimulation with suppositories or contrast enema can facilitate passage of flatus, perhaps "jump-starting" bowel movements and coordination of motility of small and large intestines.

Of special interest are strategies that target the μ-opioid receptor or serotonin-receptor 5-HT$_4$. Thus, the opioid μ-receptor antagonists have been reported to reduce GI recovery time and to facilitate hospital discharge following major abdominal operations, as well as operations outside the abdomen. Agonists directed at serotonin 5-HT4 receptor are also promising in shortening the interval of ileus following abdominal operations.[40]

Along with pharmacologic measures, it should be emphasized that in otherwise routine laparotomy or laparoscopy gentle handling of tissues, meticulous attention to hemostasis, and applications of sound principles of wound management are likely to have the greatest impact on optimizing recovery from ileus and minimizing the incidence of prolonged ileus. Efforts to reduce incision size and time spent handling the intestines through the use of laparoscopic approaches clearly improve recovery from ileus in some if not all patients undergoing standardized intra-abdominal procedures such as appendectomy, and colectomy. Even in open procedures, standardization of management and effective communication help expedite clinical fast-track pathways and facilitate earlier recovery of bowel function and discharge from hospital. Currently proposed measures to minimize the prolongation of ileus are summarized in **Table 46A.7**.

Table 46A.6. Management Options for Postoperative Ileus

Treatment	Benefit	Drawback
Nasogastric tube	Possible relief of vomiting and bloating	Does not shorten duration of ileus May contribute to fever, atelectasis, and aspiration Discomfort
Early postoperative feeding	Stimulates reflex for propulsive bowel motility and enzyme secretion Stimulates immune system Reduces postoperative and posttraumatic infectious complications Reduces risk of anastomotic dehiscence, wound infection, pneumonia	Patients may not tolerate feeding
Opioid μ-receptor antagonists	Peripheral acting FDA approved to hasten postoperative ileus following partial large or small bowel resection with primary anastomosis	Possible cardiovascular or neoplastic risk Currently restricted to inpatient use only
5-HT$_4$ receptor agonists	Peripheral acting Cisapride: FDA approval rescinded Prucalopride: FDA approved for chronic constipation	Contraindicated in structural or inflammatory conditions of intestine such as UC and Crohn's; also to be monitored closely for suicidal ideation in patients with depression Not currently FDA approved outside clinical trials for ileus or pseudo-obstruction
Laparoscopic procedures	Earlier return of bowel function and discharge from hospital Minimal skin incision, minimal mechanical bowel manipulation	Not all patients and procedures are amenable to the laparoscopic approach
Epidural anesthetics/ analgesics	Reduced duration of ileus vs. systemic opioid Increases splanchnic blood flow Anti-inflammatory	Risks associated with epidural catheter placement
Gum chewing	May shorten duration of ileus Simple and inexpensive	Limited data
Laxatives	May shorten duration of ileus Inexpensive	Limited data on efficacy
Nonsteroidal anti-inflammatory drugs (COX-2 inhibitors)	Decreases opioid needed for pain control May increase motility by acting as an anti-inflammatory	Possible increased risk of postoperative bleeding Other adverse effects

Colonic Pseudo-Obstruction (Ogilvie Syndrome)

Etiologic Factors

11 Acute pseudo-obstruction of the colon,[41] also known as Ogilvie syndrome,[42] is a paralytic ileus of the large bowel, characterized by rapidly progressive abdominal distention, often painless. Although the distention of the colon is not due to mechanical obstruction, the wall of the bowel, particularly that of the cecum, can become sufficiently distended so that its blood supply is compromised. Gangrene, perforation, peritonitis, and shock can follow. Less than 5% of the cases occur in the absence of any inciting condition or event.

Major risk factors for development of Ogilvie syndrome include traumatic injury (11%), infections such as pneumonia, sepsis (10%); obstetric/gynecologic conditions (10%); myocardial infarction and congestive heart failure (10%); abdominal and pelvic surgery (9%); neurologic conditions such as Parkinson disease, spinal cord injury, multiple sclerosis, and Alzheimer disease (9%); orthopedic procedures (7%); other medical conditions including metabolic imbalances, for example, hypokalemia, hypocalcemia, hypomagnesemia (32%); other surgical conditions (12%). Evidence suggests that Ogilvie syndrome is thought to be related, at least in part, to sympathetic nervous overactivity or interference with sacral parasympathetic efferents. It is postulated that the distal colon becomes atonic due to interruption of the S2 to S4 parasympathetic nerve fibers. Other theories about the pathophysiologic causes include autonomic dysfunction, reduced colonic ganglion cells, and loss of intrinsic nitric oxide activity, but the cause remains unknown.

Diagnosis

This syndrome is commonly encountered in patients hospitalized for over 3 to 7 days, often in men greater than 60 years of age. Primary manifestations variably include gastrointestinal symptoms such as nausea, vomiting, abdominal pain, constipation, and diarrhea. Labored breathing caused by abdominal distention may be observed as part of the clinical picture. Other than distention, there are no characteristic physical or laboratory findings for this syndrome. On percussion, the abdomen is resonant due to the presence of air in dilated segments of small intestine and colon.

Laboratory findings associated with this syndrome may include hypokalemia, hypocalcemia, hypomagnesemia, and hypophosphatemia, which are implicated as etiologic factors.

Table 46A.7. Opportunities to Prevent Prolonged Ileus

Opportunities to Prevent Prolonged Ileus
Minimization of trauma to tissues; using proper technique in the operating room with gentle handling of bowel during surgery
Minimal use of narcotics for analgesia, for any route of administration (intravenous, intramuscular, epidural)
Perioperative Dexamethasone (8 mg IV) reduces nausea and vomiting; may shorten duration of ileus; lidocaine infusions shorten ileus by reducing inflammatory response
Use of opioid antagonists that target the enteral mu-receptor
Generous use of midthoracic epidural anesthesia with local anesthetic use
Use of nonsteroidal anti-inflammatory (COX-2 inhibitors) agents for analgesia
Early feeding
Correction of any electrolyte or metabolic imbalances
Early recognition of septic complications (eg, abdominal abscess, pneumonia, central line sepsis) that may contribute to prolongation beyond the expected period for ileus

Leukocytosis, elevation of sedimentation rate, or C-reactive protein is also present if systemic inflammation is present or perforation is impending.

The diagnosis is usually apparent from plain films (**Fig. 46A.12**). Radiographs of the abdomen may reveal air in the small bowel and distention of discrete segments of the colon (ie, cecum or transverse colon often up to splenic flexure) or the entire abdominal colon. Haustral markings disappear with increasing distention. CT scan is currently the standard method for identifying colon pseudo-obstruction and excluding alternative diagnoses, including toxic megacolon and mechanical obstruction. Mechanical obstruction of the colon, occurring in volvulus or obturator obstructions from cancer or diverticular disease, presents with acute pain along with distention. Patients with toxic megacolon may typically manifest with symptoms such as fever, tachycardia, abdominal tenderness, bloody diarrhea, or other manifestations of severe colitis.

Management[43,44] (Algorithm 46A.3)

Once diagnosis is confirmed and distal obstruction or toxic megacolon is ruled out, colonic pseudo-obstruction is treated with attention to underlying neurologic or metabolic disturbances. Minimization of narcotics and utilization of μ-opioid receptor antagonists can also be helpful. Use of neostigmine and decompressive colonoscopy is dependent on clinical context but may be utilized in stepwise fashion. In many cases, a nonoperative course of therapy can be continued safely for several days, with resolution of acute colonic pseudo-obstruction in 70% to 90% of patients. Serial abdominal radiographs should be followed to assess bowel size and evaluate for concerning signs. A nasogastric tube is helpful if the patient is vomiting and will prevent swallowed air from passing distally. Surgery is reserved for patients with evidence of ischemic bowel, perforation, peritonitis, or clinical deterioration.

Colonoscopic decompression is a commonly employed treatment strategy in appropriate patients and should only be performed by experienced endoscopists. Endoscopic decompression is successful in 60% to 90% of cases, but the condition can recur in up to 40% of patients. This rate of recurrence may be decreased by placement of a decompressive tube. Recurrence requires repeat colonoscopic decompression in approximately 40% of cases after initial successful decompression. The placement of a decompression tube with the aid of a guidewire at the time of colonoscopy may reduce the need for repeated colonoscopic decompression. Rectal tubes are ineffective as primary modalities in managing distention of the proximal colon.

Neostigmine, a parasympathomimetic, is used in the treatment of acute colonic pseudo-obstruction. Decompression with this drug has been achieved in 80% to 100% of patients, with a recurrence rate of 5%. Neostigmine has expected cardiovascular side effects such as bradycardia, hypotension, and dizziness; and is excreted via the kidneys. Thus there are few but serious relative contraindications to its use in treatment of acute colonic pseudo-obstruction, including significant cardiac disease, a

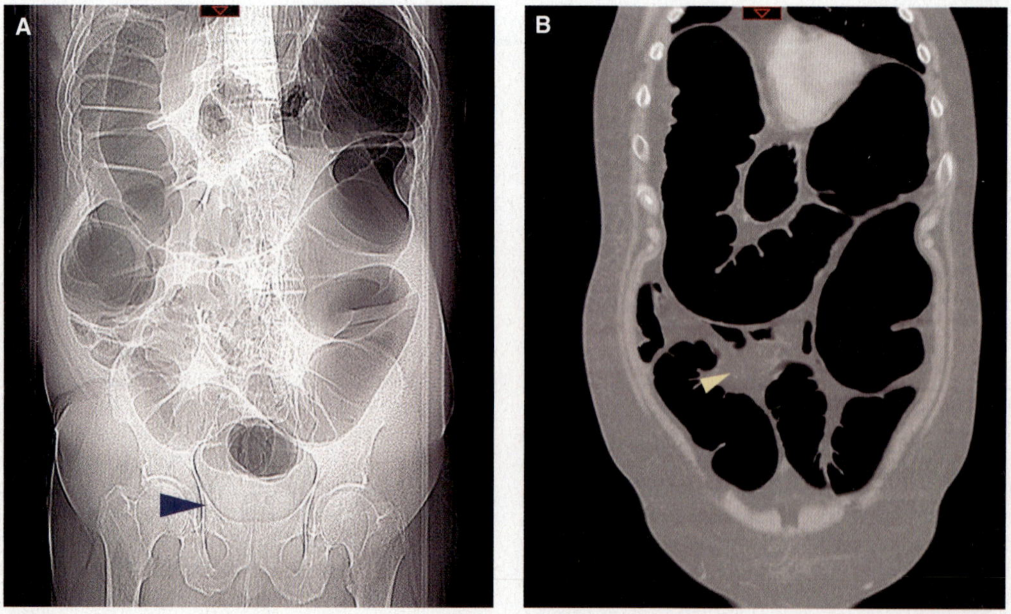

Figure 46A.12. Acute Colonic pseudo-obstruction, "Ogilvie" syndrome, recognized on plain films and CT scan. Panel **A:** Plain radiograph showing diffuse dilation of colon and no evidence of air in the area of the rectum (*dark arrowhead*). Panel **B:** Coronal CT image showing that the small bowel (*light arrowhead*) is decompressed between distended loops of colon. (Images courtesy of Dr. Frank Brennan, VA Medical Center, White River Junction, VT).

Algorithm 46A.3

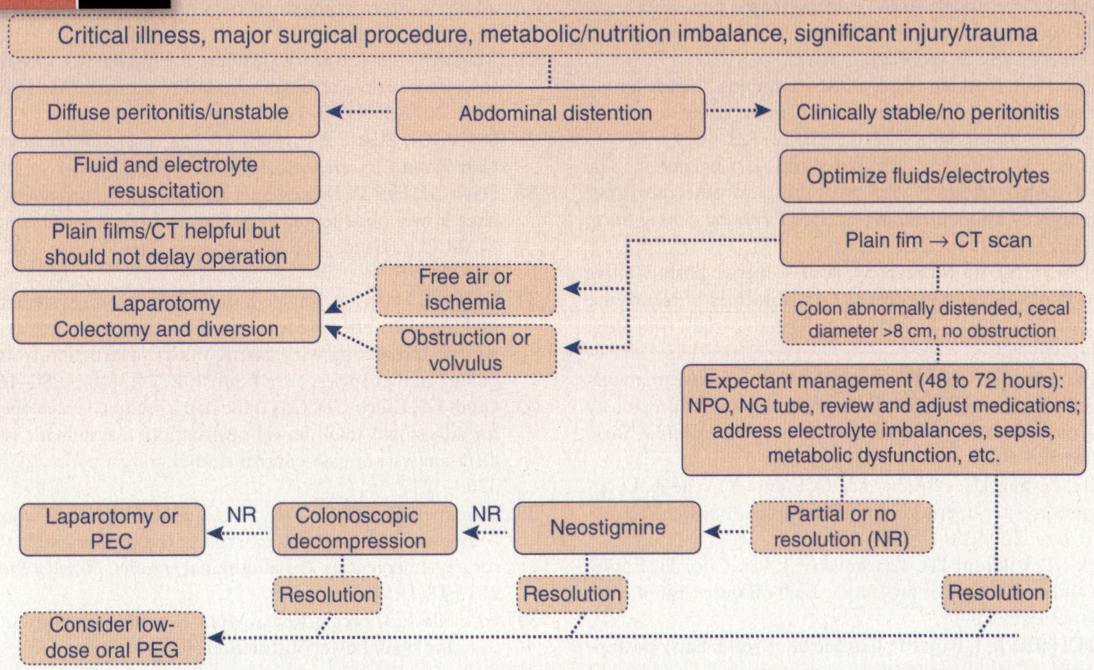

Algorithm 46A.3. Evaluation and decisions in diagnosis and management of acute colonic pseudo-obstruction (Ogilvie syndrome). Note that PEC is not endorsed by some societies and can only be recommended when performed by experienced proceduralists. NR, no resolution; PEC, percutaneous endoscopic cecostomy; PEG, polyethylene glycol (laxative regimen).

baseline heart rate of less than 60 beats/min or systolic blood pressure of less than 90 mm Hg; active bronchospasm requiring medication; a history of colon cancer or partial colonic resection; active gastrointestinal bleeding; pregnancy; or a serum creatinine concentration of more than 3 mg/dL (265 μmol/L). Other side effects include mild-to-moderate crampy abdominal pain, excessive salivation, and vomiting. Side effects, such as increasing airway secretions and bronchospasm, can be reduced by concomitant use of glycopyrrolate without reduction of colonic response. Some institutions may require more intensive level of care prior to usage of neostigmine, given the risks and side effects involved. Updated guidelines recommend use of neostigmine therapy initially in the sequence of therapeutic intervention, ahead of colonoscopy, but clinical context may drive the order in which these are done. After resolution of the acute distension by pharmacologic agents or endoscopic decompression, there may be benefit in a short course of a gentle laxative regimen, using oral polyethylene glycol.

Patients should undergo immediate exploration if they exhibit signs of clinical deterioration or bowel perforation (peritoneal signs on physical examination or free air on radiographs). Surgery is also considered for patients not responding to medical and endoscopic management. For example, if the clinical picture is worsening and the cecal diameter increases beyond 10 to 12 cm or if it persists for more than 48 hours, intervention is recommended. The duration of distention may be more important than the absolute size of the cecum with respect to the likelihood of spontaneous perforation. The extent of colonic resection will depend on intraoperative findings, but often at the very least requires right hemicolectomy, with further colonic resection depending on clinical context and any signs of colonic ischemia. In the majority of these patients, end ileostomy will be required, though in certain clinical circumstances, temporary abdominal closure postresection with return to the operating room in 24 to 48 hours may allow for primary anastomosis. In cases where resection and end ileostomy are performed, a mucus fistula may be helpful to decompress the downstream colon if there are ongoing concerns about motility in this segment. In the past, decompression through cecostomy procedures (ostomy or tube) was performed in frail or hemodynamically unstable patients who might not tolerate a full laparotomy. In some cases, the procedure could be performed without full general anesthesia. Operative cecostomy in any form was not well tolerated and fell out of favor. Recent reports suggest that there may be benefit from colonoscopically placed tubes that are smaller and better tolerated, and before the colon becomes so dilated that patchy ischemia and perforation are imminent.[45]

ACKNOWLEDGMENT

We gratefully acknowledge the contributions of previous edition author, Amanda B. Cooper, as portions of those chapters have been retained in this revision.

References

1. ten Broek RP, Issa Y, van Santbrink EJ, et al. Burden of adhesions in abdominal and pelvic surgery: systematic review and met-analysis. *BMJ*. 2013;347:f5588.
2. Eskelinen M, Ikonen J, Lipponen P. Contributions of history-taking, physical examination, and computer assistance to diagnosis of acute small-bowel obstruction. A prospective study of 1333 patients with acute abdominal pain. *Scand J Gastroenterol*. 1994;29(8):715–721.
3. Maglinte DD, Howard TJ, Lillemoe KD, Sandrasegaran K, Rex DK. Small-bowel obstruction: state-of-the-art imaging and its role in clinical management. *Clin Gastroenterol Hepatol*. 2008;6(2):130–139.
4. Feister K, Konstantinoff K, Hamade M, Mellnick V. Pearls and pitfalls of imaging small bowel obstruction. *Can Assoc Radiol J*. 2024;75(3):631–643.
5. Fonseca AL, Schuster KM, Maung AA, Kaplan LJ, Davis KA. Routine nasogastric decompression in small bowel obstruction: is it really necessary? *Am Surg*. 2013;79(4):422–428.
6. Zielinski MD, Haddad NN, Cullinane DC, et al. Multi-institutional, prospective, observational study comparing the Gastrografin challenge versus standard treatment in adhesive small bowel obstruction. *J Trauma Acute Care Surg*. 2017;83(1):47–54.

7. Ten Broek RPG, Krielen P, Di Saverio S, et al. Bologna guidelines for diagnosis and management of adhesive small bowel obstruction (ASBO): 2017 update of the evidence-based guidelines from the world society of emergency surgery ASBO working group. *World J Emerg Surg*. 2018;13:24.
8. Diaz A, Ricci KB, Rushing AP, et al. Re-examining "Never letting the sun rise or set on a bowel obstruction" in the era of acute care surgery. *J Gastrointest Surg*. 2021;25(2):512–522.
9. Harmankaya M, Oreskov JO, Burcharth J, Gogenur I. The impact of timing of antibiotics on in-hospital outcomes after major emergency abdominal surgery. *Eur J Trauma Emerg Surg*. 2020;46(1):221–227.
10. Duron JJ, Silva NJ, du Montcel ST, et al. Adhesive postoperative small bowel obstruction: incidence and risk factors of recurrence after surgical treatment: a multicenter prospective study. *Ann Surg*. 2006;244:750–757.
11. Jeong WK, Lim SB, Choi HS, Jeong SY. Conservative management of adhesive small bowel obstructions in patients previously operated on for primary colorectal cancer. *J Gastrointest Surg*. 2008;12(5):926–932.
12. Fevang BT, Fevang J, Lie SA, Soreide O, Svanes K, Viste A. Long-term prognosis after operation for adhesive small bowel obstruction. *Ann Surg*. 2004;240(2):193–201.
13. ten Broek RP, Bakkum EA, Laarhoven CJ, van Goor H. Epidemiology and prevention of postsurgical adhesions revisited. *Ann Surg*. 2016;263(1):12–19.
14. Ellozy SH, Harris MT, Bauer JJ, Gorfine SR, Kreel I. Early postoperative small-bowel obstruction: a prospective evaluation in 242 consecutive abdominal operations. *Dis Colon Rectum*. 2002;45:1214–1217.
15. Lee SY, Park KJ, Ryoo SB, Oh HK, Choe EK, Heo SC. Early postoperative small bowel obstruction is an independent risk factor for subsequent adhesive small bowel obstruction in patients undergoing open colectomy. *World J Surg*. 2014;38(11):3007–3014.
16. Yamada T, Okabayashi K, Hasegawa H, et al. Meta-analysis of the risk of small bowel obstruction following open or laparoscopic colorectal surgery. *Br J Surg*. 2016;103(5):493–503.
17. Hamdan K, Somers S, Chand M. Management of late postoperative complications of bariatric surgery. *Br J Surg*. 2011;98(10):1345–1355.
18. Gabrielli M, Jarry C, Hurtado S, et al. Small bowel obstruction following laparoscopic Roux-en-Y gastric bypass: is it always necessary to operate? A 5-year, high volume center experience. *Langenbecks Arch Surg*. 2021;406(6):1839–1846.
19. Saeter AH, Fonnes S, Li S, Rosenberg J, Andresen K. Mesh versus non-mesh for emergency groin hernia repair. *Cochrane Database Syst Rev*. 2023;11(11):CD015160.
20. Tastaldi L, Krpata DM, Prabhu AS, et al. Emergent groin hernia repair: a single center 10-year experience. *Surgery*. 2019;165(2):398–405.
21. Rosen MJ, Krpata DM, Petro CC, et al. Biologic vs synthetic mesh for single-stage repair of contaminated ventral hernias: a randomized clinical trial. *JAMA Surg*. 2022;157(4):293–301.
22. Pawlak M, East B, de Beaux AC. Algorithm for management of an incarcerated inguinal hernia in the emergency settings with manual reduction. Taxis, the technique and its safety. *Hernia*. 2021;25(5):1253–1258.
23. Halabi WJ, Kang CY, Ketana N, et al. Surgery for gallstone ileus: a nationwide comparison of trends and outcomes. *Ann Surg*. 2014;259(2):329–335.
24. Inukai K. Gallstone ileus: a review. *BMJ Open Gastroenterol*. 2019;6(1):e000344.
25. Thatipalli N, Gattani R, Nayak K, Sudabattula K. Bouveret syndrome: etiology, clinical presentation, differential diagnosis, complications, and treatment options. *Cureus*. 2024;16(7):e64754.
26. Honjo H, Mike M, Kusanagi H, Kano N. Adult intussusception: a retrospective review. *World J Surg*. 2015;39(1):134–138.
27. Rea JD, Lockhart ME, Yarbrough DE, Leeth RR, Bledsoe SE, Clements RH. Approach to management of intussusception in adults: a new paradigm in the computed tomography era. *Am Surg*. 2007;73:1098–1105.
28. Marsicovetere P, Ivatury SJ, White B, Holubar SD. Intestinal intussusception: etiology, diagnosis, and treatment. *Clin Colon Rectal Surg*. 2017;30(1):30–39.
29. Soybel DI, Bliss DP Jr, Wells SA Jr. Colon and rectal carcinoma. *Curr Probl Cancer*. 1987;11(5):257–356.
30. Davis M, Hui D, Davies A, et al. Medical management of malignant bowel obstruction in patients with advanced cancer: 2021 MASCC guideline update. *Support Care Cancer*. 2021;29(12):8089–8096.
31. Cobb W, Harris S, Xavier J, de la Fuente SG. Systematic review of long-term effectiveness of endoscopic gastrojejunostomy in patients presenting with gastric outlet obstruction from periampullary malignancies. *Surg Endosc*. 2024;38(8):4680–4685.
32. Quah GS, Eslick GD, Cox MR. Laparoscopic versus open surgery for adhesional small bowel obstruction: a systematic review and meta-analysis of case-control studies. *Surg Endosc*. 2019;33(10):3209–3217.
33. Sermonesi G, Tian B, Vallicelli C, et al. Cesena guidelines: WSES consensus statement on laparoscopic-first approach to general surgery emergencies and abdominal trauma. *World J Emerg Surg*. 2023;18(1):57.
34. Farinella E, Cirocchi R, La Mura F, et al. Feasibility of laparoscopy for small bowel obstruction. *World J Emerg Surg*. 2009;4:3.
35. O'Connor DB, Winter DC. The role of laparoscopy in the management of acute small-bowel obstruction: a review of over 2,000 cases. *Surg Endosc*. 2012;26(1):12–17.
36. Chapman SJ, Thorpe G, Vallance AE, Harji DP, Lee MJ, Fearnhead NS; Association of Coloproctology of Great Britain and Ireland Gastrointestinal Recovery Group. Systematic review of definitions and outcome measures for return of bowel function after gastrointestinal surgery. *BJS Open*. 2019;3(1):1–10.
37. Rebmann E, Paisant A, Delestre M, et al. Use of gastric point-of-care ultrasonography to evaluate postoperative ileus. *Br J Surg*. 2024;111(10):znae274.
38. Nelson R, Edwards S, Tse B. Prophylactic nasogastric decompression after abdominal surgery. *Cochrane Database Syst Rev*. 2007;2007(3):CD004929.
39. Emile SH, Horesh N, Garoufalia Z, Gefen R, Ray-Offor E, Wexner SD. Strategies to reduce ileus after colorectal surgery: a qualitative umbrella review of the collective evidence. *Surgery*. 2024;175(2):280–288.
40. Talwar G, Sharma S, McKechnie T, et al. Prucalopride and bowel function post gastrointestinal surgery: systematic review and meta-analysis of randomized controlled trials. *Am Surg*. 2024;90(6):1682–1701.
41. Arthur T, Burgess A. Acute colonic pseudo-obstruction. *Clin Colon Rectal Surg*. 2022;35(3):221–226.
42. Ogilvie H. Large-intestine colic due to sympathetic deprivation; a new clinical syndrome. *Br Med J*. 1948;2(4579):671–673.
43. Naveed M, Jamil LH, Fujii-Lau LL, et al. American Society for Gastrointestinal Endoscopy guideline on the role of endoscopy in the management of acute colonic pseudo-obstruction and colonic volvulus. *Gastrointest Endosc*. 2020;91(2):228–235.
44. Alavi K, Poylin V, Davids JS, et al. Prepared on behalf of the Clinical Practice Guidelines Committee of the American Society of Colon and Rectal Surgeons. The American Society of Colon and Rectal Surgeons clinical practice guidelines for the management of colonic volvulus and acute colonic pseudo-obstruction. *Dis Colon Rectum*. 2021;64(9):1046–1057.
45. Vanek P, Urban O, Falt P. Percutaneous endoscopic cecostomy for management of Ogilvie's syndrome: a case series and literature review with an update on current guidelines (with video). *Surg Endosc*. 2023;37(10):8144–8153.

46B

Small Intestine: Normal Anatomy, Physiology, and Pathophysiology of Obstruction and Ileus Syndromes

David I. Soybel

Key Points

1. The normal adult anatomy of the small intestine results from a program of embryologic events leading to 270 degrees of counterclockwise rotation of the bowel around its axis and fixation of the small and large intestines to the retroperitoneum. Failure of this program results in a spectrum of surgically significant intestinal malformations and may be associated with clinically important abnormalities in other organ systems.
2. Principle functions of the small intestine include: (a) breakdown of food to simple nutrient units that can be absorbed; (b) regulation of absorption of water, macronutrients (eg, fat, carbohydrate, protein), and micronutrients (eg, vitamins, minerals); (c) endocrine signaling to adjacent regions of the alimentary tract, liver and pancreas, and distant organs such as kidney and brain; (d) interface with commensal and symbiotic microorganisms, and defense mechanisms against pathogens. Disturbances in these principal functions can complicate the course of surgical illnesses and interfere with recovery from major surgical procedures.
3. Proper digestion of food and extraction of nutrients requires coordinated motor movements within the small intestines with regions that are upstream (mouth, stomach, esophagus) and downstream (colon, rectum, anus).
4. Increasingly it is clear that epithelial, endocrine, neural and motor components interact, with each other and with luminal nutrients and intestinal microflora to maintain nutritional equilibrium and support homeostasis in the human organism as a whole.
5. The pathophysiology of syndromes of intestinal obstruction, ileus, and colonic pseudo-obstruction (Ogilvie syndrome) each reflect, in different ways, the causes and consequences of interrupting normal flow of intestinal contents and disrupting luminal ecology.

This chapter provides an overview of normal anatomy and physiology of the small intestine. Cellular-level physiology is reviewed where relevant to understanding the contributions of the alimentary canal to fluid and electrolyte balance, nutrition and metabolism, elimination of waste, microbial ecology, and defense against pathogenic organisms. A framework such as this should lead to a more complete understanding of the pathogenesis of conditions such as obstruction and ileus of the small intestine and pseudo-obstruction of the colon, also known as Ogilvie syndrome. In addition, such a framework is critical for recognizing the symptoms, signs and natural history of these conditions, as well as the indications and timing for surgical intervention.

ANATOMY AND PHYSIOLOGIC FUNCTIONS OF THE SMALL INTESTINE

1 Gross Anatomy

The normal small intestine begins at the pylorus and terminates at the ileocecal valve. Three distinct regions are recognized: the duodenum, the jejunum, and the ileum. In live adults, the length of the small intestine measures between 4 and 6 m, varying somewhat with demographics and methods of measurement.

Duodenum

The duodenum is the most proximal segment of the small intestine: it begins at the pylorus and ends at the ligament of Treitz, where it joins the jejunum. The length of the duodenum is just over 20 cm, with four distinct regions (**Fig. 46B.1**).

The first region (D1), the bulb is perhaps 2.5 to 4 cm in length, projecting laterally and superiorly to the right. Tethered to the liver by the hepatoduodenal ligament, it lies cephalad to the pancreatic head. The bulb lies intimately anterior to the gastroduodenal artery (GDA) and less intimately to the common bile duct, which themselves are anterior to the portal vein (PV). Viewed through the endoscope or a duodenotomy at operation, the mucosa of the duodenum is almost smooth and flat, with occasional low ridges (**Fig. 46B.2**).

The second region (D2) is recognized externally as the descending segment and the presence of mucosal folds, known as Kerckring folds or "plica circulares" (**Fig. 46B.2**). This segment passes lies posterior to the right colon and hepatic flexure and in front of the right renal vessels and the inferior vena cava. It lies lateral to the pancreatic head and is pierced medially in its mid-portion for entry of the common bile duct and the major pancreatic duct (Wirsung) at the ampulla of Vater and a separate upstream entry of the minor pancreatic duct (Santorini) at the minor papilla (**Fig. 46B.2**). On its exterior,

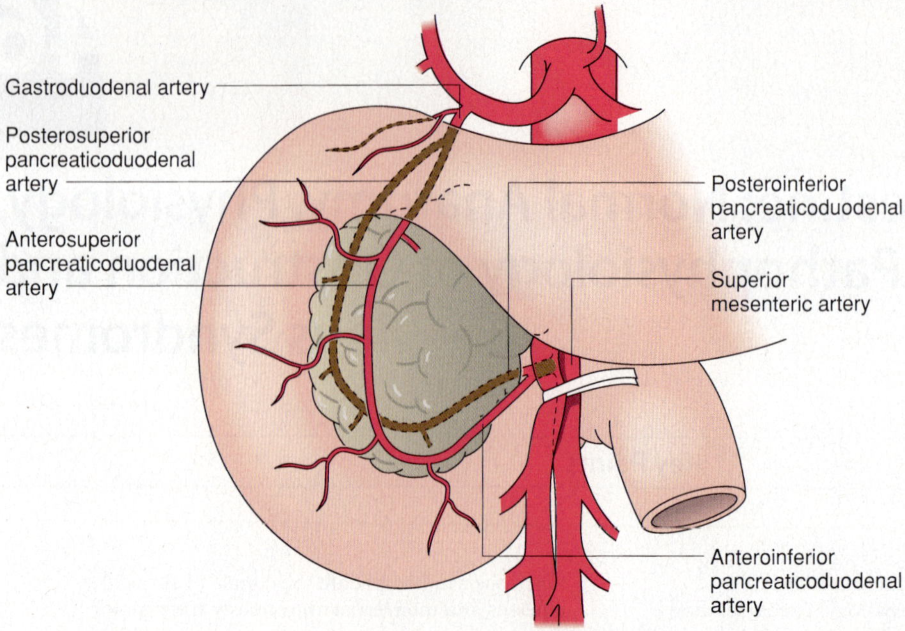

Figure 46B.1. Arterial blood supply to the duodenum.

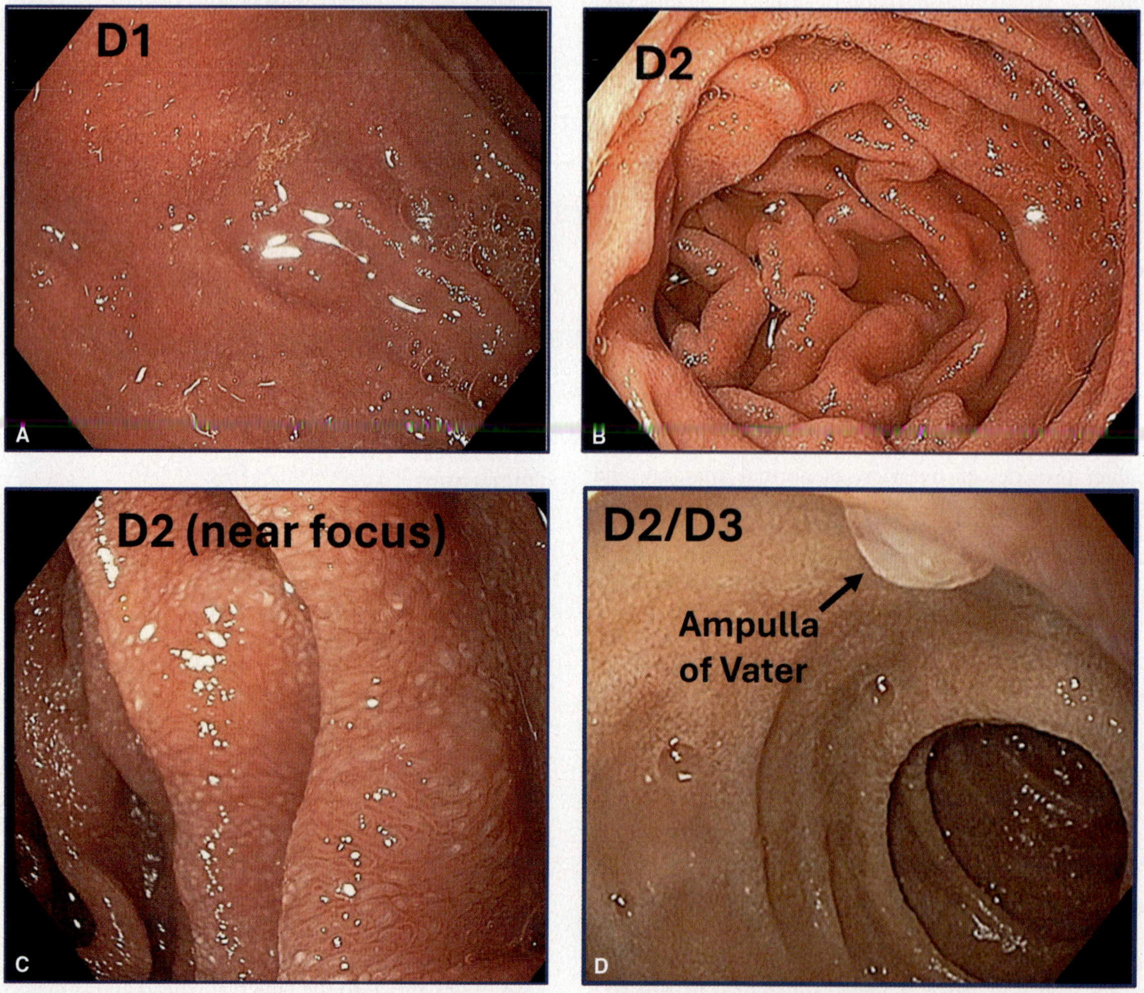

Figure 46B.2. Endoscopic views of the duodenal bulb (D1), the descending segment (D2), and transverse segment (D3) and the ampulla of Vater (junction of segments D2 and D3), which transmit bile and pancreatic secretions from duct of Wirsung: Top left (**A**): endoscopic image of region of the duodenal bulb (D1), with low-profile mucosal folds. Top right (**B**), endoscopic image of the descending segment (D2), showing more numerous and higher profile mucosal folds than in segment D1. Lower left (**C**), endoscopic image of the descending segment (D2) in higher magnification, demonstrating the outline of individual duodenal glands in relief; lower right (**D**), providing a view of the junction of the descending segment (D2) and the transverse segment (D3), with the Ampulla of Vater in the view. (Images courtesy of David Klibansky MD, Gastroenterology Section, VA Medical Center, White River Junction VT.)

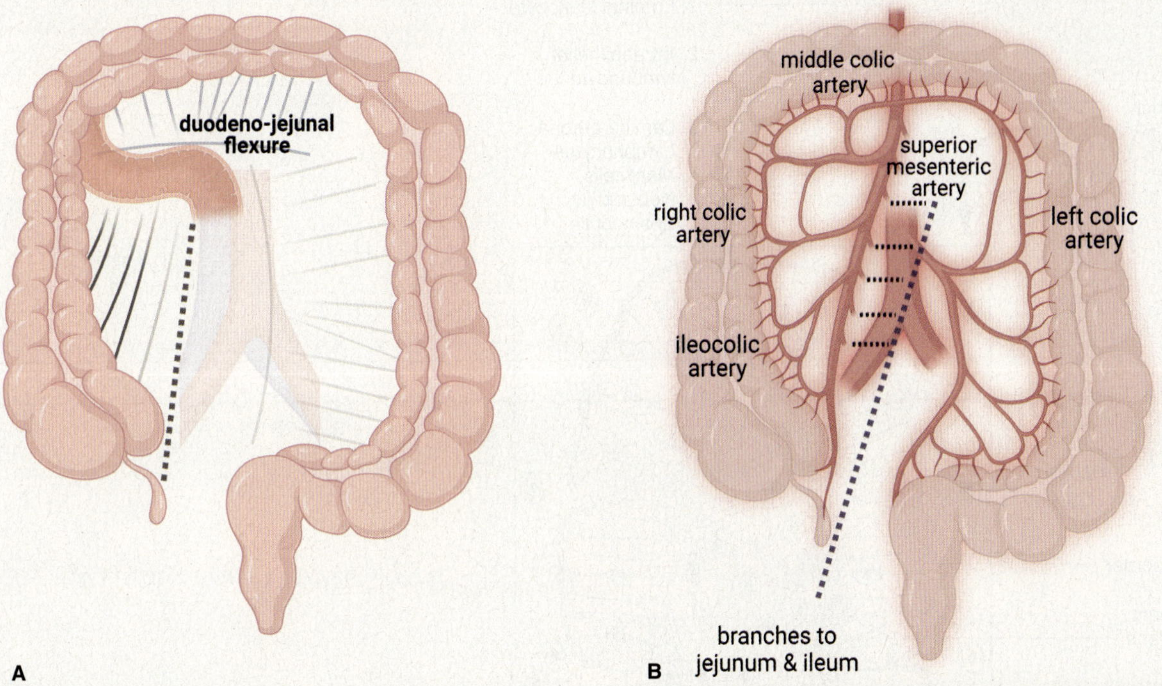

Figure 46B.3. Relationships between the root of the mesentery and the vasculature of the small and proximal large intestines. **A:** The "root" is comprised of parallel leaves covered by peritoneum traveling inferiorly to the right lower quadrant of the abdomen, from the base of the duodeno-jejunal flexure (ligament of Treitz) and encasing the vascular supply of the jejunum, ileum, and ascending colon. **B:** The superior mesenteric artery is the source of arterial blood flow to the jejunum and ileum, as well as the blood supply to the appendix and proximal two-thirds of the colon. (Created in BioRender. Soybel, D. 2024. https://BioRender.com/x43s536)

the duodenal bulb (D1) is enveloped by peritoneum, D2 is covered anteriorly by peritoneum otherwise lies behind the peritoneum. Intraoperatively, release of the lateral and posterior peritoneal attachments (Kocher maneuver) is important for access to the portal structures and in performing resections of the duodenum and pancreas.

The third (transverse) and fourth (ascending) segments complete the duodenal sweep (**Fig. 46B.1**). The third portion (D3) courses from right to left; crossing the midline anterior to the spine, aorta, and inferior vena cava; and is closely attached to the uncinate process of the pancreas. The superior mesenteric artery (SMA) and vein (SMV) course anterior to the transverse duodenum to provide blood supply to the gut. The SMA forms an acute angle as it originates from the aorta and crosses over the duodenum, marking the transition to the fourth portion. An abnormally narrow angle can result in obstruction of the duodenum. The ascending duodenum (D4) is about 5 cm in length, coursing upward and obliquely to the ligament of Treitz, which marks the end of the duodenum and the return of the small bowel to the peritoneal cavity.

2 Jejunum and Ileum

The ligament of Treitz is a fibrous remnant of skeletal muscle arising superiorly from the right crus of the diaphragm and smooth muscle arising inferiorly from the duodenum. These fibrous remnants merge with connective tissues that surround the celiac artery, creating a fibrous bundle that passes between the pancreas and the left renal vein, separating duodenum from jejunum. The anatomic boundary between jejunum and ileum is not sharp. The names "jejunum" and "ileum" date back to the 2nd-century physician Galen and his 14th-century Latin translators, and were assigned before rigorous anatomic methods were developed by Vesalius in the 16th century.[1]

Following its emergence past the ligament of Treitz, the intestine is suspended within the peritoneal cavity by a thin, broad-based mesentery attached to the posterior abdominal wall with all surfaces covered by peritoneum. In its normal position, the root of the mesentery is anchored by attachments to the retroperitoneum at the ligament of Treitz and extending inferiorly and to the right, ending at the complex of terminal ileum, cecum, and appendix (**Fig. 46B.3A**). The jejunum is wider (~25 cm) than the proximal ileum (~20 mm) and distal ileum (~19 mm), which is narrowest a few centimeters proximal to the ileocecal valve. The mucosa of the jejunum is also thicker, characterized by prominent plicae circulares that become shorter and less frequent in the ileum. The mesentery of the jejunum is often thinner and less adipose than that of the ileum. The mesentery of the terminal ileum is often broadly based, so that the superior and posterior surfaces are more retro- than intraperitoneal.

Blood Supply, Lymphatics, and Extrinsic Innervation

The duodenum shares its blood supply with the head and uncinate process of the pancreas through the superior pancreaticoduodenal arteries that originate from the GDA as it passes posterior to the first segment of the duodenum; and the inferior pancreaticoduodenal arteries, which take their source from the SMA (SMA), as it emerges in front of the fourth portion of the duodenum (**Fig. 46B.1**). Venous tributaries travel alongside the arteries: of note, there is not a gastroduodenal vein but only smaller tributaries that drain eventually to the PV. Considerable variation occurs in the branching and course of the GDA which usually travels inferiorly to the left of the common bile duct and in front of the PV. The PV is formed by the confluence of the SMV and splenic artery, enveloped on three sides by the head of the pancreas, superior to uncinate process. Awareness of variations of these structures is essential for safe management of lesions of the duodenum, the pancreas, bile ducts, and liver—whether the interventions be endoscopic, image-based, or operative.[2,3]

The arterial supply and venous drainage of the jejunum is provided by the SMA and the SMV, respectively (**Fig. 46B.3B**). The SMA branches into smaller arcades of vessels. The vasa recta, intestinal arterial branches, enter into the intestinal wall

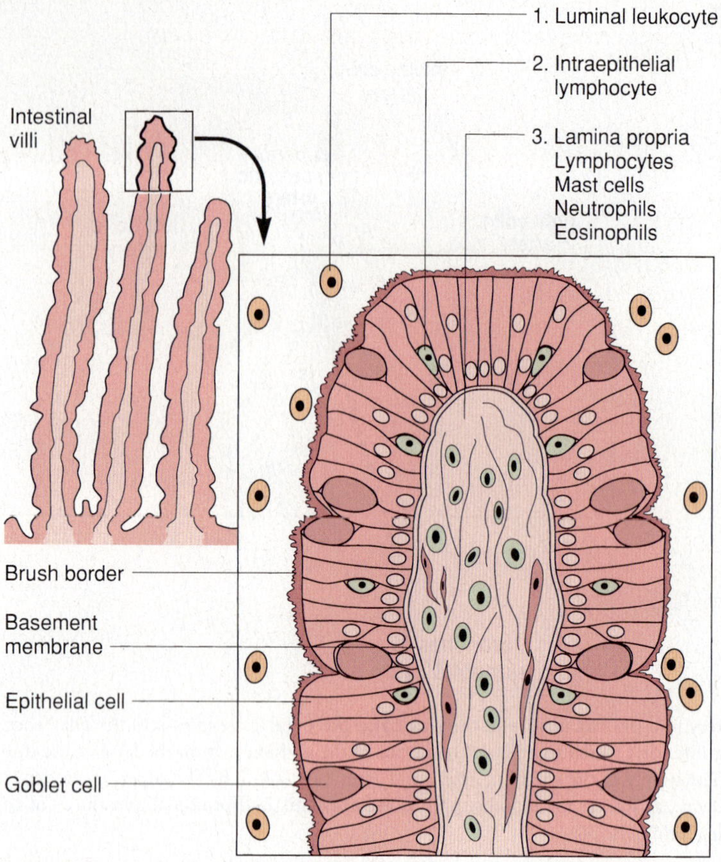

Figure 46B.4. Small intestinal villus with associated immunologic cells.

without anastomosing (**Fig. 46B.4**). The vasa recta of the jejunum are straight and long, in contrast to those of the ileum, which are shorter with greater arborization. The venous and lymphatic drainage follow the arterial supply. The main venous outflow is through the SMV. Lymphatics may be visible endoscopically in the intestinal wall or intraoperatively through the veil of the mesentery after patients have ingested fatty foods or cream (to form chylomicrons); they can also be visualized using synthesized macromolecules or nanoparticles absorbed through the mesothelial serosa.[4] Acute and chronic impediments to flow may occur in any one or all three systems—arterial, venous, or lymphatic—with consequences for viability of the intestine as well as resistance to injury and infection.

The small intestine receives afferents and sends efferent innervation through branches of the vagus nerve (parasympathetic) and the splanchnic nerves (sympathetic) that connect through the celiac ganglion and plexus located in front of the aorta and crura of the diaphragm at the level of the first lumbar vertebra, near the orifices of the celiac trunk, SMA, and renal arteries. Small nerve branches follow the paths of the arteries into the wall of the intestine. The celiac ganglion has proven useful as a target for injection of anesthetic or ablative agents to mitigate intractable visceral pain associated with upper abdominal cancers, chronic pancreatitis, and conditions such as median arcuate syndrome.[5]

Microscopic Anatomy

The wall of the small intestine is composed of four distinct layers—mucosa, submucosa, muscle, and serosa. The role of the mucosa is absorption and secretion. On the luminal mucosal surface are formed the circular folds ("plicae circulares") that are normally present in all segments of the small intestine distal to the first portion of the duodenum. The submucosa contains an elaborate network of blood vessels, lymphatics, and nerves (Meissner plexus). The muscular portion of the wall includes outer longitudinal and inner circular muscle layers. Between the muscle layers lies the myenteric (Auerbach's) plexus. The muscular layers are responsible for coordinating peristaltic movements. The outermost layer, the serosa, is composed of a thin layer of mesothelial cells overlying loose connective tissue. The serosa covers the surfaces of the small bowel and the investing mesentery, leaving dorsal surfaces that are retroperitoneal.

Mucosa

The mucosa lines the luminal surface of the small intestine (**Fig. 46B.5**). Key functions of this barrier include facilitation of nutrient absorption and beneficial associations with commensal organisms. Specialized cell types and a healthy mucus layer protect underlying cells and tissue integrity from pathogens, parasites, irritants, and toxins.[6,7]

The mucosa consists of three layers: epithelial cells, lamina propria, and a narrow layer of smooth muscle, the muscularis mucosae. The basic structural unit of the mucosa consists of villus and crypt. Villi are finger-like projections of extending into the intestinal lumen that have a columnar epithelial surface and a cellular connective tissue core of lamina propria. Each villus contains a central lacteal (lymphatic), and a vascular network consisting of a small artery, vein, and capillaries. Ninety percent of the cells of the villi are columnar epithelial cells responsible for absorption and secretion; individual enterocytes appear, die, and are replaced in as little as 5 days. Crowning the apices of the columnar cells are microvilli, that are produced by numerous folds in the apical membrane and account for the brush border appearance. Densely glycosylated proteins (mucins) are essential components of the mucus layer that forms above and around the villus tips, including glycosylated proteins rooted in the cell membrane "glycocalyx" and gel-forming mucins that are not structural but are strongly tethered together to form a mucus barrier. Other cell types located within the villus mucosa include enteroendocrine cells (EECs) and mucus-secreting goblet cells. In addition present in

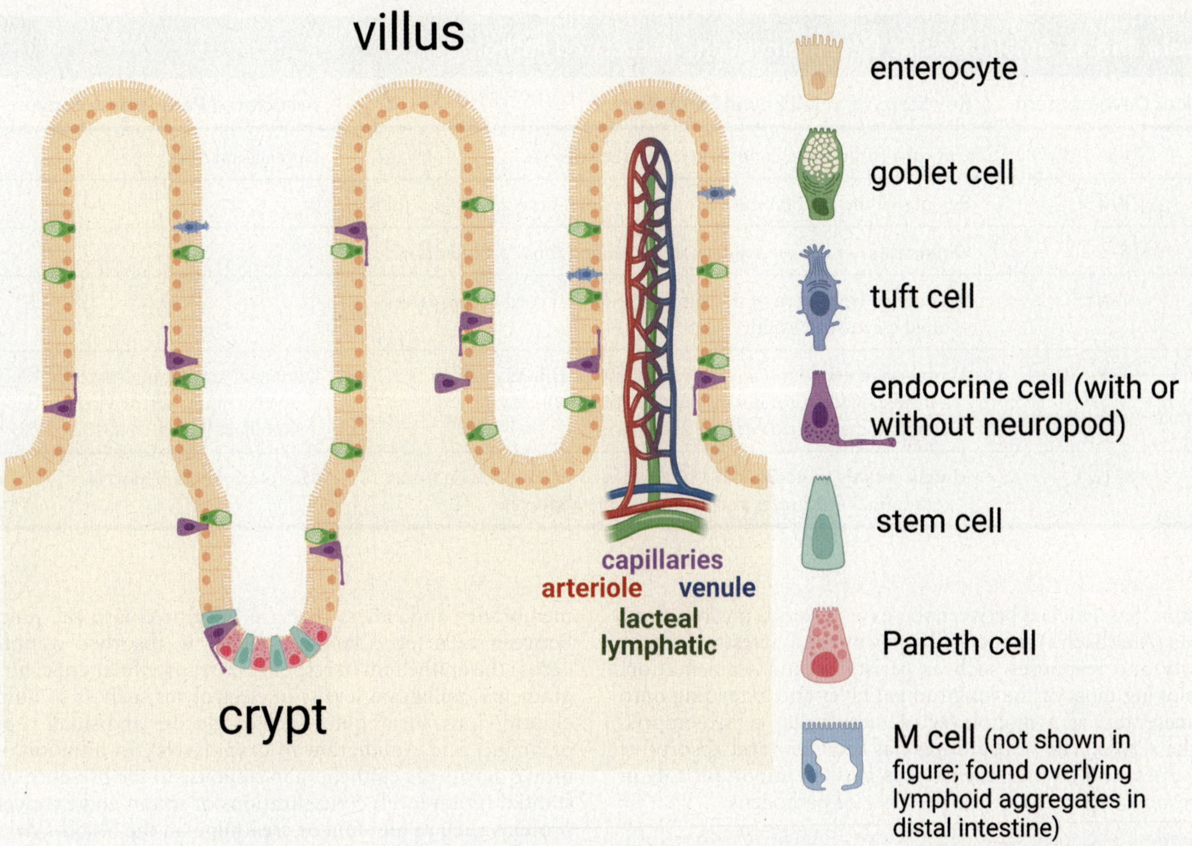

Figure 46B.5. The adult intestinal epithelium is arranged in crypt-villus units. The villus projects into the lumen, and is comprised of mostly of water and solute absorbing enterocytes, as well as enteroendocrine cells and goblet cells, as well as other cell types such as Tuft cells and M-cells (not shown). Deep in the crypts of Lieberkühn harbor (transit amplifying [TA] zones), are rapidly proliferating stem cells which differentiate into the different cell types as they ascend to the villus and ultimately undergo programmed cell death (apoptosis) and detach to become detritus. At the bases of the crypts are the Paneth cells, which (along with goblet cells, M cells, and Tuft cells) play an important role in intestinal defenses against luminal organisms and microbiota. (Created in BioRender. Soybel, D. 2024. https://BioRender.com/c15i460)

the villus is the rare "tuft" cell, characterized by an extensive intracellular tubulovesicular network and an apical bundle of microfilaments anchoring a "tuft" of microvilli projecting into the lumen.

About three-quarters of the distance from the tip of the gland to its base, the villus forest transitions to the crypts of Lieberkühn. Stem cells within the crypts of Lieberkühn are the source of the four major types of differentiated epithelial cells, including: the absorptive enterocyte, mucin-secreting goblet cells, hormone-secreting EECs, and Paneth cells. About 90% of the cells along the crypt-villus axis are enterocytes and their absorptive progenitor cells. The lateral membranes of neighboring enterocytes are connected by tight junctions, an apparent fusion of adjoining plasma membranes just below the level of the brush border. Movement of ions and water can occur by either a transmembrane or a paracellular route through tight junctions, which behave as selective pores. Goblet cells secrete gel-forming mucins, which support the lubrication and barrier functions of the mucus layer while permitting selective absorption of nutrients. EECs secrete hormones and other bioactive amines that may regulate proliferation, differentiation, and functions of adjacent or distant tissues. At the bases of the crypts are Paneth cells, which secrete antimicrobial peptides that play a key role in host microbiome interactions.[8] In addition they support the environment for maintaining a stem cell niche. As stem cells divide, they pass out of the crypt, moving along signaling gradients triggering differentiation to the mature epithelial cell types populating the crypt-villus continuum. In histologic sections, a normal relationship between the height of the villi and the depth of the crypts is between 3:1 and 5:1.

Submucosa

The submucosa is a dense connective tissue layer with a rich network of blood vessels, nerves, and lymphatics. It provides the blood flow, microenvironment of connective tissue and growth factors, and the mechanical strength[9] that supports healing after injuries or surgical procedures such as anastomosis or placement of tubes for enteral access. Worth noting is the presence of important functional structures within the submucosal layer in different regions of the intestine. In the duodenum, unique glandular structures known as Brunner glands[10] that secrete a bicarbonate-and mucin-rich mélange thought to support duodenal defenses against acidic gastric content. In the distal ileum, the submucosa also supports secondary immune-defense structures known as Peyer patches, which are localized collections of lymphoid follicles. Peyer patches are thought to play an important role in adaptive immunity to allergens, commensals, and pathogens.[11] These disparate observations suggest that harbored within the submucosa is a certain plasticity, enhancing the resilience of the mucosal layer that is exposed to a diverse set of challenges that include caustic internal secretions such as bile acids, toxins, irritants, and pathogens. In line with these observations, isolated patches of small intestine submucosa from humans and sterilized/de-immunized animal tissues have found a place in applications that promote wound healing and other forms of tissue engineering.

Muscularis Propria and Serosa

Lying exterior to the mucosa and submucosa are two layers of smooth muscle: the inner layer of muscle has a circular orientation, while the outer layer orients along the axis of the small

Table 46B.1. Small Intestine Development and Associated Pathology

Wk of Development	Key Steps in Small Bowel Formation	Associated Pathophysiology
3	Gut tube forms from endoderm lining the yolk sac	Duplication cysts
3–4	Regions of the gut become more defined as embryo grows and folds	
5–6	Obliteration of intestinal lumen due to endodermal proliferation	
7–8	Physiologic herniation of midgut into umbilical cord accompanies rapid increase in length	
7–9	Apoptosis of endoderm and growth of mesoderm recanalizes gut tube. Midgut rotates 90 degrees counterclockwise. Omphalomesenteric/vitelline duct closes	Duodenal atresia; malrotation; Meckel diverticulum, patent vitelline duct, umbilical hernia
8–12	Midgut rotates an additional 180 degrees counterclockwise (total rotation: 270 degrees) as it returns to the abdomen	Malrotation; omphalocele

intestine. Sandwiched between these two layers is the myenteric plexus (Auerbach's) that coordinates intrinsic intestinal motor activity and responses such as peristalsis and segmentation. Enveloping most of the longitudinal layer and extending onto the mesentery is a monolayer of mesothelial cells, comprising the serosa. The serosal layer has secretory and absorptive properties, and its mesothelial cells play an important role in the response to injury or the presence of pathogens.

Embryologic Considerations

The gastrointestinal (GI) tract is formed from the endodermal layer of the developing embryo. The duodenum develops from the embryologic foregut, while the embryologic midgut gives rise to the jejunum, ileum, and proximal and two-thirds of the transverse colon. In the timeline of fetal development relevant to surgically relevant pathologic anatomy, a number of milestones are prominent (**Table 46B.1**), helping to explain the appearance of congenital conditions such as duplication cysts, duodenal atresia, Meckel diverticulum, rotational abnormalities with risk of midgut volvulus, patent vitelline duct, omphalocele, and umbilical hernia. Conditions such as Meckel diverticulum and rotational abnormalities are not common, but neither are they so rare in the average abdominal surgeon's practice (see Chapter 98: Pediatric Abdomen).

Physiology: Intestinal Absorption and Secretion

The small intestine serves as the principal organ of digestion and absorption of dietary components, including water, simple electrolytes (sodium, chloride, potassium), macronutrients (carbohydrates, proteins, fat), and micronutrients (vitamins, minerals). The intestinal mucosa provides a barrier supported by diverse defense secretory functions to neutralize and flush toxins and pathogenic organisms. Coordinating absorption and secretion are humoral mechanisms and feedback loops, mediated by hormones and neurotransmitters released locally from endocrine cells and neurons embedded in the intestine, as well from distant organs. Through its specialized cells and structures of immune sensing and responses, the small intestine exercises homeostatic control over microbial communities that invested in the luminal surfaces and crevices of the villi and crypts. Increasingly appreciated is the influence of the gut and its microbiome on the functions of distant organs, including neurologic functions of the brain such as cognition, memory, and mood.[12]

Absorption: Water, Simple Electrolytes, Macronutrients, and Micronutrients

Water

Cellular mechanisms of water absorption in the GI tract include both water channels (eg, aquaporins) that are embedded in cell membranes and others that are integrated into the junctions between cells (eg, Claudins). Water is absorbed osmotically across the epithelium in response to transcellular concentration gradients (milligram-levels) of electrolytes such as sodium and chloride ions, metabolites such as glucose and small peptides, or amino acids (milligram to gram-levels). In addition, water moves across the epithelium in response to the presence of substantial (gram-level) concentrations of serum and extracellular proteins such as albumin or creatinine on the blood-side of the mucosa or synthetic solutes in the lumen such as polyethylene glycol used as laxatives or contrast agents such as amidotrizoate (gastrografin) used in radiologic imaging.

Simple Electrolytes

Physiologically relevant monovalent electrolytes include sodium (Na^+), chloride (Cl^-), potassium (K^+), and bicarbonate (HCO_3^-). Sodium ions (Na^+) are transported through channels or selective transport proteins in the apical cell membranes of the cells in the brush border of the villus. The force motivating transport is a large gradient between extracellular Na^+ (up to 140 mEq/L) and intracellular Na^+ (<10 mEq), maintained by a Na^+-K^+-ATPase that pumps Na^+ ions out of the cell in exchange for K^+ ions into the cell. The same pump maintains a much higher concentration of K^+ ions inside the cell (~90 mEq/L) as compared to extracellular or luminal concentrations (5 to 15 mEq/L). Absorption of K^+ ions from diet thus requires considerable energy if the cellular route is used and must be coupled to the transport of other ions with highly favorable gradients, such as Na^+, Cl^-, H^+, or HCO_3^-. Absorption of luminal Cl^- may be coupled to the absorption of Na^+ (symport Na^+:Cl^-) or to exchange with another anion such as bicarbonate (antiport, Cl^-:HCO_3^-). Gradients of HCO_3^- are maintained by a combination of cell-based mechanisms, including its generation from CO_2 and water, catalyzed by carbonic anhydrase. These gradients are highly influenced by H^+ ion concentrations (pH) on either side of the mucosa and within the epithelial cells themselves, conforming to the Henderson–Hasselbach relationship.

Macronutrients

Macronutrients provide large quantities of basic components (sugars, lipids, amino acids) for the body to assemble its own proteins and nucleic acids and to build and store energy sources such as complex carbohydrates and fats. To obtain macronutrients in large (gram-level) quantities the digestive process begins with mastication in the mouth and exposure to enzymes in the saliva that begin the digestion of starch into less complex carbohydrates. The process continues in the stomach with the transformation of food and liquid into a slurry known as chyme (from the Greek *khumos* meaning "juice").

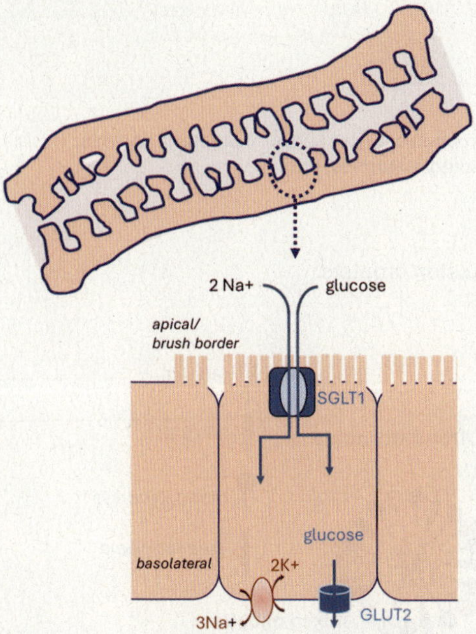

Figure 46B.6. Intestinal absorption of dietary glucose and disposition of glucose from the enterocyte. Uptake from the lumen across the apical membrane occurs predominantly through the sodium-coupled glucose transporter (SGLT1), while transport to the capillary side occurs though GLUT2, a carrier protein that facilitates diffusion across the basolateral membrane to the subepithelial spaces. Courtesy of Dr. David I. Soybel.

Continued processing of the chyme continues in the stomach with secretion of hydrochloric acid (H^+Cl^-) and trituration in the presence of acid-activated enzymes that lyse peptide bonds (pepsinogen) and complex lipids (lipases). A preliminary partitioning of the meal's contents occurs in the stomach, such that the components to enter the duodenum initially tend to be carbohydrates and peptides, followed by lipids. The density and composition of the meal influence the rate of gastric emptying across the pylorus: iso-osmolar liquids containing simple sugars and peptides move rapidly into the duodenum within minutes, while hyperosmolar and lipid-rich food slows gastric emptying to hours. What flows out (and when) through the pylorus plays a major role in determining timing, magnitude, and integration of neuroendocrine responses in the small intestine and pancreas. Macronutrient digestion, availability, and absorption are regulated by two other luminal actors: bile and fiber.

Carbohydrates. Carbohydrates provide a major source of daily caloric intake in Western diets and are present in three main digestible forms: complex plant-based starches such as amylopectin, disaccharides such as sucrose and monosaccharides. Digestion of complex starches will normally have been completed in the stomach, resulting in the formation of triglycerides which are further digested by brush border saccharidases in the jejunum. The brush border of the small bowel contains specific enzymes (amylase, sucrase, isomaltase) that hydrolyze oligo- and disaccharides into monosaccharides such as glucose, galactose, and fructose. Monosaccharides glucose and galactose are transported (**Fig. 46B.6**) across the apical (lumen-side) cell membrane via a sodium ion-dependent hexose transporter, SGLT-1, which utilizes the energy of the Na^+ gradient generated by the Na^+-K^+-ATPase located on the basolateral (serosal-side) membrane of the villus epithelial cell. In contrast, fructose is transported across the apical membrane through a carrier (GLUT5) depending on concentration gradients in a process known as facilitated diffusion. The monosaccharides are then transported across the basolateral membrane by the carrier GLUT2. This hexose transporter allows for the diffusion of all three monosaccharides into the extracellular space and ultimately into the portal blood flow. A small portion of these monosaccharides may be used by the enterocyte for its own energy needs.

Protein. Protein provides an important caloric energy source as well as the essential building blocks for production of new proteins. A nearly equal amount of protein is ingested daily from dietary sources (70 to 100 g) as is provided by endogenous proteins (50 to 60 g of protein per day) in the small intestine from secreted enzymes, desquamated cells, and plasma protein leakage. Similar processes of digestion occur for both dietary and endogenous sources of protein.

Although digestion of protein begins in the stomach, most protein digestion occurs in the small intestine by pancreatic peptidases and proteases. Pancreatic enzymes flow through the major (duct of Wirsung) and minor papillae (duct of Santorini) into the duodenum, initiating the dominant phase of protein digestion. Pancreatic proteases are initially released as proenzymes (zymogens), similar to pepsinogen in the stomach. In the presence of neutral pH and enterokinase in the brush border of the duodenal mucosa, trypsinogen is converted to trypsin which activates the other zymogens into their active endopeptidases (trypsin, chymotrypsin, and elastase). By means of these enzymes and exopeptidases such as (caroxypeptidase A and B) proteins are fully digested to short oligopeptides, di- and tripeptides, and single amino acids. Cellular uptake of these smaller molecules occurs through energy-dependent co-transport, carriers, and diffusion. Of note, the transport of di-and tripeptides occurs in conjunction with H^+ ions through a transporter PEPT-1, which is important for the absorption and bioavailability of peptide-like agents that include anticancer drugs, antihypertensives, and antibiotics.

Fat. Forty percent of the average daily caloric intake (60 to 90 g) in a Western diet is in the form of fat. Ninety percent of these ingested fats are triglycerides, while the remainder is comprised of cholesterol and phospholipids. Enzymes from the pancreas are important in the process of fat digestion, examples including lipase which breaks down triglycerides to fatty acid and monoglycerides, cholesterol esterase which hydrolyzes cholesterol ester compounds to cholesterol and free fatty acid, and phopholipase A2 which hydrolyzes phospholipids thereby generating—among other products—arachidonic acid that is a precursor to potent lipid mediators of inflammation. An additional and important component of dietary fat includes the fat-soluble vitamins including vitamin A and carotenoids, vitamin D, vitamin E, and one form of vitamin K (**Fig. 46B.7**).

Bile Salts. Bile salts mix with hydrolyzed lipids, cholesterol, and fat-soluble vitamins, forming small aggregates called micelles that associate with the cell membrane and brush border to facilitate uptake of micellar components by the intestinal villi. Diverse mechanisms of uptake are present in the brush border and apical cell membranes to handle each component. An important downstream event is that fatty acids and monoglyceride are transported into the endoplasmic reticulum, where endogenous triglyerides are formed and assembled—along with cholesterol, lipoproteins, and other lipids—into chylomicrons (**Fig. 46B.7**). Chylomicrons are transported into the central lacteal of the villus, where they pass to the larger lymphatics, thence to the bloodstream, and then distributed to metabolically active organs such as liver, kidney, heart, and muscle.

Fiber. Fiber is composed of nondigestible long and often branched polymers of carbohydrates, and in nature includes antioxidant and other biologically active compounds that nourish or protect the intestinal epithelium. These "co-passengers" include polyphenols, carotenoids, plant sterols, lignans, terpenoids, and

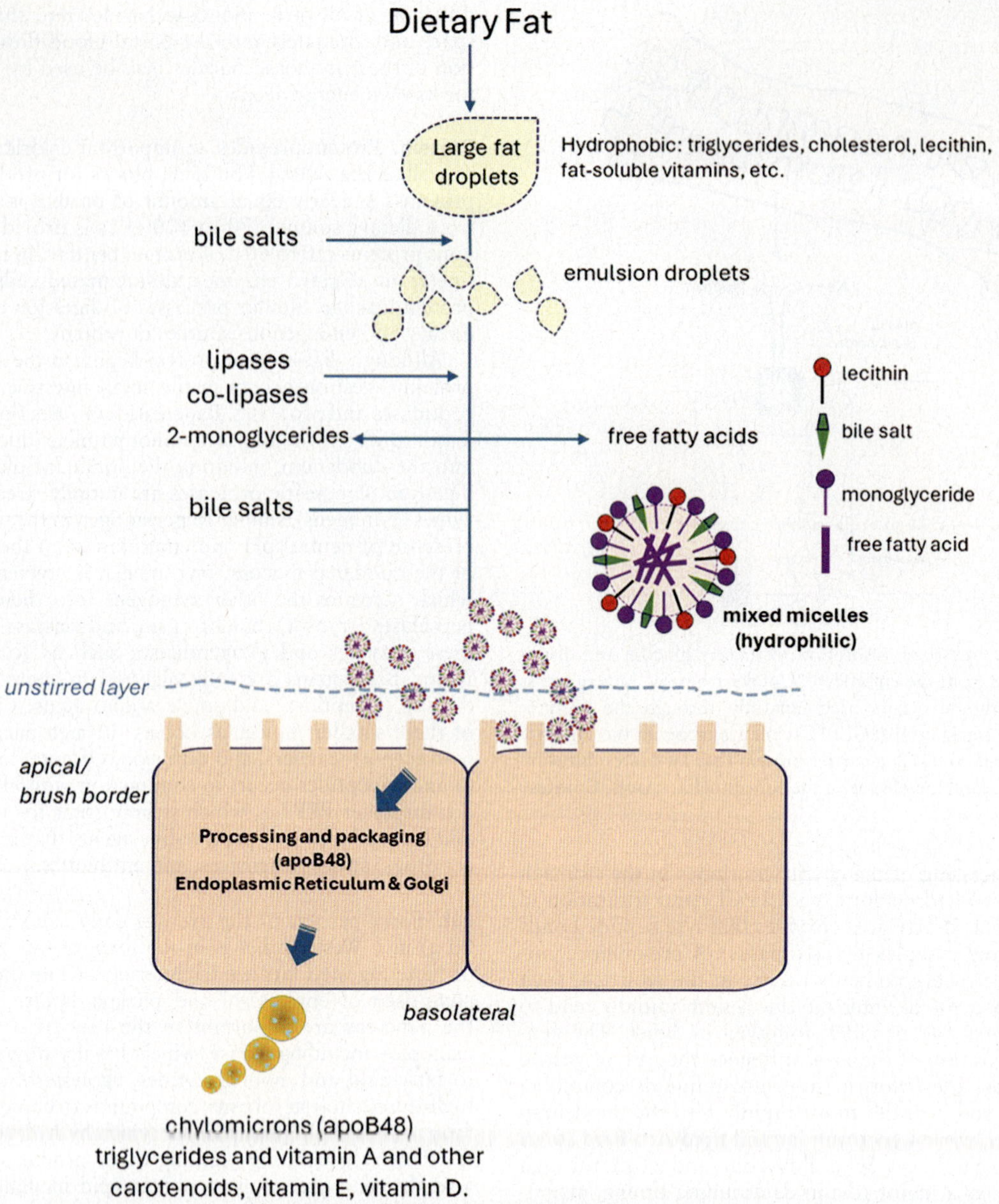

Figure 46B.7. Intestinal absorption of lipids and fat-soluble vitamins. Dietary fat includes triglycerides and other phospholipids, cholesterol, lecithin; as well the lipid component includes pro-vitamin A and other carotenoids (lycopene, lutein), pro-vitamin D, and vitamin E (tocopherols). As these components are separated by the action of different lipases, they reconvene within mixed micelles that are stable in aqueous environments, and thus capable of crossing the unstirred aqueous layer to be taken up by the enterocyte for processing, packaging, and extrusion in chylomicrons that travel in the lymph to the circulation and eventually to the liver. Courtesy of Dr. David I. Soybel.

sulfated polysaccharides. Fiber plays a significant role modulating intestinal motility, the enteroendocrine response to chyme, and "probiotic" properties of the microbiome in the distal small intestine and the colon. Fiber can be classified as "soluble," referring to dispersal in water to become a soluble gel; and "insoluble" referring to capacity to absorb water but maintain structure. In general, soluble forms are more fully fermented than insoluble forms and are considered more influential on body metabolism; in contrast, insoluble fiber is linked to coordination of motor activity throughout the alimentary tract. For the average adult taking in 2,000 calories per day, the recommended intake includes 25 g of fiber.[13]

Micronutrients

Micronutrients serve as cofactors in the processes that maintain molecular structures and energy stores, promote growth and homeostasis, and support immune function and tissue repair (**Table 46B.2**). In the micronutrient category are included minerals, metals, and inorganic compounds such as ionized magnesium (Mg^{2+}), calcium (Ca^{2+}), Iron ($Fe^{2+/3+}$), and phosphate (PO_4^{3-}); "trace" elements such as copper (Cu^{2+}), zinc (Zn^{2+}), iodide (I^-), and fluoride (F^-); and "ultra-trace" elements such as molybdenum (Mo), boron (B), nickel (Ni), and arsenic (As) which are often found in multivalent associations with complex organic compounds. Minerals and trace metals are absorbed preferentially in the duodenum and proximal intestine and luminal conditions in the upper intestine are important in optimizing their bioavailability and absorption by the small intestine. This is especially true for gastric acid (HCl), which enters the duodenum with chyme and is not neutralized immediately by duodenal and pancreatic sources of bicarbonate (HCO_3^-). Acidic gastric juice is present long enough in the duodenum to facilitate absorption of polyvalent cations such Ca^{2+} and Zn^{2+}. Gastric acid also plays an important role in duodenal absorption of heme-bound iron, which requires an acid environment for conversion from its nonabsorbable ferric (Fe^{3+}) form to its ferrous (Fe^{2+}) form. For Fe^{3+} that is bound to nonheme proteins, reduction to Fe^{2+} utilizes ascorbic acid

Table 46B.2A. Small Intestine Absorption of Minerals (Cations/Cation Complexes)[a]

Mineral	Recommended Adult Daily Intake (Male/Female)[a]	Dietary Sources	Site(s) of Absorption	Unique Functions/Sites of Action
Magnesium	350 mg/265 mg	Nuts, seeds, legumes, leafy greens, whole grains	Jejunum/ileum	Bone, protein, muscle, excitable membranes, ATP
Calcium	800/800–1000 mg	Milk, dairy, leafy greens, fortified soy and flour	Duodenum	Bone, teeth, muscle, excitable membranes, signal transduction
Iron	6 mg/5 mg–8 mg	Red meat, fish, poultry, shellfish, egg, legumes	Duodenum/proximal jejunum	Hemoglobin, mitochondria, oxidative stress, and scavenging
Zinc	9.4 mg/6.8 mg	Meat, nuts, shellfish	Duodenum/proximal jejunum	Enzymes, genetic material structure, stability of secretory granules, wound healing
Copper	700 mg/700 mg	Vegetables, grains, legumes, meat, fish, poultry	Stomach/duodenum/jejunum	Enzyme structure and cofactor
Manganese	2.3 mg/1.6 mg	Grains, dried fruit, vegetables	Small intestine	Enzyme structure and cofactor
Selenium	55 mcg/55 mcg	Shellfish, kidney, liver	Small intestine	Enzyme structure and cofactor; folate synthesis
Chromium	30–35 mcg/20–25 mcg	Grains, cereals, vegetables, fruits	Small intestine	Cofactor with insulin to regulate glucose homeostasis
Molybdenum	45 mcg/45 mcg	Legumes, cereal grains, leafy vegetables, beef liver	Small intestine	Enzyme structure and cofactor
Cobalt	ultra-trace element (unclear RDA)	Milk, dairy, fish, shellfish	Small intestine	Vitamin B12 cofactor; production of RBCs

[a]Data taken from Byrd-Bredbenner C, Moe G, Berning J, Kelley D, (Eds.). *Wordlaw's Perspectives in Nutrition*. McGraw Hill Education; 2019. Appendix J.

(vitamin C) which is then restored from its oxidized state after absorption in the small intestine and a complex recycling pathway through the stomach and also requiring gastric acidity. Pharmacologic inhibition of gastric acid secretion, through histamine receptor type-2 (H_2) or proton pump inhibitors (PPIs) are known to cause disturbances in intestinal absorption of minerals such as Ca^{2+}, Zn^{2+}, and $Fe^{3+/2+}$ as well as vitamin B12. Similar consequences were well recognized historically following operations that remove or disable the acid-secreting portion of the stomach; and they are recognized following bariatric procedures when the gastric body and fundus are excluded from the digestive pathway, in some cases differently in different populations.[14]

Also included in the micronutrient category are organic compounds: the vitamins. Vitamins are subdivided into those that are water soluble and fat soluble. Water soluble include the B-vitamins and ascorbate (vitamin C), which are absorbed preferentially in the upper intestine. The case of vitamin B12 (cyanocobalamin) is complicated.[15] Cyanocobalamin is present in animal foods (liver, fish, shellfish, dairy products) but absent in plants or unfortified plant-based foodstuffs. As the process of digestion begins to break down these food sources,

Table 46B.2B. Small Intestine Absorption of Minerals (Anion/Anion Complexes)

Mineral	Recommended Adult Daily Intake (Male/Female)[a]	Dietary Sources	Site(s) of Absorption	Unique Functions/Sites of Action
Sulfur	2–3 g (with amino acids)	Meats, poultry, fish, eggs, milk, legumes, leafy green vegetables, nuts, beer, wine, coffee	Jejunum	Enriched proteins (cysteine, methionine)
Phosphorus	580 mg/580 mg	Meats, fish, poultry, eggs, milk, nuts, seeds, legumes, grains, processed foods (soda)	Jejunum	Bone and teeth health; acid–base balance; energy (ATP)
Iodine/Iodide	95 mcg/95 mcg	Seafood, vegetables, fortified water, and salt	Stomach/proximal intestine	Thyroid hormone
Fluoride	4 mg/3 mg	Seafood, fortified toothpaste, and water	Stomach/small intestine	

[a]Data taken from Byrd-Bredbenner C, Moe G, Berning J, Kelley D, (Eds.). *Wordlaw's Perspectives in Nutrition*. McGraw Hill Education; 2019. Appendix J.

Table 46B.2C. Small Intestine Absorption of Water-Soluble Vitamins

Water-Soluble Vitamin	Recommended Adult Daily Intake (Male/Female)[a]	Dietary Source	Route of Absorption	Resultant Deficiency Recognized in
Vitamin C	90 mg/75 mg	Citrus; tomato; cantaloupe, strawberry	Carrier-mediated Na dependent	Scurvy
Vitamin B7 (Biotin)	30 mg/30 mg	Liver, egg yolks, soybeans, milk, meat	Carrier-mediated Na dependent	Seborrheic dermatitis, alopecia, myalgia, paresthesia
Vitamin B12 (Cobalamin)	2.4 mcg/2.4 mcg	Meats, fish, poultry, and eggs	Sequential chaperones and ileal absorption	Megaloblastic anemia (also due to lack of gastric intrinsic factor [IF] deficiency in atrophic gastritis)
Vitamin B9 (Folic Acid)	400 mg/400 mg	Vegetables, liver, oranges, cantaloupes, fortified breads	Specific folate carriers once unconjugated	Neural tube defects/Spinal bifida; megalobastic anemia (alone or in conjunction with B12 deficiency)
Vitamin B3 (Niacin)	16 mg/14 mg	Milk, eggs, meat, fish, whole grains	Specific carrier	Pellagra (skin inflammation, diarrhea, cognitive dysfunction)
Vitamin B6 (Pyridoxal-5´-phosphate)	1.7 mg/1.5 mg	Meats, fish, potatoes, fruits, gut bacteria	Dephosporylation (intestinal alkaline phosphatase) and passive absorption	Irritability, depression, dermatitis, glossitis, cheilosis, peripheral neuritis, microcytic
Vitamin B2 (Riboflavin)	1.3 mg/1.1 mg	Dairy, eggs, meats, green leafy vegetables	Riboflavin transporters	Glossitis, corneal vascularization, and poor growth
Vitamin B1 (Thiamine)	1.2 mg/1.1 mg	Whole grains, nuts, dried legumes	Thiamine transporters	Megaloblastic anemia, encephalopathy

[a]Data taken from Byrd-Bredbenner C, Moe G, Berning J, Kelley D, (Eds.). *Wordlaw's Perspectives in Nutrition*. McGraw Hill Education; 2019. Appendix J.

two binding proteins become important in protecting B12 from hostile chemical conditions and microbial consumption: haptocorrin (also known as R-protein), a glycoprotein secreted by the salivary glands; and intrinsic factor (IF), also a glycoprotein produced by parietal cell subpopulations in the stomach, and secreted concurrently with the activation of secretion of hydrochloric acid (HCl). Orally ingested B12 becomes bound to haptocorrin that shields B12 from the acidic environment of the stomach. Downstream, the haptocorrin-cynocobalamin complex is broken down by pancreatic enzymes, releasing cobalamin in the pH-alkaline environment of the duodenum and now frees to bind with IF, a secretory product of the gastric parietal cells. Protected from intestinal microorganism, the IF-B12 complex is taken up through a process of receptor-mediated endocytosis. Cellular processing in lysosomes releases B12, which is then transported across the basolateral membrane, to the bloodstream where it binds to transcobalamin and eventually to store in the liver. Of interest, some of this stored B12 is released in bile and participates in the enterohepatic circulation.

Fat-soluble vitamins include vitamin A as well as other carotenoids, vitamin E (tocopherols), and vitamin D precursors (cholecalciferols) which are absorbed with other components of dietary fat throughout the jejunum and ileum. Also in the fat-soluble class is vitamin K, which has two forms: vitamin K1 (phylloquinone) which is found in green leafy vegetables and vitamin K2 (menaquinone), which is sourced from the fat fraction of dairy products. Both K1 and K2 forms may be absorbed by jejunum and ileum.[16] In the distal intestine, luminal conditions are equally important in optimizing

Table 46B.2D. Small Intestine Absorption of Fat-Soluble Vitamins

Fat-Soluble Vitamins	Route of Absorption	Daily Intake[a]	Dietary Source	Result of Deficiency
Vitamin A	Small intestine micelles	3000 IU	Meat, cheese, milk, fruit, vegetable	Night blindness (early), blindness (late), keratinization, infection, impaired wound healing
Vitamin D	Small intestine micelles	600–800 IU	UVB	Fatigue, depression, rickets (childhood), osteomalacia (adults)
Vitamin E	Ileum (micelles and localized transporters)	15 mg	Sunflower oil, nuts	Peripheral neuropathy, immunodeficiency, weakness, impaired vision
Vitamin K	Small intestine micelles	100–120 μg	Coagulation, bone formation	Bleeding diathesis (factors II, VII, IX, X)

[a]Data taken from Byrd-Bredbenner C, Moe G, Berning J, Kelley D, (Eds.). *Wordlaw's Perspectives in Nutrition*. McGraw Hill Education; 2019. Appendix J.

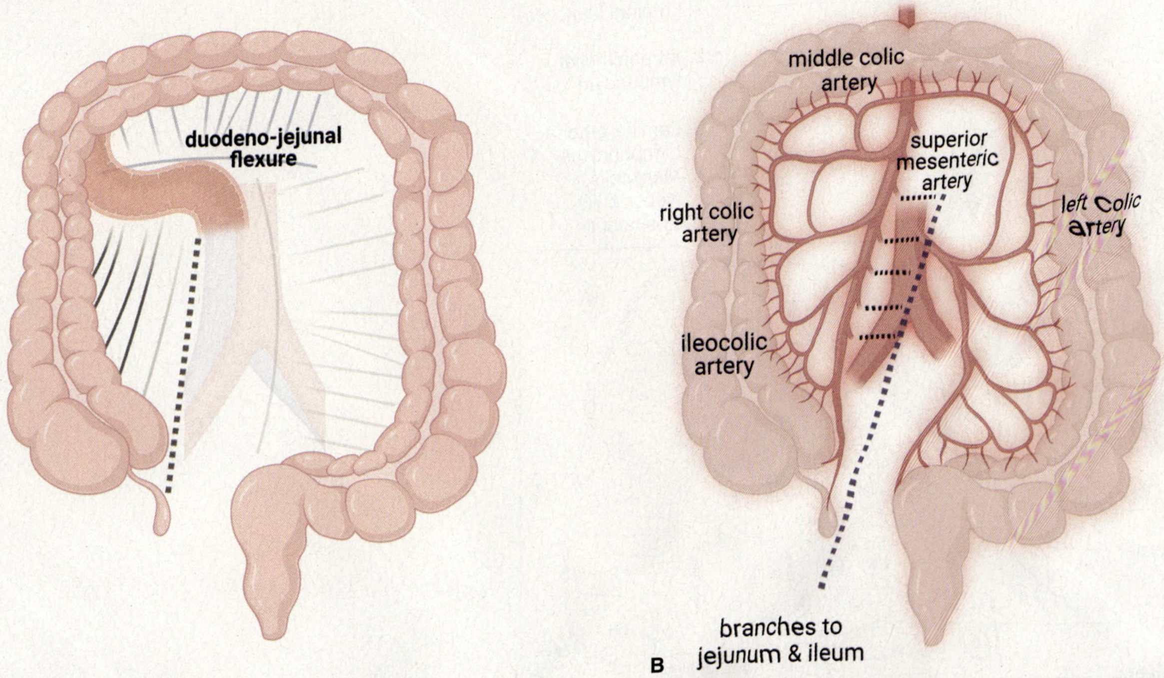

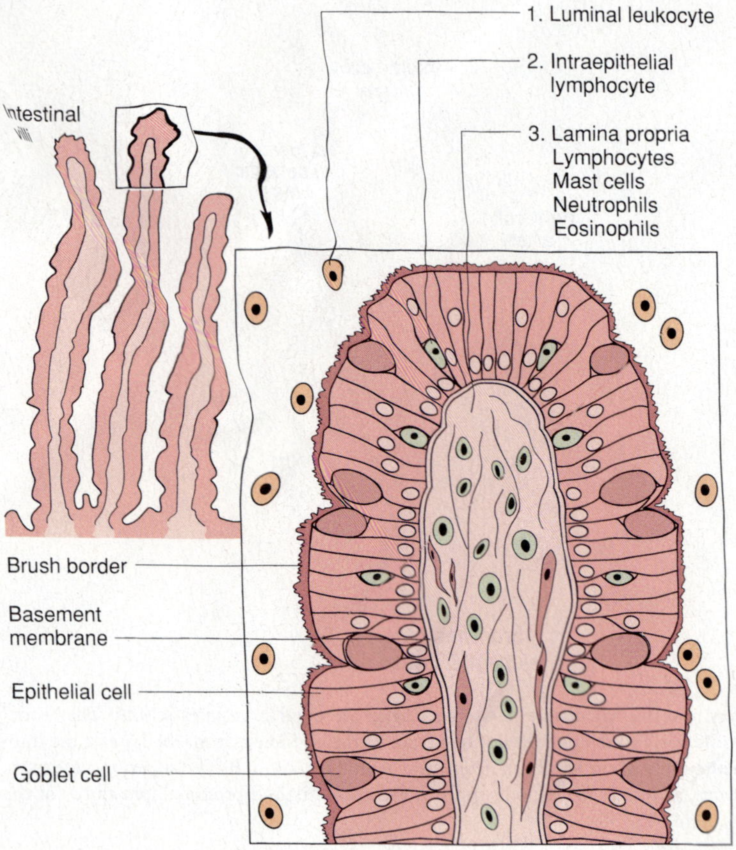

bioavailability and absorption of the fat-soluble vitamins as well as vitamin B12. Micelles formed from the aggregation of bile salts, cholesterol, and other lipids carry vitamins A, E, D (as well as vitamin K forms) to the brush border of the intestinal epithelial cells where they are absorbed by diverse molecular mechanisms. Extended loss of luminal bile salts, for example in obstructive jaundice or external biliary diversion, can result in depletion of any of these vitamins. As discussed below, microbial communities normally present at the mucosal surface themselves acquire, metabolize, and alter the availability of almost any energy source, protein, or micronutrient. In pathologic circumstances, systemic micronutrient disturbances have been described as the result of bacterial overgrowth in nonsurgical and postsurgical circumstances. Such deficiencies may include vitamin B12, folate, and the fat-soluble vitamins such as vitamin K with clinical consequences such as anemia, coagulation disturbance, decreased bone density and osteoporosis, neuropathy, and coagulopathy.[17]

Table 46B.3. Average Daily Intestinal Secretions

Anatomic Source	Intraluminal Secretion (mL)	Fluid Reabsorption (mL)
Oral intake	2000	—
Oropharyngeal	1500	—
Stomach	5000	—
Liver	1000	—
Pancreas	1000	—
Small intestine	2000	8000
Large intestine	200	1250

Secretion of Water, Electrolytes, and Specialized Constituents

As summarized in **Table 46B.3**, each segment of the GI tract secretes fluids of varying composition. It may seem paradoxical that an organ charged with absorption of 8 L of fluid each day should also have need of actively secreting 2 L of fluid. Such secretions are responses to three functional concerns. The first is to provide controlled hydration and osmolarity for specialized electrolyte secretions coming from goblet cells that secrete mucus and secretions from deeper in the mucosa, such as the bicarbonate and protein-rich secretions of submucosal Brunner glands in the duodenum[18] and proteinaceous and cytokine-rich secretions of Paneth cells at the bases of the crypts in the mucosa of the jejunum and ileum. The second is to provide lubrication and a controlled electrolyte content to the mucus layer, providing protection against abrasive and sheer forces as chyme and undigested content such as fiber come into contact during peristalsis and segmentation. The third is to provide for rapid detachment and flushing of pathogens.

The principal driver for water and electrolyte secretion involves Cl^- transport by secretory cells at the bases of the intestinal crypts (**Fig. 46B.8**). The secretory mechanism involves uptake of Cl^- ions across the basolateral membrane through energy-dependent uptake of 2 Cl-ions (coupled with single Na^+ and K^+ ions) across the basolateral membrane. Secretion occurs through a channel in the apical membrane, CFTR (cystic fibrosis transmembrane regulator), which propels Cl-ions into the lumen in response to favorable chemical and electrical gradients. Sodium (Na^+) ions and water accompany Cl^- secretions passively, through paracellular pathways and tight junctions, maintaining electroneutrality and osmotic equilibrium. This is a cellular-level mechanism by which diseases caused by bacteria such as *Vibrio cholera* and enterotoxigenic *Escherichia coli*, through their toxins, elicit profound diarrhea, and states of electrolyte disturbance.

As noted above specialized constituents of intestinal secretion come from sources such as Brunner glands, Goblet cells, and Paneth cells. Each of these cell types can be recognized

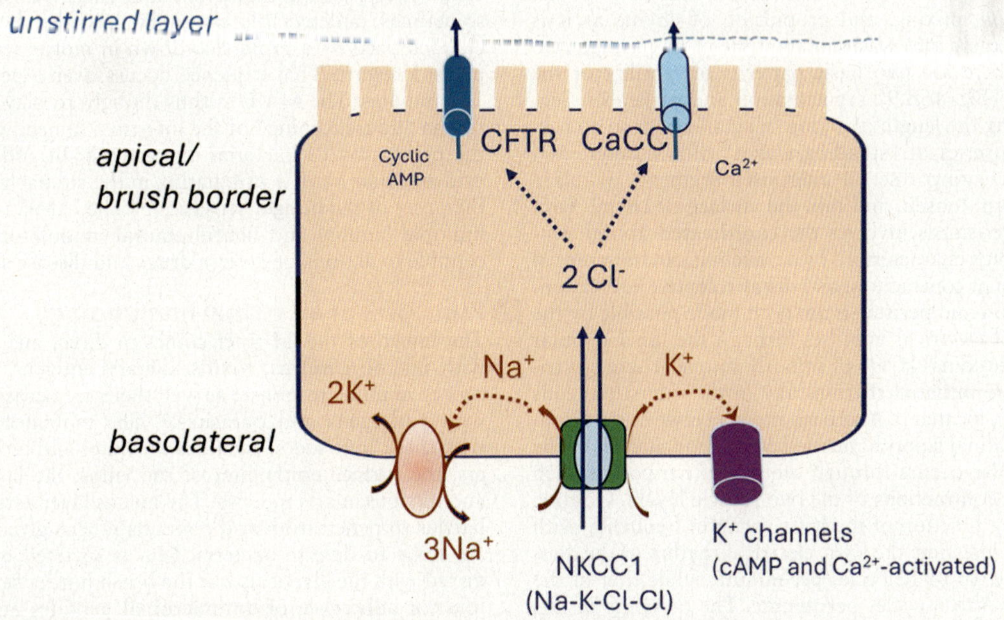

Figure 46B.8. Cellular level control of anion (chloride) secretion in crypts and submucosal glands of the small intestine. Secretion of chloride drives responses to intestinal pathogens and toxins and is accomplished at the apical membrane through both cAMP-activated channels (CFTR, cystic fibrosis transmembrane regulator) and Ca^{2+}-activated calcium channels (CaCCs). Not shown are movements of sodium ions, which pass through intercellular junctions; and those of water molecules, which pass through both intercellular junctions and possibly water channels in the apical membrane (aquaporins). (From Keely SJ, Barrett KE. Intestinal secretory mechanisms and diarrhea. *Am J Physiol Gastrointest Liver Physiol.* 2022;322(4):G405–G420. Figure 1.)

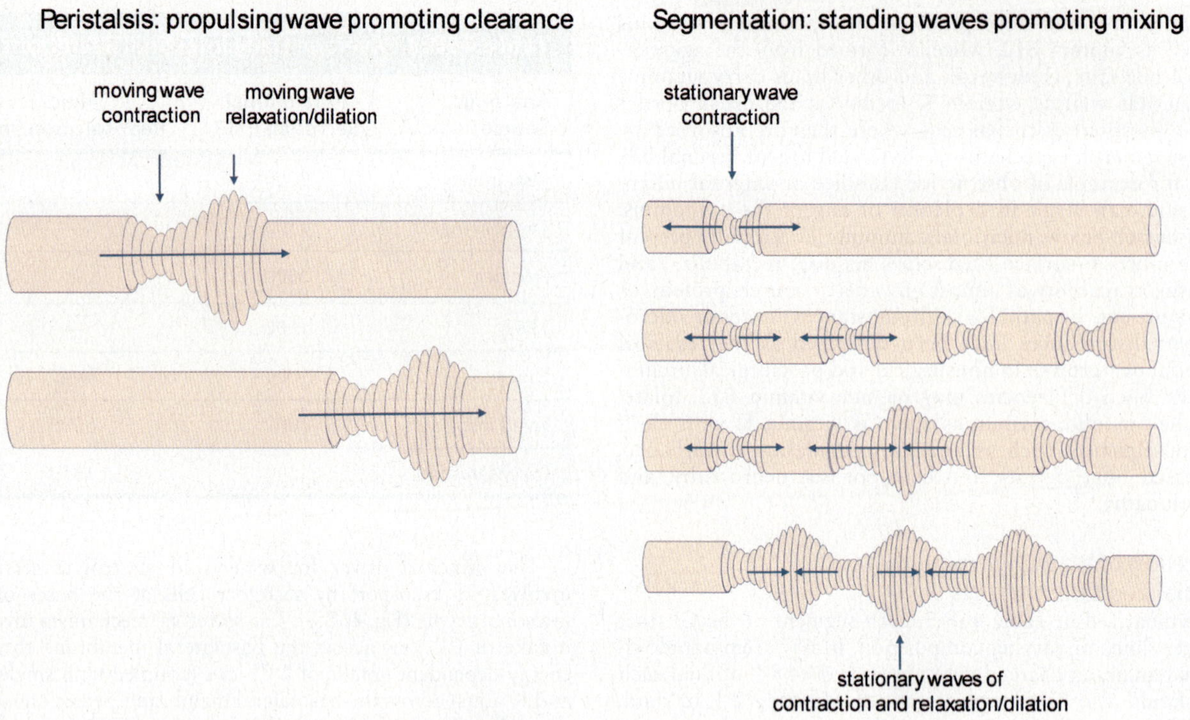

Figure 46B.9. Schematic illustration of the two basic patterns of motility of the small intestine. Peristalsis is a migrating wave of propulsion, which also creates a wake of negative pressure that pulls liquid *succus* in addition to pushing forward solid matter. Segmentation permits mixing of intestinal content with the mucosal surface, thereby enhancing absorption of nutrients and clearing debris from the mucosal surface. Courtesy of Dr. David I. Soybel.

by defining anatomic and unique secretions. In their unique locations within the mucosa, each demonstrate capacities for nourishing adjacent cells through luminal contact and communication, and promoting mucosal defenses against luminal irritants, toxins, and pathogens. These considerations underscore the energy-dependence of intestinal fluid and electrolyte transport, and other defense mechanisms.

3 Physiology: Motility of the Small Intestine

Coordinated movements of the GI tract are necessary for the proper digestion, mixing, and propulsion of chyme as it is transformed largely into waste by the time of its passage into the colon.[19] There are two basic patterns of motility of the small intestine (**Fig. 46B.9**): segmentation and peristalsis. Segmentation along the length of a loop of small intestine is characterized by a series of "standing waves" of circumferential contractions, creating a set of interposed segments of relaxation that churn, loosen, and mix the surface of chyme with the mucosa. Peristalsis involves the coordinated aboral propulsion of a bolus characterized by a traveling, circumferential wave of proximal contraction, and distal receptive relaxation.

Segmentation and peristalsis are both made possible by the transmission of electrical impulses through the inner circular and outer longitudinal layers of smooth muscle. These electrical impulses are initiated rhythmically in the interstitial cells of Cajal (ICCs), located in Auerbach plexus between the circular and longitudinal smooth muscle layers. Propagation of the electrical impulse occurs through the neural network, which coordinate the contractions of the two muscle layers. Of note, the pacemaking function of the ICCs varies in frequency with location in the intestine: the basic electrical rhythm of the duodenum is about 10 to 12 cycles per minute, while that of the ileum is about 4 to 6 cycles per minute. The outcome of this gradient, for both patterns of digestive activity, is more active churning and mixing of chyme in the proximal intestine, with a general propulsion of the luminal contents in the direction of the ileocecal valve.

Between cycles of feeding and digestion, the intestine in the fasting state goes through a cyclic motility pattern known as the migrating motor complex (MMC). The MMC is initiated in the stomach and proximal intestine and has three well-described phases: phase I is a period of relative quiescence; phase II is a period of accelerated irregular electrical spiking and muscular activity; phase III is a series of high-amplitude rapid electrical spikes corresponding to rhythmic gut contractions. Phase III contractions propagate along the length of the stomach and small intestine, and are thought to sweep clean the intestine of debris left over from digestion, dead cells, loosened mucus, and nonadherent microorganisms. A short and sometimes undetectable phase IV has also been described, characterized by a rapid slowdown in motor activity prior to phase I restart. This sequence occurs over a period of 90 to 120 minutes. The MMC is thus thought to play an important role in "housekeeping" of the intestinal lumen, which includes the prevention of bacterial overgrowth. In addition, there is evidence that MMCs originating in the stomach play a role in the onset of the hunger sensation.[20] The MMC is regulated by multiple luminal and neurohumoral modulators, and is susceptible to actions of diverse drugs and disease states.[20]

4 Principles of Intestinal Immunology

The lumen of the GI tract comes in direct and daily contact with microorganisms, toxins, dietary antigens, and modulators of immune response; as well there are occasional contacts with pathogens and parasites.[21] The immunologic interface with these "outsiders" includes the outer and inner mucus layers, the surface epithelium of the villus, the lamina propria, and the muscularis mucosa. The mucus layer acts as a physical barrier to penetration and contains mucus glycoproteins that are toxic to diverse bacteria. Mucus secreted by goblet cells mixed with the glycocalyx at the brush border serves as a scaffold for adherence of antimicrobial peptides and antibodies. At the tips of the villi, a deeper physical barrier is made up of the surface epithelial cells and other intercalated specialized cell types: EECs, goblet cells, and tuft cells—all connected by tight junctions and collectively serving as a physical barrier to penetration. The surface epithelial cells of the gut mucosa have developed features that make the intestinal epithelium an active immunologic as well as anatomic barrier. For example, these nonclassical immune cells express major histocompatibility complex (MHC) class I and II molecules, consistent with their ability to participate in adaptive immune recognition of pathogenic bacteria. Intestinal epithelial cells also express toll-like receptors (TLRs) on their apical surface that enables them to detect bacterial products and to initiate an innate immune response.

At the base of the intestinal crypts are Paneth cells, which are terminally differentiated, strikingly long-lived in comparison to their surface epithelial cousins, and morphologically distinguished by their apically situated zinc-rich secretory granules. Paneth cells play a critical role in regulating the ecology of the intestinal lumen through release of large secretory granules that contain antimicrobial proteins (eg, α-defensin, lysozyme, and Reg-IIIγ). They also release cytokines such as interleukins, tumor necrosis factor, and regenerating islet-derived protein IIIγ (REGIIIγ) in response to danger signals such as TLRs and other proinflammation cytokines. Lastly, Paneth cells secrete growth factors crucial for normal functioning of the stem cells responsible for replenishing cell populations of the crypts and the villus. In experimental studies, depletion of Paneth cell populations is also associated with microbial dysbiosis and exacerbation of acute and chronic inflammation states such as Crohn disease, suggesting an important role in initial, innate immunologic response to pathogenic microorganisms.[8,22]

The epithelial layer also harbors resident and migrant T-lymphocytes, also called intraepithelial lymphocytes (IELs). IELs have the capability of performing innate immune effector functions such as production of cytokines and clonally expanding in response to antigens encountered previously. Together the epithelium and their immune cell companions play a major role in the ability to distinguish between benign and danger signals.[23] Underneath the surface epithelium, in the lamina propria, are nonaggregated, diffusely distributed and different types of immune cells. B cells in the lamina propria undergo cytokine-induced differentiation to become active producers of immunoglobulin A (IgA) that is secreted into the gut lumen. Mast cells and eosinophils are also present in the lamina propria in small numbers. They exhibit an important role in allergic and hypersensitivity reactions as well as defense against parasites. Parasites, including worms, are initially recognized by the Tuft cells which have chemosensory capabilities—"taste" receptors—that initiate a response leading to tagging with immunoglobulin E (IgE) and killing by toxic proteins secreted by eosinophils.[24]

Within the submucosa of the ileum are aggregates of lymphoid tissue, Peyer patches. Out of Peyer patches, the nonaggregated lymphoid tissue of the lamina propria, and other specialized cells of immune response such as dendritic cells, is formed an immune-response network known as Mucosa-Associated Lymphoid Tissue (MALT) or Gut-Associated Lymphoid Tissue (GALT). The network is important in the processing of antigens presented by ingested food, toxins, and microorganisms. Such antigens are detected and processed for presentation by dendritic cells that push pseudopods up between epithelial cells without disrupting intercellular junctions. In addition, antigens are processed by the so-called microfold (M) cells, which overlie the lymphoid follicles and are capable of antigen endocytosis, with subsequent transport into the underlying tissue and uptake by local dendritic cells and macrophages. Dendritic cells and macrophages that receive antigens from M cells present them to T cells in the GALT, leading ultimately to appearance of IgA-secreting plasma cells in the mucosa. B-lymphocyte precursors proliferate in germinal centers within the Peyer patches. About 70% of the body's lymph cells are located in the intestine and its mesenteric lymph nodes, reflecting the enormous burden of distinguishing between the benign and nourishing components of food and fiber and the danger signals associated with pathogens and parasites in the gut lumen.

The Intestinal Microbiome

The term "microbiome" seems to have originated in 2001 with the Nobel laureate Joshua Lederberg, to signify *"the ecological community of commensal, symbiotic, and pathogenic microorganisms that literally share our body space and have been all but ignored as determinants of health and disease."*[25] With respect to the evolving understanding of this community and its connections to human health and disease, several foundational concepts have emerged. The first is that the food humans eat influences the kinds of bacteria that are found in the intestines and throughout the body. Conversely, the microbiome profile of the human modulates the absorption of energy sources and influences the host's metabolic pathways and machinery that metabolizes these sources. Such influences are connected: first, to direct influences of bacteria on breakdown of complex carbohydrates, proteins, and lipids as well as the bioavailability of their simple subunits when released by digestion; second, to physiologic modulation of motor and endocrine responses that drive motility and regulate cellular nutrient transport of small sugars, peptides and lipids[26]; and, third, to modifications of endogenously released bile acids, especially in the colon, that exert profound metabolic effects directly on metabolic activities of the intestinal epithelium and indirectly after passage into the portal system on the liver and other more distant tissues.[27] In addition, much influence is connected to the inflammatory response to shifts in microbial species that occur with diets rich in processed foods. Thus, the microbial profile of the intestine is seen as a marker and driver of metabolic disease, including complications of obesity that include diabetes, fatty infiltration of the liver and steatohepatitis,[28] as well as inflammation-associated conditions affecting diverse organs such as heart and brain.[12,29]

A second concept is that by assisting in the breakdown and fermentation of chyme's components, the bacteria of the intestine are instrumental in the synthesis, release, and bioavailability of micronutrients and nutrients that maintain gut health. This includes vitamin B12 and vitamin K where bacteria play a direct role in metabolizing plant sources of precursor compounds. In addition, microbes are critical in the formation of short-chain fatty acids (SCFAs) from fiber that in turn are important energy sources for the surface epithelium of the colon. Recent studies,[30] however, have also underscored the role of bacterial enzymes, phytases, that release mineral micronutrients ($Fe^{2+/3+}$, Ca^{2+}, Mg^{2+}, Zn^{2+}) as well as phosphate. Also increasingly appreciated is the role that intestinal microorganisms may play in the synthesis and release for mucosal absorption of other B-vitamins (thiamine, biotin, folate, niacin, panthothenic acid, pyridoxine, riboflavin, etc.). It is difficult to determine, under stable conditions, to what extent bacterial metabolism contributes to bioavailability of any one micronutrient. It is increasingly clear, however, that pathologic states can drive new imbalances or exacerbate preexisting imbalances in the body's stores of micronutrients, especially when coupled to underlying genetic variation in the ways such micronutrients are taken in and metabolized.[30]

A third concept is the importance of the intestinal microbiome on the immune health of different regions of the gut and immune protection of the human organism generally. The oral cavity has an abundant microbiota, made up of over 770 bacterial species distributed in specialized habitats of the mouth and oropharynx.[31] The upper GI tract has much fewer microorganisms due to the rapid flow of food content and the acidic pH of the stomach, as well as the secretory properties of the stomach and duodenum. The number of bacteria in the free lumen of a healthy stomach is quite low, perhaps as low as 10 CFU/mL; although the microbial profiles in these regions can be radically altered by conditions or drugs that impair secretion of acid. Descending in the alimentary canal, the number of resident microorganisms gradually increases and their profile changes. In the duodenum and jejunum, there are about 10^3 to 10^4 organisms per mL, dominated by *Bacteroides,*

Lactobacillus, and *Streptococcus* species. In the ileum, the number reaches as much as 10^8 per mL of luminal content, dominated by species of the genera *Bacteroides, Clostridium, Enterococcus, Lactobacillus,* and *Veilonella*, as well as those of the order Enterobacterales. The slower passage of food content in the large intestine favors the establishment of semistable communities of microorganisms. Their number is perhaps 10^{11} per mL of luminal contents, representing about 800 species. The dominant phyla are *Firmicutes, Bacteroidetes, Actinobacteria, Proteobacteria, Fusobacteria,* and *Verrucomicrobia*.[31,32] Together, the phyla *Firmicutes* and *Bacteroidetes* account for perhaps 90% of gut microbiobe population.

These foundational ideas have led to the concept of "dysbiosis," a condition in which the balance of the different species is unhealthy, thereby exacerbating underlying diseases or permitting conditions that open the door to colonization and diseases caused by pathogenic bacteria.[33] The plasticity of the microbiome reflects a number of factors, including the competition among bacteria for habitat and nutrients. In addition, experimental and clinical investigations have provided increasingly convincing evidence that acute and chronic conditions and stresses, modify and are modified by the microbiome of the alimentary tract. Increasingly, there is also evidence that diet, dietary and micronutrient supplements, and medications can influence the ecology of the gut, sometimes favoring beneficial commensals such as lactobacillus or bifidobacteria, but sometimes opening the door to potential pathogens. Mechanisms and implications of interactions between the gut microflora and the small intestinal microenvironment remain incompletely understood. In this regard an emerging concept is the integration of the intestinal microbiome with other systems in the body, including the central nervous system functions as diverse as the experience of chronic pain and addiction, inflammatory conditions such as multiple sclerosis, and neurodegenerative syndromes such as Alzheimer disease. Such communications are bidirectional, and likely have implications for the patient's experience of surgical illness and recovery from major operations.[34]

Endocrine, Paracrine, and Neurocrine Communication Pathways of the Intestine

The suffix "crine" in the words endocrine, exocrine, neurocrine, paracrine, apocrine, and holocrine is derived from the Greek " κρινω" or "krino," which translates as "I separate from" or "I secrete" and seems to have been proposed in 1893 by the French physiologist, Édouard Laguesse, a result of studying the islets of Langerhans.[35] The term "hormone" (from the Greek όρμάω or hormáō, "to set in motion, to urge on") was coined by the English physiologist Ernest Starling. In 1901, with his colleague (and brother-in-law) William Bayliss, Starling demonstrated the existence of a peptide which he called "secretin" that is released internally by duodenal mucosa in response stimulation by hydrochloric acid and leads to exocrine secretions by the pancreas that lead back to the intestine. In 1905 Starling proposed the word "hormone" to describe "the chemical messengers which speeding from cell to cell along the blood stream, may coordinate the activities and growth of different parts of the body."[36] Since the introduction of these terms, it has been documented that EECs comprise about 1% of the mucosal cell population, thereby recognizing the alimentary tract as the largest repository of hormone-secreting cells in the human body. More than twenty bioactive agents are produced and released by cells of the small intestine. These agents respond to stimuli from the gut that include nutrients, products of microbial metabolism, alterations in states of nutrition and metabolism, and other neurohumoral signals. It is also evident that epithelial and immune cells of the mucosa produce internal secretions in response to injury or stress that also influence local responses in the intestine, regional responses in organs such as pancreas and liver, and even activities of the brain and neurologic system.[37–39]

A comprehensive review of endocrine, paracrine, and neurocrine attributes of the intestine lies beyond the scope of this chapter. At the same time, some attention is required to the details of individual hormones and neurotransmitters that influence key functions of the small intestine and that may initiate or exacerbate its disorders. **Table 46B.4** provides a compilation of selected hormones produced by EECs of the alimentary tract, including some relevant hormones secreted by neuroendocrine elements of the stomach and colon. Outlined in the table are their sites of production, the principal stimuli leading to their production and release, and their physiologically significant influences.

From classic studies of endocrine, paracrine, and neurocrine capabilities of the small intestine, three general concepts have emerged. The first is that, broadly characterized, EECs are divided into those that respond to mechanical stimuli, irritants and toxins—these are the enterochromaffin cells that secrete serotonin; and those that respond to nutrients that are in the lumen and/or after being absorbed—these are the peptide secreting hormones. A second concept is the considerable redundancy of endocrine functions within individual regions of the small intestine, arising in part from similarities in the amino acid sequences and tertiary structures of specific groups hormones and their receptors; and in part from the presence of hormones in different regions that influence the same receptors. A third concept is the influence of such hormones on organ systems outside the alimentary tract itself including: (1) influences on pancreatic endocrine secretions from the islets of Langerhans (insulin, glucagon, etc.) and exocrine, digestive enzyme-rich secretions from pancreatic acini and bicarbonate-rich fluid and electrolyte sections from the pancreatic ducts; (2) conjoined influences with pancreatic endocrine secretions on intermediary metabolism in the liver and secretions of bile from the gallbladder; (3) and conjoined influences with pancreatic endocrine secretion and on metabolism in visceral and somatic adipose issues; and (4) signaling of hunger and satiety in the central nervous system (**Fig. 46B.10**).

From recent investigations, one other concept has emerged: that there are gut hormones not derived from EECs, but from epithelial cells within the villus-crypt unit. Such hormones include the guanylin peptides (GPs), guanylin and uroguanylin, which are small peptides (15 to 19 amino acid residues) in the natriuretic hormone family because of their ring structures and demonstrated influence on sodium and water excretion not only in the GI tract but in the kidney. Production of GPs occurs mainly in the intestine by a wide variety of cell types, including Paneth cells, the goblet cells, the colonic Paneth-like cells, the epithelial cells, and the somatostatin-secreting D-cells of the small intestine and colonic mucosa. Drivers of secretion depend on the specific region of intestine: luminal pH driving secretion of uroguanylin in the duodenum and proximal jejunum, luminal salt content influencing secretion of both GPs throughout the intestine.[40] Recent studies have also indicated that Paneth cells also secrete hormones such as Peptide YY, which exhibit antimicrobial properties with unsuspected implications for supporting commensal microbes and resisting hostile forms.[41]

PATHOPHYSIOLOGY OF INTESTINAL OBSTRUCTION, ILEUS, AND
5 PSEUDO-OBSTRUCTION OF THE COLON

Pathophysiology of Intestinal Obstruction

The sequence of events in intestinal obstruction was described in a classic series of clinical and experimental investigations in the early- and mid-1900s by Owen Wangensteen at the University of Minnesota[42]: a segment of intestine becomes obstructed, subsequent pathophysiologic events in upstream regions include (1) the accumulation of gas and fluid; (2) luminal stasis in association with release of microbe-generated toxins that impair mucosal secretion and absorption,

Table 46B.4. Intestinal Hormones

Hormone	Site of Secretion	Cell Type	Regulation: Stimulation/Inhibition	Principal Function	Clinical Relevance/Applications
Gastrin	Stomach, duodenum	G	Vagus, amino acids, gastric distention	Enhances histamine-induced gastric acid secretion; trophic	Target of peptic ulcer operations; gastrin analogs useful in diagnosis of neuroendocrine tumors (medullary carcinoma)
Ghrelin	Stomach	X	Fasting	Actives appetite and GI motility	Target of bariatric operations; potential target for appetite suppression
Secretin	Duodenum, jejunum	S	Vagal stimulation, acid pH, fatty acids, bile salts	Exocrine pancreas duct secretion	Stimulation test for gastrinoma; useful in MRI pancreatography
Cholecystokinin	Duodenum, jejunum	I	Vagal stimulation, fatty acids	Exocrine pancreas acinar cell secretion; gallbladder motility	Infusion used in tests of gallbladder filling/emptying; diagnosis of cholecystitis
GIP	Duodenum, jejunum	K	Carbohydrate, protein, fat, bile acids	Glucose-dependent insulin secretion	Cooperates with GLP-1 to regulate insulin response to glucose and lipid metabolism in adipose tissue.
Motilin	Duodenum, jejunum	Mo/ECL	Interdigestive interval, alkaline pH	Phase III Migrating Myoelectric Complex	Actions mimicked by macrolides (eg, erythromycin) in treatment of gastroparesis
Glucagon-like peptide-1	Jejunum, ileum, colon, rectum	L	Carbohydrate, protein, fat	Glucose-dependent insulin secretion	Agonists suppress appetite and improve glucose control (incretin mimetic class) in diabetics
Glucagon-like peptide P-2	Jejunum, ileum, colon, rectum	L	Carbohydrate, protein, fat	Intestine stem cell expansion and crypt cell proliferation, and intestinal growth	Agonists are trophic (stimulating mucosal hypertrophy) and improve absorption of nutrients, electrolytes, and water. Treatment of severe short bowel syndrome
Somatostatin	Stomach, duodenum, jejunum, ileum	D	Nutrient detection and low pH, simulation by other GI hormones	Suppresses exocrine and endocrine secretions, reduces portal blood flow	Agonists used to moderate exocrine secretions of the intestine, suppress endocrine hypersecretion in carcinoid syndromes, reduce bleeding in portal hypertension. Rare hyperfunctioning tumor
Vasoactive intestinal polypeptide	Enteric nerves	Neurons	Vagal stimulation	Stimulates water and electrolyte secretion	Rare hyperfunctioning tumors cause secretory diarrhea syndrome
Serotonin	Duodenum, jejunum, ileum, colon, rectum	Enteroch-romaffin	Luminal nutrients; mechanical/irri-tant stimulation of intestine	Stimulates water and electrolyte secretion, complex effects on motility	Rare serotonin-secreting tumors cause secretory diarrhea syndrome and GI motility disturbance. Serotonin-agonists useful in irritable bowel syndromes
Beta-endorphin	Enteric nerves	Neurons, immune cells	Inflammation	Slows GI motility (opioid mu-receptor); enhances salt and water absorption	Medications to treat diarrhea; exogenous opioids major risk factors for constipation, including postoperatively.
Cannabinoids	Enteric nerves	Neurons, immune cells	Inflammation	Slow gastric emptying	Cannabis hyperemesis syndrome in chronic, long-term users of the drug

From Prior Edition of Mulholland Chapter 48 and Bakar, et al. 2023.
From Bakar RB, Reimann F, Gribble FM. The intestine as an endocrine organ and the role of gut hormones in metabolic regulation. *Nat Rev Gastroenterol Hepatol.* 2023;20(12):784–796.

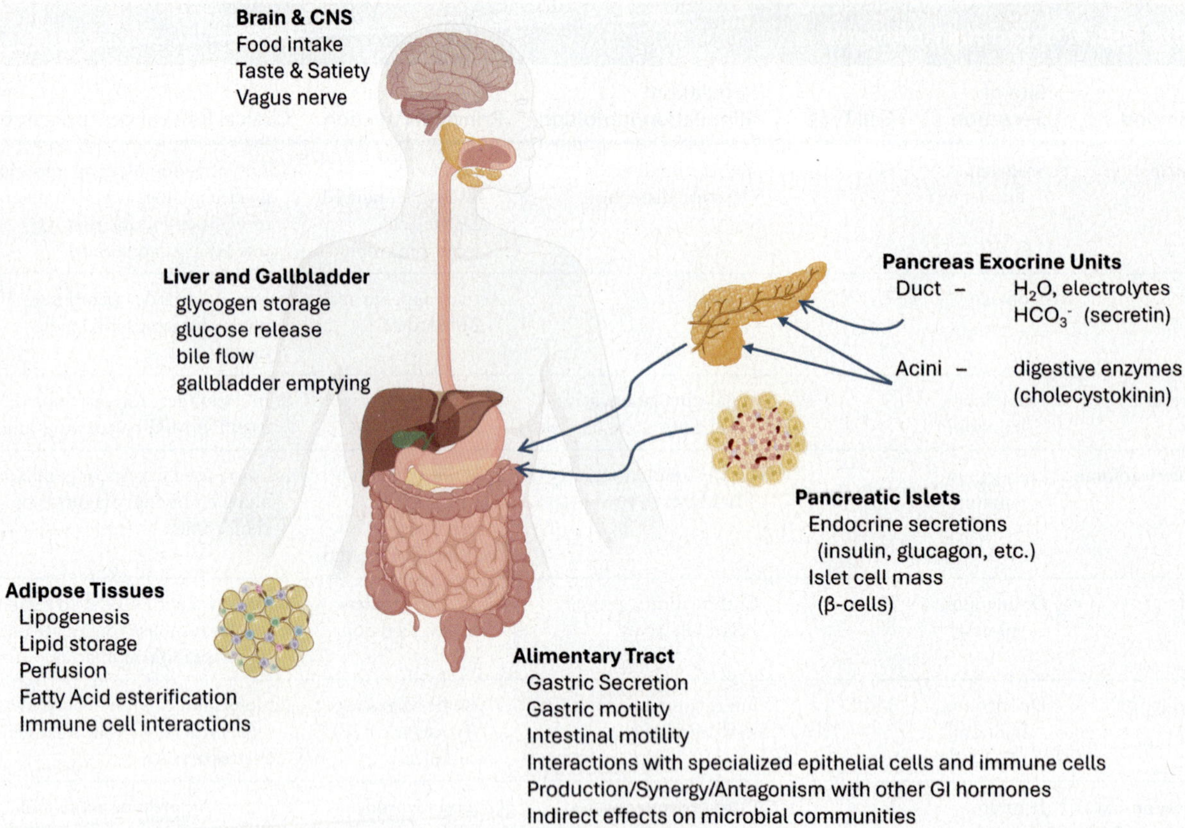

Figure 46B.10. Processes regulated by gut hormones throughout the body. Gastrointestinal tract hormones integrate physiologic processes in secretory and metabolically active tissues, including the pancreas, liver, adipose tissues, the central nervous system, and within the alimentary tract itself. Emerging evidence suggests bi-directional influences between gut hormones and other luminal actors, including nutrients, bile acids, and intestinal microbial communities. (Created in BioRender. Soybel, D. 2024. BioRender.com/f10b518)

as well as translocation of bacteria to the gut wall, lymphatics, and systemic circulation; (3) a series of adaptive changes in intestinal motor function—at first relaxation to keep luminal pressures low, then hyperperistalsis in the effort to clear the blockage, and finally loss of organized motility patterns; and (4) alterations in blood flow to the mucosa and the gut wall, resulting not in ischemia, loss of mucosal integrity, inflammation, edema, and ultimately gangrene. Ultimately it is the confluence of these disturbances that determines how quickly a simple obstruction evolves to cause symptoms or a closed-loop obstruction progresses to gangrene and perforation.[42,43]

A simple, acute "open-loop" obstruction is most commonly associated with a kink, stricture, or obturator (eg, a gallstone or foreign body) that leads to a mechanical blockage of the lumen at one site in the intestine, preventing passage of luminal content downstream. Proximal obstruction is characterized by vomiting and loss of gastric, pancreatic, and biliary secretions, with resulting electrolyte disturbances. These disturbances—occurring more commonly in patients who are elderly, diabetic, and frail–include dehydration, metabolic alkalosis, hypochloremia, hypokalemia, hyponatremia, and acute kidney injury (AKI).[44] In contrast, obstructions of the distal ileum may lead only to a slowly progressing distention of the small intestine, with accommodation by intestinal myoelectrical function and minor alterations in fluid and electrolyte balances.

A closed-loop obstruction usually refers to a twisting, or volvulus, of the bowel around the axis of its mesentery induced by an adhesive band or due to incarceration in a hernia (internal or external). Reflex hyperperistalsis and twisting of the mesentery occur early and are associated with intense pain and reflex nausea and vomiting. In a relatively short segment of intestine, and depending on region involved, continued secretion of mucus to high intraluminal pressures, stasis, bacterial overgrowth, mucosal disruption, and elevation of luminal pressures convert intermittent cramps to constant and worsening pain. Ischemia caused by the twist itself results initially from obstruction of venous outflow, with back-pressure build up in the intestinal wall. When luminal pressure exceeds mural venous pressure and then capillary perfusion pressures, inflammatory cells are recruited from surrounding peritoneal structures. This sequence of events leads to intense inflammation, release of exudate and the first localization of pain from the umbilicus to the area of peritoneum lying nearest the involved segment of intestine. Peritoneal findings (localized tenderness, involuntary guarding, rebound or referred tenderness) and fevers appear. Gangrene and perforation follow and, if not contained by surrounding structures, free perforation leads to release of intestinal fluid containing toxic microbes as well as the influx of fluid from the circulation due to intense peritoneal inflammation. Toxins from necrotic intestinal tissue and bacterial overgrowth are released, leading to circulatory collapse and shock.

Pathophysiology of Ileus

An *ileus* or *"eileos"* (from classical Greek for "twisting") reflects a loss of forward peristalsis and coordination of the motility of the different regions of the GI tract causing a functional obstruction. Ileus is a consequence of systemic disturbances such as sepsis or ketoacidosis, activation of reflexes after injury to the central nervous system, direct contact of bowel with noxious conditions or toxins, metabolic derangements, and contamination with noxious agents (blood, urine, intestinal succus, bacteria) in the retroperitoneum due to perforation, pancreatitis, aneurysm rupture, or pelvic fracture.[45]

Implicated in the pathogenesis of ileus is a diverse array of circulating peptides and neurotransmitters, some that enhance GI motility and others that inhibit myoelectric function. Among them are acetylcholine, calcitonin gene–related peptide (CGRP), Substance P released through vagal pathways (activate motor function), and catecholamines released by sympathetic neurons and the adrenal medulla (dampen motor function). Among the most clinically consequential are the opioids, both synthetic and endogenous, which delay gastric emptying and promote nonperistaltic contractions that increase intraluminal pressure along the length of the GI tract.

Also implicated, through experimental and clinical investigations, are inflammatory cells and mediators of inflammation in the development of prolonged ileus.[46] Surgical intervention results in activation of mast cells and macrophages within the gut wall, leading to release of proinflammation cytokines and activation of their receptors, including interleukins 1, 6, and 10; activation of cyclooxygenase isoform-2 (COX-2) and inducible nitric oxide (iNOS). Thus, the hypothesis has evolved that focal manipulation of the bowel results in a panenteric inflammation and modulation of the enteric nervous system, resulting in postoperative ileus. Nutritional imbalances may exacerbate ileus by impairing the capabilities of the immune system.[47]

Pathophysiology of Colonic Pseudo-obstruction (Ogilvie Syndrome)

Acute pseudo-obstruction of the colon, also known as Ogilvie syndrome, is a paralytic ileus of the large bowel, characterized by rapidly progressive abdominal distention reflecting accumulation of air and secretions within the lumen. As has been observed for ileus of the small intestine, a combination of neurogenic, hormonal, metabolic, and inflammation-driven disturbances are associated with a loss of normal motor function that is the cause of Ogilvie syndrome. The suddenness with which the colon dilates seems driven largely by postsynaptic sympathetic stimulation directed at the intramuscular ganglia (Auerbach plexus and ICCs).[48] The dominance of the central neurogenic drive is suggested by the effectiveness of interventions such as neostigmine, which targets acetylcholinesterase in the presynaptic space of the autonomic nerves. The result of neostigmine therapy is to block the breakdown of acetylcholine before it interacts with postsynaptic membrane cholinergic receptors, thereby restoring the balance between parasympathetic and sympathetic influences on the intrinsic nervous system. Additional supporting pieces of evidence include anecdotal observations that Ogilvie syndrome can be reversed with spinal sympatholytic anesthesia.[49]

CLOSING COMMENTS

With respect to the care of the surgical patient, the importance of anatomy and physiology of the small intestine continues to increase in relevance. Embryologic considerations are crucial for understanding congenital conditions such as atresias, duplications, rotational abnormalities, and Hirschprung disease; in addition, they form the basis for understanding the classification, location and progression of abdominal pain, and clinical signs connected to illnesses such as intestinal obstruction, motility disorders, and inflammatory diseases such as Crohn disease.

The mucosa of the small intestine serves as a gateway for selective absorption of macro- and micronutrients as well as medications, and has specialized features permitting recycling of facilitating carriers such as chylomicrons. In different segments of the intestine, the mucosa serves as barrier to noxious agents and microorganisms, and displays enzymatic properties that inactivate toxins and poisons and control the bacterial populations living commensally in close proximity to the mucosal surface. Specialized cell sensors within the mucosa have been identified that monitor the presence of microorganisms and potential pathogens, while specialized lymphoid structures in the distal intestine continuously sample the microflora and provide friend-or-foe information to the mechanisms controlling cellular and innate immunity. Increasingly it is becoming clear that promoting homeostasis within the intestinal lumen can avoid turning commensals into combatants.[50]

The neuromotor functions of the intestine facilitate mixing of luminal content with digestive enzymes and facilitating structures for optimal absorption of nutrients; as well as mechanisms for downstream disposal of nonabsorbable dietary components in anticipation of future digestive needs. Together the specialized secretory and motor functions of the intestine coordinate to prevent stasis, bacterial overgrowth, and accumulation of pathogens. The microcirculation within the gut wall serves as a conduit for delivery of oxygen, nutrients and buffers against build-up of acid and other metabolic toxins; while both the microcirculation and lymphatics serve as conduits for transfer of absorbed nutrients to the liver and systemic circulation, respectively. The neuroendocrine functions of the small intestine have become increasingly relevant to the development of therapeutics (such as agonists of GLP-1 and inhibitors of GIP) that target appetite, obesity, diabetes, and intermediary metabolism; and those (targeting receptors for somatostatin, opioids, and the autonomic nervous system) that support palliation of secretory and motor disturbances such as obstruction, ileus, and diarrheas.

ACKNOWLEDGMENTS

We gratefully acknowledge the contributions of previous edition authors, Joslin Cheverie, Jared S. Matson, and Sonia L. Ramamoorthy, as portions of those chapters have been retained in this revision.

References

1. Sakai T, Masayuki F. Manners of terminology and description in Galen's anatomy in the ancient Rome and their historical consequences up to the modern time. *Anat Sci Int*. 2024;99(4):348–356.
2. Desai GS, Pande PM. Gastroduodenal artery: single key for many locks. *J Hepatobiliary Pancreat Sci*. 2019;26(7):281–291.
3. Ostrowski P, Bonczar M, Gliwa J, et al. The arterial anatomy of the posterior duodenum – A computed tomography angiography analysis with implications for abdominal surgery. *Clin Anat*. 2023; 36(8):1116–1126.
4. Parungo CP, Soybel DI, Colson YL, et al. Lymphatic drainage of the peritoneal space: a pattern dependent on bowel lymphatics. *Ann Surg Oncol*. 2007;14(2):286–298.
5. Vorenkamp K, Yi P, Kemp A. Sympathetic blocks for visceral pain. *Phys Med Rehabil Clin N Am*. 2022;33(2):475–487.
6. Kolev HM, Kaestner KH. Mammalian intestinal development and differentiation-the state of the art. *Cell Mol Gastroenterol Hepatol*. 2023;16(5):809–821.
7. Sheng YH, Hasnain SZ. Mucus and mucins: The underappreciated host defence system. *Front Cell Infect Microbiol*. 2022;12:856962.
8. Salzman NH, Bevins CL. Dysbiosis–a consequence of Paneth cell dysfunction. *Semin Immunol*. 2013;25(5):334–341.
9. Egorov VI, Schastlivtsev V, Turusov RA, Baranov AO. Participation of the intestinal layers in supplying of the mechanical strength of the intact and sutured gut. *Eur Surg Res*. 2002;34(6): 425–431.
10. Krause WJ. Brunner's glands: A structural, histochemical and pathological profile. *Prog Histochem Cytochem*. 2000;35(4):259–367.
11. Reboldi A, Cyster JG. Peyer's patches: Organizing B-cell responses at the intestinal frontier. *Immunol Rev*. 2016;271(1):230–245.
12. Shaik L, Kashyap R, Thotamgari SR, Singh R, Khanna S. Gut-brain axis and its neuro-psychiatric effects: A narrative review. *Cureus*. 2020;12(10):e11131.
13. Slavin J. Fiber and prebiotics: Mechanisms and health benefits. *Nutrients*. 2013;5(4):1417–1435.
14. Jawara D, Ufearo DM, Murtha JA, et al. Racial disparities in selected micronutrient deficiencies after bariatric surgery: A systematic review. *Surg Obes Relat Dis*. 2024;20(3):283–290.

15. Green R, Allen LH, Bjorke-Monsen AL, et al. Vitamin B(12) deficiency. *Nat Rev Dis Primers*. 2017;3:17040.
16. Paulus MC, Drent M, Kouw IWK, Balvers MGJ, Bast A, van Zanten ARH. Vitamin K: a potential missing link in critical illness-a scoping review. *Crit Care*. 2024;28(1):212.
17. Achufusi TGO, Sharma A, Zamora EA, Manocha D. Small intestinal bacterial overgrowth: comprehensive review of diagnosis, prevention, and treatment methods. *Cureus*. 2020;12(6):e8860.
18. Collaco AM, Jakab RL, Hoekstra NE, Mitchell KA, Brooks A, Ameen NA. Regulated traffic of anion transporters in mammalian Brunner's glands: a role for water and fluid transport. *Am J Physiol Gastrointest Liver Physiol*. 2013;305(3):G258–G275.
19. Deloose E, Janssen P, Depoortere I, Tack J. The migrating motor complex: control mechanisms and its role in health and disease. *Nat Rev Gastroenterol Hepatol*. 2012;9(5):271–285.
20. Deloose E, Tack J. Redefining the functional roles of the gastrointestinal migrating motor complex and motilin in small bacterial overgrowth and hunger signaling. *Am J Physiol Gastrointest Liver Physiol*. 2016;310(4):G228–G233.
21. Mowat AM, Agace WW. Regional specialization within the intestinal immune system. *Nat Rev Immunol*. 2014;14(10):667–685.
22. Podany AB, Wright J, Lamendella R, Soybel DI, Kelleher SL. ZnT2-mediated zinc import into Paneth cell granules is necessary for coordinated secretion and Paneth cell function in mice. *Cell Mol Gastroenterol Hepatol*. 2016;2(3):369–383.
23. Lockhart A, Mucida D, Bilate AM. Intraepithelial lymphocytes of the intestine. *Annu Rev Immunol*. 2024;42(1):289–316.
24. Coutry N, Gasmi I, Herbert F, Jay P. Mechanisms of intestinal dysbiosis: new insights into tuft cell functions. *Gut Microbes*. 2024;16(1):2379624.
25. Lederberg J, McCray AT. Ome sweet 'omics–a genealogical treasury of words. *The Scientist*. 2001;15(7):8–8.
26. Krajmalnik-Brown R, Ilhan ZE, Kang DW, DiBaise JK. Effects of gut microbes on nutrient absorption and energy regulation. *Nutr Clin Pract*. 2012;27(2):201–214.
27. Fogelson KA, Dorrestein PC, Zarrinpar A, Knight R. The gut microbial bile acid modulation and its relevance to digestive health and diseases. *Gastroenterology*. 2023;164(7):1069–1085.
28. Hartmann P, Schnabl B. New developments in microbiome in alcohol-associated and nonalcoholic fatty liver disease. *Semin Liver Dis*. 2021;41(1):87–102.
29. Ronen D, Rokach Y, Abedat S, et al. Human gut microbiota in cardiovascular disease. *Compr Physiol*. 2024;14(3):5449–5490.
30. Barone M, D'Amico F, Brigidi P, Turroni S. Gut microbiome-micronutrient interaction: The key to controlling the bioavailability of minerals and vitamins? *Biofactors*. 2022;48(2):307–314.
31. Kunath BJ, De Rudder C, Laczny CC, Letellier E, Wilmes P. The oral-gut microbiome axis in health and disease. *Nat Rev Microbiol*. 2024;22(12):791–805.
32. Sender R, Fuchs S, Milo R. Revised estimates for the number of human and bacteria cells in the body. *PLoS Biol*. 2016;14(8):e1002533.
33. Winter SE, Baumler AJ. Gut dysbiosis: Ecological causes and causative effects on human disease. *Proc Natl Acad Sci U S A*. 2023;120(50):e2316579120.
34. Kurdi M, Bajwa SJS, Sharma R, Choudhary R. Gut microbiota and probiotics in perioperative management: A narrative review. *Cureus*. 2024;16(9):e68404.
35. Goet JP. Gustave Edouard Laguesse; his demonstration of the significance of the Islands of Langerhans. *Diabetes*. 1953;2(4):322–324.
36. Starling EH. The Croonian lectures. I. On the chemical correlation of the functions of the body. *The Lancet*. 1905;166:339–341.
37. Bany Bakar R, Reimann F, Gribble FM. The intestine as an endocrine organ and the role of gut hormones in metabolic regulation. *Nat Rev Gastroenterol Hepatol*. 2023;20(12):784–796.
38. Bildstein T, Charbit-Henrion F, Azabdaftari A, Cerf-Bensussan N, Uhlig HH. Cellular and molecular basis of proximal small intestine disorders. *Nat Rev Gastroenterol Hepatol*. 2024;21(10):687–709.
39. Yip JLK, Balasuriya GK, Spencer SJ, Hill-Yardin EL. The role of intestinal macrophages in gastrointestinal homeostasis: heterogeneity and implications in disease. *Cell Mol Gastroenterol Hepatol*. 2021;12(5):1701–1718.
40. Della Corte V, Pacinella G, Todaro F, Pecoraro R, Tuttolomondo A. The natriuretic peptide system: A single entity, pleiotropic effects. *Int J Mol Sci*. 2023;24(11):9642.
41. Pierre JF, Peters BM, La Torre D, et al. Peptide YY: A Paneth cell antimicrobial peptide that maintains Candida gut commensalism. *Science*. 2023;381(6657):502–508.
42. Wangensteen OH. *Intestinal Obstructions*. 3rd ed. Charles C. Thomas; 1955.
43. Ellis H. *Intestinal Obstruction*. Appleton Crofts; 1982.
44. Sun D, Wang L, Liu S. Clinical features and influencing factors of acute kidney injury in patients with intestinal obstruction: A meta-analysis. *Altern Ther Health Med*. 2024;30(9):250–255.
45. Wattchow D, Heitmann P, Smolilo D, et al. Postoperative ileus-An ongoing conundrum. *Neurogastroenterol Motil*. 2021;33(5):e14046.
46. Sui C, Tao L, Bai C, et al. Molecular and cellular mechanisms underlying postoperative paralytic ileus by various immune cell types. *Front Pharmacol*. 2022;13:929901.
47. Phillips BE, Goletzke AK, Smith PB, et al. Impaired recovery from peritoneal inflammation in a mouse model of mild dietary zinc restriction. *Mol Nutr Food Res*. 2016;60(3):672–681.
48. Arthur T, Burgess A. Acute colonic pseudo-obstruction. *Clin Colon Rectal Surg*. 2022;35(3):221–226.
49. Mashour GA, Peterfreund RA. Spinal anesthesia and Ogilvie's syndrome. *J Clin Anesth*. 2005;17(2):122–123.
50. Alverdy JC. The role of dietary prehabilitation on anastomotic healing. *Curr Opin Clin Nutr Metab Care*. 2023;26(5):470–475.

Crohn Disease

Olga Lavryk and Scott R. Steele

Key Points

1 Crohn disease can affect the entire gastrointestinal (GI) tract from mouth to anus in skip areas with characteristic skip lesions rather than continuous involvement of bowel and is likely from a multifactorial etiology.

2 Crohn disease patients experience flares and remissions during the disease course.

3 Crohn disease may manifest in the GI tract in one or more disease patterns—fistulizing, inflammatory, and fibrostenotic—resulting in fistulas, abscesses/phlegmons, and/or obstruction, respectively.

4 Crohn disease is associated with an increased long-term risk of developing colorectal cancer compared to the general population. Patients should be screened accordingly, and surgical treatment is typically more aggressive in the setting of underlying microscopic colorectal dysplasia or dysplastic lesions.

5 Several classes of medications are available for Crohn disease, depending on the spectrum of disease. These range from topicals and aminosalicylates to steroids, immunosuppressants, and/or biologic agents.

6 Treatment for Crohn disease is multifactorial. Medical treatment is focused on mucosal healing and symptom reduction, while surgery is key in treating complications such as stenosis, perforation, fistula, and abscess.

7 Surgery for Crohn disease is not curative but instead aimed at symptom control. Thus, bowel-preserving surgery is crucial for Crohn disease, given the high need for future resections and the potential for diseased/nonfunctioning bowel.

8 The decision to embark on surgical intervention must account for the patient's clinical presentation, concomitant medical therapy, underlying continence, anatomy, and overall nutritional status.

9 Anorectal conditions in Crohn patients must be managed with special considerations given the potential for poor wound healing, incontinence, and worsened quality of life with aggressive surgical intervention.

10 Treating perianal Crohn disease consists of controlling perianal sepsis with adequate drainage and systemic control of inflammation with biologic therapy.

Crohn disease is a chronic, inflammatory condition of the alimentary tract. The disease was first described by Crohn, Ginzburg, and Oppenheimer in 1932. The disease's underlying mechanism is unknown, and it can manifest with a broad spectrum of presentations and severity. Several Crohn patients may respond well to medications, while others are recalcitrant to multiple high-dose biologics or steroids. Therefore, treatment options must be individualized for each patient with Crohn disease. Basic tenets of Crohn disease include that it may occur anywhere along the alimentary tract, has no "curative" operation, and is hallmarked by periods of flares and quiescent disease. Despite improvements in medical therapy, upward of 75% of patients will still require at least one operation during their lifetime to treat complications associated with the disease or nonresponsiveness to medical therapy.[1] As such, careful consideration must be given to each patient's future function when weighing therapeutic options to resolve the current problem. Surgeons must be exceedingly aware of the indications, surgical options, and expected outcomes for patients with Crohn disease. To maximize the latter, it is crucial also to have a thorough understanding of not only the principles guiding surgical treatment, but also the medical therapies that may either allow avoidance of surgery altogether. This chapter will cover the clinical presentation, diagnostic evaluation, medical therapies, and surgical treatment for Crohn disease.

EPIDEMIOLOGY

1 The age of onset of Crohn disease follows a bimodal distribution, either in the second to fourth decades of life or in the sixth decade.[2] Systematic reviews have found an annual incidence of Crohn disease ranging from 20.2 per 100,000 person-years in North America and 12.7 per 100,000 person-years in Europe to 5.0 person-years in Asia and the Middle East.[2] Males and females tend to be affected equally, though Whites and certain ethnic groups such as Ashkenazi Jewish descent have higher overall rates.[3] Given the geographic and temporal variation in the epidemiology of Crohn disease, recent research has focused on environmental and genetic factors that may be driving these shifts.

ETIOLOGY

Despite tremendous progress in the overall understanding of the disease and advancements in comprehension of various phenotypical manifestations, the exact etiology of Crohn disease remains unknown. The development of the disease is thought to be a result of environmental triggers acting upon a combination of genetic and intestinal factors that drive the growth of compromised intestinal immune response followed by mucosal inflammation. Immune cells like CD-4 T cells, CD-8 T cells, B cells, CD 14 monocytes, and natural killers are involved in the process as they infiltrate the gut in

Crohn disease and create an out-of-proportion inflammatory reaction.

Genetics plays an essential role in the disease pathophysiology. Approximately 2% to 14% of patients report a family history of Crohn disease, which is higher in those of Jewish ancestry.[4] The concordance rate for monozygotic twins ranges from 20% to 50%, suggesting that genetics plays a role and the disease is not entirely dependent on environmental and/or acquired factors.[5] Over 200 alleles have been associated with inflammatory bowel disease (IBD), though only 37 are specific for Crohn disease. Several genes involved and linked to Crohn disease are related to the host's ability to sense bacterial or control innate immunity and Th17-cell function, and can result in an altered mucus layer of the GI tract.[6] Attention has revolved around the NOD2 (formerly CARD15) gene on chromosome 16, a region involved in host interactions with bacterial lipopolysaccharide to activate NF-κB, which correlates to Crohn disease phenotype.[7] Genome-wide association studies have provided insight that polymorphisms in genes such as ATG16L1 and IRGM play a role in autophagy in Crohn patients. This process involves the regulation of cell development and differentiation, senescence, and ultimately, the inflammatory system response to what the body deems normal and abnormal.[8] Impaired recognition and processing in this aspect results in deregulation and disease pathogenesis. In addition, other genes such as TLR4, HLA, and IRF5 that are involved in the innate and adaptive immune system response are seen to be altered in Crohn patients.

Theories regarding a host–microbiome connection have evolved over the past few decades. The gut microbiome is the largest reservoir of microbes in the entire body and functions in digestion, immunity, and suppression of harmful organisms. Various elements, including genetics, age, geography, hygiene, diet, drugs, smoking, and many others influence the state of an individual's microbiome.[9] An interplay between the immune system and the microbiome has been identified in IBD, and various microbes may be either protective against or increase susceptibility to the development of the disease. *Escherichia coli*, particularly the adherent-invasive strains, have been found in higher concentrations in patients with ileal Crohn disease and can induce granuloma formation—a pathognomonic feature of Crohn disease.[10] Conversely, evidence suggests that certain microbes are protective in IBD. *Bacteroides* and *Clostridium* have been shown to reduce intestinal inflammation by upregulating regulatory T cells and regulating NF-kB activation to decrease mucosal inflammation. *Bifidobacterium*, *Lactobacillus*, and *Faecalibacterium* are protective against mucosal inflammation through the downregulation of inflammatory cytokines and upregulation of IL-10.[11–13] Alternations of the microbiome may also increase the risk of later disease recurrence of patients in remission, what represents a promising target for drug therapy. In addition, inflammation itself can disrupt the stability of microbiota.

Recently increased intestinal permeability has been evidenced to determine later Crohn disease development. The viable bacteria and their products, such as outer membrane vesicles, lipopolysaccharides, peptidoglycans, and bacterial DNA, migrate from the lumen through the mucosa to normally sterile tissue such as mesenteric lymph nodes, mesenteric adipocytes, and are referred to as bacterial translocation. Bacterial translocation represents a bacterial reservoir stimulating visceral fat production for CRP production and promoting inflammatory response.

Although the beneficial effects of antibiotics in the treatment of Crohn disease provide indirect evidence for a bacterial etiology, no distinct organism has been identified to date. Similarly, several viruses, such as EBV, CMV, and measles, have been postulated to have an association with the development of Crohn disease; however, multiple reports have found little evidence to support this notion.[14] Other causative immune factors have included overexpression and dysregulation of tumor necrosis factor, an imbalance between proinflammatory and anti-inflammatory cytokines, and an impaired mucosal susceptibility in sampling gut antigens.[15] Combined, these all contribute to regulatory mechanisms that may be altered and play a role in the pathogenesis of Crohn disease.

Environmental factors may also play a role, highlighted by the well-established link between smoking and an increased susceptibility to Crohn disease as well as a worsened clinical course with higher recurrence rates. While patients with Crohn disease frequently have concomitant food intolerances, the role of dietary habits remains debatable.[16] Taken together, rather than a causative effect, it is felt that the microbiome in the human gastrointestinal (GI) tract is heavily influenced by dietary intake, leading to a local environment ripe to foster susceptibility to Crohn disease. This remains an area of increasing discovery and rapid change that is certain to evolve as the etiology and underlying reasons for such wide variability in phenotypical manifestations and clinical course in this disease are explored.

The pathogenesis of perianal Crohn disease is poorly understood. One of the hypotheses is related to inflammation causing the superficial ulcer, which afterward extends to a deeper ulcer into the deeper structure by stool exposure and the pressure of defecation. The second hypothesis implies infection of the anal glands with penetration of infection beyond the intersphincteric space.

DIAGNOSTIC EVALUATION

Crohn disease and ulcerative colitis both fall under the umbrella of IBD, and no specific tests at present permit a definitive diagnosis of either condition. The diagnosis is established using a combination of history and physical examination, laboratory values, radiographic, and endoscopic findings. Even so, 5% to 15% of patients with ulcerative colitis are eventually diagnosed with Crohn disease or indeterminate colitis when new concerning symptoms arise.[17] There are several classification schemes available for Crohn disease. Classification based on phenotypic manifestations includes fibrostenotic disease (stricturing), fistulizing disease (penetrating), and inflammatory disease (phlegmonous). Patients may have one, two, or all three, as evidenced by the high rate of strictures with proximal fistulas. Location is also frequently used to classify disease, with the distal ileum having the highest rate of disease incidence (**Fig. 47.1**). Localized inflammation in the ileocecal region occurs in approximately 45% of patients, colonic in 25% to 33%, proximal small-bowel disease in 25%, <10% will have isolated upper GI or isolated perianal disease, with

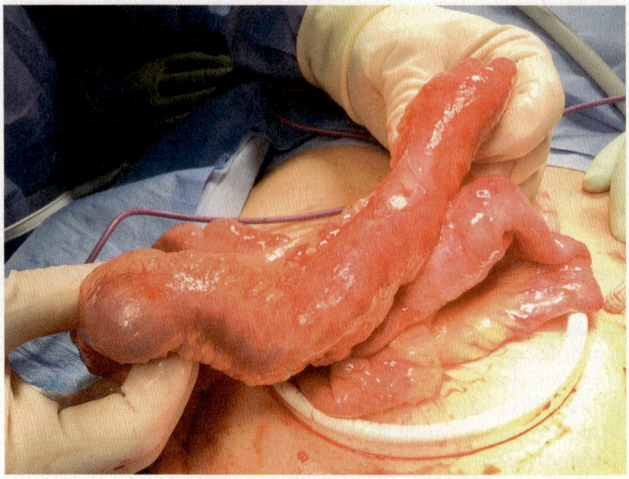

Figure 47.1. Terminal ileitis.

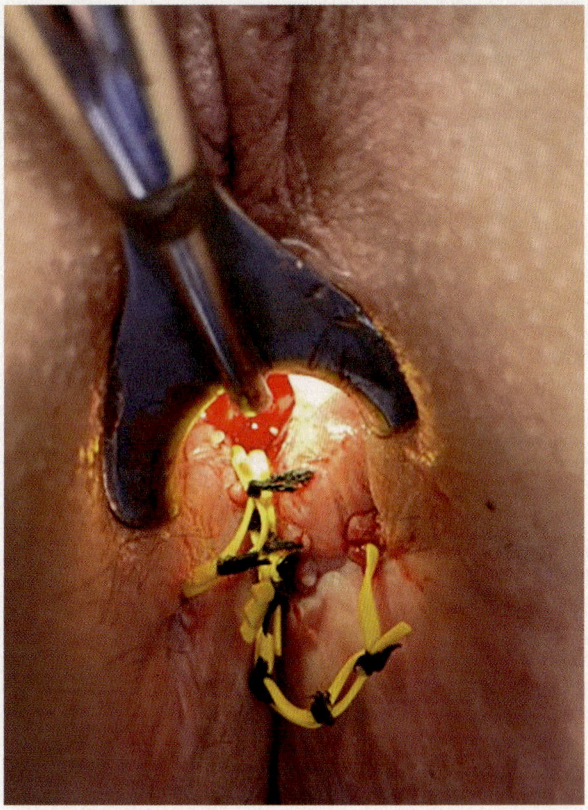

Figure 47.2. Perianal fistulas.

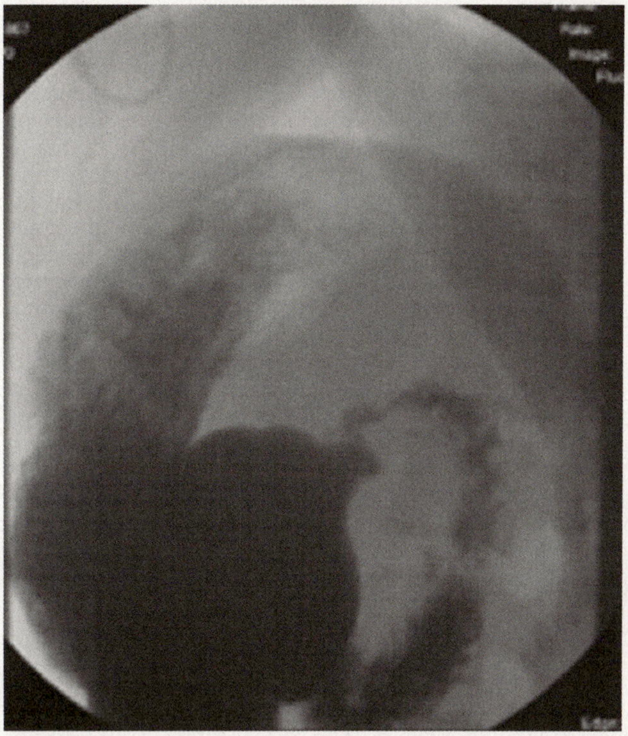

Figure 47.3. Upper GI contrast study demonstrating a stricture in the duodenum.

many patients having disease in more than one location. In general, patients with concomitant perianal disease tend to have a more severe clinical course, and perianal disease in the setting of Crohn may precede abdominal manifestations in up to 45% (**Fig. 47.2**).[18] Identification of suspicious perianal disease should prompt an investigation into more proximal disease.

2 Due to the chronic and heterogeneous nature of the disease, different classification manifestations may occur independently, concomitantly, or even vary along the longitudinal course of the disease. Fibrostenotic pattern may appear in any location, though most commonly occurs in the terminal ileal region, where patients present with obstructive-type symptoms such as nausea, vomiting, and decreased oral intake. More proximal diseases (eg, gastroduodenal) can often present with obstructive-type symptoms such as nausea, vomiting, and early satiety. Inflammatory disease may present with a wide range of symptoms such as abdominal pain, fever, an abdominal mass, change in bowel habits, and/or weight loss. Finally, penetrating or fistulizing disease may be completely asymptomatic (eg, entero–entero fistula of adjacent bowel), present with anorectal abscesses and/or fistulas, or more commonly complain of symptoms depending on the involvement of the secondarily involved organ; for example, recurrent urinary tract infections, pneumaturia, vaginal discharge, or diarrhea.

CLINICAL EVALUATION

Upper Gastrointestinal

Gastroduodenal Crohn disease is rare, occurring in only 0.5% to 4% of all Crohn patients and typically asymptomatic. Yet up to 40% of these patients will demonstrate early subclinical evidence of Crohn disease on radiologic or endoscopic evaluation.[19] When present, symptoms typically represent a gastric outlet obstruction and include epigastric abdominal pain, nausea, vomiting, early satiety, bloating, weight loss, and anorexia. Crohn disease of the esophagus is exceedingly rare, involving <0.5% of patients, and extraesophageal disease is nearly always present. A high index of suspicion should lead to diagnostic testing such as contrast imaging (eg, fluoroscopic upper GI, small-bowel follow-through) and endoscopy that will confirm the diagnosis (**Fig. 47.3**).

Small Bowel

3 The distribution of disease and phenotypic classification dictate the clinical presentation, with ileocecal disease being the most commonly affected site. Patients with disease in this location will classically present with a slow onset of right lower quadrant abdominal pain, fatigue, nausea, vomiting, abdominal mass, and pain with hip extension from psoas muscle involvement. Obstructive symptoms may also occur in patients with either fibrostenotic or acute inflammation (**Fig. 47.4**). Diarrhea tends to be nonbloody. However, heme-positive stools may occur, and gross blood is rarely a manifestation of a small-bowel source.

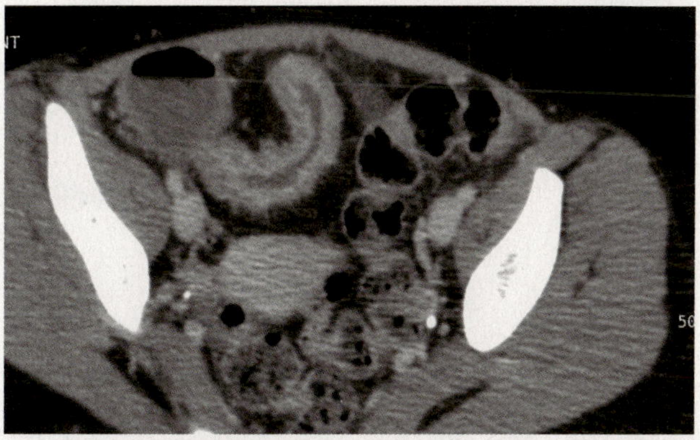

Figure 47.4. CT enterography demonstrating terminal ileal disease resulting in obstructive symptoms.

Colonic

Colonic involvement may occur in isolation in approximately 25% of patients. However, it is often seen concomitantly with perianal (associated with left-sided colonic inflammation) or terminal ileal (associated with cecal and ascending colon inflammation) disease.[20] Within the colon, the distribution is somewhat variable, with approximately one-third of patients having total colonic involvement, 40% showing segmental disease, and left-sided only in up to 30%. Patients with colonic involvement may experience abdominal pain, mucus drainage, and malnutrition regardless of location within the large intestine. Unlike ulcerative colitis, rectal bleeding is not routine, and bowel movements are often nonbloody, except in those with moderate-to-severe colitis. Diarrhea is often of smaller volume and may be from malabsorptive (eg, salt/water and bile acid malabsorption), infectious (eg, CMV superinfection), or from an enterocolonic fistula.[21] In addition to disease in the small bowel, patients can experience hip or back pain from fistulas, cramping, and obstructive symptoms. Patients with penetrating disease may also experience symptoms with associated involvement of the secondary organ (eg, feculent vaginal drainage from a colovaginal fistula, pneumaturia or fecaluria from bladder involvement, or skin drainage from an enterocutaneous fistula).

Anorectal

Perianal Crohn disease is a manifestation of often overlapping conditions such as skin tags, fissures, fistulas, ulcers, abscesses, anorectal strictures, and anorectal cancer. Isolated perianal disease is the presenting symptom in 5% to 15% of Crohn patients, though upward of 25% to 80% may experience symptoms at some point. Perianal involvement is more common in those with concomitant rectal or colonic disease. In addition, active disease in the perineum is felt to act as a harbinger of an overall more virulent course.[22]

Patients with Crohn disease may also have "traditional" anorectal complaints, the most common being perianal skin tags. These tend to be large, flat, with a bluish hue, and classically described as an "elephant ear" appearance. Perianal abscesses, fistulae, and fissures that do not follow the typical pattern of cryptoglandular disease should raise suspicion for a diagnosis of Crohn disease. Fissures tend to be deeper, off the midline, and much more painful than routine hypertonic associated fissures (**Fig. 47.5**). Patients presenting with perianal findings consistent with or concerning for Crohn disease should undergo a thorough physical examination and complete endoscopic and radiologic evaluation. Finally, patients with long-standing Crohn may develop anal stenosis or an anal stricture at the verge secondary to repeated bouts of chronic inflammation.

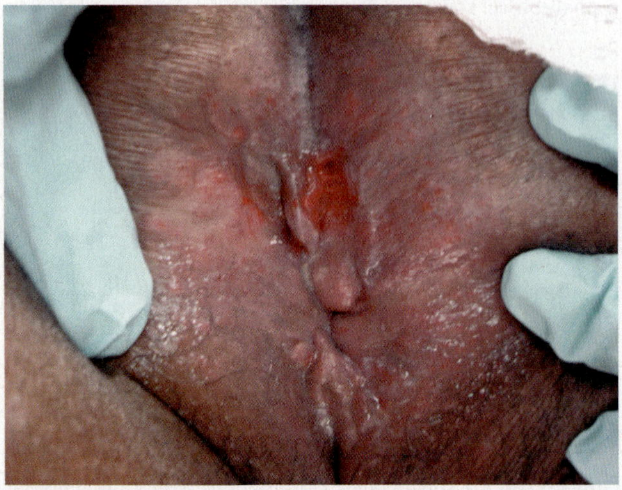

Figure 47.5. Anal fissure in Crohn disease.

Table 47.1. Differential Diagnosis of Crohn Disease

Ulcerative colitis
Irritable bowel syndrome
Acute appendicitis
Diverticulitis
Malignancy
Infectious colitides (CMV, *Yersinia*, *Escherichia coli*, *Salmonella*, etc.)
Clostridium difficile colitis
Ischemic colitis
Pancreatitis
Meckel diverticulum
Tuberculosis
Radiation enteritis
Behçet disease

DIFFERENTIAL DIAGNOSIS

The differential diagnosis for Crohn disease is comprehensive and includes both benign and malignant processes (**Table 47.1**). Crohn disease has certain traits that are highly suggestive of its presence (eg, noncontiguous multisite disease, fistulas, creeping fat) versus other disorders. Yet, a variety of abdominal processes may mimic Crohn disease. For example, ileocolic Crohn disease can be misdiagnosed as acute appendicitis, right-sided diverticulitis, an infectious process, or a perforated malignancy. Radiologic studies may demonstrate patterns of bowel inflammation consistent with Crohn disease, and laboratory examination may reveal elevated CRP and/or white blood cell count. Careful consideration of the differential diagnosis must be taken both preoperatively and intraoperatively.

When the disease is isolated to the colon, the primary differentiation involves distinguishing Crohn colitis from ulcerative colitis, though other infectious and inflammatory colitis remain in the differential. Both diseases share common histopathologic traits, which contribute to the diagnostic dilemma.

Perianal Crohn disease differential diagnosis includes traditional cryptoglandular abscess and fistulas, skin tags may mimic routine hemorrhoids, and/or tags, and infectious causes such as HIV, syphilis, and tuberculosis may share phenotypical manifestations with Crohn. Ultimately, it is the entire evaluation of the individual disease presentation, including information taken from history, laboratory, pathologic, endoscopic, radiologic, and clinical examinations, that will help clarify the picture and aid in diagnosis.

Extraintestinal Disease

Similar to ulcerative colitis, patients with Crohn disease may have manifestations from the disease process that extend outside of the GI tract (**Table 47.2**). Extraintestinal disease (EID) has been reported in 6% to 47% of patients with IBD. It has an increased concordance among siblings and first-degree relatives, suggesting a genetic component that has been linked to the major histocompatibility complex (MHC) on chromosome 6.[23] EID occurs secondary to the systemic inflammatory process associated with the underlying disease and affects a wide range of organ systems. While the GI tract may be the primary source, the dysfunction in immune regulation incites a pathologic response that may occur in nearly every location in the body simultaneously with, preceding, or following GI manifestations. Overall, rheumatologic/joint problems (eg, peripheral or sacroiliac arthritis, arthralgias) are the most common, occurring in up to one-third of patients. Other more frequent sites of involvement include the skin, eyes, and hepatobiliary system, while the renal, pulmonary, nervous, and coagulation systems are involved to a lesser extent. It is important to distinguish between manifestations that parallel bowel disease activity (episcleritis, peripheral arthritis,

Table 47.2. Classification of Extraintestinal Manifestations of Crohn Disease

Organ System	Extraintestinal Manifestation
Musculoskeletal	Arthralgias, peripheral arthritis, ankylosing spondylitis, sacroiliitis, myopathy, metabolic bone disorders
Ocular	Uveitis, iritis, episcleritis, conjunctivitis, optic neuritis
Renal	Glomerulonephritis, amyloidosis, urolithiasis
Skin/Mucocutaneous	Erythema nodosum, pyoderma gangrenosum, aphthous ulcers
Hematologic	Thromboembolic disease, anemia
Pulmonary	Bronchitis, pleuritis, tracheal stenosis
Hepatobiliary	Hepatitis, primary sclerosing cholangitis, primary biliary cirrhosis, pancreatitis, cirrhosis, cholangiocarcinoma, portal vein thrombosis
Cardiac	Pericarditis, myocarditis
Neurologic	Demyelinating disease, neuritis

erythema nodosum) from those that do not (ankylosing spondylitis, pyoderma gangrenosum, primary sclerosing cholangitis) (**Fig. 47.6**). In these cases, EID may flare before the bowel (or in the setting of asymptomatic active bowel disease) and necessitate adjustments in medical management. Conversely, surgical intervention directed at the bowel may occasionally be required for recalcitrant EID that may go into remission following bowel resection.

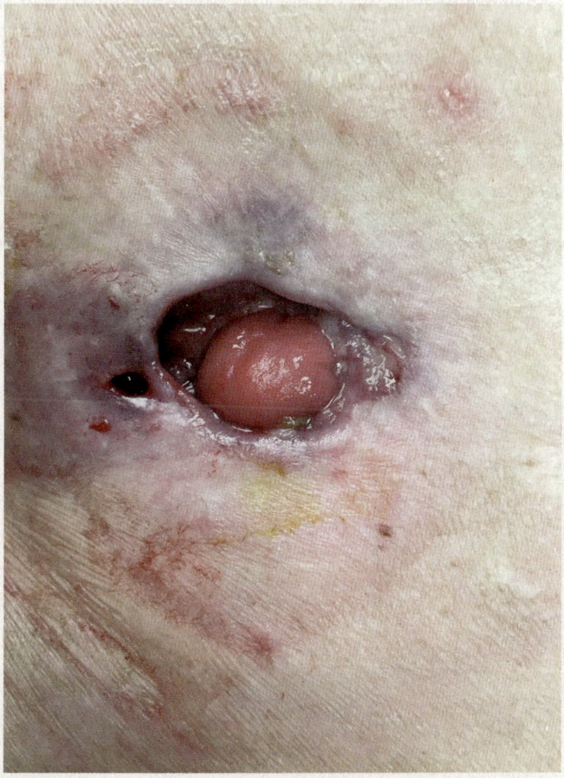

Figure 47.6. Pyoderma gangrenosum surrounding an ileostomy.

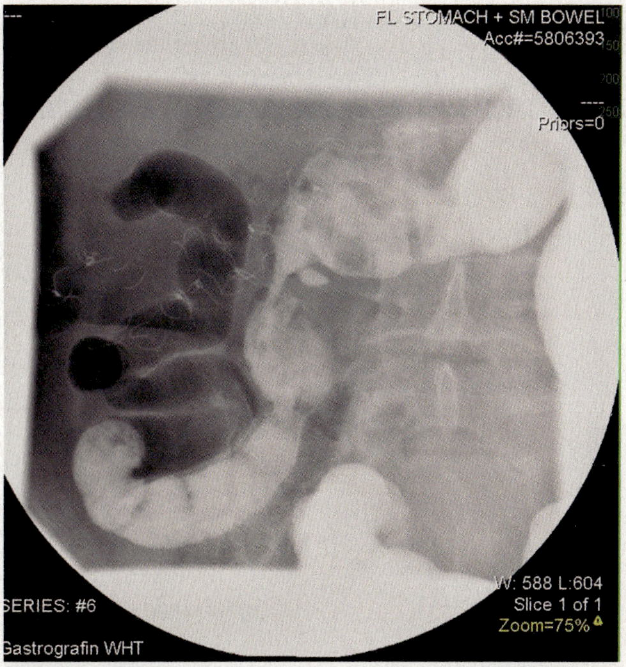

Figure 47.7. Contrast study demonstrating Crohn stricture.

DIAGNOSTIC METHODS

Radiology

Over recent years, the radiographic assessment of Crohn disease has developed dramatically. Previously, fluoroscopic imaging, including small-bowel follow-through or retrograde contrast studies, with barium or gastrograffin contrast was essential. These studies were used to identify ulcerations that create cobblestone and nodular patterns, mucosal granularity, loss of villous morphology, skip lesions, strictures, and fistulas (**Fig. 47.7**). Contrast studies can still provide a wealth of information regarding anatomy and aid in operative planning. Over the years, the utilization of computed tomography enterography (CTE) and magnetic resonance imaging enterography (MRE) has become the most effective method for the evaluation of Crohn disease, and these imaging modalities have been shown to alter treatment course and evaluate response to treatment (**Figs. 47.8** and **47.9**). Both modalities have high sensitivity (>90%) and specificity (>90%) for diagnosing active small-bowel disease. Regarding identifying and quantifying small-bowel disease activity, CTE and MRE are equally sensitive and specific, although CTE has the advantage of better-quality images. MRE is radiation free, which is important for young patients requiring multiple imaging during their lifetime. It is superior to CTE in identifying fistulas and strictures

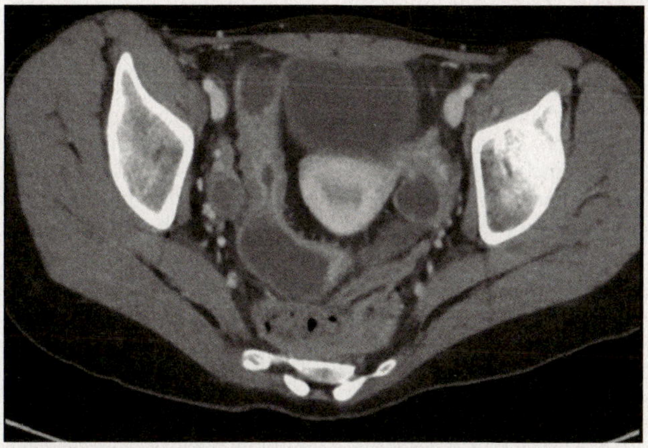

Figure 47.8. CT enterography demonstrating small-bowel stricture.

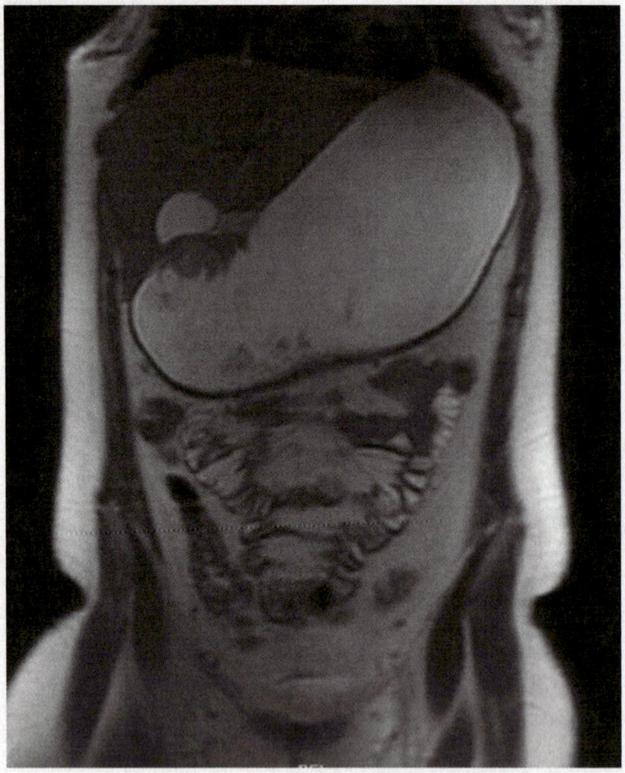

Figure 47.9. MR enterography demonstrating terminal ileal disease in the setting of multifocal disease. This patient also has a duodenal stricture resulting in marked gastric dilation.

and allows real-time imaging to assess peristalsis in segments of suspected disease. Diffusion-weighted imaging can reveal active inflammation without IV contrast. The multiplanar CT or MR enterography distends the bowel with water and neutral contrast agent (VoLumen) and IV contrast bolus, resulting in multiplanar reconstruction. In the acute phase, the hyperenhancing inner mucosa is seen, a density middle ring representing the submucosa edema, engorged vasa recta known as Comb sign, and mesenteric lymphadenopathy.[21] The radiographic findings of transmural healing on CTE and MRE have been shown to correspond to mucosal healing on endoscopic examination in most settings.[25] Although CTE and MRE will include imaging of the pelvis and sphincter complex, if imaging is deemed necessary for perianal fistula or abscess, a standard pelvic MRI should be obtained. Positron emission tomography (PET) and PET-MRI are other modalities that have shown some promise for the evaluation of Crohn disease, though not currently used routinely.

Endoscopy

Endoscopy is an indispensable tool used to identify the extent and severity of the disease and perform biopsies to aid in diagnosis. Endoscopic evaluation of the entire colon, including the terminal ileum, along with appropriate biopsies, is required in patients suspected of Crohn disease. Early changes in the mucosa include aphthous ulcerations, erosions, and serpiginous ulcers that occur in a skip-type pattern. As the full-thickness inflammatory cycle continues, these ulcerated areas progressively enlarge and coalesce, forming a cobblestone-type pattern. Rectal sparing and active terminal ileal disease may help differentiate Crohn disease from ulcerative colitis. However, the latter may demonstrate similar characteristics due to medical therapy and backwash ileitis.[26] Finally, strictures or associated masses may indicate the need for surgical or therapeutic intervention (Fig. 47.10).

4 Patients with Crohn disease should undergo more aggressive malignancy surveillance compared to the general population.

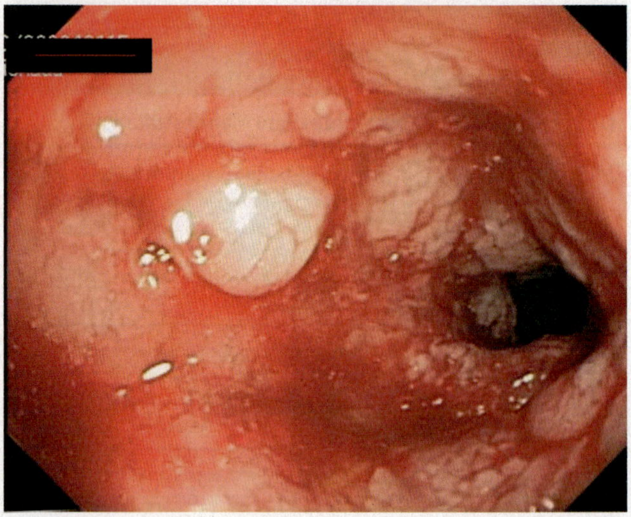

Figure 47.10. Endoscopic view of terminal ileal stricture.

Screening colonoscopy should start 8 to 10 years after the onset of colitis and have repeat examinations every 1 to 2 years.[27] Previous recommendations supported routine biopsies in four quadrants every 10 cm throughout the colon. While high-definition white light endoscopy remains the current recommendation for neoplasia screening in IBD, recently, there has been a shift toward using chromoendoscopy. Compared to white light endoscopy, chromoendoscopy using methylene blue or indigo carmine demonstrates higher rates of both adenoma and dysplasia detection.[28] Narrow-band imaging (NBI) can be helpful for adenoma detection in a healthy colon; however, due to the presence of background inflammation in the setting of Crohn disease, NBI is not recommended as an adjunct for endoscopic surveillance in these patients.[29] Patients with chronic disease may demonstrate pseudopolyps on endoscopic examination (**Fig. 47.11**). Pseudopolyps are masses of scar tissue representing the formation of granulation tissue resulting from alternating cycles of ulceration and regeneration. In general, they are benign and do not warrant intervention, but will make for increasing difficulty with screening for colorectal cancer with more severe incidence.

Esophagogastroduodenoscopy (EGD) also plays a role for patients with suspected or known proximal disease and can identify ulcers, fistulas, and strictures that may be responsible for various upper GI symptoms. In addition, therapeutic interventions (eg, dilation, needle-knife) can be performed through the scope. Overall, both upper and lower endoscopy are relatively safe procedures, with complications in IBD patients

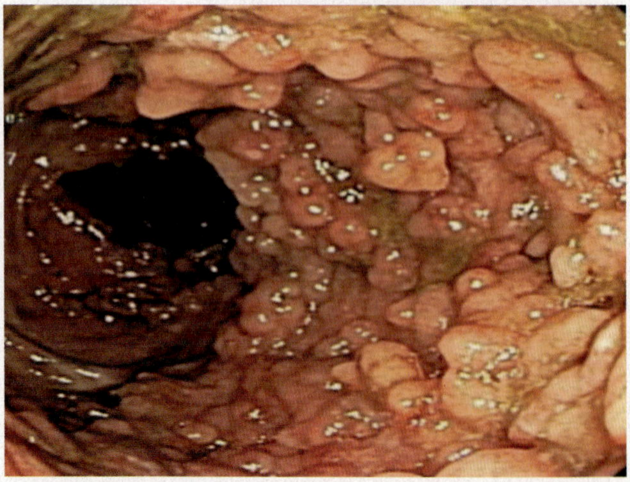

Figure 47.11. Colonic pseudopolyps.

Table 47.3. Clinical Endoscopic Scoring Systems for Crohn Disease

Simple Endoscopic Score for Crohn Disease (SES-CD)

Severity	0	1	2	3
Size of ulcers	None	<0.5 cm	0.5–2 cm	>2 cm
Ulcerated surface	None	<10%	10–30%	>30%
Inflamed surface	None	<50%	50–75%	>75%
Stenosis	None	Single, passable	Multiple, passable	Not passable
Each segment of bowel is assigned values for all four severity variables.				

Crohn Disease Endoscopic Index of Severity

	Rectum	Sigmoid and Left Colon	Transverse Colon	Right Colon	Ileum	Total
Deep ulceration (0 = absent; 12 = present)						1
Superficial ulceration (0 = absent; 6 = present)						2
Surface involved by the disease (cm)						3
Ulcerated surface measured (cm)						4
Total 1 + total 2 + total 3 + total 4 =						A
Number (n) of segments explored =						n
Total A divided by n						B
Ulcerated stenosis anywhere: 0 = absent, 3 = present						C
Nonulcerated stenosis anywhere: 0 = absent; 3 = present						D
Total score = B + C + D						CDEIS

including bleeding, though perforation remains a minimal risk of every endoscopic procedure. Additionally, endoscopic evaluation provides an ability to track and quantify disease activity by use of scoring systems such as the Crohn Disease Endoscopic Index of Severity (CDEIS) or Simple Endoscopic Score for Crohn Disease (SES-CD) (**Table 47.3**).[30]

The detection of small-bowel Crohn disease presents its own challenge when the disease is beyond the reach of a gastroscope or colonoscope. Enteroscopy is helpful in assessing mucosal disease in real-time, identifying abnormal mucosa, and undertaking therapy with pneumatic balloon dilation.

Video capsule endoscopy uses wireless technology to capture continuous images of the upper GI tract mucosa to help determine disease presence and activity beyond endoscopy's reach and the limitations of traditional small-bowel imaging. While the diagnostic yield may not be as high, it is comparable to ileocolonoscopy and better than small-bowel follow-through for detecting small-bowel inflammation. Furthermore, negative predictive values range from 96% to 100%, essentially ruling out the diagnosis of Crohn disease when the results are normal. Of note, it is imperative to exclude moderate–severe strictures before their use, as their presence can result in bowel obstruction from the capsule lodged at the stenosis point (**Fig. 47.12**).[31]

Pathology

The presence of noncaseating granulomas on pathologic examination is pathognomonic of Crohn disease. However, they are only found in 25% to 42% of patients and may be a marker of more virulent disease. Also, a small subset of long-standing ulcerative colitis patients may have granulomas on biopsy.[32] Routine depth endoscopic biopsies may miss granulomas; often, they are only visible on resected full-thickness specimens. Other histologic evidence of Crohn disease includes architectural distortion of the crypts (size, shape, symmetry), ulcerations, pseudopolyps, and skip areas—some of which may also be found in ulcerative colitis (**Fig. 47.13**). Other discriminating features of Crohn disease on gross examination include the potential for full-thickness involvement of the bowel wall and the presence of "creeping fat," where the mesenteric fat extends over the serosal surface of the bowel wall—"creeping"

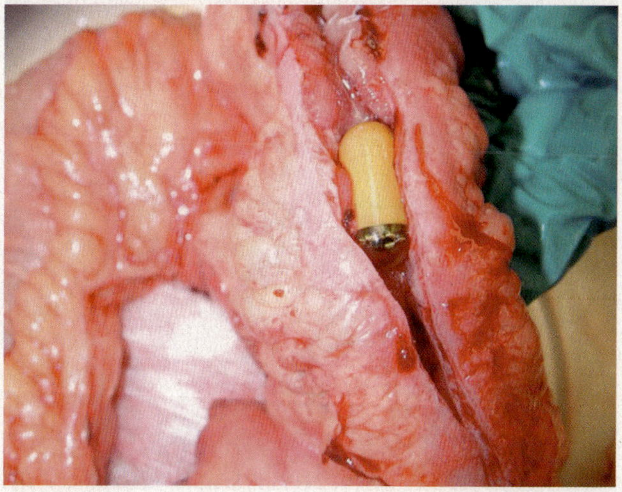

Figure 47.12. Capsule endoscopy pill lodged in small-bowel stricture.

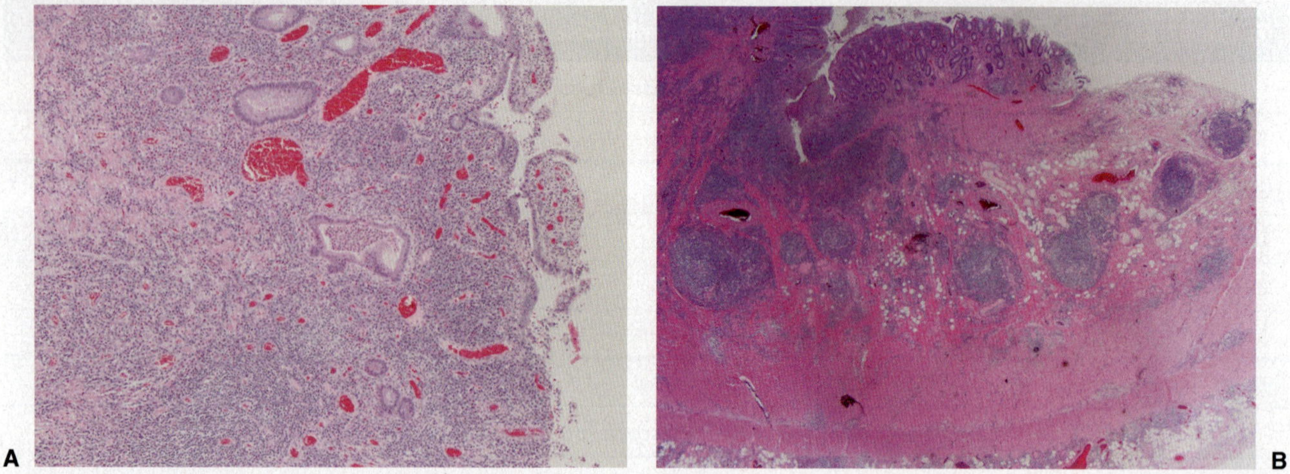

Figure 47.13. **A:** Active colitis with crypt abscess formation and atypical regenerative features consistent with chronic crypt-destructive colitis. (Courtesy of George Leonard, MD.) **B:** Full-thickness involvement of chronic inflammatory infiltrate from mucosa to serosa and pseudopolyp formation. (Courtesy of George Leonard, MD.)

over the ordinarily distinct mesenteric/bowel wall interface (**Fig. 47.14**). Furthermore, gross pathologic examination of Crohn disease specimens may range from acutely inflamed, edematous, hyperemic bowel to thickened, fibrotic, and "woody." Finally, the mesentery is classically thickened, with increased edema, friability, and vascularity.

Laboratory Analysis

No single laboratory examination will provide a definitive diagnosis of Crohn disease, yet there are tests available to help discriminate between Crohn and other processes. Though not recommended for routine use, serum measurements of perinuclear antineutrophil cytoplasmic antibodies (p-ANCAs) and antisaccharomyces cerevisiae antibodies (ASCAs) can be used to help differentiate Crohn disease from ulcerative colitis. The former is a known marker associated with ulcerative colitis, whereas elevated levels of ASCA are associated with Crohn disease. Unfortunately, only 30% to 50% of Crohn patients will test positive for ASCA, and up to 10% of healthy individuals will also have elevated serum levels.[33]

C-reactive protein is a nonspecific marker for inflammation that has been useful in tracking disease activity and response to treatment. More recently, fecal biomarkers such as fecal calprotectin, lactoferrin, and neopterin are used to monitor intestinal inflammation and have been shown to reliably correlate with endoscopic disease activity and response to anti-TNF therapy. While nonspecific, elevations in fecal biomarkers have also been shown to correlate with higher levels of recurrence following surgical resection.[34]

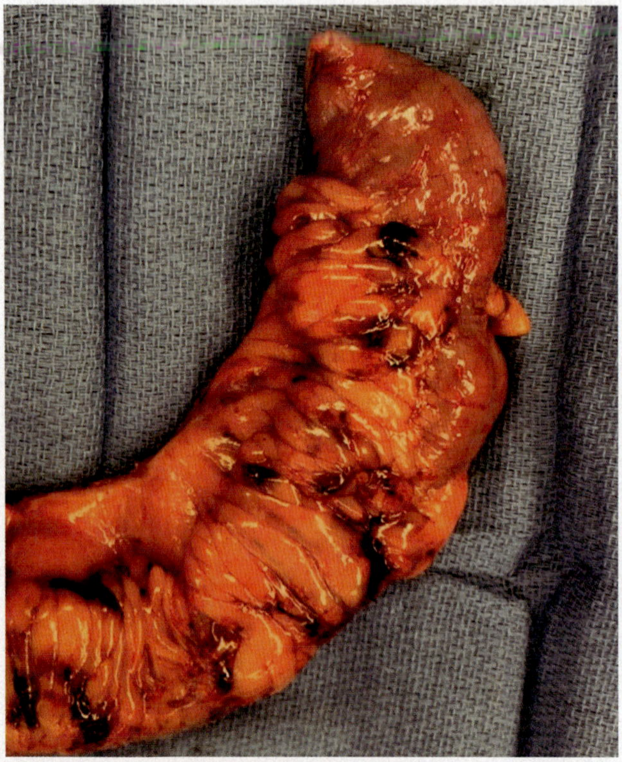

Figure 47.14. Creeping fat along terminal ileum.

TREATMENT

Medical Management

Nutritional Management

5 While an in-depth discussion of the medical management of Crohn disease is beyond the scope of this chapter, a few points are worth noting. First, despite the spectrum of disease presentations, Crohn remains one hallmarked by inflammation (ie, abdominal pain) and diarrhea. Supportive care that includes antidiarrheal and antimotility agents, along with a bland diet, is a good first-line approach to providing symptomatic control. It is important to exclude the concomitant presence of "superinfections" such as cytomegalovirus or *C. difficile* infection, as antimotility medications may result in the onset of toxic megacolon and a rapidly progressive clinical deterioration. Endoscopic biopsies can rule these out in addition to stool studies. Simple over-the-counter, readily available medications such as loperamide and bismuth, along with prescription medications such as diphenoxylate, codeine, and tincture of opium, often provide tremendous relief from abdominal pain, cramping, and loose stools.

Nutritional support in all patients with Crohn disease is paramount. Ideally, preservation of oral feeding in any form is crucial for maintaining the absorptive and protective mechanisms provided by the GI mucosal lumen villi and microvilli. Exclusive enteral nutrition involves an entirely liquid diet using formula per nasal tube or orally for 6 to 8 weeks, followed by slow reintroduction of other foods. This is the first-line therapy for the treatment of Crohn disease in pediatric patients, as it avoids growth suppression associated with steroids and has been shown to result in complete mucosal healing in adults as well. When enteral intake is impossible, parenteral nutrition is invaluable in preserving nutritional stores, maintaining positive nitrogen balance, preventing weight loss, and improving perioperative outcomes. This must be weighed against the potential complications of intravenous routes, including infectious complications and thromboembolic events.[35]

Table 47.4. Available Medications for Crohn Disease

Class of Medication	Examples	Role in Therapy
Antibiotics	Metronidazole	Induction of remission Treatment of infection
5-ASA	Mesalamine Olsalazine Sulfasalazine	Maintenance of remission in mild cases
Steroids	Budesonide[a] Methylprednisolone Prednisone Prednisolone	Induction of remission
Immunomodulators	6-Mercaptopurine Azathioprine Cyclosporine[b] Methotrexate Tacrolimus	Induction and maintenance of remission
Biologics	Adalimumab Certolizumab Infliximab Natalizumab Ustekinumab Vedolizumab	Induction and maintenance of remission
Small molecules	Tofacitinib Upadacitinib Filgotinib Deucravacitinib Ozanimod Brepocitinib Cobitolimod	

[a]Budesonide is taken enterally and has only topical effect, no systemic effect.
[b]Cyclosporine can be used as rescue therapy/induction in refractory cases, but has not been supported by evidence in the treatment of Crohn disease.

Pharmacologic Management

6 As there is no cure for Crohn disease, medical management aims to achieve symptom control and remission. Many medications are approved for the treatment of Crohn disease. Medical management can be classified based on disease phenotype and severity. Disease severity can be mild, moderate, severe, or medically refractory. There are several classes of medications used to treat Crohn disease, including probiotics, antibiotics, 5-aminosalicylate (5-ASA) compounds, glucocorticoids, immunomodulators, and biologic agents with differing mechanisms of action and purpose of use (**Table 47.4**).

Patients with mild-to-moderate disease can be treated with sulfasalazine agents or mesalamine (Pentasa, Asacol). Multiple trials demonstrated the benefits of sulfasalazine for ileal, ileocolonic, and colonic diseases. 5-ASA compounds are released at various locations along the digestive tract and control apoptosis, cell proliferation, inflammation, and metabolite function. These drugs must be taken with folic acid supplementation. Previously, these drugs were the standard therapy for the treatment of Crohn disease; however, several trials have not shown benefit over placebo. There is no role for 5-ASA drugs in the induction of remission in Crohn disease. Side effects of 5-ASA compounds include GI upset, headache, bone marrow suppression, hemolytic anemia, hepatitis, fever, hypersensitivity reactions, pancreatitis, pneumonia, and rash. Patients with mild disease may still be useful as frontline agents.[36]

In contrast, corticosteroids are more effective in managing active Crohn disease and remission induction. Glucocorticoids are frequently used for moderate-to-severe disease. They function by modulating the immune response, inhibiting the expression of adhesion molecules, and decreasing inflammatory cells infiltrating the intestine. The side effect profile of these drugs limits their use to acute episodes. Budesonide is an oral glucocorticoid with minimal systemic absorption that works topically in the terminal ileum and proximal colon. Remission induction is achieved at a dose of 9 mg daily for 8 weeks and then tapered to a maintenance dose of 6 mg/d. Prednisone is a systemically absorbed glucocorticoid that can be used for induction of remission at a dose of 40 to 60 mg/d and tapered down after 2 to 6 weeks until discontinuation of the medication. Side effects include acne, hyperglycemia, hypertension, mood disruption, moon facies, weight gain, glaucoma, cataracts, insomnia, osteonecrosis, osteoporosis, and adrenal suppression. Patients should be closely monitored for symptom response as they may develop "steroid-resistant" or "steroid-dependent" disease and should be considered for additional therapies, including surgery. Alternatives to steroid therapy for inducing remission are azathioprine and 6-mercaptopurine.

Immunomodulators, such as thiopurines and methotrexate, are another class of medications used for induction and maintenance of remission. The addition of these medications can also allow for tapering of glucocorticoids. Thiopurines, 6-MP and its precursor, azathioprine, interfere with nucleic acid metabolism, and a clinical improvement can typically be seen 6 to 12 weeks following initiation of therapy. Before starting therapy, thiopurine methyltransferase (TMPT) levels should be measured, and the drug should not be given if levels are deficient. Side effects include nausea, vomiting, an increase in liver enzymes, pancreatitis, leukopenia, and lymphoma. A complete blood count should be monitored routinely. Methotrexate is a folic acid analog used for both induction and maintenance of remission that has inhibitory activity against enzymes in the metabolic pathway of folic acid. This leads to decreased production of inflammatory mediators via accumulation of adenosine through thymidylate, purine, and methionine inhibition. Patients must take folic acid supplementation along with the medication. Side effects include GI upset, stomatitis, leukopenia, hepatic fibrosis, hypersensitivity reactions, and pneumonitis.

When considering the treatment strategy for patients with Crohn disease, it is crucial to keep in mind the goals of treatment, which include resolution of current inflammation and resultant symptoms and prevention of the risk of long-term complications. With these goals at the forefront, it is necessary to consider several patient-specific factors such as age, extent of inflammation, severity of symptoms, nutritional status, and long-term function.

A new era of biologic medical therapy started in 1998 after the FDA approved infliximab. Antitumor necrosis factor (TNF) monoclonal antibodies have shown induction of remission of active luminal disease, relapse of quiescent luminal disease, healing, and prevention of fistula in Crohn disease. The anti-
5 TNF agents infliximab, adalimumab, and certolizumab are the most widely used and are now considered first-line agents in the treatment of Crohn disease. Infliximab is given by intravenous infusion with a loading dose followed by biweekly or monthly maintenance doses. Adalimumab and certolizumab are given as subcutaneous injections. All three drugs have similar response rates. Drugs should be monitored closely as side effects, and the development of antibodies can occur. Side effects of these medications include a risk of infection, tuberculosis autoimmune reactions, liver dysfunction, heart failure, lymphoma, and multiple sclerosis. Before starting these medications, patients should be tested for tuberculosis and hepatitis.[37]

Additional biologic agents have been developed for patients with loss of response or contraindications to anti-TNF class. These include target integrins (natalizumab, vedolizumab) and interleukin-12/23 (ustekinumab, risankizumab). Both drugs are useful for the induction and maintenance of remission. These drugs must also be monitored closely. Natalizumab is FDA approved for the treatment of Crohn disease after the failure of anti-TNF agents. This medication has been shown to have the potential for progressive multifocal leukoencephalopathy and should be monitored closely. Vedolizumab is an anti-inflammatory drug that works through inhibition of cell adhesion molecules. This medication is well tolerated and has been shown not to have an increased risk of infectious complications or lymphoma. Ustekinumab, an inhibitor of IL-12 and IL-23, has been shown to have efficacy in the induction and maintenance of disease with a limited side effect profile. The infection profile of this medication is like that of placebo, and the risk of malignancy mirrors that of the general population.[38]

Recently, small-molecule agents were introduced. These can be administered orally and include JAK-kinase inhibitors, such as tofacitinib, filgotinib, and upadacitinib.

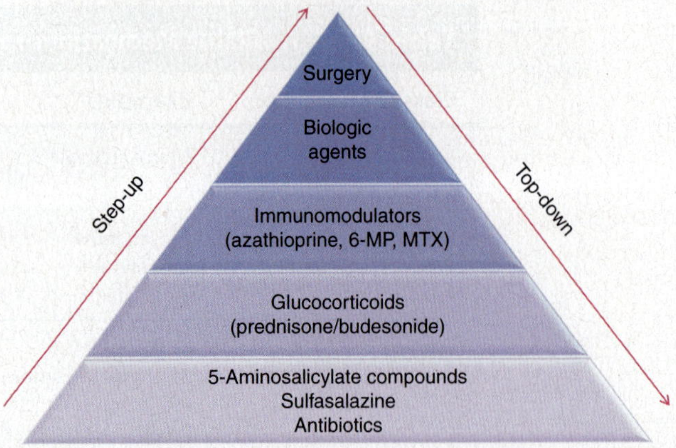

Figure 47.15. Step-up and top-down treatment strategies for Crohn disease.

Initially, biologic agents were only administered to patients with severe disease requiring surgery for disease complications. However, multiple randomized trials have found that overall remission rates were higher with biologics when administered to patients within 2 years of diagnosis. With that, biologics are given before developing strictures and for patients at higher risk for disease-related complications. As more classes of biologic therapy are approved, patients now often prefer to receive alternative classes of biologic agents rather than going to surgery. Furthermore, patients now more often present to the operating room with more advanced diseases and longer duration of immunosuppression. Importantly, in the prebiologic era, up to 30% of patients who underwent surgery would require another operation within 10 years. In biologics, only 10% will need another operation 8 years after the first surgery.[39]

Probiotics, which are typically not harmful, may have the effect of altering the gut microbiome; however, no randomized control trials or meta-analyses have demonstrated this consistently. The influence of antibiotics on the remission of Crohn disease remains unclear. Though there currently are no antibiotics approved by the Federal Drug Administration specifically for the treatment of inflammation in Crohn disease, they may aid in remission and decrease relapse. Metronidazole can be used for the treatment of symptoms of perianal Crohn disease, and there are some data to suggest that rifaximin may be beneficial in maintaining remission.

There are two general approaches to the treatment of Crohn disease (**Fig. 47.15**). Traditionally, a "step-up" approach was taken where less effective medications are started first with an incremental increase to more effective medications, which are potentially riskier (**Table 47.5**). The other approach is a

Table 47.5. Medications for the Induction of Remission of Crohn Disease

	Ileum	Colon	Upper GI
Mild	Budesonide	Sulfasalazine Systemic steroids	Systemic steroids Immunomodulators
Moderate	Budesonide or systemic steroid or antibiotics if sepsis Consider anti-TNF	Systemic steroids If relapse: anti-TNF ± immunomodulators Discuss surgery	Systemic steroids If relapse: anti-TNF ± immunomodulators Discuss surgery
Severe	Systemic steroids If relapse: anti-TNF ± immunomodulators Discuss surgery Infrequent relapse: steroid + immunomodulator	Systemic steroids If relapse: anti-TNF ± immunomodulators Discuss surgery	Systemic steroids + immunomodulators If relapse: anti-TNF ± immunomodulators

"top-down" approach, in which the more aggressive medications are initiated despite the potential for greater risk. There are advantages and disadvantages to both approaches, and they must be individually weighed for each patient with close monitoring for safety. This may include monitoring serum drug levels of biologic agents, which has recently become clinically helpful in guiding therapy. Drug levels of adalimumab >8.5 μg/mL are associated with decreased levels of serum CRP, fecal calprotectin levels, and endoscopic mucosal healing.[40] Multidisciplinary management and close discussion with medical colleagues, primarily gastroenterology, nutrition therapy, radiology, and medical psychology, are extremely useful in this aspect, especially when patients may require surgical treatment while on certain medications that could affect decision making and outcomes. Before all the medical options are exhausted, the patient should have a surgical consultation about the risks and benefits of operation versus continuation with medical therapy.

PREOPERATIVE CONSIDERATIONS

Total parenteral nutrition may be indicated in severe malnutrition, with more than 5% of body weight loss in 1 month and 10% in 6 months, BMI less than 19 kg/m^2, and albumin less than 3 g/dL. Appropriate nutrition status is paramount in achieving wound and anastomosis healing. Preoperative TPN significantly reduces noninfectious complications. Traditional teaching was that immunosuppressive medications are detrimental for anastomotic healing and are associated with a higher risk of infectious complications. A meta-analysis has shown that infliximab increases the rate of postoperative complications, especially postoperative infections, and thus, the timing of surgery was related to the most recent dose of biologic treatment. Patients with penetrating intra-abdominal disease should be drained nonoperatively with interventional radiology prior to the operating room. Adequate preoperative drainage minimizes the intra-abdominal inflammation, allowing for a more limited bowel resection. Finally, preoperative discussion about temporary or permanent stoma is paramount before proceeding with surgery. Early patients' education and setting of clear preoperative expectations are crucial.[41]

OPERATIVE MANAGEMENT

Indications for Surgery

Surgery is not curative for CD but rather targeted for symptom control, and all efforts should be taken to preserve the bowel length. The basic tenet in the management of Crohn disease is that surgery is typically reserved either for disease refractory to medical therapy or complications from the disease. Refractory disease is still the most common reason for surgery in patients with Crohn disease. Complications resulting in a potential need for operative intervention include fistula, abscess, obstruction (stricture), growth retardation, perforation, EID, bleeding, and malignancy. Of note, hemorrhage in Crohn disease is a rare event and is more commonly seen in ulcerative colitis or diverticular disease. Despite improvements in medical therapy, over 70% of all Crohn patients will require surgery at some point in their lives, with almost half of those requiring additional procedures. Therefore, having a firm understanding of the general principles and technical specifics is vital for surgeons who care for these patients.

General Principles

7 Certain overarching principles guide the planning and operative management. First, Crohn disease is a process marked by lifelong potential for recurrence; therefore, preservation of intestinal length is paramount during the planning phase. During the first operation, a detailed description of the remaining bowel length should be described. The margins of surgical resection should be done to grossly normal bowel and not microscopic. The recurrence of CD is not affected if microscopic CD is present at the margins.

This translates to not only maximizing bowel length, but also ensuring functional bowel. Next, the extent of resection versus intestinal sparing procedures is dependent on multiple factors, including location and duration of disease, indication for surgery, ability to exclude malignancy, and prior resections that may have resulted in shortened small bowel.

8 In addition, as the stools tend to be loose, consideration must be given to rectal compliance and sphincter function during surgical planning to avoid a "perineal colostomy," whereby continuity is preserved. Still, the patient has no sphincter control, significantly affecting quality of life. Furthermore, unlike ulcerative colitis, where removal of the entire colon and rectum is a curative operation, in Crohn disease, a segmental resection for both small and large bowel is often sufficient with ileocolonic, colocolonic, and rectal anastomoses, all playing a role in avoiding a permanent stoma while maximizing functional bowel. Crohn patients with pancolitis may undergo a total abdominal colectomy with ileorectal anastomosis (for those with rectal sparing) or total proctocolectomy with end ileostomy. While there are select patients with Crohn disease whose manifestations are more on the spectrum of ulcerative colitis and may do well with a total proctocolectomy with ileal pouch–anal anastomosis, this is typically discouraged, and is normally the result of an initial misdiagnosis of ulcerative colitis.[42]

Technical tips also come into play when planning for Crohn resections. For example, when performing a proctectomy, it is important to consider the potential for a delayed or nonhealed perineal wound. An intersphincteric dissection, which maximizes the amount of healthy muscle/tissue remaining, helps avoid this complication. Some patients will require more extensive procedures such as flaps (ie, gracilis, myocutaneous thigh), and may require plastic surgeon involvement (**Fig. 47.16**). As with small-bowel resection, the length of the resection margin does not influence the risk of relapse, and resection to a grossly normal bowel is all that is required. Finally, diversion is more commonly used due to both the presence of active disease as well as the potential negative healing effects of the Crohn medications.

In the case of suspected acute appendicitis in a patient with unknown Crohn disease, careful consideration should be paid to the extent of resection–ileocectomy versus appendectomy alone. Traditional teaching recommends performing an appendectomy alone if the cecum is normal or withholding resection and undergoing medical treatment only. Performing an appendectomy in the setting of cecal inflammation leaves the patient at risk of developing a perforation and/or fistula at that site.

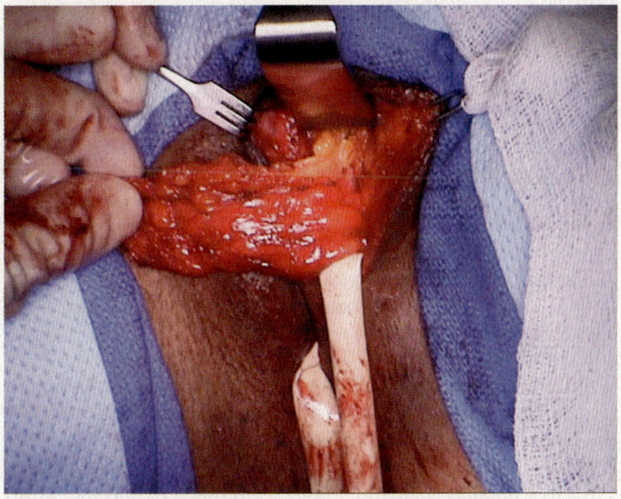

Figure 47.16. Bulbocavernosus flap for rectovaginal fistula (Martius flap).

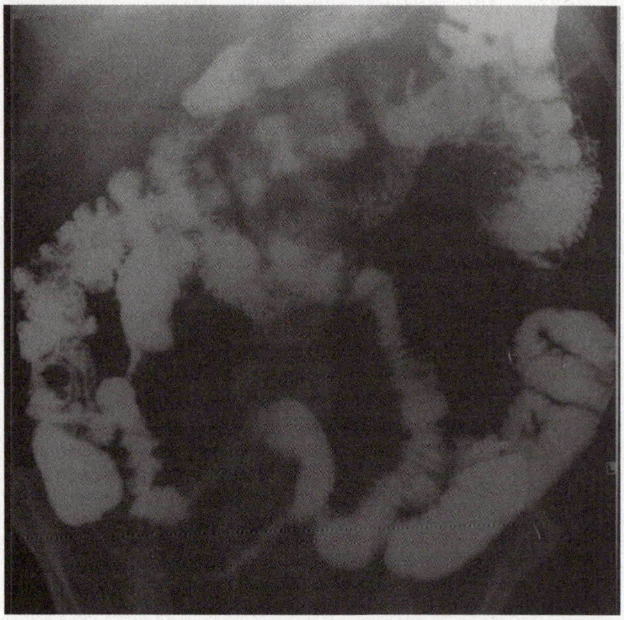

Figure 47.17. Multiple strictures demonstrated on small-bowel follow-through.

However, ileocolonic resection for isolated disease may be in the patient's long-term best interests, with one series reporting that almost half of patients required no further surgery, compared to 92% of those undergoing appendectomy only. A complete evaluation of the GI tract should be performed at the time of surgery.

Strictures in Crohn disease most commonly occur in the terminal ileum, but may arise anywhere along the GI tract (**Fig. 47.17**). Due to the transmural inflammation, it is not uncommon to have luminal narrowing within the bowel, especially with repeated flares. However, the underlying cause of obstruction may be from external compression from a phlegmonous/inflammatory process or secondary to the fibrostenotic pattern of disease. In the former, medical management may be successful by decreasing the inflammation and resolving the compression on the bowel wall, though surgery may still be required if symptoms are refractory to medical therapy. Patients with fibrotic strictures typically have little to no response to medical management and most often require surgery. Emerging evidence suggests that early treatment of strictures with aggressive biologic therapy may aid in preventing the onset of fibrosis, especially in patients under.[40]

Strictures also differ based on their location. The rate of colonic strictures has been reported to be as high as 7% to 17%. Generally, these benign strictures are responsive to medical management and endoscopic dilation for moderate- to high-grade stenosis. EGD and push enteroscopy allow for therapeutic intervention, such as dilation, for those with gastric outlet obstruction. Inflammatory strictures tend to have an ulcer in the mucosal surface at the mesenteric side of the bowel and have the risk of bleeding. Strictures of the small bowel have been reported in 20% to 40% of Crohn patients.[43] Treatment typically consists of medical management, though depending on the severity of obstructive symptoms, many patients will require intervention. Small-bowel strictures are often amenable to dilation if accessible via double-balloon enteroscopy. Symptomatic relief occurs in 75% to 90% following the first dilation, while approximately 30% to 40% will require repeated intervention. For those with initial success, the cumulative dilation-free rate at three years is 40% to 50%. Overall, complications occur in 10% to 15% (<5% significant complications), and include pain, fistula, fevers, bleeding, and perforation. Despite this success, many will require operative intervention when symptoms fail to resolve, repeated bouts occur, or when a stricture is associated with a nonresolving inflammatory process, malnutrition, immunosuppression, or fistula. Surgical options then include stricturoplasty or resection, the latter required in the presence of a malignant stricture in the setting of Crohn disease (**Fig. 47.18**).[44]

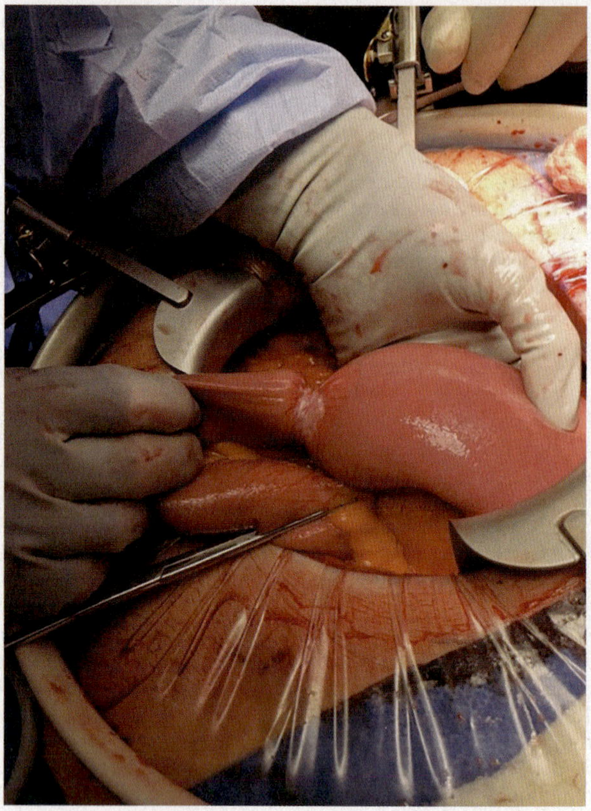

Figure 47.18. Malignant stricture in setting of Crohn disease.

Stricturoplasty can be performed to address fibrostenotic disease in the absence of inflammation and acts to preserve bowel length by avoiding resection altogether (**Fig. 47.19**). There are several surgical techniques based on the length of the stricture. The Heineke–Mikulicz method involves a longitudinal incision along the antimesenteric border of the bowel with a transverse closure and is useful for shorter bowel segments. The Finney stricturoplasty, classically used for longer strictures of 7 to 15 cm in length, involves a longitudinal enterotomy along the length of the diseased segment of the intestine. The bowel is then folded upon itself, creating a full-thickness anastomosis. Finally, for longer strictures, the Michelassi stricturoplasty involves dividing the stricture and

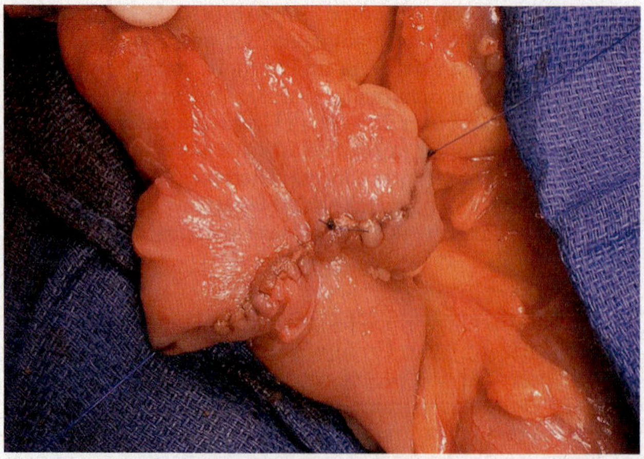

Figure 47.19. Small-bowel stricturoplasty.

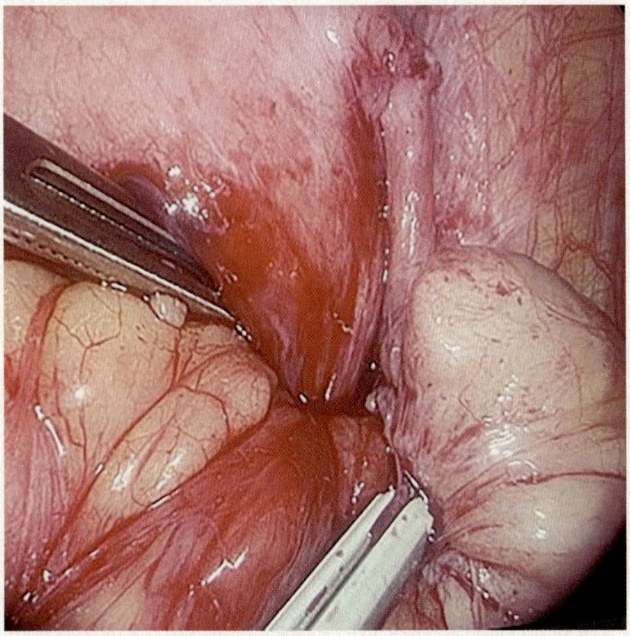

Figure 47.20. Ileouterine fistula.

its associated mesentery in the middle of the length of the stricture. The intestine overlaps in an isoperistaltic fashion, and longitudinal enterotomies are created along the length of the strictured bowel and anastomosed. Complications have been reported in 4% to 15% of large series and include obstruction, bleeding, sepsis, perforation, and death. Contraindications to stricturoplasty include malnutrition, presence of a phlegmon/perforation/fistula at the site, multiple strictures within a small segment, and suspicion of a malignancy.

Recurrence of stricture may occur at the prior stricturoplasty site, in particular just proximal to it. Strictures at prior anastomotic sites may occur from recurrent disease or secondary to technical problems. They are often amenable to dilation, yet failure is high, thus requiring resection for symptomatic strictures. There are some data to suggest that side-to-side stapled ileocolic anastomoses have a decreased rate of postoperative complications, including leak, recurrence, and reoperation, when compared to hand-sewn end-to-end anastomoses.[45]

Intra-abdominal fistulas may arise from small or large bowel and affect any adjacent structure. It is important to determine the site of origin of the fistula, as this section of the bowel will typically require a formal resection. On the other hand, the adjacent organ may be involved in the process secondarily without primary disease involvement. Therefore, it is important to evaluate the adjacent organ, when possible (such as the colon in an ileosigmoid fistula), to ensure there is no active disease that will need to be addressed (**Fig. 47.20**). The preferred treatment is to take the fistula down, resect the diseased segment of bowel, and primarily repair the adjacent site. If there is concern for active disease in the adjacent site, such as in the above example with the ileosigmoid fistula, the preferred strategy would be to perform a concomitant colonic resection. Transmural bowel inflammation and communication can also occur with the skin, bladder, uterus, ureter, or vagina. Once again, the bowel is the offending organ and should be resected, while ligation of the fistula and closure of the secondarily involved organ is adequate treatment. These organs do not have the potential for active Crohn disease, and they can often be repaired. If the inflammatory process is severe or there is a concern for concomitant malignancy, the entire process should be resected en bloc with appropriate reconstruction. Finally, asymptomatic enteroenteric or enterocolonic fistulas do not require surgery and medical treatment, especially with biologic agents that have relatively good success.[46]

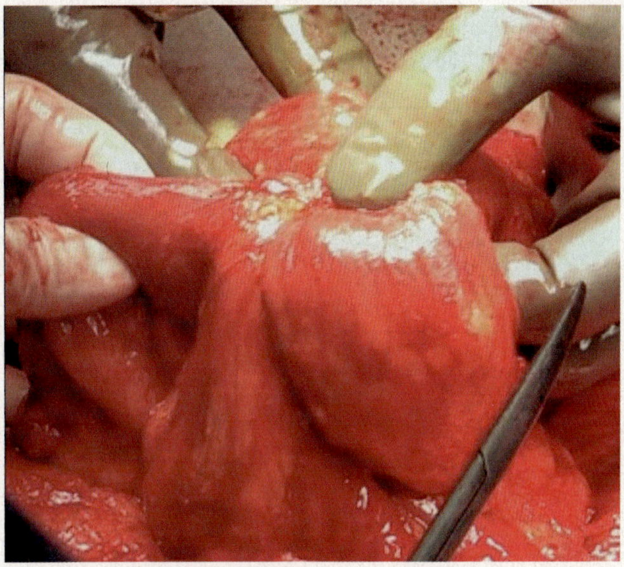

Figure 47.21. Colonic stricture.

Treatment for malignancy in Crohn patients is similar to that of the general population, with resection following standard oncologic principles. As synchronous and metachronous lesions have been reported in up to 10%, consideration should be given to a subtotal colectomy with ileorectal anastomosis in the absence of rectal lesions. However, segmental colectomy has been well described in Crohn disease.

Malignancy is present in approximately 7% of all colonic strictures, and Crohn disease carries an increased risk of colorectal cancer above the general population. It is challenging to differentiate malignant from benign strictures clinically therefore all colonic strictures should typically undergo endoscopic evaluation and biopsy. If malignancy is suspected, a standard oncologic resection should be performed (**Fig. 47.21**). For those that are benign and nonresponsive to medical management, endoscopic dilation has been shown to provide symptomatic relief in over 80% of patients, with most patients with colonic strictures requiring repeated dilations.

SPECIFIC CONSIDERATIONS

Ileocolic and Small-Bowel Disease (Algorithm 47.1)

Following resection, consideration should be given to the patient's nutritional status, medications, and overall physiologic state, as diverting stoma may be required to minimize the incidence and consequences of an anastomotic leak. As the rate of perioperative complications tends to be higher in this population, a minimally invasive approach has been associated with improved short-term outcomes in Crohn disease patients, including decreased morbidity and shorter length of stay for both primary and recurrent disease (**Table 47.6**).

The mesentery in active Crohn disease always presents a particular challenge for surgeons. Traditionally, the mesentery is thick, edematous in nature, with increased neovascularization, and was felt to be a bystander of the disease. At the same time, recent studies elucidated the phenomenon of creeping fat to be related to gut microbiota translocation into mesenteric lymph nodes and adipose tissue. Extended mesenteric excision was described and is associated with decreased surgical recurrence compared to historic controls (40% vs 2.9%, $P < .0003$.) Dr. Kono described the exclusion of mesentery by constructing supporting columns. SuPREME-CD randomized trial demonstrated that Kono-S is independently associated with decreased endoscopic recurrence.[47]

Safe mesenteric division involves techniques such as overlapping clamps with mass and individual vessel suture ligation where appropriate. Minimally invasive approaches typically

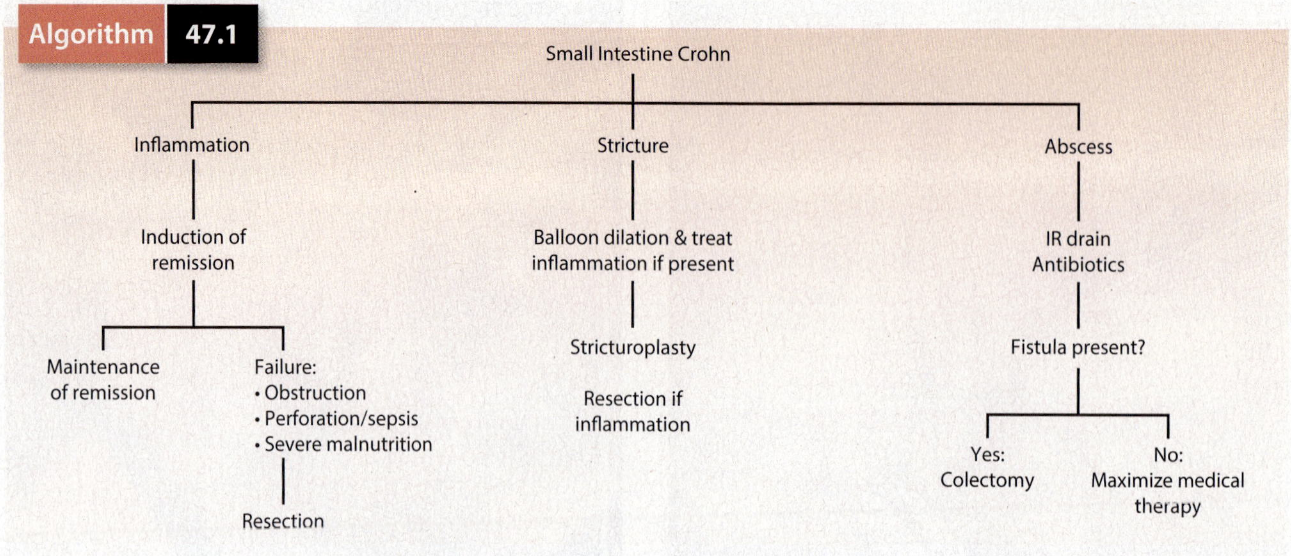

Algorithm 47.1. Management of small-bowel disease in Crohn disease.

rely on advanced vessel-sealing devices for hemostasis. However, they may be inadequate in Crohn disease patients, and conversion to an open procedure may be necessary to control hemorrhage. Avoiding mesenteric hematomas is crucial, as these may result in continued bleeding and compromise the blood supply to the healthy remaining bowel. Recently, wide resection of the mesentery in Crohn disease, similar to that of an oncologic resection, has been shown to decrease the need for reoperation and decrease future recurrence of Crohn disease.

The recommended type of anastomosis used to restore continuity following resection is variable. Options include stapled or handsewn, antiperistaltic, isoperistaltic, end-to-end, and end-to-side. The Kono-S–type anastomosis is a novel antimesenteric end-to-end handsewn anastomosis thought to prevent the recurrence of Crohn disease (**Fig. 47.22**).

Colorectal Conditions

Toxic colitis may occur in Crohn disease patients, similar to those with ulcerative colitis (**Algorithm 47.2**). Following resuscitation and intravenous steroids or immunosuppressants, emergent surgical intervention is required for those with recalcitrant disease, perforation, or a deteriorating clinical state. The operative procedure of choice is a subtotal colectomy with end ileostomy. Debate exists regarding the handling of the rectal stump. However, options include a distal mucus fistula with remnant sigmoid, implantation into the subcutaneous space, local reinforcement of the stump, and short stump with intra-abdominal drain. Proctocolectomy should be avoided in this situation due to the prolonged operative time and increased risk of morbidity and mortality.[48]

An ileoanal pouch in the patient with Crohn disease is most commonly encountered in the setting of an initial diagnosis of ulcerative colitis, with manifestations of Crohn disease at a later stage.[49] While specific expert centers may advocate total proctocolectomy and ileal pouch construction for highly select patients with Crohn disease, in general, this is to be discouraged. Retrospective studies have reported 35% to 93% of patients will have Crohn-related complications such as pouchitis, abscesses, and pouch–anal fistulas, with another 10% requiring pouch excision or permanent diversion. Cumulative Kaplan Meier 5-year pouch survival was 80% versus 60% in index and redo IPAA ($P < .0001$), at 10 years 74% versus 38%, respectively ($P < .0001$).

Furthermore, roughly half of patients will experience urgency or continence issues. Of those patients with a

Table 47.6. Perioperative Complications of Bowel Resection in Crohn Patients[a]

Complication[a]	Incidence (%)
Bleeding	1–5
Anastomotic leak	1.3–17[b]
Anastomotic stricture	6–13
Anastomotic recurrence of disease	15–39
Bowel obstruction/ileus	5–23
Abscess/intra-abdominal sepsis (excluding leak)	2.1–15
Surgical site infection	10–33
Venous thromboembolic event	1.4–3.3

[a]Risk factors: malnutrition, obesity, emergent surgery, immunosuppressant use, smoking, older age, open approach, stoma surgery.
[b]Depending on location and definition (clinical vs radiologic).

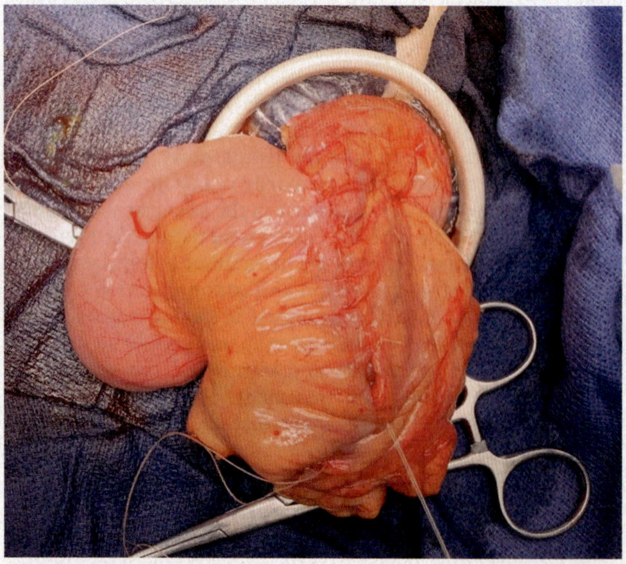

Figure 47.22. Kono-S–type anastomosis.

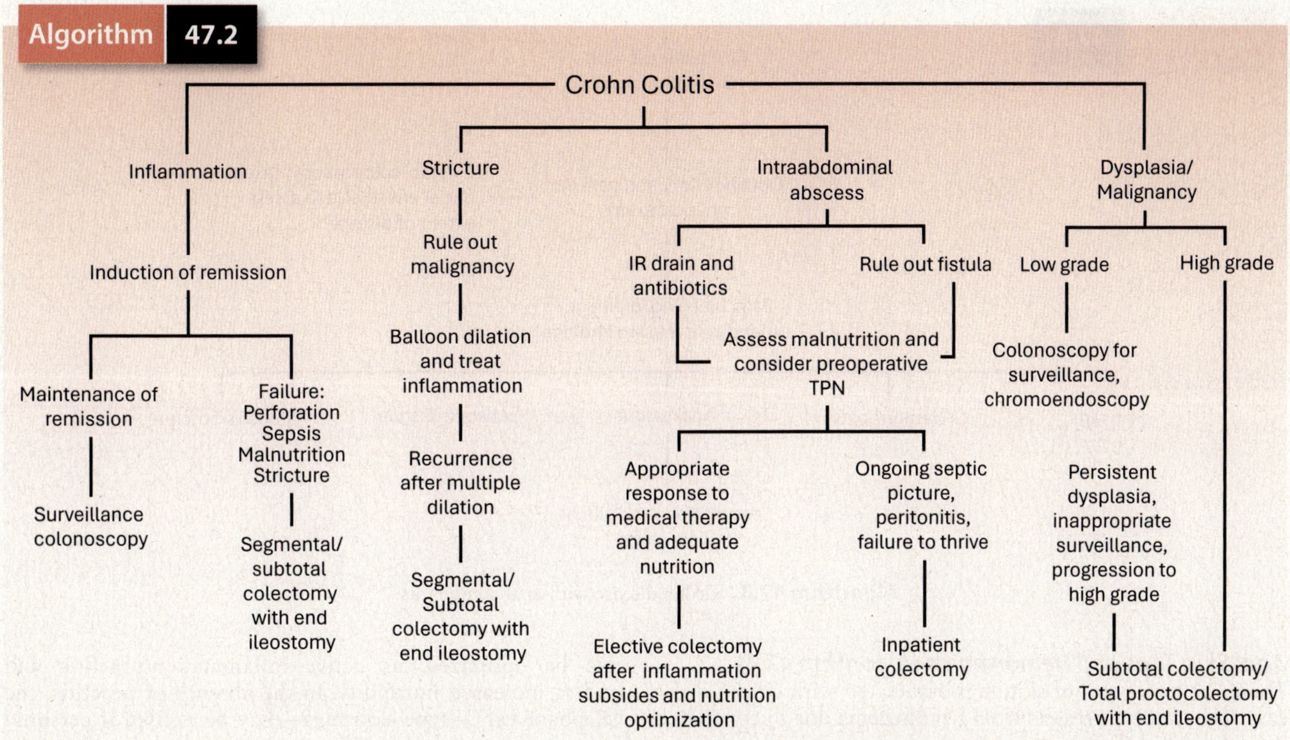

Algorithm 47.2. Management of colitis in Crohn disease.

functioning pouch, over half will continue to require medication to treat active Crohn disease.

Colorectal Malignancy

The risk of developing malignancy is elevated in the setting of Crohn disease, and the management of dysplasia and invasive cancer remains controversial. In the IBD setting, the lesion type must be considered, and a sporadic adenoma is managed differently than a nonadenomatous dysplasia–associated lesion or mass (DALM). Traditional sporadic adenomas can be managed with polypectomy and surveillance. A DALM is a raised dysplastic lesion that does not resemble a conventional sporadic adenoma. A DALM generally considers total proctocolectomy, given the high incidence of synchronous nonvisible dysplastic lesions and metachronous colorectal cancers. Absolute indications for surgery include high-grade dysplasia, multifocal dysplasia, and invasive cancer. Low-grade dysplasia and high-grade dysplasia are both risk factors for invasive cancer, as they are associated with the identification of synchronous cancer in 19% and 42% of cases, respectively. In the setting of invasive cancer, the extent of resection is controversial—segmental colectomy can be considered for select patients with Crohn disease, although total proctocolectomy remains the traditional recommendation. Ileoanal pouch anastomosis can be regarded as in only highly selected patients.[50]

Influence of Immunosuppressive Medications on Surgical Outcomes

There has been intense interest in whether preoperative immunosuppression with biologics increases perioperative complications. A strong consideration when operating on patients with Crohn disease is the potential for adverse postoperative outcomes in patients on immunosuppressive medications such as steroids and biologic agents. Patients undergoing colectomy for IBD have been shown to have higher rates of infections when compared to those undergoing colectomy for cancer. The main postoperative complications of concern are anastomotic leak, superficial surgical infection, and deep-organ space infection. Currently, no strict guidelines exist regarding the preoperative management of steroids and biologic agents. Several studies have demonstrated that anti-TNF agents are associated with higher surgical site infection rates but not higher rates of anastomotic leak, and newer biologic agents are still under investigation. Recently, a PUCCINI trial showed that preoperative anti-TNF drugs were not an independent risk factor for postoperative infections. Data on the impact of newer biologics such as vedolizumab, ustekinumab, and tofacitinib are emerging. Patients with lower levels of vedolizumab had lower rates of ileus but no difference in infection complications, SSI, reoperation, or readmission. Data on ustekinumab and tofacitinib remains sparse but so far has not shown evidence of adverse perioperative outcomes.

Historically, the administration of immunosuppressive medications was taken into consideration in terms of surgical intervention. Anti-TNF agents are held for 4 weeks preoperatively, vedolizumab for 4 to 8 weeks, and ustekinumab for 4 weeks preoperatively. In current practice, the biologics are continued on their regular schedule, and it is generally recommended to schedule surgery as far from the last dose of medication, around the time of the next scheduled dose.

However, a combination of biologic medications, steroids, and malnutrition must be considered intraoperatively, potentially leading to higher rates of diversion.

Venous Thromboembolism Prophylaxis

Patients undergoing surgery for IBD experience higher rates of postoperative venous thromboembolism (VTE). The rate of postoperative VTE in patients with Crohn disease ranges from 0% to 4.9%. Seventy-four percent of patients who experience VTE present during the initial postoperative hospitalization, and 61% within the first 2 weeks postoperatively. Standard perioperative VTE prophylaxis should be administered while patients are hospitalized, and patients should be considered for extended prophylaxis upon discharge.

Treatment of Anorectal Conditions (Algorithm 47.3)

9 A distinguishing characteristic of the surgical treatment for anorectal Crohn disease is to first consider whether or not they are symptomatic. As a follow-up principle, aggressive intervention in the asymptomatic patient is unwarranted and potentially dangerous.

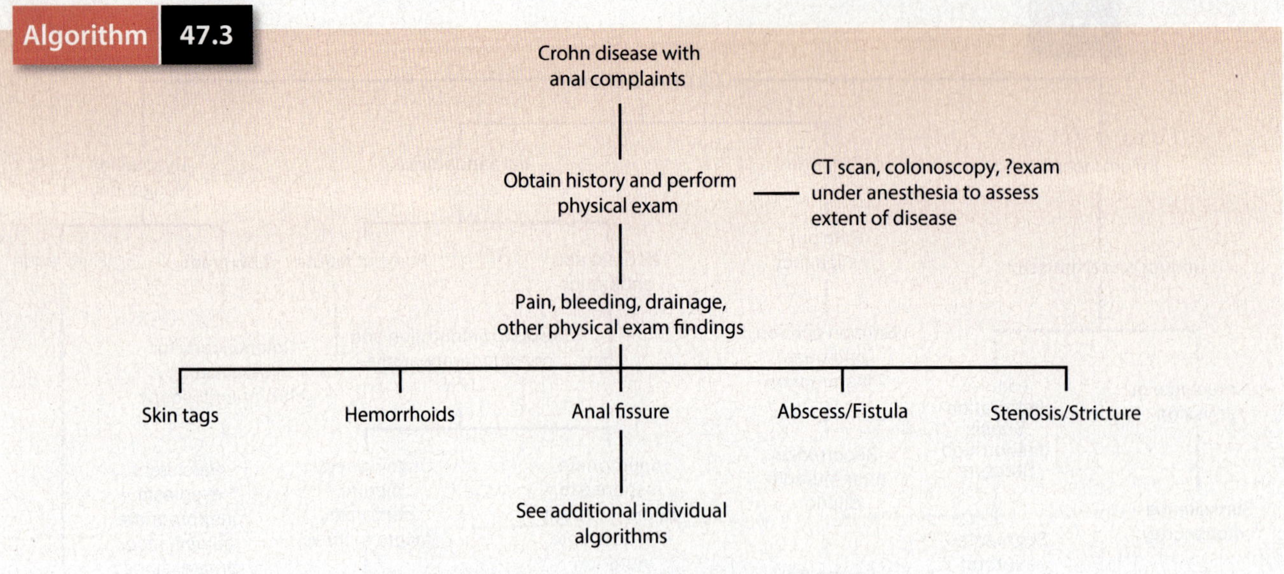

Algorithm 47.3. Crohn disease with anal complaints.

Anal Skin Tags and Hemorrhoids (Algorithm 47.4)

There are two types of skin tags associated with Crohn disease. The first type results from lymphedema due to concomitant intestinal disease and is hard, blue-colored, edematous, and tender (**Fig. 47.23A**). The other type is often referred to as "elephant ear" skin tags and are broad-based, soft, and painless (**Fig. 47.23B**). When considering surgical intervention for these tags, it is essential to keep in mind that Crohn disease patients have the propensity for poor healing, especially in the face of diarrhea. Patients should be counseled about the risk of nonhealing wounds, continence problems, and mucus drainage. An initial attempt at conservative treatment with warm sitz baths and diarrhea control is warranted. During this time, medical therapy for Crohn disease should also be optimized, as active inflammation/proctitis will lead to increased morbidity. In the absence of proctitis, the "elephant ear"—type skin tags—may be excised if personal hygiene is particularly bothersome, and wound healing can usually ensue.

Internal hemorrhoids are not common in the setting of Crohn disease, and patients who present with rectal bleeding should initially be evaluated for a flare of the underlying disease. However, if present, in the absence of proctitis and/or active perianal disease, they may be treated similarly as a patient without Crohn disease, with conservative management of proper bowel hygiene, fiber supplementation, and band ligation, reserving surgical management as a last resort after failure of nonsurgical treatment.

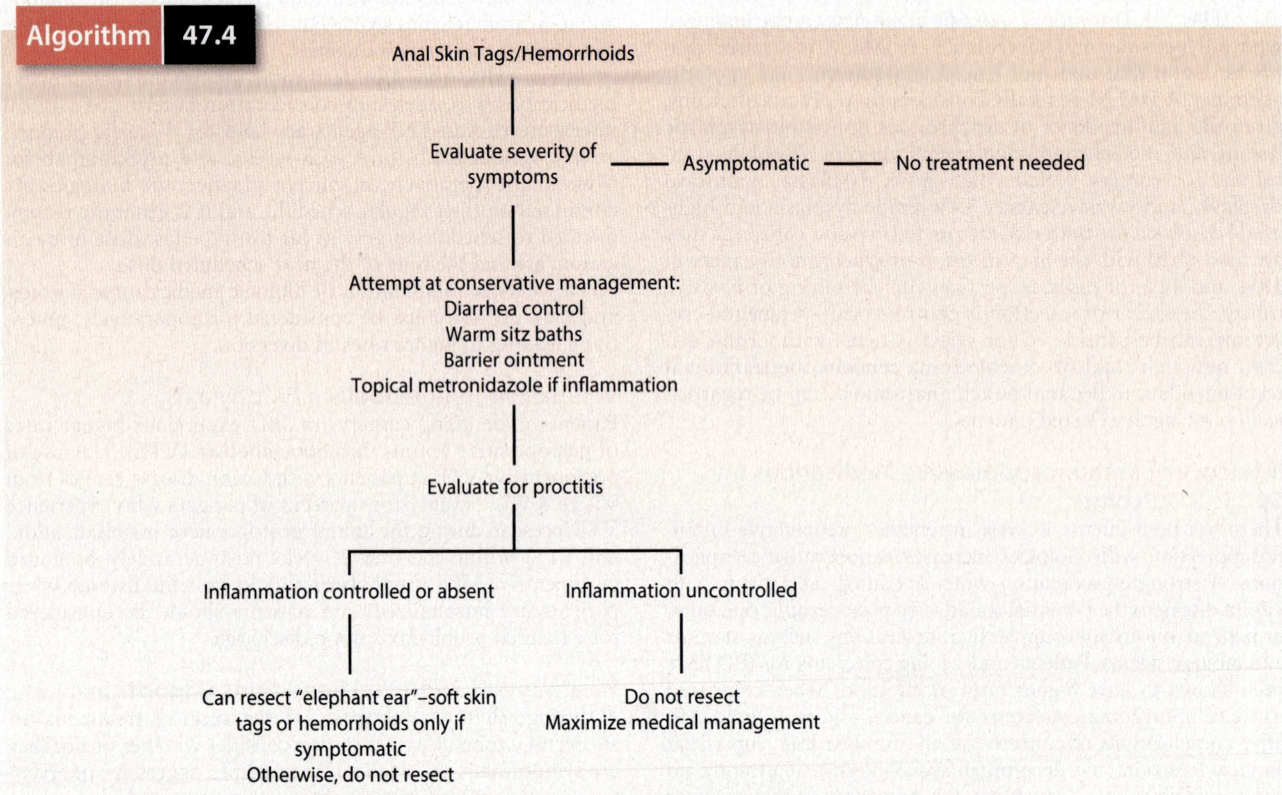

Algorithm 47.4. Management of anal skin tags and hemorrhoids in Crohn disease.

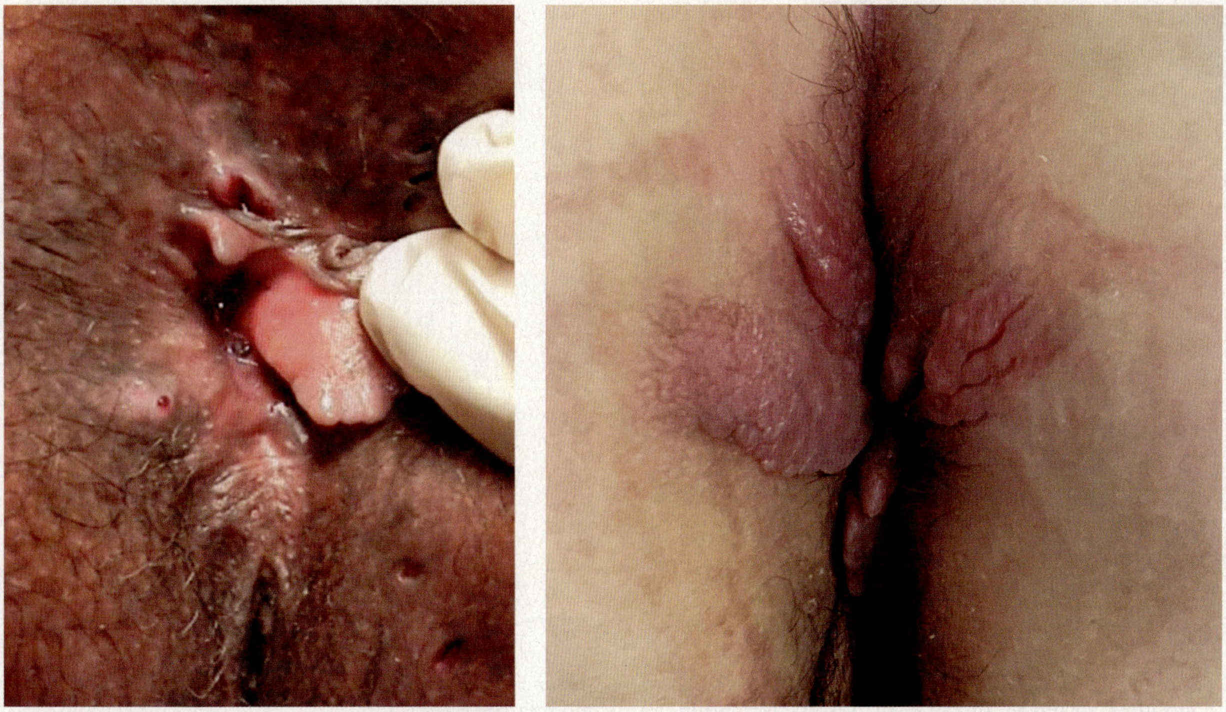

A B

Figure 47.23. **A:** Crohn skin tags: elephant ear–type skin tags. **B:** Type of Crohn skin tags that should not be excised.

Anorectal Abscess/Fistula (Algorithm 47.5)

More than 30% of patients with Crohn disease will develop perianal abscess or fistula, and the treatment remains controversial. Perianal abscesses and fistulas in the setting of active perianal Crohn disease do not typically follow the traditional patterns of routine cryptoglandular-based disease (**Fig. 47.24**). The primary goal of treatment is the same, however, to control sepsis and maintain continence. The best treatment course depends on the individual patient and the patient's fistula characteristics.

When presenting initially as an abscess, incision and drain-
10 age are indicated, and it is essential to place the incision as close to the anal verge as possible while still achieving adequate drainage, considering the possibility of fistula development. Alternatively, a small mushroom-tipped catheter may be placed in the cavity close to the anal verge, thus evacuating the abscess and allowing the cavity to close around the catheter while allowing continued drainage.

If there is suspicion of a fistula, determining the anatomy of the tract is required, and attention must be paid to the presence of proctitis, the status of the sphincter, prior anal operations, and the potential for chronic diarrhea. In the setting of a fistula, a seton should be placed initially until further workup

Algorithm 47.5

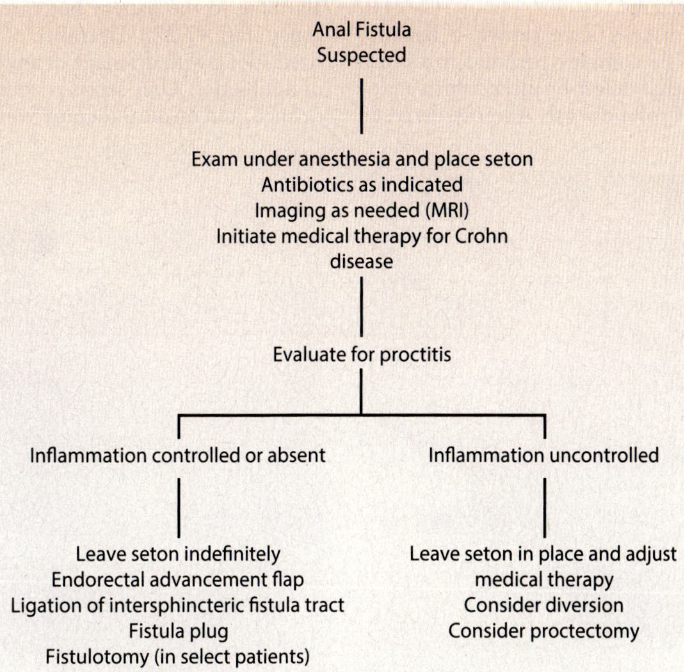

Algorithm 47.5. Management of anal fistula in Crohn disease.

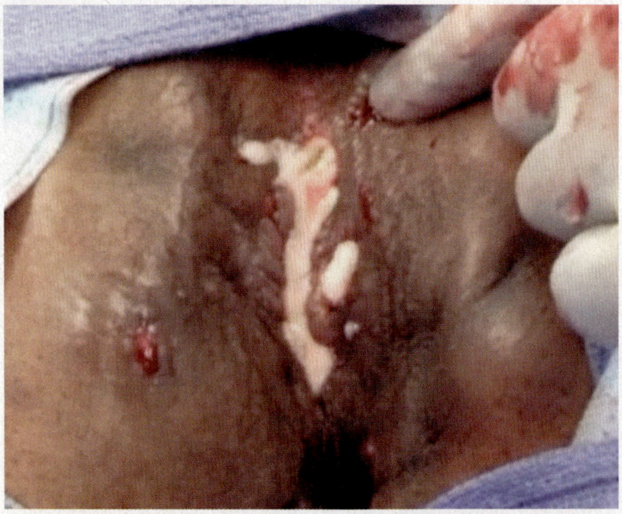

Figure 47.24. Perianal fistulas in Crohn disease with "watering-can perineum." Hydrogen peroxide is injected through an external opening, with bubbles coming from multiple other openings.

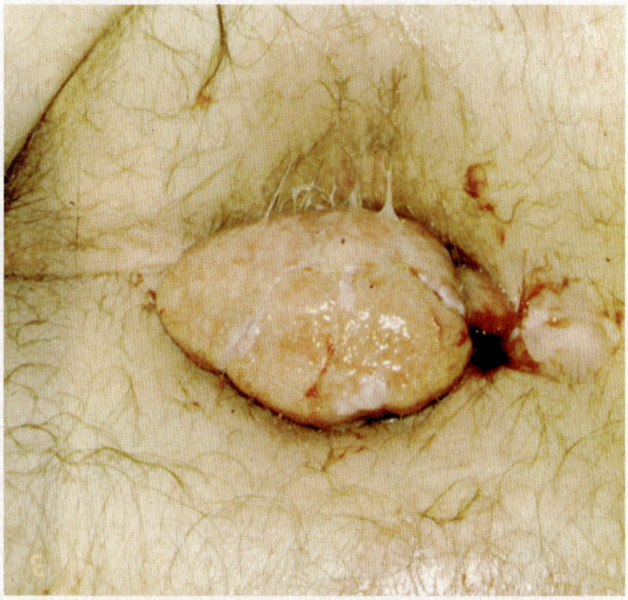

Figure 47.26. Anal cancer arising in perianal Crohn disease.

can be completed (**Fig. 47.25**). The goal of the seton is to allow for continuous drainage and prevent abscess formation. In addition, it can potentially turn a chronic inflammatory tract into a more chronic fibrotic one. After handling the acute situation, patients should be evaluated thoroughly for intestinal disease and considered for medical treatment.

In the absence of proctitis, treatment is determined based on the characteristics of the fistula. A low-lying fistula in the absence of overt proctitis can often be treated safely with a fistulotomy. Care must be given, even in these situations, as decreased continence may still ensue. When the fistula is higher or more complex, the initiation of anti-TNF agents has been reported to heal fistulas in up to 60% of patients. Other treatment options include fibrin glue (not recommended), fistula plugs (success rates <20%), endorectal advancement flaps, or the LIFT procedure (ligation of the intersphincteric fistula tract). Meta-analysis of endorectal advancement flap versus LIFT procedure for Crohn disease demonstrates no difference in healing rates, with both procedures achieving success in approximately 50% to 60% of cases.

Recently, mesenchymal stem cells have shown a beneficial effect on fistula healing. The complex perianal fistula is thought to arise from an epithelial defect or ulcer, which may be caused by inflammation in Crohn disease. Adipose-derived mesenchymal stem cells have anti-inflammatory and immunomodulatory effects.

In the presence of active proctitis, the best course of action is typically to place a seton and initiate medical therapy. Setons can remain indefinitely, but patients should be periodically reexamined to ensure adequate drainage and to screen for the development of squamous cell carcinoma and adenocarcinoma arising in a fistulous tract (**Fig. 47.26**).

Unfortunately, fistulas and fistula procedures all vary in their outcomes, with healing rates ranging from 15% to 97% and morbidity rates from 3% to 78%, making it difficult to compare results accurately. As such, consideration should be given to a diverting stoma for recurrent or complex fistulas, and upward of 68% of patients may require permanent diversion or even proctectomy.

Rectovaginal/Anovaginal Fistula

Rectovaginal fistulas are particularly problematic in Crohn disease patients. Passage of air and/or stool from the vagina can be alarming to the patient but rarely constitutes a surgical emergency (**Fig. 47.27**). Clearance of active sepsis should be prioritized, along with drainage of any abscess and the administration of antibiotics. After sepsis is controlled, the anatomy should be defined, and medical therapy with immunologic and/or biologic

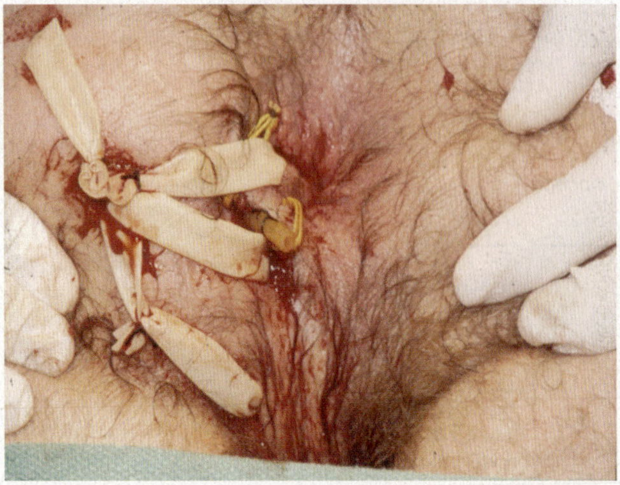

Figure 47.25. Seton drains made of Penrose drains placed through fistula.

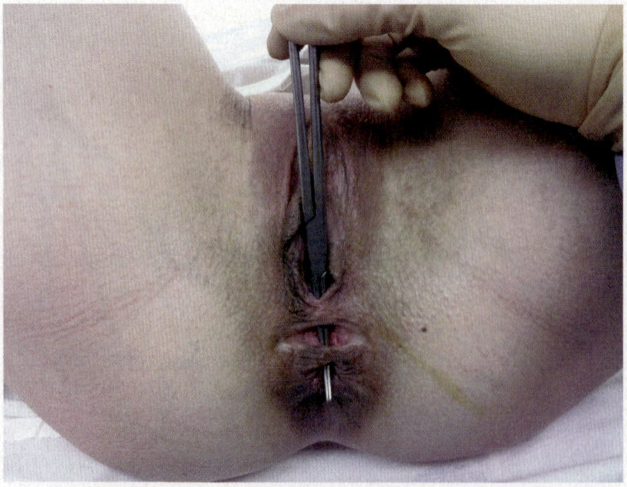

Figure 47.27. Rectovaginal fistula.

Algorithm 47.6

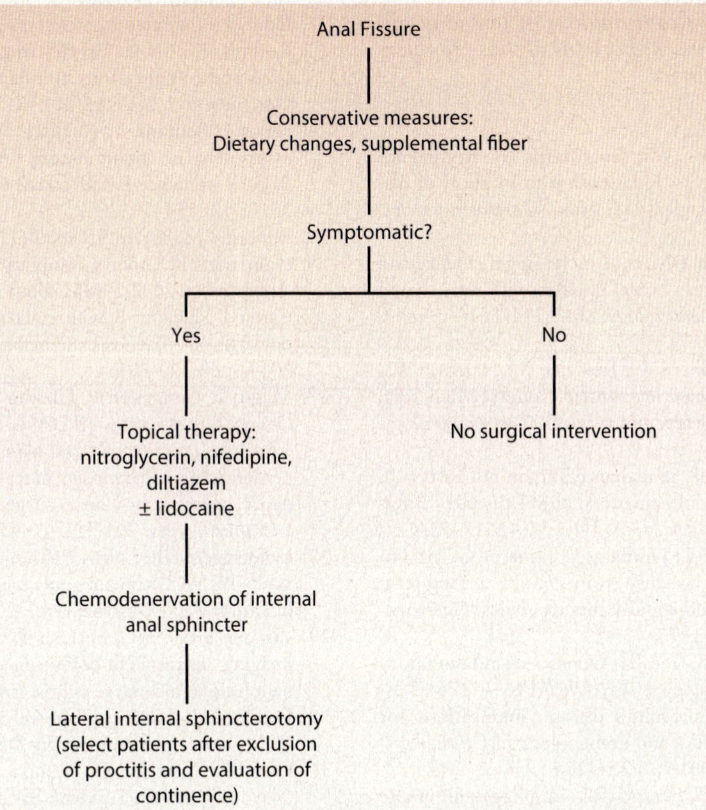

Algorithm 47.6. Management of anal fissure in Crohn disease.

therapy should be initiated. The mainstay of management of these patients is medical therapy, with surgical treatment taken into consideration with caution. Recurrence rates are high, and even with optimal treatment, upward of 20% of patients will eventually require proctectomy with permanent stoma. Surgical options include fistula plug, endorectal advancement flap, LIFT procedure, episioproctotomy, sphincteroplasty, tissue interposition, and proctectomy. Diversion is used liberally to improve healing. In certain situations, a lifelong seton may be necessary.

Anal Fissure (Algorithm 47.6)

Patients with Crohn disease can present with routine typical fissures associated with anal sphincter hypertonicity versus atypical fissures that are the result of the Crohn disease itself. All patients should be evaluated for the extent and severity of active intestinal Crohn disease. Excessive pain should raise the suspicion of an underlying abscess and prompt an examination under anesthesia.

Routine typical fissures without active perianal disease can be treated in the standard fashion. Bowel habit management with a high-fiber diet, stool softeners, fiber supplementation, and topical calcium channel blocker ointment are first-line treatments. Botulinum toxin injection and sphincterotomy can also be considered if medical therapy fails, though sphincterotomy should minimize the wound as much as possible.

Crohn disease–associated fissures are hallmarked by deep, burrowing, off the midline, and sometimes multiple wounds. Many anal fissures are, fortunately, painless and require no intervention. Initial attempts at conservative therapy with topical metronidazole, smooth muscle relaxants, and local anesthetics may be attempted to alleviate symptoms and help heal. For particularly symptomatic fissures, botulinum toxin has also been used. In contrast, other authors have advocated a more aggressive surgical approach in Crohn disease patients, with one report citing 67% of patients who were treated surgically with either lateral internal sphincterotomy or fissurectomy ultimately healed. Given the continence risks associated with surgery, medical management directed toward Crohn disease is the preferred initial therapy in patients with Crohn-related fissures. Surgical intervention with a tailored lateral internal sphincterotomy should be reserved for those patients with minimal active anorectal inflammation who fail all reasonable conservative therapy, and still, sphincter muscle division should be kept to a minimum.

Anorectal Malignancy

Risk factors in patients with Crohn disease include the presence of chronic inflammation, long-standing open wounds, and the use of immunosuppressant medication. Both squamous cell carcinoma (Marjolin ulcer) and adenocarcinoma and their variants may occur. Patients, especially those with long-term indwelling setons, should be periodically examined at least annually to exclude the presence of malignancy or other pathology. All suspicious lesions should undergo biopsy, and any malignancy identified should undergo proper staging and treatment.

SUMMARY

Crohn disease remains a complex disease process with many different manifestations in the GI tract and extraintestinal locations. Although advances in medical therapy continue to evolve and significantly alter the way patients are managed, surgeons still play a large role in the medical and surgical therapy of the disease, though multidisciplinary care with gastroenterologists is crucial to achieve optimal therapy. Due to its recurring nature, providers must adhere to the principles of preventing and managing disease complications versus aiming for a cure. By focusing on the maximization of functional outcomes, surgeons can optimize outcomes through a multimodal approach and minimize additional complications.

ACKNOWLEDGMENT

We gratefully acknowledge the contributions of previous edition author, Anuradha R. Bhama, as portions of those chapters have been retained in this revision.

References

1. Whelan G, Farmer RG, Fazio VW, Goormastic M. Recurrence after surgery in Crohn's disease. Relationship to location of disease (clinical pattern) and surgical indication. *Gastroenterology.* 1985;88(6):1826–1833.
2. Molodecky NA, Soon IS, Rabi DM, et al. Increasing incidence and prevalence of the inflammatory bowel diseases with time, based on systematic review. *Gastroenterology.* 2012;142(1):46–54.e42; quiz e30.
3. Loftus J, Silverstein MD, Sandborn WJ, Tremaine WJ, Harmsen WS, Zinsmeister AR. Crohn's disease in Olmsted County, Minnesota, 1940–1993: incidence, prevalence, and survival. *Gastroenterology.* 1998;114(6):1161–1168.
4. Yang H, McElree C, Roth MP, Shanahan F, Targan SR, Rotter JI. Familial empirical risks for inflammatory bowel disease: differences between Jews and non-Jews. *Gut.* 1993;34(4):517–524.
5. Halfvarson J, Bodin L, Tysk C, Lindberg E, Järnerot G. Inflammatory bowel disease in a Swedish twin cohort: a long-term follow-up of concordance and clinical characteristics. *Gastroenterology.* 2003;124(7):1767–1773.
6. McGovern DP, Kugathasan S, Cho JH. Genetics of inflammatory bowel diseases. *Gastroenterology.* 2015;149(5):1163–1176.e2.
7. Cho JH. The Nod2 gene in Crohn's disease: implications for future research into the genetics and immunology of Crohn's disease. *Inflamm Bowel Dis.* 2001;7(3):271–275.
8. Muzes G, Tulassay Z, Sipos F. Interplay of autophagy and innate immunity in Crohn's disease: a key immunobiologic feature. *World J Gastroenterol.* 2013;19(28):4447–4454.
9. Blaser MJ, Falkow S. What are the consequences of the disappearing human microbiota? *Nat Rev Microbiol.* 2009;7(12):887–894.
10. Ryan P, Kelly RG, Lee G, et al. Bacterial DNA within granulomas of patients with Crohn's disease—detection by laser capture microdissection and PCR. *Am J Gastroenterol.* 2004;99(8):1539–1543.
11. Kelly D, Campbell JI, King TP, et al. Commensal anaerobic gut bacteria attenuate inflammation by regulating nuclear-cytoplasmic shutting of PPAR-γ and RelA. *Nat Immunol.* 2004;5(1):104–112.
12. Llopis M, Antolin M, Carol M, et al. Lactobacillus casei downregulates commensals' inflammatory signals in Crohn's disease mucosa. *Inflamm Bowel Dis.* 2009;15(2):275–283.
13. Sokol H, Pigneur B, Watterlot L, et al. Faecalibacterium prausnitzii is an anti-inflammatory commensal bacterium identified by gut microbiota analysis of Crohn disease patients. *Proc Natl Acad Sci U S A.* 2008;105(43):16731–16736.
14. Wagner J, Sim WH, Lee KJ, Kirkwood CD. Current knowledge and systematic review of viruses associated with Crohn's disease. *Rev Med Virol.* 2013;23(3):145–171.
15. Wallace KL, Zheng LB, Kanazawa Y, Shih DQ. Immunopathology of inflammatory bowel disease. *World J Gastroenterol.* 2014;20(1): 6–21.
16. Cabré E, Domènech E. Impact of environmental and dietary factors on the course of inflammatory bowel disease. *World J Gastroenterol.* 2012;18(29):3814–3822.
17. Yantiss RK, Odze RD. Diagnostic difficulties in inflammatory bowel disease pathology. *Histopathology.* 2006;48(2):116–132.
18. Dias CC, Rodrigues PP, da Costa-Pereira A, Magro F. Clinical prognostic factors for disabling Crohn's disease: a systematic review and meta-analysis. *World J Gastroenterol.* 2013;19(24): 3866–3871.
19. Isaacs KL. Upper gastrointestinal tract endoscopy in inflammatory bowel disease. *Gastrointest Endosc Clin N Am.* 2002;12(3): 451–462, vii.
20. Farmer RG, Hawk WA, Turnbull RB. Clinical patterns in Crohn's disease: a statistical study of 615 cases. *Gastroenterology.* 1975; 68(4 Pt 1):627–635.
21. Wenzl HH. Diarrhea in chronic inflammatory bowel diseases. *Gastroenterol Clin North Am.* 2012;41(3):651–675.
22. Satsangi J, Grootscholten C, Holt H, Jewell DP. Clinical patterns of familial inflammatory bowel disease. *Gut.* 1996;38(5):738–741.
23. Rothfuss KS, Stange EF, Herrlinger KR. Extraintestinal manifestations and complications in inflammatory bowel diseases. *World J Gastroenterol.* 2006;12(30):4819–4831.
24. Panes J, Bouhnik Y, Reinisch W, et al. Imaging techniques for assessment of inflammatory bowel disease: joint ECCO and ESGAR evidence-based consensus guidelines. *J Crohns Colitis.* 2013;7(7):556–585.
25. Minordi LM, Bevere A, Papa A, Larosa L, Manfredi R. CT and MRI evaluations in Crohn's complications: a guide for the radiologist. *Acad Radiol.* 2022;29(8):1206–1227.
26. Carter D, Eliakim R. Current role of endoscopy in inflammatory bowel disease diagnosis and management. *Curr Opin Gastroenterol.* 2014;30(4):370–377.
27. Magro F, Gionchetti P, Eliakim R, et al. European Crohn's and Colitis Organisation [ECCO]. Third European evidence-based consensus on diagnosis and management of ulcerative colitis. Part 1: definitions, diagnosis, extra-intestinal manifestations, pregnancy, cancer surveillance, surgery, and ileo-anal pouch disorders. *J Crohns Colitis.* 2017;11(6):649–670.
28. Lichtenstein GR, Loftus EV, Isaacs KL, Regueiro MD, Gerson LB, Sands BE. ACG clinical guideline: management of Crohn's disease in adults. *Am J Gastroenterol.* 2018;113(4):481–517.
29. van den Broek FJC, Fockens P, van Eeden S, et al. Narrow-band imaging versus high-definition endoscopy for the diagnosis of neoplasia in ulcerative colitis. *Endoscopy.* 2011;43(2):108–115.
30. Vucelic B. Inflammatory bowel diseases: controversies in the use of diagnostic procedures. *Dig Dis.* 2009;27(3):269–277.
31. Hall BR, Leinicke JA, Armijo PR, Smith LM, Langenfeld SJ, Oleynikov D. No survival advantage exists for patients undergoing loop ileostomy for clostridium difficile colitis. *Am J Surg.* 2019;217(1):34–39.
32. Mahadeva U, Martin JP, Patel NK, Price AB. Granulomatous ulcerative colitis: a re-appraisal of the mucosal granuloma in the distinction of Crohn's disease from ulcerative colitis. *Histopathology.* 2002;41(1):50–55.
33. Smids C, Horjus Talabur Horje CS, Groenen MJM, van Koolwijk EHM, Wahab PJ, van Lochem EG. The value of serum antibodies in differentiating inflammatory bowel disease, predicting disease activity and disease course in the newly diagnosed patient. *Scand J Gastroenterol.* 2017;52(10):1104–1112.
34. Abraham BP, Kane S. Fecal markers: calprotectin and lactoferrin. *Gastroenterol Clin North Am.* 2012;41(2):483–495.
35. Ashton JJ, Gavin J, Beattie RM. Exclusive enteral nutrition in Crohn's disease: evidence and practicalities. *Clin Nutr.* 2019;38(1): 80–89.
36. Ford AC, Kane SV, Khan KJ, et al. Efficacy of 5-aminosalicylates in Crohn's disease: systematic review and meta-analysis. *Am J Gastroenterol.* 2011;106(4):617–629.
37. Leone GM, Mangano K, Petralia MC, Nicoletti F, Fagone P. Past, present and (foreseeable) future of biological anti-TNF alpha therapy. *J Clin Med.* 2023;17;12(4):1630.
38. Morita Y, Imaeda H, Nishida A, et al. Association between serum adalimumab concentrations and endoscopic disease activity in patients with Crohn's disease. *J Gastroenterol Hepatol.* 2016; 31(11):1831–1836.
39. Wolff BG. Resection margins in Crohn's disease. *Br J Surg.* 2001; 88(6):771–772.
40. Zittan E, Kabakchiev B, Milgrom R, et al. Higher adalimumab drug levels are associated with mucosal healing in patients with Crohn's disease. *J Crohns Colitis.* 2016;10(5):510–515.
41. Solitano V, Facciorusso A, Jess T, et al. Comparative risk of serious infections with biologic agents and oral small molecules in inflammatory bowel diseases: a systematic review and meta-analysis. *Clin Gastroenterol Hepatol.* 2023;21(4):907–921.e2.
42. Tekkis PP, Purkayastha S, Lanitis S, et al. A comparison of segmental vs subtotal/total colectomy for colonic Crohn's disease: a meta-analysis. *Colorectal Dis.* 2006;8(2):82–90.
43. Govani SM, Stidham RW, Higgins PDR. How early to take arms against a sea of troubles? The case for aggressive early therapy in

Crohn's disease to prevent fibrotic intestinal strictures. *J Crohns Colitis.* 2013;7(11):923–927.

44. Hirai F, Beppu T, Takatsu N, et al. Long-term outcome of endoscopic balloon dilation for small bowel strictures in patients with Crohn's disease. *Gastroenterol Endosc.* 2017;59(5):1344–1351.
45. He X, Chen Z, Huang J, et al. Stapled side-to-side anastomosis might be better than handsewn end-to-end anastomosis in ileocolic resection for Crohn's disease: a meta-analysis. *Dig Dis Sci.* 2014;59(7):1544–1551.
46. Poritz LS, Rowe WA, Koltun WA. Remicade® does not abolish the need for surgery in fistulizing Crohn's disease. *Dis Colon Rectum.* 2002;45(6):771–775.
47. Luglio G, Rispo A, Imperatore N, et al. Surgical prevention of anastomotic recurrence by excluding mesentery in Crohn's disease: the SuPREMe-CD study – a randomized clinical trial. *Ann Surg.* 2020;272(2:210–217.
48. Stewart D, Chao A, Kodner I, Birnbaum E, Fleshman J, Dietz D. Subtotal colectomy for toxic and fulminant colitis in the era of immunosuppressive therapy. *Colorectal Dis.* 2009;11(2):184–190.
49. Lavryk OA, Hull TL. Comparison of long-term outcomes of primary and redo IPAA for patients with Crohn's disease. *Int J Colorectal Dis.* 2019;34(11):1945–1951.
50. Guagnozzi D, Lucendo AJ. Colorectal cancer surveillance in patients with inflammatory bowel disease: what is new? *World J Gastrointest Endosc.* 2012;4(4):108–116.

48

Small Intestinal Neoplasms

James W. Fleshman and Steven G. Leeds

Key Points

1 Primary tumors: (a) Adenoma, adenocarcinoma, neuroendocrine tumors (NETs), lymphoma, sarcoma (all layers of the intestine) and (b) surgical resection is necessary for all except lymphoma (indication is obstruction and bleeding).

2 Rising incidence of NETs globally.

3 Majority of small intestinal neoplasms are asymptomatic: Symptoms are related to size and location within the length of the intestine.

4 Diagnostic tools: (a) capsule endoscopy, (b) small bowel enteroscopy, (c) device-assisted enteroscopy (DAE), (d) deep enteroscopy, (e) enterography (CT or MR).

5 Metastatic disease is related to the size of the primary tumor.

6 Metastases are detected by CT, MRI, MR enterography, octreotide scan (DOTA-TATE).

7 Recurrence of NET detected by serial chromogranin A blood levels.

8 Gastrointestinal stromal tumors (GISTs) arise in interstitial cells of Cajal (pacemaker of intestine) cured by surgical resection.

9 GIST mutations: c-kit—protooncogene of tyrosine kinase gene, responds to long-term tyrosine kinase inhibitors.

10 Melanoma: most common metastatic lesion to the small intestine.

11 Treatment: (a) endoscopic resection of small adenomas and hamartomas and (b) small bowel resection after localization for all large benign lesions unreachable by endoscopy, benign lesions >4 cm in size, possible undiagnosed malignancy, and GIST, NET, or metastatic disease.

Small intestinal neoplasms represent less than 5% of cancers in the entire intestinal tract. They are not listed as a major tumor site in the American Cancer Society Cancer Facts and Figures publication for 2024.[1]

The most common small intestine malignancy is now the neuroendocrine tumor (NET) (incidence 6.98/100,000 US population).[2]

1 Rates for types of malignancy in small bowel neoplasms:

- Adenocarcinoma 40%
- Sarcoma or gastrointestinal (GI) stromal 32%
- Lymphoma 17%
- Neuroendocrine 10%

Metastatic cancer of the small intestine is rare (melanoma, breast, colon) and presents most often as carcinomatosis with direct invasion to the outer surface of the small intestine, which is usually not amenable to complete resection.

EPIDEMIOLOGY

2 Estimated 12,440 new cases and 2090 deaths due to small intestine cancer in 2024 by the American Cancer Society.[3]

PATHOGENESIS

The cause of the low cancer rate and the presumed protective nature of the small intestine are due to:

1. Small bowel contents are liquid and alkaline with decreased chemical and mechanical damage to the mucosal lining.
2. Rapid transit results in shortened carcinogenic exposure (1½-hour transit through intestine to cecum).
3. Rapid turnover of epithelium outpaces growth of neoplastic cells.
4. Fewer anaerobes in the lumen cause less carcinogenesis
5. Epithelium detoxifies carcinogenic products.
6. Lymphoid tissue producing IgA may provide immunologic protection and modulate tumor growth.

3 7. Numerous different genomic alterations exist in small intestinal adenocarcinoma compared to colonic adenocarcinoma indicating different pathways and targets for therapy (**Table 48.1**).

PREDISPOSITION TO SMALL BOWEL ADENOCARCINOMA

Individuals with significant genetic and clinical factors predisposing them to a higher likelihood of small bowel cancer can be identified based on the existence of other disease processes (**Table 48.2**).

1. Familial adenomatous polyposis: Diffuse adenomatous polyps develop in the entire GI tract which can transition to adenocarcinoma over time, especially in the periampullary region of the duodenum.[4]
2. Crohn disease: Chronic inflammation in the distal jejunum and ileum in a male patient with fistulizing-type disease creates a relative risk (OR 33) of developing cancer in a stricture.[5]
3. Celiac disease: Lymphomas (T cell and non-Hodgkin) are 10 to 13 times more likely to occur in patients with longstanding disease.[6]

Table 48.1. Mutational Complexity of Small Bowel Adenocarcinoma

p53	58.4%
KRAS	53.6%
APC	26.8%
SMAD4	17.4%
PIK3CA	16.1%[a]
CDKN2A	14.5%
ERBB2	9.5%[a]
HER2	
BRAF	9.1%[a]
ATM	7.6%[a]
FBW7	6.9%[a]
ERBB3	6.3%[a]
NFI	6.0%[a]
MDM2	5.7%[a]
PTEN	5.7%[a]
CTNNB1	5.7%[a]

[a]Targetable genetic alterations.

4. Peutz–Jeghers syndrome: Genetic syndrome due to STK11 (serine/threonine kinase 11) mutation produces small intestine hamartomatous polyps and mucocutaneous melanin pigmentation with a relative risk of small bowel cancer (OR 520).[7]
5. Lynch syndrome: Mutation in the mismatch repair gene (M1SH2) results in the development of adenocarcinoma of the colon and small intestine (OR 100).[8]
6. Multiple endocrine neoplasia (MEN): MEN-1, von Hippel–Lindau syndrome, and neurofibromatosis type 1—all produce small bowel adenocarcinoma.[9]
7. Lifestyle: Cigarette smoking, obesity, low-fiber diet, alcohol intake, biliary disease, organic solvent, and nuclear exposure are all modifiable factors predisposing to developing small bowel cancer (**Table 48.3**).

Table 48.2. Genetic Syndromes Predisposing for Small Bowel Adenocarcinoma

Familial adenomatous polyposis (FAP)
Crohn disease
Celiac disease
Peutz–Jeghers syndrome
Lynch syndrome
Multiple endocrine neoplasia type 1 (MEN-1)
Von Hippel–Lindau syndrome
Neurofibromatosis type 1

Table 48.3. Modifiable Risk Factors for Small Bowel Adenocarcinoma

Diet (high fat, low fiber)
Alcohol
Smoking
Obesity
Biliary tract disease
Occupational exposure (organic solvents, nuclear waste)
Vitamin D deficiency
Sedentary lifestyle

From Barsouk A, Rawla P, Barsouk A, Thandra KC. Epidemiology of cancers of the small intestine: trends, risk factors, and prevention. *Med Sci (Basel).* 2019;7(3):46.

CLINICAL PRESENTATION OF SMALL BOWEL NEOPLASMS (TABLE 48.4)

1. Tumors less than 4 cm in maximum dimension are usually asymptomatic.
2. Presenting symptoms: weight loss (30% to 50%), nausea, vomiting, anemia, pain
3. Metastasis present in 50%, bleeding, perforation, obstruction, intussusception, bleeding ulceration, volvulus, carcinoid syndrome (liver metastases from NET).[10]

DIAGNOSTIC OPTIONS

The small intestine is only easily accessed by endoscopy at the proximal and distal ends. Intubation of the ileocecal valve and distal ileum during colonoscopy gives one a view of the terminal 25 cm of the ileum. Even this is not possible in up to 10% of patients.[11] Only rarely can an upper endoscope be pushed past the ligament of Trietz into the most proximal jejunum. Injury to the duodenum is a real risk during this maneuver.

Table 48.4. Complications Resulting from Small Bowel Tumors

Complication	Details
Weight loss	30–50% of patients History and physical examination of the patient
Nausea/vomiting	Nonspecific finding
Obstruction	Include in differential for patients never undergoing an abdominal surgery Diagnosis made with radiographs or CT scan
Ulceration/bleeding	Commonly with lymphoma Mass can be seen on CT scan, but ulceration and bleeding found with capsule endoscopy or deep endoscopy
Perforation	Emergent surgical management May see free air on radiographs or CT scan
Metastasis	50% metastasis with incidence of malignant small bowel tumors at time of diagnosis

Other techniques for evaluating the small intestine are available:

4 1. Small bowel enteroscopy uses balloon or spiral motion to fix and pull the scope forward through the intestine and allows forceps biopsy of lesions.
   a. Device-assisted enteroscopy (DAE) (double-balloon enteroscopy) can reach 140 cm.
   b. Single-balloon enteroscopy, with over tube, using fluoroscopy
   c. Spiral enteroscopy, with external spiraled grooves on the endoscope, allows the scope to advance to more than 150 cm.[12]
   d. Balloon-guided enteroscopy, with sequential inflation of two balloons on the outer surface of the scope[13]
   e. Capsule endoscopy with video transmission of images does not allow biopsy.[14]
2. Imaging with 3D reconstruction of cross-sectional images to give a three-dimensional image and allow spatial determination of the tumor relative to bowel length.[15]
   a. CT enterography
   b. MRI enterography
3. Laparoscopic exploration of the abdomen for[16]:
   a. Identification of the lesion, evaluation of the mesentery and lymphatic tissue
   b. Biopsy of the lesion
   c. Oncologic resection of the lesion with clear margins and complete lymph node evaluation

MANAGEMENT OF BENIGN SMALL INTESTINAL LESIONS

Endoscopic resection of benign lesions is only possible in the duodenum and terminal ileum (**Table 48.5**). Snare (cold) with a loop through the upper endoscope and the colonoscope are the safest approaches. Bleeding can be controlled after the resection with snare cautery localized to the bleeding vessel. If the snare cautery is used to resect, there is a high possibility of burning a hole in the bowel wall. This is difficult to manage without an exploratory laparotomy. Symptomatic or large benign lesions will usually require a wider resection with associated small intestine to allow a safe complete removal and avoid a partial resection of a hidden malignancy. Preoperative localization with CT or MRI enterography (or angiography for a hemangioma) is helpful.

After endoscopic resection of any lesion, it is helpful to place an indelible ink tattoo to mark the resection site for future follow-up. During the procedure to identify a small lesion, an intravenous single dose of 3 mL of indocyanine green may guide the endoscopist or surgeon to the tumor.

Table 48.5. Benign Lesions: Required Approach for Removal

Lesion	Endoscopic Resection	Small Bowel Resection
Adenoma <4 cm	Y	N
Hamartoma <4 cm	Y	N
Adenoma >4 cm	N	Y
Hamartoma >4 cm	N	Y
Hemangioma	N	Y
GIST any size	N	Y
Neuroendocrine tumor	N	Y

MANAGEMENT OF MALIGNANT SMALL INTESTINAL TUMORS

Small intestinal cancers account for 5% of all gastrointestinal cancers. These are divided into neuroendocrine tumors (NETs) (40%), adenocarcinomas (40%), lymphoma/GISTs/sarcoma (20%).

NEUROENDOCRINE TUMORS

Neuroendocrine tumors (NETs) are formerly known as carcinoids.

Pathogenesis

1. Arise from secretory enterochromaffin cells in the small intestine, can be benign or very aggressive.
2. NETs have increased in individuals over 65 years of age (3.56/100,000 gastropancreatic and 1.02/100,000 small intestinal) according to Surveillance, Epidemiology, and End Results (SEER) Database Data.[17]
3. Serotonin is released from NETs and causes the symptoms of diarrhea, flushing, bronchospasm, cutaneous vasomotor symptoms, and right heart valvular dysfunction—all part of the carcinoid syndrome.
4. Serotonin is a derivative of tryptophan. It is rapidly inactivated in the liver to 5-hydroxyindolacetic acid (5-HIAA) which is secreted by the kidney and detectable as a marker in the urine.
5. Only tumors outside the portal venous system drainage (tumors in the liver or tumors drained by peripheral veins) produce enough serotonin in the systemic circulation to result in the carcinoid syndrome.
6. Large NETs can cause intestinal obstruction due to size, sclerotic changes in the bowel mesentery as a reaction to local serotonin release which creates constriction of the bowel lumen, or as a lead point in intestinal intussusception. NETs frequently result in diffuse tumor implants throughout the peritoneal cavity and invade locally to cause symptoms.

5 7. Metastasis is related to NET size. A tumor >2 cm in size has a rate of distant metastasis = 5% and nodal metastasis = 12%.
8. Prognosis is related to numerous factors (**Table 48.6** general factors and **Table 48.7** pathologic factors).

Table 48.6. Prognostic Factors Influencing Overall Survival (OS) in NETs

Good Prognosis (OS)	Poor Prognosis (OS)
Localized to bowel	Distant spread
30+ y	1 y
Grade 1	Grade 4
16.2 y	0–1 y
Rectum	Pancreas
25 y	3.6 y
Appendix	Small intestine
30 y	14 y
Well differentiated	Poorly differentiated
Size <1 cm	Size >2 cm

Table 48.7. Pathologic Classification of Neuroendocrine Tumors[18]

Differentiation	Grade	Criteria
Well differentiated	Low (typical)	<2 mitoses/10 HPF and ≤2% Ki67 index
Intermediate (atypical)	2–20 mitoses/10 HPF or 3–20% Ki67 index	
Poorly differentiated	High	>20 mitoses/10 HPF or >20% Ki67 index

Diagnosis and Clinical Staging

6 1. CT and MR enterography provide evidence of local and systemic tumor.
2. CT angiography adds information on liver metastases.
3. TNM staging of small intestine NETs is based on tumor size, number of lymph nodes involved with tumor metastases, and the presence of distant metastatic disease.[19]
4. Octreotide scan or fluorodeoxyglucose (FDG) positron emission tomography (PET) scanning can confirm and increase sensitivity for detecting metastatic disease.
5. DOTA-TATE scanning (Tetraxetan-tyrosine 3 octreotate ^{64}Cu) based on somatostatin receptors (especially SSTR-2 with ^{177}Lu) gives a clear picture of disease extent and provides theranostic evidence that peptide receptor radionuclide therapy (PRRT) may be of benefit for nonoperative therapy. Subtype 2 of SSTR is the most common for small intestine NET.[19]
6. Survival rates at 5 years depend on location in the bowel and stage of disease (**Table 48.8**).

Treatment and Survival (Algorithm 48.1)

1. Complete surgical resection of primary NET tumor and local nodal metastasis is the only chance for cure of localized disease.[20]
2. Survival after resection and treatment has been improving over the last 10 years. Palliation with somatostatin analogs to inhibit secretion of serotonin has been successful in reducing the effects of carcinoid syndrome.
3. Debulking of tumor by at least 90% improves symptoms in patients with peritoneal disease.
4. Radiofrequency ablation of liver lesions decreases release of serotonin and contributes to reduction of carcinoid symptoms.[21]
5. Transarterial chemoembolization (TACE) reduces symptoms of nonresectable disease in the liver.
6. SSTR 2 and 5 exist in 70% to 90% of NETs and allow SSTR-based scanning for diagnosis, staging, and therapy.
7. SSTR-positive NETs can respond to PRRT. The European Association of Nuclear Medicine created guidelines for detection and treatment of NETs in 2017. Radionuclides utilized include ^{177}Lu, ^{68}Ga, ^{64}Cu.[22]
8. SSTR PET/CT scan should be used for[23]:
   a. Detection of primary occult site primary in patients with demonstrated neuroendocrine metastasis or increased specific tumor markers, with negative conventional imaging for primary lesions.
   b. Characterization, staging, and restaging of foregut and midgut NETs (when 18F-DOPA PET is unavailable or inconclusive).
   c. Indications for SSTR-PET/CT
      i. Staging and restaging of residual or recurrent disease
      ii. Prognosis based on SSTR-positive tumors responding to targeted somatostatin analog therapy
      iii. Assessment of eligibility for PRRT (with ^{177}Lu or ^{90}Y DOTA-peptides)
      iv. Therapy response monitoring after surgical or radiopharmaceutical treatment
      v. DOTA-TATE or DOTA-TOC (Tetraxetan [Tyr-3]-Octreotate or Tetraxetan [Tyr-3]–Octreotide) attached to ^{64}Cu.
7 vi. Elevated serum chromogranin A blood levels.

SMALL BOWEL ADENOCARCINOMA

The second most common malignancy in the small bowel—30% of small bowel cancer.

1. 7.3/million lives worldwide.[24]
2. More common in developed countries[25]
3. Age-adjusted incidence: Black > White > Hispanic > Asian/Pacific Islander
4. Symptoms
   a. Abdominal pain: 45% to 76%
   b. Nausea and vomiting
   c. Weight loss
   d. Fatigue
   e. Anemia
   f. Occult GI bleeding
5. Diagnosis requires high index of suspicion.[26]
   a. Mean duration of symptoms 10 months
   b. Carcinoembryonic antigen (CEA) and carbohydrate antigen 19-9 (CA 19-9) elevated in 30% to 40%.[27]
   c. Upper gastrointestinal (UGI) small bowel follow-through or enteroclysis detects mass but not metastasis.
   d. CT enterography (sensitivity 84.7% and specificity 96.9%) and can find metastasis.
   e. Magnetic resonance enterography (sensitivity 91% and specificity 95%)[28]
   f. DAE (balloon assisted) indicated for anemia
6. Treatment (**Algorithm 48.2**)
   a. Surgical resection[29]

Table 48.8. 5-Year Survival Rates by Neuroendocrine Tumor Location (1973–1997)[a]

Site	All Stages (%)	Local Stage (%)	Regional Stage (%)	Distant Stage (%)
Stomach	75.1/55.3	90.2/69.6	40.4/27.2	18.0/9.0
Small bowel	76.1/54.6	94.5/70.4	84.4/64.1	51.2/32.4
Appendix	76.3/65.0	95.6/87.8	80.0/67.6	37.5/26.8
Colon	69.5/41.8	94.1/77.1	72.5/35.3	27.8/4.1
Rectum	87.5/77.8	94.9/86.2	53.7/42.1	14.6/13.1

Survival rates are all age-adjusted to standard 2000 population.
[a]Cancer-specific survival/relative overall survival.
From Maggard MA, O'Connell JB. Updated population-based review of carcinoid tumors. *Ann Surg.* 2004;240(1):117–122, with permission.

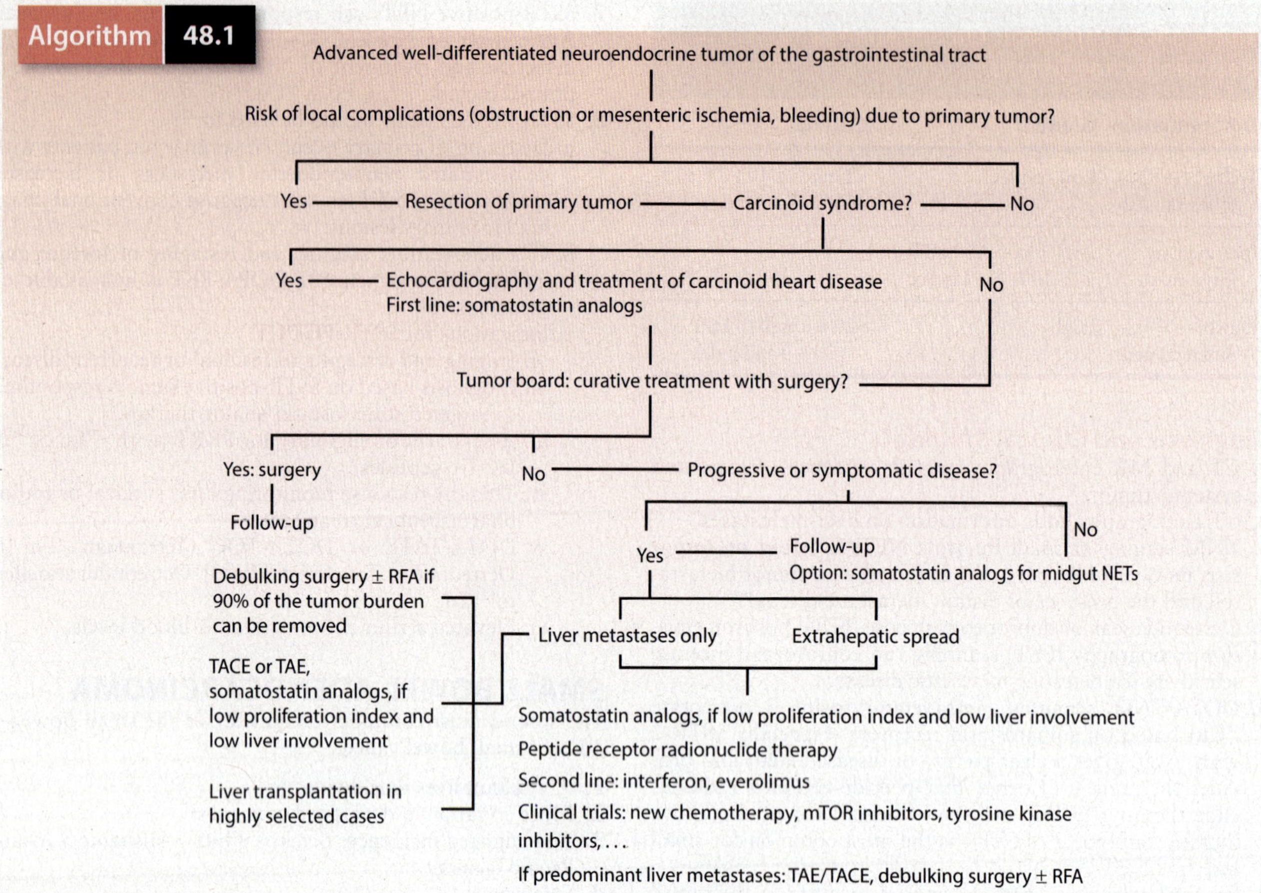

Algorithm 48.1. Management algorithm for patients with advanced neuroendocrine tumors (NETs) of the gastrointestinal tract. mTOR, mammalian target of rapamycin; RFA, radiofrequency ablation; TAE, transarterial embolization; TACE, transarterial chemoembolization. (From Walter T, Brixi-Benmansour H, Lombard-Bohas C, et al. New treatment strategies in advanced neuroendocrine tumours. *Dig Liver Dis*. 2012;44[2]:95–105.)

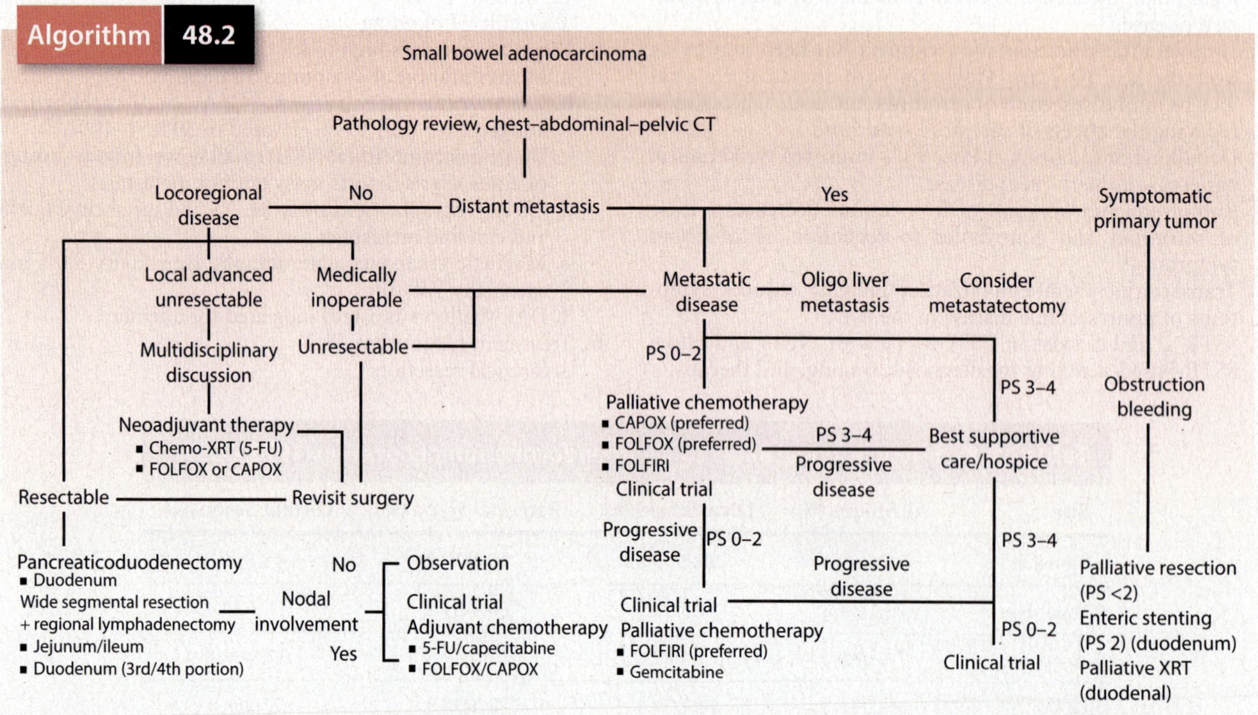

Algorithm 48.2. Algorithm showing the management of patients with small bowel adenocarcinomas. The treatment strategy depends on disease stage and involves en bloc resection for locoregional disease and systemic chemotherapy for metastatic disease. All current recommendations are based on case series, retrospective reviews, or nonrandomized prospective trials because of an absence of any randomized data. 5-FU, 5-fluorouracil; CAPOX, capecitabine and oxaliplatin; FOLFIRI, folinic acid, 5-fluorouracil, and irinotecan; FOLFOX, folinic acid, 5-fluorouracil, and oxaliplatin; PS, performance status; XRT, radiation therapy. (From Elias D, Lefevre JH, Duvillard P, et al. Hepatic metastases from neuroendocrine tumors with a "thin slice" pathological examination: they are many more than you think. *Ann Surg*. 2010;251[2]:307–310.)

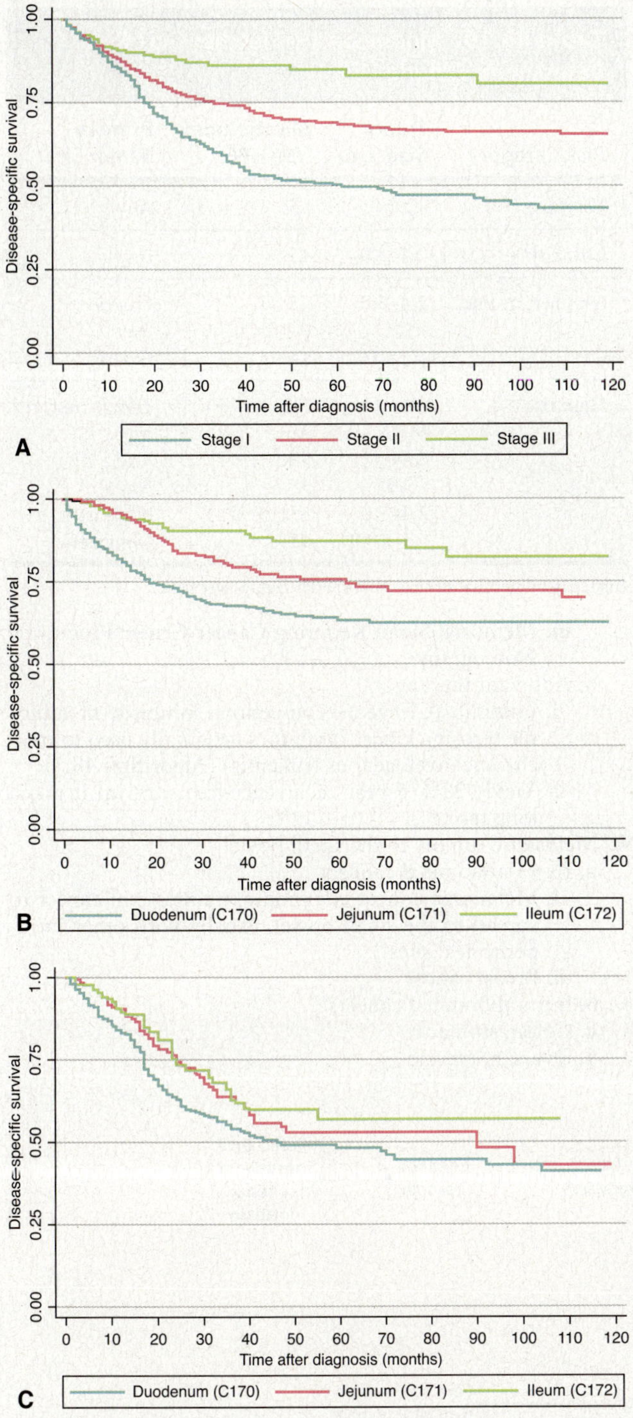

Figure 48.1. These Kaplan–Meier curves illustrate disease-specific survival for small bowel adenocarcinoma stratified by (**A**) disease stage, (**B**) subsite in the small bowel for stage I and II diseases, and (**C**) subsite in the small bowel for stage III disease. (From Codes for the duodenum (C17.0), jejunum, (C17.1), and ileum (C17.2) are from the International Classification of Diseases for Oncology and Related Health Problems, 10th Revision. (Overman MJ, Hu CY, Wolff RA, et al. Prognostic value of lymph node evaluation in small bowel adenocarcinoma: analysis of the surveillance, epidemiology, and end results database. *Cancer*. 2010;116[23]:537.)

i. Segmental wedge resection for jejunal or ileal lesion
ii. Pancreaticoduodenectomy for duodenal lesion
iii. Ileocolic resection for terminal ileal lesion
iv. At least 10 nodes resected in specimen[30]

7. Prognosis after resection (5-year survival) (**Fig. 48.1**)
   a. Duodenal cancer 56% 5-year survival (0% without resection)

Table 48.9. Disease-Specific Survival for Small Bowel Adenocarcinoma According to Disease Stage, Total Number of Lymph Nodes Assessed, and Total Number of Positive Lymph Nodes[30]

	%Cumulative 5-Y DSS		
No. of Lymph Nodes	**Stage I**	**Stage II**	**Stage III**
TLN			
0	70	44	
1–7	93	69	43
>7	95	83	56
PLN			
<3			58
>3			37
LNR[a]			
T1 (0.02–0.2)			63
T2 (0.21–0.5)			53
T3 (0.52–1)			30

[a]Stratified by tertiles.
DSS, disease-specific survival; TLN, total number of lymph nodes assessed; PLN, total number of positive lymph nodes; LNR, lymph node ratio.

   b. Jejunal and ileal based on stage and number of lymph nodes resected with and without metastasis (**Table 48.9**).
   c. Nodal involvement requires adjuvant chemotherapy.
   d. Recurrence: usually distant (59%), locoregional (19%), or both (22%)[31]
   e. Stage depends on lymph node involvement and ratio of positive to total number of nodes resected.[32]

8. Adjuvant therapy
   a. Based on 5-fluorouracil *and* oxaliplatin, irinotecan, gemcitabine, or capecitabine[77]
   b. Mismatch repair (MMR)/microsatellite instability (MSI)-positive tumors may be related to Lynch syndrome—may respond to checkpoint inhibitors rather than 5-fluorouracil–based therapy.[34]
   c. Neoadjuvant therapy can convert 90% of unresectable small bowel cancer to resectability.[35]

OTHER TUMORS FOUND IN THE SMALL BOWEL

1. Primary lymphoma: 15% to 20% of all small intestinal neoplasms[35]
   a. 60% to 65% in the ileum
   b. 20% to 25% in the jejunum
   c. 6% to 8% in the duodenum
2. Secondary lymphoma > primary lymphoma
   a. Gastrointestinal tract is the most common site for extranodal disease of any lymphoma.
   b. Most common secondary lymphoma is diffuse large B-cell lymphoma.
   c. Presentation of small bowel lymphomas
      i. Nausea/vomiting
      ii. Abdominal pain
      iii. Anemia
      iv. Weight loss
      v. Rarely: obstruction, intussusception, perforation

d. Management
   i. Surgery only for obstruction, perforation, or bleeding
   ii. Adjuvant chemotherapy is the backbone of treatment.
   iii. Specific chemotherapy for lymphoma
   iv. Antibiotic therapy for *Helicobacter Pylori*- or *Campylobacter jejuni*–induced immunoproliferative small intestinal disease (IPSID) in immunosuppressed patients (transplant)[36]
   v. Radiation and chemotherapy for recurrent lymphoma[37]

8 **3.** Gastrointestinal stromal tumor (GIST)

a. Most common mesenchymal tumor of the small bowel. Arising from the interstitial cells of Cajal which serve as the intestinal pacemakers.[38]
   i. 60% to 70% gastric
   ii. 20% to 30% small intestine
   iii. 4% to 5% duodenum

9 b. Genetic mutation associated with GIST: c-kit—protooncogene codes for tyrosine kinase inhibitor[39]

c. Presentation
   i. Vague abdominal symptoms
   ii. Abdominal pain
   iii. GI bleeding from mucosal erosion
   iv. Abdominal mass

d. Detection
   i. Endoscopy shows extraluminal/submucosal mass.
   ii. CT scan—intestinal wall or mesenteric mass[40]

e. Management
   i. En bloc surgical resection with negative margins (not wide)
   ii. Lymphadenectomy not necessary due to rare nodal metastases

f. Prognosis
   i. Depends on tumor size, mitotic rate, tumor location, kinase mutational status, intact tumor resection
   ii. Five-year overall survival after resection—50% to 65%

g. Recurrence
   i. Modified Fletcher GIST Risk Assessment Criteria (**Table 48.10**)
   ii. Armed Forces Institute of Pathology Classification

Table 48.10. Modified NIH–Fletcher GIST Risk Assessment Criteria

Risk Category	Tumor Size (cm)	Mitotic Index (/50 HPF)	Primary Tumor Site
Very low risk	<2.0	≤5	Any
Low risk	2.1–5.0	≤5	Any
Intermediate risk	2.1–5.0	>5	Gastric
	<5.0	6–10	Any
	5.1–10.0	≤5	Gastric
High risk	Any	Any	Tumor rupture
	>10	Any	Any
	Any	>1G	Any
	>5.0	>5	Any
	2.1–5.0	>5	Nongastric
	5.1–10.0	≤5	Nongastric

GIST, gastrointestinal stromal tumor; HPF, high-power field.

   iii. Memorial Sloan Kettering Cancer Center Prognostic Nomogram

h. Adjuvant therapy
   i. Imatinib (Gleevec)—competitive inhibitor of multiple tyrosine kinase inhibitors (originally used to treat chronic myelogenous leukemia) (**Algorithm 48.3**)
   ii. Yields 98% 5-year recurrence-free survival if taken long term[18]

4. Metastatic tumors to the small bowel

a. Extra-abdominal cancers

10 i. Melanoma—most common extraintestinal cancer to spread to the small bowel, usually with other intraperitoneal sites[41]
   ii. Breast cancer

b. Intra-abdominal cancers[42]

c. Colon, stomach

d. Ovarian, uterine

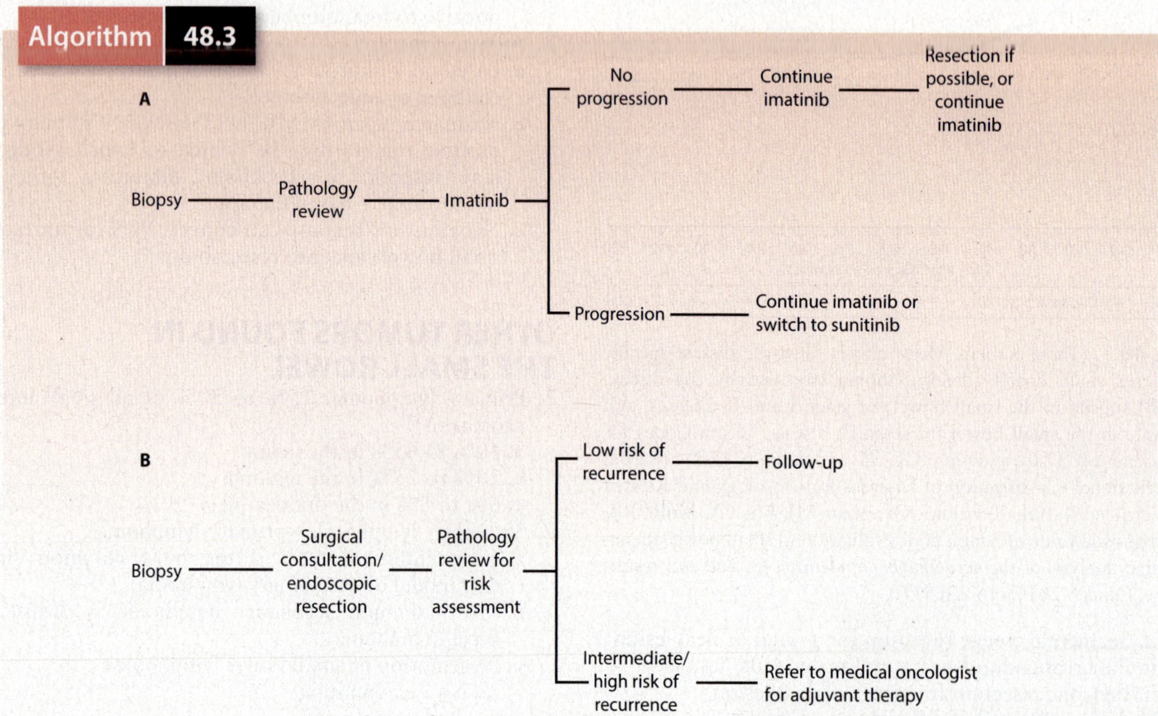

Algorithm 48.3. Treatment algorithms for patients with (**A**) advanced/metastatic gastrointestinal stromal tumor (GIST) and (**B**) resectable GIST. GIST indicates gastrointestinal stromal tumor. (From Mullady DK, Tan BR. A multidisciplinary approach to the diagnosis and treatment of gastrointestinal stromal tumor. *J Clin Gastroenterol.* 2013;47[7]:578–585.)

e. Treatment case by case
   i. Surgical resection
   ii. Intestinal bypass palliation
   iii. Endoluminal stent to relieve obstruction
   iv. Palliative systemic chemotherapy appropriate for tumor type

References

1. Barsouk A, Rawla P, Barsouk A, Thandra KC. Epidemiology of cancers of the small intestine: trends, risk factors, and prevention. *Med Sci (Basel)*. 2019;7(3):46.
2. Dasari A, Shen C, Halperin D, et al. Trends in the incidence, prevalence, and survival outcomes in patients with neuroendocrine tumors in the United States. *JAMA Oncol.* 2017;3(10): 1335–1342.
3. American Cancer Society. Surveillance and Health Equity Science, Cancer Facts and Figures. 2024;4.
4. Feldstein RC, Sood S, Katz S. Small bowel adenocarcinoma in Crohn's disease. *Inflamm Bowel Dis.* 2008;14(8):1154–1157.
5. Reynolds I, Healy P, Mcnamara DA. Malignant tumours of the small intestine. *Surgeon.* 2014;12(5):263–270.
6. Howdle PD, Jalal PK, Holmes GK, Houlston RS. Primary small-bowel malignancy in the UK and its association with coeliac disease. *QJM.* 2003;96(5):345–353.
7. Giardiello FM, Brensinger JD, Tersmette AC, et al. Very high risk of cancer in familial Peutz-Jeghers syndrome. *Gastroenterology.* 2000;119(6):1447–1453.
8. Vasen HF, Wijnen JT, Menko FH, et al. Cancer risk in families with hereditary nonpolyposis colorectal cancer diagnosis by mutation analysis. *Gastroenterology.* 1996;110(4):1020–1027.
9. Cheung DY, Choi MG. Current advance in small bowel tumors. *Clin Endosc.* 2011;44(1):13–21.
10. Lieberman DA, Faigel DO, Logan JR, et al. Assessment of the quality of colonoscopy reports: results from a multicenter consortium. *Gastrointest Endosc.* 2009;69(3 Pt 2):645–653.
11. Pennazio M, Spada C, Eliakim R, et al. Small-bowel capsule endoscopy and device-assisted enteroscopy for diagnosis and treatment of small-bowel disorders: European Society of Gastrointestinal Endoscopy (ESGE) clinical guideline. *Endoscopy.* 2015 47(4):352–376.
12. May A, Nachbar L, Ell C. Double-balloon enteroscopy (push-and-pull enteroscopy) of the small bowel: feasibility and diagnostic and therapeutic yield in patients with suspected small bowel disease. *Gastrointest Endosc.* 2005;62(1):62–70.
13. Akerman PA, Agrawal D, Chen W, Cantero D, Avila J, Pangtay J. Spiral enteroscopy: a novel method of enteroscopy by using the endo-ease discovery SB overtube and a pediatric colonoscope. *Gastrointest Endosc.* 2009;69(2):327–332.
14. Canin-Endres J, Salky B, Gattorno F. Laparoscopically assisted intestinal resection in 88 patients with Crohn's disease. *Surg Endosc.* 1999;13(6):595–599.
15. Masselli G, Di Tola M, Casciani E, et al. Diagnosis of small-bowel diseases: prospective comparison of multi-detector row CT enterography with MR enterography. *Radiology.* 2016;279:420–431.
16. Cheung DY, Kim JS, Shim KN, Choi MG; Korean Gut Image Study Group. The usefulness of capsule endoscopy for small bowel tumors. *Clin Endosc.* 2016;49(1):21–25.
17. Jann H, Roll S, Couvelard A, et al. Neuroendocrine tumors of midgut and hindgut origin: tumor-node-metastasis classification determines clinical outcome. *Cancer.* 2011;117(15):3332–3341.
18. Dematteo RP, Ballman KV, Antonescu CR, et al. Adjuvant imatinib mesylate after resection of localized, primary gastrointestinal stromal tumour: a randomized, double-blind, placebo-controlled trial. *Lancet.* 2009;373(9669):1097–1104.
19. Ambrosini V, Zanoni L, Filice A, et al. Radiolabelled somatostatin analogues for diagnosis and treatment of neuroendocrine tumors. *Cancers (Basel).* 2022;14(4):1055.
20. Walter T, Brixi-Benmansour H, Lombard-Bohas C, Cadiot G. New treatment strategies in advanced neuroendocrine tumours. *Dig Liver Dis.* 2012;44(2):95–105.
21. Gurusamy KS, Pamecha V, Sharma D, Davidson BR. Palliative cytoreductive surgery versus other palliative treatments in patients with unresectable liver metastases from gastro-entero-pancreatic neuroendocrine tumours. *Cochrane Database Syst Rev.* 2009;2009(1):CD007118.
22. Oberg K, Ferone D, Kaltsas G. ENETS Consensus guidelines for the standards of care in neuroendocrine tumors: biotherapy. *Neuroendocrinology.* 2009;90(2):209–213.
23. Lu Y, Frobom R, Lagergren J. Incidence patterns of small bowel cancer in a population-based study in Sweden: increase in duodenal adenocarcinoma. *Cancer Epidemiol.* 2012;36(3):e158–e163.
24. Raghav K, Overman MJ. Small bowel adenocarcinomas—existing evidence and evolving paradigms. *Nat Rev Clin Oncol.* 2013;10(9): 534–544.
25. Haselkorn T, Whittemore AS, Lilienfeld DE. Incidence of small bowel cancer in the United States and worldwide: geographic, temporal, and racial differences. *Cancer Causes Control.* 2005;16(7):781–787.
26. Talamonti MS, Goetz LH, Rao S. Primary cancers of the small bowel: analysis of prognostic factors and results of surgical management. *Arch Surg.* 2002;137(5):564–570, discussion 570–571.
27. Zaanan A, Costes L, Gauthier M, et al. Chemotherapy of advanced small-bowel adenocarcinoma: a multicenter AGEO study. *Ann Oncol.* 2010;21(9):1786–1793.
28. Van Weyenberg SJB, Meijerink MR, Jacobs MAJM, et al. MR enteroclysis in the diagnosis of small-bowel neoplasms. *Radiology.* 2010;254(3):765–773.
29. Nicholl MB, Ahuja V, Conway WC, Vu VD, Sim MS, Singh G. Small bowel adenocarcinoma: understaged and undertreated? *Ann Surg Oncol.* 2010;17(10):2728–2732.
30. Overman MJ, Hu CY, Wolff RA, Chang GJ. Prognostic value of lymph node evaluation in small bowel adenocarcinoma: analysis of the surveillance, epidemiology, and end results database. *Cancer.* 2010;116(23):5374–5382.
31. Tran TB, Qadan M, Dua MM, Norton JA, Poultsides GA, Visser BC. Prognostic relevance of lymph node ratio and total lymph node count for small bowel adenocarcinoma. *Surgery.* 2015;158(2):486–493.
32. Wilhelm A, Muller SA, Steffen T, Schmied BM, Beutner U, Warschkow R. Patients with adenocarcinoma of the small intestine with 9 or more regional lymph nodes retrieved have a higher rate of positive lymph nodes and improved survival. *J Gastrointest Surg.* 2016;20(2):401–410.
33. Poultsides GA, Huang LC, Cameron JL, et al. Duodenal adenocarcinoma: clinicopathologic analysis and implications for treatment. *Ann Surg Oncol.* 2012;19(6):1928–1935.
34. Markowitz SD, Bertagnolli MM. Molecular origins of cancer: molecular basis of colorectal cancer. *N Engl J Med.* 2009; 361:2449–2460.
35. Onkendi EO, Boostrom SY, Sarr MG, et al. Neoadjuvant treatment of duodenal adenocarcinoma: a rescue strategy. *J Gastrointest Surg.* 2012;16:320–324.
36. Lecuit M, Lortholary O. Immunoproliferative small intestinal disease associated with Campylobacter jejuni? *Med Mal Infect.* 2005;35(Suppl 2):S56–S58.
37. Nagashima R, Takeda H, Maeda K, Ohno S, Takahashi T. Regression of duodenal mucosa-associated lymphoid tissue lymphoma after eradication of Helicopter pylori? *Gastroenterology.* 1996;111(6):1674–1678.
38. Lai EC, Lau SH, Lau WY. Current management of gastrointestinal stromal tumors—a comprehensive review? *Int J Surg.* 2012;10(7):334–340.
39. Hirota S, Isozaki K, Moriyama Y, et al. Gain-of-function mutations of c-kit in human gastrointestinal stromal tumors. *Science.* 1998;279(5350):557–580.
40. Bumming P, Ahlman H, Andersson J, Meis-Kindblom JM, Kindblom LG, Nilsson B. Population-based study of the diagnosis and treatment of gastrointestinal stromal tumours. *Br J Surg.* 2006;93(7):836–843.
41. Coco C, Rizzo G, Manno A, Mattana C, Verbo A. Surgical treatment of small bowel neoplasms. *Eur Rev Med Pharmacol Sci.* 2010;14(4):327–333.
42. Retsas S, Christofyllakis C. Melanoma involving the gastrointestinal tract. *Anticancer Res.* 2001;21(2B):1503–1507.

49

Section G:
PANCREAS

Pancreas Anatomy and Physiology

Anays Murillo, Teviah E. Sachs, and Jennifer F. Tseng

Key Points

1. The pancreas is an endocrine and exocrine organ that lies in the retroperitoneum, whose primary functions are to regulate carbohydrate metabolism and secrete enzymes to aid in digestion.
2. Its head lies in the second and third portions of the duodenum, its body lies behind the stomach, and its tail terminates in the hilum of the spleen. It abuts several highly critical organs and blood vessels along its course.
3. Embryologically, the pancreas is derived from a ventral and dorsal bud, which rotate with the duodenum and fuse together to create a single gland. Abnormal rotation or fusion can lead to variant pancreatic anatomy, including pancreatic divisum and annular pancreas.
4. The exocrine pancreas makes up 90% of the mass of the gland, and can primarily be divided into the central acinus, which secretes fluid and enzymes for digestion, and the ductal network through which the enzymes are flushed into the duodenum.
5. The endocrine pancreas makes up 1% to 2% of the pancreatic mass but accounts for 15% of its blood flow. Its main functional units are the islets of Langerhans, which are composed of a multitude of cells, including α- (alpha) cells, which secrete glucagon, β- (beta) cells, which secrete insulin, and δ- (delta) cells, which secrete somatostatin.
6. Insulin and glucagon act opposite one another to maintain glucose homeostasis, with insulin increasing glucose uptake by cells and glucagon stimulating gluconeogenesis and glycogenolysis from the liver. Somatostatin acts on both α- and β-cells and slows intestinal transit.
7. The superior mesenteric artery (SMA) runs behind the neck of the pancreas, as does the superior mesenteric vein, which joins the splenic vein behind the pancreatic neck to form the portal vein. Understanding this anatomy and the multiple variants that exist is crucial when operating in the abdomen and retroperitoneum.

1 ▪ The pancreas is a soft, tan-colored organ found in the retroperitoneum and has two main functions: the regulation of
2 serum glucose and the production of pancreatic enzymes critical for digestion. It lies near a multitude of upper abdominal organs and major vasculature, making the understanding of its anatomy of utmost importance to the surgeon.

▪ The pancreas is considered an upper gastrointestinal organ that acts in an exocrine, paracrine, and endocrine capacity.[1,2] The exocrine portion of the gland is comprised of acinar and ductal cells and accounts for up to 95% of the mass of the pancreas. The function of these cells is to produce and secrete an array of enzymes that are essential for absorption of nutrients in the small intestine. The endocrine function of the pancreas is carried out by the islets of Langerhans, which are distinct groupings of endocrine cells found throughout the pancreas. As opposed to the exocrine portion of the gland, these cells make up less than 1% of pancreatic tissue. However, despite their diminutive volume, they receive nearly 15% of pancreatic blood flow, which substantiates their importance.[3] These cells secrete a variety of hormones, most notably insulin, glucagon, and somatostatin, in order to regulate carbohydrate metabolism.[1,4] These endocrine hormones act systemically and upon the islets themselves, in a paracrine fashion, in order to maintain glucose homeostasis.[2] The sequelae of insult to the pancreas, whether it be surgical, traumatic, or disease, can be devastating to the patient, and therefore, a thorough understanding of pancreas physiology is paramount.

EMBRYOLOGY OF THE PANCREAS

3 ▪ The pancreas develops from two distinct primordia: the dorsal and ventral pancreatic buds. These are derived from the endoderm and form at the junction of the foregut and midgut at the septum transversum. Most of the pancreas arises from the dorsal bud, to eventually include the superior aspect of the head, the neck, the body, and the tail of the pancreas. The remainder of the head of the pancreas and the uncinate process derive from the ventral bud, which arises laterally beside the growing biliary tract. As the duodenum matures and rotates, the ventral bud follows, rotating clockwise to fuse with the dorsal bud. At the junction of the ventral and dorsal buds of the pancreas, the ducts of each bud fuse, and the duct that lies in the distal and main body of the dorsal bud empties via the ventral duct through the ampulla of Vater (major papilla) and into the duodenum. The remaining proximal duct of the dorsal bud empties directly into the duodenum more proximally, via the minor papilla (**Fig. 49.1**). The main pancreatic duct (MPD) is known as the duct of Wirsung, while the accessory pancreatic duct (APD) is known as the duct of Santorini.

▪ Though the role of endocrine cells in early development is not clearly understood, endocrine function can be measured as early as 10 weeks of gestation. Glucagon-producing α-cells differentiate first, followed by δ-cells (somatostatin) and β-cells (insulin).

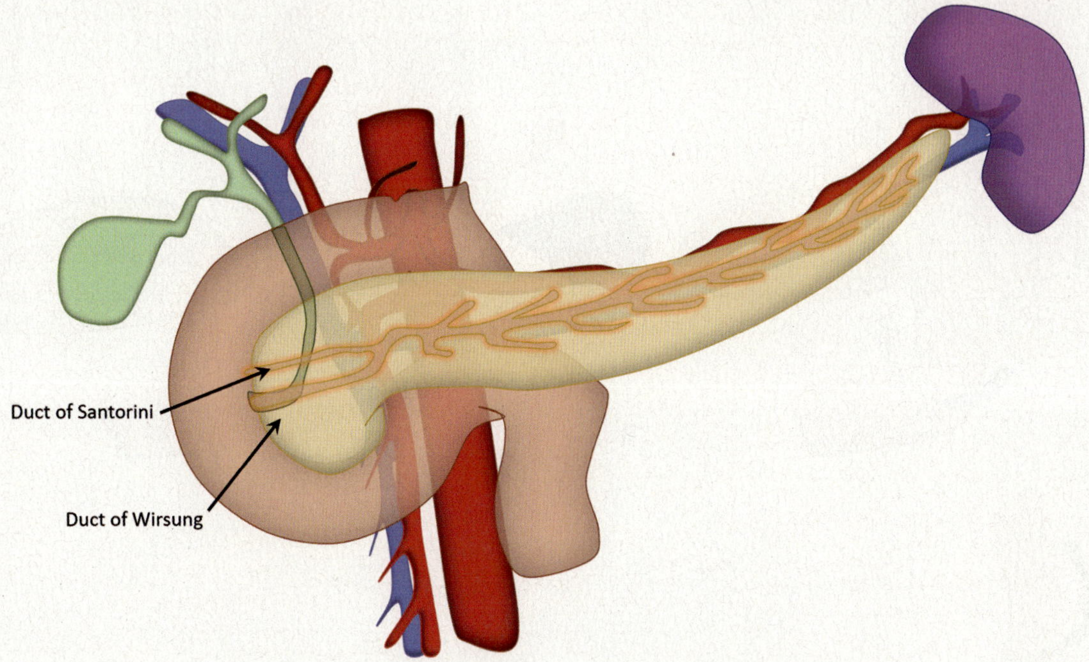

Figure 49.1. Pictorial demonstration of normal pancreatic ductal anatomy.

VARIANT EMBRYOLOGIC ANATOMY

- The variants in anatomy that come with improper embryologic development may occur in up to 30% of patients; however, most are inconsequential.

Pancreas Divisum and other MPD Variants

- Pancreas divisum is the incomplete fusion of the ventral and dorsal pancreatic buds, hence, the intrapancreatic ducts also fail to fuse. This variant occurs in less than 5% of patients, and only about 5% of those affected will develop symptoms.[5] There are three types of pancreatic divisum: type (1) the complete separation between the dorsal and ventral pancreatic ducts where the MPD drains into the minor papilla of the duodenum (MiP) and the APD opens into the major papilla of the duodenum (MP); type (2) a single MPD drains into the MiP with an absent APD; and type (3) an indirect communication between the MPD and the APD via a small branch. While pancreatic divisum is most commonly associated with pancreatitis, causality is still unclear.[6]
- Ansa pancreatica consists of an S-shaped APD that is either patent or nonpatent.
- Other MPD variants described in a recent review include: (1) bifid dual duct configuration with the MPD draining into the MP and the APD opening into the MiP, (2) bifid configuration with the MPD opening into the MiP and the APD either draining into the MP or not opening into or not reaching the MiP, and (3) the MPD draining into the MP with or without communication with the APD.
- Aside from pancreas divisum, the clinical significance of other MPD variants is minimal.[6]

Pancreaticobiliary Junction Variants

- These types of congenital malformations occur when the common bile duct (CBD) and the MPD either join or separate before entering the duodenum. A nationwide study in Japan noted high rates of biliary tract carcinogenesis of these variants, likely due to persistent pancreatic juice refluxing into the biliary tract.[7]

Annular Pancreas

- Annular pancreas may occur when a bifid or dual ventral bud forms (**Fig. 49.2A**). These two ventral buds may rotate in opposite directions (**Fig. 49.2B**) around the septum, leading to a circumferential ring of pancreatic tissue around the second portion of the duodenum (**Fig. 49.2C**). An annular variant is circumportal pancreas, which occurs when pancreatic tissue surrounds the portal vein or its immediate tributaries. Annular pancreas is rare, occurs slightly more often in females, and is usually an incidental finding in adults.[8] When symptomatic, it can cause a range of symptoms from chronic abdominal pain to acute pancreatitis in adults,[9] to very severe symptoms in neonates and children, like duodenal obstruction, usually requiring operative intervention.
- When annular pancreas is incidentally encountered in the operating room, the surgeon should take care to avoid transection of the pancreatic duct, which may lie within this tissue, as transection could lead to a pancreatic leak or fistula.
- The distal CBD can sometimes traverse the pancreas at the region of the annular pancreas in such a way that it can lead to biliary obstruction and jaundice. These cases commonly require endoscopic or operative intervention to relieve the obstruction.

Ectopic or Heterotopic Pancreas

- In ectopic or heterotopic pancreas, pancreatic tissue forms elsewhere in the gastrointestinal tract. These pancreatic rests are devoid of vascular or anatomic communication to the actual pancreas. There are four types of pancreatic heterotopia, depending on the type of tissue identified histologically (**Table 49.1**). Heterotopic pancreatic tissue can occur anywhere within the gastrointestinal tract but is most often found in the stomach followed by the duodenum, jejunum, and gallbladder. These lesions may cause symptoms ranging from abdominal pain and fullness to obstruction. In rare cases, there can be malignant degeneration where endoscopic ultrasound with biopsy is helpful in establishing a diagnosis.[10]

Hypoplasia or Agenesis

- Congenital absence of part of the pancreas is associated with exocrine pancreatic insufficiency and severe pancreatitis. A severe form is dorsal pancreatic agenesis, which is the absence of the neck, body, and tail of the pancreas derived from the dorsal bud. Though only about 100 cases

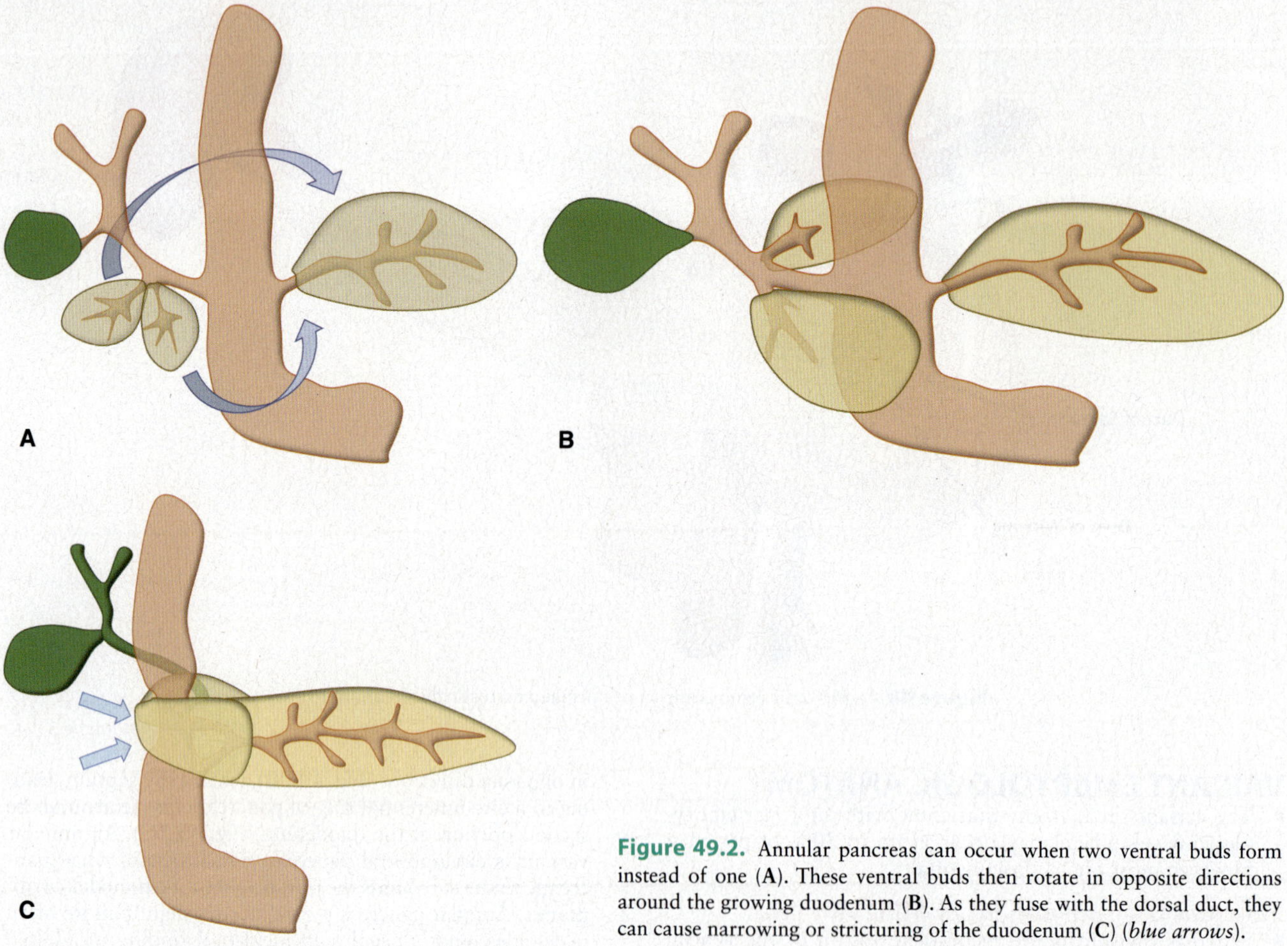

Figure 49.2. Annular pancreas can occur when two ventral buds form instead of one (**A**). These ventral buds then rotate in opposite directions around the growing duodenum (**B**). As they fuse with the dorsal duct, they can cause narrowing or stricturing of the duodenum (**C**) (*blue arrows*).

have been reported in the last century, there have been associations with nonalcoholic chronic pancreatitis and neoplasms of the residual pancreas.[11]

Congenital Pancreatic Cysts

- These fluid collections result from anomalous development of the acinar ductal network or ductal obstruction. Fluid collections are exceedingly rare but most often found in the pancreatic tail. Though benign collections can be viewed as hallmark components of genetic diseases like von Hippel–Lindau disease and autosomal-dominant polycystic kidney disease.[10]

CELLULAR ORGANIZATION OF THE PANCREAS

- The pancreas can be thought of as one gland with exocrine and endocrine functions. The cellular arrangement of the pancreas facilitates these functions. Up to 90% of the pancreatic tissue is exocrine in nature, while only 1% to 2% of the pancreas is considered endocrine. The remaining tissue consists of pancreatic stroma and vasculature.

Table 49.1. Types of Heterotopic Pancreatic Tissue as Defined by the Type of Tissue Identified on Histologic Examination

Type of Heterotopia	Distinction	Tissue Identified
I	Normal pancreas	Acini, ducts, and islet cells
II	Canalicular	Pancreatic ducts
III	Exocrine	Acini
IV	Endocrine	Islet cells

Exocrine Pancreas

4 - The exocrine pancreas has two main functions: to produce enzymes for digestion and to deliver them into the intestine. The first function is carried out by the acini, which produce all the enzymes and zymogens necessary to break down proteins, carbohydrates, and lipids for absorption by the small intestine. The acinus is the functional unit of the exocrine pancreas and consists of clusters of between 30 and 40 pyramidal cells that are arranged circumferentially around a central lumen, with their apices pointing toward the duct. These cells create the proenzymes (enzymes in their inactive form) and package them into zymogen granules for eventual secretion into the ductal network. Also important are the centroacinar cells, which secrete the fluid in which the proenzymes are delivered through the duct, and keep proenzymes in their inactive form, at an alkaline pH around 8.0. The acinar and centroacinar cells deliver their secretions into the intercalated ducts, which then coalesce to form interlobular ducts. These interlobular ducts, in turn, empty through a network of secondary ducts and eventually into the MPD for secretion into the duodenum.

Endocrine Pancreas

5 - The islets of Langerhans are the functional unit of the endocrine pancreas. These islets can contain anywhere from a few hundred to several thousand cells. The dominant cells in the islets are the β-cells, which primarily produce insulin.[2] The β-cells account for up to 70% of the mass of the

Table 49.2. Pancreatic Endocrine Cell Types

Cell Type	% Islet Cell Mass	Major Hormone Secreted	Location within Islet	Location within Pancreas	Associated Tumor Syndrome
A (α)	10%	Glucagon	Peripheral	Evenly distributed	Glucagonoma: necrolytic migratory erythema, diabetes, hypoaminoacidemia
B (β)	70%	Insulin	Central	Body/Tail	Insulinoma: hypoglycemia and associated symptoms
D	5%[a]	Somatostatin	Evenly distributed	Body/Tail	Somatostatinoma: diabetes, gallstones, steatorrhea
D_2	5%[a]	Vasoactive intestinal peptide (VIP)	Evenly distributed	Body/Tail	VIPoma: high-volume secretory diarrhea, hypokalemia, metabolic acidosis, hypochlorhydria
F	15%	Pancreatic polypeptide	Peripheral	Head/Uncinate process	Treatment directed at presenting symptoms
E/C	<1%	Substance P, serotonin	Evenly distributed	Evenly distributed	None
G	Not present in normal physiologic state	Gastrin, ACTH-related peptides	Not applicable	Head, uncinate process, duodenum	Gastrinoma: acid hypersecretion, gastric/duodenal ulcers, diarrhea

[a]Combined D and D_2 mass.

islet and are clustered toward its center. Further out from the β-cells are the α- and δ-cells, which are arranged more circumferentially around the β-cells. These cells make up as much as 20% of the pancreas.[12] The α-cells produce glucagon, which has a counter-regulatory effect on insulin. The δ-cells produce somatostatin and vasoactive intestinal peptide (VIP). F cells (also known as PP cells) produce pancreatic polypeptide (PP) and can account for 1% to 2% of the islet cell population.[13] The remaining cells include epsilon (ε) cells, which produce ghrelin, and C cells which produce substance P and serotonin.[12]

- The islets are well vascularized compared to their size, and account for 15% of pancreatic blood flow.[3] The islets have an afferent arteriole and efferent venule, between which a rich capillary bed allows for transmission of the islet hormones into circulation.
- The cellular distribution of the islets is disproportionate throughout the gland. The islets in the tail of the pancreas are dominated by β- and δ-cells, the proximal portion of the gland has more F cells, and α-cells are more evenly spread throughout the pancreas (**Table 49.2**).
- 6 The main function of the exocrine pancreas is to regulate serum glucose through the secretion of glucagon and insulin. These hormones act in a paracrine fashion on the exocrine pancreas. As serum insulin rises, exocrine functions are stimulated, leading to increased enzyme and protein synthesis and amino acid transport.[14] Glucagon acts in the opposing fashion, to downregulate pancreatic exocrine function. Somatostatin may act on β-cells and the acinar cells to downregulate pancreatic insulin secretion as well as pancreatic exocrine secretions, while VIP acts to increase water secretion in the pancreatic duct, decrease gastric secretion, and increase small intestine motility.[15]

PHYSIOLOGY OF THE PANCREAS

Exocrine Physiology

- The pancreas produces between 1.5 and 3.0 L of alkaline (pH 7.1 to 8.2) fluid per day, in which the secretory enzymes of the pancreas are delivered to the duodenum.[16] Maintaining a consistent alkaline pH is necessary for proper enzymatic function and provides a means to neutralize the acidic effluent of the stomach as it enters the duodenum.

Enzymatic Secretions

- Vagal innervation of the pancreas through cholinergic fibers acts as the primary stimulus for acinar cells to increase production and secretion of enzymes. Unlike classical synapses, neurotransmitters are released next to the islet cells, and norepinephrine and acetylcholine act on the islet cells themselves to stimulate or inhibit secretion of hormones.[17]
- Enzymes produced in the acinar cells can be grouped into those that act on carbohydrates (amylolytic), lipids (lipolytic), or proteins (proteolytic) (**Table 49.3**). Amylolytic enzymes, like amylase, break down carbohydrates into more easily digestible sugars such as maltose. Lipolytic enzymes such as lipase break down triglycerides into their main components: fatty acids and glycerols. Phospholipases break down cell membranes into arachidonic acids and phospholipids. The proteolytic enzymes (endopeptidases, exopeptidases, elastases, and nucleases) break down proteins into amino acids and nucleotides.
- Endopeptidases, like trypsinogen and chymotrypsinogen, are proenzymes, or zymogens, which are inactive forms of enzymes. They are secreted by the acinar cells via the zymogen granules and into the apical duct lumen. They are not activated until they enter the duodenum, where enterokinase is secreted by the duodenal mucosa. The enterokinase

Table 49.3. Most Common Enzymes Secreted by the Exocrine Pancreas

Enzyme	Category	Target of Action	End Product
Amylases	Amylolytic	Carbohydrates	Oligosaccharides/maltose
Lipases	Lipolytic	Lipids	Fatty acids/glycerols
Phospholipases/phospholipase B	Lipolytic	Phospholipids/cell membranes	Arachidonic acids
Cholesterol esterases	Lipolytic	Cholesterol esters	Unesterified cholesterols/fatty acids
Trypsin/chymotrypsin	Proteolytic	Peptides	Amino acids
Carboxypolypeptidase	Proteolytic	Peptides	Amino acids
Nucleases	Proteolytic	DNA/RNA	Nucleotides

then cleaves the endopeptidase, trypsinogen, initiating the proteolytic enzyme cascade where the remaining inactive precursor endopeptidases are converted into their active forms.

- The proportion of each of these groups of enzymes will fluctuate based on a variety of stimuli from neuropeptides, gastric acid secretion, and hormonal influences. Exocrine pancreatic secretion can be divided into three phases: cephalic, gastric, and intestinal (**Table 49.4**).

Bicarbonate Secretion

- Sodium bicarbonate solution is made up of water and sodium bicarbonate and is secreted by the centroacinar and terminal duct cells. The content of bicarbonate in pancreatic secretions can be as high as 145 mEq/L, as compared to bile (45 mEq/L) and serum (27 mEq/L).[18]
- When gastric acid enters the proximal duodenum, the cells of the duodenal mucosa release secretin. In addition, the presence of long-chain fatty acids and essential amino acids in the proximal small intestine leads to the release of cholecystokinin (CCK). Secretin, and to a lesser extent VIP and CCK, accelerate the uptake of bicarbonate from plasma and into the centroacinar and terminal duct cells of the acini.[19] Secretin increases cyclic AMP in these cells and activates the cystic fibrosis transmembrane conductance regulator (CFTR). The CFTR is primarily responsible for the exchange of bicarbonate for chloride, which is excreted back into the plasma to maintain anion balance.[18]
- Just as bicarbonate production by the centroacinar and terminal duct cells is activated via vagal stimulation it also inhibited by the vagus nerve via the release of atropine, and further dampened in a paracrine fashion by the hormonal effects of glucagon, PP, and somatostatin.[3,4]
- Surgical transection of vagal innervation to the upper gastrointestinal tract via truncal vagotomy can decrease the production of sodium bicarbonate solution by as much as half.[20]

Exocrine Insufficiency

- Exocrine function can be impaired by a variety of means, including loss of functional pancreatic parenchyma (surgical resection, chronic pancreatitis) or secondary loss of exocrine pancreatic function or enzymatic activity. Exocrine pancreatic insufficiency occurs when enzymatic production falls below 10% of normal.[21] Pancreatic exocrine insufficiency commonly presents with steatorrhea from insufficient lipase production.[22]
- Differentiating intestinal malabsorption from pancreatic exocrine insufficiency is the first step and can be done with a variety of tests with varying efficacy (**Table 49.5**). The most accurate tests are also the most invasive, often requiring duodenal intubation via Dreiling tube or endoscopy. Less invasive testing such as fecal fat and breath testing are easier, but less specific. In practice, when there is a high suspicion for exocrine pancreatic insufficiency, improvement with the addition of oral pancreatic enzyme replacement can be both diagnostic and therapeutic.
- Serum tests for amylase, lipase, and other enzymes are not useful in the diagnosis of pancreatic insufficiency as these enzymes are not elevated at baseline. Amylase, lipase, and trypsinogen are all useful, however, in the diagnosis of acute pancreatitis, discussed elsewhere in this book.
- The etiology of exocrine pancreatic insufficiency must be determined to treat the patient properly.

Endocrine Physiology

- The islet cells produce hormones that act in an endocrine and paracrine fashion to regulate serum glucose and affect carbohydrate metabolism. The two most important hormones are insulin (β-cells) and glucagon (α-cells), which

Table 49.4. Three Phases of Pancreatic Exocrine Secretion

Phase	Initiated by	Mediated by	Action on	Result
Cephalic	Sensory stimuli (sight, smell, taste, etc.)	Vagus nerve	Acinar cells to produce digestive enzymes	Enzymes and zymogen granules are produced in the acini
Gastric	Food within the stomach	Vagus nerve	Acinar cells to produce and secrete digestive enzymes	Enzymes and zymogens accumulate in the ductal network
Intestinal	Emptying into duodenum	Secretin and cholecystokinin	Ductal cells secrete aqueous bicarbonate solution	Enzymes and zymogen granules are washed through the ductal network and into the duodenum for activation

Table 49.5. Ways to Test Pancreatic Exocrine Insufficiency

Test Type	Item of Interest	How it is Performed	Results Consistent With Insufficiency	Other Details
Pancreatic effluent[23]	Secretin stimulation via endoscopic technique[a]	1. After overnight fasting, patient is given 0.2 μg/kg secretin bolus 2. Via endoscopic intubation, pancreatic secretions aspirated and quantified at 30- and 45-min postinjection	Peak bicarbonate concentrations <80 mmol	Gold standard Endoscopic technique requires sedation and does not yield pancreatic secretion total volume or basal rate for comparison[b]
Serum	PP	1. After overnight fasting, meal rich in carbohydrate, fat, and protein given enterally 2. Basal and postingestion serum PP values obtained	Both basal PP <100 pg/mL and response PP <250 pg/mL	Test dependent on vagal innervation; therefore prior gastric resection, truncal vagotomy, or chronic enteroneuropathic disease states can lead to false positives
Urine	BT-PABA[c]	1. 1-g bolus BT-PABA given enterally, cleaved by chymotrypsin in intestine, and PABA excreted in urine 2. PABA:BT-PABA concentration determined from 6-h urine collection	PABA concentration <60% of initial BT-PABA dose	Less invasive
Stool[22]	Qualitative "spot" analysis of stool[d]	1. At least 1-g stool sample provided 2. Fecal elastase measured	Elastase <200 mcg/g	Useful in cases of severe pancreatic insufficiency Less sensitive in mild and moderate cases
Breath[24]	Mixed triglyceride	1. Small oral bolus of C^{13} bound to corn oil given 2. CO_2 produced from enzymatic digestion and absorption quantified in patient's breath 4 h later	Cumulative recovery of C^{13} (percentage of dose given) <27%	Noninvasive Cannot differentiate between intestinal malabsorption and true pancreatic exocrine insufficiency[e]

[a]Other tests are the Lundh test (a direct measurement of enzyme secretion after a promotility agent is given) and dimethadione test (a 3-day measure of pancreatic metabolism of trimethadione to dimethadione in the setting of secretin stimulation).
[b]Historical technique was done via placing a Dreiling tube fluoroscopically and taking basal aspirates of duodenal contents.
[c]BT-PABA: N-benzoyl-1-tyrosyl paraaminobenzoic acid.
[d]Other tests are days-long stool sample collections on strict fat per day intake to calculate fat absorption. These tests are accurate but rarely performed given their level of burden.
[e]Radioactive isotope C^{14} is the original test and can differentiate between malabsorption and insufficiency but is less safe.

act in opposition to one another. Insulin activates transport of glucose into cells and inhibits the breakdown of glycogen into glucose in liver and muscle cells. It similarly inhibits the metabolism of fatty acids from adipose tissues. Glucagon acts to increase serum glucose and stimulate glycogen and fatty acid metabolism in the tissues. Somatostatin (δ-cells) causes secondary hormone activation in the intestine, and likely plays a paracrine role on the other islet cells in response to hormone.[12] Other relevant hormones include ghrelin (ε-cells) and PP (F cells) (**Table 49.6**).

Endocrine Insufficiency

- Endocrine insufficiency is generally related to insulin. A loss of β-cells, as occurs in type I diabetes, is most often due to autoimmune destruction. In these patients, the sensitivity to insulin is unaffected, and serum glucose homeostasis can be compensated with exogenous insulin. A loss of 70 to 80% of β-cells in the pancreas will generally lead to type I diabetes.[25] In type II diabetes, the islet cells produce insulin normally, but there is a loss of function or affinity for insulin on the cell surface, leading to elevated plasma glucose levels. Increased endogenous insulin stimulation, such as occurs with sulfonylureas, can be effective in type II diabetes, in addition to exogenous insulin.

PANCREATIC ANATOMY

7 ■ Understanding of the anatomic relationships of the pancreas with other organs is paramount for the surgeon.
  - Location: The pancreas is a retroperitoneal organ that runs obliquely from its head, surrounded by the second and third portions of the duodenum, to its tail, in the hilum of the spleen. Physiologically, the pancreas empties its exocrine contents from the tail, along the body and neck, and through the head, into the duodenum. However, anatomically we distinguish the head and uncinate process of the gland as proximal and the body and tail as distal.
  - Zones and Vasculature: The pancreas is often thought of as having four zones of significance: the head/uncinate process, the neck, the body, and the tail (**Fig. 49.3**). However, there is little anatomic distinction between these areas, other than their relationship to adjacent organs and vasculature. The arterial blood supply to the pancreas comes from the celiac axis (**Fig. 49.4**). Venous drainage of the pancreas follows a distribution like that of the arterial supply. In this context, it is also important to consider the relation of the pancreas to the CBD at the ampulla of Vater (**Fig. 49.5**). The zones, arterial supply, and venous drainage of the pancreas are detailed in **Table 49.7**.
  - Aberrant arterial anatomy: This type of anatomy exists in approximately 20% to 30% of patients (**Fig. 49.6**). The

Table 49.6. Important Pancreatic Hormones

Type	Precursor	How it is Stimulated	Relevance
Insulin	Preproinsulin is synthesized in the endoplasmic reticulum and then cleaved to form proinsulin Proinsulin is cleaved by a protease in the secretory vesicles, forming active insulin and C-peptide	GIP[a], GLP-1[b], CCK, and glucagon	Serum levels of exogenous insulin can be differentiated from endogenous insulin by the presence of C-peptide in bloodstream Insulin has an 8- to 10-min half-life Insulin is not metabolized by RBCs or brain cells In the liver, uptake and storage of glucose by hepatocytes can be completed independent of insulin Insulin resistance is hallmark of type II diabetes
Glucagon	Proglucagon leads to glucagon in its active form and is secreted into pancreatic venules, enters portal circulation, and acts on hepatocytes, causing increase in glycogenolysis and gluconeogenesis in the liver[17]	Hypoglycemia, with autonomic stimulation of α-cells likely being the major driver	Glucagon oversecretion, as can happen with functional pancreatic neuroendocrine tumors, can lead to profound hyperglycemia Absence of glucagon, as can happen with total pancreatectomy, can cause hypoglycemia
SST[c]	Prepro-SST is cleaved into pro-SST and then posttranslates to SST Only 5% of SST found in circulation is from the islet cells, with the remainder coming from the GI tract and hypothalamus[12]	Rising serum glucose and amino acids leucine and arginine	Majority of effects of SST are seen centrally or in the proximal GI tract, where SST inhibits gastric, pancreatic, and biliary secretion SST analogs, like octreotide, are used to slow intestinal transit, limit effects of neuroendocrine tumors, and reduce fistula output after pancreatic resection[26] SST inhibits both insulin and glucagon[12]
Ghrelin	Preproghrelin is cleaved to yield ghrelin Most circulating ghrelin is secreted by the stomach, then the small intestine, and there is only low-level ghrelin expression in islet cells	Glucagon and vagus nerve excitation	Stimulates SST thus inhibiting insulin and glucagon[27]
PP[d]	Prepro-PP precursor processed to PP in, and secreted by, islet cells	Vagus nerve excitation	Decreases glucagon, hepatic gluconeogenesis, glycogenolysis, and pancreatic/biliary secretions

[a]GIP: gastric inhibitory polypeptide.
[b]GLP-1: glucagon-like peptide-1.
[c]SST: somatostatin.
[d]PP: pancreatic polypeptide.

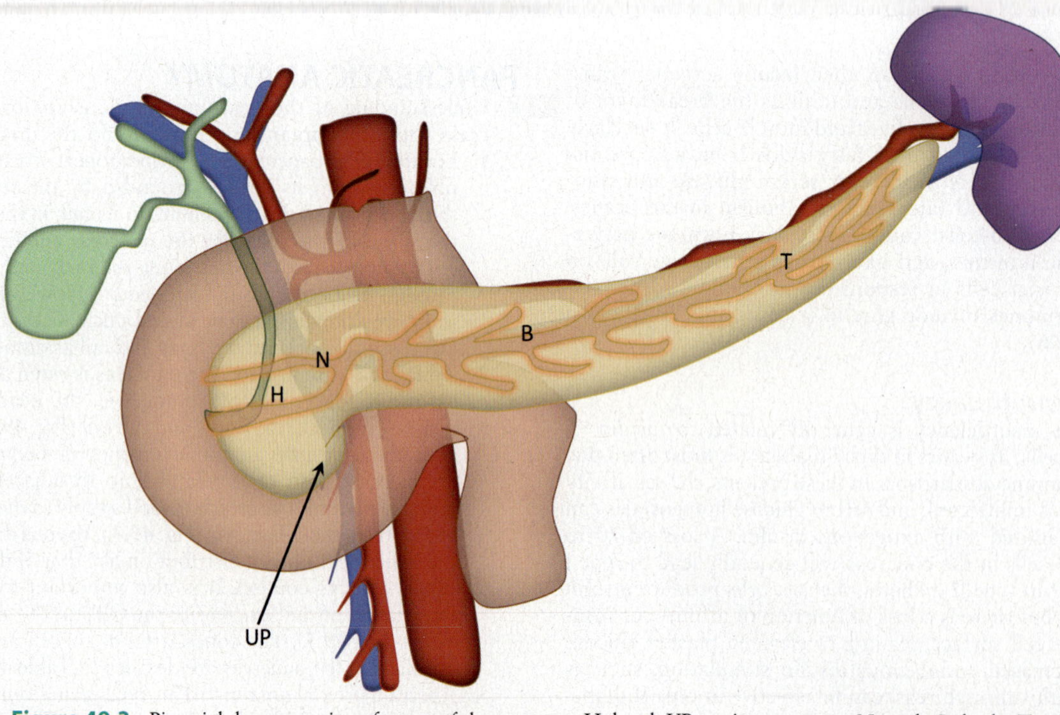

Figure 49.3. Pictorial demonstration of zones of the pancreas. H, head; UP, uncinate process; N, neck; B, body; T, tail.

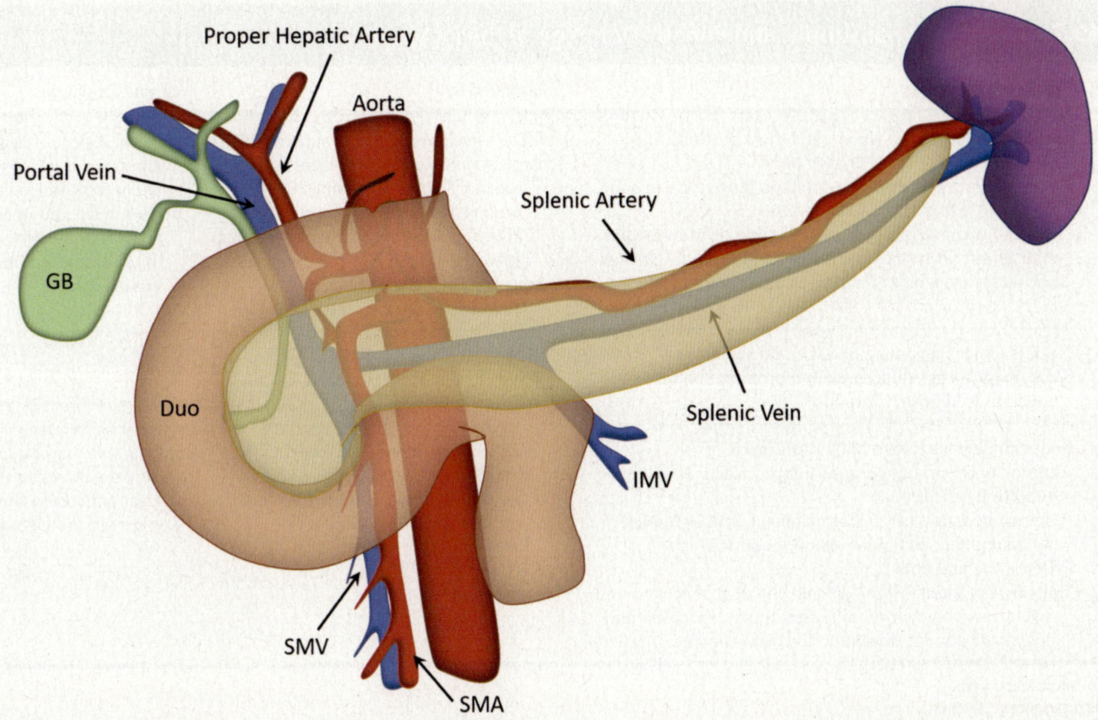

Figure 49.4. Pictorial demonstration of vasculature of the pancreas. SMV, superior mesenteric vein; SMA, superior mesenteric artery; IMV, inferior mesenteric vein; GB, gallbladder; Duo, Duodenum.

most common anomaly is a replaced or aberrant right hepatic artery arising from the superior mesenteric artery (SMA), which can occur over 20% of the time.[28] In these cases, the right hepatic artery courses posterior to the head of the pancreas and along the posterolateral aspect of the bile duct. Palpation of this border of the bile duct is paramount prior to any dissection to avoid unnecessary injury. The second most common anomaly is the replaced left hepatic artery, which most commonly is supplied by the left gastric artery. In these cases, which occur in 5% to 10% of patients, the vessel can be found along the anterior border of the caudate lobe, entering the liver between segments 3 and 4, alongside the round ligament. It should be noted that either of these anomalies can present as an accessory artery, whereby there is some degree of duplication of the arterial inflow. In some cases, the accessory artery is diminutive compared to the true artery, though care should still be taken to avoid injuring these accessory vessels as they may provide important inflow to certain segments of the liver. Less common is the replaced common hepatic artery, whereby all the inflow to the liver is supplied by a common trunk arising from the SMA. This can occur up to 5% of the time. Unlike the replaced right hepatic artery, these course more medially, between the neck and head of the pancreas, and along the posteromedial border of the CBD.

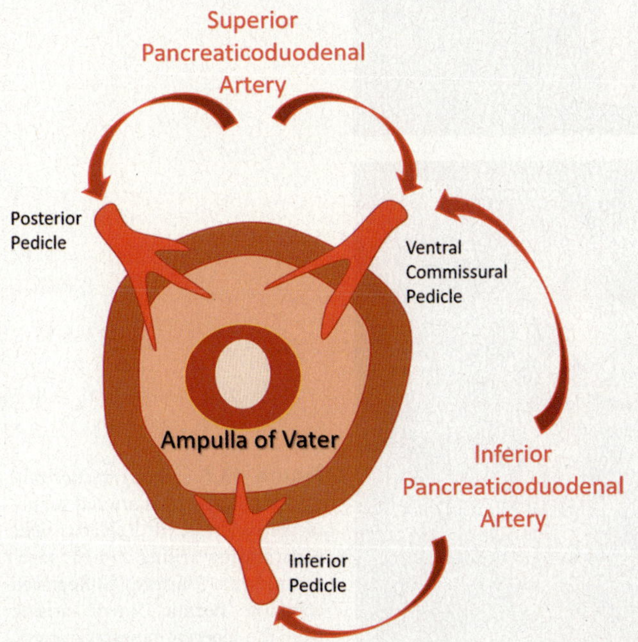

Figure 49.5. Pictorial demonstration of blood supply to the ampulla of Vater.

Lymphatics

- Due to its rich vascular supply and drainage, the pancreas has a similarly prominent lymphatic drainage. There are five major drainage patterns of the pancreas:
  - Superior: drains superior portion of pancreas head and neck
  - Inferior: drains inferior portion of pancreas head and uncinate
  - Anterior: drains prepyloric and infrapyloric regions
  - Posterior: drains portions of the head, distal CBD, and, ampulla
  - Splenic: drains pancreatic body and tail
- The 18 nodal stages as described by the Japanese Pancreas Society are presented in **Table 49.8**.

Innervation

- As previously noted, the pancreas is innervated via the vagus nerve as well as the thoracic splanchnic nerves. The sympathetic and parasympathetic nerves travel from the ganglia of the celiac axis and the proximal SMA. The sympathetic nerves inhibit exocrine and endocrine function, while the parasympathetic nerves stimulate these functions. In addition to direct stimuli, the vagal branches also have secretory neurons that secrete both stimulatory and inhibitory hormones to the islets and acini. Sensory fibers from the pancreas track toward the celiac and SMA ganglia, which can be an important focus for pain control in patients with pain from pancreatic disease.

Table 49.7. Zones, Arterial Supply, and Venous Drainage of the Pancreas

Zone	Notable Positioning	Supplied By	Venous Drainage
Head/ Uncinate Process	Head is nestled within second and third portions of duodenum, beginning right of SMV[a] Uncinate process wraps inferiorly and posteriorly around SMV and SMA[b] Head and uncinate process are fused and lie atop medial half of inferior vena cava, distal left RV[c], and right RA[d] CBD[e] runs through head and joins pancreatic duct	GDA[f] which produces the superior PDA[g] Anterior and posterior branches of superior PDA and inferior PDA (arises from proximal SMA), jointly called PDA arcade, supply proximal pancreas as well as distal CBD and duodenum Superior and inferior PDA supply ampulla of Vater	Superior aspect of head drains via superior venous arcade and into portal vein Inferior head and uncinate process drain into SMV via the anterior and inferior venous arcades
Neck	Neck is under the joining of SMV and splenic vein SMA (exits aorta behind neck and proximal body) runs medially and posterior to SMV	PDA arcade and branches of DPA[h], which arise from proximal splenic artery	Portal vein
Body/ Tail	Body/tail lie posterior to body of stomach Anterior body/tail has peritoneal layer, acting as posterior reflection of lesser sac Posterior body/tail lies in direct contact with aorta, left adrenal gland, left kidney, left RV, and RA IMV[i] lies behind body Tail variably intimate with splenic hilum; splenic vein and artery run posterior to tail; distal transverse colon and splenic flexure lie along anterioinferior border of tail	Splenic artery and its branches: DPA (supplies proximal body), great pancreatic artery (supplies midbody), and caudal pancreatic artery (supplies tail)	Splenic vein via branches: caudal pancreatic vein, great pancreatic vein, and inferior pancreatic vein

[a]SMV: superior mesenteric vein.
[b]SMA: superior mesenteric artery.
[c]RV: renal vein.
[d]RA: renal artery.
[e]CBD: common bile duct.
[f]GDA: gastroduodenal artery.
[g]PDA: pancreaticoduodenal artery.
[h]DPA: dorsal pancreatic artery.
[i]IMV: inferior mesenteric vein.

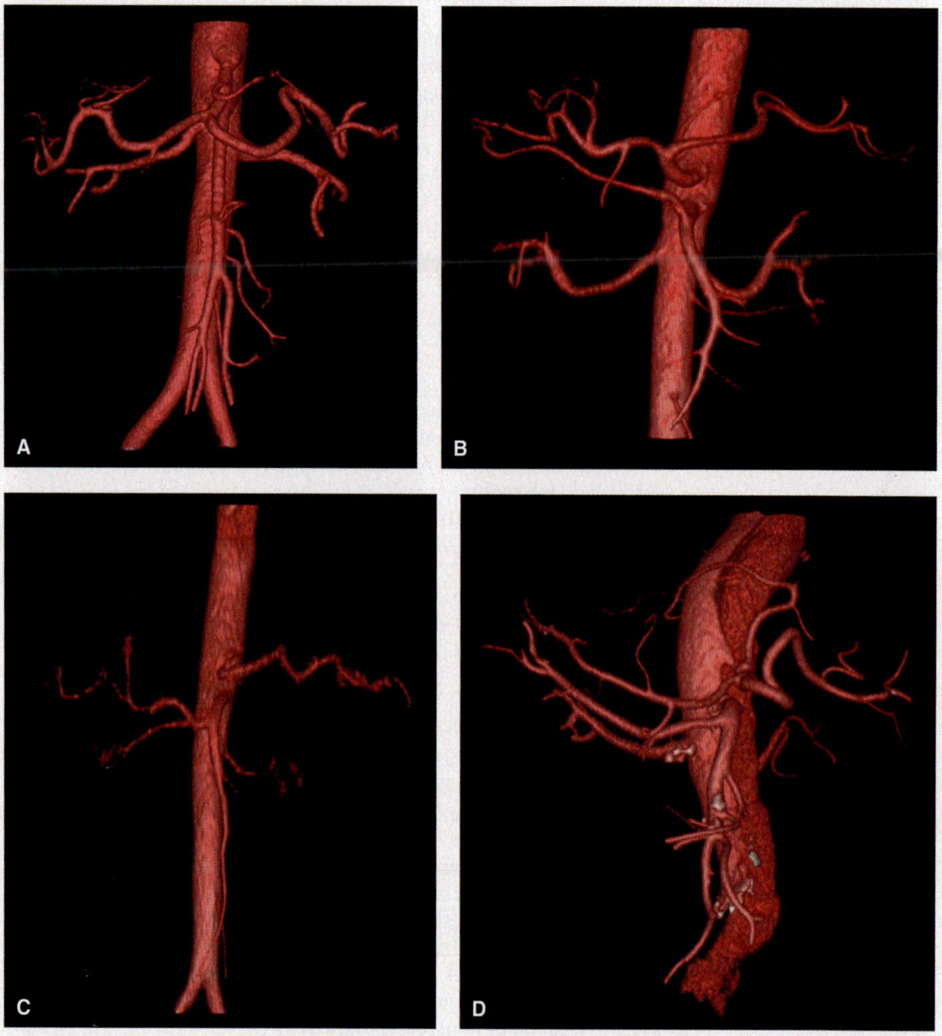

Figure 49.6. 3D CT reconstructions of (**A**) Normal arterial supply to the pancreas, (**B**) Replaced right hepatic artery arising from the superior mesenteric artery, (**C**) Replaced common hepatic artery arising from the superior mesenteric artery, and (**D**) Replaced left hepatic artery arising from the splenic artery.

Table 49.8. Japanese Lymph Node Stations

Station Number	Name	Standard	Radical
3	Gastric lesser curve	No[a]	Yes[b]
4	Gastric greater curve	No[a]	Yes[b]
5	Superior pyloric	No[a]	Yes
6	Inferior pyloric	No[a]	Yes
8	Common hepatic artery	No	No
9	Celiac origin	No	Yes[c]
12	Hepatoduodenal ligament		
12a2	Proper hepatic artery near GDA	No[d]	No[d]
12b2	Bile duct below cystic duct	Yes[e]	Yes[e]
12c	Around cystic duct	Yes	Yes
12p2	Retro portal vein below cystic duct	No[d]	No[d]
13	Posterior pancreaticoduodenal	Yes	Yes
14	SMA and SMV nodes		
14a	Origin of SMA	No	No
14b	Right side of SMA	Yes[e]	Yes[e]
14c	Anterior SMA at middle colic	No	No
14d	Left side of SMA at first jejunal branch	No	No
14v	SMV nodes	Yes[e]	Yes[e]
16	Aortocaval nodes		
16a2	Celiac to left renal vein	No	Yes[f]
16b1	Left renal vein to IMA	No	Yes
17	Anterior pancreaticoduodenal	Yes	Yes

[a]Unless a distal gastrectomy is performed as part of standard resection.
[b]Some of these nodes may accompany the distal gastrectomy specimen.
[c]Sampled only.
[d]Not formally resected.
[e]Some of these nodes may accompany the pancreaticoduodenectomy specimen.
[f]Some of these nodes, cephalad to the left renal vein, but not required to dissect the celiac axis origin.
From Yeo CJ, Cameron JL, Lillemoe KD, et al. Pancreaticoduodenectomy with or without distal gastrectomy and extended retroperitoneal lymphadenectomy for periampullary adenocarcinoma, part 2: randomized controlled trial evaluating survival, morbidity, and mortality? *Ann Surg.* 2002;236(3):355–366; discussion 366–368.

References

1. Wu D, Xu Y, Zeng Y, Wang X. Endocrine pancreatic function changes after acute pancreatitis. *Pancreas*. 2011;40(7):1006–1011.
2. Caicedo A. Paracrine and autocrine interactions in the human islet: more than meets the eye. *Semin Cell Dev Biol*. 2013;24(1):11–21.
3. Citro A, Ott HC. Can we re-engineer the endocrine pancreas? *Curr Diab Rep*. 2018;18(11):122.
4. Ballian N, Brunicardi FC. Islet vasculature as a regulator of endocrine pancreas function. *World J Surg*. 2007;31(4):705–714.
5. Ferri V, Vicente E, Quijano Y, et al. Diagnosis and treatment of pancreas divisum: a literature review. *Hepatobiliary Pancreat Dis Int*. 2019;18(4):332–336.
6. Dugic A, Nikolic S, Mühldorfer S, et al. Clinical importance of main pancreatic duct variants and possible correlation with pancreatic diseases. *Scand J Gastroenterol*. 2020;55(5):517–527.
7. Kamisawa T, Kuruma S, Tabata T, et al. Pancreaticobiliary maljunction and biliary cancer. *J Gastroenterol*. 2015;50(3):273–279.
8. Plutecki D, Ostrowski P, Bonczar M, et al. Exploring the clinical characteristics and prevalence of the annular pancreas: a meta-analysis. *HPB (Oxford)*. 2024;26(4):486–502.
9. Nagpal SJS, Peeraphatdit T, Sannapaneni SK, et al. Clinical spectrum of adult patients with annular pancreas: findings from a large single institution cohort. *Pancreatology*. 2019;19(2):290–295.
10. Ehrhardt JD, Gomez F. Embryology, pancreas. [Updated 2023 Aug 14]. In: *StatPearls [Internet]*. StatPearls Publishing; 2024.
11. Cienfuegos JA, Rotellar F, Salguero J, Benito A, Solórzano JL, Sangro B. Agenesis of the dorsal pancreas: systematic review of a clinical challenge. *Rev Esp Enferm Dig*. 2016;108(8):479–484.
12. Hartig SM, Cox AR. Paracrine signaling in islet function and survival. *J Mol Med (Berl)*. 2020;98(4):451–467.
13. Da Silva Xavier G. The Cells of the Islets of Langerhans. *J Clin Med*. 2018;7(3):54.
14. Guruswamy Damodaran R, Poussard A, Côté B, Vermette P. Insulin secretion kinetics from single islets reveals distinct subpopulations. *Biotechnol Prog*. 2018;34(4):1059–1068.
15. Verges B. Effects of anti-somatostatin agents on glucose metabolism. *Diabetes Metab*. 2017;43(5):411–415.
16. Morrison JD. Prolonged stimulation of pancreatic serous secretions by bile and sodium taurocholate in anaesthetized rats. *J Physiol Biochem*. 2012;68(4):503–520.
17. Taborsky GJ Jr. The physiology of glucagon. *J Diabetes Sci Technol*. 2010;4(6):1338–1344.
18. Case RM, Scratcherd T, Wynne RD. The origin and secretion of pancreatic juice bicarbonate. *J Physiol*. 1970;210(1):1–15.
19. Cleveland MH, Sawyer JM, Afelik S, Jensen J, Leach SD. Exocrine ontogenies: on the development of pancreatic acinar, ductal and centroacinar cells. *Semin Cell Dev Biol*. 2012;23(6):711–719.
20. Hoffmann J, Jense HE, Christiansen J, Olesen A, Loud FB, Hauch O. Prospective controlled vagotomy trial for duodenal ulcer. Results after 11–15 years. *Ann Surg*. 1989;209(1):40–45.
21. Singh VK, Haupt ME, Geller DE, Hall JA, Quintana Diez PM. Less common etiologies of exocrine pancreatic insufficiency. *World J Gastroenterol*. 2017;23(39):7059–7076.
22. Hart PA, Conwell DA. Diagnosis of exocrine pancreatic insufficiency. *Curr Treat Options Gastroenterol*. 2015;13(3):347–353.
23. Stevens T, Parsi MA. Update on endoscopic pancreatic function testing. *World J Gastroenterol*. 2011;17(35):3957–3961.
24. Lindkvist B. Diagnosis and treatment of pancreatic exocrine insufficiency. *World J Gastroenterol*. 2013;19(42):7258–7266.
25. Cnop M, Welsh N, Jonas JC, Jörns A, Lenzen S, Eizirik DL. Mechanisms of pancreatic beta-cell death in type 1 and type 2 diabetes: many differences, few similarities. *Diabetes*. 2005;54(Suppl 2):S97–S107.
26. Ma LW, Dominguez-Rosado I, Gennarelli RL, et al. The cost of postoperative pancreatic fistula versus the cost of pasireotide: results from a prospective randomized trial. *Ann Surg*. 2017;265(1):11–16.
27. Adriaenssens AE, Svendsen B, Lam BYH, et al. Transcriptomic profiling of pancreatic alpha, beta and delta cell populations identifies delta cells as a principal target for ghrelin in mouse islets. *Diabetologia*. 2016;59(10):2156–2165.
28. Shukla PJ, Barreto SG, Kulkarni A, Nagarajian MS, Nagarajan G, Fingerhut A. Vascular anomalies encountered during pancreatoduodenectomy: do they influence outcomes? *Ann Surg Oncol*. 2010;17(1):186–193.

50

Acute Pancreatitis

Lars W. A. J. VanderBroeck, Stefan A. W. Bouwense, Hjalmar van Santvoort, and Marc G. Besselink for the Dutch Pancreatitis Study Group

Key Points

1. Acute pancreatitis (AP) is one of the most common gastrointestinal disorders requiring acute hospitalization in Western countries, with a reported incidence ranging from approximately 4.5 to 100 per 100,000 persons and an increasing trend over time.
2. Although AP is mild in most patients, approximately 20% develop moderately severe or severe disease, often associated with pancreatic or peripancreatic necrosis and/or (multi)organ failure. Overall mortality of AP is approximately 4%, increasing to about 15% in sterile necrosis and up to 30% in infected pancreatic necrosis; early deaths are mainly due to organ failure, whereas late mortality is predominantly related to infected necrosis.
3. Gallstones (45%) and alcohol abuse are the most common etiologies of AP, accounting for the majority of cases, while 16% to 26% of cases remain idiopathic after standard diagnostic evaluation.
4. Severe AP can trigger an extensive inflammatory response comparable to sepsis, trauma, or burns, characterized by cytokine release, immune-cell activation, and endothelial dysfunction, leading to systemic inflammatory response syndrome (SIRS). Early SIRS is associated with worse outcomes.
5. The typical clinical presentation of AP includes sudden-onset severe abdominal pain, often accompanied by nausea and vomiting, with frequent radiation of pain to the back. The diagnosis of AP according to the 2012 Revised Atlanta Classification requires at least two of the following three criteria: (1) characteristic abdominal pain, (2) serum amylase and/or lipase levels greater than three times the upper limit of normal, or (3) imaging findings consistent with pancreatitis.
6. In the absence of curative therapy, early management of AP is supportive and consists of adequate analgesia, fluid resuscitation, and nutritional support. Balanced crystalloid solutions such as Ringer lactate are preferred for fluid resuscitation; aggressive fluid administration is associated with increased risk of fluid overload without improved outcomes. The current IAP/APA guidelines recommend a moderate infusion rate of 5 to 10 mL/kg/h until resuscitation goals are achieved. Early oral feeding as tolerated is recommended; if oral intake is insufficient, enteral nutrition is preferred over parenteral nutrition, with nasogastric or nasojejunal feeding both acceptable. Pain management should follow general pain management principles with frequent reassessment, as evidence specific to analgesic strategies in AP is limited. Prophylactic antibiotics and probiotics do not prevent infected pancreatic necrosis and are not recommended; antibiotics are indicated only in suspected or confirmed infection.
7. Approximately one-third of pancreatic and peripancreatic necrotic collections become infected, and infection is diagnosed based on clinical, laboratory, and imaging findings. Most sterile necrotic collections resolve with conservative management; invasive intervention should be avoided or delayed to reduce the risk of secondary iatrogenic infection. When intervention is required for infected necrosis, postponement until encapsulation (>4 weeks) is preferred, as early intervention is associated with increased morbidity and need for additional procedures.
8. The treatment of choice for infected necrotizing pancreatitis is the step-up approach, starting with percutaneous or endoscopic drainage and escalating to minimally invasive necrosectomy if necessary. Compared with primary open necrosectomy, the step-up approach reduces new-onset multiple organ failure, morbidity, serious adverse events, and health care costs, and has largely replaced upfront open surgery.
9. Endoscopic approaches, when technically feasible, provide outcomes comparable to surgical approaches with fewer pancreatocutaneous fistulas and shorter hospital stays. Percutaneous catheter drainage alone can be definitive in up to 56% of patients; drain upsizing improves efficacy and facilitates subsequent interventions if needed.
10. When drainage fails, minimally invasive necrosectomy, particularly video-assisted retroperitoneal debridement (VARD), is effective and associated with reduced morbidity compared with open necrosectomy.

PRESENTATION, DIAGNOSTIC ROUTE, AND TREATMENT OF ACUTE PANCREATITIS

EPIDEMIOLOGY

1 Acute pancreatitis (AP) ranks among the most prevalent gastrointestinal disorders necessitating immediate hospitalization in the Western world.[1] The annual incidence of AP fluctuates between 4.5 and 100 cases per 100,000 individuals, and reports indicate a rising trend in both Europe and the United States.[2] While global data on the incidence and prevalence of AP remain unclear due to the absence of high-quality research, an increase in related risk factors such as biliary disease, particularly in developing countries primarily driven by the increased rates of obesity, suggests that AP prevalence may also be increasing.[3,4] Although AP is typically mild in most

Table 50.1. Less Frequent Etiologies of Acute Pancreatitis[8]

Trauma	Sphincter of Oddi spasm
Neoplasms (eg, pancreatic cancer, IPMN)	Medications
Pancreas divisum	Ischemia
Hyperlipidemia/hypercalcemia	Pregnancy
Toxins Parathion Scorpion venom	ERCP, endoscopic retrograde cholangiopancreatography
Infectious agents Viruses (eg, mumps and Coxsackie B viruses; HIV) Bacteria (eg, *Salmonella* and *Shigella* species; hemorrhagic *Escherichia coli*) Biliary parasites (eg, *Ascaris lumbricoides*)	Genetic causes Cationic trypsinogen *PRSS1* mutations Pancreatic secretory trypsin inhibitor *SPINK1* mutations Cystic fibrosis transmembrane conductance regulator *CFTR* mutations
Autoimmune pancreatitis (lymphoplasmacytic sclerosing pancreatitis)	Vasculitis (eg, systemic lupus erythematosus and polyarteritis nodosa)

patients, about 20% experience a moderate to severe progression of the disease, which may include necrosis of pancreatic or peripancreatic tissue and possibly (multi-)organ failure.[5] In approximately one-third of these cases, pancreatic necrosis becomes secondarily infected, often leading to (severe) morbidity and mortality.

The overall mortality rate for AP is approximately 4%. However, in cases of severe acute pancreatitis (SAP), mortality increases significantly ranging from 15% in cases of sterile
2 necrosis to 30% among individuals with infected pancreatic necrosis.[6] Of these deaths, approximately 40% occur within the first 14 days of hospital admission, primarily due to multiorgan failure. The remaining fatalities happen after this period and are predominantly caused by complications from infected necrosis.[7]

ETIOLOGY

Gallstones (45%) and alcohol abuse (20%) are the predominant causes of AP, accounting for most of its etiologies. Other less common causes are described in **Table 50.1**.[8] In 16% to 26% of cases, the specific cause of AP remains unidentified even after standard diagnostic evaluations (see the "Diagnostics" section). These instances often necessitate further investigation through follow-up diagnostics, including repeat transabdominal ultrasounds, endoscopic ultrasounds (EUS), or magnetic resonance cholangiopancreatography (MRCP).[9] The PICUS trial demonstrated that among patients in which
3 EUS did not demonstrate a clear etiology there was a higher chance of recurrent AP compared with a proven etiology, especially among patients that had not undergone cholecystectomy presumably due to a biliary cause like microlithiasis.[10] A recent observational cohort study indicated that, among patients experiencing their first episode of AP without an identifiable cause, further diagnostic efforts uncovered ampullary or pancreatic neoplasms in 7% of cases. The likelihood to detect such neoplasms increases to 12% in patients with recurrent idiopathic AP.[9] Hence careful assessment of the underlying etiology is necessary.

PHYSIOLOGY

AP may induce acinar cell necrosis due to initial inflammation, resulting in a release of activated pancreatic enzymes (protease precursor enzymes [trypsinogen]) into the cellular interstitium, activating local vasoconstriction–dilation mechanisms. Infiltration of inflammatory cells occurs in the pancreatic parenchyma with the consequent increase of cellular necrosis.

4 In the most severe forms of AP, an extensive cellular and humoral response may develop, similar to disorders like septic shock, multiple trauma, and extensive burns. The magnitude and continuation of such events are attributed to the development of systemic inflammatory response syndrome (SIRS), which may cause organ failure.[11–15] This extensive inflammatory response consists of:

- Elevated cytokines: interleukin-1 (IL-1), IL-6, IL-8, tumor necrosis factor (TNF), and platelet activation factor (PAF) in the first 24 hours.
- Decrease in antiinflammatory cytokines: IL-2, IL-10.
- Activation of neutrophils, monocytes, lymphocytes, platelets, and endothelial cells.
- Increased expression of cell adhesion molecules and integrins in neutrophils, leading to distant organ damage, particularly in the lungs.
- Extensive tissue destruction by polymorphonuclear leukocytes.

In addition, in recent years, the "gut-lymph concept" has gained interest, as a factor contributing to (multi-)organ failure in AP mediated by an increase in the permeability of the intestinal barrier, favoring the translocation of primed neutrophils and intestinal toxic factors through circulation through the thoracic duct, in early stages, promoting multiorgan dysfunction syndrome.[16] Another aspect of this concept concerns the gut microbiota and bacterial translocation resulting from increased intestinal permeability, and their relation to infected necrosis. The POEMA trial demonstrated that colonization of the gut microbiota early in the course of necrotizing pancreatitis with Enterococcus or Staphylococcus was predictive for progression to infected pancreatic necrosis (IPN).[17]

DIAGNOSIS

Clinical Presentation

The clinical presentation of AP generally follows a consistent pattern, regardless of the underlying etiology (**Algorithm 50.1**). The typical manifestation includes sudden, severe abdominal pain, which is often accompanied by nausea and vomiting in approximately 90% of cases.[8] Among individuals with biliary pancreatitis, pain is often more pronounced in the right upper quadrant and tends to occur abruptly. Conversely, in some cases of hereditary, autoimmune, or alcoholic pancreatitis, the pain is less localized and its onset more gradual. In both scenarios, approximately 50% of patients experience pain radiating to the back.[18]

In the early phase after the onset of AP SIRS can develop because of massive inflammatory cytokine and chemokine release in the bloodstream. This process can present within hours or days after onset of initial symptoms. SIRS is directly related to the development of organ failure. Organ failure can be transient (lasting <48 hours) or persistent (>48 hours) and single, or multiple organ failure. Persistent and multiple organ failure are associated with increased mortality.[1,5,19] The most important organ systems affected (in decreasing order of percentage of patients affected) are respiratory, cardiovascular, and the renal system. Early recognition of SIRS and organ failure is important to start and/or adjust treatments and to transfer patients, when needed, to the high care department.[19]

Diagnostic Criteria

Diagnosis according to the 2012 Revised Atlanta Classification (RAC): the diagnosis of AP requires at least two of the following three criteria:

1. Abdominal pain compatible with pancreatitis
5 2. Serum amylase and/or lipase >3 times greater than the upper limit of the normal value
3. Radiologic findings consistent with pancreatitis (contrast-enhanced CT, magnetic resonance imaging [MRI], or US)

For typical clinical and laboratory findings, no additional CECT or other imaging is required to confirm the diagnosis.[1,5,18]

Severity Prediction

During admission, a three-dimensional approach is advised to predict outcome of AP combining:

- Host risk factors (eg, age, comorbidity, body mass index)
- Clinical risk stratification (eg, persistent SIRS)
- Monitoring response to initial therapy (eg, persistent SIRS, blood urea nitrogen, creatinine)

As a clinical risk stratification tool, the International Association of Pancreatology (IAP)/APA guidelines recommend the use of SIRS criteria to predict the severity of AP at 48 hours. The criteria can be found in **Table 50.2**. Persistent SIRS (>48 hours) is associated with multiorgan failure and increased mortality, making it a crucial determinant. The mortality for persistent SIRS is 25% versus 8% for transient SIRS.[1,5]

The preference for SIRS over other predictive scoring systems is due to its widespread familiarity, simplicity, and the feasibility of repetitive measurements, making it a pragmatic and effective tool in clinical settings.[1]

Classification

Most AP cases (80% to 85%) are mild and self-limiting. However, 20% of cases are moderate to severe, with mortality ranging from 15% to 30%.[5] Accurate classification is crucial for predicting SAP and identifying high-risk patients.

The most accepted classification of AP is the three-tiered RAC. An alternative is the four-tiered Determinant-Based Classification (DBC).[1,20,21]

Table 50.2. SIRS Criteria According to IAP/APA Guidelines[1]

Body temperature	≥38 of ≤36 °C
Heart frequency	≥90 beats/min
Respiratory rate or Arterial carbon dioxide tension	≥20 per minute or $PaCO_2$ <32 mm Hg (4.3 kPa)
Leucocytes or Granulocytes	>12 × 10^9/L or <4 × 10^9/L >10% increased

Table 50.3. Definition of Severity of Acute Pancreatitis According to RAC and DBC

Revised Atlanta Classification[18]
Mild AP ▪ No organ failure ▪ No local or systemic complications
Moderate severe AP ▪ Transient organ failure (<48 h) AND/OR local or systemic complications OR exacerbation of preexisting comorbidities
Severe AP ▪ Persistent organ failure (single or multiple)
Determinant-Based Classification[23]
Mild AP ▪ No organ failure ▪ No peri(pancreatic) necrosis
Moderate AP ▪ Sterile (peri)pancreatic necrosis AND/OR transient organ failure
Severe AP ▪ Infected (peri)pancreatic necrosis OR persistent organ failure
Critical AP ▪ Infected (peri)pancreatic necrosis AND persistent organ failure

Revised Atlanta Classification (RAC) (see Table 50.3)

The RAC was developed through an interactive, web-based consultation process with members of 11 pancreatic societies. It provides a comprehensive overview, including diagnostic definitions, pain onset as a reference point, and definitions for local complications and types of pancreatitis (interstitial and necrotizing). RAC classifies AP into mild, moderately severe, and severe categories based on organ failure and local complications of AP.[18]

Determinant-Based Classification (DBC) (see Table 50.3)

The DBC was developed through a global web-based survey and an international symposium involving 528 pancreatologists from 55 countries, with 240 participants from 49 countries responding. The classification was discussed at the 2011 World Congress of the International Association of Pancreatology in Kochi, India. DBC introduced a fourth severity category, "critical," based on (peri)pancreatic necrosis and organ failure.[23]

In clinical practice the RAC is most often used due to its simplicity.

Imaging

The proposed workup to assess the diagnosis of AP consists of a primary TUS to assess for underlying pathology. However, in approximately 17% to 26% of patients, the initial evaluation does not reveal an underlying etiology. For these patients, a second TUS is recommended as the best initial follow-up option. If the second TUS is inconclusive, EUS is the next preferred step, followed by MRI or MRCP. Endoscopic retrograde cholangiopancreatography (ERCP) for diagnosing a biliary cause is seldom performed due to a better diagnostic yield of EUS or MRI/MRCP.[24]

According to the IAP guidelines, an initial CT assessment in AP is warranted in specific situations: when there is diagnostic uncertainty, when confirmation of severity is needed based on clinical predictors of severe AP, or when the patient fails to respond to conservative treatment or shows signs of clinical deterioration. The optimal timing for this initial CT assessment is at least 72 to 96 hours after the onset of symptoms.[1,23]

Follow-up imaging with CT or MRI is indicated when there is no clinical improvement, if there is clinical deterioration, or particularly when invasive intervention is being considered. Important to note is that MRI can be particularly difficult to access in case of severely ill (comatose) patients admitted to the ICU. These guidelines help ensure that the use of imaging is both effective and judicious, tailored to the patient's clinical needs and the progression of the disease.[1,23]

INITIAL TREATMENT

Currently, in the absence of curative treatment, the management of the early stages of AP is based on supportive care, consisting of pain management, adequate fluid resuscitation, as well as optimal nutritional support.[25]

Fluid Resuscitation

During early pancreatitis, the systemic inflammatory response can cause significant fluid extravasation into the third space, leading to hypovolemia and subsequent organ hypoperfusion. Therefore, adequate fluid resuscitation is essential to mitigate these effects. Current literature indicates:

6
- Crystalloid solutions, such as Ringer lactate or balanced saline solutions (eg, Plasmalyte), are preferred over colloid solutions, which are associated with increased mortality.[1,5,22,25]
- A recent randomized controlled trial (RCT) revealed that aggressive fluid resuscitation (20 mL/kg bolus followed by an infusion of 3 mL/kg/h) did not result in improved outcomes compared to moderate fluid resuscitation (1.5 mL/kg/h infusion, preceded by a 10 mL/kg bolus in cases of hypovolemia). Instead, aggressive fluid resuscitation was associated with a higher incidence of fluid overload complications.[26]
- The current IAP/APA guidelines recommend a moderate infusion rate of 5 to 10 mL/kg/h until resuscitation goals are achieved.[1] Detailed resuscitation goals can be found in **Table 50.4.**

Nutrition

Appropriate nutrition is necessary to provide the patient with sufficient nutrients and energy to support itself during the enormous stress during AP. There are multiple theories on the effect of and what strategies are optimal for nutrition in AP. Current literature indicates:

- In patients with AP, it is recommended to start early (within 24 hours) oral feeding as tolerated because it helps maintain enteral nutrition (EN), protects the gut mucosal barrier, and reduces bacterial translocation, thereby lowering the risk of infected peripancreatic necrosis and other severe outcomes.[25]
- Enteral tube feeding should be the primary therapy in patients with predicted severe AP who require nutritional support. Early enteral feeding has been demonstrated to be not superior over early oral diet.[1,19]

Table 50.4. Fluid Response Criteria According to IAP/APA Guidelines[1]

Noninvasive clinical targets	▪ Heart rate <120/min ▪ Mean arterial pressure 65–85 mm Hg (8.7–11.3 kPa) ▪ Urinary output >0.5–1 mL/kg/h
Invasive clinical targets	▪ Stroke volume variation ▪ Intrathoracic blood volume determination
Biochemical targets	▪ Hematocrit 35–44%

- For patients with AP who cannot feed orally, EN is recommended over parenteral nutrition because it reduces the risk of infected peripancreatic necrosis, single organ failure, and multiple organ failure.[1,25]
- For patients with predicted severe or necrotizing pancreatitis requiring enteral tube feeding, either nasogastric (NG) or nasojejunal (NJ) routes are suggested, as no significant difference in mortality was noted between the two methods.[5,25] However, patients relatively often develop gastroparesis and therefore NJ is preferred in practice.[19]
- Intravenous administration of omega-3 fatty acid supplementation has potentially an immunomodulatory effect lowering inflammation parameters and improving patient outcomes. A Dutch randomized clinical trial with omega-3 fatty acid is performed to provide evidence on the use of omega-3 fatty acids in AP.[27,28]

Pain Management

Pain is the predominant symptom of AP and should be treated promptly and adequately. Frequent reassessment of pain scores and, if indicated, adjustment of analgesic types and/or dosages is needed to assure proper pain management.[5] Current evidence on use of analgesics in AP is limited, pain should be managed according to WHO pain ladder recommendations.

Antibiotic Prophylaxis and Interventions

Secondary infection of pancreatic and/or peripancreatic necrosis is one of the deadliest complications of AP. Bacterial translocation from the intestinal barrier is postulated as one of the mechanisms of necrosis infection. Multiple strategies have been tested to limit the development of secondary infection.[5]

- Prophylactic use of antibiotics is proven to be not effective in limiting the development of secondary infection.[1,5,25]
- Prophylactic use of probiotics is proven to be not effective in limiting the development of secondary infection and is associated with increased mortality and therefore contraindicated in AP.[1,5,29]
- Antibiotics in AP are only justified if there is a documented infection of necrosis or when there is sufficient clinical suspicion.[1,5,25]
- The use of selective digestive decontamination has shown promise in RCTs, possibly reducing the risk of infected necrosis with better patient outcomes as a result but further studies are necessary.[1,29,30]

COMPLICATIONS OF ACUTE PANCREATITIS

Local Complications of Pancreatitis

The RAC classifies local complications into two groups: collections associated with acute interstitial edematous pancreatitis and collections associated with acute necrotizing pancreatitis.[18] Over time different variations, with specific radiologic findings, can develop as depicted in **Figure 50.1**.

1. Acute Peripancreatic Fluid Collection

These are nonencapsulated fluid collections that arise within 4 weeks of AP onset. These collections are usually adjacent to the pancreas, rarely become infected, and typically resolve spontaneously. Approximately 15% will not resolve spontaneously and persist to become pancreatic pseudocysts.[18,31]

2. Pancreatic Pseudocyst

Pseudocysts are encapsulated fluid collections that form from acute peripancreatic fluid collections after at least 4 weeks.[18,31] They are not true cysts and may resolve spontaneously. On imaging, they appear round or oval with a well-defined capsule and are usually homogeneous. The

Algorithm 50.1

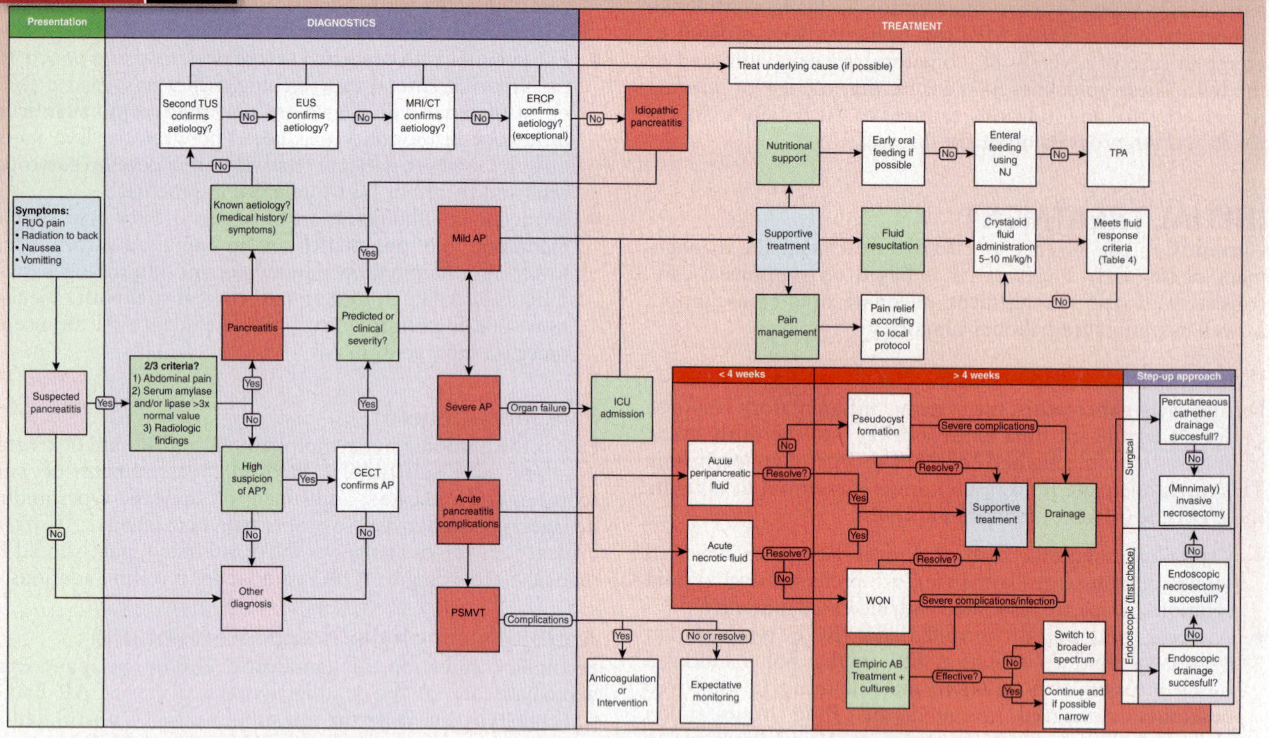

Algorithm 50.1. Flowchart of the presentation, diagnostic route and treatment of AP.

collections can be single or multiple, unilocular or multiloculated, and typically exhibit fluid density within a well-defined capsule.[31]

3. Acute Necrotic Collection

Pancreatic necrosis is observed in 5% to 10% of patients with AP and is characterized by the absence of intravenous contrast uptake of the pancreatic parenchyma on abdominal tomography. The computed tomography severity index (CTSI) classifies the percentage of pancreatic parenchymal necrosis and the presence of local alterations, giving a score of 1 to 10, finding an association of higher mortality for scores between 7 and 10.[32]

Extra pancreatic necrosis (EXPN) means there is involvement of peripancreatic tissue. The presence of EXPN has a better prognosis than pancreatic parenchymal necrosis. However, in cases of EXPN infection, there is no difference in prognosis.[33]

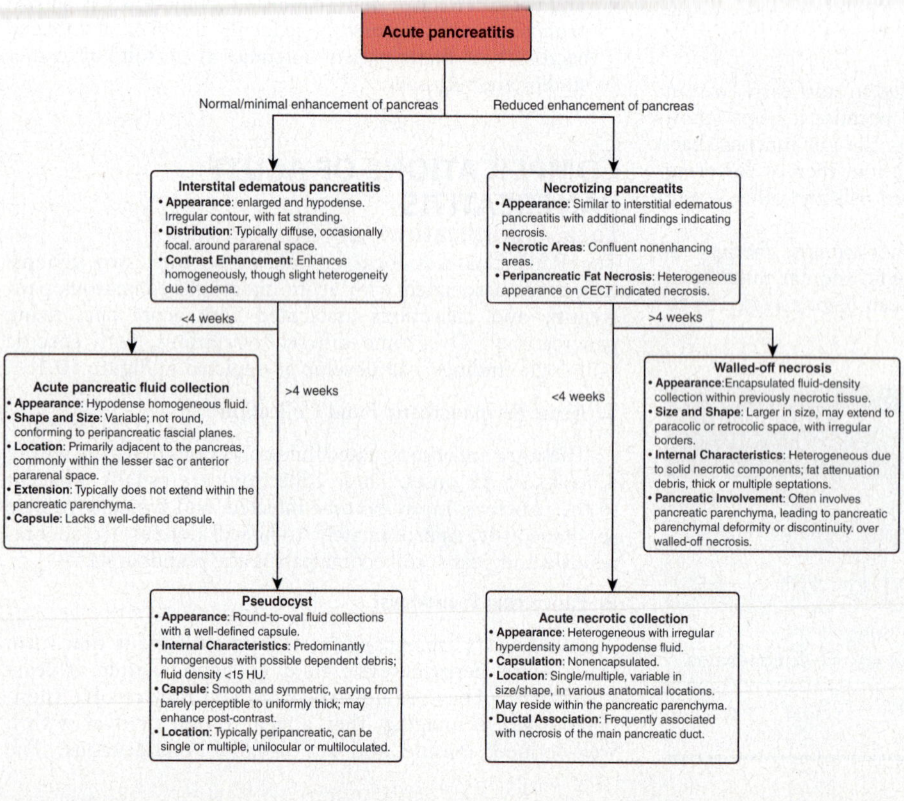

Figure 50.1. Collections associated with AP with radiologic features over time, according to revised Atlanta classification. From Banks PA, Bollen TL, Dervenis C, et al. Classification of acute pancreatitis—2012: revision of the Atlanta classification and definitions by international consensus. *Gut.* 2013;62(1):102–111. Zhao K, Adam SZ, Keswani RN, Horowitz JM, Miller FH. Acute pancreatitis: revised Atlanta classification and the role of cross-sectional imaging. *AJR Am J Roentgenol.* 2015;205:W32–W41. Balthazar EJ, Robinson DL, Megibow AJ, et al. Acute pancreatitis: value of CT in establishing prognosis. *Radiology.* 1990;174(2):331–336.

4. Walled-off Necrosis (WON)

WON develops when necrotic tissues and acute necrotic collections (ANCs) mature and form a capsule, a process that usually requires at least 4 weeks.[18] Although this is not a requirement as a recent study found that WON developed in 40% of patients in the first 3 weeks.[34] They can be distinguished from pseudocysts by their larger size, extension to the paracolic or retrocolic space, irregular border, fat attenuation debris, thick or multiple septations, and pancreatic parenchymal deformity or discontinuity.[31]

Infected Pancreatic Collections

Collections with necrosis, such as ANC and WON, become infected in about one-third of patients.[35] Infection can be diagnosed in three ways:

1. Gas configurations in the necrotic collection on imaging. Gas within a collection is the most sensitive imaging finding for infection but is only visible in 12% to 18% of cases.[31]
2. Clinical diagnosis based on signs of infection (eg, temperature >38.5 °C, rising serum inflammatory markers) or new/persistent organ failure, especially after the initial phase of SIRS.
3. Positive Gram stain or culture from a percutaneous fine-needle aspiration (FNA). However, due to the higher invasiveness, the reliability of other diagnostic methods, and the increased risk of complications with FNA, this procedure is only performed when signs are unclear and imaging options are unavailable.[1,35]

Porto-Spleno-Mesenteric Venous Thrombosis (PSMVT)

Splenic vein thrombosis occurs in approximately 23% of patients suffering from AP.[36] The development of PSMVT is associated with the presence, location, and extent of pancreatic necrosis and the severity of AP. The rate of complications related to the PSMVT over the course of AP, is low. Possible complications of PSMVT include gastric variceal bleeding, splenomegaly, and less frequently, liver failure after progression of portal vein thrombosis.[37]

MANAGEMENT OF COMPLICATIONS

Over the years, the treatment of peripancreatic collections and pancreatic necrosis has evolved. The current best practice is that conservative management should be used in most cases. There is wide acceptance that peripancreatic collections that are infected, or present symptoms that do not subside after a period of conservative treatment, should be drained and when needed debrided.[1]

Local Complications of Pancreatitis

1. Pancreatic Pseudocyst

Pancreatic pseudocysts often resolve without intervention, but treatment is required if symptoms or infections arise. Spontaneous resolution rates range from 8% to 70%, influenced by factors such as multiple locations, location in the pancreas, communication with the main pancreatic duct, and increased size during follow-up.[38–40] No absolute size mandates intervention, but cysts larger than 5 cm with no size reduction over 6 weeks are at increased risk of complications; however, due to the risk of secondary iatrogenic infection, attention should be focused on conservative treatment. Serious complications include infection, bleeding, rupture, and erosion of gastroduodenal and/or splenic arteries.

Drainage techniques—surgical, endoscopic, or percutaneous—do not demonstrate clear superiority over one another. Endoscopic transmural drainage is often preferred, particularly for perigastric or periduodenal pseudocysts, due to a lower risk of cutaneous pancreatic fistula compared to percutaneous drainage.[41–43]

2. Acute Necrotic Collection and Walled-off Necrosis

During the first 3 to 4 weeks after the appearance of ANC, it will resolve or encapsulate. Most of the necrotic collections are sterile and will resolve with conservative treatment regardless of its size.[6,44] However, in cases of infection or large-sized WON, an additional invasive intervention is usually required to limit the chance of additional morbidity and/or mortality.[45,46]

Intervention in a sterile collection carries the risk of secondary iatrogenic infection, with all its associated morbidity and mortality. A sterile necrotic collection without symptoms (eg, abdominal pain or mechanical obstruction) may require intervention; however, due to the risk of secondary iatrogenic infection, attention should be focused on conservative treatment and interventions should be delayed for 6 to 8 weeks or longer.[6]

In the first 3 to 4 weeks after an ANC appears, it will either resolve or encapsulate. Most necrotic collections are sterile and will resolve with conservative treatment, regardless of size.[6,44] However, infected or large WON often requires invasive intervention.[1,45,46]

Intervening in a sterile collection carries the risk of secondary iatrogenic infection, which is associated with substantial morbidity and mortality. In the absence of symptoms such as abdominal pain or mechanical obstruction, a sterile necrotic collection generally does not warrant immediate intervention. Instead, management should focus on conservative treatment, with any intervention preferably delayed for more than 6 to 8 weeks to minimize the risk of infection and allow walled-off necrosis (WON) to fully develop.[6]

Infected Pancreatic Collections

In almost 30% of patients, peripancreatic collections will become infected, for which the first choice of treatment is intervention according to the step-up protocol (see Step-up Approach). Regarding timing, it is preferred to wait as long as possible (>4 weeks) to allow for encapsulation of the infection. The recent POINTER trial reported that immediate intervention is not superior over postponed intervention in terms of mortality and complications. Patients undergoing postponed intervention had fewer invasive interventions during their treatment duration.[47] Secondarily, this trial noted that approximately 30% of patients could be successfully treated conservatively with antibiotics and supportive therapy. This is supported by previous studies and reviews of the literature.[47–49] The preferred antibiotics are broad-spectrum, capable of penetrating necrotic pancreatic tissue, following local antibiotic protocols. Positive cultures can guide the switch to targeted antibiotics.[1,5]

There are exceptional indications for early urgent laparotomy such as the presence of mesenteric ischemia and ACS as a direct consequence of AP, which are indications for open surgery.[50]

Porto-Spleno-Mesenteric Venous Thrombosis (PSMVT)

Most patients with splenic vein thrombosis are asymptomatic, with a 30% spontaneous recanalization rate.[51] Anticoagulation therapy should be reserved for cases in which thrombosis progresses and causes additional complications (eg, liver failure), although evidence supporting this approach is limited.[52] Identifying patients at higher bleeding risk due to esophageal varices, especially if considering anticoagulation, is crucial:

- Monitoring the drainage of the coronary vein.
- Routine endoscopy is recommended as the gold standard for detection.
- Presence of cirrhosis, which can contribute to portal hypertension.

Important to note is that a posthoc analysis of a prospective cohort in the Netherlands published in 2024 demonstrated that clinical outcomes after treatment with anticoagulants did not differ from patients that were not treated using anticoagulants in cases of PSMVT.[53]

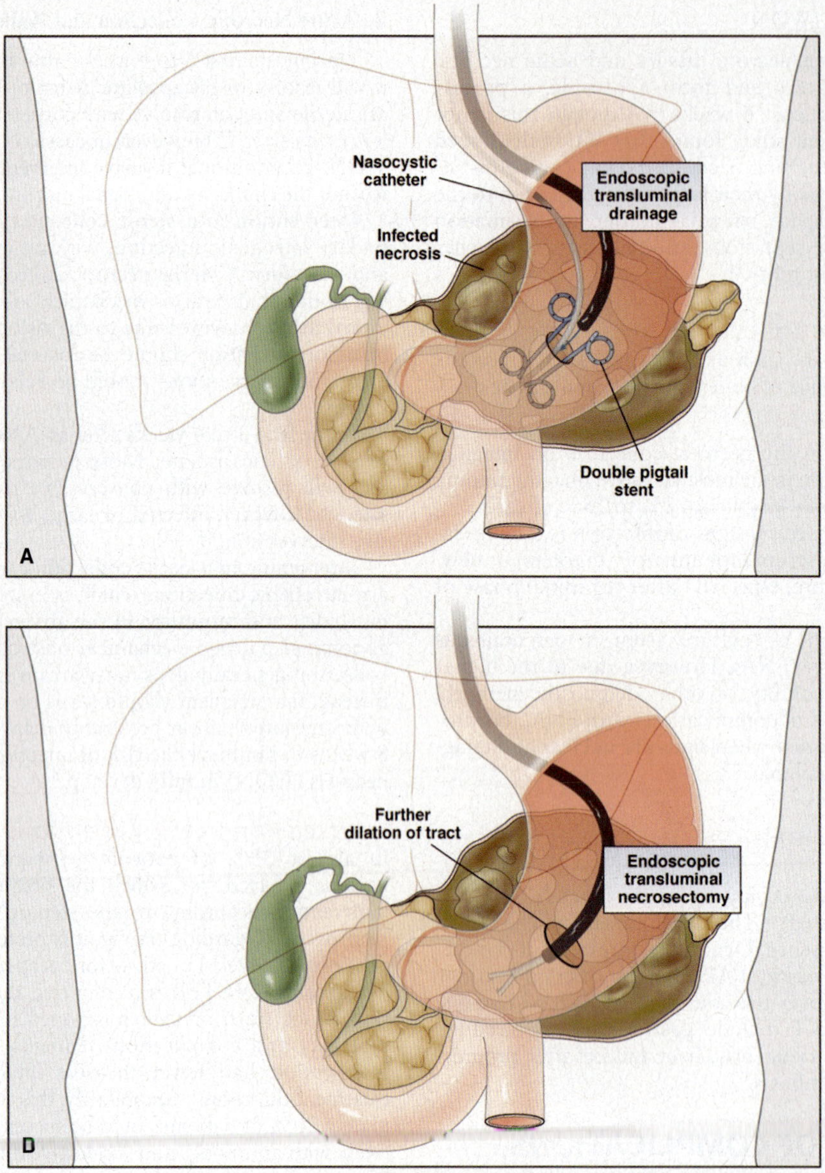

Figure 50.2. Endoscopic step-up approach. **A:** The first step of the endoscopic step-up approach is endoscopic transluminal drainage. The preferred access route for endoscopic transluminal treatment is through the posterior wall of the stomach. The necrotic collection often bulges into the stomach, facilitating endoscopic transluminal treatment. The collection is punctured through the gastric wall, followed by balloon dilatation of the tract. Two double-pigtail stents and a nasocystic catheter are placed for continuous postoperative irrigation. **B:** If necessary, the cystostomy tract is further dilated, the collection is entered by a forward-viewing endoscope, and necrosectomy is performed. (Reprinted from van Brunschot S, van Grinsven J, Voermans RP, et al. Transluminal endoscopic step-up approach versus minimally invasive surgical step-up approach in patients with infected necrotizing pancreatitis (TENSION trial): design and rationale of a randomized controlled multicenter trial [ISRCTN09186711]. *BMC Gastroenterol* 2013;13[1]:161.)

Splenomegaly is not a reliable indicator of sinistral hypertension. Routine splenectomy after splenic vein thrombosis and splenomegaly is not recommended due to the low rate of complications in this group of patients and observational management is recommended.[51]

STEP-UP APPROACH

Early intervention in necrotizing pancreatitis is associated with an increased risk of morbidity and mortality due to the additional stress it puts on a patient's body and the need for
8 extra interventions compared with a strategy until waiting for WON as shown in the POINTER trial.[47,54] It is therefore advised to wait >4 weeks to allow for WON development.[1,55]

Currently, the treatment of choice is the "step-up approach" in which the necrotic collections are drained mainly by less invasive methods (percutaneous drainage, or endoscopic drainage through stents), and in the absence of clinical improvement, there is a "step-up" toward surgical or endoscopic necrosectomy (minimally invasive initially).[56] This intensive approach reduces rates of new-onset multiple organ failure, morbidity, serious adverse events, and lower costs compared to primary open necrosectomy, which has since been largely abandoned.[57] In the step-up approach, almost half of patients can be treated with drains alone, while the other half requires additional different procedures for the final treatment, including percutaneous, endoscopic, open, or minimally invasive surgery.[47,56,58]

Endoscopic Approach

In recent decades, transmural (ie, transgastric) endoscopic management of acute necrotizing pancreatitis is increasingly
9 used. Various endoscopic techniques are used for the treatment of WON, all of which include EUS-guided transmural access to the cavity, see **Figure 50.2** EUS-guided drainage and/or necrosectomy has an advantage over the conventional transmural endoscopic approach due to greater technical success.[41,59,60]

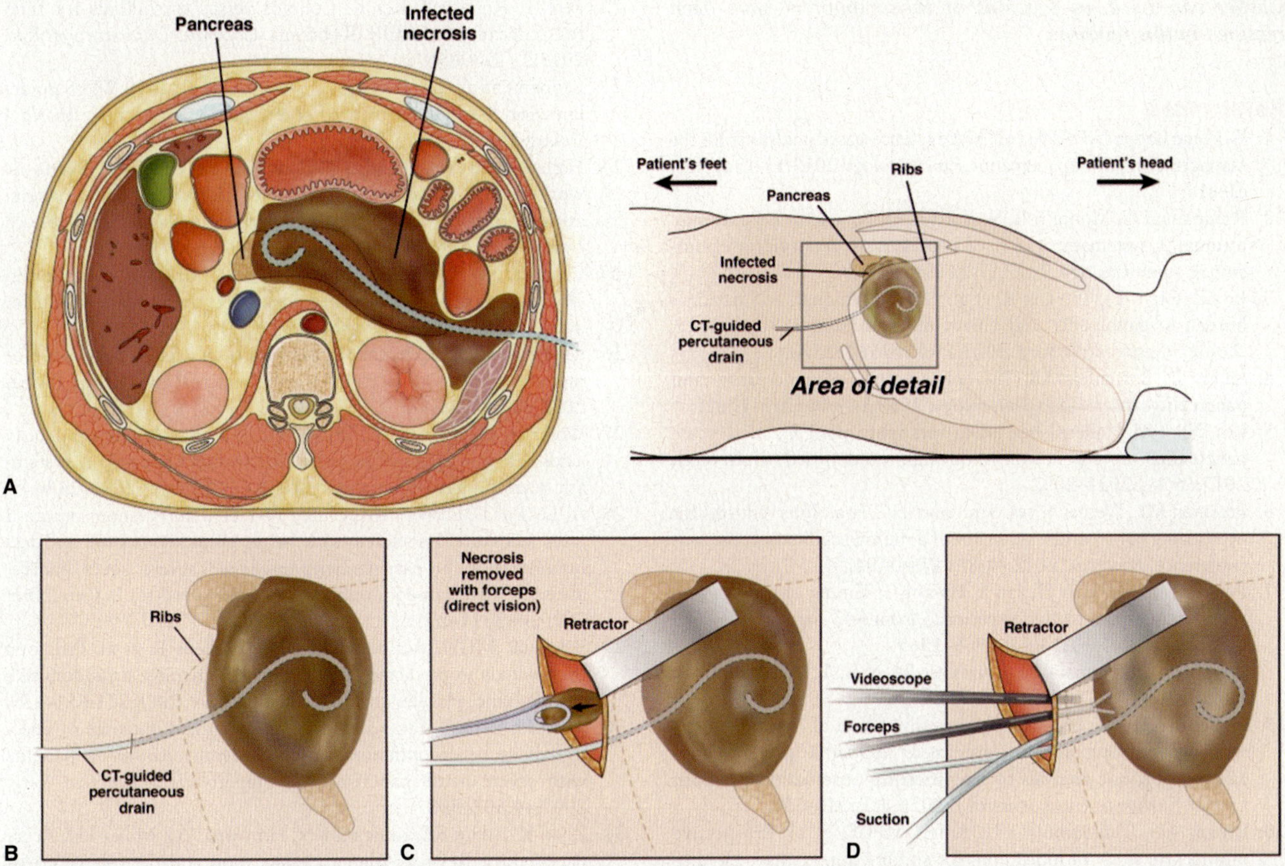

Figure 50.3. Surgical step-up approach. **A:** Cross-sectional image and torso depicting a peripancreatic collection with fluid and necrosis. The first step of the surgical step-up approach is percutaneous catheter drainage. The preferred access route is through the left retroperitoneal space between the left kidney, dorsal spleen, and descending colon. If necessary, percutaneous catheter drainage is followed by a minimally invasive surgical necrosectomy, for example, videoscopic-assisted retroperitoneal debridement. **B:** Enlargement of the area of detail shown in part A of the figure. **C:** A 5-cm subcostal incision is made, and the previously placed percutaneous drain is used as a guide into the retroperitoneum to enter the necrotic collection. The first necrosis is removed under direct vision with a long grasping forceps. **D:** Further debridement is performed under videoscopic assistance. (Reprinted from van Brunschot S, van Grinsven J, Voermans RP, et al. Transluminal endoscopic step-up approach versus minimally invasive surgical step-up approach in patients with infected necrotizing pancreatitis (TENSION trial): design and rationale of a randomized controlled multicenter trial [ISRCTN09186711]. *BMC Gastroenterol* 2013;13[1]:161.)

Endoscopic Drainage

Endoscopic drainage of infected pancreatic necrotic collection has evolved, from the use of a small plastic stent to lumen-apposing metal stent (LAMS), with a specific biflanged design that facilitates the creation of a stable and sealed fistula between the gastric or duodenal wall and the WON. The recent AXIOMA and PROMETHEUS studies demonstrate similar clinical success with similar rates of complications when comparing LAMS and plastic stents.[61,62]

Endoscopic Necrosectomy

Compared with surgical necrosectomy, an endoscopic approach significantly reduces the proinflammatory response and improves the clinical outcome (less surgical stress) among patients with acute necrotizing pancreatitis (ANP).[63] However, when used as a single-modality approach, it requires more necrosectomy sessions for definitive treatment than in combination with other interventional procedures.[64] The multicentre randomized controlled TENSION trial, compared the endoscopic step-up approach with the surgical step-approach. Both procedures were having similar mortality and morbidity. However, the endoscopic step-up group had a lower incidence of pancreatocutaneous fistula and shorter hospital stay.[65]

Percutaneous Catheter Drainage

Percutaneous catheter drainage can be a sufficiently definitive treatment in up to 56% of patients.[66] An analysis demonstrated that percutaneous drainage with antibiotics alone was a successful treatment in 50% of patients.[59] Upgrading percutaneous drains toward larger calibers (ie, upsizing) facilitates the drainage of the collection.[56] (See Infected Pancreatic Collections under Management of Complications for more information.)

Minimally Invasive Necrosectomy

If the patient with infected pancreatic necrosis does not recover
10 with drainage alone, a necrosectomy will be required. One of the most widely used techniques includes sinus tract endoscopy and video-assisted retroperitoneal debridement (VARD) (see **Fig. 50.3**).[67,68] As part of the "step-up approach," a 12- to 14-Fr percutaneous drain is placed in the pancreatic (peri)collection through the (most often left) retroperitoneum. If drainage does not lead to clinical improvement, surgical intervention is considered necessary and VARD is proposed. This technique can be considered a hybrid between pure minimal invasive retroperitoneal necrosectomy and the open translumbar approach (20-cm incision). In VARD, the small incision allows the surgeon to remove larger pieces of necrosis, with shorter operation time and less need for repetitive procedures. These minimally invasive techniques have been associated with reduced morbidity and mortality, especially in high-risk patient groups.[65]

ACKNOWLEDGMENTS

We gratefully acknowledge the contributions of previous edition authors, Elizabeth Pando Rau, Rogier Voermans, and

Casper van Eijck, as portions of those chapters have been retained in this revision.

References

1. Working Group IAP/APA. IAP/APA evidence-based guidelines for the management of acute pancreatitis. *Pancreatology.* 2013;13(4 Suppl 2):e1–e15.
2. Rompianesi G, Montalti R, Stafford A, Di Benedetto F. Pancreatic trauma: A systematic review of management strategies and outcomes. *Pancreatology*. 2017;17(2):181–193.
3. Li ZZ, Guan LJ, Ouyang R, et al. Global, regional, and national burden of gallbladder and biliary diseases from 1990 to 2019. *World J Gastrointest Surg*. 2023;15(11):2564–2578.
4. Yadav D, Lowenfels AB. The epidemiology of pancreatitis and pancreatic cancer. *Gastroenterology.* 2013;144(6):1252–1261.
5. van Dijk SM, Hallensleben NDL, van Santvoort HC, et al. Acute pancreatitis: recent advances through randomised trials. *Gut.* 2017;66(11):2024–2032.
6. Freeman ML, Werner J, van Santvoort HC, et al. Interventions for necrotizing pancreatitis: summary of a multidisciplinary consensus conference. *Pancreas.* 2012;41(8):1176–1194.
7. Fu CY, Yeh CN, Hsu JT, Jan Y, Hwang T. Timing of mortality in severe acute pancreatitis: experience from 643 patients. *World J Gastroenterol.* 2007;13(13):1966–1969.
8. Boxhoorn L, Voermans RP, Bouwense SA, et al. Acute pancreatitis. *Lancet.* 2020;396(10252):726–734.
9. Hallensleben ND, Umans DS, Bouwense SA, et al. The diagnostic work-up and outcomes of 'presumed' idiopathic acute pancreatitis: a post-hoc analysis of a multicentre observational cohort. *United European Gastroenterol J.* 2020;8(3):340–350.
10. Umans DS, Timmerhuis HC, Anten MPGF, et al. Prospective multicentre study of indications for surgery in patients with idiopathic acute pancreatitis following endoscopic ultrasonography (PICUS). *Br J Surg.* 2023;110(12):1877–1882.
11. Rinderknecht H. Activation of pancreatic zymogens. Normal activation, premature intrapancreatic activation, protective mechanisms against inappropriate activation. *Dig Dis Sci.* 1986;31(3):314–321.
12. Bialek R, Willemer S, Arnold R, Adler G. Evidence of intracellular activation of serine proteases in acute cerulein-induced pancreatitis in rats. *Scand J Gastroenterol.* 1991;26(2):190–196.
13. Luthen R, Niederau C, Grendell JH. Intrapancreatic zymogen activation and levels of ATP and glutathione during caerulein pancreatitis in rats. *Am J Physiol.* 1995;268(4 Pt 1):G592–G604.
14. Wen L, Voronina S, Javed MA, et al. Inhibitors of ORAI1 prevent cytosolic calcium-associated injury of human pancreatic acinar cells and acute pancreatitis in 3 mouse models. *Gastroenterology.* 2015;149(2):481.e7–492.e7.
15. Kruger B, Albrecht E, Lerch MM. The role of intracellular calcium signaling in premature protease activation and the onset of pancreatitis. *Am J Pathol.* 2000;157(1):43–50.
16. Fanous MY, Phillips AJ, Windsor JA. Mesenteric lymph: the bridge to future management of critical illness. *JOP.* 2007;8(4):374–399.
17. Pauw HS, van den Berg FF, Timmerhuis HC, et al. Colonization of the gastrointestinal microbiota with Enterococcus and Staphylococcus predicts infected necrosis in patients with acute pancreatitis (POEMA): a prospective multicenter study. *HPB.* 2024;26(Suppl 1):S280.
18. Banks PA, Bollen TL, Dervenis C, et al. Classification of acute pancreatitis—2012: revision of the Atlanta classification and definitions by international consensus. *Gut.* 2013;62(1):102–111.
19. Bakker OJ, van Brunschot S, van Santvoort HC, et al. Early versus on-demand nasoenteric tube feeding in acute pancreatitis. *N Engl J Med.* 2014;371(21):1983–1993.
20. Hagjer S, Kumar N. Evaluation of the BISAP scoring system in prognostication of acute pancreatitis—a prospective observational study. *Int J Surg.* 2018;54(Pt A):76–81.
21. Juneja D, Gopal PB, Ravula M. Scoring systems in acute pancreatitis: which one to use in intensive care units? *J Crit Care.* 2010;25(2):358.e9–358.e15.
22. Perel P, Roberts I, Ker K. Colloids versus crystalloids for fluid resuscitation in critically ill patients. *Cochrane Database Syst Rev.* 2013;2:CD000567.
23. Leppäniemi A, Tolonen M, Tarasconi A, et al. 2019 WSES guidelines for the management of severe acute pancreatitis. *World J Emerg Surg.* 2019;14:27.
24. Hallensleben ND, Umans DS, Bouwense SA, et al. The diagnostic work-up and outcomes of "presumed" idiopathic acute pancreatitis: A post-hoc analysis of a multicentre observational cohort. *United European Gastroenterol J.* 2020;8:340–350.
25. Crockett SD, Wani S, Gardner TB, et al. American gastroenterological association institute guideline on initial management of acute pancreatitis. *Gastroenterology.* 2018;154:1096–1101.
26. de-Madaria E, Buxbaum JL, Maisonneuve P, et al. Aggressive or moderate fluid resuscitation in acute pancreatitis. *N Engl J Med.* 2022;387:989–1000.
27. Wolbrink DRJ, Grundsell JR, Witteman B, et al. Are omega-3 fatty acids safe and effective in acute pancreatitis or sepsis? A systematic review and meta-analysis. *Clin Nutr.* 2020;39:2686–2694.
28. Al-Leswas D, Eltweri AM, Chung W-Y, et al. Intravenous omega-3 fatty acids are associated with better clinical outcome and less inflammation in patients with predicted severe acute pancreatitis: A randomised double blind controlled trial. *Clin Nutr.* 2020;39:2711–2719.
29. Besselink MGH, van Santvoort HC, Buskens E, et al. Probiotic prophylaxis in predicted severe acute pancreatitis: a randomised, double-blind, placebo-controlled trial. *Lancet.* 2008;371:651–659.
30. Sawa H, Ueda T, Takeyama Y, et al. Treatment outcome of selective digestive decontamination and enteral nutrition in patients with severe acute pancreatitis. *J Hepatobiliary Pancreat Surg.* 2007;14:503–508.
31. Zhao K, Adam SZ, Keswani RN, Horowitz JM, Miller FH. Acute pancreatitis: Revised Atlanta classification and the role of cross-sectional imaging. *AJR Am J Roentgenol.* 2015;205:W32–W41.
32. Balthazar EJ, Robinson DL, Megibow AJ, et al. Acute pancreatitis: value of CT in establishing prognosis *Radiology.* 1990;174(2):331–336.
33. Bakker OJ, van Santvoort H, Besselink MG, et al. Extrapancreatic necrosis without pancreatic parenchymal necrosis: a separate entity in necrotising pancreatitis? *Gut.* 2013;62(10):1475–1480.
34. van Santvoort HC, Bakker OJ, Bollen TL, et al. A conservative and minimally invasive approach to necrotizing pancreatitis improves outcome. *Gastroenterology.* 2011;141:1254–1263.
35. van Baal MC, Bollen TL, Bakker OJ, et al. The role of routine fine-needle aspiration in the diagnosis of infected necrotizing pancreatitis. *Surgery.* 2014;155:442–448.
36. Scott M, Ghazanfar M, Windsor J, Ramsay G, Bekheit M, Splanchnic Vein in Acute Pancreatitis Study Group. The management of splanchnic vein thrombosis in acute pancreatitis: a global DELPHI consensus study. *HPB (Oxford).* 2025;27(3):343–351.
37. Easler J, Muddana V, Furlan A, et al. Portosplenomesenteric venous thrombosis in patients with acute pancreatitis is associated with pancreatic necrosis and usually has a benign course. *Clin Gastroenterol Hepatol.* 2014;12(5):854–862.
38. Andren-Sandberg A, Dervenis C. Pancreatic pseudocysts in the 21st century. Part II: natural history. *JOP.* 2004;5(2):64–70.
39. Andren-Sandberg A, Ansorge C, Eiriksson K, Glomsaker T, Maleckas A. Treatment of pancreatic pseudocysts. *Scand J Surg.* 2005;94(2):165–175.
40. Agalianos C, Passas I, Sideris I, Davides D, Dervenis C. Review of management options for pancreatic pseudocysts. *Transl Gastroenterol Hepatol.* 2018;3:18.
41. Varadarajulu S, Bang JY, Sutton BS, Trevino JM, Christein JD, Wilcox CM. Equal efficacy of endoscopic and surgical cystogastrostomy for pancreatic pseudocyst drainage in a randomized trial. *Gastroenterology.* 2013;145(3):583.e1–590.e1.
42. Park DH, Lee SS, Moon SH, et al. Endoscopic ultrasound-guided versus conventional transmural drainage for pancreatic pseudocysts: a prospective randomized trial. *Endoscopy.* 2009;41(10):842–848.
43. Varadarajulu S, Christein JD, Tamhane A, Drelichman ER, Wilcox CM. Prospective randomized trial comparing EUS and

EGD for transmural drainage of pancreatic pseudocysts (with videos). *Gastrointest Endosc.* 2008;68(6):1102–1111.
44. Wonski M, Cebulski W, Pawlowski W, Krasnodebski IW, Slodkowski M. Walled-off necrosis: safety of watchful waiting. *Dig Dis Sci.* 2015;60(4):1081–1086.
45. Papachristou GI, Takahashi N, Chahal P, Sarr MG, Baron TH. Peroral endoscopic drainage/debridement of walled-off pancreatic necrosis. *Ann Surg.* 2007;245(6):943–951.
46. Rana SS, Bhasin DK, Sharma RK, Kathiresan J, Gupta R. Do the morphological features of walled off pancreatic necrosis on endoscopic ultrasound determine the outcome of endoscopic transmural drainage? *Endosc Ultrasound.* 2014;3(2):118–122.
47. Boxhoorn L, van Dijk SM, van Grinsven J, et al. Immediate versus postponed intervention for infected necrotizing pancreatitis. *N Engl J Med.* 2021;385(15):1372–1381.
48. Mouli VP, Sreenivas V, Garg PK. Efficacy of conservative treatment, without necrosectomy, for infected pancreatic necrosis: a systematic review and meta-analysis. *Gastroenterology.* 2013; 144(2):333.e2–340.e2.
49. Fernández-del Castillo C, Rattner DW, Makary MA, Mostafavi A, McGrath D, et al. Debridement and closed packing for the treatment of necrotizing pancreatitis. *Ann Surg.* 1998;228(5): 676–684.
50. Kirkpatrick AW, Roberts DJ, De Waele J, et al. Intra-abdominal hypertension and the abdominal compartment syndrome: updated consensus definitions and clinical practice guidelines from the World Society of the Abdominal Compartment Syndrome. *Intensive Care Med.* 2013;39(7):1190–1206.
51. Butler JR, Eckert GJ, Zyromski NJ, Leonardi MJ, Lillemoe KD, Howard TJ. Natural history of pancreatitis-induced splenic vein thrombosis: a systematic review and meta-analysis of its incidence and rate of gastrointestinal bleeding. *HPB (Oxford).* 2011;13(12):839–845.
52. Besselink MG. Splanchnic vein thrombosis complicating severe acute pancreatitis. *HPB (Oxford).* 2011;13(12):831–832.
53. Sissingh NJ, Timmerhuis HC, Groen JV, et al. Splanchnic vein thrombosis in necrotizing pancreatitis: a post-hoc analysis of a nationwide prospective cohort. *HPB (Oxford).* 2024;26:548–557.
54. Besselink MG, Verwer TJ, Schoenmaeckers EJ, et al. Timing of surgical intervention in necrotizing pancreatitis. *Arch Surg.* 2007;142(12):1194–1201.
55. Tenner S, Baillie J, DeWitt J, Vege SW. American College of Gastroenterology Guideline: Management of Acute Pancreatitis. *Am J Gastroenterol.* 2013;108:1400–1415; 1416.
56. van Santvoort HC, Besselink MG, Bakker OJ, et al. A step-up approach or open necrosectomy for necrotizing pancreatitis. *N Engl J Med.* 2010;362(16):1491–1502.
57. Gurusamy KS, Belgaumkar AP, Haswell A, Pereira SP, Davidson BR. Interventions for necrotising pancreatitis. *Cochrane Database Syst Rev.* 2016;4:CD011383.
58. Crockett SD, Wani S, Gardner TB, et al. American Gastroenterological Association Institute Guideline on Initial Management of Acute Pancreatitis. *Gastroenterology.* 2018;154(4):1096–1101.
59. Shenvi S, Gupta R, Kang M, et al. Timing of surgical intervention in patients of infected necrotizing pancreatitis not responding to percutaneous catheter drainage. *Pancreatology.* 2016;16(5):778–787.
60. ASGE Standards of Practice Committee; Muthusamy VR, Chandrasekhara V, Acosta RD, et al. The role of endoscopy in the diagnosis and treatment of inflammatory pancreatic fluid collections. *Gastrointest Endosc.* 2016;83(3):481–488.
61. Gornals JB, Velasquez-Rodriguez JG, Bas-Cutrina F, et al. Plastic pigtail vs lumen-apposing metal stents for drainage of walled-off necrosis (PROMETHEUS study): an open-label, multicenter randomized trial. *Surg Endosc.* 2024;38:2148–2159.
62. Boxhoorn L, Verdonk RC, Besselink MG, et al. Comparison of lumen-apposing metal stents versus double-pigtail plastic stents for infected necrotising pancreatitis. *Gut.* 2023;72:66–72.
63. Bakker OJ, van Santvoort HC, van Brunschot S, et al. Endoscopic transgastric vs surgical necrosectomy for infected necrotizing pancreatitis: a randomized trial. *JAMA.* 2012;307(10):1053–1061.
64. van Brunschot S, Hollemans RA, Bakker OJ, et al. Minimally invasive and endoscopic versus open necrosectomy for necrotising pancreatitis: a pooled analysis of individual data for 1980 patients. *Gut.* 2018;67(4):697–706.
65. van Brunschot S, van Grinsven J, van Santvoort HC, et al. Endoscopic or surgical step-up approach for infected necrotising pancreatitis: a multicentre randomised trial. *Lancet* 2018; 391(10115):51–58.
66. van Baal MC, van Santvoort HC, Bollen TL,et al. Systematic review of percutaneous catheter drainage as primary treatment for necrotizing pancreatitis. *Br J Surg.* 2011;98(1):18–27.
67. Carter CR, McKay CJ, Imrie CW. Percutaneous necrosectomy and sinus tract endoscopy in the management of infected pancreatic necrosis: an initial experience. *Ann Surg.* 2000;232(2):175–180.
68. Horvath KD, Kao LS, Wherry KL, Pellegrini CA, Sinanan MN. A technique for laparoscopic-assisted percutaneous drainage of infected pancreatic necrosis and pancreatic abscess. *Surg Endosc.* 2001;15(10):1221–1225.

51

Chronic Pancreatitis

Katherine A. Morgan

Key Points

1. Chronic pancreatitis (CP) is heterogeneous in etiology with an increasingly recognized role of genetic factors and smoking.
2. The most common indication for intervention in CP is severe, debilitating abdominal pain.
3. Medical and endoscopic therapies are frontline management of CP but are often unsuccessful.
4. Surgical intervention is aimed at achieving durable pain relief with least perioperative and long-term morbidity.
5. Innovative surgical therapies for CP, including minimally invasive approaches and total pancreatectomy with islet autotransplantation (TPIAT), have gained increasing enthusiasm.

The surgical management of chronic pancreatitis (CP) has evolved significantly in the modern era. The increasing recognition of genetic mechanisms for pancreatitis and the role of smoking in pathophysiology of CP have changed patient demographic as well as treatment strategies, including the surgical algorithm. Additionally, potentially field-altering research is currently being undertaken on genetics, molecular pathways, and clinical outcomes in CP.

CP is a benign inflammatory disorder of the pancreas, resulting in progressive fibrotic replacement of parenchyma. The most notable clinical presentation is severe, debilitating, and unremitting abdominal pain, often with associated nutritional failure. CP leads to progressive endocrine failure due to islet loss (type 3c diabetes mellitus)[1] and exocrine failure (malabsorption). Importantly, patients have significant impairments in quality of life.

EPIDEMIOLOGY

CP is a significant public health concern with a prevalence and annual incidence estimated at 25 to 99/100,000 and 5/100,000, respectively, in the United States and Europe.[2] The economic impact is notable, with estimated annual healthcare expenditures for pancreatitis in the United States in 2018 at $4.97 billion.[3]

ETIOLOGY

Historically, alcohol use has been the most commonly implicated etiologic factor in CP in the Western world. A more recent multi-institutional observational study by the North American Pancreatitis Study 2 (NAPS2) Group revealed a lesser contributory role for alcohol.[4] Dose and duration of alcohol consumption have been demonstrated to be contributory to CP development, although several more recent studies suggest that alcohol alone is not sufficient to cause CP. Byproducts from ethanol metabolism injure acinar cells and can activate pancreatic stellate cells (PSCs) to form extracellular matrix. One recent investigation suggested an association between alcoholic pancreatitis and a locus on the X chromosome.[5]

1 Smoking is a significant risk factor in the development of CP. Tobacco consumption has been associated with pancreatic calcifications radiographically.[6] Synergistic effects of smoking and alcohol have been described.[7] More recently, NAPS2 demonstrated that smoking is an independent risk factor for CP in a dose-dependent fashion.[4] In addition, tobacco use has been reported to be a strong risk factor for the progression of acute pancreatitis to CP, suggesting a role for smoking in pancreatic fibrogenesis.[8]

Genetic causes for pancreatitis have been a major focus of advancement in the evolving understanding of CP in the current era. In 1952, Comfort and Steinberg described hereditary pancreatitis (HP),[9] and in 1996, Whitcomb and colleagues delineated a mutation in the cationic trypsinogen gene PRSS1, which results in the inappropriate activation of trypsin and is responsible for HP.[10] HP is an autosomal dominant disorder with 80% penetrance, marked by recurrent acute pancreatitis beginning in early childhood, progression to CP in many, and a greatly (50×) increased risk of pancreatic cancer beginning in the fifth decade. Since, several other mutations in the PRSS1 gene have been identified. In addition, multiple other genetic foci have been implicated as contributing agents in CP as well, primarily related to the inappropriate activation of trypsin. Pancreas secretory trypsin inhibitor (serine protease inhibitor, Kazal type 1, and SPINK1),[11] cystic fibrosis transmembrane conductance regulator (CFTR) gene, chymotrypsin C (CRTC),[12] calcium-sensing receptor (CASR) gene,[13] and gamma-glutamyltransferase 1 (GGT1) gene[14] have all been elucidated as conferring a susceptibility to CP development. Conversely, the anionic trypsinogen gene PRSS2 may confer a protective advantage against the development of pancreatitis. Overall, the etiology of pancreatitis is variable, complex, and incompletely understood.

PATHOPHYSIOLOGY

The pathophysiology of CP is not well elucidated. A theory known as the "three-hit hypothesis" holds that (1) a stochastic event occurs, resulting in (2) inappropriate trypsin activation causing acute pancreatitis. The patient then has (3) an unfavorable immunologic response to the inflammation resulting in fibrosis and CP (**Fig. 51.1**).[15] Environmental factors (eg, alcohol) are common inciting events in the cascade, with key modulating factors being genetics and the histologic milieu.

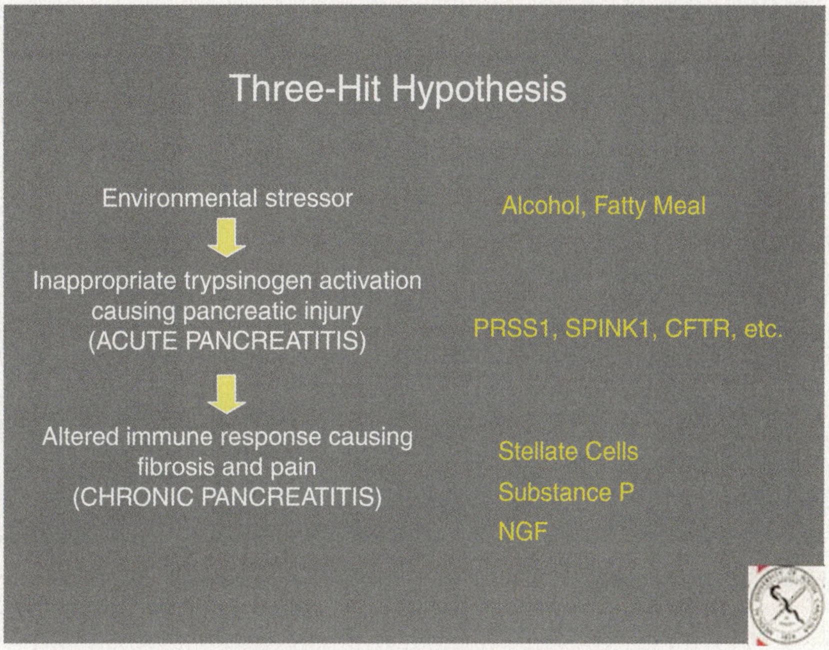

Figure 51.1. Three-hit hypothesis for pathophysiology of chronic pancreatitis. NGF, nerve growth factor. (Adapted from Whitcomb DC. Genetic risk factors for pancreatic disorders. *Gastroenterology*. 2013;144:1292–1302.)

Insights into pathophysiology of pancreatitis have occurred through advances in cellular basic science. PSCs are causative in pancreatic fibrogenesis. PSCs are residents of the healthy pancreas that become activated by inflammatory cytokines during pancreatitis to become myofibroblast-like cells, producing extracellular matrix in the interstitial space.[16] In addition, several matrix metalloproteinases have been implicated in altering extracellular matrix remodeling and collagen degradation, enhancing fibrogenesis, and irreversibly altering the organ architecture to a diseased, fibrotic pancreas.[17]

The CP pain syndrome has complex pathophysiology. Classical theory holds that pancreatic ductal obstruction due to fibrosis results in elevated intraductal and intraparenchymal pressures that cause pain. More recent theories focus on peripancreatic neuropathy. On a histologic level, peripancreatic neuronal hypertrophy as well as infiltration of the periaxonal tissue with inflammatory cells is evident.[18,19] Increased presence of the "pain neurotransmitters" is identified, including calcitonin gene-related peptide and substance P, stimulated by nerve growth factor.[20] These changes in the peripancreatic neuronal milieu may contribute to peripheral neural remodeling and central neural sensitization that make the CP pain syndrome uniquely severe and vexing to manage.

CLINICAL PRESENTATION

2 The primary presentation of CP is severe, intractable epigastric abdominal pain that radiates into the back. The classic pain is constant with periods of exacerbation. Patients often have associated gut dysfunction, with nausea, emesis, and difficulty tolerating a diet consistently, particularly during pain episodes. Patients may develop endocrine failure (pancreatogenic diabetes, type 3c) and exocrine pancreatic insufficiency (EPI) over time. Less often, patients may present with an acute complication of CP such as biliary or duodenal obstruction, a pancreatic pseudocyst, pancreatic ascites, mesenteric venous thrombosis, or mesenteric arterial pseudoaneurysm (**Table 51.1**).

On physical examination, patients generally appear malnourished. Abdominal tenderness in the epigastrium may be elicited. Laboratory values to note include chemistries to assess dehydration and acidosis, a hepatic panel to investigate biliary obstruction or malnutrition, and serum amylase and lipase, which may be elevated or may be normal in advanced disease.

RADIOGRAPHIC EVALUATION

Radiography is important in both diagnosis and management of CP. Multiphase, contrast-enhanced abdominal computed tomography (CT pancreas protocol) can show pancreatic parenchymal changes of pancreatitis, including edema, fibrosis, and atrophy. Pancreatic ductal dilation may be evident, as well as intraductal or intraparenchymal calcifications (**Fig. 51.2**). CT can be helpful to identify complications of pancreatitis such as biliary or duodenal obstruction, pseudocysts or ascites, or mesenteric vascular complications. Magnetic resonance pancreatography (MRP) can be useful in revealing parenchymal changes in enhancement and secretion (T1-weighted images) and ductal changes (T2-weighted images), particularly with the addition of secretin stimulation (**Fig. 51.3**). With increased capabilities of MR technology, MR imaging has largely replaced endoscopic retrograde cholangiopancreatography (ERCP) in diagnosis of CP. In the modern era, ERCP is utilized for therapeutic means, including endoscopic sphincterotomy, dilation, and stenting. Endoscopic ultrasound (EUS) is useful for evaluation of pancreatic parenchyma and ductal anatomy. EUS has a grading system to objectify and document pancreatitis disease severity, although the system is flawed by interobserver variability (**Table 51.2**).[21]

Table 51.1. Complications of Chronic Pancreatitis

Complication	Frequency
Pain	90%
Pseudocyst	25–30%
Biliary stricture	10–15%
Mesenteric venous thrombosis	5–10%
Duodenal stricture	4–5%
Pseudoaneurysm	2–3%
Pancreatic adenocarcinoma	2–4%[a]
Extrapancreatic malignancy	10–15%

[a]Risk of pancreatic cancer is 2% after 10 years and 4% after 20 years with chronic pancreatitis.

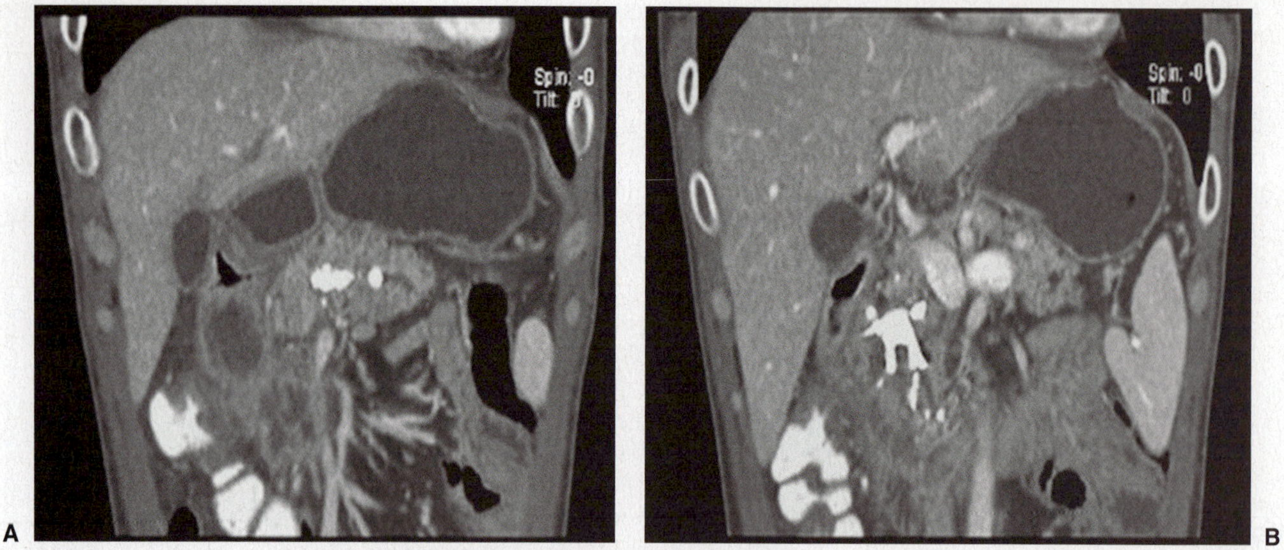

Figure 51.2. Contrasted CT scan in venous phase; coronal images showing (**A**) dilated main pancreatic duct with intraductal stones and (**B**) significant fibrotic disease burden in the head of the pancreas with intraparenchymal and intraductal calcifications.

CONSIDERATIONS IN MANAGEMENT

3 Frontline management of CP includes risk factor modification, such as alcohol and tobacco cessation. Primary medical interventions entail pain management, including adjunctive behavioral therapy, and nutritional optimization, including pancreatic enzyme replacement therapy. Behavioral therapy is a keystone of therapy in CP and is effective in modulating pain perceptions and in managing opioid misuse.[22]

ENDOSCOPIC MANAGEMENT

ERCP is the primary endoscopic modality for therapy in CP, with the goal of relieving obstructive pathology. Potential maneuvers include sphincterotomy, stone extraction, stricture dilation, and stenting.

EUS can be utilized for endoscopic pseudocyst drainage procedures and for celiac plexus neurolysis. Percutaneous and endoscopic guided celiac nerve blockade has been utilized to manage CP pain. One meta-analysis study of EUS-guided celiac plexus blockade reported short-term pain relief in about one-half of subjects.[23]

In general, the endoscopic approach is undertaken prior to consideration of surgery, given the perceived advantages of lower morbidity with a less invasive approach. Three prospective, randomized, controlled trials have compared endoscopy and surgery in patients with obstructive CP. Dite and colleagues randomized 72 patients with CP, pancreatic duct obstruction, and pain to endoscopic or surgical intervention. At 5-year follow-up, the surgical group had a greater proportion of patients who were pain free (34% vs. 15%).[24] Cahen and colleagues randomized 39 patients and noted that the surgical group had a greater proportion of patients who had pain relief (80% vs. 38%, $P = .001$), had greater improvements in quality of life, and underwent fewer procedures, despite equivalent morbidity, length of stay, and preserved pancreatic function at 5 years.[25] Most recently, the

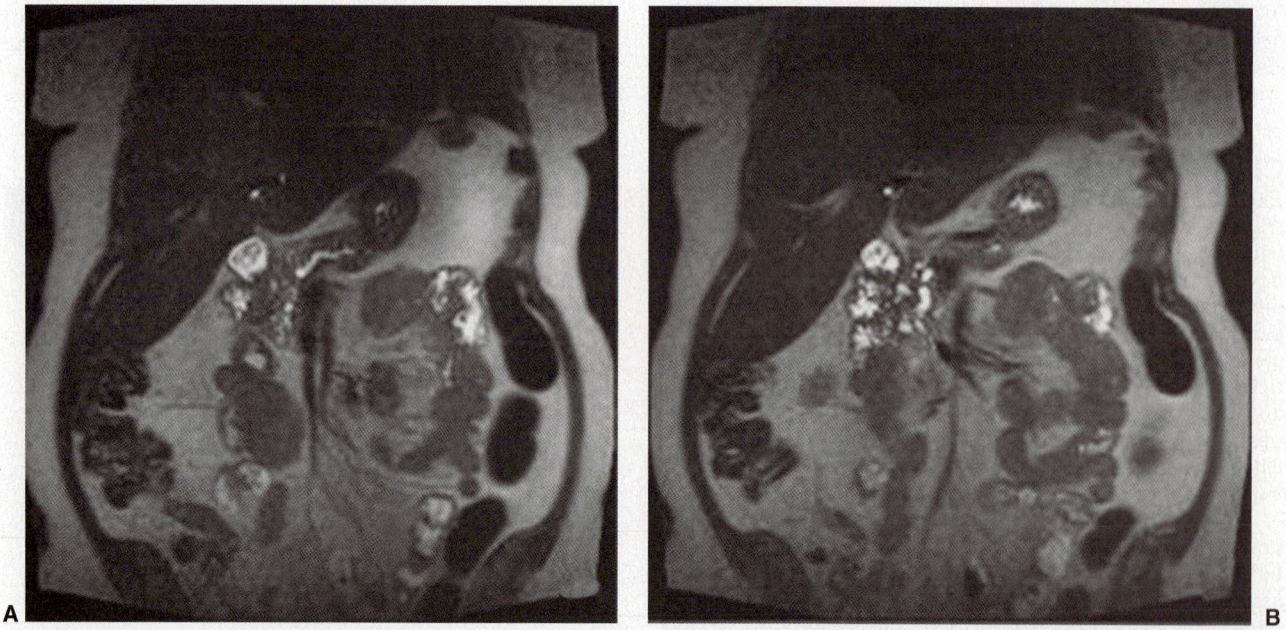

Figure 51.3. T2-weighted magnetic resonance imaging with secretin stimulation demonstrates a pathologically dilated pancreatic duct in the body of the pancreas (**A**) and cystic changes and dilated ducts in a fibrotic and inflammatory head of the pancreas (**B**).

Table 51.2. EUS Criteria for Chronic Pancreatitis
Parenchymal Criteria Hyperechoic foci Hyperechoic strands Hyperechoic lobules, foci or areas Cyst
Ductal Criteria Irregular duct contour Visible side branches Hyperechoic duct margin Dilated main duct Stone
Normal (Low Probability) 0–2 criteria present
Indeterminate (Intermediate Probability) 3–4 criteria present
High Probability 5–9 criteria present

EUS, endoscopic ultrasound.
From Wallace MB, Hawes RH, Durkalski V, et al. The reliability of EUS for the diagnosis of chronic pancreatitis: interobserver agreement among experienced endosonographers. *Gastrointest Endosc.* 2001;53:294–299.

Dutch Pancreatitis Study Group randomized 88 patients to early surgery or endoscopy first and noted that patients in the early surgery group had significantly lower Izbicki pain scores (33 vs. 51), higher patient reported pain relief (45% vs. 20%), and higher patient satisfaction (71% vs. 33%), at a mean follow up of 8 years. Notably, patients who progressed from endoscopy to surgery had a markedly lower rate of complete pain relief than individuals with early surgery first (12% vs. 55%), and the superior outcomes of early surgery were present regardless of the success of endoscopic clearance of ductal stones.[26]

SURGICAL MANAGEMENT

Approximately two-thirds of patients with debilitating pain[4]
4 from CP fail medical and endoscopic managements. The goals of surgery are to relieve pain effectively while minimizing morbidity, including minimizing perioperative complications and preserving pancreatic parenchyma. The pancreatic anatomy is the primary determinant in surgical planning. Patients with a dilated (greater than 6 to 7 mm diameter) main pancreatic duct are assumed to have obstructive pathology and are candidates for a drainage-type procedure (lateral pancreaticojejunostomy [LPJ], Frey procedure). Patients with a small-diameter main pancreatic duct are considered for resection of fibrotic and poorly drained parenchyma. Patients with head-predominant or tail-centered disease can undergo a directed partial resection. In patients with diffuse parenchymal involvement, a TP with islet autotransplantation may be appropriate (**Algorithm 51.1**). A Dutch retrospective study evaluated surgical outcomes utilizing this morphology "tailored" algorithm. Effective pain relief was reported for all procedures (69% to 83%) and 81% were opioid free, with drainage procedures being the least morbid in the short and long term.[27]

Lateral Pancreaticojejunostomy

Retrograde pancreatic drainage for relapsing pancreatitis was described by Puestow and Gillesby in 1958.[28] A modification of this original drainage procedure that more closely resembles the modern-day technique of the LPJ was reported by Partington and Rochelle in 1960.[29] LPJ is the classic operation for pancreatic drainage and entails opening the pancreatic duct anteriorly along its length, medially to the level of the gastroduodenal artery and laterally into the tail. The opened pancreatic duct is then cleared of stones, including into the head, and anastomosed to a Roux-en-Y jejunal limb for drainage.

Procedure-specific complications of note include intraoperative hemorrhage (due to splenic vein or gastroduodenal artery injury), postoperative hemorrhage (often from the gastroduodenal artery), and anastomotic leak (seen in 10% of cases).

Multiple retrospective single-institution case series have reported outcomes with LPJ, with pain-relief rates of 48% to 91%.[30–32] Morbidity is low (20% on average), and endocrine and exocrine function is often preserved.[33] LPJ is an effective and safe procedure for pain relief in many patients with dilated duct pancreatitis. Recurrent pain does occur after LPJ, however, likely due to pathology in the head of the pancreas. Intraductal stone disease in the head of the pancreas can be cleared with intraoperative pancreatoscopy and electrohydraulic lithotripsy, which has been noted to improve outcomes (reduced readmissions, increased pain-relief rates).[34] Alternatively, combining a localized head resection with LPJ can help to reduce recidivism.

Algorithm 51.1

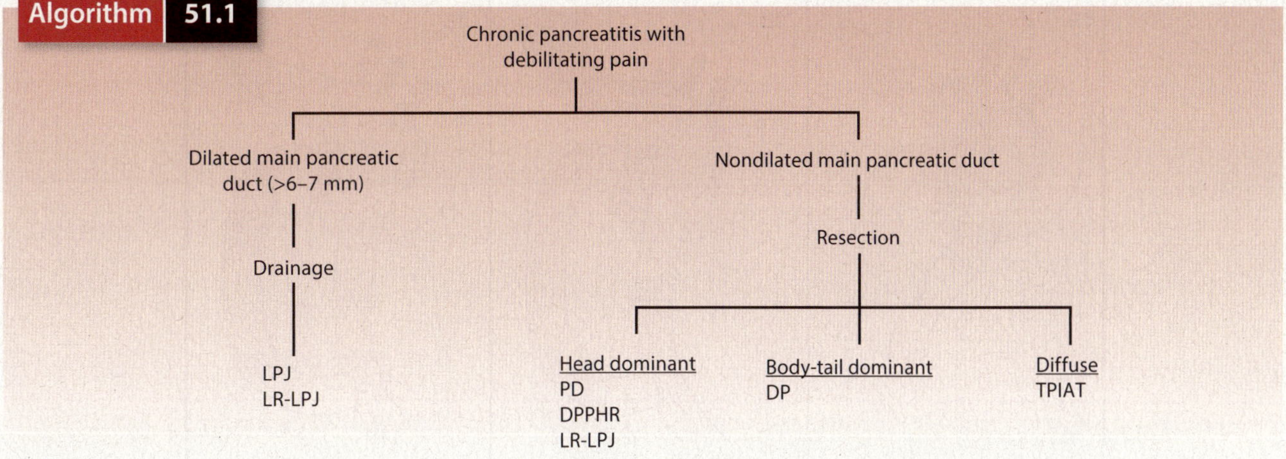

Algorithm 51.1. Algorithm for operative decision making in chronic pancreatitis. LPJ, lateral pancreaticojejunostomy; LR-LPJ, local pancreatic head resection with lateral pancreaticojejunostomy; PD, pancreatoduodenectomy; DPPHR, duodenum preserving pancreatic head resection; DP, distal pancreatectomy; TPIAT, total pancreatectomy with islet autotransplantation.

Localized Pancreatic Head Resection with Lateral Pancreaticojejunostomy

In 1987, Frey and colleagues described a local pancreatic head resection with lateral pancreaticojejunostomy (LR-LPJ) with the goal of achieving pancreatic ductal drainage, removal of damaged and poorly drained parenchyma in the head of the pancreas, and preservation of the duodenum to minimize postoperative gastrointestinal dysfunction. Frey reported initially on 50 patients, describing a morbidity of 22% and a pain-relief rate of 84%.[35] These outcomes have been validated in modern series, both at his own institution and at others, with pain-relief rates of 62% to 88%.[36,37]

Pancreatic Head Resection

Pancreatoduodenectomy (PD) for CP was described as early as 1946 by Whipple.[38] In the modern era, PD is the operation of choice for patients with complicated CP and head-dominant disease. Patients may present with duodenal or biliary obstruction as well as obstructive pancreatopathy from an inflammatory mass in the head of the pancreas. Outcomes for PD include pain relief in 70% to 89% of patients, morbidity in 16% to 53%, and mortality in less than 5% in high-volume centers.[32–39]

The pylorus-preserving pancreatoduodenectomy (PPPD) was popularized by Traverso and Longmire to maintain the physiologic benefits of a functional pylorus.[40] PPPD has been well adopted into pancreas surgery, although the purported nutritional advantages have not been evidenced.[41–43] Some authors, however, have reported improved professional rehabilitation and quality of life after PPPD versus classic PD.[44]

Duodenum-preserving pancreatic head resection (DPPHR) was developed by Beger and colleagues in the 1970s to decrease the morbidity of pancreatic head resection for CP. Pain relief is reported in 77% to 88% of patients, with professional rehabilitation rates of 63% to 69% (**Fig. 51.4**). Morbidity and mortality are acceptable at 28.5% and 1%, respectively.[45,46] The ChroPac trial, a relatively recent multicenter European trial, randomized 226 patients to PD (or PPPD) versus DPPHR. Perioperative morbidity was lower in the PD group, and at 2 years follow-up, there was no difference in the development of endocrine or exocrine failure or quality of life between the groups.[47]

Distal Pancreatectomy

In patients with CP and disease localized to the body and tail of the pancreas or in patients with a main pancreatic duct stricture in the neck or body, distal pancreatectomy (DP) can be an effective means of pain relief. Most CP patients who are candidates for DP have severe inflammatory changes in the region of the splenic hilum, making concomitant splenectomy necessary. Pain-relief rates of 57% to 84% are reported, with 15% to 32% morbidity.[48,49] Postoperative pancreatic fistula after DP is the primary morbidity of this operation and appears to be related to patient-specific factors rather than to operative technique.[49]

Total Pancreatectomy

5 TP for CP was performed as early as 1944 by Clagett at the Mayo Clinic. Perhaps tellingly, his patient died 10 weeks after surgery of a hypoglycemic event. TP can be an effective means of pain relief in patients with diffuse small-duct pancreatitis, as salvage therapy in patients who have failed lesser surgeries, and in patients with genetic pancreatitis. Brittle type 3c pancreatogenic diabetes follows TP, often with severe, potentially life-threatening hypoglycemic episodes. With TP, there is loss of not only insulin-producing beta cells but also of the alpha cells and other composite cells of the islet that produce hormones to maintain glucose homeostasis. As a result, patients may demonstrate an unpredictable response to exogenous insulin and, importantly, may develop hypoglycemic unawareness.

Total pancreatectomy with islet autotransplantation (TPIAT) was described by Sutherland and colleagues at the University of Minnesota in 1978, with the goal of ameliorating

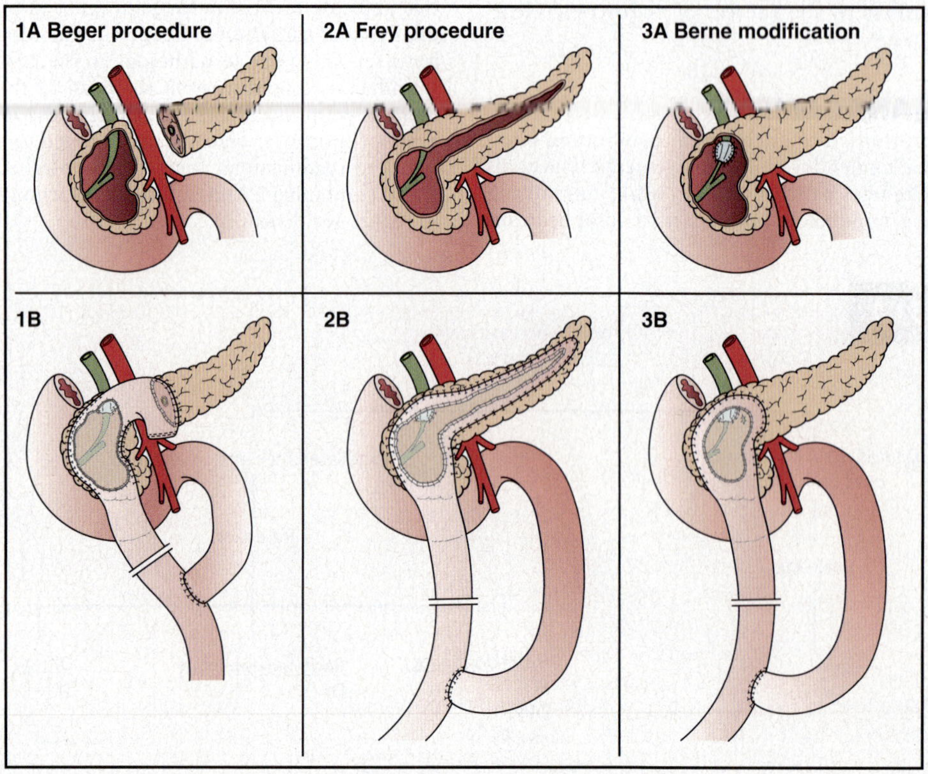

Figure 51.4. Schematic drawings of extent of resection (A) and method of reconstruction (B) for a Beger procedure (1), Frey procedure (2), and a Berne modification of the Beger procedure (3). (Reproduced from Müller MW, Freiss H, Leitzbach S, et al. Perioperative and follow-up results after central pancreatic head resection (Berne technique) in a consecutive series of patients with chronic pancreatitis. *Am J Surg.* 2008;196:364–372.)

the brittle diabetes after extensive pancreatectomy.[50] TPIAT has been increasingly accepted over the past decade, and understanding of long-term outcomes is evolving. Pain-relief rates of 72% to 86% have been reported and patients have a significantly improved quality of life. Morbidity rates of 47% to 55% are reported, with 1.4% to 6% mortality, and insulin independence in 10% to 40% long term after islet transplant.[51–53] Insulin independence after TPIAT correlates with the number of islet equivalents per kilogram harvested,[54] and transplanted islet function appears to be durable, with outcomes reported for more than 13 years.[55] Genetic pancreatitis patients have the most favorable outcomes,[53] whereas patients with alcohol-related pancreatitis fare poorly with TPIAT.[56] A multicenter Prospective Observational outcomes Study evaluating TPIAT (POST) in the United States has recently been undertaken.[57] Reported outcomes from this study have included the effective application of TPIAT in children,[58] patient serum biomarkers correlating to etiology and islet yield,[59] nutritional implications from exocrine insufficiency,[60] and preoperative HgbA1c correlates with islet yield.[61] Current study in this evolving field is focused on patient selection and approaches to improve islet survival.

Minimally Invasive Surgery for Chronic Pancreatitis

Minimally invasive pancreas surgery encompasses laparoscopic and robotic approaches. Laparoscopy began in pancreas surgery with laparoscopic staging for pancreatic cancer. The development of endoscopic stapler technology in the mid-1990s allowed for more complex pancreatic resections to emerge, and the epidemic of incidentally discovered low-grade pancreatic neoplasms allowed for the evolution of laparoscopy as the standard approach to DP. More recently, pancreatic surgeon experience with the robotic platform has increased utilization of the minimally invasive approach even further, allowing for the rising adoption of robotic DP and PD. Single and multicenter comparative studies,[62,63] and now several single and multicenter randomized controlled trials[64–66] have demonstrated the efficacy of minimally invasive pancreas surgery. Minimally invasive DP has lower blood loss, length of stay, and morbidity compared with open DP, with equivalent operative times and pancreatic fistula rates.[62,64] Minimally invasive PD has been demonstrated to have equivalent outcomes to open PD at expert centers.[63] A recent evidence-based consensus statement on minimally invasive pancreatic surgery reviewed available evidence.[67] An international survey described the prevalence of the use of minimally invasive approaches and the preferences among high-volume pancreatic surgeons worldwide. The authors reported an overall increase in the use of minimally invasive surgery (MIS) in both DP and PD, with a shift toward a preference for the robotic approach. Overall, however, open PD is still preferred over MIS PD.[68] Importantly, much of the reported experience in minimally invasive pancreas surgery is for low-grade pancreatic neoplasms and pancreatic cancer. Minimally invasive surgical approaches to CP are technically more challenging due to fibrotic distortion of anatomy and obliteration of normal tissue planes.

SUMMARY

CP is a complex disease that is challenging to manage. Notable recent progress has been made in understanding the underlying pathophysiology, including genetic causes and cellular and biochemical mechanisms, with much still to be learned. Surgery can be beneficial in many patients with debilitating pain from CP. Evolving surgical therapies, such as TPIAT and minimally invasive techniques, are promising.

References

1. Rickels MR, Bellin M, Toledo FG, et al. Detection, evaluation, and treatment of diabetes mellitus in chronic pancreatitis: recommendations from PancreasFest 2012. *Pancreatology*. 2013;13(4): 336–342.
2. Sellars ZM, McIsaac D, Yu H. Nationwide trends in acute and chronic pancreatitis among privately insured children and non-elderly adults in the United States. *Gastroenterology*. 2018;155: 469.
3. Peery AF, Crockett SD, Murphy CC, et al. Burden and cost of gastrointestinal, liver, and pancreatic disease in the United States: update 2021. *Gastroenterology*. 2022;162:621–644.
4. Coté GA, Yadav D, Slivka A, et al. Alcohol and smoking as risk factors in an epidemiology study of patients with chronic pancreatitis. *Clin Gastroenterol Hepatol*. 2011;9:266–273.
5. Whitcomb DC. Genetics of alcoholic and nonalcoholic pancreatitis. *Curr Opin Gastroenterol*. 2012;28:501–506.
6. Cavallini G, Talamini G, Vaona B, et al. Effect of alcohol and smoking on pancreatic lithogenesis in the course of chronic pancreatitis. *Pancreas*. 1994;9:42–46.
7. Maisonneuve P, Lowenfels AB, Müllhaupt B, et al. Cigarette smoking accelerates progression of alcoholic chronic pancreatitis. *Gut*. 2005;54:510–514.
8. Yadav D, Hawes RH, Brand RE, et al. Alcohol consumption, cigarette smoking, and the risk of recurrent acute and chronic pancreatitis. *Arch Int Med*. 2009;169:1035–1045.
9. Comfort MW, Steinberg AG. Pedigree of a family with hereditary chronic relapsing pancreatitis. *Gastroenterology*. 1952;21:54–63.
10. Whitcomb DC, Gorry MC, Preston RA, et al. Hereditary pancreatitis is caused by a mutation in the cationic trypsinogen gene. *Nat Genet*. 1996;14:141–145.
11. Witt H, Luck W, Hennies HC, et al. Mutations in the gene encoding the serine protease inhibitor, Kazal type 1 are associated with chronic pancreatitis. *Nat Genet*. 2000;25:213–216.
12. Szmola R, Sahin-Tóth M. Chymotrypsin C (caldecrin) promotes degradation of human cationic trypsin: identity with Rinderknecht's enzyme Y. *Proc Natl Acad Sci U S A*. 2007;104:11227–11232.
13. Felderbauer P, Hoffman P, Einwächter H, et al. A novel mutation of the calcium sensing receptor gene is associated with chronic pancreatitis in a family with heterozygous SPINK1 mutations. *BMC Gastroenterol*. 2003;3:34.
14. Brand H, Diergaarde B, O'Connell MR, Whitcomb DC, Brand RE. Variation in the gamma-glutamyltransferase 1 gene and risk of chronic pancreatitis. *Pancreas*. 2011;40:1188–1194.
15. Whitcomb DC. Genetic risk factors for pancreatic disorders. *Gastroenterology*. 2013;144:1292–1302.
16. Apte MV, Haber PS, Darby SJ, et al. Pancreatic stellate cells are activated by proinflammatory cytokines: Implications for pancreatic fibrogenesis. *Gut*. 1999;44:534–541.
17. Shek FW, Benyon RC, Walker FM, et al. Expression of transforming growth factor-beta 1 by pancreatic stellate cells and its implications for matrix secretion and turnover in chronic pancreatitis. *Am J Pathol*. 2002;160:1787–1798.
18. Bockman DE, Buchler M, Malfetheiner P, Beger HG. Analysis of nerves in pancreatitis. *Gastroenterology*. 1988;94:1459–1469.
19. Buchler M, Weihe E, Friess H, et al. Changes in peptidergic innervation in chronic pancreatitis. *Pancreas*. 1992;7:183–192.
20. Michalski CW, Shi X, Reiser C, et al. Neurokinin-2 receptor levels correlate with intensity, frequency, and duration of pain in chronic pancreatitis. *Ann Surg*. 2007;246:786–793.
21. Wallace MB, Hawes RH, Durkalski V, et al. The reliability of EUS for the diagnosis of chronic pancreatitis: Interobserver agreement among experienced endosonographers. *Gastrointest Endosc*. 2001;53: 294–299.
22. Barth KS, Balliet W, Pelic CM, et al. Screening for current opioid misuse and associated risk factors among patients with chronic nonalcoholic pancreatitis pain. *Pain Med*. 2014;15(8):1359–1364.
23. Kaufman M, Singh G, Das S, et al. Efficacy of endoscopic ultrasound-guided celiac plexus block and celiac plexus neurolysis for managing abdominal pain associated with chronic

PANCREAS

pancreatitis and pancreatic cancer. *J Clin Gastroenterol*. 2010;44(2): 127–134.
24. Dite P, Ruzicka M, Zboril V, Novotný I. A prospective, randomized trial comparing endoscopic and surgical therapy for chronic pancreatitis. *Endoscopy*. 2003;35:553–558.
25. Cahen DL, Gouma DJ, Laramee P, et al. Long-term outcomes of endoscopic vs. surgical drainage of the pancreatic duct in patients with chronic pancreatitis. *Gastroenterology*. 2011;141: 1690–1695.
26. van Veldhuisen CA, Kempeneers MA, de Rijk FEM, et al. Long term outcomes of early surgery vs. endoscopy first in chronic pancreatitis: follow-up analysis of the ESCAPE randomized clinical trial. *JAMA Surgery*. 2025;160(2):126–133.
27. Van Veldhuisen CA, Leseman CA, de Rijk FEM, et al. Nationwide outcome of tailored surgery for symptomatic chronic pancreatitis based on pancreatic morphology: validation of international guidelines. *Ann Surg*. 2025;281(4):655–663.
28. Puestow CB, Gillesby WJ. Retrograde surgical drainage of pancreas for chronic relapsing pancreatitis. *AMA Arch Surg*. 1958;76: 898–907.
29. Partington PF, Rochelle RE. Modified Puestow procedure for retrograde drainage of the pancreatic duct. *Ann Surg*. 2001;233: 793–800.
30. Nealon WH, Matin S. Analysis of surgical success in preventing recurrent acute exacerbations in chronic pancreatitis. *Ann Surg*. 2001;233:793–800.
31. Adams DB, Ford MC, Anderson MC. Outcome after lateral pancreaticojejunostomy for chronic pancreatitis. *Ann Surg*. 1994;219: 481–489.
32. Schnelldorfer T, Lewin DN, Adams DB. Operative management of chronic pancreatitis: longterm results in 372 patients. *J Am Coll Surg*. 2007;204:1039–1045.
33. Nealon WH, Thompson JC. Progressive loss of pancreatic function in chronic pancreatitis is delayed by main pancreatic duct decompression. A longitudinal prospective analysis of the modified Puestow procedure. *Ann Surg*. 1993;217:458–466.
34. Rios G, Adams DB. Does intraoperative electrohydraulic lithotripsy improve outcome in the surgical management of chronic pancreatitis? *Am Surg*. 2001;67:533–537.
35. Frey CF, Smith GJ. Description and rationale of a new operation for chronic pancreatitis. *Pancreas*. 1987;2:701–707.
36. Frey CF, Amikura K. Local resection of the head of the pancreas combined with longitudinal pancreaticojejunostomy in the management of patients with chronic pancreatitis. *Ann Surg*. 1994;220:492–504.
37. Keck T, Wellner UF, Riediger H, et al. Long term outcome after 92 duodenum preserving pancreatic head resections for chronic pancreatitis: comparison of Beger and Frey procedures. *J Gastrointest Surg*. 2010;14:549–556.
38. Whipple AO. Radical surgery for certain cases of pancreatic fibrosis associated with calcareous deposits. *Ann Surg*. 1946;124: 991–1006.
39. Sakorafas GH, Farnell MB, Nagorney DM, Sarr MG, Rowland CM. Pancreatoduodenctomy for chronic pancreatitis: long term results in 105 patients. *Arch Surg*. 2000;135:517–523.
40. Traverso LW, Longmire WP Jr. Preservation of the pylorus in pancreaticoduodenectomy. *Surg Gynecol Obstet*. 1978;146: 959–962.
41. Tran KT, Smeenk HG, van Eijck CH, et al. Pylorus preserving pancreaticoduodenectomy versus standard Whipple procedure: a prospective, randomized, multicenter analysis of 170 patients with pancreatic and periampullary tumors. *Ann Surg*. 2004;240: 738–745.
42. Seiler CA, Wagner M, Bachmann T, et al. Randomized clinical trial of pylorus-preserving duodenopancreatectomy versus classical Whipple resection—long term results. *Br J Surg*. 2005;92:547–556.
43. Iqbal N, Lovegrove RE, Tilney HS, et al. A comparison of pancreaticoduodenectomy with pylorus preserving pancreaticoduodenectomy: a meta-analysis of 2822 patients. *Eur J Surg Oncol*. 2008;34:1237–1245.
44. Ohtsuka T, Yamaguchi K, Ohuchida J, et al. Comparison of quality of life after pylorus preserving pancreatoduodenectomy and Whipple resection. *Hepatogastroenterology*. 2003;50: 846–850.
45. Beger HG, Krautzberger W, Bittner R, Büchler M, Limmer J. Duodenum-preserving resection of the head of the pancreas in patients with severe chronic pancreatitis. *Surgery*. 1985;97:467–475.
46. Beger HG, Schlosser W, Friess HM, Büchler MW. Duodenum-preserving head resection in chronic pancreatitis changes the natural course of the disease: a single-center 26-year experience. *Ann Surg*. 1999;230:512–519.
47. Diener MK, Hüttner FJ, Kieser M, et al. Partial pancreatoduodenectomy versus duodenum-preserving pancreatic head resection in chronic pancreatitis: the multicenter, randomized, controlled, double-blind ChroPac trial. *Lancet*. 2017;390:1027–1037.
48. Sakorafas GH, Sarr MG, Rowland CM, Farnell MB. Postobstructive chronic pancreatitis: results with distal resection. *Arch Surg*. 2001;136:643–648.
49. Schnelldorfer T, Mauldin PD, Lewin DN, Adams DB. Distal pancreatectomy for chronic pancreatitis: risk factors for postoperative pancreatic fistula. *J Gastrointest Surg*. 2007;11:991–997.
50. Sutherland DE, Matas AJ, Najarian JS. Pancreatic islet cell transplantation. *Surg Clin North Am*. 1978;58:365–382.
51. Chinnakotla S, Bellin MD, Schwartzenberg SJ, et al. Total pancreatectomy and islet autotransplantation in children for chronic pancreatitis: indication, surgical techniques, postoperative management, and long-term outcomes. *Ann Surg*. 2014;97: 1286–1291.
52. Morgan K, Owczarski SM, Borckardt J, Madan A, Nishimura M, Adams DB. Pain control and quality of life after pancreatectomy with islet autotransplantation for chronic pancreatitis. *J Gastrointest Surg*. 2012;16:129–133.
53. Morgan KA, Lancaster WP, Owczarski SM, Wang H, Borckardt J, Adams DB. Patient selection for total pancreatectomy with islet autotransplantation in the surgical management of chronic pancreatitis. *J Am Coll Surg*. 2018;226:446–451.
54. Rilo HR, Ahmad SA, D'Alessio D, et al. Total pancreatectomy and autologous islet cell transplant as a means to treat severe chronic pancreatitis. *J Gastrointest Surg*. 2003;7:978–989.
55. Robertson RP, Lanz KJ, Sutherland DE, Kendall DM. Prevention of diabetes for up to 13 years by autoislet transplantation after pancreatectomy for chronic pancreatitis. *Diabetes*. 2001;50: 47–50.
56. Dunderdale J, McAuliffe JC, McNeal SF, et al. Should pancreatectomy with islet cell autotransplantation in patients with chronic alcoholic pancreatitis be abandoned? *J Am Coll Surg*. 2013;216: 591–596.
57. Bellin MD, Abu-El-Haija M, Morgan K, et al. A multicenter study of total pancreatectomy with islet autotransplantation (TPIAT): POST (Prospective observational study of TPIAT). *Pancreatology*. 2018;18:286–290.
58. Nathan JD, Yang Y, Eaton A, et al. Surgical approach and short term outcomes in adults and children undergoing total pancreatectomy with islet autotransplantation: a report from the prospective observational study of TPIAT. *Pancreatology*. 2022;22: 1–8.
59. Vasu S, Yang JM, Hodges J, et al. Circulating miRNA in patients undergoing total pancreatectomy with islet autotransplantation. *Cell Transplantation*. 2021;30:963689721999330.
60. Downs EM, Eaton A, Witkowski P, et al. Nutritional risks in patients undergoing total pancreatectomy with islet autotransplantation in the POST consortium. *J of Gastrointest Surg*. 2023;27: 1893–1902.
61. Mattke J, Eaton A, Wijkstrom M, et al. Islet isolation outcomes in patients undergoing total pancreatectomy with islet autotransplantation in the POST consortium. *Transplantation*. 2025; 109(1):207–216.
62. Kooby DA, Gillespie T, Bentrem D, et al. Left-sided pancreatectomy: a multicenter comparison of laparoscopic and open approaches. *Ann Surg*. 2008;248:438–446.

63. Zureikat AH, Postlewait LM, Liu T, et al. A multi-institutional comparison of perioperative outcomes of robotic and open pancreatoduodenectomy. *Ann Surg*. 2016;264:640–649.
64. de Rooij T, van Hilst J, van Santvoort H et al. Minimally invasive versus open distal pancreatectomy (LEOPARD): a multicenter patient-blinded randomized controlled trial. *Ann Surg*. 2019;269:2–9.
65. Poves I, Burdio F, Morato O, et al. Comparison of perioperative outcomes between laparoscopic and open approaches for pancreaticoduodenectomy: the PADULAP randomized controlled trial. *Ann Surg*. 2018;268:731–739.
66. Palanivelu C, Senthilnathan P, Sabnis SC, et al. Randomized controlled trial of laparoscopic versus open pancreaticoduodenectomy for periampullary tumors. *Br J Surg*. 2017;104:1443–1450.
67. Asbun HJ, Moekotte AL, Vissers FL, et al. The Miami International Evidence-Based Guidelines on minimally invasive pancreas resection. *Ann Surg*. 2020;271:1–14.
68. van Ramshorst TM, van Hilst J, Bannone E, et al. International survey on opinions and use of robot assisted and laparoscopic minimally invasive pancreatic surgery: 5 year follow up. *HPB*. 2024;26:63–72.

52

Neoplasms of Exocrine Pancreas

Jin He

Key Points

1. Recent evidence supports that pancreatic ductal adenocarcinoma (PDAC) arises from precursor lesions referred to as pancreatic intraepithelial neoplasia (PanIN).
2. Intraductal papillary mucinous neoplasms (IPMNs) are intraductal mucin-producing tumors that range from low-grade dysplasia to high-grade dysplasia to invasive carcinoma.
3. Pancreas protocol contrast-enhanced computed tomography (CT) or magnetic resonance (MRI) is the preferred imaging test for diagnosing and staging pancreatic tumors.
4. Perioperative mortality following pancreatoduodenectomy (PD) is below 1% in high-volume centers, although perioperative complications occur in approximately 40% of patients.
5. Adjuvant chemotherapy can prolong the overall survival of patients following R0 resection of PDAC.
6. Survival after pancreatectomy for PDAC depends on the tumor biology, such as CA19-9 response to preoperative chemotherapy, tumor size reduction on imaging, and lymph node metastasis status.
7. Endoscopic palliation of patients with incurable pancreatic cancer located in the head includes biliary and duodenal stenting, nonanatomical biliary enteric anastomosis, and gastrojejunostomy.
8. Patients found to be unresectable at laparotomy for head of pancreas cancer should be considered for biliary bypass, gastrojejunostomy, and chemical splanchnicectomy to palliate the symptoms of jaundice, duodenal obstruction, and pain, respectively.

Pancreatic cancer is the fourth leading cause of cancer-related death in the United States and second only to colorectal cancer as a cause of gastrointestinal cancer-related death. In 2024, an estimated 66,440 new cases of pancreatic cancer will be diagnosed in the United States, and 51,750 people will die from the disease. The overall 5-year survival for patients with pancreatic cancer has improved to 13%.[1] This improvement is likely due to better early detection and clinical management. Studies with long-term follow-up suggest that individuals at high risk for pancreatic cancer because of genetic predisposition or strong family history can benefit from annual surveillance with endoscopic ultrasound (EUS) and/or MRI.[2] Significant advances have been made in recent years in our understanding of the pathogenesis and clinical management of pancreatic cancer. This chapter will review the epidemiology and risk factors associated with pancreatic cancer and discuss recent updates on the current clinical management of pancreatic cancer.

EPIDEMIOLOGY AND RISK FACTORS

Environmental and dietary factors have been implicated as risk factors for the development of pancreatic cancer. The most consistently observed environmental risk for the development of pancreatic cancer is cigarette smoking. It has been estimated that cigarette smoking can increase the risk of pancreatic cancer between one and a half and five times.[3] The use of smokeless tobacco also increases risk. Other risk factors include type 2 diabetes, chronic pancreatitis, obesity, and a family history of pancreatic cancer.

Most cases of pancreatic cancer have no obvious predisposing genetic factors. However, it is believed that between 5% and 10% of pancreatic cancers arise because of familial predisposition. Six genetic syndromes have been associated with an increased risk for the development of pancreatic cancer (**Table 52.1**). These include hereditary nonpolyposis colon cancer (Lynch syndrome), familial breast cancer associated with the BRCA2 mutation, Peutz–Jeghers syndrome (PJS), ataxia–telangiectasia syndrome, familial atypical multiple mole–melanoma syndrome, and hereditary pancreatitis.

Molecular Genetics

The most common somatic gene alterations in PDAC are KRAS, CDKN2A, TP53, and SMAD4. More than 90% of PDAC contain KRAS mutations. KRAS (Kirsten rat sarcoma viral oncogene homolog) mutations often occur in codons 12, 13, or 61. Point mutations of the KRAS oncogene result in an activated protein that promotes the mitogen-activated protein kinase (MAPK) cascade. Inactivation of cyclin-dependent kinase inhibitor 2A gene (CDKN2A) leads to the loss of cell cycle checkpoint and unchecked proliferation. TP53 mutations inactivate a DNA-binding protein and lead to the loss of control of cell growth. SMAD4 (SMAD family member 4 gene) is a tumor-suppressor gene that encodes a transcription factor that mediates signaling of the transforming growth factor-β (TGF-β) superfamily. For pancreatic cancer diagnosis, SMAD4 mutations are more specific than p53 or p16 mutations.

The most common germline gene alterations in PDAC are BRCA2 and CDKN2A, and less frequently in BRCA1, PALB2, and ATM. Patients with germline gene alterations have a higher risk of developing PDAC. For example, the inactivation of BRCA2, which encodes a protein involved in DNA damage repair, is associated with an up to 10-fold increased risk of pancreatic cancer, as well as breast and ovarian cancer.

Pathology

The most common neoplasms of the exocrine pancreas are ductal adenocarcinomas. Grossly, they are poorly defined and hard masses that often obstruct the distal common bile

Table 52.1. Genetic Syndromes Associated With Hereditary Pancreatic Cancer

Syndrome	Mode of Inheritance	Gene	Fold Increase in Risk	Manifestation of Pancreatic Cancer
Peutz–Jeghers	AD	*STK11*	140×	Hamartomatous polyps of the gastrointestinal tract; mucocutaneous melanin macules
Hereditary pancreatitis	AD	*PRSS-1*	60×	Recurrent episodes of severe pancreatitis starting at a young age
Familial pancreatic cancer	Unknown	Unknown	18×	At least one pair of first-degree relatives with pancreatic cancer
FAMMM	AD	*CDKN2A*	20×	Multiple nevi, atypical nevi, and melanomas
Familial breast cancer 2	AD	*BRCA2*	10×	Breast, ovarian, and pancreatic cancer
HNPCC	AD	*MLH1*, *MSH2*, *MSH6*, or *PMS2*	Unknown	Colonic, endometrial, and gastric cancers; mutator phenotype

AD, autosomal dominant; FAMMM, familial atypical multiple mole melanoma; HNPCC, hereditary nonpolyposis colorectal cancer.

duct or main pancreatic duct. They are often associated with a desmoplastic reaction that causes fibrosis and chronic pancreatitis. Microscopically, they contain infiltrating glands of varying sizes and shapes surrounded by dense, reactive fibrous tissue. The epithelial cells sometimes form papillae and cribriform structures, frequently containing mucin. The nuclei of the cells can show marked pleomorphism, hyperchromasia, loss of polarity, and prominent nucleoli. Ductal adenocarcinomas tend to infiltrate into vascular, lymphatic, and perineural spaces. At the time of resection, most ductal adenocarcinomas have already metastasized to regional lymph nodes. In addition to the lymph nodes, PDAC frequently metastasizes to the liver (80%), peritoneum (60%), lungs and pleurae (50% to 70%), and adrenal glands (25%). They can also directly invade the duodenum, stomach, transverse mesocolon, colon, spleen, and adrenal glands.

The histologic examination of a pancreas resected for cancer frequently reveals the presence of precursor lesions in the pancreatic ducts adjacent to the cancer. Like colon cancer, which arises from benign adenomas, pancreatic cancer may also demonstrate progression to malignant from benign precursor lesions. These precursor lesions are referred to as pancreatic
1 intraepithelial neoplasia (PanIN). PanIN-1 are proliferative lesions without remarkable nuclear abnormality that have a flat and papillary architecture, respectively. PanIN-3 is associated with severe architectural and cytonuclear abnormalities, but invasion through the basement membrane is absent. The older term for PanIN-3 includes carcinoma in situ (CIS). PanIN-2 is an intermediate category between PanIN-1 and PanIN-3 and is associated with a moderate degree of architectural and cytonuclear abnormality. Three-dimensional (3D) mapping techniques demonstrated a stepwise transformation from mild dysplasia to severe dysplasia in pancreatic duct lesions.[4] PanINs have some of the same genetic changes seen in infiltrating adenocarcinomas, most notably activating point mutations in codon 12 of KRAS and mutations in TP53 tumor-suppressor genes.

Other types of neoplasms of the exocrine pancreas are briefly described here.

Solid Epithelial Tumors

Adenosquamous Carcinomas[5]

Adenosquamous carcinoma is a rare variant of ductal adenocarcinoma that demonstrates both glandular and squamous differentiation (>30% component). This variant appears to have more aggressive biologic behavior than ductal adenocarcinoma, with earlier dissemination and worse survival.

Acinar Cell Carcinomas

Acinar cell carcinomas account for less than 1% of pancreatic exocrine tumors. Acinar tumors are typically smooth, fleshy, lobulated, hemorrhagic, or necrotic. Immunohistochemical staining demonstrates the expression of trypsin, lipase, chymotrypsin, or amylase. These tumors are more common in males, with a male-to-female predominance of approximately 3:1. The age of diagnosis is usually in the fifth to seventh decades. These tumors tend to be larger than ductal adenocarcinomas. Patients with acinar cell carcinoma have a slightly better prognosis than patients with ductal carcinoma. Therefore, surgical resection is the treatment of choice.

Pancreatoblastoma

Pancreatoblastomas occur primarily in children and contain both epithelial and mesenchymal elements. The epithelial component appears to arise from acinar cells. The tumors are typically large and often contain areas of degeneration and hemorrhage. If the tumor can be resected, the prognosis appears to be more favorable than that for typical ductal adenocarcinoma.

Giant Cell Carcinomas

Giant cell carcinomas account for less than 1% of nonendocrine pancreatic cancers. They tend to be large, with average diameters greater than 15 cm. Microscopically, they contain large, uninucleated or multinucleated pleomorphic tumor cells. The nuclei contain prominent nucleoli and numerous mitotic figures. Giant cell carcinomas are associated with a poorer prognosis than ductal adenocarcinomas. A variant of giant cell carcinoma is called giant cell carcinoma with osteoclast-like giant cells. These lesions are well-circumscribed with nonpleomorphic giant cells and are less aggressive than standard giant cell carcinomas.

Cystic Epithelial Tumors

Cystic neoplasms also arise from the exocrine pancreas. Cystic neoplasms are less common than ductal adenocarcinomas.

The most common benign pancreatic and peripancreatic cysts are inflammatory pseudocysts. It is important to identify cystic neoplasms because their management is very different from that of nonneoplastic cysts. With advancements in imaging technology, cystic lesions of the pancreas are being detected with increased frequency. Although many of these cystic neoplasms are small and asymptomatic, they can have malignant potential. Therefore, managing these patients is complex, and knowledge of pancreatic cyst natural history and predictors of malignant transformation is important.

Serous Cystic Neoplasms (SCN)

Serous cysts are epithelial neoplasms composed of uniform cuboidal glycogen-rich cells that usually form numerous small cysts containing serous fluid. Serous cystadenomas or microcystic adenomas are more common in women than in men (3:1 preponderance). Although most patients with SCNs are asymptomatic, large SCNs can cause obstructing symptoms such as epigastric pain, dyspepsia, nausea, or vomiting. Serous cystadenomas can be located anywhere in the pancreas and do not communicate with the pancreatic ducts. SCN on computed tomography (CT) shows a honeycomb pattern of micro lacunae, with thin septa separating different segments. SCNs can also have a sunburst pattern of central calcification, which is seen in 10% to 30% of cases. Grossly, they appear as spongy, well-circumscribed, multiloculated cysts. von Hippel-Lindau (VHL) mutation detected in the cyst fluid is diagnostic for SCN. Most SCNs are benign and indolent; rare malignant behaviors, such as liver or lymph node metastases from malignant serous cystadenocarcinoma have been reported. Telomerase reverse transcriptase (TERT) promoter alterations were associated with the fast growth of SCNs. Symptomatic SCNs should undergo surgical excision.

Mucinous Cystic Neoplasms[6]

Mucinous cystic neoplasms (MCNs) are neoplasms composed of mucin-producing epithelial cells associated with an ovarian-type stroma. These cysts do not communicate with the main pancreatic duct. MCNs account for almost 30% of all cystic neoplasms. The mean age at diagnosis is between 40 and 50 years. MCNs are more common in women with a female-to-male ratio of 9:1. Most patients with MCNs present with a lesion in the body or tail of the pancreas, and only a minority (10% to 30%) involve the head of the gland. Microscopically, the cysts are lined by tall columnar mucin-producing epithelium. The walls of the cysts contain a very distinctive "ovarian-type" stroma. This stroma comprises densely packed spindle cells with sparse cytoplasm and uniform elongated nuclei. All MCNs are premalignant lesions and should be completely resected to prevent progression to malignancy.

Invasive mucinous cystadenocarcinomas are MCNs associated with an invasive carcinoma. The extent of invasive and in situ carcinomas in MCNs can be very focal. Therefore, a benign diagnosis cannot be established on biopsy alone, and the lesions should be completely resected. The prognosis for patients with resected benign tumors is excellent. Patients with mucinous cystadenocarcinoma tend to do better than patients with ductal adenocarcinoma, with a 5-year survival of approximately 50%.

Intraductal Papillary Mucinous Neoplasms

Intraductal papillary mucinous neoplasms (IPMNs) are intraductal mucin-producing neoplasms, the most common mucinous neoplasm in the pancreas. These neoplasms extensively involve the main pancreatic ducts and/or side branches. Unlike MCNs, IPMNs lack the ovarian stroma. IPMNs can progress from low-grade dysplasia to invasive carcinoma. Microscopically, they consist of papillary projections lined by columnar mucin-secreting cells. They show varying degrees of cellular atypia. The noninvasive IPMNs are classified into low-grade and high-grade dysplasia. Invasive IPMNs are either colloid or tubular, with the latter having a worse prognosis. Further histologic subtyping of epithelial differentiation is based on the cell lineage, papillae morphology, and immunophenotype and includes classification into intestinal, gastric, pancreaticobiliary, and oncocytic subtypes.

2 IPMNs are clinically subclassified as main-duct or branch-duct type or mixed type, containing elements of both. Main-duct IPMN is characterized by the involvement of the duct of Wirsung or Santorini, which is dilated to more than 5 mm in diameter. Branch-duct IPMN originates in the side branches of the pancreatic ductal system and appears as a multilobular cystic lesion communicating with a nondilated main pancreatic duct.

IPMNs are usually found in elderly individuals. Some patients may experience symptoms that include: abdominal pain, steatorrhea, weight loss, jaundice, diabetes, and chronic pancreatitis. A substantial number of these lesions are also detected as incidental findings on cross-sectional imaging studies performed for other indications. IPMNs can be found diffusely throughout the whole gland. CT scans will typically reveal a cystic mass in the head of the pancreas that appears to communicate with the pancreatic ductal system. On endoscopy, mucin can be seen oozing from the ampulla of Vater. Endoscopic retrograde cholangiopancreatography (ERCP) can be used to confirm that the cysts communicate with the pancreatic ducts.

Two morphologic features distinguish IPMNs from MCNs: IPMNs communicate with ducts, MCNs do not; the presence of ovarian stroma is diagnostic for MCNs. IPMNs represent a continuum of disease from benign to malignant. In a series of resected IPMNs from the Johns Hopkins Hospital, the prognosis for the benign forms of the disease appears to be significantly better than for invasive IPMNs, with 1-, 2-, and 5-year actuarial survival of 97%, 94%, and 77%, respectively.[7] Although invasive IPMNs are associated with disease progression and death, the prognosis remains markedly better than for invasive ductal carcinoma of the pancreas with survival of 72%, 58%, and 43% at 1, 2, and 5 years, respectively. It is unclear if this fact is due to earlier presentation or differences in tumor biology.

International consensus for the management of IPMNs has been developed.[8] CT or MRI with MRCP is recommended for imaging IPMNs. IPMNs are classified as having either "high-risk stigmata" or "worrisome features." High-risk stigmata include obstructive jaundice in the setting of a cyst in the head of the pancreas, a main duct >10 mm, or a cyst with a solid enhancing component >5 mm in the wall. Worrisome features include cyst >3 cm, thickened enhanced cyst walls, nonenhanced mural nodules, main duct size between 5 and 9 mm, abrupt change in the MPD caliber with distal pancreatic atrophy, and lymphadenopathy. All cysts with "worrisome features" and cysts of >3 cm without "worrisome features" should undergo endoscopic ultrasonography (EUS), and all cysts with "high-risk stigmata" should be resected (**Algorithm 52.1**).

The goal of surgical therapy for invasive IPMNs should be a complete surgical resection yielding negative margins of cancer or high grade dysplasia (HGD). However, the surgery for noninvasive IPMNs is prophylactic. Except for patients with a strong family history of PDAC or genetic risk factors, a prophylactic total pancreatectomy should be avoided. Unlike those patients with completely resected noninvasive MCNs (who are routinely cured), patients with completely resected noninvasive and invasive IPMNs should undergo careful follow-up and surveillance for the development of recurrent disease or new PDAC lesions.

Solid-Pseudopapillary Tumor

Solid-pseudopapillary tumors (SPTs), also termed Hamoudi or Frantz tumors, occur primarily in young females. Radiologically, they present as a well-demarcated heterogeneous mass with solid and cystic components. EUS-guided fine needle aspiration (FNA) or core biopsy is often diagnostic, demonstrating uniform cells forming microadenoid structures, branching, and papillary clusters with delicate fibrovascular cores. Most SPTs exhibit a benign behavior. However, a small percentage of SPTs (<5%) have vascular or perineural invasion, lymph node involvement, or liver metastases. The overall 5-year survival is close to 97% in patients undergoing R0 surgical resection.

CLINICOPATHOLOGIC STAGING OF PDAC

Accurate pathologic staging of pancreatic cancer is important to provide patients with prognostic information and comparing the results of various therapeutic trials. The 8th edition of the American Joint Committee on Cancer (AJCC) staging for

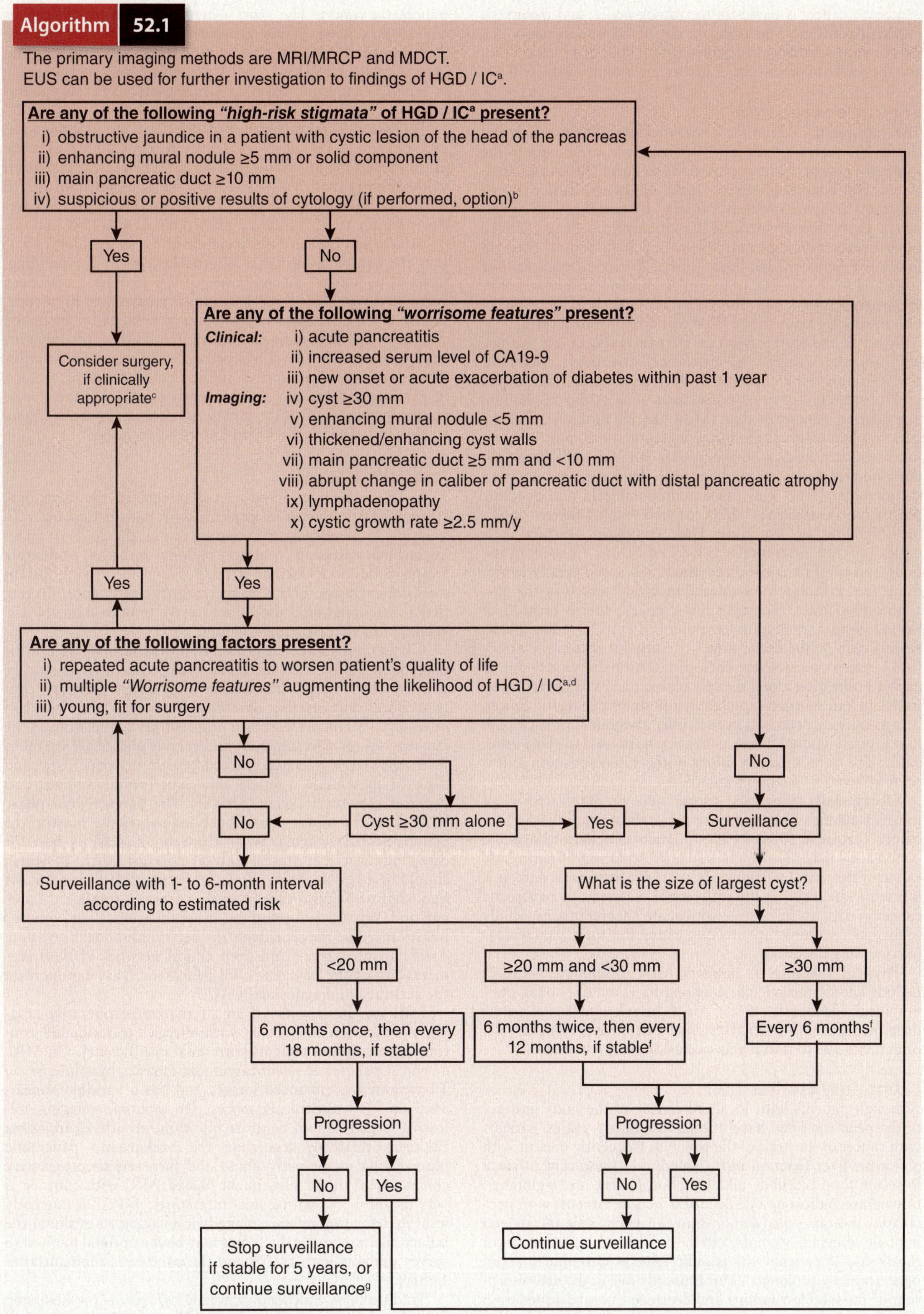

Algorithm 52.1. International evidence-based Kyoto guidelines for the management of intraductal papillary mucinous neoplasm of the pancreas. From Ohtsuka T, Fernandez-Del Castillo C, Furukawa T, et al. International evidence-based Kyoto guidelines for the management of intraductal papillary mucinous neoplasm of the pancreas. *Pancreatology*. 2024;24:255–270.

pancreatic cancer is based on the tumor, nodes, and metastasis (TNM) classification, including the size of the primary tumor (T), the presence or absence of regional lymph node involvement (N), and the presence or absence of distant metastatic disease (M).[9]

Clinical Presentation

The nonspecific symptoms associated with early pancreatic cancer, the inaccessibility of the pancreas to examination, the aggressiveness of the tumors, and the technical difficulties associated with pancreatic surgery make pancreatic cancer one of the most challenging diseases treated by surgeons and oncologists. Early diagnosis of PDAC remains a challenge. Unlike other cancer types (breast, colon, and lung cancer), the US Preventive Services Task Force (USPSTF) recommends against screening for pancreatic cancer in asymptomatic adults. However, surveillance of high-risk individuals may lead to the detection of smaller, lower-stage PDACs and improved survival.

Most of the early symptoms of pancreatic cancer, including anorexia, weight loss, abdominal discomfort, and nausea, are nonspecific. Specific symptoms are often associated with obstruction of nearby structures such as the duodenum, bile duct, or pancreatic duct. Most cancers in the head of the pancreas can obstruct the intrapancreatic portion of the common bile duct, leading to progressive jaundice, acholic stools, darkening of the urine, and pruritus. They can also obstruct the pancreatic duct and cause abdominal pain and exocrine pancreatic insufficiency (EPI), or new-onset diabetes mellitus (NODM), or worsening DM. Duodenal obstruction is typically a late symptom of advanced PDAC. Cancers in the body and tail of the pancreas often lack specific early symptoms until invading the surrounding blood vessels or the gastrointestinal tract, including the stomach, fourth portion of the duodenum, and transverse colon. PDAC invading blood vessels such as the celiac artery or superior mesentery artery (SMA) often causes severe back pain. This pain is likely due to cancer infiltration along the splanchnic plexus in the retroperitoneum. Pain is a common late symptom of pancreatic cancer. The pain usually starts as vague upper abdominal or back pain that is often ignored by the patient or attributed to some other cause. The pain is usually worse in the supine position and is often relieved by leaning forward.

Occasionally, pancreatic cancer may be discovered in an unusual manner. The new onset of diabetes may be the first clinical feature in 10% to 15% of patients. An episode of acute pancreatitis may also be the initial presentation of pancreatic cancer if the tumor partially obstructs the pancreatic duct. It is important to consider the differential diagnosis of pancreatic cancer in patients presenting with acute pancreatitis, especially individuals without an obvious cause for their pancreatitis (alcohol or gallstones).

Physical findings in patients with disseminated cancer include left supraclavicular adenopathy (Virchow node), periumbilical adenopathy (Sister Mary Joseph node), and pelvic drop metastases (Blumer shelf). Ascites can be present in 15% of patients due to portal vein occlusion or carcinomatosis.

Laboratory Studies

Although patients with localized cancer of the body and tail of the pancreas often have normal laboratory values, patients with cancer of the head of the pancreas frequently present with abnormal liver function tests, including a significant increase in serum total bilirubin, alkaline phosphatase, and γ-glutamyl transferase, indicating bile duct obstruction. Patients with pancreatic cancer may also demonstrate normochromic anemia and hypoalbuminemia secondary to the nutritional consequences of the disease. In patients with jaundice, the prothrombin time can be abnormally prolonged. This is usually due to the malabsorption of fat-soluble vitamins and decreased hepatic production of vitamin K-dependent clotting factors.

A wide variety of serum tumor markers have been proposed for use in the diagnosis and follow-up of patients with pancreatic cancer. The most extensively studied of these is CA 19-9, a Lewis blood group-related mucin glycoprotein. Approximately 5% of the population lacks the Lewis gene and cannot produce CA 19-9. DUPAN-2, only approved for testing in Japan, is a glycoprotein that can be useful in PDAC patients unable to synthesize CA 19-9.[10]

When a normal upper limit of 37 U/mL is used, the accuracy of the CA 19-9 level to identify patients with pancreatic adenocarcinoma is only about 80%. When a higher cutoff value of more than 90 U/mL is used, the accuracy improves to 85%, and increasing the cutoff value to 200 U/mL increases the accuracy to 95%. The combined use of CA 19-9 and CT, or MRCP, can improve the accuracy of the individual tests so that the combined accuracy approaches 100% for the diagnosis of pancreatic cancer. Levels of CA 19-9 have also been correlated with prognosis and tumor recurrence. In general, higher CA 19-9 values before surgery indicate an increased chance of occult distant metastases. In addition, the dynamic change of CA 19-9 level has been used to monitor the effectiveness of neoadjuvant and adjuvant chemotherapy therapy in patients. Increasing CA 19-9 levels usually indicate recurrence or progression of the disease, whereas stable or declining levels were associated with an improved prognosis.

Radiologic Studies

Radiologic imaging plays a crucial role in the diagnosis, staging, and follow-up of patients with pancreatic cancer. In addition to identifying the primary tumor, the goals of imaging include assessing local and regional invasion, evaluating lymph nodes and vascular structures, and identifying distant metastatic disease. EUS, CT, and magnetic resonance imaging (MRI) are commonly used noninvasive tests in patients suspected of having pancreatic cancer.

3 CT scanning is the most used noninvasive imaging test for diagnosing pancreatic cancer. Pancreas protocol CT should be performed with rapid injection of intravenous iodinated contrast. Slices with overlap should be reconstructed at less than or equal to 3 mm. At least two postcontrast acquisitions in the late arterial (or parenchymal) and venous phases are useful to assess the arteries (celiac, common hepatic, peripancreatic, and superior mesenteric arteries) and veins (portal, splenic, and superior mesenteric veins [SMVs]). The parenchymal phase best shows the tumor as an ill defined hypodense mass in the pancreatic parenchyma, while the venous phase is best for detecting liver metastases. Enteral contrast, such as water, should be given since this allows for better identification of the duodenal wall and results in artifact-free reformations. Coronal and sagittal reformations in both arterial and venous phases increase the sensitivity for determining local invasion. Artificial intelligence and deep neural network (DNN) segmentation of the pancreas with pancreatic mass can increase the accuracy in diagnosing PDAC.[11]

MRI can be considered an alternative preoperative staging examination in patients with allergies to iodinated contrast agents and in patients with renal insufficiency. On MRI, a typical pancreatic adenocarcinoma appears hypointense on T1-weighted unenhanced images and has a variable appearance on T2-weighted sequences. On dynamic imaging following a gadolinium contrast injection, an adenocarcinoma enhances relatively less than the background pancreatic parenchyma in the early phase and then reveals progressive enhancement in the subsequent phases. MRI with contrast is very useful in evaluating liver metastases. MRCP is currently indicated for noninvasive diagnostic imaging to evaluate the biliary and pancreatic ducts and may be the optimal method to survey patients with IPMN and the pancreatic remnant after surgery.

Traditionally, endoscopic cholangiography is the next step in evaluating the jaundiced patient. The endoscopic approach with biliary stent placement will help control the jaundice. The strengths of EUS techniques for pancreatic cancer are the clarification of small lesions (<2 cm) when CT findings are questionable or negative, detection of malignant lymphadenopathy, detection of vascular involvement, and the ability to perform EUS-guided FNA for histologic diagnosis and staging. This is essential in patients for whom a tissue diagnosis is required (poor operative candidates or undergoing neoadjuvant therapy). This approach may avoid the risks of tumor seeding from percutaneous biopsy. Percutaneous FNA of pancreatic masses is rarely helpful. The reasons for not using percutaneous biopsy in potentially resectable lesions are twofold. First, even after repeated sampling, a negative result does not exclude malignancy; in fact, the smaller and likely more curable tumors are likely to be missed by the needle. The second concern is the potential for tumor seeding, either along the needle tract or with intraperitoneal spread.

Preoperative Staging

At the time of diagnosis, only 10% of PDAC patients have tumors confined to the pancreas, 40% have locally advanced disease, and more than 50% have distant spread. The goal of preoperative staging of pancreatic cancer is to determine the feasibility of surgery with negative margins and the optimal treatment sequence for each individual patient. Specific anatomy-based CT or MRI criteria can stratify patients into four distinct groups (**Table 52.2**): (1) resectable, (2) borderline, (3) locally advanced, or (4) metastatic. The extent of further staging to be performed depends on the individual patient and the surgeon's preference. Historically, patients with resectable imaging criteria were offered surgery first approach, followed by adjuvant chemotherapy. Recent advances in the efficacy of systemic chemotherapy agents have further supported the hypothetical benefits of preoperative neoadjuvant chemotherapy, even for resectable tumors. Patients with borderline or locally advanced pancreatic cancer based on CT criteria should receive preoperative induction chemotherapy or chemoradiotherapy. Ideally, patients in these high-risk disease categories should be offered enrollment in clinical trials investigating novel treatment agents. The multidisciplinary approach of patients with pancreatic cancer after complete staging and determination of resectability based on imaging findings is always preferred.

Staging Laparoscopy

The use of diagnostic laparoscopy in pancreatic cancer remains controversial. With the recent improvements in CT imaging, the rate of unsuspected positive peritoneal findings approaches 10% to 15% for all patients. Proponents of staging laparoscopy believe that laparoscopy can identify a substantial number of patients with peritoneal or liver metastases and, therefore, should be uniformly applied to all patients with potentially resectable tumors.[12] On the other hand, opponents believe that the inherent cost of such a practice outweighs the benefit to the small number of patients for whom diagnostic laparoscopy is useful in upstaging. Selective use of staging laparoscopy should be considered for patients at high risk of occult metastatic disease. The information gained from preoperative staging provides the basis for planning therapy for each individual patient. If the results of preoperative staging with CT/MRI and laparoscopy show localized disease, resectability rates are over 90% for tumors in the head of the pancreas at the high-volume centers.

Table 52.2. Preoperative Staging Based on CT or MRI Findings

Metastatic Evidence of metastatic spread (typically to the liver, peritoneum, or lung)
Resectable No evidence of extrapancreatic disease Patent SMV/PV Normal tissue plane between tumor and the celiac, CHA, or the SMA.
Borderline resectable Patent SMV/PV, or short segment occlusion if reconstructable Evidence of tumor abutment (<180 degree or 50% vessel circumference) against celiac, CHA, or SMA
Locally advanced SMV/PV occlusion with no option for reconstruction Arterial encasement (>180 degree or 50% vessel circumference) of celiac, CHA, or SMA

SMV, superior mesentery artery, PV, portal vein; CHA, common hepatic artery; SMA, superior mesentery artery.

SURGICAL RESECTION OF PANCREATIC CARCINOMA

Carcinoma of the Head, Neck, or Uncinate Process

In 1935, Whipple et al. described a two-stage surgery technique for resection of a periampullary carcinoma. In 1954, Stafford et al reported the first one-stage resection of carcinoma of pancreatic head.[13] Surgical resection offers the only chance for long-term cure. Five-year survival after pancreaticoduodenectomy (PD) with negative margins is about 40% for node-negative disease.

The operative management of pancreatic cancer consists of two phases: first, excluding occult liver metastases or peritoneal carcinomatosis, and assessing whether the tumor resectability is consistent with the preoperative imaging. Local factors that preclude resection include retroperitoneal extension of the tumor to involve the inferior vena cava or aorta, or direct involvement or encasement of the superior mesenteric artery, hepatic artery, and celiac axis. Involvement of the SMV, or portal vein can be managed with venous resection and reconstruction in select cases. All those factors can be assessed with high-quality pancreas protocol CT or MRI. If the tumor is resectable, PD should include an R0 resection and reconstruction of pancreaticojejunostomy, hepaticojejunostomy, and gastrojejunostomy. Regional lymph nodes, including those along the SMA and celiac artery, should be resected to achieve the triangle dissection.[14]

Many techniques have been published regarding SMV and SMA dissection. For example, during this extensive Kocherization, the first structure that one encounters anterior to the third portion of the duodenum is the SMV. Alternatively, the SMV may also be identified by tracing either the middle colic vein or the right gastroepiploic vein back to the SMV. Depending on the tumor location and invasion, SMA can be approached anteriorly, posteriorly, from left or right, above or below the mesocolon.[15]

"Arterial divestment" is a recent description of periadventitial lymphoneural dissection of the hepatic artery, celiac trunk, suprarenal aorta, and superior mesenteric artery. This technique is useful for patients with locally advanced PDAC after induction chemotherapy. Intraoperative exploration revealed that, although abutting or encasing the artery on CT imaging, the arterial tunica media often is not invaded. This allows for resection of the tumor within the tunica adventitia and the attached neural plexus on top of the arterial wall through dissection within the arterial periadventitial plane. With this technique, arterial resection and reconstruction can be spared while achieving a macroscopically margin-free resection (commonly R0, sometimes R1 with tumor cells within a 1 mm margin). Arterial divestment can be associated with neurogenic diarrhea, which needs to be treated carefully with peristalsis-reducing agents (eg, loperamide, tincture of opioid).[16]

We routinely check the neck margin for frozen analysis since another resection of the body of the pancreas can be achieved for most patients. A total pancreatectomy should only be considered if the neck margin is positive when (1) young patients have a strong family history of PDAC; and (2) artery resection/reconstruction was performed. Leaving a small tail of pancreas without pancreaticojejunostomy is safe as it may help pancreatic endocrine function.

There are several techniques for restoring gastrointestinal continuity after a pancreaticoduodenal resection. Our preferred technique is to bring the end of the divided jejunum through the ligament of Treitz defect or the transverse mesocolon and perform an end-to-side pancreaticojejunostomy. The anastomosis is begun by placing a series of interrupted 3-0 silk sutures between the side of the jejunum and the posterior capsule of the end of the pancreas. A small enterotomy is then made in the jejunum to match the size of the pancreatic duct, and an inner layer of interrupted 5-0 absorbable monofilament sutures is used to create a duct-to-mucosa anastomosis. We prefer to stent this anastomosis with a short pediatric feeding tube. The anastomosis is completed with an outer layer of 3-0 silk sutures placed between the anterior pancreatic capsule and the jejunum. We rarely use the invagination technique for pancreaticojejunostomy. The biliary–enteric anastomosis is performed at 5 to 10 cm distal to the pancreaticojejunostomy. This is an end-to-side hepaticojejunostomy with a single interrupted layer of 4-0 or 5-0 absorbable synthetic suture material. No T-tube or stent is generally necessary. Approximately 40 cm distal to the biliary–enteric anastomosis, a side-to-side gastrojejunostomy is performed in an antecolic manner with an inner continuous layer of 3-0 absorbable synthetic suture material and an outer interrupted layer of 3-0 silk.

Advances in minimally invasive surgery continue to pave the way for improved oncologic outcomes. A recent multicenter randomized controlled trial showed robotic PD for patients with pancreatic cancer was associated with shorter postoperative length of hospital stay in the modified intention-to-treat (mITT) analysis. Robotic PD was safe and feasible for surgeons who had passed the learning curve.[17]

Several technical aspects of PD remain controversial. These controversies include: (1) whether or not a radical lymph node dissection is necessary, (2) whether a pylorus-preserving PD is associated with long-term outcomes, and (3) whether there is a role for minimally invasive PD. Decades of studies have shown that extended lymph node dissections are not beneficial. Preserving antral and pyloric function, the pylorus-preserving Whipple procedure reduces the incidence of postgastrectomy symptoms but is associated with a higher incidence of delayed gastric emptying. No difference appears to be found in survival among patients treated with the pylorus-sparing Whipple procedure and those managed by the traditional Whipple resection.

Carcinoma of the Body and Tail

The surgical management of adenocarcinoma of the body and tail of the pancreas is much more limited than that of the head of the pancreas because of the extent of the disease usually present at the time of symptomatic presentation. Most patients with resectable PDAC of the body and tail of the pancreas are candidates for a minimally invasive approach. Distal pancreatectomy with splenectomy is the standard choice. The resection should be extended as proximally as possible, with the transected pancreas oversewn with nonabsorbable sutures. If the pancreatic duct is identified on the cutting surface, it should be closed with a 5-0 suture in a purse-string fashion.

Postoperative Results

4 The current operative mortality following PD in high-volume centers is in the range of 1% to 3%. Although the operative mortality rates for pancreatic cancer have improved significantly, the complication rates remained around 40%. Pancreatic fistula remains the most frequent serious complication following PD, with an incidence ranging from 5% to 15%. Although the incidence of pancreatic fistula following PD remains stable, the overall associated mortality rate has diminished owing to improved management of parenteral nutrition and controlling the pancreatic leak with percutaneous or intraoperative drainage.

ADJUVANT AND NEOADJUVANT THERAPY FOR PATIENTS WITH LOCALIZED PDAC

Despite advances in surgery and perioperative care that have resulted in markedly reduced postoperative mortality after pancreatectomy, the median survival for pancreatic cancer patients has not changed significantly over the past three decades. Most patients with resected pancreatic cancer will ultimately recur and die of their recurrent disease. These outcomes suggest that systemic control with effective chemotherapy remains the critical component of the multidisciplinary approach. The results of the most important randomized prospective trials of adjuvant therapy for pancreatic cancer are summarized in **Table 52.3.**

5 The ESPAC-1 trial published in 2004 analyzed 289 patients recruited from 53 hospitals in a 2 × 2 factorial design. The four study groups included (1) surgery only (n = 69); (2) chemotherapy only (n = 73) consisting of 5-FU, 425 mg/m^2, and leucovorin, 20 mg/m^2, given daily for 5 days every 4 weeks for six cycles of treatment; (3) radiation therapy and 5-FU given (n = 75); and (4) both treatments (n = 73, chemoradiation followed by chemotherapy). The major study conclusions were that the 5-year overall survival comparisons between patients who received chemotherapy versus individuals who did not (21% vs. 8%, P = .009) and those who received radiation therapy versus those who did not (10% vs. 20%, P = .05). Adjuvant chemotherapy had a beneficial effect in resected pancreatic cancer, whereas chemoradiation had a deleterious effect.[18]

The CONKO-1 trial, conducted in Germany and Austria, represented a randomization of 368 patients following R0 or R1 resection to either observation or an experimental arm of gemcitabine. After a median follow-up time of 53 months, the median disease-free survival was 13.9 months in the gemcitabine arm versus 6.9 months in the observation arm (P < .001). There was no difference in overall survival for the gemcitabine arm versus the control group—median survival was 22 versus 20 months. Although survival was not different, gemcitabine significantly delayed the development of recurrent disease after complete resection of pancreatic cancer compared with observation alone.[19]

The current 5-year survival for patients undergoing R0 resection for adenocarcinoma of the head of the pancreas and adjuvant chemotherapy was reported to be in the range of 50%.[20] This French study compared the efficacy and safety of a modified FOLFIRINOX regimen with gemcitabine as adjuvant therapy in patients with resected pancreatic cancer. Four hundred and ninety-three patients with resected PDAC were randomized to receive a modified FOLFIRINOX regimen (20% decreased irinotecan) or gemcitabine for 24 weeks. At a median follow-up of 33.6 months, the median disease-free survival was 21.6 months in the modified-FOLFIRINOX group and 12.8 months in the gemcitabine group (P < .001). The median overall survival was 54.4 months in the modified-FOLFIRINOX group and 35.0 months in the gemcitabine group (P = .003). Adjuvant chemotherapy of a modified FOLFIRINOX regimen led to significantly longer survival than gemcitabine among patients with resected pancreatic cancer, at the expense of a higher incidence of toxic effects.

Neoadjuvant chemotherapy offers several potential benefits, including: (1) delivery of treatment to well-oxygenated tissue, which enhances the efficacy of chemotherapy, (2) downstaging can enhance the ability to achieve a negative-margin resection and thereby reduce local recurrence; and (3) avoidance of surgery in patients with rapidly progressive disease.

Table 52.3. Contemporary Adjuvant Chemotherapy Trials in Resectable PDAC

Study Group	Years	Setting	N	Treatment	Control	Endpoint	Results
ESPAC-1[18]	1994–2000	ADJ	548	5-FU alone CRT alone 5-FU CRT	Surgery alone	OS	No benefit with adjuvant CRT (15.5 vs. 16.1 mo, $P = .24$); Survival better with chemo alone (19.7 vs. 14.0 mo, $P < .01$)
CONKO-001[19]	1998–2004	ADJ	368	Gemcitabine	Surgery alone	DFS	DFS better with gemcitabine (13.4 vs. 6.7 mo, $P < .01$) OS slightly better with gemcitabine (22.8 vs. 20.2 mo, $P = .01$)
ESPAC-3[21]	2000–2007	ADJ	1088	5-FU	Gemcitabine	OS	No difference in survival between gemcitabine and 5-FU (23 vs. 26 mo, $P = .39$); lesser toxicity with gemcitabine
JASPAC-1[22]	2007–2010	ADJ	385	S-1	Gemcitabine	OS	5-y OS better with S-1 (44.1% vs. 24.4%, $P < .01$)
ESPAC-4[23]	2008–2014	ADJ	732	Gemcitabine/ Capecitabine	Gemcitabine	OS	Survival better with gem/cap (28 vs. 25 mo, $P = .03$)
PRODIGE-24[24]	2012–2016	ADJ	493	mFFX	Gemcitabine	DFS	DFS better with mFFX (21.6 vs. 12.8 mo, $P < .001$); OS better with mFFX (54.4 vs. 35.0 mo, $P = .003$).
APACT[25]	2014–2016	ADJ	866	GNP	Gemcitabine	DFS	No difference in DFS with GNP vs. gem 5-y OS better with GNP (41.8 vs. 37.7 mo, $P = .02$)

ADJ, adjuvant; DFS, disease-free survival; CRT, chemoradiotherapy; GNP, gemcitabine/nab-paclitaxel; mFFX, modified FOLFIRINOX; NAT, neoadjuvant; OS, overall survival; RCT, randomized controlled trial.

Neoadjuvant therapy can be completed without increasing the subsequent morbidity and mortality of surgical resection.

Although many retrospective studies suggested the improved outcome of patients with resectable PDAC undergoing neoadjuvant chemotherapy, the recent international RCT (NORPACT-1 trial) did not show a survival benefit from neoadjuvant fluorouracil, leucovorin, irinotecan, and oxaliplatin (FOLFIRINOX) in resectable PDAC compared with upfront surgery[26] (Table 52.4).

The Dutch group reported positive findings in the PREOPANC trial. This multicenter, randomized, phase III study randomized 248 patients with both resectable or borderline resectable cancer to either preoperative gemcitabine-based chemoradiation or upfront surgery. Both arms received adjuvant gemcitabine after surgery. The primary endpoint of median overall survival (OS) was initially not improved with preoperative chemoradiation compared to surgery (16.0 vs. 14.3 months, $P = .096$), but disease-free survival was slightly prolonged (8.1 vs. 7.7 months, $P = .032$) and R0 resection rates were significantly higher (72% vs. 40%; $P < .001$) in the preoperative chemoradiation group. Furthermore, upon long-term follow-up of this study, there was a significant 5 year overall survival advantage in the chemoradiation arm compared to surgery alone (21% vs. 7%). Neoadjuvant chemoradiation was associated with improvements in secondary outcomes, such as increased adherence to treatment, improved resection rates, and superior local disease control.[27]

Table 52.4. Neoadjuvant Therapy Trials for Resectable and Borderline Resectable PDAC

Study Group	Years	N	Treatment	Control	Endpoint	Results
Jang et al.[28]	2012–2014	50	Gemcitabine CRT	Upfront surgery	OS	Survival better with neoadjuvant CRT (21 vs. 12 mo, $P = .03$)
ESPAC-5[29]	2014–2018	90	Gemcitabine/ Capecitabine mFFX 5-FU CRT	Upfront surgery	R0 rate	No difference in R0 resection rate between four arms 1-y OS better with any NAT vs. upfront surgery (77% vs. 40%, $P < .001$)
PREOPANC[27,30]	2013–2017	248	Gemcitabine CRT	Upfront surgery	OS	No difference in median OS 5-y OS better with CRT on long-term follow up (21% vs. 7%)
A021501[31]	2017–2019	126	mFFX-SBRT	mFFX	OS	Survival better with chemo alone (67% vs. 48%)
NORPACT-1[26]	2017–2021	123	FFX	Upfront surgery	OS	No difference in median OS 23 vs. 34 mo; $P = .058$

CRT, chemoradiotherapy; SBRT, stereotactic body radiation therapy.

Ongoing trials on neoadjuvant chemotherapy are addressing the following questions: (1) What is the best regimen, GNP versus mFFX? (2) What is the appropriate duration of neoadjuvant chemotherapy? (3) How do we predict the response to chemotherapy? (4) Is there any role of chemotherapy regimen switch before surgery? Advances in understanding tumor biology and development of novel biomarkers such as ctDNA may
6 help improve patient selection for appropriate neoadjuvant chemotherapy.

CHEMOTHERAPY AND RADIATION FOR UNRESECTABLE OR METASTATIC PDAC

Specific antitumor therapies in patients with advanced PDAC have shown a marginal improvement in survival, often with relatively high toxicity rates and a negative impact on quality of life. Recently, both FOLFIRINOX and nab-paclitaxel/gemcitabine were proven superior to gemcitabine alone in patients with metastatic pancreatic cancer, leading to improvement in response rate (RR), progression-free survival (PFS), and OS. Objective RRs have improved by nearly fivefold with these newer systemic regimens (**Table 52.5**).

With better understanding of tumor microenvironment of PDAC, future progress will likely come from combining standard chemotherapy with *KRAS* inhibitors or personalized *KRAS* vaccines.

PALLIATION

The optimal palliation of symptoms to maximize quality of life is of primary importance in most patients with advanced pancreatic cancer. Both operative and nonoperative options are available for the palliation of pancreatic cancer.

Jaundice

Obstructive jaundice can result in progressive liver dysfunction, hepatic failure, and early death. In addition, the pruritus associated with obstructive jaundice can be debilitating and usually does not respond to medication. When patients undergo exploration for possible cure and are found to have unresectable disease, a biliary bypass should be performed if patients do not have a functional metal biliary stent. Traditionally, surgeons have performed either hepaticojejunostomy or choledochojejunostomy to relieve malignant biliary obstruction.[32]

The surgical palliation of jaundice can be accomplished safely, with a mortality rate of less than 3% and an overall morbidity rate of 30% to 40%.[38] In recent years, nonoperative palliation has become available as an option for managing patients who are deemed unresectable by preop staging. Plastic or metal stents can be placed across the biliary obstruction by either an endoscopic or a percutaneous technique. For pancreatic cancer, the endoscopic approach is usually preferred with a low procedure-related morbidity. Endoscopic nonanatomic biliary drainage is another option in experienced
7 centers when ERCP cannot be performed.[39] Nonoperative palliation appears to be associated with lower complication rates, lower procedure-related mortality rates, and shorter initial periods of hospitalization compared to surgical palliation.[40,41] Therefore, nonoperative palliation should be offered to patients with advanced disease or poor performance status.

Duodenal Obstruction

At the time that pancreatic cancer is diagnosed, approximately one-third of patients have symptoms of nausea or vomiting. Although true mechanical obstruction of the duodenum seen by radiologic or endoscopic examination is much less frequent, duodenal obstruction develops in almost 20% of patients before they die as the disease progresses.[42] Duodenal obstruction can be caused in the C-loop by cancers of the head or at the ligament of Trietz by cancers of the body and tail. In patients with evidence of duodenal obstruction or impending obstruction, a gastrojejunostomy is indicated for palliation. This is typically performed as an antecolic, isoperistaltic loop gastrojejunostomy with a loop of jejunum 20 to 30 cm distal to the ligament of Trietz.

In patients with unresectable pancreatic cancer who do not have symptoms of gastric outlet obstruction, whether or not to perform a prophylactic gastric bypass at the time of biliary bypass is a matter of debate. Data from a prospective, randomized trial of prophylactic gastrojejunostomy in patients with unresectable cancer do not support this view.[43] In this study, 44 patients were randomized to a gastrojejunostomy, and 43 did not undergo gastric bypass. No mortality occurred in either group. No difference was observed in either the complication rate or the postoperative length of stay. However, late duodenal obstruction developed in 19% of the patients who did not undergo bypass. A recent multicenter prospective randomized controlled trial has confirmed these results.[44] Therefore, we believe that a prophylactic gastrojejunostomy should be performed in patients undergoing surgical palliation
8 for unresectable pancreatic carcinoma.

Table 52.5. Chemotherapy Trials in Locally Advanced and Metastatic Pancreatic Cancer

Study Group	Years	Stage	N	Treatment	Control	Endpoint	Results
LAP-07[33]	2008–2011	LA	223	Gem/Erlotinib (± CRT)	Gem (± CRT)	OS	No survival benefit adding erlotinib (11.9 vs. 13.6 mo, $P = .09$) No survival benefit with CRT (15.2 vs. 16.5 mo, $P = .83$)
NEOLAP[34]	2014–2018	LA	130	Nab-paclitaxel/ Gem	mFFX	R0 rate	No difference in R0 resection rate between gem/abraxane and mFFX (36% vs. 44%, $P = .38$)
PRODIGE 35[35]	2005–2009	M	342	mFFX	Gem	OS	Survival better with FFX (11.1 vs. 6.8 mo, $P < .001$)
MPACT[36]	2009–2012	M	861	Nab-paclitaxel/ Gem	Gem	OS	Survival better with addition of nab-paclitaxel (8.5 vs. 6.7 mo, $P < .001$)
NAPOLI3[37]	2020–2021	M	770	NALIRIFOX	Nab-paclitaxel/ Gem	OS	Median OS better with NALIRIFOX (11·1 vs. 9·2 mo, $P = .036$)

LA, locally advanced; M, metastatic.

Pain

Tumor-associated pain can be incapacitating in patients with unresectable pancreatic cancer. The postulated causes of tumor-associated pain are many and include tumor infiltration into the celiac plexus, increased parenchymal pressure caused by pancreatic duct obstruction, pancreatic inflammation, gallbladder distention resulting from biliary obstruction, and gastroduodenal obstruction. The management of pain in patients dying of carcinoma of the pancreas is one of the most important aspects of their care. The appropriate use of oral agents can be successful in most patients. Patients with significant pain should receive their medication on a regular schedule and not on an "as-needed" basis. The use of long-acting morphine derivative compounds appears to be best suited for such treatment. Percutaneous neurolytic block of the celiac axis, performed under either fluoroscopic or CT guidance, is also successful in the majority of patients at eliminating pain.[45] Patients with unresectable localized PDAC at the time of surgical exploration should receive a chemical splanchnicectomy, with 20 mL of 50% alcohol injected on either side of the aorta at the level of the celiac axis.

The decision to perform nonoperative versus surgical palliation for pancreatic cancer is influenced by several factors, including the patient's symptoms, overall health status, predicted procedure-related morbidity and mortality, and projected survival. Surgical palliation can be completed with acceptable perioperative morbidity and mortality and postoperative length of stay. The avoidance of late complications of recurrent jaundice, duodenal obstruction, and disabling pain would strengthen the argument in favor of surgical palliation in those patients expected to survive 6 months or more.[46] Nonoperative methods of palliation should be considered for patients in whom preoperative staging suggests distant metastatic disease or a locally unresectable tumor, patients who are not candidates for operative intervention, and those not expected to survive more than 3 months.[47]

References

1. 2024 ACSCFFAACS. https://www.cancer.org/cancer/types/pancreatic-cancer/detection-diagnosis-staging/survival-rates.html
2. Blackford AL, Canto MI, Dbouk M, et al. Pancreatic cancer surveillance and survival of high-risk individuals. *JAMA Oncol.* 2024;10:1087–1096.
3. Chari ST, Leibson CL, Rabe KG, Ransom J, de Andrade M, Petersen GM. Probability of pancreatic cancer following diabetes: a population based study. *Gastroenterology.* 2005;129:504–511.
4. Braxton AM, Kiemen AL, Grahn MP, et al. 3D genomic mapping reveals multifocality of human pancreatic precancers. *Nature.* 2024;629:679–687.
5. Kaiser J, Hinz U, Mayer P, et al. Clinical presentation and prognosis of adenosquamous carcinoma of the pancreas – Matched-pair analysis with pancreatic ductal adenocarcinoma. *Eur J Surg Oncol.* 2021;47:1734–1741.
6. Griffin JF, Page AJ, Samaha GJ, et al. Patients with a resected pancreatic mucinous cystic neoplasm have a better prognosis than patients with an intraductal papillary mucinous neoplasm: a large single institution series. *Pancreatology.* 2017;17:490–496.
7. He J, Cameron JL, Ahuja N, et al. Is it necessary to follow patients after resection of a benign pancreatic intraductal papillary mucinous neoplasm? *J Am Coll Surg.* 2013;216:657–665; discussion 665–657.
8. Ohtsuka T, Fernandez-Del Castillo C, Furukawa T, et al. International evidence-based Kyoto guidelines for the management of intraductal papillary mucinous neoplasm of the pancreas. *Pancreatology.* 2024;24:255–270.
9. Chun YS, Pawlik TM, Vauthey JN. 8th Edition of the AJCC Cancer Staging Manual: pancreas and hepatobiliary cancers. *Ann Surg Oncol.* 2018;25:845–847.
10. Ando Y, Dbouk M, Yoshida T, et al. Using tumor marker gene variants to improve the diagnostic accuracy of DUPAN-2 and carbohydrate antigen 19-9 for pancreatic cancer. *J Clin Oncol.* 2024;42:2196–2206.
11. Kawamoto S, Zhu Z, Chu LC, et al. Deep neural network-based segmentation of normal and abnormal pancreas on abdominal CT: evaluation of global and local accuracies. *Abdom Radiol (NY).* 2024;49:501–511.
12. Gudmundsdottir H, Yonkus JA, Alva-Ruiz R, et al. Yield of staging laparoscopy for pancreatic cancer in the modern era: analysis of more than 1,000 consecutive patients. *J Am Coll Surg.* 2023;237:49–57.
13. Stafford ES, Trimble IR, Classen JN. Results of treatment of carcinoma of pancreas. *Ann Surg.* 1954;139:800–803; discussion 803–805.
14. Hackert T, Strobel O, Michalski CW, et al. The TRIANGLE operation – radical surgery after neoadjuvant treatment for advanced pancreatic cancer: a single arm observational study. *HPB (Oxford).* 2017;19:1001–1007.
15. Kinny-Koster B, Habib JR, van Oosten F, et al. Conduits in vascular pancreatic surgery: analysis of clinical outcomes, operative techniques, and graft performance. *Ann Surg.* 2023;278:e94–e104.
16. Diener MK, Mihaljevic AL, Strobel O, et al. Periarterial divestment in pancreatic cancer surgery. *Surgery.* 2021;169:1019–1025.
17. Liu Q, Li M, Gao Y, et al. Effect of robotic versus open pancreaticoduodenectomy on postoperative length of hospital stay and complications for pancreatic head or periampullary tumours: a multicentre, open-label randomised controlled trial. *Lancet Gastroenterol Hepatol.* 2024;9:428–437.
18. Neoptolemos JP, Dunn JA, Stocken DD, et al. Adjuvant chemoradiotherapy and chemotherapy in resectable pancreatic cancer: a randomised controlled trial. *Lancet.* 2001;358:1576–1585.
19. Oettle H, Neuhaus P, Hochhaus A, et al. Adjuvant chemotherapy with gemcitabine and long-term outcomes among patients with resected pancreatic cancer: the CONKO-001 randomized trial. *JAMA.* 2013;310:1473–1481.
20. Conroy T, Hammel P, Hebbar M, et al. FOLFIRINOX or gemcitabine as adjuvant therapy for pancreatic cancer. *N Engl J Med.* 2018;379:2395–2406.
21. Neoptolemos JP, Moore MJ, Cox TF, et al. Effect of adjuvant chemotherapy with fluorouracil plus folinic acid or gemcitabine vs observation on survival in patients with resected periampullary adenocarcinoma: the ESPAC-3 periampullary cancer randomized trial. *JAMA.* 2012;308:147–156.
22. Uesaka K, Boku N, Fukutomi A, et al. Adjuvant chemotherapy of S-1 versus gemcitabine for resected pancreatic cancer: a phase 3, open-label, randomised, non-inferiority trial (JASPAC 01). *Lancet.* 2016;388:248–257.
23. Neoptolemos JP, Palmer DH, Ghaneh P, et al. Comparison of adjuvant gemcitabine and capecitabine with gemcitabine monotherapy in patients with resected pancreatic cancer (ESPAC-4): a multicentre, open-label, randomised, phase 3 trial. *Lancet.* 2017;389:1011–1024.
24. Conroy T, Castan F, Lopez A, et al. Five-year outcomes of FOLFIRINOX vs gemcitabine as adjuvant therapy for pancreatic cancer: a randomized clinical trial. *JAMA Oncol.* 2022;8:1571–1578.
25. Tempero MA, Pelzer U, O'Reilly EM, et al. Adjuvant nab-paclitaxel + gemcitabine in resected pancreatic ductal adenocarcinoma: results from a randomized, open-label, phase III trial. *J Clin Oncol.* 2023;41:2007–2019.
26. Labori KJ, Bratlie SO, Andersson B, et al. Neoadjuvant FOLFIRINOX versus upfront surgery for resectable pancreatic head cancer (NORPACT-1): a multicentre, randomised, phase 2 trial. *Lancet Gastroenterol Hepatol.* 2024;9:205–217.
27. Versteijne E, van Dam JL, Suker M, et al. Neoadjuvant chemoradiotherapy versus upfront surgery for resectable and borderline resectable pancreatic cancer: long-term results of the Dutch randomized PREOPANC trial. *J Clin Oncol.* 2022;40:1220–1230.
28. Jang JY, Han Y, Lee H, et al. Oncological benefits of neoadjuvant chemoradiation with gemcitabine versus upfront surgery in patients with borderline resectable pancreatic cancer: a prospective, randomized, open-label, multicenter phase 2/3 trial. *Ann Surg.* 2018;268:215–222.
29. Ghaneh P, Palmer D, Cicconi S, et al. Immediate surgery compared with short-course neoadjuvant gemcitabine plus capecitabine, FOLFIRINOX, or chemoradiotherapy in patients with borderline resectable pancreatic cancer (ESPAC5): a four-arm,

multicentre, randomised, phase 2 trial. *Lancet Gastroenterol Hepatol*. 2023;8:157–168.

30. Versteijne E, Suker M, Groothuis K, et al. Preoperative chemoradiotherapy versus immediate surgery for resectable and borderline resectable pancreatic cancer: results of the Dutch randomized phase III PREOPANC trial. *J Clin Oncol*. 2020;38:1763–1773.
31. Katz MHG, Shi Q, Meyers J, et al. Efficacy of preoperative mFOLFIRINOX vs mFOLFIRINOX plus hypofractionated radiotherapy for borderline resectable adenocarcinoma of the pancreas: the A021501 phase 2 randomized clinical trial. *JAMA Oncol*. 2022;8:1263–1270.
32. Arshad SA, Phuoc VH. Surgical palliation of biliary obstruction: bypass in the era of drainage. *J Surg Oncol*. 2019;120:65–66.
33. Hammel P, Huguet F, van Laethem JL, et al. Effect of chemoradiotherapy vs chemotherapy on survival in patients with locally advanced pancreatic cancer controlled after 4 months of gemcitabine with or without erlotinib: the LAP07 randomized clinical trial. *JAMA*. 2016;315:1844–1853.
34. Kunzmann V, Siveke JT, Algul H, et al. Nab-paclitaxel plus gemcitabine versus nab-paclitaxel plus gemcitabine followed by FOLFIRINOX induction chemotherapy in locally advanced pancreatic cancer (NEOLAP-AIO-PAK-0113): a multicentre, randomised, phase 2 trial. *Lancet Gastroenterol Hepatol*. 2021;6:128–138.
35. Dahan L, Williet N, Le Malicot K, et al. Randomized phase II trial evaluating two sequential treatments in first line of metastatic pancreatic cancer: results of the PANOPTIMOX-PRODIGE 35 trial. *J Clin Oncol*. 2021;39:3242–3250.
36. Philip PA, Lacy J, Portales F, et al. Nab-paclitaxel plus gemcitabine in patients with locally advanced pancreatic cancer (LAPACT): a multicentre, open-label phase 2 study. *Lancet Gastroenterol Hepatol*. 2020;5:285–294.
37. Wainberg ZA, Melisi D, Macarulla T, et al. NALIRIFOX versus nab-paclitaxel and gemcitabine in treatment-naive patients with metastatic pancreatic ductal adenocarcinoma (NAPOLI 3): a randomised, open-label, phase 3 trial. *Lancet*. 2023;402:1272–1281.
38. Eisenberg I, Gaidhane M, Kahaleh M, Tyberg A. Drainage approach for malignant biliary obstruction: a changing paradigm. *J Clin Gastroenterol*. 2023;57:546–552.
39. Giri S, Seth V, Afzalpurkar S, et al. Endoscopic ultrasound-guided versus percutaneous transhepatic biliary drainage after failed ERCP: a systematic review and meta-analysis. *Surg Laparosc Endosc Percutan Tech*. 2023;33:411–419.
40. Scheufele F, Schorn S, Demir IE, et al. Preoperative biliary stenting versus operation first in jaundiced patients due to malignant lesions in the pancreatic head: a meta-analysis of current literature. *Surgery*. 2017;161:939–950.
41. Moss AC, Morris E, Leyden J, MacMathuna P. Malignant distal biliary obstruction: a systematic review and meta-analysis of endoscopic and surgical bypass results. *Cancer Treat Rev*. 2007;33:213–221.
42. Perinel J, Adham M. Palliative therapy in pancreatic cancer-palliative surgery. *Transl Gastroenterol Hepatol*. 2019;4:28.
43. Lillemoe KD, Cameron JL, Hardacre JM, et al. Is prophylactic gastrojejunostomy indicated for unresectable periampullary cancer? A prospective randomized trial. *Ann Surg*. 1999;230:322–328; discussion 328–330.
44. Van Heek NT, De Castro SM, van Eijck CH, et al. The need for a prophylactic gastrojejunostomy for unresectable periampullary cancer: a prospective randomized multicenter trial with special focus on assessment of quality of life. *Ann Surg*. 2003;238:894–902; discussion 902–895.
45. Nagels W, Pease N, Bekkering G, Cools F, Dobbels P. Celiac plexus neurolysis for abdominal cancer pain: a systematic review. *Pain Med*. 2013;14:1140–1163.
46. Committee ASoP, Jue TL, Storm AC, et al. ASGE guideline on the role of endoscopy in the management of benign and malignant gastroduodenal obstruction. *Gastrointest Endosc*. 2021;93:309–322e304.
47. Canakis A, Irani SS. Endoscopic treatment of gastric outlet obstruction. *Gastrointest Endosc Clin N Am*. 2024;34:111–125.

53

Neoplasms of the Endocrine Pancreas

Jordan M. Cloyd and George A. Poultsides

Key Points

1 Pancreatic endocrine neoplasms (PENs) are heterogeneous tumors arising from pancreatic islet cells. While still relatively uncommon, they are diagnosed with increasing incidence worldwide.

2 Consistent with other neuroendocrine neoplasms, the World Health Organization uses the combination of a proliferative index (Ki-67), mitotic rate, and morphologic features (degree of differentiation) to classify PENs as well-differentiated neuroendocrine tumors (NETs) of low (G1), intermediate (G2), or high (G3) grade or poorly differentiated neuroendocrine carcinomas (NECs).

3 PENs can be classified as either nonfunctional or functional based on their ability to secrete hormones characteristic of well-recognized clinical syndromes. While most PENs are sporadic, some may occur as part of inherited syndromes.

4 The best initial imaging technique for a PEN is a high-quality contrast-enhanced multiphasic computed tomography (CT) scan. NET-specific positron emission tomography (PET) (eg, ^{68}Ga-DOTATATE) scans provide important diagnostic and staging information for well-differentiated tumors while FDG-PET is indicated for poorly differentiated carcinomas.

5 Most localized well-differentiated PENs exhibit an indolent course, and size is an important factor that guides treatment. Asymptomatic nonfunctional PENs <1 to 2 cm may undergo active surveillance, whereas surgical resection is generally recommended for tumors >2 cm.

6 Insulinomas may present with either neuroglycopenic and/or other hypoglycemic-induced symptoms, 90% being solitary, 90% sporadic, and 90% benign, with their location evenly distributed throughout the pancreas. Ten percent are familial, typically associated with multiple endocrine neoplasia type 1 (MEN-1) syndrome, and commonly multifocal in the pancreas.

7 Most gastrinomas are located in the gastrinoma triangle. Most (75%) are sporadic, while 25% are associated with MEN-1 syndrome. They typically have malignant behavior including locally invasive growth and metastatic spread.

8 The liver is the most common site of distant metastasis for PENs. Cytoreductive surgery for neuroendocrine liver metastases is recommended when feasible. Liver-directed therapies including transarterial embolization or ablation may be considered for patients with hepatic metastases that are not amenable to resection.

9 Numerous systemic therapies exist for patients with metastatic PENs including somatostatin analogs, traditional chemotherapy such as temozolomide and capecitabine, targeted therapies such as everolimus or sunitinib, and peptide receptor radionuclide therapy (PRRT).

EPIDEMIOLOGY

Pancreatic endocrine neoplasms (PENs) are relatively rare tumors that account for 3% of pancreatic neoplasms and 7% of all neuroendocrine tumors (NETs).[1] Their incidence is steadily increasing largely due to the increased use of cross-sectional imaging, availability of endoscopic ultrasonography (EUS), and improved awareness among pathologists and clinicians.[2]
1 PENs were first described by Nicholls in 1902 as a tumor arising from pancreatic islet cells. These "islet cell adenomas" were long thought to arise from the islets of Langerhans, although currently it is felt that PENs more likely originate from multipotent stem cells in pancreatic ductules. As a result, the older terms *islet cell tumor* and *islet cell carcinoma* have largely been replaced by the accepted terms *PENs, pancreatic NETs, pancreatic neuroendocrine neoplasms,* or *pancreatic endocrine tumors*

CLASSIFICATION

Traditionally, PENs were classified according to their size and the mitotic rate of the tumor. This system placed PENs into one of three categories: pancreatic endocrine microadenomas, well-differentiated PENs, and poorly differentiated or high-grade endocrine carcinomas. PENs less than 0.5 cm in diameter were classified as pancreatic endocrine microadenomas. Oncologically, they are considered to be benign lesions. Their prevalence is estimated to be as high as 10% of the population in autopsy series·

In 2017, the World Health Organization (WHO) updated their classification of PENs into well-differentiated NETs and poorly differentiated neuroendocrine carcinomas (NECs) based on tumor morphology with further stratification based
2 on tumor grade as measured by the Ki-67 proliferation index and mitotic rate (**Table 53.1**).[3] While well-differentiated neuroendocrine tumors may be classified as either low (G1), intermediate (G2), or high grade (G3), by definition all NECs are high grade (G3). By convention, the tumor is assigned the higher grade if the Ki-67 index and mitotic rate differ.

Well-differentiated PENs can also be classified as **functional** or **nonfunctional** based on the presence or absence of a clinically recognizable syndrome (**Table 53.2**). Functional PENs are less common than nonfunctional tumors. Functional

Table 53.1. 2017 World Health Organization Classification of Pancreatic Neuroendocrine Neoplasms

	Ki67 Index	Mitotic Index
Well-Differentiated NENs		
G1 NET	<3%	<2/10 HPF
G2 NET	3–20%	2–20/10 HPF
G3 NET	>20%	>20/10 HPF
Poorly Differentiated NENs		
NEC G3	>20%	>20/10 HPF
Small Cell Type		
Large Cell Type		

NEN, neuroendocrine neoplasm; NET, neuroendocrine tumor; NEC, neuroendocrine carcinoma; HPF, high-power fields.

syndromes are the result of the secretion of biologically active hormones by the tumors and are confirmed by measurable elevations of the hormones in the blood. The most common functional PENs include insulinomas, gastrinomas, vasoactive intestinal polypeptide-omas (VIPomas), glucagonomas, and somatostatinomas. The incidence of these lesions ranges from 1 per 1 million for insulinomas to 1 per 40 million for somatostatinomas. Even less common PENs secreting calcitonin, parathyroid hormone–related protein, growth hormone–releasing factor, and adrenocorticotropic hormone have been reported. Nonfunctional PENs are classified as such due to their lack of an associated clinical syndrome, although many secrete elevated amounts of hormones, such as chromogranin A or pancreatic polypeptide.

3

MOLECULAR GENETICS

Whole-Exome Sequencing of PENs

In 2011, a seminal whole-exome sequencing study of 68 sporadic PENs[4] identified frequent somatic mutations in *MEN-1* as well as the chromatin-remodeling complex, *DAXX* (death-domain–associated protein) and *ATRX* (alpha thalassemia/mental retardation syndrome X linked). A subset of samples had mutations in genes involved in the mammalian target of rapamycin (mTOR) pathway including phosphatase and tensin homolog (PTEN), tuberous sclerosis complex 2 (TSC2), and phosphatidylinositol-4,5-bisphosphate 3-kinase, catalytic subunit α (PIK3CA). Other studies have correlated *DAXX* and *ATRX* mutations, activation of alternative lengthening of telomeres, and global chromosomal alterations with pathologic features and outcomes. A more recent whole-exome sequencing of 102 PENs samples has clarified four distinct signaling pathways in which somatic mutations were commonly found: (1) chromatin remodeling, (2) DNA damage repair, (3) mTOR signaling, and (4) telomere maintenance.[5]

Familial Syndromes

The majority of PENs are sporadic. Some of them, however, occur as part of inherited familial syndromes such as MEN-1, von Hippel–Lindau (VHL) syndrome, neurofibromatosis (NF-1), and tuberous sclerosis (TS) (**Table 53.3**).

MEN-1 is an autosomal dominant disorder caused by germline mutations in the tumor suppressor gene *MEN-1*. Although more than 20 endocrine tumors have been associated with MEN-1 syndrome, the most common include tumors of the parathyroid, anterior pituitary, and endocrine pancreas.

Less frequently than MEN-1, PENs may be associated with **VHL** syndrome. VHL syndrome is another autosomal dominant inheritance disease that includes many clinical disorders, including retinal hemangioblastomas, cerebellar and medullary hemangioblastomas, and PENs. PENs are found in a small percentage of patients with VHL syndrome, although pancreatic cysts are commonly encountered.

NF-1 (von Recklinghausen disease) is an autosomal dominant disorder that produces a well-described clinical syndrome characterized by café-au-lait spots and neurofibromas. These patients may develop pancreatic somatostatinomas, often near the ampulla of Vater. The NF-1 gene is a tumor suppressor gene located on 17q11.2 that encodes for neurofibromin, a regulator of the mTOR pathway.

TS is a rare autosomal dominant disorder associated with mutations in *TSC1* or *TSC2,* which encode the protein tuberin. It is a neurocutaneous disorder associated with characteristic skin lesions, central nervous lesions including hamartomas, and rarely PENs. Note that patients may also develop pancreatic angiomyolipomas.

DIAGNOSTIC EVALUATION

Presentation

Patients with PENs can present in several distinct ways: (1) the incidental discovery of a mass in the pancreas during cross-sectional imaging, (2) symptoms secondary to the mass effect of a lesion in the pancreas (ie, obstructive jaundice or pain), or (3) symptoms related to hormone production from a functional PEN.

Biochemical

If a nonfunctional PEN is suspected, baseline serum levels of chromogranin A and pancreatic polypeptide should be measured prior to surgical resection as these markers can be used

Table 53.2. Classification of Functional Pancreatic Endocrine Tumors

Tumor (Syndrome)	Clinical Features	Extrapancreatic Location	Malignancy Rate
Insulinoma	Hypoglycemia	Rare	10%
Gastrinoma (Zollinger–Ellison)	Peptic ulcer Diarrhea	Frequent	50%
VIPoma (Verner–Morrison; WDHA; Pancreatic Cholera)	Watery diarrhea hypokalemia achlorhydria/acidosis	10%	Most
Glucagonoma	Hyperglycemia Dermatitis	Rare	Most
Somatostatinoma	Hyperglycemia Steatorrhea Gallstones	Rare	Most

WDHA, watery diarrhea, hypokalemia, and either achlorhydria or acidosis.

Table 53.3. Familial Genetic Syndromes Associated with Pancreatic Endocrine Neoplasms

Syndrome	Chromosomal Location	Gene Product	PEN Type
MEN-1	11q13	Menin	Gastrinoma Nonfunctional
VHL	3p25-26	VHL	Various
NF-1	17q11.2	Neurofibromin	Somatostatinoma
TS	9q34 (TSC1) 16p13.3 (TSC2)	Tuberin	Various

MEN-1, multiple endocrine neoplasia 1; VHL, von Hippel–Lindau; NF, neurofibromatosis; TS, tuberous sclerosis; TSC, tuberous sclerosis complex.

during surveillance. Neuron-specific enolase is another tumor marker that is elevated in approximately 50% of PENs, most commonly in patients with pulmonary metastases. For those in whom a functional PEN is suspected, confirmatory testing of the relevant serum hormone should be performed. Assays are readily available for measuring insulin, gastrin, VIP, and glucagon. Assays for somatostatin, pancreatic polypeptide (PP), prostaglandins, and other hormonal markers are less commonly available but can be obtained from certain laboratories. Genetic testing may be indicated for those in whom a clinical syndrome is suspected, both for diagnostic confirmation but also to guide subsequent personal and family screening.

Computed Tomography

Cross-sectional imaging with thin-cut multiphasic computed tomography (CT) or magnetic resonance imaging (MRI) is typically indicated for all patients with confirmed or suspected PENs. The accuracy of CT in detecting primary PENs ranges from 64% to 82% and depends largely on the size of the tumor.[6] PENs are typically hyperdense on arterial phases of imaging. Lesions that are obvious during the early arterial phase can
4 become isodense on later phases of imaging. Therefore, a multiphase approach is typically recommended. CT is useful in assessing size and location of the primary tumor, proximity to visceral vessels, peripancreatic lymph node involvement, and the presence or absence of liver metastases (**Fig. 53.1**).

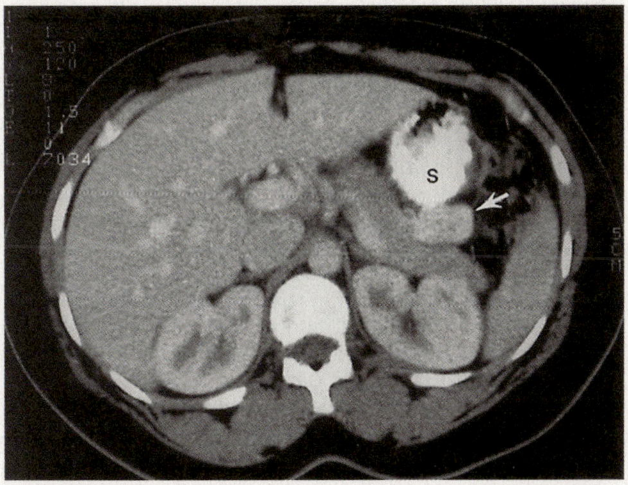

Figure 53.1. Computed tomography with oral and intravenous contrast in a patient with biochemical evidence of insulinoma. The neoplasm (*arrow*) is seen as a contrast-enhancing structure, 3 cm in diameter, in the tail of the pancreas posterior to the stomach (S). (From Yeo CJ. Islet cell tumors of the pancreas. In: Niederhuber JE, ed. *Current Therapy in Oncology*. Mosby; 1993:272, with permission.)

Magnetic Resonance Imaging

MRI is increasingly used in the detection of PENs, particularly small lesions. They are especially well visualized on T1- and T2-weighted images with fat suppression. MRI has the advantage of increased soft tissue contrast without the administration of intravenous contrast when compared to CT. PENs characteristically have high signal intensity on T2-weighted images. On dynamic contrast-enhanced T1-weighted images, the tumors show the same typical enhancement pattern as on CT scan. The sensitivity of MRI has been reported to be between 74% and 100%.[6] MRI is particularly useful to evaluate for neuroendocrine liver metastases.

Somatostatin Receptor Scintigraphy

Somatostatin receptor scintigraphy (SRS) also plays an important role in imaging patients with PENs given that over 90% of NETs express somatostatin receptors. Traditionally, the octapeptide analog of somatostatin (octreotide) labeled with indium-111 (known as Octreoscan) was the standard method of staging and characterizing NETs (**Fig. 53.2**).

This imaging modality has been largely replaced by positron emission tomography (PET)–based techniques. The most common used today is gallium Ga-68 DOTATATE which

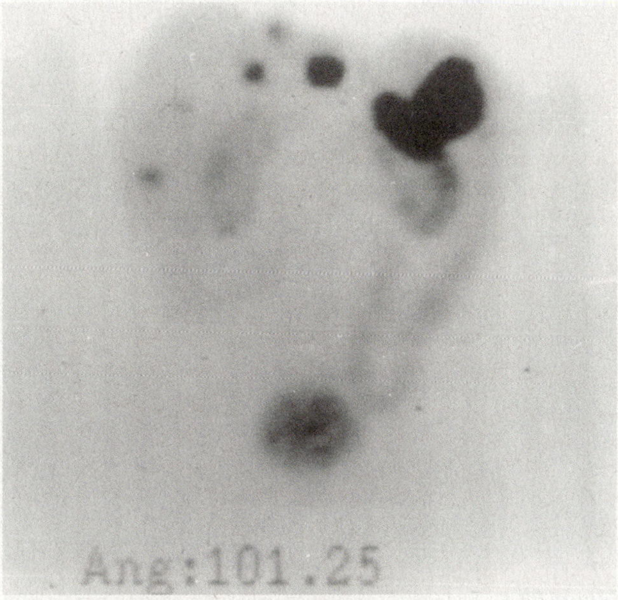

Figure 53.2. Octreotide scan (*anterior view*) in a patient with a large endocrine tumor in the tail of the pancreas (large dark mass, upper right) and several hepatic metastases (upper left quadrant). A small amount of the tracer is seen in the bladder (lower midline).

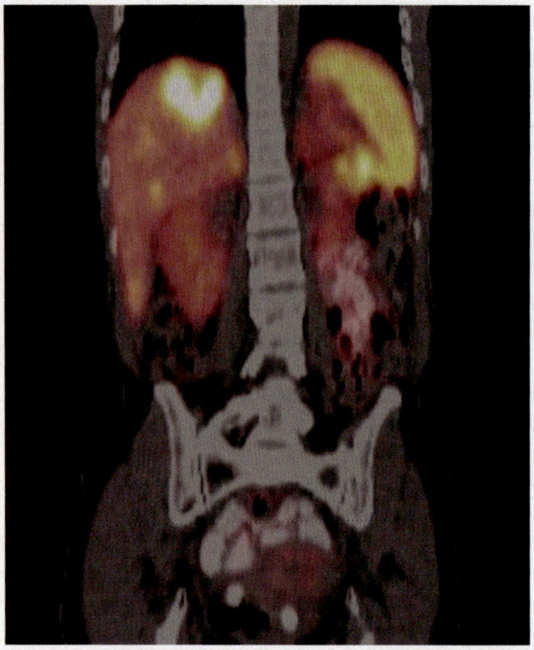

Figure 53.3. Gallium 68 dotatate PET/CT scan of a patient with a pancreatic endocrine tumor with several bulky hepatic metastases.

was approved by the FDA in 2016 and offers several benefits compared to traditional Octreoscan including improved sensitivity, less radiation, and enhanced convenience given the shorter scanning time required (**Fig. 53.3**). This method of SRS utilizes 3D PET fused with contrast-enhanced CT to provide improved spatial resolution and better sensitivity. In one seminal prospective study, the addition of Ga-68 DOTATATE to CT/MRI and Octreoscan led to a clinically significant change in management among 33% of the patients.[7]

Consensus guidelines generating appropriate use criteria have suggested that SRS-PET should replace in-pentetreotide scintigraphy for essentially all indications in which the latter was previously being used.[8]

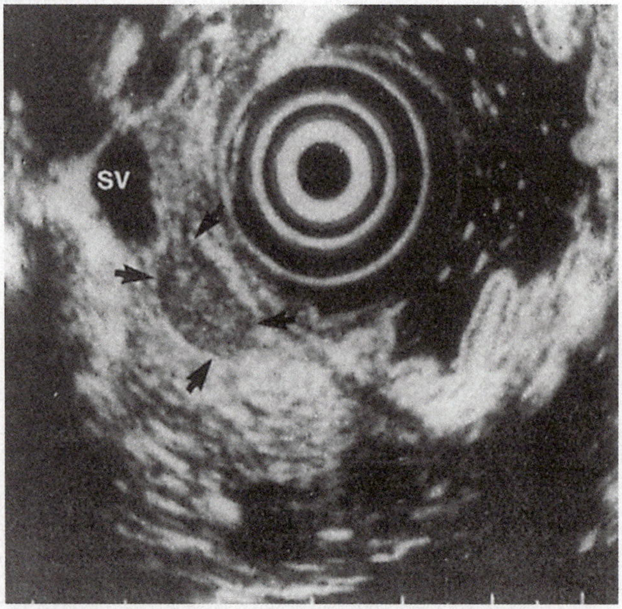

Figure 53.4. Endoscopic ultrasonographic image from a patient with an insulinoma (*arrows*) in the body of the pancreas. SV, splenic vein. (From Rösch T, Lightdale CJ, Botet JF, et al. Localization of pancreatic endocrine tumors by endoscopic ultrasonography. *N Engl J Med*. 1992;326(26):1721–1726, with permission.)

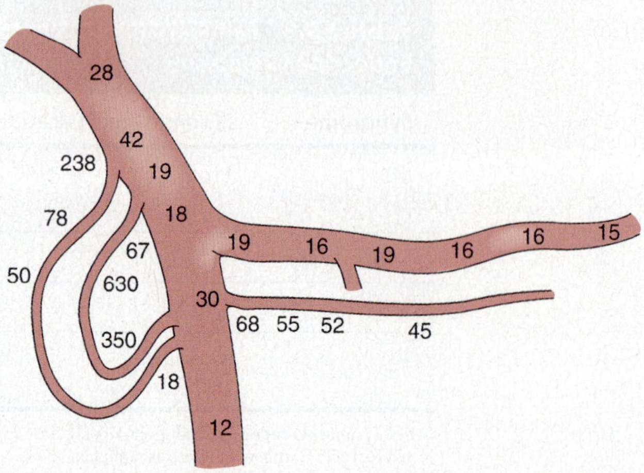

Figure 53.5. Schematic depiction of data from percutaneous transhepatic portal venous sampling (PTPVS) in a patient with an insulinoma. Insulin levels are given in microunits per milliliter. These data localize the neoplasm to the head of the pancreas. (Adapted from Norton JA, Sigel B, Baker AR, et al. Localization of an occult insulinoma by intraoperative ultrasonography. *Surgery*. 1985;97:381–384.)

Endoscopic Ultrasound

EUS is an important adjunct in the evaluation and localization of PENs. EUS provides detailed information about pancreatic neoplasms (eg, size, location, adjacency to structures), as well as the ability to perform fine needle aspiration and biopsy. EUS may also be used to localize a functional PEN after biochemical testing is suggestive of a hormonal abnormality consistent with functional syndrome (eg, gastrinoma). Proye et al.[9] evaluated preoperative EUS and SRS in 41 patients with insulinoma and gastrinoma. The sensitivity and positive predictive value of EUS were 77% and 94%, respectively, for pancreatic tumors; 40% and 100%, respectively, for duodenal gastrinomas; and 58% and 78%, respectively, for metastatic lymph nodes (**Fig. 53.4**).

Venous Sampling

Percutaneous transhepatic portal venous sampling (PTPVS) and arterial stimulation with venous sampling (ASVS) are two techniques that are rarely used today but can be helpful in localizing functional PENs when CT, MRI, SRS, and EUS are unsuccessful. Specifically, when insulinoma or gastrinoma are suspected, PTPVS may help in localizing the occult neoplasm. The technique involves placing a catheter percutaneously through the liver into the portal vein and then sequentially sampling for hormone levels in the splenic vein, superior mesenteric vein, and portal vein, thereby regionalizing the location of hormone production (**Fig. 53.5**). ASVS involves the selective visceral arterial injection of secretin or calcium with concurrent hepatic venous sampling for either gastrin or insulin. Gastrinoma cells are known to respond to secretin by releasing gastrin, and insulinoma cells are known to respond to calcium by releasing insulin. The provocative secretogogue is serially injected through an arterial catheter into at least three sites—the splenic, gastroduodenal, and inferior pancreaticoduodenal arteries. Samples are drawn from a hepatic vein catheter before and immediately after each injection. The arterial supply to the occult tumor can then be deduced based on which selective secretogogue injection is followed by a large increase in hepatic vein hormone concentration (**Fig. 53.6**).

SURGICAL EXPLORATION

Surgical exploration without preoperative tumor localization was historically described for patients with an occult but suspected functional PEN based on biochemical work-up (eg, insulinoma) but with modern diagnostic tools is now rarely needed.

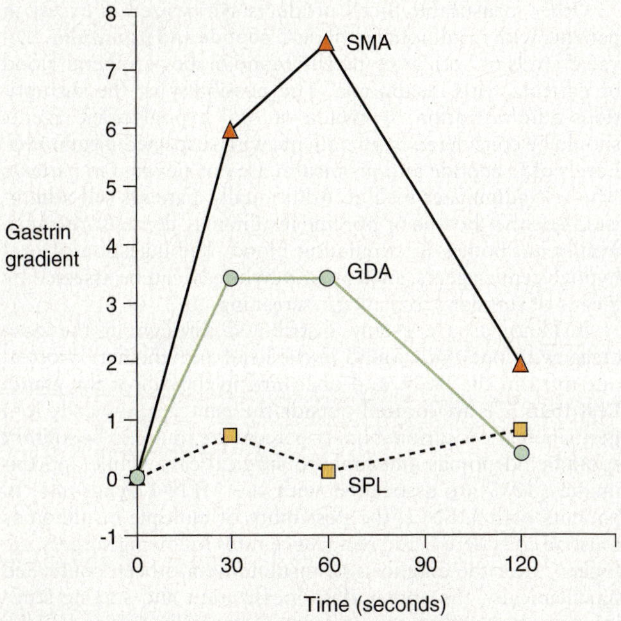

Figure 53.6. Graphic depiction of the results of arterial stimulation with venous sampling (ASVS) in a patient with gastrinoma.The rise in hepatic vein gastrin concentration (gastrin gradient) is plotted on the y-axis, and basal values are plotted on the x-axis: 1, 100% rise; 2, 200% rise; and so forth. A rise in the hepatic vein gastrin concentration observed after the injection of secretin into the superior mesenteric artery (SMA) and gastroduodenal artery (GDA) localizes the neoplasm to the head of the pancreas or duodenum. SPL, splenic artery. (Adapted from Thom AK, Norton JA, Doppman JL, et al. Prospective study of the use of intra-arterial secretin injection and portal venous sampling to localize duodenal gastrinomas. *Surgery*. 1992;112:1002–1028; discussion 1008–1009.)

Regardless, when surgical exploration for PEN is indicated, a complete evaluation of the pancreas and peripancreatic regions is performed. The body and tail of the pancreas are exposed by dividing the gastrocolic ligament and entering the lesser sac. This portion of the pancreas can be partially elevated out of the retroperitoneum by dividing the inferior retroperitoneal attachments to the gland. After the second portion of the duodenum has been elevated out of the retroperitoneum by means of the Kocher maneuver, the pancreatic head and uncinate process are palpated bimanually. The liver is carefully assessed for evidence of metastatic disease. Intraoperative pancreatic and hepatic ultrasound can be helpful in identifying occult primaries or metastatic disease with sensitivities reported between 75% and 90%.

NONFUNCTIONAL PANCREATIC ENDOCRINE NEOPLASMS

Surgical Resection

Well-differentiated nonfunctional PENs are clinically heterogeneous with some exhibiting indolent behavior while others have a more aggressive course with strong predilection for lymph node and distant metastases. Overall, the 5-year survival rate for PENs after resection remains only 65%, with a 10-year survival of 45%.[10] Size is an important determinant of outcome
5 and can be used to guide surgical decision making. PENs <1 cm typically have low malignant potential and can be safely observed, while PENs >2 cm have higher risks for lymph node and hepatic metastases that warrant resection. PENs between 1 and 2 cm are controversial and require individualized decision making regarding resection or observation.[11] Preliminary results of the ASPEN trial, a multicenter nonrandomized prospective study, found that an initial strategy of active surveillance was safe and effective for most patients with asymptomatic nonfunctional PENs <2 cm in size.[12]

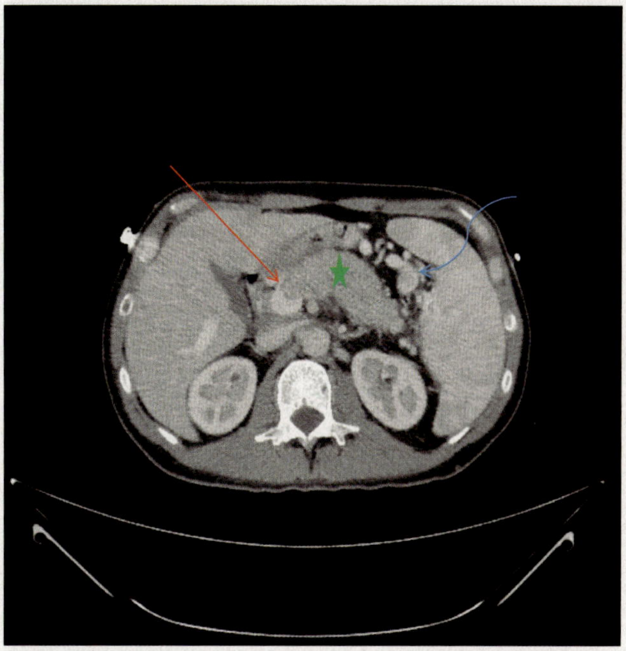

Figure 53.7. Computed tomography of a patient with a large PEN (*green star*) replacing the pancreatic body and tail, with splenic vein occlusion, perigastric varices (*blue arrow*), and tumor thrombus (*red arrow*) growing into the portal vein. This patient underwent a distal pancreatectomy, splenectomy, and partial portal vein resection with tumor thrombectomy, with complete surgical extirpation of the malignancy.

In general, when surgical resection is pursued, formal resection via either pancreaticoduodenectomy or distal pancreatectomy, depending on tumor location, is recommended. Pancreatic enucleation may be appropriate for patients with small tumors in which the lesion is far from the pancreatic duct to minimize the risks of pancreatic fistula.[13] Central pancreatectomy may be a consideration for pancreatic neck and proximal body tumors that are not amenable to enucleation in order to preserve exocrine and endocrine function.[14] Increasingly, experienced surgeons are utilizing a minimally invasive approach for patients with PENs. Both laparoscopic and robotic pancreatectomy are now performed on a routine basis with good results.[15] Patients with locally advanced disease involving the mesenteric vasculature may be candidates for radical mesenteric vascular resection (**Fig. 53.7**) or can be treated with neoadjuvant therapies in an attempt to downstage to resectability. Following resection of PENs, there is no established role for adjuvant therapy, and routine surveillance is recommended for 5 to 10 years.

Lymphadenectomy

The role of lymphadenectomy for PENs remains controversial. PENs frequently metastasize to regional lymph nodes and therefore a lymph node dissection at the time of surgical resection provides important prognostic information as well as local disease control. The rate of lymph node involvement also correlates with tumor size.[16] While consensus guidelines are lacking, most recommend performing a regional lymphadenectomy at the time of resection for most PENs.[17–19]

INSULINOMA

6 Insulinoma is the most common functional neoplasm of the endocrine pancreas (**Table 53.4**). Patients typically present with the following features, known as **Whipple triad:**

1. Symptoms of hypoglycemia during fasting
2. Documentation of hypoglycemia, with a serum glucose level typically below 50 mg/dL
3. Relief of hypoglycemic symptoms following administration of exogenous glucose

Table 53.4. Insulinoma

Parameter	Description
Symptoms	Neuroglycopenia causes confusion, personality change, coma Catecholamine surge causes trembling, diaphoresis, tachycardia Anabolic state: weight gain
Diagnostic tests	Monitored fast Insulin-to-glucose ratio
Anatomic localization	Evenly distributed throughout pancreas

Autonomous insulin secretion in insulinomas leads to spontaneous hypoglycemia, with symptoms that can be classified into two groups. Neuroglycopenic symptoms include confusion, seizure, obtundation, personality change, and coma. Hypoglycemia-induced symptoms, related to a surge in catecholamine levels, include palpitations, trembling, diaphoresis, and tachycardia. In most cases, patients consume carbohydrate-rich meals and snacks to relieve or prevent these symptoms and typically gain weight.

Insulinoma is most reliably diagnosed by means of a **monitored fast** (via the withholding of exogenous glucose). During a monitored fast, blood is sampled for glucose and insulin determinations every 4 to 6 hours and when symptoms appear. Hypoglycemic symptoms typically occur when glucose levels are below 50 mg/dL, with concurrent serum insulin levels often exceeding 25 microunits/mL. Additional support for the diagnosis of insulinoma comes from the calculation of the insulin-to-glucose ratio at different times during the monitored fast. Healthy individuals have insulin-to-glucose ratios below 0.3, whereas patients with insulinoma typically demonstrate insulin-to-glucose ratios above 0.4 after a prolonged fast.

Other measurable β-cell products synthesized in excess in patients with insulinoma include **C peptide** and **proinsulin.** Elevated levels of both are typically found in the peripheral blood of patients with insulinoma. The possibility of the surreptitious administration of insulin or oral hypoglycemic agents should be considered in all patients with suspected insulinoma. Levels of C peptide and proinsulin are not elevated in patients who self-administer insulin. Additionally, patients self-administering either bovine or porcine insulin may demonstrate anti-insulin antibodies in circulating blood. The ingestion of oral hypoglycemic agents, such as sulfonylureas, can be assessed by means of standard toxicologic screening.

Insulinomas are evenly distributed throughout the pancreas, with one-third found in the head and uncinate process, one-third in the body, and one-third in the tail of the gland. Less than 3% are located outside the pancreas, typically in a peripancreatic location. Ninety percent are found to be solitary **sporadic** adenomas amenable to surgical cure, while approximately 10% are associated with the **MEN-1 syndrome.** In patients with MEN-1, the possibility of multiple insulinomas must be considered, and recurrence rates following surgery are higher. After the diagnosis of insulinoma has been confirmed biochemically, the appropriate localization and staging studies described earlier are performed (typically CT and EUS). Once the lesion has been localized, surgical resection is recommended. As the risk of lymph node metastases is minimal, small tumors that are not close to the main pancreatic duct can be removed by enucleation (**Fig. 53.8**). Larger tumors in the neck or proximal body may be resected via central pancreatectomy. In the body and tail of the pancreas, insulinomas more than 2 cm in diameter and those close to the pancreatic duct are most commonly removed via distal pancreatectomy. Large lesions in the head or uncinate process of the gland may not be amenable to local resection and may occasionally require pancreaticoduodenectomy for complete excision.

Approximately 10% of insulinomas are malignant, presenting with lymph node or liver metastases. In the presence of hepatic metastases, resection of the primary tumor and

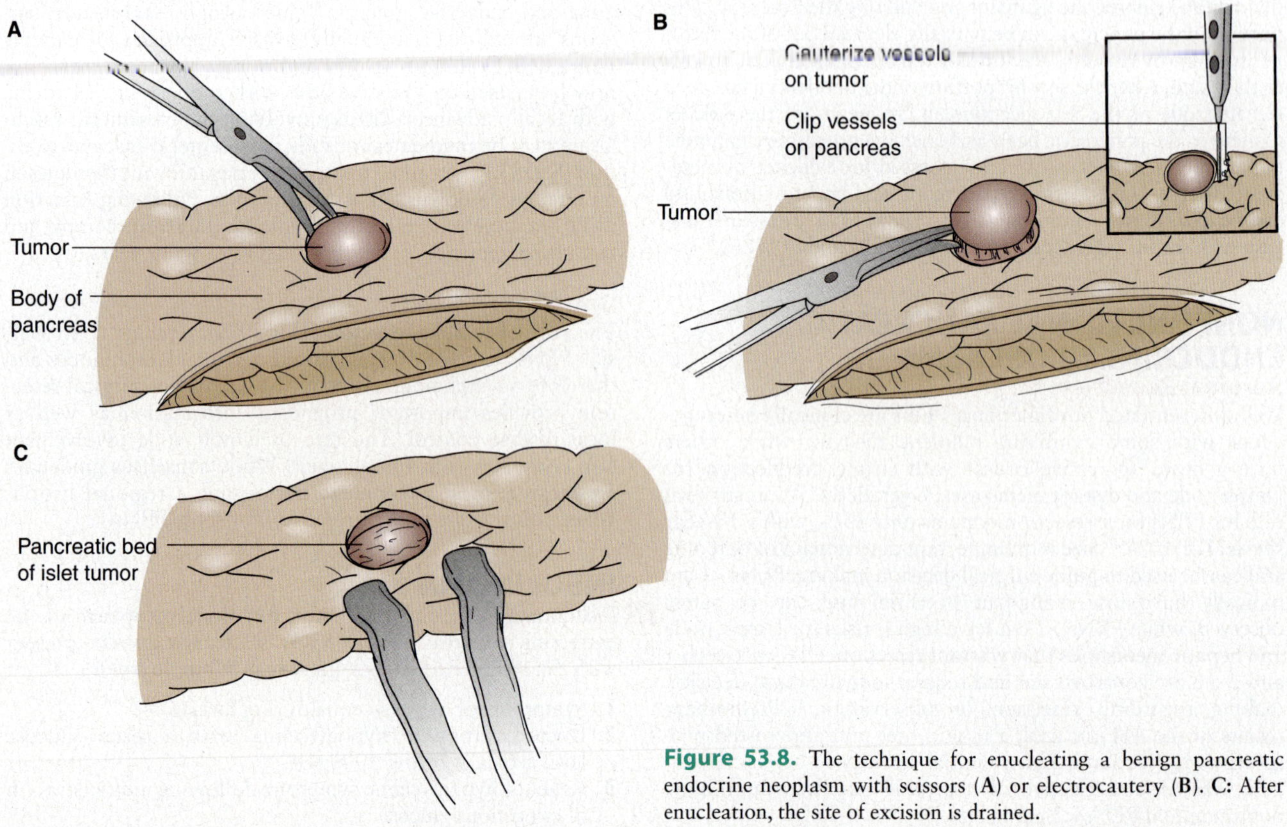

Figure 53.8. The technique for enucleating a benign pancreatic endocrine neoplasm with scissors (A) or electrocautery (B). C: After enucleation, the site of excision is drained.

Table 53.5. Gastrinoma

Parameter	Description
Symptoms	Peptic ulcer disease Diarrhea Esophagitis
Diagnostic tests	Serum gastrin measurement Gastric acid analysis (or pH testing) Secretin stimulation test
Anatomic localization	Duodenum and head of pancreas (gastrinoma triangle)

metastases should be considered to reduce hypoglycemic symptoms and improve long-term survival. In patients with unresectable disease, medications such as diazoxide and octreotide can be used to reduce insulin secretion from the tumor, minimizing hypoglycemia. Furthermore, the mTOR inhibitor everolimus, in addition to its antiproliferative effects, may improve glycemic control for patients with metastatic insulinoma. Dietary manipulations, including judicious spacing of carbohydrate-rich meals and the consumption of night-time snacks, can also reduce the number of hypoglycemic episodes. Multiple chemotherapeutic regimens have been used including streptozocin, dacarbazine, doxorubicin, and 5-fluorouracil. Combination chemotherapy has yielded the highest response rates but has not been shown to be curative.

GASTRINOMA (ZOLLINGER–ELLISON SYNDROME)

In 1955, Zollinger and Ellison described two patients with severe peptic ulcer disease and pancreatic endocrine tumors and postulated that an ulcerogenic agent originated from the
7 pancreatic tumor.[20] It has been estimated that approximately 1 in 1000 patients with primary duodenal ulcer disease and 2 in 100 patients with recurrence after peptic ulcer surgery harbor gastrinomas. While 75% of gastrinomas occur sporadically, 25% are associated with the MEN-1 syndrome. Historically, the majority of gastrinomas were found to be malignant, with metastatic disease present at the time of initial workup. With increased awareness and screening for hypergastrinemia, a higher percentage of patients present with earlier-stage and potentially curable neoplasms.

The **clinical symptoms** of patients with gastrinoma are a direct result of increased levels of circulating gastrin (**Table 53.5**). Abdominal pain and peptic ulceration of the upper gastrointestinal (UGI) tract are seen in up to 90% of patients. Diarrhea is seen in 50% of patients, with 10% having diarrhea as their only symptom. Esophageal symptoms or endoscopic abnormalities resulting from gastroesophageal reflux are seen in up to half of patients. The diagnosis of gastrinoma should be suspected in several clinical settings, including the initial diagnosis of peptic ulcer disease, recurrent ulcer after medical or surgical therapy, postbulbar ulcer, family history of ulcer disease, ulcer with diarrhea, prolonged undiagnosed diarrhea, MEN-1 kindred, nongastrinoma pancreatic endocrine tumors (high association of secondary hormone elevations), and prominent gastric rugal folds on UGI examination.

In most patients with gastrinoma, the **fasting serum gastrin** level is greater than 200 pg/mL. Gastrin levels greater than 1000 pg/mL in the setting of documented hyperacidity and ulcer disease are virtually pathognomonic for gastrinoma. Because hypergastrinemia can occur in other pathophysiologic states (**Table 53.6**), fasting hypergastrinemia alone is not sufficient for the diagnosis of gastrinoma. **Gastric acid analysis** (or at least **gastric pH testing**) is critical in differentiating between

Table 53.6. Disease States Associated with Hypergastrinemia

Nonulcerogenic causes (normal to low gastric acid secretion) Atrophic gastritis Pernicious anemia Previous vagotomy Renal failure Short-gut syndrome
Ulcerogenic causes (excess gastric acid secretion) Antral G-cell hyperplasia or hyperfunction Gastric outlet obstruction Retained excluded gastric antrum Zollinger–Ellison syndrome

ulcerogenic (high levels of acid) and nonulcerogenic (low levels of acid) causes of hypergastrinemia. To obtain an accurate gastric acid analysis, patients must not be taking antisecretory medications including histamine (H_2)-receptor antagonists or proton pump inhibitors (PPIs). The diagnosis of gastrinoma is supported by a basal acid output above 15 mEq/h in nonoperated patients, a basal acid output exceeding 5 mEq/h in patients with previous vagotomy or ulcer operations, or a ratio of basal acid output to maximal acid output exceeding 0.6.

After documenting that hypergastrinemia and excessive acid secretion exist, provocative testing with secretin may be performed to differentiate between gastrinoma, antral G-cell hyperplasia or hyperfunction, and the other causes of ulcerogenic hypergastrinemia. This is achieved with a **secretin stimulation test** (**Fig. 53.9**). A baseline gastrin level is drawn. The patient is then stimulated with 2 units/kg of secretin as an intravenous bolus, and subsequent gastrin samples are collected at 5-minute intervals for 30 minutes. An increase in the gastrin level by more than 200 pg/mL above the basal level supports the diagnosis of gastrinoma.

After the biochemical diagnosis of gastrinoma has been made, the gastric acid hypersecretion should be pharmacologically controlled. PPIs are now considered the drug of choice for this purpose. The dose is adjusted to achieve a nonacidic pH during the hour immediately before the next dose of the drug. Typically, PPI doses needed for acid control exceed usual dosing levels. After the initiation of antisecretory therapy, all patients should undergo imaging studies to localize the primary tumor and to assess for metastatic disease.

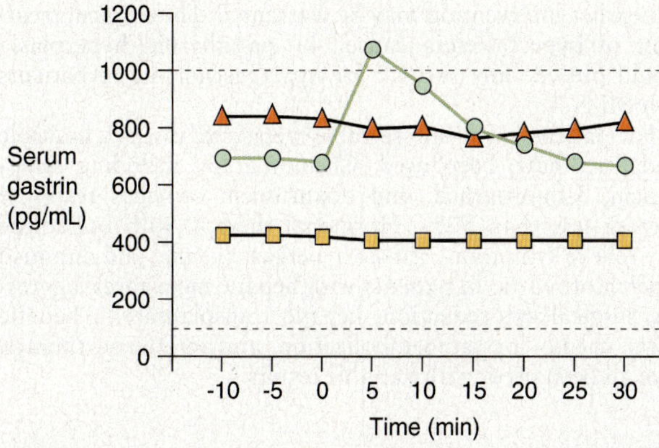

Figure 53.9. Results of intravenous secretin stimulation tests in patients with atrophic gastritis (*triangles*), gastric outlet obstruction (*squares*), and gastrinoma (*circles*). A positive test result, consistent with the presence of gastrinoma, is indicated by an increase over basal serum gastrin levels of at least 200 pg/mL. (Adapted from Wolfe MM, Jensen RT. Zollinger-Ellison syndrome: current concepts in diagnosis and management. *N Engl J Med.* 1987;317:1200–1209.)

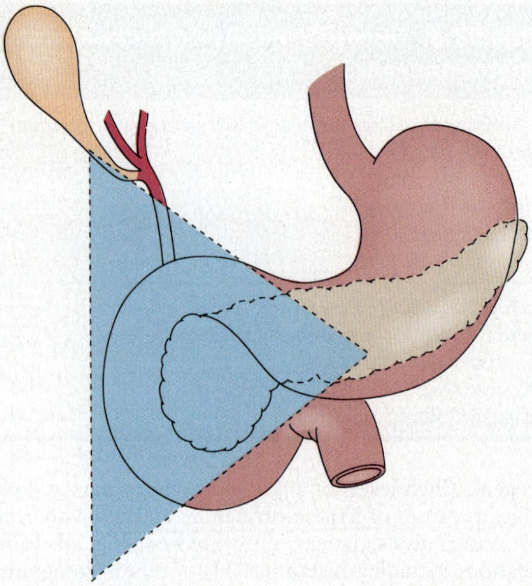

Figure 53.10. Most gastrinomas are found within the gastrinoma triangle.

For patients with resectable disease, surgical exploration with curative intent should be offered. On exploration, the entire abdomen should be assessed for areas of extrapancreatic and extraduodenal gastrinomas. Most gastrinomas are found in the **gastrinoma triangle** (**Fig. 53.10**). **Transillumination** of the duodenum may help identify small duodenal gastrinomas. If the tumor is still not identified, a longitudinal **duodenotomy** may be performed at the level of the second portion of the duodenum in search of duodenal wall microgastrinomas, which can be palpated between two fingers. Small gastrinomas in the duodenal wall can be locally resected with primary closure of the duodenal defect.[21] In a small percentage of patients, gastrinoma is found only in peripancreatic lymph nodes, with these lymph nodes harboring the apparent primary tumor.

The management of **gastrinoma in MEN-1** is not as clear given the multifocality of these lesions. Patients with sporadic gastrinomas tend to experience significantly improved disease-free survival following resection compared to those with MEN-1. In patients with MEN-1, gastrin-secreting tumors are often multicentric and associated with lymph node metastases. Although some groups have favored resection only when MEN-1 gastrinoma tumors exceed 3 cm, some have posited that earlier intervention may be warranted. The surgical **treatment of hypercalcemia** caused by parathyroid hyperplasia should precede any surgery for hypergastrinemia in patients with MEN-1.

For patients with unresectable metastatic disease, multiple modalities have been used. Chemotherapy including streptozocin, 5-fluorouracil, and doxorubicin provides response rates of less than 50%. Hormonal therapy with octreotide may relieve symptoms, reduce hypergastrinemia, and diminish hyperchlorhydria. In patients with hepatic metastases, aggressive surgical cytoreduction, hepatic transplantation, hepatic artery chemo- or radioembolization, and interferon therapy have all been used, with variable results.

VIPOMA (VERNER–MORRISON SYNDROME)

Synonyms for VIPoma include WDHA syndrome (watery diarrhea, hypokalemia, and either achlorhydria or acidosis) and pancreatic cholera syndrome (**Table 53.7**). Verner and Morrison characterized this secretory diarrheal syndrome in a 1958 report.[22] Patients characteristically present with intermittent severe, watery diarrhea averaging up to 5 L/d. Hypokalemia results from fecal loss of large amounts of potassium. Low serum potassium levels lead to lethargy, muscle weakness, and nausea. A metabolic acidosis may be present, due to loss of bicarbonate in the diarrhea. Half of the patients may have hyperglycemia or hypercalcemia, and cutaneous flushing can be observed in a minority. The diagnosis of VIPoma is made after other common causes of diarrhea have been excluded (**Table 53.8**) and an elevated serum VIP level is documented.

VIP secretion can be episodic, so repeated fasting levels should be measured if there is a strong clinical suspicion. Preoperative tumor localization is critical, because 10% of patients may have extrapancreatic tumors located in the retroperitoneum or chest. Most tumors are located in the distal pancreas where they are amenable to resection via distal pancreatectomy. In most cases, hepatic metastases accompany the primary tumor. Therapies directed at these metastases, such as resection or ablative strategies, are appropriate.

Table 53.7. VIPoma

Parameter	Description
Symptoms	Watery diarrhea Weakness Lethargy Nausea
Diagnostic Tests	Hypokalemia Achlorhydria Metabolic acidosis Serum VIP levels elevated
Anatomic Localization	Most in body and tail of pancreas, with liver metastases

VIP, vasoactive intestinal peptide.

Table 53.8. Differential Diagnosis of Verner–Morrison Syndrome

Entity	Workup
Villous Adenoma	Lower GI endoscopy
Laxative Abuse	Stool examination for phenolphthalein
Celiac Disease	Fecal fat measurement D-xylose tolerance test Small bowel biopsy
Parasitic and Infectious Diseases	Stool culture Ovum and parasite analysis *Clostridium difficile* toxin assay
Inflammatory Bowel Disease	Lower GI endoscopy Upper GI and small bowel series
Carcinoid Syndrome	Urinary 5′-HIAA Upper GI and small bowel series Abdominal CT Serum serotonin measurement
Gastrinoma	Serum gastrin measurement Gastric acid analysis Secretin stimulation test

CT, computed tomography; GI, gastrointestinal; 5′-HIAA, 5′-hydroxyindoleacetic acid.

Table 53.9. Glucagonoma

Parameter	Description
Symptoms	Dermatitis manifested as necrolytic migratory erythema Stomatitis Catabolic state: weight loss
Diagnostic tests	Hyperglycemia Hypoproteinemia Serum glucagon measurement Serum amino acid profile
Anatomic localization	Most in body and tail of pancreas, with liver metastases

Table 53.10. Somatostatinoma

Parameter	Description
Symptoms	Steatorrhea Right upper quadrant pain
Diagnostic tests	Hyperglycemia Hypochlorhydria Gallstones Serum somatostatin level
Anatomic localization	Most in head or uncinate process of pancreas; often periampullary

Surgical excision is appropriate in nearly all patients with VIPoma. Prior to surgery, fluid and electrolyte imbalances must be corrected. Octreotide can serve as a treatment adjunct, reducing the levels of circulating VIP, with a resultant decrease in the volume of diarrhea. Octreotide is also useful for symptom control in the setting of unresectable disease. Chemotherapy specific for this disease has not been well studied.

GLUCAGONOMA

The most common findings in the glucagonoma syndrome are severe dermatitis, mild diabetes, stomatitis, anemia, and weight loss (**Table 53.9**). The dermatitis manifests as a characteristic skin rash termed **necrolytic migratory erythema.** This rash exhibits cyclic migrations, and it has been theorized that the hypoaminoacidemia accompanying glucagonoma is the cause.

The diagnosis of glucagonoma is suggested by the clinical presentation and biopsy of the skin lesions but is secured by the documentation of high fasting levels of serum glucagon. Most glucagonomas are located in the body and tail of the gland. These tumors are typically large and bulky, and surgical resection requires distal pancreatectomy (**Fig. 53.11**). Metastases are found in most patients and safe debulking of these should be considered. As in patients with VIPoma and insulinoma, octreotide can be useful in controlling the signs and symptoms (hyperglycemia and dermatitis) associated with incurable glucagonoma.

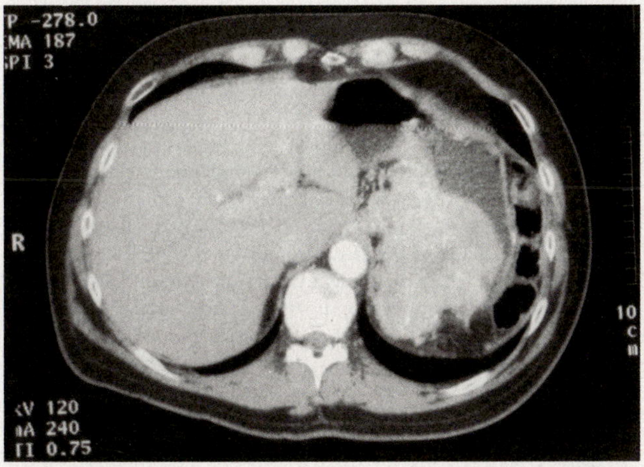

Figure 53.11. Computed tomography with oral and intravenous contrast in a patient with a glucagonoma. The large tumor appears to be posterior to the stomach and to the right of the aorta from the viewer's perspective.

SOMATOSTATINOMA

The somatostatinoma syndrome is the least common of the five generally accepted functional PEN syndromes, occurring in less than 1 in 40 million people. The clinical features are nonspecific, including steatorrhea, diabetes, hypochlorhydria, and cholelithiasis (**Table 53.10**). Fasting plasma somatostatin levels of greater than 100 pg/mL can be used to confirm the diagnosis.

Most somatostatinomas are located in the pancreatic head or periampullary region. Tumors are of variable size and are often easily localized. Metastatic disease may be present at the time of diagnosis. Safe resection of the primary tumor (often via pancreaticoduodenectomy) and careful debulking of hepatic metastases are indicated.

METASTATIC PANCREATIC ENDOCRINE TUMORS

Liver-Directed Therapies

At least one-third of patients with malignant PENs present with synchronous liver metastases at the time of diagnosis.[23] A
8 subset of these patients remain asymptomatic and experience prolonged survival even without aggressive therapy. However, the overall 5-year survival of patients with liver metastases is less than 50%. Cytoreductive surgery has been associated with excellent symptom control for patients with carcinoid syndrome as well as improved overall survival even if only 70% to 90% of the tumor burden can be resected.[24] Nevertheless, liver metastases will recur in the vast majority of patients, and multimodality treatments will be subsequently required. As a result, over the last two decades, orthotopic liver transplantation for patients with liver-only unresectable metastatic disease, no extrahepatic disease, and overall indolent tumor biology has been utilized in a small fraction of highly selected patients with promising results.

Those with unresectable disease to the liver may also be candidates for a variety of liver-directed therapies for locoregional control and symptom palliation. Transarterial embolization (TAE), chemoembolization (TACE), or radioembolization (TARE) with yttrium-90 are the most frequently used. For patients with solitary or oligometastatic disease, percutaneous or surgical ablation, either with radiofrequency or microwave ablation techniques, are good options.[25]

Somatostatin Analogs

Since the majority of NETs express somatostatin receptors, somatostatin analogs (SSAs) are widely used for patients with metastatic PENs. SSAs not only lead to effective symptom control of carcinoid syndrome, they are also associated with improved progression-free survival (PFS). Both the PROMID and CLARINET trials were prospective randomized controlled trials demonstrating PFS superiority of long-acting SSAs to

Table 53.11. Seminal Randomized Controlled Trials of Systemic Therapies for Patients with Neuroendocrine Tumors

Trial	Intervention	Mechanism of Action	Control	Population	Median PFS Improvement (Mo)
Promid[27]	Octeotide LAR	SSA	Placebo	Midgut NET (n = 84)	14.3 vs. 6.0
Clarinet[26]	Lanreotide	SSA	Placebo	GEP-NET (n = 204)	38.5 vs. 18.0
Radiant-3[29]	Everolimus	mTOR inhibitor	Placebo	PEN (n = 420)	11.0 vs. 4.6
Raymond et al.[28]	Sunitinib	TKI	Placebo	PEN (n = 171)	11.4 vs. 5.5
Netter-1[31]	^{177}Lu-DOTATATE	PRRT	Octreotide LAR (60 mg)	Midgut NET (n = 230)	NA vs. 8.4

PFS, progression-free survival; SSA, somatostatin analog; NET, neuroendocrine tumor; GEP, gastroenteropancreatic; PEN, pancreatic endocrine neoplasm; mTOR, mammalian target of rapamycin; TKI, tyrosine kinase inhibitor; PRRT, peptide receptor radionuclide therapy.

placebo among patients with metastatic well-differentiated gastroenteropancreatic NETs.[26,27] Based on these results and the indolent nature of well-differentiated PENs, SSAs are often the initial treatment for patients with slow-growing metastatic NETs. Newer, more broadly binding SSAs are being investigated but have not shown superiority compared to traditional SSAs.

Systemic Therapies

A number of systemic therapies have been developed over the
9 past decade for patients with metastatic PENs (**Table 53.11**). While historically only streptozocin-based chemotherapy regimens were available, advances in the molecular understanding of PENs have led to newer targeted therapies which offer improved response rates with better side effect profiles. For example, both **sunitinib malate**, an oral, small molecule, multitargeted tyrosine kinase inhibitor initially approved for the treatment of advanced renal cell carcinoma and refractory gastrointestinal stromal tumors, as well as **everolimus**, an oral inhibitor of the mTOR, are specifically approved for use in metastatic PENs.[28,29] More recently, the VEGF receptor inhibitor cabozantinib demonstrated improved outcomes in previously treated patients with PENs compared to placebo in the CABINET trial. Within traditional cytotoxic chemotherapy, the combination regimen of **temozolomide and capecitabine** has relatively high response rates and often used as first line treatment for PENs.[30] In addition, **peptide receptor radionuclide therapy (PRRT)** is an exciting therapy recently approved for use in the United States which binds radionuclides to SSAs. The NETTER-1 and NETTER-2 trials, demonstrated that first-line PRRT using ^{177}Lu-DOTA^{0},Tyr^{3}octreotate led to improved response rates and progression free survival among patients with metastatic advanced well-differentiated NETs regardless of tumor grade.[31] Ongoing research is currently investigating novel radiopharmaceuticals as well as targeted therapies, checkpoint inhibitors, and oncocytic viruses.[32]

References

1. Lawrence B, Gustafsson BI, Chan A, Svejda B, Kidd M, Modlin IM. The epidemiology of gastroenteropancreatic neuroendocrine tumors. *Endocrinol Metab Clin North Am*. 2011;40(1):1–18, vii.
2. Dasari A, Shen C, Halperin D, et al. Trends in the incidence, prevalence, and survival outcomes in patients with neuroendocrine tumors in the United States. *JAMA Oncol*. 2017;3(10):1335–1342.
3. Weltgesundheitsorganisation, Lloyd RV, Osamura RY, Klöppel G, Rosai J, International Agency for Research on Cancer, eds. *WHO Classification of Tumours of Endocrine Organs*. 4th ed. International Agency for Research on Cancer; 2017.
4. Jiao Y, Shi C, Edil BH, et al. DAXX/ATRX, MEN1, and mTOR pathway genes are frequently altered in pancreatic neuroendocrine tumors. *Science*. 2011;331(6021):1199–1203.
5. Scarpa A, Chang DK, Nones K, et al. Whole-genome landscape of pancreatic neuroendocrine tumours. *Nature*. 2017;543(7643):65–71.
6. Ichikawa T, Peterson MS, Federle MP, et al. Islet cell tumor of the pancreas: biphasic CT versus MR imaging in tumor detection. *Radiology*. 2000;216(1):163–171.
7. Sadowski SM, Neychev V, Millo C, et al. Prospective study of 68Ga-DOTATATE positron emission tomography/computed tomography for detecting gastro-entero-pancreatic neuroendocrine tumors and unknown primary sites. *J Clin Oncol*. 2016;34(6):588–596.
8. Hope TA, Bergsland EK, Bozkurt MF, et al. Appropriate use criteria for somatostatin receptor PET imaging in neuroendocrine tumors. *J Nucl Med*. 2018;59(1):66–74.
9. Proye C, Malvaux P, Pattou F, et al. Noninvasive imaging of insulinomas and gastrinomas with endoscopic ultrasonography and somatostatin receptor scintigraphy. *Surgery*. 1998;124(6):1134–1143; discussion 1143–1144.
10. de Wilde RF, Edil BH, Hruban RH, Maitra A. Well-differentiated pancreatic neuroendocrine tumors: from genetics to therapy. *Nat Rev Gastroenterol Hepatol*. 2012;9(4):199–208.
11. Cloyd J, Poultsides G. The landmark series: pancreatic neuroendocrine tumors. *Ann Surg Oncol*. 2021;28(2):1039–1049.
12. Partelli S, Massironi S, Zerbi A, et al. Management of asymptomatic sporadic non-functioning pancreatic neuroendocrine neoplasms no larger than 2 cm: interim analysis of prospective ASPEN trial. *Br J Surg*. 2022;109(12):1186–1190.
13. Crippa S, Bassi C, Salvia R, Falconi M, Butturini G, Pederzoli P. Enucleation of pancreatic neoplasms. *Br J Surg*. 2007;94(10):1254–1259.
14. Goudard Y, Gaujoux S, Dokmak S, et al. Reappraisal of central pancreatectomy a 12-year single-center experience. *JAMA Surg*. 2014;149(4):356–363.
15. Asbun HJ, Moekotte AL, Vissers FL, et al. The Miami International Evidence-based guidelines on minimally invasive pancreas resection. *Ann Surg*. 2020;271(1):1–14.
16. Dong DH, Zhang XF, Poultsides G, et al. Impact of tumor size and nodal status on recurrence of nonfunctional pancreatic neuroendocrine tumors ≤2 cm after curative resection: a multi-institutional study of 392 cases. *J Surg Oncol*. 2019;120(7):1071–1079.
17. Falconi M, Bartsch DK, Eriksson B, et al. ENETS Consensus Guidelines for the management of patients with digestive neuroendocrine neoplasms of the digestive system: well-differentiated pancreatic non-functioning tumors. *Neuroendocrinology*. 2012;95(2):120–134.
18. Howe JR, Merchant NB, Conrad C, et al. The North American Neuroendocrine Tumor Society consensus paper on the surgical management of pancreatic neuroendocrine tumors. *Pancreas*. 2020;49(1):1–33.
19. Mansour JC, Chavin K, Morris-Stiff G, et al. Management of asymptomatic, well-differentiated PNETs: results of the Delphi consensus process of the Americas Hepato-Pancreato-Biliary Association. *HPB (Oxford)*. 2019;21(5):515–523.

20. Zollinger RM, Ellison EH. Primary peptic ulcerations of the jejunum associated with islet cell tumors of the pancreas. *Ann Surg.* 1955;142(4):709–723; discussion, 724–728.
21. Norton JA, Alexander HR, Fraker DL, Venzon DJ, Gibril F, Jensen RT. Does the use of routine duodenotomy (DUODX) affect rate of cure, development of liver metastases, or survival in patients with Zollinger-Ellison syndrome? *Ann Surg.* 2004;239(5):617–625; discussion 626.
22. Verner JV, Morrison AB. Islet cell tumor and a syndrome of refractory watery diarrhea and hypokalemia. *Am J Med.* 1958;25(3): 374–380.
23. Cloyd JM, Wiseman JT, Pawlik TM. Surgical management of pancreatic neuroendocrine liver metastases. *J Gastrointest Oncol.* 2020;11(3):590–600.
24. Scott AT, Breheny PJ, Keck KJ, et al. Effective cytoreduction can be achieved in patients with numerous neuroendocrine tumor liver metastases (NETLMs). *Surgery.* 2019;165(1):166–175.
25. Cloyd JM, Ejaz A, Konda B, Makary MS, Pawlik TM. Neuroendocrine liver metastases: a contemporary review of treatment strategies. *Hepatobiliary Surg Nutr.* 2020;9(4):440–451.
26. Caplin ME, Pavel M, Ćwikła JB, et al. Lanreotide in metastatic enteropancreatic neuroendocrine tumors. *N Engl J Med.* 2014;371(3): 224–233.
27. Rinke A, Müller HH, Schade-Brittinger C, et al. Placebo-controlled, double-blind, prospective, randomized study on the effect of octreotide LAR in the control of tumor growth in patients with metastatic neuroendocrine midgut tumors: a report from the PROMID Study Group. *JCO.* 2009;27(28):4656–4663.
28. Raymond E, Dahan L, Raoul JL, et al. Sunitinib malate for the treatment of pancreatic neuroendocrine tumors. *N Engl J Med.* 2011;364(6):501–513.
29. Yao JC, Lombard-Bohas C, Baudin E, et al. Daily oral everolimus activity in patients with metastatic pancreatic neuroendocrine tumors after failure of cytotoxic chemotherapy: a phase II trial. *J Clin Oncol.* 2010;28(1):69–76.
30. Kunz PL, Graham NT, Catalano PJ, et al. Randomized study of temozolomide or temozolomide and capecitabine in patients with advanced pancreatic neuroendocrine tumors (ECOG-ACRIN E2211). *J Clin Oncol.* 2023;41(7):1359–1369.
31. Strosberg J, El-Haddad G, Wolin E, et al. Phase 3 Trial of 177Lu-dotatate for midgut neuroendocrine tumors. *N Engl J Med.* 2017;376(2):125–135.
32. Cloyd JM, Konda B, Shah MH, Pawlik TM. The emerging role of targeted therapies for advanced well-differentiated gastroenteropancreatic neuroendocrine tumors. *Expert Rev Clin Pharmacol.* 2019;12(2):101–108.

54

Section H: HEPATOBILIARY AND PORTAL VENOUS SYSTEM

Hepatobiliary Anatomy

Alice C. Wei

Key Points

1 Couinaud classification divides the liver into eight anatomic segments based on hepatic portal inflow and hepatic vein outflow.

2 Classic hepatic arterial anatomy is present in only approximately 50% of patients, with a replaced or accessory right hepatic artery arising from the superior mesenteric artery (SMA) and a replaced or accessory left hepatic artery arising from the left gastric artery as the most common variants.

3 The modern Calot triangle (hepatocystic triangle) is bounded by the common hepatic duct (CHD) on the left, the cystic duct inferiorly, and the undersurface of the liver, superiorly. The cystic artery can be identified in this triangle during cholecystectomy.

4 There are three major hepatic veins; most patients have a right hepatic vein that joins the right anterior wall of the inferior vena cava (IVC) and middle and left hepatic veins that converge into a common trunk before joining the IVC.

5 Multiphase computed tomography (CT) with intravenous contrast is the mainstay for preoperative liver imaging. CT scans provide anatomic details of the hepatic vasculature and characterize many hepatic lesions, often without the need for biopsy.

6 Magnetic resonance cholangiopancreatography (MRCP) can be used to visualize intra- and extrahepatic biliary anatomy and provides complimentary information to a CT for indeterminant liver lesions.

7 Intraoperative ultrasonography is used liberally to confirm the anatomy of the hepatic vessels and biliary system and localize lesions during surgery.

8 The steps in major hepatectomy include exposure, vascular inflow control, vascular outflow control, and parenchymal transection.

Liver anatomy is complex; variations in the hepatic vessels and biliary tree are regularly encountered that may not be apparent on cursory inspection of the liver. Surgeons must have a thorough understanding of each patient's unique liver anatomy and the relationship of lesions to major structures prior to any operation.

TOPOGRAPHIC AND SURFACE ANATOMY

The liver is a large, wedge-shaped organ situated in the right upper quadrant of the abdomen ventral to the inferior vena cava (IVC). Most of the liver sits in the subcostal space and is bounded superiorly, laterally, and posteriorly by the diaphragm and retroperitoneum, and anteriorly by the abdominal wall. The liver lies anterior to the stomach, gallbladder, hepatoduodenal ligament, and duodenum, and its lower extent lies adjacent to the hepatic flexure of the colon, right adrenal gland, and kidney (**Fig. 54.1**). On the liver's inferior aspect, the gallbladder sits in the gallbladder fossa, and the hepatic portal structures enter the liver via the hepatoduodenal ligament. Rouviere sulcus on the right inferior aspect delineates the border between the anterior and posterior right liver. On the left inferior aspect, Arantius cleft runs between the base of the left portal vein and the vena cava, separating the caudate lobe from the left liver. Within the Arantius cleft, the ligamentum venosum (obliterated left umbilical vein) lies between the left portal vein at the base of the falciform ligament and the left hepatic vein.

The visceral peritoneum invests most of the liver surface apart from the posterior bare area and the gallbladder fossa. The bare area is bound by the right triangular and coronary ligament (**Fig. 54.2**). In addition to these ligaments, the left triangular and the falciform ligament, which extends from ligamentum teres to the suprahepatic vena cava, connect the liver to the anterior abdominal wall. The gastrohepatic ligament connects to the ligamentum venosum (obliterated ductus venosus) in Arantius cleft. These ligaments, as well as the hepatoduodenal ligament, which arises between the pancreatic head to the liver hilum (known as the porta hepatitis), comprise the ligamentous attachments of the liver. The hepatoduodenal ligament contains the portal vein, hepatic arteries, extrahepatic bile duct and portal lymphatics (**Fig. 54.3**).

MORPHOLOGIC AND FUNCTIONAL ANATOMY

1 Over the past 100 years, a variety of anatomic models of the liver have been developed. The Couinaud classification of liver segments is the most often used by hepatobiliary surgeons (**Fig. 54.4**).[1,2] In this classification, eight segments of the liver are delimited by portal inflow and hepatic venous outflow. The right and left hemilivers are divided by a plane through the middle hepatic vein and the IVC (**Fig. 54.5**) along Cantlie line. The left and right hepatic veins subdivide their respective hemilivers each into two sectors (alternatively called sections). The sectors are further divided into segments by portal pedicles. This results in the left liver segments II, III, IVa, and IVb and right liver segments V, VI, VII, and VIII. Segment I, the caudate lobe, arises posterior to the portal pedicle and anterior to the IVC. Segment I receives inflow from both the left and right portal vessels, and caudate veins drain directly into the IVC.

The Glissonean capsule is the connective tissue that invests the hepatic arteries, portal vein, bile duct, nerves, and

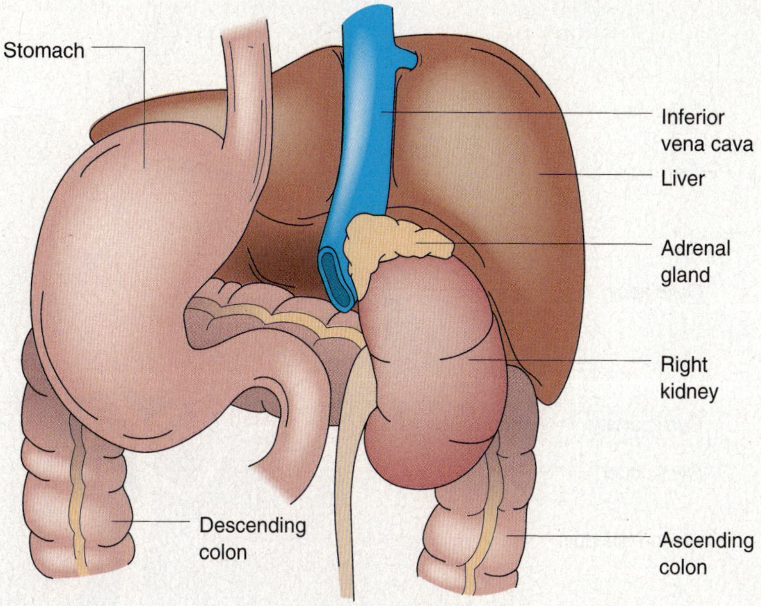

Figure 54.1. Posterior view of the liver, showing organs that produce impressions on its inferior surface.

lymphatics. The structures within the Glissonean capsule enter the liver centrally at the porta hepatis via the hepatoduodenal ligament.

Variations from the canonical anatomy occur frequently; hepatic artery variation is most common, followed by biliary tract and portal vein variants.[2] Variations often occur concomitantly. When anatomic variation is seen in one of the portal structures, the surgeon should be aware that variation in other structures may be present, and additional investigation to confirm anatomy may be indicated.

HEPATIC ARTERIES

The common hepatic artery arises from the celiac axis and becomes the proper hepatic artery as it turns cephalad in the hepatoduodenal ligament after giving off the right gastric and gastroduodenal artery branches. It lies ventral and medial in the hepatoduodenal ligament and gives off the right and left hepatic arteries. Variations in hepatic artery anatomy are common in up to 40% of individuals (**Fig. 54.6**).[3–5] This variation can be in the origin, branches, or course of the hepatic artery vasculature. Replaced or accessory right and left hepatic arteries occur in 13% and 11% of patients, respectively.[4] Typically, accessory right hepatic arteries arise from the superior mesenteric artery (SMA) and travel posterior to the common bile duct and lateral to the portal vein. Left accessory or replaced hepatic arteries most often arise from the left gastric artery and course to the liver via the gastrohepatic ligament. The cystic artery can arise either directly from the common hepatic artery or from the right hepatic artery. Variations in the take-off, size, and number of small vessels, including the cystic artery (**Fig. 54.7**), are common and must be considered when operating. Further, the location, relationship between the hepatic artery branches and other portal and/or biliary structures, and vessel of origin vary in the anterior and posterior planes with some regularity.

2

PORTAL VEINS

The main portal vein is formed by the confluence of the superior mesenteric and splenic veins. The coronary vein (left gastric vein) joins the portal vein, which travels in the posteriomedial aspect of the hepatoduodenal ligament to enter the liver. At the porta hepatis, the main portal vein splits into the right and left portal branches which enter the parenchyma of their respective hemilivers at its first division (**Fig. 54.8**). The short right portal vein enters the liver obliquely and at its second division, gives of the anterior pedicle which supplies Segments V and VIII, and a posterior pedicle which supplies Segments VI and VII. The longer left portal vein courses outside the liver and turns to lie in the umbilical fissure prior to giving off branches into the left liver. The left second division gives off segment

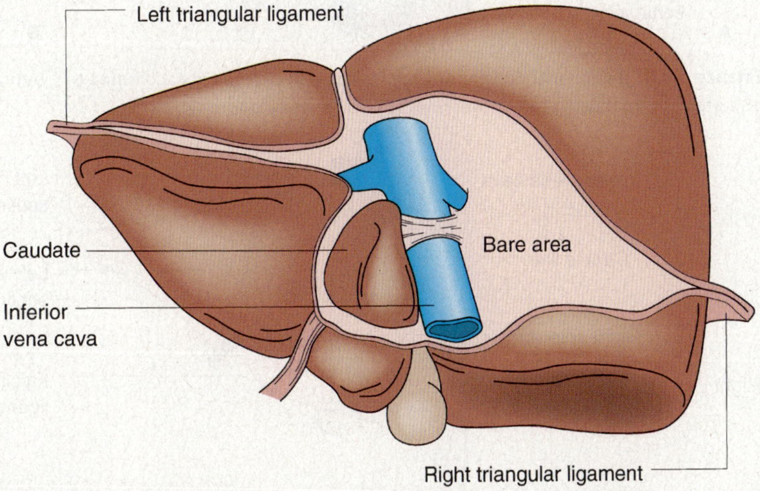

Figure 54.2. Posterior view of the liver, showing the level of peritoneal reflections.

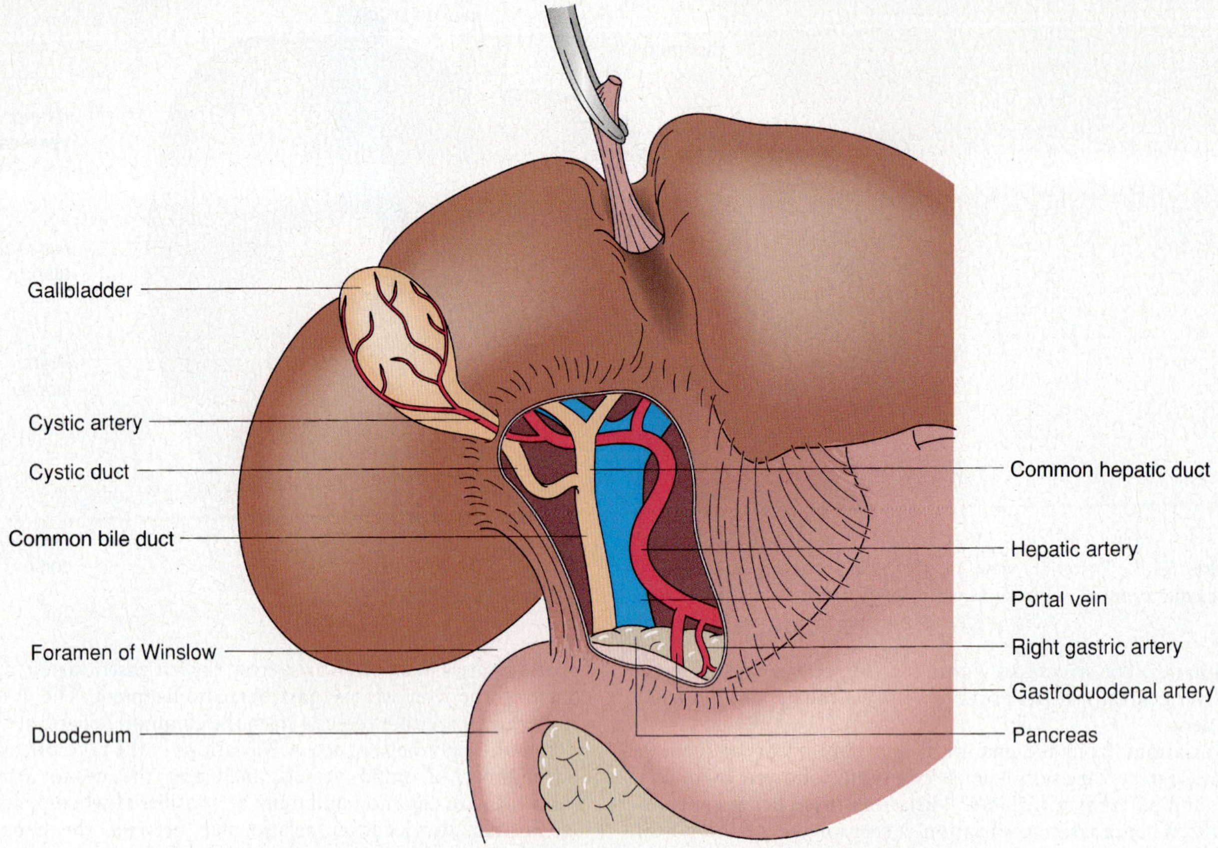

Figure 54.3. Relationship of structures within the hepatoduodenal ligament.

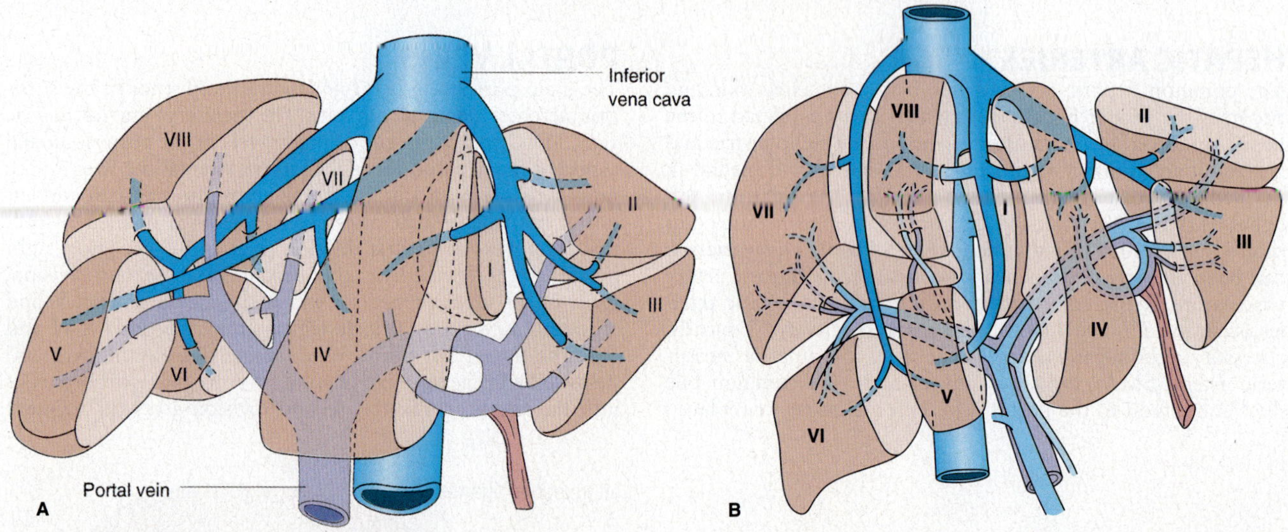

Figure 54.4. Functional divisions of the liver and liver segments according to Couinaud nomenclature with the liver in the natural position (**A**) and after it is mobilized (**B**).

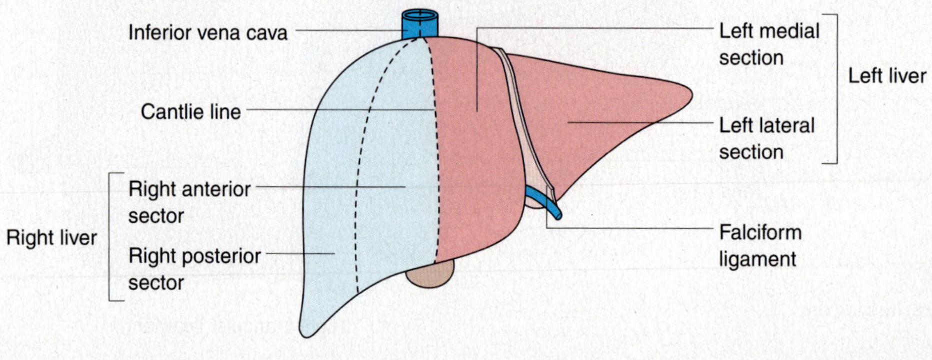

Figure 54.5. Anatomic division of the liver into right and left halves by a plane extending from the gallbladder fossa posteriorly to the inferior vena cava.

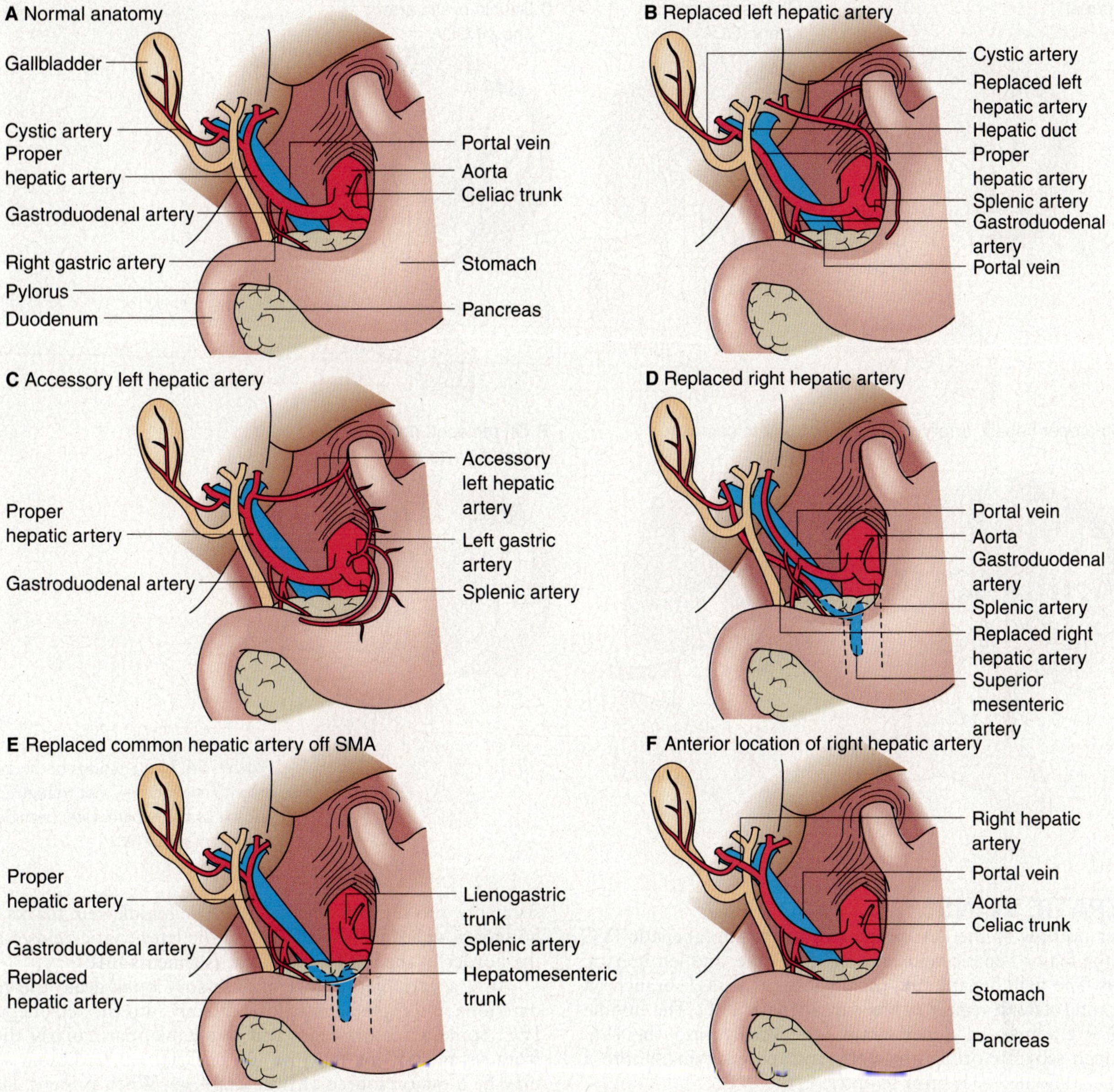

Figure 54.6. Variations in hepatic arterial anatomy.

IV branches, also known as the "recurrent branches"; the segment II and III branches supply the left lateral section of the liver (to the left of the falciform ligament). The terminal end of the left portal vein merges with the ligamentum teres as the obliterated umbilical vein. Both the right and left portal veins give off small branches to supply segment I.

BILIARY SYSTEM AND GALLBLADDER

The common bile duct lies ventral and lateral in the hepatoduodenal ligament. The right and left liver drain their respective hemilivers into right and left bile ducts, which merge to form the common hepatic duct (CHD) extrahepatically in the liver hilum (**Figs. 54.9** and **54.10**). Variations in the confluence of the biliary system occur with regularity. Common variants include a right posterior (segments VI/VII) duct draining directly into the CHD, or a right posterior system draining into the left bile duct.

The gallbladder is a pear-shaped organ that lies on the undersurface of the liver and drains into the cystic duct. The cystic duct usually runs parallel to the CHD for a variable distance before joining the CHD to form the common bile duct, which then travels through the pancreatic head and terminates at the ampulla of Vater. The cystic duct can vary in length, and when long, can take a circuitous route, either anterior or posterior, to the common bile duct prior to its insertion on either the lateral or medial side of the common bile duct (**Fig. 54.11**).

Calot triangle was originally described in 1891 as a triangle bound inferiorly by the cystic duct, medially by the CHD, and superiorly by the cystic artery. In the modern era, the working definition of Calot triangle differs from the original description.
3 tion.[2,3] The modern Calot triangle, should be referred to as the hepatocystic triangle, which is delineated by the cystic duct inferiorly, the CHD medially, and the undersurface liver superiorly.[3] In this larger triangle, the cystic artery can usually be found. This triangle is an important landmark when performing cholecystectomies. Variability in the origin, number, and location of the cystic artery is common (**Fig. 54.7**).

The surgeon should be aware of potential variations when operating in the porta hepatis, regardless of whether the procedure is a simple cholecystectomy or a complex procedure, such as a living-donor liver transplant. Preoperative and/or intraoperative cholangiography may help to avoid inadvertent injury to the biliary radicals.

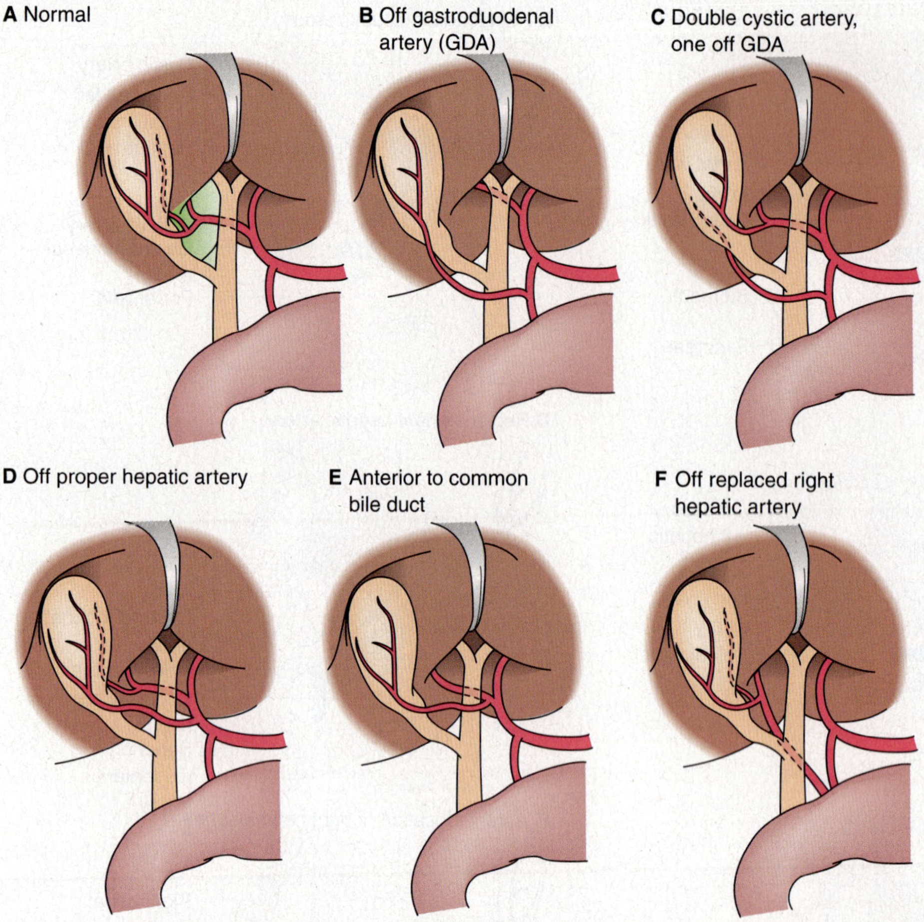

Figure 54.7. Variations of the cystic artery. The modern Calot triangle (also known as the hepatocystic triangle) is marked in green (A).

HEPATIC VEINS

Liver outflow to the IVC progresses to the suprahepatic IVC via the major hepatic veins, the right, middle, and left hepatic
4 veins. The right hepatic vein usually joins as a single branch on the anterolateral aspect of the suprahepatic IVC. The middle and left veins can either drain individually into the IVC through separate orifices or merge intraparenchymally into a short, conjoined vein prior to entering the IVC.

The hepatic veins divide the liver into sectors and drain their respective parenchyma. The right hepatic vein separates the posterior sector of the liver (segment VI/VII) from the anterior sector (segments V/VIII) and drains blood from these segments into the IVC (**Fig. 54.12**). The middle vein marks the boundary of segment IVa/IVb, and the left hepatic veins mark the border of the left lateral sector (segments II/III).

Also, a variable number of accessory veins drain the caudate lobe and right hepatic lobe directly into the retrohepatic IVC. Some accessory veins can be sizable, particularly those from segment VI of the liver. On occasion, an accessory vein may be a major source of liver drainage. When present, large accessory veins must be considered in any planned procedure. For example, in living-donor liver transplantation, major accessory veins may require implantation, and for major liver resections that involve the outflow tract, the presence of a

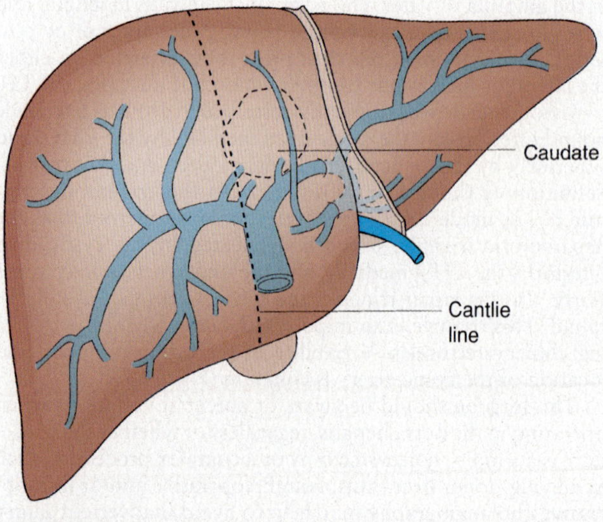

Figure 54.8. Intrahepatic divisions of the portal vein.

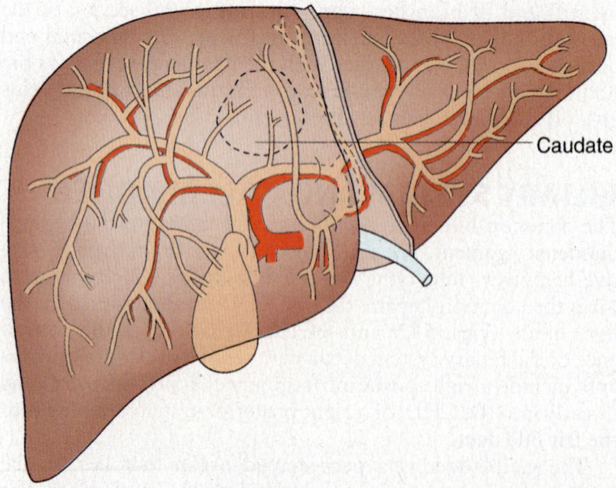

Figure 54.9. Intrahepatic divisions of the bile ducts and hepatic arteries.

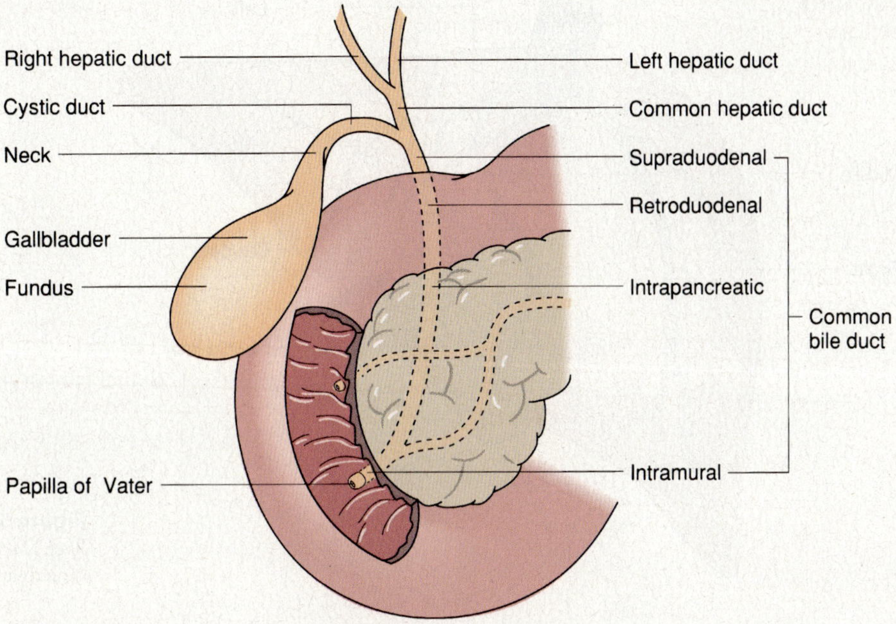

Figure 54.10. Anatomy of the extrahepatic biliary tree and pancreatic duct.

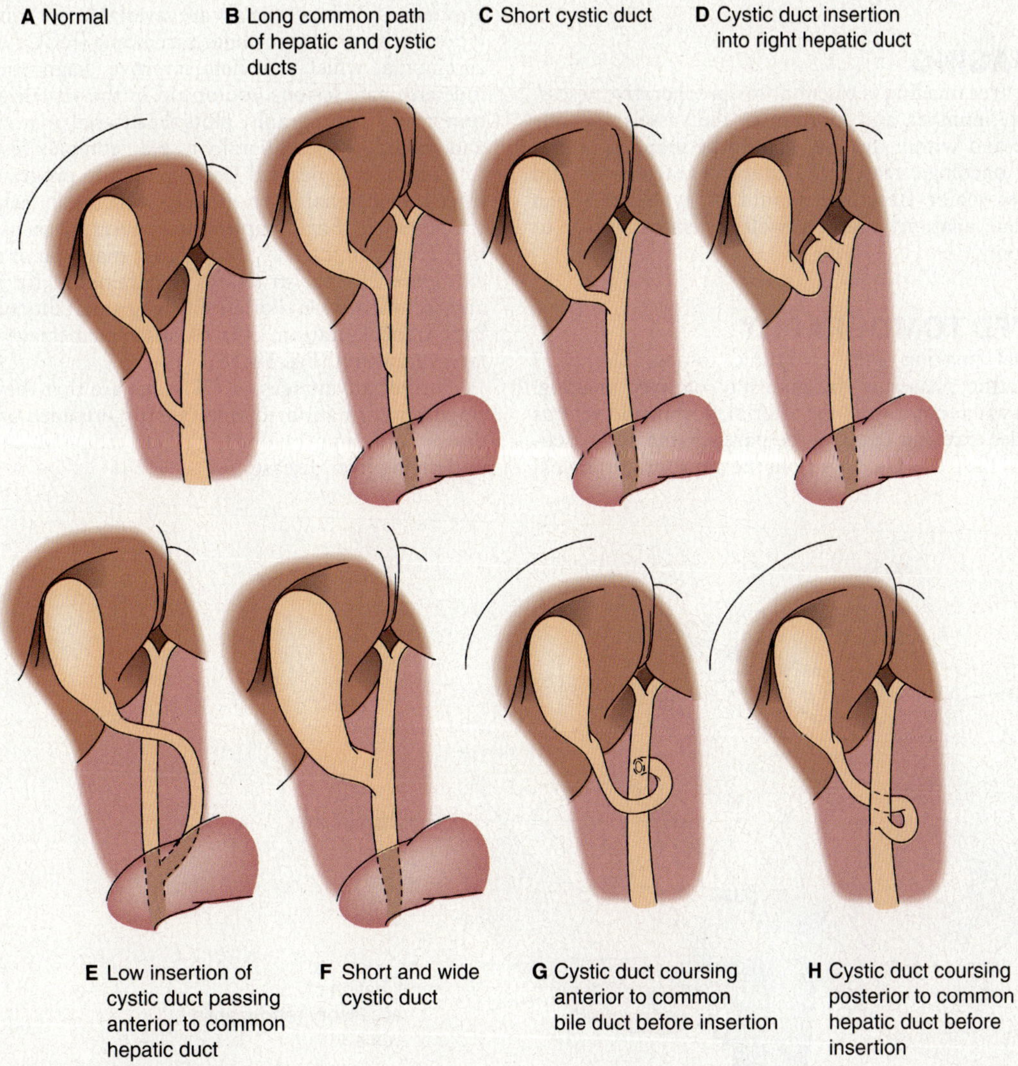

Figure 54.11. Variations in the junction of the cystic duct and common hepatic duct.

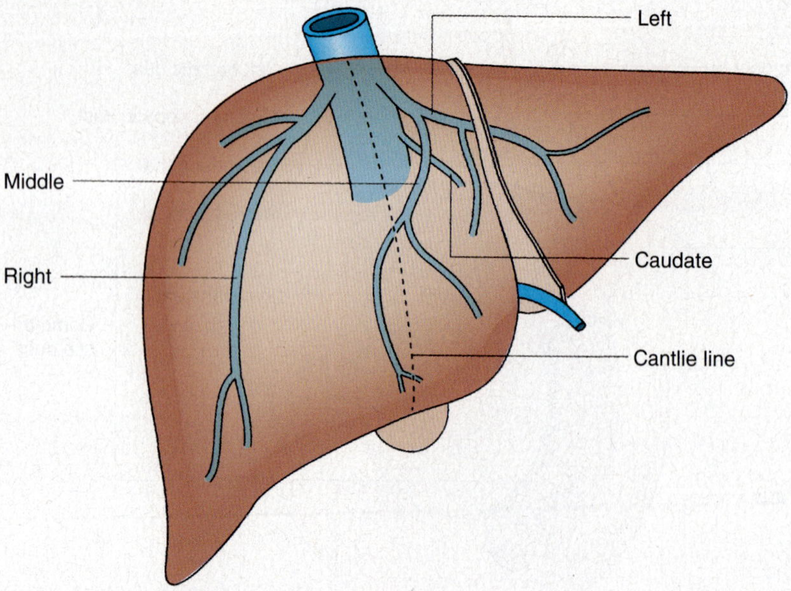

Figure 54.12. Three major hepatic veins drain the liver.The caudate segment of the liver usually drains directly into the inferior vena cava.

sizeable accessory segment VI vein may permit a nonstandard resection (**Fig. 54.13**).

LIVER IMAGING

High-quality liver imaging is essential for preoperative assessment. The size, number, and location of the vessels and bile ducts outside and within the liver should be mapped preoperatively. For oncologic resections, tumor characteristics and relationship to major structures should be evaluated. Each patient's unique anatomy must be well-understood prior to any hepatectomy.

COMPUTED TOMOGRAPHY

Cross-sectional imaging with computed tomography (CT) with liver-specific phases is the mainstay of liver imaging. 5 Well-timed vascular contrast in the arterial, portal, and venous phases provides excellent detail of the parenchyma and vascular anatomy of the liver (**Fig. 54.14**). In the appropriate clinical context, morphologic and contrast features of the tumor can be diagnostic without the need for liver biopsy (**Fig. 54.15**). Specialized CT protocols are available for different tumor types, such as hepatocellular carcinoma (HCC) and cholangiocarcinoma, which can help improve diagnostic accuracy of indeterminate lesions and/or aid in the visualization of small tumors. CT angiography plots the arterial anatomy of the liver and should be used liberally to plan complex resections.

Computer-generated liver simulation programs can render three-dimensional liver models, which can help with surgical planning. For complex procedures, such as living-donor liver resection, careful preoperative mapping of the intra- and extraparenchymal structures is paramount for safe resection and reconstruction. For establishing suitability of living-donor liver transplantation, 3-D reconstructed images are particularly important (**Fig. 54.16**).

Further advantages of CT scans are that they can provide staging information to rule out the presence of extrahepatic disease and can provide insight into the presence or absence of underlying liver disease.

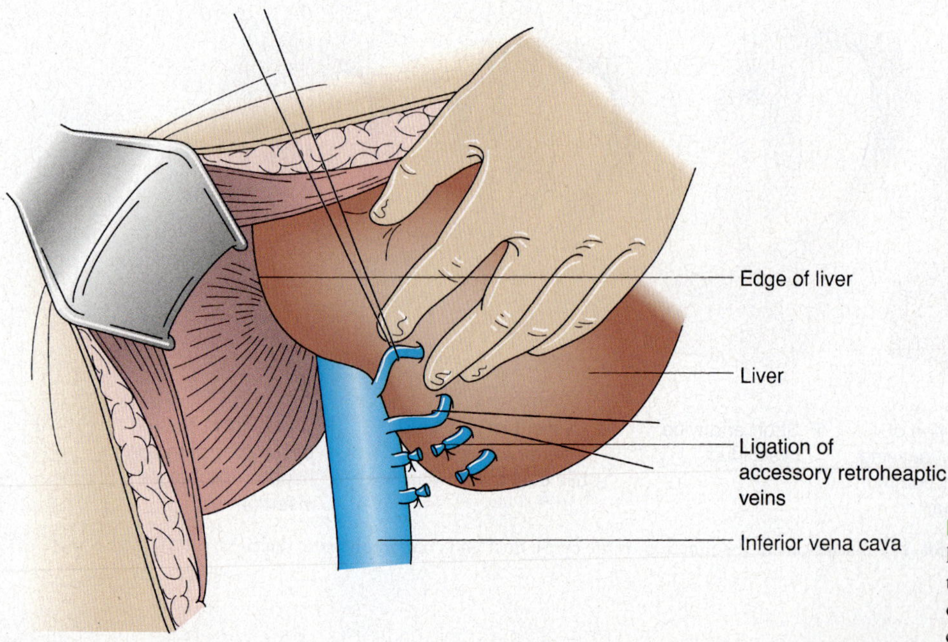

Figure 54.13. Retraction of right liver medially exposes small venous tributaries that drain the right liver directly into the retrohepatic vena cava. Several branches are ligated.

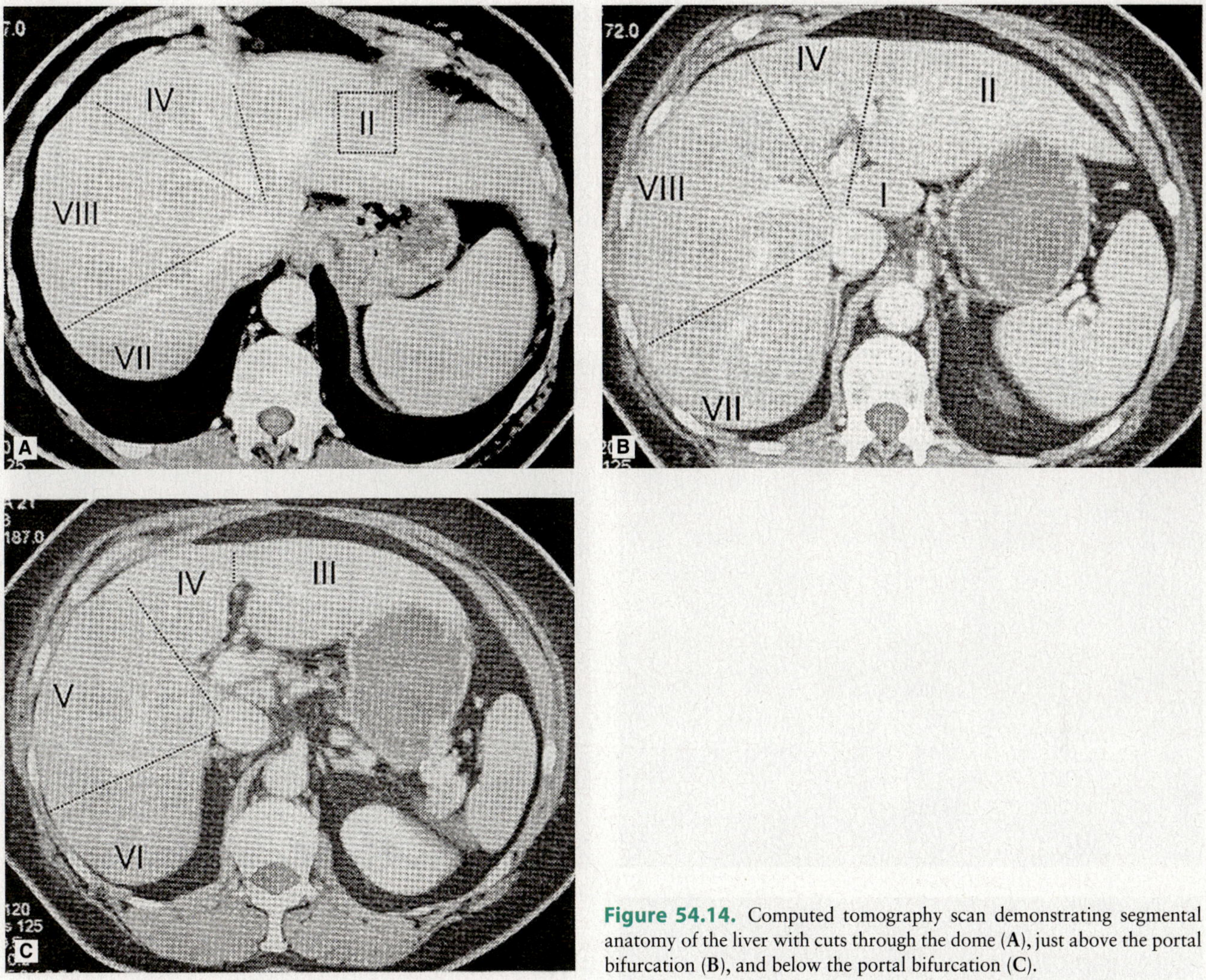

Figure 54.14. Computed tomography scan demonstrating segmental anatomy of the liver with cuts through the dome (**A**), just above the portal bifurcation (**B**), and below the portal bifurcation (**C**).

MAGNETIC RESONANCE IMAGING/ MAGNETIC RESONANCE CHOLANGIOPANCREAOTOGRAPHY

Magnetic resonance imaging (MRI) is a complementary imaging modality to CT and can provide additional information for small or indeterminant liver tumors (**Fig. 54.15**). In particular, MRI with gadolinium-based vascular or hepatobiliary contrast agents has improved sensitivity and specificity for characterizing many liver lesions. Benign lesions, such as hemangiomas, focal nodular hyperplasia, and liver cysts, can often be definitively characterized by MRI. MRI can have higher sensitivity in detecting small tumors in patients with hepatic steatosis or underlying liver disease, particularly if hepatobiliary contrast agents are used.

6 Unlike conventional CT scans, magnetic resonance cholangiopancreatography (MRCP) using T2-weighted imaging has high sensitivity for biliary structures and has largely replaced endoscopic retrograde cholangiopancreatography (ERCP) for diagnostic evaluation of the biliary tree (**Fig. 54.17**). MRCP is noninvasive and can resolve both intra- and extrahepatic biliary structures.

The disadvantages of MRI include the extended time required to obtain the scans, which can be difficult for patients who have claustrophobia or who are unable to lie still for long periods of time; the inability to fully stage the other organs in the thoracoabdominal region in the same scan; and the associated additional costs. As a result, MRI should be reserved to provide complementary information that is not obtainable by CT scan.

ULTRASOUND AND INTRAOPERATIVE LIVER ASSESSMENT

Transcutaneous ultrasound (US) can be used as a screening test for liver disease and may be an option for noninvasive surveillance of liver lesions. Routine use of transcutaneous US for preoperative assessment has been supplanted by CT and/or MRI scans.

Intraoperative US is an important modality for real-time
7 assessment of liver anatomy (**Fig. 54.18**). US at the time of laparoscopy and/or laparotomy is used in combination with visual inspection and palpation to evaluate the liver. Intraoperative US should be used liberally throughout the procedure for diagnostic purposes, to localize lesions and map intraparenchymal structures, and confirm vascular patency.

Newer modalities, including near-infrared visualization of indocyanine green (ICG) fluorescence, are increasingly being used to provide real-time imaging guidance of anatomic structures, most commonly the extrahepatic bile duct. ICG may be particularly useful in minimally invasive liver resection, as palpation and visual inspection are more limited.

PREOPERATIVE EVALUATION OF HEPATIC RESERVE

Evaluation of hepatic reserve is imprecise. For patients with underlying liver disease, a variety of different scores and tests have been developed that measure either static or dynamic liver function (**Table 54.1**). However, no single test is able to confidently predict the hepatic reserve of the future liver

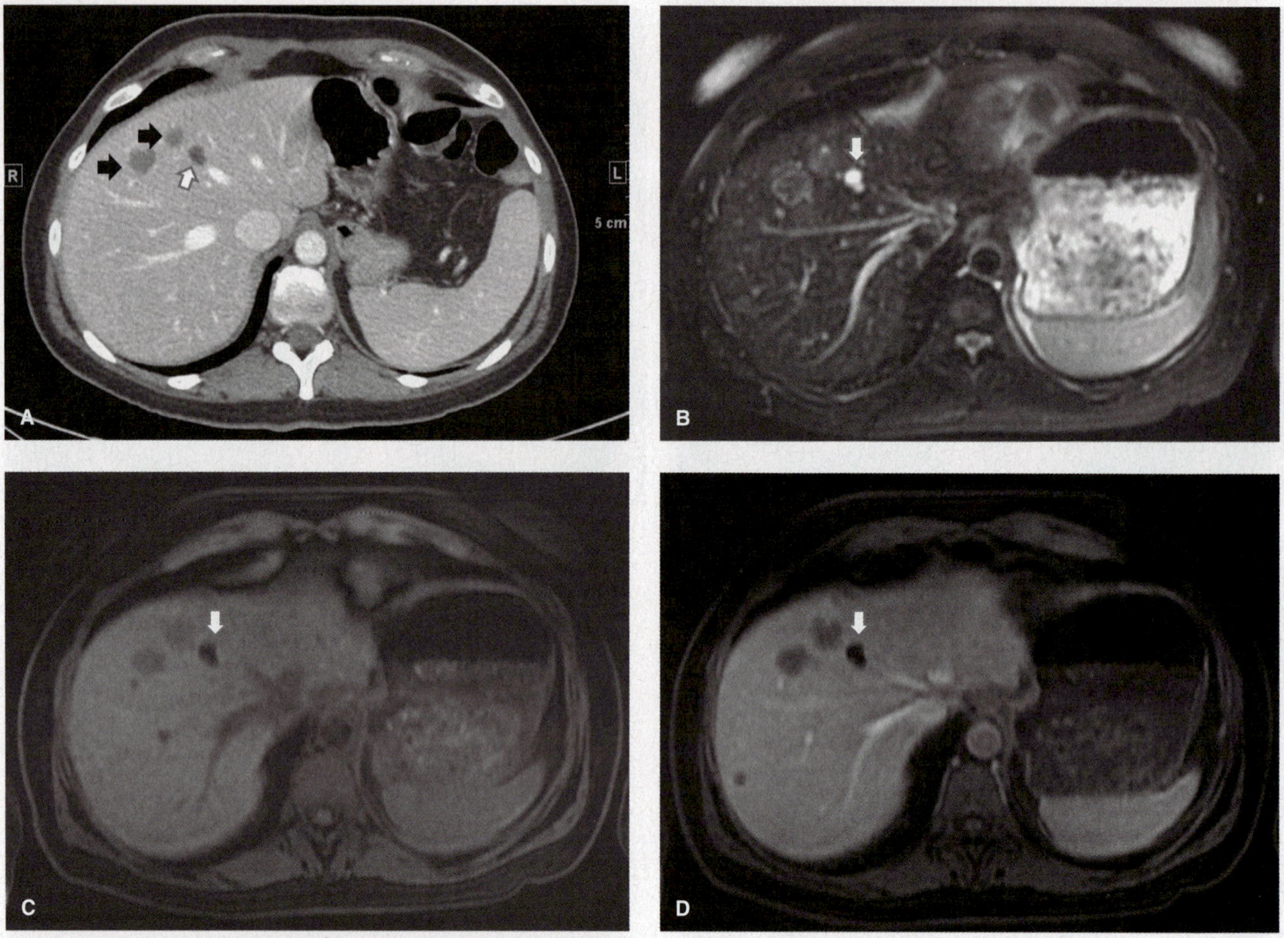

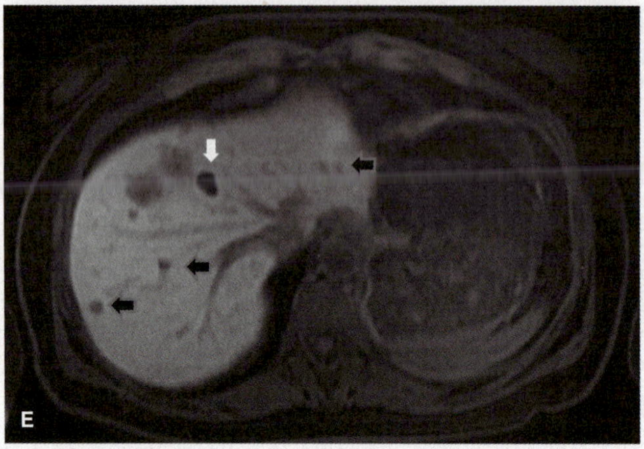

Figure 54.15. Cross-sectional imaging for a patient with colorectal liver metastases and hepatic cysts. The CT scan in portal venous phase (**A**) demonstrates two irregular hypoattenuated lesions consistent with metastases (*black arrows*). A third lesion adjacent to middle hepatic vein (*white arrow*), lower in attenuation compared to the liver metastases is noted and indeterminant. MRI imaging of the same patient in different phases (**B–E**). MRI with fat suppressed T2 weighted imaging (**B**), and precontrast fat suppressed T1 weighted imaging (**C**). Same cyst as prior CT (*white arrows*), with markedly T2 bright signal and low T1 signal. MRI with postcontrast fat suppressed T1 weighted imaging during the portal venous phase (**D**) and delayed hepatobiliary phase with Gd-EOB-DTPA (Eovist) contrast agent (**E**). Same cyst as prior CT (*arrows*). Note the subcentimeter liver metastases now visible on delayed hepatobiliary phase in segment 2 and 7/8 (*black arrows*).

remnant (FLR) that will remain following liver resection in a patient with impaired liver function.

Liver function and volume of the FLR are the most commonly used methods to evaluate hepatic reserve in North America. For cirrhotic patients, the Child–Pugh score incorporates albumin, bilirubin, International Normalized Ratio (INR), as well as the presence or absence of ascites and/or encephalopathy as a measure of hepatic reserve (**Table 54.2**). Only Child–Pugh score A and highly selected B patients are candidates for liver resection. The presence of portal hypertension, manifested by splenomegaly, varices, ascites, or thrombocytopenia, is an independent predictor of postoperative liver failure, and patients with these comorbidities are not candidates for liver resection. Other scores of liver function, including the Model of End-Stage Liver Disease (MELD) score, have limited use for predicting liver failure following resection and are not routinely used to determine suitability for liver resection (**Table 54.3**). For patients with liver

Table 54.1. Strategies to Predict Hepatic Reserve

- Child–Pugh score (Table 54.2) to assess synthetic ability (albumin, prothrombin time, and ascites), bile conjugation and excretory function (total bilirubin), and metabolic function (changes in mental status from ammonia retention)
- Model for end-stage liver disease (MELD) score estimates 3-mo mortality in patients with chronic liver disease (Table 54.3)
- Clearance of galactose or organic anionic dyes, such as indocyanine green (ICG)
- Volumetric measurements of the liver and prediction of liver remnant after resection based on three-dimensional reconstructions from computed tomography and magnetic resonance imaging

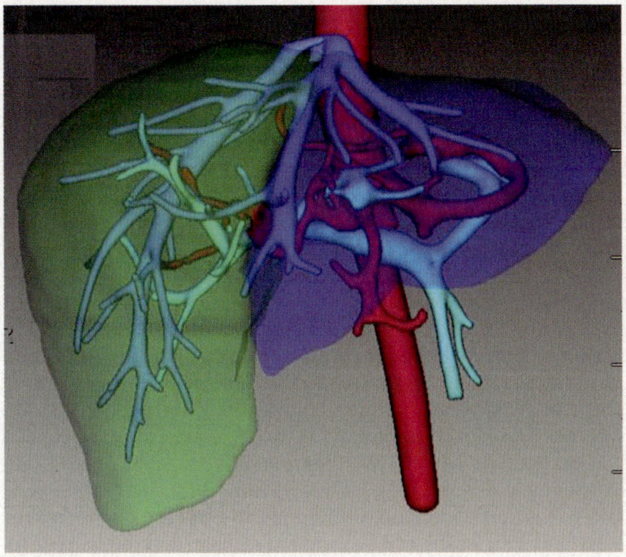

Figure 54.16. Three-dimensional reconstruction of the hepatic vasculature.

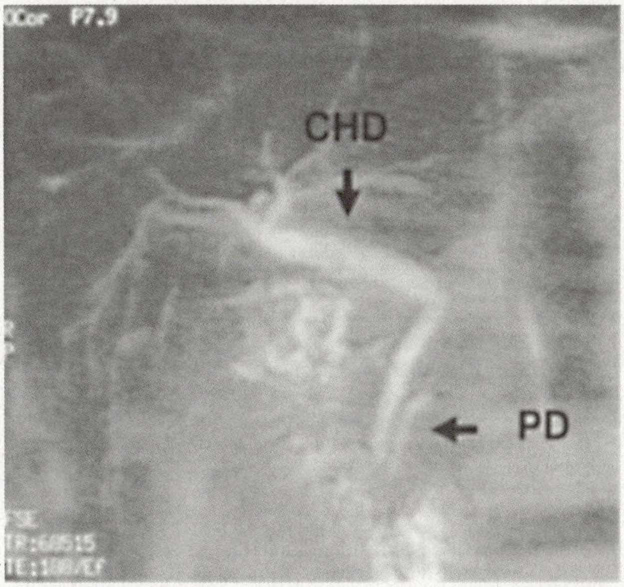

Figure 54.17. Magnetic resonance cholangiopancreatography (MRCP) of a patient after cholecystectomy with mild dilation of common hepatic duct (CHD). The pancreatic duct (PD) is also visible.

cancer or end-stage liver disease, the MELD score is useful for establishing eligibility for liver transplant, and MELD is currently used by the United Network for Organ Sharing (UNOS) for prioritizing organ allocation for liver transplants.

Worldwide, ICG retention is a common dynamic test of hepatic reserve. ICG is a tricarbocyanine protein-bound dye that is rapidly eliminated by the liver. Impaired liver function results in slower elimination times, and thus ICG retention provides a dynamic measure of liver function. In a normal liver, ICG retention at 15 minutes (ICG-R15) is 1% to 10%.

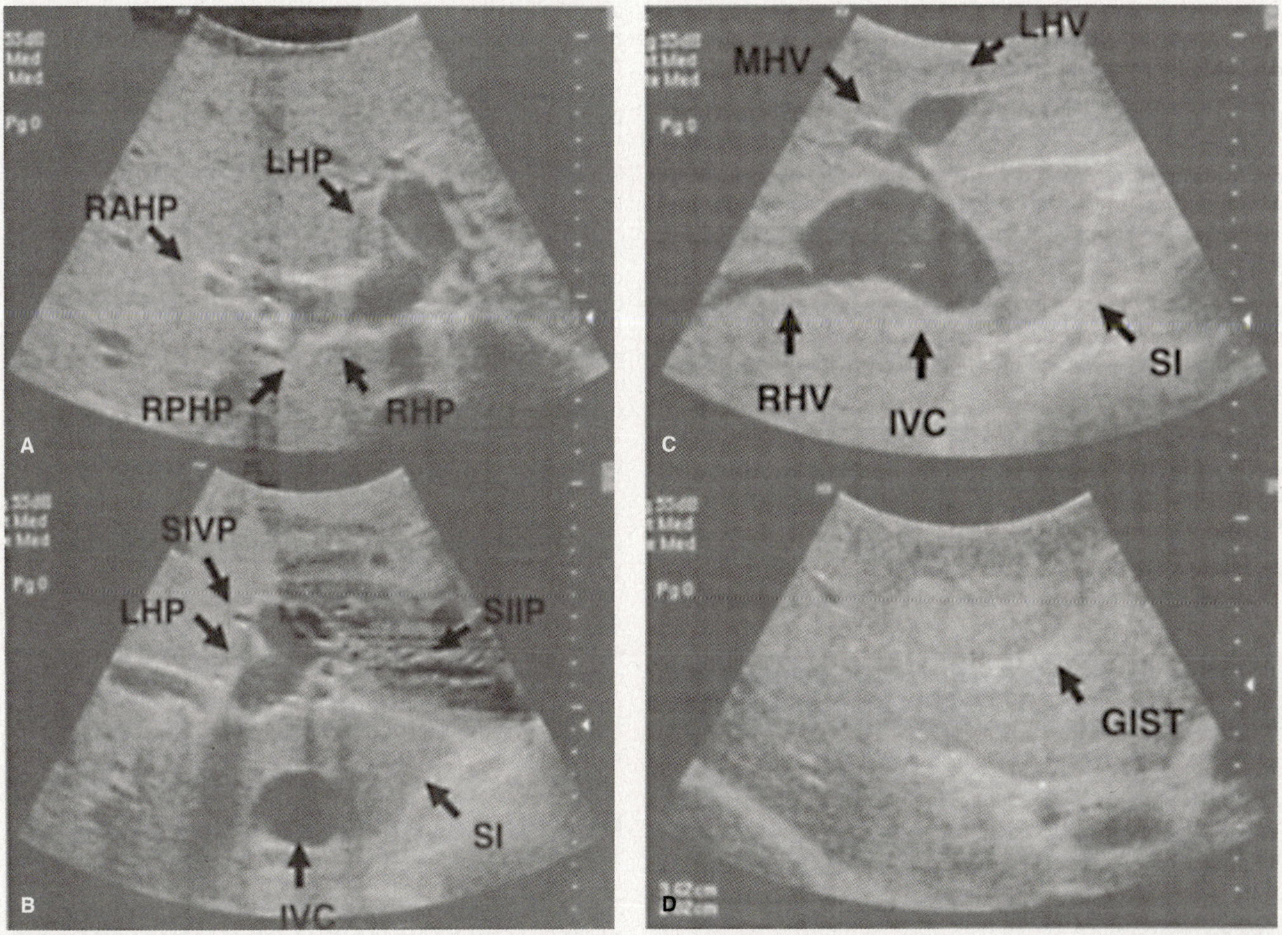

Figure 54.18. **A, B:** Intraoperative ultrasound images of liver demonstrating right hepatic pedicle (RHP), right anterior sector pedicle (RASP), right posterior sector pedicle (RPSP), left hepatic pedicle (LHP), segment II pedicle (SIIP), segment IV pedicle (SIVP), segment I (SI), and inferior vena cava (IVC). **C, D:** Intraoperative ultrasound images of liver demonstrating inferior vena cava (IVC), right hepatic vein (RHV), middle hepatic vein (MHV), left hepatic vein (LHV), segment I (SI), and a metastatic gastrointestinal stromal tumor lesion straddling segments IV and V of the liver.

Table 54.2. Child–Pugh Classification

	1 Point	2 Points	3 Points
Bilirubin (mg/dL)	<2	2–3	>3
Albumin (g/dL)	>3.5	2.8–3.5	<2.8
Ascites	Absent	Moderate	Severe
Encephalopathy	Absent	Moderate	Severe
Prothrombin time			
Seconds prolonged	<4	4–6	>6
INR	<1.7	1.7–2.3	>2.3

INR, international normalized ratio; Child–Pugh Class A: 5–6 points; Class B: 7–9 points; Class C: 10–15 points.

ICG-R15 of <10% is considered adequate hepatic reserve for major liver resection in cirrhotic patients. The acceptable ICG-R15 must be combined with additional clinical information, including the extent of the planned liver resection, the Child–Pugh score, and the presence or absence of portal hypertension, to estimate the risk of postoperative liver failure for an individual patient.

The volume of the expected FLR is associated with the risk of postoperative liver failure. For patients with normal background liver, an FLR >25% is adequate, as long as inflow/outflow and biliary drainage are preserved. For patients with liver disease, including cirrhosis, cholestasis, fatty liver disease, or prior chemotherapy, the threshold suggested for adequate FLR should be higher, closer to 40%. However, the exact threshold is not agreed upon by all surgeons. For patients with small predicted FLR and/or in cases where there is underlying hepatic dysfunction, augmentation of the FLR is possible. Liver augmentation strategies such as portal vein embolization, liver deprivation therapy (portal vein embolization and hepatic vein embolization), or associating liver and portal vein ligation for staged hepatectomy (ALPPS) can be used to induce hypertrophy in the FLR prior to hepatectomy. Portal vein embolization is performed on the side of the liver to be resected 3 to 4 weeks prior to planned resection to induce compensatory hypertrophy. Liver deprivation therapy is a newer strategy, which combines portal vein embolization with hepatic vein embolization to further promote FLR hypertrophy. ALPPS combines operative portal vein ligation with parenchymal transection to induce rapid FLR hypertrophy. This is followed by planned early hepatectomy, days after ALPPS, once FLR volume is deemed adequate. The ALLPS approach has higher rates of morbidity and perioperative mortality compared to percutaneous portal vein embolization. In turn, ALLPS is reserved for highly selected situations.

Table 54.3. MELD Score

MELD = 3.78 × ln[serum bilirubin (mg/dL)] + 11.2 × ln[INR] + 9.57 × ln[serum creatinine (mg/dL)]
40 or more—71.3% 3-mo mortality
30–39—52.6% 3-mo mortality
20–29—19.6% 3-mo mortality
10–19—6.0% 3-mo mortality
<9—1.9% 3-mo mortality

INDICATIONS FOR LIVER RESECTION AND ONCOLOGIC CONSIDERATIONS

The indications for surgery include benign and malignant tumors, biliary conditions, and living-donor liver transplant. The vast majority of liver resections are performed for malignancy for curative intent. Colorectal liver metastases (CRLM) and HCC are the most common malignant indications for hepatectomy. The evaluation of patients for oncologic indications requires consideration of patient fitness for surgery, as well as oncologic and technical criteria. Oncologic principles for curative-intent surgery are that disease is limited to the liver, the resection can be performed for R0 intent, and an FLR with adequate volume/function, liver inflow, outflow, and biliary drainage can be achieved. The indications for resection and the principles of surgery remain the same regardless of whether an open or minimally invasive approach is selected.

For patients with CRLM, preoperative staging to rule out extrahepatic disease includes a CT scan of the chest, abdomen, and pelvis, and a recent colonoscopy to evaluate disease stage. MRI and PET scans are adjuvant tests that may be helpful to characterize the disease extent, but are not routinely required. Also, prognostic variables, such as timing of liver metastases (synchronous vs. metachronous), nodal status of colorectal cancer, CEA levels, and number and size of liver metastases, may guide when or if liver resection is likely to provide a survival advantage.[6] The sequence of liver resection with respect to the timing of chemotherapy and management of the primary colorectal cancer must also be incorporated into a tailored approach for each patient. The goal of resection for CRLM is to obtain an R0 margin, optimally >1 cm, using parenchymal-sparing techniques when possible.[7] The rationale for a parenchymal-sparing approach is that it will preserve liver function and allow repeat liver resection for patients who develop recurrent CRLM. For patients with multiple CRLM, ablation may be combined with resection for small, central tumors where resection is not feasible to achieve disease control.

For patients with HCC, there is an additional requirement to understand the extent of underlying cirrhosis, which is often present. Impaired liver function may preclude liver resection of otherwise technically resectable tumors due to the high risk of postoperative liver failure. As these patients may be candidates for liver transplantation, the decision for resection versus transplantation should be made in a multidisciplinary context. For patients undergoing liver resection for HCC, the optimal resection margin is controversial. However, a resection margin aimed at approximately 2 cm is associated with decreased postoperative recurrence rates and improved survival compared with a gross resection margin of 1 cm or less.[8] Some studies favor formal anatomic resections for improved outcomes.

For less common malignancies, a decision-making process analogous to those described above is applicable. Palliative debulking of liver tumors is rare but may be considered for select patients with metastatic neuroendocrine tumors, as these tumors are more indolent than most other malignancies. As a result, liver resection may provide symptomatic control, as well as a survival advantage. Liver metastasectomy for neuroendocrine metastases is based on the ability to debulk tumor volume. The threshold of tumor that needs to be removed for benefit remains controversial; generally, debulking may provide benefit if >90% tumor volume can be debulked safely.

NOMENCLATURE FOR HEPATECTOMIES

Standard terminology should be used to document the extent of liver resection performed. The International Hepato–Pancreato–Biliary Association has endorsed the Brisbane classification as the preferred nomenclature.[9] This naming system sorts liver resections based on first-, second-, or third-order divisions of the hepatic artery and bile ducts. Resections at the level of first-order divisions are termed *hepatectomies* or *hemihepatectomies* (**Fig. 54.19**). Thus, a left hepatectomy

1 *First-order division*

Anatomical Term	Couinaud segments referred to	Term for surgical resection	Diagram (pertinent area is shaded)
Right Hemiliver **OR** *Right Liver*	*Sg 5–8(+/–Sg1)*	*Right Hepatectomy* **OR** *Right Hemihepatectomy* (stipulate +/–segment 1)	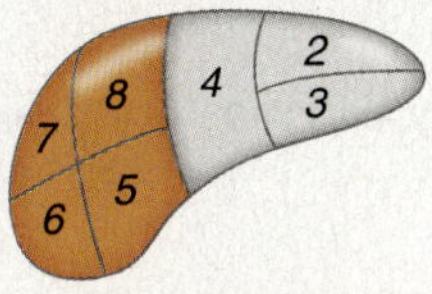
Left Hemiliver **OR** *Left Liver*	*Sg 2–4(+/–Sg1)*	*Left Hepatectomy* **OR** *Left Hemihepatectomy* (stipulate +/–segment 1)	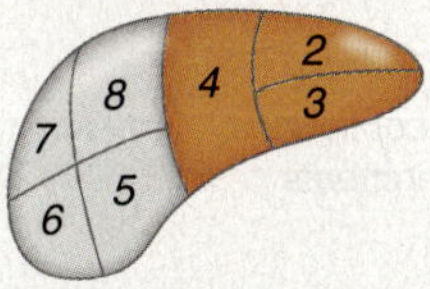

Border or watershed: The border or watershed of the first-order division which separates the two hemilivers is a plane which intersects the gallbladder fossa and the fossa for the IVC and is called the midplane of the liver.

2 *Second-order division* (second-order division based on bile ducts and hepatic artery)

Anatomical Term	Couinaud segments referred to	Term for surgical resection	Diagram (pertinent area is shaded)
Right Anterior Section	*Sg 5, 8*	Add (-ectomy) to any of the anatomical terms as in *Right anterior sectionectomy*	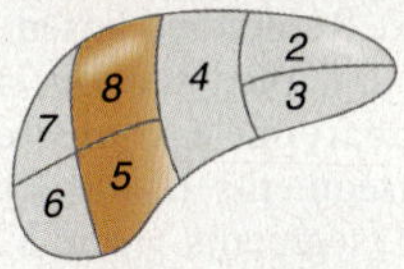
Right Posterior Section	*Sg 6, 7*	*Right posterior sectionectomy*	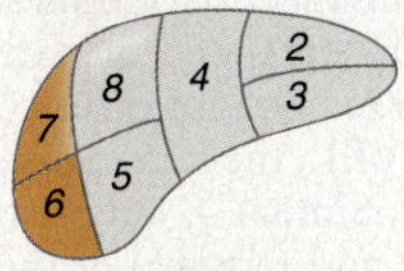
Left Medial Section	*Sg 4*	*Left medial sectionectomy* OR *Resection segment 4* (also see Third order) OR *Segmentectomy 4* (also see Third order)	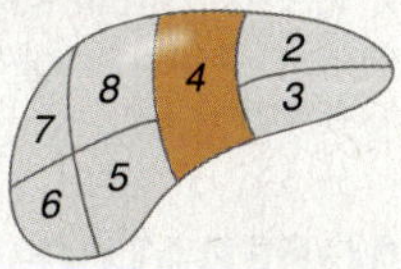
Left Lateral Section	*Sg 2, 3*	*Left lateral sectionectomy* OR *Bisegmentectomy 2, 3* (also see Third order)	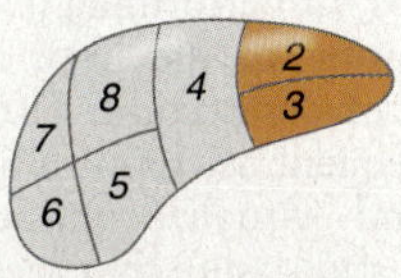

Other "sectional" liver resections

	Couinaud segments referred to	Term for surgical resection	Diagram
	Sg 4–8 (+/–Sg1)	*Right Trisectionectomy* *(preferred term)* or *Extended Right Hepatectomy* or *Extended Right Hemihepatectomy* (stipulate +/–segment 1)	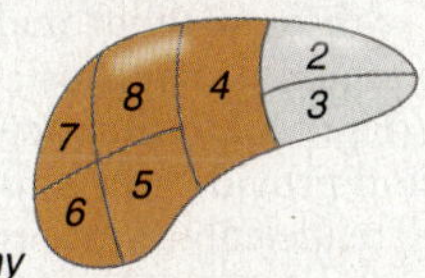
	Sg 2,3,4,5,8 (+/–Sg1)	*Left Trisectionectomy* *(preferred term)* or *Extended Left Hepatectomy* or *Extended Left Hemihepatectomy* (stipulate +/–segment 1)	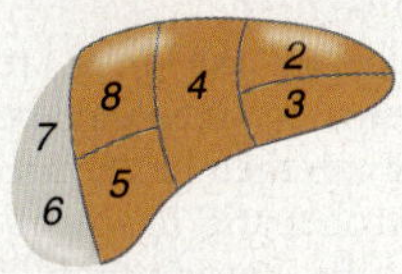

Border or watershed: The borders or watersheds of the sections are planes referred to as the *right and left intersectional planes.* The left intersectional plane passes through the umbilical fissure and the attachment of the falciform ligament. There is no surface marking of the right intersectional plane.

Figure 54.19. The Brisbane terminology of liver anatomy and resections. (Reused with permission from Strasberg SM, Belghiti J, Clavien PA, et al. The Brisbane 2000 Terminology of liver anatomy and resections. *HPB.* 2000;2(3):333–339.) *(continued)*

3	Third-order division		
Anatomical Term	**Couinaud segments referred to**	**Term for surgical resection**	**Diagram (pertinent area is shaded)**
Segments 1–9	*Any one of Sg 1 to 9*	*Segmentectomy* (eg, segmentectomy 6)	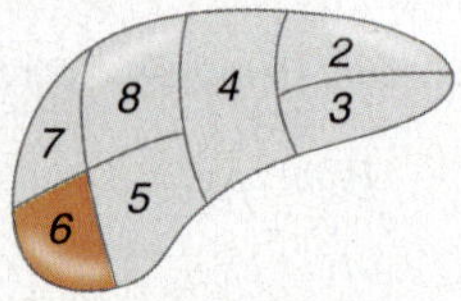
Two contiguous segments	*Any two of Sg 1 to Sg 9 in continuity*	*Bisegmentectomy* (eg, bisegmentectomy 5, 6)	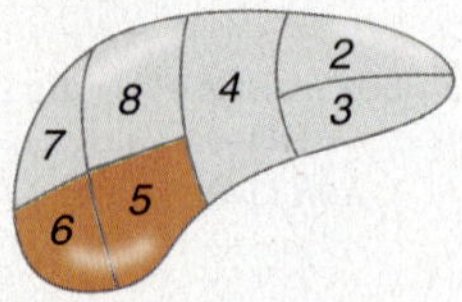

For clarity Sg. 1 and 9 are not shown. It is also acceptable to refer to ANY resection by its third-order segments, eg, right hemihepatectomy can also be called resection Sg 5–8.

Border or watershed: The border or watershed of the segments are planes referred to as intersegmental planes.

Figure 54.19. (*Continued*)

involves the removal of segments II, III, and IV, whereas a right hepatectomy involves removal of segments V, VI, VII, and VIII. Resections based on second-order divisions, which remove a named section, are termed *sectionectomies* based on the anatomic sections removed. As a result, there are left lateral (segments II and III), left medial (segment IV), right anterior (segments V and VIII), and right posterior (segments VI and VII) sectionectomies. *Trisectionectomy* is the preferred term for extended hepatectomies. Right trisectionectomy includes removal of three contiguous sections (segments IV, V, VI, VII, VIII), the right posterior, right anterior, and left medial sections. Similarly, left trisectionectomy includes a left hepatectomy and removal of the right anterior sections (segments II, III, IV, V, VIII). Single segment or two contiguous segment resections are termed *segmentectomies* and *bisegmentectomies*, respectively.

INTRAOPERATIVE CONSIDERATIONS

8 The steps for performing liver resections include exposure and mobilization of the liver, inflow and outflow control, and parenchymal resection. Throughout any hepatectomy procedure, frequent use of intraoperative US should be used to help map and visualize intraparenchymal structures, localize tumors, and ensure that the plane of parenchymal transection is appropriate.

Open hepatectomy requires unobscured access to the liver. This can be achieved with a midline incision or right subcostal incision with or without midline extension. When additional access is required, a subcostal incision can be extended to the left side (**Fig. 54.20**). Retractors are used to elevate the costal margin and provide access to the entire right upper quadrant. Reverse Trendelenburg position can improve exposure to the sub-diaphragmatic region. On occasion, when suprahepatic access is required, intrathoracic extension or midline sternotomy can be used.

Mobilizing the liver requires dividing its ligamentous attachments between the abdominal wall and retroperitoneum. The liver can then be elevated off the bare area, when required. The gastrohepatic ligament can also be divided to access the caudate lobe. During mobilization, accessory vessels should be noted and avoided. In particular, care should be taken to avoid an accessory or replaced left hepatic artery that runs in the gastrohepatic ligament. Palpation of the hepatoduodenal ligament can reveal an accessory or replaced right hepatic artery running posterior and medial to the common bile duct.

With the liver mobilized, visual inspection, palpation, and US of the liver and hepatoduodenal ligament should be performed to confirm preoperative findings and identify any new findings which may not have been noted on preoperative evaluation. This includes assessment of the background liver, as well as the number, size, and position of tumors. The location of lesions compared to the known hepatic anatomy should be assessed, and anatomic landmarks should be confirmed by US as the procedure progresses. Occasionally, operative cholangiography can supplement anatomic mapping of the biliary tree.

Safe hepatic surgery depends on the ability to minimize and control hemorrhage from the liver parenchyma during transection. The ability to obtain hepatic arterial and portal venous control is key technical step in liver resection.

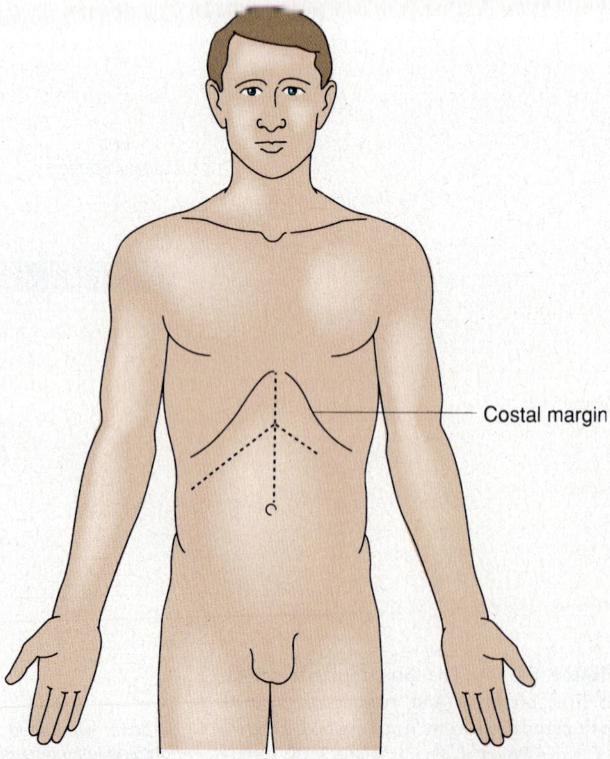

Figure 54.20. Incisions used for open hepatic resection.

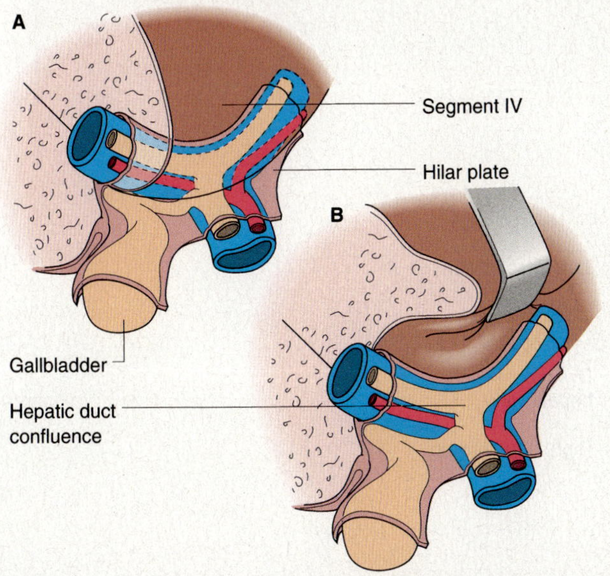

Figure 54.21. Lowering the hilar plate. **A:** The inferior border of segment IV overlies the hepatic duct confluence. **B:** Division of the connective tissue investment allows elevation of segment IV, which results in a "lower" hilar plate and surgical exposure to the hepatic duct confluence.

Temporary inflow control can be obtained using the Pringle maneuver, which is usually performed in an intermittent manner with occlusion of the hepatic artery and portal inflow with compression of the hepatoduodenal ligament. More selective inflow control can be obtained either with an intrahepatic Glissonean or an extrahepatic Glissonean approach to individual pedicles of interest.

Major hepatectomies based on first- or second-order divisions require removal of three or more segments. For these resections, exposure is obtained by taking down the liver attachments to fully mobilize and expose the lobe of interest. Permanent hepatic inflow control is obtained prior to parenchymal transection. For an intrafascial approach, the Glissonean capsule is incised to expose the hepatic artery, portal vein, and bile duct of interest. The hepatic arteries and portal veins are individually ligated and divided to obtain permanent selective inflow control. An endovascular stapler can safely and efficiently divide major vessels and biliary pedicles and should be used liberally in liver surgery. The intrafascial Glissonean approach also allows identification of the extrahepatic biliary system. Division of the biliary system can be accomplished either intra- or extrahepatically, depending on the length of the involved bile duct. Since the left biliary system has a long transverse-lying extrahepatic segment, it is usually straightforward to divide the left biliary system for a left hemihepatectomy. The right biliary system has a shorter extrahepatic component, and therefore it is sometimes necessary to divide the right bile duct within the liver parenchyma for a right hemihepatectomy. For more extensive hilar dissections, dropping the hilar plate by incising the peritoneum of the hepatoduodenal ligament at the base of segment IV may allow access to the structures at the cephalad aspect of the hepatoduodenal ligament (**Fig. 54.21**).

Some surgeons prefer an extrahepatic Glissonean pedicle approach to isolate the portal structures. In this method, the portal pedicles are accessed by performing hepatotomies near the hilar plate to encircle the portal pedicles between the Glissonean capsule and Laennec capsule, the membrane that covers the liver parenchyma (**Fig. 54.22**). There are six extrahepatic "gates" that can be accessed (**Fig. 54.22**).[10] The Glissonean pedicle approach also allows selective inflow control, either on a temporary or permanent basis. In this method, the biliary structures are divided en mass with the vascular pedicle of interest. An advantage of this approach is that variant biliary and hepatic artery anatomy lies within the Glissonean pedicle and easily controlled using this method.

Using either approach, early inflow control allows ischemic demarcation of the liver along the anatomic lines, which is helpful to guide the extent of resection required.

Outflow control is then obtained. Small veins from the caudate lobe to the IVC are individually divided to mobilize the liver off the IVC (**Fig. 54.13**). The hepatic vein of interest can then be encircled and divided with an endovascular stapler (**Figs. 54.23** and **54.24**). For left hepatectomies, formal division of the ligamentum venosum, which runs in Arantius cleft between the posterior left liver and the caudate lobe, provides easy access to the base of the left hepatic vein and facilitates control of this structure.

Parenchymal transection should be performed under low central venous pressure (CVP) conditions (<5 mm Hg) to minimize bleeding from the parenchymal surface.[11] The Pringle maneuver can also be used, either selectively or routinely, to further reduce blood loss and maintain clear visualization of the intraparenchymal structures during transection. Large intraparenchymal structures should be divided formally with sutures, clips, or staples to minimize bleeding and bile leak. A variety of techniques are used for parenchymal transection, including crush clamp, ultrasonic or waterjet dissectors, energy devices (monopolar, ultrasonic, or bipolar), and staplers. No single technique has been demonstrated to be clearly superior; thus, surgeons should be familiar with a variety of techniques.

Minor hepatectomies include resection of smaller volumes of liver, but the name is a misnomer, as these resections are often technically challenging and require a more informed understanding of the intraparenchymal structures to ensure safe resection. In the modern era, a parenchymal-sparing

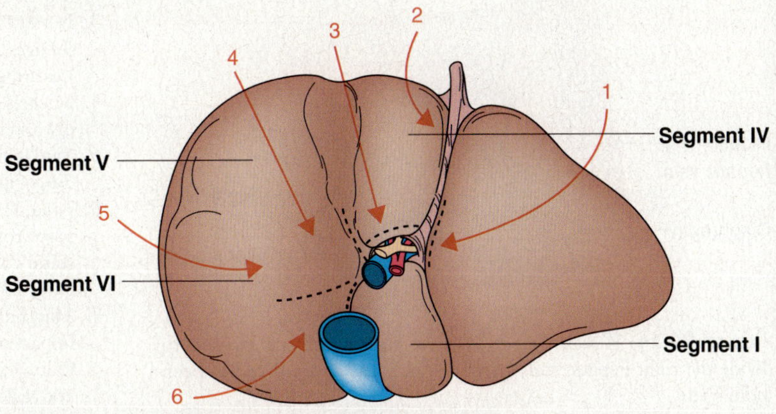

Figure 54.22. Hepatotomies to access pedicles for ligation: right hepatectomy, 4, 5, and 6; left lateral sectionectomy, 1 and 2; left hepatectomy, 1 and 3; right anterior sectorectomy, 4 and 5; and right posterior sectorectomy, 5 and 6.

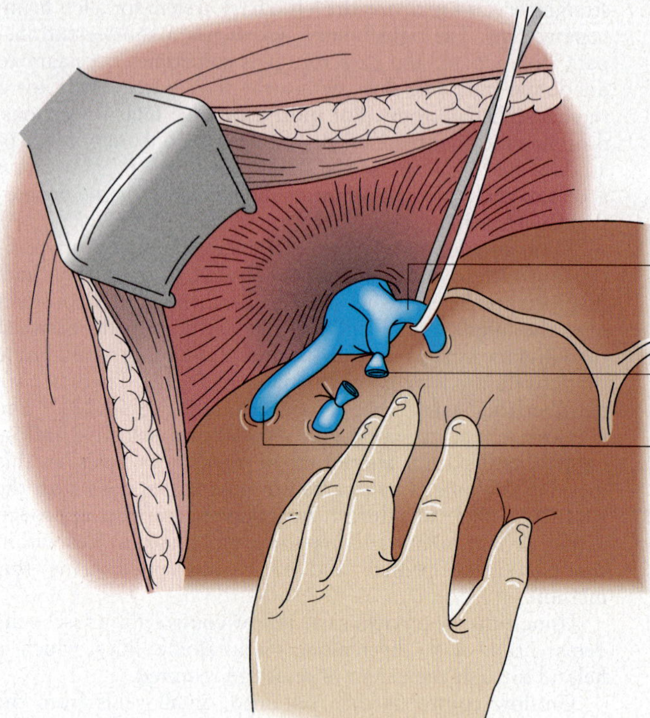

Figure 54.23. Caudal retraction of the left hepatic lobe with division of middle and left hepatic veins during left hepatic lobectomy. Often, the division of the middle and left hepatic veins is intraparenchymal.

approach is favored to preserve the FLR and allow repeat resection in the future and/or preserve liver function. In these cases, exposure and mobilization follow the same principles as discussed above, but unlike major hepatectomies, the vascular inflow and outflow structures are often within the liver. As a result, definitive inflow and outflow control is often not possible prior to parenchymal transection. Since parenchymal transection and vascular control occur concurrently, temporary inflow control with Pringle maneuver and low CVP conditions are even more important for these procedures. Parenchymal transection is performed to allow exposure and control of intrahepatic structures as they are encountered.

Once resection has been completed, the FLR and the cut edge of the liver are inspected. Any bleeding points or open biliary radicals should be oversewn, and hemostasis along the cut surface should be confirmed. The falciform ligament should be reconstructed to avoid postoperative liver torsion.

There has been major advancement in liver surgery technique with the availability of minimally invasive hepatectomy.[12]

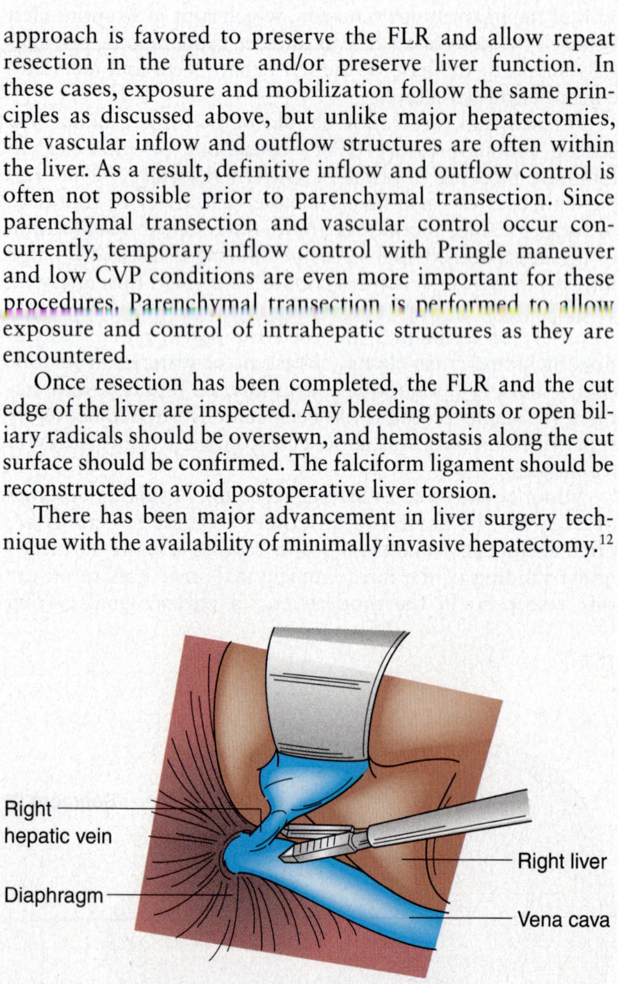

Figure 54.24. A vascular endoscopic stapling device is used to divide the right hepatic vein after the right side of the liver has been mobilized.

Minor hepatectomies in safe zone areas[13]—peripherally based lesions in segment II—VI—are performed using a minimally invasive approach at many centers. With growing experience, the use of minimally invasive techniques for formal hemihepatectomies, as well as posterior or superior lesions (segments I, IV, VII, VIII), is increasing. The minimally invasive approach provides a different anatomic view of the liver. Unlike an open procedure, which provides a ventral approach to the liver, the liver is often seen in a caudal–cranial view during minimally invasive right hepatectomy.[14] As a result, surgeons performing minimally invasive hepatectomies must be intimately familiar with how intraparenchymal structures appear from this perspective. There are several benefits of a minimally invasive approach, including improved postoperative recovery, decreased length of stay, and earlier return to full activity. Minimally invasive surgery can be approached using a pure laparoscopic, hand-assisted, hybrid, or robotic-assisted approaches.

References

1. Couinaud C, Le F. *Etudes anatomiques et chirugicales*. Massori; 1957:400–409.
2. Blumgart LH, Fong Y. *Surgery of the Liver and Biliary Tract*. 3rd ed. Vol 1. W. B. Saunders; 2000.
3. Netter FH. *The Netter Collection of Medical Illustrations. Volume 3 Digestive system. Part III. Liver, Biliary Tract and Pancreas*. Icon Learning Systems; 1957.
4. Michels NA. Newer anatomy of the liver and its variant blood supply and collateral circulation. *Am J Surg*. 1966;112(3):337–347.
5. VanDamme JP. Behavioral anatomy of the abdominal arteries. *Surg Clin North Am*. 1993;73(4):699–725.
6. Fong Y, Fortner J, Sun RL, Brennan MF, Blumgart LH. Clinical score for predicting recurrence after hepatic resection for metastatic colorectal cancer: analysis of 1001 consecutive cases. *Ann Surg*. 1999;230(3):309–318; discussion 318-21.
7. Margonis GA, Sergentanis TN, Ntanasis-Stathopoulos I, et al. Impact of surgical margin width on recurrence and overall survival following R0 hepatic resection of colorectal metastases: a systematic review and meta-analysis. *Ann Surg*. 2018;267(6):1047–1055.

8. Shi M, Guo RP, Lin XJ, et al. Partial hepatectomy with wide versus narrow resection margin for solitary hepatocellular carcinoma: a prospective randomized trial. *Ann Surg*. 2007;245(1):36–43.
9. Strasberg SM, Belghiti J, Clavien PA, et al. The Brisbane 2000 Terminology of liver anatomy and resections. *HPB*. 2000;2(3): 333–339.
10. Sugioka A, Kato Y, Tanahashi Y. Systematic extrahepatic Glissonean pedicle isolation for anatomical liver resection based on Laennec's capsule: proposal of a novel comprehensive surgical anatomy of the liver. *J Hepatobiliary Pancreat Sci*. 2017;24(1):17–23.
11. Melendez JA, Arslan V, Fischer ME, et al. Perioperative outcomes of major hepatic resections under low central venous pressure anesthesia: blood loss, blood transfusion, and the risk of postoperative renal dysfunction. *J Am Coll Surg*. 1998;187(6): 620–625.
12. Wakabayashi G, Cherqui D, Geller DA, et al. Recommendations for laparoscopic liver resection: a report from the second international consensus conference held in Morioka. *Ann Surg*. 2015;261(4): 619–629.
13. Ban D, Tanabe M, Ito H, et al. A novel difficulty scoring system for laparoscopic liver resection. *J Hepatobiliary Pancreat Sci*. 2014;21(10):745–753.
14. Soubrane O, Schwarz L, Cauchy F, et al. A conceptual technique for laparoscopic right hepatectomy based on facts and oncologic principles: the Caudal approach. *Ann Surg*. 2015;261(6): 1226–1231.

55

Hepatic Infection and Acute Liver Failure

Ola Ahmed and Maria Bernadette Majella Doyle

Key Points

1. Liver abscesses are the most common type of visceral abscess.
2. Acute liver failure (ALF) is characterized by hepatic encephalopathy and impaired coagulation (INR > 1.5) in the absence of any underlying or preexisting liver disease.
3. Liver disease etiology influences management, outcomes, and overall prognosis.
4. Viral and acetaminophen are the most common causes of ALF in adults.
5. While biologic and nonbiologic liver support systems are still under experimentation, liver transplant is the only curative treatment of choice in cases of irreversible liver failure.

PYOGENIC LIVER ABSCESS

Prevalence and Pathogenesis

Pyogenic liver abscesses result from bacterial infections and most commonly develop from intra-abdominal contamination of bowel contents, subsequently disseminating to the liver through portal circulation or contiguous spreading following biliary infections (**Fig. 55.1**). Abscesses may also occasionally arise directly from penetrating wounds or surgical procedures.
1 These specific infections account for 13% of intra-abdominal abscesses with an annual incidence of 2.3 cases per 100,000 persons with a slight predominance among male patients.[1,2] See also **Table 55.1**.[3–5]

Clinical Manifestations

See **Table 55.2**.

Diagnosis

Abdominal imaging with ultrasound (US) and computed tomography (CT) are appropriate diagnostic modalities for abscess identification, though a chest x-ray may reveal a right pleural effusion or an elevated hemidiaphragm in 50% of cases. Abdominal US can diagnose pyogenic abscesses in almost 90% of cases and can guide diagnostic or therapeutic drainage. CT is more sensitive than US (95% vs. 85%), will reveal small abscesses and further differentiate these lesions from other pathologies.[6] When CT scanning is done, intravenous contrast should be used if there are no patient contraindications. Alternative diagnostic modalities include magnetic resonance imaging (MRI) or tagged white blood cell scans, which are less common.

Blood cultures are positive in up to 50% of cases and are important diagnostic elements. These should be ideally drawn prior to antibiotic therapy. Standard serum analyses such as complete blood counts, electrolytes, renal profiles, and liver function testing are also performed to determine the degree of systemic infection and for evidence of any potential concomitant organ injury. Serologic and fecal testing of *Entamoeba histolytica* is also considered in the diagnostic workup of patients with epidemiologic risk factors.

Image-guided drainage of suspected abscesses is performed to confirm the diagnosis and the involved bacterial pathogens. Aspirate material is sent for gram staining and culture to help guide therapy.

Microbiology

Most pyogenic liver abscesses are polymicrobial, consisting of a combination of enteric and anaerobic pathogens. The most commonly identified pathogens are *Escherichia coli* and *Klebsiella pneumonia*. Streptococci species are also important causes of liver abscesses as well as *Staphylococcus aureus*. Candida coinfection can also arise in immunocompromised states.

Treatment

Multimodal treatment is essential for resolution of pyogenic liver abscesses. Drainage is both diagnostic and therapeutic and should always be considered when feasible. Drainage

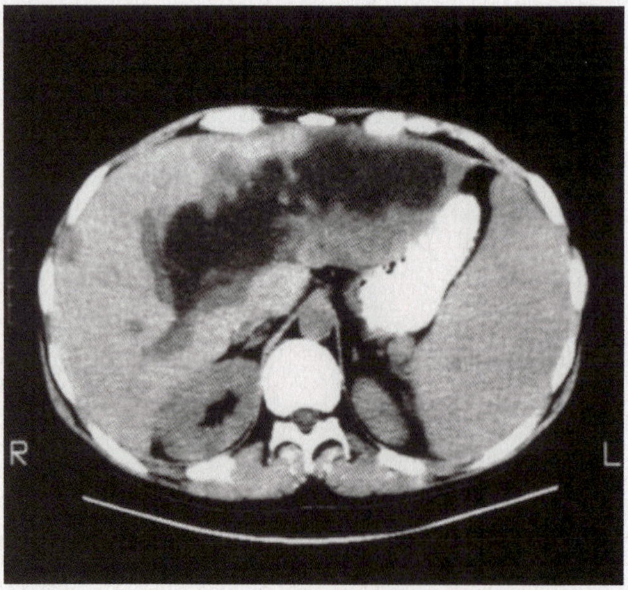

Figure 55.1. Computed tomogram of a pyogenic hepatic abscess in a liver transplant recipient with occlusion of the hepatic artery.

Table 55.1. Risk Factors: Pyogenic Liver Abscess

Risk Factors
Diabetes mellitus
Preexisting hepatobiliary or pancreatic disease
Invasive hepatic/intra-abdominal procedures
GI infections
Liver resections/transplantation
Loss of gastric acid production/atrophic gastritis
GI malignancy[3–5]

can be performed using CT/US-guided percutaneous techniques, surgically via an open or laparoscopic approach, or by endoscopic retrograde cholangiopancreatography (ERCP). Drainage catheters should remain in place until output is minimal, which is usually up to 7 days. Empiric antibiotic therapy should be administered pending microbiologic culture and sensitivity analysis. Coverage should be broad to include streptococci, enteric gram-negative bacilli, and anaerobes and guided by microbiologic expertise. Once culture and sensitivity results are available, directed therapy should be initiated, and duration is based on clinical response. A typical course is 14 days of parenteral therapy followed by oral medication for a total of 6 weeks.[7]

AMEBIC LIVER ABSCESS

Prevalence and Pathogenesis

Amebic liver abscesses are the most common extraintestinal manifestations of amebiasis caused by the protozoan *E. histolytica* (**Fig. 55.2**). Amebiasis is most prevalent in tropical and subtropical regions with poor sanitation, and fecal–oral transmission is the most common route of infection. In developed countries, it can occur in migrants from endemic areas. Most infections are asymptomatic, but amebic dysentery and pulmonary, cardiac, and brain involvement can occur, along with hepatic abscess formation.

Men are affected 10 times more commonly than women, with peak incidence in the third to fifth decade of life, and corticosteroid usage is a risk factor.[8] Ingested cysts pass through the stomach and reach the intestine. There, the cyst wall is degraded and trophozoites are released. These infective particles multiply in the colonic lumen and then may enter mesenteric veins and eventually the liver. Amebic trophozoites then

Table 55.2. Clinical Manifestations: Pyogenic Liver Abscess

Symptoms	Signs	Biochemical Findings
Fever, chills, rigors	Guarding	Leukocytosis
RUQ pain	Rebound tenderness	Transaminitis
Jaundice	Hepatomegaly	Hyperbilirubinemia
Nausea	Cachexia	Hypoalbuminemia
Anorexia		Anemia
Malaise/fatigue		
Weight loss		

RUQ, right upper quadrant.

cause obstruction of venules, thrombosis, and infarction of hepatic parenchyma, with resultant abscess formation.

Risk Factors

Risk factors predisposing to amebic liver abscesses are unclear, although immunocompromised states such as HIV may increase the likelihood of invasive disease. See **Table 55.3**.

Clinical Manifestations

Clinical presentation usually occurs within 8 to 20 weeks following return from endemic areas. See **Table 55.4**.

Diagnosis

Several imaging modalities can be utilized, specifically US, CT, or MRI. Amebic abscesses are more common in the right lobe and tend to be singular. US typically demonstrates a round, well-defined, hypoechoic mass while lesions may show a low-density mass with an enhancing rim. Abscesses appear with a low-signal intensity on T1-weighted images and high signal intensity on T2-weighted images. Elevation of the right hemidiaphragm is evident on 50% of chest radiographs. *E. histolytica* is not found in stool specimens of infected patients, but diagnostic antibodies are present in the serum 7 to 10 days after the onset of symptoms in over 90% of patients.[9] Needle aspiration with imaging modalities can be both diagnostic and therapeutic for large-sized abscesses. Abscess content is typically described as having an "anchovy paste" consistency and is acellular and proteinaceous in substance. Aspirates can be considered for antigen or Polymerase Chain Reaction (PCR) testing.

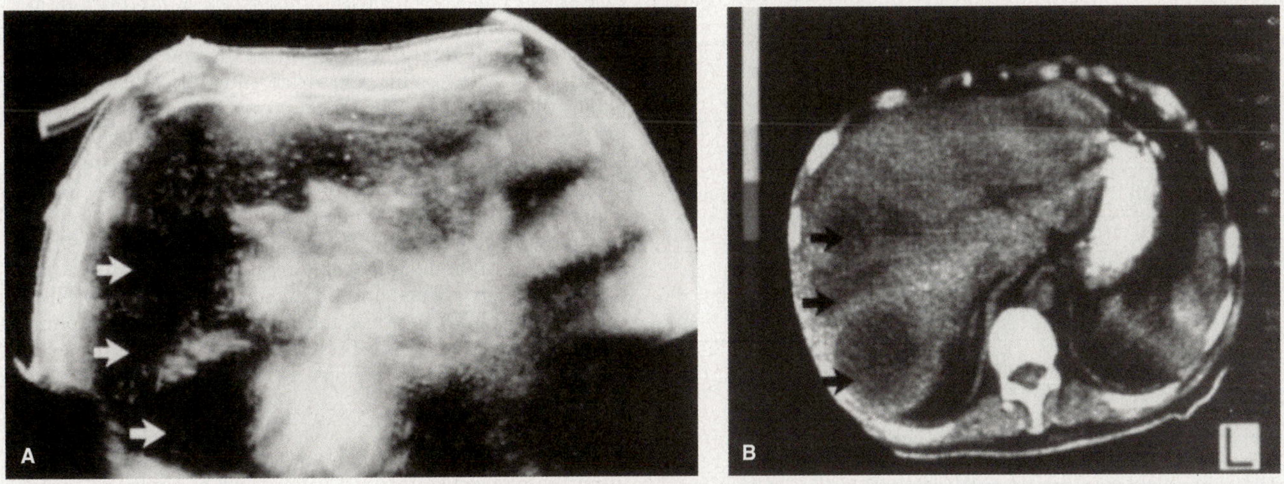

Figure 55.2. Sonogram (**A**) and computed tomogram (**B**) in a patient with multiple amebic abscesses (*arrows*).

Table 55.3. Risk Factors: Amebic Liver Abscess

Males
Endemic areas—India, Africa, Mexico, Central and South America
HIV immunosuppresion

Treatment

Treatment is based on amebicidal drugs to eliminate liver organisms and a luminal agent to eradicate intraluminal cysts. Treatment can be initiated empirically pending further evaluation. Metronidazole 500 mg to 750 mg, three times a day, for 7 to 10 days, is typically first line. Tinidazole 2 g orally for 5 days is an alternative treatment that is oftentimes better tolerated. To eradicate intraluminal cysts, the following regimens can be used: paromomycin (25 to 30 mg/kg/d orally three times a day for 7 days), diiodohydroxyquin (650 mg orally three times a day for 20 days), or diloxanide furoate (500 mg orally three times daily for 10 days for adults). Amebic abscesses can almost always be treated with medical therapy alone, and abscess drainage can be considered in large abscesses or cases of a low or absent clinical response.

ECHINOCOCCUS (HYDATID DISEASE)

Prevalence and Pathogenesis

Echinococcal infection, also called hydatid disease, is a parasitic infection due to echinococcal tapeworms including *Echinococcus granulosus* or *E. multilocularis* in humans. The liver is most commonly affected by *E. granulosus,* but this is typically asymptomatic. Dogs are the definitive host, and the life cycle of the organism is such that when the canine host ingests infected viscera (from sheep or cattle), scoleces released in the intestine develop into adult worms. Humans, an intermediate host, acquire echinococcal eggs by ingestion of contaminated foods or with infected animals. The echinococcal egg is digested in the duodenum and yields an embryo (oncospheres). Embryos invade the intestinal wall and reach the liver via the portal circulation. Surviving embryos lodge in the hepatic capillaries and develop into hydatid cysts. *E. multilocularis* is more commonly associated with alveolar disease.

Risk Factors

The disease is commonly associated with dog and sheep ownership and increasing age.[10]

Table 55.4. Clinical Manifestations: Amebic Liver Abscess

Symptoms	Signs	Biochemical Findings
Fever, chills, rigors, diaphoresis	Guarding	Leukocytosis
RUQ pain	Rebound tenderness	Transaminitis
Cough/hiccough	Hepatomegaly	Hyperbilirubinemia
Sweating	Peritonitis	Elevated alkaline phosphatase
Anorexia		
Malaise/fatigue		
Weight loss		
Diarrhea		

RUQ, right upper quadrant.

Clinical Manifestations

Liver involvement with echinococcal cyst can lead to venous obstruction, portal hypertension, sepsis, and cholangitis. The right lobe is involved in most cases (60% to 85%), and symptoms typically develop when the cyst measures at least 10 cm. This can manifest as hepatomegaly, right upper quadrant pain, nausea, and vomiting. Cysts may grow at an annual rate of around 1 to 3 cm/y. Enlarging cysts can cause symptoms of abdominal pain, biliary obstruction, and jaundice, or less commonly portal hypertension, resulting from mass or pressure effects. Occasionally, cysts may rupture into the peritoneal cavity, causing abdominal pain and anaphylaxis

Diagnosis

Hydatid cysts can be visualized using the previously mentioned imaging techniques: US, CT, and MRI. US reaches a sensitivity of 90% to 95%[11] and typically demonstrates a smooth, anechoic, round cyst with a "hydatid sand" on patient movement.[12] CT imaging has an advantage over US through its ability to demonstrate intraperitoneal rupture and concurrent infection, while MRI may further delineate the cyst capsule.[13] Serologic testing is also used during the initial diagnosis. Antibody testing with ELISA appears to be the most sensitive modality.[14]

Treatment

Surgical resection is the treatment of choice for large or complicated hydatid cysts (rupture, fistulae, compression). Surgical extirpation aims to remove the cyst intact without spillage of cyst contents. Aspiration of cyst contents prior to resection may minimize the result of any cyst spillage. After aspiration injection with ethyl alcohol or 20% sterile saline is undertaken to kill remaining scoleces. In cases where the aspirate is bilious and a communication with the biliary tree is thus suspected, the cyst should be resected without alcohol injection to prevent the occurrence of sclerosing cholangitis. Surgical excision can be performed through open or laparoscopic techniques depending on cyst features and location. Albendazole should be started 4 days prior to surgery and generally continued for at least 4 weeks postoperatively.[15] Mebendazole may be used as an alternative therapy, but is less well absorbed and continued use for at least 3 months postsurgery is advised.[16]

SCHISTOSOMA

Prevalence and Pathogenesis

Schistosoma mansoni, S. japonicum, S. haematobium, and *S. mekongi* are species of the trematode fluke that infect humans in endemic areas or visitors to these sites. Liver disease is especially severe with *S. mansoni, S. japonicum,* and *S. mekongi.* The life cycle of *Schistosoma* species alternates between sexual reproduction in humans and asexual multiplication in water snails. Cercariae enter the human host by penetrating the skin. An irritating maculopapular rash that lasts for several days is an early manifestation of infection. Schistosomes live in the intestinal lumen and eggs reach the liver via the portal circulation, where they cause an inflammatory reaction manifesting as an inflammatory granuloma surrounding a schistosomal egg. The pathogen is most prevalent in central and subtropical areas of sub-Saharan Africa, the Middle East, India, and Southeast Asia.[17] Hepatocellular carcinoma (HCC), colon cancer, and follicular lymphoma of the spleen have been reported in association with hepatic schistosomiasis.[18]

Risk factors

Acute schistosomiasis is seen typically in poor and rural communities exposed to infested waters and nonimmune visitors to endemic areas.

Table 55.5. Classification of Viral Hepatitis

	The Viral Hepatitides				
Virus	**Hep A Picornavirus (RNA)**	**Hep B Hepadnavirus (DNA)**	**Hep C Flavivirus (RNA)**	**Hep D Viroid (RNA)**	**Hep E Calicivirus (RNA)**
Transmission	Fecal–oral	Parenteral	Parenteral	Parenteral	Fecal–oral
Acute disease	Common	Common	Uncommon	Common	Yes
Evolution to chronic disease	Never	Infrequent in adults	Frequent (70%)	Yes	Described in organ transplant recipients
New cases/y	1,400,000	22,100	44,300	Unknown, found in approximately 5% of cases of HBV infection	300
# Infected (United States)	6700	862,000	2,400,000		Unknown, uncommon
Treatment	None	Lamivudine Adefovir Entecavir	Interferon + Ribavirin	Treatment of HBV	Mainly sanitary preventative
Prophylaxis	Vaccine and Ig	Vaccine and Ig	None	Vaccinate against HBV	In development
Fulminant failure	Rare	Yes	Never	With HBV, as coinfection or superinfection	Especially in pregnant women

HBV, hepatitis B virus; Hep, hepatitis; Ig, immunoglobulin.

Clinical Manifestations

While hepatocellular functioning may not be impaired, physical examination may reveal a firm, nodular liver, and features of portal hypertension such as splenomegaly and gastric varices.[19] It is usually asymptomatic until manifestations of portal hypertension declare themselves.

Diagnosis

Diagnosis requires serologic, microscopic and biochemical analysis to detect infection and parasitic burden coupled with standard imaging modalities. Stool (Kato–Katz smears) and urine analysis can allow for microscopic egg detection while antigen testing can be performed on urine analysis to characterize parasitic burden. Serum transaminases are typically normal. Tissue biopsies are useful in the setting of inconclusive diagnostic tools and will show prominent granuloma formation and severe portal fibrosis. Imaging studies are not typically useful in the diagnosis of acute infection. In chronic cases, US may show portal vein wall thickening.[20] Hypertrophy of the left lobe, splenomegaly, and engorged venous collaterals may all be observed as well. CT and MRI may show fibrosis around portal vein branches as well as low-attenuation rings through the liver parenchyma.[21]

Treatment

Preferred treatment of schistosomiasis is praziquantel, with a cure efficacy of around 90%. Follow-up stool or urine microscopy should be performed at 6 weeks in endemic areas and 3 to 6 months following treatment in nonendemic areas. Repeat treatment with praziquantel may be warranted in persistent egg detection.

Viral Hepatitis

Viral hepatitis represents an important cause of acute and chronic liver disease, cirrhosis, and hepatocellular cancer, accounting for more than half of acute hepatitis cases in the United States. In the United States, the most common viral hepatitis are hepatitis A, B and C. Hepatitis C is a leading indication for liver transplant in the United States, and its recurrence has been the most common cause for graft loss after transplant.[22]

The mechanism of liver injury is largely a host inflammatory response to the virus. **Table 55.5** summarizes the current understanding and characteristics of the five viruses most commonly associated with clinical hepatitis, their modes of transmission, and the consequences of infection.

HEPATITIS A VIRUS

Epidemiology/Risk Factors for Transmission

Hepatitis A is generally self-limiting with no risk of chronic infection. This is usually transmitted via the fecal–oral route. Common risk factors for transmission include international travel, consumption of contaminated food and water, and intravenous drug use. The disease can occur sporadically or in epidemic form, and outbreaks are not uncommon. However, incidence in the United States has declined with effective vaccination.

Clinical Features

Fulminant hepatic failure occurs in less than 1% of cases and mostly occurs in patients with underlying liver disease or coinfection. Symptoms are uncommon in children less than 6 years of age and more commonly manifest in adults, occurring in up to 70% of those infected. The incubation period is typically 28 days, ranging from 15 to 50 days (**Fig. 55.3**). See also **Table 55.6**.

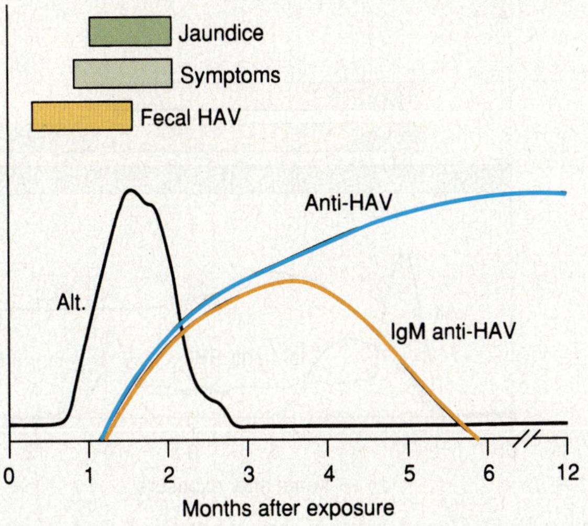

Figure 55.3. Clinical course of hepatitis A infection.

Table 55.6. Clinical Manifestations: Hepatitis A Virus

Symptoms	Signs	Biochemical Findings
Fever	Guarding	Leukocytosis
RUQ pain		Transaminitis
Vomiting		Hyperbilirubinemia
Malaise/fatigue		Elevated alkaline phosphatase
Anorexia		
Jaundice		
Acholic Stools		

RUQ, right upper quadrant.

Treatment

Treatment is mainly supportive, and infection control measures such as hand washing and isolation should be a top priority to prevent the spread of virus. Complete recovery typically occurs at 6 months in all patients. Vaccine protection for specific patient groups is warranted prior to hepatitis A exposure: all children at age one, individuals traveling to endemic areas, those with chronic disease, and HIV.

HEPATITIS B VIRUS

Epidemiology/Risk Factors for Transmission

It is estimated that nearly 2 billion people worldwide were previously or currently infected with hepatitis B, and 248 million are chronic carriers.[23] In the developing world, mother-to-child infection is the most common mode of transmission. In the United States, transmission is primarily through sexual exposure. Infection from intravenous drug use and occupational infections due to percutaneous exposure may also occur. Liver injury is due to the resultant host immune response (Fig. 55.4).

Clinical Features

The incubation period for HBV can last from 1 to 4 months. Clinical features of the virus vary in acute and chronic disease. During the initial acute stage of disease, symptoms can range from subclinical to anicteric hepatitis. Icteric hepatitis occurs in 30 percent of patients while only 0.1% to 0.5% develop fulminant hepatic failure. The presence of serum hepatitis B surface antigen (HBsAg) may precede jaundice. Acute infection is associated with detectable serum HBV DNA, hepatitis B early antigen (HBeAg), and IgM to hepatitis B core. HBeAg is a useful marker of viral replication except in patients with mutant viruses where it may be undetectable despite active replication. In such cases, detection of HBV DNA is diagnostic. The risk of liver failure is proportional to antibody titers of HBcAg and HBsAg. Serum anti-HBc IgM becomes detectable with the onset of jaundice. In most patients, when HBV does not develop into chronic hepatitis, anti-HBc IgM becomes undetectable after 6 months. Chronic hepatitis can be asymptomatic but may ultimately progress to decompensated cirrhosis and other extrahepatic manifestations of disease such as skin rashes, arthralgias, and glomerular disease (Fig. 55.5).

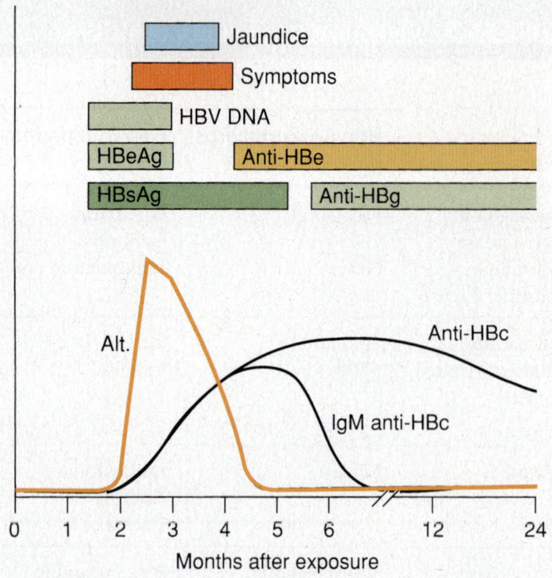

Figure 55.4. Clinical course of acute hepatitis B infection.

Treatment

Treatment for acute HBV is mainly supportive. Further efforts should be taken to prevent exposure and transmission to other individuals. Vaccinations can be offered to high-risk individuals such as health care workers, visitors to highly endemic areas, men who have sex with men, sex workers, and intravenous drug users. The hepatitis B vaccine is given as a series of three intramuscular doses and has almost 100% efficacy

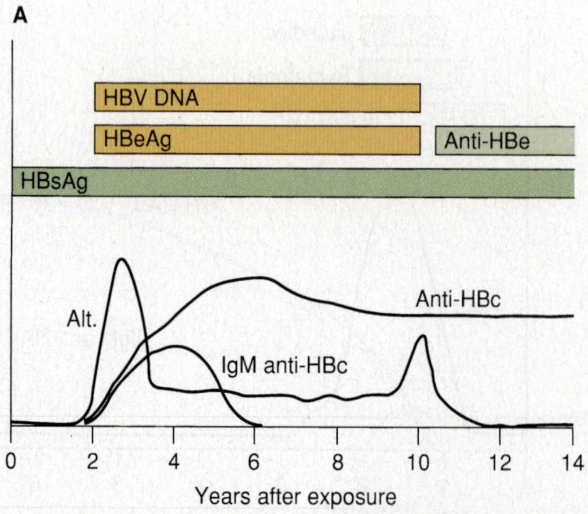

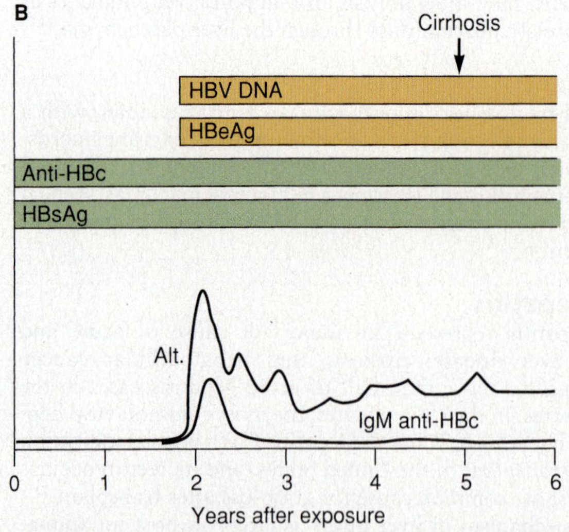

Figure 55.5. Clinical course of chronic hepatitis B. **A:** A benign chronic carrier has continued production of hepatitis B surface antigen, but there is an absence of serum markers of viral replication. **B:** A pattern of continuing liver injury and serum markers of active viral replication.

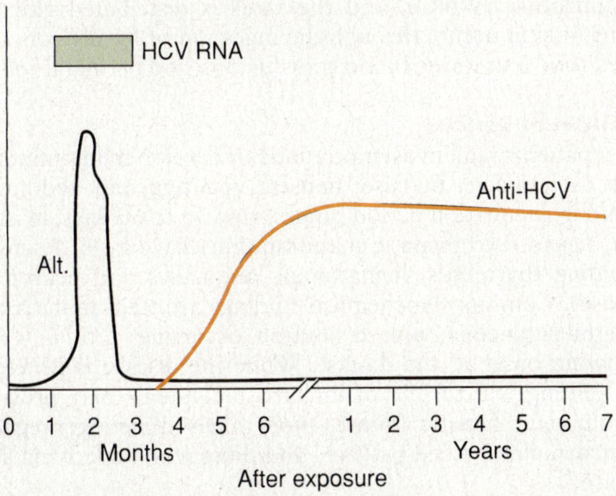

Figure 55.6. Clinical course in acute hepatitis C.

among immunocompetent persons. Hepatitis B immune globulin has a reported efficacy of 90% in the prevention of newborn infections and approximately 75% in cases of needle sticks or sexual infections in people exposed to the virus with no prior immunity. It is administered as soon as possible after exposure together with the first dose of the hepatitis B vaccine series.

Additional treatment options include antiviral therapies such as lamivudine, adefovir dipivoxil, or entecavir as monotherapy. Therapy is usually directed at HBeAg-positive cases that have an increased risk of cirrhosis and HCC. HBeAg-negative patients with a high viral load may also benefit from treatment. Treatment can be stopped following negative identification of HBsAg on two consecutive tests four weeks apart.

Liver transplantation is offered in cases progressing to cirrhosis. Recurrence of viral infection in the allograft can be as high as 80% in HBeAg-positive cases where no postoperative prophylaxis is administered.

HEPATITIS C VIRUS

Epidemiology/Risk Factors for Transmission

The estimated prevalence of hepatitis C worldwide is 177.5 million, almost 2.5% of the population.[24] In the United States alone, 44,300 new infections arise per year with an estimated 2.4 million people infected. Common risk factors are intravenous drug use, homelessness, incarceration, and sexual contact. In addition, the recent opioid epidemic has resulted in an increase in hepatitis C virus (HCV) incidence as well as unhygienic and unsafe tattooing and body piercing (**Fig. 55.6**).

Clinical Features

The HCV incubation period ranges from 15 to 150 days with symptoms commonly developing 5 to 12 weeks following exposure. Up to 80% of cases are asymptomatic. Nonspecific symptoms are seen in the remaining patients, including nausea, diarrhea, abdominal pain, myalgia, and weight loss. Extrahepatic manifestations may arise in a subset of patients, including glomerular disease, autoimmune disorders, and dermatologic conditions.[25] Initial laboratory findings may reveal elevated ALT levels (500 to 1000 IU/mL) and high HCV RNA titers. Between 50% and 85% of patients remain chronically infected, of which 5% to 30% progress to cirrhosis in the following two or three decades. Cirrhotic patients are at a further risk of developing HCC and decompensated failure (**Fig. 55.7**).

The diagnosis of chronic hepatitis C is based on the serologic demonstration of persistent HCV RNA and HCV antibodies. HCV RNA can be detected weeks earlier than antibodies, which typically appear 2 to 8 weeks after the initial infection.

Treatment

Similar to hepatitis B, treatment approaches include preventative measures for further hepatitis C transmission. Individuals

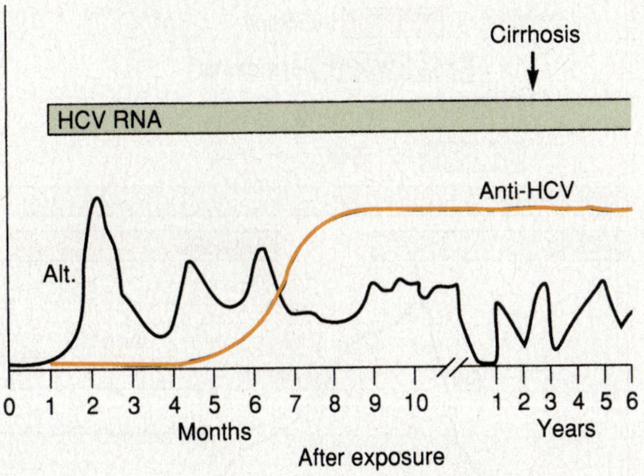

Figure 55.7. Clinical course in chronic hepatitis C.

are advised not to donate blood or share toothbrushes, take part in substance-abuse treatment facilities, and are counseled regarding safer drug injection practices. Various antiviral treatment regimens are available depending on the viral phenotype and patient risk factors and should be considered in all patients with chronic HCV infection and a detectable HCV viral level for more than 6 months. Eradication is based on achieving a sustained virologic response (SVR) 12 weeks following the completion of therapy.

Interferon (IFN) has long been considered the drug of choice for hepatitis C treatment with its ability to reduce the rate of fibrosis progression. This can be used in combination with ribavirin for either 24- or 48-week courses, depending on the genotype present. SVR rates range from 29% to 62%. Direct acting antivirals (DAAs) have also been designed to specifically inhibit HCV proteins. These agents, including simeprevir, ombitasvir and elbasvir, can be taken orally for 8 to 12 weeks with SVR rates approaching 90%.

Hepatitis C cirrhosis is a common indication for liver transplantation. However, reinfection and graft failure are almost inevitable if the virus is untreated during the pre- or posttransplant period. Five-year survival varies between 60% and 80%.

HEPATITIS D VIRUS

Epidemiology/Risk Factors for Transmission

Due to its dependence on HBV, patients with hepatitis D are always coinfected with hepatitis B. Transmission is similar to that of HBV, via parenteral or sexual exposure to blood or body fluids, and HDV only occurs in HBsAg-positive patients (**Fig. 55.8**).

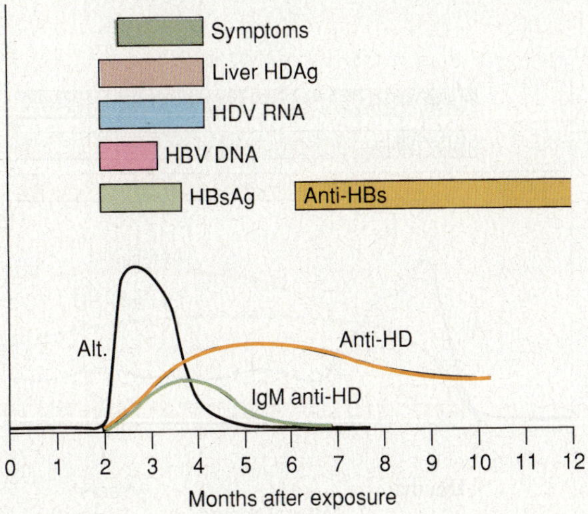

Figure 55.8. Synchronous infection with hepatitis B virus and hepatitis D virus.

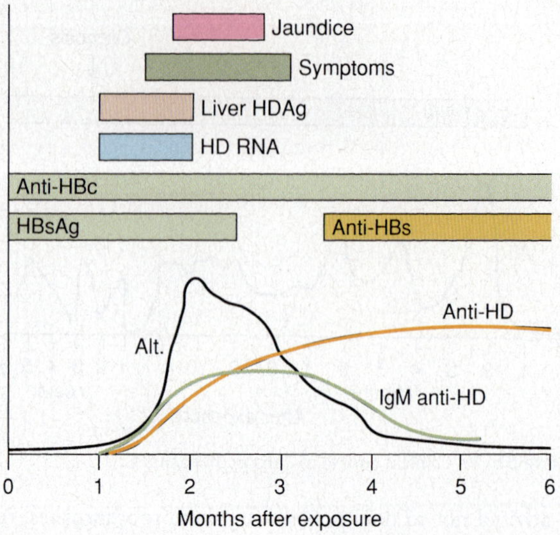

Figure 55.9. Superinfection of chronic hepatitis B carrier with hepatitis D.

Clinical Features

Acute infection is diagnosed by the presence of anti-HDV IgM. Coinfection with HBV generally produces a clinically indistinguishable disease with clinical features similar to the acute hepatitis B infection. Anti-HBc IgM distinguishes coinfection from superinfection which may manifest as a severe form of hepatitis or exacerbation of chronic HBV (**Fig. 55.9**). The diagnosis in patients with chronic liver disease is made by the presence of HBsAg and antibodies against HDV in the serum and confirmed by the presence of HDV antigen in the liver or HDV RNA in the serum. Cirrhosis may develop in up to 80% of coinfected patients compared to 15% to 30% of patients solely infected with HBV (**Fig. 55.10**).

Treatment

Treatment and prevention of HDV mirror that seen with HBV and HCV. IFN is the treatment of choice and may be administered for up to 12 months. Mainstay prevention is dependent on HBV vaccination.

HEPATITIS E VIRUS

Epidemiology/Risk Factors for Transmission

Hepatitis E is one of the least diagnosed etiologies of acute viral hepatitis. There are an estimated 20 million new infections diagnosed every year according to the World Health Organization (WHO), and the virus is distributed globally. Transmission occurs through the ingestion of fecally contaminated food and water, blood transfusions, and perinatal routes.

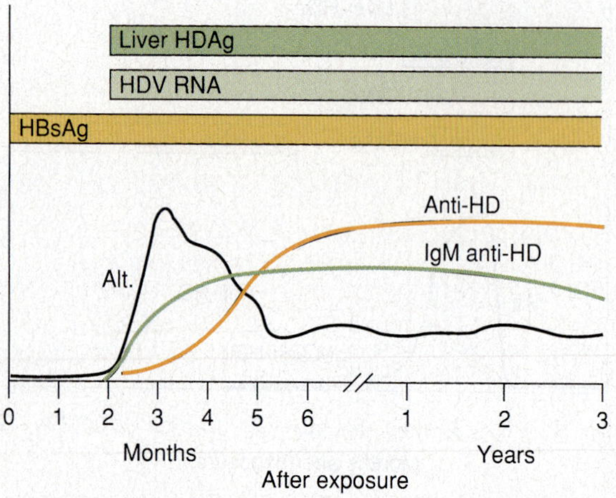

Figure 55.10. Clinical course of chronic hepatitis D infection.

Clinical Features

Most patients remain asymptomatic or develop mild symptoms such as jaundice, malaise, nausea, vomiting and abdominal pain. The incubation period ranges from 15 to 60 days. In addition, several extrahepatic manifestations have been described including thyroiditis, hematologic anomalies and neurologic diseases. Common biochemical findings are transaminitis and hyperbilirubinemia with resolution occurring 1 to 6 weeks following onset of the disease. While the disease is generally self-limiting, 0.5 to 4% of infected individuals may progress to fulminant hepatic failure, more likely affecting pregnant women, malnourished patients, and those with underlying liver disease.[26]

Treatment

Management of HEV is mainly supportive, particularly in the acute phase. The disease may persist in immunocompromised patients (transplant recipients), and a 12-week course of antiviral therapy (ribavirin) can be considered. General precautions should be taken when traveling to endemic regions. A vaccine has been developed with a 96% protective efficacy over 12 months; however, this is not widely available.[27]

Cytomegalovirus

Cytomegalovirus (CMV) is a generally asymptomatic disease causing mild nonspecific symptoms in immunocompetent persons. Transmission can occur through close and/or sexual contact, blood exposure and infected transplanted organs. Hepatic manifestations include mild hepatitis presenting as subclinical transaminitis in infected hosts and may progress to acute liver failure (ALF) in immunosuppressed persons. Viral seroprevalence ranges from 30% to 100% and is dependent on age and ethnicity.[28] Infection is lifelong due to the latency of the virus and can be detected in up to 70% of individuals in US cities. The diagnosis is confirmed by the identification of CMV specific antibodies in serum samples. However, one limitation of this diagnostic technique is that IgM specific CMV antibodies may be present for up to 6 months making it difficult to distinguish current infection from prior exposure. In addition, CMV antigenemia and PCR to detect CMV DNA have made diagnosis rapid. Histopathologic analysis with a liver biopsy may be necessary to further establish hepatitis.

Treatment

- Based on clinical course and viral load
- Largely self-limiting
- Immunocompromised patients—ganciclovir or valganciclovir
- Minimum 2 to 3 weeks or 2 to 3 months in high-risk patients[28]

Epstein–Barr Virus

Epstein–Barr virus (EBV) is largely known as an important agent in infectious mononucleosis, but most infections are asymptomatic. The disease is spread through close contact, and global seroprevalence rates are over 90%.[29] Deranged liver function tests are not uncommon and are generally self-resolving. In rare instances, acute symptomatic hepatitis occurs as a sequelae of infectious mononucleosis. The presence of jaundice may reflect either more severe hepatitis or an associated hemolytic anemia and is present in less than 5% of infected persons.[30] Leukocytosis is usually present, with the presence of atypical lymphocytes being a hallmark. Detection of heterophile antibodies, or the "monospot test" is highly specific but can be negative during the first week of clinical illness. This can be repeated at a later date; however, if the test remains negative, the diagnosis can be further investigated through EBV-specific antibody testing.

Treatment

- Supportive to alleviate symptoms
- Largely self-limiting

Herpes Simplex Virus

Acute hepatitis is a rare complication of HSV infection, although both HSV-1 and HSV-2 have been described as causative agents. Hepatic involvement commonly occurs in immunocompromised patients, neonates, pregnant women, and patients taking steroids. The prevalence of antibodies to HSV-1 is around 75% in most populations and around 20% to HSV-2. Clinical manifestations include high fever, anorexia with nausea, abdominal pain, leucopenia, and coagulopathy.[31] Mortality rates over 70% have been described when the condition occurs and male gender, age over 40 years, coagulopathy, encephalopathy, and the absence of viral treatment are considered increased risks.[32] The diagnosis can be confirmed on histopathology demonstrating diffuse eosinophilic intranuclear inclusion bodies, multinucleated cells, widespread necrosis, and inflammation.

Treatment

- Supportive to alleviate symptoms
- Intravenous acyclovir

Varicella Zoster Virus

Varicella Zoster virus (VZV) infection is common and frequently presents as primary varicella in children. Hepatitis secondary to VZV infection is rare but can be deadly, especially in immunocompromised individuals. In these individuals, clinical manifestations include fever, abdominal pain, and rash.[32] Fulminant liver failure may ensue. Reye syndrome may also develop from VZV infection in children, leading to progressive encephalopathy and hepatic dysfunction. The diagnosis of VZV hepatitis can be distinguished from other diagnoses and confirmed on a liver biopsy. Disseminated VZV requires prompt treatment with antiviral medication usually in the form of acyclovir to decrease the high mortality rate.

Treatment

- Strict contact precautions
- Immunocompromised/pregnant patients—VZV immunoglobulin

ACUTE LIVER FAILURE

Definition

2 ALF is a generally uncommon condition consisting of a rapid deterioration in liver function in the form of coagulopathy and hepatic encephalopathy in the absence of preexisting liver disease. Three specific time frames are applied to categorize and distinguish the different forms of ALF; hyperacute (<7 days), acute (7 to 21 days), or subacute (21 days to 26 weeks). The European Association for the Study of the Liver (EASL) characterizes disease duration beyond 28 weeks and before the onset of encephalopathy as chronic liver disease.[33] The most recent definition in hepatic failure nomenclature is "acute-on-chronic" liver failure, which is characterized by an acute deterioration in liver function in patients with underlying chronic liver disease[34,35]

Diagnosis

A series of standard tests are considered in every patient, and when the diagnosis still remains unclear, a liver biopsy is performed, provided there are no absolute contraindications (**Table 55.7**).

Etiology

3 The cause of liver failure influences the management approach and prognosis, and for this reason, every effort is made to establish the correct underlying cause. ALF can arise from a
4 variety of causes. In the United States, United Kingdom, and Australia, acetaminophen overdose is the most common cause, accounting for 45.7% to 65.4% of all cases. In Asia, viral hepatitis contributes to the majority of cases.[36] The cause is unclear in 15% of patients.

Table 55.7. Management in Acute Liver Failure: Initial Laboratory Evaluations

Serum chemistries Sodium, potassium, chloride, bicarbonate, calcium, magnesium, phosphate, glucose, BUN, creatinine, amylase, lipase
Hepatic panel AST, ALT, alkaline phosphatase, total bilirubin, albumin
Prothrombin time/INR
Complete blood count
Arterial blood gas, lactate, ammonia
Toxicology screen
Viral hepatitis serologies Anti-HAV IgM, Hep B surface Ag, Anti-HBV core IgM, anti-HCV, anti-HEV IgM (if indicated)
Anti-VZV IgM, Anti-HSV IgM
Autoimmune markers ANA, ASMA, IgG levels, SPEP
Pregnancy test
Serum ceruloplasmin level and 24-hr urine copper collection (if Wilson disease is suspected)

Ag, antigen; ALT, alanine aminotransferase; ANA, antinuclear antibody; ASMA, antismooth muscle antibody; AST, aspartate aminotransferase; BUN, blood urea nitrogen; HAV, hepatitis A virus; HBV, hepatitis B virus; HCV, hepatitis C virus; HEV, hepatitis E virus; HSV, herpes simplex virus; IgM, immunoglobulin M; INR, international normalized ratio; SPEP, serum protein electrophoresis; VZV, varicella zoster virus.

Drug-Induced Liver Injury

Acetaminophen hepatotoxicity occurs in a dose-dependent manner, which can occur following consumption of a single dose or staggered over multiple time points.[37] ALF more commonly develops in malnourished patients, a history of alcoholism, or in late-presenting cases.[37] Full hepatic recovery is seen in 93% of patients, and patients are less likely to proceed to poor outcomes than in instances of nonparacetamol-related hepatic failure.[38]

In contrast to the dose-dependent interactions of acetaminophen, idiosyncratic drug reactions are dose-independent and generally occur within 6 months of drug treatment.[39] Stevens–Johnson syndrome caused by phenytoin, amoxicillin-clavulanate, carbamazepine, or halothane is a form of hypersensitivity idiosyncratic responses, while isoniazid, valproate, and amiodarone mainly cause metabolic idiosyncratic reactions.

Viral Hepatitis

Hepatitis A virus infection is generally mild, accounting for less than 3% of ALF cases. Up to 70% of cases recover completely with little to no intervention, and a better overall outcome is seen than in other causes of viral hepatitis.[40,41] Hepatitis B virus accounts for 8% of all cases of ALF in Europe and the United States.[42] The majority of cases of hepatitis B are caused by new infection, while the remaining cases of ALF may develop following reactivation of previously inactive disease.[42,43] Hepatitis C does not confer a significant risk of ALF in the absence of hepatitis

Table 55.8. Clinical Manifestations: Acute Liver Failure

Symptoms	Signs	Biochemical Findings
Malaise/fatigue	Encephalopathy	Thrombocytopenia
RUQ pain	Jaundice	Transaminitis
Vomiting	Altered mental status	Hyperbilirubinemia
Nausea	Disturbed sleep	Elevated prothrombin time
Anorexia		Acute kidney injury
		Hypophosphatemia
		Hypokalemia
		Hypomagnesemia
		Hypoglycemia

B coinfection.[44] Similarly, hepatitis D virus infection can lead to ALF in the setting of concurrent hepatitis B coinfection or preexisting chronic hepatitis B infection.[45,46] Hepatitis E virus is a worldwide infection and can cause fulminant hepatic failure in specific high-risk groups.[47] Hepatitis E infection accounts for 20% to 40% of ALF cases in developing countries but is a rare case in Western societies.[48,49] VZV, HSV, and CMV are other rare viral causes (see previous sections).

Other

Other causes of ALF include heat stroke, pregnancy-related injuries [Hemolysis, Elevated Liver enzymes and Low Platelets syndrome (HELLP)], metabolic/autoimmune diseases, and hepatic ischemia.[37,42]

Clinical Features

See **Table 55.8** for additional details.

Management and Treatment

General management of patients should be in specialist units with liver transplantation services. Up to 40% of patients recover spontaneously. Serial biochemical and serum analysis are essential to monitor the patient's course and for any complications. Hemodynamic stability needs to be accurately followed, and deviations need prompt responses. Intravascular volume depletion and a low systemic vascular resistance are likely the result of decreased oral intake and fluid extravasation. Hypotension can usually resolve with normal saline, and in cases of acidosis, half-normal saline can be considered.[39] In cases of hypoglycemia, dextrose can be added to carefully titrated fluid regimens, avoiding the risk of overhydration that may worsen cerebral edema. Mean arterial pressure should be maintained at least 75 mm Hg, and if this is not achievable with sole fluid management, norepinephrine with or without vasopressin can be used.[50]

Acetaminophen toxicity can be treated with the administration of *N*-acetylcysteine, which may also be beneficial in other causes of ALF.[51] Patients with grade III or IV encephalopathy (**Table 55.9**) are at a high risk for developing cerebral edema, and intracranial pressure monitoring could be utilized to guide treatment. Elevating the head of the bed and prophylactic hypertonic saline should be considered in high-risk patients. In cases of elevated intracranial pressure, mannitol therapy is typically first-line treatment to maintain intracranial pressures below 20 to 25 mm Hg and cerebral perfusion pressures above 50 to 60 mm Hg.[52] Hyperventilation can be considered in patients, although the clinical benefits are transient.

Table 55.9. Stages of Hepatic Encephalopathy

Stage	Clinical Signs
I	Mild confusion, slurred speech, disordered sleep
II	Moderate confusion, lethargy, disorientation
III	Marked confusion, sleeping but arousable, slurred speech
IV	Coma

It may, however, be effective in patients with impending herniation. Coagulopathy should be monitored, and patients should receive stress ulcer prophylaxis to reduce potential gastrointestinal bleeding.

Liver Transplantation

5 Liver transplantation is the only definitive cure in the setting of irreversible liver failure. Identifying which patients are likely to benefit from liver transplantation and which are likely to spontaneously recover is an important and challenging step. Spontaneous recovery depends on several factors including patient age, degree of encephalopathy, and disease etiology. The King's College Criteria is an effective tool applied to determine prognosis in acetaminophen-induced fulminant hepatic failure and is used to predict survival outcomes for alternative etiologies and as an adjunct to prediction tools when proposing candidacy for liver transplantation.[53] Positive predictive values for acetaminophen and nonacetaminophen-induced ALF are 84% and 98%, respectively. Negative predictive values are 86% and 82% for acetaminophen and nonacetaminophen-induced ALF[53] (**Table 55.10**). The model for end-stage liver disease (MELD) system is another validated scoring system commonly used for chronic liver disease severity scoring. In terms of ALF, The King's College criteria appear more specific while the MELD score is more sensitive in predicting mortality.

Life Support Systems

Artificial liver support systems have been proposed in an effort to delay or preclude the need for transplantation. The two major categories are biologic and nonbiologic support systems. The most commonly investigated systems are the molecular adsorbents recirculating system (MARS) and the Prometheus system. Both systems are based on the removal of albumin-bound toxins. Results in ALF have been variable, and the devices are not widely available outside of clinical trials.

Similarly, bioartificial systems have yet to break into routine clinical practice. In this setting, a patient's blood is perfused through a bioreactor of human or porcine hepatocytes and undergoes detoxification.[54]

Table 55.10. Staging: King's College Criteria of Poor Prognostic Indicators

Acetaminophen-induced ALF: Arterial pH <7.3 irrespective of coma grade *OR all of the following:* INR >6.5, creatinine >3.4 mg/dL (300 µmol/L), grade III/IV Encephalopathy
Non–acetaminophen-induced ALF: INR >6.5 *OR any three of the following:* Age <10 or >40, drug toxicity or undetermined etiology, jaundice >7 d before encephalopathy, INR >3.5, bilirubin >17 mg/dL (300 µmol/L)

ALF, acute liver failure; INR, international normalized ratio.

Prognosis

Overall survival rates for ALF are greater than 60% and up to 55% can survive without transplantation.[55] Hepatic encephalopathy development and progression is a key prognostic indicator. However, prognosis can vary between etiologic agents and appears more favorable in acetaminophen-associated toxicity than alternative causes. Mortality also increases with the occurrence of cerebral edema, renal failure, coagulopathy, infection, and mechanical ventilation. Additional indicators of poor prognosis have been further developed in King's College in London to include the presence of three of the following; age less than 11 and greater than 40 years, jaundice present longer than 1 week before encephalopathy occurrence, serum bilirubin greater than 300 μmol/L, prothrombin time greater than 50 seconds, fulminant hepatitis secondary to non–A-, B-, or C-virus, idiosyncratic drug reactions and halothothane hepatitis.[56]

References

1. Mohsen AH, Green ST, Read RC, McKendrick MW. Liver abscess in adults: ten years experience in a UK centre. *QJM*. 2002;95(12): 797–802.
2. Huang CJ, Pitt HA, Lipsett PA, et al. Pyogenic hepatic abscess. Changing trends over 42 years. *Ann Surg*. 1996;223(5):600–607; discussion 607–609.
3. Lai HC, Lin CC, Cheng KS, et al. Increased incidence of gastrointestinal cancers among patients with pyogenic liver abscess: a population-based cohort study. *Gastroenterology*. 2014;146(1): 129–137.e1.
4. Huang WK, Chang JW, See LC, et al. Higher rate of colorectal cancer among patients with pyogenic liver abscess with Klebsiella pneumoniae than those without: an 11-year follow-up study. *Colorectal Dis*. 2012;14(12):e794–e801.
5. Kao WY, Hwang CY, Chang YT, et al. Cancer risk in patients with pyogenic liver abscess: a nationwide cohort study. *Aliment Pharmacol Ther*. 2012;36(5):467–476.
6. Lin AC, Yeh DY, Hsu YH, et al. Diagnosis of pyogenic liver abscess by abdominal ultrasonography in the emergency department. *Emerg Med J*. 2009;26(4):273–275.
7. Chen YW, Chen YS, Lee SS, et al. A pilot study of oral fleroxacin once daily compared with conventional therapy in patients with pyogenic liver abscess. *J Microbiol Immunol Infect*. 2002;35(3): 179–183.
8. Acuna Soto R, Maguire JH, Wirth DF. Gender distribution in asymptomatic and invasive amebiasis. *Am J Gastroenterol*. 2000; 95(5):1277–1283.
9. Katzenstein D, Rickerson V, Braude A. New concepts of amebic liver abscess derived from hepatic imaging, serodiagnosis, and hepatic enzymes in 67 consecutive cases in San Diego. *Medicine (Baltimore)*. 1982;61(4):237–246.
10. Wang Q, Huang Y, Huang L, et al. Review of risk factors for human echinococcosis prevalence on the Qinghai-Tibet Plateau, China: a prospective for control options. *Infect Dis Poverty*. 2014;3(1): 3–3.
11. Dhar P, Chaudhary A, Desai R, Agarwal A, Sachdev A. Current trends in the diagnosis and management of cystic hydatid disease of the liver. *J Commun Dis*. 1996;28(4):221–230.
12. Pant CS, Gupta RK. Diagnostic value of ultrasonography in hydatid disease in abdomen and chest. *Acta Radiol*. 1987;28(6):743–745.
13. Kervancioglu R, Bayram M, Elbeyli L. CT findings in pulmonary hydatid disease. *Acta Radiol*. 1999;40(5):510–514.
14. Ortona E, Riganò R, Buttari B, et al. An update on immunodiagnosis of cystic echinococcosis. *Acta Trop*. 2003;85(2):165–171.
15. Bildik N, Cevik A, Altintaş M, Ekinci H, Canberk M, Gülmen M. Efficacy of preoperative albendazole use according to months in hydatid cyst of the liver. *J Clin Gastroenterol*. 2007;41(3):312–316.
16. Guidelines for treatment of cystic and alveolar echinococcosis in humans. WHO Informal Working Group on Echinococcosis. *Bull World Health Organ*. 1996;74(3):231–242.
17. Elbaz T, Esmat G. Hepatic and intestinal schistosomiasis: review. *J Adv Res*. 2013;4(5):445–452.
18. El-Tonsy MM, Hussein HM, Tel-S H, Tawfik RA, Koriem KM, Hussein HM. Schistosoma mansoni infection: is it a risk factor for development of hepatocellular carcinoma? *Acta Trop*. 2013;128(3): 542–547.
19. Andrade ZA. Schistosomal hepatopathy. *Mem Inst Oswaldo Cruz*. 2004;99(5 Suppl 1):51–57.
20. Abdel-Wahab MF, Esmat G, Farrag A, el-Boraey YA, Strickland GT. Grading of hepatic schistosomiasis by the use of ultrasonography. *Am J Trop Med Hyg*. 1992;46(4):403–408.
21. Bezerra AS, D'Ippolito G, Caldana RP, Cecin AO, Ahmed M, Szejnfeld J. Chronic hepatosplenic schistosomiasis mansoni: magnetic resonance imaging and magnetic resonance angiography findings. *Acta Radiol*. 2007;48(2):125–134.
22. Yang JD, Larson JJ, Watt KD, et al. Hepatocellular carcinoma is the most common indication for liver transplantation and placement on the waitlist in the United States. *Clin Gastroenterol Hepatol*. 2017;15(5):767–775.e3.
23. Schweitzer A, Horn J, Mikolajczyk RT, Krause G, Ott JJ. Estimations of worldwide prevalence of chronic hepatitis B virus infection: a systematic review of data published between 1965 and 2013. *Lancet*. 2015;386(10003):1546–1555.
24. Petruzziello A, Marigliano S, Loquercio G, Cozzolino A, Cacciapuoti C. Global epidemiology of hepatitis C virus infection: an up-date of the distribution and circulation of hepatitis C virus genotypes. *World J Gastroenterol*. 2016;22(34):7824–7840.
25. Cacoub P, Renou C, Rosenthal E, et al. Extrahepatic manifestations associated with hepatitis C virus infection. A prospective multicenter study of 321 patients. The GERMIVIC. Groupe d'Etude et de Recherche en Medecine Interne et Maladies Infectieuses sur le Virus de l'Hepatite C. *Medicine (Baltimore)*. 2000;79(1):47–56.
26. Aggarwal R. Hepatitis E: clinical presentation in disease-endemic areas and diagnosis. *Semin Liver Dis*. 2013;33(1):30–40.
27. Zhu FC, Zhang J, Zhang XF, et al. Efficacy and safety of a recombinant hepatitis E vaccine in healthy adults: a large-scale, randomised, double-blind placebo-controlled, phase 3 trial. *Lancet*. 2010;376(9744):895–902.
28. Jensen KO, Angst E, Hetzer FH, Gingert C. Acute cytomegalovirus hepatitis in an immunocompetent host as a reason for upper right abdominal pain. *Case Rep Gastroenterol*. 2016;10(1):36–43.
29. Schechter S, Lamps L. Epstein-Barr virus hepatitis: a review of clinicopathologic features and differential diagnosis. *Arch Pathol Lab Med*. 2018;142(10):1191–1195.
30. Crum NF. Epstein Barr virus hepatitis: case series and review. *South Med J* 2006;99(5):544–548.
31. Norvell JP, Blei AT, Jovanovic BD, Levitsky J. Herpes simplex virus hepatitis: an analysis of the published literature and institutional cases. *Liver Transpl*. 2007;13(10):1428–1434.
32. Norvell JP, Blei AT, Jovanovic BD, Levitsky J. Herpes simplex virus hepatitis: an analysis of the published literature and institutional cases. *Liver Transpl*. 2007;13(10):1428–1434.
33. Wendon J, members P, Cordoba J, et al. EASL clinical practical guidelines on the management of acute (fulminant) liver failure. *J Hepatol*. 2017;66(5):1047–1081.
34. Hernaez R, Solà E, Moreau R, Ginès P. Acute-on-chronic liver failure: an update. *Gut*. 2017;66(3):541–553.
35. Jalan R, Gines P, Olson JC, et al. Acute-on chronic liver failure. *J Hepatol*. 2012;57(6):1336–1348.
36. Lee WM. Etiologies of acute liver failure. *Semin Liver Dis*. 2008; 28(2):142–152.
37. Bernal W, Wendon J. Acute liver failure. *N Engl J Med*. 2013; 369(26):2525–2534.
38. Koch DG, Speiser JL, Durkalski V, et al. The natural history of severe acute liver injury. *Am J Gastroenterol*. 2017;112(9):1389–1396.
39. Goldberg E, Chopra S. *Acute Liver Failure in Adults: Management and Prognosis*. 2016; UpToDate.
40. Van Damme P, Pintó RM, Feng Z, et al. Hepatitis A virus infection. *Nat Rev Dis Primers*. 2023;9(1):51.
41. Taylor RM, Davern T, Munoz S, et al. Fulminant hepatitis A virus infection in the United States: incidence, prognosis, and outcomes. *Hepatology*. 2006;44(6):1589–1597.

42. Stravitz RT, Lee WM. Acute liver failure. *Lancet.* 2019;394(10201):869–881.
43. Dao DY, Hynan LS, Yuan HJ, et al. Two distinct subtypes of hepatitis B virus-related acute liver failure are separable by quantitative serum immunoglobulin M anti-hepatitis B core antibody and hepatitis B virus DNA levels. *Hepatology.* 2012;55(3):676–684.
44. Chu CM, Yeh CT, Liaw YF. Fulminant hepatic failure in acute hepatitis C: increased risk in chronic carriers of hepatitis B virus. *Gut.* 1999;45(4):613–617.
45. Smedile A, Farci P, Verme G, et al. Influence of delta infection on severity of hepatitis B. *Lancet.* 1982;2(8305):945–947.
46. Caredda F, d'Arminio Monforte A, Rossi E, et al. Prospective study of epidemic delta infection in drug addicts. *Prog Clin Biol Res.* 1983;143:245–250.
47. Wedemeyer H, Pischke S, Manns MP. Pathogenesis and treatment of hepatitis E virus infection. *Gastroenterology.* 2012;142(6):1388–1397.e1.
48. Manka P, Bechmann LP, Coombes JD, et al. Hepatitis E virus infection as a possible cause of acute liver failure in Europe. *Clin Gastroenterol Hepatol.* 2015;13(10):1836–1842.e2.
49. Parkash O, Mumtaz K, Hamid S, Ali Shah SH, Wasim Jafri SM. MELD score: utility and comparison with King's College criteria in non-acetaminophen acute liver failure. *J Coll Physicians Surg Pak.* 2012;22(8):492.
50. Stravitz RT, Kramer DJ. Management of acute liver failure. *Nat Rev Gastroenterol Hepatol.* 2009;6(9):542–553.
51. Lee WM, Hynan LS, Rossaro L, et al. Intravenous N-acetylcysteine improves transplant-free survival in early stage non-acetaminophen acute liver failure. *Gastroenterology.* 2009;137(3):856–864, 864.e1.
52. Nath F, Galbraith S. The effect of mannitol on cerebral white matter water content. *J Neurosurg.* 1986;65(1):41–43.
53. Renner EL. How to decide when to list a patient with acute liver failure for liver transplantation? Clichy or King's College criteria, or something else? *J Hepatol.* 2007;46(4):554–557.
54. Demetriou AA, Brown RS Jr, Busuttil RW, et al. Prospective, randomized, multicenter, controlled trial of a bioartificial liver in treating acute liver failure. *Ann Surg.* 2004;239(5):660.
55. Reuben A, Tillman H, Fontana RJ, et al. Outcomes in adults with acute liver failure between 1998 and 2013: an observational cohort study. *Ann Intern Med.* 2016;164(11):724–732.
56. O'Grady JG, Alexander GJ, Hayllar KM, Williams R. Early indicators of prognosis in fulminant hepatic failure. *Gastroenterology.* 1989;97(2):439–445.

56

Cirrhosis and Portal Hypertension

Russell N. Wesson and Andrew M. Cameron

Key Points

1. Chronic injury and inflammation due to ongoing oxidative stress is a common pathway leading to cirrhosis, regardless of etiology. Removal of the inciting agent can halt progression of disease.
2. Acetaldehyde mediates injury in alcohol-induced liver disease.
3. Metabolic dysfunction–associated steatotic liver disease (MASLD) is associated with obesity, hyperlipidemia, and non–insulin-dependent diabetes. It is increasing in incidence and results in a spectrum of change from fatty infiltration to inflammation (MASH) and cirrhosis (MASH cirrhosis), and may coexist with alcohol-associated liver disease (MetALD). Effective therapeutics are emerging.
4. Viral hepatitis is the most common cause of cirrhosis worldwide, accounting for at least 50% of cases. All genotypes of Hepatitis C can now be cured with direct-acting antivirals (DAAs). Hepatitis B is treatable with antivirals.
5. Budd–Chiari syndrome (BCS) is a rare disease characterized by obstruction of the hepatic veins by webs or membranes (commonly in Asia and Africa) or thrombosis secondary to hypercoagulable states and neoplasms (commonly in the West).
6. Hepatorenal syndrome acute kidney injury (HRS-AKI) is a complication of cirrhosis, associated with ascites, characterized by progressive renal failure in the absence of intrinsic renal disease.
7. Hepatic encephalopathy is a neuropsychiatric syndrome occurring in the setting of liver disease. It is characterized by variable clinical manifestations ranging from subtle personality changes and sleep pattern derangement to confusion, lethargy, and coma.
8. Portal hypertension is defined as a portal pressure elevated above the normal range of 5 to 8 mm Hg. It is an important complication of cirrhosis (intrahepatic) and can also occur after portal vein thrombosis (prehepatic), or hepatic venous obstruction (posthepatic). Portal hypertension is responsible for the development of gastroesophageal varices and bleeding. Early use of nonspecific beta blockade in clinically significant portal hypertension (CSPH) can decrease the risk of decompensation, with carvedilol the preferred nonspecific β-adrenergic blockade (NSBB).
9. Important scoring systems include the Child–Turcotte–Pugh (CTP) score, which incorporates clinical and laboratory data to assess the functional status of the liver, estimate hepatic reserve, and predict morbidity and mortality of liver disease. The model for end-stage liver disease-sodium (MELD-3.0) score is a highly reliable prognostic marker for cirrhosis, is calculated from standard laboratory tests and criteria, and has replaced the CTP score in liver transplant candidate stratification.
10. Transjugular intrahepatic portosystemic shunt (TIPS) has become first-line therapy for refractory or recurrent bleeding esophageal varices.
11. Surgical interventions for the treatment of variceal bleeding include liver transplantation, shunt procedures, and rarely performed devascularization procedures. Liver transplantation is the definitive treatment for decompensated cirrhosis.
12. Spontaneous bacterial peritonitis (SBP) is a potentially lethal infectious complication of cirrhosis with ascites. It occurs in up to 10% of patients.

CIRRHOSIS

Background and Definition

Cirrhosis is a late stage of progressive liver fibrosis that is associated with complications that carry a high mortality. It constitutes the fifth leading cause of adult deaths and ranks eighth in economic cost among the major illnesses in the United States.[1] A majority of adults with cirrhosis are unaware they have liver disease. The concept of compensated advanced chronic liver disease is a recent paradigm shift away from the requirement of a histologic or radiologic diagnosis of cirrhosis for initial patient risk stratification.[2]

Described in the Greek myth of Prometheus, the ability of the liver to regenerate is legendary. The development of cirrhosis marks a turning point in the ability of the liver to function effectively and recover from insults. Cirrhosis is the pathologic end result of repeated, chronic injury and repair. This results grossly in a scarred, distorted nodular cirrhotic liver, and microscopically, this continued cycle causes massive derangement of the organized hepatic architecture. Cirrhosis is defined histologically by bridging fibrosis, destruction of vascular and biliary elements with regeneration, and nodule formation (**Fig. 56.1**). Clinically, cirrhosis presents in two main categories: compensated and decompensated cirrhosis. Decompensation is defined by the development of consequences of portal hypertension, that is, encephalopathy, ascites, and variceal bleeding. Median survival is quite different, with that of compensated cirrhotics at 12 years, versus 1.5 years for patients with decompensated cirrhosis (**Table 56.1**).[2] Portal hypertension is due to increased resistance at the pre-, intra-, or posthepatic position. Importantly, the chronic, ongoing inflammation resulting in cirrhosis is carcinogenic, and hepatocellular carcinoma (HCC) may arise in livers affected by cirrhosis. HCC

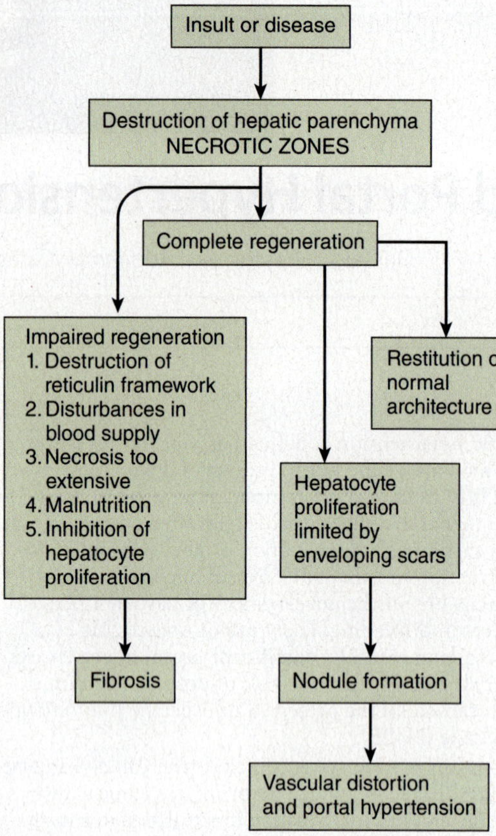

Figure 56.1. Evolution of cirrhosis. Fibrosis develops in nonregenerative necrotic areas, producing scars. The pattern of nodularity and scars reflects the type of response to injury (eg, uniform vs. nonuniform necrosis) and the extent of injury.

CLASSIFICATION

Table 56.2. Causes of Cirrhosis

Most Common Causes (Developed Countries)
Alcohol
Chronic viral hepatitis (hepatitis B and C)
Hemochromatosis
Metabolic dysfunction–associated liver disease
Less Common Causes
Primary and secondary biliary cirrhosis
Primary sclerosing cholangitis
Veno-occlusive disease
Wilson disease
Autoimmune hepatitis
Infection (brucellosis, syphilis, echinococcosis)
Drugs and toxins (eg, methotrexate, isoniazid)
α_1-Antitrypsin deficiency
Cystic fibrosis
Glycogen storage disease
Other metabolic diseases
Sarcoidosis
Copper
Small-bowel bypass
Right-sided heart failure
Hereditary hemorrhagic telangiectasia
Idiopathic

may occur in the absence of cirrhosis. The complications and causes of cirrhosis may be managed medically or via interventional radiologic techniques, and this may halt progression, improve quality of life, and increase survival. Liver transplantation, however, is the only definitive cure for decompensated cirrhosis at the current time.

1 Pathophysiology

Chronic injury with fibrosis is a central component in the development of cirrhosis. Cirrhosis does not result when injury to the liver is acute and not sustained. Cirrhosis is caused by chronic injury in a range of pathologic entities. These include viral hepatitis, alcohol, metabolic disorders, drug toxicity, and biliary obstruction, among others (**Table 56.2**). These lead to injury, hepatocyte death, chronic inflammation, fibrosis, and subsequent loss of architectural integrity and structural distortion. Injury and fibrosis occur initially in areas where injury from the etiologic agent is most severe (eg, perivenular, also known as pericentral, in the case of alcohol), progressing to panlobular and bridging fibrosis. Progression of fibrosis to cirrhosis usually occurs over years. Exceptions with rapid progression include biliary obstruction, fibrosing cholestatic hepatitis, and veno-occlusive disease. Cellular and molecular mechanisms underlying the shift from physiologic recovery to pathologic distortion after healing continue to be studied, and pathways of hepatic fibrogenesis and cirrhosis remain a central area of investigation in liver biology.[3]

Oxidative stress and chronic inflammation appear to be the final common pathway in the development of fibrosis and cirrhosis. As the liver becomes fibrotic, significant qualitative and quantitative changes occur in the extracellular matrix. The overall collagen content increases dramatically, and there is a change from the low-density basement membrane type matrix present within the subendothelial space to replacement by a high-density, interstitial type matrix. Changes in proteoglycans and glycoproteins also occur. Ultimately, the normal function of hepatocytes, **hepatic stellate cells** (HSCs), and endothelial cells is impaired. The high-density matrix activates HSCs, leading to loss of hepatocyte microvilli and disappearance of endothelial fenestrations decreases solute transport from sinusoid to hepatocyte.[4] Matrix alteration alters cellular behavior via cell membrane receptors. These, including integrins, cadherins, and selectins, may be future therapeutic targets.

HSCs (previously called the lipocytes, Ito, fat-storing, or perisinusoidal cells) play a central role in fibrogenesis and development of cirrhosis and become the primary fibrogenic cell in the injured liver. These cells are located in the space of Disse between hepatocytes and sinusoidal endothelial cells (**Fig. 56.2**). HSCs, which are normally quiescent and store vitamin A, appear to be the key mediator in the development of fibrosis and are the primary source of extracellular matrix both in the normal and fibrotic liver. Activation of HSCs occurs with ongoing inflammation, leading to an increase in expression of "fibril-forming" collagen types I, III, and V as well as heparan, dermatan, chondroitin sulfate, laminin, and fibronectin.[5] Stellate cells with fibrogenic potential are not confined to the liver and have been identified in other organs

Table 56.1. Major Complications of Cirrhosis

Portal hypertension and variceal hemorrhage
Ascites and volume overload
Spontaneous bacterial peritonitis
Hepatic encephalopathy
Hepatocellular carcinoma
Hepatorenal syndrome
Hepatopulmonary syndrome

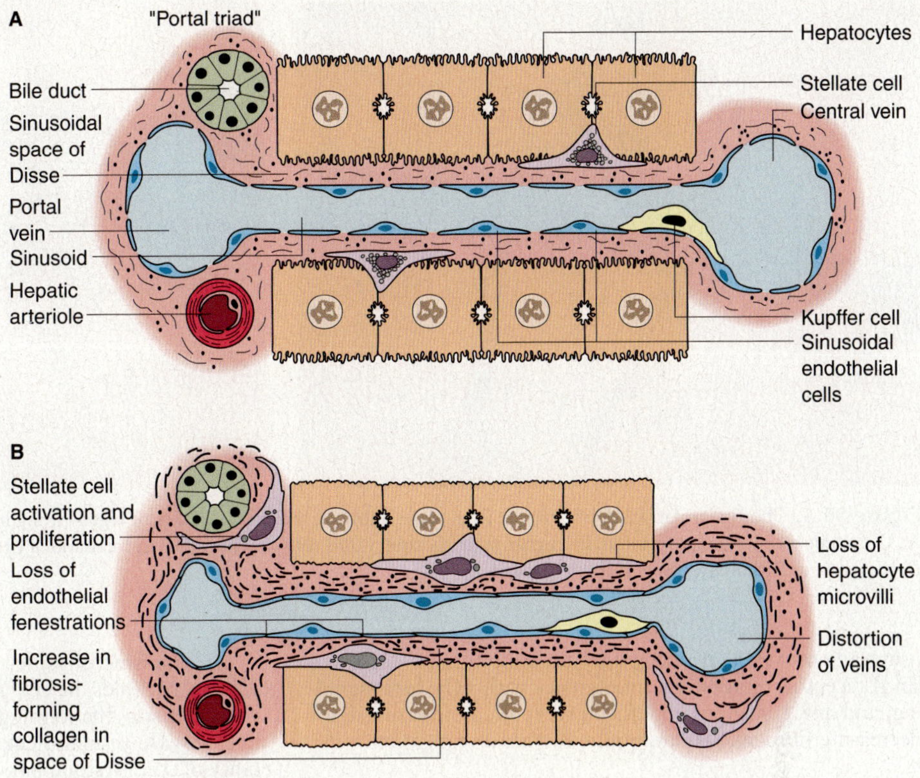

Figure 56.2. Matrix and cellular alterations in hepatic fibrosis. **A:** In normal liver, a modest amount of low-density matrix is present in the subendothelial space of Disse. **B:** In the fibrotic liver, the accumulation of fibril-forming matrix in this region leads to "capillarization" of the sinusoid and functional changes in all neighboring cell types.

and may contribute to primary or metastatic cancers as cancer-associated fibroblasts.[6]

A number of different stimuli initiate and perpetuate activation of HSCs.[7] Paracrine stimulation by neighboring sinusoidal endothelial cells, Kupffer cells, hepatocytes, and platelets *initiates* activation. Soluble mediators include the classic transforming growth factor beta-1 (TGF-β1), platelet-derived growth factor (PDGF), and epidermal growth factor (EGF). Apoptotic bodies (derived from hepatocytes) activate HSCs and Kupffer cells, as do reactive oxygen species (ROS), which are generated through lipid peroxidation of hepatocytes, macrophages, HSCs, and other cells. In alcoholic and metabolic dysfunction–associated steatohepatitis (MASH), ROS generation in hepatocytes results from the induction of cytochrome P450 2E1, leading to pericentral, zone 3 injury.

Activation of HSCs leads to further elaboration of the proinflammatory and profibrogenic cytokines TGF-β1 and PDGF, creating a self-sustaining cycle. TGF-β1 is derived from both paracrine and autocrine sources and remains the classic fibrogenic cytokine, with downstream signaling converging on Smad proteins resulting in HSC activation.[8] Roles for inflammasomes, toll-like receptors (TLR4) are emerging, while direct effects of hepatitis C on HSCs, and indirect effects of hepatitis B on immune cells contribute to HSC activation. Cannabinoids and the cannabinoid receptors CB1 and CB2 are involved in fibrogenesis and have emerged as a possible pathway for inhibiting hepatic fibrosis. Sinusoidal endothelial cells also contribute to early fibrosis, and immune cells such as CD8 and macrophages can influence activation, while regression of fibrosis can occur under the influence of certain macrophage subsets as well as dendritic cells. Regression may occur, for instance, in the setting of treatment of HCV via direct-acting antivirals (DAAs).[9] An increasing understanding of the role of inflammatory and immunomodulatory cells in liver disease may have led the way to new therapies.[10]

Ultimately fibrosis causes architectural and functional disruption of the hepatic acinus. Collagen deposition and extracellular matrix synthesis leads to thickening of the space of Disse. "Capillarization" develops with loss of the fenestrated architecture of the sinusoidal endothelium which may prevent the normal flow of nutrients to hepatocytes and increasing vascular resistance.[11] In addition, endothelial and stellate cells produce endothelin-1, a potent vasoconstrictor, causing contraction of the myofilaments within HSCs, influencing blood flow to injured areas and contributing to portal hypertension.

Treatment of Fibrosis

The point at which fibrosis becomes inexorable is unknown. Dense cirrhosis with nodule formation, portal hypertension, and early liver failure is irreversible, but less-advanced lesions can improve if injury is removed or possibly with therapy. In studies of hepatitis B, hepatitis C, and MASH, up to 70% of patients had reversal of early cirrhosis and fibrosis following successful antiviral therapies, and improvements in MASH and fibrosis after bariatric surgery.[9,12–14] Growing attention has been given to approaches that might disconnect hepatic injury from the inexorable path of fibrosis. Targeting HSCs and mediators of fibrogenesis may complement therapies that treat the inciting factors of liver injury. **Removal of injurious stimuli** is most effective when initiated early. Examples include the removal of excess iron or copper in hemochromatosis or Wilson disease, respectively. The potential success of treatment of HBV with **adefovir or entecavir**, treatment of delta hepatitis with interferon therapy, and the success of **direct-acting antiviral** (DAA) therapy against HCV and management of MASLD with GLP-1 receptor agonists, as well as thyroid hormone receptor beta agonists (eg, resmetirom) and vitamin E are additional examples.[15,16]

Suppression of hepatic inflammation has a role to play in some settings and is an active area of investigation. **Corticosteroids** are useful in many inflammatory liver diseases, in particular autoimmune hepatitis. Duration of use is limited by the extensive side effects associated with prolonged use. **Ursodeoxycholic** acid and **obeticholic** acid (a PPAR agonist) have clear efficacy in primary biliary cirrhosis.[17,18]

N-acetylcysteine, metformin, and silymarin (a natural component of milk thistle that belongs to a group of flavonoid compounds) have been explored without clear evidence of clinical efficacy. Interruption of the renin–angiotensin system

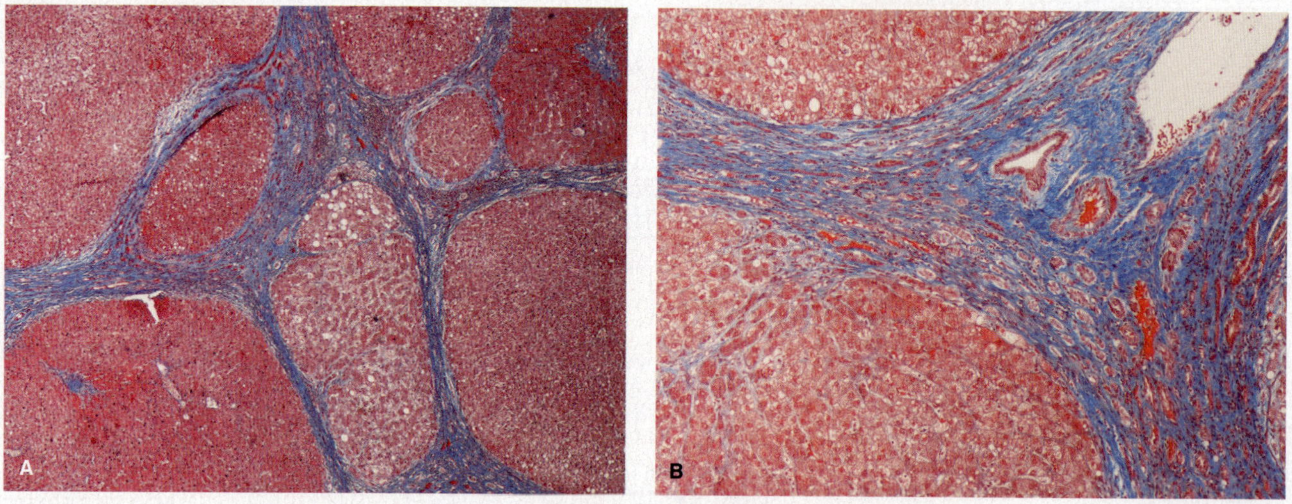

Figure 56.3. Photomicrographs A of cirrhotic liver tissue, showing irregular nodules of regenerating hepatocytes surrounded by dense fibrosis. **A:** Trichrome stain 2× magnification. **B:** Higher magnification (10×) showing portal triad surrounded by fibrosis. (Courtesy of Dr Robert Anders, Department of Pathology, Johns Hopkins Hospital.)

using angiotensin-converting enzyme inhibitors or angiotensin II receptor antagonists, interference with TGF-beta signaling, and antagonism of endothelin receptors hold promise for decreasing fibrogenesis but require further investigation.

Etiology

Historically, cirrhosis has been divided into micronodular, macronodular, and mixed patterns. However, this World Health Organization (WHO) classification (created in 1977) has little utility in terms of defining etiology due to its low specificity (**Fig. 56.3**).

Alcohol

Some patients who chronically abuse alcohol develop liver disease. This can manifest as alcohol-associated steatosis, steato-
2 hepatitis, fibrosis, and cirrhosis. Alcohol abuse is common, with an estimated prevalence globally of over 100 million individuals.[19] Alcohol-associated liver disease accounts for the most common diagnosis among waitlisted patients awaiting liver transplant, with 37.5% in the United States in 2022, and accounting for 19% of liver transplants in Europe.[20,21] Once hepatic decompensation develops, the expected 5-year transplant-free survival rate is approximately 60% for those who stop drinking alcohol and 30% if drinking continues. Cirrhosis develops in 10% to 30% of heavy drinkers. Advanced disease carries a poor prognosis, with more than half of alcoholics with cirrhosis and two-thirds of patients with alcoholic hepatitis and cirrhosis dying within 4 years of diagnosis.

An active area of investigation, alcohol injures the liver via various mechanisms. Alcohol is metabolized via several pathways, primarily to acetaldehyde and nicotinamide adenine dinucleotide (NAD) via the enzyme alcohol dehydrogenase (ADH). Acetaldehyde is metabolized via ALDH. ADH and ALDH are located predominantly within the cytoplasm of hepatocytes. The microsomal ethanol–oxidizing system (MEOS) cytochrome P450 2E1 (CYP2E1) is also responsible for approximately 10% of ethanol oxidation to acetaldehyde. Although alcohol may directly activate HSCs, **the key mediator in alcohol-induced liver disease is acetaldehyde**. CYP2E1 is largely in the perivenular/centrilobular zone 3 of the hepatic acinus. Zone 3 is also an area of relative **hypoxia** due to its distance from portal venous and hepatic arterial inflow, and levels of antioxidants such as glutathione are lowest in this zone. Activity of aldehyde dehydrogenases is also lower in zone 3. These factors contribute to the characteristic perivenular location of injury and histologic changes present in alcohol-induced liver disease.

Mechanisms of injury of acetaldehyde include the peroxidation of lipids in cell membrane. Macrosteatosis and the characteristic "ballooning degeneration" of alcohol-induced liver disease results. Acetaldehyde also increases the permeability of the intestinal barrier,[22,23] allowing delivery of bacterial endotoxin (LPS) to the liver. Kupffer cell activation by LPS via TLR4 may set off the inflammatory cascade responsible for the development of alcoholic liver disease.[24] The pathogenesis of alcoholic liver disease continues to be investigated, with roles for tumor necrosis factor alpha (TNF-α), cyclooxygenase 2, dietary fat, oxidative stress, development of antigenic adducts (acetaldehyde binding to proteins creating antigenic adducts) among others being explored. Ultimately, continued alcohol-induced injury results in progression of fibrosis to cirrhosis.

Diminished ability to oxidize fatty acids and increased lipogenesis from impaired beta oxidation and impaired tricarboxylic acid cycle activity contribute to steatosis. Genetic polymorphisms (eg, polymorphisms in PNPLA3 alleles) may impact who develops steatosis. The innate immune system is increasingly implicated in a proinflammatory response to alcohol, and inflammasome activation has been shown to mediate signaling from injury. Neutrophil infiltration and activation are a nearly pathognomic characteristic of alcohol-associated hepatitis. Endotoxin is elevated in alcohol use disorder and appears to stimulate inflammatory cytokines. Increased levels of proinflammatory cytokines (IL-1, IL-6, TNF) are also demonstrated in patients with alcohol use disorder and correlate with disease severity and histologic findings. IL-8, IL-17, and macrophage migration inhibitory factor (MIF) are other cytokines and chemokines implicated in the pathogenesis. Further, the "leaky gut" hypothesis with progressively reduced intestinal barrier function to bacterial products implicates the microbiome in a propensity and susceptibility to alcohol-associated liver disease ("a cirrhosis dysbiosis ratio") with increased delivery of endotoxin to the liver.[25]

Histologic findings: Classically, micronodular cirrhosis, the histology of alcoholic liver disease typically begins with the appearance of macrosteatosis of fatty liver disease. This progresses to alcoholic steatohepatitis when inflammation (neutrophil infiltration, generally in association with an elevated peripheral neutrophil count) and necrosis are present. Megamitochondria and Mallory–Denk bodies (eosinophilic accumulations of intermediate filaments with cytokeratin proteins, previously termed Mallory hyaline or Mallory bodies) are also characteristic. As disease duration and toxin exposure progress, fibrosis and architectural distortion occur.

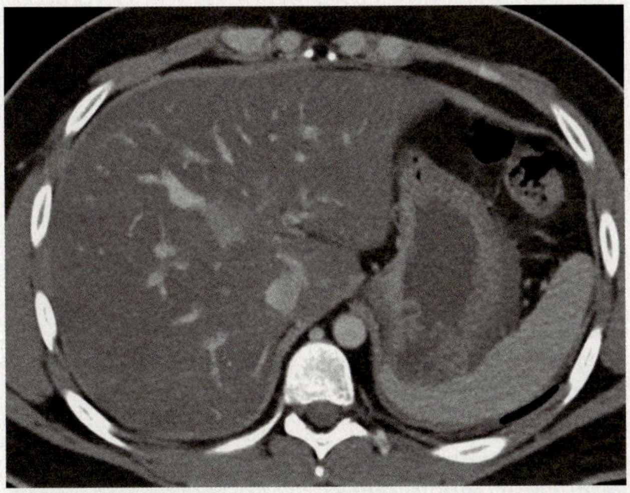

Figure 56.4. Venous-phase contrast-enhanced CT scan demonstrating a hypodense steatotic (fatty) liver. The liver is hypodense relative to the spleen. (Image courtesy of Dr. Ihab Khamel, Department of Radiology, Johns Hopkins Hospital.)

Metabolic Dysfunction–Associated Steatotic Liver Disease

3 Obesity and metabolic syndrome may produce hepatic injury and potentiate the effects of viral injury. Metabolic dysfunction–associated steatotic liver disease (MASLD, formerly known as nonalcoholic fatty liver disease [NAFLD]) describes the presence of hepatic steatosis (**Fig. 56.4**) when no other causes for secondary hepatic fat accumulation (eg, heavy alcohol consumption) are present. MASLD may progress to steatohepatitis with inflammation and apoptosis (MASH), fibrosis, and cirrhosis. MASH is the leading cause of cryptogenic cirrhosis.

This disease is a major health problem in Westernized populations and, in particular, in the United States. Steatosis has been found to present in over 50% of Americans, and MASLD is now the most common cause of chronic liver disease in the United States, affecting up to 30% of the population. Men are particularly vulnerable and the disease occurs in patients with at least one metabolic risk factor.[26] It is second only to alcohol as an indication for liver transplant.[20] Initially, the liver becomes infiltrated with fat, with subsequent lobular inflammatory infiltrate and hepatocyte apoptosis. Pathologic features are shared with alcohol-induced liver injury (**Fig. 56.5A,B**). MASLD patients have at least one metabolic risk factor, including obesity, dyslipidemia, hypertension, and type 2 diabetes, and the presence of multiple risk factors indicates increased risk of progression to MASH.[27] Ninety percent of MASLD patients have at least one of these risk factors and 30% have three or more.[28] MASLD is also a major risk factor for primary liver cancer (HCC) and in addition to hepatitis virus infection, accounts for the rapid rise in the incidence of HCC in Western countries. More broadly considered, obesity is a major risk factor for cancer deaths, with a 4.5-fold increase in the relative risk for liver cancer in obese subjects.[29]

The current understanding of MASLD involves steatosis progressing to MASH, 20% of whom will progress to cirrhosis. Insulin resistance is central and leads to hepatic steatosis. A second hit, oxidative injury, has been proposed to lead to inflammation, necrosis, and fibrosis. Genetic variants (eg, PNPLA3 and others) appear to predispose to (others are protective) progression, and other injurious agents, including iron, intestinal hormones, and the microbiome contribute. Ongoing hepatic insults lead to activation of the inflammasome and secretion of the proinflammatory cytokines to which endotoxin contributes.

Therapy for MASH centers on lifestyle modification and avoidance of ongoing or additional injury, and treating insulin resistance. General measures include avoiding other hepatotoxins, including alcohol and maintaining appropriate vaccinations against viral hepatitis, as well as other standard vaccinations (such as against pneumococcus and influenza). Modification of cardiovascular disease risk factors is important. Modest weight loss of 5% to 10% is associated with significant histologic improvements in disease severity.[28] Weight loss may be achieved via bariatric surgery if exercise fails. Fatty acid synthase inhibitors have been shown to reduce liver fat and improve proinflammatory and fibrosis markers.[30] In patients without diabetes, vitamin E and thyroid hormone receptor beta agonists (Resmetirom) have a therapeutic role.[31] In diabetics, pioglitazone and GLP-1 receptor agonists have efficacy in treating MASH. Atorvastatin, omega-3 fatty acids, and aspirin also have a role. The composition of gut microflora plays a role in the progression of disease and contributes to oxidative injury and fibrosis.

Guidelines exist for the follow-up of patients with MASLD to evaluate fibrosis progression, cardiovascular risk, and progression to cirrhosis. Patients should be followed clinically with serial noninvasive assessment of their liver fibrosis score (**Table 56.3**) if biopsy-proven MASH is present.

Viral Hepatitis

4 Viral hepatitis is the most common cause of cirrhosis worldwide, accounting for at least 50% of cases. Hepatitis A, B, C, D, and E have all been proven to cause acute hepatitis, and viral

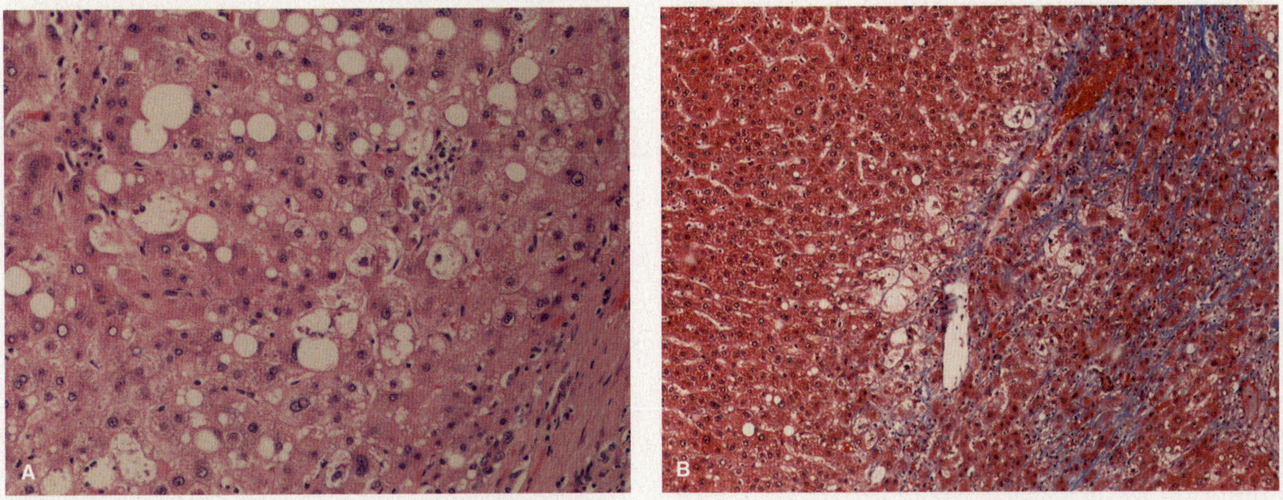

Figure 56.5. **A:** Steatohepatitis 20× magnification. Macrosteatosis, an inflammatory infiltrate, and Mallory–Denk bodies are seen. **B:** Trichrome stain demonstrating steatohepatitis and fibrosis (10× magnification). (Images courtesy of Dr. Robert Anders, Department of Pathology, Johns Hopkins Hospital.)

Table 56.3. Comparability of Terms in Three Simple Systems for Histologic Grading and Staging of Chronic Hepatitis: IASL, Metavir, and Batts–Ludwig

IASL	Metavir	Batts–Ludwig
Grade (Activity, Inflammation)		
Minimal chronic hepatitis	A1	Grade 1
Mild chronic hepatitis	A1	Grade 2
Moderate chronic hepatitis	A2	Grade 3
Severe chronic	A3	Grade 4
Stage (Fibrosis)		
Mild—portal fibrosis	F1	Stage 1
Moderate—periportal fibrosis or portal–portal septa	F1	Stage 2
Severe—bridging fibrosis (few)	F2	Stage 3
Severe—bridging fibrosis (many)	F3	Stage 3
Cirrhosis	F4	Stage 4

IASL, International Association for the Study of the Liver.
Adapted from Rockey DC, Caldwell SH, Goodman ZD, Nelson RC, Smith AD; American Association for the Study of Liver Diseases. Liver biopsy. *Hepatology.* 2009;49:1017–1044.

hepatitis, due to HBV and HCV, is the seventh leading cause of death worldwide. Histology is characterized by lymphocytic parenchymal and portal inflammation, focal necrosis, ballooning degeneration, and cholestasis. Kupffer cell and macrophage hypertrophy and hyperplasia are present with lobular disarray. Hepatitis B, C, and D may progress to chronic hepatitis, defined by persistent (>6 months) liver cell necrosis and inflammation.

Hepatitis B Virus: Less than 5% of patients who experience acute HBV infection develop chronic infection, and approximately 10% to 20% of chronically infected persons develop cirrhosis. Hepatitis B remains a major public health problem, particularly in Asia and Africa, where up to 10% of the population show evidence of chronic infection. Globally, the WHO estimates there are 254 million people living with chronic HBV in the world, with 1.1 million deaths in 2022 from HBV-related liver disease.[illegible] Vaccines and antiviral therapies are safe and effective. Antiviral medications effective against hepatitis B suppress viral replication and may reverse fibrosis and even early cirrhosis. Treatment suppresses viral replication; however, HBV DNA remains incorporated into the host genome and HCC can still develop in the noncirrhotic liver. Public health strategies with systematic vaccination of newborns are able to substantially decrease the incidence of new infections.

Hepatitis C Virus: In contrast, HCV poses a much higher risk of chronic infection: 50% to 85% of persons exposed become chronically infected, and chronic hepatitis develops in 60% of these patients. HCC develops in approximately 20% with cirrhosis due to HCV, twice that of HBV. Historically, HCV was treated with pegylated interferon and ribavirin (a therapy associated with a high rate of adverse events that limited completion of therapy), with sustained viral response (SVR) rates of up to 80% in patients with genotypes 2 and 3, but much less effective for the more common genotype 1. The discovery of DAAs has revolutionized the treatment of HCV. Choice of antivirals has evolved rapidly and depends on multiple factors, including genotype, treatment history, comorbidities, presence and stage of cirrhosis, and potential drug interactions. Multiple effective drug combinations exist. Some combinations are effective against multiple HCV genotypes, and a few combinations have pangenotypic activity. Treatment recommendations and guidelines for DAA use are published by the American Association for the Study of Liver Diseases (AASLD) and the Infectious Disease Society of America (IDSA), among others (European Association for the Study of the Liver [EASL], and the WHO).

In patients who respond to antiviral therapy, progression to cirrhosis is eliminated, however for those with fibrosis or cirrhosis ongoing surveillance for HCC is required.

Hepatitis D Virus (the delta virus—HDV): HDV is a defective RNA virus and requires coinfection with HBV to be pathogenic. Superinfection of HBV-positive patients with HDV may lead to a more rapid progression to cirrhosis and a greater risk of HCC.

Cholestasis

Cholestasis may be caused by intrahepatic or extrahepatic biliary obstruction or defects in the ability of hepatocytes to excrete bile. Important causes are biliary atresia, primary sclerosing cholangitis (PSC), and primary biliary cholangitis (PBC—previously known as primary biliary cirrhosis) (**Table 56.4**). Prolonged extrahepatic

ETIOLOGY

Table 56.4. Causes of Cholestasis

Causes
Extrahepatic
Common bile duct stones
Cancers
Pancreas
Ampulla of Vater
Bile duct
Cysts
Pancreatic
Choledochal
Infections
Parasites
Acquired immunodeficiency syndrome
Chronic pancreatitis
Bile duct strictures
Benign
Ischemic
Hodgkin disease
Biliary atresia
Intrahepatic
Primary biliary cholangitis
Space occupying lesions
Primary or metastatic hepatic tumors
Lymphoma
Amyloidosis
Vanishing bile duct syndrome
Allograft rejection
Graft vs host disease
Alagille syndrome
Idiopathic adult ductopenia
Primary sclerosing cholangitis
Hodgkin disease
Cystic fibrosis
Hepatocellular Cholestasis
Genetic
α-Antitrypsin deficiency
Benign recurrent intrahepatic cholestasis
Byler syndrome
Cholestasis of pregnancy
Abnormal bile acid synthesis
Porphyrias
Acquired
Viral hepatitis
Drugs
Alcoholic hepatitis
Bacterial infections
Total parenteral nutrition
Renal carcinoma
Hodgkin disease
Postoperative cholestasis

obstruction leads to proliferation of bile ducts, formation of bile lakes, fibrosis as a result of the direct toxic effects of bile salts on hepatobiliary elements, and eventually secondary biliary cirrhosis.

Primary Biliary Cholangitis

Several diseases characterized by cholestasis seem to be caused by underlying autoimmune or inflammatory disorders affecting either small (PBC) or large (PSC) bile ducts. PBC is a chronic, progressive autoimmune cholestatic disease that most commonly affects middle-aged women who are almost all positive for antimitochondrial antibodies, while most are also positive for antinuclear antibodies. Family members are at a greatly increased risk of the disease. PBC is characterized by a T-lymphocyte–mediated attack on small intralobular bile ducts and the biliary epithelium. Portal inflammation and destruction of intrahepatic bile ducts ultimately result in cirrhosis. Patients may be asymptomatic, or present with fatigue, jaundice, and pruritus. PBC progresses in the majority of patients, with median survival of 10 to 15 years in asymptomatic patients and 7 years in symptomatic patients.

Therapy for PBC includes the exogenous bile acid ursodeoxycholic acid. Ursodeoxycholic acid may reduce the expression of HLA class 1 antigens by hepatocytes and lessen the toxicity of retained naturally occurring bile acids. Complete response, as evidenced by normalization of liver enzymes without histologic progression, is seen in up to 30% of patients and may result in a normal life expectancy. Obeticholic acid (a farnesoid X receptor ligand) is recommended if the response to ursodeoxycholic acid is inadequate. Liver transplantation is required in those who progress to decompensated cirrhosis.

Primary Sclerosing Cholangitis

PSC is a chronic, progressive cholestatic liver disease of uncertain etiology characterized by diffuse segmental intrahepatic and/or extrahepatic biliary strictures with associated fibrosis and inflammation. The disease has no cure and leads to secondary biliary cirrhosis, portal hypertension, and hepatic failure. PSC carries a risk of cholangiocarcinoma. Median transplant-free survival ranges from 10 to 20 years. PSC is strongly associated with ulcerative colitis (less commonly Crohn disease) likely due to a common underlying mechanism involving mucosal autoimmunity to the gastrointestinal (GI) tract. Around 70% of patients with PSC have ulcerative colitis whereas only approximately 5% of patients with ulcerative colitis have symptomatic PSC. Autoantibodies and an increased expression of human leukocyte antigen (HLA) class II molecules on biliary epithelial cells are present.[33] As opposed to PBC, in PSC two-thirds of patients are male and younger than 45 years of age at the time of diagnosis. Presentation is variable with some completely asymptomatic and only abnormal liver function tests (GGT and ALP) while others may have signs of advanced disease at the time of diagnosis. Endoscopic retrograde cholangiopancreatography (ERCP) may be diagnostic for workup of the abnormal LFTs although MRCP is preferred and will show characteristic multifocal beaded intrahepatic ducts due to stricturing disease, and extrahepatic strictures may be present. Symptomatic patients have a waxing and waning course and may present with complaints of fatigue (75%), pruritus (25% to 70%), jaundice, abdominal pain and weight loss. Patients may have episodes of acute cholangitis and may progress to cirrhosis.

Pathologically, bile ductular proliferation, periductal fibrosis ("onion skin pattern")and inflammation, ductopenia, and, less commonly, obliterative fibrous cholangitis may be present. Like ulcerative colitis and colon cancer, PSC confers a significant risk of malignant transformation of the biliary mucosa. Cholangiocarcinoma develops in 1% to 2% of patients per year after the diagnosis of PSC, with an overall lifetime risk of 10% to 15%. PSC is a risk factor for both intra- and extrahepatic cholangiocarcinoma as well as gall bladder cancer. HCC risk is increased when cirrhosis is present. Surveillance for cancer with ultrasound, computed tomography (CT), or MRCP, and serum testing of CA19-9 has been recommended. When a dominant stricture, worsening symptoms or cholestasis is present, ERCP with brush cytology and fluorescence in situ hybridization (FISH) may be useful to increase sensitivity of cancer detection.

Multiple immunosuppressive and anti-inflammatory therapies have been used against PSC although none have been proven effective. Clinical trials of ursodeoxycholic acid are underway. Therapies are directed toward the complications of the disease, including biliary obstruction, cirrhosis, and cholangiocarcinoma. Dominant strictures, defined as stenosis less than 1.5 mm in the common bile duct or less than 1 mm in the hepatic duct, are readily treated endoscopically by means of dilation and/or stent placement. A dominant stricture should raise concern for the development of cholangiocarcinoma. Transplantation should be performed before cancer develops. Historically, the presence of cholangiocarcinoma was an absolute contraindication to transplantation because of poor outcomes. However, in highly selected patients with localized tumors, liver transplantation may be achieved with an acceptable survival rate after intensive preoperative therapy, radiation, and chemotherapy, as proposed by Shaw and implemented on a larger scale by the Mayo group.[34]

Metabolic and Genetic Disorders

A description of all the metabolic and genetic disorders causing liver disease is beyond the scope of this chapter. Some of these diseases are listed in **Table 56.2**.

Hereditary Hemochromatosis: This is an autosomal recessive, inborn error of metabolism, most commonly due to mutations in the hereditary hemochromatosis gene *HFE*, which results in increased intestinal absorption of iron and subsequent total-body iron overload. Iron accumulates in the periportal regions of the liver and results in hepatotoxicity via lipid peroxidation. Kupffer cells subsequently phagocytose necrotic hepatocytes and activate stellate cells. Over time, the reaction progresses to bridging fibrosis and eventually cirrhosis. Cardiac, endocrine, neurologic, cutaneous, and other systemic manifestations occur. Treatment includes reduction of iron intake, repeated phlebotomy, and liver transplantation. As with other types of cirrhosis, there is a risk of HCC.[35]

Wilson Disease: Wilson disease is an autosomal recessive disease caused by a mutation in the Wilson disease protein, resulting in deficient hepatocyte transport of copper into bile. The disease is characterized by a low serum ceruloplasmin level and manifests clinically as Kayser–Fleischer rings (corneal pigmentation), neuropsychiatric disease, and hepatic cirrhosis. Liver manifestations of Wilson disease vary widely from asymptomatic biochemical abnormalities and steatosis to acute fulminant hepatic failure, chronic hepatitis, and cirrhosis. As copper accumulates in the liver, periportal inflammation develops that leads to piecemeal and lobular necrosis, bridging fibrosis, and ultimately a mixed micronodular–macronodular cirrhosis. A scoring system has been developed to assist with the diagnosis. Treatment options include chelating agents, such as D-penicillamine, trientine, zinc salts, and orthotopic liver transplantation.

Impaired Venous Outflow or Venous Outflow Obstruction

Cirrhosis may also result from chronic obstruction of the hepatic venous outflow. Causes include chronic right-sided heart failure due to severe tricuspid regurgitation, the Budd–Chiari syndrome (BCS), and the sinusoidal obstructive syndrome (hepatic veno-occlusive disease).

Any cause of right sided heart failure can cause hepatic congestion. Sinusoidal congestion occurs and results in perivenular atrophy, hemorrhagic necrosis, distortion, and enlargement of sinusoidal fenestrations with ascites developing. Pathologically, the "nutmeg" appearance is classic with areas of hemorrhage interspersed by normal parenchyma. Perivenular fibrosis progresses to bridging fibrosis that spares portal regions. Portal sparing is characteristic of "cardiac cirrhosis."

ETIOLOGY

Table 56.5. Etiologic Factors in Budd–Chiari Syndrome

Idiopathic
Hematologic disorders Polycythemia vera Paroxysmal nocturnal hemoglobinuria Myeloproliferative disorders Antithrombin III deficiency Circulating lupus anticoagulants
Oral contraceptives
Pregnancy and postpartum
Tumors Hepatocellular carcinoma Renal cell carcinoma Adrenal carcinoma Leiomyosarcoma of the inferior vena cava
Vena caval webs
Infections Amebic abscess Aspergillosis Hydatid cyst
Phlebitis
Trauma
Veno-occlusive disease

5 **Budd–Chiari Syndrome** (see section on portal hypertension below) is a rare disease more common in women in their third or fourth decade of life. Hepatic venous obstruction (**Table 56.5**) anywhere from the terminal hepatic veins, major hepatic veins, or vena cava occurs and may be caused by obstructing webs or membranes (more commonly in Africa and Asia) or thrombosis secondary to hypercoagulable states or neoplasms (more commonly in the West).

The range of presentation is wide and characterized by duration of onset and severity: acute (fulminant) *with* acute liver failure; acute *without* acute liver failure; subacute; and finally chronic (with cirrhosis).[36] Variation in symptoms and presentation is related to the severity and rate of progression of hepatic outflow obstruction. Classically, presentation is with abdominal pain, hepatomegaly, and ascites. Duplex Doppler ultrasonography is highly sensitive in establishing the diagnosis and identifies collateral vessels to subscapular or intercostal vessels. CT and magnetic resonance imaging (MRI) (**Fig. 56.6**) delineate vascular anatomy and plan intervention. In the chronic form, the liver atrophies. Classically, the caudate lobe is spared and will hypertrophy. This is a hallmark of the disease due to the preserved caudate venous outflow into the vena cava. The hypertrophied caudate lobe narrows the retrohepatic vena cava it surrounds. This may be completely obliterated with total obstruction of blood flow.

An underlying cause is present in ~80% of cases (inherited or acquired thrombophilias, systemic factors, and hormonal causes).[37] Medical management consists of anticoagulation and management of symptoms. Interventional radiologic procedures have now taken the forefront in management of BCS, in which fresh clot can be treated with thrombolysis or strictures angioplastied or stented. If hepatic venous outflow cannot be reestablished, transjugular intrahepatic portosystemic shunting (TIPS) is able to decompress both the inferior vena cava (IVC) and

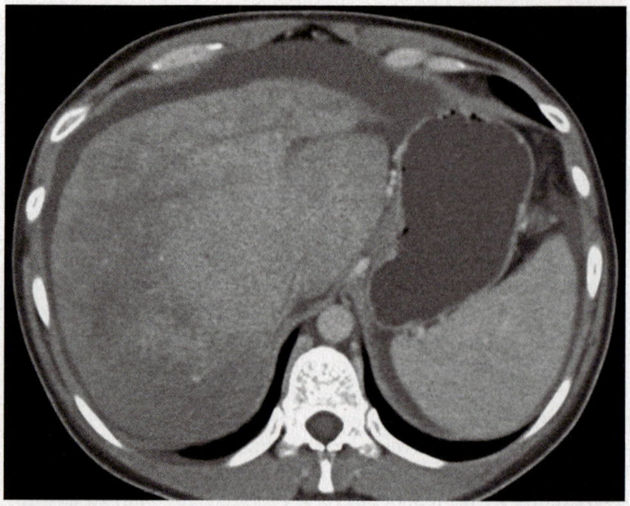

Figure 56.6. Contrast-enhanced CT of a patient with Budd–Chiari syndrome. This patient experienced an unprovoked thrombotic event, which was found to be due to a myeloproliferative neoplasm positive for *JAK2 V617F mutation.* Massively hypertrophied caudate lobe is demonstrated. Also visible is ascites, compressed IVC, and splenomegaly. This patient was successfully treated with TIPS and lifelong anticoagulation and continued to have excellent hepatic function. (Image courtesy of Dr. Ihab Khamel, Department of Radiology, Johns Hopkins Hospital.)

the portal system. In patients with fulminant BCS or decompensated cirrhosis, liver transplantation is lifesaving.

Diagnosis

Although cirrhosis can be asymptomatic, a careful history will elicit nonspecific symptoms (anorexia, weight loss, weakness, fatigue). A history of chronic alcohol abuse, hepatitis, or risk factors for virus transmission, jaundice, toxin or drug exposure, upper GI bleeding, enlarging hemorrhoids, infections, and alteration in mental status suggests the possibility of liver disease and decompensated cirrhosis. In women, chronic anovulation is common; in men, hypogonadism may develop. Physical findings are listed in Table 56.6. In

DIAGNOSIS

Table 56.6. Physical Findings in Cirrhosis

Physical Findings	Incidence (%)
Palpable liver	96
Jaundice	68
Ascites	66
Spider angiomas	49
Dilated abdominal wall veins (caput medusae)	47
Palpable spleen (splenomegaly)	46
Testicular atrophy	45
Palmar erythema	24
Noninfectious fever	22
Hepatic coma	18
Gynecomastia	15
Dupuytren contractures	5

addition, fetor hepaticus, purpura and bruising, decreased body hair, and white nails (Muehrcke and Terry nails) are common. As cirrhosis progresses, a decrease in blood pressure is often present and contributes to the development of hepatorenal syndrome (HRS). Parotid enlargement may be present in alcoholics.

Laboratory tests of liver function may be normal, or may show elevated levels of bilirubin, aspartate aminotransferase, alanine aminotransferase, and alkaline phosphatase. These are not specific for liver pathology, and may be normal even in cirrhosis. Low platelets are caused by hypersplenism and portal hypertension. The platelet growth factor thrombopoietin, which is produced by the liver, is decreased in patients with cirrhosis, and this deficit contributes.

Definitive diagnosis of cirrhosis may require imaging, biopsy, either percutaneous or operative, or gross inspection during laparoscopy or laparotomy. At biopsy, the specimen should be large enough (2 to 3 cm) and contain at least 11 portal tracts that need to be assessed. Several staging systems exist for the grading of fibrosis and cirrhosis, including the International Association for the Study of the Liver (IASL), Batts–Ludwig, and Metavir systems. The AASLD recommends use of the Batts–Ludwig or Metavir systems due to their simplicity (**Table 56.3**).[38]

Imaging classically reveals an atrophic, nodular liver and an enlarged spleen. Ultrasound is well tolerated, widely available, and noninvasive. Criteria for cirrhosis include demonstration of multiple nodular irregularities on the ventral liver surface separate from the anterior abdominal wall. Parenchymal texture is altered in the setting of fibrosis. These criteria have a sensitivity, specificity, and accuracy of approximately 90% in the diagnosis of cirrhosis.

CT imaging provides similar information. Portal phase intravenous contrast can demonstrate the presence of portosystemic collaterals (if portal hypertension is present) and assess patency of the portal vein. MRI provides similar information and may contribute to information about liver stiffness when elastography is performed. Contrast-enhanced CT and MRI are important in the characterization of the malignant potential of masses within the liver using LiRADS criteria.

Measures of liver stiffness offer a noninvasive approach to assessing fibrosis. Elastography estimates liver stiffness by applying mechanical waves and measuring their propagation speed through tissue. Modalities include ultrasound and MRI, among others. Ultrasound-based transient elastography (TE), a measure of liver stiffness, is playing an increasingly large role in the noninvasive assessment of fibrosis, with some studies demonstrating a 95% area under the receiver operating characteristic curve (AUROC) for diagnosing grade IV fibrosis (cirrhosis). MR elastography (MRE) interrogates the whole liver (unlike ultrasound-based TE) and has a higher technical success rate and better diagnostic accuracy than ultrasound-based TE.

Several laboratory indices have been found to correlate well with histologic grade of fibrosis. The NAFLD (*MASLD*) fibrosis score, for example, consists of age, BMI, diabetes, platelet count, albumin level, and AST/ALT ratio. The FibroSure (LabCorp) is a patented panel of biomarkers consisting of GGT, haptoglobin, bilirubin, apolipoprotein A1, and α-2-macroglobulin. Indirect evidence of cirrhosis includes endoscopically discovered varices of the esophagus and the presence of splenomegaly detected by CT or MRI.

Complications

The occurrence of major complications of cirrhosis signifies the occurrence of decompensated cirrhosis (**Table 56.1**).

Multiple factors can predispose to decompensation in a patient with cirrhosis. Risk factors for decompensation include bleeding, infection, alcohol intake, medications, dehydration, and constipation. Obese patients are at increased risk of decompensation. Once decompensation has occurred, patients should be assessed for liver transplantation.

Renal

Renal complications in cirrhosis are due to functional dysregulation of vascular tone throughout the body. This is characterized by sodium retention despite normo- or hypervolemia, dilutional hyponatremia secondary to free water overload, ascites, and ultimately renal failure and the HRS. Central to the pathophysiology of HRS is paradoxical arterial vasoconstriction of the renal arterial bed.[39] Among the complications of cirrhosis, HRS confers the highest risk of mortality. Although HRS is the most dramatic renal complication of liver failure, renal dysfunction in patients with advanced liver disease is generally multifactorial.

Splanchnic arterial vasodilatation, triggered by portal hypertension, plays a central role in the hemodynamic changes and the decline in renal function in cirrhosis. Observations that support a functional or "secondary effect" theory include the lack of anatomic renal abnormalities in patients with cirrhosis-related renal dysfunction, the normal function of previously dysfunctional kidneys transplanted into otherwise healthy recipients, and resolution of renal abnormalities after successful hepatic transplantation. Clinical trials have defined the critical role of optimizing colloid balance and regulating renal blood flow using agents such as terlipressin, octreotide, and midodrine in counteracting the deranged vascular tone, raising mean arterial pressure and improving renal perfusion counteracting the pathophysiology present in cirrhotic patients.[40]

Sodium Retention

Patients with cirrhosis who do not have ascites have relatively normal sodium-handling capabilities. Patients in whom ascites develops have a marked inability to excrete sodium. Because of this deficit, sodium intake in excess of renal excretion contributes to fluid overload (and a net natriuresis achieves volume removal with diuretics in treatment). The most accepted explanation for this development is the "arterial vasodilation hypothesis." Splanchnic arterial vasodilation leads to relative peripheral hypovolemia with activation of the renin–angiotensin–aldosterone and sympathetic nervous systems. Antidiuretic hormone is released with sodium and water retention and an increase in circulating volume, with subsequent edema and ascites.[41]

Nitric oxide and prostaglandins are key mediators and are elevated in both animal and human studies, and inhibitors of nitric oxide production have been shown to reduce vasodilatation and enhance renal hemodynamics.

Water Retention and Hyponatremia

Water excretion is usually normal in patients with cirrhosis before the development of ascites. Patients with cirrhosis and ascites may have a markedly impaired ability to handle free water. Increased ADH, decreased delivery of fluid to the diluting segments of the nephron, and reduced renal production of prostaglandins all contribute to water retention and subsequent hyponatremia. Symptoms include nausea, vomiting, lethargy, and seizures. Severity of hyponatremia correlates with mortality and is captured in the prognostic Na-MELD score.

Hepatorenal Syndrome

6 Patients with refractory ascites are at risk for acute kidney injury (AKI). Early diagnosis of AKI is imperative because therapy impacts survival. AKI in cirrhosis can be caused by prerenal azotemia (PRA), HRS, or acute tubular necrosis (ATN) and occurs in more than half of hospitalized patients with cirrhosis. Diagnosis of AKI can be challenging given that patients with cirrhosis often have sarcopenia and a lower baseline creatinine. Criteria for AKI in cirrhosis were revised in

Table 56.7. International Club of Ascites (ICA-AKI) Definitions for the Diagnosis and Management of AKI in Patients with Cirrhosis (KDIGO)

Definition of AKI	Increase in sCr ≥0.3 mg/dL (≥26.5 μmol/L) within 48 h; or a percentage increase sCr ≥50% from baseline, which is known, or presumed, to have occurred within the prior 7 d, and/or urine output ≤0.5 mL/kg for 6 h		
Staging of AKI	Stage 1: increase in sCr ≥0.3 mg/dL (26.5 μmol/L) or an increase in sCr ≥1.5-fold to 2-fold from baseline Stage 2: increase in sCr >2- to 3-fold from baseline Stage 3: increase of sCr ≥3-fold from baseline or sCr ≥4.0 mg/dL (353.6 μmol/L) with an acute increase ≥0.3 mg/dL (26.5 μmol/L) or initiation of renal replacement therapy		
Progression of AKI	Progression: Progression of AKI to a higher stage and/or need for RRT		Regression: Regression of AKI to a lower stage
Response to treatment	No response: No regression of AKI	Partial response: Regression of AKI stage with a reduction of sCr to ≥0.3 mg/dL (26.5 μmol/L) above the baseline value	Full response: Return of sCr to a value within 0.3 mg/dL (26.5μmol/L) of the baseline value

sCr, serum creatinine.

Adapted from Angeli P, Gines P, Wong F, et al. Diagnosis and management of acute kidney injury in patients with cirrhosis: revised consensus recommendations of the International Club of Ascites. *Gut.* 2015; 64:531–537, and from Nadim MK, Kellum JA, Forni L, et al. Acute kidney injury in patients with cirrhosis: Acute Disease Quality Initiative (ADQI) and International Club of Ascites (ICA) joint multidisciplinary consensus meeting. *J Hepatology.* 81(1):163–183.

2023 by the International Ascites Club (IAC) (**Table 56.7**) and are consistent with KDIGO criteria.[42] HRS is a phenotype of AKI that is a complication of cirrhosis characterized by progressive renal failure in the absence of intrinsic renal disease. It has also been described as occurring in acute liver failure. In patients with cirrhosis and ascites, HRS occurs in up to 20% of patients at 1 year and 40% at 5 years. Two forms of HRS are described. HRS-AKI (previously known as type 1 HRS) is a rapidly progressive decline in renal function with a high mortality. It is defined as occurring in cirrhotics with ascites, with AKI criteria (**Table 56.7**) and no improvement over 24 hours with adequate volume resuscitation. No other cause of AKI should be present. HRS-non-AKI (previously type 2) is a chronic form of renal dysfunction that evolves over weeks to

Table 56.9. International Ascites Club (IAC) Diagnostic Criteria for Hepatorenal Syndrome Acute Kidney Injury (HRS-AKI)

1. Cirrhosis with ascites
2. Increase in sCr ≥0.3 mg/dL within 48 h; or a percentage increase sCr ≥50% from baseline, which is known, or presumed, to have occurred within the prior 7 d, and/or urine output ≤0.5 mL/kg for 6 h
3. Absence of improvement in serum creatinine and or urine output within 24 h following adequate volume resuscitation (when clinically indicated)
4. Absence of strong evidence for an alternative explanation as the primary cause of AKI[a]

[a]HRS-AKI may be superimposed upon or coexist with other causes of AKI.

Adapted from Nadim MK, Kellum JA, Forni L, et al. Acute Kidney injury in patients with cirrhosis: Acute Disease Quality Initiative (ADQI) and International Club of Ascites (ICA) joint multidisciplinary consensus meeting. *J Hepatology.* 2024;81(1):163–183.

months. The development of HRS is a poor prognostic indicator: If liver transplantation cannot be performed, patients with HRS usually die within months of the development of severe disease. Distinguishing HRS-AKI from other causes of AKI is important because treatment differs.

The pathogenesis of HRS is due to renal cortical vasoconstriction induced by the activity of the renin–angiotensin–aldosterone system. The powerful endothelium-derived vasoconstrictor endothelin-1, combined with decreased renal production of vasodilator prostaglandins, also contributes. HRS is usually precipitated by an inciting event. Infection, use of nonsteroidal anti-inflammatory drugs, variceal hemorrhage, or excessive diuretic use may precipitate HRS with progressive oliguria, rising creatinine, increased cardiac output, and decreased arterial pressure.

Differential Diagnosis of HRS: This includes other causes of AKI and PRA. Excessive diuresis may lead to a rise in serum creatinine difficult to distinguish from HRS. A failure to respond to cessation of diuretics and fluid challenge suggests HRS. The disease, however, is virtually indistinguishable by laboratory testing from prerenal uremia. Both prerenal uremia and HRS are characterized by extremely low sodium concentrations in the urine, high urine osmolality, high urine-to-plasma ratios of creatinine, and normal urinary sediment (**Table 56.8**). Criteria for the diagnosis of HRS are listed in **Table 56.9**. Additional diagnostic biomarkers under study include urinary and serum neutrophil gelatinase–associated lipocalin (NGAL), urinary IL-18, urinary kidney injury molecule 1 (KIM-1), and fractional excretion of sodium (FeNa), among others.

Management of HRS: Often there is a precipitating event that requires treatment, most commonly spontaneous bacterial peritonitis (SBP) and infection. Diuretics should be stopped to prevent further injury. Volume contraction from multiple etiologies, including GI bleeding or the excessive treatment of

Table 56.8. Differential Diagnosis of Acute Azotemia in Patients with Liver Disease

	Prerenal Azotemia	Hepatorenal Syndrome	Acute Renal Failure
Urinary sodium	<10 mEq/L	<10 mEq/L	>30 mEq/L
Urine/plasma creatinine ratio	>30:1	>30:1	<20:1
Urine osmolality	100 mOsm, or more than plasma osmolality	100 mOsm, or more than plasma osmolality	Equal to plasma osmolality
Urine sediment	Normal	Normal	Casts: cellular debris

ascites, is another major precipitator. HRS is treated with volume expansion with albumin (**Table 56.9**) and empiric antibiotics until cultures are negative.

Vasoconstrictors treat splanchnic vasodilatation and can be combined with albumin to significantly improve renal function. Norepinephrine, terlipressin, or if unavailable octreotide with midodrine may be used with efficacy. A meta-analysis of all RCTs of vasopressor use in the treatment of HRS has found a reduction in all-cause mortality when vasopressors are utilized.[43] Medical therapy may reverse HRS in some patients; however, many will ultimately require liver transplantation or combined liver–kidney transplantation.

Pulmonary

Many pathologic processes in patients with cirrhosis affect pulmonary function. Some diseases affect both hepatic and pulmonary systems (ie, cystic fibrosis, α_1-antitrypsin deficiency); others are primary pulmonary processes, such as interstitial lung disease, primary pulmonary hypertension (portopulmonary hypertension [PPHTN]), and obstructive airway disease. Three important pulmonary manifestations of cirrhosis are discussed: Ascites and effusion reduce diaphragmatic excursion and total lung capacity. Intrapulmonary shunting is less common and is known as the hepatopulmonary syndrome. PPHTN is another cause of respiratory insufficiency.

Ascites and Hepatic Hydrothorax: Massive ascites can compromise diaphragmatic excursion due to raised intra-abdominal and intrapleural pressures. Hepatic hydrothorax (usually right-sided pleural effusion) may occur via transdiaphragmatic lymphatic communication. Compression of lung parenchyma by the effusion impairs gas exchange and results in ventilation–perfusion mismatch with hypoxemia. Decreased functional residual and total lung capacity result. Volume removal, either via diuresis, large-volume paracentesis, or thoracentesis, treats the problem. TIPS or indwelling pleural catheter placement are useful, although liver transplant is definitive.[44]

Hepatopulmonary Syndrome. HPS is characterized by arterial hypoxemia caused by intrapulmonary vascular dilatations (sometimes direct arteriovenous shunts) in the setting of liver disease or portal hypertension. It occurs in patients with mild to severe hepatic disease and, depending on criteria and population studied, is present in approximately 4% to 47% of patients with chronic liver disease.[45,46] Symptoms include dyspnea, platypnea (dyspnea with movement from a supine to an erect position), and orthodeoxia (decreased oxygen tension from supine to erect). The basis for these symptoms is an increasing shunt within dilated capillaries at the basal lung that occurs with standing. Spider nevi, clubbing, and cyanosis, as well as evidence of impaired oxygenation (peripheral oxygen saturation <96% on room air), may be present on examination. Degree of hypoxemia describes the severity and diagnostic criteria for HPS in patients with cirrhosis and includes: (1) PaO_2 <80 mm Hg (<70 mm Hg in patients over the age of 65 years) or (2) alveolar–arterial gradient ≥15 mm Hg (≥20 mm Hg over the age of 65 years).

Although the underlying mechanism of hypoxemia in these patients is right-to-left intrapulmonary shunting, ventilation–perfusion mismatch and impaired hypoxic vasoconstriction also play a role. Patients usually present with dyspnea and worsening hypoxemia without evidence of a primary pulmonary process. Initial diagnostic tools include pulse oximetry and arterial blood gas analysis. Pulmonary function testing excludes obstructive or restrictive airway disease as a cause of hypoxemia. A definitive diagnosis can be obtained by the use of contrast-enhanced echocardiography (bubble study) or technetium-labeled macroaggregated albumin (MAA) scanning, which will confirm the presence of intrapulmonary vascular dilation. Contrast echocardiography is sensitive and intrapulmonary vascular dilation is demonstrated by the late appearance of microbubbles in the left heart three to six cardiac cycles after injection.[47] MAA scanning revealing a shunt of >6% suggests HPS as the major contributor to hypoxemia. The only effective therapy for this disease is orthotopic liver transplantation, and those with HPS and with a PaO_2 <60 mm Hg receive priority at listing.

PPHTN refers to *pulmonary arterial hypertension* that is associated with *portal hypertension*. It is a complication of portal hypertension due to either chronic liver disease or extrahepatic causes. It is defined at right heart catheterization as a mean pulmonary arterial pressure of >20 mm Hg at rest; normal or low pulmonary artery occlusion pressure <15 mm Hg at rest; and pulmonary vascular resistance >240 dyn/s/cm^{-5} in the setting of documented portal hypertension. It is a relatively uncommon complication of cirrhosis with prevalence rates of 2% in those with chronic liver disease, to rates of 16% in those listed for transplant. When severe, it carries a substantial risk of mortality and is a contraindication to liver transplantation.[47] Doppler echocardiography will suggest elevated right heart pressures (ie, elevated peak tricuspid regurgitant velocity [TRV] >2.8 m/sec, or those with lower peak TRV but other signs of pulmonary hypertension), which is confirmed by right heart catheterization. The exact pathophysiology behind PPHTN is unknown, but portal hypertension is a necessary component of the disease process. The hyperdynamic state in portal hypertension may be the main contributory factor, although the severity of PPHTN does not correlate with the severity of portal hypertension. Although the high flow state present in cirrhosis elevates right-sided pressures, the fixed obstruction present in the pulmonary microcirculation is highly lethal and is not likely to improve with liver transplantation.

Treatment is nearly identical to that for other types of pulmonary arterial hypertension. Beta blockers should be avoided (worsen right heart failure and increase PVR). TIPS can increase preload and worsen heart failure and should be used with caution if indicated for other reasons. Prolonged IV infusion of prostaglandins (eg, epoprostenol) improves pulmonary hemodynamics and function, but does not prolong survival.[48] The oral endothelin receptor antagonists such as bosentan and ambrisentan may be used (adverse effects include liver toxicity). Phosphodiesterase-5 inhibitors (sildenafil and tadalafil) are also prescribed. As above, severe PHTN (mPAP >50 mm Hg) is an absolute contraindication to liver transplantation. For patients in whom medical therapy can maintain mPAP under 35 mm Hg and PVR less than 400 dyn/s/cm^{-5}, MELD exception points for transplant are granted.

Hepatic Encephalopathy

Etiology

7 Hepatic encephalopathy is a neuropsychiatric syndrome due to liver disease that is characterized by variable alterations in mental status. The manifestations (see clinical features below) range from subtle deficits detectable only by detailed psychometric tests to confusion, lethargy, and ultimately frank coma. Encephalopathy may present due to progression of acute hepatic failure, as a consequence of cirrhosis, or after the creation of a surgical portosystemic shunt and develops in 30% to 45% of patients with cirrhosis and in 10% to 50% of patients with TIPS. A precipitating event, such as acute variceal hemorrhage, infection, deterioration in renal function, drugs (eg, benzodiazepines), or constipation, can be found.

Ammonia has been heavily implicated in the development of this condition. However, an elevated serum ammonia is not required for diagnosis, nor is it specific. Normally, ammonia is produced by bacterial catabolism of nitrogenous sources (protein) in the intestine, after which it is absorbed into the portal circulation to undergo degradation in the liver. Ammonia and other bacterial degradation products access the peripheral circulation as a result of poor hepatic metabolism and portosystemic shunting. In cirrhotics, brain permeability to ammonia is also increased. Other agents implicated include γ-aminobutyric acid (GABA), endogenous benzodiazepines, branched-chain amino acids (BCAAs such as tryptophan), neurotoxic short-chain fatty acids, mercaptans, phenols, and endogenous opiates.

Clinical Features

A wide range of neurologic symptoms may occur in patients with hepatic dysfunction. Subtle changes may include changes in personality, memory loss, alterations in diurnal sleep variation, and minor decreases in intellectual function. The West Haven criteria describe the range of clinical stages. Neuromuscular impairment present may result in bradykinesia, asterixis, slurred speech and ataxia, and ultimately decerebrate posturing of coma. With progression, asterixis may occur. Stigmata of liver disease are usually evident, including fetor hepaticus and spider angiomas. The combination of asterixis, elevated ammonia levels, and altered mental status in a patient with known liver disease strongly suggests the diagnosis. Electroencephalographic changes are nonspecific and may occur in patients with a variety of other conditions.

Treatment

Treatment options for hepatic encephalopathy include correction of the precipitating factors where possible. Treatments to reduce bacterial load of ammonia from the intestine are also instituted. A search for precipitating infection is extremely important. Pulmonary, urinary, and ascitic infections should be sought via appropriate cultures and ascitic fluid analysis. An assessment of overall volume status and drug history as well as a search for variceal bleed can be made (**Table 56.10**).

Treatment depends on severity. Mild encephalopathy can be managed as an outpatient, whereas comatose patients may require ICU admission. Supportive care (resuscitation and volume expansion) as well as appropriate nutrition and correction of electrolyte abnormalities. *Hypokalemia*, in particular, needs correction as low potassium levels and the concurrent metabolic alkalosis increase NH4+ levels.

TREATMENT

Table 56.10. Treatment of Hepatic Encephalopathy

Identify and treat precipitating factors: Disordered carbohydrate metabolism Drugs (benzodiazepines, barbiturates) Infection (spontaneous bacterial peritonitis, other) Hypotension Hypoxia Excess exogenous protein Gastrointestinal bleeding Electrolyte abnormalities Alkalosis Constipation
Supportive therapy: Eliminate dietary nitrogen Purge gastrointestinal tract to remove blood and other nitrogenous compounds Nonabsorbable antibiotics (Rifaximin) Lactulose (or lactitol)
Dopamine receptor agonists: L-dopa and bromocriptine[a]
Branched-chain amino acid[b]
Temporary liver support
Orthotopic liver transplantation

[a]Arousal effect in selected patients may be secondary to enhanced renal function.
[b]High cost and equivocal benefits of intravenous amino acid mixtures make it difficult to justify routine use.

The removal of enteric nitrogenous compounds from the small and large bowel is critical in decreasing ammonia and other toxic substances present in blood. Lactulose is the most used and most effective agent in achieving this (see below). Orally administered *cathartics* and enemas can reduce protein and the source of ammonia. However, dietary restriction of protein is not recommended as it contributes to the skeletal muscle loss and malnutrition associated with cirrhosis. Oral *L-ornithine-L-aspartate* has been shown to be useful in cirrhosis and increases metabolism of ammonia to glutamine. Dietary supplementation with *branched-chain amino acids* (only necessary in those intolerant of protein) improves the relative deficit of these compared to aromatic amino acids and improves encephalopathy, and allows for higher dietary protein. *L-carnitine* supplementation improves cognitive deficits and reduces ammonia.

Lactulose is a nonabsorbable disaccharide cathartic when administered orally and is a mainstay of therapy. A dose of 45 to 90 g/d divided into two to four doses is generally effective and adjusted to produce two to three bowel movements per day. Lactulose reaches the distal ileum and colon, where it is metabolized by intestinal bacteria and enhances the bacterial uptake of ammonia. Hourly doses of 30 to 45 mL of lactulose can be administered to induce rapid improvement during the initial phase of therapy, and symptoms may abate within 24 to 48 hours. Side effects include flatulence, diarrhea, and electrolyte abnormalities.

Nonabsorbable antibiotics have also been used to decrease ammonia-forming bacteria in the gut. *Rifaximin* is a minimally absorbed macrolide antibiotic. The addition of rifaximin to lactulose has been shown to result in a higher proportion of patients experiencing complete reversal of hepatic encephalopathy and may also decrease mortality compared to lactulose alone. Based on current evidence, the treatment of hepatic encephalopathy should consist of the treatment of any precipitating factors, followed by lactulose administration. Rifaximin should be added for patients without improvement in the first 24 hours. Following an episode of overt hepatic encephalopathy, maintenance therapy with lactulose with or without rifaximin should be administered indefinitely as secondary prophylaxis.

Other antibiotics that have been explored with some mixed results include neomycin , metronidazole, and vancomycin. However, side effects including nephrotoxicity, ototoxicity, and bacterial resistance have precluded their use.

PORTAL HYPERTENSION

8 Portal hypertension is defined as a portal vein pressure above the normal range of 5 to 8 mm Hg. It may also be defined by a hepatic vein–portal vein pressure gradient (HVPG) greater than 5 mm Hg. Pressures in the portal venous system are measured by subtracting the free hepatic vein pressure from the wedged hepatic vein pressure, similar to the technique used to determine pulmonary capillary wedge pressure by pulmonary arterial (Swan–Ganz) catheterization. It is caused by an increase in resistance to portal venous flow, followed by an increase in portal venous inflow. The site of resistance classifies portal hypertension as pre-, intra- or posthepatic

Current guidelines classify cirrhosis into compensated and decompensated stages. Decompensated cirrhotics are those with clinically significant portal hypertension (CSPH), defined by the presence of hepatic venous wedge pressure of 10 mm Hg or more. Gastroesophageal varices and portosystemic collaterals on imaging are surrogates of CSPH, and defining the presence of CSPH is important because it defines prognosis and treatment. Among patients with CSPH who develop successive complications, including recurrent bleeding, refractory ascites, recurrent infections, jaundice, and HRS, the term "further decompensation" applies. These patients have a much higher mortality.[2]

Anatomy

The venous anatomy of the portal system is relatively constant, with the "usual" anatomy present in 98% of the population. The portal vein is formed by the confluence of the superior mesenteric and splenic veins behind the neck of the pancreas. The inferior mesenteric vein most often joins the splenic vein before the portal vein is formed. A third of people have the inferior mesenteric vein joining the superior mesenteric vein. Occasionally, the superior mesenteric vein is absent and the portal vein is formed by multiple smaller mesenteric branches that join the splenic vein.

Portosystemic Collaterals

As portal hypertension develops, portal pressure rises in tributaries of the portal vein. This elevated pressure results in the expansion and dilation of these tributaries as well as of the portosystemic collateral venous communications. The sites of portosystemic communication have important clinical consequences. Dilation of and increased flow through the coronary or left gastric vein becomes highly significant in portal hypertension. The increased blood flow through the veins of the lesser curve of the stomach and esophagus leads to esophageal and gastric varices as well as portal hypertensive gastropathy. The inferior mesenteric vein communicates with rectal branches that form hemorrhoids; the umbilical vein remnant communicates with the left portal vein and dilates to carry blood through the ligamentum teres of the falciform ligament to veins of the abdominal wall. This is visible on examination as the "*caput medusae*." Splenic venous flow increases and dilates the short gastric veins further contributing to gastric varices. Retroperitoneal collaterals (**Fig. 56.7**) form and can create large splenorenal shunts that decompress the portal system but are associated with severe encephalopathy.

Pathophysiology

Increased resistance to portal flow occurs at different levels: within the liver (intrahepatic) secondary to cirrhosis, prehepatic in situations of portal vein thrombosis, or posthepatic in hepatic venous obstruction. Normally, the porous hepatic venous sinusoids of the liver offer little resistance to portal flow. As discussed, distorted architecture due to fibrosis and regenerative nodule formation creates the increased resistance present at the intrahepatic level in cirrhosis. Consequent is splanchnic vasodilatation and increased splanchnic flow with ensuing clinical complications.

The increased blood flow through collateral vessels and subsequently increased venous return causes the characteristic hemodynamic features of portal hypertension. An increased venous return via collateral vessels results in an increase in cardiac output and total blood volume and a fall in systemic vascular resistance. Initially, blood pressure is normal; however, with disease progression, blood pressure falls.

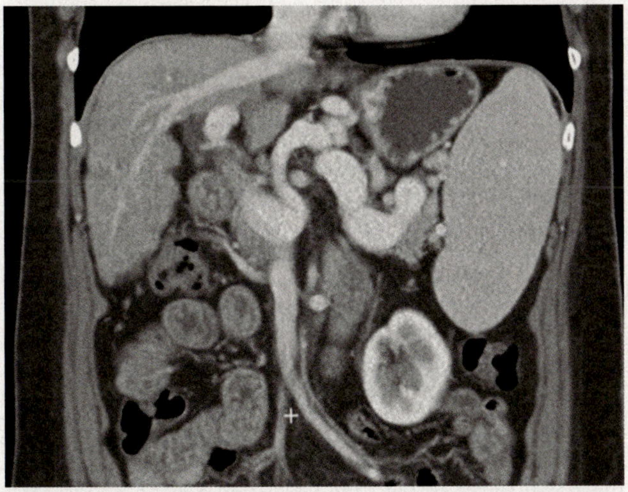

Figure 56.7. Coronal CT of a cirrhotic patient. Portal venous phase is shown, demonstrating retroperitoneal collaterals and splenomegaly. (Image courtesy of Dr. Ihab Khamel, Department of Radiology, Johns Hopkins Hospital.)

Nitric oxide, a potent vasodilator, as well as other vasodilators (prostacyclin, endotoxin, and glucagon), are elevated in patients with cirrhosis and portal hypertension.

Etiology

Different pathologic processes cause portal hypertension (**Table 56.11**).

Table 56.11. Common Causes of Portal Hypertension

Prehepatic
Congenital atresia
Extrinsic compression
Schistosomiasis
Portal, superior mesenteric, or splenic vein thrombosis
Splanchnic arteriovenous fistula
Intrahepatic (Presinusoidal)
Schistosomiasis
Idiopathic noncirrhotic portal hypertension (including nodular regenerative hyperplasia)
Primary biliary cholangitis (PBC)
Sarcoidosis
Congenital hepatic fibrosis
Primary sclerosing cholangitis
Adult polycystic liver disease
Vinyl chloride toxicity
Neoplastic occlusion of portal vein
Intrahepatic (Sinusoidal)
Arsenic poisoning
Vinyl chloride toxicity
Drugs (eg, amiodarone, methotrexate)
Chronic–Cirrhotic
MASLD
Hepatitis B, C
Alcohol
α_1-Antitrypsin deficiency
Cryptogenic
Cystic fibrosis
Hemochromatosis
Wilson disease
Chronic–Noncirrhotic
Congenital hepatic fibrosis
Focal regenerative hyperplasia
Hepatic veno-occlusive disease
Gaucher disease
Amyloid or light chain deposition in the space of Disse
Mastocytosis
Sarcoidosis
Intrahepatic (Postsinusoidal)
Budd–Chiari syndrome
Sinusoidal obstruction syndrome (veno-occlusive disease)
Chronic radiation injury
Vitamin A toxicity
Epithelioid hemangioendothelioma
Sarcoidosis
Posthepatic
Cardiac disease (Chronic heart failure, constrictive pericarditis)
IVC obstruction (eg, Budd–Chiari syndrome)
Vena cava webs

Budd–Chiari Syndrome and Veno-Occlusive Disease

Budd described the *classic* presentation of BCS—abdominal pain, ascites, and hepatomegaly. Chiari described the pathologic characteristics of the liver. Venous obstruction and hepatic venous occlusion cause an increase in pressure in the central veins with centrilobular congestion, necrosis, fibrosis, and cirrhosis with portal hypertension.

Common causes in Western populations are hypercoagulable states associated with polycythemia vera, myeloproliferative disorders, paroxysmal nocturnal hemoglobinuria, and hypercoagulable disorders. In Eastern countries, the major causes of obstruction of the vena cava and hepatic veins are membranous webs that directly occlude the vessels. The etiology of these webs is unknown. Veno-occlusive disease is characterized by obliterative endophlebitis of the intrahepatic veins. Causes of veno-occlusive disease include medications, toxins, and pyrrolizidine alkaloids (naturally occurring alkaloids in some plant species). BCS presentation is described above.

Although the diagnosis can be made by ultrasonographic evaluation of the liver and its vasculature with a sensitivity of 85% to 95%, cross-sectional imaging assists in staging and planning therapy. Duplex ultrasound may reveal the location of the obstruction and characterize flow within the vena cava and hepatic, portal, mesenteric, and splenic veins. Other common findings consistent with BCS include a lack of visualization of the hepatic veins, an enlarged caudate lobe with compressed vena cava, enlarged intrahepatic collaterals, splenomegaly, and ascites. Thrombus within the hepatic veins or IVC may be seen.

Because the vascular obstruction is usually well established at the time of presentation, anticoagulation alone is rarely sufficient. Historically, major open operations, including mesoatrial shunting and liver transplantation, were favored. However, minimally invasive approaches are now preferred, with percutaneous portacaval shunting effective in achieving decompression of the portal system, reducing mortality, and bridging to transplant.[49]

Creation of a mesoatrial shunt at surgery (described by Cameron and Maddrey) has been used to achieve decompression in the past in situations when bridging fibrosis was not present and transplant was not indicated. This involved decompressing the portal system by bypassing the hepatic veins and the narrowed IVC. After abdominal incision, the superior mesenteric vein flow is directed via graft to the right atrium and appendage. This graft is anastomosed first to the superior mesenteric vein and subsequently the right atrial anastomosis is completed.

Today, decompression of the portal system is achieved percutaneously via TIPS procedure. Contrary to TIPS in other settings of cirrhosis and portal hypertension, the rates of postprocedural encephalopathy are usually not increased in patients with BCS, because they have functionally healthy livers that are able to recover fully if decompression is achieved early, prior to the establishment of cirrhosis. If BCS results in fibrosis and cirrhosis, liver transplantation may be necessary. Postoperatively, patients require long-term anticoagulation to prevent recurrent thrombosis.

As noted, TIPS may be used as first-line therapy, and it has supplanted surgical shunting in the modern era with very good long-term outcomes. Shunt occlusion does occur; however, further angiographic intervention and anticoagulation can maintain patency.

Portal Vein Thrombosis

Portal vein thrombosis is commonly associated with advanced cirrhosis and may herald the occurrence of HCC. In children, portal vein thrombosis in the absence of cirrhosis is the most common cause of portal hypertension. However, this spontaneous portal venous thrombosis is uncommon in adults. In contrast to patients with cirrhosis, these patients have normal liver function and are not susceptible to the development of complications such as encephalopathy. Causes of portal vein thrombosis include umbilical vein infection (the most common cause in children), coagulopathies (protein C and antithrombin III deficiency), hepatic malignancy, myeloproliferative disorders, inflammatory bowel disease, pancreatitis, trauma, and previous splenorenal shunt. In patients with cirrhosis, a rebalanced hemostasis system prone to hypercoagulability can also contribute. This is mostly due to decreased levels of protein C and elevated levels of factor VIII.[50] Most cases in adults are idiopathic.

Imaging shows an echogenic lesion in the lumen of the portal vein and an absence of portal venous flow on duplex examination. With time, cavernous transformation of the portal vein may occur, recanalizing portal vein. CT and MRI are also useful in establishing the diagnosis. Portal vein thrombosis in a noncirrhotic patient may manifest initially with variceal bleeding. Splenomegaly is an important clinical sign.

The initial therapeutic option for the control of variceal hemorrhage caused by portal vein thrombosis is endoscopic esophageal variceal ligation. If unsuccessful, the distal splenorenal shunt has been the traditional surgical treatment for patients with isolated portal vein thrombosis. In patients whose intrahepatic portal vein is patent (most commonly children), a shunt may be created between the superior mesenteric vein and the patent left portal vein within the parenchyma of the liver (Rex shunt). This may be performed with internal jugular vein and may be the optimal therapeutic procedure for reestablishing physiologic portal flow.[22] This solution reduces portal pressure by restoring blood flow to the liver, preventing chronic hepatic atrophy and dysfunction, which would otherwise occur. Many consider the Rex shunt to be the first-line treatment, with splenorenal shunting reserved for patients who have no remnant intrahepatic portal system to receive the shunted blood.

Splenic Vein Thrombosis

Splenic vein thrombosis is often caused by disorders of the pancreas, including acute and chronic pancreatitis, trauma, malignancy, and pancreatic pseudocyst. This is due to the proximity of the splenic vein posterior to and abutting the pancreas. Other causes of thrombosis include retroperitoneal masses, abscesses, and inflammatory bowel disease; the remaining are idiopathic. Thrombosis results in isolated "sinistral" or "left-sided" portal hypertension. This increased venous pressure causes the development of gastric varices, which are present in approximately 80% of patients, and esophageal varices in 30% to 40%. Patients have normal liver function, and splenectomy is curative. The main indication for splenectomy is variceal hemorrhage.

Complications of Portal Hypertension

9 The most important, potentially lethal complication of portal hypertension is bleeding secondary to esophageal and gastric varices. Ascites and hepatic encephalopathy are other debilitating complications. Recently, there has been a shift to recognize compensated advanced chronic liver disease, away from the requirement of a radiologic or histologic diagnosis of cirrhosis for initial risk stratification.[2] The mortality risk associated with portal hypertension is primarily related to the functional status of the cirrhotic liver. In 1964, Child and Turcotte introduced a scoring system of liver function for the purposes of assessing prognosis after portosystemic shunt surgery in patients with cirrhosis. This has been subsequently modified several times to the Child–Turcotte–Pugh (CTP) score (**Table 56.12**). These indices incorporate clinical and laboratory data assessing the functional status of the liver, estimating hepatic reserve, and predicting morbidity and mortality. These criteria were initially adopted by the United Network for Organ Sharing (UNOS) as a tool for stratifying pretransplant mortality risk for patients on the waiting list for liver transplantation. Over the last

CLASSIFICATION

Table 56.12. Child–Turcotte Criteria for Hepatic Functional Reserve

Criterion	Class A	Class B	Class C
Encephalopathy	None	Minimal	Advanced
Ascites	None	Easily controlled	Poorly controlled
Bilirubin (mg/dL)	<2	2–3	>3
Albumin (g/gL)	>3.5	3–3.5	<3
Nutrition	Excellent	Good	Poor, "wasting"
Child–Turcotte–Pugh Grading of Severity of Liver Disease			
Score	**1**	**2**	**3**
Encephalopathy	None	1 or 2	3 or 4
Ascites	None	Mild	Moderate
Bilirubin (mg/dL)	1–2	2.1–3	≥3.1
Albumin (g/dL)	≥3.5	2.8–3.5	≤2.7
Prothrombin time (s)	1–4	4.1–6	≥6.1
or INR	<1.7	1.7–2.3	>2.3
Grade A, 5–6; grade B, 7–9; grade C, 10–15			

INR, international normalized ratio.
Adapted from Pugh RN, Murray-Lyon IM, Dawson JL, Pietroni MC, Williams R. Transection of the oesophagus for bleeding oesophageal varices. *Br J Surg.* 1973;60(8):646–649, with permission.

decade, the use of these criteria in transplant has been replaced by the model for end-stage liver disease (MELD) score, which uses serum bilirubin, creatinine, and the international normalized ratio (INR) to produce a robust prediction of 90-day mortality for patients with cirrhosis on the transplant list.[23] Subsequently, the inclusion of serum sodium to create the MELD-Na score was introduced in 2016, and the calculation was further adjusted to include patient sex and albumin with the introduction of the MELD 3.0 score currently in use.

While the MELD score was initially developed to determine prognosis of patients after undergoing TIPS, the CTP score has had long-standing use as a reliable predictor of mortality risk for shunt surgery and mortality risk of patients with cirrhosis undergoing other types of abdominal surgery. Patients with normal function, "Child A," have adequate hepatic reserve and survival rates similar to those of noncirrhotic patients, whereas Child C patients have mortality rates in excess of 50% and may not tolerate any intervention.

Varices

One of the most life-threatening complications of portal hypertension is bleeding from esophageal varices. Esophageal varices are dilated veins most commonly found in the distal 5 cm of the esophagus. In the normal esophagus, a venous plexus is located within the submucosa; distally, it is more superficial within the lamina propria. This anatomy is the reason for the incidence of bleeding from distal esophageal varices. In addition, patients with portal hypertension may have gastric varices.

As portal venous system pressure increases, varices are more likely to develop. Varices generally do not develop in persons with HVPGs less than 12 mm Hg. Pressure gradients above 12 mm Hg are invariably present in patients with varices, but this pressure does not necessarily produce varices in all patients. Gastroesophageal varices are present in 40% of patients with Child A cirrhosis, and in up to 85% of patients with Child C cirrhosis.

Esophageal varices are the cause of upper GI bleeding in approximately 10% of all patients presenting with acute bleeding. Conversely, cirrhotic patients bleed from sources *other than varices* (eg, peptic ulcer disease) in up to 40% of cases. Risk of variceal bleeding increases with duration present and variceal size. Approximately half of patient with cirrhosis have esophageal varices, and one-third of all patients with varices will develop variceal hemorrhage with the highest risk during the first year after diagnosis. Patients with large varices are at the greatest risk for an initial bleed. Variceal bleeding ceases without intervention in up to 40% of patients, although the risk of mortality and recurrent bleeding remain high. Of patients who survive an episode of bleeding, 30% rebleed within 6 weeks, and 70% at 1 year. Mortality from bleeding varies, from 5% for Child's A, less than 25% for Child's B, and more than 50% for Child C patients, respectively.[24]

When combined with clinical data such as the presence of active alcohol consumption, certain endoscopic characteristics of varices have been correlated with initial episodes of bleeding. Variceal size, Child–Pugh class, and the presence of red wale markings (longitudinal dilated venules) are contributing factors. Measurements of portal pressure predict the likelihood of bleeding, with hemorrhage occurring only in patients with gradients above 12 mm Hg.

Diagnosis of Varices and Prevention of Initial Variceal Bleeding

Noninvasive methods to diagnose and follow CSPH exist. Imaging includes CT, MRI and ultrasound that demonstrate ascites, recanalized umbilical veins and portosystemic shunts as well as splenomegaly and hepatofugal portal flow. *Liver stiffness measurement* and *TE* can reliably predict the presence of CSPH. Platelet count generally around under 150 k/mm^3 contributes to the predictive value.

Esophagogastroduodenoscopy (EGD) is the gold standard for the diagnosis of gastroesophageal varices and is indicated upon the initial diagnosis of cirrhosis and after 2 to 3 years if none are present. If small (<5-mm) varices are present, EGD is repeated in 1 to 2 years, and if patients have decompensated cirrhosis, *yearly* endoscopic screening is recommended by the AASLD. After diagnosis of varices, primary and secondary bleeding prophylaxis is implemented and includes control of the underlying cause of cirrhosis (ie, alcohol consumption or HCV treatment) and pharmacologic and surgical interventions to lower portal pressure.

Primary Prophylaxis for Prevention of Variceal Bleeding. In early-stage cirrhosis prior to the development of CSPH, treatment aims to prevent progression, decompensation, and potentially allow for regression of cirrhosis. Elimination of the etiologic agent (eg, alcohol, virus) at the current time is the mainstay of this strategy.

Beta Blockade: The use of nonspecific β-adrenergic blockade (NSBB) for the prevention of variceal bleeding has been studied extensively in RCTs. There is no evidence that NSBB prevents the development of varices in patients without CSPH. NSBB achieves β_1- and β_2-adrenergic blockade, which decreases cardiac output and increases splanchnic vasoconstriction due to diminished β_2-adrenergic mediated dilation. The end result is a decrease in portal blood flow and portal pressure (**Table 56.13**). Carvedilol is an NSBB with intrinsic anti–alpha-1-adrenergic activity and allows for a greater decrease in HVPG than traditional NSBB such as propranolol and nadolol. Carvedilol is better tolerated, more effective, and easier to use, and therefore, the preferred NSBB for management of PH.[2] Absolute and relative contraindications to beta blockade exist.

Table 56.13. Primary Prophylaxis: Management for Patients with Varices that Have Not Bled

Drug	Dose	Therapy Goals	Maintenance/Follow-up
Propranolol	▪ 20–40 mg bid adjusted every 2–3 d to a maximum of 320 mg/d in patients without ascites (160 mg/d in patients with ascites)	▪ Resting HR of 55–60 bpm ▪ Systolic BP should not decrease <90 mm Hg	▪ Monitor HR to ensure on target at every outpatient visit ▪ Continue indefinitely ▪ No need for follow-up EGD
Nadolol	▪ 20–40 mg orally once daily adjusted every 2–3 d to maximum of 160 mg/d in patients with ascites (80 mg/d in patients without ascites)		
Carvedilol	▪ Start with 6.25 mg once a day ▪ After 3 d, increase to 6.25 mg twice a day ▪ Maximum dose 12.5 mg/d	▪ Systolic BP should not decrease <90 mm Hg	▪ Continue indefinitely ▪ No need for follow-up EGD
Endoscopic variceal ligation	▪ Every 2–8 wk until the eradication of varices	▪ Variceal eradication	▪ First EGD 3–6 mo after eradication and every 6–12 mo thereafter

HR, heart rate; BP, blood pressure.
Adapted from Kaplan DE, Ripoli C, Thiele M, et al. AASLD Practice Guidance on risk stratification and management of portal hypertension and varices in cirrhosis. *Hepatology*. 2024;79:1180–1211.

Whether portal hypertension is due to prehepatic, intrahepatic, or posthepatic conditions, these drugs are effective in pressure reduction. The goal of therapy is to reduce the HVPG to less than 12 mm Hg or to more than 20% below baseline. Meeting these goals decreases bleeding risk as well as the risk of developing ascites, SBP, and death. Beta blockade with propranolol or nadolol has been clearly demonstrated to prevent initial bleeding. In patients with cirrhosis, both with and without ascites, who responded to lowering of portal pressure, NSBB has also been shown to reduce events (ascites, variceal hemorrhage, SBP, HRS, encephalopathy), reduce mortality and requirement for liver transplantation. Side effects of beta blockers may limit use, and it has been shown that they do not prevent the formation of varices in patients who do not yet have them.

Endoscopic Sclerotherapy and Variceal Ligation. Endoscopic sclerotherapy (ES) as primary prevention of variceal bleeding is no longer practiced due to incidence of esophageal and pulmonary complications. Endoscopic variceal ligation (EVL) may be used in patients with medium or large varices. Alternatively, beta blockade with NSBB or carvedilol as primary prophylaxis. Patients with cirrhosis with small, high-risk varices (ie, presence of red whale markings or occurring in a CTP-C patient) should be managed with beta-blocker prophylaxis.

Esophageal Variceal Bleeding

Initial Management. Esophageal variceal bleeding (**Table 56.14**) is a life-threatening emergency requiring intensive care. Patients who recover from the first episode of variceal hemorrhage have a high rebleeding risk (60% in the first year) with a mortality of up to 33%.

Initial management is similar to any other emergency due to hemorrhage: The airway is immediately secured, attention is given to ensuring adequate oxygenation and ventilation, and secure large-bore IV access is obtained. Laboratory studies aiding resuscitation include measurement of hemoglobin and hematocrit, coagulation status, liver function, electrolytes, and renal function.

Resuscitation begins with administration of packed red blood cells (PRBCs), platelets, and fresh frozen plasma as well as intravenous crystalloid as appropriate, and care is transitioned to an intensive care setting. Transfusion using a restrictive strategy (initiating PRBC transfusion at a hemoglobin threshold of 7 g/dL and maintaining it at 7 to 9 g/dL) is associated with a significant decrease in mortality compared to a "liberal" transfusion strategy (initiating PRBC transfusion at a hemoglobin threshold of 9 g/dL and maintaining it at 9 to 11 g/dL). Lower rebleeding and mortality rates were seen in cirrhotic patients randomized to the restrictive strategy.[51] Transfusion and volume expansion in the individual patient should consider factors such as age, cardiovascular disorders, ongoing bleeding, and hemodynamic status. It should also be noted that INR is not a reliable indicator of coagulation status in the setting of cirrhosis. There are currently no recommendations regarding administration of platelets or administration

Table 56.14. Guidelines for Management of Patients Presenting with an Acute Bleed
Resuscitation, intravenous access, endotracheal intubation, and ICU care as indicated
Performance of endoscopic evaluation within 12 h of bleed, and if variceal hemorrhage is suspected, variceal ligation should be performed
Intravenous vasoactive drugs should be initiated and continued for 2–5 d with addition of nonselective beta blockade once these are discontinued
Preemptive TIPS is indicated in patients with CTP class B score >7 and active bleeding on endoscopy or CTP class C score 10–13. This should occur within 72 h, ideally within 24 h of initial endoscopy unless contraindicated.
Covered expandable esophageal stents or balloon tamponade can bridge to TIPS in uncontrolled acute variceal hemorrhage
TIPS should be considered in patients with uncontrolled acute variceal hemorrhage ("salvage" TIPS) or who rebleed despite vasoactives and variceal ligation ("rescue" TIPS)
Prophylactic antibiotics (ceftriaxone) should be initiated

Adapted from Kaplan DE, Ripoli C, Thiele M, et al. AASLD Practice Guidance on risk stratification and management of portal hypertension and varices in cirrhosis. *Hepatology*. 2024;79:1180–1211.

Table 56.15. Vasoactive Agents Used in the Management of Acute Variceal Hemorrhage

Octreotide (somatostatin analog)	50-mcg IV bolus (can be repeated in first hour for ongoing bleeding), followed by 25–50 mcg/h continuous infusion	2–5 d
Vasopressin (with nitroglycerin)	0.2–0.4 U/min can be increased to 0.8 U/min. It should always be accompanied by nitroglycerin IV at a starting dose of 50 mcg/min (max 400 mcg/min) titrated to maintain SBP at approximately 90 mm Hg	24 h
Somatostatin	Initial IV bolus of 250 mcg (can be repeated in first hour if ongoing bleeding) Continuous IV infusion of 250–500 mcg/h	2–5 d
Terlipressin (Vasopressin analog)	Initial 24–48 h: 2 mg IV every 4–6 h until control of bleeding Maintenance: 1 mg IV every 4–6 h	2–5 d

Adapted from Garcia-Tsao G, Abraldes JG, Berzigotti A, et al. Portal hypertensive bleeding in cirrhosis: risk stratification, diagnosis, and management: 2016 Practice Guidance by the American Association for the study of liver diseases. *Hepatology*. 2017;65(1):310–355; and from Kaplan DE, Ripoli C, Thiele M, et al. AASLD Practice Guidance on risk stratification and management of portal hypertension and varices in cirrhosis. *Hepatology*. 2024;79:1180–1211.

of coagulation factors, while RCTs examining the effect of administration of factor VIIa have not shown benefit.

Cirrhotic patients who bleed are at a high risk of developing bacterial infections, including SBP. RCTs have shown that the use of antibiotic prophylaxis leads to a decrease in the development of infections, recurrent bleeding, and death. A brief period of intravenous antibiotics (eg, ceftriaxone 1 g every 24 hours) is recommended.

Pharmacologic Therapy. The administration of vasoactive medications should be commenced if variceal bleeding is suggested (**Table 56.15**). A meta-analysis of 30 RCTs shows that the use of vasoactive agents in acute variceal hemorrhage is associated with lower 7-day all-cause mortality and lower transfusion requirements.[52] Vasoactives decrease the rate of bleeding and enhance the endoscopist's ability to visualize the site of bleeding.

Vasopressin (antidiuretic hormone) has potent splanchnic vasoconstrictive properties that decrease portal and collateral blood flow. Continuous intravenous administration of vasopressin has been shown to reduce variceal bleeding, an observation initially made in 1962 and confirmed since. Compared to placebo, vasopressin stopped bleeding in 52% versus 18% of patients. However, rates of rebleeding as high as 45% were noted. Vasopressin should be used in combination with a vasodilator, such as nitroglycerin, to protect against coronary artery constriction, decrease cardiac events, and decrease intrahepatic and collateral resistance.

Somatostatin and octreotide, its longer-acting eight-amino acid derivative, have been used extensively for the treatment of variceal bleeding. These agents decrease splanchnic blood flow indirectly rather than by direct vasoconstriction. The effects of somatostatin are limited to the splanchnic circulation, so that side effects are minimized. In multiple studies, somatostatin and octreotide have proved to be as effective as vasopressin, sclerotherapy, and balloon tamponade.[53,54] A meta-analysis showed octreotide to be more effective than vasopressin in achieving hemostasis.[52] Octreotide is therefore the drug of choice in the United States. Dosing typically consists of a bolus of 50 μg followed by an infusion of 50 μg/h, to be initiated as soon as variceal bleeding is suspected and continued for 3 to 5 days after the diagnosis has been verified.

Endoscopic Interventions. Esophageal variceal ligation is performed at urgent endoscopy when varices are the source of bleeding. Signs of bleeding at endoscopy include: a visualized actively bleeding varix, a "white nipple" sign, and blood in the stomach within 24 hours of a bleed without any other evident cause. The endoscopist proceeds to suction the varix into the lumen of a plastic channel, and a rubber band is fired over the varix to complete ligation (**Fig. 56.8**). The varix and bleed are controlled, and the tissue sloughs after 1 to 3 days, leaving a shallow ulcer.

Success rates for variceal ligation range from 80% to 100%. Ligation compares favorably to sclerotherapy. Sclerotherapy can be used if bleeding is profuse and visualization is difficult.

Balloon Tamponade. Up to 20% of variceal hemorrhage episodes may be refractory to standard therapy, and in these circumstances balloon tamponade (**Fig. 56.9**) can bridge to a definitive therapy such a TIPS. Tamponade has high success rate in controlling bleeding but is also associated with a high rate of serious adverse events and a mortality rate near 20%. Tamponade entails the placement of a specialized nasogastric tube (the Sengstaken–Blakemore and Minnesota tubes) with two balloons that can be inflated separately to different pressures. These balloons compress varices present at the gastroesophageal junction and the esophagus. Once the mainstay in the initial management of variceal bleeding, use of these tubes is rare, and the techniques involved in placing them are becoming a lost art. Incorrect use may cause fatal complications due to esophageal injury. The Sengstaken–Blakemore tube consists of a gastric and an esophageal balloon with a sump port for gastric suctioning. The Minnesota tube has an

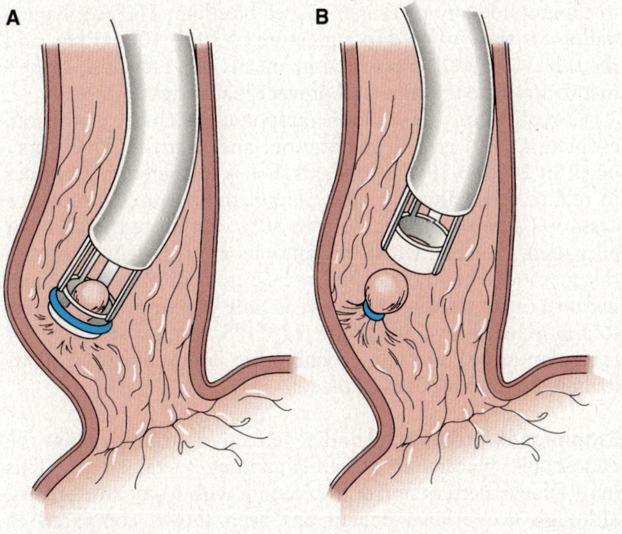

Figure 56.8. Endoscopic ligation of esophageal varices. The device used for ligation is based on the standard Barron-type ligator for the treatment of anal hemorrhoids. The esophageal varix is drawn up into the ligating device with suction (**A**), and the base of the varix is ligated with an O-ring (**B**). Up to six varices can be treated at a single session.

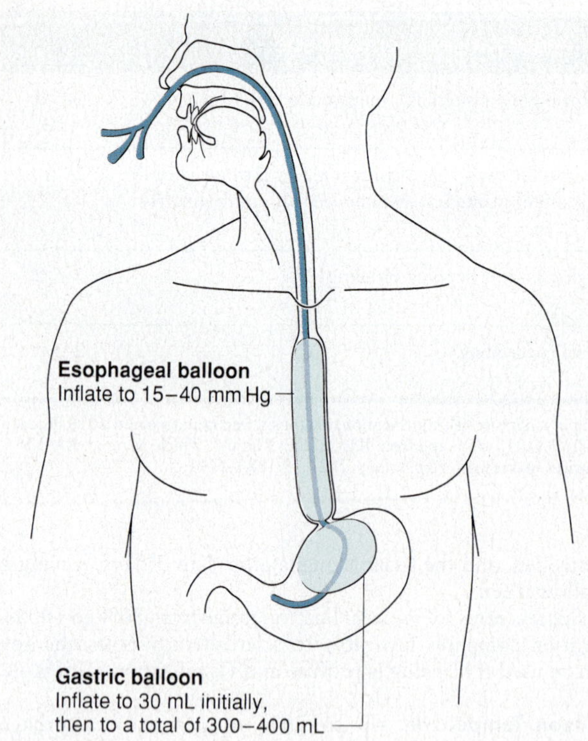

Figure 56.9. The Sengstaken–Blakemore tube is used to tamponade acutely bleeding gastroesophageal varices. The tube has three lumina—one to aspirate the stomach, another to inflate the gastric balloon, and a third to inflate the esophageal balloon. Patients treated with balloon tamponade should be in an intensive care unit, and endotracheal tubes should be placed in almost all to prevent aspiration.

additional port above the esophageal balloon for aspiration of saliva and other material.

Prior to tube placement, patients undergo endotracheal intubation to maintain a safe airway. The tube is then passed through the nose and into the stomach. Imaging confirms placement of the tip of the tube in the stomach before balloon inflation. This is critical to avoid inflation of the gastric balloon within the esophagus and subsequent esophageal perforation. The gastric balloon is inflated with 200 mL of air and firmly pulled backward against the gastroesophageal junction to tamponade any proximal gastric bleeding. The esophageal balloon is then inflated to a pressure of 30 to 40 mm Hg, and the tube is secured in position by means of a facemask or helmet to stabilize the tube and prevent inadvertent removal.

Complications of balloon tamponade include aspiration, esophageal and gastric perforation, and necrosis. These may occur in 10% to 20% of patients. Use is restricted to 24 hours to reduce the chance of these complications. Success rates for cessation of bleeding are 70% to 80%, but more than half of all patients rebleed when the balloons are deflated. Although this method is highly effective in the initial control of bleeding, because of its transient effect, it is only a temporizing bridge to a more definitive procedure (eg, TIPS, surgical shunting, or transplantation) and is used only after endoscopic and pharmacologic therapies have failed.

Esophageal Stenting. Another effective technique is the endoscopic placement of self-expanding metal stents. This may achieve better control of bleeding with fewer side effects, although no survival benefit has been shown compared to balloon tamponade. A major advantage of stenting is that the stent can stay in place for up to 7 days until definitive therapy.

Transjugular Intrahepatic Portosystemic Shunt. The mortality rate associated with failure to control active or recent bleeding is very high, and further, surgical shunts in this setting have a high morbidity and mortality. For patients who are high risk with bleeding (CTP class B with active bleeding, or CTP class C), early TIPS within the first 24 to 72 hours has data supporting efficacy. Historically, surgical shunts were performed to bypass the high-pressure hepatic vascular bed.

10 TIPS (**Figs. 56.10** and **56.11**) has become first-line treatment for bleeding esophageal varices when the aforementioned attempts fail to stop uncontrolled hemorrhage (salvage TIPS) or in those who rebleed despite vasoactives and EVL (Rescue TIPS).[2] Absolute contraindications to TIPS include congestive heart failure, uncontrolled sepsis, multiple hepatic cysts, severe pulmonary hypertension, and uncontrolled biliary obstruction. Relative contraindications include HCC, hepatic vein obstruction, severe coagulopathy or thrombocytopenia, and moderate pulmonary hypertension. After ultrasonographic confirmation of patency of the portal vein, the procedure is performed in the interventional radiology suite, where a stent (8 to 12 mm in diameter) is placed percutaneously over a wire into the jugular vein. The wire is then guided through the superior vena cava, right atrium, and IVC into a hepatic vein, after which the catheter traverses the hepatic parenchyma and connects the hepatic vein to a portal vein (usually the right portal vein). This connection creates a side-to-side portacaval shunt. Success rates in the cessation of variceal bleeding are as high as 90% to 100%, with few recurrent bleeds.[55]

The ideal portosystemic shunt lowers the portal pressure without critically reducing liver perfusion. This avoids causing hepatic dysfunction, which would accelerate the progression of cirrhosis. It is possible to measure the portal pressure during TIPS, and this can guide optimal management of the TIPS to balance control of bleeding with hepatic perfusion. To control bleeding, the therapeutic goal is to reduce the hepatic venous pressure gradient (HVPG) to below 12 mm Hg. TIPS reduces the HVPG to a mean of approximately 9 to 15 mm Hg (average, 10 mm Hg) or to around half of baseline. A residual HVPG less than 5 mm Hg has been associated with a deleterious impact on hepatic flow. Since well-validated instruments predict the survival of patients after TIPS, the procedure should be used with caution in patients with high MELD scores, though TIPS has been used successfully to bridge to transplant. The use of TIPS in massive variceal bleeding in a patient with a high MELD score who has contraindications to liver transplant should be regarded as a palliative intervention.

As with all portosystemic shunts, a significant complication of TIPS is the development of hepatic encephalopathy. The rate of encephalopathy following TIPS is 34%, compared to 19% following EVL for acute variceal bleeding, although the use of covered TIPS stents has reduced the rate of post-TIPS encephalopathy from when bare metal stents were used primarily. Early series showed stenosis or occlusion of the TIPS stent developing in up to 50% to 60% of patients in the first year. Long-term patency is now maintained by ongoing surveillance of the shunt with redilatation, thrombolysis, or replacement as required. Current shunts are lined with polytetrafluoroethylene (PTFE) and have a much higher patency than the original permeable wall stents. Primary patency rates are 76% to 89% with shunt dysfunction occurring in 15% of patients at 1 year. Patients are usually followed at 6-month intervals by ultrasonography to assess the patency of the shunt and for HCC screening. At 6 months of follow-up, 92% of patients had no episodes of rebleeding, and 82% were free of hemorrhage at 1 year. TIPS has become the standard procedure used to halt bleeding in patients who fail medical therapy. The ability to effectively decompress the portal circulation without open surgery in these critically ill patients has transformed clinical hepatology. Patients who become stable can be evaluated for transplantation electively.

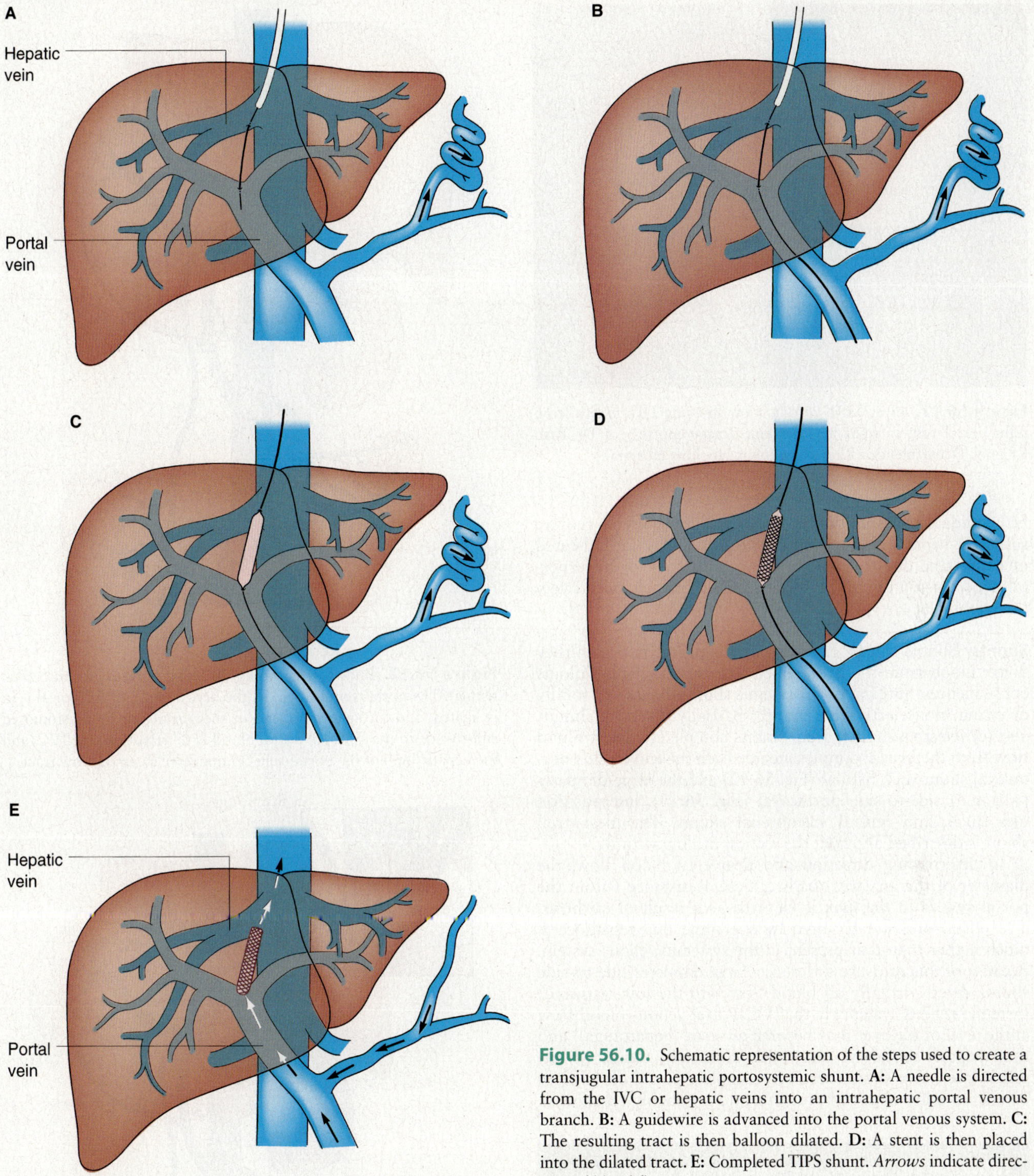

Figure 56.10. Schematic representation of the steps used to create a transjugular intrahepatic portosystemic shunt. **A:** A needle is directed from the IVC or hepatic veins into an intrahepatic portal venous branch. **B:** A guidewire is advanced into the portal venous system. **C:** The resulting tract is then balloon dilated. **D:** A stent is then placed into the dilated tract. **E:** Completed TIPS shunt. *Arrows* indicate direction of blood flow.

Patients Who Have Recovered From an Episode of Acute Variceal Hemorrhage

Patients who recover from the first episode of variceal bleeding have a 60% chance of rebleeding in the first year, with a mortality of up to 33%. Prevention of rebleed is key (**Table 56.16**). First-line therapy in these patients is the combination of NSBB and variceal ligation. TIPS has a lower rebleeding rate, although no difference in survival, but is associated with encephalopathy.

In medically treated patients, the lowest rebleeding rates are observed in patients on secondary prophylaxis who are HVPG responders (defined as a reduction in HVPG below 12 mm Hg or >20% from baseline) on pharmacotherapy. However, TIPS has been shown to lower rates of rebleeding but without differences in survival and with a higher incidence of encephalopathy.

11 *Surgical Decompression*

Background. Orthotopic liver transplantation is the definitive treatment for portal hypertension caused by cirrhosis. As discussed above, most patients with bleeding esophageal varices are managed by TIPS or variceal band ligation and NSBB. The introduction and increased use of TIPS has virtually eliminated the need for emergency surgical portosystemic shunting. There is a small group of patients with portal hypertension whose bleeding cannot be controlled by endoscopy, who may

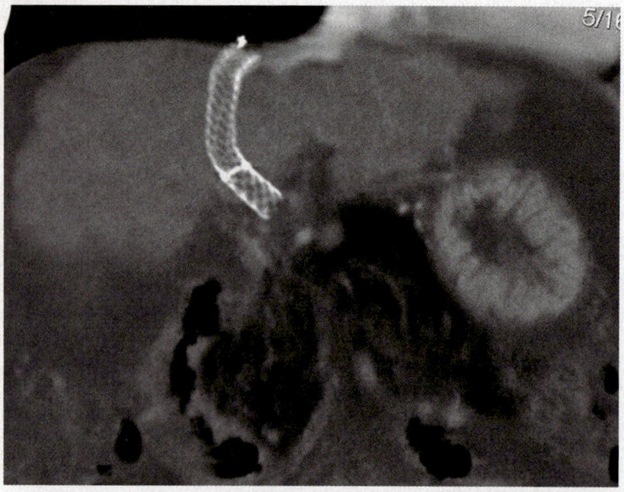

Figure 56.11. Liver MRI, coronal view showing TIPS in situ from right portal vein to right hepatic vein. (Image courtesy of Dr. Ihab Khamel, Department of Radiology, Johns Hopkins Hospital.)

be candidates for shunting procedures. These patients require sufficient hepatic reserve that liver transplant is not indicated or achievable due to inability to access a liver, or have portal hypertension due to prehepatic conditions (eg, portal vein thrombosis).

Shunts. Shunts can be classified by the degree to which they divert blood from the liver, which has important physiologic consequences. Surgical portosystemic shunts include (a) totally diverting (nonselective) shunts, (b) partially diverting shunts, and (c) selective shunts. Total shunts completely divert blood flow from the liver. Examples include both the end-to-side portacaval shunt (Eck fistula) (**Fig. 56.12**) and the large-diameter (>10-mm) side-to-side portacaval (**Fig. 56.13**), interposition mesocaval, and central splenorenal shunts. The mesoatrial shunt is described above in the section dealing with BCS.

In determining direction and degree of blood flow, the diameter of the anastomosis is critical. Resistance within the portal system in the liver is elevated as a result of cirrhosis. The portal pressure required to overcome this resistance is much higher than that present in the systemic venous system. Because of this pressure difference, large diameter side-to-side shunts divert virtually all blood flow into the low-resistance systemic venous system via the IVC. Portal venous blood flow at the level of the liver may become reversed (hepatofugal) and total hepatic perfusion decreased. Ultimately, totally diverting, nonselective shunts result in complete portal blood flow diversion, a lower portal pressure, and are highly effective in

Table 56.16. Secondary Prophylaxis: Guidelines for Prevention of Rebleeding after Variceal Hemorrhage

Maximal tolerated dosing of nonselective beta blockade with serial EVL until all varices are obliterated is performed, unless TIPS has been placed
Patients should then undergo surveillance EGD every 6–12 mo to evaluate for recurrent varices
Those patients who are candidates should be referred to a transplant center for timely evaluation

Adapted from Garcia-Tsao G, Abraldes JG, Berzigotti A, et al. Portal hypertensive bleeding in cirrhosis: risk stratification, diagnosis, and management: 2016 practice guidance by the American Association for the study of liver diseases. *Hepatology.* 2017;65(1):310–355.

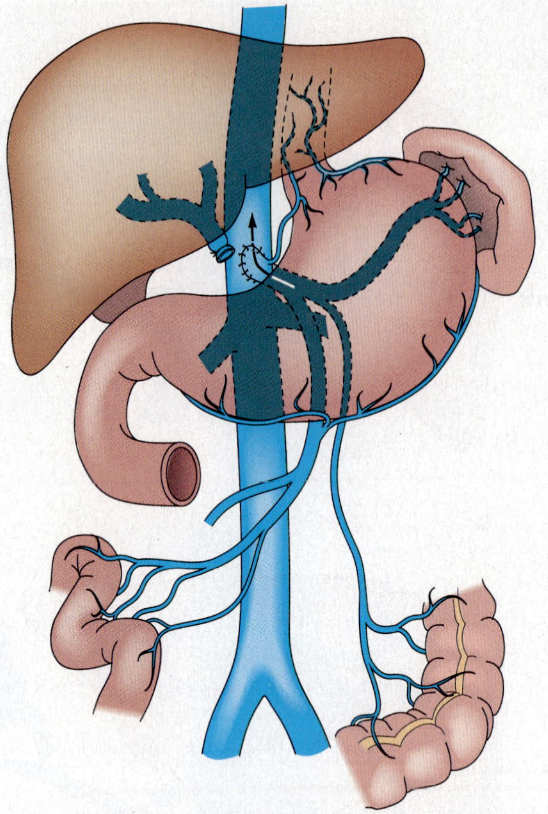

Figure 56.12. End-to-side, totally diverting portacaval shunt (Eck fistula). The portal vein is divided, the hepatic limb of the portal vein is ligated, and the splanchnic end of the portal vein is anastomosed end-to-side to the IVC. All portal blood is diverted into the IVC, and the hepatic limb of the portal vein cannot serve as an outflow tract.

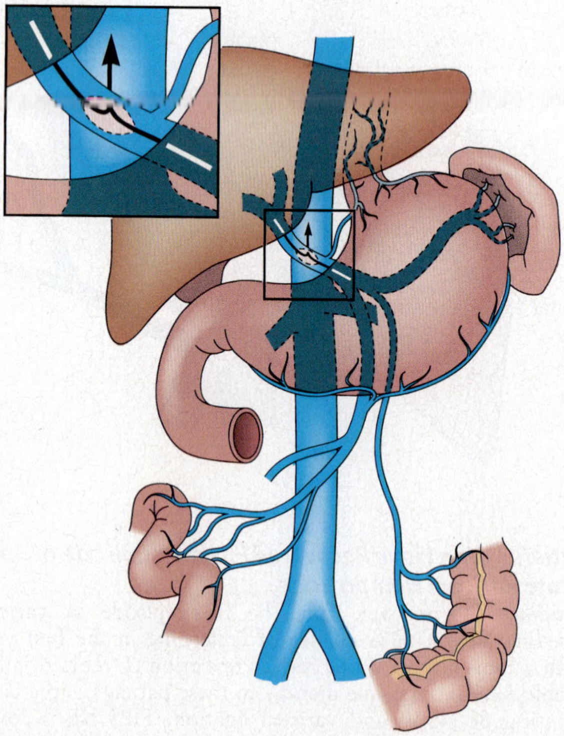

Figure 56.13. Side-to-side portacaval shunt.An anastomosis is made between the side of the portal vein and the side of the inferior vena cava. With a shunt of standard diameter, almost all splanchnic blood is diverted around the liver into the low-pressure vena cava. The hepatic limb of the portal vein serves as an outflow tract from the liver toward the low-pressure vena cava.

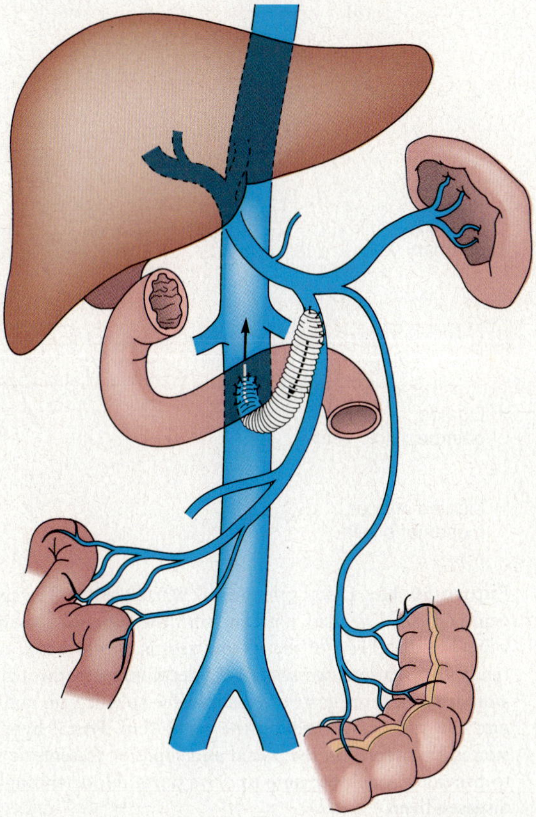

Figure 56.14. Interposition mesocaval shunt. A plastic prosthesis or an autogenous internal jugular vein is used for the shunt. One end is anastomosed to the inferior vena cava, and the other end is anastomosed to the trunk of the superior mesenteric vein. The shunt curves around the lower edge of the third portion of the duodenum and is sometimes called a C-shunt.

treating bleeding varices. They may however *accelerate* hepatic decompensation via both diminished hepatic flow and removal of hepatotrophic substances present in mesenteric venous flow. Nonselective shunting also leads to encephalopathy but may be used to treat ascites.

When initially proposed, it was suggested that **partially diverting shunts** decompressed the portal venous system sufficiently while maintaining prograde, hepatopetal portal flow into the liver. This contention has been debated extensively. Initial shunts were created with a diameter larger than 10 mm, which maintained some antegrade hepatic flow. After shunt creation, however, in most instances, complete or total shunting occurred over time as the shunt dilated and the gradient between portal pressure and IVC pressure disappeared. Smaller shunts were therefore created. Small-diameter (8-mm) side-to-side mesocaval (**Fig. 56.14**) and portacaval (Sarfeh or interposition "H" graft) (**Fig. 56.15**) shunts are performed with an interposition graft made of either expanded PTFE or dacron. The interposition "H" portacaval shunt involves ligation of portosystemic collaterals. The umbilical vein within the falciform ligament, the coronary (left gastric), the gastroepiploic along the greater curve of the stomach, and the inferior mesenteric veins are usually ligated. Bleeding from varices resolves in more than 90% of patients. This smaller-diameter shunt has a higher resistance than the larger shunt, is synthetic and therefore does not dilate, can maintain hepatic perfusion, and is associated with a lower incidence of hepatic encephalopathy. Portal pressure gradients are reduced and hepatopetal flow is maintained. Shunt thrombosis may occur in up to 16% of patients but can be treated angiographically.[56]

Selective shunts are designed to create two separate drainage systems within the portal venous network. High pressure is maintained within the mesenteric system, and a low pressure is created in the esophagogastric system by shunting blood from these varices into the systemic circulation without decompressing the mesenteric network. The most traditional and favored selective shunt is the distal splenorenal shunt. This technically

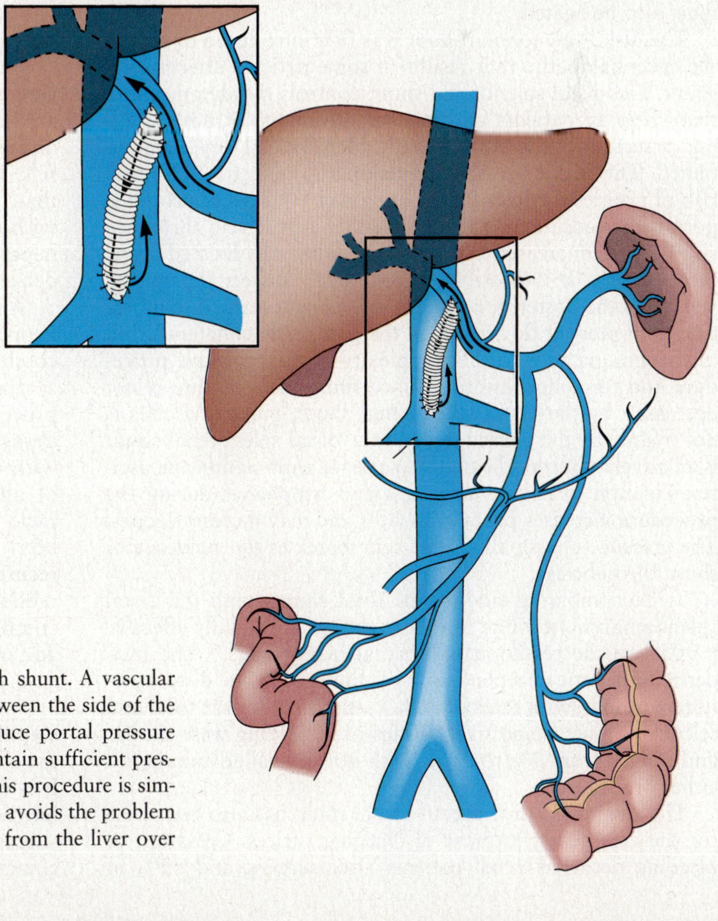

Figure 56.15. Small-diameter interposition portacaval Sarfeh shunt. A vascular prosthesis measuring 8 to 10 mm in diameter is interposed between the side of the vena cava and the side of the portal vein. The goal is to reduce portal pressure partially and thereby prevent variceal hemorrhage but still maintain sufficient pressure to permit the prograde flow of portal blood to the liver. This procedure is simpler to perform than that for the Warren shunt and theoretically avoids the problem of diversion of an increasing proportion of portal blood away from the liver over time, as occurs with the Warren shunt.

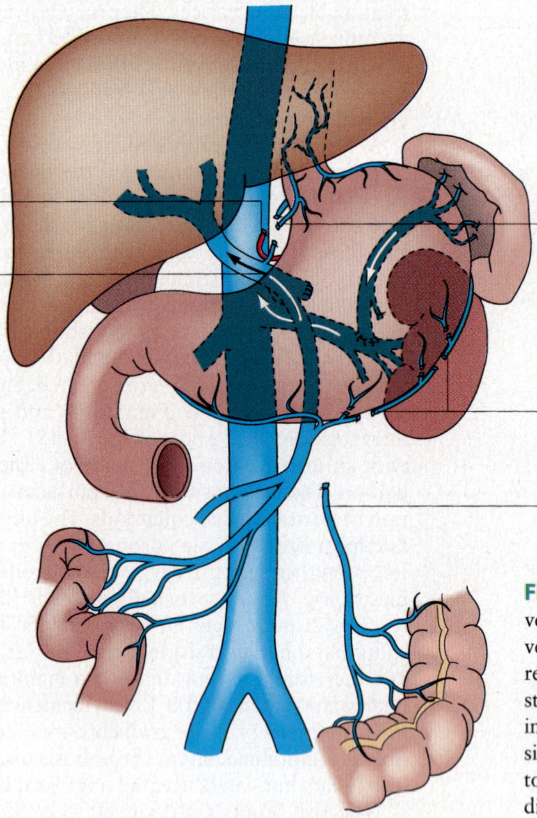

Figure 56.16. Distal splenorenal Warren shunt. The splenic vein is divided near its junction with the superior mesenteric vein. The distal end of the splenic vein is anastomosed to the renal vein. Varices are selectively decompressed through the stomach and short gastric veins into the splenic vein and then into the vena cava through the renal vein. Portal hypertension is maintained in the portal and superior mesenteric veins to provide enough pressure to drive portal blood through the diseased liver.

demanding shunt (**Fig. 56.16**) decompresses the gastroesophageal venous system through an anastomosis between the distal splenic vein and the side of the renal vein. Decompression occurs through the vasa brevia (short gastric veins), which are in continuity with the splenic vein. Collateral veins (as above) must also be ligated.

The distal splenorenal shunt was first introduced to reduce the encephalopathy that results in some patients after a total shunt. The distal splenorenal shunt controls bleeding in more than 90% of patients and has the advantage of not requiring dissection of the porta hepatis. Hepatopetal flow is maintained. The incidence of encephalopathy (5% to 24%) and risk of progressive liver failure are lower.[57,58] Loss of prograde portal flow occurs as a result of either portal vein thrombosis (10%) or increased flow through collaterals located along the pancreas. It is possible to completely dissect the splenic vein from the posterior pancreas (splenopancreatic disconnection) and prevent flow through the pancreatic collaterals, but this technique adds to the complexity of the operative procedure and to complications.[59] Since sinusoidal pressure is not decreased by the distal splenorenal shunt, massive ascites is not treated by the procedure, and the distal splenorenal shunt is relatively contraindicated in patients with significant ascites. Ligation of collateral vessels and lymphatics during the procedure increases portal pressures and may increase ascites. The presence of a small splenic vein increases the incidence of shunt thrombosis.

Trials comparing side-to-side total shunts with the distal splenorenal shunt found that both groups are equally effective (>90%) in the cessation of variceal hemorrhage.[60] The incidence of hepatic encephalopathy is lower after the distal splenorenal shunt, with rates of 36% versus 15% for the total and selective shunts, respectively. Rates of rebleeding were similar and ranged from 0% to 30%, with no survival advantage for either procedure.

The side-to-side nonselective total shunt has also been used for the emergent treatment of bleeding varices. Cessation of bleeding occurred in all patients after surgery, and 99% of patients were completely free of episodes of rebleeding. The 5-year survival was approximately 80%, most deaths occurring during the first year after surgery due to progressive hepatic failure. Hepatic encephalopathy requiring treatment occurred in 8% of patients. Of note, most of these patients had alcoholic liver disease, which shows some improvement on cessation of alcohol.

Devascularization Procedures. Devascularization procedures are techniques in which the venous drainage of the stomach and esophagus is disconnected from the liver and intestinal vessels. These procedures are relatively less technically demanding than shunting procedures and can be performed in patients with extensive portal thrombosis. They do not interfere with hepatopetal blood flow and therefore do not increase the incidence of hepatic encephalopathy.

A range of procedures of varying complexity is possible. Esophageal transection with end-to-end reanastomosis (EEA) combined with ligation of the coronary vein (**Fig. 56.17**) is a relatively simple procedure. More complex is the Sugiura procedure (**Fig. 56.18**). This procedure involves splenectomy, devascularization of the proximal stomach and esophagus with esophageal transection and reanastomosis, and ligation of all gastroesophageal collaterals via abdominal and thoracic incisions.[61] A single abdominal incision procedure has been described.[62] Japanese researchers describe bleeding as recurring in fewer than 5% of patients in Japan, but rates of rebleeding are higher and range from 10% to 54% in other countries. Operative mortality rates range from 10% to 35% and outcomes are certainly related to the severity of liver disease. Devascularization procedures are rarely performed today.

Hepatic Transplantation. Orthotopic liver transplantation is the definitive therapy for portal hypertension and cirrhosis. It is indicated for management of end-stage liver disease and has no role in the control of acute variceal bleeding. When successful, transplantation treats the underlying disease and complications of end-stage liver disease.

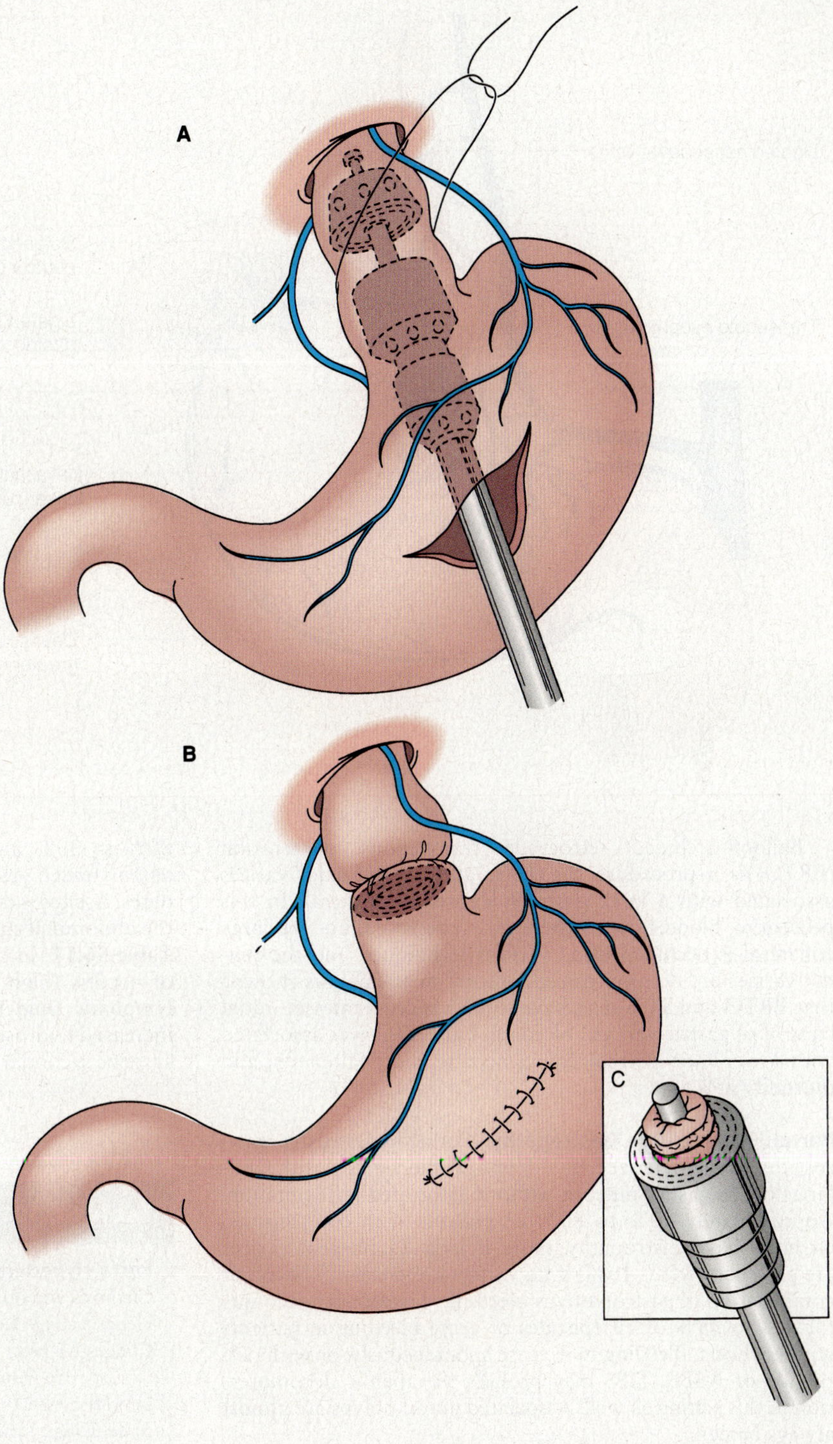

Figure 56.17. Transection and reanastomosis of the distal esophagus with the stapling device to control variceal hemorrhage. **A:** A stapling device is inserted through a small gastrotomy incision. **B:** When the device is fired, the esophagus is simultaneously transected and reanastomosed with staples. **C:** If the device fires correctly, a complete ring of esophageal tissue is excised.

In conclusion, open surgical intervention short of liver transplantation for patients with cirrhosis and portal hypertension is rare. With the advent of TIPS, surgical shunts are less often indicated. While reintervention may be required after TIPS, the overwhelming efficacy and safety of this procedure has essentially removed almost all need for open portal decompressive procedures.

Gastropathy and Gastric Varices

Approximately 20% of patients with cirrhosis have gastric varices, although their association is greater with prehepatic portal hypertension, and when present, thrombosis of the splenic and portal systems needs to be excluded. The most commonly used classification for risk stratification and management of gastric varices is the Sarin classification. Varices located along the lesser curve have a natural history similar to esophageal varices. When present along the cardia and greater curve of the fundus, varices bleed less frequently than esophageal varices but have a worse prognosis in terms of treatment failure, rebleeding, and mortality.[2] Bleeding from gastric varices occurs in approximately 25% of affected patients. In general, data is not robust in this population. NSBB is recommended to be used to prevent bleeding from gastric varices. Sclerotherapy and EVL are also effective. Other emerging endoscopic tools, such as endoscopic ultrasound-guided insertion of coils or cyanoacrylate injection, remain to be evaluated. Balloon tamponade may temporize. TIPS is highly effective as primary therapy for controlling gastric varices in patients who fail or cannot receive endoscopic therapy, with initial hemostasis rates of over 90% reported. The distal splenorenal shunt is reserved for the rare patient who cannot receive TIPS.

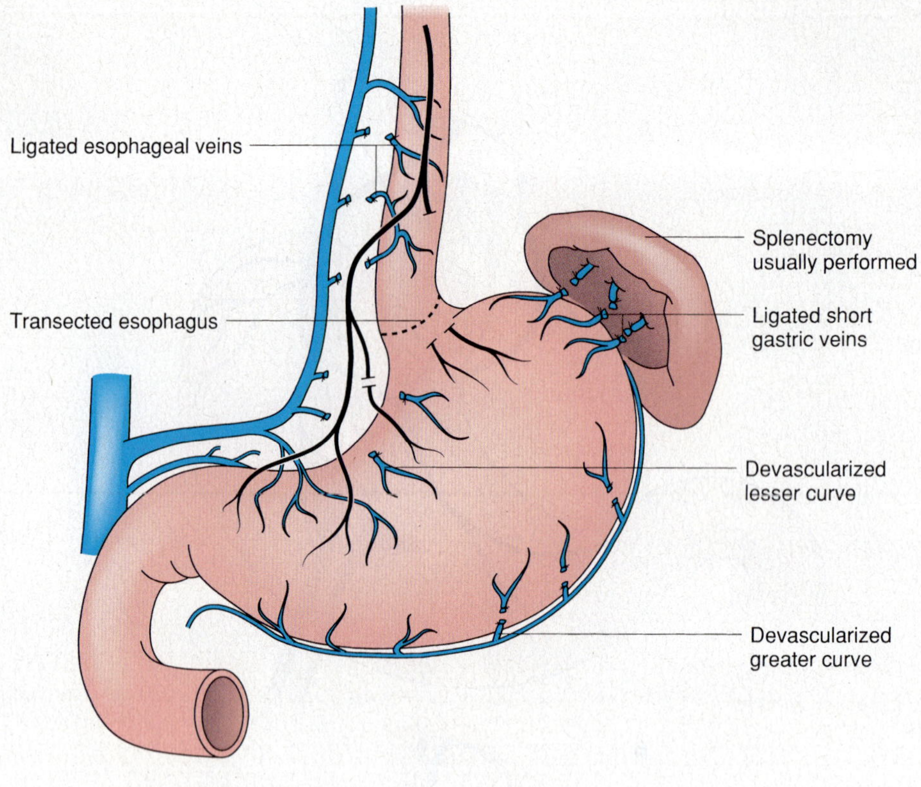

Figure 56.18. Sugiura esophageal transection and devascularization operation.

Balloon-occluded retrograde transvenous obliteration (BRTO) is a procedure for the treatment of fundal varices associated with a large gastro/splenorenal collateral. In this procedure, blood flow to the liver is preserved, but the large collateral is occluded using various techniques, and the fundal varices are decompressed. A recent meta-analysis showed that BRTO and TIPS may have similar success rates in initial control of gastric variceal bleeding, but BRTO was associated with lower rates of rebleeding, hepatic encephalopathy, and mortality at 1 year.

Portal Hypertensive Gastropathy. Portal hypertensive gastropathy is characterized by dilation of the venules and capillaries of the gastric mucosa without associated inflammation. Approximately 50% to 80% of patients with compensated cirrhosis have gastropathy, more if large esophageal varices are present, fewer (~10%) if no varices are present. The major complication of gastropathy is bleeding; gastropathy accounts for 4% to 38% of all episodes of acute bleeding in patients with cirrhosis. Bleeding may cease spontaneously, or with octreotide or NSBB. TIPS may provide therapeutic decompression in this setting as well. Associated antral polyps are almost always benign.

Ectopic Varices. Bleeding from ectopic varices is rare in cirrhotic patients, but more common in patients with prehepatic portal hypertension. Location and anatomy are variable, such that case-by-case assessment and management are necessary. Contrasted CT with portal venous phase imaging and large-volume diluted oral contrast assist with diagnosis and delineation of anatomy. Sites of ectopic variceal bleeding are surgically created stomas, duodenum, jejunoileum, and colon. A multidisciplinary approach to management is needed. Endoscopy, TIPS, and BRTO may be useful. Superficial stomal varices may be amenable to injection of cyanoacrylate or sclerosants.

Ascites

One of the first, most frequent, and important consequences of cirrhosis and portal hypertension is ascites. The development of ascites is associated with a decrease in survival from 80% to 30% at 5 years. Unfortunately, it does not lead to any increased priority in organ allocation for transplant candidates. Ascites is defined as the accumulation of free fluid within the abdominal cavity (normally <150 mL). Causes are listed in **Table 56.17**. In cirrhosis, fluid is derived from a combination of hepatic (high in protein) and splanchnic (low in protein) lymphatic fluid that cannot be absorbed as a result of the increased hydrostatic pressures within the liver and splanchnic systems secondary to cirrhosis and capillarization of the space

DIAGNOSIS

Table 56.17. Differential Diagnosis of Ascites

Portal Hypertension
Cirrhosis and other intrahepatic diseases
Hepatic congestion
Congestive heart failure
Constrictive pericarditis
Inferior vena cava obstruction
Budd–Chiari syndrome
Portal vein occlusion
Hypoalbuminemia
Nephrotic syndrome
Protein-losing enteropathy
Malnutrition
Miscellaneous Disorders
Myxedema
Ovarian disease (Meigs syndrome, struma ovarii)
Peritoneal carcinomatosis
End-stage renal disease
Chylous ascites
Bile ascites
Urine ascites

From Sleisenger MH, Fordran JS. *Gastrointestinal disease: Pathophysiology. Diagnosis and Management*. 4th ed. WB Saunders; 1989:433.

of Disse. Because of the loss of sinusoidal fenestrations and a subsequent decrease in their permeability, splanchnic lymph is more abundant than hepatic lymph in patients with advancing cirrhosis, so that the protein content of ascitic fluid is relatively low. The main underlying pathophysiology in the development of ascites is renal sodium and water retention, which leads to fluid overload.

Clinical and Laboratory Features

Ascites may be present in patients with cirrhosis who have no other overt signs or symptoms. Examination reveals shifting dullness to percussion (1.5 L of ascitic fluid), fluid waves (10 L), and bulging flanks. Respiratory status may be compromised secondary to increased intra-abdominal pressure and pleural effusion (usually right). The progression may be slow or precipitated after an inciting event, such as a bleed or infection. Fluid filled umbilical and inguinal hernias may form and be present on examination.

Diagnostic Paracentesis

The differential diagnosis of ascites is presented in **Table 56.17**. Analysis of ascitic fluid from patients with cirrhosis shows it to be straw colored and clear; measurements of protein (usually <2 g/dL), quantitative cell counts, and microbiologic culture and determination of pH, amylase, glucose, and albumin levels should be obtained. The serum-to-ascitic fluid albumin gradient (SAAG) is calculated by subtracting the albumin concentration in ascites from the serum and is helpful in determining the cause of ascites: high values (>1.1 g/dL) indicate portal hypertension, whereas lower levels are associated with other disorders, including malignancy.

Treatment

Initial management includes treating or removing the inciting factor. Where alcohol, autoimmune, or HBV-related liver disease is present, ascites can resolve with treatment of these causes. In cirrhotics, lower blood pressure is associated with worse survival. Due to the central role of the renin–angiotensin–aldosterone axis in the pathogenesis of the hemodynamic disturbances of cirrhosis, angiotensin-converting enzyme inhibitors and angiotensin II receptor blockers should be avoided. In addition, propranolol may decrease survival in patients with refractory ascites. NSAIDs inhibit prostaglandin synthesis and impair renal function.

Therapy is directed at renal sodium and water retention. A low-sodium diet is a critical part of the management of patients with cirrhosis (an upper limit of 2000 mg/d or 45 to 90 mEq/d). Fluid restriction (1000 to 1500 mL of fluid/d) is also an essential component of therapy in patients in whom hyponatremia (sodium <125 mEq/L) develops. Most patients do not respond to fluid and salt restriction alone, and diuresis is indicated (**Table 56.18**). Loop diuretics (furosemide) and potassium-sparing diuretic (spironolactone) are the two most widely used agents. They are often required in combination. A ratio of 40-mg furosemide to 100-mg spironolactone generally maintains potassium homeostasis. Diuresis of approximately 500 mL/d is the goal for patients with mild ascites and up to 1 to 2 L/d for patients with both ascites and peripheral edema. More than 90% of patients respond to dietary manipulation and diuretics. Analysis of 24-hour urinary sodium excretion or spot urine Na/K ratio can guide diuresis. Torsemide or bumetanide may be helpful if furosemide is not sufficient.

Important adverse effects of spironolactone include gynecomastia in males, hyperkalemia, and metabolic acidosis. Complications of furosemide include prerenal uremia, which occurs in approximately 20% of patients due to excessive diuresis, and hypovolemia. Additional complications include hyponatremia and encephalopathy.

Large-volume paracentesis (removal of 4 to 6 L of ascitic fluid per day) is performed for patients who are symptomatic

Table 56.18. Treatment of Ascites

Bed rest
Sodium restriction 1–2 g/d (45–90 mEq/d)
Fluid restriction 1–1.5 L/d
Diuretics Spironolactone 50 mg PO q8h Maximum of 100 mg q6h Furosemide 40–370 mg/d Torsemide or bumetanide may also be useful
Antibiotics Cefotaxime 2 g IV q12h Ofloxacin 400 mg PO q12h Prophylaxis Norfloxacin 400 mg/d while hospitalized Ciprofloxacin 750 mg PO weekly Norfloxacin 400 mg/d for 6 mo Trimethoprim/sulfamethoxazole One double-strength tablet five times a week

due to massive ascites and who do not respond to diuretics. Patients requiring paracentesis usually have severe underlying liver disease and a 1-year survival of 25%. Large-volume paracentesis involves placing a catheter into the abdominal cavity, either in the lower midline or in one of the lower quadrants. Entry lateral to the rectus muscle avoids the inferior epigastric artery. Albumin (6 to 8 g/L of ascites removed) is infused intravenously in the form of 25% albumin (12.5 g/50 mL). Patients who have less than 5 L of ascitic fluid removed do not usually require albumin replacement. Repetitive large-volume paracentesis can be safely performed.

Historically, peritoneovenous shunts (LeVeen and Denver shunts) were surgically placed tubes that connect the peritoneal cavity with the superior vena cava via the internal jugular vein. A one-way valve allowed unidirectional movement of ascitic fluid from the peritoneal cavity into the systemic circulation. Major complications and high failure rates have led to the cessation of use of these, especially with the advent of the TIPS procedure.

TIPS is highly effective in treating ascites and leads to resolution in around 80% of patients. In addition, renal function may improve. TIPS, however, is associated with an increase in encephalopathy. Patients with a MELD of 18 or more and other risk factors (advanced age, cardiopulmonary insufficiency, and sarcopenia) are not candidates for TIPS. Recurrence of ascites post-TIPS should prompt assessment of TIPS patency.

12 SBP is a potentially lethal complication of portal hypertension with ascites that occurs in up to 10% of patients. While the cause of SBP is unclear, antecedent GI hemorrhage is common, and SBP in this setting may be related to bacterial translocation from the gut. Deficits in immune function, both systemically and within the abdomen, including depressed reticuloendothelial function, low ascitic protein concentration, and deficient ascitic opsonic activity likely play a role. Patients often present with abdominal pain and fever, but some cases are discovered on routine paracentesis. Patients

Table 56.19. Bacteria Isolated from Ascitic Fluid in 519 Patients with Spontaneous Bacterial Peritonitis

Organisms	Percentage of Total
Escherichia coli	43
Klebsiella pneumoniae	11
Streptococcus pneumoniae	9
Other Streptococci	19
Pseudomonas	1
Enterobacteriaceae	4
Staphylococci	3
Miscellaneous	10

Adapted from McHutchison JG, Runyon BA. Spontaneous bacterial peritonitis. In: Surawicz CM, Owen RL, eds. *Gastrointestinal and Hepatic Infections*. WB Saunders; 1995:455.

may present with other signs not clearly related to SBP, including worsening encephalopathy and AKI, and workup for SBP in these settings should be performed. Diagnosis is made by examination of the ascitic fluid obtained by paracentesis. An elevated absolute polymorphonuclear (PMN) cell count (>250/mm^3) is diagnostic. The majority of cases are caused by a single species of organism, most commonly a gram-negative enteric bacteria (**Table 56.19**). If more than one organism is present, the diagnosis of SBP should be questioned, and a search for intra-abdominal disease (secondary peritonitis), such as a perforated viscus or diverticulitis, should be performed.

The treatment of SBP consists of supportive care and broad-spectrum antibiotics. Cefotaxime, a third-generation cephalosporin, is commonly used as empiric therapy, however, with the emergence of third multidrug-resistant organisms, broader spectrum antibiotics should be considered in the appropriate setting. Other antibiotics with proven efficacy include fluoroquinolones. A follow-up paracentesis at 48 hours will show decline in PMN count, indicating successful treatment. Duration is usually 5 to 7 days. Beta blockers should be discontinued at presentation and should not be restarted as they are associated with worse outcomes in patients with a history of SBP. Albumin infusion has been shown to significantly reduce mortality in patients with SBP and to reduce acute renal failure, and is complementary to other interventions. It is especially useful in patients with renal dysfunction and in those with severe hepatic dysfunction. Infection-related mortality is low with appropriate treatment, but high if renal failure or septic shock develops, and worse with delay in therapy.

Prophylactic antibiotics are indicated for three groups of patients with cirrhosis with ascites: (a) those with GI hemorrhage, (b) those with low ascitic fluid protein (<1.5 g/dL) and either liver failure (defined as CTP score greater than or equal to 9 or a bilirubin above 3 mg/dL) or impaired renal function (creatinine greater than or equal to 1.2 mg/dL or a BUN greater than or equal to 25, or a sodium below 130 mEq/L), and (c) those who have survived one or more episodes of SBP (recurrence rates are almost 70% at 1 year). The preferred antibiotics to be initiated in patients with hemorrhage are 7 days of intravenous ceftriaxone. Norfloxacin, ciprofloxacin, rifaximin, and trimethoprim–sulfamethoxazole are oral alternatives once intravenous therapy is no longer required. These prophylactic antibiotics reduce the incidence of SBP and improve survival.

Hernias and Ascites

Hernias of the anterior abdominal wall occur in up to 20% of patients with cirrhosis due to increased intra-abdominal pressure and nutritional deficits, with muscular wasting and thinning of the anterior abdominal wall fascia. Complications include incarceration, rupture, strangulation, and leakage. Patients with hernias and decompensated cirrhosis need to be evaluated for liver transplantation. In patients with stable liver function, hernias should be treated electively, with pre- or intraoperative paracentesis to decrease intra-abdominal pressure. No increase in complication rates was noted in a study comparing the outcome of umbilical hernia repair in patients with and without ascites. A longer hospital stay and a significantly higher recurrence occur in patients with ascites. Intra-abdominal drains may be used to remove ascites until the incision has healed, preventing ascites from leaking through the wound. Meticulous fluid management is essential during the postoperative period to prevent early reaccumulation of ascites.

In patients with severe ascites, TIPS may be performed before hernia repair to ensure a good result. Emergency repair of hernias complicated by skin breakdown with ascites leak, incarceration, or strangulation is managed in a similar fashion with preoperative large-volume paracentesis and aggressive control of ascites postoperatively.

References

1. Scaglione S, Kliethermes S, Cao G, et al. The epidemiology of cirrhosis in the United States: a population-based study. *J Clin Gastroenterol*. 2015;49(8):690–696.
2. Kaplan DE, Ripoll C, Thiele M, et al. AASLD practice guidance on risk stratification and management of portal hypertension and varices in cirrhosis. *Hepatol Baltim Md*. 2024;79(5):1180–1211.
3. Diehl AM, Chute J. Underlying potential: cellular and molecular determinants of adult liver repair. *J Clin Invest*. 2013;123(5):1858–1860.
4. McGuire RF, Bissell DM, Boyles J, Roll FJ. Role of extracellular matrix in regulating fenestrations of sinusoidal endothelial cells isolated from normal rat liver. *Hepatology*. 1992;15(6):989–997.
5. Friedman SL. Liver fibrosis in 2012: convergent pathways that cause hepatic fibrosis in NASH. *Nat Rev Gastroenterol Hepatol*. 2013;10:71–72.
6. Cogliati B, Yashaswini CN, Wang S, Sia D, Friedman SL. Friend or foe? The elusive role of hepatic stellate cells in liver cancer. *Nat Rev Gastroenterol Hepatol*. 2023;20(10):647–661.
7. Czaja AJ. Hepatic inflammation and progressive liver fibrosis in chronic liver disease. *World J Gastroenterol*. 2014;20(10):2515–2532.
8. Breitkopf K, Godoy P, Ciuclan L, Singer MV, Dooley S. TGF-β/smad signaling in the injured liver. *Z Für Gastroenterol*. 2006;44(1):57–66.
9. Rockey DC, Friedman SL. Fibrosis regression after eradication of hepatitis C virus – from bench to bedside. *Gastroenterology*. 2021;160(5):1502–1520.e1.
10. Pellicoro A, Ramachandran P, Iredale JP, Fallowfield JA. Liver fibrosis and repair: immune regulation of wound healing in a solid organ. *Nat Rev Immunol*. 2014;14(3):181–194.
11. Reeves HL, Friedman SL. Activation of hepatic stellate cells—a key issue in liver fibrosis. *Front Biosci*. 2002;7:d808–d826.
12. Marcellin P, Gane E, Buti M, et al. Regression of cirrhosis during treatment with tenofovir disoproxil fumarate for chronic hepatitis B: a 5-year open-label follow-up study. *Lancet*. 2013;381(9865):468–475.
13. D'Ambrosio R, Aghemo A, Rumi MG, et al. A morphometric and immunohistochemical study to assess the benefit of a sustained virological response in hepatitis C virus patients with cirrhosis. *Hepatology*. 2012;56(2):532–543.
14. Lassailly G, Caiazzo R, Buob D, et al. Bariatric surgery reduces features of nonalcoholic steatohepatitis in morbidly obese patients. *Gastroenterology*. 2015;149(2):379–388.

15. Harrison SA, Bedossa P, Guy CD, et al. A phase 3, randomized, controlled trial of resmetirom in NASH with liver fibrosis. *N Engl J Med*. 2024;390(6):497–509.
16. Sanyal AJ, Chalasani N, Kowdley KV, et al. Pioglitazone, vitamin E, or placebo for nonalcoholic steatohepatitis. *N Engl J Med*. 2010; 362(18):1675–1685.
17. Nevens F, Andreone P, Mazzella G, et al. A placebo-controlled trial of obeticholic acid in primary biliary cholangitis. *N Engl J Med*. 2016;375(7):631–643.
18. Hirschfield GM, Mason A, Luketic V, et al. Efficacy of obeticholic acid in patients with primary biliary cirrhosis and inadequate response to ursodeoxycholic acid. *Gastroenterology*. 2015;148(4): 751–761.e8.
19. GBD 2016 Alcohol and Drug Use Collaborators. The global burden of disease attributable to alcohol and drug use in 195 countries and territories, 1990–2016: a systematic analysis for the Global Burden of Disease Study 2016. *Lancet Psychiatry*. 2018;5(12):987–1012.
20. Kwong AJ, Kim WR, Lake JR, et al. OPTN/SRTR 2022 annual data report: liver. *Am J Transplant*. 2024;24(2S1):S176–S265.
21. Adam R, Karam V, Cailliez V, et al. 2018 Annual Report of the European Liver Transplant Registry (ELTR)–50-year evolution of liver transplantation. *Transpl Int*. 2018;31(12):1293–1317.
22. De Goyet JDV, Alberti D, Falchetti D, et al. Treatment of extrahepatic portal hypertension in children by mesenteric-to-left portal vein bypass: a new physiological procedure. *Eur J Surg*. 1999; 165(8):777–781.
23. Brown R, Kumar KS, Russo MW, et al. Model for end-stage liver disease and Child-Turcotte-Pugh score as predictors of pretransplantation disease severity, posttransplantation outcome, and resource utilization in United Network for Organ Sharing status 2A patients. *Liver Transpl*. 2002;8:278–284.
24. Garcia-Tsao G, Groszmann RJ, Fisher RL. Portal pressure, presence of gastroesophageal varices and variceal bleeding. *Hepatology*. 1985;5:419–424.
25. Llopis M, Cassard AM, Wrzosek L, et al. Intestinal microbiota contributes to individual susceptibility to alcoholic liver disease. *Gut*. 2016;65(5):830–839.
26. Williams CD, Stengel J, Asike MI. Prevalence of nonalcoholic fatty liver disease and nonalcoholic steatohepatitis among a largely middle-aged population utilizing ultrasound and liver biopsy: a prospective study. *Gastroenterology*. 2011;140:124–131.
27. Younossi ZM, Koenig AB, Abdelatif D, Fazel Y, Henry L, Wymer M. Global epidemiology of nonalcoholic fatty liver disease-Meta analytic assessment of prevalence, incidence, and outcomes. *Hepatology*. 2016;64(1):73–84.
28. Schuppan D, Schattenberg JM. Non-alcoholic steatohepatitis: pathogenesis and novel therapeutic approaches. *J Gastroenterol Hepatol*. 2013;28(suppl 1):68–76.
29. Abdelmalek MF, Suzuki A, Guy C. Increased fructose consumption is associated with fibrosis severity in patients with nonalcoholic fatty liver disease. *Hepatology*. 2010;51:1961–1971.
30. Loomba R, Mohseni R, Lucas KJ, et al. TVB-2640 (FASN Inhibitor) for the treatment of nonalcoholic steatohepatitis: FASCINATE-1, a randomized, placebo-controlled phase 2a trial. *Gastroenterology*. 2021;161(5):1475–1486.
31. Harrison SA, Bedossa P, Guy CD, et al; MAESTRO-NASH Investigators. A phase 3, randomized, controlled trial of resmetirom in NASH with liver fibrosis. *N Engl J Med*. 2024;390(6):497–509.
32. World Health Organization. Hepatitis B. Accessed September 14, 2024. https://www.who.int/news-room/fact-sheets/detail/hepatitis-b
33. Liu JZ, Hov JR, Folseraas T, et al. Dense genotyping of immune-related disease regions identifies nine new risk loci for primary sclerosing cholangitis. *Nat Genet*. 2013;45:670–675.
34. De Vreede I, Steers J, Burch P. Prolonged disease-free survival after orthotopic liver transplantation plus adjuvant chemoirradiation for cholangiocarcinoma. *Liver Transpl*. 2000;6:309–316.
35. Adams PC, Jeffrey G, Ryan J. Haemochromatosis. *Lancet Lond Engl*. 2023;401(10390):1811–1821.
36. Gavriilidis P, Marangoni G, Ahmad J, Azoulay D. State of the art, current perspectives, and controversies of Budd-Chiari syndrome: a review. *J Clin Med Res*. 2022;14(4):147–157.
37. Northup PG, Garcia-Pagan JC, Garcia-Tsao G, et al. Vascular liver disorders, portal vein thrombosis, and procedural bleeding in patients with liver disease: 2020 practice guidance by the American Association for the Study of Liver Diseases. *Hepatol Baltim Md*. 2021;73(1):366–413.
38. Rockey DC, Caldwell SH, Goodman ZD, Nelson RC, Smith AD; American Association for the Study of Liver Diseases. Liver biopsy. *Hepatology*. 2009;49:1017–1044.
39. Angeli P, Merkel C. Pathogenesis and management of hepatorenal syndrome in patients with cirrhosis. *J Hepatol*. 2008;48(suppl 1): S93–S103.
40. Biggins SW, Angeli P, Garcia-Tsao G, et al. Diagnosis, evaluation, and management of ascites, spontaneous bacterial peritonitis and hepatorenal syndrome: 2021 practice guidance by the American Association for the Study of Liver Diseases. *Hepatology*. 2021;74(2): 1014–1048.
41. Garcia-Tsao G, Parikh CR, Viola A. Acute kidney injury in cirrhosis. *Hepatology*. 2008;48(6):2064–2077.
42. Nadim MK, Kellum JA, Forni L, et al. Acute kidney injury in patients with cirrhosis: Acute Disease Quality Initiative (ADQI) and International Club of Ascites (ICA) joint multidisciplinary consensus meeting. *J Hepatol*. 2024;81(1):163–183.
43. Gluud LL, Christensen K, Christensen E. Systematic review of randomized trials on vasoconstrictor drugs for hepatorenal syndrome. *Hepatology*. 2010;51:576–584.
44. Porcel JM. Management of refractory hepatic hydrothorax. *Curr Opin Pulm Med*. 2014;20:352–357.
45. Hopkins WE, Waggoner AD, Barzilai B. Frequency and significance of intrapulmonary right-to-left shunting in end-stage hepatic disease. *Am J Cardiol*. 1992;70:516–519.
46. Younis I, Sarwar S, Butt Z, Tanveer S, Qaadir A, Jadoon NA. Clinical characteristics, predictors, and survival among patients with hepatopulmonary syndrome. *Ann Hepatol*. 2015;14(3): 354–360.
47. Machicao VI, Balakrishnan M, Fallon MB. Pulmonary complications in chronic liver disease. *Hepatology*. 2014;59: 1627–1637.
48. Swanson KL, Wiesner RH, Nyberg SL. Survival in portopulmonary hypertension: Mayo Clinic experience categorized by treatment subgroups. *Am J Transpl*. 2008;8:2445–2453.
49. Rautou PE, Moucari R, Escolano S. Prognostic indices for Budd-Chiari syndrome: valid for clinical studies but insufficient for individual management. *Am J Gastroenterol*. 2009;104: 1140–1146.
50. Intagliata NM, Caldwell SH, Tripodi A. Diagnosis, development, and treatment of portal vein thrombosis in patients with and without cirrhosis. *Gastroenterology*. 2019;156(6):1582–1599.
51. Villanueva C, Colomo A, Bosch A, et al. Transfusion strategies for acute upper gastrointestinal bleeding. *N Engl J Med*. 2013;368(1): 11–21.
52. Wells M, Chande N, Adams P, et al. Meta-analysis: vasoactive medications for the management of acute variceal bleeds. *Aliment Pharmacol Ther*. 2012;35(11):1267–1278.
53. Burroughs AK, McCormick PA, Hughes MD. Randomized, double-blind, placebo-controlled trial of somatostatin for variceal bleeding. Emergency control and prevention of early variceal rebleeding. *Gastroenterology*. 1990;99:1388–1395.
54. Jaramillo JL, Mata M, Mino G. Somatostatin versus Sengstaken balloon tamponade for primary haemostasia of bleeding esophageal varices. A randomized pilot study. *J Hepatol*. 1991;12: 100–105.
55. Miller-Catchpole R. Diagnostic and therapeutic technology assessment. Transjugular intrahepatic portosystemic shunt (TIPS). *JAMA*. 1995;273:1824–1830.
56. Rosemurgy AS, Goode SE, Zwiebel BR. A prospective trial of transjugular intrahepatic portasystemic stent shunts versus small-diameter prosthetic H-graft portacaval shunts in the treatment of bleeding varices. *Ann Surg*. 1996;224:378–384.
57. Orozco H, Mercado MA, Granados GJ. Selective shunts for portal hypertension: current role of a 21-year experience. *Liver Transpl Surg*. 1997;3:475–480.

58. Henderson JM, Warren WD, Millikan WJ. Distal splenorenal shunt with splenopancreatic disconnection. A 4-year assessment. *Ann Surg*. 1989;210:332–339.
59. Jin G, Rikkers LF. Cause and management of upper gastrointestinal bleeding after distal splenorenal shunt. *Surgery*. 1992;112:719–725.
60. Orloff MJ, Orloff MS, Orloff SL. Three decades of experience with emergency portacaval shunt for acutely bleeding esophageal varices in 400 unselected patients with cirrhosis of the liver. *J Am Coll Surg*. 1995;180:257–272.
61. Sugiura M, Futagawa S. Esophageal transection with paraesophagogastric devascularizations (the Sugiura procedure) in the treatment of esophageal varices. *World J Surg*. 1984;8:673–679.
62. Wexler MJ, Stein BL. Nonshunting operations for variceal hemorrhage. *Surg Clin North Am*. 1990;70:425–448.

57

Hepatic Neoplasms

Shishir K. Maithel

Key Points

1 Diagnostic principles and key imaging characteristics of benign, premalignant, and malignant hepatic neoplasms will be discussed.

2 General management principles and a histology-specific guide to treating these neoplasms are provided.

3 The three tenets of surgical management of malignant hepatic neoplasms include assessing oncologic appropriateness, understanding the host condition, and determining technical resectability.

4 Techniques to expand and/or optimize resectability are reviewed.

5 Basic anatomy and classification systems of liver anatomy are discussed and illustrated.

6 A step-by-step approach to five common procedures is detailed.

Improved access to and use of cross-sectional imaging have led to the more frequent discovery of hepatic tumors. In order to differentiate benign, potentially malignant, and malignant histologies, the most up-to-date imaging must be utilized. A complete clinical case analysis is required in order to determine an optimal strategy for patient treatment.

DIFFERENTIAL DIAGNOSIS

1 The most commonly diagnosed benign liver masses are listed at the top of **Table 57.1**. Most incidentally discovered liver masses in otherwise healthy individuals are benign. The most commonly diagnosed neoplasms include cavernous hemangiomas, focal nodular hyperplasia (FNH), hepatocellular adenomas (HCAs), and cystic disease. Cavernous hemangiomas are benign vascular lesions and are the most frequently seen benign liver neoplasms found in all age groups. Most patients are asymptomatic, despite their often large size, with the risk of rupture and hemorrhage being negligible. FNH is the second most common benign lesion and has a predilection in women between the ages of 30 and 50 years. In general, FNH is viewed as a hyperplastic but not neoplastic lesion that does not have malignant potential. The third most common, HCAs are also typically found in women between 30 and 50 years. They can enlarge, particularly with the use of oral contraceptives or during pregnancy. Both situations are associated with estrogen hormone stimulation. Although usually benign at diagnosis, HCAs do have the potential for malignant conversion and hemorrhage. It is this potential that guides indications for resection. While most cysts in the liver are simple, benign, and usually asymptomatic, mucinous cystic neoplasms (MCNs) and intraductal papillary neoplasms of the bile duct (IPNB) do have malignant potential. These cysts are similar to intraductal papillary mucinous neoplasms of the pancreas (IPMN).

Although the majority of liver masses are benign, the possibility of malignancy should be considered as well. These include both primary tumors, namely hepatocellular carcinoma (HCC) and intrahepatic cholangiocarcinoma (IHC), as well as the more commonly seen tumors that have metastasized to the liver. With respect to the most common primary tumor, HCC is the third most common cause of cancer-related death worldwide. Cirrhosis underlies the development of HCC in nearly 90% of cases, with an annual HCC incidence of 3% to 4% in cirrhotic patients. Chronic infections from hepatitis B and hepatitis C viruses contribute to HCC development, albeit via distinct mechanisms. Excess alcohol consumption also frequently contributes to cirrhosis-related HCC. Nonalcoholic fatty liver disease (NAFLD) is increasingly becoming a risk factor for HCC, particularly in the West, with NAFLD now being the most common reason for liver transplantation in the United States. Patients with human immunodeficiency virus (HIV) represent a higher-risk population, as they have higher rates of HCC that occur at younger ages, and tend to be more frequently symptomatic, progress more rapidly, and are associated with worse outcomes compared to HCC in non-HIV patients.

Table 57.1. Differential Diagnosis of Hepatic Neoplasms

Benign Liver Tumors
Cavernous hemangioma
Focal nodular hyperplasia (FNH)
Hepatocellular adenoma
Hepatic cysts
Intrahepatic abscess
Focal fat sparing
Primary Liver Malignancies
Hepatocellular carcinoma
Intrahepatic cholangiocarcinoma
Hilar cholangiocarcinoma
Gallbladder cancer
Metastatic Liver Malignancies
Colorectal cancer
Neuroendocrine tumors
Other (breast cancer, reproductive tract cancers, melanoma, adrenocortical carcinoma, renal cell carcinoma, sarcoma)

IHC is the second most common primary liver tumor, and its incidence has been steadily rising in European and North American countries over the last 30 years from 0.1 to 0.6 cases per 100,000. Most patients who present with IHC are asymptomatic and have no known risk factors, which often contribute to its late-stage presentation. Several risk factors have been identified, some of which are common to HCC. Chronic inflammation of the biliary epithelia is the final common pathway among them. These inflammatory conditions include primary sclerosing cholangitis, parasitic hepatic infections, hepatolithiasis, congenital biliary cystic disease, and cirrhosis. Other, more general risk factors for IHC include diabetes, obesity, biliary-enteric bypass, and tobacco use.[1]

Metastatic liver tumors can originate from a variety of primary cancers and should always be considered when evaluating a liver mass, as these are more common than a primary hepatic malignancy. The most common metastatic liver tumor originates from a primary colorectal cancer (CRC). The liver is the most common site for hematogenous spread from CRC. Roughly 25% of CRC patients present with synchronous liver metastases, and nearly 50% of CRC patients develop metachronous liver metastases after resection of their primary tumor. Neuroendocrine tumors (NETs) also commonly metastasize to the liver, usually originating from the midgut (small bowel or appendix) or pancreas, and are the second most common source of metastatic liver tumors. Over 80% of patients with metastatic NETs have liver involvement. Noncolorectal, non-NET liver metastases represent a small, but important, group of liver tumors. These most commonly include primary breast cancer, reproductive tract cancers, melanoma, adrenocortical carcinoma, renal cell carcinoma, and sarcoma.

Workup

The algorithm for the evaluation of a patient with a liver mass can be complex. Laboratory evaluation includes a complete blood count, coagulation studies, hepatitis panel, liver function tests, and tumor markers (CEA, AFP, CA 19-9, chromogranin A).

Imaging is a critical part of the workup for liver masses, and various modalities may be used. These include right upper quadrant ultrasound (US), computed tomography (CT) scan, magnetic resonance imaging (MRI), positron emission tomography (PET) scan, and somatostatin receptor (SSR) scintigraphy. Although US can be useful in differentiating a cystic or solid liver lesion, it is rarely sufficient in isolation to accurately characterize the lesion and make a diagnosis. A CT scan with a triphasic protocol that includes precontrast, arterial, and early and delayed venous images can identify and accurately characterize the majority of liver lesions.

A comprehensive MRI is the most sensitive and specific imaging modality to characterize liver lesions. The various series include fat-suppressed T1 pre- and postcontrast (arterial, portal venous, and 3- to 5-minute delay), T2 with and without fat suppression, MRCP, balanced-gradient sequence, dual-gradient echo in-phase and opposed-phase sequences, and diffusion-weighted images with a high B-value of approximately 800. The sensitivity for detecting small lesions on MRI can be enhanced by using hepatobiliary-specific contrast agents, such as gadoxetate sodium, and the specificity of MRI can be optimized with an extracellular agent. PET scan and SSR scintigraphy have limited use in the initial workup of incidental liver masses and are most helpful for assessing tumor burden, particularly extrahepatic, when metastases from PET-sensitive primary tumors and/or NETs are suspected.

If the diagnosis remains uncertain, a percutaneous core liver biopsy can be obtained. Biopsy should be performed only when the results will change management and should be avoided if HCC is suspected based on patient history and imaging characteristics. If a metastatic lesion is confirmed on biopsy, it is important to identify the primary tumor histology, as prognosis and the role of liver resection will vary greatly depending on tumor origin.

Table 57.2. Radiographic Features of Hepatic Neoplasms on Cross-Sectional Imaging (CT and MRI)

Precontrast Hypoattenuation
Hemangioma
Adenoma
Arterial Enhancement
Hepatocellular carcinoma (HCC)—with venous washout
Neuroendocrine tumors
Melanoma
Renal cell carcinoma
Focal nodular hyperplasia (FNH)
Colorectal cancer (slight)
± Hepatocellular adenoma
Early Venous Enhancement
Hemangioma (peripheral nodular enhancement)
Colorectal cancer (slight)
Delayed Venous Enhancement
Cholangiocarcinoma
Hemangioma (diffuse filling)
Colorectal cancer (increasing)
Other Notable Features
Central scar—FNH
Telangiectatic components—inflammatory adenoma

Diagnostic Principles

Upon obtaining adequate imaging, a thorough review of all diagnostic studies should be performed. This will allow for the most accurate diagnosis and determine resectability, both from an anatomic and biologic standpoint. Benign lesions are most often associated with normal lab values and low serum tumor markers. Laboratory blood tests—such as elevated bilirubin, LFTs, and INR, as well as a low platelet count—are more suggestive of primary liver tumors that often develop in the background of underlying liver dysfunction and can cause biliary obstruction. Similarly, both primary and metastatic liver tumors can be associated with elevated tumor markers. However, laboratory studies and tumor markers primarily play a supportive role in the diagnosis of incidental liver masses, and normal values do not exclude the possibility of a malignancy.

General imaging characteristics of liver tumors are shown in **Table 57.2.** Imaging is an integral part of the evaluation of hepatic neoplasms. The combination of radiologic characteristics and clinical features can often identify the etiology without the need for percutaneous biopsy. Specifically, for HCC, the diagnosis with imaging in the correct clinical context is widely accepted and is sufficient to initiate both noninvasive and invasive treatments. Alternatively, if adenocarcinoma is detected on biopsy, further staining for specific markers, including TTF-1 (lung), ER/PR (breast), CK-20 (colon), and CK-7 (pancreatobiliary), can help identify the likely site of origin. If the diagnosis remains indeterminate after high-quality imaging and biopsy, excisional biopsy with resection may be necessary, although this is rarely required.

GENERAL TREATMENT GUIDELINES

2 Once a diagnosis is confirmed, an appropriate treatment plan should be developed. When determining the resectability of hepatic lesions, several key considerations should be addressed: the operative/oncologic indication, the surgical fitness of the patient, and the technical resectability of the tumor. In asymptomatic individuals, most benign lesions require no therapy, although this depends on the exact histology. If pain is the only symptom from a benign liver tumor, in-depth discussion with

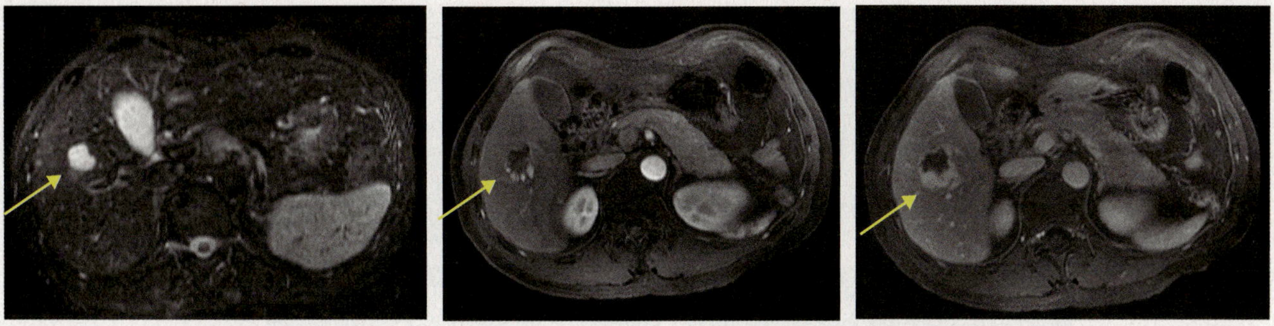

Figure 57.1. Hemangioma demonstrating bright appearance on T2 sequences and progressive peripheral nodular enhancement on delayed venous phase.

the patient and careful patient selection are critical before proceeding with resection for this indication. The management of adenomas, however, is generally more aggressive than other benign lesions because rupture and hemorrhage have been reported to occur between 10% and 30%, and malignant transformation into HCC in up to 10% of lesions.

For malignant liver tumors, operative indication is ultimately governed by tumor biology, which refers to the oncologic appropriateness of resection. For HCC and IHC, tumor size, multifocality, and vascular invasion should all be considered when determining resectability, however, specific cutoffs are inconsistent, and guidelines are variable. HCC tumors, particularly in the background of cirrhosis, that meet the Milan Criteria (MC) should be considered for transplant evaluation. For colorectal liver metastases, hepatic resection has largely become the optimal treatment modality, although only feasible in 20% to 25% of patients. Determining oncologic appropriateness for resection involves balancing synchronous liver disease, primary tumor node status and histology, number and size of liver tumors, CEA level, and disease-free interval. However, there is no perfect stratification system. Liver-directed therapy with hepatic arterial infusion should be considered in appropriate circumstances. Liver transplantation protocols are emerging for patients with unresectable colorectal liver metastases, although the optimal selection criteria are still evolving. Liver resection for NETs may be associated with symptom improvement and prolonged progression-free survival, although its role is in flux with the continued expansion and increased efficacy of other management strategies. The role of liver resection for other metastatic tumors, such as breast cancer, melanoma, and sarcoma, is unclear and should be individualized to each clinical scenario. Regardless of the liver tumor being primary or metastatic, the presence of extrahepatic disease can be an indicator of aggressive tumor biology, and the value of resection should be questioned. In any case where the oncologic appropriateness of resection is in question, a course of preoperative systemic or liver-directed therapy may help select more biologically favorable tumors prior to subjecting a patient to hepatic resection.

BENIGN/PREMALIGNANT LESIONS

Hemangioma

The prevalence ranges from 3% to 20% in the general population and has a female predominance.[2,3] As stated earlier in the introduction, these are most often "incidental" findings during an examination for some other etiology. Regardless of size, it is important to recognize and understand that most hemangiomas are *not* symptomatic. Even if patients undergo imaging for "pain," the etiology of that pain is usually due to something entirely different. This pain could be a result of biliary colic disease, dyspepsia, ulcer disease, or other similar upper GI ailments.[4] Rarely, a hemangioma can be symptomatic with compression of nearby structures, most commonly the stomach from a large hemangioma in the left lateral sector or diaphragmatic irritation from those located in the dome of the liver. Kasabach–Merritt syndrome, consisting of intravascular coagulation, clotting, and fibrinolysis within the hemangioma leading to systemic fibrinolysis and thrombocytopenia, is an exceptionally rare occurrence.[5]

The diagnosis of hemangioma relies on high-quality multiphase imaging, with a high-quality MRI representing the gold standard of care.[6] Most hemangiomas display "peripheral nodular enhancement with delayed central enhancement" with each progressive phase as the imaging progresses from arterial to venous to delayed venous phase (**Fig. 57.1**).[7] A "flash-filling" hemangioma can occur with small hemangiomas, usually measuring <2 cm, making it difficult to accurately and reliably distinguish from an arterial-enhancing tumor. Regardless, biopsy is not indicated and should be avoided, as imaging is usually diagnostic.

Given their benign, indolent, and asymptomatic nature, observation is the usual treatment strategy for patients with hemangioma. If "pain" is the primary patient complaint, efforts must be made to accurately assign the etiology of that pain and not assume that it is related to the incidentally discovered hemangioma. Most often, the presence of a hemangioma is actually unrelated to the pain.[8] If intervention is required, surgical resection remains the standard of care. Depending on the anatomic considerations of each individual case, both anatomic or nonanatomic resection and enucleation remain viable options.[9] Other liver-directed therapies, including radiation, ablation, and arterial embolization have been reported, but the lack of data supporting their efficacy makes it impossible to support their routine utilization.[10–12]

Focal Nodular Hyperplasia

FNH is the second most common benign lesion, is typically found in women between the ages of 30 and 50 years, and has a strong predilection in women compared to men, approaching 9:1.[13,14] The vast majority of these are asymptomatic and are incidentally found on imaging ordered for some other pathology. Like hemangiomas, even when patients endorse abdominal pain, the etiology is usually something other than the incidental finding of an FNH. In the rare event that an FNH does cause pain, it is usually associated with a left-sided lesion resulting in pressure on the stomach. Alternatively, a lesion near the surface of the liver can exert pressure on Glisson capsule, or a pedunculated lesion may be susceptible to intermittent torsion of the pedicle.[15]

FNH is considered to be a hyperplastic reaction from an arterial malformation in the liver that in essence, hyperperfuses the local surrounding hepatic parenchyma leading to hepatocellular hyperplasia.[16] This phenomenon is usually isolated

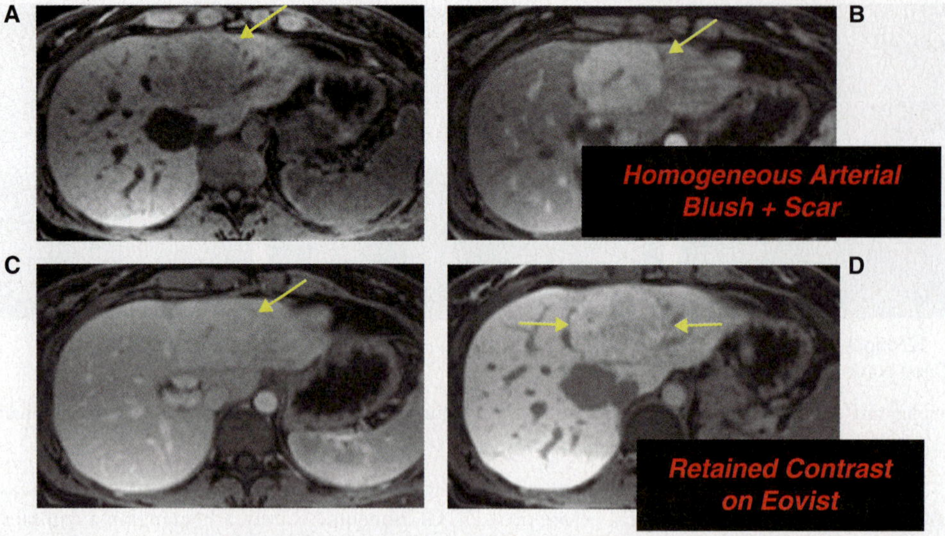

Figure 57.2. Typical appearance of FNH. **A:** Hypointense on precontrast phase. **B:** Bright with central scar on arterial phase. **C:** Homogeneous and isointense appearance to liver background on venous phase. **D:** Retained contrast on delayed images with Eovist.

and thus most frequently presents as a solitary FNH, however, multifocal FNH can occur in up to 20% of cases. FNH can also coexist with other benign lesions such as hemangioma or adenoma. Even though they do express estrogen receptors, tumor growth is not associated with oral contraceptive use or pregnancy.[17]

Obtaining the correct imaging is paramount to differentiate an FNH from an adenoma, which is a commonly encountered clinical scenario and mandates potentially very different treatment strategies. Replacing the historic sulfur-colloid scan, an MRI with a hepatobiliary contrast agent (eg, gadoxetate disodium [Eovist®]) is the standard of care to diagnose an FNH. Importantly, these contrast agents can exclude an adenoma. The retention of biliary elements in an FNH is a key distinguishing feature from adenomas that enables this typical imaging characteristic, consisting of being hypointense on precontrast T1, isointense on T2, and becoming hyperintense on venous phase T1 images with progressive fading (**Fig. 57.2**).[18] Contrast-enhanced US is another modality that, although rarely utilized, has good diagnostic capability for FNH, particularly for small lesions.[19]

Given the lack of potential for malignant transformation, hemorrhage, or other complications, the treatment for FNH is observation. Patients should be reassured of their indolent nature and be counseled that serial imaging is not necessary. In the exceptionally rare instance of a symptomatic FNH, resection or other liver-directed therapy such as transarterial bland embolization or ablation can be pursued.[20]

Hepatocellular Adenoma

HCA is a rare benign liver neoplasm and similar to FNH; it has a strong tendency to form in women (female/male ratio—9:1).[21] Given this predominance of occurrence in females, the association of HCA with estrogen stimulation has long been studied. While most believe them to be linked, there is no data to support a "causal" relationship between the two.[22] Regardless, decreased size and spontaneous regression have been repeatedly observed in HCAs with cessation of hormonal therapy. This observation has led to cessation still being the first recommendation in patients with HCA. Although the association with estrogen stimulation is believed to be true, studies have demonstrated that most HCAs remain stable during pregnancy. As such, uniform recommendations to avoid pregnancy for risk of growth, bleeding, and rupture are not warranted.[23] Importantly, the association of HCA with obesity and nonalcoholic steatohepatitis (NASH) has increasingly become more apparent. Obesity/metabolic syndrome is emerging as the dominant risk factor for HCA as opposed to oral contraception.[24,25] HCAs are also strongly associated with some rare genetic disorders, such as glycogen storage disease, maturity-onset diabetes of the young type 3, and McCune–Albright syndrome.[21]

Adenomas of the liver represent a heterogeneous disease as our molecular understanding of these lesions continues to evolve. There are four main subtypes, each of which carries its own profile of radiologic characteristics, typical host, and risk of hemorrhage and malignant transformation. The four subtypes include: HNF1α-mutated (HNF1A), inflammatory (telangiectatic—IHCA), β-catenin-mutated (b-HCA), and unclassified.[26] HNF1A has marked steatosis, IHCA is characterized by clusters of small arteries surrounded by extracellular matrix and inflammatory infiltrates, b-HCA contains pseudoglandular formations and cellular atypias such as enlarged, irregular, and hyperchromatic nuclei. Unclassified adenomas include those not having a characteristic histologic pattern.[24,27]

The best diagnostic test, aside from a difficult-to-interpret tissue biopsy, is a high-quality MRI. As mentioned above, MRI with a hepatobiliary contrast agent will usually reliably distinguish an adenoma from an FNH. HNF1A adenomas are homogeneous and will demonstrate significant fat content. IHCA displays a strong hyperintense signal on T2-weighted images and often has persistent enhancement on the delayed venous phase. The other two types, b-HCA and unclassified, have less distinct imaging features, but usually resemble other hepatocellular tumors with arterial enhancement and venous washout (**Fig. 57.3**).[28,29] Tissue biopsy is best utilized if molecular characterization will inform management.

The management of HCA is closely linked to the potential for complications—namely hemorrhage and/or malignant transformation. The risk assessment for the likelihood of these complications is mainly based on size, gender, and histologic type.[24] Importantly, the number of adenomas is not associated with an increased risk of complications. In general, 5 cm is the accepted "cutoff" for intervention, as the risk for bleeding and malignancy tends to increase with greater size.[24,30] However, these risks are still relatively low—hemorrhage occurs in less than 25% and malignant transformation in approximately 5%. Adenomas in males carry a significantly higher risk of malignant transformation and are most often the b-HCA subtype. As such, although uncommon, adenomas diagnosed in male patients should be treated, preferably with resection.[24] When factoring in the histologic subtype, the HNF1A type is very indolent and rarely symptomatic, and almost never transforms to HCC. IHCAs have a higher tendency to bleed. Other risk factors for bleeding include visualization of arteries on

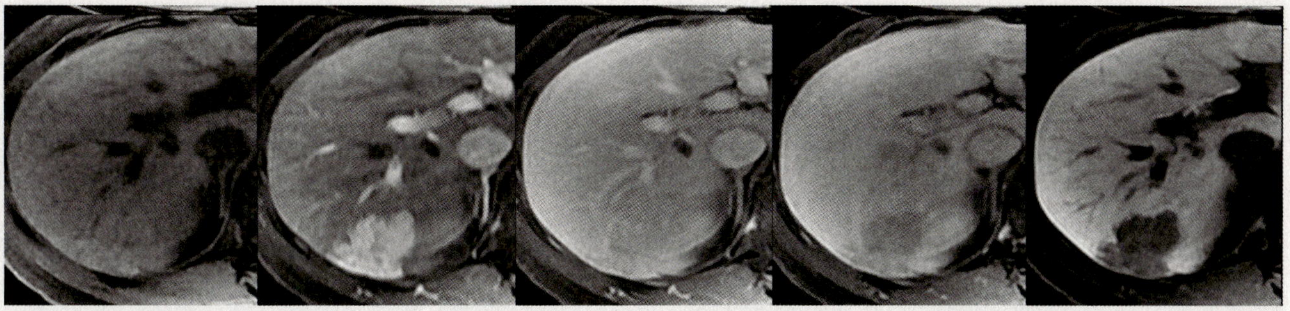

Figure 57.3. Series of images demonstrating the typical appearance of hepatocellular adenoma through the progressive phases of contrast-enhanced imaging.

imaging, location in the left lateral sector of the liver, and an exophytic growth pattern. The b-HCA subtype is characterized by a much higher risk of malignant transformation, particularly when >5 cm in size.[21,24] In general, size and gender are the main guiding principles for management, with greater than 5 cm and male gender requiring intervention.[24] The histologic subtype can help guide decision making, particularly in a borderline situation, where either resection or observation is equally being considered. For example, a 4-cm b-HCA would likely undergo resection while a 5.5-cm HNF1A could likely safely be observed.

In terms of management, if relevant, the first step is cessation of oral contraception. Weight loss can be associated with spontaneous regression of adenomas as well.[24] When indicated, the standard of care for treatment is surgical resection. Bland arterial embolization is another option, particularly in difficult-to-resect lesions or in patients with significant comorbidities.[9,31] Liver transplantation, although previously considered in patients with adenomatosis, has recently fallen out of favor as the risk of complications is not increased with multiple compared to solitary adenomas, and these lesions are most often the indolent HNF1A subtype. Instead, isolated treatment of lesions >5 cm can be undertaken, and the other smaller adenomas can be observed, often displaying spontaneous regression.[24]

Simple Cysts

Simple cysts of the liver, originally believed to be quite rare, are visualized in up to 25% of patients who undergo MRI evaluation (**Fig. 57.4**). They are cystic formations that contain serous fluid and are lined by a single layer of cuboidal or columnar epithelial cells that resemble biliary epithelium, yet they do not have any direct communication with the biliary tree. Although they can be solitary, most of the time they are multiple. Prior to even considering any intervention, a simple cyst must be differentiated from polycystic liver disease (with or without autosomal dominant polycystic kidney disease—ADPKD), mucinous cysts (discussed below), and infectious etiology (hydatid cysts or echinococcal cysts). All of these other conditions have distinct management strategies that differ from those of simple cysts.

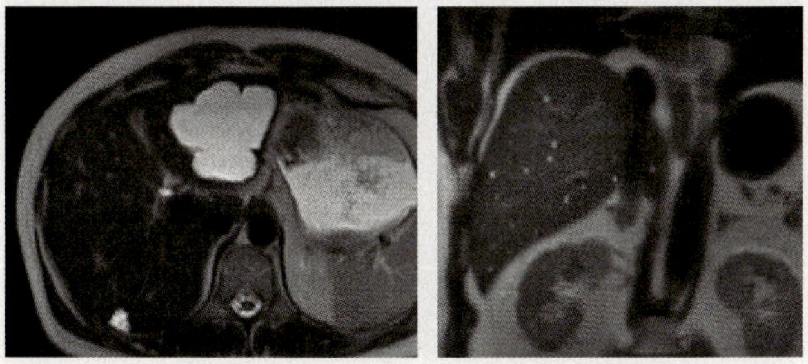

Figure 57.4. Typical appearance of a simple hepatic cyst on MRI T2 sequences.

While most simple cysts are demonstrated in females, large, complicated, and symptomatic cysts are almost exclusively seen in women over the age of 50.[32] Outside of this demographic, most simple cysts are asymptomatic and are incidentally discovered during imaging for some other pathology. A carefully detailed history must be obtained in order to exclude other etiologies of pain. Large cysts located in the left lateral sector can compress the stomach. Large exophytic cysts can apply pressure on the liver capsule and/or diaphragm, and sometimes vascular structures and/or bile ducts can be compressed radiographically. The latter is rarely an indication for intervention as the radiographic appearance of compression is not usually clinically apparent or relevant. A trial of cyst fluid aspiration can be utilized to determine if the cyst is truly symptomatic, during which the symptoms should resolve temporarily. However, they will recur as the cyst refills with fluid.[33] Acute hemorrhage into the cyst can be accompanied by severe acute pain that usually resolves over a few days. Simple cysts do not have any malignant potential.

If truly deemed to be symptomatic, management of simple cysts can be pursued with either sclerotherapy or cyst fenestration. Sclerotherapy is most frequently accomplished with a 95% ethanol solution. After the cyst is percutaneously accessed and all the fluid is drained, it is vital to first inject contrast to ensure that no direct biliary or vascular communication is present.[34] Next, approximately 100 mL of 95% ethanol is infused into the cyst cavity, and the patient is rolled in different positions to expose the alcohol to the entire cyst surface.[35] The procedure can be quite painful and blood alcohol levels can rise, thus underscoring the importance of limiting the amount of ethanol that is infused. Although the literature is sparse with reports of long-term follow-up after sclerotherapy, the symptomatic recurrence rate requiring additional treatment is believed to be low—less than 5%.[9] Although a viable option, sclerotherapy is rarely pursued.

If intervention is deemed appropriate, laparoscopic cyst fenestration is typically more commonly employed than sclerotherapy.[36] Although the procedure is simple and straightforward with good results, it should only be utilized when needed. It should not lower the threshold for intervention. The procedure can be likened to taking the "ice cream off the cone." The ice cream represents the protruding cyst from the liver surface, presenting as the interface of the ice cream and the rim of the cone. Importantly, it is not necessary to remove the cyst lining that is embedded within the liver parenchyma. In fact, attempts to do this will greatly increase the risk of complications such as bleeding and bile leak, as these structures are often being compressed just below the cyst wall. Rather, the cyst should be opened approximately 1 cm above the liver surface. The fluid is drained out, and then the cyst wall that is exterior to the liver parenchyma is removed with

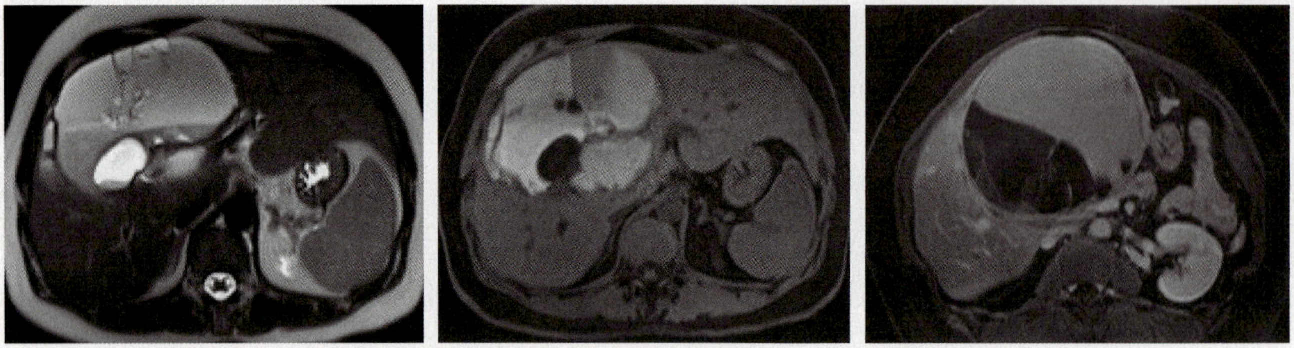

T2 Bright but has heterogeneous contents with septations and nodularity

Figure 57.5. T2 sequences of an MRI demonstrating the bright appearance of mucinous cystic neoplasms that highlight the heterogeneous contents, septations, and nodularity that distinguish them from simple cysts.

either an energy source or vascular staplers, leaving a crater of sorts. The epithelium should be carefully cauterized, and often an omental flap is created to place inside the cyst cavity. Any persistent fluid secreted from the base of the cyst wall is readily absorbed by the peritoneum and poses no risk to other organs. Success rates are high with this procedure, and if done correctly, reintervention rates are low—less than 10%.[37]

Mucinous Cysts (MCN and IPMN-B)

While neoplastic mucinous lesions of the liver are exceedingly rare, it is paramount to differentiate them from simple or infectious cysts. They may have malignant potential and thus, generally mandate complete resection. It is important to note that the terminology for these neoplastic cysts has evolved. The previous terminology of "cystadenoma" has been abandoned as the pathophysiologic understanding of these cysts has improved. As such, these cysts in the liver are believed to mirror those in the pancreas with similar rates of malignant potential. The term cystadenoma has been replaced with MCN and intraductal papillary mucinous neoplasm of the bile duct (IPMN-B).[38,39]

Much like MCN of the pancreas, MCNs of the liver are almost always solitary, occurring uniformly in younger women, and do not communicate with the biliary tree. They are histologically defined as being lined with ovarian stroma.[40,41] The embryologic descent of the right ovary explains why most MCNs are found in segment IV of the liver, just as they are nearly always found in the body/tail of the pancreas due to the path of decent of the left ovary. Although many are asymptomatic and diagnosed incidentally, most are discovered during a workup of vague epigastric pain. If it reaches a large size, an MCN can progress to cause biliary obstruction and jaundice in the minority of cases.

A good-quality MRI is the best way to radiographically distinguish MCN from other cystic lesions of the liver. Most MCNs present as fluid-containing multilocular cysts with homogeneous low- or isosignal intensity on T1-weighted images and homogeneous high signal intensity on T2-weighted images (**Fig. 57.5**).[42] Nodularity of the cyst wall may be present as well. Unlike MCN of the pancreas, cyst fluid analysis of the hepatic counterpart is not well defined. Specifically, there is no characteristic profile of CA 19-9 or CEA levels, partly since hepatic cyst fluid analysis is uncommonly obtained. If suspected, given its malignant potential, complete resection is warranted, as cyst wall fenestration is not appropriate management.[43] Resection can consist of partial hepatectomy or enucleation, as there is often a dissection plane between the MCN and normal hepatic parenchyma.

IPMN-B may macroscopically be divided into two variants: ductectatic type and cystic type. The ductectatic type can resemble main duct IPMN of the pancreas, while the cystic type is analogous to side-branch IPMN.[44] The main distinguishing feature from MCN is that IPMN-B directly communicates with the biliary tree. This can often be visualized on MRI (**Fig. 57.6**) or on cholangiography. Given the mucin secretion into the biliary tree, IPMN-B can present with transient obstruction of the bile ducts. Unlike MCN, it is equally diagnosed in both genders and usually presents in the sixth decade of life. Given its malignant potential, resection is indicated.[39] Unlike the guidelines for resection of IPMN of the pancreas, no such detailed guidelines exist for IPMN-B. Even if malignant transformation has occurred, the prognosis is usually better than after resection of de novo intrahepatic or hilar cholangiocarcinoma.

MALIGNANT LESIONS

3 Determining resectability of hepatic malignancies relies on three key concepts: oncologic appropriateness, host condition, and technical resectability.

Oncologic Appropriateness

Tumor biology dictates oncologic appropriateness. Adequately defining the extent of disease and understanding the nature of the tumor is critical before pursuing operative intervention. The surgeon's first responsibility is to determine those patients most likely to benefit from an operation, which is ultimately governed by tumor biology.

Host Condition

Host condition refers not only to the general health and surgical fitness of the patient, but also to the condition and functional status of the liver. In most patients, this can be successfully evaluated through a careful history and physical examination. Other useful tools to further risk-stratify patients include indicated adjunct laboratory values and imaging.

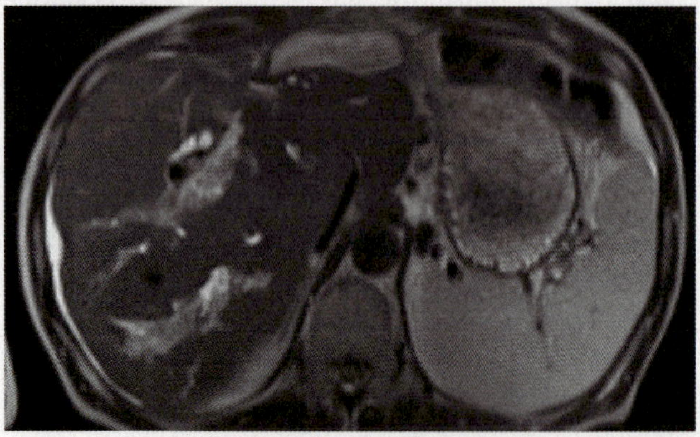

T2 Bright but communicates with the biliary tree

Figure 57.6. T2 sequences of an MRI demonstrating the biliary communication of IPMN-B.

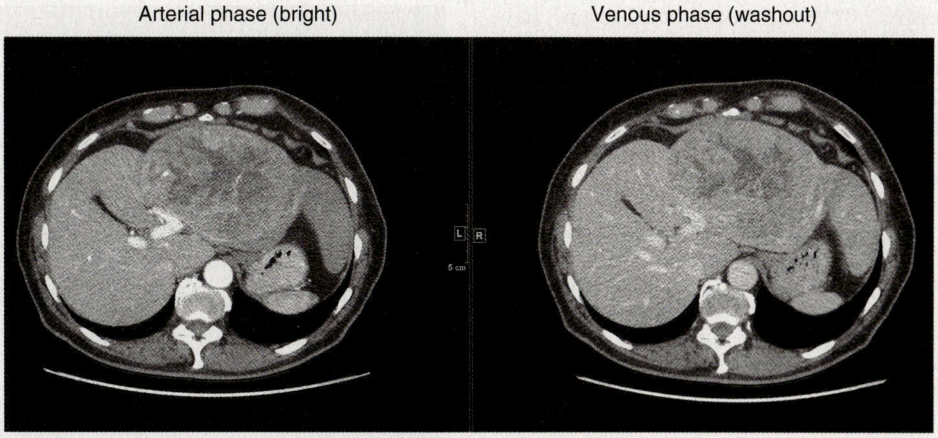

Figure 57.7. Hepatocellular carcinoma (HCC) has a bright appearance on arterial phase and tends to washout on venous phase.

Technical Resectability

Before pursuing any extent of hepatic resection, the remnant liver should be determined to have sufficient inflow, outflow, biliary drainage, and be of adequate quantity and quality to sustain hepatic function postoperatively during the regenerative period.

If surgery is determined to be reasonable from an oncologic perspective, the patient is deemed fit for surgery, and the extent of planned resection leaves an adequate functional liver remnant (FLR); nearly all patients should be candidates for liver resection. These three concepts will be elaborated upon within the context of specific liver tumors, both primary and metastatic, as well as discuss ways by which resectability rates can be potentially increased.

ONCOLOGIC APPROPRIATENESS

Determining resectability of a tumor from an oncologic perspective is paramount and should be the first consideration of any surgeon faced with a cancer patient prior to assessing technical resectability. This is based on the concept of nonmalfeasance, or "first, do no harm." When performed with curative intent, the value of surgery for malignancy is measured by its survival benefit and improvement in quality of life. Tumor biology, however, ultimately dictates patient outcome. Thus, a thorough preoperative evaluation should be performed to assess the extent of spread, which, among other tumor-specific factors, can help predict the nature of disease. Whether a primary or metastatic liver tumor, extrahepatic spread is an indicator of aggressive tumor biology. While not always a preclusion of surgery,[45] the benefit of resection in these cases should be questioned. Improvements in imaging technology and, in appropriately selected patients, staging laparoscopy have increased our ability to identify those patients unlikely to benefit from surgery and avoid unnecessary hepatectomy. In certain cases where the oncologic appropriateness of surgery is in question, a trial of preoperative systemic or liver-directed therapy may help biologically select more favorable tumors for resection.

Preoperative Evaluation

Preoperative evaluation should focus on characterizing the lesion in question, defining the extent of disease, and determining its biologic behavior. Imaging modalities include a staging chest radiograph or chest CT, and either a CT or MRI of the abdomen and pelvis, with preference depending on the type of tumor being evaluated, institutional expertise, and patient-related factors. In many cases, however, both CT and MRI may be necessary.[46] PET scan can be a useful and important tool in evaluating the extent of disease in FDG-avid tumors, particularly when assessing for extrahepatic disease.[47–50] Preoperative biopsy for certain tumor types is often not necessary and should only be pursued in select cases where the information gained will alter the treatment plan, such as administering preoperative therapy.

Despite advances in various high-quality imaging modalities, still roughly 9% to 36% of patients are found to have occult metastatic disease at the time of surgery.[51–55] Staging laparoscopy has been advocated by some to identify peritoneal metastases not detected on cross-sectional imaging, thereby avoiding unnecessary laparotomy.[54–58] However, its routine use is subject to debate, and may only be of benefit in patients already identified as high risk for having subradiographic metastatic disease.[59–61]

Hepatocellular Carcinoma

HCC is the most common primary liver tumor (**Fig. 57.7**) and the third most common cause of cancer-related death worldwide.[62] Although various nonoperative treatment options exist, surgery remains first-line therapy, with the choice between resection and transplantation generally dictated by the degree of underlying liver dysfunction and tumor burden.[63,64] From an oncologic perspective, four major clinical prognostic indicators have been identified—tumor size, multifocality, vascular invasion, and extrahepatic spread. These indicators serve as the basis for the Tumor–Node–Metastasis (TMN) staging system.[65,66] Since the widespread adoption of the MC, which utilized a selection cutoff using these clinical indicators, the identification of cirrhotic patients with HCC for transplantation has been simplified with consistently favorable results.[67,68] However, translating these clinical indicators into oncologic criteria for resection has proven difficult.

Other clinical staging systems have been proposed using different clinicopathologic parameters with varying success in applicability, cancer-specific focus, and prognostic value.[69–71] One commonly used system is the Barcelona Clinic Liver Cancer (BCLC) staging system. Stratification under BCLC is based on tumor stage, liver function, and performance status, therefore, staging patients with HCC into four categories—early, intermediate, advanced, and terminal—making treatment recommendations for each.[72,73] According to this staging system, hepatic resection is only indicated in patients with early-stage HCC (single tumor ≤5 cm or ≤3 tumors all <3 cm, without vascular invasion or extrahepatic spread; satisfactory liver function; and performance score of 0) with the oncologic appropriateness of resection mirroring that of MC.[67,72] While the BCLC system has gained increasing acceptance to guide resection, it continues to be controversial, as conflicting data regarding the prognostic value of these clinical indicators emerge.[74–80]

Historically, tumor size in HCC has been an important predictor of outcome following surgery. Readily measured preoperatively and shown to be inversely correlated with survival, tumors larger than 5 cm and 10 cm in diameter are particularly biologically aggressive.[76,81–84] However, several groups have demonstrated more acceptable and durable long-term survival following resection for large HCC, questioning the prognostic significance of tumor size alone.[77,80,85–87] Furthermore, when controlling for other factors, such as multiple tumors and presence of vascular invasion, size has demonstrated little impact on survival, even in tumors >10 cm in diameter.[65,80,88–90] In fact, the AJCC eighth edition staging classification does not use tumor size alone to stratify patients.[65,66] Increasingly, however, studies focusing on the link between tumor size and vascular invasion have shown that the frequency of microscopic and macroscopic vascular invasion drastically increases as tumor size increases.[78,80,91] This suggests that tumor size, rather than being an independent prognostic indicator, may serve as a surrogate marker for vascular invasion. Thus, while size alone should not dictate treatment, recognizing the link between size and more aggressive tumor biology is critical when discussing the oncologic appropriateness of resection in patients with HCC.

The presence of multiple tumors is another important independent prognostic factor in patients with HCC. The pathogenesis of multifocal HCC is thought to be due to at least two very different biologic mechanisms—multicentric hepatocarcinogenesis, meaning multiple de novo tumors of independent origin, and intrahepatic metastasis, meaning multifocal dissemination of a common clonal origin.[92–94] While our ability to differentiate between these two pathways may have significant implications for understanding tumor biology and guiding management, reliable biomarkers are lacking, and clinical applicability is not yet clear. However, as a whole, multifocal HCC incurs a worse prognosis than equally matched solitary tumors; this is reflected in the current AJCC staging system.[66,89,90] Although acceptable rates of survival have been shown following resection for multifocal HCC ≤5 cm in diameter, the oncologic benefit in patients with larger multifocal HCC is still subject to debate, and a trial of preoperative therapy may be prudent prior to selecting these patients for resection.[65,89,90,95]

In multiple studies, vascular invasion has been shown to be one of the best predictors of outcome following surgery for HCC.[65,73,76–80,89–91] Patients presenting with macroscopic or major vascular invasion, defined as tumor involving a major branch of the portal or hepatic vein, have particularly dismal outcomes. This finding is associated with increased risk of intrahepatic and systemic metastases, and poor overall survival.[65,89,90,96–98] Left untreated, the reported median survival of patients with HCC and major vascular invasion is 9 to 10 weeks.[96,97] Several studies have reported an overall 5-year survival of only 10% to 11%, even after hepatic resection for HCC when major vascular invasion was present.[79,89,99,100] Although a small subset of patients may have more favorable outcomes than those previously reported,[79] the benefit of resection in patients with major vascular invasion remains doubtful and controversial, and should be pursued in only highly selected patients. Microscopic vascular invasion has also been shown to be a strong predictor of outcome, with its presence associated with earlier tumor recurrence, metastatic spread, and decreased overall survival.[76–78,80,91] Unfortunately, microscopic vascular invasion is difficult to anticipate and, in isolation, is of little use in preoperatively determining resectability. The value of incorporating immunotherapy in the perioperative setting is under investigation.

In patients with HCC, extrahepatic spread, including regional lymph node involvement and distant metastases, is considered stage IV disease. With few exceptions, it is a contraindication to resection in patients with HCC.[64,66,101]

Intrahepatic Cholangiocarcinoma

The second most common primary liver tumor is intrahepatic cholangiocarcinoma (ICC) (**Fig. 57.8**), with a rising incidence seen in both European and North American countries.[102,103] Despite the rising occurrence in these countries, no currently

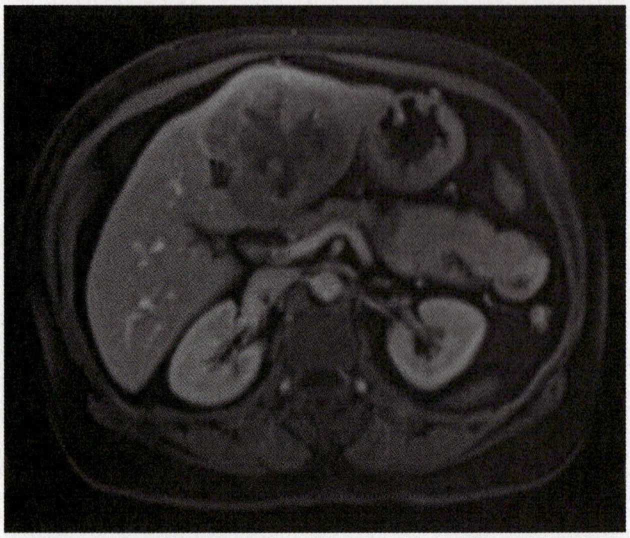

Delayed enhancement on venous phase

Figure 57.8. Cholangiocarcinoma typically depicts enhancement on delayed venous imaging.

available locoregional or systemic therapies have shown generalized therapeutic benefit for all comers, although advances in immunotherapy, targeted therapy, and liver-directed therapy show great promise for select patients. Still, surgical resection remains the only potentially curative treatment for patients with ICC.[104] When the seventh edition AJCC staging system was developed, TMN staging for ICC was based on the same major prognostic criteria of HCC including tumor size, multifocality, vascular invasion, and extrahepatic spread.[105] Given its distinct tumor biology, underlying risk factors, and clinical behavior compared to HCC, several nomograms and staging systems have been developed. These is an attempt to differentiate relevant prognostic indicators and more accurately predict survival in patients with ICC.[106–111] The eighth and ninth versions of the AJCC staging system are unique to ICC and do not merely parallel that of HCC.

The utilization of tumor size in patients with ICC as a prognostic indicator to stratify patients has been controversial. While used in previous versions of the AJCC staging system, the prognostic value of tumor size was refuted in one of the earliest proposed staging systems for ICC.[107] Supported by several groups, these authors found no independent association between tumor size and survival in ICC.[1,106,112,113] Indeed, tumor size is notably absent in the staging system proposed by Nathan et al., as well as in the seventh edition AJCC staging system addressing ICC independently.[106,110] On the other hand, the Liver Cancer Study Group of Japan (LCSGJ) found a worse prognosis in patients with ICC >2 cm in diameter. This size is used as a cutoff value in their commonly used staging system.[109] Similarly, others have shown a significant negative effect on recurrence and survival with increasing tumor size, particularly in tumors >5 cm and >7 cm. This is reflected by the fact that tumor size has been incorporated in two of the newer proposed nomograms.[108,111,114–116] More recently, increasing tumor size has been found to be associated with an increased incidence of nodal involvement, multiple tumors, vascular invasion, and poorly differentiated tumors.[117,118] The suggestion would be that larger tumor size may be indicative of more aggressive tumor biology. Though perhaps subtle, the role of size in determining resectability should not be entirely discounted. Accordingly, tumor size has been incorporated in the eighth and ninth versions of the AJCC staging system.

Multifocal intrahepatic disease is considered one of the most dominant clinicopathologic factors affecting survival in ICC. The pathophysiology of multiple ICC tumors, similar to

HCC, is thought to be due to either satellitosis, multicentric hepatocarcinogenesis, or intrahepatic metastases. Although the clinical significance of each of these is unclear, there is no debate that patients with ICC presenting with multiple tumors face a grim prognosis, particularly with ≥3 tumors.[1,108,111,114–117] While most patients with multifocal disease never reach resection, the median survival for the minority that do ranges from 12 to 19 months, with one study observing no survival benefit over patients treated nonoperatively.[1,114,116] Thus, in patients with multiple intrahepatic ICC tumors, nonoperative therapy consisting of mostly systemic therapy, sometimes combined with liver-directed therapy should be the first consideration. Resection should be reserved for only highly selected cases.

The presence of vascular invasion is often cited as an important risk factor for disease recurrence and decreased survival in patients with ICC.[1,106,108,113] Its utility as an independent prognostic indicator, however, is less clear. Indeed, when taking into account other factors, such as positive lymph node status and multiple tumors, vascular invasion frequently failed to maintain significance.[1,112,114,117,119] Furthermore, microscopic vascular invasion is difficult to identify on preoperative imaging, giving it little value in determining resectability. Even when faced with major vascular invasion, however, several groups have advocated a more aggressive surgical approach, citing increased resectability rates and comparable or better overall survival when major vascular resection was performed in order to obtain negative margins.[117,119,120] Thus, hepatic resection in the setting of major vascular invasion can be oncologically appropriate in select patients with ICC, particularly after a favorable response to a course of preoperative therapy.

Extrahepatic disease is considered stage IV, and these tumors should be deemed unresectable, except in highly select cases. Regional lymph node disease, in the latest edition of the AJCC staging system, is deemed stage IIIB as opposed to previously being designated stage IV disease. As our understanding of the role of immunotherapy and targeted therapy for actionable mutations in patients with early-stage resectable disease evolves, it is plausible that the threshold and indications for resection may change too. Specifically, the sequencing of therapy may change to incorporate neoadjuvant therapy more frequently and push resection to later in the treatment regimen.

Colorectal Liver Metastases

CRC is the most common cancer worldwide and the second most common cause of cancer-related death in the United States.[62] Approximately 25% of patients with CRC present with metastatic disease, and 50% will eventually develop metastases, with the majority being located in the liver (**Fig. 57.9**).[121,122] In patients with metastases confined only to the liver, hepatic resection is the goal, with a 5-year survival of approximately 50% in most modern series and a 10-year disease-free survival (ie, cure) reaching nearly 20%.[123,124] Unfortunately, resection is only possible in 20% to 25% of patients.

Selecting patients for resection who are likely to achieve these survival benchmarks, however, has been challenging. Several risk factors have been identified and used in various combinations to develop clinical risk scoring systems to predict long-term survival and guide therapy in patients with colorectal liver metastases. Examples of these factors include synchronous liver disease, primary tumor node status and histology, number and size of liver tumors, CEA level, disease-free interval, and the presence of extrahepatic disease.

While most studies agree as to the general importance of these factors and their cumulative effect on survival, there is little standardization in their individual cutoff values and prognostic strengths, and no one factor has unanimously been shown to affect outcomes.[125–129] In fact, one study focusing on patients cured of disease at 10 years showed that well over half of them originally had at least one, and 43% had at least three,

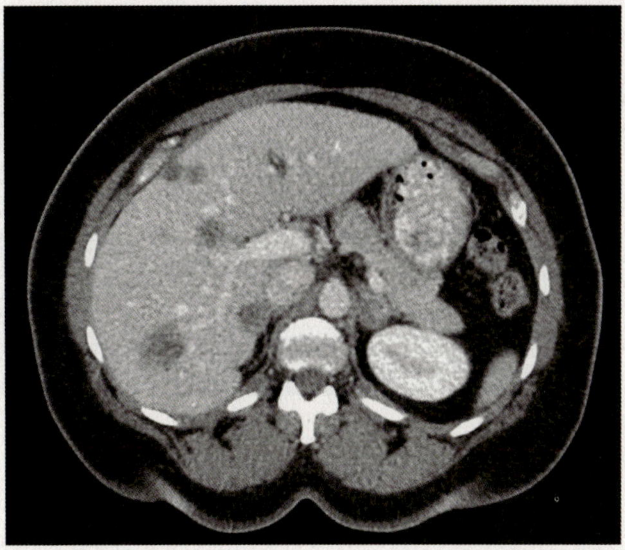

Figure 57.9. Typical appearance of colorectal cancer liver metastases on venous phase imaging.

of these poor prognostic factors—synchronous disease (7%), node-positive primary (51%), CEA >200 (7%), disease-free interval <12 months (37%), multiple hepatic tumors (40%), and size of hepatic tumor >5 cm (36%).[124] Even in the setting of extrahepatic disease, a scenario traditionally considered a contraindication to resection, acceptable 5-year survival rates up to 28% have been shown in select patients undergoing hepatic resection.[130–132] Certainly, there is little question that patients with many risk factors do worse than patients with few to none. However, the line that separates the biologically resectable from the biologically unresectable patients with colorectal liver metastases continues to evade us. Although other factors like KRAS and BRAF mutations may inform a worse prognosis after resection, they are not absolute contraindications to resection. For the minority of patients who have microsatellite unstable disease, initiation of immunotherapy prior to resection is usually recommended.

Neuroendocrine Liver Metastases

Although a rare tumor, when metastatic, the liver is involved in the majority of cases, with midgut (small bowel and appendiceal) and pancreatic location being the primary sites of disease.[133] Before considering liver resection, the full extent of disease burden must be evaluated. This can be accomplished with high-quality cross-sectional imaging (**Fig. 57.10**), usually in combination with SSR scintigraphy. While Indium-111 (octreotide scan) is useful, the Gallium-68 Dotatate scan offers greater sensitivity for detecting small-volume disease and is the preferable modality. Indications for resection include not only eradication of disease, but also control of symptoms related to the carcinoid syndrome. Surgical cytoreduction of disease, on the order of 70% to 90%, has been deemed adequate to be associated with improved survival and/or symptom relief.[134,135] As the medical and nonoperative liver-directed therapy armamentarium (including transarterial embolization, ablation, and transarterial radioembolization) for treating advanced NETs continues to evolve and expand, the role and benefit of resection must be carefully weighed against its potential morbidity. Furthermore, with the FDA approval of Peptide Receptor Radionuclide Therapy (PRRT) with Lutetium 177 Dotatate in January 2018 based on the results of the Netter-1 trial, the role of hepatic resection has been called into question, especially in patients with extrahepatic disease.[136] That being said, liver resection should always be discussed and considered in multidisciplinary tumor boards when determining the therapeutic plan for each individual patient.

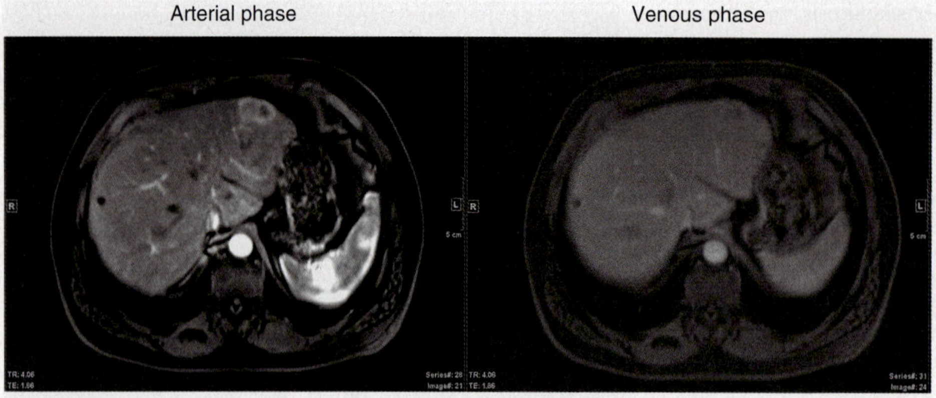

Figure 57.10. Neuroendocrine liver metastases are typically bright on arterial phase imaging and tend to wash out during the venous phase.

Noncolorectal, Nonneuroendocrine Liver Metastases

This group of patients represents a small minority of patients who are candidates for and undergo liver resection. Primary histologies that comprise this cohort of patients include melanoma, renal cell carcinoma, sarcoma, breast cancer, lung cancer, and gynecologic malignancies. Each individual scenario must be evaluated thoroughly in a multidisciplinary setting, as there are no general guidelines that dictate the appropriateness of hepatic resection for this group of patients. One must weigh the magnitude of resection and its potential morbidity, the extent of hepatic and extrahepatic disease, the systemic therapy options and their projected efficacy, and the anticipated survival of the patient.[137]

HOST CONDITION

A patient's general health status and their ability to tolerate surgery, or surgical fitness, is a critical component of determining resectability of hepatic malignancies. A thorough history and physical examination, and any other indicated adjunct workup, should be performed preoperatively on all patients. Because determining the surgical candidacy of a patient is often subjective, several risk indices have been developed to aid in patient assessment, decision making, and provide a more objective way to risk-stratify patients. Those commonly used by anesthesiologists and surgeons include the American Society of Anesthesiologists (ASA) scale, the Eastern Cooperative Oncology Group (ECOG) Performance Status, the Charlson Comorbidity Index (CCI), and the Revised Cardiac Risk Index (RCRI).[138–141] More recently, the concept of frailty has been introduced as an important surgical risk assessment tool and forms the basis of the Hopkins Frailty Score, which was later validated in a large multidisciplinary prospective study examining outcomes of patients undergoing major intra-abdominal surgery.[142,143]

TECHNICAL RESECTABILITY

4 In liver surgery, the technical resectability of a tumor is defined not only by what can be removed, but more importantly by what is subsequently left behind. Thus, hepatic arterial and portal venous inflow, venous outflow, biliary drainage, and the quantity and quality of the future liver remnant (FLR) should all be deemed adequate to sustain function and support regeneration in the postoperative period. Patients with underlying liver dysfunction pose a unique challenge when considering hepatic resection, and understanding the degree of dysfunction and its effect on prognosis is crucial. In select patients, the use of remnant-optimizing techniques and staged procedures can increase resectability and should be considered whenever possible.

Vascular Inflow/Outflow and Biliary Drainage

One of the major dilemmas in determining the technical resectability of liver tumors is balancing the appropriate operation required in order to completely remove the tumor and obtain negative margins while maintaining adequate vascular inflow, outflow, and biliary drainage of the FLR. Thus, mapping out the tumor location in relation to the patient's hepatic vascular and biliary anatomy is critical. In most patients, this can be done successfully with good-quality cross-sectional imaging, including a CT scan, MRI, or both. Even with centrally located tumors, which more frequently involve major vascular structures close to the hilum, improvements in high-quality cross-sectional imaging have allowed for better visualization and characterization of tissue planes. When biliary obstruction is suspected, cholangiography may help delineate biliary involvement, and can be done endoscopically, percutaneously, or using MRI. Given the advances in imaging, invasive cholangiography is rarely necessary.

Historically, tumor involvement of the portal vein or inferior vena cava has been considered a contraindication to surgery, as resection of these tumors incurred significant perioperative morbidity and mortality risk. However, improvements in surgical technique and perioperative management have expanded our definition of resectability. Indeed, several studies have demonstrated that in select patients, hepatectomy combined with major vascular resection or thrombectomy can be safe, with low postoperative morbidity and mortality, and that major vascular or biliary involvement should not necessarily preclude resection.[79,120,144–148] In highly select patients whose tumor involves the IVC, the hilum, or the confluence of the IVC and hepatic veins, and would otherwise be considered unresectable by any other resection techniques, ex vivo resection with autotransplantation may be an option.[149–153] However, data regarding this approach is sparse, limited to case reports and small series, and the survival benefit is unclear.

FLR QUANTITY AND QUALITY

Volumetric Assessment of the Liver

As the liver has a tremendous capacity for functional compensation and regeneration, healthy livers, without cirrhosis, can tolerate resection of up to 80% of their parenchymal volume. However, the segmental distribution of the liver's functional capacity is not uniform. It can vary from person to person, thus making it difficult to estimate the volume of the FLR needed to sustain function based on traditional anatomic nomenclature.[154] Preoperative volumetric analysis can be an important tool to assess the actual volume and predict the function of the FLR. This is particularly important when considering major and extended hepatic resections.

In the most basic sense, the FLR is standardized to total liver volume (TLV) and is expressed as the percentage of the TLV that is to be left unresected. Various methods for measuring liver volume have been proposed. One method is using CT and three-dimensional CT volumetry. This has been shown to be accurate and reproducible in calculating TLV and FLV values.[155–157] However, direct measurement of TLV on imaging can be problematic as large tumors, biliary dilatation, and underlying liver disease may affect the accuracy of the measurements. In addition, accurately measuring TLV requires that the tumor volume be excluded or subtracted, which can be particularly difficult in the setting of multiple tumors and can lead to user discrepancies and mathematical error.

An alternative approach is to estimate the TLV using a mathematical formula based on body surface area (TLV [cm^3] = −794.41 + 1267.28 × body surface area [m^2]), which has been validated in a meta-analysis and found to be superior to other similar formulas.[158,159] An FLR volume ≤20% has been found to be the strongest independent predictor of postoperative liver insufficiency, as well as a significant risk factor for postoperative liver failure and death.[160–162] Thus, an FLR volume >20% has been proposed as a cutoff for safe hepatic resection in healthy, noncirrhotic livers.

However, many patients undergoing liver resection do not have healthy livers. Although the exact pathogenesis is not entirely understood, liver injury is a known risk of chemotherapy, and increasing duration of preoperative treatment has been shown to increase the risk of postoperative complications.[163–169] Longer durations of preoperative chemotherapy (>12 weeks) have been associated with higher rates of liver injury and postoperative hepatic insufficiency.[167,170] In patients who receive short-duration preoperative chemotherapy, it has been suggested that an FLR of at least 20% to 30% is sufficient to undergo hepatic resection.[170,171] However, those receiving long-duration (>12 weeks) preoperative chemotherapy should have an FLR volume of at least 30%, although some suggest that an FLR of 40% is necessary to prevent postoperative hepatic insufficiency.[170,172,173] In patients with hepatic fibrosis or cirrhosis, the FLR volume is suggested to be at least 40% to 50% of TLV.[174,175]

Functional Assessment of the Liver

One of the most important assessments when determining resectability of liver malignancies involves the preoperative evaluation of liver function. The perioperative morbidity and mortality risk has been shown to increase with worsening degree of hepatocellular compromise in cirrhotic patients undergoing hepatic resection.[176–179] Although a long list of functional studies, imaging techniques, and serum markers exists, the multiple and diverse functions of the liver make comprehensive evaluation difficult, and no single study has been consistently proven to be the best measurement of preoperative liver function or predictor of postoperative hepatic insufficiency and failure prior to resection.

The model for end-stage liver disease (MELD) is one of two major clinical scoring systems frequently used to evaluate liver function in cirrhotic patients. MELD is based on a patient's bilirubin, international normalized ratio (INR), and creatinine.[180] Traditionally used to predict survival in cirrhotic patients awaiting liver transplantation, the utility of the MELD score has been expanded to a variety of clinical settings, including the assessment of patients being considered for partial hepatectomy.[180–183] For patients with cirrhosis undergoing hepatic resection, a MELD score ≥9 has been shown as an independent predictor of perioperative complications and mortality.[182,183] As such, a MELD score <9 can be considered reasonably safe for hepatic resection.

The other frequently used clinical scoring system, the Child–Turcotte–Pugh (CTP) score, can be used to predict liver-related mortality in cirrhotic patients. CTP takes into account both clinical measures and laboratory values, including presence of ascites, encephalopathy, total serum bilirubin, INR, and serum albumin.[184] An elevated CTP score has been associated with increased morbidity and mortality following liver resection.[177,179,185] In fact, a Child B classification (score 7 to 9) is considered a relative contraindication to resection, particularly for major hepatectomy. A Child C designation is an absolute contraindication, even for most minor resections.[186] In addition, the presence of encephalopathy, independent of the other factors, is generally considered a contraindication to resection.

An additional method of identifying cirrhotic patients at risk for postoperative complications involves an assessment for the presence of portal hypertension. Splenomegaly and/or varices present on imaging are both reliable signs of portal hypertension. However, they are rarely present in patients being considered for resection; therefore, reliance on radiographic evidence of these signs is inadequate. Portal venous wedge pressure can be used for the direct measurement of portal pressure. However, the routine use of this invasive technique is impractical. Alternatively, for patients with underlying liver dysfunction, thrombocytopenia has been shown to be a good surrogate marker for the presence of portal hypertension. It tends to be indicative of increased platelet sequestration due to portal hypertension–induced hypersplenism. Although portal hypertension is not an absolute contraindication to hepatic resection, thrombocytopenia has been associated with increased morbidity and mortality in patients undergoing resection.[187–190] Specifically, a preoperative platelet count <150/nL has been independently associated with major postoperative complications, postoperative hepatic insufficiency, and 60-day mortality in patients with HCC undergoing hepatic resection.[185] In fact, a modified Child score based on this data has been proposed, which replaces encephalopathy in the traditional CTP scoring system with preoperative platelet count. This modified Child score was found to be independently associated with major postoperative complications and 60-day mortality, and the only factor independently associated with postoperative hepatic insufficiency.[185] This modified scoring system is particularly clinically relevant as the presence of encephalopathy is uniformly a contraindication to resection and thus does not contribute greatly to a preoperative risk scoring system. Rather, a simple lab value such as the platelet count can give insight into the presence of portal hypertension. Bone marrow suppression from chemotherapy leading to a decreased production of platelets must also be considered when interpreting the meaning of thrombocytopenia.

Indocyanine green (ICG) clearance is another assessment tool used preoperatively to evaluate liver function in cirrhotic patients being considered for hepatic resection. ICG is an anionic organic dye that is selectively taken up by hepatocytes and excreted in bile. It is usually measured as a percent serum clearance at 15 minutes and indirectly reflects hepatocyte blood flow and functional capacity.[191] An ICG cutoff of <10% at 15 minutes has been reported to be safe for extended resection, a cutoff of 10% to 20% for hemihepatectomy, 20% to 30% for segmentectomy, and only enucleation for those with >40% ICG clearance.[192] However, the utility of ICG clearance over other well-established functional measures is debated, and it is rarely used in the United States.[188,193]

INCREASING TECHNICAL RESECTABILITY

Portal Vein Embolization

Portal vein embolization (PVE) is a percutaneous procedure performed preoperatively in select patients as a means to increase the volume of the anticipated FLR, which has been shown to subsequently improve liver function, thereby decreasing the risk of postoperative complications associated with small FLR size.[194–197] The portal vein of the intended specimen is embolized and occluded to induce a hypertrophic response in the FLR. The efficacy of PVE has been well documented, with a reported average increase of 12 ± 5% in FLR volume following PVE.[160,161,172,197] In fact, FLR growth due to PVE has been shown to increase resectability in almost 60% of patients who previously would have been considered unresectable due to inadequate FLR size.[171,198] Furthermore, it has been demonstrated that those patients whose FLR growth following PVE enabled them to undergo resection had no difference in postoperative morbidity and mortality compared to those who underwent resection upfront without the need for PVE.[160,198,199] Overall and disease-free survival has also been shown to be similar among these two groups in patients undergoing resection for colorectal liver metastases.[172,198] Thus, it does not seem that increasing technical resectability utilizing PVE sacrifices adherence to the principle of biologic selection.

More recent studies have found the kinetic growth rate of the FLR following PVE to be a strong predictor of postoperative liver insufficiency, liver failure, and death.[200,201] Using cutoff values of ≥2% and >2.66% FLR growth per week, patients in this group from both studies had significantly lower postoperative morbidity, and none developed liver failure or suffered liver-related death. This suggests that growth rate of the FLR, rather than the absolute standard volumetric measurements, may be a better marker for determining resectability of liver tumors following PVE, although further evaluation is still needed.

Although its application is not standardized, studies have warned against the routine use of PVE, citing a large percentage of patients in whom PVE had no effect on morbidity or mortality following hepatic resection.[171,199] Furthermore, PVE is not entirely without risk. Between 2% and 20% of patients fail to demonstrate remnant hypertrophy following PVE, and roughly 10% of patients suffer adverse events following the procedure.[197,202] Tumor progression following PVE may also be a concern and has been documented in 17% to 25% of patients with colorectal liver metastases.[198,203]

Therefore, it has been suggested that PVE be reserved for an FLR volume ≤20% of TLV in patients without underlying liver dysfunction.[160,171,198,204] Among patients with or at high risk for liver injury (eg, those who have received extensive preoperative systemic chemotherapy), PVE is recommended for an FLR volume ≤30% of TLV.[160,172,204] In patients with severe hepatic fibrosis or cirrhosis, an FLR ≤40% is the suggested cutoff value for performing PVE.[174,175,204]

Two-Stage Hepatectomy

Initially described by Adam et al. in 2000, a two-stage hepatectomy (TSH) is a potentially curative operative strategy in patients with multiple bilobar colorectal liver metastases that traditionally would be considered unresectable via a single operation, even in conjunction with systemic and local therapies.[205] The first stage of the procedure consists of resection of metastases from only one hemiliver, which is the designated FLR after the second stage is complete. Thus, it is important that parenchymal-sparing techniques be used during the first operation. In most patients, PVE of the contralateral liver is performed following the first stage. During the second-stage operation, all remaining metastases in the contralateral hemiliver are then resected, most often with a hemihepatectomy of the side that had undergone PVE. Although data examining TSHs are limited to single-institution studies with small patient cohorts and widely variable patient selection criteria, a recent meta-analysis found that in select patients with initially unresectable colorectal liver metastases, TSH resulted in low postoperative morbidity and mortality and acceptable survival outcomes.[206] In particular, these patients fared significantly better than their counterparts who received systemic chemotherapy alone. In one study examining long-term outcomes following TSH, despite higher postoperative morbidity, comparable 5-year survival was seen between patients undergoing completed TSH and those who underwent a single-stage hepatectomy during the same time period.[207]

Associating Liver Partition with Portal Vein Ligation for Staged Hepatectomy

Associating liver partition with portal vein ligation for staged hepatectomy (ALLPS) is a relatively aggressive and disputed approach to managing traditionally unresectable liver tumors. More specifically, it was developed to overcome several limitations of PVE, including the potential for disease progression during the 4- to 6-week waiting period, and inadequate FLR hypertrophy following PVE. The procedure involves in situ splitting of the liver with portal vein ligation during the first stage, inducing rapid FLR hypertrophy, followed by a short-interval (<7 days) second stage in which the hemiliver containing the tumor is removed.[208,209] While several case series have reported its technical feasibility, complications can be high. Long-term data is minimal but emerging, and its use remains controversial and debated.[210–216]

ANATOMY AND CLASSIFICATION

5 In order to perform partial hepatectomy, precise knowledge and mastery of the surgical anatomy of the liver, blood vessels, and biliary channels are essential. The liver is divided into sectors that comprise liver segments, each supplied by branches of the portal triads and drained by hepatic veins. Partial hepatectomy involves removal of one or more segments by isolation of the relevant portal venous and arterial inflow, severance of the relevant hepatic veins and biliary drainage channels, and removal of the associated liver tissue.

The anatomic division between the right and left hemiliver follows a line projected through a plane found at the principal plane or Cantlie line—running from the medial margin of the gallbladder bed to the left of the IVC posteriorly, not at the falciform ligament.[217] Each hemiliver is then subdivided into sectors, sections, and segments.

The Brisbane terminology dictates that the hepatic veins form the boundaries between the different sectors of the liver.[218] Specifically, the medial margin of the right posterior sector is the right hepatic vein and comprises segments VI and VII. The right anterior sector is bordered by the right hepatic vein laterally and middle hepatic vein medially, coursing along the principal plane, comprising segments V and VIII. These are also termed the right posterior *section* and right anterior *section* according to Brisbane terminology. Based on this same terminology system, the area of liver that comprises segments IVa, IVb, and III forms the left medial sector as it is bound by the middle and left hepatic veins. Segment II forms the left lateral sector, because the left hepatic vein divides segment II from III. From a clinically relevant perspective, however, en bloc resection of segments III, IVa, and IVb cannot be performed since this area of liver encompasses the umbilical fissure where the left portal vein is situated. Thus, according to Brisbane terminology, segment IVa/b is referred to as the *left medial section*, and it is bordered by the middle hepatic vein and umbilical fissure. The left lateral sector, according to the slightly modified terminology that is being presented here, is comprised of segments II and III. This represents the portion of liver to the left of the ligamentum teres and falciform ligament and is termed the *left lateral section* according to Brisbane terminology. Essentially, the left liver is divided into a medial and lateral sector along the line of insertion of the ligamentum teres and the falciform ligament. This modified terminology will be utilized for the remainder of this chapter as it is clinically relevant and applicable. The term "section" will not be used. The portal venous and hepatic arterial branches conform to the segmental organization and run within the segments, and the draining hepatic veins converge posteriorly toward the inferior vena cava (**Fig. 57.11**).

6 Practically, five types of hepatic resections are performed relatively routinely. The five different resections include (1) right hepatectomy, (2) left hepatectomy, (3) left lateral sectorectomy, (4) right posterior sectorectomy, and (5) segmentectomy/nonanatomic resection. A simple step-by-step algorithm for performing these procedures is detailed in **Tables 57.3 to 57.7**. The portal vein and hepatic artery divide into major right and left branches outside the liver parenchyma below the hilus. Here, when the overlying peritoneum is incised, it is usually possible to dissect each major branch beyond its bifurcation,

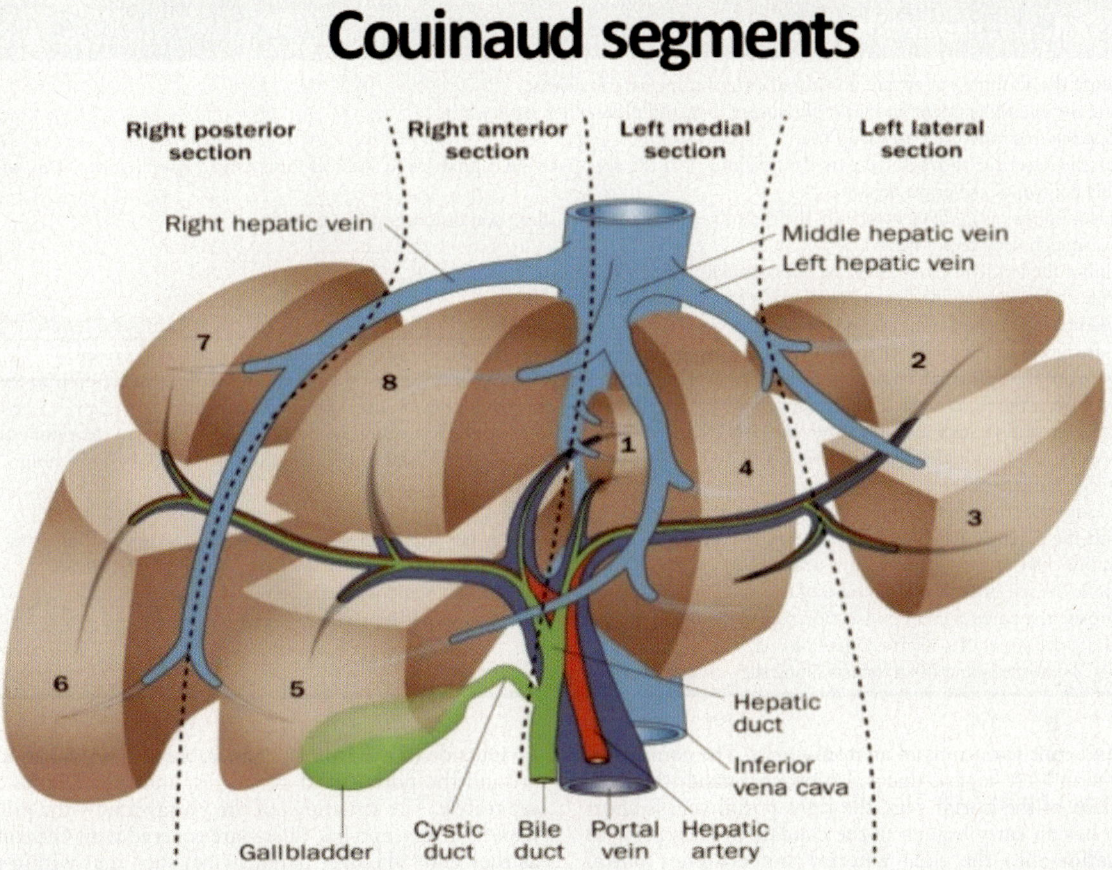

Figure 57.11. Segmental anatomy of the liver utilizing the Brisbane terminology of "sections."

Table 57.3. Right Hepatectomy (Segments V–VIII)

1. Explore the abdomen to ensure no subradiographic metastatic disease.
2. Ligate the round ligament and leave the suture long and place a hemostat on it.
3. Divide the falciform back toward IVC, staying about 1 cm off the surface to enable resuspension of the left liver.
4. Open the lesser sac through the pars flaccidum and clear the area over the caudate lobe and feel for enlarged lymph nodes. This will enable control of the porta hepatis.
5. Ultrasound the entire liver, especially the left liver remnant, to ensure no subradiographic disease.
6. Perform a cholecystectomy, but leave a long tie on the cystic duct stump. This will facilitate a safe dissection in the porta hepatis.
7. Mobilize the right liver. The right phrenic vein will mark the location of the right hepatic vein.
   a. Incise the right anterior coronary ligament.
   b. When visualization becomes difficult, incise the inferior attachments to the liver to drop the kidney and adrenal gland. Stay just lateral to the IVC.
   c. Incise the triangular ligament.
   d. This will give good exposure to retract the right liver toward the left and incise the right posterior coronary ligament.
   e. Do not divide the left coronary/triangular ligament to prevent kinking of the left inflow and outflow vessels postoperatively.
8. Ligate and divide the venous tributaries to the IVC from the caudate lobe to expose and clear off the anterior aspect of the IVC.
   a. Clips, energy devices, or staplers can be used for this depending on the size of the veins.
9. Divide the caval (caudate) ligament with a vascular load stapler.
10. Find and develop the "notch" at the dome of the liver to find space between the right and middle hepatic vein. This will facilitate extrahepatic control of the right hepatic vein.
11. With the cystic duct stump retracted medially to the left, dissect out and control the right hepatic artery. Test clamp to ensure good left hepatic arterial flow before dividing. It can either be tied or stapled.
12. Once artery is divided, dissect out the right portal vein. Test clamp to ensure the left portal vein is intact with US. Place an umbilical tape around the right portal vein and retract to the left to protect the left portal vein. Divide with an endovascular stapler.
13. Now that inflow is controlled, divide the right hepatic vein outflow with an endovascular stapler.
14. Mark out the line for parenchymal transection along Cantlie line, staying just right of the middle hepatic vein.
15. Divide the hepatic parenchyma down to the right bile duct.
16. Encircle the right bile duct intrahepatically, making sure to stay to the right of the cystic duct stump and biliary hilum to avoid injury to the contralateral biliary system. Divide the right bile duct with an endovascular stapler.
17. Complete the parenchymal transection.
18. Hydrate the patient to a status of euvolemia.
19. Ensure hemostasis and biliary stasis along the cut surface of the liver.
20. Resuspend the left liver by sewing the falciform ligament to the diaphragm with interrupted figure-of-eight 2-0 Vicryl sutures.

Table 57.4. Left Hepatectomy (Segments II–IV)

1. Explore the abdomen to ensure no subradiographic metastatic disease.
2. Ligate the round ligament and leave the suture long and place a hemostat on it.
3. Divide the falciform back toward IVC.
4. Open the lesser sac through the pars flaccida and clear the area over the caudate lobe and feel for enlarged lymph nodes. This will enable control of the porta hepatis.
5. Ultrasound the entire liver, especially the right liver remnant, to ensure no subradiographic disease.
6. Perform a cholecystectomy.
7. Mobilize the left liver by incising the left coronary and left triangular ligaments.
   a. Place a laparotomy pad over the stomach and spleen to avoid injury.
   b. Do not injure the diaphragm or left phrenic vein.
8. Divide the entire length of the lesser omentum, being careful to ligate a replaced or accessory left hepatic artery if present.
9. Dissect out the left hepatic artery at the medial aspect of the porta hepatis at the base of the umbilical fissure. Test clamp it to ensure good flow in the right hepatic artery. Divide the left hepatic artery either with ties or an endovascular stapler.
10. Dissect out and control the left portal vein at the base of the umbilical fissure. Test clamp it and ensure good flow in the right portal vein using US. Divide the left portal vein with an endovascular stapler. Divide it distal to the takeoff of caudate lobe branches to preserve caudate inflow.
11. Mark out the plane of transection, staying left of the middle hepatic vein.
12. Divide the parenchyma. Make sure to curve to the left as the transection plane approaches the porta hepatis to prevent injury to the right bile duct or right-sided inflow structures.
13. Encircle the left bile duct at the base of the umbilical fissure and divide it with an endovascular stapler.
14. Complete the parenchymal transection superiorly by dividing the left hepatic vein with an endovascular stapler.
15. Hydrate the patient to a status of euvolemia.
16. Ensure hemostasis and biliary stasis along the cut surface of the liver.

unless significant variations in anatomy exist. The confluence of the right and left hepatic ducts also occurs outside the liver. At the hilum of the portal vein, the right portal vein is short and often has an early branch to the caudate process prior to its bifurcation into the right anterior and posterior portal veins. In contrast, the left branch of the portal vein and the left hepatic duct pursue a longer, more horizontal extrahepatic course beneath segment IV and are more easily dissected free along their length.

The ligamentum teres (round ligament) runs into the umbilical fissure of the liver, at the base of which the main vascular and biliary pedicles branch to the segments of the left liver (II, III, IVa, IVb). After entering the umbilical fissure, the left branch of the portal vein curves caudally and gives branches not only to the left lateral sector (segments II and III) but together with branches of the left hepatic artery, it also supplies the left medial sector—segments IVa and IVb of the left liver, also known as the *quadrate lobe*. These branches course from left to right, starting in the umbilical fissure and supplying segments IVa/IVb.

Outside of the liver substance, there is no a distinct sheath around the portal triad structures, and they can be dissected separately. The structures of the portal triad—the portal vein, hepatic artery, and bile duct—are covered with Glisson capsule as they enter the liver parenchyma, such that within the liver, they are contained in well-formed branching fibrous sheaths often referred to as *pedicles*, each containing a vein, artery, and bile duct. Pedicles are strong structures that contain the constituents of the portal triad, and intrahepatic dissection of these pedicles enables isolation and control of vascular and biliary elements without the need to individually expose each structure outside the liver.

The liver straddles the IVC immediately below the diaphragm, and the hepatic veins have a short extrahepatic course to empty into the vena cava. This superior portion of the vena cava, with the draining hepatic veins, is covered with a fold of peritoneum that extends from the cephalad aspect of the falciform ligament to the right and left triangular ligaments. This fold of peritoneum comprises the anterior and posterior coronary ligaments, which converge to form the right and left

Table 57.5. Left Lateral Sectorectomy (Segments II–III)

1. Explore the abdomen to ensure no subradiographic metastatic disease.
2. Ligate the round ligament and leave the suture long and place a hemostat on it.
3. Divide the falciform back toward IVC.
4. Open the lesser sac through the pars flaccida and clear the area over the caudate lobe and feel for enlarged lymph nodes. This will enable control of the porta hepatis.
5. Ultrasound the entire liver, especially the right liver remnant and segment IV, to ensure no subradiographic disease.
6. Perform a cholecystectomy. This is not absolutely necessary to perform a left lateral sectorectomy, but it is conventional to perform at the time of liver resection.
7. Mobilize the left liver by incising the left coronary and left triangular ligaments.
   a. Place a laparotomy pad over the stomach and spleen to avoid injury.
   b. Do not injure the diaphragm or left phrenic vein.
8. Mark out the line of parenchymal transection just left of the falciform ligament and umbilical fissure.
9. Divide the parenchyma.
10. Encircle the segment III pedicle as it is exposed during parenchymal transection. Divide it with an endovascular stapler.
11. Encircle the segment II pedicle as it is exposed during parenchymal transection. Divide it with an endovascular stapler.
12. Complete the parenchymal transection superiorly by dividing the left hepatic vein with an endovascular stapler.
13. Hydrate the patient to a status of euvolemia.
14. Ensure hemostasis and biliary stasis along the cut surface of the liver.

Table 57.6. Right Posterior Sectorectomy (Segments VI–VII)

1. Explore the abdomen to ensure no subradiographic metastatic disease.
2. Ligate the round ligament and leave the suture long and place a hemostat on it.
3. Divide the falciform back toward IVC, staying about 1 cm off the surface to enable resuspension of the left liver, should it be necessary.
4. Open the lesser sac through the pars flaccida and clear the area over the caudate lobe and feel for enlarged lymph nodes. This will enable control of the porta hepatis.
5. Ultrasound the entire liver, especially the left liver remnant and right anterior sector, to ensure no subradiographic disease.
6. Perform a cholecystectomy.
7. Mobilize the right liver. The right phrenic vein will mark the location of the right hepatic vein.
    a. Incise the right anterior coronary ligament.
    b. When visualization becomes difficult, incise the inferior attachments to the liver to drop the kidney and adrenal gland. Stay just lateral to the IVC.
    c. Incise the triangular ligament.
    d. This will give good exposure to retract the right liver toward the left and incise the right posterior coronary ligament.
    e. Do not divide the left coronary/triangular ligament to prevent kinking of the left inflow and outflow vessels postoperatively.
8. Divide the caval (caudate) ligament with a vascular load stapler.
9. Find and develop the "notch" at the dome of the liver to find space between the right and middle hepatic vein. This will facilitate extrahepatic control of the right hepatic vein. This step is not always necessary, depending on the location of the tumor and whether or not the right hepatic vein needs to be divided to obtain a negative margin.
10. Mark out the line for parenchymal transection along the right hepatic vein using US. The line of transection will be either to the right or left of the right hepatic vein depending on whether or not it needs to be ligated to obtain a negative margin resection. The line of transection is along a transverse plane of the liver.
11. Divide the hepatic parenchyma down to the right posterior sector pedicle.
12. Encircle the right posterior pedicle and test clamp it and ensure preservation of flow in the right anterior pedicle with US. Divide the right posterior pedicle with an endovascular stapler. Extrahepatic control and division of the right posterior portal vein and right posterior hepatic artery are also feasible and commonly performed.
13. If necessary for the procedure, divide the right hepatic vein with an endovascular stapler.
14. Complete the parenchymal transection.
15. Hydrate the patient to a status of euvolemia.
16. Ensure hemostasis and biliary stasis along the cut surface of the liver.
17. If necessary, resuspend the left liver by sewing the falciform ligament to the diaphragm with interrupted figure-of-eight 2-0 Vicryl sutures. Given that the right anterior sector is left in situ, this step is often not necessary.

triangular ligaments, respectively. The right hepatic vein usually enters the vena cava separately. By contrast, the left hepatic vein runs in the left scissura between segments II and III and is often joined by the middle hepatic vein, which occupies the principal scissura, before entering the vena cava. Thus, the middle and left hepatic veins most often empty into the IVC as a common trunk. The right and left phrenic veins, which are easily visible on the surface of the diaphragm, empty into the right and left hepatic veins, respectively, and serve as a reliable landmark to mark the location of the right and left hepatic veins. Several smaller veins from the posterior surface of the liver and the caudate lobe drain directly into the IVC, termed the short hepatic veins or "caudate veins."

Table 57.7. Partial Hepatectomy/Segmentectomy

1. Explore the abdomen to ensure no subradiographic metastatic disease.
2. Ligate the round ligament and leave the suture long, and place a hemostat on it.
3. Divide the falciform back toward IVC.
4. Open the lesser sac through the pars flaccida and clear the area over the caudate lobe and feel for enlarged lymph nodes. This will enable control of the porta hepatis.
5. Ultrasound the entire liver, especially the future liver remnant, to ensure no subradiographic disease.
6. Perform a cholecystectomy.
7. Depending on what segment or what area of the liver is to be removed, the right or left liver should be mobilized as described in Tables 57.3 and 57.4.
8. Mark out the line for parenchymal transection using US to ensure an adequate margin. If a segmentectomy is to be performed, US should be utilized to define the inflow and outflow.
9. Divide and complete the hepatic parenchyma. It is helpful to use US to guide the resection to ensure a negative margin and remnant inflow during the dissection.
10. Complete the parenchymal transection.
11. Hydrate the patient to a status of euvolemia.
12. Ensure hemostasis and biliary stasis along the cut surface of the liver.

The umbilical vein runs beneath the falciform ligament and empties into the left hepatic vein. This vein is important in right-sided resections that remove segment IVa because it provides drainage of segment IVb if the procedure mandates ligation of the middle hepatic vein.

OPERATIVE PROCEDURES

Patient Positioning and Incision (Open Hepatectomy)

For open procedures, the patient should be positioned supine with both arms extended at a right angle to the body. It is not necessary to place the patient in a lateral decubitus position, as adjusting the operating table allows for adequate exposure during the operation. This exposure is adequate for most hepatic resections. The abdomen should be widely exposed from midaxillary line to midaxillary line to allow adequate space for a bisubcostal incision, should one be necessary or preferred. It is the author's preference to do all resections through a simple upper-midline laparotomy incision. A self-retaining retractor to elevate the costal margin provides ample visualization and exposure to complete the procedure safely.

Ultimately, the incision depends on body habitus and tumor location, and the surgeon should not hesitate to extend or enlarge the wound to gain adequate access. For most hepatic resections, a midline incision will suffice with appropriate costal margin and side-wall retraction. A midline incision is often most comfortable for the patient. An extended right subcostal or a bilateral subcostal with a vertical extension are other common incision choices. A slight variation of these incisions that affords excellent exposure for most resections is an upper-midline incision from the xiphoid process to approximately 2 to 3 cm above the umbilicus with right lateral extension toward a point midway between the inferior costal margin and anterior superior iliac spine. A small upper-midline incision may be made first to allow preliminary manual and visual exploration to exclude obviously unresectable disease or the presence of extrahepatic spread. Particularly for left-sided resections, a midline incision is adequate. Large tumors of the right side of the liver, especially those lying posteriorly and involving the IVC, may require a right thoracoabdominal approach, but this is rarely necessary. This can usually be avoided with either right lateral extension of an upper-midline incision with good costal margin retraction or a generous midline incision.

Exposure, Mobilization, and Assessment

After the abdomen is opened, the entire peritoneal cavity should be explored to assess for evidence of subradiographic metastatic disease. In particular, periportal lymph nodes along the hepatic artery, celiac axis, or in the portacaval groove should be assessed. Exploration of the lower abdomen through an upper abdominal incision may be difficult in patients who have had previous pelvic surgery. When direct access is limited, palpation in conjunction with preoperative cross-sectional imaging (CT or MRI) and/or PET scans is sufficient.

Prior to exploration of the liver, the ligamentum teres (round ligament) is divided near the umbilicus, and the falciform ligament is incised and separated from the anterior abdominal wall. The falciform ligament is divided as far cephalad as the subdiaphragmatic IVC. Vessels running within the falciform ligament are usually controlled with bovie electrocautery. When performing a major right-sided resection, the transection plane of the falciform ligament should be approximately 1 cm off the surface of the liver to enable resuspension of the left liver remnant should it be necessary. A long suture should be left on the round ligament to act as a handle during subsequent exploration and dissection for manipulating the liver.

Elevation of the round ligament facilitates examination of the undersurface of the liver, the porta hepatis, and umbilical fissure. Bimanual palpation should be performed, as lesions located deep within the parenchyma may be missed or underestimated with simple surface examination. The transparent tissue of the lesser omentum, or pars flaccida, should be incised to facilitate manual palpation of the caudate lobe (segment I) and the celiac lymph node basin. If the gastrohepatic ligament needs to be further divided to facilitate an adequate evaluation, attention should be directed to the possible presence of an accessory or replaced left hepatic artery. Complete assessment and palpation of the right lobe requires mobilization of the right liver from the diaphragm and retroperitoneum. This may be delayed until US examination of the liver in conjunction with initial palpation indicates that the lesions are resectable.

Mobilization of the right liver begins with complete division of the falciform ligament and identification of the right hepatic vein as the right coronary ligament is incised. As the falciform ligament fibers begin to splay at the back, one must be careful, as the hepatic vein confluence is in close proximity. Early identification of the right hepatic vein prevents subsequent injury during the lateral and inferior mobilization. The location of the right hepatic vein is marked by the right phrenic vein insertion. Once the right vein is visualized, the anterior and posterior coronary ligaments are incised to expose the entire bare area of the liver until the depth of the posterior ligament prevents adequate visualization. At this point, the inferior peritoneal attachments to the liver are incised, which is usually met with a rush of air, in order to separate and drop the adrenal gland. Releasing the inferior attachments facilitates leftward retraction of the liver and exposure of the triangular ligament. The triangular ligament is incised. With the right hepatic vein already visualized, the dissection can now safely proceed medially to complete the division of the posterior coronary ligament toward the inferior vena cava in order to fully mobilize the right hemiliver.

Next, the short retrohepatic veins draining directly from the caudate lobe to the IVC are serially divided, progressing from the inferior aspect up toward the hepatic veins. Complete exposure of the IVC and right hepatic vein requires division of the fibrous tissue, or the vena caval ligament, which usually obscures the right side or the upper part of the retrohepatic vena cava. This division can be done with an energy device or an endoscopic gastrointestinal anastomosis vascular stapler (Endo GIA; US Surgical, Norwalk, CT). It is the author's practice to routinely divide this ligament with a stapler in order to seal the blood vessels contained within this structure. The vena caval, also called caudate, ligament extends behind the vena cava posteriorly as a fibrous extension from the caudate lobe on the left. Rarely, the caudate lobe circumferentially wraps around the IVC such that the vena cava runs through a tunnel of liver parenchyma. Although this thin plate of liver tissue can be a source of difficulty, it can similarly be divided to expose the IVC completely with minimal consequence. Dividing this ligament is a necessary step in order to safely gain extrahepatic control of the right hepatic vein.

Similarly, for a planned left-sided resection, the left coronary and triangular ligaments are incised to mobilize the left lateral sector. Care must be taken not to damage the stomach and spleen at the far left of the triangular ligament, and placing a laparotomy pad under the ligament helps to protect these structures while incising the ligament. Extrahepatic control of the middle/left hepatic vein confluence is a challenging maneuver. The ligamentum venosum must be divided near its attachment to the left hepatic vein in order to expose the anterior surface of the IVC just proximal to the hepatic vein confluence. The notch in between the right and middle vein is developed, and this plane is carefully extended to exit anterior to the IVC at the level of where the ligamentum venosum was divided. Placing an umbilical tape through this space controls the middle/left hepatic vein confluence extrahepatically. This maneuver should only be performed if the location of the tumor mandates extrahepatic division of these veins to facilitate an oncologic margin-negative resection.

Intraoperative Ultrasound

Intraoperative ultrasound (IOUS) is an integral and necessary component for planning and performing hepatic resections. It is used to confirm what was seen on preoperative imaging and to assess for other lesions that may not have been seen previously or have developed in the interval time period between imaging and resection. IOUS also further delineates the exact anatomic relationship of lesions with the major vascular and biliary structures within the liver parenchyma. US guidance is also utilized to perform a needle biopsy of small, deeply placed lesions and for ablative procedures. Examination is carried out with a B-mode, real-time system and a T-shaped probe is the most ergonomic for direct application of the probe to the liver surface and in the author's opinion, provides the best images. Examination should be carried out in a systematic fashion, starting with assessing the outflow and inflow vessels, the biliary tree, and then finally the hepatic parenchyma. In case of doubt, further examination may be done after mobilization of the right or left liver, particularly for posteriorly located tumors. The probe also may be placed on the inferior surface of the liver. IOUS can help plan and guide large segmental resections traversing narrow planes between the tumor edge and major vascular structures. Thus, it is paramount that the surgeon has the ability to use and interpret IOUS in order to safely maneuver inside the liver.

GENERAL PRINCIPLES OF HEPATIC RESECTIONS

All hepatic resections mandate control of the inflow and outflow vasculature and biliary drainage to the portion of liver to be resected, with preservation of adequate hepatic arterial and portal venous blood supply and intact biliary drainage to the liver remnant. Depending on the type of resection being performed, the inflow and outflow can be controlled either outside the liver substance or within the liver parenchyma. Launois and Jamieson have historically advocated for control of the intrahepatic pedicles when oncologically feasible in order to avoid contralateral injury.[219] In practice, most surgeons use a combination of techniques in hepatic resection, doing both pedicle ligation within the liver and extrahepatic dissection to expose the individual corresponding artery and portal vein. Biliary drainage from the remnant liver must be preserved without injury, including both leakage and stricture, to the biliary tract. The hepatic venous outflow should be controlled after inflow division, and the liver parenchyma must be transected to provide tumor adequate clearance in cases of malignancy.

Inflow Control and Preservation of the Integrity of the Biliary Tree

The hepatic arterial and portal venous blood supply to the portion of liver to be removed can be controlled and ligated either by extrahepatic dissection or by transecting the relevant pedicles within the liver parenchyma. Extrahepatic vascular dissection may be accompanied by extrahepatic dissection and control of the relevant biliary radicles as well. However, this is associated with a higher risk of biliary injury, particularly during dissection on the right side, where anatomic variations in biliary anatomy are common. Thus, the right hepatic artery and right portal vein are typically divided utilizing an extrahepatic dissection for vascular control of right-sided lesions, while the corresponding biliary structures are divided within the pedicles at the time of hepatic parenchymal transection. This is not possible, however, for tumors that are close to the hilar structures, such as hilar cholangiocarcinoma. In these cases, extrahepatic biliary dissection is required, as making an intrahepatic approach would be impossible without compromising tumor clearance. For left-sided resections, although a pedicle approach is possible, dissection is most often carried out within or at the base of the umbilical fissure, and far left of the hilar bifurcation. Typically, the left hepatic artery and left portal vein are isolated and individually divided and the left bile duct is divided at the base of the umbilical fissure, thus minimizing the risk of injury to the right liver biliary drainage into the common duct.

Outflow Control

When performing a right hepatectomy, intrahepatic control of the right hepatic vein during parenchymal transection is feasible and acceptable for tumors that allow clearance superiorly with adequate tumor margins and with safe intrahepatic access to these vessels. However, extrahepatic control of the right hepatic vein is also safe and provides the added benefit of controlling the main outflow and disconnecting the specimen from the vena cava prior to parenchymal transection. This can potentially help reduce blood loss during parenchymal transection. For the difficult tumors lying high and posteriorly, extrahepatic control and ligation also facilitates an adequate oncologic margin. Because the middle hepatic vein usually merges with the left hepatic vein prior to draining to the IVC, the middle hepatic vein is usually taken within the liver substance when performing an extended right hepatectomy. During an extended left hepatectomy for a superiorly situated tumor, the middle and left hepatic veins are often controlled as a single unit outside the liver. For a standard left hepatectomy, the middle hepatic vein is preserved and the left hepatic vein is divided within the liver, often as the last step of parenchymal transection. If isolated extrahepatic left hepatic vein control is needed, a small hepatotomy is usually needed to dissect the plane between the middle and left hepatic veins. This is seldom needed or performed.

Parenchymal Transection

Once the inflow and outflow are controlled, parenchymal transection ensues. It is important to maintain a state of low central venous pressure (CVP) in order to minimize bleeding. Central venous access for CVP monitoring is not necessary as long as intravenous fluids are tightly restricted. Several methods may be used to transect the liver parenchyma. The author's preference has been to use a simple crushing technique where Glisson capsule is scored with diathermy along the line of proposed transection, and a Kelly clamp is used to crush the liver tissue and expose small vessels, biliary channels, and larger pedicles. These structures can then be secured and divided using a variety of techniques. The simplest and economical method is to use clips and suture ligation. However, a variety of energy devices can be used that include (1) computer-controlled bipolar cautery (LigaSure; Valleylab, Boulder, CO); (2) a saline-linked radiofrequency ablation monopolar device (TissueLink; TissueLink Medical, Dover, NH), or a bipolar variation (Aquamantys, TissueLink Medical); (3) a Harmonic Scalpel (SonoSurg; Olympus Key Med, New York, NY). All of these devices have been used with success by a variety of investigators.[220–222] They have also been used successfully in the performance of laparoscopic partial hepatectomy. Larger structures can be controlled with sutures or vascular staplers.

The technique of using a Kelly clamp to crush the tissue is rapid and efficient. Although some surgeons choose to apply intermittent inflow occlusion to control blood flow to the remnant, this is most often not necessary if low CVP is maintained.[223] Should inflow occlusion still be necessary, intermittent 15-minute periods of occlusion, interspersed by 5-minute periods of relief to allow perfusion of the remnant and decompression of the bowel, is usually a safe technique. Prolonged occlusion during hepatic resection in patients with jaundice or cirrhosis should be avoided. Prolonged portal inflow occlusion is unnecessary, and for major hepatic resections, complete parenchymal transection is usually accomplished in 20 to 30 minutes. During the short breaks between applications of the Pringle maneuver, the argon beam coagulator (Force GCU System; Valleylab) can be used to control small vessel oozing on the side of the remnant. Avitene (Davol, Warwick, RI), Surgicel (Ethicon, Somerville, NJ), or fibrin sealants also may be applied to the cut surface of the liver to achieve final hemostasis after transection is complete.

Alternate options for the Kelly clamp technique to expose the intrahepatic vascular and biliary anatomy include an ultrasonic dissector or a water-jet dissector.[224] The ultrasonic dissector has some advantages in dissecting liver parenchyma away from delicate vascular and biliary structures, particularly when a margin-negative resection is dependent on the precise dissection of that area. A disadvantage of the ultrasonic dissector is that it can be time consuming and offers no apparent advantage during the majority of parenchymal transection. No published data are available to indicate that any one technique is associated with decreased blood loss.

Some have described the use of broad coagulation devices, an example of which is the Habib 4X (AngioDynamics, Latham, NY). It uses radiofrequency energy to coagulate liver parenchyma widely along the planned transection plane with or without the use of vascular staplers; this method does not clearly expose the internal structures of the liver. The author does not advocate for such an approach and strongly believes that parenchymal transection should be a controlled dissection to avoid serious damage to the liver remnant and minimize bleeding and risk of bile leak.

The basic steps to performing common hepatic resection procedures are listed in **Tables 57.3** to **57.7**.

SUMMARY

The nuances of determining resectability for liver tumors can be difficult to master, owing to the variety of primary and secondary malignancies involving the liver, the diversity of patient-specific factors to consider, and the hepatic anatomic and functional variability that represents the norm. The basic principles, however, are simple—if surgery is deemed appropriate from an oncologic standpoint, the patient is in reasonably good health and can withstand the operation, and the tumor can be safely removed without compromising the viability of the future remnant, nearly all patients will be candidates for resection. However, as our understanding of tumor biology improves, diagnostic and operative techniques evolve, and systemic and local therapies improve, the selection of patients for resection will continue to both expand and simultaneously be refined.

References

1. de Jong MC, Nathan H, Sotiropoulos GC, et al. Intrahepatic cholangiocarcinoma: an international multi-institutional analysis of prognostic factors and lymph node assessment. *J Clin Oncol.* 2011;29(23):3140–3145.
2. Semelka RC, Sofka CM. Hepatic hemangiomas. *Magn Reson Imaging Clin N Am.* 1997;5(2):241–253.
3. Choi BY, Nguyen MH. The diagnosis and management of benign hepatic tumors. *J Clin Gastroenterol.* 2005;39(5):401–412.
4. Yoon SS, Charny CK, Fong Y, et al. Diagnosis, management, and outcomes of 115 patients with hepatic hemangioma. *J Am Coll Surg.* 2003;197(3):392–402.
5. Concejero AM, Chen CL, Chen TY, Eng HL, Kuo FY. Giant cavernous hemangioma of the liver with coagulopathy: adult Kasabach-Merritt syndrome. *Surgery.* 2009;145(2):245–247.
6. Itai Y, Ohtomo K, Furui S, Yamauchi T, Minami M, Yashiro N. Noninvasive diagnosis of small cavernous hemangioma of the liver: advantage of MRI. *AJR Am J Roentgenol.* 1985;145(6):1195–1199.
7. Nino-Murcia M, Olcott EW, Jeffrey RB Jr, Lamm RL, Beaulieu CF, Jain KA. Focal liver lesions: pattern-based classification scheme for enhancement at arterial phase CT. *Radiology.* 2000;215(3):746–751.
8. Farges O, Daradkeh S, Bismuth H. Cavernous hemangiomas of the liver: are there any indications for resection? *World J Surg.* 1995;19(1):19–24.
9. Erdogan D, Busch OR, van Delden OM, et al. Management of liver hemangiomas according to size and symptoms. *J Gastroenterol Hepatol.* 2007;22(11):1953–1958.
10. Gaspar L, Mascarenhas F, da Costa MS, Dias JS, Afonso JG, Silvestre ME. Radiation therapy in the unresectable cavernous hemangioma of the liver. *Radiother Oncol.* 1993;29(1):45–50.
11. Reading NG, Forbes A, Nunnerley HB, Williams R. Hepatic haemangioma: a critical review of diagnosis and management. *Q J Med.* 1988;67(253):431–445.
12. Gao J, Ke S, Ding XM, et al. Radiofrequency ablation for large hepatic hemangiomas: initial experience and lessons. *Surgery.* 2013;153(1):78–85.
13. Chandrasegaram MD, Shah A, Chen JW, et al. Oestrogen hormone receptors in focal nodular hyperplasia. *HPB (Oxford).* 2015;17(6):502–507.
14. Vilgrain V. Focal nodular hyperplasia. *Eur J Radiol.* 2006;58(2):236–245.
15. Buetow PC, Pantongrag-Brown L, Buck JL, Ros PR, Goodman ZD. Focal nodular hyperplasia of the liver: radiologic-pathologic correlation. *Radiographics.* 1996;16(2):369–388.
16. Wanless IR, Mawdsley C, Adams R. On the pathogenesis of focal nodular hyperplasia of the liver. *Hepatology.* 1985;5(6):1194–1200.
17. Mathieu D, Kobeiter H, Maison P, et al. Oral contraceptive use and focal nodular hyperplasia of the liver. *Gastroenterology.* 2000;118(3):560–564.
18. Hussain SM, Terkivatan T, Zondervan PE, et al. Focal nodular hyperplasia: findings at state-of-the-art MR imaging, US, CT, and pathologic analysis. *Radiographics.* 2004;24(1):3–17; discussion 18–19.
19. Kim TK, Jang HJ, Burns PN, Murphy-Lavallee J, Wilson SR. Focal nodular hyperplasia and hepatic adenoma: differentiation with low-mechanical-index contrast-enhanced sonography. *AJR Am J Roentgenol.* 2008;190(1):58–66.
20. Hedayati P, VanSonnenberg E, Shamos R, Gillespie T, McMullen W. Treatment of symptomatic focal nodular hyperplasia with percutaneous radiofrequency ablation. *J Vasc Interv Radiol.* 2010; 21(4):582–585.
21. Nault JC, Bioulac-Sage P, Zucman-Rossi J. Hepatocellular benign tumors-from molecular classification to personalized clinical care. *Gastroenterology.* 2013;144(5):888–902.
22. Jeannot E, Poussin K, Chiche L, et al. Association of CYP1B1 germ line mutations with hepatocyte nuclear factor 1alpha-mutated hepatocellular adenoma. *Cancer Res.* 2007;67(6):2611–2616.
23. Cobey FC, Salem RR. A review of liver masses in pregnancy and a proposed algorithm for their diagnosis and management. *Am J Surg.* 2004;187(2):181–191.
24. Dokmak S, Paradis V, Vilgrain V, et al. A single-center surgical experience of 122 patients with single and multiple hepatocellular adenomas. *Gastroenterology.* 2009;137(5):1698–1705.
25. Brunt EM, Wolverson MK, Di Bisceglie AM. Benign hepatocellular tumors (adenomatosis) in nonalcoholic steatohepatitis: a case report. *Semin Liver Dis.* 2005;25(2):230–236.
26. Zucman-Rossi J, Jeannot E, Nhieu JT, et al. Genotype-phenotype correlation in hepatocellular adenoma: new classification and relationship with HCC. *Hepatology.* 2006;43(3):515–524.
27. Farges O, Ferreira N, Dokmak S, et al. Changing trends in malignant transformation of hepatocellular adenoma. *Gut.* 2011; 60(1):85–89.
28. Laumonier H, Bioulac-Sage P, Laurent C, et al. Hepatocellular adenomas: magnetic resonance imaging features as a function of molecular pathological classification. *Hepatology.* 2008;48(3): 808–818.
29. Ronot M, Bahrami S, Calderaro J, et al. Hepatocellular adenomas: accuracy of magnetic resonance imaging and liver biopsy in subtype classification. *Hepatology.* 2011;53(4):1182–1191.
30. Deneve JL, Pawlik TM, Cunningham S, et al. Liver cell adenoma: a multicenter analysis of risk factors for rupture and malignancy. *Ann Surg Oncol.* 2009;16(3):640–648.
31. Huurman VA, Schaapherder AF. Management of ruptured hepatocellular adenoma. *Dig Surg.* 2010;27(1):56–60.
32. Moreaux J, Bloch P. Solitary biliary cysts of the liver. *Arch Fr Mal App Dig.* 1971;60(4):203–224.
33. Saini S, Mueller PR, Ferrucci JT Jr, Simeone JF, Wittenberg J, Butch RJ. Percutaneous aspiration of hepatic cysts does not provide definitive therapy. *AJR Am J Roentgenol.* 1983;141(3):559–560.
34. Tikkakoski T, Makela JT, Leinonen S, et al. Treatment of symptomatic congenital hepatic cysts with single-session percutaneous drainage and ethanol sclerosis: technique and outcome. *J Vasc Interv Radiol.* 1996;7(2):235–239.
35. Nakaoka R, Das K, Kudo M, Chung H, Innoue T. Percutaneous aspiration and ethanolamine oleate sclerotherapy for sustained resolution of symptomatic polycystic liver disease: an initial experience. *AJR Am J Roentgenol.* 2009;193(6):1540–1545.
36. Antonacci N, Ricci C, Taffurelli G, Casadei R, Minni F. Systematic review of laparoscopic versus open surgery in the treatment of non-parasitic liver cysts. *Updates Surg.* 2014;66(4): 231–238.
37. Tan YM, Chung A, Mack P, Chow P, Khin LW, Ooi LL. Role of fenestration and resection for symptomatic solitary liver cysts. *ANZ J Surg.* 2005;75(7):577–580.
38. Zen Y, Fujii T, Itatsu K, et al. Biliary papillary tumors share pathological features with intraductal papillary mucinous neoplasm of the pancreas. *Hepatology.* 2006;44(5):1333–1343.
39. Zen Y, Jang KT, Ahn S, et al. Intraductal papillary neoplasms and mucinous cystic neoplasms of the hepatobiliary system: demographic differences between Asian and Western populations,

and comparison with pancreatic counterparts. *Histopathology.* 2014;65(2):164–173.
40. Buetow PC, Buck JL, Pantongrag-Brown L, et al. Biliary cystadenoma and cystadenocarcinoma: clinical-imaging-pathologic correlations with emphasis on the importance of ovarian stroma. *Radiology.* 1995;196(3):805–810.
41. Devaney K, Goodman ZD, Ishak KG. Hepatobiliary cystadenoma and cystadenocarcinoma. A light microscopic and immunohistochemical study of 70 patients. *Am J Surg Pathol.* 1994;18(11): 1078–1091.
42. Lewin M, Mourra N, Honigman I, et al. Assessment of MRI and MRCP in diagnosis of biliary cystadenoma and cystadenocarcinoma. *Eur Radiol.* 2006;16(2):407–413.
43. Thomas KT, Welch D, Trueblood A, et al. Effective treatment of biliary cystadenoma. *Ann Surg.* 2005;241(5):769–773; discussion 773–775.
44. Nakanuma Y, Sasaki M, Ishikawa A, Tsui W, Chen TC, Huang SF. Biliary papillary neoplasm of the liver. *Histol Histopathol.* 2002;17(3):851–861.
45. Maithel SK, Ginsberg MS, D'Amico F, et al. Natural history of patients with subcentimeter pulmonary nodules undergoing hepatic resection for metastatic colorectal cancer. *J Am Coll Surg.* 2010;210(1):31–38.
46. Dewhurst C, Rosen MP, Blake MA, et al. ACR Appropriateness Criteria pretreatment staging of colorectal cancer. *J Am Coll Radiol.* 2012;9(11):775–781.
47. Ramos E, Valls C, Martinez L, et al. Preoperative staging of patients with liver metastases of colorectal carcinoma. Does PET/CT really add something to multidetector CT? *Ann Surg Oncol.* 2011;18(9):2654–2661.
48. Petrowsky H, Wildbrett P, Husarik DB, et al. Impact of integrated positron emission tomography and computed tomography on staging and management of gallbladder cancer and cholangiocarcinoma. *J Hepatol.* 2006;45(1):43–50.
49. Selzner M, Hany TF, Wildbrett P, McCormack L, Kadry Z, Clavien PA. Does the novel PET/CT imaging modality impact on the treatment of patients with metastatic colorectal cancer of the liver? *Ann Surg.* 2004;240(6):1027–1034; discussion 1035–1036.
50. Wiering B, Krabbe PF, Jager GJ, Oyen WJ, Ruers TJ. The impact of fluor-18-deoxyglucose-positron emission tomography in the management of colorectal liver metastases. *Cancer.* 2005;104(12):2658–2670.
51. Figueras J, Valls C, Rafecas A, Fabregat J, Ramos E, Jaurrieta E. Resection rate and effect of postoperative chemotherapy on survival after surgery for colorectal liver metastases. *Br J Surg.* 2001;88(7):980–985.
52. Jarnagin WR, Conlon K, Bodniewicz J, et al. A clinical scoring system predicts the yield of diagnostic laparoscopy in patients with potentially resectable hepatic colorectal metastases. *Cancer.* 2001;91(6):1121–1128.
53. Jarnagin WR, Fong Y, Ky A, et al. Liver resection for metastatic colorectal cancer: assessing the risk of occult irresectable disease. *J Am Coll Surg.* 1999;188(1):33–42.
54. Rahusen FD, Cuesta MA, Borgstein PJ, et al. Selection of patients for resection of colorectal metastases to the liver using diagnostic laparoscopy and laparoscopic ultrasonography. *Ann Surg.* 1999;230(1):31–37.
55. Goere D, Wagholikar GD, Pessaux P, et al. Utility of staging laparoscopy in subsets of biliary cancers: laparoscopy is a powerful diagnostic tool in patients with intrahepatic and gallbladder carcinoma. *Surg Endosc.* 2006;20(5):721–725.
56. Biondi A, Tropea A, Basile F. Clinical rescue evaluation in laparoscopic surgery for hepatic metastases by colorectal cancer. *Surg Laparosc Endosc Percutan Tech.* 2010;20(2):69–72.
57. Gholghesaei M, van Muiswinkel JM, Kuiper JW, Kazemier G, Tilanus HW, Ijzermans JN. Value of laparoscopy and laparoscopic ultrasonography in determining resectability of colorectal hepatic metastases. *HPB (Oxford).* 2003;5(2):100–104.
58. Jarnagin WR, Bodniewicz J, Dougherty E, Conlon K, Blumgart LH, Fong Y. A prospective analysis of staging laparoscopy in patients with primary and secondary hepatobiliary malignancies. *J Gastrointest Surg.* 2000;4(1):34–43.
59. Grobmyer SR, Fong Y, D'Angelica M, Blumgart LH, Jarnagin WR. Diagnostic laparoscopy prior to planned hepatic resection for colorectal metastases. *Arch Surg.* 2004;139(12): 1326–1330.
60. Mann CD, Neal CP, Metcalfe MS, Pattenden CJ, Dennison AR, Berry DP. Clinical Risk Score predicts yield of staging laparoscopy in patients with colorectal liver metastases. *Br J Surg.* 2007;94(7):855–859.
61. D'Angelica M, Fong Y, Weber S, et al. The role of staging laparoscopy in hepatobiliary malignancy: prospective analysis of 401 cases. *Ann Surg Oncol.* 2003;10(2):183–189.
62. Jemal A, Bray F, Center MM, Ferlay J, Ward E, Forman D. Global cancer statistics. *CA Cancer J Clin.* 2011;61(2):69–90.
63. Forner A, Llovet JM, Bruix J. Hepatocellular carcinoma. *Lancet* 2012;379(9822):1245–1255.
64. Jarnagin W, Chapman WC, Curley S, et al. Surgical treatment of hepatocellular carcinoma: expert consensus statement. *HPB (Oxford).* 2010;12(5):302–310.
65. Vauthey JN, Lauwers GY, Esnaola NF, et al. Simplified staging for hepatocellular carcinoma. *J Clin Oncol.* 2002;20(6): 1527–1536.
66. Edge SB, Byrd DR, Compton CC, et al., eds. Liver. In: *AJCC Cancer Staging Manual.* 7th ed. Springer; 2010:191–194.
67. Mazzaferro V, Regalia E, Doci R, et al. Liver transplantation for the treatment of small hepatocellular carcinomas in patients with cirrhosis. *N Engl J Med.* 1996;334(11):693–699.
68. Mazzaferro V, Bhoori S, Sposito C, et al. Milan criteria in liver transplantation for hepatocellular carcinoma: an evidence-based analysis of 15 years of experience. *Liver Transpl.* 2011; 17(Suppl 2):S44–S57.
69. A new prognostic system for hepatocellular carcinoma: a retrospective study of 435 patients: the Cancer of the Liver Italian Program (CLIP) investigators. *Hepatology.* 1998;28(3):751–755.
70. Okuda K, Ohtsuki T, Obata H, et al. Natural history of hepatocellular carcinoma and prognosis in relation to treatment. Study of 850 patients. *Cancer.* 1985;56(4):918–928.
71. Tateishi R, Yoshida H, Shiina S, et al. Proposal of a new prognostic model for hepatocellular carcinoma: an analysis of 403 patients. *Gut.* 2005;54(3):419–425.
72. Bruix J, Llovet JM. Prognostic prediction and treatment strategy in hepatocellular carcinoma. *Hepatology.* 2002;35(3):519–524.
73. Llovet JM, Fuster J, Bruix J. Prognosis of hepatocellular carcinoma. *Hepatogastroenterology.* 2002;49(43):7–11.
74. Befeler AS, Di Bisceglie AM. Hepatocellular carcinoma: diagnosis and treatment. *Gastroenterology.* 2002;122(6):1609–1619.
75. Hassoun Z, Gores GJ. Treatment of hepatocellular carcinoma. *Clin Gastroenterol Hepatol.* 2003;1(1):10–18.
76. Nathan H, Schulick RD, Choti MA, Pawlik TM. Predictors of survival after resection of early hepatocellular carcinoma. *Ann Surg.* 2009;249(5):799–805.
77. Ng KK, Vauthey JN, Pawlik TM, et al. Is hepatic resection for large or multinodular hepatocellular carcinoma justified? Results from a multi-institutional database. *Ann Surg Oncol.* 2005;12(5):364–373.
78. Pawlik TM, Delman KA, Vauthey JN, et al. Tumor size predicts vascular invasion and histologic grade: implications for selection of surgical treatment for hepatocellular carcinoma. *Liver Transpl.* 2005;11(9):1086–1092.
79. Pawlik TM, Poon RT, Abdalla EK, et al. Hepatectomy for hepatocellular carcinoma with major portal or hepatic vein invasion: results of a multicenter study. *Surgery.* 2005;137(4):403–410.
80. Pawlik TM, Poon RT, Abdalla EK, et al. Critical appraisal of the clinical and pathologic predictors of survival after resection of large hepatocellular carcinoma. *Arch Surg.* 2005;140(5): 450–457; discussion 457–458.
81. The Liver Cancer Study Group of Japan. Predictive factors for long term prognosis after partial hepatectomy for patients with hepatocellular carcinoma in Japan. *Cancer.* 1994;74(10): 2772–2780.

82. Belghiti J, Panis Y, Farges O, et al. Intrahepatic recurrence after resection of hepatocellular carcinoma complicating cirrhosis. *Ann Surg*. 1991;214(2):114–117.
83. Lai EC, Ng IO, Ng MM, et al. Long-term results of resection for large hepatocellular carcinoma: a multivariate analysis of clinicopathological features. *Hepatology*. 1990;11(5):815–818.
84. Minagawa M, Ikai I, Matsuyama Y, Yamaoka Y, Makuuchi M. Staging of hepatocellular carcinoma: assessment of the Japanese TNM and AJCC/UICC TNM systems in a cohort of 13,772 patients in Japan. *Ann Surg*. 2007;245(6):909–922.
85. Lee NH, Chau GY, Lui WY, King KL, Tsay SH, Wu CW. Surgical treatment and outcome in patients with a hepatocellular carcinoma greater than 10 cm in diameter. *Br J Surg*. 1998;85(12): 1654–1657.
86. Poon RT, Fan ST, Wong J. Selection criteria for hepatic resection in patients with large hepatocellular carcinoma larger than 10 cm in diameter. *J Am Coll Surg*. 2002;194(5):592–602.
87. Zhou XD, Tang ZY, Ma ZC, et al. Surgery for large primary liver cancer more than 10 cm in diameter. *J Cancer Res Clin Oncol*. 2003;129(9):543–548.
88. Kosuge T, Makuuchi M, Takayama T, et al. Long-term results after resection of hepatocellular carcinoma: experience of 480 cases. *Hepatogastroenterology*. 1993;40(4):328–332.
89. Poon RT, Fan ST. Evaluation of the new AJCC/UICC staging system for hepatocellular carcinoma after hepatic resection in Chinese patients. *Surg Oncol Clin N Am*. 2003;12(1):35–50, viii.
90. Lei HJ, Chau GY, Lui WY, et al. Prognostic value and clinical relevance of the 6th Edition 2002 American Joint Committee on Cancer staging system in patients with resectable hepatocellular carcinoma. *J Am Coll Surg*. 2006;203(4):426–435.
91. Tsai TJ, Chau GY, Lui WY, et al. Clinical significance of microscopic tumor venous invasion in patients with resectable hepatocellular carcinoma. *Surgery*. 2000;127(6):603–608.
92. Li Q, Wang J, Juzi JT, et al. Clonality analysis for multicentric origin and intrahepatic metastasis in recurrent and primary hepatocellular carcinoma. *J Gastrointest Surg*. 2008;12(9): 1540–1547.
93. Morimoto O, Nagano H, Sakon M, et al. Diagnosis of intrahepatic metastasis and multicentric carcinogenesis by microsatellite loss of heterozygosity in patients with multiple and recurrent hepatocellular carcinomas. *J Hepatol*. 2003;39(2):215–221.
94. Yamamoto T, Kajino K, Kudo M, et al. Determination of the clonal origin of multiple human hepatocellular carcinomas by cloning and polymerase chain reaction of the integrated hepatitis B virus DNA. *Hepatology*. 1999;29(5):1446–1452.
95. Cheng CH, Lee CF, Wu TH, et al. Evaluation of the new AJCC staging system for resectable hepatocellular carcinoma. *World J Surg Oncol* 2011;9:114.
96. Llovet JM, Bustamante J, Castells A, et al. Natural history of untreated nonsurgical hepatocellular carcinoma: rationale for the design and evaluation of therapeutic trials. *Hepatology*. 1999;29(1):62–67.
97. Pawarode A, Voravud N, Sriuranpong V, Kullavanijaya P, Patt YZ. Natural history of untreated primary hepatocellular carcinoma: a retrospective study of 157 patients. *Am J Clin Oncol*. 1998;21(4):386–391.
98. Vauthey JN, Klimstra D, Franceschi D, et al. Factors affecting long-term outcome after hepatic resection for hepatocellular carcinoma. *Am J Surg*. 1995;169(1):28–34; discussion 34–35.
99. Ikai I, Yamamoto Y, Yamamoto N, et al. Results of hepatic resection for hepatocellular carcinoma invading major portal and/or hepatic veins. *Surg Oncol Clin N Am*. 2003;12(1):65–75, ix.
100. Poon RT, Fan ST, Ng IO, Wong J. Prognosis after hepatic resection for stage IVA hepatocellular carcinoma: a need for reclassification. *Ann Surg*. 2003;237(3):376–383.
101. Uka K, Aikata H, Takaki S, et al. Clinical features and prognosis of patients with extrahepatic metastases from hepatocellular carcinoma. *World J Gastroenterol*. 2007;13(3):414–420.
102. McGlynn KA, Tarone RE, El-Serag HB. A comparison of trends in the incidence of hepatocellular carcinoma and intrahepatic cholangiocarcinoma in the United States. *Cancer Epidemiol Biomarkers Prev*. 2006;15(6):1198–1203.
103. Shaib YH, Davila JA, McGlynn K, El-Serag HB. Rising incidence of intrahepatic cholangiocarcinoma in the United States: a true increase? *J Hepatol*. 2004;40(3):472–477.
104. Dodson RM, Weiss MJ, Cosgrove D, et al. Intrahepatic cholangiocarcinoma: management options and emerging therapies. *J Am Coll Surg*. 2013;217(4):736–750.e4.
105. Greene FL, Fleming ID, Fritz AG, et al., eds. Liver. In: *AJCC Cancer Staging Manual*. 6th ed. Springer-Verlag; 2002.
106. Nathan H, Aloia TA, Vauthey JN, et al. A proposed staging system for intrahepatic cholangiocarcinoma. *Ann Surg Oncol*. 2009;16(1):14–22.
107. Okabayashi T, Yamamoto J, Kosuge T, et al. A new staging system for mass-forming intrahepatic cholangiocarcinoma: analysis of preoperative and postoperative variables. *Cancer*. 2001; 92(9):2374–2383.
108. Wang Y, Li J, Xia Y, et al. Prognostic nomogram for intrahepatic cholangiocarcinoma after partial hepatectomy. *J Clin Oncol*. 2013;31(9):1188–1195.
109. Yamasaki S. Intrahepatic cholangiocarcinoma: macroscopic type and stage classification. *J Hepatobiliary Pancreat Surg*. 2003; 10(4):288–291.
110. Edge SB, Byrd DR, Compton CC, et al., eds. Intrahepatic bile ducts. In: *AJCC Cancer Staging Manual*. 7th ed. Springer; 2010: 201–204.
111. Hyder O, Marques H, Pulitano C, et al. A nomogram to predict long-term survival after resection for intrahepatic cholangiocarcinoma: an Eastern and Western experience. *JAMA Surg*. 2014;149(5):432–438.
112. Choi SB, Kim KS, Choi JY, et al. The prognosis and survival outcome of intrahepatic cholangiocarcinoma following surgical resection: association of lymph node metastasis and lymph node dissection with survival. *Ann Surg Oncol*. 2009;16(11): 3048–3056.
113. Inoue K, Makuuchi M, Takayama T, et al. Long-term survival and prognostic factors in the surgical treatment of mass-forming type cholangiocarcinoma. *Surgery*. 2000;127(5):498–505.
114. Endo I, Gonen M, Yopp AC, et al. Intrahepatic cholangiocarcinoma: rising frequency, improved survival, and determinants of outcome after resection. *Ann Surg*. 2008;248(1):84–96.
115. Weber SM, Jarnagin WR, Klimstra D, DeMatteo RP, Fong Y, Blumgart LH. Intrahepatic cholangiocarcinoma: resectability, recurrence pattern, and outcomes. *J Am Coll Surg*. 2001; 193(4):384–391.
116. Spolverato G, Kim Y, Alexandrescu S, et al. Is hepatic resection for large or multifocal intrahepatic cholangiocarcinoma justified? Results from a multi-institutional collaboration. *Ann Surg Oncol*. 2015;22(7):2218–2225.
117. Ribero D, Pinna AD, Guglielmi A, et al. Surgical approach for long-term survival of patients with intrahepatic cholangiocarcinoma: a multi-institutional analysis of 434 patients. *Arch Surg*. 2012;147(12):1107–1113.
118. Spolverato G, Ejaz A, Kim Y, et al. Tumor size predicts vascular invasion and histologic grade among patients undergoing resection of intrahepatic cholangiocarcinoma. *J Gastrointest Surg*. 2014;18(7):1284–1291.
119. Konstadoulakis MM, Roayaie S, Gomatos IP, et al. Fifteen-year, single-center experience with the surgical management of intrahepatic cholangiocarcinoma: operative results and long-term outcome. *Surgery*. 2008;143(3):366–374.
120. Ali SM, Clark CJ, Zaydfudim VM, Que FG, Nagorney DM. Role of major vascular resection in patients with intrahepatic cholangiocarcinoma. *Ann Surg Oncol*. 2013;20(6):2023–2028.
121. Manfredi S, Lepage C, Hatem C, Coatmeur O, Faivre J, Bouvier AM. Epidemiology and management of liver metastases from colorectal cancer. *Ann Surg*. 2006;244(2):254–259.
122. Weiss L, Grundmann E, Torhorst J, et al. Haematogenous metastatic patterns in colonic carcinoma: an analysis of 1541 necropsies. *J Pathol*. 1986;150(3):195–203.

123. House MG, Ito H, Gönen M, et al. Survival after hepatic resection for metastatic colorectal cancer: trends in outcomes for 1,600 patients during two decades at a single institution. *J Am Coll Surg*. 2010;210(5):744–752, 752–755.
124. Tomlinson JS, Jarnagin WR, DeMatteo RP, et al. Actual 10-year survival after resection of colorectal liver metastases defines cure. *J Clin Oncol*. 2007;25(29):4575–4580.
125. Fong Y, Fortner J, Sun RL, et al. Clinical score for predicting recurrence after hepatic resection for metastatic colorectal cancer: analysis of 1001 consecutive cases. *Ann Surg*. 1999; 230(3):309–318; discussion 318–321.
126. Kato T, Yasui K, Hirai T, et al. Therapeutic results for hepatic metastasis of colorectal cancer with special reference to effectiveness of hepatectomy: analysis of prognostic factors for 763 cases recorded at 18 institutions. *Dis Colon Rectum*. 2003; 46(10 Suppl):S22–S31.
127. Nordlinger B, Guiguet M, Vaillant JC, et al. Surgical resection of colorectal carcinoma metastases to the liver. A prognostic scoring system to improve case selection, based on 1568 patients. Association Francaise de Chirurgie. *Cancer*. 1996;77(7): 1254–1262.
128. Rees M, Tekkis PP, Welsh FK, O'Rourke T, John TG. Evaluation of long-term survival after hepatic resection for metastatic colorectal cancer: a multifactorial model of 929 patients. *Ann Surg*. 2008;247(1):125–135.
129. Wei AC, Greig PD, Grant D, Taylor B, Langer B, Gallinger S. Survival after hepatic resection for colorectal metastases: a 10-year experience. *Ann Surg Oncol*. 2006;13(5):668–676.
130. Carpizo DR, Are C, Jarnagin W, et al. Liver resection for metastatic colorectal cancer in patients with concurrent extrahepatic disease: results in 127 patients treated at a single center. *Ann Surg Oncol*. 2009;16(8):2138–2146.
131. Elias D, Liberale G, Vernerey D, et al. Hepatic and extrahepatic colorectal metastases: when resectable, their localization does not matter, but their total number has a prognostic effect. *Ann Surg Oncol*. 2005;12(11):900–909.
132. Elias D, Ouellet JF, Bellon N, Pignon JP, Pocard M, Lasser P. Extrahepatic disease does not contraindicate hepatectomy for colorectal liver metastases. *Br J Surg*. 2003;90(5):567–574.
133. Rindi G, Capella C, Solcia E. Cell biology, clinicopathological profile, and classification of gastro-enteropancreatic endocrine tumors. *J Mol Med (Berl)*. 1998;76(6):413–420.
134. Chambers AJ, Pasieka JL, Dixon E, Rorstad O. The palliative benefit of aggressive surgical intervention for both hepatic and mesenteric metastases from neuroendocrine tumors. *Surgery*. 2008;144(4):645–651; discussion 651–653.
135. Mayo SC, de Jong MC, Pulitano C, et al. Surgical management of hepatic neuroendocrine tumor metastasis: results from an international multi-institutional analysis. *Ann Surg Oncol*. 2010;17(12):3129–3136.
136. Strosberg J, El-Haddad G, Wolin E, et al. Phase 3 trial of (177) lu-dotatate for midgut neuroendocrine tumors. *N Engl J Med*. 2017;376(2):125–135.
137. Adam R, Chiche L, Aloia T, et al. Hepatic resection for noncolorectal nonendocrine liver metastases: analysis of 1,452 patients and development of a prognostic model. *Ann Surg*. 2006; 244(4):524–535.
138. Saklad M. Grading of patients for surgical procedures. *Anesthesiology*. 1941;2:281–284.
139. Oken MM, Creech RH, Tormey DC, et al. Toxicity and response criteria of the Eastern Cooperative Oncology Group. *Am J Clin Oncol*. 1982;5(6):649–655.
140. Charlson ME, Pompei P, Ales KL, MacKenzie CR. A new method of classifying prognostic comorbidity in longitudinal studies: development and validation. *J Chronic Dis*. 1987;40(5):373–383.
141. Goldman L, Caldera DL, Nussbaum SR, et al. Multifactorial index of cardiac risk in noncardiac surgical procedures. *N Engl J Med*. 1977;297(16):845–850.
142. Makary MA, Segev DL, Pronovost PJ, et al. Frailty as a predictor of surgical outcomes in older patients. *J Am Coll Surg*. 2010;210(6):901–908.
143. Revenig LM, Canter DJ, Taylor MD, et al. Too frail for surgery? Initial results of a large multidisciplinary prospective study examining preoperative variables predictive of poor surgical outcomes. *J Am Coll Surg*. 2013;217(4):665–670.e1.
144. Nuzzo G, Giordano M, Giuliante F, et al. Complex liver resection for hepatic tumours involving the inferior vena cava. *Eur J Surg Oncol*. 2011;37(11):921–927.
145. Hemming AW, Reed AI, Langham MR Jr, et al. Combined resection of the liver and inferior vena cava for hepatic malignancy. *Ann Surg*. 2004;239(5):712–719; discussion 719–721.
146. Shi J, Lai EC, Li N, et al. Surgical treatment of hepatocellular carcinoma with portal vein tumor thrombus. *Ann Surg Oncol*. 2010;17(8):2073–2080.
147. Wu CC, Hsieh SR, Chen JT, et al. An appraisal of liver and portal vein resection for hepatocellular carcinoma with tumor thrombi extending to portal bifurcation. *Arch Surg*. 2000;135(11): 1273–1279.
148. Pesi B, Ferrero A, Grazi GL, et al. Liver resection with thrombectomy as a treatment of hepatocellular carcinoma with major vascular invasion: results from a retrospective multicentric study. *Am J Surg*. 2015;210(1):35–44.
149. Gruttadauria S, Marsh JW, Bartlett DL, Gridelli B, Marcos A. Ex situ resection techniques and liver autotransplantation: last resource for otherwise unresectable malignancy. *Dig Dis Sci*. 2005;50(10):1829–1835.
150. Oldhafer KJ, Lang H, Schlitt HJ, et al. Long-term experience after ex situ liver surgery. *Surgery*. 2000;127(5):520–527.
151. Sugimachi K, Shirabe K, Taketomi A, et al. Successful curative extracorporeal hepatic resection for far-advanced hepatocellular carcinoma in an adolescent patient. *Liver Transpl*. 2010;16(5): 685–687.
152. Hemming AW, Cattral MS. Ex vivo liver resection with replacement of the inferior vena cava and hepatic vein replacement by transposition of the portal vein. *J Am Coll Surg*. 1999;189(5): 523–526.
153. Lodge JP, Ammori BJ, Prasad KR, Bellamy MC. Ex vivo and in situ resection of inferior vena cava with hepatectomy for colorectal metastases. *Ann Surg* 2000;231(4):471–479.
154. Abdalla EK, Denys A, Chevalier P, Nemr RA, Vauthey JN. Total and segmental liver volume variations: implications for liver surgery. *Surgery*. 2004;135(4):404–410.
155. Heymsfield SB, Fulenwider T, Nordlinger B, Barlow R, Sones P, Kutner M. Accurate measurement of liver, kidney, and spleen volume and mass by computerized axial tomography. *Ann Intern Med*. 1979;90(2):185–187.
156. Saito S, Yamanaka J, Miura K, et al. A novel 3D hepatectomy simulation based on liver circulation: application to liver resection and transplantation. *Hepatology*. 2005;41(6):1297–1304.
157. Yamanaka J, Saito S, Fujimoto J. Impact of preoperative planning using virtual segmental volumetry on liver resection for hepatocellular carcinoma. *World J Surg*. 2007;31(6):1249–1255.
158. Vauthey JN, Abdalla EK, Doherty DA, et al. Body surface area and body weight predict total liver volume in Western adults. *Liver Transpl*. 2002;8(3):233–240.
159. Johnson TN, Tucker GT, Tanner MS, et al. Changes in liver volume from birth to adulthood: a meta-analysis. *Liver Transpl*. 2005;11(12):1481–1493.
160. Abdalla EK, Barnett CC, Doherty D, Curley SA, Vauthey JN. Extended hepatectomy in patients with hepatobiliary malignancies with and without preoperative portal vein embolization. *Arch Surg*. 2002;137(6):675–680; discussion 680–681.
161. Ribero D, Abdalla EK, Madoff DC, Donadon M, Loyer EM, Vauthey JN. Portal vein embolization before major hepatectomy and its effects on regeneration, resectability and outcome. *Br J Surg*. 2007;94(11):1386–1394.
162. Vauthey JN, Pawlik TM, Abdalla EK, et al. Is extended hepatectomy for hepatobiliary malignancy justified? *Ann Surg*. 2004;239(5):722–730; discussion 730–732.
163. Karoui M, Penna C, Amin-Hashem M, et al. Influence of preoperative chemotherapy on the risk of major hepatectomy for colorectal liver metastases. *Ann Surg*. 2006;243(1):1–7.

164. Nakano H, Oussoultzoglou E, Rosso E, et al. Sinusoidal injury increases morbidity after major hepatectomy in patients with colorectal liver metastases receiving preoperative chemotherapy. *Ann Surg*. 2008;247(1):118–124.
165. Pawlik TM, Olino K, Gleisner AL, et al. Preoperative chemotherapy for colorectal liver metastases: impact on hepatic histology and postoperative outcome. *J Gastrointest Surg*. 2007;11(7): 860–868.
166. Vauthey JN, Pawlik TM, Ribero D, et al. Chemotherapy regimen predicts steatohepatitis and an increase in 90-day mortality after surgery for hepatic colorectal metastases. *J Clin Oncol*. 2006;24(13):2065–2072.
167. Kishi Y, Zorzi D, Contreras CM, et al. Extended preoperative chemotherapy does not improve pathologic response and increases postoperative liver insufficiency after hepatic resection for colorectal liver metastases. *Ann Surg Oncol*. 2010;17(11):2870–2876.
168. Nordlinger B, Sorbye H, Glimelius B, et al. Perioperative chemotherapy with FOLFOX4 and surgery versus surgery alone for resectable liver metastases from colorectal cancer (EORTC Intergroup trial 40983): a randomised controlled trial. *Lancet*. 2008;371(9617):1007–1016.
169. Cleary JM, Tanabe KT, Lauwers GY, et al. Hepatic toxicities associated with the use of preoperative systemic therapy in patients with metastatic colorectal adenocarcinoma to the liver. *Oncologist*. 2009;14(11):1095–1105.
170. Shindoh J, Tzeng CW, Aloia TA, et al. Optimal future liver remnant in patients treated with extensive preoperative chemotherapy for colorectal liver metastases. *Ann Surg Oncol*. 2013;20(8):2493–2500.
171. Kishi Y, Abdalla EK, Chun YS, et al. Three hundred and one consecutive extended right hepatectomies: evaluation of outcome based on systematic liver volumetry. *Ann Surg*. 2009;250(4): 540–548.
172. Azoulay D, Castaing D, Krissat J, et al. Percutaneous portal vein embolization increases the feasibility and safety of major liver resection for hepatocellular carcinoma in injured liver. *Ann Surg*. 2000;232(5):665–672.
173. Narita M, Oussoultzoglou E, Fuchshuber P, et al. What is a safe future liver remnant size in patients undergoing major hepatectomy for colorectal liver metastases and treated by intensive preoperative chemotherapy? *Ann Surg Oncol*. 2012;19(8):2526–2538.
174. Shirabe K, Shimada M, Gion T, et al. Postoperative liver failure after major hepatic resection for hepatocellular carcinoma in the modern era with special reference to remnant liver volume. *J Am Coll Surg*. 1999;188(3):304–309.
175. Clavien PA, Petrowsky H, DeOliveira ML, et al. Strategies for safer liver surgery and partial liver transplantation. *N Engl J Med*. 2007;356(15):1545–1559.
176. Bruix J, Castells A, Bosch J, et al. Surgical resection of hepatocellular carcinoma in cirrhotic patients: prognostic value of preoperative portal pressure. *Gastroenterology*. 1996;111(4):1018–1022.
177. Franco D, Capussotti L, Smadja C, et al. Resection of hepatocellular carcinomas. Results in 72 European patients with cirrhosis. *Gastroenterology*. 1990;98(3):733–738.
178. Teh SH, Nagorney DM, Stevens SR, et al. Risk factors for mortality after surgery in patients with cirrhosis. *Gastroenterology*. 2007;132(4):1261–1269.
179. Schroeder RA, Marroquin CE, Bute BP, Khuri S, Henderson WG, Kuo PC. Predictive indices of morbidity and mortality after liver resection. *Ann Surg*. 2006;243(3):373–379.
180. Kamath PS, Wiesner RH, Malinchoc M, et al. A model to predict survival in patients with end-stage liver disease. *Hepatology*. 2001;33(2):464–470.
181. Wiesner RH, McDiarmid SV, Kamath PS, et al. MELD and PELD: application of survival models to liver allocation. *Liver Transpl*. 2001;7(7):567–580.
182. Teh SH, Christein J, Donohue J, et al. Hepatic resection of hepatocellular carcinoma in patients with cirrhosis: Model of End-Stage Liver Disease (MELD) score predicts perioperative mortality. *J Gastrointest Surg*. 2005;9(9):1207–1215; discussion 1215.
183. Cucchetti A, Ercolani G, Vivarelli M, et al. Impact of model for end-stage liver disease (MELD) score on prognosis after hepatectomy for hepatocellular carcinoma on cirrhosis. *Liver Transpl*. 2006;12(6):966–971.
184. Pugh RN, Murray-Lyon IM, Dawson JL, et al. Transection of the oesophagus for bleeding oesophageal varices. *Br J Surg*. 1973;60(8):646–649.
185. Maithel SK, Kneuertz PJ, Kooby DA, et al. Importance of low preoperative platelet count in selecting patients for resection of hepatocellular carcinoma: a multi-institutional analysis. *J Am Coll Surg*. 2011;212(4):638–648; discussion 648–650.
186. Manizate F, Hiotis SP, Labow D, et al. Liver functional reserve estimation: state of the art and relevance for local treatments: the Western perspective. *J Hepatobiliary Pancreat Sci*. 2010;17(4): 385–388.
187. Cucchetti A, Ercolani G, Vivarelli M, et al. Is portal hypertension a contraindication to hepatic resection? *Ann Surg*. 2009; 250(6):922–928.
188. Jarnagin WR, Gonen M, Fong Y, et al. Improvement in perioperative outcome after hepatic resection: analysis of 1,803 consecutive cases over the past decade. *Ann Surg*. 2002;236(4):397–406; discussion 406–407.
189. Poon RT, Fan ST, Lo CM, et al. Improving perioperative outcome expands the role of hepatectomy in management of benign and malignant hepatobiliary diseases: analysis of 1222 consecutive patients from a prospective database. *Ann Surg*. 2004;240(4):698–708; discussion 708–710.
190. Kaneko K, Shirai Y, Wakai T, et al. Low preoperative platelet counts predict a high mortality after partial hepatectomy in patients with hepatocellular carcinoma. *World J Gastroenterol*. 2005;11(37):5888–5892.
191. Caesar J, Shaldon S, Chiandussi L, Guevara L, Sherlock S. The use of indocyanine green in the measurement of hepatic blood flow and as a test of hepatic function. *Clin Sci*. 1961;21: 43–57.
192. Imamura H, Seyama Y, Kokudo N, et al. One thousand fifty-six hepatectomies without mortality in 8 years. *Arch Surg*. 2003;138(11):1198–1206; discussion 1206.
193. Bennett JJ, Blumgart LH. Assessment of hepatic reserve prior to hepatic resection. *J Hepatobiliary Pancreat Surg*. 2005;12(1): 10–15.
194. Ijichi M, Makuuchi M, Imamura H, Takayama T. Portal embolization relieves persistent jaundice after complete biliary drainage. *Surgery*. 2001;130(1):116–118.
195. Uesaka K, Nimura Y, Nagino M. Changes in hepatic lobar function after right portal vein embolization. An appraisal by biliary indocyanine green excretion. *Ann Surg*. 1996;223(1):77–83.
196. Hirai I, Kimura W, Fuse A, Suto K, Urayama M. Evaluation of preoperative portal embolization for safe hepatectomy, with special reference to assessment of nonembolized lobe function with 99mTc-GSA SPECT scintigraphy. *Surgery*. 2003;133(5):495–506.
197. Abdalla EK, Hicks ME, Vauthey JN. Portal vein embolization: rationale, technique and future prospects. *Br J Surg*. 2001;88(2): 165–175.
198. Shindoh J, Tzeng CW, Aloia TA, et al. Portal vein embolization improves rate of resection of extensive colorectal liver metastases without worsening survival. *Br J Surg*. 2013;100(13):1777–1783.
199. Farges O, Belghiti J, Kianmanesh R, et al. Portal vein embolization before right hepatectomy: prospective clinical trial. *Ann Surg*. 2003;237(2):208–217.
200. Shindoh J, Truty MJ, Aloia TA, et al. Kinetic growth rate after portal vein embolization predicts posthepatectomy outcomes: toward zero liver-related mortality in patients with colorectal liver metastases and small future liver remnant. *J Am Coll Surg*. 2013;216(2):201–209.
201. Leung U, Simpson AL, Araujo RL, et al. Remnant growth rate after portal vein embolization is a good early predictor of post-hepatectomy liver failure. *J Am Coll Surg*. 2014;219(4):620–630.
202. Di Stefano DR, de Baere T, Denys A, et al. Preoperative percutaneous portal vein embolization: evaluation of adverse events in 188 patients. *Radiology*. 2005;234(2):625–630.

203. Hoekstra LT, van Lienden KP, Doets A, Busch OR, Gouma DJ, van Gulik TM. Tumor progression after preoperative portal vein embolization. *Ann Surg*. 2012;256(5):812–817; discussion 817–818.
204. Abdalla EK, Adam R, Bilchik AJ, Jaeck D, Vauthey JN, Mahvi D. Improving resectability of hepatic colorectal metastases: expert consensus statement. *Ann Surg Oncol*. 2006;13(10):1271–1280.
205. Adam R, Laurent A, Azoulay D, Castaing D, Bismuth H. Two-stage hepatectomy: a planned strategy to treat irresectable liver tumors. *Ann Surg*. 2000;232(6):777–785.
206. Lam VW, Laurence JM, Johnston E, Hollands MJ, Pleass HC, Richardson AJ. A systematic review of two-stage hepatectomy in patients with initially unresectable colorectal liver metastases. *HPB (Oxford)*. 2013;15(7):483–491.
207. Wicherts DA, Miller R, de Haas RJ, et al. Long-term results of two-stage hepatectomy for irresectable colorectal cancer liver metastases. *Ann Surg*. 2008;248(6):994–1005.
208. Schnitzbauer AA, Lang SA, Goessmann H, et al. Right portal vein ligation combined with in situ splitting induces rapid left lateral liver lobe hypertrophy enabling 2-staged extended right hepatic resection in small-for-size settings. *Ann Surg*. 2012;255(3): 405–414.
209. Alvarez FA, Ardiles V, Sanchez Claria R, Pekolj J, de Santibañes E. Associating liver partition and portal vein ligation for staged hepatectomy (ALPPS): tips and tricks. *J Gastrointest Surg*. 2013;17(4):814–821.
210. Aloia TA, Vauthey JN. Associating liver partition and portal vein ligation for staged hepatectomy (ALPPS): what is gained and what is lost? *Ann Surg*. 2012;256(3):e9; author reply e16–e19.
211. Li J, Girotti P, Konigsrainer I, Ladurner R, Königsrainer A, Nadalin S. ALPPS in right trisectionectomy: a safe procedure to avoid postoperative liver failure? *J Gastrointest Surg*. 2013;17(5):956–961.
212. Vennarecci G, Laurenzi A, Levi Sandri GB, et al. The ALPPS procedure for hepatocellular carcinoma. *Eur J Surg Oncol*. 2014; 40(8):982–988.
213. Vennarecci G, Laurenzi A, Santoro R, et al. The ALPPS procedure: a surgical option for hepatocellular carcinoma with major vascular invasion. *World J Surg*. 2014;38(6):1498–1503.
214. Andriani OC. Long-term results with associating liver partition and portal vein ligation for staged hepatectomy (ALPPS). *Ann Surg*. 2012;256(3):e5; author reply e16–e19.
215. de Santibanes E, Clavien PA. Playing Play-Doh to prevent postoperative liver failure: the "ALPPS" approach. *Ann Surg*. 2012; 255(3):415–417.
216. Ratti F, Schadde E, Masetti M, et al. Strategies to increase the resectability of patients with colorectal liver metastases: a multicenter case-match analysis of ALPPS and conventional two-stage hepatectomy. *Ann Surg Oncol*. 2015;22(6):1933–1942.
217. Couinaud C. Anatomic principles of left and right regulated hepatectomy: technics. *J Chir (Paris)*. 1954;70(12):933–966.
218. Strasberg SM, Phillips C. Use and dissemination of the Brisbane 2000 nomenclature of liver anatomy and resections. *Ann Surg*. 2013;257(3):377–382.
219. Launois B, Jamieson GG. The importance of Glisson's capsule and its sheaths in the intrahepatic approach to resection of the liver. *Surg Gynecol Obstet*. 1992;174(1):7–10.
220. Clavien PA, Emond J, Vauthey JN, Belghiti J, Chari RS, Strasberg SM. Protection of the liver during hepatic surgery. *J Gastrointest Surg*. 2004;8(3):313–327.
221. Sakamoto Y, Yamamoto J, Kokudo N, et al. Bloodless liver resection using the monopolar floating ball plus ligasure diathermy: preliminary results of 16 liver resections. *World J Surg*. 2004; 28(2):166–172.
222. Strasberg SM, Drebin JA, Linehan D. Use of a bipolar vessel-sealing device for parenchymal transection during liver surgery. *J Gastrointest Surg*. 2002;6(4):569–574.
223. Pringle JH. V. Notes on the arrest of hepatic hemorrhage due to trauma. *Ann Surg*. 1908;48(4):541–549.
224. Hanna SS, Nam R, Leonhardt C. Liver resection by ultrasonic dissection and intraoperative ultrasonography. *HPB Surg*. 1996; 9(3):121–128.

58

Calculous Biliary Disease

Salila S. Hashmi, Rebecca L. Buttar, and Elijah Dixon

Key Points

1. Gallstones are classified by their cholesterol content: cholesterol (70% to 80%) or pigmented (20% to 30%) with pigmented stones further classified as black or brown.
2. The pathogenesis of cholesterol gallstones is multifactorial involving: (a) cholesterol supersaturation in bile, (b) crystal nucleation, (c) gallbladder dysmotility, and (d) gallbladder absorption/secretion.
3. Prophylactic cholecystectomy is generally not indicated in patients with asymptomatic gallstones.
4. Laparoscopic cholecystectomy is a safe procedure even when performed for acute cholecystitis.
5. Choledocholithiasis (common bile duct [CBD] stones) can have an asymptomatic course or may present along the spectrum of mild biliary colic to fulminant sepsis from acute cholangitis, biliary pancreatitis, or hepatic abscesses.
6. Endoscopic cholangiography (ERCP) with sphincterotomy allows for the diagnosis of CBD stones in most cases and allows for therapeutic intervention if stones are identified. ERCP with stone extraction is effective in removing stones in 85% to 95% of cases but is associated with postprocedural complications (pancreatitis and cholangitis).
7. CBD exploration may be required to remove stones that cannot be removed via ERCP.

1 There are two types of gallstones—cholesterol or pigmented stones. Cholesterol stones are most common, accounting for 70% to 80% of gallstones. The pathogenesis of cholesterol stones is multifactorial, involving: (a) cholesterol supersaturation in bile, (b) crystal nucleation around a calcium salt core, (c) gallbladder dysmotility, and (d) gallbladder absorption/
2 secretion. The pigmented stones can be black or brown and are made up of calcium bilirubinate. Black stones are exclusively found in the gallbladder, whereas brown stones can also be found in the biliary tree (both intra and extrahepatic).

RISK FACTORS FOR GALLSTONE FORMATION

Cholelithiasis results from an interplay between genetic and environmental factors.

Age: The incidence of gallstones increases with age. Most pediatric patients with gallstone disease have an associated hemolytic disease.

Gender: Females are at a higher risk—this is secondary to hormonal effects of estrogen, oral contraceptive use, or hormonal therapy after menopause. Pregnancy increases the risk of biliary sludge formation.

Genetics: Genetic components have been implicated in up to 30% of patients in some population studies. Cholesterol stones occur in ratios of 3:1 in family members. Genetic mutations have been identified in hepatic cholesterol metabolism. Patients with conditions that upregulate hemolysis have higher stone formation

Physical activity: Obesity is a risk factor for gallstone development.

Diet: Patients receiving parenteral nutrition are at risk of developing biliary stasis and gallstones.

Other disease processes/medications: Cirrhosis can induce gallstone formation in about 25% to 30% of patients. Inflammatory bowel disease, ileal resection, and cystic fibrosis interfere with bile reabsorption and can lead to cholelithiasis. Medications including estrogens, synthetic hormones (lanreotide), and thiazide diuretics increase biliary cholesterol secretion, whereas ceftriaxone can also induce biliary stasis and therefore, gallstone formation. Glucagon-like peptide-1 receptor agonist use is also associated with an increased risk of gallbladder and biliary diseases.

NATURAL HISTORY OF GALLSTONES

Eighty percent of people with cholelithiasis will remain asymptomatic, with 2% to 3% per year of individuals with known gallstones developing symptoms and 1% to 2% developing complications such as cholecystitis, pancreatitis, or cholangitis annually. Symptoms can be described as postprandial right upper quadrant (RUQ) pain (usually after a fatty meal). Half of the patients with symptoms will develop a second symptomatic episode within a year. These symptoms correspond to intermittent impaction of gallstones at the gallbladder neck as the gallbladder contracts to deliver bile into the common bile duct (CBD).

GALLSTONES AND GALLBLADDER CANCER

There are limited data to suggest that inflammation with large gallstones (>3 cm) increases the risk for gallbladder cancer. Therefore, there is no role for prophylactic cholecystectomy
3 for asymptomatic cholelithiasis to decrease cancer risk except for certain populations in which the incidence of gallbladder cancer is unusually high (Chileans, Pakistani women, Pima Indians). Calcification of gallbladder (porcelain gallbladder) is encountered in <1% of patients. It can be complete intramural calcification or selective/focal mucosal type. The rate of

Table 58.1. Criteria for Diagnosis of Acute Cholecystitis on Other Imaging Modalities[1–3]

Imaging Modality	Findings	Advantages	Disadvantage
Transabdominal US	▪ Gallbladder wall thickening >4 mm ▪ Enlarged gallbladder (long axis ≥8 cm, short axis ≥4 cm) ▪ Pericholecystic fluid ▪ Presence of gallstones/sludge ▪ Murphy sign	▪ Sensitivity and specificity 80–85% ▪ Quick, readily available ▪ Inexpensive ▪ No radiation exposure	▪ User dependent
Biliary scintigraphy (HIDA)	▪ Lack of visualization of gallbladder implies obstructed cystic duct ▪ Ejection fraction <35%—signifies biliary pathology	▪ Sensitivity 95–98% and specificity 90% ▪ Diagnostic yield is higher than US	▪ False positive after prolonged fasting or after a heavy meal ▪ Not readily available ▪ Radiation exposure
CT	▪ Gallbladder wall thickening ▪ Presence of gallstones ▪ Complications of cholecystitis—gangrenous cholecystitis, liver abscess/perforation		▪ Typically, less helpful for diagnosis of acute cholecystitis ▪ Radiation exposure
MRI/MRCP	▪ Gallbladder wall thickening ▪ Stones in the common bile duct	▪ Sensitivity 86% and specificity 82% ▪ As accurate as abdominal US	▪ Overestimate the presence of gallbladder inflammation ▪ Quality of images depends on patient's cooperation to hold their breath ▪ Radiation exposure

gallbladder malignancy was 6% versus 1% in a matched cohort of patients without gallbladder wall calcification.[4] Reports suggest an association between gallbladder calcification and gallbladder cancer more in focal calcification rather than complete calcification. Previously, laparoscopic cholecystectomy was recommended for all patients; now, factors like symptoms, calcification patterns, and age/comorbidities need to be considered prior to making that decision.[5]

CHOLECYSTITIS

Cholelithiasis begets cholecystitis, which can present as acute inflammation or ongoing, intermittent inflammation leading to chronic cholecystitis.

Acute Cholecystitis

Acute cholecystitis develops when bile flow is obstructed secondary to an impacted gallstone in the gallbladder neck (infundibulum) or in the cystic duct. This leads to biliary stasis, gallbladder wall edema, venous obstruction, and, in extreme cases, eventual arterial obstruction causing necrosis of the gallbladder wall. Acute inflammation may be complicated by secondary biliary infection with gram negative bacteria such as *Klebsiella* and *Escherichia coli*.

Clinical Manifestations

Clinical course can vary from mild epigastric/RUQ pain with fever/chills to frank sepsis secondary to perforation or development of emphysematous/gangrenous cholecystitis. Inflammation results in midepigastric or RUQ pain with localized peritoneal irritation. Murphy sign, defined by cessation of inspiration secondary to pain, due to the presence of an inflamed gallbladder during deep abdominal palpation at the midclavicular line of the RUQ, is pathognomonic for acute cholecystitis.

Imaging

According to the Tokyo guidelines and the World Society of Emergency Surgery, ultrasound (US) is recommended as the first-choice imaging method for the morphologic diagnosis of acute cholecystitis.[6,7] US findings of gallbladder wall thickening >4 mm, enlarged gallbladder, pericholecystic fluid, presence of gallstones, and/or positive sonographic Murphy sign are consistent with acute cholecystitis.

Criteria for diagnosis of acute cholecystitis on other imaging modalities are listed in **Table 58.1.**

Diagnosis

Criteria for diagnosis of acute cholecystitis are listed in **Table 58.2.** Compared with pathologic samples, the diagnostic accuracy of clinical criteria is between 94% and 60%. The World Society of Emergency Surgery guidelines for acute calculous cholecystitis recommend the combined use of clinical, laboratory, and imaging findings for diagnosis.[7]

Three grades of severity have been described with grade III (severe) acute cholecystitis causing systemic symptoms due to organ damage as listed in **Table 58.3.** These grades have been validated in multiple studies and are significantly associated with prognosis, length of hospital stay, conversion to open surgery, and medical costs.[8–10] However, these grades do not predict surgical complexity.

Treatment

Initial medical treatment involves parenteral hydration and antibiotics with coverage against enteric bacteria. Cholecystectomy is the standard surgical therapy for patients with acute cholecystitis.[11] Despite symptom resolution, the patient should undergo cholecystectomy as the definitive treatment, given that the likelihood of a second biliary-related complication is high.

Table 58.2. Tokyo Guidelines for Diagnosis of Acute Cholecystitis[6,12]

A. Local signs of inflammation (1) Murphy sign (2) RUQ mass/tenderness
B. Systemic signs of inflammation (1) Fever (2) elevated C-reactive protein (CRP) (3) elevated white blood cell (WBC) count
C. Imaging findings characteristic of acute cholecystitis
<u>Suspected diagnosis</u>: one item in A + one item in B
<u>Definite diagnosis</u>: one item in A + one item in B, and C

Table 58.3. Grades of Acute Cholecystitis (Tokyo Guidelines)

Grade I	Grade II	Grade III
No organ dysfunction and mild inflammatory gallbladder changes	Elevated WBC RUQ tenders/ palpable tender mass Duration of complaints >72 h Marked local inflammation (gangrenous cholecystitis, pericholecystic abscess, hepatic abscess, biliary peritonitis, emphysematous cholecystitis) Duration of complaints >72 h	Cardiovascular dysfunction requiring vasopressor support Neurologic dysfunction—decreased level of consciousness Respiratory dysfunction—PaO_2/FiO_2 ratio <300 Renal dysfunction—oliguria, Cr > 2 Hepatic dysfunction Hematologic dysfunction platelets <100,000/mm^3

Laparoscopic cholecystectomy has become standard of care. The timing of the cholecystectomy (early vs. delayed—after 6 weeks) has been much debated. Early cholecystectomy removes the pathologic source resolves the acute inflammatory response, potentially making the surgery safer with fewer complications and morbidity. No significant differences in patient outcomes between early and delayed surgeries with respect to bile duct injuries, bleeding, laparoscopic-to-open conversions, postoperative infection, and patient death have been reported.[8]
4 However, 23% of delayed patients presented with complications requiring emergent cholecystectomy. In addition, total length of stay in the hospital, including the index admission and subsequent admission either for biliary complications and/or later cholecystectomy, was significantly longer for these patients. A 2013 Cochrane Review included six randomized trials with 488 patients; this study compared early (within 7 days of presentation) to late (>6 weeks after initial treatment) cholecystectomy and reported similar results.[13] Multiple studies demonstrate that *early* should be within the index admission and the 72-hour limit is a relative rule given improved skills of surgeons with laparoscopic surgery. Tokyo guidelines recommend early (within 7 days, within 72 hours even better) laparoscopic cholecystectomy for grade I patients. In grade II (moderate) patients, consider urgent/early laparoscopic cholecystectomy if patient performance status is good. If the patient's condition is poor, urgent/early biliary drainage and delayed/elective cholecystectomy should be considered. In grade III (severe) patients with high surgical risk, urgent/early biliary drainage should be performed. In selected patients with no negative predictive factors (total bilirubin ≥2, neurologic dysfunction, respiratory dysfunction) or with cardiovascular or renal system failure that is rapidly reversible after admission early laparoscopic cholecystectomy can be considered.[14]

CHRONIC CHOLECYSTITIS

Cholelithiasis is the cause of chronic cholecystitis in most (>90%) of patients. It leads to episodes of cystic duct obstruction manifesting as recurrent biliary colic. These recurrent attacks lead to scarring and a nonfunctioning, noncontracting gallbladder. Chronic cholecystitis presents similarly to biliary colic. Diagnosis is accomplished with an US showing circumferential thickened gallbladder wall with gallstones in the setting of recurrent episodes of RUQ abdominal pain. In some patients the gallbladder may be shrunken and small. Chronic cholecystitis is treated with cholecystectomy. A subtype of chronic cholecystitis is xanthogranulomatous cholecystitis which can present as gallbladder mass. Inflammation of the gallbladder wall leads to permeation of bile within the wall. The bile is engulfed by macrophages and the resulting lipid-laden macrophages lead to a chronic granulomatous inflammatory response. Histology shows diffuse or focal mural changes with xanthoma cells (foamy histiocytes containing lipids and bile pigment), giant multinucleate histiocytes, and acute or chronic inflammatory cells. Micro abscesses may also form in the gallbladder wall and a fibrous reaction may lead to adhesions with the adjacent liver, duodenum, and transverse colon.[15] Studies have shown that contrast enhanced US may be a better modality for differentiating xanthogranulomatous cholecystitis from gallbladder cancer.[16]

ACUTE ACALCULOUS CHOLECYSTITIS

Acute acalculous cholecystitis is significantly higher in intensive care unit patients. It is associated with increased bile stasis and decreased gallbladder emptying and function, which leads to bile being inspissated, forming biliary sludge. The diagnosis requires a high index of clinical suspicion, given that most critically ill patients are sedated and mechanically ventilated, which makes reliable physical examination difficult. Late or missed diagnosis may lead to gallbladder ischemia, progression to gangrene, and eventual perforation, resulting in a mortality rate of up to 15% to 30%. Diagnosis may be made using bedside ultrasonography following similar criteria for acute calculous cholecystitis, minus the presence of calculi. The sensitivity of US in this setting ranges from 50% to 100% with a specificity of 90% to 94%. A hepatobiliary iminodiacetic acid (HIDA) scan with morphine amplification can be used to increase bile secretory pressure, which allows bile to reflux through a contracted gallbladder neck, thereby decreasing false-positive rates, providing sensitivity rates of 67% to 100% and specificity rates of 69% to 100%. A negative US in a patient with a high clinical suspicion for acute acalculous cholecystitis may benefit from an HIDA scan to improve diagnostic yield. Treatment includes a percutaneous cholecystostomy (PC) tube in critically ill and/or unstable patients and a cholecystectomy for a stable patient. PC tube may be the definitive treatment for acute acalculous cholecystitis, given that there is no mechanical obstruction secondary to cholelithiasis.

OTHER CONDITIONS

Gangrenous Cholecystitis

Gangrenous cholecystitis is most often found in diabetic patients. As the fundus is the furthest from blood supply, it is the most common site for necrosis. Usually, patients with gangrenous cholecystitis have full-thickness necrosis, however, this does not necessarily result in perforation. CT findings include irregular thickening of the gallbladder wall, poor enhancement of the wall (interrupted rim sign), increased density of fatty tissue around the gallbladder, gas in the gallbladder lumen or wall, membranous structures within the lumen (intraluminal flap or intraluminal membrane), and perigallbladder abscess.[17] Contrast-enhanced CT or MRI are recommended for diagnosing gangrenous cholecystitis, as these findings may be underappreciated on US.[18]

Emphysematous Cholecystitis

Emphysematous cholecystitis results from gas-forming bacteria in the bile. This can lead to perforation, intra-abdominal abscesses, generalized peritonitis, and necrotizing fasciitis of the abdominal wall. Given that intramural gas can be difficult to identify on US, CT is recommended for diagnosis and can assess presence of perforation and/or intra-abdominal abscess formation. Treatment includes antibiotic coverage for

Clostridium, and a cholecystostomy tube placement for unstable patients or a cholecystectomy for stable patients.[7]

Of note, the Tokyo guidelines classify both gangrenous and emphysematous cholecystitis as moderate severity.

Mirizzi Syndrome

Biliary obstruction secondary to cholecystitis is called Mirizzi syndrome. Type I involves compression of the CBD secondary to an impacted stone in the infundibulum or cystic duct. Type II involves a cholecystocholedochal fistula. Open cholecystectomy was the standard of care, but laparoscopic/robot-assisted approach is not prohibitive. Given the degree of inflammation, a subtotal cholecystectomy or a biliary reconstruction may also be required.

Cholecystoenteric Fistulae

Approximately 1% to 2% of all patients with cholecystitis develop choelecystoenteric fistula. During an episode of cholecystitis, the gallbladder will fistulize into a bowel loop (usually the duodenum or transverse colon). Gallstone Ileus is when a large gallstone may pass into the bowel and cause a mechanical bowel obstruction, usually distally in areas of narrow caliber, such as the ileocecal valve or sigmoid colon. The initial management involves removal of the gallstone through a proximal enterotomy with possible bowel resection. Decision to proceed with resection of the biliary enteric fistula and cholecystectomy at the time of index operation depends on patient's clinical condition and the degree of tissue inflammation. An association between gallbladder cancer and cholecystoenteric fistula has been suggested, and this situation requires a high clinical suspicion for malignancy.

CHOLECYSTECTOMY

Laparoscopic cholecystectomy was first performed in 1985. Minimally invasive technique (laparoscopic or robot assisted) is the gold standard operative technique, given significant increase in patient comfort, decreases in operative time, length of stay, and overall costs. Contraindications to laparoscopic cholecystectomy may include (i) patient inability to tolerate pneumoperitoneum, (ii) bleeding diatheses, (iii) decompensated cirrhosis with ascites and varices.

TECHNIQUE—LAPAROSCOPIC CHOLECYSTECTOMY

The abdomen is typically entered near the umbilicus with an open Hasson or a closed Veress needle technique. We prefer using an open Hasson and recommend a finger sweep before inserting the Hasson port. This helps to clear away any adhesed bowel. The abdomen is then insufflated with CO_2. If the patient has had a previous midline surgery, or there is suspicion of significant adhesions in the midline, consider entering the peritoneal cavity under direct vision using an Optiview technique in the right or left upper quadrant, and then place the other ports under direct vision.

The patient should be placed in reverse Trendelenburg with right side up.

Three additional operating ports are placed under direct visualization: one 5-mm port in the epigastric/subxiphoid area, one 5-mm port in the RUQ in the anterior axillary line, in a position to grasp the fundus of the gallbladder and retract it cephalad, and another 5-mm port in the right midclavicular line in a position to grasp the infundibulum. Care should be taken to place ports at least a hand's breadth away from each other to avoid instrument interference.

Typically, the fundus is retracted cephalad (10 o'clock position) by an assist; however, depending on the length of the gallbladder, you may need to apply this retraction below the fundus. The infundibulum is grasped with the operator's left hand and retracted toward the right lower quadrant to expose the triangle of Calot/hepatobiliary triangle

A few minutes should be spent orienting oneself to the patient's anatomy. Sometimes the inferior portion of the gallbladder is not visible secondary to adhesions. The dissection of the triangle should be performed above the Sulcus of Rouviere to avoid any injury. A pulsation may help guide visualization of the hepatic artery, especially left hepatic artery. Usually, a portion of the bile duct can also be seen. If the dissection will be below the umbilical fissure, this means that one is too far out to the left in the porta, and retraction must be adjusted.

Dividing the peritoneum on either side of the gallbladder with electrocautery aids in exposure of the triangle. We recommend doing this before dissecting deep into the triangle. Hook cautery is used for dissection in the triangle to gently separate the lymphatic and fatty tissue. The blunt tip of the laparoscopic suction device is also a useful tool, especially in an inflamed field, allowing for simultaneous dissection and suctioning of blood. The goal is to identify two distinct structures entering the underside of the gallbladder (the cystic artery and cystic duct), creating the Strasberg critical view of safety. This is done with a combination of hook cautery, suction catheter, and Maryland forceps. Sometimes the artery is very anterior to the triangle and may need to be clipped to complete the dissection before the cystic duct can be clipped and divided confidently (especially if the dissection is difficult secondary to inflammation). This should be done with extreme caution and only in select cases. We recommend placing two clips on the stay side of both the artery and the duct and one clip toward the gallbladder and then dividing between.

The peritoneum surrounding the gallbladder is then incised further using electrocautery, and the gallbladder is then taken off the cystic plate. If bleeding is encountered, electrocautery should be used to control it immediately before visibility is lost once the gallbladder has been taken off the cystic plate. Inadvertent excursion into the deep plane at this point can lead to bleeding from tributaries of the middle hepatic veins.[19]

Once the gallbladder is free, it is placed in an impermeable bag and removed through the umbilical port site, which may need to be enlarged in the setting of large calculi.

Refer to **Figure 58.1** for suggestions regarding port placement and **Table 58.4** for some tips, tricks, and common pitfalls

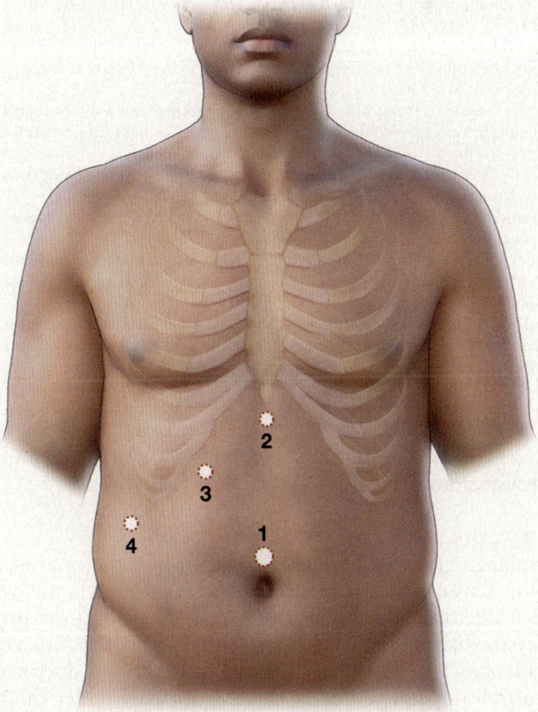

Figure 58.1. Suggestions for port placement for laparoscopic, robot-assisted cholecystectomy.

HEPATOBILIARY AND PORTAL VENOUS SYSTEM

Table 58.4. Laparoscopic Cholecystectomy: Key Technical Steps, Pearls, and Potential Pitfalls

Key Technical Steps: ■ Laparoscopic access, insufflation, patient positioning, port placement ■ Anatomy orientation—identify landmarks B-SAFE (Bile duct, the Sulcus of Rouviere, the left hepatic Artery pulsation, the umbilical Fissure, and the duodenum [enteric]) ■ Traction on the Hartmann pouch can create kinking of the bile duct and can produce an illusion of the porta hepatis being the hepatobiliary triangle ■ Establish critical view of safety to identify cystic duct and artery ■ Clip cystic artery and duct and divide them ■ Dissection of the gallbladder from the cystic plate
Pearls ■ Take time to orient yourself to the anatomy, the bottom of the gallbladder is a poor landmark ■ Incise the peritoneum posteriorly in the safe triangle (above the sulcus of R Rouviere) and carry the dissection upward to open the hepatobiliary triangle completely ■ Use intraoperative cholangiogram and/or laparoscopic ultrasound if any difficulty obtaining critical view of safety ■ If critical view of safety cannot be clearly defined, consider subtotal cholecystectomy
Pitfalls ■ Common bile duct, right, right anterior/posterior sectoral duct injury ■ Bleeding from accessory right hepatic artery ■ Bleeding from the cystic plate ■ Using hook cautery rather than blunt dissection with suction catheter for difficult gallbladder

Safe Cholecystectomy Guide:

From Brunt LM, Deziel DJ, Telem DA, et al. Safe Cholecystectomy Multi-society Practice Guideline and State of the Art Consensus Conference on prevention of bile duct injury during cholecystectomy. *Ann Surg*. 2020;272(1):3–23.

Greene B, Tsang M, Jayaraman S. The inferior boundary of dissection as a novel landmark for safe laparoscopic cholecystectomy. *HPB (Oxford)*. 2021;23(7):981–983.

Gupta V. How to achieve the critical view of safety for safe laparoscopic cholecystectomy: technical aspects. *Ann Hepatobiliary Pancreat Surg*. 2023;27(2):201–210.

Deng SX, Greene B, Tsang ME, Jayaraman S. Thinking your way through a difficult laparoscopic cholecystectomy: technique for high-quality subtotal cholecystectomy. *J Am Coll Surg*. 2022;235(6):e8–e16.

Hugh TB. New strategies to prevent laparoscopic bile duct injury–surgeons can learn from pilots. *Surgery*. 2002;132(5):826–835.

Sutherland F, Ball CG, Schendel J, Dixon E. Is an optical illusion the cause of classical bile duct injuries? *Can J Surg*. 2021;64(1):E1–E2.

Schendel J, Ball C, Dixon E, Sutherland F. Prevalence of anatomic landmarks for orientation during elective laparoscopic cholecystectomies. *Surg Endosc*. 2020;34(8):3508–3512

de'Angelis N, Catena F, Memeo R, et al. 2020 WSES guidelines for the detection and management of bile duct injury during cholecystectomy. *World J Emerg Surg*. 2021;16:30; www.tvasurg.ca/lapchole

with regard to the anatomy and technique of performing a cholecystectomy.

Intraoperative Cholangiogram

A cholangiogram is a useful adjunct when the anatomy is unclear. This can be performed laparoscopically via the cystic duct. A ductotomy is made on the anterior wall of the proximal cystic duct. The duct proximal to this is ligated with a clip. A cholangiocatheter is then threaded through this ductotomy, and a radio-opaque contrast agent is injected under fluoroscopy. The role of routine cholangiography in prevention of bile duct injury is controversial. An adequate cholangiogram includes identification of the cystic duct, visualization of both the right and left hepatic ducts, a smooth tapering of the CBD, and presence of contrast into the duodenal lumen.

Newer techniques of fluorescent-assisted biliary system identification using systemically injected near-infrared dyes, such as indocyanine green, may assist in identification of the critical structures without requiring intraoperative catheter placement. Fluorescent imaging requires a special camera system and allows for continuous intraoperative biliary mapping. Intraoperative US is another adjunct that can be utilized to define anatomy.

OTHER APPROACHES TO CHOLECYSTECTOMY

Single-Incision Laparoscopic Approach

The desire for minimally invasive surgery led to the development of the single-incision approach to laparoscopic cholecystectomy (SILS). This is generally performed by placing a multiport access device through the umbilical incision and inserting various instruments through the single port. The safety of SILS in elective cholecystectomies has been proven in various clinical trials, though there have been reports of increased operative time and hernia rates.

Robotic Cholecystectomy

Robotic cholecystectomy has been increasingly used as robot-assisted surgery in general gains popularity. Studies have shown that this is a safe approach with comparable outcomes between robotic and laparoscopic approaches. However, the cost to the healthcare system continues to be under investigation

Open Cholecystectomy

Open cholecystectomy is now a rare operation used when there is another concurrent procedure or when a laparoscopic cholecystectomy is converted to an open procedure. Conversion may be due to an inability to identify anatomy or an inadvertent injury. In the setting of acute cholecystitis, converting to an open cholecystectomy is not protective of bile duct injury. Open cholecystectomy can be performed through either an upper midline or right subcostal (Kocher) incision. Typically, dissection is performed in a top-down fashion, from the fundus toward Calot triangle with identification of the cystic artery and duct at the gallbladder neck. Dissection can still be started in the triangle as described above to obtain the critical view. Duct and artery can be divided between clips or sutures. The gallbladder is then removed from the cystic plate using electrocautery either in a top-down approach or from the infundibulum upward.

SUBTOTAL CHOLECYSTECTOMY

Subtotal cholecystectomy (either minimally invasive or open) is used to avoid biliary tract injury in cases where anatomy is unclear or when there is an impaction of a large stone at the cystic duct. The gallbladder is opened above the neck, and all stones are removed, leaving the neck of the gallbladder in situ to protect the critical structures. The posterior wall of the gallbladder may be left attached to the liver bed as well. The neck of the gallbladder may be closed with suture or stapler (reconstituting technique) or left open (fenestrating technique). Omentum can be placed within the neck of the gallbladder as well. While the reconstitution can lead to stone reformation and recurrent symptoms, fenestration has a higher likelihood of bile leak or biliary fistula. A similar proportion of patients have been shown to require reintervention after reconstituting versus fenestrating subtotal cholecystectomy (26% vs 32%). More completion cholecystectomies were required after a fenestrating procedure (9% vs 4%). A closed suction drain is placed in the gallbladder fossa after a subtotal cholecystectomy to evacuate any bile leak, which generally resolves spontaneously.

Table 58.5. Indications for Prophylactic Cholecystectomy

Pediatric gallstones associated with sickle cell disease
Congenital hemolytic anemia
Gallbladder polyp >10 mm
Calcifications
Acalculous cholecystitis/biliary dyskinesia
Concern for gallbladder malignancy
Cholelithiasis and no/ infrequent access to medical care

Percutaneous Drains After Cholecystectomy

There is no current evidence in support of leaving drains after an uncomplicated cholecystectomy (minimally invasive or open). Drain placement should be generally deferred, but can be considered in cases with gallbladder necrosis or those at higher risk for postoperative bile leak (subtotal cholecystectomy). In these situations, drains are not preventative but may assist in the early diagnosis of bile leaks.[20,21]

COMPLICATIONS OF CHOLECYSTECTOMY

The associated mortality rate of cholecystectomy is <0.3%. The most feared complication is a biliary duct injury with the incidence following laparoscopic cholecystectomy being between 0.3% and 0.6% (vs 0.2% and 0.3% for open surgery). A leak from the cystic artery stump is rare and occurs when the clips are dislodged. Due to their close anatomic relationship, major vascular injuries, especially to the right hepatic artery, may occur in association with bile duct injuries. During laparoscopy, spillage of stones into the peritoneal cavity occurs in 5% to 40% of cases. Intra-abdominal abscesses, subcutaneous abscesses, and fistulation of stones through the abdominal wall have all been described; therefore, every attempt should be made to remove spilled stones and suction bile spills.

Asymptomatic cholelithiasis can be managed expectantly without surgical intervention. Prophylactic cholecystectomy is indicated in certain circumstances (**Table 58.5**). Patients who have a higher risk of malignancy in the setting of gallbladder disease, presence of large gallstones (>2.5 cm), or calcification of gallbladder wall (porcelain gallbladder) are commonly offered prophylactic cholecystectomy. Patients who are more likely to have recurrent symptoms or complications secondary to gallstones may also undergo prophylactic cholecystectomy. For example, those with hereditary spherocytosis, sickle cell disease, and other hemoglobinopathies.

PERCUTANEOUS CHOLECYSTOSTOMY

PC tubes can be used as a bridge to cholecystectomy or as a definitive management of acute cholecystitis in critically ill patients or those who are poor surgical candidates.[22] There is no data to suggest a difference in outcomes for placement of transhepatic versus transperitoneal tubes.[23] The technical success for radiologically guided tubes is 98% to 100%. Potential complications include: pericholecystic abscess, intrahepatic hematoma, biliary peritonitis, and biliary pleural effusion. After clinical improvement, a cholangiogram is performed to rule out obstruction at the level of the cystic duct. If there is evidence of obstruction, the tube can be clamped for 10 to 14 days to ensure that the patient will tolerate removal. If clamping is tolerated, the tube is removed. If clamping is not tolerated, a cholecystectomy should be considered, or the tube may need to be left for a longer duration.[24] Patients with a persistent obstruction who are poor surgical candidates may need tube upsizing and/or percutaneous/endoscopic removal of stones.

It is recommended to delay laparoscopic cholecystectomy by at least 8 weeks after placement of PC tube. Early cholecystectomy (less than 8 weeks) has been associated with a higher risk of complications and longer hospital length of stay.[25,26] This may be due to maximal medical optimization preoperatively.[27] When doing a laparoscopic cholecystectomy in a patient with a PC tube, it is recommended to remove the cholecystostomy tube at the outset of the operation so that the fundus can be easily retracted. The suction catheter can be used to drain the bile from the gallbladder to prevent leakage of bile, stones, and sludge. Alternatively, a clip can be placed at the site where the tube was entering the gallbladder, or a grasper can be used to both cover the hole and retract the fundus cephalad. The rate of CBD injury during a laparoscopic cholecystectomy after PC tube may be higher than in the general population.[24] However, there is no difference in risk of CBD injury in the early cholecystectomy versus late group after placement of PC tube.

Other Therapies

Ursodeoxycholic acid (ursodiol) is thought to decrease the frequency of biliary colic attacks by dissolving cholesterol crystals, decreasing hepatic secretion of biliary cholesterol, thereby decreasing stone formation. Unfortunately, most stones recur (>50% at 5 years), and in a prospective randomized study of ursodiol therapy, it did not decrease the number of attacks nor gallstone-related complications during the waiting period for cholecystectomy. Extracorporeal shock wave lithotripsy (ESWL) uses high energy waves to disintegrate stones by non invasive technique. ESWL can dissolve small stones by converting them into sand like structure or decrease the size of larger calculi in the CBD or distal cystic duct and make them potentially extractable by percutaneous or endoscopic techniques. It is a safe procedure with rare complications, including hematomas (biliary or otherwise), bowel perforation, and necrotizing pancreatitis.

SPECIAL CONSIDERATIONS

Gallstone Pancreatitis

Gallstone pancreatitis is the most common form of acute pancreatitis and is due to obstruction of the ampulla by a stone, causing reflux of bile into the pancreatic duct. In most cases, the obstruction is transient. Patients should undergo cholecystectomy following clinical resolution of pancreatitis. No data support any differences between early endoscopic retrograde cholangiopancreatography (ERCP) and conservative management of pancreatitis regardless of severity. However, in patients with continuous biliary obstruction or concurrent cholangitis, early ERCP reduced mortality and systemic complications.[28]

Gallbladder Cancer

An incidental gallbladder cancer is found in 0.2% to 2% of all laparoscopic cholecystectomies. If cancer is suspected preoperatively, a staging workup with CT of chest, abdomen/pelvis, or CT chest and MR abdomen/pelvis should be completed before cholecystectomy, and the patient should be referred to a hepatobiliary surgery specialist. Bile spillage should be avoided during surgery, as this is associated with worse outcomes if cancer is found on final pathology.[29,30] If the preoperative malignancy suspicion is very high, then an en bloc hepatic resection (parts of segment 4b and 5) is recommended. This can be done with laparoscopic or robotic energy (Harmonic, Ligasure, vessel sealer) devices. The gallbladder is taken en bloc with the attached cystic plate, to ensure a negative margin. A portal lymphadenectomy is also done at the same time for appropriate staging. The gallbladder with en bloc liver should be extracted in an impermeable bag to reduce the risk of seeding the peritoneum and/or port sites. If a gallbladder cancer is incidentally discovered on pathology, the patient should be referred to hepatobiliary surgery for further hepatic resection, portal lymphadenectomy, and possible bile duct resection (if the cystic duct margin is positive). The optimal time interval for re-resection for incidentally discovered gallbladder cancer is between 4 and 8 weeks after the initial cholecystectomy.

Cholecystitis During Pregnancy

It is now recognized that complications to both mother and fetus may be increased if cholecystectomy is postponed to the postpartum period. Nonoperative management may be pursued for biliary colic. Cholecystectomy is recommended for acute cholecystitis regardless of trimester of pregnancy.[31,32] If the fetus is viable, then obstetrical consultation is indicated with intraoperative fetal monitoring. The periumbilical port site may need to be adjusted based on the gestational age. It is recommended to position the mother in the partial left lateral decubitus position to minimize pressure from the gravid uterus on the inferior vena cava.

Cholecystitis and Cirrhosis

Cholecystitis in the presence of liver cirrhosis should generally be treated with PC tube placement. Selected patients (typically Child's A/B) may undergo cholecystectomy if they do not have varices. Laparoscopic approach is associated with shorter operative time, reduced length of stay, and reduced complication rates compared to open approach.[33–35] Higher Model for End Stage Liver Disease (MELD) score, increased operative time, intraoperative blood loss, lower platelet count, and high INR all lead to higher morbidity in patients with cirrhosis.[36,37] Therefore, patient selection is of utmost importance. Elective surgery in patients with varices and ascites should be avoided. They should be treated with PC tubes if they develop acute cholecystitis. If varices are found on the gallbladder wall intraoperatively, subtotal cholecystectomy and stone retrieval are recommended to avoid bleeding.

CHOLEDOCHOLITHIASIS

Choledocholithiasis is defined as the presence of stones in the extrahepatic biliary tree. CBD stones are classified as primary or secondary stones based on where they originate. Primary CBD stones form within the bile duct in conditions with bile stasis: (i) benign biliary strictures, (ii) bile duct cysts (choledochal cysts), or (iii) sphincter of Oddi dysfunction. They can
5 also occur in patients with congenitally absent gallbladders or those whose CBD was clear at the time of previous cholecystectomy. They are predominantly brown-pigment stones. Secondary stones are more common and form in the gallbladder and migrate into the bile duct. Most of these stones are cholesterol stones. Of patients with symptomatic gallstones, 10% to 15% will have choledocholithiasis and most patients with secondary CBD stones will have cholelithiasis.[38]

Clinical Presentation

Clinical presentation of choledocholithiasis can vary from an asymptomatic course to biliary colic (the most common presentation), jaundice, cholangitis, and pancreatitis. CBD stones can pass into the duodenum without clinical consequence. The incidence and frequency with which this occurs are unknown. In patients who are nonjaundiced with nondilated bile ducts on US, the incidence of CBD stones at the time of cholecystectomy is approximately 5%. One-third of these patients pass the stone spontaneously. Intermittent obstruction of CBD and passage of stones can cause varying fluctuations in bilirubin and liver enzymes. Persistent CBD obstruction can lead to cholangitis and present as Charcot triad—fever/rigors, jaundice, RUQ pain, or Reynaud pentad—hypotension and mental status changes in addition to Charcot triad. Pancreatitis is the second most common presentation of choledocholithiasis, with 50% of patients with pancreatitis having CBD stones, depending on the timing of the cholangiography.

Diagnosis

Without clinical signs (cholangitis or pancreatitis), the diagnosis is made radiologically and biochemically. Although liver biochemical tests have a strong negative predictive value (97%), they only have a positive predictive value of 15% to 50% when they are abnormal in patients with suspected CBD stones. (ϒ-glutamyltransferase has been suggested to be the most sensitive and specific of the liver enzymes.)[37] Transabdominal US alone has a poor sensitivity of 22% to 60% in detecting choledocholithiasis and is highly operator dependent. Presence of gallstones or CBD diameter greater than 6 mm can be predictive of choledocholithiasis. Computed tomography (CT) scans also have a low sensitivity. Magnetic resonance cholangiopancreatography (MRCP) is the gold standard noninvasive imaging modality to detect duct stones with a sensitivity of 81% to 100% and specificity of 92% to 100%. Small stones less than 5 mm can still be missed with MRCP, though its accuracy is comparable to ERCP and an intraoperative cholangiogram (IOC). Laparoscopic intraoperative US using a high-frequency probe allows for evaluation of the CBD with a sensitivity of detecting CBD stones of 71% to 100%. In addition, laparoscopic US, like EUS, allows for the adequate evaluation of the distal bile duct for stones. Certain treatment algorithms recommend an endoscopic ultrasound (EUS) as the first approach prior to ERCP in patients at intermediate risk of choledocholithiasis, or in patients with severe gallstone pancreatitis. If no stones are seen on EUS, an ERCP can be avoided. Given the invasive nature of ERCP and the risks of bleeding, perforation, ascending cholangitis, and postprocedure pancreatitis, it is now reserved as a therapeutic measure rather than a diagnostic test. When routine IOC was being performed at the time of open cholecystectomy, choledocholithiasis was discovered in 10% to 15% of patients, and those that were clinically significant were even less. Use of IOC at the time of laparoscopic cholecystectomy has yielded similar results. It has been shown that only 2.2% of patients with positive IOC required ERCP 6 weeks postcholecystectomy for symptomatic choledocholithiasis.[39]

The American Society for Gastrointestinal Endoscopy has proposed a risk stratification scheme to detect duct stones based on common predictive factors (**Table 58.6**).[40] This has

Table 58.6. The American Society for Gastrointestinal Endoscopy Predictors of Choledocholithiasis[40]

Predictors of Choledocholithiasis	
Very strong	
CBD stone on transabdominal US	
Ascending cholangitis	
Bilirubin >4 mg/dL	
Strong	
Dilated CBD (>6 mm) on US	
Bilirubin elevated (1.8–4 mg/dL)	
Moderate	
Abnormal liver biochemical test (other than bilirubin)	
Age >55	
Clinical gallstone pancreatitis	
Likelihood	
Presence of any very strong predictor	High
Presence of both strong predictors	High
No predictors	Low
All other patients	Intermediate

Table 58.7. ERCP Prior to Cholecystectomy Versus CBD Exploration for Choledocholithiasis

ERCP prior to cholecystectomy for suspected choledocholithiasis	▪ High-risk group, especially those needing decompression for cholangitis ▪ Severe gallstone pancreatitis and persistent choledocholithiasis
Common bile duct exploration at the time of cholecystectomy	▪ Large, impacted stones ▪ Multiple failed endoscopic attempts ▪ Anatomy precluding endoscopy such as previous gastric bypass ▪ Intermediate preoperative risk for choledocholithiasis with IOC confirming choledocholithiasis

ERCP, endoscopic retrograde cholangiopancreatography; CBD, common bile duct; IOC, intraoperative cholangiogram.

been validated in a large cohort of multi-institutional patient cohort.

Management

Management of choledocholithiasis includes endoscopic, surgical (open and/or laparoscopic), and percutaneous approaches. The sequence of events for management varies depending on local expertise (surgery, gastroenterology, and radiology).[41] For acutely ill patients with cholangitis or severe gallstone pancreatitis and persistent choledocholithiasis, ERCP prior to cholecystectomy is recommended.

Table 58.7 provides the timing and sequence of interventions based on clinical scenario.

There is evidence to support a single-stage laparoscopic cholecystectomy with IOC and CBD exploration versus preoperative ERCP followed by laparoscopic cholecystectomy. Prospective randomized trials have shown equivalent duct
6 clearance rates, morbidity, but shorter length of stay with
7 single-stage procedure.[42] This is dependent on the surgeon's comfort level with CBD exploration. Management of patients with high and low risk of choledocholithiasis is generally agreed upon. It is the management of patients with intermediate risk that poses a challenge. A randomized clinical trial has shown shorter length of stay and decrease in morbidity with upfront single-stage cholecystectomy and IOC compared to preoperative ERCP and subsequent ERCP.[43]

Endoscopic Approach

After biliary cannulation, a cholangiogram is performed to define anatomy and confirm choledocholithiasis. Endoscopic sphincterotomy is performed. Balloon baskets and Fogarty balloon catheters are employed for stone extraction. Large stones may also mandate dilatation of the papilla using endoscopic balloon dilators, mechanical lithotripsy, or intracorporeal lithotripsy with laser or electrohydraulic probes to reduce stone size. ERCP is successful in about 90% of cases, with failure rates increasing with stone size >15 mm. Complications of ERCP include: cholangitis, sphincterotomy bleeding, acute pancreatitis, and perforation (duodenal and biliary).

Percutaneous Approach

There are two common approaches. A rendezvous procedure involves passage of a guidewire percutaneously through the bile ducts and into the duodenum. This guidewire is then used by endoscopists for an ERCP. This is useful in patients with altered anatomy (Bilroth II) or large duodenal diverticulum precluding ERCP. In a complete percutaneous approach, a transhepatic fistula is created, allowed to mature for 7 to 8 days, then used for stone retrieval.

Table 58.8. Different Techniques for Common Bile Duct Exploration[44–47]

	Transcystic	Transcholedochal
Success	80–90%	83–96%
Morbidity	Bile leak 1% Acute pancreatitis 0.5% Cystic duct rupture 6.8%	Bile leak 14% Pancreatitis 7.3% Reoperation 7.3% Mortality 1%

SURGICAL TECHNIQUES FOR CHOLEDOCHOLITHIASIS

Laparoscopic Surgical Approach

Laparoscopic Common CBD Exploration (LCBDE)

Concomitant LCBDE at the time of laparoscopic cholecystectomy is ideal for patients with CBD stones incidentally identified at the time of IOC. LCBDE can be performed via a transcystic (small stones less than 1 cm) or transcholedochal technique (**Table 58.8**). Usually, the same port sites as a laparoscopic cholecystectomy can be used, with potentially an additional 5-mm port along the left midclavicular line. The gallbladder is left in situ for retraction. A cystic ductotomy is made, and a guidewire is advanced. To relax the Sphincter of Oddi, 1 mg of glucagon is administered intravenously, and after 3 minutes, a cholangiocatheter is advanced from the ductotomy into the CBD and then saline irrigated to flush small stones and debris out of the bile duct under fluoroscopic guidance. A choledochoscope can be used for direct visualization, with stone extraction accomplished with the use of a basket. The ampulla may need dilatation, which can be performed with a long ureteral balloon over a guide wire. This technique can also be used for cystic duct dilatation if needed. Upon completion, the cystic duct can be ligated using an Endoloop, clips, or suture.

The transcholedochal technique is performed for larger stones when the CBD is >1 cm in diameter. An anterior longitudinal choledochotomy below the cystic duct is made between two stay sutures on the CBD using fine absorbable sutures. The same techniques as mentioned above are used for stone retrieval. If all the stones are removed and CBD is clear, the choledochotomy is primarily closed. However, if there is concern for recurrent/retained stones, the choledochotomy should be closed over a T-tube (see below).

Laparoscopic Biliary Enteric Bypass

If there is a distal biliary stricture (malignancy excluded) or a risk of recurrent stones, a choledochoduodenotomy or a Roux-en-Y hepaticojejunostomy should be considered. In the past, there were concerns for sump syndrome with choledochoduodenotomy, which implied food debris blocking the bile flow. This is now thought to be a technical error secondary to a narrow anastomosis. This anastomosis allows for easy endoscopic access to the biliary tree if needed. In cases where duodenum cannot be mobilized secondary to inflammation, a Roux-en-Y hepaticojejunostomy should be performed. Future direct endoscopic access to the biliary tree is not achievable with this anastomosis.

Laparoscopic-Assisted Endoscopic Retrograde Cholangiopancreatography

Accessing the ampulla in patients who have had previous Roux-en-Y gastric bypass can be difficult even with balloon endoscopy. Laparoscopic access to the gastric remnant is an alternative. The stomach is brought up to the abdominal wall; a gastrostomy is made; and a radially dilating trocar is placed through the gastrostomy. An endoscope is then passed down through this trocar to perform ERCP.[48] On completion of

ERCP, the gastrostomy can be closed with sutures or an endoscopic stapler.

Open Surgical Approach

Open Common Bile Duct Exploration

In the current era, open CBD exploration is infrequently performed. It is commonly reserved for the presence of large, impacted stones causing Mirizzi syndrome, and patients in whom anatomy precludes endoscopic treatment (such as prior gastric resection/bypass, duodenal diverticula, or presence of biliary enteric fistula.

A wide Kocher maneuver is performed to allow for exposure of the entire bile duct. A supraduodenal longitudinal choledochotomy is made as distally along the duct as possible between two fine, absorbable stay sutures. This allows for: creation of an anastomosis if needed, leaves a maximal amount of CBD for additional future procedures, and allows the use of a rigid choledoscope since it measures about 7 cm. Fogarty cannulation is performed, passing the catheter into the duodenum. The balloon is then carefully inflated while the catheter is being retracted against the papilla to clear the stones from the duct. Care is taken to avoid passage of stones into the proximal duct. This can be done for stones in the proximal duct as well. Inflation of the balloon needs to be precise—underinflation can miss stones, and overinflation can lead to duct damage. After a choledochotomy is made, a choledoscope (rigid or flexible) can also be used to remove stones. Use of rigid instruments, including grasping forceps, should be avoided as they can damage the bile duct and lead to strictures. The duct should be flushed with saline; this allows for clearance of small stones and sludge.

Use of T-tubes has fallen out of favor due to concerns with bile leak and persistent biliary fistulas, with a Cochrane Review in 2013 calling for more randomized trials to be conducted with low risk of bias and assessing the risk–benefit effect of these tubes.[49] Therefore, the choledochotomy can be closed with interrupted fine absorbable sutures, but if needed (high-risk patients), a 12-French T-tube can be left in place and secured with interrupted fine absorbable sutures, taking care not to catch the tube with the sutures.

To prepare a T-tube for insertion, cut the two limbs and remove half the diameter of the part that will be in the CBD. This will prevent bile duct obstruction and allow easy removal. Once the T-tube is placed, completion cholangiography is performed to assess for CBD patency. The T-tube is left for straight drainage until postoperative day 5 to 7, when a T-tube cholangiogram is performed. If no obstruction is present, the tube can be clamped and pulled after 4 to 6 weeks after tract maturation. T-tubes do not prevent bile leakage and should be used with a closed suction drain in proximity. If retained stones are identified, the biliary tree can be accessed percutaneously via the T-tube once the tract has matured, and the stones can be removed.

Transduodenal Sphincteroplasty

Patients with impacted stones at the ampulla or with primary bile duct stones, recurrent stones, intrahepatic stones, or a benign distal bile duct stricture may require an open biliary drainage procedure, such as a transduodenal sphincteroplasty. This involves a Kocher maneuver followed by a lateral duodenotomy. A transcystic Fogarty can be helpful in identify the papilla if not readily visible. The Fogarty can be passed through the papilla to be used as a guide for the sphincteroplasty. The sphincteroplasty is then performed for 4 to 5 mm at the 11 o'clock position superiorly to avoid the duct of Wirsung which is present medially; this is done with sharp electrocautery. Sphincteroplasty in then extended to allow instrumental exploration of the CBD with forceps for stone extraction. Sutures are placed on the outer wall between the duodenal mucosa and the CBD wall, taking care to avoid the duct of Wirsung. Stones can also be removed using Fogarty, saline irrigation, and a choledoscope. Closure is with choledochoduodenostomy or Roux-en-Y Hepaticojejunostomy with the consideration for one versus the other being the same as described above in the laparoscopic biliary enteric bypass section.

Table 58.9. Classification of Intrahepatic Stones

Japanese Classification	Takada Classification
Type I: Intrahepatic stones alone	Type I: No stricture, mild biliary dilatation
Type IE: Intra- and extrahepatic ductal stones	Type II: Distal CBD/ ampullary stricture
Type L: Left-sided intrahepatic ductal stones	Type III: Hilar stricture
Type R: Right-sided intrahepatic ductal stones	Type IV: Unilateral hepatic duct stricture
Type C: Caudate stones	Type V: Multiple bilateral strictures

INTRAHEPATIC STONES

Hepatolithiasis or intrahepatic stones are defined as stones present above the confluence of the left and right hepatic ducts. These can occur secondary to chronic biliary stasis and in the presence of choledochal cysts, biliary strictures, and/or biliary parasites. Most of these patients (70%) do not have gallstones. The two most common classifications, listed in **Table 58.9**, are based on distribution of stones and presence of biliary stricture.

Most patients with hepatolithiasis present with cholangitis. Diagnosis is made with US, CT, or MRCP. Endoscopic and percutaneous cholangiography are invasive and therefore, used less readily. Initial management for symptomatic patients includes resuscitation and treatment for cholangitis. Biliary drainage can be performed via percutaneous or endoscopic technique, depending on the location of stricture and distribution of stones. Definitive treatment may require hepatectomy, especially if there is concern for cholangiocarcinoma, which has been reported to be 5% to 10%. Depending on the location of strictures, hepatectomy and hepaticojejunostomy with anchoring jejunal limb to the abdominal wall may also be performed. This allows for percutaneous access in the future if stone retrieval is needed. Recurrence rates are high (0% to 50.8%) even when intrahepatic stones are completely removed and depend on presence of bile duct strictures and treatment modality.

References

1. Kiewiet JJ, Leeuwenburgh MM, Bipat S, et al. A systematic review and meta-analysis of diagnostic performance of imaging in acute cholecystitis. *Radiology.* 2012;264:708–720.
2. Kaoutzanis C, Davies E, Leichtle SW, et al. Abdominal ultrasound versus hepato-iminodiacetic acid scan in diagnosing acute cholecystitis—what is the real benefit? *J Surg Res.* 2014;1:44–52.
3. Rodriguez LE, Santaliz-Ruiz LE, De La Torre-Bisot G, et al. Clinical implications of hepatobiliary scintigraphy and ultrasound in the diagnosis of acute cholecystitis. *Int J Surg.* 2016;35:196–200.
4. Schnelldorfer T. Porcelain gallbladder: a benign process or concern for malignancy? *J Gastrointest Surg.* 2013;17:1161–1168.
5. Morimoto M, Matsuo T, Mori N. Management of porcelain gallbladder, its risk factors, and complications: a review. *Diagnostics (Basel).* 2021;11(6):1073.
6. Yokoe M, Hata J, Takada T, et al. Tokyo Guidelines 2018 diagnostic criteria and severity grading of acute cholecystitis (with videos). *J Hepatobiliary Pancreat Sci.* 2018;25(1):41–54.
7. Pisano M, Allievi N, Gurusamy K, et al. 2020 World Society of Emergency Surgery updated guidelines for the diagnosis and treatment of acute calculus cholecystitis. *World J Emerg Surg.* 2020;15:61.
8. Paul Wright G, Stilwell K, Johnson J, et al. Predicting length of stay and conversion to open cholecystectomy for acute cholecystitis

using the 2013 Tokyo Guidelines in a US population. *J Hepatobiliary Pancreat Sci.* 2015;22:795–801.
9. Hayasaki A, Takahashi K, Fujii T, et al. Factor analysis influencing postoperative hospital stay and medical costs for patients with definite, suspected or unmatched diagnosis of acute cholecystitis according to the Tokyo guidelines 2013. *Gastroenterol Res Pract.* 2016;2016:7675953.
10. González-Muñoz JI, Franch-Arcas G, Angoso-Clavijo M, et al. Risk-adjusted treatment selection and outcome of patients with acute cholecystitis. *Langenbecks Arch Surg.* 2017;402(4):607–614.
11. Gutt CN, Encke J, Köninger J, et al. Acute cholecystitis: early versus delayed cholecystectomy, a multicenter randomized trial (ACDC Study, NCT00447304). *Ann Surg.* 2013;258:385–391.
12. Naidu K, Beenen E, Gananadha S, et al. The yield of fever, inflammatory markers and ultrasound in the diagnosis of acute cholecystitis: a validation of the 2013 Tokyo Guidelines. *World J Surg.* 2016;40:2892–2897.
13. Gurusamy KS, Davidson C, Gluud C, et al. Early versus delayed laparoscopic cholecystectomy for people with acute cholecystitis. *Cochrane Database Syst Rev.* 2013;6:CD005440.
14. Mayumi T, Okamoto K, Takada T, et al. Tokyo Guidelines 2018: management bundles for acute cholangitis and cholecystitis. *J Hepatobiliary Pancreat Sci.* 2018;25(1):96–100.
15. Singh VP, Rajesh S, Bihari C, et al. Xanthogranulomatous cholecystitis: what every radiologist should know. *World J Radiol.* 2016;8(2):183–191.
16. Bo X, Chen E, Wang J, et al. Diagnostic accuracy of imaging modalities in differentiating xanthogranulomatous cholecystitis from gallbladder cancer. *Ann Transl Med.* 2019;7(22):627.
17. Patel NB, Oto A, Thomas S. Multidetector CT of emergent biliary pathologic conditions. *Radiographics.* 2013;33:1867–1888.
18. Yeh DD, Cropano C, Fagenholz P, et al. Gangrenous cholecystitis: deceiving ultra-sounds, significant delay in surgical consult, and increased postoperative morbidity. *J Trauma Acute Care Surg.* 2015;79:812–816.
19. Ball CG, MacLean AR, Kirkpatrick AW, et al. Hepatic vein injury during laparoscopic cholecystectomy: the unappreciated proximity of the middle hepatic vein to the gallbladder bed. *J Gastrointest Surg.* 2006;10(8):1151–1155.
20. Gurusamy KS, Samraj K, Mullerat P, et al. Routine abdominal drainage for uncomplicated laparoscopic cholecystectomy. *Cochrane Database Syst Rev.* 2007;(4):CD006004.
21. Prevot F, Fuks D, Cosse C, et al. The value of abdominal drainage after laparoscopic cholecystectomy for mild or moderate acute calculous cholecystitis: a post hoc analysis of a randomized clinical trial. *World J Surg.* 2016;40:2726–2734.
22. Loozen CS, Van Santvoort HC, Van Duijvendijk P, et al. Laparoscopic cholecystectomy versus percutaneous catheter drainage for acute cholecystitis in high risk patients (CHOCOLATE): multicentre randomised clinical trial. *BMJ.* 2018;363:k3965.
23. Beland MD, Lakir P, Ahn SH, et al. Image-guided cholecystostomy tube placement: short- and long-term outcomes of transhepatic versus transperitoneal placement. *AJR Am J Roentgenol.* 2019;212(1):201–204.
24. Park JK, Yang JI, Wi JW, et al. Long term outcome and recurrence factors after percutaneous cholecystostomy as a definitive treatment for acute cholecystitis. *J Gastroenterol Hepatol.* 2019;34(4):784–790.
25. Altieri MS, Bevilacqua L, Yang J, et al. Cholecystectomy following percutaneous cholecystostomy tube placement leads to higher rate of CBD injuries. *Surg Endosc.* 2019;33:2686–2690.
26. Altieri MS, Yang J, Yin D, et al. Early cholecystectomy (≤8 weeks) following percutaneous cholecystostomy tube placement is associated with higher morbidity. *Surg Endosc.* 2020;34(7):3057–3063.
27. Khasawneh MA, Shamp A, Heller S, et al. Successful laparoscopic cholecystectomy after percutaneous cholecystostomy tube placement. *J Trauma Acute Care Surg.* 2015;78(1):100–104.
28. Tse F, Yuan Y. Early routine endoscopic retrograde cholangiopancreatography strategy versus early conservative management strategy in acute gallstone pancreatitis. *Cochrane Database Syst Rev.* 2012;(5):CD009779.
29. Blakely AM, Wong P, Chu P, et al. Intraoperative bile spillage is associated with worse survival in gallbladder adenocarcinoma. *J Surg Oncol.* 2019;120(4):603–610.
30. Horkoff MJ, Ahmed Z, Xu Y, et al. Adverse outcomes after bile spillage in incidental gallbladder cancers: a population-based Study. *Ann Surg.* 2021;273(1):139–144.
31. Pearl JP, Price RP, Tonkin AE, et al. Guidelines for the use of laparoscopy during pregnancy. *SAGES Guidelines Committee.* 2011;1–33
32. American College of Obstetricians and Gynecologists' Committee on Obstetric Practice and the American Society of Anesthesiologists. *Non Obstetric Surgery During Pregnancy.* 2019; Committee Opinion Number 775.
33. Laurence JM, Tran PD, Richardson AJ, et al. Laparoscopic or open cholecystectomy in cirrhosis: a systematic review of outcomes and meta-analysis of randomized trials. *HPB (Oxford).* 2012;14(3):153–161.
34. Gad EH, Kamel Y, Alsebaey A, et al. Laparoscopic cholecystectomy in patients with liver cirrhosis: 8 years experience in a tertiary center. A retrospective cohort study. *Ann Med Surg (Lond).* 2020;51:1–10.
35. Strömberg J, Hammarqvist F, Sadr-Azodi O, et al. Cholecystectomy in patients with liver cirrhosis. *Gastroenterol Res Pract.* 2015;2015:783823.
36. Mancero JMP, D'Albuquerque LAC, Gonzalez AM, Larrea FIS, De Oliveira E Silva A. Laparoscopic cholecystectomy in cirrhotic patients with symptomatic cholelithiasis: a case-control study. *World J Surg.* 2008;32(2):267–270.
37. Perkins L, Jeffries M, Patel T. Utility of preoperative scores for predicting morbidity after cholecystectomy in patients with cirrhosis. *Clin Gastroenterol Hepatol.* 2004;2(12):1123–1128.
38. Peng WK, Sheikh Z, Paterson-Brown S, et al. Role of liver function tests in predicting common bile duct stones in acute calculous cholecystitis. *Br J Surg.* 2005;92(10):1241–1247.
39. Collins C, Maguire D, Ireland A, et al. A prospective study of common bile duct calculi in patients undergoing laparoscopic cholecystectomy: natural history of choledocholithiasis revisited. *Ann Surg.* 2004;239(1):28–33.
40. Maple JT, Ben-Menachem T, Anderson MA, et al. The role of endoscopy in the evaluation of suspected choledocholithiasis. *Gastrointest Endosc.* 2010;71(1):1–9.
41. Dasari BVM, Tan CJ, Gurusamy KS, et al. Surgical versus endoscopic treatment of bile duct stones. *Cochrane Database Syst Rev.* 2013;(9):CD003327.
42. Rogers SJ, Cello JP, Horn JK, et al. Prospective randomized trial of LC+LCBDE vs ERCP/S+LC for common bile duct stone disease. *Arch Surg.* 2010;145(1):28–33.
43. Iranmanesh P, Frossard JL, Mugnier-Konrad B, et al. Initial cholecystectomy vs sequential common duct endoscopic assessment and subsequent cholecystectomy for suspected gallstone migration: a randomized clinical trial. *JAMA.* 2014;312(2):137–144.
44. Kroh M, Chand B. Choledocholithiasis, endoscopic retrograde cholangiopancreatography, and laparoscopic common bile duct exploration. *Surg Clin North Am.* 2008;88(5):1019–1031, vii.
45. Verbesey JE, Birkett DH. Common bile duct exploration for choledocholithiasis. *Surg Clin North Am.* 2008;88(6):1315–1328, ix.
46. Paganini AM, Guerrieri M, Sarnari J, et al. Thirteen years' experience with laparoscopic transcystic common bile duct exploration for stones. Effectiveness and long-term results. *Surg Endosc.* 2007;21(1):34–40.
47. Nathanson LK, O'Rourke NA, Martin IJ, et al. Postoperative ERCP versus laparoscopic choledochotomy for clearance of selected bile duct calculi: a randomized trial. *Ann Surg.* 2005;242(2):188–192.
48. Schreiner MA, Chang L, Gluck M, et al. Laparoscopy-assisted versus balloon enteroscopy-assisted ERCP in bariatric post-Roux-en-Y gastric bypass patients. *Gastrointest Endosc.* 2012; 75(4):748–756.
49. Gurusamy KS, Koti R, Davidson BR. T-tube drainage versus primary closure after open common bile duct exploration. *Cochrane Database Syst Rev.* 2013;(6):CD005640.

59

Biliary Injury, Strictures, and Sclerosing Cholangitis

Joshua Kong and D. Rohan Jeyarajah

Key Points

1 Bile duct injury remains a common complication of cholecystectomy.

2 The method and timing of bile duct injury repair depend on the location and extent of the injury, the presence of concomitant vascular injury, the presence of biloma or sepsis, the timing of recognition, and the technique used for the index case (MIS or open).

3 Management of benign biliary strictures is dependent on etiology. Treatment strategies include medical management, endoscopic stenting, and surgical bypass or resection.

While the etiology of injuries and acquired or autoimmune-based strictures of the bile ducts are diverse (see **Table 59.1**), a basic understanding of biliary anatomy and physiology as well as its impact on liver homeostasis can guide management decisions. The recognition and initial management of biliary injury and stricture are important skills for general surgeons, as appropriate initial therapeutic approaches can significantly impact the outcome of definitive management. Based on the published frequency of biliary injuries and the ubiquitous nature of cholecystectomy, the majority of general surgeons will see a biliary injury in their practice over the course of their careers.[1] While the acute and chronic nature of injuries and strictures, respectively, impacts their presentation, the principles of management remain similar: (1) control any associated infection/sepsis (due to intraperitoneal leak or cholangitis); (2) restoration of biliary drainage (internally or externally); (3) assessment of malignant potential; (4) timely definitive management; and (5) continue appropriate surveillance and reintervention. Superior outcomes have been demonstrated using a multidisciplinary approach involving an interventional radiologist, gastroenterologist, and experienced HPB surgeon.[1–3]

BILE DUCT INJURY

1 Traumatic injury to the bile duct is rare. Most bile duct injuries are iatrogenic and occur during a cholecystectomy. Less well recognized is the potential for bile duct injury during other operations including distal gastric/proximal duodenal procedures and liver resection. The likelihood of bile duct injury during laparoscopic cholecystectomy has been decreased since its adoption. The incidence has remained steady between 0.2% and 0.6% over the last decade, approaching that of open cholecystectomy at 0.1% to 0.2%.[4,5] In comparison, robotic-assisted cholecystectomy, which is rapidly being adopted in practice in the United States, has been associated with an equivalent or slight increased risk of bile duct injury with an up to 0.4% incidence.[5,6] While devastating to the patient medically and financially, bile duct injury also causes dramatic distress, moral injury, and legal-financial burden to the surgeon. Nevertheless, good long-term outcomes have been reported, especially when the injury is repaired by an experienced HPB surgeon.[7]

This chapter will focus on cholecystectomy as the initiating factor; however, the workup and management listed can be applied regardless of the index operation. For cholecystectomy, factors implicated as elevating the risk of associated injuries include obesity, acute inflammation, and anatomic abnormalities, among others (**Table 59.2**). The etiology of bile duct injuries is variable but generally falls into one of two categories: (1) misinterpretation/misidentification of pertinent anatomy[8] or (2) aberrant anatomy.

In the "classic" case, the distal common bile duct is mistaken as the cystic duct, and the common hepatic duct is transected as the surgeon takes the gallbladder off the liver bed (**Fig. 59.1**). In effect, this results in a "resection" of the bile duct, not a transection. The surgeon must recognize that the blood supply to the bile duct has been altered; therefore, primary repair is not preferred, even if technically feasible. Injury resulting from aberrant biliary anatomy often occurs due to the cystic duct inserting low or traveling parallel to the common bile duct. Alternatively, an accessory posterior right hepatic duct can be encountered in up to 6% of patients (**Fig. 59.2**).[4] Finally, other mechanisms, such as traction injury or inadvertent dissection into the common hepatic duct, have been described more commonly with open procedures and a "top-down" approach. Aiming toward the patient's feet, as soon as the fundus of the gallbladder has been dissected, rather than aiming toward the porta, can help avoid this injury (**Fig. 59.3**).

Independent of the underlying etiology, classification systems for bile duct injury have been developed. The most utilized classification used historically to describe location rather than extent (**Table 59.3**).[5] Practically speaking, the classification of biliary injuries is important only when the ultimate definitive management depends on the injury pattern. A special category of injury is combined vascular and biliary injury, typically termed vasculobiliary injuries.[6] These most commonly involve stricture or occlusion of the right hepatic artery, although portal vein injuries are also described. Most often, the surgeon encounters bleeding from the right hepatic artery, lays clips into the bile duct, and causes an injury in the process. The surgeon must remember that the bile duct receives preferential blood supply from the arterial circuit, and therefore, an arterial injury can increase the risk of a biliary stricture.

Several strategies for mitigating the risk of bile duct injury have been proposed, including obtaining the "critical view of safety," intraoperative cholangiogram, and various forms of subtotal cholecystectomy. The critical view of safety describes

Table 59.1. Causes of Benign Biliary Strictures
Postoperative Strictures
Post-Biliary Surgery/Intervention
Laparoscopic Cholecystectomy
▪ Transection/resection
▪ Occlusion (w/ clip)
▪ Laceration
▪ Thermal injury
Open Cholecystectomy
▪ Traction injury
Transection/Resection/Laceration
Common Bile Duct Exploration
ERCP
Injury During Other Procedures
Liver Resection
▪ Ischemic/thermal injury
▪ Post biliary leak
▪ Stapler/ligation of major biliary structures
Gastrectomy
Portal–Caval Shunt
Trauma-Blunt/Penetrating
Vascular/Ischemic
▪ Secondary biliary cirrhosis
Postradiation
Stricture of Biliary–Enteric or Biliary–Biliary Anastomosis
Strictures Secondary to Inflammatory Conditions
Cholecystitis, Choledocholithiasis, Mirrizzi Syndrome
Primary Sclerosing Cholangitis
Primary Biliary Cirrhosis
Stricture/Stenosis of Sphincter of Oddi
Duodenal Ulcer
Crohn Disease
Autoimmune (IgG4-cholangiopathy)
Viral
Drug

the view obtained following clearance of tissue within the triangle of Calot such that only two structures (cystic duct and artery) are connecting the gallbladder to the central hepatoduodenal structures. An important aspect in obtaining this view is initiating dissection on the infundibulum of the gallbladder, not on the triangle of Calot itself. It is our practice to identify the hepatic artery through its pulsation in the hepatoduodenal ligament as the first step of cholecystectomy. Visual

Table 59.2. Factors Associated with Intraoperative Bile Duct Injury
Chronic Inflammation
Anatomic Abnormalities ▪ Low insertion of right posterior duct ▪ Short cystic duct
Narrowing of the Angle between GB and Falciform
Long Parallel Cystic Duct
Obesity
Emergency Surgery
Previous Upper Abdominal Surgery
Failure to Identify the Cystic Duct/Critical View
Intraoperative Hemorrhage

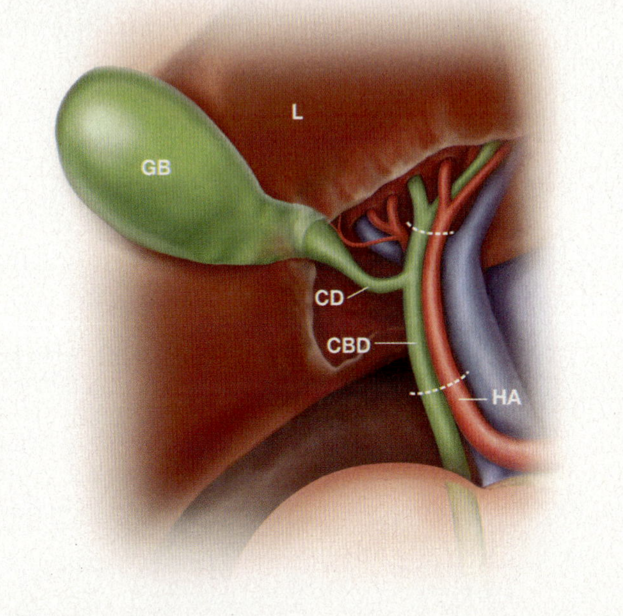

Figure 59.1. Classic laparoscopic bile duct injury. The common bile duct is mistaken for the cystic duct and resected (marked by the *dotted line*). A variable extent of the extrahepatic biliary tree is resected with the gallbladder. L, liver; GB, gallbladder; CD, cystic duct; CBD, common bile duct; HA, hepatic artery. *, Fusion of the CD and common hepatic duct.

identification of this structure allows the surgeon to be aware of the bile duct, which lies to the patient's right of the pulsation. Dissection should not be immediately adjacent to the artery. In the case of an inflamed gallbladder, the triangle of Calot may be obliterated, and the spared plane is between the common

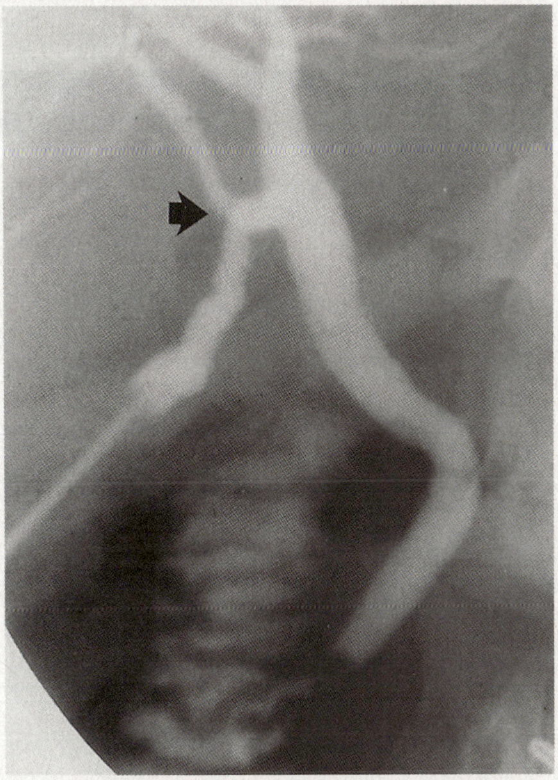

Figure 59.2. Operative cholangiogram demonstrating a right lobe segmental bile duct entering the cystic duct (*arrow*). Division of the cystic duct proximal to this insertion can result in a bile leak or obstruction of bile flow from a significant segment of the liver.

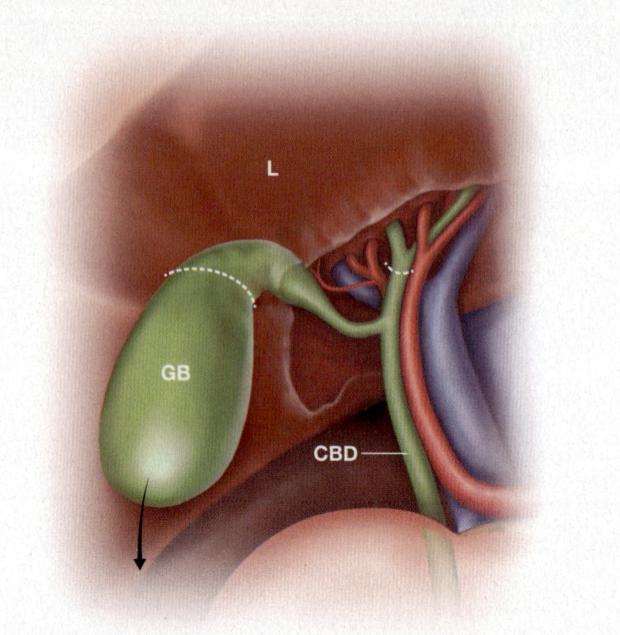

Figure 59.3. "Top-down" approach with retraction of gallbladder fundus toward the patient's feet (*arrow*), away from porta to avoid bile duct injury (*dotted line* highlights potential injury sites). L, liver; GB, gallbladder; CBD, common bile duct.

bile duct and hepatic artery. Some general surgeons practice routine use of IOC during cholecystectomy. Population-based data would suggest that routine IOC does not impact the incidence of bile duct injury but may be beneficial for selected use.[9–11] However, identification of a biliary injury is facilitated at the index operation when IOC is performed, which may expedite management and reduce morbidity.[12] The entirety of the bile duct, intrahepatic ducts, and duodenal filling must be seen to call the cholangiogram normal. Most commonly, either distal filling with no intrahepatic filling or the opposite is interpreted as a normal study in the setting of a bile duct injury. More recently, fluorescent imagining with indocyanine green, which enables real-time intraoperative identification of extrahepatic biliary anatomy, has been suggested to lower the risk of bile duct injury and conversion to open surgery.[13] Finally, while conversion to an open procedure should be considered in all patients in whom anatomic landmarks cannot be clearly defined, this may not provide a significantly reduced risk of biliary injury if the operating surgeon is not accustomed to routine open cholecystectomy. In this scenario, it may be reasonable to place a drain and transfer the patient to an experienced HPB surgeon. Two alternative strategies have been described: the perforating and fenestrating partial cholecystectomy.[14] Partial cholecystectomy has gained acceptance as an alternative to conversion for surgeons less comfortable in open gallbladder surgery who are confronted with significant portal inflammation and difficulty identifying relevant structures. The risk of postoperative biliary fistula is relatively low, and emphasis should be placed on clearing all stones to prevent recurrent symptoms.

Table 59.3. Strasberg Classification of Bile Duct Injury

A Cystic Duct Stump Leak or Minor Leak from Gallbladder Fossa
B Right Posterior Sectoral Duct Occlusion
C Right Posterior Sectoral Duct Leak
D Main Duct Leak with Intact Duct
E1 Transected Main Duct with Stricture >2 cm from Confluence
E2 Transected Main Duct with Stricture <2 cm from Confluence
E3 Stricture of Common Hepatic Duct with Right and Left Hepatic Ducts Still in Communication
E4 Stricture of Common Hepatic Duct with Right and Left Hepatic Ducts Separated
E5 Stricture of the Common Hepatic Duct and Right Posterior Sectoral Duct Occlusion

Clinical Presentation

Based on timing, the presentation of biliary injuries can be classified into acute (days) and delayed (usually after a week). Acutely, biliary injuries are often identified intraoperatively from visualization of unexpected bile leaks, which can be confirmed through an intraoperative cholangiogram. However, most patients present in a subacute setting (weeks) with symptoms associated with biloma or cholangitis due to bile leak or stricture, respectively, including right upper quadrant abdominal pain, fever, or jaundice. Patients with a significant delay in diagnosis (months) can present with biliary cirrhosis from chronic obstruction and the sequelae of advanced liver disease, including portal hypertension and cirrhosis. This presentation occurs as repeated bouts of cholangitis can lead to chronic liver disease.[15] In the case of vasculobiliary injury to the right posterior branch of the bile duct and the hepatic artery, patients can present with recurring liver abscesses to the right posterior section of the liver. Alternatively, the affected sector of the liver may atrophy.

Evaluation

Intraoperatively, once bile duct injury is suspected or identified, the operating surgeon should control the bile leak by placing a percutaneous drain in the right upper quadrant of the abdomen, closing the abdomen, and immediately transferring to the nearest HPB surgery center. Evaluation of the patient begins with a focused history and physical examination. Intraoperative details of the index operation, including approach, structures identified, placement of clips, and hemostatic techniques, should be clearly documented and, ideally, confirmed with the primary surgeon through direct communication.

Identifying any signs of sepsis, such as fever, tachycardia, hypotension, or altered mental status, is critical. Complete blood count and liver function tests should be obtained, including alkaline phosphatase, total bilirubin, and coagulation parameters. To evaluate for undrained fluid collection or blockage of the bile duct, a triple-phase CT scan with IV contrast should be obtained, which can also help evaluate potential concurrent arterial and venous vasculobiliary injuries. In the acute setting without intra-abdominal sepsis, cholangitis, or active bleeding that requires immediate intervention and in the subacute setting, MRI/MRCP with a hepatocyte-selective contrast agent, such as gadoxetate disodium (primovist or eovist) that are taken up and excreted by hepatocytes through the bile ducts can help identify the site of injury.[3] ERCP and PTC are additional diagnostic modalities to identify the site of injury with potential therapeutic capabilities.

If delayed repair is planned and undrained collections are present, then image-guided drainage should be performed first, prior to ERCP, to reduce the risk of postprocedural sepsis, ideally via a percutaneous route. If a tangential injury is suspected, then ERCP has the advantage of providing diagnostic information and the ability to intervene. If a complete transection/occlusion is suspected, then ERCP will have little diagnostic value and has the disadvantage of being an invasive modality. On the other hand, PTC is associated with the risk of cholangitis and is technically challenging in the acute setting as the intrahepatic bile ducts are often not dilated.

Treatment

2 Typically, intraoperative or early (within 48 hours) identification of bile duct injury, followed by immediate repair by an HPB specialist, leads to the best outcome.[16,17] In theory, early repair precludes clinical deterioration, leading to lower hospital length of stay and cost.[18,19] However, the optimal timing of surgical repair for bile duct injury is debated. The most recent systemic review and meta-analysis, which compared early (<14 days), intermediate (14 days to 6 weeks), and late (>6 weeks) hepaticojejunostomy, reported that intermediate repair was associated with the highest morbidity and delayed repair had a lower stricture rate. Mortality was not different between the three timings.[20]

At our institution, the decision as whether to proceed with repair is based on a scoring system and four criteria (manuscript in review):

1. The index surgery approach (MIS vs open),
2. Concurrent vascular injury,
3. The presence of biloma, and
4. Sepsis requiring pressor support.

A score is assigned to each category (**Table 59.4**) to stratify patients into a low-risk (≤4 points) or high-risk (>4 points) group. Patients in the low-risk group should proceed with immediate surgery. In contrast, individuals in the high-risk group should follow the principles of delayed management:

1. Control sepsis/drain undrained collections,
2. Establish biliary drainage, and
3. Definitive management/surgical repair once sepsis and inflammation resolve.

As noted above, patients with undrained fluid collections in the porta hepatitis should have image-guided drainage often after initiating fluid resuscitation and broad-spectrum antibiotics targeting enteric organisms.

Bile leak due to minor injury such as a cystic stump or accessory injury (Strasberg type A) can be managed endoscopically with ERCP, sphincterotomy with or without stent placement in >90% of the time. For more severe lateral bile duct injuries (Strasberg type C), the success rate is approximately 85% to 89%.[21] Percutaneous biliary drainage is required for complete transection +/– occlusion with delayed presentation. PTC cannulation of unobstructed ducts can be challenging when the duct is not occluded. However, injecting the biloma drain can help fill the bile duct and aid the interventional radiologist in placing the biliary drain. If the duct can be cannulated, ideal management would be to span the defect with a PTC. Otherwise, external drainage of the duct alone can improve the control of bile flow and sepsis. If the duct is occluded, external drainage is established with a catheter secured at or above the level of the injury.

For biliary strictures that can be endoscopically stented, a series of stent exchanges every 3 to 4 months may be performed with a 74% to 89% success rate.[21] If an ongoing bile leak is present, this will most typically stop following biliary drainage. The biloma drainage catheter can be removed while continuing external drainage of the biliary tree via PTC. The patient must be instructed on caring for the biliary drainage catheter. Furthermore, the patient must be cautioned about the risk of volume depletion and instructed to increase oral fluid intake while the external drain is in place. The timing of definitive management typically can be considered from 6 to 12 weeks following control of the local sepsis. Concomitant vascular injury (up to 40% of the time), delayed presentation, and previous repair (~30% of the time) complicate management and often require a multidisciplinary approach, with 10% of patients requiring liver resection.[21]

Definitive surgical management typically involves a biliary–enteric anastomosis, most commonly with a Roux-en-Y hepaticojejunostomy. Hepaticoduodenostomy is an alternative option. The blood supply to the distal common bile duct is often disrupted in these settings, however, leading to an increased risk of postanastomotic stricture. Perioperative planning and optimization considerations include the potential for nutritional deficiencies with extended external biliary drainage, including vitamin K deficiency, which may impact the risk of perioperative hemorrhage.

The first step to the repair is to remove all visualized clips, followed by identification of the bile duct. Routine intraoperative ultrasound is performed to identify the bile duct and hepatic artery, as well as patency of intrahepatic arterial and venous vessels. The position of the right hepatic artery in relation to the bile duct must be noted as this typically runs posterior to the duct; it can course anteriorly and, in this position, is at high risk for injury during subsequent definitive operative repair as the porta hepatis can be scarred and the structures obscured. If a PTC catheter is present, it can facilitate the process of identifying the duct. Otherwise, a small gauge needle and a syringe with aspiration of bile can also be used to identify the duct. After identification, the anterior wall of the duct can be opened longitudinally as the arteries run at the 3 and 9 o'clock positions laterally. An intraoperative cholangiogram is also performed to ensure that all segments of the liver are drained.

Without thermal injury, a partially transected bile duct may be repaired primarily with sutures with or without a T-tube. If the injury is near or at the biliary confluence (Strasberg type E3 and 4), the Hepp-Couinaud technique can be performed using a right angle, or a probe can be inserted into the bile duct and the ductotomy extended onto the left hepatic duct to provide for a larger anastomosis.[22] We perform an end-to-side anastomosis using 5-0 absorbable monofilament suture, typically PDS (**Fig. 59.4**). When a biliary drain is in place, we typically cut the coiling string and place it across the anastomosis, effectively stenting this and ensuring that the back wall is not caught in the suture. Again, optimal long-term outcomes are obtained when the repair of bile duct injuries is undertaken by a surgeon with significant hepatobiliary training, as this index surgery will carry the risk of future stricture.[12,13]

The management of concomitant biliary and vascular injury requires special consideration. The most common concomitant

Table 59.4. Risk Stratification Characteristics for Bile Duct Injury

Characteristics	Score
Index Surgery approach	
Laparoscopic	1
Open	2
Laparoscopic converted to open	2
Vascular Injury	
Yes	3
No	1
Biloma	
Yes	2
No	1
Sepsis	
Yes	3
No	1

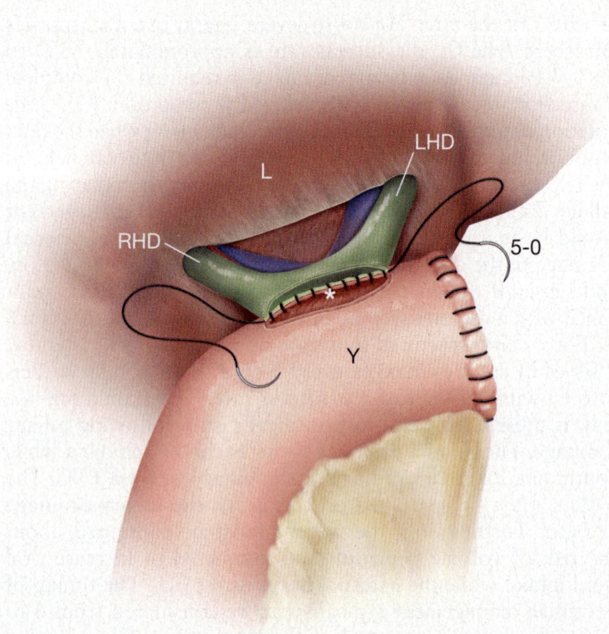

Figure 59.4. Hepaticojejunostomy at the confluence of right and left hepatic duct using absorbable suture. L, liver; RHD, right hepatic duct; LHD, left hepatic duct; 5-0, suture; Y, Y-limb of jejunum; *, back row anastomosis.

vascular injury is to the right hepatic artery, with injury to the hepatic artery proper and portal vein less common. Of note, arterial collaterals exist through the hepatic duct confluence so that arterial supply to the right biliary tree may be maintained in the presence of the right hepatic artery injury if the confluence is not disrupted. Repair of associated vascular injury (artery or portal vein) is rarely indicated unless identified at the time of injury. If the vascular integrity of the biliary system is in question, delayed repair is preferred and, in the most dramatic cases, may require hepatic resection.

Outcomes

Several retrospective series have reported the short- and mid-term outcomes of definitive operative repair.[23,24] Repair failure is typically defined as diagnosed stricture or the need for imaging/intervention secondary to suspected stricture/cholangitis. Early referral to a hepatobiliary surgeon was associated with decreased postoperative complications and biliary stricture.[25]

Biliary-enteric anastomotic stricture is an important measure of long-term outcome. The incidence ranges from 4% to 69%, with most studies in the 10% to 20% range. Strictures develop most commonly between 11 and 30 months, with 90% presenting within 7 years following repair. Untreated strictures can lead to recurring cholangitis, secondary biliary cirrhosis, and death.[26]

Early recognition and repair are associated with decreased cost and hospital length of stay.[27] Among patients undergoing hepaticojejunostomy, later repair (> 90 days following bile duct injury) has been associated with a decreased risk of anastomotic stricture compared with repair performed within 14 to 90 days of injury.[28] This finding may be potentially explained by the full demarcation of devascularization of the bile duct, allowing for repair at the appropriate level on the bile duct, which usually has better blood supply proximally.

Follow-Up

Following definitive repair, the patients are at risk long-term for stricture of the anastomosis. Although the incidence of postanastomotic stricture is relatively low, the consequences can be devastating. We recommend annual liver function testing to assess for the development of strictures, which may be associated with a rising alkaline phosphatase level. Early identification of strictures is essential and can typically be dilated percutaneously prior to the development of secondary biliary cirrhosis and liver failure.

BILIARY STRICTURE

The etiology of benign biliary strictures includes iatrogenic/postoperative and various other infectious/inflammatory conditions (**Table 59.1**). Postoperative biliary strictures due to bile duct injuries have been addressed above. The approach to nonneoplastic biliary strictures depends on the etiology and location within the biliary tree, and the need to rule out a neoplastic process is a vital component of the evaluation.

Clinical Presentation

Patients with benign biliary strictures often present with either cholangitis or jaundice, yet can also be asymptomatic with only incidental findings on imaging. Patients with cholangitis typically present with some combination of fever, right upper quadrant pain, and jaundice. Patients with sepsis secondary to cholangitis will have hypotension, tachycardia, and altered mental status at presentation. This may be in the setting of known predisposing factors such as recurrent pancreatitis, stone disease, previous biliary surgery, and primary sclerosing cholangitis (PSC). Alternatively, patient may present without any known risk factors. In the setting of a biliary stricture, the surgeon should ensure that the appropriate tests are done to rule out a possible malignancy.

Evaluation

Similar to patients with bile duct injury, evaluation begins with a focused history and physical examination with special attention to predisposing factors, including a history of biliary intervention/surgery, recurrent pancreatitis, and a history of inflammatory bowel disease. Laboratory evaluation includes complete blood count, liver function testing, and coagulation profile. Biochemically, there is usually a cholestatic pattern of elevated alkaline phosphatase and total bilirubin. However, if >25% of the liver drains bile appropriately, patients may have isolated alkaline phosphatase elevation while the level of total bilirubin remains normal. IgG4 levels should be considered. Negative results do not rule out this as a diagnosis, as tissue IgG4 levels are far more sensitive than serum levels for diagnosis.

For patients with signs and symptoms of cholangitis and/or sepsis, fluid resuscitation and broad-spectrum antibiotics should be initiated as part of the evaluation, and the remainder of the workup should be performed while hospitalized. Patients without infection/sepsis can be evaluated as an outpatient. Typically, the next step in evaluation includes a CT scan of the abdomen with IV contrast. MRCP and MRI with diffusion-weighted sequence can delineate a mass well. The presence of a mass must raise a high suspicion for malignancy and requires further evaluation. Without an obvious mass, the typical next step is a combination of ERCP, EUS, and biliary endoscopy (if available). ERCP is initially performed to relieve jaundice. EUS is used to biopsy a mass or the site of stricture when extrahepatic; alternatively, EUS can target a suspicious lymph node or liver lesion, particularly in the left liver. Brushings and intrabiliary endoscopy can be utilized to obtain tissue from the area of a stricture. Brushings should be evaluated by cytology and, if available, fluorescence *in situ* hybridization (FISH). If endoscopic stenting with drainage of as many relevant hepatic segments as possible cannot be achieved, percutaneous biliary drainage (PTC) should be considered. In general, drainage of intrahepatic and perihilar strictures through the right hepatic duct is favored, as targeting the left hepatic duct increases the risk of injury to the hilar structures. ERCP is the preferred modality for the drainage of extrahepatic strictures.[29]

Treatment

3 The etiology of benign biliary stricture dictates treatment, which ranges from medical management to endoscopic and/or

operative management. For instance, an inflammatory stricture secondary to an autoimmune disease such as IgG4 cholangiopathy can be treated with corticosteroids.

Patients with pancreatitis-related biliary strictures may be managed with stenting if the stricture is related to acute inflammation. For patients with chronic inflammatory changes or fibrotic stricturing, definitive management may require operative intervention. Endoscopic ultrasound is beneficial for indeterminant biliary strictures to differentiate malignant and benign biliary strictures and guide clinical management.[30] In the absence of a convincing history of pancreatitis or a clear PSC/autoimmune diagnosis, a concern for malignancy must be high.

Two options for benign strictures are possible:

1. Whipple pancreaticoduodenectomy or
2. Biliary bypass, typically to a Roux limb.

The choice of approach depends on whether there is head-dominant pancreatitis, which would likely benefit from resection, and the ability to safely perform such an operation. A resective approach should be considered if malignancy cannot be excluded or if there is concurrent stricturing of the pancreatic duct, chronic pain, or gastric outlet obstruction. Pancreaticoduodenectomy relieves all these obstructive symptoms but is a higher-risk surgery than a bypass. PSC represents a unique situation that will be discussed in detail in the next section. Postoperative biliary strictures can be balloon dilated and stented successfully in select patients. However, definitive management will often require operative bypass, which can be accomplished by biliary-enteric anastomosis as described above.

Outcomes

The data regarding successful outcomes following endoscopic management of biliary strictures reports variable rates depending on retrospective versus prospective evaluation, plastic versus fully covered self-expanding metal, and etiology (most commonly pancreatitis vs posttransplant anastomotic stricture vs post cholecystectomy). A meta-analysis comparing long-term stricture resolution rates between different treatment options for benign biliary strictures noted that surgery (hepaticojejunostomy or duodenojejunostomy) had the highest stricture resolution rate (84%), followed by PTC (81%), multiple plastic stents (79%), and covered self-expanding metal stents (76%), albeit the difference was not statistically significant.[31] The only significant finding was that single plastic stent placement was inferior (23%) and, therefore, not recommended.[32] Similarly, another meta-analysis also demonstrated fewer ERCPs required with metal stenting and a stricture recurrence rate of 16%.[33]

Follow-Up

Patients undergoing endoscopic stenting +/– balloon dilation for biliary stricture may require repeated procedures, the timing of which typically will be dictated by the choice of plastic versus covered metal stenting. In general, annual ultrasound and liver function testing are recommended for patients undergoing biliary-enteric bypass, as discussed above.

SCLEROSING CHOLANGITIS

Sclerosing cholangitis is a nonspecific finding of chronic cholestasis, leading to inflammation, fibrosis, and stricturing of the bile duct.[34] Stricturing can be related to primary (PSC) or secondary to another cause (**Table 59.5**), which leads to scarring and strictures.[35] Management of the underlying etiology is required for the treatment/prevention of secondary sclerosing cholangitis and may include medical, endoscopic, or operative intervention based on the etiology. In contrast, PSC is an autoimmune disease, often associated with ulcerative colitis (approximately two-thirds of patients with PSC will have ulcerative colitis) and carries a markedly increased risk of cholangiocarcinoma (400- to 1,000-fold increase compared to the general population).[21] PSC can present with intra- or extrahepatic ductal strictures, or with cholestatic small duct disease. A finding of diffuse strictures throughout the biliary tree is pathognomonic of the disease (although segmental involvement is possible), and progressive disease often leads to chronic cholestasis and eventual liver failure requiring transplant. The presence of a dominant stricture with or without an associated mass in a patient with PSC requires a workup to rule out cholangiocarcinoma. Surgical intervention on the biliary tree other than transplant or cholecystectomy is uncommon, while endoscopic management is the mainstay of therapeutic and surveillance strategies.

Table 59.5. Causes of Secondary Sclerosing Cholangitis

Infectious
Recurrent pyogenic cholangitis (RPC)
Toxic
Hepatic arterial thrombosis
Ischemic-type biliary lesions (liver transplant recipients)
Critical illness (ie, hypoperfusion)
Systemic vasculitis
Hematologic disorders (ie, sickle cell disease and paroxysmal nocturnal hemoglobinuria)
Radiation therapy
Immunologic
IgG4-related
Inflammatory pseudotumor
Eosinophilic
Congenital
Caroli disease
Cystic fibrosis
Miscellaneous
Choledocholithiasis
Chronic pancreatitis
Sarcoidosis
Amyloidosis
Malignancy

Content adapted from Ludwig DR, Anderson MA, Itani M, Sharbidre KG, Lalwani N, Paspulati RM. Secondary sclerosing cholangitis: mimics of primary sclerosing cholangitis. *Abdom Radiol (NY)*. 2023;48(1):151–165.

Clinical Presentation

Clinical presentation is a spectrum from incidental findings (alkaline phosphatase/bilirubin elevations and/or imaging changes) to painless jaundice, to cholangitis, sepsis and biliary cirrhosis. The initial diagnosis of PSC may be at the time of cholangiocarcinoma diagnosis.

Evaluation

The initial evaluation is similar to those noted above for biliary stricture, with a focused history and physical examination, followed by bloodwork, resuscitation as indicated, and imaging studies. Diagnosis of PSC is made based on clinical presentation and elevated alkaline phosphatase, gamma glutamyl transferase, and transaminitis, with multifocal structuring of intrahepatic and/or extrahepatic bile ducts on either ERCP or MRCP. Although not necessary for diagnosis of large-duct PSC, classic percutaneous biopsy demonstrates periductal concentric fibrosis.[35] Imaging characteristics of cirrhosis and/or portal hypertension should also be assessed. ERCP allows stenting and brushing/biopsy of any dominant strictures. Adjunctive studies such as FISH specifically evaluating the specimens for polysomy is recommended. A high index of suspicion should be maintained for malignancy in these patients and surveillance should be undertaken at a specialized center.

Treatment

For secondary cholangitis, treatment is targeted at the underlying etiology. In this setting, endoscopic and/or operative intervention on the liver/biliary tree may be undertaken. For example, in patients with recurrent pyogenic cholangitis (RPC), there often is selective involvement of the left lateral sector of the liver with progressive sclerosis and recurrent episodes of cholangitis secondary to intraductal stone formation.[35] Resection of the involved liver segments can provide durable management. For other indications, such as IgG4 cholangiopathy, the treatment is medical. For PSC, the treatment modality for symptomatic strictures is endoscopic dilation, brushing, and stenting with close surveillance, the timing of which is dictated by the findings on cytology and FISH. Progressive liver failure or cholangiocarcinoma is treated with liver transplant in appropriately selected patients with PSC, although recurrence of PSC in the transplanted liver is possible.

ACKNOWLEDGMENTS

We gratefully acknowledge the contributions of previous edition authors, Rory L. Smoot and Sean P. Cleary, as portions of those chapters have been retained in this revision.

References

1. Goykhman Y, Kory I, Small R, et al. Long-term outcome and risk factors of failure after bile duct injury repair. *J Gastrointest Surg*. 2008;12(8):1412–1417.
2. Flum DR, Cheadle A, Prela C, Dellinger EP, Chan L. Bile duct injury during cholecystectomy and survival in Medicare beneficiaries. *JAMA*. 2003;290(16):2168–2173.
3. de'Angelis N, Catena F, Memeo R, et al. 2020 WSES guidelines for the detection and management of bile duct injury during cholecystectomy. *World J Emerg Surg*. 2021;16(1):30.
4. Fletcher R, Cortina CS, Kornfield H, et al. Bile duct injuries: a contemporary survey of surgeon attitudes and experiences. *Surg Endosc*. 2020;34(7):3079–3084.
5. Kalata S, Thumma JR, Norton EC, Dimick JB, Sheetz KH. Comparative safety of robotic-assisted vs laparoscopic cholecystectomy. *JAMA Surg*. 2023;158(12):1303–1310.
6. Strosberg DS, Nguyen MC, Muscarella P, Narula VK. A retrospective comparison of robotic cholecystectomy versus laparoscopic cholecystectomy: operative outcomes and cost analysis. *Surg Endosc*. 2017;31(3):1436–1441.
7. Perera MT, Silva MA, Hegab B, et al. Specialist early and immediate repair of post-laparoscopic cholecystectomy bile duct injuries is associated with an improved long-term outcome. *Ann Surg*. 2011;253(3):553–560.
8. Way LW, Stewart L, Gantert W, et al. Causes and prevention of laparoscopic bile duct injuries: analysis of 252 cases from a human factors and cognitive psychology perspective. *Ann Surg*. 2003;237(4):460–469.
9. Lilley EJ, Scott JW, Jiang W, et al. Intraoperative cholangiography during cholecystectomy among hospitalized Medicare beneficiaries with non-neoplastic biliary disease. *Am J Surg*. 2017;214(4):682–686.
10. Sheffield KM, Riall TS, Han Y, Kuo YF, Townsend CM, Goodwin JS. Association between cholecystectomy with vs without intraoperative cholangiography and risk of common duct injury. *JAMA*. 2013;310(8):812–820.
11. Törnqvist B, Strömberg C, Akre O, Enochsson L, Nilsson M. Selective intraoperative cholangiography and risk of bile duct injury during cholecystectomy. *Br J Surg*. 2015;102(8):952–958.
12. Rystedt JM, Montgomery AK. Quality-of-life after bile duct injury: intraoperative detection is crucial. A national case-control study. *HPB (Oxford)*. 2016;18(12):1010–1016.
13. Dip F, Lo Menzo E, White KP, Rosenthal RJ. Does near-infrared fluorescent cholangiography with indocyanine green reduce bile duct injuries and conversions to open surgery during laparoscopic or robotic cholecystectomy? – A meta-analysis. *Surgery*. 2021;169(4):859–867.
14. Strasberg SM, Pucci MJ, Brunt LM, Deziel DJ. Subtotal cholecystectomy-"Fenestrating" vs "Reconstituting" subtypes and the prevention of bile duct injury: Definition of the optimal procedure in difficult operative conditions. *J Am Coll Surg*. 2016;222(1):89–96.
15. Hilscher MB, Kamath PS, Eaton JE. Cholestatic liver diseases: A primer for generalists and subspecialists. *Mayo Clin Proc*. 2020;95(10):2263–2279.
16. Seeras K, Qasawa RN, Kashyap S, Kalani AD. Bile duct repair. In: *StatPearls [Internet]*. StatPearls Publishing; 2024.
17. Perera MT, Silva MA, Shah AJ, et al. Risk factors for litigation following major transectional bile duct injury sustained at laparoscopic cholecystectomy. *World J Surg*. 2010;34(11):2635–2641.
18. Dageforde LA, Landman MP, Feurer ID, Poulose B, Pinson CW, Moore DE. A cost-effectiveness analysis of early vs late reconstruction of iatrogenic bile duct injuries. *J Am Coll Surg*. 2012;214(6):919–927.
19. Elser H, Bergquist JR, Li AY, Visser BC. Determinants, costs, and consequences of common bile duct injury requiring operative repair among privately insured individuals in the United States, 2003–2020. *Ann Surg Open*. 2023;4(1):e238.
20. Manivasagam SS, Chandra JN, Khera D, Aradhya PS, Hiremath AM. Optimal timing of surgical repair after bile duct injury: A systematic review and meta-analysis. *Cureus*. 2024;16(2):e53507.
21. Schreuder AM, Busch OR, Besselink MG, et al. Long-term impact of iatrogenic bile duct injury. *Dig Surg*. 2020;37(1):10–21.
22. Hepp J, Couinaud C. [Approach to and use of the left hepatic duct in reparation of the common bile duct]. *Presse Med (1893)*. 1956;64(41):947–948.
23. Sahajpal AK, Chow SC, Dixon E, Greig PD, Gallinger S, Wei AC. Bile duct injuries associated with laparoscopic cholecystectomy: timing of repair and long-term outcomes. *Arch Surg*. 2010;145(8):757–763.
24. Walsh RM, Henderson JM, Vogt DP, Brown N. Long-term outcome of biliary reconstruction for bile duct injuries from laparoscopic cholecystectomies. *Surgery*. 2007;142(4):450–456; discussion 456–457.
25. Wang X, Yu WL, Fu XH, Zhu B, Zhao T, Zhang YJ. Early versus delayed surgical repair and referral for patients with bile duct injury: A systematic review and meta-analysis. *Ann Surg*. 2020;271(3):449–459.
26. Ahmad H, Zia HH, Salih M, Naseer M, Khan NY, Bhatti ABH. Outcomes of hepaticojejunostomy for post-cholecystectomy bile duct injury. *J Int Med Res*. 2023;51(3):3000605231162444.
27. Savader SJ, Lillemoe KD, Prescott CA, et al. Laparoscopic cholecystectomy-related bile duct injuries: a health and financial disaster. *Ann Surg*. 1997;225(3):268–273.
28. Booij KAC, Coelen RJ, de Reuver PR, et al. Long-term follow-up and risk factors for strictures after hepaticojejunostomy for bile duct injury: An analysis of surgical and percutaneous treatment in a tertiary center. *Surgery*. 2018;163(5):1121–1127.
29. Elmunzer BJ, Maranki JL, Gómez V, et al. ACG clinical guideline: Diagnosis and management of biliary strictures. *Am J Gastroenterol*. 2023;118(3):405–426.
30. Tang RSY. Endoscopic evaluation of indeterminate biliary strictures: Cholangioscopy, endoscopic ultrasound, or both? *Dig Endosc*. 2024;36(7):778–788.
31. Coté GA, Slivka A, Tarnasky P, et al. Effect of covered metallic stents compared with plastic stents on benign biliary stricture resolution: A randomized clinical trial. *JAMA*. 2016;315(12):1250–1257.
32. Huszár O, Kokas B, Mátrai P, et al. Meta-analysis of the long term success rate of different interventions in benign biliary strictures. *PLoS One*. 2017;12(1):e0169618.
33. Khan MA, Baron TH, Kamal F, et al. Efficacy of self-expandable metal stents in management of benign biliary strictures and comparison with multiple plastic stents: a meta-analysis. *Endoscopy*. 2017;49(7):682–694.
34. Lawson KL, Wang HL. Primary sclerosing cholangitis, small duct primary sclerosing cholangitis, IgG4-related sclerosing cholangitis, and ischemic cholangiopathy: Diagnostic challenges on biopsy. *Surg Pathol Clin*. 2023;16(3):533–548.
35. Ludwig DR, Anderson MA, Itani M, Sharbidre KG, Lalwani N, Paspulati RM. Secondary sclerosing cholangitis: mimics of primary sclerosing cholangitis. *Abdom Radiol (NY)*. 2023;48(1):151–165.

60

Biliary Neoplasms

Sharon Weber, Kaitlyn J. Kelly, and Yuman Fong

Key Points

1 Biliary malignancies represent uncommon malignancies with a poor prognosis because of their insidious onset, propensity for local invasion, and rapid disease progression.

2 The only curative option in patients with biliary malignancies is complete surgical resection.

3 There is an increasing role of multidisciplinary therapy for biliary tract malignancies.

4 Nonoperative palliative biliary decompression can be accomplished with percutaneous or endoscopic stenting, depending on the level of obstruction.

INTRODUCTION

Tumors arising in the gallbladder and biliary tree are rare, with approximately 10,650 cases per year in the United States and 140,000 per year worldwide.[1,2] These tumors are often asymptomatic until late in the course of the disease. Consequently, these tumors commonly present in an advanced, unresectable stage. Surgery remains the only curative option for biliary malignancies. Complete resection of biliary neoplasms often requires radical resection and complex biliary reconstruction that should only be performed at specialized, high-volume centers. Both the late diagnosis and the complex operative techniques required for potentially curative resection contribute to the challenge of these cases. This chapter reviews the incidence, diagnosis, and therapy of these malignancies as well as the outcomes of treatment.

GALLBLADDER CARCINOMA

1 Gallbladder cancer is a rare malignancy with a dismal prognosis because of its insidious onset, propensity for local invasion, and rapid disease progression. Overall, most series report a 5-year survival of less than 5%.

Incidence

Gallbladder cancer is the most common, and arguably most aggressive, biliary tract malignancy. There are only 6000 to 7000 new cases diagnosed in the United States each year but there are high incidence pockets in Japan, Korea, Eastern Europe, and South America. This tumor occurs more frequently in women (female:male ratio = 3:1), and peak incidence is in the seventh decade. There is a tremendously increased risk of gallbladder cancer in particular indigenous populations, including Mapuche Indians in South America (12.3 cases/100,000 males and 27.3/100,000 females), and Native Americans in New Mexico (8.9 cases/100,000 people), and Alaska natives.[3]

The increased risk of gallbladder cancer with cholelithiasis is well established; 70% to 90% of all patients with carcinoma also have gallstones. However, less than 0.5% of patients with gallstones are found to have gallbladder cancer, so routine cholecystectomy for asymptomatic gallstones because of concern for gallbladder cancer is not warranted. In recent series of patients undergoing elective cholecystectomy for gallstones, gallbladder cancer is found incidentally in <0.5% of patients.[4] The association of gallstones with carcinoma is probably related to chronic inflammation. Larger stones (>3 cm) are associated with a 10-fold increased risk of cancer.[4,5]

In the past, the finding of a calcified gallbladder wall, called "porcelain gallbladder" (**Fig. 60.1**), was associated with a high risk of cancer, in some series ranging from 25% to 60%.[6] Thus, the recommendation was for all patients with porcelain gallbladder to undergo open cholecystectomy, even if asymptomatic. Recent series evaluating this issue suggest that the risk of gallbladder cancer in patients with porcelain gallbladder has likely been greatly overestimated, and is more likely on the order of 7% to 15%, therefore changing the recommendation to prophylactic laparoscopic cholecystectomy for these patients.[6,7]

Patients with choledochal cysts have an increased risk of carcinoma developing anywhere in the biliary tree, but the incidence is highest in the gallbladder. This risk increases with age. Therefore, cholecystectomy is recommended for all patients with choledochal cysts at the time of diagnosis. Additional risk factors include gallbladder polyps that are >1 cm in size or documented to be growing, inflammatory bowel disease, primary sclerosing cholangitis, and chronic typhoid.

Pathology and Staging

More than 80% of gallbladder cancers are adenocarcinomas; there are several histologic subtypes, including papillary, nodular, and tubular. Papillary tumors, which grow predominantly into the gallbladder lumen, have an improved prognosis compared with the other subtypes. Poor prognostic signs in gallbladder cancer include high grade, and vascular invasion.[3] The most important prognostic factor may be lymph node status, although 5-year survivors with nodal involvement have been documented. Less than 5% of cases are squamous cell carcinomas, with the remaining 10% being anaplastic lesions.

Gallbladder cancer spreads via lymphatic and venous drainage. Because of drainage pattern of cholecystic veins directly into the adjacent liver, these tumors often involve hepatic parenchyma, most commonly portions of segments IV and V. Lymphatic spread occurs first to the cystic duct (Calot) node, then to pericholedochal and hilar nodes, and finally to peripancreatic, duodenal, periportal, celiac, and superior mesenteric artery nodes. Nodal disease in the porta hepatis

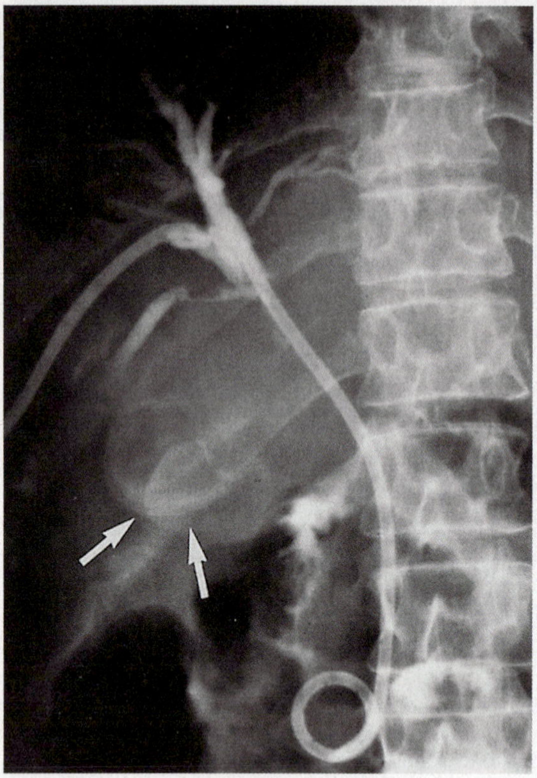

Figure 60.1. Unresectable gallbladder cancer demonstrating palliative transhepatic percutaneous stent placed to relieve jaundice. Porcelain gallbladder is present (*arrows*).

often causes common bile duct (CBD) obstruction and resultant jaundice, which is the first clinical symptom in 30% of patients. Jaundice may also be caused by tumors arising in the infundibulum, which may spread directly to the cystic duct and common hepatic duct. Although peritoneal metastases are frequent, distant extraperitoneal metastases are not.

Limited information exists regarding the genetic changes in gallbladder cancer. Recently reported gene abnormalities associated with gallbladder cancer include K-ras, ERBB2, ARID1A, and PI3 kinase pathway aberrations.[8,9] The finding that patients with an anomalous pancreaticobiliary junction have a greater frequency of K-ras mutations has led investigators to believe that reflux of pancreatic enzymes into the biliary tree may contribute to the development of cancer. Because of our limited knowledge of the sequence of molecular changes, there are no known detectors of early disease or of risk assessment. Clearly, this is an area that needs improvement, particularly in endemic areas.

The gallbladder differs histologically from the rest of the gastrointestinal tract in that it lacks a muscularis mucosa and submucosa. The gallbladder wall is composed of (a) a single layer of columnar cells, the mucosa, and lamina propria; (b) a fibromuscular layer; (c) a perimuscular, subserosal layer containing lymphatics and neurovascular structures; and (d) a serosal surface, except where the gallbladder is embedded in the liver. Because lymphatics are present in the subserosal layer only, tumors invading less than the full thickness of the muscular layer have minimal risk of nodal spread. Thus, disease invading into, but not through, the muscular layer of the gallbladder is T1b disease (stage I), whereas invasion into the perimuscular connective tissue is T2 (stage IIa or b). If on the peritoneal side, it is T2a, and if on the hepatic side, T2b. Stage III disease includes tumors that have perforated the serosa or have directly invaded the liver or other surrounding structures (T3), which are clearly more advanced but still potentially resectable. Tumors that invade the main portal vein, hepatic artery, or two or more extrahepatic organs/structures are classified as T4 (stage IVA) and are typically unresectable. Lymph node metastasis to one to three regional nodes is N1, and to four or more regional nodes is N2. N1 nodal metastasis is classified as stage IIIB and N2 as stage IVB. In line with other pancreaticobiliary malignancies, the stage III grouping refers to locally advanced disease and stage IV indicates locally advanced unresectable or metastatic disease.

Clinical Findings and Diagnosis

Most patients are found to have gallbladder cancer during workup or treatment of cholelithiasis or choledocholithiasis. In patients with symptoms, abdominal pain consistent with biliary colic or acute cholecystitis is most common. Patients also present with jaundice, weight loss, anorexia, or an increase in abdominal girth secondary to ascites. Physical findings may include right upper quadrant tenderness or a palpable mass, hepatomegaly, and ascites. Laboratory investigation, if abnormal, is most often consistent with biliary obstruction. Because of its nonspecific presentation and the lack of reliable screening tests, gallbladder cancer is not diagnosed preoperatively in more than half the cases.

Imaging evaluation often starts with ultrasound or CT and reveals a thickened gallbladder wall or a mass within or replacing the gallbladder on ultrasound examination. Because polyps, asymmetric wall thickening from cholecystitis (especially xanthogranulomatous type), and carcinoma can have an echogenicity similar to the gallbladder wall, these lesions are often difficult to distinguish.[10,11] This is even more difficult when inflammation is present from gallstones.

Improvements in MRI technology, diffusion-weighted imaging, and magnetic resonance cholangiopancreatography (MRCP) have evolved into a single, noninvasive imaging modality that allows complete assessment of biliary, vascular, hepatic, parenchymal, and nodal involvement, as well as involvement of adjacent organs (**Fig. 60.2**). In patients who are jaundiced, direct cholangiography may be useful to delineate

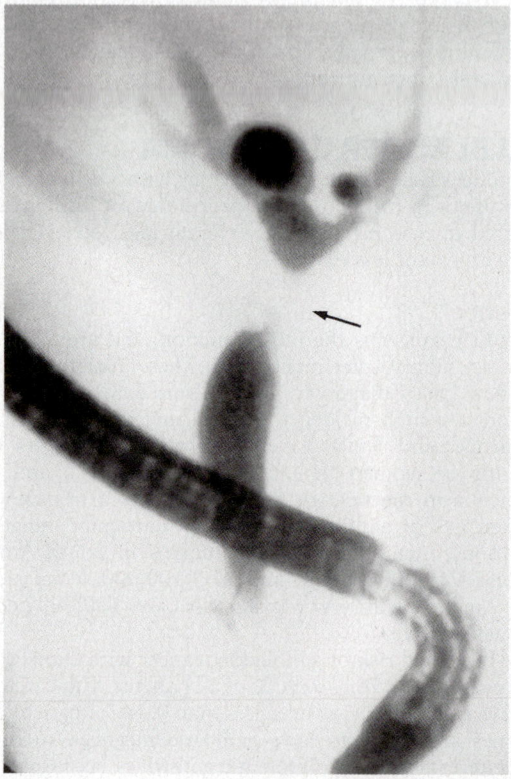

Figure 60.2. Endoscopic retrograde cholangiopancreatogram obtained from a patient with gallbladder cancer. Mid–bile duct obstruction (*arrow*) is caused by direct extension of tumor to the cystic and common hepatic duct.

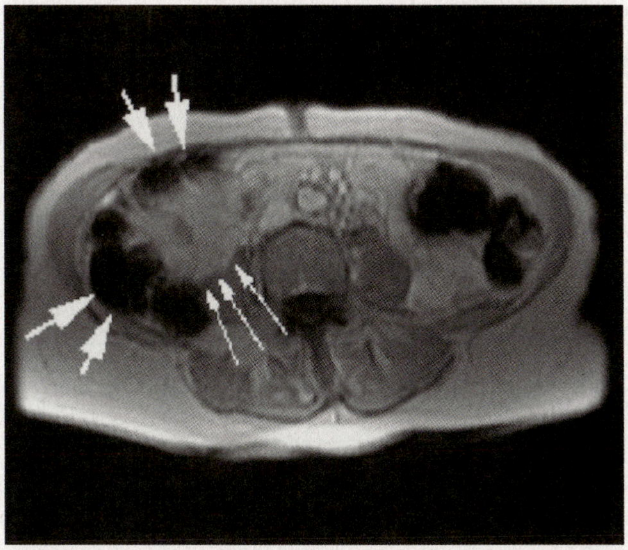

Figure 60.3. T1-weighted magnetic resonance imaging scan of a patient with gallbladder cancer (*small arrows*) with extension into the duodenum and the hepatic flexure of colon (*large arrows*).

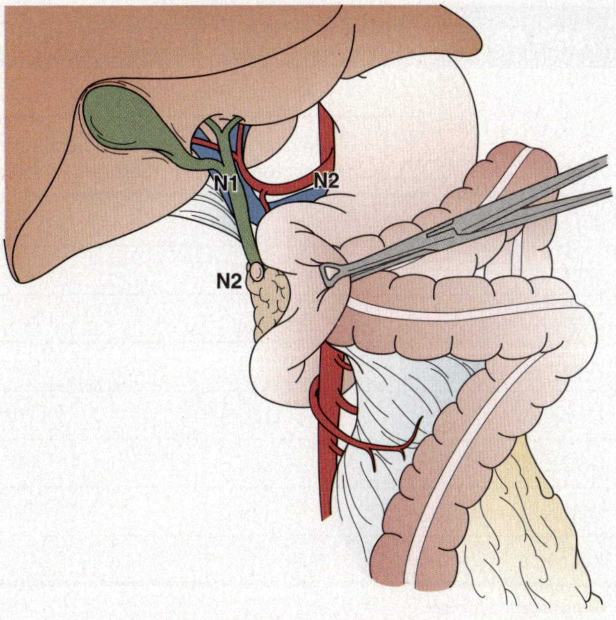

Figure 60.4. Illustration of the highest peripancreatic lymph node.

the extent of biliary involvement as well as to palliate symptoms of biliary obstruction. A mid–bile duct obstruction not caused by gallstones is gallbladder cancer until proved otherwise (**Fig. 60.3**).

In patients who present with incidentally discovered gallbladder cancer following cholecystectomy, staging should be performed with high-quality CT of the chest, abdomen, and pelvis. Recent data suggest there may also be a role for PET/CT in this setting.[12]

Surgery

2 The curative option for patients with gallbladder cancer is complete surgical resection. It is essential for optimal patient care that patients with gallbladder cancer be recognized before laparoscopic cholecystectomy is performed, because of the risk of bile spillage, with its potential for subsequent carcinomatosis.

Role of Staging Laparoscopy

Because gallbladder cancer has such a propensity to spread intraabdominally, this tumor is ideal for detection of intraabdominal metastases with laparoscopy. This is demonstrated by the fact that up to 23% of patients are found to have unresectable disease at the time of laparoscopy, and this yield is >50% in patients with locally advanced disease.[13] These patients can begin other forms of systemic therapy earlier and may undergo the procedure as an outpatient. Particularly because patients with unresectable disease have a median survival of only 6 months, the impact on quality of life, including decreased length of stay in the hospital, cannot be overemphasized.

Cholecystectomy with or without Partial Hepatectomy

The results of treatment, as well as the scope of operation, are related to depth of tumor penetration. For tumors limited to the muscular layer of the gallbladder (T1), there is near-universal agreement that simple cholecystectomy is adequate. T1 tumors have not yet invaded the subserosal layer, which contains lymphatics, and therefore lymphadenectomy is not required. Attesting to the fact that early gallbladder carcinoma is completely curable, simple cholecystectomy has resulted in 90% to 100% survival when early cancer is an incidental finding after elective cholecystectomy.[14]

The extent of surgical resection for T1b tumors is more controversial, with recommendations historically ranging from simple cholecystectomy to radical excision, including hepatectomy. The current consensus for these tumors when found incidentally after laparoscopic cholecystectomy, for medically fit patients, is to proceed with re-resection to determine with certainty if there was residual disease and to ensure negative margins. In a series of 135 patients who underwent reexploration following laparoscopic cholecystectomy, 61% of all and 36% of those with T1b primary tumors were found to have residual disease.[14] For T1b or greater tumors, extended resection with cholecystectomy combined with resection of liver segments IVb and V and portal lymphadenectomy is recommended.[14–17]

There is currently no international consensus on the extent of lymphadenectomy that is appropriate for gallbladder cancer. Extensive lymphadenectomy including para-aortic nodes is advocated in the East, but is not universally accepted. Recently, a technique of intraoperative nodal staging was proposed that entails sampling the highest peripancreatic lymph node for frozen section. This is the lymph node situated between the N1 and N2 nodal stations at the junction of the bile duct and the superior border of the head of the pancreas (**Fig. 60.4**). Metastatic disease to this node has been shown to be a poor prognostic factor.[18]

Dissection of lymph nodes should include all tissues from the bifurcation of the hepatic ducts to the distal CBD. Proponents of this approach advocate liver resection on the basis that it is the only way to obtain an adequate margin on the hepatic side of the gallbladder and resection of the regional nodes allows the best chance for complete tumor clearance. For all of these reasons, simple cholecystectomy is inadequate for T2 or greater tumors. When larger anatomic hepatic resections have been performed in patients with T2 tumors, it has increased the 5-year survival from 25% to 40% after simple cholecystectomy to 70% to 100% after radical resection.[19]

For T3 and T4 lesions, there is a high likelihood of intraperitoneal and hematogenous spread and significant morbidity from the radical procedures that are often necessary for excision of local disease. Recent series, however, support an aggressive approach to resection of these large tumors, particularly if no indication of nodal involvement is found and negative margins can be achieved. For T3 and resectable T4 tumors, a minimal resection includes segments IVb and V. Extended right hepatectomy (segments IV, V, VI, VII, and VIII) may be necessary to obtain complete resection; recent data suggest that this procedure should not be done empirically if it is not necessary to obtain negative margins due to increased

Table 60.1. Five-Year Survival after Resection for Gallbladder Cancer Stratified by T Stage

	T1 or T2 Tumors		T3 or T4 Tumors	
Author	**Simple Cholecystectomy (%)**	**Radical Cholecystectomy or Segmental Resection (%)**	**Simple Cholecystectomy (%)**	**Radical Cholecystectomy or Segmental Resection (%)**
Kai et al.	25	60 (T2)	—	—
Jensen et al.	29	42	—	—
Mayo et al.	16	53	8	11
Balakrishnan et al.	71	80	18	23
Jung et al.	48 (T2)	78 (T2)	—	—
Goel et al.	—	80	—	12
D'Angelica et al.	—	79[b]		30
Roos et al.	—	—	—	37

[a]No significant difference.
[b]10 patients (10%) with simple cholecystectomy included.

morbidity and lack of survival benefit.[20,21] With aggressive resection, long-term survival can be achieved even for patients with these more advanced tumors. **Table 60.1** summarizes recent studies reporting outcomes after surgical resection of gallbladder cancer relative to different T stages.[21–26]

Surgical exploration should be performed for all patients without medical contraindications. If a T1 tumor is suspected, a cholecystectomy and biopsy of regional nodes should be performed after thorough examination of the abdominal cavity for any signs of tumor dissemination. The pathology and depth of penetration should be confirmed by frozen section, and the procedure terminated if a T1 tumor with negative margins is confirmed. For T2 lesions, a radical cholecystectomy (with resection of segments IVb and V) with lymphadenectomy should be performed. For T3 lesion and resectable T4 lesions, a segment IVb and V resection or extended right hepatectomy is performed if needed to obtain negative margins. Similarly, bile duct resection should only be performed if necessary to achieve negative margins.

Complete regional lymphadenectomy should be performed, skeletonizing the CBD, hepatic artery, and portal vein. Short-term postoperative outcomes following resection of gallbladder cancer have remained relatively stable over time, with postoperative morbidity occurring in 30% to 40% of patients, and mortality occurring in <5%.[23,26]

Neoadjuvant and Adjuvant Therapy

Very few randomized trials have been completed to inform the role of neoadjuvant and adjuvant therapy for gallbladder cancer. Given the relative rarity of these malignancies in the United States, large-scale, randomized trials are feasible only in the context of a multiinstitutional or cooperative group
3 setting. Consensus guidelines state that neoadjuvant therapy should be considered for patients with gallbladder cancer who have jaundice, although there is little data supporting any one regimen. Commonly used regimens include combinations of gemcitabine with oxaliplatin, cisplatin, or capecitabine, or 5-fluorouracil–based regimens. A meta-analysis published in 2019 identified 474 patients with gallbladder cancer treated in eight studies with neoadjuvant therapy and surgery or surgery alone and concluded that data were insufficient for routine use of neoadjuvant therapy, but it is recommended for patients presenting with jaundice.[27] These patients have particularly poor outcomes with surgery alone and have been shown to have response rates >50% to neoadjuvant therapy.[28]

A multicenter phase II trial of adjuvant capecitabine and gemcitabine followed by concurrent capecitabine and radiation therapy was conducted by the Southwest Oncology Group for patients with resected gallbladder cancer or extrahepatic cholangiocarcinoma. The results of this study were published in 2015 and showed promising findings of 65% 2-year survival.[29] These studies suggest that patients with gallbladder cancer with high risk for recurrence (T2 or greater, node-positive, or margin-positive), who did not receive neoadjuvant therapy, should be considered for adjuvant treatment with systemic chemotherapy or chemoradiation.

Prognosis

The 5-year survival rate for all patients with gallbladder cancer is less than 5% in most series, with a median survival of 6 months. This is primarily because most patients present with unresectable disease. Of those patients undergoing resection, survival is dependent on depth of penetration and nodal status. Nearly 100% survival is reported after simple cholecystectomy for T1a disease, whereas patients with T2 and T3 tumors without nodal disease have a 5-year survival greater than 50%. Node positivity is an ominous finding, with few series reporting 5-year survivors. **Table 60.2** summarizes results of modern series of curative intent treatment of gallbladder cancer, with 5-year overall survival ranging from 32% to 66%.[20,23,24,26,30–33]

Table 60.2. Results of Modern Series of Multimodality, Curative-Intent Treatment of Gallbladder Cancer

Author	Number Resected	Mortality (%)	5-Year Survival (%)
Kai et al.	90	2	40
Jensen et al.	443	—	42
Creasy et al.	255	—	43
Romatoski et al.	299	—	38
Goel et al.	172	5	44
Das et al.	161	—	66
Ozturk et al.	94	—	32

Follow-Up after Resection for Gallbladder Cancer

The most common sites of recurrence after resection of gallbladder cancer include carcinomatosis, intrahepatic metastases, or nodal recurrence in the retroperitoneum. For most tumors, local recurrence is found synchronously with diffuse intraabdominal spread. When jaundice or cholangitis is the presenting symptom of possible recurrence, a nonsurgical palliative approach using percutaneous transhepatic cholangiogram (PTC) or endoscopic retrograde cholangiopancreatography (ERCP) with stenting is usually favored unless a benign postsurgical stricture is suspected. Because of the rapid growth of tumor in patients with recurrence, the hospitalization and recovery time from a surgical bypass is usually not justified for recurrences resulting in biliary obstruction.

The routine follow-up of a patient after resection of gallbladder cancer includes office visits every 3 months with physical examination and measurement of liver function tests, and cross-sectional imaging every 3 to 6 months for the first 2 years. In patients who remain free of disease at 2 years, follow-up should be every 6 to 12 months for up to 5 years. CA 19-9 may be followed if it was elevated at baseline. If recurrence is identified, molecular profiling should be performed and options of systemic therapy, clinical trial, or best supportive care discussed.

Issues for the Future

Clearly, improving our ability to recognize early gallbladder cancer in high-risk geographic areas would have an important impact on outcome in these patients. This will likely require implementation of screening programs in high-risk areas, which could result in prophylactic cholecystectomy. In addition, standardization of minimum pathologic assessment of gallbladder specimens in high-risk areas is important to allow for accurate diagnosis, staging, and treatment of patients.

Studies on characterization of molecular aberrations in gallbladder cancer by next-generation sequencing have led to the discovery of targetable mutations and the development of novel therapies, and these studies should continue into the future to identify new targets. In addition, there is a role for neoadjuvant therapy for patients with locoregionally advanced gallbladder cancer given their poor prognosis following surgery and clinical trials are needed.

CHOLANGIOCARCINOMA

Cholangiocarcinoma may arise within the liver (intrahepatic cholangiocarcinoma [ICC] or peripheral cholangiocarcinoma), at the liver hilum (hilar cholangiocarcinoma or Klatskin tumor), or in the extrahepatic bile duct (extrahepatic cholangiocarcinoma [ECC]). While all arise from the biliary epithelium, the location of these tumors affects prognosis as well as the potential for curative resection.

Resection of biliary neoplasms, particularly hilar cholangiocarcinoma, often requires radical resections and complex biliary reconstructions that should be performed only at high-volume, experienced centers. There is also a role for surgery in palliation for these cancers by providing biliary bypass for jaundiced patients with unresectable tumors. Because disease is often diagnosed late in the course and because complex operative techniques are required for potentially curative resection, these tumors represent one of the greatest challenges for definitive treatment.

INCIDENCE

The incidence of ICC in the United States is approximately 0.7/100,000 with a similar mortality. During the last 30 years, it appears that both the incidence and mortality in the United States are increasing.[34] The overall incidence of hilar cholangiocarcinoma, the most common type, is 1.0/100,000 per year in the United States, although rates are higher in other geographic regions such as Israel and Japan. Using the Surveillance, Epidemiology, and End Results (SEER) Medicare databases, Welzel et al. noted hepatitis C virus infection, chronic nonalcoholic liver disease and obesity, and smoking being associated only with ICC and not ECC, possibly explaining the divergent trends in incidence.[35] Cholangiocarcinomas arise slightly more often in males, with a male-to-female ratio of 1.3:1 and an average age of 50 to 70 years.

Known risk factors for cholangiocarcinoma include primary sclerosing cholangitis, ulcerative colitis, choledochal cysts, and biliary tract infection, either with *Clonorchis* or in chronic typhoid carriers. Some industrial chemicals (eg, nitrosamines, dioxin, asbestos, and polychlorinated biphenyls) have also been implicated in the pathogenesis of cholangiocarcinoma.[35]

Pathology and Staging

More than 90% of bile duct cancers are adenocarcinomas. They are morphologically described as nodular, which is the most common, scirrhous, diffusely infiltrating, or papillary. Histologic subtypes include acinar, ductular, trabecular, alveolar, and papillary. Papillary tumors have an improved outcome. Much less common types of bile duct tumors include cystadenocarcinomas, intraductal papillary neoplasms of the bile duct (IPNBs), hemangioendotheliomas, and mucoepidermoid carcinomas. In patients with ICC, negative prognostic signs include vascular invasion, multiple tumors, and lymph node metastases.[34]

Historically, ECCs have been classified according to their location in the upper (60%), middle (15% to 20%), or lower third (15% to 20%) of the bile duct. Middle-third lesions arise between the cystic duct and the superior border of the duodenum. Lower-third lesions are found below the superior border of the duodenum but above the ampulla. The problem with this classification is that the anatomic landmarks are somewhat arbitrary and not clinically useful. A more useful classification is to divide these lesions into upper-half or lower-half tumors, based on the location of the cystic duct as it enters the common duct (in the case of normal anatomy). The usefulness of this classification scheme is that it allows the surgeon to delineate whether a hepatic or pancreatic resection will be required for clearance of tumor.

While the American Joint Commission on Cancer (AJCC) follows tumor node metastasis (TNM) staging for bile duct cancers, other staging systems have been created that attempt to incorporate clinically important indicators of resectability for hilar cholangiocarcinoma that are defined preoperatively, including hepatic lobe atrophy or portal vein involvement.[36] With the increasing acceptance of major hepatic resection for these tumors, this preoperative staging system attempts to define whether there is ipsilateral involvement alone, because tumors with bilateral extension past the primary biliary radicles are not resectable.

Clinical Findings and Diagnosis

The presentation of patients with cholangiocarcinoma is variable. Patients with hilar or extrahepatic tumors most commonly present with painless jaundice. Symptoms of mild right upper quadrant pain, pruritus, anorexia, malaise, and weight loss may also be reported. Cholangitis is the presenting symptom in 10% to 30% of patients. Some patients, particularly those with ICC may be asymptomatic and have their tumors discovered incidentally or on evaluation for abnormal liver function tests. Many of these patients will present to the surgeon with a biopsy showing adenocarcinoma without a known primary tumor. The standard evaluation in these patients should include tumor markers including carcinoembryonic antigen (CEA) or α-fetoprotein (AFP); upper and lower endoscopy to evaluate for a gastrointestinal source; CT scan to assess for a primary tumor in the gastrointestinal tract or pancreas; and, in women, a mammogram. If no site of primary disease is found, in most patients, the diagnosis is ICC.

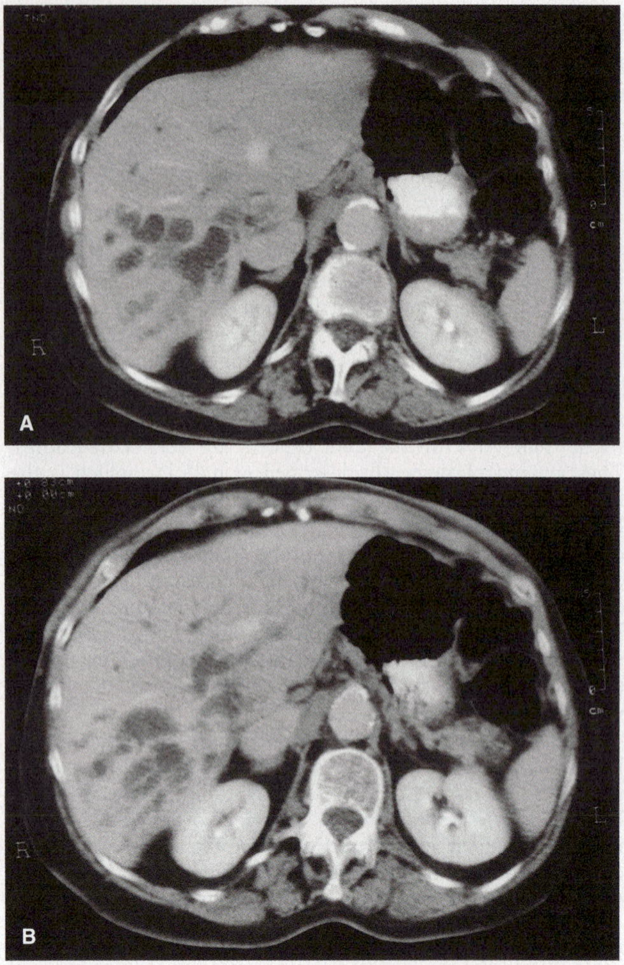

Figure 60.5. Computed tomography scan in a patient with hilar cholangiocarcinoma, demonstrating dilated intrahepatic ducts in the right lobe (**A:** predominantly posterior sector, **B:** both anterior and posterior sectors) but inability to directly visualize tumor.

On CT, cholangiocarcinomas most often appear as hypodense masses with irregular margins on precontrast phase images, with peripheral rim enhancement on arterial phase, followed by progressive hyperattenuation on venous and delayed phases. Intrahepatic lesions often exhibit associated capsular retraction and segmental/lobar atrophy and ductal dilatation. Hilar and proximal extrahepatic lesions demonstrate dilated intrahepatic biliary ducts with a normal, collapsed gallbladder, and, depending on the level of the tumor, a nondilated or partially dilated extrahepatic biliary tree (**Fig. 60.5**). While conventional CT is useful for assessment for extrahepatic, metastatic disease and perihilar adenopathy, high-resolution CT and/or MRI are required for accurate assessment of the tumor and for determination of resectability (**Figs. 60.6** and **60.7**). Portal vein patency can be determined with ultrasound, CT, or MRI. Particularly for hilar tumors, signs of hepatic lobar atrophy should be carefully sought because this indicates ipsilateral portal vein involvement by tumor. MRCP offers the potential of evaluating parenchymal, vascular, biliary, and nodal involvement with a single noninvasive examination.

In most centers, direct cholangiography is used to evaluate the extent of biliary involvement and provide palliation for jaundice. ERCP has little role to play in high biliary obstruction because opacification of the proximal biliary tree is difficult. ERCP, however, can be effectively used to image more distal lesions.

In many cases, it is difficult to obtain pathologic confirmation of cholangiocarcinoma, even with the use of biliary brushings and cytology obtained at the time of direct cholangiography. In these cases, patients may be offered surgical therapy based on clinical suspicion and radiographic appearance.

Surgery

Surgical excision of cholangiocarcinoma is the treatment of choice, with no other potentially curative therapy available. Mortality is high and often occurs within a year of diagnosis without treatment. The immediate causes of death are most commonly hepatic failure or cholangitis related to tumor growth and inadequate drainage of the biliary tree. The goals of surgery are complete removal of tumor with R0 margins while leaving a sufficient liver remnant, and establishing adequate biliary drainage. Patients with ICC require additional consideration. Those patients with multifocal, and especially bilobar intrahepatic tumors, even if technically resectable with negative margins and adequate remnant liver, should not be considered for resection. These patients have very poor prognosis. What remains controversial is whether peritumoral satellite lesions also represent metastatic disease. Because this is unknown and surgery is the only potentially curative therapy for these patients, satellite lesions are not currently considered an absolute contraindication to resection.

Hilar cholangiocarcinoma is often unresectable due to local factors. These include invasion of the main portal vein or both the right and left portal veins and hepatic arteries and tumor extension into second-order biliary radicals of both right and left hepatic lobes. By contrast, tumors extending into second- or third-order biliary radicles on one side of the liver without vascular involvement can be resected for cure. It has become

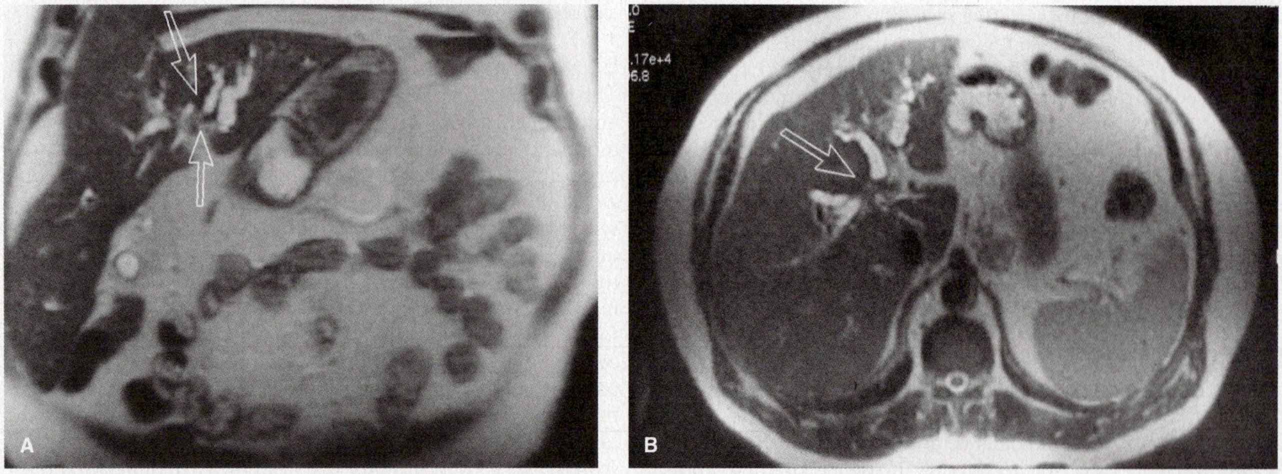

Figure 60.6. Coronal (**A**) and axial (**B**) magnetic resonance imaging in a patient with hilar cholangiocarcinoma. Dilated intrahepatic ducts are present with a soft tissue density consistent with tumor (*arrows*).

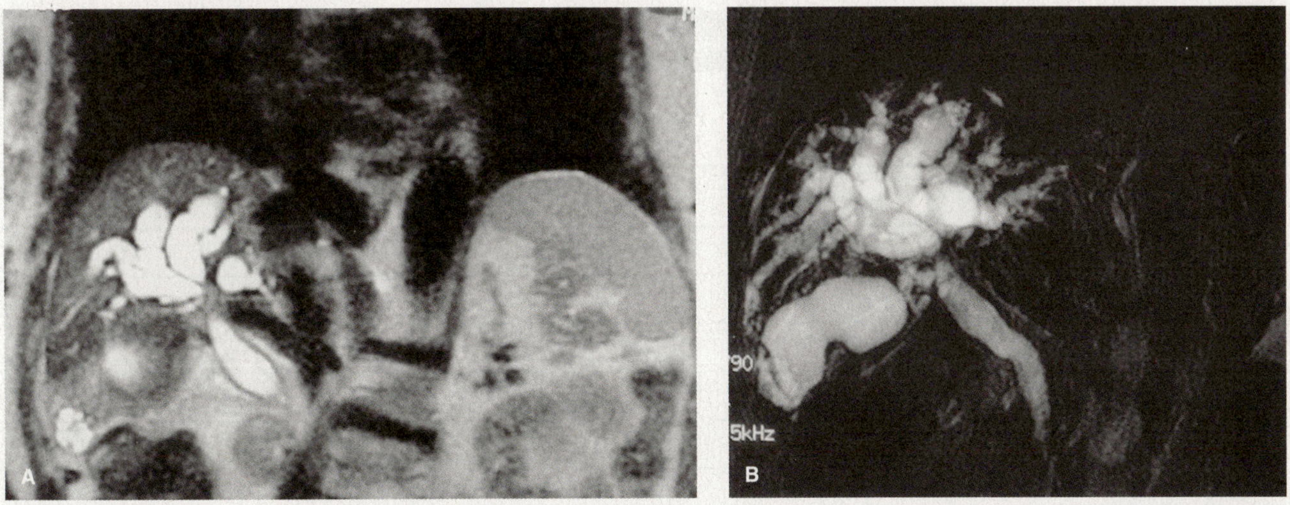

Figure 60.7. Coronal (**A**) magnetic resonance imaging and magnetic resonance cholangiopancreatography (**B**) in a patient with hilar cholangiocarcinoma, demonstrating dilated intrahepatic ducts narrowing at the area of obstruction.

clear over the last three decades that curative treatment for patients with tumors of the hilum or those involving the upper half of the bile duct depends on aggressive excision that often requires a major liver resection. Historically, treatment of hilar cholangiocarcinoma was associated with mortality as high as 30%. With major improvements in the safety of these operations at high-volume centers, resection of hilar tumors now results in mortality of less than 10%, even when liver resections are required.[37]

Role of Staging Laparoscopy

Because of the potential morbidity of a laparotomy that has no therapeutic benefit, staging laparoscopy has been advocated to save patients from unnecessary laparotomy. In patients with hilar cholangiocarcinoma, 45% will benefit from staging laparoscopy because of detection of occult extrahepatic disease.[38] Laparoscopy is a very sensitive means to detect peritoneal metastases or additional intrahepatic disease through the use of laparoscopic ultrasound but is less sensitive in detecting nodal metastases or locally invasive tumors.

Partial Hepatectomy with or without Bile Duct Resection

The extent of hepatectomy required for resection of cholangiocarcinoma is dependent on the tumor location in relation to the portal inflow and venous outflow of the liver. Intraoperative ultrasound is a useful adjunct for assessment of tumor extent and for small satellite lesions that may not be apparent on cross-sectional imaging.

Small ICCs may be removed by nonanatomic wedge resection, but these tumors are often large and require extended right or left hepatectomy. For hilar and proximal hepatic duct lesions, complete resection usually requires combined biliary and hepatic resection with or without major vascular reconstruction. In addition, caudate resection may be required due to direct extension into caudate biliary radicles or parenchyma. Resection of the extrahepatic bile duct with Roux-en-Y hepaticojejunostomy to the remnant duct is required in these cases but is not recommended unless necessary for margin negative resection. Intraoperative assessment of the bile duct resection margin should be performed if additional duct can potentially be taken. If not, assessment on permanent sectioning is sufficient.

Lymphadenectomy

Regional lymphadenectomy is essential for accurate staging of cholangiocarcinoma, and may be important for locoregional disease control, but has historically been underperformed for intrahepatic and hilar tumors. Recent data have shown that lymph node metastases are present in 30% to 40% of patients.[39–41] Regional lymph nodes include those along the porta hepatis, the hepatoduodenal ligament, the hepatic artery for essentially all patients. In addition, for those with primary tumors of the right hemiliver, retropancreatic nodes should be removed. For those with primary tumors of the left hemiliver, perigastric lesser curve nodes (levels 1, 3, and 5) should be removed.[37] A recent study utilizing the SEER database noted that removal of at least six lymph nodes is recommended for accurate staging of ICC.[41]

Pancreaticoduodenectomy

For cholangiocarcinoma of the lower half of the extrahepatic bile duct, pancreaticoduodenectomy is requiring for complete tumor extirpation. The proximal bile duct margin should be assessed by frozen section to ensure tumor clearance. Regional lymphadenectomy is inherent in this procedure.

Liver Transplantation for Hilar CC and the Mayo Protocol

Orthotopic liver transplantation (OLT) was thought to hold promise for patients with hilar CC, because of the ability to achieve adequate margins by complete hepatectomy. Unfortunately, when used as a single treatment modality, results have been poor. Three- and 5-year survival rates have been reported at 25% to 30%.[42] Because of this poor outcome, Mayo Clinic developed a protocol combining neoadjuvant therapy with liver transplant, based on a strategy initially developed by the University of Nebraska. This protocol uses high-dose neoadjuvant 5-fluorouracil and 4000 to 4500 cGy external beam radiation, followed by transcatheter iridium-192 brachytherapy with a target dose of 2000 to 3000 cGy and then liver transplantation.[43] 5-FU is given during radiation and capecitabine following this until transplantation. Inclusion criteria include (i) locally advanced unresectable disease with either positive intraluminal brush cytology, biliary aneuploidy by digital image analysis (DIA) and fluorescent in situ hybridization, positive intraluminal biopsy, or CA19-9 ≥100 in the setting of a radiographic malignant stricture; (ii) primary sclerosing cholangitis with resectable disease; and (iii) absence of medical contraindications for OLT. If a mass lesion is seen, it must be <3 cm. Exclusion criteria include (i) extrahepatic disease including regional lymph node involvement; (ii) uncontrolled infection; (iii) prior attempt at resection; (iv) prior treatment with radiation or chemotherapy; and (v) previous malignancy within 5 years. Prior to transplantation, patients undergo a staging laparotomy, at which time biopsy of perihilar lymph nodes as well as any lymph nodes or nodules suspicious for

Table 60.3. Results after Resection for Hilar Cholangiocarcinoma

Author	*N*	Percent Resected	Postoperative Mortality (%)	5-Year Survival (%)	Survival (Months)	
					Mean	Median
Jarnagin et al.	225	71	10	27		35
Rea et al.	46		9	26		28
Jang et al.	48		0	48		
Konstadoulakis et al.	73	81	7	35		
Yubin et al.	115	100	2	22		40
Roos et al.	135	100	15	30		42
Zhang et al.	159	100	6	40		49
Zeng et al.	282	100	6	30	—	28
Ahmad Al-Saffar et al.	73	100	10	—	—	29

tumor is performed. Only patients with negative staging operations remain eligible for transplantation.[43]

The prolonged course of neoadjuvant therapy, staging laparotomy, and time on the OLT waiting list provides an opportunity to exclude patients demonstrating disease progression. This highly rigorous selection bias in favor of patients with biologically favorable disease is reflected in the early outcomes published from the Mayo group. In a recent review of 71 patients enrolled in this transplant protocol, only 38 underwent transplantation (38%). These patients were compared to 26 patients (of 54 explored, 48%) who underwent successful resection. When compared to those undergoing resection (some with node-positive disease), patients undergoing transplantation were younger ($p < .001$) and more likely to have inflammatory bowel disease ($p < .03$) and primary sclerosing cholangitis (PSC) ($p < .001$). It is important that only 38% of patients had histologically proven cancer. In these highly disparate groups, 5-year survival was 82% after transplantation (38 patients) compared to 21% after resection of 26 patients ($p = .022$).[44] There were also fewer recurrences in the transplant patients (13% vs 27%), and recurrences occurred later after transplantation than after resection (mean 40 months vs 21 months). Direct comparisons are difficult with this study given the differences between groups. A recent meta-analysis of patients with unresectable hilar cholangiocarcinoma reported 5-year overall survival of 65% for those who underwent neoadjuvant therapy followed by transplantation, versus 32% for those who had transplantation alone.[45]

At present, OLT cannot be considered a standard form of therapy for hilar cholangiocarcinoma for patients with resectable disease, with the exception of tumors arising in the setting of PSC, but it does offer a potential option for those with unresectable tumors who fit the rigorous inclusion and exclusion criteria of these protocols.

Prognosis after Resection

Results of modern studies on resection of hilar cholangiocarcinoma are summarized in **Table 60.3**. In patients amenable to curative resection, the median survival is 28 to 49 months with a 5-year survival rate of 22% to 45%.[33,46–52] Surgical resection provides both improved survival and improved quality of life. The greatest risk factors for recurrence include the presence of positive margins, and node-positive tumors.

In patients with ICC, recent studies have shown 3-year survival rates as high as 60% have been reported, with 5-year survival rates of 30% to 40%.[53–56] A recent meta-analysis has suggested that anatomic resection is superior to nonanatomic wedge resection for ICC.[54] Patients with unresectable disease have a median survival of 12 months. Thus, completely resected ICC appears to have an improved prognosis over proximal (hilar) cholangiocarcinoma. Patients with cholangiocarcinoma arising in the distal bile duct have both an increased resectability rate and improved prognosis over those with hilar cholangiocarcinomas. Patients with resectable distal bile duct cancer have a 5-year survival rate of 30% to 50% in modern series, with a decreased survival if nodes are involved with tumor.[55]

Unresectable Cholangiocarcinoma

4 For patients with unresectable hilar cholangiocarcinoma, biliary drainage is necessary. Nonoperative palliative biliary decompression can be accomplished with percutaneous or endoscopic stenting, depending on the level of obstruction. Proximal lesions are usually approached percutaneously with placement of expandable stents or drainage catheters (**Fig. 60.8**). Internal stents result in fewer electrolyte abnormalities and improvement in patient comfort, although morbidity and mortality occurs in up to 30% of patients and stent occlusion is common. Newer techniques to perform external biliary stenting without crossing the ampulla appear to be associated with a lower risk of cholangitis and should be considered, as recurrent uncontrolled sepsis from cholangitis due to undrained liver segments is a frequent cause of demise in unresectable patients. Systemic therapy options have improved for patients with advanced, unresectable disease. In 2022, the TOPAZ-1 trial reported an estimate 24-month overall survival of nearly 25% for patients treated with durvalumab plus chemotherapy.[57,58] This study, along with the KEYNOTE-966 study which utilized pembrolizumab, le to the FDA approval of immune checkpoint inhibitors for biliary tract cancers.[57,59]

Palliative surgical bypass such as a segment III bypass (**Fig. 60.9**) can also be performed, however is less often necessary with current availability of advanced endoscopic and percutaneous techniques.

Liver-directed therapies such as transarterial chemoembolization (TACE), transarterial radioembolization (TARE), and ablation (microwave ablation, stereotactic body radiation therapy) are also potential treatment options for patients with ICC who are not candidates for resection. These therapies have not been evaluated in a randomized prospective

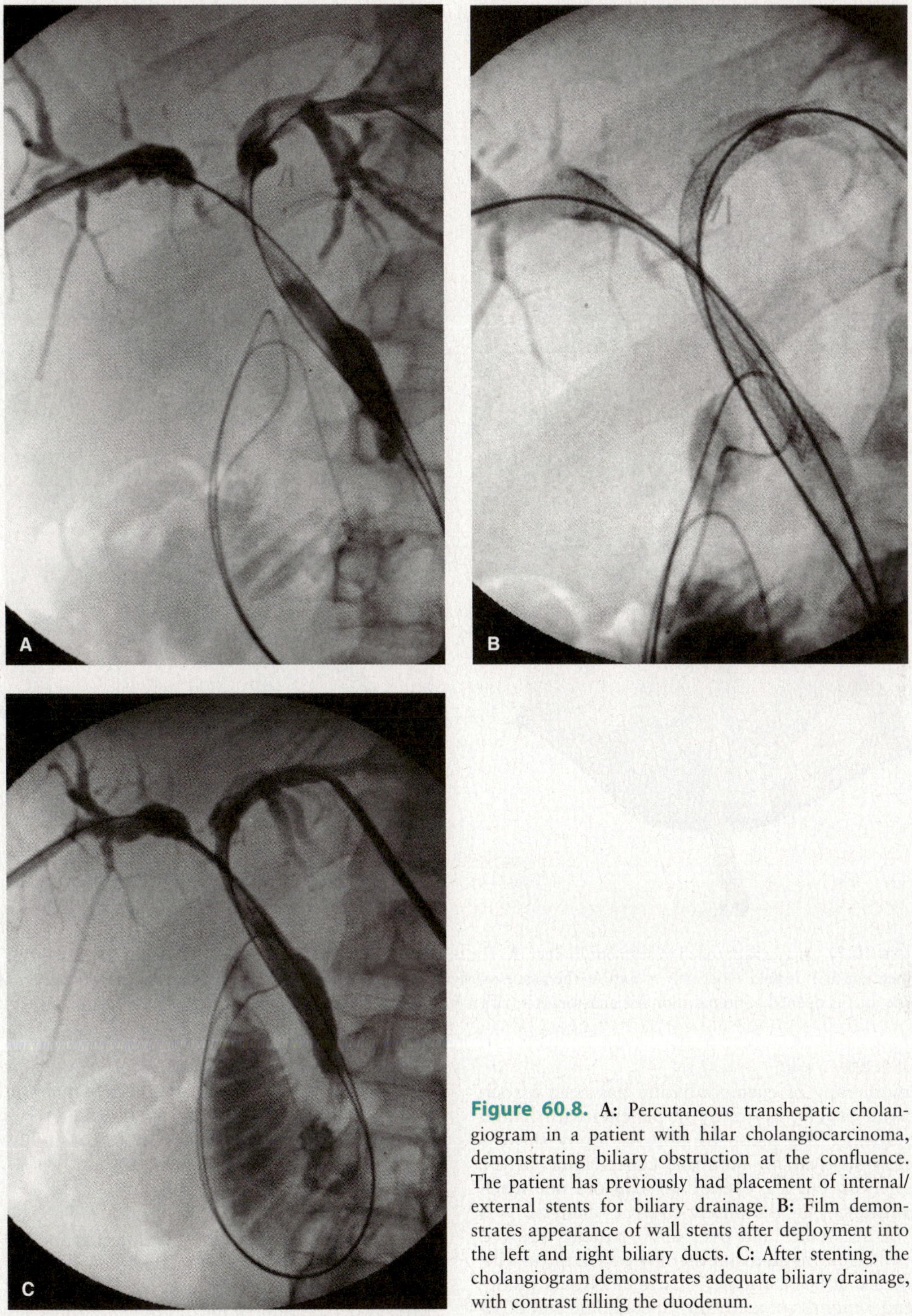

Figure 60.8. **A:** Percutaneous transhepatic cholangiogram in a patient with hilar cholangiocarcinoma, demonstrating biliary obstruction at the confluence. The patient has previously had placement of internal/external stents for biliary drainage. **B:** Film demonstrates appearance of wall stents after deployment into the left and right biliary ducts. **C:** After stenting, the cholangiogram demonstrates adequate biliary drainage, with contrast filling the duodenum.

trial, but have shown promising results in both retrospective and early-phase prospective studies.[55]

Hepatic Arterial Chemotherapy

In patients with unresectable ICC, 70% die from advanced liver disease, thus the focus becomes controlling the liver disease. Increasing data demonstrate efficacy for floxuridine (FUDR) delivered by hepatic artery pump, with many early studies from Memorial Sloan Kettering Cancer Center (MSKCC) and a recent multicenter phase II study from the Netherlands showing improved OS compared to historical controls receiving gemcitabine/cisplatin, with OS of 22.1 months, despite 2/3 having multifocal disease.[60–62] Moreover, 8% were ultimately resected after downstaging. These results mirror several phase II MSKCC studies.[61,62] Hepatic arterial infusion (HAI) FUDR can also be followed by consolidative radiotherapy which allows further control of liver disease.

Neoadjuvant Therapy

There are limited clinical trial data to define a standard regimen or definitive benefit, and thus clinical trial participation is encouraged. Clinically, neoadjuvant therapy is considered in patients with more advanced disease, such as ICC patients with grossly involved porta hepatis nodes, or when downstaging may result in improved ability to achieve complete resection. When utilized, systemic regimens are extrapolated from results in the metastatic setting such as durvalumab + gemcitabine + cisplatin or pembrolizumab + gemcitabine + cisplatin or other standard chemotherapy combinations without immunotherapy.

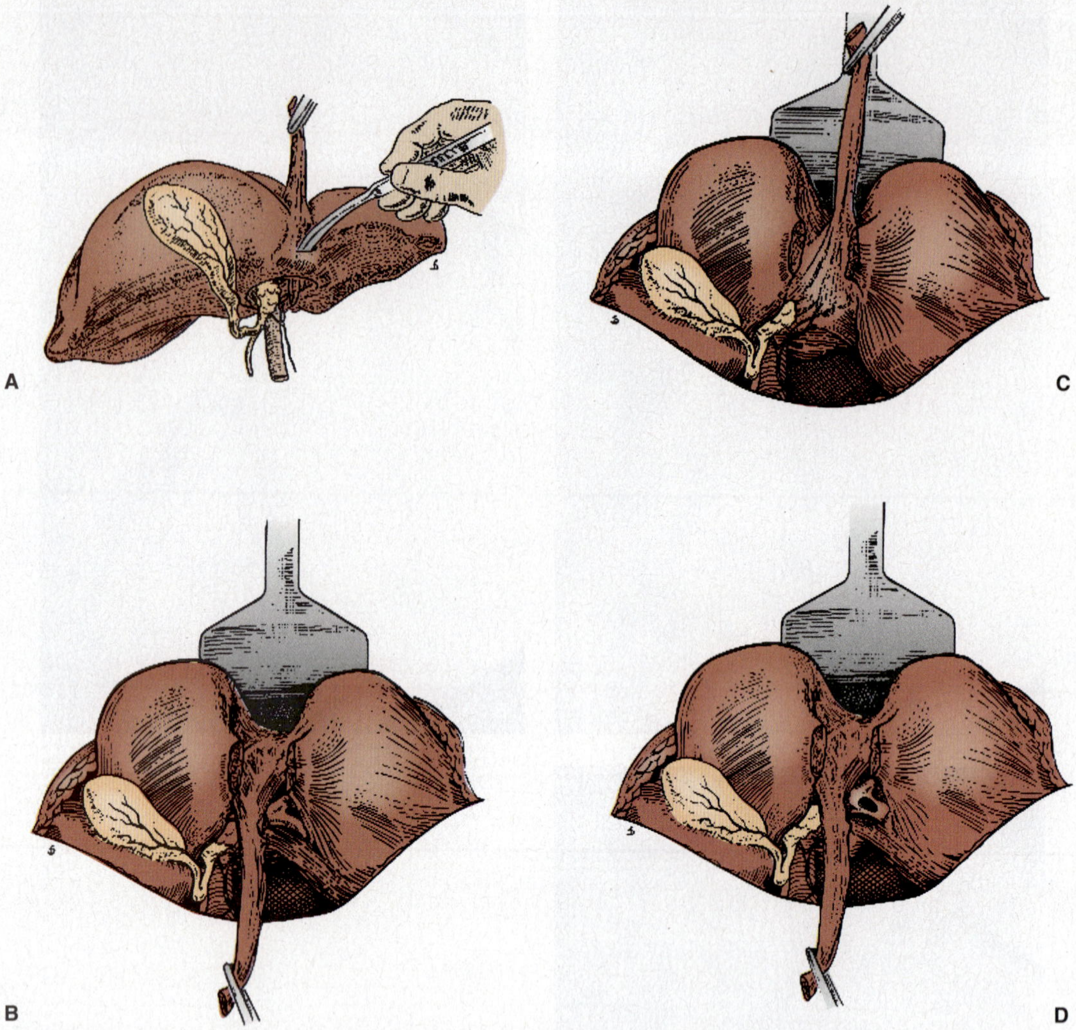

Figure 60.9. Surgical approach to segment III duct. **A:** The bridge of tissue present at the base of the liver is divided. **B:** The ligamentum teres is held superiorly to expose the tissue overlying the segment III duct. **C:** The segment III duct is exposed. **D:** The duct is opened in preparation for anastomosis with a Roux-en-Y jejunal limb. (Courtesy of Dr. L. H. Blumgart.)

Adjuvant Therapy

Adjuvant chemotherapy or chemoradiation has been associated with survival benefit, especially in patients with lymph node–positive disease. The phase III BILCAP study showed improved overall survival for adjuvant capecitabine in the per-protocol analysis, but the overall survival did not reach statistical significance in the intent-to-treat analysis.[63] A meta-analysis of 20 studies and over 6500 patients showed that the greatest benefit for adjuvant therapy was in those with LN-positive disease and R1 disease.[64] Current NCCN guidelines recommend 6 months of adjuvant capecitabine and 2019 ASCO guidelines agree with the recommendation, but also recommend that chemoradiotherapy (CRT) should be offered for R1 margin.[65]

Follow-Up after Resection of Cholangiocarcinoma

Recurrence following resection of ICC is within the liver in 60% of patients. The most likely site of recurrence after resection of hilar cholangiocarcinoma is locoregionally within the bile duct, regional lymph nodes, or liver. Therapy for recurrence is palliative and consists of doublet chemotherapy (gemcitabine/cisplatin) with or without immunotherapy. The main symptoms of recurrence that demand palliation are pruritus or cholangitis associated with jaundice, and can usually be managed by ERCP or PTC, depending on the level of obstruction.

Routine follow-up consists of office visits every 3 months with physical examination and measurement of liver function tests. Surveillance cross-sectional imaging is recommended every 3 to 6 months for the first 2 years following resection and then every 6 to 12 months for up to 5 years.

Issues for the Future

Further studies are needed to develop effective neoadjuvant therapies for cholangiocarcinoma. Continued assessment of novel drugs and radiosensitizers, and biologic agents is warranted. A better understanding of the molecular pathogenesis and genetics of bile duct cancers may lead to new therapeutic strategies and possibly preventive strategies for high-risk populations.

BENIGN GALLBLADDER NEOPLASMS

Incidence

Benign tumors of the biliary tract are rare, but have been reported more frequently as imaging modalities (eg, ultrasound and CT scan) have come into widespread and frequent use. In patients undergoing cholecystectomy, the reported incidence of benign gallbladder tumors is less than 3%.[7]

Pathology

Polyps and Pseudotumors

Benign gallbladder tumors are most frequently polyps or polypoid lesions. The incidence of polyps in asymptomatic

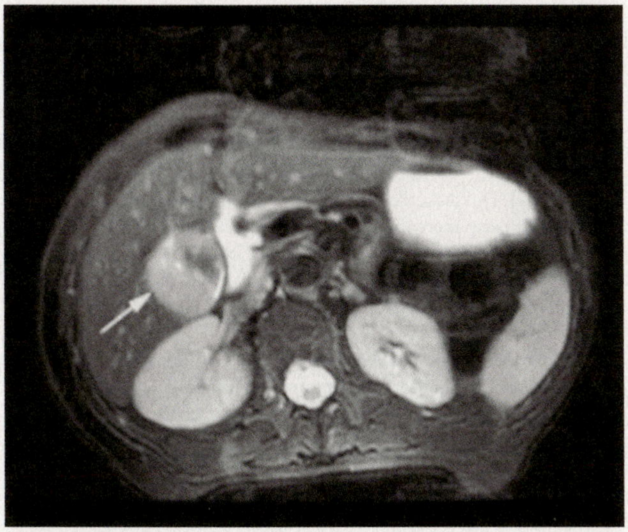

Figure 60.10. T2-weighted magnetic resonance imaging scan showing a sessile polyp within the gallbladder (*arrow*) that was malignant on histologic examination.

patients is about 5%. Cholesterol polyps (cholesterolosis), accounting for half of all gallbladder polypoid lesions, result from epithelium-covered, cholesterol-laden macrophages in the lamina propria. These lesions are likely a result of an error in cholesterol metabolism. They extend from the mucosa on a narrow stalk, grossly appearing as yellow spots on the mucosal surface. Nearly all are multiple, and most are less than 10 mm in size. When a polyp is pedunculated, it is benign in most cases; alternatively, sessile "polyps" are more often malignant (**Fig. 60.10**). Inflammatory polyps result from chronic inflammation and extend by a narrow vascularized stalk into the gallbladder lumen. These lesions are considered benign.

Adenomas

Gallbladder adenomas are found infrequently. They may be tubular or papillary, both arising from the epithelial layer of the gallbladder. Multiple papillary adenomas, or papillomas, are called *papillomatosis*. A direct association between benign adenoma, adenoma containing carcinoma in situ, and invasive carcinoma has been demonstrated; thus these lesions are considered premalignant. Malignant transformation, however, has only rarely been reported, primarily from large adenomas. Because of the frequency of biliary polyps, guidelines have been published that dictate workup and interval imaging.[66]

Adenomyomatosis

Adenomyomatosis of the gallbladder is characterized by localized or diffuse hyperplastic extensions of the mucosa into, and often beyond, a hypertrophied gallbladder muscular layer. Hyperplasia occurs at outpouchings of the mucosa of the gallbladder through the wall (Rokitansky–Aschoff sinuses) and through the crypts of Luschka. This can result in focal thickening of the gallbladder wall, resembling gallbladder adenocarcinoma. The etiology is unknown. These are considered benign and do not need follow-up unless there is diagnostic uncertainty.

Other Benign Gallbladder Tumors

Other benign lesions include tumors arising from the tissue of the gallbladder wall, such as leiomyomas, lipomas, hemangiomas, granular cell tumors, and heterotopic tissue, including gastric, pancreatic, or intestinal epithelium.

Clinical Findings

Patients with benign gallbladder tumors may present with symptoms consistent with choledocholithiasis, including right upper quadrant pain, fatty food intolerance, and nausea, and then discovered at the time of evaluation for these symptoms. Many benign gallbladder lesions are discovered incidentally after elective cholecystectomy. Most lesions, however, are asymptomatic and are discovered incidentally following imaging.

Diagnosis

Diagnosis of benign gallbladder polyps is usually made when an ultrasound study is obtained to evaluate a patient for symptoms consistent with gallstones. On ultrasound, a filling defect that does not change with position is likely a polyp or carcinoma and not a gallstone. Cholesterol polyps are typically small, submucosal, multiple, and hyperechoic on ultrasound because of their high cholesterol content. Other than this typical appearance and the fact that malignant polyps are usually more than 1 cm in size, it is difficult to differentiate benign from malignant polyps.

Both intravenous contrast-enhanced and unenhanced CT or MRI are helpful in distinguishing benign from malignant polyps.

Treatment

Large polyps, greater than 10 mm, have the greatest malignant potential. Without the evidence of invasion or metastatic disease, however, no radiologic test can reliably differentiate benign from malignant lesions. Therefore, if large (>1 cm) polyps are present, even in asymptomatic patients without stones, cholecystectomy is warranted. In addition, resection is recommended for smaller pedunculated lesions with evidence of a vascularized stalk. Small pedunculated lesions with the gross characteristics of a benign cholesterol polyp may be observed. Follow-up would be performed as outlined in Society of Radiologists in Ultrasound (SRU) guidelines.[66]

BENIGN BILE DUCT NEOPLASMS

Incidence

Benign bile duct tumors, at times clinically resembling hilar cholangiocarcinoma occur in less than 1% of patients.[4]

Pathology

The most common benign tumors of the extrahepatic biliary tree arise from the glandular epithelium lining the ducts; about two-thirds of benign tumors are polyps, adenomatous papilloma, or bile duct adenomas. Most are found in the periampullary region, but they can be distributed throughout the entire biliary tree (**Fig. 60.11**). Multiple papillomas also have been

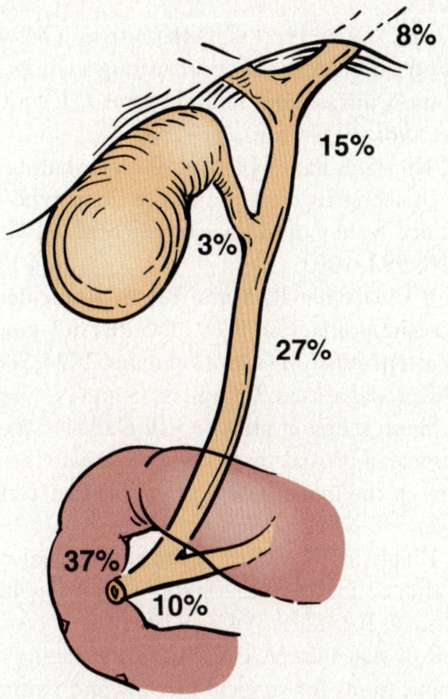

Figure 60.11. Distribution of papillomas and adenomas of the biliary tree. The ampulla and common bile duct are the most frequent sites.

reported throughout the intrahepatic and extrahepatic biliary tree, termed *multiple biliary papillomatosis*. Although local recurrence and progression to death from obstructive jaundice and cholangitis occur frequently in these rare cases, these tumors have little, if any, malignant potential. Other benign tumors (eg, cystadenoma, granular cell myoblastoma, leiomyoma, heterotopic tissue) have also been reported.

One condition that deserves consideration is the case of "malignant masquerade," an inflammatory, fibrotic lesion clinically resembling hilar cholangiocarcinoma, but pathologically consisting only of extensive fibrosis and inflammatory cells without evidence of dysplasia or preneoplastic change. Many of these cases likely represent IgG4-related autoimmune cholangiopathy, which can occur in isolation but can be associated with autoimmune pancreatitis. IgG4-related disease is now recognized as a systemic disorder that can affect multiple organs, including the biliary system. Ischemic cholangiopathy (ISC) is characterized by transmural lymphoplasmacytic infiltration in the walls of the biliary tree and peribiliary tissue with associated fibrosis. The epithelium is typically normal (unlike in PSC). Differentiating these strictures from PSC or malignancy is exceedingly difficult and requires an experienced team.

References

1. Siegel R, Ma JM, Zou ZH, Jemal A. Cancer Statistics, 2014. *Ca-Cancer J Clin*. 2014;64(1):9–29.
2. Wistuba, II, Gazdar AF. Gallbladder cancer: lessons from a rare tumour. *Nat Rev Cancer*. 2004;4(9):695–706.
3. Hundal R, Shaffer EA. Gallbladder cancer: epidemiology and outcome. *Clin Epidemiol*. 2014;6:99–109.
4. Andrea C, Enzo A. Cholesterol gallstones larger than 3 cm appear to be associated with gallbladder cancer: identification of a high risk group of patients that could benefit from preventive cholecystectomy. *Ann Surg*. 2016;263(3):e56.
5. Mathur SK, Duhan A, Singh S, et al. Correlation of gallstone characteristics with mucosal changes in gall bladder. *Trop Gastroenterol*. 2012;33(1):39–44.
6. Stephen AE, Berger DL. Carcinoma in the porcelain gallbladder: a relationship revisited. *Surgery*. 2001;129(6):699–703.
7. Schnelldorfer T. Porcelain gallbladder: a benign process or concern for malignancy? *J Gastrointest Surg*. 2013;17(6):1161–1168.
8. Javle M, Rashid A, Churi C, et al. Molecular characterization of gallbladder cancer using somatic mutation profiling. *Hum Pathol*. 2014;45(4):701–708.
9. Jiao Y, Pawlik TM, Anders RA, et al. Exome sequencing identifies frequent inactivating mutations in BAP1, ARID1A and PBRM1 in intrahepatic cholangiocarcinomas. *Nat Genet*. 2013;45(12): 1470–1473.
10. Bang SH, Lee JY, Woo H, et al. Differentiating between adenomyomatosis and gallbladder cancer: revisiting a comparative study of high-resolution ultrasound, multidetector CT, and MR imaging. *Korean J Radiol*. 2014;15(2):226–234.
11. Kang TW, Kim SH, Park HJ, et al. Differentiating xanthogranulomatous cholecystitis from wall-thickening type of gallbladder cancer: added value of diffusion-weighted MRI. *Clin Radiol*. 2013;68(10):992–1001.
12. Krishnaraju VS, Kumar R, Mittal BR, et al. Incidentally detected gallbladder carcinoma: Can F-18 FDG PET/CT aid in staging and prognostication? *Nucl Med Mol Imaging*. 2024;58(3):104–112.
13. Agarwal AK, Kalayarasan R, Javed A, Gupta N, Nag HH. The role of staging laparoscopy in primary gall bladder cancer–an analysis of 409 patients: a prospective study to evaluate the role of staging laparoscopy in the management of gallbladder cancer. *Ann Surg*. 2013;258(2):318–323.
14. Butte JM, Kingham TP, Gonen M, et al. Residual disease predicts outcomes after definitive resection for incidental gallbladder cancer. *J Am Coll Surg*. 2014;219(3):416–429.
15. Ito H, Ito K, D'Angelica M, et al. Accurate staging for gallbladder cancer: implications for surgical therapy and pathological assessment. *Ann Surg*. 2011;254(2):320–325.
16. Lee SE, Jang JY, Lim CS, Kang MJ, Kim SW. Systematic review on the surgical treatment for T1 gallbladder cancer. *World J Gastroenterol*. 2011;17(2):174–180.
17. Widmann B, Warschkow R, Beutner U, et al. Effect of lymphadenectomy in curative gallbladder cancer treatment: a systematic review and meta-analysis. *Langenbecks Arch Surg*. 2020;405(5): 573–584.
18. Kelly KJ, Dukleska K, Kuk D, et al. Prognostic significance of the highest peripancreatic lymph node in biliary tract adenocarcinoma. *Ann Surg Oncol*. 2014;21(3):979–985.
19. Fuks D, Regimbeau JM, Le Treut YP, et al. Incidental gallbladder cancer by the AFC-GBC-2009 Study Group. *World J Surg*. 2011;35(8):1887–97.
20. Creasy JM, Goldman DA, Gonen M, et al. Evolution of surgical management of gallbladder carcinoma and impact on outcome: results from two decades at a single-institution. *HPB (Oxford)*. 2019; 21(11):1541–51.
21. D'Angelica M, Dalal KM, DeMatteo RP, Fong Y, Blumgart LH, Jarnagin WR. Analysis of the extent of resection for adenocarcinoma of the gallbladder. *Ann Surg Oncol*. 2009;16(4):806–816.
22. Balakrishnan A, Barmpounakis P, Demiris N, et al. Surgical outcomes of gallbladder cancer: the OMEGA retrospective, multicentre, international cohort study. *EClinicalMedicine*. 2023;59:101951.
23. Goel S, Aggarwal A, Iqbal A, Talwar V, Mitra S, Singh S. Multimodality management of gallbladder cancer can lead to a better outcome: Experience from a tertiary care oncology centre in North India. *World J Gastroenterol*. 2021;27(45):7813–7830.
24. Jensen EH, Abraham A, Habermann EB, et al. A critical analysis of the surgical management of early-stage gallbladder cancer in the United States. *J Gastrointest Surg*. 2009;13(4):722–727.
25. Jung W, Jang JY, Kang MJ, et al. Effects of surgical methods and tumor location on survival and recurrence patterns after curative resection in patients with t2 gallbladder cancer. *Gut Liver*. 2016;10(1): 140–146.
26. Kai M, Chijiiwa K, Ohuchida J, Nagano M, Hiyoshi M, Kondo K. A curative resection improves the postoperative survival rate even in patients with advanced gallbladder carcinoma. *J Gastrointest Surg*. 2007;11(8):1025–1032.
27. Hakeem AR, Papoulas M, Menon KV. The role of neoadjuvant chemotherapy or chemoradiotherapy for advanced gallbladder cancer—A systematic review. *Eur J Surg Oncol*. 2019;45(2):83–91.
28. Chaudhari VA, Ostwal V, Patkar S, et al. Outcome of neoadjuvant chemotherapy in "locally advanced/borderline resectable" gallbladder cancer: the need to define indications. *HPB (Oxford)*. 2018;20(9):841–847.
29. Ben-Josef E, Guthrie KA, El-Khoueiry AB, et al. SWOG S0809: A phase II intergroup trial of adjuvant capecitabine and gemcitabine followed by radiotherapy and concurrent capecitabine in extrahepatic cholangiocarcinoma and gallbladder carcinoma. *J Clin Oncol*. 2015;33(24):2617–2622.
30. Das SC, Ghosh J, Kanta S, et al. Outcomes of resectable gallbladder cancer: a retrospective analysis from a tertiary care centre in India. *Cureus*. 2024;16(7):e65735.
31. Ozturk NB, Dadamyan A, Jamil LH. A single-center analysis of patient characteristics and overall survival in patients with resectable gallbladder cancer. *Healthcare (Basel)*. 2024;12(20):2091.
32. Romatoski KS, Chung SH, Sawhney V, et al. Factors associated with surgical management in gallbladder cancer-a surveillance, epidemiology, and end results medicare-based study. *J Surg Res*. 2024;304:9–18.
33. Roos E, Strijker M, Franken LC, et al. Comparison of short- and long-term outcomes between anatomical subtypes of resected biliary tract cancer in a Western high-volume center. *HPB (Oxford)*. 2020;22(3):405–414.
34. Endo I, Gonen M, Yopp AC, et al. Intrahepatic cholangiocarcinoma: rising frequency, improved survival, and determinants of outcome after resection. *Ann Surg*. 2008;248(1):84–96.
35. Welzel TM, Mellemkjaer L, Gloria G, et al. Risk factors for intrahepatic cholangiocarcinoma in a low-risk population: a nationwide case-control study. *Int J Cancer*. 2007;120(3):638–641.

36. Matsuo K, Rocha FG, Ito K, et al. The Blumgart preoperative staging system for hilar cholangiocarcinoma: analysis of resectability and outcomes in 380 patients. *J Am Coll Surg*. 2012;215(3): 343–355.
37. Nathan H, Pawlik TM, Wolfgang CL, Choti MA, Cameron JL, Schulick RD. Trends in survival after surgery for cholangiocarcinoma: a 30-year population-based SEER database analysis. *J Gastrointest Surg*. 2007;11(11):1488–1496; discussion 1496–1497.
38. Cho A, Yamamoto H, Kainuma O, et al. Laparoscopy in the management of hilar cholangiocarcinoma. *World J Gastroenterol*. 2014;20(41):15153–15157.
39. de Jong MC, Nathan H, Sotiropoulos GC, et al. Intrahepatic cholangiocarcinoma: an international multi-institutional analysis of prognostic factors and lymph node assessment. *J Clin Oncol*. 2011;29(23):3140–3145.
40. Ito K, Ito H, Allen PJ, et al. Adequate lymph node assessment for extrahepatic bile duct adenocarcinoma. *Ann Surg*. 2010; 251(4):675–681.
41. Zhang XF, Xue F, Dong DH, et al. Number and station of lymph node metastasis after curative-intent resection of intrahepatic cholangiocarcinoma impact prognosis. *Ann Surg*. 2021;274(6): e1187–e1195.
42. Meyer CG, Penn I, James L. Liver transplantation for cholangiocarcinoma: results in 207 patients. *Transplantation*. 2000;69(8): 1633–1637.
43. Sudan D, DeRoover A, Chinnakotla S, et al. Radiochemotherapy and transplantation allow long-term survival for nonresectable hilar cholangiocarcinoma. *Am J Transplant*. 2002;2(8):774–779.
44. Rea DJ, Heimbach JK, Rosen CB, et al. Liver transplantation with neoadjuvant chemoradiation is more effective than resection for hilar cholangiocarcinoma. *Ann Surg*. 2005;242(3):451–458; discussion 8–61.
45. Cambridge WA, Fairfield C, Powell JJ, et al. Meta-analysis and meta-regression of survival after liver transplantation for unresectable perihilar cholangiocarcinoma. *Ann Surg*. 2021;273(2): 240–250.
46. Jang JY, Kim SW, Park DJ, et al. Actual long-term outcome of extrahepatic bile duct cancer after surgical resection. *Ann Surg*. 2005;241(1):77–84.
47. Jarnagin WR, Fong Y, DeMatteo RP, et al. Staging, resectability, and outcome in 225 patients with hilar cholangiocarcinoma. *Ann Surg*. 2001;234(4):507–517; discussion 17–9.
48. Konstadoulakis MM, Roayaie S, Gomatos IP, et al. Aggressive surgical resection for hilar cholangiocarcinoma: is it justified? Audit of a single center's experience. *Am J Surg*. 2008;196(2):160–169.
49. Rea DJ, Munoz-Juarez M, Farnell MB, et al. Major hepatic resection for hilar cholangiocarcinoma: analysis of 46 patients. *Arch Surg*. 2004;139(5):514–523; discussion 23–5.
50. Yubin L, Chihua F, Zhixiang J, et al. Surgical management and prognostic factors of hilar cholangiocarcinoma: experience with 115 cases in China. *Ann Surg Oncol*. 2008;15(8):2113–2119.
51. Zeng D, Wang Y, Wen N, Li B, Cheng N, Lu J. Short-term and long-term clinical outcomes of combined caudate lobectomy for intrahepatic cholangiocarcinoma involving the hepatic hilus: a propensity score analysis. *Gut Liver*. 2025;19:438–453.
52. Zhang XF, Bagante F, Chen Q, et al. Perioperative and long-term outcome of intrahepatic cholangiocarcinoma involving the hepatic hilus after curative-intent resection: comparison with peripheral intrahepatic cholangiocarcinoma and hilar cholangiocarcinoma. *Surgery*. 2018;163(5):1114–1120.
53. Bagante F, Spolverato G, Weiss M, et al. Defining long-term survivors following resection of intrahepatic cholangiocarcinoma. *J Gastrointest Surg*. 2017;21(11):1888–1897.
54. Berardi G, Risi L, Muttillo EM, et al. Anatomic versus non-anatomic liver resection for intrahepatic cholangiocarcinoma: a systematic review and patient-level meta-analysis. *Ann Surg Oncol*. 2024;31: 9170–9182.
55. Elias C, Rahman A, Mial-Anthony J, et al. Advancements in cholangiocarcinoma: evolving strategies for diagnosis, treatment, and palliation over three decades. *Chin Clin Oncol*. 2024;13:70.
56. Ahmad Al-Saffar H, Jansson H, Danielsson O, Moro CF, Sturesson C. Different biliary tract cancers, same operation: importance of cancer origin in patients with hilar-invading tumors. *Scand J Surg*. 2025;114:35–43.
57. Oh DY, He AR, Bouattour M, et al. Durvalumab or placebo plus gemcitabine and cisplatin in participants with advanced biliary tract cancer (TOPAZ-1): updated overall survival from a randomised phase 3 study. *Lancet Gastroenterol Hepatol*. 2024;9(8): 694–704.
58. Oh DY, Ruth He A, Qin S, et al. Durvalumab plus gemcitabine and cisplatin in advanced biliary tract cancer. *NEJM Evid*. 2022;1(8):EVIDoa2200015.
59. Kelley RK, Ueno M, Yoo C, et al. Pembrolizumab in combination with gemcitabine and cisplatin compared with gemcitabine and cisplatin alone for patients with advanced biliary tract cancer (KEYNOTE-966): a randomised, double-blind, placebo-controlled, phase 3 trial. *Lancet*. 2023;401(10391):1853–1865.
60. Franssen S, Holster JJ, Jolissaint JS, et al. Gemcitabine with cisplatin versus hepatic arterial infusion pump chemotherapy for liver-confined unresectable intrahepatic cholangiocarcinoma. *Ann Surg Oncol*. 2024;31(1):115–124.
61. Cercek A, Boerner T, Tan BR, et al. Assessment of hepatic arterial infusion of floxuridine in combination with systemic gemcitabine and oxaliplatin in patients with unresectable intrahepatic cholangiocarcinoma: a Phase 2 Clinical Trial. *JAMA Oncol*. 2020;6(1):60–67.
62. Jarnagin WR, Schwartz LH, Gultekin DH, et al. Regional chemotherapy for unresectable primary liver cancer: results of a phase II clinical trial and assessment of DCE-MRI as a biomarker of survival. *Ann Oncol*. 2009;20(9):1589–1595.
63. Primrose JN, Fox RP, Palmer DH, et al. Capecitabine compared with observation in resected biliary tract cancer (BILCAP): a randomised, controlled, multicentre, phase 3 study. *Lancet Oncol*. 2019;20(5):663–673.
64. Horgan AM, Amir E, Walter T, Knox JJ. Adjuvant therapy in the treatment of biliary tract cancer: a systematic review and meta-analysis. *J Clin Oncol*. 2012;30(16):1934–1940.
65. Shroff RT, Kennedy EB, Bachini M, et al. Adjuvant therapy for resected biliary tract cancer: ASCO Clinical Practice Guideline. *J Clin Oncol*. 2019;37(12):1015–1027.
66. Kamaya A, Fung C, Szpakowski JL, et al. Management of incidentally detected gallbladder polyps: society of radiologists in ultrasound consensus conference recommendations. *Radiology*. 2022;305(2):277–289.

Anatomy and Physiology of the Colon, Rectum, and Anus

Melanie S. Morris

Key Points

1. The mesorectum is enclosed by the fascia propria of the rectum.
2. The ileocolic branch of the superior mesenteric artery supplies the right colon and the proximal transverse colon.
3. The inferior mesenteric artery supplies the distal transverse colon, sigmoid colon, and rectum.
4. The inguinal lymph nodes drain the lymphatics from the anal canal below the dentate line.
5. The microbiomes are colonic flora which promote mucosal immunity, digest complex nutrients, protect against pathogenic organisms, and may play a role in disease.
6. Understanding colorectal anatomy and physiology is essential for safe and effective colorectal surgical judgment and technique.

The main functions of the colon, rectum, and anus are to serve as a reservoir and conduit for stool. However, it also plays a role in the digestion and absorption of complex carbohydrate and protein residue, fueling colonic bacteria, and lubricating stool for transit. Understanding the anatomy and physiology of the colon, rectum, and anus is important to appropriately treat the pathology associated with it.

EMBRYOLOGY

Knowledge of embryologic origins explains gastrointestinal function and allows surgeons to identify appropriate planes of dissection and prevent injury to surrounding structures. The primitive gut is derived from endoderm and is divided into three segments (foregut, midgut, and hindgut) by the third week of gestation. The small intestine distal to the ampulla of Vater and the colon proximal to the splenic flexure are formed from the midgut, while the remaining colon (distal to the splenic flexure), rectum, and anal canal (proximal to the dentate line) are formed from the hindgut. This has implications for arterial blood supply, as structures formed by the midgut are supplied by the superior mesenteric artery, while structures formed by the hindgut are supplied by the inferior mesenteric artery.

The midgut undergoes a three-stage process of rotation and fixation starting in the 6th week of gestation. In the first stage, the midgut elongates over the superior mesenteric artery, herniates out of the abdominal cavity through the umbilical cord, and then rotates 90 degrees in a counterclockwise direction. In the second stage, which starts in the 10th week of gestation, the midgut returns to the abdominal cavity while continuing to rotate an additional 180 degrees counterclockwise around the superior mesenteric artery. This results in the colon lying anterior to the duodenum. In the third stage, the cecum migrates inferiorly to the right lower quadrant, and then fixation of the ascending and descending colon begins. Major anomalies of rotation typically occur during the second stage, and include nonrotation, malrotation, reversed rotation, omphalocele, and internal hernia.

The terminal end of the hindgut is termed the cloaca. During development, the intestinal and urogenital tracts are joined at the cloaca until the urorectal septum migrates caudally, dividing the cloaca into the urogenital plate anteriorly and the anal plate posteriorly. The dentate line represents the fusion plane of the endodermal and ectodermal tubes, with the anal transition zone referring to the cloacal part of the anal canal which includes both endodermal and ectodermal components.[1]

GROSS ANATOMY

The colon is a tubular organ measuring on average 150 cm, though overall length is highly variable. Typically, the colonic diameter decreases over its course, with the cecum measuring about 7.5 to 8.5 cm and the distal sigmoid colon about 2.5 cm. As described above, the ascending and descending colon are fixed to the lateral peritoneal wall, with the posterior aspects fused to the retroperitoneum. In contrast, the transverse and sigmoid colon are intraperitoneal structures.

The colon is distinguished from the rest of the gastrointestinal tract by three unique anatomic features: taeniae coli, haustra, and appendices epiploicae (**Fig. 61.1**). The three taeniae coli are continuous condensations of the outer longitudinal muscle layer of the colon and are named according to their attachments: taenia mesocolica (posteromedial, attached to the mesocolon), taenia omentalis (posterolateral, attached to the greater omentum), taenia libera (anterior, no attachments). The three taeniae originate at the base of the appendix, course along the length of the colon, and then converge at the rectosigmoid junction, marking the anatomic beginning of the rectum. They are one-sixth shorter than the rest of the bowel wall, resulting in outpouchings between the taenia called sacculations or haustra, which are separated by the plicae semilunares. The appendices epiploicae are antimesenteric fat appendages that protrude from the colonic serosa and vary in size.

The colon begins in the right lower quadrant with the cecum. The cecum extends approximately 6 to 8 cm below the

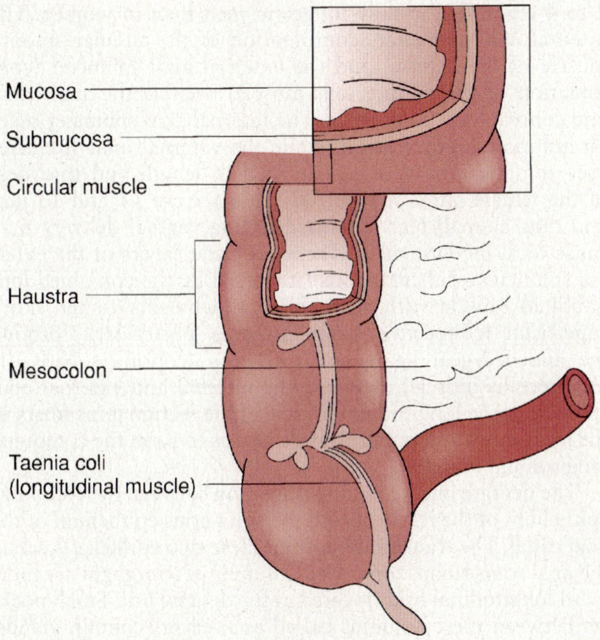

Figure 61.1. Layers of the colonic wall.

ileocecal valve, which is located at posteromedial aspect of the cecum (**Fig. 61.2**). The ileocecal valve is formed by angulation between the ileum and cecum via the superior and inferior ileocecal ligaments and prevents reflux of stool back into the ileum.[2] The cecum is the widest portion of the colon, has the thinnest wall, and is entirely enveloped by peritoneum.

The origin of the appendix can be identified by following the converging taeniae at the most proximal portion of the cecum. In the vast majority of people (85% to 95%), the appendix lies posterior to the cecum, lateral and in line to the terminal ileum. Other variants in position include retrocecal (toward the psoas muscle), pelvic, and retroileal.[3] Visualization and documentation of the appendiceal orifice and ileocecal valve is important for ensuring complete colonic examination during colonoscopy.

From the cecum, the right colon ascends approximately 15 cm to the hepatic flexure, which is anterior to the inferior pole of the right kidney and overlies the second portion of the duodenum. When the right colon and mesentery are mobilized during a colectomy, care must be taken to visualize and avoid injury to the underlying duodenum and right ureter. Only the anterior surface of the right colon is invested with peritoneum; laterally, the white line of Toldt marks the extent of the peritoneal covering and serves as an important landmark during surgical mobilization of the colon.

The transverse colon stretches from the hepatic flexure to the splenic flexure and is the longest segment of colon (between 30 and 60 cm). The transverse colon is suspended by the transverse mesocolon and is completely intraperitoneal. It is the most mobile portion of the colon and may descend to the level of the iliac crests or deep into the pelvis. The greater omentum descends from the greater curve of the stomach in front of the transverse colon and then ascends to attach to the transverse colon on its anterosuperior edge. To mobilize the transverse colon or enter the lesser sac, the fusion plane of the omentum to the transverse colon must be dissected.

The splenic flexure is situated high in the left upper quadrant, more cephalad than the hepatic flexure, and abuts the lower pole of the spleen. There are attachments from the colon to the diaphragm at the level of the 10th and 11th ribs and spleen (phrenocolic and splenocolic ligaments), and these must be carefully divided during mobilization of the flexure to avoid splenic injury.

The descending colon is approximately 25 cm long and courses from the splenic flexure to its junction with the sigmoid colon at the pelvic brim. It lies anterior to the left kidney and, like the right colon, the anterior, lateral, and medial portions of the descending colon are covered by peritoneum.

The sigmoid colon extends from the pelvic brim to the sacral promontory, where it continues as the rectum and generally measures 15 to 50 cm in length. It is completely invested by peritoneum. The sigmoid colon is extremely mobile and has a generous mesentery that extends along the pelvic brim from the iliac fossa across the sacroiliac joint to the second or third sacral segment. Because of its mobile mesentery, the sigmoid colon can twist, forming a volvulus which causes obstruction. The left ureter runs in the intersigmoid fossa, which is at the base of the mesosigmoid. When a high ligation of the inferior mesenteric artery is performed during a cancer operation or the sigmoid colon is being mobilized along the white line of Toldt, the left ureter should be identified to avoid injury.

At the sacral promontory, the colon becomes the rectum. The rectosigmoid junction is marked by the convergence of the colonic taenia. The outer layer of the rectal wall is composed

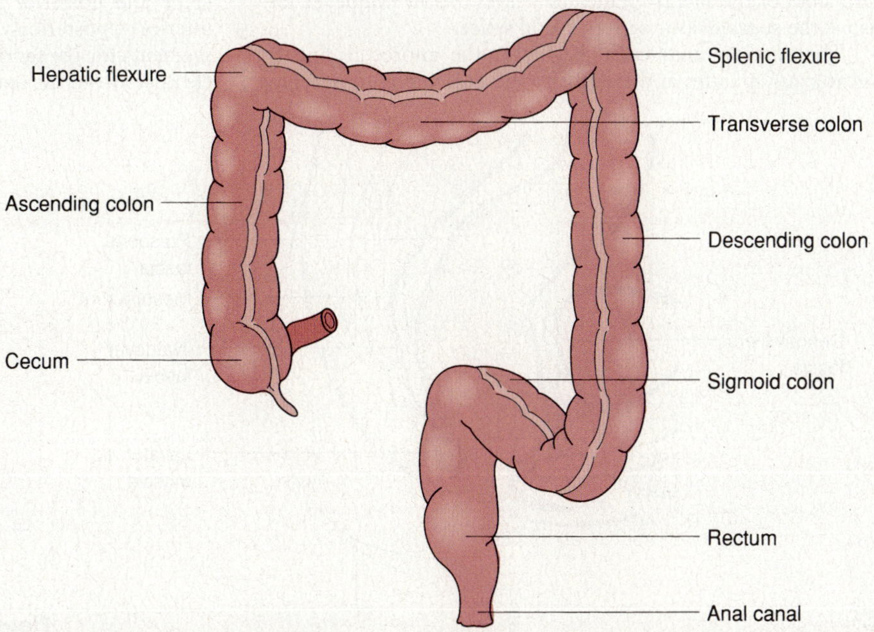

Figure 61.2. General anatomic components of the colon.

of the longitudinal muscle, where the three teniae splay. The rectum measures 12 to 15 cm in length. It proceeds posterior and caudal along the curvature of the sacrum and coccyx, passing through the levator ani muscles, at which point it turns abruptly caudal and posteriorly at the anorectal ring, becoming the anal canal. Anterior to the rectum are the uterine cervix and posterior vaginal wall in women, and the bladder and prostate in men. Posteriorly, the rectum occupies the sacral concavity where the median sacral vessels, presacral veins, and sacral nerves run, all of which are invested in the presacral fascia. The rectum is marked by three curves. The upper and lower curves are convex and to the right, while the middle is convex and to the left. Within the lumen, these correspond to the valves of Houston, which separate the lower third, middle third, and upper third of the rectum—important landmarks when the location of a rectal abnormality is established endoscopically (the lower rectal valve is at 7 to 8 cm from the anal verge, middle rectal valve at 9 to 11 cm, and upper rectal valve at 12 to 13 cm).[4] The valves do not contain all layers of the bowel wall and thus biopsy at this location carries minimal risk of perforation. The middle valve of Houston is the internal landmark corresponding to the anterior peritoneal reflection. The anterior and lateral surfaces of the upper third of the rectum are intraperitoneal, whereas only the anterior surface of the middle third of the rectum is intraperitoneal in location. The lower third of the rectum is entirely extraperitoneal. The
1 mesorectum is the term used to describe the areolar tissue surrounding the rectum that contains nerves, lymphatics, and terminal branches of the superior hemorrhoidal branch of the inferior mesenteric artery. Although it invests the rectum circumferentially, the mesorectum is most prominent posterior to the rectum. It is invested by the fascia propria of the rectum, a continuation of the parietal endopelvic fascia (**Fig. 61.3**). The fascia propria (investing fascia) includes the distal two-thirds of the posterior rectum and the distal one-third of the anterior rectum, where it is no longer intraperitoneal. A total mesorectal excision, which is critical to obtain negative radial margins in rectal cancer resections, entails removal of the entire rectum without violating the fascia propria of the rectum. This is accomplished by mobilizing the rectum using the plane between the fascia propria of the rectum and the presacral fascia. Anterior to the investing fascia (fascia propria) is a delicate layer of connective tissue known as Denonvilliers fascia, which separates the rectum from its anterior structures. Waldeyer fascia (rectosacral fascia) is the presacral fascia that is an extension of the parietal pelvic fascia from the periosteum of sacral segment four to the posterior wall of the rectum. It contains branches of the sacral splanchnic nerves. Below Waldeyer fascia is the supralevator or retrorectal space.

The surgical anal canal begins at the anorectal ring or levator ani muscles and extends to the anal verge. It measures 2 to 4 cm and is usually longer in men than in women. The internal anal sphincter (continuation of the circular smooth muscle of the rectum) and the external anal sphincter (continuation of the puborectalis muscle) encircle the anal canal and control fecal continence. The internal anal sphincter relies on autonomic innervation, while the external anal sphincter uses somatic innervation. The median length and thickness of the female anterior external sphincter are 11 and 13 mm and thus a small tear sustained during vaginal delivery may cause fecal incontinence.[5] There are three layers of the external sphincter—subcutaneous (traversed by the conjoined longitudinal muscle with some fiber attachments to the skin), superficial (connective tissue attaches posteriorly, forming the anococcygeal ligament), and deep (continues with the puborectalis muscle). Between the internal and external anal sphincters, the longitudinal muscle of the rectum joins fibers of the levator ani and puborectalis muscles to form the conjoined longitudinal muscle.

The dentate line marks the transition between the columnar epithelium of the intestine and the squamous epithelium of the anal canal. The transition between these two epithelia is called the anal transitional zone. The Columns of Morgagni are the 6 to 14 longitudinal folds located at the dentate line. Small pockets between these columns called anal crypts contain glands, which may become obstructed with foreign material to cause perianal abscesses or fistulas. Below the dentate line is the anoderm, which extends to the anal verge and does not contain accessory skin structures, such as hair, sebaceous, and sweat glands. The autonomic nervous system innervates proximal to the dentate line and the somatic nervous system supplies the anoderm and distally. Thus, surgical procedures distal to the dentate line are painful.

Pelvic Floor

The perineal body is the tendinous insertion of the external anal sphincter, bulbocavernosus, and superficial and deep transverse perineal muscles. It supports the perineum and separates the vagina from the anus. Three striated muscles that attach to the pubic bone make up the pelvic floor or levator ani muscles: iliococcygeus, pubococcygeus, and puborectalis. The pelvic floor muscles are supplied by branches from the third sacral nerve, while the external anal sphincter is supplied by nerve fibers traveling with the pudendal nerve on the levator's undersurface.

The puborectalis originates from the back of the symphysis pubis and forms a U-shaped sling as it joins the opposite muscle posteriorly. The iliococcygeus muscle arises from the ischial spine and posterior part of the obturator fascia and travels inferiorly, posteriorly, and medially to insert into the last two segments for the sacrum and coccyx. The pubococcygeus muscle arises from the anterior half of the obturator fascia and the

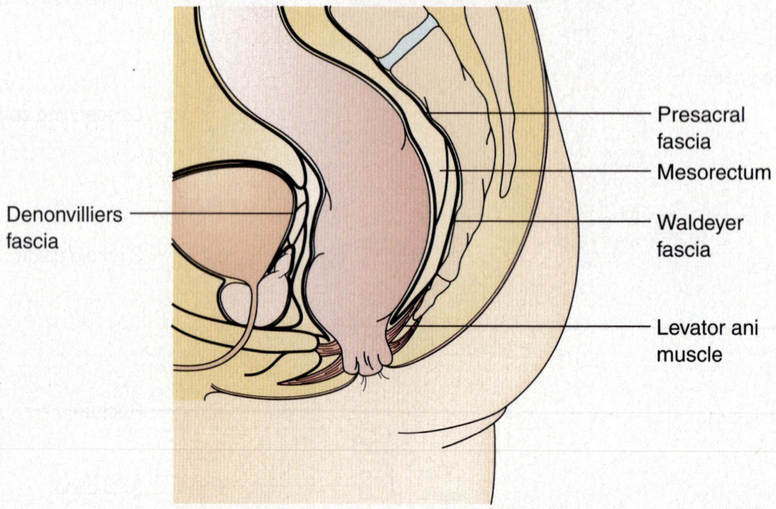

Figure 61.3. Fascial relationships of the pelvis.

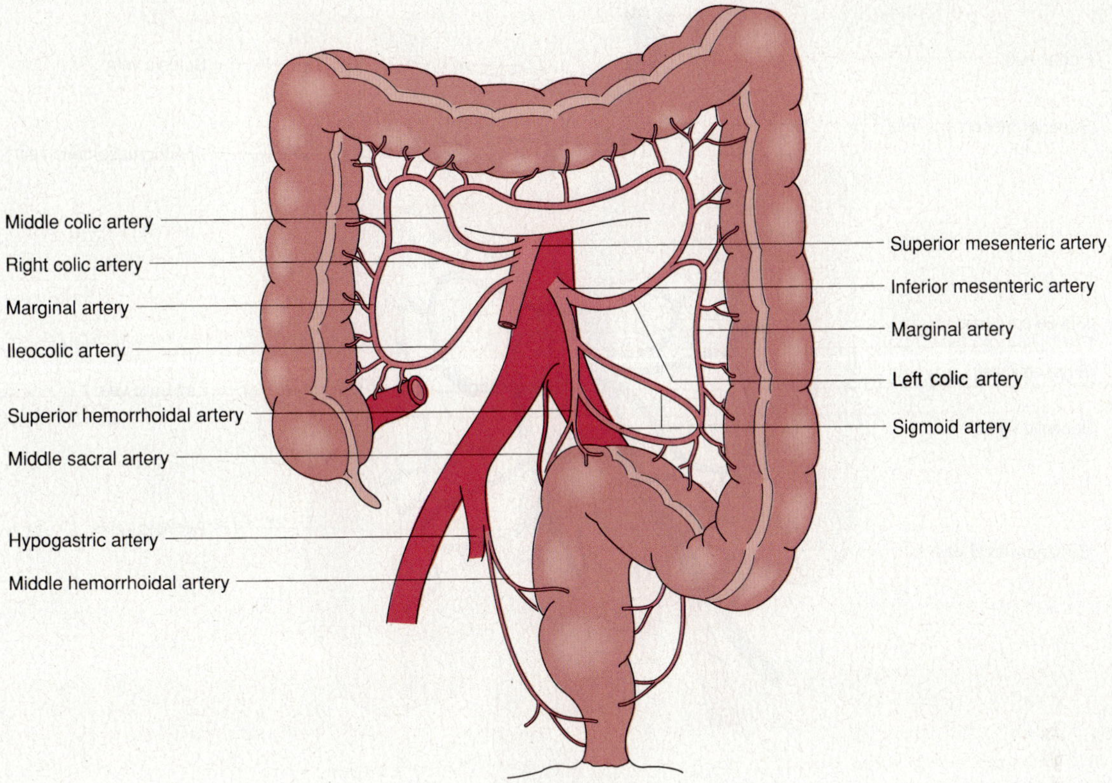

Figure 61.4. Arterial blood supply of the colon.

posterior pubis. Its fibers are directed backward, downward, and medially, where they decussate with fibers of the opposite side. The decussation is called the anococcygeal raphe.

Anorectal Spaces

The perianal space surrounds the anal canal superficially and contains the external hemorrhoidal plexus. The ischioanal space extends laterally and goes superiorly to the levator ani from the skin on the perineum. The levator ani and external sphincter muscles form the medial boundary, while the lateral wall is formed by the obturator fascia. The superficial postanal space connects the perianal spaces with each other posteriorly below the anococcygeal ligament, while the deep postanal space lies above the anococcygeal ligament. The ischioanal and perianal spaces make the ischioanal fossa. The deep postanal and ischiorectal spaces form a horseshoe configuration, which is how horseshoe abscesses may occur. Failure to adequately drain the deep postanal space may allow the horseshoe abscess to persist. Below the perianal space between the sphincter muscles is the intersphincteric space. The submucosal space contains the internal hemorrhoidal plexus and lies between the internal anal sphincter and the mucosa distal to the dentate line. Proximally, it becomes the submucosa of the rectum. Above the levator complex is the supralevator space, which extends superiorly to the peritoneum at the rectosacral fascia. The retrorectal space extends above the rectosacral fascia and lies between the upper two-thirds of the rectum and sacrum.

Arterial Blood Supply

The arterial blood supply to the colon, rectum, and anus is highly variable. The superior mesenteric artery typically arises from the aorta, runs posterior to the pancreas, and passes ante-
2 rior to the third portion of the duodenum (**Fig. 61.4**). In addition to supplying the small bowel through jejunal and ileal branches, the superior mesenteric artery gives rise to the ileocolic, right colic, and middle colic branches that supply the cecum, ascending colon, and proximal transverse colon. The right colic arterial anatomy is particularly variable and can be absent or arise from the ileocolic or the superior mesenteric artery. The middle colic artery has a right branch that supplies the hepatic flexure and the right portion of the transverse
3 colon, while the left branch supplies the left portion of the transverse colon. The inferior mesenteric artery arises from the anterior surface of the aorta, typically 3 to 4 cm above the aortic bifurcation, and supplies the distal transverse colon, descending colon, sigmoid colon, and upper rectum. The inferior mesenteric artery gives rise to the left colic artery and sigmoidal branches, then continues in the sigmoid mesentery, and after crossing the left iliac vessels, is renamed the superior rectal/hemorrhoidal artery. The inferior mesenteric artery may also function as an important collateral vessel to the lower extremities during instances of distal aortic occlusion. The superior hemorrhoidal artery descends behind the rectum and splits into right and left branches in the mesorectum. It is the main blood supply of the rectum. The middle and inferior rectal/hemorrhoidal arteries arise from either the internal pudendal arteries or the hypogastric arteries and supply the distal two-thirds of the rectum. The presence of the middle rectal artery can be variable.

Venous Drainage

The veins that drain the large intestine bear the same terminology and follow a course similar to their corresponding arteries (**Fig. 61.5**). The veins from the right colon and transverse colon, along with the veins draining the small intestine, drain into the superior mesenteric vein. The superior mesenteric vein runs slightly anterior and to the right of the superior mesenteric artery. The superior mesenteric vein courses beneath the neck of the pancreas, where it joins with the splenic vein to form the portal vein. The inferior mesenteric vein is a continuation of the superior rectal vein and drains blood from the left colon, sigmoid colon, rectum, and superior anal canal. The inferior mesenteric vein follows a course of its own, starting at the left colic artery, and ascends over the psoas muscle in a retroperitoneal plane. The vein courses under the body of the pancreas to drain into the splenic vein. During an anterior resection of

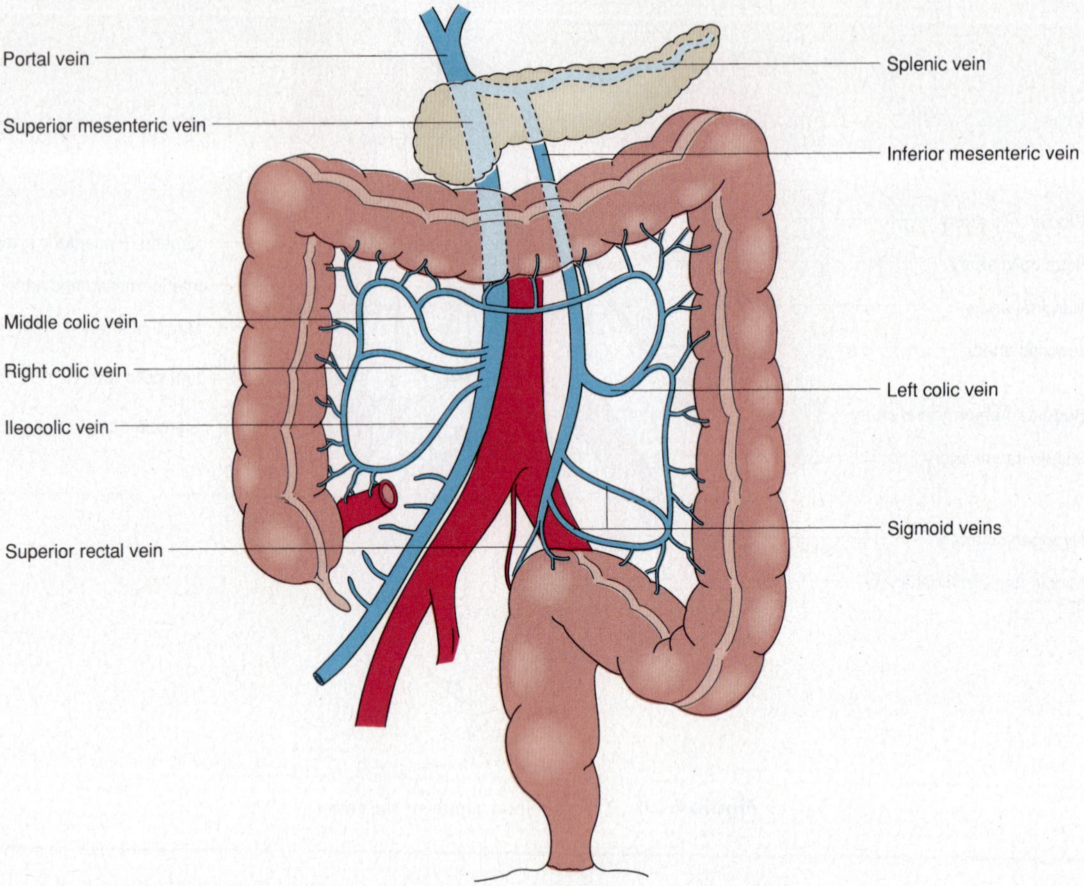

Figure 61.5. Venous drainage of the colon by the portal vein.

the rectum, division of the inferior mesenteric vein at the inferior border of the pancreas can provide additional mobility of the left colon to facilitate a coloanal anastomosis. The superior hemorrhoidal (rectal) veins drain blood from the rectum and upper part of the anal canal, where the internal hemorrhoidal plexus is situated, into the portal system via the inferior mesenteric vein. The middle hemorrhoidal (rectal) veins drain the lower part of the rectum and upper part of the anal canal into the systemic circulation via the internal iliac veins. The inferior hemorrhoidal (rectal) veins drain blood from the lower rectum and anal canal, where the external hemorrhoidal plexus is located, via the internal pudendal veins into the systemic venous circulation via the internal iliac veins. In the setting of portal hypertension, the superior, middle, and inferior hemorrhoidal veins interact to shunt venous blood from the portal system into the systemic circulation.

Lymphatic Drainage

4 Lymphatic drainage generally follows the arterial blood supply of the colon and rectum. As such, performing a high ligation of the feeding artery during oncologic segmental colon resection should ensure adequate lymph node harvest. In the anal canal, lesions above the dentate line drain into the inferior mesenteric lymph nodes while lesions below the dentate line drain into both the internal iliac lymph nodes and the inferior mesenteric lymph nodes.

Neural Components

The colon possesses extrinsic and intrinsic (enteric) neuronal systems. The extrinsic system consists of sympathetic and parasympathetic nerves that inhibit or stimulate colonic peristalsis, respectively. The sympathetic innervation to the right colon originates from the lower thoracic segments of the spinal cord and travels in the thoracic splanchnic nerves to the celiac and superior mesenteric plexuses. Postganglionic fibers emerge from here and course along the superior mesenteric artery and its branches to the right side of the colon. The parasympathetic nerves originate from the right vagus nerve and travel along with the sympathetic nerves to the right side of the colon. The left side of the colon and the rectum receive sympathetic fibers that arise from L1 through L3 segments of the spinal cord. This passes through the ganglionated sympathetic chains and leaves as a lumbar sympathetic nerve to join the preaortic plexus. It extends along the inferior mesenteric artery as the mesenteric plexus and then becomes the presacral nerve or superior hypogastric plexus. These hypogastric nerves are identified at the sacral promontory 1 cm lateral to the midline. The key zones of sympathetic nerve damage are during ligation of the inferior mesenteric artery and during initial posterior rectal mobilization adjacent to the hypogastric nerves. The parasympathetic supply to the left side of the colon and the rectum comes from S2 through S4 spinal cord segments. The sacral nerve fibers become the nervi erigentes, which join the pelvic plexus at the pelvic side walls. To prevent injury during full mobilization of the rectum, the lateral ligament should be cut close to the rectal side wall. Both the sympathetic and parasympathetic nervous systems play a role in erection. Damage to the parasympathetics can lead to erectile dysfunction, and retrograde ejaculation can occur with damage to sympathetic nerve injury.

The intrinsic, or enteric, nervous system consists of two groups of plexuses that are identified by their location within the colon wall. This system can function independently of the central nervous system and controls motility, exocrine and endocrine functions of the gut, intestinal immune regulation and inflammatory responses. The Meissner plexus is located in the submucosa between the muscularis mucosae and the circular muscle of the muscularis propria and is important in secretory control. The myenteric plexus, also known as the *Auerbach plexus*, is located between the inner circular muscle and outer longitudinal muscle layers of the colon and primarily controls intestinal motility.[4]

The internal anal sphincter is supplied by the sympathetic and parasympathetic nerves that supply the lower rectum. The parasympathetic nerves are inhibitory. The external sphincter is supplied by the inferior rectal branch of the internal pudendal nerve and the perineal branch of S4. Sensation of the anal canal is from the inferior rectal nerve, which is a branch of the pudendal nerve.

PHYSIOLOGY

The primary function of the colon is to store and transport stool. However, it also absorbs water, electrolytes (sodium and chloride), undigested starches, and bile salts. The physiologic control of colonic water and electrolyte transport requires careful integration of neural, endocrine, and paracrine components. Although colonic epithelium does not actively absorb glucose or amino acids as the small-intestinal epithelium does, the colon does absorb short-chain fatty acids and vitamins that are produced by bacterial breakdown of nonabsorbed carbohydrates and amino acids. These short-chain fatty acids, which include acetate, butyrate, and propionate, are absorbed in a concentration-dependent fashion. They are a major energy substrate for colonic epithelial cells and represent the major fecal anions.[6]

Approximately 1,500 mL of ileal effluent reaches the cecum in a 24-hour period, 90% of which is reabsorbed in the colon. The colon has a tremendous capacity that allows it to absorb as much as 5 to 6 L of water within a 24-hour period. When colonic capacity is exceeded, diarrhea results.[7] Normally formed feces consist of 70% water and 30% solid material. Almost half of the solid material is made up of bacteria and the other half is composed of undigested food material and desquamated epithelium. Water absorption in the colon is a passive process that depends primarily on the osmotic gradient established by the active transport of sodium across the colonic epithelium.[8] The composition of ileal effluent and luminal flow rates also plays an important role in water absorption. Upsetting the balance of these three factors results in diarrhea. The absorptive capacity is not the same throughout each segment of the colon. Salt and water absorption is greatest in the right colon.[9] Patients undergoing a right hemicolectomy should therefore be counseled preoperatively that they may experience loose bowel movements in the early postoperative period. Patients should also be reassured that this will resolve with time as the remaining colon adapts.

Colonic Flora

The bacterial flora of the colon is established soon after birth
5 and is largely dependent on dietary and environmental factors. The colon is populated by approximately 10^{13} commensal bacteria.[10] The vast majority of the normal colonic flora consists of anaerobic bacteria, with *Bacteroides* species being most prevalent, particularly *Bacteroides fragilis*.[11] Aerobic colonic bacteria are mainly coliforms and enterococci, with *Escherichia coli* being the most predominant coliform. The colonic flora is important for (a) digestion and absorption of complex macromolecules, (b) protecting the colon against invasion by noncommensal bacteria, and (c) development of mucosal immunity. Fermentation of carbohydrates generates short-chain fatty acids, including acetic acid, propionic acid, and butyrate, which is the primary nutrient for the colonic mucosa. Colonic bacteria also produce certain vitamins, such as vitamins K and B_{12}, which are absorbed by the host. The enterohepatic circulation of bilirubin and bile acids depends on bacterial enzymes produced by fecal flora. The degradation of bile pigments by colonic bacteria gives stool its characteristic brown color. Colonic bacteria also play an important role in preventing infection by controlling the growth of potentially pathogenic bacteria such as *Clostridium difficile*. Host and colonic flora have a mutualistic relationship; however, disturbances of this coexistence can lead to human disease.[12] Changes in diet and use of antibiotics can dramatically alter the microbiome. The microbiome of colonic flora is suspected to play a role in the pathogenesis of inflammatory bowel disease, obesity, and other diseases.

Colonic Motility

6 Motor activity varies greatly throughout the colon. There are two patterns of colonic motility: segmental contractions, which are single or clustered contractions, and propagated activity, which is either high-amplitude (>100 mm Hg) propagated contractions (HAPCs) or low-amplitude (<60 mm Hg) propagated contractions (LAPCs). *Segmental contractions* are intermittent contractions of the longitudinal and circular muscles that result in the segmented appearance of the colon.[13] These contractions propel luminal contents in a back-and-forth pattern over short distances, slowing aboral transit and allowing for water reabsorption.[14] *Propagated activity* consists of strong, propulsive contractions of the smooth muscle that involve a long segment of colon.[15] The LAPCs move luminal contents forward at a rate of 0.5 to 1.0 cm/s and typically last for 20 to 30 seconds.[13] HAPCs occur three to four times per day, primarily after awakening, exercise, and after meals.

The orderly progression of colonic luminal contents from cecum to anus requires the coordination of smooth muscle contractions. Calcium-dependent cyclic depolarization and repolarization of the colonic smooth muscle cell membrane generates a basic electrical pattern of slow-wave activity. This activity allows each smooth muscle cell to control its own contraction and to couple with adjacent smooth muscle cells.[16] The extrinsic (autonomic) and intrinsic (enteric) neuronal systems also interact to influence colonic motility.

Defecation

When fecal matter enters the rectum, the internal anal sphincter relaxes, which is called the rectoanal inhibitory reflex, or RAIR. Then, the external anal sphincter contracts to maintain continence. Distention of the rectum in this setting is the primary stimulus for defecation to begin. At this point, the urge to defecate may be suppressed by conscious contraction of the external anal sphincter. Receptive relaxation of the rectal ampulla accommodates the fecal mass and the urge to defecate passes unless the volume of feces is extremely large or the sphincter mechanism is impaired. If the subject voluntarily agrees to the urge to defecate, a Valsalva maneuver occurs, which increases the intra-abdominal pressure to overcome the resistance of the external anal sphincter. Relaxation of the pelvic muscles causes the pelvic floor to descend and the anorectal angle to straighten. Conscious inhibition of the external anal sphincter then allows passage of the feces. On completion, the pelvic floor returns to its resting position and the anal sphincter muscles return to their resting activity, closing the anal canal. Under normal circumstances, this process occurs once every 24 hours; however, the interval between bowel movements may vary between 8 and 12 hours and 2 to 3 days in normal subjects.

Anal Continence

There are varying degrees of anal continence, with a spectrum from complete control to complete lack of control. Maintaining continence is complex, as both voluntary and involuntary mechanisms play a role in anal continence. The most important mechanisms involve the internal anal sphincter, which contributes 52% to 85% of the pressure generated to maintain continence.[17,18] The remaining anal basal pressure is comprised of the external anal sphincter (30%) and the hemorrhoidal cushions (15%). The internal sphincter is supplied by dual extrinsic innervation: sympathetic outflow (S5) via the hypogastric nerve provides motor supply and parasympathetic outflow (S1 to S3) provides inhibition. The external sphincter nerve supply is dependent on the pudendal nerve (S2 to S4) and maintains tonic activity at rest. When stool enters the rectum, the contents of the rectum are sampled by sensors in the anal canal to determine whether the contents are solid, liquid, or gas. By discriminating between the consistency of the stool, the pelvic floor and sphincter muscles are able to coordinate a complex mechanism through angulation of the pelvic floor and contraction of the anal sphincter muscles. Other mechanisms contributing to continence include stool consistency and volume.

SUMMARY

Understanding colorectal anatomy and physiology is essential for safe and effective colorectal surgical judgment and technique.

ACKNOWLEDGMENTS

We gratefully acknowledge the contributions of previous edition authors, Elise H. Lawson and Elizabeth C. Wick, as portions of those chapters have been retained in this revision.

References

1. Gordon PH, Nivatvongs S, eds. *Principles and Practice of Surgery for the Colon, Rectum, and Anus.* 3rd ed. Informa Healthcare USA, Inc.; 2007.
2. Kumar D, Phillips SF. The contribution of external ligamentous attachments to function of the ileocecal junction. *Dis Colon Rectum.* 1987;30(6):410–416.
3. Wakeley CP. The position of the vermiform appendix as ascertained by an analysis of 10,000 cases. *J Anat.* 1933;67(Pt 2):277–283.
4. Jorge JMN, Habr-Gama A, eds. *Anatomy and Embryology of the Colon, Rectum, and Anus.* Springer; 2007.
5. Morren GL, Beets-Tan RG, van Engelshoven JM. Anatomy of the anal canal and perianal structures as defined by phased-array magnetic resonance imaging. *Br J Surg.* 2001;88(11):1506–1512.
6. Latella G, Caprilli R. Metabolism of large bowel mucosa in health and disease. *Int J Colorectal Dis.* 1991;6(2):127–132.
7. Szmulowicz UM, Hull TL. *Colonic Physiology. The ASCRS Textbook of Colon and Rectal Surgery.* Springer; 2011.
8. Grady GF, Duhamel RC, Moore EW. Active transport of sodium by human colon in vitro. *Gastroenterology.* 1970;59(4):583–588.
9. Giller J, Phillips SF. Electrolyte absorption and secretion in the human colon. *Am J Dig Dis.* 1972;17(11):1003–1011.
10. Hooper LV, Gordon JI. Commensal host-bacterial relationships in the gut. *Science.* 2001;292(5519):1115–1118.
11. Cho I, Blaser MJ. The human microbiome: at the interface of health and disease. *Nat Rev Genet.* 2012;13(4):260–270.
12. Rescigno M. The pathogenic role of intestinal flora in IBD and colon cancer. *Curr Drug Targets.* 2008;9(5):395–403.
13. Ritchie JA. Movement of segmental constrictions in the human colon. *Gut.* 1971;12(5):350–355.
14. Husebye E. The patterns of small bowel motility: physiology and implications in organic disease and functional disorders. *Neurogastroenterol Motil.* 1999;11(3):141–161.
15. Hertz AF, Morton CJ, Cook F, et al. The passage of food along the human alimentary canal. *Guys Hosp Rep.* 1907;61:389–427.
16. Daniel EE. Symposium on colonic function. Electrophysiology of the colon. *Gut.* 1975;16(4):298–306.
17. Cali RL, Blatchford GJ, Perry RE, Pitch RM, Thorson AG, Christensen MA. Normal variation in anorectal manometry. *Dis Colon Rectum.* 1992;35(12):1161–1164.
18. Frenckner B, Euler CV. Influence of pudendal block on the function of the anal sphincters. *Gut.* 1975;16(6):482–489.

62

Gastrointestinal Bleeding

Eric M. Pauli

Key Points

1 Gastrointestinal bleeding is classified as upper, lower, or small bowel bleeding based on the accessibility of the bleeding site to endoscopic identification and intervention.

2 Esophagogastroduodenoscopy is the initial diagnostic and therapeutic procedure of choice in almost all cases of upper gastrointestinal bleeding.

3 Radiologic examinations play a major role in the diagnosis and therapy of gastrointestinal bleeding and are complementary to endoscopic evaluation.

4 Hemodynamically stable patients with hematochezia should undergo colonoscopy after resuscitation and bowel preparation.

5 As many as 15% of hemodynamically unstable patients presenting with hematochezia will be bleeding from an upper gastrointestinal source.

6 About 70% of patients with overt gastrointestinal bleeding in whom endoscopy failed to identify a site of hemorrhage will be bleeding from the small intestine.

7 Video capsule endoscopy is the diagnostic test of choice for hemodynamically stable patients suspected to have small bowel bleeding.

8 Multimodal endoscopic therapy significantly reduces the rate of recurrent bleeding and the need for urgent surgical intervention in patients with high-risk lesions.

9 Bleeding from lesions not amenable to endoscopic therapy or who fail repeat endoscopic therapy should be managed by angiographic embolization or surgery.

NOMENCLATURE

Bleeding from the gastrointestinal (GI) tract is classified as overt or occult based on the presence or absence of visible signs of blood loss. Patients with overt GI bleeding (GIB) may present with hematemesis (vomiting blood), melena (black, tarry stools), or hematochezia (passage of fresh blood per anus). Patients with occult GIB may present with iron deficiency anemia or a positive fecal occult blood test. This chapter focuses on the clinical features, evaluation, and management of patients with overt GIB. Although advanced endoscopic and interventional radiologic techniques have dramatically reduced the role of surgery in the management of GIB, collaboration between interventionist and surgeon is still critical for many patients.

1 GIB is classified as upper, lower, or small bowel based on the location of the bleeding relative to anatomic landmarks; upper GIB (UGIB) originates proximal to the duodenal–jejunal junction (ie, the ligament of Treitz), lower GIB (LGIB) originates distal to the ileocecal valve (ie, colon and rectum), and small bowel GIB (SBGIB), previously referred to as obscure GIB, originates within the jejunum and ileum.

EPIDEMIOLOGY

Bleeding is the fifth most common GI symptom prompting an ambulatory visit (after abdominal pain, vomiting, nausea, and diarrhea) and is responsible for >1.5 million annual visits.[1] Of hospitalized patients with overt GIB, about 40% to 60% have UGIB, 25% to 32% have LGIB, 5% to 10% have SBGIB, and 29% to 35% have an unknown source.[1–4] The most common causes of overt GIB and their relative frequencies are shown in **Table 62.1**.

Bleeding is the most common indication for hospital admission (and readmission) for GI diseases in the United States (US). In 2018, GIB caused >530,000 hospitalizations, >84,000 readmissions (17.4%), 1.3 million days of hospitalization, $3.6 billion in aggregate costs, and >8,100 deaths (2.4% mortality).[1]

The incidence of UGIB in the United States is about 67 cases per 100,000 population, with a 21% declining incidence over the last 30 years, largely due to decreased bleeding from peptic ulcer disease (PUD) and gastritis.[5] The incidence of LGIB (as traditionally defined) is about 33 cases per 100,000 population, with significant decrease in the incidence of hospitalization over time.[1] Some of this decrease represents better reporting of SBGIB as its own entity, no longer categorized as LGIB. Although overt GIB can occur at any age, it is particularly prevalent in the elderly. The median age of patients hospitalized for upper and LGIB is 67 and 74 years, respectively.[1,5,6] UGIB is slightly more common in males (55%), and LBIG is slightly more common in females (52%).[5,6]

CLINICAL PRESENTATION

A thorough medical history, physical examination, and basic laboratory tests provide important information regarding the location and cause of bleeding, risk factors for GIB, and the severity of bleeding. Clinical scenarios associated with various causes of GIB are shown in **Table 62.2**.

Site and Cause of Bleeding

Patients with UGIB will usually present with hematemesis or melena. Hematemesis is the vomiting of bright red blood or dark heme-positive material, termed "coffee-ground emesis." The latter is blood that has been partially degraded, suggesting that bleeding has stopped. The vomiting of bright red blood suggests recent and/or ongoing bleeding. Melena is the passage of black, tarry stools with a characteristic pungent odor. It is caused by bacterial degradation of blood and can occur with

Table 62.1. Causes of Overt Gastrointestinal Bleeding and Their Relative Frequencies[1–6]

Upper GI Bleeding	Relative Frequency (%)
Peptic ulcer disease	20–50
Erosive disease (gastritis, esophagitis, duodenitis)	8–15
Mallory–Weiss tear	8–15
Varices	5–10
Vascular lesions (Dieulafoy lesion, gastric antral vascular ectasia)	5
Esophageal/gastric neoplasm	3–5
Hemobilia, hemosuccus pancreaticus, aortoenteric fistula, Cameron lesion	Uncommon—rare
Small Bowel GI Bleeding	**Relative Frequencies Poorly Defined**
Age ≤ 40 y	Age ≥40 y
Small bowel diverticulum (jejunal, Meckel's)	NSAID-related ulcers
Inflammatory bowel disease	Angioectasia
Polyposis syndromes	Neoplasm
Neoplasm	Dieulafoy lesion
Dieulafoy lesion	
Lower GI Bleeding	**Relative Frequency (%)**
Diverticular bleeding	26–31
Internal hemorrhoids	14–19
Neoplasm	6–20
Colon ischemia	6–12
Postpolypectomy bleeding	3–8
Inflammatory bowel disease	2–9
Angioectasias	1–6
Infectious colitis, NSAID colopathy, radiation colitis/proctitis, stercoral ulcer, Dieulafoy lesions	Uncommon—rare

GI, gastrointestinal; NSAID, nonsteroidal anti-inflammatory drug.

Table 62.2. Clinical Scenarios Associated with Overt Gastrointestinal Bleeding

Upper GI Bleeding

Peptic ulcer disease
Prolonged epigastric pain, hematemesis/melena in a person taking aspirin or NSAIDs

Esophagitis/esophageal ulceration
Hematemesis/melena, history of gastroesophageal reflux, pyrosis, or dysphagia

Mallory–Weiss tear
Vomiting/retching followed by hematemesis/melena

Gastroesophageal varices
Painless, large-volume bleeding, history of cirrhosis or alcoholism

Aorta–GI fistula (generally duodenal or esophageal)
Large-volume bleeding (hematemesis/hematochezia), history of open aortic implant graft

Small Bowel GI Bleeding

Angioectasias
Recurrent GIB in an elderly patient with chronic renal failure or aortic stenosis

Meckel diverticulum
Painless, large-volume rectal bleeding in a child or young adult

Lower GI Bleeding

Diverticular bleeding
Painless, intermittent large-volume hematochezia, history of colonic diverticulosis

Internal hemorrhoids
Intermittent low-volume bleeding, bright red blood on toilet tissue or in toilet water

Colonic angiodysplasia
Intermittent low-volume bleeding, history of aortic stenosis, LVAD, or nephropathy

Colon ischemia
Abdominal pain, hematochezia in an elderly patient with cardiovascular disease
Bloody diarrhea shortly after abdominal aortic aneurysm repair

LVAD, left ventricular assist device.

as little as 50 mL of blood. Clinical findings most suggestive of a UGIB include melena, nasogastric (NG) lavage fluid containing blood or coffee grounds, and a serum urea nitrogen-to-creatinine ratio of more than 30.

Hematochezia is the passage of bright red blood, maroon-colored blood, or blood clots per anus. Although it is generally associated with bleeding from the colon or rectum, 15% of patients with hematochezia will have severe UGIB bleeding source.

Risk Factors for GI Bleeding

Important risk factors for overt GIB include advanced age, smoking, *Helicobacter pylori* (*H. pylori*) infection, nonsteroidal anti-inflammatory drug (NSAID) and/or aspirin (ASA) use, antiplatelet and/or anticoagulant use, and the presence of chronic illnesses, especially kidney, liver, and cardiac disease.[5,6] Risk factors have a synergistic effect; the combination of NSAIDs and anticoagulants doubles the risk of UGIB compared with NSAID or anticoagulant use alone. GIB commonly complicates hospitalizations for other common illnesses such as sepsis, neurologic injuries (stroke, trauma), myocardial infarction, renal failure, cirrhosis, and cancer.[6]

Severity of Bleeding

GIB varies from minor, self-limited episodes of blood loss to massive hemorrhage with shock. The medical history, physical examination, and basic laboratory tests provide important information regarding the severity of bleeding. Basic laboratory tests should include a complete blood count, basic metabolic panel, liver function tests, coagulation profile, and blood type and crossmatch. Patients with GIB may present with symptoms and physical exam features of acute blood loss; light-headedness, dizziness, syncope or near syncope, shortness of breath, tachycardia, tachypnea, clammy/mottled skin, oliguria, and hypotension. Advanced age, chronic illnesses, and medications may obscure normal signs of shock.

RISK ASSESSMENT AND TRIAGE

The severity of GIB and the patient's hemodynamic response guide triage for diagnostic studies and therapeutic interventions. Fortunately, most overt GIB will stop spontaneously. Minor, self-limited bleeding in stable patients may be managed in an ambulatory setting, whereas patients with ongoing or severe bleeding require intensive care and urgent endoscopic intervention. Patients with persistent GIB or who rebleed are likely to require endoscopic, angiographic, or surgical intervention and are at higher risk of morbidity and mortality.

Risk Assessment Tools for Upper GI Bleeding

UGIB risk scores are divided into two groups: preendoscopic and postendoscopic. Preendoscopic risk scores do not depend

Table 62.3. Variables Used in Risk Assessment Tools for Patients with Upper GI Bleeding

Glasgow-Blatchford Score (predicts inpatient treatment need)	Rockall Score (predicts mortality)	AIMS65 Score (predicts mortality, LOS and cost)	ABC Score (predicts 30-d mortality for UGIB and LGIB)
Systolic BP and HR	Systolic BP and HR	Systolic BP	Age
Blood urea nitrogen	Age	Age	Blood Tests: Urea Albumin Creatinine
Other Admission Findings: Melena at presentation Syncope at presentation Hepatic disease Cardiac failure	Comorbidities: Cardiac Renal Liver failure Disseminated malignancy	International normalized ratio	Comorbidities: Altered mental state Liver cirrhosis Disseminated malignancy ASA Classification
Hemoglobin	Endoscopic diagnosis	Albumin	
	Endoscopic findings of recent hemorrhage	Mental status	

on endoscopic visualization of bleeding and can be calculated soon after admission. Examples include the Glasgow–Blatchford score (GBS), the AIMS65 score, and the ABC score. Notably, the ABC score was designed for utilization in both UGIB and LGIB. The Rockall score is the most commonly used postendoscopic assessment tool.[7] The variables used in these risk assessment tools are shown in **Table 62.3**.

Risk Assessment Tools for Lower GI Bleeding

The best studied LGIB predictive model, the Oakland score, utilizes clinical variables alone (age, gender, prior LGIB, blood on rectal exam, heart rate, systolic blood pressure, and hemoglobin). Meta-analysis of nine studies suggests the Oakland score is the best available LGIB tool to predict safe discharge, the need for transfusion and the likelihood of major bleeding.[8]

RESUSCITATION

Airway Management

Patients with severe GIB who are inadequately ventilating or who are unable to protect their airway should undergo endotracheal intubation; however prophylactic endotracheal intubation is not indicated as it is associated with cardiopulmonary complications such as pneumonia.

Volume Resuscitation

Volume resuscitation with two large-bore intravenous (IV) canulae and isotonic saline solution is all that is required in most patients. The decision to transfuse blood or blood products depends on the specific needs of the patient. Randomized controlled trials support a restrictive transfusion strategy withholding packed red blood cells (PRBC) until a hemoglobin threshold of 7.0 to 8.0 g/dL is reached.[9] A higher threshold (8 to 10 g/dL) is used for patients with ischemic cardiac disease. Patients with massive GIB should receive a balanced hemorrhagic resuscitation regimen (eg, a 1:1:1 ratio of PRBC, fresh frozen plasma, and platelets). Patients must be appropriately resuscitated prior to endoscopy as inadequate resuscitation is associated with adverse outcomes, including in-hospital mortality.[10]

Hemodynamic Monitoring

Patients with evidence of active bleeding, those who have sustained significant blood loss, and those with risk factors for adverse outcomes should be admitted to an intensive care unit (ICU). The placement of a urinary catheter and frequent monitoring of heart rate, blood pressure, oxygen saturation, and mental status are minimum necessary to monitor patients who have suffered significant GIB. The presence of comorbidities such as cardiac, renal, or hepatic disease may necessitate invasive cardiac monitoring in order to optimize intravascular volume replacement therapy.

Gastric Emptying Interventions

The routine placement of an NG tube in patients with suspected GIB is not recommended. Prokinetic agents (erythromycin and metoclopramide) improve gastric visualization during endoscopy by emptying the study of blood clot and residual food. A meta-analysis of randomized controlled trials concluded that patients who receive erythromycin were more likely to have adequate endoscopic visualization and were less likely to need a second endoscopy, which resulted in a shorter hospital stay.[11] However, there were no differences in transfusion requirements, the duration of endoscopy, or the need for surgical intervention to manage bleeding.[11]

Acid Suppression

All patients with signs of clinically significant UGIB (hematemesis, hematochezia, melena), regardless of blood transfusion requirements or hemodynamic stability, should be started on IV proton pump inhibitor (PPI) therapy while undergoing initial evaluation and resuscitation.

Management of Antithrombotic Drugs

Twenty-nine percent to 44% of patients with severe GIB are taking antithrombotic drugs (antiplatelet agents and/or anticoagulants).[6] Management strategy must balance the effect of the antithrombotic agent, the severity of bleeding, the risk of thromboembolic events, and the speed at which reversal is needed. The treatment of patients who develop GIB while receiving antithrombotic medications is the subject of numerous consensus guidelines, including those promulgated by the American Society for Gastrointestinal Endoscopy.[12] A full summary of these guidelines is beyond the scope of this work.

DIAGNOSTIC ALGORITHMS

Upper GI Bleeding

2 The initial diagnostic test in almost all cases of UGIB is esophagogastroduodenoscopy (EGD). This procedure is diagnostic

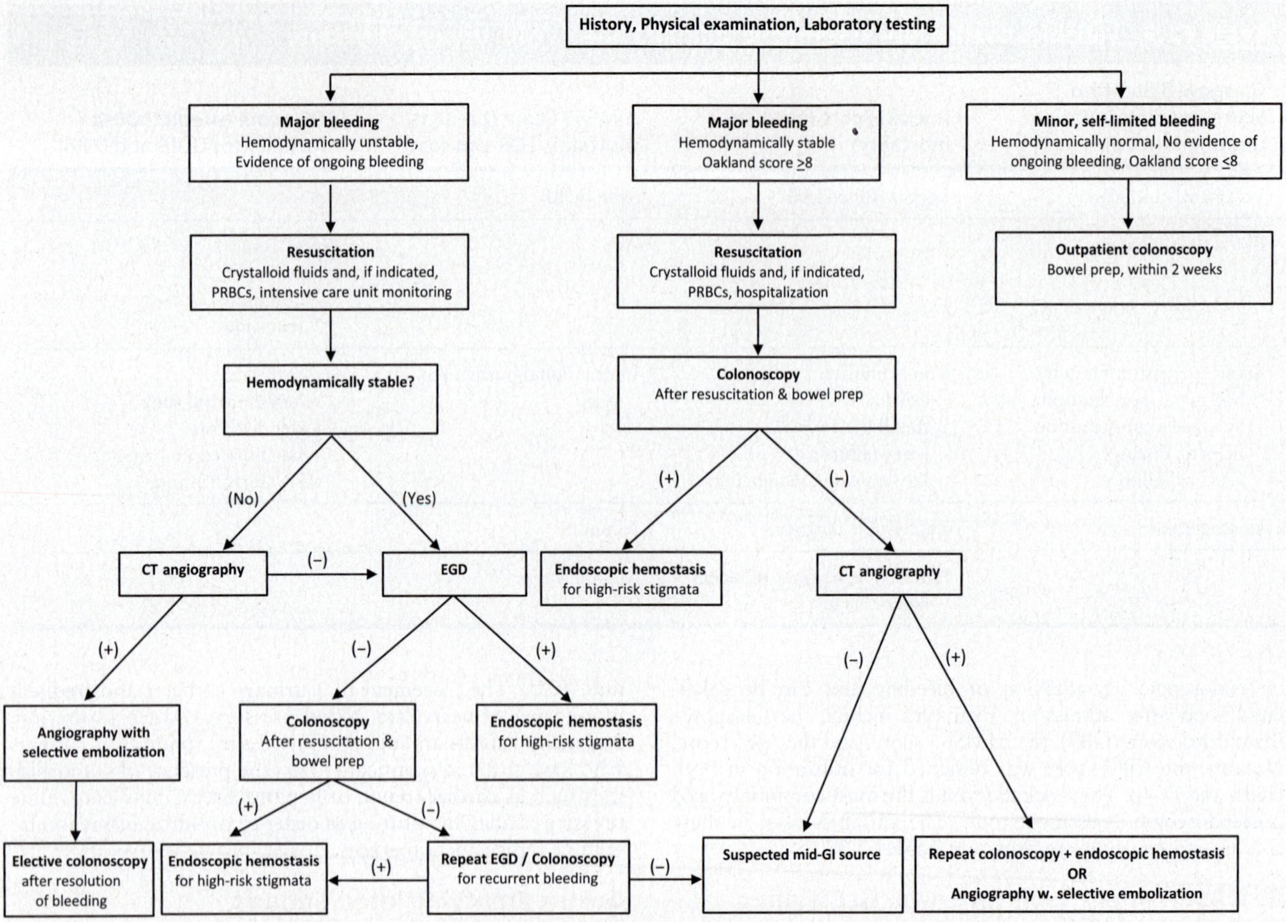

Figure 62.1. Diagnostic algorithm for patients presenting with hematochezia. PRBCs, packed red blood cells; EGD, esophagogastroduodenoscopy; GI, gastrointestinal; CT, computed tomography; (+), diagnostic; (–), nondiagnostic.

in 95% of cases, permits immediate therapy, and allows assessment of rebleeding risk. Endoscopy also facilitates discharge of low-risk patients, improves outcomes for high-risk patients, and reduces resource utilization. Following appropriate resuscitation, patients should undergo EGD within 24 hours. Patients with cirrhosis and suspected variceal bleeding or refractory hemodynamic instability from bleeding should undergo EGD within 12 hours. If no source of UGIB is identified, a colonoscopy should be considered (in patients without hematemesis) to evaluate for LGIB. For example, a patient with melena and a negative EGD may have a right-sided colonic lesion identified.

If no source of bleeding can be identified on EGD and subsequent colonoscopy, consideration should be given to computed tomographic angiography (CTA). CTA can be performed expeditiously, detects bleeding rates as low as 0.3 mL/min, and iden-
3 tifies sources outside the reach of a standard endoscope. In actively bleeding patients, CTA has an 85% sensitivity and a 92% specificity.[13]

Visceral angiography is indicated when a site of active bleeding is not amenable to endoscopic hemostasis. In this setting, visceral angiography has a high diagnostic accuracy and is effective in achieving hemostasis with catheter-based embolization techniques in about 80% of cases.[13] Visceral angiography will detect bleeding at rates of 0.5 to 1.0 mL/min, a rate of bleeding that correlates with the need for ongoing volume resuscitation to maintain hemodynamic stability. If the bleeding has stopped or is intermittent, the bleeding site will not be visualized by angiography.

Lower GI Bleeding

The timing and manner of diagnostic studies for patients with LGIB depend upon the severity of bleeding and the hemodynamic status of the patient. A diagnostic algorithm for the evaluation of patients with LGIB is shown in **Figure 62.1**. Patients with minor self-limited episodes of bleeding and no other indication for hospitalization (eg, Oakland score ≤10) may be discharged from the emergency department and evaluated by colonoscopy in an outpatient
4 setting.[14] Hemodynamically stable patients with suspected LGIB should undergo inpatient colonoscopy. The timing of the procedure is controversial because the literature is conflicted regarding the benefits of colonoscopy within 24 hours versus more delayed evaluation. Patients should undergo bowel preparation prior to colonoscopy in order to optimize visualization of the colonic mucosa. Unprepped colonoscopy is reserved for LGIB known (or highly suspected) to be in the anorectal region.

CTA is indicated when colonoscopy documents evidence of bleeding but is unable to identify the source. Additionally, hemodynamically unstable patients with hematochezia unresponsive to volume resuscitation should undergo CTA as the initial diagnostic test since these patients are unlikely to tolerate the bowel preparation necessary for colonoscopy. If a source of bleeding is identified by CTA, the patients should undergo visceral angiography with superselective emboliza-
5 tion. If a source of bleeding is not identified by CTA, an EGD should be performed, given the 15% chance of UGIB in unstable patients presenting with hematochezia.

SMALL BOWEL GI BLEEDING

6 About 70% of patients with overt GIB with a negative EGD and colonoscopy are bleeding from the small intestine.[15] Hemodynamically stable patients should first undergo repeat EGD and/or colonoscopy, which will identify a site of bleeding in

30% to 40% of patients. This is especially true if the initial endoscopic examination was suboptimal (eg, poor bowel prep). With significant GIB requiring ongoing transfusion, visceral angiography or CTA can be performed to identify the site of bleeding and guide subsequent endoscopic or angiographic hemostasis.

For stable patients who have undergone adequate EGD and colonoscopy, wireless video capsule endoscopy (VCE) is the
7 next test of choice. VCE examines the complete small bowel in 80% to 90% of cases and has a diagnostic yield of 80% in patients with suspected SBGIB, especially if performed <72 hours after bleeding.[15] Recurrent bleeding after a negative VCE is infrequent (6% to 11%).[15] Patients with suspected SBGIB and obstructive symptoms should not undergo VCE as capsule retention occurs in about 1% of examinations, typically at the site of a small bowel stricture.

Additional imaging studies may be used if VCE is unavailable. Multiphase CT enterography uses IV contrast and large-volume oral contrast to detect small bowel inflammatory lesions, neoplasms, and vascular abnormalities with a diagnostic yield of 40% to 57% in patients with SBGIB.[16] Technetium-99m pertechnetate scintigraphy identifies ectopic gastric mucosa in patients suspected to be bleeding from a Meckel diverticulum, which results in a focus of abnormal radioactivity in the right lower abdomen. The diagnostic accuracy of pertechnetate scintigraphy is greater than 90% in children but is less than 50% in adults.[17] Small bowel enteroscopy (SBE, sometimes referred to as device-assisted enteroscopy) is a broad term that includes spiral, single-, and double-balloon enteroscopy (DBE). These labor-intensive procedures utilize specially designed overtubes that accommodate a thin, flexible enteroscope. DBE is the most widely studied method for the diagnosis and management of SBGIB; it can identify the source of bleeding in most patients (78%), with a higher likelihood of identification with performed <30 days after the suspected SBGIB (84% vs 57%).[18] DBE also permits therapy in patients identified to have an SBGIB on VCE, CT enterography, or CTA.

ENDOSCOPIC OPTIONS FOR ACUTE BLEEDING MANAGEMENT

Endoscopic tools have been utilized to manage GIB since the mid-1970s. It should be noted that many early innovations in the endoscopic hemostasis armamentarium were invented or coinvented by surgical endoscopists who recognized the advantages of endoscopic therapy over traditional open surgical management of GIB. Endoscopic modalities of acute hemostatic control are broadly defined by their mechanism of action: electrosurgical, injection, mechanical, topical (see **Table 62.4**). A variety of other endoscopic tools (cryotherapy, radiofrequency ablation) are available for the management of chronically bleeding lesions, but will not be discussed here.

Electrosurgical Energy Devices (Fig. 62.2)

Contact Devices

The endoscopic application of electrosurgical energy to seal a bleeding vessel (coaptive hemostasis) is a principle familiar to surgeons and is fundamentally no different than the surgical application of energy. The most commonly utilized device, a bipolar probe, is applied to an area of bleeding (or a visible nonbleeding vessel) with enough force to tamponade the bleeding. Applied current moves from one portion of the probe to another, resulting in local tissue effect that seals the vessel through protein coagulation.

Alternatively, a hemostatic grasping forceps can be utilized. These monopolar devices were originally designed to coagulate small vessels encountered during endoscopic mucosal resection, but have since been utilized to perform coapitve hemostasis on actively bleeding lesions. The vessel is grasped within the jaw (providing mechanical tamponade), and a low-voltage energy is applied. The low voltage is effective at hemostasis without tissue effect at a deeper level or carbonization of tissue.[19]

Noncontact Devices

Argon plasma coagulation (APC) probes deliver a stream of inert argon gas that is subsequently converted into plasma

Table 62.4. Endoscopic Options for the Management of Gastrointestinal Bleeding

Category	Type	Common Application	Limiting Factors
Electrosurgical Energy	Bipolar probe	Actively bleeding or visible vessel in ulcer base	Tissue effect can spread, more common in thin-walled locations
	Coagulation grasper	Actively bleeding or visible vessel in ulcer base	Jaw size and tissue rigidity may limit ability to grasp vessels
	Argon plasma coagulation	Focal of diffuse mucosal based vascular malformations	High volume argon gas causes distension, superficial coagulation only
Injection	Epinephrine	Initial step of multimodal therapy for bleeding PUD	Less effective as monotherapy for high-risk lesions
Mechanical	Through the scope clips	Wide bleeding applications	Difficult to apply to woody or fibrotic tissue
	Over-the-scope clips	Wide bleeding applications	Requires endoscopic removal and application
	Endoscopic suturing	Wide bleeding applications	Requires endoscopic removal and application, requires advanced endoscopic skillset
	Endoloop	Temporize bleeding tumors or polyps	Requires tumor to be small enough to fit into the loop
	Band ligation	Variceal and hemorrhoidal bleeding	Requires endoscopic removal and application, work poorly on woody or fibrotic tissue
Topical	TC-325	Actively bleeding lesions	Commonly forms clogs in the delivery catheter
	Endoclot	Actively bleeding lesions	Not approved for Forrest 1a bleeding

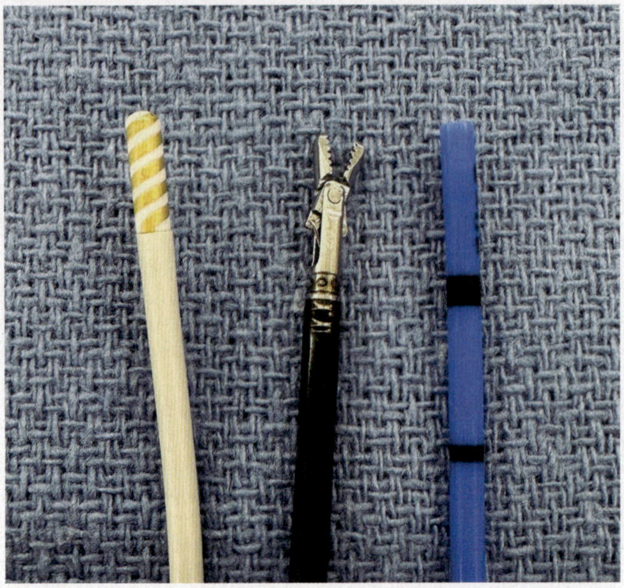

Figure 62.2. Electrosurgical energy devices for hemostasis (left to right) bipolar probe, hemostatic grasping forceps, forward shooting argon plasma coagulation probe.

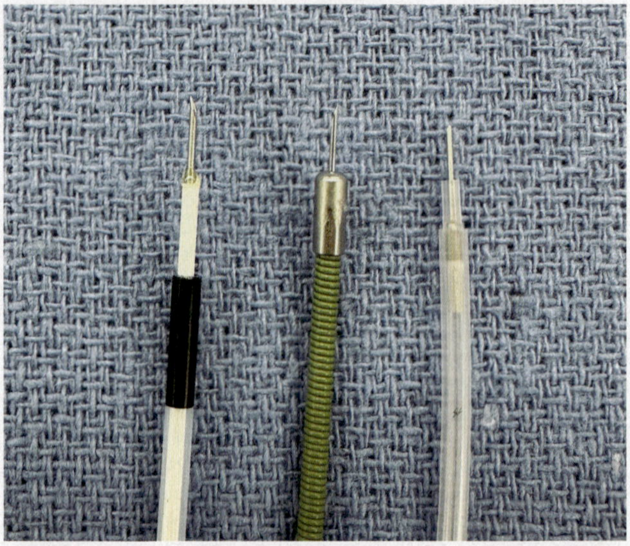

Figure 62.4. Endoscopic needles capable of performing injection therapy for GI bleeding.

(ionized argon) by a monopolar electrode located at the tip of the device. The probe tip is placed near (approximately 5 mm) away from the intended target, allowing a high-frequency current to induce coagulation as it is conducted through the gas. Placing the probe against the tissue reduces the effectiveness of therapy and risks introducing pressurized gas into the submucosa. APC catheters are available with a variety of distal tips (eg, forward, side, circumferential) that alter the shape and direction of the gas flow to alter the direction of therapy. APC works best on superficial lesions like bleeding vascular malformations, because the coagulation effect is extremely superficial (**Fig. 62.3**). Additionally, it is commonly applied to diffusely bleeding GI tract tumors.[20]

Injection Therapy

Endoscopic needles can be used to deliver a variety of agents around an area of bleeding or directly into blood vessels themselves. After the injection catheter is advanced though the working channel of the endoscope, a needle is extended to a preset distance (**Fig. 62.4**). The needle is then pushed into the intended target and a syringe is used to deliver a liquid agent. Filling the surrounding tissues with a liquid results in tamponade and/or the agent may have some direct effect on bleeding as well (eg, vasoconstriction, thrombogenesis).

The most commonly utilized agent is dilute epinephrine (1;10,000) which is injected circumferentially around an area of bleeding to permit the application of a second form of hemostasis (generally a contact electrosurgical method or a clip application). Epinephrine monotherapy has been demonstrated to result in higher rates of rebleeding for high-risk lesions, and as such, it generally should not be used as an isolated method of hemorrhage control. Some agents, such as cyanoacrylate, thrombin, or fibrin glue, can be injected directly into blood vessels (generally gastric or esophageal varices) to form an immediate stable clot and thrombose the vessel. These therapies have higher rates of complications and remote embolization and should not be attempted by inexperienced endoscopists.

Mechanical Therapy

The term mechanical therapy is applied to a wide array of devices that provide durable tissue compression that tamponades bleeding, directly occludes blood flow and permits vascular thrombosis through stasis.

Through the Scope Clip

Through the scope (TTS) clips are metal tissue compression devices mounted on the end of a catheter passed through the working channel of the endoscope. They are widely available in endoscopy units worldwide and are made by most manufacturers of endoscopic disposable tools. TTS clips vary greatly in physical profile and functional properties, including jaw opening distance, the ability to open and close repeatedly, tooth characteristics, rotatability, compression strength, jaw

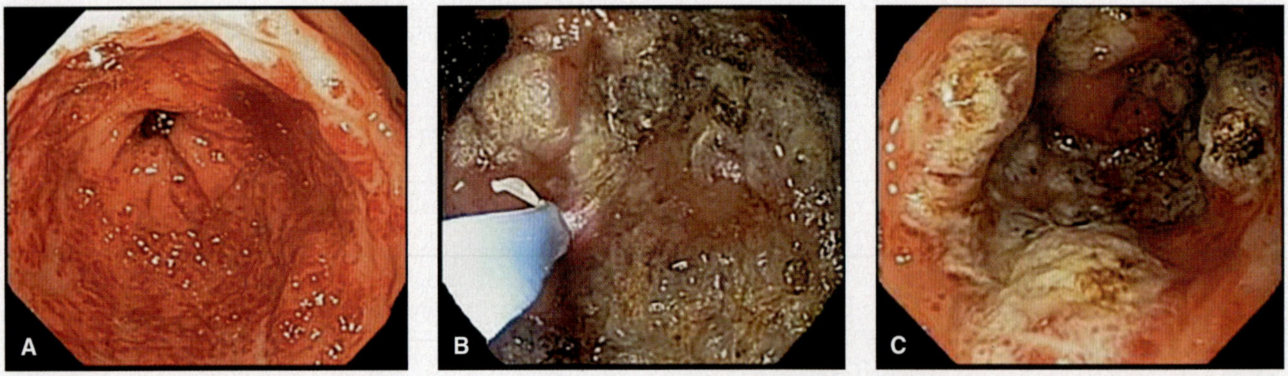

Figure 62.3. **A:** Endoscopic view of bleeding gastric antral vascular ectasias in an anticoagulated patient. **B:** APC application. **C:** Endoscopic view of the gastric antrum after APC therapy.

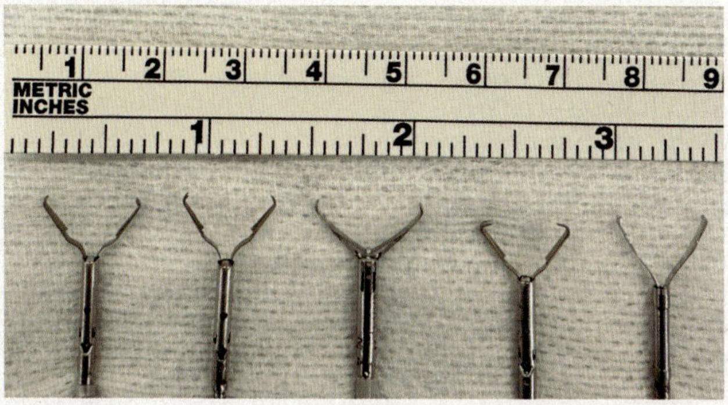

Figure 62.5. Through the scope clips from various manufacturers demonstrated a variety of jaw opening widths, tooth types, and jaw thickness.

deformation force, deployed length/stem height and price (**Fig. 62.5**). While each of these characteristics may theoretically influence the type of clip an endoscopist chooses to use, practically most endoscopy units carry a limited selection of clips from one manufacturer. Endoscopists should be familiar with the strengths and weaknesses of the specific clips they have access to.

When employed for bleeding, the jaws of the clip are opened and then closed to capture tissue around the source of bleeding to provide mechanical compression. This may be particularly challenging when the bleeding source is surrounded by woody or fibrotic tissue (such as at the base of an ulcer) or when the bleeding is in a difficult-to-access location (such as the posterior duodenal wall). Despite these issues, their wide availability and deployment of TTS make them a valuable tool for endoscopic management of GIB. The latter point is particularly important; the endoscope does not need to be removed and readvanced to the site of bleeding to permit TTS clip therapy. As soon as bleeding has been slowed with injection therapy or contact thermal methods, a TTS clip can be rapidly deployed as a component of multimodal therapy.

Over-the-Scope Clips

Over-the-scope (OTS) clips are large, nitinol alloy devices that are cap-mounted onto the distal endoscope in an "open" position (**Fig. 62.6**). They are navigated into position, affixed to the endoscope, and deployed onto tissue from the cap. Because of their large size, they are capable of addressing bleeding in areas of large tissue defects (eg, large ulcers), and because of the elastic properties of nitinol, they are able to apply compression force even when tissues are fibrotic or woody. OTS clips are presently available from two manufacturers and come in a variety of diameters, depths, and tooth characteristics.

OTS clips have been demonstrated to be effective as both first-line therapy for bleeding and salvage therapy for rebleeding in nonvariceal GIB.[19] When compared to traditional multimodal therapy (epinephrine plus contact electrosurgical energy or TTS clips), OTS clip monotherapy demonstrated significantly lower rates of persistent bleeding (6% vs 42%, respectively).[19] The overall success rate of OTS clips for GIB management is as high as 85% in large series.[19] Despite their advantages, OTS clip use requires the endoscope to be removed after the bleeding source had been identified in order for the cap-mounted clip to be applied. The endoscope must subsequently be readvanced into position with a large diameter rigid cap on the distal tip. This can be problematic in smaller patients or those with GI tract strictures that may not accommodate the outer diameter of the device.

Endoscopic Suturing

Endoscopic suturing devices have been commercially available in the United States for more than a decade and have been applied to a wide array of GIB applications. Initially available

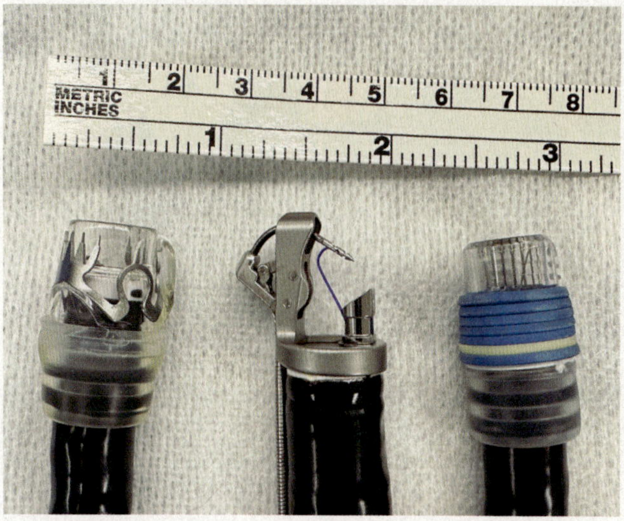

Figure 62.6. Cap-based methods of mechanical compression for hemostasis (left to right); over-the-scope clip mounted on the end of a single-channel therapeutic gastroscope, endoscopic suturing device mounted on the end of a double-channel therapeutic gastroscope, band ligation device mounted on the end of a diagnostic gastroscope. Note the difference in endoscope diameter, cap diameter, and cap length between the devices.

only for use with a double-channel endoscope, newer versions of endoscopic suturing devices are able to mounted on the end of a standard gastroscope (**Fig. 62.6**). Suturing devices are capable of taking full-thickness bites of the GI tract and are therefore capable of capturing large amounts of tissue with each bite.

Unfortunately, despite the conceptual simplicity of "suture the bleeding," these devices are challenging to use. They require the endoscope to be removed to affix the device, they have to be navigated to the site of bleeding, they are available only on gastroscopes (which limits their utility in the more proximal colon), they have a large outer diameter and may not fit in smaller patients or across GI tract strictures, they require working space for the suturing arm to open, they work poorly in a fully retroflexed position and suture tangles can prolong the procedure time and/or prevent appropriate tissue compressing when the suture is cinched.

Band Ligation

Elastic band ligation of internal hemorrhoids was first performed in the 1950s and was subsequently adapted for the management of esophageal varices in the 1980s. Band ligation devices mount onto the end of a diagnostic gastroscope with a small, rigid cap that holds multiple (4 to 10) bands stretched over the cap (**Fig. 62.6**). After tissue is drawn into the cap with suction, a rubber band is deployed from the cap, which compresses the base of the captured tissue. Band ligation is the most widely accepted therapy for acute variceal bleeding but has been applied to other bleeding sources including diverticular, hemorrhoidal, vascular malformations, Dieulafoy lesions, Mallory–Weiss tears, and postpolypectomy bleeding. One disadvantage of band ligation is the need to remove the scope to mount the device. This is less of a concern with variceal bleeding, as the endoscope and slim cap can easily be readvanced into position nearly universally. Band ligation works poorly in woody or fibrotic ulcers because this tissue cannot be drawn up into the cap to create a "neck" of tissue for the band to affix to. As such, they are rarely applied to PUD-related UGIB.

Endoloop Ligation

Endoloops are detachable nylon snares that are commonly utilized as prophylaxis against GIB when removing a polyp or tumor with a large, thick stalk. The loop is deployed at the base

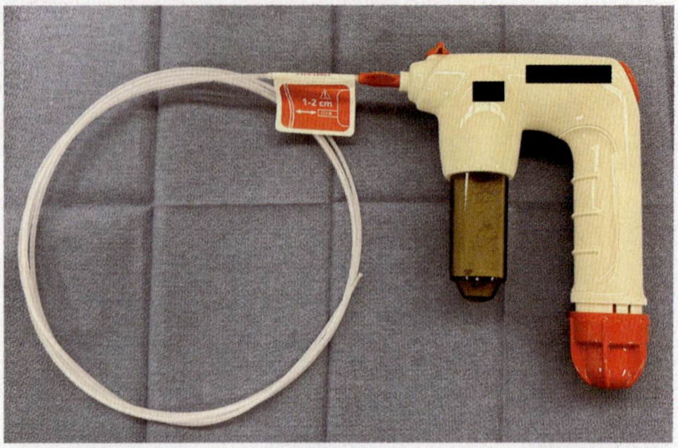

Figure 62.7. Topical hemostatic agent TC-325 granular mineral delivery system; catheter attached to a disposable carbon dioxide (CO_2) cannister.

of the polyp to compress the blood supply running through the stalk prior to endoscopic removal. The same technique of loop ligation has been applied to bleeding from angiodysplasia and a variety of bleeding tumors (fibrovascular polyps, GI stromal tumors, metastatic tumor implants).[19,20]

Topical Therapy

Hemostatic agents designed specifically for endoscopic applications have been available in the United States for less than a decade. They require active bleeding to be effective, but require little endoscopic targeting because they have a wide area of distribution. Although they have been applied as both first-line therapy and rebleeding therapy, they also have a high reported rate of rebleeding (19%).[21] They may also be considered as a temporizing measure, allowing bleeding to be controlled enough to transfer a patient to a facility capable of managing the bleeding endoscopically or to arrange for angiographic or surgical management of bleeding.

TC-325

TC-325 is a granular mineral delivered through a catheter attached to a disposable carbon dioxide (CO_2) cannister (**Fig. 62.7**). When applied to active bleeding, the agent absorbs water from the blood, which provides mechanical tamponade and concentrates factors to activate the clotting cascade.[21] The product can be difficult to deliver because liquid present in the delivery catheter or instrument channel can cause aggregation of the mineral and resultant clogging. Deployment of the agent inside the scope can result in channel clogging, necessitating formal endoscope repair to unclog it.

Starch Polysaccharide

Plant starch-derived polysaccharide powder is delivered through a catheter attached to a pressurized room air compressor. When applied to active bleeding, the agent absorbs water from the blood, resulting in high concentration of platelets, red blood cells, and coagulation factors.[21] The created matrix is highly adhesive and not degradable by human enzymes, which results in a protective coating over the applied area for several days. Notably, the product is not approved for Forrest 1a bleeding (see below).

UPPER GASTROINTESTINAL BLEEDING

Peptic Ulcer Disease

Even in an era of widely available acid suppression medication, PUD remains the most common cause of UGIB, accounting for about 50% of cases. *H. pylori* infection and gastroerosive drugs (commonly NSAIDs and ASA), are independent and synergistic risk factors for PUD-related UGIB in 80% of cases. NSAIDs also potentiate other risk factors for UGIB, such as advanced age, anticoagulants, corticosteroids, and selective serotonin reuptake inhibitors. About 30% of patients present with bleeding as the initial symptom of their PUD, and about 50% of patients will have antecedent upper abdominal pain.

The Forrest classification of PUD-related UGIB was initially developed to improve communication among endoscopists about ulcer description, but has since become a risk assessment tool for bleeding, rebleeding, and mortality.[22,23] **Table 62.5** reviews the Forrest classification type and commonality, treatment recommendations, and the risk of rebleeding. In general, high-risk endoscopic stigmata include active ulcer bleeding and a nonbleeding visible vessel. Low-risk endoscopic stigmata include ulcers with flat pigmented spots or clean ulcer base.

Multiple types of endoscopic therapy have been utilized to control PUD-related UGIB, but few prospective studies have been performed. Patients should be managed with multimodal therapy, most commonly with electrosurgical energy and TTS endoscopic clips with/without epinephrine injection (**Figs. 62.8 and 62.9**). A meta-analysis of studies evaluating bleeding control in high-risk ulcers concluded that epinephrine injection alone had a higher rate of rebleeding compared to other monotherapies (electrosurgical energy, TTS clip application) or epinephrine injection followed by another modality.[23] TTS clip application and electrosurgical energy use are equally effective as monotherapy.[23] OTS clips appear to achieve higher

Table 62.5. Forrest Classification of Peptic Ulcers and Management Recommendations[3,22]

Forrest Class	Endoscopic Stigmata	Prevalence (%)	Endoscopic Management	Medical Management	Rebleeding Risk (%)
Ia	Active arterial bleeding	12	Endoscopic hemostasis	High-dose PPI (bolus + continuous infusion) for 72 h	55
Ib	Oozing without visible vessel		Endoscopic hemostasis	High-dose PPI (bolus + continuous infusion) for 72 h	
IIa	Nonbleeding visible vessel	8	Endoscopic hemostasis	High-dose PPI (bolus + continuous infusion) for 72 h	43
IIb	Adherent clot	8	Clot removal + endoscopic hemostasis	High-dose PPI (bolus + continuous infusion) for 72 h	22
IIc	Flat spot	16	None indicated	Daily oral PPI	10
III	Clean ulcer base	55	None indicated	Daily oral PPI	5

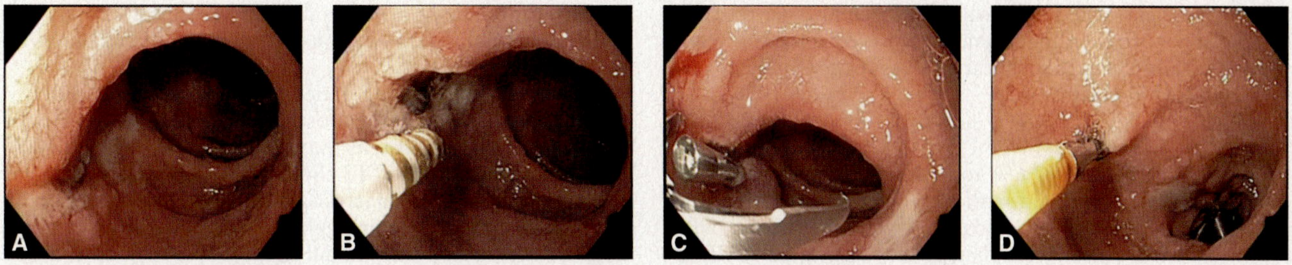

Figure 62.8. Multimodal management of a duodenal peptic ulcer; (**A**) Forrest class IIa ulcer, (**B**) electrosurgical energy applied with a bipolar probe, (**C**) TTS clip application, and (**D**) duodenal biopsy performed to evaluate for *H. pylori*.

rates of initial hemostasis and lower rates of 30-day rebleeding with shorter procedure times.[19] When patients rebleed after standard multimodal endoscopic therapy, OTS clips are more effective at controlling than repeating standard interventions (85% vs 42% success rate).[24] Consequently, some experts suggest that OTS clips be utilized as first-line therapy for high-risk ulcers.

Patients with high-risk ulcers should also receive high-dose PPI therapy administered as an IV bolus followed by continuous infusion for 72 hours postendoscopy. This regimen has been demonstrated to reduce rebleeding, the need for surgery, and mortality. Daily oral PPI therapy is then continued for 4 to 8 weeks. Patients with low-risk lesions (clean base, flat spot) should receive oral PPIs once a day from the time of diagnosis. All patients should be tested for *H. pylori* in the acute setting, and 14-day bismuth quadruple therapy initiated if *H. pylori* is detected.

Patients who rebleed following initial endoscopic control should undergo an attempt at repeat endoscopic hemostasis. Endoscopic retreatment controlled bleeding in 73% of patients and has a lower rate of adverse events compared with surgery.[25] If the bleeding is unable to be controlled at the second endoscopy or if the patient rebleeds, the patient should undergo angiographic embolization or surgery. In such cases, placement of a radiopaque TTS clip at the time of endoscopy can assist in identifying the location of the bleeding at subsequent angiographic or surgical intervention. Meta-analyses comparing embolization to surgery found higher rates of rebleeding with embolization but a trend toward higher mortality rates with surgery.[26]

9 The type of surgery performed depends on the location, the patient's medical status, and the experience of the surgeon. For favorably located gastric ulcers, such as those along the greater curvature, excision of the ulcer with closure of the gastrotomy will suffice. If the ulcer is unfavorably located, for example, near the gastroesophageal junction, simple oversewing of the bleeding vessel may adequately control the hemorrhage. In cases without ulcer resection, biopsy of the ulcer margin, either at the time of operation or at follow-up endoscopy in 4 to 8 weeks, is important to rule out malignancy. Extensive gastric resections (eg, subtotal or total gastrectomy) are generally not performed in these medically complex and unstable patients. Liberal use of intraoperative endoscopy can guide ulcer oversewing or permit on-table leak testing following gastrotomy closure.

Most bleeding duodenal ulcers requiring surgical control are large, posterior lesions. A longitudinal incision in the anterior wall of the duodenal bulb will allow visualization of the bleeding gastroduodenal artery in the base of the ulcer, which should be oversewn proximally and distally to the bleeding site with figure-of-eight stitches. An additional U-stitch placed underneath the bleeding site controls the transverse pancreatic artery entering the gastroduodenal artery posteriorly. The performance of a vagotomy and drainage procedure (usually a Heineke–Mikulicz pyloroplasty) is associated with a lower mortality than oversewing the ulcer alone. Operations for PUD, including vagotomy and pyloroplasty, are described in detail in Chapter 43.

Stress Ulceration

Stress ulceration is characterized by erosions and superficial ulcers in the stomach, and to a lesser extent the duodenum, of critically ill patients as a result of disruption of the gastroduodenal mucosal barrier. Critical illness or injury reduces gastric blood flow and causes mucosal ischemia and reperfusion injury. This, in turn impairs mucosal barrier defenses and ultimately disrupts mucosal integrity. The clinical spectrum varies from asymptomatic, superficial erosions to deep mucosal/submucosal ulcerations with overt UGIB and hemodynamic instability. The incidence of overt UGIB in critically ill, hospitalized patients is between 0.9% and 5.0%. Patients requiring mechanical ventilation, renal replacement therapy, and extracorporeal life support are at higher risk.

For patients with stress-related UGIB, endoscopy should be performed within 12 to 24 hours of presentation, depending on the severity of the bleeding. The presence of high-risk endoscopic stigmata identifies lesions that may be amenable to endoscopic hemostasis. When bleeding is diffuse and no individual targets for therapy exist, consideration should be given to the broad application of a topical hemostatic agent. High-dose PPI therapy is the mainstay of treatment for patients whose lesions are not appropriate for endoscopic hemostasis,

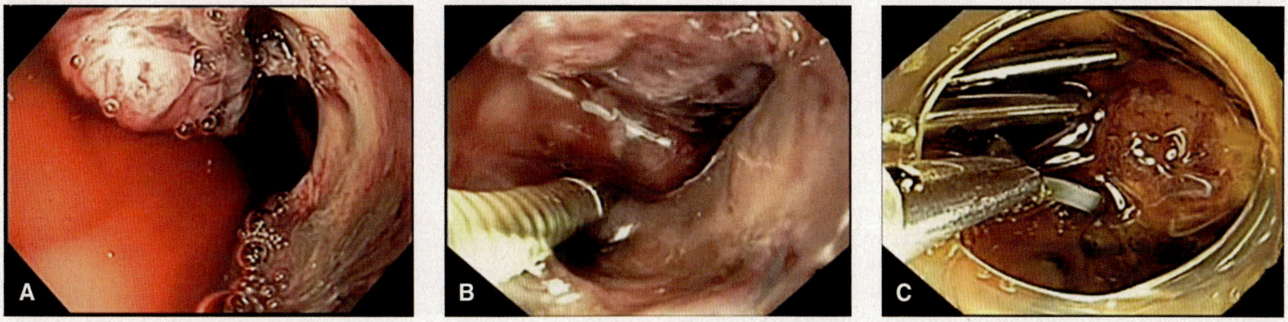

Figure 62.9. Multimodal management of a duodenal peptic ulcer; (**A**) Forrest class Ib ulcer, (**B**) injection of epinephrine, and (**C**) TTS clip application.

as well as patients who undergo successful endoscopic therapy. The need for surgical management of severe bleeding from stress ulceration is extremely rare. Stress-related UGIB is further discussed in Chapter 43.

Esophagitis

Severe esophagitis causes 6% to 15% of UGIB cases and is most commonly associated with gastroesophageal reflux disease (GERD).[5] Fungal (Candida) and viral (herpes simplex, cytomegalovirus [CMV]) esophagitis may also cause UGIB in immunocompromised individuals. GERD and esophagitis are further discussed in Chapter 41. Notably, a minority (23% to 38%) of these patients will have symptomatic GERD.[27] UGIB from esophagitis generally presents as hematemesis (43% to 86%) and/or melena (38% to 52%) with hematochezia (2%) and hemodynamic instability (5%) being uncommon. Patients with bleeding from esophagitis have more stable vital signs, higher blood counts, lower Rockall scores, lower risk of rebleeding, and a lower mortality than patients with other causes of UGIB.[27] Consequently, most patients respond well to PPI therapy and few require endoscopic hemostasis measures (3%). Many patients with bleeding from esophagitis can be triaged to early discharge once the diagnosis is made endoscopically.

Mallory–Weiss Syndrome

Mallory–Weiss syndrome is a longitudinal partial-thickness laceration of the distal esophagus and/or proximal stomach after vomiting, retching, coughing, or straining. Similar tears can be seen following esophageal instrumentation (eg, NG tube, EGD, transesophageal echocardiogram). Extension of the laceration into the submucosa disrupts vasculature and results in 8% to 15% of UGIB cases. Risk factors for Mallory–Weiss syndrome include the presence of a hiatal hernia and a history of heavy alcohol (both noted in 40% to 80% of cases). Most Mallory–Weiss related lacerations occur in patients <40 years old. Characteristically, patients describe nonbloody emesis, retching, or coughing followed by subsequent hematemesis. This "classic" presentation occurs in slightly more than 50% of cases. About 10% of patients present with melena in the absence of hematemesis. The amount of bleeding is variable, with more severe bleeding occurring in patients with portal hypertension.

The mortality rate of Mallory–Weiss related UGIB is about 5%. Risk factors for poor outcomes include advanced age, medical comorbidities, and active bleeding at the time of endoscopy.[28] Patients should receive high-dose PPIs, regardless of whether bleeding requires endoscopic control. Mallory–Weiss related UGIB can be managed with epinephrine injection, electrosurgical methods, or endoscopic clips. As with PUD, epinephrine should not be used as a monotherapy due to high rates of rebleeding.[28,29] Care must be exercised with the application of electrosurgical energy to the thin-walled, partly torn esophagus (that lacks a serosa), as high energy and high tamponade force risks transmural injury and/or delayed perforation. Surgical oversewing the bleeding site through an anterior gastrotomy or under endoscopic guidance is rarely necessary.

Dieulafoy Lesion

A Dieulafoy lesion is an abnormally enlarged artery that courses through the submucosa of the stomach (70%), duodenum (15%), esophagus (8%), colon (2%), rectum (2%), or small intestine (1%).[30] Severe bleeding results when the arterial wall erodes through a small defect in the overlying mucosa. Dieulafoy lesions typically (90%) occur in patients >60 years of age. Males are affected more commonly than females, and medical comorbidities are common. The use of NSAIDs, ASA, or anticoagulants is also common among patients with bleeding Dieulafoy lesions.[30] Patients present with hematemesis and melena, and most are actively bleeding at presentation. One-third of patients are hemodynamically unstable and two-thirds require blood transfusions. Recurrent bleeding occurs in about 20% of patients.[30]

Greater than 90% of patients with bleeding Dieulafoy lesions can be managed endoscopically, although it should be noted that most studies have evaluated foregut Dieulafoy lesions. Endoscopic TTS clip application is more effective at achieving initial hemostasis and at reducing the risk of rebleeding compared to epinephrine monotherapy, and many authors advocate multimodal endoscopic therapy. Band ligation and OTC clips have also been utilized to manage bleeding Dieulafoy lesions. Recurrent bleeding after initially successful endoscopic hemostasis is managed with repeat endoscopic therapy.

Patients who fail endoscopic hemostasis are treated with angiographic embolization or surgery. The operative management of gastric Dieulafoy lesions is laparoscopic or open wedge resection of the lesion after preoperative endoscopic localization. Lesions in the small bowel or colon are treated with resection of the involved bowel, and lesions in the rectum are managed by oversewing the bleeding vessel.

Gastroesophageal Varices

Of the 50% of patients with cirrhosis that develop gastroesophageal varices (GEV), 10% to 15% will bleed yearly (**Fig. 62.10**). Each variceal UGIB carries up to a 20% mortality rate.[31] Up to 85% of patients with decompensated cirrhosis will have GEV compared with 30% to 40% of compensated patients with compensated cirrhosis.[31] The risk of variceal bleeding depends on the severity of liver disease, the size of the varices, and the presence of specific endoscopic findings suggesting recent or impending bleeding; a red wale mark is a longitudinal red streak, a cherry-red spot is a circular red dot, and a white nipple sign is a platelet–fibrin plug. Importantly, as many as one-third of UGIB in patients with cirrhosis will be unrelated to portal hypertension, the most common of which is PUD.

Patients with variceal bleeding present with effortless (nonforceful), recurring hematemesis of large volumes of dark red blood. The history and physical examination will identify risk factors for cirrhosis and its associated physical findings (eg, jaundice, ascites, spider angiomas, portosystemic collaterals in the abdominal wall). Laboratory tests may demonstrate hepatic synthetic dysfunction (prolonged prothrombin time, hypoalbuminemia, hyperbilirubinemia) and/or hypersplenism and bone marrow suppression (thrombocytopenia, leukopenia).

Acute variceal bleeding is a medical emergency requiring prompt, intensive care. A restrictive PRBC transfusion strategy (described earlier) is associated with lower rates of early rebleeding and mortality compared to more liberal transfusion

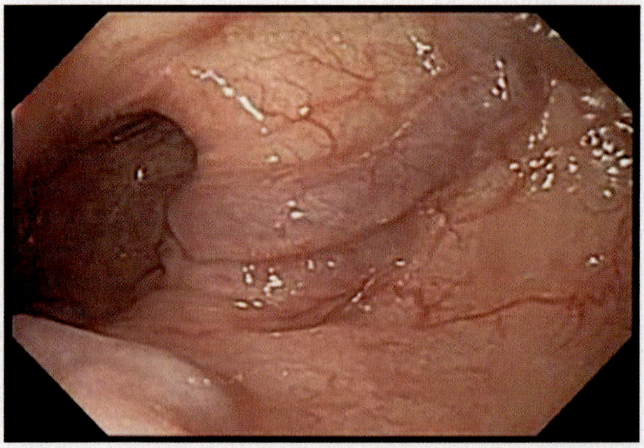

Figure 62.10. Esophageal varices in a patient with cirrhosis and a bleeding duodenal ulcer undergoing diagnostic endoscopy.

strategies. Patients with cirrhosis and UGIB are at a high risk of developing bacterial infections (eg, urinary tract infections, bacterial peritonitis). The administration of 7 days of prophylactic antibiotics (generally, IV ceftriaxone transition to oral ciprofloxacin) decreases the risk of infections, rebleeding, and death.[32] The IV infusion of vasoactive medication should be started as soon as possible in patients with suspected GEV UGIB; even before confirmatory EGD. Vasoactive medications (vasopressin, somatostatin, octreotide, and terlipressin) significantly improved control of acute variceal bleeding, and reduced transfusion requirements, hospital length of stay, and early mortality.

Uncommonly, patients with bleeding EGV may require balloon tamponade to temporarily control the UGIB while the patient is stabilized and a definitive management plan is enacted. Balloon tamponade therapy has a widely variable rate of success in controlling initial bleeding (30% to 90%) and may not be available in every location or have staff capable of placing or managing the balloon.

Endoscopy should be performed as soon as possible following resuscitation and not more than 12 hours after presentation. Once endoscopy confirms bleeding EGV, endoscopic variceal ligation (EVL) with a cap-based elastic banding device should be performed as first-line therapy. Endoscopic sclerotherapy (injection of ethanolamine or sodium morrhuate) can be used as a fallback method should EVL fail. EVL therapy is preferred to sclerotherapy because of a similar success rate but a lower overall complication rate. Endoscopic therapy for bleeding EGV has a success rate of around 90%.[33]

Following EVL, performing a transjugular intrahepatic portosystemic shunt (TIPS) lowers treatment failure and mortality rates in high-risk patients. For patients in whom early TIPS is not performed, IV vasoactive medications should be continued for 2 to 5 days, and nonselective beta blockers (eg, propranolol) should be started once the vasoactive drugs have been discontinued. Rescue TIPS is indicated in those patients in whom hemorrhage cannot be controlled by vasoactive drug infusion and EVL, or if bleeding recurs.

Following a first variceal bleed, patients have a 60% chance of rebleeding in the first year and a mortality rate of up to 33%. If a TIPS was performed during the initial bleeding episode, no additional therapy is required, but the patient should be referred for liver transplant evaluation. Patients rebleeding while on a nonselective beta blocker should undergo TIPS. A multicenter randomized controlled trial comparing TIPS to EVL plus nonselective beta blockers found that TIPS was associated with a significantly lower rate of rebleeding, a higher rate of early encephalopathy, and no differences in survival.[34] The evaluation and surgical management of patients with complications of cirrhosis is discussed in Chapter 56.

Clinical Outcomes for Upper GI Bleeding

The overall mortality rate for patients with UGIB is 2% to 2.5%.[5] The mortality rate for patients bleeding from GEV is three to five times higher than from nonvariceal causes.[31] Hospitalized patients who develop UGIB have a mortality rate three to four times higher than that of patients who present to the hospital with GIB.

LOWER GASTROINTESTINAL BLEEDING

Colonic Diverticulosis

Diverticular disease is the most common cause of LGIB, accounting for about 30% of cases.[6] The cumulative incidence of LGIB in patients with colonic diverticulosis is 2.2% at 5 years.[35] Diverticular bleeding most commonly originates from the right colon despite the fact that in diverticular disease predominantly affects the left colon. Bleeding is caused by perforation of a blood vessel located at the neck or apex of the diverticulum (**Fig. 62.11**). The *vasa recta* penetrate the colon wall through obliquely oriented connective tissue septa.

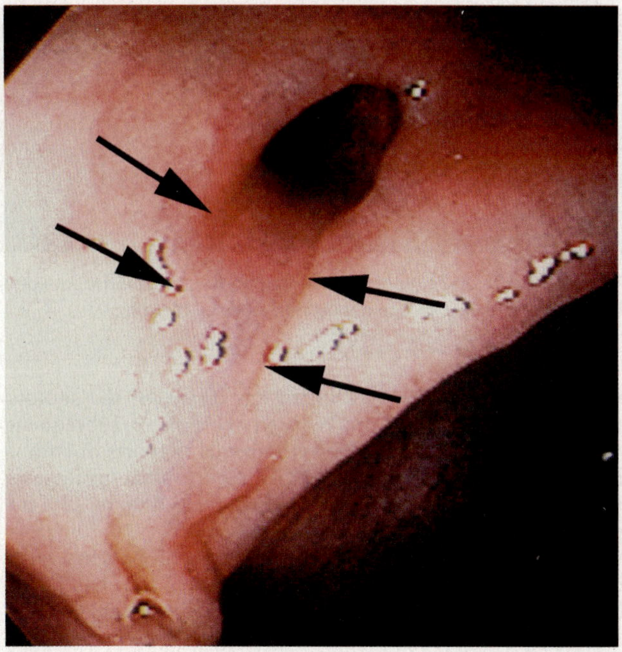

Figure 62.11. Endoscopic view of a colonic diverticulum showing the blood supply underneath the colonic mucosa at the neck of the diverticulum (*arrows*).

Protrusion of the mucosa and submucosa through this tissue plane forms the diverticulum and causes apposition of the colonic mucosa and the underlying blood supply. Ulceration of the mucosa of the diverticulum and disruption of the arterial wall causes luminal hemorrhage.

Patients with diverticular bleeding present with painless, intermittent, large-volume hematochezia. The color of the blood varies from dark maroon to bright red blood clots depending on the location and intensity of the bleeding. Patients with diverticular bleeding do not typically exhibit small amounts of bleeding. Important risk factors for diverticular bleeding are age greater than 70 years, pancolonic disease, the use of NSAIDs, ASA, or anticoagulants, and a previous episode of diverticular bleeding.[35] Although most (75% to 80%) diverticular bleeding will stop spontaneously, rebleeding is common (15%). Recurrent bleeding is more common in older individuals and those taking antiplatelet agents. If a person has had two prior episodes of diverticular bleeding, the annual risk of recurrent hemorrhage is about 11%.[35]

About 25% of patients with diverticular bleeding will require an intervention to stop the bleeding. Endoscopic therapy is effective for patients with active bleeding and high-risk endoscopic stigmata (eg, nonbleeding visible vessel), but requires that the bleeding be localized to a specific diverticulum during endoscopy. The subsequent method of endoscopic therapy applied depends upon the location of the bleeding, the ability to access the site, the operator's experience, and available endoscopic tools.[36] Utilization of TTS endoscopic clips (with or without epinephrine injection) reduces the possibility of transmural thermal injury and perforation associated with electrosurgical energy use, especially in the thin-walled right colon or within the diverticulum itself.[36] A meta-analyses of endoscopic treatment options (including band ligation, clip application, and electrosurgical energy) reported a 99% to 100% initial hemostasis rate.[37] Emerging literature suggests that OTS clips are also highly effective (100%) in stopping diverticular bleeding with a 0% adverse event rate and a low rate of rebleeding (8.3%).[19]

Patients with severe bleeding who cannot tolerate colonoscopy should undergo CTA to identify the site of bleeding, followed by selective visceral angiography. Superselective embolization with microcoils, polyvinyl alcohol particles, or

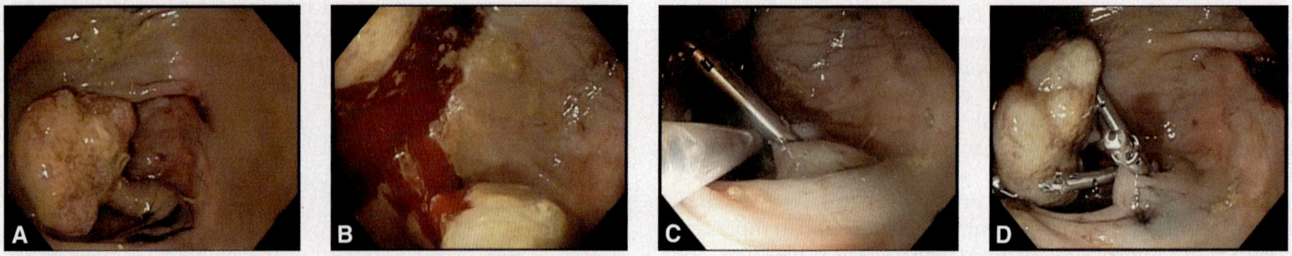

Figure 62.12. A: Pedunculated, benign polyp in a pediatric patient undergoes accidental cold snare polypectomy. B: Resultant postpolypecotmy bleeding. C and D: TTS clip application stops all bleeding.

water-insoluble gelatin (gel foam) has improved the success rate of this procedure and reduced the risk of subsequent adverse events, specifically bowel ischemia. Reports of embolization as first-line therapy for LGIB report initial hemostasis in 85% to 96% of patients, with early rebleeding in 22% of patients.[38]

The indications for surgical treatment of patients with diverticular hemorrhage include: (1) bleeding that has failed endoscopic and angiographic therapy, (2) recurrent bleeding refractory to endoscopic and angiographic therapy, and (3) massive hemorrhage unresponsive to resuscitation. Preoperative localization of the bleeding site is critical to limit the extent of resection, reduce the likelihood of rebleeding, and improve short- and long-term outcomes. A subtotal colectomy is indicated in rare instances in which the site of bleeding cannot be localized. The rate of recurrent bleeding after a subtotal colectomy is less than 4% but the perioperative mortality rate is 2% to 6%. The surgical management of complications of diverticular disease is discussed in Chapter 67.

Postpolypectomy Bleeding

LGIB following colonoscopic polypectomy occurs at a rate of 9.8% and is divided into immediate or delayed postpolypectomy bleeding (PPB) based on whether the patient has been discharged from the endoscopy unit.[39] Risk factors for PPB include antithrombotic agent use, right-sided polyps that are flat and >2 cm or pedunculated with thick stalk (Fig. 62.12). Management of PPB depends on the severity of bleeding, its location, and endoscopist's experience. Commonly used methods include epinephrine injection, electrosurgical energy, TTS clip application, or polyloop placement. Delayed PPB is the result of mucosal scab slough or spread of a thermal injury zone of necrosis if a hot polypectomy was performed. Patients should be stabilized and undergo a bowel preparation with plans for a colonoscopy within 24 hours. If bleeding stops, colonoscopy is not required. Patients with ongoing PPB can undergo standard endoscopic therapy for LGIB.

Internal Hemorrhoids

Hemorrhoids are normal, dilated submucosal arteriovenous channels located in the anal canal above (internal hemorrhoids) or below (external hemorrhoids) the dentate line. Although usually asymptomatic, patients with hemorrhoids may present with painless, recurrent episodes of bleeding that cause coating or streaking of the stool with bright red blood, blood dripping into the toilet, or blood staining on toilet tissue. Hemorrhoidal bleeding requiring transfusion is uncommon except in patients taking anticoagulants and those with portal hypertension.

Mild hemorrhoidal bleeding can be successfully managed with diet and lifestyle modification. Dietary changes include fiber supplementation and increased water consumption with the goal of reducing straining during defecation. Other lifestyle modifications include the avoidance of prolonged sitting or straining on the toilet, improved perianal hygiene, and avoiding triggers of constipation or diarrhea.

Anoscopy can identify internal hemorrhoids as the cause of rectal bleeding, but colonoscopy is still necessary to exclude another more serious source of LGIB. Band ligation (endoscopic or surgical) is effective in controlling hemorrhoidal bleeding in more than 90% of patients. Patients who have failed banding or other forms of endoscopic treatment, those with symptomatic combined internal/external hemorrhoids, and patients who are coagulopathic may require operative treatment. Although more effective than banding, operative treatment is associated with a higher rate of complications such as anal stenosis and postoperative bleeding. The management of complications of hemorrhoids is discussed in Chapter 68.

Colon Ischemia

Colon ischemia (or ischemic colitis) is an acute condition caused by transient ischemia and reperfusion of a segment of the colon that leads to localized inflammation, mucosal ulceration, and bleeding. The vascular watershed areas of the colon, such as the splenic flexure and the sigmoid colon, are particularly susceptible to ischemia. The severity of the injury ranges from reversible localized inflammation to transmural infarction and necrosis. Colon ischemia accounts for 7% to 12% of US hospital admissions for LGIB, most commonly affecting the left colon in older, often female (57% to 76%) patients.[40]

Patients note sudden cramping, mild, left lower abdominal pain, an urgent desire to defecate, and the passage of bright red or maroon-colored blood or bloody diarrhea. Physical examination demonstrates tenderness and voluntary guarding over the affected segment of colon. Peritonitis suggests full-thickness ischemia, perforation, or an alternate diagnosis. The acute onset of symptoms is an important feature of colon ischemia and distinguishes it from other causes of colitis in which the onset of symptoms is more gradual. Most episodes of colon ischemia are benign, self-limited, and cause mild rectal bleeding. Severe bleeding is also more commonly associated with gangrenous colon ischemia (10%) and fulminant pancolitis (2%).[40]

Risk factors for the development of colon ischemia include cardiovascular and pulmonary diseases, irritable bowel syndrome, diabetes mellitus, and collagen vascular diseases. Surgical procedures, especially those that require ligation or occlusion of the inferior mesenteric artery, are also associated with the colon ischemia. The rate of colon ischemia following abdominal aortic aneurysm repair is about 2%.[41]

Patients with suspected colon ischemia should initially undergo CT with IV and oral contrast to identify the affected colon segment and exclude other diagnoses. CT findings (segmental wall thickening, mucosal thumbprinting, and pericolonic fat stranding) are not specific enough to differentiate colon ischemia from other causes of colitis, and so colonoscopy within 48 hours is still indicated. Patients with peritonitis or evidence of irreversible ischemic injury should not undergo colonoscopy.

The colonoscopy should be performed with low-volume CO_2 insufflation to avoid a distension-related colon perforation.

On endoscopic examination, the colonic mucosa will appear erythematous, edematous, ulcerated, and friable. In instances of gangrene, the muocsa will appear dusky with blue–black nodules.[40] The mucosa should be biopsied except in instances of gangrene. Endoscopic therapy can be administered for focal areas of bleeding (colonic ulcers) or delivered more broadly using hemostatic posers.[21]

Colon ischemia generally resolves spontaneously without specific treatment. Patients with more significant clinical findings require hospitalization for supportive measures (fasting, IV fluid resuscitation, and broad-spectrum antibiotics). Surgical management is required in about 14% of patients due to peritonitis, clinical deterioration, fulminant colitis, or endoscopic evidence of bowel necrosis.[40] The mortality rate for patients needing operative management is 37% to 47%.[40]

Inflammatory Bowel Disease

Clinically significant LGIB is rare in patients with inflammatory bowel disease (IBD), but is more common in Crohn disease (CD, 1.2%) than ulcerative colitis (UC, 0.1%).[42] In patients with CD, bleeding is equally distributed between the small bowel, ileocolonic region, and colon. Severe bleeding from UC is usually caused by pancolitis.[42] Very early–onset IBD (children <6 years old) is more likely to present with rectal bleeding (33%) than children diagnosed later.

Colonoscopy will identify bleeding areas of active inflammation or ulcerations in 60% to 80% of cases.[42] Fluid resuscitation and medical treatment of IBD address the majority of cases (89%), and only 10% to 15% of bleeding is amenable to endoscopic therapy.[42] Surgery for initial or recurrent bleeding control is common in patients with CD (20%) and uncommon for patients with UC.[42] The clinical presentation, diagnostic evaluation, and management of complications of IBD are discussed in Chapters 47 and 63.

Infectious Colitis

Overt LGIB (often as bloody diarrhea and fever) can occur with infections caused by *Campylobacter*, *Salmonella*, *Shigella*, Shiga toxin–producing *Escherichia coli*, CMV, or *Clostridium difficile*. Immunocompromised patients (eg, chemotherapy or immunosuppressants) are particularly susceptible to CMV colitis. Treatment consists of fluid resuscitation and targeted antibiotics or antiviral agents.

SMALL BOWEL GASTROINTESTINAL BLEEDING

The differential diagnosis of SBGIB is strongly influenced by the patient's age and medical history. Bleeding is vascular (24%), inflammatory (16% to 18%), or neoplastic (11%) in etiology.[2] Recurrent bleeding occurs in about one-third of patients. Patients <40 years old are more likely to be bleeding from CD or a Meckel diverticulum, whereas patients >40 years old are more likely to be bleeding from angioectasias and NSAID ulcers. A history of a bleeding diathesis, medication usage (NSAIDs, antithrombotic agents), valvular heart disease, chronic renal disease, and cirrhosis are important risk factors for SBGIB.

Meckel Diverticulum

Meckel diverticulum is the most common congenital GI anomaly, occurring in 0.3% to 2.9% of the population.[43] About 4% of Meckel diverticula are symptomatic, and 25% to 35% of those present with GIB.[43] Bleeding occurs when acid produced by heterotopic gastric oxyntic glands within the diverticulum cause peptic ulceration of adjacent small bowel mucosa. As noted above, technetium-99m pertechnetate scintigraphy identifies ectopic gastric mucosa in patients suspected of bleeding from a Meckel diverticulum. Alternatively, retrograde enteroscopy (commonly DBE) is performed through the terminal ileum. Recent studies suggest that DBE has a higher diagnostic yield than other traditional imaging modalities, identifying the diverticulum in 90% to 100% of cases and permitting immediate endoscopic therapy for hemorrhage control.[44] Small bowel resection (including the diverticulum and the ulcer) with primary enteroenterostomy is the surgical therapy of choice.

Small Bowel Diverticula

Diverticular disease of the small intestine is an uncommon cause of GIB. Small bowel diverticula are pseudodiverticula (like colonic diverticula) and may be complicated by diverticulitis, obstruction, and bleeding. About 80% of small bowel diverticula are located in the jejunum, and multiple diverticula are common (67%). The pathogenesis of overt SBGIB is the same as that of colonic diverticulum; erosion of a blood vessel through the diverticular wall.

Patients present with melena or hematochezia, depending on the location of the diverticulum and the intensity of bleeding. CTA can localize the site of active bleeding, and subsequent enteroscopy or visceral angiography will facilitate hemostasis. Small bowel resection with primary enteroenterostomy is the surgical therapy of choice if endoscopy and angiography fail to control hemorrhage.

SOURCES OF BLEEDING THROUGHOUT THE GI TRACT

Angioectasia

Angioectasias, the most common vascular abnormality of the GI tract, are characterized by abnormal, ectatic, dilated, and tortuous small blood vessels within the mucosa and submucosa. They are most commonly located in the jejunum (80%), duodenum (51%), stomach (23%), and right colon (11%), but 60% of patients will have lesions in multiple sites.[45]

The majority of angioectasias are asymptomatic and incidentally discovered during routine endoscopy in patients >60 years old. Risk factors include advanced age, chronic renal disease, and cardiovascular disease.[45] Bleeding from angioectasias in patients with aortic stenosis (Heyde syndrome) is postulated to result from an acquired von Willebrand factor deficiency. Symptomatic patients generally present with chronic, well-compensated occult blood loss. Less commonly, patients present with hematemesis, melena, or hematochezia depending on the location of the lesion and the intensity of the hemorrhage.

VCE is the first-line diagnostic test for patients with suspected SBGIB. Patients with active bleeding on VCE should undergo SBE (generally via DBE) with APC application.[2] Octreotide reduces the transfusion requirements of bleeding angioectasias. Unfortunately, recurrent bleeding is common (34% to 45%). Risk factors for recurrent bleeding include the number of angioectasias, age >65 years, jejunum location, cardiac valvular disease, chronic renal disease, use of anticoagulants, and the need for transfusion.[45]

Hemodynamically unstable patients with active bleeding should undergo CTA. Subsequent angiography and superselective embolization will control the bleeding in 70% to 80% of cases, with recurrent bleeding in about 12% of cases.[46] Surgical management is reserved for failed endoscopic and angiographic hemostasis. Laparotomy or laparoscopy with intraoperative enteroscopy will identify the site of bleeding in patients with overt hemorrhage and facilitate endoscopic or surgical hemostasis. Aortic valve replacement reduces the risk of bleeding from angioectasias in patients with Heyde syndrome.

Gastrointestinal Stromal Tumors

Gastrointestinal stromal tumors (GISTs) are infrequent causes of overt GIB. GISTs occur most commonly in the stomach (50%), small intestine (25%), colon (10%) duodenum (5%), or esophagus (1%).[47] The median age of patients with a GIST is 65 years, with a slight predominance in females. About

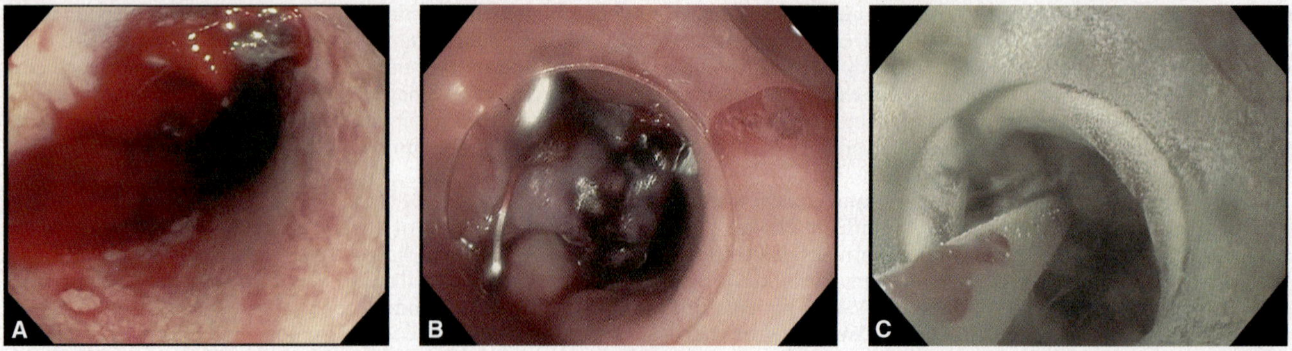

Figure 62.13. **A:** Actively bleeding esophageal ulcer as a result of an aortic endograft erosion. **B:** OTS clip application performed after aortic bleeding was ruled out. **C:** Application of topical hemostatic agent TC-325 to manage ongoing slow ooze.

one-third of patients with a GIST will present with overt evidence of GIB.[20] Fewer patients will present only with signs of occult blood loss. Cross-sectional imaging or endoscopy is diagnostic in the majority of cases. The specific diagnostic modality depends upon the GIST location and the magnitude of hemorrhage. Endoscopic hemostasis can be achieved with electrosurgical energy, mechanical compression (TTS clips, OTS clips, endoloops), injection therapy, or hemostatic spray.[20] The choice of therapy depends on the type of bleeding encountered, available endoscopic tools, and endoscopist experience. Patients should subsequently undergo surgical resection of the GIST with a grossly negative margin. Postoperative tyrosine kinase inhibitor therapy with imatinib is useful for patients at high risk of recurrence. The molecular biology, clinical presentation, and management of patients with GISTs are discussed in detail in Chapter 45.

Aortoenteric Fistulae

Communication between the aorta and the GI tract may occur as a result of aneurysmal disease, infectious aortitis (*primary aortoenteric fistula*) or more commonly from the erosion of a prosthesis (vascular or enteral stent) through the GI tract wall (*secondary aortoenteric fistula*). The incidence of aortoenteric fistula following open or endovascular aortic reconstructive surgery is about 1%. Fistulae between the aorta and the esophagus, stomach, duodenum, small bowel, and colon have all been reported.[48] The disease is most commonly described as erosion of the proximal portion of an abdominal aortic graft into the distal duodenum, were the intestine is in contact with the graft suture line. Patients may present with massive GIB and exsanguination. Others may have an initial episode of GIB (herald bleed) that is subsequently followed in hours/days/weeks by catastrophic hemorrhage. Patients may also complain of back or abdominal pain and less commonly have fever or signs of sepsis from graft infection or GI tract perforation.

The diagnosis of an aortoenteric fistula must be considered in any patient with an aortic or enteral prosthesis or an abdominal aortic aneurysm who presents with GIB (**Fig. 62.13**). If the patient is hemodynamically stable, CTA may demonstrate evidence of an aortoenteric fistula or signs of perigraft infection. If CTA is negative or nondiagnostic, endoscopy should be urgently performed to identify evidence of the aortoenteric fistula (such as the blood, clot, or exposed graft or aortic wall) or to identify and manage other causes of GIB. No attempt at endoscopic therapy should be made, and care should be taken to avoid dislodging fresh thrombus overlying the fistula as this can induce exsanguinating hemorrhage (**Fig. 62.14**). Emergency laparotomy with exposure of the fistula location should be undertaken. Surgical management requires repair of the GI tract defect, removal of infected prosthetic material, and (generally) an extra-anatomical bypass procedure.[48] The complications of abdominal aortic operations, including aortoduodenal fistulas and their management, are discussed in Chapter 92.

Postoperative Staple Line Bleeding

Surgical staplers are commonly used during GI surgery for both extirpative and reconstructive purposes. Although they are highly reliable devices, postoperative complications such as leak, ischemia, and bleeding are widely reported. Technical errors (eg, stapler misfire) and cognitive errors (eg, selected staple height is too high for the tissue thickness) play an important role in the risk of bleeding and the need for transfusion.[49] For bariatric surgical interventions, the rate is as high as 3% to 5.8% while rates of 6.5% have been reported for low anterior colorectal resections.[49] Most bleeding will be extraluminal (ie, intra-abdominal). Intraluminal staple line bleeding may present as hematemesis, bowel obstruction (from thrombus), hematochezia, or melena and may occur with or without hemodynamic instability, depending on the severity and ongoing nature of the bleeding.

Endoscopy in the early postoperative period is safe and does not risk anastomotic or staple line perforation if conducted by an experienced team under low-flow CO_2 insufflation.[50] To reduce the risk of ischemia to the staple line, epinephrine injection and electrosurgical energy application should be utilized only with bleeding that cannot be effectively controlled with mechanical compression from a TTS or OTS clip (**Fig. 62.15**). Most anastomotic bleeding is from a focal source and responds well to mechanical compression.[50] Diffuse staple line ooze resulting from a coagulopathic state can be broadly treated with hemostatic spray or judicious APC application and correction of the coagulopathy when possible.

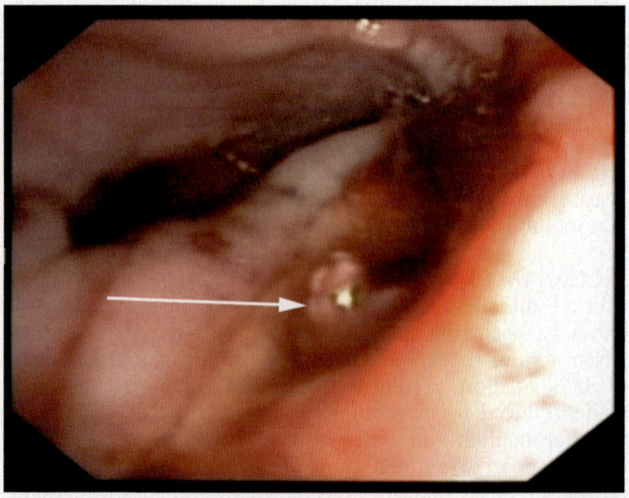

Figure 62.14. Visibly ulcerated aorta (*arrow*) in a patient with a long-standing esophageal stent that had chronically eroded into the mediastinum.

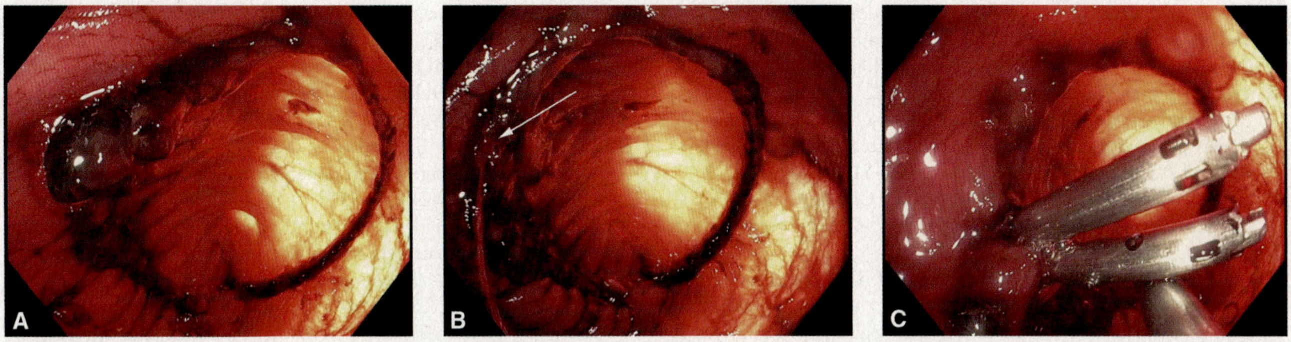

Figure 62.15. Postoperative anastomotic bleeding; (A) fresh clot seen at a new ileocolic anastomosis of a patient with hematozecia and hypotension on postoperative day one. **B:** Removal of the clot demonstrates active arterial hemorrhage (*arrow*). **C:** TTS clip application results in cessation of bleeding.

ACKNOWLEDGMENTS

We gratefully acknowledge the contributions of previous edition authors, Richard H. Turnage and Benjamin L. Davis, as portions of those chapters have been retained in this revision.

References

1. Peery AF, Crockett SD, Murphy CC, et al. Burden and cost of gastrointestinal, liver, and pancreatic diseases in the United States: update 2021. *Gastroenterology.* 2022;162(2):621–644.
2. Gerson LB, Fidler JL, Cave DR, et al. ACG clinical guideline: diagnosis and management of small bowel bleeding. *Am J Gastroenterol.* 2015;110(9):1265–1287.
3. Laine L, Yang H, Chang SC, et al. Trends for incidence of hospitalization and death due to GI complications in the United States from 2001 to 2009. *Am J Gastroenterol.* 2012;107(8):1190–1195.
4. Mujtaba S, Chawla S, Massaad JF. Diagnosis and management of non-variceal gastrointestinal hemorrhage: a review of current guidelines and future perspectives. *J Clin Med.* 2020;9(2):402.
5. Wuerth BA, Rockey DC. Changing epidemiology of upper gastrointestinal hemorrhage in the last decade: a nationwide analysis. *Dig Dis Sci.* 2018;63(5):1286–1293.
6. Oakland K, Guy R, Uberoi R, et al. Acute lower GI bleeding in the UK: patient characteristics, interventions and outcomes in the first nationwide audit. *Gut.* 2018;67(4):654–662.
7. Rockall TA, Logan RF, Devlin HB, Northfield TC. Risk assessment after acute upper gastrointestinal hemorrhage. *Gut.* 1996;38(3):316–321.
8. Almaghrabi M, Gandhi M, Guizzetti L, et al. Comparison of risk scores for lower gastrointestinal bleeding: a systematic review and meta-analysis. *JAMA Netw Open.* 2022;5(5):e2214253.
9. Teutsch B, Veres DS, Pálinkás D, et al. Potential benefits of restrictive transfusion in upper gastrointestinal bleeding: a systematic review and meta-analysis of randomised controlled trials. *Sci Rep.* 2023;13:1730123.
10. Laursen SB, Leontiadis GI, Stanley AJ, et al. Relationship between timing of endoscopy and mortality in patients with peptic ulcer bleeding: a nationwide cohort study. *Gastrointest Endosc.* 2017;85(5):936–944.
11. Rahman R, Nguyen DL, Sohail U, et al. Pre-endoscopic erythromycin administration in upper gastrointestinal bleeding: an updated meta-analysis and systematic review. *Ann Gastroenterol.* 2016;29(3):312–317.
12. ASGE Standards of Practice Committee; Acosta RD, Abraham NS, Chandrasekhara V, et al. The management of antithrombotic agents for patients undergoing GI endoscopy. *Gastrointest Endosc.* 2016;83(1):3–16.
13. Singh-Bhinder N, Kim DH, Holly BP, et al. ACR Appropriateness Criteria nonvariceal upper gastrointestinal bleeding. *Am J Radiol.* 2017;14(5S):S177–S188.
14. Oakland K, Kothiwale S, Forehand T, et al. External validation of the Oakland score to assess safe hospital discharge among adult patients with acute lower gastrointestinal bleeding in the US. *JAMA Netw Open.* 2020;3(7):e209630.
15. ASGE Standards of Practice Committee; Gurudu SR, Bruining DH, Acosta RD, et al. The role of endoscopy in the management of suspected small-bowel bleeding. *Gastrointest Endosc.* 2017;85(1):22–31.
16. Agrawal JR, Travis AC, Mortele KJ, et al. Diagnostic yield of dual-phase computed tomography enterography in patients with obscure gastrointestinal bleeding and a non-diagnostic capsule endoscopy. *J Gastroenterol Hepatol.* 2012;27(4):751–759.
17. Irvine I, Doherty A, Hayes R. Bleeding Meckel's diverticulum: a study of the accuracy of pertechnetate scintigraphy as a diagnostic tool. *Eur J Radiol.* 2017;96:27–30.
18. Shinozaki S, Yamamoto H, Yano T, et al. Long-term outcome of patients with obscure gastrointestinal bleeding investigated by double-balloon endoscopy. *Clin Gastroenterol Hepatol.* 2010;8(2):151–158.
19. Naseer M, Lambert K, Hamed A, Ali E. Endoscopic advances in the management of non-variceal upper gastrointestinal bleeding: a review. *World J Gastrointest Endosc.* 2020;12(1):1–16.
20. Ofosu A, Ramai D, Latson W, Adler DG. Endoscopic management of bleeding gastrointestinal tumors. *Ann Gastroenterol.* 2019;32(4):346–351.
21. Alali AA, Moosavi S, Martel M, et al. Topical hemostatic agents in the management of upper gastrointestinal bleeding: a meta-analysis. *Endosc Int Open.* 2023;11(4):E368–E385.
22. Forrest JA, Finlayson ND, Shearman DJ. Endoscopy in gastrointestinal bleeding. *Lancet.* 1974;2(7877):394–397.
23. Laine L, Jensen DM. Management of patients with ulcer bleeding. *Am J Gastroenterol.* 2012;107(3):345–360.
24. Schmidt A, Gölder S, Goetz M, et al. Over-the-scope clips are more effective than standard endoscopic therapy for patients with recurrent bleeding of peptic ulcers. *Gastroenterology.* 2018;155(3):674–686.e6.
25. Lau JYW, Sung JJY, Lam YH, et al. Endoscopic retreatment compared with surgery in patients with recurrent bleeding after initial endoscopic control of bleeding ulcer. *N Engl J Med.* 1999;340(10):751–756.
26. Tarasconi A, Baiocchi GL, Pattonieri V, et al. Transcatheter arterial embolization versus surgery for refractory non-variceal upper gastrointestinal bleeding: a meta-analysis. *World J Emerg Surg.* 2019;14:3.
27. Guntipalli P, Chason R, Elliott A, et al. Upper gastrointestinal bleeding caused by severe esophagitis: a unique clinical syndrome. *Dig Dis Sci.* 2014;59(12):2997–3003.
28. Ljubicic N, Budimir I, Pavic T, et al. Mortality in high-risk patients with bleeding Mallory-Weiss syndrome is similar to that of peptic ulcer bleeding. Results of a prospective database study. *Scand J Gastroenterol.* 2014;49(4):458–464.
29. Lee S, Ahn JY, Jung HY, et al. Effective endoscopic treatment of Mallory-Weiss syndrome using Glasgow-Blatchford score and Forrest classification. *J Dig Dis.* 2016;17(10):676–684.
30. Kanth R, Mali P, Roy PK. Outcomes in Dieulafoy's lesion: a 10-year clinical review. *Dig Dis Sci.* 2015;60(7):2097–2103.

31. Kovalak M, Lake J, Mattek N, et al. Endoscopic screening for varices in cirrhotic patients: data from a national endoscopic database. *Gastrointest Endosc.* 2007;65(1):82–88.
32. Chavez-Tapia NC, Barrientos-Gutierrez T, Tellez-Avila F, et al. Meta-analysis: antibiotic prophylaxis for cirrhotic patients with upper gastrointestinal bleeding-an updated Cochrane review. *Aliment Pharmacol Ther.* 2011;34(5):509–518.
33. Poza Cordon J, Froilan Torres C, Burgos García A, et al. Endoscopic management of esophageal varices. *World J Gastrointest Endosc.* 2012;4(7):312–322.
34. Holster IL, Tjwa ETTL, Moelker A, et al. Covered transjugular intrahepatic portosystemic shunt versus endoscopic therapy + beta-blocker for prevention of variceal rebleeding. *Hepatology.* 2016;63(2):581–589.
35. Vajravelu RK, Mamtani R, Scott FI, et al. Incidence, risk factors, and clinical effects of recurrent diverticular hemorrhage: a large cohort study. *Gastroenterology.* 2018;155(5):1416–1427.
36. Standards of Practice Committee, American Society for Gastrointestinal Endoscopy; Pasha SF, Shergill A, Acosta RD, et al. The role of endoscopy in the patient with lower GI bleeding. *Gastrointest Endosc.* 2014;79(6):875–885.
37. Ishii N, Omata F, Nagata N, Kaise M. Effectiveness of endoscopic treatments for colonic diverticular bleeding. *Gastrointest Endosc.* 2018;87(1):58–66.
38. Khanna A, Ognibene SJ, Koniaris LG. Embolization as first-line therapy for diverticulosis-related massive lower gastrointestinal bleeding: evidence from a meta-analysis. *J Gastrointest Surg.* 2005;9(3):343–352.
39. Reumkens A, Rondagh EJ, Bakker CM, et al. Post-colonoscopy complications: a systematic review, time trends, and meta-analysis of population-based studies. *Am J Gastroenterol.* 2016;111(8):1092–1101.
40. Brandt LJ, Feuerstadt P, Longstreth GF, et al. ACG clinical guideline: epidemiology, risk factors, patterns of presentation, diagnosis, and management of colon ischemia. *Am J Gastroenterol.* 2015;110(1):18–44.
41. Perry RJT, Martin MJ, Eckert MJ, et al. Colonic ischemia complicating open vs endovascular abdominal aortic aneurysm repair. *J Vasc Surg.* 2008;48(2):272–277.
42. Pardi DS, Loftus EV, Tremaine WJ, et al. Acute major gastrointestinal hemorrhage in inflammatory bowel disease. *Gastrointest Endosc.* 1999;49(2):153–157.
43. Hansen CC, Soreide K. Systematic review of epidemiology, presentation, and management of Meckel's diverticulum in the 21st century. *Medicine (Baltimore).* 2018;97(35):e12154.
44. Chou JW, Chung CS, Huang TY, et al. Meckel's diverticulum diagnosed by balloon-assisted enteroscopy: a multicenter report from the Taiwan Association for the Study of Small Intestinal Diseases (TASSID). *Gastroenterol Res Pract.* 2021;2021:9574737.
45. Bollinger E, Raines D, Saitta P. Distribution of bleeding gastrointestinal angioectasias in a western population. *World J Gastroenterol.* 2012;18(43):6235–6239.
46. Hongsakul K, Pakdeejit S, Tanutit P. Outcome and predictive factors of successful transarterial embolization for the treatment of acute gastrointestinal hemorrhage. *Acta Radiol.* 2014;55(2):186–194.
47. Parab TM, DeRogatis MJ, Boaz AM, et al. Gastrointestinal stromal tumors: a comprehensive review. *J Gastrointest Oncol.* 2019;10(1):144–154.
48. Mauriac P, Francois MO, Marichez A, et al. Adjuncts to the management of graft aorto-enteric erosion and fistula with in situ reconstruction. *Eur J Vasc Endovasc Surg.* 2021;62(5):786–795.
49. Chekan E, Whelan R. Surgical stapling device–tissue interactions: what surgeons need to know to improve patient outcomes. *Med Devices (Auckl).* 2014;7:305–318.
50. Ryou SH, Bang KB. Endoscopic management of postoperative bleeding. *Clin Endosc.* 2023;56(6):706–715.

63

Ulcerative Colitis

Aaron J. Dawes and Arden M. Morris

Key Points

1. Ulcerative colitis (UC) is a form of inflammatory bowel disease (IBD) characterized by mucosal and submucosa inflammation of the colon and rectum. This process is contiguous and homogeneous, beginning in the rectum, and extending proximally for a variable distance.
2. Intestinal and some extraintestinal manifestations of UC resolve after complete removal of the colon and rectum.
3. The acute indications for surgical intervention include acute severe UC, toxic megacolon, perforation, and uncontrolled bleeding. Medically refractory disease, dysplasia, and cancer are indications for elective surgery.
4. Current surgical options depend on the acuity of presentation of the disease; minimally invasive methods should be employed when clinically indicated and technically feasible.
5. Ileal pouch-anal anastomosis (IPAA) can provide patients with a continent reservoir for stool; however, permanent end ileostomy remains a viable option for patients who do not qualify or do not wish to undergo pouch construction.
6. Although perioperative and late complications after IPAA are common, the vast majority of patients enjoy a high quality of life after surgery.

UC is a chronic, idiopathic inflammatory disorder affecting over 1 million Americans of both sexes and all age groups, although peak onset occurs between the second and fourth decades of life.[1] Unlike Crohn disease (CD)—a related, but distinct form of IBD affecting the entire gastrointestinal (GI) tract—UC primarily affects the mucosa and submucosa of the colon and rectum through recurrent episodes of inflammation, ulceration, and healing. While chronic UC increasingly has been managed successfully via medical and biologic therapy, surgery continues to play a role in the treatment of acute severe disease, medically refractory disease, dysplasia, and cancer.

EPIDEMIOLOGY

Although exact numbers remain difficult to determine, several epidemiologic trends have emerged. First, the worldwide incidence of UC is increasing, primarily due to newly industrializing countries in Asia (0.68 to 6.5 per 100,000 person-years), South America (0.19 to 6.8 per 100,000 person-years), and Africa (3.3 per 100,000 person-years).[2] In contrast, the incidence of UC in developed nations appears to have stabilized or even begun to decline since the beginning of the 21st century. Second, the prevalence of UC has increased dramatically over time, likely due to earlier detection, better disease control, and lower mortality. The prevalence of UC continues to be the highest among industrialized nations in Europe (505 per 100,000 people in Norway), North America (286 per 100,000 in the United States), and Oceania (196 per 100,000 in Australia), but is expected to climb in developing nations as a result of the rising incidence of disease.[2] Finally, the age-specific incidence of UC appears to be bimodal with the largest peak between 15 and 40 years old followed by a separate, smaller peak at 50 to 75 years old (**Fig. 63.1**). There appears to be no sexual predominance in either incidence or prevalence of UC.

ETIOLOGY AND RISK FACTORS

The etiology of UC remains unknown, but is likely multifactorial. Current models focus on genetic susceptibilities that are unmasked by environmental triggers resulting in dysregulation of the immune system, chronic intestinal inflammation, and mucosal damage.

Genetics

Although familial clustering has been identified since the earliest descriptions of UC, most patients who are diagnosed with UC will have no family history of IBD. Between 10% and 15% of UC patients have a family member with IBD, particularly UC as opposed to CD, further suggesting that the two diseases represent separate clinical entities.[3] Interestingly, parent–child and sibling–sibling pairings appear to be more common than pairings involving more distant relatives despite no clear Mendelian inheritance pattern. Monozygotic twin concordance varies, but has been reported to be between 10% and 19%.[4,5] In addition, certain ethnic groups, particularly Ashkenazi Jewish populations, have significantly higher rates of UC compared to geographic controls.[6] Overall, first-degree relatives of patients with UC have a fourfold increase in their risk of developing the disease.[7]

Over 200 separate gene loci have been associated with an increased risk of developing IBD. The vast majority are located in genes involved in inflammatory signaling or mucosal barrier function and confer a risk for both UC and CD, although several disease-specific relationships have been identified.[8] For example, alterations in certain human leukocyte antigen haplotypes and in cell–cell junction signaling appear to be more associated with UC than CD.[9,10] Although a promising area for future research, currently identified genetic features explain only 7.5% of disease variance in UC and most patients who carry IBD-associated risk alleles do not go on to develop IBD.[11]

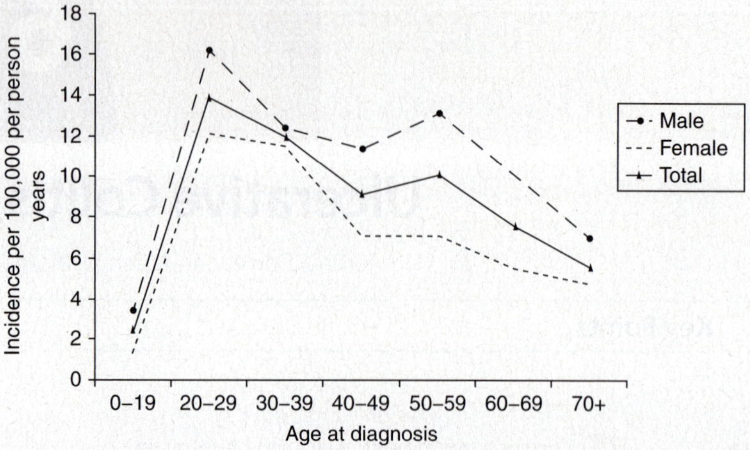

Figure 63.1. Age-specific incidence of UC in Midwestern US population. (Adapted from Loftus CG, Loftus EV Jr, Harmsen WS, et al. Update on the incidence and prevalence of Crohn's disease and ulcerative colitis in Olmsted County, Minnesota, 1940–2000. *Inflamm Bowel Dis.* 2007;13[3]:254–261.)

Environment

Diets high in fat (particularly trans-unsaturated and omega-6 fatty acids), red meat, and refined sugar appear to be associated with an increased risk of developing UC.[12,13] Interestingly, the increasing incidence of UC within developing countries appears to parallel the increasing exposure to a Western diet, which tends to be high in fat, red meat, and refined sugar. Although higher levels of dietary fiber are associated with a lower risk of developing CD, there is no consistent evidence for UC. Breast milk does appear to be protective against the development of both UC and CD, including a dose-dependent response with the lowest rates among children who were breastfed for at least 12 months compared to 3 or 6 months.[14] Although exposure to antibiotics in childhood was once considered a risk factor for developing IBD, multiple more recent studies have failed to demonstrate a consistent relationship, especially for UC. Tobacco smokers appear to have a lower incidence of UC compared to nonsmokers, although the underlying mechanism is poorly understood. Interestingly, smoking cessation is associated with an increase in the incidence of UC as well as disease severity. Appendectomy may be protective against developing UC, with up to a 40% risk reduction based on a recent meta-analysis.[15] The mechanism remains unknown, but has been hypothesized to be related to "priming" the immune system toward appropriate self-regulation.

Microbiome

Failure of the normal homeostasis between the intestinal immune system and the colonic microbiome undoubtedly contributes to the pathogenesis of UC; how this process occurs and whether changes in the microbiome of patients with UC are primary or secondary effects of the disease; however, remains debated. Colonocytes from patients with UC demonstrate impaired mucin production, which is thought to contribute to epithelial injury, increased mucosal permeability to luminal pathogens, and increased stimulation of the innate immune system.[16] Patients with UC have also been shown to have a decreased diversity of colonic bacteria ("microbial dysbiosis"), including lower densities of *Clostridia* and *Bacteroides* species, which produce short-chain fatty acids that serve as an important energy source for colonocytes. Unlike in CD, however, no study has been able to demonstrate *in vivo* loss of tolerance to gut microbiota in UC nor has any study shown an impact of antibiotics on disease activity, both of which call into question the microbiome as a direct cause of UC. Patients with UC also have fewer autoantibodies to bacterial antigens than do patients with CD and do not appear to share any of the genetic–microbiotal relationships previously identified in CD, such as the association between NOD2, proinflammatory bacteria, and disease phenotype.[17] Research into the microbiome of patients with IBD continues with the ultimate goal of opening a new frontier of microbiotal and immunologic therapies.

CLINICAL FEATURES

1 Symptoms of UC are dynamic and typically parallel the severity of disease. Inflammation classically begins in the rectum and extends proximally in a homogeneous and continuous fashion. The degree of colonic involvement is variable, ranging from the rectum alone (proctitis) to the rectosigmoid (proctosigmoiditis) to the entire colon and rectum (pancolitis) in approximately 20% of patients. Unlike in CD, the small intestine is spared, aside from the final few inches of the terminal ileum, which can experience a reversible "backwash ileitis" from the reflux of diarrheal stool (**Table 63.1**). Heterogeneous inflammation, rectal sparing, significant ileal disease, or the presence of a fistula raise the concern for CD and warrant further evaluation.

The classic symptoms of UC are diarrhea and rectal bleeding, although patients may present anywhere along the spectrum from chronic low-grade disease to fulminant colitis. The diarrhea is typically small volume, consisting of mostly blood

Table 63.1. Clinicopathologic Features of Ulcerative Colitis Versus Crohn Disease

Common Clinicopathologic Characteristics of IBD

Manifestation	UC	CD
Bleeding	Common	Rare
Crypt abscesses	Common	Rare
Rectal involvement	Common	Rare
Small bowel involvement	Rare	Common
Transmural inflammation	Rare	Common
Bowel wall fissures	Rare	Common
Fibrosis	Rare	Common
Fistulas	Rare	Common
Perianal disease	Rare	Common
Ulcers	Rare	Common
Cobblestoning	None	Common
Pattern of involvement	Continuous, mucosal/submucosal, distal to proximal	Skip lesions, transmural

Table 63.2. Mayo Clinic Score

Mayo Clinic Score
Stool Frequency (3-day average)
(Total number of stools/d)
0 = Normal number of stools for this patient
1 = 1–2 stools/d more than normal for this patient
2 = 3–4 stools/d more than normal for this patient
3 => 5 stools/d more than normal for this patient
Rectal Bleeding (3-day average)
0 = No blood seen
1 = Streaks of blood with <50% of stools
2 = Obvious blood seen with >50% of stools
3 = Blood alone passed
Physician's Global Assessment (PGA)
0 = Normal
1 = Mild disease
2 = Moderate disease
3 = Severe disease
Finding of Flexible Proctosigmoidoscopy (Endoscopic Subscore)
0 = Normal or inactive disease
1 = Mild disease (erythema, decreased vascular pattern, mild friability)
2 = Moderate disease (marked erythema, absent vascular pattern, friability, erosions)
3 = Severe disease (spontaneous bleeding, ulceration)

and mucus, and can be as frequent as every 1 to 2 hours. Paradoxically, patients with isolated rectosigmoid disease may experience constipation and incomplete evacuation (tenesmus) as a result of rectal spasm. The bleeding is also typically a slow, low-volume ooze from diseased mucosa rather than the massive hemorrhage that can be seen with vessel injury. Many patients experience diffuse, crampy abdominal pain, especially in the left lower quadrant, that is relieved or improved by defecation. Persistent or severe pain is uncommon and should raise concern for severe disease with inflammation extending to the serosa.

Disease severity is typically calculated using the Mayo score, the partial Mayo score (ie, without the Endoscopic Subscore), or the two-question Patient-Reported Outcomes subscore (PRO2; calculated based on stool frequency and degree of rectal bleeding alone) (**Table 63.2**). Worsening abdominal distention along with signs of systemic involvement, including fever, tachycardia, and leukocytosis, are worrisome for fulminant colitis or toxic megacolon and require immediate surgical evaluation. Chronic signs of illness, including weight loss, fatigue, anemia, and anorexia, must be identified and addressed as a part of a comprehensive treatment plan, ideally prior to surgical intervention.

Extraintestinal Manifestations

Approximately 30% of patients with UC will develop at least one extraintestinal manifestation of their disease, which can occur in almost any organ system but most commonly affect the
2 joints, skin, and eyes.[18] Many extraintestinal manifestations parallel disease activity, increasing in severity as GI symptoms worsen. Others have an independent disease course that may or may not improve with medical therapy or even colectomy. For 25% of UC patients, an extraintestinal manifestation will be the initial presentation of their disease.[19] Specific treatments depend on the extraintestinal manifestation, although most benefit from treatment of the underlying UC and require active and coordinated therapy with the appropriate medical subspecialists.

Musculoskeletal

Arthritis is the most common extraintestinal manifestation of UC, affecting over 20% of patients. True peripheral and axial spondyloarthropathies are less common, but can be particularly debilitating.[20] In general, peripheral arthritis is acute, affects a limited number of joints (≤4), and parallels colonic disease activity while axial disease is more widespread and follows an independent course. Patients with a family history or the HLA-B27 haplotype are at higher risk of developing axial disease, including severe forms such as ankylosing spondylitis. NSAIDs and exercise programs remain the mainstays of management, although tumor necrosis factor (TNF)-α antagonists can be used in more severe cases.

Cutaneous

Erythema nodosum is the most common cutaneous manifestation of IBD, occurring among 4% to 6% of patients.[18] Patients experience the sudden onset of symmetric, warm, tender, and red-violet nodules on the extensor surfaces of the lower limbs, especially the anterior tibial area. The number and severity of lesions tightly parallels colonic disease activity and persistence can be interpreted as a sign of inadequate disease control. Treatment typically involves supportive care for mild disease and systemic corticosteroids in severe cases. Pyoderma gangrenosum is a neutrophilic dermatosis that occurs less frequently than erythema nodosum, but is more difficult to treat and does not reliably parallel disease activity. Lesions begin as painful erythematous papules that rapidly progress to deep ulcers with granulated bases and undermined, "gun-metal gray" borders (**Fig. 63.2**). Pyoderma gangrenosum can occur

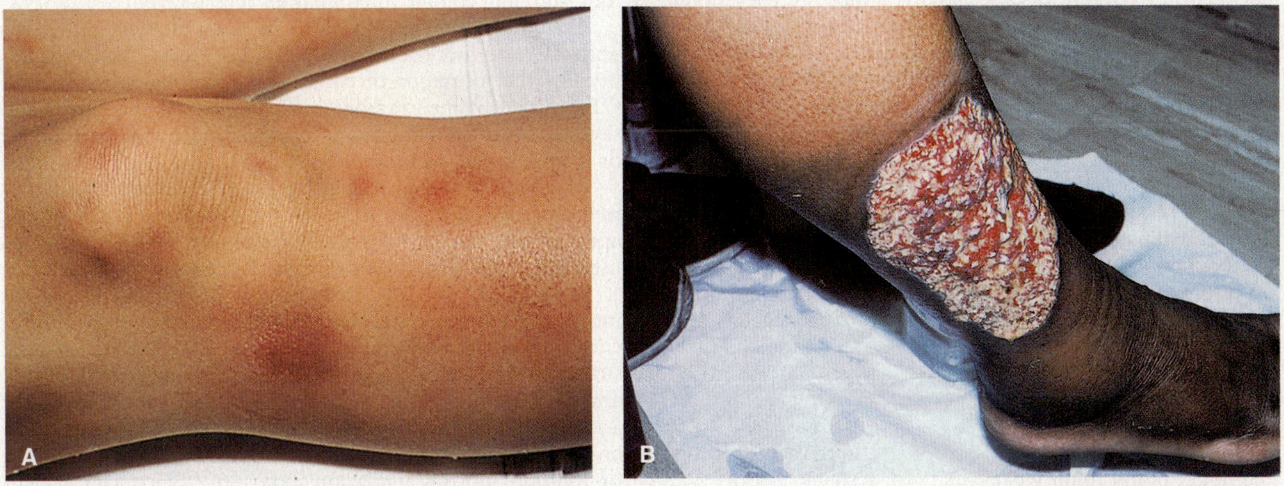

Figure 63.2. **A:** Erythema nodosum. **B:** Pyoderma gangrenosum. (Reproduced with permission from Goodheart HP. *A Photoguide of Common Skin Disorders: Diagnosis and Management*. Lippincott Williams & Wilkins; 1999.)

Table 63.3. Extraintestinal Manifestations of UC by Disease Activity

Parallel Disease Activity	Independent of Disease Activity	Variable Course
Erythema nodosum	Polyarticular peripheral arthritis/ arthropathies	Primary sclerosis cholangitis
Pauciarticular peripheral arthritis/ arthropathies	Axial arthropathies (sacroiliitis, ankylosing spondylitis)	Pyoderma gangrenosum
Acute synovitis	Uveitis/iritis	
Episcleritis	Aphthous ulceration	

Adapted from Vavricka SR, Schoepfer A, Scharl M, et al. Extraintestinal manifestations of inflammatory bowel disease. *Inflamm Bowel Dis.* 2015;21(8):1982–1992.

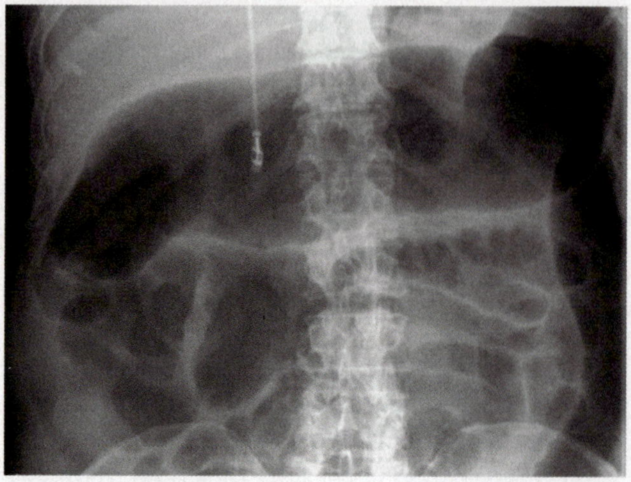

Figure 63.3. Abdominal x-ray of megacolon.

anywhere on the body, but most commonly affects the legs, peristomal skin, and sites of previous trauma ("pathergy"). Although small or superficial lesions can be treated with topical medications, most require systemic corticosteroids and/or steroid sparing agents, especially TNF-α antagonists in the setting of IBD.[21] Peristomal lesions can be particularly difficult to treat. Although occasionally necessary, re-siting should be performed with caution as lesions are known to recur at the new stoma site.

Ocular

Although UC patients frequently report ophthalmologic symptoms, fewer than 10% actually develop ocular inflammation, including episcleritis, iritis, and uveitis.[22] Episcleritis is the most common and is characterized by redness without vision changes. Both iritis and uveitis are less common, but can produce pain, blurry vision, and eventually blindness if not treated promptly with steroids or immunomodulatory medications.[23]

Hepatobiliary

Asymptomatic transaminitis is the most common hepatobiliary abnormality in UC, affecting nearly 50% of patients. Although much less common—occurring in only 3% to 7% of UC patients—primary sclerosing cholangitis (PSC) is the most concerning hepatobiliary manifestation of UC since there is no effective therapy short of liver transplantation. PSC is independent of colonic disease activity; it may precede colonic symptoms of UC by up to 7 years and persists even after proctocolectomy (**Table 63.3**). In addition, patients with PSC have four to five times higher risk of developing colorectal cancer than patients with UC alone; as such, they require more intensive endoscopic surveillance.[24]

DIAGNOSIS

Physical examination is often nonspecific, although worsening abdominal distention and generalized abdominal pain are indicators of severe disease. As with other septic conditions, the triad of tachycardia, fever, and leukocytosis suggests systemic toxicity and should prompt rapid resuscitation and early surgical evaluation.

Laboratory Testing

There is no specific diagnostic test for UC. In the acute setting, a complete blood count will evaluate for systemic toxicity and anemia. Serum albumin and prealbumin provide a measure of protein loss and malnutrition. Erythrocyte sedimentation rate (ESR) or C-reactive protein (CRP) levels can be drawn and followed as markers of disease activity. Stool studies and a *Clostridium difficile* assay should be sent to rule out bacterial and parasitic infections.

Calprotectin, a calcium-binding protein expressed by neutrophils, can be measured in the stool as a marker of colonic mucosal inflammation. Meta-analyses report an 80% to 95% sensitivity and a 76% to 96% specificity for distinguishing IBD from non-IBD diagnoses, including irritable bowel syndrome.[25,26] In fact, patients with fecal calprotectin levels <50 μg/g have only a 1% to 4% chance of having IBD. Fecal calprotectin levels also appear to correlate with endoscopic findings, degree of mucosal healing, and risk of relapse at 3 and 6 months.[27]

Serum antibodies, such as anti–*Saccharomyces cerevisiae* antibody (ASCA) and atypical perinuclear antineutrophil cytoplasmic antibody (pANCA), are often elevated in IBD, but do not reliably distinguish UC from CD or predict disease activity in UC.

Imaging

Conventional plane film x-rays are quick and can be useful in the rare case of frank perforation or toxic megacolon. Classically, barium enema was performed in the diagnosis of chronic UC, although it has largely been replaced by more modern imaging modalities. Colonic foreshortening, loss of haustral markings, and linear, "collar button ulcers" are signs of long-standing colonic inflammation (**Fig. 63.3**).

Computed tomography (CT) of the abdomen and pelvis with IV and occasionally oral and/or rectal contrast has become the technique of choice in evaluating acute disease. CT can be obtained rapidly, can demonstrate the extent and severity of inflammation, and can rule out extraintestinal air or other signs of perforation.

Magnetic resonance imaging (MRI), especially specialized enterographic protocols involving biphasic oral contrast agents (magnetic resonance enterography [MRE]), is often used for evaluating chronic disease (**Fig. 63.4**).

Both MRE and CT enterography (CTE) can assess for intra- and extramucosal disease activity, including the presence of fistulae, phlegmons, masses, or abscesses that might suggest a disease process other than UC. Importantly, MRE and CTE are both 90% to 95% sensitive for small bowel CD, a diagnosis that must be excluded, if at all possible, prior to any elective surgical intervention.[28,29] MRE has the advantage of limiting ionizing radiation exposure, which can benefit younger patients who may require multiple imaging studies over their lifetime.

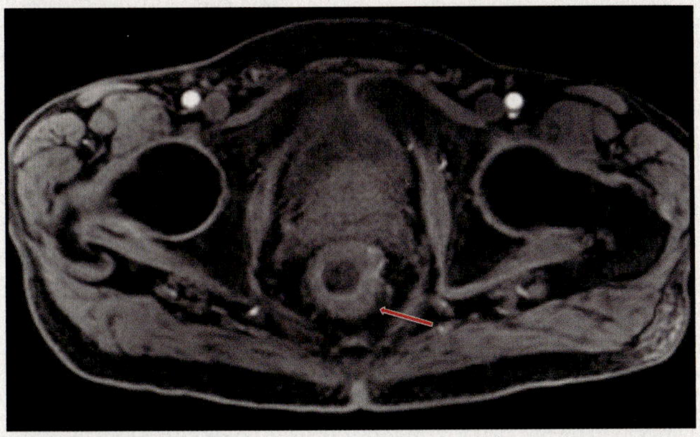

Figure 63.4. MRI demonstration of active UC with rectal wall thickening, increased vascularity, and inner layer hyperenhancement. (Courtesy of Dr. William Reed.)

Endoscopy

Endoscopy with biopsies remains the gold standard for the diagnosis of UC. Limited evaluation with flexible sigmoidoscopy or rigid proctoscopy is often sufficient given the near universal involvement of the rectum and may be safer in the setting of acute inflammation when full colonoscopy poses an increased risk of perforation. Mucosal inflammation is typically graded on the Mayo Endoscopic Subscore (MES), a component of the Mayo score (**Table 63.3**), which has demonstrated a strong correlation with microscopic findings and good interrater reliability.[30] Biopsies should also be taken to confirm histologic evidence of IBD, rule out concomitant cytomegalovirus (CMV) infection, and evaluate for dysplasia.

Surveillance and management of dysplasia in IBD has evolved in recent years. In short, surveillance colonoscopy should begin within 8 to 10 years of the onset of symptoms and should be performed every 1 to 2 years. Patients with a family history of colorectal cancer or PSC should be surveilled more frequently. At least 32 random biopsies must be performed throughout the colon—typically eight each in the right, transverse, left, and sigmoid colon—to achieve a 90% sensitivity for ruling out dysplasia.[31] Any polyps that are discovered should be removed endoscopically, if possible, and biopsies should be taken of the surrounding tissue to rule out persistent dysplasia.[32]

Pathology

Macroscopic Appearance

UC starts in the rectum and progresses proximally in a continuous fashion, with the most severe inflammation typically occurring in the rectum (**Fig. 63.5**). Inflamed mucosa generally appears granular, friable, and congested when viewed endoscopically. This pattern can dissipate either gradually or

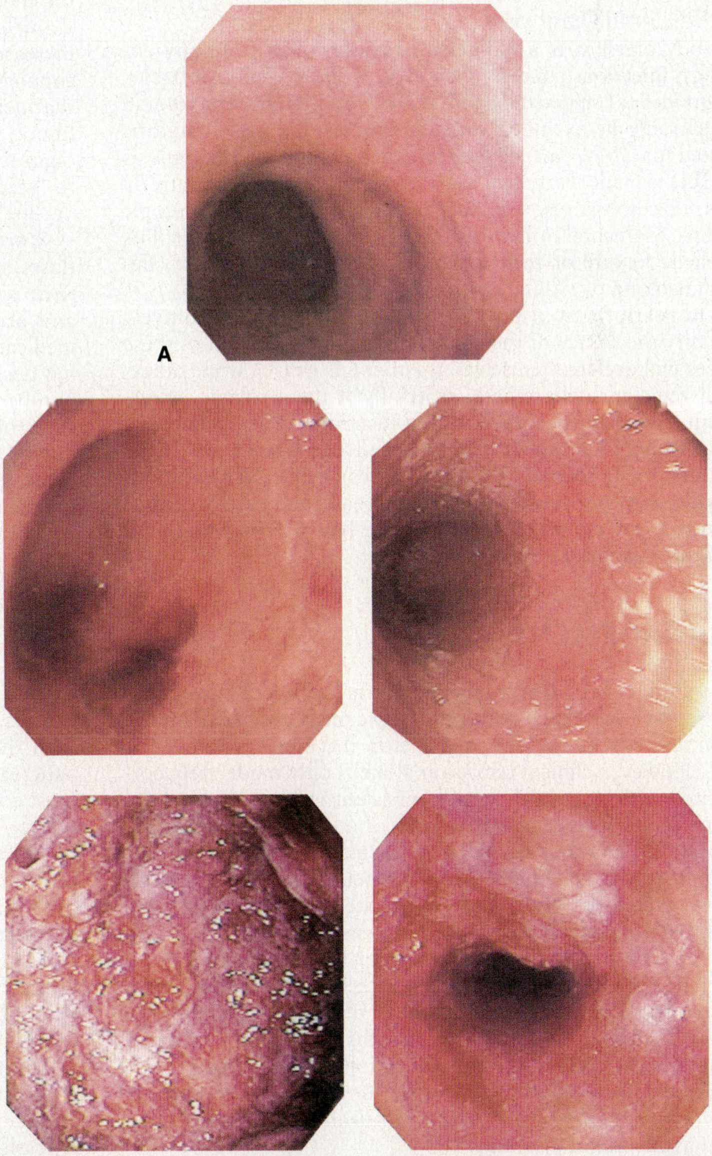

A B C D E

Figure 63.5. UC endoscopic findings with (**A**) Loss of normal vascular pattern. **B:** Contact bleeding. **C:** Granularity. **D:** Ulceration and friability. **E:** Colonic stricture. (Reproduced with permission from Corman ML. *Colon and Rectal Surgery.* 5th ed. Lippincott Williams & Wilkins; 2005.)

COLON AND RECTUM

abruptly as one moves proximally, but is never interrupted by areas of normal mucosa ("skip lesions"). Rectal mucosa in UC may be "burned out" or may demonstrate local treatment effect, but it is never spared, as it can be in CD.

Ulcers, superficial fissures, and pseudopolyps may be present in more severely inflamed areas, however, unlike in CD, fibrosis and strictures are uncommon (**Table 63.2**). In fact, the presence of stricturing disease in suspected UC should raise concern for malignancy until proven otherwise, especially if symptomatic, proximal to the splenic flexure, or late in the course of the disease. As noted previously, the presence of fistulizing disease suggests CD rather than UC.

Microscopic Appearance

Histology should confirm evidence of both inflammation and chronicity. Inflammation is typically evidenced by neutrophils within the surface epithelium, lamina propria, and crypts. Neutrophilic infiltration of the crypts ("cryptitis") can lead to aggregation ("crypt abscesses") and eventually ulceration (**Table 63.2**). As these findings are also present in acute non-IBD colitis, additional evidence of chronicity (eg, irregularities in crypt size, shape, and spacing) or regeneration (mucin depletion, hyperchromatic nuclei, Paneth cell metaplasia) is required to make the diagnosis of UC. Although inflammation in UC is traditionally confined to the mucosa and submucosa, the colon wall can be inflamed transmurally in the setting of acute severe disease, mimicking CD.

Differential Diagnosis

Bloody diarrhea is a hallmark of acute colitis from any etiology. Infectious sources, such as *C. difficile,* Campylobacter, Salmonella, *Escherichia coli* 0157:H7, and Entamoeba, should specifically be excluded via stool studies. Biopsies should be tested for CMV, regardless of whether an underlying diagnosis of IBD is made. Persistent diarrhea with a normal or relatively normal colonoscopy warrants biopsies to rule out microscopic colitis. Segmental inflammation may be due to ischemic colitis (splenic flexure or rectosigmoid) or diverticular disease (sigmoid colon).

In nearly 10% of the cases, it is impossible to definitively classify the source of the colitis. Over time, a portion of these cases will declare themselves as either CD or UC, while others will remain indeterminate, especially if the serologic assessment is inconclusive. As has been mentioned throughout, distinguishing UC from CD can be a challenge, particularly in the setting of CD colitis (25% of CD cases). Upper GI symptoms, small bowel involvement, perianal disease, and patchy colonic involvement should elicit some pause before proceeding with definitive surgical interventions.

MANAGEMENT

Medical Management

Resolution of rectal bleeding and normalization of bowel habits are well correlated with endoscopic measures of inflammation and can be useful end points in the initial treatment of UC. However, clinical remission alone is only moderately correlated with deep healing and persistent inflammation at the microscopic level increases the risk of relapse, hospitalization, colectomy, and dysplasia–even in asymptomatic or minimally symptomatic individuals. Modern societal recommendations have therefore increasingly advocated a "treat-to-target" approach in which treatment is intensified until predefined therapeutic goals have been met.[33] For UC, short-term targets include *clinical response* (defined as a decrease in the partial Mayo score of 2 points) and *clinical remission* (partial Mayo score ≤1), ideally within 6 to 12 months of induction. Intermediate targets include the normalization of biomarkers (CRP, ESR, and fecal calprotectin) while long-term targets include *endoscopic healing* (MES ≤1), normalization of quality of life, and avoidance of disability.[34]

Treatment is generally based on disease severity. Patients with mild-to-moderate colitis are treated in the outpatient setting with oral and/or rectal medications while patients with fever, tachycardia, or significant abdominal tenderness are admitted to the hospital for intravenous resuscitation and steroids.

Mild-to-Moderate Colitis

Aminosalicylates continue to be the first-line treatment of mild UC and can be used both for induction and maintenance of remission. Mesalamine (5-ASA) is the active compound, but is metabolized by proximal intestinal cells and requires either specialized coating or azo bonding to another compound to reach more distal disease. Alternatively, oral and rectal preparation can be used concomitantly.[35] Noncompliance with 5-ASA maintenance therapy is associated with a fivefold increase in disease recurrence.[36] Occasionally, budesonide, a topical corticosteroid, may be required to help achieve remission; however, it appears to be less effective as monotherapy than 5-ASA alone and is typically weaned in favor of other immunomodulatory medications during maintenance.[37]

Moderate-to-Severe Colitis

Patients with more severe disease (Mayo 6 to 12 or MES 2 to 3) are at higher risk of failure, recurrence, and colectomy, if remission cannot be achieved and maintained. Early age at onset (<40 years old), more extensive disease, deep ulcers on endoscopy, steroid dependence, and infection with either *C. difficile* or CMV have all been identified as predictors of increased 3-month colectomy rates.[38] The lack of evidence supporting the use of 5-ASA in severe UC and the concern that delays in achieving remission may increase both the likelihood and risks of surgery have shifted the treatment paradigm toward earlier use of biologics ("top down" as opposed to "step up") with the goal of preventing further physiologic decline.[39]

Corticosteroids remain the primary treatment of acute UC flares, with remission rates approaching 70%.[40] In the outpatient setting, oral prednisone doses of 40 mg/d are common and are typically tapered as symptoms improve and other medications are introduced. Overall, the use of corticosteroids has decreased in recent years, largely due to the increase in the number and effectiveness of available biologic agents. Corticosteroids should not be used for maintenance of remission due to their side-effect profile, including osteoporosis, diabetes, glaucoma, and an increased risk of infection and even mortality.[41]

Thiopurines, including 6-mercaptopurine and its prodrug azathioprine, have been used extensively in the treatment of moderate-to-severe UC; however, their slow onset of action makes them more appropriate for maintenance therapy rather than induction. In fact, azathioprine was found to be superior to 5-ASA in maintenance of remission and may be equivalent to some biologics, although no head-to-head trials exist.[42] Skin cancers, lymphoma, and severe infections have been reported with the use of these medications. Liver enzyme elevations, pancreatitis, and cholestasis have also been seen, although the most commonly reported side effects are headaches, hypersensitivity, and abdominal pain.

Infliximab, a chimeric mouse–human monoclonal antibody targeting TNF-α, was approved for the treatment of CD in 1998 and for UC in 2005. Infliximab successfully induced remission in over 60% of patients in the ACT 1 and 2 trials and significantly increases the likelihood of mucosal healing.[43] Extended follow-up has demonstrated that 15% of patients who initially respond to infliximab subsequently have to discontinue therapy due to side effects or loss of efficacy.[44] Newer TNF-α antagonists, including adalimumab, certolizumab, and golimumab, have also been shown to induce and maintain remission in UC, although none seem as effective at inducing remission as infliximab. Vedolizumab, a monoclonal antibody targeting integrin α4β7, prevents neutrophilic translocation in intestinal capillaries, thereby modulating the immune response in a gut-specific fashion. In head-to-head trials, vedolizumab was more successful than adalimumab at inducing clinical remission, at least among biologic naïve patients.[45] There was no difference among patients who had previously been treated with a TNF-α antagonist. Based on this evidence, the American Gastroenterological Association recommends initial biologic treatment with either infliximab or vedolizumab followed by either ustekinumab, a monoclonal antibody targeting IL-12 and IL-23, or tofacitinib, a small molecule Janus kinase inhibitor, in primary nonresponders.[39]

Overall, biologic agents are well tolerated. Infection, including reactivation of dormant mycobacterial and fungal infections, as well as certain autoimmune reactions remains a persistent concern. The data regarding malignancy risk with TNF-α antagonists are mixed, although there appears to be a small increase in the risk of lymphoma and nonmelanoma skin cancers.[46] More recently, biologics have been used in combination with either thiopurines or methotrexate as "dual therapy" in order to improve their pharmacokinetics (higher drug levels) and decrease their immunogenicity (lower rates of antidrug antibodies). Dual therapy may be more effective by mitigating antibody formation to biologic agents. A multiarmed randomized controlled trial found no difference in corticosteroid-free remission or mucosal healing between azathioprine and infliximab monotherapy, but did find significantly better rates among patients receiving both medications.[47] Patient selection is key, however, as combination therapy also appears to increase the rate of adverse drug reactions.

Acute Severe Ulcerative Colitis

Patients with acute severe UC require hospitalization for bowel rest, fluid resuscitation, pain control, and intravenous immunosuppression. IV corticosteroids, such as methyl-prednisolone, are first-line therapy with daily doses of 40 to 60 mg being common. There is no evidence to support any particular steroid preparation, dose, or dosing strategy over another. Antibiotics are not required unless there is evidence of perforation. All patients with IBD are at substantively increased risk for venous thromboembolism and should be treated during a flare with prophylactic heparinoids unless contraindicated.

Failure to improve within 48 to 96 hours of appropriate medical therapy should prompt reevaluation with either the addition of a second-line "rescue" medication or surgery. As mentioned previously, infliximab induces remission in roughly 60% of patients and may allow up to 90% of steroid-refractory patients to avoid colectomy in the urgent setting.[48] Cyclosporine can also be used as a second-line medication and may be more effective that steroids alone, however, serial lab draws to determine levels and close monitoring for toxicity is required. Two randomized controlled trials demonstrated no difference in short-term colectomy rates for steroid-refractory patients treated with infliximab versus cyclosporine.[49,50] Both medications have mean response times of 5 to 7 days, after which surgery should strongly be considered as sequential "rescue" therapy is ineffective.

Surgical evaluation should take place early in the course of the hospitalization to ensure that important discussions regarding the risks and benefits of surgery are not rushed. If available, an enterostomal therapist should also meet with patients to answer questions, discuss stoma care, and begin the adjustment process.

SURGERY

3 Indications

Approximately 20% to 30% of UC patients will ultimately require surgery. While the short-term colectomy rate appears to have decreased in the era of biologic medications,[51] the long-term colectomy rate remains roughly the same, suggesting that current medical therapies may be more successful at shifting surgery to an elective setting than at obviating it completely. Two population-based studies report conflicting data regarding changes in the indication for surgery in the current era, with one study from Japan suggesting a relative increase in surgery for dysplasia and cancer and one study from Finland finding no significant differences over time.[52,53]

Exposure to prednisone doses >10 mg/d increases the risk of perioperative infection, anastomotic leak, and pelvic sepsis and generally represents a contraindication to proctectomy or IPAA. Despite an initial concern for higher rates of infectious and anastomotic complications, more recent studies using large prospective cohorts have found no association between preoperative exposure to TNF-α antagonists and postoperative complication rates.[54] Similarly, multiple studies involving vedolizumab and at least one large study involving ustekinumab demonstrate no clear evidence for differences in postoperative complications. Based on these data, most high-volume IBD surgeons choose not to stop or even alter the dosing of biologic medications in the perioperative period. Still, given the accelerating development of new biologic medications and the lack of a national consensus, patients should make individualized decisions about their medications in combination with their surgeon and IBD gastroenterologist.

Fulminant Colitis and Toxic Megacolon

Fulminant colitis, as defined by Truelove and Witts, is an aggressive form of acute severe colitis characterized by fever, tachycardia, abdominal tenderness, greater than 10 bloody bowel movements per day, anemia requiring transfusion, elevated ESR, and colonic dilatation on radiography.

Megacolon is defined as dilation of the transverse colon beyond 6 cm (**Fig. 63.3**); toxic megacolon refers to the combination of megacolon and severe sepsis or even septic shock that can occur as a result of significant colonic inflammation, loss of mucosal integrity, and bacteria translocation. Toxic megacolon is not specific to UC and can occur in the setting of colitis from other sources, including infection and ischemia. Toxic megacolon from UC is seen most often in new diagnoses, but can occur during acute exacerbations of chronic disease. As with fulminant colitis, patients experience severe colonic and systemic inflammation, as demonstrated by high fevers, tachycardia, severe abdominal pain, and leukocytosis or leukopenia.

Aggressive resuscitation and broad-spectrum antibiotics should be started immediately. All opiates and antidiarrheal agents should be discontinued to avoid worsening colonic distention. Steroids should be started as soon as an infectious source is ruled out. Primary nonoperative treatment should not be prolonged due to high risk of perforation and decompensation. In one study, patients experiencing more than eight stools per day or three to eight stools per day with a CRP >45 mg/mL after 3 days of rescue therapy had an 85% chance of requiring colectomy during their hospitalization.[55] Moreover, early surgical intervention is associated with a decrease in the mortality rate among patients failing medical therapy.

Uncontrolled Bleeding

Less than 5% of UC patients have life-threatening GI bleeding. In this rare circumstance, a total abdominal colectomy is necessary to remove the inflamed and friable mucosa. Operations for bleeding represent only 10% of emergent colectomies performed in UC patients.

Dysplasia and Cancer

Patients with UC are at an increased risk of developing colorectal cancer compared to the general population, with younger patients and patients with pancolitis, longer disease duration, family history of IBD, or PSC at the highest risk. Meta-analyses report 10-, 20-, and 30-year rates of colorectal cancer at 2%, 8%, and 18%, respectively,[56] although newer

Table 63.4. Staged Approaches to Total Proctocolectomy in UC

Approach	Steps	Considerations
Three stage	1. Total abdominal colectomy with end ileostomy 2. Completion proctectomy, IPAA, and DLI 3. Loop ileostomy takedown	Patients who require urgent colectomy, who are nutritionally depleted, or on steroids at the time of their first procedure. Longer time to restoration of continuity.
Traditional two stage	1. Total proctocolectomy, IPAA, and DLI 2. Loop ileostomy takedown	Patients who can tolerate pelvic surgery at the time of their first procedure (eg, dysplasia in otherwise quiescent disease).
Modified two stage	1. Total abdominal colectomy with end ileostomy 2. Completion proctectomy and IPAA	Uncommon. Patients who undergo urgent colectomy, but are medically and nutritionally optimized at the time of their second operation. Requires IPAA creation without diversion.
One stage	Total proctocolectomy, IPAA	Rare. Patients who are ideal surgical candidates at the time of their first operation. Unable to confirm pathology prior to IPAA creation. Requires IPAA creation without diversion.

DLI, diverting loop ileostomy; IPAA, ileal pouch anal anastomosis.

population-based cohorts suggest that the actual risk may be slightly lower.[57]

Cancer in the setting of UC appears to have the same stage-specific prognosis, but is often detected at a later stage than in the general population. In fact, nearly 20% of colorectal carcinomas in the setting of UC are unresectable at the time of diagnosis.[58] Given the fact that patients with UC undergo colonoscopy more frequently than the general population, such a pattern of disease indicates that cancer development in UC patients may be accelerated or may follow a different progression from dysplasia to carcinoma.

As mentioned above, the guidelines have changed in response to growing evidence that the majority of dysplasia is visible and potentially resectable, even in the setting of IBD. The traditional recommendation for total proctocolectomy in the setting of dysplasia was based on elevated risk of malignant transformation throughout the colon or rectum. Under the new guidelines, visible polypoid lesions that are completely removed endoscopically with biopsies of the surrounding tissue that demonstrate no evidence of dysplasia can be managed as they would in patients without IBD.[32] In addition, rather than mandating colectomy, "invisible" dysplasia on random biopsies may instead be followed using close-interval chromoendoscopy or high-definition white light, which have demonstrated higher detection rates and lower incidence of metachronous colorectal cancer when compared to standard-definition white light endoscopy. Still, any dysplasia in the setting of UC warrants further evaluation by a specialist and may still prompt total proctocolectomy, if surveillance is not feasible or in the setting of unresectable or multifocal disease.

Medically Refractory Disease

Inability to fully control UC symptoms or to do so without the chronic use of steroids remains the most common indication for surgery. Proctocolectomy can also improve many of the extracolonic manifestations of UC and can be considered in particularly debilitating or recalcitrant cases of erythema nodosum, large joint arthritis, aphthous ulceration, or episcleritis.

Surgical Management

Unlike for CD, surgery with total proctocolectomy is considered curative in UC. Multiple surgical options are available and the ultimate choice of operation should be determined by the indication, urgency, continued need for immunosuppressive medications, and medical and nutritional condition of the patient (**Table 63.4**). In general, the decisions regarding colectomy, proctectomy, and IPAA should be made independently, given that proctectomy can often be postponed safely after abdominal colectomy and that patients with permanent end ileostomy have both lower long-term complication rates and can have equivalent quality of life to those with a restorative IPAA.[59]

Total Abdominal Colectomy with End Ileostomy

For urgent indications, including fulminant colitis, toxic megacolon, uncontrolled bleeding, and perforation, the operation of choice is a total abdominal colectomy with preservation of the rectum and creation of an end ileostomy (**Table 63.5** and

Table 63.5. Total Abdominal Colectomy: Key Technical Steps, Pearls, and Potential Pitfalls

Key Technical Steps

1. Abdominal entry either via laparoscopic port placement or midline laparotomy
2. Mobilize right colon and divide ileocolic pedicle
3. Open the entire gastrocolic ligament to enter the lesser sac and expose the transverse mesocolon
4. Divide the lateral attachments of the sigmoid colon, left colon, and splenic flexure
5. Make a window in the mesentery and divide the distal sigmoid or rectosigmoid
6. Divide the remaining transverse, left, and sigmoid mesocolon
7. Extracorporealize the colon through an extraction site or the planned ileostomy trephine
8. Create an end ileostomy

Pearls

- There is no set order to removing the colon; move to another area of the colon and come back if dissection is proving difficult
- Unless there is concomitant cancer or dysplasia, plan to divide the mesentery along the border with the colon, which requires less mobilization and can prevent disorientation
- Do not divide the superior rectal artery or inferior mesenteric artery to prevent retraction of the rectal stump and a more complex second stage operation

Potential Pitfalls

- Bleeding from the middle colic or short gastric vessels
- Injury to the ureters, pancreas, spleen, or duodenum
- Avulsion of the terminal ileal mesentery while extracorporealizing the specimen
- Twisting the mesentery of the ileostomy during creation

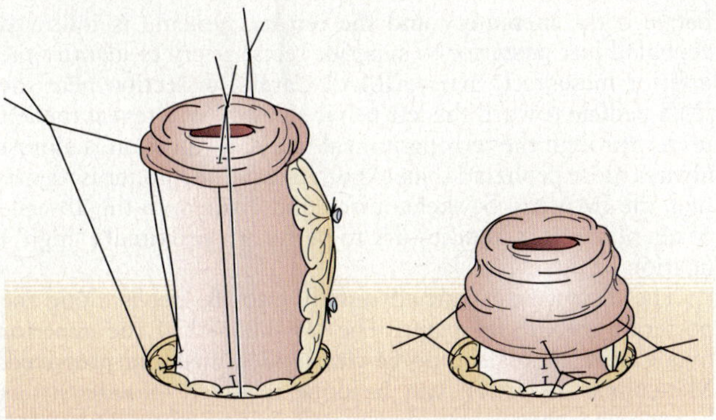

Figure 63.6. Brooking ileostomy.

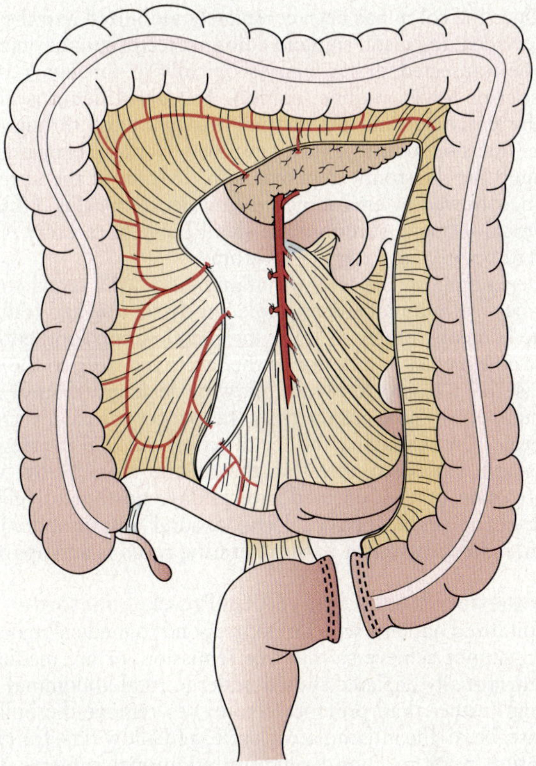

Figure 63.8. Mobilized colon with vessels divided, and stapled at the rectum. This specimen is ready for extraction; the ileum can be transected intracorporeally, or after specimen is extracorporealized.

Fig. 63.6). Resection of the rectum in the urgent setting should be avoided, if possible, to both allow for continent reconstruction at a later time and to avoid a pelvic dissection under suboptimal clinical conditions. Mobilizing the rectum unnecessarily disrupts the mesorectal planes, making subsequent reconstruction more difficult. In addition, active inflammation and anasarca can obscure dissection planes, putting the ureters and pelvic nerves at unnecessary risk. In addition, consideration should be given to the level of ileal transection proximally, keeping in mind that pouch reach is dependent on the available bowel and the length of its mesentery. Under certain circumstances, the ileocolic artery must be preserved to allow for back filling of the arcades if the superior mesenteric artery must be divided to enable the ileal pouch to reach the anus.

Stoma marking by an enterostomal therapist should take place preoperatively, if possible. Managing a poorly placed stoma is a major source of preventable morbidity and frustration for patients. If there is concern regarding visualization of the ureters, stents should be placed prior to beginning the operation. Although they do not reduce the rate of ureteral injury, they do aid in intraoperative identification of any injury and can help facilitate prompt repair.

4 A minimally invasive approach should be attempted, if the patient is stable and the surgeon is sufficiently comfortable with the technique. After establishing pneumoperitoneum and placing additional ports, the colon is mobilized systematically in either a medial-to-lateral or lateral-to-medial fashion (**Figs. 63.7** and **63.8**). Although the sequence of the operation varies from surgeon to surgeon (eg, right colon first vs left colon first), a systematic technique should be employed. Unless there is concern for cancer, the vessels can be transected close to the bowel wall to avoid the risks of high ligation. Particular attention should be paid to the splenic flexure, as a splenic tear will unnecessarily complicate the operation.

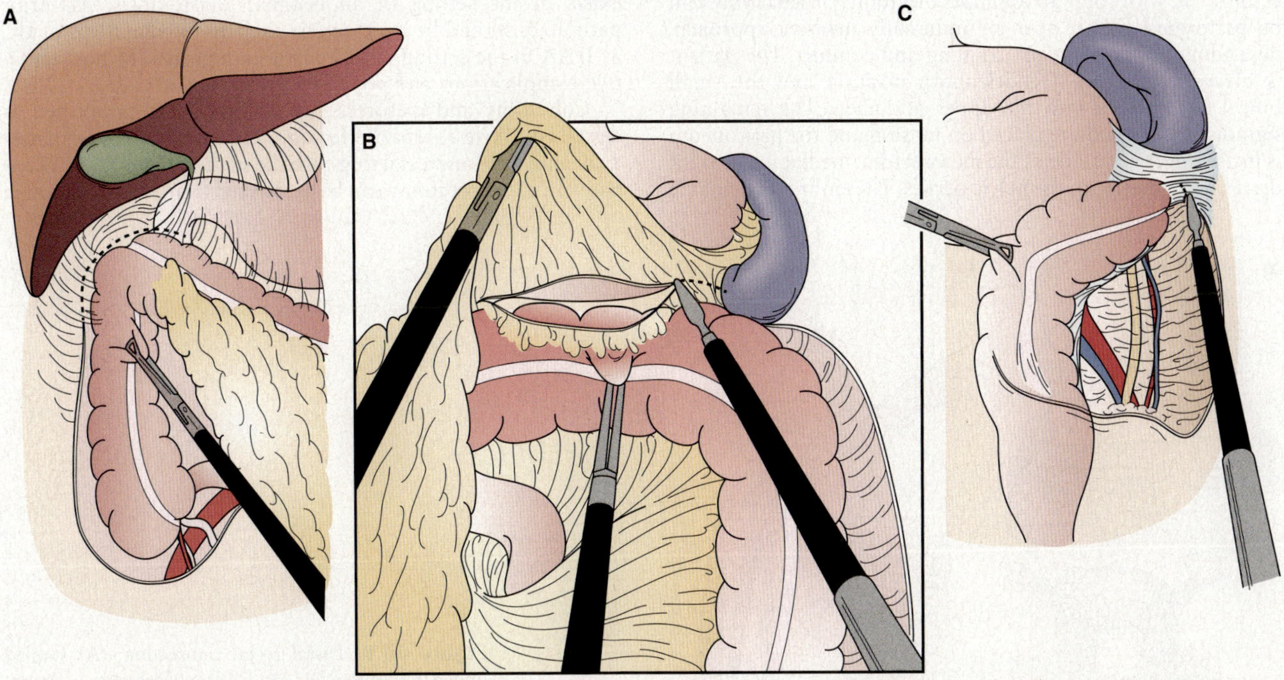

Figure 63.7. Colon mobilization. A: right colon. B: transverse colon. C: left colon.

Once the colon has been completely mobilized and the vessels divided, the distal sigmoid colon or rectosigmoid junction can be transected, either laparoscopically or through a Pfannenstiel or lower midline incision. The distal ileum is either similarly divided and the specimen is extracted through the lower incision or the entire specimen is extracorporealized through the ileostomy trephine, with division of the terminal ileum, followed by creation of an end ileostomy (**Fig. 63.6**). It is critical to make sure that the small bowel mesentery is not twisted before maturing the ileostomy.

Depending on the level of inflammation, the rectal stump may be at substantial risk of staple line disruption and leakage. Some surgeons prefer to leave the rectal stump long enough to be able to tack it anterior to the fascia but deep to the skin in case of a stump blowout, allowing leakage of stool into subcutaneous tissue rather than the peritoneal cavity. Other strategies for managing the rectal stump include oversewing the staple line, decompressing the rectum from below with a soft drain that is removed several days postoperatively, or purse-stringing the proximal end around a transabdominal drain, if an early return to the operating room is anticipated.

Completion Proctectomy/Total Proctocolectomy

Hospitalized patients who do not respond to medical management, cannot achieve steroid-free remission, or are medically or nutritionally depleted should undergo total abdominal colectomy (rather than proctocolectomy) to remove the bulk of disease, break the inflammatory cycle, and allow time for rehabilitation prior to considering any additional surgery. After recovery, patients who either have persistent rectal symptoms (pain, tenesmus, bleeding, discharge) or desire restoration of continuity can proceed with completion proctectomy. Short of persistent symptoms requiring steroids, an inability to perform surveillance of the rectum, or evidence of dysplasia/cancer, proctectomy is not mandatory and patients can live full lives with a permanent ileostomy and their remaining rectum in place, as long as they continue surveillance. Unfortunately, proctectomy is required for restoration of continuity as ileorectal anastomosis has not demonstrated favorable outcomes in UC and should be avoided outside of specific clinical situations (eg, palliation and young women considering future pregnancy).

Abdominal colectomy is performed as above, either at a prior operation or during the initial phase of total proctocolectomy. As with total abdominal colectomy, proctectomy can be performed via an open or minimally invasive approach, depending on the surgeon's training and comfort. The patient is placed in a steep Trendelenburg position and the small bowel is displaced into the upper abdomen. The remaining sigmoid and rectum are placed on tension and the peritoneum is incised over right side of the mesorectum, medial to the right ureter, and anterior to the pelvic nerves. The embryologic plane between the mesentery and the retroperitoneum is followed cephalad just posterior to superior rectal artery to identify the inferior mesenteric artery (IMA). Careful dissection near the IMA pedicle toward the left pelvic sidewall will reveal the left ureter through the retroperitoneal fascia; its location is almost always more cephalad than expected. After the ureter is identified, the IMA can be skeletonized and divided. In the absence of neoplasia, it is unnecessary to perform a proximal ("high") ligation of the IMA.

The dissection is carried distally into the pelvis along the posterior mesorectal plane. The "wishbone" of the superior hypogastric plexus should be clearly identified and protected. Meticulous dissection can be done relatively bloodlessly as long as one stays in the correct embryologic plane. Dissection posteriorly through the presacral fascia risks injuring the presacral veins, which can result in troublesome and sometimes life-threatening bleeding. All effort should be made to complete the dissection posteriorly, prior to dividing the anterior peritoneal reflection and entering either the rectovaginal or rectoprostatic plane. Denonvilliers fascia should not be violated in order to avoid contributing to sexual dysfunction in men.

Once the dissection is carried down to the pelvic floor circumferentially, the distance from the anal verge can be assessed via digital rectal examination. In patients undergoing IPAA, the rectum is transected using a stapler and removed from the field. In patients undergoing proctectomy and permanent ileostomy, a perineal dissection is begun, either in the lithotomy or prone position. Unlike an abdominoperineal resection for cancer, the perineal dissection begins in the intersphincteric groove and extends proximally in the relatively bloodless plane between the sphincters until the abdominal cavity is entered. Performing an intersphincteric dissection leaves the external sphincter in situ, allowing it to be incorporated into a layered perineal closure to improve wound healing.

Ileal Pouch-Anal Anastomosis

Total proctocolectomy with IPAA is the most commonly performed elective operation for UC, typically in the setting of
5 persistent mild-to-moderate disease or dysplasia. While higher than end ileostomy, IPAA has an acceptable morbidity rate (20% to 30%) and produces a quality of life that approaches normal controls. IPAA is not appropriate in patients with poor anal sphincter function, a history of anorectal disease, or an inability to tolerate the increased risk of pelvic sepsis that exists in the setting of an ileoanal anastomosis. All prior pathology should be reviewed to confirm the diagnosis of UC as IPAA in the setting of CD carries a high risk of postoperative complications and pouch failure.

Colectomy and mesorectal mobilization are performed as described above except the rectum is transected approximately 1 cm above the anorectal ring with the stapler (**Fig. 63.9A**). Alternatively, a mucosectomy can be performed from below, although

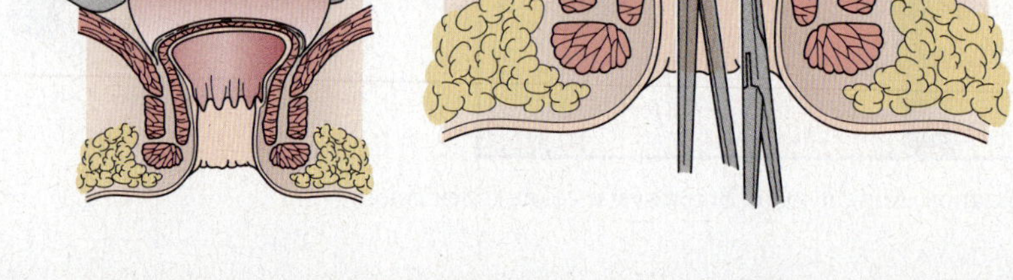

Figure 63.9. Distal rectal transection, (**A**) stapled above the dentate line, or (**B**) a mucosectomy in preparation for a hand-sewn anastomosis.

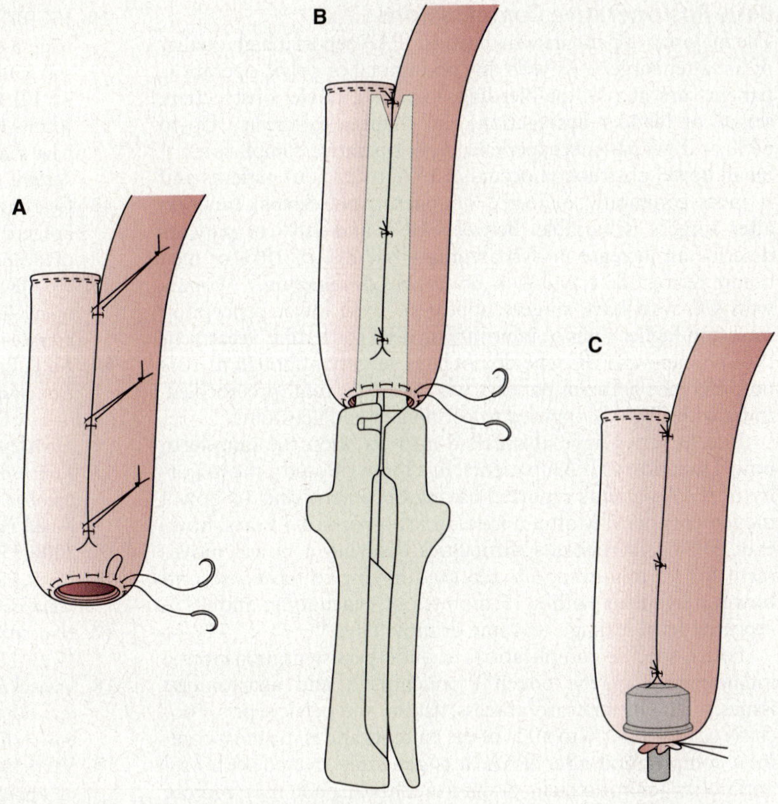

Figure 63.10. IPAA construction and anastomosis, (**A**) terminal ileum alignment for (**B**) common channel creation. **C:** EEA anvil attachment at the apex of the pouch.

this necessitates a hand-sewn ileoanal anastomosis (**Fig. 63.9B**). Overall, there is no difference in perioperative complications between double-stapled and hand-sewn IPAA anastomoses.[60] Some studies suggest leaving a small rectal cuff improves defecatory function, although any residual rectal mucosa poses some risk of dysplasia or recurrent proctitis ("cuffitis").

After the proctectomy has been completed, a pouch is fashioned from the terminal ileum. Multiple pouch configurations exist; although there is no evidence to support one over another, the double-loop J-pouch configuration is the most popular in the United States (**Fig. 63.10**). A portion of the distal or terminal ileum is pulled toward the anus to align the bowel in a "J" configuration. Before committing to pouch formation, it is necessary to confirm that the apex will reach the rectal cuff or anus without tension, which is typically done by stretching the apex slightly beyond the pubic symphysis. Multiple maneuvers can be performed to "lengthen" the reach of the pouch, if necessary, and are beyond the scope of this discussion. Once the apex location is decided on, the two limbs of the ileum are aligned with interrupted suture to create a pouch of 15 to 20 cm in length. An enterotomy is made at the apex of the pouch and a GIA stapler is used to fashion a common channel between the two limbs. The pouch can then be anastomosed to the distal segment either by using an EEA stapler (placing the anvil in the J pouch and firing pin through the rectal pouch) or via a hand-sewn anastomosis (**Fig. 63.11**).

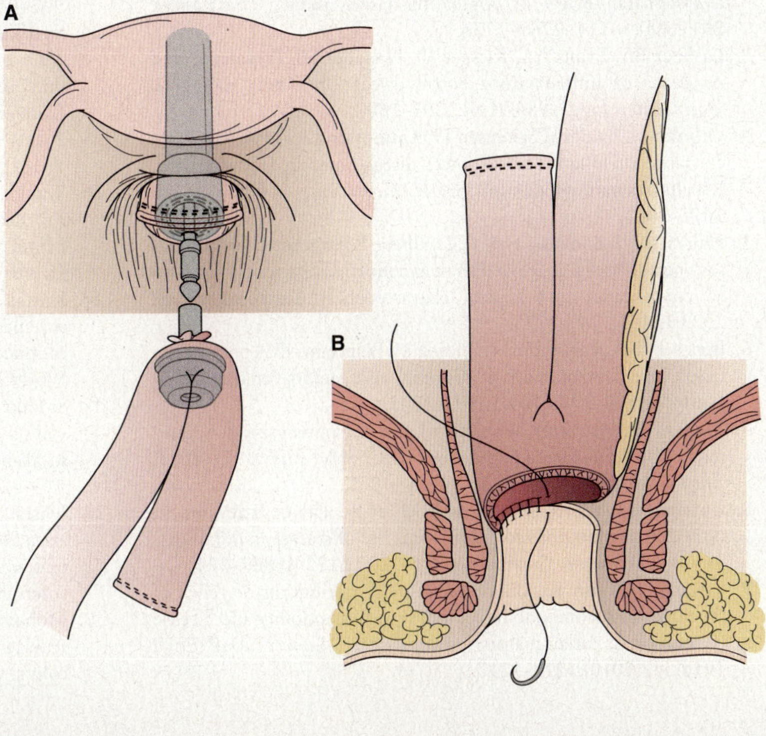

Figure 63.11. Anastomosis of the J-Pouch with (**A**) stapled anastomosis and (**B**) hand-sewn anastomosis.

IPAA-Postoperative Complications

6 The majority of patients who have an IPAA report a high quality of life after surgery. As with any abdominal or pelvic operation, patients are at risk for bleeding, infection, bowel obstruction, sexual or bladder dysfunction, and changes to fertility. Up to 60% of IPAA patients experience a perioperative complication.[61] Small bowel obstruction occurs in 15% to 20% of patients and is most commonly managed nonoperatively. Sexual function after surgery is variable. Between 10% and 20% of patients describe an increase in dyspareunia while 2% to 19% of men report retrograde ejaculation or erectile dysfunction.[62] Women with UC who have surgery appear to have lower conception rates and higher rates of infertility or need for fertility treatment than women with UC who do not have surgery, although there is no difference between patients who undergo total proctocolectomy with IPAA as opposed to permanent end ileostomy.[63]

Recent series have also called into question the long-term bowel function of IPAA patients. In a large US study, the majority of IPAA patients reported having between 6 and 10 bowel movements per day after a median follow-up of 4 years, however, 90% still reported difficulties delaying a bowel movement for 15 minutes, 56% reported having to have a second bowel movement within 15 minutes of evacuating, and 19% reported fecal leakage on some or most days.[61]

Pouch-specific complications include persistent, nonspecific inflammation of the pouch ("pouchitis"), and anastomotic issues, including stricture, abscess, fistula, and pelvic sepsis. Pouchitis occurs in 40% to 50% of the patients and is the most common complication after IPAA. It is generally treated with oral antibiotics (ciprofloxacin or metronidazole), but may require evaluation with endoscopy and biopsy, if symptoms persist. Other medications that have been shown to help treat pouchitis include corticosteroids, budesonide, 5-ASA, and allopurinol. Up to 10% of IPAA patients experience a frank anastomotic leak and 12% develop a persistent fistula tract. Antibiotics, drainage, and salvage procedures can be performed; however, between 7% and 8% of patients will eventually require pouch excision.

References

1. Ye Y, Manne S, Treem WR, Bennett D. Prevalence of inflammatory bowel disease in pediatric and adult populations: recent estimates from large national databases in the United States, 2007–2016. *Inflamm Bowel Dis.* 2020;26(4):619–625.
2. Ng SC, Shi HY, Hamidi N, et al. Worldwide incidence and prevalence of inflammatory bowel disease in the 21st century: a systematic review of population-based studies. *The Lancet.* 2017;390(10114):2769–2778.
3. Lashner BA, Evans AA, Kirsner JB, Hanauer SB. Prevalence and incidence of inflammatory bowel disease in family members. *Gastroenterology.* 1986;91(6):1396–1400.
4. Orholm M, Binder V, Sørensen TI, Rasmussen LP, Kyvik KO. Concordance of inflammatory bowel disease among Danish twins. Results of a nationwide study. *Scand J Gastroenterol.* 2000;35(10): 1075–1081.
5. Halfvarson J, Bodin L, Tysk C, Lindberg E, Järnerot G. Inflammatory bowel disease in a Swedish twin cohort: a long-term follow-up of concordance and clinical characteristics. *Gastroenterology.* 2003;124(7):1767–1773.
6. Bernstein CN, Rawsthorne P, Cheang M, Blanchard JF. A population-based case control study of potential risk factors for IBD. *Am J Gastroenterol.* 2006;101(5):993–1002.
7. Moller FT, Andersen V, Wohlfahrt J, Jess T. Familial risk of inflammatory bowel disease: a population-based cohort study 1977–2011. *Am J Gastroenterol.* 2015;110(4):564–571.
8. Cuthbert AP, Fisher SA, Mirza MM, et al. The contribution of NOD2 gene mutations to the risk and site of disease in inflammatory bowel disease. *Gastroenterology.* 2002;122(4):867–874.
9. Satsangi J, Welsh KI, Bunce M, et al. Contribution of genes of the major histocompatibility complex to susceptibility and disease phenotype in inflammatory bowel disease. *Lancet Lond Engl.* 1996;347(9010):1212–1217.
10. UK IBD Genetics Consortium, Barrett JC, Lee JC, et al. Genome-wide association study of ulcerative colitis identifies three new susceptibility loci, including the HNF4A region. *Nat Genet.* 2009; 41(12):1330–1334.
11. Jostins L, Ripke S, Weersma RK, et al. Host–microbe interactions have shaped the genetic architecture of inflammatory bowel disease. *Nature.* 2012;491(7422):119–124.
12. Geerling BJ, Dagnelie PC, Badart-Smook A, Russel MG, Stockbrügger RW, Brummer RJ. Diet as a risk factor for the development of ulcerative colitis. *Am J Gastroenterol.* 2000;95(4):1008–1013.
13. Hou JK, Abraham B, El-Serag H. Dietary intake and risk of developing inflammatory bowel disease: a systematic review of the literature. *Am J Gastroenterol.* 2011;106(4):563–573.
14. Xu L, Lochhead P, Ko Y, Claggett B, Leong RW, Ananthakrishnan AN. Systematic review with meta-analysis: breastfeeding and the risk of Crohn's disease and ulcerative colitis. *Aliment Pharmacol Ther.* 2017;46(9):780–789.
15. Koutroubakis IE, Vlachonikolis IG. Appendectomy and the development of ulcerative colitis: results of a metaanalysis of published case-control studies. *Off J Am Coll Gastroenterol ACG.* 2000;95(1):171.
16. Du L, Ha C. Epidemiology and pathogenesis of ulcerative colitis. *Gastroenterol Clin North Am.* 2020;49(4):643–654.
17. Danese S, Fiocchi C. Ulcerative colitis. *N Engl J Med.* 2011;365(18): 1713–1725.
18. Vavricka SR, Brun L, Ballabeni P, et al. Frequency and risk factors for extraintestinal manifestations in the Swiss inflammatory bowel disease cohort. *Am J Gastroenterol.* 2011;106(1):110–119.
19. Vavricka SR, Rogler G, Gantenbein C, et al. Chronological order of appearance of extraintestinal manifestations relative to the time of IBD diagnosis in the Swiss Inflammatory Bowel Disease Cohort. *Inflamm Bowel Dis.* 2015;21(8):1794–1800.
20. Ossum AM, Palm Ø, Lunder AK, et al. Ankylosing spondylitis and axial spondyloarthritis in patients with long-term inflammatory bowel disease: results from 20 years of follow-up in the IBSEN study. *J Crohns Colitis.* 2018;12(1):96–104.
21. Agarwal A, Andrews JM. Systematic review: IBD-associated pyoderma gangrenosum in the biologic era, the response to therapy. *Aliment Pharmacol Ther.* 2013;38(6):563–572.
22. Cloché V, Buisson A, Tréchot F, et al. Ocular symptoms are not predictive of ophthalmologic inflammation in inflammatory bowel disease. *Dig Liver Dis Off J Ital Soc Gastroenterol Ital Assoc Study Liver.* 2013;45(3):195–199.
23. Jaffe GJ, Dick AD, Brézin AP, et al. Adalimumab in patients with active noninfectious uveitis. *N Engl J Med.* 2016;375(10): 932–943.
24. Soetikno RM, Lin OS, Heidenreich PA, Young HS, Blackstone MO. Increased risk of colorectal neoplasia in patients with primary sclerosing cholangitis and ulcerative colitis: a meta-analysis. *Gastrointest Endosc.* 2002;56(1):48–54.
25. Ayling RM, Kok K. Fecal Calprotectin. *Adv Clin Chem.* 2018;87: 161–190.
26. Waugh N, Cummins E, Royle P, et al. Faecal calprotectin testing for differentiating amongst inflammatory and non-inflammatory bowel diseases: systematic review and economic evaluation. *Health Technol Assess Winch Engl.* 2013;17(55):xv–xix, 1–211.
27. Kostas A, Siakavellas SI, Kosmidis C, et al. Fecal calprotectin measurement is a marker of short-term clinical outcome and presence of mucosal healing in patients with inflammatory bowel disease. *World J Gastroenterol.* 2017;23(41):7387–7396.
28. Siddiki HA, Fidler JL, Fletcher JG, et al. Prospective comparison of state-of-the-art MR enterography and CT enterography in small-bowel Crohn's disease. *AJR Am J Roentgenol.* 2009;193(1): 113–121.
29. Jensen MD, Ormstrup T, Vagn-Hansen C, Østergaard L, Rafaelsen SR. Interobserver and intermodality agreement for detection of small bowel Crohn's disease with MR enterography and CT enterography. *Inflamm Bowel Dis.* 2011;17(5):1081–1088.
30. Mohammed Vashist N, Samaan M, Mosli MH, et al. Endoscopic scoring indices for evaluation of disease activity in ulcerative colitis. *Cochrane Database Syst Rev.* 2018;1(1):CD011450.

31. Rubin CE, Haggitt RC, Burmer GC, et al. DNA aneuploidy in colonic biopsies predicts future development of dysplasia in ulcerative colitis. *Gastroenterology*. 1992;103(5):1611–1620.
32. Laine L, Kaltenbach T, Barkun A, et al. SCENIC international consensus statement on surveillance and management of dysplasia in inflammatory bowel disease. *Gastroenterology*. 2015;148(3): 639–651.e28.
33. Peyrin-Biroulet L, Sandborn W, Sands BE, et al. Selecting Therapeutic Targets in Inflammatory Bowel Disease (STRIDE): Determining therapeutic goals for treat-to-target. *Am J Gastroenterol*. 2015;110(9):1324–1338.
34. Turner D, Ricciuto A, Lewis A, et al. STRIDE-II: An update on the Selecting Therapeutic Targets in Inflammatory Bowel Disease (STRIDE) Initiative of the International Organization for the Study of IBD (IOIBD): Determining therapeutic goals for treat-to-target strategies in IBD. *Gastroenterology*. 2021;160(5):1570–1583.
35. Ford AC, Achkar JP, Khan KJ, et al. Efficacy of 5-aminosalicylates in ulcerative colitis: systematic review and meta-analysis. *Am J Gastroenterol*. 2011;106(4):601–616.
36. Kane S, Huo D, Aikens J, Hanauer S. Medication nonadherence and the outcomes of patients with quiescent ulcerative colitis. *Am J Med*. 2003;114(1):39–43.
37. Sherlock ME, MacDonald JK, Griffiths AM, Steinhart AH, Seow CH. Oral budesonide for induction of remission in ulcerative colitis. *Cochrane Database Syst Rev*. 2015;2015(10):CD007698.
38. Dias CC, Rodrigues PP, da Costa-Pereira A, Magro F. Clinical predictors of colectomy in patients with ulcerative colitis: systematic review and meta-analysis of cohort studies. *J Crohns Colitis*. 2015;9(2):156–163.
39. Feuerstein JD, Isaacs KL, Schneider Y, et al. AGA clinical practice guidelines on the management of moderate to severe ulcerative colitis. *Gastroenterology*. 2020;158(5):1450–1461.
40. Faubion WA Jr, Loftus EV, Harmsen WS, Zinsmeister AR, Sandborn WJ. The natural history of corticosteroid therapy for inflammatory bowel disease: a population-based study. *Gastroenterology*. 2001;121(2):255–260.
41. Lichtenstein GR, Feagan BG, Cohen RD, et al. Serious infection and mortality in patients with Crohn's disease: more than 5 years of follow-up in the TREAT™ registry. *Am J Gastroenterol*. 2012;107(9):1409–1422.
42. Ardizzone S, Maconi G, Russo A, Imbesi V, Colombo E, Bianchi Porro G. Randomised controlled trial of azathioprine and 5-aminosalicylic acid for treatment of steroid dependent ulcerative colitis. *Gut*. 2006;55(1):47–53.
43. Rutgeerts P, Sandborn WJ, Feagan BG, et al. Infliximab for induction and maintenance therapy for ulcerative colitis. *N Engl J Med*. 2005;353(23):2462–2476.
44. Reinisch W, Sandborn WJ, Rutgeerts P, et al. Long-term infliximab maintenance therapy for ulcerative colitis: the ACT-1 and -2 extension studies. *Inflamm Bowel Dis*. 2012;18(2):201–211.
45. Sands BE, Peyrin-Biroulet L, Loftus EV Jr, et al. Vedolizumab versus adalimumab for moderate-to-severe ulcerative colitis. *N Engl J Med*. 2019;381(13):1215–1226.
46. Mariette X, Tubach F, Bagheri H, et al. Lymphoma in patients treated with anti-TNF: results of the 3-year prospective French RATIO registry. *Ann Rheum Dis*. 2010;69(2):400–408.
47. Panaccione R, Ghosh S, Middleton S, et al. Combination therapy with infliximab and azathioprine is superior to monotherapy with either agent in ulcerative colitis. *Gastroenterology*. 2014;146(2): 392–400.e3.
48. Aratari A, Papi C, Clemente V, et al. Colectomy rate in acute severe ulcerative colitis in the infliximab era. *Dig Liver Dis Off J Ital Soc Gastroenterol Ital Assoc Study Liver*. 2008;40(10):821–826.
49. Laharie D, Bourreille A, Branche J, et al. Ciclosporin versus infliximab in patients with severe ulcerative colitis refractory to intravenous steroids: a parallel, open-label randomised controlled trial. *Lancet Lond Engl*. 2012;380(9857):1909–1915.
50. Williams JG, Alam MF, Alrubaiy L, et al. Infliximab versus ciclosporin for steroid-resistant acute severe ulcerative colitis (CONSTRUCT): a mixed methods, open-label, pragmatic randomised trial. *Lancet Gastroenterol Hepatol*. 2016;1(1):15–24.
51. Barnes EL, Jiang Y, Kappelman MD, et al. Decreasing colectomy rate for ulcerative colitis in the united states between 2007 and 2016: a time trend analysis. *Inflamm Bowel Dis*. 2020;26(8): 1225–1231.
52. Uchino M, Ikeuchi H, Hata K, et al. Changes in the rate of and trends in colectomy for ulcerative colitis during the era of biologics and calcineurin inhibitors based on a Japanese nationwide cohort study. *Surg Today*. 2019;49(12):1066–1073.
53. Kolehmainen S, Lepistö A, Färkkilä M. Impact of anti-TNF-alpha therapy on colectomy rate and indications for colectomy in ulcerative colitis: comparison of two patient cohorts from 2005 to 2007 and from 2014 to 2016. *Scand J Gastroenterol*. 2019;54(6):707–711.
54. Cohen BL, Fleshner P, Kane SV, et al. Prospective cohort study to investigate the safety of preoperative tumor necrosis factor inhibitor exposure in patients with inflammatory bowel disease undergoing intra-abdominal Surgery. *Gastroenterology*. 2022;163(1):204–221.
55. Travis SPL. Predicting outcome in severe ulcerative colitis. *Dig Liver Dis Off J Ital Soc Gastroenterol Ital Assoc Study Liver*. 2004;36(7):448–449.
56. Eaden JA, Abrams KR, Mayberry JF. The risk of colorectal cancer in ulcerative colitis: a meta-analysis. *Gut*. 2001;48(4):526–535.
57. Bernstein CN, Blanchard JF, Kliewer E, Wajda A. Cancer risk in patients with inflammatory bowel disease: a population-based study. *Cancer*. 2001;91(4):854–862.
58. van Heerden JA, Beart RW Jr. Carcinoma of the colon and rectum complicating chronic ulcerative colitis. *Dis Colon Rectum*. 1980;23(3):155–159.
59. Jimmo B, Hyman NH. Is ileal pouch-anal anastomosis really the procedure of choice for patients with ulcerative colitis? *Dis Colon Rectum*. 1998;41(1):41–45.
60. Reilly WT, Pemberton JH, Wolff BG, et al. Randomized prospective trial comparing ileal pouch-anal anastomosis performed by excising the anal mucosa to ileal pouch-anal anastomosis performed by preserving the anal mucosa. *Ann Surg*. 1997;225(6):666–676; discussion 676–677.
61. Lee GC, Cavallaro PM, Savitt LR, et al. Bowel function after j-pouch may be more complex than previously appreciated: a comprehensive analysis to highlight existing knowledge gaps. *Dis Colon Rectum*. 2020;63(2):207–216.
62. Berndtsson I, Oresland T, Hultén L. Sexuality in patients with ulcerative colitis before and after restorative proctocolectomy: a prospective study. *Scand J Gastroenterol*. 2004;39(4):374–379.
63. Waljee A, Waljee J, Morris AM, Higgins PDR. Threefold increased risk of infertility: a meta-analysis of infertility after ileal pouch anal anastomosis in ulcerative colitis. *Gut*. 2006;55(11):1575–1580.

64

Colorectal Polyps and Hereditary Colorectal Cancer Syndromes

Emily Steinhagen and Matthew F. Kalady

Key Points

1 Colonic polyps are common and range from benign growths to malignancy. Clinical significance varies according to their histology with broad classification including adenomatous, serrated, hyperplastic, or inflammatory. Dysplasia is inherent to adenomas.

2 Colorectal cancer may develop in polyps via the classical adenoma-to-carcinoma pathway driven by *APC* gene mutations, the mutator or microsatellite instability pathway, or the CpG island methylation pathway.

3 Screening and surveillance decrease the risk of colorectal cancer by detecting and removing polyps before they develop into cancer. Colonoscopy is the preferred method of screening as it is highly effective and allows for intervention.

4 Patients with hereditary polyposis syndromes require screening and surveillance for both colonic and extracolonic malignancies as they have increased risks that vary by genetic syndrome.

5 Prophylactic surgery in hereditary polyposis syndromes plays an important role and should be individualized based on the syndrome and the patient.

Polyps occur frequently in the colon and rectum and may represent precursor lesions to colorectal cancer (CRC). As such, identification and removal of these lesions may decrease an individual's risk of developing CRC. There are three main pathways through which CRC can develop, and each involves a precursor lesion. The classical adenoma-to-carcinoma pathway, characterized by chromosomal instability, is most common and consists of adenomas developing progressive mutations, including *KRAS*, *APC*, and *p53*, eventually leading to CRC. The mutator or microsatellite instability (MSI) pathway and hypermethylation pathways occur due to failure to repair DNA replication errors. Precursor lesions in the methylator pathway are frequently serrated polyps (**Fig. 64.1**).

Approximately 5% of CRCs arise within a hereditary syndrome.[1] For patients and families with a hereditary predisposition to CRC, there are typically other at-risk organ systems for neoplasia, and progression to cancer may occur more quickly compared to sporadic cases. Recognition of these syndromes enables appropriate screening and surveillance.

Polyps may be classified by their shape as well as their histology. Polyps may be sessile, protruding directly from the bowel wall with a broad base; pedunculated, on a fibrovascular stalk; or flat, which may be the most difficult to recognize endoscopically (**Fig. 64.2**). Polyps may also be considered as neoplastic, with malignant potential, or nonneoplastic. Neoplastic polyps typically include adenomas and serrated polyps. Nonneoplastic polyps include hyperplastic polyps (HPs), hamartomatous polyps such as juvenile polyps or inflammatory polyps. Submucosal lesions such as lipomas, leiomyomas, lymphoid aggregates, or other lesions may appear polypoid as well.

COLORECTAL POLYPS

Adenomatous Polyps

1 Adenomas are epithelial lesions that typically appear smooth but may become nodular and irregular as they grow and develop advanced histology. They are generally asymptomatic and are found in up to half of individuals who undergo screening colonoscopy. By definition, adenomas have potential for malignant transformation, although only a smaller percentage actually become cancer. Removing adenomas via screening and surveillance colonoscopy is a major factor in the decreasing incidence of CRC in the United States.

Epidemiology

Traditionally, adenoma rates have been higher in the United States and Western countries compared to parts of Asia, South America, and Africa. However, as the "Western" lifestyle has spread, the incidence of adenoma and CRC has increased in these regions. Studies evaluating the incidence of adenomas on screening or surveillance colonoscopies suggest that the rate may approach 50%.[2] The incidence of adenomas increases with age in all populations. It is estimated that in a patient with an adenoma, there is a 30% to 50% chance that they have at least one additional adenoma.[3]

Even outside of defined hereditary syndromes that predispose to polyps and CRC, heredity plays a role in adenoma and CRC risk. There is a two- to threefold risk of CRC among those with a first-degree relative who has adenomas or CRC. The more affected family members, the higher the risk. However, the risk may be impacted by the shared environment as well as shared genetics.

It was previously thought that adenomas were uniformly distributed throughout the colon, but the majority of colorectal adenomas are located in the left colon and rectum, which also mirrors the distribution of CRC.

Histology

Adenomatous polyps are characterized by their physical features, size, glandular structure, and degree of dysplasia. Tubular adenomas consist of at least 80% dysplastic tubules that are arranged in a tightly packed network and extend toward

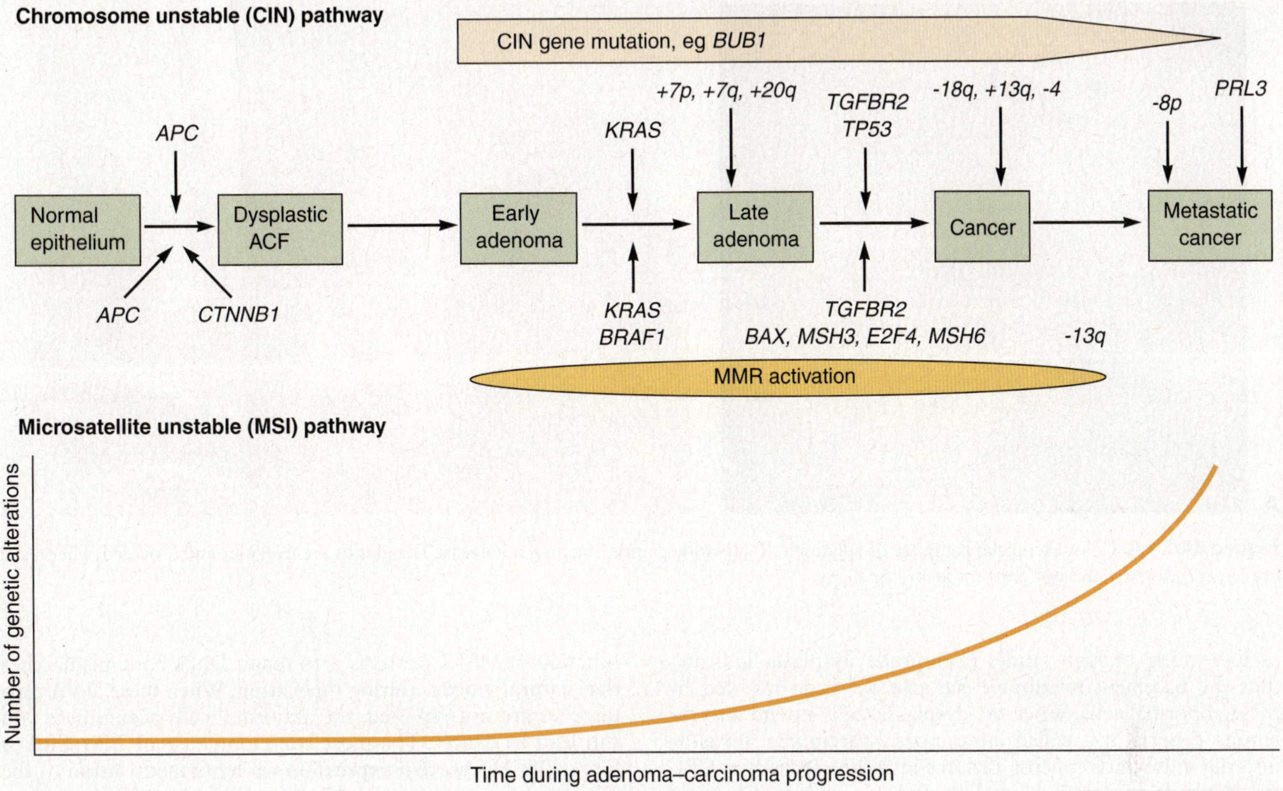

Figure 64.1. Proposed sequence of genetic events in the development of colon cancer. Carcinomas arise from an accumulation of events whose sequence has been defined for two of the carcinogenesis pathways. Tumors progress through the adenoma-to-carcinoma sequence along pathways marked by chromosomal instability (CIN) or microsatellite instability (MSI). At least one more pathway, characterized by promoter methylation of tumor-suppressor genes, serrated polyps, and cancers with variable degrees of microsatellite instability, is incompletely understood, and not shown here. ACF, aberrant crypt focus; TGF, transforming growth factor.

the normal lamina propria. Villous adenomas have at least 80% villous fronds that consist of a core of lamina propria surrounded by adenomatous epithelium; these fronds are elongated crypts. Tubulovillous adenomas have features of both.

Adenomas are, by definition, dysplastic. The degree of dysplasia depends on the degree of abnormality in the crypt architecture as well as the appearance of the nuclei. Abnormalities in crypt architecture may be described as irregular branching, crowding, or "back-to-back" configurations (Fig. 64.3). Signs of nuclear atypia include larger size, pleomorphism, and hyperchromatic appearance. There may be multiple mitoses and pseudostratification within the cells. Dysplasia is graded

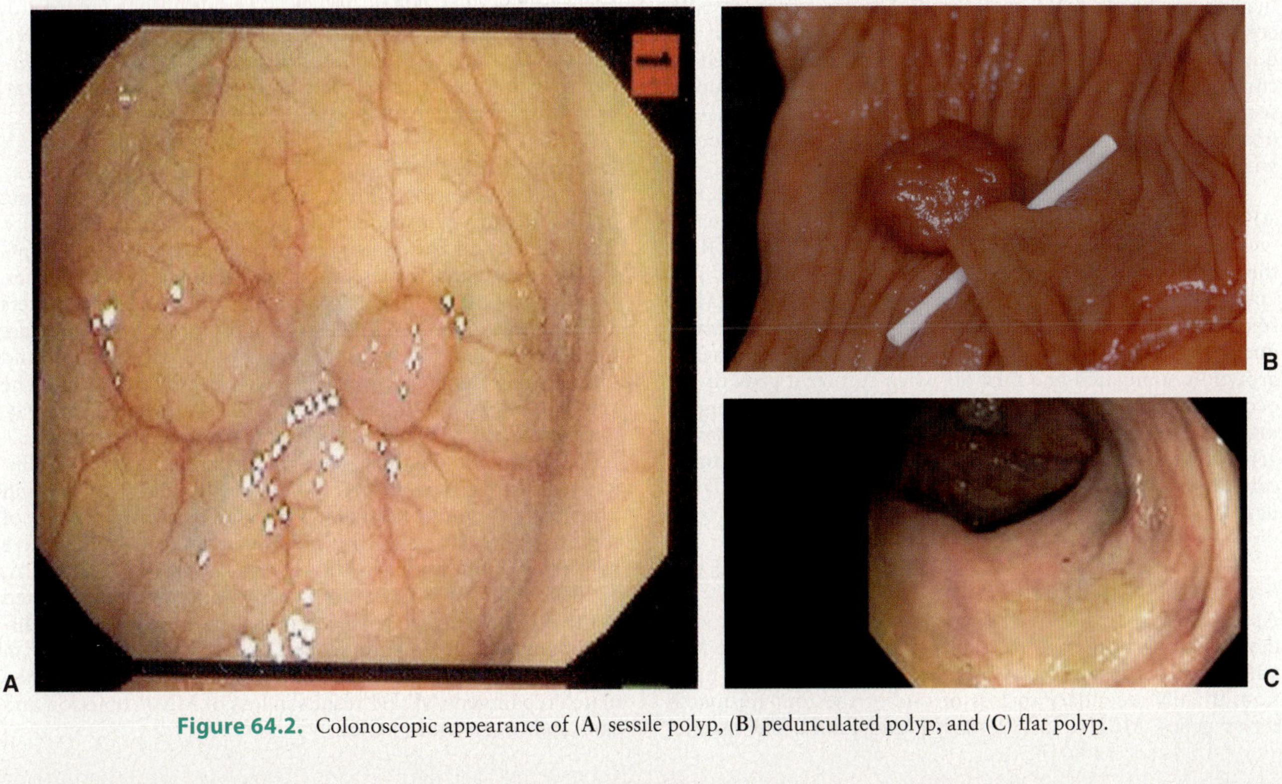

Figure 64.2. Colonoscopic appearance of (A) sessile polyp, (B) pedunculated polyp, and (C) flat polyp.

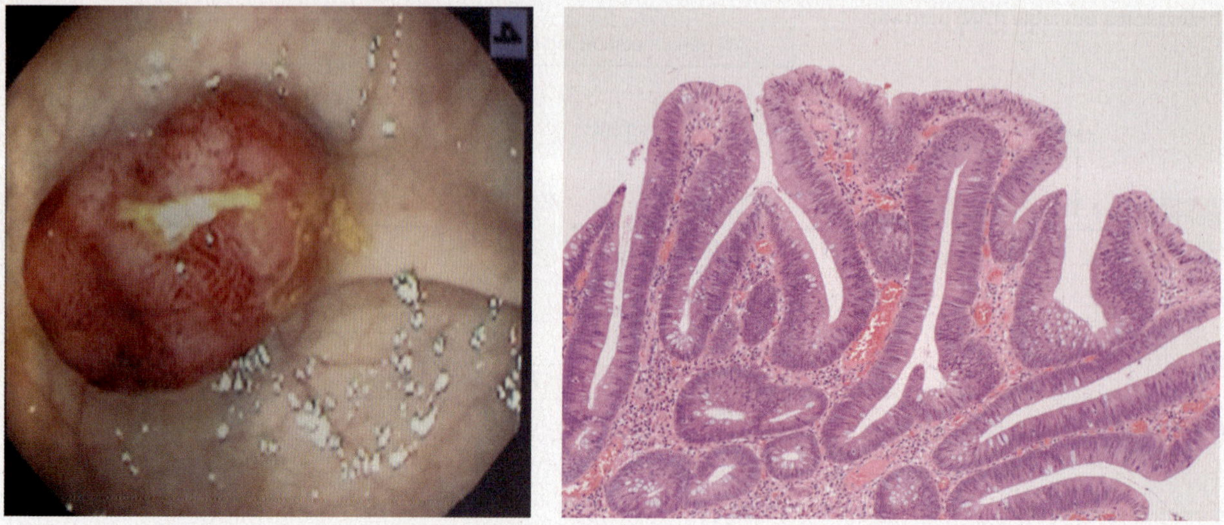

Figure 64.3. **A:** Colonoscopic appearance of adenoma. **B:** Histologic appearance of adenoma. The glands are irregular and crowded. The nuclei are hyperchromatic and not uniform in size or shape.

as low grade or high grade. High-grade dysplasia indicates that the basement membrane has not yet been invaded by these abnormal cells. When the dysplastic cells extend into the lamina propria, it is called intramucosal carcinoma. Invasion into the muscularis mucosa denotes invasive carcinoma. CRC risk depends on size and histology. Patients with an advanced adenoma defined as size at least 1 cm, high-grade dysplasia, or tubulovillous or villous histology are at a significantly increased risk of developing CRC.

Etiology/Molecular Pathways

Classical Pathway

2 Adenomas develop through a progressive sequence of genetic and molecular alterations that lead to proliferation, cellular accumulation, and atypia. The vast majority of CRCs develop along this chromosomal instability, or classical adenoma-to-carcinoma pathway, during which there is a process of multistep carcinogenesis. In sporadic cases (those not associated with a hereditary mutation), there are spontaneous changes that occur during DNA replication. The frequency of CRC compared with other types of cancer is likely a result of frequent cell turnover. Mutation of the *APC* gene, located on chromosome 5q, is an early event in the adenoma-to-carcinoma sequence. This tumor suppressor gene can act as a gatekeeper of sorts, and once it is mutated, cellular proliferation can occur without regulation.

The protein produced by the *APC* gene is β-catenin. Once *APC* is mutated, there is a loss of phosphorylation of β-catenin, which is important for crypt proliferation. Mutations in *KRAS*, the prototypical oncogene in CRC, are frequently seen in polyps as well. In more advanced adenomas, *KRAS* mutation frequency increases. Proto-oncogenes function in signal transduction to regulate normal cell growth. They turn on when growth is stimulated and turn off when sufficient growth has occurred. When mutated, there is unregulated growth signaling and excessive cellular proliferation. The tumor suppressor gene *p53* must be inactivated to transition from adenoma to carcinoma. The *p53* gene typically prevents cells with DNA damage from replicating by stopping mitosis progression from the G1 to S phase.

Microsatellite Instability Pathway

Approximately 15% to 20% of adenomas and carcinomas develop along a different molecular pathway; labeled the MSI pathway. This results from a loss of mismatch repair function, usually secondary to loss of one of the four mismatch repair genes: *MLH1, MSH2, MSH6,* and *PMS2*. The normal function of MMR proteins is to repair DNA base mismatches that naturally occur during replication. When these DNA mismatches are not repaired, the abnormal cells accumulate and can lead to cancer. The most common cause of MSI CRC is loss of MLH1 protein expression via hypermethylation of the gene promoter region, which leads to silencing of its transcription. MSI CRC can also develop from a germline pathogenic variant in any of the mismatch repair genes, which is the cause of Lynch syndrome (LS). Since DNA mismatches tend to occur in repeating areas of DNA sequences called microsatellites, these tumors are called MSI high, or MSI-H.

There are specific genes that can be affected by loss of MMR function. An example is *transforming growth factor B receptor II (TGF-BII)* that maintains normal cellular behavior. When TGF-β receptors are inactivated, cells no longer have normal growth regulation control. One of the more notable features of the MSI pathway is that the progression may occur more rapidly (1 to 2 years) compared to the classical pathway. Cancers that develop along this pathway are more likely to occur on the right side of the colon, with histology notable for poor differentiation, signet ring or mucinous tumor subtypes, and an abundance of tumor-infiltrating lymphocytes. Compared with tumors developing along the classical pathway, MSI CRC has better prognosis.

CpG Island Methylation Pathway

The CpG island methylator pathway (CIMP) describes a subset of CRC that develops along a pathway of epigenetic instability. The hallmark of this mechanism is hypermethylation of CpG islands, which inactivates tumor suppressor and other genes. More than half of human genes are regulated by promoters and CpG islands represent one type of promoter. When they are hypermethylated, the genes are inappropriately silenced, and this can deregulate key genes involved in carcinogenesis. The CIMP pathway, also called the methylator or serrated pathway, is associated with *BRAF* mutations and serrated polyps.

Cancers with a high degree of methylation represent a clinically distinct group of tumors with a different histology and potentially different behavior. Typically, promoter regions of tumor suppressor genes are involved. Tumors notably have high rates of mutations in *BRAF*, and loss of *p16, CDKN2A, THBS1,* and *HPP1*. These tumors are more commonly located in the proximal colon, have mucinous features, are poorly differentiated, occur at an older age, and are more frequent in female patients.[4] As discussed above, methylation of the mismatch repair gene MLH1 results in loss of MMR function and can result in an MSI-H CRC.

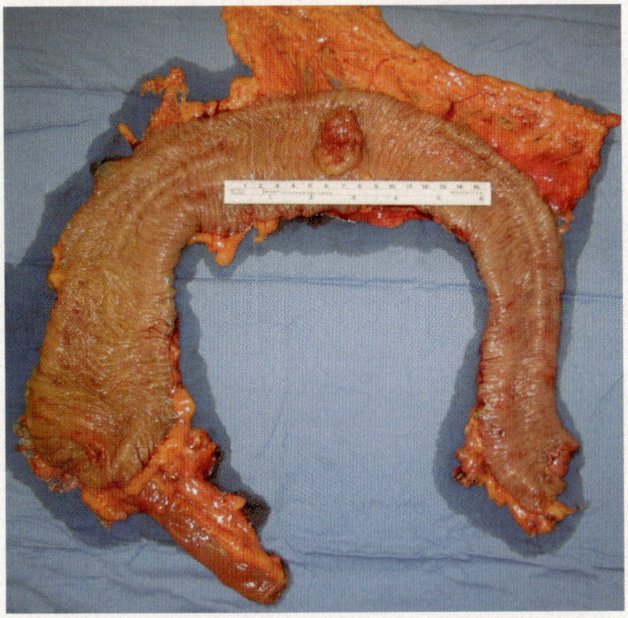

Figure 64.4. Large polyp harboring invasive carcinoma as seen in a resected colon.

Progression to Cancer

Though nearly all CRCs originate from adenomas or serrated lesions, most polyps do not develop into cancer. Malignant potential is related to size and histology, with larger size and villous components in adenomas representing higher-risk lesions for progression. Adenomas that are 0.5 cm or less very rarely contain severe dysplasia or carcinoma (<0.5%), and only 1% to 2% of adenomas less than 2 cm contain carcinoma. In autopsy studies, up to 40% of adenomas >2 cm harbor an associated cancer (**Fig. 64.4**). The risk of cancer in adenomas larger than 1 cm, with villous components, and high-grade dysplasia estimated at 3%, 17%, and 37%, respectively, but may increase with age. The rate of transition to cancer is estimated at 2.6% in patients aged 55 to 59, and 5.1% in those over 80.[5] It is generally estimated that it takes 5 to 10 years to go from normal mucosa to cancer. This explains the findings of The National Polyp Study, which demonstrated the protective effect of screening colonoscopy for at least 10 years.

Clinical Features

Most patients with adenomatous polyps are asymptomatic. However, hematochezia may be present when larger polyps are in the distal colon or rectum, and right-sided polyps may cause melanotic stools. In addition, iron deficiency anemia (with or without associated systemic signs and symptoms) can result from occult bleeding related to polyps. Polyp size is directly related to bleeding risk and volume. Those less than 2 cm typically lose less than 1 mL of blood daily. Secretory diarrhea may be associated with large, villous adenomas in the distal colon and rectum and can also be associated with hypokalemia and hypochlorhydria. When polyps are particularly large, they can also lead to obstructive symptoms or alterations in bowel function.

Serrated Polyps

Incidence

Serrated polyps have different histologies and include sessile serrated lesions (SSLs) (also called sessile serrated adenomas [SSA] or polyps) with and without dysplasia, traditional serrated adenomas, and HPs. The prevalence of serrated polyps is about 20% to 30% in average-risk individuals. The vast majority of serrated polyps (about 75%) are hyperplastic and are not considered to have malignant potential. HPs are most commonly seen in the sigmoid colon and rectum (**Fig. 64.5**). Sessile serrated lesions account for nearly 25% of serrated polyps, have malignant potential, and are more than 80% located in the proximal colon. Approximately 4% to 8% of SSLs have dysplasia. Sessile serrated lesions are found in approximately 15% of average risk individuals. These often occur more frequently on the right side of the colon and are frequently flat and covered with a mucous cap, which can make them difficult to identify endoscopically (**Fig. 64.5**). Traditional serrated adenomas are rare, located distally, and can progress to CRC.

Histology

Serrated polyps are characterized by colonic crypt saw-tooth pattern and nuclear atypia. The crypt base is serrated and dilated, and the proliferative zone has migrated to the side of the crypt rather than the base. SSAs represent 3% to 20% of

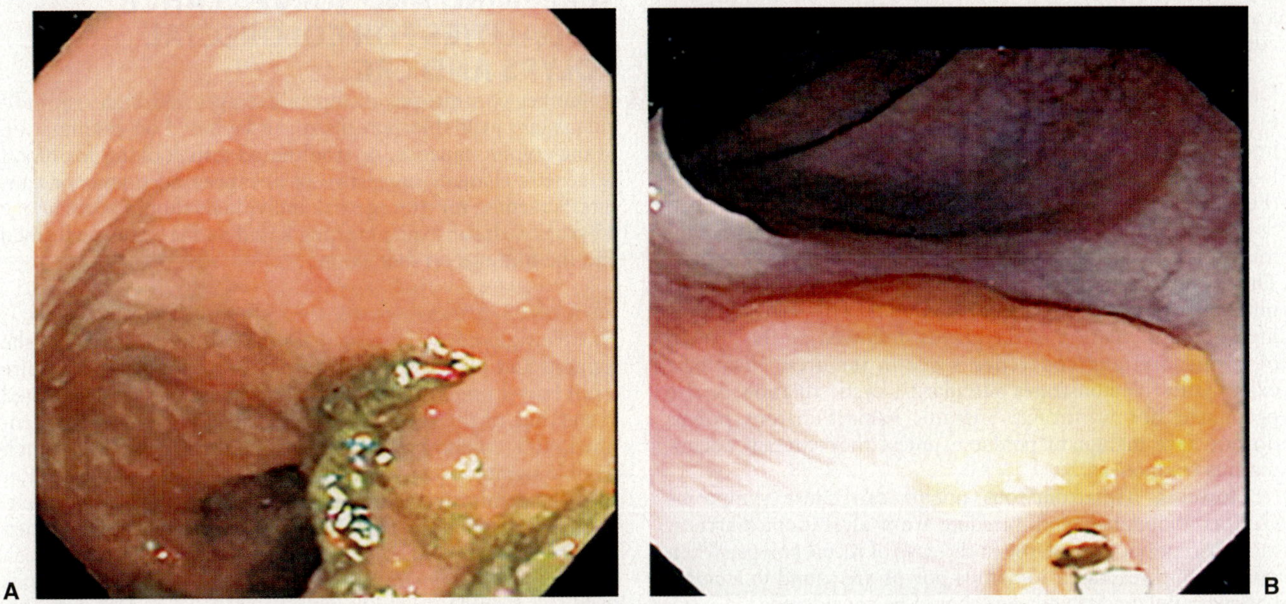

Figure 64.5. Typical appearance of small hyperplastic polyps that are commonly seen in the rectum and sigmoid colon (**A**). Sessile serrated adenomas (**B**) are often flat lesions that have a bonze a mucous cap. These flatter polyps may be difficult to visualize on colonoscopy.

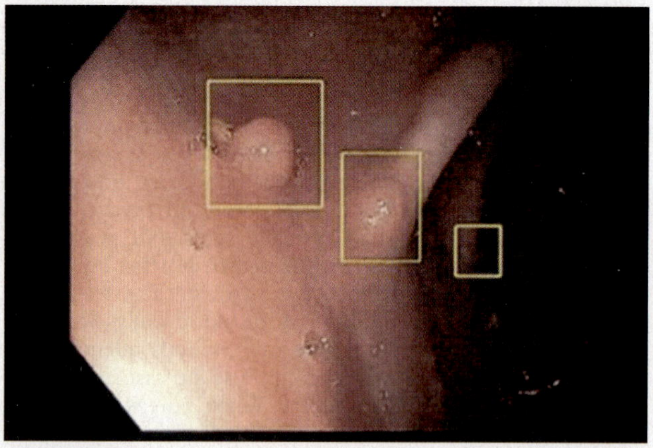

Figure 64.6. Colonoscopic appearance of hamartomatous polyps from a patient with a PTEN mutation.

serrated polyps. The two most frequent serrated polyps, traditional serrated adenomas and SSAs, are associated with *BRAF* mutations and the CIMP or MSI pathways. Histologically, these lesions are characterized by elongated, nonbranching mucosal crypts and hyperplasia without atypia. They arise from faulty epithelial maturation and a failure of apoptosis. Sessile serrated lesions are usually larger than HPs and have a distorted architecture of the serrated crypts. They are characterized by horizontal growth along the muscularis mucosa, dilation of the crypt base, serrations that extend into the crypt base, and asymmetrical proliferation. Serrated dysplasia characterized by eosinophilic cytoplasm and tightly packed small glands with more pronounced nuclear atypia. Traditional serrated adenomas display distorted villous or tubulovillous architecture along with serrated features.

Progression to Cancer

Serrated lesions have malignant potential, and serrated or methylated CRC is a defined molecular subtype. Approximately 15% of all CRCs arise via this pathway based on histologic features. There is an accumulation of genetic and epigenetic changes that is usually initiated by a mutation in a gene that regulates mitogen-activated protein kinase pathway, such as *BRAF*. *BRAF* mutations then lead to broad methylation, including CpG islands, that cause loss of *MLH1* expression and resultant MSI-H lesions. The time for this transformation is believed to be shorter or similar to the adenoma-to-carcinoma sequence.

Hamartomatous Polyps

Hamartomatous polyps are localized overgrowths of mature intestinal epithelial cells. They appear as smooth, pedunculated lesions with intact-appearing mucosa on endoscopy (**Fig. 64.6**).

They are usually lined with normal epithelium over a submucosal core that does not involve the muscularis mucosa. The pathogenesis is thought to be a mucosal ulceration or inflammation that blocks colonic glands. This leads to proliferation and dilation of the glands, followed by the growth of granulation and connective tissue in the area. Histologic examination demonstrates vascularity, cystic dilation, and a prominent fibrous stroma. Sporadic hamartomatous polyps do not have malignant potential unless they contain adenomatous components.

However, hamartomatous polyps can cause symptoms such as abdominal pain, bleeding from ulceration, diarrhea, intussusception, or prolapse in the case of rectal polyps. When more than three hamartomatous polyps are found in a single patient, a polyposis syndrome should be considered.

Juvenile polyps can occur sporadically or as part of a syndrome. They are made up of dilated mucous-filled glands with abundant lamina propria. Unlike other polyps, these typically occur in children under age 10. Most frequently, a child will have a single pedunculated polyp with a smooth surface. They are thought to occur in about 2% of children. They often present with hematochezia due to their vascular nature. If they occur distally, they may prolapse (**Fig. 64.7**). More proximal lesions can cause intussusception. They have no malignant potential and are removed when symptomatic.

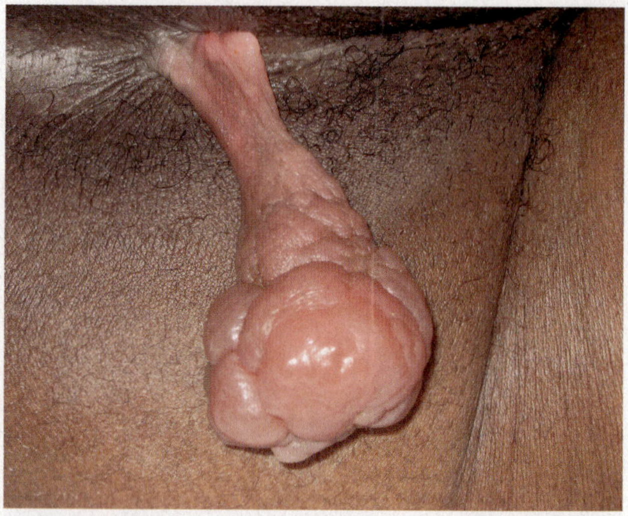

Figure 64.7. Prolapsed hamartomatous polyp protruding through the anus.

Inflammatory Polyps

Inflammatory polyps are sometimes referred to as pseudopolyps, occurring in areas of mucosal damage and repair. They are most frequently found in patients with inflammatory bowel disease, but may be found in other types of colitis as well. Inflammatory polyps are uniform in width from the base to the head and consist of islands of inflamed regenerating mucosa surrounded by ulceration. Since they arise in areas of inflammation, multiple inflammatory polyps may develop in the affected area. The polyps themselves require no specific treatment and do not need to be removed unless there is uncertainty about the diagnosis.

SCREENING AND SURVEILLANCE MODALITIES FOR COLORECTAL POLYPS AND CRC

3 A number of strategies to screen average- and high-risk individuals are available. Screening can be based on examination of the colonic mucosa, or stool-based tests looking for blood or genetic changes suggestive of advanced adenomas or cancers. Screening for average-risk individuals should begin at age 45 years with subsequent testing based on the exam performed and the findings on that exam.

Flexible Sigmoidoscopy

Flexible sigmoidoscopy visualizes the rectum and parts of the sigmoid and descending colon. In general, it does not require a full bowel preparation, and polypectomy may be completed at the time of the procedure. If precancerous polyps are identified, full colonoscopy is typically recommended. Though flexible sigmoidoscopy does not visualize all at-risk mucosa, it has been demonstrated to reduce mortality from CRC approximately 26% to 31% compared to no screening.[6] Even when performed once at age 60, a 33% reduction in CRC has been observed.[7] Screening protocols for average risk individuals include a flexible sigmoidoscopy every 5 years. Although this test does not evaluate the proximal colon, it provides benefit over no screening.

Colonoscopy

Colonoscopy involves direct visualization of the entire colorectal mucosa while facilitating synchronous removal of polyps, biopsies of larger polyps/masses, and has been demonstrated to reduce CRC mortality. Colonoscopic polypectomy is associated with a 53% reduction in CRC mortality.[8] A SEER-Medicare database study also confirmed via case-control study that colonoscopy is associated with a significant reduction in CRC-related death. The association was stronger with left-sided cancers, which is consistent with other European and Canadian studies.[9] These findings suggest that right-sided lesions are not detected as frequently and/or that they grow at different rates. Colonoscopy remains the gold standard test for detecting adenomas and CRC. Colonoscopy requires patients to complete a bowel preparation with cathartics and sedation and carries risks such as bleeding or perforation. After a normal colonoscopy with an adequate bowel preparation, the recommended interval for the next colonoscopy is 10 years.

CT Colonography

CT colonography, also referred to as "virtual colonoscopy," involves high-resolution cross-sectional images of the abdomen and pelvis. It is a rapid and safe method of evaluating the colon. The National CT Colonography Trial, a multicenter study that compared CT colonography with same-day colonoscopy in 2,600 patients, found that the sensitivity of CT colonography for polyps >10 mm was 90% and the negative predictive value was 99%. However, patients still require mechanical bowel preparation for the test, and those with abnormal findings then typically need to undergo colonoscopy for biopsy or polypectomy. One area of concern is the ability to detect serrated lesions, which are typically flat and more likely to be located in the right colon. As a screening test, this should be performed every 5 years.

Stool-Based Tests

Stool-based tests are noninvasive screening modalities that detect blood or shed cellular debris from polyps or cancer. Patients can often complete these tests at home and avoid the risks of sedation, and the potential discomfort or risks of an invasive procedure. While they do not require mechanical bowel preparation, some dietary changes in the days leading up to the test may be necessary for optimal results.

Fecal occult blood test (FOBT) assesses for the presence of peroxidase in stool. It is a qualitative test that can be altered by the presence of peroxidase from red meat, certain fruits and vegetables, or inactivated by high doses of vitamin C. Patients must comply with dietary restrictions for several days prior to testing to improve the accuracy of the results and typically three samples are utilized to complete the test with appropriate sensitivity and specificity. This screening test is recommended annually. Importantly, only 15% of polyps <1 cm are detected with this modality, while 80% of polyps >2 cm result in a positive FOBT. Annual or biannual testing reduces CRC-related deaths by 15% to 30%.[10]

Fecal immunohistochemical test (FIT) is an immunohistochemical, semiquantitative test that measures hemoglobin in a stool sample. The premise is that adenomas and cancers are prone to minor bleeding, and therefore, the presence of blood in the stool may suggest their presence. Compared to FOBT, FIT test is quantitative. It has improved sensitivity and specificity compared to FOBT. However, FIT tests are less effective at detecting adenomas as compared to carcinomas. FIT testing is intended to be repeated every year. If the test is positive, colonoscopy is recommended. The sensitivity of FIT is estimated at 79%, with a specificity of 94%, though depending on the threshold for a positive test, these numbers can vary.[1] There is no high-quality evidence evaluating the impact of FIT testing on CRC mortality in the United States.

Stool DNA testing (multitarget stool DNA, MT-sDNA, Cologuard®) is a noninvasive screening test. The sensitivity for CRC is 92.3% and 42.4% for adenomas. Stool DNA testing generally has higher sensitivity but lower specificity compared to FIT. Use of these tests is recommended every 3 years. A positive test warrants a colonoscopy for further evaluation.

While colonoscopy remains the gold standard for screening and surveillance for CRC, many patients do not wish to undergo this procedure, and the best screening test is the one that the patient will have. A number of societies offer evidence-based guidelines that are updated regularly to enable practitioners to counsel patients about the appropriate age to screen for CRC and the suggested interval depending on the patient and modality utilized.

POLYPOSIS SYNDROMES

There are several syndromes associated with colorectal polyps and an increased risk of CRC (**Table 64.1**). Importantly, nearly all patients with a polyposis syndrome are at risk of extracolonic manifestations and require heightened screening and surveillance. The syndromes can be broadly classified according to the type of predominant polyp: adenomas, hamartomas, or serrated polyps. The adenomatous polyposis syndromes include familial adenomatous polyposis (FAP) as well as the attenuated form, aFAP; *MUTYH*-associated polyposis (MAP), and the extremely rare polymerase proofreading adenomatous polyposis (PPAP) and NTHL1 adenomatous polyposis (NAP). Hamartomatous polyposis syndromes are characterized by gastrointestinal hamartomas, and include juvenile polyposis syndrome (JPS), Peutz–Jeghers syndrome (PJS), and *PTEN* hamartoma syndromes (Cowden disease and Bannayan–Riley–Ruvalcaba syndrome [BRRS]). Hereditary mixed polyposis syndrome is characterized by both hamartomatous and adenomatous polyps of the gastrointestinal tract. Serrated polyposis is defined by clinical criteria and characterized by either large or numerous serrated polyps. Although LS is a hereditary CRC syndrome, it is generally not associated with polyposis.

4 Patients with polyposis or who are suspected of having a hereditary syndrome should be referred to a medical geneticist, genetic counselor, or another health care professional with specialized expertise and experience in cancer genetics for consideration of counseling and genetic testing. If there is a family history of a CRC syndrome, the decision to refer is straightforward. In addition, patients with 10 or more adenomas, two or more hamartomas, and five or more serrated polyps proximal to the sigmoid should also be considered for further evaluation. The reason for referral prior to testing is to take a more detailed family history, to provide risk counseling, psychosocial assessment and support, education, and a detailed discussion about genetic testing prior to obtaining informed consent.

Adenomatous Polyposis Syndromes

Familial Adenomatous Polyposis/Attenuated FAP

Incidence

FAP is an autosomal dominantly inherited syndrome that occurs in 1 in 10,000 births. The penetrance and presentation can vary even within the same family who share a mutation. It accounts for less than 1% of all CRCs. Importantly, approximately 25% of cases of FAP are *de novo* mutations, meaning that there is no family history of the syndrome. It is the second most common inherited CRC syndrome. FAP is characterized by hundreds to thousands of polyps throughout the colorectum (**Fig. 64.8**) as well as a variety of extracolonic manifestations. The median age for adenoma development in patients with classical FAP is 17 years. Untreated patients develop CRC at a median age of 40, with death at a mean age of 44.

Genetics/Molecular Pathways

The *APC* gene is located on chromosome 5q21. Its most well-described function is in the Wnt signaling pathway, in which the APC protein forms a complex with c-myc, GSK3, axin, and casein that allows the degradation of β-catenin.

Table 64.1. Summary of Hereditary Colorectal Cancer Syndromes

	Gene/Chromosome	Inheritance Pattern	Colorectal Phenotype	Extracolonic Features
Familial adenomatous polyposis (FAP)	*APC* 5q21	Autosomal dominant	Dozens to hundreds of polyps Early-age CRC onset	Upper GI neoplasia, hepatoblastoma, thyroid cancer, desmoid tumors, supranumerary teeth, osteomas, fibromas, cysts
Lynch syndrome	*MLH1, MSH2, MSH6, PMSH2*	Autosomal dominant	Increased risk CRC, early age of onset of CRC	Small bowel cancer, urothelial cancer, endometrial and ovarian cancer, gastric cancer Sebaceous cancers
MUTYH-associated polyposis (MAP)	*MUTYH* 1p35	Autosomal recessive	Dozens to hundreds of polyps Early age of onset of CRC	Upper GI neoplasia
Peutz–Jeghers syndrome	*LKB1/STK11* 19p13.3	Autosomal dominant	Hamartomatous polyps Increased CRC risk	Small bowel polyps, mucocutaneous pigmentation; cancers of bowel, pancreatic cancer, ovarian cancer, cervical cancer, breast cancer
Juvenile polyposis	*SMAD4, BMPR1A, ENG* 10q21.1, 10q22.3, 9134.11	Autosomal dominant	Hamartomatous polyps; few to hundreds. 10–50% risk of CRC	15% with malrotation, heart or brain abnormalities, cleft palate, polydactyly, genitourinary tract abnormalities
Bannayan–Riley–Ruvalcaba	*PTEN* (60% of cases) 10q23 Unknown	Autosomal dominant	Hamartomas, increased risk of CRC	Macrocephaly, macrosomia at birth, genital freckling in males, developmental delay/intellectual disability, hemangiomas, hypotonia
Cowden syndrome	*PTEN* 10q23 Unknown	Autosomal dominant	Hamartomas, increased risk of CRC	Hamartomas of mucous membranes, breast cancer, thyroid cancer, endometrial cancer, renal cancer, melanoma (all early onset)
Serrated polyposis	*RNF43* Unknown	Presumed autosomal dominant	Few to hundreds of hyperplastic and serrated polyps; increased risk of CRC	Multiple other cancers reported; not enough data to conclusively determine
Hereditary mixed polyposis	*GREM1* 15q13.3	Autosomal dominant	Adenomas, hyperplastic polyps, hamartomas, serrated polyps	Unknown

When APC is nonfunctional, β-catenin accumulates and enters the nucleus, where it induces transcription of cellular growth factors. Cell proliferation, enhanced cell-to-cell adhesion, and cell migration result. The APC protein also stabilizes microtubules and helps organize cell migration; it also binds cytoskeletal regulators and when not present, mis-segregation of chromosomes during mitosis can occur.

A number of different mutations in the *APC* gene can lead to FAP. There are truncating mutations that lead to a dysfunctional protein, as well as missense mutations. When there is a germline mutation in one copy of the *APC* gene, it creates a situation where there is loss of heterozygosity in which a so-called "second-hit" leads to the classical adenoma-to-carcinoma sequence. While there are correlations between specific genetic mutations and phenotypic features, the phenotype can still vary between individuals with the same mutation, even within the same family (**Fig. 64.9**). These differences may be a result of other genes, environmental influences, or other factors. When the *APC* gene mutation occurs in the "mutation cluster" region of exon 15, it predicts a more virulent form of FAP with thousands of colonic polyps and an earlier age of onset of CRC. Mutations at the 3′ end of the gene, in contrast, tend to have a milder phenotype.

Diagnosis

FAP is diagnosed by the existence of a germline pathogenic variant in *APC*. Many patients are diagnosed after screening

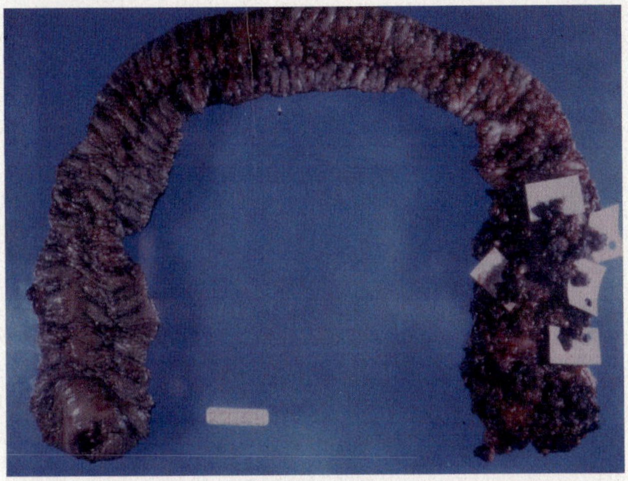

Figure 64.8. Colon resection from a patient with FAP with thousands of polyps throughout the colon.

or genetic testing, prompted by a family history of FAP. Each child of an affected patient with FAP has a 50% chance that they will inherit the mutation and therefore develop the manifestations of disease.

Some patients without a family history may also be referred for testing based on colorectal polyposis or extracolonic findings such as supranumerary teeth, osteomas, or congenital hypertrophy of the retinal pigment epithelium (CHRPE). Others present with symptoms from polyposis that may include bleeding, change in bowel habits, and abdominal pain. FAP can be diagnosed on a clinical basis when more than 100 colonic adenomas are identified, even if an *APC* pathogenic variant is not identified. Up to 90% of individuals with a suggestive clinical phenotype will have a mutation identified.

Genetic counseling is an important part of genetic testing for FAP and other hereditary syndromes. Screening panels can sometimes identify one or more mutations of uncertain significance that must be interpreted. Patients may also misunderstand their results and subsequent cancer risk, as well as the implications for family members. There are frequently psychosocial implications with testing both affected and unaffected family members that should be considered and addressed. With the frequent availability of panel-based testing, more than one gene alteration may be identified. Therefore, informed counseling is critical and should be performed by an experienced genetic counselor.

Colon Cancer Risks and Surveillance

Nearly all patients with classical FAP will develop CRC if untreated. The incidence of CRC rises dramatically after age 30. Typically, risk-reducing surgery is recommended once an individual reaches physical and emotional maturity in their late teens or early 20s. However, polyp burden or symptoms may necessitate earlier intervention. If the number of polyps can be controlled via colonoscopy, it is reasonable to continue surveillance.

Patients with known or suspected FAP, or those in families with a known *APC* mutation who have not undergone genetic testing, should undergo annual colonoscopy at ages 10 to 15 years. Most patients with FAP will develop polyps by their early 20s. Flexible sigmoidoscopy may be an option, but it would miss the onset of polyps in the right side of the colon, where they are more likely to occur in attenuated cases.[11]

Extracolonic Features

Gastroduodenal polyps. More than 90% of FAP patients will have upper GI lesions. The most frequent finding is fundic gland polyps, which are benign and have no malignant potential (**Fig. 64.10**). Histologically, they are hamartomatous. However, gastric adenomas and carcinomas may be found, particularly in Japanese and Korean patients.[12] In Western populations, the risk of gastric cancer is less than 1%. Factors associated with an increased risk include carpeting of the stomach, larger polyp size (>20 mm), polypoid appearing mounds, and adenomas.[13] Duodenal and periampullary polyps and carcinoma are also a common feature in FAP patients; the lifetime risk of duodenal cancer is 3% to 5% and half of all duodenal adenomas occur in the periampullary location. The duodenal adenomas tend to occur later than the colonic lesions, and there tend to be fewer polyps compared to the more diffuse colonic polyposis. Duodenal adenomas are classified by the Spigelman system (**Table 64.2**), which estimates the risk of carcinoma and determines the appropriate surveillance protocol.[14] It is based on the number, size, and histologic features of the polyps.

CHRPE is a common and completely benign feature present in some FAP patients. The lesions are well demarcated and gray–brown or oval; they are sometimes described as "bear claws." While small, isolated lesions occur in the retinal epithelium of nonaffected patients, the presence of multiple or bilateral lesions is highly suggestive of FAP. CHRPE lesions can be seen on slit lamp examination but are otherwise not seen on routine ophthalmologic examinations. Mutations between codons 543 and 1309 of the *APC* gene are associated with a higher incidence of CHRPE. In some families, the presence of CHRPE can be used to identify affected family members.

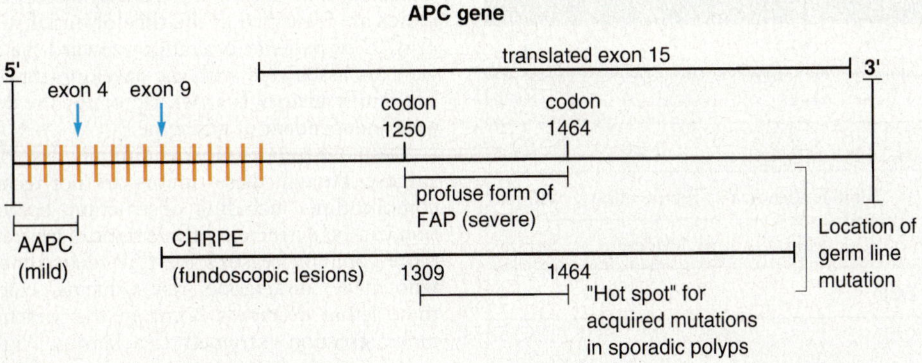

Figure 64.9. This scheme of the *APC* (adenomatous polyposis coli) gene illustrates the genotype–phenotype correlations. Most mutations of APC result in premature stop codons; therefore, the site of the mutation usually indicates the relative length of the mutant protein product. Mutations at the 5′ end of the gene produce "attenuated" FAP, a milder form of the disease. The retinal lesions (congenital hypertrophy of retinal pigmented epithelium [CHRPE]) occur when the mutations are between exons 9 and 15. The portion of the *APC* gene that binds to other cytoskeletal elements in the cell is represented at the 3′ end of the 15th exon. Mutations in a hot spot immediately downstream from the β-catenin–binding site (between codons 1250 and 1464) result in a more virulent, profuse form of familial adenomatous polyposis. This site is also the location of most of the acquired mutations in sporadic colorectal neoplasms.

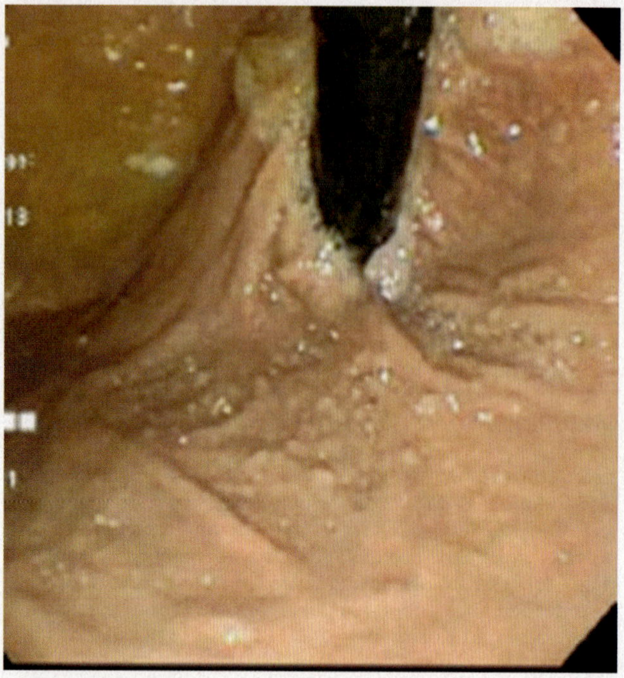

Figure 64.10. Endoscopic appearance of fundic gland polyps from a patient with FAP.

Osteomas and fibromas are benign, slow-growing neoplasms of the bone. The classical description in FAP is in the jaw or skull, but they can be present in any bone. They may be detected on physical examination if they are large, or on x-rays, particularly those done for dental indications. Osteomas are associated with a subtype of FAP known as Gardner syndrome and they may precede the development of gastrointestinal polyposis. Other manifestations of Gardner syndrome include epidermoid cysts, supernumerary teeth, and desmoids. In addition, other benign lesions such as epidermoid cysts, fibromas, and lipomas occur much more frequently in the FAP population. Epidermoid cysts occur in mid to late adolescence and often occur in atypical locations such as the face, scalp, and extremities. Supernumerary teeth, dentigerous cysts, and secondary retention of teeth are all associated with FAP. Supernumerary teeth are usually present before age 10 and should be removed only if they impede the development of normal dentition. Dentigerous cysts develop from the epithelium of the enamel organ and develop before teeth erupt from the jaw. They can grow and occupy a significant portion of the jaw.

Table 64.2. Spigelman Classification for Duodenal Adenomas in FAP

Points	1	2	3
Polyp number	1–4	5–20	>20
Polyp size (mm)	1–4	5–20	>20
Histology	Tubular adenoma	Tubulovillous	Villous
Dysplasia	Mild	Moderate	Severe
Interval to next EGD			
Stage 0 (0 points)	5 y		
Stage I (1–4 points)	5 y		
Stage II (5–6 points)	3 y		
Stage III (7–8 points)	1–2 y		
Stage IV (9–12 points)	EUS or surgery		

Thyroid cancer has been recognized at increased rates in FAP patients. The rates range from 1% to 12% and more frequently affects female patients. Thyroid cancer is diagnosed at a mean age of 27 years. In most cases, the histology is papillary, but the cribriform-morular variant is closely associated with FAP. Multicentric thyroid cancer is more frequent in FAP patients compared to sporadic cases. As with sporadic thyroid cancer, outcomes are excellent and treatment is similar. Screening for thyroid cancer is now typical for FAP patients.

Hepatoblastoma. Unlike other FAP-associated cancers which typically occur in adulthood, hepatoblastoma tends to occur in young children. The incidence in FAP patients is 1.6% and is more common in males. Screening can be performed using ultrasound as well as alpha-fetoprotein levels every 3 to 6 months from birth until 5 or 10 years of age. However, genetic testing is usually deferred until adolescence in individuals from FAP families; in order to decide about screening for hepatoblastoma, genetic testing must be performed in infancy to determine if the child is at risk.

Desmoids are slow-growing mesenchymal tumors made of well-differentiated fibroblasts and myofibroblasts with abundant collagen. Up to one-third of FAP patients develop desmoids, at a rate of more than 1,000 times the rate in nonaffected populations. While the tumors are technically benign and do not metastasize, they do tend to be locally aggressive and infiltrate surrounding tissues. Additionally, recurrence rates are high after removal. Desmoids may occur in any part of the body, but the intra-abdominal desmoids tend to be most clinically significant. As many as 80% of FAP-related desmoids are found in the mesentery, with the remainder occurring primarily in the abdominal wall (**Fig. 64.11**). In addition to mass-like desmoids, flat-white desmoplastic plaques may also be found. They can affect the mesentery and lead to ischemic bands or obstructions.

The clinical presentation of desmoids range from asymptomatic plaques or masses discovered incidentally on imaging or during prophylactic surgery, or with nonspecific symptoms. Large or locally aggressive desmoids may lead to abdominal pain, bowel obstruction, ischemia, venous thrombosis via compression, motor or sensory deficits from nerve compression, ureteric obstruction, enteric fistula, and gastrointestinal hemorrhage.

Risk factors for desmoid development include surgical trauma, female gender, the presence of other extraintestinal manifestations of FAP, and a family history of desmoids.[15] Desmoids are identified at the time of initial surgical intervention in <5% of patients. Mutations toward the 3′ end of the *APC* gene are associated with the development of desmoid tumors, but family history is a risk factor for the development of disease, independent of genotype.

Desmoid tumors most commonly develop after abdominal surgery. Though these tumors are not technically malignant, complications including obstruction, necrosis, and fistulization can be extremely problematic. They represent one of the more common reasons for FAP-related mortality in patients who have undergone risk-reducing colectomy. Typically, these lethal desmoids occur in the mesentery and this can make resection extremely treacherous. High recurrence rates are observed after attempted excision. The risk of desmoids is less after laparoscopic surgery compared with open, and is less after colectomy and ileorectal anastomosis compared to total proctocolectomy and ileal pouch anal anastomosis.[16] In particular, colectomy rather than total proctocolectomy has been proposed for women who are concerned about desmoids affecting fertility but will ultimately require completion proctectomy.

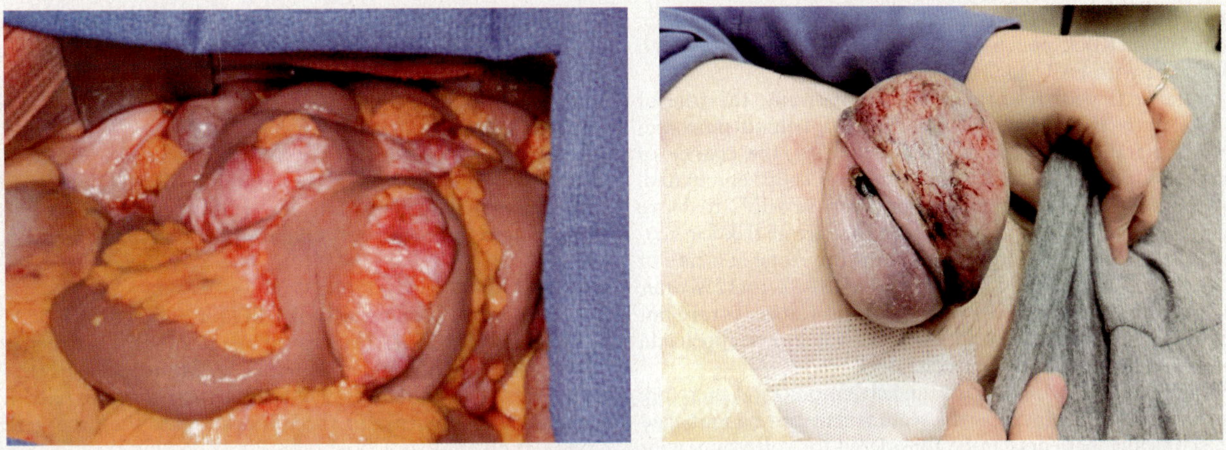

Figure 64.11. **A:** Mesenteric desmoids may limit the ability to perform colon resection or to create a pouch that reaches the pelvis for a restorative procedure. **B:** Abdominal wall desmoid in a young woman with FAP. This is a source of significant morbidity for the patients despite the nonmalignant nature of the desmoid tumor.

Intra-abdominal desmoid staging takes into account tumor size, symptoms, behavior, and the presence of complications.[17] This can help in evaluating desmoids over time and determining treatment options. Stage I desmoids are asymptomatic and not growing. They are usually found incidentally at the time of surgery or CT scan performed for other reasons. Stage II tumors are symptomatic and 10 cm or less, but not growing. These tumors may require treatment because of symptoms. Stage III desmoids are symptomatic tumors that are 11 to 20 cm in size, or asymptomatic and slow growing. Treatment may also be recommended for these large desmoid tumors. Finally, Stage IV desmoids are symptomatic and more than 20 cm in size, display rapid growth, or cause significant complications. Tumors that cause life-threatening complications such as sepsis, free bowel perforation, or massive bleeding require urgent treatment. Other important features that may guide management include their shape (mass, nodular, or flat), the number of tumors present, the location, whether they occur before or after operative intervention, and hormone receptor status.

Management of desmoid disease in FAP can be quite challenging. Asymptomatic desmoids are often observed or treated with nonsteroidal anti-inflammatory drugs (NSAIDs) such as sulindac. Antiestrogens, primarily tamoxifen and raloxifene may be used for small symptomatic desmoids. The management of more symptomatic or growing desmoid disease is changing and includes tyrosine-kinase inhibitors such as sorafenib or pazopanib.[18] Recently published data on the gamma secretase inhibitor nirogacestat has demonstrated promise with significant disease regression in 41% of patients.

Surgery for intra-abdominal desmoids may not be feasible when they are in their common location in the root of the mesentery. In addition, high recurrence rates following resection limit the utility of surgery to carefully selected cases. Often, the characteristic infiltrating growth pattern makes complete resection impossible without extensive small bowel resection. Major complications have been reported in up to 50% of patients with intra-abdominal desmoids treated with surgical resection. In addition, extensive resection may lead to short bowel syndrome and its attendant management challenges. Abdominal wall desmoids may be treated with surgical resection, including 1-cm margins. Reconstruction with prosthetic mesh or a myocutaneous flap may be required for larger tumors.

Surveillance Protocols

Patients with FAP should undergo annual colonoscopy starting at ages 10 to 12. Upper endoscopy with a side-viewing endoscope to optimize visualization of the ampulla is performed by ages 20 to 25. Subsequent intervals depend on findings and are typically based on the Spigelman classification. Annual thyroid examination should be performed. Many experts recommend that FAP patients undergo thyroid ultrasound in the late teenage years, and that the examination be repeated potentially up to every 3 years, particularly for women. There is no particular screening protocol for desmoids, but once desmoids are diagnosed, surveillance may include imaging with either CT or MRI, or ultrasound if dictated by personal or family history. There is no specific protocol for evaluating the small bowel beyond the duodenum in FAP. There is no evidence supporting routine enterography or video capsule endoscopy. In cases where screening for hepatoblastoma is desired, AFP levels can be measured every 3 to 6 months for the first 5 years of life and along with abdominal ultrasound and palpation (**Table 64.3**).

Surgical Treatment of FAP

Patients with classical FAP are destined to develop CRC unless they undergo risk-reducing colectomy. Surgical options depend on the number and distribution of polyps. Timing also depends on the number and size of polyps, symptoms, patient age, and maturity. Ideally, surgery should occur when patients have reached physical maturity as well as the ability to cope psychologically with their diagnosis and consequences of surgical treatment.

Total proctocolectomy is appropriate for patients with diffuse polyposis involving the colon and rectum, as well as those with primary colonic disease who prefer a more definitive operation. Patients may choose to have a permanent ileostomy, but restorative proctocolectomy with ileal pouch-anal anastomosis

Table 64.3. Summary of Surveillance Guidelines for FAP Patients

Organ System	Surveillance Test	Frequency
Colorectal	Colonoscopy	Annually
Stomach/duodenum	EGD	At least every 3 y depending on findings
Thyroid	Ultrasound	Annually
Liver (hepatoblastoma) [a]Controversial	Ultrasound and alpha-fetoprotein	Every 6 mo until 5–10 y of age

[a]This is to note that surveillance of the liver is a controversial recommendation.

(IPAA) is typically performed in suitable candidates. Continent ileostomy, or Kock pouch, may also be an option in selected individuals with FAP.

In the setting of restorative proctocolectomy, the role of mucosectomy is debated in FAP. The idea behind mucosectomy is that by removing all at-risk mucosa, the chance of polyps and cancer developing is theoretically eliminated. However, even with a mucosectomy, it is possible to leave behind microscopic islands of mucosa that are at risk for neoplasia. Adenomas occur in the anal transition zone at a rate of 28% to 51% after stapled anastomosis and 10% to 22% after mucosectomy with hand-sewn anastomosis. Cancer is rare but does occur at a rate of 1% to 2% following either approach, so continued surveillance is necessary.

When polyp distribution is primarily colonic and there are less than 20 to 30 polyps in the rectum that can be managed endoscopically, patients can be considered for colectomy with IRA. With appropriate patient selection, the risk of subsequent proctectomy is less than 10%.

Patients must have regular surveillance of either their ileorectal anastomosis (IRA) or ileal pouch following risk-reducing surgery. It is generally recommended than an IRA be evaluated with flexible endoscopy every 6 to 12 months, depending on the rectal polyp burden. Pouchoscopy with evaluation of the anal transition zone should be performed every 1 to 3 years.

Attenuated FAP

Attenuated FAP (aFAP) is a milder phenotype of FAP. It is characterized by fewer colonic polyps with a later age of onset and a lower risk of CRC. The typical range of polyps in aFAP is 10 to 100 adenomas. The distribution is more likely to be right sided than pan-colonic compared to FAP, usually with relative rectal sparing. The onset of CRC tends to occur later in life compared to classic FAP, but the risk of cancer may be up to 80% by age 70. Routine colonoscopy and polypectomy may decrease the risk. The extracolonic tumor spectrum is similar to FAP and therefore screening and surveillance regimens are also similar.

Some patients with mild, attenuated FAP may be managed endoscopically and avoid colectomy. If their colon and rectum can be endoscopically cleared of polyps and they are willing to submit to frequent follow-up, they may be able to forego surgery. Most patients with aFAP are well suited to colectomy with IRA.

MUTYH-Associated Polyposis (MAP)

MAP is an autosomal recessive polyposis syndrome caused by mutations in the base-excision repair gene, *MUTYH*. Patients tend to have a milder form of colonic polyposis compared to FAP. Most patients have fewer than 100 adenomas. Other polyp types such as hyperplastic or serrated lesions may also be present. Because of the autosomal recessive inheritance pattern, the family history may not be as obvious as in FAP. Polyps typically develop in the third to sixth decades of life.

Incidence

Between 1% and 2% of the Caucasian population carry a single-mutated copy of the *MUTYH* allele. The most frequent alterations are *Y179C*, *G396D*, and *E480X*. The *Y179C* variant is less active than *G396* and therefore represents the most severe phenotype. For non-European descent individuals, the genetic alterations may be different and occur at different frequencies, but this has not yet been well described.

Genetics/Molecular Pathways

Germline mutations in *MUTYH* permit excess number of acquired mutations in the *APC* gene, which is why MAP is phenotypically similar to FAP. The *MUTYH* gene encodes a specific DNA glycosylase excision repair protein that is responsible for excising adenine nucleotides that are mismatched with 8-oxo-guanine, which is a product of oxidative damage to DNA. The mutations are typically G:C → T:A transversions. MAP is an autosomal recessive syndrome, so the individual must inherit two mutated alleles of the gene.

Extracolonic Features

The spectrum of extracolonic features and cancers in MAP is similar to FAP. However, they occur less frequently and are not as well characterized in this syndrome. Consequently, the surveillance protocols are similar in the two syndromes.

Cancer Risks

The estimated lifetime risk of CRC for patients with MAP is approximately 75%. The typical age of onset is between ages 45 and 59, slightly older than in FAP. Monoallelic carriers of *MUTYH* gene mutations may be at increased risk of CRC. The estimated risk is two to three times higher than the general population.[19]

Surveillance Protocols and Management

Patients with MAP should undergo colonoscopy every 1 to 2 years with polypectomy as indicated. Surveillance should be initiated by ages 25 to 30. Those with unresectable polyps or a large polyp burden should be referred for surgical consideration. Similar to those patients with FAP, the extent of surgery (total abdominal colectomy with IRA vs. total proctocolectomy) depends on the polyp burden in the rectum. In a patient with an IRA, the rectum should be surveyed with flexible sigmoidoscopy every 6 to 12 months. Monoallelic carriers of *MUTYH* mutations should also have colonoscopies every 5 years beginning at age 40, or 10 years prior to the earliest diagnosis of CRC in the family.

Because of the risk of upper GI neoplasia, baseline upper endoscopy including visualization of the ampulla of Vater should be performed by ages 30 to 35. Surveillance examination interval is determined by the Spigelman stage in the same way it is used for FAP. The overall risk of duodenal cancer in MAP is approximately 5%.

Rare Adenomatous Polyposis Syndromes

With advances in genetic testing, a number of additional, very rare syndromes have been described. Polymerase proofreading-associated polyposis (PPAP) is an autosomal dominant syndrome characterized by mutations in the polymerase proof reading genes *POLE* and *POLD1*, which results in a highly penetrant syndrome of tens to hundreds of polyps and a high risk of CRC. The carcinomas are microsatellite stable, follow the chromosomal instability or classical pathway to development from adenomas, and are a result of unrepaired DNA replication errors. Patients may have family histories suggestive of LS. Female patients may be at increased risk for endometrial, breast, and ovarian cancers. There are also descriptions of small bowel cancer and brain tumors associated with this syndrome.

The *NTLH1* gene, which encodes for a base excision repair protein, has been implicated in an autosomal recessive syndrome that is similar to MAP. It has been described in a cluster of Dutch families with a single founder mutation. The suspected carrier frequency in that population is 1 in 75,000. In a different individual with two separate mutations in the gene, the constellation of CRC, carcinoma of the bladder, meningioma, breast carcinoma, intradermal nevi, and basal cell carcinoma has been described. This suggests that the range of DNA lesions affected by this protein is broader than in MAP. The phenotype in affected families is consistent with an attenuated colorectal polyposis.

A mixed polyposis syndrome is described in patients with mutations to the *CRAC1* gene. Polyps may be serrated, hamartomatous, and adenomatous. CRC risk appears to be elevated. This gene is described in the Ashkenazi Jewish population. The gene was identified via linkage analysis and appears to be a single, founder mutation.

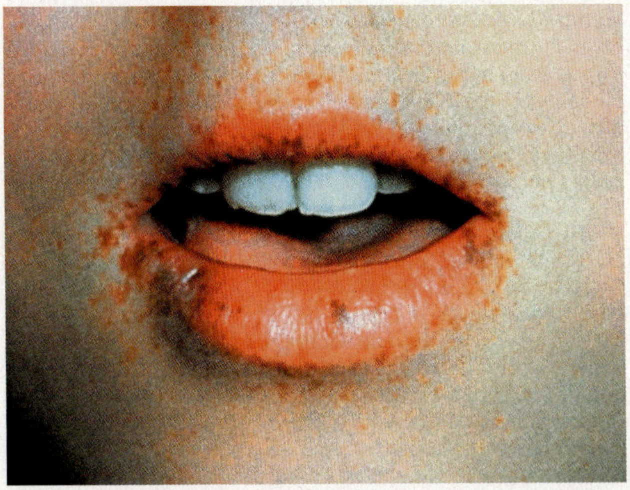

Figure 64.12. Perioral hyperpigmentation associated with PJS.

Because these syndromes are still being delineated in small groups and clusters of families, the phenotype is not well defined. There is insufficient evidence for specific screening, surveillance, or surgical treatment. As in cases without an identifiable genetic mutation, the individual and family phenotype should guide treatment decisions.

Hamartomatous Polyposis Syndromes

Peutz–Jeghers Syndrome (PJS)

PJS is an autosomal dominant syndrome associated with GI polyps and characteristic skin pigmentation. There are two genetic alterations associated with PJS, *LKB1* and *STK11*, both of which encode serine/threonine kinase.

The GI polyps in PJS are hamartomatous. They are nonneoplastic but histologically distinct from other hamartomatous polyps such as juvenile polyps. They may be found in the stomach, small intestine, or colon. Polyps may cause bleeding, intussusception, or obstruction.

PJS is also characterized by distinctive cutaneous manifestations. The dark, macular lesions on the mouth and buccal mucosa (**Fig. 64.12**) as well as on the nose, lips, hand, feet, genitals, and anus tend to be more prominent early in life and then less obvious by puberty They are different than typical freckles in that they are present at birth and the buccal mucosa may be involved in PJS; the lesions also extend within the vermilion border of the lips.

Patients with PJS are at increased risk of cancers within and outside the gastrointestinal tract. At-risk organs include the stomach, small intestine, colorectum, breast, pancreas, and biliary tree. Ovarian cysts, sex cord tumors, and Sertoli cell testicular tumors may also be present. Small bowel cancer and CRC are relatively rare in PJS.

Management of PJS is aimed toward removal of polyps in the GI tract. Traditional upper and lower endoscopy are utilized, but more advanced techniques such as double balloon or push enteroscopy may also be required. Surgery is utilized in cases where endoscopic management is not feasible or if symptoms develop. Combined laparoscopy and endoscopy may also be useful to enable treatment of the entire small bowel. There is no prophylactic surgery recommended for PJS.

Juvenile Polyposis Syndrome

JPS has been described with three distinct phenotypes: JPS limited to the colon, JPS limited to the stomach, and JPS throughout the GI tract. There are two genetic alterations associated with the syndrome, involving the *SMAD4* and *BMPR1A* genes. Each are thought to account for 20% of JPS cases. The remainder of the cases have an unknown genetic etiology. When JPS occurs in conjunction with hereditary hemorrhagic telangiectasia, it is typically associated with *SMAD4*. In addition, some *PTEN* mutations have also been linked to JPS, but this is rare.

Clinical manifestations include bleeding, intussusception, obstruction, and autoamputation of polyps that then pass through the GI tract. Rarely, protein-losing enteropathy may develop. Approximately 15% of patients with JPS have other abnormalities such as malrotation, heart or brain abnormalities, cleft palate, polydactyly, or genitourinary tract abnormalities.

Management of PJS is aimed toward removal of polyps in the GI tract. Advanced techniques such as double balloon or push enteroscopy may also be required. Surgery is utilized in cases in which endoscopic management is not feasible. Combined laparoscopy and endoscopy may also be useful to enable treatment of the entire small bowel using the "clean sweep" to clear all small bowel polyps, and thus reducing the risk of future symptoms.[20]

Cowden Syndrome

Cowden syndrome, also known as PTEN hamartoma tumor syndrome, is associated with a mutation on chromosome 10q23.3. Mutations are found in about 85% of patients diagnosed with Cowden syndrome. The *PTEN* gene is a tumor suppressor gene that acts as a negative regulator of the Akt/PKB signaling pathway, which in turn regulates levels of phosphoinositol triphosphate. It is also involved in regulating cell cycle, apoptosis, and angiogenesis. While intestinal polyps are important features, the extracolonic manifestations are more prominent. Though hamartomatous intestinal polyps occur in 30% to 85% of cases, there is no strong evidence of an increased risk for CRC from the hamartomatous polyps related to this syndrome. Patients may also have benign hamartomas and malignant tumors of the breast, thyroid, uterus, brain, and mucocutaneous tissue.

Diagnosis is based on meeting pathognomonic major and minor criteria developed in consensus guidelines. Testing should be offered to patients who have a family history of the syndrome if they meet the diagnostic criteria or if they have Lhermitte–Duclos disease. Major criteria include breast cancer, endometrial cancer, follicular thyroid cancer, multiple GI hamartomas or ganglioneuromas, macrocephaly, macular pigmentation of the glans penis, or mucocutaneous lesions including trichilemmoma, palmoplantar keratoses, multifocal or extensive oral mucosal papillomatosis, or multiple cutaneous facial papules. Minor criteria include autism spectrum disorder, CRC, more than three esophageal acanthoses, lipomas, intellectual disability, certain forms of thyroid cancers or benign lesions, renal cell carcinoma, single GI hamartoma or ganglioneuroma, testicular lipomatosis, or vascular malformation. In an individual with a relative who meets the clinical diagnosis criteria but who has not been tested, testing is appropriate if they meet any "major" or two "minor" criteria.

Breast cancer rates in women with Cowden syndrome are between 30% and 50%; men are also at risk. Benign breast conditions are also common in Cowden syndrome. Thyroid abnormalities including goiter, thyroglossal duct cysts, and thyroid cancer are an important feature of Cowden syndrome. Renal cell cancer has also been described.

Because of the broad spectrum of tumors, patients with Cowden syndrome are recommended to undergo surveillance of their breast, endometrium, kidney, and thyroid. In terms of CRC risk, it is recommended that colonoscopy be started at age 35 or 5 to 10 years prior to the first known CRC in the family. Patients should undergo colonoscopy at least every 5 years for surveillance.

Bannayan–Riley–Ruvalcaba Syndrome

BRRS is a hamartomatous polyposis syndrome that also includes a constellation of macrocephaly, hypotonia, developmental delays in about half of all cases, pigmented speckling of the penis in men, hypermobile joints, and lipomas and hemangiomas in addition to the hamartomas of the intestine. More than two-thirds of patients with BRRS have a mutation in the *PTEN* gene. It is a rare disorder with dozens of cases reported in the literature, but it may be underdiagnosed in milder phenotypes. The incidence of gastrointestinal polyps is 45%.[21] The cancer risks associated with this syndrome are not well defined, but many authors consider it analogous to Cowden syndrome. Most authors suggest considering individuals with BRRS at higher than average risk for malignancy, similar to Cowden syndrome.[22]

Serrated Polyposis Syndrome

Serrated polyposis syndrome (SPS) is a clinical diagnosis based on the presence of many or large serrated polyps in the colorectum. It appears to have an autosomal dominant inheritance pattern, although the genetic cause is not well defined. Overall, 40% of first-degree relatives of SPS patients also have serrated polyps.

Genetics

Some patients who meet the clinical criteria for SPS have pathogenic variants in the *RNF43* gene, but the majority of patients do not have an identifiable genetic mutation. The *RNF43* gene regulates *AMTIATR* (ataxia-telangiectasia mutated/ataxia-telangiectasia and Rad3-related protein) response to DNA damage.

Diagnosis

The diagnosis of SPS is based on World Health Organization criteria and includes at least five serrated polyps proximal to the sigmoid colon with at least two greater than 10 mm in size, or more than 20 serrated lesions or polyps of any size that are distributed throughout the colorectum, with at least five proximal to the rectum.[23]

Cancer Risk

Individuals with SPS are at higher-than-average risk for CRC, with a range of 15% to 30%.

Surveillance

If endoscopic management is feasible, all polyps 5 mm or greater in size should be removed. Subsequently, patients should undergo surveillance colonoscopies at 1- to 3-year intervals. If the number and/or size of polyps renders endoscopic management impossible, or CRC develops, patients should be referred for surgery. Total colectomy is recommended for CRC or high polyp burden of polyps that is not able to be effectively managed endoscopically. Because most patients do not have an identifiable genetic mutation, management of their relatives presents a challenge. It appears that first-degree relatives, even those without an SPS phenotype, have an increased risk of CRC.[24] Consensus guidelines recommend that first-degree relatives should be screened at the youngest age of onset of SPS in the family, 10 years earlier than the diagnosis of CRC, or by age 40—whichever is earliest in the case of an individual family. Colonoscopy should be repeated at least every 5 years and more frequently if indicated by findings.

Lynch Syndrome (LS)

LS is an autosomal dominant condition defined by a pathogenic variant in one of the MMR genes: *MLH1, MLH2, MSH6*, and *PMS2*. Patients with LS are at increased risk for a number of cancers including CRC, endometrial, urothelial, and small bowel. The risk varies based on which gene is mutated.

Incidence

LS accounts for approximately 3% of all CRCs, though the frequency may be higher in younger patient groups. The incidence is 1 in 279 individuals.

Genetics/Molecular Pathways

LS is an autosomal dominant syndrome with varying penetrance. It is caused by a pathogenic variant in an MMR gene. LS-associated CRC develops via the MSI pathway. Additionally, deletions in the *EPCAM* gene cause hypermethylation of the *MSH2* promoter, which leads to silencing of the gene and causes LS. Rarely, if two parents carry mutations to the same MMR gene, their offspring will be at risk of constitutional MMR deficiency (CMMRD). The cancer risk in CMMRD is extremely elevated and cancers can occur in childhood.

Diagnosis

LS is a genetic diagnosis defined by a germline pathogenic variant in one of the mismatch repair genes as discussed earlier. This should be distinguished from clinical criteria such as Amsterdam criteria or Bethesda criteria, which can identify individuals who should undergo LS testing. These criteria are neither sensitive nor specific and although individuals who meet those criteria are at increased risk of CRC, the germline variant defines the syndrome and defines the risk of colorectal and extracolonic malignancies. Correct diagnosis of LS is important because of the high risk of metachronous cancers, and because it enables affected family members to benefit from potentially lifesaving early detection or prevention of the characteristic cancers.

Most pathology labs will routinely do testing on the resected CRC or diagnostic biopsy to evaluate if that patient should undergo germline testing for LS. There are two main options for tumor-based testing for LS: immunohistochemistry (IHC) and PCR-based MSI testing. IHC uses antibodies to stain for the four most common MMR proteins. The lack of expression of any one of these MMR proteins is suggestive of LS. It is important to note that *MLH1* expression is more commonly lost via hypermethylation of the promoter region of *MLH1*. These cases develop as sporadic CRCs along the methylator pathway. Absence of *MLH1* on staining should trigger assessment for the *BRAF* V600E variant that accounts for nearly all of these sporadic cases. MSI testing uses PCR to assess for five microsatellites. If three or more are unstable, the tumor is considered MSI-high and suggestive of LS. There is high concordance between the two techniques. Neither IHC nor MSI is sufficient to diagnose LS and germline testing is necessary for definitive diagnosis. Multigene panel testing for LS and other syndromes is commonly employed for diagnosis and should be considered for all patients with CRC.

Colorectal Cancer Risks

Not all patients with LS will develop CRC; the overall lifetime risk is between 8% and 56%, but varies by mutation and gender.[25] The cumulative incidences by age 75 in men and women with pathogenic *MLH1* mutations is 56% and 4%, respectively; similarly it is 56% and 43% for *MSH2* carriers but substantially lower for men and women carriers of *MSH6* mutations at 16% and 17%, and even for those with *PMS2* mutations, the risk is 32% and 9% by gender. It appears that aspirin may decrease the risk of CRC in patients with LS; the benefit may also extend to other LS-associated cancers.[9] The optimal dose and duration of treatment are not yet clear.

CRC Surveillance

Patients with LS are at high risk for a large number of malignancies and therefore require complex surveillance regimens. Colonoscopy should begin at ages 20 to 25 (or 2 to 5 years younger than the earliest family member with CRC), with surveillance intervals of 1 to 2 years. This approach has been demonstrated to decrease the risk of CRC in LS patients.

Extracolonic Cancers and Surveillance

Patients with LS are at high risk for extracolonic malignancies compared with the general population. Surveillance is

Table 64.4. Summary of Surveillance Guidelines for Lynch Syndrome Patients

Organ System	Surveillance Test	Frequency
Colorectum	Colonoscopy	Every 1–2 y
Skin	Skin exam	Annually
Gynecologic	Endometrial biopsy Consider TVUS, CA-125	Annually
Small bowel	Capsule endoscopy	No consensus; consider every 2–3 y
Stomach	EGD	Every 1–3 y
Urologic	Urinalysis	Consider annually in select patients

warranted and varies by organ, as described below. Recommendations for surveillance are given in **Table 64.4**.

Gynecologic Cancers. The lifetime risk of endometrial cancer may be even higher than CRC in some cases. While the risk of endometrial cancer in the general population is about 3%, for women with LS, it is approximately 37% for those with an *MLH1* mutation, 44% for *MSH2* mutations, 45% for *MSH6* mutations, and 21% for those with *PMS2* mutations. The mean age at endometrial cancer diagnosis in women with LS is 46 to 54 years, compared with a mean age of 60 years otherwise. Up to 20% of Lynch-associated endometrial cancers are diagnosed before age 40. Similar to sporadic cases, endometrial cancer in LS tends to be diagnosed early and have a good prognosis. Women with LS who have atypical bleeding should be evaluated promptly. In addition, endometrial biopsy should be performed every 1 to 2 years for surveillance as it is highly sensitive and specific. Transvaginal ultrasound in postmenopausal women may also be used, although supportive evidence is generally lacking.

The lifetime risk of ovarian cancer for women with LS is 7% to 24%, again varying by mutation. The mean age at diagnosis is 43 to 50 years compared to 60 years in the general population. It is not clear that screening for ovarian cancer reduces the morbidity or mortality of ovarian cancer in women with LS, as also observed with sporadic cases.

Based on the high risk of gynecologic malignancies, hysterectomy with or without salpingo-oophorectomy should be considered in women who have completed childbearing and are fit for surgery.

Small Bowel Cancer. The risk of small bowel carcinoma in LS is highest in those with *MSH2* and *MSH6* mutations, who have a lifetime risk between 0.6% and 7%. Tumors are found throughout the small intestine at a median age of 39 to 53 years. There are no specific guidelines for routine screening. The use of enteroscopy as well as video capsule endoscopy have not been demonstrated to decrease rates of small bowel cancer in LS patients. While there are no clear data to support screening for small bowel cancer, esophagogastroduodenoscopy (EGD) with visualization at the duodenum at the time of colonoscopy every 3 to 5 years starting at age 40 is suggested by consensus guidelines.

Gastric Cancer. Some studies have estimated the lifetime risk of gastric cancer in LS to be as high as 13% in Asian populations. But the lifetime risk in North America and Western Europe is likely closer to 5%; the mutation with the highest frequency is *MSH2*. A carefully conducted time-trend study of gastric cancer found an 8.0% and 5.3% lifetime risk of this malignancy in males and females with MMR gene mutation, respectively, and a lack of familial clustering.[11] There are no studies that have evaluated the effectiveness of screening and surveillance for gastric cancer in LS patients, but EGD with gastric antrum biopsy every 3 to 5 years starting at age 40 is considered reasonable. If *Helicobacter pylori* is detected, it should be treated.

Urothelial Cancer. Patients with LS, particularly *MSH2* and *MSH6* mutations, are at increased risk of urothelial cell cancer at a rate of 20 times the general population, or a lifetime risk of 0.4% to 20%. The median age at diagnosis is 56 years. Although screening is suggested, none of the currently available tests, such as urinalysis or urine cytology, has proven to be sensitive or specific. Patients with an *MSH2* pathogenic variant, male gender, and family history of urothelial cancer are at the highest risk. Some experts recommend annual cystoscopy or CT urogram for this subset of patients starting at ages 30 to 35 years.

Prostate Cancer. The relative risk of prostate cancer is 3.6 times the general population, but there are no specific screening guidelines or evidence to suggest earlier onset or higher stage at diagnosis compared to average-risk populations.

Breast Cancer. While there is an increased risk of breast cancer in LS patients, there is insufficient evidence to support increased screening above the recommendations for average-risk individuals.

CNS Cancer. Other than annual physical examination and neurologic examination beginning at 25 to 30 years, no additional testing is recommended.

Surgical Treatment of CRC in LS

When LS is suspected preoperatively, testing should be considered to diagnose or rule out LS unless there are compelling reasons for urgent surgery. There is clear evidence that patients with LS who have colon cancer should be offered total abdominal colectomy with ileorectal anastomosis to decrease the risk of metachronous colon cancer. After segmental resection, the rates of metachronous adenomas and carcinomas are 33% and 25% even with excellent follow-up, compared to 11% and 8% after total abdominal colectomy.[26] There is a clear benefit in terms of cost effectiveness, probability of being alive and cancer free, and quality-of-life years with more extensive surgery in many circumstances.[27] For LS patients with rectal cancer, decisions are individualized, based on patient and tumor factors. In women with LS, it is recommended that they undergo prophylactic hysterectomy and bilateral salpingo-oophorectomy by age 40. When women have completed childbearing earlier than age 40, it is reasonable to contemplate prophylactic surgery. In addition, when women with LS who still have their uterus, tubes, and ovaries undergo surgery for CRC, synchronous prophylactic hysterectomy and salpingo-
5 oophorectomy are recommended.

Familial CRC Type X

Families that meet the Amsterdam I criteria but do not have a pathogenic variant in an MMR gene identified are referred to as familial CRC Type X. These patients have a two-fold increased risk of CRC compared to the general population, but lower than those with LS. Colonoscopy should start at age 45, or 10 years younger than the youngest CRC in that family. If colonoscopy is normal, it should be repeated every 5 years. For FCC X patients who develop CRC, a segmental rather than total colectomy is recommended as the risks of metachronous CRC are not as well defined and there is an absence of evidence that extended resection reduces cancer risk. In contrast to LS, patients with FCC X do not have a well-defined an increased risk of extracolonic malignancy and no specific surveillance is recommended, but should be tailored to the family history.

Undefined Syndromes

There are patients who phenotypically meet criteria for a hereditary syndrome and/or have a family history that is extremely suggestive, but do not have an identifiable genetic mutation. Management, therefore, is based on phenotype. Those individuals with dozens to hundreds of polyps should be managed in the same way as FAP patients, though their risk of extracolonic features may be less. The more common scenario, however, is a patient with 11 to 20 polyps. These patients are managed individually based on specifics of the phenotype and clinical judgment. The patient must be willing to undergo frequent surveillance at 1- to 3-year intervals and polypectomy should be performed to clear the colon. If it becomes impossible to safely survey the colon endoscopically or advanced lesions are found, colectomy is appropriate.

SUMMARY

Polyps are an extremely common finding on colonoscopy, particularly as individuals age. Screening and surveillance with polypectomy have the potential to decrease both the risk and the mortality related to CRC. Hereditary CRC syndromes are complex clinical problems that require coordinated care from multiple specialists. Patients are at increased risk of developing colorectal and extracolonic cancers and these develop at an earlier age than the general population. Optimal care is given in the context of a registry or organized program to ensure that all screening and surveillance guidelines are followed.

ACKNOWLEDGMENT

We gratefully acknowledge the contributions of previous edition author, Neil Hyman, as portions of those chapters have been retained in this revision.

References

1. Xue L, Williamson A, Gaines S, et al. An update on colorectal cancer. *Curr Probl Surg*. 2018;55:76–116.
2. Raju GS, Vadyala V, Slack R, et al. Adenoma detection in patients undergoing a comprehensive colonoscopy screening. *Cancer Med*. 2013;2:391–402.
3. Winawer SJ, Zauber AG, Ho MN, et al. Prevention of colorectal cancer by colonoscopic polypectomy. The National Polyp Study Workgroup. *N Engl J Med*. 1993;329:1977–1981.
4. Issa J.P. CpG island methylator phenotype in cancer. *Nat Rev Cancer*. 2004;4:988–993.
5. Brenner H, Hoffmeister M, Stegmaier C, Brenner G, Altenhofen L, Haug U. Risk of progression of advanced adenomas to colorectal cancer by age and sex: estimates based on 840,149 screening colonoscopies. *Gut*. 2007;56:1585–1589.
6. Atkin W, Wooldrage K, Parkin DM, et al. Long term effects of once-only flexible sigmoidoscopy screening after 17 years of follow-up: the UK Flexible Sigmoidoscopy Screening randomised controlled trial. *Lancet*. 2017;389:1299–1311.
7. Zauber AG, Winawer SJ, O'Brien MJ, et al. Colonoscopic polypectomy and long-term prevention of colorectal-cancer deaths. *N Engl J Med*. 2012;366:687–696.
8. Baxter NN, Warren JL, Barrett MJ, Stukel TA, Doria-Rose VP. Association between colonoscopy and colorectal cancer mortality in a US cohort according to site of cancer and colonoscopist specialty. *J Clin Oncol*. 2012;30:2664–2669.
9. Burn J, Gerdes AM, MacRae F, et al. Long-term effect of aspirin on cancer risk in carriers of hereditary colorectal cancer: an analysis from the CAPP2 randomised controlled trial. *Lancet*. 2011;378: 2081–2087.
10. Issa IA, Noureddine M. Colorectal cancer screening: an updated review of the available options. *World J Gastroenterol*. 2017;23: 5086–5096.
11. Syngal S, Brand RE, Church JM, et al. ACG clinical guideline: genetic testing and management of hereditary gastrointestinal cancer syndromes. *Am J Gastroenterol*. 2015;110:223–262.
12. Sasaki K, Kawai K, Nozawa H, et al. Risk of gastric adenoma and adenocarcinoma in patients with familial adenomatous polyposis in Japan: a nationwide multicenter study. *J Gastroenterol*. 2024;59:187–194.
13. DelSignore M, Jeong T, Denmark G, et al. Incidence and natural history of gastric high-grade dysplasia in patients with familial adenomatous polyposis syndrome. *Gastrointest Endosc*. 2023;97: 25–34.e6.
14. Spigelman AD, Williams CB, Talbot IC, Domizio P, Phillips RK. Upper gastrointestinal cancer in patients with familial adenomatous polyposis. *Lancet*. 1989;2:783–785.
15. Elayi E, Manilich E, Church J. Polishing the crystal ball: knowing genotype improves ability to predict desmoid disease in patients with familial adenomatous polyposis. *Dis Colon Rectum*. 2009;52: 1762–1766.
16. Sommovilla J, Liska D, Jia X, et al. IPAA is more "desmoidogenic" than ileorectal anastomosis in familial adenomatous polyposis. *Dis Colon Rectum*. 2022;65:1351–1361.
17. Church J, Lynch C, Neary P, LaGuardia L, Elayi E. A desmoid tumor-staging system separates patients with intra-abdominal, familial adenomatous polyposis-associated desmoid disease by behavior and prognosis. *Dis Colon Rectum*. 2008;51:897–901.
18. Gounder MM, Mahoney MR, Van Tine BA, et al. Sorafenib for advanced and refractory desmoid tumors. *N Engl J Med*. 2018;379: 2417–2428.
19. Win AK, Cleary SP, Dowty JG, et al. Cancer risks for monoallelic MUTYH mutation carriers with a family history of colorectal cancer. *Int J Cancer*. 2011;129:2256–2262.
20. Oncel M, Remzi FH, Church JM, Connor JT, Fazio VW. Benefits of "clean sweep" in Peutz-Jeghers patients. *Colorectal Dis*. 2004;6: 332–335.
21. Manfredi M. Hereditary hamartomatous polyposis syndromes: understanding the disease risks as children reach adulthood. *Gastroenterol Hepatol (N Y)*. 2010;6:185–96.
22. Chen HM, Fang JY. Genetics of the hamartomatous polyposis syndromes: a molecular review. *Int J Colorectal Dis*. 2009;24:865–874.
23. Nagtegaal ID, Odze RD, Klimstra D, et al; WHO Classification of Tumours Editorial Board. The 2019 WHO classification of tumours of the digestive system. *Histopathology*. 2020;76:182–188.
24. Boparai KS, Reitsma JB, Lemmens V, et al. Increased colorectal cancer risk in first-degree relatives of patients with hyperplastic polyposis syndrome. *Gut*. 2010;59:1222–1225.
25. Dominguez-Valentin M, Sampson JR, Seppälä TT, et al. Cancer risks by gene, age, and gender in 6350 carriers of pathogenic mismatch repair variants: findings from the Prospective Lynch Syndrome Database. *Genet Med*. 2020;22:15–25.
26. Kalady MF, McGannon E, Vogel JD, Manilich E, Fazio VW, Church JM. Risk of colorectal adenoma and carcinoma after colectomy for colorectal cancer in patients meeting Amsterdam criteria. *Ann Surg*. 2010;252(3):507–511.
27. Jiang B, Ofshteyn A, Idrees JJ, et al; University Hospitals Research in Surgical Outcome & Effectiveness (UH-RISES). Total abdominal colectomy is cost-effective in treating colorectal cancer in patients with genetically diagnosed Lynch syndrome. *Am J Surg*. 2019;218(5):928–933.

Colorectal Cancer

Valentine Nfongen Nfonsam

Key Points

1. Over the last several decades, the overall incidence and mortality for colorectal cancer (CRC) has declined especially among individuals aged 65 years or older, likely due to increased screening and improvement in treatment modalities. However, during that same time there has been a significant increase in the incidence of CRC among younger individuals less than 50 years old. The etiology of this increase in early-onset CRC is unknown but likely multifactorial.
2. Recent advances in molecular biology have led to better understanding of the CRC disease process, identification of disease biomarkers and personalization of CRC treatment.
3. Improvement in treatment paradigm including Total Neoadjuvant Treatment for rectal cancer has led to higher percentage of complete clinical response and higher adoption of watch-and-wait treatment option.
4. Use of laparoscopic and robotic surgical techniques in combination with enhanced recovery programs has accelerated patient recovery, reduced hospital length of stay and postoperative complications.
5. While long-term survival for patients with stage IV disease remains low, median survival for these patients has improved significantly in recent years, probably due to more effective chemotherapy and more aggressive surgery.
6. A multidisciplinary approach to the treatment of CRC enhances better outcomes and quality of life in patients.

The incidence of colorectal cancer (CRC) has been declining over the years. However, CRC remains a deadly disease with about 50,000 deaths a year in the United States. CRC is one of the most curable malignancies when diagnosed at an early stage. Identification of populations at risk and screening of asymptomatic patients are therefore crucial imperatives. This chapter provides a comprehensive overview of the disease, including epidemiology, risk factors, molecular characteristics, progression, staging, screening, diagnosis, and treatment.

EPIDEMIOLOGY

CRC is the third most common malignancy and the second most common cause of cancer death in the United States. The American Cancer society estimates that in 2024 a total of 152,810 people will be diagnosed with CRC in the United States—106,590 new colon cancers and 46,220 new rectal cancer cases. An estimated 53,010 people died from the disease in 2024.[1] Approximately 1 in 24 Americans will be diagnosed with CRC in their lifetime. The incidence and mortality of CRC have been decreasing since the mid-1980s. This decrease is likely due to increased awareness, more robust screening initiatives and mitigating lifestyle-related risk factors. Most recently, however, there has been a deceleration in the decline of CRC incidence and mortality (**Fig. 65.1**).[2]

1 The incidence and mortality rates for CRC vary with age. The median age at colon cancer diagnosis is 67 years in men, and 71 years in women; for rectal cancer, 62 years in men and 63 years in women.[2] Over the last several decades, the overall incidence and mortality of CRC has trended down. During the same period, there has been an alarming increase in younger patients (<50 years old) (**Fig. 65.2**). This change in trend is especially worrisome, as the incidence is occurring in patients younger than the recommended screening age.[2] Both, the incidence and mortality for CRC are 30% to 40% higher in men than in women. The reasons for these differences are not completely understood but probably reflect an interaction between risk factors and hormonal differences. There are also gender differences in the distribution of CRC, with a higher proportion of proximal tumors in women.

Marked ethnic and racial disparities exist in the incidence and mortality of CRC. Both are highest for African Americans and lowest for Asians/Pacific Islanders, but the differences in mortality are proportionally larger compared with the differences in incidence.

CRC is the third most common cancer in men and the second most common cancer in women worldwide, with an estimated 1.9 million new cases diagnosed in 2020 (WHO).[3] It is responsible for 9% of cancer deaths worldwide. The age-standardized incidence of CRC varies significantly by country. It is decreasing in developed countries that have implemented screening programs (United States, Israel, and Japan) or have modified factors known to be associated with increased risk of CRC (Australia and New Zealand). By 2040 the burden of CRC will increase to 3.2 million new cases per year (an increase of 63%) and 1.6 million deaths per year (an increase of 73%). However, the incidence rates are increasing in both developed and developing countries with changes in unfavorable risk factors such as adoption of a western diet, obesity, and smoking. Despite the increase in incidence, mortality for CRC is decreasing in many countries, most likely because of improvements in both screening and treatment.[3]

CRC RISK FACTORS

Several modifiable and nonmodifiable risk factors are associated with CRC (**Table 65.1**). Information about individual risk factors can be used to reduce incidence and mortality through behavior

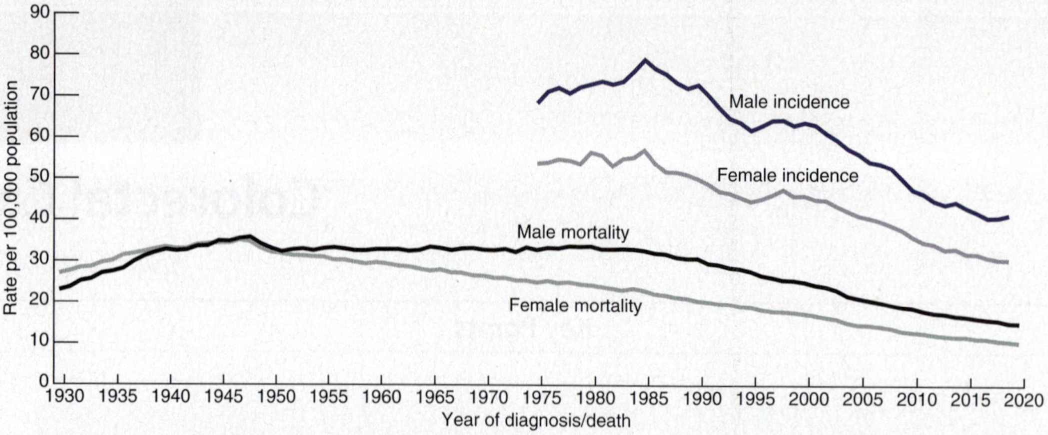

Due to changes in International Classification of Diseases (ICD) coding for mortality, numerator information has changed over time. All rates are age adjusted to the 2000 US standard population. Incidence rates are adjusted for reporting delays and exclude appendix.

Sources: Incidence: Surveillance, Epidemiology, and End Results (SEER) Program, SEER 8 registries, National Cancer Institute, 2022. Mortality: US Mortality Volumes 1930 to 1968, US Mortality Data 1969-2020, National Center for Health Statistics, Centers for Disease Control and Prevention, 2022.

Figure 65.1. Long-term Trends in Colorectal Cancer Incidence (1975–2019) and Mortality (1930–2020) by Sex, US. In men and women combined, the age-standardized CRC incidence rate has decreased from 66.2 per 100,000 at its peak in 1985 to 35.5 per 100,000 in 2019, an overall decline of 46%, because of changing patterns in risk factors (eg, declines in smoking) and the uptake of screening. Declines in incidence, earlier detection, and improvements in treatment have resulted in a 57% drop in the overall CRC death rate from 1970 (29.2 per 100,000) to 2020 (12.6 per 100,000). The pace of these declines has slowed from 3% to 4% annually during the 2000s to 1% annually for incidence and 2% annually for mortality during the past decade, at least in part because population screening is approaching saturation and rates are increasing or stable in middle-aged and younger individuals. (From American Cancer Society. *Cancer Facts and Figures 2023–2025*. American Cancer Society, Inc.)

modification and screening programs.[4] Except for the relatively uncommon hereditary syndromes with known patterns of inheritance, the relative contribution of inherited and environmental factors to the development of CRC is controversial. Analysis of cohorts of twins from Scandinavian countries suggests a significant but relatively minor contribution of hereditary factors to the development of sporadic CRC; the environment seems to play a larger role in the development of sporadic cancers.[5]

The list of behavioral or modifiable factors that increase CRC risk includes obesity, smoking, diet, and alcohol intake. More than half (55%) of CRCs in the United States are attributable to potentially modifiable risk factors.[3] Physical activity and dairy products reduce CRC risk.[2] Obesity is associated with increased risk of developing CRC in both men and women.[6] Abdominal obesity, measured as waist size, seems to be more important than excess weight, particularly in men. Being overweight increases the risk of CRC, independent of the level of physical activity. The most physically active people have a 25% lower risk of developing CRC, compared to the least active people. Both recreational and occupational physical activity reduces CRC risk, and sedentary people who become physically active later in life do reduce their CRC risk.[7] An increased risk of CRC has been associated with high consumption of red or processed meats.[8] On the other hand, the risk of CRC is inversely correlated with the intake of fiber and whole grains, fruits and vegetables, dairy products and calcium, vitamin D, and folates.[8] Heavy alcohol consumption (more than 3 drinks/day) is associated with the development of CRC, and the effect seems to be dose dependent. The risk seems to be higher for men than for women. There is no difference in the effect regarding the type of alcohol.[9] Smoking increases the incidence and mortality from CRC, and in particular, rectal cancer.[10,11]

The majority of CRC (75%) occurs in people who do not have any particular predisposing factors, and are therefore considered to be at average risk. This presentation is termed sporadic CRC. The remaining 25% of patients have hereditary risk factors that predispose them to the development of CRC: either a well-defined hereditary CRC syndrome (5%) or a close relative who has been diagnosed with the disease (20%). People with one or more first-degree relatives with CRC have between a 1.9 and 4.4 relative risk of developing CRC compared with the average population. The risk is higher when the affected relative was diagnosed at an early age, or when several relatives have been affected.[12,13] Recent population-based studies have noted a greater familial aggregation of early-onset CRC among first-degree relatives diagnosed before the age of 40, compared to patients diagnosed after the age of 41. This age-of-onset effect could not be attributed solely to known hereditary CRC syndromes.[14] CRC survivors have four times the lifetime risk of developing a new (metachronous) CRC, compared with people at average risk. The estimated mean annual incidence of metachronous CRC is 0.3%, with a cumulative incidence of 3.1% at 10 years.[15] A personal history of adenomatous colorectal polyps also increases the risk of CRC, in particular for patients with larger or multiple polyps and an early age at diagnosis.[16]

Patients with chronic inflammatory bowel disease, both ulcerative colitis and Crohn disease, are at increased risk of developing CRC.[17] The risk increases with the duration of the disease. It is estimated that, after 10 years of disease, the risk of developing CRC increases by around 1% each year. Thus, it is estimated that patients with 30 years of inflammatory bowel disease have an 18% risk of developing CRC. The risk is higher for patients diagnosed with inflammatory bowel disease at an early age and with disease extending proximal to the splenic flexure. A high cumulative burden of inflammation, that takes into consideration the intensity and the duration of inflammation, has been associated with a higher risk of colorectal neoplasia.[18] However, the incidence of CRC in patients with ulcerative colitis seems to be decreasing. A recent meta-analysis of population-based cohort studies reported a 1.7 increased risk of CRC among inflammatory bowel disease patients, compared with the general population, after adjusting for age, gender, and duration of disease.[19] These changes are probably due to more effective treatments and the efficacy of surveillance programs.[20]

Patients with type II diabetes have a higher risk of developing CRC compared to the nondiabetic individual, even when adjusting for factors such as obesity and sedentary lifestyle.[21] In addition, CRC survival rates are lower for diabetic patients compared to nondiabetic patients.[22] The relationship between diabetes and CRC seems to be stronger for men than for women.

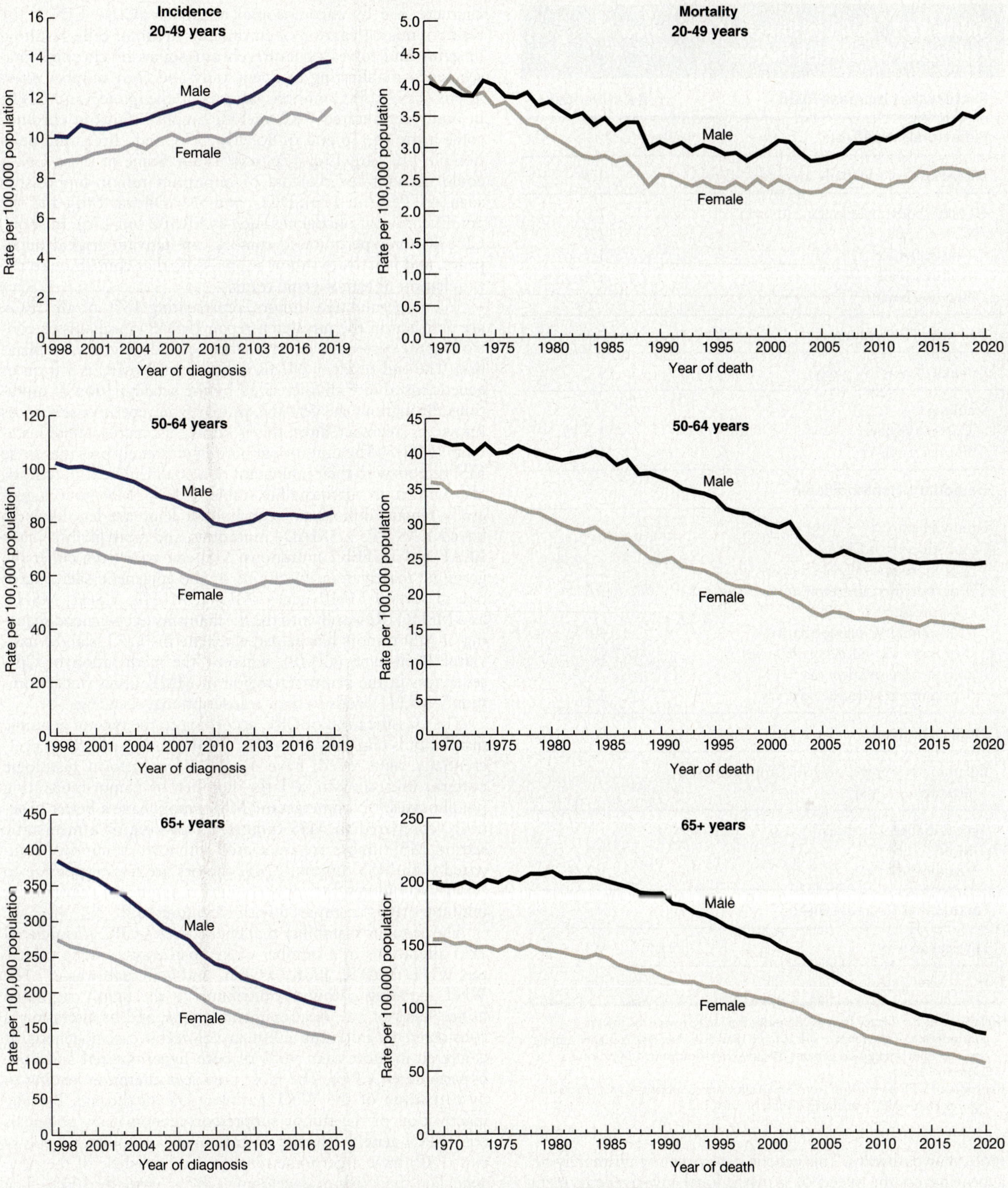

Rates are age adjusted to the 2000 US standard population. Incidence rates are adjusted for reporting delays and exclude appendix.

Sources: Incidence: North American Association of Central Cancer Registries, 2022. Mortality: National Center for Health Statistics, Centers for Disease Control and Prevention, 2022.

Figure 65.2. Trends in Colorectal Cancer Incidence (1998–2019) and Mortality (1970–2020) by Age and Sex, US. (From American Cancer Society. *Cancer Facts and Figures 2023–2025*. American Cancer Society, Inc.)

MOLECULAR CHARACTERISTICS

Elucidating and understanding the molecular characteristics of CRC has been a major advancement in developing personalized treatments. The traditional model of CRC tumor development is often represented as a linear and sequential progression from normal epithelium to small adenoma, to large adenoma, to invasive carcinoma, and finally to metastatic disease.[23] This so-called adenoma–carcinoma sequence has been deemed the result of the progressive accumulation of alterations in the genome. Our understanding of CRC tumorigenesis has been informed by whole genome sequencing. Every CRC has a multitude of distinct genetic alterations that perturb a number of

Table 65.1. Relative Risks for Established Colorectal Cancer Risk Factors

Factors that Increase Risk:	Relative Risk[a]
Behavioral, Modifiable	
Heavy alcohol use (daily average >3 drinks)	1.3
Obesity (body mass index ≥30 kg/m^2)	1.3
Colon, male	1.5
Colon, female	1.1
Rectum, male	1.3
Rectum, female	1.0
Red meat (100 g/day)	1.1
Processed meat (50 g/day)	1.2
Smoking	
Current vs never	1.5
Former vs never	1.2
Hereditary, Nonmodifiable	
Family History	
Family history of CRC	
1 or more first-degree relatives	2.2
1 or more first-degree relatives diagnosed before age 50	3.6
2 or more first-degree relatives	4.0
1 or more second-degree relatives	1.7
Family history of adenoma	
1 or more first-degree relatives	2.0
Medical History	
Inflammatory bowel disease (Crohn disease, ulcerative colitis)	1.7
Type 2 diabetes mellitus	
Male	1.4
Female	1.2
Factors that Decrease Risk:	
Physical activity	0.7
Dairy (400 g/day)	0.9

[a]Relative risk for dietary factors compares the highest with the lowest consumption. If the relative risk is more than 1.0, then risk is higher among exposed than unexposed persons. Relative risks less than 1.0 indicate a protective effect.

Reproduced with permission from American Cancer Society. *Cancer Facts and Figures 2020–2022*. American Cancer Society, Inc.

molecular pathways. This genetic heterogeneity ultimately has a bearing on the speed of growth, local invasiveness, meta-
2 static potential, and response to therapy.

The most comprehensive molecular analysis of CRC to date has been conducted by The Cancer Genome Atlas (TCGA) Consortium.[24] They have used state-of-the-art technology to elucidate the mutational spectrum, the chromosomal and subchromosomal changes, the epigenetic regulation and transcriptional alterations in a large number of CRCs. A key finding that has helped frame our molecular understanding of CRC is the wide variation in the number of somatic mutations present in most tumors. According to the number of mutations, CRC can be effectively classified as hypermutated, harboring a median of 728 nonsilent mutations per tumor, and nonhypermutated, with a median of 58 nonsilent mutations (**Fig. 65.3**). Nonhypermutated tumors comprise 84% of CRCs, and are characterized by chromosomal instability (CIN). CIN is the result of missegregation of chromatids in tumor cells, resulting in gains and losses of entire chromosomes or chromosomal segments; manifesting as aneuploidy and copy number alterations (CNAs).[25] Common patterns of aneuploidy and CNAs in nonhypermutated CRC include amplifications in chromosome arms 1q, 7p and q, 8q, 13q, 17q, and 20p/q, and deletions in 8p, 14q, 15q, 17p, and 18p/q. Some of these CNAs could account for the loss of important tumor suppressors such as TP53 (on 17p), DCC, and SMAD4 (on 18q), and the amplification of oncogenes such as ERBB2 (on 17q). In short, CIN in nonhypermutated tumors can activate critical oncogenes, and inactivate tumor suppressors that contribute to the acquisition of tumorigenic traits.

The hypermutated tumors, representing 16% of all CRCs, are deficient in the mismatch-repair (MMR) mechanisms controlling the correction of errors that occur during DNA replication. The end result of MMR deficiency (dMMR) is a form of genetic instability characterized by the accumulation of mutations throughout the genome, primarily in repetitive sequences known as microsatellites; this is known as microsatellite instability (MSI).[26] The mutational burden ultimately provides these MSI tumors with their malignant potential. Unlike CIN tumors, also known as microsatellite stable or MSS, MSI tumors generally remain diploid or near-diploid. They are less likely to have KRAS, TP53, SMAD4 mutations, and more likely to have BRAF and TGFBR2 mutations. MSI can arise from either the germline inactivating mutations or the epigenetic silencing of one of several MMR genes (MLH1, MLH3, MSH2, MSH3, and MSH6). Research into the mechanisms of epigenetic silencing of MSI tumors has helped elucidate the CpG Island Methylator Phenotype (CIMP), whereby the methylation of CpG sequences in the promoter region of MMR genes (most commonly MLH1) leads to their transcriptional silencing.

The classification of CRC according to the type of genomic instability is clinically relevant.[27] MSI tumors tend to be preferentially right sided, have a solid or cribriform histologic pattern, and contain a large number of tumor-infiltrating lymphocytes.[28] Nonmetastatic MSI tumors have a better prognosis, compared to MSS tumors.[29] However, in a metastatic setting, MSI tumors are associated with a worse survival compared with MSS tumors.[30] MSI tumors are less responsive to fluoropyrimidines, but most responsive to immune checkpoint inhibitors (ICIs) compared with MSS tumors.[31]

The genomic instability that characterizes CRC is associated with alterations in a number of key pathways; among others, the WNT, MAPK, PI3K, TGF-β, and p53 pathways.[24] The WNT signaling pathway contributes to the tightly regulated homeostasis of intestinal epithelial crypts, and its alteration is considered an initiating event in colorectal carcinogenesis. It is altered in more than 90% of both hypermutated and nonhypermutated CRCs. The most prevalent alteration leading to dysregulation of the WNT pathway occurs through biallelic inactivation of the tumor suppressor adenomatous polyposis coli (APC) gene.[32] Patients with familial adenomatous polyposis (FAP) have a germline mutation in one allele of the APC gene, and their risk of developing CRC is virtually 100%. The WNT pathway is also commonly altered as a result of stabilizing mutations of the CTNNB1 gene coding for β-catenin, a protein normally targeted for degradation by APC. The accumulation of β-catenin as a result of APC loss or stabilizing CTNNB1 mutations leads to its translocation to the nucleus, where it interacts with transcription factors of the TCF/LCF family, turning them into transcriptional activators. The end result is an increase in the transcription of genes that are normally important for stem cell renewal and differentiation but, when inappropriately expressed at high levels, can cause cancer.

Mutational inactivation of the TGF-β pathway, important in regulating cell growth arrest and apoptosis, is a common event in CRC.[33] Downstream effectors of this pathway such as the transcription factor SMAD4, and associated proteins

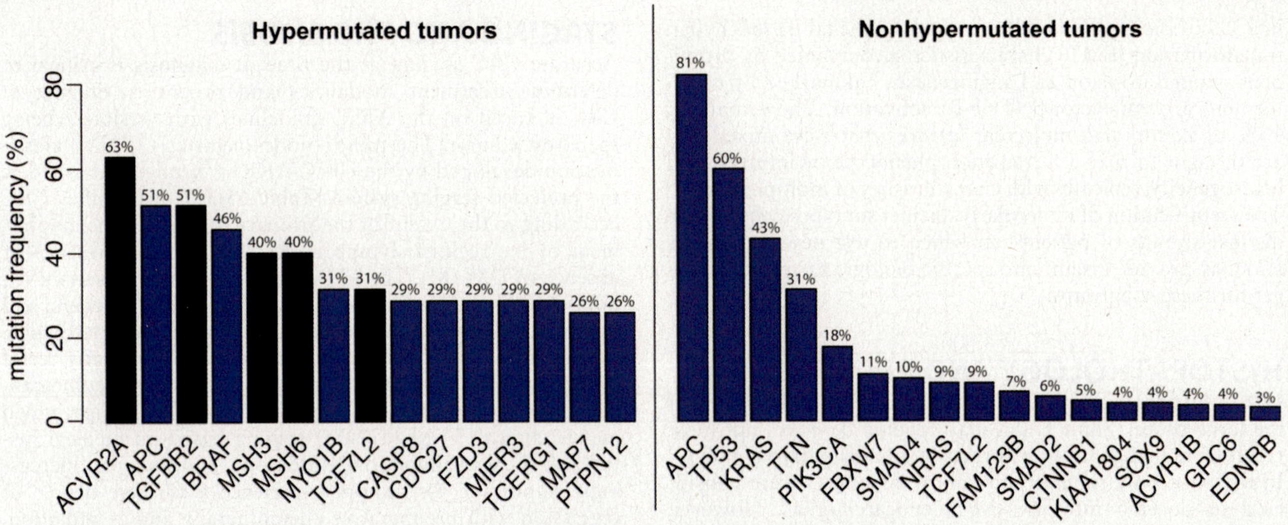

Figure 65.3. Mutation frequencies in hypermutated and nonhypermutated tumors in CRC. *Blue bars* represent genes identified by MutSig and genes in *black bars* are identified by manual examination of sequence data. (Reproduced with permission from Comprehensive molecular characterization of human colon and rectal cancer. *Nature*. 2012;487(7407):330–337.)

SMAD2 and SMAD3, are also inactivated by mutation or homozygous deletion of chromosomal segment 18q. Another member of this pathway, deleted in CRC (DCC), is also commonly inactivated by deletion of chromosome 18q.

A common theme of the WNT and TGF-β signaling pathways is the increased activity of c-Myc, a regulator gene that codes for a multifunctional transcription factor which plays a role in cell cycle progression, apoptosis, and cellular transformation. c-Myc seems to play a central role in colorectal carcinogenesis.[34]

The TP53 gene is a member of a pathway of regulators of cell cycle arrest and cell death in response to a variety of genotoxic stresses. Mutations in the TP53 tumor suppressor gene occur in more than half of nonhypermutated CRCs. In most tumors, both alleles of the gene are inactivated by a combination of a mutation in one allele, and loss of the second allele by deletion of the chromosomal segment 17p. Loss of the TP53 tumor suppressor gene is generally considered an early event that plays a role in the transition from adenoma to invasive carcinoma.[35] In hypermutated tumors, the TP53 pathway may be attenuated by mutations in other genes, such as the proapoptotic BAX.

The MAPK pathway consists of a cascade of tightly coordinate kinases that work together to regulate cell division and proliferation. KRAS, a protooncogene that becomes constitutively activated by mutation, resulting in uncontrolled cell proliferation, is mutated in 37% of CRC. Interestingly, a number of studies from model organisms reveal that KRAS mutation by itself is not sufficient to initiate tumorigenesis; in order to have oncogenic potential it requires a previous APC mutation. The MAPK pathway is the molecular pathway that has successfully been therapeutically targeted in CRC. Inhibition of this pathway using antibodies against the epidermal growth factor receptor (EGFR) reduces progression in wild-type KRAS/NRAS metastatic CRC.[36] Activating mutations of BRAF, also an effector member of the MAPK pathway downstream of KRAS, are seen in 13% of CRC. The BRAF mutation is associated with poor prognosis, specifically in MSI tumors.[37]

The PI3K/AKT/mTOR signaling pathway, with important roles in cell proliferation and apoptosis, is abnormally activated in nearly half of all CRCs. Moreover, in the TCGA cohort, PI3K and RAS pathways are simultaneously affected by mutations in one-third of all CRCs, suggesting that simultaneous inhibition of both pathways may be required to achieve a therapeutic effect.[38]

Gene expression has been linked to tumor phenotype and biologic behavior in CRC. Recently, an international consortium of six groups that examined shared, large-scale high-throughput gene expression data was able to create a transcriptomic-based molecular classification of CRC. This novel classification distinguishes four consensus molecular subtypes (CMS) of CRC, with distinct genomic and clinical features (**Fig. 65.4**).[39] The CMS group classification is currently considered the most robust molecular system connected to distinct biologic and clinical characteristics and serves as a framework for molecularly targetable interventions. CMS2 was named the canonical subtype that made up 37% of all clusters observed and exhibited epithelial characteristics with marked WNT and MYC activated pathway signaling. CMS1 made up 14% of the categorized molecular clustering and displayed MSI along with significant immune activation and hypermutated features. The CMS3 subtype made up 13% of the molecular clustering and showed features of epithelial and metabolic dysregulation. The CMS4 subtype was found

CMS1 MSI immune	CMS2 Canonical	CMS3 Metabolic	CMS4 Mesenchymal
14%	37%	13%	23%
MSI, CIMP high, hypermutation	SCNA high	Mixed MSI status, SCNA low, CIMP low	SCNA high
BRAF mutations		*KRAS* mutations	
Immune infiltration and activation	WNT and MYC activation	Metabolic deregulation	Stromal infiltration, TGF-β activation, angiogenesis
Worse survival after relapse			Worse relapse-free and overall survival

CIMP, CpG island methylator phenotype; MSI, microsatellite instability; SCNA, somatic copy number alterations.

Figure 65.4. The consensus molecular subtypes. CMS1 displays subtype clusters that involve hypermutation and microsatellite instability along with increased immune cell infiltrates consisting of Th1 lymphocyte, cytotoxic T cell, NK cell infiltration, and upregulated immune checkpoints such as PD-1. CMS2 clustering involves the upregulation of canonical pathways including WNT and MYC downstream targets. CMS3 clustering is defined by dysregulation of metabolic pathways including carbohydrate and fatty acid oxidation and the loss of TH17 cells. CMS4 clustering is referred to as a mesenchymal subtype that involves the upregulation of EMT pathways. CMS4 clustering also shows elevated TGF-β signaling, matrix remodeling, angiogenesis, complement activation as well as integrin-β3 upregulation, stromal infiltration, immune upregulation, and platelet signatures. (Reproduced with permission from Guinney J, Dienstmann R, Wang X, et al. The consensus molecular subtypes of colorectal cancer. *Nat Med*. 2015;21(11):1350–1356.)

in 23% of the molecular clusters with epithelial mesenchymal transformation (EMT) characteristics accompanied by prominent stromal invasion and angiogenesis, hallmarked by transforming growth factor-β (TGF-β) activation. The remaining 13% of tumors had molecular features that were mixed and are thought to reflect a transition phenotype or intratumoral heterogeneity, typically with characteristics of multiple CMS.[40] The identification of molecularly distinct subtypes can provide distinct subsets of patients on which to test new treatments and may provide insight into specific biologic pathways to target for these subgroups.

HISTOPATHOLOGY AND PROGRESSION

CRC is an adenocarcinoma arising from the epithelial lining of the large bowel. Some CRCs may develop de novo, but most result from malignant transformation of adenomatous polyps. In the past, only tubular and villous adenomas were considered to develop into invasive adenocarcinomas. However, recent evidence suggests that serrated polyps can also develop into CRCs. Polyps arise from normal mucosa and gradually increase in size. Some polyp characteristics—size larger than 1 cm, tubulovillous or villous histology, multiple occurrences—are associated with a high risk of malignant transformation. Most screening programs are designed to recognize the presence of polyps, or early malignant change in polyps or the surrounding mucosa.

Most CRCs are typically adenocarcinomas that form glandular structures resembling the normal colonic epithelium. However, there are several histologic types of adenocarcinoma (**Table 65.2**). Colorectal adenocarcinomas are assigned to one of four histologic grades according to their histologic resemblance to the normal colonic epithelium. The histologic grade is associated with oncologic outcome independent of other risk factors including tumor staging.

CRC is locally invasive, potentially spreading through the full thickness of the bowel wall into adjacent tissues. From the primary site, CRC often extends to the regional lymph nodes and to other organs. CRC can metastasize to almost any organ, but the most common sites are the liver and lungs. Approximately 20% to 34% of patients have metastases at the time of diagnosis, and another 30% of those initially treated with curative intent will subsequently develop distant metastases (DMs). Other sites of DM are the brain and bones, but these are unusual in the absence of liver metastases. Patients may also develop peritoneal spread, with the formation of malignant ascites. The risk of nodal metastasis increases with the depth of tumor invasion into the bowel wall, and the risk of DM is higher for patients with nodal metastasis.

Table 65.2. Histopathologic Types of Colorectal Cancer

Carcinomas
Adenocarcinoma
Medullary carcinoma
Mucinous adenocarcinoma (greater than 50% mucinous content)
Signet ring cell carcinoma (greater than 50% signet ring cells)
Neuroendocrine adenocarcinoma
Squamous cell carcinoma
Adenosquamous carcinoma
Small cell carcinoma
Undifferentiated carcinoma
Other Tumors
Carcinoid
Lymphoma
Sarcomas

STAGING AND PROGNOSIS

Accurate CRC staging at the time of diagnosis is critical to determine treatment modalities and prognosis. Staging of CRC is based on the AJCC guidelines with version 9 being the latest edition. The tumor–node–metastasis (TNM) classification developed by the UICC/AJCC is firmly established as the preferred staging system (**Table 65.3**).[41] It classifies CRC according to the extent of the primary tumor (T), the involvement of the regional lymph nodes (N), and the presence or absence of DM (M). The TNM classification is important for both clinical and pathologic staging. Most colon cancers, and many rectal cancers, are staged after surgery and pathologic examination of the surgical specimen (pTNM). Many rectal cancer patients, and a small but growing number of colon cancer patients, do not receive surgery as the initial therapy, which makes clinical TNM (cTNM) staging based on medical history, physical examination, endoscopy, and imaging, increasingly important. As tumors experience a variable degree of regression with preoperative chemotherapy and/or radiation, it is important that patients receiving neoadjuvant therapy are assigned an accurate cTNM stage before starting treatment. For patients who have received neoadjuvant therapy, a modified pathologic staging is generated after surgical resection, annotated by the prefix y (ypTNM). The 9th version of the AJCC Cancer Staging Manual incorporates a four-tier tumor regression grading (TRG) system for patients receiving neoadjuvant therapy. In this grading system TRG 0 represents Complete Response, no viable tumor cells or complete pathologic response (pCR); TRG 1, Near-complete Response; TRG 2, Partial Response; and TRG 3, Poor Response. Tumor regression seems to correlate closely with prognosis and long-term oncologic outcome.[41]

Relative survival in CRC patients decreases according to the depth of tumor penetration into the bowel wall and number of lymph nodes involved, but the presence of DM is the single most important predictor of survival in these patients (**Table 65.3**). Other tumor and treatment-related prognostic factors, in addition to the TNM stage, are listed in **Table 65.4**.

Quantitative parameters of lymph node evaluation—number of positive lymph nodes, total number of lymph nodes examined, and lymph node ratio—have prognostic implications in CRC. The number of nodes involved by tumor is included in the N category of the TNM system. The current staging system recommends examining a minimum of 12 lymph nodes for adequate staging.[41] The total number of lymph nodes retrieved is lower in rectal cancer patients treated with preoperative chemotherapy and radiation, but the minimal number of nodes required for adequate staging in these patients is unknown. The total number of nodes examined has an important impact on outcome in patients with colon and rectal cancer; in patients with all T and N combinations, the probability of survival increases linearly with the number of lymph nodes examined. The lymph node ratio, defined as the number of positive lymph nodes divided by the total number of retrieved nodes, has also been considered an independent predictor of survival.[42] However, the results have not been extensively validated, and the lymph node ratio is not currently included in staging. Irregular tumor deposits in the mesocolon or mesorectum without surrounding lymph node tissue, are considered peritumoral tumor deposits; they are not counted as lymph nodes but are classified as N1c, and contribute to stage III.[41] These are considered to represent large vessel or perineural invasion. The significance of micrometastasis detected by immunohistochemistry (usually with anticytokeratin antibodies) in H&E negative nodes of patients with stage II disease is controversial. Although some studies have reported an association between micrometastasis, increased recurrence and reduced survival, the detection of micrometastasis has not been incorporated into clinical practice, and at the present time should be considered investigational.[43]

Table 65.3. American Joint Committee on Cancer (AJCC) TNM Staging Classification for Colorectal Cancer[a]

Definitions for T, N, M

T Primary Tumor	
TX	Primary tumor cannot be assessed
T0	No evidence of primary tumor
Tis	Carcinoma in situ: intramucosal carcinoma (involvement of lamina propria with no extension through muscularis mucosae)
T1	Tumor invades the submucosa (through the muscularis mucosae but not into the muscularis propria)
T2	Tumor invades muscularis propria
T3	Tumor invades through muscularis propria into the pericolorectal tissues
T4	Tumor invades the visceral peritoneum or invades or adheres to adjacent organ or structure
T4a	Tumor invades through the visceral peritoneum (including gross perforation of the bowel through tumor and continuous invasion of tumor through areas of inflammation to the surface of the visceral peritoneum)
T4b	Tumor directly invades or adheres to adjacent organs or structures
N Regional Lymph Nodes	
Nx	Regional lymph nodes cannot be assessed
N0	No regional lymph node metastasis
N1	1–3 regional lymph nodes are positive (tumor in lymph nodes measuring ≥0.2 mm), or any number of tumor deposits are present and all identifiable lymph nodes are negative
N1a	1 regional lymph node is positive
N1b	2–3 regional lymph nodes are positive
N1c	No regional lymph nodes are positive, but there are tumor deposits in the subserosa, mesentery, or nonperitonealized pericolic or perirectal/mesorectal tissues
N2	4 or more regional lymph nodes are positive
N2a	4–6 regional lymph nodes are positive
N2b	7 or more regional lymph nodes are positive
M Distant Metastasis	
M0	No distant metastasis by imaging etc.; no evidence of tumor in distant sites or organs
M1	Metastasis to one or more distant sites or organs or peritoneal metastasis is identified
M1a	Metastasis to one organ or site (eg, liver, lung, ovary, nonregional lymph node) is identified without peritoneal metastasis
M1b	Metastases to two or more sites or organs or metastasis to one organ or site (eg, liver, lung, ovary, nonregional lymph node) is identified without peritoneal metastasis
M1c	Metastasis to the peritoneal surface is identified alone or with other site or organ metastases

Prognostic Groups

Stage	T	N	M
0	Tis	N0	M0
I	T1	N0	M0
	T2	N0	M0
IIA	T3	N0	M0
IIB	T4a	N0	M0
IIC	T4b	N0	M0
IIIA	T1–T2	N1/N1c	M0
	T1	N2a	M0
IIIB	T3–T4a	N1/N1c	M0
	T2–T3	N2a	M0
	T1–T2	N2b	M0
IIIC	T4a	N2a	M0
	T3–T4a	N2b	M0
	T4b	N1-N2	M0
IVA	Any T	Any N	M1a
IVB	Any T	Any N	M1b
IVC	Any T	Any N	M1c

Note: cTNM is the clinical classification, pTNM is the pathologic classification. The y prefix is used for those cancers that are classified after neoadjuvant pretreatment (eg, ypTNM). Pathologic complete response ypT0N0cM0 may be similar to Stage 0 or I. The prefix r is to be used for those cancers that have recurred after disease-free interval (rTNM).

[a]**Disclaimer:** *The [chapter] Content does not reflect the views or interpretations of the American College of Surgeons.*

Table 65.4. Colorectal Cancer Prognostic Factors[a]

Pathologic Features
TNM stage
Total number of nodes examined
Extramural non-nodal tumor deposits
Tumor location
Circumferential resection margin
Local residual disease (R status)
Tumor regression after neoadjuvant therapy
Lymphovascular invasion
Perineural invasion
Histologic type, grade, and presence of mucin
Host immune response (presence of tumor-infiltrating lymphocytes within tumor)
Clinical Features
Preoperative serum CEA levels
Bowel obstruction and/or perforation
Molecular Features
Microsatellite instability
KRAS mutation
BRAF mutation

Used with permission of the American College of Surgeons. The original source for this information is the *AJCC Cancer Staging Manual*. Copyright © 2017 American College of Surgeons.

[a]**Disclaimer:** *The [chapter] Content does not reflect the views or interpretations of the American College of Surgeons.*

The location of the tumor has prognostic implications. In general, patients with right-sided tumors tend to be older, more frequently women, have more advanced histologic grade and more advanced disease stage at diagnosis. Right-sided tumors are more likely to be MSI and have more BRAF mutations. Stage I and II right-sided cancers have better cancer-specific survival compared to left-sided tumors, but stage III and specially stage IV right-sided tumors have worse specific survival compared to left-sided tumors.[44] In patients with rectal cancer, tumors located in the distal rectum have worse prognosis compared with tumors located in the upper rectum.

The quality of the surgery and the completeness of tumor resection also provide important prognostic information. The distance of tumor to the circumferential resection margin (CRM)—defined as the surgically dissected nonperitonealized surface of the specimen—provides important prognostic information in both colon and rectal cancers.[45,46] The CRM is considered positive if tumor is within 1 mm of the resection margin (rather than 0 mm). In rectal cancer patients, involvement of the CRM (ie, the margin created by the surgeon around the rectum and mesorectal fat) occurs most frequently anteriorly, where the mesorectum is at its thinnest. The presence of tumor at the CRM, because of advanced stage or inadequate resection, is associated with a high rate of recurrence and decreased probability of survival.[47]

The AJCC has established codes for completeness of the resection, which should be reported for each procedure.[41] A resection is defined as R0 when the entire tumor is resected and the margins are histologically negative; R1 when the margins are grossly uninvolved but histologically positive; and R2 when the tumor is not completely resected, and there is gross residual tumor at the primary site, regional lymph nodes, or metastatic sites.

Other factors associated with worse outcomes include elevated CEA levels before surgery, high histologic grade, signet ring cell and small cell histopathologic type, lymphatic and blood vessel invasion, and perineural invasion.[41] Vascular invasion is considered a sign of aggressive behavior in CRC and has been associated with a higher risk of disease progression and poor prognosis. Capillary invasion is often associated with lymphatic invasion, and these are commonly designated as lymphovascular invasion. Large vessel invasion, detectable on magnetic resonance imaging (MRI), has been shown to be an adverse risk factor in rectal cancer.[48]

While the TNM staging system provides important prognostic information, it is inadequate for individual prognostication. Outcomes for individual patients within each tumor stage are variable. Recently, nomograms using a number of clinical and pathologic characteristics have been designed to improve prediction and survival beyond TNM staging in patients with colon or rectal cancer, particularly in the setting of stage II tumors (**Fig. 65.5**).[49] In addition to providing prognostic information, nomograms may potentially guide clinical decisions, such as the use of adjuvant chemotherapy or the regularity of surveillance. However, nomograms have not been routine part of clinical decision making.

Several molecular markers such as MSI, 18q loss of heterozygosity, KRAS, and BRAF, among others, have been associated with prognosis in CRC patients. In addition, some of these markers are now used to make treatment decisions, particularly in metastatic CRC. For example, MSI tumors are likely to respond to PD-1 blockade, KRAS wild-type tumors are likely to respond to anti-EGFR therapy, and BRAF V600E mutant tumors are likely to respond to a combination of BRAF, MEK, and EGFR inhibitors.[50–53]

Increasing evidence demonstrates that the evolution of cancer is strongly dependent on the complex tumor microenvironment in which it develops, comprised of a variety of elements including fibroblasts, lymph vessels, and cells of the immune system. The presence of tumor infiltrating lymphocytes (TILs), usually seen in MMRd patients, is associated with good prognosis in patients with CRC, regardless of MMR status.[54] Quantification of lymphocyte populations, in particular CD3- and CD8-positive T cells, has led to the development of a score referred to as Immunoscore, a score highly reproducible across institutions, with increasing score correlating with longer patient survival.[55]

Based on recent advances in the molecular characterization of CRC, several multigene molecular signatures (Oncotype DX, Coloprint, and ColDx) have been designed as prognosticators of recurrence and outcomes. While these molecular signatures seem to determine risk of recurrence independent of other well-established risk factors, they have not been fully incorporated into clinical practice.[56–58]

SCREENING AND PREVENTION

Most CRC develops slowly from a benign polyp to an invasive cancer. This sequence provides a window of opportunity for the detection and removal of premalignant adenomatous polyps and early-stage cancers. Removal of adenomatous polyps reduces the incidence of cancer, and the diagnosis of CRC at earlier stages reduces mortality.[59,60] Several prospective studies have proven that screening for colorectal polyps and cancer using a variety of methods reduces CRC mortality, and the reduction in mortality persists long-term after screening.[61–64] Screening has certainly contributed significantly to the drop in CRC mortality rates over the years. Screening for CRC is cost-effective, in terms of the quality-adjusted life-years gained, compared to nonscreening. In the United States, screening for CRC is recommended for men and women over age 50, although the guidelines are currently changing due to the recent rise in young onset CRC. While overall uptake of CRC screening is improving, it remains relatively low among individuals with lower socioeconomical status and without a usual source of healthcare.[65]

Screening Tests

Numerous screening methods for CRC have been used over the years (**Tables 65.5 and 65.6**). These fall into one of two categories: stool tests, which detect the presence of blood or

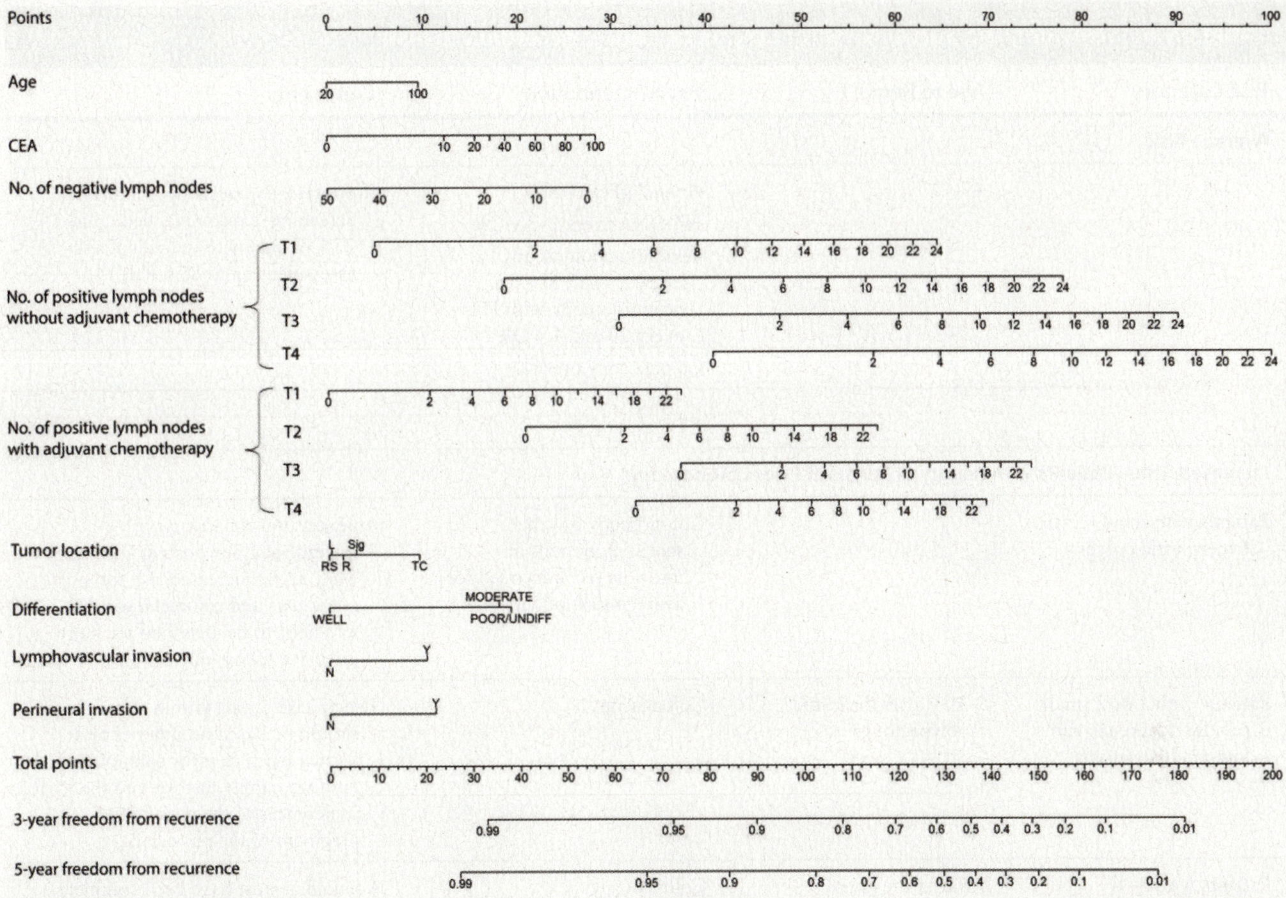

Figure 65.5. Colon cancer nomogram for freedom from recurrence. Locate the patient's preoperative level of carcinoembryonic antigen (in nanograms per milliliter) on the CEA axis. Draw a straight line up to the Points axis to determine how many points toward recurrence the patient should receive. Repeat this process for each of the remaining axes, drawing a straight line each time to the Points axis. Sum the points received from each prognostic variable and locate this number on the Total points axis. Draw a straight line from the total points down to the 3- or 5-year freedom from recurrence axis to ascertain the patient's specific risk of remaining free from recurrence for either 3 or 5 years. CEA, carcinoembryonic antigen; L, left colon; R, right colon; RS, rectosigmoid colon; Sig, sigmoid colon; TC, transverse colon. (Reproduced with permission from Konishi T, Shimada Y, Hsu M, et al. Contemporary validation of a nomogram predicting colon cancer recurrence, revealing all-stage improved outcomes. *JNCI Cancer Spectr*. 2019;3(2):pkz015.)

altered DNA in the stool; and structural tests, which identify polyps and cancers. Efficacy in detecting CRC, cost-effectiveness as a screening tool, supporting evidence, and patient acceptability vary for each of these tests.[66]

Stool Tests

CRCs and polyps bleed more than the normal mucosa and detecting occult blood in the stool is the basis of the most widely used screening tests. Blood is detected by searching the stool for hemoglobin using chemical or immunologic methods; patients found to have blood in the stool should then undergo colonoscopy. The original fecal occult blood tests (FOBTs) relied on guaiac-based detection of the pseudoperoxidase activity of hemoglobin. However, as pseudoperoxidase activity is not specific to human hemoglobin, foods such as red meat can produce false positives. Additionally, medications, such as aspirin and nonsteroidal anti-inflammatory drugs, and foods, such as those rich in vitamin C, should be avoided due to the risk of an inaccurate test. These drugs and foods should be avoided 2 to 3 days prior to the FOBT. As most tumors bleed slowly and intermittently, the sensitivity of this test remains low. Rehydration of the test cards increases sensitivity, at the cost of reducing specificity. The sensitivity of the test increases with the number of samples tested; testing two samples per stool on three consecutive bowel movements is recommended. Several prospective, randomized trials have demonstrated that screening by FOBT, followed by total colonic evaluation with colonoscopy in individuals with a positive test, reduces mortality from CRC.[67–70]

Table 65.5. Tools for Colorectal Cancer Screening

a. Fecal tests—detect primarily cancer
Guaiac-based fecal occult blood test (gFOBT)
Fecal immunochemical test (FIT)
Stool DNA test (sDNA)
b. Structural examinations—detect polyps and colorectal cancer
Flexible sigmoidoscopy (FSIG)
Optical-colonoscopy (OC)
Double–contrast barium enema (DCBE)
Computed tomography colonoscopy (CTC)

Fecal immunochemical tests (FITs) rely on antibodies that are specific to human hemoglobin, and the analysis of samples by automated quantification methods. FITs are as sensitive as the guaiac-based tests, but more specific in detecting human hemoglobin in stool. As this avoids the false-negative results in the presence of vitamin C and false-positive results in the presence of red meat, the test does not require any dietary modification prior. As with any fecal test, a positive result with FIT requires a complete colonoscopic examination. FIT has better screening performance, compared to FOBT.[71–75] As an additional consideration, FIT may be more easily implemented as a screening regimen, compared with sole usage of colonoscopy.[76] Based on this evidence, a number of countries have introduced screening programs utilizing these tools.

Table 65.6. Screening and Surveillance for Colorectal Cancer According to Risk[a]

Risk Category	Age to Begin	Recommendation	Comment
Average Risk			
	45–50	Annual gFOBT/FIT/ FIT-DNA every 1–3 y OR flexible sigmoidoscopy every 5 y OR flexible sigmoidoscopy with FIT every 10 and 1 y OR Colonoscopy every 10 y OR CTC every 5 y	If positive, colonoscopy is indicated. Screening is recommended up to 75 y of age (with individual risk assessment up to 85 y old)
Increased Risk—Patients with History of Polyps at Prior Colonoscopy			
Patients with small rectal hyperplastic polyps	—	Colonoscopy or other screening options at intervals recommended for average-risk individuals	An exception is patients with a hyperplastic polyposis syndrome. They are at increased risk for adenomas and colorectal cancer and need to be identified for more intensive follow-up
Patients with 1 or 2 small tubular adenomas with low-grade dysplasia	5–10 y after the initial polypectomy	Colonoscopy	The precise timing within this interval should be based on other clinical factors (such as prior colonoscopy findings, family history, and the preferences of the patient and judgment of the physician)
Patients with 3–10 adenomas, 1 adenoma ≥1 cm, or any adenoma with villous features or high-grade dysplasia	3 y after the initial polypectomy	Colonoscopy	Adenomas must have been completely removed. If the follow-up colonoscopy is normal or shows only 1 or 2 small tubular adenomas with low-grade dysplasia, then the interval for the subsequent examination should be 5 y (7–10 y for 3–4 small adenomas)
Patients with ≥10 adenomas on a single examination	1 y after the initial polypectomy	Colonoscopy	Consider the possibility of an underlying familial syndrome
Patients with adenomas (≥20 mm) that are removed piecemeal	2–6 mo to verify complete removal	Colonoscopy	Once complete removal has been established, subsequent surveillance needs to be individualized based on the endoscopist's judgment. Completeness of removal should be based on both endoscopic and pathologic assessments
Increased Risk—Patients with Colorectal Cancer			
Patients with colon and rectal cancer should undergo high-quality perioperative clearing	3–6 mo after cancer resection, if no previous colonoscopy, and if no unresectable metastases are found during surgery; alternatively, colonoscopy can be performed intraoperatively	Colonoscopy	In the case of nonobstructing tumors, this can be done by preoperative colonoscopy. In the case of obstructing colon cancers, CTC with intravenous contrast or DCBE can be used to detect neoplasms in the proximal colon

Table 65.6. Screening and Surveillance for Colorectal Cancer According to Risk (*Continued*)

Risk Category	Age to Begin	Recommendation	Comment
Patients undergoing curative resection for colon or rectal cancer	1 y after the resection (or 1 y following the performance of the colonoscopy that was performed to clear the colon of synchronous disease)	Colonoscopy	This colonoscopy at 1 y is in addition to the perioperative colonoscopy for synchronous tumors. If the examination performed at 1 y is normal, then the interval before the next subsequent examination should be 3 y. If that colonoscopy is normal, then the interval before the next subsequent examination should be 5 y. Following the examination at 1 y, the intervals before subsequent examinations may be shortened if there is evidence of HNPCC or if adenoma findings warrant earlier colonoscopy. Periodic examination of the rectum for the purpose of identifying local recurrence, usually performed at 3–6-mo intervals for the first 2 or 3 y, may be considered after low anterior resection of rectal cancer
Increased Risk—Patients with a Family History			
Either colorectal cancer or adenomatous polyps in a first-degree relative before age 60 y or in 2 or more first-degree relatives at any age	Age 40 y, or 10 y before the youngest case in the immediate family	Colonoscopy	Every 5 y
Either colorectal cancer or adenomatous polyps in a first-degree relative age 60 or older or in 2 second-degree relatives with colorectal cancer	Age 40 y. Screening options at intervals recommended for average-risk individuals	Screening options at intervals recommended for average-risk individuals	Screening should be at an earlier age, but individuals may choose to be screened with any recommended form of testing
High Risk			
Genetic diagnosis of FAP or suspected FAP without genetic testing evidence	Age 10–12 y	Annual FSIG to determine if the individual is expressing the genetic abnormality and counseling to consider genetic testing	If the genetic test is positive, colectomy should be considered
Genetic or clinical diagnosis of HNPCC or individuals at increased risk of HNPCC	Age 20–25 y, or 10 y before the youngest case in the immediate family	Colonoscopy every 1–2 y and counseling to consider genetic testing	Genetic testing for HNPCC should be offered to first-degree relatives of persons with a known inherited MMR gene mutation. It should also be offered when the family mutation is not already known, but one of the first three of the modified Bethesda criteria is present
Inflammatory bowel disease, chronic ulcerative colitis, and Crohn colitis	Cancer risk begins to be significant 8 y after the onset of pancolitis or 12–15 y after the onset of left-sided colitis	Colonoscopy with biopsies for dysplasia	Every 1–2 y; these patients are best referred to a center with experience in the surveillance and management of inflammatory bowel disease

[a]Summary estimation of published guidelines.

gFOBT, guaiac-based fecal occult blood test; FIT, fecal immunochemical test; FIT-DNA, multi targeted stool DNA test; CRC, colorectal cancer; CTC, computed tomographic colonography; DCBE, double-contrast barium enema; FAP, familial adenomatous polyposis; FSIG, flexible sigmoidoscopy; HNPCC, hereditary nonpolyposis colon cancer; MMR, mismatch repair.

Detection of altered DNA from exfoliated tumor cells has been investigated as a screening test for CRC for years. Like the detection of hemoglobin, detection of altered DNA triggers patient referral for colonoscopy. Large, prospective studies of this test show fair sensitivity in detecting CRC and low sensitivity in detecting large adenomas, compared with colonoscopy.[77,78] Two recent studies found stool DNA testing sensitivity to be at the high end of the reported FIT range, but at the low end of the typical FIT range for specificity in detecting CRC and advanced precancerous lesions.[79,80] The most recent United States Preventive Task Force (USPTF) guidelines have included stool DNA testing as a screening option; however, they caution about the potential for overly intensive surveillance due to clinician and patient concerns in patients with a negative colonoscopy after an abnormal stool DNA test.[81]

Structural Tests

Two-thirds of CRCs and polyps are in the sigmoid colon and rectum and can be reached with a 60-cm flexible sigmoidoscope. Flexible sigmoidoscopy is safe, fast, does not always require sedation, and allows the biopsy of suspicious lesions. It has a minimal risk of perforation (approximately 1 in 20,000). The effectiveness of flexible sigmoidoscopy as a screening modality requires examination to at least 40 cm from the anal verge. The main limitations of flexible sigmoidoscopy are discomfort which can deter some patients from undergoing future examinations and that it is does not examine the entire colon. However, the presence of distal adenomatous polyps increases the probability of finding additional polyps or cancers in more proximal segments of the large bowel. If an adenomatous polyp is found during flexible sigmoidoscopy, the patient should undergo complete colonoscopy. Due to differences in the distribution of colorectal neoplasia in patients of different age, gender, and racial groups, the efficacy of flexible sigmoidoscopy may vary. Several case-control studies have demonstrated that screening by sigmoidoscopy reduces mortality from CRC by two-thirds in the setting of tumors located within reach of the sigmoidoscope.[82,83] More recently, several prospective studies have demonstrated that screening with flexible sigmoidoscopy reduced CRC incidence and mortality by approximately 25%.[84–86] Furthermore, at least two prospective trials demonstrated a reduction in CRC incidence and mortality with only one flexible sigmoidoscopy screening between 55 and 64 years of age.[86,87] The long-term follow-up of these trials (15 to 17 years) demonstrated sustained reduction in CRC mortality.[88–90] The optimal testing frequency is still controversial. The USPTF currently recommends repeating surveillance every 5 years.[81]

The evidence for combining stool tests (FIT or FOBT) and flexible sigmoidoscopy is mixed. Some studies have shown that the combination of these two screening methods is more effective in detecting colorectal neoplasia than each method used individually, whereas one prospective study looking at flexible sigmoidoscopy with and without FOBT found no benefit in detection, but improvement in CRC mortality.[85,91] This screening strategy may be of benefit to patients who desire direct endoscopic visualization but wish to avoid a full colonoscopy.[81]

Colonoscopy is considered the most accurate test for the early diagnosis and prevention of CRC. It allows direct visualization of the mucosa of the entire colon and rectum, simultaneously allowing the biopsy or removal of suspicious lesions. Colonoscopy is also used to evaluate patients who have tested positive on other screening tests. However, colonoscopy is inconvenient, requires dietary modification and bowel preparation beforehand, is usually performed under conscious sedation, and carries a risk of complications of 1–2 per 1000. Colonoscopy is also more expensive compared to other screening methods. Overall, patient acceptability of colonoscopy seems to be higher compared to other invasive screening methods, and it is now the most used screening method in the United States. There is evidence to suggest that colonoscopy reduces CRC mortality.[91–95] Comparative studies show that colonoscopy is more effective in detecting advanced colonic neoplasia, in both men and women, than a single FOBT combined with sigmoidoscopy. Colonoscopy is more likely to detect preneoplastic polyps, but just as likely to detect invasive CRC as FITs. In addition, colonoscopy provides the protective benefit of screening the proximal colon.[96] Several randomized control trials to assess long-term outcomes of CRC site-specific incidence and mortality for colonoscopy are currently underway.

Computed tomography colonography (CTC), also referred to as virtual colonoscopy, involves thin-section, multidetector, helical CT, and three-dimensional viewing for interpretation.[97] It has largely replaced double-contrast barium enema as it has been shown to be superior.[98,99] A meta-analysis of studies looking at CTC compared to colonoscopy found CTC to have a high sensitivity for adenomas ≥10 mm with somewhat lower sensitivity for adenomas ≥6 mm.[100] Besides the challenge of identifying small lesions, CTC has been shown to be less accurate with flat lesions and sessile serrated polyps.[101,102] CTC obviates some of the drawbacks of colonoscopy, such as the need for sedation and recovery time. However, it still requires standard bowel preparation and gaseous distension of the colon. New methods of tagging and subtracting residual stool are trying to obviate the need for bowel preparation. Furthermore, patients found to have lesions on CTC still require full visualization of the colon with colonoscopy. CTC has downstream consequences including radiation exposure and detection of incidental extracolonic findings that may trigger expensive and, sometimes, unnecessary diagnostic tests.

Risk Categories

Patients with symptoms of CRC should undergo the appropriate diagnostic studies; they are not candidates for screening. Screening recommendations for the general population are based on individual risk assessment. Based on the past medical history and family history of CRC or polyps, individuals are assigned to one of three risk categories, with different screening recommendations (**Table 65.6**).[103] Several different groups provide guidelines for CRC screening including the USPTF, American Cancer Society, United States Multi-Society Task Force, and National Comprehensive Cancer Network.[81,99,104,105]

Average Risk

Most guidelines define average risk as asymptomatic, without family history of CRC or familial CRC syndromes, without personal history of CRC or adenomatous polyps or IBD, and at the age of 50. However, in response to the increase in young onset CRC, the American Cancer Society has recently changed the age to start screening to 45. Furthermore, most recommend cessation of screening at 75 years old, with the option of screening up to 85 years based on comorbidities, life expectancy, and individualized discussion with each patient, as the benefit of early detection of and intervention declines after age 75 years. Acceptable forms of screening include FIT, FOBT, stool DNA testing, flexible sigmoidoscopy, CTC, or colonoscopy. The most recent American Cancer Society and USPTF guidelines do not offer a preferred or ranked order of screening strategies, but rather offer various choices, with the goal to maximize overall screening uptake. Digital rectal examination (DRE) should be performed at the time of sigmoidoscopy or colonoscopy in all individuals. People found to be positive on stool testing, CTC, or flexible sigmoidoscopy should undergo entire colon and rectum examination by colonoscopy.

Increased Risk

Family History

Individuals with a first-degree relative (parent, sibling, or child) with CRC or adenomatous polyps diagnosed before 60 years of age or two first-degree relatives diagnosed at any age should start screening with colonoscopy at 40 years of age or 10 years younger than the earliest diagnosis in their family, whichever comes first. The test should be repeated every 5 years. Individuals with one first-degree relative with CRC or adenomatous polyp diagnosed at 60 years of age or older, or with two or more second-degree relatives (grandparent, grandchild, aunt, uncle, niece, nephew, half-sibling) with CRC or adenomatous polyps at any age, should undergo screening as average-risk individuals—but starting at 40 years of age. Patients with one second-degree relative or one or more third-degree relatives (first cousin) affected are at average risk.

History of Polyps at Previous Colonoscopy

Patients undergoing endoscopic excision of 1 to 2 small (<1 cm) adenomatous polyps should have the entire colon examined at the time of the polypectomy. Colonoscopy should be repeated 7 to 10 years later. If the test is negative, they should then follow the screening recommendations for average risk.[106]

Patients with more than three small adenomas (<10 mm), adenomas with villous features or high-grade dysplasia, or a large adenomatous polyp (>1 cm) who have the entire colon examined at the time of polypectomy, should undergo complete colonoscopy 3 years later—and, if normal, every 5 years thereafter (except in patients with more than three small adenomas—they can go back to 10 years).

A complete colonic examination should be carried out before surgery in any patient undergoing a planned curative resection for CRC. The colonoscopy should be repeated at 1 year to exclude metachronous lesions. If the examination at 1 year is normal, it should be repeated after 3 years, and every 5 years thereafter if the previous one was normal.

Patients with Colorectal Cancer

Patients with colon and rectal cancer should undergo high-quality perioperative clearing of polyps with colonoscopy 3 to 6 months after resection, if not performed before surgery. Surveillance after curative resection is described in detail in Surveillance after Curative Resection for Colon and Rectal Cancer section.

High Risk

This category includes individuals from families diagnosed with hereditary forms of CRC.[107] At-risk members of families with hereditary cancer syndromes should be informed about the benefits and limitations of genetic counseling and genetic testing.

Familial Adenomatous Polyposis

Individuals with a family history of FAP (first-degree relatives of FAP patients) should undergo genetic counseling and screening for FAP between the ages of 10 and 12 years to identify carriers of the *APC* gene mutation. Once the diagnosis of FAP is established, the patient should undergo colectomy, or a yearly colonoscopy until colectomy. Upper gastrointestinal endoscopy should be performed regularly at intervals of 6 months to 4 years based on the extent of the duodenal polyposis. Siblings and children of a patient with FAP should start surveillance by flexible sigmoidoscopy at puberty.

MYH-Associated Polyposis

Depending on the individual, age of presentation, and number and size of polyps, the patient may be advised to undergo a prophylactic colectomy or yearly colonoscopy beginning at 25 years of age. Upper gastrointestinal surveillance should be performed following the guidelines for patients with FAP.

Lynch Syndrome

Individuals from families fitting the Amsterdam criteria for HNPCC should have a colonoscopy at 21 years of age, then every 2 years until 40 years of age, and yearly thereafter. Genetic counseling and testing should be considered.

Consequences of Screening

The full spectrum of clinical consequences of screening, other than the prevention of deaths from CRC, is difficult to predict because every screening strategy initiates a cascade of events, each one with uncertain probability. The rate of false-positive tests, the number of colonoscopies performed, the complications of the screening and diagnostic tests, and the number of patients who may require surveillance because of screening, are complex factors that arise at different times over several decades. However, cost-effectiveness analysis in the United States has demonstrated that screening for CRC in average-risk patients, according to the strategies outlined above, compares favorably with other healthcare interventions such as mammography or treatment of mild hypertension.[108,109] It is important to understand that screening does not completely eliminate the risk of CRC. Up to 9% of CRCs are diagnosed within 6 to 36 months after a screening colonoscopy.[110,111] These interval cancers tend to be preferentially located in the proximal colon. This may be related to failure to reach the proximal colon, residual stool obscuring the view in the proximal colon, or different characteristics of the proximal lesions that makes them more difficult to detect or remove.

Implementation of Guidelines

The general population has limited awareness of the risks of CRC or its symptoms; as a result, the number of individuals participating in screening programs has been low. The dissemination of information to patients is an essential part of the screening program. Primary care physicians have a responsibility to inform their patients about their risk of CRC, the benefits of screening and different screening strategies, and to set up a system for implementing these guidelines.[109,112,113] Through such efforts, the proportion of adults 50 to 75 years of age having colonoscopy has increased steadily over the past decades: from 19.1% in 2000 to 55% in 2010, and to 68.8% in 2018.[114]

DIAGNOSIS

The differential diagnosis of CRC includes diverticulitis, irritable bowel syndrome, inflammatory bowel disease, ischemic colitis, and benign anorectal conditions such as hemorrhoids or rectal mucosal prolapse.

While the proportion of CRCs diagnosed through screening is increasing, most are still diagnosed after patients become symptomatic. CRC can cause a myriad of symptoms, many of which are nonspecific and highly prevalent among healthy individuals. Therefore, the diagnosis of colorectal carcinoma often requires a high index of suspicion.

Symptoms and Signs

The most common symptoms in patients with CRC are abdominal pain, change in bowel habits, rectal bleeding, anemia, anorexia, and weight loss. The clinical manifestations of CRC differ depending on the location and stage of the tumor.

Abdominal pain is nonspecific; it may be localized to any quadrant of the abdomen or may be diffuse. When the pain is persistent and colicky, it is more likely to represent obstructive symptoms resulting from a left-sided lesion. More localized tenderness with signs of localized peritonitis indicates local invasion of the adjacent peritoneum or perforation. It can be difficult to distinguish the pain associated with diverticular disease from that due to a carcinoma in the sigmoid or descending colon. Patients with diverticular disease may also have an underlying carcinoma. Abdominal pain may occasionally be related to extensive metastatic disease in the liver or retroperitoneal lymph nodes. Rectal cancer can also cause perineal discomfort and is often associated with tenesmus, the sensation of incomplete defecation. A locally advanced rectal cancer (LARC) can also cause sacral or sciatic pain.

An unexplained change in bowel habits lasting more than 2 weeks requires investigation for CRC. Constipation associated with colicky abdominal pain is a common manifestation of partially obstructing tumors. Abdominal pain, constipation, and abdominal distension suggest a complete colonic obstruction, which is more common in tumors located in the sigmoid colon and rectum. Some patients with sigmoid or rectal cancer may also complain of diarrhea, which may sometimes be bloody.

Bleeding from tumors in the sigmoid colon and rectum is often wrongly attributed to hemorrhoids or other benign anal conditions. However, blood from hemorrhoids is usually bright red and is accompanied by anal discomfort; the bleeding is intermittent and splashes the toilet pan. Anal fissure is also a common cause of rectal bleeding; the blood is often bright, occurring after defecation, and is typically associated with sharp anal pain triggered by defecation. Painless defecation with rectal blood that is darker in color and mixed in with stool is more likely to be secondary to an underlying carcinoma. Rectal bleeding, particularly when associated with tenesmus, requires a thorough diagnostic investigation to exclude an underlying rectal tumor.

The development of nonspecific anemia of unknown origin is a common manifestation in patients with a carcinoma in the proximal colon. There should be a very high suspicion for CRC in patients with unexplained microcytic anemia. These patients should be examined initially with colonoscopy and not just prescribed iron pills. Anorexia and weight loss frequently accompany CRC and are often associated with advanced disease. The differential diagnosis in these patients is a gastric carcinoma, but when investigations are negative it is important to exclude a large-bowel malignancy. As the bowel lumen is larger and the stools overall looser in the proximal colon, obstructive symptoms are uncommon; therefore, patients with tumors proximal to the splenic flexure often present with advanced disease.

CRC can also be identified incidentally during investigations for other pathologies such as gallstones, gynecologic, or urinary conditions. A complete family history, with emphasis on past history of CRC or polyps, is essential to diagnose some hereditary cancer syndromes. A family history of endometrial, gastric, urologic, or other HNPCC-associated cancers is also important because it may help in diagnosing Lynch II syndrome.

The evaluation of patients suspected of CRC requires a complete physical examination. Features that should arouse suspicion of malignancy include pallor, palpable abdominal mass, and a palpable mass on DRE. Hepatomegaly indicates advanced disease with extensive liver metastases, and consequently a very poor prognosis. A hard mass in the pouch of Douglas felt on DRE may indicate peritoneal carcinomatosis (PC). Other signs of an underlying CRC include pneumaturia, ischiorectal or perineal abscesses, or even deep venous thrombosis.

Diagnostic Evaluation

Patients with symptoms suggesting CRC should have a colonoscopy to evaluate the entire colon (**Fig. 65.6**). The examination should be complete, as up to 4% of patients with CRC have synchronous cancers and many more have colorectal polyps.[115,116] Up to one-third of these synchronous cancers are in locations requiring a different surgical resection, further emphasizing the importance of complete colonoscopy. As many patients undergo minimally invasive surgery (MIS), the endoscopist should mark the vicinity of the tumor with India ink to help locate the lesion intraoperatively. CT colonography and DCBE are less effective in investigating patients with symptoms suggestive of CRC, but they are useful in patients with partially obstructive tumors, in whom colonoscopy cannot be completed. In patients with obstructive lesions, the proximal colon can be examined either by preoperative imaging studies such as PET-CT, or intraoperatively by direct palpation of the colon. In any case, patients with a complete colonoscopy before surgery should have a surveillance colonoscopy 6 months after surgery.

Staging of the disease after diagnosis is important as it informs treatment decisions. A CT scan of the chest, abdomen, and pelvis with intravenous and oral contrast is important in

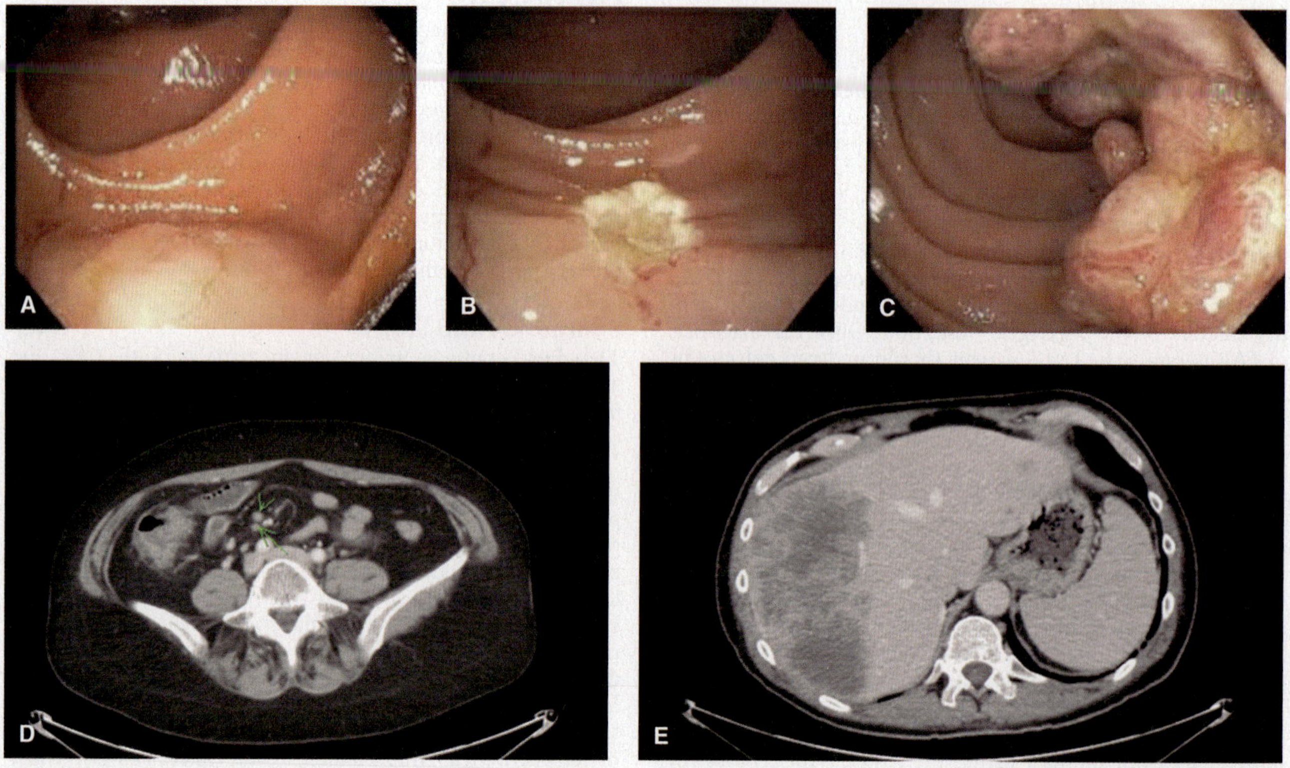

Figure 65.6. Staging modalities for colorectal cancer. **A:** Sessile polyp. **B:** Polyp removed at colonoscopy with hot snare technique. **C:** Sigmoid colon cancer at colonoscopy. **D:** Circumferential ascending colon tumor with regional lymphadenopathy (*arrowheads*). **E:** Liver metastases of colorectal origin.

3 order to locate the tumor, detect mesentericnodes, and exclude liver metastasis and gross PC (**Fig. 65.6**). In addition, preoperative imaging helps the surgeon plan the resection. In patients with iodine allergy, and in patients with undetermined lesions on CT, a PET-CT, or an abdominopelvic MRI may provide additional information. Pelvic MRI, and less often rectal ultrasound, is increasingly being used for staging of rectal cancer.

Laboratory evaluation includes complete blood cell count, coagulation parameters, and chemistry panel. Preoperative CEA should be measured because it provides prognostic information and can be useful during patient surveillance.

TREATMENT

Surgery is the primary treatment for CRC, but surgery is not the initial form of treatment for many patients and some individuals do not require surgery at all. As data emerge, there is an increasing tendency to adopt a "watch-and-wait" approach in the treatment for rectal cancer. Treatment is different for colon than for rectal cancer and depends also on the clinical stage of the tumor. Treatment decisions must also consider the patient's performance status, comorbidities, hereditary CRC predisposition, as well as desires and expectations.

Preoperative Preparation

Appropriate perioperative assessment and preparation are very important to minimize perioperative complications. Surgical site infection (SSI) is the most common complication after colon and rectal cancer resection, occurring in 4% to 26% of cases.[117,118] In addition to causing patient suffering, SSIs lengthen hospital stay and increase costs.[119] The institutional rate of SSI after colorectal surgery is now an important quality metric for several benchmarking programs. Several federal and state-wide initiatives aimed at improving surgical care recommend implementing measures to reduce the rate of SSI and other complications in patients undergoing elective colorectal surgery.[120,121]

The necessity for bowel preparation prior to surgery has been debated for decades. The colon has the largest concentration of bacteria in the human body. A gram of feces contains 10^{11} polymicrobial bacteria, mostly gram negatives and anaerobes.[122] Oral mechanical bowel preparation using polyethylene glycol to reduce the bacterial load and risk of intraoperative fecal spillage has been considered an axiom in colon and rectal surgery. However, a number of prospective trials have failed to demonstrate benefit from mechanical bowel cleansing in preventing SSIs.[123,124] Combination of mechanical bowel preparation with oral antibiotics, usually neomycin and erythromycin, may be more effective than mechanical bowel preparation alone. A large retrospective study of more than 27,000 patients undergoing elective colorectal resection compared the use mechanical bowel preparation with and without oral antibiotics, oral antibiotics alone, or no preparation. Dual preparation was associated with lower rates of SSI, organ space infection, wound dehiscence and anastomotic leak compared to no preparation, and lower rates of SSI than antibiotic bowel preparation alone. Dual preparation was not associated with an increased risk of *Clostridium difficile* infection.[125]

High-quality evidence indicates that antibiotics covering aerobic and anaerobic bacteria, delivered orally or intravenously (or both) prior to elective colorectal surgery, reduce the risk of postoperative surgical wound infection by as much as 66%.[126] For patients without penicillin allergy, a second-generation cephalosporin (cefotetan or cefoxitin) is often administered intravenously within 30 minutes of the surgical incision, with redosing during the procedure as required according to the half-life of the drug and the duration of surgery. For penicillin-allergic patients, metronidazole or clindamycin combined with either ciprofloxacin or gentamicin is acceptable, as are aztreonam and fluoroquinolones.[127] Ertapenem, a long-acting carbapenem active against gram negatives and anaerobes, is an accepted alternative to second-generation cephalosporins for prophylaxis in CRC. Ertapenem has a long life and does not require redosing in prolonged procedures but has been associated with increasing risk of *C. difficile* infection.[128] Other measures that prevent SSI include tight glucose control in diabetic patients, smoking cessation, clipping rather than shaving the skin of the abdominal wall, and maintaining normothermia and adequate oxygenation during anesthesia.[129]

Patients undergoing surgery for CRC are also at risk of venous thromboembolism (VTE) and should have thromboembolic prophylaxis with unfractionated heparin or low–molecular-weight heparin during the peri- and postoperative periods.[130] The American Society of Clinical Oncology (ASCO) has published evidence-based clinical practice guidelines which include the recommendation for prophylaxis starting before surgery and continuing for at least 7 to 10 days following surgery. Extended prophylaxis for up to 4 weeks following surgery should be given to patients undergoing major abdominal and pelvic surgery.[131]

An evaluation of patient comorbidities and performance status should be made prior to surgery. Some patients should to be referred to their primary care provider and their modifiable risk factors optimized before surgery. Comorbidities can impact decision-making and affect short- and long-term outcomes. Fertility options should be discussed with all individuals of child-bearing potential.

Patients who may require a stoma should be seen before surgery by an enterostomal therapist. Adequate marking of the site improves outcomes for patients requiring a stoma. Preoperative teaching shortens the time patients require to become proficient managing the stoma, and reduces hospital stay.[132]

The Enhanced Recovery After Surgery (ERAS) protocols were introduced in open colorectal surgery in the 1990s, with the aim of speeding patient recovery, improving patient outcomes and satisfaction, shortening hospitalization, and reducing healthcare costs.[133] ERAS protocols span the entire perioperative period, and attempt to minimize surgical stress and postoperative ileus through patient education, preoperative hydration and carbohydrate loading, goal-directed intraoperative fluid management, narcotic sparing for intraoperative and postoperative pain control, and early mobilization and oral feeding in the postoperative period. A number of prospective trials have indicated that the implementation of ERAS protocols reduces length of hospital stay, compared to conventional recovery in patients undergoing open or minimally invasive surgery for CRC.[134,135] A recent systematic review and a meta-analysis confirmed that ERAS protocols resulted in a shorter length of stay (LOS) and a reduction in overall complications, with no difference in mortality and surgical complications.[136,137] Similar results have recently been reported from an international registry.[138]

Principles of Surgical Treatment

The goal for any curative-intent surgery is to remove the tumor-bearing segment of the bowel with adequate margins, along with en bloc excision of the mesentery containing the feeding vessels and regional lymph nodes. The location of the primary tumor determines lymphatic drainage and dictates the extent of the resection. Lymphatic capillaries are primarily located in the submucosal and subserosal layers of the bowel wall. The lymphatic flow in the colon is primarily circumferential, with longitudinal spread along the bowel wall thought to be less than 1 cm in each direction. Therefore, a 5-cm margin of normal bowel on either side of the primary tumor is considered sufficient to avoid anastomotic recurrence. The length of the terminal ileum resected in patients with right colon cancer does not influence the risk of anastomotic recurrence. In the rectum, where the longitudinal lymphatic flow is primarily upward, cancer cells rarely spread distally along the bowel wall farther than 1 cm from the macroscopic distal end of the tumor. Consequently, a 2-cm margin of normal bowel distal

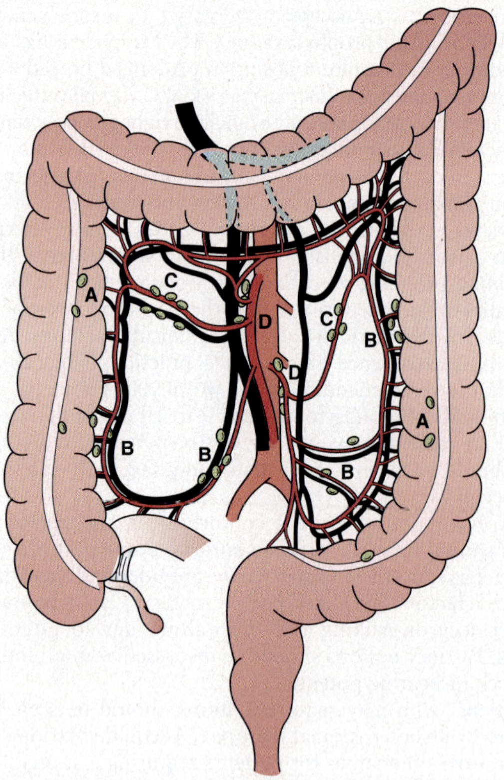

Figure 65.7. Anatomy of the colon. *A*, Epicolic lymph nodes. *B*, Paracolic lymph nodes. C, Intermediate lymph nodes. *D*, Apical-central lymph nodes.

to the tumor, or even less in patients treated with neoadjuvant therapy, is considered appropriate to an oncologically safe resection.[139]

The lymphatic channels in the bowel wall drain to the regional nodes, which are classified in different groups according to their proximity to the bowel and its blood supply (**Fig. 65.7**). The "epicolic" nodes are in the bowel wall under the peritoneum, usually close to the epiploic appendices. The "paracolic" lymph nodes are located along the marginal vessels. Next, the "intermediate" nodes are positioned in the middle of the mesentery. Finally, the "central" or "apical" lymph nodes are located close to the root of the mesentery, near the origin of the named vessels. While CRC generally spreads sequentially from the paracolic to the central or apical lymph nodes, nodal metastases skipping one of the groups are common.[140]

The extent of the mesenteric resection is determined by the need to remove all the lymph nodes draining the corresponding segment of bowel, including the central lymph nodes located at the origin of the named feeding blood vessels. As most tumors are located between two named vascular pedicles, both of these should be resected at their origin. When suspected of being involved by tumor, the central nodes should be marked on the specimen, as they have negative prognostic information. Other lymph nodes located away from the feeding vessels and suspected of tumor involvement during surgery, should be removed and analyzed, because in some patients the lymphatic drainage does not follow an orderly pattern.[141,142] If residual metastatic lymph nodes remain after sampling, the resection should be considered incomplete.

While achieving safe oncologic margins and adequate lymphadenectomy are the main considerations when performing a surgical resection for CRC, ensuring an adequate blood supply to the bowel ends, and maintaining tension-free anastomosis, are also important in order to avoid anastomotic complications.

Locally advanced tumors attached to other organs should be removed en bloc with contiguously involved structures. As it is impossible to distinguish clinically or radiographically between inflammatory adhesions and tumor infiltration, it is preferable to perform an en bloc resection of any organ attached to the primary tumor, rather than spilling cancer cells by separating structures infiltrated by tumor. Intraoperative tumor perforation has negative prognostic implications. It is important to report the completeness of the resection (R0, R1, or R2), combining clinical and pathologic information, to determine risk of locoregional recurrence (LRR) and long-term prognosis.

The concept of the no-touch technique, with initial control of the vascular supply before manipulation of the tumor to avoid releasing cancer cells into the blood stream, has not been shown to be associated with improved outcomes.[143] However, early vascular control with medial-to-lateral dissection of the mesentery, before mobilization of the colon, is the preferred approach during minimally invasive colorectal surgery, because it helps identify all vascular and retroperitoneal structures.

Proper surgical technique is crucial in achieving optimal results in CRC patients. The removal of the rectum along with its mesorectal envelope, using sharp dissection along normal anatomical planes—an operation called total mesorectal excision (TME), or TME—is associated with a reduced risk of local tumor recurrence.[144,145] Conversely, application of the same surgical principles to colon cancer, including the removal of all the lymph node-bearing mesentery to the origin of the named blood vessels—an operation called complete mesocolic excision or CME—has not been universally adopted due to conflicting evidence of the association of CME with improved survival and concern for higher complication rates in CME.[146–148] Published studies on CME are difficult to evaluate and compare because of inconsistent definitions, unclear description of the extent of dissection, and absence of randomization.[149] Often, the radicality of resection is self-reported by the surgeons. Confirmation of correct extent of resection should be validated by pathologists.[150] Prospective clinical trials should provide more conclusive evidence to the efficacy of CME.

TREATMENT OF LOCALIZED COLON CANCER

Malignant Colonic Polyps

Malignant polyps are classified based on the level of tumor invasion. The identification of a focus of invasive carcinoma in a polyp removed by snare excision during colonoscopy represents a surgical dilemma. These types of polyps are often referred to as "malignant polyps," to distinguish them from lesions that are almost exclusively invasive adenocarcinoma with exophytic or polypoid morphology. Malignant polyps are now encountered more often because tumors are diagnosed at an earlier stage, as a result of screening programs. Although there are some lymphatic channels in the lamina propria, tumors superficial to the muscularis mucosa (also known as intramucosal carcinoma, carcinoma in situ, or Tis) are considered to carry no risk of lymph node metastasis. When the malignant cells penetrate beyond the muscularis mucosa they can access the lymphatic channels of the submucosa and metastasize to the regional lymph nodes. This risk of nodal metastasis depends on the morphology of the polyp, the depth of the invasive component, the presence of unfavorable histologic features (grade 3 or 4, lymphovascular invasion, perineural invasion) and the margin of resection.[151] Imaging studies are usually of no help in these patients, except to exclude DMs (which are uncommon). In pedunculated polyps with focus of invasive cancer located in the head, neck, or stalk of the polyp, with favorable histologic features, resected with negative margins, the risk of nodal metastasis is small (**Fig. 65.8**). In these circumstances additional surgery is considered unnecessary, as the risk of surgery may outweigh the risk of residual tumor in the bowel wall or nodal metastasis.

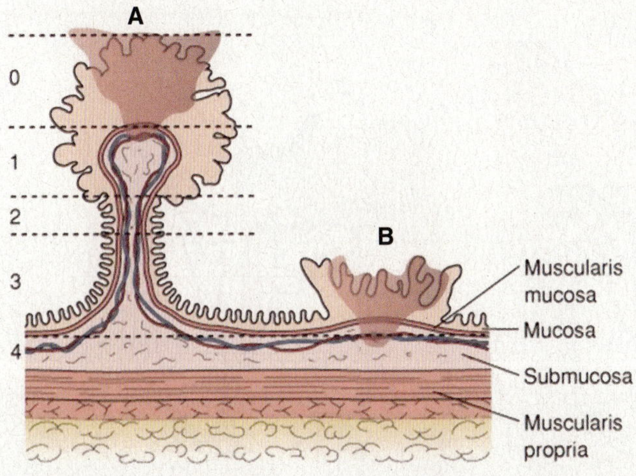

Figure 65.8. Malignant polyp. Haggitt levels of invasion. Level 0, Noninvasive, severe dysplasia; Level 1, Invading through muscularis mucosa but limited to the head of pedunculated polyp; Level 2, Invading the neck of pedunculated polyp; Level 3, Invading the stalk of pedunculated polyp; Level 4, Invading into submucosa of the bowel wall below the stalk of a pedunculated polyp and all sessile polyps.

On the other hand, patients with pedunculated polyps with focus of invasive adenocarcinoma reaching the base of the polyp, sessile polyps with focus of invasive adenocarcinoma, the presence of adenocarcinoma at the resection margin, and malignant polyps with unfavorable histologic features, are at risk of regional nodal metastasis, and should be offered surgical resection.[152,153] Other factors such as the location of the polyp in the colon or rectum, the patient's comorbidities and performance status, and the patient's desires, should be taken into consideration.[154] Therefore, a final decision should only be made after full review of the pathology reports, and disclosure to the patient of the risks and benefits of each approach.

Surgery for Localized Colon Cancer

Patients with biopsy-proven adenocarcinoma of the colon without evidence of DM, and without contraindications to major surgery, should be treated with surgical resection. The extent of a colon cancer resection is dictated by the location of the primary tumor. Tumors in the cecum and ascending colon require a right hemicolectomy that implies division of the ileocolic, right colic (if present), and the right branch of the middle colic vessels (**Fig. 65.9**). The portion of the omentum attached to the removed segment of colon should be resected en bloc with the colon and mesentery. Tumors located at the hepatic flexure and in the right side of the transverse colon require an extended right colectomy that, in addition to the ileocolic and right colic vessels, requires division of the middle colic vessels at their origin (**Fig. 65.9**). Tumors in the mid portion of the transverse colon can be treated with an extended right colectomy, or a transverse colectomy. A transverse colectomy involves division of the middle colic vessels only but often requires mobilization of both the hepatic and splenic flexure to ensure a tension-free anastomosis (**Fig. 65.9**). Tumors located in the distal transverse colon, splenic flexure, and proximal descending colon can be treated with a left hemicolectomy, which requires division of the left branch of the middle colic and left colic artery at its branch point from the inferior mesenteric artery (**Fig. 65.9**). Locally advanced tumors located in the transverse colon can metastasize to the regional lymph nodes located along the greater omentum and gastroepiploic arcades, leading some surgeons to recommend removal of the omentum with the gastroepiploic arcade. In these patients, an omentectomy with division of the gastroepiploic vessels at their origin may be necessary for complete nodal control.[155] However, the benefit of such an extended lymphadenectomy is debated. Sigmoid tumors require sigmoid colectomy, which includes the superior rectal artery and its takeoff from the inferior mesenteric artery (**Fig. 65.9**).

Patients with synchronous tumors, which occur in up to 5.3% of patients with CRC, should be investigated for hereditary CRC syndromes or other predisposing conditions. Patients with sporadic synchronous cancers can be treated with separate resections, or an extended resection incorporating both lesions, depending on the location of the primaries.[156] When performing a segmental resection, it is important to preserve the blood supply to the intermediate segment of colon in order to avoid ischemia, which can lead to perioperative complications. A subtotal or total colectomy should be considered for HNPCC patients with synchronous tumors or other risk factors as inflammatory bowel disease.

The COST trial and several other well-conducted prospective trials have proved that laparoscopic colectomy for cancer is associated with short-term benefits and equivalent long-term oncologic outcomes, compared with the traditional open surgical approach.[157] Patients treated laparoscopically have less postoperative pain, earlier return of bowel function, shorter hospital stay, and a decreased rate of complications. However, laparoscopic surgery is technically challenging and has a long learning curve. Laparoscopy may be particularly difficult in patients with multiple adhesions from previous surgery, in obese patients, and in patients with locally advanced disease. Late conversion from laparoscopic to open surgery (also known as reactive conversion) is associated with higher complication rates compared to open surgery, while early or preemptive conversion is associated with complication rates similar to open surgery.[158]

The introduction of robotic platforms, which enhance the visualization and dexterity of the surgeon, has added a new dimension to minimally invasive colon cancer surgery. The evidence accumulated so far indicates that robotic colon resection is associated with lower conversion rates, similar complication rates, and higher costs, compared to conventional laparoscopic colon resection.[159]

Postoperative Adjuvant Therapy for Localized Colon Cancer

Certain patients with what appears to be localized colon cancer at the time of diagnosis develop recurrence after a curative-intent surgery. These recurrences could be attributed to micrometastases that are already present, but clinically undetectable, at the time of diagnosis, or inadequate surgical technique. Postoperative adjuvant chemotherapy aims to improve survival by eradicating micrometastatic disease. Numerous chemotherapeutic agents are now considered for adjuvant therapy, mostly based on their efficacy as observed in the setting of metastatic colon cancer. However, the mainstays of adjuvant therapy following resection of localized colon cancer remain fluoropyrimidines (5-fluorouracil [5-FU] and capecitabine) and oxaliplatin.

5-FU, a member of the family of antimetabolites, is a pyrimidine analog that works by irreversible inhibition of thymidylate synthase (TS), the rate-limiting enzyme in pyrimidine nucleotide synthesis, and by incorporation of its metabolites into RNA and DNA. 5-FU can only be delivered intravenously and is commonly administered with leucovorin, a reduced folate that is thought to stabilize fluorouracil's interaction with the enzyme TS. Capecitabine is an oral prodrug of fluorouracil that is absorbed intact through the gastrointestinal mucosa and undergoes enzymatic conversion to fluorouracil. Response rates to fluoropyrimidine, as first-line therapy alone for metastatic CRC, are only around 10% to 20%. Neutropenia, stomatitis, and diarrhea are the most common side effects of 5-FU. The toxicity profile for capecitabine is similar to 5-FU, with hand-foot syndrome being more frequent. Oxaliplatin produces cytotoxic effects by forming both inter- and intrastrand cross links leading to disruption of DNA replication and apoptosis. As a single agent, oxaliplatin has limited effect

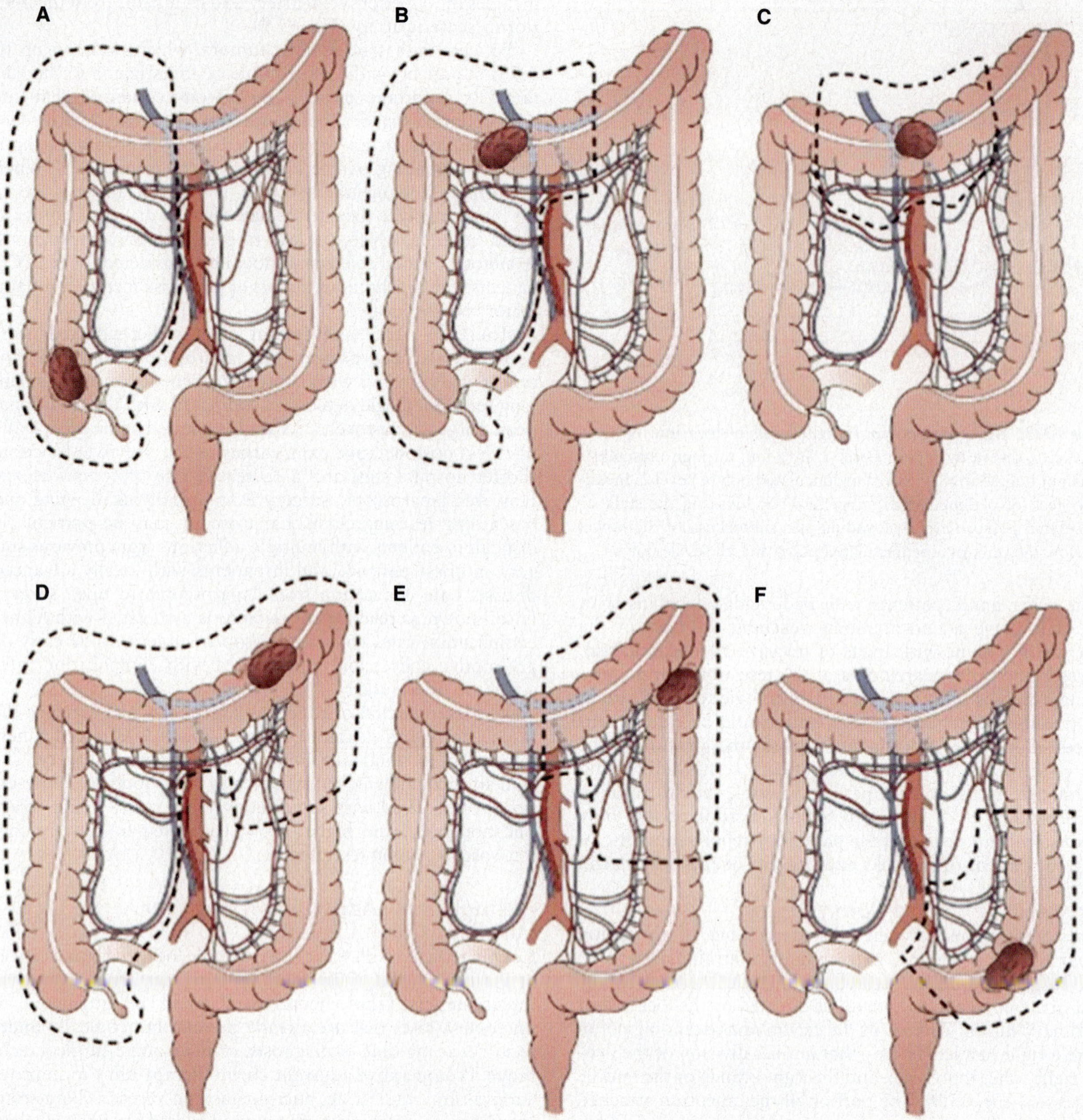

Figure 65.9. Segmental colonic resections. A: Right colectomy. B: Extended right colectomy to transverse colon. C: Transversectomy. D: Right colectomy extended to splenic flexure. E: Left colectomy. F: Sigmoidectomy.

in CRC; but in combination it enhances the cytotoxic effect of fluoropyrimidines, possibly through downregulation of TS. The most relevant side effect of oxaliplatin is a progressive and often irreversible peripheral neuropathy. Other chemotherapy agents commonly used in patients with metastatic CRC have not shown proven benefit in the adjuvant setting.

The use of adjuvant therapy for stage III colon cancer was first shown to provide measurable benefit in the National Cancer Institute (NCI) Cooperative Intergroup trial INT-0035. Patients who received 5-FU and levamisole for 1 year after surgical resection had a 33% risk reduction in death or recurrence, compared to those who underwent surgery alone.[160,161] Since then, we have come to recognize that levamisole is overall an inactive agent; therapeutic combinations have evolved and have been tested rigorously.[162] A number of multi-institutional prospective, randomized trials have demonstrated a survival advantage with postoperative chemotherapy in selected patients after curative-intent surgery, compared to surgery alone. Pooled analyses of these trials have reported an approximately 30% reduction in recurrence, and 26% improvement in survival, in patients with stage III colon cancers treated with 6 months of postoperative fluoropyrimidine-based chemotherapy.[163,164] More recently, the landmark MOSAIC (Multicenter International Study of oxaliplatin, fluorouracil, and leucovorin in the Adjuvant Treatment of Colon Cancer) trial, which randomized 2246 stage II/III colon cancer patients to 5-FU/leucovorin with or without oxaliplatin, reported an additional 20% reduction in recurrence and 5% improvement in 5-year disease-free survival (DFS; 73.3% vs 67.4%; $p = .003$) in patients treated with 5-FU/leucovorin plus oxaliplatin, compared to 5-FU/leucovorin alone.[165,166] Based on these results, the current recommendation for patients with stage III colon cancer following curative-intent surgery consists of 6 months of 5-FU/leucovorin and oxaliplatin (FOLFOX), or capecitabine and oxaliplatin (CAPEOX).

Investigation into adjuvant therapy for stage III colon cancer was conducted in the scope of the International Duration Evaluation of Adjuvant Chemotherapy (IDEA) collaboration;

it included six different prospective trials conducted in different countries, and randomized patients after curative resection to either 6 months, or 3 months of postoperative fluoropyrimidine- and oxaliplatin-based adjuvant chemotherapy. An expert panel interpretation of the results recommends 6 months of postoperative adjuvant chemotherapy for patients at high risk of recurrence (T4 or N2). For low-risk patients (T1–3/N1), 3 or 6 months of adjuvant chemotherapy is considered equivalent. Based on these results, a shared decision-making approach between the patient and the provider is recommended when deciding duration of adjuvant chemotherapy in patients with resected stage III colon cancer, taking into consideration the patient's comorbidities and performance status, the completeness of the surgical resection, the number of lymph node retrieved, and the histopathologic characteristics of the tumor.[167]

Several studies have proven that the addition of irinotecan—a topoisomerase I inhibitor that is effective in metastatic CRC—to standard fluoropyrimidines is not superior to fluorouracil/leucovorin combinations alone in stage III colon cancers.[168] Similarly, bevacizumab (anti–VEGF-A) and cetuximab (anti-EGFR), two biologic agents that have shown efficacy in metastatic disease, do not improve survival, compared to FOLFOX alone.[169–171] Therefore, at the present time irinotecan, bevacizumab, and cetuximab are not recommended in the adjuvant treatment of nonmetastatic CRC.

The use of adjuvant chemotherapy after curative resection for stage II CRC has been controversial for more than a decade. Three prospective, randomized trials have addressed the subject using 5-FU–based regimens, all of them failing to show a clear benefit of adjuvant treatment over observation alone.[161,172,173] The addition of oxaliplatin to the adjuvant regimen does not seem to improve the results of pyrimidine-based regimens for stage II. Most of the evidence for adjuvant treatment in stage II CRC comes from pooled analyses, in which stage II and III CRC patients, undergoing different chemotherapy regimens and controls, are analyzed. The most influential study, including 37 trials and 11 meta-analyses, found a significant improvement in DFS for 5% to 10%, favoring adjuvant chemotherapy; nevertheless, no difference in OS was observed.[174] Therefore, postoperative adjuvant chemotherapy is still not routinely recommended after curative resection for stage II CRC. However, there is evidence that some node-negative patients at high risk for recurrence may benefit from postoperative adjuvant chemotherapy. Determining which patients are at high risk has most commonly included consideration of features such as tumor perforation, T4 category tumors, poorly differentiated histology, lymphovascular or perineural invasion, and patients with fewer than 12 nodes in the surgical specimen (who are considered inadequately staged).[175] At the present time, the use of adjuvant therapy for stage II disease ought to be weighed carefully by a multidisciplinary team, with adequate counseling of the patient. As mentioned earlier, some predictive nomograms may help stratify risk in patients with stage II disease, enabling us to more effectively select those more likely to benefit from adjuvant therapy; however, these tools have not been widely incorporated into clinical practice.

The search for molecular prognosticators aimed at stratifying stage II patients according to the risk of relapse, is an active area of research. MMR deficiency has been associated with an improved prognosis, but a decreased benefit from fluoropyrimidine-based adjuvant therapies, in patients with stage II disease.[31] Because of this, MMR/MSI testing is recommended for patients with stage II disease. Current guidelines recommend no use of single-agent fluoropyrimidine treatment for patients with stage II tumors exhibiting MSI or MMR deficiency. The discovery that ICIs are effective in MMRd CRC has revolutionized the treatment of locally recurrent and metastatic MMRd CRC.[176,177] Immune checkpoint blockade is currently not recommended in nonmetastatic MMRd CRC, but clinical trials are investigating the efficacy of ICI in nonmetastatic dMMR/MSI CRC.[178] The multigene molecular signatures discussed previously were developed, in large part, to stratify risk in patients with stage II CRC, and to identify those most likely to benefit from adjuvant chemotherapy.[56–58] While initial results are promising, there is insufficient evidence to recommend their use in selecting adjuvant therapy for patients with stage II CRC.

TREATMENT OF LOCALIZED RECTAL CANCER

The treatment of rectal cancer is challenging compared with colon cancer. Given the location of the rectum within the narrow bony pelvis surrounded by the urogenital organs, large blood vessels, and autonomic nerves, and its proximity to the anal sphincters, rectal cancer surgery is technically challenging, potentially associated with perioperative complications, and often followed by loss of urinary, sexual, and bowel function that permanently impairs quality of life. In addition, rectal cancer has been associated with a higher rate of local recurrence after curative-intent surgery, compared to colon cancer. But the extraperitoneal location of most of the rectum and its proximity to the anal orifice make it accessible to explorations (DRE, endorectal ultrasound [ERUS]) and interventions (external-beam radiation therapy [RT], brachytherapy, and local excision [LE]) not currently available for colon cancer.

The selection of the best treatment option for each rectal cancer patient is a complex process and requires consideration of the clinical tumor stage, location of the tumor within the rectum, the impact of treatment upon anorectal and genitourinary function, and the consequences for the patient in terms of prognosis and quality of life. Some rectal cancers can be treated with LE. Others require a TME, with or without sphincter preservation. Finally, many rectal cancer patients require chemotherapy and radiation to reduce the risk of local recurrence and DM.

Anatomy of the Rectum

The rectum represents the distal portion of the large bowel, extending from the rectosigmoid junction—the area where the tenia coli (characteristic of the sigmoid colon) splay and become the longitudinal muscular layer of the rectum—to the anorectal ring, a palpable anatomical landmark that corresponds to the imprint of the puborectalis muscle on the bowel wall. The anal canal extends from the anorectal ring to the anal verge, the palpable groove between the distal edge of the internal sphincter and the subcutaneous portion of the external sphincter (**Fig. 65.10**). For practical purposes and standardization, the rectum is defined in terms of distance in centimeters from the anal verge. The distance of a tumor from the anal verge is best measured using a rigid proctoscope, which allows the simultaneous visualization of the anal verge and the centimeter marks on the outside of the scope. In European countries, tumors with the distal edge located within the last 15 cm of the large bowel are considered rectal cancers; in the United States, the limit is 12 cm. The location of tumor in relation to the peritoneal reflection and the sacral promontory, and its distance from the anal verge, can also be determined by MRI, particularly in sagittal views.

The mesorectum is the visceral mesentery of the rectum containing the terminal branches of the superior rectal vessels and the rectum's lymphatic drainage. The upper portion of the rectum, located above the anterior peritoneal reflection, is covered with peritoneum in the front and on both sides. In this upper portion of the rectum, the mesorectum which is a continuation of the mesentery of the sigmoid colon, covers the rectum only posteriorly and is attached to the concavity of the sacrum. Below the peritoneal reflection the rectum is completely extraperitoneal and fully surrounded by the mesorectum. The mesorectum is covered by a thin, glistening membrane called the mesorectal fascia (MRF). Posteriorly,

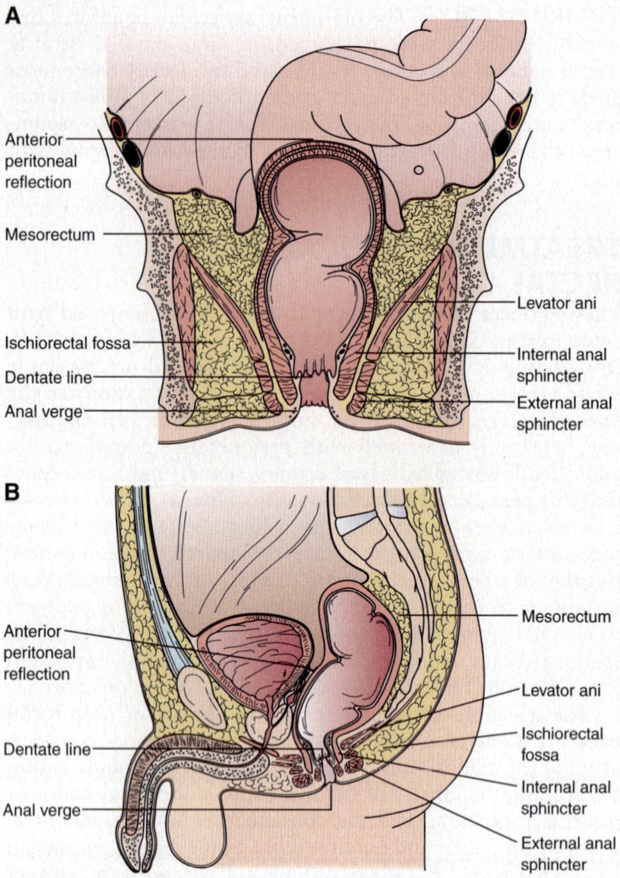

Figure 65.10. Anatomy of the rectum. **A:** Coronal pelvis. **B:** Sagittal pelvis.

the mesorectum is separated from the presacral fascia by an avascular plane of loose areolar tissue that is the natural plane of dissection during a radical proctectomy. Anteriorly, the mesorectum is separated from the urogenital organs by a remnant of the fusion of two layers of the embryologic peritoneal cul-de-sac known as Denonvilliers fascia—an important anatomical landmark in rectal cancer surgery. Below the peritoneal reflection, the lateral rectal ligaments or "lateral stalks" connect the mesorectum to the pelvic sidewall. The mesorectum tapers off distally as the rectum funnels toward the anorectal ring, where the longitudinal layer of the muscularis propria becomes the internal anal sphincter.

The blood supply of the rectum comes primarily from the superior rectal artery, which is the terminal branch of the inferior mesenteric artery after it gives off the left colic artery. The superior rectal vein has a parallel course to its homonymous artery and joins the left colic vein to form the inferior mesenteric vein draining into the splenic vein. The lower portion of the rectum and the anal canal also receive blood supply from the internal iliac vessels through the middle rectal artery, an inconsistent branch of the inferior vesical artery. The inferior rectal artery is a branch of the pudendal artery. The middle and inferior rectal vessels anastomose with the upper rectal vessels, supplying enough blood to the entire rectum. As in other locations, the middle and inferior rectal veins follow the course of the homonymous arteries, draining into systemic circulation through the internal iliac veins.

The anatomy of the autonomic pelvic nerve system is very important when operating in the rectum, because of its proximity to the plane of dissection during different parts of the operation. Damage to these nerves can result in urinary and/or sexual dysfunction. The hypogastric plexus, located in front of the aorta, contains predominantly preganglionic sympathetic fibers originating from the lumbar sympathetic trunk. The fibers of the hypogastric plexus converge at the level of the aortic bifurcation into well-defined hypogastric nerves, which course laterally and anteriorly over the internal iliac vessels toward the lateral pelvic sidewall. There they join the splanchnic pelvic nerves, containing primarily postganglionic parasympathetic fibers from the anterior rami of S2, S3, and S4, to form the pelvic plexus. Branches of the pelvic plexus provide innervation to the distal ureter, the vas deferens, the seminal vesicles, urinary bladder, and prostate. Branches of the pelvic plexus also provide innervation to the distal rectum, passing through the lateral stalks. Finally, distal to the lateral stalks, the distal pelvic plexus forms the urogenital neurovascular bundles that pass close to the posterolateral aspect of the seminal vesicles or the vagina, extending toward the apex of the prostate and the neck of the bladder.

Clinical Staging of Rectal Cancer

The preoperative evaluation of the rectal cancer patient follows the same principles as that of the colon cancer patient, but the wider spectrum of therapeutic options for rectal cancer patients requires accurate information about the location and stage of the tumor. The clinical stage is important in making treatment decisions, such as the intent of the treatment (palliative or curative), the need for neoadjuvant therapy, or even the extent of the surgery (LE vs TME).

Patients with rectal cancer should undergo a complete colonoscopy because synchronous polyps are present in up to 30% of patients, and synchronous cancers in up to 5.3% of patients. They also require a CT scan of the chest, abdomen, and pelvis to exclude DM, which is present in 20% of patients at the time of diagnosis.

The preoperative locoregional staging of rectal cancer follows the clinical TNM system, based on depth of tumor penetration in the rectal wall and the presence of regional lymph nodes. However, the preoperative assessment of rectal cancer goes beyond determination of clinical tumor stage; it includes the distance of tumor from the anal verge, its relationship to the sphincter complex and the levator muscles, the proximity of tumor to the MRF, and the presence of extramural venous invasion (EMVI). This information is essential in planning treatment and surgery. Gross morphologic features such as size, morphology, and ulceration have been associated with prognosis. However, when stratified by stage, these characteristics have not appeared to contribute independently to oncologic outcomes, and therefore they are not incorporated into treatment decisions.

DRE and proctoscopy provide the surgeon with the first direct impression of the tumor. Tumor mobility on DRE provides a gross estimation of the tumor depth of invasion. There is a four-category clinical classification of rectal tumors, based on mobility on DRE, which supposedly corresponds to the four T categories of the TNM system. However, the correlation between the clinical and pathologic T classifications is not very accurate and varies significantly with the experience of the examiner. In general, DRE can distinguish between mobile tumors, most likely limited to the bowel wall, and tethered or fixed tumors, likely penetrating beyond the bowel wall. However, DRE fails to identify more than 50% of pathologically proven involved nodes. Finally, only very distal tumors are within reach of the examining finger. Therefore, pretreatment clinical staging requires imaging studies including ERUS, high-quality rectal MRI, as well as CT scan of the chest, abdomen, and pelvis with intravenous contrast.

Ultrasound with an endorectal rotating probe is the imaging modality that best depicts the different layers of the bowel wall and is most useful for staging early rectal cancer (**Fig. 65.11**).[179] But ERUS has a relatively short focal range, and cannot depict important anatomical structures such as the MRF. CT scans provide accurate images of the rectum, adjacent pelvic structures, and even the MRF, but have lower tissue resolution compared to MRI. A CT scan of the chest, abdomen,

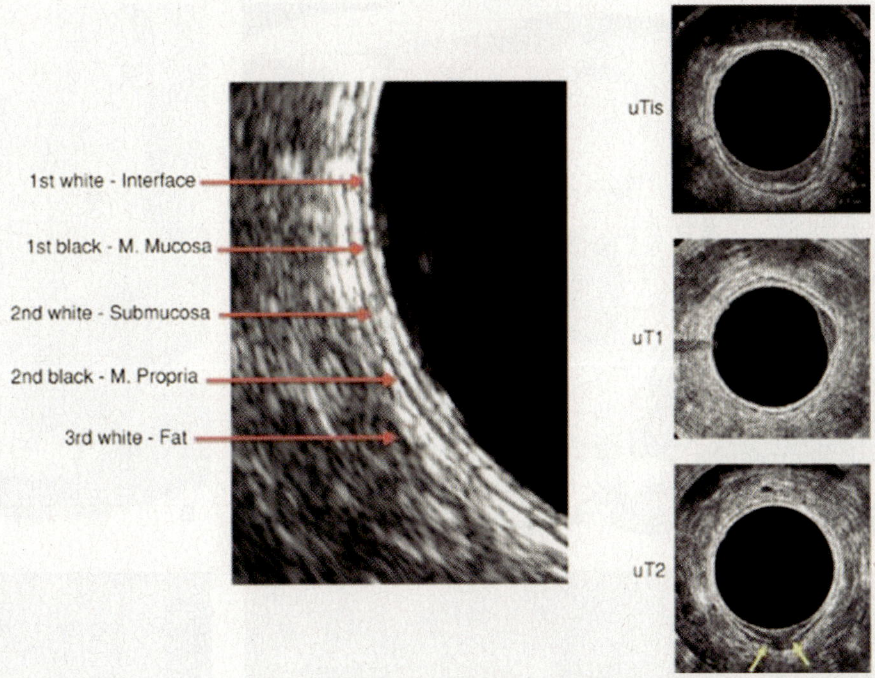

Figure 65.11. Endorectal ultrasound in rectal cancer staging. The sonographic five-layer structure of the rectal wall consists of three hyperechoic layers (interface, submucosa, perirectal fat and serosa) separated by two hypoechoic layers (muscularis mucosa and muscularis propria). Lesions are T staged as uT0/uTis when the mass is within the hypoechoic M. mucosa layer. Tumors staged as uT1 are invading the hyperechoic submucosal layer. Lesions with a distinct break of the submucosal layer and invasion into the hypoechoic muscularis propria layer are staged as uT2 (*yellow arrows*).

and pelvis should be performed in every rectal cancer patient to exclude DMs. MRI with a surface phased-array coil has become the preferred imaging modality for locoregional staging of rectal cancer. Using various sequences and multiple planes, MRI provides high-tissue resolution and excellent anatomical depiction of the rectum, the mesorectum, the MRF, the levator muscles, and other pelvic structures, relative to tumor location (**Fig. 65.12**).[180] The addition of new contrast agents and advanced functional sequences such as diffusion-weighted imaging (DWI) and dynamic contrast enhancement (DCE) permit the quantification of tumor biologic processes such as microcirculation, vascular permeability, and tissue cellularity. DWI images in particular are useful for assessment of rectal cancer response to neoadjuvant therapy.[181,182]

Tumor distance from the MRF—the CRM when performing TME surgery—has prognostic implications for local recurrence and patient survival, and has become one of the most important parameters in the preoperative evaluation of rectal cancer patients.[47] MRI is the most accurate imaging modality in determining the distance of the tumor to the MRF, and predicting CRM involvement. The MERCURY trial, a prospective observational study assessing the accuracy of MRI in predicting a curative resection in rectal cancer, reported 92% specificity in predicting a negative CRM.[183] Other important tumor features accurately assessed by MRI, and associated with patient outcomes, are extramural spread, EMVI, involvement of the peritoneal reflection, and distance of tumor from the levator muscle and sphincter complex.[184,185] Using information on these parameters for patients registered to the MERCURY trial, clinicians are able to stratify rectal cancer patients with good prognosis (eg, clear CRM, no evidence of EMVI, T2 or T3 <5 mm and not involving the intersphincteric plane) with a 3% LR rate and an 85% 5-year DFS after treatment with surgery alone.[186] In European and Scandinavian countries, the information gained from imaging, rather than clinical TNM staging, is used to determine treatment in patients with rectal cancer.[187]

3 Tumor response to neoadjuvant therapy has prognostic value, and restaging after neoadjuvant therapy is becoming increasingly important in reassessing treatment options and planning the surgical procedure. Some patients with a clinical complete response, a subjective assessment that no viable tumor remains based on DRE, endoscopy with or without biopsy, and MRI, are now offered alternatives to rectal resection, such as "watch and wait," in the context of clinical trials.[188–190] In the investigation of the accuracies of DRE, endoscopy, and MRI in predicting complete response, endoscopy is the most accurate.[191] This is true despite the fact that MRI can provide both morphologic and functional information regarding the tumor that can be seen in T2-weighted and diffusion-weighted sequences, respectively. When all three modalities (DRE, endoscopy, and MRI) are consistent with absence of residual tumor, the accuracy of predicting complete response can be as high as 98%. Clinical and radiologic modalities underestimate response to neoadjuvant treatment. DRE underestimates response in 78% of patients, relative to response in pathologic specimens.[192] Nearly three-quarters of patients with pCR have a residual mucosal abnormality that would have led to their being categorized as having had an incomplete clinical response.[193] Of patients for whom DRE, endoscopy, and MRI all indicate the possible presence of residual tumor, 15% still experience a complete response.[191]

Local Excision for Early-Stage Rectal Cancer

Selected patients with stage I rectal cancer, those with tumors localized to the bowel wall (T1 or T2) and without involvement of the mesorectal nodes (N0), can be hypothetically cured with an LE of the portion of the rectal wall containing the tumor. This operation spares most of the mortality, morbidity, and bowel, urinary and sexual dysfunction associated with TME. However, the success of LE requires meticulous patient selection. With LE, the mesorectum is not inspected for pathologic nodal staging. Therefore, LE should only be offered to patients with a low risk of nodal metastasis. The selection criteria for LE include: tumor should be located in the lower rectum, within 8 cm from the anal verge, tumor size smaller than 3 cm, involving less than 30% of the circumference of the rectum, mobile on DRE, localized to the submucosa on ERUS, without evidence of metastatic lymph nodes on ERUS and CT or MRI, and no high-risk histologic features (ie, grade 3 or 4, lymphovascular or perineural invasion).[194]

With the advancement of surgical technology including the use of endoscopic instrumentation and large operating proctoscopes (TEM, Richard Wolf Medical Instruments Corp., Vernon Hills, IL; TEO, Karl Storz Corp., El Segundo, CA) or single-port devices (TAMIS, Trans-Anal Minimally Invasive Surgery), LE can now be easily performed for tumors located in the mid and upper rectum. However, the benefit of LE is more

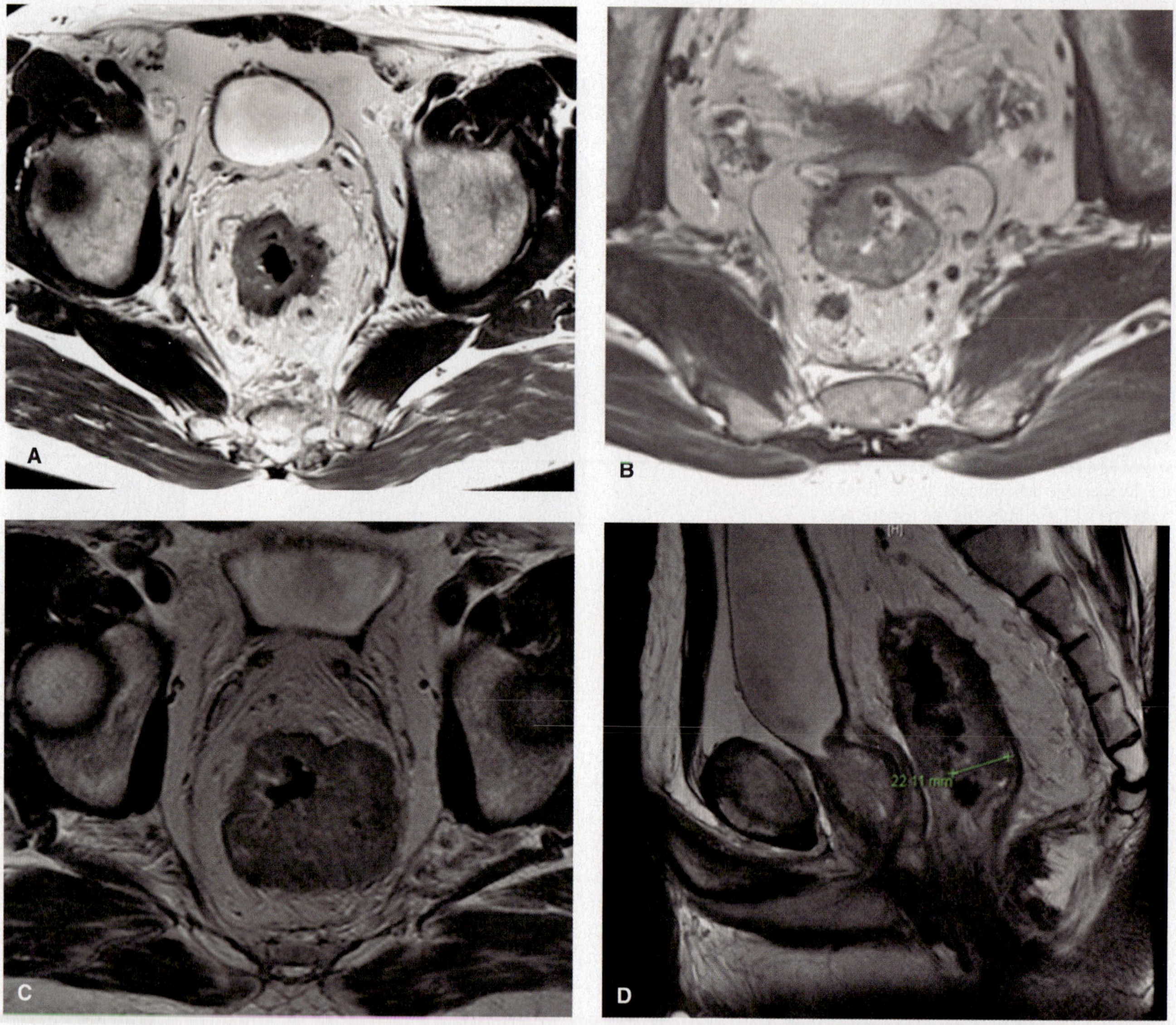

Figure 65.12. Magnetic resonance imaging in rectal cancer staging. Routine use of rectal MRI in the context of a multidisciplinary assessment of rectal cancer has been used to plan neoadjuvant therapy and surgery, and has been shown to reduce the incidence of positive circumferential margins. **A:** Rectal tumor with mesorectal lymph nodes suspicious for metastatic disease. **B:** Locally advanced rectal cancer threatening the mesorectum anteriorly. **C:** Rectal cancer invading the mesorectum in left lateral position. **D:** Sagittal view of a bulky locally advanced rectal cancer.

significant for very distal tumors that otherwise would require a low anastomosis or a permanent stoma. The real benefit of LE for tumors located in the upper rectum is a matter of debate.

Independent of the approach, a full-thickness excision of the portion of the bowel wall involved by tumor, with a 1-cm negative margin is required to avoid local recurrence. The final decision regarding the suitability of LE is made after the pathologic evaluation of the surgical specimen. If the resection margins are positive, depth of invasion is beyond the submucosa (T stage ≥2), or the histology reveals high-risk features (grade 3 or 4, lymphovascular or perineural invasion), the patient should be offered immediate salvage TME.

Even in patients with tumors meeting all selection criteria, LE is associated with a higher rate of LR compared to TME. The recurrence rates for T1 tumors treated with LE have been described as up to 23%.[195–197] While some patients who develop LR after a failed LE are candidates for salvage TME, only half of these patients are ultimately cured of their tumors. Recurrences after LE generally present as more advanced tumors, often requiring extended pelvic dissection.[198,199] The oncologic outcome for these patients is worse than those treated originally with TME; this reinforces the importance of patient selection for this strategy.

A systematic review of one small randomized trial and 12 observational studies, including a total of 2855 patients with T1N0M0 rectal cancer treated by LE (TAE/TEM-TEO) versus TME, showed that LE was associated with lower perioperative mortality (relative risk 0.31, 95% CI 0.14–0.71), major postoperative complications (relative risk 0.20, 95% CI 0.10–0.41), and need for a permanent stoma (relative risk 0.17, 95% 0.09–0.30). The LR rate was higher for patients treated with LE, and overall survival significantly lower, compared to patients treated with TME. The relative risk of dying after LE was 1.46 (95% CI 1.19–1.77), which corresponds to 72 more deaths per 1000 patients at 5 years. Meta-regression showed that the difference in overall survival observed between groups could be explained by the higher use of LE for tumors located in the lower third of the rectum, which is associated with worse prognosis. Survival was similar between groups when only tumors located in the distal rectum were included in the analysis.[200]

Several studies have compared the outcomes of different techniques—conventional transanal excision, TEMS, TEO, and TAMIS—for LE of rectal cancer, with most comparisons limited to conventional TAE and TEMS. A recent meta-analysis of 6 retrospective case series including 927 procedures, reported that TEMS was associated with less specimen fragmentation, less positive resection margins, and lower LR rates. No difference was observed in complication rate.[201]

In summary, the literature suggests that LE may be an alternative to TME for patients with small, distal T1N0 rectal cancers, without high-risk histologic features, that would otherwise require a CAA or an APE. Transanal endoscopic techniques may be superior to conventional transanal excision. Patients considering LE should be informed about the potential gains in improved quality of life, but also about the higher risk of LR and the need for salvage surgery.

Patients with T2N0 tumors are not candidates for treatment by LE alone, independent of tumor histologic features. The rate of LR for these patients when treated with LE alone ranges from 13% to 47%, significantly higher compared to similar stage tumors treated with TME. Five-year overall survival is also significantly lower for patients with T2N0 tumors treated with LE (65% to 67.6%) compared to TME (76.7% to 81%).[202] A recent survey of the NCDB found that patients with T2N0 tumors treated with LE alone had a higher hazard ratio for death compared to similar patients treated with TME (1.535, 95% CI 1.283–1.835).[203] Similar results have been reported in an independent cohort from the SEER database.[204] Based on this evidence, LE alone cannot be recommended as an alternative to RS for patients with T2N0 tumor treated with curative intent.

RT has been used to reduce the rate of LR in patients with T2N0 rectal cancer treated with LE. A number of retrospective case series have reported 15% to 21% LR rates and 66% to 76.1% 5-year survival rates with LE followed by radiation or chemoradiation for T2N0 tumors.[205–207] The CALGB 8984 trial investigated the role of LE followed by 5-FU–based adjuvant chemoradiation for patients with T2N0 cancers, reporting a 66% (95% CI, 51% to 84%) overall survival and 64% (95% CI, 51% to 80%) DFS.[208] The trial compared the survival curves of patients with similar stage tumors treated with TME, concluding that LE and postoperative chemoradiation may be an alternative for patients with T2N0 tumors. However, 32% of the patients initially accrued for this trial were ultimately excluded from analysis due to tumor size, inaccurate staging, surgical specimen fragmentation, high-grade histologic features, or involved resection margins. Therefore, the conclusion is applicable only for properly staged early rectal cancers penetrating only into the muscularis propria (pT2), with full-thickness excision negative resection margins, and no high-risk histologic features.

The results of several retrospective studies have suggested that chemoradiation before LE reduces the risk of recurrence to rates similar to those observed in similar stage patients treated with TME alone.[209,210] However, these studies are limited by small sample size, variable clinical staging criteria and imaging modalities, and the use of different CRT regimens. A retrospective study using the SEER database showed that patients who had undergone neoadjuvant CRT and LE had equivalent oncologic outcomes compared to patients who had a radical resection/TME.[204] One prospective trial found that patients with ERUS-staged T2N0 rectal cancer treated with neoadjuvant CRT had similar recurrence and survival rates when randomized to LE or TME. More than one in four patients in the TME arm required a permanent colostomy, and a similar number required a temporary ileostomy.[211] Two single-arm prospective studies have shown that CRT followed by LE for early-stage distal rectal cancers is associated with local recurrence and DFS rate equivalent to similar tumors treated with TME.[212,213] However, this treatment approach is associated with bowel dysfunction and impairment in quality of life, particularly in patients with very distal tumors.[212,214] The GRECCAR-2 trial randomized patients with T2 or T3 distal rectal cancer that responded to CRT to either LE or TME. Local recurrence rates, DFS, and fecal incontinence were similar for patients treated in both treatment arms.[215] In summary, the standard treatment of T2N0 rectal cancer is TME. Neoadjuvant CRT followed by LE may be an alternative for patients with very distal T2N0 tumors interested in organ preservation, who otherwise would require a permanent colostomy.

LE and other forms of local therapy, such as endocavitary radiation, brachytherapy, or electrofulguration, have been used for palliation in patients who have more advanced tumors or are unfit for a major surgical procedure.

Transabdominal Resection for Rectal Cancer

Patient preparation for rectal cancer surgery is similar to that for colon cancer surgery. Stoma marking is particularly important in these patients, as many will require a temporary or permanent stoma. In addition to discussing fertility options with all individuals of child-bearing potential, female patients receiving neoadjuvant radiation who are interested in preserving fertility should consult their gynecologist regarding the possibility of ovarian transposition. Mechanical bowel preparation, antibiotic and thromboembolic prophylaxis are similar to those described for colon cancer patients. Many surgeons recommend a rectal washout immediately before surgery to eliminate exfoliated cancer cells that could potentially implant in the anastomosis and cause LR. In fact, a recent meta-analysis with 5012 patients found that this practice is associated with a lower incidence of LR.[216] On the operative table, the patient should be placed in lithotomy with the legs in stirrups to provide the surgeon with simultaneous access to the abdomen and perineum. It is important to avoid pressure on the bony prominences, which might cause peroneal nerve compression. Patients requiring prolonged Trendelenburg position during surgery are at risk of compartment syndrome, in particular obese patients and those with peripheral vascular disease. These patients require monitoring of the peripheral pulses, and position changes, to prevent compartment ischemia.

Principles of Total Mesorectal Excision

TME is the standard surgical treatment for rectal cancer. This operation requires dissection under direct vision along the areolar tissue plane situated between the MRF and the presacral fascia with the goal of not just removing the primary tumor, but also the lymphatic drainage. A sharp dissection along this plane is associated with a higher probability of achieving a negative CRM, lower risk of bleeding from inadvertent tearing of the presacral veins, and reduced risk of injuring the hypogastric nerves.

Adequate lymphadenectomy requires division of the lymphovascular pedicle at the origin of the superior rectal vessels, caudal to the branching of the left colic artery from the inferior mesenteric artery. In patients with clinically suspicious nodes at the origin of the inferior mesenteric artery, the lymphovascular control should be extended proximally by dividing the inferior mesenteric artery close to the origin (high ligation). In both cases the sigmoidal branches are included in the surgical specimen; therefore, the proximal division of the bowel should ideally be performed at the junction of the descending and the sigmoid colon, incorporating most of the sigmoid colon in the surgical specimen.[217] As distal tumor extension along the rectal wall is limited, a distal margin of 2 cm of normal bowel wall is considered adequate for most tumors. However, distal spread in the mesorectum may extend farther than intramural spread. Not infrequently, mesorectal deposits are found 3 to 4 cm distal to the lower edge of the tumor. Therefore, for tumors of the upper rectum, the mesorectal excision should be extended to 5 cm distal to the lower edge of the tumor. In these patients the mesorectum should be divided perpendicular to the axis of the rectum. As some of the distal mesorectum is left in the pelvis along with the distal rectal stump, this operation is known as tumor-specific TME (TSME), to distinguish it from the TME performed with dissection carried to the pelvic floor, the rectum divided distal to the end of the mesorectum, and the entire mesorectum included in the surgical specimen.

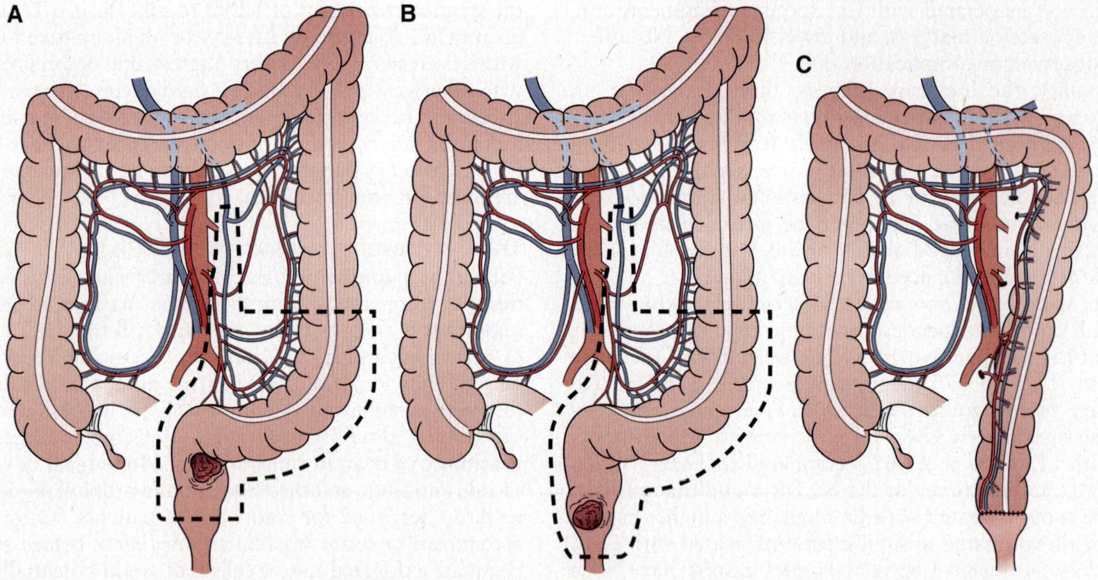

Figure 65.13. A: Low anterior resection, section in the distal third of the rectum, candidate for colorectal anastomosis. B: Low anterior resection, section above the sphincteric complex, candidate for coloanal anastomosis. C: Colorectal anastomosis.

Sphincter Saving Procedures

A TSME or a TME is compatible with sphincter preservation by anastomosing the divided end of the descending or the sigmoid colon to the rectal stump. This operation is known as a low anterior resection or LAR (**Fig. 65.13**). In this operation the rectum is divided distal to the tumor using a stapling device that simultaneously staples and divides the rectum, leaving a short rectal stump. The anastomosis is completed with a circular stapler that brings together the end of the colon to the rectal stump. The reestablishment of the large bowel's continuity by suturing the colon to the anal canal, working through the anus, is known as coloanal anastomosis or CAA (**Fig. 65.13**). The connection of the colon to the rectum or anal canal can be performed by an end-to-end or a side-to-end connection, or with the creation of a J-pouch reservoir. A tension free, well vascularized low colorectal or coloanal anastomosis requires a complete mobilization of the entire left colon with take-down of the splenic flexure, including division of the inferior mesenteric vein close to the ligament of Treitz. Following ligation of the IMA, the blood supply to the entire left colon is based on the left branch of the middle colic vessels through the marginal artery.

Many patients undergoing a sphincter-saving procedure report high bowel frequency, urgency, soiling, and inability to defer defecation for 15 minutes.[218] This constellation of symptoms is commonly known as low anterior resection syndrome (LARS) or clustered defecation.[219] The frequency and severity of these symptoms is variable and depends, to some degree, on the location of the tumor and the anastomosis, the patient's prior bowel function, and the use of neoadjuvant or adjuvant therapy.[220] Pelvic irradiation, before or after surgery, increases significantly the risk of bowel dysfunction.[221,222] The anatomical and physiologic factors that contribute to LARS are not completely understood. Anal sphincter pressures are not different in patients with or without LARS. What appears to be different is an exaggerated anal sphincter relaxation to even small volumes of stool within the neorectum.[223] Surgeons have tried to overcome this low capacitance of the neorectum—which results from an end-to-end anastomosis—by creating a colonic reservoir: either a colonic J-pouch, or a side-to-end anastomosis. A number of studies have compared the functional outcomes after straight end-to-end anastomosis and a colonic J-pouch. A systematic review of reconstructive techniques after LAR identified 9 trials that randomized a total of 473 rectal cancer patients to either colonic J-pouch or straight end-to-end anastomosis, reporting that short-term bowel function was better for J-pouch compared to straight anastomosis.[224] Frequency and urgency were less prevalent in patients with a colonic J-pouch, but the rate of fecal incontinence was similar in both groups. The only two trials that followed patients for more than 118 months found minimal or no long-term differences between groups. Although the methodology of these studies was very heterogeneous, they do indicate that a colonic J-pouch is associated with a short-term improvement in frequency and urgency, but no apparent long-term benefit, compared to end-to-end anastomosis. The same systematic review found no differences in anastomotic leak rate, or other complications, between groups. Of note, almost one-third of patients with colonic J-pouches often complained of long-term difficulty emptying the rectum, requiring use of laxatives or suppositories.[225,226] These symptoms are more prevalent when larger pouches are created; therefore, pouch size should be limited to 5 to 6 cm.[227,228]

The side-to-end anastomosis (created by inserting the anvil of a circular stapler 3 to 4 cm from the end of the mobilized descending colon) can also potentially increase the reservoir capacity of the anastomosis. It has similar functional results but is easier to construct than the colonic J-pouch; although it, too, is associated with defecatory problems.[229] The creation of a transverse coloplasty proximal to an end-to-end anastomosis is another option used to increase the capacity of the neorectum, but is associated with a higher anastomotic leak rate.[224]

In summary, colonic reservoirs are associated with a temporary improvement in bowel frequency and urgency, but have the risk of long-term defecatory problems. In general, the authors prefer an end-to-end anastomosis using the larger descending colon, rather than the sigmoid colon, for creation of the neorectum.

Management of Low Anterior Resection Syndrome (LARS)

First-line treatment for patients suffering from LARS symptoms is dietary modification. The patients should avoid foods that will cause their stool to be soft (eg, caffeine, spicy food, alcohol and fat).[230–232] Patients are encouraged to consume high-fiber foods to increase the stool bulk and solid stool consistency, thus improving symptoms of incontinence due to diarrhea. The Nurses' Health Study of 58,330 women demonstrated that women with the highest intake of fibers (25 g/day) had a 31% lower risk for fecal incontinence (mainly due to liquid stool) compared with women with the lowest intake.[230]

An important treatment modality for LARS is medical. Loperamide is the most commonly used drug and medication therapy often focuses on the reduction in colonic motility and reduction of defecation episodes.[230,231] Loperamide also increases the anal resting tone due to possible activation of the internal anal sphincter. In addition, 5-HT3 antagonists and bile acid sequestrants have demonstrated promising results.[233]

Pelvic floor rehabilitation is another treatment modality for LARS. A few studies have studies have evaluated the efficacy of rehabilitative treatment of patients with LARS, mostly dealing with symptoms of "incontinence" and "stool frequency."[231,234] One study demonstrated a decrease in incontinence and number of defecation episodes in 19 patients who underwent biofeedback and home exercises for 4 weeks as a treatment for functional problems after various colorectal surgical procedures.[231,232]

Surgery and/or radiotherapy can lead to the denervation of the autonomic nervous system and consequently to an impairment of sympathetic as well as parasympathetic nerve fiber activity[232] leading to fecal incontinence. In turn, sacral nerve stimulation (SNS) can improve fecal incontinence by stimulating S2 or S3.

The integrity of the anastomosis should be tested intraoperatively with a pneumatic test, or by endoscopy, with distension of the bowel while submerging the anastomosis in water. Air leaks thus detected may be treated with suture repair, redo of the anastomosis, and/or the creation of a proximal diverting stoma. Testing the integrity of the anastomosis during surgery has been associated with a lower risk of clinical postoperative anastomotic leak.[235]

Low colorectal and coloanal anastomoses have a risk of leakage ranging from 3% to 34%, depending on the patient population, the use of neoadjuvant radiation, the distance of the anastomosis from the anal verge, and the surgical technique.[236,237] An anastomotic leak can cause pelvic sepsis, which may not only preclude sphincter preservation, but may also be associated with an increased risk of local recurrence and poorer survival, although more recent data have questioned this association.[238–240] To prevent these possible complications, a diverting stoma is recommended for patients having a TME, and for patients receiving neoadjuvant radiation.[241] Diverting stomas do not prevent complications, but mitigate the consequences of a leak and reduce the need for urgent reoperation in patients developing a leak.[242,243] A loop ileostomy is preferred over a transverse loop colostomy because it is easier to create and close.[244] However, loop ileostomies are associated with postoperative dehydration and electrolyte abnormalities requiring hospital readmission.[245,246] Prevention of these complications requires adequate patient education and training about stoma management.

Abdominoperineal Excision

For many cancers located in the distal rectum, particularly those infiltrating the levator muscles or the anal sphincter, an oncologically safe circumferential and/or distal resection margin is not compatible with sphincter preservation. In these patients an R0 resection requires a TME with en bloc excision of the levator muscles and the anal canal, and the creation of a permanent end colostomy. This operation is known as abdominoperineal excision of the rectum or APE (**Fig. 65.14**). As the name indicates, the APE has two parts: an abdominal part and a perineal part. During the abdominal part, the proximal lymphovascular control, division of the colon, and dissection along the mesorectal plane are similar to those in LAR, except that the mesorectal dissection should stop at the upper level of the levators, to avoid disturbing the portion of the rectum resting on the levator muscles. During the perineal part, the anal canal with the sphincter complex and the levator muscles are dissected off the ischiorectal fat, all the way to the apex of the ischiorectal fossa. The levators are divided close to their insertion in the white line near the obturator internus and coccygeus muscles. The levator muscles are left attached to the rectum, and the resulting surgical specimen has a cylindrical appearance; therefore, this procedure is called cylindrical APE or extralevator APE (ELAPE) (**Fig. 65.14**).[247] However, some surgeons question the need to entirely remove both levator muscles in every rectal cancer patient, and recommend removing only the portion of the levators required to clear the tumor. This operation has been called the standard APE (SAPE).[248] The choice between an ELAPE and SAPE is controversial. The potential oncologic benefit of larger tissue removal needs to be weighed against the increased morbidity potentially associated with a larger perineal defect, particularly in patients treated with neoadjuvant therapy.[249] A recent meta-analysis with 949 patients from 1 randomized trial, 1 prospective case-control study, and 6 retrospective case series, indicated that ELAPE is associated with lower intraoperative rectal perforation, lower positive CRM, and lower risk of local recurrence, but with similar complication rates, compared to SAPE.[250] At the present time, the hypothetical benefit of the ELAPE over the SAPE has not been proven conclusively. It is possible that both techniques—the total or the tumor-specific excision of the levator muscles—may be equivalent as long as an R0 resection, with an intact rectal specimen, is achieved.

Many surgeons will perform both parts of the APE operation with the patient in modified lithotomy, also known as the Lloyd–Davis position. It provides relatively good access to the perineum and allows two teams to work simultaneously—one in the abdomen, and one in the perineum. Others perform the abdominal part in the supine position, and the perineal part with the patient prone over a hip roll and padding of the bony prominences. The prone position, also known as jackknife position, provides better exposure of the perineum, and facilitates assistance and teaching. It requires turning the patient, which takes time, and does not allow a two-team approach. Results seem to be similar with both approaches, and the selection is based on surgeon preference.[251]

Minimally Invasive Surgery for Rectal Cancer

Over the last several decades, there has been a significant shift from open surgery for rectal cancer to minimally invasive approaches. The goal of MIS in rectal cancer is to reduce the size of the abdominal incision, thus expediting recovery, without compromising the completeness of the mesorectal excision or the oncologic outcomes. However, the adoption of MIS for rectal cancer has been slow due to the difficulty of working in the relatively deep and narrow pelvic space using long, rigid, nonarticulated laparoscopic instruments. According to a number of retrospective case series and small randomized controlled trials, laparoscopic TME is associated with less
4 postoperative pain, less surgical morbidity, and shorter length of hospital stay, but equivalent completion of the mesorectal excision, CRM positivity, and even LR, compared to open TME.[252–254] While these studies have shown that laparoscopic TME is feasible, less than 25% of all rectal cancer operations are performed laparoscopically in the United States.[255]

Five large multi-institutional prospective, randomized trials have compared open and laparoscopic TME for rectal cancer (**Table 65.7**).[256–260] The combined experience of these trials indicates that laparoscopic TME results in longer operative time, less blood loss, faster bowel recovery, and shorter hospital stay compared to open TME. Operative mortality and intra- and postoperative complications were not different between groups. When investigating successful oncologic resection comprised of positive distal margin, positive circumferential margin and completeness of TME, ALACART and Z6051 both failed to demonstrate noninferiority of laparoscopic resection. In addition, although not all of them powered to demonstrate differences in oncologic outcomes, these five studies have shown that LR, DM, and survival were not different between groups. The combined experience of these studies suggests that with the noninferiority margin for the

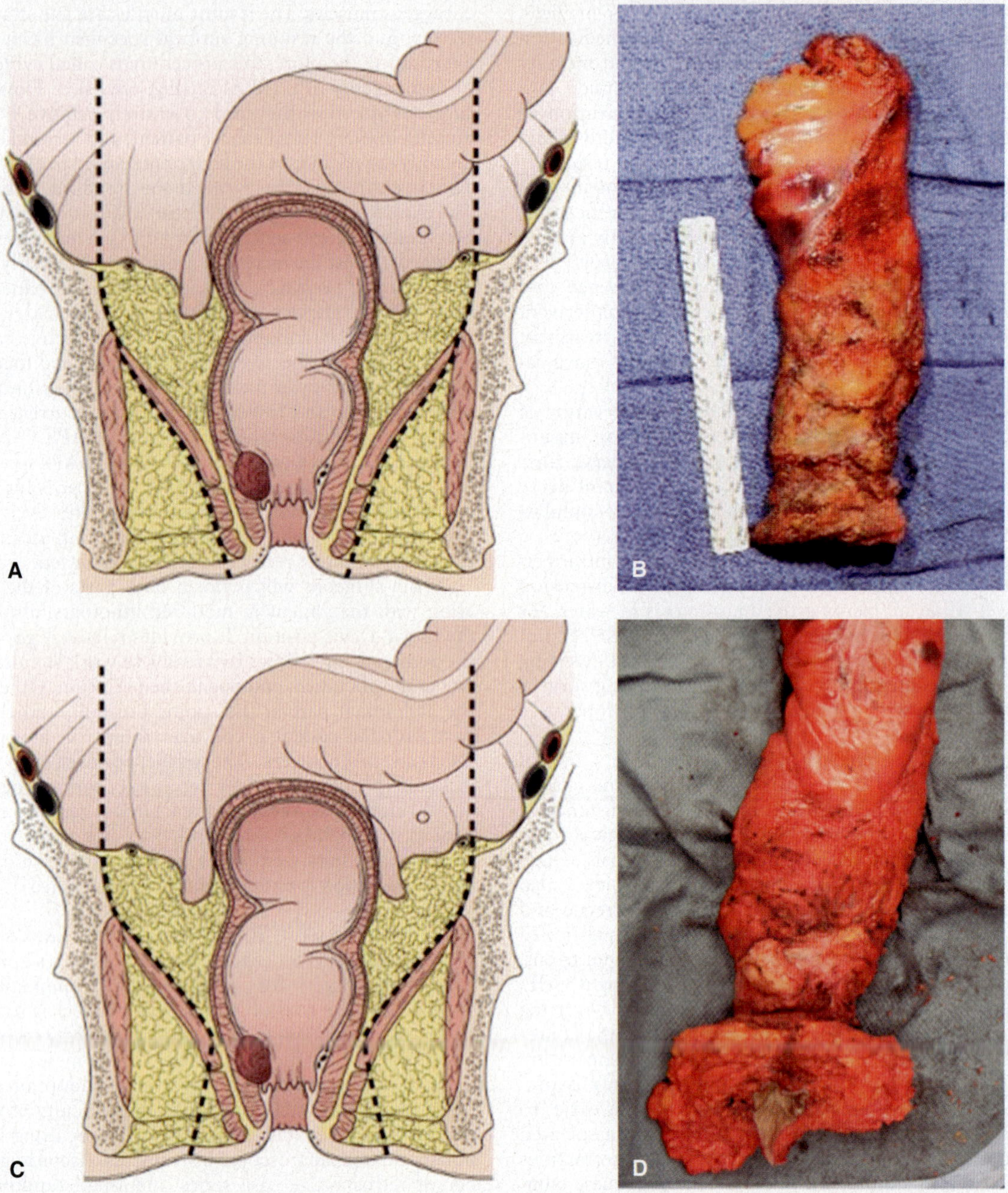

Figure 65.14. Total mesorectal excision. Following correct anatomical planes and avoiding entry into the mesorectum or sphincter muscles (extralevator approach) results in a surgical specimen that has a cylindrical appearance with no mesenteric "waist" or narrowing. **A:** Planes of dissection for ELAPE. **B:** ELAPE specimen. **C:** Planes of dissection for SAPE. **D:** SAPE specimen with mesenteric "waist."

quality of the surgical resection in some studies, the long-term oncologic outcomes are equivalent for patients treated with open or robotic TME. However, patients in these trials were treated at high-volume centers and operated by surgeons experienced in minimally invasive techniques. Whether similar results can be achievable in the community is still debatable.

Robotic surgery for rectal cancer has gained increasing adoption over the last two decades. MIS has led to improved recovery time, shorter hospital LOS, and decreased postoperative pain. Robotic surgery enhances elements to MIS including improved ergonomics causing less physical demand to the surgeon, better visualization with three-dimensional imaging, additional dexterity through flexible surgical instruments, and ability to navigate in narrow spaces such as the pelvis. The experience accumulated thus far—based on retrospective institutional case series—suggests that robotic TME is equivalent to laparoscopic TME in terms of completeness of the mesorectal excision, CRM positivity, and short-term oncologic outcomes. Conversion rates appear to be lower compared to laparoscopic TME, but hospital charges are higher.[261] A prospective, randomized study comparing laparoscopic and robotic TME—the Robotic Versus Laparoscopic Resection for Rectal Cancer (ROLARR) trial—demonstrated no difference in conversion or circumferential margin positivity between the two surgical approaches.[262] However, as laparoscopy has not become standard in LARC, it is likely that the controversy regarding the benefit of robotic TME will continue for years.

The transanal–total mesorectal excision (TaTME), or down-to-up TME, is a transanal, minimally invasive approach for the dissection of the distal rectum in patients with a narrow pelvis.[263,264] With this approach, lymphovascular control, the entire colonic mobilization, and dissection of the upper rectum are performed using conventional transabdominal laparoscopy. The dissection of the distal rectum is performed

Table 65.7. Open versus Laparoscopic Rectal Resections: Results of the Most Representative Series

Open/Laparoscopic	CLASICC (2005–2007–2010–2013)	COLOR II (2013)	COREAN (2010–2014)	ALaCaRT (2015–2019)	ACOSOG-Z6051 (2015–2019)
N	381	1103	340	473	462
Rectal cancers included	All	T1–3 (>2 mm from endopelvic fascia) Upper-mid-low	Mid-low cT3NX	T1–3 (>2 mm from endopelvic fascia) Upper-mid-low	Stage II and III, Upper-mid-low
Neoadjuvant CRT (%)	0	34/32	100/100	48/50	91.2/95
Operative time (min)	135/180[a]	188/240 $p < .001$	197/224.9 $p < .001$	190/210 $p = .007$	221/266 $p < .001$
Blood loss (mL)	NR	400/200 $p < .001$	217.5/200 $p < .006$	150/100 $p = .002$	318/256 $p = .004$
TME (%)	67/79	67/60 $p = .120$	100/100	92/87	90.5/84.6 $p = .05$
APR (%)	27/25	23/29	14.1/11.2 $p = .708$	10/11	23.8/22.7
Conversion (%)	34	17	1.2	9	11
Positive CRM (%)	14/16 $p = .8$	10/10 $p = .850$	4.1/2.9 $p = .770$	3/7 $p = .06$	7.7/12.1 <1 mm
Lymph nodes (n)	13.5/12	14/13 $p = .085$	18/17 $p = .085$	NR	16.5/17.9
First bowel movement (days)	6/5	3/2 $p < .001$	5.12/4.02 $p < .001$	2/2	3/2 $p = .04$
Hospital stay (days)	13/10	9/8 $p = .036$	9/8 .056	8/8	7/7.3
Morbidity (%)	13/14	37/40 $p = .42$	23.5/21.1 $p = .603$	25/20	54.1/53.8
Local recurrence (%)	10.1/9.7 $p = .96$	5/5[a,c]	4.9/2.6 $p = .42$	3.1/5.4	4.5/4.6
Systemic recurrence (%)	18.6/16.4 $p = .74$	20.1/19.1[a,c]	17/15 $p = .42$	17.3/19.6	16.7/14.6
DFS (%)	52.1/53.2 $p = .953$[a]	70.8/74.8[a,c]	72.5/79.2[b]	82/80	83.2/79.5
OS (%)	52.9/60.3 $p = .132$[a]	83.6/86.7[a,c]	90.4/91.7[b]	93/94	86.5/85

[a]3-year survival.
[b]5-year survival.
[c]Difference <5% calculated for noninferiority.

through the anus, using either conventional transanal equipment for very distal tumors, or endoscopic equipment (TEMS, TEO, TAMIS) for higher tumors. The rectal wall is incised circumferentially, distal to the tumor, and the MRF is identified. The lumen of the colon is closed with a purse-string suture to avoid contamination. The dissection is carried cephalad in the proper plane until the abdominal field is reached. The specimen is then removed, and the anastomosis performed through the anus. This approach is particularly useful for patients with very distal rectal cancers treated with chemoradiation therapy, in which the surgeon has no anatomical cues about where to transect the rectum in order to achieve a negative distal margin. The transanal approach allows the surgeon to choose precisely the point for transecting the rectum while visualizing the distal edge of the tumor. The benefit of the down-to-up approach for higher rectal cancers that could be treated with a conventional transabdominal dissection and a double-stapled anastomosis are uncertain. A multicenter-matched comparison of robotic resection and TaTME of 730 patients with mid to distal rectal cancer did not show differences in specimen quality or conversion rate between these surgical approaches.[265] Outcomes of all patients that underwent TaTME in Norway were compared to outcomes of patients that underwent TME in a national database. TaTME patients experienced more local recurrences and anastomotic leaks. These reports were alarming enough to halt all TaTME in Norway.[266] TaTME is technically challenging, has a long learning curve and should be considered a treatment option for rectal cancer only in very experienced hands.

Adjuvant and Neoadjuvant Radiation and Chemotherapy for Locally Advanced Rectal Cancer

Several randomized, controlled trials conducted in the pre-TME era demonstrated that RT given before or after surgery reduced the rate of LR, compared to surgery alone.[267–269] However, the relevance of these trials was later questioned because surgery was not standardized and the LR rates reported in the control arms—approximately 25%—were considered too high compared with patients treated in later years with surgery alone according to TME principles. The efficacy of RT in the setting of quality TME surgical resection was investigated in the Dutch Colorectal Cancer Group trial, which randomized 1861 patients with resectable disease to TME alone or short-course RT (SCRT) (5 Gy a day × 5 days, for a total dose of 25 Gy), followed by TME within 2 to 7 days. The study showed that SCRT reduced the rate of LR in resectable rectal cancer treated by TME, compared to TME alone; however, SCRT did not provide a significant survival benefit.[270] This trial proved that preoperative RT decreases the rate of LR in LARC patients treated with TME surgery.

The benefit of combining chemotherapy with RT was proven by several randomized trials that compared postoperative RT combined with 5-FU, administered as a bolus or as continuous venous infusion (CVI), to postoperative RT alone, in patients with pathologic stage II and III rectal cancers.[271,272] The results proved that combined 5-FU and radiation was more effective than radiation alone in reducing the risk of LR, and that CVI 5-FU was associated with lower toxicity compared to bolus 5-FU.

The European Organization for Research and Treatment of Cancer (EORTC) protocol 22921 was developed to assess the effect of adding chemotherapy to preoperative RT, and the subsequent value of postoperative chemotherapy in rectal cancer patients.[273] At the 5-year mark, LR was significantly lower in all three arms receiving any chemotherapy (pre- or postoperative) compared to preoperative RT alone, indicating a benefit of chemotherapy in reducing the risk of LR, regardless of when it was administered. The addition of chemotherapy to RT did not impact survival. Additional work by the Federation Francophone de la Cancerologie Digestive corroborated these findings.[274] These studies showed that, similar to what was found using postoperative radiation, adding chemotherapy to preoperative RT also reduced the rate of LR, compared to preoperative RT alone.

The German Rectal Cancer Group (CAO/ARO/AIO 94) compared preoperative versus postoperative CRT in 823 patients with clinical T3–4/N+ rectal cancer.[275] RT in this trial consisted of 50.4 Gy in 25 fractions with bolus 5-FU as a radiosensitizer. In the preoperative treatment group, surgery was performed 6 weeks after completion of CRT. Both groups had surgery according to TME principles and received postoperative adjuvant chemotherapy. The preoperative CRT group had less toxicity and lower 5-year LR rates compared to the postoperative CRT group (6% vs 13%). This study found no differences in the rates of DR, DSS, or OS. The NSABP R-03 study also compared the use of preoperative versus postoperative 5-FU/LV, using 45 Gy in 25 fractions in T3/4, N+ patients, to evaluate differences in DFS, LR, or OS.[276] Despite stopping the study early due to limited accrual, the R-03 study reported better DFS in the preoperative CRT group, compared to the postoperative group, with a near-significant difference (p = .065) in OS and no difference in LR. The results of these two trials established preoperative CRT as the preferred treatment for LARC in both Europe and the United States.

Capecitabine has been demonstrated to be noninferior to infusional 5-FU as a radiosensitizer for LARC, in both the NSABP R-04 trial and the German Cancer Research Center multi-center trial.[277,278] Several large, prospective trials have failed to prove that the addition of oxaliplatin to a fluoropyrimidine (5-FU or capecitabine) is superior to fluoropyrimidine alone as a radiosensitizer in patients with LARC.[278–281] Therefore, based on the current evidence, oxaliplatin is not recommended as a radiosensitizer added to a fluoropyrimidine in patients with LARC.

As an alternative to the standard hypofractionation (180 to 200 cGy a fraction) commonly delivered during the standard long-course CRT over a 6-week period, RT may be delivered as short course (SCRT) using fewer, larger fractions (5 Gy daily fractions for 5 consecutive days and a total dose of 25 Gy). In these patients, surgery is performed within 7 days of completion of the radiation. Both schemes are biologically equivalent in eradicating cancer cells, but SCRT has the potential benefits of shorter duration of treatment, more efficient utilization of resources, and reduced cost compared to CRT. However, higher dose per fraction increases the risk of delayed toxicity, and tumor regression is lower with SCRT. Two prospective, randomized trials comparing SCRT with CRT have reported equivalent local tumor control with both regimens, and the selection between CRT and SCRT is based on doctor and patient preferences.[282,283] In general, tumor regression is lower with SCRT when surgery is performed within 7 days of the last dose of radiation. For that reason, CRT has been the preferred radiation modality in the setting of large tumors that may benefit from maximal tumor regression before surgery. However, recent data suggest that the tumor response rate increases if surgery is delayed for 6 to 8 weeks after SCRT.[284]

Current guidelines recommend CRT or SCRT with the aim of reducing the risk of LR for all patients with stage II and III rectal cancers. However, the risk of LR depends on the distance of the tumor from the anal verge, the risk being lower for tumors located in the upper rectum compared to those in the lower rectum. It is possible that some patients with high rectal cancers, specifically those with T3N0 tumors and a clear CRM, may not actually benefit from preoperative radiation but may simply be exposed to radiation-associated toxicity. The PROSPECT trial sought to assess the benefit of preoperative radiation for rectal cancer.[285] This study concluded that FOLFOX chemotherapy with selective use of 5FUCRT is noninferior to 5FUCRT for neoadjuvant treatment of LARC prior to low anterior resection with TME.

Chemotherapy for Locally Advanced Rectal Cancer

In the past, LR was the dominant problem in patients with LARC, but in the modern era more patients develop DM than LR. Consequently, patients with LARC treated with neoadjuvant CRT and TME are recommended for postoperative adjuvant chemotherapy, with the aim of reducing DM and improving survival. However, the data supporting this recommendation are limited, and based heavily on experience using adjuvant therapy for resected colon cancers. A meta-analysis of 21 controlled trials in patients receiving potentially curative surgery, including a total of 4854 patients randomized to surgery plus fluoropyrimidine-based postoperative chemotherapy, and 4367 patients to surgery and observation, has shown a significant reduction in the risk of death (17%) (HR = 0.83, CI: 0.76–0.91) and a reduction in the risk of DR (25%) (HR = 0.75, CI: 0.68–0.83) among patients undergoing adjuvant chemotherapy, compared to those undergoing observation.[286] A review of the experience of a large national database suggests that there is a survival benefit for rectal cancer patients receiving chemotherapy after CRT and TME.[287] On the other hand, a pooled analysis of four prospective randomized trials suggests a minimal improvement in DFS from postoperative 5-FU–based adjuvant chemotherapy in patients with rectal cancer treated with preoperative chemoradiation.[288] Despite these conflicting results, current guidelines recommend 4 months of postoperative adjuvant chemotherapy (5-FU or capecitabine plus oxaliplatin) for patients with LARC treated with neoadjuvant chemoradiation and TME surgery.

Total Neoadjuvant Therapy

Total neoadjuvant therapy (TNT) is now recognized as the preferred standard for the treatment of LARC. With this treatment approach, all chemotherapy and radiation are given upfront before surgical intervention. This approach avoids potential delay or abandonment of adjuvant chemotherapy due to postsurgical complications. Delivering systemic chemotherapy before surgery has the potential advantages of increasing treatment compliance, treating micrometastatic disease early, enhancing the response of the primary tumor, and shortening the time to temporary ileostomy reversal. Patients treated with TNT generally have a higher primary tumor response compared with patients treated with standard chemoradiation and surgery; however, a beneficial effect in terms of survival has not been demonstrated.[289–292] The two most important studies evaluating the effect of TNT are the RAPIDO and PRODIGE-23 trials.

In the RAPIDO trial, 912 patients were randomized to receive preoperative treatment consisting of SCRT followed by chemotherapy (6 cycles of CAPOX or 9 cycles of FOLFOX) and TME versus standard-of-care treatment. All patients enrolled had high-risk stage II and III rectal cancer, defined as having at least one of the following criteria on MRI staging: cT4a, cT4b, extramural vascular invasion (EMVI), cN2 (metastasis in four or more locoregional lymph nodes), involved MRF, or enlarged lateral lymph nodes. The primary endpoint was 3-year disease-related treatment failure (DrTF), which included locoregional failure, DM, new primary colon tumor, or treatment-related death. Patients receiving TNT demonstrated a decreased DrTF rate of 23.7% compared with 30.4% in the control arm (HR 0.75, $p = .019$). The experimental arm also had double the pCR rate (28.4% vs 14.3%) and significantly lower incidence of DMs (20.0% vs 26.8%, $p = .005$). However, in the neoadjuvant phase, the use of TNT was associated with higher rates of grade ≥3 adverse events (48% vs 25%, respectively) leading to treatment discontinuation in 15% versus 9% of patients, respectively. Given the longer systemic treatment delivery in the standard-of-care arm, the global rates of severe adverse events were 63% compared with 48% in the control arm. Recent update of RAPIDO, with a median follow-up of 5.6 years, demonstrated that the experimental treatment was associated with an increased risk of LRR compared with standard of care (12% vs 8%, respectively, $p = .007$), while the reduction in DrTF and DMs was sustained. The 5-year OS was 81.7% versus 80.2%, respectively.

The PRODIGE-23 trial randomized 461 patients with rectal adenocarcinoma and high-risk features, such as cT3/cT4 disease, to receive 6 cycles of mFOLFIRINOX, followed by LCRT, TME, and a further 6 cycles of adjuvant mFOLFOX versus long-course standard LCRT, followed by TME and 12 cycles of mFOLFOX6 or 8 cycles of capecitabine. The primary endpoint of the PRODIGE-23 trial was DFS, whereas toxicity, pCR, metastasis-free survival (MFS), OS, and quality of life were secondary endpoints. Patients receiving TNT had an improved 3-year DFS of 76% versus 69% in the standard-of-care group ($p = .034$). The experimental arm also had two-fold higher pCR rate (27.8% vs 12.1%) and increased 3-year MFS (79% vs 72%).[293] In total, 98% of patients in the TNT group received mFOLFIRINOX, and 92% managed to complete the preplanned six cycles. The overall incidence of grade 3 or higher adverse events in these patients was 46%, which is similar to the control arm. The reduced duration of adjuvant chemotherapy in the TNT group led to less severe toxicity, including peripheral sensory neuropathy. The regimen appeared to be better tolerated than in previous studies that analyzed FOLFIRINOX in metastatic setting due to the omission of fluorouracil bolus and the inferior dose of fluorouracil in continuous infusion. The 7-year results of PRODIGE-23 indicated that the TNT arm achieved a 7-year DFS rate of 67.6% compared with 62.5% in the standard-of-care arm. Increases in MFS, cancer-specific survival, and OS were also observed. Among patients with metastatic relapses, the median OS was 44.4 months in the neoadjuvant arm compared with 39.4 months in the standard-of-care arm ($p = .062$).[293]

Outcomes of Multimodality Treatment in Patients with Locally Advanced Rectal Cancer

There are expected complications that could arise from the treatment of patients with LARC. Every step should be taken to mitigate and reduce treatment complications. Perioperative mortality in patients undergoing multimodality therapy, including TME for LARC, ranges from 1% to 3.5%, and between 23% and 48% of patients develop perioperative complications.[294] Sepsis is the most common complication after rectal cancer surgery. A recent systematic review of the literature, including 53 prospective cohort studies and 45 randomized trials, found a 2% postoperative death rate, 7% rate of surgical wound infection, 11% rate of anastomotic leakage, and a 12% rate of pelvic sepsis.[295] In addition to pelvic sepsis, perineal wound dehiscence is the most common complication after APE. In a large systematic review of 45 studies, the rate of perineal wound complication after SAPE was 15.3% for patients treated with surgery alone, and 32% in those treated with surgery and RT.[296] Many of these patients also had pelvic sepsis. The proportion of patients with perineal complications was similar for those who had ELAPE: 14.8% for surgery alone and 37.6% for surgery and radiation. The rate of perineal hernia was also similar for patients treated with SAPE and ELAPE: 1.8% versus 2%. Other common postoperative complications include urinary retention, pneumonia, and thromboembolic disease.

Surgery for rectal cancer, particularly when combined with CRT or SCRT, has iatrogenic long-term consequences including urinary, sexual, and bowel dysfunction. Up to 39% of patients develop urinary complications, 45% sexual dysfunction, and even a larger proportion, bowel dysfunction.[297,298] A recent population based study found a 26% rate of moderate bowel problems, 17% urinary dysfunction, and 25% severe problems with sexual function among patients treated for rectal cancer. Patients with a stoma were more likely to have difficulty with body image and sexual activity compared to patients with no stoma. Less than 30% of rectal cancer patients reported perfect health; rectal cancer patients were more likely to report problems, compared to patients with colon cancer. A follow-up study of the Dutch TME trial reported that these treatment-related symptoms persist 14 years after treatment; they reported increased sexual dysfunction, and a small decrease in overall functioning, as measured by a variety of quality-of-life questionnaires distributed to the general population.[299]

Contemporary cohorts of stage II and III rectal cancers treated with neoadjuvant CRT, TME, and postoperative chemotherapy have mostly reported 5-year LR rates between 5% and 10%, 5-year DFS of around 60%, and 5-year OS around 70%.

Treatment Selection in Patients with Localized Rectal Cancer

Patients with rectal cancer have multiple treatment options depending on the clinical stage of the tumor, as determined by DRE, proctoscopy, and imaging studies, on the distance of tumor from the anal verge, and on patient performance status and expectations.

The standard treatment for patients with stage I rectal cancer (T1N0 or T2N0) is TME, but LE has increasingly been chosen as a reasonable and acceptable alternative for patients with distal T1N0 tumors. CRT and LE may also be considered as an alternative to TME in patients with T2N0 tumors

Algorithm 65.1

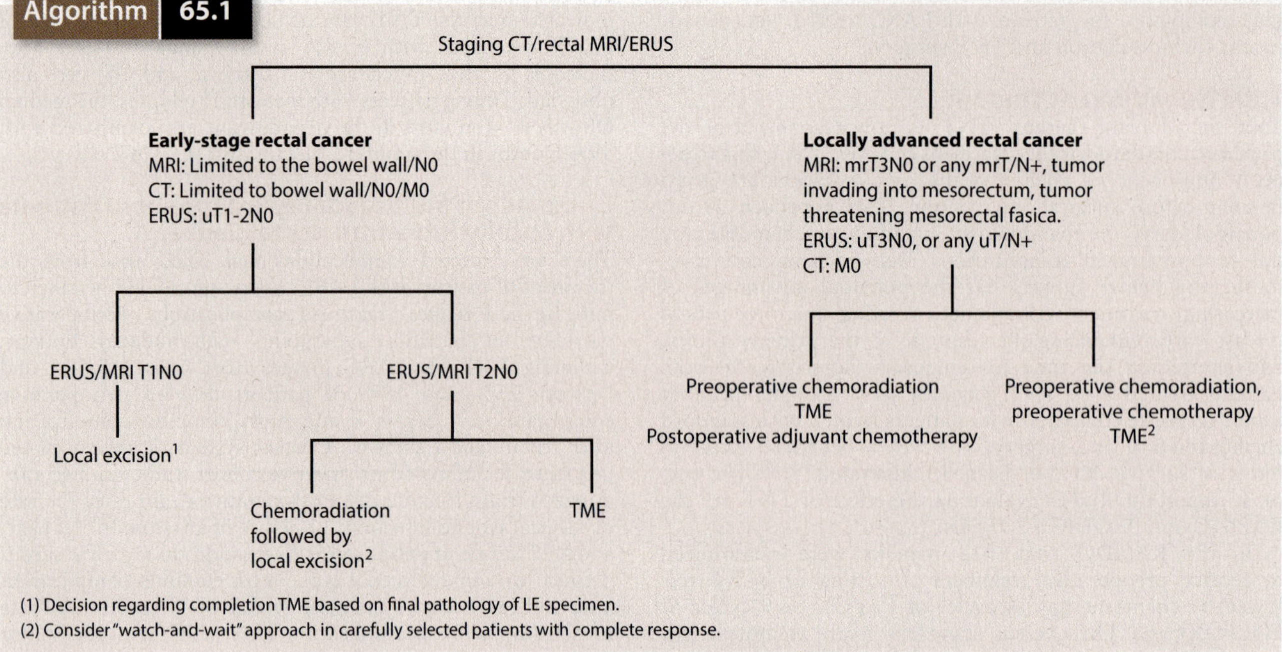

Algorithm 65.1. Approach to rectal cancer according to clinical staging.

interested in sphincter preservation, in whom a TME would require a permanent colostomy.

More advanced tumors—those penetrating beyond the muscularis propria (T3–4, any N) and/or involving the regional lymph nodes (any T, N+), and without evidence of DM—have several treatment options. In the United States and many other countries, where decisions regarding the treatment of rectal cancer are based on clinical TNM staging, patients with locally advanced disease are treated with 5-FU or capecitabine-based CRT, followed by TME, with consideration given to FOLFOX prior to CRT as an acceptable option (**Algorithm 65.1**).

In Europe and Scandinavia, where rectal cancer patients are stratified into different risk categories based on MRI features, patients are recommended for different treatment approaches according to their individual risk category (**Algorithm 65.2**). The MRI-based risk stratification system uses a number of features, such as the proximity of the primary tumor to the MRF, the depth of tumor penetration into the mesorectum, the presence of large venous invasion, and the presence of metastatic lymph nodes. Based on these features, they have developed a three-tier classification scheme that includes low risk (the good), intermediate risk (the bad), and high risk (the ugly); each group has a different risk of relapse, and therefore requires different treatment strategies.[187,300] The low-risk group is recommended TME alone. The intermediate-risk group is recommended SCRT followed by TME, while the high-risk group is recommended neoadjuvant CRT followed by TME. This treatment approach, guided by MRI risk categorization, is based mainly on results of prospective observational studies conducted in institutions with significant expertise in rectal cancer, but has not yet been tested in prospective, randomized trials.

For patients requiring a TME, the decision between an APE and a sphincter-preserving low anterior resection depends on the relationship of the tumor with the anal sphincter and the levator muscle. In general, an APE is required when the tumor directly involves these structures, or is so close to the sphincter that

Algorithm 65.2

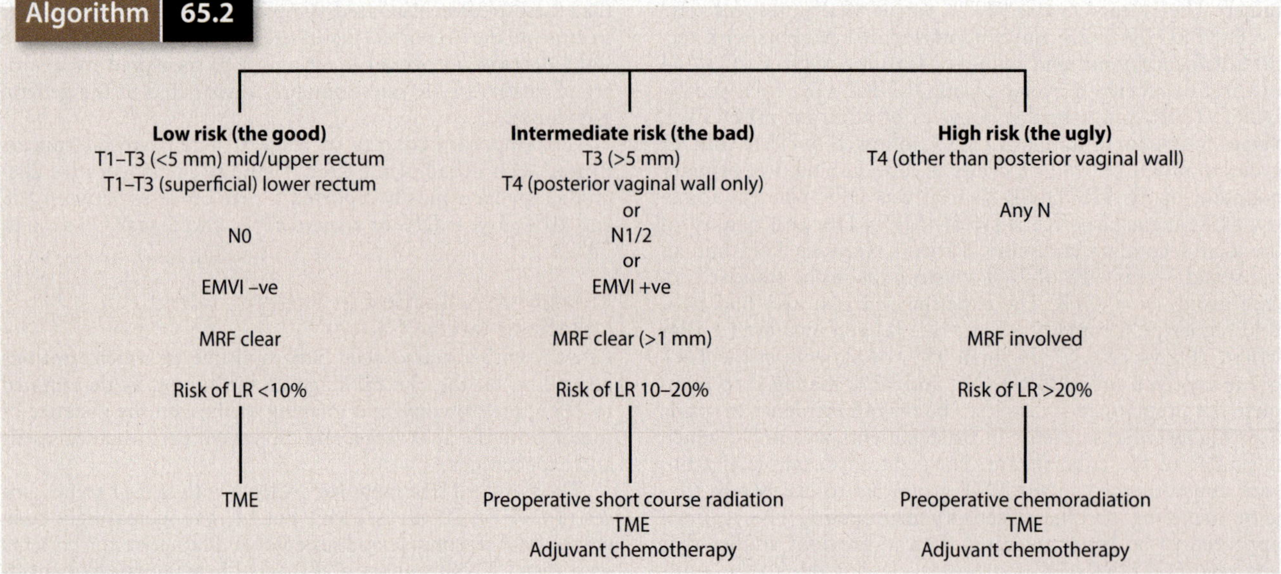

Algorithm 65.2. Approach to locally advanced rectal cancer based on a three-tier risk stratification system ("the good, the bad, and the ugly").

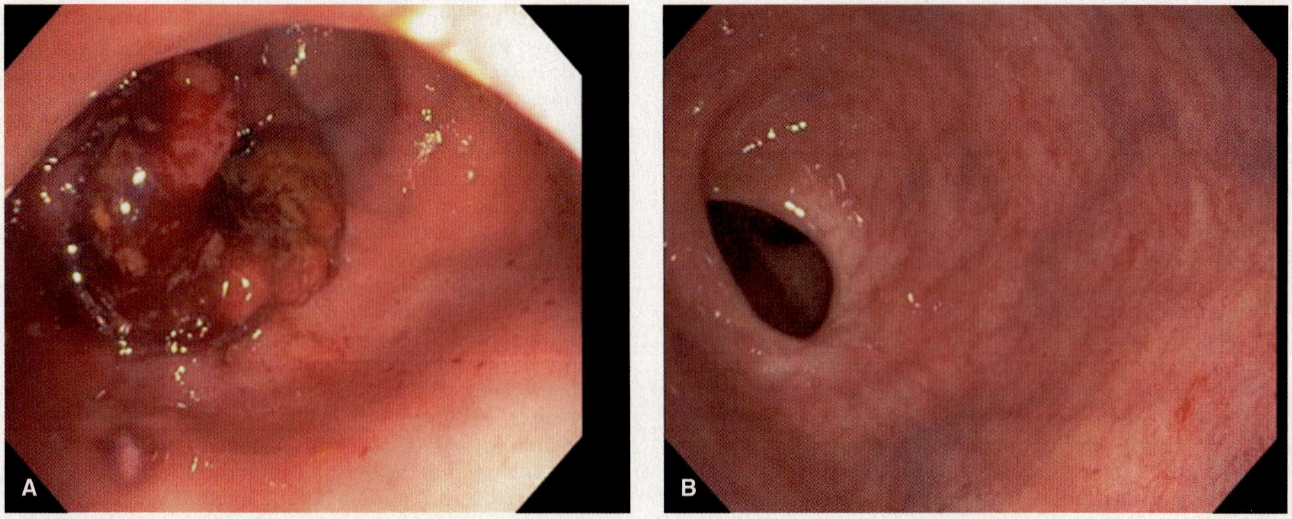

Figure 65.15. Neoadjuvant treatment including chemoradiation and chemotherapy in rectal cancer can lead to a complete response, and selected patients with such response can potentially avoid surgery. This nonoperative management strategy is referred to as the "watch-and-wait" approach. Recent data suggest that watch-and-wait can be a reasonable option in carefully selected and closely followed patients. **A:** Low rectal cancer invading sphincter muscles, proctectomy would require a permanent stoma. **B:** No evidence of tumor regrowth, 3 years after completion of neoadjuvant therapy the patient remains cancer free with a rectum-preserving watch-and-wait approach.

resection with a negative resection margin will result in a loss of sphincter function. In borderline cases, baseline anal sphincter and bowel function, as well as patient wishes and desires should be taken into consideration. The patient should be counseled about LR rates and expected long-term surgical outcomes.

Watch and Wait

In recent years, the proportion of patients being treated with "watch and wait" has increased significantly with the adaption of TNT, which has improved the percentage of patients with complete pathologic response. Rectal adenocarcinomas display a variable degree of response to radiation and chemotherapy. A significant proportion of patients undergoing neoadjuvant chemotherapy and radiation have no viable cancer cells in the rectal specimens after TME surgery. Patients with such a pathologic complete response, have a low risk of tumor recurrence and excellent long-term survival.[301] Based on this observation, surgeons are now questioning the need for TME surgery in patients without apparent residual viable tumor based on DRE, endoscopy, and MRI.[302] Patients with such a clinical complete response are now followed in a close surveillance protocol known as watch and wait (**Fig. 65.15**). While some patients have developed local tumor regrowth requiring TME surgery, some have achieved long-term organ preservation. This approach is particularly appealing to patients with distal rectal cancer who otherwise will require an abdominoperineal excision of the rectum and an end colostomy. Retrospective institutional case series have supported the watch-and-wait strategy for patients with a clinical complete response to neoadjuvant CRT.[303] Previous studies have also suggested that watch and wait may be safe, but it should be considered an experimental approach deserving further investigation.[190] However, with the significant rise in the treatment of rectal cancer with TNT, a stronger case is being made for watch and wait.[301–303]

TUMOR-RELATED EMERGENCIES

Between 15% and 30% of all CRC patients present as surgical emergencies, obstruction (78%) being the most common presentation, followed by perforation (10%) and bleeding (4%).[304–306] Chronic bleeding leading to severe anemia is common, particularly in right-sided tumors; but acute hemorrhage requiring surgical or endovascular intervention is infrequent. Obstruction is the presenting symptom in more than 15% of patients diagnosed with CRC, and CRC is responsible for more than 50% of all cases of acute colonic obstruction.[307] Rectal cancers seldom present as an emergency (5.9%); this is much more likely with colon cancers (21.7%), most of which are in the left colon where the feces are solid, the lumen is smaller, and tumors are more likely to be annular.[305] Large-bowel obstruction may be secondary to other conditions such as diverticular disease and volvulus, which are the differential diagnosis of CRC.

The obstructed bowel undergoes significant changes in motility, secretion, and blood flow, which are responsible for the clinical manifestations. Progressive distension in the presence of a competent ileocecal valve results in a closed-loop obstruction. The increase in intraluminal pressure can compromise the mucosal blood flow and lead to irreversible ischemia. Tension in the wall of the distended bowel increases in proportion to the fourth power of the radius; the risk of ischemia and subsequent perforation is therefore high, particularly in the cecum, the segment of colon with the largest diameter.[308] The risk of perforation is related not only to the caliber of the colon, but also to the onset of obstruction (higher risk when acute) and the duration of the obstruction. Mucosal ischemia has been implicated as the cause of a nonspecific form of colitis that, in some patients, develops proximally to the site of obstruction. The presence of ischemia, which can only be diagnosed at the time of surgery, should influence the extent of resection.

Acute colonic obstruction manifests as abdominal discomfort or frank pain (depending on the onset of the obstruction), reduction or complete cessation of the passage of flatus and feces, and progressive abdominal distension. Abdominal tenderness, particularly if associated with fever and leukocytosis, requires immediate evaluation to exclude perforation or ischemia. DRE reveals an empty rectum in most patients with large-bowel obstruction.

Colonic obstruction must be distinguished from pseudo-obstruction. While the symptoms are similar, colonic pseudo-obstruction often presents in a specific clinical setting (patient immobilization, use of opioids, electrolyte imbalance), is still associated with passage of small amounts of stool and flatus, and is not associated with tenderness.[309] However, definitive diagnosis often requires specific radiologic tests, such as CT and MRI.

A plain abdominal film demonstrates colonic distension, with air-fluid levels, and a cut-off at the site of obstruction.

The absence of small-bowel distension indicates a competent ileocecal valve, with an increased risk of cecal perforation. The presence of gas in the small bowel and rectum raises the possibility of ileus or colonic pseudo-obstruction, but radiologic findings can be misleading. The presence of intramural gas indicates advanced ischemia. A chest radiograph should always be obtained to exclude the presence of pneumoperitoneum.

A water-soluble contrast enema may help to determine the degree and level of obstruction. The flow of contrast to the cecum and the absence of mucosal abnormalities suggest pseudo-obstruction. The osmotic effect of the water-soluble contrast material may have a therapeutic effect in decompressing the colon in these patients.[310] The mucosal detail at the site of obstruction may help to define the cause of obstruction. However, endoscopy is a better alternative to contrast enema when confirming the presence of cancer. CT of the chest, abdomen, and pelvis often locates the transition point between the distended bowel above the obstruction and the collapsed bowel distal to that point. It also helps define the cause of the obstruction and, if malignant obstruction is confirmed, it is useful in staging the tumor.[311]

When compared with elective surgery, patients requiring emergency surgery tend to have more advanced disease. Even when stratified by stage, however, survival is worse for patients undergoing emergency surgery.[305,312] Also, an R1 or R2 resection is 10 times more likely for patients receiving emergency surgery.[313]

Patients presenting with obstructing CRC have higher operative mortality and morbidity and a poorer long-term prognosis than patients undergoing elective resection.[306,314] Perioperative mortality is three times higher in surgery performed for obstruction, compared with elective surgery.[306] Cardiopulmonary complications and abdominal sepsis are the major causes of in-hospital mortality and morbidity. The aim of surgery is therefore to minimize morbidity while obtaining functional results similar to those obtained for patients undergoing elective resection.

Patients with colonic obstruction are often dehydrated, and require preoperative fluid resuscitation and correction of electrolyte imbalances before surgery. A urinary catheter facilitates fluid management. Unstable patients should be monitored appropriately in the intensive care unit. A nasogastric tube prevents accumulation of swallowed air. Given the large fecal load proximal to the point of obstruction, antibiotic prophylaxis with a second-generation cephalosporin or a combination of an aminoglycoside and metronidazole should be given at the time of surgery.

The surgical management depends on the location of the obstruction. Lesions proximal to the splenic flexure are commonly treated by an extended right hemicolectomy, with primary anastomosis between the terminal ileum and the nonobstructed colon distal to the lesion. This is a single procedure that removes the entire segment of distended and potentially ischemic bowel and eliminates the risk of leaving a synchronous tumor in the obstructed colon. Some of these patients develop mild diarrhea, which is usually temporary.

The management of a lesion located distal to the splenic flexure is more controversial. The earlier described three-stage procedure (1—Diverting colostomy, 2—Tumor resection and anastomosis, 3—Colostomy closure) is rarely used today. A safe choice is the two-stage procedure, with initial resection of the segment containing the tumor, closure of the rectal stump as a Hartmann pouch, and construction of an end colostomy, followed by bowel anastomosis at a later date. However, the cumulative mortality and morbidity of both procedures is significant, and at least 30% of patients are left with a permanent colostomy.[315] In most tertiary centers, this operation is now limited to situations in which a primary anastomosis is contraindicated (eg, extensive peritoneal contamination and/or severe sepsis).

The goal of surgery today is to relieve the obstruction and treat the cancer in a single operative procedure. Options include: (1) self-expanding metallic stents (SEMS) as a bridge to elective segmental colon resection, (2) subtotal colectomy and ileorectal anastomosis, (3) segmental colon resection, intraoperative colonic lavage, and primary anastomosis.

The rationale for the use of SEMS is temporary relief of the obstruction, avoiding the morbidity associated with an emergency operation, allowing medical stabilization, full staging work-up, one-stage surgery with primary anastomosis, and a minimally invasive approach. Most of the experience with this method comes from retrospective case-series studies; the success in relieving the obstruction ranges from 40% to 100%.[316] SEMS also has associated complications, such as reobstruction (12%), migration (11%), and perforation (4.5%).[316]

Several randomized, controlled trials comparing SEMS with emergency surgery have been published, with conflicting results.[317–321] Overall, the clinical success rate of relieving obstruction with SEMS ranges from 40% to 97%. It is important to recognize that the overall complication rate across these trials is variable (8.3% to 35%) and a recent prospective trial conducted in the Netherlands was stopped prematurely, due to an increased number of colonic perforations in the SEMS arm.[321] Perforation from the use of stents may result in a shorter DFS.[322] A Dutch population-based cohort study compared decompressing stoma and SEMS as a bridge to surgery for left-sided obstructive colon cancer and found no difference in intermediate-term oncologic outcomes and similar complication rate.[323]

A subtotal colectomy with ileorectal anastomosis is a quick operation in which nondistended bowel is used for the anastomosis. This procedure minimizes the risk of fecal spillage, eliminates the risk of missing a synchronous tumor in the obstructed portion of the colon, and facilitates surveillance. The disadvantages, however, include a higher incidence of bowel obstruction after ileorectal anastomosis and the development of postoperative diarrhea, which may become incapacitating in elderly patients.[324]

A segmental resection with intraoperative colonic lavage and primary anastomosis avoids the risk of postoperative diarrhea, but carries a risk of fecal spillage and missing synchronous tumor. In addition, it requires using previously obstructed bowel for the construction of the anastomosis. Surgical tradition has condemned the performance of an anastomosis in an unprepared colon. Experience accumulated from the management of patients with civilian colon trauma has demonstrated that, under specific circumstances, a primary anastomosis can be performed safely in an unprepared colon, provided the bowel appears healthy and there is no extensive soiling in the peritoneal cavity. This experience has been transferred to the treatment of malignant colonic obstruction. Therefore, a segmental resection with colonic lavage and primary anastomosis is a viable option, as long as the colon is not ischemic and there is no spillage during the operation. The use of a temporary diverting ileostomy may be necessary, but when the safety of a primary anastomosis is questionable, a staged procedure with a segmental resection, a Hartmann pouch, and an end colostomy, may be preferable.[325]

SURVEILLANCE AFTER CURATIVE RESECTION FOR COLON AND RECTAL CANCER

Recurrence of CRC after curative treatment is a dreaded sequelae and outcomes with further treatment is dependent on how early the recurrence is identified. About one-third of patients with CRC treated with curative intent will develop recurrence of disease or a second colorectal primary. The majority of recurrences arise within 3 years of the initial treatment, and almost all arise within 5 years. Recurrences are usually diagnosed at an advanced stage and have an ominous prognosis. Therefore, surveillance regimens are critical to identify recurrences before they become symptomatic, and while they are still potentially resectable.[326,327] Several meta-analyses of prospective, randomized trials comparing intensive or minimal surveillance after curative resection in patients with stage I to III CRC suggest that recurrences were diagnosed earlier and surgical salvage was more likely in patients undergoing intensive surveillance.[328] The survival benefit can only be partly attributed to the improved ability to resect recurrences; other elements such as increased psychological support, behavior modifications, and better treatment of comorbid conditions that accompany intensive surveillance regimens are also thought to contribute to improved survival. Based on this evidence, cancer organizations have established guidelines for surveillance after curative resection of CRC. All of them include a combination of regular history and physical examination, determination of CEA level, endoscopy, and imaging of the chest, abdomen, and pelvis. Some clinicians recommend surveillance for stage II and III diseases, while others also include stage I. In the future, surveillance will be risk adapted, targeting patients more likely to benefit from intensive surveillance based on clinical and molecular prognostic factors. Despite these recommendations, a recent population-based cohort study of 57 patients concluded that 70% were diagnosed between scheduled examinations.[327]

TREATMENT OF STAGE IV COLON AND RECTAL CANCER

Between 20% and 34% of all CRC patients are metastatic at the time of diagnosis; these are known as synchronous metastases. Another one-third of patients will develop metastasis sometime after undergoing treatment of the primary disease; this is known as metachronous metastasis. Synchronous metastases are usually more extensive and, in general, carry a worse prognosis compared to metachronous metastases.

The liver is the most common site of CRC metastasis, and liver metastasis is the most common cause of cancer death in patients with CRC. Autopsy studies have revealed that 50% of patients dying from CRC have liver metastasis and, in one-third of them, the liver is the only site of metastatic disease.[329] Some patients with liver-only metastatic disease are resectable at the time of diagnosis. Others are not resectable, due to the involvement of critical structures by large volume of metastatic disease. The treatment of stage IV CRC patients is complex, and requires consideration of the number of organs involved, the number and size of the metastasis, the location, the symptoms related to the primary in the colon or rectum, whether the tumor is resectable or not, and the patient's performance status. Treatment decisions should be made after discussion in a multidisciplinary tumor board.[330] A simplified algorithm for the treatment of patients with stage IV CRC is presented in **Algorithm 65.3**. The discussion is centered on patients with liver metastases, but these principles are equally applicable to patients with lung metastasis. Surgery is the only curative treatment for patients with colorectal metastases. Other forms of local therapy, such as RT or ablation, may improve survival. Most patients with metastatic disease benefit from systemic chemotherapy, either as adjuvant treatment to surgery or as the sole form of treatment.

Treatment of the Primary Tumor in Stage IV CRC

In the past, all patients presenting with synchronous metastasis were recommended to have resection of the primary tumor, to avoid complications such as obstruction or perforation during treatment of the metastatic disease. However, recent data suggest that patients with unresectable metastasis and an asymptomatic primary are unlikely to develop complications related to the primary tumor that require surgical intervention while the patient is receiving systemic chemotherapy. Currently, primary tumor resection is recommended for patients undergoing curative-intent resection of all metastatic disease, or for patients with unresectable metastasis and a symptomatic primary tumor. The treatment of patients with unresectable metastasis and an asymptomatic primary tumor is controversial. The benefit of avoiding complications related to tumor progression should be balanced against the mortality and morbidity associated with a noncurative resection, and the delay in starting systemic chemotherapy.

Observational studies and secondary analysis of prospective trials have reported an association between primary

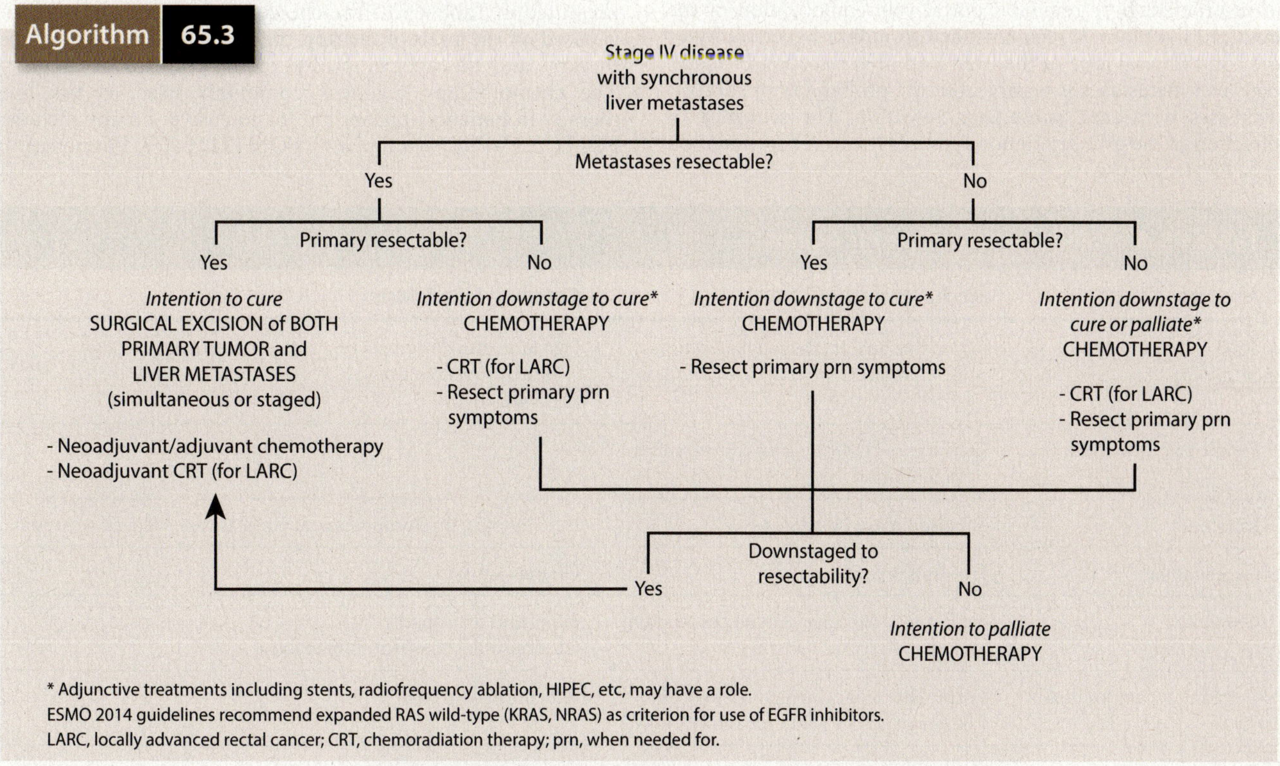

Algorithm 65.3. Stage IV rectal cancer treatment algorithm.

tumor resection and improved survival. A recent meta-analysis found a difference of 6.4 months in survival in patients undergoing resection.[331] However, these studies are limited by strong patient selection bias and outdated chemotherapy regimens. Patients undergoing resection are more likely to have liver-only disease, single metastasis, and tumors located in the colon. Rectal cancer patients are less likely to undergo primary tumor resection compared to patients with colon cancer, probably due to the higher complexity of rectal surgery, the possibility of using palliative CRT, and the fear of a colostomy.

Resection of asymptomatic tumors in stage IV disease has not consistently shown improvements in survival, nor does it necessarily reduce the risk of complications.[332] A recent analysis of the SEER database revealed that the proportion of patients with stage IV CRC undergoing primary tumor resection has been progressively decreasing in the last decade.[333] Despite this decrease in primary tumor resection, relative survival has been increasing during the same period of time. The improvement in survival has coincided with the introduction of more effective chemotherapy agents. However, the relative contribution of the declining rate of primary resection and the more active chemotherapeutic agents is unknown. In this SEER data analysis, more than half of patients diagnosed with stage IV CRC in 2009 had resection of the primary tumor, suggesting that current treatment practice lags behind evidence-based treatment guidelines. These data lend support to current guidelines that do not recommend primary tumor resection in asymptomatic patients with unresectable metastases.[334]

Surgical Treatment of Colorectal Metastases

The prognosis of patients with liver metastases has improved over the last several decades with 5-year survival ranging from 40% to 60% for many patients. Patients with a single, isolated liver metastasis have 5-year overall survival rates as high as 70% to 80%. Liver metastases are considered resectable with curative intent if all disease can be removed with negative resection margin while preserving adequate liver reserve. Incomplete resection or tumor debulking is not recommended because it is associated with morbidity without impacting survival. The size of the metastasis is not a contraindication for surgery. When a curative liver resection may potentially result in insufficient liver remnant, portal vein embolization of the involved liver lobe is recommended to induce hypertrophy of the contralateral lobe of the liver. Repeated resection of recurrent liver metastases is feasible, but the probability of survival decreases with each subsequent resection. The sequence of resection of the primary tumor and liver lesion is dependent on several factors. Simultaneous liver and colon resection is safe and efficient in a selected group of patients. Overall complication rate and hospital stay are lower as a second laparotomy can be avoided.[335,336]

The role of nonsurgical liver-directed therapy for the treatment of liver-only or liver-dominant metastatic disease is controversial. Tumor ablation is indicated in patients who are amenable to local therapy but are not candidates for surgical resection due to comorbidities. It can also be combined with surgery in patients with mixed resectable and unresectable lesions due to their anatomical location or insufficient liver remnant.[337] Other liver-directed therapies for which there is no consensus regarding efficacy are transarterial hepatic chemoembolization/radioembolization, liver-directed radiation, and hepatic arterial infusion (HAI) therapy. HAI was first developed over 45 years ago and has shown to be appropriate adjuvant treatment for patients with liver-dominant metastatic disease.[338] Patients with liver metastases refractory to all standard lines of chemotherapy may respond to HAI with 5-fluorodeoxyuridine (5-FUDR).[339] Additionally, selected patients with strictly defined unresectable CRLM can experience enough response after combination treatment with HAI and systemic therapy to become resectable.[340]

Colorectal lung metastases can also be surgically removed following the same principles outlined for liver metastasis. Resection must be complete, based on the anatomic location of the disease, and with maintenance of adequate respiratory function. Resection of both liver and lung metastases is feasible in selected cases, but resection in the presence of nonhepatic extrapulmonary disease should be reserved for carefully selected patients. Ablation and radiation are also options for patients with nonresectable lung metastases.[334]

Chemotherapy for Metastatic Disease

Principles of Chemotherapy

A number of antineoplastic agents such as 5-FU or capecitabine, oxaliplatin, and irinotecan, and new biologic agents, such as bevacizumab, ziv-aflibercept, cetuximab, panitumumab, and regorafenib, are currently used in combination or as single agents in patients with metastatic CRC. The putative mechanism of action and the toxicity profile of each drug are presented in Table 65.8. The choice of the treatment regimen is based on the goals of therapy, the type and time of previous therapy, and the toxicity profile of the constituent drugs.[334] The chemotherapy regimens commonly used as first-line therapy in patients appropriate for intensive therapy include: FOLFOX (5-FU/LV/oxaliplatin), FOLFIRI (5-FU/LV/irinotecan),

Table 65.8. Main Chemotherapeutic Agents

Agents	Mechanism	Common Side Effects
5-FU	Pyrimidine analog, thymidylate synthase (TS) inhibitor	Hematologic: thrombocytopenia. GI: mucositis. Hepatic steatosis (yellow liver). Photosensitivity
Folinic acid (leucovorin)	Enhances 5-FU effects and contributes to TS inhibition	—
Irinotecan	Topoisomerase I inhibitor	Hematologic: myelosuppression. GI: diarrhea. Hepatic steatosis
Capecitabine	Pro-drug of 5-FU	GI: mucositis
Oxaliplatin	Platinum-based agent, DNA cross-linking	Peripheral neuropathy GI: sinusoidal congestion (blue liver)
Cetuximab/panitumumab	Anti-EGFR monoclonal antibody (for use with KRAS wild-type tumors only)	Acneiform skin rash
Bevacizumab	Anti-VEGF monoclonal antibody	Compromised wound healing

CapeOx (capecitabine/oxaliplatin), infusional 5-FU/LV, capecitabine as a single agent, or FOLFIRINOX (5-FU/LV/oxaliplatin/irinotecan). Cetuximab or bevacizumab can be added to first-line therapy in patients with KRAS/NRAS wild-type CRC, and other combinations such as FOLFOXIRI with bevacizumab have shown promising results.[341,342] The role of maintenance therapy after first-line therapy, and treatment after progression of metastatic disease on first-line therapy, is beyond the scope of this chapter. Median survival of patients with unresectable metastatic CRC, which previously rarely exceeded 12 months, now exceeds 30 months when these agents are used. Increasing evidence suggests that the selection of chemotherapeutic agents will continue to be guided by molecular and genomic characterizations. Early reports have indicated that combined therapy with BRAF and EGFR inhibitors may be effective in treating BRAF V600E metastatic CRC specifically.[343]

Adjuvant Chemotherapy in Resectable Disease

Most patients who undergo resection for CRC liver metastasis ultimately relapse in the liver. It is theorized that the addition of systemic therapy provides treatment of occult micrometastatic disease, reducing the risk of relapse. A number of randomized controlled trials have found a modest improvement in RFS, but not in OS, with chemotherapy delivered before or after liver resection, compared with resection alone. The optimal timing of chemotherapy remains unknown.[344] The potential advantages of preoperative therapy include earlier treatment of micrometastatic disease, evaluation of tumor responsiveness, and the possibility of avoiding resection in patients with tumor progression during therapy. The main disadvantages of preoperative chemotherapy are the progression of nonresponsive tumors that become unresectable during systemic chemotherapy, and the increase in perioperative morbidity due to chemotherapy-induced liver toxicity. The EORTC Intergroup Trial—the only randomized trial evaluating the role of perioperative FOLFOX (3 months before and 3 months after liver surgery) in the management of resectable liver metastases—demonstrated an absolute increase of 7.3% in 3-year progression-free survival in the combined treatment group, compared with the resection-alone group.[345,346] This trial demonstrated an increased rate of postoperative complications in the chemotherapy group (25%) compared with surgery alone (16%), specifically showing a doubling in biliary fistula and hepatic failure rates. The study concluded that perioperative chemotherapy may improve cancer-specific outcomes, but at the cost of increased rates of postoperative complications, including liver dysfunction. Long-term follow-up has revealed the same benefit in progression-free survival, but no difference in OS with the addition of perioperative chemotherapy. The chemotherapy regimens used in the adjuvant setting are the same as those used in first-line therapy. However, bevacizumab can be added as long as it is discontinued at least 6 to 8 weeks before surgery and not restarted for 8 weeks after surgery, because it interferes with wound healing.[347] Cetuximab and panitumumab have been added to first-line regimens in patients with KRAS/NRAS wild type, but the benefits have been inconsistent. In fact, recent data suggest these could even be detrimental; therefore, they are not recommended at this time.[348]

Chemotherapy in Borderline Resectable Disease

A few patients present with liver-only metastases that are not amenable to a complete resection, due to close proximity to essential anatomical structures. Systemic chemotherapy in this setting aims to convert an unresectable patient to resectable status. The duration of treatment in these patients is important. There is a need to balance the minimum time required to achieve a response that will make the patient resectable, while avoiding hepatotoxicity from the chemotherapeutic agents. Both FOLFOX and FOLFIRI increase resectability in 12.5% to 40% of patients initially considered unresectable. A study has shown that adding irinotecan to FOLFOX (FOLFIRINOX) in patients with initially unresectable metastasis increased the resection rate compared to FOLFOX alone.[349] Adding EGFR inhibitors to FOLFOX or FOLFIRI increased the resectability rate in patients with wild-type KRAS/NRAS tumors and initially unresectable liver metastasis.[350,351] Angiogenesis inhibitors combined with FOLFIRI modestly increase resectability of initially unresectable liver metastasis compared to FOLFIRI alone, but have no effect when combined with oxaliplatin-containing regimens.[352,353] To limit FOLFOX- and FOLFIRI-associated toxicity, patients receiving systemic chemotherapy to increase resectability should be evaluated for response every 2 months, and undergo surgery as soon as they become resectable.

Treatment of Peritoneal Carcinomatosis

PC represents the dissemination of cancer cells throughout the lining of the abdominal cavity. Despite advances in cytotoxic chemotherapy and targeted therapy for CRC, these therapies remain less effective for CRC PC. Most patients with PC have widespread metastatic disease and are treated with systemic chemotherapy. The treatment of patients with the peritoneum as the only site of metastasis is controversial.[354,355] Complete cytoreductive surgery (CRS), with removal of all visible abdominal and pelvic disease, and hyperthermic intraperitoneal chemotherapy (HIPEC) are now commonly used in patients with peritoneum-only metastatic CRC. Patient selection is critical for the treatment of PC with cytoreductive surgery and HIPEC. The most commonly used drug for intraperitoneal chemotherapy is mitomycin C, which is minimally active against CRC. As experimental data do not support any biologic benefit from the hyperthermia component, the role of HIPEC has been questioned. Oxaliplatin, irinotecan, doxorubicin, paclitaxel, and carboplatin have also been tested. Comparative studies have not shown a conclusive advantage of mitomycin C over oxaliplatin.[356] This aggressive treatment is associated with significant mortality (0.9% to 5%) and morbidity (12% to 52%), with the most common complications being SSI, hematologic toxicity, and intestinal fistula. Many single-institution case series have reported improved survival in patients treated with CRS and HIPEC followed by systemic chemotherapy, compared to systemic chemotherapy alone. A recent review of 19 studies conducted from 1999 to 2009 reported a median survival of 33 months for patients treated with CRS and HIPEC versus 12.5 months for patients undergoing palliative surgery and/or systemic chemotherapy.[357] These studies have been criticized because of strong patient selection bias favoring peritoneum-only disease in the CRS/HIPEC group, an undefined role for palliative treatment, and suboptimal chemotherapy in the nonsurgical group. One prospective trial randomized patients to 5-FU/LV with palliative surgery versus CRS, HIPEC, and postoperative 5-FU/LV. OS was 12.6 months in the standard arm versus 22.2 months in the HIPEC group.[358] This study has been criticized because it also included patients with pseudomyxoma peritonei of appendiceal origin, and because it was conducted before most of the drugs currently used in metastatic disease were available. In the French PRODIGE-7 randomized trial, CRS-HIPEC showed no overall survival benefit over CRS alone and suggests that HIPEC should be abandoned in patients with resectable PC.[359] However, this study has been criticized because of its small sample size and for using oxaliplatin as a HIPEC regimen. In spite of this criticism, CRS and HIPEC are commonly performed regimens for patients with peritoneum-only colorectal metastases.[360]

The selection criteria for this complex and potentially morbid treatment are not well defined. The most important prognostic factors in patients undergoing CRS and HIPEC are the Peritoneal Cancer Index (PCI), a grading of tumor burden at the time of surgery, and the completeness of cytoreduction (CC) score. Unfortunately, the determinants of these scores are only available at the time of abdominal exploration during surgery. Therefore, they have not been useful in selecting those patients more likely to benefit from CRS and HIPEC. Recently, a Peritoneal Surface Disease Severity Score (PSDSS) that includes patient symptoms, extent of peritoneal dissemination, and primary tumor histology has been developed to stratify patients at the time of diagnosis, without the need of an operation.[361] The PSDSS score system has been found to be an independent prognostic factor in multivariate analysis, not only for patients undergoing CRS and HIPEC, but also for patients treated with systemic chemotherapy. This score may help eliminate selection bias in future comparisons of different treatments, in patients with peritoneum-only metastatic CRC. Complete resectability of the disease is considered an important factor for HIPEC to have the greatest chance of success. Other factors that play a role in the decision to use HIPEC include responsiveness to chemotherapy, extent of disease, and overall tumor biology.

Immunotherapy for CRC

An important part of the immune system is its ability to keep itself from attacking the body's normal cells. To do end, the immune system uses "checkpoints"—proteins on immune cells that need to be turned on (or off) to start an immune response. CRC cells sometimes use these checkpoints to avoid being attacked by the immune system. Drugs that target these checkpoints help to restore the immune response against CRC cells. For people with either early- or advanced-stage colorectal cancer, immunotherapy is now a cornerstone of treatment if the tumor has findings of dMMR (deficient mismatch repair) or MSI-H (microsatellite instability-high). In the last few years immune checkpoint inhibition—targeting inhibitory signal that tumors use to scape immune recognition—has become new treatment modality for MMRd/MSI-H metastatic CRC.[362] Antibodies targeting PD1 (pembrolizumab, nivolumab, dostarlimab), PDL1 (atezolizumab), and CTL4 (ipilimumab) are now used in clinical practice in patients with metastatic disease and in the adjuvant setting for nonmetastatic MMRd/MSI-H colon and rectal cancers, alone or in combination with other chemotherapy agents and RT.[177,363–367] While highly effective in achieving durable responses, immune checkpoint inhibition is also associated with specific toxicity such as diarrhea and colitis, skin rashes, elevation of liver enzymes and fatigue. Other side effects of these drugs include cough, nausea, loss of appetite, constipation, joint pain, and itching. With more advances in the understanding of the intersection between host immune surveillance and tumorigenesis, immunotherapy will continue to play an important role in the treatment of CRC.

TREATMENT OF LOCALLY RECURRENT CRC

LR after curative-intent surgery is defined as a relapse of tumor in the surgical field of the initial procedure, including the anastomosis, regional nodes, surgical scars, and drain tracts.[365] Intraluminal recurrence at the site of the anastomosis is most likely due to inadequate resection margins at the index operation. Recurrence outside of the lumen of the bowel at the site of the vicinity of the anastomosis is likely due to micrometastasis form unresected lymph nodes. While most patients with LR also have DM, a few have isolated LR. A complete surgical resection is the only curative option for patients with isolated locally recurrent CRC, but is associated with considerable morbidity and mortality.[368]

The risk of LR is higher for rectal cancer compared to colon cancer, for advanced stage tumors (T4), for tumors with high-risk histologic features (lymphovascular and perineural invasion, grade III or IV, signet ring cell histology), perforating or obstructing tumors, and patients with close or involved CRM. Most local recurrences present within 3 years after primary surgery, but LR tends to occur later in patients treated with CRT and surgery, compared to those treated with surgery alone. In the Dutch TME trial, 10% of LRs occurred more than 3 years after surgery in patients treated with TME, versus 31% in patients treated with preoperative RT and TME.[369]

While some LRs are detected though surveillance, while asymptomatic, most are diagnosed after they become symptomatic. This presentation underscores the importance of routine surveillance and vigilance. Symptoms of local recurrence include bowel obstruction, abdominal distension, rectal or vaginal bleeding, and urinary problems.[370] Pelvic pain is common, and is a predictor of reduced long-term survival.[371] A common manifestation of recurrence in patients who have had abdominoperineal resection (APR) is a nonhealing perineal wound. Whenever symptoms suggestive of recurrence arise, a detailed history and complete physical examination must be done. This includes DRE in patients who have undergone sphincter-preserving surgery, and a pelvic examination in females. If recurrent tumor is identified, endoscopy and imaging studies will help assess extent of disease and surgical risk. A complete colonoscopy should be performed if possible. Intraluminal recurrences are easily diagnosed with endoscopy and biopsy. Cystoscopy is required for patients who present with urogenital symptoms, as these strongly indicate tumoral invasion of the ureters and bladder.[372] CEA is routinely measured during follow-up surveillance after primary rectal cancer resection. Elevation of this tumor marker is frequently the first sign of recurrence.[373] However, elevated CEA is present in only about 50% of patients. Patients with elevated CEA should undergo further work-up with imaging studies.

A CT scan of the chest, abdomen, and pelvis is the primary imaging modality used in these patients, and it is especially helpful in identifying metastases in the liver, lung, and peritoneum, and evaluating regional adenopathy.[374] MRI is more accurate than CT in detecting and staging pelvic LR[375]; although it has been ineffective when added to routine follow-up, ERUS may be useful in diagnosing LR after LE of distal rectal cancer.[376] Positron emission tomography (PET) using the glucose analog fluorodeoxyglucose (FDG), particularly when combined with a CT scan, is helpful in distinguishing between postsurgical changes and tumor recurrence. In a meta-analysis comparing FDG-PET, FDG-PET/CT, CT, and MRI in the detection of recurrent CRC in patients with high suspicion of recurrent disease, based on symptoms or elevated CEA, FDG-PET and FDG-PET/CT performed more accurately than CT scan.[377] PET/CT also demonstrated greater accuracy than MRI in identification of lymph node recurrence in a lesion levels analysis.[378] Overall accuracy of FDG-PET/CT is slightly higher than FDG-PET: 92.3% (94% sensitivity, 77.2% specificity) versus 89% (90.3% sensitivity, 80% specificity).[379] However, lesions measuring less than 1 cm in diameter are more difficult to detect with PET scanning, as are mucinous tumors, due to poor FDG uptake. Finally, FDG-PET cannot be used to detect or evaluate LR if there is residual inflammation of the tumor bed secondary to chronic leaks. Regardless of the imaging studies used to help diagnose LR, histologic confirmation is imperative. Anastomotic recurrences should be biopsied endoscopically; extraluminal recurrences can usually be biopsied percutaneously, under radiologic (CT) guidance.

The treatment of locally recurrent CRC should be discussed in a multidisciplinary setting, since it often involves colorectal
6 surgical oncologists, radiation oncologists, medical oncologists, and other specialists. Patients with multifocal LR should be treated with systemic chemotherapy, as in metastatic disease. Only patients with localized LR and good performance status are candidates for surgical resection. Even these patients may benefit from additional systemic chemotherapy or chemoradiation, if they did not receive it at the time of treatment of the primary tumor.[380] Some patients with recurrent rectal cancer treated initially with standard doses of radiation (50.4 Gy in 180 cGy fractions, or biologically equivalent total dose) can be reirradiated to the gross tumor volume using small fractions (180 to 200 cGy), with or without sensitizing chemotherapy.[380] In turn, these patients should be discussed in a multidisciplinary tumor board. Reirradiation seems to increase the possibility of an R0 resection in patients with resectable

disease or provides good palliation in unresectable patients. Following preoperative chemotherapy and/or radiotherapy, restaging should be done to exclude interim development of DM and to ascertain the extent of the LR.

Surgery is the only curative option for patients with locally recurrent rectal cancer. Without treatment, median survival is typically 6 to 7 months[381]; systemic chemotherapy can prolong survival, similar to patients with systemic recurrence. Only patients with good performance status, with recurrences that, based on anatomical location, are amenable to an R0 resection, should be considered surgical candidates. A resection with gross positive margins (R2) should not be attempted, because it provides no oncologic advantage to the patient and is associated with significant morbidity. Patients found to have microscopic positive margins (R1) may benefit from intraoperative radiation. However, this modality is only available at some institutions and requires preoperative planning. Therefore, the treatment of locally recurrent CRC should be limited to institutions with appropriate expertise and equipment.

Only about one-third of patients with isolated locally recurrent CRC are candidates for surgical salvage with curative intent. In the Intergroup Study 0114, which investigated several chemotherapy regimens in patients with LARC, only 159 (35%) of the 448 patients with single-site first recurrences in the liver, lung, or pelvis had curative-intent surgery.[370] The proportion of patients undergoing resection was similar for liver, lung, or local recurrences. OS differed significantly between the resected and nonresected groups, with 5-year OS of 27% and 6%, respectively ($p < .001$). The 5-year DFS was in the range of 30% for patients undergoing resection of tumors in solitary sites of the liver or lung, and 20% for those undergoing resection of LRs. Retrospective case series from institutions with experience in the treatment of locally recurrent CRC report 5-year survival rates close to 35% for patients with R0 resections, compared to 21% for patients with R1 resections.

Even with all the advances in treatment modalities, not every patient with a recurrent disease can be treated with curative intent. Palliation is an important aspect of the treatment of these patients. Malignant bowel obstruction often requires palliative surgery, stomas, endoluminal stents, or percutaneous gastrostomy tubes. Urinary obstruction is common, requiring stents or percutaneous nephrostomies. Pain is a common symptom in these patients, often requiring the assistance of pain specialists and specialists in palliative care. Carefully selected rectal cancer patients who are unable to or unwilling to undergo palliative resection due to extensive comorbidity, can be treated with aggressive palliative radiation.[382–384]

ACKNOWLEDGMENTS

We gratefully acknowledge the contributions of previous edition authors, Julio Garcia-Aguilar and Emmanouil P. Pappou, as portions of those chapters have been retained in this revision.

References

1. Siegel RL, Miller KD, Jemal A. Cancer statistics, 2019. *CA Cancer J Clin.* 2019;69(1):7–34.
2. Siegel RL, Miller KD, Goding Sauer A, et al. Colorectal cancer statistics, 2020. *CA Cancer J Clin.* 2020;70(3):145–164.
3. American Cancer Society. *Global Cancer Facts & Figures.* 4th Edition. https://www.cancer.org/. 2018.
4. Chan AT, Giovannucci EL. Primary prevention of colorectal cancer. *Gastroenterology.* 2010;138(6):2029–2043.e2010.
5. Lichtenstein P, Holm NV, Verkasalo PK, et al. Environmental and heritable factors in the causation of cancer—analyses of cohorts of twins from Sweden, Denmark, and Finland. *N Engl J Med.* 2000;343(2):78–85.
6. Xue K, Li FF, Chen YW, Zhou YH, He J. Body mass index and the risk of cancer in women compared with men: a meta-analysis of prospective cohort studies. *Eur J Cancer Prev.* 2017;26(1):94–105.
7. Boyle T, Keegel T, Bull F, Heyworth J, Fritschi L. Physical activity and risks of proximal and distal colon cancers: a systematic review and meta-analysis. *J Natl Cancer Inst.* 2012;104(20):1548–1561.
8. Vieira AR, Abar L, Chan DSM, et al. Foods and beverages and colorectal cancer risk: a systematic review and meta-analysis of cohort studies, an update of the evidence of the WCRF-AICR Continuous Update Project. *Ann Oncol.* 2017;28(8):1788–1802.
9. McNabb S, Harrison TA, Albanes D, et al. Meta-analysis of 16 studies of the association of alcohol with colorectal cancer. *Int J Cancer.* 2020;146(3):861–873.
10. Liang PS, Chen TY, Giovannucci E. Cigarette smoking and colorectal cancer incidence and mortality: systematic review and meta-analysis. *Int J Cancer.* 2009;124(10):2406–2415.
11. Parajuli R, Bjerkaas E, Tverdal A, Le Marchand L, Weiderpass E, Gram IT. Cigarette smoking and colorectal cancer mortality among 602,242 Norwegian males and females. *Clin Epidemiol.* 2014;6:137–145.
12. Butterworth AS, Higgins JP, Pharoah P. Relative and absolute risk of colorectal cancer for individuals with a family history: a meta-analysis. *Eur J Cancer.* 2006;42(2):216–227.
13. Henrikson NB, Webber EM, Goddard KA, et al. Family history and the natural history of colorectal cancer: systematic review. *Genet Med.* 2015;17(9):702–712.
14. Heikkinen SMM, Madanat-Harjuoja LM, Seppä KJM, et al. Familial aggregation of early-onset cancers. *Int J Cancer.* 2020; 146(7):1791–1799.
15. Mulder SA, Kranse R, Damhuis RA, Ouwendijk RJ, Kuipers EJ, van Leerdam ME. The incidence and risk factors of metachronous colorectal cancer: an indication for follow-up. *Dis Colon Rectum.* 2012;55(5):522–531.
16. Martinez ME, Baron JA, Lieberman DA, et al. A pooled analysis of advanced colorectal neoplasia diagnoses after colonoscopic polypectomy. *Gastroenterology.* 2009;136(3):832–841.
17. Beaugerie L, Itzkowitz SH. Cancers complicating inflammatory bowel disease. *N Engl J Med.* 2015;372(15):1441–1452.
18. Choi CR, Al Bakir I, Ding NJ, et al. Cumulative burden of inflammation predicts colorectal neoplasia risk in ulcerative colitis: a large single-centre study. *Gut.* 2019;68(3):414–422.
19. Lutgens MW, van Oijen MG, van der Heijden GJ, Vleggaar FP, Siersema PD, Oldenburg B. Declining risk of colorectal cancer in inflammatory bowel disease: an updated meta-analysis of population-based cohort studies. *Inflamm Bowel Dis.* 2013; 19(4):789–799.
20. Andersen NN, Jess T. Has the risk of colorectal cancer in inflammatory bowel disease decreased? *World J Gastroenterol.* 2013;19(43):7561–7568.
21. Ma Y, Yang W, Song M, et al. Type 2 diabetes and risk of colorectal cancer in two large U.S. prospective cohorts. *Br J Cancer.* 2018;119(11):1436–1442.
22. Becker DJ, Iyengar AD, Punekar SR, et al. Diabetes mellitus and colorectal carcinoma outcomes: a meta-analysis. *Int J Colorectal Dis.* 2020;35(11):1989–1999.
23. Fearon ER, Vogelstein B. A genetic model for colorectal tumorigenesis. *Cell.* 1990;61(1):759–767.
24. Cancer Genome Atlas Network. Comprehensive molecular characterization of human colon and rectal cancer. *Nature.* 2012;487(7407):330–337.
25. Negrini S, Gorgoulis VG, Halazonetis TD. Genomic instability—an evolving hallmark of cancer. *Nat Rev Mol Cell Biol.* 2010; 11(3):220–228.
26. Vilar E, Gruber SB. Microsatellite instability in colorectal cancer—the stable evidence. *Nat Rev Clin Oncol.* 2010;7(3):153–162.
27. Rodriguez-Salas N, Dominguez G, Barderas R, et al. Clinical relevance of colorectal cancer molecular subtypes. *Crit Rev Oncol Hematol.* 2017;109:9–19.
28. Jenkins MA, Hayashi S, O'Shea AM, et al. Pathology features in Bethesda guidelines predict colorectal cancer microsatellite instability: a population-based study. *Gastroenterology.* 2007;133(1):48–56.
29. Popat S, Hubner R, Houlston RS. Systematic review of microsatellite instability and colorectal cancer prognosis. *J Clin Oncol.* 2005;23(3):609–618.

30. Venderbosch S, Nagtegaal ID, Maughan TS, et al. Mismatch repair status and BRAF mutation status in metastatic colorectal cancer patients: a pooled analysis of the CAIRO, CAIRO2, COIN, and FOCUS studies. *Clin Cancer Res*. 2014;20(20):5322–5330.
31. Ribic CM, Sargent DJ, Moore MJ, et al. Tumor microsatellite-instability status as a predictor of benefit from fluorouracil-based adjuvant chemotherapy for colon cancer. *N Engl J Med*. 2003;349(3):247–257.
32. Nathke I. Cytoskeleton out of the cupboard: colon cancer and cytoskeletal changes induced by loss of APC. *Nat Rev Cancer*. 2006;6(12):967–974.
33. Colak S, Ten Dijke P. Targeting TGF-β signaling in cancer. *Trends Cancer*. 2017;3(1):56–71.
34. Ben-David E, Bester AC, Shifman S, Kerem B. Transcriptional dynamics in colorectal carcinogenesis: new insights into the role of c-Myc and miR17 in benign to cancer transformation. *Cancer Res*. 2014;74(19):5532–5540.
35. Naccarati A, Polakova V, Pardini B, et al. Mutations and polymorphisms in TP53 gene an overview on the role in colorectal cancer. *Mutagenesis*. 2012;27(2):211–218.
36. Segelov E, Chan D, Shapiro J, et al. The role of biological therapy in metastatic colorectal cancer after first-line treatment: a meta-analysis of randomised trials. *Br J Cancer*. 2014;111(6):1122–1131.
37. Taieb J, Le Malicot K, Shi Q, et al. Prognostic value of BRAF and KRAS mutations in MSI and MSS stage III colon cancer. *J Natl Cancer Inst*. 2016;109(5):djw272.
38. Francipane MG, Lagasse E. mTOR pathway in colorectal cancer: an update. *Oncotarget*. 2014;5(1):49–66.
39. Guinney J, Dienstmann R, Wang X, et al. The consensus molecular subtypes of colorectal cancer. *Nat Med*. 2015;21(11):1350–1356.
40. Menter DG, Davis JS, Broom BM, Overman MJ, Morris J, Kopetz S. Back to the colorectal cancer consensus molecular subtype future. *Curr Gastroenterol Rep*. 2019;21(2):5.
41. American College of Surgeons, Amin MB, Edge SB, Greene FL, et al., eds. *AJCC Cancer Staging Manual*. 8th ed. Springer; 2017.
42. Ozawa T, Ishihara S, Nishikawa T, et al. Prognostic significance of the lymph node ratio in stage IV colorectal cancer patients who have undergone curative resection. *Ann Surg Oncol*. 2015;22(5): 1513–1519.
43. Sloothaak DAM, van der Linden RLA, van de Velde CJH, et al. Prognostic implications of occult nodal tumour cells in stage I and II colon cancer: the correlation between micrometastasis and disease recurrence. *Eur J Surg Oncol*. 2017;43(8):1456–1462.
44. Li Y, Feng Y, Dai W, Li Q, Cai S, Peng J. Prognostic effect of tumor sidedness in colorectal cancer: a SEER-based analysis. *Clin Colorectal Cancer*. 2019;18(1):e104–e116.
45. Goffredo P, Zhou P, Ginader T, et al. Positive circumferential resection margins following locally advanced colon cancer surgery: risk factors and survival impact. *J Surg Oncol*. 2020;121(3):538–546.
46. Birbeck KF, Macklin CP, Tiffin NJ, et al. Rates of circumferential resection margin involvement vary between surgeons and predict outcomes in rectal cancer surgery. *Ann Surg*. 2002;235(4):449–457.
47. Nagtegaal ID, Quirke P. What is the role for the circumferential margin in the modern treatment of rectal cancer? *J Clin Oncol*. 2008;26(2):303–312.
48. Chand M, Siddiqui MR, Swift I, Brown G. Systematic review of prognostic importance of extramural venous invasion in rectal cancer. *World J Gastroenterol*. 2016;22(4):1721–1726.
49. Konishi T, Shimada Y, Hsu M, et al. Contemporary validation of a nomogram predicting colon cancer recurrence, revealing all-stage improved outcomes. *JNCI Cancer Spectr*. 2019;3(2):pkz015.
50. Yiu AJ, Yiu CY. Biomarkers in colorectal cancer. *Anticancer Res*. 2016;36(3):1093–1102.
51. Le DT, Durham JN, Smith KN, et al. Mismatch repair deficiency predicts response of solid tumors to PD-1 blockade. *Science*. 2017;357(6349):409–413.
52. Kopetz S, Grothey A, Yaeger R, et al. Encorafenib, binimetinib, and cetuximab in BRAF V600E-mutated colorectal cancer. *N Engl J Med*. 2019;381(17):1632–1643.
53. De Roock W, Claes B, Bernasconi D, et al. Effects of KRAS, BRAF, NRAS, and PIK3CA mutations on the efficacy of cetuximab plus chemotherapy in chemotherapy-refractory metastatic colorectal cancer: a retrospective consortium analysis. *Lancet Oncol*. 2010;11(8):753–762.
54. Kong JC, Guerra GR, Pham T, et al. Prognostic impact of tumor-infiltrating lymphocytes in primary and metastatic colorectal cancer: a systematic review and meta-analysis. *Dis Colon Rectum*. 2019;62(4):498–508.
55. Pagès F, Mlecnik B, Marliot F, et al. International validation of the consensus immunoscore for the classification of colon cancer: a prognostic and accuracy study. *Lancet*. 2018;391(10135): 2128–2139.
56. You YN, Rustin RB, Sullivan JD. Oncotype DX(®) colon cancer assay for prediction of recurrence risk in patients with stage II and III colon cancer: a review of the evidence. *Surg Oncol*. 2015;24(2):61–66.
57. Kopetz S, Tabernero J, Rosenberg R, et al. Genomic classifier ColoPrint predicts recurrence in stage II colorectal cancer patients more accurately than clinical factors. *Oncologist*. 2015;20(2): 127–133.
58. Niedzwiecki D, Frankel WL, Venook AP, et al. Association between results of a gene expression signature assay and recurrence-free interval in patients with stage II colon cancer in cancer and Leukemia Group B 9581 (Alliance). *J Clin Oncol*. 2016;34(25):3047–3053.
59. Winawer SJ, Zauber AG, Ho MN, et al. Prevention of colorectal cancer by colonoscopic polypectomy. The National Polyp Study Workgroup. *N Engl J Med*. 1993;329(27):1977–1981.
60. Lieberman DA. Clinical practice. Screening for colorectal cancer. *N Engl J Med*. 2009;361(12):1179–1187.
61. Zauber AG, Winawer SJ, O'Brien MJ, et al. Colonoscopic polypectomy and long-term prevention of colorectal-cancer deaths. *N Engl J Med*. 2012;366(8):687–696.
62. Shaukat A, Mongin SJ, Geisser MS, et al. Long-term mortality after screening for colorectal cancer. *N Engl J Med*. 2013;369(12):1106–1114.
63. Loberg M, Kalager M, Holme O, Hoff G, Adami HO, Bretthauer M. Long-term colorectal-cancer mortality after adenoma removal. *N Engl J Med*. 2014;371(9):799–807.
64. Doubeni CA, Corley DA, Quinn VP, et al. Effectiveness of screening colonoscopy in reducing the risk of death from right and left colon cancer: a large community-based study. *Gut*. 2018;67(2): 291–298.
65. Hall IJ, Tangka FKL, Sabatino SA, Thompson TD, Graubard BI, Breen N. Patterns and trends in cancer screening in the United States. *Prev Chronic Dis*. 2018;15:E97.
66. Lin JS, Piper MA, Perdue LA, et al. Screening for colorectal cancer: updated evidence report and systematic review for the US Preventive Services Task Force. *JAMA*. 2016;315(23):2576–2594.
67. Mandel JS, Bond JH, Church TR, et al. Reducing mortality from colorectal cancer by screening for fecal occult blood. Minnesota Colon Cancer Control Study. *N Engl J Med*. 1993;328(19): 1365–1371.
68. Jorgensen OD, Kronborg O, Fenger C. A randomised study of screening for colorectal cancer using faecal occult blood testing: results after 13 years and seven biennial screening rounds. *Gut*. 2002;50(1):29–32.
69. Lindholm E, Brevinge H, Haglind E. Survival benefit in a randomized clinical trial of faecal occult blood screening for colorectal cancer. *Br J Surg*. 2008;95(8):1029–1036.
70. Scholefield JH, Moss SM, Mangham CM, Whynes DK, Hardcastle JD. Nottingham trial of faecal occult blood testing for colorectal cancer: a 20-year follow-up. *Gut*. 2012;61(7): 1036–1040.
71. Brenner H, Tao S. Superior diagnostic performance of faecal immunochemical tests for haemoglobin in a head-to-head comparison with guaiac based faecal occult blood test among 2235 participants of screening colonoscopy. *Eur J Cancer*. 2013;49(14):3049–3054.
72. Hol L, van Leerdam ME, van Ballegooijen M, et al. Screening for colorectal cancer: randomised trial comparing guaiac-based and immunochemical faecal occult blood testing and flexible sigmoidoscopy. *Gut*. 2010;59(1):62–68.

73. Guimarães DP, Fregnani JH, Reis RM, et al. Comparison of a new-generation fecal immunochemical test (FIT) with guaiac fecal occult blood test (gFOBT) in detecting colorectal neoplasia among colonoscopy-referral patients. *Anticancer Res*. 2019;39(1): 261–269.
74. Hassan C, Giorgi Rossi P, Camilloni L, et al. Meta-analysis: adherence to colorectal cancer screening and the detection rate for advanced neoplasia, according to the type of screening test. *Aliment Pharmacol Ther*. 2012;36(10):929–940.
75. Robertson DJ, Lee JK, Boland CR, et al. Recommendations on fecal immunochemical testing to screen for colorectal neoplasia: a consensus statement by the US Multi-Society Task Force on Colorectal Cancer. *Gastroenterology*. 2017;152(5):1217–1237.e1213.
76. Quintero E, Castells A, Bujanda L, et al. Colonoscopy versus fecal immunochemical testing in colorectal-cancer screening. *N Engl J Med*. 2012;366(8):697–706.
77. Ahlquist DA, Sargent DJ, Loprinzi CL, et al. Stool DNA and occult blood testing for screen detection of colorectal neoplasia. *Ann Intern Med*. 2008;149(7):441–450, w481.
78. Lidgard GP, Domanico MJ, Bruinsma JJ, et al. Clinical performance of an automated stool DNA assay for detection of colorectal neoplasia. *Clin Gastroenterol Hepatol*. 2013;11(10): 1313–1318.
79. Imperiale TF, Ransohoff DF, Itzkowitz SH, et al. Multitarget stool DNA testing for colorectal-cancer screening. *N Engl J Med*. 2014;370(14):1287–1297.
80. Redwood DG, Asay ED, Blake ID, et al. Stool DNA testing for screening detection of colorectal neoplasia in Alaska Native people. *Mayo Clin Proc*. 2016;91(1):61–70.
81. Bibbins-Domingo K, Grossman DC, Curry SJ, et al. Screening for colorectal cancer: US Preventive Services Task Force recommendation statement. *JAMA*. 2016;315(23):2564–2575.
82. Selby JV, Friedman GD, Quesenberry CP Jr, et al. A case-control study of screening sigmoidoscopy and mortality from colorectal cancer. *N Engl J Med*. 1992;326(10):653–657.
83. Newcomb PA, Norfleet RG, Storer BE, et al. Screening sigmoidoscopy and colorectal cancer mortality. *J Natl Cancer Inst*. 1992;84(20):1572–1575.
84. Schoen RE, Pinsky PF, Weissfeld JL, et al; PLCO Project Team. Colorectal cancer incidence and mortality with screening flexible sigmoidoscopy. *N Engl J Med*. 2012;355(25):2345–2357.
85. Holme Ø, Løberg M, Kalager M, et al. Effect of flexible sigmoidoscopy screening on colorectal cancer incidence and mortality: a randomized clinical trial. *JAMA*. 2014;312(6):606–615.
86. Segnan N, Armaroli P, Bonelli L, et al. Once-only sigmoidoscopy in colorectal cancer screening: follow-up findings of the Italian Randomized Controlled Trial—SCORE. *J Natl Cancer Inst*. 2011;103(17):1310–1322.
87. Atkin WS, Edwards R, Kralj-Hans I, Wooldrage K, et al; UK Flexible Sigmoidoscopy Trial Investigators. Once-only flexible sigmoidoscopy screening in prevention of colorectal cancer: a multicentre randomised controlled trial. *Lancet*. 2010;375(9726): 1624–1633.
88. Atkin W, Wooldrage K, Parkin DM, et al. Long term effects of once-only flexible sigmoidoscopy screening after 17 years of follow-up: the UK Flexible Sigmoidoscopy Screening randomised controlled trial. *Lancet*. 2017;389(10076):1299–1311.
89. Holme Ø, Løberg M, Kalager M, et al. Long-term effectiveness of sigmoidoscopy screening on colorectal cancer incidence and mortality in women and men: a randomized trial. *Ann Intern Med*. 2018;168(11):775–782.
90. Miller EA, Pinsky PF, Schoen RE, et al. Effect of flexible sigmoidoscopy screening on colorectal cancer incidence and mortality: long-term follow-up of the randomised US PLCO cancer screening trial. *Lancet Gastroenterol Hepatol*. 2019;4(2):101–110.
91. Segnan N, Senore C, Andreoni B, et al. Randomized trial of different screening strategies for colorectal cancer: patient response and detection rates. *J Natl Cancer Inst*. 2005;97(5):347–357.
92. Rutter CM, Savarino JE. An evidence-based microsimulation model for colorectal cancer: validation and application. *Cancer Epidemiol Biomarkers Prev*. 2010;19(8):1992–2002.
93. Brenner H, Stock C, Hoffmeister M. Effect of screening sigmoidoscopy and screening colonoscopy on colorectal cancer incidence and mortality: systematic review and meta-analysis of randomised controlled trials and observational studies. *BMJ*. 2014;348:g2467.
94. Nishihara R, Wu K, Lochhead P, et al. Long-term colorectal-cancer incidence and mortality after lower endoscopy. *N Engl J Med*. 2013;369(12):1095–1105.
95. Brenner H, Chang-Claude J, Jansen L, et al. Reduced risk of colorectal cancer up to 10 years after screening, surveillance, or diagnostic colonoscopy. *Gastroenterology*. 2014;146(3): 709–717.
96. Sharaf RN, Ladabaum U. Comparative effectiveness and cost-effectiveness of screening colonoscopy vs. sigmoidoscopy and alternative strategies. *Am J Gastroenterol*. 2013;108(1):120–132.
97. de Haan MC, Pickhardt PJ, Stoker J. CT colonography: accuracy, acceptance, safety and position in organised population screening. *Gut*. 2015;64(2):342–350.
98. Halligan S, Wooldrage K, Dadswell E, et al. Computed tomographic colonography versus barium enema for diagnosis of colorectal cancer or large polyps in symptomatic patients (SIGGAR): a multicentre randomised trial. *Lancet*. 2013;381(9873): 1185–1193.
99. Rex DK, Boland CR, Dominitz JA, et al. Colorectal cancer screening: recommendations for physicians and patients from the U.S. Multi-Society Task Force on Colorectal Cancer. *Am J Gastroenterol*. 2017;112(7):1016–1030.
100. de Haan MC, van Gelder RE, Graser A, et al. Diagnostic value of CT-colonography as compared to colonoscopy in an asymptomatic screening population: a meta-analysis. *Eur Radiol*. 2011;21(8):1747–1763.
101. Ijspeert JEG, Tutein Nolthenius CJ, Kuipers EJ, et al. CT-colonography vs. colonoscopy for detection of high-risk sessile serrated polyps. *Am J Gastroenterol*. 2016;111(4):516–522.
102. Sakamoto T, Mitsuzaki K, Utsunomiya D, et al. Detection of flat colorectal polyps at screening CT colonography in comparison with conventional polypoid lesions. *Acta Radiol*. 2012;53(7):714–719.
103. Levin B, Lieberman DA, McFarland B, et al. Screening and surveillance for the early detection of colorectal cancer and adenomatous polyps, 2008: a joint guideline from the American Cancer Society, the US Multi-Society Task Force on Colorectal Cancer, and the American College of Radiology. *Gastroenterology*. 2008;134(5):1570–1595.
104. Wolf AMD, Fontham ETH, Church TR, et al. Colorectal cancer screening for average-risk adults: 2018 guideline update from the American Cancer Society. *CA Cancer J Clin*. 2018;68(4): 250–281.
105. Provenzale D, Gupta S, Ahnen DJ, et al. NCCN guidelines insights: colorectal cancer screening, version 1.2018. *J Natl Compr Canc Netw*. 2018;16(8):939–949.
106. Gupta S, Lieberman D, Anderson JC, et al. Recommendations for follow-up after colonoscopy and polypectomy: a consensus update by the US Multi-Society Task Force on Colorectal Cancer. *Gastroenterology*. 2020;158(4):1131–1153.e1135.
107. Gupta S, Provenzale D, Llor X, et al. NCCN guidelines insights: genetic/familial high-risk assessment: colorectal, version 2.2019. *J Natl Compr Canc Netw*. 2019;17(9):1032–1041.
108. Pignone M, Saha S, Hoerger T, et al. Cost-effectiveness analyses of colorectal cancer screening: a systematic review for the U.S. Preventive Services Task Force. *Ann Intern Med*. 2002;137(2): 96–104.
109. Maciosek MV, Coffield AB, Edwards NM, et al. Priorities among effective clinical preventive services: results of a systematic review and analysis. *Am J Prev Med*. 2006;31(1):52–61.
110. Singh S, Singh PP, Murad MH, et al. Prevalence, risk factors, and outcomes of interval colorectal cancers: a systematic review and meta-analysis. *Am J Gastroenterol*. 2014;109(9):1375–1389.
111. Samadder NJ, Curtin K, Tuohy TM, et al. Characteristics of missed or interval colorectal cancer and patient survival: a population-based study. *Gastroenterology*. 2014;146(4):950–960.

112. Lairson DR, Dicarlo M, Deshmuk AA, et al. Cost-effectiveness of a standard intervention versus a navigated intervention on colorectal cancer screening use in primary care. *Cancer*. 2014;120(7):1042–1049.
113. Gupta S, Halm EA, Rockey DC, et al. Comparative effectiveness of fecal immunochemical test outreach, colonoscopy outreach, and usual care for boosting colorectal cancer screening among the underserved: a randomized clinical trial. *JAMA Intern Med*. 2013;173(18):1725–1732.
114. Joseph DA, King JB, Dowling NF, et al. Vital signs: colorectal cancer screening test use—United States, 2018. *MMWR Morb Mortal Wkly Rep*. 2020;69(10):253–259.
115. Mulder SA, Kranse R, Damhuis RA, et al. Prevalence and prognosis of synchronous colorectal cancer: a Dutch population-based study. *Cancer Epidemiol*. 2011;35(5):442–447.
116. Latournerie M, Jooste V, Cottet V, et al. Epidemiology and prognosis of synchronous colorectal cancers. *Br J Surg*. 2008;95(12):1528–1533.
117. Eagye KJ, Nicolau DP. Deep and organ/space infections in patients undergoing elective colorectal surgery: incidence and impact on hospital length of stay and costs. *Am J Surg*. 2009;198(3):359–367.
118. Cima R, Dankbar E, Lovely J, et al. Colorectal surgery surgical site infection reduction program: a national surgical quality improvement program–driven multidisciplinary single-institution experience. *J Am Coll Surg*. 2013;216(1):23–33.
119. Urban JA. Cost analysis of surgical site infections. *Surg Infect (Larchmt)*. 2006;7(Suppl 1):S19–S22.
120. Cataife G, Weinberg DA, Wong HH, et al. The effect of Surgical Care Improvement Project (SCIP) compliance on surgical site infections (SSI). *Med Care*. 2014;52(2 Suppl 1):S66–S73.
121. The American College of Surgeons. ACS National Surgical Quality Improvement Program (ACS NSQIP®). https://www.facs.org/quality-programs/acs-nsqip.
122. Stephen AM, Cummings JH. The microbial contribution to human faecal mass. *J Med Microbiol*. 1980;13(1):45–56.
123. Contant CM, Hop WC, van't Sant HP, et al. Mechanical bowel preparation for elective colorectal surgery: a multicentre randomised trial. *Lancet*. 2007;370(9605):2112–2117.
124. Jung B, Pahlman L, Nystrom PO, et al. Multicentre randomized clinical trial of mechanical bowel preparation in elective colonic resection. *Br J Surg*. 2007;94(6):689–695.
125. Klinger AL, Green H, Monlezun DJ, et al. The role of bowel preparation in colorectal surgery: results of the 2012–2015 ACS-NSQIP data. *Ann Surg*. 2019;269(4):671–677.
126. Nelson RL, Gladman E, Barbateskovic M. Antimicrobial prophylaxis for colorectal surgery. *Cochrane Database Syst Rev*. 2014;5:CD001181.
127. Bratzler DW, Dellinger EP, Olsen KM, et al. Clinical practice guidelines for antimicrobial prophylaxis in surgery. *Am J Health Syst Pharm*. 2013;70(3):195–283.
128. Itani KM, Wilson SE, Awad SS, et al. Ertapenem versus cefotetan prophylaxis in elective colorectal surgery. *N Engl J Med*. 2006;355(25):2640–2651.
129. Poggio JL. Perioperative strategies to prevent surgical-site infection. *Clin Colon Rectal Surg*. 2013;26(3):168–173.
130. Kakkos SK, Caprini JA, Geroulakos G, et al. Combined intermittent pneumatic leg compression and pharmacological prophylaxis for prevention of venous thromboembolism in high-risk patients. *Cochrane Database Syst Rev*. 2008(4):CD005258.
131. Lyman GH, Bohlke K, Khorana AA, et al. Venous thromboembolism prophylaxis and treatment in patients with cancer: American Society of Clinical Oncology Clinical Practice Guideline Update 2014. *J Clin Oncol*. 2015;33(6):654–656.
132. Danielsen AK, Burcharth J, Rosenberg J. Patient education has a positive effect in patients with a stoma: a systematic review. *Colorectal Dis*. 2013;15(6):e276–283.
133. Bardram L, Funch-Jensen P, Jensen P, et al. Recovery after laparoscopic colonic surgery with epidural analgesia, and early oral nutrition and mobilisation. *Lancet*. 1995;345(8952):763–764.
134. Serclova Z, Dytrych P, Marvan J, et al. Fast-track in open intestinal surgery: prospective randomized study (Clinical Trials Gov Identifier no. NCT00123456). *Clin Nutr*. 2009;28(6):618–624.
135. Yang D, He W, Zhang S, et al. Fast-track surgery improves postoperative clinical recovery and immunity after elective surgery for colorectal carcinoma: randomized controlled clinical trial. *World J Surg*. 2012;36(8):1874–1880.
136. Zhuang CL, Ye XZ, Zhang XD, et al. Enhanced recovery after surgery programs versus traditional care for colorectal surgery: a meta-analysis of randomized controlled trials. *Dis Colon Rectum*. 2013;56(5):667–678.
137. Spanjersberg WR, Reurings J, Keus F, et al. Fast track surgery versus conventional recovery strategies for colorectal surgery. *Cochrane Database Syst Rev*. 2011;(2):CD007635.
138. ERAS Compliance Group. The impact of enhanced recovery protocol compliance on elective colorectal cancer resection: results from an international registry. *Ann Surg*. 2015;261(6):1153–1159.
139. Monson JR, Weiser MR, Buie WD, et al; Standards Practice Task Force of the American Society of Colon and Rectal Surgeons. Practice parameters for the management of rectal cancer (revised). *Dis Colon Rectum*. 2013;56(5):535–550.
140. Shiozawa M, Akaike M, Yamada R, et al. Clinicopathological features of skip metastasis in colorectal cancer. *Hepatogastroenterology*. 2007;54(73):81–84.
141. Toyota S, Ohta H, Anazawa S. Rationale for extent of lymph node dissection for right colon cancer. *Dis Colon Rectum*. 1995;38(7):705–711.
142. Saha S, Johnston G, Korant A, et al. Aberrant drainage of sentinel lymph nodes in colon cancer and its impact on staging and extent of operation. *Am J Surg*. 2013;205(3):302–305; discussion 305–306.
143. Wiggers T, Jeekel J, Arends JW, et al. No-touch isolation technique in colon cancer: a controlled prospective trial. *Br J Surg*. 1988;75(5):409–415.
144. Heald RJ. The 'Holy Plane' of rectal surgery. *J R Soc Med*. 1988;81(9):503–508.
145. MacFarlane JK, Ryall RD, Heald RJ. Mesorectal excision for rectal cancer. *Lancet*. 1993;341(8843):457–460.
146. Hohenberger W, Weber K, Matzel K, et al. Standardized surgery for colonic cancer: complete mesocolic excision and central ligation—technical notes and outcome. *Colorectal Dis*. 2009;11(4):354–364; discussion 364–365.
147. Olofsson F, Buchwald P, Elmståhl S, et al. No benefit of extended mesenteric resection with central vascular ligation in right-sided colon cancer. *Colorectal Dis*. 2016;18(8):773–778.
148. Bertelsen CA, Neuenschwander AU, Jansen JE, et al. 5-year outcome after complete mesocolic excision for right-sided colon cancer: a population-based cohort study. *Lancet Oncol*. 2019;20(11):1556–1565.
149. Alhassan N, Yang M, Wong-Chong N, et al. Comparison between conventional colectomy and complete mesocolic excision for colon cancer: a systematic review and pooled analysis: a review of CME versus conventional colectomies. *Surg Endosc*. 2019;33(1):8–18.
150. Garcia-Granero A, Pellino G, Giner F, et al. A proposal for novel standards of histopathology reporting for D3 lymphadenectomy in right colon cancer: the mesocolic sail and superior right colic vein landmarks. *Dis Colon Rectum*. 2020;63(4):450–460.
151. Nivatvongs S. Surgical management of malignant colorectal polyps. *Surg Clin North Am*. 2002;82(5):959–966.
152. Haggitt RC, Glotzbach RE, Soffer EE, et al. Prognostic factors in colorectal carcinomas arising in adenomas: implications for lesions removed by endoscopic polypectomy. *Gastroenterology*. 1985;89(2):328–336.
153. Butte JM, Tang P, Gonen M, et al. Rate of residual disease after complete endoscopic resection of malignant colonic polyp. *Dis Colon Rectum*. 2012;55(2):122–127.
154. Okabe S, Shia J, Nash G, et al. Lymph node metastasis in T1 adenocarcinoma of the colon and rectum. *J Gastrointest Surg*. 2004;8(8):1032–1039; discussion 1039–1040.

155. Kessler H, Hohenberger W. Extended lymphadenectomy in colon cancer is crucial. *World J Surg*. 2013;37(8):1789–1798.
156. Nosho K, Kure S, Irahara N, et al. A prospective cohort study shows unique epigenetic, genetic, and prognostic features of synchronous colorectal cancers. *Gastroenterology*. 2009;137(5): 1609–1620.e1601–1603.
157. Clinical Outcomes of Surgical Therapy Study Group; Nelson H, Sargent DJ, Wieand HS, et al. A comparison of laparoscopically assisted and open colectomy for colon cancer. *N Engl J Med*. 2004;350(20):2050–2059.
158. Yang C, Wexner SD, Safar B, et al. Conversion in laparoscopic surgery: does intraoperative complication influence outcome? *Surg Endosc*. 2009;23(11):2454–2458.
159. Zhang X, Wei Z, Bie M, et al. Robot-assisted versus laparoscopic-assisted surgery for colorectal cancer: a meta-analysis. *Surg Endosc*. 2016;30(12):5601–5614.
160. Laurie JA, Moertel CG, Fleming TR, et al. Surgical adjuvant therapy of large bowel carcinoma: an evaluation of levamisole and the combination of levamisole and fluorouracil. *J Clin Oncol*. 1989;7:1447–1456.
161. Moertel CG, Fleming TR, Macdonald JS, et al. Intergroup study of fluorouracil plus levamisole as adjuvant therapy for stage II/Dukes' B2 colon cancer. *J Clin Oncol*. 1995;13(12): 2936–2943.
162. Porschen R, Bermann A, Loffler T, et al. Fluorouracil plus leucovorin as effective adjuvant chemotherapy in curatively resected stage III colon cancer: results of the trial adjCCA-01. *J Clin Oncol*. 2001;19(6):1787–1794.
163. Mamounas E, Wieand S, Wolmark N, et al. Comparative efficacy of adjuvant chemotherapy in patients with Dukes' B versus Dukes' C colon cancer: results from four National Surgical Adjuvant Breast and Bowel Project adjuvant studies (C-01, C-02, C-03, and C-04). *J Clin Oncol*. 1999;17(5):1349–1355.
164. Sargent DJ, Goldberg RM, Jacobson SD, et al. A pooled analysis of adjuvant chemotherapy for resected colon cancer in elderly patients. *N Engl J Med*. 2001;345(15):1091–1097.
165. Andre T, Boni C, Mounedi-Boudiaf L, et al. Oxaliplatin, fluorouracil, and leucovorin as adjuvant treatment for colon cancer. *N Engl J Med*. 2004;350:2343–2351.
166. Andre T, Boni C, Navarro M, et al. Improved overall survival with oxaliplatin, fluorouracil, and leucovorin as adjuvant treatment in stage II or III colon cancer in the MOSAIC trial. *J Clin Oncol*. 2009;27(19):3109–3116.
167. Grothey A, Sobrero AF, Shields AF, et al. Duration of adjuvant chemotherapy for stage III colon cancer. *N Engl J Med*. 2018;378(13):1177–1188.
168. Van Cutsem E, Labianca R, Bodoky G, et al. Randomized phase III trial comparing biweekly infusional fluorouracil/leucovorin alone or with irinotecan in the adjuvant treatment of Stage III colon cancer: PETACC-3. *J Clin Oncol*. 2009;27:3117–3125.
169. Allegra CJ, Yothers G, O'Connell MJ, et al. Bevacizumab in stage II-III colon cancer: 5-year update of the National Surgical Adjuvant Breast and Bowel Project C-08 trial. *J Clin Oncol*. 2013;31(3):359–364.
170. de Gramont A, Van Cutsem E, Schmoll HJ, et al. Bevacizumab plus oxaliplatin-based chemotherapy as adjuvant treatment for colon cancer (AVANT): a phase 3 randomised controlled trial. *Lancet Oncol*. 2012;13(12):1225–1233.
171. Alberts SR, Sargent DJ, Nair S, et al. Effect of oxaliplatin, fluorouracil, and leucovorin with or without cetuximab on survival among patients with resected stage III colon cancer: a randomized trial. *JAMA*. 2012;307(13):1383–1393.
172. Schippinger W, Samonigg H, Schaberl-Moser R, et al. A prospective randomised phase III trial of adjuvant chemotherapy with 5-fluorouracil and leucovorin in patients with stage II colon cancer. *Br J Cancer*. 2007;97(8):1021–1027.
173. Gray R, Barnwell J, McConkey C, et al. Adjuvant chemotherapy versus observation in patients with colorectal cancer: a randomised study. *Lancet*. 2007;370(9604):2020–2029.
174. Figueredo A, Charette ML, Maroun J, et al. Adjuvant therapy for stage II colon cancer: a systematic review from the Cancer Care Ontario Program in evidence-based care's gastrointestinal cancer disease site group. *J Clin Oncol*. 2004;22(16):3395–3407.
175. Marshall JL. Risk assessment in stage II colorectal cancer. *Oncology (Williston Park)*. 2010;24(1 Suppl 1):9–13.
176. Le DT, Kim TW, Van Cutsem E, et al. Phase II open-label study of pembrolizumab in treatment-refractory, microsatellite instability-high/mismatch repair-deficient metastatic colorectal cancer: KEYNOTE-164. *J Clin Oncol*. 2020;38(1):11–19.
177. Overman MJ, Lonardi S, Wong KYM, et al. Durable clinical benefit with nivolumab plus ipilimumab in DNA mismatch repair-deficient/microsatellite instability-high metastatic colorectal cancer. *J Clin Oncol*. 2018;36(8):773–779.
178. Lau D, Kalaitzaki E, Church DN, et al. Rationale and design of the POLEM trial: avelumab plus fluoropyrimidine-based chemotherapy as adjuvant treatment for stage III mismatch repair deficient or POLE exonuclease domain mutant colon cancer: a phase III randomised study. *ESMO Open*. 2020;5(1):e000638.
179. Garcia-Aguilar J, Pollack J, Lee SH, et al. Accuracy of endorectal ultrasonography in preoperative staging of rectal tumors. *Dis Colon Rectum*. 2002;45(1):10–15.
180. Beets-Tan RG, Lambregts DM, Maas M, et al. Magnetic resonance imaging for the clinical management of rectal cancer patients: recommendations from the 2012 European Society of Gastrointestinal and Abdominal Radiology (ESGAR) consensus meeting. *Eur Radiol*. 2013;23(9):2522–2531.
181. Heijnen LA, Lambregts DM, Martens MH, et al. Performance of gadofosveset-enhanced MRI for staging rectal cancer nodes: can the initial promising results be reproduced? *Eur Radiol*. 2014;24(2):371–379.
182. Hotker AM, Garcia-Aguilar J, Gollub MJ. Multiparametric MRI of rectal cancer in the assessment of response to therapy: a systematic review. *Dis Colon Rectum*. 2014;57(6):790–799.
183. MERCURY Study Group. Diagnostic accuracy of preoperative magnetic resonance imaging in predicting curative resection of rectal cancer: prospective observational study. *BMJ*. 2006;333(7572):779.
184. Brown G, Radcliffe AG, Newcombe RG, et al. Preoperative assessment of prognostic factors in rectal cancer using high-resolution magnetic resonance imaging. *Br J Surg*. 2003;90(3): 355–364.
185. Taylor FG, Quirke P, Heald RJ, et al. Preoperative magnetic resonance imaging assessment of circumferential resection margin predicts disease-free survival and local recurrence: 5-year follow-up results of the MERCURY study. *J Clin Oncol*. 2014;32(1):34–43.
186. Taylor FG, Quirke P, Heald RJ, et al. Preoperative high-resolution magnetic resonance imaging can identify good prognosis stage I, II, and III rectal cancer best managed by surgery alone: a prospective, multicenter, European study. *Ann Surg*. 2011;253(4):711–719.
187. Blomqvist L, Glimelius B. The 'good', the 'bad', and the 'ugly' rectal cancers. *Acta Oncol*. 2008;47(1):5–8.
188. Habr-Gama A, Perez RO, Nadalin W, et al. Operative versus nonoperative treatment for stage 0 distal rectal cancer following chemoradiation therapy: long-term results. *Ann Surg*. 2004;240(4):711–717; discussion 717–718.
189. Maas M, Beets-Tan RG, Lambregts DM, et al. Wait-and-see policy for clinical complete responders after chemoradiation for rectal cancer. *J Clin Oncol*. 2011;29(35):4633–4640.
190. Smith JJ, Chow OS, Gollub MJ, et al. Organ Preservation in Rectal Adenocarcinoma: a phase II randomized controlled trial evaluating 3-year disease-free survival in patients with locally advanced rectal cancer treated with chemoradiation plus induction or consolidation chemotherapy, and total mesorectal excision or nonoperative management. *BMC Cancer*. 2015;15:767.
191. Maas M, Lambregts DM, Nelemans PJ, et al. Assessment of clinical complete response after chemoradiation for rectal cancer with digital rectal examination, endoscopy, and MRI: selection for organ-saving treatment. *Ann Surg Oncol*. 2015;22(12):3873–3880.
192. Guillem JG, Chessin DB, Shia J, et al. Clinical examination following preoperative chemoradiation for rectal cancer is

not a reliable surrogate end point. *J Clin Oncol.* 2005;23(15): 3475–3479.
193. Smith FM, Wiland H, Mace A, et al. Clinical criteria underestimate complete pathological response in rectal cancer treated with neoadjuvant chemoradiotherapy. *Dis Colon Rectum.* 2014;57(3):311–315.
194. National Comprehensive Cancer Network (NCCN). *NCCN Clinical Practice Guidelines in Oncology—Rectal Cancer.* www.nccn.org. 2020.
195. Garcia-Aguilar J, Mellgren A, Sirivongs P, et al. Local excision of rectal cancer without adjuvant therapy: a word of caution. *Ann Surg.* 2000;231(3):345–351.
196. Paty PB, Nash GM, Baron P, et al. Long-term results of local excision for rectal cancer. *Ann Surg.* 2002;236(4):522–529; discussion 529–530.
197. Madbouly KM, Remzi FH, Erkek BA, et al. Recurrence after transanal excision of T1 rectal cancer: should we be concerned? *Dis Colon Rectum.* 2005;48(4):711–719; discussion 719–721.
198. Weiser MR, Landmann RG, Wong WD, et al. Surgical salvage of recurrent rectal cancer after transanal excision. *Dis Colon Rectum.* 2005;48(6):1169–1175.
199. Friel CM, Cromwell JW, Marra C, et al. Salvage radical surgery after failed local excision for early rectal cancer. *Dis Colon Rectum.* 2002;45(7):875–879.
200. Kidane B, Chadi SA, Kanters S, et al. Local resection compared with radical resection in the treatment of T1N0M0 rectal adenocarcinoma: a systematic review and meta-analysis. *Dis Colon Rectum.* 2015;58(1):122–140.
201. Clancy C, Burke JP, Albert MR, et al. Transanal endoscopic microsurgery versus standard transanal excision for the removal of rectal neoplasms: a systematic review and meta-analysis. *Dis Colon Rectum.* 2015;58(2):254–261.
202. Mellgren A, Sirivongs P, Rothenberger DA, et al. Is local excision adequate therapy for early rectal cancer? *Dis Colon Rectum.* 2000;43(8):1064–1071; discussion 1071–1074.
203. Stitzenberg KB, Sanoff HK, Penn DC, et al. Practice patterns and long-term survival for early-stage rectal cancer. *J Clin Oncol.* 2013;31(34):4276–4282.
204. Bhangu A, Brown G, Nicholls RJ, et al. Survival outcome of local excision versus radical resection of colon or rectal carcinoma: a Surveillance, Epidemiology, and End Results (SEER) population-based study. *Ann Surg.* 2013;258(4):563–571.
205. Minsky BD, Enker WE, Cohen AM, et al. Local excision and postoperative radiation therapy for rectal cancer. *Am J Clin Oncol.* 1994;17(5):411–416.
206. Bouvet M, Milas M, Giacco GG, et al. Predictors of recurrence after local excision and postoperative chemoradiation therapy of adenocarcinoma of the rectum. *Ann Surg Oncol.* 1999;6(1): 26–32.
207. Benson R, Wong CS, Cummings BJ, et al. Local excision and postoperative radiotherapy for distal rectal cancer. *Int J Radiat Oncol Biol Phys.* 2001;50(5):1309–1316.
208. Greenberg JA, Shibata D, Herndon JE 2nd, et al. Local excision of distal rectal cancer: an update of cancer and leukemia group B 8984. *Dis Colon Rectum.* 2008;51(8):1185–1191; discussion 1191–1194.
209. Kim CJ, Yeatman TJ, Coppola D, et al. Local excision of T2 and T3 rectal cancers after downstaging chemoradiation. *Ann Surg.* 2001;234(3):352–358; discussion 358–359.
210. Nair RM, Siegel EM, Chen DT, et al. Long-term results of transanal excision after neoadjuvant chemoradiation for T2 and T3 adenocarcinomas of the rectum. *J Gastrointest Surg.* 2008;12(10):1797–1805; discussion 1805–1806.
211. Lezoche E, Baldarelli M, Lezoche G, et al. Randomized clinical trial of endoluminal locoregional resection versus laparoscopic total mesorectal excision for T2 rectal cancer after neoadjuvant therapy. *Br J Surg.* 2012;99(9):1211–1218.
212. Stijns RCH, de Graaf EJR, Punt CJA, et al. Long-term oncological and functional outcomes of chemoradiotherapy followed by organ-sparing transanal endoscopic microsurgery for distal rectal cancer: the CARTS study. *JAMA Surg.* 2019;154(1):47–54.
213. Garcia-Aguilar J, Renfro LA, Chow OS, et al. Organ preservation for clinical T2N0 distal rectal cancer using neoadjuvant chemoradiotherapy and local excision (ACOSOG Z6041): results of an open-label, single-arm, multi-institutional, phase 2 trial. *Lancet Oncol.* 2015;16(15):1537–1546.
214. Lynn PB, Renfro LA, Carrero XW, et al. Anorectal function and quality of life in patients with early stage rectal cancer treated with chemoradiation and local excision. *Dis Colon Rectum.* 2017;60(5):459–468.
215. Rullier E, Rouanet P, Tuech JJ, et al. Organ preservation for rectal cancer (GRECCAR 2): a prospective, randomised, open-label, multicentre, phase 3 trial. *Lancet.* 2017;390(10093):469–479.
216. Rondelli F, Trastulli S, Cirocchi R, et al. Rectal washout and local recurrence in rectal resection for cancer: a meta-analysis. *Colorectal Dis.* 2012;14(11):1313–1321.
217. Lange MM, Buunen M, van de Velde CJ, et al. Level of arterial ligation in rectal cancer surgery: low tie preferred over high tie. A review. *Dis Colon Rectum.* 2008;51(7):1139–1145.
218. Zotti P, Del Bianco P, Serpentini S, et al. Validity and reliability of the MSKCC Bowel Function instrument in a sample of Italian rectal cancer patients. *Eur J Surg Oncol.* 2011;37(7):589–596.
219. Emmertsen KJ, Laurberg S. Low anterior resection syndrome score: development and validation of a symptom-based scoring system for bowel dysfunction after low anterior resection for rectal cancer. *Ann Surg.* 2012;255(5):922–928.
220. Emmertsen KJ, Laurberg S. Bowel dysfunction after treatment for rectal cancer. *Acta Oncol.* 2008;47(6):994–1003.
221. Lundby L, Krogh K, Jensen VJ, et al. Long-term anorectal dysfunction after postoperative radiotherapy for rectal cancer. *Dis Colon Rectum.* 2005;48(7):1343–1349; discussion 1349–1352; author reply 1352.
222. Chen TY, Wiltink LM, Nout RA, et al. Bowel function 14 years after preoperative short-course radiotherapy and total mesorectal excision for rectal cancer: report of a multicenter randomized trial. *Clin Colorectal Cancer.* 2015;14(2):106–114.
223. Lewis WG, Martin IG, Williamson ME, et al. Why do some patients experience poor functional results after anterior resection of the rectum for carcinoma? *Dis Colon Rectum.* 1995;38(3): 259–263.
224. Brown CJ, Fenech DS, McLeod RS. Reconstructive techniques after rectal resection for rectal cancer. *Cochrane Database Syst Rev.* 2008(2):CD006040.
225. Parc R, Tiret E, Frileux P, et al. Resection and colo-anal anastomosis with colonic reservoir for rectal carcinoma. *Br J Surg.* 1986;73(2):139–141.
226. Seow-Choen F, Goh HS. Prospective randomized trial comparing J colonic pouch-anal anastomosis and straight coloanal reconstruction. *Br J Surg.* 1995;82(5):608–610.
227. Hida J, Yasutomi M, Fujimoto K, et al. Functional outcome after low anterior resection with low anastomosis for rectal cancer using the colonic J-pouch. Prospective randomized study for determination of optimum pouch size. *Dis Colon Rectum.* 1996;39(9):986–991.
228. Lazorthes F, Gamagami R, Chiotasso P, et al. Prospective, randomized study comparing clinical results between small and large colonic J-pouch following coloanal anastomosis. *Dis Colon Rectum.* 1997;40(12):1409–1413.
229. Machado M, Nygren J, Goldman S, et al. Functional and physiologic assessment of the colonic reservoir or side-to-end anastomosis after low anterior resection for rectal cancer: a two-year follow-up. *Dis Colon Rectum.* 2005;48(1):29–36.
230. Staller K, Song M, Grodstein F, et al. Increased long-term dietary fiber intake is associated with a decreased risk of fecal incontinence in older women. *Gastroenterology.* 2018;155: 661–667.
231. Harji D, Fernandez B, Boissieras L, et al. A novel bowel rehabilitation programme after total mesorectal excision for rectal cancer: the BOREAL pilot study. *Colorectal Dis.* 2021;23:2619–2626
232. Bazzell A, Madsen LT, Dains J. Clinical management of bowel dysfunction after low anterior resection for rectal cancer. *J Adv Pract Oncol.* 2016;7:618–629.

233. Itagaki R, Koda K, Yamazaki M, et al. Serotonin (5-HT3) receptor antagonists for the reduction in symptoms of low anterior resection syndrome. *Clin Exp Gastroenterol*. 2014;7:47–52.
234. Ho KK, Sik YC, Sik YY, Nam YS, Seok-Byung L, Cheon KJ. Effectiveness of biofeedback therapy in the treatment of anterior resection syndrome after rectal cancer surgery. *Dis Colon Rectum*. 2011;54:1107–1113.
235. Daams F, Wu Z, Lahaye MJ, et al. Prediction and diagnosis of colorectal anastomotic leakage: a systematic review of literature. *World J Gastrointest Surg*. 2014;6(2):14–26.
236. Jones OM, John SK, Horseman N, et al. Low anastomotic leak rate after colorectal surgery: a single-centre study. *Colorectal Dis*. 2007;9(8):740–744.
237. Eberl T, Jagoditsch M, Klingler A, et al. Risk factors for anastomotic leakage after resection for rectal cancer. *Am J Surg*. 2008;196(4):592–598.
238. McArdle CS, McMillan DC, Hole DJ. Impact of anastomotic leakage on long-term survival of patients undergoing curative resection for colorectal cancer. *Br J Surg*. 2005;92(9):1150–1154.
239. den Dulk M, Marijnen CA, Collette L, et al. Multicentre analysis of oncological and survival outcomes following anastomotic leakage after rectal cancer surgery. *Br J Surg*. 2009;96(9):1066–1075.
240. Smith JD, Paty PB, Guillem JG, et al. Anastomotic leak is not associated with oncologic outcome in patients undergoing low anterior resection for rectal cancer. *Ann Surg*. 2012;256(6):1034–1038.
241. Matthiessen P, Hallbook O, Andersson M, et al. Risk factors for anastomotic leakage after anterior resection of the rectum. *Colorectal Dis*. 2004;6(6):462–469.
242. Tan WS, Tang CL, Shi L, et al. Meta-analysis of defunctioning stomas in low anterior resection for rectal cancer. *Br J Surg*. 2009; 96(5):462–472.
243. Machado M, Hallbook O, Goldman S, et al. Defunctioning stoma in low anterior resection with colonic pouch for rectal cancer: a comparison between two hospitals with a different policy. *Dis Colon Rectum*. 2002;45(7):940–945.
244. Rondelli F, Reboldi P, Rulli A, et al. Loop ileostomy versus loop colostomy for fecal diversion after colorectal or coloanal anastomosis: a meta-analysis. *Int J Colorectal Dis*. 2009;24(5):479–488.
245. Chun LJ, Haigh PI, Tam MS, et al. Defunctioning loop ileostomy for pelvic anastomoses: predictors of morbidity and nonclosure. *Dis Colon Rectum*. 2012;55(2):167–174.
246. Fish DR, Mancuso CA, Garcia-Aguilar JE, et al. Readmission after ileostomy creation: retrospective review of a common and significant event. *Ann Surg*. 2017;265(2):379–387.
247. Marr R, Birbeck K, Garvican J, et al. The modern abdominoperineal excision: the next challenge after total mesorectal excision. *Ann Surg*. 2005;242(1):74–82.
248. Perdawood SK, Lund T. Extralevator versus standard abdominoperineal excision for rectal cancer. *Tech Coloproctol*. 2015; 19(3):145–152.
249. Musters GD, Buskens CJ, Bemelman WA, et al. Perineal wound healing after abdominoperineal resection for rectal cancer: a systematic review and meta-analysis. *Dis Colon Rectum*. 2014; 57(9):1129–1139.
250. Yu HC, Peng H, He XS, et al. Comparison of short- and long-term outcomes after extralevator abdominoperineal excision and standard abdominoperineal excision for rectal cancer: a systematic review and meta-analysis. *Int J Colorectal Dis*. 2014;29(2):183–191.
251. de Campos-Lobato LF, Stocchi L, Dietz DW, et al. Prone or lithotomy positioning during an abdominoperineal resection for rectal cancer results in comparable oncologic outcomes. *Dis Colon Rectum*. 2011;54(8):939–946.
252. Lujan J, Valero G, Hernandez Q, et al. Randomized clinical trial comparing laparoscopic and open surgery in patients with rectal cancer. *Br J Surg*. 2009;96(9):982–989.
253. Ng KH, Ng DC, Cheung HY, et al. Laparoscopic resection for rectal cancers: lessons learned from 579 cases. *Ann Surg*. 2009;249(1):82–86.
254. Greenblatt DY, Rajamanickam V, Pugely AJ, et al. Short-term outcomes after laparoscopic-assisted proctectomy for rectal cancer: results from the ACS NSQIP. *J Am Coll Surg*. 2011;212(5): 844–854.
255. Addae JK, Gani F, Fang SY, et al. A comparison of trends in operative approach and postoperative outcomes for colorectal cancer surgery. *J Surg Res*. 2017;208:111–120.
256. Jayne DG, Thorpe HC, Copeland J, et al. Five-year follow-up of the Medical Research Council CLASICC trial of laparoscopically assisted versus open surgery for colorectal cancer. *Br J Surg*. 2010;97(11):1638–1645.
257. Jeong SY, Park JW, Nam BH, et al. Open versus laparoscopic surgery for mid-rectal or low-rectal cancer after neoadjuvant chemoradiotherapy (COREAN trial): survival outcomes of an open-label, non-inferiority, randomised controlled trial. *Lancet Oncol*. 2014;15(7):767–774.
258. van der Pas MH, Haglind E, Cuesta MA, et al. Laparoscopic versus open surgery for rectal cancer (COLOR II): short-term outcomes of a randomised, phase 3 trial. *Lancet Oncol*. 2013;14(3): 210–218.
259. Stevenson AR, Solomon MJ, Lumley JW, et al. Effect of laparoscopic-assisted resection vs open resection on pathological outcomes in rectal cancer: the ALaCaRT randomized clinical trial. *JAMA*. 2015;314(13):1356–1363.
260. Fleshman J, Branda M, Sargent DJ, et al. Effect of laparoscopic-assisted resection vs open resection of stage II or III rectal cancer on pathologic outcomes: the ACOSOG Z6051 randomized clinical trial. *JAMA*. 2015;314(13):1346–1355.
261. Xiong B, Ma L, Zhang C, et al. Robotic versus laparoscopic total mesorectal excision for rectal cancer: a meta-analysis. *J Surg Res*. 2014;188(2):404–414.
262. Jayne D, Pigazzi A, Marshall H, et al. Effect of robotic-assisted vs conventional laparoscopic surgery on risk of conversion to open laparotomy among patients undergoing resection for rectal cancer: the ROLARR randomized clinical trial. *JAMA*. 2017;318(16):1569–1580.
263. de Lacy AM, Rattner DW, Adelsdorfer C, et al. Transanal natural orifice transluminal endoscopic surgery (NOTES) rectal resection: "down-to-up" total mesorectal excision (TME)—short-term outcomes in the first 20 cases. *Surg Endosc*. 2013;27(9):3165–3172.
264. Rouanet P, Mourregot A, Azar CC, et al. Transanal endoscopic proctectomy: an innovative procedure for difficult resection of rectal tumors in men with narrow pelvis. *Dis Colon Rectum*. 2013;56(4):408–415.
265. Lee L, de Lacy B, Gomez Ruiz M, et al. A multicenter matched comparison of transanal and robotic total mesorectal excision for mid and low-rectal adenocarcinoma. *Ann Surg*. 2019;270(6): 1110–1116.
266. Wasmuth HH, Faerden AE, Myklebust T, et al. Transanal total mesorectal excision for rectal cancer has been suspended in Norway. *Br J Surg*. 2020;107(1):121–130.
267. Gastrointestinal Tumor Study Group. Prolongation of the disease-free interval in surgically treated rectal carcinoma. *N Engl J Med*. 1985;312(23):1465–1472.
268. Gerard A, Buyse M, Nordlinger B, et al. Preoperative radiotherapy as adjuvant treatment in rectal cancer: final results of a randomized study of the European Organization for Research and Treatment of Cancer (EORTC). *Ann Surg*. 1988;208: 606–614.
269. Fisher B, Wolmark N, Rockette H, et al. Postoperative adjuvant chemotherapy or radiation therapy for rectal cancer: results from NSABP protocol R-01. *J Natl Cancer Inst*. 1988;80:21–29.
270. Kapiteijn E, Marijnen CA, Nagtegaal ID, et al. Preoperative radiotherapy combined with total mesorectal excision for resectable rectal cancer. *N Engl J Med*. 2001;345(9):638–646.
271. O'Connell MJ, Martenson JA, Wieand HS, et al. Improving adjuvant therapy for rectal cancer by combining protracted-infusion fluorouracil with radiation therapy after curative surgery. *N Engl J Med*. 1994;331(8):502–507.
272. Smalley SR, Benedetti JK, Williamson SK, et al. Phase III trial of fluorouracil-based chemotherapy regimens plus radiotherapy in postoperative adjuvant rectal cancer: GI INT 0144. *J Clin Oncol*. 2006;24(22):3542–3547.

273. Bosset JF, Calais G, Mineur L, et al. Fluorouracil-based adjuvant chemotherapy after preoperative chemoradiotherapy in rectal cancer: long-term results of the EORTC 22921 randomised study. *Lancet Oncol*. 2014;15(2):184–190.
274. Gerard JP, Conroy T, Bonnetain F, et al. Preoperative radiotherapy with or without concurrent fluorouracil and leucovorin in T3-4 rectal cancers: results of FFCD 9203. *J Clin Oncol*. 2006;24(28):4620–4625.
275. Sauer R, Becker H, Hohenberger W, et al. Preoperative versus postoperative chemoradiotherapy for rectal cancer. *N Engl J Med*. 2004;351(17):1731–1740.
276. Roh MS, Colangelo LH, O'Connell MJ, et al. Preoperative multimodality therapy improves disease-free survival in patients with carcinoma of the rectum: NSABP R-03. *J Clin Oncol*. 2009;27(31):5124–5130.
277. O'Connell MJ, Colangelo LH, Beart RW, et al. Capecitabine and oxaliplatin in the preoperative multimodality treatment of rectal cancer: surgical end points from National Surgical Adjuvant Breast and Bowel Project trial R-04. *J Clin Oncol*. 2014;32(18):1927–1934.
278. Hofheinz RD, Wenz F, Post S, et al. Chemoradiotherapy with capecitabine versus fluorouracil for locally advanced rectal cancer: a randomised, multicentre, non-inferiority, phase 3 trial. *Lancet Oncol*. 2012;13(6):579–588.
279. Gerard JP, Azria D, Gourgou-Bourgade S, et al. Comparison of two neoadjuvant chemoradiotherapy regimens for locally advanced rectal cancer: results of the phase III trial ACCORD 12/0405-Prodige 2. *J Clin Oncol*. 2010;28(10):1638–1644.
280. Rodel C, Liersch T, Becker H, et al. Preoperative chemoradiotherapy and postoperative chemotherapy with fluorouracil and oxaliplatin versus fluorouracil alone in locally advanced rectal cancer: initial results of the German CAO/ARO/AIO-04 randomised phase 3 trial. *Lancet Oncol*. 2012;13(7):679–687.
281. Aschele C, Cionini L, Lonardi S, et al. Primary tumor response to preoperative chemoradiation with or without oxaliplatin in locally advanced rectal cancer: pathologic results of the STAR-01 randomized phase III trial. *J Clin Oncol*. 2011;29(20):2773–2780.
282. Bujko K, Nowacki MP, Nasierowska-Guttmejer A, et al. Long-term results of a randomized trial comparing preoperative short-course radiotherapy with preoperative conventionally fractionated chemoradiation for rectal cancer. *Br J Surg*. 2006;93(10):1215–1223.
283. Ngan SY, Burmeister B, Fisher RJ, et al. Randomized trial of short-course radiotherapy versus long-course chemoradiation comparing rates of local recurrence in patients with T3 rectal cancer: Trans-Tasman Radiation Oncology Group trial 01.04. *J Clin Oncol*. 2012;30(31):3827–3833.
284. Erlandsson J, Holm T, Pettersson D, et al. Optimal fractionation of preoperative radiotherapy and timing to surgery for rectal cancer (Stockholm III): a multicentre, randomised, non-blinded, phase 3, non-inferiority trial. *Lancet Oncol*. 2017;18(3):336–346.
285. Schrag D, Shi Q, Weiser MR, et al. Preoperative treatment of locally advanced rectal cancer. *N Engl J Med*. 2023;389(4):322–334.
286. Petersen SH, Harling H, Kirkeby LT, et al. Postoperative adjuvant chemotherapy in rectal cancer operated for cure. *Cochrane Database Syst Rev*. 2012;3:CD004078.
287. Xu Z, Mohile SG, Tejani MA, et al. Poor compliance with adjuvant chemotherapy use associated with poorer survival in patients with rectal cancer: an NCDB analysis. *Cancer*. 2017;123(1):52–61.
288. Breugom AJ, Swets M, Bosset JF, et al. Adjuvant chemotherapy after preoperative (chemo)radiotherapy and surgery for patients with rectal cancer: a systematic review and meta-analysis of individual patient data. *Lancet Oncol*. 2015;16(2):200–207.
289. Fernández-Martos C, Pericay C, Losa F, et al. Effect of aflibercept plus modified FOLFOX6 induction chemotherapy before standard chemoradiotherapy and surgery in patients with high-risk rectal adenocarcinoma: the GEMCAD 1402 randomized clinical trial. *JAMA Oncol*. 2019;5(11):1566–1573.
290. Cercek A, Goodman KA, Hajj C, et al. Neoadjuvant chemotherapy first, followed by chemoradiation and then surgery, in the management of locally advanced rectal cancer. *J Natl Compr Canc Netw*. 2014;12(4):513–519.
291. Marco MR, Zhou L, Patil S, et al. Consolidation mFOLFOX6 chemotherapy after chemoradiotherapy improves survival in patients with locally advanced rectal cancer: final results of a multicenter phase II trial. *Dis Colon Rectum*. 2018;61(10):1146–1155.
292. Fokas E, Allgäuer M, Polat B, et al. Randomized phase II trial of chemoradiotherapy plus induction or consolidation chemotherapy as total neoadjuvant therapy for locally advanced rectal cancer: CAO/ARO/AIO-12. *J Clin Oncol*. 2019;37(34):3212–3222.
293. Conroy T, Castan F, Etienne PL, et al. Total neoadjuvant therapy with mFOLFIRINOX versus preoperative chemoradiotherapy in patients with locally advanced rectal cancer: long-term results of the UNICANCER-PRODIGE 23 trial. *Ann Oncol*. 2024;35(10):873–881.
294. Marijnen CA, Kapiteijn E, van de Velde CJ, et al. Acute side effects and complications after short-term preoperative radiotherapy combined with total mesorectal excision in primary rectal cancer: report of a multicenter randomized trial. *J Clin Oncol*. 2002;20(3):817–825.
295. Paun BC, Cassie S, MacLean AR, et al. Postoperative complications following surgery for rectal cancer. *Ann Surg*. 2010; 251(5):807–818.
296. Foster JD, Tou S, Curtis NJ, et al. Closure of the perineal defect after abdominoperineal excision for rectal adenocarcinoma—ACPGBI Position Statement. *Colorectal Dis*. 2018;20(Suppl 5):5–23.
297. Peeters KC, van de Velde CJ, Leer JW, et al. Late side effects of short-course preoperative radiotherapy combined with total mesorectal excision for rectal cancer: increased bowel dysfunction in irradiated patients—a Dutch Colorectal Cancer Group study. *J Clin Oncol*. 2005;23(25):6199–6206.
298. Hendren SK, O'Connor BI, Liu M, et al. Prevalence of male and female sexual dysfunction is high following surgery for rectal cancer. *Ann Surg*. 2005;242(2):212–223.
299. Wiltink LM, Chen TY, Nout RA, et al. Health-related quality of life 14 years after preoperative short-term radiotherapy and total mesorectal excision for rectal cancer: report of a multicenter randomised trial. *Eur J Cancer*. 2014;50(14):2390–2398.
300. Smith N, Brown G. Preoperative staging of rectal cancer. *Acta Oncol*. 2008;47(1):20–31.
301. Maas M, Nelemans PJ, Valentini V, et al. Long-term outcome in patients with a pathological complete response after chemoradiation for rectal cancer: a pooled analysis of individual patient data. *Lancet Oncol*. 2010;11(9):835–844.
302. Habr-Gama A, São Julião GP, Fernandez LM, et al. Achieving a complete clinical response after neoadjuvant chemoradiation that does not require surgical resection: it may take longer than you think! *Dis Colon Rectum*. 2019;62(7):802–808.
303. van der Valk MJM, Hilling DE, Bastiaannet E, et al. Long-term outcomes of clinical complete responders after neoadjuvant treatment for rectal cancer in the International Watch & Wait Database (IWWD): an international multicentre registry study. *Lancet*. 2018;391(10139):2537–2545.
304. Scott NA, Jeacock J, Kingston RD. Risk factors in patients presenting as an emergency with colorectal cancer. *Br J Surg*. 1995; 82(3):321–323.
305. Wong SK, Jalaludin BB, Morgan MJ, et al. Tumor pathology and long-term survival in emergency colorectal cancer. *Dis Colon Rectum*. 2008;51(2):223–230.
306. McArdle CS, Hole DJ. Emergency presentation of colorectal cancer is associated with poor 5-year survival. *Br J Surg*. 2004; 91(5):605–609.
307. Yeo HL, Lee SW. Colorectal emergencies: review and controversies in the management of large bowel obstruction. *J Gastrointest Surg*. 2013;17(11):2007–2012.
308. Lopez-Kostner F, Hool GR, Lavery IC. Management and causes of acute large-bowel obstruction. *Surg Clin North Am*. 1997;77(6):1265–1290.
309. Batke M, Cappell MS. Adynamic ileus and acute colonic pseudo-obstruction. *Med Clin North Am*. 2008;92(3):649–670, ix.
310. Dachman AH. What are the indications for use of water-soluble contrast agent enemas in colon distension? *AJR Am J Roentgenol*. 1996;166(4):988.

311. Maddu KK, Mittal P, Arepalli CD, et al. Colorectal emergencies and related complications: a comprehensive imaging review—noninfectious and noninflammatory emergencies of colon. *AJR Am J Roentgenol*. 2014;203(6):1217–1229.
312. Bass G, Fleming C, Conneely J, et al. Emergency first presentation of colorectal cancer predicts significantly poorer outcomes: a review of 356 consecutive Irish patients. *Dis Colon Rectum*. 2009;52(4):678–684.
313. Metcalfe MS, Norwood MG, Miller AS, et al. Unreasonable expectations in emergency colorectal cancer surgery. *Colorectal Dis*. 2005;7(3):275–278.
314. Tekkis PP, Kinsman R, Thompson MR, et al. The Association of Coloproctology of Great Britain and Ireland study of large bowel obstruction caused by colorectal cancer. *Ann Surg*. 2004;240(1):76–81.
315. Deans GT, Krukowski ZH, Irwin ST. Malignant obstruction of the left colon. *Br J Surg*. 1994;81(9):1270–1276.
316. Watt AM, Faragher IG, Griffin TT, et al. Self-expanding metallic stents for relieving malignant colorectal obstruction: a systematic review. *Ann Surg*. 2007;246(1):24–30.
317. Cheung HY, Chung CC, Tsang WW, et al. Endolaparoscopic approach vs conventional open surgery in the treatment of obstructing left-sided colon cancer: a randomized controlled trial. *Arch Surg*. 2009;144(12):1127–1132.
318. Alcantara M, Serra-Aracil X, Falco J, et al. Prospective, controlled, randomized study of intraoperative colonic lavage versus stent placement in obstructive left-sided colonic cancer. *World J Surg*. 2011;35(8):1904–1910.
319. Pirlet IA, Slim K, Kwiatkowski F, et al. Emergency preoperative stenting versus surgery for acute left-sided malignant colonic obstruction: a multicenter randomized controlled trial. *Surg Endosc*. 2011;25(6):1814–1821.
320. Ghazal AH, El-Shazly WG, Bessa SS, et al. Colonic endolumenal stenting devices and elective surgery versus emergency subtotal/total colectomy in the management of malignant obstructed left colon carcinoma. *J Gastrointest Surg*. 2013;17(6):1123–1129.
321. van Hooft JE, Bemelman WA, Oldenburg B, et al. Colonic stenting versus emergency surgery for acute left-sided malignant colonic obstruction: a multicentre randomised trial. *Lancet Oncol*. 2011; 12(4):344–352.
322. Sloothaak DA, van den Berg MW, Dijkgraaf MG, et al. Oncological outcome of malignant colonic obstruction in the Dutch Stent-In 2 trial. *Br J Surg*. 2014;101(13):1751–1757.
323. Veld JV, Amelung FJ, Borstlap WAA, et al. Comparison of decompressing stoma vs stent as a bridge to surgery for left-sided obstructive colon cancer. *JAMA Surg*. 2020;155(3):206–215.
324. The SCOTIA Study Group. Single-stage treatment for malignant left-sided colonic obstruction: a prospective randomized clinical trial comparing subtotal colectomy with segmental resection following intraoperative irrigation. *Br J Surg*. 1995;82(12):1622–1627.
325. Sasaki K, Kazama S, Sunami E, et al. One-stage segmental colectomy and primary anastomosis after intraoperative colonic irrigation and total colonoscopy for patients with obstruction due to left-sided colorectal cancer. *Dis Colon Rectum*. 2012;55(1):72–78.
326. Tjandra JJ, Chan MK. Follow-up after curative resection of colorectal cancer: a meta-analysis. *Dis Colon Rectum*. 2007; 50(11):1783–1799.
327. Baca B, Beart RW Jr, Etzioni DA. Surveillance after colorectal cancer resection: a systematic review. *Dis Colon Rectum*. 2011;54(8):1036–1048.
328. Jeffery M, Hickey BE, Hider PN. Follow-up strategies for patients treated for non-metastatic colorectal cancer. *Cochrane Database Syst Rev*. 2007(1):CD002200.
329. Welch JP, Donaldson GA. The clinical correlation of an autopsy study of recurrent colorectal cancer. *Ann Surg*. 1979;189(4):496–502.
330. Siriwardena AK, Mason JM, Mullamitha S, et al. Management of colorectal cancer presenting with synchronous liver metastases. *Nat Rev Clin Oncol*. 2014;11(8):446–459.
331. Clancy C, Burke JP, Barry M, et al. A meta-analysis to determine the effect of primary tumor resection for stage IV colorectal cancer with unresectable metastases on patient survival. *Ann Surg Oncol*. 2014;21(12):3900–3908.
332. Cirocchi R, Trastulli S, Abraha I, et al. Non-resection versus resection for an asymptomatic primary tumour in patients with unresectable stage IV colorectal cancer. *Cochrane Database Syst Rev*. 2012;8:CD008997.
333. Hu CY, Bailey CE, You YN, et al. Time trend analysis of primary tumor resection for stage IV colorectal cancer: less surgery, improved survival. *JAMA Surg*. 2015;150(3):245–251.
334. National Comprehensive Cancer Network (NCCN). NCCN Clinical Practice Guidelines in Oncology—Colon Cancer. www.nccn.org. 2020.
335. Martin R, Paty P, Fong Y, et al. Simultaneous liver and colorectal resections are safe for synchronous colorectal liver metastasis. *J Am Coll Surg*. 2003;197(2):233–241; discussion 241–242.
336. Silberhumer GR, Paty PB, Denton B, et al. Long-term oncologic outcomes for simultaneous resection of synchronous metastatic liver and primary colorectal cancer. *Surgery*. 2016;160(1):67–73.
337. Wong SL, Mangu PB, Choti MA, et al. American Society of Clinical Oncology 2009 clinical evidence review on radiofrequency ablation of hepatic metastases from colorectal cancer. *J Clin Oncol*. 2010;28(3):493–508.
338. Kemeny N, Daly J, Oderman P, et al. Hepatic artery pump infusion: toxicity and results in patients with metastatic colorectal carcinoma. *J Clin Oncol*. 1984;2(6):595–600.
339. Cercek A, Boucher TM, Gluskin JS, et al. Response rates of hepatic arterial infusion pump therapy in patients with metastatic colorectal cancer liver metastases refractory to all standard chemotherapies. *J Surg Oncol*. 2016;114(6):655–663.
340. D'Angelica MI, Correa-Gallego C, Paty PB, et al. Phase II trial of hepatic artery infusional and systemic chemotherapy for patients with unresectable hepatic metastases from colorectal cancer: conversion to resection and long-term outcomes. *Ann Surg*. 2015;261(2):353–360.
341. Loupakis F, Cremolini C, Masi G, et al. Initial therapy with FOLFOXIRI and bevacizumab for metastatic colorectal cancer. *N Engl J Med*. 2014;371(17):1609–1618.
342. Jones C, Taylor MA, McWilliams B. The role of cetuximab as first-line treatment of colorectal liver metastases. *HPB (Oxford)*. 2013;15(1):11–17.
343. Yaeger R, Cercek A, O'Reilly EM, et al. Pilot trial of combined BRAF and EGFR inhibition in BRAF-mutant metastatic colorectal cancer patients. *Clin Cancer Res*. 2015;21(6):1313–1320.
344. Araujo R, Gonen M, Allen P, et al. Comparison between perioperative and postoperative chemotherapy after potentially curative hepatic resection for metastatic colorectal cancer. *Ann Surg Oncol*. 2013;20(13):4312–4321.
345. Nordlinger B, Sorbye H, Glimelius B, et al. Perioperative chemotherapy with FOLFOX4 and surgery versus surgery alone for resectable liver metastases from colorectal cancer (EORTC Intergroup trial 40983): a randomised controlled trial. *Lancet*. 2008;371(9617):1007–1016.
346. Nordlinger B, Sorbye H, Glimelius B, et al. Perioperative FOLFOX4 chemotherapy and surgery versus surgery alone for resectable liver metastases from colorectal cancer (EORTC 40983): long-term results of a randomised, controlled, phase 3 trial. *Lancet Oncol*. 2013;14(12):1208–1215.
347. Scappaticci FA, Fehrenbacher L, Cartwright T, et al. Surgical wound healing complications in metastatic colorectal cancer patients treated with bevacizumab. *J Surg Oncol*. 2005;91(3):173–180.
348. Primrose J, Falk S, Finch-Jones M, et al. Systemic chemotherapy with or without cetuximab in patients with resectable colorectal liver metastasis: the New EPOC randomised controlled trial. *Lancet Oncol*. 2014;15(6):601–611.
349. Ychou M, Rivoire M, Thezenas S, et al. A randomized phase II trial of three intensified chemotherapy regimens in first-line treatment of colorectal cancer patients with initially unresectable or not optimally resectable liver metastases. The METHEP trial. *Ann Surg Oncol*. 2013;20(13):4289–4297.
350. Bokemeyer C, Bondarenko I, Makhson A, et al. Fluorouracil, leucovorin, and oxaliplatin with and without cetuximab in the first-line treatment of metastatic colorectal cancer. *J Clin Oncol*. 2009;27:663–671.

351. Van Cutsem E, Köhne CH, Hitre E, et al. Cetuximab and chemotherapy as initial treatment for metastatic colorectal cancer. *N Engl J Med*. 2009;360:1408–1417.
352. Fuchs CS, Marshall J, Mitchell E, et al. Randomized, controlled trial of irinotecan plus infusional, bolus, or oral fluoropyrimidines in first-line treatment of metastatic colorectal cancer: results from the BICC-C Study. *J Clin Oncol*. 2007;25(30):4779–4786.
353. Saltz LB, Clarke S, Diaz-Rubio E, et al. Bevacizumab in combination with oxaliplatin-based chemotherapy as first-line therapy in metastatic colorectal cancer: a randomized phase III study. *J Clin Oncol*. 2008;26:2013–2019.
354. Cercek A, Saltz L. Factors dictating outcomes in patients with colorectal cancer and peritoneal carcinomatosis: selection, resection, or convection? *J Clin Oncol*. 2012;30(3):226–228.
355. Franko J, Shi Q, Goldman CD, et al. Treatment of colorectal peritoneal carcinomatosis with systemic chemotherapy: a pooled analysis of North Central Cancer Treatment Group phase III trials N9741 and N9841. *J Clin Oncol*. 2012;30(3):263–267.
356. Hompes D, D'Hoore A, Wolthuis A, et al. The use of oxaliplatin or mitomycin C in HIPEC treatment for peritoneal carcinomatosis from colorectal cancer: a comparative study. *J Surg Oncol*. 2014;109(6):527–532.
357. Chua TC, Esquivel J, Pelz JO, et al. Summary of current therapeutic options for peritoneal metastases from colorectal cancer. *J Surg Oncol*. 2013;107(6):566–573.
358. Verwaal VJ, Bruin S, Boot H, et al. 8-year follow-up of randomized trial: cytoreduction and hyperthermic intraperitoneal chemotherapy versus systemic chemotherapy in patients with peritoneal carcinomatosis of colorectal cancer. *Ann Surg Oncol*. 2008;15:2426–2432.
359. Quenet F, Elias D, Roca L, et al. A UNICANCER phase III trial of hyperthermic intra-peritoneal chemotherapy (HIPEC) for colorectal peritoneal carcinomatosis (PC): PRODIGE 7. *J Clin Oncol*. 2018;36:abstr LBA3503.
360. Cao C, Yan TD, Black D, et al. A systematic review and meta-analysis of cytoreductive surgery with perioperative intraperitoneal chemotherapy for peritoneal carcinomatosis of colorectal origin. *Ann Surg Oncol*. 2009;16(8):2152–2165.
361. Pelz JO, Stojadinovic A, Nissan A, et al. Evaluation of a peritoneal surface disease severity score in patients with colon cancer with peritoneal carcinomatosis. *J Surg Oncol*. 2009;99(1):9–15.
362. Ganesh K, Stadler ZK, Cercek A, et al. Immunotherapy in colorectal cancer: rationale, challenges and potential. *Nat Rev Gastroenterol Hepatol*. 2019;16(6):361–375.
363. Le DT, Kavan P, Kim TW, et al. KEYNOTE-164: pembrolizumab for patients with advanced microsatellite instability high (MSI-H) colorectal cancer. *J Clin Oncol*. 2018;36(15 suppl):abstr 3514.
364. Andre T, Lonardi S, et al. Nivolumab + ipilimumab combination in patients with DNA mismatch repair-deficient/microsatellite instability-high (dMMR/MSI-H) metastatic colorectal cancer (mCRC): first report of the full cohort from CheckMate-142. *J Clin Oncol*. 2018;36(4 suppl):abstr 553.
365. Bendell JC, Bang Y, Chee C, et al. A phase Ib study of safety and clinical activity of atezolizumab (A) and cobimetinib (C) in patients (pts) with metastatic colorectal cancer (mCRC). *J Clin Oncol*. 2018;36(suppl 4S):abstr 560.
366. Shahda S. A multi-center, single arm, phase II study of pembrolizumab (MK-3475) in combination with chemotherapy for patients with advanced colorectal cancer: HCRN GI14-186. ClinicalTrials.gov: NCT02375672.
367. Segal N. single arm phase II study to assess the efficacy of pembrolizumab plus radiotherapy or ablation in metastatic colorectal cancer patients. ClinicalTrials.gov: NCT02437071.
368. Bozzetti F, Bertario L, Rossetti C, et al. Surgical treatment of locally recurrent rectal carcinoma. *Dis Colon Rectum*. 1997;40(12):1421–1424.
369. van Gijn W, Marijnen CA, Nagtegaal ID, et al. Preoperative radiotherapy combined with total mesorectal excision for resectable rectal cancer: 12-year follow-up of the multicentre, randomised controlled TME trial. *Lancet Oncol*. 2011;12(6):575–582.
370. Tepper JE, O'Connell M, Hollis D, et al. Analysis of surgical salvage after failure of primary therapy in rectal cancer: results from Intergroup Study 0114. *J Clin Oncol*. 2003;21(19):3623–3628.
371. Hashiguchi Y, Sekine T, Sakamoto H, et al. Intraoperative irradiation after surgery for locally recurrent rectal cancer. *Dis Colon Rectum*. 1999;42(7):886–893; discussion 893–895.
372. Balbay MD, Slaton JW, Trane N, et al. Rationale for bladder-sparing surgery in patients with locally advanced colorectal carcinoma. *Cancer*. 1999;86(11):2212–2216.
373. Tan E, Gouvas N, Nicholls RJ, et al. Diagnostic precision of carcinoembryonic antigen in the detection of recurrence of colorectal cancer. *Surg Oncol*. 2009;18(1):15–24.
374. Chau I, Allen MJ, Cunningham D, et al. The value of routine serum carcino-embryonic antigen measurement and computed tomography in the surveillance of patients after adjuvant chemotherapy for colorectal cancer. *J Clin Oncol*. 2004;22(8):1420–1429.
375. Lambregts DM, Cappendijk VC, Maas M, et al. Value of MRI and diffusion-weighted MRI for the diagnosis of locally recurrent rectal cancer. *Eur Radiol*. 2011;21(6):1250–1258.
376. de Anda EH, Lee SH, Finne CO, et al. Endorectal ultrasound in the follow-up of rectal cancer patients treated by local excision or radical surgery. *Dis Colon Rectum*. 2004;47(6):818–824.
377. Maas M, Rutten IJ, Nelemans PJ, et al. What is the most accurate whole-body imaging modality for assessment of local and distant recurrent disease in colorectal cancer? A meta-analysis. *Eur J Nucl Med Mol Imaging*. 2011;38(8):1560–1571.
378. Schmidt GP, Baur-Melnyk A, Haug A, et al. Whole-body MRI at 1.5 T and 3 T compared with FDG-PET-CT for the detection of tumour recurrence in patients with colorectal cancer. *Eur Radiol*. 2009;19(6):1366–1378.
379. Lu YY, Chen JH, Chien CR, et al. Use of FDG-PET or PET/CT to detect recurrent colorectal cancer in patients with elevated CEA: a systematic review and meta-analysis. *Int J Colorectal Dis*. 2013;28(8):1039–1047.
380. Vermaas M, Nuyttens JJ, Ferenschild FT, et al. Reirradiation, surgery and IORT for recurrent rectal cancer in previously irradiated patients. *Radiother Oncol*. 2008;87(3):357–360.
381. Garcia-Aguilar J, Cromwell JW, Marra C, et al. Treatment of locally recurrent rectal cancer. *Dis Colon Rectum*. 2001;44(12):1743–1748.
382. Lutz ST, Jones J, Chow E. Role of radiation therapy in palliative care of the patient with cancer. *J Clin Oncol*. 2014;32(26):2913–2919.
383. Lin AY, Dinning PG, Milne T, Bissett IP, O'Grady G. The "rectosigmoid brake": review of an emerging neuromodulation target for colorectal functional disorders. *Clin Exp Pharmacol Physiol*. 2017;44:719–728.
384. Garcia-Aguilar J, Patil S, Gollub MJ, et al. Organ preservation in patients with rectal adenocarcinoma treated with total neoadjuvant therapy. *J Clin Oncol*. 2022;40:2546–2556.

Diverticular Disease

Paul E. Wise

Key Points

1 The prevalence of diverticulosis varies greatly across global populations but is essentially ubiquitous in older adults in North America and Europe.

2 Although a minority of patients become symptomatic, the high prevalence of diverticulosis leads to a large and growing burden of diverticular disease including acute diverticulitis (both complicated and uncomplicated), recurrent diverticulitis, and diverticular hemorrhage.

3 The etiology of diverticulosis and diverticular disease is incompletely understood but includes both inherent and environmental risk factors.

4 Diverticulitis can be effectively diagnosed, and its severity classified, with cross-sectional imaging, especially CT imaging.

5 Acute uncomplicated diverticulitis may often be treated in outpatient settings, and antibiotics may be omitted in some patients.

6 Acute complicated diverticulitis may be successfully treated with nonoperative management, percutaneous abscess drainage, or require urgent laparotomy and colectomy depending on disease severity and patient factors.

7 Anastomosis (with or without diversion) at the time of urgent colectomy may be an option for well-selected patients.

8 The decision to operate electively for secondary prevention of diverticulitis should be individualized based on patient- and disease-specific factors.

9 Clinical guidelines for the treatment of diverticular disease, including acute diverticulitis, have changed significantly, reflecting improving understanding of the natural history of the disease.

Diverticular disease is one of the most common colorectal conditions evaluated and treated in the United States. The precursor lesion, diverticulosis, is ubiquitous, and its most common resultant pathology, diverticulitis, causes millions of outpatient visits, tens of thousands of operations, and results in billions of dollars in expense every year. Patient presentations vary, including mild, self-limited disease, life-threatening abdominal sepsis, chronic complications, and recurrent disease. Improved understanding of diverticulitis has meaningfully changed clinical guidelines as traditional dogmas have fallen under increased scientific scrutiny. Today, diverticulitis patients may avoid antibiotics, are less likely to require inpatient admission or emergency operations, more likely to be anastomosed when urgent operation is required, less likely to undergo elective colectomy, and more likely to have percutaneous procedures and minimally invasive surgery. However, much remains to be discovered about optimal treatment for diverticular disease.

TERMINOLOGY AND ANATOMY

Diverticulosis coli describes the presence of colonic pseudodiverticula ("false diverticula"), discrete sacs of mucosa and submucosa herniating through the circular muscle adjacent to penetrating mesenteric vessels ("vasa recta"), emerging between the tenia coli on the antimesenteric aspect of the colon (**Fig. 66.1**).[1] With rare exception, diverticulosis is an acquired condition of adults that increases in frequency with advancing age.[2] Incidental diagnosis of this asymptomatic lesion can be made at the time of colonoscopy (**Fig. 66.2**), contrast enema, or cross-sectional imaging. In Europe and North America, diverticulosis is most prominent in the sigmoid colon, effected in 95% of patients with the disease,[3] while the disease in Asia and Africa is, for unknown reasons, predominantly in the right colon and comprised more frequently of "true diverticula" (containing all layers of the bowel wall).[4] Isolated sigmoid diverticulosis in the United States is present in 60% of cases, and the pattern of involvement progresses proximally with 10% of cases presenting as total colonic diverticulosis. Much less common than colonic diverticulosis, small bowel and rectal diverticula will not be addressed in this text.

The two most common colonic diverticular diseases (ie, when diverticulosis becomes symptomatic) are diverticulitis (inflammation of the diverticula and its sequelae) and diverticular hemorrhage. Two less common manifestations include segmental colitis associated with diverticulosis (SCAD) and symptomatic uncomplicated diverticular disease (SUDD) which have clinical overlap with inflammatory bowel disease (IBD) and irritable bowel syndrome (IBS), respectively.

EPIDEMIOLOGY

1 Diverticulosis is nearly ubiquitous in older adults in Western Europe and North America with notably lower rates in Africa and Asia. Endoscopic studies indicate that >50% of individuals in the United States over age 60 have diverticula.[3] Incidence increases with age, demonstrates a male predominance under age 60 and a female predominance thereafter,[4] with some stud-
2 ies showing equal sex distribution after age 50.[5] Although only 4% of patients with incidentally discovered diverticulosis develop diverticular disease,[2] the high prevalence of diverticulosis leads to a substantial burden of disease. Over 200,000 inpatient admissions and over 600,000 emergency room visits annually in the United States are attributed to diverticular

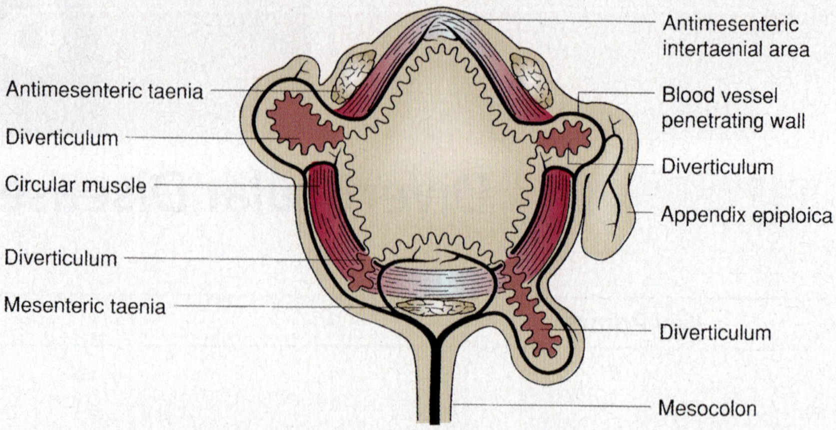

Figure 66.1. Cross section of the colon illustrating the relation of diverticula to the blood vessels penetrating the circular muscle layer, the taeniae, and the appendices epiploicae.

disease, resulting in billions of dollars in expense.[6] Diverticulitis is considered a disease of older adults in industrialized societies, but even within the modern era, incidence continues to increase rapidly, particularly among young adults under age 50.[4,5] Prevalence of diverticulitis is highest in white women (312/100,000) and Hispanic men (188/100,000), with women overall having a lower odds of complicated disease, while the prevalence of diverticular bleeding is highest in both Black women (72/100,000) and men (54/100,000) with the pathophysiology of the sex and race differences being unclear.[6] Epidemiologic differences in the United States may further impact disparities in diverticular disease costs and outcomes associated with race.[7] Globally, while Africa and Asia have population rates of diverticulosis of 2% to 9.4% and 8% to 28.5%, respectively, their rates are increasing, presumably due to adopting "westernized lifestyles."[5]

ETIOLOGY

3 The causes of diverticulosis and the triggers that produce diverticulitis and diverticular bleeding are multifactorial and incompletely understood, but compelling associations between inherent and environmental risk factors have been observed (Table 66.1), with many challenges to being able to test the causal relationships of these factors.

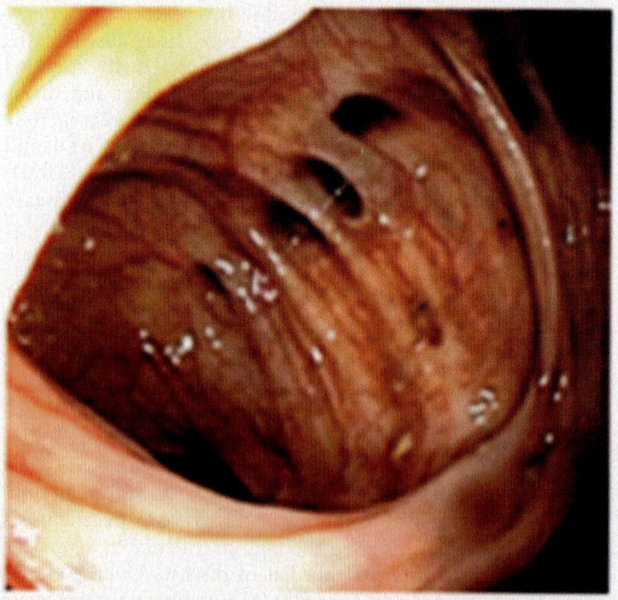

Figure 66.2. Endoscopic image of diverticulosis coli. Multiple diverticula are visible without evidence of inflammation or bleeding.

Inherent Risk Factors: Genetics

In addition to inherent factors like age and sex, an individual's genetics is estimated to be associated with approximately 40% to 50% of the cases of diverticular disease.[5] Twin and sibling studies have identified increased disease concordance between monozygotic twins as compared to dizygotic twins and three-time higher rates in siblings than the general population.[8] Disease concordance was higher for more severe disease. In addition, family history has been recognized as an independent risk factor for recurrence and complications.[9] Multiple genome-wide association studies have shown diverticular disease to be associated with the genes linked with connective tissue and extracellular matrix disorders (eg, Ehlers–Danlos), neuromuscular function and motility disorders, vascular alterations, and immunity,[5] in addition to growing data about the use of polygenic risk scores from biobank studies on the odds of more severe diverticular disease that might inform care decisions in the future.[10] These data suggest that, like most common diseases, diverticular disease is a complex trait with both environmental and genetic risk factors, and thus research in this area is growing exponentially as technology advances.

Inherent Risk Factors: Colonic Structure and Function

The acquired, age-related nature of diverticulosis and diverticular disease, in addition to the noted genetic associations, has led to the belief that connective tissue is involved in its pathophysiology. Observed associations with rare connective

Table 66.1. Inherent and Environmental Risk Factors Associated with Diverticular Disease

Risk Factors Associated with Diverticular Disease	
Inherent	**Environmental**
▪ Age ▪ Genetic background *Family history, ethnicity* ▪ Sex ▪ Mendelian syndromes *Ehler–Danlos syndrome, Marfan syndrome, polycystic kidney disease, Williams syndrome* ▪ Acquired connective tissue disorders *Aneurysm, rectal prolapse, hernia, collagen cross-linking* ▪ Altered colonic motility	▪ Diet *Low fiber, high red meat intake* ▪ Lifestyle factors *Obesity, smoking, physical inactivity* ▪ Geography *Country of birth, country of residence, Northern latitude, urban environment* ▪ Microbiome ▪ Other *Medication use, UV light exposure, vitamin D*

tissue disorders such as Ehlers–Danlos, Marfan, and Williams syndromes support this, as does the association of diverticular disease with more common acquired connective tissue traits such as hernia, rectal prolapse, and aneurysm.[5,10,11] At the histologic level, cross-linking of collagen fibrils has been associated with rigidity and strength loss associated with diverticulosis. Increased elastin deposition and smooth muscle alterations are observed in the longitudinal muscles of the tenia coli, leading to the thick bowel walls appreciated in diverticulitis patients.[5]

The Western predominance of diverticulosis in the relatively narrow noncompliant sigmoid colon led to the theory of diverticula being secondary to increased intraluminal pressure. Motility studies have demonstrated increased contractility in patients with diverticulosis compared to controls.[12] Studies comparing patients with diverticular disease to controls and patients with varying degrees of diverticulitis have noted alterations in nerve function as well as alterations in serotonin, growth factors, immune mediators, histamine, and cytokines, but it is unknown if these alterations are causal, correlated, or reactive to the disease state.[5]

Environmental Risk Factors: Diet and Lifestyle

Multiple modifiable lifestyle risk factors have been associated with diverticular disease. Dietary fiber was first identified in the 1960s. Working in Uganda, Painter and Burkitt observed the high-fiber diets and low disease prevalence among Africans compared to their British counterparts.[13] More recent work is predominantly supportive of high-fiber diets (especially with fruit consumption) and diets low in red meat being associated with significantly lower risk of symptomatic diverticular disease, and seeds and nuts as an inciting factor clearly having been disproven. Central obesity, smoking, alcoholism, and physical inactivity are associated with the incidence of, as well as more complicated, diverticulitis. Other associations including low vitamin D levels, low UV light exposure, hypertension, type 2 diabetes, medication use (eg, nonsteroidal antiinflammatories, corticosteroids, opioids), and others have been observed, but whether these relationships are causal or correlative is not yet clear.[5,8,14]

Environmental Risk Factors: Microbiome

The microbiome clearly has an important role in gut health, but its role in diverticular disease is a topic of ongoing research. The colonic microbiome may link diet and disease through the bacteria that process dietary fiber into the short-chain fatty acids critical for intestinal epithelial proliferation and barrier function, in addition to gut motility and hypersensitivity.[14,15] Western diet is associated with both decreased diversity of the gut microbiome as well as diverticular disease, but associations between the two are mixed other than a strong relationship between the microbiome and SUDD. Despite the limited associations, changes in the microbiome have been observed in patients with a history of diverticulitis, but it is unknown whether these changes predate or follow the disease state. Modulation of the microbiome through fiber intake, probiotics, and medications (eg, rifaximin, mesalamine) have been used to mitigate diverticular symptoms, but the impact of microbiome alterations remains a compelling area of research.[5,14]

ACUTE DIVERTICULITIS

Presentation

Acute diverticulitis presents with local inflammatory symptoms (eg, pain, tenderness, bowel habit changes) and systemic inflammatory symptoms (eg, fevers) depending on the severity
4 of disease. The modified Hinchey classification (**Table 66.2**) provides ordinal categorization to the severity of acute inflammatory diverticulitis correlated with associated CT findings.[16–18] Initial treatment strategy is guided by Hinchey stage. Stage 0–I disease typically presents with predominantly local inflammatory symptoms and signs. Patients complain of left lower quadrant pain, fever, altered bowel habits, malaise, and may have nausea/vomiting or urinary symptoms. Duration of symptoms on presentation is typically 12 to 48 hours. When taking a history, patients should be asked about bowel habits and continence as well as prior abdominal operations and endoscopies, family history of colorectal cancer (CRC) or polyps. Review of systems should ascertain the presence or absence of fecaluria, pneumaturia, frequent urinary tract infections, foul vaginal discharge, and/or stool per vagina which suggest the presence of a fistula.

History should also seek evidence of other etiologies. Profuse diarrhea and history of travel, sick contacts, or suggestive food exposures should prompt consideration and evaluation of gastroenteritis. Chronic abdominal pain, weight loss, subacute change in bowel habits, and history of melena or hematochezia are not typical of acute diverticulitis and should arouse suspicion for an alternative diagnosis such as IBD or CRC. Because diverticular hemorrhage is typically painless, acute diverticulitis with hematochezia is unusual, so other causes such as IBD, malignancy, or ischemic or infectious colitis should be considered and assessed with sigmoidoscopy or other diagnostic modalities.

Physical examination in stage 0–II disease reveals focal tenderness or local peritonitis, usually in the left lower quadrant. Rectal examination may demonstrate pelvic tenderness. Fever may be present, but hypotension, tachycardia, and signs of septic physiology are typically absent in early stages. Stage III and IV disease frequently presents with diffuse peritonitis and attendant septic physiology, which may range from fever and tachycardia to septic shock with multisystem organ failure. Differential diagnosis is broad at these stages and includes perforation (eg, peptic ulcer disease, appendicitis, CRC), acute ischemic colitis, pancreatitis, and IBD flare.

Diagnosis

Standard laboratory investigations of abdominal pain should include complete blood count, basic serum chemistries, amylase, lipase, pregnancy testing, and urinalysis. Nonspecific inflammatory markers including C-reactive protein (CRP), fecal calprotectin, and procalcitonin are frequently elevated in diverticulitis, more so in severe disease. Studies have demonstrated the potential of these markers to discriminate the clinical severity of the diverticulitis, but this has yet to be incorporated into many routine diagnostic algorithms.[16,17,19]

Standard radiographic imaging is mandatory to confirm the diagnosis. While ultrasound and MRI have diagnostic uses to limit ionizing radiation and where CT may be unavailable or contraindicated,[16] CT scan remains the most common and effective test for acute diverticulitis.[14] Ideally performed with intravenous (± oral) contrast, CT sensitivity and specificity for diverticulitis are greater than 95% even without contrast media.[18] CT scan findings can stratify patients into Hinchey stages and exclude mimicking pathology (although may not always distinguish inflammatory from malignant pathology). Typical CT findings vary based on Hinchey stage (**Table 66.2**). In addition to staging, CT can predict the likelihood of antibiotic failure based on size and location of diverticular abscesses, guide percutaneous abscess drainage, and predict recurrent abscess formation. Air in the bladder or vagina may suggest an occult fistula. CT scan can also be useful for operative planning in evaluating the degree of inflammation, particularly adjacent to pelvic sidewall structures and ureters, and gauging the colon redundancy and height of the splenic flexure. In the setting of peritonitis, abdominal x-ray showing pneumoperitoneum may prompt urgent operation without further diagnostic testing. Endoscopy is not a routine part of the acute diagnostic algorithm but should be judiciously used when other diagnoses are seriously considered, such as malignancy, IBD, and ischemia.

Table 66.2. Modified Hinchey Classification, Expected CT Imaging Findings, and Likely Initial Treatment Strategy for Increasingly Severe Presentations of Diverticulitis

Modified Hinchey Classification	CT Findings	Initial Treatment
0 Mild clinical diverticulitis	Diverticuli, colonic wall thickening	Supportive care, possible antibiotic treatment
Ia Pericolic inflammation	Diverticuli, wall thickening, pericolic soft tissue changes, small extraluminal gas locules	Supportive care, possible antibiotic treatment
Ib Pericolic or mesocolic abscess	Ia Changes with local fluid collection(s)	<3 cm abscess: antibiotics >3 cm abscess: antibiotics and percutaneous drainage
II Pelvic, retroperitoneal, distant abscess	Ia Changes with remote fluid collection(s)	<3 cm abscess: antibiotics >3 cm abscess: antibiotics and percutaneous drainage
III Purulent peritonitis	Pneumoperitoneum, ascites, peritoneal thickening, possible extravasation of oral contrast	Operative exploration, antibiotics, potential need for critical care
IV Feculent peritonitis	Same as III	Same as III

Modified from Klarenbeek BR, de Korte N, van der Peet DL, et al. Review of current classifications for diverticular disease and a translation into clinical practice. *Int J Colorectal Dis.* 2012;27(2):207–214.

Treatment

Acute Uncomplicated Diverticulitis

5 Included in the Hinchey 0–Ia stages, "uncomplicated diverticulitis" refers to inflammation limited to the colon and pericolic tissues without abscess or perforation. Traditional treatments of uncomplicated diverticulitis were inpatient admission, bowel rest, and antibiotics. More modern approaches to uncomplicated diverticulitis include expanded use of outpatient treatment[20] with failure rates <5%,[4] most prudently applied to otherwise healthy, stable, reliable individuals with relatively mild local symptoms. Immunocompromised patients (eg, corticosteroids, chemotherapy) and/or patients with significant comorbidities are more likely to require inpatient care and possibly early surgical intervention.[16,21] That said, the majority of uncomplicated cases in the United States are now managed in the outpatient setting.[16]

Antibiotics have long been standard of care medical therapy for acute diverticulitis, but recent randomized controlled trials (RCTs) and systematic reviews have failed to demonstrate a benefit (**Table 66.3**).[22–24] In 2020, the American Society of Colon and Rectal Surgeons incorporated these data into its clinical practice guidelines, including omission of antibiotics as a strong treatment recommendation in otherwise healthy patients with early diverticulitis.[14] Dietary recommendations during an attack of acute diverticulitis have also varied, but typically involve a liquid diet until symptoms have improved, followed by transition to a low-residue/low-fiber diet and then high-fiber diet, all based on dogma with little evidentiary support.[21]

Following resolution of a first episode of diverticulitis, 10% to 30% of patients will recur.[2] Physicians commonly recommend adoption of lifestyle modifications associated with reduced incident diverticulitis, including weight loss, high-fiber diet, and smoking cessation, although it is unknown if these measures actually prevent recurrence. Patients with uncomplicated diverticulitis harbor a low risk for occult colorectal neoplasia compared to those with complicated diverticulitis, but colonoscopy is generally recommended for both groups after resolution of a first episode,[14,16] especially if the patient is not up-to-date on screening colonoscopy, and should be strongly considered if CT imaging demonstrates lymphadenopathy or colonic wall "shouldering," the patient's symptoms are suggestive of malignancy, or complete recovery is not achieved with nonoperative management.

Acute Complicated Diverticulitis

Intraabdominal Abscess

Diverticular abscess is present in 10% to 20% of hospitalized diverticulitis patients. Best confirmed on imaging, abscesses may be intramural, pelvic, pericolic, intra- or perihepatic, or retroperitoneal (**Fig. 66.3**). The underlying etiology is assumed to be contained diverticular perforation and associated flora are enteric in nature. Small abscesses (<3 cm) may often be treated successfully with antibiotics alone, but larger collec-
6 tions fail medical management up to 44% of the time.[25] Image-guided percutaneous drainage by interventional radiology (IR) is the mainstay of therapy. Unilocular collections are more likely to be successfully managed with percutaneous drainage than multifocal or loculated abscesses, and transabdominal routes are more likely to be successful than transgluteal, transvaginal, or transrectal routes that are often painful and poorly tolerated. Overall, initial nonoperative therapy is successful in >90% of cases,[14,21] but more urgent surgical intervention is indicated if septic symptoms fail to improve or worsen.

Following recovery from an episode of complicated diverticulitis, patients should undergo colonoscopy, as noted above, due to the risk of occult malignancy in up to 8%.[16] In the recent past, surgical guidelines advised elective colectomy

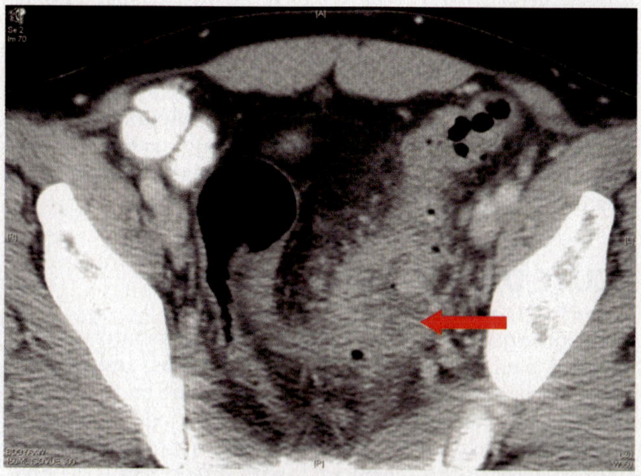

Figure 66.3. Sigmoid diverticulitis with pericolic abscess (*arrows*).

Table 66.3. Randomized Controlled Trials for Diverticulitis, Grouped Thematically

Trial Name	DIVER	AVOD	DIABOLO	DINAMO	DIRECT	COSMID	LASER
Year(s)[a]	2014	2012/2019	2017/2018	2021	2017/2019	2019[b]	2021/2023
Interventions	Outpatient versus inpatient management of acute uncomplicated diverticulitis	Antibiotics or no antibiotics for acute uncomplicated diverticulitis	Antibiotics or no antibiotics for first episode acute uncomplicated diverticulitis	Antibiotics or no antibiotics for acute uncomplicated diverticulitis	Nonoperative management or elective lap sigmoidectomy for recurrent diverticulitis	Nonoperative management or elective lap sigmoidectomy, assessing patient-related outcomes	Nonoperative management or elective laparoscopic sigmoidectomy
Conclusions	Outpatient management safe and feasible as no difference in readmission or mortality	Antibiotics should be reserved for complicated cases of diverticulitis only (no differences after 11 yrs for recurrences or GI-specific QOL)	Antibiotics do not improve time to recovery, readmission, adverse events, ongoing and recurrent disease, sigmoid resection, or mortality (short-and long-term)	Antibiotics do not decrease risk of readmission, return to emergency room, pain control, or need for operation at 90 d	Higher QOL in resection group, even at 5 yrs, with higher risk of short-term complications	Results pending ClinicalTrial.gov NCT04095663	Higher QOL in resection group, even at 2 yrs, but higher risk of short-term complications (18% nonop group required sigmoidectomy)
Trial Name	LADIES (LOLA)	SCANDIV	DILALA	ColonPerfRCT	DIVERTI	LADIES (DIVA)	DIVERTI2
Year(s)[a]	2015/2022	2015/2021	2016/2018	2012	2017/2021	2019	2022[b]
Interventions	Laparoscopic lavage, HP, or sigmoidectomy and anastomosis	Laparoscopic lavage or resection	Laparoscopic lavage or HP	HP or resection and anastomosis with DLI in Hinchey III/IV	HP or resection and anastomosis (with or without diversion) for Hinchey III/IV	HP or resection and anastomosis for Hinchey III/IV	Resection and anastomosis with or without diverting stoma for Hinchey III/IV
Conclusions	Lap lavage not superior to sigmoidectomy, study terminated early due to event rate in lavage group, but 3-yr outcomes were equivalent (45% of lavage group needed resection)	Lap lavage is not superior to sigmoidectomy, severe outcomes were the same, high mortality in both, and at 5 yrs, 30% lavage group needed resection, (missed cancers in lavage group)	No difference in morbidity or mortality, time in hospital, or readmissions; 42% vs 68% had ≥1 subsequent operation and 7% vs 23% a stoma (lavage vs HP groups at 2 yrs)	No difference in overall complications, but 90% DLI reversal vs 57% colostomy reversal; and lower LOS, costs, OR time, serious complications in the group with anastomosis/DLI	No difference in mortality, higher rate of stoma reversal in those with anastomosis and diversion; QOL worse after HP which also had higher hernia rates	No difference in short-term morbidity or mortality, 12-mo stoma-free survival higher in the resection and anastomosis group	Results pending ClinicalTrial.gov NCT04604730

[a]Includes the year of the original trial and long-term follow-up publication date, if any; citation is latest trial publication.
[b]Year enrollment started.
DLI, diverting loop ileostomy; HP, Hartmann procedure; LOS, length of stay; QOL, quality of life; LADIES trials: DIVA, perforated diverticulitis: sigmoid resection with or without anastomosis; LOLA, laparoscopic lavage.
Adapted from Kodadek LM, Davis KA. Current diagnosis and management of acute colonic diverticulitis: What you need to know. *J Trauma Acute Care Surg*. 2024;97(1):1–10.

after any episode of complicated diverticulitis, but reported rates of recurrent complicated disease ranges from 12% to 46%.[14,21] These data, however, are heterogeneous, retrospective, and mostly from single institutions with limited numbers and follow-up, but most (including meta-analyses) suggest that while recurrence rates of diverticulitis may be high after a successfully treated episode of complicated diverticulitis, most can be managed nonoperatively with few requiring urgent operations or colostomy ("first episode tends to be the worst episode"). Given the observation that recurrence and surgery are not inevitable consequences of diverticular abscess, however, has led to a relaxation of guidelines from advising colectomy to advising *consideration* of colectomy after a complicated attack.[14] Patients should be seen in consultation with a surgeon and the risks of recurrence balanced against patient preferences and patient factors impacting operative tolerance and morbidity/mortality risks. When counseling patients on risk of recurrence and need for operative intervention, it should be noted that large abscesses (>5 cm), regardless of location, and pelvic abscesses are more likely to recur.

Perforated Diverticulitis with Peritonitis

Emergent/urgent operation is required in 1% of diverticulitis patients overall but may be required in 15% to 32% of hospitalized patients.[14,21] Hinchey III and IV disease presents with peritonitis and requires urgent operative intervention. Patients should be given broad-spectrum antibiotics, rapidly hemodynamically stabilized as needed, and explored. The goal of the operation is to achieve infectious source control by evacuating intraperitoneal purulence and/or feces and, usually (see "lavage" below), resecting the affected bowel. Emergency colectomy for diverticulitis is morbid, potentially fatal, and care of unstable, elderly, or frail patients should be rapid and meticulous. Overall, 30-day mortality is 5.1%. Patients >80 years of age, with serum creatinine >1.2 mg/dL, ASA class 4/5, or albumin <2.5 g/dL are increased risk of mortality, and patients with four of these predictors have a 30-day mortality rate >50%.[14]

The most common approach to Hinchey III and IV diverticulitis is a Hartmann procedure (HP), which means resection of the diseased bowel to soft, compliant proximal colon, stapled or suture closure of the distal rectal or sigmoid stump, and creation of an end colostomy. The major downside of this approach is the need for a second major operation to restore intestinal continuity, assuming the patient is even a candidate. HP reversal most often requires repeat laparotomy (although minimally invasive approaches are feasible in some patients), can entail a challenging lysis of adhesions and pelvic dissection to "dig out" the rectal stump, and is associated with significant operative morbidity. Because of this, "temporary" urgent colostomies may become permanent in up to 45% of
7 patients.[14,21] Therefore, creation of a primary anastomosis with or without diverting loop ileostomy (DLI) is an attractive alternative, as has been assessed in multiple RCTs comparing this to HP (**Table 66.3**).[26–29] These trials have reached similar conclusions: morbidity and mortality of the primary operation were the same between the two approaches, but stoma-free survival was higher with primary anastomosis. HP at the initial operation led to greater morbidity at the time of ostomy takedown. Although compelling, these results have not changed clinical practice. In the United States >90% of urgent colectomies for diverticulitis are still performed with end colostomy.[30] In clinical practice, the surgeon should decide to perform HP or an anastomosis on an individual basis, evaluating patient stability and comorbidities (including baseline continence and mobility), the quality of the tissues, and the degree of contamination.

An alternative approach in Hinchey III diverticulitis, laparoscopic lavage (LL) garnered serious clinical and academic interest as a potential alternative to resection. With LL, the patient undergoes laparoscopic irrigation and drainage of intraperitoneal contamination without mobilization or resection of the colon. After early enthusiasm from retrospective data, RCTs of LL versus HP (**Table 66.3**) did demonstrate some advantages of LL, including shorter operative times and lower stoma rates.[31–33] However, while short- and long-term mortality rates were equivalent, missed adenocarcinomas and high disease recurrence rates and need for subsequent operations in 30% to 45% after LL tempered the enthusiasm for this as an alternative to resection. Overall, colectomy remains the preferred approach to Hinchey III/IV diverticulitis, but LL may be appropriate for well-selected, healthy Hinchey III patients.[14,34]

Surgical Technique—Urgent Operation for Perforated Diverticulitis

Preoperatively, the patient should be marked bilaterally for a potential ostomy while sitting up, if possible, avoiding skin folds, creases, and bony prominences. Operative approach may be open or minimally invasive considering the condition of the patient, anticipated severity of contamination, and skill of the operating surgeon. Lithotomy position is favored to allow creation of a circular stapled anastomosis, if possible; perform colonoscopy, if necessary; and assist in identification of structures in the inflamed pelvis or allow for ureteral stent placement, if needed. After clearing fecal/purulent material from the operative field, purulent rinds and adhesions may be broken up bluntly, but not at the expense of further bowel injury. Areas of perforation may be oversewn to control contamination. The colon is divided just proximal to the diseased area and dissection carried to just above the sacral promontory, if possible. Sidewall structures are identified (**Fig. 66.4**) and dissection is kept close to the inflamed colon to minimize risk to surrounding structures. The distal noninflamed sigmoid or upper rectum is transected, and the specimen passed from the field. Any remaining contamination is irrigated to clear. If the patient is unstable after contamination is controlled, it is reasonable to stop at this point, pack the abdomen open with the bowel in discontinuity, and proceed to the intensive care unit for stabilization. However, if the patient is stable, the colon is mobilized for either creation of a colostomy or anastomosis. Due to inflammatory foreshortening of the mesentery, either approach may require takedown of the splenic flexure (**Fig. 66.5**), division of the inferior mesenteric artery (IMA), and possibly division of the inferior mesenteric vein (IMV) to achieve adequate reach for a tension-free anastomosis or appropriately matured colostomy. If the patient

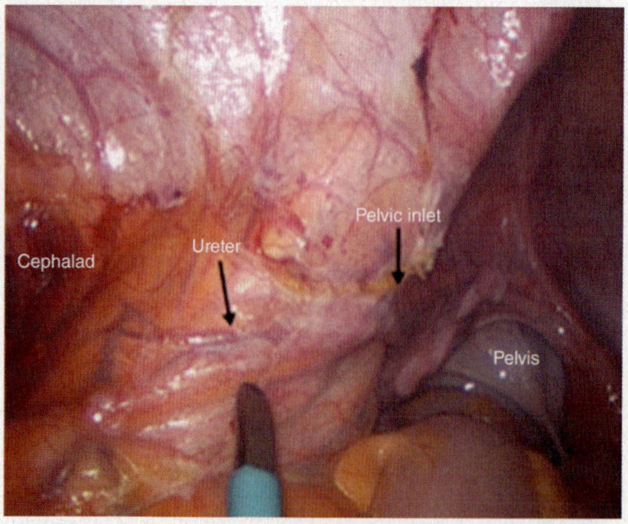

Figure 66.4. Surgical view of the left-sided pelvic sidewall structures demonstrating the ureter and iliac vessels.

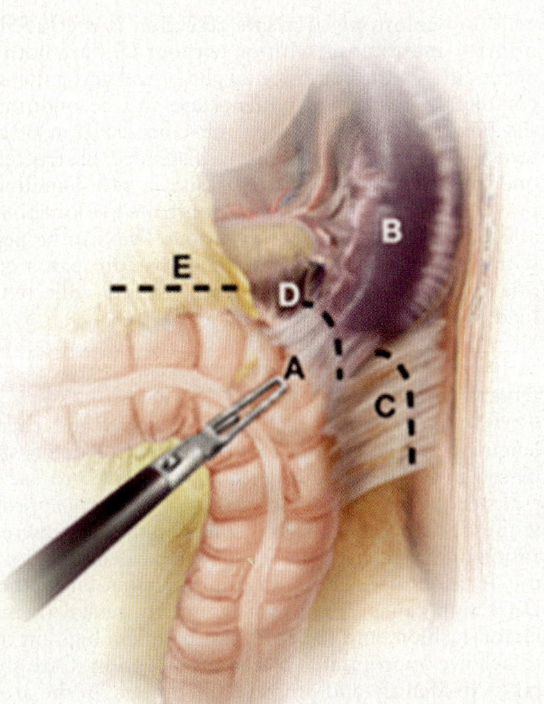

Figure 66.5. Illustration of the relationship of the splenic flexure of the colon (A) to the spleen (B). Full mobilization requires division of the abdominal (C), lienocolic/splenocolic (D), and omental (E) attachments.

and bowel are suitable for an anastomosis (with or without DLI), full mobilization and careful assessment should allow the anastomosis to be tension-free and perfused, and leak test should be performed.

If, at the index operation, a primary anastomosis was performed with DLI, the patient should typically be allowed to recover for 2 to 3 months, the anastomosis evaluated with water-soluble contrast enema and/or sigmoidoscopy, and the DLI reversed electively. If an HP was performed and subsequent reversal is desired, the patient should be allowed to recover for at least 3 to 6 months from their acute illness and optimize their functional status through management of comorbid conditions, increased physical activity, smoking cessation, nutritional support, and weight loss, as necessary. Thorough review of the initial operative note is key to understand the handling of the rectal stump and mesenteric vasculature. Colonoscopic screening should be updated, if necessary, and cross-sectional imaging (with or without rectal contrast) and/or hypaque enema may better delineate anatomy. Preoperative continence should be queried and can be evaluated formally by manometry and defecography, or informally by examination and asking the patient to hold an enema in the rectum. Preoperative ureteral stents should be considered but are not mandatory. HP reversal can be undertaken by an open or minimally invasive approach. The rectal stump should be freshened to healthy, compliant rectum and any residual sigmoid removed. The stump may be foreshortened and shrunken with disuse, so placement of an EEA sizer per anus may assist in identification and dilation.

RECURRENT DIVERTICULITIS AND CHRONIC PRESENTATIONS

Recurrent Diverticulitis

After recovering from acute, uncomplicated diverticulitis, 13% to 33% of patients will have recurrent attacks.[2] For decades, the assumption that every uncomplicated diverticulitis attack added up incrementally to an individual's risk of subsequent free perforation led to the recommendation for elective sigmoid colectomy for secondary prevention after two attacks of diverticulitis (and after one attack in young patients). However, improved understanding of the natural history of the disease has demonstrated that the risk of subsequent complicated diverticulitis is <5%[35] and that the likelihood of needing a subsequent emergent operation for diverticulitis is 1 in 2,000 patient years (i.e., 18 elective colectomies would be needed to prevent 1 emergent operation).[14]
8 Therefore, colectomy should not be routinely performed to prevent free perforation and colostomy after uncomplicated diverticulitis. That said, there have been two RCTs comparing elective sigmoid resection with nonoperative management for recurrent diverticulitis that support improved quality of life (QOL) after resection, although with greater complication risks (**Table 66.3**),[36,37] and the COSMID trial hopes to look at this issue in the context of patient-reported
9 outcomes.[38] Current practice guidelines recommend a case-by-case decision for each recurrent diverticulitis patient.[14] Patient factors influencing the decision might include frequency and severity of episodes, missed work and activities, health care expense, access to care, persistent symptoms between attacks, and antibiotic intolerance. These should be balanced against surgical candidacy, likelihood of operative morbidity, and predicted postoperative functional outcome using a framework of shared decision making. Online and educational decision aids may help facilitate patient and clinician recommendations.[35]

Surgical Technique—Elective Sigmoid Colectomy for Recurrent Diverticulitis

Sigmoid colectomy may be performed open or minimally invasively with laparoscopy, hand-assisted laparoscopic techniques, or robotics. As with other abdominal operations, particularly when coupled with enhanced recovery pathways, minimally invasive approaches can shorten length of stay, decrease pain, decrease blood loss, and minimize wound complications.[14,21] Resections for diverticulitis, including for complicated disease, urgent indications, and ostomy reversals are increasingly performed laparoscopically. National trends indicate use of laparoscopy for elective diverticulitis surgery increased from 48% to 70% between 2006 and 2013.[39] While laparoscopy is almost ubiquitous, robotic approaches have gained favor in the United States as robotics has also become more available. Comparisons between laparoscopic and robotic approaches show similar conversion rates to open (between 0% and 18%), depending on the extent of the disease. Robotic approaches typically also show similar or slightly better length of stay and patient outcomes, but increased operative time and costs in some studies.[14,40] Overall, as resources and surgical expertise allows, a minimally invasive approach has several advantages and is preferred when possible.

Regardless of approach, the goal of the operation is not to remove *all* diverticula but all affected bowel. The proximal colonic margin should be soft, pliable, and noninflamed bowel while the distal margin should be at the upper rectum, identified by splaying of the tenia coli and loss of haustral folds (and no diverticula or inflammation). Leaving distal sigmoid behind can be associated with up to a 12.5% risk of recurrent diverticulitis postoperatively.[21] Dissection may proceed from medial to lateral or vice versa based on surgeon preference. The retroperitoneal structures and ureter should be clearly seen and protected. The lateral attachments and mesentery of the colon should be divided and mobilized until a tension-free anastomosis is created. Typically, this requires high ligation of the IMA (which is not mandatory as level of IMA division does not impact function or QOL[41]) and mobilization of the splenic flexure. Occasionally, division of the IMV and release of the greater omentum may be required

COLON AND RECTUM

for colon conduit reach. The anastomosis is created in a hand-sewn or stapled fashion according to the principles of a tension-free, straight, viable, and patent anastomosis (and surgeon's preference).

Fistulas and Stenosis/Obstruction

Fistula is a rare complication of diverticular disease occurring in 2% of cases and occurs when a contained diverticular perforation erodes into an adjacent viscera or the abdominal wall. Some patients have a provocative presentation of building abdominal pressure followed by relief and discharge of gas and/or pus via the bladder (eg, pneumaturia, fecaluria), vagina, or skin. Although the fibrotic inflammation found at operation speaks to chronic inflammation, presentation of a fistula is not necessarily preceded by recurrent attacks of diverticulitis.

Colovesical fistulas are the most common type of diverticular fistula (65%) and are more common in men than women.[21] They can present with pneumaturia, fecaluria, frequent urinary tract infections, renal impairment, and/or urosepsis. "Dirty" urinalysis and gas in the urinary bladder are appreciated on imaging and essentially pathognomonic for the diagnosis. Differential diagnosis includes emphysematous cystitis and rectourethral fistulas, particularly in patients who have had prostatectomy or pelvic radiation. Cystoscopy and colonoscopy should be considered to exclude a locally advanced colonic or bladder malignancy.

Colovaginal fistulas are the next most common (25%) and present with foul vaginal discharge and gas per vagina, typically in women who have had a hysterectomy. Many patients are referred from gynecologists, and an area of inflammation and granulation tissue at the vaginal cuff is commonly seen on speculum or vaginoscopic examination. Colonoscopy should be performed to exclude malignancy. Differential diagnosis includes vaginal infection, anovaginal fistulas, and erosion of pelvic mesh in women with a history of rectopexy or sacrocolpopexy. Rare diverticular fistula types include colouterine, coloenteric, and colocutaneous. Principles of surgical repair for all fistulas broadly are resection of the diseased colon as per the principles described above, repair of the attached normal organ (when possible), and separation of the two repairs with healthy tissue, when possible.

Colonic stenosis and large bowel obstruction can occur as sequelae of chronic diverticular inflammation. Patients may present urgently with a large bowel obstruction or with subacute symptoms including cramping pain, change in bowel habits, and bloating. Obstruction can be secondary to inflammatory phlegmon or abscess and therefore may respond to antibiotics, percutaneous drainage, and observation, obviating the need for emergent operation. However, completely obstructing fibrotic strictures risk proximal perforation and usually require surgical intervention. Interval endoluminal stent placement as a bridge to surgery can be considered, but they can make subsequent colectomy more challenging due to reactive inflammation, so early resection after decompression is recommended. Of note, successful stent placement is less likely in diverticular disease than CRC and has a reported perforation rate in benign strictures of 6% to 13%.[42] Endoluminal stent placement as definitive treatment should only be considered in very poor surgical candidates. Urgent presentation of large bowel obstruction may preclude preoperative endoscopic assessment, and the degree of inflammation can make differentiating diverticular strictures from malignancy difficult, thus oncologic principles at the time of urgent resection should be considered. The cecum should always be assessed for viability as a first step in the operation, especially with a competent ileocecal valve causing a closed-loop large bowel obstruction up to the stricture. Inflammatory fibrotic strictures and tensely dilated colon may make for prohibitively challenging urgent pelvic operations. Surgical options include diversion with a loop or end-loop colostomy if a safe resection is precluded. HP or primary anastomosis with or without DLI are both options depending on the condition of the bowel and patient. Often, completely obstructed patients are too deconditioned and the bowel too dilated to permit consideration of an anastomosis. In the case of tensely distended obstructed colon, on-table decompression may assist in safe handling of the bowel, decrease chances of uncontrolled stool spillage, and allow for more bowel preservation. This can be performed with saline lavage via the appendix or through a colotomy (ideally in a segment to be resected) and collected off the field.

Surgical Technique—Operation for Diverticular Fistula

Chronic inflammation can alter anatomy and create challenging pelvic dissections in these patients. Patients should be placed in lithotomy and consideration given to use of ureteral stents. Minimally invasive approaches are appropriate if within the skillset of the surgeon. Minimally invasive mobilization of the splenic flexure is particularly useful as it reduces the incision needed to appropriately mobilize the colon. Dissection can proceed in a lateral to medial or medial to lateral fashion, and the IMA can be taken high on the aorta to achieve appropriate colonic mobilization. Care should be taken to identify and preserve the ureters. In the area of the fistula, woody inflammation often makes laparoscopic or robotic dissection complex, although use of hand-assisted techniques, sponge sticks, or suction may well mimic manual blunt dissection. In the open technique, the colon can be bluntly pinched apart from the bladder or vagina. Ideally malignancy is preoperatively excluded in these patients to avoid "cracking through" a locally advanced malignancy that requires a multivisceral resection. After fistula separation, colonic dissection is carried to the top of the rectum and sometimes lower, if necessary, to identify soft pliable bowel. The colon anastomosis is typically carried out with a circular stapling device and leak test performed. Colovesical fistulas are typically to the dome of the bladder, but urologic help is advisable if they involve the trigone. Repair of the vagina or bladder is typically unnecessary, but wider defects or tissues that allow closure despite the inflammation can be repaired primarily. Ideally, a flap of viable omentum or peritoneal flap can be interposed between anastomosis and bladder or vagina, and a pelvic drain should be considered. DLI may be required if anastomosis quality is not ideal. Postoperatively after colovesical fistula repair, a urinary catheter is typically left in place for 7 to 10 days and a cystogram performed prior to removal, although duration of postoperative Foley remains debated,[43] thus should be based on surgeon preference and experience.

Less Common Presentations of Diverticular Disease

Segmental Colitis–Associated Diverticulosis (SCAD) and Symptomatic Uncomplicated Diverticular Disease (SUDD)

Chronic conditions related to diverticular disease, SCAD and SUDD are more frequently described in the literature as impacting patients' QOL, and both warrant further research. SCAD impacts 2% to 11% of patients with diverticulosis and is characterized on endoscopy by edema and/or erythema of the interdiverticular mucosa of the sigmoid colon, some even with ulcers or erosions, with the diverticula themselves free of inflammation (and rectum and right colon spared) and can overlap with IBD histologically. Symptoms include bleeding and diarrhea as well as left lower abdominal pain without systemic evidence of inflammation.[44] Radiographic studies may show segmental sigmoid thickening with diverticulosis but no diverticulitis, and treatment is usually nonoperative with fiber, antibiotics, and/or salicylates. Sigmoidectomy may be rarely required for persistent disease and symptoms.[21]

SUDD impacts 1% to 7% of diverticulosis patients. Although definitions vary, it is characterized by left lower quadrant abdominal pain, bowel habit changes (eg, diarrhea, constipation, bloating) that can overlap with IBS, and local inflammation (eg, elevated fecal calprotectin) without evidence of systemic inflammation or radiographic changes to suggest diverticulitis. Colonoscopy should rule out other pathology, and treatment involves probiotics, fiber diet, rifaximin, and/or mesalamine, and, for significant cases with persistent QOL declination despite nonoperative management, sigmoid colectomy.[14,45]

Giant Diverticula

Giant diverticula are rare and described as diverticula >4 cm in diameter, are commonly found in the sigmoid colon, and have been described to grow to 40 cm.[21] The etiology is unknown, but hypotheses include physical air trapping and gaseous overproduction by bacteria. Symptoms may cause mass effect, but asymptomatic presentation is common. Treatment is by sigmoid colectomy and can be done minimally invasively.[46]

Right-Sided Diverticulitis

Right-sided diverticulitis is rare among European-ancestry populations (≤5% incidence), but more common in Asia and in Asian immigrants (up to 76%).[21] Clinical presentation includes right-sided pain, fevers, chills, and gastrointestinal distress. Given the location, the differential diagnosis includes terminal ileitis, cholecystitis, typhlitis, epiploic appendagitis, mesenteric adenitis, genitourinary pathology, and, of course, appendicitis, which may be clinically indistinguishable and radiologically confusing. Like sigmoid diverticulitis, patients with uncomplicated inflammation and a clear diagnosis can be managed nonoperatively.[16,21] Recurrent disease, unclear diagnoses, and perforation should be treated with right hemicolectomy, much like sigmoid diverticulitis.[47]

Diverticular Hemorrhage

Diverticular hemorrhage is a noninflammatory diverticular pathology caused by erosion of the mesenteric vessels by an adjacent diverticulum and occurs in up to 5% of patients with diverticulosis.[21] Diverticular bleeding is the most common source of lower GI hemorrhage (accounting for up to 42%), especially in older patients on anticoagulant medications, presenting classically as bright red, painless, and brisk bleeding.[48] Differential diagnosis includes rapid upper GI hemorrhage, arteriovenous malformations, neoplasm, ischemic or inflammatory colitis, and anorectal hemorrhage. Patients should be stabilized, blood made available, nasogastric lavage considered (or upper endoscopy to rule out upper GI source), and a rectal examination performed to exclude distal pathology. Localization should include CT angiography as recommended by GI societies to then guide IR or colonoscopy treatments,[17] depending on patient stability and ability to receive intravenous contrast. Bleeding ceases spontaneously in most cases, but when a bleeding diverticulum is seen on colonoscopy, treatments include epinephrine injection, cautery, and/or clips,[48] and treatments with IR include embolization of the offending vessel (with risk of ischemia). Rebleeding occurs in a minority of patients and surgery is rarely required. In one large cohort of almost 15,000 patients with diverticular hemorrhage, almost 1,400 had a second episode, but only 64 required colectomies.[49] Segmental resection may be necessary in diverticular hemorrhage that is massive, recurrent, or fails endoscopic control, and total colectomy (with ileostomy if unstable or not a candidate for anastomosis) may be needed if localization is not able to pinpoint an offending colonic segment.

SUMMARY

Diverticular disease is a common colorectal condition with a spectrum of presentations, treatments, and prognoses. Due to its high incidence, the practicing general, colorectal, or acute care surgeon is likely to see multiple manifestations throughout their career. Diverticulitis is a complex trait with both environmental and inherent risk factors, especially genetic factors, although its exact pathophysiology remains incompletely understood. Diagnosis is frequently suspected based on symptoms and signs and confirmed with CT imaging. Treatment parallels the Hinchey classification system. Current treatment guidelines have changed with improving understanding of the disease. Uncomplicated disease may be treated without antibiotics in appropriate circumstances. Indications for elective surgery have changed and minimally invasive approaches adopted. Complex presentations including recurrence, free perforation, fistula, and obstruction remain challenges for the surgeon to pick the right operation for the right patient at the right time. Scientific understanding of diverticular disease is progressing, but many questions remain about global variations of the disease, triggers for diverticulitis and its associated conditions, and decision aids to predict disease recurrence and establish best treatments.

ACKNOWLEDGMENT

We gratefully acknowledge the contributions of previous edition author, Lillias H. Maguire, as portions of that chapters have been retained in this revision.

References

1. Slack WW. The anatomy, pathology, and some clinical features of diverticulitis of the colon. *Br J Surg.* 1962;50(220):185–190.
2. Strate LL, Morris AM. Epidemiology, pathophysiology, and treatment of diverticulitis. *Gastroenterology.* 2019;156(5):1282–1298.e1.
3. Peery AF, Keku TO, Martin CF, et al. Distribution and characteristics of colonic diverticula in a United States screening population. *Clin Gastroenterol Hepatol.* 2016;14(7):980–985.
4. Bharucha AE, Parthasarathy G, Ditah I, et al. Temporal trends in the incidence and natural history of diverticulitis: A population-based study. *Am J Gastroenterol.* 2015;110(11):1589–1596.
5. Humphrey HN, Sibley P, Walker ET, et al. Genetic, epigenetic and environmental factors in diverticular disease: systematic review. *BJS Open.* 2024;8(3):zrae032.
6. Zheng NS, Ma W, Shung DL, Strate LL, Chan AT. Sex, race, and ethnicity differences in patients presenting with diverticular disease at Emergency Departments in the United States: A national cross-sectional study. *Gastro Hep Adv.* 2023;3(2):178–180.
7. Uwumiro FE, Olakunde T, Fagbenro A, et al. Trends in diverticular disease hospitalizations and racial disparities in outcomes across the United States. *Cureus.* 2024;16(7):e65572.
8. Peery AF, Shaukat A, Strate LL. AGA clinical practice update on medical management of colonic diverticulitis: Expert review. *Gastroenterology.* 2021;160(3):906–911.e1.
9. Almalki T, Garfinkle R, Kmiotek E, et al. Family history is associated with recurrent diverticulitis after an episode of diverticulitis managed nonoperatively. *Dis Colon Rectum.* 2020;63(7):944–954.
10. Ueland TE, Mosley JD, Neylan C, et al. Multiancestry transferability of a polygenic risk score for diverticulitis. *BMJ Open Gastroenterol.* 2024;11(1):e001474.
11. Broad JB, Wu Z, Clark TG, et al. Diverticulosis and nine connective tissue disorders: epidemiological support for an association. *Connect Tissue Res.* 2019;60(4):389–398.
12. Bassotti G, Battaglia E, Spinozzi F, Pelli MA, Tonini M. Twenty-four hour recordings of colonic motility in patients with diverticular disease: evidence for abnormal motility and propulsive activity. *Dis Colon Rectum.* 2001;44(12):1814–1820.

13. Painter NS, Burkitt DP. Diverticular disease of the colon: A deficiency disease of Western civilization. *Br Med J.* 1971;2(5759):450–454.
14. Hall J, Hardiman K, Lee S, et al; Prepared on behalf of the Clinical Practice Guidelines Committee of the American Society of Colon and Rectal Surgeons. The American Society of Colon and Rectal Surgeons Clinical Practice Guidelines for the treatment of left-sided colonic diverticulitis. *Dis Colon Rectum.* 2020;63(6):728–747.
15. Makki K, Deehan EC, Walter J, Bäckhed F. The impact of dietary fiber on gut microbiota in host health and disease. *Cell Host Microbe.* 2018;23(6):705–715.
16. Kodadek LM, Davis KA. Current diagnosis and management of acute colonic diverticulitis: What you need to know. *J Trauma Acute Care Surg.* 2024;97(1):1–10.
17. Williams S, Bjarnason I, Hayee B, Haji A. Diverticular disease: update on pathophysiology, classification and management. *Frontline Gastroenterol.* 2023;15(1):50–58.
18. Tiralongo F, Di Pietro S, Milazzo D, et al. Acute colonic diverticulitis: CT findings, classifications, and a proposal of a structured reporting template. *Diagnostics (Basel).* 2023;13(24):3628.
19. Schena CA, Covino M, Laterza V, et al. The role of procalcitonin as a risk stratification tool of severity, prognosis, and need for surgery in patients with acute left-sided colonic diverticulitis. *Surgery.* 2024;176(1):162–171.
20. Biondo S, Golda T, Kreisler E, et al. Outpatient versus hospitalization management for uncomplicated diverticulitis: a prospective, multicenter randomized clinical trial (DIVER Trial). *Ann Surg.* 2014;259(1):38–44.
21. Hawkins AT, Wise PE, Chan T, et al. Diverticulitis: an update from the age old paradigm. *Curr Probl Surg.* 2020;57(10):100862.
22. Isacson D, Smedh K, Kikberg M, Chabok A. Long-term follow-up of the AVOD randomized trial of antibiotic avoidance in uncomplicated diverticulitis. *Br J Surg.* 2019;106(11):1542–1548.
23. van Dijk ST, Daniels L, Ünlü C, et al. Long-term effects of omitting antibiotics in uncomplicated acute diverticulitis. *Am J Gastroenterol.* 2018;113(7):1045–1052.
24. Mora-López L, Ruiz-Edo N, Estrada-Ferrer O, et al; DINAMO-study Group. Efficacy and safety of nonantibiotic outpatient treatment in mild acute diverticulitis (DINAMO-study): A multicentre, randomised, open-label, noninferiority trial. *Ann Surg.* 2021;274(5):e435–e442.
25. Vaghiri S, David SO, Sultani AB, Safi SA, Knoefel WT, Prassas D. Clinical relevance of the 3-cm threshold in sigmoid diverticulitis with abscess: consensus or quandary? *Int J Colorectal Dis.* 2024;39(1):106.
26. Oberkofler CE, Rickenbacher A, Raptis DA, et al. A multicenter randomized clinical trial of primary anastomosis or Hartmann's procedure for perforated left colonic diverticulitis with purulent or fecal peritonitis. *Ann Surg.* 2012;256(5):819–826.
27. Loire M, Bridoux V, Mege D, et al. Long-term outcomes of Hartmann's procedure versus primary anastomosis for generalized peritonitis due to perforated diverticulitis: follow-up of a prospective multicenter randomized trial (DIVERTI). *Int J Colorectal Dis.* 2021;36(10):2159–2164.
28. Lambrichts DPV, Vennix S, Musters GD, et al; LADIES trial collaborators. Hartmann's procedure versus sigmoidectomy with primary anastomosis for perforated diverticulitis with purulent or faecal peritonitis (LADIES): a multicentre, parallel-group, randomised, open-label, superiority trial. *Lancet Gastroenterol Hepatol.* 2019;4(8): 599–610.
29. Pinson J, Tuech JJ, Ouaissi M, et al. Role of protective stoma after primary anastomosis for generalized peritonitis due to perforated diverticulitis-DIVERTI 2 (a prospective multicenter randomized trial): rationale and design (NCT04604730). *BMC Surg.* 2022;22(1):191.
30. Cho NY, Le NK, Kim S, et al. Trends in the adoption of diverting loop ileostomy for acute complicated diverticulitis in the United States. *Surgery.* 2024;176(1):38–43.
31. Hoek VT, Edomskis PP, Stark PW, et al. Laparoscopic peritoneal lavage versus sigmoidectomy for perforated diverticulitis with purulent peritonitis: three-year follow-up of the randomised LOLA trial. *Surg Endosc.* 2022;36(10):7764–7774.
32. Azhar N, Johanssen A, Sundström T, et al; SCANDIV Study Group. Laparoscopic lavage vs primary resection for acute perforated diverticulitis: Long-term outcomes from the Scandinavian Diverticulitis (SCANDIV) Randomized Clinical Trial. *JAMA Surg.* 2021;156(2):121–127.
33. Kohl A, Rosenberg J, Bock D, et al. Two-year results of the randomized clinical trial DILALA comparing laparoscopic lavage with resection as treatment for perforated diverticulitis. *Br J Surg.* 2018;105(9):1128–1134.
34. Kollatos C, Sköldberg F, Graf W. Evaluation of laparoscopic peritoneal lavage for perforated diverticulitis: a national registry-based study. *Br J Surg.* 2024;111(5):znae109.
35. Hawkins AT, Fa A, Younan SA, et al. Decision aid for colectomy in recurrent diverticulitis: Development and usability study. *JMIR Form Res.* 2024;8:e59952.
36. Bolkenstein HE, Consten ECJ, van der Palen J, et al; Dutch Diverticular Disease (3D) Collaborative Study Group. Long-term outcome of surgery versus conservative management for recurrent and ongoing complaints after an episode of diverticulitis: 5-year follow-up results of a multicenter randomized controlled trial (DIRECT-Trial). *Ann Surg.* 2019;269(4):612–620.
37. Santos A, Mentula P, Pinta T, et al. Quality-of-life and recurrence outcomes following laparoscopic elective sigmoid resection vs conservative treatment following diverticulitis: prespecified 2-year analysis of the LASER randomized clinical trial. *JAMA Surg.* 2023;158(6):593–601.
38. https://www.clinicaltrials.gov/study/NCT04095663 accessed November 10, 2024.
39. Papageorge CM, Kennedy GD, Carchman EH. National trends in short-term outcomes following non-emergent surgery for diverticular disease. *J Gastrointest Surg.* 2016;20(7):1376–1387.
40. Larkins K, Mohan H, Apte SS, et al. A systematic review and meta-analysis of robotic resections for diverticular disease. *Colorectal Dis.* 2022;24(10):1105–1116.
41. Mari G, Montroni I, Origi M, et al. Functional and short-term outcomes in elective laparoscopic colectomy for symptomatic diverticular disease with either low ligation or inferior mesenteric artery preservation: A randomized trial. *Surg Laparosc Endosc Percutan Tech.* 2020;31(1):40–43.
42. Walayat S, Johannes AJ, Benson M, et al. Outcomes of colon self-expandable metal stents for malignant vs benign indications at a tertiary care center and review of literature. *World J Gastrointest Endosc.* 2023;15(4):309–318.
43. Holland C, Vabi BW, Sheny PP, et al. Removal of indwelling urinary catheter two days after colovesical fistula repair: A single-arm prospective trial. *J Gastrointest Surg.* 2022;26(12):2597–2599.
44. Sbarigia C, Ritieni C, Annibale B, Carabotti M. Common diagnostic challenges and pitfalls in segmental colitis associated with diverticulosis (SCAD). *J Clin Med.* 2023;12(18):6084.
45. Calini G, Abd El Aziz MA, Paolini L, et al. Symptomatic Uncomplicated Diverticular Disease (SUDD): Practical guidance and challenges for clinical management. *Clin Exp Gastroenterol.* 2023;16:29–43.
46. Bachelani AM. Natural history and surgical treatment of a giant colonic diverticulum: A case report. *World J Clin Cases.* 2024;12(17): 3151–3155.
47. Lee YF, Tang DD, patel SH, Battaglia MA, Shanker BA, Cleary RK. Recurrence of acute right colon diverticulitis following nonoperative management: A systematic review and meta-analysis. *Dis Colon Rectum.* 2020;63(10):1466–1473.
48. Jensen DM. Endoscopic diagnosis and treatment of colonic diverticular bleeding. *Gastrointest Endosc Clin N Am.* 2024;34(2): 345–361.
49. Vajravelu RK, Mamtani R, Scott FI, Waxman A, Lewis JD. Incidence, risk factors, and clinical effects of recurrent diverticular hemorrhage: a large cohort study. *Gastroenterology.* 2018;155(5): 1416–1427.

67

Anorectal Disorders

Amy L. Halverson

Key Points

1. The most common manifestation of internal hemorrhoids is painless, bright red rectal bleeding associated with bowel movements. A high-fiber diet supplemented with bulk-forming agents may reduce symptoms of hemorrhoids and is ideal for first- and second-degree hemorrhoids.
2. Rubber band ligation is suitable for symptomatic first- and second- and some third-degree internal hemorrhoids that do not respond to bulk-forming agents. Hemorrhoidectomy is required in only a few patients with symptomatic hemorrhoids.
3. Anal fissure is an ischemic ulcer in the lower portion of the anal canal. Treatment, both medical and surgical, involves relaxing the internal anal sphincter.
4. The basic principles of anal fistula treatment are to limit the access fecal contents into the tract while preserving the anal sphincter.
5. Pilonidal disease results from hair in the subcutaneous tissue as the nidus for a chronic foreign-body reaction. Treatment aims to remove the offending tuft of hair.
6. Rectal prolapse results from intussusception that extends beyond the anal verge. Fit patients are best treated with transabdominal rectopexy. A perineal approach is an option for individuals who are considered too high risk for general anesthesia.
7. Surveillance and treatment of high-grade dysplasia can decrease progression to invasive anal cancer in high-risk individuals.
8. Palpable lesions of the anal canal are not hemorrhoids and may be cancers; examination under anesthesia and biopsy allow for correct diagnosis.

ANATOMY AND PHYSIOLOGY

The rectum descends along the curvature of the sacrum and passes through the levator ani muscles, where it becomes the anal canal (**Fig. 67.1**). The anal canal is the terminal portion of the intestinal tract (**Fig. 67.2**). It continues from the rectum 3 to 5 cm through the pelvic floor musculature to the hair-bearing skin of the anal margin. Understanding the various types of anal epithelium is important for diagnosis of both benign and malignant conditions. The rectum is lined with columnar epithelium which transitions to squamous epithelium at the dentate line. The endoderm in the first 1 to 2 cm proximal to the dentate line is called the transition zone and represents a gradual change from squamous epithelium to the columnar epithelium lining the rectum. The dentate line represents the true division between embryonic endoderm and ectoderm. Distal to the dentate line, the anal canal is lined with anoderm,

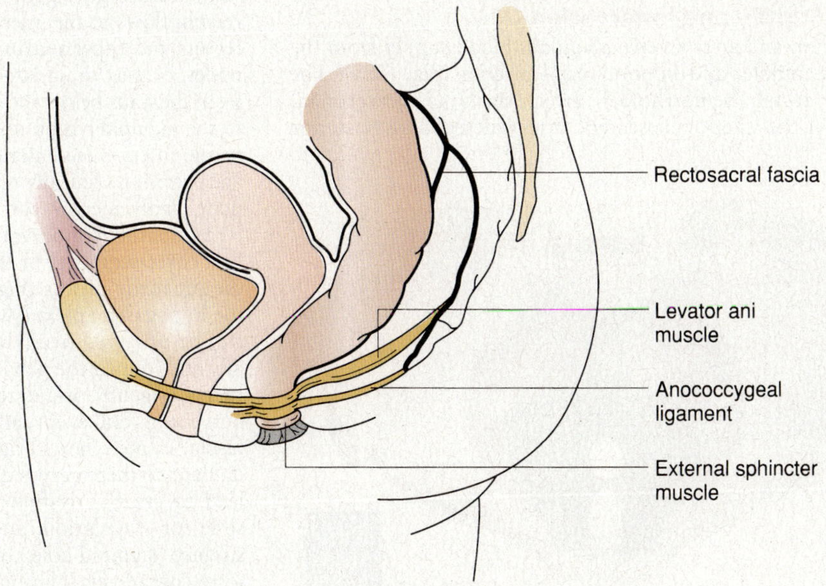

Figure 67.1. Pelvic anatomy.

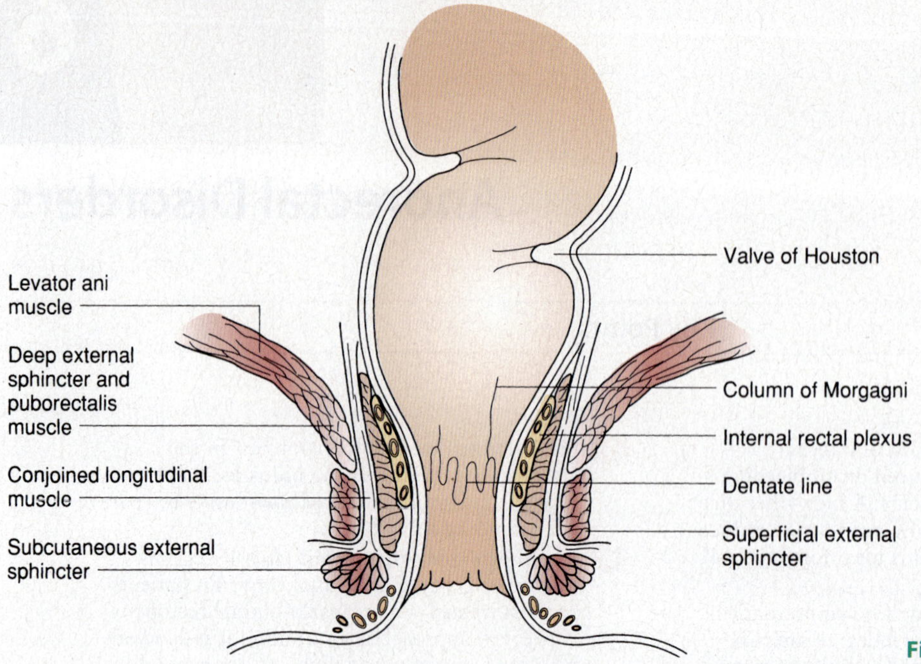

Figure 67.2. Anatomy of the anal canal.

a squamous epithelium without hair. The anoderm transitions to skin at the anal verge. Folds of tissue at the dentate line form anal papillae. Between the papillae lie the anal crypts, which house the anal glands. These structures are important because anal abscesses and fistula may originate from these glands.

The muscularis propria of the rectum continues distally to form a ring of smooth muscle around the anal canal, the internal anal sphincter. The pelvic floor is composed of the levator ani muscle (which has three parts: puborectalis, pubococygeus, and ileococcygeous) and external anal sphincter. These muscles and their connections are responsible for both continence and defecation. The puborectalis muscle forms a sling that extends from the posterior pubis around the rectum and maintains an acute angle at the anorectal junction, which serves as an importance continence mechanism (**Fig. 67.3**). The external anal sphincter is a striated muscle that surrounds the internal anal sphincter. It is contiguous with the levator ani and attaches to the coccyx with the anococcygeal ligament. The configuration of the muscles and ligaments results in several distinct spaces (**Fig. 67.4**).

Blood Supply and Innervation

The rectum and anus receive abundant blood supply from the superior, middle, and inferior rectal arteries (**Fig. 67.5**). The superior rectal (hemorrhoidal) artery starts as the terminal branch of the inferior mesenteric artery, descending posterior

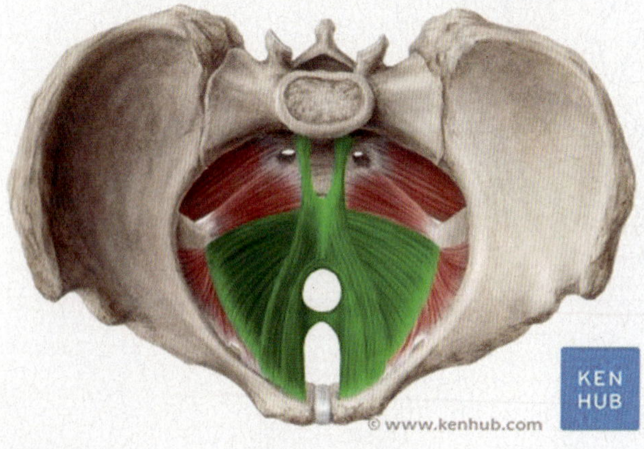

Figure 67.3. Muscles of the pelvic floor.

to the rectum where it bifurcates to supply the rectum and upper anal canal. The middle rectal arteries (present as a distinct vessel in <15% of people) arise from the internal pudendal or inferior gluteal arteries (branches of the internal iliac artery). The inferior rectal arteries also arise from the internal pudendal arteries to supply the anal sphincters and anal canal. The venous drainage of the anus is via both the portal and systemic venous systems. The superior rectal vein drains the rectum and upper anal canal into the portal venous system through the inferior mesenteric vein. The middle and inferior rectal veins drain into the systemic venous system via the internal iliac veins (**Fig. 67.6**). Because of the rich communication between these veins, patients with portal hypertension may develop portosystemic shunts resulting in bleeding rectal varices. Hemorrhoids are submucosal sinusoids that contain both arterial (typically terminal branches of superior hemorrhoidal artery) and venous (usually superior, middle, and inferior hemorrhoidal veins) supply. Sinusoids differ from veins in that histologically the walls of these vascular structures do not contain muscles.

Lymphatic drainage of the rectum and anus mirrors the venous drainage (**Fig. 67.7**). Drainage from the upper and middle rectum flows to the inferior mesenteric lymph nodes. The lower rectum and upper anal canal may drain to the inferior mesenteric nodes, or may drain laterally to the internal iliac nodes. Lymph from the anus below the level of the dentate line typically drains to the inguinal lymph nodes; however, drainage may also occur to the inferior mesenteric and internal iliac nodes. This drainage pattern is clinically relevant when identifying regional lymph node involvement in patients with distal rectal or anal cancer.

Sympathetic innervation of the rectum originates from the first three segments of the lumbar spinal cord and synapse at the preaortic plexus (**Fig. 67.8**). The nerves bifurcate to form the hypogastric plexus which, during a low anterior resection, can be observed overlying the sacrum before extending laterally and joining the pelvic plexus. Parasympathetic innervation (nervi erigenti) originates from the 2nd, 3rd, and 4th sacral nerve roots and eventually extends medially along Denonvillier fascia. In men, nervi erigenti are responsible for erection, and damage to these nerves during rectal or prostate surgery would lead to erectile dysfunction. Sympathetic nerves are responsible for ejaculation, and damage to these structures during surgery (sigmoid colectomy or anterior resection) would lead to retrograde ejaculation. Injury to the pelvic nerves may also lead to bladder dysfunction. In women, dysfunction following nerve injury is less well understood; however, some patients

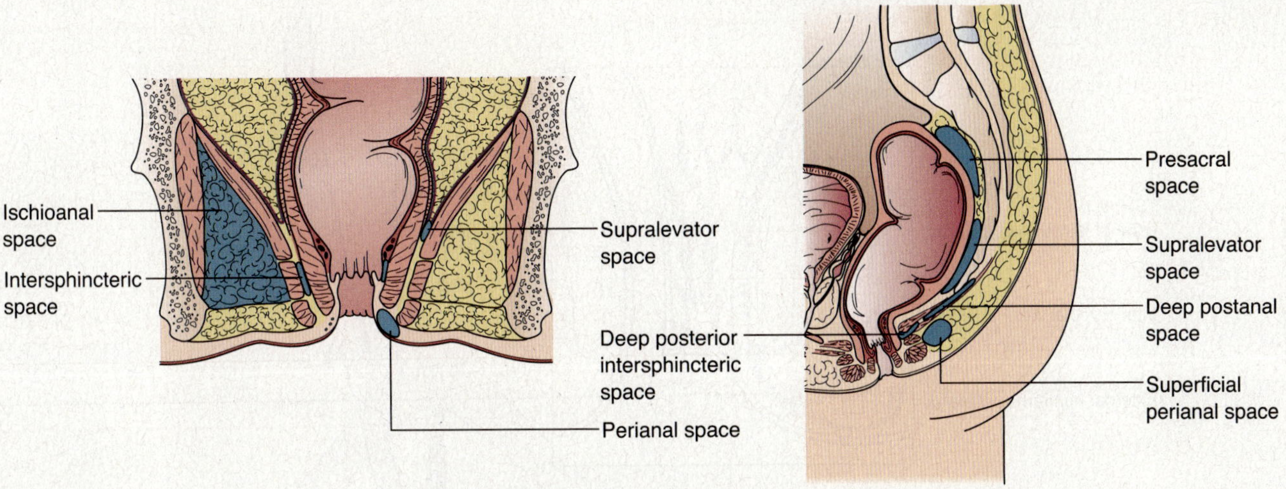

Figure 67.4. Anorectal spaces.

do report dyspareunia and decreased lubrication during intercourse following pelvic surgery.[1,2]

The internal anal sphincter receives both sympathetic and parasympathetic innervation and maintains tonic contraction at rest. The external anal sphincter is innervated by the inferior rectal branch of the pudendal nerve and perineal branch of the 4th sacral nerve. The inferior rectal nerve also carries sensory information from the anal canal. The majority of sensory nerve endings within the anal canal are located distal to the dentate line, making the anoderm exquisitely sensitive. This has clinical implications in diagnosing pathology and counseling patients regarding pain during and after anorectal procedures.

Physiology

The main function of the rectum is to serve as a distensible reservoir for stool. The principal function of the anus and pelvic floor is the maintenance of continence and regulation

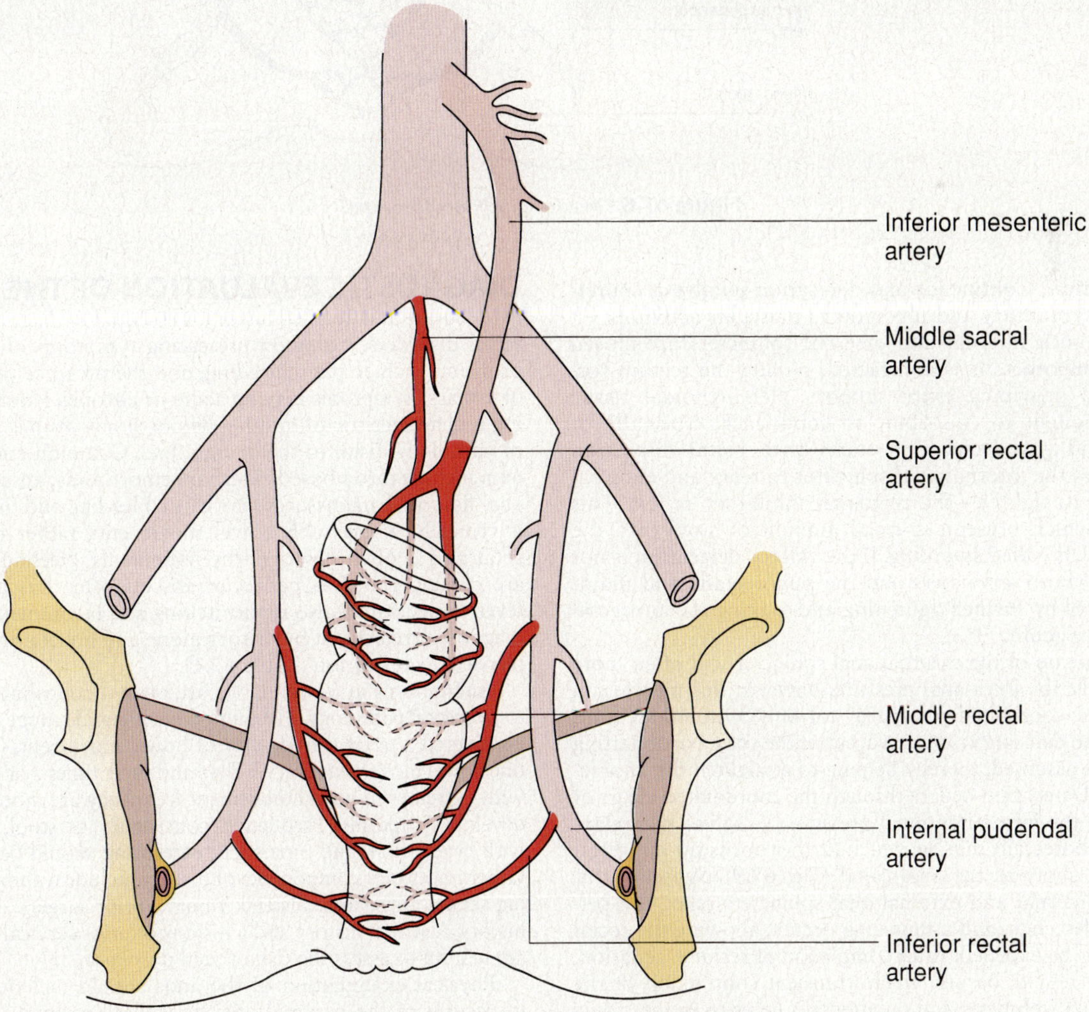

Figure 67.5. Arterial supply of the rectum.

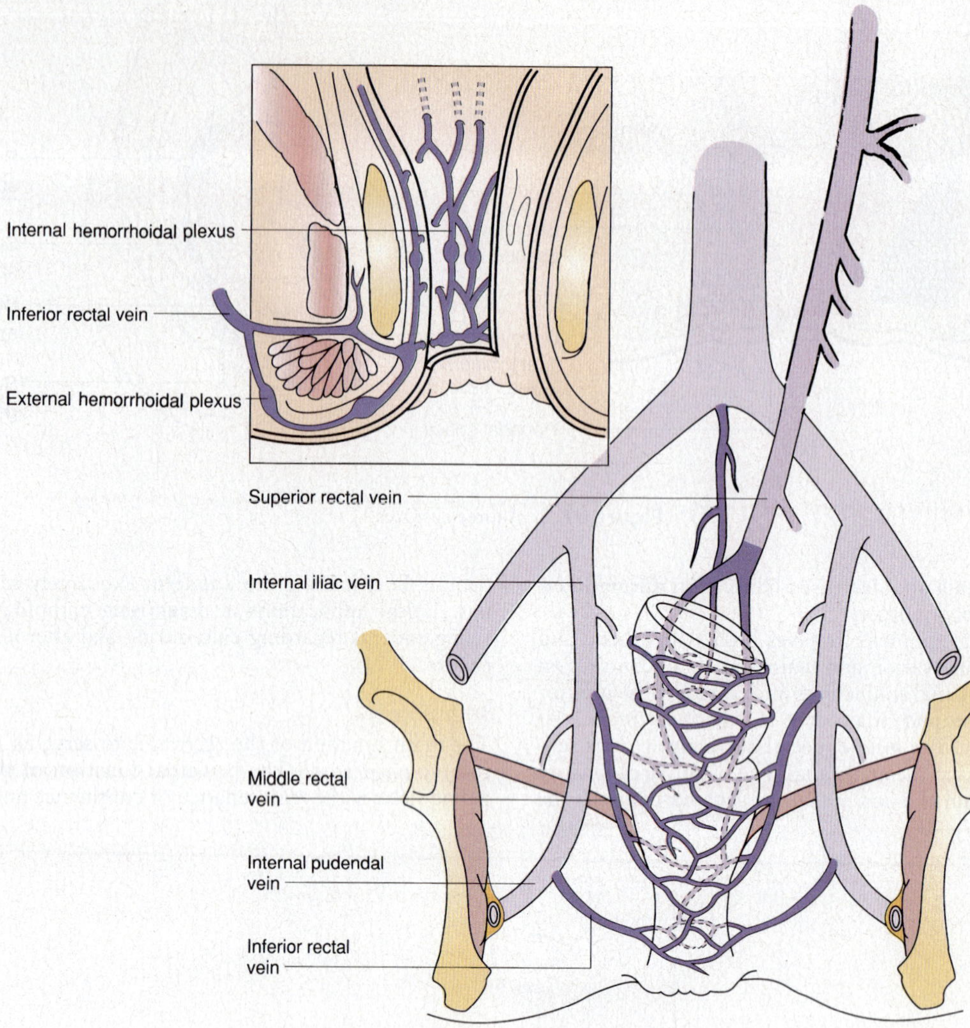

Figure 67.6. Venous supply of the rectum.

of defecation. Continence and defecation involve a combination of voluntary and involuntary muscular activities. At baseline, both internal and external sphincters are closed and the puborectalis is contracted, pulling the rectum forward and providing extra support. Hemorrhoidal tissue is also thought to contribute to continence, especially of mucus and gas. Defecation starts with rectal distention that causes the internal anal sphincter to relax and external sphincter to tighten—the rectoanal inhibitory reflex. This process, which presents a small amount of stool into the anal canal, is called *sampling*. If the call for defecation is not answered, both sphincters and the puborectalis will maintain control by further tightening and making the anorectal angle more acute.

Contraction of the external anal sphincter will often more than double the intra-anal pressure; however, this muscle can typically be contracted voluntarily for only 30 to 60 seconds. If the call to defecate is answered, either the sitting or squatting position is assumed, thereby helping to straighten the anorectal angle. Defecation occurs through the coordinated effort of increasing the intra-abdominal pressure (Valsalva) and relaxing the puborectalis muscle, which further opens the anorectal angle and shortens the anal canal (**Fig. 67.9**). Subsequently, both the internal and external anal sphincters relax, the pelvic floor descends, and a funneling occurs, allowing the rectal contents to be expelled. After completion of rectal evacuation, a "closing reflex" occurs, where transient contraction of the external anal sphincter and puborectalis helps to restore tonic contracture of the internal anal sphincter.

DIAGNOSTIC EVALUATION OF THE ANUS

An accurate and detailed history is essential to diagnosing anorectal disorders. Common presenting symptoms of anorectal problems include pain, bleeding, and the presence of prolapse or a mass. Symptoms may be acute or chronic. Painless bleeding is characteristic of internal hemorrhoids. Pain is indicative of pathology distal to the dentate line. Common etiologies of pain include thrombosed external hemorrhoids, abscesses, and anal fissures. Anal fissures may cause bleeding and fissure pain is typically worse with bowel movements rather than constant and is often described by patients as, "feeling like they are passing glass." A perirectal abscess often has associated fever. Patients may also report itching and incontinence. Many diagnoses are evident by history alone and are confirmed with physical examination (**Table 67.1**).

Alternations in bowel habits are often a contributing factor to anorectal pathology. Although there is a wide range of what is considered a normal frequency of bowel movements—between one bowel movement every 3 days and three times a day, patients with extremes in bowel movement frequency are more likely to develop symptoms. Frequency, consistency of stool, straining with evacuation, and time spent defecating should be assessed. Other important components of history include trauma (including sexual abuse and obstetric injury), prior surgery, and travel history. A sexual history and a history of prior cervical dysplasia are helpful to assess the risk of anal dysplasia.

Physical examination of the anus should include a visual inspection of the perianal area as well as a digital examination (**Table 67.2**). Patients may be examined in either the

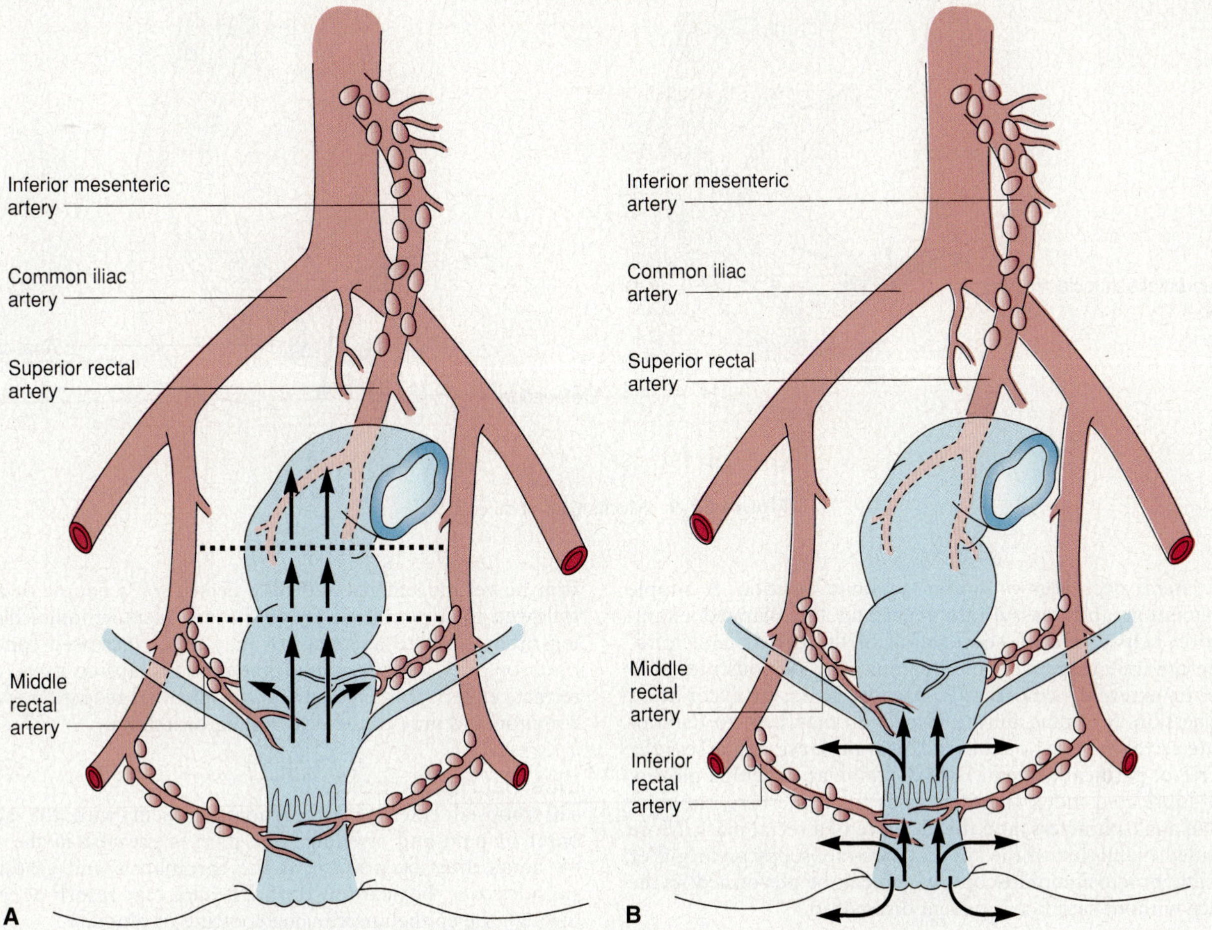

Figure 67.7. A: Lymphatic drainage of the rectum. B: Lymphatic drainage of the anal canal.

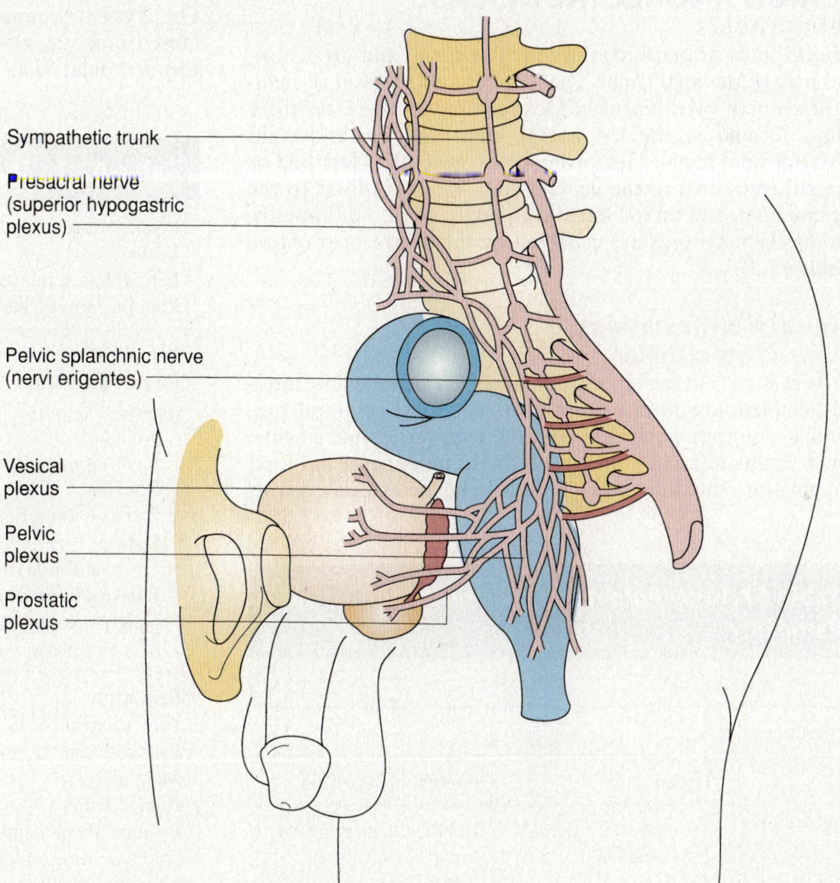

Figure 67.8. Innervation of the rectum.

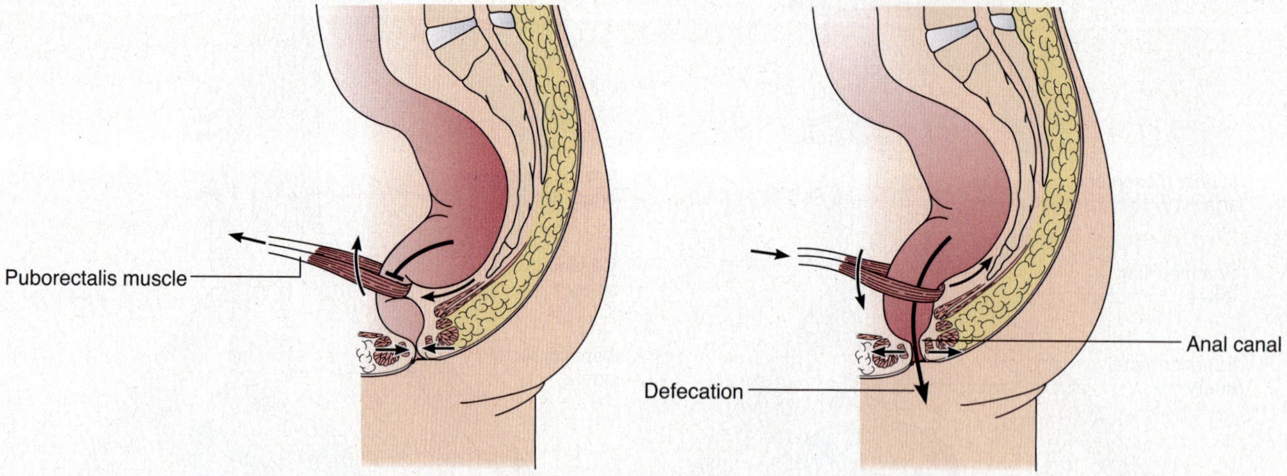

Figure 67.9. Mechanism of defecation.

left lateral decubitus or prone jackknife position. A simple explanation and reassurance regarding the planned examination help to ensure cooperation of the patient and minimize anxiety. Inspection of the anus may demonstrate skin tags or external hemorrhoids, fissures, scars, or excoriation of the skin. Straining during inspection may help to demonstrate rectal mucosal or full-thickness prolapse and assess the degree of perineal descent. Digital examination with a gloved, well-lubricated index finger assesses for tenderness, the tone of the anal sphincters, and the presence of a rectal mass. More detailed evaluation of the anus includes anoscopy and rigid or flexible proctosigmoidoscopy, which can be performed in the office without significant patient discomfort.

BENIGN ANORECTAL DISEASE

1 Hemorrhoids

Hemorrhoids are cushions of vascular tissue and are a normal part of the anal canal. The number and location of hemorrhoids may vary, however. Most commonly there are three pillars located in the left lateral, right anterior, and right posterior anal canal. Hemorrhoids are generally classified as internal (proximal to the dentate line), external (distal to the dentate line), and mixed (most commonly seen). Additionally, internal hemorrhoids are classified by the degree of prolapse (**Table 67.3**).

Clinical Manifestations

Internal Hemorrhoids

As there is no somatic innervation above the dentate line, internal hemorrhoids do not cause pain. The most common presenting symptom is painless bleeding with bowel movements, which can manifest as either blood on the toilet paper to blood dripping into the toilet bowl. Bleeding may be associated with firm bowel movements and may persist for a couple of days followed by a period of no symptoms. Hemorrhoidal bleeding rarely leads to anemia, but may be of increased concern in chronically anticoagulated patients. Prolapsing tissue that retracts either spontaneously or with manual reduction is also common and may cause fecal soiling or itching.

External Hemorrhoids

Thrombosed external hemorrhoids present with the acute onset of pain and swelling. The pain is greatest in the first 48 hours after occurrence of the thrombosis and gradually subsides over the next few days. The clot may resorb or erode through the epithelium causing spotting of blood.

Evaluation

On physical examination hemorrhoids may present with prolapsed mucosa, as edematous external tags or soft, residual hemorrhoidal skin tags. Thrombosed external hemorrhoids

Table 67.1. Symptoms of Common Benign Pathology

	Pain	
Bleeding	+	–
+	Fissure	Internal hemorrhoid
–	Thrombosed external hemorrhoid Abscess	Residual hemorrhoidal tag Condyloma

Table 67.2. The Complete Rectal Examination

Preparation
Enema
Left lateral decubitus or prone jackknife position
Lighting, gloves, lubrication, anoscope
Visualization
Retract the buttocks
Inspect for:
Soiling
Excoriation or abrasion
Scarring
Patulous anus, deformity or flattening of folds
Fissure
External fistula opening
External hemorrhoids
Condyloma lesion
Mucosal prolapse
Palpation
Slow insertion of lubricated, gloved finger
Pain with digital examination
Mass
Anal stricture
Prostate abnormalities (men) or anterior rectocele (women)
Sphincter tone at rest and voluntary squeeze
Puborectalis relaxation with strain

Table 67.3. Hemorrhoid Classification

Degree	Description
First	Hemorrhoids bleed but do not prolapse
Second	Hemorrhoids prolapse on straining and reduce spontaneously
Third	Hemorrhoids prolapse on straining and require manual reduction
Fourth	Prolapsed hemorrhoids cannot be manually reduced

appear as tender, firm, and often bluish masses. Having patients strain may be useful to demonstrate hemorrhoid prolapse. Digital exam allows for assessment of sphincters (important to document if surgery is considered at some point) and masses. Anoscopy is used to inspect internal hemorrhoids and assess the appropriateness of office-based treatment. Colonoscopy should be performed when patients have bleeding that is not consistent with physical exam findings, or when symptoms do not respond to initial treatment. Hematochezia is a common presenting symptom of other disorders including colitis, diverticulosis, and cancer.

Treatment

Treatment should be tailored to the patient's symptoms, which may not correlate with physical exam findings. One should clarify the patient's goals in seeking treatment. Patients may only want evaluation and reassurance that their condition is benign. Treatment of internal hemorrhoidal bleeding may not satisfy patients who are bothered by residual hemorrhoidal tags. Treatment options include nonoperative measures alone, office-based procedures, or operative procedures.

Nonoperative Management

Excessive straining during defecation or prolonged sitting on the toilet, for example, while reading, contribute to hemorrhoidal problems. Symptoms can be reduced or eliminated in many patients by altering their dietary intake and bowel habits. Increasing fiber and fluid intake eliminates a large proportion of problems with grade I and II hemorrhoids and can significantly improve symptoms with higher-grade hemorrhoids. Fiber can be either dietary or supplemental and works by increasing bulk and moisture in the stool. Various suppositories and topical medications may provide symptomatic relief. Long-term use of medications containing steroids, analgesics, and emollients can cause allergic reactions or sensitization. Sitz baths soothe symptoms, but do not address the underlying cause of the problem. However, in patients with external hemorrhoid problems, using water for cleaning can be a useful adjunct to improving itching and avoiding overcleaning.

2 Office-Based Treatments

Office-based procedures include rubber band ligation, infrared coagulation, and sclerotherapy. These procedures are quick and usually painless alternatives to surgery.

Rubber band ligation can be performed through an anoscope in the office without the use of anesthesia. It is important to clarify expected outcomes to the patient: rubber band ligation does not address external hemorrhoidal tags and may require more than one treatment to achieve adequate symptom improvement. The band is placed around the hemorrhoid 2 to 3 cm above the dentate line, causing localized ischemia of the intervening tissue. Placement of the band too close to the dentate line will result in intolerable pain (**Fig. 67.10**). Placing more than two bands at once may increase discomfort and

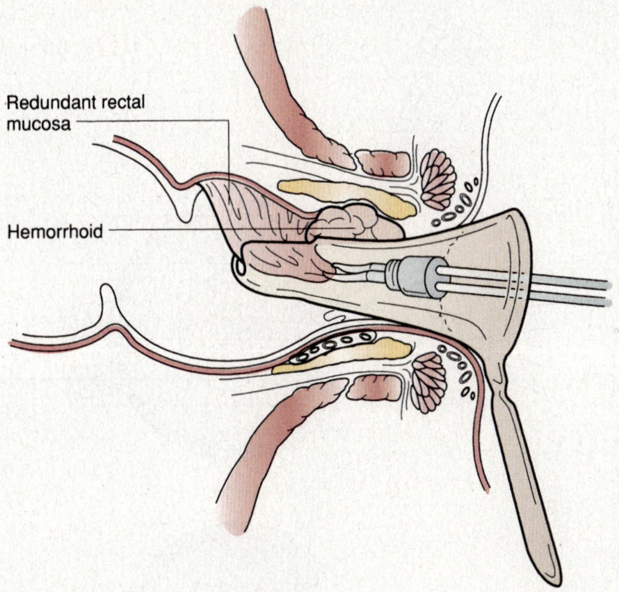

Figure 67.10. Rubber band ligation.

is generally not recommended. Approximately 1 to 2 weeks after rubber band placement, the hemorrhoid tissue will slough, and the patient may experience spotting of blood. Fibrosis that occurs at the site of the banding causes fixation of the remaining hemorrhoidal tissue, which helps to prevent further prolapse and bleeding. Improvement or resolution of symptoms may be achieved in more than 80% of individuals.[3] Complications are rare and include pain and thrombosis. Significant bleeding requiring urgent intervention may occur following <1% of procedures. Rare cases of pelvic sepsis have been reported.

Sclerotherapy involves the injection of a sclerosing agent (such as 5% phenol solution) into the submucosa that leads to fibrosis of the surrounding tissue. Injection is performed through an anoscope, and may be an option for symptomatic hemorrhoids that are too small to band. Recent studies evaluating pilodocanol foam sclerotherapy (PFS) have shown outcomes comparable to rubber band ligation. Infrared coagulation uses infrared energy applied to the hemorrhoid tissue that causes tissue necrosis and subsequent scarring to decrease bleeding and prolapse.

Operative Treatment

Excisional hemorrhoidectomy is the most definitive treatment for hemorrhoid-related symptoms and is indicated in patients who fail conservative or office-based procedures. Hemorrhoidectomy is typically an outpatient procedure, and in most cases performed under monitored anesthesia care (MAC) and local or regional (spinal) anesthesia. The patient is placed in the prone jackknife position with the buttocks taped apart. Initial ligation of the apex of the hemorrhoidal tissue helps to decrease bleeding during dissection. The skin is incised at the distal extent of the hemorrhoid and the hemorrhoidal tissue is carefully separated off of the underlying internal sphincter. The dissection may be undertaken with the use of a scalpel, scissors, electrocautery, or controlled electrical energy such as ultrasonic shears or a bipolar vessel sealing device (**Fig. 67.11**). Vessel sealing devices should be used with caution so as to not excise too much tissue. It is critical to preserve the underlying internal anal sphincter muscle. The wound may be left open or closed with absorbable suture. When closing the mucosa and anoderm, the dentate line should be reapproximated to avoid mucosal ectropion. Additionally, limiting intravenous fluids to <700 cc may help to decrease postoperative urinary retention, which occurs after approximately 15% of procedures.[4] Excisional hemorrhoidectomy is superior to office-based therapies

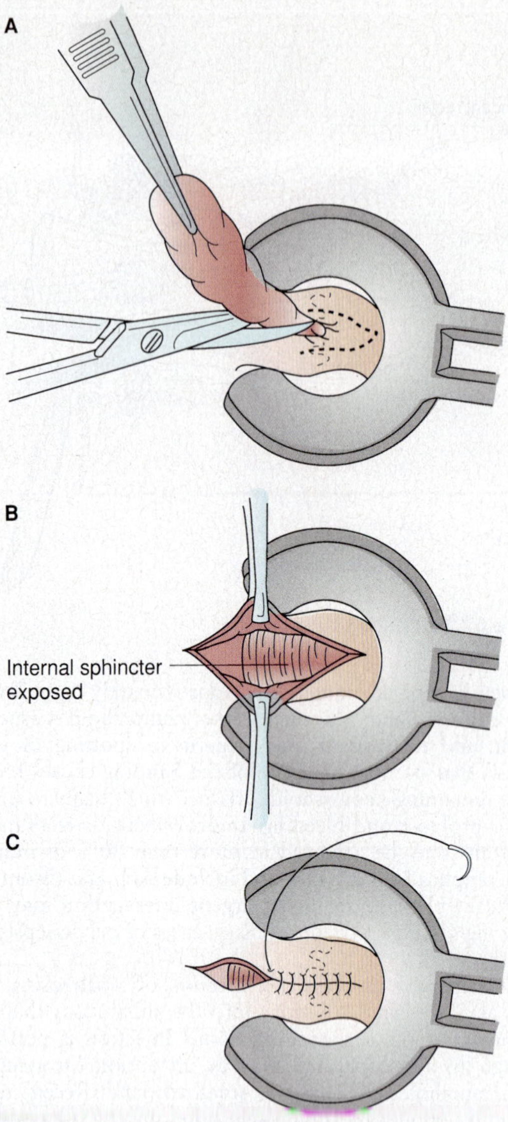

Figure 67.11. Technique of closed hemorrhoidectomy.

in achieving complete remission; however, is associated with significant postoperative pain. Multimodal analgesia including acetaminophen, NSAIDs, tramadol, and gabapentin helps to minimize opiate use.

Thrombosed External Hemorrhoids

Thrombosed external hemorrhoids are a relatively common complication of hemorrhoidal disease. The exact etiology is unknown; however, their occurrence is often associated with physical exertion or straining as well as diarrhea. Patients typically present with a painful, tender mass in the perianal area. Pain peaks at 48 to 72 hours and subsides over 3 to 5 days. This condition is self-limited and will resolve over a few weeks without lingering symptoms, although some patients will have residual skin tags. Treatment options include nonoperative therapy with analgesia and stool softeners. Incision and thrombectomy may be performed in the office with a local anesthetic. After administration of local anesthetic (typically lidocaine with epinephrine), an incision is made in the anoderm overlying the thrombus and the clot is evacuated with gentle pressure.[5,6]

Anal Fissure

An anal fissure is a linear tear in the anoderm of the distal anal canal. Although more commonly found in younger patients, fissures can occur at any age and equally afflict male and females. Fissures can be classified as acute (present for <6 weeks) or chronic based on the duration of symptoms Fissures occur most commonly in the posterior midline and less frequently in the anterior midline. Lateral fissures are less common and should alert the clinician to the possibility of infection, HIV, Crohn disease, or malignancy. Fissures may occur with trauma from passing hard stool or from diarrhea. Hypertonicity of the underlying internal sphincter muscle is thought to contribute to localized ischemia, thereby inhibiting wound healing.

Clinical Manifestations

Anal fissures typically present with sharp pain during defecation, often described as feeling like, "passing glass." Some individuals experience a persistent throbbing pain lasting from minutes to hours after defecation. Rectal bleeding is typically minimal and limited to spotting on toilet paper.

Patients with an acute fissure will not tolerate a rectal exam. Gently retracting the buttocks may allow visualization of the distal aspect of the fissure, often with an associated anal skin tag. Fibers of the internal anal sphincter can often be seen at the base of the chronic fissure. If there is a concern for other issues, the patient should be taken to the operating room to be examined under anesthesia or return to clinic within 6 to 8 weeks after treatment is initiated to allow for a more thorough exam. Some patients will have superficial fissuring on the perianal skin, often accompanied with itching after bowel movement. These fissures associated with perianal irritation/dermatitis are more distal, superficial, and often multiple.

3 Management

Medical Management

Treatment of anal fissures concentrates on symptom relief. The presence of a fissure without any symptoms (once other causes have been ruled out) is not an indication for treatment. Most patients will experience improvement or complete disappearance of symptoms with a bowel management program consisting of increased dietary fiber, oral liquid intake, and stool softeners. Topical application of 0.2% to 1% nitroglycerin ointment or a calcium channel blockers, such as 2% nifedipine or diltiazem, can also facilitate healing fissures. All formulations are applied superficially and have similar success rates of 50% to 60%. An adverse side effect of headache is reported by nearly 30% of individuals treated with topical nitroglycerine.[7]

Botulinum Toxin injection

Injection of endopeptidase blocks acetylcholine release thus causing temporary paralysis of the muscle. Effects last for up to 3 months. Technique, dose, and success rate vary widely in the literature. Generally, 100 units of botulinum toxin are injected directly into the internal sphincter in four to five aliquots. Recent studies show similar effectiveness between botox and topical nitrates.[8] Treatment with botox may result in short-term incontinence to gas or rarely infection from the injection itself. No significant long-term complications have been reported. This can be a good option for patients with continence problems, when use of a more definitive procedure is associated with higher chance of complications. Although this can be done in the office, if the patient cannot tolerate anoscopy and diagnosis is uncertain, then anoscopy with sedation should be undertaken.

Surgical Management

Lateral internal sphincterotomy is considered the gold standard for treatment of anal fissures and has a 98% success rate. This is an outpatient procedure associated with only minimal postoperative discomfort. It can be performed in open fashion by incising the anoderm overlying the internal sphincter and sharply dividing the internal sphincter muscle extending cephalad with electrocautery under direct vision. In the closed technique, a scalpel is inserted in the intersphincteric groove, turned toward the anal canal, and a portion of the muscle is

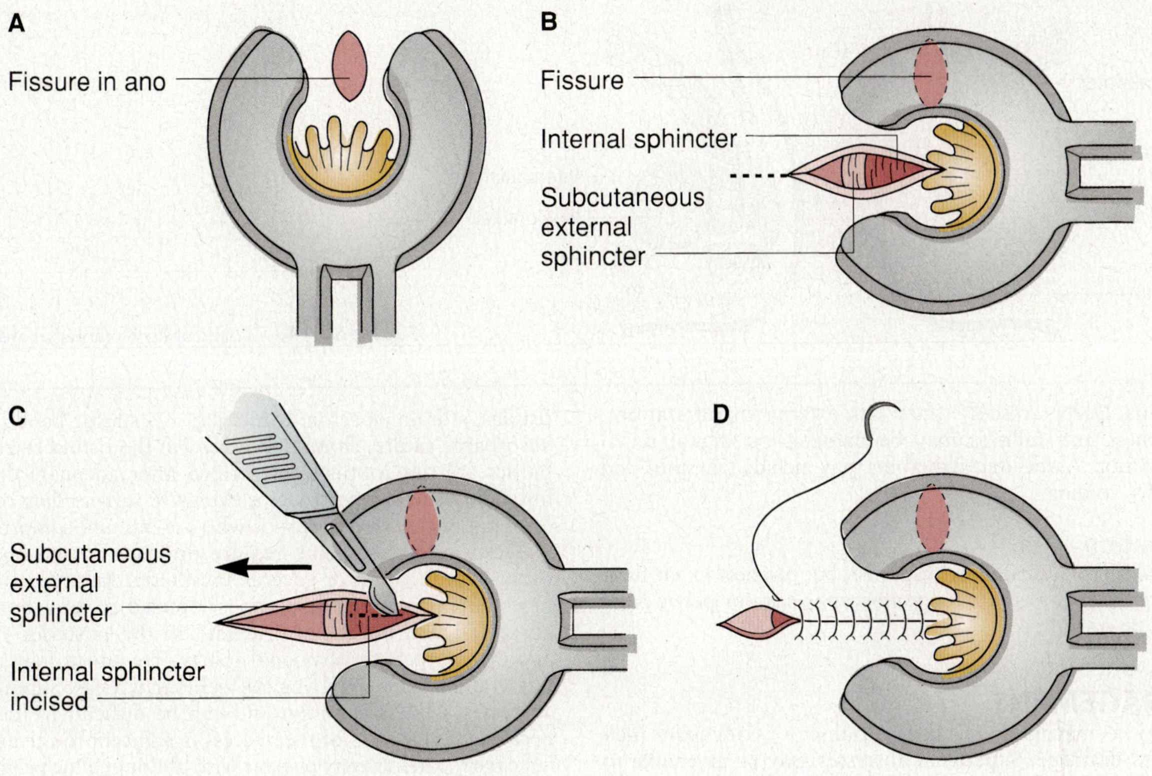

Figure 67.12. Technique of lateral internal sphincterotomy.

divided toward, but not including the anoderm. With both approaches, a divot in the internal sphincter should be easily palpated afterward. The defect in the perianal skin is closed with absorbable suture (**Fig. 67.12**). The amount of sphincter muscle divided should be limited to the length of the fissure (tailored sphincterotomy). This decreases the chance of incontinence afterward without significantly compromising the success rate. Recent reported incontinence rates following sphincterotomy are range from 2% to 17%.[9] This procedure should not be offered to patients with baseline continence problems. Sphincterotomy should not be performed in the anterior or posterior midline since this can result in a keyhole deformity leading to leakage of mucus and stool. If sphincterotomy is not successful, one may proceed with a repeat lateral sphincterotomy on the opposite side. In patients with resistant fissures or continence problems, advancement flaps such as house or V–Y flaps can be performed alone or in conjunction with sphincterotomy. Healing rates following sphincterotomy combined with advancement flap have been reported to be comparable to those following sphincterotomy with lower rates of incontinence.[10]

Anorectal Abscess

Anorectal abscesses typically occur as a result from infection of the glands that empty into the anal crypts, located between anal papilla at the dentate line. The crypts may extend into the perianal tissue. These glands can become clogged resulting in an abscess. The infection originates within the anal space and may extend to other perianal spaces (**Figs. 67.13** and **67.14**).

Clinical Manifestations

Abscesses present with acute onset of perianal pain, often accompanied by fever. Superficial perianal or ischiorectal abscesses may have associated induration, fluctuance, or

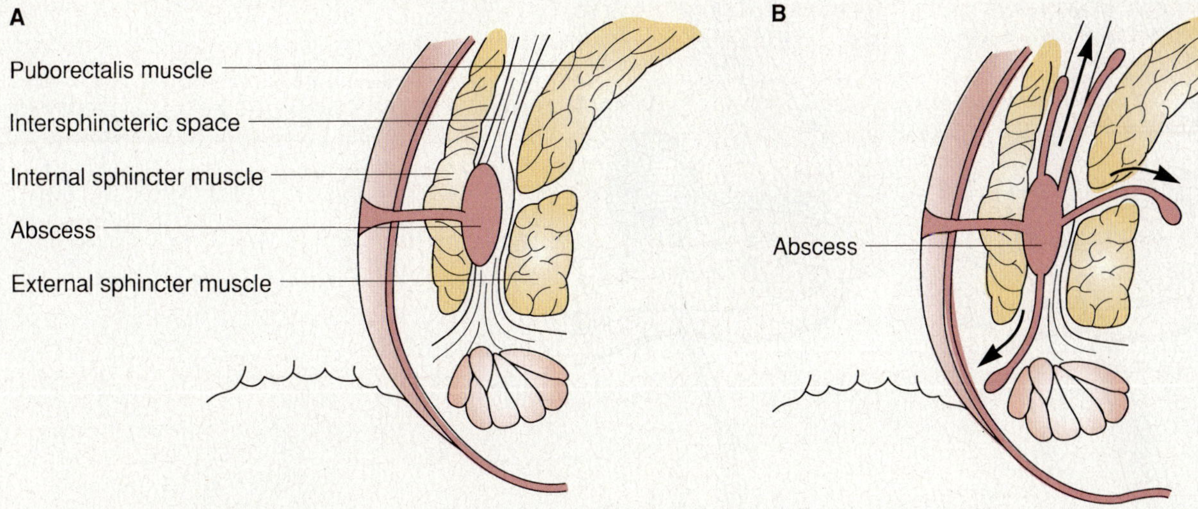

Figure 67.13. Pathways of infection.

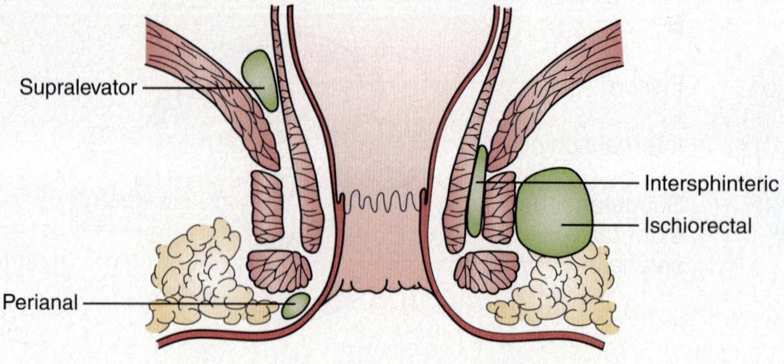

Figure 67.14. Classification of anorectal abscesses.

erythema. Deeper abscesses may lack external manifestations. Tenderness and fullness may be palpable on digital rectal examination. Associated symptoms may include tenesmus and difficulty voiding.

Evaluation

When a perianal abscess is suspected, but physical exam findings are limited, a computed tomography scan or pelvic MRI should be considered.

MANAGEMENT

The key to managing an anorectal abscess is adequate incision and drainage. Superficial abscesses may be amenable to drainage in the outpatient setting. One approach to draining an abscess is to make a 1-cm incision over the abscess cavity at the most tender or fluctuant point. When choosing the site for incision, consider the potential for subsequent fistula formation. An external fistula opening may occur at the site of the incision site. Therefore, one should choose an incision site as close as possible to the anal verge that will still allow adequate drainage. A 10F to 16F drainage catheter (Pezzer or Malecot) is inserted through the incision into the abscess cavity (**Fig. 67.15**). Alternatively, a larger elliptical or cruciate incision may be made over the abscess cavity. If using a cruciate incision, the skin edges should be excised to allow ongoing drainage. Patients should irrigate or soak the wound and cover with dry gauze. Anoscopy with examination of the dentate line may reveal an internal fistula opening. Probing to identify a fistula tract at the time of abscess drainage should be done with caution as aggressive probing may create a false tract. A superficial fistula tract identified at the time of abscess drainage may be treated with primary fistulotomy. For deeper fistulas, a draining seton, consisting of a silastic band or nonabsorbable suture, should be placed in the fistula tract. Antibiotics are not routinely prescribed after adequate drainage but are indicated when there is extensive surrounding cellulitis or in patients with diabetes or who are immunocompromised.

Deeper abscesses may require drainage in the operating room with sedation or general anesthesia. An abscess involving bilateral ischioanal spaces is referred to as a horseshoe abscess. These infections originate in the posterior midline and extend to both ischioanal spaces. Treatment may require bilateral incisions overlying the ischioanal areas. Supralevator abscesses are less common and can be difficult to diagnose. Because the location of the abscess is adjacent to the abdominal cavity, patients may present with abdominal or pelvic pain. Digital examination may demonstrate induration, or a tender mass located in the distal rectum above the level of the anorectal ring. The etiology of a supralevator abscess dictates its management. These abscesses may result as an extension of an intersphincteric abscess, extension of an ischioanal abscess, or may result from an intra-abdominal abscess from perforated diverticulitis, appendicitis, or Crohn disease. A supralevator abscess secondary to extension from an ischioanal abscess should be drained through the ischioanal area. A supralevator abscess secondary to extension from an intersphincteric abscess should be drained into the rectum, as drainage through the ischioanal area may result in a complex suprasphincteric fistula. Percutaneous, image-guided, drainage may be an option in patients with a supralevator abscess secondary to an intra-abdominal source. After adequate drainage, approximately half of patients will heal. Alternatively, patients may experience a recurrent abscess or develop an anal fistula.[11]

Rarely, anorectal abscesses can result in necrotizing infection and death, a condition referred to as Fournier gangrene. This

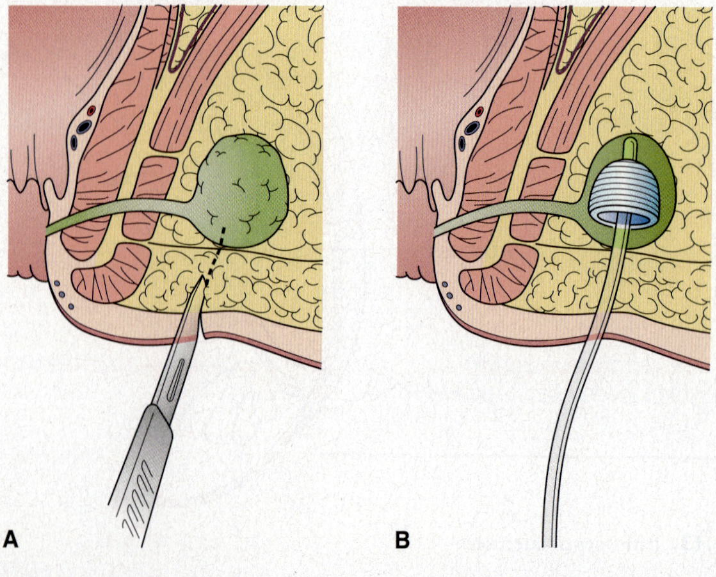

Figure 67.15. Abscess drainage with drain placement.

situation may result from a delay in diagnosis and management of an anorectal abscess, infection with a highly virulent organism, or may be due to patient factors such as diabetes or compromised immune function. The infection superficially spreads around the perineum, causing necrosis of the skin and underlying muscle and fascia. Treatment includes empiric broad-spectrum intravenous antibiotics and prompt surgical debridement of the necrotic tissue until healthy tissue is encountered.

Anal Fistula

Clinical Manifestations

A recurrent abscess is usually indicative of a cryptoglandular fistula arising from the glands in the anal crypts. Fistulas may occur without a prior history of an abscess. Fistulas present as a perianal nodule, often with persistent or intermittent purulent drainage. On physical examination, there may be an external opening with granulation tissue. Sometimes the external opening will close over superficially, making the fistula more difficult to identify.

The differential diagnoses of cryptoglandular fistulae include hydradinitis, which is inflammation of the apocrine sweat glands with resulting subcutaneous fistula tracts. In hydradinitis, the fistulae are superficial and do not extend into the anal canal. A second differential is pilonidal disease. The origin of inflammation of pilonidal disease is a tuft of hair in the gluteal cleft creating a foreign-body reaction.

Evaluation

A thorough history should include information about the duration of symptoms, a history of prior anorectal surgery, sphincter function, and associated urogenital symptoms. Additionally, one should inquire about a change in bowel habits or abdominal symptoms that may suggest Crohn disease.

Goodsall rule states that if an imaginary line is drawn transversely across the anus, an external fistula opening seen posterior to this line will originate from an internal opening in the posterior midline, whereas an opening anterior to this line will originate from the closest anal crypt (**Fig. 67.16**). Locating the internal opening is not always possible with a fistula probe, and in this situation, other diagnostic maneuvers may be necessary. Injection of the external opening with hydrogen peroxide either with or without the use of endoanal ultrasound may help identify smaller fistulas. For patients with complex fistulas, including multiple fistulas, recurrent fistula and fistulas associated with Crohn disease, ultrasound, MRI, or fistulography with a water-soluble contrast and fluoroscopy may help to delineate a fistula tract (**Box 67.1**).

Management

The first step in treating a fistula is to identify the entire length of the fistula tract. During an exam under anesthesia with the patient under MAC in the prone or lithotomy position, a probe is passed along the course of the fistula tract and assessed relative to the degree of sphincter muscle proximal and distal

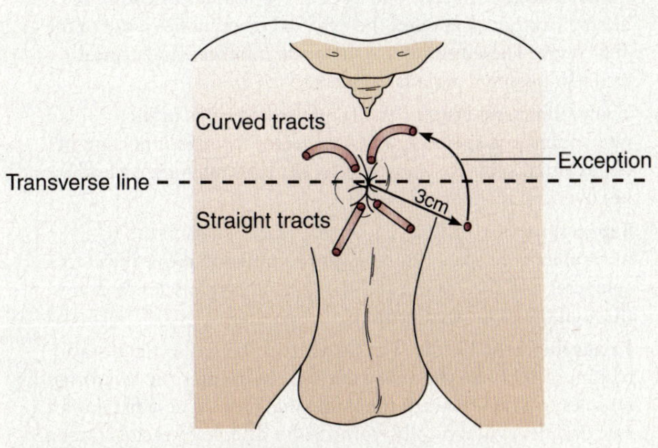

Figure 67.16. Goodsall rule.

to the fistula tract. The fistulotomy, unroofing of the fistula tract, is performed for the portion of the fistula peripheral to the anal sphincter. Simple, superficial fistulas may be treated with primary sphincterotomy. In general, involvement of less than 30% of the sphincter muscle is considered amenable to primary sphincterotomy. In women, the anterior anal canal is shorter and one should be cautious about performing an anterior fistulotomy. Primary fistulotomy is associated with fistula healing rates as high as 90%. Fistulas involving more sphincter muscle that is prudent to divide should be treated with seton placement and an interval definitive procedure.

4 There are numerous options for treating fistulas. Regardless of technique, the goal is to obliterate the fistula tract while preserving sphincter function. Treatment options include primary fistulotomy, seton placement, advancement flaps, and ligation of intersphincteric fistula tract (LIFT). Instillation of fibrin glue or use of a fistula plug are associated with high recurrence rates and are no longer recommended as primary treatment for fistulas.

After initial placement, a seton may be sequentially tightened at 2- to 4-week internals to form a "cutting" seton where the seton gradually erodes through the sphincter muscle. When the seton is deemed to be superficial enough, a second stage fistulotomy is performed to remove the seton. The cutting seton is associated with success rates as high as 94%. The disadvantage of using a cutting seton is the risk of compromise of the sphincter function. The reported rates of incontinence after using a cutting seton range from 0% to 67%. This variability is related to the type of fistulas treated and criteria for assessing anal incontinence.[11] Despite the risks, the cutting seton may be used selectively.

Endoanal advancement flap is a sphincter sparing procedure that involves raising a flap of the rectal wall (**Fig. 67.17**). The fistula tract is curetted, and the internal fistula tract opening is sutured closed with absorbable suture. The raised flap of tissue is placed over the internal opening and sutured in place. The success rate of the advancement flap ranges from 66% to 87%.[11] In the case of a failed advancement flap, one may perform a repeat flap repair after an interval to allow for resolution of inflammation.

Another treatment for an anal fistula is the LIFT procedure (**Fig. 67.18**). After a seton has been in place long enough for fibrosis around the seton to form, the fistula tract is ligated and divided. An incision is made over the intersphincteric groove and deepened down to the fistula tract. Both ends of the exposed length of fistula tract are ligated and the tract is sharply divided. Reported success rates after the LIFT procedure range from 40% to 95%.[12]

Anal Fistula and Crohn Disease

Anal fistulas occur in 13% to 54% of individuals with Crohn disease.[13] Asymptomatic fistulas in the setting of Crohn disease do not need to be treated.[14] Crohn-related fistulas may be complex with more than one external opening. The initial treatment of these fistulas is to unroof the branching tracts to create a single tract at the internal opening. Once a single fistula without inflammation is achieved, the techniques for treating fistulas described previously are applicable to patients with Crohn-related fistula. Prior to attempting a fistula repair procedure, examination should assess for anal canal fibrosis and acute mucosal inflammation. Crohn-related anal fistulae may be controlled with long-term seton placement and medical management of the Crohn disease. Temporary diversion may facilitate fistula healing, and proctectomy may be necessary for severe perianal disease.[15]

Anovaginal and Rectovaginal Fistulae

Clinical Manifestations

A rectovaginal fistula is a communication between the anterior anus or rectal wall and the posterior vagina. Such fistulae can be debilitating due to passage of gas or stool into the vagina resulting in incontinence and skin excoriation. An anovaginal

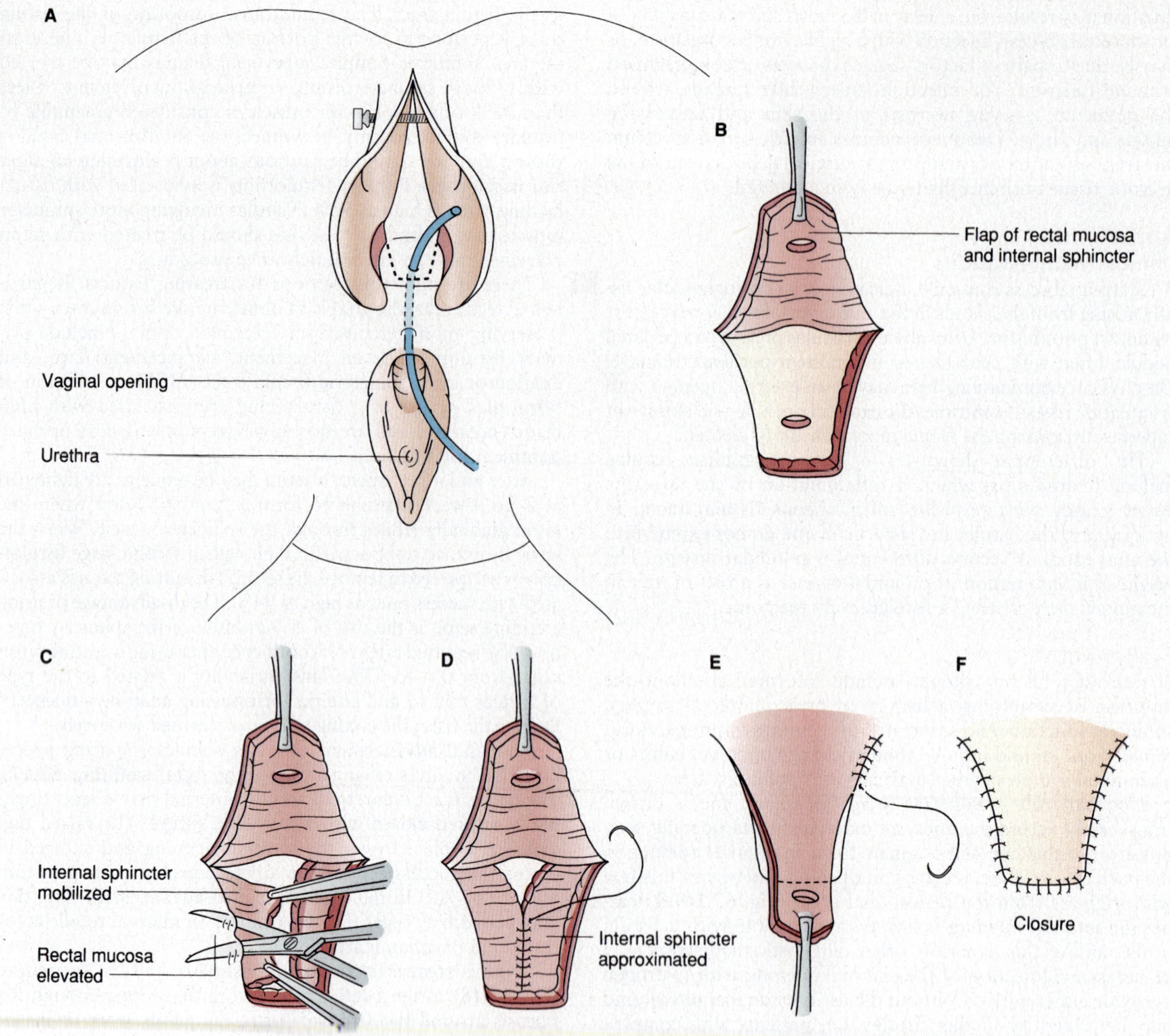

Figure 67.17. Technique of mucosal advancement flap.

fistula may occur as a complication from cryptoglandular disease with or without associated Crohn disease. Anovaginal fistulae may also result from obstetric injury, iatrogenic injury, or other perineal trauma.

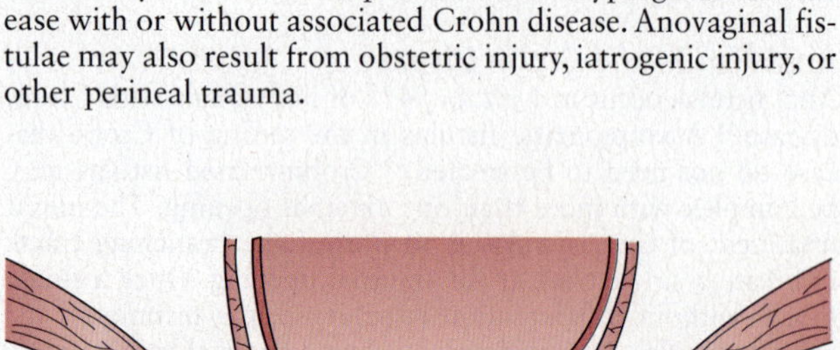

Figure 67.18. Ligation of intersphincteric fistula.

Evaluation

The clinician should ask about the patient's obstetric and surgical history. Obstetric injury may result in a fourth degree (full thickness) tear of the rectovaginal septum. In addition

Box 67.1 Classification of Anal Fistulas

Intersphincteric Fistula. The tract of the fistula lies within the intersphincteric space and the external opening lies close to the anal verge. These fistulas are the most common, and typically result following a perianal abscess.

Transsphincteric Fistula. The fistula tract begins in the intersphincteric space and then traverses through a portion of the external sphincter muscle. The external opening typically lies over the ischioanal fossa.

Suprasphincteric Fistula. The fistula tract begins in the intersphincteric space and then passes upward above the external sphincter and then perforates the levator ani muscles to drain through the ischioanal fossa.

Extrasphincteric Fistula. The fistula tract begins in the distal rectum rather than the anal canal and perforates the levator ani muscles to drain through the ischioanal fossa. These fistulas are rare and develop typically from Crohn disease or rectal trauma.

to leakage of stool per the vagina, individuals may experience anal incontinence due to sphincter compromise. Physical examination should include inspection of the perianal skin and introitus. Digital rectal exam will assess the thickness of the perineal body and may palpate a defect. Anoscopy may be helpful in visualizing the opening in low fistulas, while proctoscopy or flexible sigmoidoscopy may be required in mid or high fistulas. If a rectovaginal fistula is suspected clinically but no defect can be visualized, a rectal enema of saline or water with methylene blue may be administered after vaginal tampon insertion. Staining on the tampon is indicative of a fistula. A contrast enema under fluoroscopy may be needed in more complex cases to identify the fistula. In the setting of a low fistula occurring after obstetric injury, evaluation should include assessment of the anal sphincter using ultrasound.

Management

In patients with small fistulas and minimal symptoms, medical treatment with bulk agents such as fiber may be sufficient in controlling symptoms. Repair of fistulas that occur in patients as a result of an obstetric injury should be delayed 3 to 6 months to allow for resolution of inflammation. Similarly, repeat surgery after a prior failed repair should be delayed 3 to 6 months following the prior repair.

Treatment of low rectovaginal or anovaginal fistulas with an intact sphincter may be accomplished by endorectal advancement flap or vaginal advancement flap. Most colorectal surgeons prefer to perform an advancement flap transanally rather than vaginally as the repair is to the high-pressure side. The opening in the vagina may be left open to drain. Success rates of endorectal advancement flaps for simple low rectovaginal fistulas are as high as range from 41% to 78%.[11]

If a low rectovaginal fistula is associated with incontinence secondary to a defect in the anal sphincter, repair with an overlapping sphincter repair has been shown to have good results. Episioproctotomy (perineoproctotomy) involves dividing the tissue distal to the fistula. The rectal mucosa is then repaired followed by an overlapping sphincter repair to form a buttress between the rectal and vaginal defects. Finally, the vaginal mucosa and anoderm are reapproximated. Hull and colleagues compared the outcomes of 50 women with rectovaginal fistulas treated with episioproctotomy and 37 who underwent rectal advancement flap for anovaginal fistulas. The success rates for fistula healing were similar for both procedures—78% for episioproctotomy and 62% for mucosal advancement flap. Episioproctotomy was associated with significantly better fecal continence ($P < .001$) and sexual ($P = .04$) function.[16]

High rectovaginal fistulas are treated with an abdominal procedure based on the etiology of the fistula and the condition of surrounding tissues. The principles of fistula repair include identifying healthy, well vascularized tissue, and utilizing interposition grafts, such as omentum or rectus muscle, to decrease the risk of recurrent fistulization.

Pilonidal Disease

Clinical Manifestations

Pilonidal disease is subcutaneous inflammation caused by imbedded hair resulting in a foreign-body reaction. Pilonidal disease may present as an acute abscess with pain, induration, erythema, or fluctuance adjacent to the gluteal cleft. Pilonidal disease may also manifest as a series of one or more chronic sinus tracts or "pits" in the gluteal cleft.

Evaluation

Physical examination is usually adequate for evaluation of the pilonidal sinus tract. MRI may be helpful to differentiate a pilonidal sinus from a cryptoglandular fistula.

5 Management

An acute pilonidal abscess is managed by incision and drainage. Definitive treatment of chronic pilonidal disease involves excising the nidus of infection, commonly with excision of the

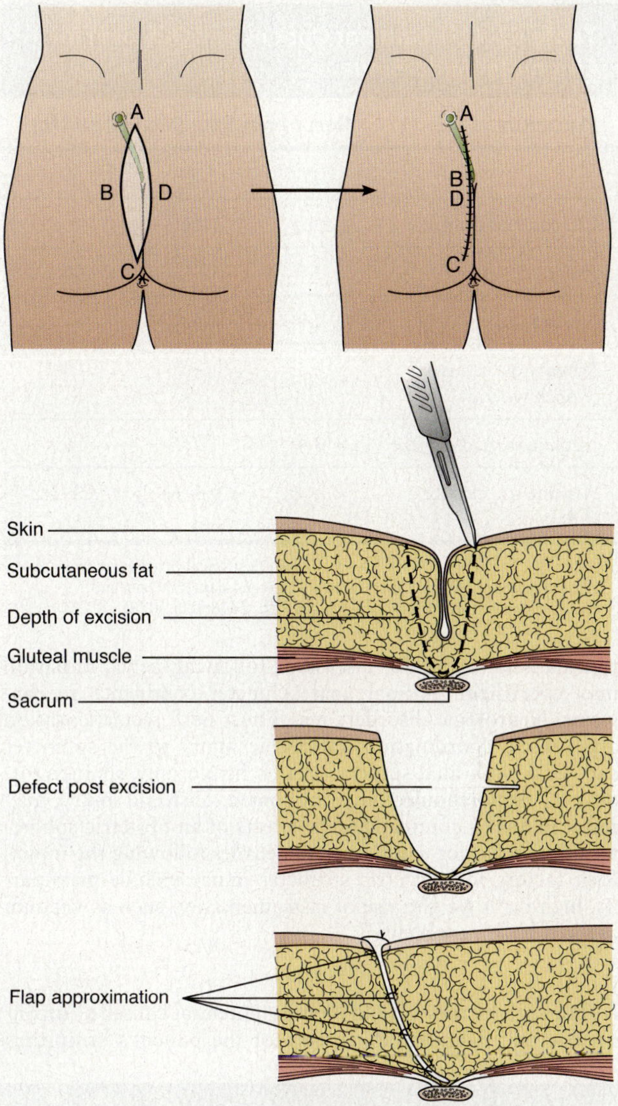

Figure 67.19. Technique of pilonidal sinus excision with primary closure.

skin and subcutaneous tissue to incorporate all of the residual pits. The wound can then be left open or closed. There are various described techniques for wound closure.

Midline closure is associated with a relatively high recurrence rate.[17] The alternative closure techniques involve incision placement lateral to the gluteal cleft and skin advancement or rotational flaps that result in an asymmetric closure off of the midline (**Fig. 67.19**). Less invasive techniques including pit excision alone using a punch biopsy and phenol instillation to obliterate the sinus tract, are associated with higher recurrence rates (**Table 67.4**).[18]

Anal Incontinence

Clinical Presentation

Anal incontinence is the uncontrolled passage of feces or flatus. The severity of incontinence may range from minor soiling to complete incontinence of solid stool. Fecal incontinence affects approximately 8% of the population and is more prevalent in older individuals.[19]

Anal continence depends on the reservoir function of the rectum, the individual's ability to sense the presence of stool in the rectum and the coordinated function of the anal sphincters and pelvic floor (see Physiology). Fecal incontinence is a symptom that may result from a variety of clinical conditions. Alterations in stool consistency or changes in rectal compliance due

Table 67.4. Treatment Options and Outcome for Chronic Pilonidal Sinus

Procedure	Recurrence Rate (Mo Follow-Up)		
	12	24	60
Incision and drainage	10.4	25.9	40.2
Phenol	1.9	14.1	40.4
Pit excision	2.7	6.5	15.6
Primary excision and open wound	1.5	4.2	13.1
Midline wound closure	3.4	7.0	16.8
Asymmetric closure ± flap	0.2–1.0	0.6–1.6	3.2–5.2

Stauffer VK, Luedi MM, Kauf P, et al. Common surgical procedures in pilonidal sinus disease: a meta-analysis, merged data analysis, and comprehensive study on recurrence. *Sci Rep*. 2018;8(1):3058.

to inflammatory bowel disease or following pelvic radiation may overwhelm normal anal sphincter continence mechanisms. Neurologic disorders may affect both rectal sensation and muscle coordination. Iatrogenic injury to the sphincter can occur with anal surgery such as fistulotomy, sphincterotomy, or hemorrhoidectomy. In women, obstetric injury, may result in anal incontinence. The effects of an obstetric sphincter injury may not manifest until decades following the injury. Risk factors for obstetric sphincter injury include primiparity, high birth weight, use of instrumentation such as vacuum assisted birth or forceps.[20]

Evaluation

A thorough history should identify potential causes of incontinence and delineate the nature of the patient's symptoms including frequency of bowel movements, the presence of tissue prolapse with bowel movements as well as the frequency of incontinence episodes and whether the incontinence is to flatus, liquid stool, or solid stool. The initial evaluation should also assess the extent to which a patient's symptoms affect their quality of life. When evaluating a patient with incontinence, it is important to differentiate between incontinence related to a compromised sphincter, soiling due to mucosal prolapse, or overflow incontinence related to underlying constipation. Fecal incontinence in the absence of urgency or incontinence to flatus is suggestive of soiling related to mucosal prolapse. Straining with bowel movements or a sensation of incomplete evacuation raises the suspicion of pelvic floor dysfunction.

Physical examination should include inspection of the perianal skin for scars from previous surgery or obstetrical injury, and excoriation from chronic soiling. Separation of the buttocks may demonstrate gaping of the anus in individuals with a compromised sphincter. Digital examination can provide a gross assessment of both resting tone and squeeze effort. Anoscopy may identify mucosal inflammation or enlarged internal hemorrhoids.

The structural integrity of the anal sphincters is commonly assessed using endoanal ultrasound. Transperineal ultrasound or MRI can also assess sphincter anatomy. Anal sphincter and pelvic floor muscle function may be assessed with defecography and anal manometry. Manometry measures anal pressure using a transducer catheter placed in the anal canal. Pressures are recorded with the patient at rest, when squeezing, and during simulated defecation. Evaluation of rectal sensation is performed by placing a balloon catheter above the anorectal ring and then gradually inflating the balloon with air (**Table 67.5**).

Management

Bowel Management Program

Patients with loose stool may benefit from a bowel management program that includes increased dietary fiber to bulk the stool and absorb excess liquid, making the stool easier to

Table 67.5. Anal Manometric Parameters

Measurement	Definition	Normal Range
High-pressure zone	The length of the anal canal with resting pressures ≥30% higher than rectal pressure	3–5 cm
Resting pressure	The pressure in the high-pressure zone at rest after a period of stabilization	40–70 mm Hg
Maximum voluntary pressure	The highest pressure recorded above the baseline (0) at any level of the anal canal during maximum squeeze effort by the patient	>70 mm Hg
Squeeze pressure	Calculated difference between the maximum voluntary pressure and the resting pressure	>100 mm Hg
Sphincter endurance	The length of time that the patient can maintain a squeeze pressure above the resting pressure	>10 s
Rectal pressure	Pressure generated by the rectum with rest, squeeze, and push	60–70 mm Hg
Sensory threshold	The minimum rectal volume perceived by the patient	20–40 mm Hg
Urge sensation	*Sensation* is the volume associated with the initial urge to defecate	80–140 mm Hg
Maximum tolerated volume	The volume at which the patient experiences discomfort and an intense desire to defecate	130–150 mm Hg
Balloon expulsion test	Evaluates the ability of the patient to expel a balloon inflated with 50–60 mL of water	Patients with normal anorectal function are expected to expel the balloon

Lee GC, Kunitake H, Milch H, et al. What is the risk of anal carcinoma in patients with anal intraepithelial neoplasia III? *Dis Colon Rectum*. 2018;61:1350–1356.

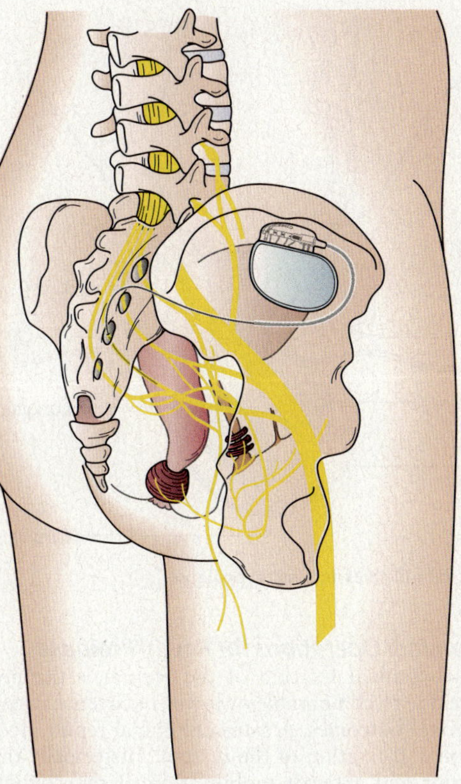

Figure 67.20. Position of sacral nerve stimulator.

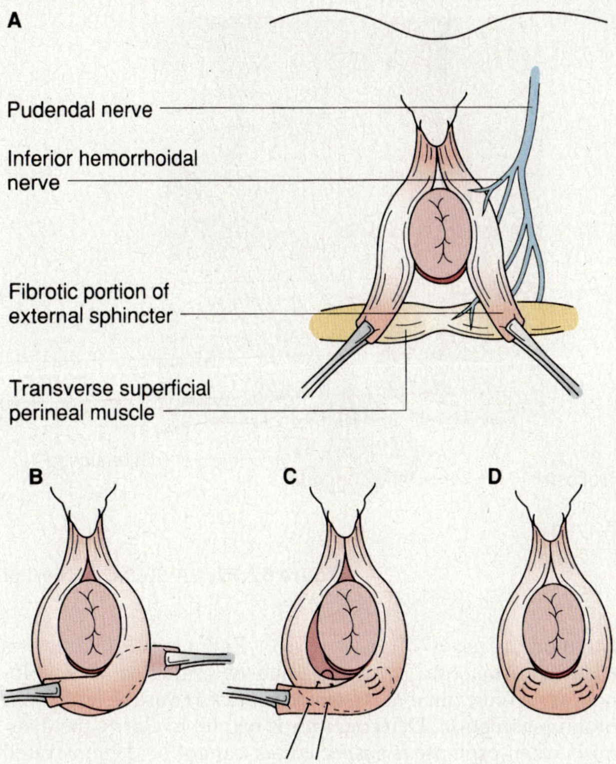

Figure 67.21. Technique of overlapping sphincteroplasty.

sense and control. Medical management may include constipating agents such as loperamide or diphenoxylate atropine. Bile acid binders can also thicken the stool and decrease stool frequency. Taking an enema after a bowel movement helps to empty the rectum thereby decreasing the leakage between bowel movements.

Pelvic Floor Physical Therapy

Pelvic floor physical therapy helps to optimize sphincter and pelvic floor function. Therapy is targeted to the patient's need and may include sphincter strengthening, coordination of pelvic floor relaxation during defecation and improving rectal sensation. Biofeedback typically employs the use of a pressure-sensitive probe placed into the anal canal to measure the strength and coordination of the anal sphincter and pelvic floor musculature. The data from the probe are then transmitted to a monitor, where the patient is able to watch the manometric tracings. Through a series of coached exercises and visual feedback, patients can improve pelvic muscle control. Reported rates of improvement with biofeedback range from 50% to 90%.[21] Successful therapy depends, in part, on the knowledge and skills of therapist and patient motivation.

Sacral Neuromodulation

Interventions to treat fecal incontinence include bowel management program, neuromodulation and sphincter repair or augmentation. Sacral neuromodulation involves stimulation of a sacral nerve with an implantable stimulator (**Fig. 67.20**). The exact mechanism of this technique is not known. Studies have demonstrated improvement in symptoms even with an existing sphincter defect. This technique involves placing an electrode into the foramen of the sacral vertebrae, most commonly S3. The electrode is initially connected to an external neurostimulator. If the patient experiences improvement in function, a long-term neurostimulator is placed subcutaneously. Complications following neurostimulator implantation include infection, pain, either at the stimulator site or painful stimulation, and loss of efficacy over time.

Sphincter Repair and Augmentation

Overlapping sphincter repair is an option for patients with significant external sphincter defects. The fibrotic scar tissue at the site of the defect is divided and the two ends of the sphincter muscle are identified and are mobilized laterally. The ends of the muscle are sutured in an overlapping fashion (**Fig. 67.21**). While this procedure is associated with an initial success rate of greater than 80%, the durability of the repair is limited with nearly half of patients developing recurrent incontinence after long-term follow-up.[22]

Rectal Prolapse

Clinical Manifestation

Rectal prolapse is the full-thickness protrusion of the rectum through the anal canal. Rectal prolapse occurs in approximately 0.5% of the general population and is more common in women.[23] Although typically seen in women over age 50 years old, rectal prolapse may be seen in younger individuals with developmental delay or psychiatric comorbidities. Rectal prolapse may be associated with chronic constipation in up to 50% of individuals.[23] The chronic traumatic stretch of the anal sphincter results in fecal incontinence in the majority of patients.

Evaluation

Patients report protrusion of tissue that occurs with defecation or, in more advanced prolapse, may occur with moderate activity such as ambulating. The prolapse may reduce spontaneously or require manual reduction. Patients may experience fecal soiling and symptoms of incontinence. A complete history should include information about bowel habits and any associated genitourinary dysfunction such as urinary incontinence or vaginal vault prolapse. On digital rectal examination there is usually decreased sphincter tone. An enterocele appears as smooth prolapse limited to the anterior rectal wall. It is important to differentiate full-thickness rectal prolapse, with concentric folds of tissue from mucosal prolapse, with radial folds of tissue. Examination of the prolapsed tissue is facilitated by having the patient Valsalva while seated on a

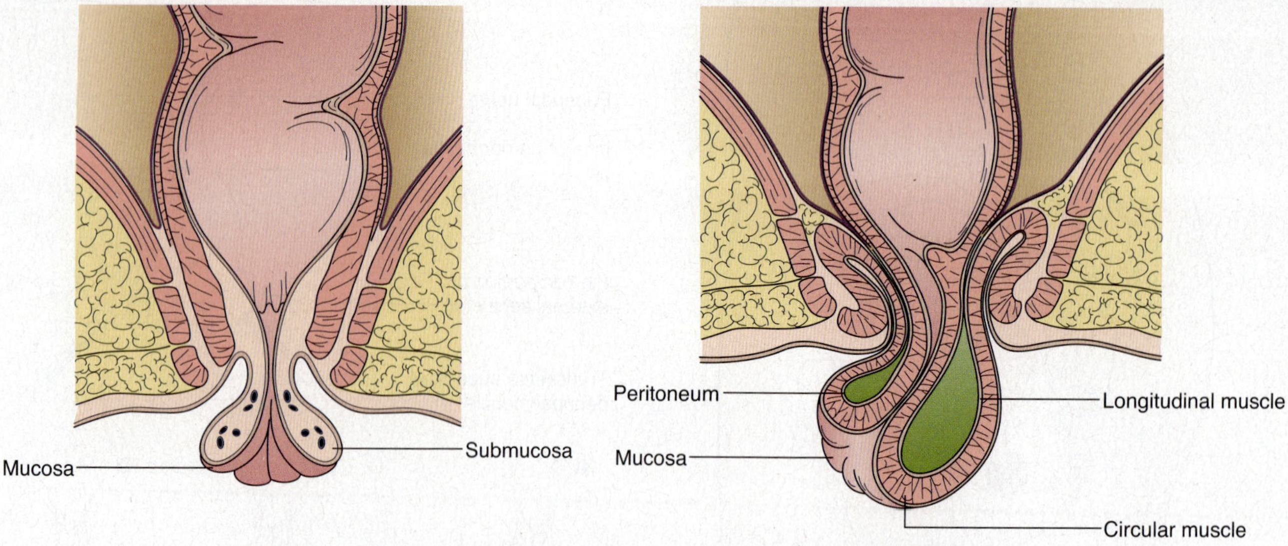

Figure 67.22. (A) Rectal mucosal prolapse and (B) full-thickness rectal prolapse.

commode (**Figs. 67.22 and 67.23**). Endoscopy often shows edematous mucosa. Patients should be evaluated with colonoscopy to rule out a mass, which could serve as the lead point of intussusception. Defecography is helpful to clarify the diagnosis when prolapse is suspected but cannot be demonstrated on exam. Additionally, defecography can reveal intussusception and concomitant pathology such as enterocele and pelvic floor dysfunction. Anorectal manometry may also be useful to evaluate for associated pelvic floor dyssynergia.

Patients may present with full-thickness rectal prolapse that is not reducible. If the prolapsed bowel appears viable, then application of table sugar directly to the exposed mucosa may facilitate manual reduction. If the prolapsed tissue has advanced ischemia, then prompt, transperineal resection is indicated.

6 Management

Treatment of rectal prolapse requires surgical intervention. The choice of procedure depends on a history of previous procedures and the patients overall medical condition.

Abdominal Operations for Rectal Prolapse

Transabdominal fixation of the rectum is the procedure of choice due to comparable or lower recurrence rates and better functional outcomes. A transabdominal repair involves mobilization and fixation of the rectum. Historically this involved posterior and anterior mobilization of the rectum and fixation of the rectum to the sacral promontory, with or without concomitant sigmoid colon resection. One problem with this approach is that posterior mobilization of the rectum may worsen constipation. In one report 50% of individuals with baseline constipation reported worsening constipation and 15% of patients reported denovo constipation.[24] In theory, the increased constipation could be related to disruption of rectal innervation. A newer technique involves only anterior mobilization of the rectum and fixation of the rectum to the sacrum with synthetic or biologic mesh. Early reported outcomes of this anterior rectopexy technique indicated improvement in patients with preoperative constipation and no patients reporting new constipation (**Fig. 67.24**). Subsequent studies

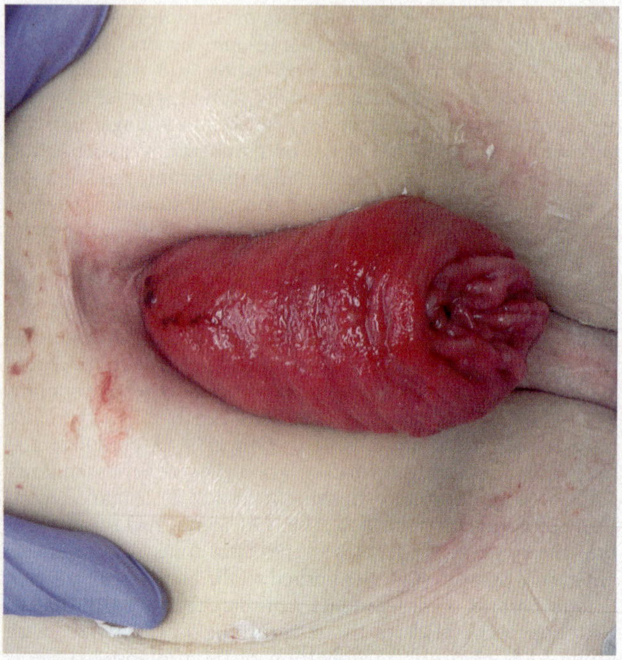

Figure 67.23. Photo of full-thickness rectal prolapse.

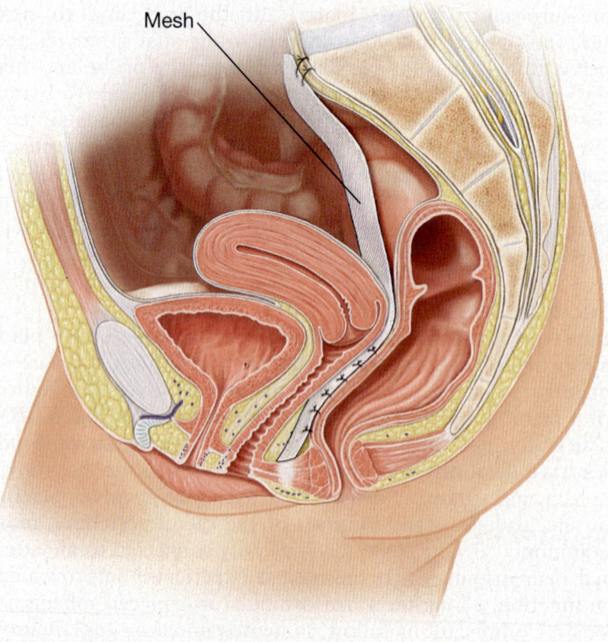

Figure 67.24. Ventral rectopexy. Mesh is sutured to the anterior rectum and sacral promontory.

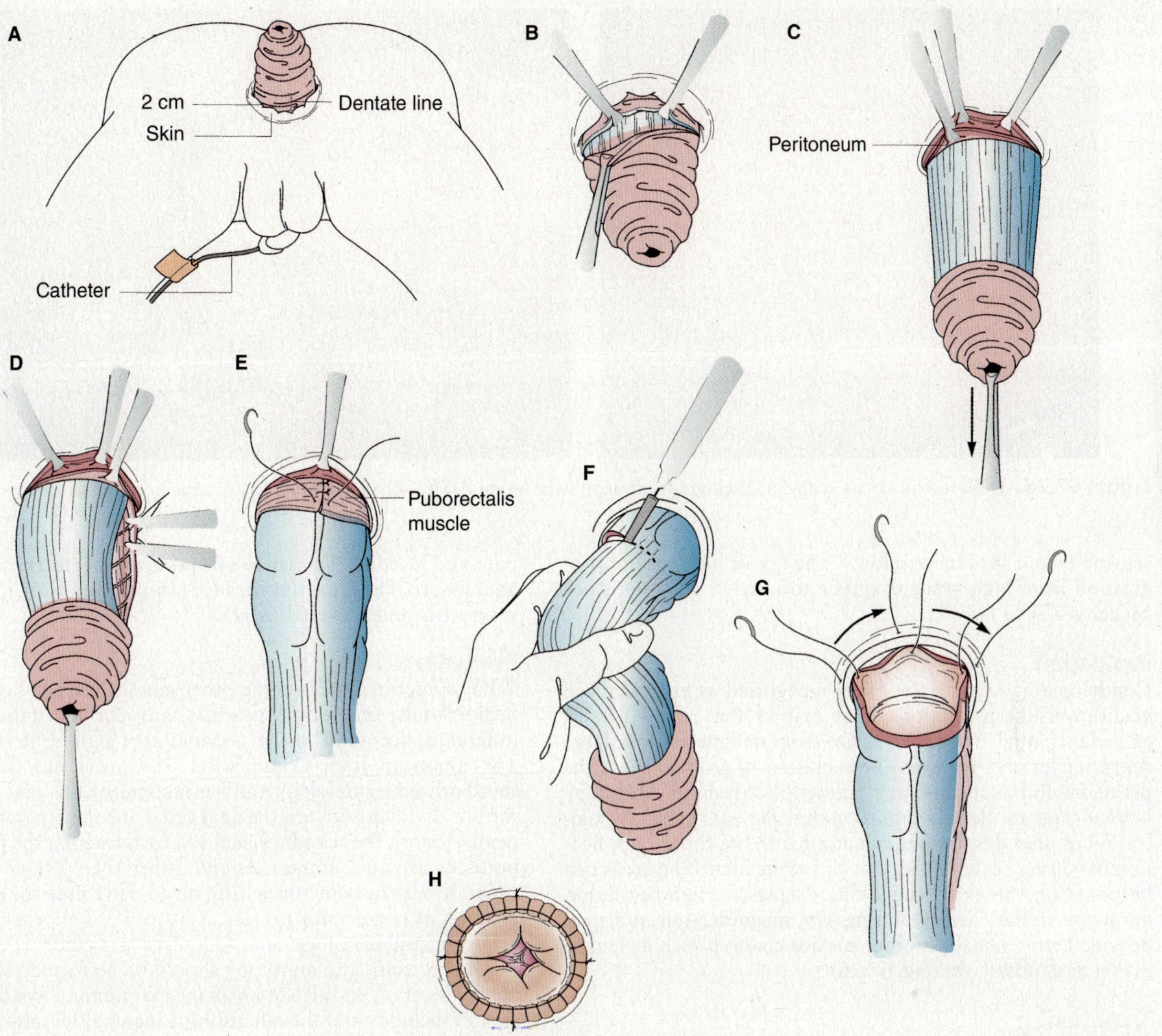

Figure 67.25. (A–H) Perineal proctosidmoidectomy.

reported recurrence rates up to 14% and denovo constipation was reported in 6%.[25,26]

Perineal Operations for Rectal Prolapse

A transperineal approach for rectal prolapse is indicated for ischemic, nonreducible prolapse. This approach has the advantage that it may be performed under regional anesthesia. The patient is placed in the prone position. Excess rectum is excised and the colon is anastomosed to the distal rectum just proximal to the dentate line (**Fig. 67.25**). Levator muscle imbrication prior to colonic anastomosis may ameliorate postoperative incontinence. The Delorme procedure is an alternative perineal approach that is appropriate for individuals with limited prolapse of 5 cm or less. This procedure involves stripping the mucosa of the prolapsed rectum from the muscularis propria, followed by plication of the muscularis propria and reanastomosis of the mucosa. This technique has a high recurrence rate but has very low associated morbidity, and may therefore be useful in frail, older patients.

ANAL NEOPLASIA

7 Condyloma Acuminata and Squamous Intraepithelial Lesions

Anal condylomata acuminata or "warts" are caused by the human papilloma virus (HPV). HPV is a papovirus of which more than 130 subtypes of HPV have been identified. The estimated prevalence among adults aged 18 to 59 in the United States is 43%.[27] Inoculation of the anal epithelium allows entry of the HPV into the basal cell layers. As these cells proliferate, viral replication occurs in the nucleus. The basal cells then migrate toward the surface and infective particles are released in the form of visible warts.

HPV changes are classified into three grades of dysplasia: condyloma (no dysplasia), low-grade squamous intraepithelial lesions (LSILs) and high-grade squamous intraepithelial lesions (HSILs). Select serotypes are implicated in oncogenic cellular transformation; HPV serotype 16 is associated with 89% of anal squamous cell cancers.[28] Individuals at increased risk for anal dysplasia include women with a history of cervical neoplasia, men who have sex with men (MSM), and individuals who are immunosuppressed. The mechanism for oncogenesis involves inactivation of the P53 tumor suppressor gene by viral proteins.

Clinical Manifestations

Patients with anal dysplasia may experience, pain, bleeding, or pruritus, although the majority of patients are asymptomatic.[29]

Anal Dysplasia Surveillance

Since HPV and anal dysplasia are often asymptomatic, individuals with at increased risk for anal dysplasia should be evaluated. Surveillance with anal cytology (anal Papanicolaou [Pap] test) smears every 1 to 2 years can be used, although

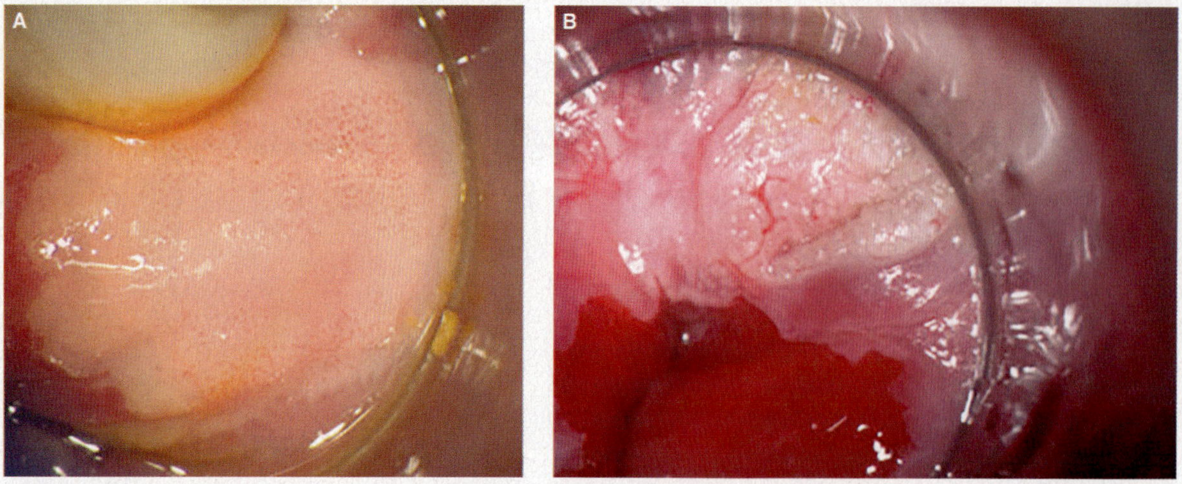

Figure 67.26. High-resolution anoscopy. **A:** High-grade intraepithelial lesion (HSIL). **B:** Superficial invasive squamous cell cancer.

sensitivity and specificity is low.[30] The 5-year incidence of progression from high-grade dysplasia to invasive squamous cell cancer is 2% to 6%.[31]

Evaluation

Condyloma acuminata are easily recognized as epithelialized cauliflower-like projections. They may be flat, raised, sessile, or pedunculated, and range in size from millimeters to a large fungating lesions. They may be in clusters or grow to cover the perineum and anal canal in a "carpet-like" fashion. Anoscopy is important to identify lesions within the anal canal. Visualization of anal dysplasia is enhanced with the topical application of 4% acetic acid. Irregular and white blanching areas can be noted on the exam suggesting dysplasia. High-resolution anoscopy (HRA) involves using 10× magnification and may provide better visualization of surface changes such as leukoplakia and mosaicism (**Fig. 67.26**).

Treatment

Treatment is indicated for gross condyloma lesions or when HSIL is identified on surveillance anoscopy with biopsy. Treatment is variable and includes tangential excision, fulgaration, cryotherapy, infrared coagulation, laser, or chemical therapy (trichroloacetic acid). Treatment of larger or multiple condylomatous lesions or extensive HSIL identified by anoscopy and biopsy, may be facilitated with sedation, which allows for placement of a larger anoscope and better visualization of the anal canal. A recent prospective randomized study comparing treatment of HSIL to active monitoring found that treatment of HSIL reduced the progression to anal cancer by 57%.[32]

Topical agents such as podofilox, imiquimod, and flurouracil applied by the patient on the perianal skin and in the anal canal have been shown to slow progression of the disease and decrease the need for reintervention.[33] Vaccination against more virulent strains of condyloma (Gardesil) is currently available. The vaccine is effective in reducing progression of anal dysplasia.[34] High-volume centers have reported recurrence rates of 66% to 70%. Therefore, ongoing surveillance is warranted.

Squamous Cell Carcinoma

Historically anal cancer was most common in women aged 50 to 70. Over the past three decades, the incidence of anal cancer has increased in women and at an even higher rate in MSM. Recent data shows that the rate per 100,000 is 1.6 for men and 2.2 for women.[35] Fewer than half of patients present with localized disease.[35]

8 Clinical Manifestations

Squamous cell carcinoma may occur on the perianal skin and in the anal canal. Patients often present with symptoms of pain and bleeding, similar to symptoms of hemorrhoids or an anal fissure. The gross appearance is typically a firm, ulcerated mass with rolled, everted edges.

Evaluation

While symptoms may mimic other conditions such as fistula, hemorrhoids, or chronic pruritus, any chronic unhealed or indurated ulceration in the perianal area should be biopsied. The American Joint Commission on Cancer has developed standardized terminology and has recognized the anal verge as the line dividing between the anal canal and anal margin. Practically, lesions that can be visualized by retracting the patient's buttocks are anal margin lesions rather than lesions of anal canal. It may be sometimes difficult to determine the primary location of large, bulky tumors. A history of symptoms, physical exam, and histology can often serve as a guide.

Digital exam and anoscopy should be performed to evaluate the location and size of an anal canal tumor. Physical exam should include careful evaluation of inguinal lymph nodes as most common sites of loco regional disease. Suspicious nodes may be evaluated further with fine needle aspiration. Staging should be done with a CT scan of the chest and abdomen along with CT or MRI of the pelvis. Additional work-up includes HIV testing and evaluation for cervical dysplasia in women. Also, one should discuss fertility preservation in appropriate patients.

Treatment

Anal Margin Tumors

T1 (<2 cm) and T2 (2 cm to 5 cm) well-differentiated lesions that do not invade the sphincter muscle may be treated with local excision with a 1-cm margin. More advanced lesions are treated with a combination of 5-fluorouracil, mitomicin C, and radiation. Patients generally receive 50.4 Gr with additional boost to inguinal lymph nodes if lymph node metastases are suspected. Abdominoperineal resection (APR) is indicated for persistent or recurrent disease and in the setting of significant functional issues related to tumor or consequences of treatment (incontinence). This surgery may require excision of a large portion of the perineum and closure with a myocutaneous flap.

Anal Canal Tumors

The standard treatment for anal canal lesions is chemotherapy with 5-flurouracil and mitomycin C and radiation. In select patients where superficially invasive squamous cell cancer is identified in a biopsy or incidentally, such as in a hemorrhoidectomy specimen, and there are negative margins, local excision with close observation is acceptable. APR (usually with myocutaneous flap closure of the perineum) is reserved for

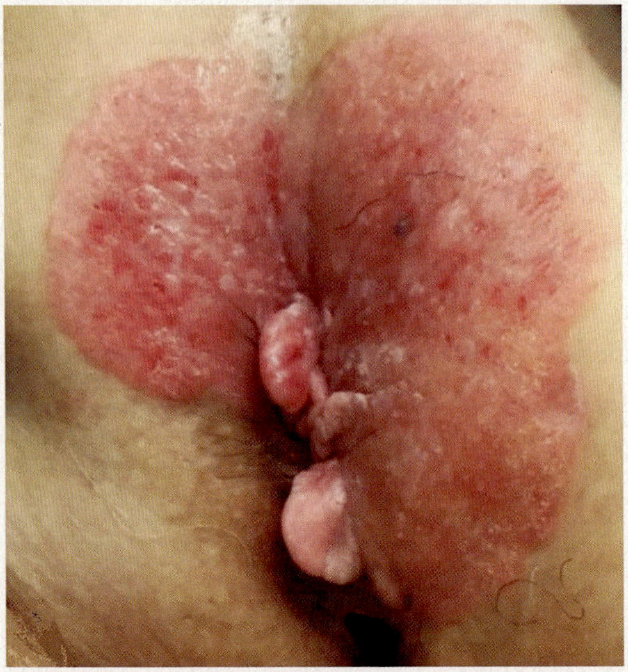

Figure 67.27. Perianal Paget disease.

patients with persistent or recurrent disease. As long as there is no evidence of tumor progression, tumors response to treatment should be monitored for up to 6 months as persistent disease may continue to regress even at 26 weeks.[36]

Paget Disease

Extramammary Paget disease (EMPD) is a rare adenocarcinoma found in the skin of the axilla and anogenital regions. Primary EMPD arises from the skin rich in apocrine glands whereas secondary EMPD results from the cutaneous spread of an underlying internal malignancy. Perianal Paget disease begins as a benign in situ neoplasm but may eventually become invasive as an adenocarcinoma. Paget disease occurs most commonly in individuals aged 50 to 80 years.

Clinical Manifestations

The typical appearance is an erythematous, sometimes sharply demarcated rash that may ooze or scale (**Fig. 67.27**). Pruritus is present in about 40% of patients.[37] Paget disease must be differentiated from other dermatologic conditions such as eczema, lichen sclerosis, and hyperkeratosis; these conditions tend to present in a circumferential pattern, whereas Paget disease tends to be unilateral.

Evaluation

Physical examination should include palpation of regional lymph nodes. The diagnosis is made by biopsy, which demonstrates the presence of cells with hyperchromatic nuclei and abundant pale-staining cytoplasm. Depth of invasion is the most important prognostic factor. Patients with Paget disease should also undergo a colonoscopy, as proximal visceral neoplasms may occur in 20% of individuals.[38] Further evaluation includes CT scan of the chest, abdomen, and pelvis.[37]

Treatment

The treatment options for perianal Paget disease include topical therapy or surgical resection. Topical therapy with Imiquimod has a 73% response rate.[39] The recommended surgical is Mohs micrographic surgery or surgery with complete circumferential peripheral and deep margin assessment. Patients with underlying cancer are generally treated based on the type of cancer identified.

Melanoma

Melanoma occurs most commonly in the skin and eyes, but can also develop from the transitional epithelium within the anal canal or the anoderm at the anal verge. This tumor is more common in females than in males and is relatively rare, accounting for less than 4% of all anal malignancies.[40]

Clinical Manifestations

Symptoms include pain, pruritus, and bleeding. Anal melanomas may not contain pigment and can be difficult to differentiate from SCC. Anal canal melanomas spread submucosally into the rectum, but do not typically invade other organs. Lymphatic spread to mesenteric lymph nodes is present in up to 35% of patients at the time of diagnosis, and hematogenous spread to distant sites is common as well.

Evaluation

Initial evaluation should include CT of the chest and abdomen and MRI of the pelvis. Careful evaluation of lymph nodes and anal sphincter involvement should be done by physical exam and imaging. Further genetic analysis of tumors can identify specific mutations in molecular pathways that can be targeted by systemic therapies.

Treatment

Melanomas of the anal canal do not respond to chemotherapy or radiation, making surgery the only chance for cure. Options include wide local excision or APR; however, the prognosis is poor and recurrences are common. A recent review by Smith and colleagues found that overall survival and relapse-free survival did not differ between the local excision and APR.[41] Consideration should be given to palliation of symptoms and maintaining adequate function. If the presenting lesion is not amenable to local excision without sacrificing function, then APR is warranted. Recent studies using targeted systemic therapy and immunomodulators have shown prolonged survival in patients with cutaneous melanoma; however, data on their effects on mucosal melanomas is still lacking.[42]

ACKNOWLEDGMENT

We gratefully acknowledge the contributions of previous edition author, Vitaliy Y. Poylin, as portions of those chapters have been retained in this revision.

COLON AND RECTUM

References

1. Lindsey I, Guy RJ, Warren BF, Mortensen NJ. Anatomy of Denonvilliers' fascia and pelvic nerves, impotence, and implications for the colorectal surgeon. *Br J Surg*. 2000;87(10):1288–1299.
2. Church JM, Raudkivi PJ, Hill GL. The surgical anatomy of the rectum–a review with particular relevance to the hazards of rectal mobilisation. *Int J Colorectal Dis*. 1987;2(3):158–166.
3. Iyer VS, Shrier I, Gordon PH. Long-term outcome of rubber band ligation for symptomatic primary and recurrent internal hemorrhoids. *Dis Colon Rectum*. 2004;47(8):1364–1370.
4. Toyonaga T, Matsushima M, Sogawa N, et al. Postoperative urinary retention after surgery for benign anorectal disease: potential risk factors and strategy for prevention. *Int J Colorectal Dis*. 2006;21(7):676–682.
5. Greenspon J, Williams SB, Young HA, Orkin BA. Thrombosed external hemorrhoids: outcome after conservative or surgical management. *Dis Colon Rectum*. 2004;47(9):1493–1498.
6. Hawkins AT, Davis BR, Bhama AR, et al; Clinical Practice Guidelines Committee of the American Society of Colon and Rectal Surgeons. The American Society of colon and rectal surgeons clinical practice guidelines for the management of hemorrhoids. *Dis Colon Rectum*. 2024;67(5):614–623.
7. Lund JN, Scholefield JH. Glyceryl trinitrate is an effective treatment for anal fissure. *Dis Colon Rectum*. 1997;40(4):468–470.
8. Sahebally SM, Meshkat B, Walsh SR, Beddy D. Botulinum toxin injection vs topical nitrates for chronic anal fissure: an updated

systematic review and meta-analysis of randomized controlled trials. *Colorectal Dis.* 2018;20(1):6–15.

9. Jin JZ, Bhat S, Park B, et al. A systematic review and network meta-analysis comparing treatments for anal fissure. *Surgery.* 2022; 172(1):41–52.
10. Davids JS, Hawkins AT, Bhama AR, et al. The American Society of Colon and Rectal Surgeons clinical practice guidelines for the management of anal fissures. *Dis Colon Rectum.* 2023;66(2):190–199.
11. Gaertner WB, Burgess PL, Davids JS, et al. The American Society of Colon and Rectal Surgeons clinical practice guidelines for the management of anorectal abscess, fistula-in-ano, and rectovaginal fistula. *Dis Colon Rectum.* 2022;65(8):964–985.
12. Emile SH, Khan SM, Adejumo A, Koroye O. Ligation of intersphincteric fistula tract (LIFT) in treatment of anal fistula: an updated systematic review, meta-analysis, and meta-regression of the predictors of failure. *Surgery.* 2020;167(2):484–492.
13. Gionchetti P, Dignass A, Danese S, et al. 3rd European evidence-based consensus on the diagnosis and management of Crohn's disease 2016: part 2: surgical management and special situations. *J Crohns Colitis.* 2017;11(2):135–149.
14. Vogel JD, Johnson EK, Morris AM, et al. Clinical practice guideline for the management of anorectal abscess, fistula-in-ano, and rectovaginal fistula. *Dis Colon Rectum.* 2016;59(12):1117–1133.
15. Steinhart AH, Panaccione R, Targownik L, et al. Clinical practice guideline for the medical management of perianal fistulizing Crohn's disease: the Toronto consensus. *Inflamm Bowel Dis.* 2018;25(1):1–13.
16. Hull TL, El-Gazzaz G, Gurland B, Church J, Zutshi M. Surgeons should not hesitate to perform episioproctotomy for rectovaginal fistula secondary to cryptoglandular or obstetrical origin. *Dis Colon Rectum.* 2011;54(1):54–59.
17. Johnson EK, Vogel JD, Cowan ML, Feingold DL, Steele SR; Clinical Practice Guidelines Committee of the American Society of Colon and Rectal Surgeons. The American Society of Colon and Rectal Surgeons' clinical practice guidelines for the management of pilonidal disease. *Dis Colon Rectum.* 2019;62(2):146–157.
18. Stauffer VK, Luedi MM, Kauf P, et al. Common surgical procedures in pilonidal sinus disease: a meta-analysis, merged data analysis, and comprehensive study on recurrence. *Sci Rep.* 2018;8(1):3058.
19. Ditah I, Devaki P, Luma HN, et al. Prevalence, trends, and risk factors for fecal incontinence in United States adults, 2005–2010. *Clin Gastroenterol Hepatol.* 2014;12(4):636–643.e1–e2.
20. Andre K, Stuart A, Kallen K. Obstetric anal sphincter injuries-maternal, fetal and sociodemographic risk factors: a retrospective register-based study. *Acta Obstet Gynecol Scand.* 2022;101(11): 1262–1268.
21. Richter HE, Jelovsek JE, Iyer P, et al. Characteristics associated with clinically important treatment responses in women undergoing nonsurgical therapy for fecal incontinence. *Am J Gastroenterol.* 2020;115(1):115–127.
22. Zutshi M, Tracey TH, Bast J, Halverson A, Na J. Ten-year outcome after anal sphincter repair for fecal incontinence. *Dis Colon Rectum.* 2009;52(6):1089–1094.
23. Bordeianou L, Paquette I, Johnson E, et al. Clinical practice guidelines for the treatment of rectal prolapse. *Dis Colon Rectum.* 2017;60(11):1121–1131.
24. Aitola PT, Hiltunen KM, Matikainen MJ. Functional results of operative treatment of rectal prolapse over an 11-year period: emphasis on transabdominal approach. *Dis Colon Rectum.* 1999; 42(5):655–660.
25. Franceschilli L, Varvaras D, Capuano I, et al. Laparoscopic ventral rectopexy using biologic mesh for the treatment of obstructed defaecation syndrome and/or faecal incontinence in patients with internal rectal prolapse: a critical appraisal of the first 100 cases. *Tech Coloproctol.* 2015;19(4):209–219.
26. Postillon A, Perrenot C, Germain A, et al. Long-term outcomes of robotic ventral mesh rectopexy for external rectal prolapse. *Surg Endosc.* 2020;34(2):930–939.
27. McQuillan G, Kruszon-Moran D, Markowitz LE, Unger ER, Paulose-Ram R. Prevalence of HPV in adults aged 18–69: United States, 2011–2014. *NCHS Data Brief.* 2017;(280):1–8.
28. Amin M. *AJCC Cancer Staging Manual.* American College of Surgeons; 2017.
29. Hicks CW, Wick EC, Leeds IL, et al. Patient symptomatology in anal dysplasia. *JAMA Surg.* 2015;150(6):563–569.
30. Stewart DB, Gaertner WB, Glasgow SC, Herzig DO, Feingold D, Steele SR; Prepared on Behalf of the Clinical Practice Guidelines Committee of the American Society of Colon and Rectal Surgeons. The American Society of Colon and Rectal Surgeons clinical practice guidelines for anal squamous cell cancers (revised 2018). *Dis Colon Rectum.* 2018;61(7):755–774.
31. Arens Y, Gaisa M, Goldstone SE, et al. Risk of invasive anal cancer in HIV-infected patients with high-grade anal dysplasia: a population-based cohort study. *Dis Colon Rectum.* 2019;62(8):934–940.
32. Palefsky JM, Lee JY, Jay N, et al. Treatment of anal high-grade squamous intraepithelial lesions to prevent anal cancer. *N Engl J Med.* 2022;386(24):2273–2282.
33. Megill C, Wilkin T. Topical therapies for the treatment of anal high-grade squamous intraepithelial lesions. *Semin Colon Rectal Surg.* 2017;28(2):86–90.
34. Goldstone SE, Giuliano AR, Palefsky JM, et al. Efficacy, immunogenicity, and safety of a quadrivalent HPV vaccine in men: results of an open-label, long-term extension of a randomised, placebo-controlled, phase 3 trial. *Lancet Infect Dis.* 2022;22(3): 413–425.
35. National Cancer Institute. Cancer stat facts: anal cancer. [cited 2020 1/28] https://seer.cancer.gov/statfacts/html/anus.html
36. Glynne-Jones R, Sebag-Montefiore D, Meadows HM, et al. Best time to assess complete clinical response after chemoradiotherapy in squamous cell carcinoma of the anus (ACT II): a post-hoc analysis of randomised controlled phase 3 trial. *Lancet Oncol.* 2017;18(3):347–356.
37. Kibbi N, Owen JL, Worley B, et al. Anatomic subtype differences in extramammary Paget disease: a meta-analysis. *JAMA Dermatol.* 2024;160(4):417–424.
38. Lee GC, Kunitake H, Stafford C, Bordeianou LG, Francone TD, Ricciardi R. High risk of proximal and local neoplasms in 2206 patients with anogenital extramammary Paget's disease. *Dis Colon Rectum.* 2019;62(11):1283–1293.
39. Shah RR, Shah K, Wilson BN, et al. Extramammary Paget disease. Part II. Evidence-based approach to management. *J Am Acad Dermatol.* 2024;91(3):421–430.
40. Matsuda A, Miyashita M, Matsumoto S, et al. Abdominoperineal resection provides better local control but equivalent overall survival to local excision of anorectal malignant melanoma: a systematic review. *Ann Surg.* 2015;261(4):670–677.
41. Smith HG, Glen J, Turnbull N, et al. Less is more: a systematic review and meta-analysis of the outcomes of radical versus conservative primary resection in anorectal melanoma. *Eur J Cancer.* 2020;135:113–120.
42. Griewank KG, Scolyer RA, Thompson JF, Flaherty KT, Schadendorf D, Murali R. Genetic alterations and personalized medicine in melanoma: progress and future prospects. *J Natl Cancer Inst.* 2014;106(2):djt435.

68

Appendiceal Diseases

Ana C. De Roo

Key Points

1 Recent data indicate an immune-related role for the appendix as a repository for beneficial bacteria of the microbiome.

2 Acute appendicitis, one of the most common urgent abdominal conditions in high-income countries, is considered to be the result of obstruction due to appendicolith, inflammation of lymphoid aggregates, or other blockage of the appendiceal lumen.

3 Signs and symptoms of appendicitis may be especially vague in the early stages, due to autonomic innervation, and become more pronounced with progressive inflammation of the somatically innervated parietal peritoneum.

4 An abdominal computed tomography (CT) scan is the imaging test of choice among patients with clinical signs of appendicitis.

5 Complicated appendicitis refers to the presence of abscess or perforation and occurs in about 10% of cases in the United States.

6 Controversy persists about the role of interval appendectomy among patients with complicated appendicitis. Adults with complicated appendicitis who do not undergo interval appendectomy should at least undergo a follow-up CT scan and/or colonoscopy to rule out other pathology.

7 Substantial randomized controlled trial data support using antibiotics first among patients with uncomplicated appendicitis, absence of appendicolith, and the ability to follow up; still, about 30% of patients can expect to fail nonoperative management in the 90 days after diagnosis, increasing to 40% at 1 year, and 46% at 2 years.

8 Appendicitis is the most common nonobstetrical abdominal condition of pregnancy and should be treated by appendectomy due to high risk for premature delivery or fetal demise.

ANATOMY AND PHYSIOLOGY

The vermiform appendix is a finger-like, antimesenteric projection of bowel, approximately 6 mm in diameter and up to about 9 cm long, attached at the cecum as a closed tube. It sits adjacent to the ileocecal valve at the proximal convergence of the taeniae coli. Its free end is mobile and can extend in any direction. In a postmortem analysis of 10,000 cases in England,[1] Wakeley described its location primarily in relation to the cecum and ileum: retrocecal, 65.3%; pelvic, 31%; subcecal, 2.3%; preileal (anterior), 1%; and right paracolic gutter and postileal (posterior), 0.4%. As with the small intestine and colon, the wall of the appendix consists of mucosa, submucosa, muscularis externa, and serosa. The appendix is innervated by the autonomic nervous system and thus lacks somatic pain fibers. The appendiceal artery, a branch of the ileocolic artery, provides the blood supply, and is encased in the mesoappendix, a short extension of ileal mesentery. Similar to the terminal ileum, the submucosa harbors numerous lymphoid follicles.

Most nonhuman mammals have no appendix, which was considered support for the long-standing theory that it was a vestigial organ that may have assisted with cellulose digestion
1 but had no current function. More recently, however, investigators have proposed an immune-related role as a repository for beneficial bacteria of the microbiome and a site of defense against pathogens.[2] Theoretically, if an enteric pathogen were to destroy the colonic microbiome, the size and shape of the appendix would facilitate a protected space for normal flora that could then repopulate the colon.

APPENDICITIS

Etiology and Pathophysiology

At more than 270,000 cases annually, acute appendicitis is one of the most common urgent abdominal conditions in the United
2 States with a lifetime risk of 6% to 9%.[3] Due to its unique structure, inflammation of the appendix or acute appendicitis generally is considered the result of a closed loop obstruction, either by a foreign body such as an appendicolith or alternatively by inflammation of lymphoid aggregates, effectively blocking the appendiceal lumen. The ensuing bacterial entrapment causes further activation of lymphoid cells, cytokines, and edema; all the while, mucus accumulates contributing to luminal pressure. The resultant dilation leads to increased mural pressure, venous congestion, ischemia, and ultimately necrosis and perforation. This convenient etiologic explanation is likely accurate in many cases. The common finding of an appendicolith could explain the higher prevalence of appendicitis among persons who consume a Western diet.[4] The finding of lymphoid hyperplasia could explain the higher prevalence of appendicitis among persons between the ages of 10 and 20, who have substantially more lymphoid tissue in the appendiceal submucosa. In older adults, appendicolith or mass are more common sources of obstruction and appendicitis.

Although appendicitis traditionally was thought to progress steadily until perforation, a more recent theory posits that complicated (perforated) and uncomplicated appendicitis may have different etiologies, suggesting that they should be treated as different entities. An analysis of the National Hospital Discharge Survey between 1975 and 2006 described outbreaks and

Table 68.1. Signs of Acute Appendicitis on Physical Examination

Name	Description	Implication
McBurney Sign	Pain with pressure to McBurney point	Right lower quadrant inflammation
Dunphy Sign	Right lower quadrant abdominal pain with abdominal wall flexion, for example, cough	Inflammation of the parietal peritoneum
Rovsing Sign	Referred pain at the right lower quadrant after pressure to the left lower quadrant abdomen	Right lower quadrant inflammation
Psoas Sign	Right lower quadrant abdominal pain upon tapping the right heel	Retrocecal inflammation
Obturator Sign	Pain with internal and external rotation of the right hip	Pelvic inflammation

seasonal variation in the diagnosis of uncomplicated appendicitis,[5] supporting an infectious etiology, and noted epidemiologic similarities between uncomplicated appendicitis and influenza that were not identified for *perforated* appendicitis.[6]

Diagnosis

History and Physical Examination

3 Vague periumbilical pain, the most common symptom of early appendicitis, can be attributed to the embryologic origin of autonomic fibers in the midgut. As the appendix becomes increasingly inflamed, it activates somatic pain fibers in the parietal peritoneum. Most often, this will be at McBurney point, one-third of the distance from the anterior superior iliac spine to the umbilicus. The numerous potential locations of the middle and tip of the appendix can result in a confusing array of possible symptoms, as reflected by the variety of signs associated with different anatomic sites (**Table 68.1**). The most common symptoms, in addition to periumbilical pain that migrates to the right lower quadrant, are anorexia, nausea, and vomiting. Further symptoms can include diarrhea, constipation, and even burning with urination, although all are unlikely to be as severe or as progressive as pain.

Physical examination signs can be just as ambiguous as the clinical history. Patients may have a low-grade fever that is rarely higher than 102 °F and may or may not have mild tachycardia. Although tenderness to pressure at McBurney point is highly suggestive, it is not entirely reliable, especially among women who may be experiencing ovarian torsion or cystic disease. Conversely, cervical motion tenderness during a pelvic examination may indicate an inflamed pelvic appendix rather than a gynecologic condition. Rebound tenderness and involuntary guarding, or contraction of the abdominal wall in response to pressure, can help to clarify peritoneal irritation. To establish retrocecal appendicitis, stimulating the iliopsoas muscle by tapping the heel or extending the right hip may be helpful.

Laboratory and Imaging Studies

The white blood count and a urine analysis are the most important laboratory values in the diagnosis of appendicitis. While the white blood count may be normal, it is more likely to be in the slightly high range from 10 to 14,000 white blood cells per mL. Urine analysis may show increased leukocytes or microscopic hematuria. In the setting of a suspicious history and physical examination, a C-reactive protein level >10 mg/mL is suggestive of acute appendicitis and >50 mg/mL suggests complicated appendicitis.

Given the imprecision of clinical history, physical examination, and laboratory signs, several authors have proposed grading schemes to assist with diagnosis (**Table 68.2**). The rationale for a scoring system rather than simply relying on imaging is based on concerns for radiation associated with CT scan, especially among children and the inaccuracy and operator dependency of ultrasound. In a retrospective study of 747 consecutive children who presented to a Dutch hospital with symptoms concerning for appendicitis, a head-to-head comparison of the three grading schemes was performed. Thirty-six percent of patients overall were diagnosed with acute appendicitis. The area under the receiver–operator curve of the appendicitis inflammatory response (AIR) score was 0.90, the Alvarado score was 0.87, and the pediatric appendicitis score was 0.82.[7] The AIR outperforms the Alvarado score in adults as well.[8]

Ideally, imaging studies should be sufficiently accurate to help the clinician balance timeliness of treatment with a reduction in unnecessary operations. Ultrasound, while operator dependent and not reliably accurate, is still favored among children as a means to spare radiation exposure. Signs of appendicitis by ultrasound include a target lesion (thick-walled, noncompressible lumen), peritoneal fluid, or abscess. For adults with suspected appendicitis, helical CT with thin-
4 cut slices and intravenous contrast is standard. Signs of appendicitis on CT scan include appendicolith, mesenteric fat stranding, diameter >10 to 13 mm, appendiceal wall thickening >3 mm, and phlegmon (**Fig. 68.1**); complicated or perforated appendicitis can be identified through periappendiceal gas or abscess. Because radiation exposure is an increasing concern with CT scan, a single-institution randomized controlled trial powered for noninferiority compared low-dose and standard-dose CT scans among 891 adults with suspected appendicitis.[9] The study demonstrated similar rates of negative appendectomy (3.2% and 3.5%) and similar rates of perforation (26.5% and 23.3%), concluding that low-dose CT is not inferior to standard-dose CT for the diagnosis of appendicitis in young adults. Although uptake of a low-dose protocol has been slow, additional randomized controlled trials have supported these findings.[10] While magnetic resonance imaging (MRI) has high sensitivity and specificity, it is currently an expensive and uncommon approach for diagnosing appendicitis, and is more commonly used to diagnose appendicitis during pregnancy to spare the fetus from radiation.

Differential Diagnosis

The differential diagnosis must be considered during the preliminary workup and should include enteritis, pyelonephritis, nephrolithiasis, gynecologic issues such as ovarian torsion or cyst, tubo-ovarian abscess or tubal pregnancy, small bowel or cecal obstruction or perforation, Meckel diverticulitis, inflammatory bowel disease, and cecal diverticulitis or cancer. Clinical examination, laboratory studies, and CT scan can help to distinguish most but not all of these conditions as demonstrated by a low but ongoing negative appendectomy rate.

Management

Complicated Appendicitis

Traditional management of appendicitis has focused on performance of surgical resection as rapidly as possible after diagnosis, and appendectomy remains the most common urgent abdominal operation in the United States. Much of the rationale for urgent surgery was related to a perceived risk of impending perforation and a desire to avoid sepsis. Complicated appendicitis refers to

Table 68.2. Grading Schemes to Assess Risk of Acute Appendicitis

Scoring System	Symptoms (Points)	Signs (Points)	Laboratory Values (Points)	Score (Sum of Points)	Recommendation
Alvarado Score	Migration of pain (1) Anorexia (1) Nausea/ vomiting (1)	Right lower quadrant tenderness (2) Rebound pain (1) Elevated temperature ≥37.3 °C or 99 °F (1)	Leukocytes ≥10,000 (2) Differential ≥75% polymorphonuclear cells (1)	5–6 7–8 9–10	Compatible with appendicitis; observation Probable appendicitis; surgery High probability of appendicitis; surgery
Pediatric Appendicitis Score (PAS)	Migration of pain (1) Anorexia (1) Nausea/ vomiting (1)	Right lower quadrant tenderness (2) Cough/hopping/ percussion/tenderness in the right lower quadrant (2) Elevated temperature ≥37.3 °C or 99 °F (1)	Leukocytes ≥10,000 (2) Differential ≥75% polymorphonuclear cells (1)	≤5 ≥6	Not appendicitis; observation Appendicitis; surgery
Appendicitis Inflammatory Response Score (AIR)	Nausea/ vomiting (1)	Right lower quadrant tenderness (1) Rebound tenderness (1, 2, 3) Elevated temperature ≥38.5 °C	Leukocytes 10,000–15,000 (1); ≥15,000 (2) Differential polymorphonuclear cells 70–84% (1); ≥85% (2) C-reactive protein 10–49 mg/mL (1); ≥50 mg/mL (2)	0–4 5–8 9–12	Low probability of appendicitis Indeterminate group; in-hospital observation with additional imaging or diagnostic laparoscopy High probability of appendicitis; surgery

Adapted from Macco S, Vrouenraets BC, de Castro SMM. Evaluation of scoring systems in predicting acute appendicitis in children. *Surgery.* 2016;160(6):1599–1604.

appendicitis accompanied by gangrene, abscess, or phlegmon, indicating micro- and macroperforation, and occurs in up to
5 10% of acute appendicitis cases.

In the setting of complicated appendicitis, there are essentially three management options: urgent appendectomy, interval (delayed) appendectomy, or nonoperative management. The second management option entails controlling infection and reducing inflammation using antibiotics, percutaneous drainage if possible, and supportive measures such as bowel rest and intravenous hydration. After a 6- to 12-week interval, laparoscopic or open appendectomy is performed. The rationale for interval appendectomy rather than urgent appendectomy is that nearby structures are less likely to be injured when inflammation has subsided. Interval appendectomy was first described in the mid-20th century and gained traction in the early 2000s as preoperative CT scans became common practice, enabling preoperative identification of appendiceal abscesses.

As interval appendectomy became an accepted management strategy, surgeons began to question the need for any appendectomy, thereby giving rise to the third treatment option for complicated appendicitis: antibiotics, drainage if possible, and supportive measures followed by no appendectomy. Proponents of nonoperative management cite a low rate of previously unrecognized pathology, low rate of recurrent appendicitis, and a high operative complication rate. By contrast, advocates of interval appendectomy for complicated appendicitis cite the concern for possible cystadenoma or malignancy, early recurrence, and low complication rate. The complication rate is generally less than 10% and complications are often limited to wound infection or abdominal abscess; the sheer volume of appendectomies, however, makes the absolute complication rate higher than many other types of operations.[11] The Peri-Appendicitis Acuta (peri-APPAC) trial,[12] in which patients with complicated appendicitis who had been treated with antibiotics and drainage if necessary were randomized 3 months later to appendectomy versus MRI and colonoscopy. This study was terminated prematurely on ethical grounds due to 20% rate of malignancy, about 10-fold higher than expected from a meta-analysis of 61 studies.[13] Regardless, adult patients with perforated appendicitis who do not undergo an immediate or interval appendectomy must be evaluated with a follow-up CT and/or colonoscopy in order to ascertain the absence of other pathology, such as Crohn disease
6 or cancer.

Surgical Approaches

The classic open appendectomy operation starts over McBurney point with an oblique incision of the skin in Langerhans lines, incision of the external oblique aponeurosis, and a muscle-splitting incision before opening the peritoneum. If the appendix is not immediately apparent, the terminal ileum is grasped and followed to the cecum. At times, depending on the location of the appendix and the patient's body habitus, it may be necessary to mobilize the cecum laterally to locate the appendiceal base. If the base is obscured by substantial inflammation, following the teniae proximally can be helpful. The appendiceal artery is divided and the appendiceal base is ligated usually with a stapler or suture. The appendix is amputated just distal to ligation and removed. Previously, the appendiceal stump was inverted with suture to prevent mucocele formation or fistula, but there are no data to support this step. The peritoneum and pelvis then should be irrigated, and the abdominal wall is closed in layers. The key steps of appendectomy are listed in **Table 68.3**.

Laparoscopic appendectomy is essentially the same operation as open appendectomy, usually performed through three laparoscopic ports instead of an open incision. With the exception of the laparoscopic-specific procedures such as insufflation of the abdomen, each step is the same, and the major

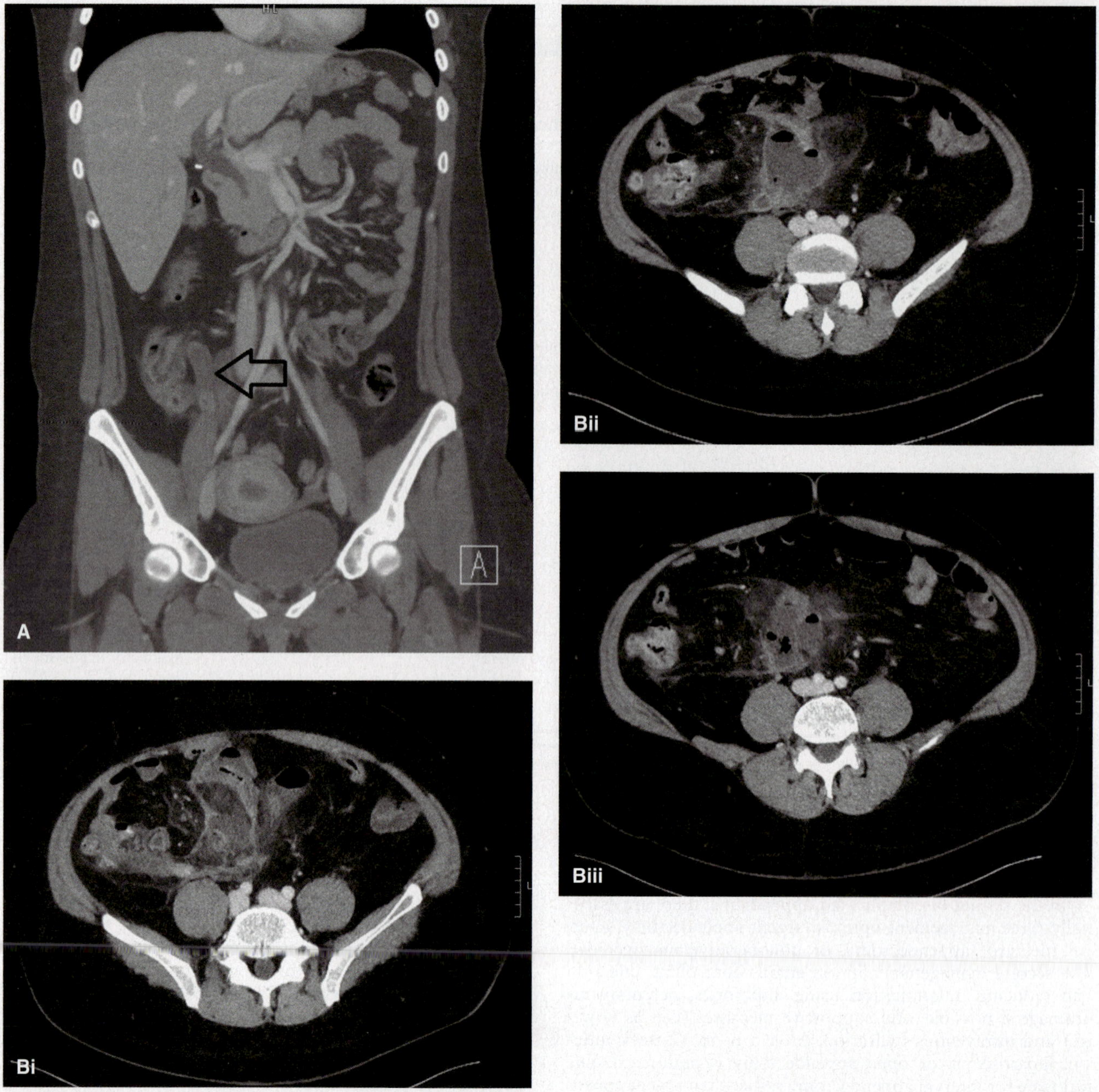

Figure 68.1. Computed tomography displaying (**A**) nonperforated appendicitis with a distended, thick-walled appendix; (**B**) perforated appendicitis with an adjacent abscess.

potential risk categories (bleeding, abscess, wound infection, damage to nearby structures) are also the same. Compared with open appendectomy, the laparoscopic approach leads to fewer wound infections, reduced hospital stay, and reduced pain, and is an advantageous approach in the setting of uncertainty or unexpected operative findings with a normal appendix.[14] Both randomized trials and case series have demonstrated that the laparoscopic approach confers about 35% higher odds of organ space surgical site infection than the open approach, but the risk remains well under 10%.

Single-incision laparoscopic surgery (SILS), in which a single port site scar is hidden in the umbilicus, has garnered interest for it is a cosmetic advantage over conventional laparoscopic appendectomy. Although case duration and expense can be much higher, the single-incision approach in pediatric surgery is increasingly accepted. A large single-institution cohort study found that the need for conversion to conventional laparoscopy was associated with obesity, male sex, or complicated appendicitis.[15]

In the event that an open or laparoscopic operation is performed and a normal appendix is identified, a search for other pathology should be conducted. Specifically, the surgeon should examine the terminal ileum for evidence of Crohn disease or more proximally a Meckel diverticulum, the cecum, or redundant sigmoid, for diverticulitis, Crohn disease, or neoplasm, and in a woman, the adnexal structures for evidence of cysts, inflammation, infection, neoplasm, or other mass. A major advantage of the laparoscopic approach is the ease of examination of and potentially intervention on nonappendiceal structures.

Nonoperative Management of Uncomplicated Appendicitis

Traditional surgical management of appendicitis has been based on the poorly supported hypothesis that surgically untreated appendicitis leads to perforation and pelvic abscess. Even in the best case scenario, an appendectomy is painful and requires several weeks of recovery (3 to 4 weeks

Table 68.3. Key Technical Steps for Appendectomy

Key Steps

1. Gain access to the abdomen
2. Identify the appendix
3. Dissect free the base of the appendix
4. Divide the base of the appendix
5. Control and divide the appendiceal artery and mesoappendix
6. Remove the appendix from the abdomen
7. Close the abdomen

Pearls

1. If the appendix is challenging to identify, follow the confluence of the taenia coli, or grasp the ligament of Treves for assistance mobilizing the terminal ileum and cecum. It may be necessary to mobilize the cecum from the retroperitoneum to locate a retrocecal appendix
2. If the base of the appendix is compromised, staple across a small portion of healthy appearing cecum just beyond the base of the appendix
3. If the base is obscured by inflammation, it may be helpful to divide the mesoappendix first with an energy device

Potential Pitfalls

1. Incorporating terminal ileum or cecum into the staple line inadvertently
2. Rupturing the appendix—spilling infection or mucinous neoplasm

for laparoscopic and 4 to 6 weeks for open surgery) before return to usual activity. Recovery time is especially pertinent because appendicitis is more common among active young adults[16] who are more likely than their older counterparts to hold physically demanding jobs, have a high deductible health insurance plan, and lack paid sick leave. Appendectomy also has a complication rate from 3% to 21%[11,16] and is costly at a median charge per case of $33,000 in 2012.[17]

Noting circumstances in which delayed or omitted appendectomy has *not* resulted in peritonitis, or even in progression of disease, many surgical investigators have proposed that nonoperative management is a viable option among selected patients.[18] Thus far, six randomized trials suggest that broad-spectrum antibiotics may change what was perceived as the natural history of acute appendicitis and that many adult
7 patients can be treated with antibiotics alone.[19–24] The Comparison of Outcomes of Antibiotic Drugs and Appendectomy (CODA) trial compared 10 days of antibiotic therapy, including at least 24 hours of intravenous administration, with appendectomy and found that among 776 adults with CT confirmed uncomplicated appendicitis who were treated with antibiotics, 29% underwent appendectomy by 90 days, 41% of those with an appendicolith and 25% of those without.[23] The complication rate was higher in the antibiotics group, but this was driven by the high complication rate in patients with appendicoliths. In longer-term follow-up, 40% of patients initially managed with antibiotics required appendectomy, and 46% underwent appendectomy by 2 years.[25] The trial was designed as a noninferiority trial, meaning that it was powered to detect whether nonoperative management with antibiotics was inferior to the gold standard of appendectomy, when evaluating the primary outcome, which was the European Quality of Life-5 Dimensions (EQ-5D) questionnaire. The study team powered the study to assess for a difference in 0.05 points in the EQ-5D score. That is, if nonoperative management was less than 0.05 points lower, it would be deemed noninferior to appendectomy. The CODA trial found antibiotics were noninferior to appendectomy with a mean difference of 0.01 points (95% confidence interval, 0.001–0.03). Patients treated with antibiotics, as compared to surgical patients, had a higher rate of repeat hospitalization within 90 days (24% vs 5%) and emergency department visits (9% vs 4%), but reported fewer days of missed work (5.26 vs 8.73). These trends were maintained when analysis was limited to patients without appendicoliths. The rate of incidental neoplasm was 0.6%, in line with other series' reports.[26] Of the 12 patients diagnosed with a neoplasm, 5 underwent initial management with antibiotics, and were diagnosed with a neoplasm at a mean time of 91 days (range 36 to 232 days).

There is one aspect of nonoperative management upon which all agree, however: no studies to date support a nonoperative approach for every patient who presents with signs and symptoms of acute appendicitis. Identifying appropriate patients for nonoperative management—and importantly, those for whom such an approach is likely to fail—is an area of keen interest among surgical researchers. Among the currently open questions are how to compare the relative benefits, harms, and costs of each treatment option and under what circumstances they differ. The risk of postoperative complications, for example, varies widely by patient age, comorbid disease, and clinical presentation. Moreover, the potential harms of broad-spectrum antibiotics, radiation exposure, and appendicitis recurrence are not easily quantified.

Special Populations

Pregnancy

Appendicitis is the most common nonobstetrical urgent abdominal condition among pregnant women, followed closely by
8 cholecystitis. Both can be difficult to diagnose, especially in late pregnancy, due to common pregnancy symptoms of general nausea, mild leukocytosis, and compression or relocation of structures by the enlarging uterus. Consequently, appendicitis in pregnancy is associated with late presentation, maternal morbidity, and fetal mortality. In a cohort analysis of 3,133 pregnant women who underwent appendectomy,[27] fetal loss and preterm delivery occurred in 6% and 11% of those with complicated appendicitis compared with 2% and 4% of those with uncomplicated appendicitis. Given the risk, nonoperative management is not considered an acceptable option among pregnant women. While there has been some debate about the safety of a laparoscopic versus open approach, data indicate that in experienced hands, there is no elevated risk of fetal loss or preterm labor based on surgical approach and guidelines recommend laparoscopy while the fundus is lower than the umbilicus.[28]

Older Adults

The diagnosis of appendicitis in frail or older adult patients may be challenging and is often delayed. Older adults are much more likely to present with complicated and specifically perforated appendicitis. In contrast to younger patients, a precipitous leukopenia may be identified rather than leukocytosis. In addition to perforation, the rate of unexpected malignancy is substantially higher as patient age increases. In the Peri-APPAC trial noted above,[12] all cases of malignancy occurred in patients aged >40 years. Among older adults with apparently perforated appendicitis, antibiotic treatment alone is inadequate and a planned resection should follow. In the setting of suspected cancer, a very conservative approach traditionally would include open appendectomy through a midline incision.

APPENDICEAL NEOPLASMS

Patients with appendiceal neoplasms are at increased risks of synchronous colonic pathology, therefore should be evaluated with colonoscopy (CPG).[29]

Neuroendocrine Tumors

About two-thirds of all appendiceal neoplasms originate from neuroendocrine tissue and about half of all neuroendocrine neoplasms in the gut are located within the appendix. Neuroendocrine tumors of the appendix are usually diagnosed incidentally after appendectomy. Most are low grade, confined to the appendix, without synchronous neuroendocrine tumors, and small at the time of diagnosis. Appendiceal neuroendocrine tumors <2 cm in size and without the advanced features of high mitotic index (>2 mitoses per high-power field), Ki-67 >3%, mesoappendiceal invasion, or positive margin can be managed by appendectomy alone.[30,31] Follow-up right colectomy is recommended for neuroendocrine tumors with advanced features or size ≥2 cm due to concern for lymphatic spread. Hematogenous metastasis to the liver is also possible but extremely rare. The so-called goblet cell carcinoid tumors have been reclassified as adenocarcinoma as they are not of neuroendocrine origin.[32]

Appendiceal Mucinous Neoplasms

Low-grade appendiceal mucinous neoplasms (LAMNs) and high-grade appendiceal mucinous neoplasms (HAMNs) are characterized by a dilated, mucus-filled appendiceal lumen. The term mucocele is no longer considered a pathologic diagnosis. LAMN and HAMN do not metastasize hematogenously or lymphatically and rarely invade structures; instead, in a phenomenon known as "pushing invasion," the wall of the appendix is dissected by acellular mucin, which can then spread over surfaces.[32] An appendix in which LAMN is entirely contained without spillage into the peritoneal cavity can be treated with appendectomy alone. In the presence of intraperitoneal spillage, however, intraperitoneal mucinous deposits, or pseudomyxoma peritonei, can develop, filling the, paracolic gutters, diaphragmatic peritoneum, pelvic peritoneum, and omentum. HAMN contains high-grade dysplasia but no infiltrative features. As a newly characterized diagnosis, its behavior is not well understood, but it is believed to be more likely to contribute to aggressive peritoneal disease than LAMN. Mucinous adenocarcinomas are similar to HAMN but also infiltrate surrounding structures and histologically display tumor budding surrounded by desmoplastic stroma. In the setting of peritoneal disease, cytoreductive surgery and hyperthermic intraperitoneal chemotherapy (HIPEC) can be considered.

Adenocarcinomas

Adenocarcinomas of the appendix are extremely rare and are characterized like those of the colon. Appendiceal adenocarcinoma should be treated by a right colectomy, unless identified incidentally after appendectomy and showing only low-risk features: T1, low grade, and no lymphovascular invasion. Goblet cell adenocarcinomas have been recently reclassified, as noted above, and can exhibit a range of tumor biology, including transmural spread. These tumors can be hard to distinguish pathologically from signet cell carcinoma. In both cases, aggressive treatment with right colectomy and a search for transmural, lymphatic, and hematogenous spread is warranted.

ACKNOWLEDGMENT

We gratefully acknowledge the contributions of previous edition author, Arden M. Morris, as portions of those chapters have been retained in this revision.

References

1. Wakeley CP. The position of the vermiform appendix as ascertained by an analysis of 10,000 cases. *J Anat*. 1933;67(Pt 2):277–283.
2. Kooij IA, Sahami S, Meijer SL, Buskens CJ, te Velde AA. The immunology of the vermiform appendix: a review of the literature. *Clin Exp Immunol*. 2016;186(1):1–9.
3. Kozak LJ, DeFrances CJ, Hall MJ. National hospital discharge survey: 2004 annual summary with detailed diagnosis and procedure data. *Vital Health Stat 13*. 2006;(162):1–209.
4. Ferris M, Quan S, Kaplan BS, et al. The global incidence of appendicitis: a systematic review of population-based studies. *Ann Surg*. 2017;266(2):237–241.
5. Livingston EH, Woodward WA, Sarosi GA, Haley RW. Disconnect between incidence of nonperforated and perforated appendicitis: implications for pathophysiology and management. *Ann Surg*. 2007;245(6):886–892.
6. Alder AC, Fomby TB, Woodward WA, Haley RW, Sarosi G, Livingston EH. Association of viral infection and appendicitis. *Arch Surg*. 2010;145(1):63–71.
7. Macco S, Vrouenraets BC, de Castro SMM. Evaluation of scoring systems in predicting acute appendicitis in children. *Surgery*. 2016;160(6):1599–1604.
8. de Castro SMM, Ünlü C, Steller EP, van Wagensveld BA, Vrouenraets BC. Evaluation of the appendicitis inflammatory response score for patients with acute appendicitis. *World J Surg*. 2012;36(7):1540–1545.
9. Kim K, Kim YH, Kim SY, et al. Low-dose abdominal CT for evaluating suspected appendicitis. *N Engl J Med*. 2012;366(17): 1596–1605.
10. Sippola S, Grönroos J, Sallinen V, et al. A randomised placebo-controlled double-blind multicentre trial comparing antibiotic therapy with placebo in the treatment of uncomplicated acute appendicitis: APPAC III trial study protocol. *BMJ Open*. 2018;8(11):e023623.
11. Scott JW, Olufajo OA, Brat GA, et al. Use of national burden to define operative emergency general surgery. *JAMA Surg*. 2016; 151(6):e160480.
12. Mällinen J, Rautio T, Grönroos J, et al. Risk of appendiceal neoplasm in periappendicular abscess in patients treated with interval appendectomy vs follow-up with magnetic resonance imaging: 1-year outcomes of the peri–appendicitis acuta randomized clinical trial. *JAMA Surg*. 2019;154(3):200–207.
13. Andersson RE, Petzold MG. Nonsurgical treatment of appendiceal abscess or phlegmon: a systematic review and meta-analysis. *Ann Surg*. 2007;246(5):741–748.
14. Jaschinski T, Mosch CG, Eikermann M, Neugebauer EA, Sauerland S. Laparoscopic versus open surgery for suspected appendicitis. *Cochrane Database Syst Rev*. 2018;11(11):CD001546.
15. Gates NL, Rampp RD, Koontz CC, Holcombe JM, Bhattacharya SD. Single-incision laparoscopic appendectomy in children and conversion to multiport appendectomy. *J Surg Res*. 2019;235:223–226.
16. Wray CJ, Kao LS, Millas SG, Tsao K, Ko TC. Acute appendicitis: controversies in diagnosis and management. *Curr Probl Surg*. 2013;50(2):54–86.
17. Hsia RY, Kothari AH, Srebotnjak T, Maselli J. Health care as a "market good"? Appendicitis as a case study. *Arch Intern Med*. 2012;172(10):818–819.
18. Livingston E, Vons C. Treating appendicitis without surgery. *JAMA*. 2015;313(23):2327–2328.
19. Hansson J, Körner U, Khorram-Manesh A, Solberg A, Lundholm K. Randomized clinical trial of antibiotic therapy versus appendicectomy as primary treatment of acute appendicitis in unselected patients. *Br J Surg*. 2009;96(5):473–481.
20. Styrud J, Eriksson S, Nilsson I, et al. Appendectomy versus antibiotic treatment in acute appendicitis. A prospective multicenter randomized controlled trial. *World J Surg*. 2006;30(6):1033–1037.
21. Turhan AN, Kapan S, Kütükçü E, Yiğitbaş H, Hatipoğlu S, Aygün E. Comparison of operative and non operative management of acute appendicitis. *Ulus Travma Acil Cerrahi Derg*. 2009;15(5):459–462.
22. Vons C, Barry C, Maitre S, et al. Amoxicillin plus clavulanic acid versus appendicectomy for treatment of acute uncomplicated appendicitis: an open-label, non-inferiority, randomised controlled trial. *Lancet*. 2011;377(9777):1573–1579.
23. Collaborative C, Flum D, Davidson G, et al. A randomized trial comparing antibiotics with appendectomy for appendicitis. *N Engl J Med*. 2020;384(9).
24. Salminen P, Paajanen H, Rautio T, et al. Antibiotic therapy vs appendectomy for treatment of uncomplicated acute appendicitis: the APPAC randomized clinical trial. *JAMA*. 2015;313(23):2340–2348.
25. CODA Collaborative; Davidson GH, Flum DR, Monsell SE, et al. Antibiotics versus appendectomy for acute appendicitis – longer-term outcomes. *N Engl J Med*. 2021;385(25):2395–2397.
26. Writing Group for the CODA Collaborative. Appendiceal neoplasms in patients treated with antibiotics for acute appendicitis:

secondary analysis of the CODA randomized clinical trial. *Br J Surg*. 2023;110(12):1659–1662.

27. McGory ML, Zingmond DS, Tillou A, Hiatt JR, Ko CY, Cryer HM. Negative appendectomy in pregnant women is associated with a substantial risk of fetal loss. *J Am Coll Surg*. 2007;205(4):534–540.
28. Kumar SS, Collings AT, Wunker C, et al. SAGES guidelines for the use of laparoscopy during pregnancy. *Surg Endosc*. 2024;38(6): 2947–2963.
29. Glasgow SC, Gaertner W, Stewart D, et al. The American Society of Colon and Rectal Surgeons, clinical practice guidelines for the management of appendiceal neoplasms. *Dis Colon Rectum*. 2019;62(12):1425–1438.
30. Hrabe J. Neuroendocrine tumors of the appendix, colon, and rectum. *Surg Oncol Clin N Am*. 2020;29(2):267–279.
31. Ricci C, Ingaldi C, Alberici L, et al. Histopathological diagnosis of appendiceal neuroendocrine neoplasms: when to perform a right hemicolectomy? A systematic review and meta-analysis. *Endocrine*. 2019;66(3):460–466.
32. Carr NJ. Updates in appendix pathology: the precarious cutting edge. *Surg Pathol Clin*. 2020;13(3):469–484.

69

Section J: HERNIA AND SPLEEN

Abdominal Wall Hernias

Jenny M. Shao

Key Points

1 The concept of the "abdominal core" aims to capture the complex relationships of the circumferential soft tissues of the diaphragm superiorly, abdominal wall and flanks anterolaterally, and pelvic floor inferiorly. Maintenance of abdominal core health may include surgical (eg, hernia repair) and nonsurgical interventions (eg, physical therapy) with an emphasis on maximizing core stability and function. Major risk factors for the development of abdominal wall hernias include inadequate hernia prevention techniques during open abdominal surgery, disease processes increasing intra-abdominal pressure, connective tissue disorders, and any condition that prevents adequate wound healing.

2 Inguinal hernias constitute approximately 75% of abdominal wall hernias, with femoral hernia accounting for 5%. Femoral hernias are more common in women, but a woman with a groin hernia is still five times more likely to have an inguinal hernia (usually indirect) than a femoral hernia.

3 Watchful waiting is an acceptable alternative to routine repair for male inguinal hernia patients with minimal symptoms and those who are high-risk surgery candidates. This does not apply to females because of the higher risk of needing an emergent repair. Patients in the watchful waiting group should be aware of the likelihood of long-term crossover into treatment group. The literature dealing with groin hernia in women is insufficient making management decisions difficult. In general, a minimally invasive approach is recommended if expertise is available to avoid missing an occult femoral hernia.

4 Incisional, umbilical, and epigastric hernias account for 15%, and miscellaneous hernias make up the other 5% of all abdominal wall hernias. For ventral hernias, abdominal wall dynamics are better addressed with muscles reapproximated, contributing to improved quality of life and patient satisfaction.

5 Carefully consider decision making to select the appropriate operation by evaluation, patient, hernia, and risk factors. Tailoring the surgical approach to the patient disease process is important. Complex abdominal wall reconstruction and myofascial release (separation of an abdominal wall fascial layer from a muscular layer) are useful tools in the armamentarium of the hernia surgeon.

6 The goal is the to perform the least abdominal wall manipulation possible while still achieving tension-free fascial defect closure and providing a durable hernia repair. Hernia disease is a chronic condition; therefore, it makes sense to reserve last resort techniques for the larger and more complex hernias to avoid burning future bridges for repair.

One of the most frequently performed operations by general surgeons worldwide is the repair of an abdominal wall hernia. According to the National Institute of Diabetes and Digestive and Kidney Diseases (NIDDK), in the years 2009–2010, abdominal wall hernias were responsible for 3.6 million ambulatory care visits, 380,000 hospitalizations, and 1322 deaths in the United States.[1] As our understanding of the complexities of the abdominal wall and how it relates to abdominal core function continues to evolve, hernia surgery has started to evolve into its own subspecialty. Increasing academic interest, advancement in our understanding of abdominal wall manipulation, bolstered by technology and device development has resulted in significant changes to many hernia surgeons' practices.[2,3] In this chapter, we have provided detailed abdominal wall anatomy, an overview of general hernia prevention, treatment principles, descriptions of the different types of hernias, diagnosis, surgical decision making, hernia surgery techniques, possible pitfalls, and discussion of new advancements in the field of hernia surgery.

1 ANATOMY OF THE ABDOMINAL CORE

The concept of the "abdominal core" aims to capture the complex relationships of the circumferential soft tissues of the diaphragm superiorly, abdominal wall and flanks anterolaterally, and pelvic floor inferiorly. Maintenance of abdominal core health includes exercise, physical therapy, medical therapy (including compression garment/truss use), alternative medical therapies, surgical intervention (eg, hernia repair), and measures to prevent disease (eg, hernia prophylaxis). Most pertinent to abdominal core surgeons, the anatomy of the abdominal wall and the inguinal region are presented, first from the viewpoint of the surgeon using open techniques (anterior approach) and subsequently from the perspective of the surgeon utilizing a minimally invasive approach (posterior approach). Anatomic terms for which synonyms and eponyms are commonly used are listed in **Table 69.1**. Specific anatomic nomenclature can now be found in *Terminologia Anatomica*.

The abdominal wall is made of thin sheets of muscle and aponeurosis connective tissue in a laminar fashion. Despite the individually thin nature, lamination of the abdominal wall creates abdominal wall strength, and the weak spots of the abdominal wall most prone to hernia formation are found between areas of lamination in which only peritoneum and fascia exist. Understanding these potential areas of weakness forms the bases for both hernia prevention and repair.

Table 69.1. Anatomic Terms with Common Synonyms and Eponyms

Term; Synonyms and Eponyms
Fascial Structures/Spaces
Fatty layer of superficial fascia; panniculus adiposus; Camper fascia
Investing fascia of external abdominal oblique; fascia innominata
Membranous layer of superficial fascia; Scarpa fascia
Retroinguinal space; space of Bogros
Retropubic space; space of Retzius
Ligamentous Structures
Iliopectineal ligament; iliopectineal arch
Iliopubic tract; Thompson ligament (band)
Inguinal ligament; Poupart ligament
Lacunar ligament; Gimbernat ligament
Pectineal ligament; Cooper ligament
Aponeurosis-Derived Structures
Arcuate line; semicircular line; linea semicirculars; line of Douglas
Falx inguinalis (often incorrectly referred to as *conjoined tendon*)
Reflected inguinal ligament; reflex ligament; Colles ligament
Semilunar line; linea semilunaris

Diaphragm

The diaphragm forms the cranial "ceiling" of the abdominal core and separates the thoracic cavity from the abdominal cavity. The skeletal muscle of the diaphragm originates from the caudal aspect of the sternum, lower ribs, and vertebrae forming a dome-shaped structure with a central membranous tendon. Unlike most other skeletal muscles, several vital structures pass through openings within the diaphragm including the esophagus, aorta, and inferior vena cava. The main arterial supply to the diaphragm includes the musculophrenic and inferior phrenic arteries; venous drainage is obtained via the superior and inferior phrenic veins. Generally, vasculature of the diaphragm projects radially from the hiatal openings. The right and left phrenic nerves, originating from cervical roots C3–C5, enter the diaphragm mostly medially and branch radially outward. The esophageal hiatus has particular significance as it is a common site of herniation of intra-abdominal contents into the mediastinal space. The muscular right crus of the diaphragm, a critical landmark in hiatal hernia repair, has two components: a right and left pillar that form the esophageal hiatus itself. The left crus of the diaphragm itself typically does not encircle the esophagus. Functionally, the diaphragm is critical to breathing. As the diaphragm contracts, the thoracic cavity increases in volume, enabling inspiration. As the diaphragm relaxes, the recoil of the lungs and thorax allows for expiration. The diaphragm is also critical to forced expiratory functions such as coughing and sneezing.

Anterior Abdominal Wall and Flanks

Superficial Fascia, Vessels, and Nerves

The anterior abdominal wall consists of layers of muscle, aponeurosis, and adipose tissue. The most superficial fascial layer or *Camper fascia* continuous inferiorly with the outer layer of fascia covering the perineum and genitalia, also contains the dartos muscle fibers of the scrotum. The major blood vessels of the superficial fatty layer are the superficial epigastric vessels and superficial circumflex iliac vessels, which are tributaries of the femoral vessels. The superficial fascia is also replete with lymphatic vessels that drain into the inguinal lymph nodes inferior to the umbilicus. These lymphatic structures cross the inguinal ligament, so that they are potentially placed in the surgical field during open herniorrhaphy.

A second fascial layer in the superficial abdominal wall is the deep fascia of Scarpa and consists of compressed fibrous components of the superficial fascia. The superficial fascia also fuses with the layer of fascia (fascia innominata) investing the external abdominal oblique muscle. This fascia is bound inferiorly to the inguinal ligament and pubis before continuing onto the thigh, where it blends with the fascia lata to seal the space beneath and inferior to the inguinal ligament, which is the inferior portion of the myopectineal orifice. This portion of the inguinal region includes Hesselbach (inguinal) triangle superiorly and therefore constitutes the weakest aspect of the groin.

The skin of the anterior abdominal wall is segmentally innervated in the familiar dermatome pattern. The nerve branches to this area are derived from the anterior and lateral cutaneous branches of the ventral rami of the 7th to 12th intercostal nerves and from the ventral rami of the first and second lumbar nerves. Disruption of one of these nerves is rarely noted by the postoperative patient because the dermatome fields overlap significantly. The anterior and lateral cutaneous branches reach the subcutaneous layer by coursing between the flat lateral muscles and by piercing the sheath of the rectus abdominis.

Anterior Musculature and Ligaments

The division of the wall into anterior and posterior segments is somewhat artificial because the anterior muscles, with the exception of the rectus abdominis, arise posteriorly and also form part of the posterior wall.

The three muscles of the lateral aspect of the anterior abdominal wall (**Fig. 69.1**) are composed of a variable amount of muscle with a large aponeurosis. The aponeurosis is the tendon of insertion for the lateral muscles, and it also forms the sheath of the rectus abdominis. The midline decussation of the three aponeuroses forms the linea alba. Fibrous tissue layers are of great importance to the hernia surgeon because of their ability to support sutures. *Fascia* and *aponeurosis* are terms commonly used to describe these fibrous structures, but are often confused and used interchangeably. In this chapter, an aponeurosis is defined as the non–muscle-fiber-containing portion of a muscle usually present at insertion points. Muscle fibers are said to "give way" to the corresponding aponeurosis. Fascia, on the other hand, is the fibrous tissue that lines or envelops muscles.

External Abdominal Oblique Muscle and Associated Ligaments

The external abdominal oblique muscle (**Figs. 69.1** and **69.2A,B**) is the most superficial of the three lateral abdominal muscles. The external abdominal oblique arises from the posterior aspects of the lower eight ribs and interdigitates with both the serratus anterior and the latissimus dorsi at its origin. The direction of the muscle fibers varies from nearly horizontal in its upper portion to oblique in the middle and lower portions. The mostly horizontal fibers, which originate posteriorly, insert onto the anterior portion of the iliac crest. The obliquely arranged anteroinferior fibers of insertion fold on themselves to form the inguinal ligament. The remaining portion of the aponeurosis inserts into the linea alba after contributing to the anterior portion of the rectus abdominis sheath. Some fibers cross the linea alba to reinforce further the anterior rectus sheath of the opposite side.

The more medial fibers of the aponeurosis of the external oblique divide into a medial and a lateral crus to form the external or superficial inguinal ring. The spermatic cord (or round ligament) and branches of the ilioinguinal and genitofemoral nerves pass through this opening. The *inguinal ligament* (**Fig. 69.3**) is worthy of special consideration because of its important role as both a landmark and an integral component of many groin hernia repairs. The inguinal ligament is formed by obliquely oriented anteroinferior aponeurotic fibers of the external abdominal oblique. The ligament is

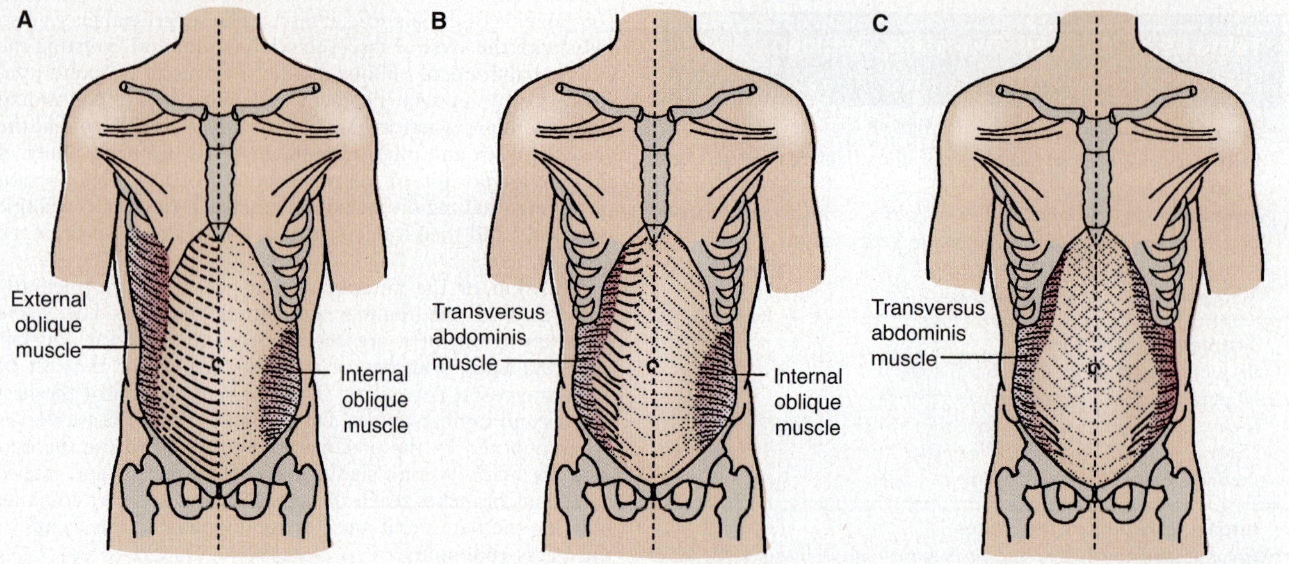

Figure 69.1. Pattern of crossing of the aponeurotic fascicles of the abdominal wall musculature. **A:** Fascicles from the right external oblique and anterior lamina of the left internal oblique. **B:** Fascicles from the right transversus abdominis and posterior lamina of the left internal oblique. **C:** Fascicles between the right and left transversus abdominis muscles.

formed when the aponeurosis folds beneath itself. Its lateral attachment is to the anterior superior iliac crest; its medial insertion is primarily on the pubic tubercle.

The medial insertion of the inguinal ligament in most persons is dual. One portion runs along the superior surface of the pubic tubercle and symphysis to form (or at least reinforce) the superior pubic ligament. The other portion is fan shaped and spans the distance between the inguinal ligament proper and the pectineal line of the pubis. This fan-shaped portion of the ligament is called the *lacunar ligament* (**Fig. 69.3**). It blends laterally with the pectineal (Cooper) ligament.

Internal Abdominal Oblique Muscle and Aponeurosis

The middle layer of the lateral abdominal group is the internal abdominal oblique muscle (**Figs. 69.1** and **69.2B,C**). This muscle primarily arises from the iliac fascia along the iliac crest and forms a band of iliac fascia fused with the inguinal ligament. The uppermost fibers course obliquely toward the distal ends of the lower three or four ("floating") ribs. The muscle fibers of the internal oblique fan out following the shape of the iliac crest so that the lowermost fibers are directed inferiorly. These fibers arch over the round ligament, or spermatic cord. Some of the lower muscle bundles in the male join fibers of the transversus abdominis to form the cremaster muscle. The aponeurosis of the internal oblique (**Fig. 69.4A**) above the level of the umbilicus splits to envelop the rectus abdominis, reforming in the midline to join and interweave with the fibers of the linea alba. Below the level of the umbilicus (**Fig. 69.4B**), the aponeurosis does not split but rather runs anterior to the rectus muscle, continues medially as a single sheet, joins the anterior rectus sheath, and finally contributes to the linea alba. The aponeurotic portion of the internal oblique is widest at the level of the umbilicus.

Transversus Abdominis Muscle and Aponeurosis

The transversus abdominis muscle (**Figs. 69.1** and **69.2C**) arises from the fascia along the iliac crest and inguinal ligament and from the lower six costal cartilages and ribs, where it interdigitates with the lateral diaphragmatic fibers. The muscle bundles of the transversus abdominis for the most part run horizontally. The lower medial fibers, however, may continue in a more inferomedial course toward the site of insertion on the crest and pecten of the pubis.

The aponeurosis of the transversus abdominis joins the posterior lamina of the internal abdominal oblique, forming above the umbilicus a portion of the posterior rectus sheath. Below the umbilicus, the transversus abdominis aponeurosis is a component of the anterior rectus sheath. The gradual termination of aponeurotic tissue on the posterior aspect of the rectus abdominis forms the arcuate line (of Douglas) (**Fig. 69.5**). The transversus abdominis muscle and aponeurosis extend medial to the semilunar line. The medial aponeurotic fibers of the transversus abdominis insert on the pecten pubis and the crest of the pubis to form the falx inguinalis. These fibers infrequently are joined by a portion of the internal oblique aponeurosis; only then is a true conjoined tendon formed.[4]

The arch formed by the termination of the aponeurotic fibers of the transversus abdominis is called the *aponeurotic arch* (**Fig. 69.5**). The area beneath the arch varies. A high arch may be a predisposing factor in direct inguinal hernia. Contraction of the transversus abdominis causes the arch to move down toward the inguinal ligament in a kind of shutter mechanism, which reinforces the weakest area of the groin when intra-abdominal pressure is raised.

Rectus Abdominis

The rectus abdominis (**Figs. 69.2D** to **69.4**) forms the central and anchoring muscle mass of the anterior abdomen. The rectus muscle arises from the fifth to the seventh costal cartilages and inserts on the pubic symphysis and pubic crest. Each rectus muscle is segmented by tendinous intersections at the levels of the xiphoid process and the umbilicus and at a point midway between these two. The principal blood supply reaches the muscle from the superior and inferior epigastric arteries (**Fig. 69.4**), which anastomose just superior to the umbilicus. Other vessels are anterior branches of the intercostal arteries; these reach the muscle by entering the lateral aspect of the rectus sheath. The innervation of the muscle is from the 7th to the 12th intercostal nerves, which laterally pierce the aponeurotic sheath of the muscle. The lateral edge of the muscle is demarcated by a slight depression in the aponeurotic fibers coursing toward the muscle; this depression is the *semilunar line*.

The small pyramidalis muscle (**Fig. 69.2D**) accompanies the rectus abdominis at its origin in a minority of people. The pyramidalis arises from the pubic symphysis. It lies within the rectus sheath and tapers to attach to the linea alba, the conjunction of the two rectus sheaths and the major site of insertion of three aponeuroses from all three lateral muscle layers.

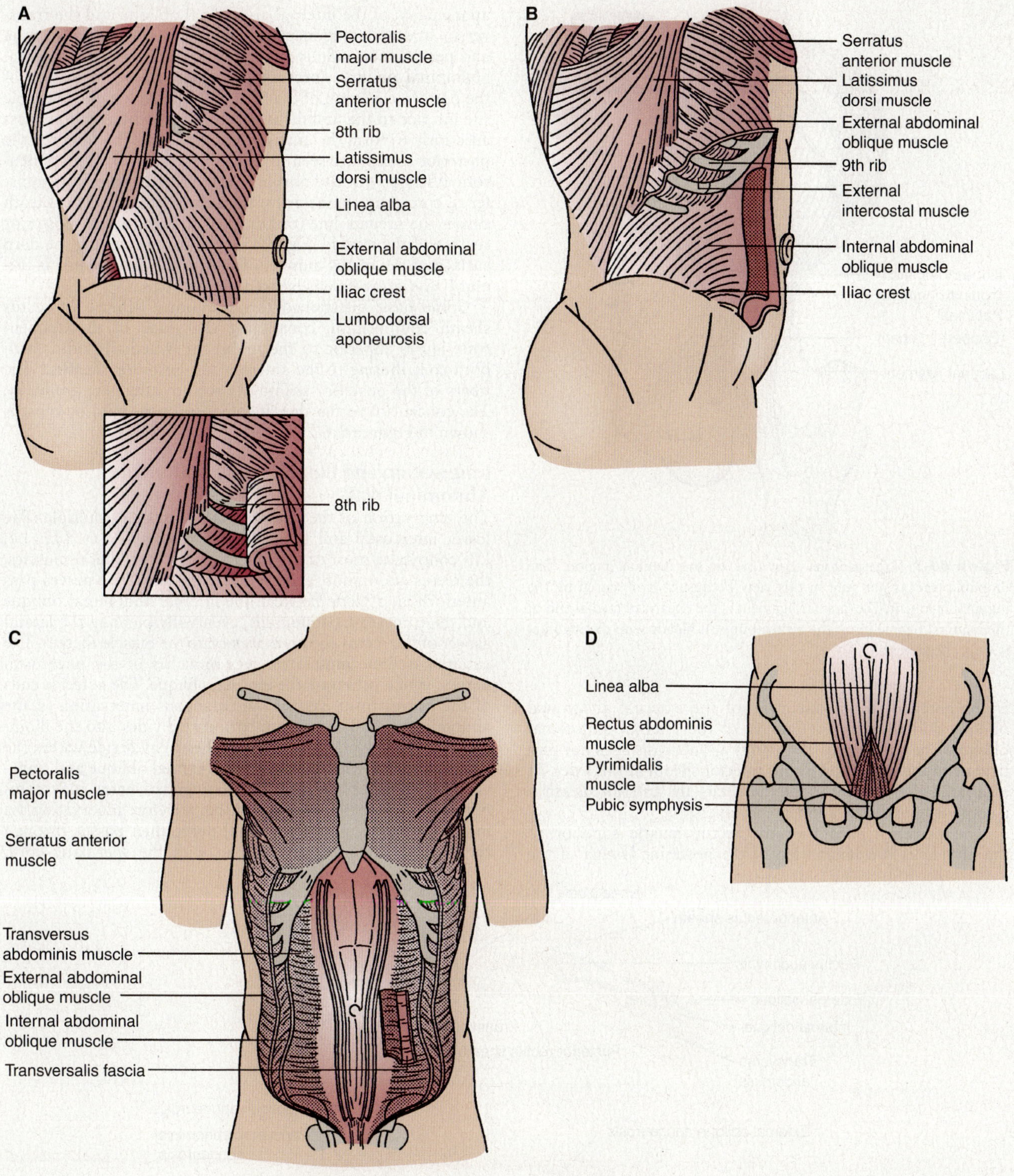

Figure 69.2. A: External oblique muscle and aponeurosis. B: Internal oblique muscle and aponeurosis. C: Transversus abdominis muscle and aponeurosis. D: Lower rectus abdominis and pyramidalis muscle. The linea alba is formed by the intermeshed fibers of the aponeuroses of the lateral muscle layers; it is tensed by the pyramidalis, which inserts into it.

Rectus Sheath

Although the components of the rectus sheath individually have been discussed in relation to the three lateral abdominal muscles, it should also be considered as a distinct entity. Three features of the rectus muscle and its sheath can be observed even topographically in well-muscled or very thin subjects:

1. The semilunar line is a slight depression in the aponeurotic fibers corresponding to the lateral edge of the rectus muscle. It marks the site of initial lateral insertion of the aponeurotic tendons of the lateral abdominal muscles.
2. The tendinous inscriptions divide each muscle into three parts.[5] These are the basis of the expression "six pack," popularized by bodybuilders.
3. The linea alba is the midline confluence of the aponeuroses of the rectus muscles and also the internal and external oblique muscles.

The composition of the rectus sheath varies depending on the level sampled. The anterior sheath superior to the umbilicus

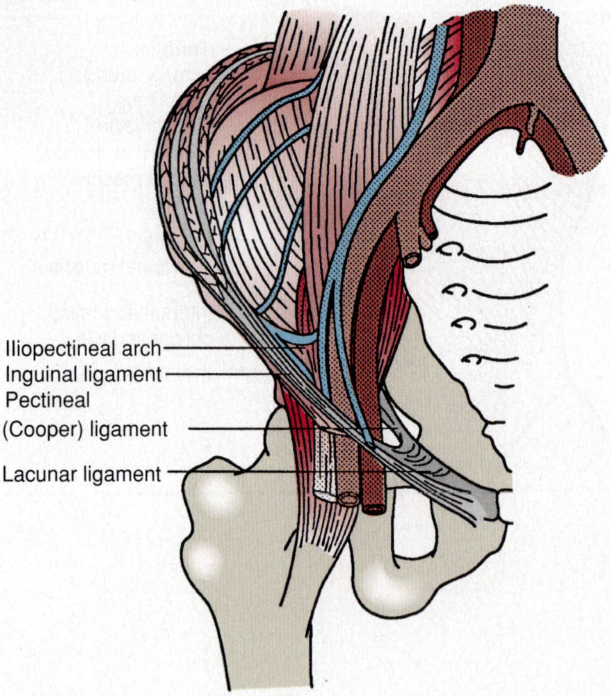

Figure 69.3. Ligamentous structures of the inguinal region. The iliopubic tract is not seen in this view because it is obscured by the inguinal ligament. The lacunar ligament is the expanded medial end of the inguinal ligament; on the pecten pubis, it blends with the inguinal (Cooper) ligament.

is composed of the aponeurosis of the external abdominal oblique and the anterior lamina of the internal abdominal oblique. The transversus abdominis aponeurosis does not participate in the formation of the anterior sheath at this level. At a variable level inferior to the umbilicus, the anterior sheath is a composite of all the aponeurotic layers.

The posterior sheath of the rectus muscle superior to the umbilicus is a lamination of the posterior lamina of the aponeurosis of the internal abdominal oblique and the transversus abdominis aponeurosis, while the transversalis fascia and peritoneum underly the aponeurotic layers. The external abdominal oblique does not participate in the formation of the posterior portion of the rectus sheath. At a highly variable site inferior to the umbilicus, all the aponeurotic tendons pass anteriorly to form the anterior rectus sheath. The fibers of the posterior sheath are seen to attenuate gradually. The aponeurotic fibers do not end abruptly at the arcuate line. This transfer of connective tissue away from the posterior rectus sheath causes the arcuate line (of Douglas) to form on the posterior surface of the muscle (**Fig. 69.5**). The tissue covering the deep surface of the rectus muscle inferior to the arcuate line is primarily the transversalis fascia and peritoneum.

Some have questioned this traditional scheme of rectus sheath composition, contending that each of the aponeurotic layers superior to the umbilicus is actually bifid, with both contributing to the anterior and posterior sheaths.[6] The fibers of the posterior sheath are seen to attenuate gradually. The concept of rectus sheath composition favored by most is shown in **Figure 69.6**.[7]

Innervation and Blood Supply of the Anterior Abdominal Wall

The innervation of the anterior wall muscles is multiple. The lower intercostal and upper lumbar nerves (T7 to T12, L1, L2) contribute most of the innervation to the lateral muscles, the rectus abdominis, and the overlying skin. The nerves pass anteriorly in a plane between the internal abdominal oblique and the transversus abdominis, eventually piercing the lateral aspect of the rectus sheath to innervate the muscle therein. The external oblique muscle receives branches of the intercostal nerves, which penetrate the internal oblique. The anterior ends of the nerves form part of the cutaneous innervation of the abdominal wall. The first lumbar nerve divides into the ilioinguinal and iliohypogastric nerves. These may divide within the psoas major muscle or between the internal oblique and transversus abdominis muscles. The ilioinguinal nerve may communicate with the iliohypogastric nerve before innervating the internal oblique. The ilioinguinal nerve then passes through the external inguinal ring to run with the spermatic cord,

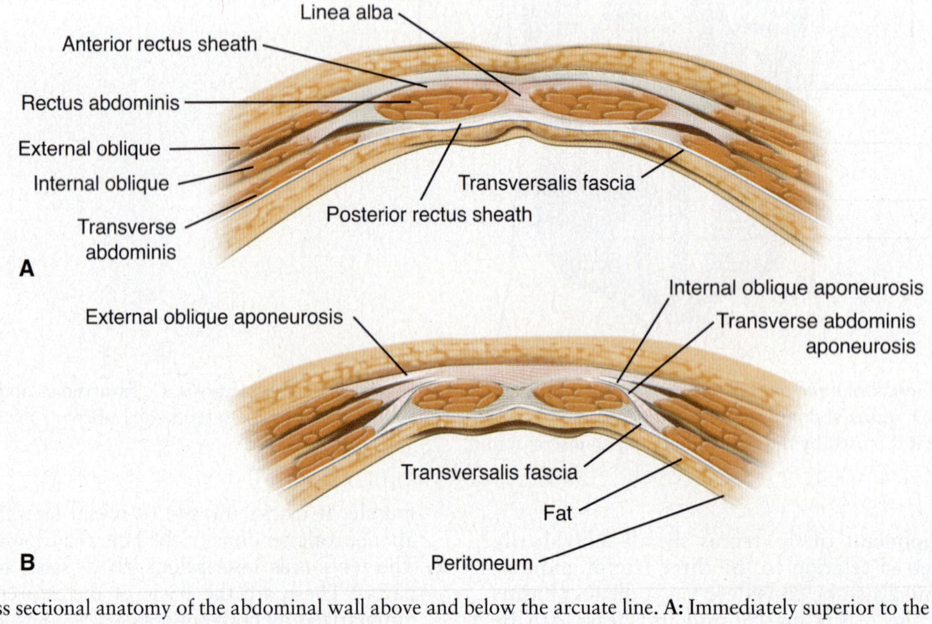

Figure 69.4. Cross sectional anatomy of the abdominal wall above and below the arcuate line. **A:** Immediately superior to the umbilicus, the rectus sheath consists of anterior and posterior components. The anterior sheath is composed of the aponeuroses of the external and internal abdominal oblique muscles, and the posterior sheath consists of the posterior aponeurotic lamina of the internal oblique and the aponeurosis of the transversus abdominis muscle. **B:** The rectus sheath inferior to the arcuate line (of Douglas) consists of an anterior portion made up of fibers from all aponeurotic layers; the posterior portion at this point comprises only transversalis fascia covered internally by peritoneum. (From Varvares M. The total hard palate defect: Rectus abdominis free flap. In: Genden E, ed. *Master Techniques in Otolaryngology – Head and Neck Surgery: Reconstructive Surgery*. Wolters Kluwer; 2015:169–175. Fig. 21.2.)

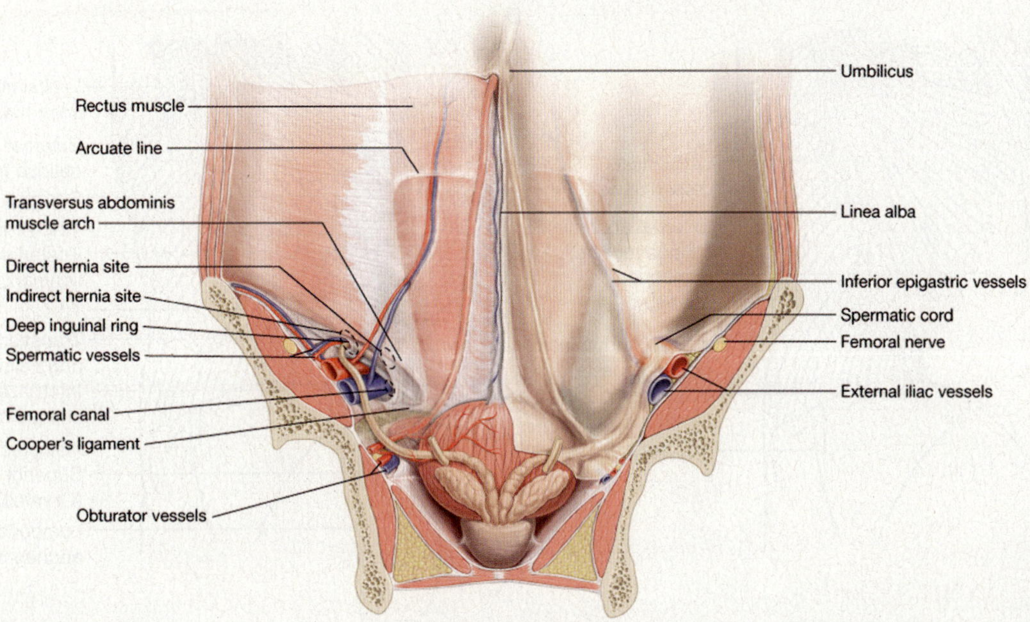

Figure 69.5. The deep inguinal region, pelvis, and anterior abdominal wall from the viewpoint of a surgeon using a laparoscopic technique. The anterior wall folds upward approximately at the iliopubic tract in this illustration. (From Hawn MT, Mulholland MW, eds. *Operative Techniques in Foregut Surgery*. Wolters Kluwer; 2015. Fig. 34.1.)

whereas the iliohypogastric nerve pierces the external oblique to innervate the skin above the pubis. The cremaster muscle fibers, which are derived from the internal oblique muscle, are innervated by the genitofemoral nerve (L1, L2).

The blood supply of the lateral muscles of the anterior wall is primarily from the lower three or four intercostal arteries, the deep circumflex iliac artery, and the lumbar arteries. The rectus abdominis has a complicated blood supply derived from the superior epigastric artery (a terminal branch of the internal thoracic, or internal mammary, artery), the inferior epigastric artery (a branch of the external iliac artery), and the lower intercostal arteries. The latter arteries enter the sides of the muscle after traveling between the oblique muscles. The superior and inferior epigastric arteries enter the rectus sheath and anastomose near the umbilicus.

Posterolateral (Lumbar) Abdominal Wall

The posterolateral or lumbar portion of the abdominal wall (**Fig. 69.7**) is often overlooked in discussions of abdominal hernia, perhaps because of the much more common occurrence of groin and femoral hernias. The configuration of the muscle layers in the lumbar area also predisposes to hernia formation. For the purposes of this discussion, the lumbar portion of the abdominal wall is defined as the area bounded superiorly by the

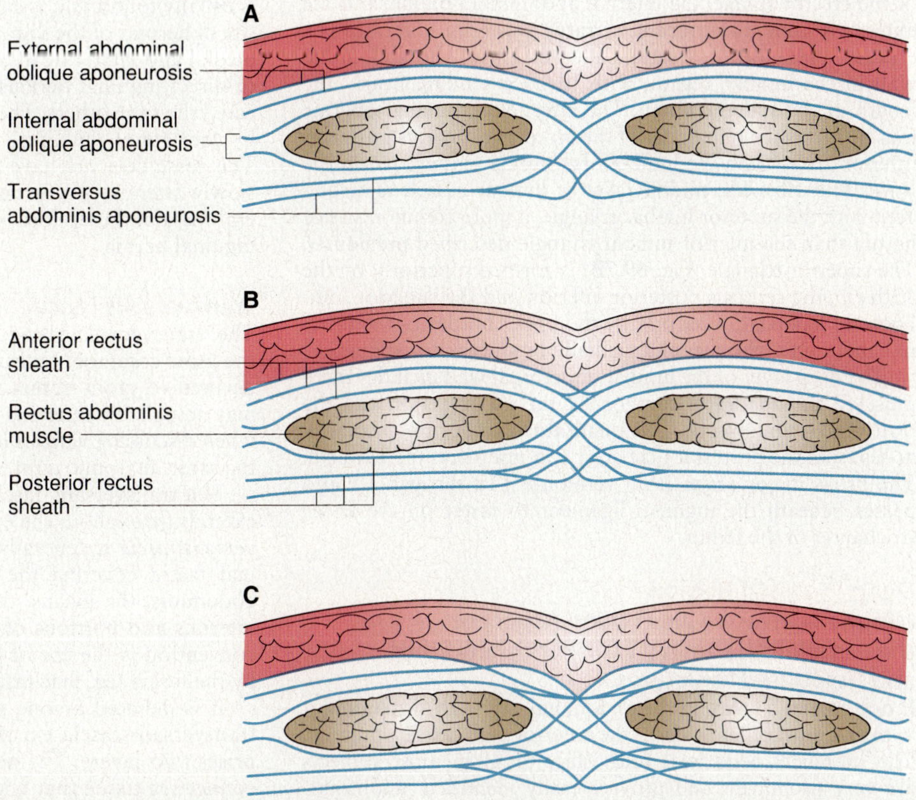

Figure 69.6. Patterns of midline decussation of the aponeuroses. **A:** Single anterior and posterior lines of decussation. **B:** Single anterior and triple posterior lines of decussation. **C:** Triple anterior and posterior lines of decussation.

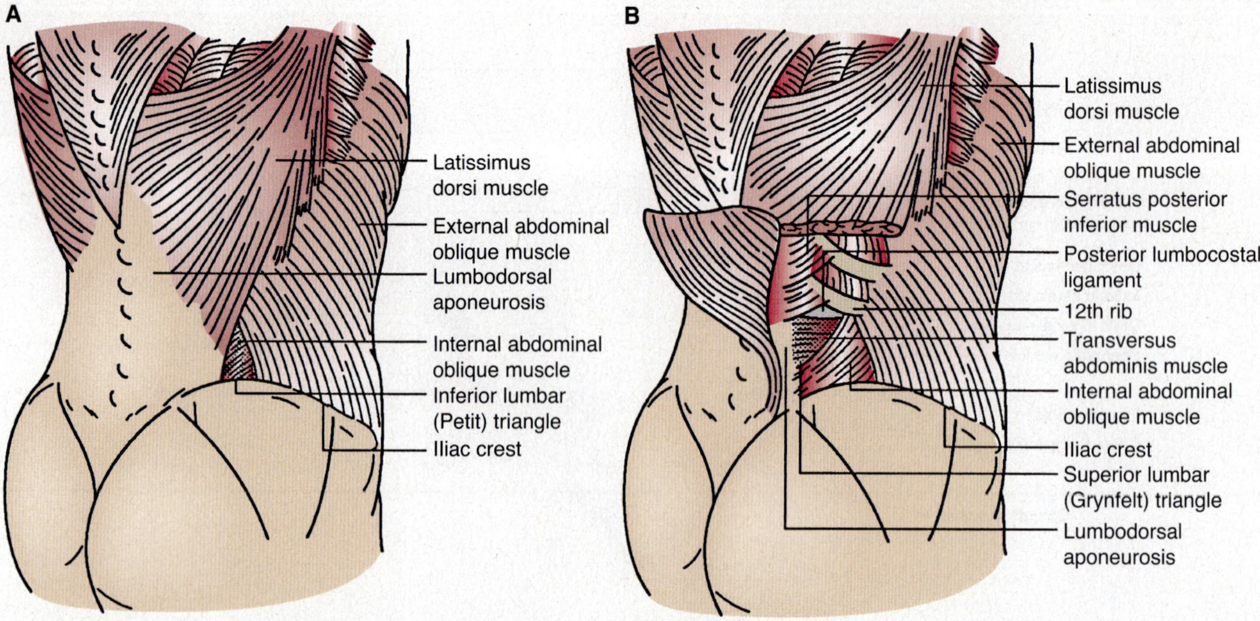

Figure 69.7. The lumbar abdominal wall with the inferior lumbar triangle (**A**) and the superior lumbar triangle (**B**).

12th rib, inferiorly by the iliac crest, and medially by the erector spinae group. Eight muscles arrayed in three layers constitute the posterolateral or lumbar portion of the abdominal wall.

The most superficial layer is composed of the external abdominal oblique muscle, which arises from the posteroinferior portion of the lower ribs and inserts in part along the posterior iliac crest. Closely associated with the external oblique in this area is the latissimus dorsi, which arises from the posterior iliac crest, the spinous processes of the sacrum and lumbar vertebrae, and the lumbodorsal fascia. The muscle courses obliquely toward its insertion on the medial aspect of the intertubercular groove of the humerus. The triangular space formed by the two muscles just described and the iliac crest is called the *inferior lumbar (Petit) triangle* (**Fig. 69.7A**).

The middle layer of lumbar abdominal muscles consists of the erector spinae, the internal abdominal oblique, and the extremely thin insignificant serratus posterior inferior. The erector spinae forms a significant portion of the abdominal wall in the lumbar region, with fibers extending nearly the length of the spinal column. The internal abdominal oblique muscle forms the remainder of the layer. The serratus posterior inferior arises from the lumbodorsal fascia and inserts on the lower four ribs. The middle layer of lumbar muscle is associated with the superior lumbar triangle, a more common site of hernia than the inferior lumbar triangle described previously. The superior triangle (**Fig. 69.7B**) is formed superiorly by the 12th rib, the serratus posterior inferior, and the superior lumbocostal ligament; inferiorly by the upper border of the internal abdominal oblique; and medially by the erector spinae.

The deep layer of the lumbar abdominal wall includes three muscles: the quadratus lumborum, the psoas major, and the transversus abdominis. The quadratus lumborum primarily arises from the posterior iliac crest and inserts on the 12th rib. The psoas major arises from vertebrae T12 through L5 and passes beneath the inguinal ligament to insert on the lesser trochanter of the femur.

Deep Inguinal Region

Minimally Invasive View: Deep Aspect of the Anterior Abdominal Wall, Peritoneal Folds, and Associated Structures

If one creates a space in the abdominal cavity by distending it with gas, an excellent view of the anterior wall can be obtained. The umbilical peritoneal folds (**Fig. 69.8**) in most subjects are very prominent and provide easily identified landmarks. The folds (ligaments) primarily exist because the peritoneum covers underlying structures.

The single median umbilical fold extends from the umbilicus to the urinary bladder and covers the urachus, the fibrous remnant of the fetal allantois. The urachus may be patent for a short distance in adults or may open into the umbilical scar in newborns. The medial umbilical fold is formed by the underlying obliterated portion of the fetal umbilical artery. This normally cordlike structure, like the urachus, may be patent for a portion of its length. Indeed, the proximal, patent portion of the artery normally supplies the superior vesicular arteries to the bladder. The lateral fold covers the inferior epigastric arteries as they course toward the posterior rectus sheath, which they enter approximately at the level of the arcuate line.

Between the median and the medial ligaments, a depression is usually found that is called the *supravesical fossa*. This is the site of hernias of the same name. The fossa formed between the medial and lateral ligaments is the medial fossa; this is the site of direct inguinal hernias. The lateral fossa is less well delineated than the others. The medial border of the fossa is formed by the lateral umbilical ligament and the rectus abdominis. This fossa does not have a lateral border; rather, the concavity slowly attenuates. The deep inguinal ring is located in the lateral fossa and therefore is the site of the congenital or indirect inguinal hernia.

Transversalis Fascia

The transversalis fascia (endoabdominal fascia) is perhaps the most commonly misunderstood structure in the literature devoted to groin hernia. Confusion results because surgeons may actually be referring to very different anatomic structures when discussing various hernia repairs; however, each may use the same anatomic term.

The transversalis fascia proper is a continuous sheet that extends throughout the extraperitoneal space. The term *transversalis fascia* is generally defined as the deep or endoabdominal fascia covering the internal surface of the transversus abdominis, the iliacus, the psoas muscles, and the obturator internus and portions of the periosteum. One variant of this convention is the use of terms specific to the muscle covered by the fascia (eg, iliac fascia).

It is debated among surgeons whether only one layer of transversalis fascia exists, or if the transversalis fascia comprises two layers. The posterior lamina is a layer of fibrous connective tissue that widely varies in density and continuity

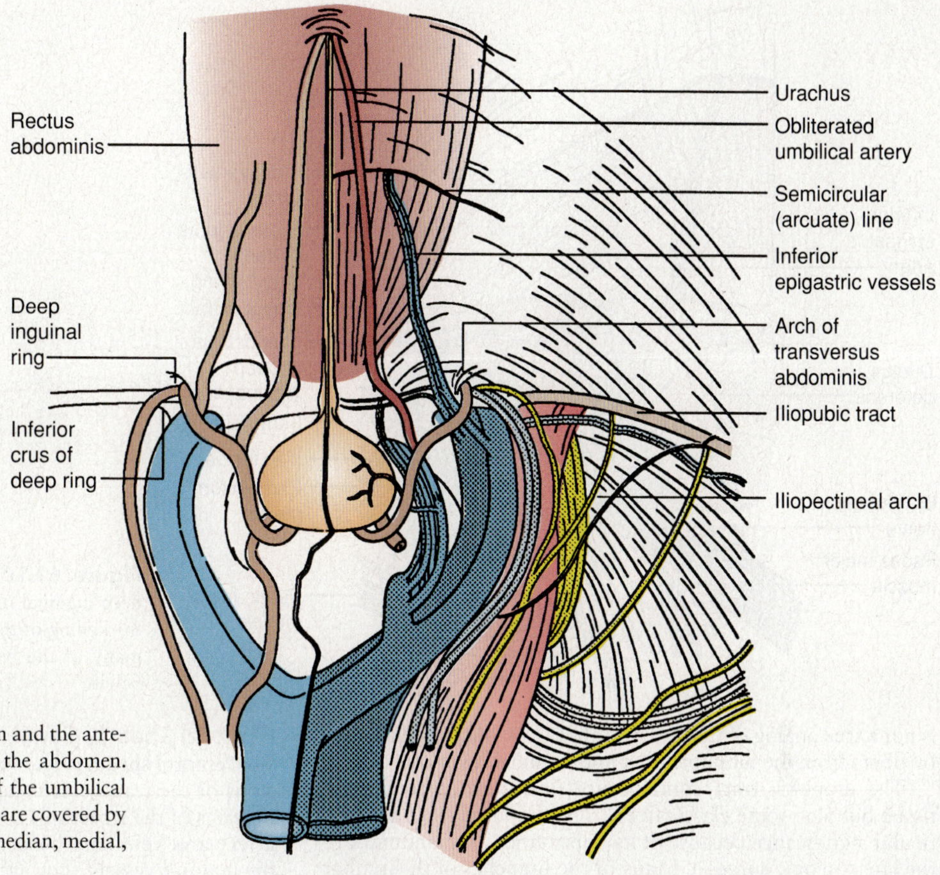

Figure 69.8. The deep inguinal region and the anterior abdominal wall seen from within the abdomen. The urachus, the obliterated portion of the umbilical artery, and the inferior epigastric vessels are covered by peritoneal folds, respectively called the median, medial, and lateral umbilical folds.

and is interspersed with adipose tissue, as seen in **Figure 69.9.** This layer is often referred to simply as the *preperitoneal fascia.* The anterior lamina is more uniform and is adherent to the deep surface of the transversus abdominis and the rectus abdominis. The posterior lamina is contained within the preperitoneal space, which is defined as the space between the peritoneum and the anterior lamina of the transversalis fascia. The inferior epigastric vessels are enclosed by, or interspersed with, the adipose tissue and the fibrous tissue of the posterior lamina of the transversalis fascia. The vessels are in contact anteriorly with the anterior lamina of the transversalis fascia as they course upward to enter the rectus abdominis sheath.

Transversalis Fascia Derivatives

The transversalis fascia analogs or derivatives are the iliopectineal arch, iliopubic tract, and crura of the deep inguinal ring. The superior and inferior crura form a transversalis fascia sling, a structure shaped like a "monk's hood," around the deep inguinal ring (**Fig. 69.8**). The transversalis fascia also contributes the internal spermatic fascia to the spermatic cord at this point. This "sling" has functional significance; when the transversus abdominis contracts, the crura of the ring are pulled upward and laterally, which results in a valvular action that helps to prevent the indirect formation of a hernia.

The iliopubic tract (**Figs. 69.8** to **69.10**) has become an increasingly important landmark for surgeons as the use of laparoscopic technology has increased.[8,9] The iliopubic tract is the thickened band of transversalis fascia formed at the zone of transition between the deep surfaces of the iliac and transversus abdominis muscles. The structure courses parallel to the more superficially located inguinal ligament, is attached to the iliac crest laterally, and inserts on the pubic tubercle medially. The tract forms along its course a portion of the inferior crus of the deep inguinal ring and then contributes to the anterior and medial walls of the femoral sheath. The tract fuses with the inguinal ligament to form a component of the inferior wall of the inguinal canal. At its insertion on the pubic tubercle, it curves backward slightly to blend with Cooper pectineal ligament. The pectineal ligament is actually a condensation of periosteum and

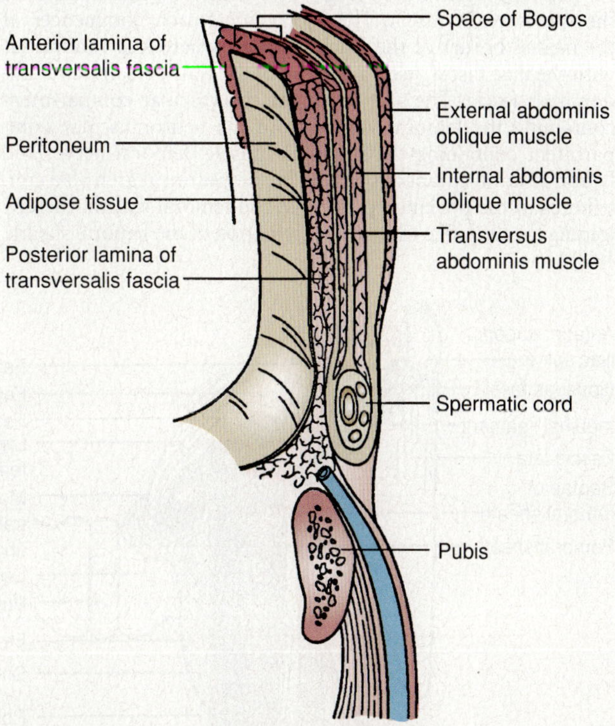

Figure 69.9. A parasagittal section through the layers of the anterior abdominal wall and groin. Observe that the transversalis fascia is depicted as a bilaminar structure.

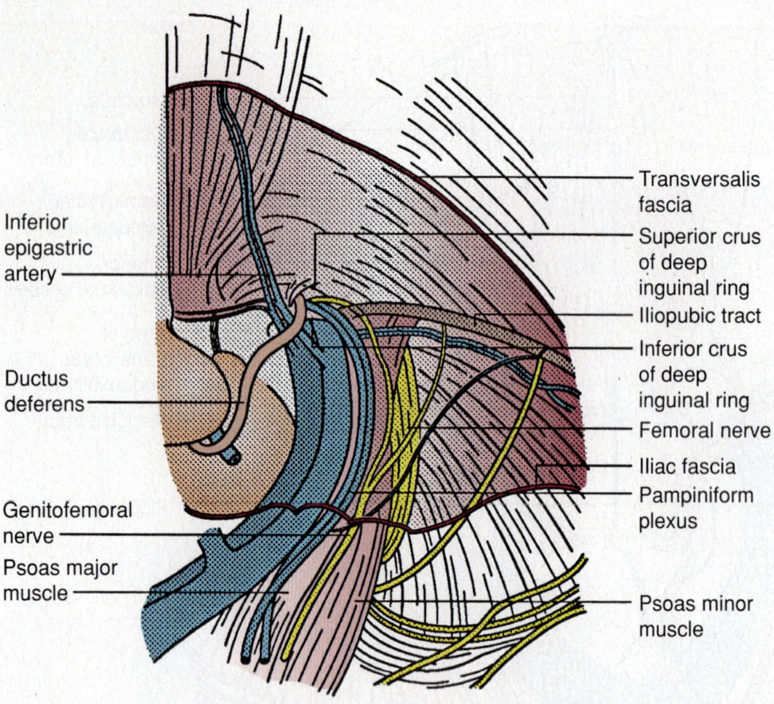

Figure 69.10. A schematic representation of the deep inguinal region. The iliopubic tract is shown as a thickening of the transversalis fascia, inferior to which many of the branches of the lumbar plexus exit the pelvis.

is not a true analog of the transversalis fascia, but it is reinforced by fibers from the iliopubic tract and inguinal ligament.

The iliopubic tract contains not only fibrous connective tissue but also some elastic fibers. The iliopubic tract has particular significance because of its importance as a landmark to the laparoscopic surgeon. Many of the branches of the lumbar plexus run inferior to the tract, and damage to these nerves may be the result of aggressive dissection or the placement of tacks or staples to affix a prosthesis below this structure. The tract is not obviously visible in every patient from a laparoscopic view, but its location should always be immediately known to the surgeon because of its constant relationship to the other landmarks in this area.

The iliopectineal arch (**Fig. 69.8**) is also a condensation of the transversalis fascia. The iliopectineal arch commences at the medial border of the iliacus muscle, where it is continuous with the iliac fascia, itself a portion of the transversalis (endoabdominal) fascia. The arch separates the vascular compartment containing the femoral vessels from the neuromuscular compartment containing the iliopsoas muscle, femoral nerve, and lateral femoral cutaneous nerve. The iliopectineal arch also contributes to the proximal portion of the femoral sheath, thereby joining the iliopubic tract in the formation of the femoral sheath.

Femoral Sheath, Canal, and Ring

The femoral sheath (**Fig. 69.11**) is primarily composed of extensions of the transversalis fascia. The sheath is best understood in terms of the structures contained within. As the external iliac artery and vein pass beneath the inguinal ligament to become the femoral vessels, they are covered anteriorly by the transversalis fascia proper. This fascial layer is posteriorly and laterally joined by portions of the iliopsoas fascia, which themselves are continuations of the transversalis fascia. At the inguinal ligament, the iliopsoas fascia forms the iliopectineal arch. This arch divides the vascular compartment (lacuna vasorum), containing the femoral vessels, from the muscular portion (lacuna musculorum), which contains the iliopsoas muscle, femoral nerve, and lateral femoral cutaneous nerve. The vascular lacuna is further divided by septa into compartments for the vessels and the femoral branch of the genitofemoral nerve.

The medial border of the femoral sheath follows the transversus abdominis aponeurosis to its insertion just lateral to that of the lacunar ligament and extends inferiorly to fuse eventually with the medial septum and adventitia of the femoral vein. The resultant cone-shaped cul-de-sac is the femoral canal. The canal normally contains only wisps of connective tissue and small lymphatic nodes. The wider proximal part of

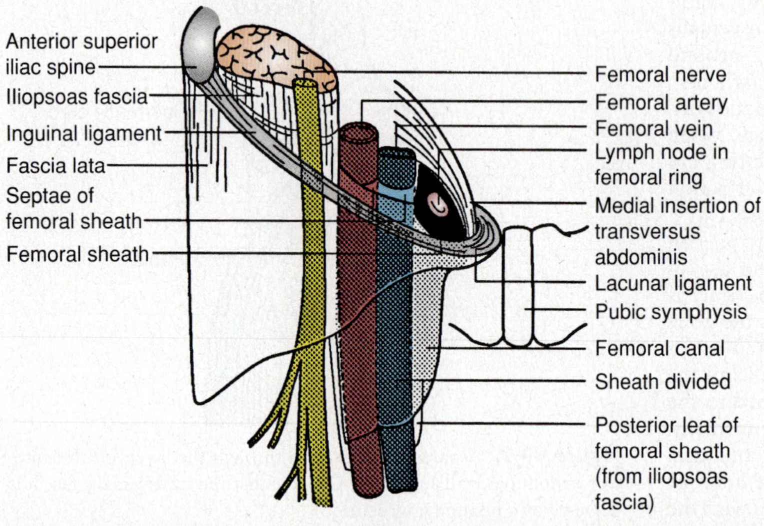

Figure 69.11. Schematic view of the femoral sheath, ring, and canal. The transversalis fascia forms the anterior portion of the sheath, and the iliopsoas fascia forms the posterior portion. Septae separate the vessels from each other and the vein from the femoral canal. The femoral ring contains a lymph node. The ring is formed medially by the aponeurosis of the transversus abdominis aponeurosis, anteriorly by the inguinal ligament, posteriorly by the pubic bone, and laterally by the femoral sheath.

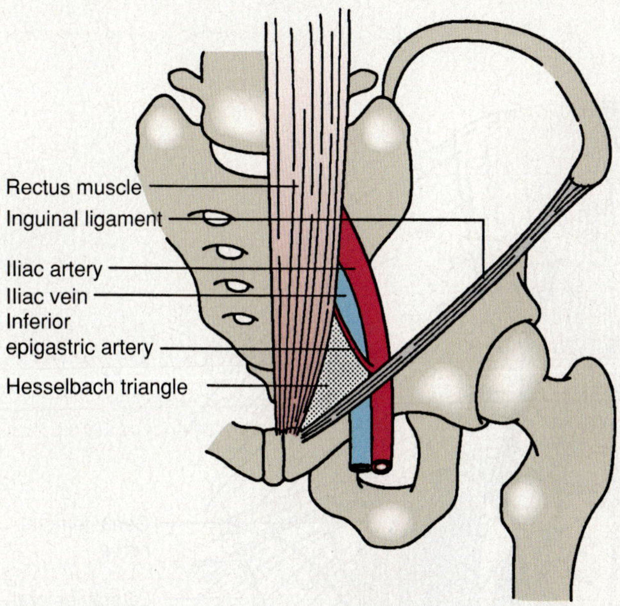

Figure 69.12. The inguinal (Hesselbach) triangle.

the canal, the femoral ring, contains a large node, which is often referred to as *Cloquet node*.

The femoral ring is the extraperitoneal opening of the canal. The boundaries of the ring are formed medially by the curved edge of the transversus abdominis aponeurosis, not the lacunar ligament, which inserts more medially.[10] Laterally, the ring is bounded by the connective tissue septum and the adventitia that is interposed between it and the femoral vein. The anterior boundary is the inguinal ligament; posteriorly, the ring is reinforced by the iliopubic tract and iliopectineal ligament. The canal is not in direct communication with the pelvic cavity. The transversalis fascia is not a component of the roof of the canal because it is diverted at this point to form the femoral sheath. This weakened area is therefore quite prone to hernia formation, especially in female subjects.

Inguinal (Hesselbach's) Triangle

The inguinal triangle is the site of direct inguinal hernias. This triangle is most often described from the anterior aspect (**Fig. 69.12**), in which case the inguinal ligament forms the base of the triangle, the rectus abdominis forms the medial border, and the inferior epigastric vessels form the superolateral border. The triangle as originally described by Hesselbach had the pectineal ligament as its base. The latter description is quite useful to the surgeon viewing the abdomen from within because the inguinal ligament cannot be seen from this viewpoint. When the inguinal triangle is transilluminated, the thinness and translucency of the area of abdominal wall within the triangle underscores its importance in hernia development and repair. In the most translucent area, little or no muscle is present. Only the peritoneum and the transversalis fascia cover the triangle here. The aponeurotic arch of the transversus abdominis crosses the triangle just below the apex in most people. A high aponeurotic arch affords less reinforcement to the triangle and may therefore predispose a person to the formation of a direct inguinal hernia.

Components of the Cord Structures for Men and Women

In men, the spermatic cord (**Figs. 69.10** to **69.13**) is closely associated with the deep inguinal ring. The spermatic cord is most appropriately described at this point because the deep ring itself is formed by derivatives of transversalis fascia, as is the innermost covering layer of the spermatic cord, the internal spermatic fascia. The middle covering layer is called the *cremasteric fascia* and contains the cremasteric muscle bundles; both are derived from the internal abdominal oblique muscle and fascia. The outermost covering of the spermatic cord is the external spermatic fascia, which is continuous with the investing fascia of the external abdominal oblique muscle.

The tunica vaginalis is initially a component of the cord, but normally it atrophies and closes early in neonatal life. This structure is an evagination of peritoneum. The testicle descends retroperitoneally in fetal life and is merely in contact with the posterior aspect of the tunica. An indirect congenital hernia enters the patent tunica vaginalis.

The cord structures enclosed by the coverings described earlier are the ductus (vas) deferens, the pampiniform venous plexus, the testicular artery, and the genital branch of the genitofemoral nerve, a branch of the lumbar plexus (**Figs. 69.8, 69.10,** and **69.14**).

In women, the cord consists of the round ligament. The round ligament of the uterus consists of a fibromuscular connective tissue connecting the superolaterally to the uterus and runs through the deep internal ring and exits the superficial inguinal ring and attaches to the pubis within the labia majora. The round ligament often runs next to the genital branch of the genitofemoral nerve and its relationship to the nerve is very closely intertwined at the deep inguinal ring and provides sensory innervation to the mons pubis[11] (**Fig. 69.15**).

Branches of the Lumbar Plexus

The nerves crossing the iliac fossa are some of the most variable in the body. This variability may be the cause of frequent intraoperative injury to the fragile nerves. The lumbar plexus is formed by roots from the 12th thoracic nerve and the 1st through 4th lumbar nerves. Cutaneous territories innervated by branches of the lumbar plexus are seen in **Figure 69.14A**.

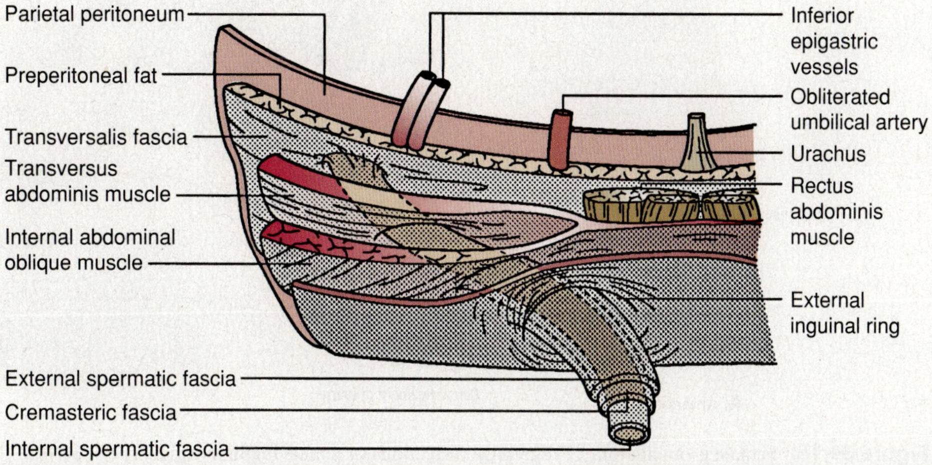

Figure 69.13. The component layers covering the contents of the spermatic cord.

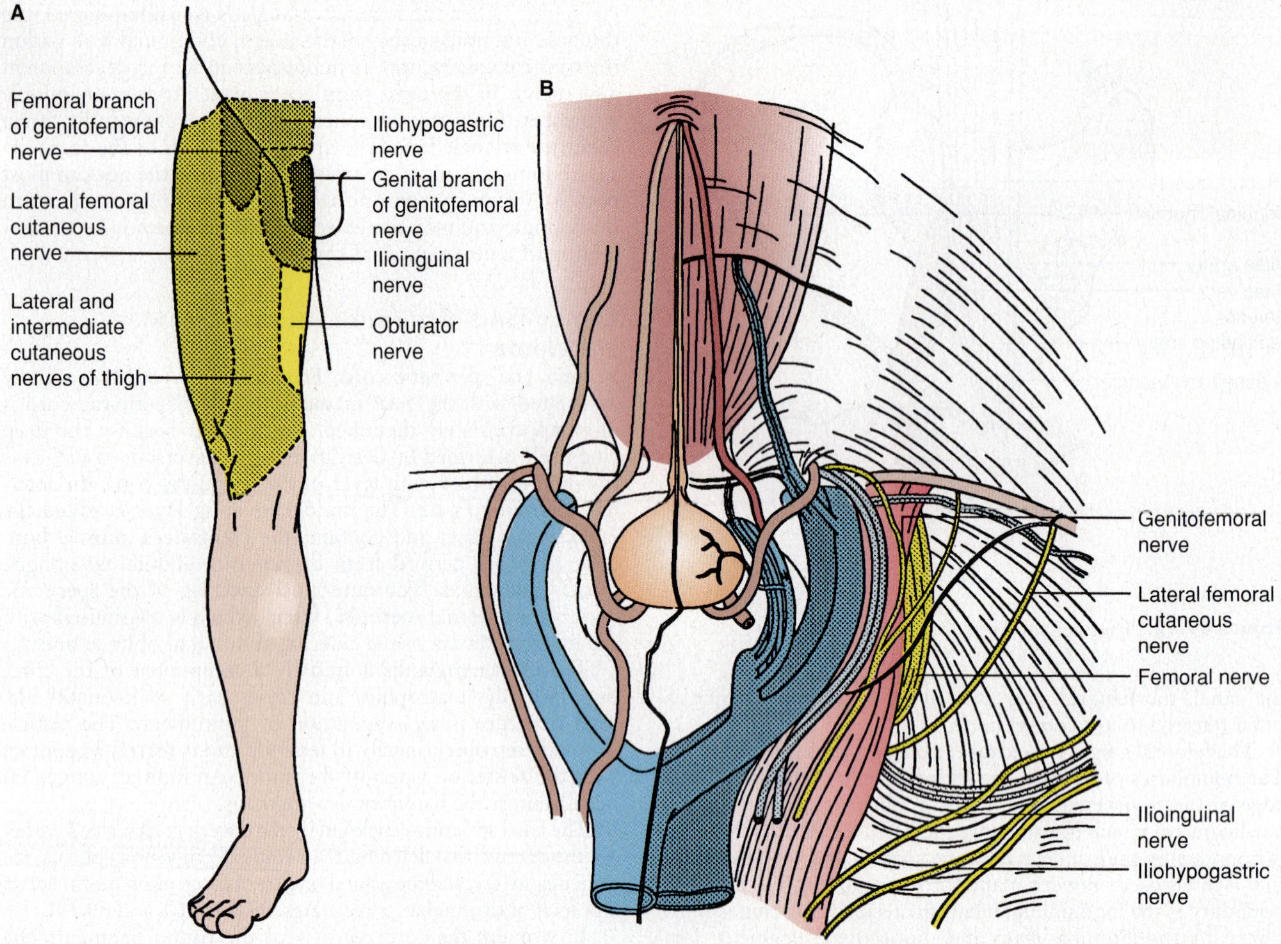

Figure 69.14. A: The cutaneous territories innervated by several branches of the lumbar plexus. B: Some of the branches of the lumbar plexus seen from within the abdomen.

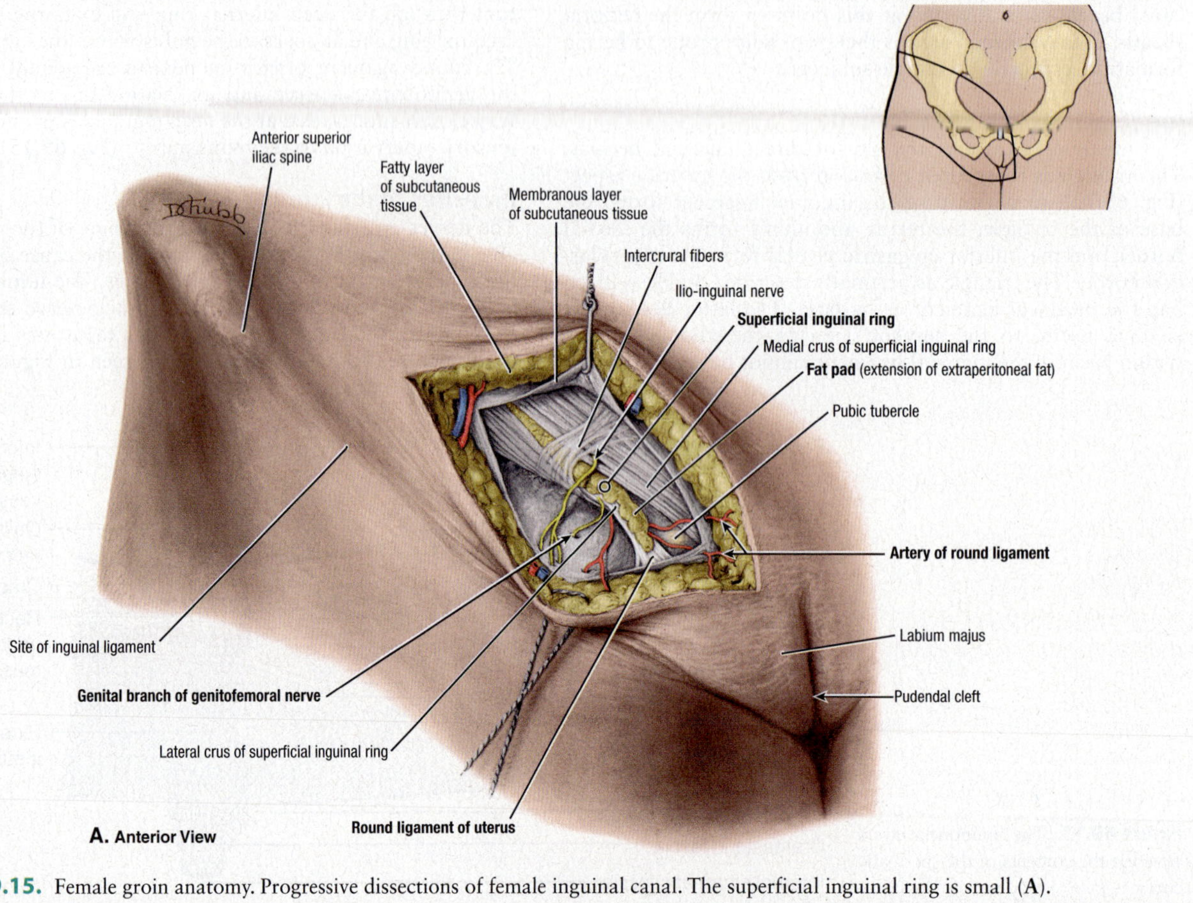

Figure 69.15. Female groin anatomy. Progressive dissections of female inguinal canal. The superficial inguinal ring is small (A).

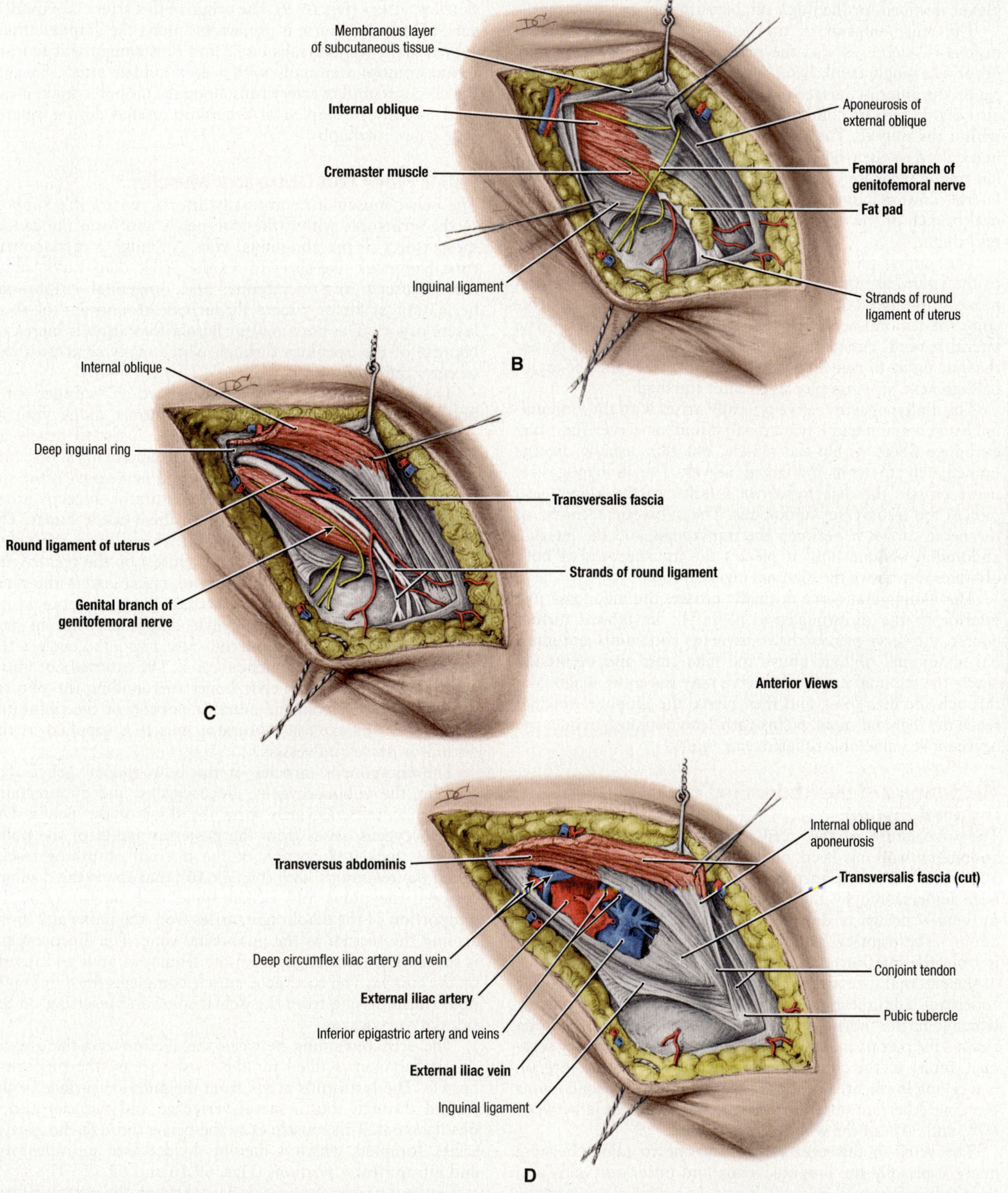

Figure 69.15. (*Continued*) Passing through the superficial inguinal ring are the round ligament of the uterus, a closely applied fat pad, the genital branch of the genitofemoral nerve, and the artery of the round ligament of the uterus (B). The round ligament breaks up into strands as it leaves the inguinal canal and approaches the labium majus. The ilio-inguinal nerve may also pass through the superficial inguinal ring (C). The external iliac artery and vein are exposed deep to the inguinal canal by excising the transversalis fascia (D). (From Abdomen. In: AMR, Dalley AF II. *Grant's Atlas of Anatomy.* 15th ed. Wolters Kluwer; 2021:291–389. Fig. 4.15.)

The five terminal branches commonly encountered in laparoscopic herniorrhaphy can be discerned in many people as they course across the iliacus muscle covered by peritoneum and the iliac fascia (a portion of the transversalis–endopelvic fascia). The nerves form within or deep to the psoas major muscle (**Fig. 69.14B**), often ramifying with other nerves within or close to the muscle. The nerve branches initially lie within the so-called triangle of pain,[12] bordered medially by the psoas muscle, anteriorly and inferiorly by the iliopubic tract, and laterally by the iliac crest. With the exception of the genital branch of the genitofemoral nerve, the branches of the lumbar plexus destined for the thigh run beneath the iliopubic tract.

The most anterior of the nerves encountered, the genitofemoral nerve, is also the most variable. This nerve may occur as a single trunk lying deep to the peritoneum and fascia on the anterior surface of the psoas muscle. The nerve may also divide into its component genital and femoral branches within the muscle. The genital branch travels with the spermatic cord or the round ligament, entering at the deep inguinal ring; it ultimately innervates the cremaster muscle and the lateral scrotum in men or the mons pubis in women. The femoral branch of the nerve innervates the skin of the proximal mid-thigh.

The lumbar plexus branch encountered immediately deep to the lateral aspect of the psoas muscle is the large femoral nerve. Although not routinely encountered during laparoscopy, the femoral nerve has been injured in some cases.[13] The lateral femoral cutaneous nerve crosses the iliac fossa under the iliac fascia to run deep to the iliopubic tract and the inguinal ligament, which it pierces to enter the thigh.

The iliohypogastric nerve typically arises with the ilioinguinal by a common trunk from the first lumbar nerve. They may exchange fibers within the muscle, but they usually diverge immediately to form individual nerves. The iliohypogastric nerve crosses the iliac fossa just inferior to the kidney and pierces the transversus abdominis. The subsequent course of the nerve carries it between the transversus and the internal abdominal oblique until it pierces the aponeuroses of both obliques just above the external inguinal ring.

The ilioinguinal nerve normally crosses the iliac fossa just inferior to the iliohypogastric nerve. In its typical further course, the nerve pierces the transversus abdominis and internal abdominal oblique above the iliac crest and eventually enters the inguinal canal. The nerve may run more diagonally through the iliac fossa and then pierce the iliopubic tract to reach the inguinal canal.[14] This path "can obviously render the nerve more vulnerable to iatrogenic injury."

Vasculature of the Abdominal Wall and Deep Inguinal Region

The vasculature of the deep inguinal region and anterior abdominal wall has been analyzed by surgeons for well over 100 years. The importance and variability of these vessels have been underscored by the ominous mnemonics used to refer to them—"crown of death" (*corona mortis*) and "triangle of doom." The primary blood supply to the deep anterior wall is from the inferior epigastric artery. This artery is a branch of the external iliac artery. In many cases, an artery called the "aberrant" obturator artery arises from the inferior epigastric, which joins the "normal" obturator artery and thereby forms a circle—the corona mortis—before entering the obturator foramen. Injury to the circle, usually sustained while the surgeon is working in the area of the Cooper ligament, causes copious bleeding. Aberrant obturator vessels can be present in between 60% and 90% of the whole pelves studied.[15,16]

The veins in this area are also prone to injury because many, especially the iliopubic veins and obturator veins and their tributaries, may be much larger than their accompanying arteries. One network of veins in the area is situated on the inferior deep surface of the rectus muscles. The veins of this network, which anastomose with the pubic branches discussed earlier, have been called the *rectusial veins*.[17]

The vessels in the vascular compartment of the deep inguinal region are the external iliac artery and vein. They arise within a triangular area bordered laterally by the gonadal vessels and medially by the ductus deferens. The primary continuations of the external iliac vessels are the femoral artery and vein. The inferior epigastric artery is a branch of the external iliac. The obturator artery may arise from either of these arteries as a replacement or accessory to the obturator branch of the internal iliac artery.

A final vessel to consider in this review is the deep circumflex iliac artery (**Fig. 69.9**). The origin of this artery is extremely variable, but its course is predictable along the iliopubic tract. It pierces the transversalis fascia and runs along the iliac fossa to anastomose eventually with a deep lumbar artery. Because the deep circumflex artery runs along the iliopubic tract, it can inadvertently be stapled or otherwise injured during laparoscopic herniorrhaphy.

Pelvic Floor and Obturator Muscles

The pelvic musculature normally affords remarkable support to the structures within the true pelvis and form the caudal most aspect of the abdominal core. Although a myoaponeurotic hammock-like sheet forms the pelvic diaphragm, obturator muscles and membrane, and urogenital diaphragm, herniation of fat or viscera through or around any of these layers occurs. The potential for hernia formation is increased because of the openings through which many structures exit or enter the pelvis.

The Latin term *obturator* is translated as "stopper for a bottle." The aptly named obturator internus, along with its membrane and the obturator externus, closes off nearly all the large obturator foramen. The small superolateral aperture through which the obturator vessels and nerve pass is the site where obturator hernias form. The obturator internus arises from the deep surface of parts of all three pelvic bones. The muscle fibers converge on a tendon, which leaves the pelvis through the lesser sciatic foramen to insert on the greater trochanter. The dense internal obturator fascia covers the muscle and is thickened to form the arcuate ligament, from which the levator ani muscles (the pelvic diaphragm) are in part suspended. The obturator internus fascia splits to enclose the pudendal vessels in the pudendal canal. The external obturator muscle arises from the pelvic bones surrounding the obturator foramen and from the anterior portion of the obturator membrane. The external obturator muscle is supplied by the obturator nerve and vessels.

The component muscles of the bowl-shaped pelvic diaphragm, the pubococcygeus, iliococcygeus, and puborectalis, along with the coccygeus form the floor of the pelvis. The pubococcygeus arises from the posterior aspect of the pubis and the thickened portion of the internal obturator fascia, called the *tendinous arch* (**Fig. 69.16**), that spans the distance between the pubis and ischial spine. The puborectalis, the midportion of the diaphragm, arises from the pubis and loops around the rectum as the puborectal sling. The iliococcygeus is suspended at its origin from the tendinous arch and inserts on the coccyx. The coccygeus muscle completes the diaphragm posteriorly, arising from the ischial spine and inserting on the sides of the coccyx.

The area remaining between the sacrum and the greater sciatic foramen is filled for the most part by the piriformis muscle. The piriformis arises from the anterior surface of the second through fourth sacral vertebrae and the sacrotuberous ligament. This muscle exits the pelvis through the greater sciatic foramen, which is thereby divided into suprapiriform and infrapiriform portions (**Figs. 69.16** and **69.17**). The superior gluteal nerves and vessels pass through the suprapiriform foramen, whereas the inferior gluteal nerves and vessels in company with the sciatic nerve pass through the infrapiriform foramen.

The most pronounced deficit in the pelvic diaphragm is situated anteriorly, where an aperture must allow the urogenital structures to pass out of the pelvis. This area is reinforced by the urogenital diaphragm, a structure primarily consisting of the superficial and deep transverse perineal muscles. The deep transverse perineal muscle is enclosed by a weak superior fascia and a sturdier inferior perineal fascia. The urogenital diaphragm has been shown to be more funnel shaped than sandwich like, and exists only in humans because the human pelvic outlet faces inferiorly, unlike that of quadrupeds.

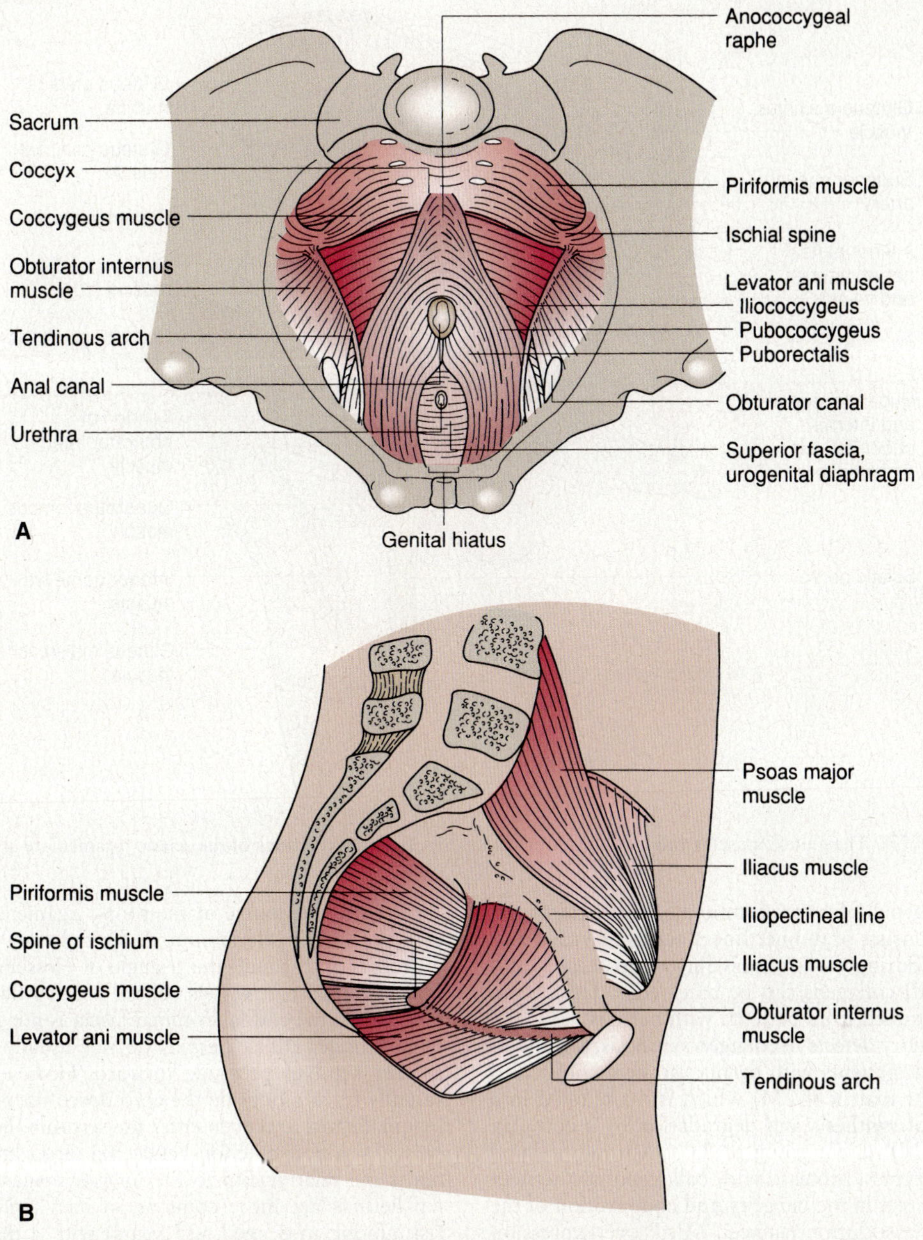

Figure 69.16. **A:** The pelvic diaphragm (levator ani and the piriformis) and the urogenital diaphragm viewed from within the pelvis. **B:** Hemisection of the pelvis revealing the levator ani, piriformis, obturator internus, and psoas muscles.

WHY DO HUMAN BEINGS DEVELOP ABDOMINAL WALL HERNIAS?

The most common hernias develop at sites where the abdominal wall has areas of natural weakness or openings such as the internal inguinal ring, the umbilicus, and the esophageal hiatus. Previous surgical incisions (incisional hernia) are also common areas where hernias develop. Factors that increase the intra-abdominal pressure, such as obesity, heavy lifting, coughing with chronic lung disease, straining during a bowel movement or urination, and ascites, can also play a role in hernia formation. Other major risk factors for the development of an abdominal wall hernias include connective tissue disorders (aneurysms, collagen vascular disease, matrix metalloproteinase [MMP] abnormalities, etc.), and any disease process that inhibits wound healing (smoking, immunosuppression, chronic illness, etc.).

There is minimal evidence that vigorous abdominal wall activity or heavy lifting is an independent risk factor for abdominal wall hernia development. Studies have demonstrated that increasing cumulative exposure to daily lifting activities and prolonged standing or walking at work was associated with an increased risk of having an indirect inguinal hernia repair.[18,19] This may be due to the fact that a patent processus vaginalis may be more susceptible to changes in intra-abdominal pressures, whereas in a direct hernia, other mechanisms may be involved in connective tissue degradation and weakening of the transversalis fascia. Still, the role of mechanical activity in the development of abdominal wall hernia is not completely clear, and further research is needed to determine if inguinal hernias can be prevented and if the postoperative prognosis can be improved by reducing occupational mechanical exposures.

Familial predisposition and the role of connective tissue diseases play in hernia development is slowly becoming better understood. Family history of hernia formation as it has been reported to increase the risk of developing a hernia by up to eight times. Various connective tissue disorders, such as osteogenesis imperfecta, Marfan syndrome, Ehlers–Danlos syndrome, and congenital hip dislocation, are also associated with hernia formation. Imbalances in collagen, the basic building block of the abdominal wall, contribute to hernia disease.

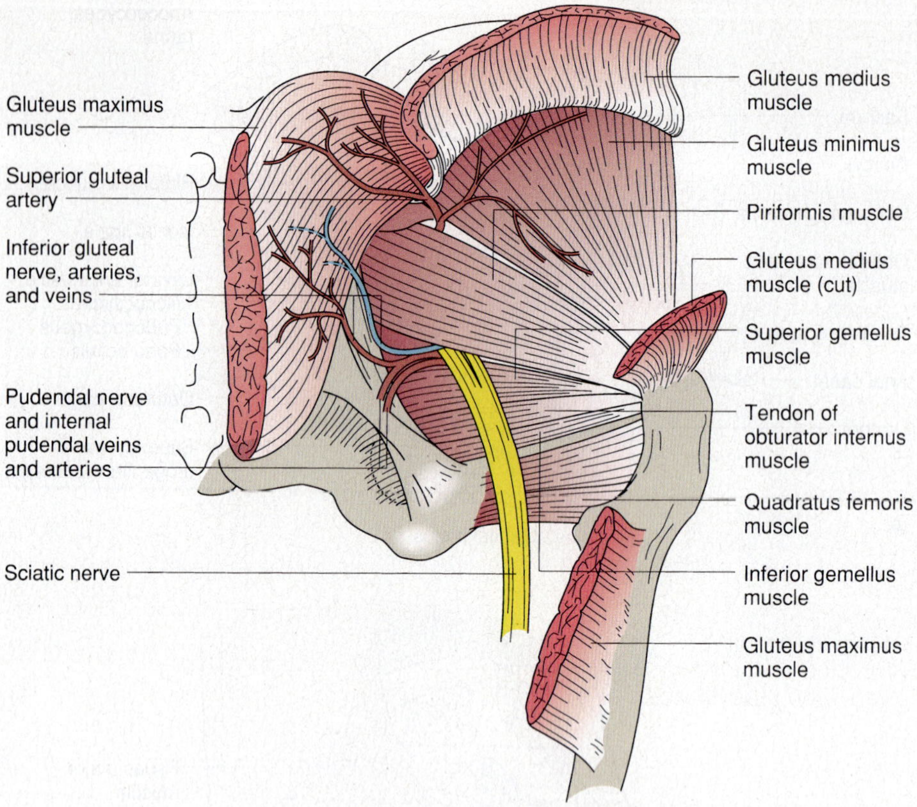

Figure 69.17. The gluteal muscles and lateral rotators of the hip. External relations of the sciatic foramen are also evident.

While type I collagen confers predominantly tensile strength, type III collagen consists of thinner fibers and is regarded as a temporary matrix during tissue remodeling. A decreased ratio of type I to type III collagens can be detected in fascial and skin specimens obtained from patients with hernias.

Aside from primary defects in collagen synthesis, the imbalances in collagen in patients with hernia can be attributed to altered extracellular matrix (ECM) which is maintained in a dynamic balance of synthesis and degradation by a complex set of enzymes. MMPs are a group of 23 structurally related zinc-dependent enzymes, protease with collagenolytic activity and have a pivotal role in the integrity and composition of the ECM. There is an association between MMP overexpression and endogenous regulators, the most important of which are the tissue inhibitors of MMP (TIMPs), and abdominal wall hernia formation.[20] Despite the increasing knowledge regarding MMPs in incisional and inguinal hernia, the exact role of MMPs in the pathogenesis of hernia formation remains unclear. In addition to MMPs and TIMPs, factors that have been implicated in hernia development include deficiency of the elastic fiber system of the transversalis fascia, decreased tropoelastin and lysyl oxidase-like 1 synthesis, elastase overexpression, and TGF-beta1 overexpression. It remains unclear whether these alterations in hernia patients are a part of the "cause-or-effect" phenomenon.

GROIN HERNIAS

Groin hernias are described as inguinal and femoral, with inguinal hernias being further subdivided into direct and indirect hernias (some authorities refer to these as medial and lateral hernias, respectively). Groin hernias may be primary or recurrent. An indirect hernia occurs as a protrusion of abdominal contents through the internal ring, lateral to the inferior epigastric vessels, into the inguinal canal. Indirect inguinal hernias (lateral hernias) are situated within the inguinal canal and follow the course of the spermatic cord and therefore may extend into the scrotum. In female patients, an indirect hernia can follow the course of the round ligament and may present as a swelling in the labium. A direct hernia (medial hernia) is a protrusion through the triangle of Hesselbach medial to the inferior epigastric vessels. These hernias develop through an area where the endoabdominal fascia is not protected by overlying muscle. Direct hernias do not usually involve the cord, as they tend to protrude forward. However, they can occasionally track alongside the cord down the entire length of the inguinal canal and even enter the scrotum. For this reason, the only absolute distinction between a direct and an indirect hernia is the relationship to the inferior epigastric vessels. Inguinal hernias are more common in men (with a 15% lifetime risk among men aged >25 years) with a male-to-female age-adjusted ratio of 7.5:1.[21] A femoral hernia protrudes through the femoral canal, which is bordered by the inguinal ligament superiorly, the lacunar ligament medially, Cooper ligament inferiorly, and the femoral vein laterally. This hernia presents below the inguinal ligament (**Fig. 69.18**). In a sliding hernia, part of the sac is formed by the viscera, on the left side the sigmoid colon or bladder, and on the right side the cecum or bladder (**Fig. 69.19**).

2 Epidemiology

Inguinal hernias occur in persons of all ages, from the neonate to the elderly. Inguinal hernias constitute approximately 75% of abdominal wall hernias, with femoral hernia accounting for 5%. Femoral hernias are more common in women, but a woman with a groin hernia is still five times more likely to have an inguinal hernia (usually indirect) than a femoral. The lifetime risk of developing a groin hernia is approximately 25% in males and 5% in females. Inguinal hernias are more common on the right than the left and are 10 times more likely in males than in females.[22] Indirect inguinal hernias are twice as common as direct hernias. The reported prevalence of inguinal hernia in the general population varies widely in the literature primarily due to a lack of a consistent reporting mechanism. The most reliable data use hernia repair as a surrogate for the prevalence. There is typically a bimodal incidence pattern

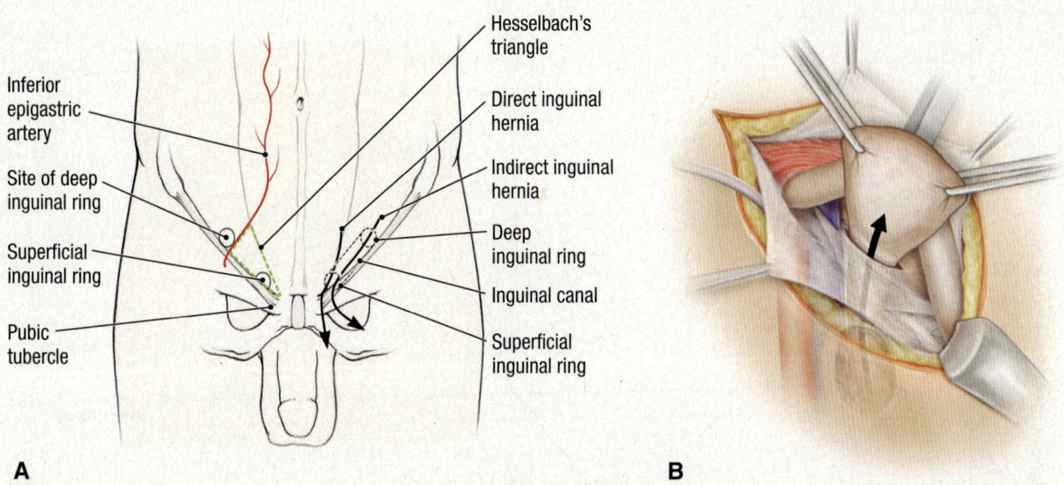

Figure 69.18. Location of groin hernias. **A:** Inguinal hernia. This presents above the inguinal ligament and extends below it. (From The Abdomen. In: Detton AJ. *Grant's Dissector*. 16th ed. Wolters Kluwer; 2017:99–140. Fig. 4.12.) **B:** Femoral hernia. This presents below the inguinal ligament. When addressing a femoral hernia, the sac is opened and its contents inspected prior to reduction of the sac. (From Itani KMF, Sbayi S. Inguinal hernia: open approaches. In: Hawn MT, ed. *Operative Techniques in Surgery.* 2nd ed. Wolters Kluwer; 2023:163–175. Fig. 2.1.13.)

peaking at the extremes of life with an initial peak at 0 to 5 years followed by a second peak at 70 to 80 years[23] as shown in **Figure 69.20**.

Generally right-sided inguinal hernias are more common than left due to the later involution of the patent processus vaginalis in men on the right side. In men, indirect inguinal hernias outnumber direct by about 2:1, with femoral hernias making up a much smaller proportion. The literature dealing with groin hernia in women is insufficient making management decisions difficult. For females, indirect inguinal hernias are the most common which are five times more common than femoral hernias. In contrast, femoral hernias account for fewer than 10% of all groin hernias and the prevalence is higher in females than in males. Femoral hernias are especially dangerous as 40% of all femoral hernias present as emergencies, with incarceration or strangulation and need emergency repair which is associated with high mortality. Femoral recurrences are particularly common in women in whom the diagnosis at the time of the primary repair was an inguinal hernia, strongly suggesting a missed femoral hernia at the original procedure. Femoral hernias are also more common in older patients and in those who have previously undergone inguinal hernia repair. Risk factors for the development of an inguinal hernia are listed in **Table 69.2**.

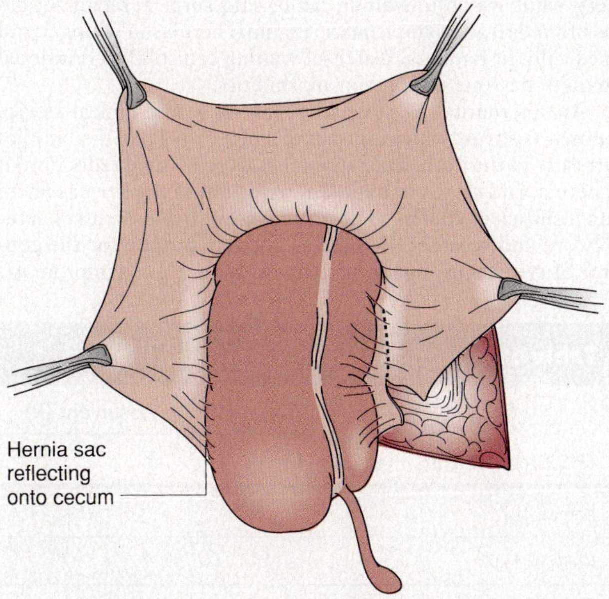

Figure 69.19. Sliding hernia (right indirect inguinal).

Classification

The primary purpose of a classification system for any disease is to stratify for severity so that reasonable comparisons can be made between various treatment strategies.[24] However, with the multiplicity of operative techniques and approaches for repair of groin hernias, no one classification system has been accepted by all practitioners. The reason why it is so difficult to develop a classification system that all surgeons can agree on is that in the final analysis, the physical examination represents an important component, and no one has been able to eliminate its subjectivity. The European Hernia Society (EHS), Nyhus, Gilbert, Schumpelick, Harkins, Casten, Halverson and McVay, Lichtenstein, Bendavid, Stoppa, Alexandre, and Zollinger have developed groin hernia classification systems. The EHS classification is a simple system using three variables, location (M = medial, L = lateral, and F = femoral), size of the defect (1 [≤1 finger], 2 [1 to 2 fingers], and 3 [≥3 fingers]), and status (P = primary, R = recurrent, and X = unknown) (**Table 69.3**).[25] The Nyhus system which is shown in **Table 69.4** remains popular among many surgeons in the Unites States.

Clinical Diagnosis

Groin hernias present with a bulge upon valsalva. With indirect hernias, the bulge may extend down into the scrotum. If the bulge goes away when the patient lies down or is typically not present in the morning when they first wake up, indicates that the patient has a reducible inguinal hernia. Most patients will indicate that they have a groin bulge that is associated with pain, often worse when standing for long periods of time, or with increasing physical activity. On physical exam, applying pressure over the superficial ring externally with the fingertip will control an indirect hernia and prevent it from protruding when the patient strains. A direct hernia will typically be palpable slightly higher and medial. It should be noted that the accuracy of this clinical assessment is questioned by many authorities. A femoral hernia presents as a swelling below the inguinal ligament and just lateral to the pubic tubercle (**Fig. 69.18**).

Differential Diagnosis

The clinical presentation of a groin hernia, especially when large, is frequently obvious to the examiner. A thorough history

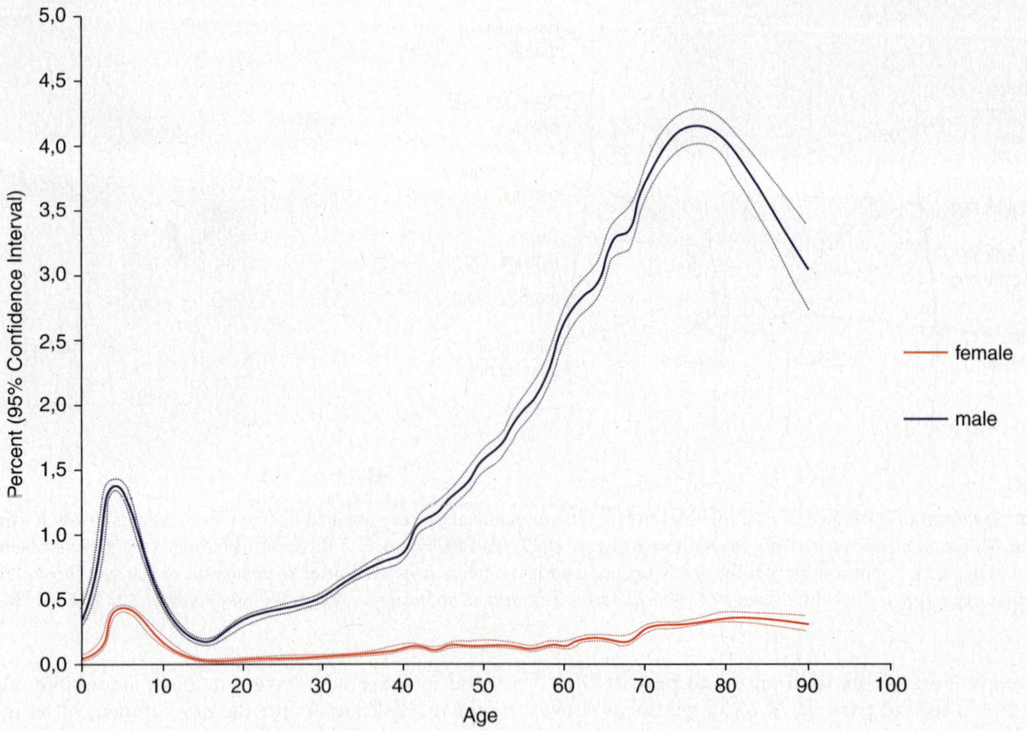

Figure 69.20. Prevalence of combined inguinal and femoral hernia repair (ie, all groin hernias), stratified by age and gender. The results indicate the percentage of persons at a given age in the population who were operated for a groin hernia during the study period. Example: 4.19% CI 4.04% to 4.34% of all males aged 75 to 80 years in Denmark were operated for a groin hernia at least once during the study period. (From Burcharth J, Pedersen M, Bisgaard T, et al. Nationwide prevalence of groin hernia repair. *PLoS One*. 2013;8(1):e54367, with permission.)

is critical as patients can often times present with groin pain the absence of a noticeable groin bulge on physical exam. In those patients, additional confirmatory imaging is needed to confirm the diagnosis. Groin pain can also be from other non–hernia-related etiologies such as musculoskeletal injuries (ie, athletic pubalgia), hip pain, etc. Occasionally a groin bulge can be mistaken for a hernia, when in fact it can from a number of different conditions (**Table 69.5**). If the history and physical exam are not consistent, cross-sectional imaging should be obtained to make a definitive diagnosis.

Table 69.2. Risk Factors for the Development of an Inguinal Hernia

Male sex
Increased age
COPD
Smoking
Low body mass index
High intra-abdominal pressure
Collagen vascular disease
History of abdominal aortic aneurysm
History of thoracic aortic aneurysm
Patent processus vaginalis
History of an open appendectomy
Peritoneal dialysis
Family history

3 Surgical Indications

Historically, surgeons have recommended repair of inguinal hernias at diagnosis unless specific contraindications are present. This concept was challenged for asymptomatic or minimally symptomatic male patients based on several randomized controlled trials which demonstrated that watchful waiting for minimally symptomatic inguinal hernias was safe.[26] However, long-term follow-up from these randomized controlled trials have demonstrated a crossover rate of over 70% by 7.5 years for patients in the watchful waiting group. Patients who opt for this strategy should be informed that it may be safe to delay surgery, but increasing symptoms will more than likely make them choose to have their hernia repaired over the next 5 to 10 years. Given the high rate of eventually needing surgery, while watchful waiting can be safe, surgical repair should be offered to all asymptomatic inguinal hernias in younger and medically fit patients. Watchful waiting can still be considered in older patients with major morbidities.

An alternative to surgical repair is a mechanical device known as a truss which consists of a belt with a pad that applies pressure to the groin after spontaneous or manual reduction of a hernia, and serves to maintain reduction of the hernia. There are insufficient studies to determine how effective trusses actually are and whether they are as good as surgery for the control of symptoms, but some patients do achieve symptomatic

Table 69.3. EHS Classification of Groin Hernias

		Primary (P)		Recurrent (R)	
EHS Groin Hernia	**0**	**1**	**2**	**3**	**x**
Lateral (L)					
Medial (M)					
Femoral (F)					

Table 69.4. Nyhus Classification of Groin Hernias

Type	Description
I	Indirect hernia Normal-sized internal ring Typically in infants, children, small adults
II	Indirect hernia Dilated internal ring Posterior wall intact Inferior epigastric vessels not displaced Does not extend to the scrotum
III	Posterior wall defect
IIIA	Direct hernia Size not taken into account
IIIB	Indirect hernia Dilated internal ring encroaching on Hesselbach triangle (massive scrotal, sliding, or pantaloon type)
IIIC	Femoral hernia
IV	Recurrent hernia
IVA	Direct
IVB	Indirect
IVC	Femoral
IVD	Combined

relief. This may be a good option for patients who are prohibitively high risk for surgery due to existing comorbidities. **Table 69.6** summarizes the International Guidelines for Groin Hernia Management.[27]

Preoperative Considerations

Most elective groin hernias can be repaired on outpatient basis. Typically for both open and minimally invasive inguinal hernia repairs, general anesthesia is utilized. With the newer anesthesia reversal agents, urinary retention is infrequent. For patients who cannot tolerate general anesthesia, local anesthesia with or without supplemental intravenous sedation can be utilized during open inguinal hernia repairs. Any minimally invasive hernia repair requires general anesthesia and can only be performed in patients who can safely tolerate general anesthesia and pneumoperitoneum. There is no clear evidence that antibiotic prophylaxis is necessary, except in patients with high risk for infection. Despite lack of evidence, it is routinely used in the United States because prosthesis placement.

Surgical Treatment of Groin Hernias

Four developments in the latter half of the 20th century significantly decreased morbidity and favorably influenced the recurrence rate to the currently accepted level of less than 2%: (a) the routine use of prosthetic materials, (b) the widespread acceptance of the "tension-free" concept, (c) the realization that the preperitoneal space can be used for hernia repair, and (d) minimally invasive surgery techniques (**Algorithms 69.1** and **69.2**). These concepts are discussed in this section; the treatment strategies are divided between an open approach in the anterior space and a posterior or preperitoneal approach, which can be done either open or minimally invasively. Surgical decision making for inguinal hernia surgery approach can be nuanced for complex patients. Deciding which surgical approach to employ depends on patient factors, hernia factors, and surgeon familiarity with different procedure types.

Patient and Procedure Selection

Generally, a minimally invasive approach has become the more favored approach for an initial nonrecurrent uncomplicated inguinal hernia. Recent studies from the Danish and Swedish Hernia Registries have demonstrated that almost 40% of female patients undergoing an inguinal hernia surgery for recurrence were found to have an occult femoral hernia that was likely missed at the index operation. It is the recommended method of repair for female groin hernias to minimize risk of missing a femoral hernia.[28]

This posterior preperitoneal approach has many advantages which includes the ability to evaluate the contralateral inguinal region, reinforcement of the posterior abdominal wall, and the ability to completely visualize all potential defect spaces in the myopectineal orifice to fix an indirect, direct, or femoral hernia. This can be done using two primary methods: a total extraperitoneal (TEP) or transabdominal preperitoneal (TAPP) approach. Both methods place a large piece of mesh in the preperitoneal plane to cover all three potential defect spaces—the difference lies in how the preperitoneal

Table 69.5. Differential Diagnosis of a Groin Hernia

Male-Specific Pathology
Hydrocele
Encysted hydrocele of the cord
Varicocele
Epididymo-orchitis
Torsion of the testis
Undescended/Ectopic testis
Testicular tumor
Female-Specific Pathology
Canal of Nuck cyst (hydrocele)
Leiomyoma
Endometriosis
Bartholin cyst
Varicocele of the round ligament
Non–Sex Specific Pathology
Inguinal lymphadenopathy
Psoas abscess
Cutaneous lesions (eg, sebaceous cyst and skin tumor)
Pseudohernia
Femoral artery aneurysm
Saphena varix
Lipoma
Neoplasm

Table 69.6. Summarizes the International Guidelines for Groin Hernia Management

Grade 3/4

- Mesh-based repair is recommended for adult inguinal hernias.
- Flat mesh Lichtenstein technique is recommended over 3-dimensional implants.
- Laparo-endoscopic (TEP or TAPP) technique is suggested for male primary unilateral hernias.
- Shouldice technique is recommended in nonmesh repair.

Grade 4/4

- Antibiotic prophylaxis is not recommended in average-risk cases.
- Local anesthesia is recommended for reducible open repair.
- Timely repair, laparoendoscopic technique, and consideration of femoral hernias are recommended in female groin hernias.
- Minimizing spermatic cord trauma reduces orchialgia.
- Laparoendoscopic repair is recommended after failed anterior repair.
- Anterior repair is recommended after a failed posterior repair.
- Considering cost-effectiveness, day-case laparoendoscopic repair is recommended.

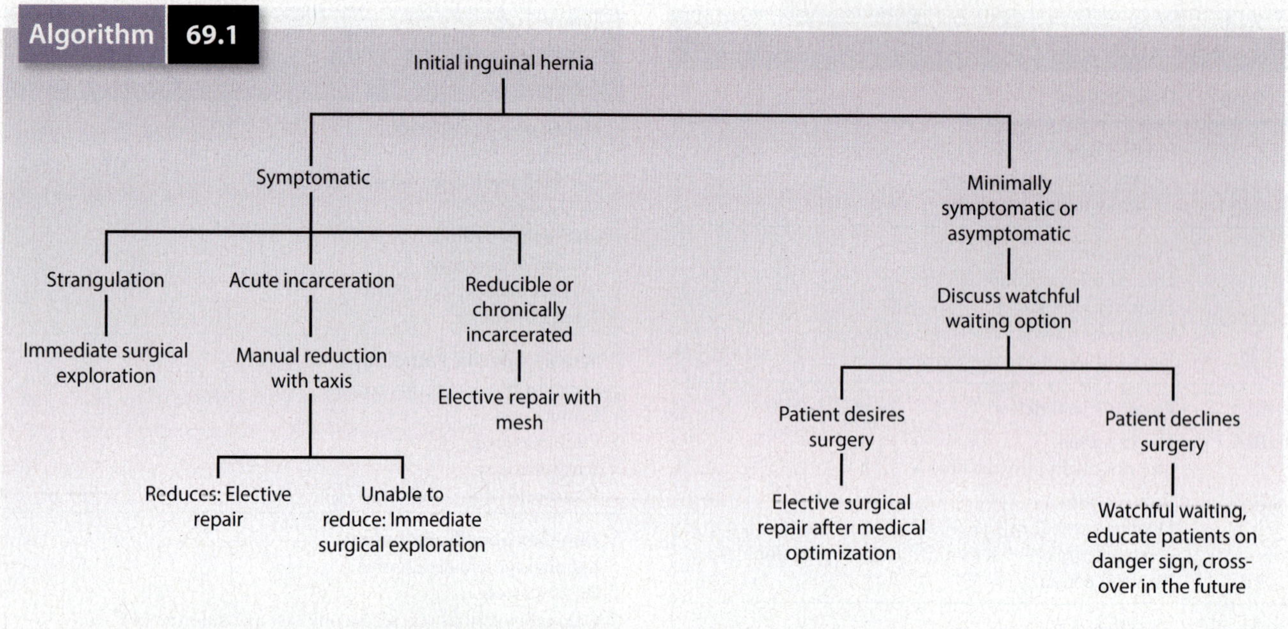

Algorithm 69.1. Management of initial inguinal hernia.

space is accessed. In the TEP approach, most often the space is accessed bluntly using a balloon dissector, and this is done by taking advantage of the anatomic landmarks of the posterior rectus sheath and the end of the arcuate line by directly accessing the space of Retzius and Bogros. In the TAPP approach, the surgeon starts intra-abdominally and then creates a large preperitoneal flap through careful dissection.

Each method has its unique advantages, but the TAPP approach can be universally used for almost all inguinal hernia dissections as it allows the surgeon to accomplish the following that may not always be possible using the TEP technique including: (1) Reduction of incarcerated hernia contents under direct visualization, especially if bowel is involved or if there are adhesions in the hernia sac preventing reduction prior to surgery; (2) Controlled dissection in the preperitoneal space, especially in cases of reoperative lower abdominal or pelvic surgery in which a blunt balloon dissection is not feasible (recurrent inguinal hernia, lower midline laparotomy, prior prostatectomy, bladder sling, etc.), and potentially minimizes bleeding risk for patients on anticoagulation or antiplatelet therapy; (3) Possibility of inguinal sac abandonment especially in the setting of a large inguinoscrotal hernia, this is potentially harder to do from the preperitoneal space; (4) Ease of dissection for patients with higher BMI or have very short or

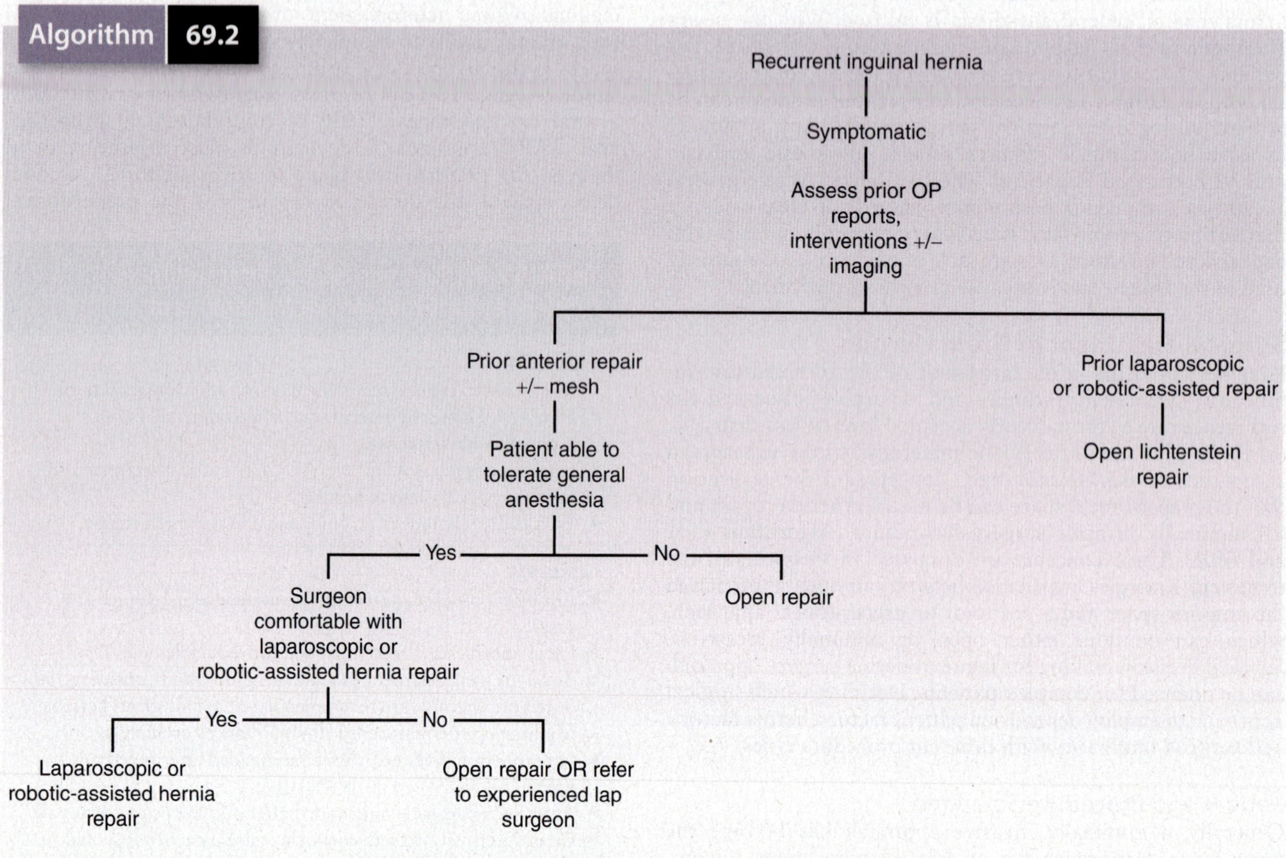

Algorithm 69.2. Management of recurrent inguinal hernia.

narrow pelvis that may limit TEP incisions for dissection. One of the disadvantages of the TAPP technique is that the peritoneal flap must then be reapproximated either with tacks, peritoneal staples, or suturing which can add to the operative time. Generally, a TEP is a great approach for small inguinal hernias that are reducible on exam, in relatively thin patients without prior pelvic or abdominal surgery.

An open approach to inguinal hernia surgery can either be done as an open anterior abdominal wall repair or a preperitoneal repair. Patients may be a better candidate for open repair if they have a recurrence after a prior minimally invasive repair, hostile abdomen from prior abdominal surgery, high-risk comorbidities that prohibit general anesthesia, anticoagulation, or large inguinoscrotal hernias. Due to the nature of the inguinal hernia defect, sometimes in very large defects, posterior placement of mesh against a large abdominal wall defect without plication of the muscle or closure of the defect and lead to mesh eventration and recurrence. In these cases, an open repair may lead to increased abdominal wall stabilization and decreased risk for recurrence and eventration. For very large inguinoscrotal hernias, a drain may be placed in the scrotal sac to help decrease seroma formation. In loss of domain inguinoscrotal hernias, with a large abdominal wall defect and scrotal component, the surgeon can consider preoperative counseling of the patient for prophylactic orchiectomy to completely close the abdominal wall defect to minimize risk of hernia recurrence or testicular torsion postoperatively. One benefit of an open repair is the ability to perform a tissue-based repair without mesh, which is not generally feasible for a preperitoneal repair, as this repair relies on a posterior mesh patch.

Depending on the clinical situation, patient comorbidities, hernia characteristics, and surgeon familiarity with certain techniques, one approach may be favored over the other. Randomized controlled trials as well as meta-analysis of pooled data several trials have shown that on average, patients undergoing laparoscopic herniorrhaphy have less pain initially than open, tension-free herniorrhaphy, return to normal activities sooner with a lower incidence of wound infection, hematoma, and less incidence of chronic pain/numbness.[27,29] These advantages of laparoscopic hernia repair must be interpreted in light of potential disadvantages, which include higher learning curve for mastery of technique, potential complications related to the laparoscopy such as bowel perforation, bladder, or major vascular injury, interparietal hernias at sites of peritoneal violation, the need for a general anesthetic, and increased cost due to the laparoscopic or robotic equipment. Conversely, the open operation can be performed under local anesthesia with minimal risk of intra-abdominal injury and lower cost. Ultimately, these decisions should be tailored for each individual patient based on each unique circumstance. In general, regardless of approach, a mesh repair is recommended because of its dramatic decrease in recurrence rate when compared to tissue repair. There are specialty centers performing pure tissue repairs with reported outcomes equaling a mesh repair, but these similar outcomes may be hard to achieve and generalizable. The next sections describe both the minimally invasive and open approaches in technical detail.

Preperitoneal Approach

The preperitoneal space is situated between the transversalis fascia and the peritoneum. The final common denominator in all groin hernias is failure of the transversalis fascia to retain the intra-abdominal contents. Repairs performed in this space make the distinction between direct, indirect, and femoral irrelevant because the repair is accomplished behind the defective transversalis fascia, addressing the entire myopectineal orifice. This repair can be approached minimally invasively or using a lower midline open approach.

Minimally Invasive Approach

A minimally invasive hernia repair can be done either laparoscopically or robotically. Specifically, the two most common

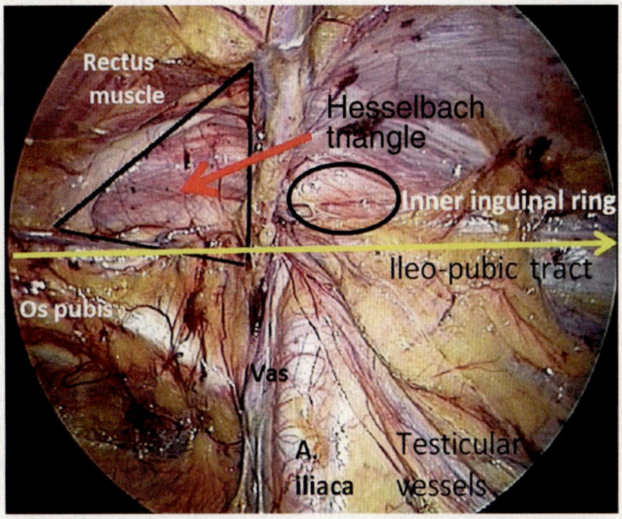

Figure 69.21. The myopectineal orifice. Superior to the inguinal ligament, this area includes the inguinal (Hesselbach) triangle. Inferior to the ligament, the orifice transmits the iliopsoas muscle, the femoral nerve and vessels, and the femoral canal and sheath. (From Bates AT, Pechman DM. Robotic inguinal hernia repair. In: Hawn MT, ed. *Operative Techniques in Surgery*. 2nd ed. Wolters Kluwer; 2023:186–189. Fig. 2.3.4.)

techniques are the *transabdominal preperitoneal repair* (TAPP repair) (**Fig. 69.21**) or *totally extraperitoneal laparoscopic repair* (TEP repair). An intraperitoneal onlay mesh technique is not used for inguinal hernia repair due to high recurrence rates and need for mesh fixation laterally which can cause chronic pain. A robotic technique can be employed and usually if done robotically, a TAPP approach is favored, although a TEP approach has been described, but is less widely adopted. There have been several inconclusive evaluations comparing a robotic-assisted approach to inguinal hernia repair to a laparoscopic approach. Representative retrospective studies have not shown significant benefit to robotic repair over laparoscopy. In terms of clinical and patient reported outcomes when examining recurrence, postoperative pain, quality of life, mobility, wound morbidity, or cosmesis, the transabdom inal laparoscopic inguinal repair (RIVAL) study did not show a significant difference between any of these outcomes.[30] But there may be some unique advantages that a robotic repair can provide over a laparoscopic repair, and this is seen most distinctly in larger, complex, acutely incarcerated, inguinoscrotal, recurrent, or reoperative settings in which the improved visualization, endowrist articulation, and suturing can facilitate dissection and flap reapproximation for the surgeon. Robotic surgery may also increase minimally invasive surgery access for surgeons who did not do training primarily in laparoscopy, and can potentially increase the prevalence of those who can offer patients a minimally invasive repair. Ultimately the best approach is the one the surgeon feels most confident in to do the best repair for the patient.

Operative Techniques

Transabdominal Preperitoneal Repair (TAPP)

The TAPP repair can be performed either via robotic-assisted or laparoscopic approach. Preprocedure the patient will usually void prior to surgery to avoid using a Foley catheter. Both arms should be padded and tucked at the patient side. The procedure is begun by gaining access to the abdominal space and establishing pneumoperitoneum. Generally, a diagnostic laparoscopy is done to inspect for unexpected pathology, and then the patient is placed in Trendelenburg as attention is turned to the pelvis to carefully inspect both myopectineal orifices. Two additional cannulas are placed just lateral to the rectus sheath on either side of the midline (**Fig. 69.22B**).

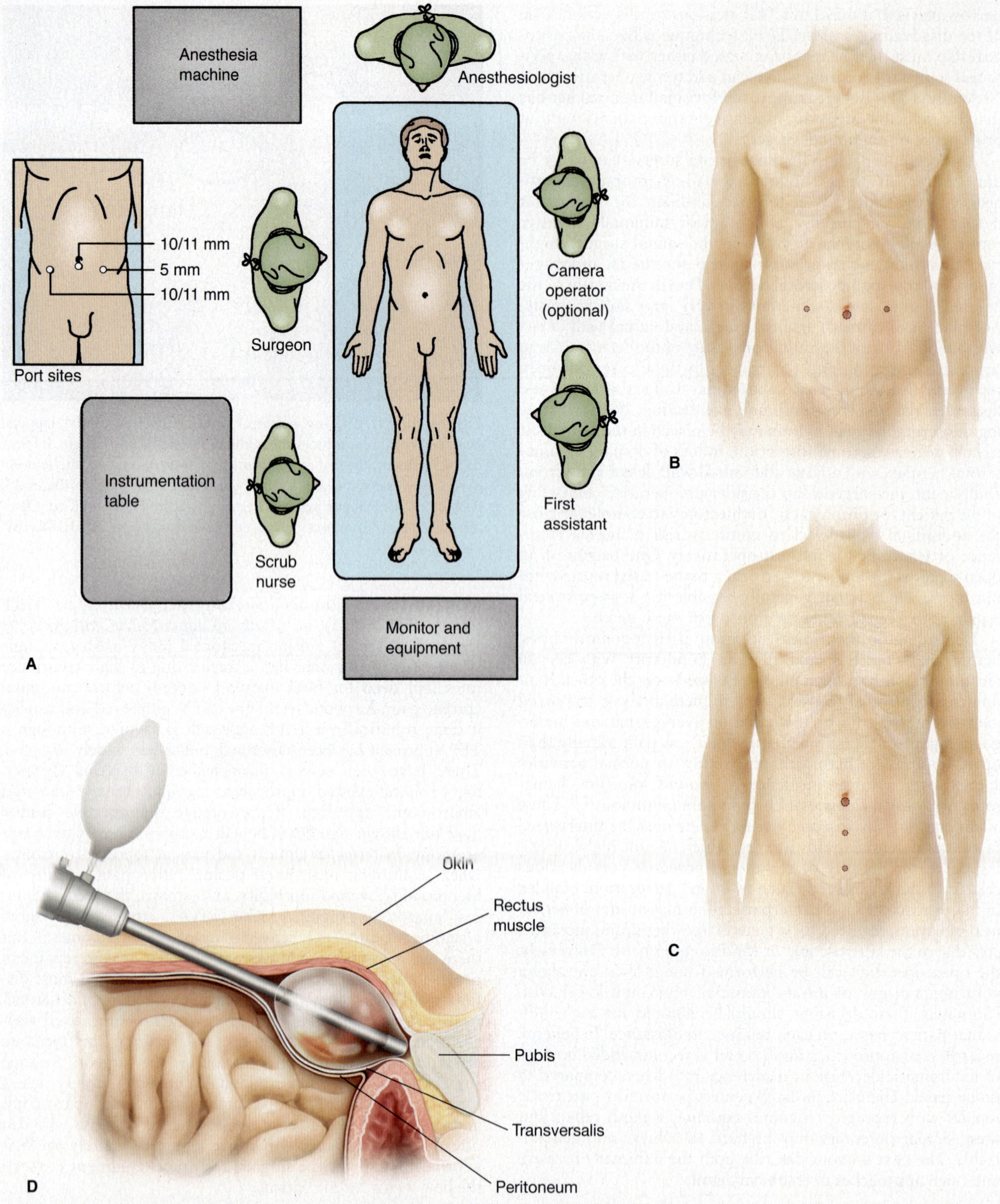

Figure 69.22. Transabdominal preperitoneal (TAPP) versus totally extraperitoneal (TEP). **A:** Typical operative setup and cannula site selection for a TAPP laparoscopic inguinal herniorrhaphy. **B, C:** Port placement. **B:** For TAPP, ports are placed at the umbilicus and lateral to the linea semilunaris at the level of the umbilicus. **C:** TEP ports are placed in the midline at the umbilicus, 2 cm above the symphysis pubis, and the final in between the first two, at least 4 cm cranial to the second port. **D:** Endoscopic balloon dissector, TEP. The balloon dissector is inserted into the retrorectus space, advanced toward the pubic symphysis, and fully insufflated for 2 minutes to allow adequate hemostasis. (From Poulose BK, Holzman MD, Baucom RB. Inguinal hernia: laparoscopic approaches. In: Mulholland MW, ed. *Operative Techniques in Surgery.* Wolters Kluwer; 2015:281–288. Figs. 2.2.2 and 2.2.9.)

For a unilateral hernia, a transverse incision is begun at the lateral side of the medial umbilical ligament and extended to the anterior superior iliac spine to create a large peritoneal flap. It is important to enter the true preperitoneal plane and not the retromuscular plane (anterior to the transversalis fascia). Conversely, the retromuscular plane can be preferentially entered in situations where previous pelvic operations have been performed (ie, prostatectomy, Pfannenstiel incision, rectal surgery, open appendectomy) or if the peritoneal layer is exceedingly thin. Knowing which

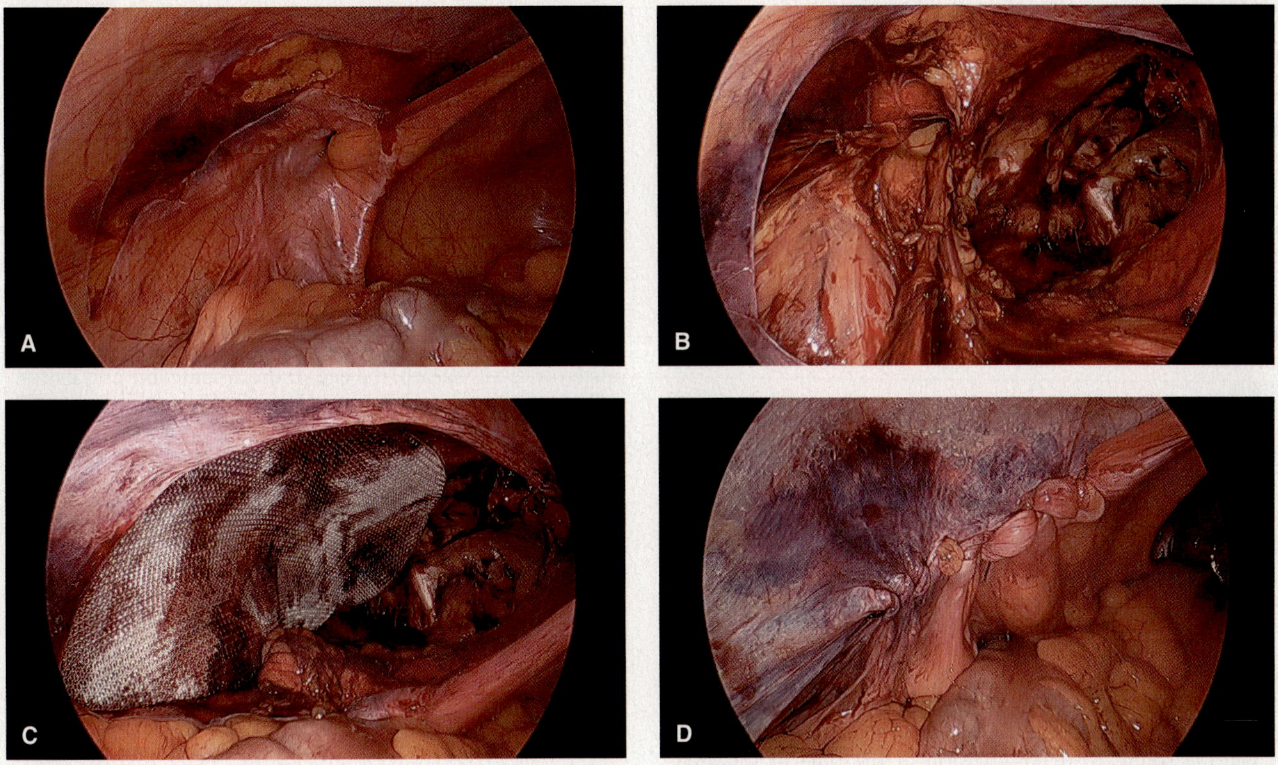

Figure 69.23. Transabdominal preperitoneal (TAPP) repair. **A:** The peritoneal incision during a laparoscopic TAPP repair. **B:** The exposed myopectineal orifice after hernia completed dissection during a TAPP repair. **C:** Mesh placement to cover the entire myopectineal orifice. **D:** Sutured peritoneal closure at the end of a TAPP repair. (From Gunter RL, Greenberg JA. Symptomatic primary inguinal hernia. In: Dimick JB, ed. *Clinical Scenarios in Surgery*. 2nd ed. Wolters Kluwer; 2019:3–8. Figs. 1.3 to 1.6.)

plane the dissection is occurring is critical in this step. A combination of blunt and electrocautery dissection is utilized to create this preperitoneal space and to minimize bleeding. The surgeon should obtain the critical view of the myopectineal orifice as described by Jorge Daes and Edward Felix.[31] Typically, the first landmark to be identified is Cooper ligament and the medial border of the dissection. This dissection should cross the midline and extend at least 2 cm below the Cooper ligament and the bladder. Then the dissection takes place lateral to the deep ring along the lateral abdominal wall, taking care to stay along the curve of the peritoneal flap, and avoiding deeper dissection to the abdominal wall fat, musculature, to preserve lateral abdominal wall nerves. The ipsilateral inferior epigastric vessels, Cooper ligament, and iliopubic tract are identified (**Figs. 69.23 and 69.24**). Once these structures are visualized, the type of hernia is

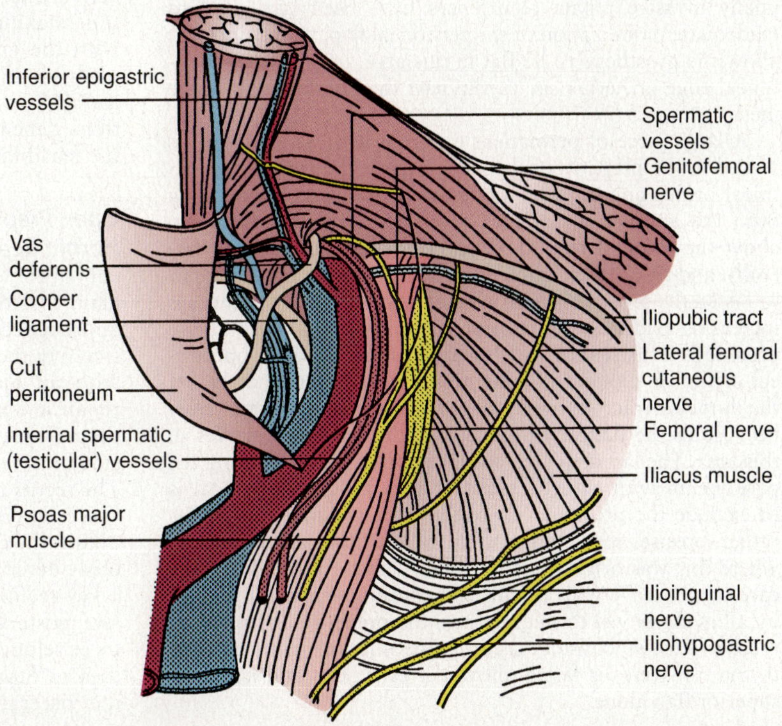

Figure 69.24. Important structures that must be identified after a preperitoneal dissection: inferior epigastric vessels, Cooper ligament, spermatic vessels, vas deferens, iliopubic tract, genitofemoral nerve, femoral nerve, lateral femoral cutaneous nerve, ilioinguinal nerve, iliacus muscle, and psoas major muscle.

well defined by its relationship to the inferior epigastric vessels.

In male groins, an indirect hernia can be reduced by stripping the cord structures off the hernia sac, which are typically medial. In very large inguinoscrotal hernia sacs, this may be abandoned and the peritoneum of the hernia sac reapproximated. Once the cord structures are mobilized, it is critical to make sure the peritoneal flap is dissected as inferiorly as possible off the cord structures and that the peritoneal flap is dissected well proximal to the bifurcation of the vas deferens and the internal spermatic vessels. After completing this step, surgeons should also check for a cord lipoma at the time of surgery as a missed lipoma can be a potential source for recurrent pain or the sense that the hernia has recurred after hernia repair.

In female groins, an indirect hernia dissection of the round ligament should be done with care. Often times, there is more scarring of the peritoneum around the area of the round ligament. While there are certain studies to suggest that routine division of the round ligament does not increase risk of chronic pain or complications, there is still a lack of data to support whether or not this should be routinely done. Most surgeons opt to divide the round ligament away from the deep ring to avoid injuring branches of the genitofemoral or ilioinguinal nerve. This allows for flatter mesh placement especially if the ligament lies in an orientation that is unfavorable for mesh placement. In general, there are no large-scale female-specific studies assessing the long-term impact of routine round ligament division at the time of inguinal hernia surgery on recurrence, chronic pain, quality of life, childbearing, etc.

Then the direct, femoral and obturator spaces should also be examined for potential hernias, and the last portion of the dissection should occur around the femoral vessels to decrease risk of potential injury. If the hernia defect is very large, there can be a risk for mesh eventration, as this repair is at its core a bridging repair. For direct defects, plicating or tacking down the hernia sac to Cooper ligament can help create a healing shelf to prevent eventration. For large indirect hernia defects, because of the uncertain relationship to the nerves, plication is not generally recommended. In this case, achieving posterior overlap toward the psoas muscles by further mobilizing the peritoneum inferiorly can help. Otherwise, an anterior counter incision to plicate the floor may be considered. For any minimally invasive repair, recurrences have been attributed to inadequate mobilization of the peritoneal flap, which does not allow the prosthesis to lie flat in this area, or allows the peritoneal edge or hernia sac to slip past the inferior edge of the mesh.

A large piece of permanent mesh (at least 15 × 10 cm) is placed in the preperitoneal space to cover the entire myopectineal orifice and all three potential hernia spaces, extending onto the anterior abdominal wall superiorly at least 2 cm above the hernia defect, to the anterior superior iliac spine laterally, and to Cooper ligament medially. Most surgeons prefer to fasten the prosthesis with sutures, tacks, or glue but there is increasing evidence that fixation is not necessary when a large prosthesis is used that widely overlaps the entire myopectineal orifice. If fixation is done, this should never place below the iliopubic tract when lateral to the internal spermatic vessel because of the danger of damage to the important nerves in this area. The last step is to cover the prosthesis by closing the peritoneum with sutures, tacks, staples, or glue. The goal is to exclude the prosthesis from the intra-abdominal contents rather precise approximation of the peritoneal edges from where this was originally transected. The closure should take care to not leave gaps as this can cause interparietal hernias by allowing bowel to migrate into the preperitoneal space. If there is tension, consider securing the inferior peritoneal flap to the transversalis fascia above the prosthesis and leave the superior flap alone.

For bilateral inguinal hernias, two different approaches are commonly used. The existing peritoneal flap can be either extended or a separate peritoneal flap can be created similar to a unilateral approach. The advantage of this is easier handling of the peritoneal flap closure. For a bilateral approach, the symphysis pubis is completely exposed so that both preperitoneal dissections communicate with each other.

Totally Extraperitoneal Repair (TEP)

This repair differs from a TAPP repair in the way the preperitoneal space is accessed. Instead of bringing down a preperitoneal flap from inside the abdomen, the preperitoneal space is directly accessed by using the anatomic relationship of the posterior rectus sheath, the end of the arcuate line and its connection to the space of Retzius. For a TEP repair, a periumbilical incision is made and the anterior rectus sheath is opened on one side and the rectus muscle is bluntly retracted laterally to expose the posterior rectus sheath. To open this posterior space, either blunt dissection can be done or a balloon dissector can be inserted and insufflated. If a balloon dissector is used, the camera can be inserted to directly visualize the dissection planes as the space is created. For a unilateral hernia repair, the contralateral space can be compressed to prevent dissection of the space. Once the space is large enough, two additional cannulas are placed in the midline, one approximately 5 cm above the symphysis pubis and the other midway between the umbilicus and the symphysis pubis. Then using similar operative principles to the TAPP dissection, the critical view of the myopectineal orifice can be achieved, and mesh can be placed.

The presumed advantages of a TEP over a TAPP procedure are that the inherent complications of entering the peritoneal cavity, such as intra-abdominal organ injury, postoperative bowel obstruction secondary to adhesions or trocar site herniation, can be avoided. But complications such as missed peritoneal tears or inadvertent bowel injury can still occur from the dissection. There can also be inadvertent injury to the inferior epigastric vessels if they are dropped posteriorly during the balloon dissection. If that occurs, care should be taken to lift the vessels anteriorly toward the abdominal wall and the plane accessed posterior and lateral to the epigastrics. Additionally, for a TEP procedure there are still technical differences from a TAPP that arise from the difference in view, the limited operative space, thus making the learning curve required to become familiar with the anatomy from this perspective is high. As previously mentioned, this technique may not be used universally for all hernias and there may be some relative contraindications depending on patient or hernia factors that will limit the feasibility of this approach.

Open Preperitoneal Approach to Inguinal Hernia Repair

An open preperitoneal repair is typically reserved for giant loss of domain inguinoscrotal hernias that cannot be approached using an inguinal incision or minimally invasively in the preperitoneal space. This can also be combined with an open retrorectus or preperitoneal ventral hernia repair in a patient that has a concurrent inguinal hernia. The preperitoneal space can be entered via a lower midline incision or a transverse incision placed slightly higher than usual. The rectus muscle is retracted medially and the preperitoneal space entered. A similar hernia dissection is completed to obtain the critical view of the myopectineal orifice, as previously described. For very large loss of domain hernia repairs, a key technicality of this repair is the need for more extensive posterior dissection extending to the retroperitoneum to envelope the visceral contents and this is often referred to as a Stoppa repair, or giant prosthetic reinforcement of the visceral sac (GPRVS).[32] A large prosthesis is used that extends far beyond the margins of the myopectineal orifice and envelops the visceral sac. The mesh is held in place by intra-abdominal pressure, which pushes outward toward the undersurface of the transversalis fascia. If the hernia sac is large, it is amputated or inverted beneath a purse-string suture to smooth the external surface of the visceral sac. The distal peritoneal sac is left in place, undissected, and attached to the cord. With a sliding indirect hernia, the sac is easily dissected away from the cord. For a bilateral repair, one large chevron-shaped mesh can be used for both sides as described by Stoppa. One disadvantage of this technique is the need for a larger incision and substantial amount of dissection, associated pain, and higher morbidity.

Another approach is to take advantage of both the preperitoneal space and the conventional anterior space using a bilayered prosthesis in which a cylinder of prosthetic material connects the two layers through the hernia defect or the internal ring using the Prolene Hernia System (PHS) where both an onlay and sublay mesh is placed.[33] This technique has largely fallen out of favor because of its violation of both the anterior and posterior preperitoneal planes, which makes any hernia recurrence more difficult to repair. Other less commonly performed preperitoneal repairs include the Kugel procedure, Trans Rectus sheath Pre Peritoneal technique, the Trans Inguinal Pre Peritoneal, the Onstep technique, and the Ugahary technique.[34] A detailed description of each of these operations is beyond the scope of this chapter.

Open Anterior Approach to Inguinal Hernia Repair

Open anterior inguinal hernia repair approaches can be grouped into two broad categories: tissue-based repair and mesh-based repair. Most operations will have two separate phases, the first focuses on dissecting out the hernia sac while preserving the cord structures, the second focuses on reconstruction and repair of the defect.

Hernia Sac Dissection

For the simplest Nyhus type I indirect inguinal hernias, which include most inguinal hernias in children, are adequately treated by obliteration of the congenital patent processus vaginalis alone. Since the inguinal floor is otherwise normal, reconstruction is not required. Classically, the hernia sac is dissected from the cord structures, ligated, and removed at its origin at the internal ring, the so-called high ligation of the sac, thus the term *herniotomy.* A herniotomy alone is rarely utilized in adults.

Stepwise, the external landmarks of the pubic tubercle and the anterior superior iliac spine and palpated and marked out. The skin incision starts at the pubic tubercle and is extended laterally. The external oblique aponeurosis is opened in the line of its fibers through the external ring and the lower leaf is freed from the spermatic cord. The spermatic cord is freed from the floor of the inguinal canal and the pubic tubercle. Mobilization of the cord structures is completed by means of blunt dissection, and a Penrose drain is placed around them so that they can be retracted during the procedure. In a female patient the round ligament can be similarly mobilized.

The genital branch of the genitofemoral nerve and the spermatic vessels are included with the cord or round ligament. The ilioinguinal and iliohypogastric nerves are usually preserved and can be identified once the external oblique aponeurosis is opened (**Fig. 69.25**). There is no evidence for routine transection of the ilioinguinal nerve, although if it is injured during the dissection, it can be tied off, sharply transected, and then buried within the underlying muscle. The cremasteric fibers are separated, and the hernia sac is dissected from the cord structures to a point proximal to the internal ring. Ligation can be performed at this point (high ligation), followed by division of the neck of the sac or just reduction into the abdominal cavity. Prior to this, the sac can be opened to allow a digital examination of the abdominal cavity and femoral ring.

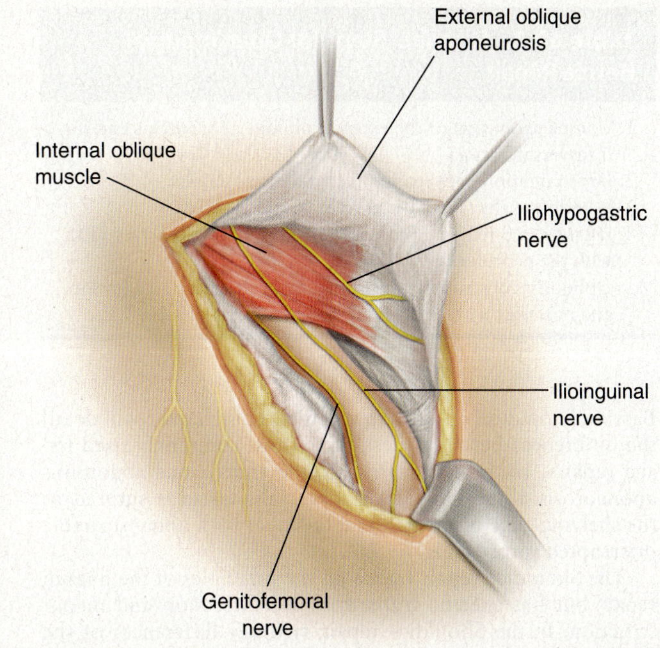

Figure 69.25. Open inguinal hernia repair. Location of the ilioinguinal and genitofemoral iliohypogastric nerves. (From Itani KMF, Sbayi S. Inguinal hernia: open approaches. In: Hawn MT, ed. *Operative Techniques in Surgery*. 2nd ed. Wolters Kluwer; 2023:163–175. Fig. 2.1.3.)

Inguinal Floor Reconstruction

The terms *herniorrhaphy* or *hernioplasty* are used when a procedure to reconstruct the inguinal floor is added. For indirect hernias, the sac is first dealt with in an identical manner as for a herniotomy. The only exception is large indirect inguinal scrotal hernias where complete removal of the sac might result in too high of an incidence of cord and testicular complications because of the extensive dissection required to completely separate them from the cord. For these cases, the sac can be abandoned and transected at the midpoint of the canal, and the distal sac is left in situ. Direct hernia sacs are almost never removed but instead are dissected from surrounding structures and reduced into the preperitoneal space. Dividing the transversalis fascia circumferentially at the neck (base) of the sac will aid in this reduction in some cases. The defect may be closed primarily at this point to maintain the reduction while a formal repair is being performed, but it may not be necessary. The latter is considered a matter of convenience and adds nothing to the strength of the final outcome.

The next step is to reconstruct the inguinal floor. There are two ways to do this. The first is a tissue repair, so named because only the patient's native tissue is used without foreign prosthetic material. The second is the tension-free repair (TFR), which implies the use of a prosthesis or mesh to repair the weakened inguinal floor, eliminating the need to reapproximate tissues that were not in apposition naturally. Edoardo Bassini (1844–1924) is considered the father of modern inguinal hernia surgery because in the latter part of the 19th century he introduced the first tissue repair based on solid anatomic principles, which became the "gold standard" for inguinal hernia repair for most of the 20th century. His scientific approach led to the development of several distinct steps essential for the procedure (**Table 69.7**). Before Bassini's achievements, elective herniorrhaphy was almost never recommended because the results were unfavorable.

Open Anterior Tissue–Based Repair

Today, there are at least 70 named tissue repairs described in the literature. Most are relatively minor modifications of the

Table 69.7. Essential Steps for Open Inguinal Hernia Repair

1. Complete division of the external oblique aponeurosis and the transversalis fascia
2. Differentiation between indirect and direct defects
3. Isolation of the spermatic cord or round ligament
4. Ligation and removal of the sac at the deep inguinal ring flush with the peritoneum
5. Oblique reconstruction of the inguinal canal with an anterior and posterior wall and an internal and external ring

Bassini, Shouldice, and McVay repairs. This chapter will detail the differences between these three most commonly used tissue repairs. In the Bassini repair, the transversus abdominis aponeurosis along with the transversalis fascia is sutured to the shelving edge of the inguinal ligament with nonabsorbable interrupted sutures (**Fig. 69.26**).

The Shouldice repair builds on the principles of the Bassini repair but has specific framework for dissection and reconstruction. In the Shouldice repair, two key differences of the dissection are management of the cremasteric muscle and the incision in the transversalis fascia. The cremasteric muscle is intentionally separated from the cord structures and then intentionally tied and transected, with the distal end resuspended later. An indirect hernia sac is dissected off the cord structures and reduced into the internal ring, and the floor is palpated for a direct defect. Any cord lipoma found can be excised. Then the floor or transversalis fascia is opened and divided from the internal ring to the pubic tubercle and the femoral space and Cooper ligament is interrogated. The musculofascial elements laterally are then sutured to different levels of the inferior flap of the external oblique aponeurosis with four rows of running sutures (**Fig. 69.27**). The first row is started medially with approximation of the transversalis fascial to the ligament of Henle (medial border of the rectus sheath) and transitions to the underside of the transversus abdominis toward the internal ring with a tightening of the ring and incorporation of the proximal end of the cremasteric stump. Then the same suture transitions in the lateral direction in the second row with approximation of the conjoined tendon to the shelving edge of the inguinal ligament. A key step in this operation is to make sure the medial portion of this second suture line goes past the pubic tubercle before it is tied to the original suture to decrease the risk of a medial recurrence. The third row starts laterally at the internal ring and takes the conjoined again to the external oblique aponeurosis just above the shelving edge, the fourth line then duplicates this in reverse to complete the four-layer closure.

Although the suture material originally used for this repair was stainless steel wire, other nonabsorbable materials, such as Prolene, are now used. The McVay repair (**Fig. 69.28**) addresses both inguinal and femoral hernias. The central attenuated portion of the inguinal floor is excised. Cooper ligament must be clearly identified. The inguinal floor is then repaired by approximating the transversus abdominis aponeurosis and transversalis fascia to Cooper ligament between the pubic tubercle and the femoral vein. A so-called transition stitch is then necessary between the transversalis fascia, Cooper ligament, and inguinal ligament to bring the repair above the femoral vessels. The repair is then continued laterally along the inguinal ligament.

A relaxing incision may be necessary for repairs of large indirect hernias and whenever the McVay repair is used. Failure to make a relaxing incision has been implicated in a greater incidence of recurrence. The relaxing incision is made in the anterior rectus sheath in a vertical direction and is extended 3 to 4 cm above the pubis to a level opposite the internal ring (**Fig. 69.28**). The resulting defect in the sheath is protected posteriorly by the body of the rectus muscle, which prevents herniation at that site.

Open Anterior Mesh-Based Repair

As population-based studies began to supplant personal series, it became obvious that the recurrence rate for tissue repairs approached 10% to 15%. In the 1990s, widespread adoption of the routine use of prosthesis (usually a mesh material) in a tension-free manner was popularized by Lichtenstein, and decreased recurrence rates to 1% to 2%. The Lichtenstein operation is considered the "gold standard" operation for open inguinal hernia repairs with mesh (**Fig. 69.29**).[35] The initial dissection is identical to the tissue repairs described in the previous sections. If a femoral hernia is present, the inguinal floor is incised, exposing the preperitoneal fat, femoral space, and Cooper ligament, and the mesh can be modified to cover

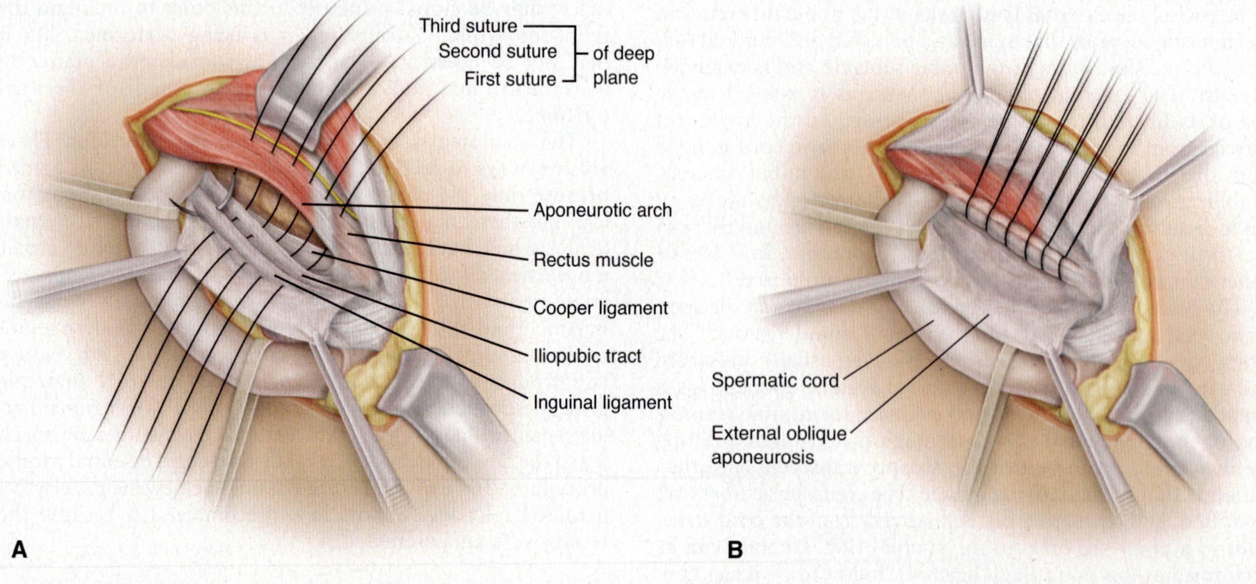

Figure 69.26. Bassini repair. **A:** If the transversalis fascia is opened in a Bassini repair, the iliopubic tract may be incorporated into the lateral stitch. **B:** The Bassini repair is carried lateral until the internal ring is re-created. (From Itani KMF, Sbayi S. Inguinal hernia: open approaches. In: Hawn MT, ed. *Operative Techniques in Surgery*. 2nd ed. Wolters Kluwer; 2023:163–175. Figs. 2.1.7 and 2.1.8.)

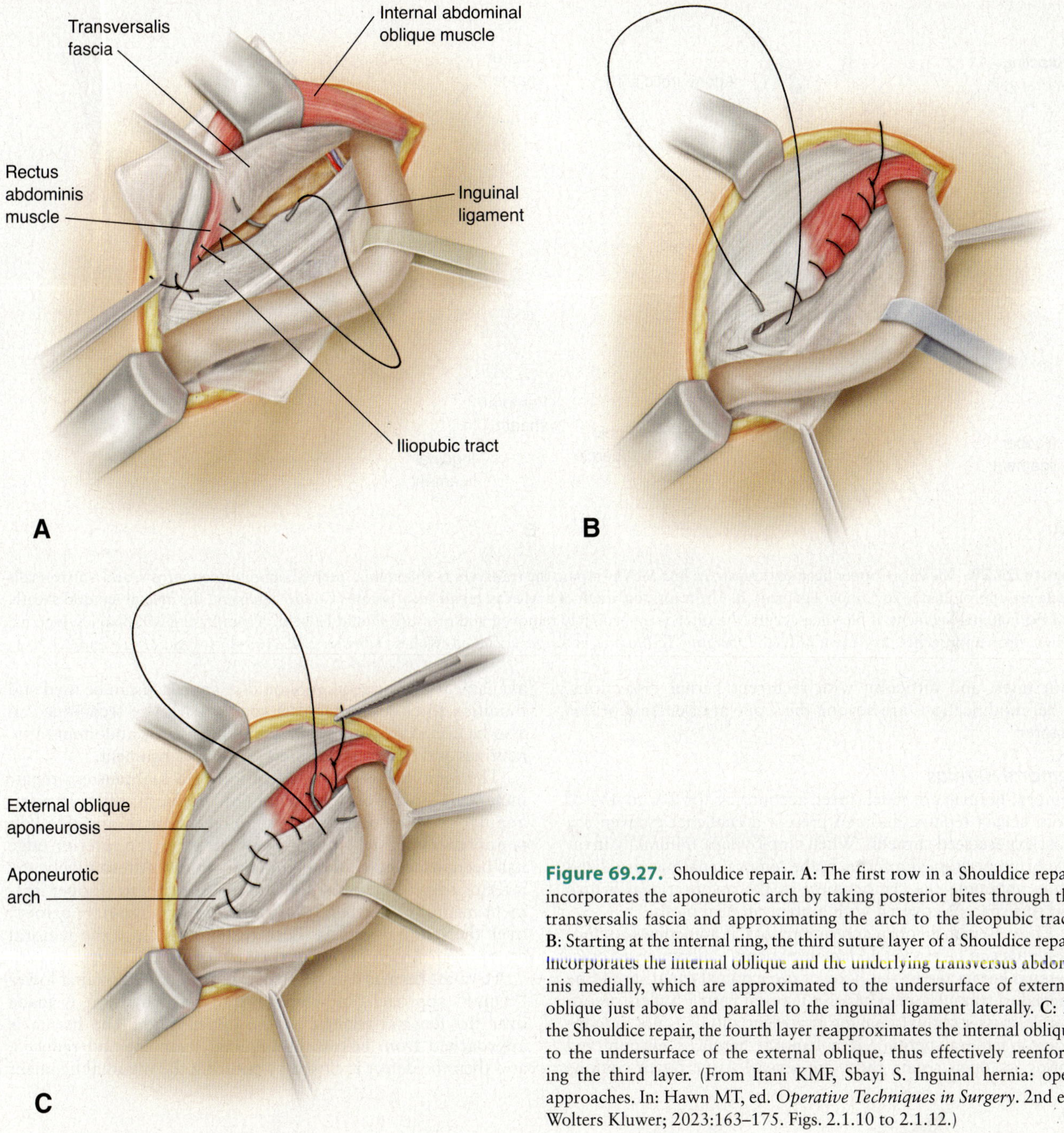

Figure 69.27. Shouldice repair. A: The first row in a Shouldice repair incorporates the aponeurotic arch by taking posterior bites through the transversalis fascia and approximating the arch to the ileopubic tract. B: Starting at the internal ring, the third suture layer of a Shouldice repair incorporates the internal oblique and the underlying transversus abdominis medially, which are approximated to the undersurface of external oblique just above and parallel to the inguinal ligament laterally. C: In the Shouldice repair, the fourth layer reapproximates the internal oblique to the undersurface of the external oblique, thus effectively reenforcing the third layer. (From Itani KMF, Sbayi S. Inguinal hernia: open approaches. In: Hawn MT, ed. *Operative Techniques in Surgery*. 2nd ed. Wolters Kluwer; 2023:163–175. Figs. 2.1.10 to 2.1.12.)

this femoral space (see Femoral Hernias Section). Once the sac has been dealt with and any sizable cord lipoma resected, a 15 cm by 7 cm sheet of mid-weight or heavy-weight polypropylene mesh is used, the medial end of which is rounded to the shape of the medial corner of the inguinal canal. This medial end is allowed to extend 2 cm medial to the pubic tubercle. The first running permanent suture starts by anchoring the medial portion of the mesh to the pubic tubercle, and then continues by approximating the inferior aspect of the mesh to the shelving edge of the inguinal ligament. This is continued just proximal to the internal ring and tied to itself. Next, superior absorbable sutures are placed in an interrupted fashion approximating the mesh to the conjoined tendon, taking care to avoid the iliohypogastric nerve.

A slit is cut in the lateral end of the mesh and the cord or round ligament is positioned between the two tails. The two tails are placed over each other in a so-called shutter valve stitch placed just lateral to the cord including the inferior surface of the superior tail, the inferior surface of the inferior tail, and the inguinal ligament. The tails are then tucked under the external oblique aponeurosis to the level of the anterior superior iliac spine. The external oblique aponeurosis is closed to recreate the external ring.

In female patients undergoing open inguinal hernia repair, there is limited evidence for preserving or dividing the round ligament. Because the genital branch of the genitofemoral nerve and the ilioinguinal nerve can run along with the ligament, it is recommended that this structure be preserved if possible and treated very similarly to the cord structures in a male patient.

Several modifications to the Lichtenstein operation exist, the most popular of which includes a prosthetic mesh plug in addition to a mesh patch. There is considerable debate among hernia experts about the potential issues with a mesh plug and it has largely fallen out of favor for the following reasons: violation of the preperitoneal plane, potential increase in chronic

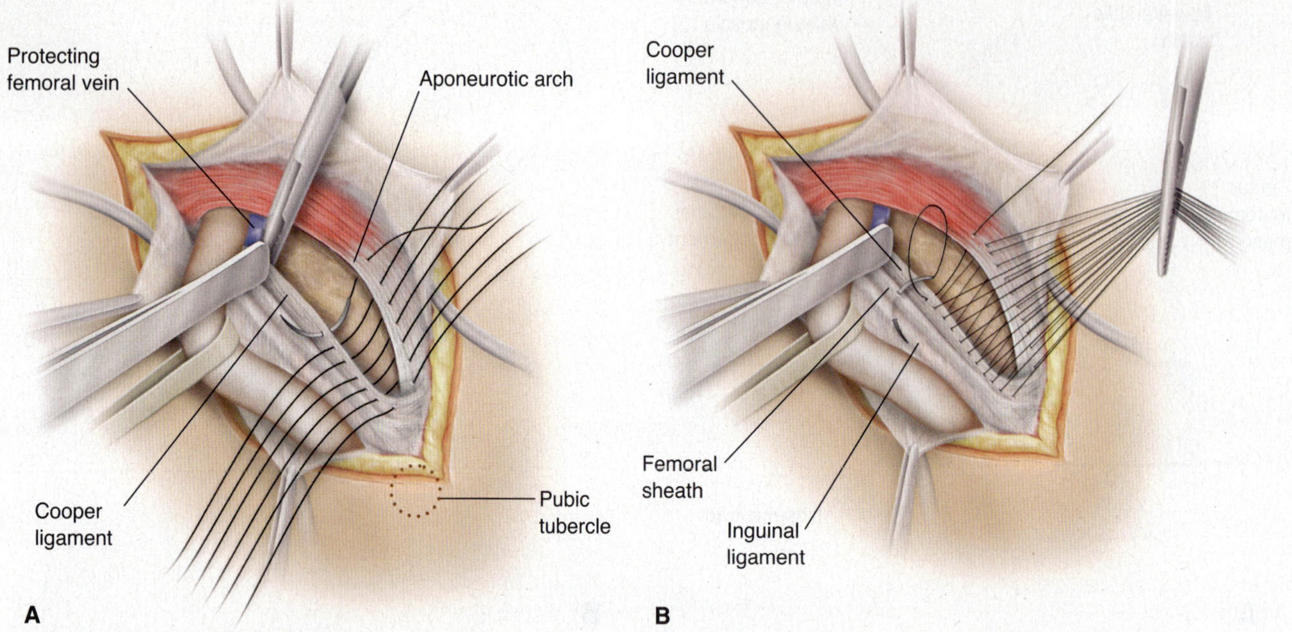

Figure 69.28. McVay (Cooper ligament) repair. **A:** In a McVay repair, the transversus abdominis, internal oblique aponeurosis, and transversalis fascia are approximated to Cooper ligament. **B:** The transition stitch of a McVay repair incorporates Cooper ligament, the medial femoral sheath, and the inguinal ligament. If bleeding occurs, the stitch is immediately removed and pressure should be held. (From Itani KMF, Sbayi S. Inguinal hernia: open approaches. In: Hawn MT, ed. *Operative Techniques in Surgery*. 2nd ed. Wolters Kluwer; 2023:163–175. Figs. 2.1.14 and 2.1.15.)

pain rates, and difficulty with recurrent hernia dissections. Other modifications are beyond the scope of discussion of this chapter.

Femoral Hernias

Femoral hernias are much rarer, accounting for 2% to 4% of groin hernia repairs, and can present a challenge to even the most experienced surgeon. When employing a minimally invasive or preperitoneal approach, the femoral space is visualized while obtaining the critical view of the myopectineal orifice and this space is covered with a preperitoneal mesh.

Conversely in an open anterior approach, sometimes a femoral hernia can be missed. In female patients undergoing an open inguinal hernia repair the floor of the inguinal canal should be opened to routinely inspect for a femoral hernia (unless preoperative cross-sectional imaging is present and does not demonstrate a femoral hernia). If a femoral hernia is encountered during an open repair, there are several tissue repair options available to the surgeon. A Shouldice approach can be used and modified to close the femoral space. A McVay technique can also be utilized to approximate the transversus abdominis aponeurosis and transversalis fascia to Cooper ligament.

The femoral hernia modification of a Lichtenstein repair includes a posterior "extension" of the mesh, often in a triangular configuration, when shaping the mesh and this flap is approximated to Cooper ligament after the inferior edge has been attached to the inguinal ligament. Alternatively, the inferior edge of the prosthesis is sewn directly to Cooper ligament medially and then transitioned to the inguinal ligament over the femoral vessels. Both techniques close the femoral canal.

Femoral hernias can alternatively be repaired from a lower "crural" approach, in which a transverse incision is made over the femoral triangle in the upper thigh. The hernia is approached from below the inguinal ligament and reduced, and then the defect is closed by suturing the inguinal ligament

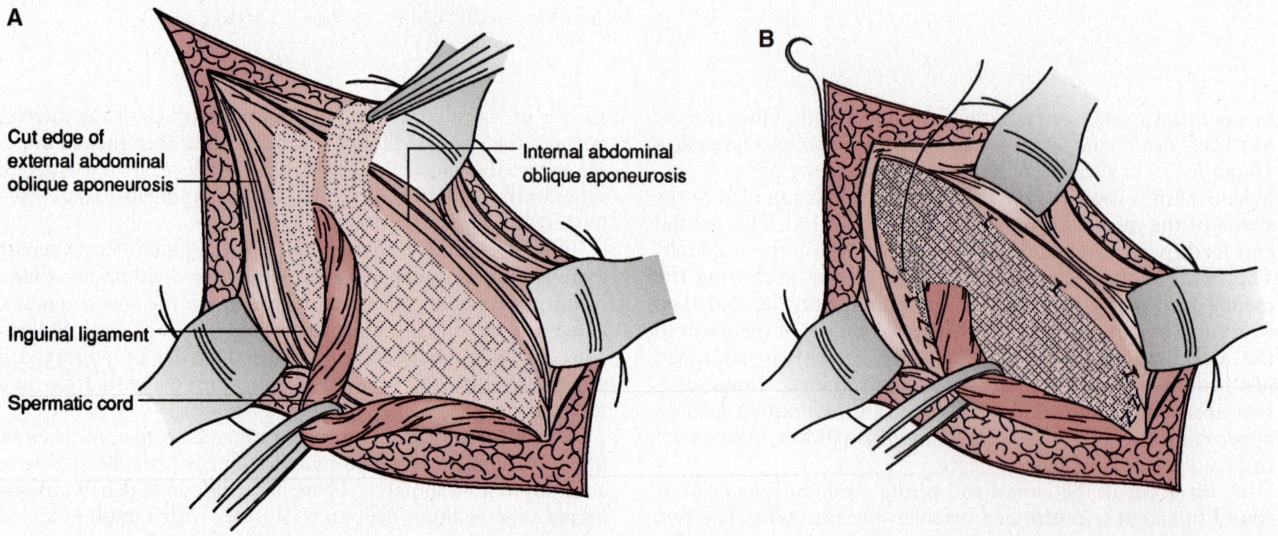

Figure 69.29. The Lichtenstein hernioplasty. **A:** Showing placement of the mesh. **B:** Suture placement for mesh fixation.

to Cooper ligament from below. An alternative is to insert a small mesh plug into the defect and suture the periphery to the inguinal ligament and Cooper ligament. If this technique is used, it is important to leave a layer of adventitial tissue between the femoral vein and the plug. The femoral vein should not be skeletonized. The repair can also be carried out from above via an inguinal approach, as in the McVay repair. In the setting of an incarcerated femoral hernia, it can be difficult to reduce the hernia at surgery, and it is not uncommon to have to divide the inguinal ligament to obtain greater freedom to perform this reduction. As previously discussed in female patients undergoing a groin hernia repair, a minimally invasive approach is preferred to decrease risk of missing an femoral hernia.

Unusual Groin Hernias

Obturator Hernia

This hernia is the result of abdominal contents protruding through the obturator canal in the pelvis. This canal is the opening in the superior part of the obturator membrane covering the foramen formed by the union of the pubic bone and ischium, through which the obturator nerve, artery, and vein pass from the pelvic cavity into the thigh. A recent history of profound asthenia and weight loss is not unusual, which is most likely due to the loss of the protective fat in the obturator canal. This may account for the fact that women, more often than men, are afflicted with this hernia because their broader pelvis results in a larger obturator canal. The diagnosis of an obturator hernia is difficult because it is rare and physical examination is rarely helpful because the associated mass is concealed beneath the adductor muscles of the thigh. The main symptom is intermittent pain, however, this will classically present as bowel obstruction in the elderly patient in the absence of prior abdominal surgery. A helpful physical examination maneuver is the Howship–Romberg sign where inner thigh pain is experienced with internal rotation of the thigh. During repair, the defect is approached transperitoneally; the hernia is reduced, and mesh placed over the defect. Depending on the expertise of the responsible surgeon, either a conventional open or laparoscopic operation is reasonable, though laparoscopy offers the optimal visualization and ease of repair.

Littre and Amyand Hernia

Littre hernia is a groin hernia containing a Meckel diverticulum. If the diverticulum is symptomatic or strangulated, then it is mandatory to resect it at the time of the hernia repair. An Amyand hernia is a groin hernia containing the appendix. If the appendix is inflamed or acute appendicitis occurs, an appendectomy may need to be performed at the time of hernia repair. Rarely an ovary can also be incarcerated in a groin hernia and need to be reduced.

Pediatric Inguinal Hernias

Given the high incidence of indirect inguinal hernias due to a patent processus vaginalis in pediatric patients, hernia repairs are completed using a high ligation technique. Concerns exist with the use of mesh in adolescents with respect to effect on fertility, long-term groin pain, and infection risk.[36,37] Post pubertal males have a similar anatomy to the adult population with a larger inguinal ring diameter and variations on transverse fascia defects. It is unclear as to which age/size does a child become an adult with respect to principles of hernia repair. Longitudinal studies comparing different hernia repair techniques in adolescents are needed before we can determine optimal treatment for adolescents especially those with weak inguinal floors and direct hernias.

Complications of Inguinal Hernia Repair

Incidence of complications after inguinal hernia repair is generally low and range around 1% to 5%. The most common tend to be seromas and hematomas. These are more likely to occur in patients with large hernia sacs or on anticoagulation. In patients with very large inguinoscrotal sacs, a prophylactic drain at the time of surgery can be considered. If one develops, most resolve with no interventions, as the fluid or blood eventually resorbs over time. For those patients who are symptomatic, aspiration of the fluid can be performed. Those with large hematomas noted immediately post op can be taken back to the OR for evacuation of the hematoma. This is not recommended for hematomas that are longstanding and discovered several weeks after surgery.

Bruising of the groin or testicles can also often occur, and most will resolve fairly quickly within 1 to 2 weeks after surgery. Bleeding is overall unlikely, but in those who had a minimally invasive repair, a bleed can often be more occult in the extraperitoneal space and difficult to identify on physical exam. Patients can develop a large hematoma in the space of Retzius and if it is stable can be managed with transfusions and nonoperative intervention as the venous bleeding will tamponade. For larger symptomatic hematomas patients may require reintervention to drain the hematoma whether that is surgically or with consultation to interventional radiology. Here cross imaging will be important, if the hematoma displaces your inguinal hernia mesh, reoperation is the best option.

Wound infections rarely occur after minimally invasive hernia operations. It is more common after an open operation, but the overall incidence is still low (<5%) and can be depended on patient-specific risk factors that may predispose someone to infection. Overall, the mesh infection rate for inguinal hernia repairs is very low (<2%), with an even lower risk of mesh explantation. The risk for a delayed mesh infection after the patient has an uncomplicated immediate postoperative recovery course is very unlikely to happen.

Like all hernia surgeries that employ a prosthetic material, there can be mesh-related complications. For all prosthetic materials, there can changes to that material overtime, especially contraction and shrinkage. To what degree this impacts chronic pain rates, recurrence, and quality of life is largely unknown. Mesh implant illness is rare, but has been reported, and this mesh sensitivity is not well understood, but more likely to occur in thin females with other autoimmune pathology. Occasionally mesh will have to be explanted due to erosion, meshoma, chronic pain, recurrence, or infection, and this nuanced discussion is beyond the scope of this chapter.

Some complications related to the postop recovery such as urinary retention and ileus have showed decreased incidence in recent years due to novel paralytic reversal agents. Other technical complications are related to inadvertent injury to structures around the hernia dissection, which can lead to things such as bowel, bladder, vascular, testicular cord, etc. injuries. Injury to the vas deferens or testicle can result in infertility, while injury to the cord vessels may result in ischemic orchitis and atrophy of the testicle over time. This ischemia can manifest as postoperative pain and swelling of the testicle. The management of a patient with ischemic orchitis is usually conservative with elevation and anti-inflammatory medication. Usually due to collateralization of blood supply, an orchiectomy is rarely needed. Occasionally after inguinal hernias, a hydrocele of the testicle can develop.

Chronic Groin Pain

Chronic postoperative groin pain, defined as groin pain persisting >3 to 6 months after surgery can be a challenging problem to address (**Algorithm 69.3**). While the incidence of postop chronic groin pain at about 6 months after surgery is about 10% to 15%, studies have shown that for the majority of people this pain may continue to diminish over time. Postoperative predictor for chronic pain includes preoperative pain. While some may blame the placement of a prosthesis as the cause to chronic pain, limited evidence indicates that rates of chronic pain after inguinal hernia operation are similar whether or not mesh is used.

Algorithm 69.3

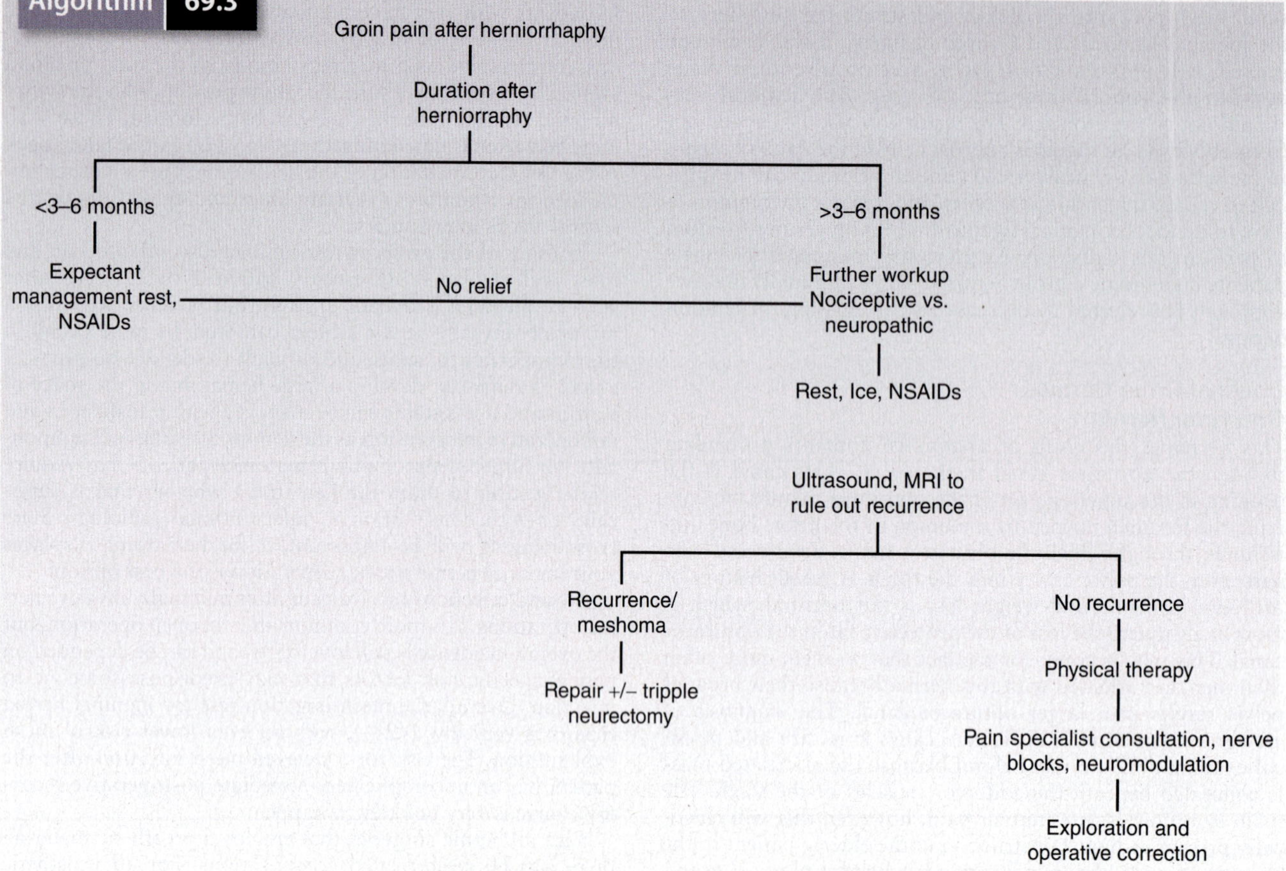

Algorithm 69.3. Management of groin pain after herniorrhaphy.

Perhaps the most important determination for patients with chronic postherniorrhaphy pain is to obtain an accurate history and physical exam. This physical exam should exclude hernia recurrence and systematically map out pain, numbness, and loss of sensation. Understanding when the pain started, if it is constant, and if it has improved over time are some important questions to ask. If this pain is the same pain as prior to surgery without an accompanying bulge, additional imaging can be obtained to rule out other pathology that may have been concurrent with an inguinal hernia. There are a variety of conditions that cause groin pain that are not hernia related (**Table 69.8**) and making the correct diagnosis is important and should be done ideally prior to surgery. Ultrasonography, CT, and MRI all have their place in the evaluation of these patients and imaging should be obtained to rule out recurrence or other pathology. If a recurrence is found, typically a hernia repair is offered. If there is no recurrence, investigation of other etiologies is important. MRI is perhaps the most beneficial because of its ability to differentiate between muscle tear, osteitis pubis, bursitis, and stress fracture. Strain of the adductor muscle complex (adductor longus, brevis, magnus, and gracilis muscles) is commonly overlooked in this group.

True postherniorrhaphy groin pain should be divided into two types: (a) nociceptive pain, which is caused by tissue damage, is further subdivided into somatic and visceral pain, and (b) neuropathic pain due to direct nerve damage. Somatic pain is the most common and is usually caused by damage to ligaments, tendons, and muscles. Visceral pain refers to that which is related to a specific visceral function such as urination or ejaculation (see dysejaculation syndrome, later). Neuropathic pain is much less common but is important to recognize because surgical treatment is possible if the cause is incorporation of a nerve in staples or suture material. The nerves that are usually involved are the ilioinguinal nerve, the iliohypogastric nerve, both the genital and femoral branches of the genitofemoral nerve, and the lateral cutaneous nerve of the thigh. The former two are especially prone to injury during a conventional herniorrhaphy, whereas the latter are most likely damaged during laparoscopy. A femoral nerve injury is extremely rare and is usually the result of a gross technical misadventure. Pain

Table 69.8. Conditions Other Than a Hernia Associated with Groin Pain

- Nerve entrapment
- Adductor tenoperiostitis
- Pelvic stress fractures
- Osteitis pubis
- Symphysis syndrome
- Gilmore groin (groin disruption)
- Iliopsoas bursitis
- Tendinopathies
- Posterior inguinal wall insufficiency or avulsion fractures
- Synovitis
- Osteoarthritis
- Legg–Calvé–Perthes disease
- Slipped femoral capital epiphysis
- Osteochondritis dissecans or avascular necrosis of the femoral head
- Acetabular labral tears
- Prostatitis
- Epididymitis
- Nephrolithiasis
- Urinary tract infection
- Lymphadenitis

and/or paresthesia in their distribution characterize patients' symptoms for the more common nerves. There is significant overlap of these nerves, and therefore, it is commonly difficult to sort out exactly which nerve is damaged.

Both nociceptive and neuropathic pain is best treated initially with reassurance and conservative treatment with anti-inflammatory medications and local nerve blocks because these will frequently resolve spontaneously. An exception is the patient who complains of severe pain immediately (ie, in the recovery room). This patient may be best served by immediate reexploration before scar tissue develops. When groin exploration is required, triple neurectomy and neuroma excision, adhesiolysis, and foreign-body removal (ie, mesh or suture) are options for treatment. The patients reoperated for persistent pain after hernia surgery often experience a reduction in pain, but a small percentage of patients experience no relief or even worsening of their symptoms.[38] Given the heterogeneity of the problem, further well-designed studies are necessary to identify patient population that may benefit the most from surgical intervention. It cannot be overemphasized that these complex patients should be evaluated and treated at centers with specific multidisciplinary expertise in this area.

Inguinal Hernia Recurrence

The accuracy of reported recurrence rates after inguinal hernia repair comes in to question because recurrence can occur many years after the index operation (50 years or greater) making precise follow-up impossible.[39] A lower risk for recurrence with the use of prosthetic material for the repair of an inguinal hernia has been clearly proven by meta-analysis with relatively short-term follow-up.[27] Recurrence rates of 2% or less are now routinely reported from specialty centers performing either minimally invasive or open TFRs with mesh. Minimally invasive repairs tend to recur inferiorly due to lack of adequate inferior peritoneal dissection and mesh coverage, while open repairs most commonly recur medially where the mesh is anchored to the pubic tubercle. The recurrence rates for tissue-based repairs are higher than for mesh repairs. Although the reported recurrence rate for hernia repairs is less than 1% at the Shouldice Clinic, this has not been widely reproduced elsewhere. Risk factors for recurrence include any complications during the first month after surgery, hernia factors, and likely some patient factors. From a clinical standpoint, a hernia should not be classified recurrent unless there is a visible bulge or there is unequivocal evidence of a hernia by an imaging modality such as ultrasound, CT, or MRI. This is especially important for patients who present with pain after their hernia repair because their pain is likely due to a preoperative condition other than the hernia or a postinguinal herniorrhaphy pain syndrome which might be exacerbated by further groin surgery.

The general principle for managing recurrent hernias depends on the original repair. The logical approach is to perform the herniorrhaphy in the space that has not been previously dissected. If the patient had a previous open anterior repair, then a preperitoneal repair is best. On the other hand, if the index operation was a preperitoneal one, then a repair should be performed as an open anterior repair. The dissection of the redo open groin space and preperitoneal space both offer its unique challenges and can be difficult operations with higher risk of injuring surrounding structures.

SPORTS HERNIA/ATHLETIC PUBALGIA

The term *sports hernia* is confusing because, by definition, these patients do not actually have a hernia but rather a weakness of the posterior inguinal floor. This condition has received considerable attention because of its prevalence in high-profile athletes involved in sports who require rapid changes in direction of the hip area such as soccer, football, basketball, track and field, tennis, and hockey. Alteration in the

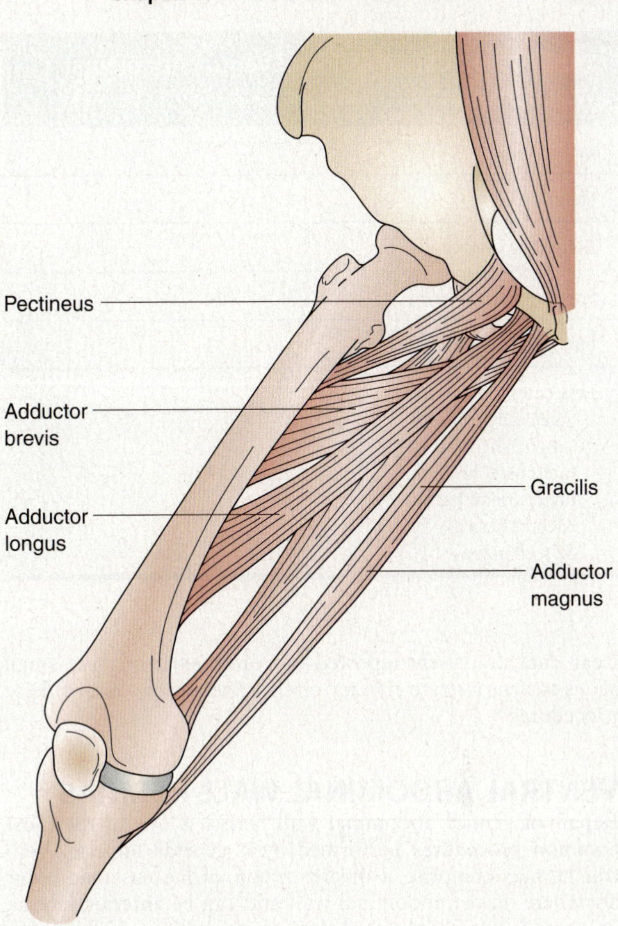

Figure 69.30. Complicated arrangement of muscle pulling in different directions that attach to the pubic bone.

complex balance that must be maintained between the lower abdominal muscles and the leg adductor muscles and tendons, all revolving around the area of the pubic bone, is the final common denominator for many of the conditions that cause groin pain in up to 5% of athletes (**Fig. 69.30**).[40] The first step in approaching these patients is to make sure that one is not dealing with a cause outside of the groin with referred pain, such as lumbosacral radiculopathic pain, prostatitis, hip disease, and a gastrointestinal cause. The differential diagnosis is listed in **Table 69.8**.

Some authorities prefer to refer to this condition as "athletic pubalgia," as this conveys the concept that the physical examination is inconclusive, and the cause of groin pain is unclear. Imaging may be performed by ultrasound, but cross-sectional imaging (CT or magnetic resonance imaging [MRI]) is the most useful diagnostic modality in the absence of a highly experienced ultrasonographer.[41] Compared to CT, MRI provides excellent overall anatomic detail especially with the development of fast imaging scanners that will allow dynamic imaging (ie, performed during straining) with or without the addition of intraperitoneal contrast agents.

The initial treatment is conservative with mandatory inactivity, elastic immobilization bandages, ice/massage, nonsteroidal anti-inflammatory analgesics, and occasional steroids (systemic and/or local). Physical therapy performed by a specialized practitioner can often improve symptoms. Surgery should be reserved after nonoperative interventions have been performed. Although lacking clear-cut anatomic justification, a mesh hernia repair similar to either an anterior Lichtenstein or a TEP laparoscopic operation is the most popular procedure, sometimes combined with a variety of muscle reattachment procedures and tenotomies. The best results are obtained with a multidisciplinary approach including a surgeon, an orthopedist, a physical therapist, and a sports medicine physician. No

Table 69.9. Classification of Ventral Abdominal Wall Hernias

Incisional
Umbilical
Epigastric
Parastomal
Flank
Less common variations Spigelian hernias Lumbar hernias Intercostal hernias Interparietal hernia Richter hernia Miscellaneous

Table 69.10. European Hernia Society (EHS) Classification of Incisional Hernia

Midline	Subxiphoid Epigastric Umbilical Infraumbilical Suprapubic	M1 M2 M3 M4 M5
Lateral	Subcostal Flank Iliac Lumbar	L1 L2 L3 L4
Recurrent incisional hernia	Yes	No
Length (cm) Width <4 cm 4–10 cm >10 cm		Width (cm) W1 W2 W3

clear data or patient-reported outcomes exist in these small series to demonstrate efficacy or effectiveness of some of these procedures.

VENTRAL ABDOMINAL WALL HERNIAS

Repair of ventral abdominal wall hernia is one of the most common procedures performed by a general surgeon. Ventral hernias comprise a diverse group of hernias that occur anywhere on the abdominal wall and can be anterior, lateral, or posterior. It is estimated that about 20% to 30% of any major open abdominal operation can result in an incisional hernia and as of data in 2006, account for about 350,000 operations per year with a total cost of 3.2 billion health care dollars spent.[42] Reducing the burden of hernia disease by both decreasing the incidence and hernia recurrence rates by just 1% can decrease this cost by up to 32 million dollars.

Epidemiology and Classification

In general, an inguinal hernia is the most common, while incisional, umbilical, and epigastric hernias account for 15% of all remaining hernias and miscellaneous hernias make up the other 5%. **Table 69.9** uses the common general terminology for classifying abdominal wall hernias.

Perhaps the most commonly used classification system was proposed by an expert panel of European Hernia Society in which incisional hernias are classified based on location, size, recurrences, and symptoms (**Table 69.10**).[43]

An additional classification scheme that can be utilized is the Ventral Hernia Working Group (VHWG)[44] (**Table 69.11**), which subdivides hernias into different classes of morbidity based on risk of postoperative surgical site occurrences (SSOs).

Clinical Diagnosis

Similar to groin hernias, ventral hernias are diagnosed both by history and physical exam. Most patients will present with abdominal wall bulging that worsens with valsalva. Sometimes these hernias as asymptomatic, other times they can be painful, cause issues with bowel function, and increase with any rise in intra-abdominal pressure. On physical exam, chronically incarcerated hernias that are not typically reducible per patient history should not be reduced on exam. There can be adhesions within the hernia sac that make this impossible, it can cause pain to the patient, and if the incarcerated contents are omentum or preperitoneal fat, reducing these contents could then allow bowel contents to incarcerate instead and result in the need for an emergent operation. If the contents are easily reducible, sometimes it is possible to palpate the fascial defect. Other things on exam should also be noted such as previous scars, crossing incisions that can compromise the blood supply to the skin, or lateral incisions that could potentially cause muscle denervation or atrophy. The physical exam should be completed in both the supine position and with valsalva to best understand abdominal wall function and true defect size and herniated contents.

Differential Diagnosis

Ventral hernias have an accompanying fascial defect should be distinguished from pseudo hernia or abdominal wall laxity which results from denervation of the abdominal wall musculature (eg, after polio or flank incisions). Rectus diastasis, or a separation of the rectus muscles after abdominal wall expansion (childbearing, obesity, etc.) can also mimic the bulge of a ventral hernia, but the key distinction is lack of a fascial defect. In both a pseudo hernia and rectus diastasis, the abdominal wall muscles bulge forward on straining and have the appearance of a hernia, but no frank fascial defect can be discerned on physical examination or cross-sectional imaging. Occasionally this can be misleading in an incisional hernia without a palpable fascial defect and what appears to be intact diastasis on imaging, but if there is an overlying incision, this bulge is in fact an incisional hernia. An abdominal wall bulge can also rarely represent an abdominal wall mass from a benign etiology (ie, lipoma), or malignant disease process (ie, primary tumor or metastatic abdominal wall lesion). In female patients who have had prior cesarean sections, hysterectomies, or endometriosis surgery, a painful bulge can also be an abdominal wall endometrioma. One defining characteristic that will separate out an abdominal wall hernia, however,

Table 69.11. Ventral Hernia Working Group (VHWG) Classification of Incisional Hernia

Grade 1	Grade 2 Comorbid	Grade 3 Potentially Contaminated	Grade 4 Infected
Low risk of complications No history of wound infections	Smoker Obese Diabetic Immunosuppressed COPD	Previous wound infection Stoma present Violation of gastrointestinal tract	Infected mesh Septic dehiscence

will be its change with abdominal wall position, pressure, and upon valsalva. Not all hernias can be reducible, but most will change and feel different than other masses.

Radiographic Imaging

Radiographic imaging should be obtained if it would provide additional information on the hernia characteristics, clarify patient anatomy, and impact how a particular hernia is surgically repaired. It is often not needed for primary nonrecurrent hernias at the umbilicus or epigastric region that are small and are felt to contain intra-abdominal or preperitoneal fat. If studies are to be obtained, ultrasounds can be utilized, but CT scans typically provide richer information that can better inform the surgeon on the hernia characteristics such as fascial defect size, quality, and size of surrounding muscle, identify prior mesh, assess for fat planes, and inform the surgeon on key patient hernia and anatomy factors that may impact choice of hernia repair. Hernia radiography is a new emerging field and in-depth assessment of CT imaging is an important tool for hernia surgeons to understand and utilize.

VENTRAL HERNIA PREVENTION

Abdominal Wall Closure

The best way to avoid a hernia operation is to prevent a hernia from occurring in the first place. There are a variety of risk factors that predispose a patient to hernia formation, as discussed earlier in this chapter, and many are outside the surgeon's control.[45] What surgeons can control are how and where incisions on the abdomen and abdominal closure techniques. General strategies to reduced incisional hernia rates include placing incisions away from known weak areas of the abdominal wall such as the umbilicus, semilunar line, through a diastasis, etc., and using off midline extraction sites such as Pfannenstiel incisions. For abdominal wall closure, it is recommended that the fascia of any port site greater than a 10-mm port should be closed. Specifically for midline abdominal wall closures, the anterior sheath should be clearly identified and cleared off, and a continuous small-bites technique using slowly absorbable sutures using a 4:1 suture to wound length ratio should be used to better distribute the tension of the closure and to promote the healing process along the entire midline.[46] The STITCH trial has demonstrated that using a small-bites technique with the appropriate suture material (smaller needle and nonlooped suture) can decrease the rates of incisional hernia formation after primary laparotomy by 50%.[47] Although this study has been criticized for a variety of different reasons including its relatively low-average BMI patient population of 25 kg/m^2, current guidelines advocate for its use in the closure of elective midline laparotomies.

Another common practice after laparotomy is to prescribe abdominal binders. Although most surgeons prescribe abdominal binders following laparotomy, there is no evidence that these devices decrease pain; improve respiratory function; or prevent incisional hernias, seroma formation, or wound complications. The use of a binder may provide some comfort in the immediate postoperative period to some patients and should be recommended for this purpose only.[45,48]

Prophylactic Mesh Placement

Recent randomized controlled trials and a recent meta-analysis have shown that prophylactic implantation to prevent incisional hernia formation can decrease the incidence of incisional hernias by about 50% in midline laparotomies in higher-risk patients.[49–51] Prophylactic mesh can also be considered when creating stomas to help decrease the incidence of parastomal hernia formation. These practice patterns are often not widely adopted due to concerns for mesh infection, adding time to a case, and experience and comfort of the surgeon with prophylactic mesh placement. Further large-scale randomized controlled trials with long-term follow-up are necessary to identify specific group of patients in whom reinforcement is essential and cost effective, and to identify the optimal mesh type and location for prophylaxis.

Hernia Repair in the Emergent Setting

Incarcerated means "trapped" or "imprisoned." Clinically, an incarcerated hernia is an irreducible hernia. An incarceration is not in and of itself a surgical emergency. Many hernias are chronically incarcerated due to adhesions of contents (eg, preperitoneal fat, omentum, bowel, ovary, etc.) to the hernia sac.

An acutely incarcerated, painful hernia must be managed carefully. An attempt at reduction is reasonable unless there are signs of strangulation, which is not always obvious by clinical examination. Immediate surgical exploration is the safest approach when the diagnosis is not clear. The advantage of reduction followed by elective repair is that edematous tissue associated with an acute incarceration can normalize prior to repair. If an attempt at reduction seems reasonable, the patient is given medications to simultaneous relax the abdominal wall muscles and provide pain relief. A slight Trendelenburg position may facilitate reduction of a groin hernia. The maneuver of taxis entails grasping the neck of the hernia with the fingers of one hand and then applying intermittent pressure on the most distal part of the hernia with the other hand while massaging the hernia back in. Taxis has the effect of elongating the neck of the hernia so that the contents of the hernia may be guided through this area back into the abdominal cavity with a rocking movement. Most hernia sacs are much larger than the neck or hernia defect itself and pushing directly on the sac can cause occlusion the hernia neck, pain, and prevent it from being reduced (**Fig. 69.31**). The maneuver of taxis should not be performed with excessive pressure or too vigorously. If the hernia is strangulated, gangrenous bowel might be reduced into the abdomen or perforated in the process. One or two gentle attempts should be made at taxis. If they are unsuccessful, this procedure should be abandoned.

Strangulation of a hernia is a serious and life-threatening condition in which the hernia contents become ischemic and nonviable. The pathogenesis of this condition involves intra-abdominal contents within the hernia sac and is pinched off at the narrower hernia neck. This pressure initially produces venous congestion, resulting in edema. Eventually, the

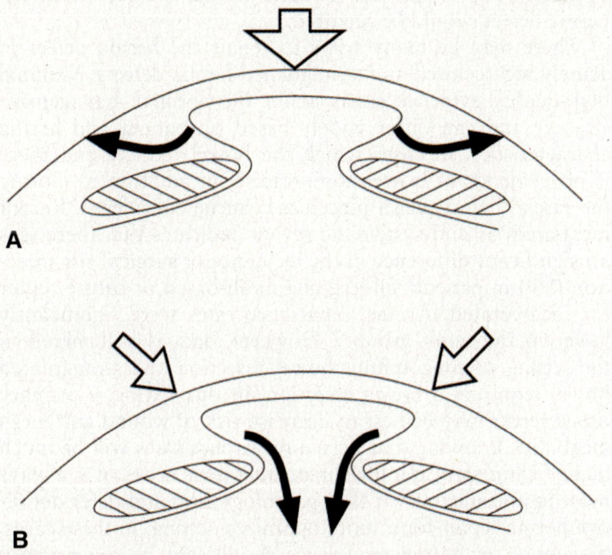

Figure 69.31. Reduction of a hernia by taxis. **A:** Applying pressure on the hernia directly occludes the neck. **B:** Elongating the neck of the hernia while applying pressure allows reduction.

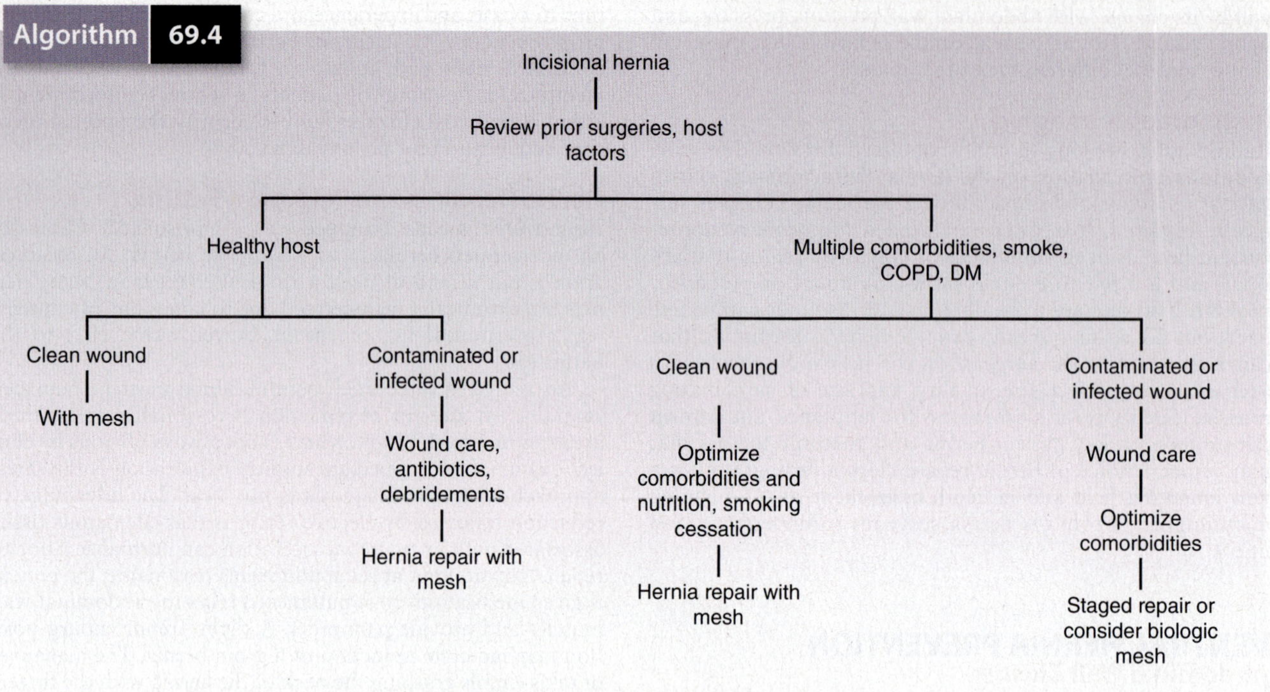

Algorithm 69.4. Management of incisional hernia.

pressure is so great that the arterial supply is obstructed, and the contents become gangrenous.

Patient management strategies include rapid resuscitation, with nasogastric tube decompression, replacement of fluids and electrolytes, and administration of antibiotics. In these instances, no attempt should be made to reduce the hernia. These patients should be taken for emergent surgery with controlled reduction of the incarcerated hernia contents and evaluation for viability of incarcerated contents. Occasionally after reduction of the bowel, it will start to pink up as it regains its blood supply. In these cases, the bowel can be observed and additional adjuncts to examine the bowel such as a Wood lamp or indocyanine green (ICG) can be used to assess for bowel viability. If there is an obvious perforation or if the bowel appears gangrenous, a bowel resection and anastomosis should be performed. This can be done both open or minimally invasively depending on the comfort level of the surgeon. Then to prevent another hernia incarceration, the hernia defect should be repaired.

There may be many ways to repair the hernia defect in acutely incarcerated and strangulated hernia defects. Minimal high-quality evidence exists about the optimal management strategy and can differ widely based on patient and hernia characteristics. In cases which the bowel reduces and there is no evidence of bowel compromise, in addition to closing the fascial defect, mesh placement can be considered. Recent meta-analysis and systematic review indicates that there was no significant difference in the incidence of surgical site infection (SSI) in patients undergoing mesh-based or suture repair for incarcerated hernias, recurrence rates were significantly lower in the mesh group.[52] However, data is still mixed in the setting of concomitant bowel resection and strangulated bowel requiring a bowel resection. In this setting, a primary tissue repair may be best to decrease risk of wound and mesh morbidity, knowing that hernia recurrence rates will be much higher. Ultimately, if a life-threatening issue arises, it is always most important to treat that pathology first and defer definitive hernia repair for a more optimized setting. In these cases, prevention of hernia recurrence should not be the primary goal of the operation. No evidence exists to recommend the usage of mesh in these cases and the judgment should be made by the operating surgeon on a case-by-case basis.

4 GENERAL PRINCIPLES FOR THE TREATMENT OF VENTRAL HERNIAS

The abdominal wall is a complex unit of the abdominal core and plays an important role in respiration, defecation, micturition, movement of the trunk, and protection of intra-abdominal organs (**Algorithm 69.4**). It has been shown that health-related quality of life improves after ventral incisional hernia repair, presumably related to improved abdominal wall function.[53] A variety of surgical techniques can be used to repair abdominal wall defects. There is considerable debate as to the gold standard for repair, in part due to the lack of prospective randomized trials comparing surgical techniques, but also due to the significant heterogeneity of both patient and hernia factors that is inherent to hernia repair. Considering the choice of surgical approach (open, laparoscopic, or robotic), the massive catalog of available mesh, the choice of position in the abdominal wall (onlay, retromuscular, preperitoneal, or intraperitoneal), and the number of mesh fixation options, combined with widely varied hernia morphology and patient comorbidities, it is no surprise the optimal repair has not yet been determined in the literature. Even so, there are key principles that all good ventral hernia repairs should accomplish if possible: tension-free approximation of the anterior sheath in the midline and mesh augmentation of the abdominal wall (for most abdominal wall defects). Different surgical approaches and management will be outlined later in this chapter.

Preoperative Preparation

Successful management of ventral hernias begins with appropriate preoperative evaluation and optimization. Many of these patients have had multiple prior surgeries, including previous attempts at hernia repair and it is important for the surgeon to obtain and review all the previous operative reports and review the preoperative imaging. Careful review of the patient history will also elucidate if additional preoperative work up or procedures need to be done prior to hernia repair. Preoperative planning may also include consultation with other specialties such as plastic surgery, infectious disease, colorectal, gynecology, interventional radiology, etc. if concurrent operations are required, or if additional adjuncts need to be performed prior to surgery.

Additional optimizing focuses on identifying modifiable patient factors and comorbidities that may impact the success of a hernia repair. Patient factors, such as smoking, obesity, COPD, and diabetes can be major contributors to failure of ventral hernia repair and perioperative complications.[44] Smoking cessation is advocated by most surgeons for at least 4 weeks prior to complex ventral hernia repair. Obesity increases both the wound complications and risk of hernia recurrence, and many surgeons may recommend some degree of weight loss prior to repair. Options include concurrent hernia repair with bariatric surgery, neoadjuvant bariatric surgery with delayed definitive repair of the abdominal wall, waiting for self-directed or medically supervised weight loss, or proceeding with a higher-risk repair for highly symptomatic patients or those at risk of needing an emergent operation. The optimal strategy for these patients is difficult, as the surgeon must weigh the patient's ability to lose weight, access to bariatric surgery, and the symptoms and risk of the hernia itself. Diabetes should be well controlled, with data showing better outcomes with preoperative HgbA1c <7.2 mg/dL. Cardiopulmonary risk stratification is often needed in high-risk patients as well. Finally, there is increased attention given to preoperative nutritional optimization prior to hernia repair, with may improve perioperative morbidity, but evidence of improved hernia outcomes is lacking.

COMMON MIDLINE VENTRAL HERNIAS

In this next section, we will describe common types of ventral hernias as well as surgical management strategies that can be applicable to treat these defects. Though there are different classifications of ventral hernias, most typical ventral hernias are though the midline and linea alba, and this first section will be dedicated toward addressing these types of defects.

Umbilical Hernias

Umbilical and periumbilical hernias are a very common type of ventral hernia. While some can be congenital, most are acquired. In pediatric patients, arrest of the normal spontaneous closure of the umbilical ring through which umbilical blood vessels pass in the developing fetus, results in a fascial defect. In infants, the fascial defect varies in size but is most commonly 1 to 2 cm. A large proportion of pediatric umbilical hernias heal spontaneously, and 80% of them close by the time the patient is 2 years old. The management of umbilical hernias is nonoperative in children up to the age of 2 or 3 years, but persistent umbilical hernias require surgery. In adult patients, umbilical hernias are typically acquired and there are several predisposing factors for the development of umbilical hernias. These risk factors for hernia formation through a preexisting weak spot of the abdominal wall involves expansion of the abdominal wall and subsequent increase in intra-abdominal pressure, and can include multiple pregnancies, obesity, cirrhosis with ascites, large abdominal tumors, etc.[44] Other periumbilical masses that can be confused with an umbilical hernia include umbilical granulomas, epidermal inclusion cysts, omphalomesenteric duct remnant cysts, and urachal cysts. Most of these hernias are less than 3 cm in size; there is no standard definition to delineate when an umbilical hernia then is termed a ventral hernia instead based on size alone, but most would consider and treat an umbilical hernia >4 cm in size similar to an incisional or ventral hernia.

Epigastric Hernias

Epigastric hernias are another variation of a midline ventral hernia that occur through a defect in the linea alba in which patients complain of a bulge in the upper midline above the umbilicus. In the majority of these patients, weakness of the linea alba may exist through anatomic variation (only a single decussation of the fibers of the linea alba is present rather than the usual triple decussation) (**Fig. 69.7**) or thinning of the linea alba due to diastasis recti. The incidence of epigastric herniation is much less common than umbilical hernias and likely represents <5% of typical hernias. Epigastric hernias can be more common in woman than men with a peak incidence of repair around age 40 years. The majority of epigastric hernias are small and contain only incarcerated preperitoneal fat without a true opening into the peritoneal cavity. If approaching these repairs minimally invasively, the preperitoneal fat must be taken down from the anterior abdominal wall to appreciate the fascial defect.

Incisional Hernias

Incisional hernias can occur anywhere where there has been a previous surgical incision, but most commonly the occur in the midline. With more than 2 million laparotomies performed yearly in the United States, the estimated incidence of incisional hernias after a midline laparotomy incision is quoted to be about 10% to 20% after major abdominal operations but can be as high as 69% depending on the patient population studied. Overall, the cumulative incidence of incisional hernias is linear, and they can present after considerable delay following the index operation. The variability in the incidence rates is due to many contributing factors including patient-related comorbidities and technical factors during the surgery. Patients with certain diseases, such as diverticulitis and abdominal aortic aneurysm (AAA), are more prone to develop an incisional hernia when they require surgical intervention.[54,55] The highest incidence of incisional hernia formation is with midline laparotomy incisions or extraction sites when compared to, transverse incisions, paramedian incisions, Pfannenstiel incisions, and laparoscopic trocar sites.[56,57] It is worth noting that off midline incisions run their own risk such as muscle denervation and atrophy if they span lateral abdominal wall nerves or completely transect a muscle and can lead to other complications of the abdominal wall.

Incisional hernias can occur for a variety of different reasons and include patient risk factors and surgical technique. Patient factors that decrease wound healing or increase risk for infection are the most typical risk factors and include things such as obesity, cigarette smoking, pulmonary disease, debilitation from cancer, chemotherapy, the use of steroids, hypoalbuminemia, emergency surgery, sepsis, open abdomen, etc. Poor surgical technique to close the abdomen, rough handling of tissues, type of suture used, closure of the abdomen under tension, are just a few of the technical causes of incisional hernia formation. Appropriate evidence-based midline closure techniques should be followed as previously outlined.

Diastasis Recti

Diastasis recti or rectus diastasis is not a true hernia, even though it can appear as a midline abdominal wall bulge. The key differentiating factor is that there is no fascial defect through which intra-abdominal contents are protruding. It appears as a bulge because of the widening of the linea alba with separation of the midline rectus muscles. While there is some debate about how far the rectus muscles have to be apart for it to be considered rectus diastasis, typically a distance of two-finger widths or 3 cm is considered a mild diastasis.[58] Even though a rectus diastasis does not cause surgical emergencies, the area of weakness can be more prone to hernia formation and be symptomatic due to lack of core function. Rectus diastasis affects abdominal core stability, which mimics a ventral hernia and can lead to functional abdominal wall issues related to core dysfunction, back pain, pelvic floor function, bowel function, etc. Currently, in the United States, many insurance companies still consider diastasis recti solely a cosmetic concern and may not reimburse a surgical intervention. Recently there has been a growing body of evidence to indicate

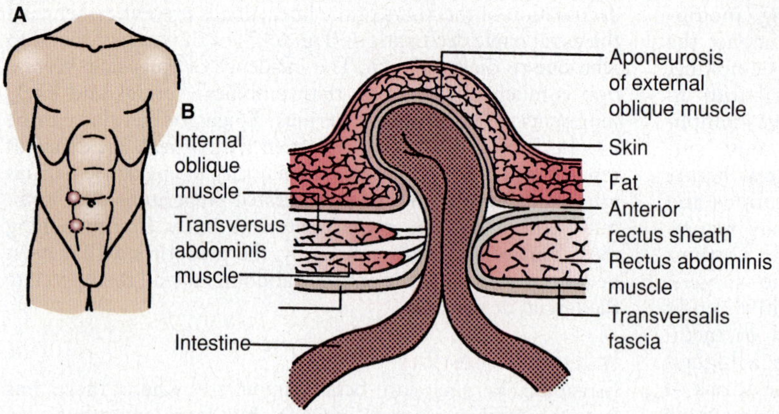

Figure 69.32. Spigelian hernia. **A:** Usual site of occurrence. **B:** Transverse section of abdominal wall showing site of defect.

that to treatment of diastasis recti, especially in conjunction with concurrent hernia repairs may decrease hernia recurrence.[59,60]

LATERAL AND FLANK HERNIAS

Spigelian Hernia

A Flemish anatomist, Adriaan van der Spieghel, first described the semilunar line, which is the lateral limit of the posterior rectus sheath. Also called the spontaneous lateral ventral hernia, a Spigelian hernia protrudes through an area of weakness just lateral to the rectus sheath most often below the arcuate line (**Fig. 69.32**). The hernia is usually interparietal, rarely penetrating the external oblique fascia, and therefore can be difficult to appreciate on physical exam. The typical presentation is lower abdominal swelling or pain just lateral to the border of the rectus muscle. Pain and tenderness may be the only signs without a true appreciable bulge. If a Spigelian hernia is suspected, a CT scan can be obtained to make the diagnosis. Surgical repair can be done either open or minimally invasively. A minimally invasive repair is preferred especially if the external oblique muscle is intact, and a TAPP mesh repair may be utilized. In an open repair, the external oblique muscle may sometimes have to be opened surgically in order the repair the deeper transversus abdominis and internal oblique defect.

Lumbar and Flank Hernias

The lumbar region is the area bounded inferiorly by the iliac crest and superiorly by the 12th rib, posteriorly by the erector spinae group of muscles, and anteriorly by the edge of the external oblique muscle as it extends from the 12th rib to the iliac crest. The three varieties of primary lumbar hernia are described in **Table 69.12** and can be from a variety of etiologies including trauma, increased intra-abdominal pressure (cough), and incisional. Understanding the etiology of the hernia can be important because it can potentially impact the type of repair you can perform. With lateral incisional hernias, denervation can occur with atrophy of the muscle, while in traumatic hernias the muscle can avulse off of bony prominences, which would require a different repair strategy. In patients who have had prior breast reconstructive surgery with a transverse rectus abdominis myocutaneous (TRAM) flap or deep inferior epigastric perforator (DIEP) flap surgery, they can have partial-thickness disruption of the posterior rectus sheath, atrophy of the rectus muscle, denervation, or complete absence of that muscle, and can impact repair.

Table 69.12. Types of Lumbar Hernia

Type	Description
Superior lumbar hernia of Grynfeltt	Occurs through a space between the latissimus dorsi, the serratus posterior inferior, and the posterior border of the internal oblique muscle
Inferior lumbar hernia of Petit	Occurs through a defect in the space bounded by the latissimus dorsi posteriorly, the iliac crest inferiorly, and the posterior border of the external oblique anteriorly
Secondary lumbar hernia	Develops as a result of trauma, mostly surgical (eg, renal surgery), or infection; lumbar hernias were encountered relatively frequently in the past in cases of spinal tuberculosis with paraspinal abscesses

These hernias require repair if they are large or symptomatic, typically with mesh. If left unrepaired, most of the time these hernias will increase in size with unopposed unilateral contraction of the muscle. They can be much easier to repair when the fascial defect is smaller and at the onset of the hernia occurrence. Options for repair include a preperitoneal and retroperitoneal dissection to facilitate mesh reinforcement in this plane below the closed defect, and can be accomplished open, laparoscopically or robotically. For partial-thickness defects, a minimally invasive approach is sometimes helpful, as the external oblique layer is intact and the defect more difficult to identify from an open approach. For eventration in the absence of true hernia, nonoperative management is appropriate in most patients. If repair is desired due to significant size, abdominal wall and core instability, or patient young age, a similar approach with wide mesh reinforcement is appropriate, ideally in a sublay preperitoneal/retroperitoneal position, with plication of the redundant and atrophied overlying oblique musculature.[61,62] For the inferior lumbar hernia, a rotation flap of the fascia lata can be considered (**Fig. 69.33**).[61,62]

PARASTOMAL HERNIAS

Parastomal hernia is among the most common complications of permanent enterostomies and can have significant effects on the patients' quality of life, physical and psychological well-being, and health care resources. The incidence of parastomal hernia varies with the type of the stoma (1.8% to 28% for ileostomy and 4% to 48% for colostomies),[63,64] but the true incidence is likely much higher given that creating an ostomy site through the abdominal wall essentially creates a controlled hernia defect. A classification system for parastomal hernias has been recommended based on the size and presence of a concomitant incisional hernia by the European Hernia Society (**Table 69.13**) which will help standardize the definition of parastomal hernias for future studies.[65]

Poor site selection or technical errors, such as location (too close to the midline, or through the semilunar line), making the fascial opening too large, excessive splitting and stretching of muscle fibers, epigastric nerve denervation,

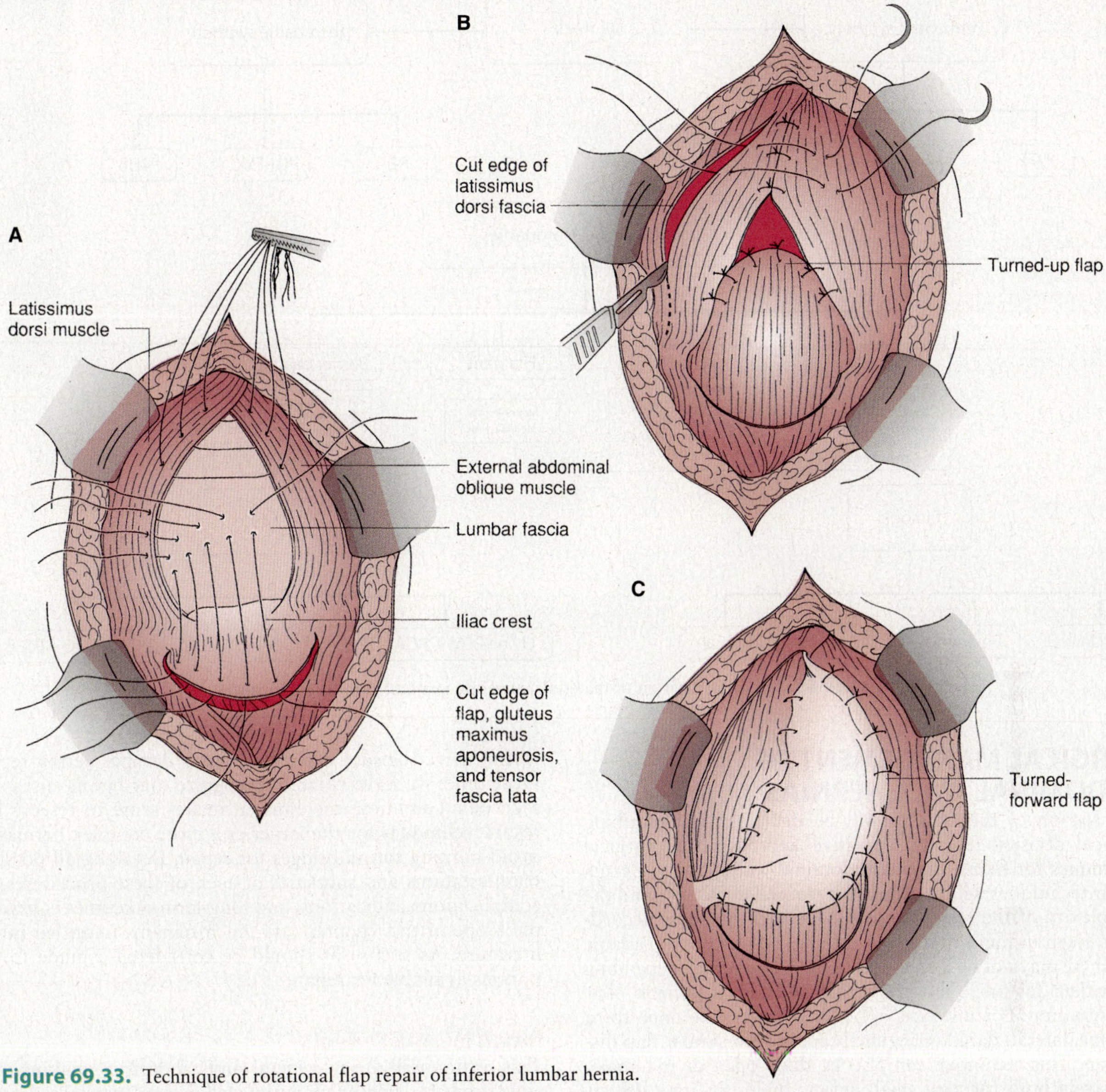

Figure 69.33. Technique of rotational flap repair of inferior lumbar hernia.

placing a stoma in an incision, or emergency rather than elective creation of stoma, can be risk factors for parastomal hernia formation. There can be other patient factors than can predispose to parastomal hernia formation such as obesity, malnutrition, advanced age, collagen abnormalities, postoperative sepsis, abdominal distention, constipation, obstructive uropathy, steroid use, and chronic lung disease also contribute. Utilizing techniques for stomal construction, such as extraperitoneal tunneling, stapled ostomy, and prophylactic mesh reinforcement for permanent colostomies especially in the posterior sublay position have been suggested to help prevent hernias from forming. Currently, only prophylactic mesh reinforcement of permanent end colostomy has significant data to clearly warrant routine use.[66–68] If a parastomal hernia is asymptomatic, a nonoperative approach can be utilized. Symptomatic parastomal hernias most commonly present with pain, obstructive symptoms, difficulty pouching due to the hernia with leakage and wound issues, and impact on quality of life (**Table 69.14**).

Table 69.13. European Hernia Society (EHS) Classification of Parastomal Hernias

EHS Classification Grid for Parastomal Hernia		Small <5 cm	Large >5 cm
Concomitant incisional hernia	No Yes	Primary	Recurrent

Table 69.14. Indications for Repair of a Parastomal Hernia

Absolute
Obstruction
Incarceration with strangulation
Relative
Incarceration
Prolapse
Stenosis
Intractable dermatitis
Difficulty with appliance management
Large size
Cosmesis
Pain

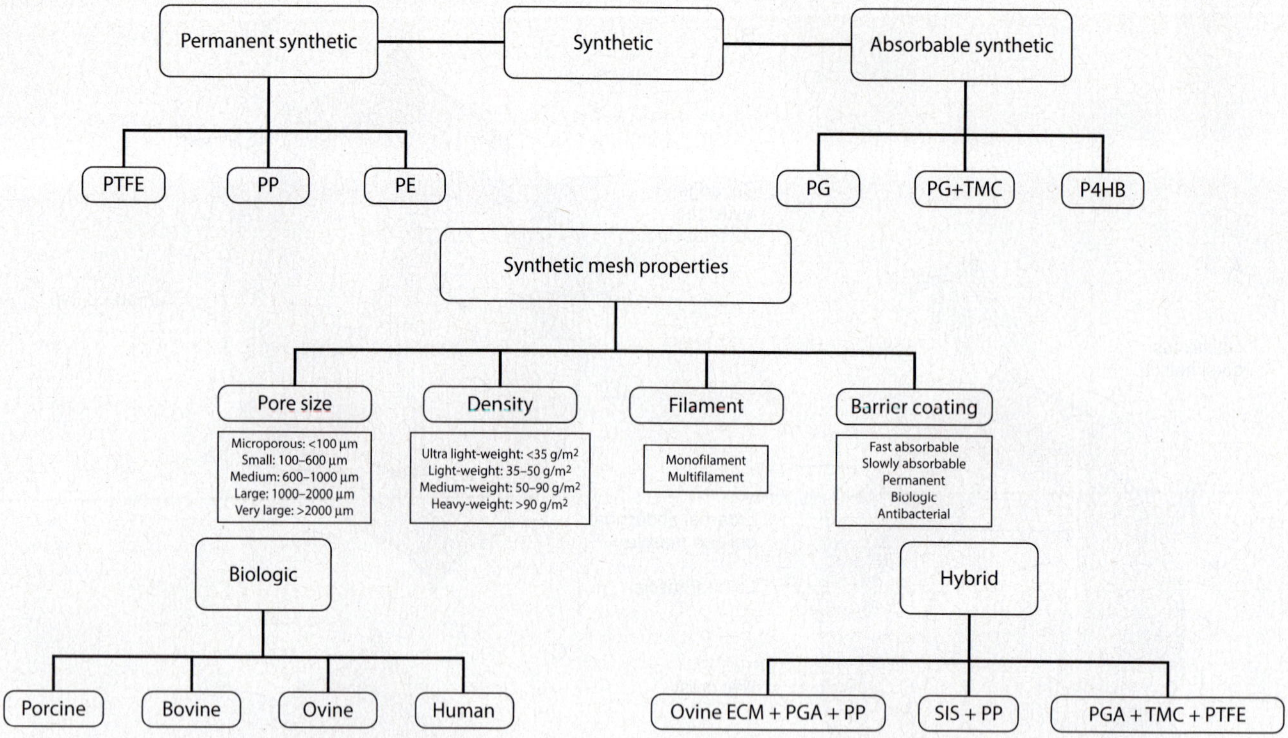

Figure 69.34. Classification of materials currently available for hernia repair.

SURGICAL MANAGEMENT OF ABDOMINAL WALL HERNIAS

The section of the chapter will be dedicated to describing surgical decision making, operative approach, and surgical techniques for fixing various abdominal wall hernias. Hernia repair techniques will be grouped by fascial defect size and the complexity of the techniques described will increase accordingly. Keep in mind that there are many techniques available and there may not be a one surgery fits all approach depending on patient factors, anatomy, hernia characteristics, and clinical situation. For instance, a TAPP repair can be done for a midline, lateral, flank, or inguinal repair, with similar flap dissection. This technique can also be done open or minimally invasively both for very small defects and very large defects depending on the clinical situation.

Mesh prosthesis can also be placed into various layers of the abdominal wall creating additional variation in surgical technique. Historically the terms onlay, inlay, sublay, and underlay have been used to describe location of mesh, but this is falling out of favor as more specific terms detailing the exact location of the mesh is used such as extraperitoneal or retrorectus instead of the more general term sublay. There are also a large variety of mesh augmentation materials available and detailing all the different available mesh types and characteristics is beyond the scope of this chapter. Broadly, there are three large categories of mesh: synthetic, absorbable synthetic, and biologic. The most widely used mesh category is synthetic and they can be characterized by properties based on material, pore size, density/mesh weight, structure, and barrier coating. Each different property will give a certain mesh a different attribute and potential indications for usage. **Figure 69.34** summarizes mesh characteristics and key properties.

Due to the various repair possibilities combined with patient and hernia factors, surgical decision making for hernia repair can be very nuanced and challenging. Keep in mind that one technique can also be applicable to other types of hernia defects depending on the clinical scenario and hernia location. Ultimately, the goal is to perform the least abdominal wall manipulation possible while still achieving tension-free fascial defect closure and providing a durable hernia repair. Over time, we have come to recognize that hernia disease is a chronic condition, therefore, it makes sense to reserve last resort techniques for the larger and more complex hernias to avoid burning future bridges for repair. Detailing all possible manifestations and subtleties of each of these procedures, its complications, indications, and long-term outcomes is beyond the scope of this chapter, and much remains unsettled in the literature. As such, this should be considered a guide to the options available for repair.

Small Hernia Defects

This section will review general surgical decision-making considerations for small abdominal wall defects (typically defined <4 cm in size) followed by technical descriptions of specific procedures. There is considerable debate about mesh augmentation and the hernia size at which mesh should be placed. The most recent European Hernia Society and American Hernia Society joint guidelines recommendations based on meta-analysis and literature review indicate that there is high-quality evidence and strongly recommend that mesh should be used for repair of umbilical and epigastric defects to reduce recurrence rates. All randomized control trials, cohort studies, and prospective observational studies demonstrate that hernia recurrence rates are lower for mesh repairs compared to suture repair without increase in complications or chronic pain.[69] For ventral hernia defects that are smaller than 1 cm in size, limited evidence exists, while the evidence indicates mesh is beneficial, long-term data is lacking. The guidelines state that it is recommended to use mesh for repair of umbilical and epigastric hernias, suture repair can be considered with shared decision making for small hernia defects are <1 cm in size.[69]

For small midline hernia defects, it is also important to note if the patient has a concurrent diastasis or other midline weakness. If a diastasis exists on physical exam or imaging, a minimally invasive repair may be favored as these patients will tend to have higher rates of Swiss cheese defects along the diastasis that is not always apparent clinically. This may also result in concurrent plication of the diastasis to decrease tension off of the fascial defect closure of the hernia defect and potentially decrease recurrence. Current evidence and long-term data for concurrent diastasis plication is limited, but increasingly recognized as a surgical issue that may need to be addressed concurrently. For off de novo midline lateral or flank hernias, carefully consider the location of the lateral abdominal wall nerves and whether all layers of the abdominal wall are intact is important. Ultimately many of these will benefit from an MIS TAPP approach with closure of the fascial defect.

Primary Suture Repair

Many primary suture repair techniques exist for small ventral hernia defects, but there is limited evidence to indicate the which surgical technique is the best. Most of these done open with an incision directly over the hernia site. Once the herniated contents are identified, the hernia sac and the incarcerated contents, if not already reduced, are reduced intra-abdominally. If there are incarcerated bowel contents, opening the hernia sac to visualize the bowel is recommended. Once that is completed, the hernia sac, or peritoneum and then be closed over the bowel. The fascial defect edges should be clearly defined with the hernia sac dissected away from the fascia to avoid catching it in the subsequent defect closure. The fascial edges should also be debrided if necessary to ensure that good tissue is being incorporated into the closure. In midline defects, be careful of concurrent or midline diastasis, if this exists, mesh augmentation or minimally invasive repair may provide better repair strategies.

Recommendations indicate that most repairs are done either slowly resorbable or nonabsorbable sutures with the technique dictated by the surgeon.[69] If permanent sutures are used, there is higher risk of possible suture sinus or granuloma formation from the knot of the suture. Simple suture repair with interrupted, running, or figure-8 sutures, either absorbable or permanent is commonplace, accounting for more than 50% of umbilical hernia repairs.[70] Other double suture row techniques such as the Mayo technique or the Keel technique has also been described. James Mayo described the classic overlapping, vest-over-pants (double-breasting or waistcoat) technique in 1901, in which the upper edge of the linea alba overlaps the lower edge (**Fig. 69.35**).

Repair With Mesh Prosthesis

Most ventral hernia defects less than 4 cm in size (including epigastric and umbilical hernias) are repaired with a mesh prosthesis. The type of approach, either open or minimally invasive (laparoscopic or robotic) will depend on hernia characteristics, location, surgeon familiarity with the technique, and location of mesh placement. The concept of prosthetic mesh repair of abdominal wall hernias has been around for over 100 years with many different materials used over this period of time. Since its inception, there has been a proliferation of different mesh products on the market, but perhaps the most commonly used synthetic material is polypropylene. The mesh material, fiber construct, pore size, fiber density and strength, barrier coating, and layer of the abdominal in which it is placed largely determine the risk of infection, mesh salvage in the event of infection, and the risk of hernia recurrence. This underlies the importance of understanding the physical properties of mesh and where it is positioned within the abdominal wall at the time of repair (**Fig. 69.36**).

Lack of high-quality data comparing optimal mesh selection, the sheer variety of options, and generally poor information and knowledge of specific mesh properties can make mesh selection quite daunting. The choice of mesh is left largely to the judgment and experience of the operating surgeon, but for elective, clean hernia repair cases, most will opt for a midweight macroporous polypropylene mesh in the extraperitoneal or retrorectus based on data and evidence demonstrating superior incorporation in this plane, lower infection rates, lower recurrence, and higher quality of life.[71]

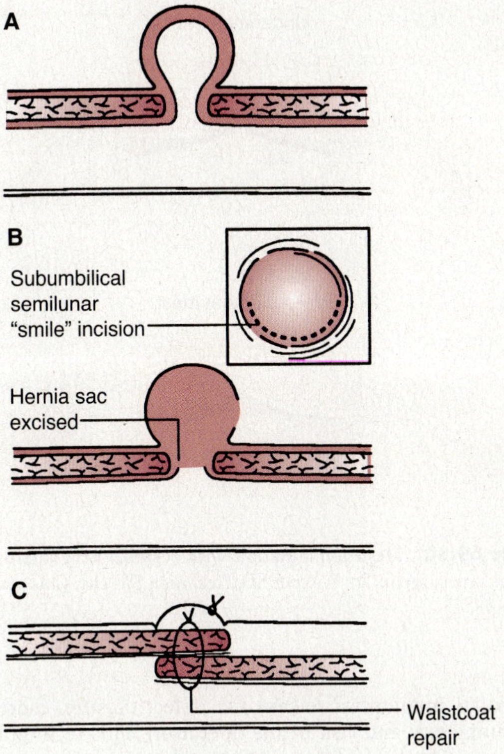

Figure 69.35. Mayo repair of an umbilical hernia. **A:** Diagram of longitudinal section through the hernia. **B:** Subumbilical "smile" incision. The hernia sac is excised. **C:** Waistcoat type of closure.

Open Approach with Mesh

For small midline defects 1 to 4 cm in size, a mesh repair technique is recommended. Once the hernia sac is reduced and dissected out, the preperitoneal space can be exploited by bluntly dissecting the peritoneum from the undersurface of the posterior rectus sheath for enough distance to be able to place an appropriate prosthesis. A mesh prosthesis is placed in the preperitoneal space and then the fascial edges defect closed. Alternatively, intraperitoneal placement using a barrier-coated mesh, but this can have its own issues including adhesions and potential bowel issues if the mesh edges are not fixated intra-abdominally. Recent results from a multicenter randomized control trial suggest a higher complication rate for intraperitoneal versus preperitoneal mesh for umbilical hernia,[72] which has been seen in some other retrospective studies of intraperitoneal mesh as well.[73–75] Optimal mesh size for overlap is not known for these small defects, but the guidelines suggest a 3-cm overlap for a 1- to 4-cm hernia defect size.[69] Others have started advocating for using a mesh suture technique for small fascial hernia defects, but very literature exists regarding this technique. Even though these are small hernias with small fascial defects, these can be challenging technically because the dissection is being completed through a small fascial defect size and small skin incision.

If a preperitoneal, or intra-abdominal technique cannot be completed, an onlay mesh repair can be considered. In this technique, the mesh is placed directly on top of the anterior sheath. The defect is closed, and mesh placed directly on the anterior rectus fascia after dissection of the subcutaneous fat away from the underlying anterior rectus fascia circumferentially around the hernia defect. Typically a noncoated permanent synthetic mesh is used, and fixation techniques vary. Technically, this is probably the simplest repair, as the tissue planes are familiar and easy to identify and has the potential advantage of not requiring entry into the abdominal cavity. However, closure of larger defects with this approach may result in excessive tension, requiring some

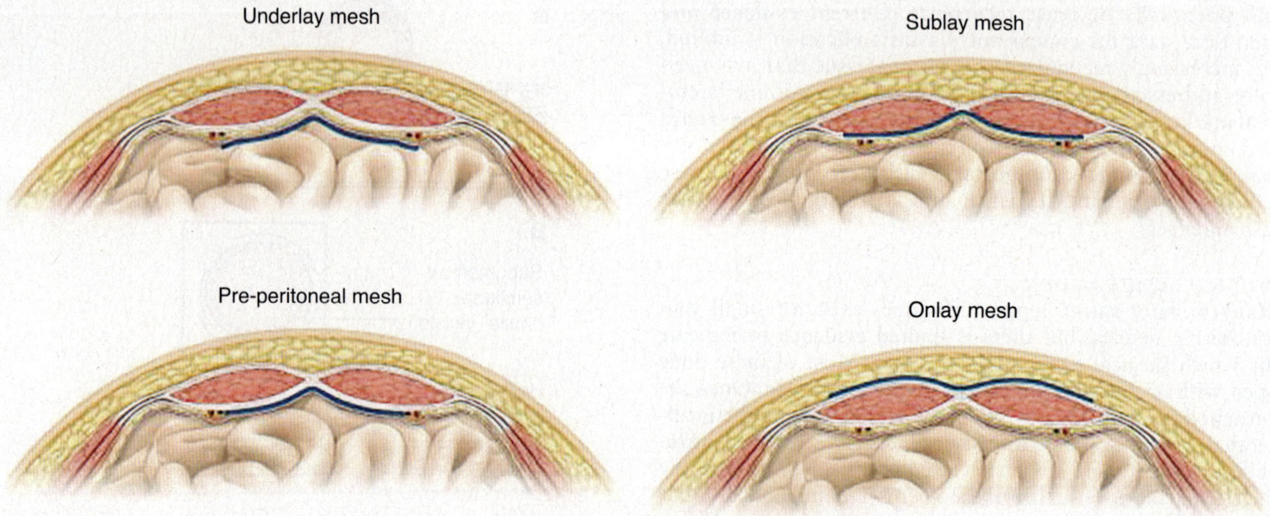

Figure 69.36. Mesh implantation with regard to the anatomy of the anterior abdominal wall. (Reprinted with permission from Leeds SG. Ventral hernia repair. In: Wexner SD, Fleshman JW, eds. *Colon and Rectal Surgery: Anorectal Operations.* 2nd ed. Wolters Kluwer; 2018:299–315. Figure 38.7.)

additional myofascial release for defect closure, increasing the complexity and risk of the operation. This technique has the highest rate of SSI and SSOs due to the subcutaneous dissection required. This space is inherently poorly vascularized, and dissection may further obliterate the periumbilical epigastric perforators, leading to increased risk of infection, seroma, or abdominal wall ischemia and necrosis. Patients should be well selected for this technique and have overall low preoperative wound risk. From a technical standpoint, care should be taken to preserve the vascular perforators in the subcutaneous space. Also, the thin layer of lymphatics immediately anterior to the fascial layer of the anterior abdominal wall should be preserved. Wound complications occur in up to 20% of traditional onlay repairs. With careful patient selection and using fibrin glue as an adjunct with midweight macroporous polypropylene, SSI and SSO rates are comparable to sublay placement of mesh.[76] Additionally, hernia recurrence appears to be higher after onlay repair. This may be explained by Pascal's law which states that pressure exerted on an enclosed fluid acts equally in all directions, and in the case of an onlay technique, this results in lifting forces against the mesh.[77] Further, SSI is a known risk factor for hernia recurrence. Though some advocate this technique, these factors should be considered.[78,79]

Minimally Invasive Approach with Mesh

A laparoscopic or robotic approach for small ventral hernias is a good option as well, particularly for patients with concurrent diastasis, concern for multiple Swiss cheese defects, obese patients, or need for large mesh overlap. There may be some benefit to this approach, including decreased operative time and faster return to normal activity compared to an open repair. The two most common techniques employed for small hernia defects are an intraperitoneal onlay/underlay mesh (IPOM/IPUM Plus) with fascial defect closure or a TAPP approach. Doing an IPOM repair without closure of the fascial defect has largely fallen out of favor as this is technically a bridging repair with high risk of recurrence. These can both be done either robotic or laparoscopically, but with the advent of robotic-assisted surgery, the fascial defect suturing for both techniques is technically easier using the robotic platform due to the wrist articulation.

For both an IPOM plus or TAPP approach, patient positioning is supine with both arms tucked. There can be a role for a slight flex or break in the bed if the patient has no preexisting back issues to allow for better access and trocar placement. The first step of the operation is gaining safe access to the abdomen, and preoperative imaging can be helpful in selecting the appropriate spot for entry away from prior incisions. This is most commonly done at Palmer point using a Veress needle or direct optiview technique, a Hasson cutdown can be completed, but often if the hernia is in the midline or at the umbilicus this approach does not always work well. Ports are placed laterally away from the hernia on the same side of the abdominal wall allowing the surgeon to work toward the location of the hernia. The first step is to reduce all incarcerated hernia contents, if this is bowel, the reduction should be done carefully to avoid bowel injury or missed traction injuries. If possible, a no touch technique should be employed to reduce the bowel. If the incarcerated contents is preperitoneal fat, this preperitoneal fat should be cleared from the anterior abdominal wall and reduced from the hernia sac.

The TAPP approach is increasingly popular, as it emulates the open preperitoneal repair in a minimally invasive fashion. In a TAPP technique a preperitoneal flap is created by taking down this peritoneal and preperitoneal fat layer, which can be contiguous with reduction of the herniated preperitoneal fat and hernia sac. Once this preperitoneal plane is developed, the hernia fascial defect can be closed with sutures, typically a slowly absorbing suture is used, barbed sutures have become increasingly popular for MIS fascial defect closure. During this fascial defect closure, care must be taken to incorporate the anterior sheath, which can sometimes be difficult because the surgeon is suturing intra-abdominally and often cannot visualize the anterior sheath. Some surgeons will also opt to imbricate the hernia sac with the fascial defect closure, and the tack down the umbilical stalk (for an umbilical midline hernia). Closure can also be performed using percutaneous transfascial sutures using a suture passer (**Fig. 69.37**) if laparoscopic or robotic suturing is not an option. After fascial defect closure, the preperitoneal flap is measured and a noncoated permanent synthetic mesh is placed into the space. It can be fixated lightly using absorbable sutures or fibrin glue—no evidence currently exists on the optimal fixation method. The preperitoneal flap is then closed and the mesh is completely excluded from the abdominal cavity.

In an IPOM/IPUM plus technique, after clearing the abdominal wall from preperitoneal fat, the fascial defect is

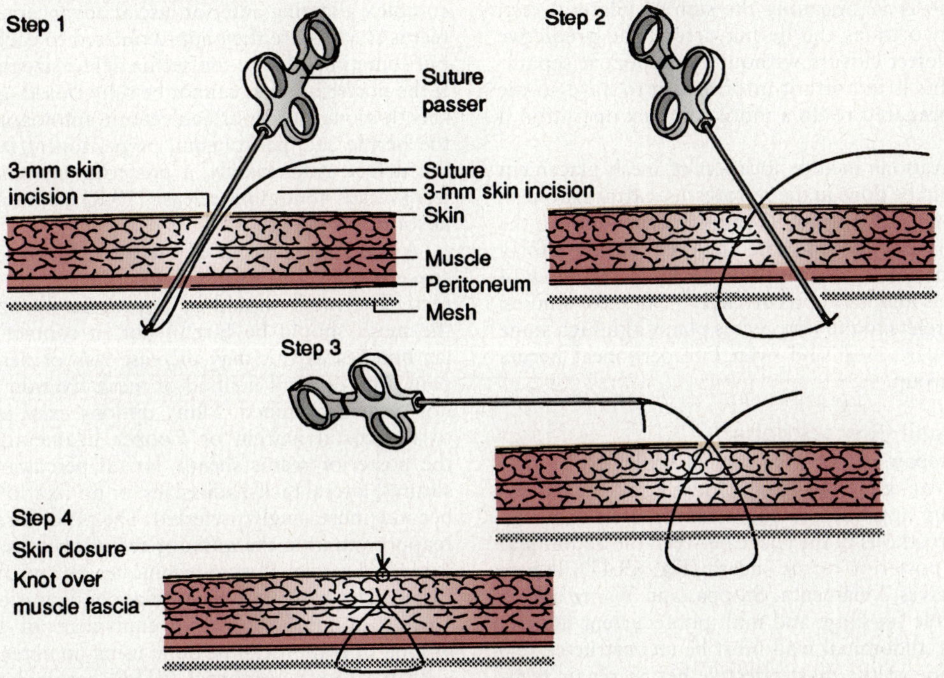

Figure 69.37. Fixation of prosthesis to the peritoneal surface of the abdominal wall with the use of a suture passer. **Step 1:** The suture passer device with a heavy nonabsorbable suture is passed through a 3-mm stab incision in the skin at an oblique angle. The device and suture traverse the entire abdominal wall and then the prosthesis. Once the peritoneal cavity is entered, the suture is released and the passer is withdrawn back into the subcutaneous tissue. **Step 2:** The device is redirected at a different angle through the abdominal wall and prosthesis and the suture is grasped. **Step 3:** The suture is pulled out of the abdominal cavity so that the two free ends are extracorporeal. **Step 4:** The suture is tied with the knot resting on the fascia. The skin is then closed.

closed with sutures similarly to the TAPP. In a true IPOM/IPUM, the fascial defect is left untouched without closure and is a bridging mesh repair. The space is then measured, and a coated synthetic mesh is brought inside the abdomen and fixated either with tacks or sutures circumferentially around the edge of the mesh to the anterior abdominal wall. Intra-abdominally placed mesh should have an antiadhesive barrier of some kind, often referred to as a tissue separating mesh, as it is in direct contact with the viscera. Several options exist as discussed in the previous sections (Fig. 69.34). The mesh should be sized after appropriately measuring the hernia defect and appropriate overlap. Ideal mesh overlap is 5 cm or greater, and likely increases with increasing defect size.[80,81] The IPOM/IPUM without fascial defect closure has largely fallen out of favor due to the fact it does not recreate abdominal core function, the risk of hernia recurrence for large, bridged defects, and due to eventration or pseudo recurrence in which the mesh bellows out across the unclosed hernia defect, mimicking a hernia recurrence. Most surgeons will opt for IPOM/IPUM with fascial defect closure (IPOM/IPUM Plus) procedure as it will recreate abdominal wall core function and reduces seroma formation. This remains a reproducible and highly reliable technique for surgeons fixing small ventral hernia defects.

The International Endohernia Society published updated guidelines on laparoscopic ventral hernia repair in 2019 and is an invaluable resource into surgical technique and the controversies in laparoscopic ventral hernia repair.[82] The greatest value of any minimally invasive hernia repair is the reduction in wound complications due to the small access incisions, lower wound infection rates, decreased hospital stay, and patient preference.[83,84] Improvements in wound infection has been consistently demonstrated, though minor SSOs such as seromas are more commonly seen with an MIS repair. However, MIS VHR has not clearly reduced hernia recurrence rates. As with any hernia repair technique, patient selection is key. This technique can be more beneficial for patients at high risk for wound complications, minimal prior abdominal surgery, and smaller- to moderate-sized defects. Relative contraindications to MIS VHR include patient intolerance of pneumoperitoneum or general anesthesia, and open abdominal wall wounds or other poor skin and soft tissue quality that requires resection. With the advent of MIS component separation techniques, larger hernia defects can also be repaired, and this will be discussed in later sections.

Medium Size Hernia Defects

Medium size abdominal wall defects (typically defined as 4 to 10 cm in size) can be treated similar to small size defects. Depending on the defect size, location, and characteristics, previously discussed techniques including open suture repair, preperitoneal, onlay, or minimally invasive IPOM/IPUM Plus or TAPP can be utilized. At a defect width of more than 4 to 6 cm depending on the patient anatomy and rectus width, typically these are not great candidates for an IPOM/IPUM Plus. Here we will add additional technical descriptions of specific procedures that may be helpful to manage larger defects. In hernias of this size (4 to 10 cm), mesh is recommended for all repairs unless there is a contraindication, as the hernia recurrence rate without mesh likely approaches 100% over time.

For medium size defects, cross-sectional imaging can be very helpful to characterize the hernia defect as well as other anatomical considerations of the abdominal wall. Assessing rectus width and integrity for a possible retrorectus repair and calculating the rectus to defect (Carbonell's) ratio can be very useful for surgical planning purposes. While other measurements and predictive tools exist, the rectus to defect ratio is easy, widely reproducible, and fast to calculate. The ratio is calculated by adding the width or both recti muscles and then dividing by the width of the hernia fascial defect width. If the ratio is >2, meaning the sum of bilateral recti is greater than two times the hernia defect, the predictive value of fascial defect closure without a component separation is 90%.[85] This is important information to have so the surgeon can be prepared to do a more complex operation if indicated.

Other considerations include location of mesh placement whether this should be done in the retrorectus, extraperitoneal, intraperitoneal, or onlay position is variable depending on the surgeon. Meta-analysis does indicate however, that the sublay repair may be superior to other locations and decrease risk of both complications and hernia recurrence.[79,86] In most studies, the sublay repair refers to the retrorectus plane, although some may group extraperitoneal and even intraperitoneal hernia repairs into this group.

Retrorectus Repair (Rives-Stoppa)

The retrorectus repair (sometimes termed sublay), was first described by Rives, and commonly known as the Rives-Stoppa repair, this approach is characterized by the placement of a large prosthesis in the space between the abdominal muscles and the posterior rectus sheath (**Fig. 69.17**). It was popularized by Rives, Velamenta, Stoppa, and Wantz and is particularly suitable for large and multiply recurrent hernias when most of the abdominal wall must be reconstructed.[87,88] It is considered one of the most effective hernia repair techniques and is widely used and reproducible. Due to the well-vascularized compartment created for mesh placement during retromuscular repair, this approach has the lowest SSI and prosthetic-related complications of any open repair.[78,79] This repair can be done open or minimally invasively using laparoscopic or robotic techniques.

The open approach may be more favored for those needing soft tissue, scar revision, or multiple prior abdominal surgeries, or those who have a hernia recurrence with prior mesh that may need resection. The procedure is begun by excising the previous scar and dissecting the peritoneal sac of the hernia to the level of the fascia. Occasionally, the sac does not have to be opened and the procedure can be performed totally extraperitoneal. Once the hernia contents have been reduced and a lysis of adhesions has been performed, the retrorectus dissection is done by incising the medial border of the posterior rectus sheath about 0.5 to 1 cm from the edge of the rectus sheath just lateral to the linea alba. The posterior sheath is then dissected away from the undersurface of the recti to the lateral edge of the rectus sheath, with care being taken to prevent damage to the perforating intercostal neurovascular bundles at the lateral side of the sheath (**Fig. 69.38**). Incising the medial border of the posterior sheath alone bilaterally has the effect of medializing the rectus-anterior sheath myofascial unit to facilitate primary fascial closure by flattening out the rectus complex allowing anterior fascial advancement. The posterior rectus sheaths are then approximated to each other primarily, but sometimes due to the hernia defect size this is not possible. If the posterior layer cannot be fully closed using the posterior sheath alone, surgeons can recruit autologous tissues such as the hernia sac, peritoneum, preperitoneal fat, to help bridge the defect. Additionally, a posterior myofascial release or a transversus abdominis release (TAR) can also be performed if absolutely necessary.

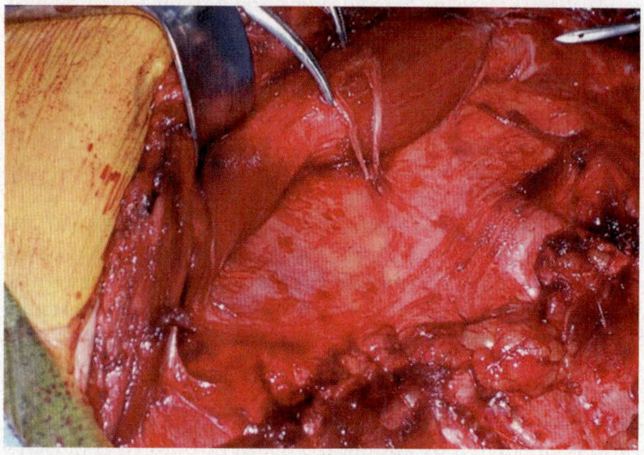

Figure 69.38. Neurovascular bundles in posterior rectus compartment supplying the rectus muscle.

A large mesh prosthesis is then placed in this retrorectus space outside the repaired posterior sheath but beneath the recti. The mesh should be appropriately sized and laterally, the mesh should be careful not to contact the neurovascular bundles as this may increase risk of nerve irritation and pain. The optimal method of mesh fixation in this space has not been determined. Many options exist including fixation to the costal margin or Cooper ligament, direct suture to the posterior rectus sheath, lateral percutaneous transfascial sutures, lateral tacks, adhesives, or no fixation at all which has become increasingly preferred. The procedure is completed by reapproximating the anterior rectus sheaths using previously described fascial closure techniques, reapproximating the rectus muscles back to their normal configuration.

The minimally invasive equivalent of the open Rives-Stoppa operation can be done using an extended or enhanced view total extraperitoneal (eTEP) hernia repair, popularized by surgeons Jorge Daes and Igor Belansky.[89] Initially described in 2018, this procedure takes advantage of the more inguinal TEP procedure and the planes that are utilized for that repair and applies those same principles to ventral hernia repair. In this procedure, the retrorectus space is directly accessed via a cutdown or direct optiview technique with a trocar, and the retrorectus space is then directly insufflated and dissected under direct visualization or using a balloon dissector. Trocars are then placed directly into the retrorectus space in a TEP manner. Then either laparoscopically or robotically, the medial border of the posterior rectus sheath is incised 1 cm away from the linea alba, and a midline crossover is achieved using the preperitoneal plane to dissect across the midline hernia sac and reduce the herniated contents, and other areas of the midline. Care is taken in this procedure not to injure the intact linea alba in other areas of the abdominal wall away from the hernia sac. Once the contralateral posterior rectus sheath is exposed, the medial border of the sheath is incised to gain access to the contralateral retrorectus space. The fascial defect is then sutured closed along the midline and any posterior defects are repaired. Once the posterior and anterior layers of the abdominal wall are intact, the retrorectus space is measured and a large pore polypropylene mesh is inserted into the retrorectus space through a trocar making sure it is sized appropriately for the space with no folds and sits away from neurovascular structures laterally. This mesh can be fixated using suture, fibrin glue, or not at all. The space is then desufflated and the trocars removed. An eTEP procedure can be technically very challenging with a steep learning curve as there are many potential pitfalls including inadequate rectus width, creating holes in the posterior layer with inadequate insufflation, potential unrecognized injury to intra-abdominal contents, inability to recognize anatomy in this space, etc. Proponents of this technique often will assess the abdominal contents intra-abdominally prior to the start or at the end of the repair to make sure there are no missed injuries.

Alternatively, a transabdominal retromuscular umbilical prosthetic repair (TARUP), can be performed.[90] Contrary to the name, this is not usually reserved for umbilical hernia repairs although initially it may have been conceived to do so. It is a minimally invasive retromuscular Rives-Stoppa repair accessing the retromuscular plane from intra-abdominally similar to a TAPP instead of direct dissection into that space (eTEP). In a TARUP, a retromuscular flap is created by detaching the lateral border of one retromuscular space, doing the midline crossover and into the contralateral space, similar to the eTEP dissection. At the end when the fascial defect is closed and mesh is placed, the retromuscular flap is sutured closed similar to a TAPP. The advantage of the TARUP is that technically it is easier and because the surgeon starts intraabdominally, there is better visualization of bowel contents and less likelihood of potential injury.

One unique complication deserves mention and is applicable to both open and MIS retrorectus repairs is an interparietal hernia. Interparietal hernias may occur due to breakdown of the posterior rectus sheath closure. This can result in herniation of the viscera into the interparietal plane between the disrupted posterior sheath and the intact mesh against the anterior abdominal wall. These often present acutely with small bowel obstruction. The surgeon must have a high index of suspicious for this complication, as it will frequently be missed as the cause of SBO by radiology. This can be identified by typical signs of SBO along with visualization of the posterior rectus sheath below the herniated bowel. Repair is necessary, and the primary goal is obliteration of the potential space between the posterior sheath and mesh in which the bowel may be incarcerated.[91] This complication can occur with any procedure involving separation and closure of the posterior sheath, including a standard Rives-Stoppa repair, TAR, or posterior component separation.

5 Large Size Hernia Defects

Large size abdominal wall defects (typically defined as >10 cm in size) usually require a complex abdominal wall reconstruction. These can be challenging hernias to repair and may require adjunct techniques including a myofascial release or component separation to achieve tension free fascial defect closure. Similar to management of medium size defects, all of these repairs require a mesh prosthesis for reinforcement of the abdominal wall, and some of the same techniques described previously can be employed in combination with a component separation or just by itself depending on the hernia characteristics. It is worthwhile noting that an anterior and posterior component separation should not be performed simultaneously as there is high risk of destabilizing the abdominal wall leading to bilateral semilunar or lateral hernia defects.

Total Preperitoneal Repair

A preperitoneal repair is not only possible for smaller hernia defects, but it can be applicable for any size defect including very large hernia defects both open and minimally invasively. The largest case series described by Todd Heniford's group details low complication rates, low hernia recurrence rates, and similar outcomes to posterior component separation.[92] The biggest advantages are preserving the retrorectus space while still utilizing the lateral extraperitoneal space which is essentially the same as the TAR plane laterally. But because the transversus muscle is preserved in this technique, it allows for completion of an external oblique release, which is not possible with a TAR, while allowing for wide mesh coverage. The drawback is the difficulty and reproducibility of the technique as it has a high learning curve. Thus, most surgeons opt for a retromuscular repair paired with a TAR instead of a total preperitoneal repair.

Myofascial Release (ie, Component Separation)

Abdominal wall reconstruction is defined as ventral hernia repair performed using a myofascial release technique. Myofascial release is defined as separation of an abdominal wall fascial layer from a muscular layer, allowing medial advancement of the separated muscle layers in order to close the hernia defect and restore native abdominal wall anatomy. Previously this has been referred to as "component separation" which is a generic term describing a variety of myofascial release techniques. The main types of myofascial release techniques currently used are described in the sections that follows.

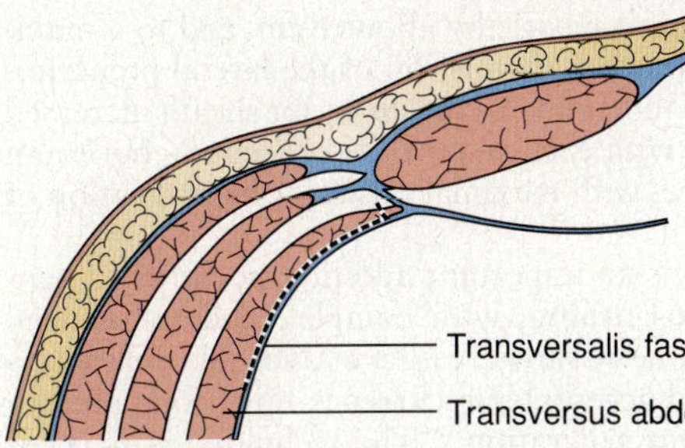

Figure 69.39. The posterior rectus sheath is incised about 0.5 to 1 cm medial to the anterior/posterior rectus sheath junction to expose the underlying transversus abdominis muscle. Note the perforator nerves that are preserved during retromuscular dissection and subsequent posterior component release.

Transversus Abdominis Release/Posterior Component Separation

The TAR allows a posterior extension of the myofascial release after initial retrorectus dissection to achieve greater fascial mobilization and overlap of mesh placement.[93] This is done by incising the first layer of the posterior rectus sheath, which is the posterior lamella of the internal oblique, just medial to the neurovascular bundles after a retrorectus dissection as previously described for a Rives-Stoppa operation. This is followed by division of the transversus abdominis muscle (in the upper abdomen) or its aponeurosis (in the mid and lower abdomen) to enter either the "pretransversalis plane" or the preperitoneal plane. The pretransversalis plane is usually more robust and is readily entered superior to the arcuate line. Utilization of this plane near the costal margin minimizes extensive defects when mobilizing the preperitoneal space alone. Inferiorly, the preperitoneal space is typically entered and mobilized. This dissection continues laterally to at least the midaxillary line but can be carried as far posteriorly as the psoas muscle. Superiorly, this can extend under the diaphragm, dissecting the peritoneum away from the central tendon of the diaphragm. Inferiorly, this can extend into the Space of Retzius, exposing the symphysis pubis and Cooper ligament. This results in the disinsertion of the transversus abdominis from the rectus sheath and releases the circumferential tension it normally applies, allowing the medialization of the rectus abdominis across the midline defect (**Figs. 69.39** and **69.40**). After closure of the posterior elements, there remains a large retromuscular space for placement of prosthetic mesh to reinforce the anterior fascial closure.

As with the Ramirez external oblique release, significant myofascial advancement is possible with each incremental step of the retrorectus + TAR approach. In a cadaver study by Majumder et al., after midline laparotomy and retrorectus dissection alone, the anterior fascia can be mobilized 4 to 7 cm, depending on the degree of tension. The addition of incision of the posterior lamella of the internal oblique, the first step in TAR, increased that release slightly, division of the

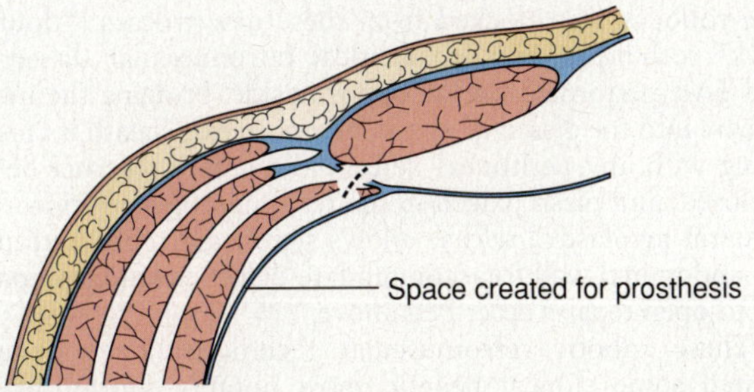

Figure 69.40. Division of the posterior rectus fascia just medial to the linea semilunaris and perforator nerves followed by division/release of the transversus abdominis muscle along its entire medial edge.

HERNIA AND SPLEEN

transversus abdominis muscle by about 1 cm, and to a maximum of 5 to 10 cm after completion of the lateral preperitoneal dissection. Mobilization of the posterior sheath increased in similar fashion with each step of the procedure, but to an even greater degree, with maximal posterior medialization of 7 to 11 cm.[94]

This technique is an important addition in the armamentarium of surgeons dealing with complex abdominal wall problems and has been shown to have favorable perioperative morbidity and acceptable recurrence rates compared to anterior component separation.[95] The technique is particularly suited for addressing recurrent hernias but should not be used simultaneously in combination with a concurrent anterior component separation. However, TAR is technically difficult because the transversalis fascia/peritoneum complex posteriorly can be extremely thin, tearing easily. In order to isolate the viscera from the prosthetic which will eventually be placed, these tears must be repaired. If this is not possible, an intervening fast absorbable mesh or biologic mesh can be used to separate the viscera from the retromuscular space. Alternatively, one of the adhesion barrier prostheses can be used.

The true benefit of robotic hernia surgery may lie in its ability to translate open hernia surgery techniques, such as preperitoneal, retromuscular, and component separation, to a minimally invasive platform. These effects may not be as apparent for smaller defects and simpler operations such as TAPP or IPOM/IPUM Plus, but for larger hernias, utilizing the robotic platform to perform complex myofascial releases, dissection, and suturing of very large defects has changed the landscape of hernia surgery. The addition of a robotic TAR allows repair of large midline hernia defects minimally invasively. While this procedure may be performed laparoscopically by experienced laparoscopists, most surgeons find that it is much easier done robotically.

For a robotic TAR, trocars are placed transabdominally in the lateral abdominal wall. After necessary adhesiolysis and hernia reduction, the contralateral rectus sheath is opened, occasionally the hernia sac or other preperitoneal tissue can be recruited. Retromuscular dissection is carried out along the length of the hernia, extending at least 5 cm above and below the defect, and continued laterally to the semilunar line. Of critical importance to this repair, as with the open approach, is the dissection of the midline above and below the hernia defect. The fascial elements coalesce to form the linea alba such that the retromuscular spaces are not continuous with each other. Thus, the midline peritoneum and preperitoneal fat must be dissected from the overlying linea alba, leaving it attached to the posterior sheath bilaterally and with care taken to avoid damage to the intact linea alba, which may result in hernia recurrence. A TAR is then performed as described above by incising the posterior lamina of the internal oblique aponeurosis, dividing the transversus abdominis muscle and aponeurosis, and extending dissection laterally in the preperitoneal plane. This continues laterally to approximately the midaxillary line, followed by placement of additional trocars in the contralateral abdomen directly into the dissected preperitoneal space. The robot is then docked from these new trocars ("double-dock" technique) and an identical retromuscular dissection and TAR performed on the opposite side, bringing the initial trocars into the dissected space. The posterior sheath is closed, along with any peritoneal defects, the anterior hernia defect is closed, and mesh placed in the retromuscular position. The bilateral myofascial release allows significant mobilization of the abdominal wall to accommodate defect closure, comparable to open repairs described above.[96–98]

These robotic retromuscular techniques have demonstrated some clinical benefit, most notably shorter length of stay and decreased pain compared to both open retromuscular repair. There remains a fairly high rate of seroma, though typically clinically irrelevant, and long-term cosmetic

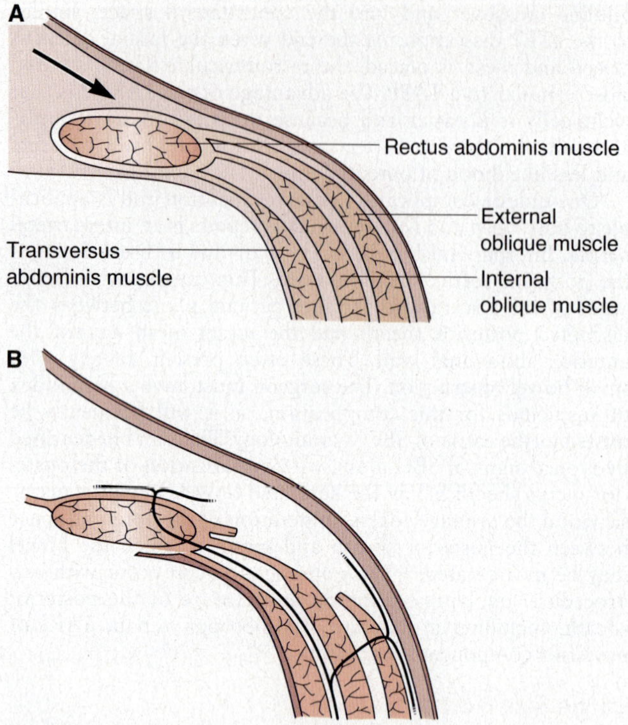

Figure 69.41. **A:** Anatomy of the anterior abdominal wall (arrow denotes plane for external oblique release). **B:** Component separation technique: External oblique release with overlay of neurovascular bundles.

outcomes can be more difficult to predict. Though there seems to be a low rate of SSI with robotic retromuscular repair, this has not yet been clearly seen in the literature.[99,100] The double-dock procedures with bilateral TAR are typically limited to large defects, that are expected to require TAR even if performed open. Patient selection is important and not all patients are great candidates for a robotic TAR with additional long-term data pending.

Anterior Component Separation

The term component separation itself was initially used to describe a technique popularized in the early 1990s by Ramirez and colleagues which is based on lateral fasciotomies that allow sliding of the muscular fascia layers toward the midline providing coverage for large midline abdominal wall defects.[101] In this technique, the skin and subcutaneous fat are dissected free from the anterior sheath of the rectus abdominis muscle and the aponeurosis of the external oblique muscle. The aponeurosis and muscle belly of the external oblique muscle are transected longitudinally lateral to the semilunar line (**Fig. 69.41**).

It is important to extend the incision inferiorly to the inguinal ligament and superiorly onto the chest wall at least 5 to 7 cm cranial to the costal margin especially for defects close to the xiphoid. The external oblique muscle is separated from the internal oblique muscle, as far laterally as possible in a relatively avascular plane, beyond the area of skin undermining toward the midaxillary line. This step is safe because the neurovascular bundle (comprising the intercostal nerves and vessels) lies deep to the internal oblique muscle. Additionally, the rectus abdominis muscle is released from its encasing posterior fascia by incising the posterior rectus sheath and separating it from the overlying rectus muscle. The result of the combined incision of the posterior rectus sheath and the external oblique release is that the internal oblique-transversus abdominis muscle and the rectus abdominis complex slide medially for up to 10 cm in the mid-abdomen, allowing closure of defects up to 20 cm. In fact, release of the posterior rectus sheath alone (note this does not refer to TAR, just the medial incision of the posterior rectus sheath) results in mobilization of 5 cm in the midabdomen. Care must be taken not to damage the neurovascular bundles that runs between the internal oblique and transversus abdominis muscle to enter the rectus sheath posterolaterally. After advancement of the rectus complex toward the midline, the fascial closure is performed followed by layered closure of the subcutaneous tissues and skin with drains. Several modifications to the original technique have been described. The technique can also be used as an adjuvant to the prosthetic repairs described next.

Unfortunately, SSO and SSI following anterior releases involving large subcutaneous dissections are significant, occurring in up to 50% of patients. This can range from simple seromas to full-thickness necrosis and loss of abdominal wall skin and soft tissue, creating potentially devastating chronic abdominal wall wounds. This results from division of the DIEPS in the periumbilical region that are divided during the massive subcutaneous dissection required for this procedure, devascularizing the mid portion of the abdominal wall. The development of posterior approaches to lateral myofascial release (previously discussed) offers an excellent alternative to the external oblique release with significantly lower wound complication rates while still gaining significant mobilization of the abdominal wall and has largely supplanted the external oblique release as the myofascial release of choice.

Several modifications of the classic Ramirez component separation have been described to mitigate some of the aforementioned wound complications. The perforator preserving technique completes the subcutaneous dissection but identifies and preserves the periumbilical perforators, significantly reducing the risk of wound complications. Endoscopic component separation utilizes laparoscopy to dissect the interparietal plane between the external and internal obliques, thus eliminating the need for subcutaneous dissection and vascular disruption. The technique involves making 2- to 4-cm incisions just below the costal margin in anterior axillary line (lateral to the attachment of the external oblique aponeurosis on the rectus sheath). The space between the external and internal oblique muscles is dissected and under camera guidance, dissector balloon is inflated which further aids blunt dissection in this layer. The external oblique aponeurosis is then divided. A balloon dissector can be used in the subcutaneous space as well. This technique can be followed by either open, laparoscopic, or robotic-assisted hernia repair.[102–105] Potential limitation might be the adequacy of the myofascial advancements using this technique. Proponents of this technique claim reduction in postoperative stay by about 50% and a distinct advantage in the setting of stomas. The primary benefit, however, is the reduction in wound complications while still achieving significant myofascial advancement (**Fig. 69.41**). Care must be taken to ensure the proper interparietal plane is dissected, as disruption of more than just the external oblique may result in lateral bulging or hernia.

Prosthetic Bridging Technique

A bridged repair is one in which the hernia defect is left unclosed, instead placing mesh across the hernia defect with wide circumferential overlap, essentially replacing the defect with prosthetic and avoiding a high-tension closure. Mesh selection depends on the approach. A barrier-coated, biologic, or absorbable synthetic mesh is required for intraperitoneal placement. If mesh is placed in an extraperitoneal position, a noncoated mesh may be used as long as there is some tissue layer between the mesh and viscera. Although this repair is theoretically attractive, it has not been as successful for incisional hernias as for inguinal hernias. The recurrence rate is especially high in obese patients and large hernia defects and is primarily used as a last resort for cases in which the fascial defect is too large, there is significant muscle missing, or atrophy of the abdominal wall that does not allow for fascial defect closure.

In the management of the open abdomen, a bridged mesh may be used to perform serial mesh excision. This is a technique whereby an open abdomen is closed by placement of a bridging mesh, with serial visits to the operating room to tighten the mesh by serially excising a strip of the midportion of the mesh, thereby eventually bringing the native fascial edges into apposition for closure. This approach allows for definitive abdominal wall closure after a mean of six visits to the operating room.[106] If fascial closure is not possible for other reasons, a bridging biologic or absorbable mesh can also be considered for stabilization of the abdominal wall accepting the eventual hernia formation for potential repair at a later time once the patient has resolved their acute life-threatening issues.

Massive Hernia with Loss of Domain

There is no consistent definition as to what constitutes a massive hernia with loss of domain. This term is often applied to very large defects in which the volume of herniated viscera exceeds the capacity of the abdominal cavity to accommodate its replacement into the visceral sac. Many of these hernias are recurrent and associated with morbid obesity, skin ulcerations, enterocutaneous fistulae, diverting stomas, and distortion of the abdominal wall from multiple prior repair attempts. Several physiologic changes such as alteration of ventilatory equilibrium and impairment of venous return results from longstanding massive hernias. Forced reduction of the hernia with replacement of contents into the abdominal cavity can increase intra-abdominal pressure considerably, resulting in respiratory insufficiency and cardiovascular compromise.[107,108] In extreme cases, it is impossible to return the contents to the abdomen and repair the hernia defect without resection of intra-abdominal contents, such as colectomy with omentectomy. Repair of massive ventral hernias with loss of domain is technically challenging and is associated with high morbidity, mortality, and recurrence rates. A good understanding of the abdominal wall anatomy and the nature of fascial defects is essential prior to repairing these ventral hernias. As complex hernia techniques have improved over time, hernia surgeons are able to tackle increasingly complex repairs. Complications of repair are higher in these patients and can include respiratory compromise, abdominal compartment syndrome, skin flap necrosis, and wound infection, in addition to the usual surgical complications. Surgeons should weigh the risk and benefits of hernia repair prior to surgery. These patients require complex abdominal wall reconstruction including preoptimization, weight loss, and advanced abdominal wall expansion techniques and should be treated in hernia centers with special interest in this area where teams have been assembled to treat complex abdominal wall pathology.

Progressive Preoperative Pneumoperitoneum

Progressive preoperative pneumoperitoneum (PPP), which was first described by Goni Moreno for repair of massive incisional hernias, is a useful technique in patients with loss of domain, from incisional or massive inguinal hernias, to expand the abdominal cavity by stretching the abdominal wall musculature and the diaphragm.[109–115] The maneuver involves injecting room air (or CO_2) via a needle or implantable catheter every 1 to 3 days for a prescribed period of time between 1 and 4 weeks. Volume of air injection varies but is most often administered to the degree the patient tolerates (development of shoulder pain, difficulty breathing, or subcutaneous emphysema). This can be performed by patients and families as outpatient but is more often performed in a hospital setting. The effect of PPP is twofold. First, there is lengthening of the abdominal musculature and expansion of the abdominal cavity volume.[114–116] While the hernia sac expands as well, often more than the abdominal cavity, if the volume expansion of the abdominal cavity is equal or greater than the original hernia sac volume, the abdomen can typically accommodate the return of the herniated contents and allow fascial closure.[117]

Second, the gradual expansion of the abdominal cavity seems to allow for physiologic adaptation that permits the massive abdominal wall reconstruction and increased abdominal pressure at the time of closure.[116]

PPP has been more commonly applied in Europe and South America with good results for large ventral hernias. Rate of fascial closure ranges from 50% to 100%, with reported recurrence rate of 3% to 37%.[115] Complications include extensive subcutaneous emphysema, SSIs, other noninfectious wound complications, abdominal wall soft tissue necrosis, venous thromboembolism (VTE), and cardiopulmonary complications. Complications tend to be higher than typical incisional hernia repairs owing to the more complex techniques usually required to achieve closure and the prolonged duration of hospitalization and/or abdominal insufflation. A variety of repair techniques are used in conjunction with PPP including external oblique release, retromuscular repair with or without additional posterior release, laparoscopic repair. Mesh reinforcement should be used due to excessively high recurrence rates with suture repair. Adjunctive measures such as chemical component separation (discussed below) may add benefit and improve the success rate of PPP.[118] Despite the relative success in reported series, this is a complex process reserved for only the most complex patients with large hernias and significant loss of abdominal domain that have little chance of closure without some ability to expand abdominal volume.

Chemical Component Separation

A newer modality for expansion of the abdominal cavity utilizes chemical paralysis of the abdominal wall by botulinum toxin A (BTA) injection into the lateral abdominal wall musculature, often termed chemical component separation. The resultant flaccid paralysis of the oblique musculature, which peaks at approximately 3 weeks after injection, has been shown to elongate and decrease the thickness of the lateral abdominal muscles, which reduces the mean hernia defect size on subsequent imaging.[119,120] This potentially improves the ability to reapproximate the hernia defect or minimize the extent of other myofascial release techniques that may increase the operative risk. Indeed, all studies to date indicate the ability to close the hernia defect in all cases. In addition to the benefits of achieving fascial closure, BTA injection seems to provide significant postoperative pain control as well.[121]

There is significant heterogeneity in the literature on the use of BTA, however. The administered dose of BTA varies between studies, ranging from 200 to 500 units with dilutions between 2 and 100 units/mL, and injections sites vary from 3 to 5 per side. Additionally, the time between injection and attempted hernia repair varies from several weeks to intraoperative injection. The complexity of incisional hernias ranges widely as well, making it difficult to discern the optimal patient that would benefit from BTA. Finally, surgical technique for hernia repair varies greatly in each study. These include simple suture repair, external oblique release (Ramirez component separation), retromuscular repair, laparoscopic repair, and concurrent PPP. There is currently no comparative data of BTA versus other modalities of abdominal wall expansion, no randomized control trials, and no clear evidence that BTA injection ultimately effects the extend of myofascial release needed for closure. Large case series demonstrates that it is safe and can increase fascial defect closure rates in very large hernia defects. Despite these drawbacks in the current literature, BTA injection appears to be quite safe and warrants further investigation to assess its efficacy in complex abdominal wall reconstruction.[119–127]

Tissue Expansion

Tissue expanders can also be used when either skin or the myofascial elements of the abdominal wall are deficient. They are implanted subcutaneously or subfascially and are gradually inflated until the desired amount of extra tissue is obtained. The limitation of the technique is the delay in definitive repair while the expansion is going on and the considerable amount of pain that patients complain of. The intra-abdominal placement of tissue expanders has also been described to address the issue of loss of domain, but this is primarily confined to the pediatric literature.

Visceral Reduction

The primary concern in hernias with loss of domain is the revisceration of the herniated contents back into the abdominal cavity. If the above measures to expand the abdominal cavity fail or are inadequate, consideration may be given to reducing the contents of the hernia itself by resection of the viscera. Options include omentectomy, colectomy, or small bowel resection. There are extremely limited data on this approach as a means to achieve fascial closure in complex hernia repair with loss of domain, and this should be considered only as a last resort in expert hands.[128,129]

Parastomal Hernia Repairs

The three general types of stomal hernia repair are fascial repair, prosthetic repair, and stomal relocation, which can be performed either laparoscopically, robotic-assisted, or open.

Fascial repair involves a local exploration around the stoma site, with primary closure of the defect. This approach is associated with up to 75% recurrence rate[130] and should be considered of historical interest only. Stoma relocation[131] is usually indicated in patients with other stomal problems, such as skin excoriation or suboptimal stomal construction. Simple relocation, however, results in risk of parastomal hernia at the nascent site of 24% to 86%, as well as up to 50% hernia recurrence at the initial site, along with risk of midline incisional hernia if a laparotomy is required. The major drawbacks of stomal relocation are the fact that a laparotomy is required, which in and of itself causes more morbidity than some of the other techniques, and that it exposes the patient to the risk of three new incisional hernias at (a) the old stoma site, (b) the laparotomy incision site, and (c) the new stoma site with reported recurrence rates ranging from 24% to 86%. Whenever possible, a prosthetic repair should be considered as this appears to be the most effective. There are several potential options for repair.

In an open onlay repair, mesh is placed anterior to the anterior rectus aponeurosis. Incision may be midline or a curvilinear incision outside the boundaries of the patient's appliance (**Fig. 69.42**).

The skin and subcutaneous tissue are then dissected from the underlying anterior fascia widely around the stoma and hernia defect. The defect is closed around the stoma, and a prosthetic onlay placed around the stoma and fixed to the underlying fascia. The problem with this approach is that the undermining of subcutaneous tissue leads to wound complications due to the relatively poor vascularity and potential disruption of perforating vessels during dissection. As with any onlay technique for ventral hernia repair, patients should be selected carefully to minimize wound risk. This approach is a reasonable one in patients with hostile abdomens and where intraperitoneal mesh is to be avoided. Recurrence rates of up to 26% have been reported with this technique with a mesh removal rate up to 23%.[132]

A retromuscular or preperitoneal repair can also be performed in which mesh is placed posterior to the rectus muscle and anterior to the posterior rectus sheath (retromuscular repair) or mesh placement between posterior rectus sheath and peritoneum (preperitoneal repair) has been described in small case series. Posterior component separation with retromuscular mesh positioning is a technique that has been described in patients with complex parastomal hernias which uses mesh to reinforce all "at-risk" areas for recurrence.[133,134] This approach allows any midline hernias to be easily addressed as well. The fascial defect is closed down around the stoma, and then mesh is placed. Mesh may be cut as a keyhole, wrapping the mesh around the stoma left in situ and subsequent closure of slit cut in the mesh. If the stoma is revised or relocated, the stoma can be brought back through the mesh directly without requiring

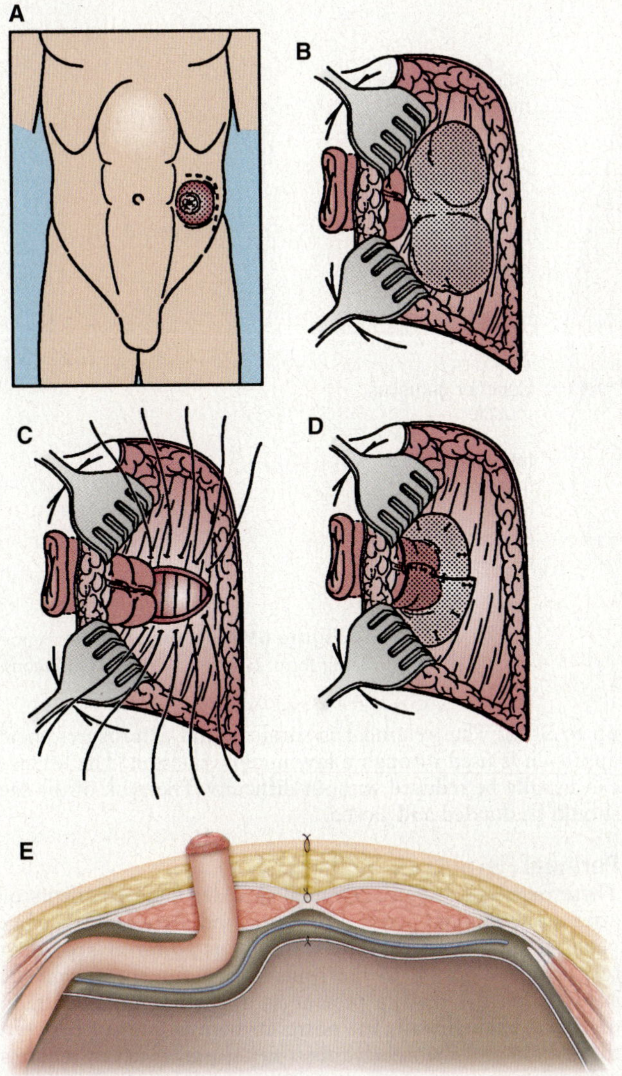

Figure 69.42. Repair of a parastomal hernia. **A:** Incision around hernia. **B:** Hernia sac is identified, the contents are reduced, and the peritoneum is closed. **C:** The edges of the fascial defect are reapproximated. **D:** The fascial repair is reinforced with polypropylene mesh, which is wrapped around the subcutaneous portion of the colon and sutured in place. **E:** Rives-Stoppa retromuscular incisional and parastomal hernia repair with unilateral transversus abdominis release (TAR) modified-Sugarbaker technique for mesh placement. (From Love W, Carbonell AM. Complex situations in abdominal wall reconstruction. In: Ellison CE, Upchurch GR Jr, eds. *Fischer's Mastery of Surgery.* 8th ed. Wolters Kluwer; 2024:2007–2011. Fig. 218.5.)

a long slit to be cut in the mesh. This can be also accomplished using a stapled technique, fixating the mesh to the posterior sheath with a circular stapler and bringing the stoma back through the mesh. An extraperitoneal Sugarbaker technique is also possible, lateralizing the stoma within the retromuscular space and placing an intact flat mesh below the stoma as described below.[135] This approach is feasible using a robotic approach, but is most often performed via midline laparotomy.

An intra-abdominal prosthetic repair is also possible, and its biggest advantage is that it eliminates the need for the abdominal wall dissection. It also enlists the mechanical advantage of placing the prosthesis on the peritoneal side of the abdominal wall.[136] The intra-abdominal approach is particularly suited for a minimally invasive approach, which provides excellent visualization. Several techniques have been described.[137] This can be performed in two ways. (1) The Sugarbaker technique in which the bowel is first lateralized along the abdominal wall. The mesh is placed over the entire fascial defect and under the lateralized bowel, and fixated circumferentially except laterally where the bowel exits to create a mesh flap valve around the stoma. (2) The Keyhole technique requires a 2- to 3-cm cutout is made in the mesh for the ostomy while widely covering the defect. This can be tricky as too small of an opening can obstruct the enterostomy while too large of an opening can result in recurrence, the mesh must be slit, then reclosed, in order to place it circumferentially around the ostomy. Recurrence rate is lower with Sugarbaker repair compared to keyhole when mesh is placed intraperitoneally.

Unusual Hernias

Richter Hernia

A special type of incarcerated hernia is a Richter hernia. It was initially described by August Gottlieb Richter in 1785. A Richter hernia is differentiated from other incarcerated hernias as only the antimesenteric border of the intestine protrudes into the hernia sac without involving the entire circumference of the intestine so that intestinal obstruction does not occur (**Fig. 69.43**). This may be difficult to palpate on physical exam and often times the diagnosis comes from imaging. The most common site is the femoral ring (36% to 88%), followed by the inguinal canal (12% to 36%), an abdominal wall incision (4% to 25%), and can also occur in other locations in which abdominal hernias occur. The surgical treatment is similar to other operations in which bowel needs to be reduced. The herniated bowel is reduced by opening the hernia sac and lysing the adhesions of the bowel to the anterior abdominal wall. Subsequently, a hernia operation is then performed.

Sciatic Hernia

A sciatic hernia is a protrusion of a peritoneal sac through the major or minor sciatic foramen (**Fig. 69.44**). These very

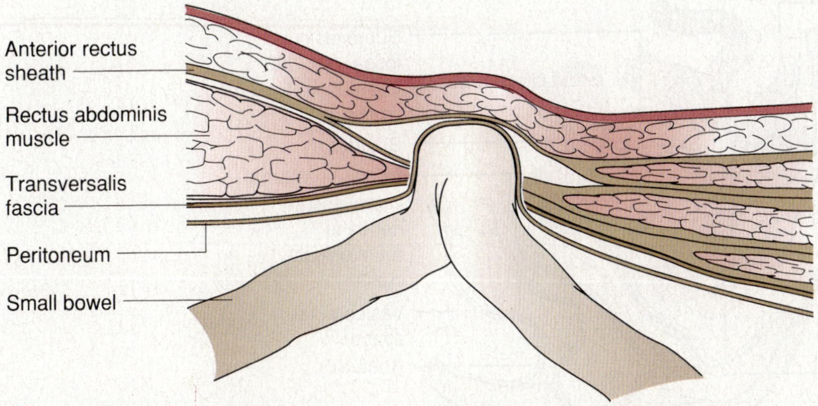

Figure 69.43. Richter hernia. Part of the bowel wall herniates through the defect in the abdominal wall.

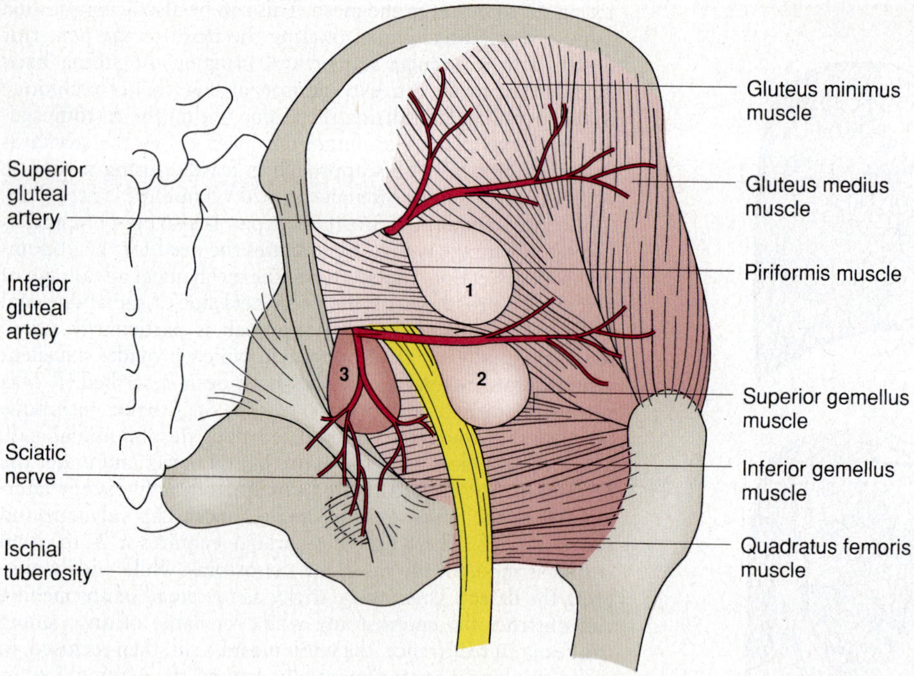

Figure 69.44. Sciatic hernia. **1:** Suprapiriform. **2:** Infrapiriform. **3:** Subspinous.

rare hernias present with a swelling on the buttock. The sciatic nerve may be involved. A ureter can become obstructed if it is included with the herniated tissues. The treatment of these hernias is surgical. Both transperitoneal and transgluteal approaches have been described. A combination of the two is sometimes used. The defect usually requires a prosthetic mesh repair.

Supravesical Hernia

This hernia is anterior to the urinary bladder and forms when the integrity of the transversus abdominis muscle and the transversalis fascia fail, both of which insert into Cooper ligament. The preperitoneal space is continuous with the retropubic space of Retzius, and the hernia sac protrudes into this area. The sac of the hernia is directed laterally, emerges at the lateral border of the rectus muscle, and presents in the inguinal, femoral, or obturator region. It can also be associated with an inguinal, femoral, or obturator hernia. Treatment of this hernia depends on recognizing it at the time of groin exploration and reinforcing the defect.

A second variety of these hernias is known as an internal supravesical hernia. They are classified according to whether they cross in front of, beside, or behind the bladder (Fig. 69.45). Bowel symptoms predominate in patients with these hernias, and urinary tract symptoms develop in up to 30%. The treatment is surgical, and a transperitoneal approach is used through a low midline incision. The hernias can usually be reduced without difficulty. The neck of the sac should be divided and closed.

Perineal Hernia

These hernias are more common in older female patients or after an abdominal perineal resection and are related to a lax pelvic floor. They are termed *anterior* or *posterior* according to their relationship to the transverse perineal muscle. The anterior hernias usually present as a swelling in the labium or lateral vaginal wall. The posterior hernias present between the rectum and the ischial tuberosity. Surgical repair requires a transperitoneal or posterior approach, and, if the opening is large, a prosthetic mesh repair is required.

Perivascular Hernia

These hernias present through defects between the inguinal ligament and the iliopubic bone. They are known by various eponyms according to their position. The hernia protruding through a defect in the lacunar ligament is *Laugier hernia*. The hernia protruding through the pectineal fascia is *Cloquet hernia*. The hernia extending anterior to the femoral vessels but behind the inguinal ligament is *Velpeau hernia*. The hernia behind the vessels is *Serafini hernia*. Lateral to

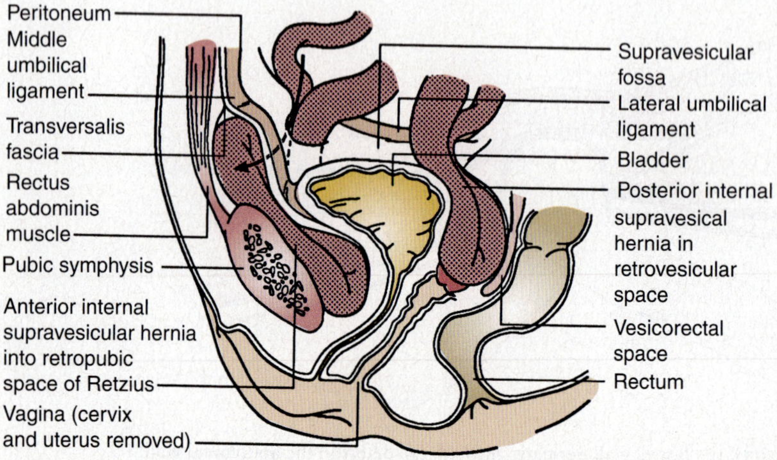

Figure 69.45. Internal supravesical hernias.

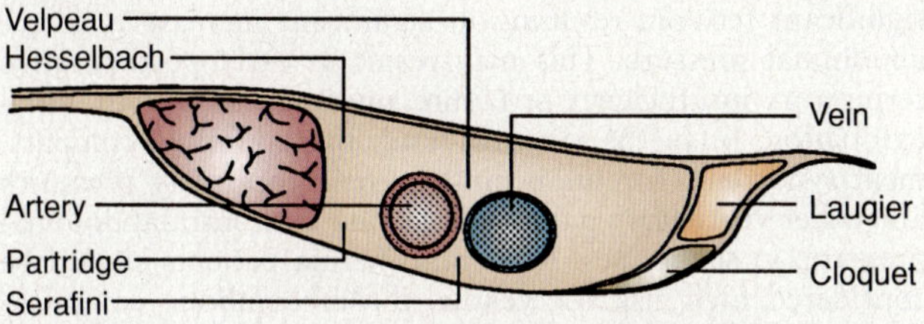

Figure 69.46. Perivascular hernias and their eponyms.

the femoral artery are two hernias, the anterior one being *Hesselbach hernia* and the more posterior one is *Partridge hernia* (Fig. 69.46).

6 HERNIA RECURRENCE

Hernia recurrence rates vary based on technique, patient factors, and hernia size, and range from as low as 5% to as high as 70% in the surgical literature. There has been increasing recognition of abdominal wall hernias as a chronic disease process. Much of the current hernia preoptimization process and evolution of hernia surgical techniques targets risk factors for hernia formation with many aimed a decreasing SSI, tension on fascial defect closure, and reinforcement strategies. Overall studies have shown that perhaps recurrent incisional hernias undergoing repairs are at higher risk of complications than prior repairs, and that with each successive repair, the recurrence rate becomes higher.[138] Therefore, surgical decision making and surgical technique have both become increasingly important in this field and selecting the appropriate operation to maximize a patient's outcomes is paramount to success.

Hernia recurrences happen over time and the true incidence of this is largely unknown as most studies follow patients for only a short time period after hernia repair. Patients presenting with recurrent bulge, pain, and symptoms similar to prior hernia symptoms should undergo in office evaluation along with cross-sectional imaging to assess the abdominal wall. If a hernia recurrence is detected, operative planning needs to consider the prior hernia repairs performed and what the next best approach may be. Often times if the prior mesh is intact, well incorporated, it may not need to be resected. If the prior mesh will interfere with the new repair, if it is compromised, infected, it will need to be excised. If a prior component separation has already been done, it can limit the options available for another repair. It is also important to consider if there are additional modifiable risk factors putting the patient at risk for hernia recurrence and if those need to be addressed prior to surgery. After careful evaluation and discussion with the patient, consider previously discussed surgical strategies for repair.

COMPLICATIONS OF VENTRAL HERNIA REPAIR

Ventral hernia repair and abdominal wall reconstruction is complex, and the incidence of complications depends on multiple factors including the complexity of the hernia repair, the technique used, mesh selection, and patient comorbidities. It is often difficult to parse and compare complications between different procedures and meshes in the literature due to the lack of comparative trials as well as nonstandardized nomenclature. The recently developed terminology of SSO, which includes both the commonly understood SSI as well as other noninfectious wound complications, provides a good framework for reporting and better comparison across hernia studies.[139] Several risk calculators are available to assist in optimizing patients for surgery, selection of the optimal surgical approach, and for informed consent. The American College of Surgeons National Surgical Quality Improvement Project (ACS NSQIP) risk calculator accounts for patient-related factors for morbidity and mortality. The Ventral Hernia Risk Score (VHRS), Hernia Wound Risk Assessment Tool (HWRAT), Ventral Hernia Working Group (VHWG), the Carolinas Equation for Determining Associated Risks (CeDAR), the Michigan Surgical Quality Collaborative (MSQC), and the Americas Hernia Society Quality Collaborative Outcomes Reporting App for Clinician and Patient Engagement (AHSQC ORACLE) are all available tools to assist the surgeon in predicting the risk of wound and general complications following VHR (**Fig. 69.47, Table 69.15**).[140,141] These scoring systems have been developed using variable methodology, primarily based on retrospective or registry-based

HERNIA AND SPLEEN

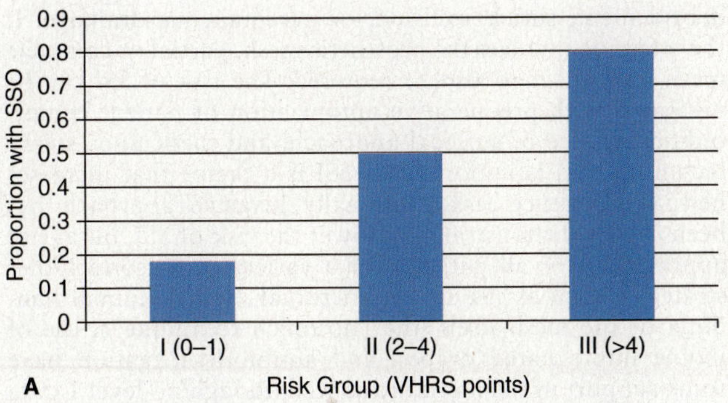

OR	VHRS for SSO Points	VHRS for SSI Points
Mesh implant	2	—
Concomitant hernia repair	2	2
Skin flaps created	2	2
ASA score ≥3	—	2
BMI ≥40	—	3
Wound class 4	9	7

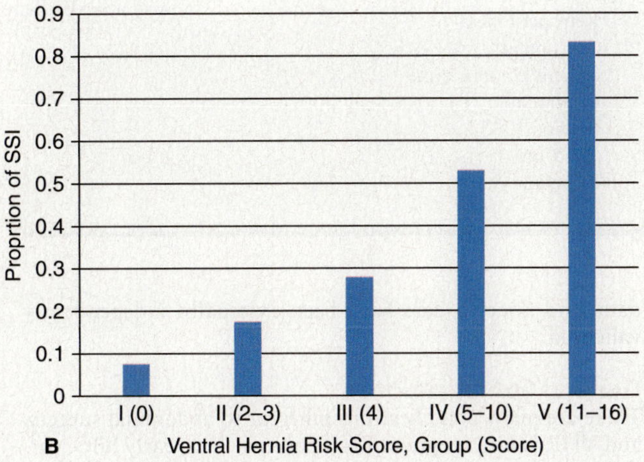

Figure 69.47. **A, B:** Ventral Hernia Risk Score (VHRS) for surgical site occurrence and surgical site infection.

Table 69.15. Complications of Herniorrhaphy

Related to Laparoscopy
Vascular injury
Intra-abdominal
Retroperitoneal
Abdominal wall
Gas embolism
Visceral injury
Bowel perforation
Bladder perforation
Trocar site complications
Hematoma
Hernia
Wound infection
Keloid
Bowel obstruction
Trocar or peritoneal closure site hernia
Adhesions
Diaphragmatic dysfunction
Hypercapnia
Related to Patient
Urinary infection
Ileus
Nausea and vomiting
Aspiration pneumonia
Cardiovascular and respiratory insufficiency
Related to Herniorrhaphy
Recurrence
Neurologic
Iliohypogastric
Ilioinguinal
Genitofemoral
Lateral cutaneous
Cord and testicular problems
Wound infection
Seroma
Hydrocele
Hematoma
Wound
Scrotal
Retroperitoneal
Osteitis pubis
Prosthetic complications
Contraction
Erosion
Infection
Rejection
Pain

data, and none to date have been externally, independently validated.

General Complications

There are many complications inherent to abdominal surgery, and VHR is no exception. Postoperative ileus, early SBO, cardiac, pulmonary, and renal complications can all occur following any VHR. These can be mitigated somewhat by choice of technique, with open repairs tending to have a higher risk of ileus, SBO, or wound complications. Cardiac arrhythmias may complicate pneumoperitoneum during laparoscopic or robotic repair. Urinary retention may occur in complex cases, particularly if dissection is required around the bladder. Pulmonary complications may be increased with some complex VHR, particularly large hernia defects and those with loss of domain. Attempting to reviscerate the herniated contents into the abdominal cavity and close the hernia defect may require significant tension, resulting in significant increase in intra-abdominal pressure. This may result in early postoperative respiratory insufficiency or failure, pneumonia, prevent initial extubation, or in the extreme result in abdominal compartment syndrome. Attention must be paid to airway pressures and other ventilatory parameters, along with intra-abdominal pressure, in such cases. All ventral hernia patients should be considered high risk for venous thromboembolic complications and be prophylaxed accordingly.

Surgical Site Infection

SSI is defined by the Center for Disease Control (CDC) and is divided into three types by the depth of the infection. Superficial SSI involves only the skin and subcutaneous tissue of the associated incision, presenting within 30 days with typical signs of infection including tenderness, swelling, erythema, or heat. Diagnosis requires one of these signs along with purulent drainage, positive culture, or deliberate opening of the surgical wound. This does not include cellulitis, stitch abscess/granuloma, or infection at stab incisions. This is the most common type of SSI with most hernia repairs. Deep SSI involves the fascia or muscle layers, also presenting with typical signs of infection. Also included in the criteria are fever, spontaneous wound dehiscence, or abscess. Infection occurring in the retromuscular compartment or preperitoneal space after abdominal wall reconstruction would be considered a deep space infection. Organ-space SSI can have differing definitions depending on the procedure performed. For the purpose of hernia repair, these occur deep the abdominal wall musculature in the intra-abdominal compartment. Diagnostic criteria include purulent drainage from organ-space drains, percutaneously placed drains in fluid collection/abscess cavity with positive culture, or intra-abdominal sepsis.

The risk of SSI increases with increasing level of contamination of the operation, with dirty or infected wounds having the highest risk of infection at around 40%. Other factors also contribute to this risk including smoking, COPD, diabetes, obesity, immune compromise, history of infection, and surgical technique. As discussed above, many of these risk factors are modifiable and should ideally be addressed prior to surgery. Most SSIs require treatment of some kind, referred to as an SSI requiring procedural intervention (SSOPI). This can include the use of antibiotics, wound opening, wound debridement, suture excision, or percutaneous drainage. If the infection involves the prosthetic mesh, partial or complete mesh removal may also be required. The risk of SSI can be mitigated with preoperative optimization of patient comorbidities, choice of surgical approach, and meticulous sterile technique and is important as SSI is a factor that increases hernia recurrence risk. Minimally invasive approach has been clearly demonstrated to lower the risk of SSI, but is not appropriate for all patients for a variety of reasons. Other strategies such as use of antimicrobial mesh, minimal handling of the mesh itself (the "no-touch technique"), use of iodine impregnated drapes, and antibiotic irrigation have some support in the literature as well, though no level 1 data currently support any of these practices.

Surgical Site Occurrence

There are a variety of wound complications that can occur as a result of hernia repair and AWR that do not meet the criteria for SSI. Current nomenclature refers to these as SSOs, though this term is sometimes used as a broader term under which SSI is included. Included under SSO are seroma or serous wound drainage hematomas, cellulitis, skin and soft tissue ischemia or necrosis, exposed prosthetic mesh, or enterocutaneous fistula. This also allows specific descriptors of the origins of some types of SSI, such as infected seroma or hematoma, infected or contaminated prosthetic mesh, or purulent wound drainage. As with SSI, intervention is sometimes necessary for treatment (SSOPI), though often simple SSOs, such as seroma, can be

Table 69.16. HW RAT Breakdown of Risk Factors for Wound Complications

Risk Grouping	Risk Factors	Risk Score
Mild risk factors (+1)	Diabetes	1
	COPD	1
	Class I obesity	1
	45–64 yrs old	1
	Intra-abdominal procedure	1
Intermediate risk factors (+2)	Smoking	2
	ASA physical status >2	2
	Panniculectomy	2
	Clean-contaminated wound	2
	Partially dependent functional status	2
	Low albumin	2
	<45 yrs of age	2
	Operative time 43–71 (min)	2
Moderate risk factors (+3)	Totally dependent functional status	3
	Inpatient operation	3
	Class III obesity	3
	Component separation	3
Severe risk factors (+4 or more)	Contaminated wound	4
	Operative time (71–117 min)	4
	Dirty/infected wound	5
	Operative time (>118 min)	6

HW-RAT	Risk Score	Number of Patients (%)	Incidence of SSO (%)
1	0–10	16,097 (59.6%)	538 (3.3%)
2	11–13	5784 (21.4%)	536 (9.3%)
3	14–16	2861 (12.3%)	472 (14.2%)
4	17–19	998 (21.7%)	217 (21.7%)
5	>19	812 (3.0%)	215 (26.5%)

managed expectantly without intervention. Noninfectious SSOs can be reduced with the use of drains, though their use does not confer protection against SSI.[142]

Mesh-Related Complications

Among the most feared complications of VHR is a complication related to the implanted prosthetic mesh. This can include mesh infection or periprosthetic infection, exposed mesh, extrusion of mesh through the skin, or enterocutaneous fistula. Mesh infection is typically reported in <1% of laparoscopic or robotic cases and <5% for open repair. The risk of mesh erosion or fistula is unknown, with data limited primarily to case reports or small case series. The risk of any of these complications and the treatment required varies greatly by presentation, mesh type, and mesh location. Generally speaking, no particular mesh seems to be a higher risk of infection when used in clean cases. However, the properties of the mesh and location within the abdominal wall seem to have significant impact on the treatment needed. Intraperitoneal mesh typically requires removal, though there are reports of salvage. Treatment of extraperitoneal mesh infection, those placed in the preperitoneal, retromuscular or onlay position, varies more by mesh type. Generally, microporous, multifilament, laminar, or composite mesh requires complete removal, whereas monofilament, large-pore mesh is salvage in the majority of cases. In the event of enterocutaneous fistula, mesh removal is generally required. Fistula can occur as an acute complication after hernia repair, typically as a result of unrecognized enterotomy, or can present late due to mesh erosion into the viscera or a subsequent abdominal operation. Mesh removal is universally required for intraperitoneal mesh in both the acute and late setting. For mesh in an extraperitoneal position, there are reports of spontaneous closure despite presence of the mesh, though partial or complete mesh removal are frequently required (**Table 69.16**).[96,143]

References

1. Digestive Disease Statistics for the United States. 2013. https://www.niddk.nih.gov/health-information/health-statistics/digestive-diseases. Accessed December 11, 2025.
2. Köckerling F, Sheen AJ, Berrevoet F, et al. The reality of general surgery training and increased complexity of abdominal wall hernia surgery. *Hernia*. 2019;23(6):1081–1091.
3. Poulose BK, Adrales GL, Janis JE. Abdominal core health—A needed field in surgery. *JAMA Surg*. 2020;155(3):185–186.
4. Condon RE. Reassessment of groin anatomy during the evolution of preperitoneal hernia repair. *Am J Surg*. 1996;172(1):5–8.
5. Milloy FJ, Anson BJ, Mcafee DK. The rectus abdominis muscle and the epigastric arteries. *Surg Gynecol Obstet*. 1960;110:293–302.
6. Askar OM. Surgical anatomy of the aponeurotic expansions of the anterior abdominal wall. *Ann R Coll Surg Engl*. 1977;59(4):313–321.
7. Cooper A. *The Anatomy and Surgical Treatment of Abdominal Hernia*. Printed for T. Cox, and sold by Messrs. Johnson, Longman and Rees; 1804.

HERNIA AND SPLEEN

8. Teoh LS, Hingston G, Al-Ali S, Dawson B, Windsor JA. The iliopubic tract: an important anatomical landmark in surgery. *J Anat.* 1999;194(Pt 1):137–141.
9. Quinn TH, Ryberg A, Annibali R, et al. Anatomy of the anterior abdominal wall and deep inguinal region from the laparoscopic surgeon's perspective. In: Lansafame RJ, ed. *Prevention and Management of Complications in Minimally Invasive Surgery.* Igaku Shoin; 1996:197.
10. Anson BJ, Morgan EH, McVay CB. Surgical anatomy of the inguinal region based upon a study of 500 body-halves. *Surg Gynecol Obstet.* 1960;111:707–725.
11. Jacob BP, Chen DC, Ramshaw B, Towfigh S, eds. *The SAGES Manual of Groin Pain.* 1st ed. Springer International Publishing; 2016.
12. Annibali R, Quinn TH, Fitzgibbons RJ Jr. Anatomy of the inguinal region from the laparoscopic perspective: critical areas for laparoscopic hernia repair. In: Bendavid R, ed. *Prostheses and Abdominal Wall Hernias.* Landes; 1994:82.
13. Annibali R, Quinn TH, Fitzgibbons RJ Jr. Avoiding nerve injury during laparoscopic hernia repair: critical areas for staple placement. In: Arregui ME, Nagan RF, eds. *Inguinal Hernia: Advances or Controversies.* Radcliffe Medical; 1994:41.
14. Brick WG, Colborn GL, Gadacz TR, Skandalakis JE. Crucial anatomic lessons for laparoscopic herniorrhaphy. *Am Surg.* 1995;61(2):172–177.
15. Gilroy AM, Hermey DC, DiBenedetto LM, Marks SC Jr, Page DW, Lei QF. Variability of the obturator vessels. *Clin Anat.* 1997;10(5):328–332.
16. Missankov AA, Asvat R, Maoba KI. Variations of the pubic vascular anastomoses in black South Africans. *Acta Anat (Basel).* 1996;155(3):212–214.
17. Bendavid R. The space of Bogros and the deep inguinal venous circulation. *Surg Gynecol Obstet.* 1992;174(5):355–358.
18. Vad MV, Frost P, Bay-Nielsen M, et al. Impact of occupational mechanical exposures on risk of lateral and medial inguinal hernia requiring surgical repair. *Occup Environ Med.* 2012;69(11): 802–809.
19. Lau H, Fang C, Yuen WK, et al. Risk factors for inguinal hernia in adult males: a case-control study. *Surgery.* 2007;141(2): 262–266.
20. Antoniou GA, Tentes IK, Antoniou SA, et al. Matrix metalloproteinase imbalance in inguinal hernia formation. *J Invest Surg.* 2011;24(4):145–150.
21. Ruhl CE, Everhart JE. Risk factors for inguinal hernia among adults in the US population. *Am J Epidemiol.* 2007;165(10):1154–1161.
22. Nilsson E, Kald A, Anderberg B, et al. Hernia surgery in a defined population: a prospective three year audit. *Eur J Surg.* 1997; 163(11):823–829.
23. Burcharth J, Pedersen M, Bisgaard T, Pedersen C, Rosenberg J. Nationwide prevalence of groin hernia repair. *PLoS One.* 2013; 8(1):e54367.
24. Prasaud P, Cemaj S, Fitzgibbons RJ. Basic features of groin hernia and its repair. In: Yeo CJ, Dempsey DT, Klein AS, eds. *Shakelford's Surgery of the Alimentary Tract.* 6th ed. Saunders; 2006.
25. Miserez M, Alexandre JH, Campanelli G, et al. The European Hernia Society groin hernia classification: simple and easy to remember. *Hernia.* 2007;11(2):113–116.
26. Schroeder AD, Tubre DJ, Fitzgibbons RJ Jr. Watchful waiting for inguinal hernia. *Adv Surg.* 2019;53:293–303.
27. Hernia Surge Group. International guidelines for groin hernia management. *Hernia.* 2018;22(1):1–165.
28. Henriksen NA, Thorup J, Jorgensen LN. Unsuspected femoral hernia in patients with a preoperative diagnosis of recurrent inguinal hernia. *Hernia.* 2012;16(4):381–385.
29. Treadwell J, Tipton K, Oyesanmi O, Sun F, Schoelles K. Surgical options for inguinal hernia: comparative effectiveness review [Internet]. Rockville (MD): Agency for Healthcare Research and Quality (US); 2012 Aug. Report No.: 12-EHC091-EF.
30. Prabhu AS, Carbonell A, Hope W, et al. Robotic inguinal vs transabdominal laparoscopic inguinal hernia repair: the RIVAL randomized clinical trial. *JAMA Surg.* 2020;155(5):380–387.
31. Daes J, Felix E. Critical view of the myopectineal orifice. *Ann Surg.* 2017;266(1):e1–e2.
32. Wantz GE. Giant prosthetic reinforcement of the visceral sac. The Stoppa groin hernia repair. *Surg Clin North Am.* 1998;78(6): 1075–1087.
33. Gilbert AI, Young J, Graham MF, Divilio LT, Patel B. Combined anterior and posterior inguinal hernia repair: intermediate recurrence rates with three groups of surgeons. *Hernia.* 2004;8(3): 203–207.
34. Andresen K, Rosenberg J. Open preperitoneal groin hernia repair with mesh: a qualitative systematic review. *Am J Surg.* 2017;213(6): 1153–1159.
35. Amid PK, Shulman AG, Lichtenstein IL. Open "tension-free" repair of inguinal hernias: the Lichtenstein technique. *Eur J Surg.* 1996;162(6):447–453.
36. Aasvang EK, Kehlet H. Chronic pain after childhood groin hernia repair. *J Pediatr Surg.* 2007;42(8):1403–1408.
37. Tekatli H, Schouten N, van Dalen T, et al. Mechanism, assessment, and incidence of male infertility after inguinal hernia surgery: a review of the preclinical and clinical literature. *Am J Surg.* 2012; 204(4):503–509.
38. Magnusson N, Gunnarsson U, Nordin P, Smedberg S, Hedberg M, Sandblom G. Reoperation for persistent pain after groin hernia surgery: a population-based study. *Hernia.* 2015;19(1):45–51.
39. Köckerling F, Koch A, Lorenz R, Schug-Pass C, Stechemesser B, Reinpold W. How long do we need to follow-up our hernia patients to find the real recurrence rate. *Front Surg.* 2015;2:24.
40. Taylor DC. Abdominal musculature abnormalities as a cause of groin pain in athletes. *Am J Sports Med.* 1991;19(4):421.
41. Bou Antoun M, Reboul G, Ronot M, Crombe A, Poussange N, Pesquer L. Imaging of inguinal-related groin pain in athletes. *Br J Radiol.* 2018;91(1092):20170856.
42. Poulose BK, Shelton J, Phillips S, et al. Epidemiology and cost of ventral hernia repair: making the case for hernia research. *Hernia.* 2012;16(2):179–183.
43. Muysoms FE, Miserez M, Berrevoet F, et al. Classification of primary and incisional abdominal wall hernias. *Hernia.* 2009; 13(4):407–414.
44. Ventral Hernia Working Group; Breuing K, Butler CE, Ferzoco S, et al. Incisional ventral hernias: review of the literature and recommendations regarding the grading and technique of repair. *Surgery.* 2010;148(3):544–558.
45. Israelsson LA, Millbourn D. Prevention of incisional hernias: how to close a midline incision. *Surg Clin North Am.* 2013;93(5): 1027–1040.
46. Henriksen NA, Deerenberg EB, Venclauskas L, Fortelny RH, Miserez M, Muysoms FE. Meta-analysis on materials and techniques for laparotomy closure: the MATCH review. *World J Surg.* 2018;42(6):1666–1678.
47. Deerenberg EB, Harlaar JJ, Steyerberg EW, et al. Small bites versus large bites for closure of abdominal midline incisions (STITCH): a double-blind, multicentre, randomised controlled trial. *Lancet.* 2015;386(10000):1254–1260.
48. Christoffersen MW, Olsen BH, Rosenberg J, Bisgaard T. Randomized clinical trial on the postoperative use of an abdominal binder after laparoscopic umbilical and epigastric hernia repair. *Hernia.* 2015;19(1):147–153.
49. Borab ZM, Shakir S, Lanni MA, et al. Does prophylactic mesh placement in elective, midline laparotomy reduce the incidence of incisional hernia? A systematic review and meta-analysis. *Surgery.* 2017;161(4):1149–1163.
50. Caro-Tarrago A, Olona Casas C, Jimenez Salido A, Duque Guilera E, Moreno Fernandez F, Vicente Guillen V. Prevention of incisional hernia in midline laparotomy with an onlay mesh: a randomized clinical trial. *World J Surg.* 2014;38(9): 2223–2230.
51. Muysoms FE, Detry O, Vierendeels T, et al. Prevention of incisional hernias by prophylactic mesh-augmented reinforcement of midline laparotomies for abdominal aortic aneurysm treatment a randomized controlled trial. *Ann Surg.* 2016;263(4): 638–645.

52. Lin YT, Weng TY, Tam KW. Effectiveness and safety of mesh repair for incarcerated or strangulated hernias: a systematic review and meta-analysis. *World J Surg*. 2020;44(7):2176–2184.
53. Bikhchandani J, Fitzgibbons RJ Jr. Repair of giant ventral hernias. *Adv Surg*. 2013;47:1–27.
54. Bosanquet DC, Ansell J, Abdelrahman T, et al. Systematic review and meta-regression of factors affecting midline incisional hernia rates: analysis of 14,618 patients. *PLoS One*. 2015;10(9): e0138745.
55. Pogacnik JS, Messaris E, Deiling SM, et al. Increased risk of incisional hernia after sigmoid colectomy for diverticulitis compared with colon cancer. *J Am Coll Surg*. 2014;218(5):920–928.
56. Shell DH 4th, de la Torre J, Andrades P, Vasconez LO. Open repair of ventral incisional hernias. *Surg Clin North Am*. 2008;88(1): 61–83, viii.
57. Kisielinski K, Conze J, Murken AH, Lenzen NN, Klinge U, Schumpelick V. The Pfannenstiel or so called "bikini cut": still effective more than 100 years after first description. *Hernia*. 2004;8(3): 177–181.
58. Reinpold W, Köckerling F, Bittner R, et al. Classification of rectus diastasis—a proposal by the German Hernia Society (DHG) and the International Endohernia Society (IEHS). *Front Surg*. 2019;6:1.
59. ElHawary H, Chartier C, Alam P, Janis JE. Open versus laparoscopic surgical management of rectus diastasis: systematic review and pooled analysis of complications and recurrence rates. *World J Surg*. 2022;46(8):1878–1885.
60. Castagneto-Gissey L, Russo MF, Palumbo P, et al. Subcutaneous versus retromuscular approach for the minimally invasive surgical treatment of rectus diastasis with concomitant ventral hernia: systematic review and meta-analysis of current techniques. *Hernia*. 2025;29(1):264.
61. Patel PP, Warren JA, Mansour R, Cobb WS 4th, Carbonell AM. Large single-center experience of open lateral abdominal wall hernia repairs. *Am Surg*. 2016;82(7):608–612.
62. Beffa LR, Margiotta AL, Carbonell AM. Flank and lumbar hernia repair. *Surg Clin N Amer*. 2018;98(3):593–605.
63. Kald A, Juul KN, Hjortsvang H, Sjödahl RI. Quality of life is impaired in patients with peristomal bulging of a sigmoid colostomy. *Scand J Gastroenterol*. 2008;43(5):627–633.
64. Carne PW, Robertson GM, Frizelle FA. Parastomal hernia. *Br J Surg*. 2003;90(7):784–793.
65. Rubin MS, Schoetz DJ Jr, Matthews JB. Parastomal hernia. Is stoma relocation superior to fascial repair. *Arch Surg*. 1994;129(4): 413–418; discussion 418–419.
66. Antoniou SA, Agresta F, Garcia Alamino JM, et al. European Hernia Society guidelines on prevention and treatment of parastomal hernias. *Hernia*. 2018;22(1):183–198.
67. Cross AJ, Buchwald PL, Frizelle FA, Eglinton TW. Meta-analysis of prophylactic mesh to prevent parastomal hernia. *Br J Surg*. 2017;104(3):179–186.
68. Brandsma HT, Hansson BME, Aufenacker TJ, et al. Prophylactic mesh placement during formation of an end-colostomy reduces the rate of parastomal hernia. *Ann Surg*. 2017;265(4):663–339.
69. Henriksen NA, Montgomery A, Kaufmann R, et al; European and Americas Hernia Societies (EHS and AHS). Guidelines for treatment of umbilical and epigastric hernias from the European Hernia Society and Americas Hernia Society. *Br J Surg*. 2020;107(3): 171–190.
70. Appleby PW, Martin TA, Hope WW. Umbilical hernia repair: overview of approaches and review of literature. *Surg Clin N Am*. 2018;98(3):561–576.
71. Orenstein SB. Permanent prosthetics: polypropylene, polyester, ePTFE, and hybrid mesh. In: Davis S Jr, Dakin G, Bates A, eds. *The SAGES Manual of Hernia Surgery*. Springer; 2019.
72. Ponten JEH, Leclerq WKG, Letinga T, et al. Mesh OR patch repair of epigastric and umbilical site (MORPHEUS Trial): a complete 2 year follow-up. *Ann Surg*. 2019;270(1):33–37.
73. Patel PP, Love MW, Ewing JA, Warren JA, Cobb WS, Carbonell AM. Risks of subsequent abdominal operations after laparoscopic ventral hernia repair. *Surg Endosc*. 2017;31(2):823–828.
74. Halm JA, de Wall LL, Steyerberg EW, Jeekel J, Lange JF. Intraperitoneal polypropylene mesh hernia repair complicates subsequent abdominal surgery. *World J Surg*. 2007;31(2):423–429.
75. Gray SH, Vick CC, Graham LA, et al. Risk of complications from enterotomy or unplanned bowel resection during elective hernia repair. *Arch Surg*. 2008;143(6):582–586.
76. Haskins IN, Voeller GR, Stoikes NF, et al. Onlay with adhesive use compared with sublay mesh placement in ventral hernia repair: was Chevrel right? An Americas Hernia Society Quality Collaborative Analysis. *J Am Coll Surg*. 2017;224(5):962–970.
77. Klinge U, Conze J, Krones CJ, Schumpelick V. Incisional hernia: open techniques. *World J Surg*. 2005;29(8):1066–1072.
78. Albino FP, Patel KM, Nahabedian MY, Sosin M, Attinger CE, Bhanot P. Does mesh location matter in abdominal wall reconstruction? A systematic review of the literature and a summary of recommendations. *Plast Reconstr Surg*. 2013;132(5):1295–1304.
79. Holihan JL, Nguyen DH, Nguyen MT, Mo J, Kao LS, Liang MK. Mesh location in open ventral hernia repair: a systematic review and network meta-analysis. *World J Surg*. 2016;40(1):89–99.
80. Tulloh B, de Beaux A. Defects and donuts: the importance of the mesh:defect area ratio. *Hernia*. 2016;20(6):893–895.
81. LeBlanc K. Proper mesh overlap is a key determinant in hernia recurrence following laparoscopic ventral and incisional hernia repair. *Hernia*. 2015;20(1):85–99.
82. Bittner R, Bain K, Bansal VK, et al. Update of Guidelines for laparoscopic treatment of ventral and incisional abdominal wall hernias (International Endohernia Society (IEHS))—Part A. *Surg Endosc*. 2019;33(10):3069–3139.
83. Flament JB, Palot JP, Burde A. Treatment of major incisional hernias. *Probl Gen Surg*. 1995;12(1):151–158.
84. Gurusamy KS, Samraj K. Wound drains after incisional hernia repair. *Cochrane Database Syst Rev*. 2007;(1):CD005570.
85. Love MW, Warren JA, Davis S, et al. Computed tomography imaging in ventral hernia repair: can we predict the need for myofascial release? *Hernia*. 2021;25(2):471–477.
86. Sosin M, Nahabedian MY, Bhanot P. The perfect plane: a systematic review of mesh location and outcomes, update 2018. *Plast Reconstr Surg*. 2018;142(3 Suppl):107S–116S.
87. Lipman J, Medalie D, Rosen MJ. Staged repair of massive incisional hernias with loss of abdominal domain: a novel approach. *Am J Surg*. 2008;195(1):84–88.
88. Temudom T, Siadati M, Sarr MG. Repair of complex giant or recurrent ventral hernias by using tension-free intraparietal prosthetic mesh (Stoppa technique): lessons learned from our initial experience (fifty patients). *Surgery*. 1996;120(4):738–743; discussion 743–744.
89. Belyansky I, Daes J, Radu VG, et al. A novel approach using the enhanced-view totally extraperitoneal (eTEP) technique for laparoscopic retromuscular hernia repair. *Surg Endosc*. 2018;32(3):1525–1532.
90. Baur J, Ramser M, Keller N, et al. Robotische Hernienchirurgie: Teil II: Robotische primär ventrale und inzisionale Hernienversorgung (rv-TAPP und r-Rives/r-TARUP). Videobeitrag und Ergebnisse einer Kohortenstudie an 118 Patienten [Robotic hernia repair: Part II: Robotic primary ventral and incisional hernia repair (rv-TAPP and r-Rives or r-TARUP). Video report and results of a series of 118 patients]. *Chirurg*. 2021;92(9):809–821. German. Erratum in: Chirurgie (Heidelb). 2022;93(Suppl 2):142.
91. Davis JR, Villareal JE, Cobb WS, Carbonell AM, Warren JA. Interparietal hernia complicating retromuscular ventral hernia repair. *Am Surg*. 2016;82(7):658–659.
92. Heniford BT, Ross SW, Wormer BA, et al. Preperitoneal ventral hernia repair: a decade long prospective observational study with analysis of 1023 patient outcomes. *Ann Surg*. 2020;271(2): 364–374.
93. Novitsky YW, Elliott HL, Orenstein SB, Rosen MJ. Transversus abdominis muscle release: a novel approach to posterior component separation during complex abdominal wall reconstruction. *Am J Surg*. 2012;204(5):709–716.
94. Majumder A, Miller HJ, del Campo LM, Soltanian H, Novitsky YW. Assessment of myofascial medialization following posterior

component separation via transversus abdominis muscle release in a cadaveric model. *Hernia.* 2018;22:637–644.

95. Hodgkinson JD, Leo CA, Maeda Y, et al. A meta-analysis comparing open anterior component separation with posterior component separation and transversus abdominis release in the repair of midline ventral hernias. *Hernia.* 2018;22(4):617–626.
96. Hope WW, Cobb WS, Adrales GL. *Textbook of Hernia.* Springer; 2017.
97. Carbonell AM, Warren JA, Prabhu AS, et al. Reducing length of stay using a robotic-assisted approach for retromuscular ventral hernia repair a comparative analysis from the Americas Hernia Society Quality Collaborative. *Ann Surg.* 2018;267(2):210–217.
98. Warren JA, Cobb WS, Ewing JA, Carbonell AM. Standard laparoscopic versus robotic retromuscular ventral hernia repair. *Surg Endosc.* 2016;31(1):324–332.
99. Bittner JG 4th, Alrefai S, Vy M, Mabe M, Del Prado PAR, Clingempeel NL. Comparative analysis of open and robotic transversus abdominis release for ventral hernia repair. *Surg Endosc.* 2018;32(2):727–734.
100. Martin-del-Campo LA, Weltz AS, Belyansky I, Novitsky YW. Comparative analysis of perioperative outcomes of robotic versus open transversus abdominis release. *Surg Endosc.* 2018;32(2):840–845.
101. Ramirez OM, Ruas E, Dellon AL. "Components separation" method for closure of abdominal-wall defects: an anatomic and clinical study. *Plast Reconstr Surg.* 1990;86(3):519–526.
102. DiCocco JM, Fabian TC, Emmett KP, Magnotti LJ, Goldberg SP, Croce MA. Components separation for abdominal wall reconstruction: the Memphis modification. *Surgery.* 2012;151(1):118–125.
103. Azoury SC, Dhanasopon AP, Hui X, et al. A single institutional comparison of endoscopic and open abdominal component separation. *Surg Endosc.* 2014;28(12):3349–3358.
104. Oviedo RJ, Robertson JC, Desai AS. Robotic ventral hernia repair and endoscopic component separation: outcomes. *JSLS.* 2017;21(3):1–6.
105. Azoury SC, Dhanasopon AP, Hui X, et al. Endoscopic component separation for laparoscopic and open ventral hernia repair: a single institutional comparison of outcomes and review of the technique. *Hernia.* 2014;18(5):637–645.
106. Alexander AM, Scott DJ. Laparoscopic ventral hernia repair. *Surg Clin North Am.* 2013;93(5):1091–1110.
107. Schlosser KA, Maloney SR, Prasad T, Colavita PD, Augenstein VA, Heniford BT. Too big to breathe: predictors of respiratory failure and insufficiency after open ventral hernia repair. *Surg Endosc.* 2020;34(9):4131–4139.
108. Van Hoef S, Dries P, Allaeys M, Eker HH, Berrevoet F. Intra-abdominal hypertension and compartment syndrome after complex hernia repair. *Hernia.* 2024;28(3):701–709.
109. Klinge U, Zheng H, Si ZY, Schumpelick V, Bhardwaj R, Klosterhalfen B. Synthesis of type I and III collagen, expression of fibronectin and matrix metalloproteinases-1 and -13 in hernial sac of patients with inguinal hernia. *Int J Surg Investig.* 1999;1(3):219–227.
110. Bittner R, Bingener-Casey J, Dietz U, et al. Guidelines for laparoscopic treatment of ventral and incisional abdominal wall hernias (International Endohernia Society (IEHS)-part 1. *Surg Endosc.* 2014;28(1):2–29.
111. Moreno IG. Chronic eventrations and large hernias; preoperative treatment by progressive pneumoperitoneum; original procedure. *Surgery.* 1947;22(6):945–953.
112. Mayagoitia JC, Suarez D, Arenas JC, Díaz de León V. Preoperative progressive pneumoperitoneum in patients with abdominal-wall hernias. *Hernia.* 2006;10(3):213–217.
113. Toniato A, Pagetta C, Bernante P, Piotto A, Pelizzo MR. Incisional hernia treatment with progressive pneumoperitoneum and retromuscular prosthetic hernioplasty. *Langenbecks Arch Surg.* 2002;387(5–6):246–248.
114. Dumont F, Fuks D, Verhaeghe P, et al. Progressive pneumoperitoneum increases the length of abdominal muscles. *Hernia.* 2009;13(2):183–187.
115. Alam NN, Narang SK, Pathak S, Daniels IR, Smart NJ. Methods of abdominal wall expansion for incisional hernia repair; a systematic review. *Hernia.* 2016;20(2):191–199.
116. Sabbagh C, Dumont F, Fuks D, Yzet T, Verhaeghe P, Regimbeau JM. Progressive preoperative pneumoperitoneum preparation (the Goni Moreno protocol) prior to large incisional hernia surgery; volumetric, respiratory, and clinical impacts. A prospective study. *Hernia.* 2012;16(1):33–40.
117. Allen JA, Warren JA, Bittle J. Volumetric analysis of patients undergoing abdominal wall reconstruction after progressive preoperative pneumoperitoneum. *Hernia.* 2018;22(Suppl 1):S51.
118. Bueno-Lledo J, Torregrosa A, Jimenez R, Pastor PG. Preoperative combination of progressive pneumoperitoneum and botulinum toxin type A in patients with loss of domain hernia. *Surg Endosc.* 2018;148(8):544–555.
119. Motz BM, Schlosser KA, Heniford BT. Chemical components separation: concepts, evidence, and outcomes. *Plast Reconstr Surg.* 2018;142:58S–63S.
120. Ibarra-Hurtado TR, Nuño-Guzmán CM, Echeagaray-Herrera JE, et al. Use of botulinum toxin type a before abdominal wall hernia reconstruction. *World J Surg.* 2009;33:2553–2556.
121. Zendejas B, Khasawneh MA, Srvantstyan B, Jenkins DH, Schiller HJ, Zielinski MD. Outcomes of chemical component paralysis using botulinum toxin for incisional hernia repairs. *World J Surg.* 2013;37:2830–2837.
122. Ibarra-Hurdato TR, Nuno-Guzman CM, Miranda-Diaz AG, Troyo-Sanromán R, Navarro-Ibarra R, Bravo-Cuéllar L. Effect of botulinum toxin type A in lateral abdominal muscles thickness and length in patients with midline incisional hernias secondary to open abdomen management. *Hernia.* 2014;18(5):647–652.
123. Zeilinski MD, Goussouss N, Schiller HJ, Jenkins D. Chemical component separation with botulinum toxin A: a novel technique to improve primary fascial closure rates of the open abdomen. *Hernia.* 2013;17(1):101–107.
124. Elstner KE, Read JW, Rodriguez-Acevedo O, Ho-Shon K, Magnussen J, Ibrahim N. Preoperative progressive pneumoperitoneum complementing chemical component relaxation in complex ventral hernia repair. *Surg Endosc.* 2017;31:1914–1922.
125. Ibarra-Hurtado TR, Nuño-Guzmán CM, Miranda-Díaz AG, Troyo-Sanromán R, Navarro-Ibarra R, Bravo-Cuéllar L. Effect of botulinum toxin type A in lateral abdominal wall muscles thickness and length of patients with midline incisional hernia secondary to open abdomen management. *Hernia.* 2014;18:647–652.
126. Zielinski MD, Goussous N, Schiller HJ, Jenkins D. Chemical components separation with botulinum toxin A: a novel technique to improve primary fascial closure rates of the open abdomen. *Hernia.* 2013;17:101–107.
127. Deerenberg EB, Shao JM, Elhage SA, et al. Preoperative botulinum toxin A injection in complex abdominal wall reconstruction-a propensity-scored matched study. *Am J Surg.* 2021;222(3):638–642.
128. Benoit O, Moszkowicz D, Milot L, et al. Right colectomy with absorbable mesh repair as a salvage solution for the management of giant incisional hernia with loss of domain: results of a bicentric study. *World J Surg.* 2020;44(6):1762–1770.
129. Qaja E, Le C, Benedicto R. Repair of giant inguinoscrotal hernia with loss of domain. *J Surg Case Rep.* 2017;11:1–3.
130. Smietanski M, Szczepkowski M, Alexandre JA, et al. European hernia society classification of parastomal hernias. *Hernia.* 2014;18(1):1–6.
131. Hansson BM, Slater NJ, van der Velden AS, et al. Surgical techniques for parastomal hernia repair: a systematic review of the literature. *Ann Surg.* 2012;255(4):685–695.
132. Allen-Mersh TG, Thomson JP. Surgical treatment of colostomy complications. *Br J Surg.* 1988;75(5):416–418.
133. Hotouras A, Murphy J, Thaha M, Chan CL. The persistent challenge of parastomal herniation: a review of the literature and future developments. *Colorectal Dis.* 2013;15(5):e202–e214.
134. Beffa LR, Warren JA, Cobb WS, Knoedler B, Ewing JA, Carbonell AM. Open retromuscular repair of parastomal hernias with synthetic mesh. *Am Surg.* 2017;83(8):906–910.

135. Pauli EM, Juza RM, Winder JS. How I do it: novel parastomal herniorrhaphy utilizing transversus abdominis release. *Hernia.* 2016;20(4):547–552.
136. Raigani S, Criss CN, Petro CC, Prabhu AS, Novitsky YW, Rosen MJ. Single-center experience with parastomal hernia repair using retromuscular mesh placement. *J Gastrointest Surg.* 2014;18(9):1673–1637.
137. Sugarbaker PH. Peritoneal approach to prosthetic mesh repair of paraostomy hernias. *Ann Surg.* 1985;201(3):344–346.
138. Holihan JL, Alawadi Z, Martindale RG, et al. Adverse events after ventral hernia repair: the vicious cycle of complications. *J Am Coll Surg.* 2015;221(2):478–485.
139. Haskins IN, Horne CM, Krpata DM, et al. A call for standardization of wound events reporting following ventral hernia repair. *Hernia.* 2018;22:729–736.
140. Fischer JP, Wink JD, Tuggle CT, Nelson JA, Kovach SJ. Wound risk assessment in ventral hernia repair: generation and internal validation of a risk stratification system using the ACS-NSQIP. *Hernia.* 2015;19(1):103–111.
141. Berger RL, Li LT, Hicks SC, Davila JA, Kao LS, Liang MK. Development and validation of a risk-stratification score for surgical site occurrence and surgical site infection after open ventral hernia repair. *J Am Coll Surg.* 2013;217(6):974–982.
142. Krpata DM, Prabhu AS, Carbonell AM, et al. Drain placement does not increase infectious complications after retromuscular ventral hernia repair with synthetic mesh: an AHSQC analysis. *J Gastrointest Surg.* 2017;21:2083–2089.
143. Warren JA, Love M, Cobb WS. Factors affecting salvage rate of infected prosthetic mesh. *Am J Surg.* 2020;220(3):751–756.

70

The Spleen

Ryan Howard and Hope T. Jackson

Key Points

1 The spleen is the second largest lymphatic organ with hematologic and immunologic function located in the left upper quadrant of the abdomen. Anatomically, it relates to the diaphragm both superiorly and laterally and spans the 9th, 10th, and 11th ribs posteriorly.

2 The normal size of the spleen is approximately 13 × 7 × 4 cm and the typical weight of a spleen is 150 to 200 g.

3 The spleen removes senescent erythrocytes, remodels abnormal red blood cells (RBCs), recycles iron, and generates B- and T-lymphocytes in response to antigens.

4 The spleen also facilitates opsonization and phagocytosis of encapsulated organisms including *Streptococcus pneumonia, Haemophilus influenzae, and Neisseria meningitidis*. Vaccines targeting encapsulated organisms can prevent overwhelming postsplenectomy infection.

5 Splenomegaly can occur as a result of neoplastic, infectious, inflammatory, congestive, infiltrative, and hematologic conditions.

6 Splenectomy remains a relevant treatment option for many conditions affecting the spleen. Indications include trauma, hematologic and malignant disorders, and cysts and infections.

7 Key operative strategy involves determining the optimal operative approach based on patient clinical factors as open, laparoscopic, and robotic approaches have all been utilized.

Understanding both the anatomy and physiology of the spleen is important to safe surgical practice. Many surgeons either directly treat or incidentally manage patients with splenic diseases, which are generally hematologic and immunologic conditions. In addition, over recent years many advances have been made in minimally invasive and spleen-preserving approaches to diseases of the spleen. In this chapter we review the spleen, including its history, anatomy, physiology, pathophysiology, indications for operative intervention, and opera-
1 tive approaches and techniques.

HISTORY

The spleen has a unique history as a mysterious organ whose function long eluded common knowledge.[1] While the origin of the word "spleen" is unclear, it is believed to have been derived from the Green "splen" and "spancknon," which means viscus.[2] Plato thought that its function was to "maintain the liver bright and pure" and Hippocrates thought the spleen was the source of "black bile" and associated with feelings of melancholy.[3] Conversely, in the Talmud the spleen is described as the source of laughter, and melancholy was thought to come from removal of the spleen. The spleen has a longstanding association with the ability to run. In ancient Greece, runners may have had their spleen ablated in an attempt to improve their speed.[4] This was ultimately studied in mice in 1922, where mice who had undergone splenectomy were in fact reported to run faster than mice who still had their spleen intact.[2]

Inquiry into the spleen advanced during the Renaissance. Mondino de Luicci identified the short gastric vessels in the 14th century, and Paracelsus questioned whether the spleen was a necessary organ in the 16th century. At that time, Versalius performed splenectomies in mice and determined it was not essential to life. However, it wasn't until 1911 that Micheli identified that the spleen was the site of red blood cell destruction in autoimmune hemolytic anemia. Shortly after, in 1916, a Czech medical student named Paul Kaznelson proposed that splenectomy may be beneficial in patients with idiopathic thrombocytopenic purpura.

The first splenectomy was reported to be performed in 1549 by Adriano Zaccaria on a woman with splenomegaly due to malaria.[3] His report noted that the spleen weighed 1,310 grams. Viard was reported to have performed the first spleen-preserving procedures in 1581 by removing a portion of the spleen that had prolapsed through an abdominal wound. The first authenticated splenectomy was performed in 1826 in Germany by Carl Frederick Quitterbaum in a patient with secondary hypersplenism due to cirrhosis, and the patient died 6 hours after the procedure. An 1877 series reported 50 splenectomies with a 70% mortality rate, and in 1900 another series reported 360 splenectomies with a 40% mortality rate. It was not until 1992 that the first laparoscopic splenectomy was described, which went on to become the accepted standard for surgical treatment of the spleen in the nontrauma setting.[5]

EMBRYOLOGY AND ANATOMY

During fetal development, the spleen derives from an outpouching of the mesogastrium during the 5th week of gestation.[6,7] Its natural location after natural rotation of the gut is the left upper quadrant, where it relates to the diaphragm superiorly and laterally and spans the 9th to 11th ribs along the left mid to posterior axillary line (**Fig. 70.1**). The ventral surface of the spleen approximates the greater curvature of the stomach as well as the tail of the pancreas, which is in contact with the splenic capsule 30%. The inferior pole of the spleen relates to the left kidney posteriorly and the splenic flexure of the colon anteriorly (see **Fig. 70.3**).

2 The spleen typically measures 13 × 7 × 4 cm in size and weighs approximately 150 to 200 g.[8] The spleen can typically

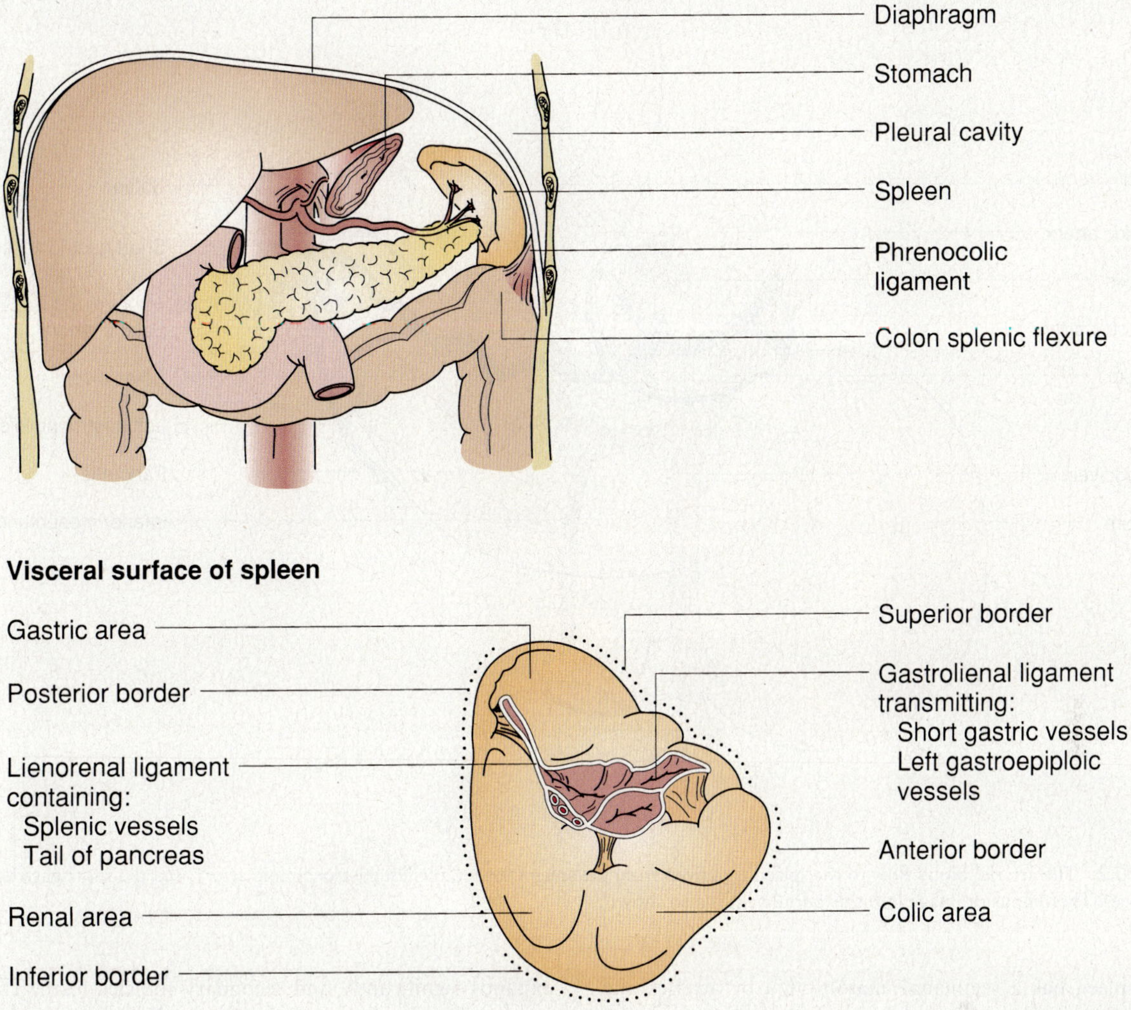

Figure 70.1. Anatomic relation of the spleen to the liver, diaphragm, pancreas, colon, and kidney. The stomach is sectioned to illustrate the anatomic relation in situ.

be palpated below the costal margin only after doubling in size to 300 to 400 g.[9] The size threshold for defining massive splenomegaly is arbitrarily set at 1,500 g, which is about 10 times the typical size in adults. Finally, the spleen can also have a natural cleft in the capsule that can be misinterpreted as splenic disruption on cross sectional imaging obtained in the setting of trauma.

The vascular anatomy of the spleen is relatively straightforward and includes the splenic artery, splenic vein, and short gastric vessels (**Fig. 70.2**).[10] Typical blood flow to the spleen is estimated to be 200 to 300 mL/min, equal to roughly 5% of cardiac output. The splenic artery is one of the major branches off the celiac trunk and has a characteristic serpentine course toward the spleen along the superior border of the pancreas with loops extending both superiorly and inferiorly. There are multiple branches along the length of the splenic artery to the body and tail of the pancreas. It then typically branches approximately 2 to 3 cm from the splenic hilum, giving off the superior polar artery. As it approaches the spleen further, the main artery then gives off three to five more branches which enter along the trabeculae of the spleen. The short gastric vessels provide additional blood supply via the left gastroepiploic artery. In cases of splenic enlargement, the spleen may develop additional blood supply directly from the omentum, diaphragm, or mesentery of the splenic flexure of the colon. The spleen's venous drainage begins with segmental venous branches that leave the trabeculae and coalesce into the main splenic vein in the hilum. The splenic vein typically travels along the posterior surface of the pancreas where additional small branches leaving the pancreas drain into it, then it joins with the superior mesenteric vein to form the portal vein. The lymphatic drainage of the spleen is located along the vasculature, with primary lymph nodes located in the hilum of the spleen and along the splenic artery and short gastric vessels.

There are multiple ligaments attached to the spleen which maintains its fixed position in the left upper quadrant (**Fig. 70.3**). These primarily include the splenogastric, splenorenal, and splenocolic ligaments. These ligaments can be absent in cases of "wandering spleen," where the spleen is found outside of the left upper quadrant.[11] The splenogastric ligament is a left-sided superior extension of the greater omentum along the greater curvature of the stomach and includes the short gastric vessels. The splenorenal ligament travels parallel to the posterolateral border of the spleen and inserts to the superior pole of Gerota fascia. Division of this ligament during mobilization of the spleen is what allows reflection of the spleen away from the tail of the pancreas. The splenocolic ligament is the last of the three major ligaments, and this is a short attachment associated with the splenic flexure of the colon that may be vascularized or not. Other minor ligaments that are variably present include the spleno-omental and splenophrenic ligaments, which are more likely to be present in cases of splenic enlargement. Attachments to the greater omentum may also be present, and it is crucial to interrogate and divide these attachments prior to exerting vigorous traction on the omentum to avoid disruption of the inferior splenic capsule.

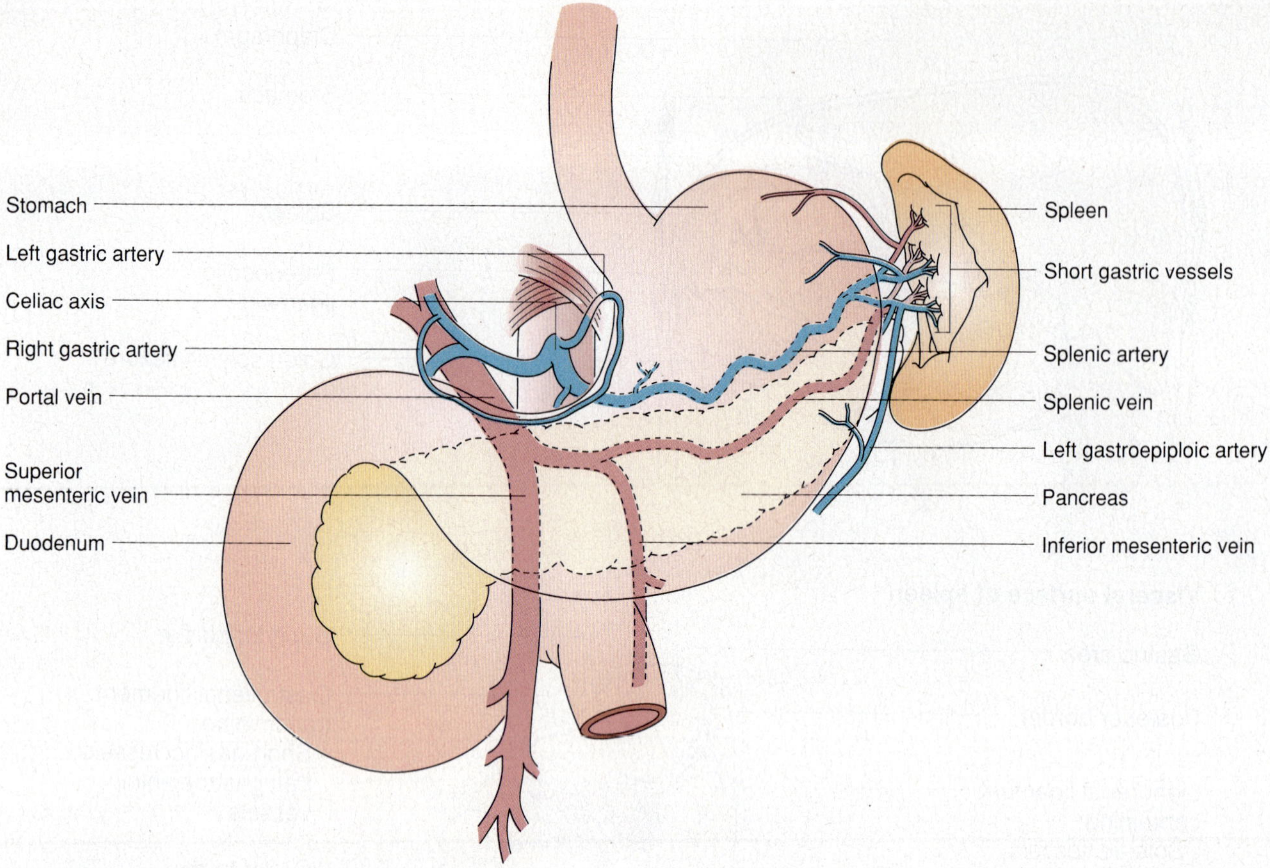

Figure 70.2. The arterial blood flow to the spleen is derived from the splenic artery, the left gastroepiploic artery, and the short gastric arteries (vasa brevia). The venous drainage into this portal vein is also shown.

The spleen has a segmental anatomy fed by arteries and drained by veins that exit via the trabecula, which are fibrous bands attached to the splenic capsule. The splenic capsule is made up of a single layer of mesothelium and several layers of fibroelastic tissue. The parenchyma of the spleen itself is made up of white pulp, which surrounds arteries, a marginal zone, and red pulp which comprises 75% of the splenic parenchyma.[12] Trabecular arteries entering the spleen are a continuation of the segmental arterial branches that form perpendicular branches and central arteries (**Fig. 70.4**).[13] These central arteries are surrounded by the periarterial lymphatic sheath composed of T lymphocytes and follicles with B cells in various stages of development. During antigenic stimulation, this area expands significantly and secondary follicles form. The marginal zone contains a combination of lymphatics and macrophages. Finally, the red pulp is composed of splenic cords and sinuses. The splenic cords, known as cords of Billroth, are a meshwork of fibroblasts and mature macrophages. The splenic sinuses are a meshwork of thin-walled red cell spaces filled with a large amount of erythrocytes.

Blood flow through the parenchyma of the spleen occurs in two ways: slow flow and fast flow.[14] Slow flow comprises roughly 90% of the splenic blood flow and involves erythrocytes traveling through the fenestrated meshwork of the red pulp. This slow flow is involved in the spleen's role in clearing senescent erythrocytes. Fast flow comprises only 10% of

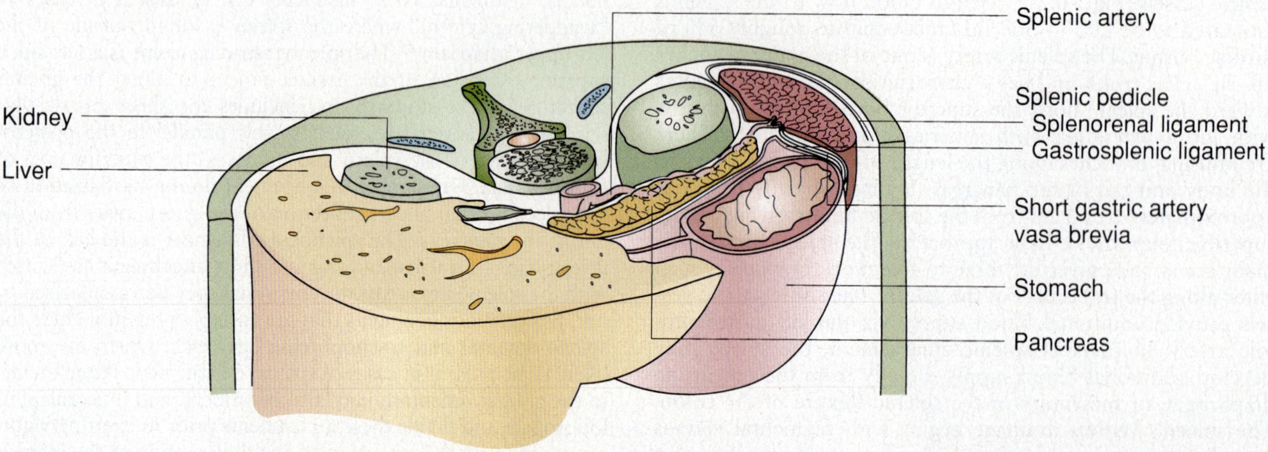

Figure 70.3. The relations of the spleen to the abdominal and retroperitoneal viscera are seen in a cross-section of the left-facing torso.

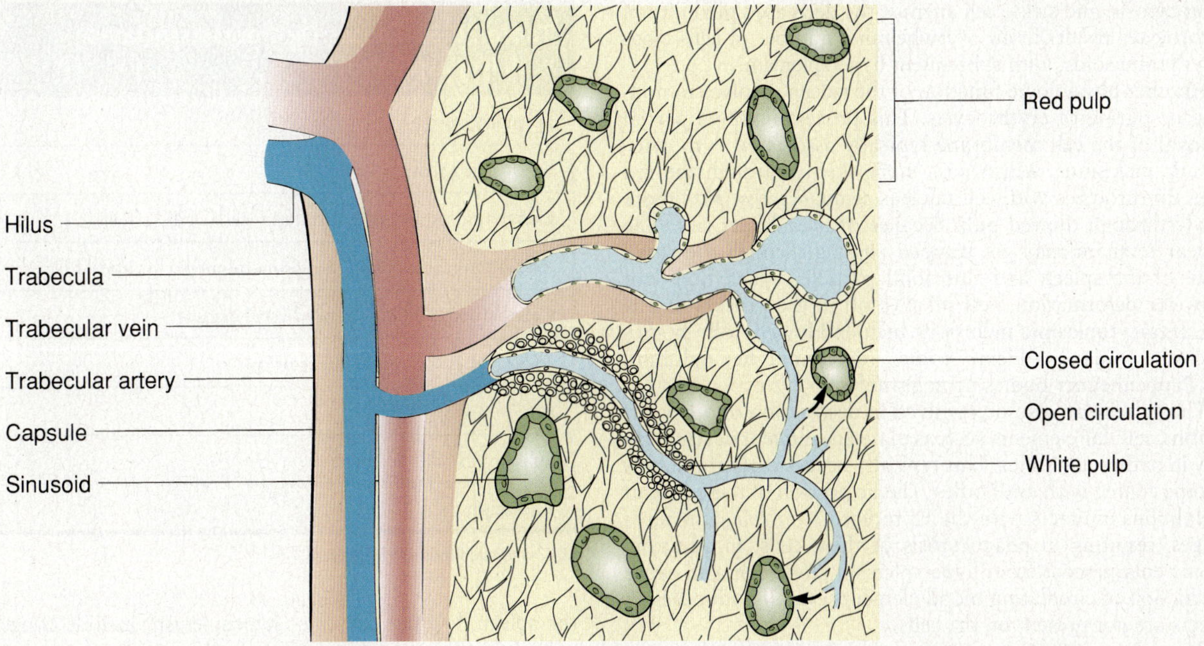

Figure 70.4. The splenic microanatomy is shown with depictions of both the open and closed circulations.

splenic blood flow, involves a greater volume of plasma and fewer erythrocytes, and involves blood traveling through splenic arteries and returning rapidly to the splenic veins.

There can also be splenic tissue that is completely independent from the main body of the spleen known as accessory spleens. These are small nodules of splenic tissue typically measuring 0.5 cm to 3–4 cm that can be found in the splenic hilum (the most common location), omentum, small bowel mesentery, or less commonly the retroperitoneum or pelvis. Accessory spleens have a reported incidence of 10% to 20%.[15] It is critical to identify any accessory spleens in the management of autoimmune splenic diseases, as long-term cure of these diseases relies upon removal of all splenic tissue. While accessory spleens can be seen on standard cross-sectional imaging, nuclear scans can also be obtained to identify accessory spleens preoperatively, or to identify residual splenic tissue in the case of persistent disease following splenectomy.[16]

PHYSIOLOGY

The two major functions of the spleen are hematologic and immunologic (**Table 70.1**).[12] Its hematologic function primarily involves destroying and clearing blood cells in circulation, as well as producing and storing blood cells, primarily platelets. Its immunologic function is to generate cellular and humor immune responses via the production of antibodies, primarily to opsonized antigens and encapsulated organisms.

Hematologic Function of the Spleen

3 In its hematologic role, the spleen removes senescent erythrocytes, remodels abnormal RBCs, and recycles iron (via splenic macrophages) (**Table 70.2**). In humans, the average lifespan of a normal erythrocyte is approximately 120 days.[17] Removal of erythrocytes is called "culling" and occurs via phagocytosis by macrophages. The unique blood flow patterns of the spleen result in hemoconcentrated erythrocyte-laden fluid entering the sinuses of the red pulp. It is here that slow flow through the sinusoid network with adjacent macrophage filled cords results in erythrocytes becoming trapped and phagocytized by macrophages. Although the exact mechanism by which senescent red cells are trapped for destruction is unclear, however one hypothesis is that over the lifespan of an erythrocyte, loss of compliance and cell membrane elements over time makes them more prone to trapping in the mesh of the sinusoids. It may also be the case that changes in specific cell surface molecules are what targets red cells for destruction. It is estimated that the spleen destroys approximately 100 billion erythrocytes daily in the red pulp. In pathologic conditions such as spherocytosis,

Table 70.1. Normal Functions of the Spleen

Hematologic
Culling or destruction of senescent erythrocytes
Pitting or removal of cytoplasm inclusive in erythrocytes
Reservoir for platelets and granulocytes
Hematopoiesis—as fetus or in conditions with bone marrow destruction
Immunologic
Filtration and trapping of circulatory antigens
Lymphocyte stimulation and proliferation
Antibody production in germinal follicles
Production of opsonin: tuftsin and properdin
Opsonins: tuftsin and properdin

Table 70.2. Hematologic Changes Postsplenectomy/Hyposplenic Condition

1. Erythrocytes
    1. Howell–Jolly bodies (nuclear fragments)
    2. Heinz bodies (hemoglobin deposits)
    3. Pappenheimer bodies (iron deposits)
    4. Target cells
    5. Spur cells (acanthocytes)
2. Platelets
    1. Transient thrombocytosis
3. Leukocytes
    1. Transient leukocytosis
    2. Persistent lymphocytosis
    3. Persistent monocytosis

elliptocytosis, and sickle cell anemia, the decreased pliability of erythrocytes results in an overwhelming number of cells clogging the sinusoids, with subsequent hypersplenism.

Another physiologic function of the spleen involves remodeling or pitting of erythrocytes. This process involves partial removal of the cell membrane typically associated with cytoplasmic inclusions, which pass more slowly through the red pulp. Erythrocytes with cell nucleus remnants also pass more slowly through the red pulp because of their larger size. The nuclear remnant may get trapped passing through the small space of the spleen and this solid particle, which does not allow for deformation, gets pinches off in the process of pitting. Intracytoplasmic inclusions include Howell–Jolly bodies (nuclear remnants), Heinz bodies (denatured hemoglobin), and Pappenheimer bodies (iron granules).

The spleen can also be involved in destruction of other circulating cellular elements such as platelets and leukocytes typically in pathologic states. This typically occurs when these cells become coated with antibodies. The Fc portion of these immunoglobulins interacts with the Fc receptors on splenic macrophages, resulting in phagocytosis of these cells. In addition, splenic enlargement from hypersplenism alone can also cause destruction of circulating blood elements even if antibodies or defects are not present on the cells.

The spleen also serves as a potential source for hematopoiesis of all cell types during gestation. The white pulp of the spleen has germinal centers that produce reactive lymphocytes. Throughout normal adult life there may also be production of lymphocytes and macrophages in the spleen. Splenic erythropoiesis and myelopoiesis can also occur in certain disease states. For example, in agnogenic myeloid metaplasia, in which the bone marrow is replaced with fibrotic scar, the spleen takes over some of the marrow's normal hematopoietic function. The spleen also serves as a reservoir of circulating blood elements. It is estimated that 30% of all platelets reside in the spleen.[18]

Immunologic Function of the Spleen

The immunologic function of the spleen is to generate an immune response to antigens that are identified and cleared from the blood. This primarily involves recognizing opsonized antigens and specific encapsulated microorganisms that become trapped in the spleen. The spleen contains all necessary cell types for generating an immune response, including phagocytic cells, dendritic cells, T cells, and B cells found in the marginal zone of the white pulp. These cellular components and the structure of the germinal follicles are similar to those found in lymphatic tissue and becomes similarly enlarged with antigenic stimulation from microbes or antigens.

The spleen is also the site of synthesis of the opsonins properdin and tuftsin, which play a role in the nonspecific immune response. Tuftsin is a small peptide that binds to the surface of granulocytes and promotes their phagocytic function.[19] Properdin is involved in initiating the alternative pathway of complement activation where abnormal cells or bacteria bound by antibodies are destroyed. Because the spleen is not the only source of these nonspecific immune-enhancing proteins, splenectomy may only lead to a modest alteration in this function.

PATHOPHYSIOLOGY

The common pathophysiology of the spleen falls into two broad categories: hyposplenism and hypersplenism. These categories provide guidelines and inform clinical decision-making when considering patients for splenectomy and when managing patient after splenectomy.

Hyposplenism

4 There are several common causes of hyposplenism (**Table 70.3**). The most common cause of hyposplenism is surgical removal of the spleen.[20] Other causes of hyposplenism include congenital asplenia or acquired destruction of splenic tissue due to autoimmune disorders and sickle cell anemia or celiac disease. Lack of functioning splenic tissue can be evaluated with a ^{99}Tc-labeled spleen scan or pitted red blood cell count. The pathophysiologic consequences of hyposplenism result from absence of the normal hematologic and immunologic functions of the spleen. Regarding its hematologic function, hyposplenism will result in an increase in Howell–Jolly bodies, Heinz bodies, and Pappenheimer bodies, as well as an increase in circulating platelets, leukocytes, and reticulocytes. The increase in platelets can range between 500,000 and one million, but is often transient given the short half-life of platelets. The increase in circulating leukocytes reflects the storage of a large proportion of these cells in the spleen, and this may also be transient. Regarding its immunologic function, patients with asplenia or hyposplenism are at increased risk of developing overwhelming sepsis by encapsulated organisms, including *Streptococcus pneumonia, Haemophilus influenzae, and Neisseria meningitidis*.[21]

Table 70.3. Causes/Disorders Associated with Hyposplenism

Splenectomy
Sickle cell anemia
Congenital asplenia (autosomal recessive disorder)
Autoimmune disorders (eg, glomerulonephritis and SLE)
Celiac disease/inflammatory bowel disease
Tumor or cystic replacement of spleen
Amyloidosis
Splenic vascular accident
Radiation

SLE, systemic lupus erythematosus.

Hypersplenism

Hypersplenism is defined by increased splenic function which manifests as a decrease in one or more circulating blood elements, related to the spleen's culling function. The criteria for hypersplenism are: (1) documented anemia, thrombocytopenia, or leukopenia; (2) normal compensatory response by the bone marrow to correct the cytopenia; and (3) correction of the cytopenia following splenectomy.[22] **Table 70.4** lists the causes of hypersplenism, which are categorized according either to the blood cells affected or by the pathology of the spleen itself. The pathophysiologic process ultimately involves destruction of a given circulating blood element within the splenic parenchyma. In cases where hypersplenism is accompanied by a significantly enlarged spleen, additional manifestations result from mass effect from the spleen. A common symptom of this mass effect is early satiety and weight loss due to the stomach being compressed by an enlarged adjacent spleen. Other causes of hypersplenism may be secondary to other conditions such as portal hypertension subsequent to cirrhosis or even splenic vein thrombosis. Hypersplenism is a common indication for elective splenectomy, which can cure the cytopenia and relieve compressive symptoms from splenomegaly.[23]

SURGICAL TREATMENT FOR DISEASES OF THE SPLEEN

Each year, approximately 25,000 splenectomies are performed in the United States.[24] Across various studies, the most common

Table 70.4. Causes of Hypersplenism

I Primary diseases of blood cells; normal spleen
- A. Congenital
  - i. Erythrocyte abnormalities
    - a. Hereditary spherocytosis
    - b. Hereditary elliptocytosis
    - c. Glucose 6-phosphate dehydrogenase deficiency
    - d. Pyruvate kinase deficiency
  - ii. Hemoglobin abnormalities
    - a. Thalassemia major
    - b. Sickle cell anemia (eventually results in splenic infarction and hyposplenism)
  - iii. Platelet abnormalities
    - a. Wiskott–Aldrich syndrome
- B. Acquired
  - i. Autoimmune hemolytic anemia
  - ii. Autoimmune neutropenia—Felty syndrome
  - iii. Immune thrombocytopenia purpura
  - iv. Thrombotic thrombocytopenia purpura

II Primary disorders of the spleen
- A. Neoplastic
  - i. Hairy cell leukemia
  - ii. Chronic lymphocytic leukemia
  - iii. Chronic myelogenous leukemia
  - iv. Non-Hodgkin lymphoma
- B. Cellular infiltrative (hematopoiesis)
  - i. Agnogenic myeloid metaplasia
  - ii. Mastocytosis
  - iii. Chediak–Higashi
- C. Metabolic infiltration
  - i. Gaucher disease
  - ii. Sarcoidosis
- D. Vascular
  - i. Splenic vein thrombosis
  - ii. Portal vein hypertension (cirrhosis)

Table 70.5. Indications for Splenectomy in Two Large Series

	Kraus et al.	Hernandez et al.
N	1,280[25]	724[26]
Dates	1986–1995	1966–2011
Trauma	167 (13%)	139 (19%)
Malignancy	386 (30%)	256 (35%)
Benign hematologic disease	219 (17%)	83 (11%)
Intraoperative iatrogenic injury or incidental	336 (26%)	90 (12%)
Other	172 (13%)	156 (22%)

indications for splenectomy include trauma (~40%), splenectomy incidental to another procedure (~25%), and splenectomy for staging purposes, such as in the case of Hodgkin disease (~20%). A report of indications for splenectomy over a 50-year period in Olmsted County, Minnesota showed that the most common indication was malignancy (35%) followed by trauma (19%).[26] Until only the last 30 years, open splenectomy was the only operation to consider in relation to diseases and trauma of the spleen. Laparoscopic splenectomy was first described in 1991 and is now considered the preferred approach. Robotic surgery has been applied to distal pancreatectomy and splenectomy since 2000.[27] Although asplenia was long thought to have no significant detriment to normal life, in recent decades spleen-preserving approaches have gained in popularity. For example, trauma splenectomy has become less common in favor of conservative management, observation, or even partial splenic embolization via radiologic procedures. A summary of the various indications for splenectomy is included in **Table 70.5**. This section discusses the specific conditions that may indicate splenectomy, including trauma, autoimmune and erythrocyte disorders, hypersplenism, vascular abnormalities, and other miscellaneous indications.

Trauma of the Spleen

The spleen is the most commonly injured abdominal organ due to blunt trauma in the United States.[28] Among the 1.5 million adults in the United States who experience blunt trauma, nearly 40,000 are diagnosed with a splenic injury.[29] Comparatively, approximately 8% of splenic injuries are due to penetrating trauma. The first splenectomy performed in the United States was undertaken by a British naval surgeon in San Francisco in 1816 when a man was stabbed resulting in herniation of the spleen through the abdominal wound.[1] Although splenic trauma was uniformly managed with total splenectomy for the first half of the 20th century, in 1962 Dr. Campos Christo of Brazil reported a partial splenectomy and splenic salvage for both penetrating and blunt trauma.[30] With subsequent advances in cross-sectional imaging techniques and refinement of trauma systems, management has shifted significantly away from mandatory splenectomy to an emphasis on splenic preservation and conservative management when feasible.

One must maintain a high suspicion for splenic injury in patients who sustain blunt abdominal trauma. The most common traumatic mechanisms leading to splenic injury or rupture are motor vehicle and bicycle accidents. Signs of splenic injury include vital sign abnormalities such as tachycardia and hypotension, left upper quadrant tenderness, peritonitis, and left-sided rib fractures, especially involving the left 9th to 11th ribs. Patients may also have referred pain to the left shoulder (Kehr sign). As with any trauma patient, assessment should proceed according to the principles of advanced trauma life support, beginning with airway, breathing, and circulation. In patients who are clinically and hemodynamically stable, the preferred modality to evaluate for splenic trauma is a computed tomography (CT) scan of the abdomen and pelvis with intravenous contrast. A CT scan allows for assessment of the presence of splenic trauma as well as grading of its severity. In the setting of splenic trauma, a CT scan may demonstrate alterations to the splenic contour, extrasplenic blood, subcapsular hematomas, or frank disruption of the splenic parenchyma.[31] The grading system of splenic trauma is summarized in **Table 70.6**. Other adjuncts to assessment for splenic trauma include a complete blood count, a chest x-ray to evaluate for rib fractures, and in settings where cross sectional imaging may not be available, peritoneal lavage, although this is now performed much less frequently.

Patients presenting with hemodynamic instability or diffuse peritonitis after blunt trauma should be taking urgently to the operating room for exploratory laparotomy.[32] Transfusion with either balanced blood products or whole blood should begin expediently while making preparations for the OR. The standard operative approach involves a generous midline laparotomy, packing of all four quadrants, then systematic inspection of the abdomen. If the spleen is identified as the source of hemorrhage, its lateral attachments should be rapidly mobilized, usually via blunt dissection, to deliver the spleen medially into the operative field. Hilar vessels should be controlled and ligated to control hemorrhage. Patients who undergo emergent splenectomy for trauma will require splenic vaccinations against encapsulated organisms in the coming days to weeks after surgery, discussed later in this chapter.

Table 70.6. Grading of Splenic Injuries

Grade	Laceration	Hematoma
I	<1-cm depth	Subcapsular <10% surface area
II	1–3 cm not involving a trabecular vessel	Subcapsular 10–50% surface area or intraparenchymal <5 cm
III	>3-cm depth or any depth involving a trabecular vessel	Subcapsular, >50% surface area or ruptured subcapsular or intraparenchymal laceration ≥5 cm
IV	Segmental or hilar vessel involvement	
V	Shattered spleen or hilar vessel disruption	

With increased recognition of the spleen's hematologic and immunologic function, as well as advances in cross sectional imaging and interventional radiologic procedures, up to 90% of patients with splenic trauma are now managed nonoperatively.[29] Recent studies demonstrate that the success rate of nonoperative management is as high as 96% and the splenic salvage rate is 88%.[33] Nonoperative management should only be undertaken for stable patients and should take place in a closely monitored setting such as an intensive care unit. This generally involves serial evaluations with abdominal examinations and complete blood counts, with an understanding that should the patient develop worsening abdominal pain, unstable vital signs, and/or a decrease in their hemoglobin, they have failed nonoperative management and should be taken for additional intervention. Although urgent transfer to the operating room is appropriate for patients who deteriorate after an attempt at nonoperative management, intervention via interventional radiology techniques is becoming increasingly common.

Specifically, splenic artery embolization is becoming increasingly common in the nonoperative management of splenic injury and hemorrhage. Over the past two decades, the use of splenic artery embolization has increased from 2.7% to 22.6%.[33] Current guidelines recommend angiographic evaluation and consideration of embolization in patients with grade III or greater injuries (which have a high failure rate with observation alone), patients with a contrast blush on their initial CT scan (suggesting active hemorrhage), patients with a moderate amount of hemoperitoneum, and patients who have evidence of ongoing splenic hemorrhage.[32] The main benefit of splenic artery embolization appears to be an increased chance of splenic preservation in patients with high-grade splenic injuries. In a recent meta-analysis of 10,000 patients with blunt splenic injury, 68% of patients were managed without surgery. In patients who did not undergo splenic artery embolization, the overall failure rate was 8.3%, however when stratifying patients according to their injury grade, the failure rate was as high as 83% for patients with a grade V injury.[34] In patients who did undergo splenic artery embolization, the overall failure rate was higher at 15.7%, however there was no increase in failure among patients with higher-grade injuries. Current utilization rates of splenic artery embolization vary significantly, from 1% to 19% among centers, and centers that more frequently utilize this technique appears to have lower failure rates for patients undergoing nonoperative management. Ultimately, the Eastern Association for the Surgery of Trauma describes splenic artery embolization as an "important adjunct to nonoperative management of splenic injuries."

Finally, the most feared complication of nonoperative management of splenic injuries is delayed splenic rupture after discharge. The vast majority of patients who fail nonoperative management do so in the first 3 to 5 days after injury, allowing for intervention during hospitalization. Although low at roughly 1%, delayed splenic rupture in the outpatient setting must be considered for patients following nonoperative management.[29]

Autoimmune and Erythrocyte Disorders

There are two categories of disease for which patients will commonly be considered for splenectomy: autoimmune disorders and erythrocyte disorders. In disorders related to autoimmunity, antibodies are inappropriately generated which lead to targeting of normal circulating cells for destruction. The most common example of this is immune thrombocytopenic purpura (ITP), in which antibodies to platelets are generated. In erythrocyte disorders, intrinsic cellular deficits of specific blood cells lead to their premature elimination in the spleen. A common example of this disease category is sickle cell disease, in which RBCs have an abnormal morphology. Alternatively, in Wiskott–Aldrich syndrome (WAS), a cellular adhesion molecule is altered leading to thrombocytopenia. This section reviews these categories of disease in which splenectomy may be considered as treatment. A summary of conditions can be found in **Table 70.7**.

Immune Thrombocytopenic Purpura

ITP is a disease characterized by autoimmune destruction of platelets leading to thrombocytopenia. It is typically diagnosed after other causes of thrombocytopenia have been ruled out. While the disorder is most often idiopathic, it can also occur secondary to conditions such as systemic lupus erythematosus, HIV/AIDS, and lymphoma. There are two common age-related peaks for diagnosis: one between the ages of 20 and 30, with

Table 70.7. Final Pathologic Diagnoses in 122 Spleens Removed for Diagnostic Purposes

Total Number of Diagnostic Splenectomies		122
Indication	**Diagnosis**	
Splenic mass		52
	Lymphomas	17
	Metastatic Cancer	14
	Carcinoma	12
	Sarcoma	2
Benign		21
	Cysts	11
	Hamartoma	3
	Hemangioma	3
	Other	4
Splenomegaly		41
	Lymphoma	24
	Benign lymphoid proliferation	5
	Benign vascular	4
	Granulomatous disease	4
	Infarction/hemorrhage	4
Categorize lymphoma		29
	Malignant (successful)	28
	Benign	1

Adapted from Kraus MD, Fleming MD, Vonderheide RH. The spleen as a diagnostic specimen: a review of 10 years' experience at two tertiary care institutions. *Cancer.* 2001;91(11):2001–2009.

females being slightly more affected than males, and another after the age of 60, where gender distribution becomes equal.[35] The pathogenesis of ITP is not fully understood, as multiple mechanisms may contribute to the clinical picture. Traditional theories suggest that antiplatelet antibodies lead to the premature destruction of platelets in the spleen, liver, or both. However, up to half of ITP patients do not exhibit these antibodies. Other proposed mechanisms include T-cell abnormalities and the involvement of CD8 cells.[35]

The primary feature of ITP is isolated thrombocytopenia (platelet count <100,000/mm³). Although life-threatening bleeding is rare (occurring in less than 5% of cases), patients typically present with symptoms such as fatigue, easy bruising, and mucocutaneous bleeding. A thorough history and physical examination are essential to rule out other potential causes of thrombocytopenia. A peripheral blood smear typically shows a reduced platelet count, with platelets appearing otherwise normal. Routine diagnostic evaluations do not generally include tests for antiplatelet antibodies or bone marrow biopsy.

Treatment for ITP is based on the severity of the clinical presentation. In cases with active bleeding, the primary goal is to control the hemorrhage. The typical treatment regimen includes platelet transfusions, corticosteroids, and intravenous immune globulin (IVIG). Since platelet destruction continues, transfusions are usually effective for only a few hours, and repeated transfusions may be needed while corticosteroids and IVIG begin to take effect. In life-threatening situations, tranexamic acid may also be beneficial. Most patients with ITP, however, do not require treatment. Severe bleeding tends to occur only when the platelet count drops below 30,000/mm³, so treatment is usually initiated at this threshold. Corticosteroids are the mainstay of therapy, although up to 70% to 90% of patients experience relapse once the corticosteroids are tapered or discontinued. Additional treatment options include IVIG and Rh0(D)-immune globulin, but, like corticosteroids, these therapies often fail to provide long-term remission.

Recently, new treatment options have become available. These include thrombopoietin-receptor agonists (eg, eltrombopag, romiplostim) and immunomodulators (eg, rituximab). Thrombopoietin-receptor agonists are indicated for patients who have not responded to other treatments. Clinical trials have shown that 70% to 95% of patients experience an increase in platelet count, with 40% to 60% maintaining this response long-term. Similarly, immunomodulatory treatments have yielded favorable results, with 40% of patients achieving a complete response and up to 60% showing some degree of improvement. However, rituximab is not yet FDA-approved for the treatment of ITP.

For patients who do not respond to corticosteroids or other therapies, or those who cannot tolerate treatment, splenectomy remains an option. Although splenectomy can be curative in most cases, up to 30% of patients may experience a relapse. With the development of more effective treatments for ITP and the risks associated with postsplenectomy sepsis, the use of splenectomy as a treatment has become less common.[36]

Thrombotic Thrombocytopenic Purpura

Thrombotic thrombocytopenic purpura (TTP), or Moschowitz syndrome, is characterized by microangiopathic hemolytic anemia and severe thrombocytopenia. The classic pentad of symptoms is fever, anemia, thrombocytopenia, renal dysfunction, and neurologic manifestations. This pentad reflects the various organ systems impacted by this microvascular process, including thrombocytopenic purpura due to microvascular disease in the skin, neurologic manifestations such as headache due to microvascular disease in the central nervous system, renal failure or hematuria due to microvascular disease of the kidney, and microvascular hemolytic anemia due to destruction of erythrocytes traveling to damaged vessels. Less common presenting symptoms can include myocardial infarction and stroke. The etiology of TTP is a severe deficiency in the ADAMTS13 protein which processes von Willebrand Factor (vWF). This deficiency can be either hereditary or, more commonly, acquired through the development of autoantibodies. Thrombocytopenia in this condition typically occurs once ADAMTS13 levels are less than 10%.[37] On peripheral blood smear, fragmented erythrocytes are seen.

For patients with hereditary TTP, treatment involves regular infusions of fresh frozen plasma to replenish deficient blood components. For patients with acquired deficiency due to autoantibodies, initial treatment can involve plasmapheresis, immunosuppressive agents such as corticosteroids, rituximab, and vincristine.[38] Antiplatelet drugs such as aspirin and dipyridamole are also used, but have been found to be less effective in preventing platelet aggregation in this condition.

Because the spleen is thought to be a site of significant ADAMTS13 autoantibody production in TTP, there is a role for splenectomy in patients who fail to respond to immunosuppressive therapy. However, while some reports demonstrate that upward of 70% of patients achieve remission following splenectomy, others have found that less than 10% of patients achieve remission.[39]

Autoimmune Hemolytic Anemia

Autoimmune hemolytic anemia results from the production of antibodies to red cell membrane proteins, leading to red cell destruction. This disease is more common in females (2:1) and typically presents after age 50. Presenting symptoms include anemia, jaundice, and fever, with enlargement of the spleen in half of patients. The two forms of autoimmune hemolytic anemia are warm autoimmune hemolytic anemia and cold autoimmune hemolytic anemia, which have distinct etiologies and treatments.

Warm autoimmune hemolytic anemia is caused by IgG antibodies to erythrocytes, which lead to removal by the spleen due to macrophage recognition of the antibody. These antibodies have a maximal binding capacity at 37 °C, thus the "warm" classification. Approximately half of cases are idiopathic, while the other half may be caused by infections (eg, mycoplasma pneumonia, viral infections, HIV/AIDS) or neoplastic processes like leukemia or lymphoma. Laboratory diagnosis will demonstrate anemia, reticulocytosis, hemolysis, and a positive direct Coombs test. Initial treatment includes blood transfusion for severe anemia, while long-term management involves immunosuppression with corticosteroids and/or rituximab. Although splenectomy has been historically performed in the management of this disease, current guidelines recommend medical management in favor of splenectomy given the variable effectiveness and long-term risks associated with splenectomy. Specifically, 1-year remission rates following splenectomy are only 50%, and a quarter of those patients will relapse within a year.[40]

In cold autoimmune hemolytic anemia, cold-reactive IgM antibodies bind to erythrocytes, which leads to complement activation, erythrocyte aggregation and clumping, and ultimately hemolysis. In this condition, the spleen has less of a pathologic role in this condition and splenectomy is not an effective treatment. Laboratory diagnosis will demonstrate hemolysis, a positive direct antiglobulin test, and elevated cold agglutinin titer. Treatment involves avoidance of cold temperatures, transfusions, and plasmapheresis. Corticosteroids and ritixumab are less effective, and splenectomy is not performed.

Autoimmune Neutropenia (Felty Syndrome)

Felty syndrome is characterized by neutropenia and splenomegaly in patients with rheumatoid arthritis. Less than 1% of individuals with rheumatoid arthritis develop this syndrome. The underlying abnormalities in Felty syndrome include reduced neutrophil production, increased neutrophil sequestration and destruction, as well as excessive margination of neutrophils. As a result, patients with Felty syndrome are at a heightened risk of infections due to neutropenia, contributing to a 5-year mortality rate of up to 36%. Initial treatment typically involves antirheumatic medications like methotrexate.[41] If this approach proves ineffective, alternative treatments may include colony-stimulating factors or splenectomy. Splenectomy can help alleviate neutropenia and reduce the frequency of recurrent infections.

Hereditary Spherocytosis

Hereditary spherocytosis, an autosomal dominant disorder, is the most common congenital hemolytic anemia, affecting approximately 1 in 2,000 individuals. The condition primarily results from defects in spectrin and ankyrin, which lead to a reduction in erythrocyte membrane surface area and decreased deformability. This loss of deformability prevents affected erythrocytes from passing through the spleen's microcirculatory channels, leading to increased destruction of the cells. Key clinical features of hereditary spherocytosis include anemia, jaundice, gallstones, reticulocytosis, splenomegaly, and the presence of spherocytes on peripheral blood smear. Diagnosis is typically made through a combination of detailed history, physical examination, and laboratory tests. Since the spleen plays a major role in the sequestration and destruction of these abnormal erythrocytes, splenectomy can be curative for most patients. Prior to surgery, patients should be evaluated for gallstones, and if present, a laparoscopic cholecystectomy is recommended.[42]

Hereditary Elliptocytosis

Hereditary elliptocytosis is a less common condition than hereditary spherocytosis, but like its counterpart, it results from defects in membrane proteins that cause erythrocytes to take on an elliptical shape, which in turn reduces their deformability. While most individuals with hereditary elliptocytosis are asymptomatic and are often diagnosed incidentally when a peripheral blood smear is performed for unrelated reasons, some may present with symptoms such as anemia, jaundice, and splenomegaly. In severe cases, splenectomy can be 5 considered; however, it is typically recommended only for patients older than 5 years of age who exhibit significant symptoms.[43]

Hereditary Nonspherocytic Hemolytic Anemia

This group of hemolytic anemias is heterogeneous, arising from inherited defects in various enzymes critical to glycolysis.[44] The most common forms are glucose-6-phosphate dehydrogenase (G6PD) deficiency and pyruvate kinase deficiency. In G6PD deficiency, many patients remain asymptomatic, with hemolytic episodes typically triggered by factors such as infection, ingestion of fava beans, or exposure to oxidative drugs. Treatment is mainly supportive, and splenectomy is generally not recommended. In contrast, pyruvate kinase deficiency often manifests with hemolysis-related symptoms, along with complications like hyperbilirubinemia and gallstones. About 80% to 85% of patients with this condition also have splenomegaly. Supportive care is the cornerstone of treatment, and splenectomy may help alleviate some symptoms and reduce the need for blood transfusions.[45]

Thalassemia

Thalassemia is an inherited disorder caused by structural defects in the globin chains. While it was once classified by the underlying molecular defect, the current system distinguishes between transfusion-dependent thalassemia (TDT) and non–transfusion-dependent thalassemia (NTDT) based on the patient's need for regular blood transfusions. These categories are clinically defined and not mutually exclusive. Patients with NTDT may occasionally require transfusions, while those with TDT typically need ongoing transfusions for survival.[46] The molecular defects in thalassemia lead to ineffective erythropoiesis and peripheral hemolysis, which contribute to symptoms such as anemia and iron overload. Ineffective erythropoiesis is also linked to complications like bone disease, organomegaly from extramedullary hematopoiesis, gallstones from hemolysis, and hypercoagulability, all of which may result in significant organ damage.

Thalassemia is diagnosed through peripheral blood smear analysis, where findings such as microcytosis, hypochromia, and variations in cell size and shape are commonly observed. The specific features can vary depending on the underlying molecular defect. Hemoglobin analysis is also essential, though it must be interpreted in the context of the patient's clinical presentation. DNA analysis is required for a definitive diagnosis.

Standard treatments for thalassemia include blood transfusions, iron chelation, and splenectomy. Transfusions not only help address anemia but also suppress ineffective erythropoiesis. Iron chelation therapy manages the iron overload resulting from either increased intestinal absorption or frequent transfusions. In TDT, splenectomy is rarely indicated, given the ease of access to safe, regular blood transfusions. In contrast, splenectomy can benefit some NTDT patients by improving anemia and lowering the risk of infection. However, this procedure can also induce a hypercoagulable state in NTDT patients, in addition to the usual risks associated with splenectomy. It is generally considered only for those who cannot receive transfusions or iron chelation therapy, or for patients experiencing hypersplenism or symptomatic splenomegaly.[47]

Sickle Cell Disease

Sickle cell disease is an inherited disorder caused by a missense mutation in the gene for sickle hemoglobin. The disease is becoming more prevalent, with over 300,000 infants diagnosed each year. It is particularly common in regions where malaria is endemic, as individuals who are heterozygous for the sickle cell mutation have some protection against malaria. The abnormal shape of the erythrocytes results in hemolytic anemia and vaso-occlusion, where blocked small blood vessels can lead to tissue ischemia, severe pain, and, in some cases, organ failure.[48]

Initially, most patients with sickle cell disease are born with normal spleens, but over time, the spleen typically develops both functional hyposplenism and splenomegaly. This is due to the spleen's role in promoting sickling, which increases erythrocyte adhesion and clearance. Although the exact mechanism is not fully understood, splenic injury begins early in most cases. As hyposplenism becomes a common feature in sickle cell patients, splenectomy is rarely necessary. While vaso-occlusive episodes often do not progress to sickle cell crisis, acute splenic sequestration can occur, where RBCs become trapped in the spleen. This leads to symptoms such as abdominal pain, distension, and signs of anemia or shock due to a rapid decrease in hemoglobin levels. Treatment for acute sequestration primarily involves blood transfusion and addressing any underlying causes, such as infection. For patients who experience recurrent sequestration, splenectomy may be considered.[49]

The treatment for sickle cell disease includes prophylactic penicillin for young children, hydroxyurea, and regular blood transfusions. While stem cell transplantation has the potential to cure the disease, it remains limited in availability. Although most patients with sickle cell disease do not require splenectomy, it may be indicated for those with hypersplenism. Laparoscopic splenectomy is the preferred approach, and partial splenectomy can be an option for young children to help preserve immune function.

Wiskott–Aldrich Syndrome

WAS is an X-linked immunodeficiency disorder characterized by a triad of recurrent infections, eczema, and bleeding tendencies.[50] While males are primarily affected, females can be carriers and, in rare cases, may also display symptoms. WAS is associated with abnormalities in both T and B cells, and it can lead to complications such as hemorrhagic episodes, autoimmune disorders, and an increased risk of lymphoma and other malignancies. The underlying cause of thrombocytopenia in WAS is not fully understood but is thought to involve both increased platelet destruction in the spleen and dysfunction of megakaryocytes.[51]

Thrombocytopenia is a hallmark of WAS, often presenting in the first year of life with symptoms such as easy bruising, spontaneous or prolonged bleeding (especially after circumcision), and petechiae. While eczema and recurrent infections are common, they are not universally present in all patients. When thrombocytopenia is observed, WAS should be suspected, but genetic testing remains the definitive method for diagnosis.

Hematopoietic stem cell transplantation or gene therapy is the curative treatment for WAS, ideally performed within the first 2 years of life. For adults who have not undergone treatment, hematopoietic stem cell transplantation may still be an option. Supportive care includes infection prophylaxis, management of thrombocytopenia, and treatment for associated autoimmune disorders or other complications. Splenectomy may be considered for patients with severe thrombocytopenia, especially when the risk of bleeding significantly affects their quality of life. This is particularly relevant for those with the milder form of WAS, known as X-linked thrombocytopenia, where the risk of infections is lower.

Hypersplenism

Hypersplenism is physical enlargement of the spleen, also known as splenomegaly. This can be categorized as neoplastic disorders, hematopoietic disorders, and metabolic or storage disorders, and the hypersplenism typically occurs later in the disease course. Symptoms are generally related to splenomegaly and include abdominal discomfort, early satiety, and bloating, as well as cytopenias due to splenic sequestration of circulating blood elements. Splenectomy in these cases can be performed for diagnosis or to relieve symptoms related to splenomegaly

Chronic Lymphocytic Leukemia

Chronic lymphocytic leukemia (CLL) is the most common leukemia in the developed world. It has a 2:1 male:female predominance and a median age at diagnosis of 72 years. The pathophysiology of CLL is clonal proliferation of mature B cells in the spleen, blood, lymph nodes, and bone marrow. Presenting symptoms include fatigue, lymphadenopathy, hepatosplenomegaly, and eventually anemia and thrombocytopenia, although many patients are diagnosed incidentally on bloodwork obtained for other reasons. Treatment is usually indicated for patients with progressive anemia or thrombocytopenia and can include steroids or other immunosuppressive therapies. The standard chemotherapy regimen is fludarabine plus cyclophosphamide, which can lead to remission in many patients.

Splenomegaly is common in CLL because of the infiltrative nature of this disease (**Fig. 70.5**). Splenectomy is typically reserved for patients with advanced CLL, refractory pancytopenia despite medical treatment, or severe mass effect from splenomegaly. Patients who undergo splenectomy can have up to an 85% resolution rate for thrombocytopenia and 100% resolution rate of anemia.[52] For nonsurgical candidates, splenic irradiation can also be considered, which has been found to reduce spleen size in 72% of patients, relieve pain in 59% of patients, and improve cytopenias in 78% of patients.[53,54]

Chronic Myelogenous Leukemia

Chronic myelogenous leukemia (CML) represents about 15% of adult leukemia cases and is most commonly associated with the Philadelphia chromosome (Ph). This chromosome results from a translocation event, leading to the formation of the BCR-ABL1 fusion gene, which produces a protein with uncontrolled tyrosine kinase activity. CML typically progresses through three stages: chronic, accelerated, and blast phases, with the majority of patients being diagnosed during the chronic phase. To diagnose CML, a thorough history and physical examination are essential, including palpation of the spleen.[55] Laboratory tests such as a complete blood count, liver function tests, and basic chemistry panels are also important. Splenomegaly, or an enlarged spleen, is a key indicator, as its size correlates with an increased risk of mortality in CML patients. In addition, confirming the presence of the BCR-ABL1 gene through a bone marrow biopsy is strongly recommended for a definitive diagnosis. Common clinical findings include leukocytosis, thrombocytosis, and splenomegaly, which occur in more than half of those affected. The cornerstone of treatment for CML involves tyrosine kinase inhibitors (TKIs), with second-generation TKIs—such as dasatinib, nilotinib, and bosutinib—demonstrating better outcomes than the first-generation drug, imatinib. However, selecting the appropriate TKI should be tailored to the specific characteristics of the patient. Though not curative, splenectomy may be considered in cases of symptomatic splenomegaly and thrombocytopenia, as it can alleviate symptoms and reduce the need for transfusions.[56]

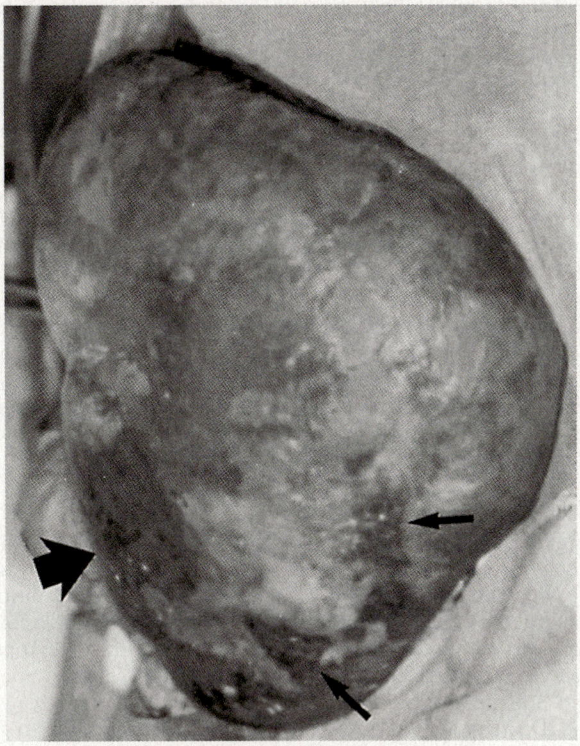

Figure 70.5. A massively enlarged, 2.2-kg spleen from a patient with chronic lymphocytic leukemia. Superficial areas of infarction are indicated by *thin arrows* and splenic infarction by the *thick arrow*.

Non-Hodgkin Lymphoma

Non-Hodgkin lymphoma is the most common cause of lymphoma and is roughly six times more common than Hodgkin disease in the United States. This heterogeneous disease arises primarily from mature B cells due to genetic mutations or infections such as the Epstein–Barr virus.[57] Patients present with lymphadenopathy, splenomegaly, and have of patients will also have B symptoms. While blood tests can aid in diagnosis, definitive diagnosis is made with a lymph node biopsy. Cross sectional imaging can be used to stage the disease and evaluate its extent. For patients with low-grade lymphoma, chemotherapy is not curative and many of these patients are observed and never require treatment. For patients with high-grade lymphoma, the R-CHOP regimen (rituximab, cyclophosphamide, doxorubicin, vincristine, and prednisolone) is standard and achieves cure in 60% to 70% of patients. Splenectomy can be considered for patients with symptoms due to the spleen's mass effect, or with progressive cytopenia.[58] Up to 80% of patients have decreased transfusion requirements following surgery, and nearly all have relief of compressive symptoms.[59]

Hairy Cell Leukemia

Hairy cell leukemia is named for the characteristic appearance of "hairy cells" (abnormal B cells) which have irregular filament projections from the cell surface. These cells infiltrate the bone marrow and spleen with almost no peripheral lymphadenopathy. The most common presenting symptoms are splenomegaly and/or cytopenia. Historically, hairy cell leukemia was known as the "surgical leukemia" since splenectomy was the primary treatment, leading to remission in roughly half of patients. Although splenectomy still has a role for patients with splenomegaly or cytopenic-related complications, medical therapy with drugs such as cladribine, pentostatin, or rituximab is now first-line.[60]

Myelodysplastic Syndrome

Myelodysplastic syndrome (MDS) is a clonal stem cell disorder primarily affecting older adults, with the median age of diagnosis ranging from 65 to 70 years.[61] The condition is marked by gene mutations and/or cytogenetic alterations that lead to ineffective hematopoiesis, resulting in cytopenias. About one-third of patients with MDS eventually progress to acute myeloid leukemia (AML). The underlying cause of MDS remains unknown in most cases and thought to be linked to environmental, occupational, or hereditary factors. Patients commonly present with nonspecific symptoms due to anemia, thrombocytopenia, and neutropenia. A peripheral blood smear will typically show a small number of circulating blasts, but bone marrow analysis is required for definitive diagnosis. Cytogenetic testing may be necessary in cases where the diagnosis is unclear and can also provide important prognostic information. The treatment approach for MDS depends largely on the patient's risk profile, as determined by the International Prognostic Scoring System (IPSS). For those with lower-risk disease, the main goals of treatment are to alleviate the effects of cytopenia, reduce transfusion dependence, and improve quality of life. Therapeutic options include erythropoiesis stimulating agents and hypomethylating agents. Transfusions may be required for certain patients to manage cytopenia. For patients with higher-risk MDS, the focus shifts to extending survival and preventing progression to AML. Treatment strategies for these individuals include allogeneic stem cell transplantation, intensive chemotherapy, and hypomethylating agents. As with other hematologic malignancies, patients with MDS can develop significant splenomegaly. While splenectomy may be considered to address symptoms, it carries a high risk of complications, and its benefits in terms of survival improvement remain unproven.

Metastatic Disease to the Spleen

Splenic metastasis occurs in roughly 2% to 7% of patients with cancer. The most common solitary splenic metastasis stem from colon and ovarian cancer, while the most common multivisceral lesions stem from breast, lung, colorectal, ovarian cancer, and melanoma. Diagnosis can be made with an image-guided tissue biopsy or magnetic resonance imaging (MRI) with gadolinium to evaluate enhancement patterns. Splenectomy is considered on an individual basis usually as part of a multidisciplinary conference, and can be performed to relieve symptoms of splenomegaly or improve long-term disease-free survival.[62]

Gaucher Disease

Gaucher disease is an autosomal recessive disease with a deficiency in lysosomal hydrolase, β-glucosidase, which is encoded by chromosome 1. It is the most common lysosomal storage disease and there is a markedly increased incidence of Gaucher disease in Ashkenazi Jews. The insufficient lysosomal enzyme activity leads to accumulation of glucosylceramide in the bone marrow, liver, and spleen. There are three subtypes of Gaucher disease. Type I comprises 99% of cases and is diagnosed in adulthood, while types II and II are typically diagnosed in infancy or childhood, and have a more severe disease course. Diagnosis is achieved by confirming insufficient enzyme activity. First-line therapy includes enzyme replacement therapy with regular infusions and substrate reduction therapy with medications that reduce the buildup of fatty substances. Although splenectomy previously played a role, enzyme replacement therapy now leads to improvement in splenomegaly in 50% to 60% of patients.[63]

VASCULAR DISORDERS OF THE SPLEEN

Vascular problems with the spleen that can lead to splenectomy include both venous and arterial problems. The most common situation would be splenic vein thrombosis and splenectomy in this setting is curative for the patient. Splenic artery aneurysms are one of the more common visceral aneurysms and can be an indication for splenectomy.

Splenic Vein Thrombosis

Splenic vein thrombosis typically occurs secondary to pancreatic disorders due to the close relationship between the splenic vein and the pancreas. It may present in up to 12% of patients with chronic pancreatitis and 22% of patients with acute pancreatitis.[64] It can also occur in cases of pancreatic cancer due to invasion of the vein. Splenic vein thrombosis leads to left-sided or "sinistral" portal hypertension. This localized area of venous hypertension can lead to the development of gastric varices (53% to 77% of patients) due to increased pressure in the gastroepiploic system. Clinically, patients with sinistral portal hypertension may present with upper gastrointestinal bleeding due to rupture of gastric varices in 4% to 12%. In the setting of acute hemorrhage, upper endoscopy may demonstrate gastric varices. The presence of gastric varices in the absence of esophageal varices is also suggestive. Various imaging techniques can then be used to confirm the thrombus within the splenic vein. Because the majority of patients do not experience acute bleeding, most patients are diagnosed via CT, MRI, or ultrasound.

For patients without acute bleeding, anticoagulation should be considered as initial therapy. Splenectomy is typically employed for patients with uncontrollable episodes of bleeding.[64] Splenectomy leads to the reduction of collateral flow, alleviating the hypertension that led to the development of gastric varices. Splenectomy was previously recommended for all patients with splenic vein thrombosis to prevent future bleeding episodes, but due to advances in imaging, antiocoagulation, and the realization that a minority of patients present with acute hemorrhage, observation is safe for most patients.[65]

Splenic Artery Aneurysm

Of all the visceral arterial aneurysms, splenic artery aneurysm is the most common and accounts for approximately 60% of such aneurysms. Most splenic artery aneurysms are asymptomatic and are diagnosed incidentally on imaging for other reasons. Women are affected four times more often than men, and there is some thought that this is potentially related to the increased frequency of abdominal ultrasound for women during pregnancy. Women also more frequently have true aneurysms, while men more frequently have pseudoaneurysms, which are more prone to rupture. Typical symptoms include abdominal pain, and aneurysmal rupture should be suspected when patients present with abdominal pain in the setting of anemia. Treatment of splenic artery aneurysms is determined by the size of the aneurysm. Risk of rupture increases substantially when the aneurysm size exceeds 2 cm. Patients who are asymptomatic and have aneurysms smaller than 2 cm can be followed with serial imaging. The special case is in women of child-bearing age who are planning pregnancy, or for women who are already pregnant. There is a high risk of rupture during pregnancy and therefore it is recommended that they be treated even if smaller than 2 cm. Reasons for the increased risk during pregnancy are thought to be related to increased levels of circulating hormones that lead to increased blood flow and pressure in the splenic artery. Pseudoaneurysms should also be repaired, regardless of size.[66]

For patients that do require treatment, there are a variety of approaches. Aneurysms can be surgically resected or ligated, and endovascular approaches that can be used as well. Splenectomy can be used as an adjunct to aneurysm resection. Both surgical and endovascular options are safe and effective, but endovascular repairs may result in a faster recovery and shorter length of stay.[67]

MISCELLANEOUS INDICATIONS FOR SPLENECTOMY

6 Less commonly encountered indications for splenectomy include cysts, abscesses, as well as the "wandering spleen." The indications are discussed here.

Cysts of the Spleen

Splenic cysts are typically classified as either parasitic or nonparasitic, as first described by Fowler in 1913. Parasitic cysts are almost always hydatid cysts caused by Echinococcus. Fewer than 5% of all patients with echinococcal infection will develop hydatid cyst of the spleen. Many patients are asymptomatic, but mass effect from an enlarging cyst can cause pain or discomfort due to mechanical displacement of other abdominal organs. Diagnosis is made through a thorough history and physical examination in conjunction with serology and imaging. Ultrasound and CT scan may demonstrate peripheral calcification, daughter cysts within the larger cavity, or additional cysts in the liver. Splenectomy is the most common treatment, and great care should be taken intraoperatively to avoid spillage from the cyst which can cause anaphylactic shock. The cyst can be carefully aspirated if it is sufficiently large to prevent adequate mobilization of the spleen. Partial splenectomy may also be considered based on the location of the cyst. Medical therapy such as albendazole is used as an adjunct.[68]

Nonparasitic cysts are classified into several different categories, often based on whether the cyst is primary or secondary. Primary cysts (20% to 30% of all nonparasitic cysts) include congenital cysts and neoplastic cysts. Neoplastic cysts include hemangiomas, lymphangiomas, and dermoid cysts. Secondary cysts (70% to 80% of all nonparasitic cysts) are either traumatic or necrotic.[69] Within the designation of nonparasitic cysts, there are many debates regarding the overall classification without a single accepted classification scheme. For asymptomatic cysts smaller than 5 cm in diameter with typical imaging findings, nonoperative treatment is recommended. Typical findings on imaging include the absence of solid components, regular appearance of the cyst wall, and lack of any contour defect. For larger or more symptomatic cysts there are several proposed approaches. Total splenectomy has historically been the most common treatment but has given way to other treatments. Total or subtotal cyst resection can prevent the need for partial or total splenectomy and laparoscopic methods are currently described both for cyst removal and partial splenectomy with good success.[70] Aspiration and marsupialization (which can lead to recurrence of the cyst) have been described but are no longer recommended.

Splenic Abscess

While uncommonly encountered, splenic abscess carries significant risk of mortality if not adequately treated. Causes of splenic abscess include: hematogenous spread of bacteria (eg, infectious endocarditis, intravenous drug use); ischemia secondary to trauma; secondary infection from adjacent organs (eg, pancreas, bowel); and in certain immunocompromised states. Commonly encountered bacteria are *Streptococcus species and Escherichia coli.* Typical symptoms include fever and left upper quadrant pain, as well as splenomegaly in some patients. Imaging such as ultrasound or CT scan will show findings of a rim enhancing fluid collection, and treatment consists of appropriate antibiotics followed by source control. While splenectomy was traditionally advocated for source control, percutaneous drainage of splenic abscess has demonstrated substantial success (67% to 100%) and should be considered first. For patients who fail percutaneous drainage, subtotal or total splenectomy is an option.[71]

Ectopic Spleen (Wandering Spleen)

Ectopic, or "wandering," spleen is a condition in which the spleen is located in the lower abdomen or pelvis, rather than the left upper quadrant. The abnormality is due to laxity of the peritoneal attachments. This condition is more commonly encountered in children and is 10 times more common in females. About half of patients with this condition are asymptomatic. Symptoms associated with wandering spleen are typically due to acute torsion, or rupture after trauma. For patients with life-threatening hemorrhage, splenectomy is recommended. For patients who are incidentally found to have wandering spleen, laparoscopic splenopexy has been described.[72,73]

INCIDENTAL SPLENECTOMY

Incidental splenectomy, or removal of the spleen during the course of another operation, is less common in more recent years with the adoption of minimally invasive techniques, but there are still operative circumstances where this may still occur. While these operations are explained in detail in other portions of this textbook, here we briefly address reasons why this may occur.

Incidental splenectomy can occur during distal pancreatectomy due to the intimate association of the splenic vein to the undersurface of the pancreas, as well as the many venous branches to the pancreatic parenchyma. With an increased understanding of the risks associated with splenectomy, there has been renewed interest in distal pancreatectomy without splenectomy. This can be achieved either through the preservation or resection of the splenic vessels. In cases where the splenic vessels are divided, the short gastric vessels are carefully preserved to maintain blood flow to the spleen. It should be noted that these approaches should only be employed when anatomically and oncologically appropriate.[74,75]

Splenectomy may also be employed in conjunction with resection of proximal gastric cancers, tumors involving the left kidney or adrenal gland, and retroperitoneal masses invading the spleen. The purpose of splenectomy in these cases is often to provide adequate exposure to dissect bulky disease posterior to the spleen. It should be recognized that despite the risk that asplenia confers to patients, the spleen can be safely removed to facilitate a complete resection.

IATROGENIC SPLENECTOMY

Because of its proximity to organs in the left upper quadrant of the abdomen, the spleen can be injured during the course of other operations, sometimes requiring removal. This scenario is not ideal, however, as the patient will be asplenic without the opportunity for prophylactic vaccines prior to the operation. While the best method to protect against this is not to injure the spleen at all, understanding the operations that put the spleen most at risk can give a sense of when to be especially cautious.

A 2019 retrospective study describing all splenectomies at a single hospital over a 17-year period in England found that the most common operation leading to iatrogenic splenectomy was elective open colon resection ($n = 12$, 46%) followed by emergency open colonic resection ($n = 7$, 27%).[67] Nearly half of all splenectomies in this study were unplanned. Of the unplanned splenectomies, 36% ($n = 26$) were iatrogenic. Of those in the iatrogenic category, 42% ($n = 11$) occurred during a procedure for benign disease and 58% ($n = 15$) during a procedure for malignant disease.[76] While the spleen can be damaged due to a variety of factors in colorectal surgery, it is especially high risk in cases where the splenic flexure must be mobilized. A 2018 report from the Cleveland Clinic reported on their series of 2,336 colorectal operations that required splenic flexure mobilization. They reported a 1.1% risk of splenic injuries, most of which (64%) were managed with topical hemostatic agents. Splenorrhaphy was used in 16%, and the remaining 20% underwent splenectomy. The rate of splenic injury was much lower in laparoscopic cases (0.25% vs 1.5%, $p = .005$), leading the authors to conclude that laparoscopic colon resection may result in fewer iatrogenic spleen injuries due to the increased visualization.[77]

Other operations that may place the spleen at risk for injury include left nephrectomy, left adrenalectomy, bariatric procedures, antireflux procedures, and colonoscopy. In a 2013 study of 4,323 patients undergoing nephrectomy at the Mayo Clinic, they reported iatrogenic splenectomy in 33 patients (0.8%). Of these patients, 94% underwent a radial open left nephrectomy. Iatrogenic splenectomy was expectedly associated with longer operative time, more blood loss, higher rate of complications, and longer hospital length of stay.[78]

DIAGNOSTIC SPLENECTOMY

Diagnostic splenectomy has historically been used in cases when a patient has a splenic mass diagnosed on imaging in which definitive diagnosis was necessary, or in cases where a patient had splenomegaly on physical examination without any clear underlying disorder. In a 2001 series of more than 1,200 patients undergoing splenectomy, diagnostic splenectomy accounted for only 9.5% of the cases.[26] In the 1980s and 1990s, splenectomy was also used to reduce tumor burden in patients with leukemia or to diagnose or stage lymphoma.[79] While most patients can be diagnosed with imaging, laboratory studies, blood smears, and in some cases less-invasive biopsy methods, in some cases of lymphoma, the diagnosis is still unclear. Furthermore, studies demonstrate that 37% to 57% of patients with idiopathic splenomegaly harbor lymphoma. In a 2019 study of 113 patients undergoing diagnostic splenectomy at the Mayo Clinic Arizona, 35 (40%) had an unknown diagnosis prior to surgery. Of these patients, 16 (46%) received a definitive diagnosis following the operation. However, more than half of these patients (56%) underwent a change in their medical management as a result of the findings, and 54% reported symptom resolution. Given these findings the authors suggest that for patients who present with equivocal findings, diagnostic splenectomy can be a useful adjunct in their evaluation.[80]

Recognizing the significant morbidity that can accompany splenectomy, less-invasive options for diagnosis such as percutaneous image guide biopsy have been developed. As with indications for diagnostic splenectomy, splenic biopsy is indicated in cases of an indeterminant splenic mass where diagnosis cannot be determined by clinical or other diagnostic methods. Splenic biopsy is successful in more than 90% of cases and is significantly less invasive compared to splenectomy.[81]

SPLENECTOMY: OPERATIVE TECHNIQUE

Splenectomy remains a relevant treatment option for many
7 conditions affecting the spleen as described earlier in this chapter. An important decision to make early on is operative approach. For example, a patient presenting in acute trauma with splenic laceration will likely require an open approach, where a patient with underlying hematologic abnormality may be a good candidate for a laparoscopic or robotic approach. Secondarily, some patients may be a good candidate for a partial splenectomy. In this section we will describe the preoperative considerations, the steps of the operation, and the postoperative care for patient undergoing splenectomy.

Preoperative Evaluation

For patients who are undergoing urgent splenectomy for hemorrhagic shock related to trauma or splenic rupture, rapid evaluation and management should follow advanced trauma life support protocols.

For all other patients, standard evaluation should include careful history and physical examination. History should include a complete medical history to determine their fitness for undergoing general anesthesia, as well as a more nuanced understanding of the indication for splenectomy. The surgeon should inquire as to prior operative history which may help determine the approach. Imaging will help determine the size of the spleen as some approaches may not be suitable for extremely large specimens. Importantly, all patients undergoing elective splenectomy should undergo routine vaccination with vaccines to prevent against overwhelming postsplenectomy sepsis from pneumococcus pneumonia, *H. influenzae* type B, meningococcus, and seasonal flu. Ideally these would be administered at least 2 weeks prior to a scheduled splenectomy, but there is debate around the optimal time frame.[24] This will be discussed in detail in the section entitled "Sequelae of Splenectomy and Hyposplenism."

Description of Procedure

Open Splenectomy—Nontraumatic

The patient is positioned supine on the operating room table. The operation begins with either a midline laparotomy incision or a left subcostal incision. Once the abdominal cavity is safely entered, a self-retaining retractor system should be employed to facilitate exposure of the spleen. Retract the stomach medially to gain access to the gastrosplenic ligament and identify an avascular space for entry into the lesser sac. Using an energy device, serially ligate the vessels in the gastrosplenic ligament to gain access to the splenic hilum. Identify the course of the splenic artery and carefully incise the overlying peritoneum to fully expose the vessel. After gaining proximal and distal control, the artery can then be ligated either with silk sutures or a vascular stapler. It is important to ligate the artery before the vein as it allows for drainage of the organ prior to removal, possibly lessening blood loss.

Continue to divide the gastrosplenic ligament to fully mobilize the spleen from the stomach. Care should be taken near the upper pole of the spleen as the stomach is in close proximity, and sometimes completely adherent, to the spleen. Continue to mobilize the spleen by dividing the posterior and lateral attachments to deliver the organ into the surgical field. Take care not to injure the capsule of the spleen as this can cause significant hemorrhage. Finally, divide the splenocolic ligament to fully mobilize the spleen. Once the hilum is visible, the vessels can be serially ligated either with clamps and ties, or with a vascular stapling device. After removing the specimen and meticulously achieving hemostasis, maintain vigilance for the possibility of an accessory spleen which must also be removed before completing the operation. A schematic of this approach is demonstrated in **Figure 70.6**.

Open Splenectomy—Traumatic

Open splenectomy for trauma takes place during an exploratory laparotomy. The patient is supine on the operating room take, prepped from neck to knees with arms extended. A generous midline laparotomy is made, immediately packing all four quadrants of the abdomen. Once any ongoing hemorrhage has been controlled, begin a thorough examination to

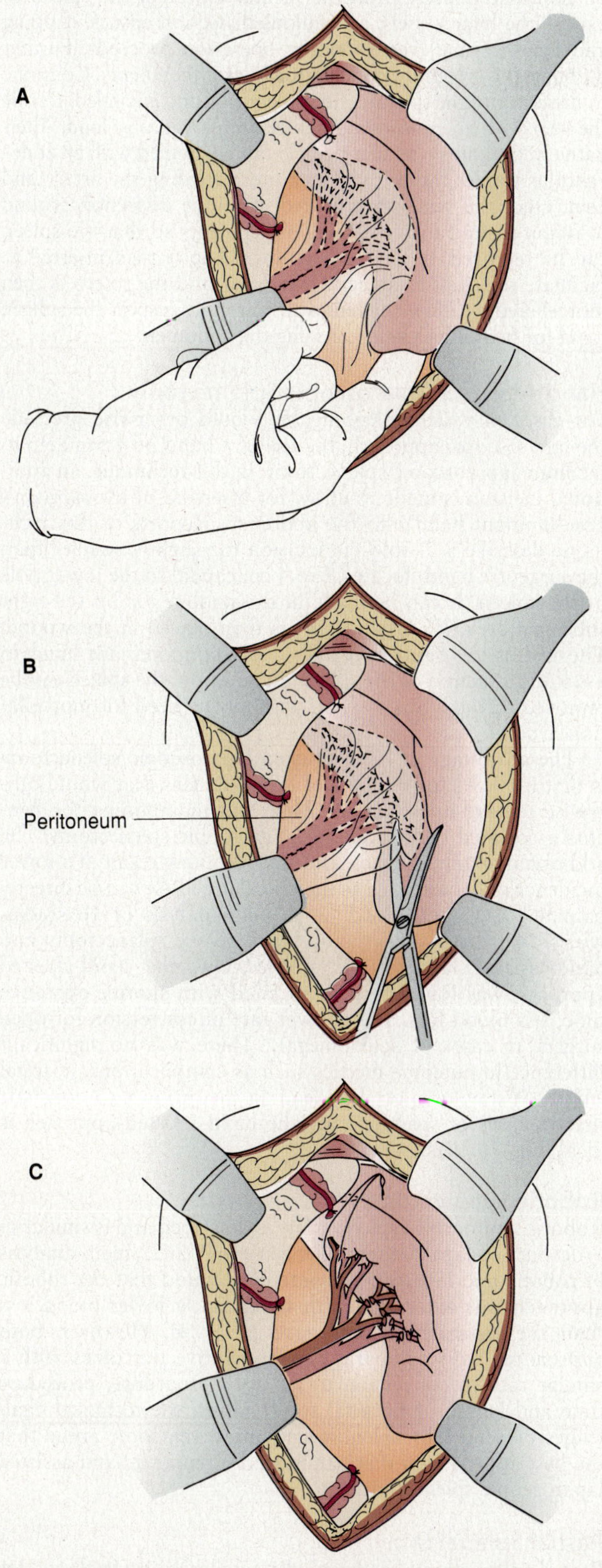

Figure 70.6. Technique for nonemergent open splenectomy. **A:** The inferior pole is reflected laterally by the assistant's fingers, exposing the lower edge of the hilar peritoneal envelope. **B:** The hilar peritoneum is opened, here shown progressing from inferior to superior. **C:** Individual vessels are identified and suture is ligated.

determine the source. If the spleen is determined to be injured and bleeding, elevate the spleen medially using a combination of rolled laparotomy packs and blunt dissection as demonstrated in **Figure 70.7**.

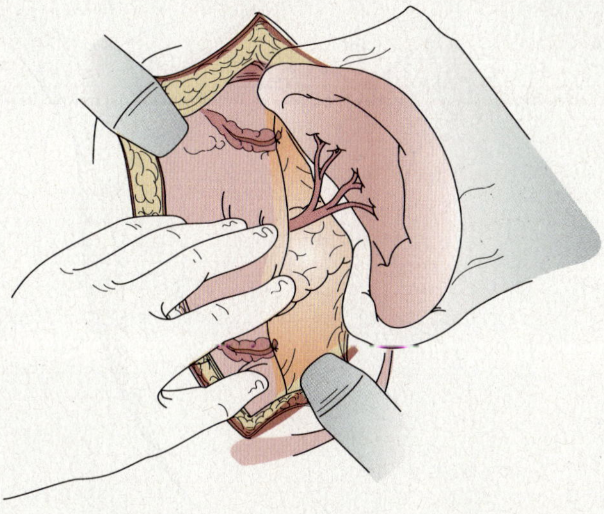

Figure 70.7. Lateral mobilization permits the spleen to reach the surface of a midline wound despite the presence of intact hilar vessels.

Once in the surgical field, serially clamp and ligate all vessels of the splenic hilum to control bleeding and remove the organ. Unlike an elective or planned splenectomy, the hemoperitoneum incurred during the initial injury has often facilitated much of the dissection. Once the organ is removed, again meticulously check for ongoing bleeding as missed bleeding from the short gastric vessels can be a significant cause of ongoing hemorrhage. A schematic of this approach is demonstrated in **Figure 70.8**. A schematic of technique to repair superficial splenic lacerations is demonstrated in **Figure 70.9**.

Laparoscopic Splenectomy

In the elective setting, laparoscopic splenectomy is the preferred approach in many centers. First introduced in the early 1990s, the laparoscopic approach was found to be associated with less blood loss intraoperatively, less pain, shorter hospital length of stay, and lower morbidity.[82] Initially, laparoscopic splenectomy was contraindicated for cases of splenomegaly but as the technology developed and surgeons gained experience it became more common. However, some of the previously cited benefits may not apply for patients with splenomegaly. In a 2019 matched case study, the authors found that for patients with moderate splenomegaly (splenic weight 500 to 1,000 g), the laparoscopic approach was associated with a significantly longer operating time and 14% conversion rate. There was no difference in length of stay, morbidity, or mortality. However, for patients with massive splenomegaly (>1,000 g), the laparoscopic approach was associated with longer operating room time, 35% conversion rate, and a higher rate of readmission compared to open surgery. The authors concluded that for patients with splenomegaly, it is not clear whether the laparoscopic approach is superior.[82]

The procedure begins with the patient in a right lateral decubitus position with a flexed table to optimally expose the left flank. Port positions and selection may vary slightly between surgeons, but a commonly described method is to place four to five ports in the left subcostal plane. Entry can be gained either via Hasson or Veress technique. The entry port is placed in either in the periumbilical location or just lateral to Palmer point. After visual inspection of the abdomen and assessment of the size of the spleen, additional ports are placed just below the left subcostal margin to allow appropriate triangulation of the spleen. Begin by mobilizing the splenic flexure of the colon using an energy device. Carry this dissection medially to enter the lesser sac and divide the short gastric vessels. As in open splenectomy, take care at the upper pole of the spleen as the stomach may be very adherent at this point. Next visualize the splenic artery to allow for dissection. As dissection continues,

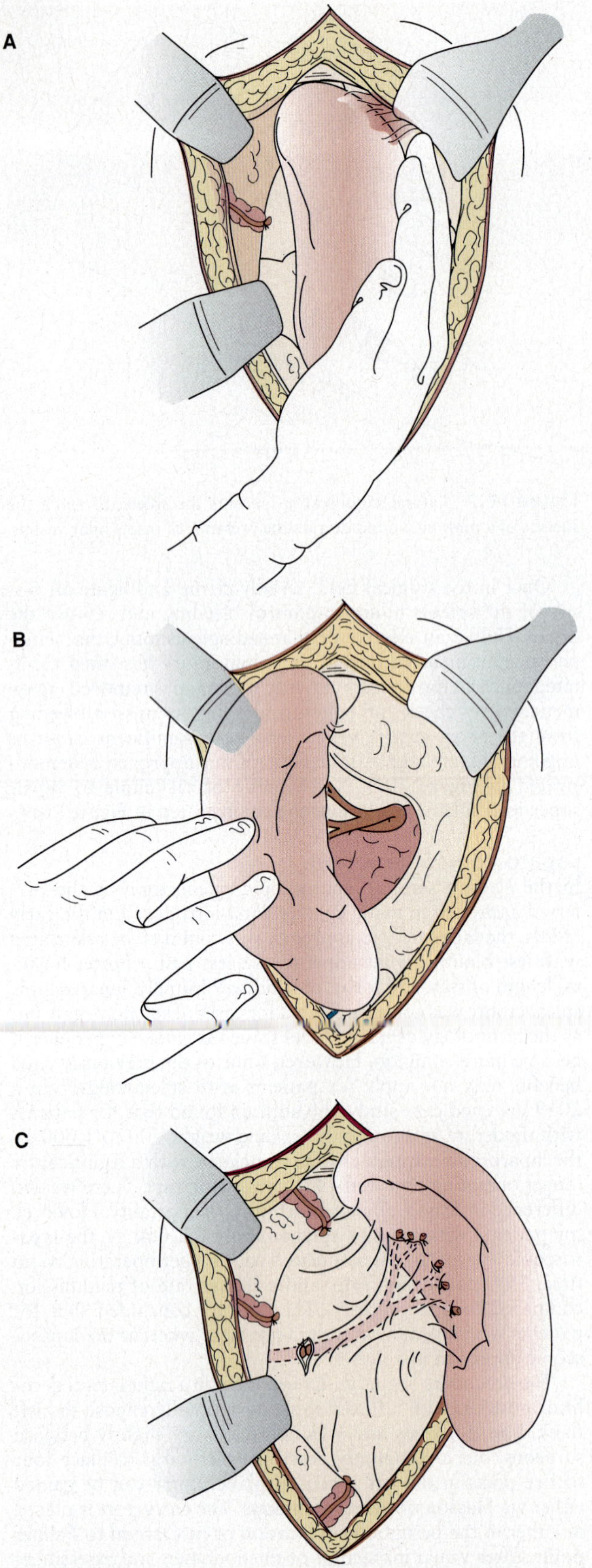

Figure 70.8. **A, B:** Rapid mobilization of a bleeding spleen can be accomplished in most patients by blunt dissection of the lateral attachments. **C:** The splenic hilum can then be quickly controlled.

small branches may be encountered that can be serially clipped and ligated. Once the splenic artery is dissected circumferentially, it is doubly clipped and ligated. Alternatively, a surgical stapling device can be used to divide the artery.

Continue dissection on the medial aspect of the spleen to expose the hilar vessels. Meticulous dissection ensues, clipping and ligating small vessels as the operation proceeds. Further mobilize the spleen by dividing the hilar attachments. Continue to dissect until the splenic vein is identified and encircled. Divide the vein with an endoscopic stapler with a vascular load. Alternatively, the entire vascular pedicle can be divided with an endovascular stapler rather than separately dividing the artery and vein. Once the vessels are ligated, continue dissection around to organ to free any remaining attachments so that the spleen can be removed. A specimen removal bag is then inserted to facilitate removal, brought to skin level, and the spleen is then morcellated to allow for removal. Carefully inspect the splenic fossa for hemostasis before closing the abdomen.

Hand-Assisted Laparoscopic Splenectomy

For cases in which splenomegaly would otherwise preclude the laparoscopic approach, the use of a hand port can help to facilitate laparoscopic splenectomy. In this technique, an additional incision is made to allow for insertion of the surgeon's nondominant hand into the abdomen. Reports of this technique describe a 7- to 8-cm incision (or slightly smaller than the surgeon's hand) located 2 to 4 cm caudal to the lower pole of the spleen. It can be made in the midline, or on the right subcostal area.[83,84] A hand port is then placed in the wound. The use of the hand port allows the nondominant hand to assist in retraction of the spleen. In addition, the spleen can be removed through this incision without the need for morcellation in some cases.

The advantage of hand-assisted laparoscopic splenectomy is that it allows for removal of larger spleens that would otherwise require open surgery while still maintaining the benefits associated with standard laparoscopic splenectomy. The additional tactile feedback afforded also may result in a lower incidence of hemorrhage as the vascular pedicle can be directly palpated and controlled.[84] In a meta-analysis of 16 studies with 754 patients undergoing laparoscopic splenectomy and hand-assisted laparoscopic splenectomy, the hand-assisted approach was found to be associated with shorter operative time, less blood loss, and a lower rate of conversion for open surgery in cases of splenomegaly. There was no significant difference in outcome metrics such as complications, hospital length of stay, or mortality, leading the authors to conclude that in cases of splenomegaly the hand-assisted approach is ideal (**Fig. 70.10**).[85]

Robotic Splenectomy

Robotic approach to splenectomy is described and is similar in procedure to laparoscopic splenectomy. A 2022 meta-analysis of robotic and laparoscopic outcomes found that the robotic approach was associated with significantly lower blood loss than the laparoscopic approach (p = .4). However, both approaches have comparable perioperative outcomes with a similar rate of conversion to an open procedure, procedure time and length of hospital stay.[86] Given the technical challenges presented by splenomegaly, however, some argue that the best approach in that circumstance remains hand-assisted laparoscopic splenectomy.[87]

Partial Splenectomy

Partial splenectomy has been advocated because it allows for removal of pathology while still preserving the immune function of the spleen and preventing overwhelming postsplenectomy sepsis. Indications for partial splenectomy include cysts, intraparenchymal lesions, hematologic disease, abscess, as well as others. The operation begins with division of the gastrocolic ligament followed by the gastrosplenic ligament to enter the lesser sac. Short gastric vessels are divided to allow visualization and temporary occlusion of the splenic artery. The spleen is then completely mobilized and segmental vascular control at the splenic hilum is achieved. Once the vessels are

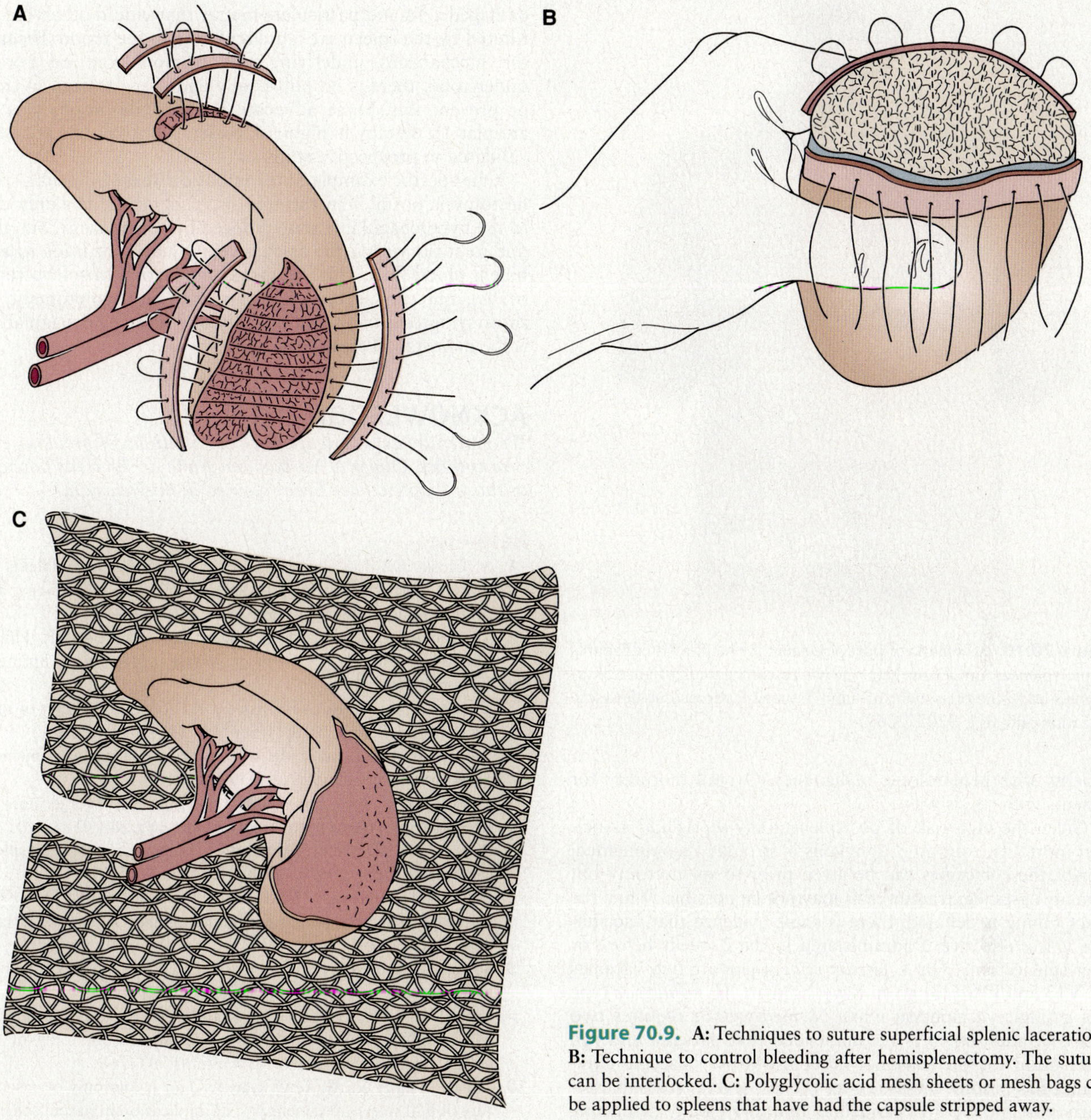

Figure 70.9. **A:** Techniques to suture superficial splenic lacerations. **B:** Technique to control bleeding after hemisplenectomy. The sutures can be interlocked. **C:** Polyglycolic acid mesh sheets or mesh bags can be applied to spleens that have had the capsule stripped away.

controlled, the splenic artery is then unclamped to allowed for visualization of the newly created ischemic zone, which can then be resected. That portion of the spleen is transected using an energy device, and subsequently removed. Given the potentially large surface area of splenic parenchyma now exposed, meticulous hemostasis must be achieved before closure. This can be accomplished with energy or hemostatic agents.[88]

SEQUELAE OF SPLENECTOMY AND HYPOSPLENISM

Postsplenectomy Sepsis

For patients who are asplenic, either due to surgical removal or functional asplenia, postsplenectomy sepsis is a significant concern. Hyposplenism, or impaired splenic function, may also occur in patients with HIV infection, chronic graft-versus-host-disease, and severe celiac disease. The spleen is the most effective organ for removal of IgG-coated bacteria and encapsulated bacteria. As these bacteria are not effectively opsonized by other methods, asplenic or hyposplenic patients are at particularly high risk of infection from encapsulated bacteria such as *Streptococcus pneumoniae* and *H. influenzae* type b. Other common high-risk organisms also include *N. meningitidis, E. coli, and Staphylococcus aureus*. It is important to remember that patients who have not undergone surgical splenectomy may be functionally asplenic due to underlying disease and thus may still be at risk for these infections.[24]

The risk of postsplenectomy sepsis depends on the indication for splenectomy. Healthy patients undergoing trauma splenectomy have the lowest risk while patients with surgical asplenia due to sickle cell disease, thalassemia, or portal hypertension are at highest risk. Patients with hereditary spherocytosis or ITP are at intermediate risk. Children, particularly infants, are at highest risk. The risk of postsplenectomy sepsis is highest in the first year following splenectomy but remains high for at least 10 years or longer. While the overall risk of postsplenectomy sepsis is low, mortality is high. Prior to the availability of effective vaccines, the incidence of postsplenectomy sepsis was 3.2% and led to death in up to two-thirds of affected patients.[24] A 2014 study of more than 20,000 splenectomized patients from 1970 to 2009 in Sweden indicated that there was a nearly six-fold higher risk of sepsis compared to the general population. As previously described, patients who underwent splenectomy for trauma has a lower risk than

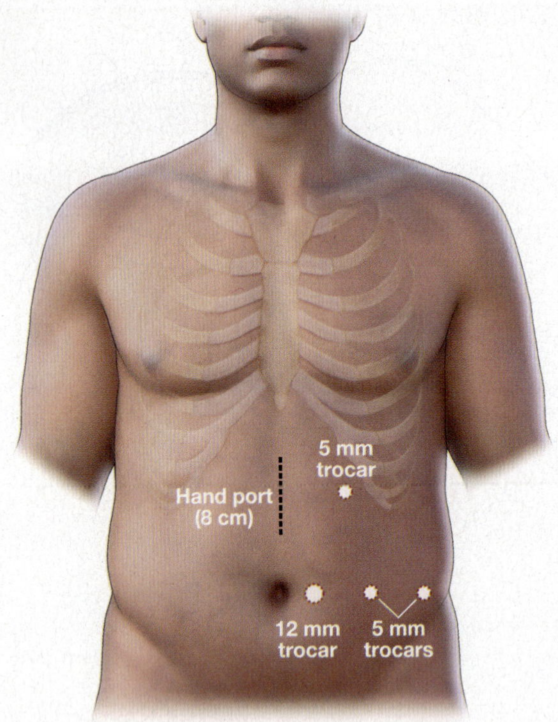

Figure 70.10. Schematic of port placement for hand-assisted laparoscopic splenectomy. From https://www.researchgate.net/figure/Skin-incision-and-port-placement-of-hand-assisted-laparoscopic-devascularization-and_fig1_320572069

patients with hematologic malignancy. Overall mortality for patients with sepsis was 17%.[89]

Given the high risk of postsplenectomy sepsis and associated mortality, routine prophylaxis is strongly recommended. Ideally, these vaccines can be given prior to splenectomy but in many cases (eg, trauma) this may not be possible. While the exact timing is debated, there is some evidence that vaccination is less effective if administered in the 2 weeks before or after splenectomy. For *S. pneumoniae,* there are two vaccines (PCV13 and PPSV23) given 8 weeks apart. *H. influenzae* type b is a single vaccination while *N. meningitidis* requires two doses. In addition, it is recommended that patients undergo vaccination for the seasonal influenza virus.[24] Vaccine compliance has become an issue over the last several years, particularly post the COVID pandemic. In a 2019 study describing vaccination rates in Minnesota over a nearly 50-year period, only 62% of patients received adequate vaccination, with only 32% receiving booster vaccines. Importantly for patient counseling, patients who did not receive appropriate vaccination more frequently presented with sepsis and developed sepsis at a shorter time interval following surgery compared to those who were vaccinated.[27]

Initial symptoms of postsplenectomy sepsis include nonspecific viral symptoms such as fever, chills, rigors, diarrhea, and vomiting. However, these symptoms can rapidly progress to fulminant sepsis in 1 to 2 days. Effective treatment begins with early recognition of patient risk so that a diagnosis can be made quickly. Treatment includes blood cultures and early initiation of broad spectrum antibiotics following standard sepsis treatment guidelines.[90]

Vascular Complications Following Splenectomy

A less commonly recognized complication following splenectomy is arterial and venous thrombosis, as well as vascular remodeling leading to pulmonary hypertension. These complications vary by indication and are most common following splenectomy for thalassemia. While the exact mechanism is not well understood, it is thought to be related to a combination of platelet activation, altered lipid profile, hypercoagulability, and changes to vascular endothelium. This may be because damaged cells and particulate matter that would otherwise be filtered by the spleen are left circulating in the blood. Because the mechanisms underlying this phenomenon are poorly understood, there is no universally endorsed strategy to treat or prevent this. Some advocate for thromboprophylaxis or antiplatelet therapy in high-risk patients, but this has not been validated in prospective studies.[91]

One specific example of thrombotic disease following splenectomy is portal vein thrombosis. This occurs not only due to the hypercoagulable state induced by splenectomy, but also due to stasis within the splenic vein stump that leads to turbulent blood flow. This is a rare complication of splenectomy (<1%), but can be fatal. Patients may be asymptomatic or show symptoms of abdominal pain and fever. Anticoagulation is the mainstay of treatment.[92]

ACKNOWLEDGMENTS

We gratefully acknowledge the contributions of previous edition authors, Oliver A. Varban and Anne P. Ehlers, as portions of those chapters have been retained in this revision.

References

1. McClusky DA 3rd, Skandalakis LJ, Colborn GL, Skandalakis JE. Tribute to a triad: history of splenic anatomy, physiology, and surgery—part 1. *World J Surg.* 1999;23(3):311–325.
2. Morgenstern L. A history of splenectomy. In: Hiatt JR, Philips EH, Morgenstern L, eds. *Surgical Diseases of the Spleen.* Springer-Verlag; 1997.
3. Dionigi R, Boni L, Rausei S, Rovera F, Dionigi G. History of splenectomy. *Int J Surg.* 2013;11(Suppl 1):S42–S43.
4. Morgenstern L. Love in the time of spleen: a personal memoir. *J Am Coll Surg.* 2006;202(2):335–339.
5. Carroll BJ, Phillips EH, Semel CJ, Fallas M, Morgenstern L. Laparoscopic splenectomy. *Surg Endosc.* 1992;6(4):183–185.
6. Patterson KD, Drysdale TA, Krieg PA. Embryonic origins of spleen asymmetry. *Development.* 2000;127(1):167–175.
7. Brendolan A, Rosado MM, Carsetti R, Selleri L, Dear TN. Development and function of the mammalian spleen. *Bioessays.* 2007;29(2):166–177.
8. Sprogøe-Jakobsen S, Sprogøe-Jakobsen U. The weight of the normal spleen. *Forensic Sci Int.* 1997;88(3):215–223.
9. Skandalakis PN, Colborn GL, Skandalakis LJ, Richardson DD, Mitchell WE Jr, Skandalakis JE. The surgical anatomy of the spleen. *Surg Clin North Am.* 1993;73(4):747–768.
10. Liu DL, Xia S, Xu W, Ye Q, Gao Y, Qian J. Anatomy of vasculature of 850 spleen specimens and its application in partial splenectomy. *Surgery.* 1996;119(1):27–33.
11. Desai DC, Hebra A, Davidoff AM, Schnaufer L. Wandering spleen: a challenging diagnosis. *South Med J.* 1997;90(4):439–443.
12. Mebius RE, Kraal G. Structure and function of the spleen. *Nat Rev Immunol.* 2005;5(8):606–616.
13. Kraus MD. Pathology of the spleen. *Introduction. Semin Diagn Pathol.* 2003;20(2):83.
14. Peters AM. Splenic blood flow and blood cell kinetics. *Clin Haematol.* 1983;12(2):421–447.
15. Dogan NU, Uysal II, Demirci S, Dogan KH, Kolcu G. Accessory spleens at autopsy. *Clin Anat.* 2011;24(6):757–762.
16. Phom H, Kumar A, Tripathi M, et al. Comparative evaluation of Tc-99m-heat-denatured RBC and Tc-99m-anti-D IgG opsonized RBC spleen planar and SPECT scintigraphy in the detection of accessory spleen in postsplenectomy patients with chronic idiopathic thrombocytopenic purpura. *Clin Nucl Med.* 2004;29(7):403–409.
17. Werre JM, Willekens FLA, Bosch FH, et al. The red cell revisited—matters of life and death. *Cell Mol Biol (Noisy-le-grand).* 2004;50(2):139–145.
18. Espersen K, Frandsen H, Lorentzen T, Kanstrup IL, Christensen NJ. The human spleen as an erythrocyte reservoir in diving-related interventions. *J Appl Physiol (1985).* 2002;92(5):2071–2079.

19. Zoli G, Corazza GR, D'Amato G, Bartoli R, Baldoni F, Gasbarrini G. Splenic autotransplantation after splenectomy: tuftsin activity correlates with residual splenic function. *Br J Surg.* 1994;81(5):716–718.
20. Feder HM Jr, Pearson HA. Assessment of splenic function in familial asplenia. *N Engl J Med.* 1999;341(3):210–212.
21. William BM, Corazza GR. Hyposplenism: a comprehensive review. Part I: basic concepts and causes. *Hematology.* 2007;12(1):1–13.
22. Lv Y, Lau WY, Li Y, et al. Hypersplenism: history and current status. *Exp Ther Med.* 2016;12(4):2377–2382.
23. Resende V, Petroianu A. Functions of the splenic remnant after subtotal splenectomy for treatment of severe splenic injuries. *Am J Surg.* 2003;185(4):311–315.
24. Rubin LG, Schaffner W. Clinical practice. Care of the asplenic patient. *N Engl J Med.* 2014;371(4):349–356.
25. Kraus MD, Fleming MD, Vonderheide RH. The spleen as a diagnostic specimen: a review of 10 years' experience at two tertiary care institutions. *Cancer.* 2019;91(11):2001–2009.
26. Hernandez MC, Khasawneh M, Contreras-Peraza N, et al. Vaccination and splenectomy in Olmsted County. *Surgery.* 2019; 166(4):556–563.
27. Giulianotti P, Sbrana F, Bianco F, et al. Robot-assisted laparoscopic pancreatic surgery: single-surgeon experience. *Surg Endosc.* 2010;24:1646–1657.
28. Harbrecht BG, Zenati MS, Ochoa JB, Puyana JC, Alarcon LH, Peitzman AB. Evaluation of a 15-year experience with splenic injuries in a state trauma system. *Surgery.* 2007;141(2):229–238.
29. Zarzaur BL, Rozycki GS. An update on nonoperative management of the spleen in adults. *Trauma Surg Acute Care Open.* 2017; 2(1):e000075.
30. McClusky DA 3rd, Skandalakis LJ, Colborn GL, Skandalakis JE. Tribute to a triad: history of splenic anatomy, physiology, and surgery—part 2. *World J Surg.* 1999;23(5):514–526.
31. Gavant ML, Schurr M, Flick PA, Croce MA, Fabian TC, Gold RE. Predicting clinical outcome of nonsurgical management of blunt splenic injury: using CT to reveal abnormalities of splenic vasculature? *AJR Am J Roentgenol.* 1997;168(1):207–212.
32. Stassen NA, Bhullar I, Cheng JD, et al; Eastern Association for the Surgery of Trauma. Selective nonoperative management of blunt splenic injury: an Eastern Association for the Surgery of Trauma practice management guideline. *J Trauma Acute Care Surg.* 2012; 73(5 Suppl 4):S294–S300.
33. Rajani RR, Claridge JA, Yowler CJ, et al. Improved outcome of adult blunt splenic injury: a cohort analysis. *Surgery.* 2006; 140(4):625–631; discussion 631–632.
34. Requarth JA, D'Agostino RB Jr, Miller PR. Nonoperative management of adult blunt splenic injury with and without splenic artery embolotherapy: a meta-analysis. *J Trauma.* 2011;71(4):898–903; discussion 903.
35. Cooper N, Ghanima W. Immune thrombocytopenia. *N Engl J Med.* 2019;381(10):945–955.
36. Bromberg ME. Immune thrombocytopenic purpura—the changing therapeutic landscape. *N Engl J Med.* 2006;355(16): 1643–1645.
37. Joly BS, Coppo P, Veyradier A. Thrombotic thrombocytopenic purpura. *Blood.* 2017;129(21):2836–2846.
38. Saha M, McDaniel JK, Zheng XL. Thrombotic thrombocytopenic purpura: pathogenesis, diagnosis and potential novel therapeutics. *J Thromb Haemost.* 2017;15(10):1889–1900.
39. Sayani FA, Abrams CS. How I treat refractory thrombotic thrombocytopenic purpura. *Blood.* 2015;125(25):3860–3867.
40. Jäger U, Barcellini W, Broome CM, et al. Diagnosis and treatment of autoimmune hemolytic anemia in adults: recommendations from the First International Consensus meeting. *Blood Rev.* 2020;41:100648.
41. Balint GP, Balint PV. Felty's syndrome. *Best Pract Res Clin Rheumatol.* 2004;18(5):631–645.
42. Perrotta S, Gallagher PG, Mohandas N. Hereditary spherocytosis. *Lancet.* 2008;372(9647):1411–1426.
43. Da Costa L, Galimand J, Fenneteau O, Mohandas N. Hereditary spherocytosis, elliptocytosis, and other red cell membrane disorders. *Blood Rev.* 2013;27(4):167–178.
44. Frank JE. Diagnosis and management of G6PD deficiency. *Am Family Physician.* 2005;72(7):1277–1282.
45. Grace RF, Mark Layton D, Barcellini W. How we manage patients with pyruvate kinase deficiency. *Br J Haematol.* 2019;184(5): 721–734.
46. Viprakasit V, Ekwattanakit S. Clinical classification, screening and diagnosis for thalassemia. *Hematol Oncol Clin North Am.* 2018;32(2):193–211.
47. Taher AT, Weatherall DJ, Cappellini MD. Thalassaemia. *Lancet.* 2018;391(10116):155–167.
48. Piel FB, Steinberg MH, Rees DC. Sickle cell disease. *N Engl J Med.* 2017;376(16):1561–1573.
49. Brousse V, Buffet P, Rees D. The spleen and sickle cell disease: the sick(led) spleen. *Br J Haematol.* 2014;166(2):165–176.
50. Corash L, Shafer B, Blaese RM. Platelet-associated immunoglobulin, platelet size, and the effect of splenectomy in the Wiskott-Aldrich syndrome. *Blood.* 1985;65(6):1439–1443.
51. Puck JM, Candotti F. Lessons from the Wiskott-Aldrich syndrome. *N Engl J Med.* 2006;355(17):1759–1761.
52. Delpero JR, Houvenaeghel G, Gastaut JA, et al. Splenectomy for hypersplenism in chronic lymphocytic leukaemia and malignant non-Hodgkin's lymphoma. *Br J Surg.* 1990;77(4):443–449.
53. Hallek M, Shanafelt TD, Eichhorst B. Chronic lymphocytic leukemia. *Lancet.* 2018;391(10129):1524–1537.
54. Zaorsky NG, Williams GR, Barta SK, et al. Splenic irradiation for splenomegaly: a systematic review. *Cancer Treat Rev.* 2017; 53:47–52.
55. Savage DG, Szydlo RM, Goldman JM. Clinical features at diagnosis in 430 patients with chronic myeloid leukaemia seen at a referral centre over a 16-year period. *Br J Haematol.* 1997;96(1):111–116.
56. Kalidas M, Kantarjian H, Talpaz M. Chronic myelogenous leukemia. *JAMA.* 2001;286(8):895–898.
57. Bowzyk Al-Naeeb A, Ajithkumar T, Behan S, Hodson DJ. Non-Hodgkin lymphoma. *BMJ (Clin Res Ed.).* 2018;362:k3204.
58. Morel P, Dupriez B, Gosselin B. Role of early splenectomy in malignant lymphomas with prominent splenic involvement (primary lymphomas of the spleen). A study of 59 cases. *Cancer.* 1993;71(1):207–215.
59. Shankland KR, Armitage JO, Hancock BW. Non-Hodgkin lymphoma. *Lancet.* 2012;380(9844):848–857.
60. Sarvaria A, Topp Z, Saven A. Current therapy and new directions in the treatment of hairy cell leukemia: a review. *JAMA Oncol.* 2016;2(1):123–129.
61. Adès L, Itzykson R, Fenaux P. Myelodysplastic syndromes. *Lancet.* 2014;383(9936):2239–2252.
62. Compérat E, Bardier-Dupas A, Camparo P, Capron F, Charlotte F. Splenic metastases: clinicopathologic presentation, differential diagnosis, and pathogenesis. *Arch Pathol Lab Med.* 2007;131(6): 965–969.
63. Grabowski GA. Phenotype, diagnosis, and treatment of Gaucher's disease. *Lancet.* 2008;372(9645):1263–1271.
64. Shatzel JJ, O'Donnell M, Olson SR, et al. Venous thrombosis in unusual sites: a practical review for the hematologist. *Eur J Haematol.* 2019;102(1):53–62.
65. Heider TR, Azeem S, Galanko JA, Behrns KE. The natural history of pancreatitis-induced splenic vein thrombosis. *Ann Surg.* 2004;239(6):876–880.
66. de Oliveira Mariúba JV. Splenic aneurysms: natural history and treatment techniques. *J Vasc Bras.* 2019;19:e20190058.
67. Zhu C, Zhao J, Yuan D, et al. Endovascular and surgical management of intact splenic artery aneurysm. *Ann Vasc Surg.* 2019; 57:75–82.
68. Culafić DM, Kerkez MD, Mijac DD, et al. Spleen cystic echinococcosis: clinical manifestations and treatment. *Scand J Gastroenterol.* 2010;45(2):186–190.
69. Mirilas P, Mentessidou A, Skandalakis JE. Splenic cysts: are there so many types? *J Am Coll Surg.* 2007;204(3):459–465.
70. Morgenstern L. Nonparasitic splenic cysts: pathogenesis, classification, and treatment. *J Am Coll Surg.* 2002;194(3):306–314.
71. Shetty M, Deme S, Mohan K, et al. Experience with splenic abscess from Southern India. *J Clin Diagn Res.* 2016;10(10): OC22–OC25.

72. Varga I, Babala J, Kachlik D. Anatomic variations of the spleen: current state of terminology, classification, and embryological background. *Surg Radiol Anat.* 2018;40(1):21–29.
73. Magowska A. Wandering spleen: a medical enigma, its natural history and rationalization. *World J Surg.* 2013;37(3):545–550.
74. Rodríguez JR, Madanat MG, Healy BC, Thayer SP, Warshaw AL, Fernández-del Castillo C. Distal pancreatectomy with splenic preservation revisited. *Surgery.* 2007;141(5):619–625.
75. Warshaw AL. Distal pancreatectomy with preservation of the spleen. *J Hepatobiliary Pancreat Sci.* 2010;17(6):808–812.
76. Dixon S, Horgan LF. The elusive spleen. *Ann R Coll Surg Engl.* 2019;101(3):176–179.
77. Isik O, Sapci I, Aytac E, et al. Laparoscopy reduces iatrogenic splenic injuries during colorectal surgery. *Tech Coloproctol.* 2018; 22(10):767–771.
78. Wang JK, Tollefson MK, Kim SP, et al. Iatrogenic splenectomy during nephrectomy for renal tumors. *Int J Urol.* 2013;20(9): 896–902.
79. Pugalenthi A, Bradley C, Gonen M, et al. Splenectomy to treat splenic lesions: an analysis of 148 cases at a cancer center. *J Surg Oncol.* 2013;108(8):521–525.
80. Hangge PT, Sheaffer WW, Neville M, et al. The diagnostic value of splenectomy in patients without a definitive preoperative diagnosis. *Am J Surg.* 2019;217(1):78–82.
81. Singh AK, Shankar S, Gervais DA, Hahn PF, Mueller PR. Image-guided percutaneous splenic interventions. *Radiographics.* 2012; 32(2):523–534.
82. Shin RD, Lis R, Levergood NR, Brooks DC, Shoji BT, Tavakkoli A. Laparoscopic versus open splenectomy for splenomegaly: the verdict is unclear. *Surg Endosc.* 2019;33(4):1298–1303.
83. Misiakos EP, Bagias G, Liakakos T, Machairas A. Laparoscopic splenectomy: current concepts. *World J Gastrointest Endosc.* 2017; 9(9):428–437.
84. Pietrabissa A, Morelli L, Peri A, et al. Laparoscopic treatment of splenomegaly: a case for hand-assisted laparoscopic surgery. *Arch Surg.* 2011;146(7):818–823.
85. Huang Y, Wang XY, Wang K. Hand-assisted laparoscopic splenectomy is a useful surgical treatment method for patients with excessive splenomegaly: a meta-analysis. *World J Clin Cases.* 2019;7(3): 320–334.
86. Bhattacharya P, Phelan L, Fisher S, Hajibandeh S, Hajibandeh S. Robotic vs. laparoscopic splenectomy in management of non-traumatic splenic pathologies: a systematic review and meta-analysis. *Am Surg.* 2022;88(1):38–47.
87. Di Franco G, Gianardi D, Bianchini M, Palmeri M, Morelli L. The role of hand-assisted laparoscopic splenectomy for mega spleens in the da Vinci era. *J Robot Surg.* 2019;13(6):791–792.
88. Borie F. Laparoscopic partial splenectomy: surgical technique. *J Visc Surg.* 2016;153(5):371–376.
89. Edgren G, Almqvist R, Hartman M, Utter GH. Splenectomy and the risk of sepsis: a population-based cohort study. *Ann Surg.* 2014;260(6):1081–1087.
90. Luu S, Spelman D, Woolley IJ. Post-splenectomy sepsis: preventative strategies, challenges, and solutions. *Infect Drug Resist.* 2019;12:2839–2851.
91. Crary SE, Buchanan GR. Vascular complications after splenectomy for hematologic disorders. *Blood.* 2009;114(14):2861–2868.
92. van't Riet M, Burger JW, van Muiswinkel JM, Kazemier G, Schipperus MR, Bonjer HJ. Diagnosis and treatment of portal vein thrombosis following splenectomy. *Br J Surg.* 2000;87(9):1229–1233.

71

Breast Disease

Julie A. Margenthaler

Key Points

1. Any clinically suspicious mass, even in the absence of an imaging abnormality, needs to be biopsied.
2. Core needle biopsy is the preferred strategy for breast cancer diagnosis. Core needle biopsy is less invasive and less expensive than excisional biopsy and facilitates definitive breast cancer treatment planning.
3. The upgrade of lobular neoplasia diagnosed on core biopsy at time of surgical excision to malignancy is 1% to 3% and as such, surgical excisional biopsy is no longer indicated if there is radiographic–pathologic concordance.
4. All women should undergo risk assessment by age 35 to determine the best approach for breast cancer screening.
5. Surgical options for the treatment of ductal carcinoma in situ (DCIS) include breast-conserving surgery as a component of breast-conservation therapy (BCT) (partial mastectomy and postoperative radiation therapy [RT]) or simple mastectomy.
6. Sentinel lymph node biopsy has largely replaced axillary lymph node dissection for axillary staging, and the therapeutic impact of axillary lymph node dissection may be limited to specific subsets of breast cancer patients.
7. Local regional management of invasive breast cancer consists of BCT (partial mastectomy with RT) or mastectomy, noting that the choice in locoregional management does not typically impact the recommendation for adjuvant medical therapy.
8. A negative surgical margin for invasive breast cancer is now defined as no tumor at the ink margins. Given the potential for gaps between lesions in DCIS, a negative surgical margin is still defined as ≥2 mm. These guidelines have significantly reduced the reexcision rate for women undergoing breast-conserving surgery.
9. Nipple-sparing mastectomy is a safe option for genetic mutation carriers (including BRCA 1 and BRCA 2).
10. Axillary RT may result in less morbidity than axillary lymph node dissection in patients with early-stage breast cancer with clinically negative axillary examinations who have ≤2 positive sentinel lymph nodes.

ANATOMY

Surgical Anatomy of the Breast

The boundaries of the mature adult breast are the 2nd rib superiorly, the 6th rib inferiorly, the sternal edge medially, and the midaxillary line laterally. Breast tissue also extends into the axilla. Posteriorly, the breast lies on top of portions of the deep investing fasciae of the pectoralis major (PM) muscle, the serratus anterior muscle, the external abdominal oblique muscles, and the upper extent of the rectus sheath (**Fig. 71.1**). The breast is composed of skin, subcutaneous tissue, and breast parenchyma. The skin overlying the breast is thin and contains hair follicles, sebaceous glands, and exocrine sweat glands. The subcutaneous tissue is composed of fat, vasculature supplying the skin, lymphatics, and nerves. The breast parenchyma consists of parenchymal components and stroma.

Breast tissue is located within the superficial fascia of the anterior thoracic wall and consists of 15 to 20 lobes of glandular tissue that are divided by connective tissue with adipose tissue filling the space between the lobes (**Fig. 71.2**). Each lobe is composed of 20 to 40 lobules, which are themselves composed of 10 to 100 alveoli. Each lobe ends in a lactiferous duct that dilates into lactiferous sinuses, which then open through constricted orifices into the nipple. The suspensory ligaments of Cooper are fibrous connective bands that extend from the deep fascia to connect to the dermis, providing the breast with both support and mobility. The upper outer quadrant of the breast contains more breast parenchyma and is the most frequent site of both benign and malignant breast disease.

The skin of the nipple and areola is highly pigmented and somewhat wrinkled, composed of stratified squamous epithelium. Deep to the nipple and areola are bundles of smooth muscle fibers that are arranged radially, circumferentially, and longitudinally, allowing for erection of the nipple from stimuli. Along the margin of the areola are sebaceous glands and sweat glands. Accessory glands known as Montgomery glands have nodular elevations (tubercles of Morgagni) that open onto the surface of the areola. The nipple and areola are highly innervated, with the nipple containing numerous free sensory nerve endings and Meissner corpuscles, whereas the areola contains both Ruffini-like endings and Krause-end bulbs. The sensory innervation of the breast is mainly the lateral and anterior cutaneous branches of the second through 6th intercostal nerves. There is also a small region of skin over the upper portion of the breast that is supplied by the anterior or medial branches of the supraclavicular nerve that arises from the cervical plexus.

The arterial blood supply to the breast consists of the internal mammary artery (perforating branches), the posterior intercostal artery (lateral branches), and several branches of the axillary artery, including the superior thoracic artery, the lateral thoracic artery, and the pectoral branches of the thoracoacromial artery. The breast's venous system parallels its arterial system, consisting of the internal mammary veins, the posterior intercostal veins, and the axillary vein tributaries.

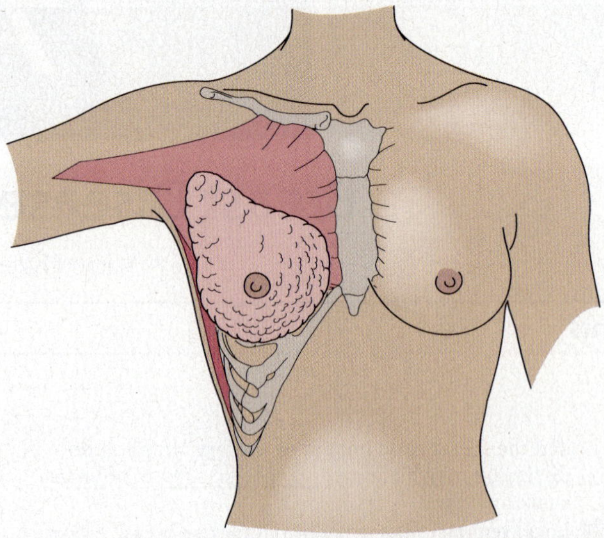

Figure 71.1. The adult female breast. The upper and medial portions of the breast rest on the pectoralis major muscle, and the inferolateral portion rests on the serratus anterior.

Lymphatic Drainage

The lymphatic flow from the breast is unidirectional through thin-walled, valveless vessels that are interconnected through three groups. The primary group of lymphatic vessels comes from within the gland in the interlobular spaces and along the lactiferous ducts. The lymphatic vessels that drain the skin, nipple/areola, and the central portion of the gland constitute the subareolar plexus. The third plexus is on the deep surface of the breast and communicates with small vessels in the deep fascia underlying the breast. More than 75% of the lymph from the breast passes to the axillary lymph nodes, whereas the remainder passes to parasternal nodes. The flow of lymph to either the axillary or the parasternal nodes is independent of the quadrant from which the lymph originated. Occasionally, lymph flow can be found outside of these three interconnected plexuses, occurring along the lateral cutaneous branches of the posterior intercostal arteries, within the rectus sheath or subperitoneal plexus by following branches of the intercostal and musculophrenic vessels, or directly to subclavicular or apical nodes.

The axilla is a pyramidal compartment between the upper extremity and the thoracic walls, which can be thought of as consisting of four walls, an apex, and a base. The anterior wall consists of the pectoralis major/minor and its associated fasciae. The subscapularis muscle, teres major muscle, latissimus dorsi muscle, and associated tendons form the posterior wall. The medial wall consists of the serratus anterior muscle and associated intercostal muscles of the upper four or five ribs. A thin strip of the humerus and the bicipital groove, which is between the insertion of the muscles of the anterior and posterior walls, forms the lateral wall. The apex is an aperture that extends into the posterior triangle of the neck through the cervicoaxillary canal, which is bounded by the clavicle anteriorly, the scapula posteriorly, and the 1st rib medially. The base of the axilla is the axillary fascia and skin.

The axillary lymph nodes have traditionally been divided into three levels, corresponding to their location relative to the pectoralis minor (**Fig. 71.3**). Level 1 nodes (external mammary, axillary vein, and scapular lymph node groups) are inferior and lateral to the pectoralis minor; level 2 nodes (central lymph node and some subclavicular lymph node groups) are behind the pectoralis minor; and level 3 nodes (subclavicular lymph node group) are medial to the pectoralis minor. The interpectoral nodes (Rotter nodes) are located between the pectoralis major and minor muscles along the lateral pectoral nerve. The supraclavicular nodes are contiguous with the apex

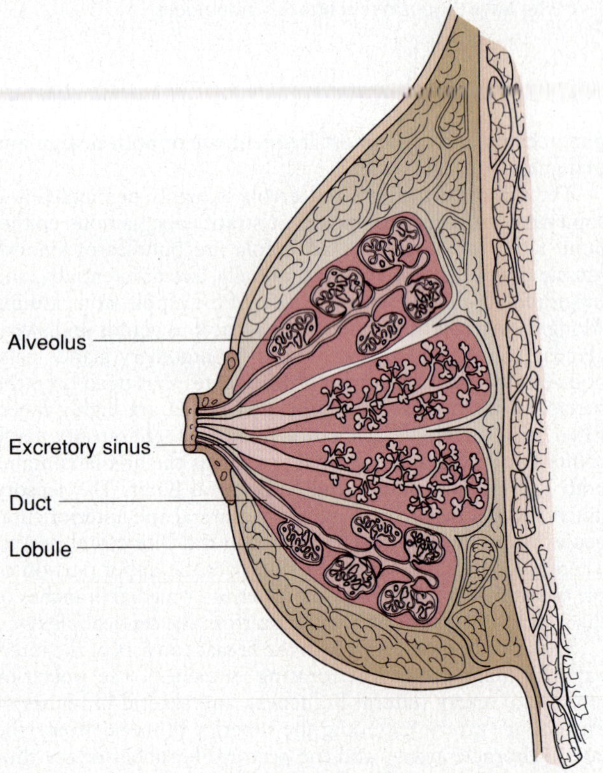

Figure 71.2. The breast consists of 15 to 20 lobes of glandular tissue. Within each lobe, the lobules are composed of branched tubuloalveolar glands. Each lobule ends in a lactiferous duct. These ducts dilate into lactiferous sinuses beneath the nipple.

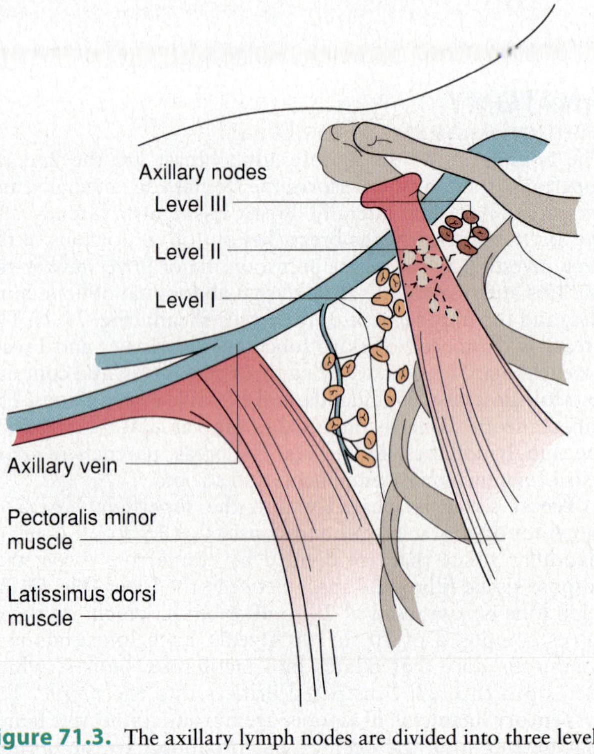

Figure 71.3. The axillary lymph nodes are divided into three levels by the pectoralis minor muscle. The level I nodes are inferior and lateral to the pectoralis minor, the level II nodes are below the axillary vein and behind the pectoralis minor, and the level III nodes are medial to the muscle against the chest wall.

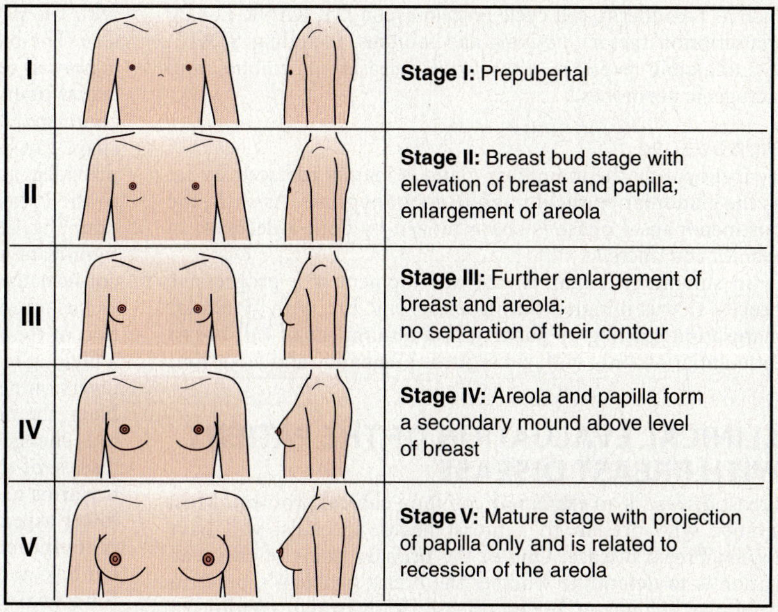

Figure 71.4. Tanner stages of breast development.

of the axilla. The internal mammary nodes are located in the first six intercostal spaces within 3 centimeters of the edge of the sternum, with the highest concentration of nodes found in the first three intercostal spaces.

BREAST PHYSIOLOGY

Breast Development

The mammary gland is a complex secretory organ consisting of multiple different cell types. Epithelial cells form the ductal network of the gland, which is embedded within a fat pad composed of adipocytes. In addition, there are vascular endothelial cells that make up the blood vessels, stromal cells including fibroblasts, and immune cells. During the three stages of mammary development (embryonic, pubertal, and pregnancy/lactation), these cells undergo an intricate series of changes under the regulation of hormones and regulatory factors, resulting in permanent changes to the mammary gland that both modify its architecture and biologic characteristics. Understanding breast development and morphology is extremely important to the study of both premalignant and malignant conditions.

In humans, mammary gland development starts in the sixth week of fetal life with the formation of bilateral milk lines or ectodermal thickenings that extend from the axilla to the groin. These ridges rapidly regress except for those of the thorax, where invagination of ectoderm cells into the mesenchyme results in mammary bud formation. In the human embryo, at about 5 months, the deep layer of the mammary bud epithelium starts to proliferate and produces about 10 to 25 secondary buds, which will later correspond to lactiferous ducts. Canalization, or the formation of lumens within the solid core of these epithelial structures, occurs later in development. By birth, six to eight of these ducts are patent and empty into the nipple. A parallel bundle of an additional 25 smaller ducts also appear and are the precursors to the milk-producing units of the breast. The subareolar lymphatic plexus also develops from the ectoderm in a similar fashion, while the nipple forms from the proliferation of the mesenchyme under the areola.

In infants, only small ductal structures are seen within the stroma, and during childhood these structures continue to grow isometrically at a rate similar to the rest of the body until puberty.

During puberty, the female glands enlarge rapidly secondary to maturation of the ductal system into a lobuloalveolar system. This is characterized by thickening of the ductal epithelium, elongating ducts, and an increasing amount of periductal connective tissue. In addition, stem cells at the tips of the ductal tree form terminal end buds, which are highly proliferative and give rise to alveolar buds. In early puberty, these alveolar buds empty into a terminal ductal lobular unit and are referred to as lobules type 1. Under the influence of ovarian hormones (estrogen and progesterone), lobules type 1 will differentiate into lobules type 2, which are characterized by smaller but more numerous buds that are noted as ductules or alveoli. It has been postulated that each menstrual cycle fosters new budding that never fully returns to the baseline of the prior cycle. In addition to estrogen and progesterone, pubertal breast development is also dependent on other hormones and regulatory factors, including prolactin, growth hormone, glucocorticoids, growth factors (hepatocyte growth factor, IGF-1, IGF-2, FGF, neuregulins, especially heregulin), vitamin D receptor, metalloproteinases, and PTEN.[1]

As these developmental events are occurring, physical changes in the breast contour and the appearance of the nipple become evident and are illustrated as the five Tanner stages of breast development (Fig. 71.4).[2]

Pregnancy and Lactation

Although the pubertal phase is marked by significant lobular development, the mammary gland does not achieve full differentiation until after pregnancy and lactation. In early pregnancy, the distal ducts continue to proliferate, resulting in more lobules and more alveoli within each lobule. However, by mid-pregnancy, proliferation of the lobules ceases and instead, alveolar cells begin to differentiate into acini by hypertrophy and the ability to secrete colostrum into the lumina of the ductules. By the third trimester, the acini become distended with colostrum, and the breast's connective tissue and fat become largely replaced by glandular proliferation. In addition, the connective tissue becomes infiltrated with plasma cells, lymphocytes, and eosinophils. There is also a marked increase in vascularity. The stage of lactogenesis, or the ability to synthesize and secrete milk, marks the final stage of maturation of the mammary gland (lobule type 4). Following lactation or during weaning, the mammary gland involutes with lobules type 4 returning to the prepregnancy state as lobules type 2 and 3.[3]

The hormones and regulatory factors that govern mammary development during pregnancy and lactation overlap with those previously discussed for pubertal breast development, with estrogen, progesterone, and prolactin playing chief roles. Other hormones and regulatory factors include intracellular signaling molecules (c-erbB, hox genes, cell–cell adhesion molecules such as E-cadherin, cell cycle protein cyclin D1, RANK-L, slug transcription factor), activins and inhibins, including STAT5, hypothalamic peptides, thyrotropic-releasing hormone, and lactogenic hormones.[4]

Menopause

By menopause, the mammary gland is mainly replaced by fat as the glandular epithelium undergoes apoptosis. As such, the postmenopausal phase is characterized by both a decrease in lobules and ducts.[5]

In summary, human breast development is a progressive process that is initiated during embryonic life, with glandular maturation starting at puberty, and attainment of full breast differentiation only with subsequent pregnancy and lactation.

CLINICAL EVALUATION OF THE PATIENT WITH BREAST DISEASE

Breast disease is an extremely common clinical problem. Most women who present to a breast health specialist will have benign breast disease. One of the primary goals of the evaluation is to determine whether the breast problem represents benign or malignant breast disease. With benign conditions, the goals are to reassure the patient and, if indicated, provide symptomatic treatment. With a malignant condition, prompt evaluation and treatment should be undertaken, typically involving a breast surgeon, medical oncologist, and radiation oncologist. In this section, clinical breast examination (CBE), diagnostic imaging studies, and biopsy procedures used to evaluate the patient with breast disease are discussed.

During the CBE, it is important to discuss with the patient whether she has any breast concerns and to elicit a gynecologic history, including menopausal status (for premenopausal patients, the time in their menstrual cycle), and the use of any hormonal therapies. If a woman has any breast problems, a thorough history needs to be obtained (**Table 71.1**).

Clinical Breast Examination

CBE is performed in both the sitting and supine positions. The patient is disrobed from the waist up and then provided a front-opening gown. Visual inspection is first accomplished with the patient sitting upright with the arms relaxed to her side. The bilateral breasts are compared for size and shape. It is normal to find slight differences in breast size, with the left breast often slightly bigger than the right. Breast shape is also contrasted. Recent changes to breast size or alterations in breast shape can be concerning signs and need to be evaluated by the provider, as tumors located superficially can cause changes to the breast contour. The skin of the breasts is inspected for dimpling, edema (peau d'orange), and/or erythema. In cases of significant erythema and peau d'orange, the provider needs to consider the diagnosis of an inflammatory breast cancer (IBC) versus an infectious etiology. This is followed by close inspection of the nipples for symmetry. Although some women have a lifelong history of nipple inversion, any new history of nipple inversion needs to be regarded with a high index of suspicion. Next, the nipple–areola complex is evaluated for any eczematous changes or ulcerations (to suggest conditions such as Paget disease of the breast [PDB]). The patient is then asked to raise her arms to allow for a more complete visual inspection of the lower aspect of the breasts bilaterally. The visual examination is completed when the patient is asked to place her hands on her hips and then to contract the pectoral muscles. This allows for a final visual assessment of breast symmetry. Furthermore, tumors deep within the substance of the breast involving Cooper ligaments can result in skin retraction and can sometimes be seen best with contraction of the pectoral muscles.

With the patient remaining in the sitting position but now with the pectoral muscles relaxed, palpation of the regional lymph nodes of the neck, clavicles (infraclavicular and supraclavicular), and axilla is then performed. To best delineate the axillary lymph nodes, the patient should be examined with the ipsilateral arm supported (**Fig. 71.5**). Attention is paid to evaluate the size, consistency (soft or firm), and characteristics (mobile or matted, tender or nontender) of the lymph nodes. Bimanual palpation of the breasts for masses and asymmetry completes the sitting examination.

The patient is then placed in the supine position with the ipsilateral arm raised above the head and the contralateral breast covered with the gown. The breast tissue is carefully palpated to evaluate for masses and asymmetry. It must be noted that generalized lumpiness is not a pathologic finding, with most normal breasts having more nodularity in the upper outer quadrants, at the inframammary ridge, and in the subareolar region. Comparing the breasts for symmetry by palpation may help discriminate benign findings from those that require additional evaluation. The area examined extends from the clavicle to the lower rib cage and medially from the sternal border to the midaxillary line. In addition, the axillary tail of the breast should be carefully palpated. The three search patterns that have been described are concentric circles, radial spoke method, and the vertical strip pattern (**Fig. 71.6**). As the first two methods can result in a less than thorough examination of the nipple–areola complex, we prefer the vertical strip pattern, as it incorporates this area. Otherwise, with the other two search patterns, a separate examination of the nipple–areola complex needs to be performed.

DIAGNOSIS

Table 71.1. Medical History of a Breast Problem

General
Age at menarche
Number of pregnancies
Number of live births
Age at first birth
Family history of ovarian cancer, gynecologic cancers, and other cancers, including affected relative, age of onset, and presence of bilateral disease
History of breast biopsies (and histologic diagnosis, if available)
Premenopausal women
- Date of last menstrual period
- Length and regularity of cycles
- Use of oral contraceptives

Postmenopausal women
- Date of menopause
- Use of hormone replacement therapy

Specific
Onset
Duration
Frequency
Severity
Relationship to menstrual cycle or use of hormone replacement therapy

Diagnostic Mammography and Breast Ultrasound

A woman who has an indeterminate or abnormal CBE will typically benefit from a diagnostic imaging evaluation, which can include mammography, targeted ultrasound, and/or MRI. 1 *It is important to note that any clinically suspicious mass, even in the absence of an imaging abnormality, needs to be biopsied as up to 15% of breast cancers are mammographically occult.*[6]

Soft tissue densities and clustered microcalcifications are two common mammographic findings suggestive of breast cancer. Soft tissue densities can appear as well-defined round/oval/lobulated masses, spiculated masses, irregular masses, or as areas of architectural distortion without an obvious mass (**Fig. 71.7**). Nearly 90% of spiculated soft tissue masses are

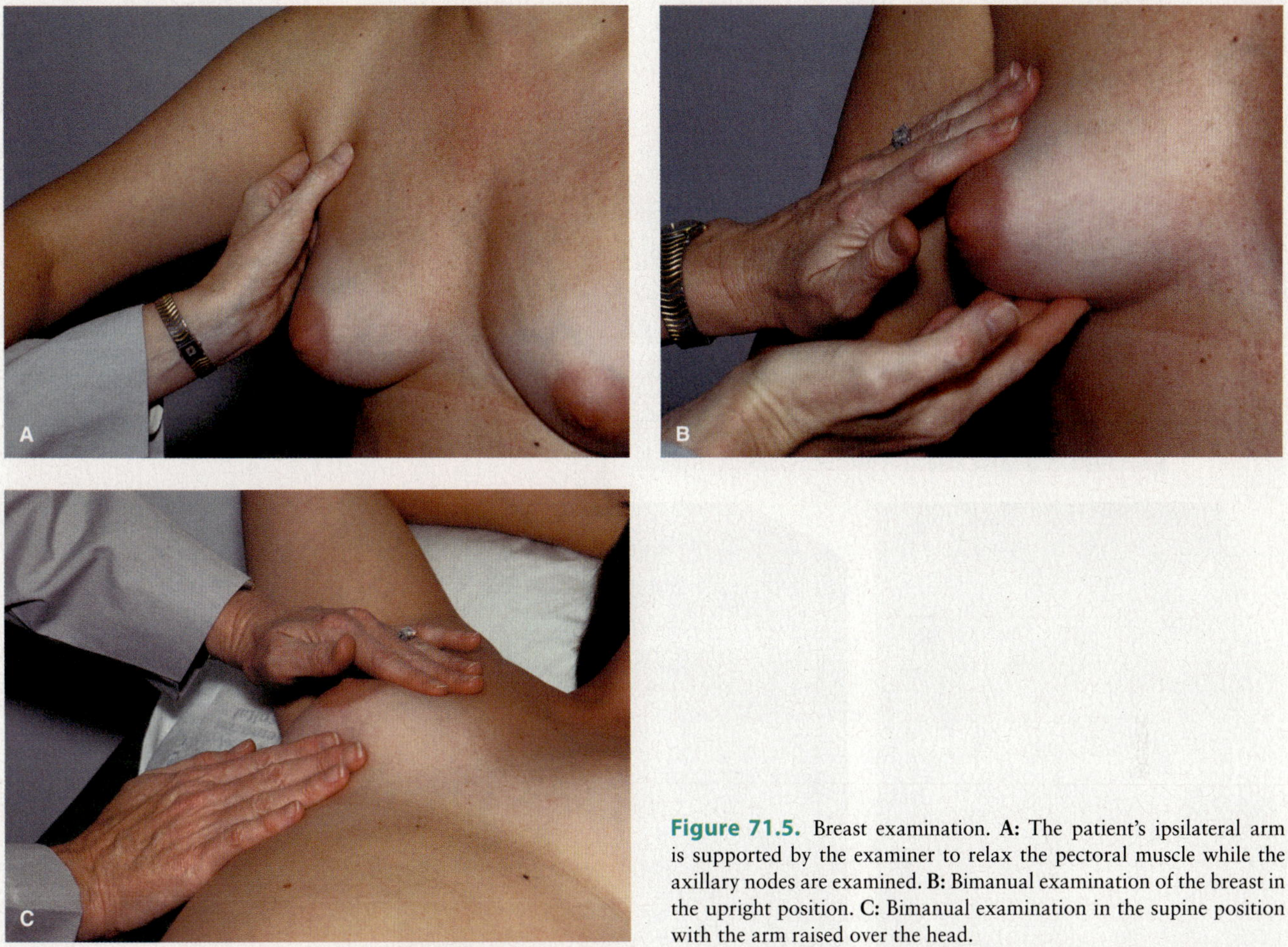

Figure 71.5. Breast examination. **A:** The patient's ipsilateral arm is supported by the examiner to relax the pectoral muscle while the axillary nodes are examined. **B:** Bimanual examination of the breast in the upright position. **C:** Bimanual examination in the supine position with the arm raised over the head.

associated with invasive cancer whereas well-defined solid masses are less commonly predictive of malignancy. Microcalcifications can have benign or malignant features, with benign calcifications often appearing rim-like, large, coarse, smooth, round, and/or oval in appearance. Calcifications that are associated with malignancy tend to be smaller in size, ranging between 0.1 to 1 mm in diameter. They are typically clustered, numbering four to five per cubic centimeter. Histologically, these represent intraductal calcifications in areas of necrotic tumor or calcifications within mucin-secreting tumors. In addition, malignant microcalcifications can often appear in a granular or linear branching pattern, with the linear branching pattern being highly associated with malignancy (**Fig. 71.8**).

Breast ultrasound is another important diagnostic imaging modality for the evaluation of breast masses and/or mammographic abnormalities. Breast ultrasound is complementary to mammography and is particularly valuable for the evaluation of breast masses. Breast ultrasound can increase the sensitivity and specificity of mammography for detection of breast cancer.[7] Ultrasound can differentiate a cystic mass from a solid one, characterize a palpable lesion that is not seen on

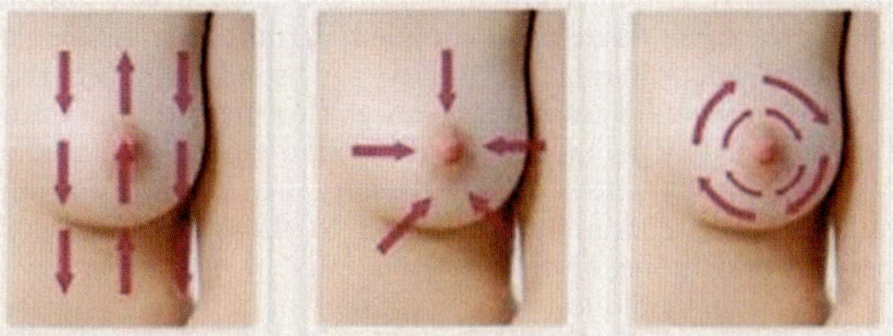

Figure 71.6. Clinical breast examination search patterns: vertical strip, radial spoke, and concentric circles.

mammography, and can assist with determining the actual size of a lesion. Ultrasonographic features that are used to characterize a lesion include shape (oval, round, lobular, irregular); margin (circumscribed, obscured, microlobulated, ill-defined, speculated); orientation (parallel or not parallel to skin); matrix echogenicity (anechoic, hypoechoic, hyperechoic); homogeneity (homogeneous, heterogeneous); and attenuation (indifferent, shadowing, enhancement).

Diagnostic MRI

Gadolinium contrast-enhanced MRI is complementary to mammography and breast ultrasound. It is not typically used for the evaluation of benign breast masses, but it does have a high sensitivity for detection of breast cancer. As such, MRI is most commonly used to evaluate the extent of disease and exclude occult breast cancers in patients with newly diagnosed breast cancer. In a meta-analysis of 44 studies, the sensitivity and specificity of diagnostic breast MRI were determined to be 90% and 72%, respectively.[8] The role of MRI in the evaluation of newly diagnosed breast cancer patients is discussed in ***Evaluation of the Patient with Breast Cancer***.

Biopsy Procedures

Breast biopsy is one of the most common general surgery procedures performed in the United States. There are multiple different types of breast biopsy, ranging from fine-needle aspiration (FNA) biopsy to excisional biopsy. The different types of breast biopsy are discussed below.

Fine-Needle Aspiration (FNA)

FNA of the breast is the least invasive breast biopsy procedure. FNA can be used for both diagnosis and treatment, and can be performed using palpation or image guidance. FNA is commonly used to sample suspicious breast and axillary lesions,

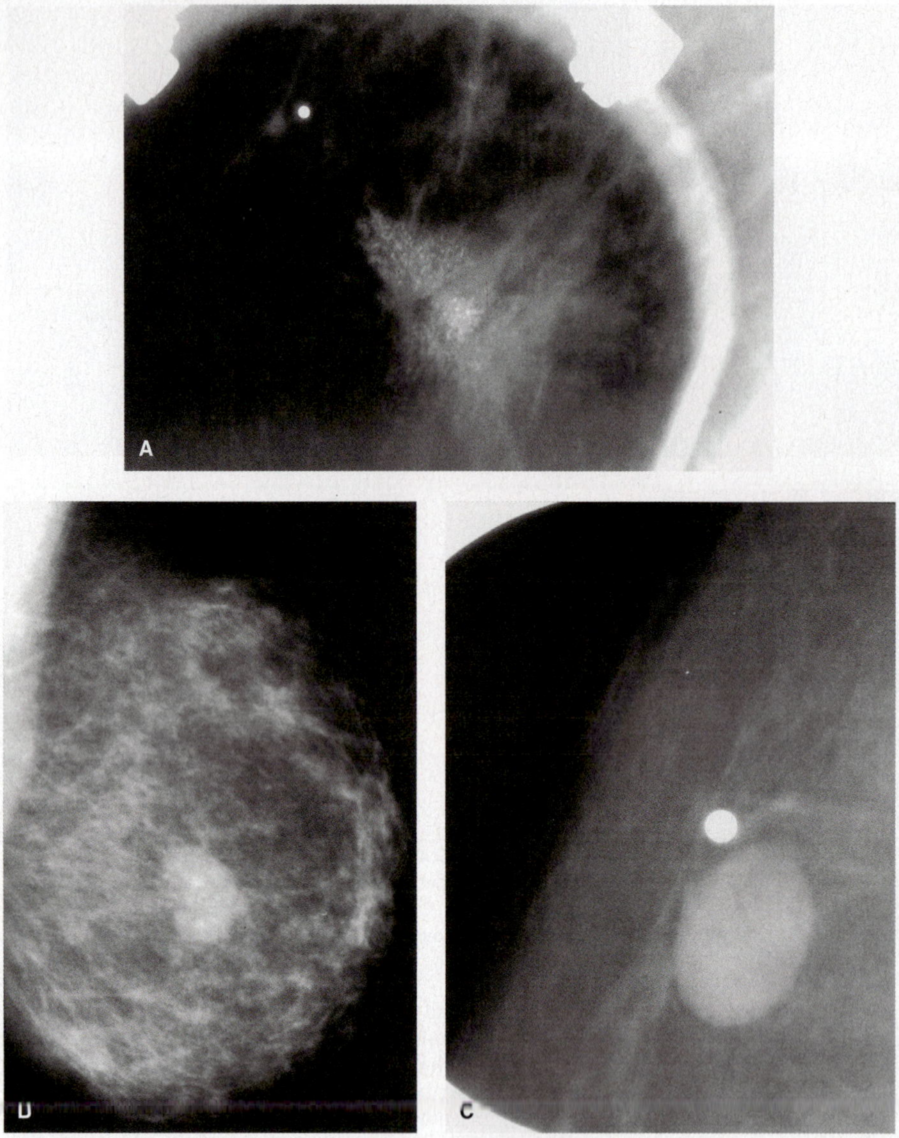

Figure 71.7. Mammographic masses. **A:** Spiculated mass with calcifications. **B:** Lobulated mass with indistinct posterior margin. **C:** Well-circumscribed mass.

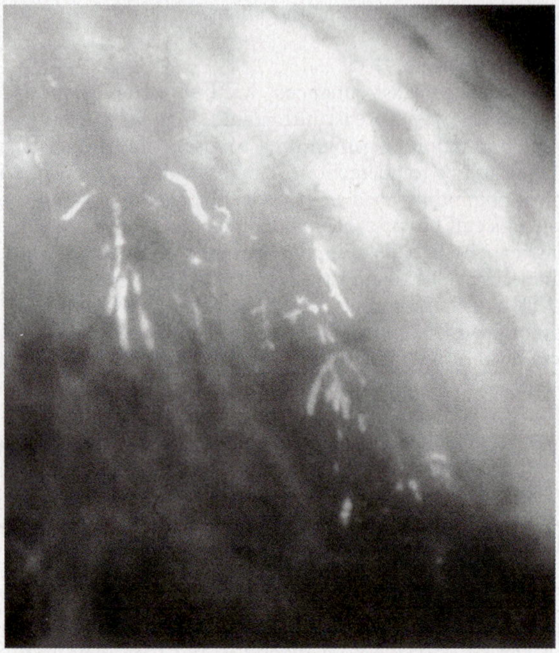

Figure 71.8. Microcalcifications. The branching, irregular appearance is classic for ductal carcinoma in situ.

especially those that are palpable. Other indications include drainage of simple cysts and small abscesses. In institutions with experienced cytopathologists, diagnostic FNA has a reported sensitivity of 98% and a specificity of 97%.[9] However, as the tissue architecture cannot be evaluated by FNA, a definitive diagnosis of invasive cancer cannot be made. In the past, FNA was commonly used to sample palpable breast masses as part of the triple test for evaluation of palpable masses. Currently, ultrasound can more accurately assess these lesions, and low-suspicion lesions are followed with serial imaging. High-suspicion lesions are best sampled by core needle biopsy to allow assessment of tissue architecture (**Fig. 71.9**).

Core Needle Biopsy

2 Core needle biopsy is also a minimally invasive strategy for breast biopsy. Given the limitations of FNA, core needle biopsy allows for more tissue to be sampled, permitting a histologic diagnosis and offering the ability to discriminate between invasive and noninvasive breast cancer. Core needle biopsy can be performed by palpation, but ultrasound-guided core needle biopsy typically offers superior results. Ultrasound imaging and patient preparation are similar to those described for patients undergoing FNA.

For nonpalpable lesions that cannot be imaged by ultrasound but are present on mammography (most commonly microcalcifications), stereotactic core biopsy can be performed. Stereotactic techniques use the principle of triangulation,

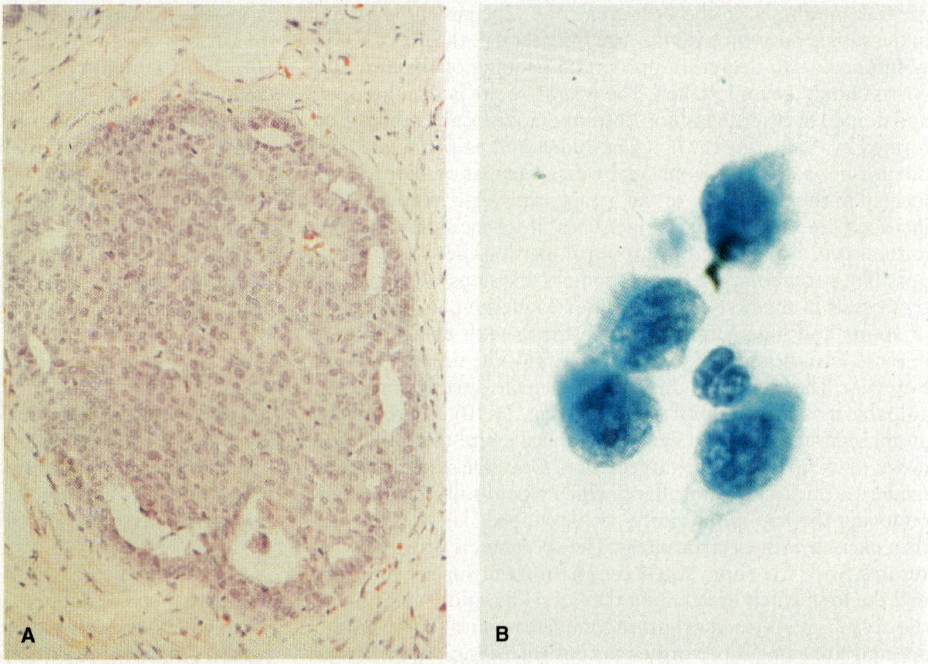

Figure 71.9. Comparison of core needle biopsy specimen (**A**) and fine-needle aspiration specimen (**B**). Only the core specimen can demonstrate the architectural detail.

which allows the precise location of a breast lesion to be determined in three dimensions.[10] The patient can be upright or prone depending on the machine. More commonly, the patient is placed in the prone position on the stereotactic table, which has an opening for the breast. A mammography unit is attached beneath the table and compresses the dependent breast. An initial scout image is obtained perpendicular to the compressed breast and evaluated. Following biopsy, repeat images are obtained to ensure the area of concern has been adequately biopsied. The procedure may be repeated to obtain additional cores. Most stereotactic core biopsies are performed with vacuum assistance, allowing for greater accuracy. If suspicious microcalcifications are biopsied, the samples can be examined with specimen imaging to ensure the presence of microcalcifications within the biopsy samples.

Failure to obtain an adequate sample can result in a false-negative diagnosis, although the false-negative rate is very low. In some instances, the results of the core biopsy may not be definitive, and a surgical excision is required. If the core biopsy demonstrates atypical ductal hyperplasia (ADH), atypical lobular hyperplasia (ALH), radial scar, or lobular carcinoma in situ (LCIS), surgical excision is required to exclude a diagnosis of malignancy. In the clinical context of persistent suspicious physical or imaging abnormalities (discordance between clinical and/or imaging findings and pathology results), surgical excision is required. Please see **Table 71.2** for indications for surgical excision after core biopsy.

INDICATIONS/CONTRAINDICATIONS

Table 71.2. Indications for Surgical Biopsy After Core Biopsy

- Atypical ductal hyperplasia
- Radial scar
- Columnar cell hyperplasia with atypia
- Papillary lesions
- Lack of concordance between appearance of mammographic lesion and histologic diagnosis
- Nondiagnostic specimen (including absence of calcifications on specimen radiograph when biopsy is performed for calcifications)

Incisional Biopsy

Incisional biopsy typically involves surgical removal of part of a large mass for diagnosis. With the advent of core needle biopsy techniques, incisional biopsy is rarely required. However, if a core needle biopsy is nondiagnostic and the mass is too large to remove without significant cosmetic compromise, an incisional biopsy can be performed for definitive diagnosis.

Excisional Biopsy

Excisional biopsy of the breast is the surgical removal of a breast lesion. Although core needle biopsy has largely obviated the need for excisional biopsy for diagnostic considerations, indications for this procedure still remain. Indications include breast lesions that are presumed to be benign but require excision, discordance between clinical evaluation/diagnostic imaging and pathology requiring further tissue sampling, high-risk lesions (including atypical hyperplasia, radial scar, papilloma, LCIS) identified on core biopsy, abnormalities that are close to the nipple or chest wall, small breasts that are not amenable to core biopsy (given the needle excursion is often 2 cm), and for patients who cannot tolerate stereotactic core needle biopsy. In addition, excisional biopsy may be considered for complex cysts, aspirated cysts that do not completely resolve, and when follow-up imaging for a lesion with previous benign pathology from a core biopsy shows an increase in size or has suspicious changes. Excisional biopsies may also be performed for likely benign lesions that are greater than 2 cm, painful, or recurring, or where the mass represents growing cysts or fibroadenomas. Patient preference for complete removal of a benign lesion may also be an indication for excisional biopsy.

For nonpalpable lesions, the abnormality can be localized preoperatively using a needle localization wire that is placed with the patient in a sitting position with the breast compressed by a labeled grid plate. Various needles used include the Kopans needle (checkmark wire), the Hawkins needle (multiple barbs and the only retractable wire for repositioning), and the Homer needle (J wire and nontransectable needle). For lesions that are superficial and can be readily imaged by ultrasound, needle localization can be performed under ultrasound guidance. Alternatively, there are other localization techniques including radioactive seeds, magnetic seeds, and radar seeds. The patient is then taken to the operative setting, where excision of the lesion can be performed under local anesthesia (mixture of short- and long-acting anesthetics with epinephrine) with sedation or general anesthesia. In the operating room, the patient is placed in the supine position with the arm ipsilateral to the index lesion positioned at 90 degrees. Appropriate padding of the arm and wrists should be undertaken. The operative site is then prepped and draped in a sterile fashion. Intraoperative localization is performed by evaluating the imaging studies and palpating the needle (for nonpalpable lesions) or by direct palpation. For lesions located in the upper half of the breast, transverse or curvilinear incisions are made along Langer lines. If an incision is needed in the lower half of the breast, radial incisions are used. When possible, periareolar or inframammary incisions are made as they result in the best cosmesis. Prior to incision, an anesthetic of short- and long-acting local anesthesia with epinephrine is injected into the skin and along the path of the needle localization wire. The incision is then typically made directly above the palpable mass or the tip of the needle (**Fig. 71.10**). Alternatively, an incision can be made next to the needle and then followed down to its tip to find the target lesion. Once the skin incision is made, the thickest possible flaps, which would still result in fully removing the lesion anteriorly, are developed. The specimen is then excised with electrocautery. The specimen is oriented with sutures, with the short stitch designating the superior margin and the long stitch designating the lateral margin. Palpation of the cavity is performed to ensure complete removal of the lesion. Specimen imaging is performed to confirm excision of the lesion of interest. Hemostasis is then achieved with electrocautery and the cavity is irrigated with saline. The cavity is examined again to confirm hemostasis. The skin is closed in two layers. The dermis is reapproximated with interrupted sutures of 3-0 Vicryl and the skin is closed with a subcuticular running stitch of 4-0 Monocryl. Cyanoacrylate tissue adhesive is then applied, allowing the patient to take a shower within 24 hours. For allergies to skin glue, adhesive strips can be applied. No pressure dressing is needed. A sports bra may be worn to stabilize the breast for the first 48 hours.

Skin Punch Biopsy

For any suspicious cutaneous lesion of the breast or chest wall, a biopsy can be obtained using a punch biopsy device, which consists of a circular blade. Punch biopsy devices are available in various sizes ranging from 1 mm to 8 mm, with the 4-mm size most commonly used in breast biopsies. The area to be biopsied is first selected. Common sites are the most abnormal-appearing site within a lesion or the edge of an actively growing lesion. The involved skin is cleansed and infiltrated with 2 to 3 mL of 1% lidocaine. The punch device is held vertically over the skin and rotated downward using a twirling motion until the subcutaneous fat or the hub of the device is reached. The specimen is then transected at the base with iris scissors. The skin is approximated with an interrupted stitch or U-stitch of 4-0 Monocryl.

COMMON CLINICAL PROBLEMS AND MANAGEMENT ALGORITHMS

The most common clinical breast problems include breast masses, breast pain, nipple discharge, and breast infections. Clinical algorithms for the evaluation of these common breast problems have been developed to facilitate optimal care.

Breast Mass

A breast mass is defined as a palpable area in the breast that may be either benign or malignant. When a woman presents with a palpable breast finding, a thorough history and physical examination needs to be performed. The history should include a thorough review of the patient's medical problems and any risk factors associated with breast cancer (see ***Management of Patients at High Risk for Breast Cancer***).

In women less than 40 years old with no family history of premenopausal breast cancer or other risk factors, a targeted ultrasound is an appropriate initial imaging approach for a breast mass that appears clinically benign (**Algorithm 71.1**). The ultrasound is used to determine if a dominant mass is indeed present, as normal glandular tissue of the breast, especially in young women, may feel nodular. In a review of 605 women younger than 40 years of age who were referred for evaluation of a breast mass, only 36% of the masses detected by patients had a surgical correlate. Furthermore, only 29% of the masses

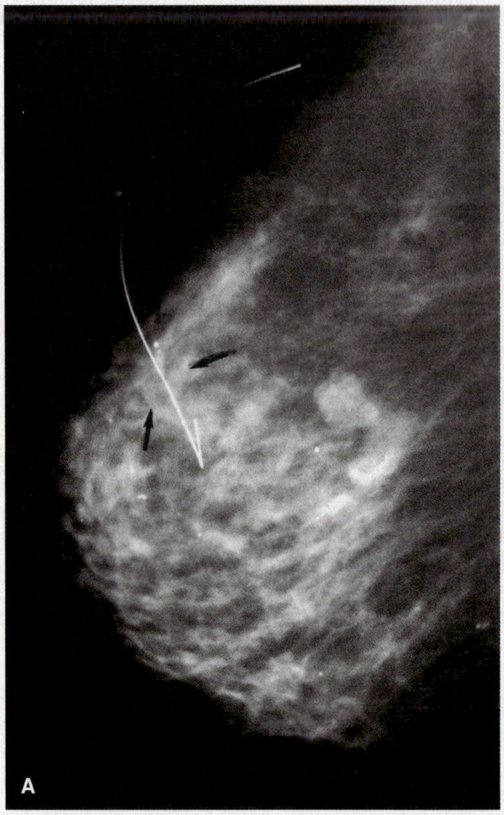

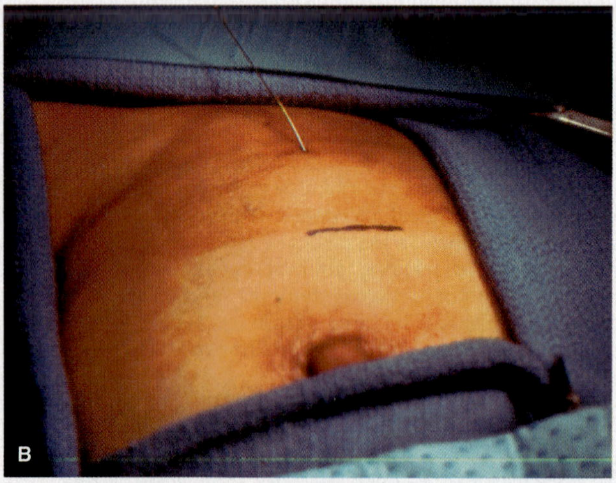

Figure 71.10. Incision placement for needle localization biopsy. **A:** The mammogram demonstrates that the lesion (*arrow*) is inferior to the point of wire entry. **B:** Incision placement inferior to wire entry to allow access to the lesion.

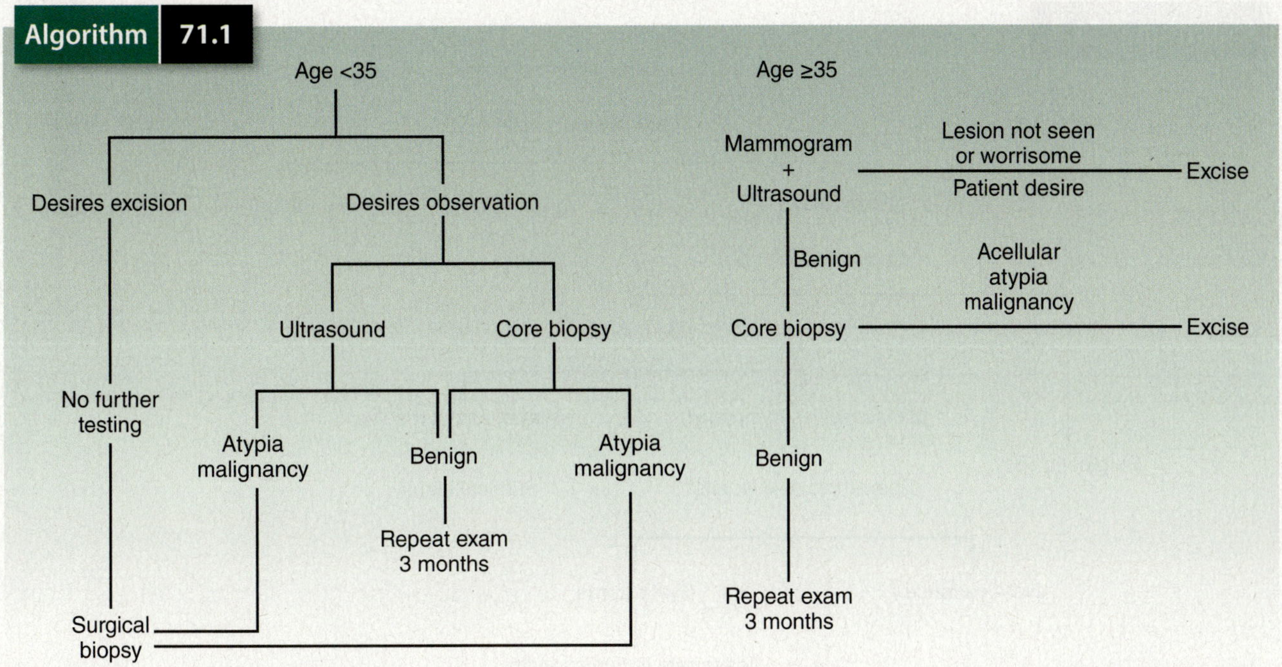

Algorithm 71.1. Diagnosis and management of the patient with a clinically benign breast mass. The use of imaging studies varies according to age because breast carcinoma is infrequent in women younger than 35 years old.

detected by primary care providers were confirmed.[11] Consideration can then be made regarding the need for additional imaging such as mammography or an MRI. In women aged 40 or older, the initial imaging approach to a palpable mass should include a mammogram and ultrasound. These studies should be obtained prior to any biopsies are performed as postbiopsy changes can distort subsequent imaging evaluation. Of note, all clinically suspicious palpable masses need to be biopsied even in the absence of imaging findings as 15% of breast cancers can be mammographically occult (**Algorithm 71.2**).[6] Ultrasound also provides important information about the etiology of a breast mass, and can further categorize the mass as either cystic or solid. Workup of a cystic lesion typically involves aspiration of the cyst, with further evaluation based on the results of the aspiration (**Algorithm 71.3**). The definitive diagnosis of a breast mass is often confirmed by a core needle biopsy, although FNA is an appropriate alternative (**Table 71.3**). Core needle biopsy is typically preferred to excisional biopsy.

Breast cysts are common causes of dominant masses in premenopausal and perimenopausal women. If a cyst is found in a

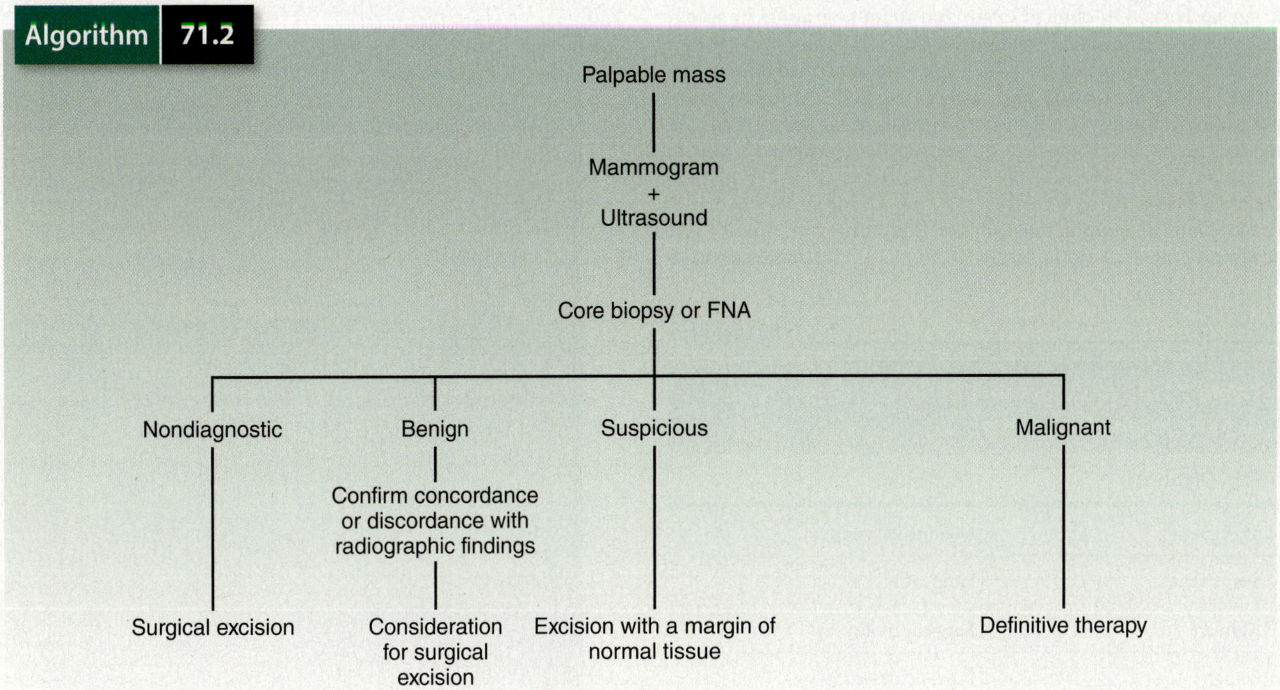

Algorithm 71.2. Diagnosis and management of the patient with a clinically indeterminate or suspicious solid breast mass. In this circumstance, imaging studies are insufficient to exclude malignancy, and tissue sampling is required.

Algorithm 71.3

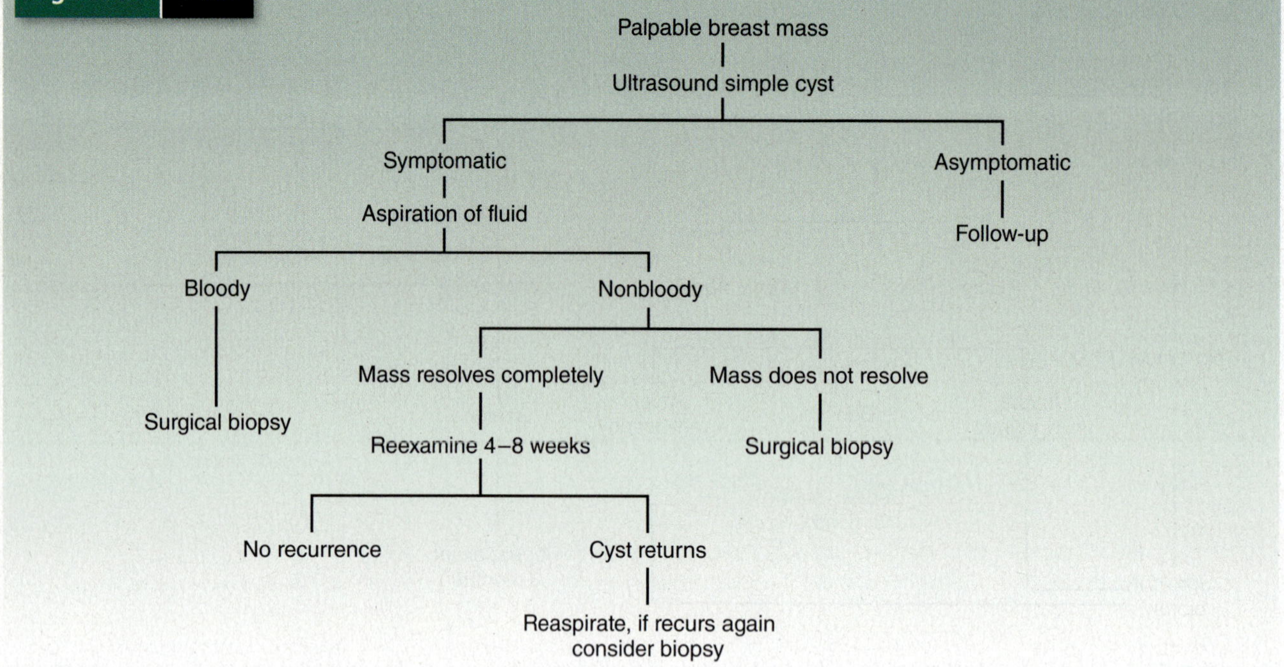

Algorithm 71.3. Diagnosis and management of the patient with a cystic lesion. Bloody fluid on aspiration, failure of the mass to resolve completely, and prompt refilling of the same cyst are indications for surgical biopsy.

postmenopausal woman in the absence of hormone therapy use, it should be regarded with a high degree of suspicion. Palpable masses that present as benign solid masses include fibroadenomas, fibrocystic disease, and fat necrosis. Fibrocystic breast disease has been used to describe a variety of benign breast disorders associated with nodular breast tissue. This term, however, should be reserved for women who have a biopsy consistent with one of the histologic components of fibrocystic change. Breast surgery, blunt trauma, injection of native or foreign substance such as fat and silicone, and radiation therapy (RT) can result in fat necrosis. On clinical exam and mammographic imaging, fat necrosis can mimic a malignancy, often leading to a biopsy. However, when oil cysts, which are circumscribed masses of mixed soft tissue density and fat with a calcified rim, are present radiographically, a definitive diagnosis of fat necrosis can be made (**Fig. 71.11**). Please see the section ***Benign Breast Disease***.

Breast Pain

Breast pain (mastalgia, mastodynia, idiopathic breast pain) is a common concern and is rarely (0.5% to 3.3%) representative of breast cancer. It is noted that some **IBCs** can present with pain. While two-thirds of patients present with cyclical breast pain, another one-third have pain that is unrelated to the menstrual cycle and more likely to be secondary to a breast or chest wall lesion.

Cyclical breast pain is associated with hormonal changes during the menstrual cycle and often occurs the week prior to the onset of menses and often dissipates once menstrual flow is established. During the menstrual cycle, the breast undergoes

TREATMENT

Table 71.3. Management of Breast Masses Based on Core Biopsy Diagnosis

FNA Diagnosis	Treatment
Malignant	Definitive therapy
Suspicious	Surgical biopsy
Atypia	Surgical biopsy
Benign	Possible observation[a]
Nondiagnostic	Surgical biopsy

[a]See discussion in text on clinical approach to the patient with a solid breast mass.

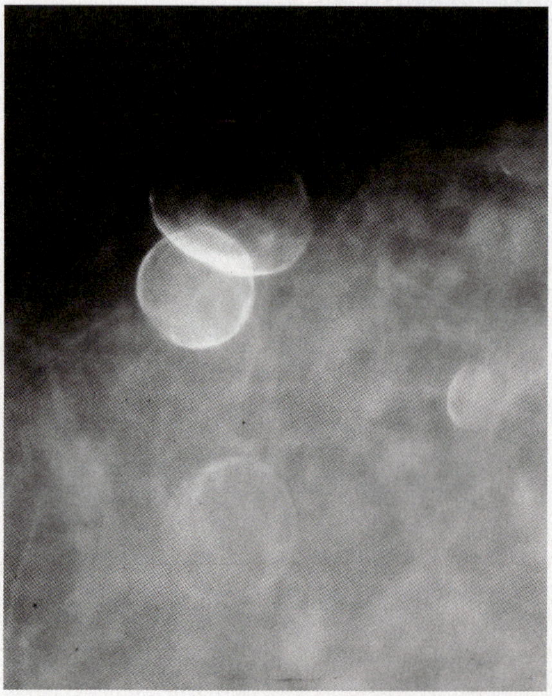

Figure 71.11. Oil cysts. The calcified rims of these cysts in a patient with a history of trauma are diagnostic.

significant histologic changes as described by Vogel.[12] During the secretory phase, luminal cells produce apocrine secretions, and the stromal cells become edematous, which may contribute to the pathogenesis of breast pain. However, the exact physiologic events are not understood completely. Furthermore, while most women do experience mild cyclical breast pain, it is not clear why others have more pronounced pain. Cyclical breast pain is typically bilateral and involves the upper outer aspect of the breasts with radiation to the axillae or down the arms.

Noncyclical breast pain is more frequently unilateral and variable in its location in the breast. Possible etiologies include large pendulous breasts with pain resulting from stretching of the Cooper ligaments, duct ectasia, macrocysts, medications (including antidepressants, hormones, and antibiotics), and infections. Thrombophlebitis of the lateral thoracic or superior thoracoepigastric vein (Mondor disease) is an uncommon presentation for breast pain characterized by a tender subcutaneous cord in the lateral aspect of the breast (**Fig. 71.12**). Mondor disease may result from trauma, radiation to the breast, and/or breast surgery. It can also occur in women with nonpalpable breast cancers, and a mammogram should be obtained when diagnosed. For symptomatic relief, a patient can use anti-inflammatory medications, although Mondor disease often resolves spontaneously without the need for a specific therapy. Referred pain to the breast from the chest wall or ribs can also occur. Spinal or paraspinal problems and medical conditions (biliary, pulmonary, esophageal, and cardiac disease) can also result in referred pain.

The workup for breast pain should include a careful history, including questions related to the menstrual cycle, a thorough physical examination, and, in women 35 years and older, a mammogram. If a malignancy is suspected, biopsy should be performed. If the CBE and diagnostic imaging studies are normal, reassurance that the symptoms are not consistent with breast cancer often provides significant relief for the patient.

Initial therapy for idiopathic breast pain includes lifestyle changes, the use of supportive garments such as a well-fitting brassiere with a steel underwire, a low-fat-high-carbohydrate diet, and elimination of caffeine and nicotine. Oral analgesics with acetaminophen or nonsteroidal anti-inflammatory drugs (NSAIDs) should be initiated. Topical analgesic gels containing diclofenac or salicylate can be applied to the affected breast areas. If a patient is on oral contraceptives or hormone replacement therapy, discontinuation of these medications may improve pain. However, in women not using oral contraceptives with cyclical breast symptoms, the initiation of this therapy has been shown to reduce breast pain severity and duration. Although inconclusive evidence exists for the role of evening primrose oil (3000 mg daily),[13] it is often part of the initial therapeutic approach. Evening primrose oil needs to be taken for at least 4 to 6 months to achieve a positive effect.

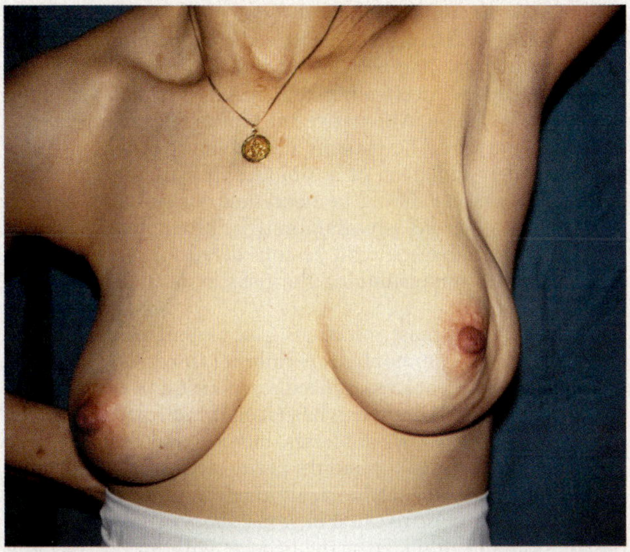

Figure 71.12. Mondor disease. Thrombophlebitis of the thoracoepigastric vein causes retraction of the lateral portion of the breast, which crosses to the midline at the inferior areolar margin and is accompanied by a palpable cord.

Approximately 5% of women will still have debilitating breast pain despite lifestyle changes and the initial therapies described above. For these women, therapies such as danazol, tamoxifen, bromocriptine, and gonadotropin-releasing hormone (GnRH) agonists can be considered. However, only danazol has been approved by the FDA for the treatment of idiopathic breast pain. Danazol (100 mg to 400 mg daily) is an antigonadotropin that results in a hypoestrogenic state. However, its use is often discontinued as it also induces a hyperandrogenic state, with most women having side effects of increased facial hair, acne, deepening of the voice, and adverse blood lipid profiles. Tamoxifen (10 mg daily) has also been shown to be effective, although side effects, including the risk of blood clots, endometrial cancer, and hot flashes, limit its use. As both danazol and tamoxifen have significant teratogenic effects, women on these therapies must be counseled to use an effective birth control method. Although bromocriptine and GNRH agonists have been studied for use in breast pain, they are not currently recommended because of significant side effects. Therapies that have been proven to be ineffective include diuretics, progesterone, and vitamins. Surgery to excise trigger spots (in the absence of an identifiable lesion) is not recommended.

Nipple Discharge

Nipple discharge is a common breast symptom that often results in surgical consultation. The most common cause of pathologic nipple discharge is an intraductal papilloma, but breast cancer can also present as a pathologic nipple discharge. The first step in evaluation of nipple discharge is to determine whether the nipple discharge is pathologic or physiologic. Physiologic discharge is nonspontaneous or is elicited by manual compression of the nipple. It often involves multiple ductal orifices in the nipple and is present in both breasts. The discharge is commonly white or clear (although it can also present as yellow, green, brown, or gray fluid) and is negative on occult blood test. In contrast, pathologic nipple discharge is spontaneous, is present in a single breast/ductal orifice, and is often positive on occult blood test. However, any nipple discharge that is spontaneous is considered pathologic. Age is also predictive of breast cancer risk in women with nipple discharge. In a study involving women with pathologic nipple discharge, breast cancer was present in 3% of women <40 years old, 10% in those 40 to 60 years old, and 32% in those over 60 years old.[14]

Clinical evaluation of nipple discharge includes a careful history and physical examination. The history includes questions regarding whether the discharge is spontaneous or elicited, unilateral or bilateral. The patient should be questioned regarding any recent trauma to the breast. The past medical history and medications are reviewed. Medications such as oral contraceptives, metoclopramide, phenothiazines, and selective serotonin reuptake inhibitors can be associated with nipple discharge. A premenopausal woman presenting with milky fluid discharge bilaterally or galactorrhea should be evaluated for endocrine disease. Hypogonadism, as suggested by amenorrhea or hot flashes/vaginal dryness, should prompt a workup for hyperprolactinemia. In addition, hypothyroidism, pituitary adenoma, and chest trauma (including thoracotomy) can result in galactorrhea. When endocrine disease is suspected, patients should undergo laboratory evaluation, including quantitative hCG, prolactin level, and thyroid function tests. The physical examination should include a visual

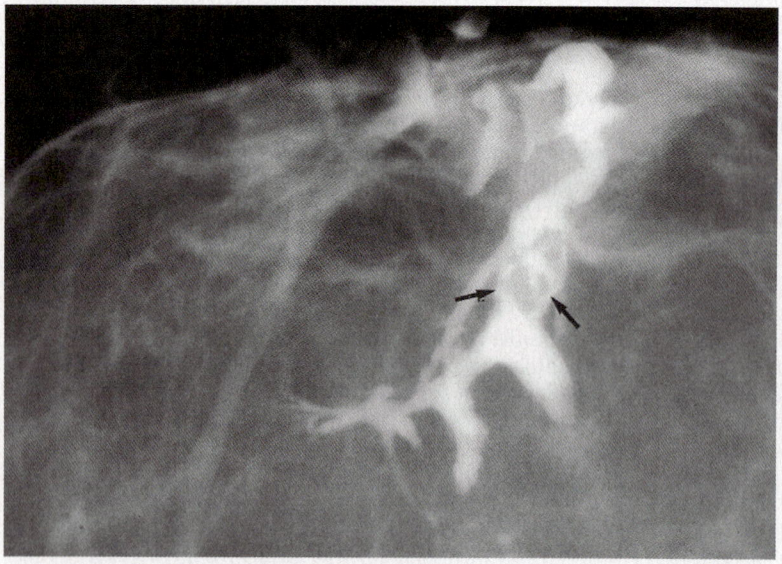

Figure 71.13. Ductogram. A large defect (*arrows*) represents an intraductal papilloma.

field test, as often these patients may show signs of bitemporal field loss or chiasmal syndrome. A careful breast examination is performed to evaluate for any dominant masses, skin changes such as eczema/infections, nipple changes such as Paget disease, or adenopathy. Each of the quadrants of the involved breast is massaged from the periphery to the nipple–areolar complex and then pressure is applied to the base of the nipple–areolar complex to elicit discharge. This will help define the involved quadrant of the breast and whether the discharge is from a single ductal orifice. The color of any nipple discharge should be noted, and an occult blood test should be performed.

After initial evaluation, no further workup is required in women who have physiologic discharge, and these women should be advised to avoid manual compression of the nipples.

Imaging evaluation is indicated for patients with pathologic nipple discharge and includes an ultrasound, mammography for patients >30 years old, and MRI. In patients with an imaging abnormality, a biopsy should be considered. Additional diagnostic tests that may be helpful include ductography and ductoscopy. Ductography is performed by instilling contrast medium into the involved duct to identify any lesions in the ductal system. Lesions will appear as either a complete ductal obstruction, irregularities in the duct wall, or as an intraductal filling defect (**Fig. 71.13**). However, the absence of a lesion on ductography does not rule out a cancer.[15] Ductoscopy is often performed in the operating room and involves the use of a small fiberoptic ductoscope that is placed into the involved duct. The benefit of ductoscopy is that it allows for direct visualization of any potential lesions, which may result in more precise excision.

The most common etiology of pathologic nipple discharge is a papilloma, which is a benign epithelial lesion with supporting stroma that grows within a duct. When a papilloma is diagnosed by core biopsy, the standard recommendation is to proceed with surgical excision, as it may be associated with atypia or ductal carcinoma in situ (DCIS). Other causes for pathologic nipple discharge include malignancy (most commonly DCIS, 5% to 15% of cases) and ductal ectasia, which is characterized by ductal dilatation with loss of elastin in the duct walls and the presence of chronic inflammatory cells. It is not known, however, whether the inflammatory cells result from a primary or secondary infection, and antibiotics are not recommended.

If a malignancy is identified as the etiology of a pathologic nipple discharge, it should be managed accordingly, with appropriate cancer surgery typically the first treatment. In the absence of a known malignancy, pathologic nipple discharge should be treated with terminal duct excision. Prior to excision, the patient should refrain from any nipple stimulation. If the involved duct can be identified intraoperatively, a lacrimal duct or instillation of methylene blue may aid with the ductal excision. Terminal duct excision is commonly performed with a circumareolar incision and involves removal of the duct from its proximal to distal extent, which is often a distance of 2 to 3 cm. Alternatively, ductoscopy can be performed as previously prescribed, and then the outer sheath of the cannula can be left in place as a guide for surgical excision of the involved duct. If there is difficulty isolating the involved duct or multiple ducts are involved, central or total terminal duct excision may be indicated. The potential risks of terminal duct excision include inability to breastfeed and hyposensitivity or hypersensitivity of the nipple.

Breast Infections

Breast infections are less common outside of the postpartum period. As such, breast infections can be classified as lactating or nonlactating infections. Lactating infections occur commonly during the initial 6 weeks of breastfeeding and during the process of weaning. In the initial stages of infection, a mastitis or cellulitis is typically found, with associated pain, erythema, induration, and fever. A woman should not be counseled to discontinue breastfeeding. Commonly, the cellulitis results from *Staphylococcus aureus*. Treatment includes pain management (acetaminophen, NSAIDs) and an antibiotic such as dicloxacillin. Alternative antibiotics include cephalexin and erythromycin. The mastitis should improve within 24 to 48 hours after initiation of antibiotics. If symptoms or fever persists, an abscess should be ruled out. For small or superficial abscesses, needle aspiration may be attempted. However, incision and drainage should be considered for large or complex abscesses, understanding the risks associated with milk fistula formation.

Nonlactating breast infections can present as periareolar abscesses or, less commonly, as peripheral abscesses. For small- or moderate-sized abscesses, needle aspiration is the first line of treatment, and a drain can be placed if indicated. However, for larger and/or deeper abscesses, incision and drainage may be indicated. This is commonly performed in the operating room under general anesthesia, although if the anterior aspect of the abscess is close to the skin, it may be possible to perform the incision and drainage at the bedside with infiltration of a local anesthetic. A preoperative ultrasound can be obtained to better evaluate the size and location of the abscess. Often, the abscess is not located directly under the area of greatest erythema, and careful breast examination should be performed to localize the area of greatest fluctuance. *Biopsy of the cavity should always be considered, as breast infection may be an unusual breast cancer presentation.* For a subareolar abscess, removal of the sinus tract as well as the segmental duct should be considered. Antibiotics, such as cephalexin 500 mg QID, are commonly prescribed for 7 to 10 days postoperatively, although once a wound is properly drained and cellulitis subsides, the patient can discontinue all antibiotics. For chronic subareolar abscesses, it may be necessary to completely excise the involved duct.

In the setting of recurrent or persistent abscess formation or inflammatory changes despite adequate surgical management, other etiologies need to be considered, including idiopathic granulomatous mastitis, Wegener granuloma, sarcoidosis, tuberculosis, and histoplasmosis.

BENIGN BREAST DISEASE

Benign breast lesions can be classified into three groups: (1) nonproliferative breast lesions, (2) proliferative breast lesions without atypia, and (3) proliferative breast lesions with atypia (**Table 71.4**).

Nonproliferative Breast Lesions

Nonproliferative breast lesions include breast cysts, papillary apocrine change, epithelial-related calcifications, and mild hyperplasia of the usual type. These lesions are not associated with an increased risk of breast cancer.[16] Papillary apocrine change is characterized by proliferation of ductal epithelial cells showing apocrine features and has eosinophilic cytoplasm. Benign calcifications found in normal ducts, lobules, breast stroma, and blood vessel walls are referred to as epithelial-related calcifications. Mild hyperplasia of the usual type occurs when the number of epithelial cells within a duct is more than two but not more than four cells in depth, and the epithelial cells do not cross the lumen of the involved space.[17]

The most common nonproliferative lesions of the breast are cysts, which often present clinically as solitary masses that can be associated with pain. They are fluid-filled, round or ovoid structures arising from the terminal duct lobular unit when fluid accumulates because of distension and obstruction of the efferent ductule. Given that cysts arise from lobular pathology, they occur mainly during lobular development, menstrual cyclic changes, and lobular involution in pre- and postmenopausal women, with peak incidence between 35 and 50 years of age.[18]

CLASSIFICATION

Table 71.4. Classification of Benign Breast Disease

Nonproliferative: No Increase in Risk
Cysts: micro or macro
Ductal ectasia
Simple fibroadenoma
Mastitis
Fibrosis
Metaplasia: squamous or apocrine
Mild hyperplasia
Proliferative: RR 1.5–2.0
Complex fibroadenoma
Papilloma
Sclerosing adenosis
Hyperplasia: moderate or severe
Proliferative With Atypia: RR 4.5–5.0
Atypical ductal hyperplasia
Atypical lobular hyperplasia

RR, relative risk.

The three types of cysts are simple, complicated, and complex. Simple cysts are well circumscribed and, on ultrasound, have posterior acoustic enhancement. In addition, they are anechoic and do not have solid components or Doppler signals. If simple cysts are diagnosed by ultrasound, they are by definition benign and do not require further intervention, although cyst aspiration can be performed if the patient is symptomatic. Alternatively, FNA can also be used to diagnose simple cysts. If the aspirated fluid is nonbloody and the palpable mass completely resolves, this is also diagnostic of a simple cyst, and no further diagnostic evaluation is required. A follow-up CBE ± ultrasound can be performed in 3 to 6 months to document stability, and the patient may resume routine breast cancer screening.

Unlike simple cysts, which are not associated with malignancy, complicated and complex breast cysts are associated with malignancy in <1% and 1% to 23%, respectively.[19] On ultrasound, complicated cysts appear as masses with homogeneous low-level internal echoes due to echogenic debris. However, there are no solid components, thick walls, or thick septa. Complex cysts are defined as cysts with solid components, thick walls, or thick septa. Complex cysts are characterized on ultrasound by the absence of posterior wall enhancement and the appearance of anechoic and echogenic components. Complicated cysts can be confirmed as benign by biopsy, either through FNA, core biopsy, or excisional biopsy. Alternatively, ultrasound imaging and mammography (if the lesion was visualized on mammography) with CBE every 6 months for 2 years can be performed to document stability. If complicated cysts develop any concerning changes, such as an increase in size or development of a solid component, biopsy should be performed per consensus guidelines. Complex cysts mandate biopsy. If no fluid is aspirated by FNA, then core biopsy under image guidance should be performed with care to biopsy the solid component. A metallic clip marking the biopsy site facilitates surgical excision if necessary and facilitates follow-up imaging. If pathology is concordant with imaging findings, then follow-up with CBE and ultrasound imaging every 6 to 12 months for 1 to 2 years can be performed to document stability. For any concerning changes in the appearance of the lesion or an increase in size, excisional biopsy should be performed. In patients who may be noncompliant with follow-up care, surgical excision should be considered for complicated and complex breast cysts per consensus guidelines.

Proliferative Breast Lesions Without Atypia

Proliferative breast lesions without atypia include ductal hyperplasia, intraductal papillomas, sclerosing adenosis, radial scars, and fibroadenomas. Ductal hyperplasia is often an incidental finding noted on biopsies obtained for mammographic abnormalities or for breast masses. Ductal hyperplasia is characterized by an increased number of cells within the ductal space; however, the cells retain the cytologic features of benign cells. Ductal hyperplasia is not associated with a significant risk for subsequent breast cancer, and no additional treatment is necessary. Women with intraductal papillomas often present with pathologic nipple discharge (see section on ***Nipple Discharge*** above). These lesions consist of a monotonous array of papillary cells that grow from the wall of a duct or cyst into its lumen. Given that intraductal papillomas can harbor areas of atypia or DCIS, surgical excision is recommended when intraductal papillomas are diagnosed by core needle biopsy. If no atypia or DCIS is found at the time of excision, then no further treatment is necessary.[20] Sclerosing adenosis typically presents as a mammographic abnormality or a mass and requires no further treatment following biopsy, as it is a benign lobular lesion resulting from increased fibrous tissue and interspersed glandular cells.[21] Complex sclerosing lesions or radial scars are often found incidentally when a breast mass or radiologic abnormality is biopsied or excised. These lesions are characterized by a fibroelastic core with radiating ducts and lobules, and radial scars can appear spiculated on mammography. When diagnosed on core biopsy, radial scars should be excised, as 8% to 17% are associated with malignancy at surgical excision.[22] If the surgical excisional confirms a radial scar, no additional treatment is needed.

Fibroadenomas typically present as well-circumscribed mobile masses that are not fixed to the surrounding breast tissue. They are benign solid tumors made of glandular as well as fibrous tissue, and are found most commonly in women between the ages of 15 and 35 years. Fibroadenomas with benign imaging characteristics can be followed with serial CBE and ultrasound imaging to ensure stability. Alternatively, core needle biopsy can be performed to confirm the diagnosis. If a fibroadenoma is asymptomatic, surgical excision is not necessary. However, if the presumed fibroadenoma is symptomatic or increases in size, excision can be performed for symptomatic relief or to rule out a malignancy such as a phyllodes tumor. Fibroadenomas that are associated with proliferative changes such as sclerosing adenosis, ductal epithelial hyperplasia, epithelial calcification, or papillary apocrine changes are referred to as complex fibroadenomas. Surgical excision of these lesions is often recommended to exclude a diagnosis of breast cancer, although this is controversial, as some advocate that these lesions can be followed similarly to simple fibroadenomas.[23]

A fibroadenoma that is greater than 10 cm in size is referred to as a giant fibroadenoma, and excision is recommended, as these lesions are hard to differentiate from a phyllodes tumor. Juvenile fibroadenomas occur in young women between the ages of 10 and 18 and can vary in size from 5 to 20 cm in diameter. Surgical excision is recommended as these lesions can be cosmetically distressing for the young patient and are difficult to differentiate from a phyllodes tumor, although risk to the prepubertal breast bud is a potential complication.

Proliferative Breast Lesions with Atypia

Proliferative breast lesions with atypia include ADH, ALH, flat epithelial atypia (FEA), and LCIS. Although these lesions are not considered premalignant, they are associated with an increase in the patient's future risk of developing breast cancer (**Fig. 71.14**).

ADH is characterized by a proliferation of uniform epithelial cells with monomorphic round nuclei filling part, but not all, of the involved duct. ADH often presents as suspicious microcalcifications seen on mammography. In contrast, ALH is often an incidental finding found on breast biopsies performed for other reasons, such as an abnormal mammogram or breast mass. ALH is characterized by a proliferation of monomorphic, evenly spaced, dyshesive cells filling part, but not all, of the involved lobule. Atypical hyperplasias are associated with an increased risk of subsequent breast cancer (relative risk 3.7 to 5.3) in both the ipsilateral and contralateral breast.[24] Atypical hyperplasias are often diagnosed on core needle biopsy, and in this clinical context, surgical excision is indicated to exclude a diagnosis of malignancy. Atypical hyperplasias are upgraded to DCIS or invasive breast cancer in 10% to 20% of cases. If the diagnosis of atypical hyperplasia is made by excisional biopsy and the area is adequately sampled, reexcision is not necessary or recommended. Instead, the patient should be counseled toward risk reduction strategies which include CBE every 6 to 12 months, annual screening mammography, and consideration for chemoprevention with a selective estrogen receptor modulator (SERM) or an aromatase inhibitor (AI) per consensus guidelines. In addition, the patient should be counseled to perform consistent breast self-examinations such that she will become familiar with her breasts and report changes promptly to her provider (please see the section on ***Management of Patients at High Risk for Breast Cancer*** below).

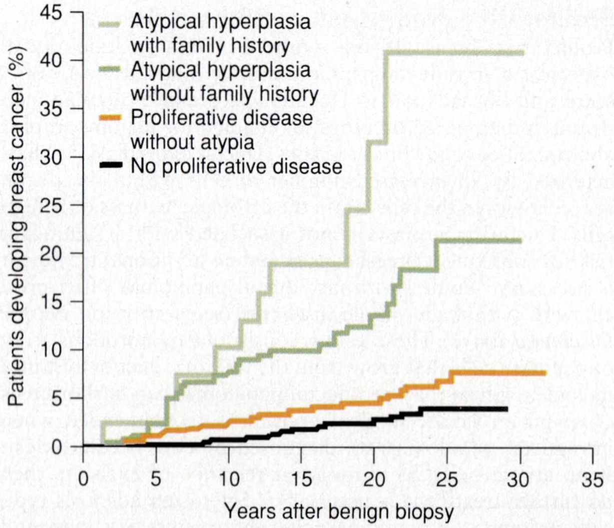

Figure 71.14. Cumulative risk for the development of invasive breast cancer after a biopsy for benign breast disease. Women with atypical hyperplasia (ductal or lobular type) are at a significantly increased risk for the development of breast cancer. (Reproduced with permission from Page DL, Dupont WD. Anatomic markers of human premalignancy and risk of breast cancer. *Cancer*. 1990;66:1326.)

Lobular Carcinoma In Situ (LCIS)

LCIS is a noninvasive lesion that arises from the lobules and terminal ducts of the breast. It is characterized by solid proliferation of small cells, with small, uniform, round-to-oval nuclei, and variably distinct cell borders. The cytoplasm of the cells is clear to lightly eosinophilic and occasionally there are intracytoplasmic vacuoles that may be large enough to produce signet ring cell forms. LCIS tends to have a very low proliferative index and are estrogen-receptor positive. LCIS is more prevalent in premenopausal women and white women.

LCIS is often diagnosed as an incidental finding on a breast biopsy that has been performed for another reason, such as
3 an area of fibrocystic change or mammographic abnormality. If LCIS is identified on core biopsy, in the past, excisional biopsy was always recommended, given the possible upgrade to DCIS or invasive cancer that was presumed to occur in 15% to 38% of patients.[25] However, more recently, this risk of an upgrade to malignancy is found to be much lower at a rate of 1% to 3% if LCIS is found as an incidental finding on core biopsy.[26] As such, if radiographic and pathologic concordance exists, a possible alternative to surgical excision is imaging and clinical follow-up. If LCIS is found on excisional biopsy, no further surgical intervention is needed. However, if *pleomorphic* LCIS is identified at a surgical margin on excisional biopsy, wide excision with negative margins is recommended, as pleomorphic LCIS can be hard to differentiate from DCIS.[27]

Although it is not a premalignant lesion, LCIS conveys a substantially increased risk for breast cancer. The relative risk of developing an invasive cancer in women with LCIS is approximately two to three times higher than for women without LCIS (**Table 71.5**).[28] LCIS also conveys an increased risk for breast cancer to the contralateral breast. Historically, women diagnosed with LCIS were treated with bilateral prophylactic mastectomies. However, this approach has been proven to be too aggressive, given that *most* women with LCIS who do not have other contributory factors (eg, family history of premenopausal breast cancer) will not develop an invasive breast cancer. Instead, a careful lifetime surveillance protocol similar to that described above for atypical hyperplasias can be followed. Chemoprevention with a SERM and/or AI can also be discussed with the patient. There are currently no randomized trials to compare the efficacy of

Table 71.5. Risk for Breast Cancer Development After Lobular Carcinoma in Situ

Study	No. of Patients	Invasive Cancer (%)	Follow-Up (yrs)	Relative Risk
Haagensen[29]	287	18	16.3	6.9
Rosen et al.[30]	99	12.5	24	9.0
Andersen[31]	47	26.4	15	12.0
Salvadori et al.[32]	80	6.3	5	10.3
Ottesen et al.[33]	69	11.6	5	11.0
Bodian et al.[34]	236	26[a]	18	5.4
Fisher et al.[35]	182	33	5	—

[a]Includes intraductal and invasive cancer.

surveillance protocol versus prophylactic mastectomy in women with LCIS.

FEA is an intraductal finding that is characterized by the replacement of native epithelial cells by a single layer, or up to three to five layers of mildly atypical cells. When diagnosed at core biopsy, the risk of upgrade to a malignancy at surgical excision is 5% to 15%. When FEA is diagnosed by excisional biopsy, no further surgery is warranted. However, if FEA is diagnosed by core needle biopsy, excisional biopsy should be considered. Alternatively, radiologic surveillance can be performed, and if there is an absence of a residual mammographic abnormality and core biopsy was felt to be adequate, no further surgery is needed. Excisional biopsy must be performed for any residual lesions seen. When FEA is found at the margins, wider excision is not needed. Although FEA is an atypia, it conveys the same risk of breast cancer that is associated with benign proliferative disease without atypia, and as such, patients should continue routine surveillance.[36] There is also no data to support the use of chemoprevention.

MANAGEMENT OF PATIENTS AT HIGH RISK FOR BREAST CANCER

Risk Factors

Breast cancer is the most common cancer in women in the United States. Approximately 200,000 women and 2000 men are diagnosed with invasive breast cancer each year. Breast cancer is the most common cancer in women of every major ethnic group, and the highest rate is among Caucasian women, with 122 newly diagnosed breast cancer cases per 100,000 women each year. Understanding the risk factors for breast cancer is important, as some of these risks can be modified to decrease a patient's risk either through lifestyle/behavioral changes and/or the use of chemoprevention.

Increasing Age

As a woman ages, her risk for breast cancer increases: birth to age 49, 1.9% probability of developing invasive breast cancer (1 in 53); age 50 to 59, 2.3% (1 in 43); age 60 to 69, 3.5% (1 in 29); age 70 and older, 6.7% (1 in 15). From birth to death, the probability of developing invasive breast cancer is 12.3% or 1 in 8.

Estrogen Exposure

A woman's lifetime exposure to estrogens appears to correlate with her risk for breast cancer. Exposure to estrogens can be approximated by age of first menarche, age of menopause, and age of first live birth, with nulliparous women who have an early menarche and a late menopause having the highest risk. Premenopausal women who undergo bilateral oophorectomy are at decreased risk. Given that high endogenous levels of estrogen are known to increase the risk of breast cancer in both premenopausal and postmenopausal women, the use of exogenous hormones and their associated risk for breast cancer has been studied and debated. The use of hormonal contraceptives does not appear to significantly increase the risk of breast cancer.[37] However, the use of hormone replacement therapy in postmenopausal women has been associated with an increased risk of breast cancer as reported in the Women's Health Initiative Estrogen Alone and Estrogen-Plus-Progestin Studies, which were stopped early secondary to this and other concerns.[38] In the Estrogen-Plus-Progestin study, the HRT used was a combined estrogen–progestin therapy (EPT) that was given to postmenopausal women with an intact uterus. The risk of breast cancer is relatively low, as EPT would result in an additional eight cases of breast cancer if 10,000 women took EPT for a year. Short-term use of less than 3 years does not appear to significantly increase the risk of breast cancer, and after the cessation of EPT use for 3 years, a woman's risk returns to baseline.

Given that lactation interrupts ovulation and modifies pituitary and ovarian hormone secretion, it has been postulated that breastfeeding can reduce breast cancer risk. This finding remains inconclusive. Limited data suggest that longer duration of lactation in premenopausal women may reduce risk. A pooled analysis consisting of over 50,000 women with breast cancer and 96,000 controls concluded that for every 12 months of breastfeeding, there was an associated 4.3% reduction in the relative risk of breast cancer.[39]

Environmental and Lifestyle Factors

Women who were subjected to ionizing radiation of the chest, such as for treatment of Hodgkin lymphoma or through exposure from nuclear plant accidents or the atomic bomb, have an increased risk of breast cancer. The prepuberty stage (age 10 to 14) appears to be the most vulnerable time for exposure, with little associated risk when exposure occurs after age of 45.[40] Alcohol use is associated with an increased risk of breast cancer and correlates with the amount of consumption, with differences noted with alcohol intake as low as three drinks per week versus those who abstain from alcohol. A meta-analysis of 110 studies shows a small but significant association (RR 1.05, 95% CI 1.02–1.08).[41] The relationship between cigarette use and breast cancer risk remains controversial because of unresolved issues of confounding and dose response, however a meta-analysis found that smoking before menarche and before the first birth was associated with an increased risk for breast cancer.[42] Furthermore, in women diagnosed with breast cancer, lifetime cigarette smoking (≥20 pack-years) was associated

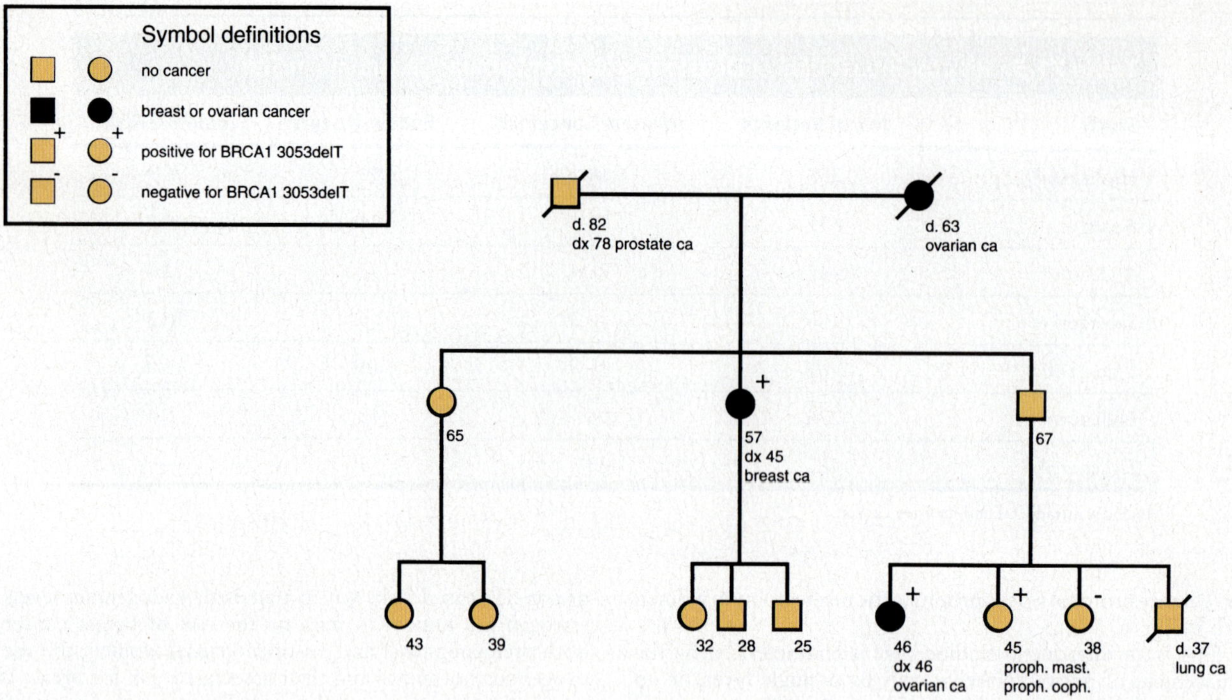

Figure 71.15. Pedigree of genetic breast cancer. The family illustrated in the pedigree carries a mutation of the BRCA1 gene; multiple relatives are affected with breast and ovarian cancer.

with an increased risk of recurrence and all-cause mortality.[42] The role of dietary factors such as fat intake, red meat and processed meat, phytoestrogens, calcium/vitamin D, and antioxidants in modifying breast cancer risk remains inconclusive. Regular physical exercise and a diet composed mainly of fruits and vegetables likely provide protection against breast cancer.

Family History

The number of first-degree relatives with breast cancer is strongly associated with a woman's risk for the future development of breast cancer. If one first-degree relative is affected, the risk of breast cancer increases by approximately twofold, and if two first-degree relatives are affected, the risk of breast cancer is increased by approximately threefold. The age at diagnosis of the first-degree relative is also important, as a women's risk is approximately threefold higher when the diagnosis occurs before age 30 but only 1.5-fold higher if the diagnosis is after age 60.[43]

When evaluating family history, it is important to note that the majority of breast cancers are caused by sporadic mutations (mutations that occur in somatic cells that cannot be inherited). When studying the family tree of women with *sporadic breast cancer*, these women typically have no family history of breast cancer through two generations, including siblings, offspring, parents, and both maternal and paternal aunts, uncles, and grandparents. Less than 10% of breast cancers are hereditary. In families with *hereditary breast cancer*, the family tree is characterized by earlier onset of breast cancer, bilateral breast cancer, a greater frequency of primary cancers such as breast and ovary, and an autosomal dominant inheritance pattern (**Fig. 71.15**).[44] For women who have first- or second-degree relatives with breast cancer but do not meet the hereditary breast cancer definition noted above, these women have *familial breast cancer* where it is likely that both genetic and environmental factors play a role in their susceptibility.[43]

The most commonly identified hereditary breast cancer mutations are in the *BRCA1* or *BRCA2* genes, which are localized to chromosome 17q21 and chromosome 13q12.3, respectively. Both serve as tumor suppressor genes and function as gatekeepers in controlling gene transcription, regulating repair of DNA damage (especially double-strand breaks during cell replication), and may play a role in the maintenance of genomic stability.[44] Founder mutations exist in the Ashkenazi Jewish population, with specific mutations in *BRCA1* (185delAG, 5382insC) and *BRCA2* (617delT).[44] Other BRCA-specific mutations have been identified in Dutch, Scandinavian, French–Canadian, and Belgian populations.[45]

The lifetime risk of breast cancer in *BRCA1* and *BRCA2* mutation carriers is estimated to be as high as 85%, which is markedly elevated from a baseline risk of 12% in the general population (**Table 71.6**). Ovarian cancer risk is higher

RESULTS

Table 71.6. Estimated Lifetime Cancer Risks for BRCA1 and BRCA2 Mutations (to Age 70)

Type of Cancer	General Population (%)	BRCA1 Carrier (%)	BRCA2 Carrier (%)
Breast cancer	8.0	40–85	40–85
Contralateral breast cancer	0.5–1/y	40–65	40–65
Male breast cancer	0.1	1–5	5–10
Ovarian cancer	1.4	30–45	10–20

Modified from Isaacs C, Peshkin BN, Lerman C. Evaluation and management of women with a strong family history of breast cancer. In: Harris JR, Lippman ME, Morrow M, et al., eds. *Diseases of the Breast*. 3rd ed. Lippincott Williams & Wilkins; 2004:316.

in *BRCA1* carriers with an estimated risk of 40% to 60% whereas *BRCA2* carriers have a risk of 15%. Among male patients with breast cancer who have a *BRCA* mutation, one-third of mutations involve *BRCA1* and two-thirds involve *BRCA2*. The risk of breast cancer in males is 1% to 5% with a *BRCA1* mutation, and 5% to 10% with a *BRCA2* mutation, versus a risk of 0.1% in the general population.[46] In addition, prostate and pancreatic cancers are more common in patients with *BRCA2* mutations.[46]

Prior to genetic testing, patients should undergo genetic counseling where the complexities of testing are discussed along with potential emotional and financial ramifications that can result from positive test results. Ideally, genetic testing should start with a family member affected with breast or ovarian cancer or both. If that individual tests negative, further testing on an unaffected relative is unlikely to be informative. Candidates for gene testing have expanded over time. This has historically included those with a known *BRCA1* or *BRCA2* gene mutation in the family, a personal history of breast cancer at age 45 or younger, a personal history of breast cancer at age 50 or younger and a family member (parent, sibling, child, grandparent, grandchild, uncle, aunt, nephew, niece or first cousin) diagnosed with breast cancer at any age, a personal history of triple-negative breast cancer (TNBC) diagnosed at age 60 or younger, a personal history of ovarian cancer, a personal or family history of male breast cancer, and Ashkenazi Jewish heritage and a personal or family history of breast or ovarian cancer per consensus guidelines. Once an individual tests positive for a mutation, she should inform her first- and second-degree relatives of their risk status and the potential for DNA testing.

It is now standard to perform panel testing on patients suspected of having hereditary breast cancer. In addition, genetic testing is considered or recommended for nearly all women newly diagnosed with breast cancer. Other breast cancer susceptibility genes that have become more commonly recognized due to panel testing procedures include *p53*, *ATM*, PALB2, CHEK2, *CDH1*, and *PTEN*. The Li–Fraumeni or sarcoma, breast, leukemia, and adrenal gland (SBLA) syndrome corresponds with *p53* mutations and includes a broad spectrum of cancers including sarcoma, breast cancer and brain tumors, lung and laryngeal cancer, leukemia, lymphoma, and adrenal cortical carcinoma.[47] The *ATM* gene mutation results in a childhood neurologic disorder referred to as ataxia-telangiectasia which is characterized by progressive cerebellar and neuromotor deterioration, telangiectasia of the conjunctivae and facial skin, and growth retardation. Females with the *ATM* mutation have a five times higher risk for developing breast cancers than the general population.[48] Females with the *CDH1* or E-cadherin gene mutation have a 70% lifetime risk for diffuse gastric cancer and a 40% risk for lobular breast cancer.[49] Distinctive mucocutaneous lesions referred to as trichilemmomas characterize Cowden disease, which is associated with an increased risk of breast, thyroid, and genitourinary tract cancers in women, resulting from the *PTEN* gene mutation.[50]

Clinical Risk Assessment

4 Through large population studies, numerous factors that can increase breast cancer risk have been identified as summarized in **Table 71.7**. In an effort to quantitate these potential risks such that preventive strategies can be better tailored, multiple risk assessment tools have been developed including the BCRAT or the Gail model 2,[51] BRCAPRO,[52] BOADICEA,[53] Tyrer–Cuzick,[54] and the Breast cancer surveillance consortium.[55] The Gail model calculates risk over a defined time interval and predicts risk accurately in groups of women 35 years of age and older who undergo annual mammography. The model is not for women who have a strong family history of breast cancer (such as genetic mutation carriers) or those with LCIS. The components of the Gail model include current age, age at menarche, age at time of first live birth, number of first-degree relatives with breast cancer, number of prior breast biopsies, prior breast biopsy with atypia, and race. A sample risk calculation is shown in **Figure 71.16**. Women are considered to be high-risk if their 5-year risk is >1.7%, or if their lifetime risk of breast cancer is at least 20%.

CLASSIFICATION

Table 71.7. Magnitude of Known Breast Cancer Risk Factors

Relative Risk <2
Early menarche
Late menopause
Nulliparity
Proliferative benign disease
Obesity
Alcohol use
Hormone replacement therapy
Relative Risk 2–4
Age >35 first birth
First-degree relative with breast cancer
Radiation exposure
Prior breast cancer
Relative Risk >4
Gene mutation
Lobular carcinoma in situ
Atypical hyperplasia

Management

All women at high risk for breast cancer should undergo genetic counseling, with education provided about the risk factors, genetics, and natural history of breast cancer. These women should be followed with enhanced surveillance, and chemoprevention or prophylactic surgery should be considered. For women who have a genetic predisposition, such as those with a *BRCA1* or *BRCA2* mutation, many experts support aggressive surveillance, including CBE biannually beginning at age 20, and annual mammography and MRI screening performed in a staggered fashion such that imaging occurs every 6 months starting at age 25. The use of screening MRI for women at high risk is supported by numerous studies. Prophylactic mastectomies can be considered at any age; many women prefer to defer this until after childbearing, as they would like to breastfeed. Ovarian cancer screening for *BRCA1* and *BRCA2* carriers includes transvaginal ovarian ultrasound, serum CA-125, and annual pelvic exams starting at age 30. When childbearing is complete, prophylactic oophorectomies should be considered. In women with a family history but no

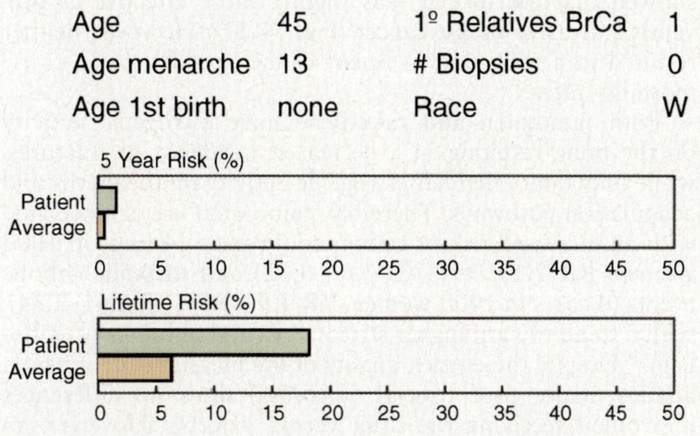

Figure 71.16. Breast cancer risk assessment according to the Gail model. This woman's 5-year risk for the development of breast cancer is 1.6%, and her lifetime risk is 18%.

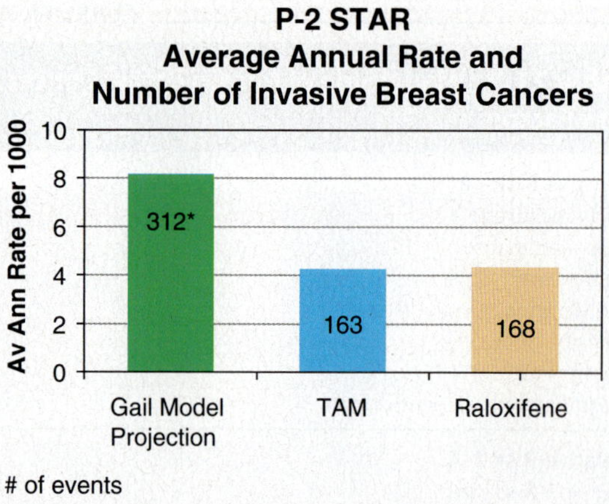

Figure 71.17. Both tamoxifen and raloxifene when taken for 5 years in the National Surgical Adjuvant Breast and Bowel Project P-2 (STAR trial) were equally effective at reducing the risk of invasive breast cancer.

known genetic abnormality, screening mammography should begin 10 years before the age of onset in the youngest diagnosed first-degree relative or at age 40. Furthermore, in the absence of a genetic abnormality, women who have a lifetime risk of breast cancer >20% should also be monitored with annual screening MRI.

In addition to its role in the treatment of breast cancer, endocrine therapy (chemoprevention) can reduce the risk of invasive and/or in situ breast cancers in women at high risk for breast cancer. Women who are known to benefit from chemoprevention include those >35 years with a history of LCIS, DCIS, or atypical proliferative lesions of the breast, women between 35 and 59 years with a Gail model risk of breast cancer >1.7% over 5 years, and women with known *BRCA1* or *BRCA2* mutations who do not undergo bilateral prophylactic mastectomies. Currently, there is no data regarding the risks and benefits of chemoprevention in male patients with breast cancer, and as such, the use of these agents in men is not recommended.

For pre- and postmenopausal women at increased risk of breast cancer, both tamoxifen and raloxifene can be used. As SERMs, both agents block the effects of endogenous estrogen on normal breast tissue and breast cancer. Using data from four trials in the 2013 US Preventive Services Task Force (USPSTF) meta-analysis, tamoxifen has been shown to reduce the risk of estrogen receptor (ER)–positive breast cancer (RR 0.70, 95% CI 0.59–0.82). Similarly, using data from two trials in the 2013 USPSTF meta-analysis, raloxifene reduced the risk of ER–positive breast cancers (RR 0.44, 95% CI 0.27–0.71).[56] In terms of the choice between tamoxifen and raloxifene, the STAR trial directly compared tamoxifen with raloxifene and showed that the former was slightly more effective at preventing invasive breast cancer (**Fig. 71.17**). However, neither resulted in a reduction in breast cancer-specific, or all-cause mortality rates.[57]

Both tamoxifen and raloxifene have estrogenic activity on the bone resulting in a decreased incidence of fractures, while only tamoxifen has estrogenic activity on the uterus and coagulation pathways. Therefore, tamoxifen use is associated with an increased risk of endometrial cancer (4 cases in 1000 women, RR 2.13, 95% CI 1.36–3.32) and thromboembolic events (4 cases in 1000 women, RR 1.93, 95% CI 1.41–2.64), with a trend toward higher stroke rates and pulmonary embolism.[35] Despite these risks, quality of life measures (depression, anxiety, major psychosocial outcomes) show no differences in women receiving the drug versus placebo. However, an increase in vasomotor symptoms, gynecologic symptoms, and problems of sexual functioning was noted.[35] As congenital anomalies have been associated with tamoxifen, women with childbearing potential must implement an effective contraceptive method. For women desiring a pregnancy, tamoxifen should be discontinued for at least 2 months prior to attempting pregnancy.

In postmenopausal women, studies show that AIs are a reasonable alternative to tamoxifen and raloxifene. AIs suppress plasma estrogen levels by inhibition of aromatase, an enzyme that converts androgens to estrogens. Although AIs are commonly used for breast cancer treatment, they are not approved in the United States for breast cancer prevention at this time. Also, while both the USPSTF and ASCO support the use of SERMs for both premenopausal and postmenopausal women, only ASCO considers the use of exemestane as a reasonable alternative to SERMs for postmenopausal women.[58] More recently, the International Breast Cancer Intervention Study (IBIS-II trial) showed that high-risk postmenopausal women who took the AI anastrozole had a 50% reduction in the number of invasive breast cancers and DCIS compared to placebo. The side effects of anastrozole include musculoskeletal problems, hypertension, vaginal dryness, and vasomotor symptoms.[59] AIs may also be associated with a loss of bone
5 density.

The decision to proceed with endocrine therapy chemoprevention must be individualized. In general, the data support the use of endocrine therapy versus observation. For premenopausal and postmenopausal women, tamoxifen or raloxifene are both reasonable options. If a woman's primary concern is breast cancer prevention, then tamoxifen should be chosen. However, if there are risk factors for uterine cancer and/or thromboembolic complications, raloxifene is a reasonable alternative. If a postmenopausal woman does not want to take a SERM, then an AI can be prescribed.

DUCTAL CARCINOMA IN SITU (DCIS)

DCIS is commonly defined as the proliferation of malignant epithelial cells within the mammary ductal system with no evidence of invasion into the surrounding stroma on routine light microscopic examination (**Fig. 71.18**). It is further categorized by its size, nuclear grade, presence and extent of comedo necrosis, and architectural pattern. Common histologic subtypes of DCIS include comedo, cribriform, micropapillary, papillary, and solid. DCIS is designated as Tis (DCIS) by the TNM staging system and considered a Stage 0 breast cancer. The incidence of DCIS increases with age and is uncommon in women younger than 30 years. In women aged 50 to 64 years, the risk is as high as 88 per 100,000 women. Among the breast cancers diagnosed in the United States, 25% are DCIS. The risk of development of metastases and/or death in women with DCIS is rare (<1%).

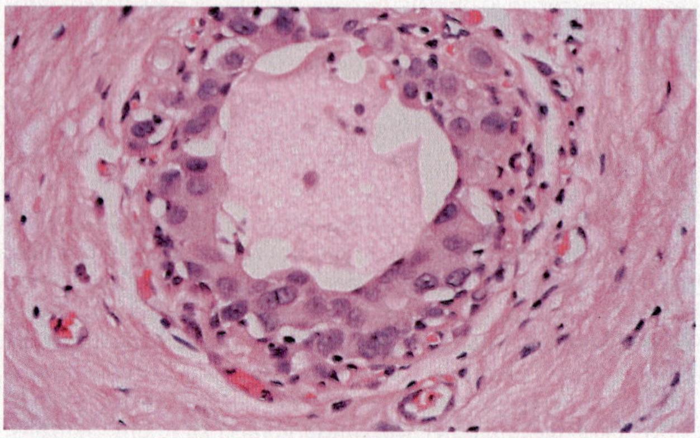

Figure 71.18. Photomicrograph of ductal carcinoma in situ. The abnormal cells do not cross the ductal basement membrane. The necrotic debris in the center of the duct is responsible for the calcification visible on mammography.

Most patients with DCIS will present with no breast-related symptoms or findings on physical examination. More than 90% of all cases of DCIS are detected on imaging studies—commonly as microcalcifications on mammography. Prior to routine screening mammography, DCIS presented as a palpable mass, in association with nipple discharge, or as Paget disease. Although most patients with DCIS have microcalcifications of indeterminate morphology, patterns that are highly suggestive of DCIS include linear branching or segmental types of pleomorphic microcalcifications.

Once an abnormal lesion is detected by diagnostic imaging, the diagnosis of DCIS is typically confirmed by breast biopsy. Of note, when DCIS is diagnosed initially by core biopsy, 15% to 20% of lesions will be upgraded to invasive cancer at the time of definitive resection. Large, high-grade DCIS lesions are more likely to have an invasive component.

Surgical options for the treatment of DCIS include breast-conserving surgery as a component of breast conservation therapy (BCT) (partial mastectomy and postoperative RT) or simple mastectomy. Although there is no randomized trial that has ever compared the treatment of DCIS by mastectomy with treatment by BCT, a large number of clinical studies have shown that the local recurrence rate of BCT is 10% to 15% after 10 years and that approximately half of the local recurrences are invasive carcinoma. Mastectomy is curative in 98% of patients with DCIS, regardless of the tumor grade or the size of the lesion. However, both surgical treatment options are associated with equivalent long-term survival as shown in both retrospective and prospective analyses. Given that partial mastectomy is a much less invasive surgical procedure, BCT is typically recommended over mastectomy. Mastectomy should be performed if BCT is contraindicated or based on patient preference. BCT is contraindicated with multicentric disease, extensive disease where resection would result in poor cosmesis, and in patients who cannot receive RT. For patients undergoing mastectomy, immediate breast reconstruction options should be reviewed.

BCT typically includes a partial mastectomy with negative surgical margins, followed by RT to eradicate any residual disease. RT is typically recommended, except in rare circumstances (see section on ***Breast Cancer in the Elderly***). Four prospective, randomized clinical trials—NSABP B-17 (1998, 2001), EORTC 10853 (2006), United Kingdom (2003), and the SweDCIS (2008) have focused on the role of RT in the treatment of DCIS (**Table 71.8**). Despite differences in study design, the results are very similar, demonstrating a 50% to 60% reduction in local recurrence with surgical excision and RT compared to surgical excision alone. Furthermore, the results of NSABP B-17 confirm that the reduction in local recurrence persists through 12 years of follow-up. However, no survival benefit from RT was observed. Patients with comedo necrosis, uncertain margins, and/or those at highest risk for recurrence appear to benefit most from RT. However, even in the most favorable subgroup (absent or slight comedo necrosis, clear margins), RT was associated with a reduction in the absolute incidence of breast recurrence by 7% at 8 years.

Given the risks, inconvenience, and cost associated with RT, attempts have been made to define a subgroup of patients with DCIS who may not require RT. The ECOG 5194 study investigated patients undergoing local excision alone in women with low-risk DCIS (low- to intermediate-grade DCIS lesions were <2.5 cm, and high-grade DCIS lesions were <1.0 cm). Margins were at least 3 mm, and a postexcision mammogram was obtained for all patients to document the adequacy of surgical resection. Tamoxifen following excision was allowed but not required. At a median follow-up of 6.7 years, the local recurrence rate at 5 years was 6.1% (95% CI 4.1% to 8.2%) for patients with low- to intermediate-grade DCIS ($n = 565$), and 15.3% (95% CI 8.2% to 22.5%) for patients with high-grade DCIS ($n = 105$). These findings suggest that local excision alone may be sufficient for select patients with low- to intermediate-grade DCIS. However, identifying these patients remains a challenge.

Other models which have attempted to predict the likelihood of local recurrence following excision alone in patients with DCIS include the Van Nuys Prognostic Index (VNPI) and its updated version, the University of Southern California Van Nuys Prognostic Index (USC/VNPI). Patients are classified into three groups based on pathologic classification: (1) non–high-grade DCIS without comedo type necrosis, (2) non–high-grade DCIS with comedo type necrosis, and (3) high-grade DCIS with or without comedo type necrosis. The USC/VNPI score (range is 4 to 12) is then calculated based on the pathologic classification score and points given for margins, tumor size, and the patient's age. The study's conclusion is that women with an overall low score (4, 5, 6) did not require RT. However, attempts to replicate and validate the USC/VNPI score in other datasets have had varying success, and as such, it is not commonly used.

Gene expression analysis has been explored in an attempt to distinguish patients who may omit postexcision RT. One such risk profile, which integrates key cancer biologic pathways and clinicopathologic factors (DCISionRT; PreludeDx, Inc., Laguna Hills, CA, USA), has previously been shown to prognosticate 10-year total and invasive breast cancer risks and also predict the benefit of adjuvant RT.[59]

Axillary lymph node involvement in DCIS is rare, and sentinel lymph node biopsy is not indicated during breast-conserving surgery. In the NSABP B-17 and B-24 trials, the axillary recurrence rates, irrespective of treatment, were 0.83 and 0.36 per 1000 patient-years of follow-up. If a patient is undergoing a mastectomy following core needle biopsy, SLN biopsy can be considered as it is possible that an occult invasive breast cancer will be identified, and SLNB is often not feasible after

SURGICAL ENDOCRINOLOGY

RESULTS

Table 71.8. Results of Randomized Trials of Radiotherapy in Ductal Carcinoma in Situ

Study	Patients (No.)	Median Follow-up (mo)	IBTR (%)	
			E	RT
NSABP B-17	813	44	40	17
EORTC 10853	1,010	126	26	15
United Kingdom	1,030	53	14	6
SweDCIS	1,046	96 (mean)	27	12

DCIS, ductal carcinoma in situ; E, excision alone; EORTC, European Organization for Research and Treatment of Cancer; IBTR, ipsilateral breast tumor recurrence; NSABP, National Surgical Adjuvant Breast Project; RT, radiation therapy.

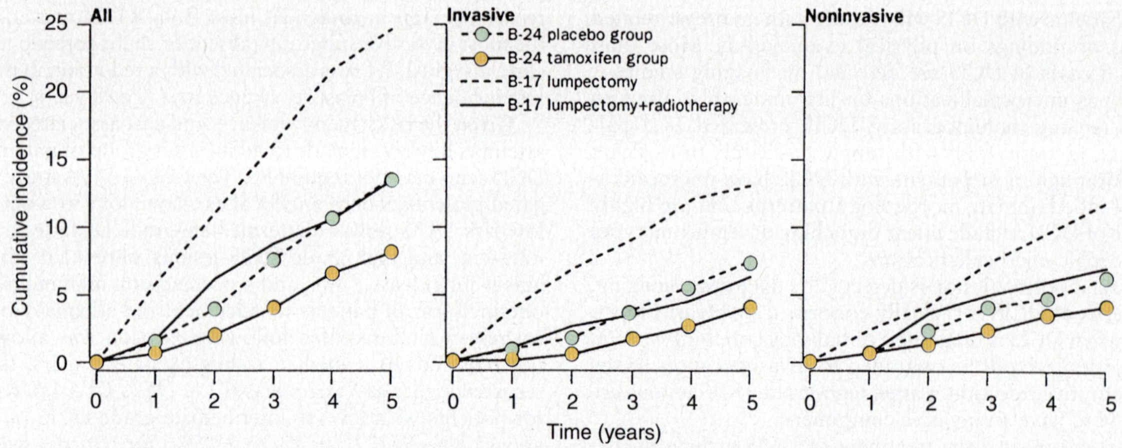

Figure 71.19. Benefits of radiation therapy and tamoxifen in ductal carcinoma in situ. The cumulative incidence of breast cancer events in the ipsilateral and contralateral breasts for patients treated in the National Surgical Adjuvant Breast and Bowel Project B-17 and B-24 trials is shown. The reduction in recurrence is greatest for patients receiving radiotherapy and tamoxifen.

mastectomy. However, techniques of delayed SLN biopsy are now possible with the use of magnetic tracer injection at the time of mastectomy.

After breast-conserving surgery, a postexcision mammogram should be considered prior to the initiation of RT to ensure that there are no persistent residual suspicious calcifications. Treatment for DCIS after breast-conserving surgery is not considered complete without adjuvant RT (see section on ***Radiation Therapy***).

There is no role for chemotherapy in DCIS. However, endocrine therapy is commonly recommended. Fifty percent to 75% of DCIS specimens express estrogen and progesterone receptors (PRs). Tamoxifen remains the standard treatment for chemoprevention in patients with a history of DCIS. The benefit of tamoxifen therapy in decreasing local recurrence rates is supported by both a meta-analysis of two randomized trials and by NSABP B-24. The meta-analysis consists of 3375 women and shows that tamoxifen after surgery for DCIS reduces recurrence of both ipsilateral DCIS (HR 0.75; 95% CI 0.61–0.92) and contralateral DCIS (HR 0.50; 95% CI 0.28–0.87) (**Fig. 71.19**). There is also a trend toward decreased ipsilateral invasive cancer (HR 0.79; 95% CI 0.62–1.01) and reduced contralateral invasive cancer (HR 0.57; 95% CI 0.39–0.83). The number needed to treat in order for tamoxifen to have a protective effect against all breast events was 15. However, there was no difference in all-cause mortality (RR 1.11; 95% CI 0.89–1.39). In a retrospective review of NSABP B-24, it was found that at 10 years of follow-up, patients ($n = 732$) with ER-positive DCIS treated with tamoxifen had significant decreases in any subsequent (invasive and/or noninvasive; ipsilateral and/or contralateral) breast cancer events compared with those who received placebo (HR 0.58, 95% CI 0.42–0.81, $P < .0015$).

Management of patients with DCIS who have not undergone bilateral mastectomies includes consideration of tamoxifen for 5 years rather than observation, recognizing that although there is an improvement in recurrence rates, there is no proven survival benefit per consensus guidelines. In women who have undergone bilateral mastectomies, the risks associated with tamoxifen use likely outweigh the benefits. Furthermore, tamoxifen is not typically recommended for patients with ER-negative DCIS.

EVALUATION OF THE PATIENT WITH BREAST CANCER

Breast cancer is a heterogeneous disease that can be characterized further based on clinical and pathologic features. Further characterization and staging of breast cancer in newly diagnosed breast cancer patients can facilitate definitive treatment. Pathologic, biologic, and anatomic characteristics are used in combination to predict prognosis and response to therapy.

AJCC TNM Staging

The American Joint Committee on Cancer (AJCC) TNM staging system for breast cancer is an internationally accepted system used to characterize the extent of disease, predict prognosis, and facilitate medical decision making. Unlike the seventh edition, this new staging system is no longer just based on anatomic findings (TNM anatomic stage groups) but now includes pathologic prognostic (TNM pathologic prognosis stage groups) and clinical prognostic (TNM clinical prognostic stage groups) factors by incorporating such things as tumor grade and receptor status (estrogen, progesterone, HER2 amplification). The system we will discuss in detail is the TNM anatomic staging system, where breast cancer is classified on the basis of the primary tumor type (invasive or in situ) and size (T), the presence or absence of regional lymph node involvement (N), and the presence or absence of distant metastases (M).

Noninvasive breast cancers are noted as Tis and further classified into Tis (DCIS) and Tis (Paget). LCIS is now considered a benign entity and, as such, not classified as Tis. T1 tumors are invasive cancers ≤20 mm; T2 tumors are >20 mm but ≤50 mm; whereas T3 tumors are >50 mm. T4 tumors are any size with direct extension to the chest wall and or the skin, resulting in nodules or ulcerations. Invasion of cancer into the dermis alone does not qualify as T4. IBC, which is defined by typical skin changes involving a third or more of the skin of the breast, is classified as T4d.

Lymph node classification criteria differ depending on whether the lymph nodes were clinically or pathologically assessed and, as such, are designated as cN or pN, respectively. When possible, pathologic classification is preferred. Regional lymph nodes are defined as those of the ipsilateral axilla, ipsilateral intramammary, internal mammary nodes, and supraclavicular nodes. Metastasis to any other lymph node, including cervical or to the contralateral axillary lymph node, is classified as distant disease (M1). In regard to the clinical classification of the regional lymph nodes, cN0 refers to no regional lymph node metastases. Mobile level I and II axillary lymph nodes containing metastases that are ipsilateral are considered cN1, whereas fixed or matted nodes are cN2. When metastases occur in the infraclavicular lymph nodes, ipsilateral internal mammary lymph nodes *and* axillary lymph nodes, or in the ipsilateral supraclavicular lymph nodes, it is classified as cN3.

In order to discuss the pathologic classification of regional lymph nodes, it is important to note that breast cancer metastases must be greater than 0.2 mm and exceed 200 cells in a single histologic lymph node cross section to be considered clinically relevant. As such pN0 refers to no regional lymph node metastases, pN1mi is used to describe micrometastases (greater than 0.2 mm or more than 200 cells, but none greater than 2.0 mm), and pN1 is used to describe metastases in one to three lymph nodes, and/or internal mammary nodes with metastases detected by SLN biopsy but not clinically detected. pN2 disease occurs when metastases are present in four to nine axillary lymph nodes or in clinically detected internal mammary lymph nodes in the absence of axillary lymph node metastases. pN3 disease includes metastases in 10 or more axillary lymph nodes, metastases to the infraclavicular (level III axillary) lymph nodes, in clinically detected ipsilateral internal mammary lymph nodes in the presence of one or more positive level I, or II axillary lymph nodes, in more than three axillary lymph nodes and in internal mammary lymph nodes with micrometastases or macrometastases detected by SLN biopsy but not clinically detected, or in ipsilateral supraclavicular lymph nodes.

Distant metastasis (M1) is defined as detectable metastases as determined by classical clinical and radiographic means and/or histologically proven larger than 0.2 mm. When no clinical or radiographic evidence of distant metastases is present, but deposits of molecularly or microscopically detected tumor cells are found in circulating blood, bone marrow or other nonregional nodal tissue that are no larger than 0.2 mm in a patient with no symptoms of metastases the designation used is cMO(i+).

The particular combination of the T, N, and M characteristics defines the overall breast cancer stage. Although the TNM staging system estimates predicted survival, it should not be used alone to dictate treatment.

Histologic Subtype and Tumor Grade

Most invasive breast cancers arise from epithelial elements and are categorized as carcinomas, consisting of several histologic subtypes. Based on the Surveillance Epidemiology and End Results (SEER) database of the National Cancer Institute between 1992 and 2001, estimated percentages of each histologic subtype of breast cancer in a series involving 135,157 women showed infiltrating ductal carcinoma (IDC) as the most common (76%), followed by invasive lobular (8%), ductal/lobular (7%), mucinous/colloid (2.4%), tubular (1.5%), medullary (1.2%), and then papillary (1%).

IDC is the most common type of invasive breast cancer. On gross pathologic evaluation, these lesions are typically firm, gray-white, gritty masses. Cytologic features of these cells range from low grade to highly malignant. Microscopically, these cancers are characterized by cords and nests of tumors cells with varying amounts of gland formation. As these cancer cells infiltrate the breast parenchyma, they induce a fibrous response, resulting in their characteristic irregular, stellate shape. Often IDC is associated with a variable amount of DCIS.

Infiltrating lobular carcinomas (ILC) are the second most common type of breast cancer. The incidence rate of lobular carcinoma is rising faster than the rate of ductal carcinoma in the United States. Furthermore, postmenopausal hormone therapy use may be more strongly associated with lobular carcinoma that ductal carcinoma. Although some ILC may appear similar to IDC macroscopically, others may not show a mass lesion with the excised tissue appearing normal or having only a slightly firm consistency. As such, the microscopic size of ILC may be much greater than what is measured grossly. Unlike IDC, ILC induces only a minimal fibrous reaction. Microscopically, these tumors are characterized by small cells that insidiously infiltrate the mammary stroma and adipose tissue individually and in a single file pattern, often growing in a target-like configuration around normal breast ducts. LCIS or DCIS may be present with ILC. There is a higher frequency of bilateral and multicentric disease with ILC than IDC. ILC are more common in older women, and are typically larger but more differentiated than IDC. ILC are almost always ER positive. The prognosis for ILC and IDC appears to be similar, however, recent reports suggest that the short-term prognosis for ILC may be more favorable. ILC tend to metastasize later than IDC and spread to unusual locations such as the peritoneum, meninges, and the gastrointestinal tract. Furthermore, lobular breast cancers have been observed in families that carry germline mutations in *CDH1*, the gene that encodes for the E-cadherin protein. The lack of E-cadherin can be used to distinguish ILC from IDC.

Mucinous (colloid) carcinoma is a less common histologic subtype that is more common in older patients. On gross examination, these tumors have a soft gelatinous appearance and tend to be well circumscribed. Microscopically, they are characterized by nests of tumor cells, with uniform and low-grade nuclei, dispersed in large pools of extracellular mucus. These lesions have a favorable prognosis. Another histologic subtype with favorable prognosis is tubular carcinoma, which is characterized by the presence of well-formed tubular or glandular structures infiltrating the stroma. The tumor cells are low grade and are often associated with low-grade DCIS. Metastatic disease is rare with tubular carcinoma.

Medullary carcinomas are well circumscribed, soft, tan masses with areas of hemorrhage and necrosis. Microscopically, the tumor cells are poorly differentiated, grow in a syncytial pattern, and have an intense lymphoplasmacytic infiltrate. These cancers occur more frequently in younger patients and are more frequent in women with *BRCA1* mutations, although the majority of breast cancers in patients with *BRCA1* mutation are not medullary. Despite, their aggressive histologic appearance, medullary carcinomas are associated with a more favorable prognosis than IDC.

Other breast cancer subtypes include macropapillary carcinomas which are highly aggressive and have a tendency for lymph node metastasis even when small in size. Also likely associated with a worse prognosis, metaplastic carcinomas are well circumscribed tumors that contain various combinations of poorly differentiated ductal adenocarcinoma, mesenchymal (sarcomatous), and other epithelial (eg, squamous cell) components. When the squamous cell component predominates, the tumors tend to be more aggressive and are frequently refractory to treatment when compared with IDC. Unlike IDC, metaplastic breast cancers tend to have fewer T1 tumors, more node-negative tumors, more poorly differentiated or undifferentiated tumors, and have fewer ER–positive tumors. Metaplastic breast cancers are treated similarly to other invasive breast cancers.

The grade of a breast cancer is determined by a combination of the architectural and cytologic features, usually assessed by utilizing the Elston–Ellis modification of the Scarff–Bloom–Richardson scoring system. This system is based on three parameters including tubule formation, nuclear pleomorphism, and mitotic activity. Each category is assigned a score of 1 to 3 and then a summation score of 3 to 9. The lowest possible score is 3 with scores of 3 to 5 defined as grade 1, 6 or 7 as grade 2, and 8 or 9 as grade 3. Cells that infiltrate the stroma as solid nests of glands and where the nuclei are relatively uniform with little or no evidence of mitotic activity are referred to as well differentiated or grade 1 tumors. When the tumor cells infiltrate as solid nests with some glandular differentiation and nuclear pleomorphism is present, the tumor is categorized as grade 2 or moderately differentiated. In addition, the mitotic activity is moderate. In poorly differentiated or grade 3 tumors, solid nests of neoplastic cells without evidence of gland formation are present. In addition, there is marked nuclear atypia and high mitotic activity.

Biomarker Profile (ER, PR, HER2)

As targeted therapies exist targeting breast cancers that express the ER, PR, and/or the HER2 protein, these biomarkers have significant treatment implications. As such, when an invasive breast cancer is diagnosed, expression of these biomarkers is determined. Using immunohistochemistry and image analysis, ER and PR are considered positive if greater than or equal to 10% of cells stain positive. The Allred score is another method to quantify ER and PR expression. The Allred score integrates the percentage of cells that stain positive, with the intensity of staining to give a score of 0 to 8. The goal of the Allred score is to quantify ER expression based on the likelihood that a breast cancer patient will respond to endocrine therapy. One of the benefits of the Allred score is that by integrating both the percentage and intensity of staining, patients with <10% staining may be identified who benefit from endocrine therapy. The receptor tyrosine kinase protein HER2 is a member of the epidermal growth factor receptor family and its amplification or overexpression has been shown to contribute to breast cancer development and progression. HER2 can now be targeted using monoclonal antibodies and small molecule inhibitors. Using immunohistochemistry and image analysis, HER2 is scored 0, 1+, 2+, and 3+. Positivity is noted as 3+, whereas scores of 0 and 1+ are considered negative. A score of 2+ is considered indeterminate and further testing for gene amplification can be performed using either FISH (fluorescence in situ hybridization) or CISH (chromogenic in situ hybridization). The HER2 FISH assay is based on the gene copy number and the ratio between the number of HER2 and chromosome enumeration probe 17 (CEP17) sequences, with positivity defined as a HER2/CEP17 ratio ≥2.0. Positivity is also defined as HER2 copy number ≥6.0 signals/cell even if the HER2/CEP17 ratio is <2.0. Alternatively, a more cost effective and comparable method to FISH testing is the HER2 CISH assay.

The Ki-67 antigen is present in all phases of the cell cycle except for the G0/resting phase and reflects of the proliferative potential of a breast cancer. Ki-67 is determined by IHC and noted as a percentage, where <10% is considered a low proliferative index, 10% to 20% is considered borderline, and >20% is considered high. The Ki-67 index can also be used to measure the response to endocrine therapy.

Molecular Subtyping

Recent advances in molecular biology, including the development of sophisticated techniques for gene expression profiling, have established a new taxonomy of breast cancer, defining molecular subtypes of breast cancer. This new taxonomy has had a profound impact on the clinical management of breast cancer, as the molecular subtypes differ markedly in prognosis and response to therapy. As gene expression profiling is not routinely performed on clinical specimens, molecular subtypes have been approximated based on expression of the ER, PR, HER2 expression, and other biomarkers. Commonly defined subtypes include luminal A (ER+, PR+, HER2−, Ki-67 < 14%), luminal B (ER+ and or PR+, HER2±, Ki-67 ≥ 14%), HER2 (ER and PR−, HER2+), and basal like (ER, PR, and HER−). Luminal A and B subtypes have ER expression, however the former group has a much better overall survival (OS). Luminal B HER2+ and HER2 subtypes benefit from targeted therapies against HER2. Furthermore, both HER2 and basal-like breast cancers are known to have higher initial responses to anthracycline-based chemotherapy than the luminal subtypes but are associated with a decreased disease-free survival.

Breast MRI

Although there is no data from prospective randomized trials demonstrating improved outcomes with the addition of MRI to the diagnostic evaluation of newly diagnosed breast cancers, the consensus guidelines suggest that diagnostic MRI should be considered in patients with newly diagnosed breast cancer when (1) the clinical extent of disease appears larger than what is observed on mammography, (2) there is concern about pectoralis muscle involvement, (3) there is no evidence of a breast primary in the presence of axillary lymph node metastases, (4) there is no disease identified on physical examination or mammography in the presence of PDB, (5) in women at very high risk for contralateral breast cancers such as those with *BRCA1/2* mutations, and (6) to help determine the extent of disease prior to treatment. Of note, MRI is associated with a high false-positive rate, and many MRI-detected abnormalities will need to be biopsied in order to meaningfully interpret the results of the MRI.

Sentinel Lymph Node Biopsy

Breast cancer spread to ipsilateral axillary lymph nodes is common, occurring in 15% to 30% of patients. The presence of axillary lymph node metastases has important prognostic implications and can impact medical, surgical, and radiation oncology decision making. However, axillary lymph node dissection (ALND) has significant risks, and the therapeutic impact of axillary surgery remains to be clearly defined. Currently, SLNB is the procedure of choice for staging of the axilla in breast cancer. Axillary ultrasound has also been used and can facilitate evaluation of patients with an equivocal physical examination (**Table 71.9**).

6 The SLN hypothesis predicts that breast cancers metastasize to one or a few lymph nodes prior to involving other lymph nodes in the corresponding lymph node basin. Prospective studies have confirmed this hypothesis, demonstrating that the pathology of the SLN accurately predicts the pathology of the corresponding axillary lymph node basin (**Table 71.10**). SLNB has significantly fewer complications than ALND, with the risk of lymphedema being significantly lower (2% after SLNB vs 13% after ALND at 12 months).

The SLNB procedure begins with localization of the SLN through injection of radioactive colloid and/or blue dye. Given that the combined use of both tracers appears to be complementary and that failed SLN identification is minimized when both tracers are used, this is our recommended approach. A systematic review by an expert panel convened by ASCO concluded that the use of both blue dye and radioactive colloid was associated with a trend toward a lower false-negative rate.

Prior to surgery, radioactive technetium sulfur colloid is injected either peritumorally, intradermally, or into the subareolar plexus. Lymphoscintigraphy can be performed to identify areas of increased radioactivity. Alternatively, a handheld gamma probe can be used to survey the axilla and identify hot spots. The patient is then brought to the operating room and positioned with the ipsilateral arm abducted up to 90 degrees. The breast, anterior chest wall, and axilla are prepped and draped in the usual standard sterile fashion. Five milliliters of blue dye (isosulfan or methylene blue dye) is injected either around the tumor periphery, at the palpable edge of the biopsy cavity, or into the subareolar plexus. Blue dye should not be injected directly into the tumor itself, as the lymphatics may be occluded by tumor. Likewise, blue dye should not be injected into the seroma cavity following breast surgery, as the seroma cavity may not have sufficient lymphatic drainage. For these reasons, we typically inject into the subareolar plexus. Breast

Table 71.9. Approach to the Axillary Nodes

Finding	Approach
Clinically negative	Sentinel lymph node biopsy
Radiographically suspicious	Fine-needle aspiration (image guided) If no metastatic disease identified, then sentinel lymph node biopsy If metastatic disease is identified, consideration for axillary lymph node dissection
Clinically suspicious	Fine-needle aspiration (image or hand guided) Follow-up management as for radiographically suspicious

Table 71.10. Results of Prospective, Multi-Institutional Studies of Lymphatic Mapping and Sentinel Node Biopsy

Study	No. of Patients	% SN Identification	% False Negative
ACOSOG Z10[60]	5,237	98.7	N/A
ALMANAC[61]	803	96.1	6.7
NSABP B-32[62]	5,611	97.1	9.8
Sentinella/GIVOM[63]	697	95	16.7

ACOSOG, American College of Surgeons Oncology Group; ALMANAC, Axillary Lymphatic Mapping Against Nodal Axillary Clearance; GIVOM, Gruppo Interdisciplinare Veneto Oncologia Mammaria; NSABP, National Surgical Adjuvant Breast and Bowel Project; SN, sentinel node.

massage is performed for 5 minutes to dilate the breast lymphatics and facilitate lymphatic drainage.

Isosulfan blue can be used for SLNB; however, anaphylaxis requiring resuscitation can occur in 0.7% to 1.1% of cases. Alternatively, methylene blue can be used. The risks associated with methylene blue include skin necrosis if injected intradermally, pain secondary to caustic reaction, and pulmonary edema. These risks can be minimized by diluting the methylene blue, with common dilutions ranging from 2:3 (2 mL of methylene blue mixed with 3 mL of saline, injecting 5 mL total) to 1:4 (1 mL of methylene blue mixed with 4 mL of saline, injecting 5 mL total). In patients taking serotonergic psychiatric medications, methylene blue should be used with caution as the dye can prevent the action of monoamine oxidase A, resulting in toxic levels of serotonin or serotonin syndrome. This is characterized by mental status changes, muscle twitching, excessive sweating, shivering, diarrhea, trouble with coordination, and/or fever.

Using a handheld gamma probe, the axilla is systematically surveyed and the skin is marked at the location of the hottest spot. A small incision is then made below the hair-bearing area of the axilla and carried down through the subcutaneous tissue. The clavipectoral fascia is incised with care to visually identify any blue lymphatics. The blue lymphatics are then followed toward the axilla to identify the sentinel lymph node. Successful SLN identification by blue dye is defined as the identification of any blue node or non–blue node with a blue afferent lymphatic. These lymph nodes are also evaluated with the gamma probe, and the associated counts are recorded. The dissection is continued until all lymph nodes associated with a blue afferent lymphatic are removed, and any remaining lymph nodes have less than 10% radioactivity compared to the most radioactive lymph node. This often results in more than one SLN being identified and removed. Finally, palpation of the axilla is performed, and any suspicious lymph nodes are also removed as gross tumor involvement can interfere with uptake of both radioactive colloid and blue dye. In the case of gross tumor involvement, the radioactive colloid and blue dye may be diverted to a lymph node other than the true SLN, giving rise to a false-negative result if palpation of the axilla and removal of suspicious lymph nodes is not performed. Once all SLNs have been identified and removed, hemostasis is obtained, and the clavipectoral fascia is reapproximated with interrupted Vicryl stitches. The deep dermal layer is reapproximated with interrupted 3-0 Vicryl stitches, and the skin is closed with a running subcuticular stitch.

TREATMENT OF THE PATIENT WITH BREAST CANCER

Breast cancer is currently treated with a multidisciplinary approach. Most patients benefit from a combination of therapies, which may include surgery, medical therapy, and RT. This multidisciplinary approach has resulted in a significant reduction in breast cancer mortality. One important consideration is optimal coordination of surgery with the other treatment modalities. In the discussion below, we will first provide an overview of how the different treatment modalities are coordinated in early-stage, locally advanced, and metastatic breast cancer. After this overview, surgery, medical therapy, and RT will be discussed in more detail.

7

Overview

Most patients with newly diagnosed breast cancer have no evidence of metastatic disease and are diagnosed with *early-stage* breast cancer. This includes patients with clinical stage I (T1N0), IIA (T1N1 or T2N0), or IIB (T2N1) disease. Local regional management often consists of BCT (partial mastectomy with RT) or mastectomy, noting that the choice in locoregional management does not typically impact the recommendation for adjuvant medical therapy. For patients with clinical T1N0 disease, surgery is typically the first treatment modality. For patients with clinical T2N0 or T2N1 disease, neoadjuvant chemotherapy or endocrine therapy is often the first treatment modality. The goal of neoadjuvant therapy is to shrink the primary breast cancer prior to surgery, facilitating BCT. For patients with a clinically suspicious axilla, an ultrasound-guided FNA may be helpful to determine whether there is metastatic spread to the axilla. If the FNA is negative, then the patient should undergo a SLNB at the time of surgery. For patients with a clinically negative axilla, an SLNB should be planned at the time of surgery with a decision about further management of the axilla, if any, pending the results of the SLNB. The decision to recommend chemotherapy for patients with early breast cancer is primarily dependent on tumor characteristics but also integrates the patient's overall health status and personal preference. Adjuvant chemotherapy is typically considered when high-risk features are present, such as high-grade tumor, large tumor size (≥1.0 cm), unfavorable biomarker profile, or lymph node involvement. However, molecular diagnostic tools, such as Oncotype DX, have become a standard tool in the decision regarding the use of adjuvant systemic therapy for patients with ER+/HER2-negative breast cancers. For patients with breast cancers that are hormone receptor positive, endocrine therapy is typically recommended postoperatively. If adjuvant chemotherapy is recommended, then endocrine therapy is given after completion of chemotherapy. For patients with TNBC, adjuvant chemotherapy is commonly given if the tumor size is ≥0.5 cm. Patients who have HER2-positive breast cancers that are ≥0.5 cm are treated with adjuvant chemotherapy plus HER2-directed therapy. Adjuvant RT is typically recommended for all patients who are treated with BCT, and a subset of patients who are treated with mastectomy (see ***Radiation Therapy***).

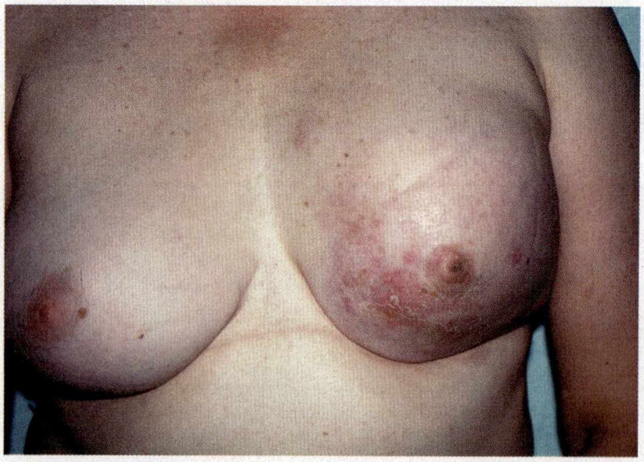

Figure 71.20. Locally advanced breast cancer. The breast is lifted and the upper half is bulging because of the large tumor. Distortion in the inferolateral contour is evident. The medial skin changes are caused by dermal tumor satellites.

Patients with *locally advanced disease* (clinical stage IIB [T3N0], or stage IIIA–IIIC [T1–T3N2 disease or T4 disease]) are at a higher risk for recurrence and distant metastases, and neoadjuvant and/or adjuvant chemotherapy and RT are typically recommended (**Fig. 71.20**). Benefits of neoadjuvant chemotherapy in this clinical context include the ability to treat any potential systemic disease immediately, and the ability to directly assess the response to treatment by physical examination and imaging, allowing for suboptimal regimens to be discontinued and other regimens to be prescribed. In patients with hormone receptor-positive disease, neoadjuvant chemotherapy or endocrine therapy can be used depending on the clinical characteristics. For patients with TNBC, neoadjuvant chemotherapy is indicated with or without immunotherapy. For patients with HER2-positive breast cancer, HER2-directed therapy with trastuzumab and pertuzumab should be given in addition to chemotherapy. Even if patients have an excellent clinical response, they should undergo surgery to remove the area of involvement. Although BCT is an option for patients with locally advanced breast cancer (LABC) who have a significant clinical response to neoadjuvant chemotherapy, mastectomy is typically recommended for those who initially present with breast cancers that are greater than 5 cm.

Approximately 5% of patients with newly diagnosed breast cancer will present with stage IV disease, and up to 30% of patients who present with early-stage breast cancer at diagnosis will develop distant metastatic disease. The approach to patients with metastatic breast cancer is focused on prolonging survival and improving quality of life by minimizing cancer-related symptoms. As such, the treatment plans for these patients are highly individualized.

For patients with hormone receptor positive, HER2-negative disease, the preference is for endocrine therapy alone. However, for patients with rapidly progressing disease, endocrine-resistant disease, or a large tumor burden involving visceral organs, chemotherapy should be considered. For patients with $HER2^+$ disease, HER2-directed therapies should be administered along with chemotherapy. For patients with TNBCs, chemotherapy is the only option for treatment of metastatic disease.

When chemotherapy is indicated, the preference is for sequential single-agent therapy, which includes taxanes and anthracyclines. Other options, especially for patients with bone-predominant ER^+ metastatic disease who have failed two trials of endocrine therapy, include capecitabine, which is derived from the antimetabolite fluorouracil. Capecitabine also may be indicated for metastatic disease to the brain as it appears to cross the blood–brain barrier. Other agents include eribulin, gemcitabine, ixabepilone, etoposide, and platinum agents.

Although combination chemotherapy conveys a higher risk of toxicity, its use is indicated when tumor burden is large or when patients have significant symptomatic disease. This includes anthracycline-containing regimens, nonanthracycline taxane-based regimens, and combination regimens incorporating platinum salts. It is important to note that no prospective study has shown that combination chemotherapy improves OS compared with single-agent sequential chemotherapy.

For women with metastatic breast cancer, data exist that extending chemotherapy duration is associated with improved progression-free and OS. However, prolonged chemotherapy can be associated with more serious toxicities such as neutropenia and neuropathy. As such, an individualized approach should be undertaken, weighing tumor response against side effects. During treatment for metastatic disease, the patient needs to be monitored for treatment failure, which includes clinical deterioration during treatment, evidence of new metastatic disease, and an increasing size of previously documented metastatic lesions.

The recommendations for adjuvant therapy are summarized in **Table 71.11**.

TREATMENT

Table 71.11. Recommendations for Adjuvant Therapy

Patient Group	Recommended Treatment
Node Negative, Low Risk	
Tumor <0.5 cm	No treatment or endocrine therapy if ER+
Special histologic types 1–2 cm, grade 1, ER+	
Node Negative, Higher Risk	
ER+	Endocrine therapy OR chemotherapy + endocrine therapy
ER−	Chemotherapy
Any HER2+	Add trastuzumab to chemotherapy
Node Positive	
ER+	
Premenopausal	Chemotherapy + endocrine therapy
Postmenopausal	Chemotherapy + endocrine therapy OR endocrine therapy alone
ER−	Chemotherapy
Any HER2+	Add trastuzumab to chemotherapy

ER+, estrogen receptor positive; ER−, estrogen receptor negative.

Surgical Therapy

Partial Mastectomy

Breast-conservation therapy (BCT) consists of breast-conserving surgery (partial mastectomy) followed by RT (**Fig. 71.21**).

The use of BCT is supported by six prospective randomized clinical trials demonstrating that partial mastectomy plus RT offers equivalent survival to mastectomy with a low rate of local recurrence (**Table 71.12**).

The local recurrence rate with BCT is 5% to 22% versus 4% to 14% with mastectomy. Of note, most recurrences after mastectomy occur within the first 3 years, but recurrences after BCT tend to occur later. Factors that increase local recurrence rate following partial mastectomy include young age, lymph node involvement, ER^- disease, and absence of RT. The American College of Surgeons, the American College of Radiology, the College of American Pathologists, and the Society of Surgical Oncology have developed consensus standards of care for BCT. Most patients can be offered BCT except for those with

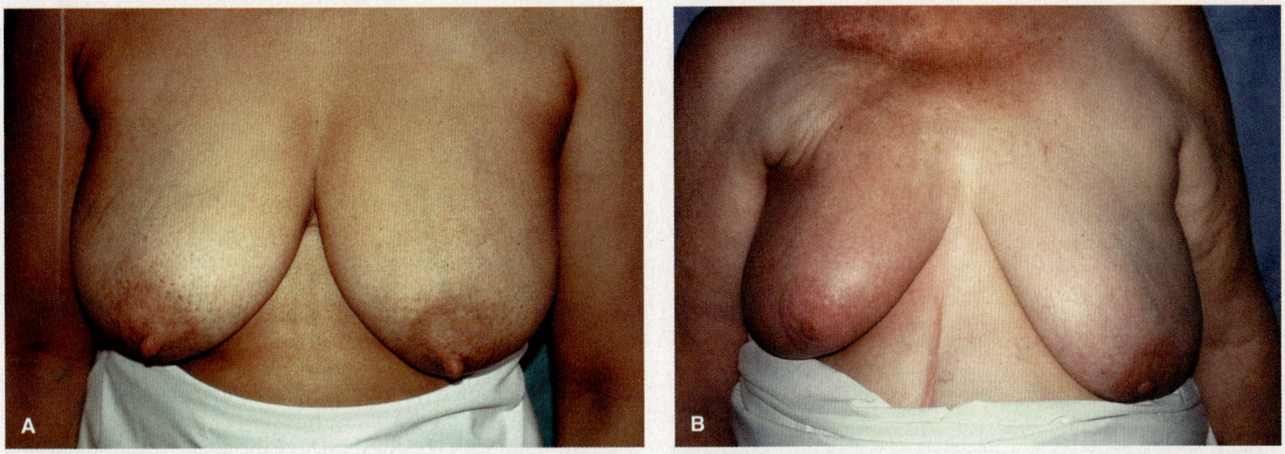

Figure 71.21. Cosmetic outcome after breast-conserving therapy with radiation. **A:** Excellent cosmetic outcome. The treated breast (**left**) is identical to the untreated breast. **B:** Fair cosmetic outcome. Significant shrinkage and loss of ptosis is evident in the treated right breast.

(1) multicentric disease, (2) diffuse suspicious microcalcifications on mammography, (3) a history of RT that includes a portion of the affected breast such that when combined with the current proposed treatment would result in an excessively high total radiation dose to the chest wall, (4) pregnancy (although if in the third trimester, partial mastectomy can be performed with planned breast irradiation deferred postpartum), (5) IBC, and (6) persistently positive margins after multiple attempts at breast-conserving surgery (**Table 71.13**).

The operative approach for a partial mastectomy is very similar to an excisional biopsy and is sometimes referred to as a wide excision, lumpectomy, or segmental mastectomy. The considerations for placement of the incision are similar to those for excisional biopsy, however it is best to keep the incision within the boundaries of a potential mastectomy incision, and the incision should be made directly over the lesion rather than at the wire insertion site to minimize tunneling. As negative margins are associated with lower rates of recurrence, many techniques have been developed to ensure negative margins at the time of the initial surgery. One common technique is to remove the breast cancer with surrounding normal tissue, and then obtain additional shave margins. Each shave margin is labeled and oriented in relationship to the primary cancer.[64–69] Approaches to evaluate intraoperative margin status include frozen section, cytologic touch prep analysis, and intraoperative ultrasound. However, no method has proven superior, and there is no established standard of care. In patients undergoing breast-conserving surgery, it is important to discuss the potential need for reexcision. A histologically positive margin is defined as a margin that has tumor present at the inked margin. Patients with a positive margin have at least a twofold increase in ipsilateral local breast cancer recurrence. As such, controversy has centered on the optimal amount of normal tissue that should be excised around the cancer to minimize
8
local recurrence risk. A recent multidisciplinary consensus panel supports the use of "tumor at ink" as the criteria for positive margin/reexcision based on a meta-analysis that included 33 studies with 28,162 patients and 1,506 ipsilateral recurrences.[70] Like most other institutions, we have adopted this new definition of a positive margin for invasive breast cancers to guide decisions about reexcision. However, given the concern for gaps between lesions or skip lesions in DCIS, we continue to define a negative margin for this pathology as ≥2 mm, understanding that this practice may evolve pending more study results.

Axillary Lymph Node Dissection

SLNB has replaced ALND for axillary staging in most women, and the therapeutic impact of ALND may be limited to specific subsets of breast cancer patients. In the American College of Surgeons Oncology Group Z0011 trial, eligible patients had T1–T2 invasive breast cancers, no palpable adenopathy, and one to two SLNs containing metastases identified by frozen section, touch preparation, or H&E staining. Patients were randomized to undergo ALND or no further axillary treatment. Systemic therapy was at the discretion of the treating

RESULTS

Table 71.12. Survival in Prospective Randomized Trials Comparing Breast-Conserving Therapy With Mastectomy

		Overall Survival		Local Recurrence	
Trial	**Follow-Up (Yrs)**	**BCT (%)**	**Mastectomy (%)**	**BCT (%)**	**Mastectomy (%)**
Institut Gustave-Roussy	15	73	65	9	14
Milan I	20	42	41	7	2
NSABP B-06	20	46	47	14	10
NCI	20	54	58	31	6
EORTC	10	65	66	20	12
Danish	6	79	82	3	4

BCT, breast-conserving therapy; EORTC, European Organization for Research and Treatment of Cancer; NCI, National Cancer Institute; NSABP, National Surgical Adjuvant Breast and Bowel Project.

INDICATIONS/CONTRAINDICATIONS

Table 71.13. Contraindications to Breast-Conserving Therapy in Invasive Carcinoma

Absolute Contraindications

- Two or more primary tumors in separate quadrants of the breast
- Persistent positive margins after reasonable surgical attempts
- Pregnancy is an absolute contraindication to the use of breast irradiation. When cancer is diagnosed in the third trimester, it may be possible to perform breast-conserving surgery and treat the patient with irradiation after delivery
- A history of prior therapeutic irradiation to the breast region that would result in retreatment to an excessively high radiation dose
- Diffuse malignant-appearing microcalcifications

Relative Contraindications

- A history of scleroderma or active systemic lupus erythematosus
- Large tumor in a small breast that would result in cosmesis unacceptable to the patient. In this circumstance, preoperative chemotherapy should be considered.
- Very large or pendulous breasts if reproducibility of patient setup and adequate dose homogeneity cannot be ensured

physician. Patients ineligible for the trial included those with matted lymph nodes, ≥3 positive nodes, gross extranodal disease, and those treated with neoadjuvant therapy.[60] After 10 years of follow-up, SLNB alone was not inferior to ALND in patients with limited sentinel lymph node involvement treated with BCT. Of note, these findings have been compared with those of the NSABP B04 trial that was conducted over a decade ago, which randomized women with clinically negative nodes to treatment with radical mastectomy, total mastectomy plus axillary radiation, or total mastectomy with delayed ALND if nodal recurrences were observed. No statistically significant survival differences were observed between any of the groups initially, or at any of the analyses up to 25 years of follow-up. These studies suggest that for contemporary women, ALND may not provide a survival benefit in patients who are clinically node negative. Currently, ALND is limited to patients with positive sentinel lymph nodes who do not meet Z0011 criteria, those with a contraindication to SLNB, such as pregnant women, those with clinically palpable pathologic lymph nodes, and patients with IBC.

The boundaries of an ALND are the axillary vein superiorly, the serratus anterior muscle and long thoracic nerve medially, and the latissimus dorsi muscle and thoracodorsal nerve laterally. Contemporary axillary dissection in breast cancer involves removal of the level 1 and 2 lymph nodes (**Fig. 71.22**).[71] Level 3 nodes are palpated, and only in the presence of gross disease is dissection performed, as removal of these nodes greatly increases the risk of lymphedema and is rarely (<1%) involved in the absence of level 1 and 2 disease.[72,73] Typically, a yield of ≥10 axillary lymph nodes is achieved with ALND.

The procedure is performed under a general anesthetic that does not include a muscle relaxant, as identification of the long thoracic and thoracodorsal nerves is critical to the dissection. Preoperative antibiotics and deep venous thrombosis prophylaxis with sequential compression devices are employed. The

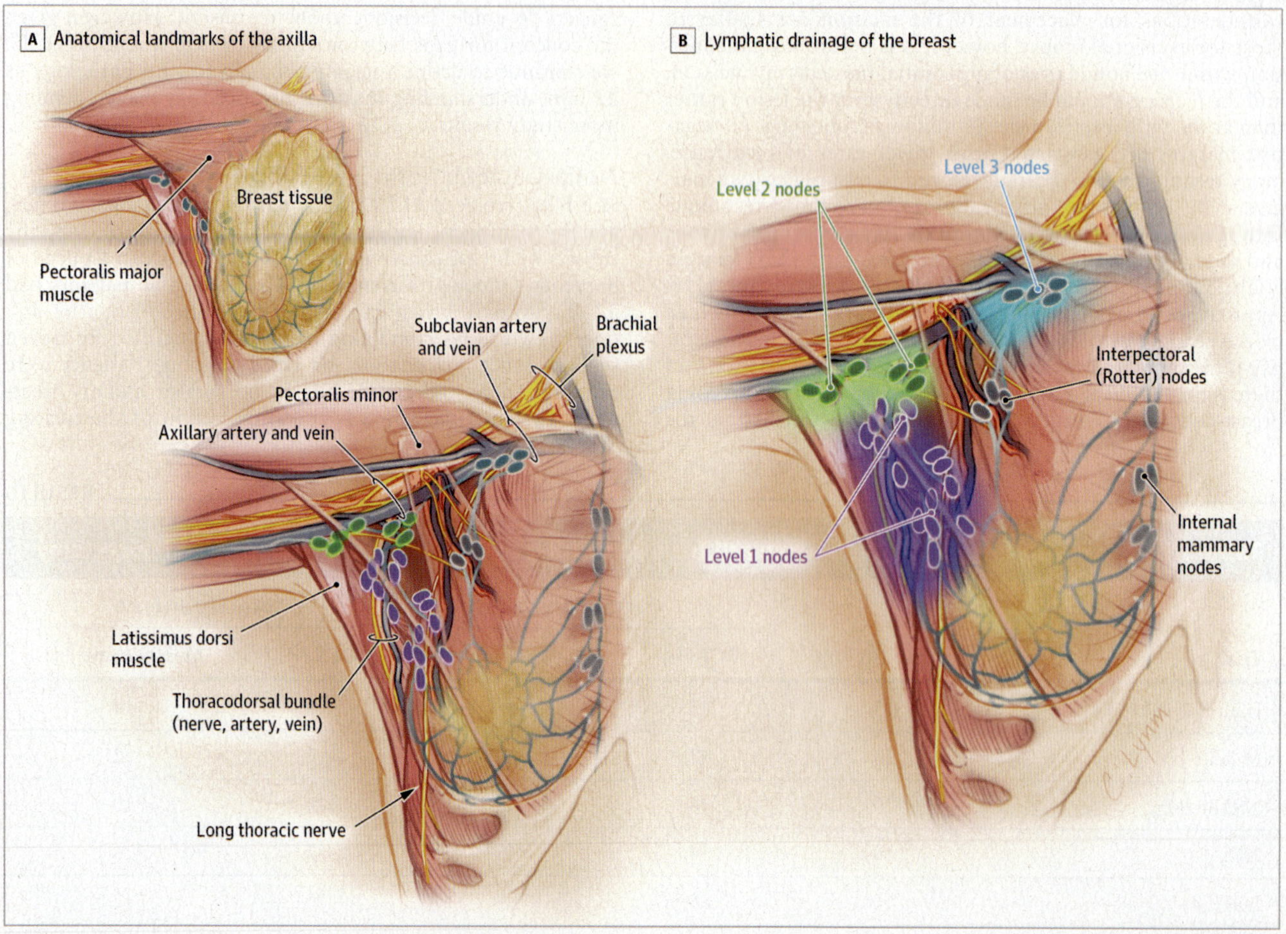

Figure 71.22. **A:** Anatomical landmarks of the axilla. The boundaries of the axillary lymph node dissection are the axillary vein superiorly, the latissimus dorsi and thoracodorsal bundle laterally, and the serratus anterior muscle and long thoracic nerve medially. **B:** Lymphatic drainage of the breast. During an axillary lymph node dissection, level 1 and 2 lymph nodes are removed.

patient is placed in the supine position with the ipsilateral arm abducted ≤90 degrees. Use of a stockinette allows for mobilization of the arm during dissection. If the ALND is performed through a mastectomy incision (modified radical mastectomy), no additional incisions are required. Also, for partial mastectomies performed in the upper outer quadrant, the partial mastectomy incision can be extended to the axilla. For palpable nodes that are close to, or have eroded the skin, it is important to take the overlying skin during the dissection.

For an ALND performed during a partial mastectomy or as a separate procedure, a curvilinear skin incision is made 1 to 2 cm below the hair-bearing area of the axilla, following Langer lines from the border of the PM muscle to the latissimus dorsi muscle. Although flaps can be developed superiorly, inferiorly, laterally, and medially, most surgeons find that this is not necessary. Once the skin incision is made, the lateral edge of the PM muscle is palpated and the PM fascia is then opened with electrocautery. The lateral edge of the PM is then retracted medially to expose the pectoralis minor (PMi) muscle, with care to avoid injury to the medial pectoral nerve, which innervates both the PM and the PMi. The tissue at the border of the PMi is then incised with care to avoid injury to the axillary vein or brachial plexus superiorly. If the arm is in a stockinette, it should be flexed medially and anteriorly to relax the PMi. The PM and PMi are then retracted and using blunt dissection, the axillary vein at the medial extent of the dissection can be identified. Further blunt dissection can be performed just below the medial aspect of the axillary vein and just lateral to the chest wall to identify the long thoracic nerve. The long thoracic nerve can also be palpated along the chest wall and once it is identified, the nerve is dissected free of surrounding tissue inferiorly to the insertion. To avoid injury, the fascial layer on the serratus anterior muscle which holds the nerve in place should not be opened. Attention is now turned to identification of the thoracodorsal nerve. Dissection is initiated midaxilla just inferior to the axillary vein. Anterior to the bundle is often the thoracoepigastric vein, which is a large superficial venous tributary arising from the axillary vein. Although the thoracoepigastric vein may need to be transected to allow for completion of the dissection, it is important to first identify the thoracodorsal nerve. The axillary fat pad/contents can then be dissected away from the thoracodorsal bundle using blunt dissection from superiorly to inferiorly with a long fine tonsil clamp. Once the long thoracic and thoracodorsal nerves are identified and dissected free of surrounding tissue, the axillary contents can be mobilized and removed. Of note, there are usually three to five intercostobrachial nerves that supply sensation to the medial–posterior aspect of the arm and run medial to lateral in the field of dissection. An attempt should be made to spare these nerves but only if they do not directly interfere with the dissection. The axillary contents are retracted inferiorly, and using electrocautery or sharp dissection, it is freed from the teres major posteriorly. The axillary contents are then sent en bloc to the pathologist. The wound is suction irrigated with sterile saline and hemostasis is achieved. A single 19 French round Blake drain can be placed above or below the bra line. However, some surgeons do not place drains for ALNDs, as in the absence of an associated mastectomy, the drainage is often scant. The skin is closed with interrupted 3-0 Vicryl sutures and a 4-0 subcuticular stitch. If a drain is placed, it is removed when drainage is less than 30 mL per 24 hours. No antibiotic prophylaxis is necessary.

The approach to axillary lymph node dissection described above is a medial to lateral approach with the long thoracic nerve, axillary vein, and thoracodorsal nerve identified in sequence. Alternatively, one can approach the dissection through a lateral to medial approach. With this method, once the clavipectoral fascia is incised to enter the true axilla, the anterior surface of the latissiumus dorsi is identified at the lateral extent of the axillary dissection. The clavipectoral fascia is then incised along the superior and medial aspects of the axilla. Dissection is then performed to first identify the thoracodorsal nerve, then the axillary vein superiorly, and then the long thoracic nerve medially. Once all the nerves and vascular structures are identified, the axillary contents are mobilized and removed.

Complications from ALND include motor and/or sensory nerve injury. Injury to the long thoracic nerve may result in winged scapula, whereas injury to the thoracodorsal nerve leads to weakness of internal rotation and extension, characterized by the functional inability to hold a book under the arm. Other risks include seroma formation, infection, and lymphedema.[74–76] The risk of lymphedema is lifelong and is as high as 30%.

Simple Mastectomy

A mastectomy is performed for patients with breast cancer who are not candidates for BCT or for patients who prefer a mastectomy. For women at high risk for the development of breast cancer, it can be performed as a prophylactic procedure. The goal of mastectomy is complete removal of the breast tissue while preserving muscle function, and viable skin flaps for primary closure. Preoperatively, the patient is examined in the holding area, where the breast is marked and the correct site of surgery is confirmed. An intravenous antibiotic that covers skin flora, such as cefazolin, given before skin incision has been shown to significantly decrease the risk of infection in patients undergoing mastectomy (relative risk 0.60, 95% CI 0.45–0.81).[77] The patient is then placed in the supine position with the arms abducted up to 90 degrees with padding placed beneath the arms and wrist to avoid brachial nerve and radial nerve injury. The skin is then cleansed with a preparation of chlorhexidine gluconate/isopropyl alcohol or betadine solution and the patient is draped in a sterile fashion. The most common skin incision used is an elliptical incision in the horizontal (Stewart incision) or diagonal plane (Orr incision), although historically a vertical plane incision for high-lying or infraclavicular lesions has also been used (**Fig. 71.23**). The medial border of this incision is 2 cm from

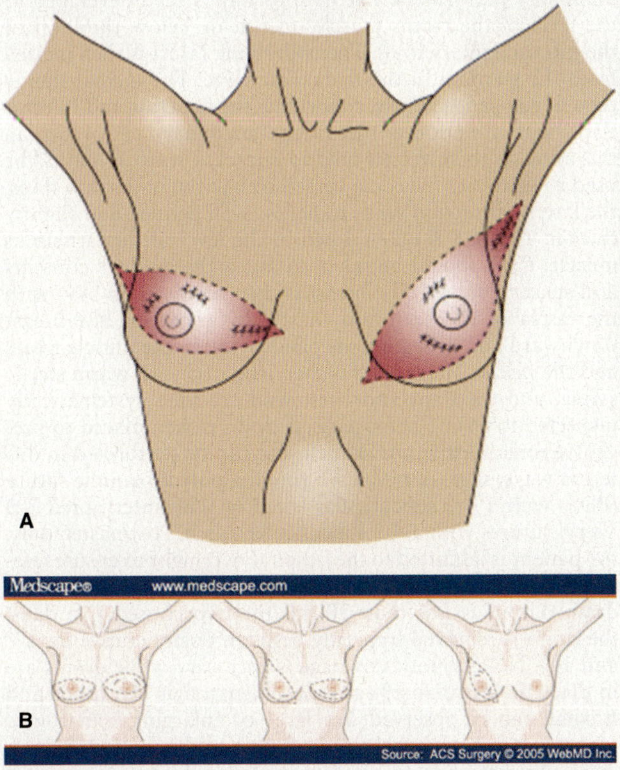

Figure 71.23. Incision placement for modified radical mastectomy. The incision should include the nipple–areola complex, biopsy scar, and excess skin of the breast.

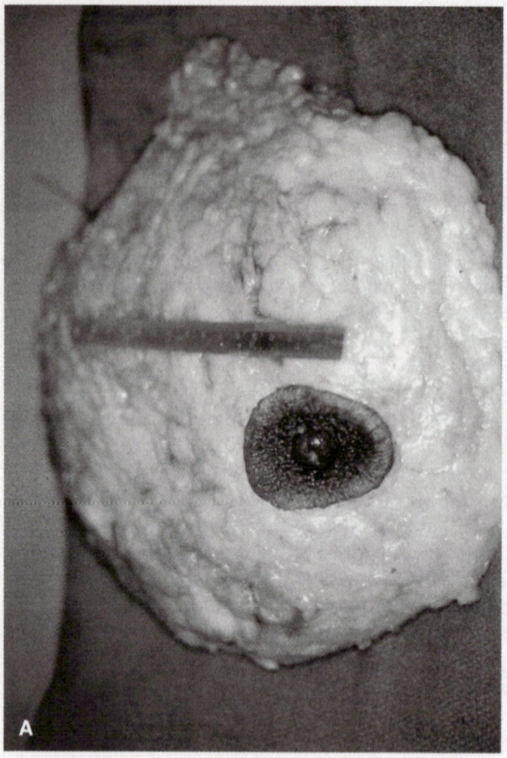

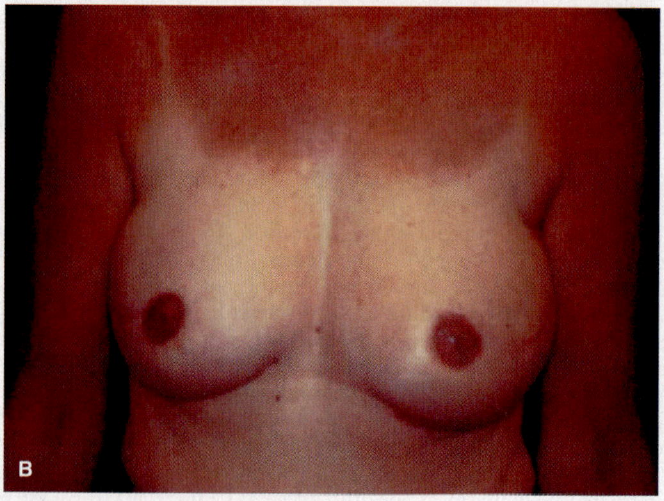

Figure 71.24. Skin-sparing mastectomy. **A:** The only skin removed was the nipple–areola complex. **B:** Cosmetic outcome after bilateral skin-sparing mastectomy and transverse rectus abdominis myocutaneous (TRAM) flap reconstruction.

the sternal edge and the lateral border is at the midaxillary line. The elliptical incision should include the skin directly over the tumor, especially if the tumor is superficial. Once the incision is made, a superior skin flap is developed in the relatively avascular plane between the skin and the breast parenchyma, to the level of the clavicle. The fascia of the PM muscle is then incised from the sternum to the edge of the lateral edge of the muscle with care to preserve the internal mammary perforators. The inferior flap is then developed to the level of the rectus muscle (just at or below the level of the inframammary fold). The underlying fascia is then incised from the sternum to the midaxillary line. The medial flap is then developed similarly, connecting the superior and inferior flaps, with attention to the internal mammary perforators in this area. As these vessels tend to retract, a stick tie should be used to ligate any bleeding vessel. Unlike the other skin flaps, the lateral dissection tends to be less well defined and slightly thicker. The flap is taken down to the level of the latissimus muscle. Care should be taken to avoid the axillary contents and sensory nerves. The breast is then removed en bloc with the fascia of the pectoralis muscle by retracting the breast downward and dissecting the plane between the muscle fibers and the fascia. The wound is then irrigated with warm sterile saline, and the flaps and chest wall are then systematically inspected to ensure hemostasis. A drain is then placed to prevent seroma formation. Skin closure can be performed in different ways, such as with a 3-0 running polydioxanone suture (PDS) with a 4-0 subcuticular stitch or with interrupted 3-0 Vicryl sutures with a 4-0 subcuticular stitch. Postmastectomy, the patient is admitted to the hospital overnight to ensure adequate pain control, and to monitor for acute bleeding. When drain output is less than 30 mL for two consecutive days, the drain is removed (typically between postoperative days 7 and 14). No antibiotic coverage is necessary while drains are in place. In less than 1% of cases, hematomas can occur and if small can be observed. For large or enlarging hematomas (encompassing greater than one-fourth of the chest wall), surgical exploration is required to evacuate the hematoma and stop any sources of bleeding. Other complications associated with mastectomy include skin flap necrosis, pneumothorax, cellulitis, neuropraxia, and lymphedema.

If immediate reconstruction is planned, a *skin-sparing* incision is made, which often consists of making either a smaller horizontal ellipse around the nipple–areola complex, a circular incision just encompassing the nipple–areola complex, or a lollipop incision (**Fig. 71.24**). In some circumstances, the patient may be a candidate for a *nipple-sparing mastectomy* if her breasts are small to moderate in size, often no larger than a C cup, with minimal ptosis, and the breast cancer is at least 2 cm from the nipple. Tumor size, histology, or lymph node status are no longer considered exclusion criteria for nipple-sparing mastectomy, and current exclusion criteria include clinical involvement of the nipple–areolar complex, PDB, bloody nipple discharge, multicentric disease[78] and/or inflammatory carcinoma.[79] Nipple-sparing mastectomies are often performed through an inframammary fold incision or a radial lateral incision. More recently, a lateral vertical incision has been described. This incision is associated with a significant reduction in hypertrophic scar formation versus the radial lateral
9 incision.[80] Intraoperatively, a biopsy of the retroareolar margin is performed and must be histologically negative for malignancy. BRCA mutation carriers are also candidates for nipple-sparing mastectomies. In a study of 26 patients with BRCA mutations undergoing prophylactic mastectomies, DCIS was identified in one patient compared with two cases of DCIS in the matched control group. There were no locoregional recurrences in the patients with BRCA mutations at 37 months of follow-up.[81] These findings support that nipple-sparing options are reasonable for patients with BRCA mutations.

Although the goal of a mastectomy is to completely remove the breast cancer and normal breast tissue, local recurrence remains a risk. The risk of local recurrence is 6% at 5 years in patients with no lymph node involvement, and 16% at 5 years in patients with one to three lymph nodes involved. With the addition of RT, the risk of local recurrence decreases to 2%. When four or more lymph nodes are involved, the risk of recurrence is 26% at 5 years, decreasing to 6% with the addition of RT.[82]

In women with a personal history of breast cancer, the absolute risk of contralateral breast cancer is estimated to be 0.5% to 1.0% per year or 5% to 10% during the 10 years following diagnosis.[83] As such, most women will not develop

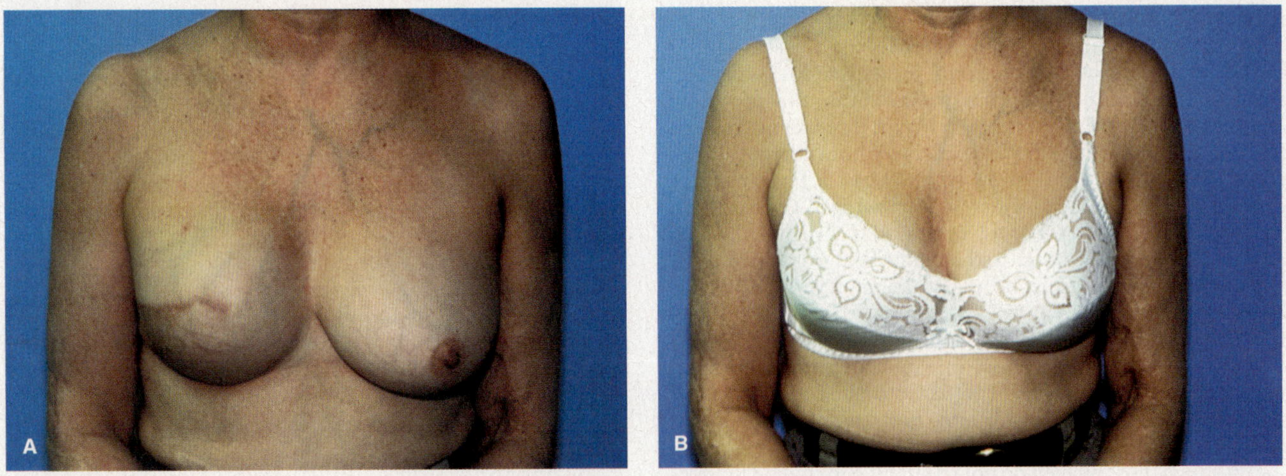

Figure 71.25. Breast reconstruction with tissue expanders. Although the breasts are not identical, this is not evident when a bra is worn.

a contralateral breast cancer. As no randomized clinical trials have been performed, it is not known if contralateral prophylactic mastectomy (CPM) is associated with a survival benefit in women with a personal history of breast cancer. However, a survival benefit for CPM has been shown for patients with a deleterious *BRCA1* or *BRCA2* mutation.[84–87] The decision to perform a CPM must be individualized with each individual patient. Of note, a twofold increased risk of major complications exists with CPM when compared with unilateral mastectomy.[88,89]

Breast Reconstruction

All patients undergoing mastectomy should be offered consultation with a plastic surgeon for consideration of breast reconstruction, recognizing that some women may choose to forego this procedure and prefer the use of breast prosthesis. The two main types of breast reconstruction include implant-based and autologous tissue breast reconstruction. Implants include silicone or saline implants. Autologous tissue techniques used for breast reconstruction often include either the transverse rectus abdominus myocutaneous (TRAM) flap or the deep inferior epigastric perforator (DIEP) flap.

Breast reconstruction can be performed immediately after a mastectomy procedure (immediate reconstruction) or at a later time (delayed reconstruction). For implant-based breast reconstruction, the most common technique involves a two-stage method with placement of a tissue expander under the PM muscle at the time of the mastectomy (**Fig. 71.25**). The tissue expander can then be filled incrementally with saline, with the first fill typically occurring 1 to 3 weeks postoperatively with additional fills every 1 to 2 weeks until the desired expansion is achieved. The tissue expander is then left in place for several months to allow for maximal skin remodeling. During the second stage, the tissue expander is removed and replaced with a silicone or saline implant. This two-stage reconstruction method is particularly beneficial for women who will need adjuvant RT, as radiation can result in flap necrosis, fibrosis, and shrinkage, resulting in poor cosmetic outcomes after immediate implant and/or tissue flap reconstruction. Instead, the tissue expander allows for skin preservation and the ability to then proceed with either an implant or autologous reconstruction at a later date. The complications associated with tissue expander placement include infection requiring removal. This occurs at a rate of 1.2%, but may be higher in women being treated with chemotherapy and/or RT.[90]

Although silicone gel implants are superior to saline implants in terms of offering a more natural contour and texture, the use of silicone implants remains controversial secondary to unsubstantiated claims of a link between silicone implants and autoimmune disease first reported in 1992. Since that time, no studies have shown a causative relationship, and the American College of Rheumatology and the FDA have concluded that there is no additional risk of connective tissue disease in patients with silicone implants.[91]

Studies determined a link between textured implants and anaplastic large cell lymphoma of the breast. Thus, the FDA recalled these textured devices, and only smooth implants are recommended currently.[92]

The primary benefit of autologous tissue breast reconstruction is that the reconstructed breast appears and feels more natural than following implant-based breast reconstruction. In addition, autologous tissue breast reconstruction may be the only option in patients who have undergone chest wall radiation, as skin fibrosis may preclude implant-based breast reconstruction. A common procedure is the free TRAM flap, which involves removing skin, subcutaneous fat, muscle, and associated blood supply from the lower abdomen. The blood supply includes the deep inferior epigastric artery and vein, which are anastomosed to the internal mammary or thoracodorsal arteries and veins. The TRAM flap is contoured to replicate the native breast. Similar to the TRAM flap, the DIEP perforator flap uses the same lower abdominal skin and subcutaneous fat but spares the rectus abdominis muscle. In both methods, the donor site is closed as a modified abdominoplasty.

Radical Mastectomy

In 1907, Halsted presented to the American Surgical Association his results of 232 patients who underwent his radical mastectomy at Johns Hopkins. Halsted's radical mastectomy involved wide excision of skin via a teardrop incision extending across the deltopectoral groove, excision of the entire PM muscle, resection of the PMi muscle to expose the axillary contents for dissection, and excision of the supraclavicular lymph nodes. In certain cases, he also removed the mediastinal nodes. Immediate skin grafting was performed to close all of the wounds.[93] With advances in breast cancer screening, adjuvant medical therapy, and RT, a concomitant evolution toward less radical surgery has ensued. A report by the American College of Surgeons Commission on Cancer demonstrated a dramatic decline in the use of the radical mastectomy from 47.9% of breast cancer cases in 1972 to 3.4% of cases in 1981.[94] Further, the **modified radical mastectomy**, which consists of a simple mastectomy and axillary lymph node dissection, was considered a satisfactory alternative to the radical mastectomy by 1980.[95] A randomized, prospective clinical study by W.A. Maddox in 1983 showed no significant differences in disease-free survival, OS, or local recurrence rates at 5 years for modified radical versus radical mastectomy. These differences are likely secondary to the routine use of chemotherapy for patients with involved axillary lymph nodes by this time period. When patients are not candidates for breast conservation and SLNB, a modified radical mastectomy is indicated. Please see the section on ***Axillary Lymph Node Dissection*** above.

Radiation Therapy

The primary indication for the use of RT in breast cancer is to reduce the risk of a locoregional recurrence following surgery, and potentially improve survival by eradicating persistent locoregional disease that may be resistant to systemic therapy.

The standard approach for patients who undergo breast-conserving surgery is to deliver whole breast RT with a dose of 50 to 60 Gy. The regimen is often given in 2 Gy fractions, 5 days a week for a total of 5 weeks. A 60 Gy regimen, which also includes a 10 Gy boost to the tumor bed, was found to be more effective for patients 45 years of age or younger, with a local relapse rate of 14% (60 Gy) compared to 28% (50 Gy) ($P < .0001$).[96] Alternative RT strategies are currently under investigation, including the use of rapid fractionation schedules, such as the delivery of 41 to 42 Gy over 15 fractions, and accelerated partial breast radiation. Early results show excellent clinical outcomes.[97–99]

Although most women do not require RT following mastectomy, postmastectomy RT is often recommended for women at high risk for locoregional recurrence, including women with four or more positive lymph nodes, tumor size greater than 5 cm, or with positive surgical margins. In these instances, postmastectomy radiation can reduce the rate of chest wall recurrence by 65% to 75%.[100–103]

Of note, optimal locoregional management of the axilla remains to be defined. Both surgery and RT can be used to treat disease in the axilla. Previously, ALND was the preferred treatment modality for prevention or treatment of axillary disease. More recent studies suggest that RT may be equally effec-
10 tive with less morbidity. The EORTC AMAROS trial randomized patients with clinical T1–T2 N0 breast cancer to ALND or RT to the axilla after a positive SLNB.[104] The two arms had comparable axillary control, but patients in the RT arm had significantly less morbidity. At 5 years, 23% of patients in the ALND arm had lymphedema compared to 11% in the RT arm. Currently, in patients with clinical T1–T2 N0 disease who undergo mastectomy with a positive SLNB, ALND is the standard approach, as these patients were not included in the Z0011 study. However, findings from the AMAROS trial suggest that in this group of patients, RT may provide similar locoregional control with less morbidity.

Chemotherapy

The role of medical therapy is to eradicate breast cancer cells at the primary tumor site, or at any other site in the body. Systemic therapies include but are not limited to chemotherapy, endocrine therapy, and targeted therapy.

The decision as to whether or not to treat breast cancer patients with chemotherapy is complex. Considerations include patient age, menopausal status, AJCC TNM stage, histologic grade, biomarker profile, proliferation index, and medical comorbidities. Fortunately, online calculators exist to estimate the risks and benefits of chemotherapy and other adjuvant therapies. Adjuvant! Online is a popular risk–benefit calculator that is based on population-wide data that focuses on recurrence risk and probability of survival. This is a web-based program that is generated from collective data from the Surveillance, Epidemiology, and End Results (SEER) database, the Early Breast Cancer Trialists Collaborative Group (EBCTCG), individual clinical trial results, and published literature. Other calculators include Cancermath.net[105] and FinProg project.[106] Molecular profiling using Oncotype DX or similar molecular assay can be used for patients with node-negative ER$^+$/HER2$^-$ breast cancers. For Oncotype DX, a score of ≥31 is associated increased risk of recurrence with a recommendation for administration of chemotherapy.

Adjuvant chemotherapy is often initiated 4 to 6 weeks after surgery. Although treatment earlier is not beneficial, a delay of greater than 12 weeks may be detrimental. If adjuvant RT is indicated, it is administered starting 3 to 4 weeks after completion of chemotherapy.

Anthracyclines (Doxorubicin, Daunorubicin, Epirubicin)

These compounds are derived from *Streptomyces* bacteria and function by inhibiting DNA and RNA synthesis by intercalating between base pairs of the DNA/RNA strand, blocking DNA transcription and replication by inhibiting topoisomerase II enzyme, generating free oxygen radicals, and by inducing histone eviction from chromatin. The main adverse effect is cardiotoxicity.

Taxanes (Paclitaxel, Docetaxel)

These compounds are derived from plants of the genus *Taxus* (yews) and function by disrupting microtubule formation and inhibiting mitosis. The main adverse effect is peripheral neuropathy. Given that these compounds are not water soluble, allergic reactions to the diluent may result.

Cyclophosphamide

This compound is a nitrogen mustard alkylating agent that functions by adding an alkyl group to the guanine base of DNA, resulting in intrastrand and interstrand DNA crosslinks and therefore interfering with DNA replication. The main adverse effects include acute myeloid leukemia, bladder cancer, hemorrhagic cystitis, and infertility.

5-Fluorouracil

This compound is an antimetabolite that works as an irreversible inhibitor of thymidylate synthase and therefore interferes with DNA synthesis. The main adverse effect is mucositis.

Methotrexate

This compound is both an antimetabolite and an antifolate that blocks dihydrofolate reductase and therefore inhibits the synthesis of folic acid, which is essential for DNA, RNA, thymidylate, and protein synthesis. The main adverse effect is ulcerative stomatitis.

Platinum Agents (Carboplatin or Cisplatin)

These compounds bind to and cause crosslinks in DNA, triggering apoptosis. The main adverse effects are nephrotoxicity, neurotoxicity, and ototoxicity.

Endocrine Therapy

Patients with all stages of breast cancer that express the ER or PR are candidates for endocrine therapy. In the premenopausal setting, the focus is on blocking ovarian function and the effects of estrogen. In postmenopausal women, the ovaries are no longer the predominant source of estrogen, but instead, estrogen is synthesized mainly from nonglandular sources such as subcutaneous fat. As such, blocking estrogen production is very effective in the postmenopausal population.

Blocking Ovarian Function (Leuprolide, Goserelin, Buserelin)

As the ovaries are the main source of estrogens in premenopausal women, ovarian ablation can be achieved either surgically by removal of the ovaries or through medical therapy with luteinizing hormone–releasing hormone (LHRH) agonists such as goserelin or leuprolide. These compounds function by binding to the GnRH receptor, resulting in initial FSH and LH release. However, with prolonged drug exposure, desensitization of the pituitary occurs, whereby the levels of LH and FSH become profoundly suppressed. This results in inhibition of the growth of ovarian follicles and steroidogenesis.

Blocking Estrogen at the Receptor (Tamoxifen, Raloxifene, Fulvestrant)

As SERMs, tamoxifen and raloxifene competitively bind to the ER and prevent estrogen from binding. As a selective ER down regulator (SERD), fulvestrant binds to the ER and targets it for destruction. Fulvestrant is used only in postmenopausal women who have hormone receptor-positive metastatic disease and who experience progression following endocrine therapy.

Blocking Estrogen Production (Anastrozole, Letrozole, Exemestane)

The enzyme aromatase converts androgenic substrates to estrogen, and therefore, its inhibition can effectively decrease plasma levels of estrogen. Nonsteroidal AIs include anastrozole and letrozole, whose binding activity can be reversed. Exemestane is a steroidal AI that irreversibly binds aromatase and permanently inactivates it.

Targeted Therapy

Targeted Therapy for HER2$^+$ Breast Cancers

Amplification or overexpression of the human epidermal growth factor receptor 2 (HER2) is present in approximately 20% of primary breast cancers. Given that effective targeted therapies exist for these patients, all newly diagnosed breast cancers are routinely tested for HER2 expression/amplification.

Trastuzumab is a monoclonal antibody that targets HER2$^+$ breast cancers by multiple mechanisms, including (1) interfering with the homo- and heterodimerization of HER2 and inhibiting mitogen-activated protein kinase (MAPK) and phosphoinositide 3-kinase (PI3K/Akt) signaling pathways, (2) immune-mediated killing of tumors that overexpress HER2 by a mechanism referred to as antibody-dependent cellular cytotoxity (ADCC), and (3) triggering HER2 internalization and degradation through promoting the activity of tyrosine kinase-ubiquitin ligase c-Cbl.

Pertuzumab is a monoclonal antibody that interferes with the dimerization of HER2 to HER3, therefore interfering with MAPK and PI3K pathway activation. It also induces ADCC.

Trastuzumab emtansine (T-DM1) is an antibody–drug conjugate that consists of trastuzumab linked with the cytotoxic agent mertansine (DM1). While trastuzumab binds to the HER2 receptor, mertansine enters the cell and destroys it by binding to tubulin. This allows toxin to be targeted specifically to the cancer cell.

Targeted Therapy for Triple-Negative Breast Cancers (Experimental Options)

Although patients with TNBC often have an excellent response to chemotherapy, overall outcomes are worse compared to patients with ER$^+$ and/or HER2$^+$ disease.[107,108] The lack of effective targeted therapies for TNBC likely contributes to this disparity in outcome. Drugs targeting TNBCs are in clinical trials and include inhibitors targeted to the epidermal growth factor receptor (cetuximab), angiogenisis (bevacizumab), DNA damage or poly adenosine diphosphate-ribose polymerase (olaparib, veliparib, iniparib), the proto-oncogene Src (dasatinib), and histone deacetylase (vorinostat). Given the heterogeneity of TNBC, multitargeted therapy will likely be needed to eradicate this disease.

Special Issues in Breast Cancer Treatment

Inflammatory Breast Cancer

A common clinical presentation for IBC is *peau d'orange*, characterized by edema, warmth, and erythema. Unlike other types of breast cancer, patients with IBC often have associated pain and tenderness with an enlarged and firm breast. The nipple can also be involved with flattening, erythema, crusting, blistering, and retraction. Despite the reference to inflammation, the skin changes are not secondary to an inflammatory process but rather secondary to tumor emboli within the dermal lymphatics.[109] As noted by Sir Charles Bell in 1812, these cancers tend to be much more aggressive—"when a purple color is on the skin over the tumor accompanied by shooting pains, it is a very unpropitious beginning."[110] By 1924, Lee and Tannenbaum described 28 cases of women presenting with a rare, rapidly progressive breast cancer with inflammatory features and introduced the term "inflammatory breast cancer."[111]

IBC is an aggressive form of LABC that affects approximately 1% to 5% of women with breast cancer.[112] It is designated as primary tumor stage T4d. The consensus-based criteria for the diagnosis of IBC was determined by an international expert panel who proposed the following features: (1) rapid onset of breast erythema, edema, and/or *peau d'orange*, and/or warm breast, with or without an underlying palpable mass, (2) duration of history no more than 6 months, (3) erythema occupying at least one-third of the breast, and (4) pathologic confirmation of invasive carcinoma.[113] Furthermore, although dermal lymphatic involvement supports the diagnosis of IBC, which can be obtained with a full-thickness skin punch biopsy, it is neither necessary nor sufficient in the absence of the classical clinical findings. The diagnosis of IBC is made with clinical exam findings, followed by breast imaging, which includes mammography and ultrasound to help detect sites within the breast that can be biopsied to confirm the breast cancer. To determine extent of disease, we routinely obtain a breast MRI. A skin punch biopsy can then be performed, but is not required for diagnosis. As IBC is a clinically and pathologically distinct form of LABC that is particularly fast growing, invasive, and angiogenic, nearly all women have lymph node involvement at the time of presentation, and approximately a third of patients will have distant metastases.[114,115] As such, all women with IBC need to undergo complete staging, including a chest/abdomen/pelvic CT scan and bone scan. Head CT should be considered if symptoms are present.

The treatment for IBC is based on multimodality treatments, similar to those described for women with LABC. However, BCT, SLN biopsy, and immediate breast reconstruction are generally considered inappropriate for patients with IBC. Treatment often consists of neoadjuvant chemotherapy that is anthracycline- and taxane-based until all signs of skin inflammation have resolved and the breast and axillary masses are deemed operable. Surgical management with a modified radical mastectomy is then performed with delayed breast reconstruction, if appropriate. Adjuvant RT follows using standard fields determined by CT planning, ensuring that the chest wall, supraclavicular, infraclavicular, and the internal mammary lymph nodes are radiated.[115] RT to the axillary bed after axillary dissection is often individualized. However, if the patient still remains inoperable after neoadjuvant chemotherapy, then RT ensues, with the goal that the patient will thereafter become operable. For ER$^+$ IBC, adjuvant endocrine therapy is given. For HER2$^+$ IBC, trastuzumab (± pertuzumab) is added to the neoadjuvant regimen, and adjuvant trastuzumab is given to complete 1 year of treatment.

Currently, there is no optimal systemic regimen (chemotherapy or targeted therapy) identified for IBC. However, patients who obtain a complete pathologic response from chemotherapy have a significantly higher disease-free survival and OS.[116,117] Despite the combination of surgery and RT improving locoregional control, there is no impact on OS.[118] Even with multimodality treatments, the prognosis for patients with IBC remains poor with 5-year disease-free survival rates of 20% to 45% and an OS of 30% to 70%.[116,118–121]

Breast Cancer in the Elderly

In the United States, approximately half of newly diagnosed breast cancers are in older women, typically defined as age ≥65 years. Older patients tend to receive less than standard therapy worldwide,[122–125] with decreased rates of surgery and use of adjuvant RT, but with increased use of primary endocrine therapy.[126] This may be secondary to more indolent tumors present in elderly women versus younger women.[127] However, after controlling for confounding factors such as comorbidity, social support, and functional status, older women are still treated less aggressively than their younger counterparts. In general, treatment approaches should not be altered for medically fit older women, except for the use of SLNB and/or RT in early ER+ disease.

The ability to omit axillary surgery without an adverse effect on outcome in older women (age ≥70 years) with favorable breast cancers has been well studied and supported by multiple randomized trials. These women had clinically negative axillary examinations, small (<2 cm) ER+ breast cancers, and were all treated with adjuvant endocrine therapy.[128–130]

The ability to omit adjuvant RT in older women who have undergone partial mastectomy for early ER+ breast cancer is supported by CALGB 9343. This phase III study involved 636 women (age ≥70 years) who had T1N0M0 ER+ breast cancer who were treated with partial mastectomy and then randomly assigned to either receive RT plus tamoxifen (317 women) or tamoxifen alone (319 women). The primary end points studied included time to local or regional recurrence, frequency of mastectomy, breast cancer-specific survival, time to distant metastasis, and OS. At 10 years, 98% of patients receiving RT plus tamoxifen compared with 90% of those receiving tamoxifen alone were free from local and regional recurrences. However, there were no significant differences in time to mastectomy, time to distant metastasis, breast cancer-specific survival, or OS between the two groups. Ten-year OS was 67% (95% CI, 62% to 72%) and 66% (95% CI, 61% to 71%), respectively.[131] This led to breast-conserving surgery and endocrine therapy alone being incorporated as a category I recommendation in the current consensus guidelines for older women.

For older women with comorbidities, functional status limitation, or frailty, the Comprehensive Geriatric Assessment (CGA) can serve as an objective measure to aid in treatment decisions. The CGA has been used in elderly cancer patients, including those with breast cancer, and range from 44 to 84 questions. The ELCAPA study looked at how the CGA could alter an initial treatment plan in 375 patients aged 70 years and older. Treatment plans were modified in 20.8% of cases, with most plans changed to decrease treatment intensity, although there were some regimens (10.8%) that were intensified.[132] Given how extensive the full CGA can be, other screening tools that have been developed include the Vulnerable Elders Survey-13, Barber Questionnaire, Geriatric 8, Cardiovascular Health Study, and the abbreviated CGA.

For medically frail patients, surgical management followed by observation is commonly offered, especially if a patient's life expectancy is limited. If surgical intervention is not an option, endocrine therapy can be offered to patients with ER+ disease and single-agent chemotherapy for those with ER− disease. In the presence of HER2+ disease, single-agent HER2-directed therapy or its addition to systemic therapy can be prescribed, understanding that the latter approach carries additive risks of toxicity. RT is not recommended unless local control of disease is needed for symptom management. Finally, palliative and supportive care services need to be offered to patients who wish to avoid both surgical and systemic therapies.

Breast Cancer during Pregnancy

Gestational breast cancer is a rare disease affecting approximately 1 in 1000 pregnancies, but it may become more common as women delay childbearing.[133–136] It is defined as breast cancer that is diagnosed during pregnancy, within the first postpartum year, or anytime during lactation. Similar to nonpregnant women, women with gestational breast cancer present most often with a breast mass or skin thickening. Any mass that persists for greater than 2 weeks needs diagnostic imaging and possible biopsy.

The breast becomes engorged and hypertrophied during pregnancy, making imaging more difficult. When women present with a mass in pregnancy, ultrasound is first obtained, which can differentiate between a simple cyst, a complex cyst, or a solid tumor. The majority of gestational breast cancers present as a focal solid mass.[137,138] In the presence of an abnormal ultrasound, a diagnostic mammogram can then be obtained to further determine the extent of disease and has been shown to be safe in pregnancy as long as abdominal shielding is used.[139] Although MRI with gadolinium has been shown to be more sensitive than mammography for detecting invasive breast cancer, gadolinium is contraindicated in pregnancy. MRI has also not been systemically studied for the evaluation of breast masses in pregnancy or lactation. All suspicious masses must be biopsied, even in the presence of normal imaging studies, through core needle biopsy, incisional biopsy, or excisional biopsy. In a patient who has a concerning axillary exam, FNA biopsy is indicated.

The most common histologic type of gestational breast cancer is IDCs that are poorly differentiated and diagnosed at an advanced stage. Compared to nonpregnant women, women with gestational breast cancers have less hormone receptor-positive breast cancers (approximately 25% vs 55% to 60%).[140,141] The association between HER2 disease and gestational breast cancer is not currently known. For pregnant or lactating women with locally advanced disease, staging evaluation is necessary. Given the large cumulative radiation dose that can be associated with CT scans and the contraindication for gadolinium use (therefore limiting the utility of MRI) in pregnancy, staging imaging for pregnant women commonly include a chest x-ray, an abdominal ultrasound of the liver, and a "low-dose" bone scan or a skeletal MRI.

For women diagnosed with breast cancer at an early gestational age, pregnancy termination is an option. However, studies have not shown better outcomes with early termination. In a study involving 176 patients, pregnancy did not directly affect the prognosis of breast cancer, instead, poor survival was related to younger age (less than 40 years old) and to the large number of ER–negative tumors (71%).[142] Multiple subsequent studies have shown that pregnancy does not have a negative impact on OS.[143–145] In 2012, a meta-analysis involving 3000 patients with gestational breast cancer who were compared to 37,100 controls, found that gestational breast cancer was associated with a higher risk of death. However, this was limited to women diagnosed in the postpartum period.[146]

The treatment for breast cancer for women diagnosed in the postpartum or lactational period does not differ from that recommended for nonpregnant patients. However, for patients receiving chemotherapy, trastuzumab, or endocrine therapy, breastfeeding is not recommended given the potential toxicity to the infant. The treatment for pregnant women does not differ significantly from established guidelines, but includes modifications to ensure the safety of the developing fetus. During any trimester of pregnancy, surgical and anesthetic risks to the fetus have been shown to be minimal.[147–150] Mastectomy can be performed and for early breast cancers, this can eliminate the need for RT as it is contraindicated in pregnancy. Typical radiation doses used for breast cancer range from 46 to 60 Gy, which has been shown to convey a first-trimester fetal dose of 0.04 to 0.15 Gy or a third-trimester dose as high as 2 Gy.[144,151] The threshold determined for prenatal radiation exposure for fetuses under 16 weeks of gestation is 0.10 to 0.20 Gy, and after 16 weeks, 0.50 to 0.70 Gy to avoid risk of congenital malformations.[152] As such breast-conserving treatment (which necessitates RT) remote from delivery is not a feasible option. Otherwise, the choice between breast-conserving surgery versus mastectomy can be guided by a patient's preference and the biology of the tumor.

Isosulfan blue dye is contraindicated in pregnant women, and methylene blue, when used in amniocentesis, has been associated with fetal complications. However, a small series of studies using methylene blue or double filtered technetium sulfur for SLNB have suggested its safety and success in pregnant women.[153–156] Given the small number of pregnant patients included in these studies, the potential risks of methylene blue and technetium sulfur to the fetus, along with the potential inaccuracy of SLNB in pregnancy, need to be discussed with the patient preoperatively.

The most common regimens used in gestational breast cancers are anthracycline based, AC (doxorubicin plus cyclophosphamide) or FAC (fluorouracil plus AC). The exposure of the fetus during organogenesis or the first trimester to chemotherapy can be detrimental and conveys risks, including congenital abnormalities, chromosomal abnormalities, and miscarriage. Although chemotherapy exposure in the second and third trimesters is not associated with organogenesis, risks of intrauterine growth restriction, lower gestational age at birth, and low–birth-weight occur in about half of exposed infants.[157–160] As such, chemotherapy is often initiated after the first trimester and given its association with transient neonatal myelosuppression, it should be avoided 3 to 4 weeks prior to delivery. When possible, timing of delivery is restricted to 34 or more weeks of gestation and requires confirmation of fetal lung maturity to minimize complications associated with prematurity. Given that gestational breast cancer can present as locally advanced disease, neoadjuvant chemotherapy can be first given, followed by surgery in the postpartum period, and if indicated, adjuvant RT and endocrine therapy can then be initiated. For women who are diagnosed late in pregnancy or the postpartum/lactational period, prior to commencement of chemotherapy, which may impair infertility, these women should be offered consultation with a reproductive endocrinologist to discuss fertility-preserving options.

Trastuzumab is contraindicated in pregnancy given its association with oligohydramnios, which can result in fetal death, pulmonary hypoplasia, and fetal developmental abnormalities.[161] The use of methotrexate and endocrine therapy are also contraindicated during pregnancy. These therapies can be initiated in the postpartum period.

Given that the majority of women diagnosed with gestational breast cancers are of reproductive age, many desire additional pregnancies. In a meta-analysis of fourteen studies, 1244 women who became pregnant following breast cancer were compared to 18,145 control patients. Pregnancy in breast cancer survivors did not convey a worse survival but suggested a protective effect. Some suggest that pregnancy may have an unknown biologic antitumor effect, although more likely this is secondary to healthier women with better prognosis choosing to reproduce over their sicker peers and therefore resulting in a bias toward improved survival. As most recurrences happen within the first 2 years after diagnosis and treatment, it is generally recommended that pregnant women wait 2 years before contemplating another pregnancy.

Breast Cancer in Men

Male breast cancer in the United States accounts for 0.5% to 1% of all breast cancers diagnosed annually.[162] Risk factors for male breast cancer include family history of breast cancer and genetic mutations including *BRCA1* and *BRCA2*. *BRCA2* is more commonly associated with male breast cancer and conveys a 6% lifetime absolute risk, which is an approximately 100-fold higher risk than in the general male population.[163] As such, all men diagnosed with breast cancer need genetic counseling and BRCA testing. Other genetic mutations include *PTEN* which is linked to Cowden syndrome, *TP53* which is associated with Li–Fraumeni syndrome, mismatch repair genes that are linked to hereditary nonpolyposis colorectal cancer (Lynch syndrome), and *PALB2* mutations.[164,165] Other risk factors include those that increase circulating estrogens such as hormonal therapies, hepatic dysfunction, obesity, marijuana use, and thyroid disease. It is also associated with Klinefelter syndrome, which is characterized by 47XXY genotype. These male patients have atrophic testes and gynecomastia. In addition, they have high serum concentrations of gonadotropins (follicular stimulating hormone, luteinizing hormone) and a low serum testosterone level, resulting in a high ratio of estrogen to testosterone. Those with Klinefelter syndrome have a 19.2- and 57.8-fold increase in the incidence of and mortality from breast cancer.[166] Primary testicular conditions (orchitis, undescended testes, testicular injury) are associated with an increased risk of male breast cancer as it can result in lower androgen production and therefore result in a higher than normal estrogen-to-androgen ratio.[167,168]

Unfortunately, men are often diagnosed with breast cancer at an advanced stage. They commonly present with a firm retroareolar mass that is painless. Workup for a suspicious breast mass in men is similar to that for a woman and includes a mammogram and biopsy. Ultrasound is typically less informative. The most common histologic subtype is invasive ductal carcinoma (90%). Lobular carcinoma is rarely diagnosed in men. DCIS is also less frequent in men versus women. Most male breast cancers are ER^+ (81.5%).[169] The staging system for male breast cancers is similar to that for women and is classified according to the TNM AJCC staging system.

The treatment for early-stage male breast cancer has generally been a modified radical mastectomy. However for a man with a clinically negative axillary exam, an expert panel from the American Society of Clinical Oncology (ASCO) considers SLN biopsy to be an "acceptable" method. It is generally accepted that in men who have no evidence of disease in the SLN biopsy, no further axillary surgery is needed. For men who have a positive SLN, given there is lack of data for men in regards to this issue, they should be treated similarly to women with positive SLN biopsies. There is limited data regarding the use of breast-conserving surgery in men. A retrospective study of seven men treated with breast-conserving therapy followed for a median of 67 months reported that there was no recurrence of disease. If men do elect for a partial mastectomy, adjuvant RT is essential and is based on results showing that adjuvant RT after breast-conserving surgery for women conveys a survival advantage.[170] For men with LABC (T3N0, N1-2, or T2N2) or IBC, treatment plans are similar to that for women. Consideration for neoadjuvant chemotherapy prior to surgery should be made. The treatment of metastatic breast cancer in males should parallel that for women.

Adjuvant chemotherapy, RT, anti-HER2 therapy, and endocrine therapy should mirror those for women. As the majority of male breast cancers are ER positive, endocrine therapy with tamoxifen should be given. In a limited study involving 39 men, those treated with tamoxifen had better 5-year actuarial survival (61% vs 44%) and disease-free survival (56% vs 28%).[171] Although there is limited data, tamoxifen appears to be superior to AIs in the adjuvant setting for male breast cancer.[172] Extrapolating from the ATLAS trial for women,[173] for men with higher-risk breast cancers, consideration toward extending tamoxifen to 10 years should be considered.

Male breast cancer patients should undergo similar post-treatment surveillance as that recommended for women. However, the role of screening mammography for the contralateral breast in these men has not been explored. It is important to recognize that male breast cancer patients are at risk for developing secondary cancers such as those of the small intestine, rectum, skin (nonmelanoma), pancreas, and prostate.[174]

Locoregional Breast Cancer Recurrence

Breast cancer recurrence can occur after both mastectomy and BCT (partial mastectomy and RT), with the median time to recurrence after mastectomy of 2 to 3 years versus 3 to 4 years after BCT.[175–177] When breast cancer reappears on the chest wall it is defined as a local recurrence. However, breast cancer that involves the lymph nodes such as the ipsilateral axillary, supraclavicular, infraclavicular or internal mammary nodes is referred to as a regional recurrence. Among patients who undergo mastectomy for an operable breast cancer, 5% to 10% of patients will have a local or regional recurrence within 10 years whereas patients who undergo BCT have a risk of 10% to 15%, and in patients who forego RT after a partial mastectomy, the risk of recurrence is as high as 35%.[178] Although BCT is associated with an increased risk of locoregional recurrence, there are no differences in OS as supported by a single institutional NIH randomized study (n = 237) and two European randomized trails (EORTC trial 10801 and DBCG trial 82-TM). The latter involved approximately 1800 patients with stage I and II breast cancer who were randomized to undergo a modified radical mastectomy or BCT. Patients who developed a local recurrence in these trials were then analyzed for survival and time to subsequent local recurrence after salvage treatment. There were no differences between the two groups in regards to survival and time to subsequent local recurrence after treatment for an early locoregional recurrence.[178]

The primary risk factors for postmastectomy recurrence include the size of the primary cancer and the number of positive axillary lymph nodes, where ≥4 involved nodes have been consistently shown to increase axillary recurrence rate to over 20%.[179] In women with four or more positive lymph nodes, tumor size greater than 5 cm, or those with positive surgical margins, postmastectomy RT is often recommended as it can reduce the rate of chest wall recurrence by 65% to 75%.[101–103] The most common presenting sign of a postmastectomy recurrence is a clinical mass or multiple small nodules on the chest wall or overlying skin in or near the mastectomy scar/skin flaps. Other signs of a recurrence can include inflammatory changes without an associated mass and painless masses found in the axilla or the supraclavicular fossa. Workup for a recurrence should also be undertaken for patients who present with lymphedema or a brachial plexopathy. When a recurrence is suspected, a core biopsy should be obtained to confirm the diagnosis and to evaluate hormone and HER2 receptor status. In addition, a metastatic workup should be performed. The 5-year survival rate for patients based on site of recurrence is 52% for chest wall alone, 50% for axilla alone, 28% for supraclavicular nodes alone, 28% for chest wall plus axilla, and 7% when both the supraclavicular nodes and chest wall/axilla are involved.[180] The subsequent treatment plan for patients with recurrent breast cancer is complex and requires a multidisciplinary team.

After BCT, the primary risk factors for recurrence are the use of RT and pathologic margin status. When an ipsilateral breast cancer is identified it is important to determine whether this is indeed a true recurrence versus a second primary cancer; a true recurrence is often found within the primary tumor site or the boost volume of the treated breast. Unlike postmastectomy recurrences, which are commonly detected on physical examination, post-BCT recurrences are often identified by surveillance mammography. However, it is important to note that any physical examination changes that occur more than 1 year after completion of RT warrant further workup, even in the presence of a normal mammogram. In this setting, consideration should be made for MRI and biopsy. For any recurrent disease, biopsy is obtained to confirm diagnosis and tumor receptor status, followed by a complete metastatic staging workup. In the absence of metastatic disease, the standard approach to a local recurrence after BCT is a mastectomy, with most patients surviving at least 10 years.[181] In the setting of more advanced recurrent disease, such as that associated with skin involvement or inflammatory changes of the skin, systemic therapy may need to be considered prior to mastectomy. The decision to proceed with axillary restaging should be considered by a multidisciplinary team. Furthermore, the management of regional recurrence after BCT is complex and should be planned with a multidisciplinary approach.

Paget Disease of the Breast

Although the presentation of breast cancer is commonly associated with a mass or a mammographic abnormality, it must be considered in the setting of chronic nipple ulceration. PDB was first noted by Sir James Paget in 1874 when he described 15 women with chronic nipple ulcerations who then developed cancer of the involved breast within 2 years.[182] The hallmark of Paget disease is a scaly, raw, vesicular, or ulcerated lesion that begins on the nipple and then spreads to the

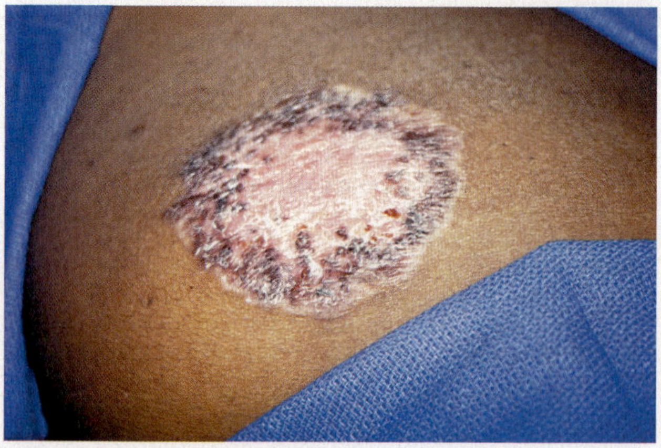

Figure 71.26. Paget disease of the nipple. Depigmentation and desquamation of the nipple and areola are evident.

areola (**Fig. 71.26**). This is often a unilateral process and can be associated with bloody nipple discharge. Symptoms which can occur prior to the development of clinically apparent disease include pain, burning, and pruritus. PDB is a rare disease accounting for only 1% to 3% of new cases of breast cancer in females in the United States.

The diagnostic workup of PDB is to first establish the diagnosis and then to identify the underlying breast cancer which is present in 85% to 88% of cases, despite often not being associated with a breast mass or a mammographic abnormality.[183] Full-thickness wedge or punch biopsy of the nipple should be performed. PBD is characterized histologically by the presence of large cells with prominent nucleoli and a pale cytoplasm (Paget cells) occurring singly or in small groups within the epidermis of the nipple. Other characteristics of Paget cells include the presence of low–molecular-weight cytokeratins such as CK7. Approximately 50% of PDB cases express hormone receptors and between 70% and 90% of cases overexpress HER2.

For patients with PDB, a physical examination including bilateral breast examination and mammography should be performed to help identify the underlying breast cancer. Approximately one-half of patients with PDB will have an associated mammographic abnormality. Interestingly, these abnormalities can occur distant from the nipple–areolar complex. If no palpable masses are found and mammography is normal, there is a greater likelihood of DCIS than an invasive cancer.[184] If mammography and breast imaging fail to locate disease, then an MRI can be obtained, recognizing that although it is highly sensitive, it is not highly specific. As such, MRI-detected lesions should be biopsied to confirm the diagnosis of a breast cancer.

The treatment for PDB is either a mastectomy or breast-conserving therapy, which includes a partial mastectomy and whole breast RT. Breast-conserving surgery includes resection of the nipple–areola complex and the underlying cancer with negative margins obtained (central lumpectomy). Given that the nipple–areola complex is removed, some women may consider this cosmetically unacceptable. Evaluation and treatment of the axilla is dependent on the underlying cancer identified. Adjuvant systemic therapy is also determined by the involved breast cancer.

Phyllodes Tumor

Phyllodes tumors are uncommon (<0.5% of all breast malignancies) fibroepithelial breast tumors first described by Johannes Muller in 1838 as *cystosarcoma phyllodes*.[185] Given that these tumors often do not have cystic components and are not true sarcomas, they are now referred to simply as phyllodes tumors (**Fig. 71.27**). The malignant potential of phyllodes tumors differ widely, with some behaving like fibroadenomas and others that can degenerate histologically into sarcomatous

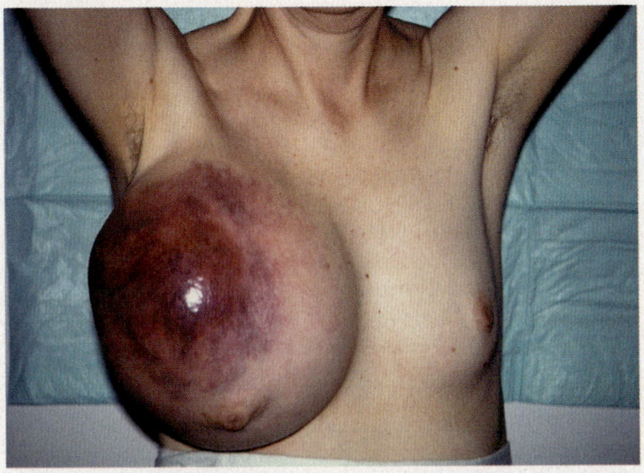

Figure 71.27. Breast asymmetry resulting from a benign phyllodes tumor. Skin changes are caused by pressure necrosis.

lesions and metastasize distantly. As such, they are histologically classified as benign (50%), borderline (25%), or malignant (25%) based upon the degree of stromal cellularity and atypia, mitotic rate, and the presence or absence of stromal overgrowth and infiltrative margins. Risk factors for phyllodes tumors are not known, aside from their association with Li–Fraumeni syndrome.[186]

Patients with phyllodes tumors present with a smooth, multinodular, well-demarcated, firm mass that is both mobile and painless. The average tumor size is 4 to 7 cm. Although palpable axillary lymphadenopathy can be found in up to 20% of patients, lymph node involvement is rare.[187] Imaging is notable for a smooth multilobulated mass that resembles a fibroadenoma. Core needle biopsy is recommended for diagnosis. However, it has a false-negative rate of 25% to 30%.[188–189] As such, in the presence of a rapidly enlarging mass, excisional biopsy should be performed.

The treatment for all phyllodes tumors is surgical excision to negative histologic margins; however, the definition of negative margins does differ between institutions ranging from no tumor at ink to 1 cm margins. As such, these cases are best addressed in multidisciplinary fashion with pathology. Even large tumors can be treated with breast-conserving surgery without compromising cancer-specific survival. Lymph node involvement is also very rare, in the SEER database, only 8 of 498 women had involved nodes.[190] As such, most surgeons do not routinely perform SLNB for phyllodes tumors. The use of adjuvant RT and chemotherapy is controversial, however in the setting of a large borderline or malignant phyllodes tumor these treatments should be considered. If systemic therapy for malignant phyllodes tumor is undertaken, it is based on guidelines for treating sarcomas. Similar to breast sarcomas, malignant phyllodes tumors can metastasize to the lungs and as such patients should undergo chest x-ray every 6 months for 2 years and then annually. Unfortunately, once metastasis develops, the mean OS is 30 months.[191]

ACKNOWLEDGMENT

We gratefully acknowledge the contributions of previous edition author, Thanh U. Barbie, as portions of those chapters have been retained in this revision.

References

1. Kleinberg DL. Early mammary development: growth hormone and IGF-1. *J Mammary Gland Biol Neoplasia.* 1997;2:49–57.
2. Russo J, Rivera R, Russo IH. Influence of age and parity on the development of the human breast. *Breast Cancer Res Treat.* 1992;23:211–218.
3. Barash I. Stat5 in the mammary gland: controlling normal development and cancer. *J Cell Physiol.* 2006;209:305–313.
4. McCarty KJ. Breast. In: Sternberg S, ed. *Histology for Pathologists.* Lippincott-Raven; 1997.
5. Helminen HJ, Ericsson JL. Studies on mammary gland involution. I. On the ultrastructure of the lactating mammary gland. *J Ultrastruct Res.* 1968;25:193–213.
6. Barlow WE, Lehman CD, Zheng Y, et al. Performance of diagnostic mammography for women with signs or symptoms of breast cancer. *J Natl Cancer Inst.* 2002;94:1151–1159.
7. Flobbe K, Bosch AM, Kessels AG, et al. The additional diagnostic value of ultrasonography in the diagnosis of breast cancer. *Arch Intern Med.* 2003;163:1194–1199.
8. Peters NH, Borel Rinkes IH, Zuithoff NP, et al. Meta-analysis of MR imaging in the diagnosis of breast lesions. *Radiology.* 2008;246:116–124.
9. Ljung BM, Drejet A, Chiampi N, et al. Diagnostic accuracy of fine-needle aspiration biopsy is determined by physician training in sampling technique. *Cancer.* 2001;93:263–268.
10. Parker SH, Burbank F, Jackman RJ, et al. Percutaneous large-core breast biopsy: a multi-institutional study. *Radiology.* 1994;193:359–364.
11. Morrow M, Wong S, Venta L. The evaluation of breast masses in women younger than forty years of age. *Surgery.* 1998;124:634–640; discussion 640–641.
12. Vogel PM, Georgiade NG, Fetter BF, et al. The correlation of histologic changes in the human breast with the menstrual cycle. *Am J Pathol.* 1981;104:23–34.
13. Pruthi S, Wahner-Roedler DL, Torkelson CJ, et al. Vitamin E and evening primrose oil for management of cyclical mastalgia: a randomized pilot study. *Altern Med Rev.* 2010;15:59–67.
14. Seltzer MH, Perloff LJ, Kelley RI, et al. The significance of age in patients with nipple discharge. *Surg Gynecol Obstet.* 1970;131:519–522.
15. Cardenosa G, Doudna C, Eklund GW. Ductography of the breast: technique and findings. *AJR Am J Roentgenol.* 1994;162:1081–1087.
16. Schnitt SJ. Benign breast disease and breast cancer risk: morphology and beyond. *Am J Surg Pathol.* 2003;27:836–841.
17. Schnitt SJ, Collins LC. Pathology of benign breast disorders. In: Harris JR, ed. *Breast Diseases.* Lippincott; 2010:69.
18. Berg WA, Sechtin AG, Marques H, et al. Cystic breast masses and the ACRIN 6666 experience. *Radiol Clin North Am.* 2010;48:931–987.
19. Dixon JM, McDonald C, Elton RA, et al. Risk of breast cancer in women with palpable breast cysts: a prospective study. Edinburgh Breast Group. *Lancet.* 1999;353:1742–1745.
20. Valdes EK, Feldman SM, Boolbol SK. Papillary lesions: a review of the literature. *Ann Surg Oncol.* 2007;14:1009–1013.
21. Jensen RA, Page DL, Dupont WD, et al. Invasive breast cancer risk in women with sclerosing adenosis. *Cancer.* 1989;64:1977–1983.
22. Linda A, Zuiani C, Furlan A, et al. Radial scars without atypia diagnosed at imaging-guided needle biopsy: how often is associated malignancy found at subsequent surgical excision, and do mammography and sonography predict which lesions are malignant. *AJR Am J Roentgenol.* 2010;194:1146–1151.
23. El-Wakeel H, Umpleby HC. Systematic review of fibroadenoma as a risk factor for breast cancer. *Breast.* 2003;12:302–307.
24. Degnim AC, Visscher DW, Berman HK, et al. Stratification of breast cancer risk in women with atypia: a Mayo cohort study. *J Clin Oncol.* 2007;25:2671–2677.
25. Margenthaler JA, Duke D, Monsees BS, et al. Correlation between core biopsy and excisional biopsy in breast high-risk lesions. *Am J Surg.* 2006;192:534–537.
26. Middleton LP, Sneige N, Coyne R, et al. Most lobular carcinoma in situ and atypical lobular hyperplasia diagnosed on core needle biopsy can be managed clinically with radiologic follow-up in a multidisciplinary setting. *Cancer Med.* 2014;3:492–499.
27. Nakhlis F, Gilmore L, Gelman R, et al. Incidence of adjacent synchronous invasive carcinoma and/or ductal carcinoma in-situ in patients with lobular neoplasia on core biopsy: results from a

prospective multi-institutional registry (TBCRC 020). *Ann Surg Oncol.* 2016;23:722–728.
28. Sneige N, Wang J, Baker BA, et al. Clinical, histopathologic, and biologic features of pleomorphic lobular (ductal-lobular) carcinoma in situ of the breast: a report of 24 cases. *Mod Pathol.* 2002;15:1044–1050.
29. Haagensen CD. Lobular neoplasia (lobular carcinoma in situ). In: Haagensen CD, Bodian C, Haagensen DE, eds. *Breast Carcinoma: Risk and Detection.* WB Saunders; 1981:238–291.
30. Rosen P, Kosloff C, Lieberman PH, et al. Lobular carcinoma in situ of the breast: detailed analysis of 99 patients with average follow-up of 24 years. *Am J Surg Pathol.* 1978;2:225–251.
31. Andersen JA. Lobular carcinoma in situ of the breast. An approach to rational treatment. *Cancer.* 1977;39:2597–2602.
32. Salvadori B, Bartoli C, Zurrida S, et al. Risk of invasive cancer in women with lobular carcinoma in situ of the breast. *Eur J Cancer.* 1991;27:35–37.
33. Ottesen GL, Graversen HP, Blichert-Toft M, et al. Lobular carcinoma in situ of the female breast. Short-term results of a prospective nation wide study. The Danish Breast Cancer Cooperative Group. *Am J Surg Pathol.* 1993;17:14–21.
34. Bodian CA, Perzin KH, Lattes R. Lobular neoplasia. Long term risk of breast cancer and relation to other factors. *Cancer.* 1996;78:1024–1034.
35. Fisher B, Costantino JP, Wickerham DL, et al. Tamoxifen for the prevention of breast cancer: current status of the National Surgical Adjuvant Breast and Bowel Project P-1 study. *J Natl Cancer Inst.* 2005;97:1652–1662.
36. Khoumais NA, Scaranelo AM, Moshonov H, et al. Incidence of breast cancer in patients with pure flat epithelial atypia diagnosed at core-needle biopsy of the breast. *Ann Surg Oncol.* 2013;20:133–138.
37. Colditz GA, Rosner B. Cumulative risk of breast cancer to age 70 years according to risk factor status: data from the Nurses' Health Study. *Am J Epidemiol.* 2000;152:950–964.
38. Collaborative Group on Hormonal Factors in Breast Cancer. Breast cancer and hormonal contraceptives: collaborative reanalysis of individual data on 53 297 women with breast cancer and 100 239 women without breast cancer from 54 epidemiological studies. *Lancet.* 1996;347:1713–1727.
39. Collaborative Group on Hormonal Factors in Breast Cancer. Breast cancer and breastfeeding: collaborative reanalysis of individual data from 47 epidemiological studies in 30 countries, including 50302 women with breast cancer and 96973 women without the disease. *Lancet.* 2002;360:187–195.
40. John EM, Kelsey JL. Radiation and other environmental exposures and breast cancer. *Epidemiol Rev.* 1993;15:157–162.
41. Bagnardi V, Rota M, Botteri E, et al. Light alcohol drinking and cancer: a meta-analysis. *Ann Oncol.* 2013;24:301–308.
42. Gaudet MM, Gapstur SM, Sun J, et al. Active smoking and breast cancer risk: original cohort data and meta-analysis. *J Natl Cancer Inst.* 2013;105:515–525.
43. Collaborative Group on Hormonal Factors in Breast Cancer. Familial breast cancer: collaborative reanalysis of individual data from 52 epidemiological studies including 58,209 women with breast cancer and 101,986 women without the disease. *Lancet.* 2001;358:1389–1399.
44. Gudmundsdottir K, Ashworth A. The roles of BRCA1 and BRCA2 and associated proteins in the maintenance of genomic stability. *Oncogene.* 2006;25:5864–5874.
45. Peelen T, van Vliet M, Petrij-Bosch A, et al. A high proportion of novel mutations in BRCA1 with strong founder effects among Dutch and Belgian hereditary breast and ovarian cancer families. *Am J Hum Genet.* 1997;60:1041–1049.
46. Frank TS, Deffenbaugh AM, Reid JE, et al. Clinical characteristics of individuals with germline mutations in BRCA1 and BRCA2: analysis of 10,000 individuals. *J Clin Oncol.* 2002;20:1480–1490.
47. Lynch HT, Mulcahy GM, Harris RE, et al. Genetic and pathologic findings in a kindred with hereditary sarcoma, breast cancer, brain tumors, leukemia, lung, laryngeal, and adrenal cortical carcinoma. *Cancer.* 1978;41:2055–2064.
48. Swift M, Chase CL, Morrell D. Cancer predisposition of ataxia-telangiectasia heterozygotes. *Cancer Genet Cytogenet.* 1990;46:21–27.
49. Berx G, Van Roy F. The E-cadherin/catenin complex: an important gatekeeper in breast cancer tumorigenesis and malignant progression. *Breast Cancer Res.* 2001;3:289–293.
50. Brownstein MH, Wolf M, Bikowski JB. Cowden's disease: a cutaneous marker of breast cancer. *Cancer.* 1978;41:2393–2398.
51. National Cancer Institute. The Breast Cancer Risk Assessment Tool: Online Calculator (The Gail Model). www.cancer.gov/bcrisktool/
52. UTSW Medical Center. https://bcrisktool.cancer.gov/
53. University of Cambridge. Centre for Cancer Genetic Epidemiology: BOADICEA. ccge.medschl.cam.ac.uk/boadicea
54. IBIS Breast Cancer Risk Evaluation Tool. www.ems-trials.org/riskevaluator/
55. BCSC. Breast Cancer Surveillance Consortium Risk Calculator. https://tools.bcsc-scc.ucdavis.edu/BC5yearRisk/#/
56. Nelson HD, Smith ME, Griffin JC, et al. Use of medications to reduce risk for primary breast cancer: a systematic review for the U.S. Preventive Services Task Force. *Ann Intern Med.* 2013;158:604–614.
57. Vogel VG, Costantino JP, Wickerham DL, et al. Update of the national surgical adjuvant breast and bowel project study of tamoxifen and raloxifene (STAR) P-2 trial: preventing breast cancer. *Cancer Prev Res (Phila).* 2010;3:696–706.
58. Cuzick J, Sestak I, Forbes JF, et al. Anastrozole for prevention of breast cancer in high-risk postmenopausal women (IBIS-II): an international, double-blind, randomised placebo-controlled trial. *Lancet.* 2014;383:1041–1048.
59. Weinmann S, Leo M, Francisco M, et al. Validation of a ductal carcinoma in situ biomarker profile for risk of recurrence after breast-conserving surgery with and without radiation therapy. *Clin Cancer Res.* 2020;26(15):4054–4063.
60. Giuliano AE, Hunt KK, Ballman KV, et al. Axillary dissection vs no axillary dissection in women with invasive breast cancer and sentinel node metastasis: a randomized clinical trial. *JAMA.* 2011;305:569–575.
61. Goyal A, Newcombe RG, Chhabra A, et al. ALMANAC Trialists Group Factors affecting failed localisation and false-negative rates of sentinel node biopsy in breast cancer—results of the ALMANAC validation phase. *Breast Cancer Res Treat.* 2006;99(2):203–208.
62. Krag DN, Anderson SJ, Julian TB, et al. National surgical adjuvant breast and bowel project. Technical outcomes of sentinel-lymph-node resection and conventional axillary-lymph-node dissection in patients with clinically node-negative breast cancer: results from the NSABP B-32 randomised phase III trial. *Lancet Oncol.* 2007;8(10):881–888.
63. Zavagno G, De Salvo GL, Scalco G, et al. GIVOM Trial lists. A randomized clinical trial on sentinel lymph node biopsy versus axillary lymph node dissection in breast cancer: results of the Sentinella/GIVOM trial. *Ann Surg.* 2008;247(2):207–213.
64. Gibson GR, Lesnikoski BA, Yoo J, Mott LA, Cady B, Barth RJ Jr. A comparison of ink-directed and traditional whole-cavity re-excision for breast lumpectomy specimens with positive margins. *Ann Surg Oncol.* 2001;8:693–704.
65. Hewes JC, Imkampe A, Haji A, Bates T. Importance of routine cavity sampling in breast conservation surgery. *Br J Surg.* 2009;96:47–53.
66. Rizzo M, Iyengar R, Gabram SG, et al. The effects of additional tumor cavity sampling at the time of breast-conserving surgery on final margin status, volume of resection, and pathologist workload. *Ann Surg Oncol.* 2010;17:228–234.
67. Tengher-Barna I, Hequet D, Reboul-Marty J, et al. Prevalence and predictive factors for the detection of carcinoma in cavity margin performed at the time of breast lumpectomy. *Mod Pathol.* 2009;22:299–305.
68. Janes SE, Stankhe M, Singh S, et al. Systematic cavity shaves reduces close margins and re-excision rates in breast conserving surgery. *Breast.* 2006;15:326–330.
69. Jacobson AF, Asad J, Boolbol SK, et al. Do additional shaved margins at the time of lumpectomy eliminate the need for re-excision. *Am J Surg.* 2008;196:556–558.

70. Moran MS, Schnitt SJ, Giuliano AE, et al. Society of Surgical Oncology-American Society for Radiation Oncology consensus guideline on margins for breast-conserving surgery with whole-breast irradiation in stages I and II invasive breast cancer. *Ann Surg Oncol.* 2014;21:704–716.
71. NIH consensus conference. Treatment of early-stage breast cancer. *JAMA.* 1991;265:391–395.
72. Veronesi U, Rilke F, Luini A, et al. Distribution of axillary node metastases by level of invasion. An analysis of 539 cases. *Cancer.* 1987;59:682–687.
73. Rosen PP, Lesser ML, Kinne DW, et al. Discontinuous or "skip" metastases in breast carcinoma. Analysis of 1228 axillary dissections. *Ann Surg.* 1983;197:276–283.
74. Yeoh EK, Denham JW, Davies SA, et al. Primary breast cancer. Complications of axillary management. *Acta Radiol Oncol.* 1986;25:105–108.
75. Lotze MT, Duncan MA, Gerber LH, et al. Early versus delayed shoulder motion following axillary dissection: a randomized prospective study. *Ann Surg.* 1981;193:288–295.
76. Ivens D, Hoe AL, Podd TJ, et al. Assessment of morbidity from complete axillary dissection. *Br J Cancer* 1992;66:136–138.
77. Tejirian T, DiFronzo LA, Haigh PI. Antibiotic prophylaxis for preventing wound infection after breast surgery: a systematic review and metaanalysis. *J Am Coll Surg.* 2006;203:729–734.
78. Spear SL, Hannan CM, Willey SC, et al. Nipple-sparing mastectomy. *Plast Reconstr Surg.* 2009;123:1665–1673.
79. Fortunato L, Loreti A, Andrich R, et al. When mastectomy is needed: is the nipple-sparing procedure a new standard with very few contraindications. *J Surg Oncol.* 2013;108:207–212.
80. Kamioka N, Mori H, Okazaki M. Significant reduction of hypertrophic scarring by lateral vertical incision in skin-sparing and nipple-sparing mastectomy. *J Med Dent Sci.* 2010;57:203–208.
81. Peled AW, Irwin CS, Hwang ES, et al. Total skin-sparing mastectomy in BRCA mutation carriers. *Ann Surg Oncol.* 2014;21:37–41.
82. Golshan M. Chapter 36: mastectomy. In: Harris JR, Lippman ME, Morrow M, et al., eds. *Diseases of the Breast.* 4th ed. Lippincott Williams & Wilkins; 2010.
83. Fowble B, Hanlon A, Freedman G, et al. Second cancers after conservative surgery and radiation for stages I-II breast cancer: identifying a subset of women at increased risk. *Int J Radiat Oncol Biol Phys.* 2001;51:679–690.
84. Bedrosian I, Hu CY, Chang GJ. Population-based study of contralateral prophylactic mastectomy and survival outcomes of breast cancer patients. *J Natl Cancer Inst.* 2010;102:401–409.
85. Lostumbo L, Carbine NE, Wallace J. Prophylactic mastectomy for the prevention of breast cancer. *Cochrane Database Syst Rev.* 2010;(11):CD002748.
86. Zeichner SB, Zeichner SB, Ruiz AL, et al. Improved long-term survival with contralateral prophylactic mastectomy among young women. *Asian Pac J Cancer Prev.* 2014;15:1155–1162.
87. van Sprundel TC, Schmidt MK, Rookus MA, et al. Risk reduction of contralateral breast cancer and survival after contralateral prophylactic mastectomy in BRCA1 or BRCA2 mutation carriers. *Br J Cancer.* 2005;93:287–292.
88. Miller ME, Czechura T, Martz B, et al. Operative risks associated with contralateral prophylactic mastectomy: a single institution experience. *Ann Surg Oncol.* 2013;20:4113–4120.
89. Osman F, Saleh F, Jackson TD, et al. Increased postoperative complications in bilateral mastectomy patients compared to unilateral mastectomy: an analysis of the NSQIP database. *Ann Surg Oncol.* 2013;20:3212–3217.
90. Spear SL, Majidian A. Immediate breast reconstruction in two stages using textured, integrated-valve tissue expanders and breast implants: a retrospective review of 171 consecutive breast reconstructions from 1989 to 1996. *Plast Reconstr Surg.* 1998;101:53–63.
91. Hennekens CH, Lee IM, Cook NR, et al. Self-reported breast implants and connective-tissue diseases in female health professionals. A retrospective cohort study. *JAMA.* 1996;275:616–621.
92. FDA. Questions and answers about breast implant-associated anaplastic large cell lymphoma (BIA-ALCL). http://www.fda.gov/medicaldevices/ProductsandMedicalProcedures/ImplantsandProsthetics/Breastimplants/ucm239995.htm
93. Halsted WSI. The results of radical operations for the cure of carcinoma of the breast. *Ann Surg.* 1907;46:1–19.
94. Anonymous. *Report by the American College of Surgeons Commission on Cancer.* American College of Surgeons; 1982.
95. Moxley JH III, Allegra JC, Henney J, et al. Treatment of primary breast cancer. Summary of the National Institutes of Health Consensus Development Conference. *JAMA.* 1980;244:797–800.
96. Omlin A, Amichetti M, Azria D, et al. Boost radiotherapy in young women with ductal carcinoma in situ: a multicentre, retrospective study of the Rare Cancer Network. *Lancet Oncol.* 2006;7:652–656.
97. Shah C, McGee M, Wilkinson JB, et al. Clinical outcomes using accelerated partial breast irradiation in patients with ductal carcinoma in situ. *Clin Breast Cancer.* 2012;12:259–263.
98. Ciervide R, Dhage S, Guth A, et al. Five year outcome of 145 patients with ductal carcinoma in situ (DCIS) after accelerated breast radiotherapy. *Int J Radiat Oncol Biol Phys.* 2012;83:e159–e164.
99. Shah C, Vicini F, Wazer DE, et al. The American Brachytherapy Society consensus statement for accelerated partial breast irradiation. *Brachytherapy.* 2018;17(1):154–170.
100. Ragaz J, Jackson SM, Le N, et al. Adjuvant radiotherapy and chemotherapy in node-positive premenopausal women with breast cancer. *N Engl J Med.* 1997;337:956–962.
101. Recht A, Edge SB, Solin LJ, et al. Postmastectomy radiotherapy: clinical practice guidelines of the American Society of Clinical Oncology. *J Clin Oncol.* 2001;19:1539–1569.
102. Harris JR, Halpin-Murphy P, McNeese M, et al. Consensus Statement on postmastectomy radiation therapy. *Int J Radiat Oncol Biol Phys.* 1999;44:989–990.
103. Favourable and unfavourable effects on long-term survival of radiotherapy for early breast cancer: an overview of the randomised trials. Early Breast Cancer Trialists' Collaborative Group. *Lancet.* 2000;355:1757–1770.
104. Donker M, van Tienhoven G, Straver ME, et al. Radiotherapy or surgery of the axilla after a positive sentinel node in breast cancer (EORTC 10981–22023 AMAROS): a randomised, multicentre, open-label, phase 3 non-inferiority trial. *Lancet Oncol.* 2014;15(12):1303–1310.
105. http://cancer.lifemath.net.
106. www.finprog.org/default.asp.
107. Rouzier R, Perou CM, Symmans WF, et al. Breast cancer molecular subtypes respond differently to preoperative chemotherapy. *Clin Cancer Res.* 2005;11:5678–5685.
108. Foulkes WD, Smith IE, Reis-Filho JS. Triple-negative breast cancer. *N Engl J Med.* 2010;363:1938–1948.
109. Robbins GF, Shah J, Rosen P, et al. Inflammatory carcinoma of the breast. *Surg Clin North Am.* 1974;54:801–810.
110. Bell C. *A System of Operative Surgery Founded on the Basis of Anatomy.* Hale and Hosmer; 1812:128.
111. Lee BJ, Tannenbaum NE. Inflammatory carcinoma of the breast: a report of twenty-eight cases from the breast clinic of Memorial Hospital. *Surg Gynecol Obstet.* 1924;39:580–595.
112. Chang S, Parker SL, Pham T, et al. Inflammatory breast carcinoma incidence and survival: the surveillance, epidemiology, and end results program of the National Cancer Institute, 1975–1992. *Cancer.* 1998;82:2366–2372.
113. Dawood S, Merajver SD, Viens P, et al. International expert panel on inflammatory breast cancer: consensus statement for standardized diagnosis and treatment. *Ann Oncol.* 2011;22:515–523.
114. Kleer CG, van Golen KL, Merajver SD. Molecular biology of breast cancer metastasis. Inflammatory breast cancer: clinical syndrome and molecular determinants. *Breast Cancer Res.* 2000;2:423–429.
115. Jaiyesimi IA, Buzdar AU, Hortobagyi G. Inflammatory breast cancer: a review. *J Clin Oncol.* 1992;10:1014–1024.
116. Harris EE, Schultz D, Bertsch H, et al. Ten-year outcome after combined modality therapy for inflammatory breast cancer. *Int J Radiat Oncol Biol Phys.* 2003;55:1200–1208.

117. Hennessy BT, Gonzalez-Angulo AM, Hortobagyi GN, et al. Disease-free and overall survival after pathologic complete disease remission of cytologically proven inflammatory breast carcinoma axillary lymph node metastases after primary systemic chemotherapy. *Cancer.* 2006;106:1000–1006.
118. Perez CA, Fields JN, Fracasso PM, et al. Management of locally advanced carcinoma of the breast. II. Inflammatory carcinoma. *Cancer.* 1994;74:466–476.
119. Smoot RL, Koch CA, Degnim AC, et al. A single-center experience with inflammatory breast cancer, 1985–2003. *Arch Surg.* 2006;141:567–572; discussion 572–573.
120. Baldini E, Gardin G, Evangelista G, et al. Long-term results of combined-modality therapy for inflammatory breast carcinoma. *Clin Breast Cancer.* 2004;5:358–363.
121. Liauw SL, Benda RK, Morris CG, et al. Inflammatory breast carcinoma: outcomes with trimodality therapy for nonmetastatic disease. *Cancer.* 2004;100:920–928.
122. Wyld L, Garg DK, Kumar ID, et al. Stage and treatment variation with age in postmenopausal women with breast cancer: compliance with guidelines. *Br J Cancer.* 2004;90:1486–1491.
123. Enger SM, Thwin SS, Buist DS, et al. Breast cancer treatment of older women in integrated health care settings. *J Clin Oncol.* 2006;24:4377–4383.
124. Lavelle K, Todd C, Moran A, et al. Non-standard management of breast cancer increases with age in the UK: a population based cohort of women > or = 65 years. *Br J Cancer.* 2007;96:1197–1203.
125. Cyr A, Gillanders WE, Aft RL, et al. Breast cancer in elderly women (>/= 80 years): variation in standard of care. *J Surg Oncol.* 2011;103:201–206.
126. Bastiaannet E, Liefers GJ, de Craen AJ, et al. Breast cancer in elderly compared to younger patients in the Netherlands: stage at diagnosis, treatment and survival in 127,805 unselected patients. *Breast Cancer Res Treat.* 2010;124:801–807.
127. Diab SG, Elledge RM, Clark GM. Tumor characteristics and clinical outcome of elderly women with breast cancer. *J Natl Cancer Inst.* 2000;92:550–556.
128. Chagpar AB, McMasters KM, Edwards MJ; North American Fareston Tamoxifen Adjuvant Trial. Can sentinel node biopsy be avoided in some elderly breast cancer patients? *Ann Surg.* 2009;249:455–460.
129. International Breast Cancer Study Group; Rudenstam CM, Zahrieh D, et al. Randomized trial comparing axillary clearance versus no axillary clearance in older patients with breast cancer: first results of International Breast Cancer Study Group Trial 10–93. *J Clin Oncol.* 2006;24:337–344.
130. Martelli G, Miceli R, Costa A, et al. Elderly breast cancer patients treated by conservative surgery alone plus adjuvant tamoxifen: fifteen-year results of a prospective study. *Cancer.* 2008;112:481–488.
131. Hughes KS, Schnaper LA, Bellon JR, et al. Lumpectomy plus tamoxifen with or without irradiation in women age 70 years or older with early breast cancer: long-term follow-up of CALGB 9343. *J Clin Oncol.* 2013;31:2382–2387.
132. Caillet P, Canoui-Poitrine F, Vouriot J, et al. Comprehensive geriatric assessment in the decision-making process in elderly patients with cancer: ELCAPA study. *J Clin Oncol.* 2011;29:3636–3642.
133. Stensheim H, Moller B, van Dijk T, et al. Cause-specific survival for women diagnosed with cancer during pregnancy or lactation: a registry-based cohort study. *J Clin Oncol.* 2009;27:45–51.
134. Salani R, Billingsley CC, Crafton SM. Cancer and pregnancy: an overview for obstetricians and gynecologists. *Am J Obstet Gynecol.* 2014;211:7–14.
135. Ventura SJ. First births to older mothers, 1970–86. *Am J Public Health.* 1989;79:1675–1677.
136. Voulgaris E, Pentheroudakis G, Pavlidis N. Cancer and pregnancy: a comprehensive review. *Surg Oncol.* 2011;20:e175–e185.
137. Liberman L, Giess CS, Dershaw DD, et al. Imaging of pregnancy-associated breast cancer. *Radiology.* 1994;191:245–248.
138. Ahn BY, Kim HH, Moon WK, et al. Pregnancy- and lactation-associated breast cancer: mammographic and sonographic findings. *J Ultrasound Med.* 2003;22:491–497; quiz 498–499.
139. Behrman RH, Homer MJ, Yang WT, et al. Mammography and fetal dose. *Radiology.* 2007;243:605; author reply: 605–606.
140. Anderson BO, Petrek JA, Byrd DR, et al. Pregnancy influences breast cancer stage at diagnosis in women 30 years of age and younger. *Ann Surg Oncol.* 1996;3:204–211.
141. Middleton LP, Amin M, Gwyn K, et al. Breast carcinoma in pregnant women: assessment of clinicopathologic and immunohistochemical features. *Cancer.* 2003;98:1055–1060.
142. Nugent P, O'Connell TX. Breast cancer and pregnancy. *Arch Surg.* 1985;120:1221–1224.
143. Clark RM, Chua T. Breast cancer and pregnancy: the ultimate challenge. *Clin Oncol.* 1989;1:11–18.
144. Gemignani ML, Petrek JA, Borgen PI. Breast cancer and pregnancy. *Surg Clin North Am.* 1999;79:1157–1169.
145. Amant F, von Minckwitz G, Han SN, et al. Prognosis of women with primary breast cancer diagnosed during pregnancy: results from an international collaborative study. *J Clin Oncol.* 2013;31:2532–2539.
146. Azim HA Jr, Santoro L, Russell-Edu W, et al. Prognosis of pregnancy-associated breast cancer: a meta-analysis of 30 studies. *Cancer Treat Rev.* 2012;38:834–842.
147. Barron WM. The pregnant surgical patient: medical evaluation and management. *Ann Intern Med.* 1984;101:683–691.
148. Mazze RI, Kallen B. Reproductive outcome after anesthesia and operation during pregnancy: a registry study of 5405 cases. *Am J Obstet Gynecol.* 1989;161:1178–1185.
149. Gianopoulos JG. Establishing the criteria for anesthesia and other precautions for surgery during pregnancy. *Surg Clin North Am.* 1995;75:33–45.
150. Duncan PG, Pope WD, Cohen MM, et al. Fetal risk of anesthesia and surgery during pregnancy. *Anesthesiology.* 1986;64:790–794.
151. Antypas C, Sandilos P, Kouvaris J, et al. Fetal dose evaluation during breast cancer radiotherapy. *Int J Radiat Oncol Biol Phys.* 1998;40:995–999.
152. CDC. Radiation and Pregnancy: Information for Clinicians. https://www.cdc.gov/nceh/radiation/emergencies/prenatalphysician.htm
153. Keleher A, Wendt R III, Delpassand E, et al. The safety of lymphatic mapping in pregnant breast cancer patients using Tc-99m sulfur colloid. *Breast J.* 2004;10:492–495.
154. Gentilini O, Cremonesi M, Trifiro G, et al. Safety of sentinel node biopsy in pregnant patients with breast cancer. *Ann Oncol.* 2004;15:1348–1351.
155. Mondi MM, Cuenca RE, Ollila DW, et al. Sentinel lymph node biopsy during pregnancy: initial clinical experience. *Ann Surg Oncol.* 2007;14:218–221.
156. Gropper AB, Calvillo KZ, Dominici L, et al. Sentinel lymph node biopsy in pregnant women with breast cancer. *Ann Surg Oncol.* 2014;21:2506–2511.
157. Berry DL, Theriault RL, Holmes FA, et al. Management of breast cancer during pregnancy using a standardized protocol. *J Clin Oncol.* 1999;17:855–861.
158. Cardonick E, Iacobucci A. Use of chemotherapy during human pregnancy. *Lancet Oncol.* 2004;5:283–291.
159. Hahn KM, Johnson PH, Gordon N, et al. Treatment of pregnant breast cancer patients and outcomes of children exposed to chemotherapy in utero. *Cancer.* 2006;107:1219–1226.
160. Zemlickis D, Lishner M, Degendorfer P, et al. Maternal and fetal outcome after breast cancer in pregnancy. *Am J Obstet Gynecol.* 1992;166:781–787.
161. Zagouri F, Sergentanis TN, Chrysikos D, et al. Trastuzumab administration during pregnancy: a systematic review and meta-analysis. *Breast Cancer Res Treat.* 2013;137:349–357.
162. White J, Kearins O, Dodwell D, et al. Male breast carcinoma: increased awareness needed. *Breast Cancer Res.* 2011;13:219.
163. Tai YC, Domchek S, Parmigiani G, et al. Breast cancer risk among male BRCA1 and BRCA2 mutation carriers. *J Natl Cancer Inst.* 2007;99:1811–1814.
164. Ding YC, Steele L, Kuan CJ, et al. Mutations in BRCA2 and PALB2 in male breast cancer cases from the United States. *Breast Cancer Res Treat.* 2011;126:771–778.

165. Boyd J, Rhei E, Federici MG, et al. Male breast cancer in the hereditary nonpolyposis colorectal cancer syndrome. *Breast Cancer Res Treat.* 1999;53:87–91.
166. Brinton LA. Breast cancer risk among patients with Klinefelter syndrome. *Acta Paediatr.* 2011;100:814–818.
167. Thomas DB, Jimenez LM, McTiernan A, et al. Breast cancer in men: risk factors with hormonal implications. *Am J Epidemiol.* 1992;135:734–748.
168. Thomas DB. Breast cancer in men. *Epidemiol Rev.* 1993;15: 220–231.
169. Chavez-Macgregor M, Clarke CA, Lichtensztajn D, et al. Male breast cancer according to tumor subtype and race: a population-based study. *Cancer.* 2013;119:1611–1617.
170. Golshan M, Rusby J, Dominguez F, et al. Breast conservation for male breast carcinoma. *Breast.* 2007;16:653–656.
171. Ribeiro G, Swindell R. Adjuvant tamoxifen for male breast cancer (MBC). *Br J Cancer.* 1992;65:252–254.
172. Eggemann H, Ignatov A, Smith BJ, et al. Adjuvant therapy with tamoxifen compared to aromatase inhibitors for 257 male breast cancer patients. *Breast Cancer Res Treat.* 2013;137:465–470.
173. Davies C, Pan H, Godwin J, et al. Long-term effects of continuing adjuvant tamoxifen to 10 years versus stopping at 5 years after diagnosis of oestrogen receptor-positive breast cancer: ATLAS, a randomised trial. *Lancet.* 2013;381:805–816.
174. Hémminki K, Scelo G, Boffetta P, et al. Second primary malignancies in patients with male breast cancer. *Br J Cancer.* 2005;92: 1288–1292.
175. van Tienhoven G, Voogd AC, Peterse JL, et al. Prognosis after treatment for loco-regional recurrence after mastectomy or breast conserving therapy in two randomised trials (EORTC 10801 and DBCG-82TM). EORTC Breast Cancer Cooperative Group and the Danish Breast Cancer Cooperative Group. *Eur J Cancer.* 1999;35:32–38.
176. Francis M, Cakir B, Ung O, et al. Prognosis after breast recurrence following conservative surgery and radiotherapy in patients with node-negative breast cancer. *Br J Surg.* 1999;86:1556–1562.
177. Dalberg K, Mattsson A, Sandelin K, et al. Outcome of treatment for ipsilateral breast tumor recurrence in early-stage breast cancer. *Breast Cancer Res Treat.* 1998;49:69–78.
178. Early Breast Cancer Trialists' Collaborative Group (EBCTCG); Darby S, McGale P, et al. Effect of radiotherapy after breast-conserving surgery on 10-year recurrence and 15-year breast cancer death: meta-analysis of individual patient data for 10,801 women in 17 randomised trials. *Lancet.* 2011;378:1707–1716.
179. Katz A, Strom EA, Buchholz TA, et al. Locoregional recurrence patterns after mastectomy and doxorubicin-based chemotherapy: implications for postoperative irradiation. *J Clin Oncol.* 2000;18:2817–2827.
180. Willner J, Kiricuta IC, Kolbl O. Locoregional recurrence of breast cancer following mastectomy: always a fatal event? Results of univariate and multivariate analysis. *Int J Radiat Oncol Biol Phys.* 1997;37:853–863.
181. Solin LJ, Fourquet A, Vicini FA, et al. Salvage treatment for local or local-regional recurrence after initial breast conservation treatment with radiation for ductal carcinoma in situ. *Eur J Cancer.* 2005;41:1715–1723.
182. Paget J. On disease of the mammary areola preceding cancer of the mammary gland. *St Bartholomew's Hosp Rep.* 1874; 10:87.
183. Chen CY, Sun LM, Anderson BO. Paget disease of the breast: changing patterns of incidence, clinical presentation, and treatment in the U.S. *Cancer.* 2006;107:1448–1458.
184. Ikeda DM, Helvie MA, Frank TS, et al. Paget disease of the nipple: radiologic-pathologic correlation. *Radiology.* 1993;189:89–94.
185. Müller J. *Uber den feineren Ban und Die Formen der Krankaften Geschwulste: Volume 1.* Greiner; 1838:54–57.
186. Birch JM, Alston RD, McNally RJ, et al. Relative frequency and morphology of cancers in carriers of germline TP53 mutations. *Oncogene.* 2001;20:4621–4628.
187. Reinfuss M, Mitus J, Duda K, et al. The treatment and prognosis of patients with phyllodes tumor of the breast: an analysis of 170 cases. *Cancer.* 1996;77:910–916.
188. Dillon MF, Quinn CM, McDermott EW, et al. Needle core biopsy in the diagnosis of phyllodes neoplasm. *Surgery.* 2006;140:779–784.
189. Lee AH, Hodi Z, Ellis IO, et al. Histological features useful in the distinction of phyllodes tumour and fibroadenoma on needle core biopsy of the breast. *Histopathology.* 2007;51:336–344.
190. Macdonald OK, Lee CM, Tward JD, et al. Malignant phyllodes tumor of the female breast: association of primary therapy with cause-specific survival from the Surveillance, Epidemiology, and End Results (SEER) program. *Cancer.* 2006;107:2127–2133.
191. Kessinger A, Foley JF, Lemon HM, et al. Metastatic cystosarcoma phyllodes: a case report and review of the literature. *J Surg Oncol.* 1972;4:131–147.

72

Thyroid Gland

Sarah B. Fisher and Elizabeth G. Grubbs

Key Points

1. Understanding of the anatomy and embryology of the thyroid gland facilitates identification and preservation of the recurrent laryngeal nerves and parathyroid glands.
2. A nonrecurrent laryngeal nerve is most common on the right and is associated with vascular developmental abnormalities (arteria lusoria), whereas a left nonrecurrent nerve (rare) may be observed with situs inversus.
3. Initial imaging for thyroid pathology includes a thorough ultrasound that encompasses the thyroid and the central and lateral neck compartments, with fine-needle aspiration (FNA) biopsy of nodules serving as the gold standard for initial diagnosis.
4. The Bethesda system uses cytopathology to risk-stratify FNA-biopsy results; molecular testing is a diagnostic adjunct for indeterminate nodules but requires an understanding of the strengths and limitations of the specific test.
5. A diagnosis of medullary thyroid cancer (MTC) should prompt a genetic evaluation, with the genotype/phenotype correlation guiding timing of care for those with hereditary syndromes (MEN2A, MEN2B, and familial MTC).
6. Anaplastic thyroid cancer (ATC) should be suspected in the patient with rapid growth and sudden onset of compressive symptoms, hoarseness, and/or dysphagia; imaging will often demonstrate invasion into local structures. These patients should be rapidly triaged to a multidisciplinary team experienced in treating ATC.
7. When deciding between lobectomy and total thyroidectomy for small well-differentiated thyroid cancers, surgical decision making should take into account the underlying disease process, the necessity of adjuvant radioactive iodine, and patient preferences.
8. Compartment-based lymph node dissection is therapeutic for patients with lymph node metastases.

Thyroid lobectomy and total thyroidectomy are both appropriate surgical options for managing thyroid conditions, with their use depending on the specific clinical scenario. Lobectomy may be sufficient for diagnostic evaluation of indeterminate nodules or managing select cases of thyroid cancer or nodular disease, while total thyroidectomy is typically preferred for more extensive disease, such as advanced thyroid cancer, certain cases of hyperthyroidism, or prophylaxis in the setting of Multiple Endocrine Neoplasia (MEN) Type 2. A concomitant compartmental anatomically based lymph node dissection is appropriate for some thyroid malignancies. An understanding of the embryology, anatomy, and physiology of thyroid disease and the technical aspects of the operation is essential to avoid complications of thyroid surgery.

EMBRYOLOGY

The thyroid is the first endocrine gland in the body to form during development, with the median thyroid component descending from the foramen cecum at the base of the tongue at around 4 weeks of gestation. The lateral portion of the thyroid develops later from the caudal pharyngeal endoderm and fourth and fifth branchial pouches; fusion with the median portion forms the tubercle of Zuckerkandl. By 6 weeks of gestation, the foramen cecum resorbs, leaving a fibrous thyroglossal duct attached to the central hyoid bone. This is clinically relevant when incomplete resorption of the tract results in a thyroglossal duct cyst, or, more commonly, persistence of the distal portion of the tract results in a pyramidal lobe. Developmental abnormalities of the aortic arch may lead to altered position of the recurrent laryngeal nerves (RLNs).[1] Embryologic anomalies and their surgical implications are summarized in **Table 72.1**.

1 ANATOMY OF THE THYROID

The thyroid is a bilobed gland that weighs between 15 and 30 g and sits anterior to the trachea, just inferior to the cricoid cartilage within the central compartment of the neck. Each lobe is approximately 4 to 5 cm in craniocaudal dimension, 2 to 3 cm anteroposterior, and 3 cm in width, although substantial variations in size exist. Laterally, the thyroid is bordered by the medial aspects of the carotid sheath. Anteriorly, the sternothyroid and sternohyoid muscles cover the gland. The trachea and the esophagus (particularly on the left side) comprise the posterior borders. The pretracheal fascia extends to form a thin layer of connective tissue that invests the thyroid; in the absence of thyroiditis or invasive malignancy, this layer represents an easily mobilized plane of dissection. The sheath condenses as the anterior suspensory ligament of the thyroid above the isthmus; posteromedially to the thyroid gland, it condenses to form the firm attachment to the trachea called the ligament of Berry. The RLN and its insertion into the larynx, behind the articulation of the thyroid and cricoid cartilages, is often intimately associated with the ligament of Berry and the RLN is most vulnerable to iatrogenic injury at this relatively fixed point.

Table 72.1. Medical and Surgical Implications of Embryologic Thyroid Anomalies

Condition	Mechanism	Presentation	Treatment
Thyroid agenesis	Failure of the thyroid anlage to form	Congenital hypothyroidism (dwarfism and irreversible brain dysfunction, or cretinism)	Early recognition allows for thyroid hormone replacement
Thyroglossal duct cyst	Failure of the thyroglossal duct to completely resorb	Midline neck mass that elevates with tongue protrusion	Sistrunk procedure: resection of the entire thyroglossal duct including the midportion of the hyoid bone
Lingual thyroid	Failure of the median portion of the thyroid to descend	Mass at the base of the tongue, often combined with the absence of thyroid tissue elsewhere	Surgical excision or radioactive iodine ablation, with awareness of the need for thyroid hormone replacement
Ectopic thyroid tissue	Embryologic rests of thyroid tissue in the *central* compartment of the neck	Ectopic thyroid mass (thyroid cancer may also develop in these rests)	Surgical excision; not to be confused with thyroid tissue in the lateral compartment, which is not an embryologic abnormality and instead represents a regional nodal metastasis of differentiated thyroid cancer
Nonrecurrent laryngeal nerve	Abnormal development of the aortic arch; most often right-sided (0.3–1.6% of patients undergoing thyroid surgery) and associated with an aberrant right subclavian artery that arises directly from the aorta and courses posterior to the esophagus. May occur on the left (0.04%) but requires a right-sided aortic arch (as in situs inversus)	Typically silent; may be associated with dysphagia lusoria (compression of the esophagus between the trachea and a retroesophageal right subclavian artery)	Preoperative imaging that suggests aberrant arterial anatomy should heighten awareness of the possibility of a nonrecurrent nerve

Vasculature

The thyroid has a rich blood supply, which is increased in certain pathologic conditions. The superior thyroid artery arises off the external carotid artery and courses inferiorly along the inferior pharyngeal constrictor muscles to the thyroid, branching into at least an anterior and posterior branch close to the superior pole of the thyroid gland. The inferior thyroid artery arises from the thyrocervical trunk, courses medially deep to the carotid artery, and branches into several smaller vessels that join the thyroid directly just inferior to the ligament of Berry near the tracheoesophageal groove. These vessels are intimately associated with the RLN, and care must be taken during ligation to avoid iatrogenic nerve injury. Careful ligation of both the superior and inferior thyroid arteries close to the thyroid capsule will allow preservation of branches that supply the parathyroid glands. A thyroid ima artery, when present (10% of patients), arises directly from the great vessels and courses anterior to the trachea to the inferior portion of the thyroid gland. The thyroid ima artery is variable in presence and size, but can represent a significant source of blood loss when unrecognized.

The venous drainage of the thyroid is comprised of a plexus of vessels that condense into three named veins: the superior and middle thyroid veins drain to the ipsilateral internal jugular vein, and the inferior thyroid vein drains into the ipsilateral brachiocephalic vein. The middle thyroid vein may be absent or duplicated; when present, medialization of the thyroid may stretch and tear this vein if unrecognized.

Lymphatics

The lymphatic plexus surrounding the thyroid gland is rich and variable. Intracapsular lymph channels in the thyroid gland provide communication across the isthmus and between lobes. The central lymph node compartment includes levels VI and VII and encompasses the prelaryngeal, pretracheal, and paratracheal lymph nodes. It extends superiorly from the hyoid bone, inferiorly to the innominate artery and is bounded laterally by the carotid sheath; level VI is distinguished from level VII at the level of the sternal notch (**Fig. 72.1**).[2] The prelaryngeal lymph nodes reside in the midline just above the anterior suspensory ligament and the isthmus of the thyroid. Also called Delphian lymph nodes after the Greek Mythology "Oracle of Delphi" for their role as a harbinger of outcome,

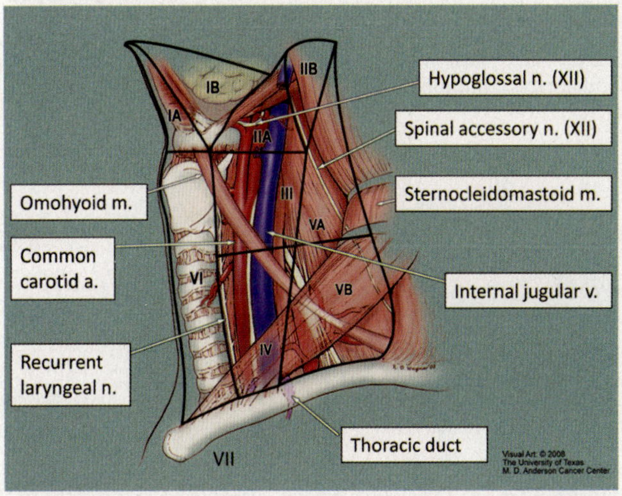

Figure 72.1. The central (VI and VII) and lateral (I to V) compartments of the neck. (Adapted from Fisher SB, Perrier ND. Chapter 15: Differentiated thyroid cancer—surgical considerations. In: *Comprehensive Clinical Oncology*. Vol English Edition. Libromed Panama; 2020, with permission from Libromed Panama, Republic of Panama. *Comprehensive Clinical Oncology, Current Practices*, English Edition, 2020.)

SURGICAL ENDOCRINOLOGY

these are frequently the first nodes encountered upon opening the midline raphe. When associated with metastasis from malignancy, these nodes are associated with adverse pathologic characteristics of the primary tumor and involvement of other central or lateral compartment lymph nodes.[3] Although most lymph node metastases from thyroid cancer occur in the central compartment before spread to the lateral compartment, "skip" metastases to the lateral compartments have been reported, particularly in tumors located in the superior poles.[4]

The lateral compartment includes the submental nodes (level I), upper jugular (level II), midjugular (level III), lower jugular (level IV), and posterior triangle (level V) (**Fig. 72.1**).[2] The role and extent of prophylactic and therapeutic node dissection for thyroid cancer is discussed later.

Nerves

The thyroid gland itself is innervated by the cervical sympathetic chain, with two nerves in close vicinity that do not directly innervate the thyroid but are of critical importance: the external branch of the superior laryngeal nerve and the RLN.

The superior laryngeal nerve arises from the vagus and bifurcates into the internal branch (which enters the larynx at the thyrohyoid membrane to provide sensory information to the superior larynx) and the external branch, which contributes to voice pitch and projection by innervating the cricothyroid muscle. The course of the external branch is variable and meticulous dissection close to the superior pole is necessary to prevent iatrogenic injury during thyroidectomy (**Fig. 72.2**).

An understanding of the course of the RLN is critical for all surgeons who operate in the neck or chest (**Fig. 72.3**).[2] Inadvertent unilateral injury results in ipsilateral vocal cord paralysis and possible hoarseness; bilateral injury often requires an emergent surgical airway due to paralysis of the vocal cords in a closed position. On the right, the RLN arises from the vagus at the level of the subclavian artery, passing underneath it before ascending into the central neck at an oblique angle. The left RLN has a more vertical trajectory, arising from the vagus nerve at the level of the aortic arch posterior to the ligamentum arteriosum and ascending in the tracheoesophageal groove. Up to 34% of RLNs will branch prior to insertion, with motor fibers carried anteriorly and sensory branches posteriorly.[5] In addition to hoarseness due to motor dysfunction, inadvertent injury to the posterior sensory fibers can result in aspiration.

2 A nonrecurrent, or direct, laryngeal nerve, is most common on the right (up to 1.6% of patients) and is typically associated with a retroesophageal right subclavian artery (**Table 72.1**). Left-sided nonrecurrent laryngeal nerves require a right-sided aortic arch (situs inversus) with an aberrant left subclavian and are less common (**Table 72.1**). When available, preoperative recognition of aberrant vasculature on cross-sectional imaging (ie, CT of the chest or upper mediastinum) should alert the surgeon to the possibility of a nonrecurrent nerve. As CT of the chest is not routinely performed for most patients undergoing thyroidectomy, thoughtful ultrasound (US) may offer a more accessible alternative. Although operator dependent, in experienced hands, US can correctly identify aberrant neck vasculature (specifically the lack of a brachiocephalic trunk) and preoperatively predict patients with nonrecurrent right-sided laryngeal nerves with minimal exam time (median 5 minutes in one study) and few false positives (associated with obesity, large goiter, or tortuous arteries).[6] Although nonrecurrent laryngeal nerves are rare, their presence is associated with increased risk of iatrogenic nerve injury (12.9%).

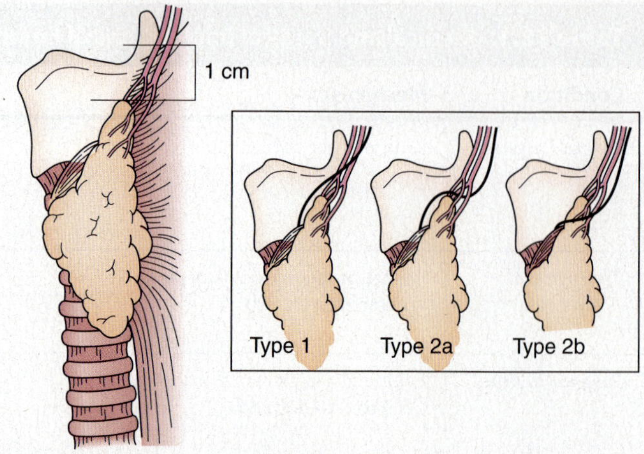

Figure 72.2. The Cernea classification of the external branch of the superior laryngeal nerve highlights the anatomic variability with progressively increasing risk of iatrogenic injury during thyroidectomy. Type I crosses the superior thyroid vessels ≥1 cm above the superior thyroid pole, type II crosses within 1 cm above the pole, and type III crosses below the superior pole.

Parathyroid Glands

The location of the parathyroid glands is variable but is often in close proximity to the thyroid, and care should be taken during thyroidectomy to preserve the parathyroid gland and its blood supply. Superior parathyroid glands are typically located superior to the tubercle of Zuckerkandl and posterior to the course of the RLN; they may be encountered adherent to the posterior thyroid capsule, within the tracheoesophageal groove, or directly adjacent to the RLN.[7] Inferior parathyroids are more variable and may be similarly adjacent to the RLN, associated with the inferolateral aspect of the thyroid, or

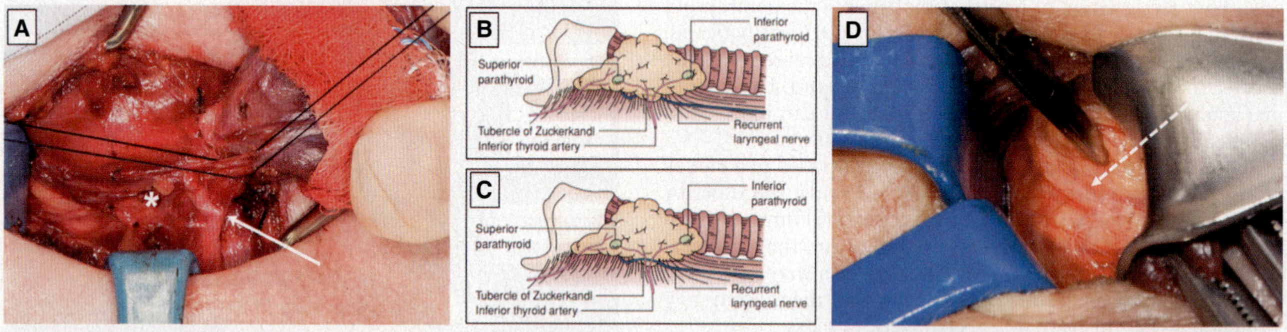

Figure 72.3. **A**: The most commonly encountered course of the right recurrent laryngeal nerve (RLN, *arrow*) with the thyroid rotated medially into the field, and the superior parathyroid preserved (*star*). The course of the nerve may vary with relation to the tracheoesophageal groove as well as the tubercle of Zuckerkandl, in which the nerve passes medial and posterior (**B**) versus (**C**), in which the RLN passes lateral to an enlarged tubercle. In the event of anomalous vasculature, the nerve will be nonrecurrent, as shown in (**D**) by the *arrow*, with the thyroid again retracted medially. (A–D: (Additional figures are adapted from Fisher SB, Perrier ND. Chapter 15: Differentiated thyroid cancer—surgical considerations. *Comprehensive Clinical Oncology*. Vol English Edition. Libromed Panama; 2020, with permission from Libromed Panama, Republic of Panama. *Comprehensive Clinical Oncology, Current Practices*, English Edition, 2020.)

within the thyrothymic ligament. True intrathyroidal parathyroids are rare. Normal parathyroids are often symmetric (80% for superior glands and 70% for inferior glands) and correct identification of their location and preservation of their blood supply is important to prevent postoperative hypocalcemia after thyroidectomy.

THYROID PHYSIOLOGY

The follicular cells of the thyroid produce thyroxine (T4) and tri-iodothyronine (T3) under the stimulus of thyrotropin (or thyroid stimulating hormone, TSH), which is secreted by the anterior pituitary. The process is dependent on dietary iodide, which in most developed regions far exceeds the daily requirement of 100 to 150 µg, with excess excreted by the kidneys. On a cellular level, thyroid follicles are comprised of epithelial cells (thyrocytes), which are organized in an ovoid structure with the interior containing iodinated thyroglobulin (colloid). The active uptake of iodide occurs via a Na+/I– symporter mediated by a Na+/K+-adenosine triphosphatase pump on the basolateral plasma membrane. After entry into the cell, thyroid peroxidase (TPO) couples iodide with tyrosine, leading to the production of T4 and T3, which are then coupled to thyroglobulin for storage (**Fig. 72.4**). The release of thyroid hormone into the circulation is mediated through micropinocytosis stimulated by TSH.

In humans, T4 is produced in excess of T3 by a ratio of 13:1 under normal physiologic conditions. A less active but more stable hormone, T4 is converted to T3 in the periphery (primarily liver and plasma) by type 1 deiodinase enzymes. The half-life of T3 is between 8 and 12 hours, whereas the half-life of T4 is approximately 7 days. The majority of circulating T4 and T3 (>99%) is bound to plasma proteins (thyroglobulin, albumin, thyroxine-binding prealbumin).

CLINICAL EVALUATION OF THE PATIENT WITH A THYROID DISORDER

A thorough history includes questions about prior thyroid-related concerns, medication use, previous thyroid biopsies, and history of head and neck or upper esophageal/thoracic surgery or radiation. Medications such as amiodarone or lithium can induce hyperthyroidism. A history of transient or permanent hypothyroidism requiring exogenous thyroid hormone should alert the clinician to the possibility of thyroiditis. Previous thyroid biopsies or the presence of known nodules on previous imaging studies provide information regarding patterns of growth and natural history that can be used to assess the risk of malignancy. Radiation exposure history (therapeutic or environmental), in addition to potentially creating fibrosis within the surgical field, is an important risk factor for later development of papillary thyroid cancer (PTC).[8] Family history of thyroid disorders or syndromic patterns that suggest an increased risk of thyroid cancer should be evaluated (eg, MEN type II, Cowden syndrome, Carney complex, familial adenomatous polyposis and/or Gardner syndrome, Werner syndrome, *DICER1* syndrome) and referral to genetic counseling considered.

Symptoms of hypo- or hyperthyroidism (**Table 72.2**) should be assessed and confirmed with laboratory testing. Mechanical symptoms such as dysphagia, dysphonia, dyspnea, compressive symptoms, and neck pain should be clarified with attention to duration, severity, and exacerbating factors. The timeline of symptom presentation provides clues to the etiology. A rapidly growing mass is concerning for thyroid lymphoma or anaplastic thyroid cancer (ATC), whereas a stable nodule over many years is less suspicious for malignancy.

The physical examination should include a thorough neck examination focusing on the thyroid (size, texture, nodularity, mobility) and evaluation for central and lateral adenopathy.

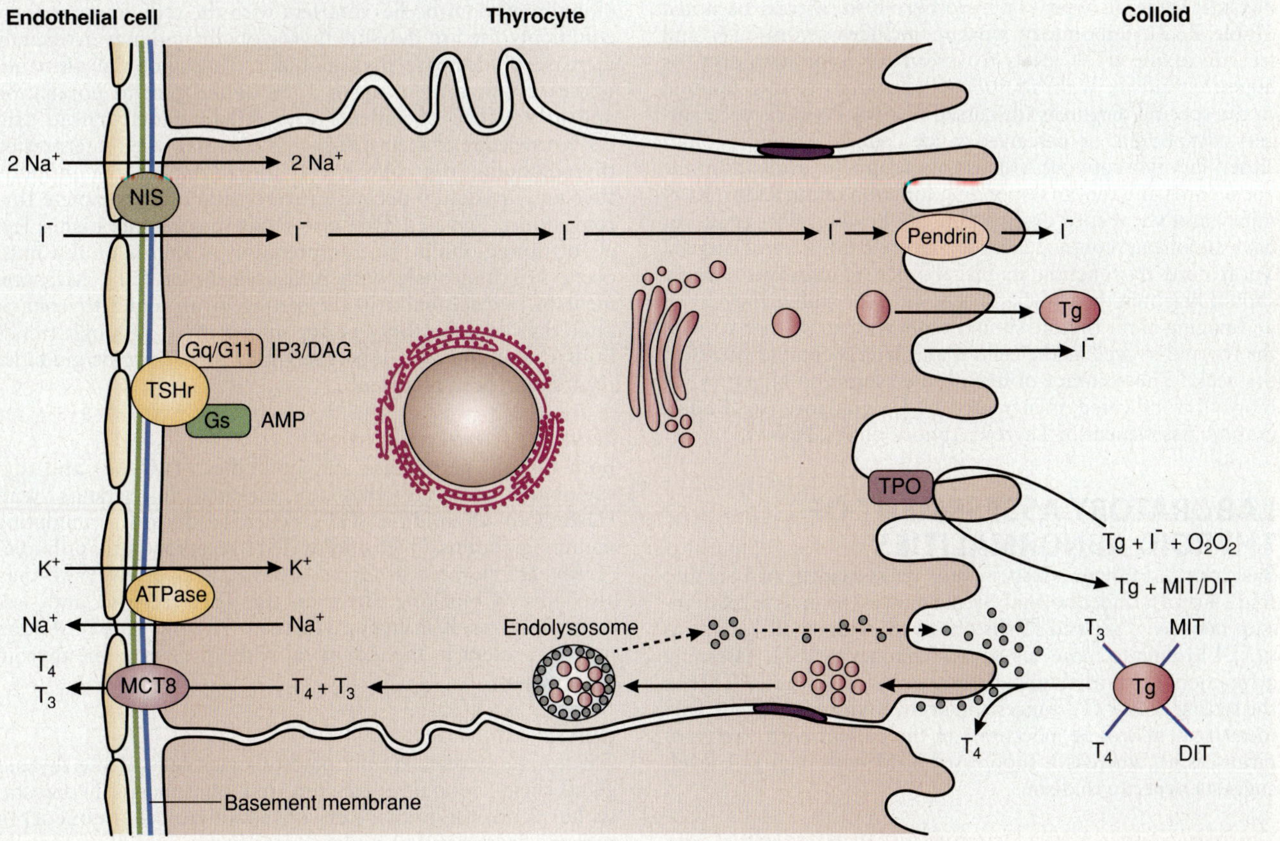

Figure 72.4. Thyroid hormone metabolism. Thyroxine (T_4) and tri-iodothyronine (T_3) are produced by the thyroid follicular cell in a complex biochemical pathway. It is dependent on the movement of circulating iodide through the follicular cell and into the intracellular colloid space. T_3 and T_4 are then bound to thyroglobulin (Tg) for eventual transport back through the follicular cell to be released into the intravascular space.

Table 72.2. Symptoms of Hypo- or Hyperthyroidism

	Hypothyroidism	Hyperthyroidism
Symptoms	Fatigue Sensitivity to cold Weight gain Dry skin/hair/nails Constipation Muscle weakness Depression	Nervousness or irritability Heat intolerance Palpitations Hyperphagia Weight loss Thin skin Diarrhea Weakness Insomnia
Signs	Puffy facies Macroglossia Bradycardia Hypermenorrhea or menorrhagia Delayed relaxation of deep tendon reflexes Hypercholesterolemia Generalized nonpitting edema	Thyromegaly ± thyroid bruit Tachycardia Sweating Oligo or amenorrhea Hyperactive deep tendon reflexes Tremor Pretibial myxedema[a] Exophthalmos[a]
Laboratory findings	Low fT4 Elevated TSH	Elevated fT4 and/or T3 Low/Suppressed TSH

[a]In patients with hyperthyroidism related to Graves disease.
fT4, serum free thyroxine; TSH, thyroid-stimulating hormone; T3, serum tri-iodothyronine.

Physical signs of hyper- or hypothyroidism should be noted (**Table 72.2**). Laboratory workup includes serum TSH and free thyroxine (fT4) levels to screen for hypothyroidism or hyperthyroidism, with additional laboratory testing tailored to the specific diagnosis (discussed below). Previous neck surgery, dysphonia, or perceived voice changes should prompt either laryngoscopy or videostroboscopy to evaluation the vocal cords and the corresponding function of the RLNs. RLN injury and vocal cord dysfunction can be clinically occult but have significant consequences for future contralateral surgery. Vocal cord dysfunction in the absence of previous surgery should heighten the clinician's suspicion for malignancy.

Imaging of the thyroid should begin with an US that assesses the thyroid as well as the central and lateral compartments of the neck.[9] The accuracy of fine-needle aspiration biopsy (FNA biopsy), if indicated, is increased by US guidance (see Radiographic Assessment of Thyroid Abnormalities, below).

LABORATORY ASSESSMENT OF THYROID ABNORMALITIES

Basic thyroid function tests include measurement of TSH and free T4 (fT4). Under normal circumstances, an inverse relationship between TSH and fT4 is observed, with small variations in fT4 leading to more substantial changes in TSH. Assuming a functional hypothalamic–pituitary axis, an elevated TSH in the setting of low fT4 suggests hypothyroidism (note that TSH measurement will be inaccurate in the patient with panhypopituitarism), whereas a suppressed TSH with high fT4 levels suggests hyperthyroidism.

Thyroid Stimulating Hormone (Thyrotropin, TSH)

Immunometric assays to measure TSH are highly sensitive and specific, making it the ideal method for detecting thyroid dysfunction in the patient with a functioning hypothalamic–pituitary axis. The range of normal is a spectrum and is usually between 0.27 mcIU/mL and 4.20 mcIU/mL, although target ranges for treatment during specific conditions (such as pregnancy or as suppressive therapy for differentiated thyroid cancer) are typically lower. Interpretation of TSH, particularly within the spectrum of normal ranges, must be considered with regard to concomitant symptoms of hypo- or hyperthyroidism (**Table 72.2**).

Free versus Total Thyroxine (T4) and Tri-iodothyronine (T3)

Levels of total T3 and T4 (defined as both free and protein bound) can vary based on variation in levels of plasma proteins. Multiple medications, including nonsteroidal anti-inflammatories, birth control pills, phenytoin, carbamazepine, furosemide, and aspirin, can alter levels of transport proteins directly or compete with T4 and T3 for binding, leading to variability in total T3 or T4 without impact on true thyroid function. Measuring free T4 improves the ability to detect true physiologic thyroid dysfunction, independent of alterations in transport proteins. Measurement of free T3, while possible, is often unreliable due to the extremely low level of circulating T3 not bound to plasma proteins. Instead, total T3 is often used as a surrogate, and is most useful when assessing hyperthyroid states—it may be elevated even when TSH and fT4 are normal. Conversely, it is also the last test to become abnormal in the hypothyroid state and thereby less useful in this setting.

Thyroglobulin and Thyroglobulin Antibodies

Thyroglobulin is a protein produced by normal thyroid tissue and differentiated thyroid cancer cells that clinically serve as a tumor marker. After complete removal of native thyroid tissue (ie, thyroidectomy), thyroglobulin should be undetectable, and, in the absence of thyroglobulin autoantibodies, a rise in thyroglobulin suggests microscopic disease recurrence. Thyroglobulin autoantibodies interfere with the radioimmunoassay commonly used to measure thyroglobulin and may artificially increase or decrease thyroglobulin. Thyroglobulin autoantibodies are present in up to 10% of the general population and up to 20% of patients with differentiated thyroid cancer. Knowledge of their presence is essential when interpreting thyroglobulin; in a patient with autoantibodies, the antibody titer may gradually decrease (over years) after complete thyroidectomy. Elevated TSH also tends to stimulate higher levels of thyroglobulin, so interpretation of thyroglobulin must occur simultaneously with measurement of TSH. Measurement of thyroglobulin in the setting of an intact thyroid or after thyroid lobectomy is not informative, although trends in thyroglobulin after lobectomy may provide some guidance regarding risk of recurrence.

Thyroid Autoantibodies

Both thyroid peroxidase autoantibodies (TPO-Ab) and thyroglobulin autoantibodies are elevated in patients with Hashimoto thyroiditis (HT), whereas thyroid stimulating immunoglobulins (TSI) and/or TSH receptor autoantibodies (TrAb) are elevated in Graves disease. Conversely TrAb may also have a blocking effect on the TSH receptor and, less commonly, result in hypothyroidism. Thyroid autoantibodies may be present in the individual without measurable thyroid dysfunction.

Calcitonin

Calcitonin, secreted by the parafollicular cells of the thyroid gland, helps modulate calcium and phosphorus homeostasis but is not the primary driver (parathyroid hormone is) in humans. It is useful as a tumor marker for medullary thyroid cancer (MTC). Given the rarity of MTC, calcitonin should not be used as a screening test for the general population, but tested only when suspicion for MTC exists.[9]

RADIOGRAPHIC ASSESSMENT OF THYROID ABNORMALITIES

US is the gold standard imaging modality for the thyroid and is advantageous in that it does not expose the patient to ionizing radiation. Other imaging modalities, including radionuclide imaging, computed tomography (CT), magnetic resonance imaging (MRI), and/or fluorodeoxyglucose positron emission tomography (FDG-PET) have specific roles in the evaluation of the patient with a thyroid complaint.

Ultrasound

3 Although user dependent, US provides information on the size, location, and radiographic characteristics of thyroid nodules, assessment of thyroid parenchyma, and evaluation of cervical lymph nodes. Regardless of the presence of other imaging, all patients with suspected structural abnormalities (thyroid nodules, thyroid cancer) should undergo a dedicated US that examines the thyroid and the central and lateral compartments of the neck. This is best performed with a high-frequency probe (7.5 to 15 mHz). Assessment of constitution (solid, cystic, spongiform, or mixed), presence of microcalcifications, and evaluation of echogenicity, shape, and borders (smooth vs irregular) is important when assessing risk for malignancy (**Fig. 72.5**).[9] Hypoechogenicity, irregular borders, and/or subtle microcalcifications are concerning for malignancy, whereas hyperechogenicity, smooth borders, and/or a "halo sign" (an anechoic rim) are more often benign. Large macrocalcifications, associated with posterior acoustic shadowing, are often benign. Combined with size, US characteristics inform the decision to perform FNA (**Table 72.3**).[10] Routinely performing FNA-biopsy on all nodules results in unnecessary procedures, whereas overly stringent criteria for biopsy may miss a clinically relevant cancer. In general, nodules above 1 cm, those with particularly concerning US characteristics, or those that are increasing in size over time merit FNA-biopsy. US should also be used to evaluate and/or FNA-biopsy lymph nodes (suspicious findings include loss of fatty hilum, microcalcifications, hyperechoic change, rounded shape, or necrosis[9]), which alters the planned operation in up to one third of patients with thyroid nodules.[2] Both the Thyroid Imaging Reporting and Data System (TI-RADS), developed by the American College of Radiology, and the American Thyroid Association (ATA) guidelines classification system are valuable ultrasonographic tools for evaluating thyroid nodules, as they aid in assessing the risk of malignancy in nodules.[11]

Radionuclide Imaging

Radionuclide uptake scans provide information regarding thyroid function but do little to delineate anatomy. The most commonly performed exam, technetium (Tc) pertechnetate scintigraphy, uses ^{99m}Tc pertechnetate, an isotope that emits primarily gamma (γ) radiation and is rapidly absorbed by the thyroid. In contrast to iodine, ^{99m}Tc is not incorporated into thyroglobulin and therefore scintigraphy must be performed within 20 to 30 minutes after injection. Normal scans demonstrate uptake of the radiotracer symmetrically across the thyroid. In patients with toxic adenoma, the uptake will concentrate at the area with the nodule (a hyperfunctioning or "hot" nodule), whereas patients with hypofunctioning nodule(s) ("cold" nodule) will demonstrate relative photopenia.[13] While a hot nodule is rarely malignant, a "cold" nodule was historically considered suspicious for malignancy. Today, with the sensitivity and specificity of FNA-biopsy, the use of scintigraphy in the evaluation for malignancy is outmoded. Thyroid scintigraphy is most useful in patients with hyperthyroidism to

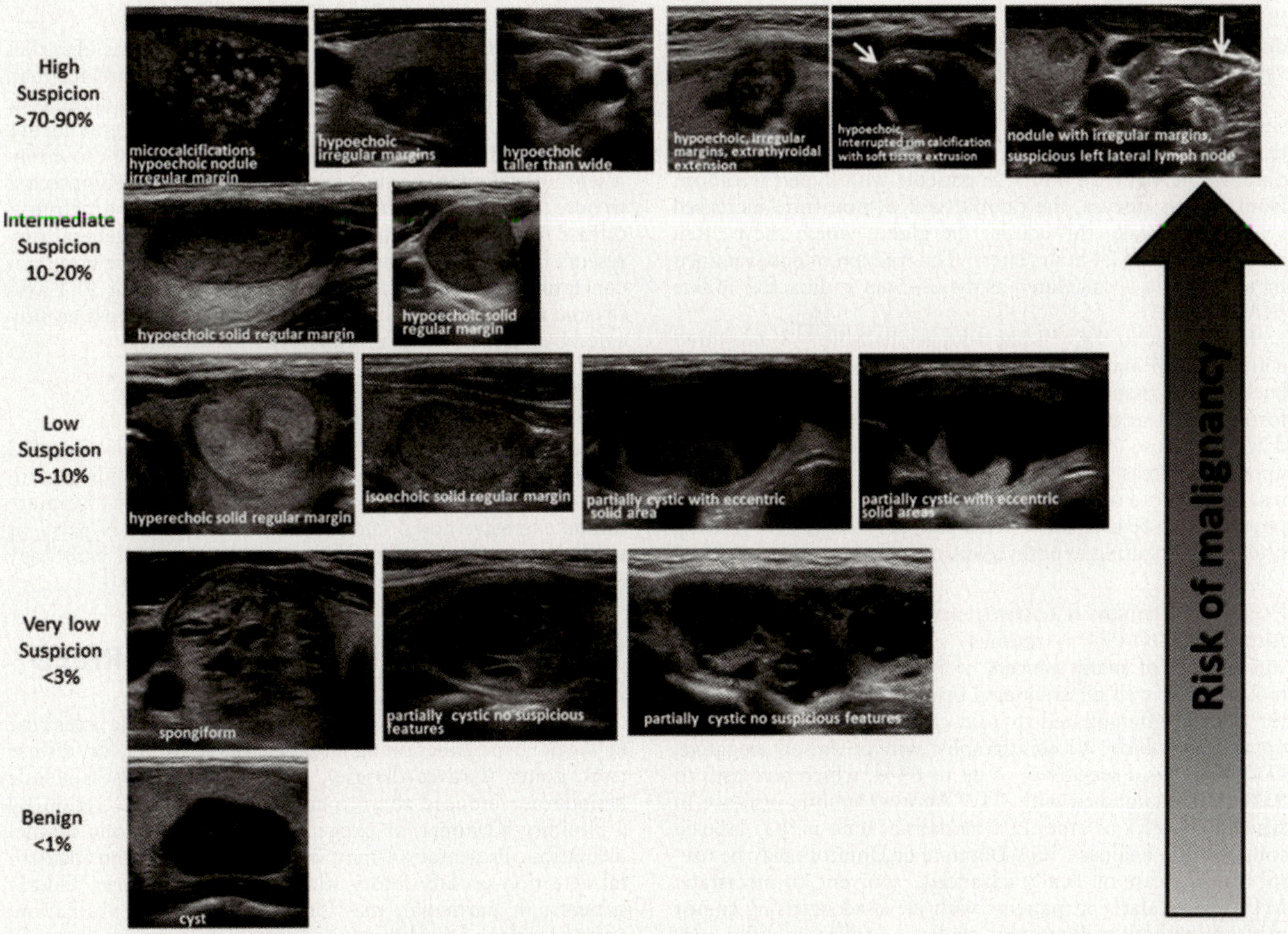

Figure 72.5. Ultrasound characteristics concerning for malignancy. (Reprinted with permission from Haugen et al.).[12]

Table 72.3. Guidelines for Fine-Needle Aspiration Biopsy of Thyroid Nodules

American Thyroid Association	National Comprehensive Cancer Network	Society of Radiologists in Ultrasound	Three-Tiered System	White Paper of the American College of Radiology
Solid hypoechoic nodules ≥1 cm with or without one or more: Irregular margins, microcalcification, taller than wide shape, rim calcifications with soft tissue extrusion, or extrathyroidal extension OR Solid isoechoic or hyperechoic nodules ≥1.5 cm without the above features OR spongiform or partially cystic nodules ≥2 cm without the above features[b]	Solid hypoechoic nodules[a] ≥1 cm with microcalcifications, infiltrative margins, or taller than wide in the transverse plane OR Solid nodules[a] without the above features ≥1.5 cm OR Spongiform nodules ≥2 cm	Solid nodules ≥1 cm with microcalcifications OR Solid nodules ≥1.5 cm OR Mixed solid-cystic nodules ≥2 cm	Solid nodules ≥1 cm with microcalcifications, hypoechoic features, increased vascularity, infiltrative margins, or taller than wide dimensions OR PET-avid nodules OR Any nodule associated with lymphadenopathy, extrathyroidal spread, lung metastases, or signs of ipsilateral vocal cord palsy	Any PET-avid nodule OR Biopsy based on US characteristics (not further specified)

[a]Or mixed solid-cystic nodules with a solid component measuring the same.
[b]May consider observation with serial ultrasound rather than biopsy if desired.
PET, positron emission tomography; US, ultrasound.
Adapted with permission from Fisher SB, Perrier ND. The incidental thyroid nodule. *CA Cancer J Clin.* 2018;68(2):97–105.

distinguish the source of overproduction (ie, a toxic adenoma vs toxic multinodular goiter [MNG] versus Graves disease).

The oral administration of ^{123}Iodine (^{123}I) allows for measurement of iodine uptake over time using the x-rays, β particles and γ rays transmitted by this radiotracer, with images obtained at 4 and 24 hours. In patients with hyperthyroidism from Graves disease, the thyroid will demonstrate increased symmetric uptake throughout the gland, which most often remains elevated 24 hours later.[13] The fraction of dose retained by the thyroid is calculated as the 24-hour radioactive iodine (RAI) uptake.

In contrast to ^{123}I, ^{131}I has a longer half-life (~8 days) and emits more β and γ radiation. It is thoroughly cleared from background tissues and is the isotope of choice when performing nuclear imaging for differentiated thyroid cancers. A diagnostic dose (1 to 5 mCi) allows for evaluation of iodine uptake, whereas therapeutic doses (30 to 150 mCi) ablate residual thyroid or thyroid cancer cells. Ablative ^{131}I scintigraphy may also be used for selected patients with Graves disease, often with resulting hypothyroidism.[14]

Positron Emission Tomography

Although FDG-PET is routinely employed for staging and surveillance of many cancers, it is not a first-line imaging modality for well differentiated thyroid cancers.[9] In contrast, for poorly differentiated thyroid cancers with loss of iodine uptake, in which ^{131}I scintigraphy will be falsely negative, FDG-PET has a sensitivity of up to 84%, which increases to 93% when combined with CT.[15] Another unique instance in which FDG-PET or other PET modalities such as ^{68}Ga-labeled somatostatin analogs (^{68}GA-Dotatate or Dotatoc) may be useful is in the case of locally advanced, recurrent, or metastatic MTC, particularly in patients with elevated or rising tumor markers without radiographic evidence of disease using conventional imaging.[16]

When an FDG-PET performed for other reasons identifies a thyroid nodule, the concern for malignancy is greater than for incidentally found nodules identified by other radiographic modalities. One systematic review of 55,000 patients identified PET-avid thyroid nodules in 1%, with 33% of those representing malignancy (most commonly PTC).[17] It is important to note that the pattern of uptake also provides information—diffuse tracer avidity within the thyroid gland in general represents benign disease, whereas uptake in a specific nodule is concerning for malignancy. Further evaluation of PET-avid thyroid nodules with US is necessary, with FNA-biopsy as indicated by characteristics on US.[9]

Computed Tomography and/or Magnetic Resonance Imaging

Cross-sectional imaging with CT (most commonly) or MRI (in select instances) is indicated for patients with findings concerning for locoregionally advanced disease (bulky primary tumor, extensive nodal metastases, concern for RLN palsy, or tracheal invasion) or for evaluation of substernal pathology (ie, MNG) not well visualized on US (**Fig. 72.6**).

THYROID DISORDERS CHARACTERIZED BY HYPERTHYROIDISM

Common causes of hyperthyroidism include toxic adenoma (a single hyperfunctioning nodule), toxic MNG, or diffuse toxic goiter (Graves disease). Less common causes include amiodarone-induced thyrotoxicosis (AIT), TSH secretion by a pituitary adenoma, or exogenous thyroid hormone supplementation. Presentation may range in severity from incidental detection on laboratory studies to thyroid storm. Elderly patients, in particular, may present with atrial fibrillation, angina, or congestive heart failure, and thyroid function should be evaluated during initial presentation of these illnesses.

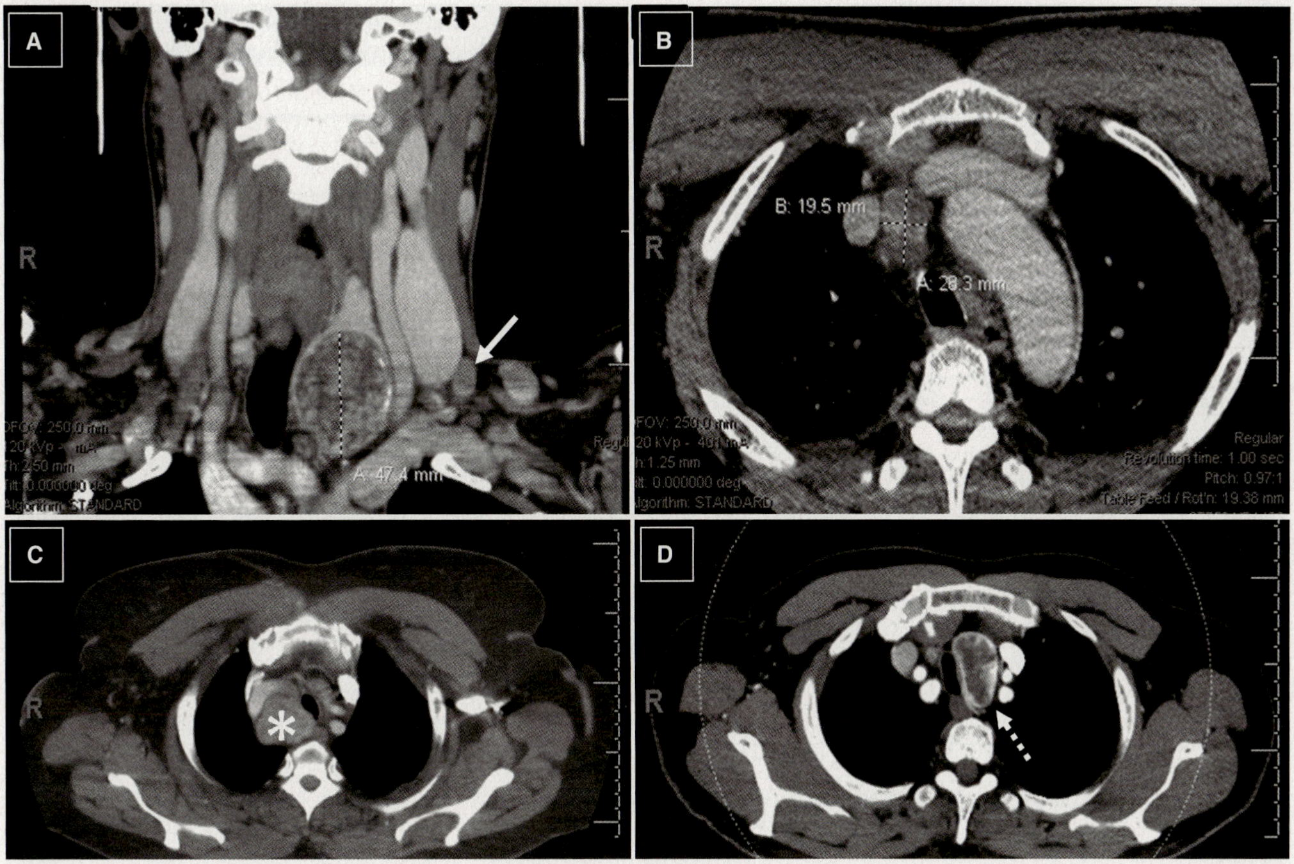

Figure 72.6. Utility of computed tomography in evaluating thyroid disease. **A:** Coronal view of a large left-sided tumor (4.7 cm) causing mild tracheal deviation and a pathologic left level IV lateral neck lymph node (*arrow*). **B:** Identification of a pathologic mediastinal/level VII lymph node (1.9 × 2.8 cm). **C:** A substernal goiter (*star*) causing tracheal compression, and **(D)** A left-sided substernal thyroid nodule (*dashed arrow*) not palpable on physical exam.

Initial treatment focuses on restoring normal physiology. Antithyroid drugs (ATDs) such as methimazole and propylthiouracil inhibit thyroid hormone synthesis with an onset of action over 2 to 6 weeks. Patients should be monitored carefully for adverse effects, including agranulocytosis (1 in 500 patients), which presents with fever and pharyngitis, and hepatotoxicity (0.3 to 0.7 per 1,000 patients). Hepatotoxicity is typically cholestatic when associated with methimazole, whereas propylthiouracil may cause hepatocellular injury and/or fulminant liver failure. Both agranulocytosis and hepatic toxicity are most common within the first 90 days of use.[14] Rash, pruritus, and arthralgias are less severe but more commonly encountered with ATDs. Beta blockade is useful in controlling tachycardia, tremors, heat sensitivity, and anxiety, and may inhibit peripheral conversion of T4 to T3 at high doses.[14] Titration of therapy should be based on T3 and fT4 levels, as TSH may remain suppressed for several months after normalization.

After stabilization, continuation of ATDs, ablation with RAI, or surgical resection offer potential definitive treatment for the patient with hyperthyroidism. The underlying etiology, patient-specific factors and preferences, and available health care infrastructure influence the optimal therapy for hyperthyroidism (**Table 72.4**).[18]

Toxic Adenoma

Typically, toxic adenomas grow to at least 2 cm in size before becoming biochemically apparent. Although RAI is a potential therapeutic option, it has several disadvantages as compared to thyroid lobectomy, including the possibility of leaving behind a palpable nodule and the probability of inducing hypothyroidism (see **Table 72.4**).[18] Thyroid lobectomy for patients with toxic adenoma has a lower rate of postoperative hypothyroidism (2% to 3%) as compared to lobectomy performed for other indications (20%). Thyroid lobectomy also has a faster return to the euthyroid state (2 to 3 days postoperatively, vs 75% response rate at 3 months for RAI) and a lower risk of disease recurrence (<1% vs 3% to 5.5% for RAI).[14]

Toxic Multinodular Goiter

Toxic MNG, in which hyperthyroidism results from more than one autonomously functioning nodules, may develop in a patient who was previously euthyroid either spontaneously or after exposure to an iodine load (Jod–Basedow phenomenon). Historically, efforts to iodinate salt or flour in iodine-deficient populations were followed by the development of toxic MNG over a time course of several years. Clinically, toxic MNG may be difficult to discern from Graves disease with nodular degeneration, however, patients with toxic MNG are more often female and older than 50 years of age, with a history of MNG. Laboratory testing demonstrates the absence of TSI and/or TrAb. Patients with toxic MNG often have concomitant indications for thyroidectomy, including compressive symptoms and/or substernal extension. While RAI remains a possible treatment option, requirement of repeated doses because of goiter size and poor iodine uptake is more common. ATDs are less likely to achieve remission in patients with toxic MNG than in Graves disease.

Graves Disease

Graves disease is an autoimmune disorder characterized by thyroid-stimulating antibodies that bind to the TSH receptor to stimulate thyroid hormone release and cause hypertrophy of the thyroid. Graves disease occurs in 20 to 50 individuals per 100,000, affecting women more frequently than men (lifetime risk 3% vs 0.5%).[19] In addition to hyperthyroidism,

Table 72.4. Comparison of Thyroidectomy, Radioactive Iodine Ablation, and Medical Therapy for Thyrotoxicosis

	Thyroidectomy	Radioactive Iodine Ablation (RAI)	Medical Therapy
Time of Onset	▪ Immediate	▪ 4–6 mo	▪ 4–6 wk
Advantages	▪ Immediately curative with quick onset ▪ May be beneficial for patients with limited access to care ▪ Lobectomy is appropriate for toxic adenoma, and may avoid iatrogenic hypothyroidism	▪ Less invasive than surgery ▪ May be more cost effective (dependent on geographic area)	▪ Noninvasive ▪ Nonablative (potential to retain native thyroid function) ▪ Achieves remission in 40–50% of patients with Graves after 12–18 mo; less likely in patients with toxic multinodular goiter
Disadvantages	▪ Typically requires medical therapy preoperatively ▪ Invasive—risk of surgical injury ▪ Results in iatrogenic hypothyroidism	▪ Requires medical therapy preprocedure in selected patients due to the risk of transient worsening of thyrotoxicosis ▪ May result in hypothyroidism (80% by 16 wk, up to 90% by 10 y) ▪ 5–15% require repeat treatment ▪ Requires isolation ▪ Avoid radioactivity in women who are pregnant or lactating ▪ 15–20% risk of inducing/aggravating Graves orbitopathy[a]	▪ Medication nonadherence ▪ Side effects Rare but serious: ▪ Agranulocytosis ▪ Hepatotoxicity ▪ Birth defects (methimazole) ▪ Vasculitis More common but less serious: ▪ Rash ▪ Arthralgias
Patient Preferences	Patients choosing surgery likely place a higher relative value on prompt and definitive control of symptoms and avoidance of radioactivity and/or side effects from medications, with less relative concern for potential surgical risks and need for lifelong hormone replacement	Patients choosing RAI likely place a higher relative value on definitive control of symptoms with avoidance of surgery and/or side effects from medications, with less relative concern for the rapid resolution of symptoms, need for lifelong hormone replacement, and worsening of Graves orbitopathy	Patients choosing medication likely place a higher relative value on the possibility of remission and avoidance of lifelong hormone replacement, and avoidance of surgery or radioactive exposure, with less relative concern for medication side effects and/or disease recurrence

[a]Exacerbation of orbitopathy may be ameliorated by concomitant steroid use.
RAI, radioactive iodine.
Adapted with permission from Fisher SB, Perrier ND, Clark O. Surgery for thyrotoxicosis. In: Wass J, Owen, K, eds. *Oxford Handbook of Endocrinology and Diabetes*. 3rd ed. Oxford University Press; 2020.

Graves disease has several distinct manifestations, including eye disease and localized dermopathy. Thyroid-associated eye disease (TED) is thought to be mediated by the accumulation of immune cells and fibroblasts within the orbit, and presentations include eyelid retraction (92%), exophthalmos (62%), extraocular muscle dysfunction (43%), ocular pain (30%), increased lacrimation (23%), and optic neuropathy (6%).[19] In the past decade, targeted molecular therapies have shown promising effects in ameliorating the symptoms of TED. Thyroid dermopathy, or thickening of the skin (most commonly observed on the shins—pretibial myxedema—but may develop elsewhere) occurs less commonly (1% to 4%) and typically in conjunction with severe TED.

Therapeutic options for patients with Graves disease include ATDs, RAI, and total thyroidectomy; lobectomy is not appropriate. Patients with a high likelihood of remission (women with mild disease, small goiters, and negative or low-titer antibodies) may benefit most from ATDs, whereas those with severe adverse reactions to ATDs, known liver disease, or medication noncompliance may favor RAI or thyroidectomy. Patients with life-limiting comorbidities, previous neck surgery or irradiation, or those without access to a high-volume thyroid surgeon may favor either RAI or ATDs. The presence of TED may be worsened by RAI, and although this effect may be ameliorated by corticosteroids,[14] thyroidectomy is often preferred in these patients. The presence of larger thyroid nodules, compressive symptoms, known or suspected malignancy, or concomitant hyperparathyroidism is an indication for thyroidectomy. Thyroidectomy is also favored for women who are pregnant, planning a pregnancy, or lactating, as RAI is contraindicated during pregnancy or lactation, and most experts recommend avoiding it within 6 months of a pregnancy. Pediatric patients are often treated initially with ATDs, but the rate of remission is lower than that observed in adults.[14] Hesitation to treat pediatric patients with RAI exists, although a definitive association with increased secondary cancer risk has not been associated with RAI as it has been with external radiation, and thyroidectomy is often favored in the pediatric patient in whom ATDs are insufficient. Thyroidectomy is appropriate in situations in which immediate control of symptoms is necessary (ie, thyroid storm or cardiovascular exacerbation refractory to medical management) as ATDs require 2 to 6 weeks and RAI may take 4 to 8 weeks to normalize thyroid function.[14]

In an elective situation, a patient with Graves disease should be rendered euthyroid prior to thyroidectomy with ATDs. Adjunct measures, which may be particularly useful for the management of the patient with severe Graves disease include beta blockade, iodine, cholestyramine, and hydrocortisone. With the exception of iodine, the specific pros and cons of each of these are outside of the scope of this chapter. Most commonly given as Lugol solution (LS, a combination of elemental iodine and potassium iodide) or saturated solution of potassium iodide (SSKI), an iodine load preoperatively suppresses thyroid hormone synthesis and release (Wolf–Chaikoff effect). The ATA supports preoperative treatment with LS or SSKI in most patients with Graves disease to reduce thyroid blood flow and vascularity,[20] although the benefits of it in the setting of modern surgical technique have been contested. While two early randomized studies demonstrated decreased blood flow on Doppler US and less operative blood loss in patients treated with LS,[21] later retrospective studies failed to identify differences in blood loss or postoperative complications.[22] It is plausible that excellent surgical technique minimizes clinically relevant blood loss and iodine supplementation is unnecessary, however, there are minimal side effects from a short course of LS or SSKI. When utilized, either may be administered as 3 to 5 drops every 8 hours for 7 to 10 days preoperatively and are most palatable dissolved in juice.

Hypoparathyroidism, either transient or permanent, is a risk after total thyroidectomy (discussed in detail below in Complications) and merits specific mention with regards to Graves disease. Retrospective studies demonstrate a higher incidence of transient hypocalcemia in patients with Graves disease as compared to euthyroid patients undergoing thyroidectomy for other reasons,[23] with rates as high as 28% in one experienced tertiary care center.[24] The specific reasons for the increased risk are not clearly defined but are thought to be related to increased complexity of the operation due to thyroid gland size and vascularity, and increased calcium metabolism and bone turnover due to hyperthyroidism.[25] Concomitant vitamin D deficiency, which may be observed at higher frequencies in patients with autoimmune thyroid disease, including Graves disease, likely also contributes to higher rates of postoperative hypoparathyroidism. When planning elective thyroidectomy, vitamin D deficiency should be corrected and selective preoperative calcium supplementation may be considered.[26]

Thyroid Storm

Thyroid storm is most often associated with uncontrolled Graves disease or amiodarone-associated thyrotoxicosis, and may be triggered by cessation of ATDs, physiologic stressors (illness or surgery), or RAI therapy (rare). The diagnosis is clinical and requires a high index of suspicion as many other critical illnesses have overlapping characteristics: thermoregulatory dysfunction (hyperpyrexia), cardiovascular instability (tachycardia, arrhythmias, congestive heart failure), central nervous system disturbance (agitation, delirium, psychosis, stupor, coma), and/or gastrointestinal dysfunction (nausea, vomiting, diarrhea, hepatic failure). Associated with a mortality of 8% to 25%, thyroid storm requires both supportive intensive care and therapy aimed at inhibiting thyroid hormone secretion and synthesis.[14] Propylthiouracil, which is typically considered second line to methimazole in treatment of *stable* patients with thyrotoxicosis, is favored in treatment of thyroid storm due to the additional inhibition of peripheral conversion of T4 to T3. Beta blockade, with its antiarrhythmic properties and inhibition of peripheral conversion is useful. Other adjuncts include steroids, which may also block peripheral conversion; cholestyramine, which enhances enterohepatic clearance of thyroid hormone; and/or iodine, which should be started after initiation of ATDs and temporarily blocks new hormone synthesis and thyroid hormone release. Supportive therapy includes cooling blankets, volume resuscitation, cardiovascular and respiratory monitoring, and invasive support as indicated, and nutritional support.

THYROID DISORDERS ASSOCIATED WITH HYPOTHYROIDISM

Hypothyroidism may be primary, arising from intrinsic thyroid disease, iatrogenic due to destruction or removal of the thyroid or administration of ATDs; or secondary due to pituitary dysfunction. Tertiary hypothyroidism, in which the hypothalamus does not produce sufficient thyrotropin-releasing hormone, is a rare cause of hypothyroidism. Treatment is largely medical with replacement of T4.

THYROIDITIS

Inflammation of the thyroid, or thyroiditis, is frequently encountered and rarely an indication by itself for surgery. Although most often associated with hypothyroidism, thyroiditis may also present with transient hyperthyroidism due to the destruction of thyroid follicles and release of preformed thyroid hormone.

Hashimoto Thyroiditis

As the most common cause of hypothyroidism in adults, HT affects up to 10% of the population and may also be called autoimmune or lymphocytic thyroiditis. It is more common in women (9:1) and most commonly presents between 30 and 50 years of age, but may occur across all age ranges. A typical presentation includes painless symmetric enlargement of the thyroid that is often characterized as rubbery and is sometimes accompanied by fullness or compressive symptoms. Laboratory studies may demonstrate a transient hyperthyroidism at the initial presentation (5% of patients), often followed by subclinical or clinical hypothyroidism; anti-TPO antibodies are typically elevated. US demonstrates a heterogeneous echotexture, and benign pseudonodules due to the autoimmune destruction of thyroid follicles and resulting architectural fibrosis and distortion may be observed. Nodular disease in a patient with HT should be evaluated with FNA-biopsy to rule out malignancy. It is not clear whether patients with HT have an increased risk of well differentiated thyroid cancer—surgical studies influenced by selection bias show a link between HT and malignancy, but population based studies do not support a relationship.[27] Patients with HT are at a higher risk for the rare thyroid lymphoma, although the overall incidence (0.37% of patients with HT) remains low.[27] Treatment is supportive, with surgery reserved for persistent severe symptoms refractory to medication.

Postpartum Thyroiditis and Painless Sporadic Thyroiditis

Postpartum thyroiditis affects up to 8% of pregnant women and is distinguished by presentation with pregnancy or during the year following pregnancy. Women with postpartum thyroiditis may demonstrate a relapsing clinical course. Care is supportive, with thyroid hormone replacement as indicated by symptoms and laboratory assessment. One-third of women will remain hypothyroid 1 year after delivery; for those with spontaneous resolution, relapse is often triggered by future pregnancies. Painless sporadic thyroiditis represents the same autoimmune process observed in postpartum thyroiditis, except it occurs independent of pregnancy or the postpartum period. Women remain more frequently affected (2:1) and it is most common between the ages of 30 and 40.

Subacute Thyroiditis

Also called de Quervain thyroiditis, giant cell thyroiditis, pseudogranulomatous thyroiditis, or subacute painful thyroiditis, subacute thyroiditis may be triggered by a virus (often coxsackievirus or echovirus, although the coronavirus pandemic in 2019 was also associated with post-infectious thyroiditis). Women are more commonly affected (5:1) and the age of onset is typically 20 to 60 years. Following a prodromal upper respiratory illness, the patient often presents with fever, malaise, and painful and firm goiter that is ultimately transient over a period of weeks to months. Pain radiating to the jaw or ears and/or associated with specific movement may be observed. Laboratory studies may demonstrate transient hyperthyroidism followed by hypothyroidism. Inflammatory markers such as erythrocyte sedimentation rate (ESR) and C-reactive protein (CRP) are often elevated. Treatment involves salicylates or nonsteroidal anti-inflammatory medications, with steroids reserved for more severe symptoms. Recurrence is rare.

Amiodarone-Induced Thyrotoxicosis or Thyroiditis

Amiodarone causes thyroid dysfunction in 15% to 20% of patients and may present as hypothyroidism or hyperthyroidism. Management of amiodarone-induced hypothyroidism is supportive; management of AIT may be more challenging. In contrast to many forms of thyroiditis, AIT is more common in men than women. Two forms of AIT exist with distinct mechanisms. In type I AIT, the iodine load from the drug itself exacerbates thyroid autonomous function, typically in the setting of a pre-existing MNG. Type I AIT is more common in iodine-deficient areas and can be treated by cessation of amiodarone (when feasible), ATDs, and/or LS or SSKI. Type II AIT is more common and develops independent of structural thyroid disease. Because type II AIT is a destructive process, ATDs are ineffective at controlling the hyperthyroidism and treatment consists of cessation of amiodarone (when feasible) and/or corticosteroids. Mixed or indefinite AIT may also occur with features of both type I and type II. Thyroidectomy is appropriate for patients with medically refractory disease, but is associated with a higher complication rate.

Acute Thyroiditis

Also called suppurative, pyogenic, bacterial, or infectious thyroiditis, acute thyroiditis is a rare condition caused by bacterial, fungal, mycobacterial, or parasitic infection. It most commonly affects children and young adults aged 20 to 40 years. Patients may experience fever, malaise, and/or pain radiating to the ear, with enlargement of the thyroid related to abscess formation. Given the rich vasculature and lymphatic drainage of the thyroid, infection is rare and is most often seen in patients who are immunosuppressed, or those with congenital abnormalities predisposing to infection, such as a pyriform sinus fistula. Thyroid function is typically within normal limits, and antithyroid antibodies are rarely present. FNA biopsy with Gram stain and culture confirms the diagnosis and guides antibiotic therapy. Thyroidectomy, particularly in resistant cases or those in which a structural abnormality predisposes, may be appropriate.[28]

Riedel Thyroiditis

Also known as fibrosing thyroiditis, this form of thyroiditis presents with a painless progressive goiter. Women are more commonly affected (3 to 4:1) and the peak age of onset is between 30 and 60 years of age. The cause is unknown. Patients are typically euthyroid but may progress to hypothyroidism over the course of the disease. Physical exam reveals a firm, fixed goiter that is best described as "woody." The fibrous process may extend to surrounding tissues and cause tracheal or esophageal compression or hypoparathyroidism. Other focally sclerotic conditions (retroperitoneal fibrosis, mediastinal fibrosis, or sclerosing cholangitis) may also occur. Surgical resection may be necessary to rule out malignancy or alleviate symptoms, but total thyroidectomy may not be feasible due to infiltration with other structures. Medical adjuncts to therapy include corticosteroids, methotrexate, and/or tamoxifen.[28]

NODULAR THYROID DISEASE

Thyroid nodules, whether clinically evident or incidentally discovered, are commonly encountered by medical providers across multiple specialties. The prevalence of thyroid nodules identified by palpation is estimated to be between 4% and 7%,[10] with up to 10 times more identified by imaging studies and identified in up to 50% to 60% of all adults on autopsy studies.[10] Women are more frequently affected (4:1), with the prevalence of thyroid nodules increasing with age to 50% in women over 70 years. Although most thyroid nodules are benign, appropriate risk-stratification and identification of patients who need further evaluation, biopsy, and/or surgical intervention is essential. In addition to assessing the risk of malignancy, evaluation should include attention to the presence or absence of related symptoms, which may be mechanical (such as dysphagia, dysphonia, or compressive symptoms) or related to autonomous production of excess thyroid hormone (*see Hyperthyroidism*).

Multinodular Goiter

Endemic goiter, or goiter due to iodine deficiency, remains a world health problem, although it is less likely in developed areas with dietary fortifications (iodination of salt, bread, flour, or vegetable oil). Thyromegaly from TSH stimulation occurs along with an adaptive response in which the thyroid shifts production of thyroid hormone from T4 to the more biologically potent T3. Therapy involves support with exogenous thyroid hormone therapy and/or iodine supplementation, which may not be practical in populations with limited access to care. Access to surgeons is similarly limited, and thyroidectomy in these areas is typically reserved for patients with very large goiters in whom symptoms have developed (compression, dyspnea, stridor, hoarseness, or dysphagia). In an iodine-deficient setting, recurrence rates are high (25% to 30%) and reoperative thyroid surgery accounts for 16% of all thyroidectomies.[29]

In iodine-replete areas of the world, goiter may occur independent of TSH stimulation, and it is unlikely to shrink with exogenous thyroid hormone or iodine. Management depends on assessment of risk of malignancy and presence of symptoms. When more than one nodule is present, each must be assessed for risk of malignancy based on physical exam, patient risk factors, US characteristics, and/or FNA-biopsy. Both benign and malignant lesions can grow over time, so change in size alone is not necessarily an indication for resection. Symptoms including a feeling of neck pressure or compression, dyspnea on exertion or at baseline or stridor thought to be related to tracheal compression, and/or dysphagia merit discussion of total thyroidectomy. Lobectomy may be appropriate for the patient with an asymmetric goiter in which the contralateral lobe is homogenous or characterized only by small, benign appearing nodules, particularly when the patient wishes to preserve native thyroid function.

Uninodular Disease

The management of a single dominant thyroid nodule is similar to that of a MNG, in that risk assessment for malignancy and evaluation of symptoms should guide therapy in the euthyroid patient. In contrast to MNG, diagnostic lobectomy (in the case of indeterminate risk of malignancy) or therapeutic lobectomy (in the case of compressive symptoms) is the first choice of surgical management.

Substernal or Intrathoracic Thyroid Nodular Disease

Accurate preoperative assessment of the inferior extent of a multi or uninodular goiter is imperative to avoid unwanted surprises in the operating room. Physical examination includes palpation of the inferior-most extent of the thyroid (or observation that it is not clearly assessable), which can be aided by neck extension and/or deglutition. Definite palpation and/or clear delineation of the inferior border on US suggests lack of a clinically meaningful intrathoracic component. In situations of uncertainty, CT of the neck and chest will clearly delineate the inferior-most extent of disease. The prevalence of substernal goiter ranges widely in the literature (2% to 19%), and sternotomy (partial or full) may be required in 5% (range 1% to 11%).[30]

Thyroid Cytopathology

FNA biopsy is the cornerstone of cytopathologic evaluation of structural thyroid abnormalities and is indicated for most solid or hypoechoic nodules greater than 1 cm in diameter, or for smaller nodules with radiographically suspicious features

(Table 72.3).[10] Image-guided techniques (most commonly US) should be used to increase the accuracy of FNA-biopsy, and onsite cytopathology can further improve diagnostic yield. In addition to increasing diagnostic accuracy, US guidance during FNA-biopsy also allows the clinician to select the most suspicious nodule, or area of the nodule, for biopsy, and to discern (and biopsy) multiple sites. With the exception of lymphoma, in which a core needle biopsy is often more appropriate, FNA biopsy is generally sufficient to yield diagnosis within the limits of cytopathology. Specific indeterminate lesions (discussed below) require evaluation of the architecture of surrounding cells, and therefore are unlikely to be definitively diagnosed on FNA-biopsy, which relies on aspiration of single cells.

Bethesda Classification

The ATA recommends that thyroid FNA-biopsy cytology should be reported using the Bethesda system for reporting
4 thyroid cytopathology, which was updated in 2023.[31] The Bethesda system includes six categories with an associated range of risk of malignancy for each (**Table 72.5**).[10] Bethesda I represents a nondiagnostic result and may be managed by repeat FNA-biopsy (with management guided by specific results), surveillance with intervention dictated by future changes, or diagnostic lobectomy in the event of persistent nondiagnostic findings in select circumstances. This should not be confused with unsatisfactory biopsy findings, which do not have enough cells to provide *any* diagnostic information. Repeat biopsy is often best performed after a short surveillance interval to allow resolution of any associated hemorrhage from the initial biopsy. Benign findings such as adenomatous change, colloid nodules, complex cysts, and hyperplastic nodules comprise the Bethesda II category. The majority of Bethesda II nodules may be safely observed with serial physical examination and US, although resection (thyroid lobectomy) remains an appropriate therapy for patients who are symptomatic. Repeat FNA-biopsy during surveillance of Bethesda II nodules is not routinely indicated and should be reserved only for significant changes in nodule characteristics (with or without accompanying change in size) that may suggest original sampling error. A higher index of suspicion may be necessary for patients with nodules greater than 3 to 4 cm in size as the risk of sampling error and false-negative results increases with nodule size (>3 to 4 cm). Retrospective surgical series of patients with initially benign cytology identified malignancy in 11% to 13% of patients with tumors greater than 3 to 4 cm, although this is influenced by selection bias and likely overestimates the rate of false-negative findings.[9]

Patients with Bethesda III nodules (atypia of undetermined significance) comprise an indeterminate category in which the findings do not clearly meet criteria for benign or malignant lesions. Repeat FNA-biopsy may yield a specific diagnosis, although molecular testing (see below) or diagnostic lobectomy are more frequently employed. In addition to removing the previously used term "follicular lesion of undetermined significance," the updated 2023 system distinguishes the intracellular pattern of atypia, with a higher risk of malignancy associated with atypia observed in nuclei vs other aspects of the cell.

Bethesda IV nodules represent follicular neoplasm, and the previously included term "suspicious for follicular neoplasm" has been discontinued due to confusion related to other categories with "suspicious" in the title. The cellular diagnostic criteria remain consistent with prior versions and also include any findings with the potential to be NIFTP (discussed later). Diagnostic lobectomy, with preoperative risk stratification aided by molecular testing at the discretion of the surgeon, is a reasonable approach. In selected cases with appropriate patient selection and counseling, molecular diagnostics and/or close observation may also be appropriate management strategies. Bethesda V and VI represent clinically suspicious (V) or overt malignancy (VI) and should be addressed surgically in most situations.

Molecular Evaluation

PTCs most commonly demonstrate mutations of the B-Raf proto-oncogene (*BRAF*, 45%), fusions involving the rearranged during transfection gene (*RET* 20%), whereas follicular thyroid cancers are characterized by mutations in the RAS proto-oncogene family (*NRAS>HRAS>KRAS*, 10%) or paired box 8-peroxisome proliferator activated receptor gamma (*PAX8-PPARγ*, 35%) rearrangements. Either may demonstrate mutations in telomerase reverse transcriptase (*TERT*) gene (10 to 12%, and higher in FTC).[32] Debate exists regarding the specific clinical implication of each mutation, and the prognostic significance of each is likely confounded by the presence of other adverse clinicopathologic factors. Mutations in *BRAF*, for example, are more frequently identified in patients with lymph node metastases and/or those with recurrence than in patients without metastases and/or recurrence, and *BRAF* mutated patients are also more likely to have concomitant extrathyroidal extension and higher stage than non-*BRAF*–mutated patients. Yet *BRAF* mutations may also be identified in a patient with an indolent microcancer, leading some to propose that specific combinations of mutations (ie, the combination of *BRAF* and *TERT*) may be more prognostic.[9,12] It is likely that improved understanding of the molecular profile of the tumor, rather than a single oncogene, will provide better prognostic information, but further studies are necessary.

As to the indeterminate nodule, molecular diagnostics aid in diagnosis when applied and interpreted thoughtfully. Currently, multiple molecular panels, the majority of which use gene expression classification with or without additional evaluation for specific mutations or fusions which may be associated with thyroid cancer, are commercially available as a tool to augment decision making regarding indeterminate thyroid nodules. The two most commonly used tests in the United States currently are Thyroseq and Afirma. When interpreting test results, it is essential to understand that positive and negative predictive values of tests depend on the underlying prevalence of disease, that is, the underlying prevalence of thyroid cancer, which may vary based on referral patterns.

Thyroseq v3 tests for point mutations, insertions/deletions, copy number variations, gene fusions, and gene expression variations across 112 proprietary genes and is built upon a series of previous versions.[33,34] Multi-institution validation showed excellent NPV (97.1%) with moderate PPV (64%) for Bethesda III and IV nodules, leading the authors to conclude that benign results on the classifier may obviate diagnostic surgery in patients with indeterminate nodules.[35] A recent prospective multi-institutional study identified a benign call rate of 72.6% in 500 consecutive patients with indeterminate nodules and 2 years of follow-up, further emphasizing the value of using Thyroseq v3 to reduce unnecessary diagnostic lobectomies.[36]

The Afirma Gene Sequencing Classifier (GSC), which builds off of the original gene expression classifier (GEC), uses a proprietary panel of mRNA expression patterns combined with mRNA classifiers (evaluating parathyroid lesions, MTC, *BRAFV600E* mutations, *RET/PTC1* or *RET/PTC3* fusions, and Hurthle cell lesions) to risk stratify indeterminate nodules, with a high negative predictive value (96.8%), making it most useful in ruling out malignancy in cytologically indeterminate nodules.[34] One recent external multi-institution study examined 834 indeterminate nodules and showed a negative predictive value of 99% for Bethesda III nodules and 98% for Bethesda IV nodules. While still overall excellent, the NPV does decrease when using only surgically confirmed cases (89% Bethesda III, 87% Bethesda IV),[37] underscoring a challenge of using molecular testing to "rule-out" malignancy. Currently, only a small percentage of patients with Afirma GEC/GSC or ThyroSeqv3 benign determinations undergo resection (6% to 13%), leading to the possibility that some of these patients may have an indolent malignancy that has not yet declared.[38] Patients electing for observation of a cytologically indeterminate nodule, with or without reassuring molecular testing,

Table 72.5. The Bethesda System for Reporting Thyroid Cytopathology with Suggested Management and Corresponding Risk of Malignancy

Diagnostic Category	Changes in Bethesda 2023 from prior version	Usual Management	Predicted Risk of Malignancy, % (range)[b]
Nondiagnostic/Unsatisfactory	Consistent	Repeat FNA with US guidance	13 (5–20)
Benign	Refers to 2022 WHO classification "follicular nodular disease" and includes colloid, hyperplastic, adenomatous, and benign follicular nodules	Clinical surveillance	4 (2–7)
Atypia of Undetermined Significance (AUS)	"Follicular lesion of undetermined significance" is no longer used. AUS is stratified into "nuclear," which has a higher ROM, and "other"	Molecular diagnostics and/or diagnostic lobectomy, with repeat biopsy or observation in select situations	22 (13–30)
Follicular Neoplasm	Discontinued use of "suspicious for follicular neoplasm" with consistent diagnostic criteria from prior versions and the inclusion of all cases suspected to be NIFTP	Molecular diagnostics and/or diagnostic lobectomy, with repeat biopsy or observation in select situations	30 (23–34)
Suspicious for Malignancy		Lobectomy or thyroidectomy[a]	74 (67–83)
Malignancy		Lobectomy or thyroidectomy[a]	97 (97–100)

[a]Based on tumor size, histopathologic characteristics, and anticipated need for postoperative radioablative iodine therapy.
[b]As predicted by the Bethesda system and based on Ali SZ, Baloch ZW, Cochand-Priollet B, Schmitt FC, Vielh P, VanderLaan PA. The 2023 Bethesda System for reporting thyroid cytopathology. *Thyroid*. 2023;33(9):1039–1044.
FNA, fine-needle aspiration; US, ultrasound; AUS, atypia of undetermined significance; ROM, risk of malignancy; FN, follicular neoplasm; NIFTP, noninvasive follicular thyroid neoplasm with papillary-like nuclear features.

should undergo regular surveillance, and the clinician employing molecular testing should understand the pros and cons of the specific testing platform utilized as well as the local cancer prevalence and the associated risk with the patient's cytology (the pretest probability of malignancy).

DIFFERENTIATED THYROID CANCER

PTC is the most common form of thyroid cancer, accounting for 85% of the estimated 43,720 new cases per year in the United States, followed by FTC (12%), poorly differentiated or insular thyroid cancer (3%), MTC (1% to 2%), and ATC (<1%).[39,40] Thyroid cancer exhibits a wide range of behavior, from the very indolent papillary thyroid microcarcinoma to the extremely aggressive ATC. Fortunately, well-differentiated thyroid cancers (PTC and FTC) form the bulk of the cancer burden with excellent long-term survival, and thyroid cancer accounts for only 0.4% of cancer deaths worldwide.[39]

Papillary Thyroid Cancer

PTC affects people of all ages with a peak incidence in the third and fourth decades and a female predominance (3:1). Microscopically, PTC is characterized by papillary architecture, calcifications, psammoma bodies, squamous metaplasia, and fibrosis. Large overlapping nuclei that are optically clear (Orphan Annie nuclei) and intranuclear grooves are common findings on cytology. Histopathologic variants include the follicular variant of PTC, which is notable for its diagnostic ambiguity on FNA biopsy. This particular form of PTC combines architectural feature of a follicular tumor and is often characterized as a follicular lesion. Clinically it behaves in the same manner as classic PTC (not to be confused with the noninvasive, or encapsulated form, discussed below). Other histopathologic variants associated with more aggressive clinical behavior include the hobnail, tall cell, columnar, and solid variants. Often, these histopathologic features are identified in the setting of other adverse factors, including larger tumor size, extrathyroidal extension, angiolymphatic invasion, lymph node metastases, and distant metastases.[41] The presence of these variants, in addition to other clinical factors, should be taken into consideration when planning extent of surgery (ie, lobectomy versus total thyroidectomy, discussed later).

Treatment for PTC localized to the thyroid and/or the cervical lymph nodes is surgical (thyroid lobectomy or thyroidectomy, with compartment-based lymph node dissection as appropriate), with selective use of adjuvant RAI to minimize risk of recurrence. Excellent long-term oncologic outcomes for most patients with PTC have allowed discussion of quality of life to factor into surgical planning. For example, the extent of thyroidectomy must be balanced between the concern for recurrence and need for RAI versus the desire to maintain native thyroid function and/or minimize extent of surgery and surgical risks. Unlike many other cancers, multifocality (within the thyroid) and/or lymph node involvement does not necessarily convey a poorer prognosis. Interestingly, the size of the tumor also does not correlate with the risk of lymph node metastases, and the incidence of metastases varies depending on the extent of lymph node dissection performed. While therapeutic lymph node dissection for clinically evident disease is standard of care, the value of prophylactic central neck dissection, which may identify micrometastases in as many as 30% of 80% is debated and will be discussed later.[42]

In a small subset of patients (1% to 8%) PTC may present with metastatic disease, most commonly with lung metastases. Thyroidectomy may be appropriate even for patients with distant metastases, as removal of native thyroid tissue will facilitate treatment with RAI therapy.

Papillary Thyroid Cancer: Nonoperative Management

In contrast to the more aggressive histologies, papillary thyroid microcarcinoma is defined as a PTC that is ≤1 cm in diameter. Often found incidentally during thyroidectomy for other reasons, these are generally not life-limiting. Ten-year disease-specific survival for patients with surgically treated papillary thyroid microcarcinoma is >99%,[43] and some have questioned the clinical impact of these cancers if left in situ. Active surveillance, which involves serial physical exam, US, and laboratory assessment, was first proposed in Japan for patients with small tumors (≤1 cm on US) located away from vital structures (RLNs, trachea, esophagus) without evidence of extrathyroidal extension or lymph node involvement, who wished to avoid surgery and its potential complications. In this highly monitored population of 1,235 patients, only 4.6% demonstrated tumor growth and 1.5% developed lymph node metastases and no patient developed distant metastases or died from thyroid cancer with over 10 years of follow up.[44] Similar studies in different populations, including North America, similarly show single-digit rates of tumor growth or development of nodal metastases (5.3% and 1.6% in one meta-analysis, respectively).[45] The success of active surveillance depends on disease factors (tumor size and location), patient factors (ability and desire to return regularly for surveillance), and health care system factors (reliability and availability of high-quality US and health care team infrastructure to minimize the risk of losing patients to follow-up).

Follicular Thyroid Cancer

Follicular thyroid cancers comprise 10% to 15% of all thyroid cancers, present with a female predominance, and are most common in the 5th decade of life. The histologic diagnosis hinges on the identification of vascular and capsular invasion, which is not readily identified on FNA-biopsy or frozen section determination. Follicular thyroid cancer tends to demonstrate hematogenous spread, and these patients have a higher lifetime risk of distant metastases (10% to 15%) and are less likely to manifest regional nodal disease (10%) than patients with PTC. Surgical planning, staging, and adjuvant therapy (RAI, to which up to 80% are sensitive) decisions should take this propensity for distant metastasis into consideration, and most patients with FTC are treated with total thyroidectomy, with therapeutic lymph node dissection as indicated by preoperative imaging.

Noninvasive Follicular Thyroid Neoplasm with Papillary-like Nuclear Features

In 2012, the National Cancer Institute recognized the public health burden of the over-diagnosis of cancer and encouraged efforts to revise terminology when data supported a more indolent classification. In 2016, the term "noninvasive follicular thyroid neoplasm with papillary-like nuclear features," or NIFTP, was introduced to describe the *encapsulated* follicular variant of PTC, which comprises 10% to 20% of all thyroid cancers in North America and is characterized by lack of capsular or vascular invasion. When meeting strict histologic criteria, NIFTP tumors should not recur or metastasize.[46] Although the goal of the noncancer nomenclature is to reduce the number of unnecessary operations, diagnosis of NIFTP currently still requires complete histologic assessment, and therefore lobectomy. Improved understanding of the molecular profile of these tumors may allow a less invasive diagnostic option, with some signal that micro RNA expression may aid in distinguishing this entity.

Oncocytic Thyroid Cancer

Renamed from Hurthle cell cancer to oncocytic thyroid cancer (OTC), these rare tumors are considered to be a separate entity from FTC or PTC and are characterized by the presence of oncocytic cells (abundant eosinophilic granular cytoplasm and hyperchromatic nuclei) and evidence of capsular and vascular invasion. Ambiguity in diagnosis exists as oncocytic adenomas have similar microscopic features without invasion and FNA-biopsy cannot adequately discriminate. The specificity of available molecular diagnostics is the lowest for oncocytic neoplasms as compared to other indeterminate nodules (specificity for Afirma GSC 59%; Thyroseq v3 internal validation specificity 69.3%),[47,48] and as such, diagnostic lobectomy is most commonly utilized for a "hurthle cell neoplasm." Frozen section analysis has similar limitations to FNA biopsy, and final histopathology must make the diagnosis of OTC. Once invasion is evident and the diagnosis of OTC is made, the extent of invasion observed in the tumor is used to further subdivide OTC into two types: minimally invasive (<4 foci of angioinvasion) and widely invasive (>4 foci). The distinction between the two is subject to interobserver variability, but is no less important given the relatively indolent behavior of the former and the more aggressive behavior of the latter. OTCs are more likely than PTC or FTC to demonstrate lymph node metastases and less likely to take up radioiodine (10% radioiodine avid), making surgery the mainstay of treatment.

MEDULLARY THYROID CANCER

MTC is rare (~1% to 3% of all thyroid cancers) and derives from the calcitonin-producing parafollicular C cells of the thy-
5 roid. In contrast to PTC, the development of nodal metastases correlates with tumor size (central and lateral compartment nodal disease are present in 14% and 11% of patients with T1 tumors, and 86% and 93% of patients with T4 tumors, respectively) and nodal and distant disease is more common. When presentation is associated with a palpable nodule, up to 70% of patients will have locoregional metastases, and 10% will have distant disease.[16]

Of the 25% of patients in whom MTC is hereditary (MEN 2A and 2B or familial MTC), germline activating point mutations of the *RET* proto-oncogene can be identified in the majority (95%). The specific mutation associated with hereditary MTC has a strong genotype-phenotype correlation and, when known, will guide timing of therapeutic interventions (**Table 72.6**).[49] Similar *RET* mutations may be identified in the remaining 75% of patients with sporadic disease, but at a lower frequency (40% to 50%), with *RAS* mutations accounting for an additional 10% to 15% and unknown or unidentified driver mutations in the remainder. Because a diagnosis of MTC may present as the initial proband in a family, any adult patient with MTC should undergo genetic counseling as well as screening for pheochromocytoma and hyperparathyroidism regardless of family history. In children, in whom genetic counseling and testing of a family member often leads to subsequent presentation and diagnosis at a young age, prophylactic thyroidectomy should be performed within the first

Table 72.6. Disease Phenotypes Associated with Medullary Thyroid Cancer

Syndrome	Clinical Features (% Penetrance)
MEN2A	MTC (>90%), pheochromocytoma (40–60%), parathyroid hyperplasia (20–30%), cutaneous lichen amyloidosis, Hirschsprung disease
MEN2B	MTC (>98%), pheochromocytoma (40–60%), intestinal and mucosal neuromas (98%), marfanoid habitus, inability to produce tears, everted eyelids and/or ptosis, prominent corneal nerves
Familial MTC	Isolated MTC with typically later age of onset and less aggressive clinical course

MEN, multiple endocrine neoplasia; MTC, medullary thyroid cancer.
Adapted with permission from Kiernan CM, Grubbs EG. Surgical management of multiple endocrine neoplasia 1 and multiple endocrine neoplasia 2. *Surg Clin North Am.* 2019;99(4):693–709.

year of life for those with RET codon *M918T* mutations (ATA highest risk) and prior to age 5 for those with RET codon *C634* or *A883F* mutations (ATA high risk). For the remaining patients with moderate risk (mutations other than those mentioned above), the timing of thyroidectomy may be influenced by patient and family preferences, the natural history of other affected family members, and serial observation may be appropriate for those with normal US findings and a normal serum calcitonin.[16] In addition, screening for pheochromocytoma and hyperparathyroidism should be considered in children above the age of 10, depending on the mutation profile, whereas it is not indicated in children under the age of 5, given the sequence of presentation.[49] Such care should occur in the context of a multidisciplinary center with providers who are familiar with the disease and its associated physiologic and psychosocial impacts.

All patients with suspected MTC should undergo a thorough neck US that includes the draining central and (bilateral) lateral nodal basins. In addition to routine thyroid function tests, both calcitonin and carcinoembryonic antigen should be evaluated. The baseline levels of these two tumor markers are valuable for assessing disease burden (calcitonin levels >400 pg/mL should prompt a metastatic workup with cross-sectional imaging, with particular attention to the liver as the most common site of metastasis) and over time yield insight into the rate of disease progression by allowing the calculation of doubling time. The ATA provides a calculator to assess the rate at which each biomarker doubles (https://www.thyroid.org/professionals/calculators/thyroid-cancer-carcinoma/). Doubling time is best calculated with at least four data points over a minimum of 2 years, and calcitonin is better correlated with outcome than CEA. Patients with a doubling time of less than 6 to 12 months most often demonstrate structural disease progression and decreased progression-free and overall survival, whereas a doubling time greater than 2 years is associated with disease stability and improved survival.

Surgical resection is the mainstay of therapy for MTC, with prophylactic thyroidectomy for patients with known hereditary syndromes, ideally performed prior to detection of disease, and total thyroidectomy with bilateral central neck dissections performed for known disease, with lateral neck dissection guided by biopsy-proven disease in the associated compartment. Postoperative radioiodine ablation is not indicated, except in the case of combination histology in which locoregional or distant metastases include a proportion of PTC or FTC. Adjuvant external beam radiation is reserved for the patient judged to be at high risk of recurrence who has exhausted all surgical options and is typically considered only after multiple operations. For those with distant metastatic disease and evidence of progression, tyrosine kinase inhibitors such as vandetinib (a RET, epidermal growth factor [EGFR], and vascular endothelial growth factor receptor [VEGFR] inhibitor), and cabozantinib (a RET, MET proto-oncogene, and VEGFR2 inhibitor) may be used as single agent therapy, or, for patients with RET fusions or mutations, selpercatinib or praseltinib.[40] Antimotility drugs and somatostatin analogs may be helpful for symptom relief of the hypersecretory diarrhea and flushing that may be seen with advanced MTC. Localized therapies (hepatic embolization strategies, surgical metastasectomy) may be employed in well-selected patients to palliate symptoms or delay disease progression. Although still in its therapeutic infancy, peptide receptor radionuclide therapy has shown promising results with improved survival in highly selected patients.[50]

ANAPLASTIC THYROID CANCER

6 ATC is a rare and aggressive malignancy which has traditionally been treated with palliative measures. All patients with ATC are classified as having stage IV disease, and half of the patients present with measurable distant metastases. The median overall survival for all patients is 3 to 5 months, with 1-year survival of 20%.

Traditionally surgical therapy for ATC has been limited to the palliation of acute airway compromise, although occasionally a small ATC limited to the thyroid or with limited extension to immediate surrounding tissues may be identified and treated aggressively with curative intent. For those with disease amenable to resection, multimodal adjuvant therapy with taxane or platinum-based chemotherapy and radiation has been associated with improved overall survival as compared to palliative care, although often with limited overall impact (1 year OS 42%).[51] Improved understanding of the molecular landscape of ATC in the past decade has dramatically altered therapeutic options.

In 2018, the dual agent BRAF/MEK inhibitors dabrafenib and trametinib became the first FDA-approved targeted agents for patients with *BRAFV600E*-mutated ATC based on the results of a small phase II open-label trial in 16 patients that showed an overall response rate of 69%.[51] Today, *BRAFV600E* mutation testing is a critical component of initial care for patients with ATC, and BRAF-directed therapy, when effective, induces rapid tumor regression, potentially converting patients with initially unresectable disease to surgical candidates and expanding the role for thyroidectomy and neck dissection in this disease. Survival for those patients who achieve a response sufficient to allow definitive surgical resection is markedly higher than historic estimates (94% at 1 year), although these results are derived from small, highly specialized single-institution series.[51]

Checkpoint inhibitors such as pembrolizumab have shown only modest results as monotherapy, but their combination with BRAF-directed therapy is more promising. In the surgical arena the evaluation of the addition of pembrolizumab to BRAF directed therapy in a neoadjuvant setting is underway[51] Other promising therapeutics include the multitargeted tyrosine kinase inhibitors Lenvatinib and pazopanib, with incorporation of other targeted agents guided by results of next generation sequencing and cell-free DNA liquid biopsy to identify less common but targetable mutations in *NTRK*, *ALK*, or *RET* fusions. Care of the patient with ATC should take place in a multidisciplinary setting with experience in management of this rare and aggressive disease.

OTHER THYROID MALIGNANCIES

Primary thyroid lymphomas are rare (<5% of thyroid cancers) and are most commonly non-Hodgkin lymphomas of B-cell origin. Patients describe a rapidly enlarging mass with compressive symptoms and may have a history of hypothyroidism with evidence of HT. Metastases to the thyroid from renal cell carcinoma, breast, lung, gastrointestinal cancers, melanoma, and sarcoma have been reported. Treatment is dictated by the primary cancer type and surgical resection is reserved for cases in which diagnostic ambiguity remains after FNA-biopsy and/or core needle biopsy, or for palliation of symptoms.

STAGING OF DIFFERENTIATED, MEDULLARY, AND ANAPLASTIC THYROID CANCER

Thyroid cancer is unique from most other cancers in that age directly impacts stage, with all patients with differentiated thyroid cancer diagnosed before age 55 classified as stage I (locoregional disease including cervical nodal metastases) or II (distant metastases), reflecting the excellent survival observed for most patients with differentiated thyroid cancer (**Table 72.7**). The last update to thyroid cancer staging occurred in 2018 with the 8th edition of the American Joint Committee on Cancer (AJCC). This edition is notable in that it raised the age dichotomization from 45 to 55, removed the

Table 72.7. Estimates of Survival for Patients with Differentiated Thyroid Cancer and Medullary Thyroid Cancer Stratified by American Joint Committee on Cancer Tumor-Node-Metastasis Stage (8th edition)

Age	Stage	Description (Tumor-Node-Metastasis Classification)	10-year Disease Specific Survival for PTC (Tam et al.[53])	Overall Survival Estimates for MTC (Adam et al.[54])
<55 y	I	Disease confined to the thyroid and/or the cervical lymph nodes ($T_{any}N_{any}M_0$)	99.8%	—[a]
	II	Distant metastases ($T_{any}N_{any}M_1$)	88.3%	—[a]
≥55 y	I	Tumors <4 cm confined to the thyroid without nodal disease or distant metastases ($T_{1-2}N_0M_0$)	99.8%	95%
	II	Tumors <4 cm confined to the thyroid with central nodal disease only, or tumors of any size with extrathyroidal invasion to the strap muscles without nodal disease, each without distant metastases ($T_{1-2}N_{1a/b}M_0$, $T_{3a/b}N_0M_0$)	88.3%	91%
	III	Tumors of any size with local invasion beyond the strap muscles, regardless of nodal status, without distant metastases ($T_{4a}N_{any}M_0$)	72.4%	89%
	IVa	Tumors of any size with invasion into the prevertebral fascia or encasement of the carotid or mediastinal vessels, regardless of nodal disease, without distant metastases ($T_{4b}N_{any}M_0$)	71.9%[b]	68%[b]
	IVb	Presence of distant metastases ($T_{any}M_{any}M_1$)	—[a]	—[a]

[a]Stage for MTC is independent of age.
[b]Analyzed as stage IV inclusively.
AJCC, American Joint Committee on Cancer; PTC, papillary thyroid cancer; MTC, medullary thyroid cancer.
Adapted from Tam S, Boonsripitayanon M, Amit M, et al. Survival in differentiated thyroid cancer: comparing the AJCC cancer staging seventh and eighth editions. *Thyroid.* 2018;28(10):1301–1310 and Adam MA, Thomas S, Roman SA, Hyslop T, Sosa JA. Rethinking the current American Joint Committee on Cancer TNM staging system for medullary thyroid cancer. *JAMA Surg.* 2017;152(9):869–876.

impact of microscopic extrathyroidal extension on staging, and reclassified central neck nodal disease such that level VII nodes no longer upstaged the nodal status. The anticipated 10-year disease-specific survival estimated by the AJCC 8th edition has been corroborated by retrospective studies (**Table 72.7**), however, further evaluations and refinements will continue to be necessary.[52,53]

For patients with MTC, the same tumor-node-metastasis (TNM) staging system is currently in use, without the stratification by age. The limitations of applying a system designed primarily for PTC to a different disease process are inherently evident. One large study combining the National Cancer Database (NCDB) and the United States Surveillance, Epidemiology, and End Results program (SEER) suggests that the current staging system upstages a large proportion of patients with MTC to stage IV and does not accurately stratify groups based on survival. The authors used recursive partitioning to propose new staging groups and demonstrated improved separation of survival curves by grouping patients with T1 and T2 tumors without nodal disease into stage I, expanding stage II to include patients with nodal disease or larger tumors without nodal disease, and limiting stage IV to only patients with distant metastases.[54] As with other rare cancers, continued refinements to a universal staging system will require assumptions based on large databases.

The ATC staging system follows the same definitions for TNM categories as PTC and MTC, however, all patients with ATC are considered to have stage IV disease, with patients with intrathyroidal surgically resectable cancers staged as IVA, those with locoregional nodal disease or invasion into local structures staged as IVB, and patients with distant metastases staged as IVC.

NONSURGICAL THERAPEUTIC ADJUNCTS FOR THYROID CANCER

TSH Suppression

Considered a trophic factor, TSH may be suppressed below physiologic levels by exogenous administration of thyroid hormone (levothyroxine) in patients with moderate to high risk differentiated thyroid cancer (papillary, follicular, and Hurthle cell cancers). The goal TSH range for patients with high, moderate, and low risk disease are <0.1 mU/L, 0.1 to 0.5 mU/L, and 0.5 to 2 mU/L, respectively.[9] The suppressive effects of TSH therapy must be balanced against the long-term health effects of occult hyperthyroidism, including the risks of arrhythmias and osteoporosis, and the degree of suppression is typically reduced in patients without evidence of disease over time.

Radioiodine Therapy

Radioiodine may be used in a dose-dependent manner to diagnose residual thyroid tissue, ablate remnant thyroid tissue, or treat residual or recurrent disease in patients with follicular-derived thyroid cancers. As thyroid cells should be adequately stimulated by TSH and deprived of iodine, the timing of postoperative RAI uptake scans and/or therapeutic administrations depends on the patient and specific sequence of therapy. Evaluation should be delayed at least 4 to 8 weeks after an iodine-rich contrasted CT scan is performed. Withdrawal of thyroid hormone replacement will allow the TSH to rise to stimulatory levels, but requires a 4 to 5 week period given the long half-life of levothyroxine and may result in significant hypothyroid symptoms. Replacement with T3 (liothyronine) during this time period allows a shorter withdrawal period of 2 weeks, or alternatively, recombinant human TSH can be administered to avoid the withdrawal period entirely.

Selection for administration of adjuvant RAI is a careful risk assessment that requires close communication between surgeon and endocrinologist. Extent of disease at presentation, histopathologic factors, and postoperative structural or biochemical evidence of disease influence the decision to administer RAI. In general, RAI is encouraged for patients with distant metastases, primary tumors >4 cm, or with gross extrathyroidal extension, and lymph node involvement.

External Beam Radiation Therapy

External beam radiation therapy (EBRT) is rarely indicated for the treatment of differentiated thyroid cancer and should only be used in the neck after all surgical options are exhausted. For poorly differentiated tumors that are anticipated to be RAI-resistant and that have invaded the trachea or esophagus, surgical awareness of the possible need for EBRT and subsequent planning with flap placement is beneficial to prevent fistula. More commonly, EBRT is employed for the palliation of distant bony metastases, which are less likely to be fully treated by RAI. Bone-directed therapeutics (ie, zoledronic acid or denosumab) may be combined with EBRT with a synergistic effect.

Metastatic Disease and Systemic Therapy

RAI therapy is a cornerstone of therapy for patients with locally advanced/unresectable or distant metastatic disease. While 5% to 15% of patients with differentiated thyroid cancer display loss of differentiation and subsequent inability to uptake iodide (RAI-refractory disease) at presentation, up to 50% of patients with metastatic disease will be RAI-refractory. Patients with RAI-refractory disease have 5-year disease-specific survival rates between 60% and 70%.[55] Significant interest exists in the potential to use targeted drugs to promote redifferentiation and restore susceptibility to RAI. Currently available literature (primarily in patients with metastatic DTC) is heterogeneous in patient and tumor characteristics, modality, and duration of therapy, but restoration of RAI uptake has been observed in 33% to 69% of patients, with partial responses in 25% to 75% of those treated with RAI, suggesting redifferentiation therapy a viable treatment that requires further study.[56]

The cornerstone of systemic therapy for thyroid cancer is based on the involved altered signaling pathways, including point mutations in *BRAF* (40%) and the *RAS* family of proto-oncogenes (38%), rearrangement of *RET/PTC* (10% to 20%), and rearrangements and mutations in anaplastic lymphoma kinase (*ALK*) or neurotrophic tropomyosin receptor kinase (*NTRK*)*1–3*.[40]

For patients with *BRAFV600E* mutated thyroid cancer, either single-agent vemurafenib or dabrafenib (BRAF inhibitors) or combination therapy with trametinib or cobimetinib (MEK inhibitors, typically combined with dabrafenib) have demonstrated partial responses and promising progression-free survival (as opposed to placebo). The addition of the MEK inhibitor blocks the paradoxical activation of MAPK signaling and the increase in cutaneous malignancies observed with single-agent BRAF inhibitors. Additionally, the combination of BRAF and MEK inhibitors is thought to promote redifferentiation—or restoration of the ability of thyroid cancer cells to uptake RAI—and has great interest as adjuvant therapy for RAI-resistant disease.[40]

Oral multitargeted tyrosine kinase inhibitors such as sorafenib, lenvatinib, and cabozantinib are FDA approved for RAI-refractory differentiated thyroid cancer. Other targeted therapies may be utilized for patients with specific mutations, such as RET fusions (selperctinib) or NTRK fusions (entrectinib or larotrectinib). As toxicity and resistance limit utilization, initiation of these drugs is typically applied in settings of progression of distant disease. The potential for use of these targeted therapies in a neoadjuvant setting, particularly for patients with locally advanced disease that is either unresectable or resectable with significant morbidity, is an area of future study.[40]

THYROID SURGERY

Shaped by contributions from Theodor Billroth, Theodor Kocher and William Halsted, modern thyroid surgery is safe and effective. Thyroid lobectomy, total thyroidectomy, and occasionally isolated thyroid isthmusectomy may be performed. Historically, subtotal thyroidectomy (the Hartley–Dunhill procedure, in which approximately 2.5 g of tissue is left on one side to avoid postoperative hypothyroidism) was performed for thyrotoxicosis, with the end objective to preserve native thyroid function. While this approach may still be useful in geographic areas in which thyroid hormone replacement is not readily available, subtotal thyroidectomy is rarely performed today. Near-total thyroidectomy, in which a conscious decision is made to leave a minor amount of thyroid tissue at the insertion of the RLN, is appropriate for patients with benign disease and anatomy such that further dissection may compromise the nerve.

Technique

The patient is placed in the semi-Fowler position with the neck gently hyperextended and a horizontal shoulder roll placed to open the surgical field. A natural skin crease one to two fingerbreadths above the clavicles and approximately 1 cm below the cricoid cartilage is made (**Fig. 72.7**) and the subcutaneous tissue and platysma are divided. Subplatysmal skin flaps may be developed, extending to the thyroid cartilage, sternal notch, and laterally to the sternocleidomastoid muscles, prior to dividing the midline raphe. As an alternative to subplatysmal skin flaps, the avascular space between the sternohyoid and sternothyroid muscles may be gently dissected after the midline raphe is divided. Attention should be paid to the presence of a pyramidal lobe (which should not be inadvertently left during a total thyroidectomy) and/or midline prelaryngeal (Delphian) lymph nodes (which should be assessed early during an operation for malignancy). The middle thyroid vein is divided, and the thyroid is rotated medially into the field, taking care to identify and dissect parathyroid glands laterally.

Normal parathyroid tissue is subtle and may be difficult to identify; it is characterized by a slight brownish color with a fine capillary vascular pattern not typically seen in adjacent lymph nodes, fat, or thymus. Knowledge of their common locations and careful dissection along the capsule of the thyroid will prevent inadvertent injury to the parathyroids or their blood supply. In the event of inadvertent resection or devascularization, the parathyroid should be confirmed with

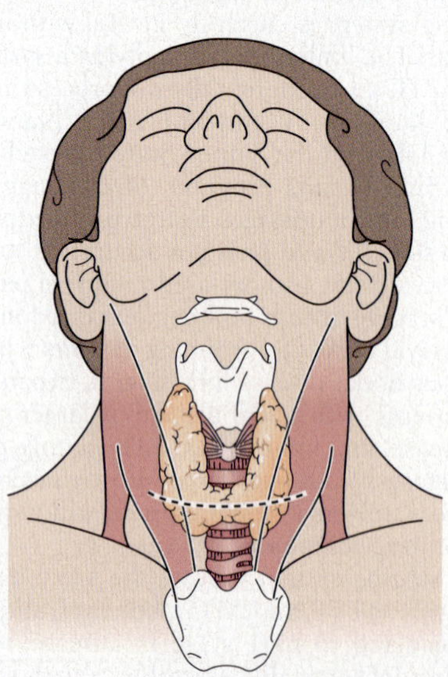

Figure 72.7. With the patient's neck extended, the *dashed line* indicates the appropriate site of incision for thyroid resection. Camouflage within an existing skin crease is often possible.

frozen section, morcelized, and reimplanted—most commonly into the sternocleidomastoid muscle. Deliberate marking of the reimplantation site with a prolene suture facilitates future exploration in the event of hyperparathyroidism, and marking the pocket with a radiopaque clip allows radiographic identification.

The superior pole is approached with close dissection along the capsule of the gland to avoid injury to the external branch of the superior laryngeal nerve. Although the external branch of the superior laryngeal nerve is not always directly visualized, in cases where it is observed, a nerve stimulator can be used to elicit contraction of the cricothyroideus muscle. The RLN should be directly visualized consistently and is often identified approximately 1.5 cm away from its insertion, facilitated by gentle traction of the surrounding tissues. Careful dissection along the anterior surface of the nerve and meticulous attention to early branches will preserve function (including attention to early branching, which may separate sensory fibers posteriorly towards the esophagus; injury of this posterior branch is associated with aspiration due to sensory dysfunction). Awareness of the possibility of a nonrecurrent laryngeal nerve (<1%), is important. More commonly found on the right side, a nonrecurrent laryngeal nerve is associated with an aberrant subclavian artery (commonly retroesophageal).[1] Following identification of the course of the RLN, the inferior thyroid pole vessels can be divided near the thyroid capsule. Careful mobilization of the thyroid to the midline continues, and Berry ligament is encountered along the anterior surface of the trachea just medial to the insertion of the RLN. The operation, as appropriate, proceeds in similar fashion on the contralateral side.

Surgical Energy Devices

There is variation in the use of specific energy devices during thyroidectomy, without a standard consensus regarding an optimal energy technique. In general, literature supports the use of energy devices with decreased operative time and similar complication rates. The surgeon should be familiar with the use of electrocautery, bipolar electrocautery, and/or surgical energy devices such as the Harmonic Scalpel or Ligasure and the heat generation and lateral thermal spread of each. Successful thyroidectomy requires knowledge of the operation and relevant anatomy and facile use of more than one technique with the ability to adapt according to need.

Intraoperative Nerve Monitoring

Intraoperative nerve monitoring (IONM) is an adjunct measure to provide dynamic functional feedback to enhance surgical decision making. It is not designed or proposed to replace surgeon familiarity with anatomy, gentle tissue handling, and meticulous dissection of the RLN. In the most commonly used form, intermittent IONM involves use of a hand-held probe to stimulate the RLN (or the vagus nerve). The transmitted signal is detected via an electrode attached to the endotracheal tube that is in contact with the vocal cords. Successful use of this system requires both the surgeon and anesthesiologist understanding of the anatomy and positioning, as well as the ability to evaluate and troubleshoot the circuit and correctly interpret the signals. When used appropriately, feedback from the system may alert the surgeon to neuropraxia not readily recognized visually, although IONM has not been shown to consistently reduce the rate of nerve injury.[57] Information from IONM may be particularly useful in high-risk patients, including patients with bulky thyroid disease, thyrotoxicosis, or extensive malignancy, patients with known unilateral vocal cord palsy, and in reoperative settings.

Extent of Operation

7 Historically, total thyroidectomy was the procedure of choice for most patients with thyroid cancer, with lobectomy reserved for very small unifocal tumors in low-risk patients. With improved understanding of the often indolent disease course of well differentiated PTC, examination of large scale datasets supports performing thyroid lobectomy for broader indications, with minimal impact on long-term survival. The ATA encourages the consideration of lobectomy for well selected younger patients (age ≤45 years) without family history or excess radiation exposure who have solitary tumors smaller than 4 cm, without evidence of extrathyroidal extension, lymphadenopathy, high-risk histopathology (ie, tall cell variant, poor differentiation), or distant metastases, as RAI is unlikely to be required in these patients, and salvage completion thyroidectomy is a tenable option in the event of locoregional recurrence.[9] The possibility of completion thyroidectomy should be discussed in any cancer patient considering lobectomy. In addition to disease-related factors, discussion should also consider patient values regarding the possibility of postoperative hormone supplementation (which is required in about 20% of patients undergoing lobectomy and is utilized more frequently in those who require TSH suppression as part of their oncologic therapy). The decision to proceed with lobectomy also mitigates the value of thyroglobulin as a postoperative tumor marker, as native thyroid tissue will also produce the protein. Health care accessibility and compliance with follow up should also be factored into the decision of lobectomy versus total thyroidectomy.

Lymph Node Dissection

Radiographically occult cervical lymph node metastases may be present in 24% to 82%[42] of patients with differentiated thyroid cancer selected for lymph node dissection, yet the prognostic value of prophylactic nodal dissection in these patients is controversial. Proponents cite the eradication of microscopic disease (that would otherwise present as persistent or potentially recurrent disease) at the initial operative setting, thereby avoiding a reoperative field. Likely due to selection bias, retrospective analyses of prophylactic central node dissection have conflicting results, with some showing improved locoregional control,[58,59] and others showing minimal if any difference.[42,60] The information gained from additional dissection increases the likelihood of receiving adjuvant RAI,[61] but also increases the risk of postoperative hypoparathyroidism[62] (3.45% vs 1.55% in one meta-analysis).[42] The
8 ATA recommends consideration of prophylactic central node dissection for patients with differentiated thyroid cancer who are most likely to demonstrate clinically relevant nodal metastases (T3/T4 tumors, extrathyroidal extension).[9] In contrast, prophylactic central node dissection should be performed for patients with known MTC.[16]

Therapeutic nodal dissection should be compartment based and performed when there is the presence of radiographic biopsy-proven disease. The anatomic boundaries of the central compartment begin superiorly at the hyoid bone, extend inferiorly to the innominate vein, and are bounded medially by the corresponding carotid artery to the midline of the trachea. The RLN should be identified and skeletonized, and care should be taken when sweeping the fibrofatty tissue to preserve the parathyroids and their blood supply.

Lateral neck dissection is most commonly performed for levels II to IV, with the decision to include levels I or V based on the presence of disease. The relevant anatomic boundaries include the belly of the digastric muscle superiorly, the sternocleidomastoid laterally, the clavicle inferiorly, the sternohyoid muscle medially, and the precervical fascia investing the scalene posteriorly. Identification and preservation of the spinal accessory, vagus, and phrenic nerves are essential. Awareness of the marginal mandibular nerve at the angle of the jaw will prevent injury (often related to pressure from a retractor). The hypoglossal nerve is less commonly seen, but the surgeon should be cognizant of it. Lymphatic channels and the thoracic duct (in the left neck), when visualized, should be carefully ligated.

COMPLICATIONS

Thyroid surgery is associated with low rates of overall morbidity (6–12%) and mortality (<1 in 10,000).[63] The most common serious complications after thyroidectomy include hypoparathyroidism, RLN injury, and/or postoperative hematoma.

Hypoparathyroidism

Hypoparathyroidism, or impaired/inadequate PTH secretion leading to hypocalcemia and hyperphosphatemia, is the most common thyroid-specific complication after thyroid surgery and may be transient or permanent. Estimates in the literature describe hypoparathyroidism in 0.33% to 68% of patients undergoing thyroid surgery.[25] This wide variability is multifactorial, influenced by differences in patient disease and risk factors, extent of the operation and surgeon experience, and a lack of consensus regarding a uniform definition of either transient or permanent hypoparathyroidism. Patients with hypoparathyroidism experience paresthesias of the hands, feet, or lips and may progress to tetany; laboratory evaluation confirms hypocalcemia. Treatment involves supplementation with oral calcium and/or calcitriol, with intravenous calcium infusion reserved for severe cases. Perioperative assessment of parathyroid hormone levels assists in the identification of patients at risk for postthyroidectomy hypoparathyroidism.

Recurrent Laryngeal Nerve Injury

Loss of function of a unilateral RLN can result in voice changes, aspiration, dysphagia, and difficulty breathing. While some patients compensate well and the injury may be silent, many experience symptoms that impair quality of life with far-reaching impacts on emotional and socioeconomic well-being. Bilateral loss of function of the RLNs results in a substantially morbid outcome, as paralysis of the cords in a paramedian position causes glottic obstruction and requires tracheotomy. Rates of VCP in the literature are variable due to differences in symptom severity, divergent practice patterns (ie, routine postoperative laryngoscopy vs symptom elicited), and lack of consensus in definition (transient vs permanent). In general, in experienced hands, the rate of permanent unilateral VCP should be <1%.

Hematoma

Postoperative hematoma can create a life-threatening airway emergency through both direct compression of the cartilaginous trachea and impaired venous and lymphatic drainage with resulting laryngopharyngeal edema. Hematoma after thyroid surgery is rare (0.7% in one national series of >19,000 patients,[64] range 0.49% to 4.3%[65]). Meticulous attention to hemostasis is essential.

Thyroid surgery is an elective and well-tolerated procedure. Surgeon experience with thyroid surgery correlates with outcomes, with patients undergoing surgery by low-volume surgeons (≤25 cases per year) more likely to experience any complication (odds ratio 1.51, $P = .002$).[63] In addition to surgeon experience, operative risk is dependent on multiple factors, including the underlying diagnosis, the impetus for and extent of surgery, and patient age and comorbidity. A thorough understanding of anatomy and careful attention to surgical technique is essential to ensuring optimal outcomes.

References

1. Toniato A, Mazzarotto R, Piotto A, Bernante P, Pagetta C, Pelizzo MR. Identification of the nonrecurrent laryngeal nerve during thyroid surgery: 20-year experience. *World J Surg.* 2004;28(7):659–661.
2. Fisher SB, Perrier ND. Chapter 15: Differentiated thyroid cancer – surgical considerations. In: Restrepo CJ, ed. *Comprehensive Clinical Oncology: Current Practices,* English Edition. Libromed Panama; 2020.
3. Iyer NG, Kumar A, Nixon IJ, et al. Incidence and significance of Delphian node metastasis in papillary thyroid cancer. *Ann Surg.* 2011;253(5):988–991.
4. Attard A, Paladino NC, Lo Monte AI, et al. Skip metastases to lateral cervical lymph nodes in differentiated thyroid cancer: a systematic review. *BMC Surg.* 2019;18(Suppl 1):112.
5. Kandil E, Abdel Khalek M, Aslam R, Friedlander P, Bellows CF, Slakey D. Recurrent laryngeal nerve: significance of the anterior extralaryngeal branch. *Surgery.* 2011;149(6):820–824.
6. Citton M, Viel G, Iacobone M. Neck ultrasonography for detection of non-recurrent laryngeal nerve. *Gland Surg.* 2016;5(6): 583–590.
7. Moreno MA, Callender GG, Woodburn K, et al. Common locations of parathyroid adenomas. *Ann Surg Oncol.* 2011;18(4): 1047–1051.
8. Ricarte-Filho JC, Li S, Garcia-Rendueles ME, et al. Identification of kinase fusion oncogenes in post-Chernobyl radiation-induced thyroid cancers. *J Clin Invest.* 2013;123(11):4935–4944.
9. Patel KN, Yip L, Lubitz CC, et al. The American Association of Endocrine Surgeons guidelines for the definitive surgical management of thyroid disease in adults. *Ann Surg.* 2020;271(3):e21–e93.
10. Fisher SB, Perrier ND. The incidental thyroid nodule. *CA Cancer J Clin.* 2018;68(2):97–105.
11. Ahmadi S, Herbst R, Oyekunle T, et al. Using the ATA and ACR ti-rads sonographic classifications as adjunctive predictors of malignancy for indeterminate thyroid nodules. *Endocr Pract.* 2019;25(9):908–917.
12. Haugen BR, Alexander EK, Bible KC, et al. 2015 American Thyroid Association Management guidelines for adult patients with thyroid nodules and differentiated thyroid cancer: The American Thyroid Association guidelines task force on thyroid nodules and differentiated thyroid cancer. *Thyroid.* 2016;26(1):1–133.
13. Rager O, Radojewski P, Dumont RA, Treglia G, Giovanella L, Walter MA. Radioisotope imaging for discriminating benign from malignant cytologically indeterminate thyroid nodules. *Gland Surg.* 2019;8(Suppl 2):S118–S125.
14. Ross DS, Burch HB, Cooper DS, et al. 2016 American Thyroid Association guidelines for diagnosis and management of hyperthyroidism and other causes of thyrotoxicosis. *Thyroid.* 2016;26(10):1343–1421.
15. Caetano R, Bastos CR, de Oliveira IA, et al. Accuracy of positron emission tomography and positron emission tomography-CT in the detection of differentiated thyroid cancer recurrence with negative (131) I whole-body scan results: a meta-analysis. *Head Neck.* 2016;38(2):316–327.
16. Wells SA Jr, Asa SL, Dralle H, et al; American Thyroid Association Guidelines Task Force on Medullary Thyroid Carcinoma. Revised American Thyroid Association guidelines for the management of medullary thyroid carcinoma. *Thyroid.* 2015;25(6):567–610.
17. Shie P, Cardarelli R, Sprawls K, Fulda KG, Taur A. Systematic review: prevalence of malignant incidental thyroid nodules identified on fluorine-18 fluorodeoxyglucose positron emission tomography. *Nucl Med Commun.* 2009;30(9):742–748.
18. Fisher SB, Perrier ND, Clark O. Surgery for thyrotoxicosis. In: Wass J, Owen, K, eds. *Oxford Handbook of Endocrinology and Diabetes.* 3rd ed. Oxford University Press; 2020.
19. Smith TJ, Hegedus L. Graves' disease. *N Engl J Med.* 2016; 375(16):1552–1565.
20. Calissendorff J, Falhammar H. Lugol's solution and other iodide preparations: perspectives and research directions in Graves' disease. *Endocrine.* 2017;58(3):467–473.
21. Whalen G, Sullivan M, Maranda L, Quinlan R, Larkin A. Randomized trial of a short course of preoperative potassium iodide in patients undergoing thyroidectomy for Graves' disease. *Am J Surg.* 2017;213(4):805–809.
22. Shinall MC Jr, Broome JT, Baker A, Solorzano CC. Is potassium iodide solution necessary before total thyroidectomy for Graves disease? *Ann Surg Oncol.* 2013;20(9):2964–2967.
23. Pesce CE, Shiue Z, Tsai HL, et al. Postoperative hypocalcemia after thyroidectomy for Graves' disease. *Thyroid.* 2010;20(11): 1279–1283.
24. Akram S, Elfenbein DM, Chen H, Schneider DF, Sippel RS. Assessing American Thyroid Association guidelines for total thyroidectomy in Graves' disease. *J Surg Res.* 2020;245:64–71.

25. Kazaure HS, Sosa JA. Surgical hypoparathyroidism. *Endocrinol Metab Clin North Am.* 2018;47(4):783–796.
26. Oltmann SC, Brekke AV, Schneider DF, Schaefer SC, Chen H, Sippel RS. Preventing postoperative hypocalcemia in patients with Graves disease: a prospective study. *Ann Surg Oncol.* 2015;22(3):952–958.
27. Resende de Paiva C, Gronhoj C, Feldt-Rasmussen U, von Buchwald C. Association between Hashimoto's thyroiditis and thyroid cancer in 64,628 patients. *Front Oncol.* 2017;7:53.
28. Pearce EN, Farwell AP, Braverman LE. Thyroiditis. *N Engl J Med.* 2003;348(26):2646–2655.
29. Gaitan E, Nelson NC, Poole GV. Endemic goiter and endemic thyroid disorders. *World J Surg.* 1991;15(2):205–215.
30. Nankee L, Chen H, Schneider DF, Sippel RS, Elfenbein DM. Substernal goiter: when is a sternotomy required? *J Surg Res.* 2015;199(1):121–125.
31. Ali SZ, Baloch ZW, Cochand-Priollet B, Schmitt FC, Vielh P, VanderLaan PA. The 2023 Bethesda system for reporting thyroid cytopathology. *Thyroid.* 2023;33(9):1039–1044.
32. Nikiforov YE. Thyroid carcinoma: molecular pathways and therapeutic targets. *Mod Pathol.* 2008;21 Suppl 2(Suppl 2):S37–S43.
33. Nikiforova MN, Mercurio S, Wald AI, et al. Analytical performance of the ThyroSeq v3 genomic classifier for cancer diagnosis in thyroid nodules. *Cancer.* 2018;124(8):1682–1690.
34. Patel SG, Carty SE, Lee AJ. Molecular testing for thyroid nodules including its interpretation and use in clinical practice. *Ann Surg Oncol.* 2021;28(13):8884–8891.
35. Steward DL, Carty SE, Sippel RS, et al. Performance of a multigene genomic classifier in thyroid nodules with indeterminate cytology: a prospective blinded multicenter study. *JAMA Oncol.* 2019;5(2):204–212.
36. Lévesque F, Payne RJ, Beaudoin D, et al. A prospective study of publicly funded molecular testing of indeterminate thyroid nodules: Canada's experience. *J Clin Endocrinol Metab.* 2025;110(4):e1031–e1037.
37. Ahmadi S, Kotwal A, Bikas A, et al. Outcomes of cytologically indeterminate thyroid nodules managed with genomic sequencing classifier. *J Clin Endocrinol Metab.* 2024;109(12):e2231–e2239.
38. Nicholson KJ, Yip L. An update on the status of molecular testing for the indeterminate thyroid nodule and risk stratification of differentiated thyroid cancer. *Curr Opin Oncol.* 2018;30(1):8–15.
39. Siegel RL, Miller KD, Wagle NS, Jemal A. Cancer statistics, 2023. *CA Cancer J Clin.* 2023;73(1):17–48.
40. Boucai L, Zafereo M, Cabanillas ME. Thyroid cancer: a review. *JAMA.* 2024;331(5):425–435.
41. Nath MC, Erickson LA. Aggressive variants of papillary thyroid carcinoma: hobnail, tall cell, columnar, and solid. *Adv Anat Pathol.* 2018;25(3):172–179.
42. Hughes DT, Rosen JE, Evans DB, Grubbs E, Wang TS, Solorzano CC. Prophylactic central compartment neck dissection in papillary thyroid cancer and effect on locoregional recurrence. *Ann Surg Oncol.* 2018;25(9):2526–2534.
43. Wang TS, Goffredo P, Sosa JA, Roman SA. Papillary thyroid microcarcinoma: An over-treated malignancy? *World J Surg.* 2014;38(9):2297–2303.
44. Chou R, Dana T, Haymart M, et al. Active surveillance versus thyroid surgery for differentiated thyroid cancer: a systematic review. *Thyroid.* 2022;32(4):351–367.
45. Cho SJ, Suh CH, Baek JH, et al. Active surveillance for small papillary thyroid cancer: a systematic review and meta-analysis. *Thyroid.* 2019;29(10):1399–1408.
46. Nikiforov YE, Seethala RR, Tallini G, et al. Nomenclature revision for encapsulated follicular variant of papillary thyroid carcinoma: a paradigm shift to reduce overtreatment of indolent tumors. *JAMA Oncol.* 2016;2(8):1023–1029.
47. Nikiforov YE, Baloch ZW. Clinical validation of the ThyroSeq v3 genomic classifier in thyroid nodules with indeterminate FNA cytology. *Cancer Cytopathol.* 2019;127(4):225–230.
48. Patel KN, Angell TE, Babiarz J, et al. Performance of a genomic sequencing classifier for the preoperative diagnosis of cytologically indeterminate thyroid nodules. *JAMA Surg.* 2018;153(9):817–824.
49. Kiernan CM, Grubbs EG. Surgical management of multiple endocrine neoplasia 1 and multiple endocrine neoplasia 2. *Surg Clin North Am.* 2019;99(4):693–709.
50. Salavati A, Puranik A, Kulkarni HR, Budiawan H, Baum RP. Peptide Receptor Radionuclide Therapy (PRRT) of medullary and nonmedullary thyroid cancer using radiolabeled somatostatin analogues. *Semin Nucl Med.* 2016;46(3):215–224.
51. Maniakas A, Zafereo M, Cabanillas ME. Anaplastic thyroid cancer: New horizons and challenges. *Endocrinol Metab Clin North Am.* 2022;51(2):391–401.
52. Tuttle RM, Haugen B, Perrier ND. Updated American Joint Committee on Cancer/Tumor-Node-Metastasis staging system for differentiated and anaplastic thyroid cancer (eighth edition): What changed and why? *Thyroid.* 2017;27(6):751–756.
53. Tam S, Boonsripitayanon M, Amit M, et al. Survival in differentiated thyroid cancer: comparing the AJCC cancer staging seventh and eighth editions. *Thyroid.* 2018;28(10):1301–1310.
54. Adam MA, Thomas S, Roman SA, Hyslop T, Sosa JA. Rethinking the current American Joint Committee on Cancer TNM staging system for medullary thyroid cancer. *JAMA Surg.* 2017;152(9):869–876.
55. Aashiq M, Silverman DA, Na'ara S, Takahashi H, Amit M. Radioiodine-refractory thyroid cancer: Molecular basis of redifferentiation therapies, management, and novel therapies. *Cancers (Basel).* 2019;11(9):1382.
56. Cabanillas ME, Busaidy NL, Sherman SI. Redifferentiation therapy-returning to our roots in a post-kinase inhibitor world. *Clin Cancer Res.* 2022;28(19):4164–4166.
57. Wang TS, Sosa JA. Thyroid surgery for differentiated thyroid cancer – recent advances and future directions. *Nat Rev Endocrinol.* 2018;14(11):670–683.
58. Barczynski M, Konturek A, Stopa M, Nowak W. Prophylactic central neck dissection for papillary thyroid cancer. *Br J Surg.* 2013;100(3):410–418.
59. Hartl DM, Al Ghuzlan A, Borget I, Leboulleux S, Mirghani H, Schlumberger M. Prophylactic level II neck dissection guided by frozen section for clinically node-negative papillary thyroid carcinoma: is it useful? *World J Surg.* 2014;38(3):667–672.
60. Zetoune T, Keutgen X, Buitrago D, et al. Prophylactic central neck dissection and local recurrence in papillary thyroid cancer: a meta-analysis. *Ann Surg Oncol.* 2010;17(12):3287–3293.
61. Viola D, Materazzi G, Valerio L, et al. Prophylactic central compartment lymph node dissection in papillary thyroid carcinoma: clinical implications derived from the first prospective randomized controlled single institution study. *J Clin Endocrinol Metab.* 2015;100(4):1316–1324.
62. Shan CX, Zhang W, Jiang DZ, Zheng XM, Liu S, Qiu M. Routine central neck dissection in differentiated thyroid carcinoma: a systematic review and meta-analysis. *Laryngoscope.* 2012;122(4):797–804.
63. Adam MA, Thomas S, Youngwirth L, et al. Is there a minimum number of thyroidectomies a surgeon should perform to optimize patient outcomes? *Ann Surg.* 2017;265(2):402–407.
64. Talutis SD, Drake FT, Sachs T, Rao SR, McAneny D. Evacuation of postoperative hematomas after thyroid and parathyroid surgery: an analysis of the CESQIP Database. *Surgery.* 2019;165(1):250–256.
65. Harding J, Sebag F, Sierra M, Palazzo FF, Henry JF. Thyroid surgery: postoperative hematoma–prevention and treatment. *Langenbecks Arch Surg.* 2006;391(3):169–173.

73

Parathyroid Glands

Carolyn D. Seib

Key Points

1. The normal parathyroid glands are flat, ovoid, and red-brown to yellow. Their dimensions are 5 to 7 mm × 3 to 4 mm × 0.5 to 2 mm, and they weigh between 30 and 50 mg each.
2. Parathyroid hormone (PTH) is the single most important hormonal regulator of calcium and phosphate metabolism in humans, with direct effects on the skeleton and kidney and indirect effects on the intestine, mediated through vitamin D.
3. A large proportion of patients with the diagnosis of primary hyperparathyroidism are minimally or seemingly asymptomatic and guidelines provide evidence-based criteria for parathyroidectomy in this setting.
4. The demonstration of an elevated plasma PTH concentration alone does not establish the diagnosis of primary hyperparathyroidism; with a simultaneous elevated serum calcium level, this finding is virtually diagnostic.
5. Preoperative imaging localization often facilitates identification of abnormal parathyroid glands prior to parathyroidectomy, allowing the surgeon to perform a focused exploration to remove a single abnormal parathyroid adenoma, using intraoperative PTH (ioPTH) measurement to confirm removal of all hyperfunctioning parathyroid tissue and that it is appropriate to conclude the operation.

ANATOMY

Typically, each person has four parathyroid glands—two superior and two inferior (**Fig. 73.1**). The normal parathyroid glands are flat, ovoid, and red–brown to yellow. They measure 5 to 7 mm × 3 to 4 mm × 0.5 to 2 mm and weigh between
1 30 and 50 mg each.[1] The lower glands are usually larger than the upper glands. The superior glands are most often embedded in the fat on the upper posterior surface of the thyroid lobe near the site where the recurrent laryngeal nerve enters the larynx. The inferior glands are usually more ventral and lie close to or within the thyrothymic ligament that extends from the inferior pole of the thyroid gland into the chest. Although this anatomy is fairly consistent, substantial variations from the usual can occur, and it is essential that the surgeon have a thorough understanding of these anatomic variations.

Variations in parathyroid gland anatomy are primarily caused by differences in patterns of embryogenesis. During the fourth and fifth weeks of fetal development, a series of four pharyngeal pouches develops. The superior parathyroid gland arises from the fourth pharyngeal pouch in conjunction with the lateral thyroid, and the inferior gland arises from the third pouch along with the thymus. The derivatives of each pouch then migrate together so that the superior parathyroid gland usually remains in close association with the upper pole of the thyroid, although it may occasionally be loosely attached by a long vascular pedicle, migrating caudad along the esophagus into the posterior mediastinum. Occasionally, a gland may be totally embedded in the thyroid parenchyma. The inferior parathyroid gland descends with the thymus, but this migration is extremely variable. Inferior glands can be found anywhere from the pharynx to the mediastinum. Regardless of their location, they usually adhere to the thymus or are within the thyrothymic ligament. Supernumerary glands can be identified in up to 15% of patients, most often in association with the thymus and more commonly in patients with secondary or tertiary hyperparathyroidism. Autopsy studies suggest that at least four parathyroid glands are virtually always present.

The arterial supply to both the superior and inferior parathyroid glands is usually from the inferior thyroid artery, although it may arise from the superior thyroid or thyroidea ima arteries, or from the rich anastomosis of vessels supplying the larynx, trachea, and esophagus. A mediastinal parathyroid gland that descended during embryonic development usually receives its blood supply from either the internal mammary artery or small arteries within the thymus; however, an enlarged parathyroid gland that grows into the mediastinum usually carries with it the corresponding branch of the inferior thyroid artery. The inferior, middle, and superior thyroid veins, which drain the parathyroid glands, empty into the internal jugular vein or the innominate vein.

Histologically, the normal adult parathyroid gland is about half parenchyma and half stroma, including fat cells (**Fig. 73.2**). In children, the gland is almost entirely composed of parenchymal chief cells. Beginning at puberty, adipocytes appear and, with age, occupy an increasing proportion of the gland. Also, with increasing age, acidophilic, mitochondria-rich oxyphil cells are present in increasing numbers and are intermixed with the glycogen-laden, polygonal, water-clear cells. Parathyroid chief cells secrete PTH. The functional significance of the water-clear cells and oxyphil cells remains unclear, but these cells are probably derived from the chief cells.

PHYSIOLOGY

The primary physiologic role of the parathyroid gland is the endocrine regulation of calcium and phosphate metabolism. Average daily exchanges of these ions from the gastrointestinal tract, bone, and kidney are shown in **Figure 73.3**.

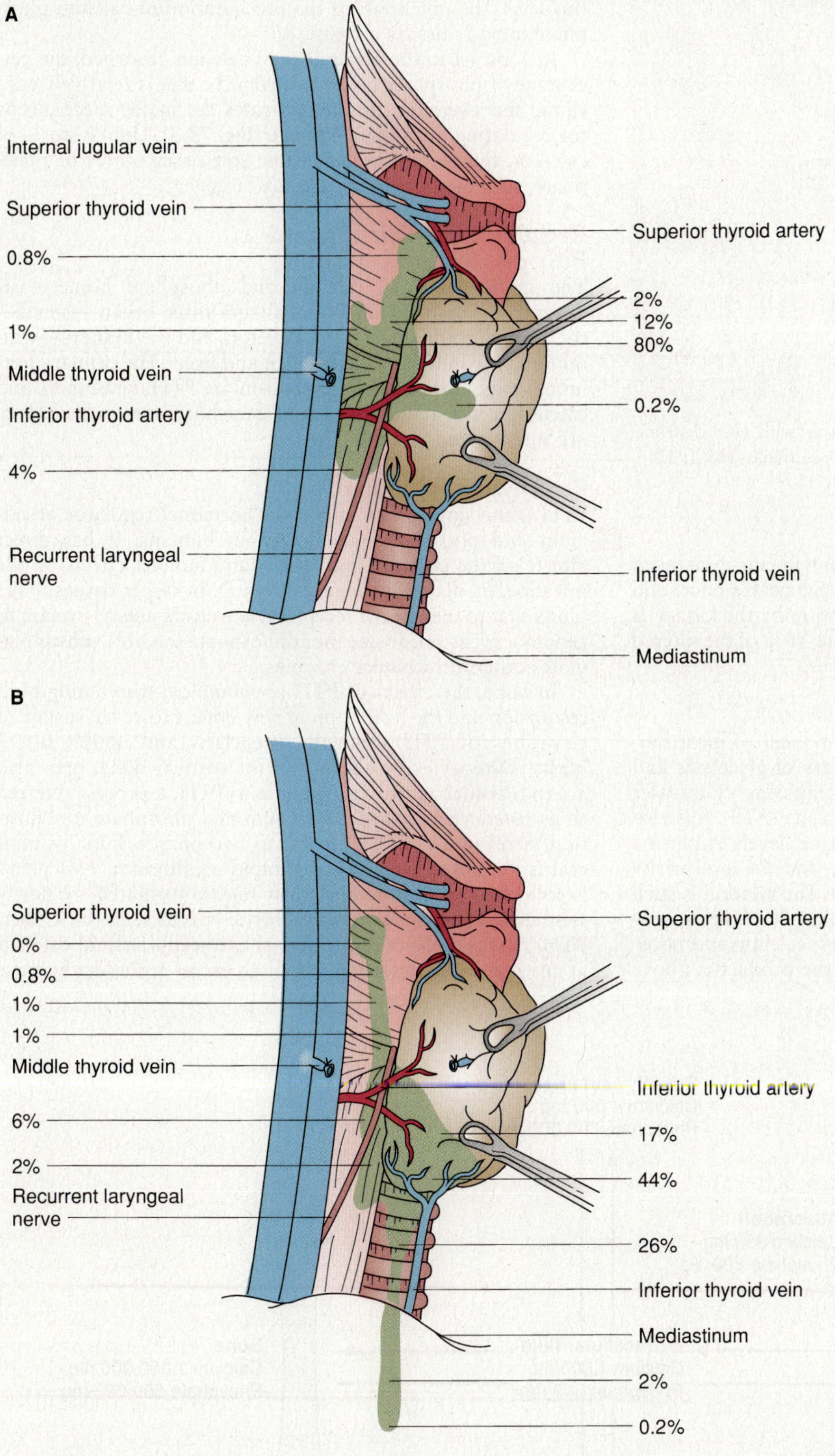

Figure 73.1. Schematic illustration of the location of the superior (**A**) and inferior (**B**) parathyroid glands from 503 autopsy studies. The more common locations are indicated by the shaded areas. The numbers represent the percentage of glands found at each location. Typically, the glands were posterolateral to the thyroid and above or below the junction of the inferior thyroid artery with the recurrent laryngeal nerve.

Calcium

Calcium ion plays a critical role in all biologic systems. It participates in enzymatic reactions and is a mediator in hormone metabolism. Calcium is intimately involved in the physiology of neurotransmission, muscle contraction, and blood coagulation. It is the major cation in bone and teeth. It represents about 2% of the average body weight, and almost all calcium is contained in the skeleton. The normal range of serum calcium is 8.5 to 10.4 mg/dL (although ranges may vary among laboratories), and the daily variation in a normal person is generally less than 10%. About half of the total serum calcium is in an ionized, biologically active form; 40% is bound to serum protein, mainly albumin, and 10% forms compounds with organic ions, such as citrate. The total serum calcium concentration is a function of the serum protein content, and because hydrogen ions compete with calcium for the same binding sites on albumin, the body fluid pH is important. In general, for every change of 1 g/dL in the serum albumin level, a direct alteration of 0.8 mg/dL occurs in the serum calcium concentration. Almost all the physiologically important activity of calcium is represented by the unbound, or free, fraction.

Calcium is absorbed in its inorganic form from the duodenum and proximal jejunum. The rate of absorption is precisely regulated according to body calcium status through vitamin D. The

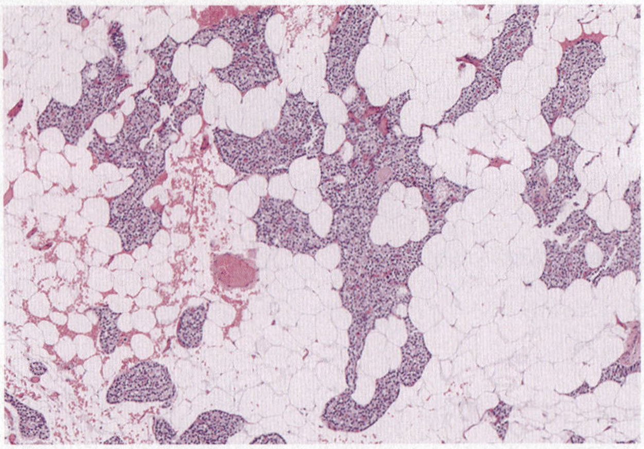

Figure 73.2. Normal adult parathyroid tissue with even distribution of chief cells and intraparenchymal adipose tissue (H&E, 10×). Image courtesy of Mobeen Rahman, MD.

calcium in the extracellular fluid is constantly being exchanged with that in the intracellular fluid, the exchangeable bone, and the glomerular filtrate. Calcium reabsorption by the kidney is closely related to that of sodium, and about 99% of the filtered load is reabsorbed under normal conditions.

Phosphate

Phosphate anion is also an integral component of most biologic systems. It is critical to the pathways of glycolysis and is the functional group for a number of high-energy transfer compounds, including adenosine triphosphate (ATP). It is also the major anion in crystalline bone. Normal levels of plasma phosphate range from 2.5 to 4.3 mg/dL, and the level varies inversely with the serum level of calcium. The relation is such that the product of plasma calcium and phosphate is relatively constant ranging between 30 and 40 (with calcium and phosphate both expressed in mg/dL). When the product is above this level, the potential for the precipitation of calcium phosphate in body tissues increases.

In contrast to the percentage of calcium absorbed, the percentage of phosphate absorbed from the diet is relatively constant, and excretion usually provides the major mechanisms for regulating phosphate balance (**Fig. 73.3**). Unlike stores of calcium, the readily exchangeable soft tissue stores of phosphate, such as those in muscle, are large.

Regulation of Calcium and Phosphate Metabolism

The maintenance of calcium and phosphate homeostasis depends on major contributions from three organ systems—the gastrointestinal tract, the skeleton, and the kidneys—with minor contributions from the skin and liver.[2] The primary hormonal regulators of this metabolism are PTH, vitamin D, and calcitonin. The actions of each of these hormones in the organs are summarized in **Table 73.1**.

Parathyroid Hormone

PTH is the single most important hormonal regulator of cal-
2 cium and phosphate metabolism in humans. It has direct effects on the skeleton and kidney and indirect effects on the intestine, mediated through vitamin D. In target tissues, PTH binds first to membrane receptors, activating adenyl cyclase to generate cyclic adenosine monophosphate (cAMP), which regulates other intracellular enzymes.

In bone, the effects of PTH are complex, stimulating both resorption and the formation of new bone. However, sustained elevations of PTH stimulate osteoclasts and inhibit osteoblasts. Osteocytes, in the matrix of cortical bone, may also act to reabsorb matrix in response to PTH, a process referred to as *osteocytic osteolysis.* Calcium and phosphate mobilization in response to PTH occurs in two phases. Initially, mineral is mobilized from areas of rapid equilibrium. This phase is followed by a more sustained release mediated by newly synthesized lysosomal and hydrolytic enzymes. In the kidney, PTH increases the reabsorption of extracellular fluid calcium at any given concentration, although excess secretion, because

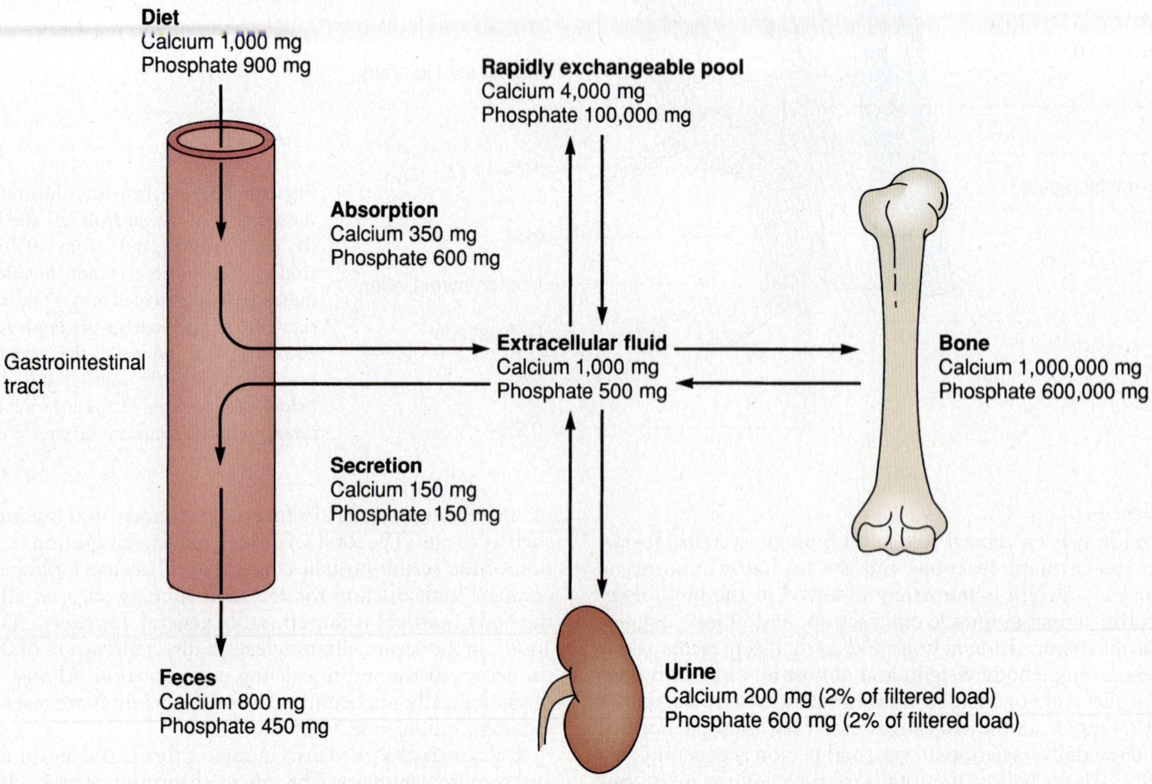

Figure 73.3. Average daily calcium and phosphate turnover in humans.

Table 73.1. Hormonal Regulation of Calcium and Phosphate Metabolism

Location	Parathyroid Hormone	Vitamin D	Calcitonin
Gastrointestinal tract	No direct effect	Stimulates calcium and phosphate absorption	No direct effect
Skeleton	Stimulates calcium and phosphate resorption	Stimulates calcium and phosphate resorption	Inhibits calcium and phosphate resorption
Kidneys	Stimulates calcium resorption	No direct effect	Inhibits calcium and phosphate resorption

of hypercalcemia, increases the net daily amount of urinary calcium excretion. Reabsorption in the proximal tubule and loop of Henle is linked with sodium transport such that factors that alter sodium transport concomitantly alter calcium reabsorption. In contrast, reabsorption in the distal nephron is independent of sodium and directly influenced by PTH. PTH also increases phosphate excretion. This action is accompanied by enhanced bicarbonate secretion. PTH probably has only indirect effects on the gastrointestinal tract, by stimulating the hydroxylation of 25-hydroxyvitamin D to 1,25-dihydroxyvitamin D in the kidney.

PTH is synthesized initially as a precursor, prepro-PTH, which is sequentially cleaved in the parathyroid gland to pro-PTH and then to PTH (**Fig. 73.4**). Secretion of this 84-amino-acid molecule is controlled by a negative feedback loop with extracellular fluid calcium, mediated by the calcium-sensing receptors (CaSR). Most PTH is secreted in this form and then cleaved in the liver into N- and C-terminal fragments. The N-terminus contains most of the biologic activity and is rapidly degraded by the liver, whereas the inactive C-terminus is slowly metabolized by the kidney.

Vitamin D

Vitamin D acts at two major sites. It increases intestinal absorption of calcium and phosphate. In addition, in the skeleton, it promotes mineralization and enhances PTH-mediated mobilization of calcium and phosphate. It has no known direct effect on the kidney.

Vitamin D_3, or cholecalciferol, is produced normally by the action of sunlight on 7-dehydrocholesterol in the skin (**Fig. 73.5**). It is then hydroxylated in the liver (25 position) and kidney (1 position) to form the active 1,25-dihydroxyvitamin D_3 (calcitriol). Vitamin D_2 is normally present in yeast and fungi but not in humans. It is the major pharmacologic source of vitamin D. Pharmaceutical preparations include vitamin D_2 (ergocalciferol), 25-hydroxycholecalciferol (calcifediol), and 1,25-dihydroxycholecalciferol (calcitriol). 1-Hydroxycholecalciferol and dihydrotachysterol are synthetic preparations that require only 25-hydroxylation for activity and so are useful for supplementation in patients with renal failure, who lack the 1-hydroxylase.

Calcitonin

Calcitonin is a 32-amino-acid protein produced by the parafollicular C (calcitonin) cells of the thyroid. The C cells are embryologically derived from the neural crest and, in lower animals, are found in the ultimobranchial bodies, which are glandular structures derived from the lowest branchial pouch. In humans, these structures are incorporated into the superior and lateral aspects of the thyroid lobes.

Total thyroidectomy, with removal of all the C cells, is well tolerated. Calcitonin is not essential for the normal control of calcium metabolism in adult humans. It does inhibit bone resorption and can produce hypocalcemia in experimental animals. It also increases urinary calcium and phosphate excretion. These effects are mediated primarily through cAMP. Several secretagogues for calcitonin have been identified, including catecholamines, gastrin, and cholecystokinin, but the most potent appear to be calcium and pentagastrin. Exogenously administered calcitonin can be useful pharmacologically to reduce serum calcium levels in the setting of severe hypercalcemia.

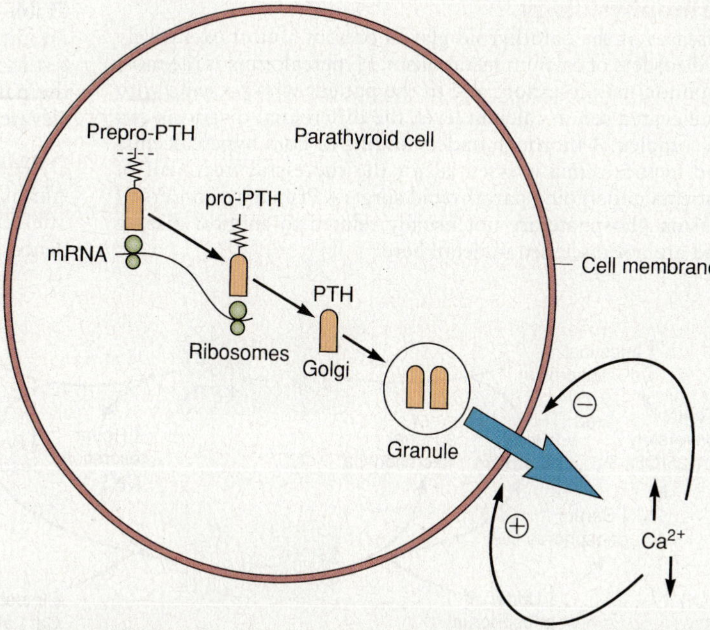

Figure 73.4. The parathyroid gland produces a precursor of PTH, prepro-PTH, that is sequentially cleaved to pro-PTH and PTH. PTH secretion is controlled by the extracellular fluid calcium concentration.

SURGICAL ENDOCRINOLOGY

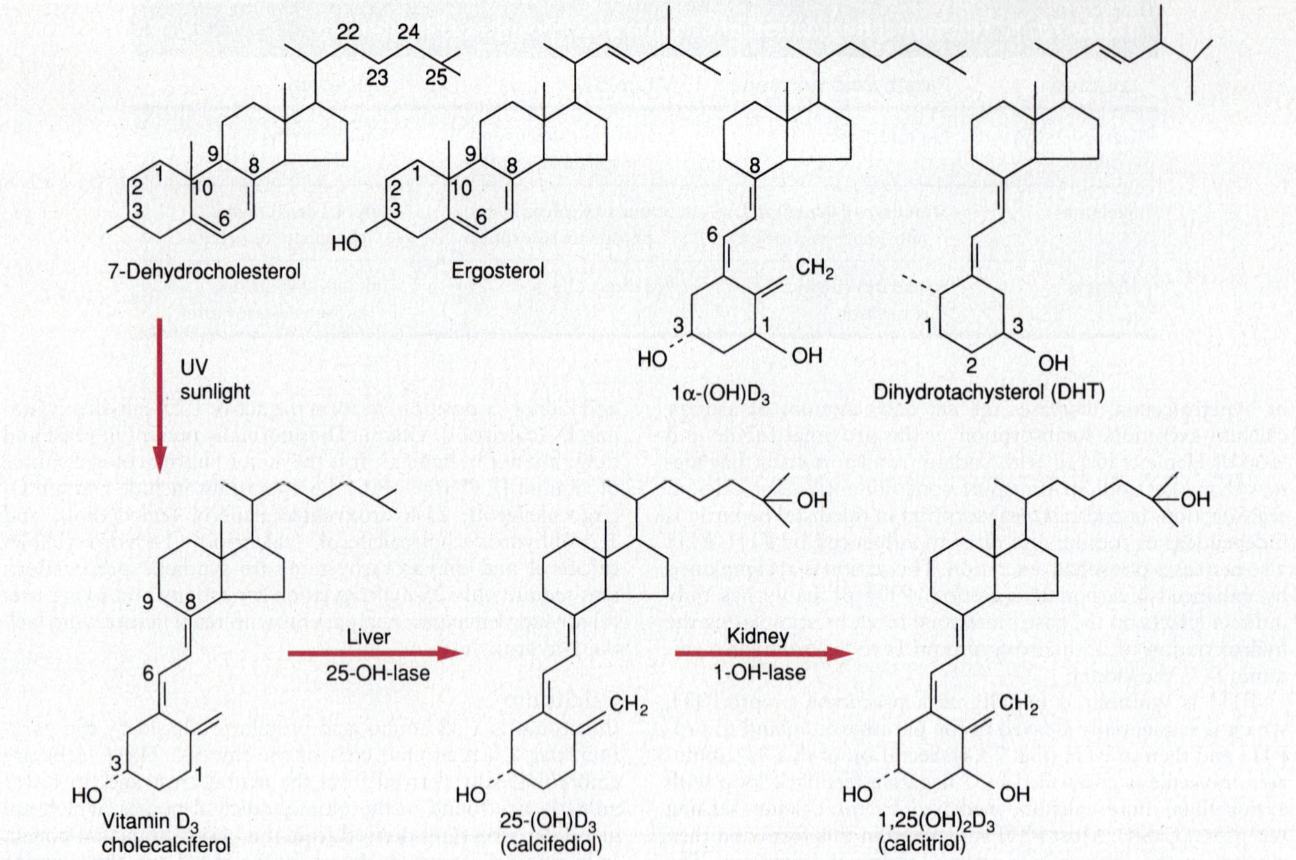

Figure 73.5. Schematic illustration of the synthesis of vitamin D_3. Ergosterol, 1-α-hydroxyvitamin D_3, and dihydrotachysterol are synthetic preparations of vitamin D.

Mineral Homeostasis

Under normal conditions, serum calcium and phosphate levels vary minimally during the course of the day. Regulation occurs primarily through PTH but also through a series of feedback loops involving vitamin D and calcitonin (Fig. 73.6). A fall in serum-ionized calcium increases PTH secretion and stimulates the production of 1,25-dihydroxyvitamin D_3. Conversely, increases in serum calcium inhibit PTH secretion and the formation of active calciferol.

Pathophysiology

Diseases of the parathyroid glands present almost exclusively as disorders of calcium metabolism. Hypercalcemia is the most common manifestation, and in the patient who presents with an elevated serum calcium level, the differential diagnosis can be complex. A thorough understanding of both hypercalcemia and hypocalcemia is essential for the successful treatment of patients undergoing parathyroid surgery. Primary disorders of plasma phosphate are not usually related to surgical disease and are not discussed in detail here.

HYPERCALCEMIA

Hypercalcemia is a relatively common clinical problem.[3–5] In the general population and in hospital outpatients, the incidence is between 0.1% and 1%. Most patients in this group have primary hyperparathyroidism. In contrast, hypercalcemia is identified in up to 3% of hospitalized patients, and nearly two-thirds of them have a malignancy.

Clinical Manifestations

The symptoms of hypercalcemia are varied and nonspecific (**Table 73.2**). Severity is a function of both the magnitude and rapidity of onset of the hypercalcemia. Many of the manifestations are subtle and are evident only in retrospect, after the patient has been successfully treated for the cause of the elevated calcium.

Differential Diagnosis

Although the diagnosis of primary hyperparathyroidism can, after appropriate investigation, be established with confidence in most patients, all causes of hypercalcemia must be

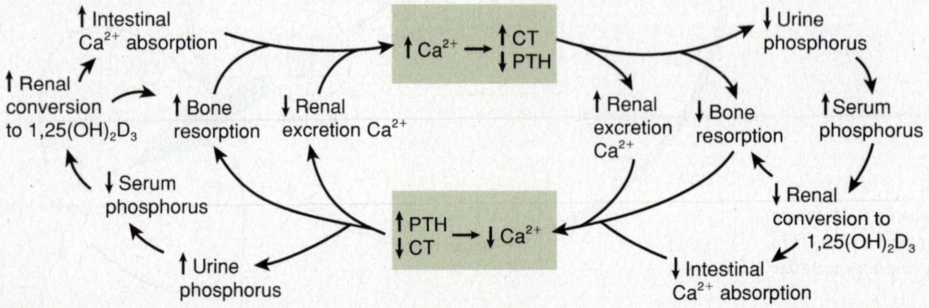

Figure 73.6. Feedback loops involved in the regulation of serum calcium and phosphorus. PTH, parathyroid hormone; CT, calcitonin.

DIAGNOSIS

Table 73.2. Clinical Features of Hypercalcemia

Neurologic
- Lethargy
- Confusion
- Coma
- Headache
- Depression
- Paranoia
- Muscle weakness
- Hyporeflexia
- Incontinence
- Memory loss
- Hearing loss
- Ataxia

Cardiovascular
- Electrocardiogram changes (short QT interval, widened T wave)
- Bradycardia
- Heart block
- Hypertension

Renal
- Polyuria
- Uremia
- Renal colic
- Nephrocalcinosis

Gastrointestinal
- Constipation
- Anorexia
- Nausea and vomiting
- Polydipsia
- Weight loss
- Pancreatitis
- Peptic ulcer
- Abdominal pain

Other
- Band keratopathy
- Conjunctivitis
- Change in vision
- Pruritus
- Thrombosis
- Myalgia

considered and excluded. The multiple causes of hypercalcemia are listed in **Table 73.3**.

Etiology

Primary Hyperparathyroidism

The diagnosis of primary hyperparathyroidism is discussed in detail later. Patients typically have elevated plasma concentrations of calcium and PTH, increased urinary excretion of calcium, and a low plasma concentration of phosphate.

Malignancy

Generally, patients with hypercalcemia and malignancy (humoral hypercalcemia of malignancy) can be classified into two groups.[6,7] Patients with solid tumors, such as lung carcinoma (25% of all cases of humoral hypercalcemia of malignancy); breast carcinoma (20%); squamous cell carcinoma of the head, neck, esophagus, or female genital tract (19%); or renal cell cancer (8%), account for three-fourths of all cases. Humoral hypercalcemia of malignancy in this setting generally appears late in the disease, with nearly all patients having known, or readily evident, malignancy. These patients have elevated levels of serum calcium, low levels of serum phosphorus, and elevated levels of urinary cAMP, consistent with increased PTH activity but normal or low-serum PTH levels. The hypercalcemia is now known to be caused by PTH-related protein secreted by the tumor, rather than by the bony metastases that many of these patients have because of the advanced nature of their cancers. In the second group, accounting for one-fourth of cases, are patients with hematologic malignancies, such as multiple myeloma, certain lymphomas, and leukemias, and a subset of patients with breast cancer. These patients have elevated levels of serum calcium, but in contrast to most patients with solid tumors and humoral hypercalcemia of malignancy, they have elevated levels of serum phosphate and low levels of urinary cAMP. These patients typically have lytic bony lesions and histologically demonstrate increased osteoclast bone resorption adjacent to tumor cells. This osteoclast-activating activity is an effect of cytokines, mainly interleukin-1 β and tumor necrosis factor-β (lymphotoxin). These cytokines promote local net bone resorption and thus produce hypercalcemia and hyperphosphatemia.

ETIOLOGY

Table 73.3. Causes of Hypercalcemia

- Hyperparathyroidism
- Malignancy
- Vitamin A or D intoxication
- Thiazide diuretics
- Hyperthyroidism
- Milk–alkali syndrome
- Sarcoidosis and other granulomatous diseases
- Familial hypocalciuric hypercalcemia
- Immobilization
- Paget disease
- Lithium therapy
- Addisonian crisis
- Idiopathic hypercalcemia of infancy

Vitamin D and Vitamin A Intoxication

When administered in excess, vitamins A and D can produce hypercalcemia. Affected patients tend to have normal or elevated serum phosphate levels associated with a low PTH level. Metastatic calcification may occur.

Thiazide Diuretics

Thiazides may increase serum calcium levels to a mild degree, primarily through hemoconcentration and decreased renal excretion. Serum phosphate may also be depressed. It often takes several weeks for the hypercalcemia to resolve after the medication is discontinued.

Hyperthyroidism

Hyperthyroidism is associated with increased bone resorption. Often, the plasma PTH is low, and a history of other thyrotoxic symptoms can be elicited. The hypercalcemia usually resolves as the patient becomes euthyroid.

Milk–Alkali Syndrome

Typically, the milk–alkali syndrome occurs in patients with peptic ulcers who consume large quantities of milk and absorbable antacids. Usually, some degree of renal failure is present. PTH levels are low. This syndrome has become much less common with the increased use of nonabsorbable antacids, histamine 2-receptor antagonists, and proton pump inhibitors as therapy for peptic ulcer disease.

Sarcoidosis and Other Granulomatous Diseases

These syndromes are associated with hypersensitivity to vitamin D. The granulomas can convert inactive vitamin D to its active form. Patients have elevated plasma globulins and low PTH levels. The administration of large doses of corticosteroids for 10 days usually reduces the hypercalcemia. Biopsy of lymph nodes or the liver may confirm the diagnosis.

Familial Hypocalciuric Hypercalcemia

This disease is an asymptomatic, autosomal dominant condition characterized by mild to moderate hypercalcemia, hypocalciuria, and normal or only slightly elevated PTH levels. It develops in people heterozygous for a mutation in the CaSR.[8–10] The mutation causes an increase in the set point for extracellular calcium concentration, so that the "normal" calcium level is higher in these people than in the normal population. No treatment is necessary, although people with this disease should receive genetic counseling. Neonatal severe hyperparathyroidism, which can be fatal, develops in children homozygous for mutations in this receptor. Management of neonates with this rare condition is challenging due to limited published evidence, but treatment with total parathyroidectomy ± autotransplantation or cinacalcet are typically considered.

Immobilization

Immobilization produces hypercalcemia by increasing the ratio of bone resorption to bone formation. These patients can usually be distinguished by history, although on laboratory evaluation, they have elevated serum levels of calcium and phosphate and a decreased serum concentration of PTH. Often, hypercalciuria is present, which may lead to the development of renal stones. Treatment is early mobilization and forced diuresis.

Other Causes

A variety of other diseases may produce hypercalcemia. For example, Paget disease of bone (osteitis deformans) typically causes mild elevations in serum calcium. Paget disease can be diagnosed on the basis of the characteristic radiographic lesion. Adrenal insufficiency may be associated with hypercalcemia, which is thought to be related to volume depletion and decreased urinary calcium excretion, although the symptoms are typically those of the primary abnormality. Lithium therapy appears to produce hypercalcemia by altering the parathyroid set point for inhibition by calcium, and, over long courses of therapy, may also be associated with hyperparathyroidism. Idiopathic infantile hypercalcemia is a rare disorder with a wide spectrum of clinical severity that is characterized by high serum and urinary calcium levels, elevated concentrations of 1,25 dihydroxyvitamin D, and suppressed PTH levels. It results from mutations in the *CYP24A1* as well as *SLC34A1* genes, which cause decreased deactivation or increased production of calcitriol, respectively.[11] Other causes include aluminum-induced renal osteomalacia and a host of analytic errors related to improper specimen collection with prolonged tourniquet times, tube contamination, and instrument drift.

Medical Treatment

Although the choice of therapy is tailored to the cause of the hypercalcemia, several general measures can prove effective (**Table 73.4**).[12,13]

For the patient with mild hypercalcemia, a trial of a decrease in dietary calcium is indicated. A reduction in intake of milk and other dairy products is suggested, along with discontinuation of thiazide diuretics and vitamin D preparations. Mobilization prevents bone demineralization.

Patients with more marked hypercalcemia (>14 mg/dL) or severe symptoms should be admitted to the hospital for treatment, with careful observation and monitoring. In the patient with severe primary hyperparathyroidism, although the definitive therapy is surgical, it is unwise to proceed with parathyroidectomy until the calcium has been reduced and is stable in a safe range. The mainstay of therapy is intravenous hydration, preferably with normal saline solution in sufficient quantities to maintain the urine output above 100 mL/h. This therapy exploits the parallel handling of calcium and sodium by the kidneys. Patients are often dehydrated before therapy, and fluid can be administered intravenously at a rate of 200 mL/h. Caution must be exercised in older patients, whose cardiac reserve may be marginal. The diuretic furosemide also increases sodium and calcium excretion, but its use is often limited in the setting of initial volume depletion. Calcitonin is a fairly weak hypocalcemic agent, but it acts rapidly and is associated with less toxicity than many of the other drugs and, as such, is often given subcutaneously in addition to hydration for acute management.[13] Bisphosphonates inhibit osteoclast activity and bone resorption directly. These agents are administered orally or parenterally and are particularly efficacious for longer-term control of hypercalcemia.[7] Treatment with glucocorticoids, which decrease intestinal calcium absorption and 1,25-dihydroxyvitamin D production, is particularly efficacious in patients with sarcoidosis and other granulomatous diseases.

TREATMENT

Table 73.4. Treatment of Hypercalcemia

Expansion of Extracellular Volume and Enhancement of Urinary Calcium Excretion
- Infusion of saline solution
- Loop diuretics (furosemide and ethacrynic acid)

Inhibition of Bone Resorption
- Calcitonin
- Glucocorticoids
- Bisphosphonates

Therapy of Primary Disease
- Tumor resection (hypercalcemia of malignancy)
- Parathyroidectomy (primary hyperparathyroidism)

Reduction of Intestinal Calcium Absorption
- Low-calcium diet
- Glucocorticoids

Other Treatments
- Dialysis
- Mobilization
- Oral phosphate
- Estrogens or progestogens (postmenopausal women with primary hyperparathyroidism)
- Chloroquine (sarcoidosis)

Modified from Attie MF. Treatment of hypercalcemia. Endocrinol *Metab Clin North Am.* 1989;18(3):807–828.

HYPOCALCEMIA

Hypocalcemia can occur as a consequence of various acquired and hereditary diseases. Generally, these disorders produce a deficiency or defect in the action of either PTH or vitamin D. It is most commonly a significant clinical problem after neck operation for thyroid disease. Chronic vitamin D deficiency is associated with compensatory PTH excess. The end result is rickets in children or osteomalacia in adults.

Clinical Features

The major signs and symptoms of hypocalcemia are a direct consequence of the reduction in plasma levels of ionized calcium, which increases neuromuscular excitability (**Table 73.5**). The earliest clinical manifestations are numbness and tingling in the circumoral area, fingers, and toes. Neuropsychiatric symptoms are also common. Patients become anxious,

DIAGNOSIS

Table 73.5. Clinical Features of Hypocalcemia

Neurologic
- Circumoral paresthesia
- Light headedness
- Depression
- Anxiety
- Confusion
- Chvostek sign
- Trousseau sign
- Irritability
- Laryngeal spasm
- Seizures

Musculoskeletal
- Tetany
- Cramps
- Involuntary twitching
- Osteomalacia

Cardiovascular
- Electrocardiogram changes (prolonged QT interval, T-wave peaking)
- Arrhythmia
- Tachycardia, hypotension

Other Features
- Lenticular cataracts

ETIOLOGY

Table 73.6. Causes of Hypocalcemia

- Hypoparathyroidism
- Vitamin D deficiency
- Pseudohypoparathyroidism
- Hypomagnesemia
- Malabsorption/Postbariatric surgery
- Pancreatitis
- Hypoalbuminemia
- Chelation of calcium
- Osteoblastic metastases
- Toxic shock syndrome
- Hyperphosphatemia

depressed, and occasionally confused. Tetany may develop, characterized by carpopedal spasm, tonic–clonic convulsions, and laryngospasm and stridor. The magnitude of symptoms at any given plasma concentration of ionized calcium varies from patient to patient. On physical examination, contraction of the facial muscles is elicited by tapping anterior to the ear, over the facial nerve (Chvostek sign), although this sign may be present in 10% of normocalcemic patients. Trousseau sign is elicited by occluding blood flow to the forearm for 3 minutes. The development of carpal spasm indicates hypocalcemia, although the test is unpleasant and clinically impractical.

Etiology

Some of the causes of hypocalcemia are listed in **Table 73.6**. The most common cause of hypocalcemia by far is excision of or damage to the parathyroid glands during thyroid surgery.

Postoperative Hypoparathyroidism

Postoperative hypoparathyroidism is the most common complication that occurs after total thyroidectomy for benign or malignant disease.[14,15] Most patients undergoing operation on the thyroid experience some alteration in serum calcium, although they often are asymptomatic; the low calcium probably represents contusion or temporary alteration of the blood supply to the parathyroid glands. The hypocalcemia is usually transient and needs not be treated unless symptoms develop. A smaller subset develops symptomatic hypoparathyroidism that may be permanent, indicating injury or removal of all functioning parathyroid tissue, requiring long-term supplementation.

Occasionally, in hyperparathyroid patients with significant related bone disease who have parathyroidectomy, a marked skeletal deposition of calcium and symptomatic hypocalcemia occurs, the so-called *hungry bone syndrome*. The plasma calcium usually reaches its nadir at 48 to 72 hours after surgery and then slowly returns to normal within several days. These patients may require calcium and vitamin D therapy for weeks or months after parathyroidectomy.

Idiopathic Hypoparathyroidism

A less common form of hypoparathyroidism is idiopathic lack of function. It occurs both sporadically and in families. In some cases, it develops as part of a polyglandular disorder and is thought to have an autoimmune basis. DiGeorge syndrome is a group of congenital disorders involving the branchial pouches that produce partial or complete agenesis of the thymus and parathyroid glands. Hypoparathyroidism can also develop in newborns as a result of prenatal suppression of the fetal parathyroid glands as a consequence of maternal hypercalcemia.[16] It is also common in otherwise normal but premature infants.

Vitamin D Deficiency

Vitamin D deficiency can occur as a result of dietary deficiency or lack of sun exposure and can result in hypocalcemia. Likewise, renal disease produces a decrease in the 1-hydroxylase activity necessary for the formation of active vitamin D. The result is a decrease in calcium absorption and an increased secretion of PTH by the stimulated parathyroid glands. Osteomalacia, abnormal fractures, and the deformities of rickets may result.

Pseudohypoparathyroidism

Pseudohypoparathyroidism describes a group of familial diseases that result from unresponsiveness to PTH. Patients with Albright hereditary osteodystrophy (type 1a pseudohypoparathyroidism) often exhibit obesity, short stature, and developmental delay. Lack of response to PTH by the kidneys results in hyperphosphatemia, hypocalcemia, and secondary hyperparathyroidism, often associated with related bone disease (osteitis fibrosa cystica).

Hypomagnesemia

This unusual deficit may result from chronic alcoholism, malabsorption, parenteral nutrition, or increased renal clearance during therapy with aminoglycosides. The deficit appears to block the physical response to PTH in addition to its release from the parathyroid gland.

Other Causes

In short-gut syndrome, after extensive small-bowel resection or bypass, or after some forms of bariatric surgery, vitamin D and calcium may be absorbed in insufficient quantities. Hypocalcemia can occur in the setting of pancreatitis as the result of fat necrosis and saponification, which allows the binding of calcium to free fatty acid complexes forming insoluble calcium soaps, in addition to cytokine release related to the systemic inflammatory response. Hypoalbuminemia causes a reduction in the total plasma calcium level, although the level of ionized calcium remains within the normal range, and patients are asymptomatic. Circulatory substances, such as the citrate used to anticoagulate banked blood and radiographic contrast media, may bind to calcium. In patients with osteoblastic metastases, particularly associated with prostate carcinoma, hypocalcemia has been attributed to increased calcium flux into the lesions. Toxic shock syndrome can be associated with hypocalcemia, but the mechanism has not been defined. Acute hyperphosphatemia, as a consequence of exogenous administration of phosphate or during the cytolytic chemotherapy of highly responsive tumors (eg, Burkitt lymphoma and acute lymphoblastic leukemia), may produce symptomatic hypocalcemia associated with soft tissue calcification.

Treatment

The treatment of hypocalcemia is summarized in **Table 73.7**. For acute, symptomatic and severe hypocalcemia, calcium should be administered intravenously. Calcium gluconate is less irritating to the veins than calcium chloride, and the calcium release is slower, without a risk for overcorrection. Usually, 20 to 30 mL of 10% solution is infused over a 15- to 20-minute period, and then 50 to 100 mL is administered over the next 12 hours in adults. A practical guide after an initial bolus dose includes 60 mL of 10% calcium gluconate in a 500-mL bag of dextrose 5% in water, infused at 1 mL/kg/h, and adjusted every 4 hours based on the serum level of calcium and patient symptoms. Bicarbonate precipitates any calcium infused through the same intravenous line, so this should be avoided. Serum magnesium should always be measured, and hypomagnesemia should be corrected if present. In patients with convulsions from advanced tetany, diphenylhydantoin (phenytoin) therapy is useful, but symptoms should never be allowed to progress to this point.

Long-term therapy is gauged on the basis of symptoms. In the postoperative patient, the continued stimulus of mild hypocalcemia to any remaining parathyroid gland tissue may prove useful. Concomitant therapy with calcium and vitamin D is

TREATMENT

Table 73.7. Treatment of Hypocalcemia

Symptom or Goal	Treatment
Symptomatic hypocalcemia	Oral calcium carbonate or intravenous calcium gluconate, and possibly active vitamin D supplements to increase the efficiency of absorption of oral supplements
Symptomatic tetany	Intravenous calcium gluconate
Correction of hypomagnesemia	Intravenous magnesium chloride
Vitamin D supplementation	Ergocalciferol, calcifediol (liver disease), calcitriol (renal disease)
Long-term therapy	Calcium carbonate; low-phosphate, low-oxalate diet; parathyroid grafting (immunosuppressed or cryopreserved autograft)

effective in a timely fashion. Oral calcium carbonate contains a higher percentage of elemental calcium (40%) compared to calcium citrate (21%) and can be given with calcitriol, an active synthetic vitamin D analog, to increase intestinal absorption. A starting dose of 2 g of oral calcium carbonate and calcitriol 0.5 to 1.0 mcg per day in divided doses is usually well tolerated. Monitoring is required to ensure patients do not develop subsequent hypercalcemia on this combined therapy.

HYPERPARATHYROIDISM

Definitions

Hyperparathyroidism is characterized by elevated PTH levels and can be primary, secondary, or tertiary. Primary hyperparathyroidism is characterized by autonomous production of PTH in the setting of elevated serum calcium levels. This category includes both benign single- and multiple-gland disease, in addition to the much rarer parathyroid carcinoma. In some cases, the disease is familial. Primary hyperparathyroidism can also be diagnosed in patients with normal calcium levels, a condition termed normocalcemic primary hyperparathyroidism, after all causes of secondary hyperparathyroidism have been ruled out.

In contrast, secondary hyperparathyroidism occurs when a defect in mineral homeostasis leads to a compensatory increase in parathyroid function. This occurs most commonly in response to kidney dysfunction but may also develop as a consequence of the hypocalcemia associated with some diseases of the gastrointestinal tract, bones, or other endocrine organs. Occasionally, with prolonged secondary stimulation, the hyperfunctioning glands are no longer physiologically responsive to an increase in ionized calcium. This autonomous state characterized by hypercalcemia and elevated PTH, referred to as tertiary hyperparathyroidism, is uncommon, affecting 1% to 5% of patients with end-stage kidney disease or after kidney transplantation, when the renal defect in calcium homeostasis is corrected.

PRIMARY HYPERPARATHYROIDISM

Incidence

The advent in the 1970s of widespread assessment of serum calcium as part of automated multichannel analysis considerably altered our understanding of the prevalence of primary hyperparathyroidism. Before that time, primary hyperparathyroidism was thought to be a relatively rare condition. Most patients presented with symptoms of disease, usually renal stones or bony manifestations. Currently, most patients are asymptomatic or have only vague symptoms or signs that can be related to hyperparathyroidism.[17,18] Occasionally, patients recognize that they had symptoms only after their well-being improves following parathyroidectomy. Incidence varies with both age and gender, but primary hyperparathyroidism is believed to develop in about 50 to 120 per 100,000 women and 20 to 50 per 100,000 men in the general population in the United States.[4,19] The incidence increases with age and varies according to race, with the disease being most common among older Black patients. Marked differences in incidence have been noted worldwide; the reasons for this variation remain unclear, although the availability of routine serum calcium and PTH measurement likely affects rates of detection.

Etiology

The cause of primary hyperparathyroidism in the majority of patients is not known. In a subset of patients, primary hyperparathyroidism can be associated with radiation exposure or genetic abnormalities. Patients with a history of head and neck irradiation are at an increased risk of primary hyperparathyroidism, which typically occurs 10 to 40 years after the exposure and in a dose-dependent manner. More recent studies have demonstrated no significant difference in the incidence of single or multigland disease among patients with and without a history of radiation exposure.[20] Primary hyperparathyroidism is most common in postmenopausal women, the population group with the highest incidence of osteoporosis and the most significant alterations in calcium and phosphate metabolism. It has been suggested that hypocalcemia due to inadequate oral intake or renal calcium leak, may stimulate the parathyroid glands and contribute to the development of primary hyperparathyroidism, but prior studies on this topic are limited.[21]

A genetic basis for primary hyperparathyroidism is identified in 10% of patients. The most common associated hereditary conditions are MEN1, MEN4, MEN-2A, and hyperparathyroid jaw tumor syndrome. In addition, familial isolated hyperparathyroidism can be due to mutations in *CASR*, *MEN1*, or *CDC73*.[22] Genetic studies of parathyroid adenomas have described an oncogene (*PRAD1*) that may be one step in the path to neoplasia in these tumors. Overexpression of the normal *PRAD1* gene, also known as *cyclin D1,* allows progression of the cell cycle from the G1 phase to the S phase, thus promoting cellular growth and division. *PRAD1* is overexpressed in 20% to 40% of parathyroid adenomas. The *MEN1* tumor-suppressor gene has also been implicated in the molecular pathogenesis of sporadic hyperparathyroidism. About 15% to 20% of sporadic parathyroid adenomas have either somatic mutation or biallelic deletion of the *MEN1* gene.[23,24]

Pathology

Single-Gland Versus Multigland Disease

Microscopically, the cell most commonly involved in primary hyperparathyroidism is the chief cell. Less frequently, the oxyphil cell is the predominant cell type in adenomas or hyperplastic parathyroid glands. Diseased glands typically have an increase in the proportion of stromal cells and a reduction in the proportion of stromal fat. Single diseased glands, or adenomas, have been classically described with a predominance of chief cells centering in a single focus, with a compressed rim of surrounding normal tissue (**Fig. 73.7**). In contrast, parathyroid hyperplasia has been characterized as a diffuse proliferation of clear cells in multiple glands, with little remaining normal tissue (**Fig. 73.8**). These criteria have proved unreliable. Although pathologic studies can usually distinguish parathyroid glands from other tissue, they may not prove useful beyond this capacity. Intraoperative decisions frequently depend on recognizing disease of one or more parathyroid glands, and in this regard, the histologic description of adenoma or hyperplasia

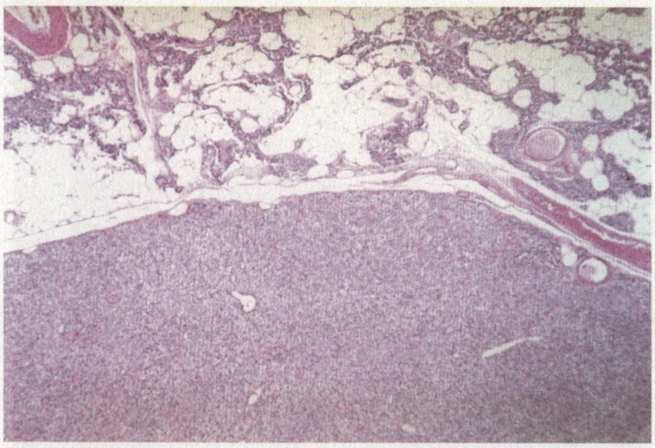

Figure 73.7. Parathyroid adenoma. The tumor consists of sheets of neoplastic chief cells and is separated from normal parenchyma by a thin capsule.

is generally unreliable in primary hyperparathyroidism, especially if only one gland is provided to the pathologist.[25]

Patients with multigland disease may have asymmetrical disease, with one gland that appears to be an adenoma and others that appears diffusely involved or even histologically normal with gross enlargement. The most reliable index of abnormality is the determination of glandular enlargement by visual inspection, in addition to darker appearance with increased turgor or firmness. The visual assessment and judgment of the experienced surgeon have proved to be an effective basis for intraoperative decisions. This approach requires that all four parathyroid glands be evaluated at the time of operation. However, ioPTH measurement provides a method to assess gland function in addition to size. The incidence of single- and multigland enlargement in 1,002 consecutive patients with primary hyperparathyroidism is shown in **Table 73.8**, describing the spectrum of disease encountered by parathyroid surgeons.

Carcinoma

Parathyroid carcinoma is a rare entity, accounting for less than 1% of all cases of primary hyperparathyroidism, and the histologic diagnosis can be exceedingly difficult. The surgeon may suspect the diagnosis when dense invasion and scarring are encountered intraoperatively, although this may also be secondary to some other inflammatory disease in the neck. Pathologic criteria include marked mitotic activity, dense fibrous stroma, and evidence of local invasion into the capsule or surrounding vessels. Malignant-appearing tumors, however, may pursue an apparently benign clinical course; the converse

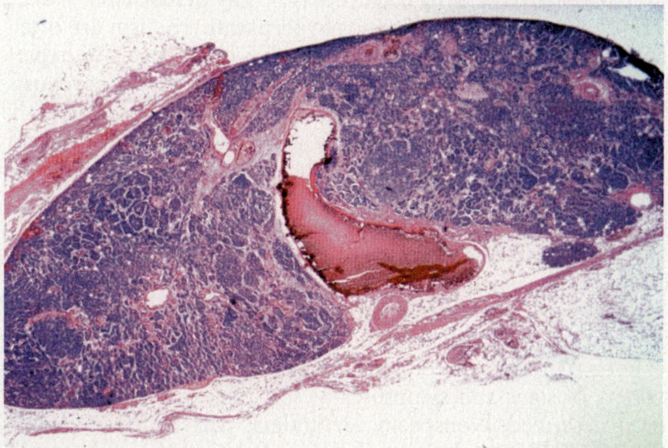

Figure 73.8. Primary parathyroid hyperplasia. The normal adipose tissue of the gland has been replaced by sheets and trabeculae of hyperplastic chief cells.

Table 73.8. Gland Enlargement in 1,002 Consecutive Patients with Primary Hyperparathyroidism

Pathology	Patient, *n*	Percentage (%)
Adenoma	788	78
Double adenoma	98	9.8
Hyperplasia	116	11.6

From Hughes DT, Miller BS, Park PB, et al. Factors in conversion from minimally invasive parathyroidectomy to bilateral parathyroid exploration for primary hyperparathyroidism. *Surgery*. 2013;154(6):1428–1434.

is less frequently true. The only reliable criteria of malignancy are metastases, most commonly to the lymph nodes, lung, or liver, and true local invasion. When review of the pathologic features of an adenoma suggests possible malignancy but are insufficient for a diagnosis of parathyroid carcinoma, these tumors are classified as atypical parathyroid tumors or atypical parathyroid neoplasms, which require clinical follow-up due to their unclear malignant potential.[26]

Clinical Presentation

The use of automated technology for determining serum calcium changed not only the estimated incidence of primary hyperparathyroidism but also the usual mode of presentation. Before screening was instituted in the 1970s, three-fourths of patients presented with kidney disease, particularly kidney stones; one-third to one-half had skeletal manifestations (including fractures), and proximal muscle weakness due to
3 neuropathy was commonly encountered. In the current day, the majority of patients diagnosed with primary hyperparathyroidism are seemingly asymptomatic at presentation, usually when hypercalcemia is detected on routine testing, and may or may not have evidence of skeletal, kidney, or other end-organ damage. Manifestations of the disease can be nonspecific and difficult to elicit in the history. As a result, there are differing opinions about the need for surgery in the asymptomatic patient and particularly for older adults or high-risk patients.[27,28]

The earliest complaints of primary hyperparathyroidism are often the vague symptoms of hypercalcemia. These vary with the magnitude of plasma calcium elevation and can include muscle weakness, anorexia, nausea, constipation, polyuria, and polydipsia. These nonspecific symptoms may or may not cause the patient to seek medical attention. Some symptomatic patients have evidence of chronic disease involving the skeleton or kidney. The goal of operative treatment for primary hyperparathyroidism is to eliminate or halt the progression of the complications of the disease.

Normocalcemic primary hyperparathyroidism is a variant of classic hypercalcemic primary hyperparathyroidism that is characterized by normal serum and ionized calcium with elevated PTH levels. All causes of secondary hyperparathyroidism must be ruled out in the diagnosis of this condition, which is often identified as the result of evaluation for osteoporosis, osteopenia, or kidney stone disease. Similar to classic hypercalcemic primary hyperparathyroidism, the normocalcemic variant can be symptomatic or asymptomatic, with or without related end-organ damage. Studies showing that almost one-fifth of patients with normocalcemic primary hyperparathyroidism will become hypercalcemic in time suggest that this variant may be a precursor to classic disease.[29]

Skeletal Manifestations

Chronic hypersecretion of PTH in primary hyperparathyroidism leads to net bone resorption over time, resulting in osteopenia and osteoporosis in a subset of patients. Low bone mineral density in primary hyperparathyroidism is most prevalent at sites comprised of a high proportion of cortical bone,

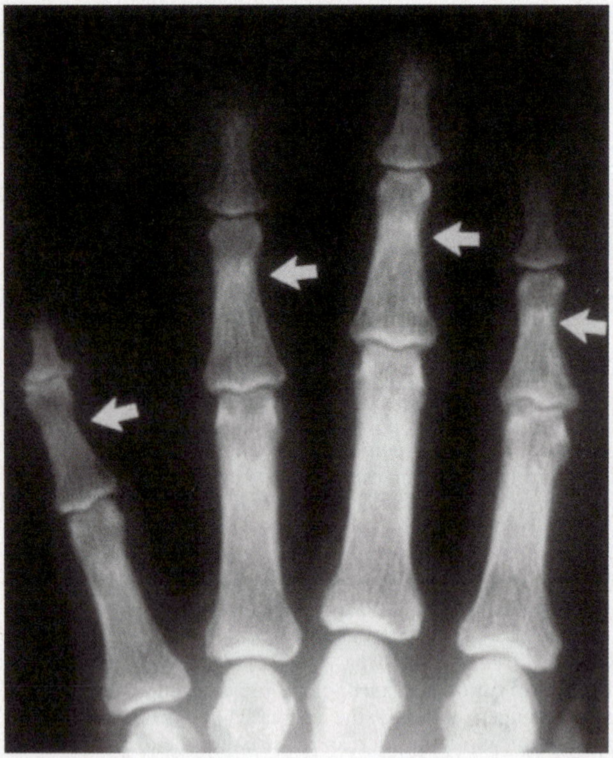

Figure 73.9. Magnification radiograph of the fingers in hyperparathyroidism. Subperiosteal cortical resorption (*arrows*) typically is most visible on the radial aspect of the middle phalanges.

which is why dual-energy X-ray absorptiometry (DXA) scans should include the one-third distal radius in this population, although other disease patterns can be seen, especially in postmenopausal women. Patients with primary hyperparathyroidism have an increased risk of asymptomatic and symptomatic fractures at multiple skeletal sites.[30]

Parathyroid bone disease in its most classic and severe form, osteitis fibrosa cystica, is seldom encountered in current practice in patients with primary hyperparathyroidism, but can be seen in patients with renal hyperparathyroidism. Five percent to 15% of patients with parathyroid bone disease present with significant symptoms of skeletal disease. Most commonly, these symptoms include bone pain and pathologic fractures. Bone changes are often demonstrable on detailed plain radiographs of the hands (**Fig. 73.9**). Characteristically, subperiosteal resorption is evident on the radial aspect of the middle phalanx of the second or third finger. Because of tufting of the distal phalanges, clubbing may be evident on physical examination. Other findings that typically involve the skull and long bones include bone cysts, "brown" tumors (ie, localized proliferations of osteoclasts), and diffuse demineralization or granularity.

Kidney Manifestations

Kidney complications develop because the hypercalcemia leads to an increase in urinary calcium excretion and because PTH increases the excretion of phosphate and produces urinary alkalosis. Both these events predispose to stone formation. Urinary stones can be treated surgically or with lithotripsy, and subsequent definitive treatment of the primary hyperparathyroidism reduces the rate of reformation. Of patients who present for the first time with renal colic, 3% to 10% are found to have primary hyperparathyroidism. Nephrocalcinosis (**Fig. 73.10**) is calcification of the renal parenchyma and occurs in 5% to 10% of patients with primary hyperparathyroidism. It causes more significant kidney damage than nephrolithiasis does. In general, the more severe the kidney damage, the less likely it is that nephrocalcinosis will regress after parathyroidectomy.

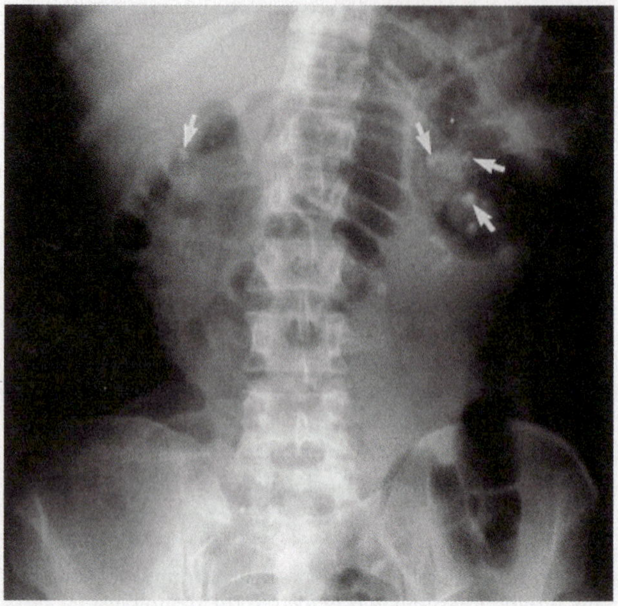

Figure 73.10. Abdominal film demonstrating nephrocalcinosis, or diffuse calcification of the renal parenchyma (*arrows*).

The incidence of hypertension in primary hyperparathyroidism increases with the degree of kidney impairment; however, it is not clear that this is a causal association.

Gastrointestinal Manifestations

Hypercalcemia is clearly associated with nonspecific gastrointestinal complaints, including nausea, vomiting, constipation, and anorexia, but attempts to demonstrate a definite relation between hyperparathyroidism and either peptic ulcer disease or pancreatitis remain unconvincing. Hypercalcemia stimulates gastric acid secretion experimentally and clinically, and has been associated with pancreatitis. Therefore, a theoretic rationale for the complex of hyperparathyroidism and gastrointestinal symptoms does exist.

Neuromuscular Manifestations

Neurologic and muscular complaints are those of hypercalcemia in general. Fatigability and proximal muscle weakness are among the most debilitating manifestations. Atrophy of type II muscle fibers, consistent with a neuropathic and not a myopathic cause, has been demonstrated. Sensory complaints include dysesthesia, a reduced vibratory sense, and stocking–glove sensory deficits.

Neurocognitive and Psychiatric Manifestations

The emotional disturbances of hyperparathyroidism are often subtle and difficult to quantify. As with other forms of hypercalcemia, they range from depression or anxiety to psychosis and coma. Patients undergoing parathyroidectomy frequently experience a sense of well-being and relief from fatigue and dullness postoperatively, even if they may have had no noticeable complaints preoperatively.

Other Manifestations

Primary hyperparathyroidism has been associated with an increased risk of cardiovascular disease and mortality, although this appears to have been most pronounced among historical cohorts with severe biochemical profiles.[31,32] In addition, a variety of signs and symptoms of soft tissue calcification have been described. Nonspecific arthralgia, particularly involving the proximal interphalangeal joints of the hands, is characteristic. The incidence of chondrocalcinosis is increased. Pruritus, vascular and cardiac calcification, and band keratopathy of the cornea have all been noted.

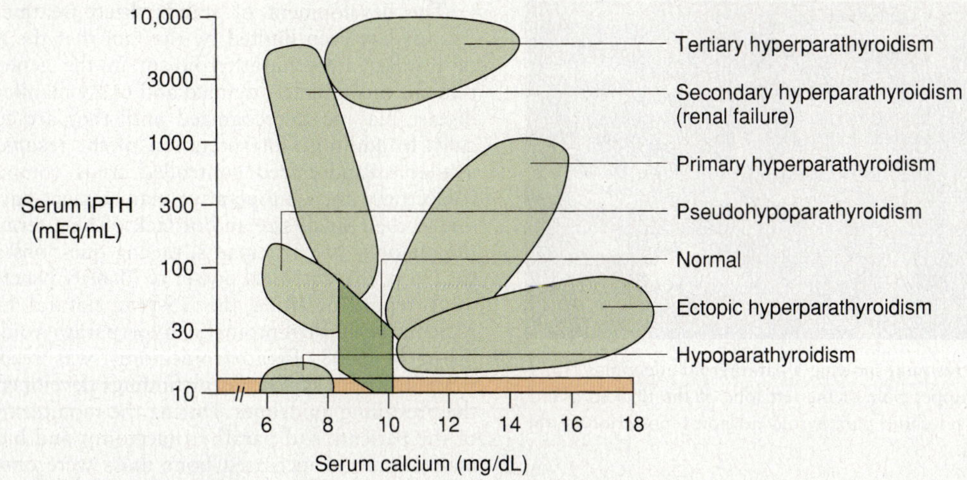

Figure 73.11. Relation between serum immunoreactive parathyroid hormone and serum calcium in patients with hypoparathyroidism, pseudohypoparathyroidism, ectopic hyperparathyroidism, and primary, secondary, and tertiary hyperparathyroidism.

Physical Findings

Except in patients with the classic deformities of advanced bone disease, physical examination is seldom helpful. Diseased parathyroid glands are infrequently palpable, except in patients with parathyroid carcinoma. A mass in the anterior neck in a patient with primary hyperparathyroidism is most commonly a thyroid nodule.

Laboratory Findings

Tests for calcium, PTH, phosphate, and urinary calcium, in addition to other laboratory tests, are useful to establish the diagnosis of hyperparathyroidism.

Calcium

Hypercalcemia is the single most important diagnostic finding; however, particularly in early or mild cases, serial analysis may show fluctuations in and out of the normal range. Coexistent hypoalbuminemia and acidosis may produce an apparently normal total serum level of calcium, even though the ionized fraction is actually elevated. Serum concentrations of ionized calcium may be helpful in patients with intermittent or mild hypercalcemia and to identify patients with the normocalcemic variant.

Parathyroid Hormone

Intact PTH measurement is an important method for establishing the diagnosis of hyperparathyroidism. The demonstration of an elevated plasma PTH concentration alone does not establish the diagnosis of primary hyperparathyroidism. With a simultaneous elevated serum calcium level, this finding is
4 virtually diagnostic (**Fig. 73.11**).

Phosphate

PTH increases renal phosphate excretion and, in about half of patients, produces hypophosphatemia. In the presence of chronic kidney disease (CKD), however, the serum phosphate levels may be normal or elevated.

Other Diagnostic Tests

Additional diagnostic tests are helpful in the evaluation of primary hyperparathyroidism. Measurement of 24-hour urinary calcium excretion is helpful in identifying patients with familial hypercalcemic hypocalciuria, in whom the rate of urinary calcium excretion is low with fractional excretion of calcium less than 0.01. Measurement of vitamin D 25OH is helpful in evaluating for coexisting secondary hyperparathyroidism due to vitamin D deficiency. Especially for patients with mild or intermittent hypercalcemia, this should be corrected prior to the biochemical diagnosis being confirmed.

Localization with Imaging Techniques

In order to try to simplify the operative approach to primary hyperparathyroidism or facilitate focused parathyroidectomy, imaging is performed to identify enlarged glands preoperatively. In the hands of an experienced surgeon, the cure rate for hyperparathyroidism at the initial operation without preoperative localization exceeds 95% with the conventional four-gland exploration. However, increasingly accurate preoperative localization with ^{99m}technetium sestamibi scintigraphy with SPECT-computed tomography (single-photon emission computerized tomography with CT), 4D-CT scans with carefully timed intravenous contrast administration, or high-resolution ultrasound, combined with intraoperative intact PTH measurement, allows termination of the operation without visualization of all four parathyroid glands. Surgeons have used these technologies in various combinations to perform focused operations and limit the extent of the neck exploration. All of the current alternative strategies, however, depend on preoperative parathyroid localization to direct the exploration.

^{99m}technetium sestamibi scintigraphy with SPECT-CT provides both functional and anatomical information on abnormal parathyroid glands (**Fig. 73.12**). Sestamibi scanning can

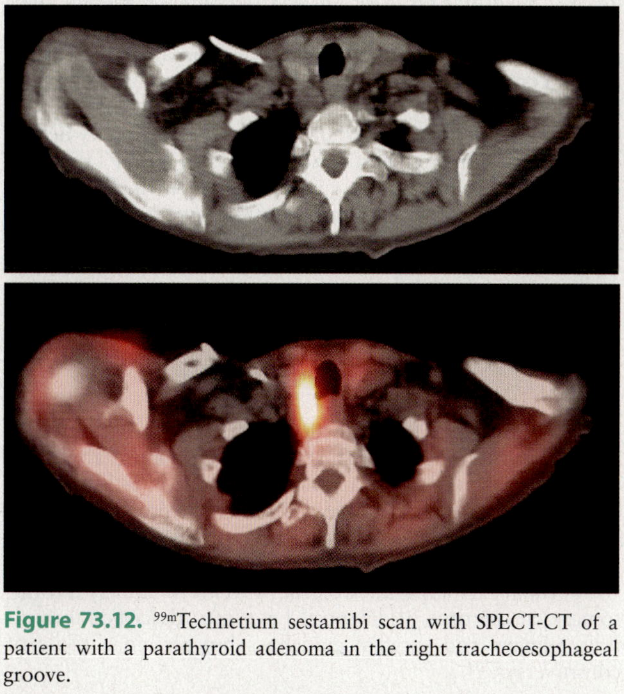

Figure 73.12. ^{99m}Technetium sestamibi scan with SPECT-CT of a patient with a parathyroid adenoma in the right tracheoesophageal groove.

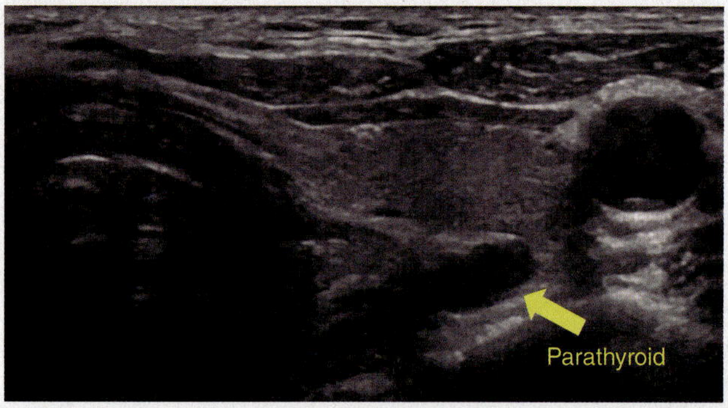

Figure 73.13. Ultrasound showing a parathyroid adenoma: Transverse image of the upper pole of the left lobe of the thyroid gland, demonstrating a hypoechoic parathyroid adenoma posterior to the thyroid parenchyma.

identify the site of abnormal tissue in 75% to 80% of patients, but has limitations in patients with small adenomas or multiple-gland disease. The availability of a CT scan with carefully timed contrast injection (4D-CT) has replaced sestamibi scan in many centers.[28] Imaging characteristics of parathyroid adenomas on 4D-CT include early and intense arterial enhancement with rapid washout relative to thyroid tissue.

High-resolution ultrasound examination of the neck is a rapid and relatively inexpensive modality that is used for localization of abnormal parathyroid tissue, particularly when it is available for use by the surgeon. The current machines scan at high frequencies (10 to 13 MHz) that allow demonstration of small abnormalities in the neck (**Fig. 73.13**). The examination is best done by a clinician in real time, as that allows the most complete assessment of the neck, rather than scans performed by a technician for later review of still pictures by the physician. The sensitivity of cervical ultrasound for abnormal parathyroid glands is about the same as for sestamibi scanning.

In patients with persistent or recurrent primary hyperparathyroidism, preoperative imaging is necessary to guide exploration in a reoperative field. High-resolution real-time ultrasonography, 4D CT, magnetic resonance imaging (MRI), and sestamibi scanning all appear to have comparable sensitivities of 50% to 60%. The results of these examinations may be less successful at centers without significant experience in their use. CT is more expensive but less operator dependent than ultrasonography. It clearly is superior in identifying deeper structures and for examining the retrosternal mediastinum. MRI is considerably more expensive than CT and has not been shown to be superior. Most surgeons prefer to have results of two or more imaging tests that confirm an abnormality before exploration in the reoperative setting.[28] FNA with PTH washout can also be helpful to guide exploration in these cases. ^{18}F-Fluorocholine positron emission tomography (PET) is an additional nuclear medicine study that can be combined with CT or MRI to localize abnormal parathyroid glands and has been shown to have high sensitivity and specificity, especially in the reoperative setting.[33]

Treatment

Indications for Surgery

The only definitive treatment for primary hyperparathyroidism is parathyroidectomy to remove one or more abnormal parathyroid glands. Operative management is indicated for all patients with symptomatic disease, including fractures, kidney stones, and neuromuscular symptoms. Indications for parathyroidectomy among the large proportion of patients with primary hyperparathyroidism who are seemingly asymptomatic at the time of diagnosis have been described in multidisciplinary and surgical guidelines but remain a topic of controversy.[27,34]

The development of standardized treatment recommendations has been limited by the fact that the natural history of primary hyperparathyroidism in the general population remains incompletely defined and many manifestations of this disease may go unrecognized until they are corrected surgically. In addition, interpretation of the results from the few available randomized controlled trials comparing parathyroidectomy and nonoperative management have been limited due to their small size and/or lack of long-term follow-up for the majority of participants, raising questions about whether they have the statistical power to identify benefits of surgery.

A report detailing the 15-year natural history of 116 patients with asymptomatic hyperparathyroidism was published in 2008. Parathyroidectomy was recommended for those in whom symptoms or findings developed, according to the prevailing guidelines. During the monitoring period, 51% of the patients had parathyroidectomy, and biochemical normalization and increased bone mass were observed in those who underwent surgery. However, the patients who did not undergo operative correction continued to have biochemical abnormalities and the cortical bone mass fell significantly. These data confirm the impression of most clinicians that mild primary hyperparathyroidism rarely takes a precipitously worsening clinical course; however, the differential bone effects that are evident by 15 years call into question how long such patients can be monitored without correction.[28]

In October 1990, a National Institutes of Health Consensus Development Conference reviewed the available evidence regarding the management of asymptomatic primary hyperparathyroidism and established evidence-based indications for operative management.[35] These have subsequently been updated four times, most recently in 2022, based on updated evidence related to the benefits of parathyroidectomy and, in the absence of data, expert consensus. Guidelines highlight the benefits of parathyroidectomy compared to nonoperative management related to improvement in bone mineral density and fracture risk reduction, which are arguably the strongest indications for operative intervention,[36,37] in addition to reducing the rate of kidney stone formation.[38] The current criteria for operative management of primary hyperparathyroidism in asymptomatic patients based on these multidisciplinary guidelines are listed in Table 73.9.

The American Association of Endocrine Surgeons (AAES) published guidelines for the definitive management of primary hyperparathyroidism in 2016 and included additional criteria that should be considered when making decisions about parathyroidectomy.[27] These included consideration for operative management in patients with neurocognitive and/or neuropsychiatric symptoms that are attributable to primary hyperparathyroidism, in addition to those with cardiovascular disease, muscle weakness, functional capacity and abnormal sleep patterns, gastroesophageal reflux, and fibromyalgia symptoms. These guidelines highlight that the complication rate of parathyroidectomy by an experienced surgeon is very low and that within a short period of time, the financial cost of medical follow-up exceeds that of treatment by operation. Based on these considerations, most patients with reasonable operative risk should be considered for and offered parathyroidectomy, and those who do not undergo operative management should be closely followed for the development of related end-organ damage. Patients who are unlikely to comply with observation protocols evaluating biochemical parameters on a yearly basis and bone mineral density every other year should be strongly considered for parathyroidectomy.

Principles of Operative Parathyroidectomy

Although neck exploration for primary hyperparathyroidism may be straightforward, it sometimes becomes an arduous procedure requiring considerable patience because of the variability in both the location and the number of diseased parathyroid glands. Persistent hyperparathyroidism and

INDICATIONS

Table 73.9. Recommendations for Surgical Management of Primary Hyperparathyroidism Based on the 5th International Workshop on the Evaluation and Management of Primary Hyperparathyroidism[34]

- Serum calcium >1 mg/dL (0.25 mmol/L) above upper limit of normal
- Skeletal features:
  - Vertebral fracture based on vertebral fracture assessment, vertebral X-ray, CT, or MRI
  - Bone mineral density by DXA with T-score <–2.5 at any site
- Renal features:
  - eGFR or CrCl <60 cc/min
  - Nephrocalcinosis or nephrolithiasis on X-ray, ultrasound, CT, or other imaging modality
- Urinary calcium excretion >250 mg/d (women) or >300 mg/d (men)
- Age <50 y

the necessity for re-exploration can usually be avoided by a meticulous initial procedure. Reoperation is predictably more difficult than the initial operation, and the risks of injury to the recurrent laryngeal nerves and hypoparathyroidism are greater in this setting.

It is essential that the surgeon be confident of the preoperative diagnosis and prospectively discusses the procedure with the patient. The potential complications of injury to either the recurrent laryngeal nerve or the superior laryngeal nerve and the development of hypocalcemia due to hypoparathyroidism require discussion. Likewise, the possibility of an unsuccessful initial operation must be explained, and the patient should recognize the risk profile of re-exploration, which in rare cases can require mediastinal access via minimally invasive approaches or, in rare cases, median sternotomy. Although focused operations are now often performed based on information from preoperative imaging localization, no patient should be explored by a surgeon who is unfamiliar with the principles and techniques of the conventional four-gland exploration.

For a four-gland exploration, the patient is placed under general anesthesia with a roll beneath the shoulders and the neck extended. The neck is opened through a transverse incision in a natural skin crease close to or overlying the thyroid isthmus, and the platysma is similarly divided. Superior and inferior flaps are developed. The strap muscles are separated in the midline and retracted laterally; division is unnecessary. One lobe of the thyroid is chosen and rotated medially. Important landmarks include the tracheoesophageal groove, the recurrent laryngeal nerve, the inferior and superior thyroid arteries, and the middle thyroid vein (**Fig. 73.14**). In most patients, the nerve lies in the tracheoesophageal groove or just laterally. Occasionally, it may be situated more anteriorly. Uncommonly, it may be nonrecurrent and originate directly from the vagus without passing around the right subclavian artery. Both of these latter variations make the recurrent nerve more susceptible to injury. The external branch of the superior laryngeal nerve, which innervates the cricothyroid muscle, usually lies medial to the superior thyroid vessels and should be carefully preserved.

During this operation, all four glands should be identified at the initial exploration because of the possibility of multigland disease. Supernumerary glands may be present and should be sought at the initial procedure if clinically relevant. Although a frozen section is not helpful in differentiating diseased from normal glands, it is generally reliable for identifying the presence or absence of parathyroid tissue, thereby confirming gland identification. Small, thin biopsy specimens are sharply incised from the gland, with extreme care taken to avoid damaging its delicate blood supply.

The upper glands are usually located far dorsally on the surface of the thyroid lobe at the level of the upper two-thirds of the gland. The lower glands are less constant and may be located anywhere from well above the thyroid to the anterior mediastinum. The lower glands are most typically in the region where the thyrothymic ligament attaches to the lower pole of the thyroid lobe. If the inferior glands cannot be localized, the thymic pedicle should be carefully examined and mobilized. Because of their common embryologic origin, the inferior gland is frequently associated with the thymic remnant. Parathyroid glands within the mediastinum sometimes can be removed by mobilizing the thymus through the cervical incision. If this technique is unsuccessful in identifying the parathyroid gland, consideration should be given for an intrathyroidal parathyroid gland. Intraoperative ultrasound examination may identify an intrathyroidal parathyroid gland, which can be confirmed with a PTH aspirate to guide thyroid lobectomy as part of a curative parathyroidectomy. If after meticulous exploration of all these areas three or four parathyroid glands have been identified, none of which is enlarged, most surgeons favor terminating the operation.

SURGICAL ENDOCRINOLOGY

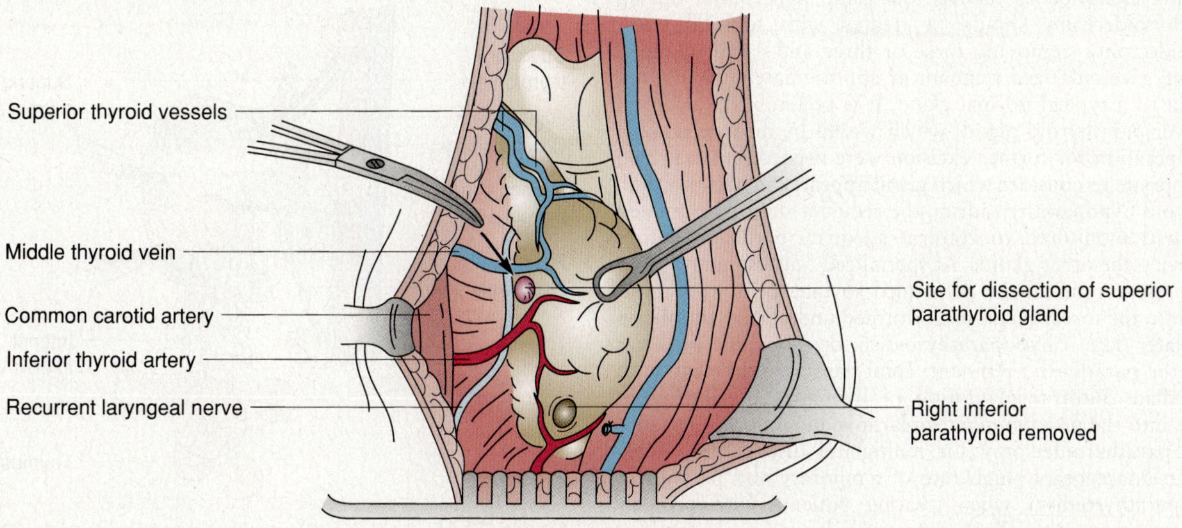

Figure 73.14. Lateral view of the right side of the neck after rotation of the thyroid lobe. The important anatomic landmarks are emphasized.

Focused Parathyroidectomy with Limited Surgical Exploration

With the availability of accurate preoperative localization methods, it has become routinely possible to identify abnormal parathyroid glands prior to operation for most patients. This allows the surgeon to perform a focused exploration to identify and remove a single abnormal parathyroid adenoma, using ioPTH measurement to confirm removal of all hyperfunctioning parathyroid tissue and that it is appropriate to
5 conclude the operation. If focused exploration does not identify a single abnormal gland or ioPTH levels do not drop after single-gland excision, the operation should be converted to a four-gland exploration. This strategy of directed, limited neck exploration is applicable to about 75% of initial parathyroid explorations, and has a similar success rate as four-gland exploration with a possible very small increase in the rates of long-term recurrence. Preoperative localization can be done by either ^{99m}technetium sestamibi SPECT-CT scan, high-resolution ultrasound, or 4D-CT. The ioPTH measurement is first assessed at the outset of the procedure, and/or immediately preceding parathyroid gland excision (the pre-excision baseline). Blood samples are obtained at time intervals after parathyroid gland resection, typically 5, 10 and maybe 20 minutes post-excision. A decrease of the PTH level by 50% from the higher of the incision or pre-excision baseline predicts long-term normocalcemia.[37] Other investigators use more sensitive criteria for the detection of multigland disease, including reduction of the PTH level into the normal range and kinetic assessments of the rate of PTH decrease.[39] This increase in sensitivity comes with the cost of decreased specificity, however. Blood samples can be obtained either centrally by the surgeon or peripherally by anesthesiology.

The limited nature of this operative approach makes it easier to perform this operation in an ambulatory setting or, in select cases, under regional or local anesthetic.[40] However, because of the possibility of multigland disease or inaccurate preoperative localization, all surgeons undertaking this approach should also be skilled in four-gland exploration.

Extent of Resection

The operative procedure performed has been based on the number of enlarged glands identified at four-gland exploration; however, with the use of ioPTH monitoring, it has become clear that not all enlarged parathyroid glands are hyperfunctioning.[41] In contrast, nearly all hyperfunctioning glands are enlarged and hypercellular. Typically, single-gland disease is treated by simple excision, whereas any combination of two- or three-gland enlargement is treated by resecting the diseased tissue and leaving the normal glands in place. Patients identified as having four-gland hyperplasia during parathyroidectomy should be treated with subtotal parathyroidectomy (removing three or three and a half glands), leaving a vascularized remnant of approximately 50 mg, the weight of a typical normal gland. It is preferable to subtotal a lower parathyroid gland, which would be more accessible if reoperation for further excision were needed, but it is also appropriate to consider which gland appears the most normal. To avoid hypoparathyroidism, the remnant should be created first and monitored to confirm adequate perfusion before removing the other glands. At specialized centers, parathyroid cryopreservation can be performed so that autotransplantation into the forearm can be performed under local anesthesia at a later date if hypoparathyroidism develops due to issues with the parathyroid remnant. Total parathyroidectomy with immediate autotransplantation of hyperplastic parathyroid tissue into the nondominant forearm is an alternative to subtotal parathyroidectomy for multigland disease, but likely has an unacceptably high rate of temporary and permanent hypoparathyroidism when treating patients with primary hyperparathyroidism. Both operations depend on meticulous identification of all parathyroid tissue for adequate results.

Special Situations

Persistent or Recurrent Hyperparathyroidism

Persistent hyperparathyroidism occurs in fewer than 5% of patients after exploration by an experienced surgeon. Most commonly, it is the result of a single diseased gland remaining in the neck or the mediastinum. Recurrent disease that develops after an interval of normocalcemia may be the result of regrowth of diseased tissue, implantation from a tumor broken at the initial procedure, or recurrent parathyroid carcinoma.

In the evaluation of these patients, it is essential to document that the initial diagnosis was correct. Familial hypocalciuric hypercalcemia should be excluded by measuring urinary calcium and creatinine excretion and calculating a calcium-creatinine clearance ratio. A value <0.01 is indicative of familial hypocalciuric hypercalcemia while a value >0.02 is suggestive of primary hyperparathyroidism.

An important consideration is whether the original operation was a focused or four-gland exploration. Reviewing the operative notes and pathology reports from the original parathyroidectomy may provide clues to the position of missed glands. The locations of parathyroid tumors not found at the initial operation but identified on subsequent exploration in one large series are shown in **Figure 73.15**.

Reoperative parathyroidectomy can be a challenging procedure. As a result, localization studies have an important role in the management of recurrent disease. Noninvasive methods are used first, including ultrasound, sestamibi with SPECT-CT, 4D-CT, MRI, and/or ^{18}F-flurocholine PET, if available. Ideally, two concordant studies are obtained. If these are unsuccessful in identifying the diseased gland, selective angiography and venous sampling for PTH can be used. The utility of these techniques varies across institutions, dependent on local experience, expertise, and preference. Venous sampling may also be helpful in some patients, although interpretation can be complicated by the alteration in venous drainage that occurs postoperatively. Because it provides no direct image but indicates the side and level of the neck where the hyperfunctioning tissue is located, it may help to direct the interpretation of other imaging studies, and the exploration to one or the other side of the neck. Both of these invasive radiographic techniques require considerable expertise. Transient cortical blindness, transverse myelitis, and cerebrovascular accidents have all been reported as complications of arteriography.

Reoperative parathyroidectomy most often involves focused exploration in the neck based on preoperative imaging localization. If a focused operation was originally performed and four-gland hyperplasia is suspected, a bilateral neck exploration,

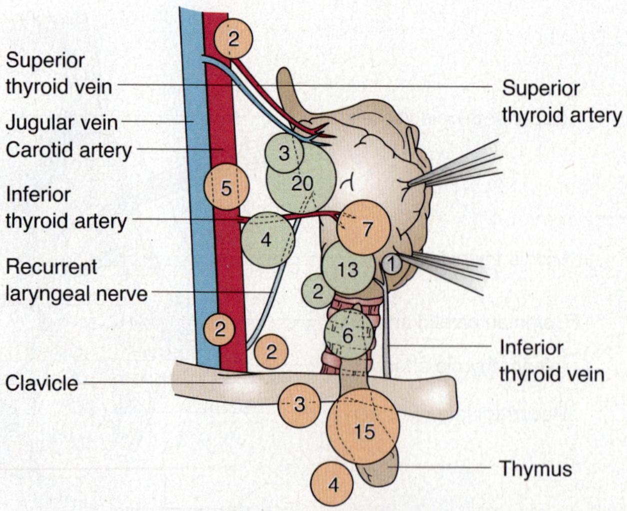

Figure 73.15. Location of parathyroid tumors missed on initial exploration but identified on subsequent operation.

focusing on nonscarred fields, may be indicated. If preoperative imaging suggests a mediastinal parathyroid adenoma, this can sometimes be accessed via a cervical incision by mobilizing the thymus. Consideration should be given for involvement of thoracic surgery for minimally invasive video-assisted or robotic-assisted thoracoscopic surgery. Median sternotomy and exploration are necessary in very few patients with primary hyperparathyroidism. Intraoperative measurement of PTH aids in documenting the adequacy of resection in patients undergoing reoperation for persistent disease.

Surgical re-exploration is successful in experienced hands in about 80% of cases. The incidence of complications is increased. Unilateral recurrent nerve injury occurs in 5% to 10% of patients postoperatively, and permanent hypoparathyroidism in 10% to 20% of patients. Cryopreservation of excised tissue may be included as a component of the management of these patients because it allows later autotransplantation if the patient becomes hypoparathyroid postoperatively. The risks of these complications must be clearly outweighed by the clinical improvement in patients with advanced disease. Reoperation in asymptomatic patients with mild disease is controversial.

Hypercalcemic Crisis

Occasionally, patients with hyperparathyroidism become acutely hypercalcemic with severe symptoms. The pathogenesis appears to involve a cycle of uncontrolled PTH secretion followed by hypercalcemia and secondary polyuria, dehydration, and reduced renal function, which exacerbate the hypercalcemia. Serum calcium concentrations may reach 16 to 20 mg/dL, and the syndrome is manifested by rapidly developing muscle weakness, nausea and vomiting, lethargy, fatigue, and even coma. Urgent medical management of hypercalcemia is pursued first. Subsequent ultrasonography, sestamibi scan, or CT scan may help to identify the enlarged gland to allow expedient correction. Definitive treatment involves resecting the diseased parathyroid tissue, which is almost always curative.

Primary Hyperparathyroidism in Pregnancy

Primary hyperparathyroidism in pregnancy is a rare disorder that not only causes hypercalcemia in the mother but can be associated with increased morbidity and mortality rates in the fetus. After delivery, the newborn is at risk for the development of hypocalcemia that can result in seizures or tetany. The outcome of pregnancies with modern management of primary hyperparathyroidism is good overall, but some data suggest that the risk of peripartum complications, including pre-eclampsia and preterm delivery, is higher for patients with primary hyperparathyroidism managed nonoperatively.[42] The general recommendation is for parathyroidectomy to be performed in the second trimester to avoid exposures during organogenesis and reduce the risk of miscarriage or preterm labor.

HYPERPARATHYROIDISM IN KIDNEY DISEASE

Secondary and Tertiary Hyperparathyroidism

Secondary hyperparathyroidism most commonly develops as a consequence of chronic renal failure, occurring in the majority of patients with CKD grade 4 and almost all patients with CKD grade 5. As kidney disease progresses, PTH hypersecretion is stimulated by phosphate retention, increased fibroblast growth factor 23 (FGF-23) concentration, decreased 1,25-dihydroxyvitamin D (calcitriol) production, and decreased ionized calcium levels. Over time, chronic elevation of PTH, which initially represents normal physiologic adaptation to CKD, becomes pathologic and contributes to renal osteodystrophy and extraskeletal calcification, including vascular calcification that is associated with increased mortality. Tertiary hyperparathyroidism is characterized by elevated PTH levels and hypercalcemia and develops when chronic PTH overproduction becomes autonomous and insensitive to plasma calcium concentration as the result of parathyroid hyperplasia. This may become evident in patients with end-stage kidney disease who undergo kidney transplantation and have persistently high PTH levels and hypercalcemia posttransplant.

Initial treatment for patients with CKD who develop secondary hyperparathyroidism is focused on controlling hyperphosphatemia with dietary restriction and phosphate binders, treating vitamin D deficiency and severe hypocalcemia, and addressing progressive PTH elevation with calcitriol or other vitamin D receptor activators, being sure to avoid the development of hypercalcemia. Therapy should be initiated carefully because metastatic soft tissue calcification can occur if patients are in a positive calcium balance for prolonged periods of time. For patients who are on dialysis with persistent elevation of PTH, calcimimetics can be initiated to reduce PTH production by increasing the sensitivity of the CaSR to calcium. Cinacalcet is an oral calcimimetic that is most commonly used, but IV etelcalcetide can be given during hemodialysis for patients with poor adherence to oral medications.

Indications for surgical therapy with parathyroidectomy include medically refractory secondary hyperparathyroidism, tertiary hyperparathyroidism with hypercalcemia that cannot be controlled medically, cortical bone fractures, proximal muscle weakness, bone or joint pain affecting quality of life, calciphylaxis or symptomatic extraskeletal calcification, intractable pruritus, and plans for kidney transplant with high risk of posttransplant hypercalcemia.[43]

The goal of operative management for hyperparathyroidism related to kidney disease is to address the source of excess PTH production while preventing morbidity related to perioperative complications, subsequent hypoparathyroidism, or recurrent hyperparathyroidism. It is important for surgeons to consider whether patients will be candidates for future kidney transplantation when planning their operation, given patients who will be on lifelong dialysis will be more susceptible to recurrent hyperparathyroidism. Subtotal parathyroidectomy is likely the optimal choice for patients with a high likelihood of kidney transplantation, while total parathyroidectomy with or without heterotopic autotransplantation may be appropriate options for patients unlikely to receive a transplant.[43] The final choice of operation should be made by the surgeon depending on their assessment of the individual patient and experience.

Preoperative risk assessment should be performed so that patients are optimized for surgery and the surgeon should communicate with the patient's nephrologist to coordinate pre- and postoperative dialysis and medication management. Preoperative treatment with oral calcium and calcitriol for 2 to 3 days can mitigate the severity of postoperative hypocalcemia and hungry bone syndrome, which develops as a result of unopposed osteoblast uptake of calcium after a postoperative decrease in PTH.

Subtotal parathyroidectomy for secondary or tertiary hyperparathyroidism involves identification of all four parathyroid glands followed by removal of 3.5 glands with preservation of a viable remnant with preserved blood supply. Bilateral cervical thymectomy should be performed to remove supernumerary glands or ectopic rests of parathyroid tissue, present in 5% to 30% of patients with hyperparathyroidism related to kidney disease. This should be done prior to gland removal in case the blood supply to the planned remnant gland is affected in this process. Typically, the most normal appearing gland is chosen for the remnant, which is created first and observed for viability before all other glands are removed. The remnant should be marked with a suture or clip to facilitate future identification as needed. Cryopreservation may be performed when available to allow for metachronous autotransplantation of parathyroid tissue in the event of long-term hypoparathyroidism.

The goal of total parathyroidectomy with autotransplantation is to remove all parathyroid tissue in the neck while providing an ongoing source of PTH production from an area that is easier to address in a reoperative setting if persistent or recurrent hyperparathyroidism develops. Bilateral cervical thymectomy is also typically performed with this operation. The presence of parathyroid tissue is confirmed via frozen section prior to autotransplantation.

Technique of Parathyroid Autotransplantation

The parathyroid gland is sliced into 15 to 20 1 × 1 × 1 mm pieces and autografted typically into the nondominant brachioradialis forearm muscle. This location permits easy subsequent access under local anesthesia if recurrent hypercalcemia develops; the grafts are easily identified by ultrasound. Function of the autograft is documented by (a) normocalcemia, with the autograft as the only source of PTH, (b) by measuring higher concentrations of hormone in the antecubital vein draining the graft bed than in the corresponding vein in the opposite arm, or (c) "transient parathyroidectomy," by placing a venous occlusive tourniquet on the arm above the graft, and measuring changes over several minutes in the PTH levels drawn from the contralateral arm.[44]

Parathyroid Carcinoma

Parathyroid carcinoma is a rare condition, accounting for less than 1% of all cases of primary hyperparathyroidism. Histologic criteria remain controversial, and the diagnosis is securely made only on the basis of local invasion or distant metastases. In comparison to patients with benign disease, these patients tend to be somewhat younger and more symptomatic. In contrast to the marked female predominance in benign disease, the male-to-female ratio in carcinoma is equal. Serum calcium, PTH, and alkaline phosphatase levels are generally more elevated, and some patients have an elevated level of human chorionic gonadotropin. Patients may have manifestations of both renal and bone disease. The affected gland is palpable in many patients.

Pathogenic variants of the *CDC73* gene (previously known as *HRPT2*) have been identified as key drivers in the development of both hereditary and sporadic parathyroid carcinoma. Hyperparathyroid-jaw tumor syndrome, a familial form of hyperparathyroidism that is inherited in an autosomal dominant manner, is caused by inactivating germline variants of *CDC73*. Patients with this condition are at an increased risk of both primary hyperparathyroidism and developing parathyroid carcinoma across their lifespan. Sporadic parathyroid carcinomas often contain *CDC73* mutations. Additional somatic drivers of parathyroid carcinoma include PI3K/AKT/MTOR pathway alterations and cyclin D1 amplification, which may be relevant clinically if considering targeted therapy for unresectable disease.

Initial treatment should include resection of the involved gland with negative margins and en bloc resection of any adjacent tissues, including the ipsilateral thyroid lobe. Ipsilateral regional lymph node dissection can also be performed if there is evidence of nodal involvement. Neither chemotherapy nor radiation therapy has shown significant benefit in patients with parathyroid carcinoma. Molecular testing may reveal tumor-specific mutations that can be addressed with novel targeted therapeutic agents. If the disease recurs, resection should be attempted because, without treatment, these patients usually succumb to uncontrolled hypercalcemia. The long-term prognosis is poor, and the opportunity for survival depends on complete initial resection.[45,46]

MULTIPLE ENDOCRINE NEOPLASIA

Although these familial disorders are typically characterized by a predisposition to the development of tumors of multiple endocrine organs, the parathyroid is characteristically involved in two of them. The disorders are all inherited in an autosomal dominant fashion, and the tumors tend to be multicentric. The tumors can be benign or malignant and can occur metachronously or synchronously. MEN-1 is characterized by the concurrence of parathyroid hyperplasia, pancreatic neuroendocrine tumors, and anterior pituitary adenomas. Classical MEN-2A consists of medullary thyroid carcinoma (MTC), pheochromocytoma, and parathyroid hyperplasia. There are three additional MEN-2A phenotypes that include variants with cutaneous lichen amyloidosis, Hirschsprung disease, and familial medullary thyroid carcinoma (FMTC). Patients with FMTC are at risk for developing MTC but not the other manifestations of MEN-2A, including parathyroid disease. MEN-2B includes MTC, pheochromocytoma, mucosal neuromas, intestinal ganglioneuromas, and a distinctive marfanoid habitus. Together these syndromes encompass much of the spectrum of endocrine neoplasia.

Pathogenesis

The genetic abnormality in MEN-1 has been identified and described in detail.[47,48] As a tumor-suppressor gene, the first mutation is inherited and becomes unmasked only when a second mutation, in some cases a deletion, develops in susceptible tissues. The resulting complete loss of the tumor suppressor allows neoplasia to develop. The occurrence of multiple second mutations explains the characteristic multicentric involvement of these diseases. Direct genetic testing is now available for some families with known mutations.

Mutations of the *RET* proto-oncogene are the cause of MEN-2A.[49] Genetic testing is now available to identify affected family members and provide the opportunity for early treatment of MTC in affected persons.

Clinical Features and Management of Multiple Endocrine Neoplasia Type 1

Characteristically, MEN-1 presents in the third and fourth decades, without any gender predilection. The syndrome is expressed with nearly complete penetrance, and autopsy studies suggest that all three organs are affected in more than 90% of patients. The phenotype varies, however, more than 90% of patients have hyperparathyroidism, but evidence of neuroendocrine tumors (30% to 80%) and pituitary tumors (15% to 50%) is less common. The cause of death in carriers of the MEN-1 mutation is related to MEN-1 in about two-thirds of patients and often caused by malignant pancreatic neuroendocrine tumors and carcinoid tumors.[50]

Parathyroid Disease

Hypercalcemia secondary to hyperparathyroidism is usually the first biochemical abnormality detected in MEN-1 and represents the best screening opportunity for members of affected kindreds until direct genetic screening is available in a specific family. Many of these patients are asymptomatic and have relatively mild hypercalcemia. Consideration should be given for genetic testing for MEN-1 in patients diagnosed with primary hyperparathyroidism who are younger than 40 years of age with multigland disease or a past medical or family history of MEN-1–related tumors.

Typically, the patients have four-gland disease, which may be particularly difficult to manage with metachronous development of multiple parathyroid adenomas. Preoperative localization may guide operative intervention, but a bilateral exploration should be planned for the index parathyroidectomy. Patients with MEN-1 are at high risk of recurrent primary hyperparathyroidism because defects in the *MEN-1* gene cause multiple parathyroid adenomas that arise independently over the life of the patient.[51] The two accepted operative approaches (subtotal parathyroidectomy and total parathyroidectomy with autograft) each have faults (as described earlier). Over time, the subtotal parathyroidectomy approach has become the preferred choice by most surgeons to avoid the risk of hypoparathyroidism. Bilateral cervical thymectomy should be performed as a part of this operation.

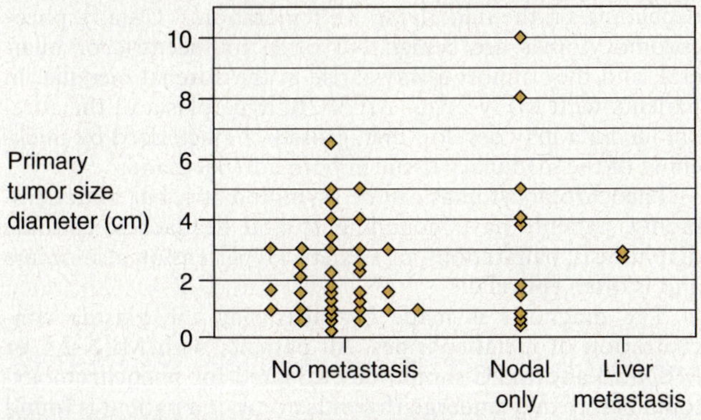

Figure 73.16. Scatter plot of largest primary tumor size versus metastatic status in 43 patients with pancreatic islet cell tumors associated with multiple endocrine neoplasia type I. Each point represents a single patient. Tumor size is not correlated with the presence of liver or lymph node metastases. (From Lowney JK, Frisella MM, Lairmore TC, et al. Pancreatic islet cell tumor metastasis in multiple endocrine neoplasia type I: correlation with primary tumor size. *Surgery.* 1998;124:1043–1049.)

Pancreatic Tumors

In MEN-1 patients with pancreatic tumors, multicentric and diffuse hyperplasia of the pancreatic islets may occur in areas distant from any grossly evident tumor. The management of these tumors is controversial because although some patients have aggressive, malignant tumors, many patients have a fairly benign course. No reliable criteria are available to detect malignant tumors. Tumor size is often cited as a useful marker of prognosis, but substantial overlap has been noted between the sizes of primary benign and malignant tumors (**Fig. 73.16**). Surgical treatment is generally recommended for patients with functional tumors and for nonfunctional tumors based on size. Gallium-68-DOTA-0-Phe1-Tyr3-Octreotate (Gallium Ga-68 DOTATATE) or Gallium-68-DOTA-0-Phe1-Tyr3-Octreotide (Gallium Ga-68 DOTATOC) PET/CT can be useful imaging techniques to demonstrate the extent of tumor.

Gastrinoma is the most common functional tumor in MEN-1; typically, a severe ulcer diathesis (Zollinger–Ellison syndrome) develops that is associated with secretory diarrhea. Serum gastrin levels are usually markedly elevated (>1,000 pg/mL); when levels are equivocal (250 to 1,000 pg/mL), provocative testing with secretin (2 m/kg) may be useful. An absolute serum gastrin increase of 200 pg/mL is diagnostic. The primary tumors are often in the submucosa of the duodenal wall and may be multifocal.

Biochemical cure of these gastrinomas is almost never possible in MEN-1, which is different than in patients with sporadic gastrinomas. Exploration and resection can reduce the need for antisecretory medications and may reduce the risk for liver metastasis. Histamine 2-receptor antagonists or proton pump inhibitors are effective in controlling acid secretion, although very high doses may be necessary; the malignant disease is often indolent.

Insulinoma is the next most common functional pancreatic neoplasm in MEN-1. Patients present with a history of sweating, dizziness, confusion, and syncope, consistent with neuroglycopenia; these symptoms are relieved by consuming carbohydrates. The diagnosis is verified by documenting fasting hypoglycemia associated with inappropriately elevated plasma insulin levels. Preoperative tumor localization is usually achieved by a combination of high-resolution CT and arteriography with selective arterial calcium stimulation and venous sampling. Calcium is injected into various pancreatic arteries and plasma insulin levels in the hepatic vein plasma are measured to detect a gradient after the injection of specific pancreatic arteries localizing the area of the pancreas containing the functional tumor. High expression of the glucagon-like peptide-1 receptor has been shown in insulinomas, with promising results from studies evaluating localization with ^{68}Gallium-DOTA-exendin-xendinCT.[52]

Because the available medical therapy for insulinoma is limited, patients are typically treated operatively to address symptoms and prevent hypoglycemia. Lesions in the tail of the gland can be enucleated if they are small; however, distal pancreatectomy carries little morbidity. Tumors of the head can usually be enucleated, so that pancreaticoduodenectomy can be avoided. In patients with malignant disease, metastases may respond to diazoxide, verapamil, or octreotide/lanreotide, which may successfully reduce insulin secretion and control symptoms. A diet of complex carbohydrates can also help stabilize serum glucose levels in the hyperinsulinemic patient.

Nonfunctional tumors are the most common pancreatic lesion in MEN-1. Their management is specific to their size and risk of malignancy, with general acceptance to operate on patients with tumors ≥2 cm in size.

Pituitary Adenomas

Prolactin-secreting tumors occur most commonly in this setting, although Cushing disease or acromegaly develops in an occasional patient. Symptoms may result from compression of the optic chiasm, which produces bitemporal hemianopsia, or from prolactin excess, which produces amenorrhea and galactorrhea in female patients and hypogonadism in male patients.

Bromocriptine inhibits prolactin secretion and shrinks many prolactinomas. Refractory tumors and those producing other hormones can be managed by pituitary ablation or radiation.

Other Tumors

MEN-1 is associated much less frequently with adrenocortical tumors and benign thyroid adenomas. Lipomas and carcinoid tumors may also occur.

Clinical Features and Management of Multiple Endocrine Neoplasia Type 2

Like MEN-1, the MEN-2 syndromes are inherited in an autosomal dominant fashion with complete penetrance but variable phenotype. Germline mutations in the *RET* (Rearranged during Transfection) oncogene are present in almost all patients with inherited forms of MTC. Bilateral MTC occurs in every affected patient. More frequently than the other syndromes, MEN-2B can arise as a new mutation that can be transmitted to subsequent generations.

Medullary Thyroid Carcinoma

MTC accounts for 1% to 2% of all thyroid malignancies, and approximately 25% of cases occur in the familial setting of MEN-2A, MEN-2B, or familial non-MEN MTC. It is usually the first tumor that develops in these patients and peak incidence is in the second or third decade. Tumors are virtually always bilateral and develop in multiple areas of the middle and upper portions of the thyroid lobe (**Fig. 73.17**). Occasionally, in young people, a diffuse proliferation of parafollicular C cells, termed *C-cell hyperplasia,* is present without frankly invasive carcinoma. This finding is highly suggestive of one of the familial MTC syndromes. Index patients typically present with a neck mass and may have hoarseness, dysphagia, or palpable cervical adenopathy. MTC most commonly produces calcitonin and carcinoembryonic antigen (CEA). The hypercalcitoninemia is often asymptomatic, although severe diarrhea can develop.

By detecting minimal elevations of plasma calcitonin, it is possible to diagnose MTC at a clinically occult stage. Basal plasma calcitonin levels in normal subjects are typically below 10 pg/mL but an increase in calcitonin occurs after

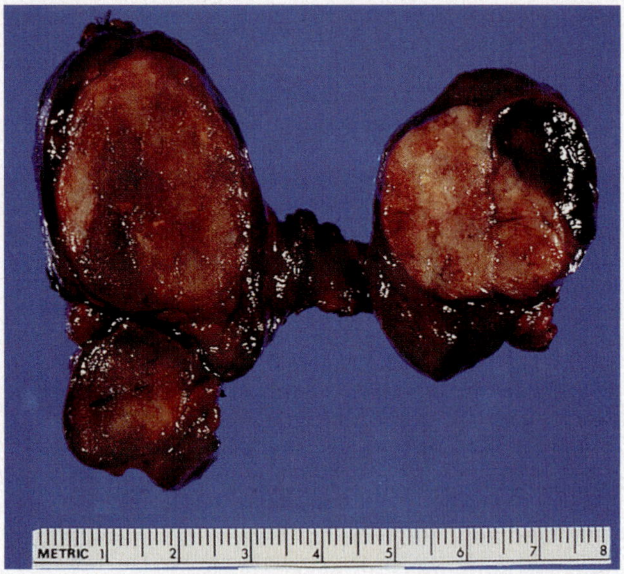

Figure 73.17. Medullary thyroid carcinoma. Coronal section of a total thyroid resection shows bilateral involvement by a firm, pale tumor.

the administration of the potent secretagogues, calcium and pentagastrin. The combined infusion of calcium and pentagastrin was the most effective screening test for familial MTC before genetic testing became available. However, pentagastrin is no longer available in the United States, so there is now more reliance on basal calcitonin level and calcium stimulation testing for screening and postoperative surveillance. Patients with occult disease may have only minimally elevated basal calcitonin levels that increase in response to pentagastrin or calcium, while patients with a more significant disease burden may show striking increases during stimulation tests. With genetic testing now widely available, prophylactic thyroidectomy to prevent the development of MTC is possible for all affected people.

The treatment of MTC is surgical resection of all suspected disease at the initial operation. Postoperatively, the presence of residual MTC can be detected by elevated basal calcitonin or provocative testing. Meticulous reoperation in patients with recurrent or persistently elevated plasma calcitonin levels, including mediastinal dissection on occasion, can normalize elevated plasma calcitonin levels and apparently cure many of them. For the patient with unresectable metastases, neither radiation nor chemotherapy is of significant benefit.[53] In recent years, targeted therapy with the selective RET tyrosine kinase inhibitors selpercatinib and pralsetinib have shown good response rates in patients with advanced MTC, with less toxicity than multikinase inhibitors, including vandetanib and cabozantinib.[54]

The clinical course of patients with the MEN-2 syndromes is determined primarily by the status of their MTC. Specific germline mutations in *RET* are associated with the aggressiveness and age of onset of MTC in these patients. This information is used to guide timing of prophylactic thyroidectomy in affected patients.[55] MTC occurs at an earlier age and is generally more aggressive in patients with MEN-2B. Patients may succumb to the disease at a young age. As a consequence of this aggressiveness, the size of kindreds with the disease is typically small, and usually only a few generations are affected.

Pheochromocytoma

Pheochromocytomas are usually detected during the initial screening or follow-up of patients in whom MTC has already been diagnosed. They typically appear in the second or third decade of life, but can be detected as early as 8 years old, depending on the underlying *RET* mutation.[55] Usually, pheochromocytomas are benign but often multicentric or bilateral, and they almost always arise in the adrenal medulla. In patients with MEN-2A or MEN-2B, hyperplasia of the adrenal medulla may develop first, grossly characterized by thickening of the medullary tissue in both adrenal glands.

Pheochromocytomas can be asymptomatic, but most commonly, patients have pounding frontal headaches, episodic diaphoresis, palpitations, or anxiety. Hypertension also occurs and is often episodic.

The diagnosis is made by measuring the plasma concentration of metanephrines. All patients with MEN-2A or MEN-2B and MTC should be evaluated for pheochromocytoma before they undergo thyroidectomy. If a patient is found to have both lesions, minimally invasive adrenalectomy after alpha blockade should be performed first, followed by neck exploration. In patients with bilateral pheochromocytomas >2 cm, consideration should be given to bilateral complete adrenalectomy, and patients should be counseled on the risks of recurrence if partial adrenalectomy is performed in this setting. In patients with MEN-2A or MEN-2B and a unilateral pheochromocytoma, only the diseased adrenal gland is removed. In about 30% of patients treated in this manner, a tumor eventually develops in the opposite gland. In the remaining patients, this approach avoids the need for glucocorticoid and mineralocorticoid replacement and the risk for adrenal crisis. After unilateral adrenalectomy, patients are carefully screened at 6-month or 1-year intervals with plasma metanephrine measurements.

Parathyroid Disease

Primary hyperparathyroidism develops in up to one-third of patients with MEN-2A, depending on the underlying *RET* mutation, although it is usually asymptomatic. Evidence suggests that patients with MEN-2A are more easily treated, with a lower incidence of recurrent hyperparathyroidism, than patients with MEN-1. Frequently, enlarged parathyroid glands are found at operation for MTC, although the patient is still normocalcemic. Multiglandular chief cell hyperplasia is the predominant histologic finding in MEN-2A, but single or double adenomas can also be identified. Significant parathyroid disease rarely develops in MEN-2B.

The surgical management of primary hyperparathyroidism in the setting of MEN-2A should take into consideration prior thyroid operations for MTC, including the number of glands identified and preserved based on operative and pathology reports. Priority should be given to avoid hypoparathyroidism. In patients with no history of cervical operations and primary hyperparathyroidism, if one or two abnormal glands are identified, these should be removed with ioPTH monitoring to confirm resection of all hyperfunctioning tissue. If four-gland disease is identified, surgical options include subtotal parathyroidectomy, leaving a vascularized remnant, or total parathyroidectomy with heterotopic autotransplantation. The latter can be considered in patients with advanced MTC, to avoid future hypoparathyroidism from parathyroid devascularization during reoperations. In normocalcemic patients with MEN-2A undergoing thyroidectomy for MTC, only abnormal appearing parathyroid glands should be removed.[55]

Nonendocrine Manifestations of Multiple Endocrine Neoplasia Type 2B

In addition to MTC and pheochromocytoma, marked abnormalities of the nervous and musculoskeletal systems develop in patients with MEN-2B. The classic phenotype is characterized by thick lips and a thin, marfanoid habitus (**Fig. 73.18A,B**). The incidence of associated skeletal abnormalities is high; these include kyphosis, pectus excavatum, pes planus or cavus, and congenital dislocation of the hip. Diffuse autonomic nervous hypertrophy is another feature. Mucosal neuromas

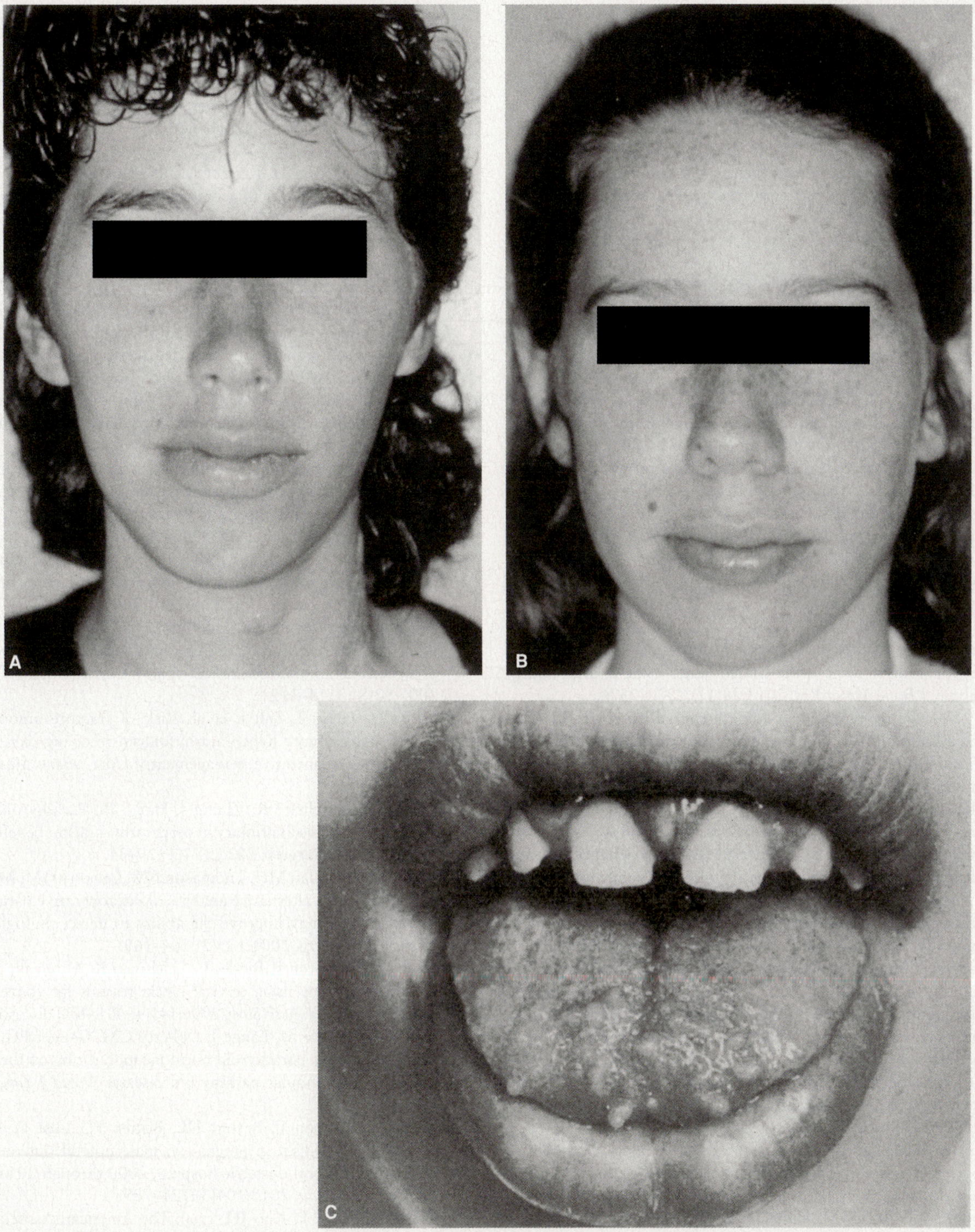

Figure 73.18. A,B: Characteristic appearance of patients with multiple endocrine neoplasia type IIB, including thick lips. C: Multiple mucosal neuromas on the tongue of a patient with MEN-2B. (From Norton JA, Froome LC, Farrell FE, et al. Multiple endocrine neoplasia type 2b: the most aggressive form of medullary thyroid carcinoma. *Surg Clin North Am.* 1979;59:109–118.)

appear on the tongue (**Fig. 73.18C**), eyelids, lips, and pharynx. Slit-lamp examination may reveal hypertrophied corneal nerves. Ganglioneuromatosis develops in the submucosal and myenteric plexuses of the gastrointestinal tract. Constipation is common, and radiographic findings may suggest megacolon or Hirschsprung disease.

ACKNOWLEDGMENT

We gratefully acknowledge the contributions of previous edition author, Gerard M. Doherty, as portions of those chapters have been retained in this revision.

References

1. Akerstrom G, Malmaeus J, Bergstrom R. Surgical anatomy of human parathyroid glands. *Surgery*. 1984;95(1):14–21.
2. Peacock M. Calcium metabolism in health and disease. *Clin J Am Soc Nephrol*. 2010;5 Suppl 1:S23–S30.
3. Endres DB. Investigation of hypercalcemia. *Clin Biochem*. 2012; 45(12):954–963.
4. Yeh MW, Ituarte PH, Zhou HC, et al. Incidence and prevalence of primary hyperparathyroidism in a racially mixed population. *J Clin Endocrinol Metab*. 2013;98(3):1122–1129.
5. Ahmad S, Kuraganti G, Steenkamp D. Hypercalcemic crisis: a clinical review. *Am J Med*. 2015;128(3):239–245.

6. Ross JR, Saunders Y, Edmonds PM, et al. A systematic review of the role of bisphosphonates in metastatic disease. *Health Technol Assess*. 2004;8(4):1–176.
7. Clines GA. Mechanisms and treatment of hypercalcemia of malignancy. *Curr Opin Endocrinol Diabetes Obes*. 2011;18(6): 339–346.
8. Pollak MR, Brown EM, Chou YH, et al. Mutations in the human Ca(2+)-sensing receptor gene cause familial hypocalciuric hypercalcemia and neonatal severe hyperparathyroidism. *Cell*. 1993;75(7):1297–1303.
9. Pollak MR, Chou YH, Marx SJ, et al. Familial hypocalciuric hypercalcemia and neonatal severe hyperparathyroidism. Effects of mutant gene dosage on phenotype. *J Clin Invest*. 1994;93(3): 1108–1112.
10. Christensen SE, Nissen PH, Vestergaard P, Mosekilde L. Familial hypocalciuric hypercalcaemia: a review. *Curr Opin Endocrinol Diabetes Obes*. 2011;18(6):359–370.
11. Lenherr-Taube N, Furman M, Assor E, et al. Mild idiopathic infantile hypercalcemia-part 2: a longitudinal observational study. *J Clin Endocrinol Metab*. 2021;106(10):2938–2948.
12. LeGrand SB, Leskuski D, Zama I. Narrative review: furosemide for hypercalcemia: an unproven yet common practice. *Ann Intern Med*. 2008;149(4):259–263.
13. Martinez-Zapata MJ, Roque M, Alonso-Coello P, Catala E. Calcitonin for metastatic bone pain. *Cochrane Database Syst Rev*. 2006;2006(3):CD003223.
14. Lo CY. Postthyroidectomy hypocalcemia. *J Am Coll Surg*. 2003; 196(3):497–498.
15. Powers J, Joy K, Ruscio A, Lagast H. Prevalence and incidence of hypoparathyroidism in the United States using a large claims database. *J Bone Miner Res*. 2013;28(12):2570–2576.
16. Ip P. Neonatal convulsion revealing maternal hyperparathyroidism: an unusual case of late neonatal hypoparathyroidism. *Arch Gynecol Obstet*. 2003;268(3):227–229.
17. Heath H 3rd. Clinical spectrum of primary hyperparathyroidism: evolution with changes in medical practice and technology. *J Bone Miner Res*. 1991;6 Suppl 2:S63–S70; discussion S83–S4.
18. Heath H 3rd, Hodgson SF, Kennedy MA. Primary hyperparathyroidism. Incidence, morbidity, and potential economic impact in a community. *N Engl J Med*. 1980;302(4):189–193.
19. Griebeler ML, Kearns AE, Ryu E, Hathcock MA, Melton LJ III, Wermers RA. Secular trends in the incidence of primary hyperparathyroidism over five decades (1965–2010). *Bone*. 2015;73: 1–7.
20. Woll M, Sippel RS, Chen H. Does previous head and neck irradiation increase the chance of multigland disease in patients with hyperparathyroidism? *Ann Surg Oncol*. 2011;18(8):2240–2244.
21. Paik JM, Curhan GC, Taylor EN. Calcium intake and risk of primary hyperparathyroidism in women: prospective cohort study. *BMJ*. 2012;345:e6390.
22. Minisola S, Arnold A, Belaya Z, et al. Epidemiology, pathophysiology, and genetics of primary hyperparathyroidism. *J Bone Miner Res*. 2022;37(11):2315–2329.
23. Arnold A, Shattuck TM, Mallya SM, et al. Molecular pathogenesis of primary hyperparathyroidism. *J Bone Miner Res*. 2002;17 Suppl 2:N30–N36.
24. Costa-Guda J, Soong CP, Parekh VI, Agarwal SK, Arnold A. Germline and somatic mutations in cyclin-dependent kinase inhibitor genes CDKN1A, CDKN2B, and CDKN2C in sporadic parathyroid adenomas. *Horm Cancer*. 2013;4(5):301–307.
25. Johnson SJ, Sheffield EA, McNicol AM. Best practice no 183. Examination of parathyroid gland specimens. *J Clin Pathol*. 2005; 58(4):338–342.
26. Erickson LA, Mete O, Juhlin CC, Perren A, Gill AJ. Overview of the 2022 WHO classification of parathyroid tumors. *Endocr Pathol*. 2022;33(1):64–89.
27. Wilhelm SM, Wang TS, Ruan DT, et al. The American association of endocrine surgeons guidelines for definitive management of primary hyperparathyroidism. *JAMA Surg*. 2016;151(10): 959–968.
28. Rubin MR, Bilezikian JP, McMahon DJ, et al. The natural history of primary hyperparathyroidism with or without parathyroid surgery after 15 years. *J Clin Endocrinol Metab*. 2008;93(9):3462–3470.
29. Lowe H, McMahon DJ, Rubin MR, Bilezikian JP, Silverberg SJ. Normocalcemic primary hyperparathyroidism: further characterization of a new clinical phenotype. *J Clin Endocrinol Metab*. 2007;92(8):3001–3005.
30. Ejlsmark-Svensson H, Rolighed L, Harslof T, Rejnmark L. Risk of fractures in primary hyperparathyroidism: a systematic review and meta-analysis. *Osteoporos Int*. 2021;32(6):1053–1060.
31. Hagstrom E, Hellman P, Larsson TE, et al. Plasma parathyroid hormone and the risk of cardiovascular mortality in the community. *Circulation*. 2009;119(21):2765–2771.
32. Yu N, Donnan PT, Flynn RW, et al. Increased mortality and morbidity in mild primary hyperparathyroid patients. The Parathyroid Epidemiology and Audit Research Study (PEARS). *Clin Endocrinol (Oxf)*. 2010;73(1):30–34.
33. Graves CE, Hope TA, Kim J, et al. Superior sensitivity of (18) F-fluorocholine: PET localization in primary hyperparathyroidism. *Surgery*. 2022;171(1):47–54.
34. Bilezikian JP, Khan AA, Silverberg SJ, et al. Evaluation and management of primary hyperparathyroidism: summary statement and guidelines from the Fifth International Workshop. *J Bone Miner Res*. 2022;37(11):2293–2314.
35. NIH Conference. Diagnosis and management of asymptomatic primary hyperparathyroidism: consensus development conference statement. *Ann Intern Med*. 1991;114(7):593–597.
36. Ambrogini E, Cetani F, Cianferotti L, et al. Surgery or surveillance for mild asymptomatic primary hyperparathyroidism: a prospective, randomized clinical trial. *J Clin Endocrinol Metab*. 2007;92(8):3114–3121.
37. Seib CD, Meng T, Suh I, et al. Risk of fracture among older adults with primary hyperparathyroidism receiving parathyroidectomy vs nonoperative management. *JAMA Intern Med*. 2022; 182(1):10–18.
38. Huang SY, Burchette R, Chung J, Haigh PI. Parathyroidectomy for nephrolithiasis in primary hyperparathyroidism: beneficial but not a panacea. *Surgery*. 2022;171(1):29–34.
39. Gauger PG, Mullan MH, Thompson NW, Doherty GM, Matz KA, England BG. An alternative analysis of intraoperative parathyroid hormone data may improve the ability to detect multiglandular disease. *Arch Surg*. 2004;139(2):164–169.
40. Carling T, Donovan P, Rinder C, Udelsman R. Minimally invasive parathyroidectomy using cervical block: reasons for conversion to general anesthesia. *Arch Surg*. 2006;141(4):401–404; discussion 404.
41. Clerici T, Brandle M, Lange J, Doherty GM, Gauger PG. Impact of intraoperative parathyroid hormone monitoring on the prediction of multiglandular parathyroid disease. *World J Surg*. 2004; 28(2):187–192.
42. Rigg J, Gilbertson E, Barrett HL, Britten FL, Lust K. Primary hyperparathyroidism in pregnancy: maternofetal outcomes at a quaternary referral obstetric hospital, 2000 through 2015. *J Clin Endocrinol Metab*. 2019;104(3):721–729.
43. Dream S, Kuo LE, Kuo JH, et al. The American Association of Endocrine Surgeons guidelines for the definitive surgical management of secondary and tertiary renal hyperparathyroidism. *Ann Surg*. 2022;276(3):e141–e176.
44. Casanova D, Sarfati E, De Francisco A, Amado JA, Arias M, Dubost C. Secondary hyperparathyroidism: diagnosis of site of recurrence. *World J Surg*. 1991;15(4):546–549; discussion 549–550.
45. Asare EA, Silva-Figueroa A, Hess KR, et al. Risk of distant metastasis in parathyroid carcinoma and its effect on survival: a retrospective review from a high-volume center. *Ann Surg Oncol*. 2019; 26(11):3593–3599.
46. Silva-Figueroa AM, Hess KR, Williams MD, et al. Prognostic scoring system to risk stratify parathyroid carcinoma. *J Am Coll Surg*. 2017;224(5):980–987.
47. Kouvaraki MA, Lee JE, Shapiro SE, et al. Genotype-phenotype analysis in multiple endocrine neoplasia type 1. *Arch Surg*. 2002;137(6):641–647.

48. Marx SJ, Goltzman D. Evolution of our understanding of the hyperparathyroid syndromes: a historical perspective. *J Bone Miner Res*. 2019;34(1):22–37.
49. Machens A, Dralle H. Multiple endocrine neoplasia type 2 and the RET protooncogene: from bedside to bench to bedside. *Mol Cell Endocrinol*. 2006;247(1–2):34–40.
50. Ito T, Igarashi H, Uehara H, Berna MJ, Jensen RT. Causes of death and prognostic factors in multiple endocrine neoplasia type 1: a prospective study: comparison of 106 MEN1/Zollinger-Ellison syndrome patients with 1613 literature MEN1 patients with or without pancreatic endocrine tumors. *Medicine (Baltimore)*. 2013;92(3):135–181.
51. Doherty GM, Lairmore TC, DeBenedetti MK. Multiple endocrine neoplasia type 1 parathyroid adenoma development over time. *World J Surg*. 2004;28(11):1139–1142.
52. Antwi K, Fani M, Heye T, et al. Comparison of glucagon-like peptide-1 receptor (GLP-1R) PET/CT, SPECT/CT and 3T MRI for the localisation of occult insulinomas: evaluation of diagnostic accuracy in a prospective crossover imaging study. *Eur J Nucl Med Mol Imaging*. 2018;45(13):2318–2327.
53. Wells SA Jr, Pacini F, Robinson BG, Santoro M. Multiple endocrine neoplasia type 2 and familial medullary thyroid carcinoma: an update. *J Clin Endocrinol Metab*. 2013;98(8):3149–3164.
54. Subbiah V, Yang D, Velcheti V, Drilon A, Meric-Bernstam F. State-of-the-art strategies for targeting RET-dependent cancers. *J Clin Oncol*. 2020;38(11):1209–1221.
55. Wells SA Jr, Asa SL, Dralle H, et al. Revised American Thyroid Association guidelines for the management of medullary thyroid carcinoma. *Thyroid*. 2015;25(6):567–610.

74

Adrenal Gland

Barbra S. Miller

Key Points

1 Hormones produced by the adrenal cortex are steroids derived from cholesterol and include glucocorticoids, mineralocorticoids, estrogens, and androgens.

2 The adrenal medulla produces epinephrine, norepinephrine, and dopamine, which are vasoactive synthetic derivatives of the amino acid tyrosine.

3 A consistent, comprehensive approach to evaluation of adrenal abnormalities is required for accurate diagnosis and optimal treatment. Evaluation includes adrenal-specific imaging and biochemical evaluation at a minimum and also may include genetic and/or other evaluation.

4 Biopsy of an adrenal neoplasm is rarely indicated, the need for which should be carefully considered in a multidisciplinary fashion and avoided if adrenocortical cancer or pheochromocytoma are in the differential and biochemical evaluation not yet completed.

5 Adrenal incidentalomas are detected by imaging in 5% to 10% of patients undergoing imaging for unrelated reasons.

6 Treatment of adrenocortical carcinoma requires careful planning and execution to ensure key technical steps are completed. Pre-, intra-, and postoperative care is critical to enabling long-term surveillance and optimal outcomes. Referral to specialized centers and enrollment in clinical trials should be considered.

7 Adrenalectomy for benign disease is most often pursued by minimally invasive means when technically feasible. Open adrenalectomy remains preferred when malignancy of primary adrenal origin cannot be excluded from the list of possible diagnoses.

ANATOMY

The adrenal glands are bilateral, retroperitoneal endocrine organs located adjacent to the superomedial aspect of the superior pole of each kidney. These glands grossly appear as thin, oblong or triangular structures, each weighing approximately 4 g. Each adrenal gland is composed of an outer cortex and an inner medulla. The adrenals are surrounded by retroperitoneal adipose tissue and can be identified by the goldenrod yellow color of the cortex and fine vessels on the surface of the gland. The right adrenal gland is bounded medially by the vena cava, the diaphragm superiorly, adipose tissue laterally, the renal vessels inferiorly, kidney inferolaterally, adipose tissue and musculature posteriorly, and Gerota fascia and the peritoneal lining anteriorly which separates most of the gland from the posterior aspect of the liver. The left adrenal gland is bounded medially by the aorta, the diaphragm superiorly, adipose tissue laterally, the kidney inferiorly, adipose tissue and musculature posteriorly, and the splenic vessels and body and tail of the pancreas anteriorly. Peritoneum separates the laterally placed spleen from the adrenal gland and is usually lateral to the adrenal gland.

Embryologically, the adrenal cortex arises from coelomic mesoderm near the urogenital ridge during the fourth to sixth weeks of gestation. Postnatally, the fetal cortex involutes, leaving only the definitive cortex to differentiate into the three adult zonae: the glomerulosa, fasciculata, and reticularis. The adrenal medulla develops from the neural crest during the fifth gestational week and migrates along paraaortic and paravertebral routes to join the developing cortex. Extra-adrenal neural crest derivatives may be found along the retroperitoneum and at the aortic bifurcation (organ of Zuckerkandl).

The outer zona glomerulosa, located just beneath the thin capsule of the adrenal gland, is the site of mineralocorticoid production. Deep to this, the zona fasciculata, composed of linear arrays of large, foamy cells with lipid inclusions, is the predominant site of glucocorticoid and adrenal sex steroid biosynthesis. The deepest layer, the zona reticularis, is the primary location of synthesis of adrenal androgens. Both the zona fasciculata and zona reticularis respond to stimulation by adrenocorticotropic hormone (ACTH).

Cells of the adrenal medulla are of neural origin (neuroendocrine) and are postganglionic cells of the sympathetic division of the autonomic nervous system. Cells are arranged in homogeneous sheets, with large, irregular, atypical-looking nuclei. The cytoplasm contains numerous secretory granules containing catecholamines, neuron-specific enolase, and chromogranin. Catecholamines originating from tyrosine (dopamine, norepinephrine, epinephrine) in these granules precipitate chromium salts, the basis for the term *chromaffin cells*.

The adrenal glands have an extensive vascular supply derived from small unnamed branches of the inferior phrenic artery superiorly, the aorta medially, and the renal artery inferiorly. Venous outflow is plentiful, with multiple small venules draining the gland in addition to the name adrenal vein. The right adrenal vein is short and empties directly into the inferior vena cava, but can have variable anatomy (emptying into a hepatic vein or being absent). The left adrenal vein either drains inferomedially into the left renal vein or into a communicating vein connecting the phrenic vein to the renal vein (**Fig. 74.1**).

BIOCHEMISTRY AND PHYSIOLOGY

Adrenal Cortex

1 Hormones produced by the adrenal cortex, derived from cholesterol extracted from plasma or synthesized intracellularly, include glucocorticoids, mineralocorticoids, estrogens, and androgens (**Fig. 74.2**).

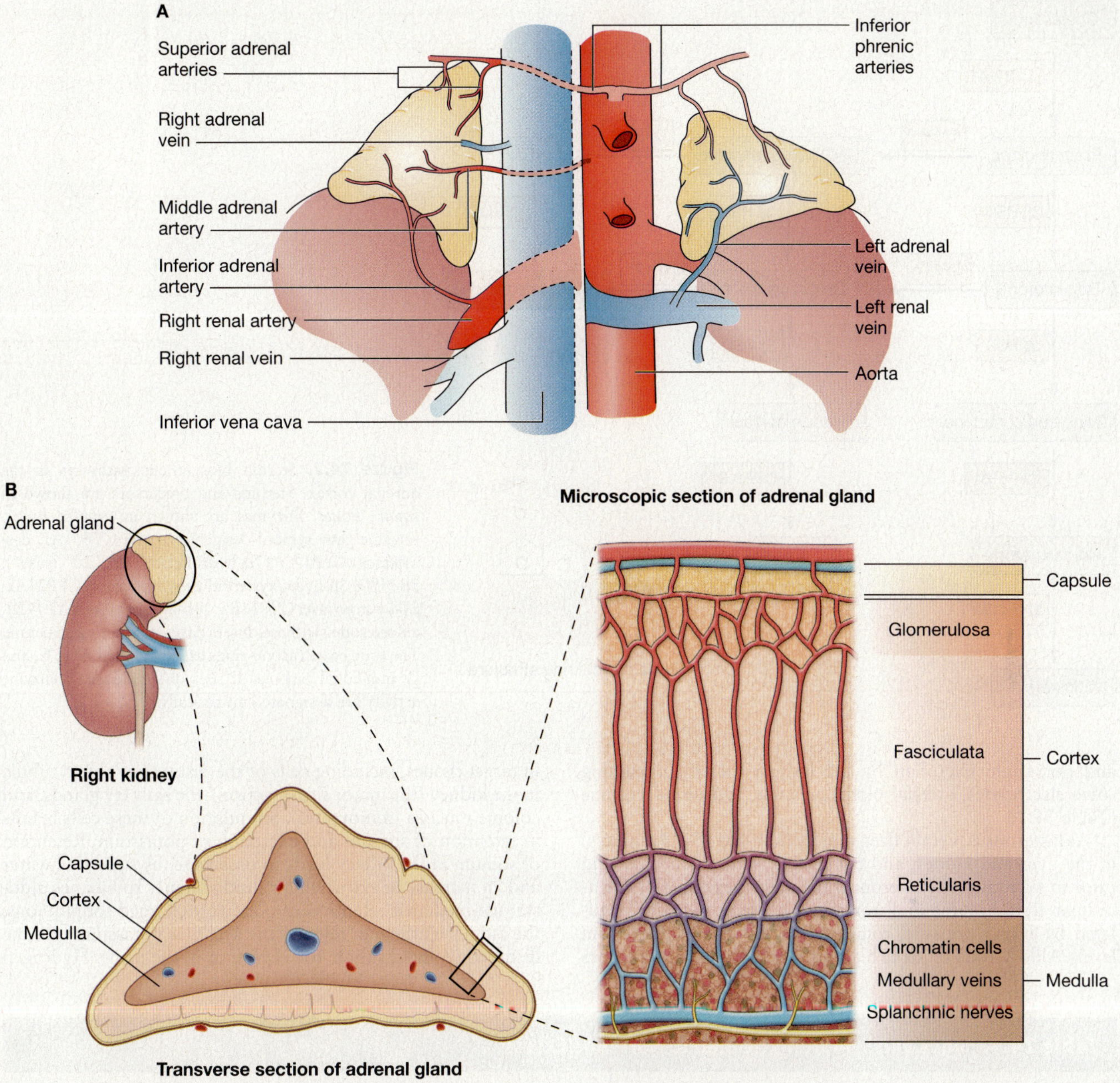

Figure 74.1. **A:** Arterial (*red*) and venous (*blue*) anatomy of the adrenal glands. **B:** Schematic showing the outer adrenal cortex and inner adrenal medulla. Examples for illustration of (**B**) adrenal cortex.

Cortisol

Cortisol is the predominant glucocorticoid in humans. The hypothalamic–pituitary–adrenal (HPA) axis is responsible for tight regulation and control of production and release of cortisol via the hypothalamus, corticotrophs of the anterior pituitary, and cells of the adrenal cortex zonae fasciculata and reticularis. Corticotrophin-releasing hormone (CRH) is secreted by the hypothalamus, and ACTH is produced by corticotrophs of the anterior pituitary. Feedback inhibition controls production.

In circulation, cortisol is bound to transcortin and albumin, with a small percentage of free cortisol available to target tissues. The half-life of cortisol in circulation is ~60 to 90 minutes but can increase dependent on the degree of cortisol excess. Cortisol is metabolized in the liver and eventually excreted in the urine. These urinary metabolites, as well as free cortisol, can be measured in the urine and play a role in differentiating benign from malignant adrenocortical tumors.

Cortisol binds to specific intracellular cytoplasmic receptors, causing translocation of activated receptor–ligand complexes to the nucleus resulting in a wide range of biologic effects such as intermediary metabolism (gluconeogenesis, lipolysis, proteolysis), immunomodulation, and regulation of intravascular volume (**Table 74.1**). Cortisol acts anabolically in vital organs to preserve glucose supply and catabolically in peripheral tissues to mobilize gluconeogenic substrates.

Aldosterone

Aldosterone is the principal mineralocorticoid in humans. Aldosterone secretion by the cells of the zona glomerulosa is regulated by the renin–angiotensin–aldosterone system and stimulated by volume depletion, hypotension, plasma sodium, and posture among other things (**Fig. 74.3**). Juxtaglomerular myoepithelial cells lining afferent arterioles of the kidney sense renal blood flow and pressure, secreting renin in response to decreased perfusion. Renin enzymatically activates angiotensinogen to angiotensin I. Angiotensin I is converted to angiotensin II by angiotensin-converting enzyme in the lung. Angiotensin II has three major effects: (a) arteriolar vasoconstriction; (b) renal sodium retention; and (c) increased aldosterone synthesis, each of which results in sodium retention

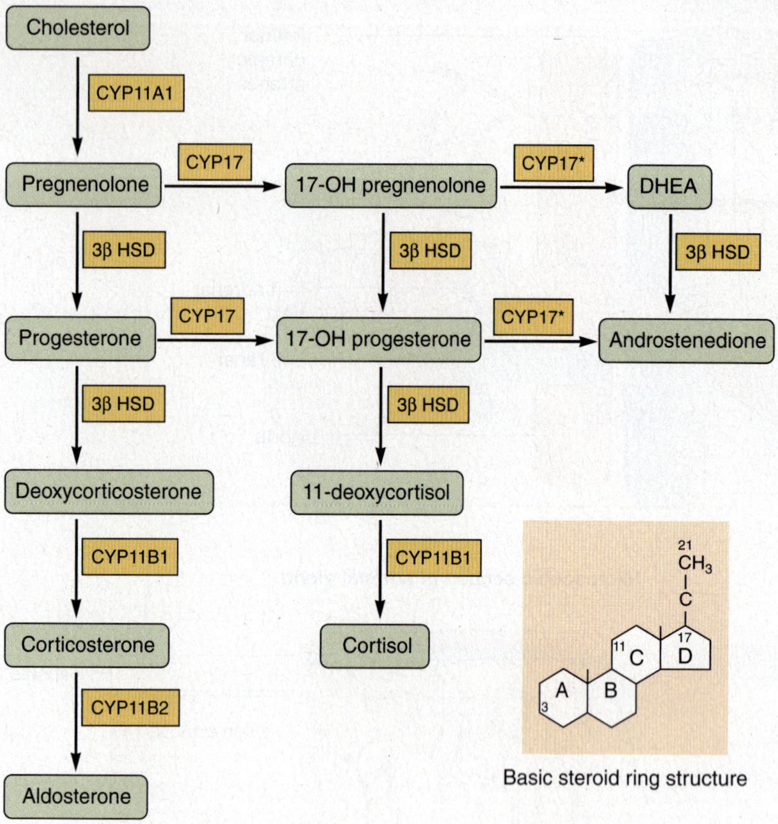

Figure 74.2. Steroid biosynthetic pathways in the adrenal cortex. Steroids and precursors are shown in *square boxes*. Enzymes are shown in *stippled boxes*. Enzyme gene symbol designations are: CYP11A1, desmolase; CYP17, 17α-hydroxylase (±17,20 lyase*); 3β-HSD, 3β-hydroxysteroid dehydrogenase; CYP21A2, 21-hydroxylase; CYP11B1, 11β-hydroxylase; CYP11B2, aldosterone synthase. Inset: Basic steroid ring structure. The four basic carbon rings are designated A, B, C, and D. Individual carbons at sites of steroidogenic enzyme activity are designated numerically.

and potassium excretion by the kidney, thereby impacting some electrolytes, arterial blood pressure, and blood volume (Table 74.1).

Aldosterone is metabolized rapidly (half-life 15–20 minutes) in the liver and kidney, and conjugated with glucuronic acid prior to excretion. Aldosterone is the major regulator of extracellular fluid volume and potassium homeostasis. It is regulated by blood pressure, total body sodium, and potassium levels. Aldosterone binds to high-affinity aldosterone receptors in target tissues, including cells of the distal convoluted tubule in the kidney (the major site of action), the salivary glands, and colonic mucosa (minor sites). Stimulation of these cells results in retention of sodium and excretion of potassium. Retention of sodium in the kidney leads to passive reabsorption of water and an increase in extracellular fluid volume. To balance aldosterone-mediated retention of positively charged sodium ions, the kidney epithelium releases intracellular potassium into the distal convoluted tubule for excretion in the urine. Hydrogen

Table 74.1. Signs and Symptoms Related to Hormone Excess

Hormone	Cortisol	Aldosterone	Sex Hormones	Catecholamines		
Side effect	Muscle wasting, decreased proximal muscle strength Hyperglycemia Peripheral fat loss Truncal obesity Increased lipids Gastric ulcers Pancreatitis Fatigue Hypertension Cardiovascular disease Bone density loss Fractures Infection Striae Bruising Thin skin Easy bleeding Anxiety, depression, suicidal ideation Decreased libido	Hypertension Positive sodium balance Hyporeninemia Hypokalemia Metabolic alkalosis Hyperglycemia Nocturia Polyuria Muscle weakness Edema Weight gain	Androgens: Acanthosis nigricans Acne vulgaris Alopecia Hirsutism Increased libido Insulin resistance Irregular or absent menses Truncal obesity Virilization	Epinephrine and Norepinephrine: β_1 β_2 α_1 α_2	 Chronotropic, inotropic Sweat glands Decreased glucose use Smooth muscle relaxation Smooth muscle contraction Gluconeogenesis Glycogenolysis Suppressed insulin effects Smooth muscle contraction	 Tachycardia Sweating Hyperglycemia Hypotension Hypertension Hyperglycemia Pallor
			Estrogens: Infertility Erectile dysfunction Hypogonadism Feminization Gynecomastia Loss of libido in males Irregular periods in women	Dopamine Atrial fibrillation Congestive heart failure Sudden onset headaches		Lowers blood pressure

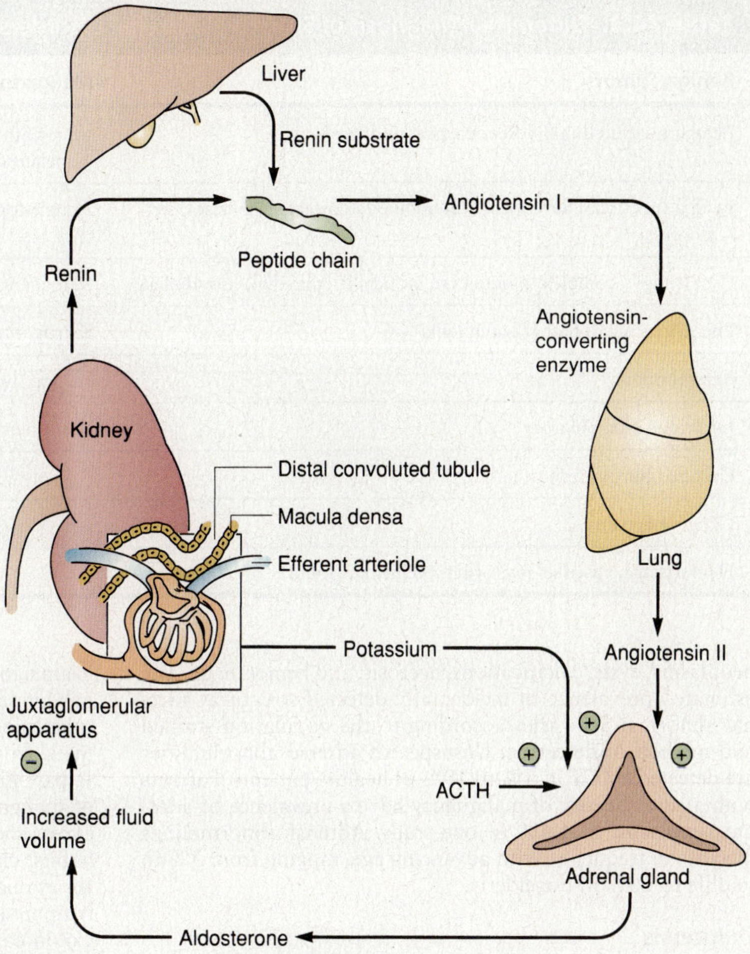

Figure 74.3. Regulatory relationships of renin, angiotensin I and angiotensin II, and aldosterone, sites of production and enzymatic conversions.

ion is also released causing acidification of the urine. In liver failure, metabolism of aldosterone is impaired, leading to elevated aldosterone levels and fluid retention.

Adrenal Androgens and Estrogens

Adrenal C-19 androngenic steroids (dehydroepiandrosterone (DHEA), DHEA-S (sulfated), androstenedione, androstenediol, testosterone, and dihydrotestosterone) are synthesized by cells of the zona reticularis. These steroids promote secondary sexual characteristics in men and virilization in women (**Table 74.1**). Unlike DHEA, DHEA-S is unique to the adrenal gland and important in differentiating hormonal syndromes originating from the gonads versus adrenal glands. Adrenal estrogens include estrone and estradiol which are converted by aromatase from androstenedione and testosterone, respectively.

Adrenal Medulla

2 Catecholamines of the adrenal medulla include epinephrine, norepinephrine, and dopamine. These vasoactive hormones are synthetic derivatives of the amino acid tyrosine. Dopamine leads to the production of epinephrine, which accounts for 80% of stored catecholamines. Tissue expression of the enzyme phenylethanolamine-N-methyltransferase (PNMT) is limited to cells of either the adrenal medulla or organ of Zuckerkandl, located near the aortic bifurcation; thus, most paragangliomas (extra-adrenal catecholamine producing tumors) produce norepinephrine rather than epinephrine.

A complex regulatory network governs synthesis and secretion of catecholamines. Factors that increase catecholamine release include splanchnic nerve stimulation, stress, and glucocorticoids. Glucocorticoids, phospholipids, cyclic adenosine monophosphate, adenosine triphosphate, protein kinase, and magnesium increase the activity of PNMT and decrease catecholamine negative feedback. Catecholamines are stored and secreted from granules within cells of the medulla in association with the matrix protein chromogranin and act on membrane-bound receptors. Chromogranin A is measurable in the blood, and its measurement can play a supporting role in the testing for and surveillance after resection of pheochromocytoma and paraganglioma, along with other functional tumors of neuroendocrine origin. Biologic effects of catecholamines are listed in **Table 74.1**.

3 EVALUATION OF ADRENAL DISORDERS

Evaluation of patients with adrenal disorders has been steadily increasing due to identification of structural abnormalities on imaging studies as well as due to an increased awareness of adverse effects of adrenal hormone excess, both overt and subclinical. Prior to the widespread use of abdominal computed tomography (CT) and magnetic resonance imaging (MRI), identification of adrenal disorders was primarily a result of clinical sequelae due to hormone excess prompting evaluation. Over the past 30 years, most adrenal evaluation has been prompted by incidental findings noted on imaging studies. Evaluation of any adrenal disorder must answer two primary questions: (1) Is the finding benign or malignant, and (2) is there evidence of hormone excess (overt or subclinical)?

Incidentally Discovered Structural Adrenal Abnormalities

Structural adrenal abnormalities identified by imaging are common. Structural abnormalities include hyperplasia, nodules/

Table 74.2. Differential Diagnosis of Structural Adrenal Disorders

Benign Tumors	Malignant Tumors
Benign nonfunctional adrenocortical nodule	Metastatic disease to the adrenal (lung, breast, renal cell, melanoma, lymphoma, colon, liver, esophageal, thyroid, other)
Benign functional adrenocortical nodule (aldosterone, cortisol, sex steroids)	Adrenocortical cancer
Cyst (simple, complex, pseudocyst, bronchial, epithelial, endothelial)	Malignant Pheochromocytoma or paraganglioma
Pheochromocytoma/paraganglioma	Retroperitoneal or inferior vena cava (IVC) sarcoma
Myelolipoma	Primary lymphoma of the adrenal
Infectious/inflammatory	Neuroblastoma
Calcified fibrous tumor	
Ganglioneuroma	
Hemorrhage, vascular malformation, hemangioma	

neoplasms, cysts, calcifications, necrosis, and hemorrhage. The estimated prevalence of incidentally detected structural adrenal abnormalities varies according to the population studied and method of detection. Unsuspected adrenal abnormalities are detected by CT in 5% to 10% of healthy patients. Patients with a prior history of malignancy have a prevalence of adrenal neoplasms in 4.4% in one study. Adrenal abnormalities increase in frequency with advancing age, ranging from 3% in midlife to 10% in the elderly.

Diagnosis

A review of 44 reports describing over 3,000 cases of adrenal incidentalomas reported that 41% were cortical adenomas, 19% were metastases from extra-adrenal malignancies, 10% were adrenocortical carcinomas, 8% were pheochromocytomas, and the remainder myelolipomas, cysts, infectious diseases, and other rare diagnoses. The differential diagnosis must also include extra-adrenal abnormalities, which may be indistinguishable from the thin adrenal (**Table 74.2**).

Each patient should undergo a consistent and comprehensive evaluation, including a thorough history and physical examination. Not all patients with hormone excess or large tumors exhibit signs or symptoms. Infectious diseases (histoplasmosis, tuberculosis, human immunodeficiency virus, etc) and metastases from extra-adrenal malignancies must be considered. A past history of malignancy as well as signs and symptoms of malignancy different from those associated with hormone excess should be elicited (fevers, weight loss, change in bowel habits, change in skin lesions, hematuria, etc) and appropriate evaluation pursued. Breast, lung, melanoma, renal cell, and lymphoma most commonly metastasize to the adrenal glands. Colon cancer metastatic to the adrenal glands is increasingly noted. A thorough family history should be sought. Family history can inform further diagnostic testing as well as the need for consideration of genetic testing (**Table 74.3**).

Biochemical Testing

Assessment of intermediary and end-products of the steroid synthesis pathway is critical to understanding the presence and cause of adrenal hormone excess. Hormones may be used as tumor markers during long-term surveillance in those diagnosed with adrenocortical carcinoma or malignant pheochromocytoma

Table 74.3. Genetic Syndromes

Syndrome	Adrenal Tumor	Gene	Mode of Inheritance
Li-Fraumeni	ACC	*TP53*	Autosomal dominant
Lynch Syndrome	ACC	*MLH1, MH2, MSH6, PMS2*	Autosomal dominant
Familial Adenomatous Polyposis	ACC	*APC*	Autosomal dominant
Beckwith Wiedemann	ACC	Defects on chromosome 11p15.5	Not applicable
Multiple Endocrine Neoplasia Type 2	Pheochromocytoma Paraganglioma	*RET*	Autosomal dominant
Von Hippel Lindau	Pheochromocytoma Paraganglioma	*VHL*	Autosomal dominant
Neurofibromatosis Type 1	Pheochromocytoma Paraganglioma	*NF1*	Autosomal dominant
Succinate Dehydrogenase	Pheochromocytoma Paraganglioma	*SDHx (A, AF2, B, C, D)*	Autosomal dominant
Protein Max	Pheochromocytoma Paraganglioma	*MAX*	Autosomal dominant
Transmembrane Protein 127	Pheochromocytoma Paraganglioma	*TMEM127*	Autosomal dominant

Table 74.4. Diagnostic Evaluation for Evaluation of Incidental Adrenal Mass

Diagnostic Evaluation	Primary	Secondary
Biochemical		
Mineralocorticoids	Metabolic panel, aldosterone, renin	24-h urine sodium, aldosterone, creatinine Saline suppression test, Captopril suppression test Urine steroids
Glucocorticoids	0800 ACTH and cortisol (not random) DHEA-S 1-mg dexamethasone suppression test unless overt signs of Cushing syndrome 24-h urine cortisol and creatinine (if abnormal 1-mg DST and/or overt clinical signs of cortisol excess) to quantify degree of cortisol excess 11-deoxycortisol (indeterminate lesions or known malignancy)	2-d low-dose DST if inadequate 1-mg DST Urine steroids
Sex steroids	17-hydroxyprogesterone Androstenedione Testosterone (in women)	17-beta-estradiol (men and postmenopausal women with indeterminate lesions or known ACC)
Catecholamines	Fractionated plasma metanephrines and normetanephrines And/or 24-h urine catecholamines, metanephrines, normetanephrines	Chromogranin A Clonidine suppression test
Imaging	Adrenal protocol CT or MRI of abdomen and pelvis	Chest CT if adrenal mass is indeterminate or malignant PET CT (FDG, DOTATATE, etc.) Bone or brain imaging if suspected skeletal or brain metastases
Adrenal biopsy	Not recommended in general Must rule out pheochromocytoma prior to biopsy if performed Ideally discuss in multidisciplinary setting prior to proceeding	Mass suspected to be a metastasis from a primary tumor of nonadrenal origin, and no other suitable metastatic site can be biopsied to guide systemic treatment Patients with possible adrenal lymphoma (often bilateral), those unfit for surgery from a medical standpoint, or those with unresectable disease when histopathologic proof is required to inform oncologic management

ACC, adrenocortical cancer; ACTH, adrenocorticotropic hormone; CT, computed tomography; DHEA-S, dehydroepiandrosterone sulfate; DOTATATE, dodecanetetraacetic acid-tyrosine-3-octreotate; DST, dexamethasone suppression test; FDG, 18F-fluoro-2-deoxy-d-glucose.

if functional. Consistent, comprehensive biochemical evaluation should be pursued as opposed to selective assessment of hormones as 25% of patients with functional adrenal tumors have no obvious clinical signs or symptoms. Significant morbidity can occur in those with "subclinical" disease, especially in the case of primary aldosteronism (PA) and mild autonomous cortisol secretion (MACS). Standard biochemical testing for hormone excess is listed in **Table 74.4** should evaluate hormones arising from the zona glomerulosa, fasciculata, and reticularis along with steroid intermediaries, and select labs originating from the pituitary, hypothalamus, other endocrine organs, and select products resulting from hormone stimulation (electrolytes, renin, etc). Intermediaries are most helpful when adrenal nodules or masses are indeterminate by imaging and a primary adrenal malignancy remains part of the differential diagnosis.
4 Biopsy of the adrenal gland is rarely indicated, may lead to needle tract seeding, and pheochromocytoma should be ruled out prior to this to avoid hypertensive crisis. Assessment for inappropriate hormone secretion can be complex as diurnal rhythms, medications, and comorbidities can lead to inaccurate results (**Table 74.5**). In many cases, repeat testing and confirmatory testing is necessary. Close collaboration with an endocrinologist is best; however, surgeons caring for patients with adrenal disorders must have a good understanding of factors impacting evaluation as well to make appropriate decisions. Imaging may also be utilized to inform biochemical testing. On occasion, a clearly benign adenoma with Hounsfield Units <10 may negate the need to test for catecholamine excess. Endocrine Society guidelines are available online and detail the biochemical evaluation and medical management of the various functional adrenal disorders.

5 Adrenal Imaging

Imaging studies usually include cross-sectional imaging in the form of either CT or MRI. CT of the abdomen (± pelvis depending on the situation) utilizing an adrenal-specific protocol is usually the best initial test for identification and characterization of most adrenal masses. Generally, further immediate imaging evaluation to differentiate benign from malignant adrenocortical tumors is unnecessary when an adrenal lesion has an attenuation of less than 10 HUs and is indicative of a benign lipid-rich adrenal adenoma. For those not meeting benign criteria, rapid washout of intravenous contrast suggests a benign process. A contrast washout percentage of >50% to 60% 10- to 15-minutes after contrast bolus is consistent with a lipid poor but still benign adenoma. There is an abundance of literature, including several guidelines, that provide recommendations for additional evaluation and management of indeterminate or obviously malignant adrenal neoplasms. Other imaging modalities may be used in a complementary fashion to differentiate benign from malignant neoplasms which is essential prior to selecting an operative

Table 74.5. Medications and Factors Impacting Biochemical Assessment of Adrenal Function and Their Effects

Cortisol			**Aldosterone**			**Pheochromocytoma**		
Medication/Factor	CBG	Cortisol	Medication/Factor	Aldosterone	Renin	Medication/Factor	NMN	MN
ACTH		++	B-blockers	–	–	Tricyclic Antidepressants (eg, amitriptyline)	+++	
Iatrogenic steroids (oral, injected, topical)			Clonidine, α-methyldopa	–	–	Phenoxybenzamine	+++	
Ketoconazole	–	–	NSAIDs	–	–	Labetalol[a]	+++	
Nephrotic syndrome	–	–	K+-wasting diuretics	nl or +	++	Monoamine oxidase inhibitors	+++	+++
Liver disease	–	–	K+-sparing diuretics	+	++	Sympathomimetics (ephedrine, pseudoephedrine, phenylephrine)	++	++
Malnutrition	+	+	ACE-inhibitors	–	++	Caffeine	+	++
Excessive alcohol		+	Angiotensin-II receptor antagonist	–	++	α-methyldopa	++	
Neuropsychiatric disorder		+	Ca^{2+} blockers (DHPs)	nl or –	+	Levodopa, carbidopa	+	
Chronic kidney disease		+	Renin inhibitors	–	– or +	Cocaine	++	
Multiple sclerosis		+	Hypokalemia	–	nl or +	Acetaminophen, sulfasalazine	++	
Obesity		+	Potassium loading	+	nl or +	Buspirone		+++
Polycystic ovarian disease		+	Sodium-restricted diet	+	++	Amphetamines, ecstasy	+	
Type 2 diabetes		+	Sodium loaded	–	–			
CYP3A4 inducers[c] (phenytoin, phenobarbitone, carbamazepine, rifampin, ethosuximide, pioglitazone, alcohol)		Falsely high after 1-mg DST	Advancing age	–	–			
CYP3A4 inhibitor[d] (Fosprepitant, itraconazole, ritonavir, fluoxetine, diltiazem, cimetidine)		Falsely low after 1-mg DST	Renal impairment	nl	–			
Metyrapone		–	Pseudohypoaldosteronism type 2	nl	–			
Mifepristone		–[b]	Pregnancy	+	++			
Osilodrostat		–	Renovascular HTN	+	++			
Oral estrogens	+							
Mitotane[e]	+	–	Malignant HTN	+	++			
Licorice[f], carbenoxolone[f] (11βHSD2 inhibitor)		+	Sleep apnea	+	–			
Carbamazepine[g]		+	Caffeine		+			
Fenofibrate[g] (LC-MS/MS)		+						
Glucocorticoids[g] (immunoassays)		+						

[a]Biochemical interference.
[b]Mifepristone blocks cortisol receptors, thereby leading to increased cortisol levels without effect. Patients may experience adrenal crisis with elevated cortisol levels when taking this medication. Effects on cortisol may be due to accelerated[c] or impaired[d] metabolism of dexamethasone, increased cortisol-binding globulin falsely elevating cortisol results[e], pharmacologic,[f] or analytical interferences.[g]
+, increase; –, decrease; DHPs, dihydropyridines; nl, normal range; NMN, normetanephrine; MN, metanephrines.

approach. Hemorrhage, evidence of necrosis, and direct invasion of adjacent organs or vasculature, and/or venous tumor thrombus are concerning for malignancy, although hemorrhage and necrosis may both be seen in those with benign conditions. Those with hemorrhage, possibly due to trauma, critical illness, or anticoagulation, should undergo short-interval follow-up scans (3 months) if there are no other reasons for immediate surgery. Others not undergoing surgery should undergo repeat imaging 6 to 12 months afterward to assess for change or growth.

Chemical shift MRI is an alternative and complementary technique to differentiate benign from malignant disease, be suggestive of pheochromocytomas, identify liver metastases in those with adrenocortical cancers (ACC) and malignant pheochromocytoma better than CT, and identify vascular invasion and tumor thrombus more accurately. Malignant masses tend to be bright on T2-weighted images because of higher fluid content. Secondary metastases to the adrenal are hypointense to liver on T1-weighted images and are brighter than liver on T2-weighted images. Metastases also typically show strong contrast enhancement. Pheochromocytomas most often have low lipid content and increased fluid, giving low T1 signal intensities and very bright T2 signal intensities.

Functional Imaging

Imaging of adrenal and other endocrine tumors utilizing radiolabeled materials have increased in the past two decades. 18FDG PET CT can be helpful in situations where malignancy is known or suspected, CT or MRI cannot confirm a benign process, and pheochromocytoma has been biochemically excluded, as well as to evaluate for metastatic disease. Standard uptake value (SUV) ratios of the tumor activity to the liver background and/or blood pool activity may be informative. Not all malignancies reveal increased 18FDG avidity, such as renal cell cancers or malignancies with significant necrosis or fluid. 11C-Metomidate PET is an additional study which may be utilized in differentiating benign from malignant adrenal tumors of cortical origin and in those with PA, although additional study is necessary.

When selecting imaging studies in indeterminate circumstances, it should be remembered that 18FDG PET CT can reveal increased uptake in both pheochromocytoma and malignant adrenocortical tumors. 68-Gallium DOTATATE CT can distinguish between malignant adrenocortical tumors and pheochromocytoma and is the most sensitive of functional imaging studies to identify tumors of neuroendocrine origin, including sites of metastatic disease. However, in some dedifferentiated and more aggressive malignant pheochromocytomas, 18FDG PET CT may be more sensitive in identifying extent of disease.

131-I MIBG can be used to evaluate for pheochromocytoma and also screen patients with pheochromocytoma for high-dose 131-I MIBG therapy. 111-In-pentetreotide scintigraphy may also be useful in identifying those with pheochromocytoma, since many neuroendocrine tumors have the appropriate receptor types (**Table 74.4**).

DISEASES OF THE ADRENAL CORTEX

Functional Disorders

Cortisol Excess

The term *hypercortisolism* refers to the physiologic state of glucocorticoid excess. The most common cause of hypercortisolism is the administration of exogenous steroids as immunosuppressive therapy for inflammatory disorders or after organ transplantation and also includes topical steroids. Endogenous hypercortisolism is caused by increased adrenal production of cortisol. This may be ACTH dependent (pituitary mediated or production of ACTH in an ectopic location leading to excess cortisol production) or ACTH-independent (mediated by abnormal intrinsic function of the adrenal gland). Excess cortisol may or may not lead to outward signs and symptoms (Cushing syndrome) and is dependent on duration of exposure and degree of excess.

Among patients with endogenous Cushing syndrome, 10% to 25% have ACTH-independent disease caused by a primary adrenal disorder. A solitary adrenal adenoma is present in the majority of these patients and often results in atrophy of adjacent and contralateral adrenocortical tissue. Bilateral macronodular adrenal hyperplasia (BMAH) accounts for additional cases of ACTH-independent hypercortisolism and is often due to a mutation in G protein-coupled receptors. Micronodular hyperplasia presents as primary pigmented nodular adrenocortical disease (PPNAD) and isolated micronodular adrenocortical disease (i-MAD). PPNAD is associated with Carney complex, phenotypically represented by endocrine and nonendocrine neoplastic disease. Rarely, other substances from glands outside the adrenal gland or tumors secrete other hormones, activating ACTH and other receptors in the adrenal gland (CRH, LH, HCG), leading to cortisol excess and Cushing syndrome with secondary adrenal hypertrophy.

Mild Autonomous Cortisol Secretion

A growing number of patients with structural disorders of the adrenal glands, as well as ~10% of patients with HTN, DM, and obesity, are found to have evidence of MACS. Formerly referred to as "subclinical" Cushing syndrome (visible features associated with Cushing syndrome are absent), the identification of MACS is rising rapidly. Overt hypercortisolism with elevated 24-hour urine cortisol levels is generally not evident. The diagnosis is most often made by identifying inadequate suppression of a 0800-cortisol level after administration of 1 mg of dexamethasone at 2300 the night prior (1-mg low-dose dexamethasone suppression test [1-mg DST]). While few with MACS go on to develop overt Cushing syndrome, those with MACS have a significantly increased risk of morbidity and mortality. Mortality is most often due to cardiovascular disease.

Presentation and Diagnosis

Clinical features of cortisol excess are listed in **Table 74.1**. The investigation of suspected hypercortisolism should answer two questions: (a) Does the patient have evidence of cortisol dysregulation? (b) What is the cause? Is this due to an abnormality involving the hypothalamus, pituitary, adrenal source, tumor, or other issue? The diagnosis of hypercortisolism is biochemical; however, a careful history and physical examination is also extremely helpful. The Endocrine Society has published excellent guidelines and algorithms for diagnosis of cortisol dysregulation (**Algorithm 74.1**).

Due to the circadian rhythm of the HPA axis, serum cortisol levels can normally vary considerably during a 24-hour period; therefore, a single random cortisol level is not helpful in establishing a diagnosis of hypercortisolism. There are multiple tests to evaluate for hypercortisolism: low-dose (1-mg or 2-day 2-mg) DST, 24-hour urinary-free cortisol excretion, and late night/bedtime salivary cortisol levels. False-positive test results occur in 10% to 15% of cases with the overnight test and can occur for multiple reasons including in those with morbid obesity, chronic alcohol use disorder, those taking estrogens, phenytoin, or other medications, 3rd shift work, and other reasons. Measurement of urinary free cortisol (not metabolites) is an alternative screening test for Cushing syndrome, but is not nearly as sensitive for identifying MACS.

Once the presence of hypercortisolism is established, one must determine if the dysregulation is ACTH dependent (pituitary or ectopic source) or ACTH independent (primary adrenal). Measurement of basal ACTH by radioimmunometric assay is the best test to make this distinction. Suppression of the absolute level of ACTH below 5 pg/mL is nearly diagnostic of an adrenocortical neoplasm. Patients with pituitary neoplasms

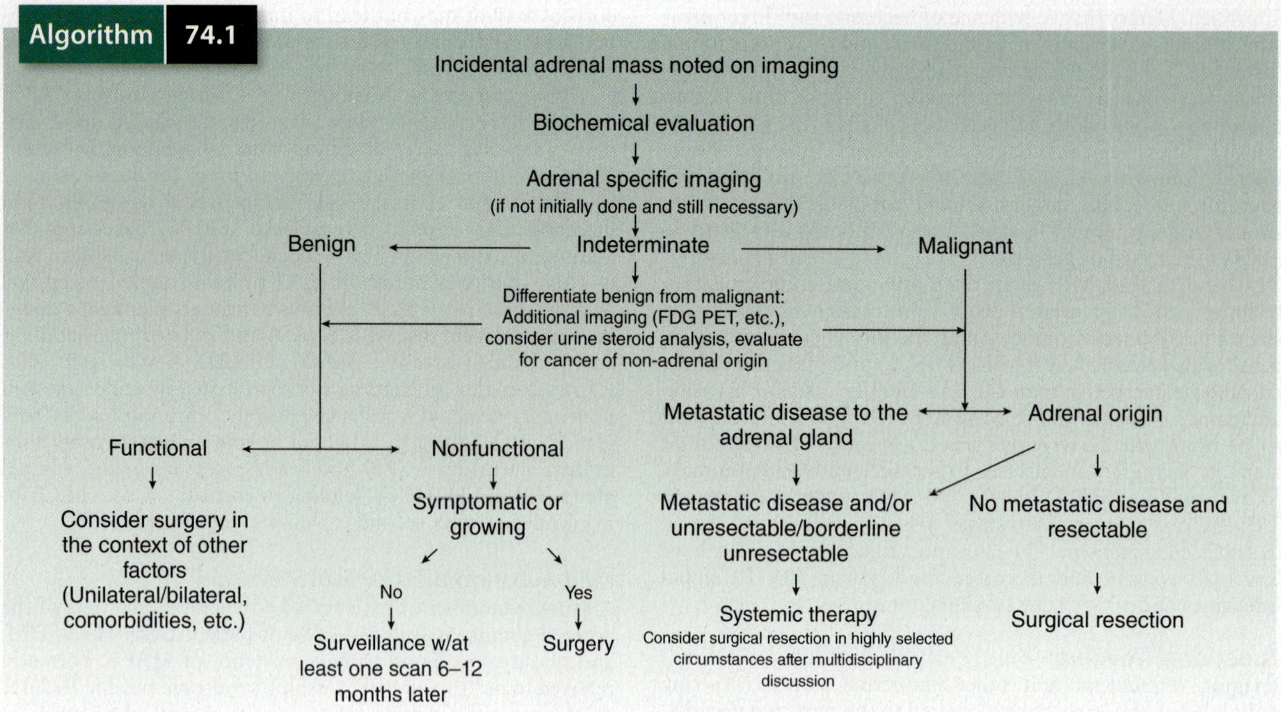

Algorithm 74.1. Evaluation of the incidental adrenal mass. PET, positron emission tomography.

and secondary bilateral adrenocortical hyperplasia have ACTH levels that may range from the upper limits of normal (15 pg/mL) to 500 pg/mL. The highest plasma levels of ACTH (more than 1,000 pg/mL) are in patients with ACTH-producing nonendocrine tumors, such as non–small-cell lung cancer.

Although 80% to 90% of patients with ACTH-dependent Cushing syndrome have Cushing disease, an 8-mg high-dose DST may be required to exclude ectopic ACTH syndrome. Hypercortisolism caused by ACTH-secreting pituitary adenomas is suppressed at least partially by high-dose dexamethasone, whereas hypercortisolism caused by adrenal tumors and ectopic ACTH-producing tumors is not suppressed. About 90% of patients with pituitary source Cushing disease have a 50% reduction in urine-free cortisol.

Biochemical confirmation of cortisol dysregulation is followed by radiologic studies. Pituitary adenomas are best imaged with gadolinium-enhanced MRI of the sella turcica, which has a sensitivity approaching 100%, although small pituitary microadenomas may be missed. Patients with ACTH-independent Cushing syndrome require thin-section CT or MRI of the adrenal, which identifies adrenal abnormalities with more than 95% sensitivity. CT or MRI of the chest may identify a source of ectopic ACTH and should be undertaken in patients with elevated ACTH and hypercortisolism that cannot be suppressed by high-dose dexamethasone. Neuroendocrine tumors may produce ACTH, and 68 Gallium DOTATATE imaging can be particularly helpful, especially to identify small tumors that may not be identified on traditional CT or MRI.

Despite the accuracy of biochemical testing and radiographic localization, inferior petrosal sinus sampling is sometimes necessary to determine the location of the tumor. An inferior petrosal sinus to peripheral plasma ACTH ratio of 2.0 at basal stimulated or of 3.0 after CRH administration is 100% sensitive and specific for pituitary adenoma. Comparison of right and left inferior petrosal sinus ratios may lateralize the adenoma if not visualized on MRI.

Treatment

ACTH-dependent Cushing syndrome is best treated by removing the source of ACTH excess. In the case of Cushing disease, transsphenoidal resection of the pituitary adenoma is successful in 80% or more of cases. If a microadenoma is not found, then hemihypophysectomy may be performed with the understanding that fertility may be impaired. Pituitary irradiation is an option when a tumor is not found or is unresectable, or cure is not achieved by transsphenoidal resection of a tumor. Treatment of ectopic ACTH syndrome involves removal of the primary lesion. Medical control may be achieved with cabergoline. Cortisol excess may be achieved in many with metyrapone or osilodrostat in inoperable cases for both pituitary and ectopic sources of ACTH, or when a tumor cannot be localized. Bilateral adrenalectomy can be considered in patients if cortisol excess cannot be well controlled medically, where severe hypokalemia, hypertension, hyperglycemia, and other sequelae become life threatening.

ACTH-independent Cushing syndrome is best treated by removal of the adrenal neoplasm. Micronodular-pigmented hyperplasia and macronodular adrenal hyperplasia may involve both adrenal glands. If medical treatment cannot control the hypercortisolism, bilateral adrenal venous sampling may detect unilateral dominance allowing for initial unilateral adrenalectomy. Bilateral adrenalectomy can be performed. This results in lifetime dependence on exogenous steroid replacement. All patients who undergo bilateral adrenalectomy should wear a medical alert bracelet warning of adrenal insufficiency and need for steroids.

Data regarding the utility of adrenalectomy in patients with MACS is evolving. Multiple series have demonstrated weight loss, an improvement in hypertension, hyperlipidemia, bone density, and glucose control following adrenalectomy for MACS, but outcomes are highly variable. Adrenalectomy is most often pursued in those with an AM cortisol >5 after 1-mg DST, in younger patients, those with suppressed plasma ACTH, and those with comorbidities attributable to cortisol dysregulation when the AM cortisol is between 3 and 5. For those with an AM cortisol 3 to 5 mg and asymptomatic or those with an AM cortisol 1.8 to 3, observation or involvement in a clinical trial is most often recommended.

Bilateral macronodular hyperplasia appears radiographically as multiple nodules within the adrenal glands. These are nearly always benign, but there theoretically is a chance of malignant transformation. Excess cortisol production, either overt or mild, may occur and is most often due to a mutation leading to constitutive activation of a G protein-coupled receptor. The surgical approach to treatment has usually been removal of the larger gland followed by reassessment of the degree of cortisol dysregulation; however, given that even small amounts of cortisol excess have adverse effects, more aggressive approaches may be taken, sometimes dependent on the amount of cortisol production and clinical sequelae, up to and including bilateral adrenalectomy. There is a growing interest in unilateral adrenalectomy with contralateral partial adrenalectomy and further surveillance over time.

Bilateral micronodular disease of the adrenal gland (nodules <1 cm) is the cause of cortisol excess in 1% to 2% of ACTH-independent cortisol excess. This is due to either isolated micronodular disease (less frequent) or PPNAD. PPNAD may be associated with Carney complex in some cases (spotty skin pigmentation, heart and skin myxomas, various endocrine tumors in addition to PPNAD). The treatment schema is similar to that for nodules in general, as well as BMAH, with bilateral adrenalectomy in those with cortisol excess again being reasonable but considered on an individual basis.

All patients who undergo adrenalectomy for overt Cushing syndrome will require postoperative glucocorticoid replacement since the contralateral gland is suppressed. For those with MACS, a lower, more customized dose may be utilized in many to minimize the time for supplementation. The duration of supplementation varies and is guided by intermittent biochemical assessment and patient symptoms.

Primary Aldosteronism

PA is the result of autonomous aldosterone secretion resulting in suppression of renin, sodium retention leading to volume excess, potassium wasting, and development of hypertension. Significant cardiovascular, renal, and other comorbidities may develop, significantly increasing the risk of morbidity and mortality caused by excess aldosterone. PA is the result of a structural disorder (nonneoplastic cell clusters and neoplasms). Secondary aldosteronism is a physiologic response of the renin–angiotensin–aldosterone system to decreased renal perfusion due to renal artery stenosis, cirrhosis, congestive heart failure, and normal pregnancy. The diagnosis of PA (no longer termed "hyper" as aldosterone levels are normal in some) is usually made between the ages of 30 and 50 years and is an important and increasingly prevalent cause of hypertension. Screening of hypertensive patients with serum aldosterone and plasma renin activity (PRA) or direct renin (DR) has suggested that PA may be the underlying cause of up to 20% of cases of essential hypertension.

PA cases are attributable to adenomas, micronodules, adenomas, hyperplasia, malignancy, or various combinations of each. PA affects men and women equally, although aldosterone-producing adenomas are the cause of PA more often in women and those of Asian and Caucasian descent. Although the cause of either adenoma or idiopathic hyperplasia is not entirely understood, basic science research has elucidated various somatic driver mutations in PA (ie, *KCNJ5*, *CACNA1D*, *ATP1A1*, *ATP2B3*, *CTNNB1*). KCNJ5 is most often responsible for PA driven by a single adenoma. Familial aldosteronism (types I to III) has been described but is rare. Rare causes of PA include adrenocortical carcinoma and ectopic aldosterone-secreting tumors. Autosomal dominant glucocorticoid-suppressible aldosteronism is another rare cause of aldosteronism resulting from the fusion of the ACTH-responsive 11-beta hydroxylase gene promoter to the aldosterone synthase gene in cells of the adrenal cortex.

Presentation and Diagnosis

Clinical manifestations are presented in **Table 74.1**. Aldosterone-mediated retention of sodium and excretion of potassium and hydrogen ions by the kidney causes moderate diastolic hypertension. Significant hypokalemia occurs in less than 40% of patients with PA and is even less frequent in cases caused by adrenal hyperplasia. PA should be suspected in hypertensive patients under age 40, those with blood pressure controlled on four or more medications, in those with uncontrolled hypertension on more than three medications, and those with hypertension and spontaneous hypokalemia at any age.

Demonstration of an elevated plasma aldosterone concentration (PAC) in the setting of suppressed PRA or DR is the classic means to establish a diagnosis of PA. More recently, it has been realized that a suppressed renin is the key to diagnosis. While a PAC of greater than 20 ng/dL and a PAC/PRA ratio of greater than 30 are diagnostic for PA with almost 90% sensitivity, there are issues with utilizing a ratio alone for diagnosis. Below this, repeat testing and confirmatory testing is recommended. Cut-offs for an inappropriate aldosterone level in the setting of a suppressed renin level are going lower and lower and are now at 10 ng/dL if renin is suppressed. It is extremely important to understand if the lab is reporting renin as DR or PRA as DR is 8 to 12 times higher than PRA and may make the PAC/renin ratio falsely low if not recognized. Before biochemical evaluation, patients should be rendered normokalemic. Medications may need to be altered or discontinued as they may affect aldosterone and renin levels. In this situation, it is key to work with the physician managing these medications to make appropriate substitutions and decisions to avoid severe hypertension during this time period (**Table 74.5**).

An elevated PAC/renin ratio alone, unless renin is suppressed and PAC is >20, does not establish the diagnosis of PA. Although there is no optimal confirmatory test or gold standard, there are four confirmatory tests approved to assist in the diagnosis of PA: oral sodium loading, saline infusion test, fludrocortisone suppression test, and captopril challenge.

Once a diagnosis is made, subtyping is important to differentiate unilateral from bilateral excess aldosterone production, as unilateral disease may be treated surgically and bilateral disease is treated medically. After the diagnosis of PA is made, imaging of the adrenal gland is indicated; however, an identified nodule does not mean the excess aldosterone production is coming from it (**Figs. 74.4** and **74.5**). Imaging correlates with the side of production about 50% of the time; therefore, additional testing is indicated in the form of adrenal vein sampling (AVS). Some believe AVS may be avoided in those less than 40 years of age; however, further data is needed to make this a firm recommendation, as excess bilateral aldosterone production has been noted in this population. MRI may be

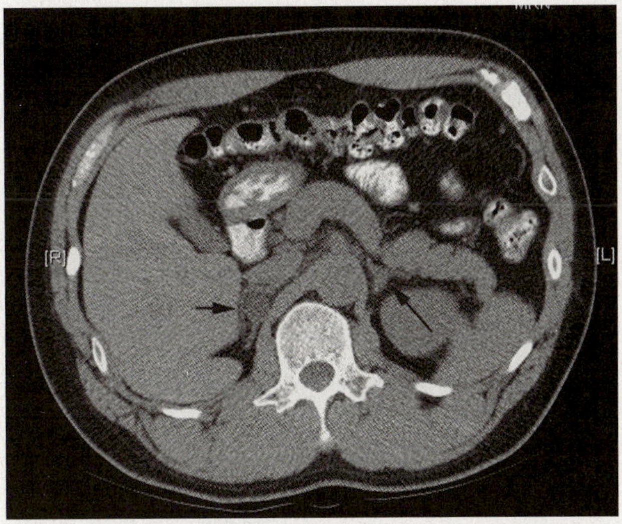

Figure 74.4. Computed tomography scan of right adrenal gland with nodule (*short arrow*). *Long arrow* reveals a morphologically normal contralateral adrenal gland.

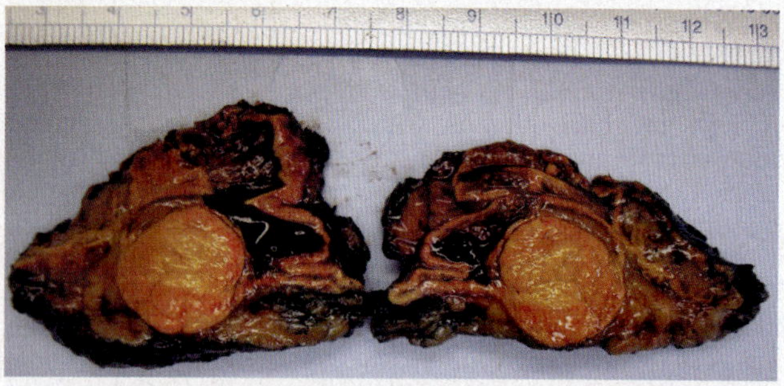

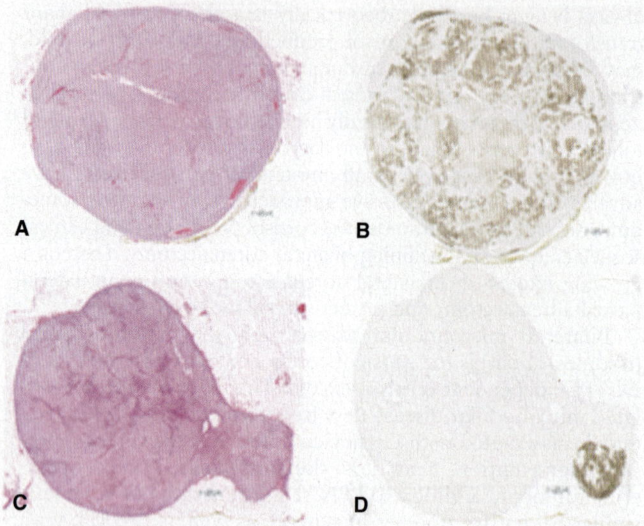

Figure 74.5. **Left:** Aldosterone-producing nodule within right adrenal gland shown in Figure 74.4. **Right:** H&E (**A,C**) and CYP11B2 stains (**B,D**): Evidence of aldosterone production from within an adenoma depicted in **B**. Separate case (**D**) with no aldosterone production (CYP11B2 negative) in larger nodule visible on imaging; however, aldosterone production is evident in small adjacent micronodule.

useful during pregnancy or in situations in which intravenous contrast medium injection is undesirable.

AVS is used to lateralize the source of excess aldosterone production. Percutaneous transfemoral cannulation of both adrenal veins is performed to allow for nearly simultaneous bilateral sampling of blood from the bilateral adrenal veins. Protocols vary between institutions. In general, it is advisable to obtain both pre- and post-ACTH (bolus plus 50 μg/h) stimulation samples. Cannulation of the right adrenal vein can be challenging. Samples from the bilateral adrenal veins and the inferior vena cava (IVC) are sent for aldosterone and cortisol levels. Most important during interpretation is to biochemically confirm catheter placement in the adrenal veins; otherwise, determining lateralization is challenging if not impossible, although strategies exist to help identify features that may be able to differentiate unilateral from bilateral disease.

Treatment

Adrenalectomy guided by AVS results in partial or complete cure of hypertension and hypokalemia in most patients. The Primary Aldosteronism Surgical Outcomes group defines cure according to both clinical and biochemical means. Minimally invasive adrenalectomy is the preferred approach to remove these tumors when benign by imaging. Aldosterone-producing adrenocortical cancers are rare and should be treated by an open approach in most situations. Life-threatening morbidity or mortality following minimally invasive procedures is rare. Postoperatively, antihypertensives, diuretics, and potassium are discontinued, and blood pressure and heart rate are followed expectantly and treated as needed. With publication of the Primary Aldosteronism Surgical Outcomes recommendations, both clinical and biochemical follow-up several times during the first year and annually thereafter is critical to understanding the long-term impact of surgery on PA. Different somatic mutations drive PA and impact surgical outcomes. Staining for aldosterone synthase may be performed by a pathologist to document the source of excess aldosterone production. If aldosterone is produced outside of an adenoma, this may suggest a similar process ongoing in the contralateral adrenal gland, regardless of AVS results.

Medical management of bilateral excess production of PA is currently treated medically with spironolactone or eplerenone. Other medications are being tested in clinical trials. Potassium-sparing diuretics may be used, including triamterene and amiloride. Exogenous administration of physiologic doses of glucocorticoids is the first-line therapy for glucocorticoid-suppressible hyperaldosteronism.

Benign Nonfunctional Adrenal Disorders

Anatomic abnormalities of the adrenal glands, which do not result in excess secretion of hormones, occur on a microscopic and macroscopic level and may be nodular or hyperplastic. In 2022, the World Health Organization revised the categorization of adrenocortical nodular disease to include five discrete entities: sporadic nodular adrenocortical disease, bilateral micronodular adrenocortical disease, bilateral macronodular adrenocortical disease, PPNAD, and I-MAD (**Fig. 74.6**).

Cysts

Whether due to trauma (pseudocyst), spontaneous development (epithelial or endothelial), or another mechanism, pure cysts can resolve over time. Those that progress can become quite large, reaching 15 cm or more. Those with a

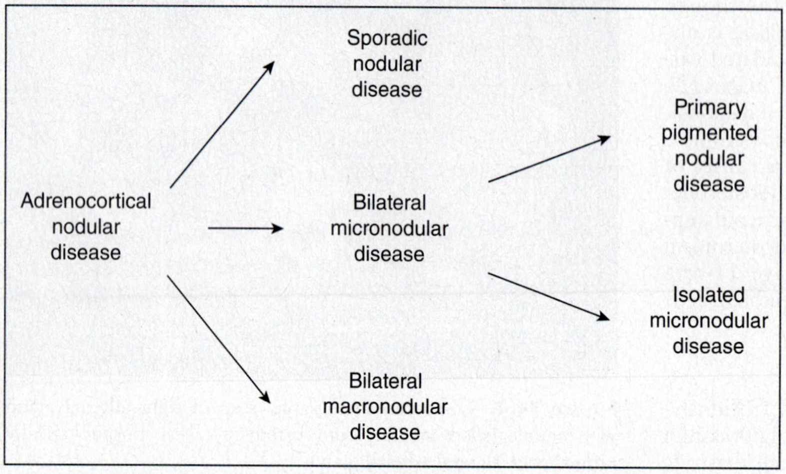

Figure 74.6. HISTALDO classification of adrenocortical nodular disease.

solid component should be treated differently, as a chance for malignancy is present. Differentiating cystic fluid from fluid due to malignancy and necrosis can be difficult. Pheochromocytomas often harbor fluid and are usually "bright" on T2 MRI images. Biochemistry or functional imaging will secure the diagnosis. Cysts with proteinaceous debris may be due to ectopic descended bronchial tissue from the chest. These occur more often on the left. Pure cysts that are small (<4 to 6 cm) and growing can be aspirated and ablated internally with ethanol as an intermediate step prior to submitting a patient to surgery. Success is lower with larger cysts.

Nodules

Benign nonfunctional nodules may be followed over time. At least one follow-up imaging study should be obtained within 6 to 12 months. Current guidelines suggest no further imaging follow-up after documentation of stability in the interim. However, each individual situation should be considered separately, as surgery may be indicated in some patients. Some will recommend future evaluation for those who are young and will live for decades, as the long-term data is not robust, and malignant transformation can occur. No recommendations for the timing of the interval between imaging studies have been made. There is debate about the need for biochemical re-evaluation on a routine basis, with some advocating for annual reassessment for 5 years or if the clinical situation suggests hormone excess. Hyperplastic glands may be treated in the same manner.

Myelolipoma

The overwhelming majority of myelolipomas are benign, nonfunctional tumors. In rare instances, they may secrete hormones, most commonly cortisol. For the most part, myelolipomas do not need to be removed if they are small, biochemically nonfunctional, and do not cause bothersome local symptoms. Extremely rare cases of malignant transformation have occurred. Growth may occur over time, and resection may ultimately be recommended. Should a myelolipoma become symptomatic or a change in operative approach increase operative risk or length of stay (open due to size instead of minimally invasive), resection can be offered.

Congenital Adrenal Hyperplasia

Congenital adrenal hyperplasia (CAH) is a genetic condition caused by a number of different mutations resulting in varying degrees of decreased cortisol, salt-wasting, and hyperandrogenism. The most common cause is due to a deficiency/absence of 21-hydroxylase. 11-beta-hydroxylase may also be affected. There are two classical and one nonclassical subtype. Classic CAH may present as simple virilizing CAH or salt-wasting CAH. These are usually diagnosed in infancy, while patients with nonclassical CAH may be asymptomatic or present with a milder form of virilization later on. Some patients do present as adults. Depending on the severity, glucocorticoids, and mineralocorticoids are often provided. Glucocorticoid administration limits excessive secretion of both CRH and ACTH, thereby minimizing the production of adrenal-derived androgens that otherwise lead to virilization in girls and precocious puberty in boys. Over time, especially in those poorly managed or noncompliant, the adrenal glands become hyperplastic, and some patients can develop myelolipomas. These can become quite large (12 to 15 cm or more), necessitating resection. Growth can be asymmetric, but most often bilateral adrenalectomy is pursued. Since they are usually already prescribed steroids, this is not a reason to avoid bilateral adrenalectomy. The decision for and timing of surgery often depends on the size of the myelolipomas that develop and the surgical approach to be pursued.

Infectious and Granulomatous Disorders

Imaging abnormalities are commonly identified in those with granulomatous disease. Changes are usually bilateral and asymmetric. Findings are nonspecific, including a mass-like appearance, cystic changes, and/or calcification. The adrenal glands can be enlarged or diminutive. Adrenal insufficiency may also result, and morning cortisol and ACTH, as well as an ACTH stimulation test may be pursued if adrenal insufficiency is a concern. In most cases, conservative treatment is all that is required. A follow-up scan may be obtained as per guidelines. Biopsy can identify the responsible organism, but should not be pursued unless malignancy has been ruled out. Often, other sites are available for biopsy. Infection of the adrenals is rare but can be seen as FDG-avid areas in cases of cryptococcus, histoplasmosis, tuberculosis, and candidiasis.

Adrenal Hemorrhage

Hemorrhage involving the adrenal gland may be visualized on imaging studies. Most often, it is due to trauma and resolves without treatment. In most cases, hemorrhage is of no clinical consequence, but in rare cases, adrenal insufficiency, cardiovascular collapse, or even death may result. Other causes may include complications of biopsy or AVS, anticoagulation or other medications, underlying structural issues including malignancy, recent surgery, or shock. Hemorrhage is contained within the adrenal gland but may result in extra-adrenal extension. Conservative management is usually sufficient, along with cessation of any anticoagulation if possible. Interventional radiology procedures may assist if the hemorrhage does not cease spontaneously. Rarely is surgical intervention required as the hematoma is contained within the retroperitoneum. Patients should undergo follow-up imaging within 6 to 12 weeks (unless indicated at a shorter interval) as up to one-third have underlying nodules/masses requiring evaluation.

Adrenal Malignancy

Adrenocortical Carcinoma

6 Adrenocortical carcinoma is a rare malignancy with an estimated incidence of 0.5 to 2 cases per million per year. Presentation peaks in the first and fifth decades of life and is more common in women. The cause of adrenocortical carcinoma is unknown; however somatic mutations in *P53*, *ERCC1*, and *IGF2* have been reported in the pathogenesis of the tumor.

Presentation and Diagnosis

Adrenocortical carcinoma is a very aggressive malignancy, and up to 75% of patients present with locoregionally advanced or distant disease. Syndromes of excess adrenal hormone production are frequent (up to 60%) and may include hypercortisolism, PA, or virilization. Patients with rapidly progressive Cushing syndrome or mixed presentations with signs of both Cushing syndrome and virilization should be suspected of having adrenocortical carcinoma. Nonfunctioning adrenocortical carcinomas present most commonly as abdominal pain or mass with vague symptoms of nausea, weight loss, and fatigue. Patients with suspected adrenocortical carcinoma should have biochemical testing to identify hormone excess (intermediaries and end-products), followed by staging investigations including cross-sectional imaging. Contrast-enhanced CT of the abdomen and chest is important to preoperatively diagnose local tumor invasion and metastatic lesions as well as to confirm a perfused contralateral kidney (**Fig. 74.7**). 18FDG PET CT may also be informative, but is not mandated in current guidelines.

Treatment

Surgical resection is the mainstay of treatment for most stages of adrenocortical carcinoma. Open resection is preferred to promote a margin-negative resection, minimize capsular penetration or tumor spillage, and prevent locoregional recurrence. Critical elements of resection have been described within the Operative Standards for Cancer Surgery developed by the Cancer Research Program and Cancer Surgery Standards Program of the American College of Surgeons

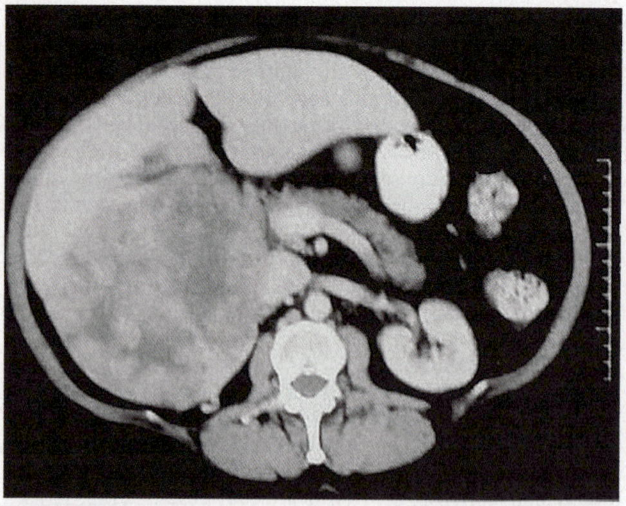

Figure 74.7. Computed tomography scan of right adrenocortical carcinoma showing invasion of liver and inferior vena cava.

(**Table 74.6**). Complete resection of a locally confined tumor is the only chance for cure from adrenocortical carcinoma. However, distant or local spread is evident in 65% of cases at presentation and a minority of patients are resectable with curative intent. Recurrence rates after surgery range from 38% to 85%, depending on stage at presentation. The AJCC system for staging is utilized, and pathology is assessed most often using the Weiss criteria for diagnosis, although other complementary criteria may be utilized. A number of subtypes of ACC exist. The oncocytic subtype has a more favorable prognosis, while the sarcomatoid subtype is associated with a more aggressive course. Other features associated with more aggressive disease and shorter survival beyond staging include high grade, angiolymphatic invasion (micro- or macroscopic), and cortisol excess.

Many patients with adrenocortical carcinoma present with metastatic disease involving the lung, lymph nodes, liver, or bone. Resection or surgical debulking of locally advanced or oligometastatic lesions at diagnosis is rarely pursued over first-line medical therapy (etoposide, doxorubicin, cisplatin [EDP] + mitotane), but in highly selected cases it may provide symptomatic relief for selected patients, especially those with low-grade, slow-growing, hormone producing cancers. Symptomatic locally recurrent or metastatic disease is best treated by resection when feasible and most often when recurrence is noted more than 12 months after initial resection, suggesting the chance for a more durable result before other metastatic disease develops. Overall median survival following diagnosis in those with metastatic disease is approximately 18 months.

Mitotane is the first and remains the only medication specifically approved for ACC. Mitotane was derived from DDT and has both anticortisol and adrenolytic actions. Mitotane is used in an adjuvant manner in patients at high risk of recurrence including those with positive margins or suboptimal tumor resection, penetration of the tumor capsule, Stage 3 disease including invasion of the periadrenal adipose tissue, microvascular or lymphatic invasion, capsular invasion, large vessel invasion or tumor thrombus, histologically high-grade disease (high Ki-67 or mitotic rate). A trial is ongoing to determine the benefit of adjuvant chemotherapy. First-line chemotherapy for those with unresectable or metastatic disease consists of EDP or carboplatin (dependent on renal function) plus mitotane. Streptozocin, tyrosine kinase inhibitors, and immunotherapeutic agents are other options for second-line treatment and beyond. Clinical trials should also be pursued. While initially found not to have much of a role in ACC, data now exists to suggest a beneficial role for adjuvant and palliative radiation therapy in many patients.

DISEASES OF THE ADRENAL MEDULLA

Pheochromocytoma

Pheochromocytomas are functional adrenal tumors that arise from neuroectodermal cells of the adrenal medulla (80% to 85%) or in certain extra-adrenal sites (paraganglioma, 15% to 20%). Paragangliomas will not be discussed further in this chapter. Pheochromocytomas are uncommon, occurring in 1% to 2% of persons, but occur with increased frequency in hypertensive populations and in those with certain heritable endocrine tumor syndromes. The peak incidence of pheochromocytoma occurs during the fourth and fifth decades of life, with men and women affected nearly equally.

Historically, the *rule of tens* was a useful way to characterize pheochromocytomas (10% bilateral, extra adrenal, familial, multicentric, malignant, and occurring in children). Recent advances have revealed that up to 40% of pheochromocytomas are hereditary, and at least 19 susceptibility genes have been identified (**Table 74.3**). Pheochromocytomas due to

Table 74.6. Operative Standards for Adrenal Cancer Surgery: Critical Elements of Resection

Resection of the primary tumor to microscopically negative margins without disruption of the tumor capsule	The primary objective of adrenalectomy is microscopically complete (R0) resection of the primary tumor. The tumor and the surrounding retroperitoneal fat, Gerota fascia, and peritoneum should be resected en bloc.
En bloc resection of adjacent organs directly invaded by cancer	If direct invasion of an adjacent organ or muscle is suspected intraoperatively, the structure(s) should be resected en bloc with the primary adrenal tumor. Creation of an artificial plane between the primary tumor and an invaded structure should not be attempted.
En bloc resection of adjacent blood vessels directly involved by primary tumor and/or tumor thrombus	If direct invasion of the inferior vena cava (IVC), renal vein, or renal artery by adrenal cancer is suspected intraoperatively, the vascular structure(s) should be resected en bloc with the primary adrenal tumor if technically feasible.
Resection of regional lymph nodes involved by metastatic adrenal cancer	If regional lymph nodes are clinically suspected to be involved by metastatic adrenal cancer, a complete, en bloc nodal dissection of the affected lymph node basin(s) should be performed. An extended prophylactic lymphadenectomy is not recommended. If en bloc dissection is not possible, any nodal tissue that is removed separately from the primary specimen should be marked and labeled as a distinct specimen for pathologic analysis. The station(s) of origin of any involved lymph nodes should be specifically noted in the operative and pathology reports.

Derived from Adrenal Cancer. In: Katz MHG, Hunt KK. Veeramachaneni N, et al., eds. *Operative Standards for Cancer Surgery, Volume 3: Sarcoma, Adrenal, Neuroendocrine, Peritoneal Malignancies, Urothelial, Hepatobiliary*. Wolters Kluwer; 2022:73–142.

inherited or de novo mutations have the potential to occur bilaterally, in synchrony or metachrony, usually have an earlier onset, and may manifest as part of a syndrome involving other tumors of different anatomic origin.

The pathologic diagnosis of malignant pheochromocytoma remains a challenge. Histologic features such as growth patterns, mitoses, and atypia of cells and nuclei correlate with malignant biologic features in pheochromocytomas and paragangliomas. However, it is difficult to predict the clinical behavior of individual tumors, and no single risk-stratification scheme is endorsed or in widespread use. In 2022, the WHO published an updated system of classification and risk stratification for pheochromocytoma and paraganglioma. The development or presence of direct invasion of adjacent organs or metastatic disease to lymph nodes or other organs is proof of a malignant pheochromocytoma or paraganglioma. The typical metastatic sites for pheochromocytoma are the lymph nodes, lung, liver, and bones.

Presentation and Diagnosis

Symptoms of pheochromocytoma are attributable to the effects of excessive circulating catecholamines on target tissues (**Table 74.1**); however, the clinical occurrence of symptoms may not always correlate with the active release of catecholamines from the tumor. The classic triad of symptoms in patients with a pheochromocytoma includes episodic headaches, sweating, and intermittent tachycardia. Hypertension is common and sustained in roughly half of patients, is paroxysmal in one-third, and absent in one-fifth. Some patients may be asymptomatic. Rarely, a tumor may be nonfunctional. This is more common with paragangliomas. Sudden death has been reported in patients with pheochromocytoma who have undergone surgical procedures or childbirth. Undiagnosed pheochromocytoma may also lead to spontaneous miscarriage.

Documentation of elevated catecholamines and their metabolites in either urine or blood is essential for the diagnosis of pheochromocytoma. Either a 24-hour urine collection for fractionated catecholamines and their metabolites (metanephrines) or plasma-fractionated metanephrines can be used to make the diagnosis. Urine catecholamines/metanephrines are the most reliable tests with a sensitivity and specificity of 98%. Plasma-fractionated metanephrines are similarly sensitive (99%), but lack specificity (85%). Measurement of plasma catecholamines should not be utilized to diagnose pheochromocytoma or paraganglioma, as levels are reflective of immediate changes in body posture, caffeine, and other stimulating factors. The only reason to send plasma catecholamines is to measure dopamine levels. Dopamine-secreting pheochromocytomas are extremely rare and often do not cause HTN but are associated with a greater risk of malignancy. Measurement of plasma chromogranin A, as with other neuroendocrine tumors, may be complementary to other tests, and can be utilized during surveillance, but is nonspecific, affected by H2 blockers and proton pump inhibitors, and is not diagnostic of a pheochromocytoma or paraganglioma on its own. Other tests exist but are not widely available.

Many medications alter or interfere with measurement of either plasma or urine catecholamines (**Table 74.5**). The decision to discontinue or change medications for the purposes of diagnosis should be done in a multidisciplinary fashion. A clonidine suppression test may be pursued as a provocative test. In some cases of diagnostic dilemma, imaging with DOTATATE-PET allows for the suggestion of a diagnosis of pheochromocytoma without discontinuation of medications to guide clinical decision making.

Biochemical confirmation of the diagnosis should be followed by radiologic evaluation to locate the tumor. Tumor localization can be done using functional or nonfunctional imaging techniques such as CT or MRI. Contrast-enhanced CT readily detects tumors 1 cm and larger and has a sensitivity of 87% to 100% for pheochromocytoma (**Fig. 74.8A**). On adrenal protocol CT, a pheochromocytoma often has attenuation values of >20 HU; however, cases of pheochromocytoma with low HU (<10) have been reported. MRI is similarly sensitive, and a T2-weighted image brightness three times greater than liver is highly specific for pheochromocytoma (**Fig. 74.8B,C**).

While iodine-131-metaiodobenzylguanidine (131-I MIBG), octreotide, and DOTATATE imaging are more specific for pheochromocytoma, these tests are not routinely required during evaluation of sporadic non-malignant appearing pheochromocytoma when supported by biochemical testing.

Treatment

Surgical resection is the only cure for pheochromocytoma. When the diagnosis of pheochromocytoma has been established and localization studies are completed, preoperative preparation of the patient focuses on blood pressure control and volume expansion (**Table 74.7**). Alpha-adrenergic blockade is initiated no later than 1 to 3 weeks before the operation. Phenoxybenzamine, a nonspecific alpha-adrenergic blocking agent, was the primary medication utilized for preoperative blockade for decades. Due to supply chain issues and often excessive cost, selective alpha blockers such as doxazosin and terazosin are more often chosen as first-line agents, increasing every few days until blood pressure reaches an acceptable target to allow ample room for inevitable increases intraoperatively. Along with alpha blockade and the expected ensuing vasodilation, liberal hydration and volume loading are encouraged to minimize orthostatic symptoms. Nasal stuffiness is expected but less common than when using dibenzyline. Some recommend liberalizing salt intake to increase volume. Beta blockers may be added if tachycardia does not resolve with fluid administration. Beta blockade should not be added until after the establishment of alpha blockade, as it can lead to heart failure. Calcium channel blockers (nifedipine and nicardipine) may be used but tend to be less effective. Metyrosine inhibits the enzyme tyrosine hydroxylase and, therefore, catecholamine synthesis, consequently depleting the supply of catecholamines in the tumor. This can be added preoperatively to alpha blockade to potentiate the control of catecholamine excess; however, it is very expensive and takes time to take effect. It should be reserved for those cases where blood pressure is not well controlled with standard therapy. Patients who have very high levels of circulating catecholamines, concern for heart failure, or have had a longstanding history of undiagnosed pheochromocytoma should undergo an echocardiogram to evaluate for catecholamine-induced cardiomyopathy. This is not uncommon and generally improves over time after surgery. Whenever available, anesthesiologists with experience in the perioperative management of pheochromocytomas should be selected for these cases. Multidisciplinary communication is key pre- and intraoperatively. Patients require active hemodynamic monitoring with preinduction arterial line placement for careful monitoring of blood pressure and arterial pH, as well as possibly a central line for vasoactive medication management, instillation of volume, and monitoring of central venous pressures.

Recurrent, malignant pheochromocytoma can include locally advanced disease or metastasis to bone, liver, lymph nodes, lungs, and the central nervous system. Treatment of malignant pheochromocytoma involves resection of metastases when feasible and medical control of hypertension. Radiation therapy may be helpful to ameliorate pain from bony metastases. Ablative therapy with 131-I MIBG or 177Lu-DOTATATE may also produce partial responses and palliation of catecholamine-induced symptoms. Radiofrequency ablation of hepatic and bone metastases can be effective in selected patients. Combination chemotherapy with cyclophosphamide, vincristine, and dacarbazine can also be effective. Overall, 5-year survival for patients with malignant pheochromocytoma ranges from 36% to 60%.

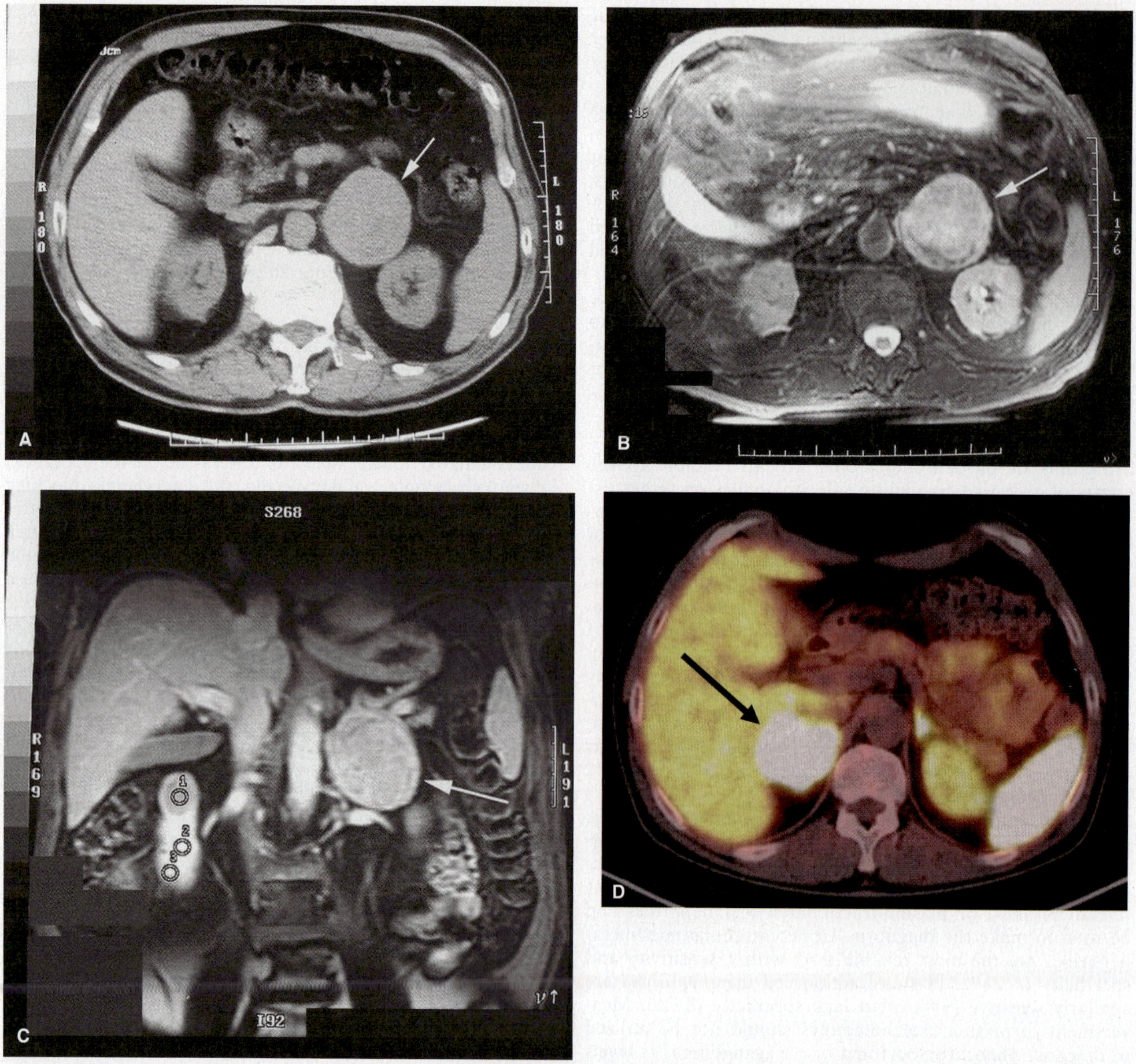

Figure 74.8. Imaging of pheochromocytoma (*arrows*). **A:** Computed tomography scan shows well-circumscribed left adrenal mass. **B:** T2-weighted magnetic resonance imaging shows the mass to be heterogeneously bright, consistent with pheochromocytoma. **C:** ^{131}I-metaiodobenzylguanine (^{131}I-MIBG) and (D) ^{68}Gallium DOTATATE scans with increased uptake in the adrenal gland compared to surrounding structures.

Neuroblastoma and Ganglioneuroma

Neuroblastomas and ganglioneuromas arise from ganglia and the adrenal medulla.

Neuroblastoma

Neuroblastomas arise from neural tissues of the sympathetic nervous system and may be benign or malignant. Neuroblastomas are the most common malignancy found in children (7% to 10% of all pediatric malignancies). It is a rare disease diagnosed in ~650 children annually in the United States, with greater prevalence in females. Most are diagnosed before the age of 5 with a median age of diagnosis of 18 months. Neuroblastoma is the most common malignant extracranial solid tumor of childhood. Sixty-five percent of neuroblastomas arise in the abdomen, with the adrenal medulla being the most common site. Surgical resection is the primary treatment when feasible. Over 50% have metastatic disease at presentation. Subjects may have paraneoplastic phenomena such as secretory diarrhea from vasoactive intestinal peptide. Chromogranin A may be utilized in diagnosis and surveillance.

Ganglioneuroma

Derived from neural crest tissue, ganglioneuromas are rare, most often arising in the retroperitoneal space or posterior mediastinum, although they can also arise in the cervical region. Most are identified incidentally on imaging, some growing to a large size before detection. In a cohort of pediatric and young adults, mean age of diagnosis was 79 months (18 months to 26 years) and ~20% were of adrenal origin. Imaging characteristics of adrenal ganglioneuromas are difficult to differentiate from other tumors of adrenal origin. Some may contain punctate calcifications (20% to 70%). They are typically non-FDG avid due to the low proliferation rate. Few are malignant, and recurrence is rare. Treatment is surgical.

Metastasis to the Adrenal Glands

The adrenal glands are frequent sites for metastases from many cancers. Carcinoma of the lung and breast account for most adrenal metastases; however, virtually any cancer, including melanoma, lymphoma, renal, colon, thyroid, and ovarian

Table 74.7. Medications for Preoperative Management of Patients with Adrenal Disorders

Target Hormone	Medication	Mechanism of Action	Starting Dose	Notes
Cortisol	Metyrapone	Inhibits 11-beta-hydroxylase	250 mg every 4 h; not to exceed 6 g/d	Current first choice for moderate to severe cortisol excess. Monitor cortisol and 11-deoxycortisol levels.
Cortisol	Ketoconazole	Inhibits 11-beta-hydroxylase, 17-hydroxylase, and 17,20-lyase	200 mg daily; goal, 600–800 mg daily	Not terribly effective for moderate to severe HC
Cortisol	Mifepristone	Cortisol receptor blocker	300 mg daily; maximum 1,200 mg daily	Cannot use cortisol level to monitor effect as receptor blockade leads to rise in cortisol. Monitor by symptoms and glucose levels.
Cortisol	Etomidate	Inhibits 11-beta-hydroxylase	0.04 mg/kg/h intravenous	Requires ICU monitoring
Cortisol	Mitotane	Inhibits cholesterol side-chain cleavage enzyme, 11-beta-hydroxylase, 18-hydroxylase, and 3b-hydroxysteroid dehydrogenase	1 g twice daily	Ineffective for moderate to severe cortisol excess; adrenolytic; requires steroid replacement in those without hormone excess; derivative of insecticide DDT
Cortisol	Osilodrostat	Inhibits 11-b-hydroxylase and aldosterone synthase	2 mg twice daily	Monitor cortisol level; titrate slowly.
Aldosterone	Spironolactone	MR antagonist	25 mg daily	Titrate according to renin level (goal >8), creatinine, blood pressure, and potassium.
Aldosterone	Eplerenone	MR antagonist	25 mg twice daily	Double the dose of spironolactone. Less side effects. Titrate according to renin, creatinine, blood pressure, and potassium.
Aldosterone	Amiloride	Potassium-sparing diuretic	5 mg daily	Monitor potassium and creatinine.
Androgens	Spironolactone	Blocks androgen receptor	25 mg daily	Monitor potassium, creatinine, blood pressure, androgen levels.
Estrogens (males)	Anastrozole	Aromatase inhibitor	1 mg daily	Assess thromboembolic risk.
Catecholamines	Phenoxybenzamine	Nonselective alpha-blocker	10 mg 2–3× daily	Titrate every few days to effect, encourage hydration. Longer ½ life better for blood pressure stability and variation in case start time
Catecholamines	Doxazosin (1/2-life 22 h) Terazosin (1/2-life 12 h) Prazosin (1/2-life 2–3 h)	Selective alpha blocker	1–2 mg nightly; 1 mg nightly; 1 mg 2–3× daily	
Catecholamines	Atenolol Propranolol Metoprolol	Beta-blocker	25 mg daily 10–20 mg 3× daily 12.5–25 mg 2× daily	Titrate to effect when volume expansion does not control heart rate adequately
Catecholamines	Nifedipine Nicardipine Amlodipine	Calcium channel blocker	30 mg daily 20 mg 3× daily 5 mg daily	Useful in patients with no or minimal preoperative hypertension or in patients who cannot tolerate alpha-blockade and can be used in combination with other antihypertensives
Catecholamines	Metyrosine	Tyrosine hydroxylase inhibitor	250 mg po qid. Increase by 250–500 mg total daily up to 4 g/d maximum	Delayed onset. Expensive, difficult to obtain. Use in rare circumstances with difficult-to-control hypertension.

carcinoma can spread to the adrenals. Autopsy series of patients with carcinoma show that the adrenal glands are involved in more than 25% of cases. Among cancer patients, 50% to 75% of newly discovered adrenal masses represent metastases. Biopsy of adrenal masses in patients with a history of carcinoma may be performed after completion of standard adrenal evaluation, especially exclusion of pheochromocytoma, but may not always be necessary. Resection of isolated adrenal metastases in select patients can be considered after multidisciplinary discussion, although subsequent extra-adrenal disease may develop. Median survival after complete resection of isolated adrenal metastases from a variety of tumors ranges from 13 to 60 months with actuarial 2- and 5-year survival of 40% and 20%, respectively.

Adrenal Lymphoma

Lymphoma may arise from or metastasize to the adrenal glands, the former being infrequent (1%). Bilateral involvement is most common, although unilateral involvement may occur and often leads to consideration of adrenocortical cancer or other metastatic disease as primary on the list of differential diagnoses. The incidence of secondary adrenal involvement in non-Hodgkin lymphoma (NHL) is 25% to 30%, including autopsies. Adrenal lymphoma is predominantly of large B-cell type. Primary adrenal lymphoma (PAL) is thought to be of hemopoietic origin in a single adrenal gland, which is then attracted to the microenvironment of the contralateral gland. HIV, EBV, immune dysfunction with past or concurrent malignancy, autoimmune disease, and mutations in p53 and c-kit genes are all thought to contribute to the development of PAL. Patients often present with bulky disease, with a mean tumor size of 8 cm in one series. Abdominal or lumbar pain, adrenal insufficiency, or "B" symptoms such as fever, weight loss, and/or night sweats are often noted. Comprehensive adrenal evaluation is pursued and includes LDH, B2 microglobulin, C-reactive protein, ferritin, tumor markers for other malignancies, and adrenal-specific biochemistry. When LDH is elevated, disease is often bilateral. LDH levels greater than twice the upper limit of normal are associated with CNS involvement. Imaging often reveals areas of necrosis and hemorrhage. These tumors are generally 18-FDG avid. Given malignancy is usually suspected, FDG-PET imaging should be pursued as additional sites of disease can be identified in ~80%. Other extranodal sites of disease can include the testicles, pituitary gland, thyroid, and eye. PAL commonly involves the vena cava, renal, and/or splenic vessels. Suspected adrenal lymphoma is one of the few circumstances in which patients benefit from biopsy of the adrenal gland. Core biopsy is preferred to allow for adequate sampling and flow cytometry. Lumbar puncture may be pursued to rule out CNS involvement. First-line therapy for primary adrenal diffuse large B-cell lymphoma is rituximab, cyclophosphamide, doxorubicin, vincristine, and prednisone (R-CHOP) chemotherapy. No survival benefit was observed in patients who underwent adrenalectomy prior to chemotherapy. CNS prophylaxis with intrathecal systemic methotrexate can be offered to patients with concern for CNS involvement. In some cases, adrenalectomy may be pursued when tissue cannot be obtained by image-guided means or there is diagnostic uncertainty after biopsy. Surgery without adjuvant chemotherapy is associated with poor long-term outcomes. The role of radiation therapy is not well defined, but can be considered in some cases. Overall 5-year survival of systemic lymphoma is 64% (73% for regional involvement, and 57% for distant disease). Prognosis of PAL is poor with 3-, 6-, and 12-month survival rates reported as 67%, 46%, and 20%, respectively.

ADRENALECTOMY

Preoperative Preparation

Care of the patient is pursued in a phased manner including preoperative, intraoperative, and postoperative phases. Multiple considerations are taken into account when planning for the successful surgical care of the patient. These considerations include multidisciplinary coordination (both surgical and medical), selection of operative approach and planning, intraoperative surgical and anesthetic conduct, pre- and rehabilitation, nutrition, optimization of comorbidities, and other items (**Table 74.8**). For those with hormone excess, an attempt to control hormone levels, correct electrolyte disturbances, and optimize blood pressure, glucose, etc, should be considered, although the time and effort to pursue this must balance the disease severity, patient condition, and risk of not doing so. A number of medications to assist in curbing excess adrenal hormone production in advance of surgery are listed in **Table 74.7**.

Surgical Approaches

7 The selection of operative approach should be determined in combination with the surgeon's skillset and familiarity with the different approaches, the patient's disease process, and anatomy. Disease considerations may include concern for malignancy, access to bilateral glands, prior surgery, medical

Table 74.8. Preoperative, Intraoperative, and Postoperative Phases of Care

Preoperative Phase	Intraoperative Phase	Postoperative Phase	Postdischarge Phase
Medical control: blood pressure, hormone excess, and glucose	Antibiotics, glucose control, blood pressure control, corticosteroids if indicated	Fluid resuscitation as needed. For large incisions, consider antibiotics for 24 h; glucose; blood pressure; corticosteroids if indicated	Physical or occupational therapy as needed
Nutrition: emphasize protein, control glucose intake	Care in positioning: skin, skeletal, nerves	Nutrition: emphasize protein	Nutrition: emphasize protein
Prehabilitation: core muscles, walking, deep breathing; physical or occupational therapy if necessary	Complete resection, follow Operative Standards for Cancer Surgery if indeterminate by imaging or known cancer.	Early mobilization, physical or occupational therapy if needed	Wean corticosteroids as indicated if unilateral adrenalectomy; ensure corticosteroids and fludrocortisone if bilateral adrenalectomy
Select operative approach	Incision care, Consider Additional mechanisms for fascial closure if cortisol excess, minimize hematoma and fluid collections	Provide information before discharge regarding signs of cortisol withdrawal, Addison disease, how to obtain medical alert bracelet	Wean diabetic and blood pressure medications if able depending on hormone status

comorbidities with limiting cardiopulmonary, hepatic, or renal issues, among others. Anatomic considerations include but are not limited to need for multivisceral resection, vascular bypass, visceral adipose tissue, rib and pelvic structure, gland position in relation to the vena cava, kidney, and renal hilum. Posterior approaches encumber additional considerations compared to anterior or lateral approaches. Surgical approaches to the adrenal glands include open, laparoscopic, retroperitoneoscopic, anterior, flank, posterior, and thoracoabdominal approaches. Minimally invasive approaches may be performed with or without hand assistance or robot assistance.

Regardless of approach, important key surgical principles must be adhered to, regardless of pathology, although this is critically important when treating tumors concerning for or known to be malignant. An open approach remains the preferred approach to malignant primary tumors of the adrenal gland. For benign disorders, unless there are anatomic or other complicating factors, a minimally invasive approach is preferred. Advantages include reduced postoperative pain, earlier resumption of oral intake, shorter hospital stay, earlier resumption of baseline activity, and superior cosmesis. Surgeons should be familiar with multiple approaches, especially open adrenalectomy, as this is the back-up approach if complications arise during minimally invasive adrenalectomy. In some, a conversion from a minimally invasive approach to a hand-assisted approach may be an appropriate intermediate step. A hand-assisted approach also may be advantageous for larger benign tumors when the incision will need to be enlarged for tumor extraction, as morcellation of an adrenal tumor should not be performed. This limits the pathologist's ability to fully assess the tumor and risks unnecessary spillage if adrenal tissue escapes the specimen bag. Various adjuncts which may be helpful to assist in identifying the gland, involvement of adjacent structures, and assessment of remnant perfusion after partial adrenalectomy, and identification of residual malignant tissue or lymph nodes include, but are not limited to, ultrasound, ICG fluorescence, autofluorescence, and radioisotope guidance.

Critical elements of resection of primary adrenal malignancies are listed in **Table 74.6**. Some of these recommendations extend to resection of benign tumors. Specifically, careful handling of the tumor and avoidance of grasping the adrenal itself, as capsular rupture of the tumor (or surface of a hyperplastic gland) can lead to recurrence of benign tumors, especially functional ones. Signs and symptoms of recurrence of hormone and clinical/biochemical sequelae can result, and even more so for those performing partial adrenalectomy, adrenalectomy for pheochromocytoma and for adrenocortical cancer.

Minimally Invasive Adrenalectomy

Laparoscopic Transabdominal Adrenalectomy

Laparoscopic transabdominal adrenalectomy may be done via anterior and lateral approaches. Patients undergo induction of general anesthesia, placement of a urinary catheter and orogastric tube, and are positioned either supine if a purely anterior approach or in a lateral decubitus position if taking a lateral approach. Exposure is facilitated by positioning of a bump and/or flexion of the operating table to enhance the space between the ribs and the iliac crest. Access to the peritoneal cavity is obtained and additional ports placed (3 to 4 on the right or 2 to 3 on the left) (**Fig. 74.9A**). The peritoneal cavity is examined visually. Right adrenalectomy begins with mobilization of the coronary and triangular ligaments of the liver. A retractable endoscopic paddle retractor aiding in mobilizing the entire right hepatic lobe from lateral to medial is particularly helpful to provide exposure of the retroperitoneal organs and vena cava while minimizing trauma to the liver, especially in those with sequelae of excess cortisol. Alternatively, some surgeons choose to retract from posterior to anterior by lifting the right lobe of the liver; however, this provides less than optimal retraction, especially if complications arise. Similarly, on the left, the spleen, pancreas, and stomach are mobilized to the hiatus. Most often, the descending colon must be mobilized to a greater extent on the left to expose the left adrenal gland than on the right, given the need to dissect along the left renal vein. An additional retractor for the spleen and pancreas may always be necessary, depending on the body habitus of the patient. The adrenal vein may be ligated at any time when encountered and convenient. The adrenal vein does not need to be ligated first, and in fact, may be less safe as opposed to dissection carefully leading to the adrenal vein. The plane between the medial kidney and adrenal gland is identified and tissue is divided with cautery or a vessel sealer. Traction and countertraction are key in developing this and other planes, as adipose tissue is divided. Great care is taken inferiorly and medially where the adrenal vein and other small veins and arteries are found. The dissection proceeds in a circumferential direction and is not proscribed. The adrenal vein may be ligated with clips, a vessel sealer, and/or in some difficult situations, an endoscopic stapler. As previously mentioned, a hand port may be placed to assist when needed. This is often placed laterally on the right and medially on the left.

Posterior Retroperitoneoscopic Adrenalectomy

Posterior retroperitoneoscopic adrenalectomy has the advantages of a minimally invasive approach while avoiding the peritoneal cavity, more direct access to the gland (no need to mobilize the liver, spleen, or pancreas), less bleeding, and, in some series, less pain. Given no risk of bowel or omental herniation through the port sites, there are no postoperative lifting restrictions, and the patient may return to normal activities as tolerated. This approach is ideal for patients with prior abdominal surgery or for bilateral adrenalectomy, as both adrenal glands can be removed without repositioning the patient. However, the posterior retroperitoneoscopic approach does not allow for multivisceral resection in the setting of malignancy or adequate access to the peritoneal cavity. It becomes more difficult in patients who have tumors larger than 6 cm and is discouraged if there is any suspicion for malignancy. Those with significant renal insufficiency may experience further worsening of their glomerular filtration rate due to the increased insufflation pressures, although in those with normal function or mild renal insufficiency, this usually resolves within 24 to 48 hours.

Patients are placed in a prone position with the knees and hips positioned at 90-degree angles to the spine and femur. Various devices exist for patients to lie upon, which allow peritoneal contents to shift away from the adrenal gland and kidney. The first port is placed just below the tip of the 12th rib; after the incision is made, the retroperitoneal space is entered in a manner similar to placing a chest tube, and a working space is created bluntly with a finger. This will become the site for the middle trocar. A blunt 5- or 10-mm trocar is placed under digital guidance just medial to the paraspinous muscle and medial to the psoas internally at a 30-degree angle from the initial port. A lateral 5-mm port is placed 4 to 5 cm lateral to the first port in a similar fashion. A blunt balloon trocar is inserted into the site of the initial incision after the other ports are placed. Pneumoretroperitoneum is initiated at 22 mm Hg to create an adequate working space. Traditionally, the videoscope is transferred from the initial middle port to the medial port for the dissection but may be moved during the case as needed. The retroperitoneal space is created bluntly and sharply, working in a medial-to-lateral fashion while pushing the retroperitoneal adipose tissue toward the floor. The lateral aspect of the superior pole of the kidney is identified and Gerota fascia entered using blunt dissection, cautery, or a vessel sealer. The upper pole of the kidney is retracted caudally, and the tissue is released from the superior aspect of the kidney. It is important not to release the tissue superior to the adrenal gland, as this tissue serves as a stabilizing handle to limit migration of the adrenal

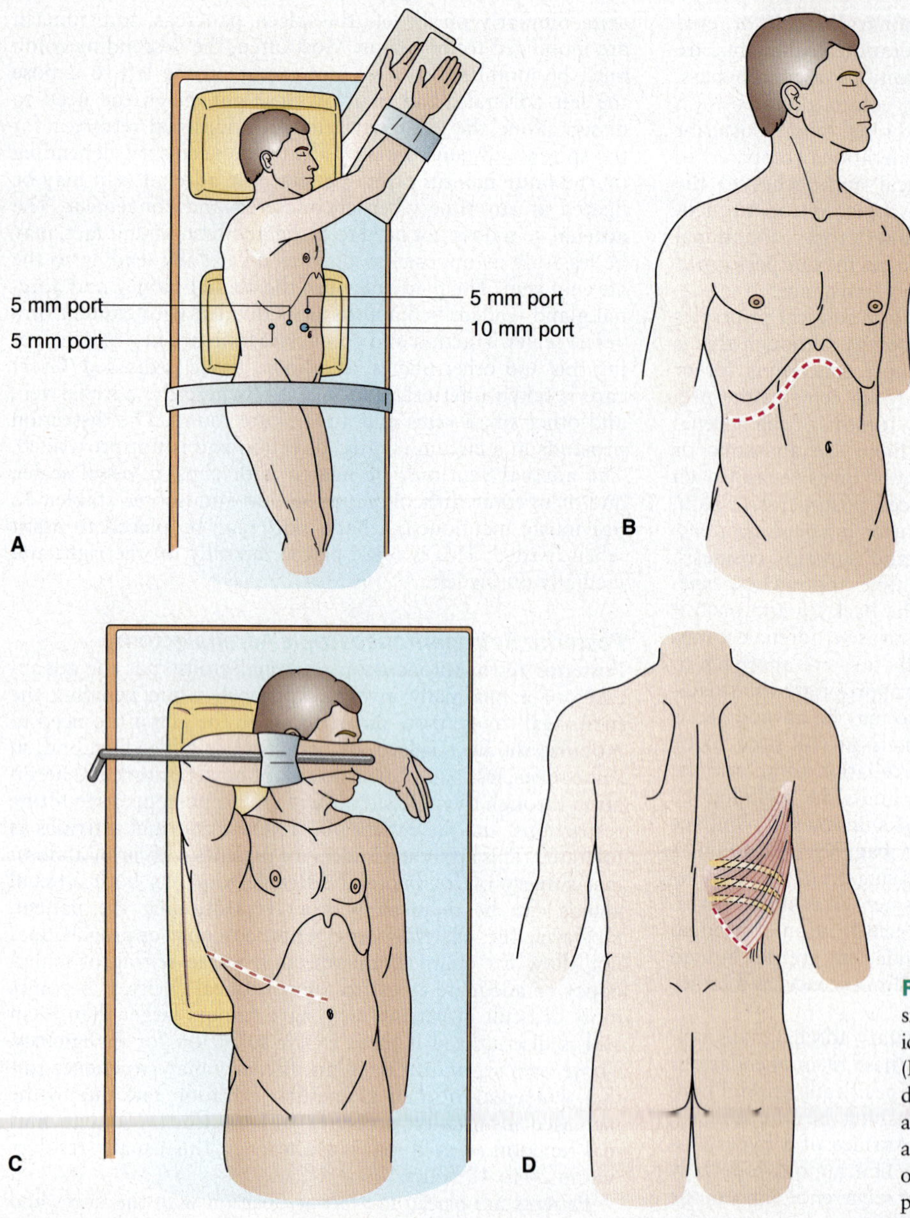

Figure 74.9. Common approaches and incisions for right adrenalectomy. Shown are typical incisions for (A) laparoscopic approach, (B) open anterior approach, (C) thoracoabdominal approach, and (D) open posterior approach. Incisions for left adrenalectomy are positioned opposite. Not shown are other approaches such as posterior retroperitoneoscopic and flank approaches.

gland toward the renal hilum. Thereafter, dissection usually proceeds along the lateral aspect of the adrenal gland, inferiorly, and then medially with ligation and division of the adrenal vein when encountered. Identification of the right adrenal vein is often easier in this approach than with the transabdominal laparoscopic approach, as the vein usually joins the vena cava posteriorly, which then becomes more anterior in a posterior approach. Due to the increased insufflation pressure, the vena cava appears flattened, and the surgeon needs to proceed with caution along the inferomedial and medial aspects of the dissection. Should bleeding be encountered, the insufflation pressure may be raised to 30 mm Hg and then decreased when appropriate. CO_2 levels should be monitored by the anesthesiologist as it can climb, and subcutaneous emphysema is not uncommonly noticed, especially in those with cortisol excess and poor tissue integrity. This resolves on its own and requires no special treatment. Once the gland is completely free, it is placed in an endoscopic specimen bag and removed. The fascia of the initial site of entry (middle port) is usually the only port site necessitating formal closure.

Lateral Retroperitoneoscopic Adrenalectomy

A combination of sorts of several approaches, and the least often utilized approach for adrenalectomy, the patient is placed in a lateral decubitus position. A 10 mm camera port is placed in the mid-axillary line, followed by two 5 mm working ports for additional instruments in the anterior and posterior axillary lines. Since access is obtained less posteriorly than in a posterior retroperitoneoscopic approach, it is important to avoid entering the peritoneal cavity. The upper pole of the kidney is mobilized and separated from the inferolateral aspect of the kidney, and the rest of the dissection performed similarly to that discussed previously. Dissection medially may be more difficult, especially on the right side, since the gland will be resting on medial structures (vena cava and aorta) more than during anterior, posterior, or lateral transabdominal cases. This particular approach has the advantage of permitting a retroperitoneal approach in patients with higher BMIs or tumors of larger size where a posterior retroperitoneoscopic is prohibitive.

Open Adrenalectomy

Anterior Open Approach

Anterior open adrenalectomy begins most often with an ipsilateral subcostal incision (**Fig. 74.9**). Often, this extends across the midline. Other incisions are possible; however, provide less access to the superior aspects of the dissection. The abdomen is opened and explored for evidence of metastatic or

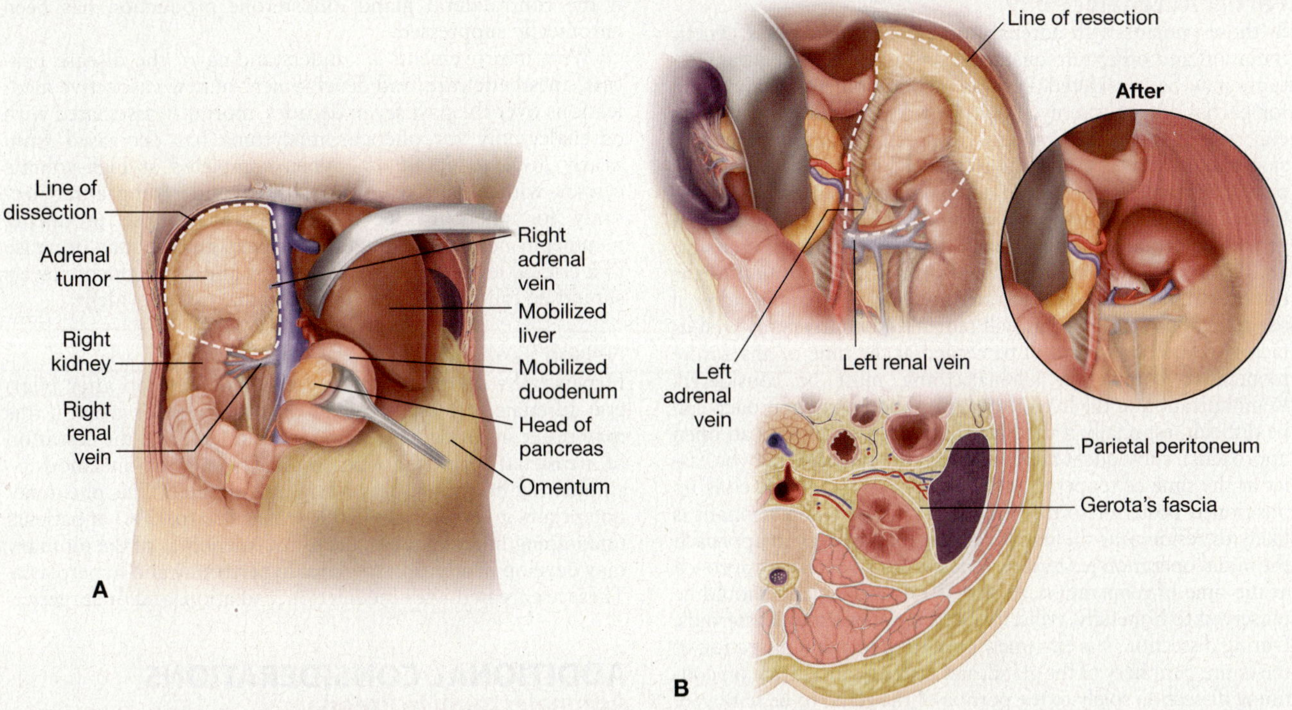

Figure 74.10. Right (A) and left (B) adrenalectomy for malignancy as per the Operative Standards for Adrenal Cancer Surgery. (Illustrations based on Adrenal Cancer. In: Katz MHG, Hunt KK. Veeramachaneni N, et al., eds. Operative Standards for Cancer Surgery, Volume 3: Sarcoma, Adrenal, Neuroendocrine, Peritoneal Malignancies, Urothelial, Hepatobiliary. Wolters Kluwer; 2022:73–142.)

other disease, including biopsy or excision of suspicious extra-adrenal lesions. Resection of the right adrenal gland proceeds with full mobilization and anteromedial retraction of the right hepatic lobe (**Fig. 74.10**). In order to expose the inferior vena cava, the liver, duodenum, and ascending colon/hepatic flexure are mobilized and retracted. A self-retaining retractor system is helpful. Critical elements of resection (**Table 74.6**) when the operation is performed out of concern for adrenocortical cancer necessitate a different approach to adrenalectomy than when done by a minimally invasive approach for benign disease. **Figure 74.10A** demonstrates the correct line of resection and includes maintaining the peritoneal lining over the tumor as the anterior margin if not invaded. It is also important, for the purposes of minimizing locoregional recurrence, correct pathologic evaluation, and survival, to include the surrounding periadrenal adipose tissue en bloc with the specimen, given that microscopic extension of malignant cells into the periadrenal adipose tissue is unrecognizable at the time of surgery in 25%.

Resection of the left adrenal gland is facilitated by mobilization of the spleen, tail of the pancreas, splenic flexure, and descending colon. With retraction medially, the left kidney, aorta, diaphragm, and adrenal are exposed (**Fig. 74.10B**). The left adrenal vein is ligated and divided at its junction with the left renal vein, although other venous tributaries are often encountered inferiorly and medially. The gland and surrounding adipose tissue are dissected out en bloc and vessels ligated and divided as encountered. Dissection should proceed from lateral to medial, and superiorly/inferiorly, where easiest. Any lymph nodes may be removed as they are encountered, but prophylactic lymph node dissection is not required if lymph nodes appear normal. There are few in the area, with most residing posterior to the renal hilum.

Open Posterior Adrenalectomy (Lumbotomy)

The open posterior approach, once a very popular approach, is rarely used anymore but remains useful in select situations, especially in those who have undergone extensive surgery in the upper abdominal quadrants where a minimally invasive approach is not possible. The patient is placed in a prone position on gel rolls under the lower chest and pelvis. A curvilinear or angled incision is made (**Fig. 74.9**) from medial to lateral over the course of the twelfth rib. The twelfth rib is removed as far medially as possible. Handheld retractors are placed medially and superiorly. The retroperitoneum is entered, and the retroperitoneal adipose tissue is swept from superior to inferior and from medial to lateral to locate the adrenal gland and prevent entry into the diaphragm. If entered, the diaphragm may be sutured closed after evacuation of air/fluid at the end of the case. The kidney is identified and retracted inferiorly with one hand while dissection around the adrenal proceeds as previously described. The wound is closed in multiple layers, making sure not to injure the neurovascular bundle of the eleventh and twelfth ribs.

Thoracoabdominal Approach

A thoracoabdominal approach to the adrenal glands is rarely needed except in a situation where access to the chest and abdomen is required in those with extensive invasive or recurrent malignant tumors, or there has been significant prior surgery in the area and an open posterior or posterior retroperitoneoscopic approach is not possible. The patient is positioned supine with the trunk rotated using a gel roll, blankets, or other items, and the abdomen/pelvis flat. The arm is extended cephalad across the chest. An incision is made in the 9th or 10th intercostal space beginning at the posterior axillary line and extended toward the midline of the abdomen (**Fig. 74.10C**). Retractors are placed, and adrenalectomy is performed. Using much the same positioning with the abdomen more rotated instead of the chest, a flank approach may also be utilized. The incision is made between the 11th and 12th rib or over the 11th rib, which can then be resected. A flank incision below the 12th rib is not advised. The incision can be carried to the midline and then taken inferiorly, similar to a thoracoabdominal incision. Reaching the superior extent of the adrenal gland can be a limiting factor, vascular control may be more difficult, and access to the contralateral side is compromised.

Partial Adrenalectomy

In those patients with adrenal tumors resulting from a genetic mutation and other infrequent circumstances, partial adrenalectomy may be considered. Patients who are potential candidates for partial adrenalectomy should be referred to a surgeon with expertise in the disease process, the specific mutation, the decision-making process, and the technical nuances of performing partial adrenalectomy. Partial adrenalectomy is most often performed in patients with pheochromocytomas resulting from a genetic syndrome to preserve cortical tissue for as long as possible and avoid the need for steroid replacement. The position of the tumor within the gland, anticipated amount of remaining adrenal tissue, venous outflow that will remain after surgery, as well as factors related to what will be needed at the time of any future reoperative completion adrenalectomy, must be considered. Remobilization of the liver after a transabdominal approach can be difficult, especially if the first operation was done as an open approach; a subsequent approach from the posterior may be easier at the time of reoperation, especially if the remnant ends up positioned posterior to the vena cava. Similarly, if a remnant is likely to reside near the renal hilum, it may be best to approach the initial operation posteriorly to allow for an anterior approach at the time of reoperation. At least 30% of the gland should be preserved to hopefully avoid the need for supplemental steroids. During dissection, it is extremely important to avoid dissection of the entire periphery of the gland, and instead concentrate on confining dissection solely to the portion of the gland to be removed, thereby avoiding disruption of small vessels providing inflow and outflow to the portion of the gland that will remain.

Considerations for postoperative care of patients undergoing adrenalectomy, regardless of approach, are listed in **Table 74.8** and are approach and disease specific. Most patients undergoing minimally invasive surgery may be discharged on postoperative day 1. Those who do not require close monitoring of electrolytes, blood pressure, or assessment of cortisol production (nonfunctional tumors) may be appropriate for same-day discharge in select circumstances. Those undergoing open approaches are usually discharged 3 to 5 days after surgery.

Complications

Surgeon volume is an important consideration in adrenalectomy, as this has been noted to decrease complications. In a nationally focused study, 82% of surgeons performing adrenalectomy completed an average of one adrenalectomy per year. Inadequate preoperative evaluation and preparation, along with limited procedural knowledge influence complication rates. Overall complications have been reported to reach 20% and vary by approach and disease process being treated. Bleeding and infection are most common. CO_2 embolism may occur with minimally invasive approaches. Cortisol excess and open approach are more often associated with wound site infection; however, this approach may be necessary to impact long-term recurrence and survival, especially for adrenocortical cancer. A longer course of postoperative antibiotics may be reasonable (24 hours vs none). Adrenal insufficiency and need for postoperative steroid supplementation is less a complication and more an expectation in patients operated on for cortisol excess, as the function of the contralateral gland is suppressed. In any patient with evidence of MACS, testing of cortisol secretion from the contralateral adrenal gland and the HPA axis should be pursued the morning after surgery. If the patient has overt Cushing syndrome, testing may be avoided as it is known that all of these patients will need full cortisol replacement for a variable period of time. For those having undergone bilateral adrenalectomy, full steroid replacement is necessary (unless there is metastatic disease with cortisol production), and fludrocortisone is usually necessary to account for mineralocorticoid function. This may be assessed according to sodium (hyponatremia), potassium (hyperkalemia), and blood pressure (relative hypotension). Patients having undergone adrenalectomy for PA may also require fludrocortisone if the contralateral gland aldosterone production has been chronically suppressed.

With improvements in understanding of the disease process, anesthetic care, and development of new vasoactive medications over the past seven decades, mortality associated with adrenalectomy for pheochromocytoma has decreased from nearly 50% to about 1% when completed at high-volume centers with expert teams. For those undergoing adrenalectomy for pheochromocytoma (especially those producing metanephrines over normetanephrines), glucose may decrease to a critical level in the first 24 hours, and serial glucose levels should be followed closely until stabilization is evident.

Nelson Syndrome

Hypertrophy of the pituitary gland may develop after bilateral adrenalectomy. Dependent on the degree of growth, this may result in headaches, vision impairment, and the cessation of menstrual periods in women. ACTH and beta-melanocyte–stimulating hormone (beta-MSH) are elevated. This phenomenon occurs in an estimated 20% (range 0% to 47%) of patients undergoing bilateral adrenalectomy. Adenomas of the pituitary may develop in addition to gland hypertrophy and hyperplasia. These are treated with medication, radiation, and/or surgery.

ADDITIONAL CONSIDERATIONS

Adrenalectomy in Pregnancy

As with other diagnoses necessitating surgery during pregnancy, it is best if adrenalectomy is delayed until after delivery. Should surgery be required, it is best performed during the second trimester. Most commonly, adrenal disorders encountered during pregnancy include pheochromocytoma, Cushing syndrome, and adrenal cortical carcinoma, all of which are extremely rare. For those with Cushing syndrome, the scant amount of literature available suggests adrenalectomy during the second trimester rather than waiting until after delivery. While surgery can be pursued during the second trimester for pregnant patients with pheochromocytoma, it is likely best to wait until the time of delivery or afterward and instead manage the patient with good alpha-, beta-, and/or calcium channel blockade. If surgery is pursued during pregnancy, to maintain adequate placental perfusion pressure, maternal systolic pressure should be maintained at or above 120 mm Hg. Should resection of a pheochromocytoma be pursued during pregnancy, surgical, anesthesia, obstetric, and neonatal teams should work closely together throughout gestation. If gestation is <32 weeks where the fetus will not be delivered, the multidisciplinary team must aggressively treat hypertensive episodes while maintaining placental perfusion pressure. Aggressive volume repletion should be pursued before and during surgery to limit significant hypotension and decreased placental perfusion once the adrenal vein is ligated, along with any other venous outflow. Additional treatment with pressors is warranted if inadequate placental perfusion is questioned. If gestation is >32 weeks, C-section can be performed with adrenalectomy performed immediately afterward. Evaluating and managing patients with indeterminate adrenal masses where adrenocortical cancer is in the differential is complicated. The full spectrum of diagnostic studies is not available, and pregnancy-associated hormones can obscure the biochemical evaluation. The critical elements of resection for surgery of known or suspected adrenocortical cancer remain in place during pregnancy. Should surgery become more urgent during the third trimester, waiting until at least 32 weeks gestation is best to allow for production of fetal pulmonary surfactant and greater maturation of the fetal lungs.

ADRENAL INSUFFICIENCY

Adrenal insufficiency reflects inadequate glucocorticoid and mineralocorticoid production by the adrenals, either secondary to suppression of the HPA axis or by destruction or

Table 74.9. Symptoms and Signs of Acute Adrenal Insufficiency

Symptoms
- Extreme fatigue, lethargy
- Confusion or disorientation
- Nausea and vomiting
- Abdominal pain
- Coma, death

Signs
- Hypotension
- Hyponatremia, hyperkalemia, azotemia
- Hypoglycemia
- Fever
- Anemia

surgical removal of the adrenal glands. The most common causes of primary adrenal insufficiency are autoimmune adrenalitis, infection, and, less commonly, gland replacement with metastatic disease. Chronic exogenous steroid use with HPA suppression and surgical resection of adrenal glands are important causes of secondary adrenal insufficiency. Clinical signs and symptoms usually do not become manifest until at least 90% of the gland is destroyed. Adrenal insufficiency usually occurs gradually unless the patient experiences stress, which may precipitate acute crisis.

Signs and Symptoms

Acute adrenal insufficiency usually manifests as shock in a patient with undiagnosed chronic adrenal insufficiency who has been subjected to physiologic stress. Similarly, patients with established adrenal insufficiency caused by exogenous steroid use may experience crisis if they do not increase glucocorticoid replacement during times of stress or illness. Symptoms of adrenal insufficiency reflect glucocorticoid and mineralocorticoid deficiencies. Signs and symptoms of acute insufficiency include fever, nausea, vomiting, refractory hypotension, and lethargy (**Table 74.9**). Acute adrenal insufficiency is a life-threatening emergency and should be suspected in stressed patients with a history of either adrenal insufficiency or exogenous steroid use. Chronic adrenal insufficiency presents more subtly, with fatigue, weight loss, anorexia, nausea and vomiting, abdominal pain, and diarrhea.

Diagnosis

Laboratory findings of adrenal insufficiency include hyponatremia, hyperkalemia, azotemia, and fasting or reactive hypoglycemia. Hypercalcemia may also be present. The ACTH stimulation test is the best test for investigating both acute and chronic adrenal insufficiency. Synthetic ACTH (250 μg) is administered intravenously, and plasma cortisol levels are measured 30 and 60 minutes later. Normal peak cortisol response should exceed 20 μg/dL. Measurement of ACTH by immunoradiometric assay (IRMA) is then used to distinguish primary from secondary and tertiary adrenal insufficiency. High plasma concentration of ACTH (>200 pg/dL) and low plasma cortisol (<10 mg/dL) are diagnostic of primary adrenal insufficiency. Low levels of plasma ACTH indicate secondary (pituitary) or tertiary (hypothalamic) adrenal insufficiency.

Treatment

Treatment of acute adrenal insufficiency may be necessary based on clinical suspicion prior to biochemical confirmation (trauma, sepsis, or presentation in extremis). Intravenous volume replacement with isotonic fluids and immediate intravenous steroid replacement therapy with 4-mg dexamethasone is essential. An ACTH stimulation test is then performed to establish the diagnosis of adrenal insufficiency after resuscitation and corticosteroid replacement. Hydrocortisone acetate is detected in laboratory measurement for cortisol, so dexamethasone should be used for replacement of glucocorticoid function until ACTH testing is complete. Thereafter, 100 mg of hydrocortisone is administered intravenously every 6 to 8 hours and is tapered to standard replacement doses as the patient's condition stabilizes. Mineralocorticoid replacement is not required until hydrocortisone doses decrease to at least less than 40 to 50 mg daily and oral intake resumes. Chronic adrenal insufficiency often requires both corticosteroid and mineralocorticoid replacement. Usual daily dosing is 12 mg/m^2 of hydrocortisone in divided doses and 0.05- to 0.10-mg fludrocortisone.

Patients who have known adrenal insufficiency or who have received supraphysiologic doses of corticosteroids recently in the period preceding surgery should receive perioperative stress–dose corticosteroids when undergoing major surgery. Administration of 100-mg hydrocortisone intravenously in the morning of major surgery, followed by 100 mg of hydrocortisone every 8 hours during the subsequent 24 hours is usually more than sufficient. Steroids may be rapidly tapered to replacement levels as the patient's condition permits. For those taking low-dose steroids undergoing procedures not expected to have significant stress responses, volume shifts, or blood loss, the patient may simply take their usual morning dose of steroids. Surgeons should take into account that the anesthesia team is often giving 4 to 8 mg of dexamethasone for nausea/vomiting prophylaxis. In certain circumstances, they may be asked to refrain from giving this if patients undergoing surgery for MACS will have a.m. cortisol levels assessed on post-operative day 1, are to receive other stress–dose steroids, or have significant hyperglycemia.

ACKNOWLEDGMENTS

We gratefully acknowledge the contributions of previous edition authors, Hadiza S. Kazaure and Sanziana A. Roman, as portions of that chapter have been retained in this revision.

Suggested Readings and Key References

Del Rivero J, Else T, Hallanger-Johnson J, et al. A review of mitotane in the management of adrenocortical cancer. *Oncologist.* 2024;29(9): 747–760.

Endocrine Society Practice Guidelines: Adrenal. Accessed 12/10/2024. https://www.endocrine.org/clinical-practice-guidelines/adrenal

Fassnacht M, Tsagarakis S, Terzolo M, et al. European Society of Endocrinology clinical practice guidelines on the management of adrenal incidentalomas, in collaboration with the European Network for the Study of Adrenal Tumors. *Eur J Endocrinol.* 2023;189(1):G1–G42.

Fleseriu M, Auchus R, Bancos I, et al. Consensus on diagnosis and management of Cushing's disease: a guideline update. *Lancet Diabetes Endocrinol.* 2021;9(12):847–875.

Katz MHG, Hunt KK, Veeramachaneni N, et al., eds. Adrenal Cancer. In: *Operative Standards for Cancer Surgery, Volume 3: Sarcoma, Adrenal, Neuroendocrine, Peritoneal Malignancies, Urothelial, Hepatobiliary*. Wolters Kluwer; 2022:73–142.

Kazaure HS, Sosa JA. Volume-outcome relationship in adrenal surgery: a review of existing literature. *Best Pract Res Clin Endocrinol Metab.* 2019;33(5):101296.

Lenders JWM, Duh QY, Eisenhofer G, et al. Pheochromocytoma and paraganglioma: an Endocrine Society Clinical Practice guideline. *J Clin Endocrinol Metab.* 2014;99(6):1915–1942.

Mete O, Asa SL, Gill AJ, Kimura N, de Krijger RR, Tischler A. Overview of the 2022 WHO classification of paragangliomas and pheochromocytomas. *Endocr Pathol.* 2022;33(1):90–114.

Mete O, Erickson LA, Juhlin CC, et al. Overview of the 2022 WHO classification of adrenal cortical tumors. *Endocr Pathol.* 2022;33(1): 155–196.

Miller BS, Auchus RJ. The evaluation and management of Cushing syndrome. *JAMA Surg*. 2020;155(12):1152–1159.

Neumann HPH, Young WF Jr, Eng C. Pheochromocytoma and paraganglioma. *N Engl J Med*. 2019;381:552–565.

Nölting S, Bechmann N, Taieb D, et al. Personalized management of pheochromocytoma and paraganglioma. *Endocr Rev*. 2022; 43(2):199–239. Erratum in: *Endocr Rev*. 2022;43(2):440. Erratum in: *Endocr Rev*. 2022;43(2):437–439.

Onuma A, Sun S, Miller BS. Partial adrenalectomy: evaluation and management—a clinical practice review. *Laparosc Surg*. 2023;7:6.

Prete A, Bancos I. Mild autonomous cortisol secretion: pathophysiology, comorbidities and management approaches. *Nat Rev Endocrinol*. 2024;20(8):460–473.

Sweeney AT, Hamidi O, Dogra P, et al. Clinical review: the approach to the evaluation and management of bilateral adrenal masses. *Endocr Pract*. 2024;30(10):987–1002.

Vaidya A, Hundemer GL, Nanba K, Parksook WW, Brown JM. Primary aldosteronism: state-of-the-art review. *Am J Hypertens*. 2022;35(12):967–988.

Williams TA, Lenders JWM, Mulatero P, et al. Outcomes after adrenalectomy for unilateral primary aldosteronism: an international consensus on outcome measures and analysis of remission rates in an international cohort. *Lancet Diabetes Endocrinol*. 2017;5(9):689–699.

Yip L, Duh Q, Wachtel H, et al. American Association of Endocrine Surgeons guidelines for adrenalectomy: executive summary. *JAMA Surg*. 2022;157(10):870–877.

75

Pituitary Surgery

Umberto Tosi, Benjamin I. Rapoport, Georgiana Alina Dobri, and Theodore H. Schwartz

Key Points

1 Clinical manifestations of sellar masses may include local mass effect and pituitary hormone excess or deficiency.

2 Pituitary adenomas account for the vast majority (>90%) of sellar lesions in surgical series, although the differential diagnosis includes a variety of pathologies.

3 Incidental sellar lesions are common findings on cranial imaging.

4 Despite recent advances in genetics and molecular biology, the pathogenesis of most sellar masses remains incompletely understood.

5 Thorough clinical, radiologic, and endocrine testing can help significantly narrow the differential diagnosis before pituitary surgery.

6 The endoscopic endonasal approach is becoming the standard of care in transsphenoidal surgical removal of pituitary adenomas.

7 Medical therapy is available for several types of hormone-secreting pituitary adenomas and is generally considered first-line treatment in patients with prolactin-secreting tumors in whom vision is not deteriorating.

8 Except for many prolactin-secreting pituitary adenomas, transsphenoidal pituitary surgery remains first-line therapy for pituitary adenomas associated with mass effect or hormone excess.

9 Medical therapy has an adjuvant role in patients with conditions caused by other types of secretory adenomas (including acromegaly and Cushing disease) when pituitary surgery is not curative.

10 Management of pituitary adenomas is most effective in a multidisciplinary setting, in which the multiple treatment options available can be individualized to a given patient. Comprehensive care of these patients routinely involves collaboration among endocrinology, ophthalmology, rhinology, and neurosurgery.

The pituitary, as the "master gland," is responsible for the control of much of the body's endocrine function. It affects the function of the thyroid, adrenals, and ovaries or testes, and regulates growth, lactation, and ovulation. Its posterior lobe helps to regulate water homeostasis, contraction during labor, and has recently been implicated with the creation of maternal–
1 neonatal bonding. Surgical disorders of the pituitary can manifest as either endocrinopathy, with syndromes of hormone hypo- or hypersecretion, or as abnormalities caused by mass effect, especially visual field deficits (classically, bitemporal hemianopsia due to compression of the optic chiasm).[1] This chapter will review the anatomy and endocrine physiology of the pituitary gland, as well as the diagnosis, imaging, and pathology of pituitary disorders, and will describe the medical and surgical management of pituitary tumors.

ANATOMY

The pituitary gland lies within the sella turcica, a bony cavity in the posterior part of the sphenoid bone. Anatomic boundaries are formed anteriorly and inferiorly by the sphenoid sinus, posteriorly by the dorsum sella and posterior clinoid processes, anterosuperiorly by the tuberculum sella, and superiorly by the diaphragm sella (a thin dural reflection over the superior margin of the gland) (**Fig. 75.1A,B**). The lateral boundaries are formed by the cavernous sinuses.[2] The gland itself is composed of anterior, intermediate, and posterior lobes (the adenohypophysis, pars intermedia, and neurohypophysis or pars nervosa, respectively). The anterior lobe consists of the pars distalis, the bulbous portion of the gland located within the sella, and the pars tuberalis, the stalk-like segment along the anterior infundibulum, which penetrates the diaphragm sella and connects the gland to the hypothalamus.[3] The vascular supply is formed by the inferior hypophyseal arteries, which arise bilaterally from the intracavernous segments of the carotid arteries and are classically described as supplying the neurohypophysis; and by the superior hypophyseal arteries, which supply the median eminence and infundibulum and also form the capillary network of the hypophyseal–portal system. Numerous bilateral collaterals render this vascular supply redundant. This portal system carries hypothalamic-releasing hormones along the infundibulum to the anterior lobe.[4] Venous drainage exits through the cavernous and superior and inferior petrosal sinuses bilaterally, and thence to the sigmoid sinuses and internal jugular veins. There is often a variably developed dural venous sinus, the circular sinus, usually at the level of the tuberculum sella, connecting the two cavernous sinuses, and there may be dural venous plexi of variable size and location beneath and posterior to the sella.

Several anatomic relationships are particularly important with regard to pathologic effects and surgical approaches. These include the cavernous sinuses, located lateral to the pituitary and containing the cavernous segments of the carotid arteries; and the suprasellar cistern, located superior to the gland and containing the optic nerves and chiasm. The cavernous sinuses are venous channels formed by dural reflections and containing venous drainage from the ophthalmic veins, middle and inferior cerebral veins, and spheno-parietal sinuses. Structures traversing the cavernous sinuses include the intracavernous segment of the carotid artery, as well as

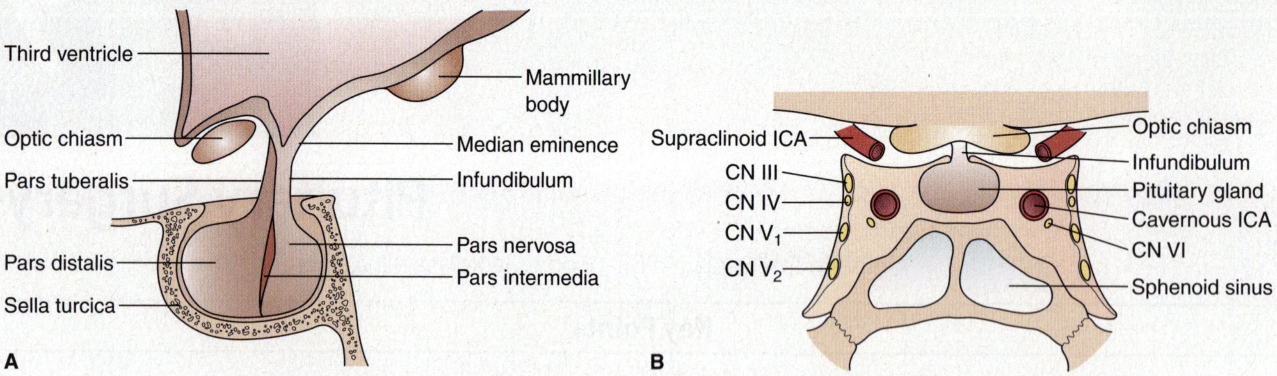

Figure 75.1. Sellar and parasellar anatomy. **A:** Sagittal view. **B:** Coronal view. ICA, internal carotid artery; CN, cranial nerve.

multiple cranial nerves, including cranial nerve III (oculomotor), cranial nerve IV (trochlear), the ophthalmic branch of the trigeminal (V1), and the maxillary branch of the trigeminal (V2). These nerves, from superior to inferior, respectively, travel in the dural reflection that forms the lateral wall of the cavernous sinus. The sixth cranial nerve (abducens) runs along the lateral aspect of the intracavernous carotid artery and is thus more susceptible to injury. Nerves III, IV, VI, and V1 exit into the superior orbital fissure, while V2 exits through the foramen rotundum. The relationship of the cavernous segment of the carotid artery to the cavernous sinus is important to understand; this segment of the artery is surrounded by the venous plexus.[5]

The optic nerves and chiasm are situated above the gland, within the suprasellar cistern. Superior extension of the sellar contents, for example, from a pituitary neoplasm, can compress the chiasm from below, leading to visual abnormalities. Axons from the nasal retinal ganglion cells (which receive input from the ipsilateral temporal visual fields) cross in the chiasm en route to the opposite occipital cortex. Compression of these crossing fibers at the level of the chiasm leads to bitemporal hemianopsia, the pathognomonic neurologic manifestation of a sellar mass.[6]

PATHOLOGY OF SELLAR LESIONS

Pituitary Adenomas

2 Pituitary neuroendocrine tumors (PitNETs), historically referred to as pituitary adenomas, are the most common tumors of the sella and most important surgical pathology of the sellar region, but the differential diagnosis of sellar lesions includes a variety of other pathologic entities (**Tables 75.1 to 75.3**).[7] The true incidence of PitNETs is difficult to determine as estimates differ depending on whether data are obtained from series of clinically significant tumors, autopsy findings, or imaging data. The prev-
3 alence of incidental sellar masses found in imaging studies is about 10% to 22%, while it is about 14% in autopsy series.[8] The original pathologic classification was based upon staining affinity for histologic dyes, that is, acidophilic, basophilic, or chromophobe. A more recent and clinically useful pathologic classification from the WHO is based upon immunocytochemistry of various hormone subtypes and cell of origin.[1] The latest WHO classification of pituitary tumors (2021) includes the use of pituitary transcription factors to further characterize the adenomas and to determine cell of origin.[3,4] Although not readily available in all centers, this new approach has led to diagnosis of more corticotroph, somatotroph, and gonadotroph adenomas and decreased the number of null cell adenomas, formerly called "null" because of weak immunocytochemistry staining. Now, high-risk features include invasion of nearby structures, rapid growth, and high proliferation, as determined by mitosis and Ki-67 staining.[9] The current WHO classification separates adenomas based on lineage; the PIT1-lineage includes somatotrophs, lactotrophs, mammosomatotroph, thyrotrophs, acidophil stem cell tumors, mixed somatotroph and lactotroph tumors, mature plurihormonal, and immature PIT1-lineage tumors. The TPIT-lineage includes corticotroph tumors. The SF1-lineage includes gonadotrophs. Tumors without distinct cell lineage include plurihormonal and null cell tumors.

Table 75.1. Tumors of the Pituitary Gland

Tumors of the Anterior Pituitary
Prolactin-producing adenoma
Growth hormone–producing adenoma
Adrenocorticotropin-producing adenoma
Gonadotropin-producing adenoma
TSH-producing adenoma
Null cell adenoma
Plurihormonal adenoma
Tumors of the Posterior Pituitary
Granular cell tumors
Pituicytoma
Spindle cell oncocytoma of the anterior pituitary
Sellar ependymoma

Modified from Lloyd RV, Osamura RY, Kloppel G, et al. *WHO Classification of Tumours of the Endocrine Organs*. 4th ed. International Agency for Research on Cancer; 2017.

Prolactinomas (Lactotroph Adenomas)

Although less important in surgical series since the advent of dopamine agonist (DA) treatment, these are one of the most common pituitary adenomas with an incidence of 6 to 10 per million per year and a prevalence of 60 to 100 cases per million.[10] Also known as lactotroph adenomas, they arise from the prolactin-secreting cells of the adenohypophysis. They are commonly microadenomas in women, but especially in men may become large and invasive. Galactorrhea is a common presenting symptom.

Growth Hormone–Secreting Adenomas (Somatotroph Adenomas)

These tumors secrete excess levels of growth hormone (GH), leading to gigantism in children and acromegaly in adults. The incidence of acromegaly is about two to four cases per million per year.[11] These tumors may sometimes coexpress prolactin (mammosomatotroph adenomas) and rarely thyroid-stimulating hormone (TSH), as these cellular subtypes appear to arise from a common stem cell origin. They are typically invasive macroadenomas.

ACTH-Secreting Adenomas (Corticotroph Adenomas)

These tumors secrete excess levels of adrenocorticotropic hormone (ACTH), leading to excess production of cortisol by the adrenal glands (Cushing disease). They are uncommon, with

Table 75.2. The 2021 WHO Classification of Pituitary Tumors

PitNET Type	Subtype	Transcription Factor	Hormone
PIT1-lineage PitNETs			
Somatotroph	Densely granulated somatotroph tumor	PIT1	GH, α-subunit
	Sparsely granulated somatotroph tumor	PIT1	GH
Lactotroph	Densely granulated lactotroph tumor	PIT1, ERα	PRL (paranuclear dot-like)
	Sparsely granulated lactotroph tumor		PRL (diffuse cytoplasmic)
Mammosomatotroph		PIT1, ERα	GH (predominant), PRL, α-subunit
Thyrotroph		PIT1, GATA3	α-subunit, βTSH
Mature plurihormonal PIT1-lineage		PIT1, ERα, GATA3	Monomorphic tumor cells with predominant GH expression and variable PRL, βTSH, and α-subunit
Immature PIT1-lineage		PIT1 (ERα, GATA3)	Monomorphic tumor cells with focal/variable staining for no hormones, or one or more of GH, PRL, βTSH, and/or α-subunit
Acidophil stem cell		PIT1, ERα	Monomorphic tumor cells with PRL (predominant) and GH (focal/variable)
Mixed somatotroph and lactotroph		PIT1, ERα	Somatotroph tumor component: GH ± α-subunit depending on tumor subtype; lactotroph tumor component: PRL (diffuse or paranuclear depending on the subtype)
TPIT-lineage PitNETs			
Corticotroph	Densely granulated corticotroph tumor	TPIT	ACTH and other POMC derivates
	Sparsely granulated corticotroph tumor		
	Crooke Cell Tumor		
SF1-lineage PitNETs			
Gonadotroph		SF1, ERα, GATA3	α-subunit, βFSH, βLH, or none
PitNETs with no distinct cell lineage			
Plurihormonal tumor		Multiple combinations	Multiple combinations in a monomorphous tumor population
Null cell tumor		None	None

Modified from Asa SL, Mete O, Perry A, Osamura RY. Overview of the 2022 WHO classification of pituitary tumors. *Endocr Pathol.* 2022;33(1):6–26.

an estimated incidence of 1.2 to 1.7 cases per million per year.[12] Pathologic diagnosis can be difficult, given that these tumors are often quite small and surgical specimens limited. Corticotroph adenomas typically exhibit loss of normal glandular architecture, with positive immunocytochemistry for ACTH.

TSH-Secreting Adenomas (Thyrotroph Adenomas)

These tumors are uncommon and typically comprise less than 1% of surgical series. Patients sometimes present with hyperthyroidism, but TSH staining without clinical hyperthyroidism is a more common scenario.[13]

Gonadotroph Adenomas

These tumors are common and comprise most of the "nonfunctioning" adenomas, as they express primarily hormone subunits, including beta-follicle stimulating hormone (FSH), luteinizing hormone (LH), or alpha subunits. They become symptomatic via mass effect, with compression of normal gland leading to pituitary hypofunction, or compression of the chiasm leading to visual field abnormalities. Very rarely, patients with these tumors may present with symptoms attributed to excess gonadal steroids, such as precocious puberty, irregular menses, or psychiatric manifestations.[14]

Table 75.3. Differential Diagnosis of Nonpituitary Sellar Lesions

Tumors
Craniopharyngioma
Meningioma
Neurohypophyseal gangliocytoma
Neurohypophyseal glioma
Granular cell tumor
Germ cell tumor
Chordomas and other soft tissue and bone tumors
Metastatic tumor
Cysts and malformations
Rathke cleft cyst
Arachnoid cyst
Epidermoid cyst
Dermoid cyst
Vascular Lesions
Saccular aneurysm
Cavernous malformation
Inflammatory Conditions (lymphocytic hypophysitis, granulomatous hypophysitis)
Infiltrative Conditions (sarcoidosis, tuberculosis, Langerhans cell histiocytosis)

Modified from Gejman R, Hedley-Whyte T. Pathology of pituitary adenomas and other sellar masses. In: Swearingen B, Biller BMK, eds. *Diagnosis and Management of Pituitary Disorders*. Humana Press; 2008.

Null Cell Adenomas

These tumors are uncommon; they manifest no clinical or immunocytochemical evidence of hormone secretion, but this may be a function of the sensitivity of the immunocytochemical technique.[15]

"Atypical" Adenomas and Pituitary Carcinomas

Pituitary carcinomas are extraordinarily rare.[16] It is defined by the presence of distant metastases or cerebrospinal fluid (CSF) dissemination. While pituitary carcinomas may demonstrate extensive pleomorphism and/or necrosis, these pathologic findings are also seen in benign adenomas. The factors correlated with aggressive clinical behavior include an elevated Ki-67 labeling index (MIB-1 fraction, proliferation index) and extensive p53 reactivity.[17] The previously used designation "atypical pituitary adenoma" has been abandoned by the current WHO classification system, in favor of "high-risk pituitary adenomas," describing their clinically aggressive behavior. This class includes the sparsely granulated somatotroph adenoma, the lactotroph adenoma in men, the Crooke cell adenoma, the silent corticotroph adenoma, and the newly introduced plurihormonal Pit-1-positive adenoma.[18]

Nonadenomatous Lesions of the Sella

Although pituitary adenomas are the most common neoplasms of the sella, a variety of other lesions can occur (Table 75.3).[19] We review them here briefly, maintaining our focus on lesions of the pituitary gland itself.

Neoplasms

Other neoplasms of the sella are uncommon but remain important in the differential diagnosis. *Craniopharyngiomas* are benign, solid, or partially cystic masses which presumably arise from remnants of Rathke pouch.[20] They occur in a bimodal distribution with peaks in childhood and in older adults. The adamantinomatous type is typical in children, and is often cystic and partially calcified. The cysts contain a "motor oil"–appearing fluid, which can produce severe chemical meningitis when in contact with the CSF. The epithelium produces keratinaceous debris and cholesterol clefts. There is often a pronounced inflammatory reaction. The papillary type is seen almost exclusively in older adults, and is now known to be closely associated with the oncogenic BRAF V600E mutation, and to respond to treatment with BRAF and MEK inhibitors.[21] Papillary craniopharyngiomas may be cystic and/or solid, and can be adherent to surrounding neural structures, especially the optic nerves and hypothalamus. Surgical resection is challenging, recurrence is particularly common in children, and multidisciplinary treatment is essential.[22] *Meningiomas* can arise anywhere along the intracranial dura, including within the sella. Meningiomas arising from the diaphragm sella or tuberculum sella can resemble pituitary adenomas and lead to endocrine dysfunction and chiasm compression.[23] *Germ cell tumors* are most common in children and young adults and occur predominantly in males. The sella is the second most common location after the pineal region, and in many cases germ cell tumors arise concurrently in both locations; the most common subtype is the germinoma followed by teratomas.[24] *Metastases* to the sella are rare.[25]

Cysts

A variety of nonneoplastic cysts can arise within the sella. Although most are incidental findings seen on routine magnetic resonance imaging (MRI), large cysts can sometimes lead to endocrine dysfunction or chiasm compression. The most common cystic structure is *Rathke cleft cyst,* arising from a remnant of Rathke pouch within the pars intermedia. Rathke cleft cysts can enlarge and may require drainage and/or resection. Most, however, are incidental findings, and require no treatment. *Epidermoid* or *dermoid cysts* arise from ectopic squamous or dermoid tissue and can fill with keratinaceous debris. They usually require resection. *Arachnoid cysts* are CSF-containing structures which may also occur within the sella, presumably arising by means of a "one-way valve" mechanism allowing CSF to enter the cyst cavity but not exit; enlarging cysts may become clinically symptomatic. These must be distinguished from Rathke cleft cysts and can be more challenging to treat. In contrast with Rathke cleft cysts, which are self-contained and may be treated with fenestration, fenestration of arachnoid cysts results in a CSF leak that must be repaired at the time of surgery.[26]

Inflammatory Lesions

Inflammatory lesions of the sella are rare. *Lymphocytic hypophysitis,* the most common, is thought to represent an immune-mediated phenomenon. It is sometimes seen in women during or after pregnancy, often in association with autoimmune disorders (Hashimoto thyroiditis, atrophic gastritis). Lymphocytic hypophysitis has also been observed with increasing frequency in patients treated with immunotherapy.[27] The stalk and gland are enlarged and infiltrated with inflammatory cells, and pituitary dysfunction may occur. *Granulomatous hypophysitis* can arise from infections, tuberculosis or fungal, or as idiopathic granulomatous inflammation, either alone or in association with sarcoidosis. Other uncommon types of hypophysitis include xanthomatous, necrotizing, and IgG4 related.

MOLECULAR PATHOGENESIS

4 The molecular pathogenesis of pituitary adenomas remains incompletely understood.[28] The majority of pituitary adenomas are monoclonal in origin, but the relative contributions of intrinsic genetic events and stimulation by hypothalamic hormones and local growth factors remain to be determined.[29] Progression to malignancy with metastasis is rare, although local invasion is common. Genetic mutations predisposing to the development of pituitary adenomas include mutations in the *AIP* gene (aryl hydrocarbon receptor interacting protein) which has been found in some familial pituitary adenoma cohorts as well as some sporadic adenomas, especially in young acromegalic patients. The *MEN1* (multiple endocrine neoplasia) gene is also associated with familial adenomas, but is uncommon in

sporadic disease, as is the *GNAS* mutation associated with McCune Albright syndrome. The *PRKAR1A* gene encodes a type 1A regulatory subunit of protein kinase A. Inactivating mutations of this gene are identified in 60% to 70% of patients with Carney complex, a condition of dominant inheritance, which may lead to acromegaly as a result of somatotroph hyperplasia or adenoma, as well as a variety of extrapituitary manifestations. Epigenetic modification has been suggested as a mechanism to influence gene expression without alteration in the underlying genome. Altered expression of genes encoding CDKN2A (cyclin-dependent kinase inhibitor), DAPK (death-associated protein kinase), FGFR2 (fibroblast growth factor receptor 2), among others, have been associated with sporadic pituitary adenomas. Loss of tumor suppressor genes may also be involved in adenoma pathogenesis. Loss of the *GADD45y* gene expression occurs in the majority of human pituitary adenomas, and products of the *AIP, PRKAR1A,* and *MEN1* genes may also act as tumor suppressors, with loss of these products in familial syndromes predisposing to the development of pituitary adenomas, in a "two-hit" model. Dysregulation of microRNAs, which can regulate translation of target mRNAs, has recently been found in pituitary adenomas, and differential expression can be associated with specific tumor subtypes. It is unclear which, if any, of these abnormalities are primary as opposed to epiphenomena in pituitary tumorigenesis.

ENDOCRINE EVALUATION

5 All patients with a sellar mass greater than 1 cm in diameter require endocrine evaluation for pituitary hypofunction, and patients with possible pituitary adenomas of any size require evaluation for hypersecretory syndromes as well.[30] This is best done in conjunction with an endocrinologist experienced in the management of pituitary disease given the numerous nuances of treatment.

Hypopituitarism

A complete history with questions targeted at change in energy, weight, appetite, thirst, urination as well as irregular menses or sexual dysfunction, along with physical examination and morning blood draw, are very important in diagnosing pituitary hypofunction. The key labs are sodium, free thyroxine (free T4) and 8 AM cortisol, especially in patients requiring surgical treatment, as unrecognized hypothyroidism or hypoadrenalism may have a profound effect on response to anesthesia and complicate recovery from surgery and can also cause hyponatremia. To avoid repeated blood draws one might add TSH, ACTH, estradiol/testosterone, LH, FSH, GH, and insulin-like growth factor 1 (IGF1) to fully characterize the pituitary axes. It is essential to recognize concomitant hypothyroidism and hypocortisolemia, as thyroid replacement may worsen hypocortisolemia by increasing hepatic metabolism of cortisol.

Central (secondary) hypothyroidism is characterized by low free T4 levels in association with inappropriately low or normal TSH. Central hypogonadism is characterized by low morning testosterone levels in men, and low estradiol levels in women, associated with inappropriately low or normal FSH and LH. Central hypoadrenalism is characterized by low morning cortisol levels in association with inappropriately low or normal ACTH. Morning serum cortisol ≤3 mcg/dL is strongly suggestive of adrenal insufficiency (in the absence of corticosteroid or opioid medications), whereas morning serum cortisol ≥18 mcg/dL assures sufficient adrenal function. Intermediate cortisol levels are indeterminate with regard to adrenocortical function and require further evaluation, including stimulation, based on clinical suspicion. GH deficiency diagnosis requires a low IGF1 in the setting of other deficient pituitary axes, or a GH stimulation test, as GH is highly pulsatile and random levels are rarely useful.

Replacement therapy, especially levothyroxine and glucocorticoid (prednisone or hydrocortisone), should be considered as soon as the diagnosis of insufficiency is confirmed, especially in those patients who require surgery. Glucocorticoid replacement should precede thyroid hormone replacement to avoid precipitating adrenal crisis. Posterior pituitary dysfunction, typically diabetes insipidus (DI), is uncommon as a presenting symptom and points away from pituitary adenoma and toward alternative etiologies, such as germ cell tumor, in the differential diagnosis of a sellar mass. DI is characterized by polyuria with polydipsia, dilute urine, and tendency to hyperosmolar dehydration if access to water is limited or thirst is deficient; confirmation may require a water deprivation test in uncertain cases.

Hypersecretory Syndromes

Pituitary adenomas may be associated with excess hormone secretion, giving rise to well-characterized clinical syndromes. It is important to recognize these preoperatively, especially since surgical treatment in some instances is not first-line therapy. In particular, patients with prolactin-secreting pituitary adenomas may be offered a trial of medical therapy, as DAs are effective in controlling tumor size and relieving mass effect.

Excess Prolactin (Prolactinomas)

Excess prolactin leads to the syndrome of amenorrhea and galactorrhea in women, and the syndrome of hypogonadism with sexual dysfunction in men. Mildly elevated prolactin levels may be related to medication effects (eg, dopamine antagonists, psychotropic medications), macroprolactin (an inactive macromolecule, prolactin bound to IgG, with no physiologic effect and requiring no intervention), a microprolactinoma (<1 cm), or "stalk effect" (**Table 75.4**). Prolactin release from

Table 75.4. Causes of Hyperprolactinemia

Physiologic	Pathologic (Pituitary)	Pathologic (Other)
Pregnancy	Prolactin-secreting adenoma	Medications (eg, antipsychotics, antidepressants, metoclopramide, verapamil, opioids, oral contraceptives)
Lactation	Growth hormone and prolactin-cosecreting tumor	Polycystic ovary syndrome
Physical stress	Any sellar mass causing "stalk effect"	Primary hypothyroidism
Sexual intercourse	Empty sella	Renal insufficiency
Nipple or breast stimulation	Hypothalamopituitary irradiation or trauma	Hepatic insufficiency (as in chronic liver disease)
Macroprolactin	Hypothalamopituitary infiltrative conditions (eg, hypophisitis, sarcoidosis, or tuberculosis)	Chest wall lesions

the anterior pituitary is, under normal circumstances, regulated by continuous inhibition; dopamine is continuously needed to inhibit the secretion of prolactin from the lactotrophs. The "stalk effect" occurs when a non–prolactin-secreting mass exerts pressure on the infundibulum and thereby diminishes the amount of dopamine that reaches the anterior pituitary (diminished inhibition), resulting in increased prolactin release. Usually the serum prolactin level associated with "stalk effect" is less than 150 ng/mL, and this must be distinguished from a prolactinoma, as the treatments are potentially different.[31] A large tumor in the setting of a mildly elevated prolactin level likely represents "stalk effect" rather than a true prolactinoma; a mildly elevated prolactin level in the setting of a microadenoma likely represents a true microprolactinoma.

Giant macroprolactinomas may secrete prolactin exuberantly, giving rise to the "hook effect," an immunoassay artifact that occurs in the presence of very high serum concentrations of prolactin, leading to substantial underreporting of prolactin levels and potentially erroneous diagnosis. To avoid this artifact, prolactin should be measured in serially diluted serum specimens.[32]

Excess Cortisol (Cushing Syndrome)

Hypercortisolemia of any cause is known as "Cushing syndrome." Patients with this condition may present with manifestations of various kinds, including metabolic (central adiposity, glucose intolerance), catabolic (muscle wasting, bone loss, skin thinning, spontaneous ecchymoses), cardiovascular (hypertension, thromboembolism, coronary artery disease), mineralocorticoid (edema, hypokalemia), hypogonadal, hyperandrogenic (hirsutism, acne), increased risk of infections, and psychiatric symptoms. Most commonly the cause is iatrogenic administration of corticosteroids; the second most common etiology is a functioning adenoma. Approximately 80% of patients with neoplastic causes of Cushing syndrome have a pituitary adenoma (Cushing disease). The remainder have adrenal tumors (adenoma, carcinoma) or ectopic tumors (nonpituitary ACTH production).[33]

The diagnosis of Cushing disease can be difficult and is best made by an endocrinologist experienced in neuroendocrine disorders. Hypercortisolemia is determined by measurement of 24-hour urine free cortisol levels, nonsuppressed serum cortisol level after low-dose dexamethasone, and elevated late-night salivary cortisol levels. These tests help establish the presence of cortisol excess and differentiate between Cushing syndrome and other states associated with high cortisol levels (**Table 75.5**). An ACTH level is the next step in investigating the source of Cushing syndrome: low ACTH levels (<5 pg/mL), implying ACTH-independent etiology, are seen with adrenal disease, as the autonomous production of excess cortisol results in normal feedback inhibition of pituitary ACTH. High or inappropriately normal ACTH levels (>15 pg/mL), implying ACTH-dependent etiology, are seen with pituitary or ectopic etiologies. ACTH levels between 5 and 15 pg/mL, although not very common, fall into a gray area and cannot clearly point toward a central or adrenal source, necessitating further dynamic testing.

If the ACTH level is elevated, an MRI of the pituitary is the next step. If no pituitary lesion is found (up to 40% of cases), or if an adenoma <6 mm is identified, further testing to confirm a pituitary source of ACTH is warranted. Bilateral inferior petrosal sinus sampling (IPSS) is the gold standard in such cases.[34] This is a catheter-based endovascular procedure in which ACTH levels obtained from the inferior petrosal sinuses (both before and after the intravenous administration of a corticotropin-releasing hormone [CRH] analog) are compared to levels obtained in the vena cava. A central-to-peripheral ACTH ratio of greater than 3:1 after the administration of CRH is considered diagnostic of a central (pituitary) source, even in the absence of tumor visualization on MRI.[35] The value of this procedure in predicting the laterality of the microadenoma is debated, but newer protocols, incorporating prolactin gradients, have improved the accuracy of lateralization predictions into the 80% range.[36] If IPSS is not available, a CRH stimulation test in combination with a high-dose dexamethasone suppression test can help to confirm a pituitary source.

Excess Growth Hormone (Acromegaly)

Excess GH secretion by a pituitary adenoma prior to epiphyseal closure leads to gigantism, while GH excess in adulthood leads to acromegaly. Adult patients typically report increased ring and shoe size, dental and jaw abnormalities with malocclusion, coarsening of facial features, headache, hoarseness, skin tags, increased sweating, carpal tunnel syndrome, arthralgias, snoring, and sleep apnea. Higher rates of hypertension, diabetes, hyperlipidemia, kidney stones, cardiomyopathy, gallstones, colon polyps, and thyroid nodules are all related to the excess of GH. Because these changes occur slowly over time, diagnosis can be delayed, and these tumors are often large and invasive at the time of detection. Acromegalic patients have a mortality risk on the order of two to three times that of the general population if GH excess is not adequately controlled. Many of these changes are reversible with successful control of the disease, but skeletal abnormalities are not.

Because GH secretion is pulsatile, random GH measurements are not useful. The diagnosis is made by an elevated serum IGF1, produced by the liver overstimulated by the excess of GH. IGF1 assays are technically challenging and require gender and age adjustment.

Table 75.5. Conditions Associated with Cortisol Excess

Cushing Syndrome	Cortisol Excess in Patients with Some Manifestations of Cushing Syndrome (but No Tumor): "Pseudo-Cushing"	Cortisol Excess in Patients without Manifestations of Cushing Syndrome
Pituitary adenoma (Cushing disease)	Depression, anxiety, obsessive–compulsive disorders	Acute illness, injury, or surgery
Ectopic ACTH secretion	Alcoholism	Hospitalization
Adrenal tumor (adenoma, carcinoma) or hyperplasia	Severe obesity	Anorexia nervosa
Iatrogenic	Poorly controlled diabetes mellitus	High corticosteroid–binding globulin (CBG) levels
Surreptitious	Polycystic ovary syndrome	
	Familial glucocorticoid resistance	

Inadequate suppression of GH after a glucose load (administered in an oral glucose tolerance test as a 75-g bolus) confirms the diagnosis when the IGF1 is less than two times upper level of normal. Whether a GH nadir cutoff of 1 mg/L, 0.4 mg/L, or even lower can be used in patients with diabetes or other comorbidities is still a matter of debate, and in these situations the patient should be referred to an endocrinologist with expertise in pituitary diseases.[37]

TSH Adenomas

While immunocytochemical staining for TSH is not uncommon, secretion of active thyrotropin leading to central hyperthyroidism is rare. The hyperthyroidism tends to be mild, with palpitations, tremor, heat intolerance, and a diffuse goiter being more frequently found at diagnosis. The majority of these tumors are macroadenomas and may therefore be associated with mass effect. Biochemically, they demonstrate a nonsuppressed (inappropriately normal or increased) TSH level. This syndrome needs to be distinguished from resistance to thyroid hormone which can lead to a similar hormone profile.[38]

Endocrine Evaluation of a Pituitary "Incidentaloma"

With the widespread availability of MRI, it is not uncommon for the radiologist to report the incidental finding of a pituitary mass. The endocrine evaluation requires screening of pituitary hormone levels to determine possible hypo- or hyperfunction, which will help to guide further therapy. Pituitary hyperplasia (which occurs when the pituitary is stimulated to produce a pituitary hormone in much higher quantity than usually) can be difficult to distinguish from a true pituitary adenoma but requires an appreciation of the clinical setting to guard against unnecessary surgical intervention. Typically, it is found in women going through puberty into early adulthood, menopause (proliferation of gonadotroph cells), pregnancy and lactation (proliferation of lactotrophs), or severe primary hypothyroidism (thyrotroph hyperplasia). Rarely, ectopic secretion of GH-releasing hormone or CRH may lead to somatotroph or corticotroph hyperplasia, respectively. All these conditions need to be distinguished from true pituitary adenomas.[26,39]

NEUROLOGIC EVALUATION IN PITUITARY ADENOMAS

The primary neurologic manifestation of a pituitary mass is ophthalmologic, from compression of the optic nerves or chiasm traveling through the suprasellar cistern. Because the ipsilateral retinal ganglion cell axons cross in the optic chiasm *en route* to the contralateral occipital cortex, the pathognomonic finding on visual field examination is bitemporal hemianopsia. The chiasm may sometimes be associated with a relatively short intracranial optic nerve segment ("prefixed") or a relatively long intracranial optic nerve segment ("post fixed"). Depending upon the relative position of the tumor and chiasm, compression may also lead to uni- or bilateral optic nerve dysfunction, or compression of an optic tract, with resulting homonymous hemianopsia. Patients may sometimes report decreased acuity, although central vision is usually preserved unless compression is severe. Painless, unilateral decrease in color vision is a sensitive sign of early optic neuropathy, as is an afferent pupillary defect (Marcus Gunn pupil). This can be demonstrated by the "swinging flashlight test," in which light shown into the affected eye leads to a paradoxical increase in pupillary size, as the ipsilateral pupillo-constrictor fibers have been damaged by ipsilateral optic nerve compression and transmit relatively decreased retinal activity. Although pituitary adenomas often invade the cavernous sinus and displace the cranial nerves within, dysfunction of cranial nerves other than the optic nerve is uncommon. When other cranial neuropathies, such as oculomotor dysfunction, are present, and especially if they are of sudden onset, one should suspect a rapidly expanding mass, that is, pituitary apoplexy, or a more aggressive tumor, for example, a malignancy. Similarly, pituitary adenomas often circumscribe but rarely constrict the cavernous carotid artery, and rarely cause neurovascular dysfunction; when neurovascular dysfunction is present an alternate pathologic diagnosis (especially meningioma) should be considered.[40]

Headaches can be part of the presentation for pituitary tumors, possibly via stretching of the surrounding dura mater, dural inflammation in apoplexy, or a form of trigeminal neuralgia. The headaches tend to be daily, retro-orbital or frontal, and throbbing. Such headaches are more frequently associated with cystic lesions and functioning adenomas (especially acromegaly), and resolve with surgery in only slightly more than 50% of patients.[41]

IMAGING OF PITUITARY ADENOMAS

Magnetic Resonance Imaging

MRI represents the standard of care in evaluating pituitary tumors. Useful sequences for imaging the sella include T1 coronal and sagittal imaging before and after gadolinium contrast administration. Other sequences (eg, T2 coronal) may be useful, especially in the evaluation of cystic structures (fluid is generally hyperintense on T2) and previous hemorrhage (which may be dark on T2). Because of the relatively decreased vascularity of adenomas compared with the normal gland, timing of scanning relative to the administration of gadolinium is important; adenomas are generally focally hypointense to normal gland. Dynamic scanning using thin-section gradient-echo sequences may improve the sensitivity of visualization with small microadenomas (eg, in Cushing disease), but gland heterogeneity may lead to decreased specificity. When preparing for surgery, it is essential to establish the location of the tumor with respect to the carotid arteries. Contrast-enhanced MRI sequences assist in assessing the extent of tumor invasion of the cavernous sinuses, and, if present, the degree of circumferential contact between the tumor and the cavernous segment of one or both carotid arteries.[42]

Computerized Tomography

Computerized tomography (CT) scanning has largely been supplanted by MRI but remains useful in the delineation of bony anatomy relevant to surgical planning and intraoperative navigation. At many centers it is common for pituitary surgery to be performed by a team comprising an otorhinolaryngologist and a neurosurgeon, the former performing the approach and the latter performing the tumor resection. Particularly when endoscopic sinus surgical approaches are used, preoperative CT is useful in defining the bony septations of the nasal sinuses, which are often poorly defined on MRI. In addition, in those few patients who cannot undergo MRI, thin-section coronal CT after contrast administration can be used to demonstrate a pituitary lesion. The presence of calcification on CT scanning can assist in the differential diagnosis; for example, a calcified cystic lesion, especially in a child, is highly likely to represent a craniopharyngioma.[43]

MRI Characteristics of Pituitary Tumors and Other Sellar Lesions

The normal gland enhances relatively homogeneously. It should be no greater than about 8 mm in coronal height in males and 10 mm in females. The infundibulum should be midline. The posterior pituitary may be bright on T1 without contrast (thought to represent secretory granules in axon terminals), although this is not a constant finding.

Pituitary adenomas should be focally hypointense relative to normal gland on T1 sequences after contrast. Microadenomas (<1 cm) may not significantly disrupt gland architecture. Macroadenomas (>1 cm) show upward bowing of the diaphragm sella associated with stalk deviation, and larger macroadenomas often demonstrate compression of the chiasm. The normal gland can be compressed, usually superiorly and posteriorly. The cavernous sinuses are variably involved; it can be difficult to distinguish invasion from compression. Lesions surrounding the cavernous carotid are obviously invasive; lesions which circumscribe less than 25% are usually compressive. It has been suggested than lesions which circumscribe less than 67% of the carotid diameter are not invasive, but this is very variable. Adenomas can also be cystic, and in such cases may show T1 bright signal before contrast consistent with high-protein fluid or hemorrhage.

Craniopharyngiomas may be cystic or solid, and intra- or suprasellar. Characteristics of the cyst fluid can vary with the protein content, with greater T1 hyperintensity associated with higher protein. The cyst wall is commonly calcified (easily verifiable on CT), especially in children. Since the tumor is often suprasellar, involving the stalk and hypothalamus, the gland is typically compressed inferiorly from above.

Pituitary cysts can demonstrate variable imaging characteristics, also depending upon their protein content. Rathke cleft cysts arise posteriorly in the sella, or sometimes along the stalk. They can be T1 hypo- or hyperintense depending on protein content and can compress the gland anteriorly or from above. The cyst wall is usually thin, with minimal enhancement. If there is a solid component or calcification, the diagnosis is more likely to represent a craniopharyngioma. Arachnoid cysts of the sella contain fluid isointense to CSF. They exhibit minimal if any enhancement of the wall, as the cyst is lined with a thin arachnoid layer. The gland is usually compressed inferiorly or anteriorly.

Germinomas usually involve the posterior gland, stalk, and/or hypothalamus. They are typically brightly enhancing, and the borders are relatively indistinct. An enhancing lesion of the posterior sella associated with a pineal mass is highly likely to represent a germinoma. Germ cell tumors may disseminate along CSF pathways, leading to enhancement around the fourth ventricle. *Meningiomas* are usually brightly enhancing, often more so than the gland itself. As they arise from the dura, they can be variably located in and around the sella. If they arise from the diaphragm, they can be difficult to distinguish from adenomas, but usually compress the gland from above.

Meningiomas are often associated with a dural "tail," which spreads out from the central mass of the tumor, sometimes with focal hyperostosis. Meningiomas of the cavernous sinus can lead to carotid constriction, whereas adenomas rarely do. This phenomenon is best seen on coronal images when comparing the transverse diameter of the intracavernous carotid arteries.

Metastases are typically locally invasive, brightly enhancing, rapidly growing, and associated with a clinical history of cancer. They can spread hematogenously to the gland, but more frequently represent focal metastases to parasellar bony structures. When invading the cavernous sinus they can lead to a cavernous sinus syndrome, whereas adenomas rarely do.

SURGICAL TECHNIQUE

6 Although the first reported pituitary operation was a craniotomy done in 1889 by Sir Vincent Horsley, the first transsphenoidal approach was described in 1907 by Hermann Schloffer, a Viennese otolaryngologist, when he reached the sphenoid via a lateral rhinotomy incision.[44] Less disfiguring approaches were devised by the American neurosurgeon Harvey Cushing, who, with William Halsted, devised the sublabial approach in 1910, and another Viennese otolaryngologist, Oscar Hirsch, who described a fully endonasal procedure.[45] Variants of these approaches remain in use today. Cushing performed over 200 transsphenoidal operations with an overall mortality rate of 5%—amazingly low given the lack of imaging, antibiotics, hormone replacement, and modern visualization—but decided in 1927 that the craniotomy was the more preferred procedure. With his decision, the transsphenoidal approach fell into relative disfavor, although kept alive by Dott in Edinburgh and Guiot in Paris, who introduced the use of intraoperative fluoroscopy as a navigation technique. Jules Hardy of Montreal described the use of the operating microscope and reported the first removal of a pituitary microadenoma in 1962, bringing pituitary surgery into the domain of microneurosurgery.[46] Since the 1990s, pituitary surgery has been reshaped by endoscopic techniques developed collaboratively by otorhinolaryngologists and neurosurgeons. With improvements in endoscope technology and compatible surgical instrumentation, purely endoscopic operations became commonplace in the field of sinus surgery, and these advances led to the use of endoscope-assisted and eventually purely endoscopic techniques for the management of pituitary adenomas and other lesions of the anterior skull base.[47]

The transsphenoidal approach is relatively noninvasive, as it employs the nasopharynx and sphenoid sinus to access the skull base, but the surgeon is constrained to operate through a narrow corridor, to a relatively deep target, surrounded by important structures (the carotid arteries and optic apparatus). The surgeon must (1) approach and navigate to the tumor, (2) visualize the pathology, and (3) maximally resect the tumor while minimizing damage to adjacent structures, including the normal gland and infundibulum.

Approach

There are two principal transsphenoidal approaches to the sella in use today, both of which are endonasal (**Fig. 75.2**). The sublabial approach, as well as the sub-frontal craniotomy, deserves mention primarily for their historical significance. The pterional craniotomy remains useful for certain sellar lesions with significant suprasellar extension.

The two endonasal approaches are limited to some degree by the width of the nasal apertures, but the advent of endoscopic systems allows contemporary surgeons access to adequate corridors for visualization and manipulation, through the nasal sinuses to the sella and anterior skull base. One endonasal approach, favored in some centers at which neurosurgeons perform both the approach and the tumor resection, uses a submucosal tunnel along the septum through an anterior mucosal incision immediately posterior to the columella. Postoperatively, nasal packing is used to reapproximate the mucosa to the septum. The direct endonasal approach, typically favored in centers at which endoscopic surgery is the norm, with the endonasal approach being performed by an otorhinolaryngologist, uses either an incision at the insertion of the septum into the face of the sphenoid, or an enlargement of the natural ostia, with a posterior septectomy. This approach facilitates bimanual surgery and operation through both nares.

Navigation

It is critical to maintain accurate orientation in the sellar approach, as the face of sella is bounded immediately laterally by the carotid protuberances, and superolaterally by the

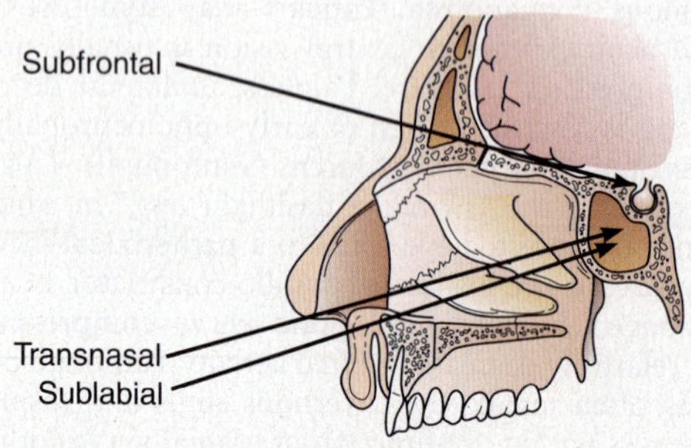

Figure 75.2. Surgical approaches to the sella.

optic canals. The insertion of the nasal septum posteriorly is usually a midline structure and can be used for orientation, while the sphenoid septations are very variable, and can be used for orientation only when correlated with preoperative imaging. Lateral intraoperative fluoroscopy was used at some centers in the era before neuronavigation. In the last two decades, neuronavigational devices have become a ubiquitous standard of care. These systems establish a three-dimensional (3D) reference frame by registering facial and bony anatomy with preoperative imaging, and they can be used to correlate intraoperative anatomy with preoperative imaging by means of a navigational "stylus" recognized by the device in real time. This gives 3D information to guide the approach, but is dependent on the accuracy of the registration, and is less valuable in determining the adequacy of resection and orientation within the tumor, as tumor anatomy can change during resection.

VISUALIZATION

Hardy introduced the use of the intraoperative microscope to pituitary surgery and it remains in widespread use today. After the introduction of the rigid endoscope to field of sinus surgery by otorhinolaryngologists, its use in transsphenoidal surgery was reported by Jankowski in 1992[48]; its utility and efficacy were confirmed in multiple studies and reviews in the ensuing two decades. In the present generation, endoscopy has replaced microscopy at many centers as the preferred mode of surgical visualization in transsphenoidal surgery. Advantages of the microscopic approach are the superb optics and binocular vision; a major disadvantage is the requirement for direct line-of-sight viewing, though for smaller tumors, including the microadenomas of Cushing disease, this disadvantage may not be significant. The endoscope affords a wider field of view and the ability to see at angles off the primary visual axis. Early endoscopes offered only monocular vision with no depth of field, though 3D endoscopes are under development.[49] Although the endoscopic technique has the potential to be less invasive, the need to provide a surgical corridor sufficient for both the endoscope and working instruments may at times require greater dissection within the nasal sinuses. Several meta-analyses have been published comparing endoscopic and microscopic techniques. The overall results for secretory tumors, where there are defined biochemical criteria for remission, appear similar, whereas endoscopy offers advantages in the setting of larger nonsecretory tumors and those invading the cavernous sinuses.[50]

Determining the Adequacy of Resection

As most pituitary tumors are removed by internal decompression allowing collapse of the tumor capsule, there may be no direct visualization of the adequacy of resection. Endoscopic inspection of the tumor capsule can sometimes provide an indication, but prolapse of the diaphragm as the capsule collapses (itself an indication of adequacy of decompression) can make thorough internal visualization difficult. Intraoperative MRI (iMRI) has been used in the determination of resection adequacy, as the technique allows the surgeon to visualize areas of residual tumor not seen with direct inspection. A number of studies have reviewed the utility of intraoperative imaging. Most report that additional tumor resection can be achieved in about 20% of cases, but this is partly a function of when, during the course of the procedure, the surgeon chooses to image, as premature imaging may bias the results in favor of iMRI.[51] In addition, intraoperative imaging can show whether the chiasm has been adequately decompressed (which correlates with postoperative visual improvement) and may assist in the avoidance of postoperative complications. The iMRI equipment is costly, however, and requires significant alterations in surgical workflow and operative time, with the small but present risk of operating in close proximity to a high-strength magnetic field. It has been debated whether resection can be better optimized with the use of the iMRI versus the endoscope, although these technologies are not mutually exclusive and are used in combination at some centers. Each approach has its adherents. In those few studies combining the use of endoscopy with the iMRI, most suggest that some degree of additional resection can be achieved after imaging.[51]

A comparison of preoperative, immediate postoperative, and 1-year postoperative MR images in a patient with a nonfunctioning macroadenoma causing elevation and compression of the optic chiasm is shown in **Figure 75.3**.

Surgical Technique

There are a number of variations in surgical technique, determined by the preference of the surgeons and the dictates of the anatomy. The patient is given antibiotics and stress-dose steroids preoperatively. Protocols for antibiotic use are not standardized, but a typical neurosurgical antibiotic regimen is almost universally extended to broad-spectrum coverage when a high-flow CSF leak is expected or encountered. A lumbar drain may be placed preoperatively if a high-flow CSF leak is anticipated, and the abdomen may be prepared for harvest of a fat graft to be used in repairing the associated skull base defect. In selected cases, intrathecal fluorescein may be administered in order to assist in the detection of small CSF leaks. Almost all patients, except for patients with Cushing disease, are given stress-dose corticosteroids. After the induction of general endotracheal anesthesia, the patient is positioned supine. The head may be turned toward the surgeon or in a neutral position if two surgeons will together be performing an endoscopic approach while standing on opposite sides of the patient. At some centers, following the endonasal approach, the otorhinolaryngologist maneuvers the endoscope while the neurosurgeon performs the tumor resection; others prefer to place the endoscope on a fixed holder during the tumor resection. The head of the patient can be held in a gel headrest or pinned using the Mayfield clamp. If neuronavigation is used, the reference fiducials or surface anatomy is registered. The area of the proposed nasal mucosal incision is infiltrated with local anesthesia with epinephrine and cocaine as vasoconstrictors.

With a direct endonasal approach the incision is made along the posterior septum, and either the septum is fractured and deviated contralaterally, or a posterior septectomy is performed.[52] The microscopic approach employs either a sublabial incision or an endonasal transseptal approach. In both cases a nasal speculum is introduced, fracturing the septum and compressing the turbinates laterally. With the endoscopic approach, the middle turbinate may require removal to increase access. The face of the sphenoid is opened, and any septations impeding access are removed. Anatomy of the sphenoid septations gleaned from preoperative imaging can be useful in guiding the approach to the midline sella, which is drilled to dura. Diamond burr drill bits are used near the dura. The dura may be lightly cauterized prior to the dural incision.

For macroadenomas, the tumor is usually immediately evident. The typical strategy involves dissecting the tumor from the dural leaflets, defining the interface between the tumor and normal gland, internally debulking the tumor with ring curettes, then completing the resection in a manner that preserves the normal gland. The normal gland can usually be distinguished by color and consistency, and in the case of macroadenomas is usually compressed posteriorly and superiorly. As the resection proceeds the diaphragm should prolapse into the operative field, particularly in cases in which the chiasm has been compressed. After tumor removal, the resection cavity is inspected for residual tumor; angled endoscopes can be useful in visualizing areas not in the direct line of sight.

When approaching microadenomas, especially those causing Cushing disease, detection can be difficult. If there is strong evidence from preoperative imaging, dissection in the indicated region may be attempted. Some surgeons approach microadenomas by dividing the gland into quadrants and

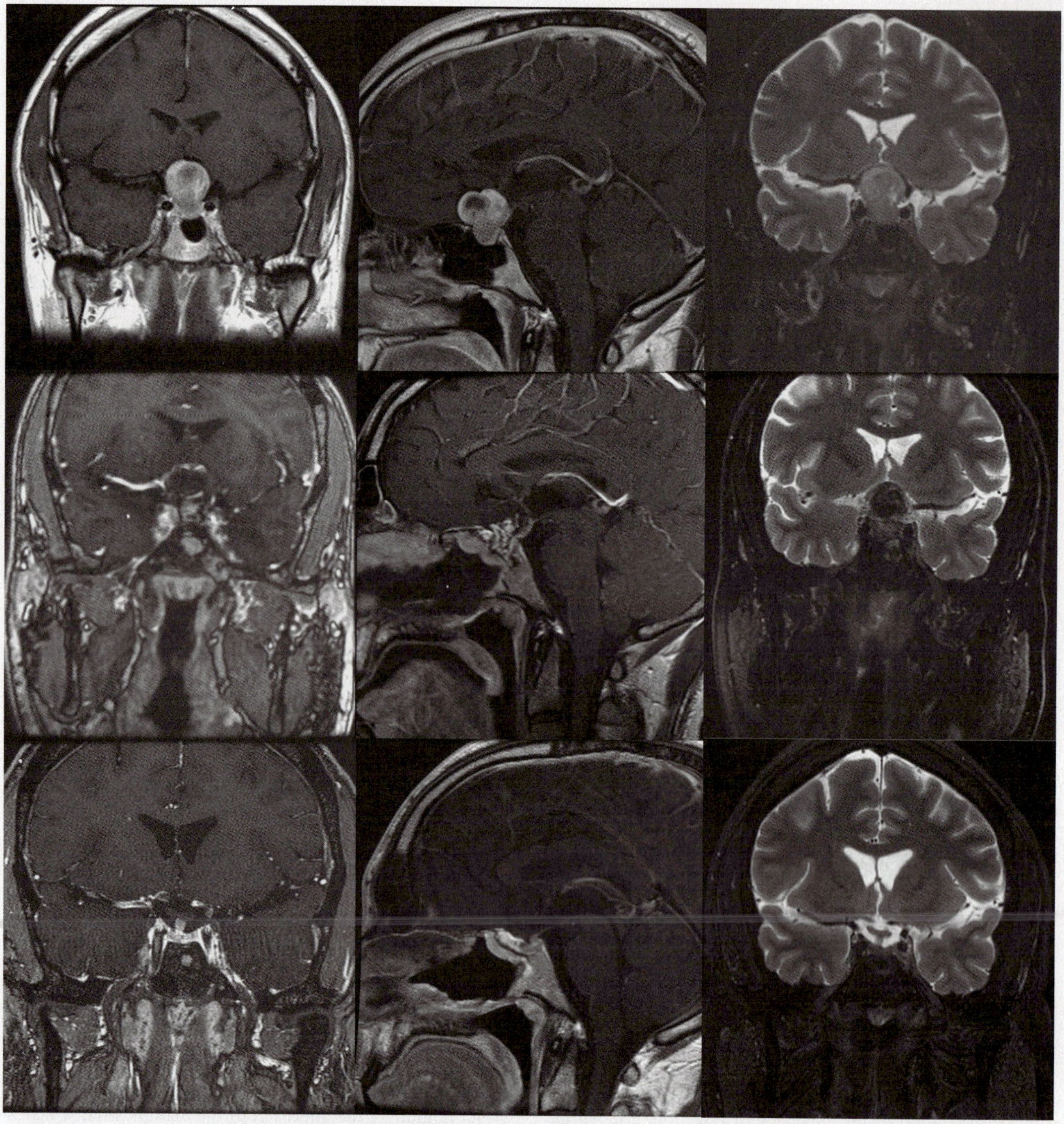

Figure 75.3. MR imaging of the sella before and after resection of a pituitary macroadenoma.

taking biopsies from each quadrant. If no tumor is found on frozen-section analysis, a hemi-hypophysectomy can be performed guided by IPSS.

Hemostasis is achieved by packing with any number of available hemostatic materials. After achieving hemostasis, many surgeons pack the tumor cavity with fat, muscle, or absorbable hemostatic material. A water-tight seal is essential if a CSF leak has been created. Many techniques have been described for achieving a water-tight reconstruction of the anterior skull base in this context. When a microscopic approach is used, a fat graft is buttressed in place and the sellar floor reconstructed with septal cartilage or bone, titanium mesh, or proprietary, commercially available materials. Fibrin glue or other sellar sealant can be used if needed. When an endoscopic approach is used, such techniques are often supplemented by rotating a vascularized nasoseptal flap over the reconstructed skull base defect, which has revolutionized the field by significantly decreasing the rate of postoperative CSF leaks.[53] Displaced turbinates and septum are then returned to their physiologic positions. With a direct endonasal approach, nasal packing is not always used. If a submucosal tunnel was created during the approach, nasal packing is placed. The use of iMRI can be timed at the discretion of the surgeon. Some surgeons maintain the sterile field and image before final closure; others complete the closure (since reopening is usually straightforward) and image prior to reversal of anesthesia.

Postoperative Management

Careful monitoring in the postoperative period is essential. Most patients require only one to two nights of hospitalization; an ICU stay is usually not necessary if a well-monitored stepdown unit is available. Potential complications include postoperative hemorrhage, CSF leakage, meningitis, epistaxis, and endocrine dysfunction (including DI, the syndrome of inappropriate antidiuretic hormone secretion [SIADH], and hypopituitarism).

1. *Cavity Hemorrhage and Visual Compromise.* Postoperative hemorrhage can occur into the tumor resection cavity with resulting visual compromise. Thus, frequent testing of postoperative acuity and confrontational field is necessary. Subjective reporting by the patient must also be taken seriously. Immediate reexploration may be required, even in the absence of convincing findings on neuroimaging.[54]
2. *Cerebrospinal Fluid Fistula.* CSF leakage can be sometimes difficult to differentiate from postoperative nasal drainage. Positional drainage (nose-down) and CT evidence of pneumocephalus are suggestive of persistent CSF leak. The classic confirmatory test to differentiate CSF from nasal drainage involves assaying collected fluid for tau protein (beta transferrin), which is found in CSF but not in nasal secretions or blood. Usually, however, these tests take days to return. Management options include the insertion of a lumbar drain to lower intracranial pressure and reduce flow through the fistula for several days, in order to allow for spontaneous closure of the leak, while maintaining antibiotic coverage. In the presence of a persistent, high-flow leak the optimal course is often reexploration and repacking of the tumor bed with closure of the fistula.
3. *Meningitis.* Infection in the immediate postoperative period is rare. Prophylactic antibiotic coverage is maintained for 24 hours, or until the nasal packing is removed. Delayed fever, especially with signs of meningitis, requires evaluation with a lumbar puncture; an occult CSF leak should be suspected. Patients may be at increased risk of sinus infection for many months.
4. *Epistaxis.* Bloody nasal secretions are common, and usually clear with nasal irrigation. Frank epistaxis is rare, usually occurs 2 or 3 weeks after surgery, and is most often caused by delayed hemorrhage from a septal branch of the sphenopalatine artery. It can sometimes be managed with nasal packing, but may require cauterization or clipping, or rarely embolization.
5. *Postoperative Endocrine Changes.* Postoperative endocrinologic changes are best managed in conjunction with an experienced endocrinologist.
   - **5.1.** *Diabetes Insipidus.* Water/sodium imbalances occur in up to 75% of the patients who undergo transsphenoidal surgery in the first 14 days after surgery, with transient DI being the most common abnormality. Transient DI usually resolves spontaneously within days and permanent DI is unlikely (1% to 2% of patients). It is important to monitor liquid intake and urine output, urine-specific gravity, and serum sodium levels in the immediate postoperative period, and to treat with hypotonic fluid and desmopressin if needed. Mild cases can be treated with ad lib fluid intake if the thirst mechanism is intact.
   - **5.2.** *Hyponatremia.* Immediate postoperative hyponatremia appearing on postoperative days (PODs) 1 to 3 tends to be mild and self-limited. Delayed hyponatremia is thought to be secondary to inappropriate release of the stored antidiuretic hormone (SIADH) following mechanical manipulation of the posterior pituitary. This syndrome typically starts between PODs 5 and 8 and can be severe (from nausea and headache to confusion and seizures). It is a significant cause of morbidity and is the leading cause of readmission after transsphenoidal surgery. More recently different regimens of fluid restriction have decreased the severity of hyponatremia and readmission (eg, 1-L daily fluid restriction started POD 4 and maintained until sodium is checked and found normal POD 5–8).[55] Mild SIADH usually responds to fluid restriction and oral salt supplements. In more severe cases furosemide, urea, or hypertonic saline need to be used. It is important not to correct the hyponatremia too quickly in order to avoid central pontine myelinolysis. The hyponatremia usually resolves within 1 week with supportive care.[56]
   - **5.3.** *Hypopituitarism.* Immediate postoperative monitoring for pituitary insufficiency, especially hypoadrenalism and hypothyroidism, is necessary. Some centers prophylactically treat with replacement steroids until adequate cortisol levels can be proven. Another approach is to check an 8 AM cortisol POD 1 to 2, at least 24 hours after any steroids have been administered, and to discharge on physiologic corticosteroid replacement only patients with cortisol below a certain level (eg, 13 to 15 mg/dL).[57] Central hypothyroidism might take longer to become evident on laboratory testing and it is recommended to check free T4 later (this test can be obtained concurrent with the sodium level required to monitor for delayed hyponatremia on POD 5 to 8). Complete postoperative hormone assessment is usually performed at 6 to 8 weeks postoperatively in order to establish remission of hormone excess and reassess pituitary function. New pituitary hormone deficiencies develop in 5% to 10% of patients, while preexisting pituitary hormone deficiencies may resolve in 30% to 40% of patients postoperatively.
   - **5.4.** *Biochemical Remission.* Patients treated for hyperfunctioning adenomas require special attention in the immediate postoperative period, especially patients with Cushing disease. Surgical remission leads to immediate lowering of ACTH and cortisol levels, and steroid replacement is required as the normal gland will remain suppressed for months. Patients can develop hypoglycemia, hypotension, tend to be hypercoagulable, and need higher doses of corticosteroid at the time of hospital discharge. Importantly, a rapid decrease in cortisol levels may be indicative of chemical cure in patients with Cushing disease; these patients are particularly vulnerable to hypocortisolemia and should be appropriately medicated. A progressive decrease in cortisol levels may similarly indicate cure; patients should be carefully monitored to avoid delayed symptoms. Patients with acromegaly in remission postoperatively may have polyuria as GH levels fall, without developing DI.

RESULTS AND COMPLICATIONS

In considering the results of pituitary surgery, the most important outcome measures relate to resolution of presenting symptoms (visual, endocrine, or other), rates of gross total tumor removal and of biochemical remission in the case of functioning adenomas, and the durability of these results. The incidence, severity, and management of each of the principal complications are also important to understand, as are considerations of cost and postoperative quality of life. Additional questions relate to whether outcomes have changed over time, and whether contemporary evidence favors particular surgical techniques. Results from a number of meta-analyses addressing these outcome measures are summarized in **Table 75.6**.

Reviews of the literature on outcomes after transsphenoidal surgery require recognition of several factors potentially affecting the interpretation of the results. Endocrine diagnostic techniques, biochemical criteria for remission for secretory tumors, and surgical techniques have changed over time, which can make comparisons difficult. Publication and reporting biases typically favor newer over older techniques, and some series may selectively report certain classes of complications. Meta-analyses can be useful but need to be interpreted with an eye to the underlying data, and with an awareness that the overwhelming majority of these analyses review retrospective case series rather than prospective or randomized controlled studies.

Table 75.6. Comparison of Outcomes and Complications in Endoscopic and Microscopic Approaches for Resection of Pituitary Adenomas

	Meta-Analyses of Retrospective Series													
Study														
Author (Yr)	Goudakos et al. (2011)		DeKlotz et al. (2012)		Ammirati et al. (2013)		Gao et al. (2014)		Li et al. (2017)		Almutairi et al. (2018)		Li et al. (2019)	
Methodologic Comments					Incomplete reporting of vascular complications in M				Only comparative odds ratios reported		Complications not assessed		Only comparative odds ratios reported	
Number of Studies Included (Total Cases)	11 (806)		38 (4,900)		38 (5,643)		15 (1,014)		23 (2,272)		70 (8,257)		17 (1,177)	
	Endoscopic	*Microscopic*	*Endoscopic*	*Microscopic*	*Endoscopic*	*Microscopic*	*Endoscopic*	*Microscopic*	*Endoscopic*	*Microscopic*	*Endoscopic*	*Microscopic*	*Endoscopic*	*Microscopic*
Endoscopic/ Microscopic Cases	369	437	2,335	2,565	2,125	3,518	487	527	Not Reported Separately	Not Reported Separately	Not Reported Separately	Not Reported Separately	582	595
Results														
Gross Total Removal	71%	69% (NSD)	**79% (favoring E*)**	**65%**	69%	64% (NSD)	**71.8% (favoring E*)**	**58.0%**	**OR 1.52 (favoring E*)**		**74.0% (favoring E*)**	**66.40%**	66.4%	66.5% (NSD)
Endocrinologic Cure (%)	66	60 (NSD)	71	71 (NSD)							75.8	75.5 (NSD)		
Visual Improvement (%)			**71 (favoring E*)**	**56**										
Recurrence									NSD					
Complications														
Overall	**RR 0.18 (favoring E*)**												**RR 1.29 (favoring E*)**	
Death (%)					0.49	0.23 (NSD)			NSD					
Cerebrospinal Fluid Leak (%)	NSD		**5 (favoring E*)**	**7**	7.00	6.34 (NSD)	12.8	12.2 (NSD)	NSD				NSD	
Meningitis (%)			1	1 (NSD)	1.11	2.08 (NSD)	1.40	2.1 (NSD)	NSD				NSD	

Transient Diabetes Insipidus (%)	15 (favoring E*)	28			9.10	10.23 (NSD)	11.30	14.0 (NSD)	NSD		
Permanent Diabetes Insipidus (%)	2 (favoring E*)	10	2	3 (NSD)	2.31	4.25 (NSD)			NSD		
Hypopituitarism (%)					8.51	11.64 (NSD)	3.00	6.1 (NSD)	NSD		
Visual Loss (%)					0.72	0.60 (NSD)					
Cranial Nerve Injury (%)					0.28	0.53 (NSD)					
Vascular Incident (%)					1.58	0.50 (favoring M*)					
Rhinologic Complications	Favoring E*		Favoring E* (<septal perforation, <epistaxis)			Favoring E* (<septal perforation)	OR 0.29 (favoring E*) (<septal perforation)			2.0% (favoring E*)	8.30%
Hospital Stay	1.5 d shorter (favoring E*)	3.3 d (favoring E*)	5.9 d			3.8 d (favoring E*)	6.3 d				
Total Cost											

Randomized Controlled or Prospective Studies

Study										
Author (Yr)	Cho et al. (2002)		Jain et al. (2007)		Enseñat et al. (2009)		Kahilogullari et al. (2013)		Little et al. (2014)	
Methodologic Comments	Prolactinomas randomized to microsublabial/ endoscopic		Randomized to microendonasal/ endoscopic		Randomized to microsublabial/endoscopic		Prospective nonrandomized		Prospective nonrandomized	
Number of Studies Included (Total Cases)	1 (44)		1 (20)		1 (50)		1 (50)		1 (166)	
	Endoscopic	*Microscopic*	*Endoscopic*	*Microscopic*	*Endoscopic*	*Microscopic*	*Endoscopic*	*Microscopic*	*Endoscopic*	*Microscopic*
Endoscopic/ Microscopic Cases	22	22	10	10	25	25	25	25	67	99

(*continued*)

Table 75.6. Comparison of Outcomes and Complications in Endoscopic and Microscopic Approaches for Resection of Pituitary Adenomas (*Continued*)

Randomized Controlled or Prospective Studies

Results									
Gross Total Removal (%)			50	50 (NSD)	**60 (favoring E*)**	35			
Endocrinologic cure (%)	66	75 (NSD)	NSD						
Visual Improvement (%)	63	60 (NSD)	NSD						
Recurrence									
Complications									
Overall	**4.5% (favoring E*)**	**27% M**	**Favoring E***		NSD				
Death									
Cerebrospinal Fluid Leak			NSD						
Meningitis									
Transient Diabetes Insipidus			NSD						
Permanent Diabetes Insipidus			NSD						
Hypopituitarism			NSD						
Visual Loss			NSD						
Cranial Nerve Injury									
Vascular Incident									
Rhinologic Complications			**Favoring E***						
Hospital Stay	**3.2 d (favoring E*)**	**5.3 d**			**3 d shorter (favoring E*)**		**0% Hyp-/0% anosmia (favoring E*)**	**52% Hyp-/25% anosmia**	
Total Cost									NSD in total hospital charges

Boldface E*/M* indicates statistically significant difference favoring endoscopic/microscopic approach.
E, endoscopic; M, microscopic; NSD, no/not significant difference; RR, risk ratio; OR, odds ratio; d, days.

Gross Total Resection. Pituitary surgery has been a mature field for decades, so an important question concerns the extent to which surgical outcomes have changed over time. A notable meta-analysis published in 2012 reviewed short-term remission and recurrence data over the preceding 25 years. No trend toward improvement in short-term remission was observed over time, but a reduced rate of tumor recurrence was noted.[58] Because of the historical time frame, the majority of series included in that analysis used a microscopic approach. In the last decade, however, a growing body of evidence has emerged suggesting that higher rates of gross total resection are being achieved with the use of endoscopy, particularly in the setting of larger tumors and those with suprasellar extension or cavernous sinus invasion.[59] In perhaps the largest meta-analysis to date comparing endoscopic and microscopic outcomes, published in 2018 and involving 70 studies and 8,257 patients, gross total removal was achieved at a rate of 74.0% for pituitary adenomas removed endoscopically as compared with 66.4% for those removed microscopically.[60]

Biochemical Remission. On the other hand, it is not clear that historical success rates for resection and biochemical remission in the management of hormone-secreting adenomas have improved over time or with the advent of endoscopic techniques.[61] The same 2018 meta-analysis found no difference in the rates of complete removal of functioning adenomas; both endoscopic and microscopic techniques achieved this endpoint at a rate of 75%. The risk of recurrence per patient year at risk has been reported to be 3.4% for prolactinomas, 0.7% in acromegaly, and 2.3% in Cushing disease, as compared with 2.2% for nonfunctioning adenomas.[58] A meta-analysis of 9 endoscopic series involving 821 patients indicated that biochemical (endocrinologic) remission was achieved in greater than 80% of cases.[62] However, it is notable that the classic pseudo-capsular resection technique pioneered by Oldfield was established using microscopic technique via a sublabial approach, and his results remain the gold standard: biochemical remission was achieved in all 261 cases of Cushing disease in which an encapsulated adenoma was identified at surgery.[63]

Visual Improvement. Visual improvement following decompression of the optic apparatus in patients with pituitary tumors causing visual field deficits is believed to depend more on the timing of the decompression than on the surgical technique. Multiple studies have suggested that microscopic and endoscopic approaches yield approximately equivalent visual outcomes.[59]

Recurrence versus Durability of Outcomes. With respect to the durability of surgical outcomes, several important findings are consistent across multiple series and meta-analyses. The most significant prognostic factors for long-term remission in functioning adenomas are low postoperative level of the relevant hormone and gross total resection.[58] In addition, even accounting for observation bias, multiple studies have suggested that most adenomas that ever recur do so within the first 5 years after surgery.

Microscopic versus Endoscopic Techniques. Multiple meta-analyses have addressed the relative efficacy of endoscopic versus microscopic techniques.[64,65] The findings of these and others are summarized and cited in **Table 75.6**. Early analyses often compared results from newer endoscopic series to results from older or historical microscopic series. In recent years these studies have begun to favor endoscopic over microscopic approaches, but it is not entirely clear whether this trend reflects publication bias. Few controlled trials have been published, and a recent meta-analysis identified only five: two randomized and three nonrandomized, involving a total of 328 patients.[66] There was no evidence for superiority of either surgical technique with respect to gross total tumor removal or biochemical control, but endoscopic pituitary surgery was associated with a significantly reduced risk of complications (RR 0.37) relative to microscopic approaches. It is important to note that this finding is consistently, though not universally, supported by multiple large meta-analyses of retrospective case series, as we will presently discuss.

Cerebrospinal Fluid Leak. CSF leak, in the early years of endoscopic pituitary surgery, was considered a major potential liability of the newer technique. This concern drew extensive attention from the surgical community, and a variety of techniques emerged and matured, including multilayer skull base reconstruction ("gasket" and "button" closures), use of vascularized nasoseptal flaps, and selective use of lumbar drainage and intrathecal fluorescein to identify small CSF leaks intraoperatively. Because many pituitary adenomas remain extraarachnoid, pituitary adenoma surgery is typically associated with fewer CSF leaks than extended approaches to nonadenomatous lesions of the sellar and parasellar region. Recent series suggest that the risk of postoperative CSF leak in pituitary adenoma surgery is approximately 1%, as compared with 1% to 3% for microscopic approaches.[59]

Meningitis, Visual Loss, and Death. The rate of postoperative meningitis, which is often a sequela associated with CSF leak, is approximately 1% to 2% following pituitary surgery and has not been shown to differ as a function of technique. Similarly, the rates of permanent new visual loss, cranial nerve injury, and death are all less than 1%, with no significant difference in complication rates between microscopic and endoscopic approaches.

Diabetes Insipidus and Hypopituitarism. The rate of postoperative endocrine dysfunction has not consistently been shown to differ significantly as a function of surgical technique. Transient DI (posterior pituitary dysfunction) occurs in approximately 10% of cases. This condition resolves in most patients, with only approximately 2% to 4% developing permanent DI. The rate of anterior pituitary dysfunction (hypopituitarism) varies more substantially across meta-analyses, with estimates ranging from 3% to 11%.

Vascular Complications. One large meta-analysis has reported a significantly higher rate of vascular complications associated with endoscopic (1.58%) as compared with microscopic (0.5%) pituitary surgery. The study incorporated 38 studies involving a total of 5,643 patients.[64] The size of the reported effect may be called into question, however, given that at least one of the included microscopic series, accounting for 592 (19.6%) of the 3,023 microscopic cases pooled for analysis, was credited with zero vascular complications even though the original series does not report on this outcome at all.[67] This finding of a difference in rates of vascular complications has not been reproduced in other meta-analyses, and no meta-analysis has suggested a difference in the rates of visual loss or surgical mortality (feared consequences of carotid artery injury) between endoscopic and microscopic approaches.

Rhinologic Complications, Hospital Stay, Cost, and Quality of Life. Rhinologic complications, including septal perforations and impaired olfaction, have consistently been shown to be less common following endoscopic pituitary surgery than following microscopic resection. This difference in the rate of common, non–life-threatening complications largely account for the observed difference in complication rates between endoscopic and microscopic approaches. Rhinologic quality-of-life outcomes favor endoscopic approaches. Hospital stay has consistently been shown to be shorter by 2 to 3 days following endoscopic surgery, though surgical and total hospitalization costs are not significantly different for endoscopic and microscopic pituitary surgery.[68]

Prolactinomas

Given the efficacy of DA treatment, surgery for prolactinomas is rarely indicated. Nonetheless, it remains effective in selected cases, especially in smaller tumors. A large surgical series reported initial remission of 91.3% in microadenomas, with a recurrence rate of 7.1%. The overall remission rate was 53.2% including giant prolactinomas.[69]

Table 75.7. Medications Used to Treat Prolactin-Secreting Pituitary Adenomas

Name	Mechanism of Action	Usual Dose Range	Adverse Effects
Bromocriptine	Dopamine receptor agonist	1.25–10 mg/d (given orally, once–twice daily)	Nausea, vomiting, dizziness, headache, nasal congestion, constipation, digital vasospasm, vivid dreams, anxiety, depression, impulsivity
Cabergoline	Dopamine receptor (D2 selective) agonist	0.5–>2.0 mg per wk (given orally several times per wk or daily)	Similar to bromocriptine (often better tolerated); high doses (>3 mg/d) have been associated with cardiac valvulopathy
Quinagolide (not available in United States)	Dopamine receptor agonist	0.075–0.9 mg/d (oral, once–twice daily)	Similar to bromocriptine. No risk of valvulopathy
Pergolide (not available in United States)	Dopamine receptor agonist	0.05–0.1 mg/d (oral, once daily)	Similar to bromocriptine. Withdrawn in United States in 2007 because of higher risk of valvulopathy

Acromegaly

Surgery remains the most effective treatment for acromegaly, despite the availability of medical therapy. Multiple surgical series in the literature report remission rates of the order of 50% to 65% for macroadenomas, and 70% to 90% for microadenomas.[70–72] It is difficult to compare results as definitions of remission have changed over time from postoperative random GH levels, to GH nadir in the setting of oral glucose challenge, to yet lower GH cutoff levels, and the assays used to measure GH levels have also changed over time. Results from specialized centers are generally better than those results reported from tumor registries.

Cushing Disease

Surgical results for Cushing disease have been reported in multiple surgical series.[58,73,74] Remission rates for microadenomas from 70% to 90% are generally reported. Neither the definition of remission of Cushing disease nor the tests used for postoperative surveillance have been standardized. These remain variable from center to center, making it difficult to compare results. In those patients not in remission after the initial procedure (reported rates range from approximately 2% to 25% per year), a second exploration is sometimes recommended, which can achieve remission in an additional 50% to 70% of patients.[58,75,76] While early as opposed to late reoperation is technically less challenging, delayed remissions have been reported, and it is important to determine that postoperative levels have plateaued at an elevated level before proceeding with reexploration.[77]

MANAGEMENT OF PITUITARY ADENOMAS BY SYNDROME

7 With the advent of medical therapy for some of the secretory tumors, surgical indications have changed, and surgical decision making needs to be considered in the context of the available treatment options.

Prolactinomas

Medical treatment with DAs is considered first-line therapy for most patients with prolactinomas, even those with large and invasive tumors.[7] Not all patients require treatment: patients with asymptomatic, stable microadenomas, who are not pursuing fertility (eg, postmenopausal women), can often be followed expectantly. The commonly used agents, bromocriptine and cabergoline, are both oral agents with excellent efficacy, are relatively inexpensive, and have minimal side effects (gastrointestinal disturbances and dizziness, although depression, anxiety, and impulsivity have been reported). Cabergoline is more effective and generally better tolerated than bromocriptine. Quinagolide is another agent similar in efficacy to cabergoline. High doses of cabergoline (>3 mg/d) have been associated with cardiac valvular dysfunction, but this does not appear to be a significant risk in the dose range usually prescribed for prolactinomas (typically 0.5 to 2.0 mg/wk, **Table 75.7**). The duration of the treatment is at least 2 years with 50% to 70% remission rate at 5 years after discontinuation; for many patients lifelong therapy is required.[78] Tumor regression in response to these agents is often dramatic. Long-standing visual dysfunction will often improve after tumor regression from medical treatment.

Surgical treatment is indicated if there is an insufficient response to medical therapy (persistent neurologic deficit in the setting of inadequate tumor shrinkage, persistently elevated prolactin even on high-dose medication, or intolerance to the medications), and in selected cases with high surgical cure rate when the patient prefers surgery over long-term or potentially lifelong medical treatment. Other indications for surgery include CSF leak and pituitary apoplexy, which may rarely complicate the treatment of large prolactinomas with DAs. Relative indications include cystic tumors, which may not shrink with medical treatment, and infertility in women who wish to become pregnant without medication. Surgical remission rate is >80% for intrasellar tumors but falls to <20% for tumors with an extrasellar component or with abnormal visual fields.[69] Radiation therapy can be recommended for tumors unresponsive to medical and surgical treatment.

Acromegaly

8 Surgery remains first-line treatment in patients who are good surgical candidates, likely to be cured by surgery, or have large macroadenomas, as debulking has been shown to improve subsequent biochemical control with medical therapy.[79,80] Surgery is rapidly effective in reducing GH levels, leads to immediate relief of symptoms from mass effect (visual loss), and has the potential to be curative, depending upon the size and degree of tumor invasiveness.

Pretreatment of surgical cases with somatostatin analogs (SSAs) both for improving postoperative remission rates and anesthetic risk have been debated without consensus. A meta-analysis, including 10 studies, both randomized and retrospective, showed a borderline positive effect with pretreatment that did not reach statistical significance, while analysis of the prospective controlled trials (with historically low pretreatment remission rates) demonstrated a statistically significant benefit.[81] Pretreatment in symptomatic acromegalic patients, especially those with cardiomyopathy and potential difficult airway management due to an enlarged tongue, is sometimes worthy of consideration as it may improve anesthetic risk.[82]

Table 75.8. Medications Used to Treat Acromegaly

Name	Mechanism of Action	Usual Dose Range	Adverse Effects
Octreotide acetate	Somatostatin receptor agonist (sstr2 and sstr5)	100–500 μg subcutaneously every 8 h	Gastrointestinal side effects, cholelithiasis, hyperglycemia, hypoglycemia, vitamin B12 deficiency, hypothyroidism, bradycardia, hair loss
Octreotide LAR	Somatostatin receptor agonist (sstr2 and sstr5)	10–40 mg intramuscularly every 4 wks	Similar to octreotide acetate
Lanreotide depot	Somatostatin receptor agonist (sstr2 and sstr5)	60–120 mg deep subcutaneously every 4 wks	Similar to octreotide acetate
Pasireotide LAR	Somatostatin receptor agonist (sstr2 and high sstr5)	20–60 mg intramuscularly every 4 wks	Same as octreotide acetate. Higher risk of hyperglycemia (50%)
Octreotide capsule	Somatostatin receptor agonist (sstr2 and sstr5)	40–80 mg orally, twice daily	Same as octreotide acetate. Needs to be taken on empty stomach
Cabergoline*	Dopamine receptor (D2 selective) agonist	0.5–7.0 mg by mouth weekly	Nausea, vomiting, dizziness, headache, nasal congestion, constipation, digital vasospasm, vivid dreams, anxiety, depression, impulsivity; high doses (>3 mg/d) have been associated with cardiac valvulopathy
Pegvisomant	Growth hormone receptor antagonist	5–40 mg subcutaneously daily	Lipohypertrophy, skin rash, hepatotoxicity

*Cabergoline is not approved by the FDA for use in acromegaly.

9 The available medical treatments include SSAs, DAs, and GH receptor antagonists.

The SSAs are usually the first line of medical treatment and are comprised of first-generation injectable agents (short-acting octreotide acetate, long-acting octreotide LAR, and lanreotide depot), second-generation injectable agents (pasireotide LAR) as well as oral agents (octreotide capsule). First-generation agents normalize IGF1 levels in 20% to 50% of cases and reduce tumor size in 50% of cases. The long-acting forms are given every 4 weeks and usually are well tolerated; the most common side effects are gastrointestinal disturbances and occasionally cholelithiasis and hyperglycemia.[80] The second-generation injectable agent pasireotide achieves better biochemical and tumor control but a majority of the patients develop hyperglycemia as a complication so it is usually used when first-generation agents fail.[83] Oral octreotide is the newest approved SSAs and is less efficacious than the injectable agents, though useful in milder acromegaly.[79]

Cabergoline, the most potent DA, is sometimes effective in acromegaly (leading to endocrine remission in up to 30% of cases), usually when the IGF1 level is not very elevated (<2.5 times the upper level of normal). It is an oral agent, well tolerated and relatively inexpensive. Its use in acromegaly is not FDA approved.[84]

The GH receptor pegvisomant blocks the peripheral action of GH and leads to dramatic lowering of the IGF1 level in 75% to 95% of patients but has no direct antitumoral effect. It is administered daily, subcutaneously, and can cause rash, insomnia, or hepatotoxicity. It can be used as monotherapy or as adjunctive to SSAs or cabergoline (**Table 75.8**).[85]

Radiation therapy is usually a third-line option for patients who are not in remission after surgery and do not respond to or tolerate medical therapy. A flowchart for the management of acromegaly is shown in **Algorithm 75.1**.

Cushing Disease

Surgical excision is generally considered to be first-line treatment for Cushing disease. Recurrent Cushing disease after initially successful surgery remains a significant problem and reexploration for recurrence is a reasonable option.

If transsphenoidal surgery is unsuccessful, a number of medications are available by acting at the level of the tumor (decreasing ACTH) and adrenals (inhibiting production of cortisol) or by blocking the cortisol receptors. Each medication has an associated set of side effects and none represents optimal therapy, but each may offer advantages in the individual patient. Combination therapy is at times used when hypercortisolemia cannot be controlled (**Table 75.9**).

Pasireotide and pasireotide LAR work at the level of the tumor as somatostatin receptor agonists, providing a modest degree of cortisol control and good tumor control, but 73% of patients develop hyperglycemia (severe in some cases). It is not usually used as first-line therapy but it is a good option for locally aggressive tumors.[83]

Cabergoline works at the level of the tumor as a dopamine receptor agonist and controls hypercortisolemia in about 30% of patients, but higher doses are needed (2 mg/wk) that increase the side effect frequency. Control may escape after 2 years of treatment. It is not FDA approved for treatment of Cushing disease.[86]

Several medications that inhibit different steps in cortisol synthesis in the adrenal are available, some FDA approved, some not. Ketoconazole normalizes cortisol levels in about 50% of patients but has a black box warning for liver failure, and a purified compound levoketoconazole is now in clinical trials.[87] Metyrapone is used off-label, and an updated compound, osilodrostat, was recently FDA approved. It achieves eucortisolemia in close to 80% of patients, with hypertension and hypokalemia as side effects to monitor.[88] Etomidate is a parenteral compound used for severe hypercortisolemia in critically ill patients with Cushing syndrome, and mitotane is very rarely used outside of adrenal cancer due to the severe side effects and adrenolytic effects.[89]

Mifepristone is a cortisol and progesterone receptor blocker FDA approved for treatment of patients with Cushing syndrome and hyperglycemia.[90] Hypertension, hypokalemia,

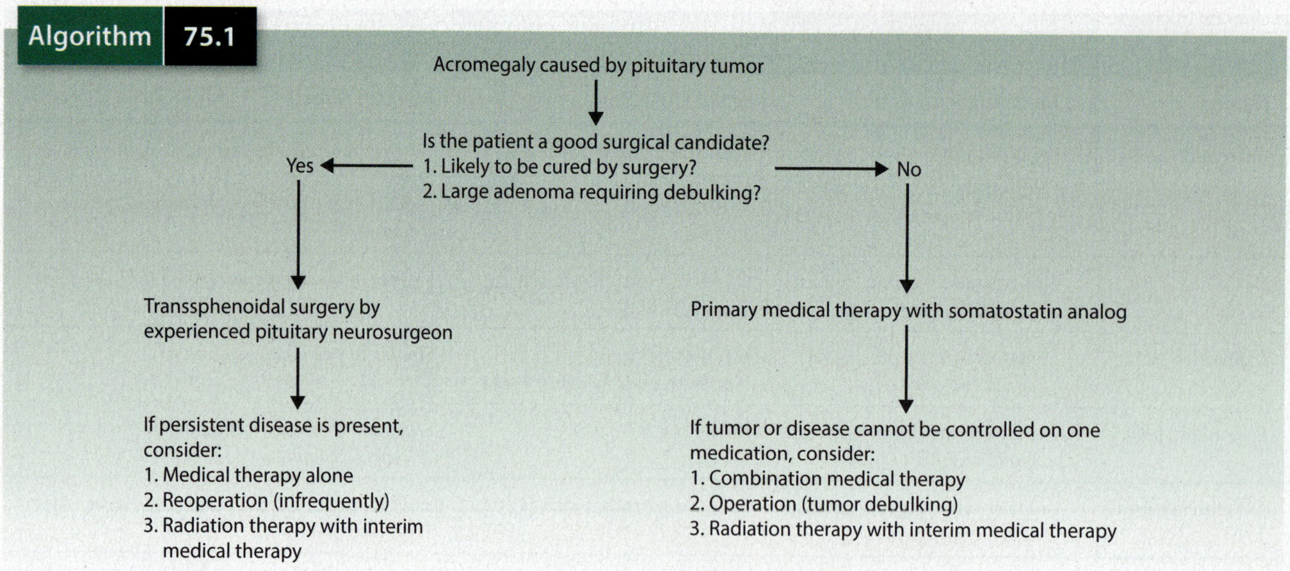

Algorithm 75.1. Treatment algorithm for acromegaly.

Table 75.9. Medications Used to Treat Cushing Disease

Name	Mechanism of Action	Usual Dose Range	Adverse Effects
Pasireotide*	Somatostatin receptor agonist (sstr1, 2, 3, and 5)	0.3–0.9 mg subcutaneously twice daily	Gastrointestinal side effects, cholelithiasis, hyperglycemia (70%), vitamin B12 deficiency, hypothyroidism, bradycardia, hair loss
Pasireotide LAR*	Somatostatin receptor agonist (sstr1, 2, 3, and 5)	10–40 mg intramuscularly every 4 wks	Similar to pasireotide
Cabergoline*	Dopamine receptor (D2 selective) agonist	0.5–7.0 mg/wk (oral, several times weekly or once per d)	Nausea, vomiting, dizziness, headache, nasal congestion, constipation, digital vasospasm, vivid dreams, anxiety, depression, impulsivity; high doses (>3 mg/d) have been associated with cardiac valvulopathy
Ketoconazole*	Adrenal steroidogenesis inhibitor	200–600 mg by mouth two to three times daily	Nausea, dyspepsia, skin rash, hepatotoxicity, hypogonadism, gynecomastia
Metyrapone*	Adrenal steroidogenesis inhibitor	250–1,000 mg by mouth three to four times daily	Nausea, dizziness, hirsutism, hypertension, edema, hypokalemia
Mitotane*	Adrenal steroidogenesis inhibitor	0.5–3.0 g by mouth three times daily	Nausea, diarrhea, dizziness, ataxia, confusion, hepatotoxicity, rash, gynecomastia, dyslipidemia, teratogenicity
Osilodrostat*	Adrenal steroidogenesis inhibitor	4–60 mg orally twice daily	Similar to metyrapone
Etomidate*	Adrenal steroidogenesis inhibitor	0.03 mg/kg intravenously as a bolus, followed by infusion: 0.1–0.3 mg/kg/h	Sedation
Mifepristone*	Glucocorticoid receptor antagonist	300–1,200 mg by mouth daily	Fatigue, headache, nausea, hypokalemia, vaginal bleeding, endometrial thickening, pregnancy termination, abnormal thyroid function tests, dyslipidemia

*Only pasireotide and mifepristone are approved by the FDA for use in Cushing disease.

Algorithm 75.2

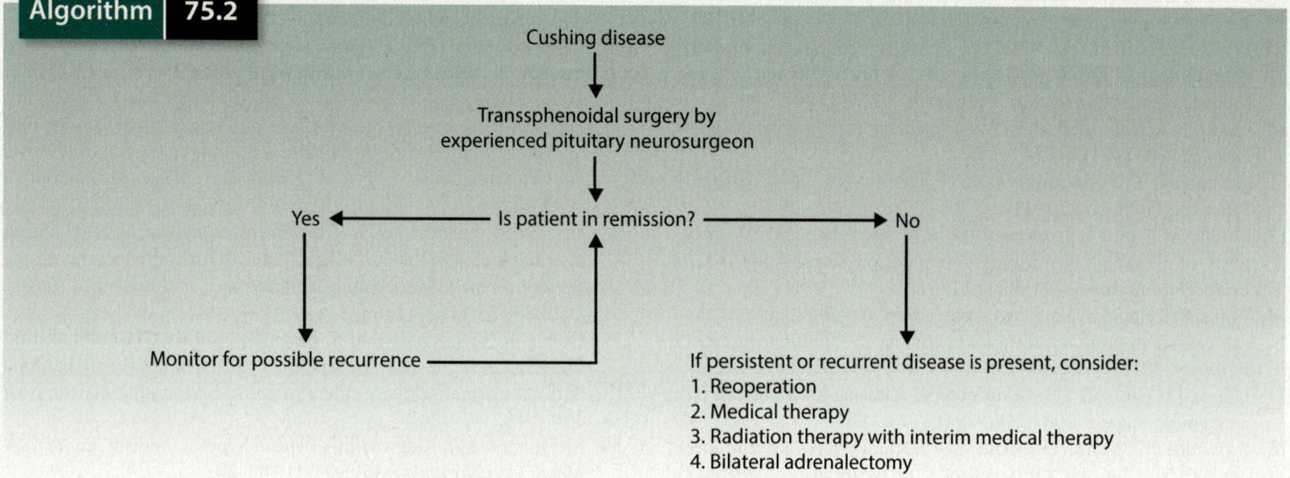

Algorithm 75.2. Treatment algorithm for Cushing disease.

and uterine hyperplasia are side effects to monitor. A purified cortisol receptor blocker is now in clinical trials.

Bilateral adrenalectomy remains a viable option, with immediate resolution of hypercortisolemia, but requires lifelong mineralocorticoid and glucocorticoid replacement. It is associated with radiographic progression of the pituitary adenoma in about half of cases, and a smaller number of patients may develop Nelson syndrome.[91]

Radiosurgery with interim medical control is often a reasonable option after unsuccessful transsphenoidal surgery; normalization of cortisol levels occurs in about 50% to 70% of patients within 2 years of treatment, but with a significant risk of anterior hypopituitarism.[92]

A flowchart for the management of Cushing disease is shown in **Algorithm 75.2.**

Nonfunctioning Tumors

Surgical removal remains first-line treatment; there are no good medical options (as the response to DAs or SSAs has been poor). Small nonfunctioning tumors (<1 cm) can be followed with serial imaging, but macroadenomas should usually be resected, especially those which are close to the chiasm or enlarging on serial scans, even without visual abnormalities. After subtotal resection it is in many cases reasonable to follow the residual tumor, with reoperation or radiation therapy reserved for those which later enlarge.[39]

Thyrotropin-Secreting Pituitary Adenomas

Pituitary surgery is first-line therapy in most cases. Patients with hyperthyroidism can be pretreated with SSAs or methimazole in order to control hyperthyroidism preoperatively, if present. After surgery, patients with residual tumors or persistent hyperthyroidism may benefit from SSA therapy, which is very effective in controlling hyperthyroidism and also affords some degree of tumor control.[93] Cabergoline can be tried if SSAs are not tolerated but efficacy seems to be low. Radiation therapy and thyroidectomy are alternative options in patients who fail to enter remission after pituitary surgery and medical therapy.

SOCIOECONOMIC CONSIDERATIONS

A number of socioeconomic considerations now affect the practice of pituitary surgery. The volume–outcome relationship, which has been shown to be manifest in a number of surgical subspecialties, holds true in pituitary surgery as well. This was originally suggested by a study showing improved outcomes for acromegaly with a dedicated pituitary surgeon.[94] Further studies have demonstrated a decrease in complication rate with increased experience, and a significant decrease in operative mortality after pituitary surgery in high-volume as opposed to low-volume centers.[95] A recent study has demonstrated that surgeon and institutional performance continue to demonstrate improvements with respect to gross total removal, biochemical remission, and complication rates, even after many hundreds of operations over more than a decade.[96] With the multiplicity of available treatment modalities, comparative cost–benefit analyses are now being performed. Treatment algorithms in acromegaly which incorporated transsphenoidal surgery were shown to be less expensive than those using medical therapy alone, and algorithms using primary surgery followed by adjunctive medical treatment as opposed to the converse approach were shown to be 30% less costly overall.[97] In Cushing disease, the economic burden of managing patient comorbidities was shown to significantly decrease after successful surgery.[98] Despite the introduction of new pharmacologic agents, it is likely that surgery will continue to play a major role in the treatment of
10 pituitary disorders; given the multiplicity of options, however, care is best individualized for a given patient in a multidisciplinary setting.

References

1. Inoshita N, Nishioka H. The 2017 WHO classification of pituitary adenoma: overview and comments. *Brain Tumor Pathol.* 2018; 35(2):51–56.
2. Rhoton AL Jr. The sellar region. *Neurosurgery.* 2002;51(4 Suppl): S335–A374.
3. Amar AP, Weiss MH. Pituitary anatomy and physiology. *Neurosurg Clin N Am.* 2003;14(1):11–23, v.
4. Le Tissier P, Campos P, Lafont C, Romanò N, Hodson DJ, Mollard P. An updated view of hypothalamic-vascular-pituitary unit function and plasticity. *Nat Rev Endocrinol.* 2017;13(5):257–267.
5. Rhoton AL Jr. The cavernous sinus, the cavernous venous plexus, and the carotid collar. *Neurosurgery.* 2002;51(4 Suppl): S375–S410.
6. Habal MB, Maniscalco JE, Lineaweaver WC, Rhoton AL Jr. Microsurgical anatomy of the optic canal: anatomical relations and exposure of the optic nerve. *Surg Forum.* 1976;27(62): 542–544.
7. Klibanski A. Clinical practice. Prolactinomas. *N Engl J Med.* 2010; 362(13):1219–1226.

8. Ezzat S, Asa SL, Couldwell WT, et al. The prevalence of pituitary adenomas: a systematic review. *Cancer*. 2004;101(3):613–619.
9. Liu X, Wang R, Li M, Chen G. Pituitary adenoma or pituitary neuroendocrine tumor: a narrative review of controversy and perspective. *Transl Cancer Res*. 2021;10(4):1916–1920.
10. Ciccarelli A, Daly AF, Beckers A. The epidemiology of prolactinomas. *Pituitary*. 2005;8(1):3–6.
11. Holdaway IM, Rajasoorya C. Epidemiology of acromegaly. *Pituitary*. 1999;2(1):29–41.
12. Lindholm J, Juul S, Jørgensen JO, et al. Incidence and late prognosis of Cushing's syndrome: a population-based study. *J Clin Endocrinol Metab*. 2001;86(1):117–123.
13. Tritos NA, Eppakayala S, Swearingen B, et al. Pathologic and clinical features of pituitary adenomas showing TSH immunoreactivity. *Pituitary*. 2013;16(3):287–293.
14. Huirne JA, Lambalk CB. Gonadotropin-releasing-hormone-receptor antagonists. *Lancet*. 2001;358(9295):1793–1803.
15. Brownlee BP, Mann D, Glenn C, McKinney KA. Nonfunctioning pituitary lesions. *Otolaryngol Clin North Am*. 2022;55(2):343–350.
16. Zada G, Woodmansee WW, Ramkissoon S, Amadio J, Nose V, Laws ER, Jr. Atypical pituitary adenomas: incidence, clinical characteristics, and implications. *J Neurosurg*. 2011;114(2):336–344.
17. Kontogeorgos G. Predictive markers of pituitary adenoma behavior. *Neuroendocrinology*. 2006;83(3-4):179–188.
18. Asa SL, Mete O, Perry A, Osamura RY. Overview of the 2022 WHO classification of pituitary tumors. *Endocr Pathol*. 2022;33(1):6–26.
19. Valassi E, Biller BM, Klibanski A, Swearingen B. Clinical features of nonpituitary sellar lesions in a large surgical series. *Clin Endocrinol (Oxf)*. 2010;73(6):798–807.
20. Larkin SJ, Ansorge O. Pathology and pathogenesis of craniopharyngiomas. *Pituitary*. 2013;16(1):9–17.
21. Brastianos PK, Santagata S. Endocrine tumors: BRAF V600E mutations in papillary craniopharyngioma. *Eur J Endocrinol*. 2016;174(4):R139–R144.
22. Brastianos PK, Twohy E, Geyer S, et al. BRAF-MEK inhibition in newly diagnosed papillary craniopharyngiomas. *N Engl J Med*. 2023;389(2):118–126.
23. Bresson D, Herman P, Polivka M, Froelich S. Sellar Lesions/Pathology. *Otolaryngol Clin North Am*. 2016;49(1):63–93.
24. Frappaz D, Dhall G, Murray MJ, et al. EANO, SNO and Euracan consensus review on the current management and future development of intracranial germ cell tumors in adolescents and young adults. *Neuro Oncol*. 2022;24(4):516–527.
25. Komninos J, Vlassopoulou V, Protopapa D, et al. Tumors metastatic to the pituitary gland: case report and literature review. *J Clin Endocrinol Metab*. 2004;89(2):574–580.
26. Giraldi E, Allen JW, Ioachimescu AG. Pituitary incidentalomas: best practices and looking ahead. *Endocr Pract*. 2023;29(1):60–68.
27. Faje AT, Sullivan R, Lawrence D, et al. Ipilimumab-induced hypophysitis: a detailed longitudinal analysis in a large cohort of patients with metastatic melanoma. *J Clin Endocrinol Metab*. 2014;99(11):4078–4085.
28. Jiang X, Zhang X. The molecular pathogenesis of pituitary adenomas: an update. *Endocrinol Metab (Seoul)*. 2013;28(4):245–254.
29. Sabatino ME, Grondona E, De Paul AL. Architects of pituitary tumour growth. *Front Endocrinol (Lausanne)*. 2022;13:924942.
30. Higham CE, Johannsson G, Shalet SM. Hypopituitarism. *Lancet*. 2016;388(10058):2403–2415.
31. Karavitaki N, Thanabalasingham G, Shore HC, et al. Do the limits of serum prolactin in disconnection hyperprolactinaemia need re-definition? A study of 226 patients with histologically verified non-functioning pituitary macroadenoma. *Clin Endocrinol (Oxf)*. 2006;65(4):524–529.
32. Serri O, Chik CL, Ur E, Ezzat S. Diagnosis and management of hyperprolactinemia. *CMAJ*. 2003;169(6):575–581.
33. Reincke M, Fleseriu M. Cushing syndrome: A review. *JAMA*. 2023;330(2):170–181.
34. Yogi-Morren D, Habra MA, Faiman C, et al. Pituitary MRI findings in patients with pituitary and ectopic ACTH-dependent Cushing syndrome: Does a 6-mm pituitary tumor size cut-off value exclude ectopic ACTH syndrome? *Endocr Pract*. 2015;21(10):1098–1103.
35. Perlman JE, Johnston PC, Hui F, et al. Pitfalls in performing and interpreting inferior petrosal sinus sampling: personal experience and literature review. *J Clin Endocrinol Metab*. 2021;106(5):e1953–e1967.
36. Sharma ST, Nieman LK. Is prolactin measurement of value during inferior petrosal sinus sampling in patients with adrenocorticotropic hormone-dependent Cushing's Syndrome? *J Endocrinol Invest*. 2013;36(11):1112–1116.
37. Dobri G, Niwattisaiwong S, Bena JF, et al. Is GH nadir during OGTT a reliable test for diagnosis of acromegaly in patients with abnormal glucose metabolism? *Endocrine*. 2019;64(1):139–146.
38. McDermott MT, Ridgway EC. Central hyperthyroidism. *Endocrinol Metab Clin North Am*. 1998;27(1):187–203.
39. Freda PU, Beckers AM, Katznelson L, et al. Pituitary incidentaloma: an endocrine society clinical practice guideline. *J Clin Endocrinol Metab*. 2011;96(4):894–904.
40. Dhandapani S, Singh H, Negm HM, Cohen S, Anand VK, Schwartz TH. Cavernous sinus invasion in pituitary adenomas: systematic review and pooled data meta-analysis of radiologic criteria and comparison of endoscopic and microscopic surgery. *World Neurosurg*. 2016;96:36–46.
41. Levy MJ, Matharu MS, Meeran K, Powell M, Goadsby PJ. The clinical characteristics of headache in patients with pituitary tumours. *Brain*. 2005;128(Pt 8):1921–1930.
42. Chapman PR, Singhal A, Gaddamanugu S, Prattipati V. Neuroimaging of the pituitary gland: practical anatomy and pathology. *Radiol Clin North Am*. 2020;58(6):1115–1133.
43. Pressman BD. Pituitary imaging. *Endocrinol Metab Clin North Am*. 2017;46(3):713–740.
44. Cucu AI, Costea CF, Perciaccante A, Donell ST, Bianucci R. The evolution of pituitary gland surgery from the ancients to the millennials. *World Neurosurg*. 2023;180:52–65.
45. Hirsch O. Endonasal method of removal of hypophyseal tumors with report of two successful cases. *JAMA*. 1910;55(9):772–774.
46. Hardy J. [Excision of pituitary adenomas by trans-sphenoidal approach]. *Union Med Can*. 1962;91:933–945.
47. Mortini P, Albano L, Barzaghi LR, Losa M. Pituitary surgery. *Presse Med*. 2021;50(4):104079.
48. Jankowski R, Auque J, Simon C, Marchal JC, Hepner H, Wayoff M. Endoscopic pituitary tumor surgery. *Laryngoscope*. 1992;102(2):198–202.
49. Tabaee A, Anand VK, Fraser JF, Brown SM, Singh A, Schwartz TH. Three-dimensional endoscopic pituitary surgery. *Neurosurgery*. 2009;64(5 Suppl 2):288–293; discussion 294–5.
50. Yu SY, Du Q, Yao SY, et al. Outcomes of endoscopic and microscopic transsphenoidal surgery on non-functioning pituitary adenomas: a systematic review and meta-analysis. *J Cell Mol Med*. 2018;22(3):2023–2027.
51. Juthani RG, Reiner AS, Patel AR, et al. Radiographic and clinical outcomes using intraoperative magnetic resonance imaging for transsphenoidal resection of pituitary adenomas. *J Neurosurg*. 2020;134(6):1824–1835.
52. Cooke RS, Jones RA. Experience with the direct transnasal transsphenoidal approach to the pituitary fossa. *Br J Neurosurg*. 1994;8(2):193–196.
53. Gstrein NA, Zwicky S, Serra C, et al. Rhinologic outcome of endoscopic transnasal-transsphenoidal pituitary surgery: an institutional series, systematic review, and meta-analysis. *Eur Arch Otorhinolaryngol*. 2023;280(9):4091–4099.
54. Younus I, Gerges MM, Dobri GA, Ramakrishna R, Schwartz TH. Readmission after endoscopic transsphenoidal pituitary surgery: analysis of 584 consecutive cases. *J Neurosurg*. 2019;133(4):1242–1247.
55. Winograd D, Staggers KA, Sebastian S, Takashima M, Yoshor D, Samson SL. An effective and practical fluid restriction protocol to

decrease the risk of hyponatremia and readmissions after transsphenoidal surgery. *Neurosurgery*. 2020;87(4):761–769.

56. Verbalis JG, Goldsmith SR, Greenberg A, et al. Diagnosis, evaluation, and treatment of hyponatremia: expert panel recommendations. *Am J Med*. 2013;126(10 Suppl 1):S1–S42.
57. Polovina TS, Kraljevic I, Solak M, et al. Early basal cortisol level as a predictor of hypothalamic-pituitary-adrenal (HPA) axis function after pituitary tumor surgery. *Exp Clin Endocrinol Diabetes*. 2020;128(11):709–714.
58. Roelfsema F, Biermasz NR, Pereira AM. Clinical factors involved in the recurrence of pituitary adenomas after surgical remission: a structured review and meta-analysis. *Pituitary*. 2012;15(1):71–83.
59. Singh H, Essayed WI, Cohen-Gadol A, Zada G, Schwartz TH. Resection of pituitary tumors: endoscopic versus microscopic. *J Neurooncol*. 2016;130(2):309–317.
60. Almutairi RD, Muskens IS, Cote DJ, et al. Gross total resection of pituitary adenomas after endoscopic vs. microscopic transsphenoidal surgery: a meta-analysis. *Acta Neurochir (Wien)*. 2018;160(5):1005–1021.
61. Dorward NL. Endocrine outcomes in endoscopic pituitary surgery: a literature review. *Acta Neurochir (Wien)*. 2010;152(8):1275–1279.
62. Tabaee A, Anand VK, Barrón Y, et al. Endoscopic pituitary surgery: a systematic review and meta-analysis. *J Neurosurg*. 2009;111(3):545–554.
63. Jagannathan J, Smith R, DeVroom HL, et al. Outcome of using the histological pseudocapsule as a surgical capsule in Cushing disease. *J Neurosurg*. 2009;111(3):531–539.
64. Gao Y, Zhong C, Wang Y, et al. Endoscopic versus microscopic transsphenoidal pituitary adenoma surgery: a meta-analysis. *World J Surg Oncol*. 2014;12:94.
65. Enseñat J, Quesada JL, Aparicio J, et al. [Prospective comparative study on 50 patients between microsurgical sublabial transsphenoidal approach and endoscopic endonasal transsphenoidal approach]. *Neurocirugia (Astur)*. 2009;20(4):335–344; discussion 344–345.
66. Bastos RV, Silva CM, Tagliarini JV, et al. Endoscopic versus microscopic transsphenoidal surgery in the treatment of pituitary tumors: systematic review and meta-analysis of randomized and non-randomized controlled trials. *Arch Endocrinol Metab*. 2016;60(5):411–419.
67. Han ZL, He DS, Mao ZG, Wang HJ. Cerebrospinal fluid rhinorrhea following trans-sphenoidal pituitary macroadenoma surgery: experience from 592 patients. *Clin Neurol Neurosurg*. 2008;110(6):570–579.
68. Bou-Nassif R, Abou-Mrad Z, El Ahmadieh TY, Tabar V, Cohen MA. Patient-reported outcomes in endoscopic endonasal skull base surgery. *Endocrinol Metab Clin North Am*. 2022;51(4):727–739.
69. Kreutzer J, Buslei R, Wallaschofski H, et al. Operative treatment of prolactinomas: indications and results in a current consecutive series of 212 patients. *Eur J Endocrinol*. 2008;158(1):11–18.
70. Shin SS, Tormenti MJ, Paluzzi A, et al. Endoscopic endonasal approach for growth hormone secreting pituitary adenomas: outcomes in 53 patients using 2010 consensus criteria for remission. *Pituitary*. 2013;16(4):435–444.
71. Starke RM, Raper DM, Payne SC, Vance ML, Oldfield EH, Jane JA Jr. Endoscopic vs microsurgical transsphenoidal surgery for acromegaly: outcomes in a concurrent series of patients using modern criteria for remission. *J Clin Endocrinol Metab*. 2013;98(8):3190–3198.
72. Wagenmakers MA, Netea-Maier RT, van Lindert EJ, Pieters GF, Grotenhuis AJ, Hermus AR. Results of endoscopic transsphenoidal pituitary surgery in 40 patients with a growth hormone-secreting macroadenoma. *Acta Neurochir (Wien)*. 2011;153(7):1391–1399.
73. Wagenmakers MA, Boogaarts HD, Roerink SH, et al. Endoscopic transsphenoidal pituitary surgery: a good and safe primary treatment option for Cushing's disease, even in case of macroadenomas or invasive adenomas. *Eur J Endocrinol*. 2013;169(3):329–337.
74. Honegger J, Schmalisch K, Beuschlein F, et al. Contemporary microsurgical concept for the treatment of Cushing's disease: endocrine outcome in 83 consecutive patients. *Clin Endocrinol (Oxf)*. 2012;76(4):560–567.
75. Patil CG, Veeravagu A, Prevedello DM, Katznelson L, Vance ML, Laws ER Jr. Outcomes after repeat transsphenoidal surgery for recurrent Cushing's disease. *Neurosurgery*. 2008;63(2):266–270; discussion 270–271.
76. Ram Z, Nieman LK, Cutler GB Jr, Chrousos GP, Doppman JL, Oldfield EH. Early repeat surgery for persistent Cushing's disease. *J Neurosurg*. 1994;80(1):37–45.
77. Valassi E, Biller BM, Swearingen B, et al. Delayed remission after transsphenoidal surgery in patients with Cushing's disease. *J Clin Endocrinol Metab*. 2010;95(2):601–610.
78. Colao A, Di Sarno A, Cappabianca P, Di Somma C, Pivonello R, Lombardi G. Withdrawal of long-term cabergoline therapy for tumoral and nontumoral hyperprolactinemia. *N Engl J Med*. 2003;349(21):2023–2033.
79. Melmed S, Popovic V, Bidlingmaier M, et al. Safety and efficacy of oral octreotide in acromegaly: results of a multicenter phase III trial. *J Clin Endocrinol Metab*. 2015;100(4):1699–1708.
80. Newman CB, Melmed S, Snyder PJ, et al. Safety and efficacy of long-term octreotide therapy of acromegaly: results of a multicenter trial in 103 patients–a clinical research center study. *J Clin Endocrinol Metab*. 1995;80(9):2768–2775.
81. Pita-Gutierrez F, Pertega-Diaz S, Pita-Fernandez S, et al. Place of preoperative treatment of acromegaly with somatostatin analog on surgical outcome: a systematic review and meta-analysis. *PLoS One*. 2013;8(4):e61523.
82. Ben-Shlomo A, Melmed S. Clinical review 154: The role of pharmacotherapy in perioperative management of patients with acromegaly. *J Clin Endocrinol Metab*. 2003;88(3):963–968.
83. Colao A, Bronstein MD, Freda P, et al. Pasireotide versus octreotide in acromegaly: a head-to-head superiority study. *J Clin Endocrinol Metab*. 2014;99(3):791–799.
84. Sandret L, Maison P, Chanson P. Place of cabergoline in acromegaly: a meta-analysis. *J Clin Endocrinol Metab*. 2011;96(5):1327–1335.
85. van der Lely AJ, Hutson RK, Trainer PJ, et al. Long-term treatment of acromegaly with pegvisomant, a growth hormone receptor antagonist. *Lancet*. 2001;358(9295):1754–1759.
86. Godbout A, Manavela M, Danilowicz K, Beauregard H, Bruno OD, Lacroix A. Cabergoline monotherapy in the long-term treatment of Cushing's disease. *Eur J Endocrinol*. 2010;163(5):709–716.
87. Pivonello R, Zacharieva S, Elenkova A, et al. Levoketoconazole in the treatment of patients with endogenous Cushing's syndrome: a double-blind, placebo-controlled, randomized withdrawal study (LOGICS). *Pituitary*. 2022;25(6):911–926.
88. Fleseriu M, Pivonello R, Young J, et al. Osilodrostat, a potent oral 11β-hydroxylase inhibitor: 22-week, prospective, Phase II study in Cushing's disease. *Pituitary*. 2016;19(2):138–148.
89. Pence A, McGrath M, Lee SL, Raines DE. Pharmacological management of severe Cushing's syndrome: the role of etomidate. *Ther Adv Endocrinol Metab*. 2022;13:20420188211058583.
90. Fleseriu M, Biller BM, Findling JW, Molitch ME, Schteingart DE, Gross C; SEISMIC Study Investigators. Mifepristone, a glucocorticoid receptor antagonist, produces clinical and metabolic benefits in patients with Cushing's syndrome. *J Clin Endocrinol Metab*. 2012;97(6):2039–2049.
91. Assié G, Bahurel H, Coste J, et al. Corticotroph tumor progression after adrenalectomy in Cushing's disease: A reappraisal of Nelson's syndrome. *J Clin Endocrinol Metab*. 2007;92(1):172–179.
92. Sheehan JP, Xu Z, Salvetti DJ, Schmitt PJ, Vance ML. Results of gamma knife surgery for Cushing's disease. *J Neurosurg*. 2013;119(6):1486–1492.
93. Kuhn JM, Arlot S, Lefebvre H, et al. Evaluation of the treatment of thyrotropin-secreting pituitary adenomas with a slow release formulation of the somatostatin analog lanreotide. *J Clin Endocrinol Metab*. 2000;85(4):1487–1491.
94. Gittoes NJ, Sheppard MC, Johnson AP, Stewart PM. Outcome of surgery for acromegaly—the experience of a dedicated pituitary surgeon. *Qjm*. 1999;92(12):741–745.
95. Barker FG, 2nd, Klibanski A, Swearingen B. Transsphenoidal surgery for pituitary tumors in the United States, 1996–2000:

mortality, morbidity, and the effects of hospital and surgeon volume. *J Clin Endocrinol Metab*. 2003;88(10):4709–4719.

96. Younus I, Gerges MM, Uribe-Cardenas R, et al. The slope of the learning curve in 600 consecutive endoscopic transsphenoidal pituitary surgeries. *Acta Neurochir (Wien)*. 2020;162(10):2361–2370.

97. Biermasz NR, Roelfsema F, Pereira AM, Romijn JA. Cost-effectiveness of lanreotide Autogel in treatment algorithms of acromegaly. *Expert Rev Pharmacoecon Outcomes Res*. 2009;9(3):223–234.

98. Swearingen B, Wu N, Chen SY, Pulgar S, Biller BM. Health care resource use and costs among patients with Cushing disease. *Endocr Pract*. 2011;17(5):681–690.

Lung Neoplasms

Robert E. Merritt

Key Points

1 Lung cancer remains the leading cause of cancer-related death in the United States.

2 Advances in the detection of somatic mutations in non–small cell lung carcinoma (NSCLC) have yielded targeted therapeutic molecular treatments for patients with metastatic lung carcinoma.

3 Non–small lung cancer is the most common lung neoplasm followed by small cell lung carcinoma (SCLC).

4 The common sites of metastatic spread include the brain, bone, adrenal glands, and liver. A metastatic evaluation includes positron emission tomography and computed tomography (PET-CT) scan, CT scan of the chest and abdomen, and a brain magnetic resonance imaging (MRI).

5 Anatomical lung resection remains the gold standard treatment for early-stage non–small cell lung carcinoma (NSCLC). Thoracoscopic and robotic-assisted approaches are increasing in utilization with similar results to thoracotomy.

6 Pulmonary carcinoid tumors are relatively indolent neoplasms of the lung that are effectively treated with surgical resection.

Lung neoplasms can be classified histologically as malignant or benign.[1] NSCLC is the most common malignant lung neoplasm
1 encountered in clinical practice. The histologic classifications of lung neoplasms are further classified as SCLC and large cell lung carcinoma (**Table 76.1**). Carcinoid and carcinoma of the salivary glands are also classified as malignant lung neoplasms. Benign lung neoplasms that are commonly encountered in clinical practice include hamartoma, adenoma, and myelolipoma (**Table 76.2**). Benign neoplasms of the lung rarely require surgical management; therefore, this chapter will focus on malignant neoplasms that require surgical removal in many cases.

Although population estimates of both the incidence and mortality of lung cancer have begun to decline, lung cancer remains second only to heart disease among all causes of mortality. With 238,340 new cases and 127,070 deaths projected for 2023, lung cancer remains the leading cause of cancer-related death in the United States. Lung cancer is second in cancer prevalence, only to prostate cancer among men and breast cancer among women, and remains the leading cause of cancer-related death for both sexes. Since 2005, both the annual incidence and mortality rates due to lung cancer have started to decrease in the United States, reflecting improvements in cancer control and prevention, particularly efforts to reduce the prevalence of smoking.[2] There is also significant regional variation in both lung cancer incidence and mortality. Among men, lung cancer mortality has decreased from 1996 through 2005 in over 80% of the 50 states and the District of Columbia, whereas among women over the same period, mortality decreased in only three states (California, New Jersey, and Texas) and has increased in 13 other states, primarily in the Midwest and South, although more recently consistent rates of decline have been noted for both men and women.[3]

The best predictor of survival for patients with lung cancer is based on staging and effective treatment strategies. Anatomical pulmonary resection remains the gold standard treatment for lung cancer, yet only approximately 37% of all patients diagnosed with lung cancer are considered surgically resectable at the time of presentation. Even among patients who have undergone complete surgical resection with curative intent for early-stage lung cancer, as determined using pathologic *T*umor–*N*ode–*M*etastasis (TNM) criteria, a substantial number will have recurrence of their cancer (**Table 76.3**).[4]

Multiple randomized clinical trials have demonstrated that adjuvant chemotherapy has improved overall survival over surgery alone for early-stage lung cancer in patients with positive lymph nodes.[5,6] In addition, lung cancer screening low-dose chest CT appears to improve early detection of resectable lung cancer with an improvement in overall survival in a high-risk population.[7–9] As understanding of molecular changes occurring in lung cancer evolves, new strategies that allow for early detection and classification of lung cancer will provide valuable information for the treatment of patients.

EPIDEMIOLOGY

Lung carcinoma is the leading cause of cancer-related death in the United States. The Surveillance, Epidemiology, and End Results (SEER) program estimated that 222,500 people were diagnosed with lung cancer in 2017, and lung cancer comprised 13.2% of all new cancer cases.[10] The prevalence of lung cancer is the Unites States is estimated to be at 408,800 people and accounted for 25.9% of cancer deaths, which is estimated to reach 155,870 cases in 2015. From 2005 to 2015, the number of lung cancer cases per 100,000 individuals has decreased from 63.0 to 54.5, and the number of lung cancer deaths has decreased from 52.9 to 45.0. Despite the improvements in the incidence and death rate for lung cancer, lung cancer still accounts for more cancer-related deaths than the combined cancer-related deaths for breast cancer, prostate cancer, colon cancer, bladder cancer, and melanoma combined. The current median age for the diagnosis of lung cancer in the United States is 70, and 30% of cases occur in patients between the ages of 65 and 74. The current survival rate for lung carcinoma is 18.1% for patients in the United States. The highest incidence of lung cancer occurs in African-American

Table 76.1. WHO Histologic Classification of Malignant Lung Neoplasms
1. Keratinizing squamous cell carcinoma
2. Nonkeratinizing squamous cell carcinoma   2.1 Basaloid

3. Adenocarcinoma
  3.1 Acinar adenocarcinoma
  3.2 Papillary adenocarcinoma
  3.3 Lepidic adenocarcinoma
  3.4 Solid adenocarcinoma
  3.5 Invasive mucinous
  3.6 Minimally invasive adenocarcinoma
  3.7 Adenocarcinoma in situ

4. Small cell carcinoma   4.1 Combined small cell carcinoma
5. Large cell neuroendocrine carcinoma
6. Adenosquamous carcinoma
7. Carcinoma with pleomorphic, sarcomatoid, or sarcomatous elements

8. Carcinoid tumor of the lung
  8.1 Atypical
  8.2 Typical

9. Carcinoma of salivary gland type
  9.1 Mucoepidermoid carcinoma
  9.2 Adenoid cystic carcinoma
  9.3 Epithelial-myoepithelial

males with 83.7 cases/100,000 persons. The incidence of lung cancer in Caucasian males is 65.9 cases/100,000 persons.

MOLECULAR TUMOR GENOMICS

The origin of carcinogenesis is caused by a series of genetic alterations in metabolic pathways in individual cells resulting in defective cell growth and differentiation served as the basis for modern molecular therapy for lung cancer.[11] The epidermal growth factor receptor (EGFR) consists of four different transmembrane kinases that regulate the cell cycle and overexpression of the EGFR receptor has been detected in NSCLC.[12] Targeted molecular therapy has been shown to have clinical
2 benefit notably for patients with advanced NSCLC. For example, among patients whose tumors are shown to carry specific somatic mutations in the EGFR gene, treatment with small-molecule tyrosine–kinase inhibitors targeting EGFR has been associated with improved progression-free survival as demonstrated by several randomized trials.[13] Whether such treatment regimens might be effective in the adjuvant setting for patients with early-stage NSCLC who have undergone curative-intent lung resection has yet to be established, but is the focus of a recently initiated cooperative group trial. The Adjuvant Lung Cancer Enrichment Marker Identification and Sequencing Trials (ALCHEMIST) will evaluate patients with resected lung adenocarcinomas (stage IB to stage IIIA). Those subjects found to have tumors carrying activating EGFR mutations or the echinoderm microtubule-associated protein-like 4 (EML4-ALK) fusion gene will be randomized to maintenance therapy with either erlotinib (EGFR) or crizotinib (ALK fusion), respectively, following completion of standard-of-care adjuvant chemotherapy with or without radiation therapy. Enrolled patients found to have neither of the targeted mutations will be followed in an observational study until tumor recurrence. These studies represent an exciting potential application of gene expression studies for use in determining patient prognosis, as well as guiding the clinical management of lung cancer and preventing the undertreatment of patients with NSCLC.

Table 76.2. WHO Histologic Classification of Benign Lung Neoplasms

1. Papillomas
  1.1 Squamous cell papilloma
  1.2 Exophytic
  1.3 Inverted
  1.4 Mixed squamous

2. Adenomas
  2.1 Sclerosing pneumocytoma
  2.2 Alveolar adenoma
  2.3 Papillary adenoma
  2.4 Mucinous cystadenoma

3. Pulmonary hamartoma
4. Chondroma
5. Teratoma

6. PEComa
  6.1 Benign
  6.2 Clear cell

3 NON–SMALL CELL LUNG CARCINOMA

Overview

Patients with suspected lung carcinoma typically present with a constellation of clinical findings.[14] In some cases, symptoms may not be present. The clinical evaluation for lung cancer includes history, physical examination, radiographic imaging studies, and risk factor assessment. The history should focus on symptoms such as cough, hemoptysis, weight loss, and cigarette smoking status. In addition, neurologic symptoms such as headache, gait imbalance, and motor weakness could indicate central nervous system involvement. The physical examination should focus on the cardiopulmonary system and the supraclavicular and cervical lymph nodes. Diagnosis and staging of lung carcinoma is typically achieved with a combination of diagnostic imaging studies, such as CT and PET. Histologic confirmation of the primary lung carcinoma may require fine-needle aspiration (FNA) with CT guidance, bronchoscopy with biopsy, or video-assisted thoracoscopic surgery (VATS). To determine the staging and extent of tumor involvement, the elements of the tumor (T), the regional and distal lymph nodes (N), and distant metastatic disease need to be elucidated. The determination of effective treatment depends on a careful evaluation of clinical staging for optimal results. Various professional medical organizations have created evidence-based clinical guidelines for the diagnosis, staging, and management of lung carcinoma.[15–18]

Diagnosis for Non–small Cell Lung Carcinoma

The diagnosis of lung carcinoma is accomplished with a combination of diagnostic tools that can determine the histologic diagnosis. Sputum cytology is a rarely used diagnostic test, but is safe and noninvasive. The diagnostic specificity of sputum cytology is 99% but the specificity is relatively low in most cases; therefore, the test is not widely utilized in the diagnostic workup for lung carcinoma.[19] Flexible fiberoptic bronchoscopy is a commonly utilized, safe, and effective diagnostic technique for the diagnosis of lung carcinoma. The overall complication rate for flexible bronchoscopy is relatively low and many diagnostic procedures can be performed. Endobronchial biopsy, brushings, bronchoalveolar lavage, and transbronchial

Table 76.3. Comparison of 8th and 7th Editions of TNM Classification for Lung Cancer

Descriptor	7th Edition TNM	8th Edition TNM
T Component		
0 cm (pure lepidic adenocarcinoma ≤3 cm in size)	T1a if <2 cm; T1b if >2–3 cm	Tis (adenocarcinoma in situ)
≤0.5 cm invasive size (lepidic predominant adenocarcinoma <3 cm total size)	T1a if <2 cm; T1b if >2–3 cm	T1 mi (minimally invasive)
≤1 cm	T1a	T1a
>1–2 cm	T1a	T1b
>2–4 cm	T1b	T1c
>3–4 cm	T2a	T2a
>4–5 cm	T2a	T2b
>5–7 cm	T2b	T3
>7 cm	T3	T4
Bronchus <2 cm from carina	T3	T2
Total atelectasis/pneumonitis	T3	T2
Invasion of diaphragm	T3	T4
Invasion of mediastinal pleura	T3	—
N Component		
No assessment, no involvement, or involvement of regional lymph nodes	NX, N0, N1, N2, N3	NX, N0, N1, N2, N3
M Component		
Metastasis within the thoracic cavity	M1a	M1a
Single extra thoracic metastasis	M1b	M1b
Multiple extra thoracic metastasis	M1b	M1b

needle aspiration can be performed with fiberoptic bronchoscopy. For central lung tumors, flexible bronchoscopy is very effective for diagnosis, and the overall sensitivity is as high as 88%.[14] Flexible bronchoscopy is most effective for lung carcinoma located in the central airways; however, peripheral lung tumors are difficult to access with standard flexible bronchoscopy. Image-guided biopsy technology such as electromagnetic navigational bronchoscopy (ENB) allows surgeons and pulmonologist to navigate to peripheral lung tumors and perform FNA biopsy. The reported sensitivity for ENB is 77% due to the limitation of not having real-time imaging available during the performance of the FNA biopsy.[20]

For the diagnosis of peripheral lung nodules, transthoracic needle aspiration (TTNA) is utilized in conjunction with CT to enhance diagnostic yield. The technique is very safe and effective; however, there is a 15% risk of postprocedure pneumothorax and 7% risk of developing a pneumothorax that requires chest tube thoracostomy.[21] The diagnostic sensitivity of TTNA is greater than 90% and the false-negative rate can be as high a 20% to 30%.[22] TTNA is very effective in obtaining a diagnosis of primary lung carcinomas, particularly for peripheral lung nodules. For patients with lung nodules that are in areas of the lung that are not accessible with TTNA, VATS offers a minimally invasive approach to perform a wedge resection. Lung nodules that are located on the outer third of the lung parenchyma are easily accessible for a diagnostic wedge excision; however, lung nodules that are located deeper in the lung parenchyma are more challenging to access with the VATS approach. Smaller lung nodules that are less than 1 cm in diameter pose a challenge to localize and perform a wedge excision for diagnostic biopsy. Needle localization, methylene blue injection, and radio-opaque fiducial marker placement can greatly enhance the ability to localize small lung nodules with the VATS technique.[23,24]

Staging of Non–Small Cell Lung Carcinoma

4 The clinical staging of lung carcinoma is paramount to determining the extent of tumor dissemination, which has implications on treatment decisions and overall prognosis. Optimal clinical staging can be determined with a careful assessment of tumor (T), node (N), and metastasis (M) utilizing invasive and noninvasive diagnostic methods. The lung cancer staging system has changed and undergone many revisions over the past several years. The original survival analysis was led by Mountain and colleagues.[25] The definitions for TNM staging system were further refined by Goldstraw and colleagues through the International Association for the Study of Lung Cancer (IASLC) staging project to develop a statistically valid foundation for the 8th edition of the TNM staging system.[26,27] The American Joint Committee on Cancer (AJCC) and the Union for International Cancer Control (UICC) utilizes the IASLC-TNM staging system recommendations into an international staging system for lung carcinoma. For the current AJCC 8th edition staging system of lung carcinoma, the IASLC collected

over 94,708 NSCLC cases from multiple institutions from multiple countries between 1990 and 2010.

The aims of the initial evaluation of a patient with NSCLC are to determine whether distant metastatic disease is present and to assess the extent of intrathoracic disease. A multidisciplinary approach, involving input from pulmonary medicine, chest radiology, medical and radiation oncology, and thoracic surgery, should be undertaken in the selection of the most appropriate diagnostic testing for any individual patient. A thorough history and physical examination, combined with a plain chest radiograph and baseline laboratory data (complete blood cell count and measurement of serum sodium, calcium, alkaline phosphatase, and lactate dehydrogenase levels), can suggest the presence of distant metastasis disease. The most common sites for metastatic for NSCLC include the brain, supraclavicular lymph nodes, bones, liver, adrenal glands, and contralateral lungs. An extensive metastatic workup is recommended and should include a CT scan of the chest and abdomen, an MRI of the brain, and a whole-body fluorodeoxyglucose (FDG)-PET scan. To confirm the histologic diagnosis, a biopsy by FNA or bronchoscopy can be performed to obtain confirmation of malignancy and to determine the extent of disease.

If the initial clinical evaluation does not demonstrate evidence of distant disease, the extent of further evaluation by additional imaging studies is controversial. Some clinicians routinely perform a complete metastatic workup with a CT scan of the chest and abdomen, CT or MRI of the brain, and FDG-PET scan. A CT scan of the chest and upper abdomen as well as FDG-PET scan have become standard to evaluate the extent of the primary tumor and the status of the mediastinal lymph nodes and to detect metastases in the contralateral lung, liver, bones, or the adrenal glands. Additional imaging studies in asymptomatic patients may detect the 5% to 10% of metastases that are occult, but these imaging studies are not clearly cost effective in patients with clinical stage I tumors. In patients who are acceptable candidates for pulmonary resection and have a suspicious solitary pulmonary nodule that is indeterminate despite appropriate evaluation, an excisional biopsy with a wedge resection and subsequent lobectomy for surgically resectable lung cancer should be pursued.[28]

The evaluation of the mediastinal lymph nodes for NSCLC is very critical for accurate staging and multimodality treatment which consists of neoadjuvant chemoradiation.[29] Chest CT scans provide only anatomic confirmation for tumor involvement of mediastinal lymph nodes based on enlarged size greater than 10 mm. A meta-analysis of over 3,400 evaluable patients demonstrated a pooled sensitivity of 57% and specificity of only 82% for CT scans. This meta-analysis also demonstrated that FDG-PET scanning appears to provide increased sensitivity of 84% and specificity of 89% in over 1,100 patients studied for the detection of mediastinal malignancy.[30] Several prospective studies have also demonstrated a superior diagnostic accuracy of FDG-PET imaging.[31–33] Although the overall sensitivity and specificity of FDG-PET mediastinal lymph node staging was 61% and 84%, respectively, there was a significant improvement with FDG-PET over chest CT scans in the detection of both hilar (N1) lymph node (42% vs 13%, $P = .0177$) and mediastinal (N2 and N3) tumor involvement (58% vs 32%, $P = .004$). Whereas FDG-PET scanning can increase the suspicion of malignancy, the negative predictive value for mediastinal lymph node metastasis does not appear to be sufficient with a false-negative rate reported as high as 13%.[34] FDG-PET evaluation of the solitary pulmonary nodule also appears to be somewhat insensitive, with a negative predictive value for benign lesions of only 57%, indicating a false-negative rate of 47%. Reliance on this modality could lead to delayed treatment for resectable early-stage NSCLC.[35]

Clinical staging for NSCLC can be accomplished by needle aspiration utilizing several approaches, including endobronchial ultrasound (EBUS) and endoscopic ultrasound (EUS). EBUS-guided transbronchial biopsy has been shown to be safe, effective, and similar in accuracy to cervical mediastinoscopy.[36] EUS with FNA (EUS-FNA) can be utilized to biopsy the mediastinal lymph nodes in the subcarinal, paratracheal, and aortopulmonary window. Cervical mediastinoscopy remains an important diagnostic modality for sampling mediastinal lymph nodes. This modality has a procedural sensitivity greater than 90%, and specificity of 100%.[37]

Treatment

Pulmonary resection remains the gold standard treatment for
5 stage I, II, and selected stage III NSCLC. The extent of resection, segmentectomy, lobectomy, bilobectomy, or pneumonectomy, is determined by the location and size of the primary tumor and also whether adjacent bronchopulmonary nodes are involved. At operation, tumor extent is evaluated by examination of the parietal pleura, pericardium, and mediastinal structures. Complete resection must achieve microscopically negative bronchial and vascular margins. If a tumor extends directly into the chest wall, diaphragm, or pericardium, an en bloc resection of the adjacent involved structures should be performed with the pulmonary resection. If there is endobronchial involvement present, the tumor can be surgically resected by lobectomy with segmental resection of the bronchus and/or pulmonary artery (bronchovascular sleeve resection), thus preserving lung function.

Patients with centrally located tumors should undergo sleeve lobectomy rather than pneumonectomy if complete resection can be achieved and such an approach is technically feasible. Several retrospective studies have demonstrated that operative mortality is reduced among patients undergoing sleeve lobectomy (0% to 5.2%) when compared with patients undergoing pneumonectomy (1.7% to 8.9%).[38–41] Moreover, overall 5-year survival is improved among patients undergoing sleeve resection, particularly among those with N0 or N1 nodal status. For peripherally located clinical stage I tumors, particularly among patients with limited pulmonary reserve or those at high risk from other comorbidities, segmental or nonanatomic wedge resection can be performed. Whether such patients are at greater risk for locoregional recurrence as suggested in earlier series, sublobar lung resection is under investigation in an ongoing multi-institutional prospective and randomized cooperative group clinical trial (CALGB 140503).[42–45]

Long-term survival after resection for NSCLC is linked to the pathologic stage of disease. The overall 5-year survival rates range from 60% to 70% for stage I tumors, from 40% to 50% for stage II tumors, and from 15% to 30% for stage IIIA tumors. Nodal involvement has the strongest adverse influence on survival. Large peripheral tumors that extend directly into the chest wall without nodal involvement (T3N0) are associated with a 5-year survival rate of 40% after complete resection, whereas involvement of mediastinal nodes is associated with only a 20% survival rate.

Some series suggest that histology also affects survival. In node-negative NSCLC, large cell neuroendocrine differentiation conferred worse survival than other types of NSCLC.[46] Different adenocarcinoma subtypes, particularly in more advanced tumors, also appear to confer worse prognosis, but the influence of histology has not been described uniformly in series to date.[47] Delineation of tumor biology by more refined histologic and molecular analyses will be needed to define which patients might be at increased risk for recurrence or treatment resistance.

The predominant sites of relapse for all stages of NSCLC after resection are distant metastases. Approximately 30% of recurrences are locoregional with tumors of both squamous and nonsquamous histology.[48] For all stages of disease, the brain is the single most common site of relapse, and brain metastases occur more frequently with nonsquamous tumors. Other common metastatic sites include bone, ipsilateral or contralateral lung, liver, and the adrenal glands.[49] At least 60% of recurrences develop in the first 2 years after operation, and virtually all recurrences related to the original primary tumor occur within 5 years after surgical resection. Even the small proportion of patients with stage II or III disease who survive 5 years are likely to survive 10 years or more postoperatively. Recurrences of the original primary tumor are uncommon after 5 years, and after that time, the occurrence of new pulmonary cancers becomes the dominant problem. The risk for development of a second lung cancer in patients with a prior history of cancer resection for NSCLC is estimated to be 2% to 3% per patient per year, with a second lung cancer developing rarely in never-smokers at the time of initial resection, and at rates of 1.8% per patient-year in former smokers and 2.7% per patient-year in current smokers.[50,51] Patients also face a consistent risk for the development of new, nonpulmonary primary cancers during the first 5 years after operation.

PULMONARY CARCINOID TUMORS

6 Carcinoid tumors, which are neoplasms with a low-grade malignant potential, account for about 2% of lung tumors in the United States. They arise from neuroendocrine stem cells of the bronchial epithelium and are classified as either typical or atypical. Histologically, typical carcinoids consist of uniform polygonal cells with round nuclei and fine granular chromatin (**Fig. 76.1**). Mitotic figures are rarely seen. Atypical carcinoids show increased mitotic activity, nuclear pleomorphism, and areas of disorganized architecture and tumor necrosis (**Fig. 76.2**).[52]

Carcinoid tumors occur equally in both sexes and at a median age of 55 years. Half of patients present with pulmonary symptoms, including hemoptysis, dyspnea, and recurrent or persistent pneumonitis because 40% of lesions are centrally located in the main or lobar bronchi. The lesions may be diagnosed by bronchoscopy, appearing as pink or purple friable endobronchial masses covered by intact epithelium. In the other half of patients, carcinoid tumors are diagnosed when radiologic abnormalities are detected on a chest roentgenogram as part of a routine examination.[53] Lymph node metastases occur in approximately 10% to 15% of patients at diagnosis, but are more frequent in atypical carcinoids. Carcinoid syndrome is associated with bronchial carcinoids in only 2% of cases, usually in patients with metastatic disease, particularly to the liver. The most common sites of metastases are lung, bone, liver, adrenals, and brain.[53]

The standard treatment for bronchial carcinoids is complete resection, regardless of the presence of nodal involvement, with mediastinal lymph node sampling or dissection. Lobectomy can be accomplished in the majority of patients with resectable disease, although parenchymal-sparing segmentectomy or nonanatomic wedge resection can be considered particularly

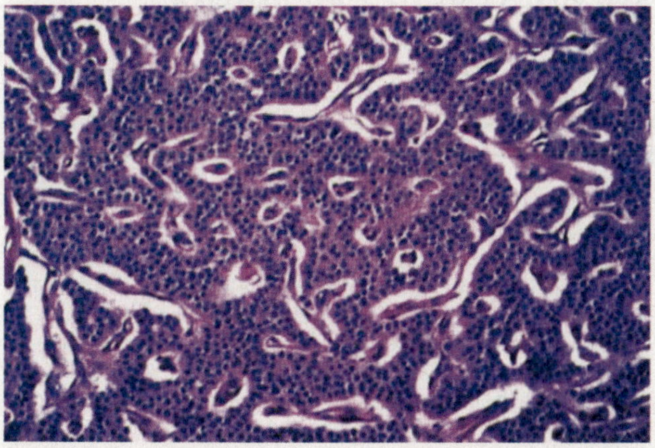

Figure 76.1. Typical carcinoid tumor of the lung. A microscopic view shows ribbons of tumor cells embedded in vascular stroma. (Reprinted with permission from Strayer DS, Saffitz JE, Rubin E. *Rubin's Pathology*. 8th ed. Wolters Kluwer; 2020. Figure 18.92.)

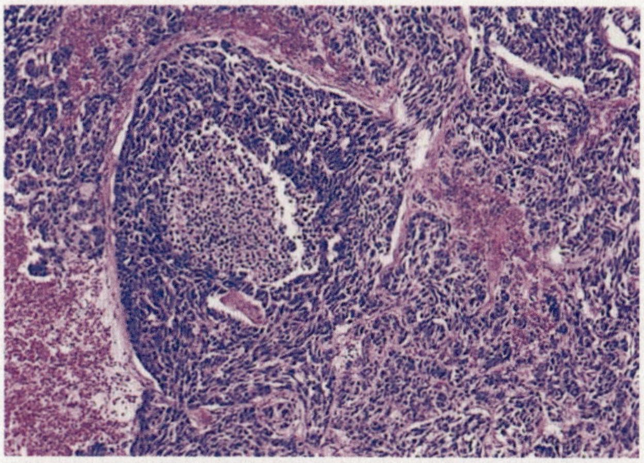

Figure 76.2. Atypical carcinoid tumor of the lung. A cellular tumor shows central necrosis and disorganized architecture. (Reprinted with permission from Strayer DS, Saffitz JE, Rubin E. *Rubin's Pathology*. 8th ed. Wolters Kluwer; 2020. Figure 18.93.)

for patients with a typical carcinoid tumor.[54] For patients who have centrally located tumors and for which pneumonectomy might be performed, bronchoplastic techniques should be considered instead.[55] Endoscopic resection is invariably associated with local recurrence and should be used only as a palliative maneuver in patients whose general medical condition precludes thoracotomy and pulmonary resection.

The long-term survival rate after resection exceeds 90% in patients with typical carcinoids, even when hilar or mediastinal nodal metastases are present. In contrast, patients with atypical carcinoids have a 5-year survival rate of 60% after complete resection. The outcome is more closely linked to histology than to tumor size, location, or nodal involvement. Recurrence is more frequent with tumors larger than 3 cm and in patients who present with lymph node metastases.[55,56]

LARGE CELL NEUROENDOCRINE CARCINOMA

Large cell neuroendocrine carcinoma is characterized by the microscopic features of neuroendocrine tumors, but the tumor cells are large, have a high mitotic rate, and frequently show necrosis (**Fig. 76.3**).[52,57] According to Travis and colleagues,

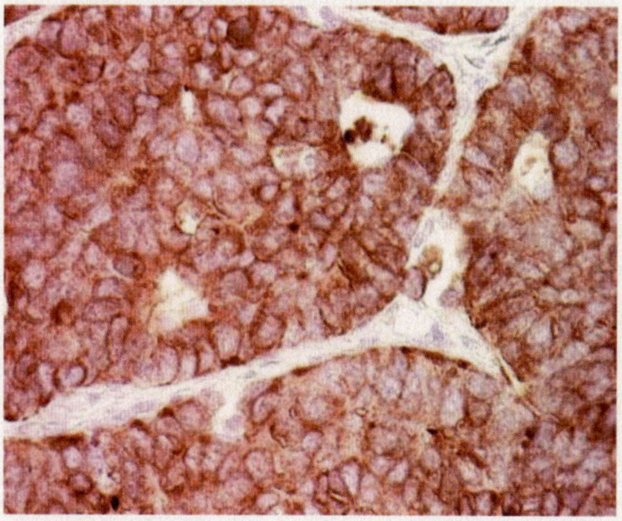

Figure 76.3. Large cell neuroendocrine carcinoma of the lung demonstrates positive immunostaining with synaptophysin antibody. (From Cagle PT. *Color Atlas and Text of Pulmonary Pathology*. Lippincott Williams & Wilkins; 2005.)

large cell neuroendocrine carcinomas are related to smoking, as is SCLC, and are high-grade tumors with 5- and 10-year survival rates of 27% and 9%, respectively, despite complete resection.[58,59] There is very minimal data available concerning adjuvant therapy. For the time being, the management of large cell neuroendocrine carcinoma is identical to that of NSCLC.[60]

SMALL CELL LUNG CARCINOMA

SCLC has the most aggressive clinical course of any type of pulmonary tumor and is often widely disseminated by the time of diagnosis. The proportion of patients with SCLC has been decreasing from 17% in the 1980s to 13% of lung cancer cases in 2002.[61] In contrast to non–small cell lung tumors, these lesions are notably responsive to chemotherapy and radiotherapy. Surgical resection is rarely indicated for SCLC since the tumor typically presents with advanced disease. The staging system for SCLC was developed by the Veterans Administration Lung Cancer Staging Group and divides patients into those with limited-stage (LS) and those with extensive-stage (ES) disease. This distinction was first based on what could be encompassed by a tolerable radiation portal. After clarification by the IASLC, LS disease includes patients with tumors confined to one hemithorax and regional lymph nodes (hilar, ipsilateral, and contralateral mediastinal nodes, and ipsilateral and contralateral supraclavicular nodes) as well as patients with ipsilateral pleural effusion, regardless of whether the cytology is positive or negative.[62] On the other hand, both pericardial and bilateral pulmonary involvement are considered ES disease.[63]

Common sites of distant metastases are bone, liver, bone marrow, and the central nervous system, and therefore the metastatic evaluation includes a bone scan, CT of the chest and abdomen, and brain MRI. Some oncologists also perform bone marrow biopsies, but because the marrow is the sole site of extensive disease in fewer than 5% of patients, biopsies are usually judged unnecessary. After the staging process, approximately 30% to 40% of patients are found to have LS disease. For patients with LS SCLC, response rates of 85% to 90% and complete response rates of 50% to 60% can be expected with the combination of etoposide and cisplatin and radiation therapy.[64] The median survival is 18 to 24 months, and the 2-year survival rates are 40% to 50%. The addition of definitive-dose thoracic radiation therapy, particularly when administered concurrently or within several weeks of completing chemotherapy confers a 5% 2- to 3-year overall survival benefit.[65–67] In ES SCLC treated with chemotherapy, response rates reach 75% to 85%, although complete response is seen in only 15% to 25% of patients. The median survival is between 7 and 11 months, with a 2-year survival less than 5%.[61] Although the prognosis in SCLC depends primarily on the anatomic extent of disease, after a review of prognostic variables in its 2,580-patient SCLC database, the Southwest Oncology Group (SWOG) determined that the two-stage system should be extended into a four-stage system, with serum lactate dehydrogenase level, age, and pleural effusion used as additional staging criteria.[68]

The small numbers of patients with SCLC evaluated by surgeons represent fewer than 10% of all patients with SCLC. These patients have peripheral tumors with no nodal involvement or only hilar nodal involvement, which would be classified as Tl–2 N0–l (stage I or II) tumors in the TNM staging system. In the past, such tumors were often diagnosed at exploratory thoracotomy for an asymptomatic coin lesion, but with the increasing use of diagnostic percutaneous needle aspiration, more patients with early-stage SCLC are now identified preoperatively. Patients with SCLC should be evaluated by a multidisciplinary team consisting of medical and radiation oncology, and surgical resection should be considered after distant disease has been excluded. For such potentially operable patients, it has been suggested that the TNM classification be used in future trials and studies.[69,70]

Retrospective series have demonstrated a 5-year survival rate of 30% to 50% after resection of T1N0 or T2N0 SCLC.[69,71,72] Because of the propensity for small cell cancers to disseminate, adjuvant chemotherapy has traditionally been given to patients, although no prospective, randomized trials have demonstrated whether this is of any benefit, due to the small numbers of patients available.[72] Relapse at the primary site, which is a problem for most patients with LS SCLC, is distinctly uncommon after complete resection of these early tumors.[73] Radiation therapy to the chest has been suggested after complete resection, but because insufficient information is available in the literature, and local relapse is uncommon, this is not considered standard treatment.[71,72] Given the propensity for patients to develop brain metastases, prophylactic cranial irradiation is recommended for patients with either LS or ES SCLC with good performance status and who have completed initial therapy with either complete or partial response.[74]

As the role of resection in patients with mediastinal nodal involvement (N2 disease) is questionable, mediastinoscopy or EBUS should be considered mandatory to exclude mediastinal nodal disease.[75] This should be performed separately from thoracotomy since it can be difficult for the pathologist to diagnose small cell cancer on a frozen section. The intraoperative management of SCLC is not significantly different from that of NSCLC, and an incomplete resection does not benefit the patient.

The addition of resection after response to induction chemotherapy has been proposed by some surgeons to cure a small number of patients with LS SCLC without mediastinal involvement.[76] Currently, the Lung Cancer Study Group (LCSG) has performed the only prospective, randomized trial evaluating the role of surgery in LS SCLC.[77] All patients enrolled in this study received induction chemotherapy followed by surgical resection. Objective responders were randomized either to lung resection followed by thoracic and cranial radiation or to radiation therapy alone. Because the survival rate was the same in both groups, with 2-year overall survival of 20%, this trial did not support the addition of pulmonary resection to the multimodality treatment of SCLC. More recently, retrospective studies suggest better long-term survival, in selected patients with stage I SCLC, of over 50% at 5 years.[70]

Finally, the occurrence of a second primary lung carcinoma after treatment for SCLC has been reported in a few patients with prolonged survival. It should not be assumed that the new tumor is of small cell histology, and these patients should be evaluated for the possibility of resection.[78] The average risk for the development of a second lung cancer in patients who survive SCLC is approximately 6% per patient per year.[79]

ADENOID CYSTIC CARCINOMA

Adenoid cystic carcinomas are slowly growing malignant tumors that arise from the submucosal glands of the trachea and main bronchi (**Fig. 76.4**). They have also been called cylindromas, adenoid cystic basal cell carcinomas, adenomyoepitheliomas, and pseudoadenomatous basal cell carcinomas. Adenoid cystic carcinomas behave much like the major and minor salivary gland tumors, to which they are microscopically identical. An important aspect of their clinical behavior is that they tend to spread in the submucosal plane along the perineural lymphatics, well beyond the obvious endoluminal component of the tumor. In a small biopsy specimen, it can be difficult to distinguish adenoid cystic carcinoma from a conventional adenocarcinoma.

Immunohistochemical stains may assist the pathologist to differentiate the two by showing the presence of the myoepithelial cell immunophenotype in adenoid cystic carcinoma.[79] Whenever possible, total excision by tracheal resection or tracheobronchial resection is the treatment of choice.[80–83] This is not always possible because of the extensive submucosal spread of tumor. In such cases, the tumor should be resected

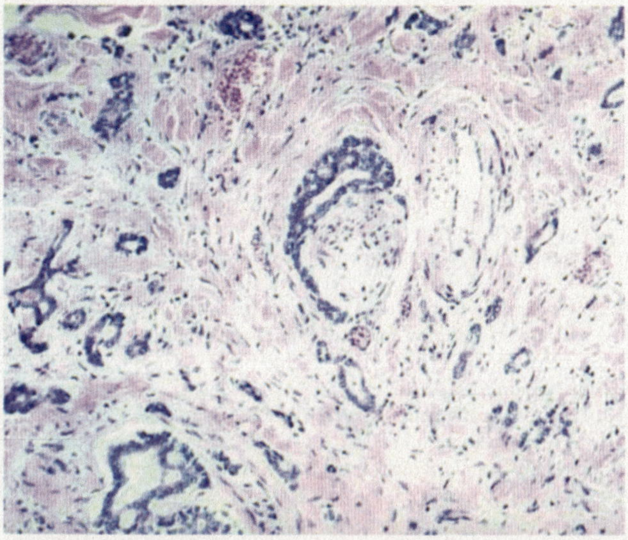

Figure 76.4. Adenoid cystic carcinoma. A photomicrograph demonstrates perineural infiltration of the tumor. (Reprinted with permission from Strayer DS, Saffitz JE, Rubin E. *Rubin's Pathology*. 8th ed. Wolters Kluwer; 2020. Figure 29.35.)

with grossly negative margins along with adjuvant radiation, since these tumors are radiation sensitive.

When resection is not feasible because of the extent of the lesion or the functional status of the patient, a palliative treatment option is endoscopic laser removal followed by radiation (brachytherapy, external beam irradiation, or both). When complete resection is possible, the prognosis is excellent. However, because of the indolent nature of adenoid cystic tumors and its responsiveness to radiation, prolonged survival is possible even with incomplete resection or palliative measures.
6 Patients frequently live 10 years or more with persistent disease, including pulmonary metastases. In such cases, repeated efforts at palliation are indicated.

MUCOEPIDERMOID CARCINOMA

Mucoepidermoid carcinomas may be low-grade or high-grade malignancies and have the same microscopic appearance as mucoepidermoid tumors of salivary gland origin. These tumors also arise in the glandular submucosa, presenting as submucosal lesions. The distinction between a low-grade and a high-grade tumor is based on mitotic activity, cellular necrosis, and nuclear pleomorphism.[84] The principles of treatment of mucoepidermoid tumors are similar to those of carcinoid tumors. The more malignant variety must be treated as a bronchogenic carcinoma. Some authors even think that adenosquamous carcinoma is the same entity as mucoepidermoid carcinoma, but arising in the periphery of the lung.[84] The prognosis for these tumors depends on the grade of malignancy and the stage of the disease. High-grade mucoepidermoid tumors have the same prognosis as bronchogenic carcinoma. Complete surgical resection with negative margins is the mainstay of treatment. Mucoepidermoid tumors are too rare to permit an evaluation of combined modality therapy for more aggressive, high-grade tumors.

References

1. Nicholson AG, Tsao MS, Beasley MB, et al. The 2021 World Health Organization classification of lung tumors: impact of advances since 2015. *J Thorac Oncol.* 2022;17:362–387.
2. Siegel RL, Miller KD, Wagle SN, Jemal A. Cancer statistics, 2023. *CA Cancer J Clin.* 2023;73:17–48.
3. Jemal A, Thun MJ, Ries LAG, et al. Annual report to the nation on the status of cancer, 1975–2005, featuring trends in lung cancer, tobacco use, and tobacco control. *J Natl Cancer Inst.* 2008;100:1672–1694.
4. Mountain CF. Staging classification of lung cancer. A critical evaluation. *Clin Chest Med.* 2002;23(1):103–121.
5. Arriagada R, Bergman B, Dunant A, Le Chevalier T, Pignon JP, Vansteenkiste J; International Adjuvant Lung Cancer Trial Collaborative Group. Cisplatin-based adjuvant chemotherapy in patients with completely resected non-small-cell lung cancer. *N Engl J Med.* 2004;350(4):351–360.
6. Douillard J-Y, Rosell R, De Lena M, et al. Adjuvant vinorelbine plus cisplatin versus observation in patients with completely resected stage IB-IIIA non-small-cell lung cancer (Adjuvant Navelbine International Trialist Association [ANITA]): a randomised controlled trial. *Lancet Oncol.* 2006;7(9):719–727.
7. The International Early Lung Cancer Action Program Investigators; Henschke CI, Yankelevitz DF, Libby DM, Pasmantier MW, Smith JP, Miettinen OS. Survival of patients with stage I lung cancer detected on CT screening. *N Engl J Med.* 2006;355(17):1763–1771.
8. National Lung Screening Trial Research Team; Aberle DR, Adams AM, Berg CD, et al. Reduced lung-cancer mortality with low-dose computed tomographic screening. *N Engl J Med.* 2011; 365(5):395–409.
9. Graham EA, Singer JJ. Successful removal of an entire lung for carcinoma of the bronchus. *CA Cancer J Clin.* 1974;24(4):238–242.
10. SEER Program. Cancer stat facts: lung and bronchus cancer. 2017. Accessed November 18, 2019. http://seer.cancer.gov/statfacts/html/lungb.html
11. Stehelin D, Varmus HE, Bishop JM, Vogt PK. DNA related to the transforming genes(s) of avian sarcoma viruses is present in normal avian DNA. *Nature.* 1976;260:170–173.
12. Rusch V, Baselga J, Cordon-Cardo C, et al. Differential expression of the epidermal growth factor receptor and its ligands in primary non-small cell lung cancers and adjacent benign lung. *Cancer Res.* 1993;53:2379–2385.
13. Lee CK, Brown C, Gralla RJ, et al. Impact of EGFR inhibitor in non-small cell lung cancer on progression-free and overall survival: a meta-analysis. *J Natl Cancer Inst.* 2013;105(9):595–605.
14. Rivera MP, Mehta AC, Wahidi MM. Establishing the diagnosis of lung cancer: diagnosis and management of lung cancer, 3rd ed: American College of Chest Physicians Evidence Based-Clinical Practice Guidelines. *Chest.* 2013;143:e142S–e165S.
15. Lim E, Baldwin D, Beckles M, et al. British Thoracic Society; Society for Cardiothoracic Surgery in Great Britain and Ireland. Guidelines on the radical management of patients with lung cancer. *Thorax.* 2010;65:1–27.
16. De Leyn P, Dooms C, Kuzdzal J, et al. Revised ESTS guidelines for preoperative mediastinal lymph node staging for non-small-cell lung cancer. *Eur J Cardiothorac Surg.* 2014;45:787–798.
17. Detterbeck FC, Lewis SZ, Diekemper R, Addrizzo-Harris D, Alberts WM. Executive summary: diagnosis and management of lung cancer, 3rd ed: American College of Chest Physicians Evidence-Based Clinical Practice Guidelines. *Chest.* 2013;143: 7S–37S.
18. Remon J, Soria JC, Peters S; ESMO Guidelines Committee. Early and locally advanced non-small cell lung cancer: an update of the ESMO Clinical Practice Guidelines focusing on diagnosis, staging, systemic and local therapy. *Ann Oncol.* 2021;32(12):1637–1642.
19. Jay SJ, Wehr K, Nicholson DP, Smith AL. Diagnostic sensitivity and specificity of pulmonary cytology: comparison of techniques used in conjunction with flexible fiber optic bronchoscopy. *Acta Cytol.* 1980;24:304–312.
20. Mahajan AK, Patel S, Hogarth DK, Wightman R. Electromagnetic navigational bronchoscopy: an effective and safe approach to diagnose peripheral lung lesions unreachable by conventional bronchoscopy in high-risk patients. *J Bronchology Interv Pulmonol.* 2011;18:133–137.
21. Wiener RS, Schwartz LM, Woloshin S, Welch HG. Population-based risk for complications after transthoracic needle lung biopsy of a pulmonary nodule: an analysis of discharge records. *Ann Intern Med.* 2011;155:137–144.
22. Gould MK, Donington J, Lynch WR, et al. Evaluation of individuals with pulmonary nodules: when is it lung cancer? Diagnosis and management of lung cancer, 3rd ed: American College

of Chest Physicians Evidence-Based Clinical Practice Guidelines. *Chest.* 2013;143:e93S–e120S.
23. Awais O, Reidy MR, Metha K, et al. Electromagnetic navigation bronchoscopy-guided dye marking for thoracoscopic resection of pulmonary nodules. *Ann Thorac Surg.* 2016;102:223–229.
24. Jackson P, Steinfort DP, Kron T, Siva S. Practical assessment of bronchoscopically inserted fiducial markers for image guidance in stereotactic lung radiotherapy. *J Thorac Oncol.* 2016;11: 1363–1368.
25. Mountain CF. Revisions in the international system for staging lung cancer. *Chest.* 1997;111:1710–1717.
26. Goldstraw P, Chansky K, Crowley J, et al. International Association for the Study of Lung Cancer Staging and Prognostic Factors Committee, Advisory Boards, and Participating Institutions; International Association for the Study of Lung Cancer Staging and Prognostic Factors Committee Advisory Boards and Participating Institutions. The IASLC Lung Cancer Staging Project: proposals for the revision of the TNM stage groupings in the forthcoming (eighth) edition of the TNM classification for lung cancer. *J Thorac Oncol.* 2016;11:39–51.
27. Detterbeck FC, Chansky K, Groome P, et al. IASLC Staging Prognostic Factors Committee, Advisory Boards, and Participating Institutions. The IASLC Lung Cancer Staging Project: methodology and validation used in the development of proposals for revision of the stage classification of NSCLC in the forthcoming (eight) edition of the TNM classification of lung cancer. *J Thorac Oncol.* 2016;11:1433–1446.
28. Rivera MP, Mehta AC; American College of Chest Physicians. Initial diagnosis of lung cancer: ACCP Evidence-Based Clinical Practice Guidelines (2nd ed.). *Chest.* 2007;132(3 suppl):131S–148S.
29. Albain KS, Swann RS, Rusch VW, et al. Radiotherapy plus chemotherapy with or without surgical resection for stage III non-small-cell lung cancer: a phase III randomised controlled trial. *Lancet.* 2009;374(9687):379–386.
30. Silvestri GA, Gould MK, Margolis ML, et al. American College of Chest Physicians. Noninvasive staging of non-small cell lung cancer: ACCP Evidenced-Based Clinical Practice Guidelines (2nd ed.). *Chest.* 2007;132(3 suppl):178S–201S.
31. Gonzalez-Stawinski GV, Lemaire A, Merchant F, et al. A comparative analysis of positron emission tomography and mediastinoscopy in staging non-small cell lung cancer. *J Thorac Cardiovasc Surg.* 2003;126(6):1900–1905.
32. Kernstine KH, Mclaughlin KA, Menda Y, et al. Can FDG-PET reduce the need for mediastinoscopy in potentially resectable non-small cell lung cancer? *Ann Thorac Surg.* 2002;73(2):394–402.
33. Vesselle H, Pugsley JM, Vallières E, Wood DE. The impact of fluorodeoxyglucose F 18 positron-emission tomography on the surgical staging of non-small cell lung cancer. *J Thorac Cardiovasc Surg.* 2002;124(3):511–519.
34. Reed CE, Harpole DH, Posther KE, et al. American College of Surgeons Oncology Group Z0050 trial. Results of the American College of Surgeons Oncology Group Z0050 trial: the utility of positron emission tomography in staging potentially operable non-small cell lung cancer. *J Thorac Cardiovasc Surg.* 2003;126(6):1943–1951.
35. Kozower BD, Meyers BF, Reed CE, Jones DR, Decker PA, Putnam JB Jr. Does positron emission tomography prevent nontherapeutic pulmonary resections for clinical stage IA lung cancer? *Ann Thorac Surg.* 2008;85(4):1166–1169.
36. Yasufuku K, Pierre A, Darling G, et al. A prospective controlled trial of endobronchial ultrasound-guided transbronchial needle aspiration compared with mediastinoscopy for mediastinal lymph node staging of lung cancer. *J Thorac Cardiovasc Surg.* 2011;142(6): 1393–1400.e1.
37. Detterbeck FC, Jantz MA, Wallace M, Vansteenkiste J, Silvestri GA; American College of Chest Physicians. Invasive mediastinal staging of lung cancer: ACCP Evidence-Based Clinical Practice Guidelines (2nd ed.). *Chest.* 2007;132(3 suppl):202S–220S.
38. Deslauriers J, Grégoire J, Jacques LF, Piraux M, Guojin L, Lacasse Y. Sleeve lobectomy versus pneumonectomy for lung cancer: a comparative analysis of survival and sites or recurrences. *Ann Thorac Surg.* 2004;77(4):1152–1156.
39. Gaissert HA, Mathisen DJ, Moncure AC, Hilgenberg AD, Grillo HC, Wain JC. Survival and function after sleeve lobectomy for lung cancer. *J Thorac Cardiovasc Surg.* 1996;111(5):948–953.
40. Okada M, Yamagishi H, Satake S, et al. Survival related to lymph node involvement in lung cancer after sleeve lobectomy compared with pneumonectomy. *J Thorac Cardiovasc Surg.* 2000;119(4 Pt 1): 814–819.
41. Merritt RE, Mathisen DJ, Wain JC, et al. Long-term results of sleeve lobectomy in the management of non-small cell lung carcinoma and low-grade neoplasms. *Ann Thorac Surg.* 2009;88(5): 1574–1581.
42. Ginsberg RJ, Rubinstein LV. Randomized trial of lobectomy versus limited resection for T1 N0 non-small cell lung cancer. Lung Cancer Study Group. *Ann Thorac Surg.* 1995;60(3):615–622; discussion 622–623.
43. Landreneau RJ, Sugarbaker DJ, Mack MJ, et al. Wedge resection versus lobectomy for stage I (T1 N0 M0) non-small-cell lung cancer. *J Thorac Cardiovasc Surg.* 1997;113(4):691–698.
44. Yano T, Yokoyama H, Yoshino I, et al. Results of a limited resection for compromised or poor-risk patients with clinical stage I non-small cell carcinoma of the lung. *J Am Coll Surg.* 1995; 181(1):33–37.
45. Altorki NK, Yip R, Hanaoka T, et al. I-ELCAP Investigators. Sublobar resection is equivalent to lobectomy for clinical stage 1A lung cancer in solid nodules. *J Thorac Cardiovasc Surg.* 2014; 147(2):754–762.
46. Robinson BM, Kennedy C, McLean J, McCaughan BC. Node-negative non-small cell lung cancer: pathological staging and survival in 1765 consecutive cases. *J Thorac Oncol.* 2011;6(10): 1691–1696.
47. Hirsch FR, Spreafico A, Novello S, Wood MD, Simms L, Papotti M. The prognostic and predictive role of histology in advanced non-small cell lung cancer: a literature review. *J Thorac Oncol.* 2008;3(12):1468–1481.
48. Martini N, Bains MS, Burt ME, et al. Incidence of local recurrence and second primary tumors in resected stage I lung cancer. *J Thorac Cardiovasc Surg.* 1995;109(1):120–129.
49. Thomas P, Rubinstein L. Cancer recurrence after resection: T1 N0 non-small cell lung cancer. Lung Cancer Study Group. *Ann Thorac Surg.* 1990;49(2):242–246; discussion 246–247.
50. Johnson BE. Second lung cancers in patients after treatment for an initial lung cancer. *J Natl Cancer Inst.* 1998;90(18):1335–1345.
51. Rice D, Kim H-W, Sabichi A, et al. The risk of second primary tumors after resection of stage I nonsmall cell lung cancer. *Ann Thorac Surg.* 2003;76(4):1001–1007.
52. Vuitch F, Sekido Y, Fong K, Mackay B, Minna JD, Gazdar AF. Neuroendocrine tumors of the lung. Pathology and molecular biology. *Chest Surg Clin N Am.* 1997;7(1):21–47.
53. McCaughan BC, Martini N, Bains MS. Bronchial carcinoids. Review of 124 cases. *J Thorac Cardiovasc Surg.* 1985;89(1): 8–17.
54. Cañizares MA, Matilla JM, Cueto A, et al. EMETNE-SEPAR Members. Atypical carcinoid tumours of the lung: prognostic factors and patterns of recurrence. *Thorax.* 2014;69(7):648–653.
55. García-Yuste M, Matilla JM, Cueto A, et al. Spanish Multi-centric Study of Neuroendocrine Tumours of the Lung for the Spanish Society of Pneumonology and Thoracic Surgery (EMETNE-SEPAR). Typical and atypical carcinoid tumours: analysis of the experience of the Spanish multi-centric study of neuroendocrine tumours of the lung. *Eur J Cardiothorac Surg.* 2007;31(2):192–197.
56. Naalsund A, Rostad H, Strøm EH, Lund MB, Strand TE. Carcinoid lung tumors—incidence, treatment and outcomes: a population-based study. *Eur J Cardiothorac Surg.* 2011;39(4): 565–569.
57. Travis WD, Linnoila RI, Tsokos MG, et al. Neuroendocrine tumors of the lung with proposed criteria for large-cell neuroendocrine carcinoma. An ultrastructural, immunohistochemical, and flow cytometric study of 35 cases. *Am J Surg Pathol.* 1991; 15(6):529–553.
58. Jiang SX, Kameya T, Shoji M, Dobashi Y, Shinada J, Yoshimura H. Large cell neuroendocrine carcinoma of the lung: a histologic

and immunohistochemical study of 22 cases. *Am J Surg Pathol.* 1998;22(5):526–537.
59. Travis WD, Rush W, Flieder DB, et al. Survival analysis of 200 pulmonary neuroendocrine tumors with clarification of criteria for atypical carcinoid and its separation from typical carcinoid. *Am J Surg Pathol.* 1998;22(8):934–944.
60. Zacharias J, Nicholson AG, Ladas GP, Goldstraw P. Large cell neuroendocrine carcinoma and large cell carcinomas with neuroendocrine morphology of the lung: prognosis after complete resection and systematic nodal dissection. *Ann Thorac Surg.* 2003; 75(2):348–352.
61. Govindan R, Page N, Morgensztern D, et al. Changing epidemiology of small-cell lung cancer in the United States over the last 30 years: analysis of the surveillance, epidemiologic, and end results database. *J Clin Oncol.* 2006;24(28):4539–4544.
62. Micke P, Faldum A, Metz T, et al. Staging small cell lung cancer: Veterans Administration Lung Study Group versus International Association for the Study of Lung Cancer—what limits limited disease? *Lung Cancer.* 2002;37(3):271–276.
63. Stahel RA, Ginsberg R, Havemann K, et al. Staging and prognostic factors in small cell lung cancer: a consensus report. *Lung Cancer.* 1989;5(4–6):119–126.
64. Shepherd FA. The role of chemotherapy in the treatment of small cell lung cancer. *Chest Surg Clin N Am.* 1997;7(1):113–133.
65. Pignon JP, Arriagada R, Ihde DC, et al. A meta-analysis of thoracic radiotherapy for small-cell lung cancer. *N Engl J Med.* 1992; 327(23):1618–1624.
66. Warde P, Payne D. Does thoracic irradiation improve survival and local control in limited-stage small-cell carcinoma of the lung? A meta-analysis. *J Clin Oncol.* 1992;10(6):890–895.
67. Fried DB, Morris DE, Poole C, et al. Systematic review evaluating the timing of thoracic radiation therapy in combined modality therapy for limited-stage small-cell lung cancer. *J Clin Oncol.* 2004; 22(23):4837–4845.
68. Albain KS, Crowley JJ, LeBlanc M, Livingston RB. Determinants of improved outcome in small-cell lung cancer: an analysis of the 2,580-patient Southwest Oncology Group data base. *J Clin Oncol.* 1990;8(9):1563–1574.
69. Inoue M, Miyoshi S, Yasumitsu T, et al. Surgical results for small cell lung cancer based on the new TNM staging system. Thoracic Surgery Study Group of Osaka University, Osaka, Japan. *Ann Thorac Surg.* 2000;70(5):1615–1619.
70. van Meerbeeck JP, Fennell DA, De Ruysscher DKM. Small-cell lung cancer. *Lancet.* 2011;378(9804):1741–1755.
71. Kreisman H, Wolkove N, Quoix E. Small cell lung cancer presenting as a solitary pulmonary nodule. *Chest.* 1992;101(1):225–231.
72. Brock MV, Hooker CM, Syphard JE, et al. Surgical resection of limited disease small cell lung cancer in the new era of platinum chemotherapy: its time has come. *J Thorac Cardiovasc Surg.* 2005; 129(1):64–72.
73. Shepherd FA, Evans WK, Feld R, et al. Adjuvant chemotherapy following surgical resection for small-cell carcinoma of the lung. *J Clin Oncol.* 1988;6(5):832–838.
74. Le Péchoux C, Dunant A, Senan S, et al. Prophylactic Cranial Irradiation (PCI) Collaborative Group. Standard-dose versus higher-dose prophylactic cranial irradiation (PCI) in patients with limited-stage small-cell lung cancer in complete remission after chemotherapy and thoracic radiotherapy (PCI 99-01, EORTC 22003-08004, RTOG 0212, and IFCT 99-01): a randomized clinical trial. *Lancet Oncol.* 2009;10(5):467–474.
75. Shah SS, Thompson J, Goldstraw P. Results of operation without adjuvant therapy in the treatment of small cell lung cancer. *Ann Thorac Surg.* 1992;54(3):498–501.
76. Shepherd FA, Ginsberg R, Patterson GA, et al. Is there ever a role for salvage operations in limited small-cell lung cancer? *J Thorac Cardiovasc Surg.* 1991;101(2):196–200.
77. Lad T, Piantadosi S, Thomas P, Payne D, Ruckdeschel J, Giaccone G. A prospective randomized trial to determine the benefit of surgical resection of residual disease following response of small cell lung cancer to combination chemotherapy. *Chest.* 1994;106(6 Suppl):320S–323S.
78. Inoue H, Iwasaki M, Ogawa J, Shohtsu A, Shioya S, Osamura Y. Surgical resection of a second primary lung carcinoma in a survivor of small cell carcinoma. *Ann Thorac Surg.* 1993;56(5):1160–1161.
79. Moran CA. Primary salivary gland-type tumors of the lung. *Semin Diagn Pathol.* 1995;12(2):106–122.
80. Webb BD, Walsh GL, Roberts DB, Sturgis EM. Primary tracheal malignant: The University of Texas, MD Anderson Cancer Center experience. *J Am Coll Surg.* 2006;202(2):237–246.
81. Gaissert HA, Grillo HC, Shadmehr MB, et al. Long-term survival after resection of primary adenoid cystic and squamous cell carcinoma of the trachea and the carina. *Ann Thorac Surg.* 2004; 78(6):1889–1896.
82. Maziak DE, Todd TR, Keshavjee SH, Winton TL, Van Nostrand P, Pearson FG. Adenoid cystic carcinoma of the airway: thirty-two-year experience. *J Thorac Cardiovasc Surg.* 1996;112(6): 1522–1531; discussion 1531–1532.
83. Chin HW, DeMeester T, Chin RY, Boman B. Endobronchial adenoid cystic carcinoma. *Chest.* 1991;100(5):1464–1465.
84. Heitmiller RF, Mathisen DJ, Ferry JA, Mark EJ, Grillo HC. Mucoepidermoid lung tumors. *Ann Thorac Surg.* 1989;47(3): 394–399.

LUNG

77

Nonneoplastic Thoracic Disease

Chigozirim N. Ekeke, Michael Pienta, and Rishindra M. Reddy

Key Points

1. Surgical intervention for chest wall tumors depends on the type of lesion and goals of surgery (resection vs diagnosis). Reconstruction varies depending on the size of the defect and location on the chest wall.
2. Thoracic outlet syndrome (TOS) may be arterial, venous, or neurogenic, and surgery for this should be performed in high-volume centers.
3. The primary treatment for a lung abscess is antibiotic therapy. Recalcitrant infection may undergo surgical treatment.
4. Massive hemoptysis is traditionally characterized as greater than 600 cc/24 hours. Asphyxiation secondary to even due to a low blood volume in the lungs can be a fatal complication of this presentation.
5. Primary spontaneous pneumothoraces may be treated with observation or drain tube placement. If pneumothoraces persist or if there are ongoing air leaks, treatment should include a thoracoscopic evaluation and possible pleurodesis.
6. Transudative pleural effusions should be treated medically, while exudative effusions may need more intervention. One-quarter of pleural effusions in a community hospital are due to malignancy.
7. Empyema ranges from parapneumonic to the organized stage. Drainage alone may be sufficient for parapneumonic, while extensive decortication is required for organized empyema.
8. Complications of tracheostomies are usually due to improper placement of the tracheostomy on the trachea (below the 3rd ring, risking a tracheoinnominate fistula) or to the use of high pressures in the cuff of the tracheostomy (causing ischemia and long-term stenosis)
9. Mediastinitis is life threatening and warrants immediate evaluation, antibiotic therapy, and surgical drainage.

The focus of this chapter is to provide an overview of thoracic-based pathology. Specifically, benign (noncardiac) and thoracic congenital diseases.

CHEST WALL ANATOMY

The chest wall is the musculoskeletal structure that contains and protects the structures of the upper trunk or thorax. There are two openings to the thorax: the superior aperture or the thoracic inlet, and the inferior aperture, which leads to the abdominal cavity. The head and arms connect to the intrathoracic structures via the inlet, whereas the diaphragm separates the thoracic and abdominal cavities at the inferior aperture. The inferior vena cava, esophagus, and aorta travel to the abdomen through the diaphragm at levels T8, T10, and T12, respectively.

The sternum is comprised of three parts: the manubrium, the sternal body, and the xiphoid. The manubrium attaches to the clavicles and the first costal cartilages. The sternal angle, also called the angle of Louis, refers to connection between the manubrium and the sternal body. The second ribs attach to the sternum at the sternal angle. The body of the sternum contains articular facets for ribs 2 to 7 and connects to the cartilaginous xiphoid inferiorly (**Fig. 77.1**).

The ribs are split into two groups; the upper 7 pairs are the true ribs, with articulations to the sternum, while the lower five are the false ribs. Ribs 8, 9, and 10 connect to each other and the upper ribs via the costal cartilage. Ribs 11 and 12 are called floating ribs as they have no anterior connection. Rib 1 is uniquely shaped as it is flat, short, and extremely curved. Ribs 2 through 10 have a more consistent configuration with the head containing articular facets for the vertebrae. Below the neck, the tubercle contains the facet for the vertebral transverse process. The costal groove along the inferior portion of the shaft houses the intercostal bundle, consisting of the nerve, artery, and vein (**Fig. 77.2**). Because of this inferior placement, most chest wall procedures, such as thoracostomy tube placement or thoracentesis, should be performed on the superior aspect of the rib to avoid injury to this bundle.

There are three intercostal muscles, the external intercostal, the internal intercostal, and the innermost intercostal muscle (**Fig. 77.3**). On the inner aspect of the chest wall, the internal thoracic (mammary) artery and vein run between the innermost intercostal muscle and the transversus thoracis muscles. The intercostal arteries have two sources, posteriorly from the descending thoracic aorta and anteriorly from the internal thoracic arteries. The intercostal nerve is a branch off the ventral ramus after it joins the sympathetic trunk. The intercostal veins follow the arteries and posteriorly drain into the azygos and hemiazygos veins. Lymphatic drainage from the posterior chest wall drains into the thoracic duct on the left and into the right lymphatic duct on the right.

The muscles of the chest wall can be divided embryologically into those from the epimeres, such as the deep back muscles, innervated by the dorsal rami, and those from the hypomeres, such as the intercostals and rectus, innervated by the ventral rami. The musculature can also be classified based on respiratory function, where the primary muscles of respiration are the intercostals and the diaphragm, and the secondary, or accessory muscles are the sternocleidomastoid, scalenes, pectoralis, serratus, and abdominal wall musculature. The major back muscles include the trapezius and latissimus dorsi

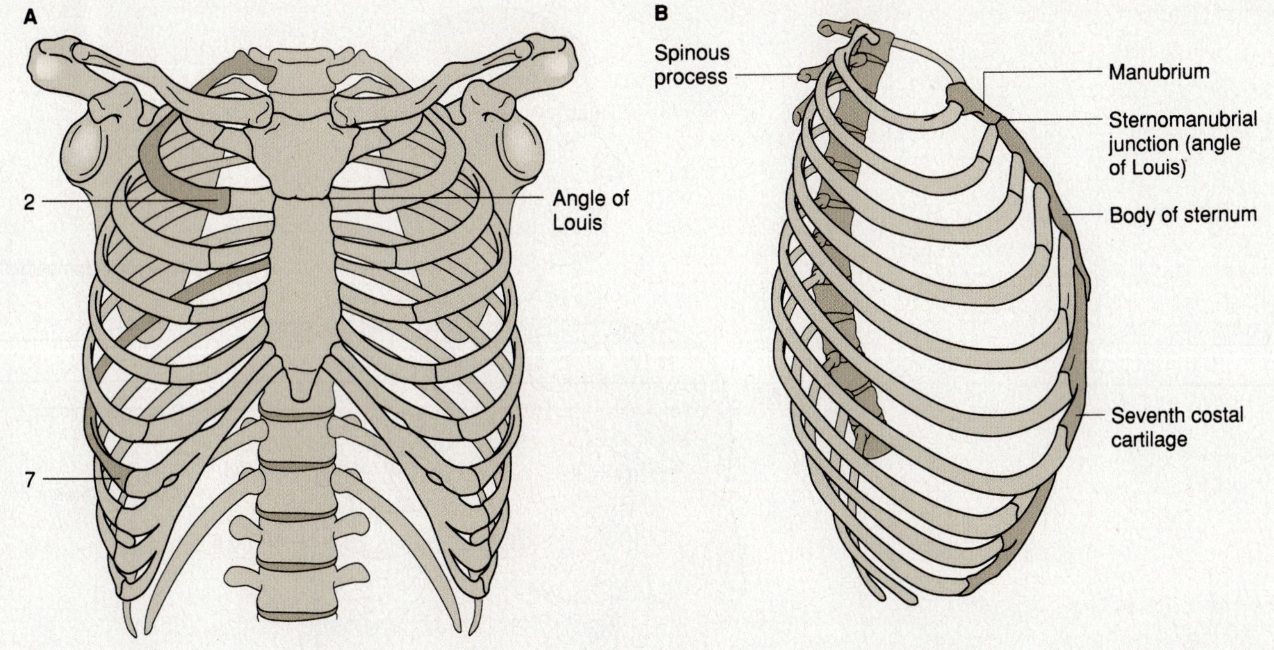

Figure 77.1. Skeletal support of the thorax. Anterior (**A**), and lateral (**B**), views. Note the anterior cartilaginous component of the upper 10 ribs, the fused costal cartilages of ribs 7 through 10, the location of the sternomanubrial junction (angle of Louis) at the level of the second rib, and the oblique course of the ribs laterally from posterior to anterior.

(**Fig. 77.4**). In normal breathing, the diaphragm performs most of the work, with the intercostals supplying about a quarter of the workload. In full inspiration, the pleura extends bilaterally down to the level of the 11th and 12th ribs (**Fig. 77.5**).

CHEST WALL NEOPLASMS

Chest wall tumors are very rare. Lesions may be divided into benign and malignant, and then further subdivided into soft tissue versus bony/cartilaginous tumors (**Table 77.1**). Most malignant tumors of the chest wall are either metastatic from carcinomas or sarcomas arising in other sites of the body, or from local extension of lung cancers or breast cancers.[1]

Almost all lesions will present as a mass, as pain, or as a combination of both. Occasionally, they will be asymptomatic and be identified on imaging for cancer surveillance or other reasons.[2] Evaluation of these lesions includes a thorough history and physical and appropriate imaging, which includes three-dimensional imaging such as a CT scan and/or MRI, as well as a PET scan for staging if clinically indicated.[1]

Surgical intervention depends on the type of lesion and the goal of surgery. Tumors may require only a needle, core, or incisional biopsy, but may also require excisional biopsies. Multidisciplinary decision making is critical as many new adjuvant therapies are available to treat primary tumors. Some

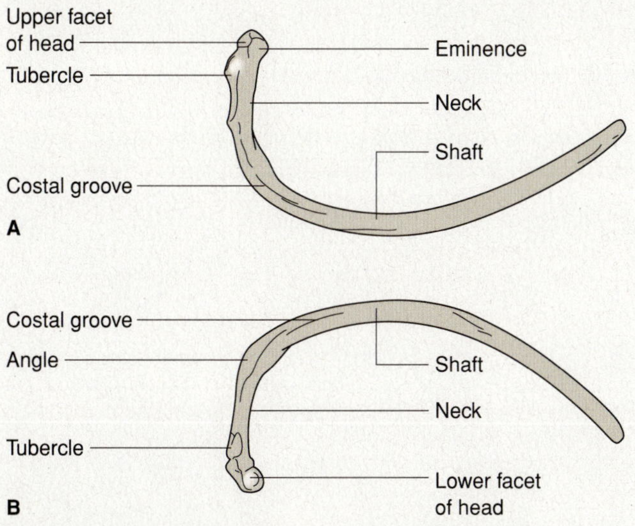

Figure 77.2. Anatomy of ribs 2 to 10 as viewed from above (**A**), and below (**B**).

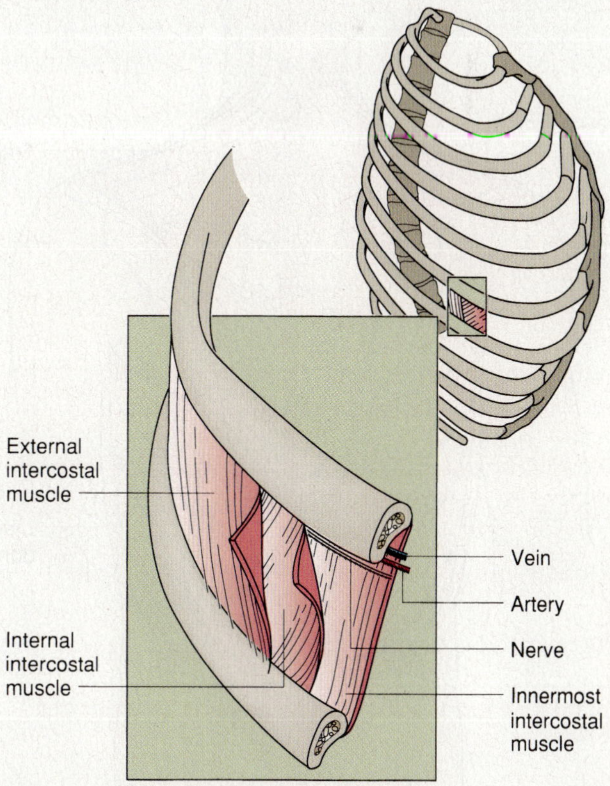

Figure 77.3. Anatomy of the intercostal space. The major intercostal muscles are the external and internal. The neurovascular bundle courses in the costal groove along the inferior aspect of the rib.

LUNG

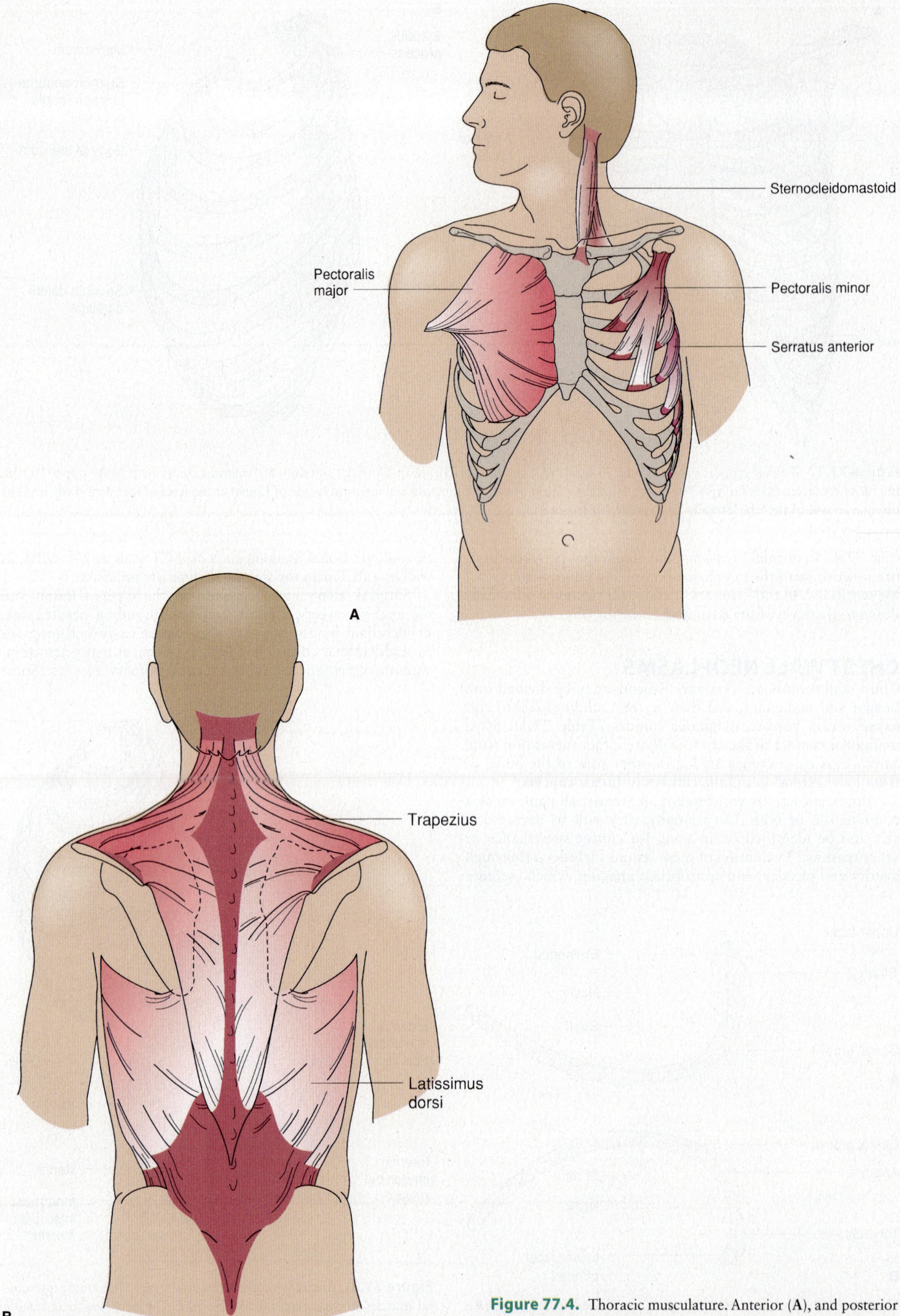

Figure 77.4. Thoracic musculature. Anterior (A), and posterior (B), views.

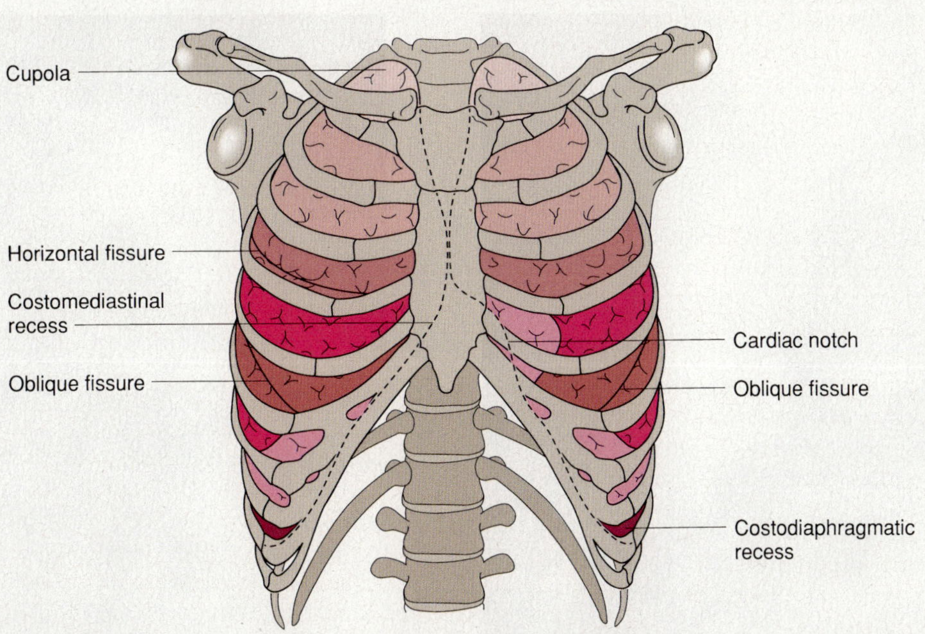

Figure 77.5. Topographic relations of the pleura to the chest wall. Laterally, the pleura extends to the level of the 11th to 12th ribs. The anterior reflection of the mediastinal and costal pleurae forms the costomediastinal recess, whereas the reflections of the costal and diaphragmatic pleurae form the costodiaphragmatic recess.

Table 77.1. Chest Wall Tumor Classification

- Benign tumors
  - Soft tissue tumors
    - Lipomas
    - Fibromas
    - Hemangiomas
    - Neurofibromas
    - Granulomas
    - Inflammatory tumor
    - Tuberculoma
  - Bony/cartilaginous tumors
    - Osteochondromas
    - Chondromas
    - Fibrous dysplasia
    - Eosinophilic granuloma
    - Osteoid osteomas
    - Osteomyelitis
    - Chondro/osteoblastomas
- Malignant tumors
  - Soft tissue tumors
    - Melanomas and other cutaneous cancers
    - Sarcomas
    - Desmoid tumors/low-grade fibrosarcomas
    - Lymphoma
    - Malignant fibrous histiocytoma
  - Bony/cartilaginous tumors
    - Chondrosarcomas
    - Osteogenic sarcomas
    - Ewing sarcomas
    - Solitary plasmocytoma
    - Lymphoma
- Metastatic tumors
  - Breast cancer
  - Lung cancer
  - Mediastinal tumors
  - Mesothelioma
  - Other sarcomas or carcinomas

low-grade malignant tumors may be underdiagnosed and considered benign if the entire specimen is not removed and examined. When resection of a primary malignant lesion is performed, wide excision is required, with margins up to 4 cm.[3]

BENIGN SOFT TISSUE TUMORS

These tumors include lipomas, fibromas, hemangiomas, and neurofibromas, among others. These can be removed by excisional biopsy and require no further treatment unless they recur. Inflammatory osteomyelitis can mimic tumors by causing pain.

BENIGN BONY/CARTILAGINOUS TUMORS

About two-thirds of benign chest wall tumors are either osteochondromas, chondromas, or fibrous dysplasia, with osteochondromas comprising almost 50% of all nonmalignant rib tumors. Osteochondromas usually present as painless masses with a male-to-female predominance of 3:1. If the lesion becomes painful, it may indicate malignant degeneration.[3] They are often found on routine radiographic examinations for other reasons and have a characteristic appearance of a pedunculated bony prominence (**Fig. 77.6**).

Chondromas account for 15% of benign rib lesions and grow from the cartilage at the sternocostal junction.[1] They have an equal male-to-female incidence. Clinically and radiographically, it is impossible to distinguish chondromas from chondrosarcomas, thus, complete excision is required to rule out malignancy.[3]

Fibrous dysplasia arises in the lateral portion or shaft of the rib and can have a "soap bubble" or "ground-glass" appearance on radiographs (**Fig. 77.7**). These lesions may become painful if they enlarge and can result in rib fractures. Surgical excision is needed for diagnosis and symptomatic relief.[4] Eosinophilic granulomas and osteoid osteomas are rare conditions that affect men more often. Patients may have multiple granulomas, including in the skull, and may benefit from radiotherapy as opposed to surgical resection. Osteomas may be symptomatic, and if so, should be resected.

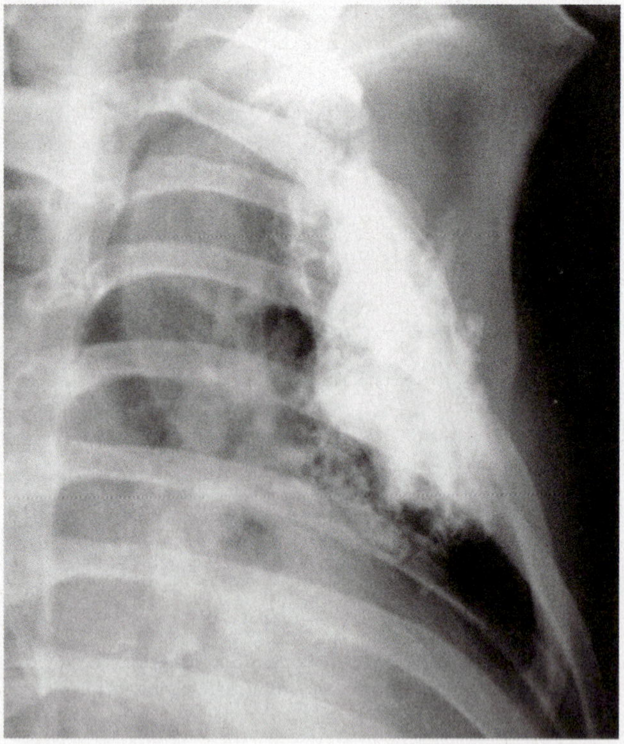

Figure 77.6. Osteochondroma of left second rib. The stippled calcification within the tumor and the intact cortex of the rib are characteristic.

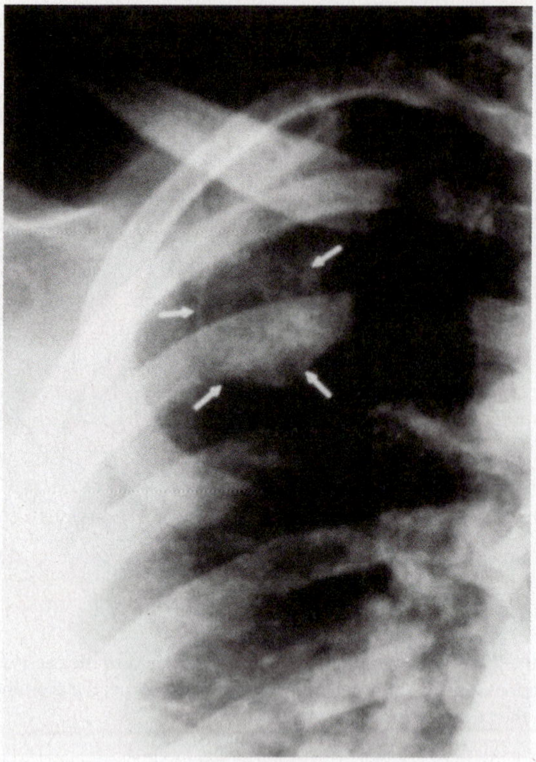

Figure 77.7. Fibrous dysplasia of the rib. Note the characteristic expansion and thinning of the cortex (*arrows*) and the central ground-glass appearance.

MALIGNANT SOFT TISSUE TUMORS

These lesions include malignant fibrous histiocytomas (MFHs; most common), rhabdomyosarcomas, leiomyosarcoma, desmoid tumors, etc.

Sarcomas also arise in the soft tissue of the chest wall, but they comprise less than 10% of all sarcomas.[2] Desmoid tumors are sometimes considered low-grade fibrosarcomas.[1] Almost half of all desmoids occur in the chest wall and shoulder, where they can encapsulate the brachial plexus, resulting in functional limitation, deformity, and refractory pain. They require wide local excision and have a high rate of local recurrence. If they encircle vital structures, they can be treated with radiotherapy after surgical excision.[3]

Combinational therapy (antiestrogen and nonsteroidal agents) has been utilized to treat desmoid fibromatosis or recurrent disease.[5] MFHs are the most common primary chest wall tumors. These tumors are more frequent in men (2:1 ratio) and generally occur after the age of 50. They are slow growing, painless, and spread along the facial planes or between muscle fibers. MFHs are unresponsive to other forms of therapy and require wide local excision. There is a high rate of recurrence following resection, and patients who have undergone resection have a 5-year survival of under 40%.[3] Rhabdomyosarcoma is the second most common soft tissue lesion of the chest wall and usually occurs in children and younger adults. It grows rapidly from the striated muscle, but is usually painless. It is treated with wide excision followed by radiation and chemotherapy, with a reported 70% survival at 5 years in children, but may be as low as 20% in adults.[3]

MALIGNANT BONY/CARTILAGINOUS TUMORS

Chondrosarcomas are the most common primary malignant bony tumors, accounting for 20% to 30% of lesions. These are well-differentiated tumors and may be difficult to distinguish from their benign counterparts on histology. Local recurrence can occur after excision, and if untreated, distant metastases can develop.[3] Osteogenic sarcomas are more common in the limbs, but also occur in the ribs. Radiographs depict a characteristic "sunburst" pattern. These tend to grow quickly and often have metastases at the time of initial presentation. Patient evaluation should include a CT scan and bone scan to check for the presence of metastatic disease. Surgery with adjuvant chemotherapy is the treatment of choice for local disease.[6] Ewing sarcomas constitute 5% to 10% of chest wall tumors. They occur in children and younger adults with a male-to-female ratio of 1.6:1. Symptoms include pain, fever, and fatigue. Radiographs show a large soft tissue mass with bony destruction-"onion peel" appearance. Patients often present with metastatic disease, and ultimately three-quarters of patients will develop metastases. Core biopsy is required prior to initiation of neoadjuvant therapy. Multimodality treatment is the key to treatment. Survival may be less than 30% at 5 years in patients with metastatic disease.[7] Askin tumor and Ewing sarcoma may present clinically and radiographically similarly. Biopsy is the key to differentiate between these two tumors.

Solitary plasmocytoma is a rare tumor of the plasma cells and can be part of a systemic disease in multiple myeloma. Lesions can be painful and usually occur in men over the age of 50. X-ray findings show cortical destruction of the rib (**Fig. 77.8**). In the setting of systemic disease, only a needle biopsy may be needed, but if the lesion is small and symptomatic, resection can be offered. For larger lesions, radiotherapy is the primary treatment.[1]

METASTATIC TUMORS

As discussed before, metastatic lesions can arise from a variety of other cancers, and treatment depends on the primary histology, time to recurrence, and goals of intervention. For isolated metastases with a long interval before recurrence, surgical resection may be warranted. Each case should be individualized and discussed within a multidisciplinary team.

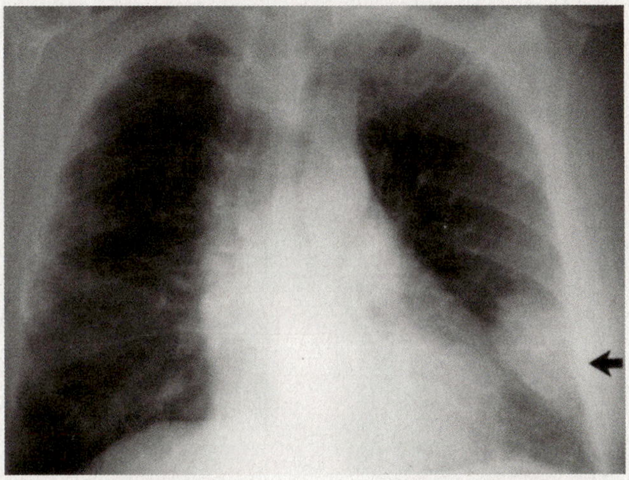

Figure 77.8. Plasmacytoma of the left seventh rib, showing characteristic cortical destruction and relatively large soft tissue component projecting into the chest.

CHEST WALL RECONSTRUCTION

Chest wall defects can result from cancer, radiation, trauma, or infection.[8] The goals of repair are to provide stabilization and protection to the thoracic cavity, to minimize 1 complications of respiration due to a flail chest, and to provide cosmetic coverage as needed. Size and location generally determine the need for chest wall stabilization. Defects less than 5 cm along the chest wall, or defects less than 10 cm on the posterior chest wall by the scapula, do not require reconstruction.[8,9] An alternative criterion is to use the number of ribs resected, and to avoid stabilization when a portion of three ribs or less has been removed.[10] Techniques for closure utilize polytetrafluoroethylene (PTFE), polypropylene methylmethacrylate (PPM) sandwich mesh, or metal plating systems combined with a composite mesh.[11] PTFE is a flexible, soft material, while the PPM sandwich mesh resembles a hardened piece of plaster between two portions of woven mesh. Different surgeons prefer different approaches, but some of the benefits cited for the PTFE repair include greater stretch and the ability to create a water-tight seal.[8] The PPM sandwich repair, on the other hand, allows the ability to mold the prosthetic and provides a firmer stabilization (**Fig. 77.9**).[11] Mortality rates from chest wall reconstruction in the setting of cancer resections have been reported at 4% in multiple series.[8,10]

Flap coverage of the soft tissue defect will almost always require the assistance of a plastic surgeon, and they should be involved preoperatively in the planning of a chest wall resection and reconstruction. The decision-making process for which flap to use depends on the location of the defect, the size of the defect, the corresponding size of the flap, and its vascular source. Pectoralis major flaps are the most common in the upper chest/neck region. Blood supply ranges from the thoracoacromial artery to intercostal perforators secondary to internal thoracic arteries (**Fig. 77.10**). The latissimus dorsi flap is also commonly used for large, ipsilateral defects. Its blood source is from the thoracodorsal artery or from perforators from the posterior intercostal vessels. It has a large arc of rotation from the thoracodorsal pedicle and can cover a wide area of the chest wall (**Fig. 77.11**). Also commonly used are rectus abdominal muscle flaps in either a vertical (VRAM) or transverse (TRAM) orientation (**Fig. 77.12**). External obliques can be used on the lower anterior chest wall, and the trapezius can be used in the midback.[12] Omental flaps are extremely useful

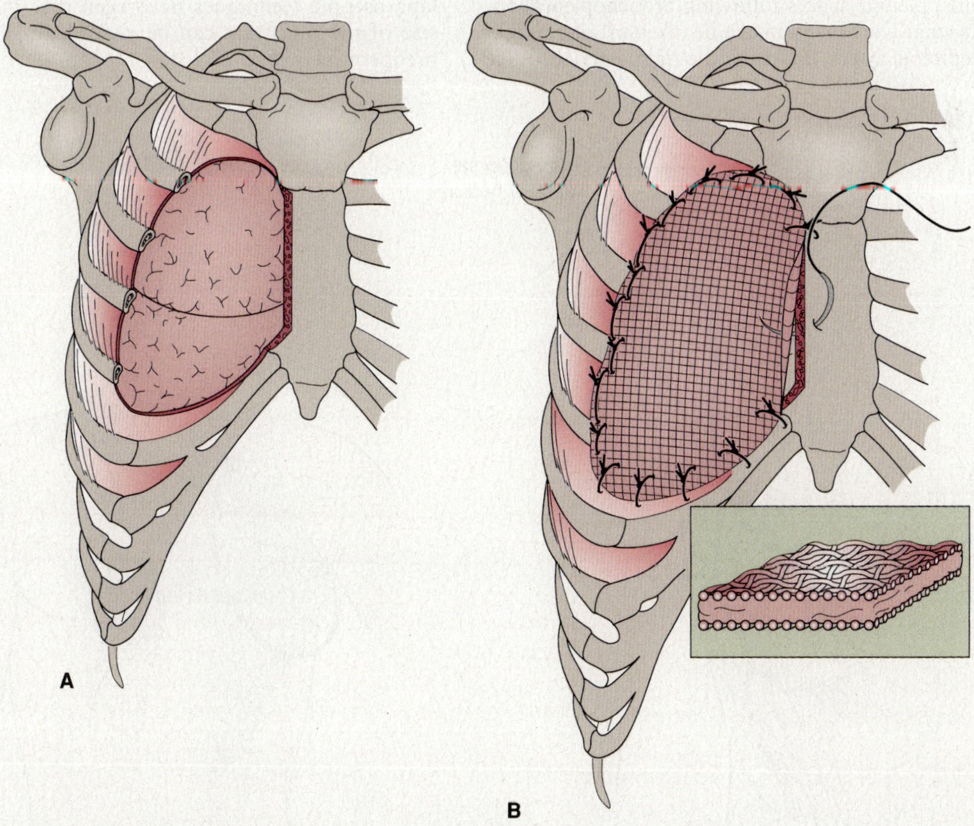

Figure 77.9. Marlex methylmethacrylate sandwich technique for chest wall reconstruction. **A:** Upper anterior chest wall defect resulting from resection of ribs 2 to 5 and a portion of sternum. **B:** Marlex methylmethacrylate prosthesis being sutured in place. Heavy, nonabsorbable sutures either encircling the ribs or passed through the sternum are used to anchor the prosthesis in place. **Inset:** Detail of prosthesis showing sandwich of hardened methylmethacrylate between two sheets of Marlex.

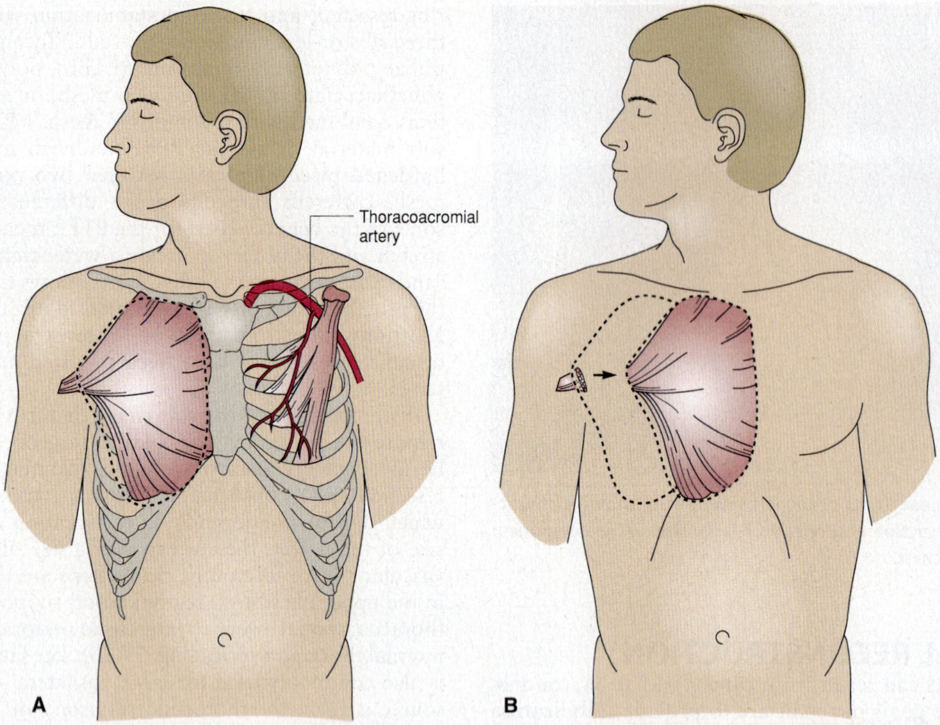

Figure 77.10. Pectoralis major muscle rotation flap. **A:** Mobilization of the flap by detaching the clavicular, sternal, and chest wall origins as well as the insertion of the muscle on the greater tubercle of the humerus. The dominant blood supply, the thoracoacromial artery, which arises from the axillary artery medial to the proximal border of the pectoralis minor muscle, is shown on the left side where the pectoralis major muscle has been removed. **B:** Medial transposition of the muscle flap, preserving the thoracoacromial neurovascular bundle.

and versatile. They can be used to cover large defects or to fill contaminated cavities, such as sternal dehiscence complicated by mediastinitis, pleural spaces following bronchopleural fistula, and empyema. The omentum can be taken off of the right or left gastroepiploic artery, but using the right arterial source allows a greater arc of rotation than from the left. The limitations of this flap are that it requires a laparotomy, although laparoscopic techniques have been described,[13] and that the size of the omentum can be variable, and difficult to assess preoperatively (**Fig. 77.13**).[12]

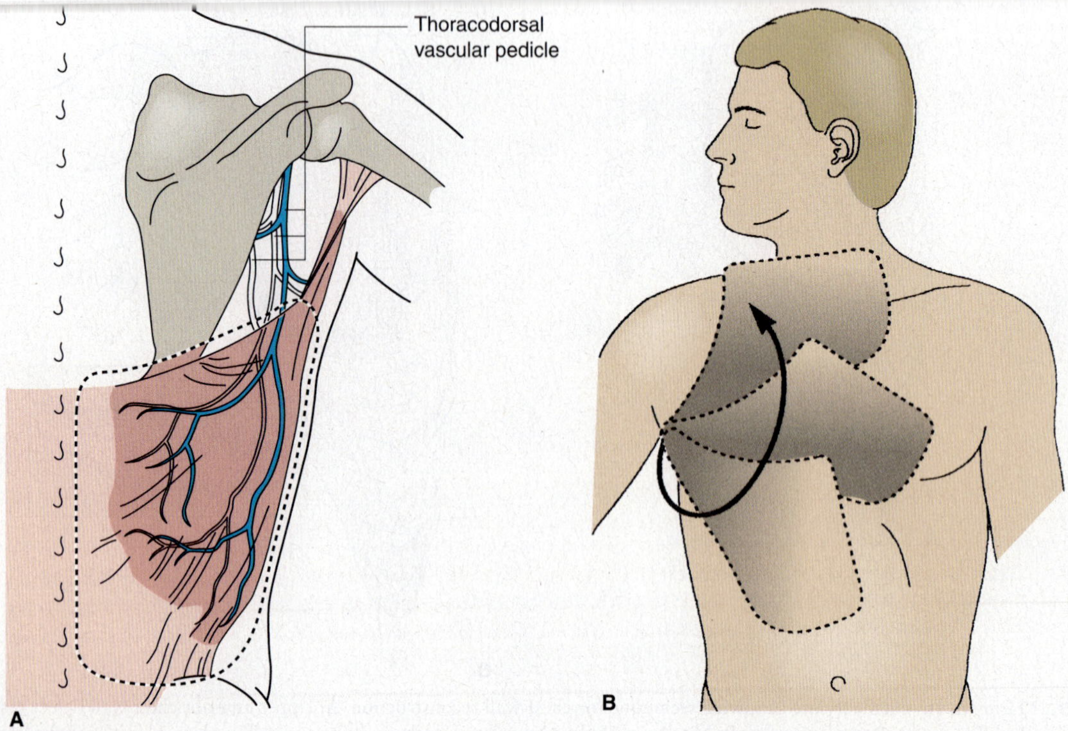

Figure 77.11. Latissimus dorsi muscle rotation flap for chest wall reconstruction. **A:** Posterior view showing detachment of the origins of the muscle. The dominant blood supply, the thoracodorsal artery, is preserved. **B:** Anterior view showing the extent to which the mobilized muscle reaches.

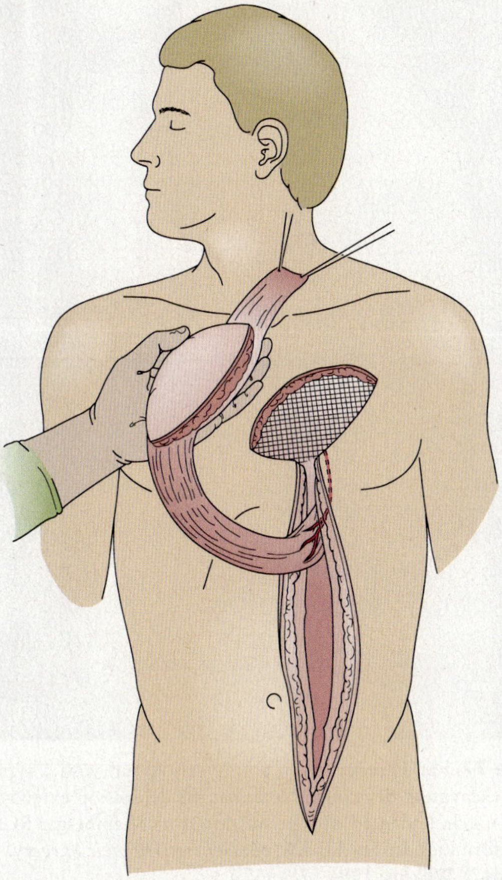

Figure 77.12. Rectus abdominis muscle rotation flap. Shown is the mobilization of the rectus abdominis muscle, which is based on the superior epigastric artery (the continuation of the internal thoracic artery), and rotation of the muscle and overlying skin to fill an anterior chest wall defect.

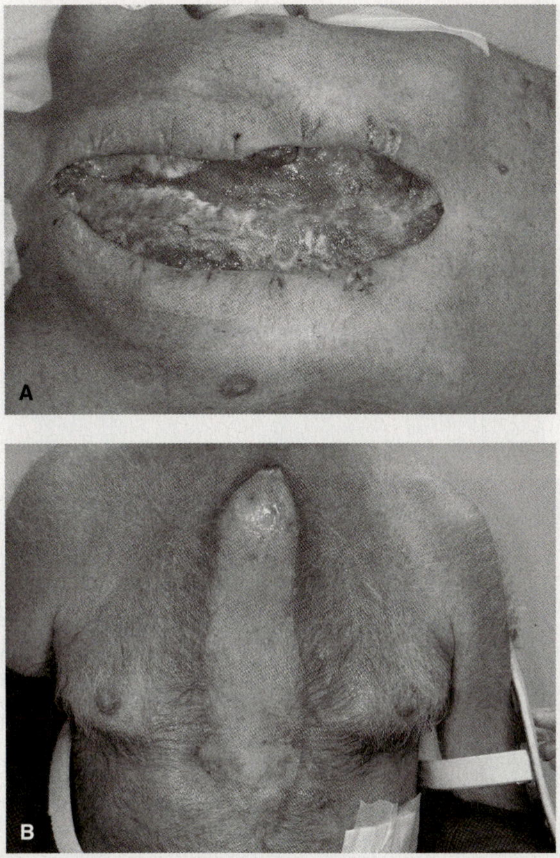

Figure 77.13. The omentum can be used to cover large defects. Shown is an open sternal wound after débridement with failed prior muscle flap (**A**), and wound 6 months after omental flap placement (**B**). (Reproduced with permission from Ghazi B, Carlson G, Losken A. Use of the greater omentum for reconstruction of infected sternotomy wounds: a prognostic indicator? *Ann Plast Surg*. 2008;60(2):169–173.)

CHEST WALL CONGENITAL ABNORMALITIES AND THORACIC OUTLET SYNDROME

Pectus Excavatum and Pectus Carinatum

Chest wall deformities occur in 1/1000 live births. They are five times more common in men than women, and up to 6% of people with these deformities will also have a connective tissue disorder. Pectus excavatum is the most common deformity and appears as a sternal depression that can be off midline. Pectus carinatum is the opposite, with a sternal protrusion, often described as a "pigeon chest" deformity. Pectus excavatum is five times more common than pectus carinatum. Scoliosis is frequently seen in this population.[14] Less common deformities include sternal clefts, which are incomplete fusions of the sternum, and Poland syndrome, where there is an absence of a pectoralis muscle and underlying bony support in the chest wall.

The techniques for surgical correction of pectus excavatum include the Ravitch and Nuss procedures. Historically, less than 15% of patients undergo surgery.[15] Most patients present as children with notable deformities. Most patients are asymptomatic, but common symptoms include fatigue, limited stamina, and cardiopulmonary limitations. The workup includes pulmonary function testing, echocardiography, and CT scans. The pectus severity index (Haller index) can be calculated by dividing the chest's transverse diameter by the depth measured from the posterior aspect of the sternum to the anterior aspect of the vertebral body (**Fig. 77.14**). Normal values are 2 to 2.2, and repair is only recommended when the index is at least greater than 3.25.[14,16] The age of the patient at which repair should be performed is also somewhat controversial, as some surgeons advocate waiting until after the age of 10, but many series have reported on a large number of patients treated at a much younger age with good outcomes.[15,17] There is a growing experience with treating adults also, as some patients seek repair at a later age (**Fig. 77.15**).[18,19]

The most commonly used open repair, first described by Dr. Ravitch, is based on removing sections of the deformed cartilage from around the sternum laterally at the ribs, while preserving the perichondrium. A stabilizing bar is placed for 6 to 24 months, usually placed in an intrathoracic position, to minimize the occurrence of flail chest and to allow the sternum to heal in an anterior position. An essential part of the procedure is a transverse sternal wedge resection through the anterior table to allow the inferior aspect of sternum to bend forward.[14,19] Incisions may be in a vertical midline over the lower half of the sternum or in an inframammary position (**Fig. 77.16**). Recurrences occur in 5% to 10% of patients, with recurrence more common in patients with connective tissue disorders.

The Nuss procedure, which utilizes a minimally invasive approach, has been described and performed. The Nuss procedure utilizes one or two stabilization bars, secured to the ribs laterally in multiple points of fixation. It routinely employs thoracoscopy, either unilateral or bilateral. Skin incisions are limited to small lateral locations at the site of the bar insertion and thoracoscopic port sites.[20] As the Nuss procedure has grown in popularity, many modifications have been made, including precise shaping of the bars and increased bar stabilization with wire fixation around the ribs to minimize bar displacement.[21]

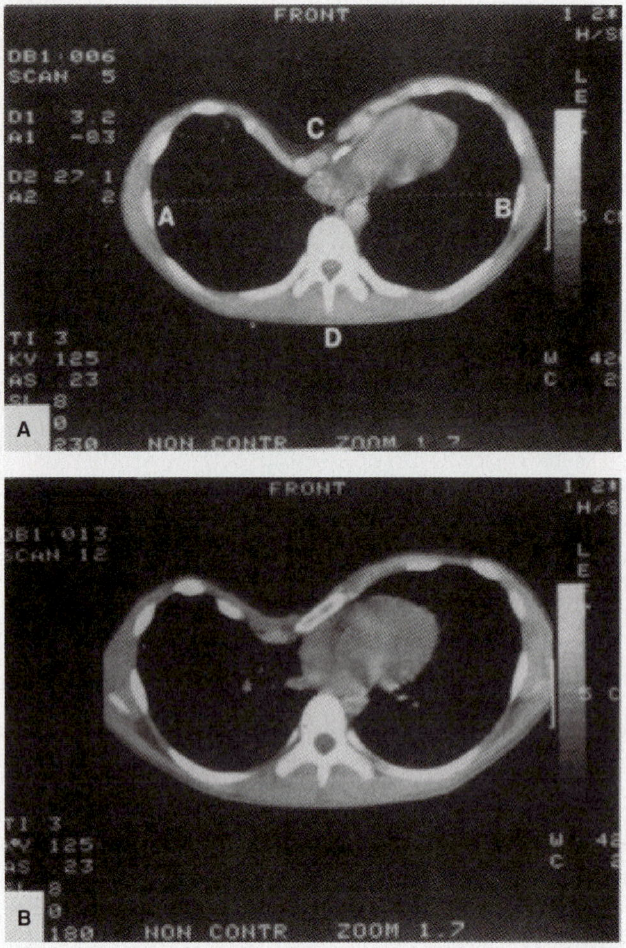

Figure 77.14. Chest CT of pectus excavatum. CT image at xiphoid with A–B (transverse diameter) and C–D (anterior–posterior diameter) indicated for the calculation of the pectus severity index A-B/C-D (**A**). CT image demonstrating angulation of the sternum to the right in the severe defect (**B**). (Reproduced with permission from Haller JA Jr, Scherer LR, Turner CS, et al. Evolving management of pectus excavatum based on a single institutional experience of 664 patients? *Ann Surg*. 1989;209(5):578–582.)

Pectus carinatum does not have the same cardiac compression concerns as pectus excavatum, but the chest is held in an enlarged position, which may limit normal respiration mechanics. Patients can have increased residual lung volumes, and their respiratory physiology can mimic emphysema physiology. This can result in breathing difficulties and limited stamina.[19] The Ravitch procedure may be performed to remove the deformed cartilage. Special attention is placed on the transverse sternal osteotomy, to depress the sternum and align it with the anterior ribs (**Fig. 77.17**).[14]

Sternal Clefts

Sternal clefts are much rarer than pectus deformity. They result from the failure of the sternum to fuse in the midline. They can vary from minor defects with the upper half of the sternum separated to complete dissociation and thoracic ectopia cordis (the heart being outside the chest wall). Upper sternal defects have a U- or V-shaped appearance and usually extend to the 4th intercostal space (**Fig. 77.18**). Repair of these defects can be easily performed by incision, complete sternotomy, oblique chondrotomies of the sternal halves, and closure. Complete sternal clefts are associated with diastasis recti and an opening between the peritoneal and pericardial cavities. Inferior clefts are associated with the pentalogy of Cantrell, a constellation of defects which include supraumbilical abdominal wall defect, lower sternal cleft, defect in the anterior diaphragm, defect in the associated pericardium, and congenital cardiac defects, often tetralogy of Fallot.[22]

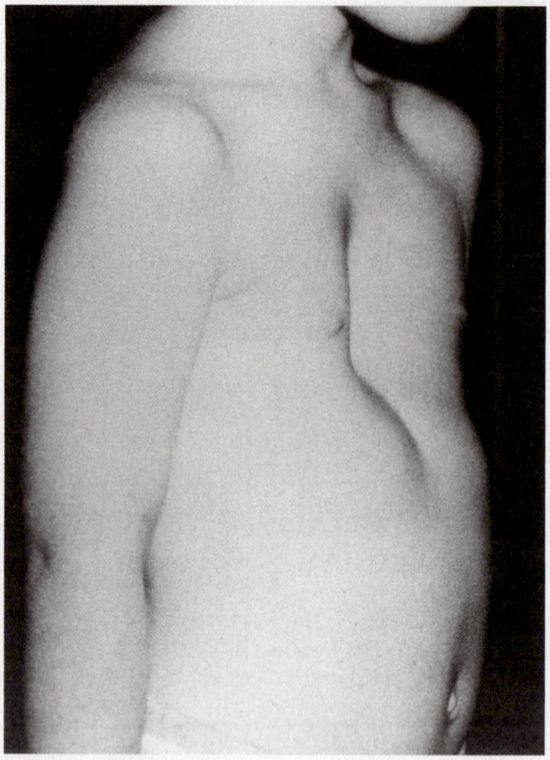

Figure 77.15. Photograph of a 4.5-year-old girl with a symmetric pectus excavatum deformity. Note that the depression extends to the sternal notch. (Adapted with permission from Shamberger RC. Chest wall deformities. In: Shields TW, ed. *General Thoracic Surgery*. 4th ed. Williams & Wilkins; 1994:529–557.)

Poland Syndrome

Poland syndrome is the clinical absence of a pectoralis muscle and underlying bony support in the chest wall, and it occurs in 1/30,000 live births. It is usually a right-sided, unilateral defect. Patients commonly have associated limb abnormalities, and may also present with renal and spinal lesions (**Fig. 77.19**). Clinical symptoms may be absent, though lung herniation can occur, requiring a more urgent repair. The surgical approach is usually multidisciplinary and ideally is deferred until after the patient has stopped growing. Repairs typically utilize mesh placement over the defect, and/or muscle flap placement.[23]

Thoracic Outlet Syndrome

The thoracic outlet in thoracic outlet syndrome (TOS) refers to the thoracic inlet, the correct anatomic term for the region of the first rib and the middle and anterior scalene muscles. Through these structures, the brachial plexus, subclavian artery, and subclavian vein travel to the upper limbs (**Fig. 77.20**). These structures may be subjected to abnormal compression by inflammation around the muscles or abnor-
2 mal bony structures such as cervical ribs, causing pain, thrombosis, and other[2] symptoms that are described as TOS. TOS can be divided into arterial, venous, or neurogenic diseases, or a combination, depending on the symptoms and clinical findings. Vascular TOS is easier to document with vascular imaging. Neurogenic TOS is more difficult to diagnose. Unfortunately for neurogenic TOS, there is no gold standard diagnostic test to confirm the syndrome. As a result, there has been significant controversy over the diagnosis and the indications for surgical treatment, especially in light of the potential for significant postoperative complications.[24,25]

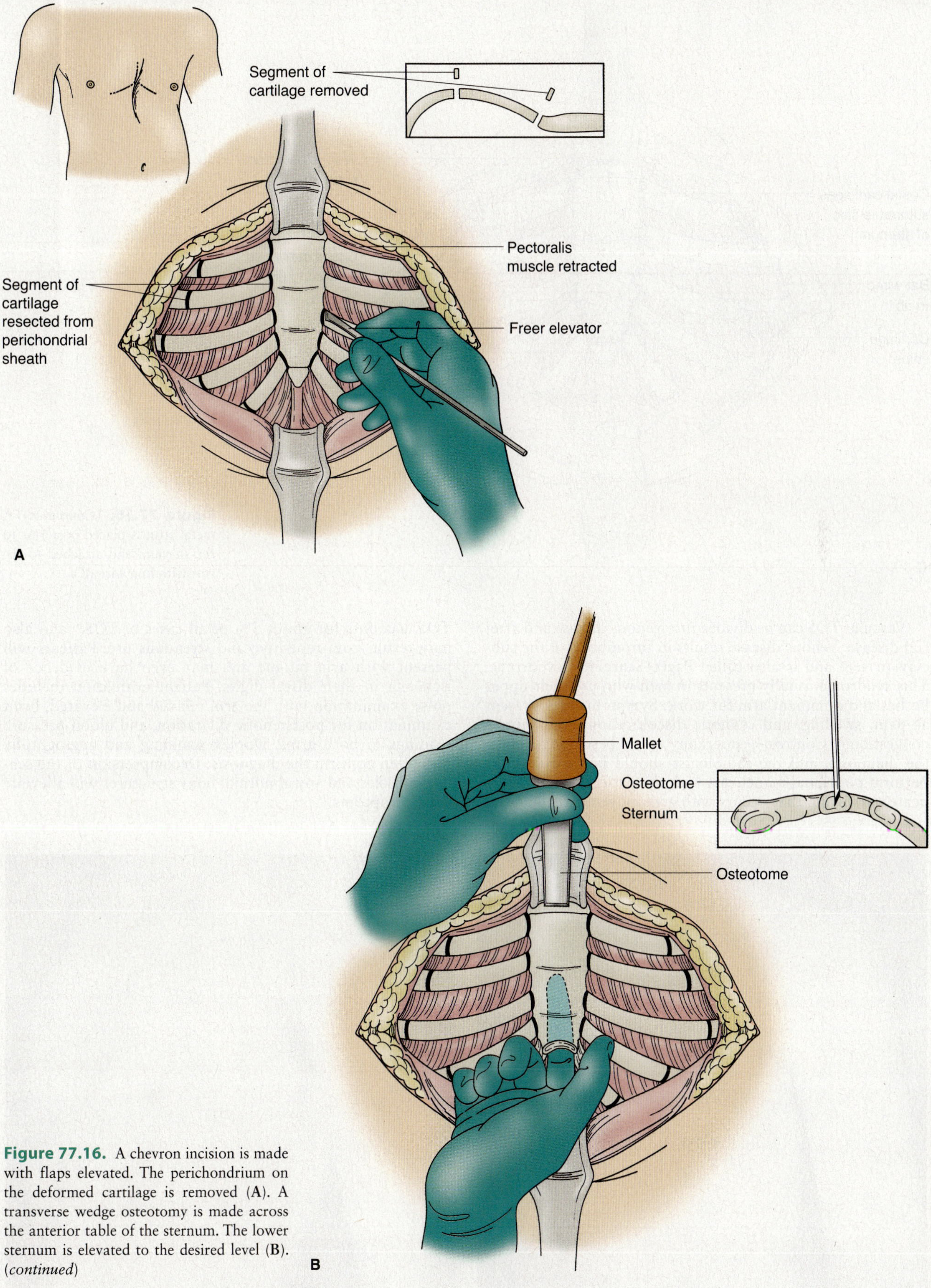

Figure 77.16. A chevron incision is made with flaps elevated. The perichondrium on the deformed cartilage is removed (**A**). A transverse wedge osteotomy is made across the anterior table of the sternum. The lower sternum is elevated to the desired level (**B**). (*continued*)

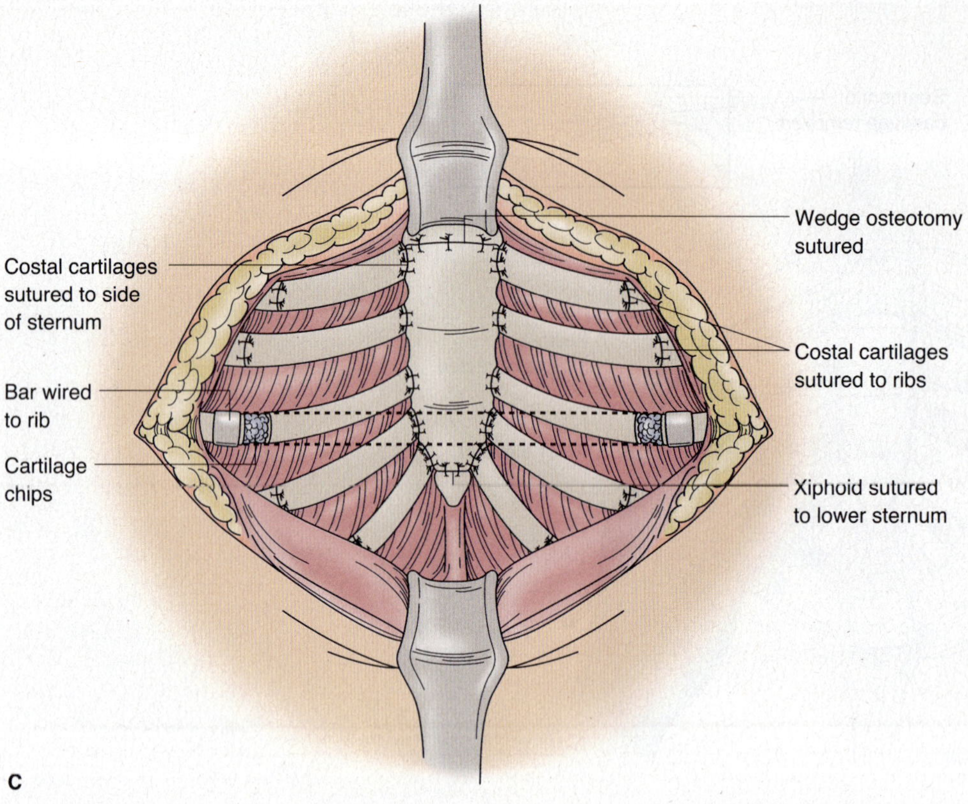

Figure 77.16. (*Continued*) A metal strut is placed posterior to the sternum and attached to the ribs with fine wire (**C**).

Vascular TOS can be divided into venous disease and arterial disease. Venous disease results in thrombosis of the subclavian vein and is also called Paget–Schroetter syndrome. This syndrome usually presents in men who use their upper bodies and dominant arm for work. Symptoms may present as pain, swelling, and cyanotic discoloration from venous congestion.[24] Contrast venography is the best test to make the diagnosis, and the radiologist should be instructed to perform positional maneuvers with the patient's arm to replicate narrowing that occurs with arm movement.[25] Arterial TOS accounts for about 5% of all cases of TOS[26] and also may result from repetitive and strenuous use. Patients will present with arm fatigue and may even have evidence of ischemia in their distal digits. Patient evaluation includes pulse examination with the arm relaxed and elevated, bruit examination for poststenotic dilatation, and blood pressure readings in both arms. Duplex scanning and angiography will often confirm the diagnosis. Decompression of the scalene muscles and any abnormal bony structures will alleviate these symptoms.[14]

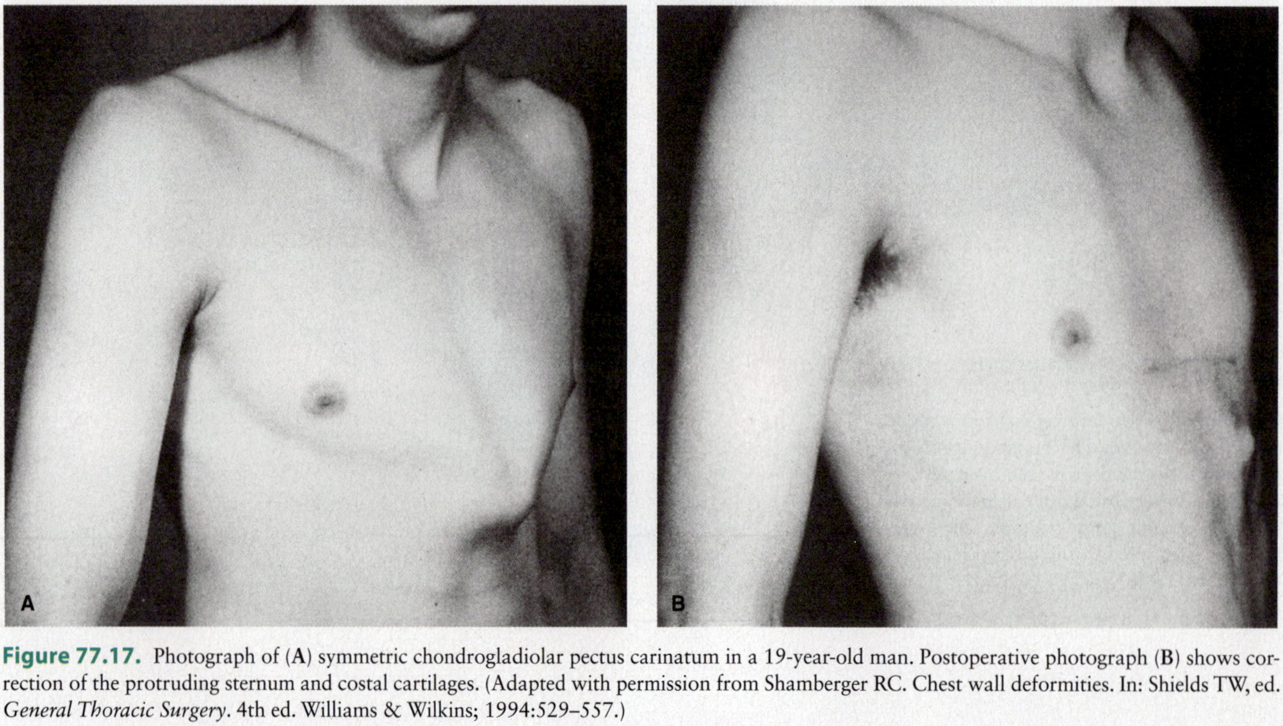

Figure 77.17. Photograph of (**A**) symmetric chondrogladiolar pectus carinatum in a 19-year-old man. Postoperative photograph (**B**) shows correction of the protruding sternum and costal cartilages. (Adapted with permission from Shamberger RC. Chest wall deformities. In: Shields TW, ed. *General Thoracic Surgery*. 4th ed. Williams & Wilkins; 1994:529–557.)

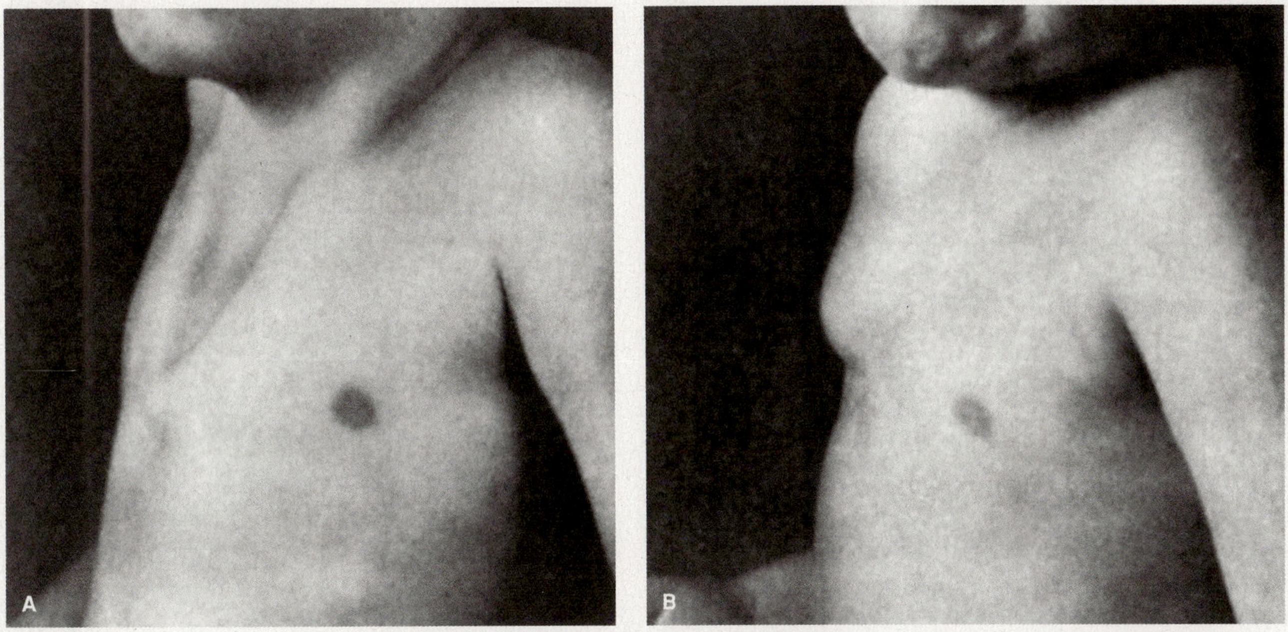

Figure 77.18. Cleft sternum at rest (**A**) and during forced expiration (**B**). Superior clefts of the sternum are variously V- or U-shaped. The appearance of the child as he cries explains the term ectopia cordis, although the heart is actually not misplaced. In the newborn, defects of this kind can be corrected by direct apposition of the sternal halves. In this child, closure of the defect was made possible by sliding chondrotomies on either side. (Reproduced with permission from Sabiston DC Jr. The surgical management of congenital bifid sternum with a partial ectopia cordis? *J Thorac Surg*. 1958;35:118.)

Neurogenic TOS presents with limb pain, numbness, or weakness. Symptoms may be bilateral, but are usually worse in the dominant arm. The distribution may not follow a peripheral nerve pattern, thus making the diagnosis confusing, but also ruling out more distal compression syndromes such as carpal tunnel in the wrist or cubital compression at the elbow. The physical examination should be focused on duplicating the patient's symptoms. The Adson maneuver may detect artery compression and is performed by palpating the affected radial pulse and having the patient take a deep inspiration while

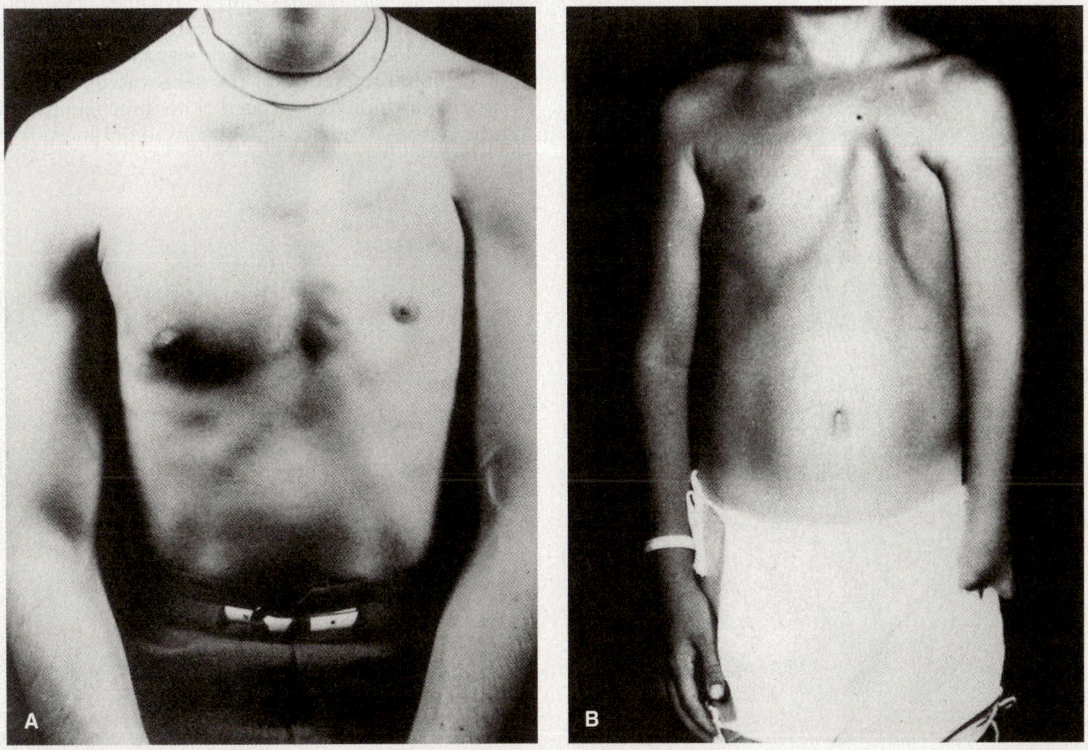

Figure 77.19. **A:** Muscular 15-year-old boy with loss of the left axillary fold, orthotopic sternum, and normal cartilages. He compensates adequately for loss of the pectoralis major and minor muscles. Surgery is not indicated in males with these findings. **B:** An 8-year-old boy with Poland syndrome. The pectoralis major and minor muscles and the serratus to the level of the fifth rib are absent. The boy has sternal obliquity, and the 3rd to 5th ribs are short, ending in points. The corresponding cartilages are absent. The endothoracic fascia lies beneath a thin layer of subcutaneous tissue. Note the hypoplastic nipple and ectromelia of the ipsilateral hand. (*continued*)

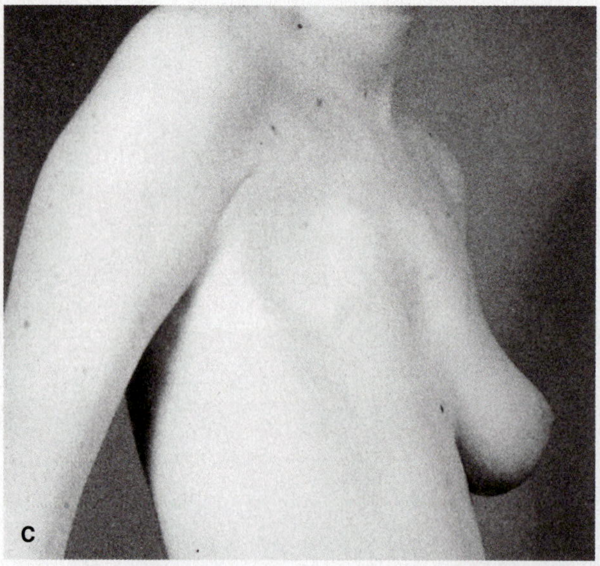

Figure 77.19. (*Continued*) **C:** A 14-year-old girl with Poland syndrome. Note the high position of the right nipple, amastia, sternal rotation, and depressed right anterior chest. The 2nd to 4th ribs and cartilages were missing, reconstructed with rib grafts. Breast augmentation will be required at full growth. (Reproduced with permission from Shamberger RC. Chest wall deformities? In: Shields TW, ed. *General Thoracic Surgery*. 4th ed. Williams & Wilkins; 1994:529–557.)

turning their head away from the affected arm (**Fig. 77.21**). High-risk anatomical variants for nTOS include accessory ribs, short costoclavicular distance, and a protuberant C7 process.[27] The test is positive if the pulse disappears, but a positive result can also be seen in asymptomatic people without TOS. Another test requires the patient to elevate their arms in a "surrender" position and open and close their hands

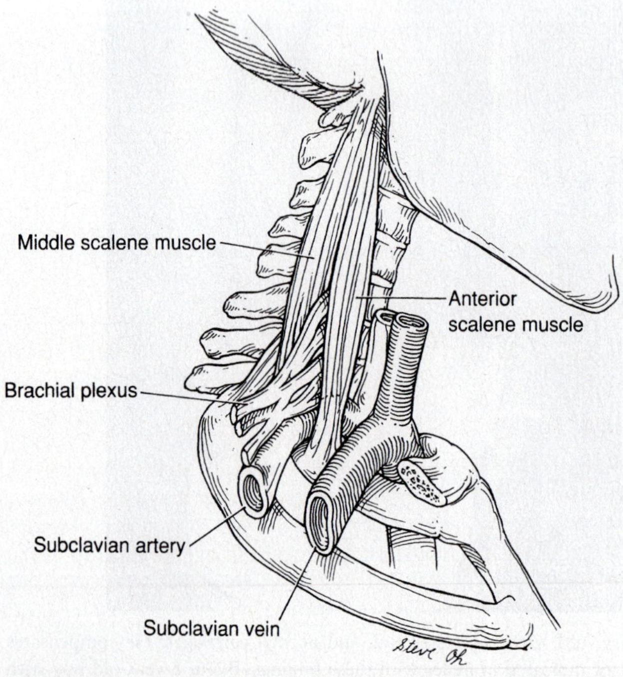

Figure 77.20. Important structures in the thoracic outlet. (Reproduced with permission from Scott-Conner CE, Dawson DL, Shirazi MK, et al. *Operative Anatomy*. 3rd ed. Lippincott Williams & Wilkins; 2008.)

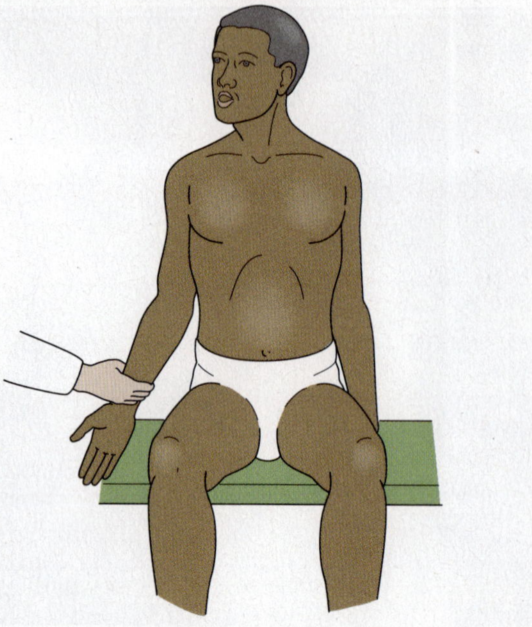

Figure 77.21. The Adson maneuver. Patient inspires and turns head away from the affected arm. The test is positive if the pulse disappears.

repeatedly. Most people with neurogenic TOS will be fatigued within a minute and be unable to continue (**Fig. 77.22**). Plain radiographs may show bony abnormalities, but no other imaging will help diagnose neurogenic TOS. Physical rehabilitation is the first step to treat patients with neurogenic TOS, and over a third of patients may get a significant improvement in their symptoms. If there is no significant improvement in symptoms, then surgical intervention is suggested.[25]

The surgical approach for TOS was traditionally a transaxillary first rib resection (**Fig. 77.23**). The approach has broadened to supraclavicular, infraclavicular, and transthoracic approaches. The transthoracic robotic approach has become popularized given the enhanced visualization of the anatomy, with minimal retraction of the neurovascular bundle, thereby limiting morbidity associated with brachial plexus injury.[26] The first rib is exposed, attachments to the anterior and middle

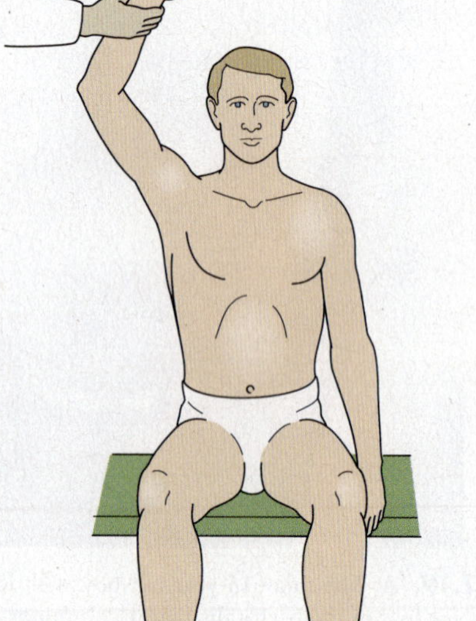

Figure 77.22. Surrender position with opening and closing of hand. Early fatigue is seen in neurogenic TOS.

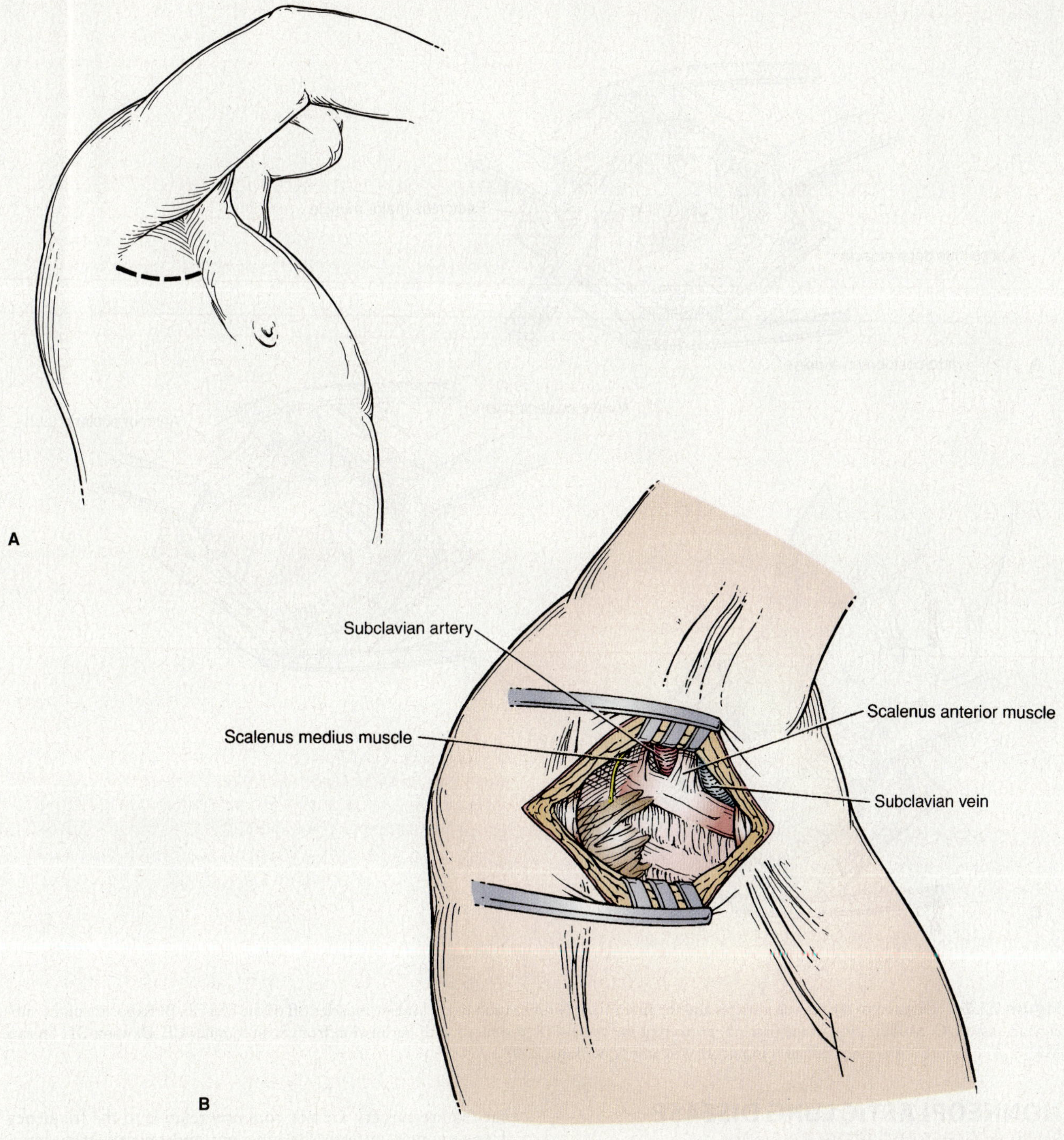

Figure 77.23. Position of the patient (**A**) and skin incision (**B**) for transaxillary approach. (Reproduced with permission from Scott-Conner CE, Dawson DL, Shirazi MK, et al. *Operative Anatomy*. 3rd ed. Lippincott Williams & Wilkins; 2008.)

scalenes are divided, and the rib is removed (**Fig. 77.24**). Special attention must be paid to the phrenic nerve lying along the anterior scalene and the axillary branches off of the brachial plexus. Small drains may be placed in the apex of the thorax if the pleural space is entered.[25,29] The supraclavicular approach also gives access to perform a cervical sympathectomy if indicated for symptoms consistent with sympathetic overactivity. In patients with arterial aneurysms, reconstruction with synthetic grafts or autologous conduits, such as an external iliac artery, can be performed. For patients with venous TOS, care should be taken to perform a circumferential venolysis and to remove the medial aspect of the first rib.[29]

Postoperative complications include pneumothorax, lymphatic leaks, especially on the left side where the thoracic duct enters the operative field, phrenic nerve palsy, and traction injury to the brachial plexus.[26] Rehabilitation and range of motion exercises should begin as soon as possible to reduce the risk of frozen shoulder.[25,29] Up to 12.5% of patients may not get any symptom relief after the surgery, and long-term physical rehabilitation is recommended.[26] Patients with combined symptoms of venous and neurogenic TOS have worse outcomes when compared to patients with only venous disease. A higher percentage of patients had persistent pain in the neurogenic group, as might be expected.[30] The treatment of this disease process requires a significant investment into the preoperative and postoperative care of these patients and should only be done in centers with a high volume and expertise in this syndrome.

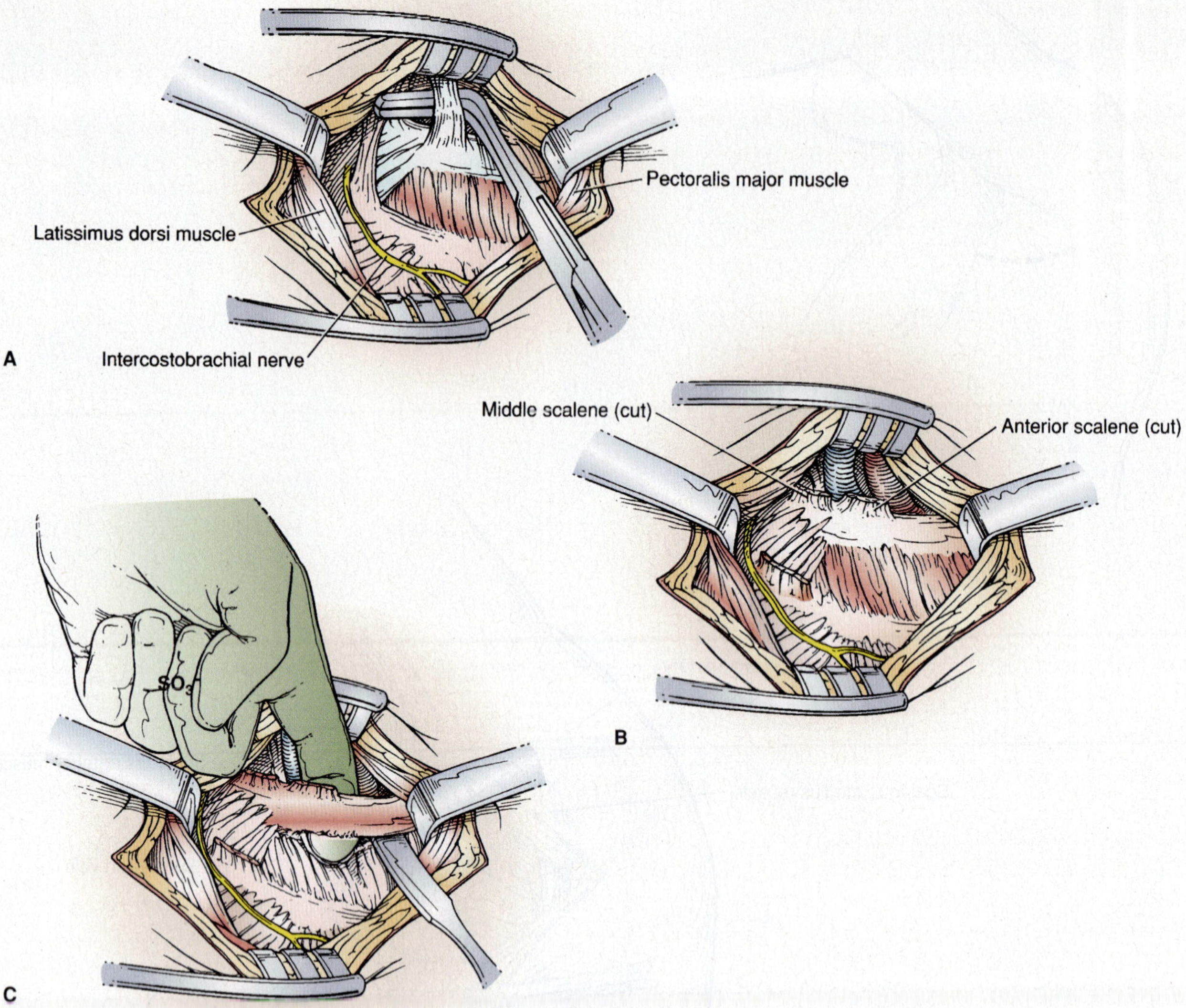

Figure 77.24. Division of the scalene muscles and the first rib. **A:** Mobilization of the scalene muscles off of the first rib. **B:** Exposure of the subclavian vessels. **C:** Mobilization of the first rib, protecting the vessels. (Reproduced with permission from Scott-Conner CE, Dawson DL, Shirazi MK, et al. *Operative Anatomy*. 3rd ed. Lippincott Williams & Wilkins; 2008.)

NONNEOPLASTIC LUNG DISEASE

Lung Abscess and Bronchiectasis

Lung abscesses can result from aspiration, bronchial obstruction, or secondary to another infectious foci (ie, endocarditis, necrotizing pneumonia, etc). Patients may present with chest pain, cough, anorexia, and fever. Radiographic studies may demonstrate an air–fluid level in the background of consolidated lung in dependent portions of the lung (posterior segment of upper lobes or superior segments).[31] Routine use of antibiotics for pneumonias has dramatically reduced the rate of lung abscess sequelae. In over 80% of cases, a pathogen can be found, and in immunocompromised patients, there are usually
3 multiple organisms involved, including *Pseudomonas aeruginosa*[3] and *Haemophilus* species. The primary treatment for lung abscesses is medical therapy with antibiotics. If a patient is clinically not improving with medical therapy alone, a guided drainage tube may be placed. A complication of this approach is the risk of a chronic air leak from a percutaneous tube placed into the lung parenchyma. Surgery may be indicated in the setting of large abscesses causing hemoptysis or other symptoms (**Algorithm 77.1**). Complications from pulmonary infections that require surgery are not common relative to the frequency of pneumonias in both the inpatient and outpatient community. However, some patients may benefit from surgical intervention to treat lung abscesses.[32]. Risk factors for medical failure include refractory infection in the setting of bronchial obstruction, large abscess (>6 cm), complicated empyema, and inability to rule out malignancy.[33]

Bronchiectasis is the abnormal dilation of bronchi/bronchioles as a result of multiple episodes of infection and inflammation. Patients can present with respiratory symptoms like dyspnea, hemoptysis, or pleuritic pain, or alternatively, may present only with systemic changes such as fatigue and weight loss.[34] Almost all patients will have a chronic cough with or without sputum production.[35] Factors contributing to the development of this disease may be genetic, anatomic, or even systemic. Genetic causes of bronchiectasis include cystic fibrosis and primary ciliary dyskinesia, which result in reduced mucus clearance and alpha-1-antitrypsin deficiency, which results in destruction of lung parenchyma.[34] Anatomic causes include postsurgical changes or acquired diseases such as chronic obstructive pulmonary disease (COPD) that lead to

Algorithm 77.1

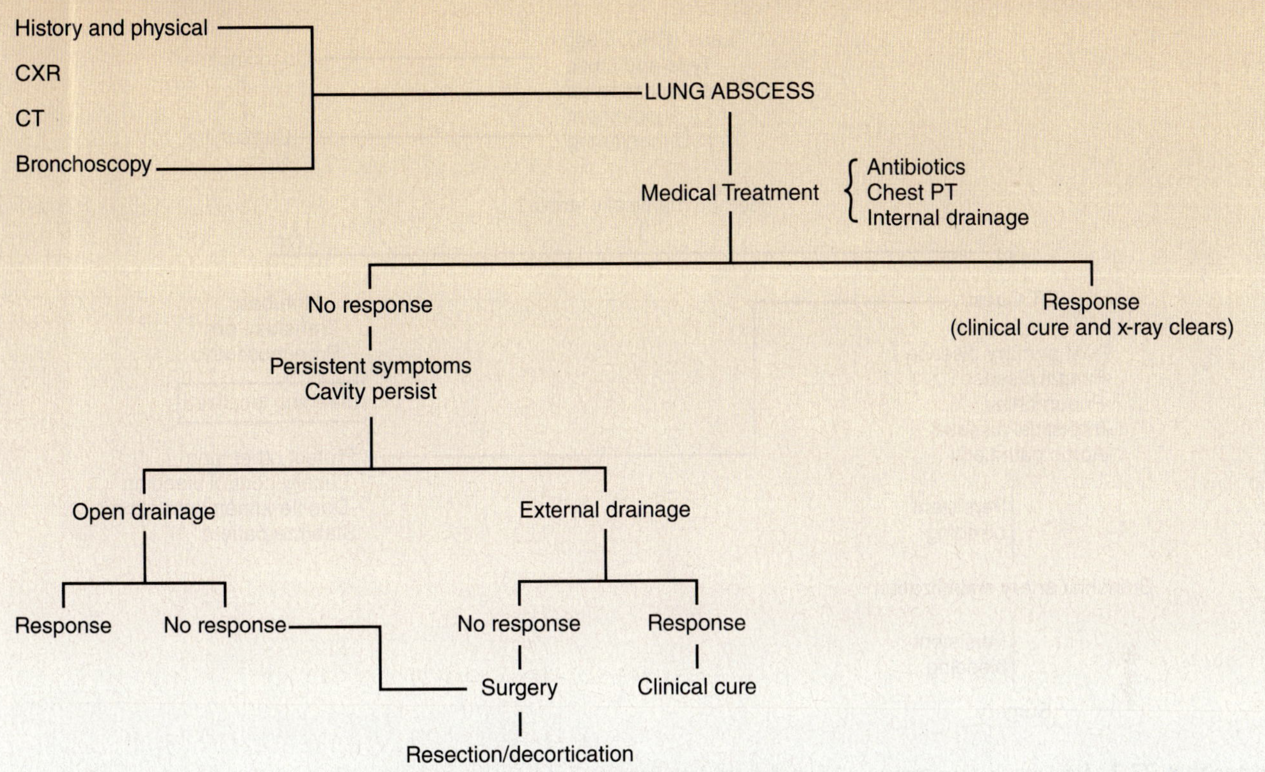

Algorithm 77.1. Algorithm for management of lung abscess. (Adapted from Shields TW, ed. *General Thoracic Surgery*. 6th ed. 2005.)

an increased risk of infection, again due to the inability to clear secretions. Autoimmune diseases such as rheumatoid arthritis and inflammatory bowel disease have been associated with increased rates of bronchiectasis.[34,35] Infectious causes include allergic bronchopulmonary aspergillosis and nontuberculous mycobacterium infections. Reflux disease is also being studied as a potential contributor. Most often, the etiology of the disease is idiopathic.[34]

There are estimated to be 110,000 patients in the United States being treated for noncystic fibrosis bronchiectasis each year. Pulmonary function tests may demonstrate moderate-to-severe airflow obstruction.[34] A chest CT scan is the optimal test to diagnose bronchiectasis (**Fig. 77.25**), and once the diagnosis is made, the search for an etiology should begin, including obtaining sputum cultures and blood tests for autoimmune markers such as rheumatoid factor.[35]

The treatment of the disease includes antibiotic therapy to control infection, the treatment of underlying diseases if they exist, reducing inflammation, improving secretion clearance, and surgery to remove focally damaged areas or transplantation if needed for more diffuse, severe disease. Antibiotic therapy includes inhaled tobramycin and gentamicin.[35] Macrolide antibiotics, like erythromycin and clarithromycin, have been increasingly studied for anti-inflammatory benefits outside their antibiotic effects. They disrupt the biofilm produced in *Pseudomonas* infections, resulting in decreased sputum volume and improved symptoms.[36] Secretion removal is also essential to improving symptoms. Standard treatments include chest physiotherapy, postural drainage, along with the use of nebulized acetylcysteine[35] and hypertonic saline[36] has been shown to improve mucus clearance.

Surgical intervention may occur at many stages of the disease process. Bronchoscopy can be useful to clear secretions or to manage hemoptysis. If the bronchiectasis is localized to a single lobe, resection can eliminate the disease and the source of chronic infection. If a patient has a genetic disease such as cystic fibrosis, a double lung transplant may be the best treatment if the patient's symptoms are severe enough.[35] Pulmonary tuberculosis can have similar indications for surgical intervention when it results in bronchiectasis or hemoptysis.[37] The rise of more multi–drug-resistant tuberculosis strains has led to the increasing need for surgical intervention.[38]

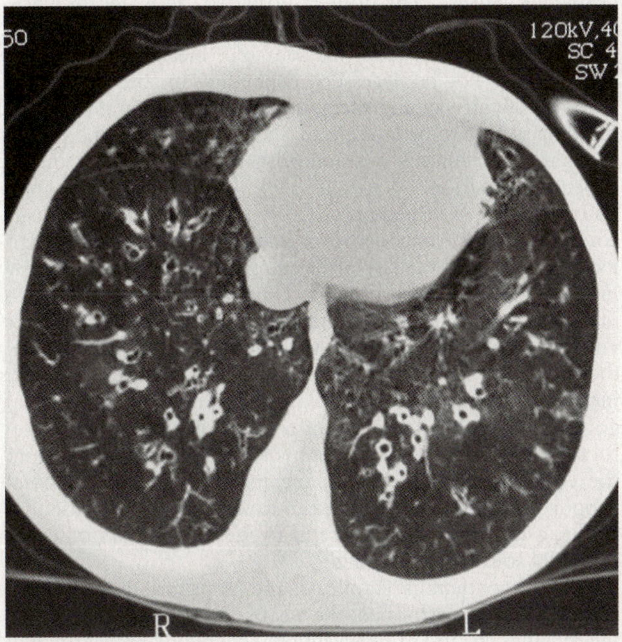

Figure 77.25. CT scan of bronchiectatic lungs. (Reproduced with permission from Shields TW, ed. *General Thoracic Surgery*, 6th ed.)

Algorithm 77.2

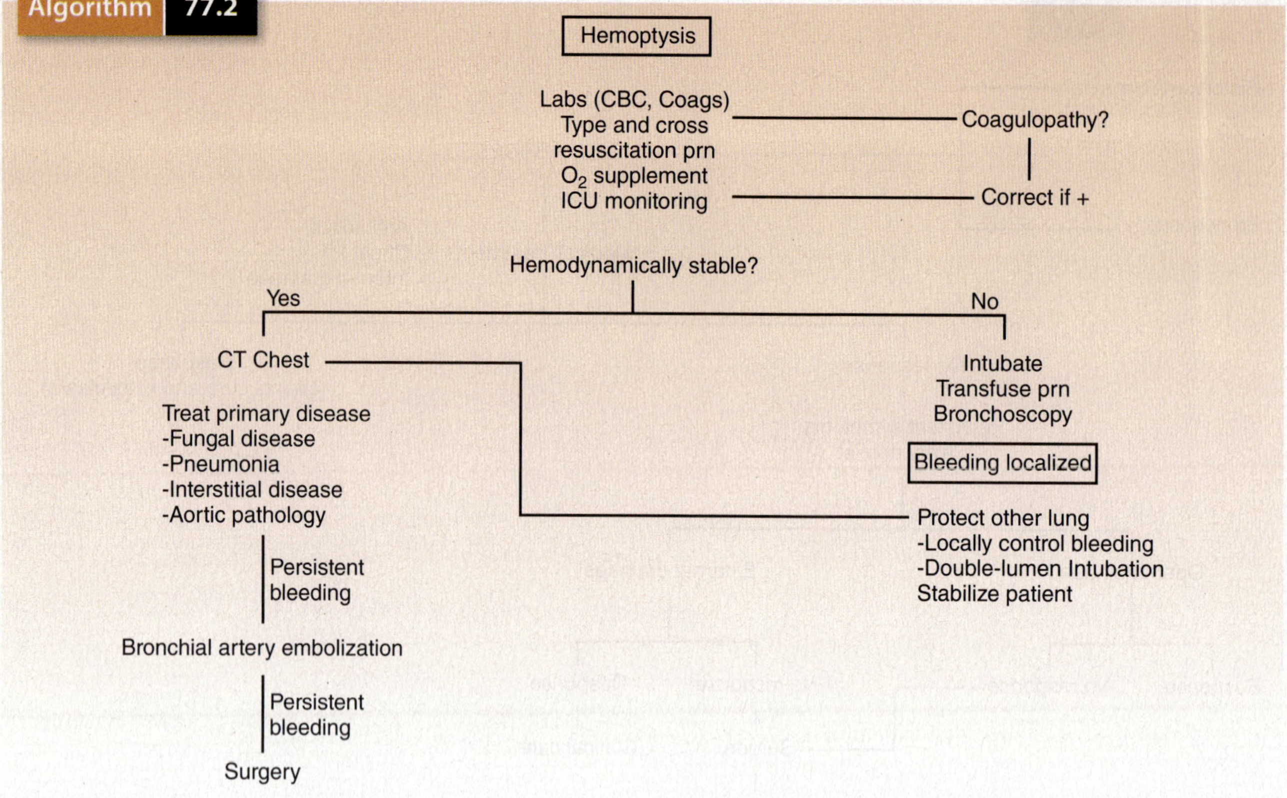

Algorithm 77.2. Hemoptysis management. (Adapted from Jean-Baptiste E. Clinical assessment and management of massive hemoptysis. *Crit Care Med.* 2000;28(5):1642–1647.)

Hemoptysis

Hemoptysis is often used to describe any blood-stained sputum following a coughing episode. True hemoptysis may only
4 be a few drops of blood, and requires investigation. Massive hemoptysis is acutely life threatening, not from blood or volume loss, but rather from asphyxiation secondary to blood in the airway. The causes of hemoptysis include, but are not limited to, cancer, infections/bronchiectasis, vascular injuries, pulmonary embolism, vasculitides, and coagulopathies, and iatrogenic causes.[39] The primary objective following presentation is to achieve airway patency, optimize oxygenation and gas exchange, and localize the source of bleeding. Intubation may or may not be necessary, depending on the volume of blood in the airway and the patient's ability to cough.[40] If the bleeding is able to be lateralized, the patient should be placed in a lateral decubitus position with the bleeding site in the dependent position.

In patients with hemoptysis, any coagulopathy should be corrected. Early bronchoscopy is essential, and the goals are to localize and treat the site of bleeding. Flexible bronchoscopy may be done, but rigid bronchoscopy is the best approach to maintain airway control, in particular in the setting of large volume hemoptysis.[40] Initial treatment may include topical therapy such as cold saline lavage, bronchial tamponade, inhaled tranexamic acid, and intubation of the contralateral good lung. Double-lumen endotracheal tubes may also be useful to isolate and protect the uninvolved lung from blood from the contralateral side obstructing its lumen. Extracorporeal support (ECMO) may be used in severe cases. If a patient is stable, a chest CT scan is useful to identify tumors or other potential sources of bleeding.[39]

Once a patient is stabilized and appropriate diagnostic tests have been performed, the treatment of continued bleeding includes the use of interventional radiology and bronchial artery embolization (BAE).[40] First introduced in 1973, BAE is the gold standard to treat massive hemoptysis, with a success rate of up to 98% within 24 hours; however, there is a recurrence rate up to 58% at 30 days.[39,40] Surgery is reserved to treat the underlying condition once the patient has been stabilized and bleeding controlled by other methods. Emergency surgery for hemorrhaging control may result in a postoperative mortality rate ranging from 38% to 59%,[39,41] particularly in the setting of malignancy. However, if a patient undergoes surgery after initial control of hemorrhage by other means, the mortality rate decreases to 4%.[40]

The patient's pulmonary reserve must be elucidated to determine surgical candidacy. A risk assessment of the benefits of surgery must be performed. In the setting of a vascular etiology of the hemoptysis, such as a ruptured aortic aneurysm, surgical repair is essential and should not be delayed once the patient is hemodynamically stable and the airway is controlled.[39] A detailed algorithm in the assessment and treatment of hemoptysis is shown in **Algorithm 77.2**.

COPD and Lung Volume Reduction

COPD includes a broad group of diseases that result in airflow obstruction and hyperinflation. Medical therapy involves smoking cessation, bronchodilator treatment, steroids, oxygen supplementation, and antibiotics as needed. Despite improvements in medical management, increased patient morbidity may be associated with exacerbations, pneumonia, or reduced functional performance due to limited exercise capacity. As a result, surgical interventions have continued to play a role in trying to ameliorate symptoms and improve survival in these patients.[42,43]

There is a more than 50-year history in the literature recording a variety of surgical approaches to help treat COPD. Interest was diminished, however, because of the high mortality associated with surgical intervention in this patient population. In the 1990s, a renewed interest in lung volume reduction surgery (LVRS) was observed following reports that this procedure was associated with a low published mortality

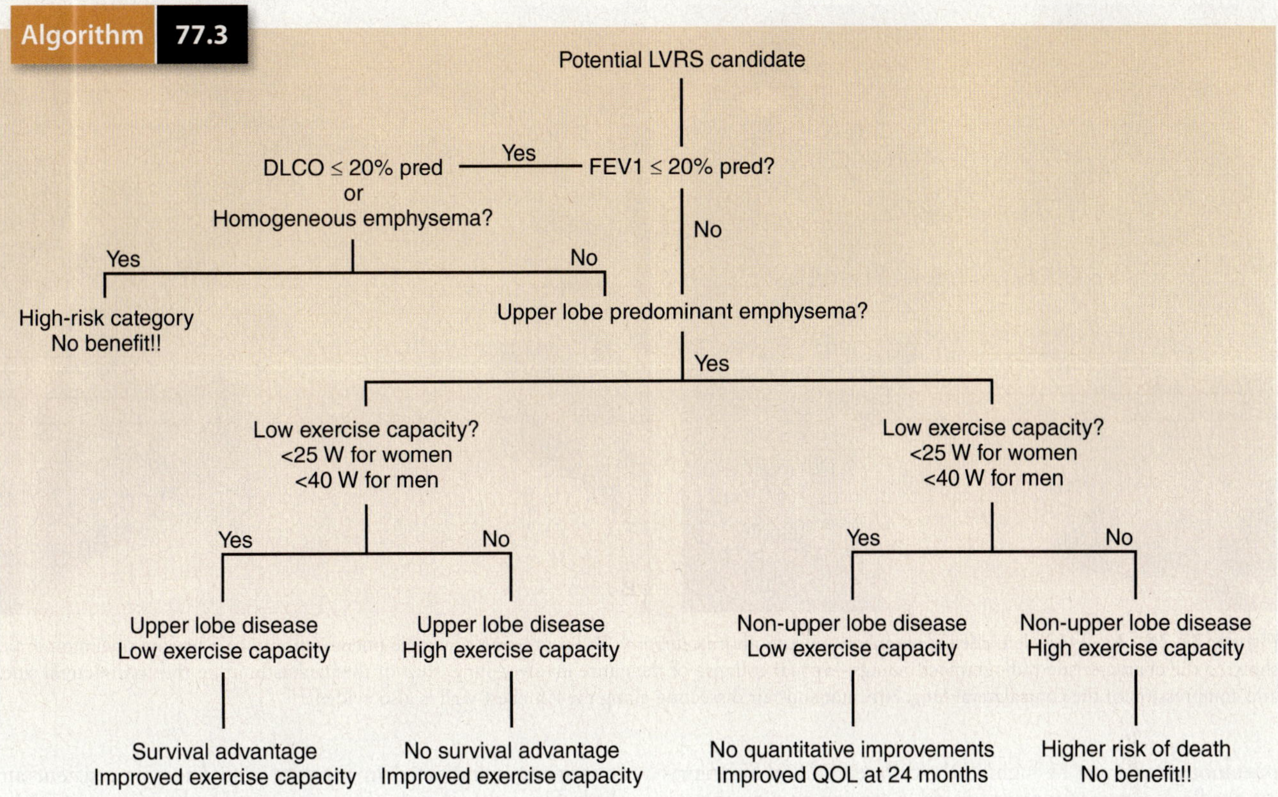

Algorithm 77.3. LVRS candidate workup. (Adapted from Martinez FJ, Chang A. Surgical therapy for chronic obstructive pulmonary disease. *Semin Respir Crit Care Med.* 2005;26(2):167–191.)

rate and a significant improvement in FEV_1 seen on pulmonary function testing. There was a national increase in interest in the procedure, as many centers began offering it. Despite continued publication of low mortality rates, evaluation of Medicare data in 1996 showed a mortality of 23% in surgically treated patients at 12 months, and Medicare reimbursement for the procedure stopped. This led to the development of the National Emphysema Treatment Trial (NETT), a prospective randomized trial to evaluate the outcomes of LVRS compared to optimal medical treatment.[42]

The goal of the NETT study was to evaluate short- and long-term survival, lung function, exercise capacity, and quality of life. Patients with upper-lobe disease and a low exercise capacity, defined as achieving less than the 40th percentile on exercise testing, 25 watts for women and 40 watts for men, showed a survival advantage and improved exercise capacity after surgery (**Algorithm 77.3**).

A new technique aimed to provide the same benefit of LVRS but without the surgical risk is the placement of one-way endobronchial valves. These are designed to allow air to escape the hyperinflated apical regions and not allow air to reenter. Endobronchial valves significantly improved pulmonary function and exercise capacity, but serious adverse events occurred in 21% of patients.[44] Endobronchial stents have been designed to cross bronchioles into hyperinflated regions of the lung and allow decompression. Other approaches being tested include the bronchoscopic introduction of biologic substances such as trypsin or thrombin into hyperinflated regions of the lung with the goal of causing local scarring and reducing the hyperinflation.[45] Other surgical procedures in the treatment of COPD include bullectomy in selected patients and lung transplants in patients with end-stage disease.[43]

Tracheobronchial Foreign Body Aspiration

Tracheobronchial foreign body (TFB) aspiration occurs most often in children, but up to 20% of cases have been reported in adults. Risk factors in adults include older age, as elderly patients have a higher incidence of neurologic disease and an impaired cough reflex. Symptoms usually involve an episode of choking, followed by a protracted cough. Fever, dyspnea, hemoptysis, and wheezing can also be present.[46] Chest x-ray may aid in the diagnosis if the aspirated TFB is radio-opaque or if there is associated air trapping, atelectasis, or pneumonia, however, the TFB is visible less than a quarter of the time, as most foods are not radio-opaque.[47] Chest CT scans are a more sensitive imaging modality, but not necessarily more specific. Bronchoscopy should be performed if TFB aspiration is suspected. Removal of the TFB can usually be accomplished by flexible bronchoscopy but may require rigid bronchoscopy in difficult cases.[46,47] A recent review found flexible bronchoscopy was successful for removal of TFB in 79% of cases.[48]

Pneumothorax

Pneumothoraces are classified as spontaneous, primary or secondary, traumatic, or iatrogenic. Primary spontaneous pneumothoraces occur in patients with no known lung disease, whereas secondary spontaneous ones occur in patients with underlying lung pathology. Iatrogenic pneumothoraces may occur in either the postsurgical or postprocedural setting, typically following central line placement or thoracentesis.[49] Traumatic pneumothoraces are covered elsewhere in this text.

Primary spontaneous pneumothoraces occur more frequently in men than women, with an incidence of 7 to 18 cases per 100,000 people for men, compared to an incidence rate of 1 to 6 cases per 100,000 people in women. Most cases occur in males younger than 30 years of age, and they rarely occur in people over the age of 40. Even though many patients with primary pneumothoraces do not have apparent lung disease, almost all are found to have subpleural bullae, the pathophysiology of which is unknown.[49] Most bullae are apical in location or located in the superior segment.[50] Patient symptoms can range from minimal to severe, and usually include pleuritic pain, dyspnea, or both. Tachycardia may also be present, and if a person is tachycardic and hypotensive, a tension

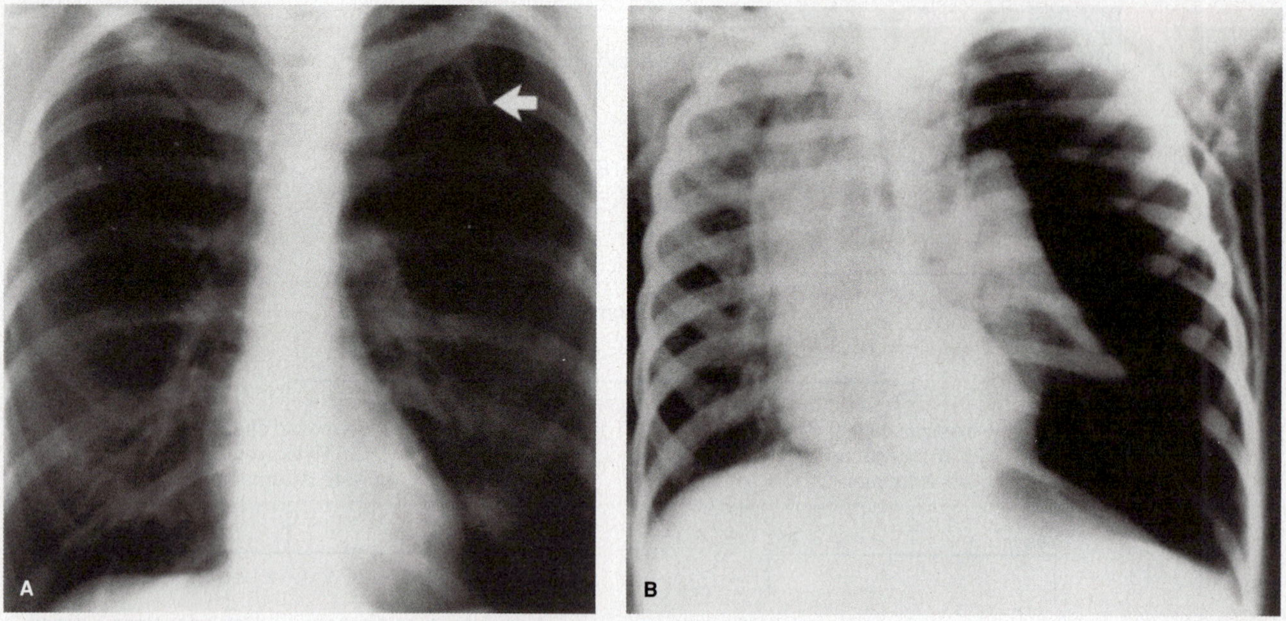

Figure 77.26. **A:** A 40% left-sided spontaneous pneumothorax (*arrow*). **B:** Progression of simple pneumothorax to a tension pneumothorax, showing the characteristic radiographic findings—virtual collapse of the entire involved lung, shift of the mediastinum to the contralateral side, and compression of the contralateral lung. Subcutaneous air dissecting along the left chest wall is also evident.

pneumothorax must be high on the differential and appropriate needle decompression considered. A tension pneumothorax occurs when air entering the pleural cavity cannot escape and the air compresses the vena cava and even the heart, resulting in hemodynamic instability (**Fig. 77.26**). Urgent needle decompression followed by chest tube placement is the preferred treatment. Most spontaneous pneumothoraces occur while patients are at rest.[49,51]

Observation is often the treatment of a stable, small pneumothorax, defined as being less than 3 cm from the apex. For a larger pneumothorax, chest tube placement is the standard
5 treatment. Most patients will have a complete resolution of their pneumothorax[6] and not need further treatment. Surgical treatment is indicated in patients who have a persistent air leak from the initial pneumothorax, high-risk occupations (pilots, scuba divers), socioeconomic insecurities, or recurrence within 2 years of initial presentation. Treatment may include chemical (ie, intrapleural doxycycline or talc infusion) or mechanical pleurodesis, in combination with thoracoscopic blebectomy (**Algorithm 77.4**).[50,51]

Secondary spontaneous pneumothoraces can occur due to a variety of lung diseases, but COPD is the most common.[52] While primary pneumothoraces can be mild clinical events, secondary ones are much more concerning because of the baseline lung disease and poor pulmonary reserve. Observation has no role in this patient population, who should undergo

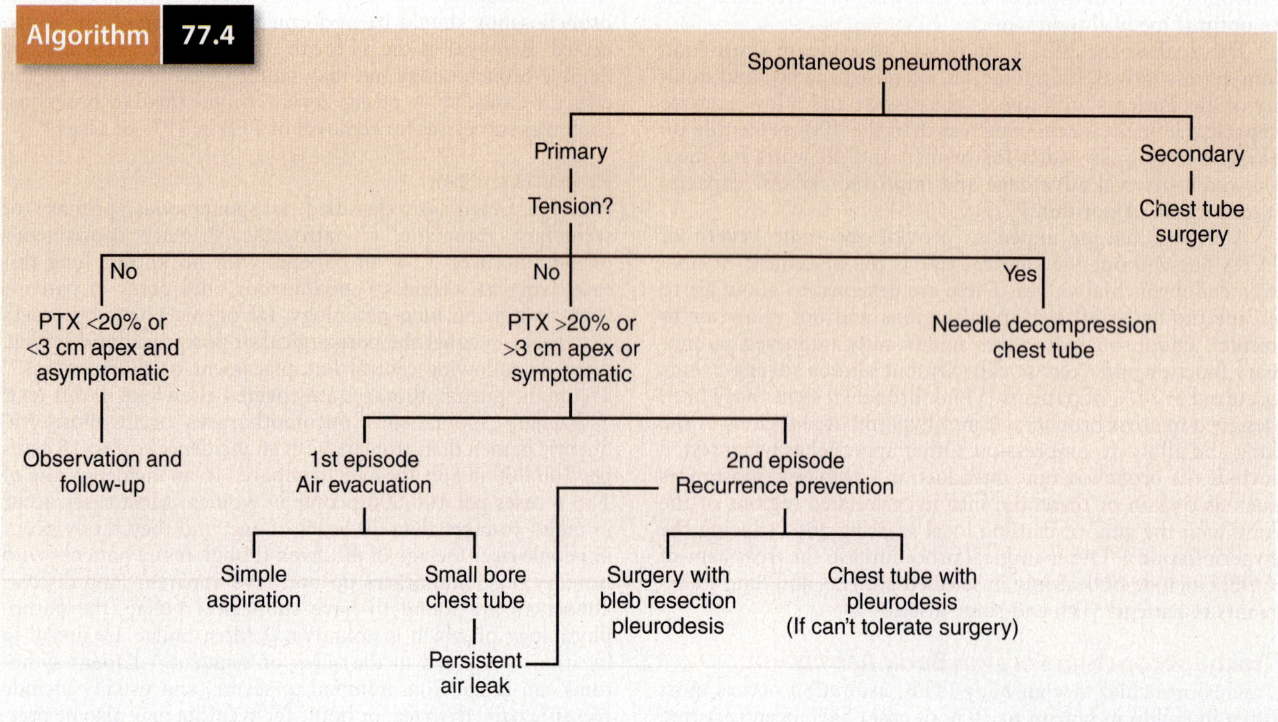

Algorithm 77.4. Algorithm to treat pneumothorax. (Adapted from Baumann MH, Noppen M. Pneumothorax. *Respirology*. 2004;9(2):157–164.)

Table 77.2. Phases of Lung Development Classification

Phase	Gestation Period	Major Developments
Embryonic	26 d to 6 wks	5 lobar bronchi
Pseudoglandular	6–16 wks	Cartilage rings, cilia form
Acinar/canalicular	16–28 wks	Type I and II pneumocytes
Saccular	28–34 wks	Distal airspace development
Alveolar	34 wks to 2 y	Alveoli proliferate from 20 to 600 million

definitive treatment to prevent a recurrence during the first event. Here, a thoracoscopic approach may be more effective in establishing an adequate pleurodesis and allow the evaluation for sources of air leaks.[51] The risk of surgery must be measured relative to physiologic performance and ability to be extubated following an operation. Iatrogenic pneumothoraces can result from transthoracic needle lung biopsies, central line placement, thoracentesis, transbronchial lung biopsies, pleural biopsies, pacemaker insertions, and positive pressure ventilation. Patients with underlying lung disease are at a higher risk of developing a pneumothorax after these procedures. Treatment should follow the same paradigm as for spontaneous pneumothoraces. Patients with a small, asymptomatic, stable pneumothorax and no underlying lung disease may be safely observed, while all others should undergo placement of a chest tube.[51] Some studies have suggested immediate aspiration of air after a CT-guided lung biopsy, resulting in a pneumothorax, with an 85% success rate in avoiding the need for chest tube placement.[50]

Congenital Lung Disease

Congenital malformations of the lung develop during fetal lung growth. They may be identified during an in utero evaluation, present as respiratory distress in the newborn, or be completely asymptomatic and found in patients as adults. They can frequently occur with other congenital malformations and may be life threatening. Lung development begins during week 3 from the foregut. It progresses through birth to approximately 2 years of age when alveolar development is complete. The five stages of lung development have been divided into the embryonic, pseuodglandular, acinar, saccular, and alveolar stages (**Table 77.2**). Malformations may occur at each step and lead to different pathologic conditions.[53] Four separate conditions will be discussed here: pulmonary sequestration, lobar emphysema, congenital cystic adenomatoid malformation (CCAM), and bronchogenic cysts.[54]

Pulmonary Sequestrations

Pulmonary sequestrations are defined as pieces of parenchymal lung separated from the respiratory tree, with the sequestration receiving its blood supply from an anomalous artery arising from the aorta, rather than having the blood supply arising from the pulmonary artery. Sequestrations have been further subdivided into extralobar and intralobar lesions, with very distinct anatomic alterations and clinical presentations. Extralobar sequestrations, which represent 25% of sequestrations, reside outside of the true pleural space. Venous drainage is usually into the azygos or hemiazygos veins. They are most often on the left side between the left lower lobe and diaphragm (**Fig. 77.27**). Up to 80% of extralobar sequestrations occur in males. Most patients present with dyspnea in the first 6 months of life. They may be diagnosed by fetal ultrasound or, after birth, by chest x-ray. Other congenital abnormalities are found in up to two-thirds of patients, with congenital diaphragmatic hernias present in a quarter of patients.[53] Intralobar lesions, which constitute the other 75% of sequestrations, reside within the normal lung and within the normal pleura. They are almost always in the lower lobes and occur on the left side just over 50% of the time. Venous drainage is usually through the pulmonary vein. It is suggested that intralobar sequestration may be an acquired disease, caused by repeated episodes of inflammation that lead to bronchiole narrowing and scarring. Ultimately, the "lobe" becomes isolated and may develop new feeding blood vessels from collateral arteries in the inferior pulmonary ligament. A complete assessment of a sequestered lesion must be performed prior to resection, and should include assessment of any potential airway or alimentary communication, determining the vascular supply of the sequestration, and determining associated congenital malformations that are more common in extralobar setting.[53]

Congenital Lobar Emphysema

Lobar emphysema is the cause of half of the episodes of newborn respiratory distress that are due to structural anomalies. Two-thirds of the cases occur in males. Distension of the distal lung occurs from obstruction of the airway, either from an intrinsic cause, such as meconium or torsion, or an extrinsic cause, such as obstructing lymph nodes. In up to half of the cases, no cause can be found. Almost all cases occur in the upper lobes, with almost equal distribution between sides. Half of the lesions will present in newborns, and the remaining 50% will reveal themselves by 6 months. Chest x-rays are diagnostic (**Fig. 77.28**).[53] Surgical resection may not be immediately necessary, and may be delayed until the child has grown, or until they develop a failure to thrive. Even after surgical resection, patients may have bronchomalacia and a tendency toward bronchospasm.[55]

Congenital Cystic Adenomatoid Malformation

CCAM lesions are the second most common cause (25%) of newborn respiratory distress, secondary to structural problems. Children will present either at birth or in early childhood with recurrent respiratory infections. The anomalies are due to an overgrowth of bronchioles, likely during the acinar phase of fetal lung development. Lesions can occur on either side and are usually isolated to one lower lobe. The classification system by Stocker (**Table 77.3**) organizes these lesions based on pathologic appearance and clinical outcome. Prenatal MRI best serves to evaluate these lesions, while postnatal chest x-ray and/or chest CT scan can be used to differentiate CCAMs from other lesions.[53] Even though lesions may be small and asymptomatic, these lesions possess the potential for malignant transformation and should be resected (**Fig. 77.29**).[55]

Bronchogenic Cysts

Bronchogenic cysts are formed from primitive foregut tissue present in the airway. They can present as single or multiple cysts in a wide variety of locations in the thorax. They usually present in young children who develop symptoms such as stridor due to airway obstruction or compression caused by the cysts.[54] Alternatively, cysts located within the lung

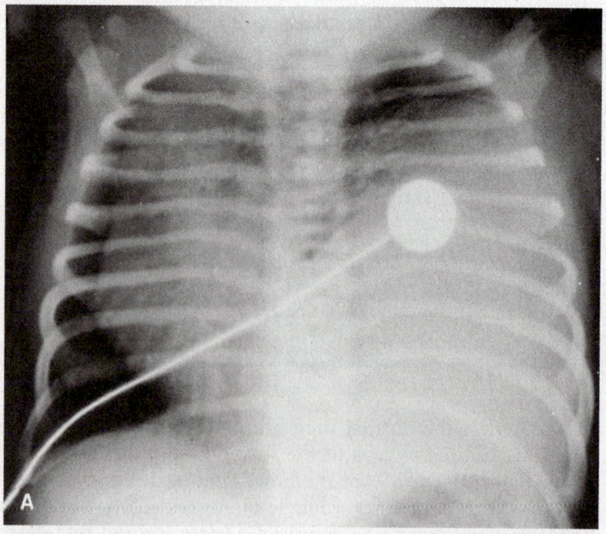

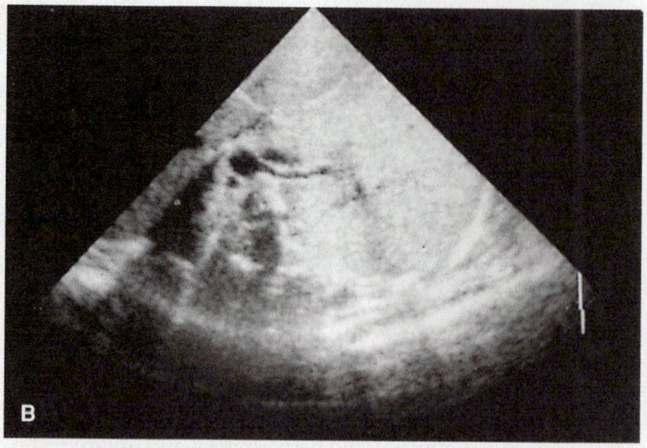

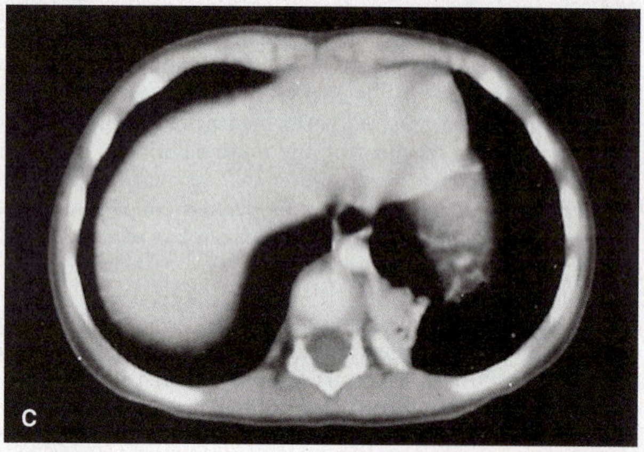

Figure 77.27. Abnormal radiograph of the chest of a newborn with respiratory distress (A). Ultrasound identified the anomalous vessel coursing through the diaphragm and entering the sequestration (B). This computed tomographic scan clearly demonstrates the anomalous artery arising from the thoracic aorta and entering the sequestered lung (C). (Reproduced with permission from Shields TW, ed. *General Thoracic Surgery*. 6th ed. 2005.)

parenchyma can become infected and present as an abscess. Therapeutic aspiration may be temporizing, but ultimately, surgery is needed.[56] Resection may have a mortality of up to 14%.[54] Most cases of congenital lung disease will present in the first 6 months of life. The main symptom is usually respiratory distress, but once children reach 1 year in age, chronic infections become the most common symptom. Diagnostic tests begin with chest x-rays, but can include ultrasound, MRI, CT scans, angiography, and bronchoscopy, depending on the lesion and location.[57] Decision making regarding the timing of surgical resection should incorporate the patient's acuity due to symptoms and their overall ability to tolerate surgery based on size.

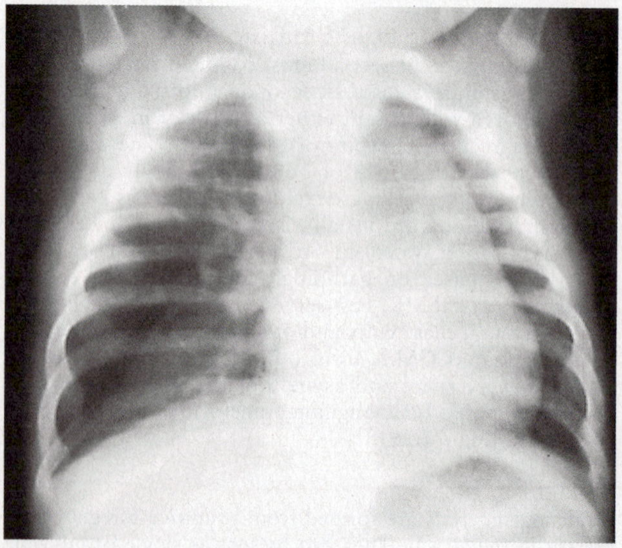

Figure 77.28. Radiograph of a newborn with lobar emphysema involving the right middle lobe. Note the compressed right lower lobe and mediastinal shift. (Reproduced with permission from Shields TW, ed. *General Thoracic Surgery*. 6th ed. 2005.)

Pleural Disease

Pleural diseases include benign complications from systemic disease, postoperative infections, local infections, and cancers from primary and metastatic sites. Pleura-based pathology leads to respiratory effort and dyspnea. Surgical intervention may be diagnostic, therapeutic, or palliative. It is imperative for the surgeon to be able to discern the pathology and communicate goals of intervention.

Table 77.3. The Stocker Classification of CCAM

Type	Features
▪ Type I	75% of lesions Few large cysts Parenchymal compression
▪ Type II	Numerous, <1 cm cysts Associated with other congenital anomalies Worse prognosis
▪ Type III	Rarest type Cysts are solid and smaller (few mm in diameter)

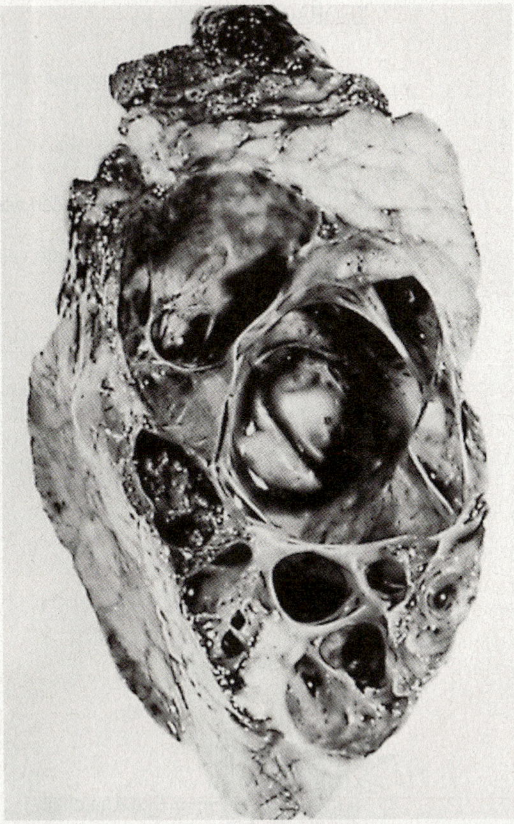

Figure 77.29. Specimen removed from an infant with a cystic adenomatoid malformation. Microscopically, there was marked proliferation of terminal bronchioles, and cartilage was lacking. (Reproduced with permission from Shields TW, ed. *General Thoracic Surgery*. 6th ed. 2005.)

PLEURAL EFFUSIONS

Pleural effusions are a common condition that elicits a surgical consult for potential drainage and even thoracoscopic intervention to assist in the diagnosis and treatment of the condition. The essential first step in the evaluation of a new effusion is to determine if it is a transudative or exudative process. A transudative fluid collection is the result of a poorly balanced hydrostatic and/or osmotic pressure across the pleural membrane, resulting in increased serum leak across the pleural barrier. Exudative processes result from inflammation or neoplastic processes that cause increased capillary leak at the pleural membrane, which results in higher protein and lactate dehydrogenase (LDH) levels in the exudative fluid compared to the transudative fluid (**Table 77.4**).[58] The Light criteria is commonly used to distinguish transudative and exudative effusions (**Table 77.5**). If one or more of the criteria are met, then the fluid is considered exudative.[59] Other tests have been evaluated, including measuring cholesterol ratios, albumin gradient, but Light criteria is highly sensitive despite low specificity.[58]

Transudative effusions are most often caused by congestive heart failure. Even if a patient does not have other symptoms of heart failure, in the setting of a transudative effusion, a complete cardiac workup should be considered. The pleural fluid concentration of N-terminal pro–B-type natriuretic peptide can accurately identify effusions due to heart failure.[60] Other causes include cirrhosis, which may or may not be associated with ascites. Isolated right- and left-sided effusions due to liver disease have been described. Effusions can be seen in more than 20% of patients with nephrotic syndrome, and so all patients with new effusions should be evaluated for the presence of proteinuria. Rarer causes include retroperitoneal urine
6 leaks or cerebrospinal[7] fluid leaks.[61] Surgical interventions, such as chest tube placement, should be avoided in transudative disease settings, as patients will continue to drain fluid

Table 77.4. Diagnosis: Differential Diagnosis of Pleural Effusions

Transudative Pleural Effusions
- Congestive heart failure
- Pericardial disease
- Cirrhosis
- Nephrotic syndrome
- Peritoneal dialysis
- Superior vena cava obstruction
- Myxedema
- Pulmonary emboli
- Sarcoidosis
- Urinothorax

Exudative Pleural Effusions
- Neoplastic diseases
  - Metastatic disease
  - Mesothelioma
- Infectious diseases
  - Bacterial infections
  - Tuberculosis
  - Fungal infections
  - Viral infections
  - Parasitic infections
  - Pulmonary embolization
- Gastrointestinal disease
  - Esophageal perforation
  - Pancreatic disease
  - Intra-abdominal abscess
  - Diaphragmatic hernia
  - Postabdominal surgery
  - Endoscopic variceal sclerotherapy
- Collagen vascular diseases
  - Rheumatoid pleuritis
  - Systemic lupus erythematosus
  - Drug-induced lupus erythematosus
  - Immunoblastic lymphadenopathy
  - Sjögren syndrome
  - Wegener granulomatosis
  - Churg–Strauss syndrome
- Postcardiac injury syndrome
- Asbestos exposure
- Sarcoidosis
- Uremia
- Meigs syndrome
- Yellow nail syndrome
- Drug-induced pleural disease
  - Nitrofurantoin
  - Dantrolene
  - Methysergide
  - Bromocriptine
  - Procarbazine
  - Amiodarone
- Trapped lung
- Radiotherapy
- Electric burns
- Urinary tract obstruction
- Iatrogenic injury
- Ovarian hyperstimulation syndrome
- Chylothorax
- Hemothorax

Table 77.5. Criteria for Exudative Effusions Based on Ratio of Pleural Fluid Protein and LDH Concentrations to Serum Concentration
Protein/serum protein >0.5
LDH/serum LDH >0.6
Pleural LDH 1.67 times normal serum LDH

LDH, lactate dehydrogenase.

from their chest until the primary cause is treated. Aspiration of fluid may help temporarily while systemic treatment is instituted, but should only be done as part of a larger treatment plan.

Exudative effusions have a number of etiologies, but infection is the most common cause.[59] Tuberculosis (TB) and fungal infections can also cause exudative effusions. Although rarer in the United States, TB is still a common etiology worldwide. If someone is suspected of having pleural TB, the pleural fluid should be evaluated for adenosine deaminase (ADA) and gamma-interferon levels, which, if low, will rule out the diagnosis of TB. If other infections are suspected, the pleural fluid should be cultured. Amylase may be tested if there is concern for esophageal perforation or a pancreatic cause.

Malignancy is the next most common cause of exudative effusions.[59] Approximately a quarter of pleural effusions in a community hospital setting have been attributed to cancer. The malignancies that cause the effusions are, in order of decreasing frequency: lung cancer, breast cancer, and hematologic cancers such as lymphoma. Other malignancies can also cause effusions, such as ovarian cancer.[62] Autoimmune processes, such as rheumatoid disease and lupus, can also cause effusions. A chylothorax may present after problems with thoracic duct lymphatic drainage leading to an accumulation of lymphatic fluid, "chyle," in one or both thoraces. The thoracic duct collects lymph from the cysterna chyli, the plexus of lymphatics in the upper abdomen, and travels anterior to the spine and just posterolateral to the aorta. It follows behind the aorta and enters the left neck, where it empties into the confluence of the left internal jugular and subclavian veins (**Fig. 77.30**). Chylous leaks are due primarily to thoracic duct injury from trauma or surgery or lymphomas resulting in obstructed lymphatics. Pleural triglyceride and chylomicrons levels will be elevated, and the fluid will have a milky color. Treatment for persistent chylothoraces may include: NPO, hyperalimentation, and, for severe cases, surgical thoracic duct ligation or thoracic duct embolization in the interventional radiology suite.[63]

The management of malignant pleural effusions includes a variety of options, but critical to the decision-making process is the knowledge of the median life expectancy in that patient due to the underlying malignancy. Chest tube drainage may be therapeutic and diagnostic, allowing fluid drainage and alleviation of symptoms of dyspnea. It will also allow determination of whether the underlying lung is able to expand. If not, it is described as a "trapped lung," and although the fluid may be gone, a persistent pneumothorax appears on chest x-rays as the lung cannot expand and fill the thorax. In these settings, an indwelling pleural drainage catheter may be the best option to intermittently drain accumulating fluid. Decortication is not recommended, as most patients with malignancy in this setting have a limited life expectancy, and the success rate is low compared to decortication in the setting of an empyema. VATS exploration may also be used to remove loculated fluid collections and to evaluate for lung reexpansion after the procedure. If the lung reexpands, further treatment includes pleurodesis, utilizing talc, doxycycline, or bleomycin. These medications will cause an inflammatory reaction between the parietal and visceral pleura, resulting in the lung being "stuck" in an expanded state. Mechanical pleurodesis can also be performed by mechanical debridement of the pleura via VATS. Chemical pleurodesis may be performed via VATS or through an existing thoracostomy tube. The goal of treatment in the setting of a malignant pleural effusion is palliation.[62] Patients treated with indwelling pleural catheters may spend fewer days in the hospital at the end of life than patients treated with pleurodesis.[64] In many cases, systemically treating the primary malignancy may obviate the need for frequent thoracentesis.[65]

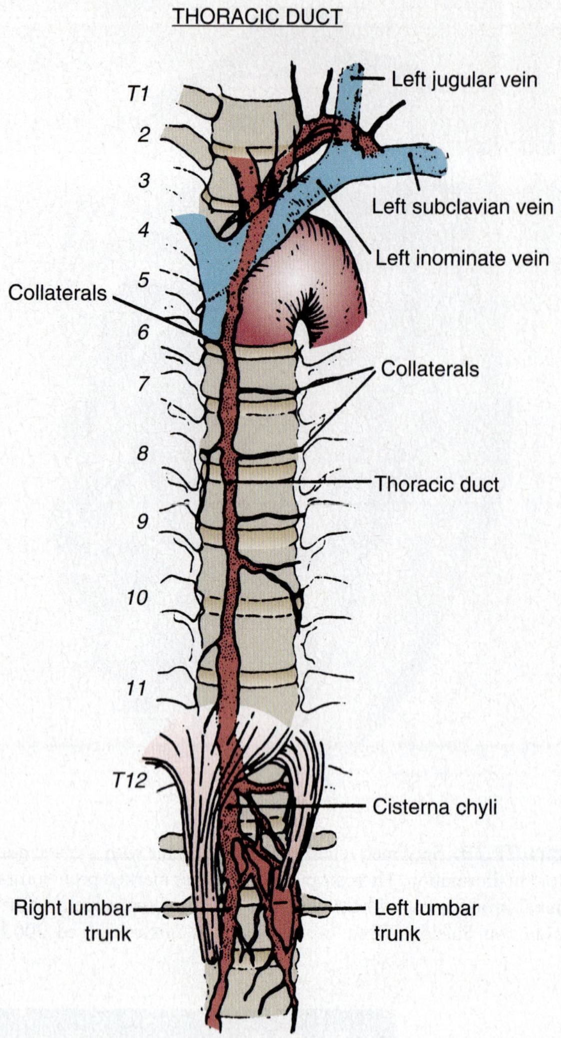

Figure 77.30. Schematic drawing of the most usual pattern and course of the thoracic duct. The single duct that enters the chest through the aortic hiatus between T12 and T10 is a relatively consistent finding and the usual site for surgical ligation.

Empyema

7 Empyema is defined as infection in the pleura space based on purulent fluid or evidence of bacterial-laden effusion.[8] This represents part of the continuum of disease that begins with simple parapneumonic effusion, where exudative fluid is not infected and not loculated. As the disease progresses, fluid becomes loculated with fibrinous septations and becomes infected, leading to pus and ultimately the development of a fibrinous peel. Up to half of pneumonias have an associated effusion, but less than 5% of cases lead to an empyema.[66] Other causes include surgical thoracotomies and/or other infections from nearby organs, such as esophageal injuries. Pleural infections have been categorized into three overlapping stages. The first is the exudative stage, where the fluid is thin, sterile, has a lower white blood cell (WBC) count and LDH levels, and the glucose level is still above 40 mg/dL

Table 77.6. Diagnostic Criteria for Pleural Fluid in Empyema

Stage	Fluid/Peel	WBC	LDH (cells/mm^3)	pH (IU)	Bacteria
Exudative	Thin/elastic	<1000	<500	>7.3	Absent
Fibrinopurulent	Purulent/inelastic	>5000	>1000	<7.1	Present
Organizing	Thick/rigid peel	Varies	Varies	<7.1	Varies

(**Table 77.6**). Treatment usually involves addressing the underlying etiology, such as pneumonia. The second stage is the fibrinopurulent stage, where the fluid becomes infected, and fibrin deposits accumulate on the pleura. The LDH and WBC count increases, and the glucose and pH levels drop. The fluid becomes thick and purulent, and the lung is often unable to expand. Chest tube drainage alone at this stage may not be effective in removing the fluid. The third stage is the organizing stage, and a thick pleural peel is created by migrating fibroblasts. At this point, a formal debridement and decortication are required to allow the lung to return to full function.[66]

Organisms causing empyemas have shifted from predominantly *Streptococcus pneumoniae* in the preantibiotic era, to anaerobic organisms in up to three-quarters of empyemas in the current era. There is also a notable difference between community-acquired and hospital-acquired empyema, with a higher prevalence of *S. aureus* and *K. pneumonia* in hospital-acquired empyemas.[67] Imaging to evaluate the presence of an empyema begins with a simple chest x-ray, but requires a chest CT to show potential loculations. After the institution of antibiotic therapy, surgical intervention depends on the stage of the disease, but may require a VATS exploration or even a thoracotomy to debride the thorax effectively and to decorticate the pleural peel off of the lung to allow reexpansion.[66] Postpneumonectomy empyemas are an especially difficult problem as there is no lung tissue to occupy the empty thorax. Risk factors in this setting include right-sided pneumonectomies (vs left), adjuvant radiation, the need for postoperative ventilation, lower starting hematocrit levels, and poor preoperative pulmonary function test results.[68,69] Treatments of these empyemas are particularly difficult and may include an open thoracostomy window (Eloessor flap) that allows for packing and granulation tissue to form in the empyema cavity.[70]

Mesothelioma

Malignant pleural mesothelioma (MPM) is a cancer of the serosal pleura, related to exposure to asbestos. Multiple hypotheses have been formed regarding how asbestos causes mesothelioma, and include the idea that asbestos fibers are inhaled deeply into the lung and penetrate the parenchymal surface, causing irritation of the pleura and repeated episodes of inflammation, ultimately leading to cancer. Other potential mechanisms include asbestos interfering with mitosis, inducing free-radical production, and induction of proto-oncogene kinases by asbestos fibers.[71] Exposure to asbestos usually occurs decades prior to presentation with mesothelioma, and has been seen in miners exposed to asbestos dust, industrial workers such as plumbers and carpenters who used asbestos products, and even in 20% of patients with no known exposure but living in industrial countries. Mesothelioma is an increasingly rare malignancy, with fewer than 5000 cases in the United States per year.[72]

Patients with mesothelioma may present with dyspnea or chest pain. Often, patients are asymptomatic, and the diagnosis is made after abnormalities are seen on a chest x-ray performed for another reason. Radiographs may show unilateral effusions and a loss of volume on the affected side, as the lung capacity is diminished due to the disease. As the disease progresses, patients may have weight loss, worsening pain, and night sweats. Prognosis is poor, with median survival as little as 1 year from the time of diagnosis.[73] Diagnostic studies include a chest CT scan or MRI to show the extent of pleural thickening as well as signs of local spread or metastasis (**Fig. 77.31**). The pathologic diagnosis almost always requires a tissue biopsy with a CT-guided biopsy, VATS, or limited thoracotomy approach. Cytologic examination of pleural fluid from a thoracentesis cannot differentiate between mesothelioma cells and other potential lung cancers. If the patient is being considered for surgical resection, a limited thoracotomy at the site of a potential later incision is optimal to limit seeding of the tumor.[73]

Mesotheliomas can be categorized into epithelial, sarcomatoid, and mixed histologies. Patients with epithelial histology have longer median survival than those with a sarcomatoid histology.[74] There are a variety of staging systems for mesothelioma, including the Butchart system, the revised Brigham and Women's Hospital system, and the TNM-based system by the International Mesothelioma Interest Group (IMIG) and International Association for the Study of Lung Cancer (IASLC) (**Table 77.7**).[75] The IMIG system allows for better reproducibility of the interpretation of local and regional lymph node spread. Laparoscopy may be useful to evaluate the patient for transdiaphragmatic spread of the tumor, differentiating between T3 and T4 tumors.[76]

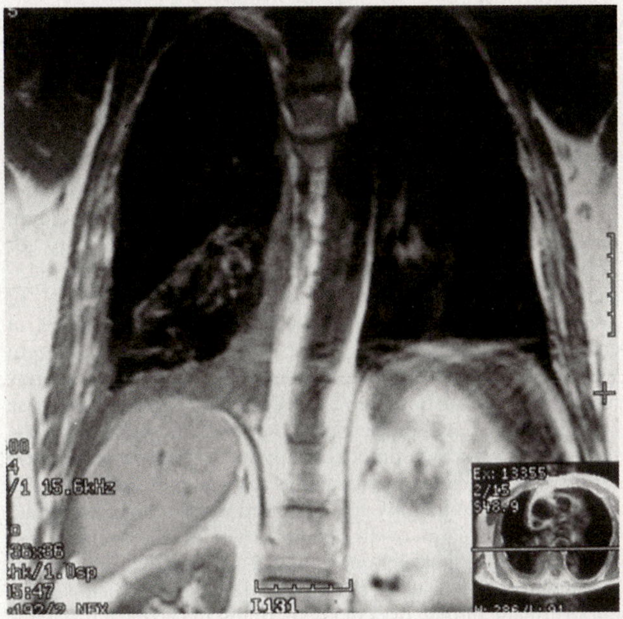

Figure 77.31. Magnetic resonance imaging of the patient in Figure 77.25 shows a large amount of tumor within the pleural space and into the diaphragmatic sulcus with no evidence of extension outside the hemithorax. (Reproduced with permission from Flores RM, Sugarbaker DJ. Malignant mesothelioma of the pleural space? *Ann Thorac Surg*. 2000;70:306.)

Table 77.7. Staging: The International Mesothelioma Interest Group (IMIG) and IASLC Staging System

T–Tumor	
T1	Tumor involving the ipsilateral parietal pleura (including mediastinal and diaphragmatic pleura) with or without involvement of visceral pleura
T2	Tumor involving each of the ipsilateral pleural surfaces (parietal, mediastinal, diaphragmatic, and visceral pleura) with at least one of the following features: Confluent visceral pleural tumor (including the fissures), involvement of diaphragmatic muscle, invasion of the lung parenchyma
T3	Locally advanced but potentially resectable tumor; tumor involving all of the ipsilateral pleural surfaces (parietal, mediastinal, diaphragmatic, and visceral pleura) with at least one of the following features: Involvement of the endothoracic fascia, extension into the mediastinal fat, solitary, completely resectable focus of tumor extending into the soft tissues of the chest wall, nontransmural involvement of the pericardium
T4	Tumor involving all of the ipsilateral pleural surfaces with at least one of the following features: Diffuse multifocal invasion of soft tissues of the chest wall, any rib involvement, invasion of the peritoneum through the diaphragm, invasion of any mediastinal organ, direct extension to the contralateral pleura, invasion of the spine or brachial plexus, transmural invasion of the pericardium (with or without pericardial effusion), or myocardium invasion
N–Lymph Nodes	
NX	Regional lymph nodes cannot be assessed
N0	No regional lymph node metastases
N1	Metastases in the ipsilateral bronchopulmonary, hilar, or mediastinal lymph nodes (including the internal mammary, peridiaphragmatic, pericardial fat pad, or intercostal lymph nodes)
N2	Metastases in the contralateral bronchopulmonary, hilar, or mediastinal lymph nodes or ipsilateral or contralateral supraclavicular lymph nodes
M–Metastases	
MX	Presence of distant metastases cannot be assessed
M0	No evidence of distant metastases
M1	Evidence of distant metastases
Stage	**Description**
I	
Ia	T1N0M0
Ib	T2N0M0, T3N0M0
II	T1N1M0, T2N1M0
IIIa	T3N1M0
IIIb	T1N2M0, T2N2M0, T3NM0
IV	Any T4
	Any M1

Used with permission of Berzenji L, Van Schil P, Carp L. The eighth TNM classification for malignant pleural mesothelioma. *Transl Lung Cancer Res.* 2018;7(5):543–549. Permission conveyed through Copyright Clearance Center. Inc.,

Treatment for mesothelioma is multimodal, including chemotherapy, radiation therapy, immunotherapy, and surgery. Surgical treatment is largely palliative, ranging from pleurodesis to maximally invasive options such as pleurectomy/decortication (P/D) for limited disease, and to the most aggressive treatment of an extrapleural pneumonectomy (EPP), with the goal of complete tumor resection. Less than a third of patients are candidates for any surgical intervention. Preoperative workup for an EPP should include a cardiac evaluation, and optimal surgical candidates have pulmonary function tests with an FEV_1 of greater than 2 L/sec and an age under 70.[76] Surgery involves an en bloc removal of the lung, pleura, pericardium, and diaphragm with reconstruction of the pericardium and diaphragm. Pleurectomy and decortication are reserved for very early-stage disease and involve removal of the pleura only with preservation of the lung parenchyma. Multimodality approaches have shown better results, with neoadjuvant chemotherapy and adjuvant radiation therapy.[77] Chemotherapy for advanced disease includes pemetrexed and cisplatin or the combination of gemcitabine and cisplatin.[78] Both have shown similar levels of palliation. Radiotherapy may also be used, but is limited by the large field requiring treatment and the risks of pneumonitis and esophagitis.[71] It is best used in combination with EPP for local control after surgery, or to treat local painful areas.[76] Immunotherapy is evolving as a first-line therapeutic option for unresectable MPM.[79] Because of the rarity of surgical cases, patients who are considered for surgery should be referred to high-volume centers where surgeons and other clinicians are comfortable treating this disease.

Trachea

A thorough knowledge of the anatomy and vascular supply of the trachea is essential to minimize complications such as postintubation tracheal stenosis and tracheoinnominate fistulas after tracheostomies.

Anatomy

The trachea is the connection from the cricoid cartilage to the carina that allows ventilation and mucous clearance from the lungs. It is oval shaped, with C-shaped cartilaginous rings creating the anterior and lateral borders. A soft tissue membrane forms the posterior wall to complete the oval shape. In the average male, the anterior–posterior dimension is 1.8 cm, while the lateral aspect is 2.3 cm. Tracheal length reaches almost 12 cm with about 2 rings per centimeter. Trachea in women are 10% to 20% smaller in size. In children, the shape is more circular, but becomes gradually more ovoid as individuals age. There is a significant amount of flexibility in the normal trachea, and remodeling can occur in chronic disease states such as emphysema. The inner lining consists of ciliated pseudostratified columnar epithelium with goblet and mucous cells interspersed. At the carina, the right and left mainstem bronchi split off. The right side is characterized by the quick takeoff of the right upper-lobe bronchus, with the bronchus intermedius continuing into the middle and lower-lobe bronchi. The left side has a longer mainstem bronchus with a split into the upper and lower lobes.[80] The blood supply begins with the inferior thyroid artery supplying the cervical trachea

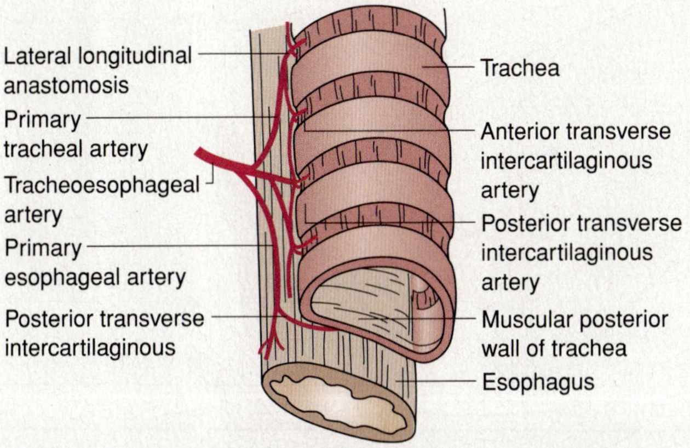

Figure 77.32. Semischematic view of the tracheal microscopical blood supply. Transverse intercartilaginous arteries derived from the lateral longitudinal anastomosis penetrate the soft tissues between each cartilage to supply a rich vascular network beneath the endotracheal mucosa.

through three tracheoesophageal branches. The lower trachea is supplied by bronchial arteries arising from the aorta. As the arteries approach the trachea, they further split to supply separate segments. Even within segments, it will branch into anterior and posterior transverse intercartilaginous arteries (**Fig. 77.32**). Because of this segmental blood supply, there should be minimal circumferential dissection around the trachea to limit impairment of the blood supply and healing in tracheal/bronchial surgery.

Surgical Airways

The most common tracheal procedure is a tracheostomy. Percutaneous tracheostomy has become the most common approach over open tracheostomy. For patients who are intubated, the indication for and timing of tracheostomy depends on a multitude of factors. The goal of a tracheostomy is to limit the risk of laryngeal stenosis caused by prolonged endotracheal intubation, to improve pulmonary toilet, and to improve oral hygiene. Generally, tracheostomy should be considered after a patient has been intubated for more than 7 days, without clear expectation for immediate extubation.[81] Ideally, patients should be on minimal ventilator settings, but tracheostomy may be performed in patients with elevated oxygen (FiO_2 of up to 60%) and ventilatory (PEEP under 10) requirements. Patients requiring more support are at high risk of decompensating if they lose their airways, even if it is just for a moment, and the decision to perform a tracheostomy should be carefully considered in this setting.[82]

Tracheostomies are performed with the neck extended. A 2-cm incision is made approximately 1 to 2 cm above the sternal notch. Dissection is carried down through the platysma, and the strap muscles are divided longitudinally. Exposure of the trachea and the 2nd and 3rd rings may require elevation of the thyroid. Lateral traction sutures may be placed around the 2nd or 3rd rings. A vertical incision is made between rings 2 and 4 and gradually dilated. A tracheostomy tube is placed under direct vision.[81,83] Percutaneous tracheostomy placement is based on the Seldinger technique. A needle is placed percutaneously into the trachea at the estimated level of the 2nd or 3rd rings with bronchoscopic visualization through a retracted endotracheal tube. A guidewire is placed into the airway, and serial dilations are performed, until a tracheostomy tube is able to be advanced over the wire.[82] Cricothyroidotomy should only be performed in the emergent setting. The cricothyroid membrane is palpated below the superior thyroid notch. A transverse incision is made to the lateral borders of the thyroid cartilage. Rapid dilation is followed by tube insertion.

Complications can vary depending on the technique and on the timing during or after the procedure (**Table 77.8**). Fistulas result from erosion of the tracheostomy tube into the innominate artery, with placement below the 3rd ring placing patients 8 at higher risk.[11] A sentinel bleed may be the initial presentation. Pressure on the fistula with immediate repair or ligation of the vessel is required (**Fig. 77.33**).[84] Postintubation stenosis (most common tracheal lesion) is usually due to necrosis caused by high-pressure cuffs, resulting in impaired blood flow to the segmental area of the trachea. This leads to the long-term loss of cartilage and narrowing of the airway. The use of low-pressure cuffs has reduced the incidence of this complication, but not eliminated it. Bronchoscopy and dilation may alleviate symptoms, but resection of the stenotic area may be needed (**Fig. 77.34**).[83]

Tracheal Tumors

Benign lesions of the trachea are less common than malignant ones. They include papillomas, chondromas, hamartomas, fibromas, and hemangiomas. Papillomas are associated with the human papillomavirus and can degenerate into malignant lesions, thus requiring resection. Chondromas arise from the cartilage and may recur after resection. Hamartomas are comprised of cartilage, epithelial, and lymphatic tissue. Recurrence

Table 77.8. Tracheostomy Complications

Immediate Complications	Early Complications	Late Complications
Hemorrhage	Hemorrhage	Tracheal Stenosis
Structural damage to trachea	Tube displacement	Granulation tissue
Failure of procedure	Pneumothorax	Tracheomalacia
Aspiration event	Pneumomediastinum	Pneumonia
Air embolism	Subcutaneous emphysema	Aspiration event
Loss of airway	Stomal infection	Tracheoarterial fistula
Death	Stomal ulceration	Tracheoesophageal fistula
Hypoxemia, hypercarbia	Accidental decannulation Dysphagia	Accidental decannulation Dysphagia

Adapted from Cheung N, Napolitano LM. Tracheostomy: epidemiology, indications, timing, technique, and outcomes. *Respir Care.* 2014;59(6):895–919.

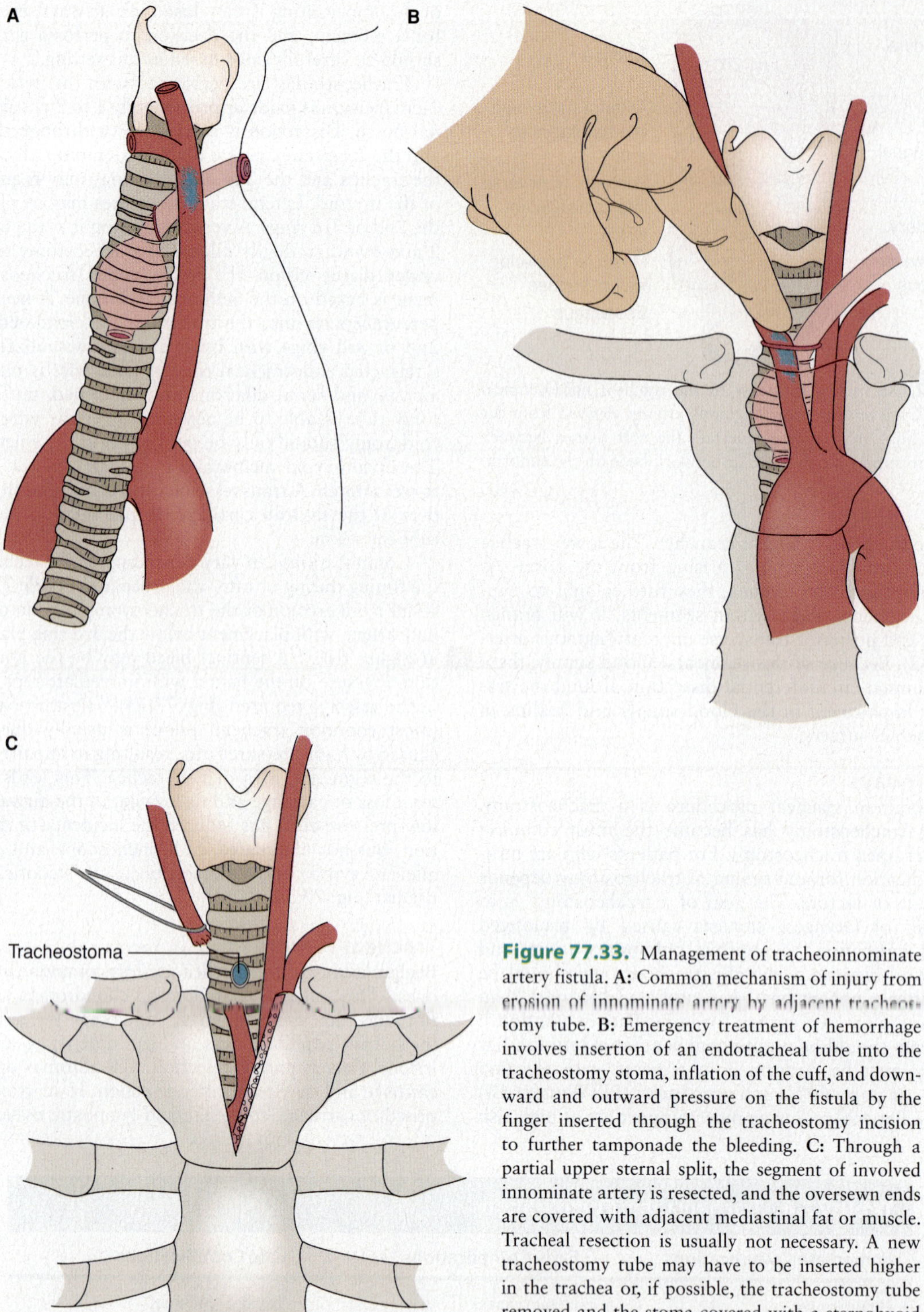

Figure 77.33. Management of tracheoinnominate artery fistula. **A:** Common mechanism of injury from erosion of innominate artery by adjacent tracheostomy tube. **B:** Emergency treatment of hemorrhage involves insertion of an endotracheal tube into the tracheostomy stoma, inflation of the cuff, and downward and outward pressure on the fistula by the finger inserted through the tracheostomy incision to further tamponade the bleeding. **C:** Through a partial upper sternal split, the segment of involved innominate artery is resected, and the oversewn ends are covered with adjacent mediastinal fat or muscle. Tracheal resection is usually not necessary. A new tracheostomy tube may have to be inserted higher in the trachea or, if possible, the tracheostomy tube removed and the stoma covered with a sternohyoid muscle flap.

is rare after resection. Fibromas can be resected via bronchoscopy. Hemangiomas are the most common pediatric tracheal mass. They may regress without treatment and can be observed if not causing obstructive symptoms. Biopsy is generally avoided due to bleeding risk. Surgery may be required if lesions persist.[85]

Although more common than benign lesions, malignant tracheal tumors are very rare, with only 600 to 700 cases in the United States per year. Lesions may be primary tracheal lesions, tumors from adjacent organs growing into the trachea, or metastatic lesions.[86] Primary tumors are most commonly squamous cell carcinomas or adenoid cystic carcinomas in the trachea, followed by carcinoids in the bronchi.[86,87] Adjacent tumors may arise in the lung, esophagus, thyroid, or mediastinum. The most common cancers that cause tracheal metastases include renal cell cancers, sarcomas, breast cancers, and colon cancers.[86] Patients will present with stridor and wheezing, and have often been recently diagnosed with adult-onset asthma and treated with inhalers and even steroids without alleviation of symptoms. Hemoptysis may also occur, though it is more common in lung cancer than in tracheal disease.[87] Patients should undergo imaging such as a neck and chest CT scan to assist in making the proper diagnosis. Bronchoscopy with a flexible or rigid endoscope is essential to aid in the evaluation of the extent of disease and to control the airway if necessary. Treatment includes tracheal resection for primary tumors if possible. For metastatic disease, palliative treatment includes endoluminal resection

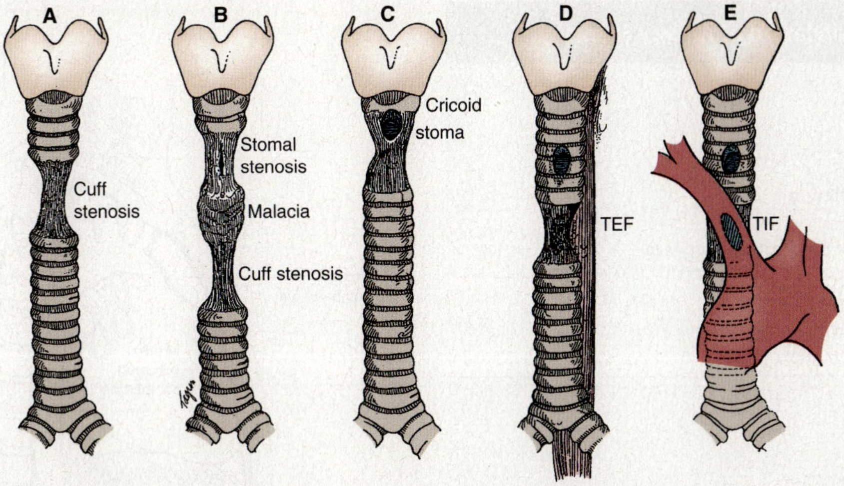

Figure 77.34. Diagrams of principal postintubation tracheal lesions. **A:** Cuff stenosis from the cuff of an endotracheal tube. **B:** Cuff stenosis from the cuff of a tracheostomy tube, usually lower in the trachea than that from an endotracheal tube. Stomal stenosis also occurs at the site of the tracheostomy itself. Malacia may occur either at the level of the cuff or in the segment between the stoma and the cuff stenosis. **C:** Cuff stenosis at the site of a high tracheostomy stoma, which has eroded into the lower margin of the cricoid cartilage. In older patients, this may erode back farther into the subglottic larynx, producing a laryngotracheal stenosis. A stoma placed in the cricothyroid membrane will, by definition, produce an intralaryngeal stenosis. **D:** Tracheoesophageal fistula (TEF) produced by pressure of the cuff against the "party wall," often abetted by an indwelling firm nasogastric tube. **E:** One type of tracheoinnominate fistula (TIF) as the result of a high-pressure cuff erosion. The more common type, but also rare, is that seen with a low-placed tracheostomy stoma, which rests against the innominate artery itself. (Reproduced with permission from Grillo HC. Surgical treatment of postintubation tracheal injuries? *J Thorac Cardiovasc Surg*. 1979;78:860–875.)

and/or radiotherapy.[87] Endoluminal treatments include mechanical core-out, laser treatment, cryotherapy, or brachytherapy. Stenting also may play a role in maintaining airway patency, either for a temporary period during radiation treatment, or in the setting of end-stage disease (**Algorithm** 77.5).[86]

Tracheomalacia and Airway Stents

Tracheomalacia occurs when the trachea loses its rigid form and the posterior membranous wall approaches the anterior wall, causing luminal narrowing and obstruction, leading to dyspnea. Patients have a characteristic seal-like cough. Chest CT scans may demonstrate this condition, and pulmonary function testing in these patients will show reduced FEV_1, FVC, and peak expiratory flow rates. Bronchoscopy is the best diagnostic test and reveals real-time airway collapse with expiration. Etiologies include congenital tracheomalacia, extrinsic compression, postintubation stenosis and inflammation, relapsing polychondritis, and COPD.[88] Surgical intervention may include resection for localized involvement, tracheobronchoplasty, or stenting.[88,89] Airway stents can be divided into two groups, silicone and metal, with each type having distinct advantages (**Table** 77.9). Newer stents being developed include covered metal stents that prevent tumor growth along the stent, but unfortunately, still allow granulation tissue to grow in at the ends.[90] Minimally invasive approaches are becoming widely adopted to treat this process, specifically laser and robotic tracheobronchoplasty.[91,92] In addition to being useful in the setting of tracheal stenosis, they can also play an essential role in palliating posttransplant bronchial stenosis.[93]

Mediastinum

The mediastinum contains a number of important structures and may be involved in different disease processes. The

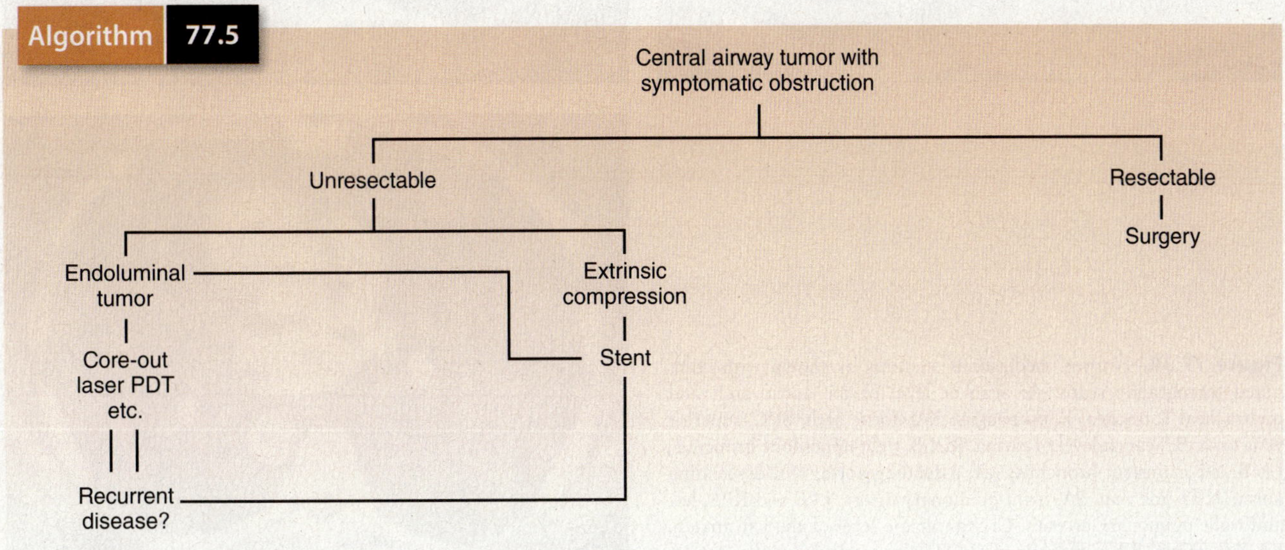

Algorithm 77.5. Algorithm for management of tracheal masses. (Adapted from Wood DE. *Surg Clin North Am*. 2002;82(3):621–642.)

Table 77.9. Classification of Airway Stents

- Silicone stents
  - Advantages
    - Adjustable
    - Removable
    - Minimal granulation
  - Disadvantages
    - Gen. anesthesia/rigid bronch to place
    - Migrates
    - Secretions adhere to stent
    - Interferes with ciliary clearance
    - Smaller inner diameter
- Metal stents
  - Advantages
    - Less migration
    - Larger inner diameter
    - Less ciliary interference
    - Flexible bronch to place
  - Disadvantages
    - May need balloon dilation
    - Difficult to remove
    - Granulation and tumor ingrowth in the stent
    - Radial force may lead to necrosis/fistula

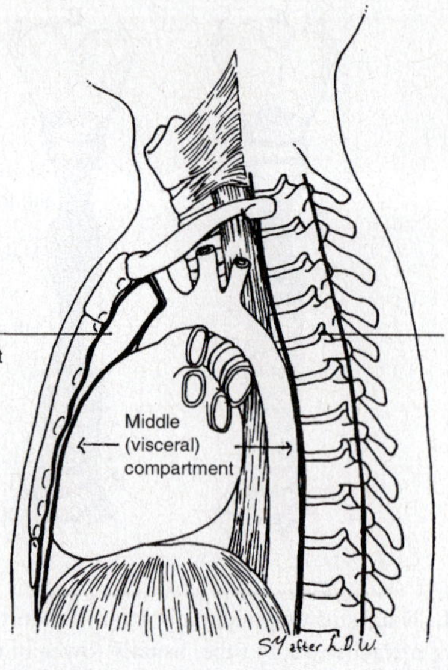

Figure 77.35. The mediastinal subdivisions. Note that the paravertebral sulcus encompasses the posterior compartment. (Reproduced with permission from Shields TW, ed. *General Thoracic Surgery*. 6th ed. 2005.)

mediastinum is divided into several compartments, including the superior, anterior, middle, and posterior regions. Sometimes the lower three compartments are extended superiorly and only three are described (**Fig. 77.35**). The anterior mediastinum includes the structures posterior to the sternum, to the anterior border of the pericardium. The middle compartment includes the pericardium, heart, aorta, and trachea. The posterior compartment includes the esophagus, sympathetic chain, and vertebral column (**Fig. 77.36**). Most lesions are found in asymptomatic patients, but presenting

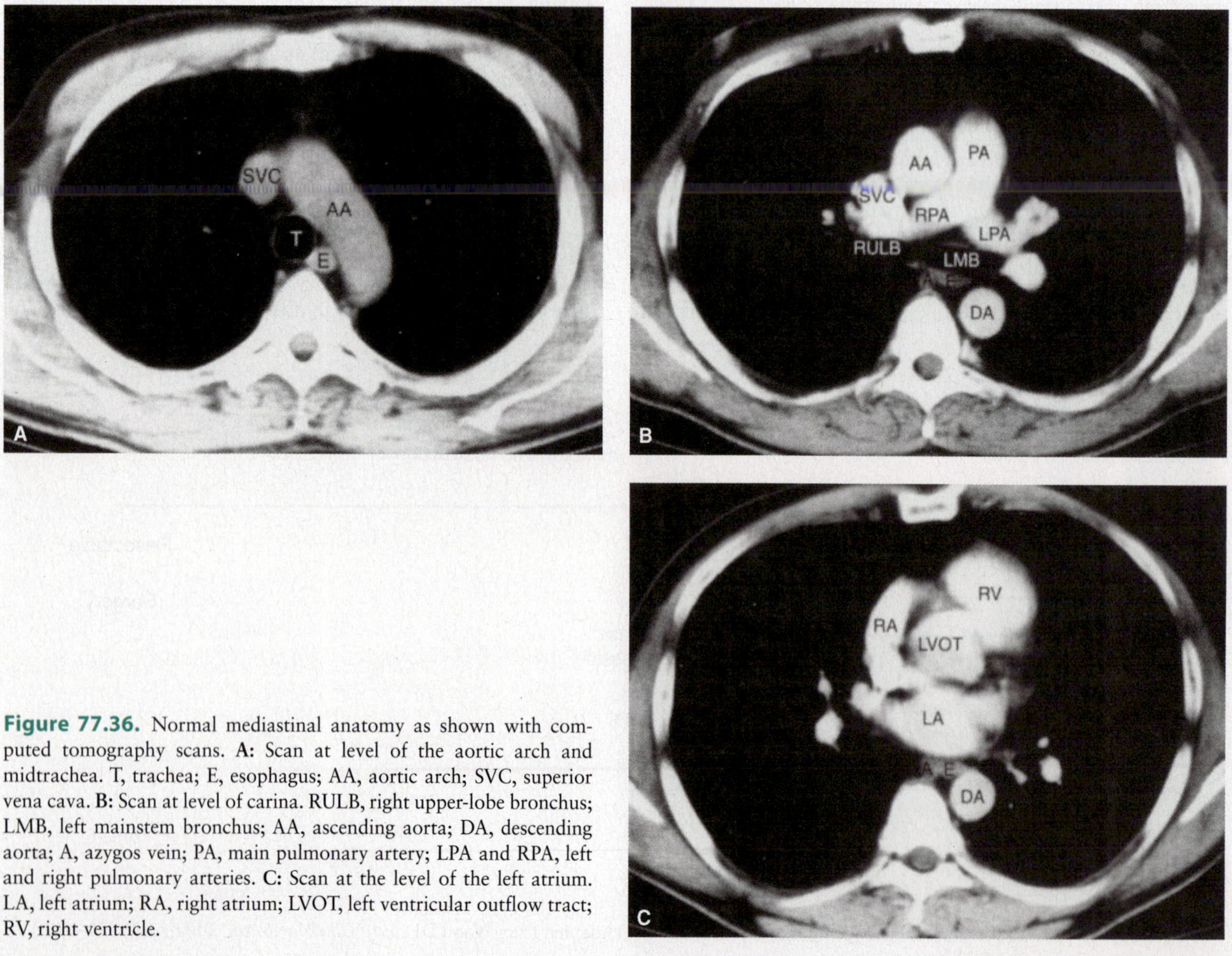

Figure 77.36. Normal mediastinal anatomy as shown with computed tomography scans. **A:** Scan at level of the aortic arch and midtrachea. T, trachea; E, esophagus; AA, aortic arch; SVC, superior vena cava. **B:** Scan at level of carina. RULB, right upper-lobe bronchus; LMB, left mainstem bronchus; AA, ascending aorta; DA, descending aorta; A, azygos vein; PA, main pulmonary artery; LPA and RPA, left and right pulmonary arteries. **C:** Scan at the level of the left atrium. LA, left atrium; RA, right atrium; LVOT, left ventricular outflow tract; RV, right ventricle.

Table 77.10. Location of Primary Mediastinal Masses in Adults and Children

Anterosuperior Mediastinum
Thymoma
Lymphoma
Germ cell tumor
Lymphangioma
Hemangioma
Lipoma
Carcinoma
Thyroid adenoma
Parathyroid adenoma
Middle Mediastinum
Pericardial cyst
Bronchogenic cyst
Lymphoma
Posterior Mediastinum
Neurogenic tumor
Enteric cyst

symptoms include dyspnea and chest pain. Symptoms may be local, related to compression on mediastinal structures, or systemic, caused by the release of cytokines or inflammatory factors, such as in lymphomas or thymomas with myasthenia gravis (MG). Imaging begins with plain radiographs, but CT scans are essential. MRI scans may be helpful to evaluate vascular or spinal involvement. PET scans are increasingly utilized as they may further aid in staging. Biopsy and/or surgical resection are required to confirm the diagnosis in most patients.[94]

Anterior Mediastinum

The anterior mediastinum can contain a variety of tumors (**Table 77.10**). Most common are thymomas, lymphomas, and germ cell tumors, in that order. Thymomas account for one-fifth of all anterior mediastinal masses in the adult population. They arise from the thymus gland and can be seen with autoimmune diseases such as MG and pure red cell aplasia. Tumors were previously classified by the Masaoka classification system, which has now been supplanted by the International Association for the Study of Lung Cancer (IASLC) TNM system (**Table 77.11**).[95] The World Health Organization (WHO) histologic criteria, which is based upon the morphology of the epithelial cells as well as the lymphocyte to epithelial cell ratio. Diagnosis is usually made by chest CT scan. Needle biopsy of a potential thymoma is not routinely recommended for fear of seeding the needle track. When thymomas are suspected, resection is the best option, via a midline sternotomy or thoracoscopic approaches (**Fig. 77.37**). Resection must take care to remove all of the tissue in the anterior compartment, including all fat and tissue around the innominate vein.

Neoadjuvant chemotherapy and radiation may be used to downstage locally invasive tumors and allow for subsequent resection. Postoperative radiation is recommended for tumors that demonstrate capsular invasion or if residual disease is present. Platinum-based chemotherapy is typically utilized in the unresectable setting.[96] MG presents with diplopia, ptosis, fatigue, and weakness. One-third to one-half of patients with thymomas have MG, but only 10% of patients with MG have thymomas. Antiacetylcholine receptor antibody levels may be measured to evaluate for MG in patients with suspected thymomas.[97] Thymic carcinomas and thymic carcinoids are other tumor types that can also arise from the thymus.

Germ cell tumors can present as benign teratomas, seminomas, and embryonal tumors, which include nonseminomatous germ cell tumors and malignant teratomas. Benign teratomas have a good prognosis, and resection is the best treatment. Seminomas comprise up to half of mediastinal germ cell malignant tumors. Patients may have symptoms from local compression or systemic symptoms such as fever, weight loss, and even gynecomastia. These tumors are radiosensitive, but in locally advanced disease, chemotherapy with later surgical resection is the favored treatment. Nonseminomatous tumors include a

Table 77.11. IASLC Staging System for Thymoma

T-Tumor	
T1a	Encapsulated or unencapsulated, with or without extension into mediastinal fat
T1b	Extension into mediastinal pleura
T2	Pericardium
T3	Lung, brachiocephalic vein, superior vena cava, chest wall, phrenic nerve, hilar (extrapericardial) pulmonary vessels
T4	Aorta, arch vessels, main pulmonary artery, myocardium, trachea, or esophagus
N–Lymph Nodes	
N0	No lymph node involvement
N1	Anterior (perithymic) nodes
N2	Deep intrathoracic or cervical nodes
M–Metastases	
M0	No metastatic pleural, pericardial, or distant sites
M1a	Separate pleural or pericardial nodule(s)
M1b	Pulmonary intraparenchymal nodule or distant organ metastasis
Stage	**Description**
I	T1N0M0
II	T2N0M0
IIIa	T3N0M0
IIIb	T4N0M0
IVa	T1-4N1M0, T1-4N0-1M1a
IVb	T1-4N2M0-1a, T1-4N0-2, M1b

Adapted from Detterbeck FC, Stratton K, Giroux D, et al. The IASLC/ITMIG Thymic Epithelial Tumors Staging Project: proposal for an evidence-based stage classification system for the forthcoming (8th) edition of the TNM Classification of Malignant Tumors. *J Thorac Oncol.* 2014;9(9)65–72.

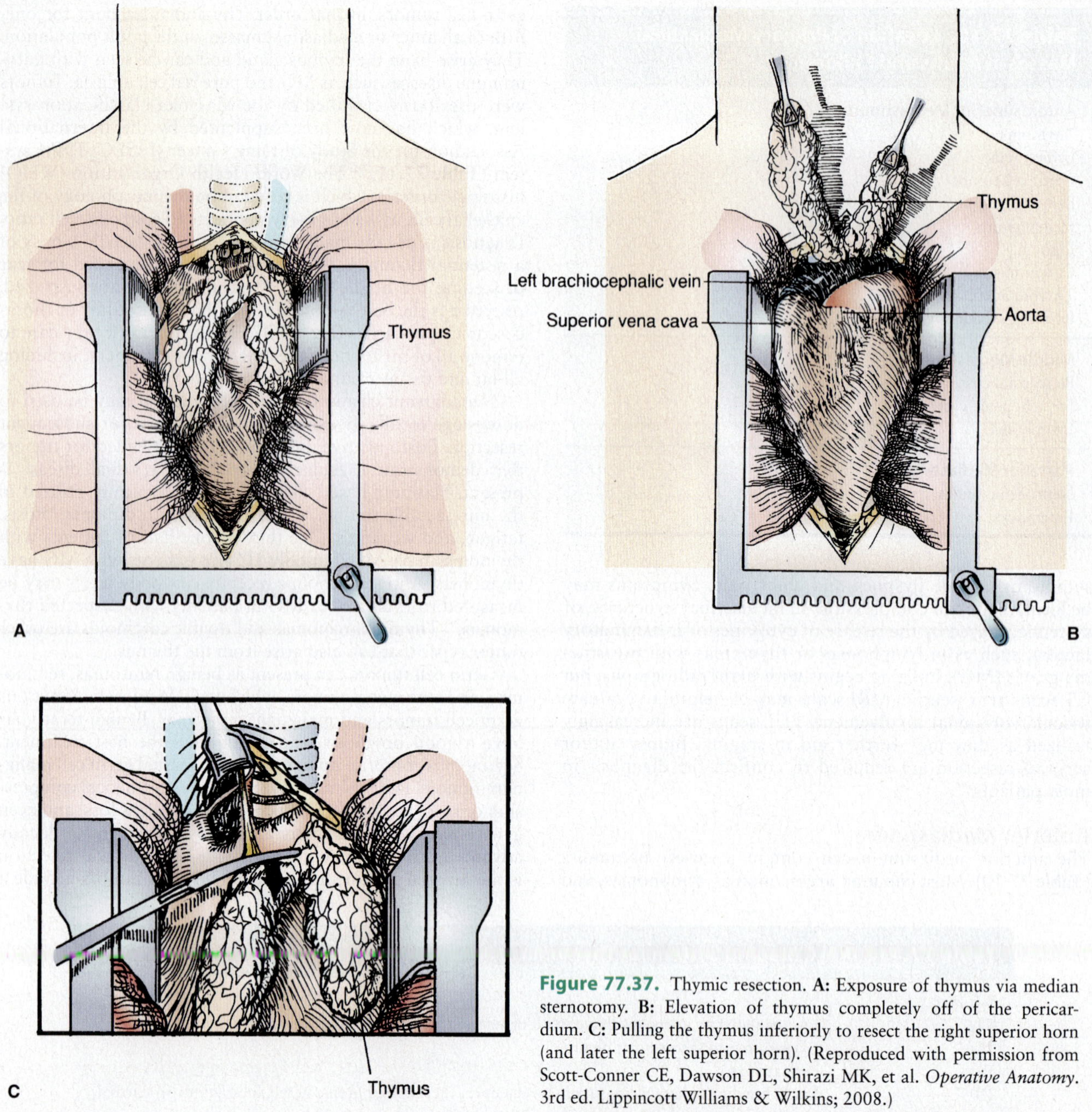

Figure 77.37. Thymic resection. **A:** Exposure of thymus via median sternotomy. **B:** Elevation of thymus completely off of the pericardium. **C:** Pulling the thymus inferiorly to resect the right superior horn (and later the left superior horn). (Reproduced with permission from Scott-Conner CE, Dawson DL, Shirazi MK, et al. *Operative Anatomy.* 3rd ed. Lippincott Williams & Wilkins; 2008.)

wide variety of histologic malignancies. They usually occur in young men and are often symptomatic (**Fig. 77.38**). Elevated alpha-fetal protein (AFP) and beta-human chorionic gonadotropin (β-hCG) levels are seen with these tumors and should be measured. Chemotherapy is the best treatment, but patients have a poorer prognosis when compared to those with seminomas. Surgery is reserved for a persistent mass in the setting of negative tumor markers. Lymphomas in the mediastinum are usually part of a wider spectrum of disease. Two-thirds of cases are Hodgkin disease. Most patients present with symptoms of fevers, night sweats, and even weight loss. Treatment is always chemotherapy-based, and surgery in the form of a biopsy is utilized only to help make the diagnosis.[97]

Middle and Posterior Mediastinum

Middle mediastinal masses include esophageal and bronchogenic cysts, pericardial cysts, lymphangiomas, and lymphomas (**Fig. 77.39**). For cystic lesions, surgical resection is the best treatment option. Posterior lesions include neurogenic tumors, which may be benign or malignant. Almost 95% of tumors come from the sympathetic chain or intercostal nerve rami. Up to two-thirds of these tumors are benign nerve sheath tumors and are usually discovered incidentally. An MRI scan may be used to evaluate intraspinal extension, "dumbbell tumors."[97] In these cases, a spine surgeon may work in combination with the thoracic surgeon to control the intraspinal component, followed by transthoracic excision of the remaining disease.

Pediatric Mediastinum

The presentation of mediastinal masses in the pediatric population varies from what is observed in adults. The rate of malignancy is slightly lower in children, and while thymomas are the most common adult masses seen, neurogenic tumors are more common in children (**Table 77.12**). Just over half of all mediastinal tumors arise in the posterior compartment.[98] Anterior masses may include the normal thymus in a young child. Teratomas are the most common germ cell tumor seen.[98] Vascular anomalies may be seen in children and include hemangiomas and cystic hygromas.[99] Middle compartment tumors are usually foregut cysts, as in the adult population.

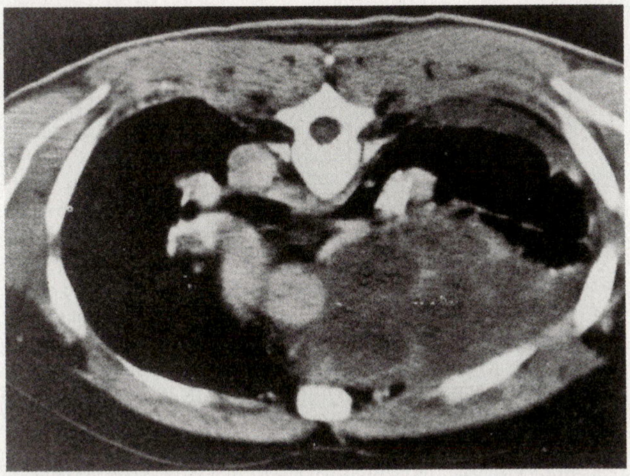

Figure 77.38. Computed tomography scan of a malignant nonseminomatous germ cell tumor of the anterior mediastinum reveals the inhomogeneous anterior mediastinal mass in contrast to the homogeneous density of a seminoma. Pleural effusion is also demonstrated in the right hemithorax. (Reproduced with permission from Shields TW. Primary lesions of the mediastinum and their investigation and treatment. In: Shields TW, ed. *General Thoracic Surgery*. Williams & Wilkins; 1994:1724–1769.)

Posterior tumors are most often malignant neurogenic tumors, compared to more benign pathology in adults.[98]

Mediastinitis

Mediastinal inflammation can arise from different sources, but it is most often infectious in nature. Acute mediastinitis is life threatening and usually results from a perforated esophagus, postcardiac procedure, or trauma. Oral infections can also result in organisms travelling through the neck into the mediastinum along fascial planes. These infections can travel as quickly as necrotizing fasciitis does in other parts of the body and should be addressed immediately. A wide variety of organisms can cause mediastinitis. Patients will have chest pain, dyspnea, and fevers. Radiographic films may show pneumomediastinum or pneumothoraces. If an esophageal perforation is suspected, an esophagogram should be performed.[9] Treatment is broad-spectrum

9

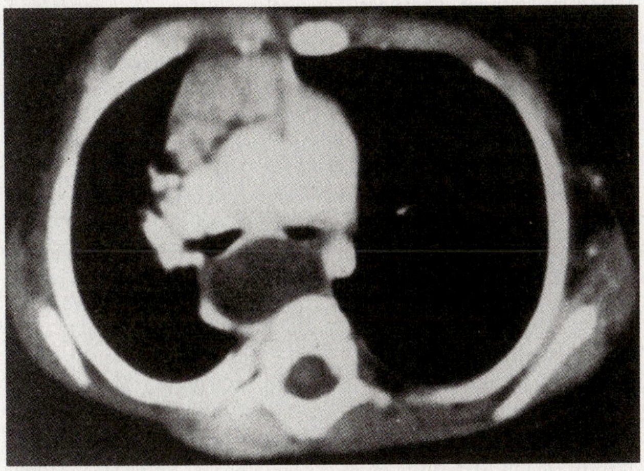

Figure 77.39. Computed tomography scan reveals a bronchogenic cyst located in the subcranial area with compression of the left mainstem bronchus with hyperinflation of the left lung, and a mediastinal shift to the right. (Reproduced with permission from Shields TW. Primary lesions of the mediastinum and their investigation and treatment. In: Shields TW, ed. *General Thoracic Surgery*. Williams & Wilkins; 1994:1764–1769.)

Table 77.12. Mediastinal Tumors in Children

Type of Tumor	Incidence Reported in Series (%)
Neurogenic	35
Lymphoma	25
Germ cell	11
Primary malignancy	2
Cysts	25

Adapted from Davis RD Jr, Oldham HN Jr, Sabiston DC Jr. The mediastinum? In: Sabiston DC Jr, Spencer FC, eds. *Surgery of the Chest*. 5th ed. WB Saunders; 1990:507.

antibiotics and surgical drainage via a cervical incision and/or thoracotomy. Quick debridement and drainage are keys to patient survival. Minimally invasive approaches to the chest may be adequate, but surgeons should have a low threshold to perform a posterolateral thoracotomy, which may give the best exposure and opportunity to debride the chest. Sternal infections after cardiac surgery can also be a serious problem requiring drainage and debridement. Ultimate repair of the defect following debridement may involve muscle or omental flaps for sternal reconstruction.

Chronic mediastinitis is a separate entity from acute mediastinitis and may arise from infectious sources or autoimmune disorders. Patients may be asymptomatic until a mass effect is seen on their mediastinal organs. CT scans are the best imaging modality to diagnose this condition, and surgery is reserved only for diagnosis or in the end stages of the disease to relieve compression on other organs. Sclerosing mediastinitis may be seen in patients with retroperitoneal fibrosis.[100]

Superior Vena Cava Syndrome

Superior vena cava (SVC) syndrome is a rare condition seen when a mediastinal mass compresses the SVC, resulting in facial and upper body edema. Only 15,000 cases per year are seen in the United States. Patients may present with cough, dyspnea, or even stridor from upper airway edema. When patients start to have symptoms, collateral venous drainage develops to drain into the azygos vein or inferior vena cava. This process usually takes weeks. Malignant tumors are the most common cause, but venous thrombosis and nonmalignant lesions cause up to one-third of cases. CT scans are the best diagnostic test. Treatment is based on supportive care and addressing the underlying condition causing the obstruction. If a malignant tumor is causing the obstruction, chemotherapy or radiotherapy may shrink the tumor and lessen symptoms. Surgical resection with SVC reconstruction may be used in specific tumors such as locally advanced thymomas. Angioplasty and stenting may be of benefit, but they are usually palliative.[101] Although it is often felt to be an emergency, most cases of SVC syndrome have a slowly progressive course. When a patient develops symptoms, supportive care, including possible intubation, will allow time for collateral venous drainage to develop and symptoms to improve without other interventions. Although the median survival is typically 6 months or less in patients with SVC syndrome from malignant obstruction, some have seen long-term survivors when the primary tumors have responded to appropriate treatment.[102] When patients present with severe symptoms, urgent surgery is not advised without a long-term plan and clear prognostication. The etiology should be elucidated, along with symptomatic management.

References

1. Incarbone M, Pastorino U. Surgical treatment of chest wall tumors. *World J Surg.* 2001;25(2):218–230.
2. Gross JL, Younes RN, Haddad FJ, Deheinzelin D, Pinto CA, Costa ML. Soft-tissue sarcomas of the chest wall: prognostic factors. *Chest.* 2005;127(3):902–908.
3. Pairolero PC. Chest wall tumors. In: Sellke FW, del Nido PJ, Swanson SJ, eds. *Sabiston and Spencer; Surgery of the Chest.* 7th ed. Elsevier Saunders; 2002:395.
4. Anderson BO, Burt ME. Chest wall neoplasms and their management. *Ann Thorac Surg.* 1994;58(6):1774–1781.
5. Choudhury H, Abidoye O. A desmoid tumor responding to systemic therapy with tamoxifen and sulindac. *Cureus.* 2023;15(3): e35723.
6. Douglas YL, Meuzelaar KJ, van der Lei B, Pras B, Hoekstra HJ. Osteosarcoma of the sternum. *Eur J Surg Oncol.* 1997;23(1):90–91.
7. Gladish G, Sabloff B, Munden R, Truong MT, Erasmus JJ, Chasen MH. Primary thoracic sarcomas. *Radiographics.* 2002;22(3):621.
8. Deschamps C, Tirnaksiz BM, Darbandi R, et al. Early and long-term results of prosthetic chest wall reconstruction. *J Thorac Cardiovasc Surg.* 1999;117(3):588–591; discussion 591–592.
9. Weyant MJ, Bains MS, Venkatraman E, et al. Results of chest wall resection and reconstruction with and without rigid prosthesis. *Ann Thorac Surg.* 2006;81(1):279–285.
10. Chang RR, Mehrara BJ, Hu QY, Disa JJ, Cordeiro PG. Reconstruction of complex oncologic chest wall defects: a 10-year experience. *Ann Plast Surg.* 2004;52(5):471–479; discussion 479.
11. Gonfiotti A, Santini PF, Campanacci D, et al. Malignant primary chest-wall tumours: techniques of reconstruction and survival. *Eur J Cardiothorac Surg.* 2010;38(1):39–45.
12. Skoracki RJ, Chang DW. Reconstruction of the chest wall and thorax. *J Surg Oncol.* 2006;94(6):455–465.
13. Acarturk TO, Swartz WM, Luketich J, Quinlin RF, Edington H. Laparoscopically harvested omental flap for chest wall and intrathoracic reconstruction. *Ann Plast Surg.* 2004;53(3):210–216.
14. Lopushinsky SR, Fecteau AH. Pectus deformities: a review of open surgery in the modern era. *Semin Pediatr Surg.* 2008;17(3): 201–208.
15. Fonkalsrud EW, Dunn JC, Atkinson JB. Repair of pectus excavatum deformities: 30 years of experience with 375 patients. *Ann Surg.* 2000;231(3):443–448.
16. Kelly RE Jr. Pectus excavatum: historical background, clinical picture, preoperative evaluation and criteria for operation. *Semin Pediatr Surg.* 2008;17(3):181–193.
17. Nuss D, Obermeyer RJ, Kelly RE Jr. Pectus excavatum from a pediatric surgeon's perspective. *Ann Cardiothorac Surg.* 2016;5(5):493–500.
18. Mansour KA, Thourani VH, Odessey EA, Durham MM, Miller JI Jr, Miller DL. Thirty-year experience with repair of pectus deformities in adults. *Ann Thorac Surg.* 2003;76(2):391–395; discussion 395.
19. Jaroszewski DE, Fonkalsrud EW. Repair of pectus chest deformities in 320 adult patients: 21 year experience. *Ann Thorac Surg.* 2007;84(2):429–433.
20. Nuss D. Minimally invasive surgical repair of pectus excavatum. *Semin Pediatr Surg.* 2008;17(3):209–217.
21. Park HJ, Lee SY, Lee CS, Youm W, Lee KR. The Nuss procedure for pectus excavatum: evolution of techniques and early results on 322 patients. *Ann Thorac Surg.* 2004;77(1):289–295.
22. Engum SA. Embryology, sternal clefts, ectopia cordis, and cantrell's pentalogy. *Semin Pediatr Surg.* 2008;17(3):154–160.
23. Moir CR, Johnson CH. Poland's syndrome. *Semin Pediatr Surg.* 2008;17(3):161–166.
24. Mackinnon SE, Novak CB. Thoracic outlet syndrome. *Curr Probl Surg.* 2002;39(11):1070–1145.
25. Thompson RW, Petrinec D. Surgical treatment of thoracic outlet compression syndromes: diagnostic considerations and transaxillary first rib resection. *Ann Vasc Surg.* 1997;11(3):315–323.
26. Maxey TS, Reece TB, Ellman PI, et al. Safety and efficacy of the supraclavicular approach to thoracic outlet decompression. *Ann Thorac Surg.* 2003;76(2):396–399; discussion 399–400.
27. Dengler NF, Pedro MT, Kretschmer T, Heinen C, Rosahl SK, Antoniadis G. Neurogenic thoracic outlet syndrome. *Dtsch Arztebl Int.* 2022;119:735–742.
28. Reyes M, Alaparthi S, Roedl JB, et al. Robotic First rib resection in thoracic outlet syndrome: a systematic review of current literature. *J Clin Med.* 2023;12(20):6689.
29. Thompson RW, Petrinec D, Toursarkissian B. Surgical treatment of thoracic outlet compression syndromes. II. Supraclavicular exploration and vascular reconstruction. *Ann Vasc Surg.* 1997;11(4):442–451.
30. Divi V, Proctor MC, Axelrod DA, Greenfield LJ. Thoracic outlet decompression for subclavian vein thrombosis: experience in 71 patients. *Arch Surg.* 2005;140(1):54–57.
31. Landay MJ, Christensen EE, Bynum LJ, Goodman C. Anaerobic pleural and pulmonary infections. *AJR Am J Roentgenol.* 1980;134(2):233–240.
32. Mansharamani NG, Koziel H. Chronic lung sepsis: lung abscess, bronchiectasis, and empyema. *Curr Opin Pulm Med.* 2003;9(3): 181–185.
33. Raymond D. Surgical intervention for thoracic infections. *Surg Clin North Am.* 2014;94(6):1283–1303.
34. O'Donnell AE. Bronchiectasis. *Chest* 2008;134(4):815–823.
35. Barker AF. Bronchiectasis. *N Engl J Med.* 2002;346(18):1383–1393.
36. Ilowite J, Spiegler P, Chawla S. Bronchiectasis: new findings in the pathogenesis and treatment of this disease. *Curr Opin Infect Dis.* 2008;21(2):163–167.
37. Naidoo R. Surgery for pulmonary tuberculosis. *Curr Opin Pulm Med.* 2008;14(3):254–259.
38. Souilamas R, Riquet M, Barthes FP, Chehab A, Capuani A, Faure E. Surgical treatment of active and sequelar forms of pulmonary tuberculosis. *Ann Thorac Surg.* 2001;71(2):443–447.
39. Jean-Baptiste E. Clinical assessment and management of massive hemoptysis. *Crit Care Med.* 2000;28(5):1642–1647.
40. Davidson K, Shojaee S. Managing massive hemoptysis. *Chest.* 2020;157(1):77–88.
41. Shigemura N, Wan IY, Yu SC, et al. Multidisciplinary management of life-threatening massive hemoptysis: a 10-year experience. *Ann Thorac Surg.* 2009;87(3):849–853.
42. Edwards M, Hazelrigg S, Naunheim K. The national emphysema treatment trial: summary and update. *Thorac Surg Clin.* 2009;19(2):169–185.
43. Martinez FJ, Chang A. Surgical therapy for chronic obstructive pulmonary disease. *Semin Respir Crit Care Med.* 2005;26(2): 167–191.
44. Klooster K, ten Hacken NHT, Hartman JE, Kerstjens HAM, van Rikxoort EM, Slebos DJ. Endobronchial valves for emphysema without interlobar collateral ventilation. *N Engl J Med.* 2015;373(24):2325–2335.
45. Shah AA, D'Amico TA. Lung volume reduction surgery for the management of refractory dyspnea in chronic obstructive pulmonary disease. *Curr Opin Support Palliat Care.* 2009;3(2):107–111.
46. Swanson KL, Edell ES. Tracheobronchial foreign bodies. *Chest Surg Clin N Am.* 2001;11(4):861–872.
47. Boyd M, Chatterjee A, Chiles C, Chin R Jr. Tracheobronchial foreign body aspiration in adults. *South Med J.* 2009;102(2):171–174.
48. Blanco Ramos M, Botana-Rial M, García-Fontán E, Fernández-Villar A, Torreira MG. Update in the extraction of airway foreign bodies in adults. *J Thorac Dis.* 2016;8(11):3452–3456.
49. Sahn SA, Heffner JE. Spontaneous pneumothorax. *N Engl J Med.* 2000;342(12):868–874.
50. Rahman NM, Davies RJ, Gleeson FV. Pleural interventions: management of acute and chronic pneumothorax. *Semin Respir Crit Care Med.* 2008;29(4):427–440.
51. Baumann MH, Noppen M. Pneumothorax. *Respirology.* 2004; 9(2):157–164.
52. Shen KR, Cerfolio R. Decision making in the management of secondary spontaneous pneumothorax in patients with severe emphysema. *Thorac Surg Clin.* 2009;19(2):233–238.
53. Mendeloff EN. Sequestrations, congenital cystic adenomatoid malformations, and congenital lobar emphysema. *Semin Thorac Cardiovasc Surg.* 2004;16(3):209–214.

54. Horak E, Bodner J, Gassner I, et al. Congenital cystic lung disease: diagnostic and therapeutic considerations. *Clin Pediatr (Phila)*. 2003;42(3):251–261.
55. Schwartz DS, Reyes-Mugica M, Keller MS. Imaging of surgical diseases of the newborn chest. Intrapleural mass lesions. *Radiol Clin North Am*. 1999;37(6):1067–1078, v.
56. Evrard V, Ceulemans J, Coosemans W, et al. Congenital parenchymatous malformations of the lung. *World J Surg*. 1999;23(11): 1123–1132.
57. Takeda S, Miyoshi S, Inoue M, et al. Clinical spectrum of congenital cystic disease of the lung in children. *Eur J Cardiothorac Surg*. 1999;15(1):11–17.
58. Heffner J. Discriminating between transudates and exudates. *Clin Chest Med*. 2006;27(2):241.
59. Feller-Kopman D, Light R. Pleural Disease. *NEJM*. 2018; 378(8):740.
60. Kolditz M, Halank M, Schiemanck CS, Schmeisser A, Höffken G. High diagnostic accuracy of NT-proBNP for cardiac origin of pleural effusions. *Eur Respir J*. 2006;28(1):144–150.
61. Light RW. The undiagnosed pleural effusion. *Clin Chest Med*. 2006;27(2):309–319.
62. Putnam J Jr. Malignant pleural effusions. *Surg Clin North Am*. 2002;82(4):867–883.
63. Johnson OW, Chick JFB, Chauhan NR, et al. The thoracic duct: clinical importance, anatomic variation, imaging, and embolization. *Eur Radiol*. 2016;26:2482.
64. Fysh ETH, Waterer GW, Kendall PA, et al. Indwelling pleural catheters reduce inpatient days over pleurodesis for malignant pleural effusion. *Chest*. 2012;142(2):394–400.
65. Murthy P, Ekeke CN, Russell KL, et al. Making cold malignant pleural effusions hot: driving novel immunotherapies. *Oncoimmunology*. 2019;8(4):e1554969.
66. Christie NA. Management of pleural space: effusions and empyema. *Surg Clin N Am*. 2010;90:919–934.
67. Lisboa T, Waterer GW, Lee YG. Pleural infection: changing bacteriology and its implications. *Respirology*. 2011;16:598–603.
68. Wright CD, Wain JC, Mathisen DJ, Grillo HC. Postpneumonectomy bronchopleural fistula after sutured bronchial closure: incidence, risk factors, and management. *J Thorac Cardiovasc Surg*. 1996;112(5):1367–1371.
69. Deschamps C, Bernard A, Nichols FC III, et al. Empyema and bronchopleural fistula after pneumonectomy: factors affecting incidence. *Ann Thorac Surg*. 2001;72(1):243–247; discussion 248.
70. Vallières E. Management of empyema after lung resections (pneumonectomy/lobectomy). *Chest Surg Clin N Am*. 2002;12(3): 571–585.
71. Robinson BW, Musk AW, Lake RA. Malignant mesothelioma. *Lancet*. 2005;366(9483):397–408.
72. Robinson BW, Lake RA. Advances in malignant mesothelioma. *N Engl J Med*. 2005;353(15):1591–1603.
73. Pistolesi M, Rusthoven J. Malignant pleural mesothelioma: update, current management, and newer therapeutic strategies. *Chest*. 2004;126(4):1318–1329.
74. Verma V, Ahern CA, Berlind CG, et al. Survival by histologic subtype of malignant pleural mesothelioma and the impact of surgical resection on overall survival. *Clin Lung Cancer*. 2018;19(6): 901–912.
75. Berzenji L, Van Schil P, Carp L. The eighth TNM classification for malignant pleural mesothelioma. *Transl Lung Cancer Res*. 2018;7(5):543–549.
76. Singhal S, Kaiser LR. Malignant mesothelioma: options for management. *Surg Clin North Am*. 2002;82(4):797–831.
77. van Ruth S, Baas P, Zoetmulder FA. Surgical treatment of malignant pleural mesothelioma: a review. *Chest*. 2003;123(2): 551–561.
78. Beebe-Dimmer JL, Fryzek JP, Yee CL, et al. Mesothelioma in the United States: a surveillance, epidemiology, and end results (SEER)-Medicare investigation of treatment patterns and overall survival. *Clin Epidemiol*. 2016;8:743–750.
79. Peters S, Scherpereel A, Cornelissen R, et al. First-line nivolumab plus ipilimumab versus chemotherapy in patients with unresectable malignant pleural mesothelioma: 3-year outcomes from CheckMate 743. *Ann Oncol*. 2022;33(5):488–499.
80. Minnich D, Mathisen D. Anatomy of the trachea, carina, and bronchi. *Thorac Surg Clin*. 2007;17(4):571.
81. Cheung N, Napolitano LM. Tracheostomy: epidemiology, indications, timing, technique, and outcomes. *Respir Care*. 2014;59(6): 895–919.
82. Angel L, Simpson C. Comparison of surgical and percutaneous dilational tracheostomy. *Clin Chest Med*. 2003;24(3):423.
83. Wain JC. Postintubation tracheal stenosis. *Chest Surg Clin N Am*. 2003;13(2):231–246.
84. Mathisen DJ. Surgery of the trachea. *Curr Probl Surg*. 1998;35(6): 453–542.
85. Mathisen DJ. Tracheal tumors. *Chest Surg Clin N Am*. 1996;6(4): 875–898.
86. Wood DE. Management of malignant tracheobronchial obstruction. *Surg Clin North Am*. 2002;82(3):621–642.
87. Gaissert H. Primary tracheal tumors. *Chest Surg Clin N Am*. 2003;13(2):247.
88. Wright CD. Tracheomalacia. *Chest Surg Clin N Am*. 2003;13(2): 349–357, viii.
89. Jaquiss RD. Management of pediatric tracheal stenosis and tracheomalacia? *Semin Thorac Cardiovasc Surg*. 2004;16(3):220–224.
90. Chin CS, Litle V, Yun J, Weiser T, Swanson SJ. Airway stents. *Ann Thorac Surg*. 2008;85(2):S792–S796.
91. Castellanos P, Mk M, Atallah I. Laser tracheobronchoplasty: a novel technique for the treatment of symptomatic tracheobronchomalacia. *Eur Arch Otorhinolaryngol*. 2017;274(3): 1601–1607.
92. Gangadharan SP, Bakhos CT, Majid A, et al. Technical aspects and outcomes of tracheobronchoplasty for severe tracheobronchomalacia. *Ann Thorac Surg*. 2011;91(5):1574–1580.
93. Mulligan MS. Endoscopic management of airway complications after lung transplantation. *Chest Surg Clin N Am*. 2001;11(4): 907–915.
94. Date H. Diagnostic strategies for mediastinal tumors and cysts. *Thorac Surg Clin*. 2009;19(1):29–35, vi.
95. Detterbeck FC, Stratton K, Giroux D, et al. The IASLC/ITMIG Thymic Epithelial Tumors Staging Project: Proposal for an Evidence-Based Stage Classification System for the Forthcoming (8th) Edition of the TNM Classification of Malignant Tumors. *J Thorac Oncol*. 2014;9(9):65–72.
96. Tomaszek S, Wigle DA, Keshavjee S, Fischer S. Thymomas: review of current clinical practice. *Ann Thorac Surg*. 2009;87(6): 1973–1980.
97. Duwe BV, Sterman DH, Musani AI. Tumors of the mediastinum. *Chest*. 2005;128(4):2893–2909.
98. Wright CD. Mediastinal tumors and cysts in the pediatric population. *Thorac Surg Clin*. 2009;19(1):47–61, vi.
99. Jaggers J, Balsara K. Mediastinal masses in children. *Semin Thorac Cardiovasc Surg*. 2004;16(3):201–208.
100. Athanassiadi KA. Infections of the mediastinum. *Thorac Surg Clin*. 2009;19(1):37–45, vi.
101. Wilson LD, Detterbeck FC, Yahalom J. Clinical practice. superior vena cava syndrome with malignant causes. *N Engl J Med*. 2007;356(18):1862–1869.
102. Yu JB, Wilson LD, Detterbeck FC. Superior vena cava syndrome—a proposed classification system and algorithm for management. *J Thorac Oncol*. 2008;3(8):811–814.

78

Section M:

VASCULAR DISEASE

Congenital Heart Disease

Douglas M. Overbey, Hiba Z. Ghandour, Seth E. M. Wolf, and Joseph W. Turek

Key Points

1 The ductus arteriosus is a fetal vascular structure that allows the movement of blood from the right ventricle (RV) directly to the systemic circulation, bypassing the high-resistance pulmonary vascular bed. Following birth, the rise in oxygen tension and a fall in prostaglandins lead to ductal closure, and the ductus becomes the ligamentum arteriosum. Failure of closure of the ductus leads to a patent ductus arteriosus (PDA).

2 Eisenmenger physiology with resulting cyanosis can occur due to worsening pulmonary vascular obstructive disease/resistance with shunt flow reversal to right-to-left.

3 Ventricular septal defects (VSDs) are the most prevalent congenital heart disease (CHD). Most VSDs close spontaneously during the first year of life (especially muscular defects). Left-to-right shunting at the ventricular level can lead to congestive heart failure (CHF) in large VSDs by 2 months of age.

4 An (ASD) is a hole in the atrial septum, accounting for 10% of the burden of CHD. Left-to-right shunting is at the atrial level and can cause right heart volume overload. Depending on the size of the ASD, it is either closed percutaneously or surgically, and not usually required until several years of age.

5 Endocardial cushion defects during cardiogenesis may result in morphologic abnormalities in the atrioventricular (AV) valves and the atrial and ventricular septa leading to atrioventricular septal defects (AVSDs or atrioventricular canal defects [AVCDs]).

6 In transposition of the great arteries (TGA), the aorta arises from the RV and the pulmonary artery (PA) from the left ventricle (ventriculoarterial discordance). Atrial level mixing (through ASD or patent foramen ovale [PFO]) and a VSD or PDA is needed for adequate systemic oxygen delivery.

7 Congenital aortic stenosis (AS) is a form of left ventricular outflow tract obstruction (LVOTO), with severe forms leading to rapid CHF. Coronary blood flow can be obstructed due to elevated left ventricular end diastolic pressure, systemic hypotension, and adherence of aortic valve leaflets depending on the subtype.

8 Tetralogy of Fallot (TOF) is the most common cyanotic CHD, occurring in 0.4 per 1,000 live births and comprising about 5% of all CHD cases. Its pathology is characterized by four components: VSD, overriding aorta, right ventricular outflow tract obstruction (RVOTO), and right ventricular hypertrophy.

9 Hypoplastic left-heart syndrome (HLHS) is characterized by underdevelopment of the left ventricle and the ascending aorta. Systemic circulation is maintained by a nonrestrictive ASD and a PDA. Staged palliation with Norwood–Glenn–Fontan is the preferred surgical management; however, many children ultimately require heart transplantation.

Congenital heart disease (CHD) is the overarching term used to describe cardiac defects present at birth. Abnormalities in the structure of the cardiac chambers, valves, and/or great vessels alter the function and subsequently the normal blood flow pattern. Many complications can ensue, including arrhythmias, valve insufficiency, and heart failure.

Surgery is the mainstay therapy for CHD, however the outcome of congenital cardiac surgery often falls into one of two categories: (1) reparative and (2) palliative. Reparative interventions improve congenital heart defects and can be curative. Curative interventions rarely leave patients with long-term complications (eg, repair of uncomplicated VSD, secundum ASD, or closure of PDA). Other reparative interventions may leave patients with lifelong sequelae and/or impairment (eg, aortic coarctation, TOF, total anomalous pulmonary venous return, transposition of the great arteries [TGA], congenital corrected transposition). Palliative interventions often do not fully repair the congenital heart defect(s), and patients often have lifelong sequelae and functional impairment (eg, HLHS, single ventricle, tricuspid atresia, Eisenmenger syndrome).

PATENT DUCTUS ARTERIOSUS

The ductus arteriosus is a fetal vascular structure that allows the movement of blood from the RV directly to the systemic circulation, bypassing the high-resistance pulmonary vascular bed. The ductus communicates between the main PA and the proximal descending thoracic aorta. Oxygen tension and prostaglandin levels vasocontrol the ductus. Following birth, the rise in oxygen tension and a fall in prostaglandins lead to ductal closure, and the ductus becomes the ligamentum arteriosum. A ductus arteriosus failing to close, or PDA, occurs in 1 out of 1,200 live births and accounts for 7% of congenital heart defects.[1]

Pathophysiology

1 The physiologic premise of a PDA is the shunting of blood across the ductus, whereby the shunt volume is determined by (1) the size of the ductus and (2) the ratio of pulmonary to systemic vascular resistance (SVR). At birth, shunting across a PDA is usually from left to right; however, excessive pulmonary blood flow (PBF) can lead to heart failure. Conversely,

in various congenital heart lesions, the PDA can maintain life-saving blood flow to either the systemic or pulmonary systems. Such cases include aortic coarctation or hypoplastic left heart syndrome, where prostaglandins (eg, prostaglandin E1 [PGE1]) are used to maintain ductal patency until operative repair can be done.

Clinical Presentation and Diagnosis

In patients with a PDA, symptoms are proportional to the shunt volume and the presence of associated defects. Left-to-right shunting produces left-sided volume overload. Physical exam findings include a widened pulse pressure and a continuous "machinery" murmur along the left upper sternal border. A plain chest film shows increased pulmonary vascular markings and left heart enlargement. Electrocardiogram (EKG) is notable for left ventricular hypertrophy and left atrial enlargement. Diagnosis is established using echocardiography.

Management

PDA closure is recommended for asymptomatic patients due to the risk of heart failure, hypertension, endocarditis, and endarteritis and performed for all symptomatic patients. Closure of the ductus may be accomplished by one of three approaches: pharmacologic, endovascular, and surgical. Indomethacin and ibuprofen are pharmacologic PDA closure agents used in premature infants. Endovascular catheter-based options use a device to occlude the ductus. The decision to manage a PDA medically, or through endovascular or open techniques largely depends on the size, patient age, hemodynamic significance of the PDA as well as the presence of complications secondary to it.

Surgical Repair and Complications

PDA closure is approached through a left posterolateral thoracotomy via the third or fourth intercostal space. After incising the pleura over the proximal descending thoracic aorta, the vagus nerve is retracted medially, and the recurrent laryngeal nerve is visualized curving behind the ductus. Care must be taken during ductal closure as it can be the largest vascular structure present and should not be confused with the aorta. Direct manipulation of ductal tissue should be minimized as it is extremely friable.

- In premature infants, the ductus is controlled with a single surgical clip.
- In older patients, occlusion of the ductus is achieved with simple silk ligature, or, preferably, by division between ligatures to minimize recurrence.

VENTRICULAR SEPTAL DEFECTS

VSDs are the most common congenital heart defect (after bicuspid aortic valve [BAV]), and they can occur in isolation or concurrently with other cardiac defects. This typically acyanotic heart disease develops from the failure of the interventricular septum to fully form. The septum is formed by two components, a muscular portion, which contains the inlet, trabecular, and infundibular segments, and a membranous portion, which is a fibrous portion of the ventricular septum that is adjacent to the central fibrous body (where the mitral, tricuspid, and aortic valve annuli make contact), and contains the AV segment (or endocardial cushions). VSDs make up 40% of congenital heart defects and are present in 4 out of every 1,000 live births.[1]

Types of VSDs

There are four types of VSDs, each classified by location in the interventricular septum (**Fig. 78.1**).

Perimembranous VSDs are most common, with an 80% incidence and are located within the membranous septum. The second most common defect is located high in the septum, adjacent to the pulmonary and aortic valves and is labeled an outlet, supracristal, infundibular or doubly committed subarterial defect, with an incidence of 10%. Inlet defects have an incidence of 5% and are located beneath the septal leaflet of the tricuspid valve (TV) and commonly associated with an AVSD. The fourth defect also has an incidence of 5% and is the muscular (or trabecular) defect, which is completely bordered by muscle.

Pathophysiology

VSDs cause increased PBF due to left-to-right shunting. This leads to volume overload on the left heart and pressure overload on the right heart. The volume of blood shunted to the right is determined by the defect's size and the ratio of pulmonary vascular resistance (PVR) to SVR (Qp/Qs). Because PVR is high at birth and slowly comes down, patients with large VSDs can be asymptomatic at birth and develop severe heart failure symptoms over the first 6 to 8 weeks of life. VSDs can be restrictive or nonrestrictive. When the cumulative size of the defect(s) is greater than or equal to the size of the aortic annulus, it is typically nonrestrictive. Babies with large, nonrestrictive VSDs with Qp/Qs greater than 2 may develop heart failure symptoms within a few months of life. Conversely, small, highly restrictive VSDs could remain asymptomatic for
2 several years. Eisenmenger physiology results when the shunt flow reverses to right to left from significant pulmonary hypertension, creating cyanosis.

Clinical Presentation and Diagnosis

Clinically, patients present with a holosystolic murmur at the left sternal border, with smaller defects accompanied by louder murmurs. A plain chest radiograph shows increased pulmo-
3 nary vascular markings and cardiomegaly. EKGs demonstrate right ventricular hypertrophy. The diagnosis of VSD is confirmed by echocardiography.

Management

The management of a patient with a VSD depends on four factors, (1) the size of the defect, (2) the type of defect, (3) the shunt volume, and (4) the PVR. Patients with large VSDs who present in heart failure should undergo early surgical repair (**Table 78.1**). If the heart failure symptoms can be suppressed by medical therapy (diuretics), then surgery may be deferred until 6 months of age. Patients with smaller VSDs may be safely followed in the absence of ventricular dilation and aortic insufficiency. Appropriate use of prophylactic antibiotics is pivotal in this population due to the low risk of endocarditis associated with VSDs. Patients with outlet VSDs have an increased risk of developing aortic insufficiency due to leaflet prolapse.[2] Certain VSDs can be closed by endovascular (catheter-based) techniques, particularly muscular defects in larger patients.

Surgical Repair and Complications

Standard approach is via a median sternotomy with aortic and bicaval cannulation for cardiopulmonary bypass. The patient is cooled to 32 °C. After aortic cross-clamping, cold cardioplegia is delivered through the aortic root. Exposure of the ventricular septum is achieved through a right atriotomy and TV leaflet retraction. This provides access to perimembranous, inlet, and some muscular VSDs. Exposure of outlet VSDs is often best achieved through a pulmonary arteriotomy. Muscular VSDs located near the ventricular apex can be difficult to expose and may require an apical ventriculotomy. After exposure, defects are closed using a variety of patch materials (Dacron, PTFE, autologous pericardium, bovine pericardium, etc.).

Pearls and Pitfalls of Repair

The AV node is an atrial structure that lies at the apex of the triangle of Koch, formed by the coronary sinus, the tendon of Todaro, and the septal attachment of the TV. The node gives rise to the bundle of His, which penetrates the AV junction

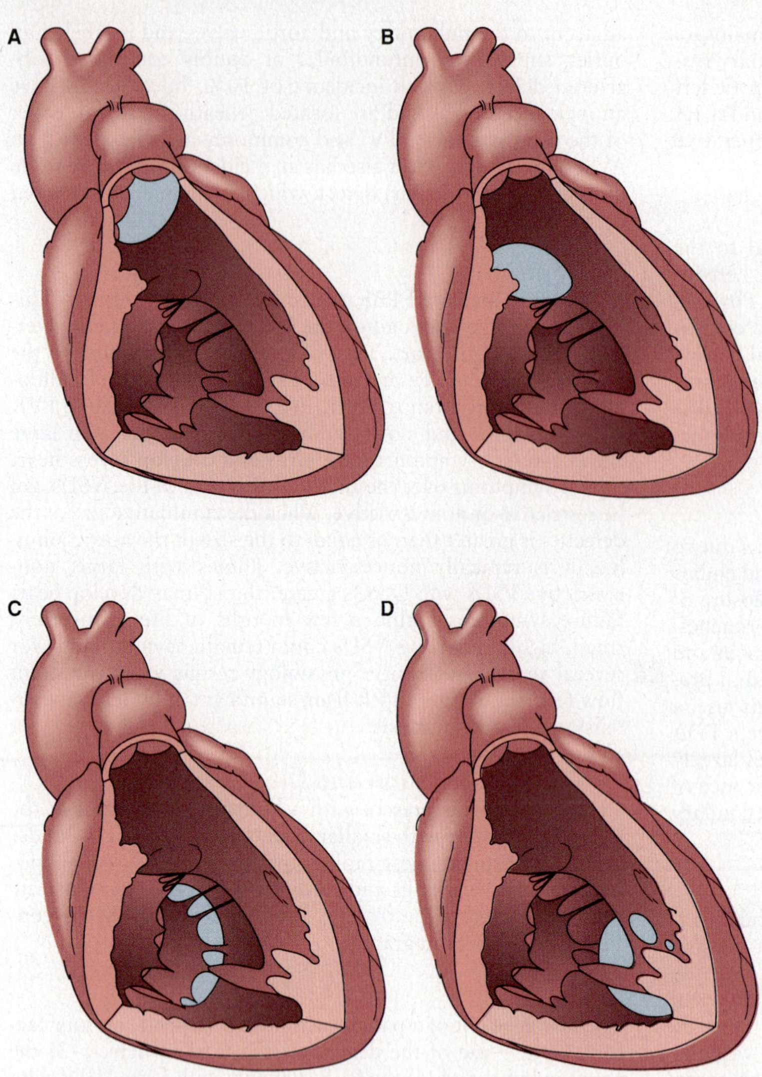

Figure 78.1. The anatomy of ventricular septal defects (VSDs) as seen through the right ventricle. **A:** Outlet, or subarterial, VSDs are generally bordered superiorly by the pulmonary valve annulus. **B:** Perimembranous VSDs are most common, extending from the membranous septum into the infundibular septum. **C:** Inlet defects are located predominantly beneath the septal leaflet of the tricuspid valve. **D:** Muscular VSDs are situated away from the valves, toward the cardiac apex.

beneath the membranous septum. The bundle of His then bifurcates into right and left bundle branches, which pass along either side of the muscular ventricular septum.

In the presence of a perimembranous VSD, the bundle of His passes along the posterior and inferior rim of the defect, generally on the left ventricular side. In this critical area, sutures must be placed superficially on the right ventricular side a few millimeters from the edge of the defect. The bundle of His also tends to run along the posterior and inferior margin of inlet VSDs. The conduction tissue is usually remote from outlet and trabecular VSDs.

OPERATIVE STEPS

Table 78.1. VSD via Sternotomy

CPB configuration	Bicaval cannulation, mild hypothermia, antegrade cardioplegic arrest
Exposure and intracardiac steps	Oblique right atriotomy, retraction of anterior and septal leaflets of tricuspid valve, inspection of ventricular septal defect and nearby aortic valve, patch closure of VSD with running suture technique
Completion	De-airing of left heart, removal of cross-clamp, primary closure of right atriotomy
Final steps	Wean off bypass, place temporary pacing wires, TEE, standard closure

CPB, cardiopulmonary bypass; VSD, ventricular septal defect; TEE, transesophageal echocardiogram.

Complications

Surgical closure of a VSD is associated with a mortality of about 1%. Potential complications include injury to the conduction tissue and injury to the tricuspid, pulmonary, or aortic valves. TV regurgitation may ensue after repair of perimembranous and inlet VSDs if the repair distorts the valve. The aortic valve can be injured in perimembranous and outlet defect repairs. Transient heart block may result postoperatively, but permanent heart block occurs in less than 1% of cases. A residual VSD is seen in about 5% of cases, and reoperation is indicated only if significant shunting persists.

ATRIAL SEPTAL DEFECTS

ASDs are defects in the atrial septum. They are the third most common congenital heart defect, occurring in 1 out of 1,000 live births and make up 10% of congenital heart defects.[1]

Embryology

Cardiac development begins during the third week of gestation and ends in the ninth week. The heart starts off as a tube with a common atrium, where the septum primum arises. The septum primum starts forming at the roof of the atrium and descends inferiorly; the opening below the inferior edge of the septum primum is the ostium primum and it gets obliterated when the septum primum fuses with the endocardial cushions. Concurrently, the ostium secundum forms in the midportion of the septum primum prior to closure of the ostium primum. The septum secundum also arises from the roof of the atrium and descends along the right side of the septum primum and covers the ostium secundum. This creates a flap valve, the foramen ovale, where blood from the inferior vena cava (IVC) may preferentially stream beneath the edge of the septum secundum and through the ostium secundum into the left atrium. PFOs are separate from ASDs due to the absence of significant shunting; however, they are clinically important due to paradoxical embolization.

Types of ASDs

There are four types of ASDs (**Fig. 78.2**). Ostium secundum is the most common ASD, representing 80% of all defects, and occurs when the ostium secundum is too large to be covered by the septum secundum or the septum primum regresses. Ostium primum ASD represents 10% of ASDs, occurs from failure of fusion of the septum primum with the endocardial cushions, and is classified as an AVSD. The sinus venosus defect is the third type and represents 10% of ASDs. It is characterized by a defect that is high in the atrial wall near the orifice of the superior vena cava (SVC) or, low in the atrial septum near the IVC. The last and least common ASD is the unroofed coronary sinus septal defect, which leads to communication between the right and left atria at the site of the coronary sinus.

Pathophysiology

ASDs lead to increased PBF secondary to left-to-right shunting. Shunting at the atrial level is determined by the size of the defect and by the relative ventricular compliance with the RV becoming more compliant gradually after birth. While this leads to volume overload on the right heart, patients are often asymptomatic. Eventually both atria and the RV can enlarge.

Clinical Presentation and Diagnosis

4 The classic physical findings in patients with ASDs include fixed splitting of the second heart sound and a systolic ejection murmur at the left upper sternal border. Chest films demonstrate cardiomegaly, with enlargement of the right atrium, RV, and PA. The EKG frequently demonstrates right-axis deviation and an incomplete right bundle branch block. Echocardiography confirms the diagnosis of ASD.

Management

Repair is recommended for all patients with symptomatic defects and in asymptomatic patients in whom the Qp/Qs is greater than 1.5. Repair can be done surgically or percutaneously. Percutaneous closure involves catheter-based devices and requires sufficient IVC and aortic rims.

Surgical Repair and Complications

Surgical repair is usually recommended for almost all ASDs, particularly large secundum defects (**Table 78.2**). Surgical repair of an ASD has minimal morbidity and a mortality approaching zero. A median sternotomy is carried out and cardiopulmonary bypass with bicaval cannulation is employed. The patient is cooled to 32 °C. After aortic cross-clamping, cold cardioplegia is delivered through the aortic root. Exposure of the atrial septum is achieved through a right atriotomy. Depending on the size, small secundum defects, or PFOs may be closed primarily by suturing the edge of the septum primum to the edge of the septum secundum. More often, larger defects are closed using a patch, as in VSD repairs. When anomalous pulmonary venous drainage is present, a baffle (an intracardiac wall or tunnel to redirect blood flow) is created to redirect the flow across the ASD. Complications seen postoperatively include supraventricular arrhythmias, with an incidence of 15% to 60% and postpericardiotomy syndrome, occurring in about 10% to 40% of cases.

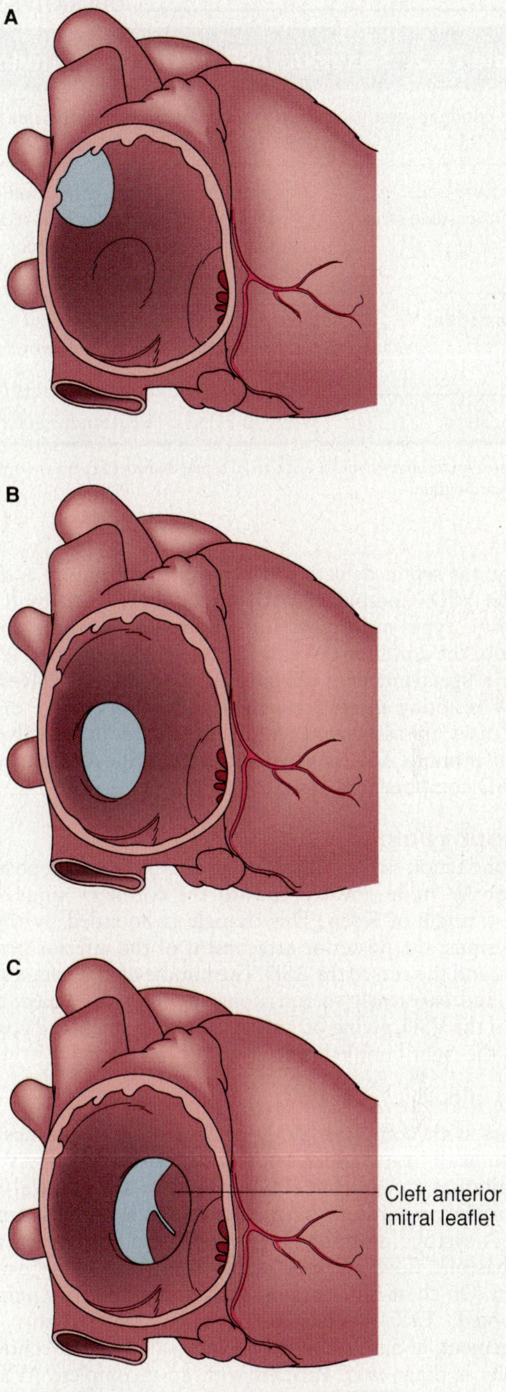

Figure 78.2. The anatomy of atrial septal defects. In the sinus venosus type (**A**), the right upper and middle pulmonary veins frequently drain to the superior vena cava or right atrium. **B:** Secundum defects generally occur as isolated lesions. **C:** Primum defects are part of a more complex lesion and are best considered as incomplete atrioventricular septal defects.

ATRIOVENTRICULAR SEPTAL DEFECTS

Endocardial cushion defects during cardiogenesis may result in morphologic abnormalities in the AV valves and the atrial and ventricular septa.

Types of AVSD

AVSDs are classified into complete and incomplete. Complete AVSD is characterized by a deficiency of endocardial cushion tissue, whereby patients are left with a common AV orifice, rather than separate mitral and tricuspid orifices, and

OPERATIVE STEPS

Table 78.2. Secundum ASD via Limited Sternotomy

CPB configuration	Bicaval cannulation, normothermia, and antegrade cardioplegic arrest
Exposure and intracardiac steps	Oblique right atriotomy, inspection of atrial septum/systemic venous return/ pulmonary venous return, patch closure of ASD
Completion	De-airing of left heart, removal of cross-clamp, primary closure of right atriotomy
Final steps	Wean off bypass, TEE, standard closure

CPB, cardiopulmonary bypass; ASD, atrial septal defect; TEE, transesophageal echocardiogram.

contiguous septal defects which result in a primum ASD and an inlet VSD. Complete AVSDs were subclassified by Rastelli into three types according to the morphology of the anterior leaflet of the common AV valve. Incomplete, or partial AVSDs, lie on a spectrum with partial fusion of the AV valves, ultimately resulting in separate right and left AV valve orifices. Most cases are associated with a cleft in the mitral valve. The ostium primum ASD is a type of incomplete AVSD in which the VSD component is absent.

Pathophysiology

The conduction tissue is displaced in an ASVD, with a posterior/inferior AV node, located toward the coronary sinus in the nodal triangle of Koch. This triangle is bounded by the coronary sinus, the posterior attachment of the inferior bridging leaflet, and the rim of the ASD. The bundle of His courses anteriorly and superiorly to run along the leftward aspect of the crest of the VSD, giving off the left bundle branch and continuing as the right bundle branch.

Clinical Presentation and Diagnosis

5 Patients with complete AVSD present early in infancy with symptoms of heart failure, with moderate–severe left AV valve regurgitation occurring in 10% of the cases. On physical examination, the precordium is hyperactive, often with a prominent thrill. A systolic murmur along the left sternal border, and a mid-diastolic flow murmur across the common AV valve is present. On chest film, cardiomegaly and pulmonary markings are noted. EKG reveals biventricular hypertrophy, atrial enlargement, and a prolonged PR interval. Doppler/echocardiography is diagnostic. Patients with an incomplete AVSD, or those with a small VSD component (transitional AVSD), generally present similarly to patients with large secundum ASDs.

Management

Operative treatment is almost always necessary when symptoms arise. If symptoms are absent, surgery is best performed before 6 months of age. These defects are commonly found in patients with Down syndrome require even sooner repair, as these patients can develop accelerated pulmonary vascular disease presenting with cyanosis.

Surgical Repair and Complications

Correcting AVSDs requires patch closure of both septal defects, and valve reconstruction (**Table 78.3**). Separate atrial and ventricular patches, a single patch or modified single patch approaches can be used. During closure of the ventricular defect, care must be taken to avoid injury to the conduction system, which passes along the posterior and inferior rim of the ventricular septum. Operative mortality depends on the

OPERATIVE STEPS

Table 78.3. Complete AVSD via Sternotomy

CPB configuration	Bicaval cannulation, mild hypothermia, antegrade cardioplegic arrest
Exposure and intracardiac steps	Oblique right atriotomy, patch closure of VSD, attachment of inferior aspect of ASD patch to superior aspect of VSD to partition the common AV valve into right and left side components, closure of left AV valve cleft, and completion of patch closure of ostium primum ASD
Completion	De-airing of left heart, removal of cross-clamp, primary closure of right atriotomy
Final steps	Wean off bypass, place temporary pacing wires, TEE, standard closure

CPB, cardiopulmonary bypass; AVSD, atrioventricular septal defects; AV, atrioventricular; VSD, ventricular septal defect; ASD, atrial septal defect; TEE, transesophageal echocardiogram.

presence of additional cardiac anomalies and postoperative left AV valve regurgitation. Mortality for repair of uncomplicated incomplete AVSDs ranges from 0% to 0.6%, and the addition of left AV valve regurgitation can increase mortality up to 10-fold.[3] For complete AVSDs, the mortality without left AV valve regurgitation is approximately 5%, and it more than doubles when significant degrees of regurgitation are present.[3]

COARCTATION OF THE AORTA

Definition, Embryology, and Epidemiology

Coarctation of the aorta is a narrowing of the proximal descending thoracic aorta distal to the origin of the left subclavian artery, near the insertion of the ductus arteriosus. The severity of coarctation is thought to be determined by the extent of luminal narrowing and the length of aorta affected. When encompassing a length of aorta proximal to the juxtaductal site, it is commonly referred to as a hypoplastic aortic arch. Coarctation likely occurs secondary to ectopic tissue from the ductus arteriosus that migrates into the wall of the aorta and constricts after birth, leading to a pressure overload on the LV. Coarctation represents 5% of congenital heart defects, occurs in 0.5 per 1,000 live births and can be associated with a BAV, PDA, and VSD.[1] The most severe form of coarctation is an interrupted aortic arch, with anatomical and luminal disruption between the ascending and descending aorta, representing 1.5% of all congenital heart defects.[4]

Clinical Presentation and Diagnosis

Infants with significant coarctation are often asymptomatic at birth but following closure of the ductus develop signs of heart failure secondary to LV pressure overload with absent lower extremity pulses, and weak upper extremity pulses. The diagnosis of coarctation is a clinical one. Plain chest films are significant for cardiomegaly and pulmonary venous congestion. EKG demonstrates a left ventricular strain pattern. Echocardiography is usually diagnostic, demonstrating aortic narrowing at the coarctation with a loss of pulsatility in the descending aorta. Older children and adults with coarctation are diagnosed on the basis of hypertension; cuff pressures highlight a pressure gradient between the arms and legs, with decreased pulses in the lower extremities. A plain chest film is notable for rib notching secondary to erosion of the inferior rib borders from the development of large intercostal collateral vessels.

OPERATIVE STEPS

Table 78.4. Repair of Coarctation of the Aorta in the Infant

Incision and exposure	Right lateral decubitus position, left third intercostal space posterolateral thoracotomy, retraction of lung anteriorly, and opening of posterior pleura
Critical steps	Exposure of left subclavian artery, aortic arch, descending thoracic aorta, and ductus; division of ductus; placement of proximal and distal clamps, excision of coarctation segment, extended end-to-end anastomosis
Completion	De-airing of anastomosis, removal of vascular clamps, assessment of pressure gradient
Final steps	Intercostal nerve block, closure of overlying pleura, and standard closure

Management

Neonates born with coarctation or an interrupted aortic arch are acutely managed medically with PGE1 for the purpose of reopening the ductus. The ultimate management of aortic coarctation and an interrupted aortic arch is with surgical repair. Older patients or those with recurrent coarctation could be amenable to interventional stenting of the narrowing.

Surgical Repair and Complications

Discrete coarctation repair is approached through a left posterolateral thoracotomy via the third or fourth intercostal space. After successful mobilization of the descending thoracic aorta, ductus (or ligamentum), transverse aortic arch, and brachiocephalic vessels, care is taken to preserve the vagus nerve and the recurrent laryngeal branch. Resection with extended end-to-end repair is the preferred surgical modality in infants and small children, especially if there is associated mild distal arch hypoplasia (**Table 78.4**). More involved aortic arch hypoplasia, an interrupted aortic arch or cases of bovine arch branching usually require a sternotomy approach with cardiopulmonary bypass for optimal repair.[5,6] In older children and adults, tension free repair may not be possible, and thus patch aortoplasty or an interposition graft may be necessary.[5,6] Endovascular repair of coarctation is a potential management option as well, for both cases of native coarctation as well as recoarctation. It is particularly used in adults and older children, allowing for minimally invasive repair and redilation as the aorta grows.

Pearls and Pitfalls

In patients without well-formed collaterals, ischemia of the spinal cord secondary to interruption of distal aortic blood flow to the anterior spinal artery may be precipitated by aortic cross-clamping, and paraplegia may result. Protective measures include induction of mild hypothermia, maintenance of a high proximal aortic pressure, minimization of cross-clamp time, and use of partial left heart bypass.

DOUBLE-OUTLET RIGHT VENTRICLE

Definition, Types, and Epidemiology

Double-outlet right ventricle (DORV) is a descriptive term that encompasses a variety of malformations. Often in DORV, both great arteries arise from the morphologic RV, with each artery having 50% or more of the valve diameter coming from the RV. DORV is almost always associated with a VSD or AVSD. There are multiple classifications of DORV, and to understand them, one must understand the importance and value of three anatomical variations in DORV: (1) the position of the VSD, (2) the position of the great arteries, and (3) the relationship between them, as well as whether the DORV is associated with pulmonic stenosis (PS) or not. One anomaly, where the aorta is on the left and the VSD is subpulmonic, is the Taussig–Bing anomaly. Double-outlet LVs can occur, however, they are extremely rare. DORV occurs in 3 to 9 out of every 100,000 live births.

Pathophysiology

The physiologic consequences of DORV depend on the associated defects. The three most important factors determining the impact on circulation are (1) the size of the VSD, (2) the presence or absence of PS, and (3) the presence and degree of left-sided obstruction. As a result, DORV may clinically resemble an isolated VSD, TOF, or TGA.

Clinical Presentation and Diagnosis

DORV is diagnosed using echocardiography, ideally prenatally, and findings vary based on the phenotypic constellation.

Management

The management of DORV is surgical. Surgical management may be univentricular, biventricular, intraventricular, or an arterial switch operation (ASO) (**Fig. 78.3**). The ASO technique may be reviewed in **Table 78.5**.

Surgical Repair

- If PS is absent: VSD size and location are important considerations in planning surgical repair. With large, nonrestrictive VSDs that are committed to the aorta, the defect can be closed with a tunnel-like patch that directs left ventricular flow into the aorta. If the VSD is restrictive, it must be enlarged to avoid creating subaortic stenosis.
- If PS is present: repair requires right ventricular outflow tract (RVOT) reconstruction with a patch or a valved allograft conduit, in addition to patch closure of the VSD.
- Taussig–Bing anomaly: there are multiple repair techniques. The most common strategy (1) is to perform an ASO thus making the VSD committed to the aorta and baffling the left ventricular outflow from the VSD to this neo-aorta. Another preferred approach, which depends on a favorable orientation of the two great vessels and VSD, would be (2) an intraventricular tunnel from the VSD to the aorta. A third approach utilizes the (3) Damus–Kaye–Stansel operation (DKS). During the DKS, the proximal PA is anastomosed end to side into the aorta. The VSD is baffled to both semilunar valves, which both connect to the aorta. An extracardiac conduit is then placed to reconstruct RV-to-PA continuity. This approach may also be useful when the VSD is doubly committed or noncommitted.

Complications

Repair of DORV with subaortic VSD has a survival of 89% at 15 years; however, the mortality increases with the caveat of a more complex repair.[6] Hospital mortality for patients getting an ASO is 2.4%.[7]

TRUNCUS ARTERIOSUS

Definition, Embryology, and Epidemiology

Truncus arteriosus is a single arterial vessel arising from the heart, overriding the ventricular septum and giving rise to the systemic, coronary, and pulmonary circulations. Persistent truncus arteriosus is the result of failed development of the aorticopulmonary septum and subpulmonary infundibulum. Failure of septation results in an infundibular VSD, a single semilunar valve, and a single arterial trunk. It accounts for 0.4% to 4% of all cases of CHD. The truncal valve leaflets

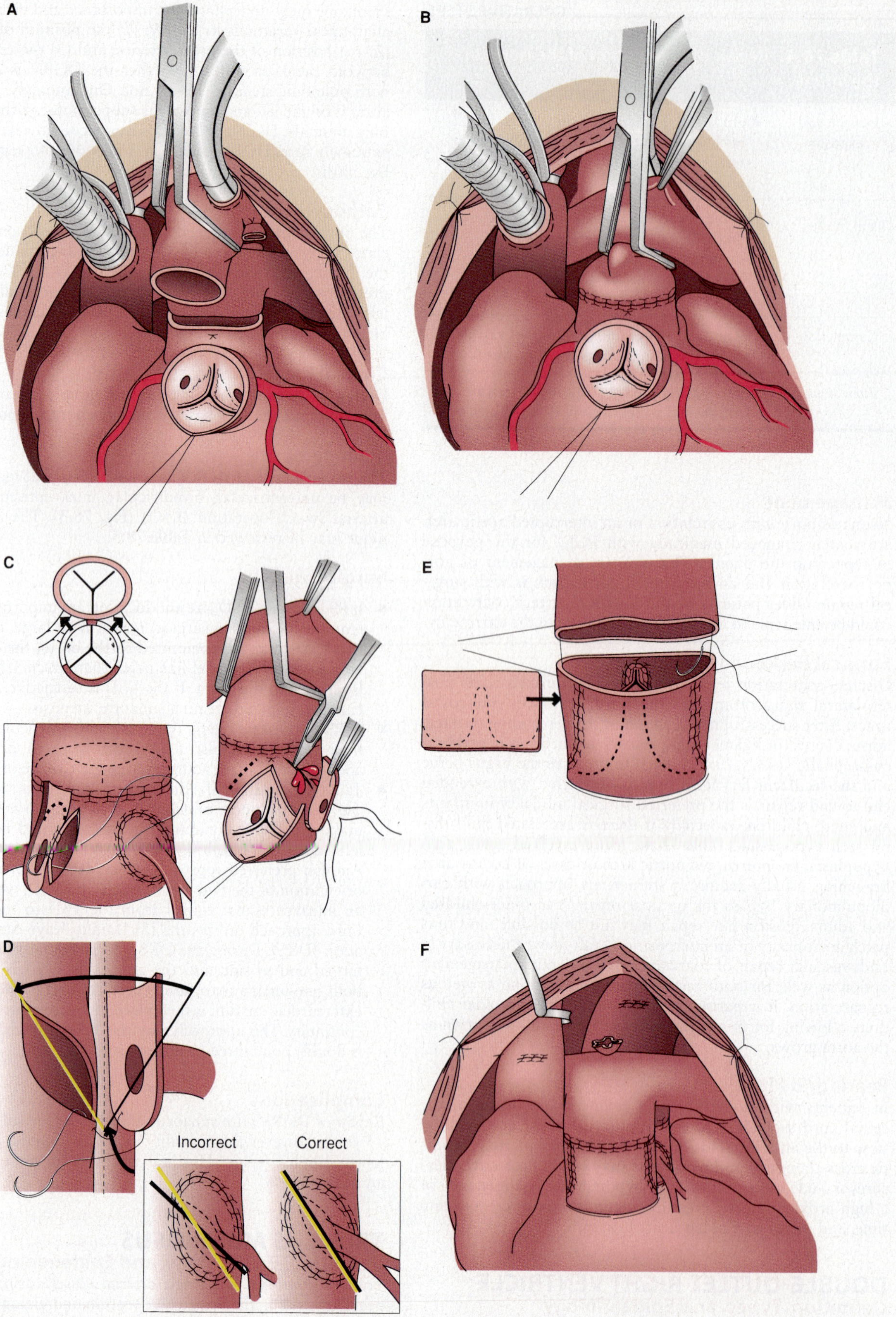

Figure 78.3. Arterial switch procedure for transposition of the great arteries. A: Division of aorta and pulmonary artery. B: LeCompte maneuver; anterior translocation of the pulmonary arteries. C: Mobilization of the coronary arteries. D: Correct orientation for coronary reimplantation. E: Placement of a pantaloon-shaped pericardial patch to reconstruct the neo-pulmonary artery. F: Completed repair.

OPERATIVE STEPS

Table 78.5. Arterial Switch Operation via Sternotomy

CPB configuration	Bicaval cannulation, mild hypothermia, antegrade cardioplegic arrest
Exposure and intracardiac steps	Division of aorta and PA, harvesting of coronary buttons, LeCompte maneuver, reconstruction of neo-aorta and positioning of coronary buttons, oblique right-atriotomy and patch closure of ASD
Completion	De-airing of left heart, removal of cross-clamp, primary closure of right atriotomy, completion of neo-pulmonary root reconstruction and reanastomosis with branch PAs
Final steps	Wean off bypass, place temporary pacing wires, TEE, standard closure

CPB, cardiopulmonary bypass; PA, pulmonary artery; ASD, atrial septal defect; TEE, transesophageal echocardiogram.

are generally dysmorphic and carry a greater degree of truncal insufficiency and mild stenosis.[8]

Types

There are two classification schemes for truncus. The Collett and Edwards classification focused on the origin of the PAs from the common arterial trunk (**Table 78.6**).[9] The Van Praagh classification system is based on the presence or absence of a VSD, the degree of formation of the aorticopulmonary septum, and the status of the aortic arch (**Fig. 78.4**).

Pathophysiology

The anatomy of truncus arteriosus results in obligatory mixing of systemic and pulmonary venous blood at the level of the VSD and truncal valve, which produces arterial saturations of 85% to 90%. The systemic arterial saturation depends on the volume of PBF, determined by the PVR. As the PVR begins to fall, excessive PBF ensues and leads to pulmonary congestion and signs and symptoms of heart failure. Truncal

Table 78.6. Collett and Edwards Classification of Truncus Arteriosus

Type	Description
I	Common arterial trunk gives rise to a main pulmonary artery and the aorta
II	Right and left pulmonary arteries arise directly and in close proximity from the posterior wall of the truncus
III	Right and left pulmonary arteries arise from more widely separated orifices on the posterior truncal wall
IV	Branch pulmonary arteries are absent. Pulmonary blood flow is derived from aorticopulmonary collaterals

valve abnormalities pose further hemodynamic changes: truncal valve regurgitation leads to ventricular dilatation and low diastolic coronary perfusion pressures which may result in myocardial ischemia, and truncal valve stenosis promotes ventricular hypertrophy, increases the myocardial oxygen demand, and limits coronary and systemic perfusion.

Clinical Presentation and Diagnosis

Neonates with truncus arteriosus present with signs of heart failure and collapsing peripheral pulses. Chest radiography shows marked cardiomegaly, pulmonary plethora, often with minimal thymus shadow, and a right aortic arch. The EKG most often depicts biventricular hypertrophy. Echocardiography is the diagnostic procedure of choice.

Management

The natural history of patients born with truncus arteriosus is early demise. The ultimate treatment of truncus arteriosus is surgical correction in the neonatal period. Medical treatment is palliative and directed toward controlling heart failure symptoms.

Surgical Repair and Complications

Complete repair entails separating the PAs from the truncus, repairing the resulting defect in the aorta, closing the VSD, and restoring the continuity of the RVOT with an extracardiac

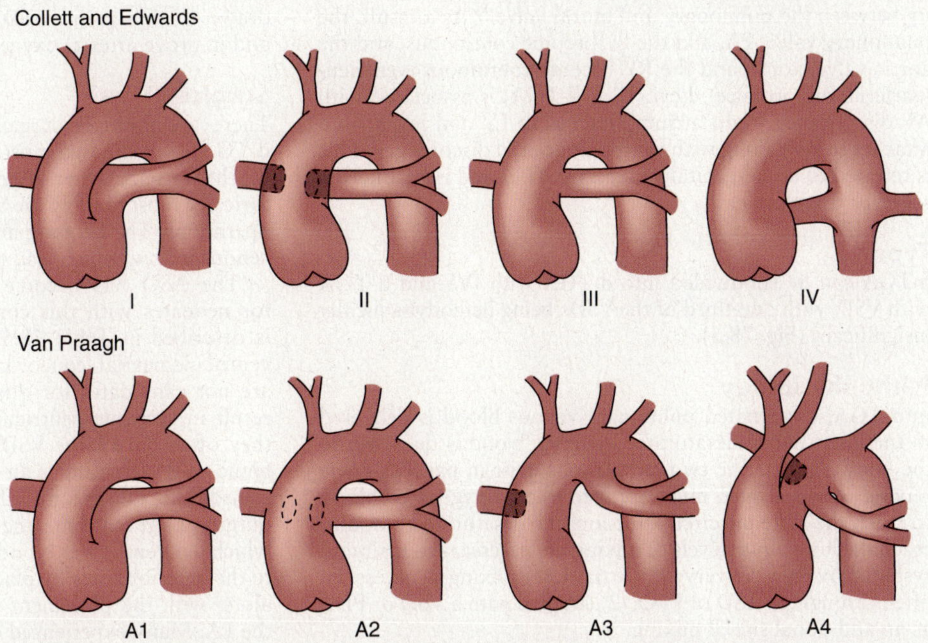

Figure 78.4. Truncus arteriosus: classification schemes as described by Collett and Edwards and by Van Praagh and Van Praagh. (Adapted from Hernanz-Schulman M, Fellows KE. Persistent truncus arteriosus: pathologic, diagnostic, and therapeutic considerations. *Semin Roentgenol.* 1985;20:121.)

OPERATIVE STEPS

Table 78.7. Repair of Truncus Arteriosus via Sternotomy

CPB configuration	Bicaval cannulation, snare PAs immediately upon commencement of CPB, mild hypothermia, antegrade cardioplegic arrest
Exposure and intracardiac steps	Division of truncal vessel and removal of PAs, repair of defect within aorta, patch closure of VSD via ventriculotomy, oblique right atriotomy and closure of ASD, restoration of continuity between RV and branch PAs with extracardiac conduit
Completion	De-airing of left heart, removal of cross-clamp, and primary closure of right atriotomy
Final steps	Wean off bypass, place temporary pacing wires, TEE, standard closure

CPB, cardiopulmonary bypass; PA, pulmonary artery; VSD, ventricular septal defect; ASD, atrial septal defect; RV, right ventricle; TEE, transesophageal echocardiogram.

conduit (**Table 78.7**). Severe truncal valve regurgitation requires truncal valve repair, if feasible.[10] Historically, patients requiring truncal valve replacement had poor prognoses, with an almost 50% hospital mortality.[10] Recently, the Turek operation, or living double root replacement, was introduced as an innovative approach to this dire condition.[11] This form of partial heart transplant could prove transformative for many other conditions in congenital heart lesions.[12]

TRANSPOSITION OF THE GREAT ARTERIES

TGA is the most common form of congenital heart disease presenting as cyanosis in the first week of life, accounting for approximately 4% of all CHDs.[1]

Embryology

In normal development, the subaortic conus is resorbed by the 5th week of gestation and allows for the usual mitral and aortic valve fibrous continuity. In dextro-TGA (d-TGA), the subpulmonary conus is resorbed, leading to fibrous continuity between the pulmonary and mitral valve.[13] As a result, the pulmonary valve, PA, and the LV become continuous, and the aortic valve, aorta, and the RV become continuous (ventriculoarterial discordance). Levo-TGA (l-TGA) is associated with AV discordance (right atrium attaches to LV and left atrium attaches to RV) along with ventriculoarterial discordance. This is referred to as congenitally corrected TGA and is beyond the scope of this chapter.

Types

d-TGA can be subdivided into d-TGA with IVS and d-TGA with VSD, with one-third of the VSDs being hemodynamically insignificant (**Fig. 78.5**).

Pathophysiology

In d-TGA, oxygenated pulmonary venous blood is delivered to the lungs, while desaturated systemic blood is delivered to the body. Because the two circulations exist in parallel, some mixing between them must occur to allow oxygenated blood to reach the systemic circulation and the desaturated blood to reach the lungs. Two levels of mixing are necessary to maintain systemic oxygen delivery: (1) Atrial level mixing is necessary, often through an ASD or PFO, (2) coupled with a VSD or PDA as an additional site of mixing.

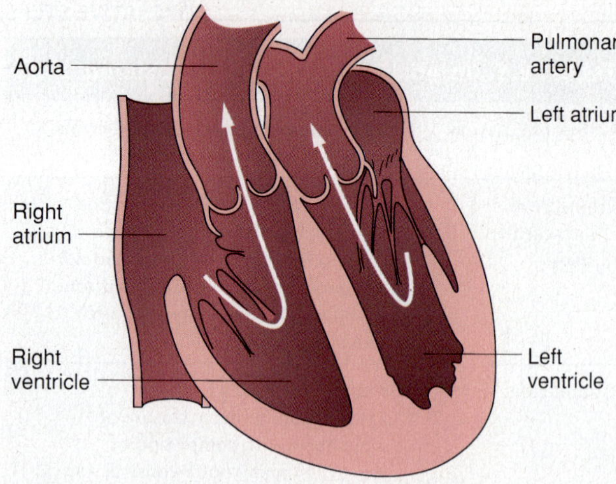

Figure 78.5. Anatomy of the most common type of transposition of the great arteries.The location of the ascending aorta is usually anterior and to the right of the pulmonary artery.

Clinical Presentation and Diagnosis

Clinical characteristics of cyanosis are dependent on the degree of mixing and the amount of PBF. Neonates with d-TGA with IVS have mixing limited to the atrial level and PDA. As the degree of mixing decreases with PDA closure after birth, the cyanosis worsens and ends with cardiovascular collapse. In d-TGA with a large VSD, there is additional opportunity for mixing and increased PBF. The neonate with d-TGA/VSD only
6 manifest mild cyanosis, with the more prominent symptoms being tachypnea and tachycardia. Auscultatory findings include a pansystolic murmur, third heart sound, mid-diastolic rumble, gallop, and narrowly split, second heart sound. The EKG demonstrates right ventricular dominance. A plain chest film demonstrates an egg-shaped heart with a narrow superior mediastinum may be seen. Echocardiography is diagnostic.

Management

Neonates born with d-TGA are acutely managed medically with PGE1 to maintain ductal patency. The ultimate management is with catheter-based interventions or surgical repair. If the patient has a restrictive ASD, an atrial septostomy is performed, where a balloon-tipped catheter is passed across the foramen ovale into the left atrium, inflated and forcibly withdrawn to enlarge the ASD and subsequently increase mixing and improve arterial oxygen saturation.

Surgical Repair

There are multiple surgical techniques employed to repair d-TGA, with the two most commonly being: (1) the ASO and (2) the Rastelli. Other surgeries were used more frequently historically, most notably the Senning and Mustard (atrial switch) operations. The Senning and Mustard focused on redirecting venous inflow, which lead to RV failure at later ages.

The ASO has become the standard surgical procedure for neonates with this condition.[14] The operative technique is described in **Table 78.5**. The arterial switch reestablishes ventriculoarterial concordance. Patients with fixed LVOTO are not candidates for this repair because correction would result in systemic ventricular outflow tract obstruction, and they often have large VSDs. Palliation early in life with systemic-to-PA shunting is an option, with definitive repair postponed until somatic growth results in cyanosis as the shunt is outgrown. At that time, the Rastelli procedure is performed, in which left ventricular blood is redirected through the VSD and to the anterior aorta by placement of an intraventricular patch along with the placement of a conduit between the RV and the PA. Many experienced centers currently recommend early

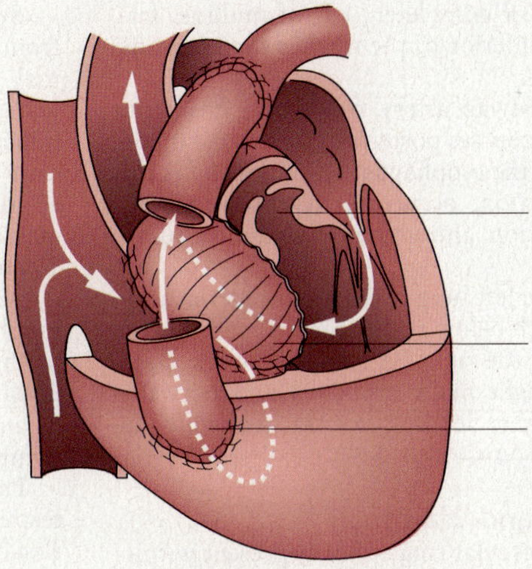

Figure 78.6. The Rastelli procedure for transposition of the great arteries with ventricular septal defect and pulmonary stenosis. A prosthetic patch placed within the right ventricle directs left ventricular blood through the defect to the aorta. The main pulmonary artery is ligated, and right ventricular blood then passes through a conduit to the distal pulmonary arteries.

complete repair using a Rastelli or Norwood–Yasui procedure (**Fig. 78.6**). Early repair eliminates the interim morbidity and mortality associated with a systemic-to-PA shunt; however, at the expense of usually a more complex postoperative course and the placement of a smaller initial conduit.

Current hospital mortality for the ASO is 2.4%. Long-term survival among perioperative survivors is excellent (approximately 97% at 25 years).[15]

PULMONARY ATRESIA WITH INTACT VENTRICULAR SEPTUM

Pulmonary atresia with intact ventricular septum (PA-IVS) is a rare congenital anomaly that accounts for less than 1% of congenital heart defects. PA-IVS patients can either have atresia of the membranous or muscular RVOT with concomitant absence of ventricular communication (intact ventricular septum). And the spectrum of disease may range from membranous PA with a normal RV to a hypoplastic RV with abnormal connections between the RV and coronary arteries.

Types

PA-IVS can be classified based on three findings: (1) membranous or muscular RVOT atresia, (2) normal or hypoplastic RV and (2) presence or absence of aberrant RV–coronary artery connections. Muscular RVOTs are usually associated with abnormal RV–coronary artery connections and incur a worse prognosis.

Pathophysiology

Secondary to high pressures in the RV, the TV is often hypoplastic or dysplastic with a malformed chordal apparatus. Patients with a normal TV often lack egress of blood, leaving the RV to become pressure overloaded, which leads to the development of abnormal connections between the RV and coronary arteries to decompress the ventricle. Secondary to this, progressive stenosis of the coronary arteries is seen, and this leads to right ventricular-dependent coronary circulation, a poor prognostic factor.

Clinical Presentation and Diagnosis

Patients often present with cyanosis and are often diagnosed using echocardiography.

Management

Neonates born with PA-IVS are acutely managed medically with PGE1 to maintain ductal patency. The ultimate management is with catheter-based interventions or surgical repair.

Surgical Repair and Complications

Surgical management of PA-IVS should be individualized based on each patient's anatomy and is dependent on the type of pulmonary atresia, TV size and function, RV size and anatomy, and coronary artery anatomy. Options range from complete repair similar to tetralogy, to single-ventricle palliation.

VASCULAR RINGS

Embryology

By the fourth week of embryonic development, six aortic (branchial) arches form between the dorsal aortae and ventral roots. Their involution and migration result in the normal or abnormal anatomy of the aorta and its branches. The first, second, and fifth arches predominantly regress. The third arch develops into the common carotid and proximal internal carotid arteries. The right fourth arch forms the proximal right subclavian artery, while the left fourth arch contributes to the aortic arch segment from the left common carotid to left subclavian arteries. The proximal right sixth arch becomes the proximal right PA, with the distal segment regressing. The proximal left sixth arch forms the proximal left PA, and the distal segment becomes the ductus arteriosus.

Anatomy and Pathophysiology

Vascular rings are a spectrum of aortic arch, PA, and brachiocephalic vessel anomalies, leading to tracheoesophageal compression. They are classified as complete or partial. Clinically significant vascular rings occur in 1% to 2% of congenital heart defects.[16]

These anomalies are frequently associated with other cardiac defects such as TOF, ASD, branch PA stenosis, coarctation, AVSD, VSD, interrupted aortic arch, and aortopulmonary window. Significant associated anomalies are present in 12% to 30% of vascular ring cases. A right aortic arch is notably linked with a higher incidence of coexisting anomalies.

Complete Rings

A double aortic arch arises when the distal right dorsal aorta fails to regress, forming a complete ring around the trachea and esophagus. In most cases, the right arch is dominant, followed by left dominance, with codominant arches being rare. The left and right carotid and subclavian arteries typically originate from their ipsilateral arches, while the ligamentum arteriosum and descending aorta usually remain on the left.

The right aortic arch forms from the involution of the left fourth arch, positioning the arch apex to the right of the trachea. Common variants include mirror-image arch branching and an aberrant retroesophageal left subclavian artery.[16] When the ligamentum arises from the descending thoracic aorta, a complete ring is formed.

Partial Rings

In innominate artery compression syndrome, the aortic arch and ligamentum are leftward positioned. But the innominate artery may arise partially or completely left of midline, traversing from left to right anterior to the trachea, and causing compression of the trachea.

An aberrant right subclavian artery, originating from the descending thoracic aorta, courses posteriorly across the mediastinum and can compress the esophagus. This anomaly is the most common arch variation, occurring in approximately 0.5% to 1% of the population, although rarely requires surgical intervention.

PA sling arises when the left lung captures its arterial supply from the right sixth arch below the tracheobronchial tree. The left PA branches from the right PA rather than the main PA, passing behind the right main bronchus and between the trachea and esophagus, leading to tracheobronchial compression.[16]

Clinical Presentation and Diagnosis

Children with a complete vascular ring typically present within the first weeks to months of life, with double aortic arch typically presenting the earliest. In younger patients, respiratory symptoms predominate, as liquids are generally well tolerated. Symptoms may include stridor, nonproductive cough, apnea, or frequent respiratory infections. These can mimic asthma, respiratory infections, or reflux, often leading to misdiagnosis. With the introduction of solid foods, dysphagia becomes more prominent.

The presentation of partial vascular rings is variable. Innominate artery compression usually presents within the first 1 to 2 years with respiratory symptoms. The aberrant right subclavian artery typically does not cause significant tracheoesophageal compression and is usually asymptomatic; when symptoms do occur, they typically arise in the seventh or eighth decade due to vessel ectasia and calcification, resulting in dysphagia lusoria from posterior esophageal impingement.

Children with PA slings often present with respiratory symptoms within the first few weeks to months, with symptoms similar to complete rings and often leading to misdiagnosis. It is associated with complete tracheal rings in 30% to 40% of cases, causing focal or diffuse tracheal stenosis, the primary source of respiratory symptoms.

Diagnosis of vascular rings is nonuniform due to variability in presentation and available diagnostic tests. A child with a presumptive diagnosis of asthma or tracheomalacia may be referred to a pulmonologist, with vascular ring suspected from chest radiograph and bronchoscopy. Diagnosis may also occur through echocardiography when assessing concurrent cardiac defects, but typically begins with a chest radiograph. Complementary studies include barium esophagogram, CT, MRI, and bronchoscopy, which are vital for defining tracheal anatomy in patients with PA slings. Echocardiography can be both diagnostic and helps exclude other cardiac anomalies.

Management and Surgical Repair

Patients with symptoms from complete or partial vascular rings require surgical correction. Repair of a double aortic arch is performed via a left, third intercostal space posterolateral thoracotomy, which allows exposure of the left subclavian artery, the double aortic arch, and the descending thoracic aorta. The procedure involves ligation and division of the ductus arteriosus and the atretic segment of the nondominant arch. If the division site is uncertain, the arches can be temporarily occluded at various points while monitoring pulses and blood pressure in each limb. Dissection around the esophagus and trachea at the ligamentum/ductus and nondominant arch facilitates retraction of vascular structures and lysis of residual obstructive adhesions.

The surgical approach for a right aortic arch with a retroesophageal aberrant left subclavian artery maximally involves ligation of the ligamentum, lysis of adhesions around the esophagus, resection of the Kommerell diverticulum and reimplantation of the vessel to the left carotid artery.

Symptoms of innominate artery compression can range from mild to severe. In cases of mild symptoms with minimal tracheal compression on bronchoscopy, observation is warranted, as symptoms may resolve with growth. Surgical indications include apnea, severe respiratory distress, significant stridor, and recurrent respiratory infections. Correction approaches for innominate artery compression syndrome include division with reimplantation more proximally on the ascending aorta, and suspension to the overlying sternum.

An aberrant right subclavian artery can compress the esophagus posteriorly but rarely causes symptoms in children. In the uncommon occasion when needed, surgical treatment involves division of the artery from the aorta and resection of any Kommerell diverticulum via a right thoracotomy and reimplantation to the right carotid or aortic arch.

Patients with PA sling, tracheobronchial compression, and respiratory symptoms should undergo surgical correction. Tracheal evaluation is essential to identify complete tracheal rings (absence of the membranous trachea). Many techniques have been described, but the current consensus favors LPA reimplantation. This procedure is performed via median sternotomy on cardiopulmonary bypass for optimal visualization, with no need for aortic cross-clamping. The left PA is divided from the right PA, translocated anterior to the trachea, and reimplanted into the main PA. Any required tracheal reconstruction is done concurrently with bronchoscopic assistance if complete tracheal rings are present.

Repair of vascular rings has been performed using video-assisted thoracoscopic surgery with or without robotic assistance. Candidates for thoracoscopic division are limited to those requiring division of nonpatent vascular structures and typically include patients over 15 kg due to instrument size limitations.

Mortality rates for vascular ring repair range from 0% to 4%, with improved survival in recent series. Most deaths are associated with other cardiac defects or respiratory infections and failure.[16]

AORTIC STENOSIS

Definition and Embryology

Development of the left ventricular outflow tract (LVOT) hinges on the proper formation of the aorticopulmonary septum and conotruncal septum. The aortic valve leaflets evolve from subendothelial swellings within the developing aorta. Anomalies in these structures, along with issues in the endocardial cushions, can lead to LVOT obstruction (LVOTO).

Types and Epidemiology

AS, a form of LVOTO, occurring at the valvar (71%), subvalvar (14%), or supravalvar (8%) levels (**Fig. 78.7**). It affects approximately 2.5% of individuals with CHD.[1] BAV is the most prevalent congenital heart anomaly, though many with BAV remain asymptomatic without stenosis or regurgitation requiring no intervention.

Valvular Aortic Stenosis

Valvar AS results from AV maldevelopment, commonly presenting with a BAV; however, tricuspid or unicuspid valves can also cause AS. In valvar AS, leaflets are often thickened and dysmorphic, with varying degrees of commissural fusion. 7 Hypoplasia of the aortic annulus may occur. About 20% of valvar AS is associated with other cardiac defects, including coarctation of the aorta, PDA, VSD, or mitral stenosis.

Clinical manifestations of valvar AS vary widely. Neonates and infants with severe AS may rapidly develop CHF, whereas older patients with milder obstruction may have a more gradual onset of symptoms.

Severe valvar AS is usually well tolerated prenatally. The RV compensates for decreased LV output and aortic valve flow by increasing output, and systemic circulation through the

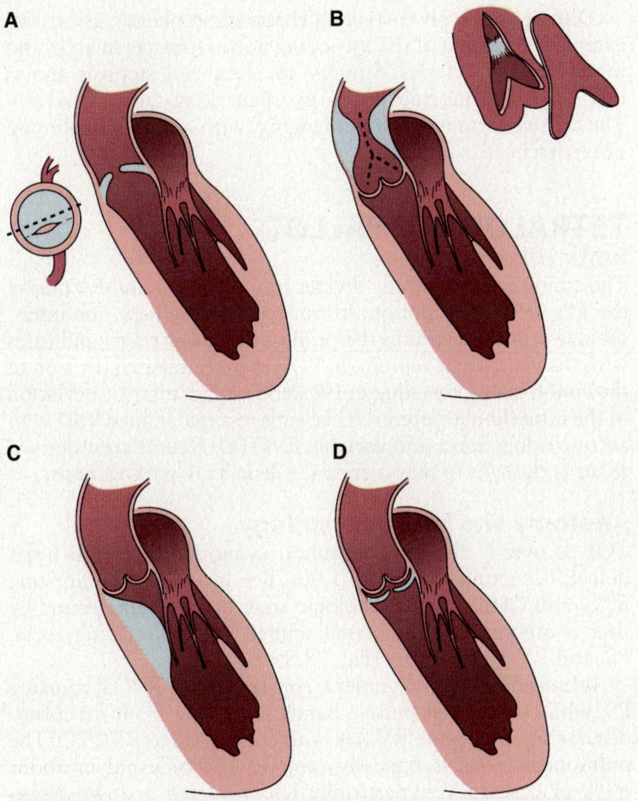

Figure 78.7. Anatomy of the types of congenital aortic stenosis. A: Valvar aortic stenosis. B: Supravalvar aortic stenosis and its repair (*inset*). C: Diffuse (tunnel) subvalvar aortic stenosis. D: Discrete subvalvar aortic stenosis.

ductus. After birth, increased venous return to the left heart exacerbates pressure load from the stenotic valve, leading to left ventricular dysfunction. Closure of the ductus postnatally may lead to systemic malperfusion, causing hypotension, acidosis, and oliguria. Elevated LV end-diastolic pressure coupled with systemic hypotension compromises coronary perfusion.

Clinical Findings and Diagnosis

Infants with critical valvar AS typically present with severe LV
7 dysfunction, classically displaying distress shortly after birth. Clinical examination reveals impaired distal perfusion with delayed capillary refill and weak pulses. In cases of severely diminished cardiac output, a systolic ejection murmur may be absent. Infants may show differential cyanosis due to lower body perfusion with deoxygenated blood shunting through the PDA. Diagnostic findings include LV hypertrophy on EKG and cardiomegaly with pulmonary congestion on chest radiography. Echocardiography is essential for confirming the diagnosis and grading the severity of valvar AS based on peak instantaneous pressure gradients: mild (<40 mm Hg), moderate (40 to 70 mm Hg), and severe (>70 mm Hg). Alternatively, catheterization classifies peak-to-peak pressure gradients: mild (<30 mm Hg), moderate (30 to 50 mm Hg), and severe (>50 mm Hg).

Fetal echocardiography enables early detection of critical valvar AS, predicting potential progression to HLHS or irreversible left ventricular dysfunction.

Management and Surgical Repair

Severe or critical valvar AS in neonates or infants is an emergency. Standard care includes endotracheal intubation, inotropic support, prostaglandin infusion to maintain ductal patency, and correction of acidosis.

For patients with adequate left-sided chambers, relief of valvar AS can be achieved through percutaneous balloon valvuloplasty, surgical valvotomy, or aortic valve replacement. Balloon valvuloplasty is preferred when the aortic valve annulus is adequate, and no additional defects are present. Closed surgical valvotomy involves passing dilators through an LV apex ventriculotomy under cardiopulmonary bypass, without aortic cross-clamping. Open surgical valvotomy offers direct visualization but does require cross-clamping. Surgical valvotomy yields improved valve gradient reduction, lower postprocedural aortic insufficiency, and excellent long-term outcomes. Goal of therapy is to reduce AS without causing excessive aortic insufficiency. Recurrence of stenosis occurs in most cases and often necessitates repeat valvotomy or eventual aortic valve replacement.

Aortic valve replacement poses challenges in neonates due to size constraints. The Ross procedure[17] with Konno aortoventriculoplasty[18] is favored in cases of hypoplastic aortic annulus or when valvuloplasty is unsuccessful. The Ross–Konno procedure offers excellent survival rates and potential for pulmonary autograft growth in the aortic position. The pulmonary valve is replaced with a cryopreserved homograft as part of the Ross procedure and homograft replacement should be anticipated as the patient grows. The introduction of "living root replacement" in the innovative partial heart transplant can be used as a growing alternative to cadaveric homografts that may preclude the need for future intervention.[11]

Select centers have performed in utero balloon dilation of the aortic valve successfully promoting left ventricular growth and function, primarily aimed at preventing HLHS rather than treating uncomplicated valvar AS.

Clinical Findings and Diagnosis in the Older Child

Unlike infants with critical AS, older children with valvular AS typically present with mild or moderate forms and are frequently asymptomatic. Symptoms such as angina, syncope, and CHF are uncommon. However, congenital valvar AS is progressive, and survival depends on the severity and progression rate of the stenosis. Sudden cardiac death is the leading cause of mortality.

Diagnosis in older children usually relies on physical examination findings. A characteristic systolic crescendo–decrescendo murmur is heard at the upper sternal border, often radiating to the neck. An ejection click may be present, and a visible apical impulse suggests significant LV hypertrophy. Severe cases may exhibit a weak and delayed pulse (pulsus tardus et parvus). EKG shows LV hypertrophy, while chest radiography is usually normal. Echocardiography is crucial for accurately assessing the level and severity of stenosis.

For severely dysplastic valves, those that develop restenosis postintervention, or those that become insufficient due to prior interventions, valve replacement may be necessary. Various options exist for valve replacement in older children, including mechanical prostheses, bioprosthetic valves, cryopreserved human allografts, and pulmonary autografts (Ross procedure). Mechanical valves are durable but require lifelong anticoagulation. Bioprosthetic valves do not necessitate long-term anticoagulation but may deteriorate over time, except for the pulmonary autograft which has the potential for growth.

Subvalvar Aortic Stenosis

Types and Pathophysiology

Subvalvar AS occurs below the aortic valve and may be discrete (80%) or diffuse (20%). Discrete or membranous subaortic stenosis rarely occurs in infants but progresses over time. It involves a crescentic or circumferential fibrous or fibromuscular membrane protruding into the LVOT. Although unclear, it is thought to develop from a congenital abnormality of the LVOT causing abnormal flow and leading to endocardial injury and fibrosis. Aortic valve leaflets are usually normal, but turbulent flow from the obstruction can thicken leaflets and cause progressive aortic insufficiency. Diffuse subaortic stenosis presents as a severe, tunnel-like obstruction and must be distinguished from hypertrophic cardiomyopathy. Both forms increase the risk of endocarditis.

Clinical Findings and Diagnosis

The clinical findings in subvalvar AS are similar to those for valvar stenosis. With a Valsalva maneuver, the intensity of the systolic murmur typically decreases in subvalvar AS. Echocardiogram remains the gold standard for evaluating the LVOT and any associated lesions.

Management and Surgical Repair

Intervention for discrete subvalvar stenosis is typically indicated when the gradient exceeds 30 to 50 mm Hg or if aortic insufficiency is present. Membrane resection via a transaortic approach is effective and durable. To minimize restenosis, concurrent septal myomectomy is recommended to reshape the LVOT. Operative mortality ranges from 0% to 3%. The reoperation rate for discrete stenosis is about 2% per year. Risks of operative intervention include heart block, iatrogenic VSD, or damage to aortic or mitral valve leaflets.

Operative indications for diffuse subaortic stenosis mirror those for valvar stenosis. In cases where there is associated hypoplasia of the aortic annulus, repair is optimally achieved through Konno aortoventriculoplasty. This procedure involves an incision across the aortic annulus and subjacent ventricular septum, with patch closure and aortic valve replacement. Alternatively, patients with an adequate aortic annulus may undergo septoplasty (modified Konno), which limits the septal incision to the immediate subvalvar area and widens the LVOT without replacing the aortic valve. Despite the technical challenges, excellent outcomes have been reported, with high survival and minimal need for reoperation.

Supravalvar Aortic Stenosis

Definition and Pathophysiology

Supravalvar AS thickens the ascending aorta wall. Localized at the sinotubular ridge (80%) forming an hourglass deformity or more diffusely (20%) into the aortic arch and branches. Abnormal aortic valve leaflets can adhere to this thickened area, potentially reducing coronary blood flow in diastole. Aortic wall thickening may also extend into the coronary ostia, further impeding blood flow. Associated cardiac lesions, especially branch PA stenoses, are common.

Supravalvar AS is genetically linked, notably with Williams syndrome due to partial chromosome 7 deletion (including the elastin gene), presenting with stenosis, intellectual disability, and distinctive facial features. Isolated elastin gene mutations can also cause familial supravalvar AS with autosomal dominant inheritance. Endocarditis is prevalent, and sudden death, often from coronary obstruction, is frequent.

Clinical Findings and Diagnosis

The signs and symptoms of supravalvar AS are similar to those in other forms of LVOTO. The diagnosis is made by echocardiography. Cross-sectional imaging with MRI or CT scan has become essential to define the aortic, coronary, and pulmonary arterial anatomy prior to surgical intervention.

Management and Surgical Repair

Operative intervention is warranted for supravalvar AS when the gradient exceeds 50 mm Hg. Several surgical approaches exist for localized supravalvar stenosis. The classic method involves a longitudinal aortotomy extended into the noncoronary sinus, with resection of the hypertrophic ridge and augmentation using an elliptical patch. Another approach uses an inverted-Y aortotomy extending into the noncoronary and right coronary sinuses, reinforced with a Y-shaped patch. The Brom repair involves transecting the ascending aorta beyond the ridge, creating incisions into each sinus of Valsalva and using triangular patches augment the incisions and relieve obstruction before reconnecting the aortic root.

Diffuse supravalvar stenosis requires circulatory arrest and extensive patching of the ascending aorta, transverse arch, and involved arch arteries. Surgery for localized stenosis shows low operative mortality and excellent long-term survival.[19] The diffuse form is more challenging, with a higher likelihood of recurrence.[19]

TETRALOGY OF FALLOT

Embryology

The conotruncus typically divides into the aorta and PA during the 5th week of gestation. In normal development, the infundibular septum separates the primitive outflow tracts and fuses with the ventricular septum. In TOF, there is unequal division of the conotruncus, resulting in PA stenosis and anterior deviation of the infundibular septum. This leads to a malaligned VSD with an overriding aorta and variable RVOTO. Neural crest-derived tissue is thought to play a critical role in TOF pathogenesis.

Anatomy and Pathophysiology

TOF is overall the most common cyanotic congenital heart defect, occurring in 0.4 per 1,000 live births and comprising 5% of all CHD cases. Pathologic anatomy is characterized by four components: anterior malaligned VSD, overriding aorta, PS, and RV hypertrophy (**Fig. 78.8**).

Infundibular malalignment constricts the RVOT, causing
8 PS, while prominent muscle bands extending from the infundibular septum to the RV free wall contribute to RVOTO. The pulmonary valve is typically stenotic and bicuspid in about 60% of cases. RV hypertrophy is considered a downstream effect of PS and RVOTO.

TOF is associated with several cardiac lesions. Pulmonary atresia occurs in 7% of cases. Branch PAs may show mild hypoplasia or discrete stenosis, commonly of the left PA at the ductal insertion. Coronary artery anomalies, such as the LAD arising from the right coronary artery (10% of cases), are clinically significant as they cross the right ventricular infundibulum and are susceptible to injury during surgery. A right aortic arch is present in 25% of TOF patients. Other associated defects include ASD, AVSD, PDA, and multiple VSDs.

Cyanosis in TOF results from right-to-left shunting across the VSD, driven by greater PVR compared to SVR. The degree of cyanosis correlates with RVOTO severity. Neonates with severe infundibular obstruction or pulmonary atresia require prostaglandin infusion to maintain ductal patency for adequate PBF and will eventually need a systemic-to-PA shunt

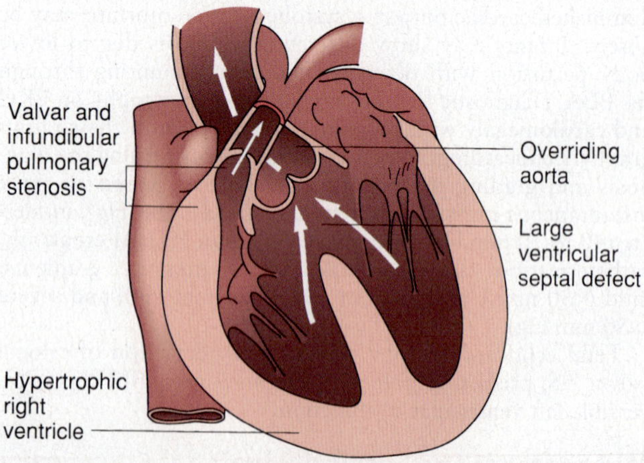

Figure 78.8. The four anatomic features of tetralogy of Fallot. The primary morphologic abnormality, anterior and superior displacement of the infundibular septum, results in a malalignment ventricular septal defect, overriding of the aortic valve, and obstruction of the right ventricular outflow. Right ventricular hypertrophy is a secondary occurrence.

or ductal stent. Most infants have sufficient antegrade PBF and can be discharged with guidance for monitoring cyanosis. Some patients exhibit mild RVOTO and present primarily with large VSD physiology, leading to left-to-right shunting and CHF without cyanosis.

Intermittent hypercyanotic spells are a hallmark of TOF, arising from transient imbalances between pulmonary and systemic blood flow. Spells can be triggered by hypovolemia or peripheral vasodilation (eg, after bathing or vigorous activity) and typically occur in infants aged 3 to 18 months. Most spells resolve spontaneously within minutes, but they can be fatal. Older children may instinctively squat to alleviate spells, as this increases SVR and enhances PBF.

Clinical Findings and Diagnosis

Auscultation typically reveals a normal first heart sound and a single second heart sound, along with a systolic ejection murmur at the left upper sternal border. Older children may develop digital clubbing from chronic cyanosis, although this is rare today. Chest radiography often shows a boot-shaped heart due to RV hypertrophy, with reduced pulmonary vascular markings. A right aortic arch may also be present. An EKG typically demonstrates RV hypertrophy. Echocardiography is definitive, and cardiac catheterization is usually unnecessary.

Management and Surgical Repair

All patients with TOF should undergo surgical repair. Early repair is indicated for neonates with severe cyanosis or infants with documented cyanotic spells. Medical management focuses on treating and preventing spells. Transfusion is warranted for anemic infants, and some centers utilize beta-blockers to reduce spell frequency. Immediate treatment during a spell includes oxygen, narcotics for sedation, and correction of acidosis. Alpha-agonists can enhance SVR, favoring PBF during refractory spells.

Single-stage repair of TOF is preferred between 4 and 6 months of age (**Table 78.8**). Initial palliation with a systemic-to-PA shunt, often modified Blalock–Taussig–Thompson, is indicated for high-risk patients, such as those with multiple anomalies, severe illness, or significant cyanosis at birth. In the absence of these factors, complete repair can be performed with lower mortality and reoperation rates.[20]

When the pulmonary valve annulus or infundibulum is severely hypoplastic, a transannular patch may be required, typically necessitating excision of the pulmonary valve. Anomalous coronary arteries crossing the infundibulum may contraindicate a transannular incision, requiring conduit placement between the RV and main PA.

OPERATIVE STEPS

Table 78.8. Complete Repair of TOF via Sternotomy

CPB configuration	Bicaval cannulation, mild hypothermia, antegrade cardioplegic arrest
Exposure and intracardiac steps	Oblique right atriotomy, retraction of septal and anterior leaflets of tricuspid valve, division of obstructing RV muscle bundles, patch closure of VSD, closure of ASD, pulmonary valvotomy or transannular patch placement as needed
Completion	De-airing of left heart, removal of cross-clamp, primary closure of right atriotomy
Final steps	Wean off bypass, place temporary pacing wires, TEE, standard closure

CPB, cardiopulmonary bypass; TOF, tetralogy of Fallot; RV, right ventricle; VSD, ventricular septal defect; ASD, atrial septal defect; TEE, transesophageal echocardiogram.

Patients with a transannular patch often develop pulmonary insufficiency, which is generally well tolerated if the TV remains competent. However, as patients age, chronic pulmonary insufficiency leads to RV dilation and potential failure. Pulmonary valve implantation may be necessary to prevent chronic volume overload. Several techniques including a left anterior mini-incision have been described to avoid redosternotomies for valve implantation.

Early mortality after complete TOF repair is about 1%. Long-term complications include recurrent RVOTO, RV dysfunction from chronic pulmonary insufficiency, aortic root dilation, and atrial arrhythmias.

The Advent of Partial Heart Transplantation

Every year thousands of children in the United States with RVOT dysfunction (eg, TOF) undergo surgical outflow tract reconstruction or replacement with a conduit. These treatment options are both temporary—RVOT reconstruction causes free pulmonary insufficiency ultimately necessitating valve replacement, while conduits (eg, homografts) are made of decellularized and cryopreserved tissue that lack growth potential and deteriorate with time. Due to these limitations, children with RVOT dysfunction face lifelong morbidity requiring repeated cardiac surgeries and major transcatheter interventions to maintain RVOT functionality.

Recently, the congenital cardiac surgery team at Duke University Hospital has pioneered "partial heart transplant" to treat RVOT dysfunction. Partial heart transplant is the first clinically successful approach to deliver growing heart valve implants.[12] This innovative approach is potentially curative because the transplanted semilunar valve has growth potential.[21]

VASCULAR DISEASE

HYPOPLASTIC LEFT-HEART SYNDROME

Definition, Embryology, and Pathophysiology

HLHS is a constellation of complex congenital cardiac anomalies characterized by severe underdevelopment of the LV and
9 ascending aorta. Systemic circulation depends on a nonrestrictive ASD with obligatory mixing of pulmonary and systemic venous blood in the right atrium and maintenance of ductal patency to maintain systemic output via the RV. Associated anomalies include aortic and mitral valve stenosis or atresia. The descending aorta is a continuation of the ductus arteriosus, while the ascending aorta and aortic arch are markedly underdeveloped. Genetics may contribute to HLHS but altered blood flow through the left heart during fetal development is a leading theory. HLHS comprises 2% to 3% of CHD cases, affecting 0.2 per 1,000 live births.[1] Survival depends on a nonrestrictive ASD allowing mixing of pulmonary and systemic venous blood in the right atrium, along with PDA to maintain systemic blood flow via the RV.

Clinical Findings and Diagnosis

HLHS is frequently diagnosed prenatally via ultrasound. Without prenatal detection, symptoms such as tachypnea, cyanosis, and cardiovascular collapse within 24 to 48 hours of birth often prompt diagnostic evaluation. Closure of the ductus arteriosus may lead to decreased pulses in the lower extremities. Auscultation reveals a single second heart sound and a soft systolic murmur at the left sternal border. EKG shows enlargement of the right atrium and hypertrophy of the RV. Chest radiograph demonstrates an enlarged heart and increased pulmonary vascular markings. Transthoracic echocardiogram is the primary diagnostic tool. While catheterization is rarely needed for diagnosis, it may be used to enlarge a restrictive ASD if present.

Management and Surgical Repair

Parents of patients with HLHS should be presented with options for staged palliation, orthotopic heart transplant or palliative care. In cases of particularly severe variants with a poor prognosis, discussing palliative care options with the family is even more crucial. Initial management involves a continuous infusion of PGE1 to maintain patency of the ductus arteriosus and correction of metabolic acidosis. Ventilatory support may be necessary to maintain a partial pressure of carbon dioxide around 40 mm Hg to prevent excessive PBF.

Heart transplantation remains a viable option for high-risk patients, particularly those with impaired RV function or severe tricuspid regurgitation, and certain centers have reported using ventricular assist devices while awaiting transplantation.[22] However, transplantation has certain challenges such as immunosuppressive risks and donor scarcity. Staged repair is generally preferred due to favorable outcomes compared to transplantation.[23]

9 The Norwood procedure remains foundational in HLHS palliation. This procedure involves four essential components: PDA ligation and division, atrial septectomy, proximal PA to aortic anastomosis (DKS amalgamation) with homograft augmentation of the aortic arch, and creation of an aortopulmonary shunt or RV to PA conduit. Hybrid stage 1 palliation has emerged as an alternative approach with use of transcatheter techniques, involving bilateral surgical PA banding or flow occluder placement and ductal stenting to optimize systemic blood flow, though it remains less commonly utilized.

The second stage involves a hemi-Fontan or bidirectional Glenn anastomosis, performed at 4 to 6 months of age after PVR has decreased. After removing the original shunt, SVC blood flow is redirected to the PA creating passive pulmonary circulation from the upper body.

The third stage, the Fontan procedure, is typically performed at 18 to 36 months. It directs IVC flow to the PA via an intraatrial baffle (lateral tunnel) or extracardiac tube conduit. Redirecting systemic venous blood flow to passively drain into pulmonary circulation and allowing oxygenated blood to enter systemic circulation through the AV valves. Strict criteria, including normal PA pressure (<20 mm Hg) and PVR (<2 Wood units/m^2), along with normal ventricular and AV valve function, are crucial for successful Fontan completion. While not truly corrective, the Fontan procedure offers substantial benefits including normalized systemic oxygen saturation and reduced ventricular volume overload.

Decades ago, HLHS was universally fatal, but advancements have significantly improved survival rates.[24] Notably, the Norwood operation remains the highest-risk stage, with select centers reporting hospital survivals exceeding 90%. Both the hemi-Fontan and Fontan procedures have demonstrated excellent survival rates, reaching up to 98% in reported cases.

Despite these advancements, outcomes vary widely across different techniques. A pivotal randomized trial, the Single-Ventricle Reconstruction trial initiated in 2005, underscored the impact of shunt type at the Norwood procedure. This study highlighted a sobering 1-year mortality rate of 30%, with risk factors including low gestational age, birth weight under 2.5 kg, and noncardiac anomalies.

CORONARY ARTERY ANOMALIES

Definition and Embryology

Coronary artery anomalies occur in 0.3% to 1.3% of the population and are classified as minor, secondary, or major based on clinical significance. Minor defects lack functional significance and are often incidental findings during cardiac catheterization. Secondary defects, while not intrinsically significant, can impact surgical management; for example, an anomalous origin of the LAD from the right coronary artery may obstruct safe transannular incisions in TOF, necessitating conduit use. Major defects are clinically significant as they adversely affect the myocardium and include coronary arteriovenous fistulae, anomalous pulmonary origin of a coronary artery, anomalous aortic origin of a coronary artery, myocardial bridging, and coronary artery aneurysm.

The embryology of congenital coronary artery anomalies remains unclear. Complex theories suggest that in utero wall tension in the right and left coronary sinuses is crucial for normal coronary development. Controversy persists regarding whether coronary arteries grow outward from the aortic root or originate from the epicardium and grow inward.

Types

Coronary Arteriovenous Fistula

Coronary arteriovenous fistula is the most common major coronary anomaly, characterized by an abnormal connection between a coronary artery (usually the right) and another vascular structure (typically a right heart chamber). Most fistulae are isolated and solitary, resulting in left-to-right shunting, which can lead to CHF. Other potential symptoms include angina, endocarditis, MI, arrhythmias, and sudden death. Diagnosis is suggested by echocardiography and confirmed through catheterization.

All symptomatic fistulae should be occluded, either surgically or via transcatheter techniques. In cases where distal flow is compromised by fistula occlusion, coronary bypass grafting may be required. The management of asymptomatic fistulae is controversial, but occlusion is recommended when significant left-to-right shunting is present. Surgical and transcatheter correction of coronary artery fistulae typically have low mortality and morbidity rates.

Coronary Artery Origin From the Pulmonary Artery

The second most common major coronary anomaly is the origin of a coronary artery from the PA, with the anomalous left coronary artery arising from the pulmonary artery (ALCAPA) being the most prevalent. Rarely, the right coronary artery or both originate from the PA. ALCAPA is typically well tolerated in utero, but postnatally, decreased pulmonary systolic pressure (following ductal closure) leads to desaturated blood perfusing the anomalous coronary. Collateral vessels may form between the normal right coronary artery and the anomalous left coronary, but coronary steal occurs due to retrograde flow into the low-pressure PA.

Most patients present between 6 weeks and 3 months of age with symptoms such as irritability, feeding difficulties, and signs of CHF. Untreated ALCAPA is almost always fatal; however, some patients may survive to adulthood, presenting with angina or sudden death. On examination, ALCAPA patients often exhibit a holosystolic murmur of ischemic mitral regurgitation, and the pulmonary component of the second heart sound may be accentuated due to pulmonary hypertension. Chest radiography typically reveals cardiomegaly and pulmonary edema, while EKG usually shows ischemia and infarction. Echocardiography is diagnostic and assesses LV dysfunction and ischemic mitral regurgitation. Catheterization may be necessary for anatomical clarification but is used less frequently due to risk of arrhythmia.

Surgical repair is indicated for all ALCAPA patients, with establishment of a two-coronary system. This is commonly achieved by reimplanting the left coronary artery and a button of adjacent PA directly into the aorta. With advances from ASO, direct reimplantation of the anomalous coronary artery is now preferred and feasible. Survival rates following ALCAPA repair have improved, with recent reports indicating an operative mortality of 6% or less. Postoperative ventricular function typically normalizes, and mitral valve function often improves, although concurrent mitral valve repair may be considered for severe mitral regurgitation. Long-term follow-up with serial imaging is essential due to the risk of lethal left ventricular scarring and subsequent failure.

Anomalous Aortic Origin of Coronary Artery

Most anomalous aortic origin of the coronary arteries (AAOCA) are minor defects; however, AAOCA can become a major anomaly when the left main coronary artery arises from the right coronary sinus and courses between the PA and aorta.

This defect is associated with cardiac symptoms and sudden death, as is the origin of the right coronary artery from the left coronary sinus, particularly in right coronary dominance. The ischemic etiology in both cases is thought to stem from the acute angle of origin and the slit-like orifice of the anomalous vessel, often with an intramural course.[25] These defects typically present in older patients.

Symptomatic patients are managed surgically by unroofing the coronary ostia into the aorta or neo-ostial creation in cases of intramural course, or, rarely, with PA translocation or coronary artery bypass grafting. Surgical correction of AAOCA is safe and effective in select patients.

Myocardial Bridging

Myocardial bridging occurs when a segment of an epicardial coronary artery, typically the LAD, takes an intramyocardial course. While this is often an incidental finding at cardiac catheterization, it can be associated with myocardial ischemia in some cases. Treatment options include division of the muscle bridge to release the coronary artery, coronary bypass beyond the bridge, or transcatheter stenting.

Coronary Artery Aneurysms

Coronary aneurysms are rare and typically associated with inflammatory conditions, such as Kawasaki syndrome, polyarteritis nodosa, Takayasu arteritis, or syphilis. They may lead to thrombosis, distal coronary stenosis, or embolization, while rupture is uncommon. Treatment options vary from antiplatelet therapy to coronary artery bypass grafting.

SUMMARY

Congenital cardiac disease is a spectrum which can range from benign conditions that are repaired at a young age with no appreciable consequences on the patient's growth and quality of life, to more serious pathologies that require frequent monitoring, surveillance and potential reoperations as the patient grows. Emphasis on the "Heart Team" model is vital, as multidisciplinary management of these complex patients is warranted.

ACKNOWLEDGMENTS

We gratefully acknowledge the contributions of previous edition authors, Vikram Sood and Jennifer C. Romano, as portions of those chapters have been retained in this revision.

References

1. Liu Y, Chen S, Zuhlke L, et al. Global birth prevalence of congenital heart defects 1970–2017: updated systemic review and meta-analysis of 260 studies. *In J Epidemiol.* 2019;48(2):455–463.
2. Blalock A, Taussig H. The surgical treatment of malformations of the heart in which there is pulmonary stenosis or atresia. *JAMA.* 1945;128:189.
3. Buratto E, McCrossan B, Galati JC, et al. Repair of partial atrioventricular septal defect: a 37-year experience. *Eur J Cardiothorac Surg.* 2015;47(5):796–802
4. Varghese R, Saheed SB, Omoregbee B, Ninan B, Pavithran S, Kothandam S. Surgical repair of interrupted aortic arch and interrupted pulmonary artery. *Ann Thorac Surg.* 2015;100(6):e139–140.
5. Turek JW, Conway BD, Cavanaugh NB, et al. Bovine arch anatomy influences recoarctation rates in the era of the extended end-to-end anastomosis. *J Thorac Cardiovasc Surg.* 2018;155(3):1178–1183.
6. Stephens EH, Feins EN, Karamlou T, et al. The Society of Thoracic Surgeons Clinical Practice Guidelines on the management of neonates and infants with coarctation. *Ann Thorac Surg.* 2024;118(3):527–544.
7. Dorobantu DM, Espuny Pujol F, Kostolny M, et al. Arterial switch for transposition of the great arteries: treatment timing, late outcomes, and risk factors. *JACC Adv.* 2023;2(5):100407.
8. Ohye RG, Sleeper LA, Mahony L, et al. Comparison of shunt types in the Norwood procedure for single-ventricle lesions. *N Engl Med.* 2010;362:1980–1992.
9. Stamm C, Friehs I, Mayer JE Jr, et al. Long-term results of the lateral tunnel Fontan operation. *J Thorac Cardiovasc Surg.* 2001;121(1):28–41.
10. Hardy WA, Kang L, Turek JW, Rajab TK. Outcomes of truncal valve replacement in neonates and infants: a meta-analysis. *Cardiol Young.* 2023;33(5):673–680.
11. Turek JW, Kang L, Overbey DM, Carboni MP, Rajab TK. Partial heart transplant in a neonate with irreparable truncal valve dysfunction. *JAMA.* 2024;331(1):60–64.
12. Rajab TK, Vogel AD, Turek JW. Partial heart transplantation: a new option for paediatric heart valve replacement. *Nat Rev Cardiol.* 2024;21(5):277–278.
13. Van Praagh R, Van Praagh S. Isolated ventricular inversion. A consideration of the morphogenesis, definition and diagnosis of nontransposed and transposed great arteries. *Am J Cardiol.* 1966:17;395–406.
14. Jatene AD, Fontes VF, Paulista PP, et al. Successful anatomic correction of transposition of the great vessels. A preliminary report. *Arq Bras Cardiol.* 1975;28(4):461–464.
15. Nellis JR, Turek JW, Aldoss OT, Atkins DL, Ng BY. Intervention for supravalvar pulmonary stenosis after the arterial switch operation. *Ann Thorac Surg.* 2016;102(1):154–162.
16. Backer CL, Mavroudis C, Rigsby CK, et al. Trends in vascular ring surgery. *J Thorac Cardiovasc Surg.* 2005;129(6):1339–1347.
17. Ross DN. Replacement of aortic and mitral valves with a pulmonary autograft. *Lancet.* 1967;2(7523):956–958.
18. Konno S, Imai Y, Iida Y, Nakajima M, Tatsuno K. A new method for prosthetic valve replacement in congenital aortic stenosis associated with hypoplasia of the aortic valve ring. *J Thorac Cardiovasc Surg.* 1975;70(5):909–917.
19. Deo SV, Burkhart HM, Schaff HV, et al. Late outcomes for surgical repair of supravalvar aortic stenosis. *Ann Thorac Surg.* 2012;94(3):854–859
20. Tamesberger MI, Lechner E, Mair R, Hofer A, Sames-Dolzer E, Tulzer G. Early primary repair of tetralogy of Fallot in neonates and infants less than four months of age. *Ann Thorac Surg.* 2008;86(6):1928–1935.
21. Rajab TK, Vogel AD, Alexander VS, Brockbank KGM, Turek JW. The future of partial heart transplantation. *J Heart Lung Transplant.* 2024;43(6):863–865.
22. Bleiweis MS, Co-Vu J, Philip J, Fudge JC, et al. Comprehensive approach to the management of patients with hlhs: analysis of 100 consecutive neonates. *Ann Thorac Surg.* 2024:119(1):169–177.
23. Andersen ND, Overbey DM, Prabhu NK, et al. Staged repair of borderline hypoplastic heart disease with early biventricular conversion. *JTCVS Tech.* 2024;24:150–163.
24. Prabhu NK, Nellis JR, Meza JM, et al. Sustained total all-region perfusion during the norwood operation and postoperative recovery. *Semin Thorac Cardiovasc Surg.* 2023;35(1):140–147.
25. Turner II, Turek JW, Jaggers J, Herlong JR, Lawson DS, Lodge AJ. Anomalous aortic origin of a coronary artery: preoperative diagnosis and surgical planning. *World J Pediatr Congenit Heart Surg.* 2011;2(3):340–345.

79

Structural Heart Disease

Barbara C. S. Hamilton, Eric P. Cantey, and Steven F. Bolling

Key Points

1. The function and competence of all heart valves are a result of the entire valvular apparatus working in harmony as a unit. Dysfunction of any one component can result in valvular incompetence.
2. Two-dimensional (2D) echocardiography with Doppler allows precise real-time analysis of valvular anatomy and function and is the study of choice for the diagnosis and management of valvular lesions.
3. Operative or procedural intervention on all heart valves is generally reserved for patients with symptomatic severe valvular dysfunction. Goal-directed medical therapy can optimize heart mechanics delaying or alleviating the need for intervention, or can serve as a bridge to valve repair or replacement.
4. Restoring the function of native valvular tissue is often in the best interest of the patient. When feasible with a good result, valve repair is generally preferred over valve replacement.

VALVULAR ANATOMY

The fibrous cardiac skeleton is the basic structural framework for the four valves of the heart: two atrioventricular valves between the atria and ventricles (the tricuspid and mitral valves), and two semilunar valves (aortic and pulmonic valves) between the ventricles and their corresponding arteries (**Fig. 79.1**). Dense connective tissue forms four rings, which are connected by the right and left trigones in a plane between the atria and the ventricles. The right fibrous trigone is between the aortic and tricuspid rings and contiguous with the membranous septum, while the left trigone and intervalvular fibrosa area between the aortic and mitral rings, forming the posterior wall of the left ventricular outflow tract (LVOT). The cardiac skeleton maintains the integrity of the valve orifices and provides points of attachment for the valve leaflets. It also serves as a partition, electrically isolating the atria and ventricles except at the atrioventricular bundle (bundle of His), which passes through the right fibrous trigone near the septal leaflet of the tricuspid valve (TV), to allow for synchronous atrioventricular contraction throughout the cardiac cycle. Normally functioning valves act as gateways between the chambers of the heart as well as the aorta and pulmonary artery, functioning in response to pressure gradients between the ventricles and atria and ventricular mechanics. Ventricular contraction, resulting in an increase in ventricular pressure, closes the atrioventricular valves (the mitral and tricuspid) while opening the semilunar valves (aortic and pulmonic). Ventricular relaxation, resulting in a decrease in ventricular pressure, will open the atrioventricular valves and, in combination with the recoil of blood from the aorta and the pulmonary artery, cause the semilunar valves to close. The function and competence of all heart valves are a result of the entire valvular apparatus working in harmony as a unit. Dysfunction
1 of any one component can result in valvular incompetence.[1]

Anatomy of the Aortic Valve

The normal aortic valve (AV) consists of three semilunar cusps projecting outward and upward into the lumen of the ascending aorta (**Fig. 79.2**). The space between the free edge of each cusp and the aorta comprises the sinuses of Valsalva, while the space between the semilunar attachments of the leaflets comprises the interleaflet triangles. Since the coronary arteries arise from two of the three sinuses, the sinuses and the respective cusps are named the right coronary, left coronary, and noncoronary (or posterior) sinuses and cusps. The AV sits within the aortic root, above the LVOT. The borders of the aortic root are from the basal attachments of the valve leaflets at the basal ring below the ventriculo-aortic junction, to the distal attachments of the leaflets to the aorta at the sinotubular junction.

The definition of the aortic annulus can be somewhat controversial.[2] For some, the crown-like semilunar attachments of the three leaflets to the aorta comprise the annulus, whereas for others, the annulus is defined as the virtual basal ring formed by connecting the nadir of each semilunar cusp. Regardless, the three key components of the aortic valvular apparatus are the aortic annulus, the AV leaflets, and the sinotubular junction. In AV dysfunction, restoration and correction of these three components restore AV competency, be it through AV repair or replacement. Variations in AV anatomy include unicuspid (fusion or absence of two of the three commissures), bicuspid (fusion or absence of one commissure) or, more rarely, quadricuspid valve.

Anatomy of the Mitral Valve

The normal mitral valve (MV) apparatus, named for its visual similarity to an Episcopal Bishop's mitre, consists of an anterior (aortic) and posterior (mural) leaflet, atrial vestibules, the atrioventricular junction, tendinous cords, and the papillary muscles supported by the inferior (diaphragmatic) wall of the left ventricle. The anterior or aortic leaflet is semicircular and deep, extending from the anteromedial aspect of the mitral annulus, and encompasses approximately one-third of the annular circumference. The posterior or mural leaflet is shallow and shaped to perfectly oppose the anterior leaflet, extending from the posterolateral aspect of the mitral annulus, and encompasses approximately two-thirds of the annular circumference. Indentations, or pleats, subdivide the posterior leaflet into three scallops which allow for competent

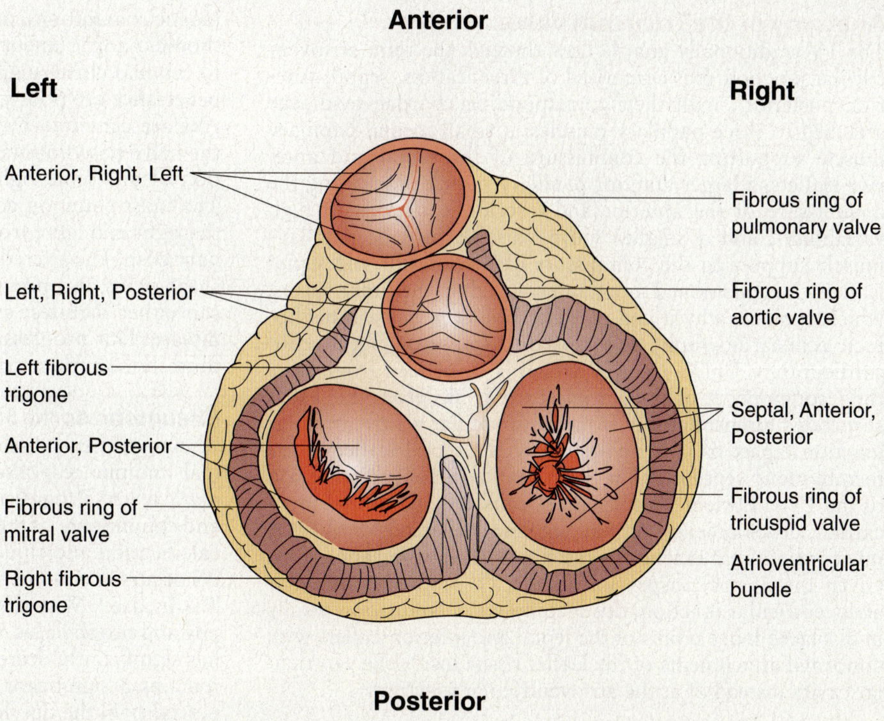

Figure 79.1. Schematic diagram of the fibrous cardiac skeleton.

coaptation of the posterior and anterior leaflets. These scallops are named P1, P2, and P3 from lateral to medial or left to right surgeon's view. Corresponding regions of the anterior leaflet are analogously referred to as A1, A2, and A3.

The leaflets are separated from one another at the annulus by the posteromedial and anterolateral commissures. The mitral annulus is formed anteriorly by the more rigid confluence of the left and right fibrous trigones and the intervalvular fibrosa and posteriorly by a less well-developed and more flexible fibrous band. In systole, the mitral annulus contracts (primarily the posterior aspect) and adopts an elliptical shape (shortening occurs perpendicular to the line of leaflet coaptation), and in diastole, it relaxes and adopts a more circular shape.[3] This dynamic motion of the annulus provides increased leaflet coaptation during systole and increased orifice area during diastole.

Two papillary muscles arise directly from the ventricular wall: the anterolateral and posteromedial papillary muscles. Importantly, the more prominent anterolateral papillary muscle is usually supplied by two coronary arteries, the left anterior descending artery and branches of the circumflex artery. The posteromedial papillary muscle is usually supplied by a single coronary artery, either from the right coronary artery or from the circumflex artery, which makes it more susceptible to rupture as a complication of myocardial infarction. The papillary muscles play an important role in the proper function of the MV, as closure and appropriate leaflet coaptation are permitted by end-diastolic and early systolic lengthening of the papillary muscles.[4]

Chordae tendineae attach the leaflets to either the papillary muscles or the ventricular wall and can be categorized by the location of the attachments. Primary chordae extend from the papillary muscle and attach to the leaflets at their free edge, ensuring proper coaptation without prolapse or flail. Secondary chordae attach to the ventricular side of the leaflets, along the line of coaptation, and are more prominent on the anterior leaflet. Tertiary chordae can arise from the papillary muscle or directly from the ventricular wall and attach to the base of the posterior leaflet. Fan-like commissural chordae attach to both leaflets and arise from either papillary muscle.

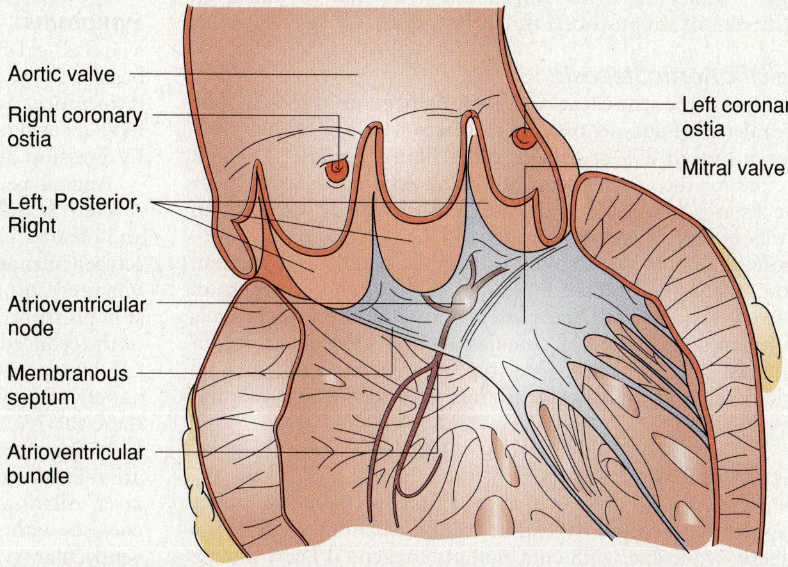

Figure 79.2. Schematic diagram of the relationship of the aortic valve to the underlying structures.

Anatomy of the Tricuspid Valve

The TV traditionally guards flow through the right atrioventricular junction. It is comprised of three leaflets (septal, anterior, posterior), with their corresponding chordae tendineae attached to three papillary muscles: a small medial papillary muscle supporting the commissure of the septal and anterior leaflets, a larger anterior papillary muscle supporting the commissure of the anterior and inferior leaflets (with high variability), and a smaller move variable inferior papillary muscle supporting the commissure of the inferior and septal leaflets. It is positioned more anteriorly than the other valves, which explains why it can often be best seen using transthoracic echocardiography as opposed to transesophageal echocardiography. Unlike the MV which is suspended from more rigid components of the fibrous cardiac skeleton, the TV is suspended almost entirely from the muscular atrioventricular junction (apart from a small area of the septal leaflet at the membranous septum).[5] The most common congenital lesion of thc TV is Ebstein malformation, caused by abnormal myocardial development with incomplete delamination of the myocardium that extends to the tricuspid valvular apparatus. Given the normal suspension of the TV from the muscular atrioventricular junction, this incomplete delamination results in displaced hinge points of the septal and inferior leaflets with abnormal attachments of the leaflet tissue inside the ventricular cavity instead of at the atrioventricular junction.[5]

Anatomy of the Pulmonic Valve

The normal pulmonic valve has many similarities to the aortic valve. The pulmonic valve is a ventriculo-arterial valve with three semilunar cusps that attach to the pulmonary artery. Like the aortic root, the pulmonic root is defined superiorly by the sinotubular junction at the level of the three commissures, and inferiorly at the nadir of the pulmonic cusps which define the virtual basal ring below the anatomic ventriculo-arterial junction.[6] The similarity between the pulmonic and AV is important when considering surgical treatment of AV disease, as the pulmonic valve can serve as an excellent replacement in young patients with AV disease, an operation known as the Ross procedure.

VALVULAR PATHOLOGY

Aortic Stenosis

Prevalence and Etiology

Aortic stenosis (AS) is the most prevalent valvular heart disease in developed countries.[7] The most common cause of AS is degenerative calcific disease, followed by congenital AS due to bicuspid valve anatomy. Rheumatic AS is becoming exceedingly uncommon in developed countries due to improved treatment of streptococcal throat infections.

Calcific Aortic Stenosis

The most frequent cause of AS is calcification of the AV. The prevalence of degenerative AS increases with age, with a prevalence rate of 2% in persons older than 65 years.[8] The risk factors for the development of calcific AS are similar to those for atherosclerotic heart disease, and include elevated serum levels of low-density lipoprotein (LDL) cholesterol and lipoprotein (a), diabetes, smoking, metabolic syndrome, hypertension, mediastinal radiation, kidney disease, and disorders of calcium metabolism.[9] Shear stress across the AV leaflets leads to inflammation, lipid accumulation, and subsequent myofibroblast differentiation. Over time this leads to fibrosis and calcification of the valvular leaflets with subsequent valvular obstruction.

Bicuspid Aortic Stenosis

Bicuspid AVs are present in approximately 1% to 2% of the population. Bicuspid AV can be seen in isolation, as part of a genetic syndrome, with concomitant congenital heart disease (aortic coarctation), or along with an aortopathy and resultant thoracic aortic aneurysm. Variable inheritance patterns lead to familial clustering, but the genetics of bicuspid AV disease penetrance are poorly understood.[10] The spectrum of bicuspid AVs are classified by the Sievers classification, which defines the valve based on the presence of raphe or ridges in the location of anatomic right, left and noncoronary commissures.[11] The most common configuration of bicuspid AV is fusion of the right and left coronary cusp, with a freestanding noncoronary cusp. The altered flow dynamics through the valve lead to shear stress and progressive degeneration of the valve, which can either manifest as stenosis, regurgitation or mixed valve disease. This progressive degeneration typically leads to symptoms in the fifth or sixth decade of life.

Rheumatic Aortic Stenosis

Rheumatic heart disease is the long-term sequelae of an abnormal immune response to streptococcal A infection (ie, rheumatic fever). Progressive inflammation, particularly at the base and commissure of the AV leaflets, leads to progressive fibrosis, calcification and clinical valvular disease. Typically, rheumatic AS occurs in conjunction with MV disease, and less commonly TV disease.[12] With the introduction of effective antibiotic therapy and prophylaxis, the prevalence of rheumatic heart disease has significantly decreased in the developed world; however, it remains a significant cause of cardiovascular morbidity and mortality in the developing world.[13]

Pathophysiology

Regardless of the etiology of AS, the cardiovascular pathophysiology is identical. Progressive narrowing of the AV leads to a pressure gradient between the LV and the aorta, and therefore a state of chronic LV pressure overload. Due to the need to maintain a consistent cardiac output and decrease LV wall tension, the LV wall remodels with subsequent myocyte hypertrophy. This has several deleterious effects, including decreased LV compliance, upstream cardiac and pulmonary vascular remodeling (left atrial dilation, pulmonary vascular remodeling and increased pulmonary hydrostatic pressure), myocardial fibrosis, increased myocardial oxygen demand and subsequent myocardial ischemia.[14] While the LV systolic function is typically preserved, in the late stages of AS the LV systolic function fails.

It should also be noted that the shear stress due to resultant turbulent flow across the stenotic AV results in an acquired von Willebrand factor deficiency, platelet dysfunction and a predisposition to small bowel angiogenesis, eponymously known as Heyde syndrome.

Diagnosis

Symptoms

The classical symptoms of AS are angina pectoris, syncope, and heart failure; however, subtle symptoms including exertional intolerance, dyspnea on exertion, fatigue and lightheadedness have an insidious onset as the compensatory mechanisms of LV pressure overload fail.[15]

Angina pectoris occurs in 30% to 50% of patients with severe AS, and is reflective of the common risk factors for AS and obstructive coronary artery disease, increased myocardial oxygen demand in the setting of LV pressure overload, and impaired coronary perfusion due to decreased coronary perfusion pressure. Exertional syncope or near syncope is reflective of the reduced cerebral perfusion and the inability to augment cardiac output in the setting of a fixed obstruction. Approximately 15% of patients present with syncope and only 50% of these survive for 3 years. Signs and symptoms of heart failure, including dyspnea on exertion, fatigue, and peripheral edema, are reflective of long-standing disease. Due to progressive left atrial dilation and subsequent remodeling, atrial fibrillation coexists with AS up to 15% of the time.[16] The loss of atrial-ventricular synchrony, and therefore LV filling can worsen

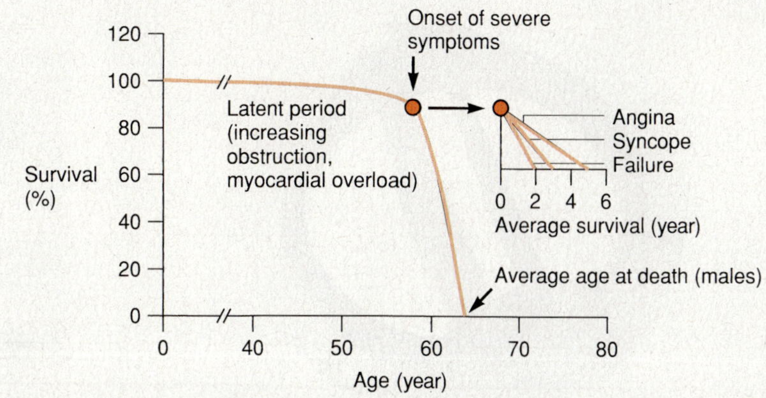

Figure 79.3. Natural history of aortic stenosis without operative treatment. Onset of symptoms identifies patients at high risk of death over the next 2 to 5 years.

symptoms. Finally, Heyde syndrome may lead to serious gastrointestinal bleeding secondary to arteriovenous malformations.

Signs

AS is frequently diagnosed by physical examination due to the loud, systolic, crescendo–decrescendo murmur best heard at the second intercostal space right of the sternum. Occasionally the murmur radiates to the carotids or the axilla, the latter of which is referred to as the Gallavardin phenomenon. As AS progresses, and the valve leaflets calcify and become immobile, the second heart sound disappears. The left ventricle must generate a significant pressure to overcome these leaflets, and therefore the systolic ejection period decreases leading to a late-peaking systolic murmur of severe AS. This can also be described as "pulsus parvus et tardus," where there is a delayed carotid impulse. Finally, in the setting of severe LV dysfunction, the cardiac output is severely depressed, and a murmur of AS may be absent. Clinical signs of heart failure, including pulmonary rales, elevated jugular venous pressure, and lower extremity edema are typically seen in this population.

Comprehensive, Multi-Modality Evaluation of Aortic Stenosis

The most common finding by electrocardiogram is signs of LV hypertrophy which is neither sensitive nor specific for the diagnosis of AS.

Echocardiography is the primary imaging modality for diagnosis and quantification of AS.[2] Echocardiography allows for visualization of the AV morphology (trileaflet, bicuspid), leaflet characteristics (calcification, thickening), and leaflet motion. It also allows for a comprehensive quantitative evaluation of concomitant valvular disease, aortic dimensions, and biventricular size and function. Doppler echocardiography allows a hemodynamic assessment of valvular stenosis severity, through calculation of the peak trans-aortic velocity, mean left ventricular aortic gradient. The latter allows the derivation
2 of the AV area.

Low-flow, low-gradient AS occurs when the left ventricle is not able to mount a stroke volume and therefore transvalvular pressure to evaluate the severity of AS. This can occur in the setting of decreased LV systolic function (classical type) or preserved LV function due to decreased compliance (paradoxical type). Dobutamine stress echocardiography helps differentiate primary valvular dysfunction from pseudostenosis.[17]

Cardiac computed tomography has evolved as a valuable tool for the evaluation of AV disease. Through ECG-gated acquisition, cardiac CT can evaluate AV morphology and leaflet tissue composition. Agaston calcium scoring, which accounts for the density and area of calcium, has been shown to be predictive of AV disease severity.[18] Cardiac CT also allows for an in depth evaluation of coronary anatomy and disease, ascending aortic dimensions, all of which in the setting of severe AS allow for therapeutic decision making.

Invasive cardiac catheterization with direct measurement of the pressure gradients across the AV is reserved for situations where the clinical presentation and noninvasive evaluation of AS severity is unclear or yields discrepant data.[17]

Natural History

The natural history of AS is marked by a prolonged latent period with few symptoms and minimal morbidity. In the presence of valvular stenosis, the AV area slowly decreases, generally by approximately 0.1 cm^2 per year.[19] The natural history of severe AS correlates well with the onset and severity of symptoms. The average life expectancy of patients with symptomatic, severe, and untreated AS is 5, 3, and 2 years for patients with angina, syncope, and heart failure, respectively (**Fig. 79.3**).[20]

Treatment

There is no effective medical therapy for the treatment or prevention of AS; therefore, medical therapy (ie, diuretics) is utilized for the treatment of LV pressure overload and subsequent pulmonary congestion. The timing of aortic valve replacement (AVR) is determined by the presence of symptoms, or the presence of LV dysfunction (LV ejection fraction <50%).[17]
3 Mechanical relief of severe AS is accomplished by surgical AV replacement (SAVR), transcatheter aortic valve replacement (TAVR), or percutaneous balloon aortic valvuloplasty (BAV).

Surgical Aortic Valve Replacement

The decision to proceed with surgical management in AS is based on disease severity and patient symptoms. Surgery is indicated in symptomatic patients with severe AS, or asymptomatic patients with severe AS and reduced LV function (<50%), progression of disease over serial studies, rapidly progressive disease, or those who fail an exercise tolerance test.[17] Patients with asymptomatic severe or moderate AS who are undergoing other cardiac surgery should also be considered for AVR at the time of the concomitant procedure.

Choice of valve prosthesis for AVR is primarily influenced by the patient's age, functional status, lifestyle, and presence of any contraindications to anticoagulation.[17] Mechanical prostheses are made of some combination of titanium, graphite, and pyrolytic carbon, require lifelong anticoagulation and are very durable (**Fig. 79.4**). Stented biologic prostheses are most commonly made of bovine pericardium or porcine valve leaflets, do not require anticoagulation, but are prone to structural valve degeneration (SVD), therefore limiting their durability (**Fig. 79.5**). All prosthetic valves, regardless of composition, are at risk for infection resulting in endocarditis and need for valve explantation. Comparisons between bioprosthetic and mechanical valves in the aortic position in patients aged 50 to 69 years show no difference in 15-year survival, but higher incidence of reoperation in the bioprosthetic group (12.1% vs 6.9%) and higher incidence of bleeding in the mechanical

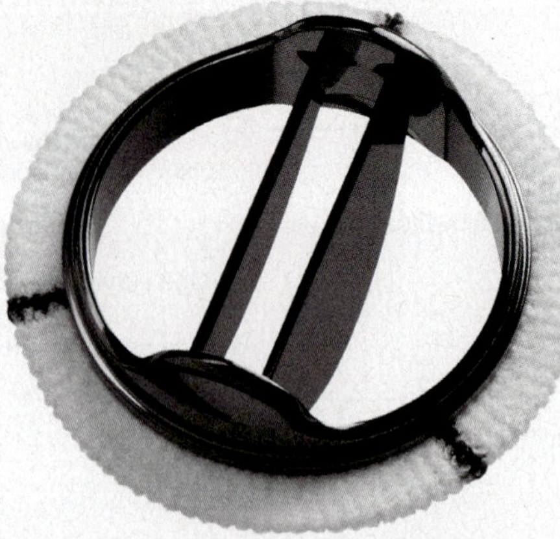

Figure 79.4. St. Jude Medical Regent Valve.

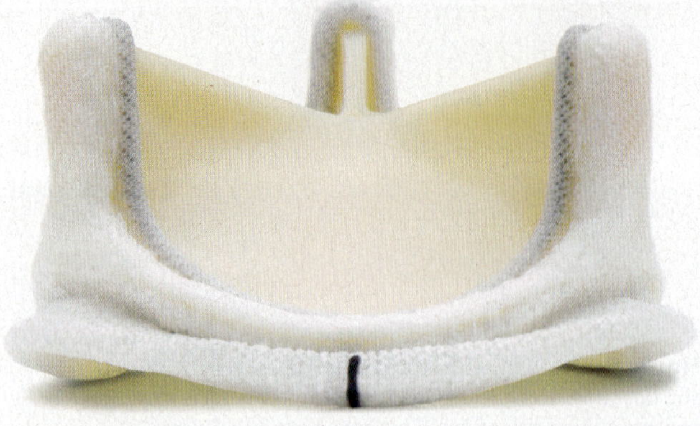

Figure 79.5. Carpentier-Edwards Magna Ease Pericardial Valve. (© 2025 Edwards Lifesciences Corporation. All rights reserved.)

prosthesis group (13.0% vs 6.6%).[21] Newer technologies in the form of tissue preservation techniques are promising in their potential to improve bioprosthetic valve longevity. Current guidelines recommend considering mechanical prostheses in patients younger than 50 years of age without contraindications to anticoagulation, although use of a pulmonary autograft for AVR (the Ross procedure) is also to be considered at advanced centers.[17] Initially introduced in 1967,[22] the Ross procedure has undergone a recent resurgence and has demonstrated excellent long-term survival with freedom from valve-related complications in young patients.[23]

Surgical AVR is performed on cardiopulmonary bypass with myocardial arrest. The traditional approach is through a full sternotomy, although minimally invasive options including a hemisternotomy or mini right anterior thoracotomy are also possible. The leaflets of the AV are resected, and sutures passed through the aortic annulus to seat the newly implanted valve. There are two structures in close proximity to the AV susceptible to injury during AV surgery (**Fig. 79.2**). The anterior leaflet of the MV is positioned under the commissure between the left and noncoronary cusps. The left bundle of His is positioned under the commissure between the right and noncoronary cusps, in the area of the membranous septum.

Transcatheter Aortic Valve Replacement

TAVR is a minimally invasive procedure that utilizes the calcified, stenotic valve as a buttress for a stented bioprosthetic valve replacement. There are two general types of TAVR valves, defined by both the properties of the stent material and location of the TAVR prosthesis in relation to the AV annulus. Self-expanding valves are supra-annular, and the stent frame is made of nitinol which retains its shape and expands in the blood pool. Balloon-expandable valves are intra-annular and are made of cobalt-chromium (**Fig. 79.6**). Due to improved lower profile of current generation devices, femoral access is typically the primary access. When femoral access is prohibitive, such as in significant peripheral arterial disease, alternative access through a surgical cutdown is utilized. These alternative options include trans-carotid, subclavian, direct aortic, trans-apical, and trans-caval.

TAVR is an approved treatment for patients with severe AS at all levels of surgical risk.[24–26] A key aspect of the care in patients with severe AS is the multidisciplinary valve team evaluation. The multidisciplinary team evaluates each individual's comorbidities, concomitant valvular and coronary artery disease, and individual anatomy to determine the surgical and percutaneous risk of AVR, and therefore, determine the best therapy for the lifetime management of the patient's aortic valve disease.[17]

Balloon Aortic Valvuloplasty

BAV is a percutaneous procedure in which a semi-compliant or noncompliant balloon is inflated across a stenotic AV in order to increase the AV area, and therefore decrease the left ventricle to aortic gradient. This procedure is a valuable tool for treatment of AS in children and young adults with congenital AS. Due to early restenosis, development of aortic insufficiency from leaflet damage, and the wide availability of TAVR, the utilization of BAV for calcific AS has decreased. Current utilization is limited to those who require a bridge to definitive AVR, or as a palliative procedure to decrease symptoms in those who are not surgical AVR or TAVR candidates.

Aortic Regurgitation

Prevalence and Etiology

Aortic regurgitation or insufficiency (AI) results from the improper coaptation of the AV leaflets due to either intrinsic leaflet abnormalities or ascending aortic or aortic root dilation. The most common causes of valvular AI include bicuspid

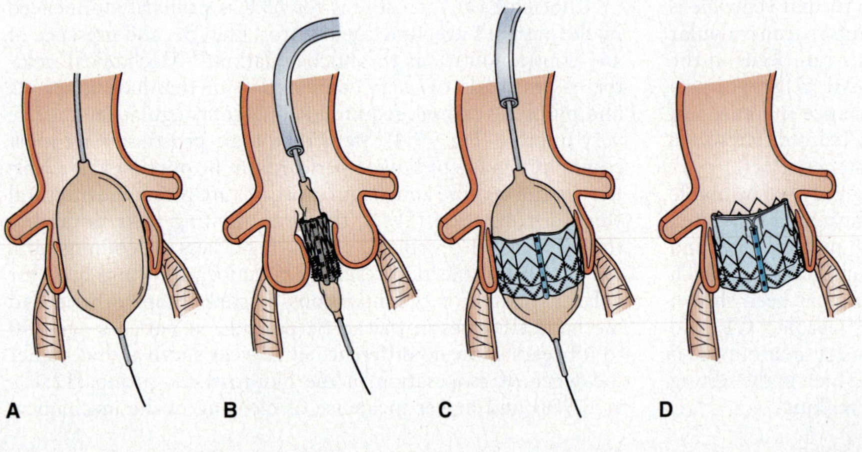

Figure 79.6. Schematic diagram of percutaneous aortic valve replacement. **A:** Balloon valvuloplasty. **B:** Balloon catheter with valve in the native diseased valve. **C:** Balloon inflation to secure the valve. **D:** Valve in place.

valve disease, calcific AV disease, rheumatic disease, and endocarditis. Bicuspid AV disease is typically due to incomplete coaptation of the leaflets, or prolapse. As above, rheumatic heart disease leads to inflammation at the base and commissures of multiple leaflets, typically leading to mixed AS and regurgitation. Endocarditis leads to destruction of the aortic leaflets either leading to prolapse or perforation. Acquired (degenerative, hypertensive), inflammatory (syphilitic, ankylosing spondylitis, giant cell arteritis) or genetic aortopathies (Marfan's, Loeys-Dietz) can lead to progressive dilation of the AV annulus and failure of leaflet coaptation.

Pathophysiology

Chronic AI leads to progressive volume overload of the left ventricle. In response to this, the left ventricle dilates and hypertrophies. This adverse remodeling leads to progressive interstitial fibrosis, decreased effective (forward) cardiac output and subsequent myocardial ischemia. In conjunction with progression of valvular dysfunction, this leads to LV pressure overload, LV failure, and clinical symptoms. It should be noted that in acute AI, which can be seen in acute aortic dissection or endocarditis, there is a rapid increase in LV volume, leading to LV pressure overload and subsequent pulmonary congestion with decreased effective forward cardiac output.

Diagnosis

Symptoms

As the left ventricle adapts to chronic volume overload through dilation and hypertrophy, chronic AI is typically well tolerated for many years. However, as the valvular disease and LV remodeling progress, individuals develop fatigue, dyspnea on exertion, angina and symptoms of heart failure—paroxysmal nocturnal dyspnea or orthopnea. As described above, acute AI, with the rapid increase in LV pressure and volume overload, typically presents with cardiogenic shock and acute pulmonary edema.

Signs

Lateral displacement of the point of maximum impulse is seen in chronic AI due to LV dilation. The classic auscultatory findings of AI are best heard at the right sternal border of the second intercostal space and include a high-pitched, blowing diastolic murmur. As aortic regurgitation progresses, the murmur will extend through diastole, and the increased cardiac output will lead to a systolic flow murmur. As LV compensatory mechanisms fail there is equalization of end-diastolic pressures between the left ventricle and aorta, and the late diastolic component of the murmur will fail.

Aortic insufficiency leads to a widened pulse pressure, which can lead to a number of peripheral exam findings, such as bounding pulses (water hammer or Corrigan pulse), pulsation of capillaries in fingernail bed (Quincke pulse), rhythmic bobbing of the head (de Musset sign), systolic and diastolic murmurs heard over the femoral artery when compressed (Duroziez sign) and pulsation of the uvula (Müller sign).[27]

Comprehensive, Multi-Modality Evaluation of AR

Echocardiography is essential for determining the mechanism of AI and the hemodynamic effect of aortic regurgitation. This is not only critical for establishing the diagnosis of AI, but for serial monitoring of aortic regurgitation severity, and left ventricle size and function. Two-dimensional echocardiography, whether by transthoracic or transesophageal acquisition, allows for assessment of the valvular apparatus to determine the etiology of aortic regurgitation (ie, calcific trileaflet AV disease, dilated aortic root with malcoaptation, leaflet prolapse). Doppler evaluation also allows for quantification of aortic regurgitation severity. This can be determined by evaluation of the Doppler flow pattern at the aortic valve—pressure half time (time for equalization of aortic and LV pressures), or diastolic flow reversal in the descending aorta; semi-quantitative measures—color Doppler jet width in the LVOT, and vena-contracta width (width of narrowest part of regurgitant jet); and quantitative measures—regurgitant volume, regurgitant fraction, and regurgitant orifice area.[28] Finally echocardiography allows for determining the extent of volume overload on the left ventricle, by measurement of LV end-diastolic volume and dimensions, as well as LV systolic function.

Tomographic imaging, particularly cardiac MRI, has evolved as a significant adjunctive imaging modality for the evaluation of aortic regurgitation. Through its high temporal and spatial resolution, cardiac MRI allows for determination of AI mechanism, quantification of AI severity, quantification of LV volumes and myocardial tissue definition (ie, late-gadolinium enhancement for the evaluation of fibrosis), as well as multiplanar evaluation of ascending aorta and aortic root dimensions.[29]

Due to the evolution of echocardiography and tomographic imaging, the use of aortography for the diagnosis and quantification of aortic regurgitation is rarely performed.

Natural History

The natural history of AI is strongly dependent on the presence of symptoms and LV dysfunction at the time of presentation. Asymptomatic patients with normal LV function develop symptoms or LV dysfunction at a rate of 6% per year. Asymptomatic patients with LV dysfunction at presentation develop cardiac symptoms at a rate of 25% per year. Finally, the mortality rate of symptomatic patients is 10% per year.[17]

Treatment

Management of patients with AI depends on the severity of symptoms and the size and function of the left ventricle. Asymptomatic patients with chronic severe AI and preserved LV size and function are treated with vasodilator medical therapy, which reduces afterload and improves forward flow.

Surgery is indicated in symptomatic patients with severe AI, asymptomatic patients with severe AI and evidence of LV dilation (LV end-systolic diameter >50 mm), LV dysfunction (ejection fraction ≤55%), progressive LV dysfunction or dilation, or patients with moderate AI undergoing other cardiac surgery.[17] Patients with acute severe AI can present in extremis and can be considered a relative surgical emergency.

The type of surgical procedure is determined by the etiology of AI, valvular characteristics, and presence of concomitant aortopathy. In individuals with isolated AV disease who are good surgical candidates, surgical management is the treatment of choice. Given the negative association of heart valve replacement on survival in young patients,[30] procedures that preserve native leaflet tissue should be considered whenever possible, including AV repair or, in patients with isolated aortic root pathology, valve-sparing root replacement (the David procedure). The method chosen for AV repair is determined by the valve pathology, with the goal of restoring adequate coap-
3 tation of the AV leaflets. Techniques include subcommissural annuloplasty, cusp repair with leaflet resection, free margin plication, resuspension, or raphe release.[31] When the valve is not amenable to preservation, considerations for prosthetic valve choice (mechanical valve, bioprosthetic valve, or pulmonary autograft) are identical to those discussed previously.
4 In mixed aortic root and valvular disease, total aortic root replacement with a prosthetic valve replacement (Bentall procedure) is performed.

In select patients with suitable anatomy, currently available commercial TAVR valves are utilized to treat individuals at prohibitive surgical risk.[32] Clinical trials are actively enrolling for AR-specific transcatheter valves.[33]

Mitral Stenosis

Prevalence and Etiology

Rheumatic fever is the leading cause of mitral stenosis worldwide; however, due to early recognition and treatment of streptococcal infections, rheumatic fever, and rheumatic mitral stenosis have nearly disappeared from the developed world. As with AV disease, inflammation of the MV apparatus occurs at the base and commissures of the MV leaflets, with progressive fibrosis and subsequent calcification of the leaflets and subvalvular apparatus. The most common etiology of mitral stenosis is due to degenerative mitral stenosis, either due to progressive mitral annular calcification. Mitral annular calcification occurs in approximately 10% of elderly patients, of which 1% to 2% develop mitral stenosis. Other risk factors for degenerative mitral stenosis include calcification, age, female sex, chronic kidney disease and LV hypertrophy. Nonvalvular obstruction of the MV leading to decrease in the MV orifice area is also possible in cases of atrial myxoma, left atrial thrombus and large vegetations from endocarditis.[34]

Pathophysiology

Progressive mitral stenosis leads to an increase in the left atrial pressure needed to transmit blood into the left ventricle during ventricular diastole. Elevated left atrial pressures lead to left atrial dilatation and fibrosis; and are transmitted the pulmonary vasculature leading to both pulmonary congestion and pulmonary vascular remodeling with pulmonary hypertension. As the right ventricle is exposed to elevated pulmonary hypertension, adverse remodeling with right ventricular dilation and subsequent tricuspid regurgitation (TR) occurs.

Due to the dependence on both passive diastolic filling and atrial contraction to maintain cardiac output, tachycardia and ectopic atrial rhythms (ie, atrial fibrillation) can worsen the transvalvular gradient and subsequent patient symptomatology. Situations that increase cardiac output and transmitral flow, such as exercise, pregnancy, anemia, or infections, can lead to an increase in the MV gradient and therefore symptomatic mitral stenosis.

Finally, mitral stenosis with subsequent left atrial dilation, fibrosis, and concomitant atrial fibrillation allows for stasis of blood within the left atrium. Because of this, patients with mitral stenosis are at higher risk for thromboembolic complications particularly in the presence of atrial fibrillation.

Diagnosis

Symptoms

As the MV orifice narrows and the transmitral gradient increases, exertional dyspnea, exercise intolerance, and lightheadedness are the most common early symptoms of mitral stenosis. Symptomatic mitral stenosis is particularly accentuated in the setting of loss of atrial contraction or situations of compensatory tachycardia to maintain cardiac output such as atrial fibrillation, pregnancy in women of childbearing age or infection. Palpitations, or worsening of previously asymptomatic mitral stenosis, can be suggestive of an underlying atrial arrhythmia.

In the advanced stages of mitral stenosis, where there is pulmonary vascular remodeling and resultant pulmonary arterial hypertension, symptoms of right heart failure may include peripheral edema and abdominal distension. Rarely, hemoptysis can occur due to pulmonary venous hypertension or rupture of bronchial arteries. Symptoms due to external compression from a dilated left atrium, including hoarseness (due to compression of the recurrent laryngeal nerve, ie, Ortner syndrome) and dysphagia (due to compression of the esophagus) can also occur.

Signs

The typical auscultatory findings of MS are best heard at the apex and include a low-pitched, rumbling mid-diastolic murmur. In the setting of rheumatic mitral stenosis, where the leaflets are fibrotic, an accentuated first sound and an opening snap can be heard; however, especially in degenerative mitral stenosis with severely calcified and immobile leaflets, this finding is not heard. Pulmonary edema, with resultant pulmonary rales, is typically not heard due to the compensation of the pulmonary venous and lymphatic drainage. A right ventricular heave and an accentuated pulmonic component of the second heart sound are suggestive of right ventricular hypertrophy and pulmonary arterial hypertension, and as the right ventricular function fails, peripheral edema, hepatomegaly, ascites, and jugular venous distension can be found.[27]

Imaging

Echocardiography is the principal tool used in the diagnosis of MS. Transthoracic and transesophageal echocardiogram, with three-dimensional reconstruction, allow for a comprehensive evaluation of the valvular apparatus. This is important for the determination of the severity of MS, mechanism of MS, and also aids in determining the ideal treatment. Echocardiographic assessment of MS allows for a comprehensive evaluation of the up-stream sequelae of MS—left atrial dilation, left atrial appendage thrombus, pulmonary hypertension, right ventricular dysfunction, and TR.

As before, the transmitral gradient is determined by both the transmitral flow and MV area. Planimetry of the MV orifice can allow for determination of the MV area. Multi-plane, three-dimensional reconstruction has substantially improved the ability to determine an accurate MV area.[17] Doppler evaluation of the MV allows for determination of the transmitral gradient, with the Doppler pattern allowing for derivation of an MV area.

Rheumatic mitral stenosis typically starts with inflammation and fibrosis of the base and commissures of leaflets, allowing for mobility of the leaflet tips and gives a classic "hockey stick" appearance of the MV leaflets. As the disease progresses, calcification of the leaflet progresses to the leaflet tips and involvement of the subvalvular apparatus occurs. Degenerative mitral stenosis typically involves the posterior leaflet with presence of mitral annular calcifications.

Exercise stress echocardiography (ESE) is used as an adjunctive tool to determine the timing of valve intervention. ESE allows objective evaluation of symptom burden and exercise capacity, while simultaneously evaluating the hemodynamic effect of MS (transmitral gradients, MV area, and pulmonary artery systolic pressure).[17] Similar to the diagnosis of other valvular heart disease, cardiac catheterization with direct pressure measurement has largely been replaced by echocardiography.

Natural History

The natural history of rheumatic heart disease is variable and of historical interest. Degenerative mitral stenosis typically appears in the setting of concomitant cardiovascular risk factors and is typically slowly progressive. Therefore the contribution of coexisting atrial fibrillation and heart failure with preserved ejection fraction are difficult to delineate purely on a patient's symptomatology. Both the presence and severity of stenosis are associated with increased mortality—with a mortality rate of 8% to 13% once symptoms of MS are present, and an 85% 5-year mortality rate with New York Heart Association class IV symptoms.[34,35]

Treatment

Medical therapy for the treatment of MS entails promotion of LV filling, decongestion of the pulmonary venous system and anticoagulation in the setting of atrial fibrillation. As before, tachycardia can impair ventricular filling, thus beta-blockers are frequently prescribed. Cautious diuresis with loop diuretics can improve pulmonary venous congestion, as overdiuresis can exacerbate hypotension. Finally, the risk of systemic thromboembolization is particularly amplified in the presence of MS and atrial fibrillation. Therefore oral anticoagulation is strongly recommended.[17]

As with AS, the treatment of MS requires relief of the mechanical obstruction, either by percutaneous balloon mitral valvuloplasty (PBMV) MV replacement, and MV repair.

Techniques in MV repair have been described in the modern era and have replaced the now historical open mitral commissurotomy.[36]

Percutaneous Balloon Mitral Valvuloplasty

PBMV requires a balloon-tipped catheter to be introduced into the left atrium via a transseptal approach and inflated across the diseased valve. In selected patients, PBMV is the standard of care with a low risk of procedural complications, and durable relief of valvular stenosis.[37] Absolute contraindications for PBMV include left atrial thrombus and moderate to severe mitral regurgitation (MR). The Wilkins score, which takes into account leaflet characteristics including thickness, mobility, and calcification along with subvalvular papillary muscle and chordae tendineae pathology, has been validated to predict valves amenable to PBMV.[38] Typically valves of rheumatic MS are more amenable to PBMV than degenerative MS.

Rheumatic Mitral Valve Repair

MV repair compared to replacement has demonstrated improved early and late patient survival.[39] Classical techniques for rheumatic MV repair include resection of diseased tissue with decalcification, as well as combinations of commissurotomy, commissuroplasty, leaflet resection, annuloplasty, and repair of the subvalvular apparatus. Additional techniques may include neochords and pericardial patches.[36]

Mitral Valve Replacement

MV replacement is necessary in symptomatic patients with severe or progressive MS when PMBV is less likely to be successful, particularly in the case of concomitant moderate to severe MR or presence of left atrial thrombus.[17] The choice of valve prosthesis for MV replacement is determined similarly to choosing the prosthesis for AVR.[17] Regardless of the prosthesis used, it is well established that preservation of the papillary muscle attachments to the annulus plays an important role in the maintenance of LV function. MV repair or replacement is performed on cardiopulmonary bypass via a full sternotomy, or a mini right lateral thoracotomy. The structures in close proximity to the MV susceptible to injury during MV surgery include the aortic valve, the atrioventricular node, and the circumflex coronary artery (**Fig. 79.7**).

Percutaneous, transcatheter MV replacement is an evolving treatment option for patients at high to prohibitive risk of surgical MV replacement. Transcatheter MV replacement in mitral annular calcification with the use of a balloon-expandable TAVR valve in the mitral position is a complex option for patients with favorable anatomy.[40] Finally, clinical trials are underway for dedicated transcatheter MV replacement valves.

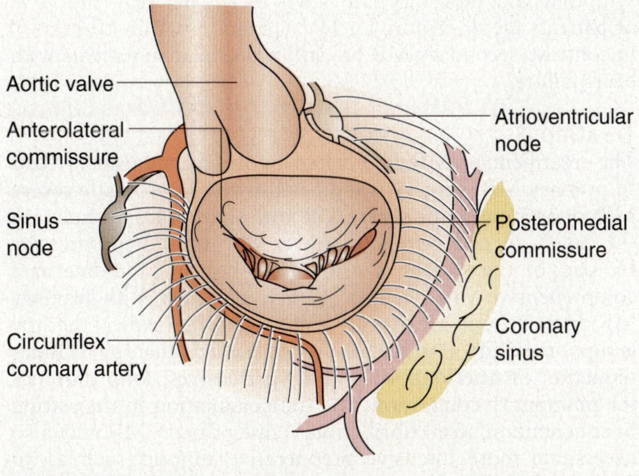

Figure 79.7. Schematic diagram of the relationship of the mitral valve to the underlying structures.

Mitral Regurgitation

Prevalence and Etiology

MR is the most common regurgitant valvular lesion.[41] There are various classification schemes to define the etiology of MR. The binary classification defines mitral pathology into primary (degenerative, ie, related to MV leaflets) and secondary MR (functional, ie, related to distortion of the coaptation plane from nonleaflet pathology).

The Carpentier classification is more comprehensive and accounts for the different mechanisms of MR (**Fig. 79.8**).[42] Type I MR, or normal leaflet motion with lack of coaptation, occurs in the setting of annular dilation from cardiomyopathy, leaflet perforation in the setting of endocarditis or congenital clefts. Excessive leaflet motion due to segmental leaflet prolapse or flail is classified as type II MR. The two main subtypes include myxomatous disease, typically seen in younger patients, and fibroelastic deficiency, typically seen in older patients. Excessive leaflet motion can also be seen in rheumatic heart disease, trauma, and endocarditis. Type III MR is seen in the setting of restricted leaflet motion and divided into two subtypes—type IIIa, restricted leaflet motion in systole and diastole, and IIIb, restricted leaflet motion in systole. Type IIIa MR is most commonly seen in rheumatic heart disease, but can also be seen in radiation heart disease, carcinoid syndrome and lupus. Type IIIb is typically seen in cardiomyopathies.

Pathophysiology

On a cellular level, myxomatous leaflets have increased cellular and extracellular matrix proliferation.[43] This leads to diffuse leaflet thickening and redundancy, chordal elongation, and annular enlargement. In contrast, fibroelastic deficiency is typically isolated to a single leaflet segment and does not lead to annular enlargement. Initially, leaflet redundancy and thickening lead to leaflet prolapse, or bowing of the leaflet tissue into the atrium. As the leaflet disease progresses, there is distortion of the MV annulus size and geometry with subsequent increase in tension on the subvalvular apparatus, the chordae tendineae can rupture culminating in a flail leaflet.

As discussed in the MS section, rheumatic heart disease leads to progressive inflammation, fibrosis and calcification of the MV leaflets and subvalvular apparatus. This can lead to ventricular tethering of the MV leaflets, and therefore malcoaptation with subsequent MR. As leaflet mobility is decreased in ventricular systole and diastole, MR frequently coexists with MS in rheumatic heart disease.

There are multiple mechanisms to functional MR (Carpentier type I and III MR). Dilation of the MV annulus can occur in atrial and ventricular myopathies, the former typically occurs in long-standing atrial fibrillation. Cardiomyopathies also lead to distortion of the subvalvular apparatus, particularly with ventricular displacement of the MV leaflets due to tethering of the papillary muscles and chordae tendineae. This can occur with a focal wall motion abnormality, particularly the inferolateral wall which supplies the posterior medial papillary muscle, in ischemic cardiomyopathy. It also can lead to tethering due to global LV dysfunction and dilation, as seen in nonischemic cardiomyopathies.[42]

Regardless of the etiology of MR, progressive MR leads to left atrial and ventricular volume overload. Left atrial dilation and subsequent fibrosis increase the risk of atrial fibrillation. As these compensatory mechanisms fail, increased left atrial pressures are transmitted to the pulmonary venous system, with pulmonary vascular remodeling and subsequent pulmonary hypertension. As with MS, this can lead to right heart dysfunction and tricuspid annulus dilation. LV volume overload leads to adverse LV remodeling through dilation, and subsequent LV pressure overload.

Acute MR, which typically occurs as a consequence of mechanical rupture of a papillary muscle in the setting of an unrevascularized myocardial infarction or rupture of a chordae

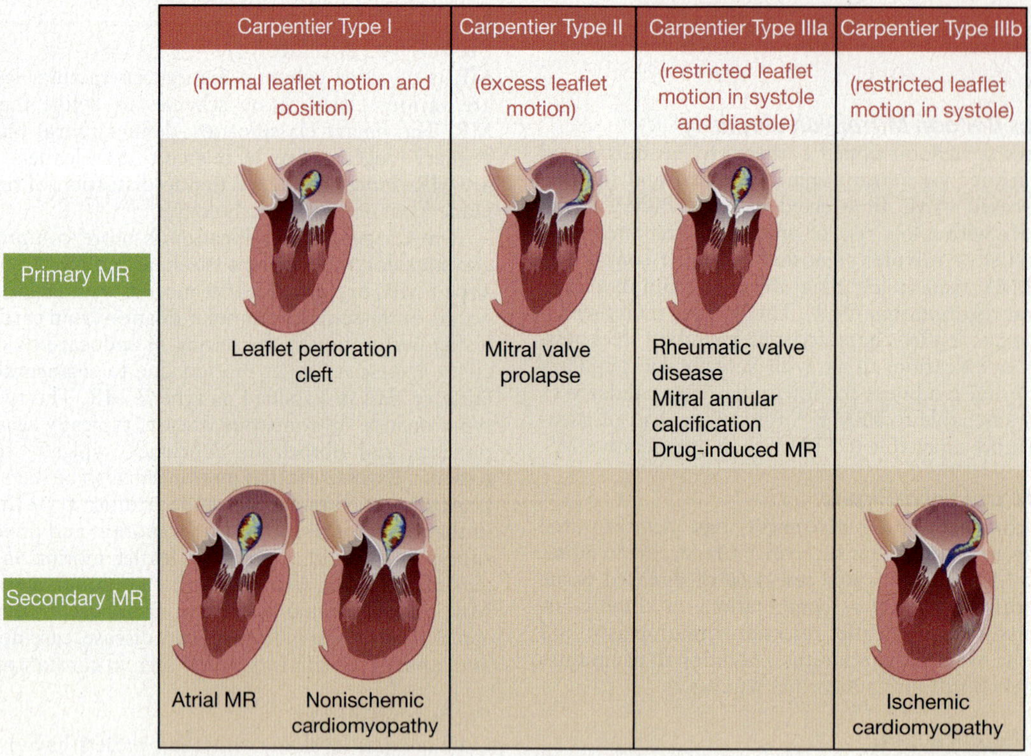

Figure 79.8. Carpentier's classification of the etiology of mitral valve disease, organized by primary versus secondary mitral regurgitation. (Reproduced with permission from El Sabbagh A, Reddy YNV, Nishimura RA. Mitral valve regurgitation in the contemporary era: insights into diagnosis, management, and future directions. *JACC Cardiovasc Imaging*. 2018;11(4):628–643.)

tendineae, is clinically and pathologically different. As there is a sudden increase in left atrial volume, the left atrium is unable to compensate and the volume is transmitted to the pulmonary vasculature with development in frank pulmonary edema. Due to a rapid decrease in the effective forward stroke volume of the left ventricle, patients with acute MR typically have cardiogenic shock with signs of end-organ hypoperfusion.

Diagnosis

Symptoms

Symptoms of chronic MR include fatigue, exertional intolerance and dyspnea on exertion. In the advanced stages of MR, development of symptoms of biventricular heart failure, including dyspnea at rest, orthopnea, paroxysmal nocturnal dyspnea, and lower extremity edema can occur. Development of atrial fibrillation is associated with palpitations. Finally, acute MR is associated with abrupt onset of symptoms, cardiogenic shock, respiratory failure, and is considered a relative surgical emergency.

Signs

The classic auscultatory findings of MR are best heard at the apex and include a blowing murmur radiating to the axilla with a diminished S1. As MR progresses, the murmur will become holodiastolic. MV prolapse typically has a midsystolic click and a late systolic ejection murmur. An S3 develops due to increased volume of blood entering the left ventricle during early diastolic filling. As the left ventricle dilates, the point of maximum impulse becomes laterally displaced. Finally, in the setting of advanced disease, signs of biventricular heart failure can be found, including pulmonary rales, and elevated jugular venous pressures.

Imaging

Due to the posterior location of the left atrium and MV apparatus, transesophageal echocardiography is the gold standard for evaluation of the mechanism of MR. TEE allows multiplanar as well as three-dimensional evaluation of the MV leaflets and subvalvular apparatus. Assessment of severity is performed by quantitative and semiquantitative variables including a ratio of regurgitant jet area:left atrial area, pulmonary vein filling patterns, effective regurgitant orifice area, regurgitant volume, and regurgitant fraction.

As with MS, exercise echocardiography can be useful in delineating the timing of intervention and differentiation between other causes of symptomatology. Additionally, magnetic resonance imaging (MRI) allows accurate quantification of regurgitant volumes, biventricular function and volumes. MRI also allows for definition of fibrosis through late-gadolinium enhancement.

Natural History

There is a significant difference in the mortality between primary and secondary MR. Patients with mild to moderate primary MR usually remain asymptomatic with little or no hemodynamic compromise for many years. At the point of symptoms, the mortality rate is 6% to 7% per year, and 90% of patients die or require an MV operation within 10 years.[44] In contrast, secondary MR has survival similar to patients with heart failure.

Treatment

The treatment of MR is dictated by the mechanism of MR. In primary MR, surgery is indicated with symptomatic severe MR, or asymptomatic severe MR with signs of LV dysfunction (EF ≤60% or end-systolic diameter ≥40 mm), or progressive LV size, or the patient is a low-risk surgical candidate at a comprehensive valve center.[17] When a patient with primary MR meets criteria for operative management, medical therapy is supportive and a bridge to surgery. Medical therapy includes reduction of afterload with antihypertensives, loop diuretics for pulmonary congestion, and anticoagulation in the setting of concomitant atrial fibrillation. Acute primary MR may also necessitate more intensive preoperative support such as an intra-aortic balloon pump, which will provide afterload reduction and increase coronary artery perfusion.

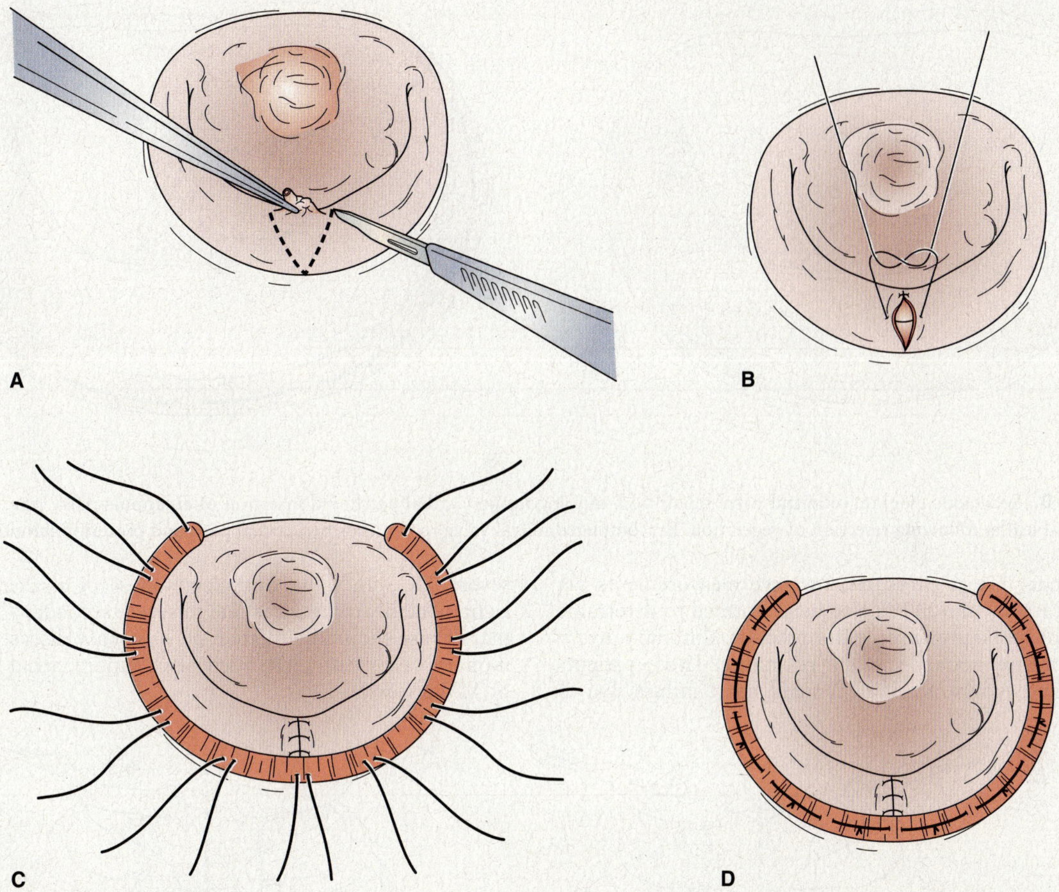

Figure 79.9. Schematic diagram of posterior mitral valve repair and insertion of annuloplasty ring. **A:** Resection of prolapsing segment. P2 triangular section. **B:** Suture reconstruction of P2 scallop. **C:** Posterior annular sutures placed through annuloplasty band. **D:** Completed mitral valve repair.

Patients with secondary (functional) MR, should undergo aggressive titration of guideline-directed heart failure therapy prior to surgical or transcatheter therapy, as medical therapy can promote reverse remodeling of the left ventricle and therefore decrease the severity of MR. Guideline-directed medical therapy (GDMT) includes renin–angiotensin–aldosterone system inhibition, beta-adrenergic blockade, mineralocorticoid receptor antagonists, and sodium-glucose cotransporter-2 inhibitors.[45] Cardiac resynchronization therapy (CRT-D) also improves ventricular synchrony and can improve ventricular remodeling.[46]

Surgery for primary MR should be performed before the onset of irreversible LV dysfunction. MV repair is the preferred surgical therapy over valve replacement, as it is low risk, durable, preserves the native valve apparatus, avoids the risk of long-term anticoagulation (as compared to mechanical valve replacement), and avoids the risk of bioprosthetic valve failure. In primary MR, valve repair has been shown to restore life expectancy to that of the general population, regardless of age.[47] Durability of repair and survival has also been linked to surgeon and institutional volume of MV repair.[48] Techniques for MV repair in primary MR include leaflet plication, leaflet resection, commissuroplasty, cleft closure, or remodeling the zone of coaptation by creating artificial chordae. Whichever repair technique is used, the goal is restoration of adequate leaflet coaptation and the repair must be supplemented by the placement of a prosthetic annuloplasty ring or band (**Fig. 79.9**).

MV repair, if possible, is also the preferred surgical therapy in patients with MV endocarditis. After thorough debridement of all infected tissue, leaflet reconstruction, if necessary, can be accomplished with the use of an autologous pericardial patch and stabilized with an annuloplasty (**Fig. 79.10**). These techniques can be performed through a variety of approaches including a full sternotomy or minimally invasive approaches: hemisternotomy, lateral right thoracotomy, or a robotic approach (**Fig. 79.11**). MV replacement is indicated when adequate MV repair cannot be accomplished. Considerations to the type of valve prosthesis are similar to those discussed in the AV section.

Surgical indications in functional MR are met only when patients with severe MR have failed GDMT and have persistent symptoms, or if they are undergoing concomitant coronary artery bypass grafting. For patients with severe functional MR who have failed GDMT, have suitable anatomy, and are at high or prohibitive surgical risk for MV repair, transcatheter edge–edge MV repair is a treatment option.[17] There is significant ongoing research and innovation in percutaneous transcatheter MV replacement, annuloplasty, and chordal repair technologies.[49]

Tricuspid Valve Disease

TV disease is less common than AV and MV disease. TR, the most common form of TV dysfunction, can occur with anatomically normal or abnormal valves. Functional TR is caused by right ventricular dilation and consequent leaflet malcoaptation in an otherwise anatomically normal valve. Right ventricular enlargement occurs in patients with pulmonary hypertension, most commonly caused by long-standing MV dysfunction. Primary TR can be caused by permanent pacemaker leads that cross through the TV, endocarditis causing leaflet destruction (most commonly occurring in intravenous drug users), or in congenital heart disease with Ebstein anomaly (discussed above). Echocardiography is used to assess the degree of TR, anatomy of the TV, right ventricular function,

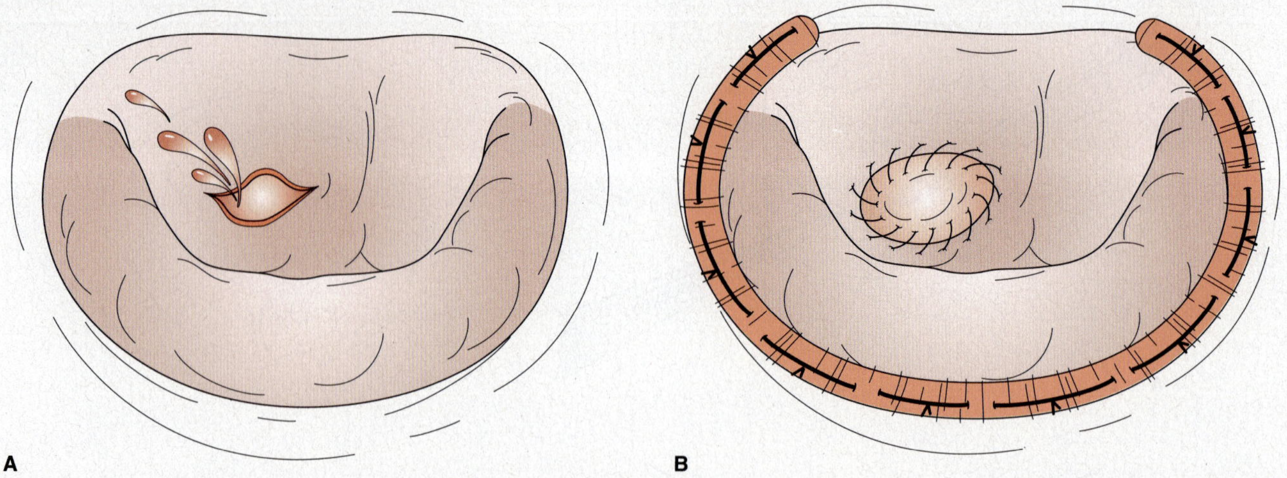

Figure 79.10. Schematic diagram of mitral valve repair with autologous pericardial patch and insertion of an annuloplasty ring. **A:** Defect in anterior mitral leaflet following resection of vegetation. **B:** Completed mitral valve repair after pericardial path and posterior annuloplasty.

and pulmonary artery pressures. Invasive measurements via right heart catheterization can also be performed to determine right-sided diastolic pressures, more precise pulmonary artery pressures, and pulmonary vascular resistance. Those patients with signs and symptoms of right-sided heart failure due to severe TR should be optimized on medical therapy. When right-sided heart failure is due to severe secondary TR, the primary cause should be treated, be it primary disease of the pulmonary vasculature, left-sided heart failure, atrial fibrillation, or MV disease.[17]

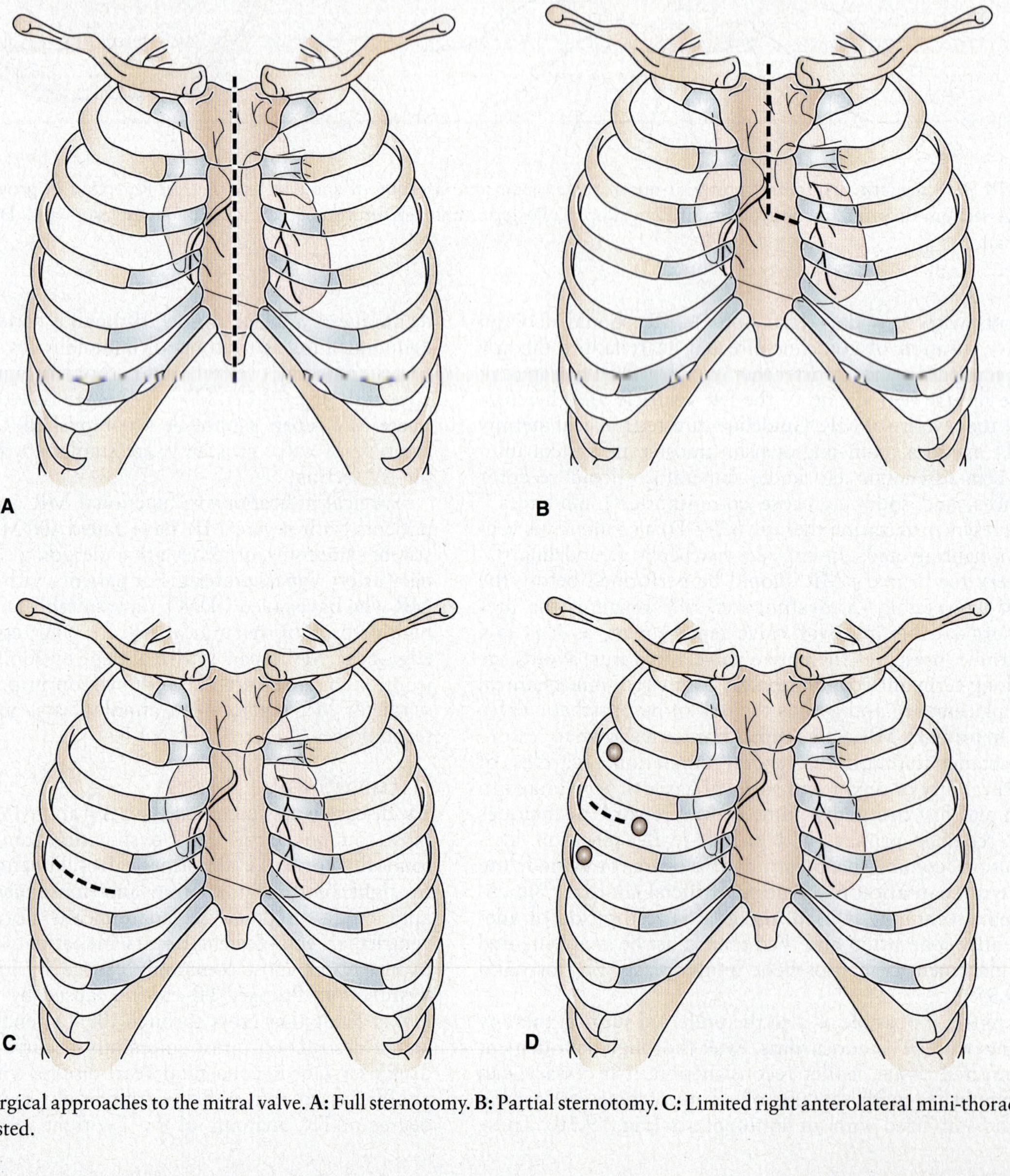

Figure 79.11. Surgical approaches to the mitral valve. **A:** Full sternotomy. **B:** Partial sternotomy. **C:** Limited right anterolateral mini-thoracotomy. **D:** Robotically assisted.

In secondary TR, mild to moderate regurgitation will often resolve following correction of the primary disease. Severe functional TR can also be corrected by reduction in the diameter of the tricuspid annulus using an annuloplasty band. Surgery is indicated in patients with severe symptomatic TR with signs or symptoms of right-sided heart failure, or progressive TR with tricuspid annular dilation >40 mm, or two prior signs and symptoms of right-sided heart failure, and who are undergoing left-sided valve surgery.[17] Severe endocarditis
4 requires complete resection of infected valve tissue, followed by TV reconstruction with pericardium or replacement with a bioprosthesis. In active drug users, insertion of a valve prosthesis may be delayed by several months following resection to decrease the risk of recurrent endocarditis.

Pulmonic Valve Pathology

Pathology of the pulmonic valve is most commonly related to congenital heart defects, and beyond the scope of this chapter. Both surgical- and catheter-based interventions are available, depending on the pathology, degree of obstruction, prior interventions, and age of the patient.[50]

ACKNOWLEDGMENTS

We gratefully acknowledge the contributions of previous edition authors, Daniel J. P. Burns, Per Wierup, and A. Marc Gillinov, as portions of those chapters have been retained in this revision.

References

1. Wells FC, Anderson RH, eds. *Mitral Valve Disease: Basic Sciences and Current Approaches to Management*. 1st ed. Springer Nature; 2021.
2. Anderson RH. The surgical anatomy of the aortic root. *Multimed Man Cardiothorac Surg*. 2007;2007(102):mmcts.2006.002527.
3. Ormiston JA, Shah PM, Tei C, Wong M. Size and motion of the mitral valve annulus in man. I. A two-dimensional echocardiographic method and findings in normal subjects. *Circulation*. 1981;64(1):113–120.
4. Marzilli M, Sabbah HN, Stein PD. Mitral regurgitation in ventricular premature contractions. The role of the papillary muscle. *Chest*. 1980;77(6):736–740.
5. Martinez RM, O'Leary PW, Anderson RH. Anatomy and echocardiography of the normal and abnormal tricuspid valve. *Cardiol Young*. 2006;16(Suppl 3):4–11.
6. Martinez RM, Anderson RH. Echocardiographic features of the morphologically right ventriculo-arterial junction. *Cardiol Young*. 2005;15(Suppl 1):17–26.
7. Aluru JS, Barsouk A, Saginala K, Rawla P, Barsouk A. Valvular heart disease epidemiology. *Med Sci (Basel)*. 2022;10(2):32.
8. Otto CM, Lind BK, Kitzman DW, Gersh BJ, Siscovick DS. Association of aortic-valve sclerosis with cardiovascular mortality and morbidity in the elderly. *N Engl J Med*. 1999;341(3):142–147.
9. Mohler ER 3rd, Gannon F, Reynolds C, Zimmerman R, Keane MG, Kaplan FS. Bone formation and inflammation in cardiac valves. *Circulation*. 2001;103(11):1522–1528.
10. Huntington K, Hunter AG, Chan KL. A prospective study to assess the frequency of familial clustering of congenital bicuspid aortic valve. *J Am Coll Cardiol*. 1997;30(7):1809–1812.
11. Sievers HH, Schmidtke C. A classification system for the bicuspid aortic valve from 304 surgical specimens. *J Thorac Cardiovasc Surg*. 2007;133(5):1226–1233.
12. Alpert JS. Aortic stenosis: a new face for an old disease. *Arch Intern Med*. 2003;163(15):1769–1770.
13. Watkins DA, Johnson CO, Colquhoun SM, et al. Global, regional, and national burden of rheumatic heart disease, 1990–2015. *N Engl J Med*. 2017;377(8):713–722.
14. Otto CM, Prendergast B. Aortic-valve stenosis–from patients at risk to severe valve obstruction. *N Engl J Med*. 2014;371(8):744–756.
15. Carabello BA. Evaluation and management of patients with aortic stenosis. *Circulation*. 2002;105(15):1746–1750.
16. Rudolph TK, Messika-Zeitoun D, Frey N, et al. Impact of selected comorbidities on the presentation and management of aortic stenosis. *Open Heart*. 2020;7(2):e001271.
17. Otto CM, Nishimura RA, Bonow RO, et al. 2020 ACC/AHA guideline for the management of patients with valvular heart disease: a report of the American college of cardiology/American heart association joint committee on clinical practice guidelines. *Circulation*. 2021;143(5):e72–e227.
18. Pawade T, Sheth T, Guzzetti E, Dweck MR, Clavel MA. Why and how to measure aortic valve calcification in patients with aortic stenosis. *JACC Cardiovasc Imaging*. 2019;12(9):1835–1848.
19. Faggiano P, Aurigemma GP, Rusconi C, Gaasch WH. Progression of valvular aortic stenosis in adults: literature review and clinical implications. *Am Heart J*. 1996;132(2 Pt 1):408–417.
20. Ross J Jr, Braunwald E. Aortic stenosis. *Circulation*. 1968; 38(1 Suppl):61–67.
21. Chiang YP, Chikwe J, Moskowitz AJ, Itagaki S, Adams DH, Egorova NN. Survival and long-term outcomes following bioprosthetic vs mechanical aortic valve replacement in patients aged 50 to 69 years. *JAMA*. 2014;312(13):1323–1329.
22. Ross DN. Replacement of aortic and mitral valves with a pulmonary autograft. *Lancet*. 1967;2(7523):956–958.
23. El-Hamamsy I, Toyoda N, Itagaki S, et al. Propensity-matched comparison of the Ross procedure and prosthetic aortic valve replacement in adults. *J Am Coll Cardiol*. 2022;79(8):805–815.
24. Reardon MJ, Van Mieghem NM, Popma JJ, et al. Surgical or transcatheter aortic-valve replacement in intermediate-risk patients. *N Engl J Med*. 2017;376(14):1321–1331.
25. Smith CR, Leon MB, Mack MJ, et al. Transcatheter versus surgical aortic-valve replacement in high-risk patients. *N Engl J Med*. 2011;364(23):2187–2198.
26. Popma JJ, Deeb GM, Yakubov SJ, et al. Transcatheter aortic-valve replacement with a self-expanding valve in low-risk patients. *N Engl J Med*. 2019;380(18):1706–1715.
27. Swartz MH. *Textbook Physical Diagnosis: History Examination*. WB Saunders Company; 2001.
28. Zoghbi WA, Adams D, Bonow RO, et al. Recommendations for noninvasive evaluation of native valvular regurgitation: a report from the American society of echocardiography developed in collaboration with the society for cardiovascular magnetic resonance. *J Am Soc Echocardiogr*. 2017;30(4):303–371.
29. Cavalcante JL, Lalude OO, Schoenhagen P, Lerakis S. Cardiovascular magnetic resonance imaging for structural and valvular heart disease interventions. *JACC Cardiovasc Interv*. 2016;9(5): 399–425.
30. Ruel M, Kulik A, Lam BK, et al. Long-term outcomes of valve replacement with modern prostheses in young adults. *Eur J Cardiothorac Surg*. 2005;27(3):425–433; discussion 433.
31. Boodhwani M, El Khoury G. Aortic valve repair. *Oper Tech Thorac Cardiovasc Surg*. 2009;14(4):266–280.
32. Yoon SH, Schmidt T, Bleiziffer S, et al. Transcatheter aortic valve replacement in pure native aortic valve regurgitation. *J Am Coll Cardiol*. 2017;70(22):2752–2763.
33. Hensey M, Murdoch DJ, Sathananthan J, et al. First-in-human experience of a new-generation transfemoral transcatheter aortic valve for the treatment of severe aortic regurgitation: the J-Valve transfemoral system. *EuroIntervention*. 2019;14(15):e1553–e1555.
34. Rowe JC, Bland EF, Sprague HB, White PD. The course of mitral stenosis without surgery: ten- and twenty-year perspectives. *Ann Intern Med*. 1960;52(4):741–749.
35. Olesen KH. The natural history of 271 patients with mitral stenosis under medical treatment. *Br Heart J*. 1962;24:349–357.
36. El Oumeiri B, Boodhwani M, Glineur D, et al. Extending the scope of mitral valve repair in rheumatic disease. *Ann Thorac Surg*. 2009;87(6):1735–1740.
37. Tomai F, Gaspardone A, Versaci F, et al. Twenty year follow-up after successful percutaneous balloon mitral valvuloplasty in a large contemporary series of patients with mitral stenosis. *Int J Cardiol*. 2014;177(3):881–885.
38. Wilkins GT, Weyman AE, Abascal VM, Block PC, Palacios IF. Percutaneous balloon dilatation of the mitral valve: an analysis

of echocardiographic variables related to outcome and the mechanism of dilatation. *Br Heart J*. 1988;60(4):299–308.

39. Moss RR, Humphries KH, Gao M, et al. Outcome of mitral valve repair or replacement: a comparison by propensity score analysis. *Circulation*. 2003;108(Suppl 1(10_suppl_1)):II90–II97.
40. Guerrero M, Vemulapalli S, Xiang Q, et al. Thirty-day outcomes of transcatheter mitral valve replacement for degenerated mitral bioprostheses (valve-in-valve), failed surgical rings (valve-in-ring), and native valve with severe mitral annular calcification (valve-in-mitral annular calcification) in the United States: data from the Society of Thoracic Surgeons/American College of Cardiology/Transcatheter Valve Therapy Registry. *Circ Cardiovasc Interv*. 2020;13(3):e008425.
41. Tsao CW, Aday AW, Almarzooq ZI, et al. Heart disease and stroke statistics-2023 update: a report from the American Heart Association. *Circulation*. 2023;147(8):e93–e621.
42. Carpentier A. Cardiac valve surgery—the "French correction." *J Thorac Cardiovasc Surg*. 1983;86:323–337.
43. Levine R, Hagége AA, Judge DP, et al. Mitral valve disease-morphology mechanisms. *Nat Rev Cardiol*. 2015;12:689–710.
44. Ling LH, Enriquez-Sarano M, Seward JB, et al. Clinical outcome of mitral regurgitation due to flail leaflet. *N Engl J Med*. 1996;335(19):1417–1423.
45. Maddox TM, Januzzi JL Jr, Allen LA, et al. 2024 ACC expert consensus decision pathway for treatment of heart failure with reduced ejection fraction: a report of the American college of cardiology solution set oversight committee. *J Am Coll Cardiol*. 2024;83(15): 1444–1488.
46. St John Sutton M, Ghio S, Plappert T, et al. Cardiac resynchronization induces major structural and functional reverse remodeling in patients with New York Heart Association class I/II heart failure. *Circulation*. 2009;120(19):1858–1865.
47. Watt TMF, Brescia AA, Murray SL, et al. Degenerative mitral valve repair restores life expectancy. *Ann Thorac Surg*. 2020;109(3): 794–801.
48. Bolling SF, Li S, O'Brien SM, Brennan JM, Prager RL, Gammie JS. Predictors of mitral valve repair: clinical and surgeon factors. *Ann Thorac Surg*. 2010;90(6):1904–1911; discussion 1912.
49. Yousef S, Arnaoutakis GJ, Gada H, Smith AJC, Sanon S, Sultan I. Transcatheter mitral valve therapies: state of the art. *J Card Surg*. 2022;37(1):225–233.
50. Stout KK, Daniels CJ, Aboulhosn JA, et al. 2018 AHA/ACC guideline for the management of adults with congenital heart disease: Executive Summary: a report of the American College of Cardiology/American Heart Association Task Force on Clinical Practice Guidelines. *Circulation*. 2019;139(14):e698–e800.

Ischemic Heart Disease

Robert B. Hawkins II and Jonathan W. Haft

Key Points

1. Because of its unique physiology, the heart is particularly susceptible to ischemic injury.
2. Atherosclerotic plaques cause ischemia from chronic flow limitations or from unstable plaque rupture.
3. Patients with coronary artery disease will present with either chronic stable angina or an acute coronary syndrome (ACS), which consists of unstable angina, a non–ST-segment myocardial infarction, or an ST-segment myocardial infarction.
4. Several well-described complications from myocardial infarctions must be anticipated and recognized early.
5. Medical treatment of coronary artery disease includes lifestyle modifications and medications to slow the progression and stabilize atherosclerotic plaques.
6. Percutaneous intervention (PCI) of coronary lesions with drug-eluting intracoronary stents continues to iteratively improve.
7. Coronary artery bypass grafting (CABG) involves creation of alternative conduits from the systemic circulation to the epicardial coronary arteries.
8. The left internal mammary artery is the superior conduit for CABG with increasing emphasis on multiple arterial conduits that may improve long-term survival.
9. CABG remains superior to both medical treatment and PCI for patients with complex multivessel disease and diabetes, left main involvement, or multivessel disease involving the left anterior descending artery with left ventricular dysfunction.

CORONARY ANATOMY AND PHYSIOLOGY

The right and left coronary arteries originate from the aorta just above the aortic valve cusps (**Fig. 80.1**). The orifices of the two arteries within the sinuses of Valsalva designate the right and left coronary cusps. The third aortic valve cusp is referred to as the noncoronary cusp. The coronary circulation is traditionally divided into three major territories: The left anterior descending (LAD) and the circumflex territories originate from the left coronary artery, and the right coronary territory usually comes from the right coronary artery.

The origin of the left coronary artery is referred to as the left main and travels posterolaterally to the left behind the pulmonary artery, where it divides into two main branches, the LAD and the circumflex coronary artery. The length of the left main coronary artery is variable, but rarely exceeds 2 cm. Atypically, the left main can be absent and the circumflex and LAD will originate from the aorta via two separate ostia.

The LAD coronary artery emerges from behind the pulmonary artery and travels inferiorly within the interventricular groove to the cardiac apex, sometimes wrapping around it onto the posterior interventricular groove. The LAD gives off two different types of branches: diagonals and septals, both of which are highly variable in size and number. The diagonals take off at acute angles and perfuse the anterolateral surface of the left ventricle. Septal branches, the first of which is typically quite prominent, emerge at a right angle from the LAD and supply the interventricular septum. The LAD is the most prominent of the three coronary territories, and carries approximately 50% of left ventricular myocardial blood flow, supplying the anterior, anterolateral, septal, and apical walls.

The circumflex coronary artery continues from the left main coronary and travels within the posterior atrioventricular groove. Branches from the circumflex are called obtuse marginal arteries, and also vary greatly in size and number. In 80% to 90% of people, the terminal branch of the circumflex supplies the posterolateral wall of the left ventricle. In the remaining 10% to 20%, the circumflex continues to the posterior interventricular septum and terminates as the posterior descending artery (PDA). This is referred to as a left dominant heart, where the left main coronary artery is supplying the posterior interventricular septum and atrioventricular node. Some patients will have a third branch of the left main referred to as the ramus intermedius, or intermediate branch. If present, this vessel is typically large, and supplies much of the anterolateral wall of the left ventricle.

The right coronary artery originates from the anterior right sinus of Valsalva and descends in the right atrioventricular groove. One or more acute marginal branches feed the right ventricular free wall. In 80% to 90% of patients, the right coronary artery continues to the posterior interventricular septum and supplies the PDA and often a variable-sized right posterolateral artery. This is referred to as a right dominant heart. Approximately 10% of patients will be considered co-dominant with both right and left sides supplying the atrioventricular node. Near the origin of the posterior descending branch, a small characteristic vessel can be seen supplying the atrioventricular node. This branch can become important in acute right coronary artery occlusions, resulting in life-threatening heart block and bradycardia. A small proximal branch of the right coronary artery supplies the sinus node on the anterolateral surface of the superior vena cava.

Anomalous origin of the coronary arteries occurs in 0.3% to 1% of the population, and their anatomy is varied and complex. Rarely, the left coronary arises from the pulmonary artery. This pathology is diagnosed in infancy, as the myocardium becomes profoundly ischemic when pulmonary

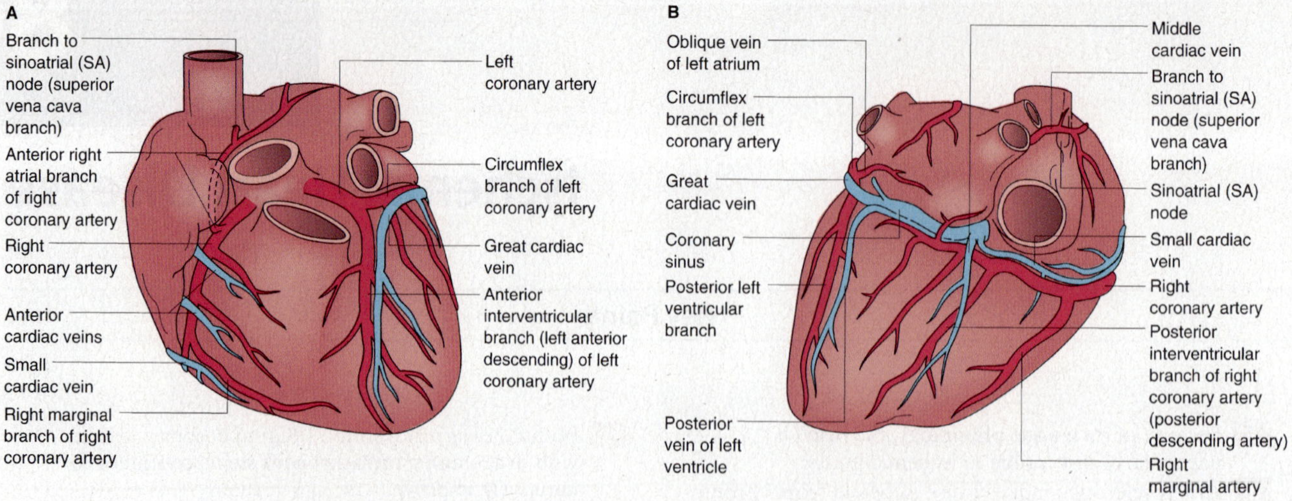

Figure 80.1. Anatomy of the cardiac circulation. **A:** Anterior view. **B:** Posterior view.

vascular resistance falls and myocardial perfusion decreases requiring surgical correction. The coronaries may also originate from atypical aortic root sinuses, and their trajectory is variable. The most worrisome problem occurs when the LAD or left main coronary artery originates from the right sinus of Valsalva. The LAD then travels posteriorly and to the left coursing between the pulmonary artery and the aortic root. This trajectory is described as "malignant" because of the potential for compression between the great vessels, particularly during exercise. Although there is little evidence, it is generally accepted that coronary unroofing or a revascularization strategy should be considered in symptomatic patients with "malignant" coronary anomalies or in asymptomatic patients with demonstrable ischemia on exercise-based noninvasive testing (eg, exercise stress echocardiogram).[1]

Venous anatomy is more predictable, and very little pathology within this system is encountered. Three named venous branches can be identified: the middle cardiac vein in the posterior interventricular groove, the posterior cardiac vein along the obtuse margin of the heart, and the great (or anterior) cardiac vein along the anterior interventricular groove. All three drain into one confluence known as the coronary sinus along the posterior atrioventricular groove (**Fig. 80.1**). The coronary sinus empties posteriorly into the right atrium between the inferior vena cava and the annulus of the tricuspid valve. A persistent left superior vena cava will typically drain into the coronary sinus posterolaterally. In addition to these identifiable named veins, the myocardium also drains directly into all chambers of the heart via thebesian veins.

1 Myocardial work consumes an enormous amount of energy substrate. In fact, only 10% to 20% of myocardial energy requirements are related to basal functions; the remainder is utilized during the continuous energy-dependent calcium mobilization and myofilament cross-linking during cyclic contraction and relaxation. Even at rest, the heart maximally extracts oxygen delivered from the bloodstream, leaving venous saturation in the coronary sinus typically 20% or less. Thus, increased energy requirements must be met with augmentation in blood oxygen delivery. When insufficient supply of oxygen is available, such as with obstructive coronary disease and increased consumption, anaerobic metabolism cannot generate enough energy substrate to perform myocardial contraction.[2] As a result, cardiac function deteriorates immediately.

The heart and its coronary circulation have a unique capacity to markedly increase blood flow, and thus oxygen delivery, during periods of increased needs.[3] While basal coronary blood flow is approximately 10 mL/kg, this can increase up to sixfold with exercise by autoregulatory mechanisms. Specifically, adenosine accumulates from the breakdown of the energy substrate adenosine triphosphate (ATP). This results in a feedback loop where adenosine receptors within the media of coronary arteries lead to vasodilation and increased blood flow to myocardial regions with increased adenosine generation. Increased myocardial activity also activates nitric oxide synthase within coronary endothelial cells, producing the powerful vasodilator nitric oxide. By immediately altering the vessel diameter and thus changing the resistance properties of epicardial vessels, these two short-acting mediators can rapidly alter coronary flow rates to meet changing energy requirements. Most coronary resistance occurs in the arterioles and not the large epicardial vessels such that the coronary microvasculature (prearterioles, arterioles, and capillaries) is largely responsible for autoregulation of blood flow.

The coronary circulation is further uniquely challenged by blood flow in the coronary arteries occurring almost entirely during diastole. During systole, increased cavitary pressure compresses intramyocardial vessels and virtually eliminates forward flow. The diastolic pressure gradient and the duration of diastole are large determinants of coronary flow. Tachycardia not only increases oxygen consumption, but also reduces the time available for myocardial perfusion, increasing the demands for epicardial flow. The rise in ventricular diastolic pressure seen in heart failure also reduces perfusion pressure at a time when heart function is often already reduced.

CORONARY ATHEROSCLEROSIS

Atherosclerosis is a progressive multifocal disease of medium and large muscular arteries of the systemic circulation. Atherosclerotic plaques or atheromas can occur anywhere in the systemic circulation but tend to present clinically in varying quantities in the coronary circulation, carotid arteries, splanchnic vessels, and lower extremities. The lesions tend to occur predominantly at vessel bifurcations, sharp curvatures, and other regions creating pressure wave reflections and recirculation.[4] All plaques consist of smooth muscle proliferation and intracellular and extracellular lipid deposition within the arterial intima (**Fig. 80.2**). The predecessor, "fatty streaks," can be seen as early as the first two decades of life as small and unobstructing. However, under certain clinical circumstances, endothelial injury from cigarette smoke, hypercholesterolemia, hyperglycemia, hypertension, or other causes of inflammation initiates a cascade of events. These include endothelial dysfunction with expression of adhesion molecules, which bind circulating inflammatory cells like monocytes. The activated

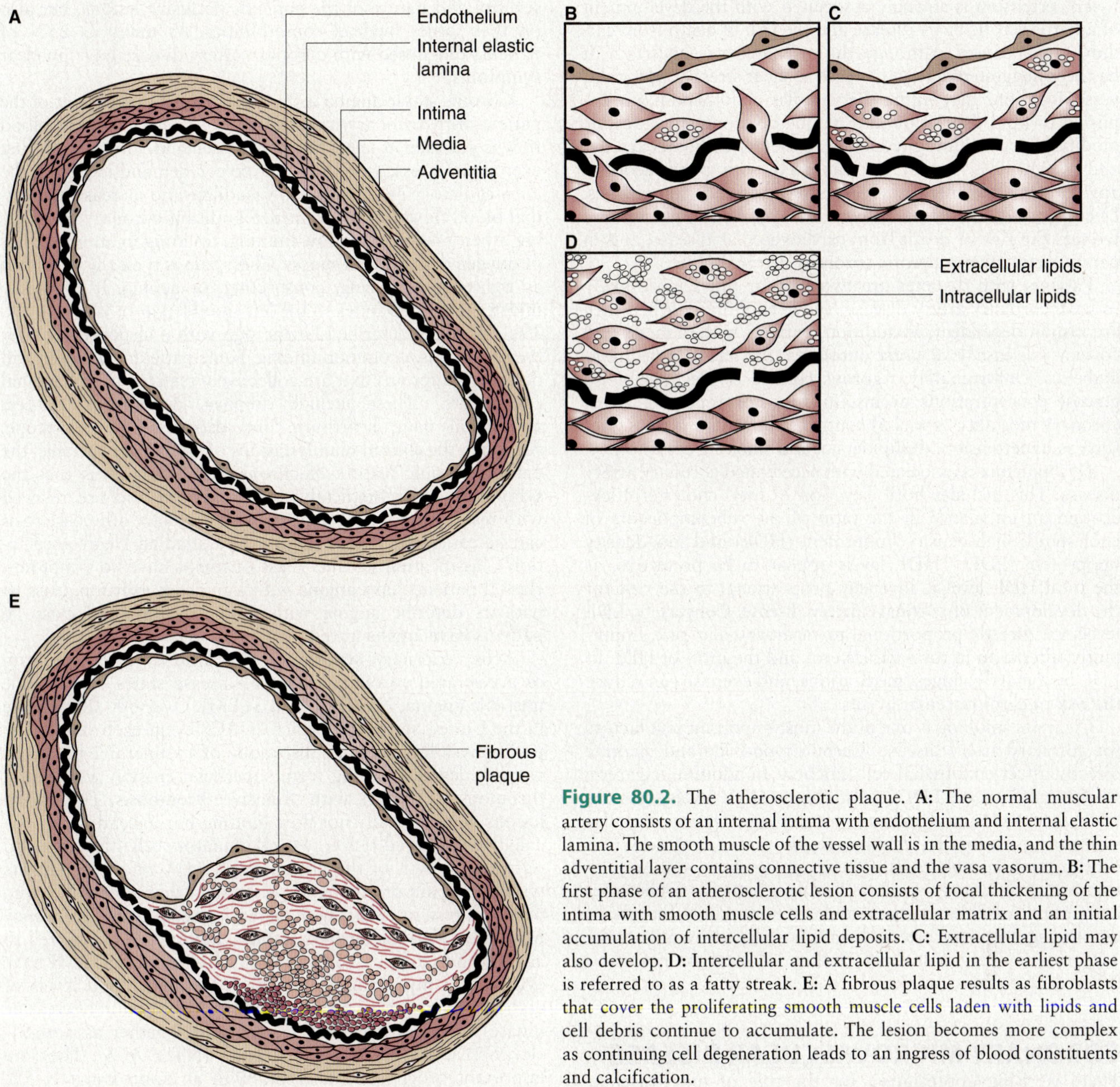

Figure 80.2. The atherosclerotic plaque. **A:** The normal muscular artery consists of an internal intima with endothelium and internal elastic lamina. The smooth muscle of the vessel wall is in the media, and the thin adventitial layer contains connective tissue and the vasa vasorum. **B:** The first phase of an atherosclerotic lesion consists of focal thickening of the intima with smooth muscle cells and extracellular matrix and an initial accumulation of intercellular lipid deposits. **C:** Extracellular lipid may also develop. **D:** Intercellular and extracellular lipid in the earliest phase is referred to as a fatty streak. **E:** A fibrous plaque results as fibroblasts that cover the proliferating smooth muscle cells laden with lipids and cell debris continue to accumulate. The lesion becomes more complex as continuing cell degeneration leads to an ingress of blood constituents and calcification.

monocyte transmigrates into the vessel wall and ingests accumulated lipids. In turn, they release cytokines, which enhance endothelial cell adhesion molecule expression and alter endothelial cell nitric oxide production promoting vasoconstriction and platelet activation and also stimulating the activation of other inflammatory cells including neutrophils and T lymphocytes. The activated monocytes accelerate further lipid accumulation and smooth muscle cell proliferation. The result is an enlarging plaque encroaching on the arterial lumen, separated from the bloodstream by a collagen-rich fibrous plaque.

2 Within the coronary circulation, atherosclerotic stenotic lesions are generally restricted to the proximal regions of the large epicardial coronary arteries. Stenoses found in the LAD and circumflex vessels are frequently isolated, short, and in the proximal segments. However, the right coronary artery often develops diffuse obstructions, although rarely extending into the posterior descending or intramural branches. For reasons that are unclear, atherosclerosis is rarely found within intramyocardial segments of the coronary arteries. Symptoms from these atherosclerotic plaques can occur from a variety of proposed mechanisms. First, the lesion can cause flow limitations, particularly when the luminal cross-sectional area is reduced by at least 75%. With this degree of obstruction, increased myocardial demand outstrips the vasodilatory reserve resulting in transient myocardial ischemia until demand returns to baseline. Symptomatically this is known as exertional angina. The atherosclerotic plaque also causes coronary ischemia when the lesion becomes unstable. The fibrous plaque can fracture or rupture, exposing the bloodstream to the highly thrombogenic internal plaque contents. This can lead to complete epicardial thrombosis, the presumed mechanism of ST-segment elevation myocardial infarction (STEMI). Additionally, subtotal plaque disruption can cause vasoconstriction, platelet activation, and embolization, resulting in ischemia without total occlusion of the epicardial vessel. This is the presumed mechanism of unstable angina (UA) and non–ST-segment elevation myocardial infarction (NSTEMI). Some plaques are more prone to rupture than others, and the composition of the fibrous cap may be an identifiable feature of an unstable lesion.

Risk factors for coronary atherosclerosis include advanced age, family history, male sex, hypertension, diabetes mellitus, dyslipidemia, and cigarette smoking. Risk factor modification and lifestyle interventions can reduce their risk of cardiac events.

Hypertension is strongly associated with the development of atherosclerotic heart disease and the risk of death from cardiovascular causes. Although the mechanism is uncertain, it has been suggested that an increase in shear stress at particular vessel locations may injure the vascular endothelium, predisposing to lipid deposition and plaque development. Lifestyle modifications including reduction in dietary sodium, exercise, and weight loss should be combined with pharmacotherapy for which numerous societies have provided guidelines. Unequivocally, reduction in elevated systolic blood pressure reduces the risk of death from cardiovascular disease, and in particular of atherosclerotic coronary artery disease.

Patients with diabetes are two to four times more likely to have coronary artery disease, and even more so when they are insulin dependent. In addition, patients with diabetes and coronary disease have worse outcomes than age-matched nondiabetics. Unfortunately, rigorous control of elevated blood glucose concentrations by insulin does not appear to affect coronary mortality as well as control of other risk factors does such as hypertension, dyslipidemia, and smoking cessation.[5]

Dyslipidemia is associated with accelerated coronary artery disease. This includes both elevation of total cholesterol levels and an imbalance in the ratio of the subcomponents of cholesterol: high-density lipoprotein (HDL) and low-density lipoprotein (LDL).[6] HDL levels appear to be protective, as the total HDL level is inversely proportional to the risk for the development of coronary artery disease. Conversely, LDL levels are directly proportional to cardiovascular risk. Importantly, alteration in total cholesterol and the ratio of HDL to LDL by dietary changes, medications, and exercise can reduce the risk of cardiovascular events.[7]

Cigarette smoking is one of the most important risk factors for coronary artery disease. Carbon monoxide and nicotine directly affect endothelial cell function. In addition, cigarette smoke can increase LDL levels, reduce HDL levels, increase fibrinogen levels, and increase platelet aggregation. Regular smokers have a four to five times higher rate of cardiovascular death than nonsmokers, and there appears to be a dose relationship, with heavier smokers having a higher prevalence of coronary disease than lighter smokers. Fortunately, the risk of developing coronary artery disease is reduced by 50% after 1 year of smoking abstinence, and at 10 years the risk is no different from never smokers.[8]

CORONARY MICROVASCULAR DISEASE

There is rising appreciation for the role of microvascular dysfunction in addition to atherosclerosis in coronary artery disease pathology. Up to 60% of patients with angina and nonobstructive coronary disease will have coronary microvascular dysfunction. Structural and functional remodeling leads to vasoconstriction and reduced vasodilatory capacity.[9] Functional changes with endothelial and vascular smooth muscle cell dysfunction impair vasodilation or cause vasospasm. Structural remodeling of the intima and media of arterioles and capillaries leads to luminal narrowing. Myocardial aspects such as left ventricular hypertrophy and diastolic dysfunction related to fibrosis also lead to reduced microvascular perfusion. Position emission tomography is the optimal method for assessment of microvascular dysfunction.[10] Risk factors overlap with traditional cardiac risk factors including hypertension, diabetes, hyperlipidemia, but also include heart failure with reduced or preserved ejection fraction. Management of these risk factors is the mainstay of therapy for coronary microvascular disease.

PATIENT PRESENTATION

The clinical manifestations of ischemic heart disease, termed angina pectoralis, occur when myocardial oxygen demand exceeds supply. The symptoms and acuity depend on the severity and nature of the patient's occlusive lesions, but also on their other medical comorbidities. As many as 25% of patients diagnosed with coronary artery disease have no clear symptoms.

3 Chronic stable angina is the most frequent complaint of the patient with coronary artery disease. At rest, coronary blood flow is adequate to meet myocardial demand. However, during exercise or stress, as myocardial oxygen demand increases, the autoregulatory mechanisms to vasodilate and increase myocardial blood flow are constrained. Significant coronary obstructing atheromas become flow limiting, resulting in an imbalance of oxygen demand and supply. Chest pain is typically described as tightness, squeezing, constricting, or aching. It is usually midsternal and radiates to the left shoulder, arm, jaw, or neck. The classically described Levine sign with a clenched fist over the sternum is a common finding. Some patients, however, will describe symptoms that are collectively referred to as "anginal equivalents." These include dyspnea, diaphoresis, nausea, abdominal pain, heartburn, and dizziness or presyncope. Although the clinical manifestations of angina are variable, the pathognomonic feature of chronic stable angina is that the symptoms occur predictably with exertion and are relieved with rest. Symptoms of patients with coronary atherosclerosis can be categorized according to the Canadian Heart Association Classification scheme. Class I patients have no symptoms, class II patients have angina with significant exertion, class III patients describe angina with mild exertion, and class IV patients have angina at rest.

Acute coronary syndromes (ACSs) refer to a spectrum of accelerated coronary occlusive disease states and include unstable angina, NSTEMI, and STEMI. Over 800,000 people in the United States experience an ACS event each year.[11] The pathophysiology includes disruption of a vulnerable plaque to varying degrees ranging from superficial erosion with mural thrombus to rupture with occlusive thrombosis. The culprit lesions were typically not flow limiting but instead were noncalcified with lipid-rich cores, inflammatory cell infiltrates, and outward growth of the arterial wall.[12] UA refers to patients with chest pain or an anginal equivalent that is new in onset, occurs at rest, or occurs with increasing severity and frequency from their baseline chronic stable symptoms, also referred to as crescendo angina. Patients who develop an NSTEMI have evidence of myocardial injury with elevated blood levels of myocardial enzymes (troponin and the MB fraction of creatine kinase). UA and NSTEMI are grouped together as non–ST-elevation acute coronary syndromes (NSTE-ACS). They are important prognostic indicators with an approximately 5% 1-year mortality rate, and NSTEMI carries the highest 2-year mortality at up to 20% of an ACS event.

STEMI represents the consequences of large epicardial vessel occlusion, typically associated with plaque rupture and occlusive thrombosis. Patients describe acute-onset chest pain that does not resolve with rest or nitroglycerine and is typically more severe than typical stable angina symptoms. Patients will often describe additional symptoms such as diaphoresis, nausea, dizziness, and epigastric pain. Although improvements in health systems have drastically increased survival from myocardial infarction, mortality for STEMI remains near 5% to 10%, with the majority of that risk isolated to the first 90 days.

COMPLICATIONS OF ACUTE MYOCARDIAL INFARCTIONS

4 STEMIs can create widespread myocyte necrosis, often resulting in catastrophic complications that require urgent intervention. Anticipation and early diagnosis can improve outcomes. These complications include cardiogenic shock, postinfarct ventricular septal defect (VSD), free wall rupture, and acute mitral valve regurgitation (**Table 80.1**). Prompt revascularization is key to preventing mechanical complications from STEMI.

Table 80.1. Complications of Acute Myocardial Infarctions

Complication	Diagnosis	Treatment
Cardiogenic shock	Echocardiography, pulmonary artery catheter	Inotropes, intra-aortic balloon pump, VAD
Ventricular septal defect	Echocardiography, cardiac catheterization	Surgical ventricular septal defect repair
Papillary muscle rupture	Echocardiography	Surgical valve replacement
Ventricular free wall rupture	Echocardiography, ventriculography	Emergent repair of ventricular defect

Cardiogenic Shock

Cardiogenic shock is a state in which cardiac output (CO) is insufficient to meet metabolic demands, despite adequate intravascular filling pressures. Between 5% and 10% of patients with acute myocardial infarctions develop cardiogenic shock. A large proportion of these patients progress to shock after arrival, typically more than 24 hours after initial presentation.[13] Overall mortality is approximately 60%, with very little improvement over recent decades. Treatments include fluids and inotropic agents to optimize myocardial contraction. Insertion of an intra-aortic balloon counterpulsation pump (IABP) can improve coronary perfusion by diastolic augmentation of perfusion pressure. This can have a profound impact by improving contractile function of peri-infarct territories. Although there is significant afterload reduction afforded by the IABP, CO typically increases by only 15% to 20%. More severe cases of shock can be treated with temporary mechanical circulatory support including percutaneous ventricular assist devices (VADs) for single-ventricle failure or extracorporeal membrane oxygenation (ECMO) for biventricular failure.[14] While these options may only be available in selected regional medical centers, durable long-term survival can be obtained in a highly selected patient population.[15] Emergent salvage revascularization can reduce mortality, with sustained benefits seen over long-term follow-up.[16]

Postinfarction Ventricular Septal Defect

A postinfarction VSD is an infrequent complication occurring after fewer than 1% of acute myocardial infarctions. The infarct is most commonly in the LAD territory, with the defect in the distal septum. Alternatively, acute right coronary occlusion can lead to a VSD in the posterobasilar septum. They typically present 5 to 10 days following initial presentation. The diagnosis should be considered in a patient in whom cardiogenic shock with refractory hypotension and pulmonary edema develops suddenly in this time frame following a myocardial infarction. On physical examination, an unmistakable holosystolic murmur can be heard over the entire precordium. The diagnosis is confirmed with echocardiography using Doppler techniques to demonstrate flow across the interventricular septum. Right heart catheterization will reveal a step-up in oxygen saturation from the right atrium to the pulmonary artery. Medical therapy involves stabilization to optimize CO and end-organ perfusion. Refractory hypotension is typical, excluding the use of afterload reducing agents. Intra-aortic balloon counterpulsation can occasionally be helpful for afterload reduction and to optimize coronary perfusion. Mechanical circulatory support can be utilized as a bridge to surgical intervention for unstable patients. Emergent surgical intervention includes revascularization and patch closure of the ventricular defect. For surgical candidates, survival rates of approximately 50% can be expected.[17]

Papillary Muscle Rupture

Severe regurgitation of the mitral valve can occur after acute myocardial infarctions, with a frequency of less than 1%. The mechanism is related to infarction of one of the papillary muscles, with resultant disruption of the mitral subvalvar apparatus and failed leaflet coaptation. Posteroinferior MIs lead to this complication two to three times more frequently than anterior infarctions, presumably because there is more collateral blood flow to the anterolateral papillary muscle compared to the posteriomedial. While chronic mitral regurgitation can be well tolerated through adaptive changes in the left atrium and pulmonary vascular bed, severe acute mitral regurgitation results in immediate heart failure, as the small left atrium offers little compliance for the massive volume overload. Papillary muscle rupture develops typically 3 to 5 days following myocardial infarction. Patients will describe acute-onset dyspnea, pulmonary edema, and possibly signs of cardiogenic shock. The diagnosis should be suspected in any patient after myocardial infarction with a new holosystolic murmur heard at the apex. Bedside surface echocardiography typically demonstrates the mitral regurgitation, and the flail leaflet may be seen. For more definitive imaging, transesophageal echocardiography (TEE) can be performed. Not only will the mitral valve pathology be clearly seen, but also alternative diagnoses such as a postinfarct VSD can be excluded. In addition to the treatments typically employed for myocardial infarctions, immediate medical therapy of ruptured papillary muscles involves afterload reduction when tolerated, with infusions of nitroglycerine or nitroprusside. If CO cannot be maintained, intra-aortic balloon counterpulsation or mechanical circulatory support can be helpful. Definitive therapy involves prompt surgical correction with mitral valve replacement, or less commonly repair, and coronary artery bypass grafting (CABG) as indicated. Surgery is associated with a high perioperative mortality rate of 20%.[18]

Ventricular Free Wall Rupture

Ventricular free wall rupture after myocardial infarction is infrequently encountered clinically, likely because of the exceedingly high mortality. The actual incidence is unknown, but may represent up to 30% of all deaths after acute myocardial infarctions. Like postinfarct VSD and papillary muscle rupture, they tend to occur between 3 and 6 days after infarction. Free wall ruptures can present in essentially one of three ways: (a) a simple full-thickness tear with catastrophic hemorrhage and death from tamponade (b) a complex serpiginous tear, partially contained leading to shock or (c) a growing pseudoaneurysm leading to heart failure. Patients with free wall rupture will typically present with cardiogenic shock and tamponade. Echocardiography will demonstrate a large pericardial effusion, frequently with echo-dense clot or ventricular wall defects. Emergent surgical intervention is required, often without coronary angiography or other time-consuming diagnostic tests. Once the pericardium is opened and cardiac tamponade is relieved, hemodynamic stability is often achieved. The site of hemorrhage is identified by the necrotic-appearing myocardium and adherent thrombus. The defect can be closed with large mattress sutures reinforced with Teflon felt strips with or without patch reinforcement. Some have advocated covering the defect with a large Teflon felt patch using biologic adhesives, avoiding sutures altogether.[19] Subacute presentation can occur months after the rupture allowing time for typical preoperative testing prior to urgent repair given unpredictable further rupture characteristics. Late presentation with a pseudoaneurysm is often stable and surgical intervention driven more by heart failure and coronary disease burden than to

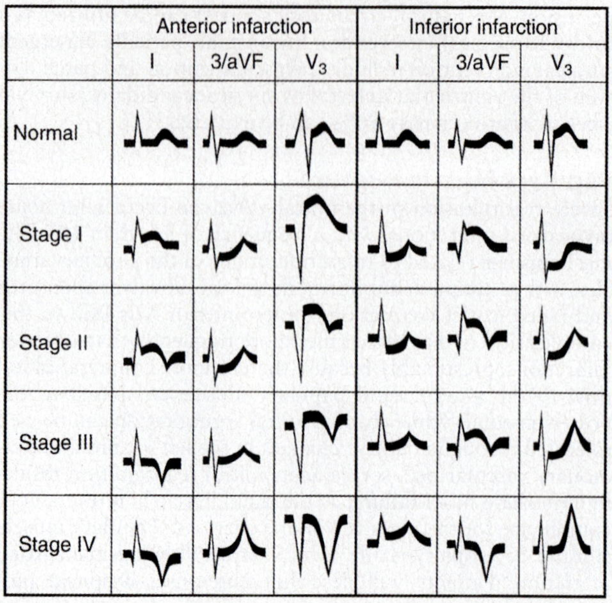

Figure 80.3. The electrocardiogram in an acute myocardial infarction.

prevent tamponade. Given that posterior ruptures are three times more common than anterior, these repairs must not only address the rupture but typically require mitral valve intervention as well.

DIAGNOSIS

The initial diagnostic tool for patients presenting with chest pain is the resting electrocardiogram (ECG). Although the majority of patients with chronic stable angina will have a normal ECG pattern, evidence of previous myocardial infarctions may be identified, either with the presence of Q waves or conduction abnormalities. Patients with an acute myocardial infarction may demonstrate ST-segment elevation (**Fig. 80.3**), prompting urgent intervention. Occasionally, more subtle ECG findings may provide clues that the chest pain is ischemic in etiology. Although nonspecific, these changes may include ST-segment depression or T-wave inversions.

During a myocardial infarction, the dying myocytes release enzymes specific to cardiac muscle into the bloodstream. These enzymes can be detected from laboratory analysis and are pathognomonic of myocardial infarction. The MB fraction of creatine kinase is cardiac specific and rises within 8 to 24 hours of infarction and returns to baseline within 2 days. Cardiac troponin has even greater specificity and serum levels rise faster than creatine kinase, improving both the speed and accuracy in the laboratory diagnosis of an acute myocardial infarction in the absence of clear ECG changes.[20]

For asymptomatic patients, or those with chronic stable angina, the most widely used diagnostic test to evaluate for coronary artery disease is exercise electrocardiography, or a "stress test." Using standardized protocols, patients are exercised on a treadmill while the 12-lead ECG is continuously recorded. Alternatively, for those patients unable to walk, a bicycle ergometer may be used. Testing is continued until patient symptoms are noted or until the development of significant downward-sloping ST-segment depression, suggesting myocardial ischemia (**Fig. 80.4**). The diagnostic accuracy of exercise stress ECG testing can be enhanced with myocardial perfusion imaging. Several radioactive tracers are used clinically, the most frequent of which is thallium-201. Because of its similarities to potassium ions, it is taken up preferentially by viable cardiac myocytes. Its distribution within the myocardium is proportional to the rate of perfusion. During stress, regions of underperfused myocardium will take up less thallium, resulting in a visible defect. Following a period of rest and reperfusion, thallium uptake normalizes, demonstrating a "reversible defect."

In some cases, patients are unable to exercise because of additional physical or psychological limitations. Pharmacologic agents can substitute for exercise by increasing myocardial oxygen demand (dobutamine) or by directly vasodilating coronary arteries (adenosine or dipyridamole), thus demonstrating regions with fixed restrictions in myocardial blood flow. Echocardiography can be used as an alternative to nuclear perfusion imaging and can be utilized with either exercise or pharmacologic protocols. Regional changes in wall motion will be observed during myocardial ischemia, followed by restoration of normal myocardial contraction after rest or discontinuation of dobutamine. Echocardiography can also identify valvular abnormalities or other conditions that may influence treatment choices.

Coronary angiography, also known as cardiac catheterization, is the definitive tool for diagnosing coronary atherosclerotic disease. Indications include symptomatic patients with typical angina refractory to medical treatments, patients with significant ischemia on exercise or pharmacologic stress testing, patients with a STEMI, or patients with an NSTE-ACS at high risk for recurrent events or persistent angina. Patients with valvular heart disease who are scheduled to undergo surgical correction should also undergo coronary angiography to identify coexisting coronary lesions, which can be addressed at the time of the valve surgery. After percutaneous access is obtained

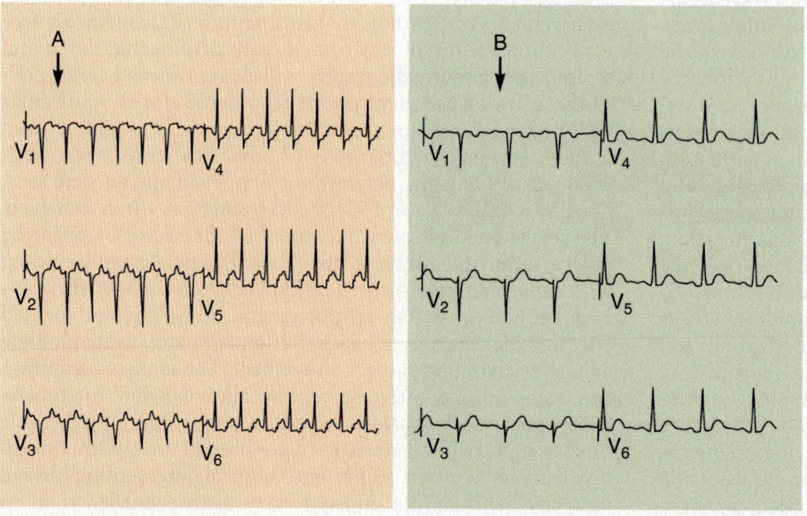

Figure 80.4. Electrocardiogram during an exercise test showing precordial leads V_1 through V_6. **A:** During exercise, depression of the ST segment and ischemia are seen in leads V_4 through V_6. **B:** These resolve after exercise is stopped.

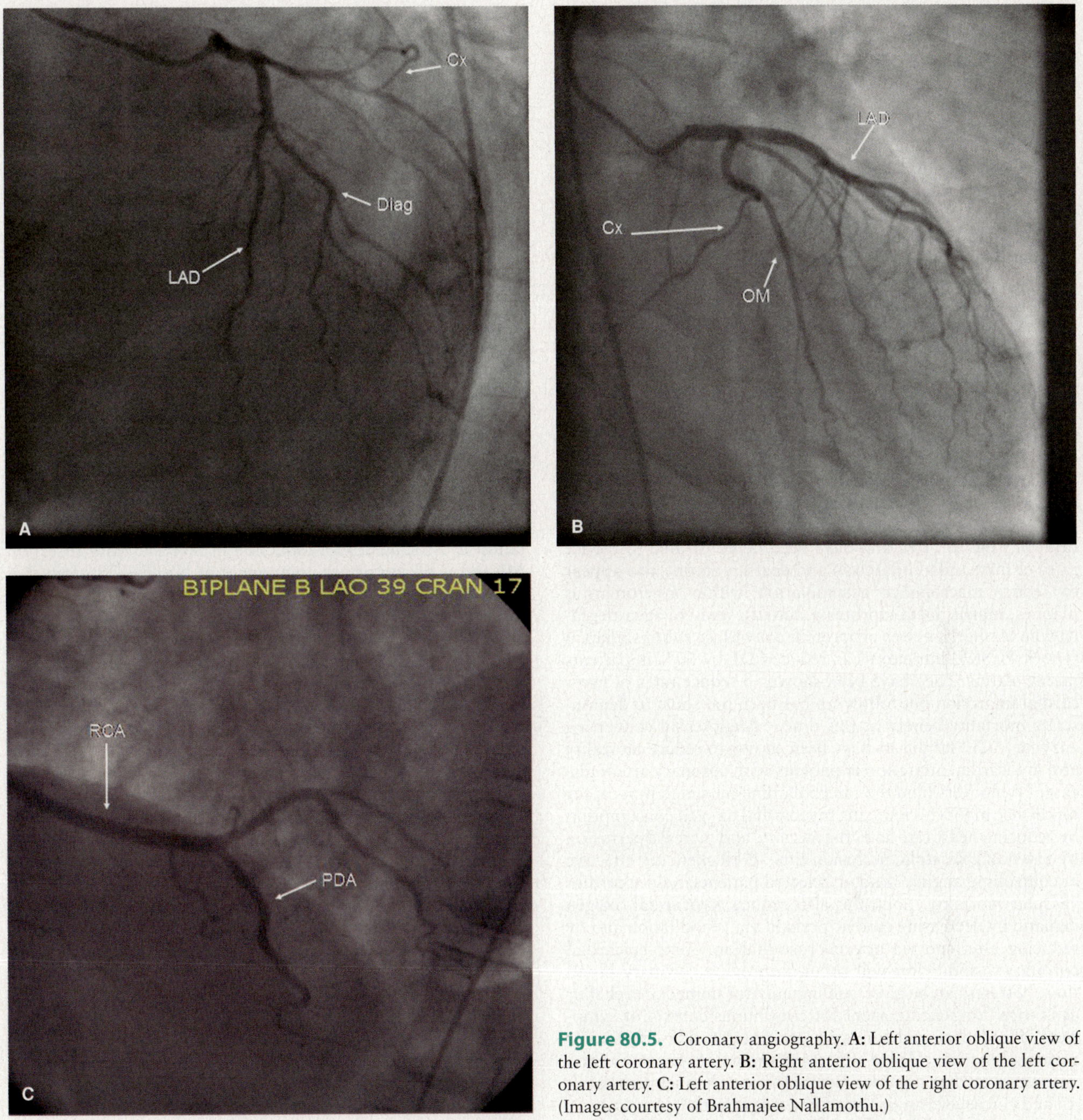

Figure 80.5. Coronary angiography. **A:** Left anterior oblique view of the left coronary artery. **B:** Right anterior oblique view of the left coronary artery. **C:** Left anterior oblique view of the right coronary artery. (Images courtesy of Brahmajee Nallamothu.)

in the femoral, brachial, or radial arteries, catheters selectively engage the ostia of the left and right coronary arteries. Radio-opaque contrast is injected with imaging of the opacified coronary artery. Standardized views are obtained of both the right and left coronary systems to provide different projections to clearly define the vascular anatomy and to quantify the severity of occlusive lesions (**Fig. 80.5**). Additionally, catheters can be inserted across the aortic valve into the left ventricular cavity, providing information about ventricular pressure throughout the cardiac cycle. Although the majority of coronary lesions are graded visually, intermediate blockages can be functionally assessed with pressure wires.[21] The general principle includes measuring aortic and distal coronary pressures, with some methods utilizing hyperemia (fractional flow reserve) while a number of nonhyperemic techniques take measurements during specific phases of the cardiac cycle. In addition, intravascular ultrasound is a helpful adjunct for assessing left main and other coronary lesions based on minimum lumen area, but also for directing stent placement and evaluating in stent restenosis.[22]

Newer imaging techniques using high-resolution multislice computed tomography (CT) scanning with three-dimensional reconstruction and magnetic resonance imaging are increasingly being utilized. These noninvasive approaches have the potential to improve the safety and convenience of coronary imaging and techniques for lesion grading and quantitative functional pressure measurements are improving; however, the standard remains coronary angiography. These techniques are often used as screening tests and are frequently followed up with traditional angiography.[23]

MEDICAL TREATMENT

5 Medical therapy of stable coronary artery disease is designed to slow the rate of progression of coronary artery atherosclerosis, to reduce the rate of complications from these lesions, and to control symptoms. Treatments are aimed at slowing plaque growth, reducing risk of plaque rupture, and reducing myocardial oxygen consumption. While advances in

pharmacologic agents have improved the treatment of atherosclerosis and reduced mortality, lifestyle modification remains the most important intervention and the most difficult to achieve. These lifestyle modifications include cessation of cigarette smoking, exercise, weight loss, dietary control of diabetes, salt restriction, and reduction in the consumption of foods high in cholesterol and fat.

Medical therapy begins with controlling risk factors that contribute to formation and destabilization of the atherosclerotic plaque. Medical treatment alone is often satisfactory for many patients with mild to moderate ischemia. The International Study of Comparative Health Effectiveness with Medical and Invasive Approaches (ISCHEMIA) trial showing no benefit to an initial invasive strategy over medical therapy alone in patients with stable coronary disease and moderate to severe ischemia.[24]

Aspirin inhibits cyclooxygenase-1 (COX-1) activity and thromboxane production, irreversibly inhibiting platelet aggregation by inhibiting platelet activity, and should be prescribed to all patients unless significant contraindications exist. Aspirin has been shown to reduce death and myocardial infarctions in patients with significant coronary artery disease. Hydroxymethylglutaryl (HMG) CoA reductase inhibitors (statins) can decrease cholesterol levels and improve the ratio of LDL to HDL and have been demonstrated to reduce rates of myocardial infarction and death.[25] Statins also appear to reduce macrophage accumulation within atheromatous plaques, matrix metalloprotease activity, and collagen degradation. Similarly, newer proprotein convertase subtilisin/kexin type 9 (PCSK9) inhibitors can reduce LDL by 60% in patients taking statins. They have been shown to reduce rates of myocardial infarction but follow-up has been too short to demonstrate mortality benefit at this time.[26] Angiotensin-converting enzyme (ACE) inhibitors have been shown to reduce mortality and myocardial infarction in patients with coronary artery disease.[27] β blockers bind the catecholamine-mediated β_1 receptor on cardiac myocytes reducing myocardial oxygen consumption by reducing heart rate and contractility, and increase perfusion by extending diastolic perfusion time. β blockers are effective at controlling angina[28] and, in selected patients, reduce cardiovascular mortality.[29] Nitrates also reduce myocardial oxygen demand by decreasing cardiac preload via venodilation and by reducing afterload via arterial vasodilation. Some epicardial coronary vasodilation will occur, improving coronary blood flow. Nitrates can be given sublingually for immediate relief or as an oral long-acting agent for continuous control of symptoms. Headaches and tolerance are notable side effects. For patients who have failed other antianginal therapies ranolazine alters cardiac myocyte membrane ion channel permeability and can relieve angina with few side effects.[30]

For patients with NSTE-ACS, laboratory testing for troponins and ECG evaluation for ST depressions differentiates UA from NSTEMI. Admission to the hospital for possible NSTE-ACS should include continuous ECG monitoring (telemetry) and capacity for emergent defibrillation given the risk for ventricular arrhythmias. For patients with unstable angina, imaging (ie, stress test) is required to determine if significant ischemia is present. If present, then UA patients can proceed with invasive coronary angiography. For patients with NSTEMI medical therapy should be continued and a risk-based determination of timing for invasive coronary angiography.

Initial medical therapy targets anti-ischemic and analgesia. This includes administration of aspirin, oxygen therapy, nitroglycerin for chest pain, morphine for pain refractory to nitrates, afterload reducing agents if left heart failure present, β blockers if no heart failure present, and a high-dose statin. Sublingual nitroglycerin can be transitioned to intravenous nitroglycerine as a continuous infusion, which is typically effective at controlling symptoms of pain and reduces myocardial strain. Small randomized trials have suggested that nitroglycerine can reduce hospital mortality, although this has not been validated in larger trials.[31] ACE inhibitors reduce mortality after acute myocardial infarctions, particularly those with decreased ventricular function.[32] Benefits are not just restricted to the afterload reduction effects, promoting ventricular remodeling of the myocardial intercellular matrix and scar formation.[33]

Antithrombotic therapy is among the most important interventions in patients presenting with an acute myocardial infarction. In addition to rapid administration of aspirin, the primary agents are the P2Y12 inhibitors including thienopyridines (clopidogrel, prasugrel) which irreversibly bind adenosine diphosphate (ADP) receptors, or cyclo-pentyltriazolopyrimidine (ticagrelor) which reversibly binds ADP receptors. There is strong evidence that the addition of clopidogrel to aspirin reduces death, myocardial infarction, and stroke in the setting of ACS.[34] Further, ticagrelor likely reduces the risk of recurrent MI compared with other P2Y12 agents.[35] Choice of agent and timing of administration should consider if the patient is undergoing an invasive strategy, and should they then proceed with surgery a delay of 3 to 7 days may be beneficial.[36] For high-risk patients, glycoprotein (Gp) IIb/IIIa inhibitors can be considered though the evidence is limited. In addition to dual-antiplatelet therapy, patients should be started on anticoagulation with either low–molecular-weight heparin or unfractionated heparin unless contraindicated. Anticoagulation is associated with reduction in mortality and recurrent MI and is an important component of NSTE-ACS given that dual-antiplatelet therapy is often delayed while determining invasive strategies.[37]

With STEMI, significant myocardium is at risk, potentially resulting in either cardiogenic shock or ventricular arrhythmias. Rapid diagnosis and treatment with recanalization of acutely occluded vessels is critical and efficacy decreases with each passing minute. Diagnosis requires both symptoms, such as chest pain or angina equivalent, dyspnea, an arrhythmia, cardiac arrest or syncope, and an ECG demonstrating ST-segment elevation, a new left bundle branch block, or another high-risk ECG finding. Reperfusion options include percutaneous intervention (PCI) or fibrinolysis. Fibrinolytic therapy was established back in the 1980s using streptokinase and demonstrated reduced mortality when it was given within 12 hours.[38] Today other agents are available with improved outcomes and should be administered if PCI is unavailable within 120 minutes, symptoms started <12 hours prior and the patient has no contraindications.

Percutaneous coronary intervention for acute STEMI is now standard practice with outcomes that are superior to fibrinolytic reperfusion.[39] Given the time sensitive nature of reperfusion there is focus on time from first medical contact to balloon inflation to salvage as much myocardium as possible. Complex interhospital and intrahospital systems are now in place to improve the efficiency and application of this treatment strategy, and PCI should be completed within 2 hours or fibrinolysis should be considered.[40]

PERCUTANEOUS CORONARY INTERVENTIONS

6 Since the inception of percutaneous transcoronary balloon angioplasty (PTCA) in 1977, catheter-directed treatment of coronary artery disease has evolved into one of the most commonly performed procedures worldwide. Advances in technology have improved outcomes and expanded the indications, particularly for the acutely ischemic heart. Using access in the radial or femoral artery catheters are advanced and engaged the coronary ostia where small steerable guide wires can be advanced through the lumen of epicardial coronary arteries. Over this wire, balloon-tipped catheters can be advanced and centered across discrete stenotic lesions and inflated to dilate the stenotic vessel (**Fig. 80.6**). Although rarely utilized today, PTCA is returning with drug-coated balloons to treat restenosis or other difficult lesions.

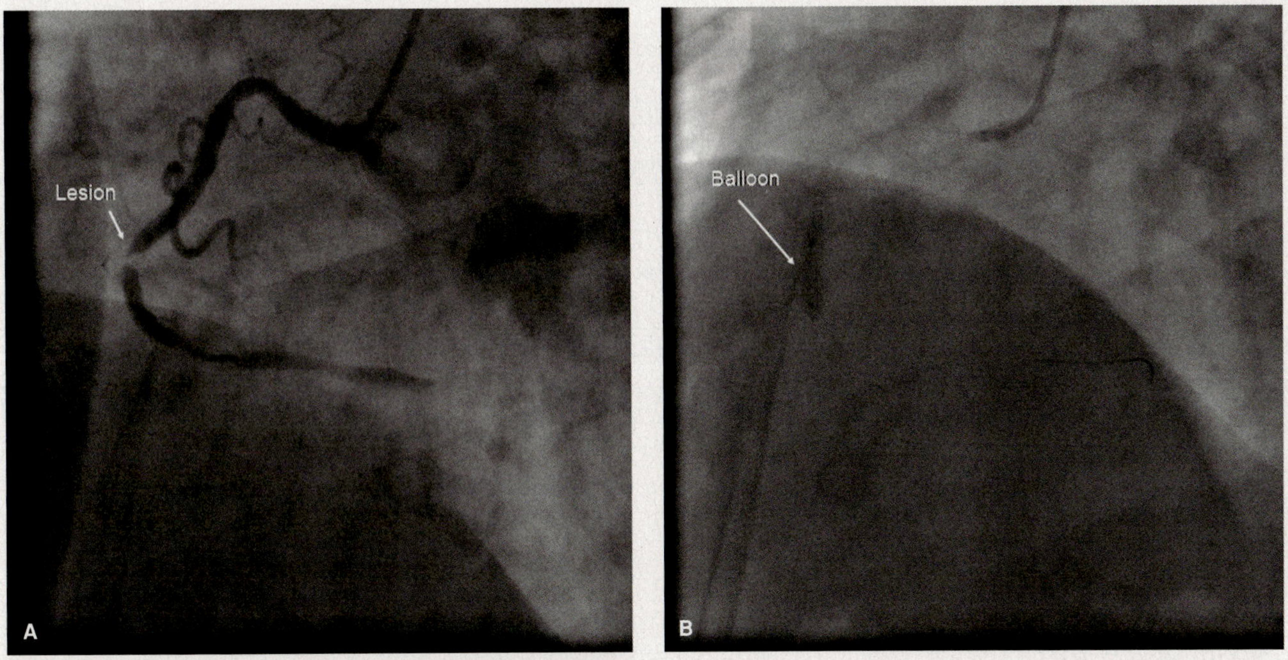

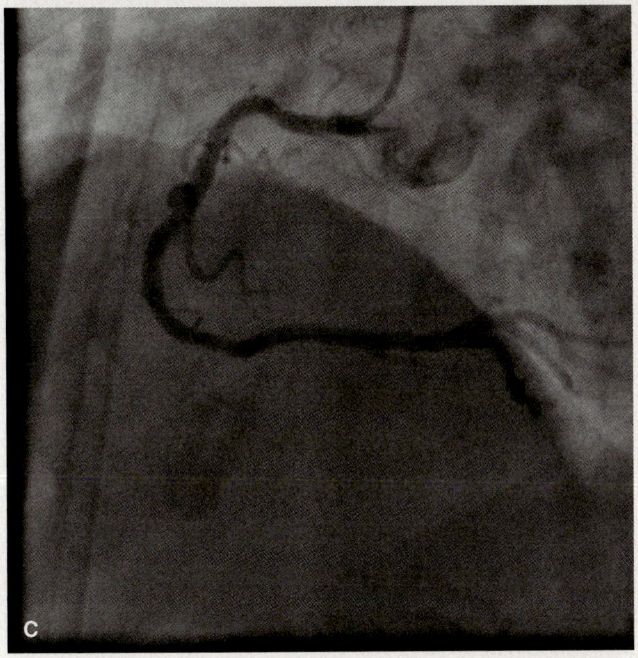

Figure 80.6. Percutaneous coronary intervention. **A:** A stenotic midright coronary artery lesion. **B:** Balloon angioplasty. **C:** Postintervention result. (Images courtesy of Brahmajee Nallamothu.)

The addition of stents, and in particular drug-eluting stents (DESs), has reduced complications and improved durability. Early complications include perforation, embolization, side branch occlusion, and stent thrombosis. Yet the procedure is safe enough to be performed without onsite cardiac surgical backup. In addition, recent generation DESs have greatly reduced restenosis rates down to less than 15%. Immunosuppressants sirolimus and paclitaxel were used for first-generation DESs, while everolimus and zotarolimus are utilized in second-generation DESs. With each iteration stents have further reduced the rate of target vessel restenosis and the need for repeat interventions.[41]

CORONARY BYPASS GRAFTING

Indications

CABG is one of the most common and most studied surgical procedures performed in the United States. Dozens of multicenter, prospective, randomized trials have been performed comparing the surgical treatment of coronary artery disease to both medical and percutaneous options. Current controversy exists related to the 2021 and 2023 revascularization guidelines due to the authors' emphasis on a diagnostic strategy trial (not revascularization strategy).[42,43] Some of the landmark studies will be discussed in detail later in the chapter, as proper understanding of these trials is important in determining appropriate treatment strategies for individual patients. In summary, these studies consistently demonstrate that CABG continues to be the best revascularization strategy, reducing the rate of myocardial infarctions, need for repeat revascularization, and mortality in patients with a broad degree of occlusive disease. Patients are generally more likely to benefit from surgical revascularization if they have worse symptoms, more severe myocardial ischemia, more extensive coronary artery occlusions, and those lesions are more complex (ie, bifurcation location, asymmetric calcification, in-stent restenosis). Recommendations can be split between stable ischemic heart disease (SIHD) and ACSs. The recommendations for SIHD are

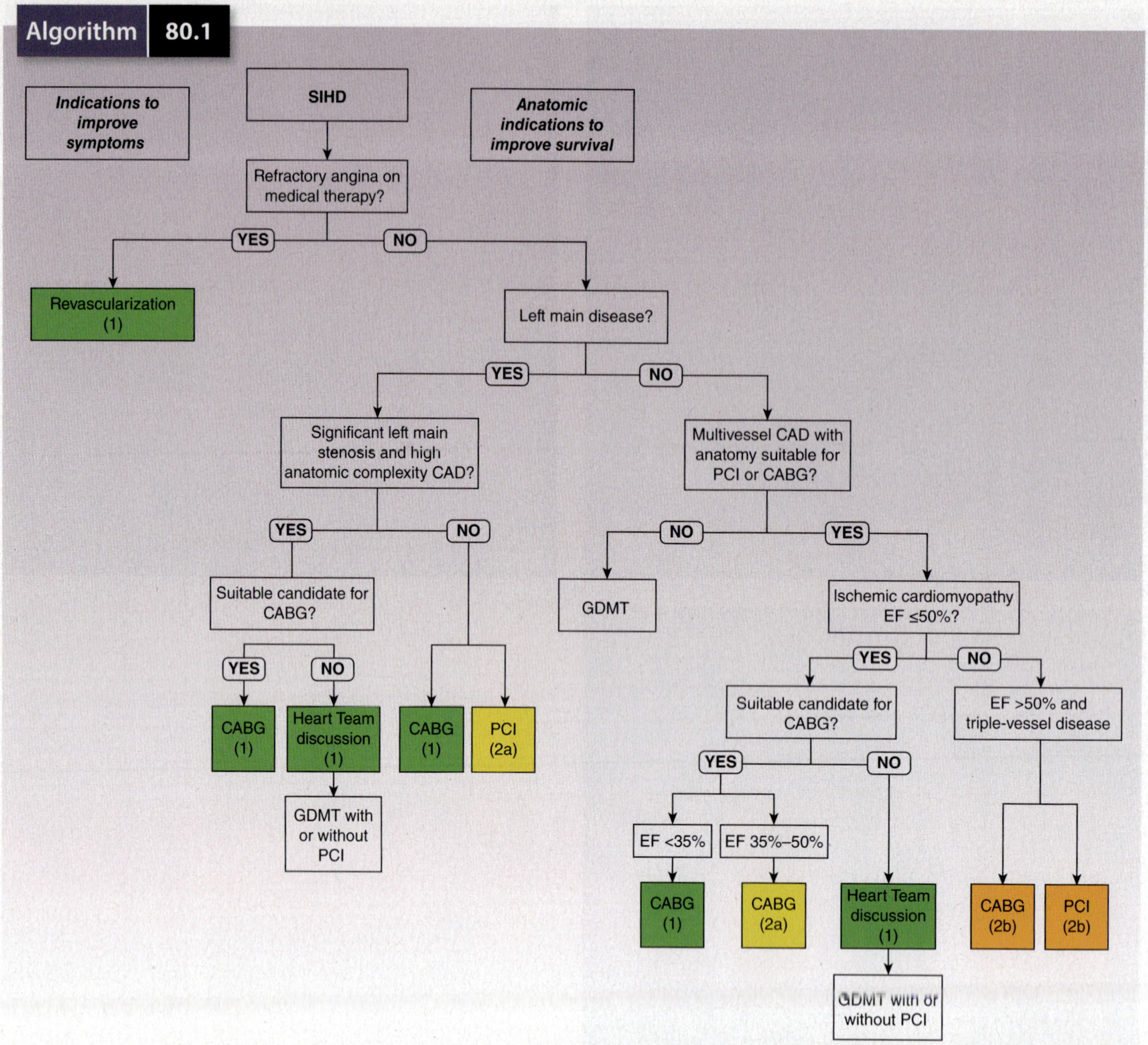

Algorithm 80.1. 2021 ACC/AHA/SCAI recommendations for revascularization in patients with stable ischemic heart disease. CABG, coronary artery bypass graft; CAD, coronary artery disease; EF, ejection fraction; GDMT, guideline-directed medical therapy; PCI, percutaneous coronary intervention; and SIHD, stable ischemic heart disease. (Reproduced with permission from Lawton JS, Tamis-Holland JE, Bangalore S, et al. 2021 ACC/AHA/SCAI guideline for coronary artery revascularization: Executive summary: a report of the American College of Cardiology/American Heart Association Joint Committee on clinical practice guidelines. *Circulation*. 2022;145(3):e4–e17.)

summarized in **Algorithm 80.1**, where recommendations are categorized based on the class of recommendation (benefit vs risk) and level of evidence (quality of primary literature).[42] Indications for revascularization with SIHD include refractory angina, left main disease, LVEF ≤50%, and three-vessel disease. Further recommendations for diabetic patients include multivessel CAD involving the LAD. Surgical societies did not endorse the guidelines due in part to downgrading the class of recommendation for CABG from I (strong recommendation) to IIa (moderate recommendation) for patients with an LVEF 35% to 50%, from I to IIb (weak recommendation) for three-vessel CAD, and a lack of recognition for the superior long-term benefits of CABG over PCI.[44,45] These recommendations are not supported by the source literature and emphasize the importance for practitioners to have a firm understanding of the underlying clinical trials.[46] The 2021 revascularization guidelines provide minimal guidance for ACS patients. For STEMI patients it is reasonable to consider CABG when PCI is not feasible in the setting of shock (Class I) or large myocardium at risk (Class IIa), at the time of repair for mechanical ischemic complications (Class I), or electively after PCI with complex multivessel CAD (Class IIa). Interestingly for NSTE-ACS patients, guidelines focus on pursuing an early invasive approach and leave the decision for type of revascularization for complex disease to a multidisciplinary heart team.

Standard Technique

7 The basic principles in coronary bypass grafting are to restore normal perfusion of ischemic myocardial territories by providing alternative routes for blood flow. Aortocoronary bypass was pioneered by Rene Favaloro at the Cleveland Clinic in the late 1960s. The technique has evolved considerably over the decades, and there remains significant variability in how this complex procedure is conducted even today.

Access to the heart is typically obtained via a median sternotomy. This incision allows exposure of the anterior surface of the heart and great vessels for initiation of cardiopulmonary

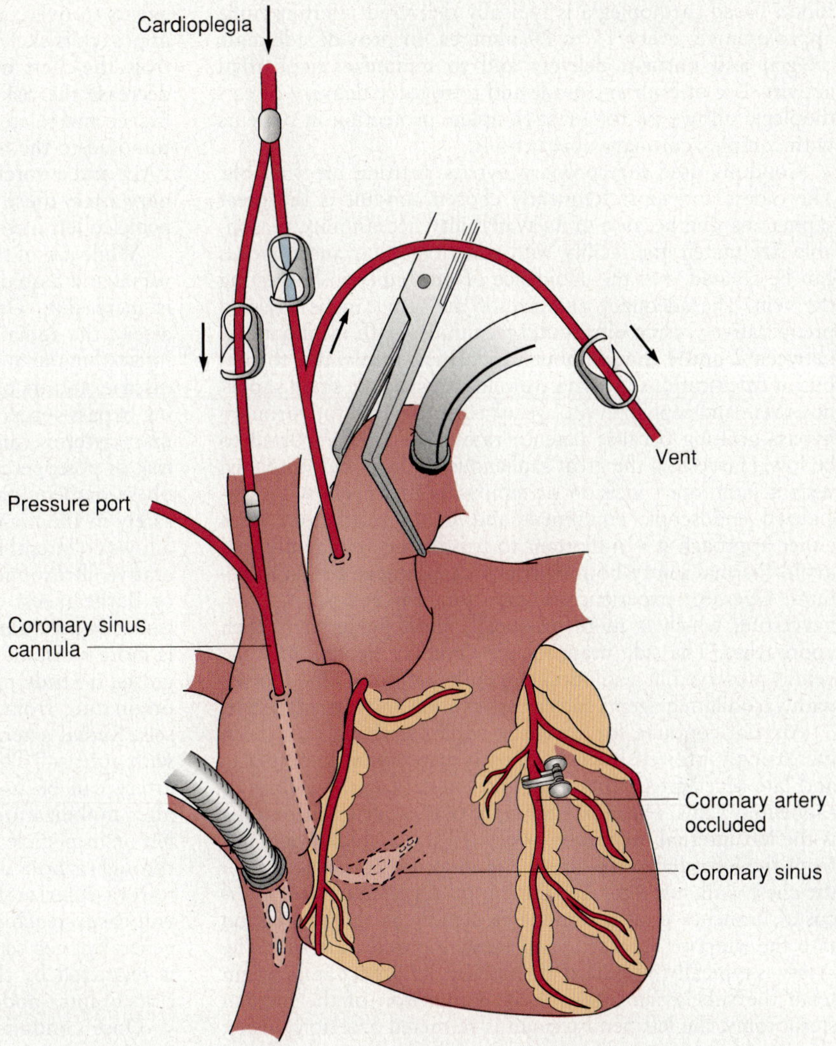

Figure 80.7. Instrumentation for cardiopulmonary bypass.

bypass (CPB), but also allows for access to the internal mammary arteries for conduit creation. Except for the severely hypertrophic heart, the entire epicardial surface can be exposed with manipulation and traction on the left ventricle. Alternatively, a left lateral thoracotomy can be used. This limits its visualization to the obtuse margin of the heart but can be advantageous, particularly if the patient has previously had a median sternotomy with dense adhesions hazarding catastrophic injury during sternal reentry. Another alternative has been a limited left anterior thoracotomy, which exposes only a small portion of the anterior wall of the left ventricle limiting revascularization to the LAD. This approach will be discussed later in the section describing minimally invasive approaches to surgical revascularization.

The key to constructing a durable and reproducible anastomosis to small diseased epicardial vessels is creation of a quiet and bloodless surgical field. The advent of CPB using extracorporeal circulation along with cardiac standstill using cardioplegia has allowed precisely this environment. The epicardial vessels are motionless and can be brought directly into the surgical field. Epicardial blood flow is eliminated, allowing direct visualization of the lumen without arterial control, avoiding potential clamp or snare injury to the fragile vessels.

After anticoagulation with intravenous heparin to achieve an activated clotting time (ACT) >480 seconds, the patient is cannulated in the distal ascending aorta. Patients may have significant atherosclerotic disease, and the cannulation site should be carefully inspected for mobile lesions using TEE and manual palpation. Use of preoperative CT scans or intraoperative epiaortic ultrasonic imaging may allow for more complete assessment but is not standard of care. After insertion, the cannula is manually deaired and connected to the arterial limb of the CPB circuit (**Fig. 80.7**). Venous drainage is accomplished with a cannula in the right atrium, typically in the atrial appendage. Bleeding from the cannulation sites is controlled by pursestring sutures around the cannulas. Bypass is initiated by venous drainage into a reservoir, emptying the heart of venous return. Blood is pumped into a membrane oxygenator and returned into the aortic cannula, typically at a blood flow rate of 2.4 L/min per m^2 of body surface area. With full flow, ventilation of the patient can be discontinued, further improving visualization and minimizing motion in the surgical field. The extracorporeal blood is cooled, creating mild hypothermia, varying from 28° to 34 °C. Systemic cooling minimizes end-organ injury from relative hypotension or hypoperfusion from nonpulsatile blood flow.

After adequate CPB is confirmed, the heart is arrested by applying a clamp across the mid-ascending aorta, proximal to the aortic cannulation site. This clamp isolates the native coronary vessels from the remainder of the systemic circulation. Cardioplegia is then delivered to the myocardium via a catheter in the aortic root and/or coronary sinus. There are a variety of cardioplegia options commercially available including both blood and crystalloid based solutions, but the most important components are cold temperature (4° to 8 °C), potassium at 15 to 30 mM/L, citrate for calcium binding, and pH buffers. The cold temperature and potassium maintain the heart in diastolic arrest, reducing myocardial oxygen consumption.

Blood-based cardioplegia is typically delivered intermittently, approximately every 15 to 20 minutes, to provide adequate oxygen and nutrient delivery and to minimize myocardial activity. Use of both antegrade and retrograde delivery of cardioplegia allows for the most complete protection in patients with complex coronary obstructions.

Conduits used for coronary bypass grafting are variable. The oldest and most frequently chosen conduit is the great saphenous vein because of its availability, accessibility, reasonable size match, the facility with which vascular anastomoses can be created, and the avoidance of morbidity in harvesting the vein. The adequacy and size of the vein can be assessed preoperatively using ultrasound techniques with ideal conduit between 2 and 4 mm without varicosities, thin walls, thrombus or calcifications. Alternative veins, such as the small saphenous vein and cephalic vein, are infrequently used for coronary bypass grafting because patency rates have been reported to be low. Harvesting the great saphenous vein can be completed with a large open incision or minimally invasively with specialized endoscopic equipment and CO_2 insufflation. With either approach it is important to handle the vein gently and avoid thermal injury both of which can damage the endothelium. Operator experience is important for endoscopic vein harvesting which is more technically challenging than open approaches. The side branches are carefully ligated, and the vein is preserved in a solution of cold heparinized blood, often with vasodilating agents such as papaverine and nitroglycerine.

8 Arterial conduits for coronary bypass grafting have been increasingly utilized because of early neointimal hyperplasia and late accelerated atherosclerosis leading to graft failure of saphenous veins. The most important of these arterial conduits is the left internal mammary artery (LIMA), which originates from the left subclavian artery and descends caudally behind the chest wall, just lateral to the sternal edge. It gives off intercostal branches until it terminates distally as the bifurcation into the superior epigastric and musculophrenic arteries. The artery is typically mobilized as a pedicle, left intact at its origin from the subclavian artery. After completion of the median sternotomy, the left hemisternum is retracted anteriorly using an elevating self-retaining retractor (**Fig. 80.8**). Under direct visualization, the mammary artery, its accompanying paired veins, and a small swath of chest-wall soft tissue are gently separated from the remaining chest wall. Intercostal branches are controlled with clips and divided sharply or with cautery. The dissection proceeds proximally to the subclavian vein and distally to the terminal bifurcation of the internal mammary. Caution must be taken during the proximal extent of the dissection, as the phrenic nerve traverses close posteriorly to the origin of the left internal mammary artery. Once fully mobilized, the internal mammary is divided at the distal bifurcation after heparinization and soaked in a solution of vasodilating agents to overcome spasm from manipulation. An alternative approach is skeletonization, with only the artery dissected free from the chest wall. This approach increases length and may decrease the risk of infection, but the rate of injury is likely higher and related to operator experience. The LIMA is anastomosed to the most important left-sided target, typically the LAD, and a notch in the pericardium to the left of the pulmonary artery must be created to allow unhindered passage of the pedicled left internal mammary artery to its distal target.

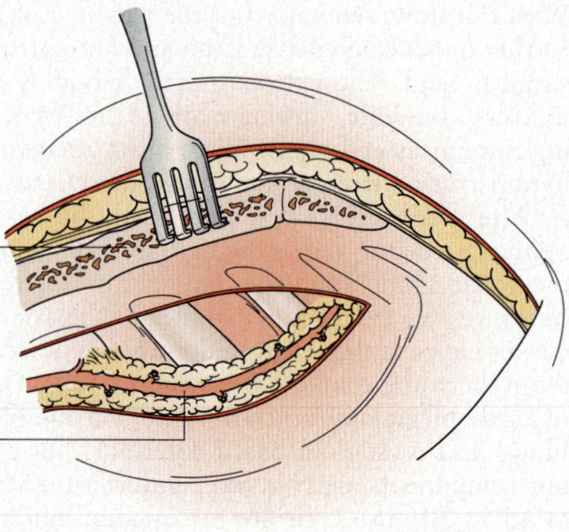

Figure 80.8. Elevation of the left hemisternum for visualization of the left internal mammary artery.

While use of the left internal mammary artery is nearly universal and a quality metric, use of additional arterial conduits is increasing. Options include the right internal mammary artery, the radial arteries, and the gastroepiploic artery. The internal mammary artery tends to be spared of atherosclerotic disease, and its patency rates are excellent many years following bypass surgery. However, utilization of both internal mammary arteries can devascularize the sternum and increase the risk of postoperative sternal wound infections, particularly in obese diabetic patients.[47] The radial artery can be harvested safely in the majority of patients, as a complete palmar arch allows collateral flow to the hand from the ulnar artery. Preoperative ultrasound in addition to a bedside-modified Allen test or Barbeau test can reliably identify patients in which hand ischemia precludes radial artery use. Although the radial artery is more resistant to late occlusions typical in saphenous vein grafts, it tends to be prone to spasm from competitive flow originating from subcritically stenosed native coronary vessels. Radial arteries should only be used on coronary targets with at least 70% proximal stenoses. The right gastroepiploic artery can be used, since it has more than adequate length after mobilization off the greater curve of the stomach. It is left on its pedicle from the gastroduodenal artery and tunneled through a hole in the diaphragm. It is most frequently used to revascularize the posterior descending coronary branch but will easily reach posterolateral branches as well. Patency has generally been reported to be excellent, but its widespread use is restricted by the additional morbidity of laparotomy and risks of intra-abdominal complications.

Once conduits have been harvested, CPB has been instituted, and cardioplegia infusion has resulted in adequate diastolic arrest, the heart is manipulated to expose the epicardial vessels of interest. Occasionally, the coronary arteries are in fact not on the epicardial surface but run within the epicardial fat or deep within the myocardium. This is common for intermediate branches and the LAD. Careful dissection is often required. If the midportion of the LAD cannot be found, the vessel can be opened at the apex and a small coronary probe can be inserted proximally and palpated to better localize the vessel. Care must be taken to ensure the target has been properly identified. Even the most seasoned cardiac surgeons have mistakenly anastomosed grafts to epicardial veins or arterial branches. When available epicardial ultrasound can be a useful adjunct but is best used when there is coronary flow. Once the target vessel is properly located, an appropriate site for anastomotic construction should be identified. It is important to have a thorough understanding of the angiographic location of significant obstructions to ensure the graft is bypassing all significant lesions. The vessel is dissected free and opened vertically in the midline. This maneuver is among the most essential and challenging and requires precision and experience. Eccentric incisions, inadvertent incisions in the posterior wall, or incisions in friable plaques can result in stenotic or leaky constructions or disruption of plaque requiring endarterectomy. The arteriotomy is extended using fine Potts scissors 3 to 5 mm in length. The conduit is beveled to the appropriate length and the anastomosis is created with a 7-0 or 8-0 continuous running polypropylene suture (**Fig. 80.9**). A well-positioned heart, motionless and dry surgical field, 2.5 to 3.5 magnifying loupes, experienced assistance, and a steady hand are essential. Some surgeons use gentle insufflation of CO_2 to clear the field of obscuring blood and to distend the coronary artery to improve

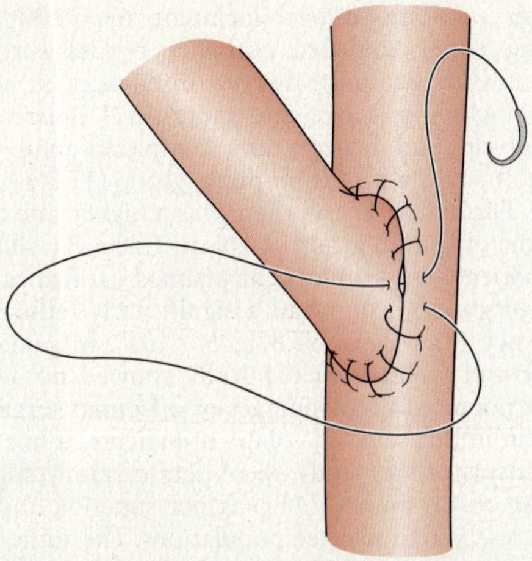

Figure 80.9. Distal coronary anastomosis with saphenous vein conduit. Excellent visualization in a quiet bloodless field is required to achieve a hemostatic and unobstructed graft.

visualization of the toe and heal. After completion of the anastomosis, saphenous vein grafts or free arterial grafts can be hand injected with cold saline to visualize patency of the vessel and competence of the construction. Antegrade cardioplegia down the grafts can assist with more complete cardiac protection. Pedicled arterial grafts can be opened, and flow down the target will be easily visualized. Use of transit time flow measurement can help assess quality of the grafts, though its use has not been verified to improve outcomes.[48]

The proximal ends of the grafts are usually connected to the ascending aorta. The grafts are cut to the appropriate length. This maneuver also requires experience, as a short graft will create tension, potentially impinging upon the distal anastomosis, and an excessively long graft may kink. The graft is distended to prevent twisting, and the aortic root is filled by infusing antegrade cardioplegia to help determine optimal graft length. Filling of the right ventricle and pulmonary artery can also be helpful. One must account for the change in geometry as the heart fills after weaning from CPB. In general, the conduits should take a straight trajectory toward their target (Fig. 80.10). An aortotomy is created using a specially designed

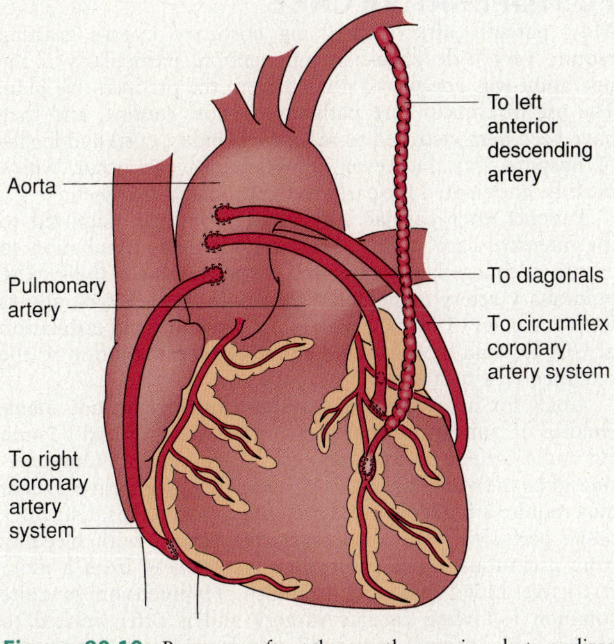

Figure 80.10. Bypass grafts take gentle curving but a direct approach to the coronary targets. The pericardium is typically left open to avoid kinking.

punch of 4 to 5 mm diameter. The grafts are beveled, and the proximal anastomosis is created with continuous running 5-0 or 6-0 polypropylene. Alternatively, the aortic cross-clamp can be removed after completion of all of the distal coronary anastomoses, and a side-biting partial aortic clamp can be placed. This technique can reduce total cardioplegia time but may increase risk of atheroembolic complications from additional aortic manipulation.

After completion of all distal and proximal anastomoses the aortic cross-clamp is removed. Once the patient has been fully re-warmed, operative hemostasis ensured, a perfusing rhythm obtained, and ventilation resumed then CPB may be weaned. The CPB flow is gradually reduced while evaluation of myocardial function and intraventricular air occurs. It is important to avoid distention of ventricular chambers, which causes unnecessary increased myocardial strain and decreased perfusion. A period of empty beating reperfusion is often helpful, particularly if the aortic cross-clamp period was prolonged or if the heart was severely ischemic preoperatively. Temporary sinus node or atrioventricular node conduction abnormalities are common, and it is standard to place temporary pacemaker leads on the ventricle, although permanent conduction abnormalities are rare without pre-existing conduction abnormalities. Although not essential for routine CABG, pulmonary artery catheters and TEE can be helpful in weaning from CPB. Excessive pulmonary artery pressures or new regional wall motion abnormalities can suggest perfusion abnormalities and should prompt careful inspection of the bypass grafts. Once satisfactory hemodynamics are achieved, the bypass cannulas are removed, and protamine is administered to reverse the anticoagulation of heparin. The pericardium is typically left open after coronary bypass grafting to avoid graft kinking or compression; however, mediastinal and thymic fat can be carefully placed over the aorta and proximal anastomoses to protect them from future sternal reentry. Drains are left within the mediastinum to collect blood, and the sternum is closed with steel wires, cables, or plates.

Off-pump Technique

While the use of CPB was essential in allowing safe and reproducible coronary anastomoses, it is now well understood that extracorporeal circulation incites a powerful inflammatory response, activating neutrophils and monocytes to release cytokines and inhibiting the clotting cascade and platelet function. Occasionally, these inflammatory changes can produce clinically relevant capillary leak, pulmonary edema, renal dysfunction, hemodynamic instability, and coagulation dysfunction. In addition, iatrogenic cardiac arrest induced by cardioplegia can infrequently result in myocardial injury and dysfunction. To avoid some of these adversities, off-pump coronary artery bypass (OPCAB) can be performed. Interestingly, CABG was originally performed without CPB in the early 1960s; however, it was largely abandoned because technically sound anastomoses could not be reliably constructed. Newer technologies are now available that have made creation of surgical bypass grafts more feasible on the full and beating heart, though still requires a high level of operator experience and skill.

The heart exposed via a median sternotomy and conduit harvested identically to the approach used for standard coronary bypass grafting with CPB. Additional sutures are placed deep within the posterior pericardium, which can be used to facilitate retraction of the heart anteriorly and rightward. A dose of heparin is administered to achieve adequate anticoagulation with an ACT >300 seconds.

Two different approaches to OPCAB focus on whether to shunt the occluded coronary and whether to start with the LIMA-LAD or most severely stenosed target vessel. A variety of approaches are acceptable but should balance minimizing regional ischemia with ease of positioning and complete revascularization. Use of bilateral internal mammary arteries, and either "I" or "Y" grafts off them, can preclude need for

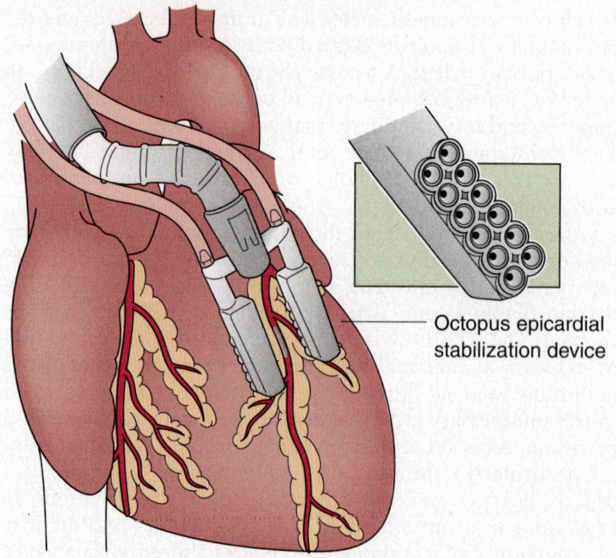

Figure 80.11. Suction-stabilizing devices allow isolation and immobilization of epicardial coronary targets.

proximal anastomoses and allow for a "no touch" technique that avoids manipulation of the ascending aorta. Should a proximal anastomosis be necessary options include either a partial occlusion clamp placed on the ascending aorta, or use of a new combined punch and sealing device. Either the proximal or distal anastomosis can be performed first, with the former allowing immediate revascularization while the later optimal graft length.

Of the potential epicardial vessels, the LAD is the easiest to expose, since it lies anteriorly. Gentle retraction on the pericardial sutures, occasionally along with a laparotomy pad placed behind the heart, will usually expose the vessel adequately. The diagonal branches are exposed with slightly further rightward retraction. The obtuse marginal vessels can be exposed with the help of a suction device placed on the apex of the heart and slowly and gently retracting the apex anteriorly and rightward. This maneuver must be performed carefully, as cardiac chamber and/or outflow tracts can become compressed. The anesthesiologist must be alerted to and familiar with these maneuvers, as temporary vasoactive infusions and fluid resuscitation to increase preload may be required. Exposure of the right coronary artery and its branches risks compression of the right ventricle with retraction superiorly. The suction apparatus placed on the acute margin can facilitate exposure, as can stiff retraction of the right-sided pericardial edges.

Once the epicardial vessel of interest is identified, a U-shaped epicardial suction stabilizing device is applied around the vessel (**Fig. 80.11**). This device can reduce myocardial motion in a small region of interest, maintaining reasonable contractility. Silastic tapes loaded on blunt needles are carefully encircled around the proximal and distal portions of the coronary artery and gently retracted for blood flow control. A variable degree of ischemia may be seen on the ECG and TEE. The vessel is dissected and opened in the same way as is done for on-pump techniques. If being used, a shunt can then be inserted and the silastic snares released to reestablish some distal flow. Use of a misted blower with CO_2 can help with visualization. The anastomosis is constructed in the same manner as on-pump CABG. Electrocardiographic normalization should be seen immediately, confirming graft patency. Once all the grafts are complete, protamine is given to at least partially reverse the anticoagulation effect of heparin. Hemostasis is confirmed and closure proceeds routinely.

Despite early enthusiasm for off-pump coronary bypass surgery, two concerns have arisen including long-term patency of grafts and completeness of revascularization. A large multicenter randomized trial including over 2000 veterans undergoing either standard coronary bypass surgery with or without CPB demonstrated no differences in short-term outcomes including stroke and mortality.[49] Importantly, the OPCAB group had fewer grafts completed than originally planned compared with the on-pump group (17.8% vs 11.1%, $P < .001$). Further, at 1 year, there was a higher rate of cardiac death in the off-pump group (2.7% vs 1.3%; $P = .03$) and for 65% of patients who underwent planned cardiac catheterization, the off-pump group had a significantly reduced rate of graft patency (82.6% vs 87.8%; $P < .01$). In summary, this important and well-conducted study showed no advantages and a few potential disadvantages of off-pump surgical revascularization in this selected cohort of patients. While there are valid criticisms of this study, these data certainly suggest that routine use of off-pump CABG is not superior, and perhaps should be reserved to selected populations. The authors use off-pump techniques for patients with a heavily calcified or atheromatous ascending aorta, severe renal or hepatic dysfunction, or in combination with minimally invasive techniques.

Minimally invasive approaches for CABG are largely limited to single-vessel bypass through a mini left thoracotomy (MIDCAB). After entering the chest in the fourth intercostal space and resecting a portion of the fourth costal cartilage, a portion of the left internal mammary artery is mobilized under direct vision. This portion of the LIMA harvest can also be accomplished using robotic assistance (RA-MIDCAB) with three ports in the left chest. Using off-pump techniques and stabilizing equipment, the internal mammary artery is anastomosed to the LAD using conventional open instruments. Given the learning curve, few centers are performing either MIDCAB or RA-MIDCAB, though outcomes appear satisfactory with excellent graft patency and complication rates.[50] Given the limited number of isolated proximal LAD stenosis cases, many MIDCAB cases are hybrid procedures involving PCI to a secondary artery ensuring patients still receive the survival benefit seen with a LIMA-LAD graft.[51] A few select surgeons have taken RA-MIDCAB a step further and are performing totally endoscopic coronary artery bypass (TECAB).[52,53] The procedure can be performed with or without CPB and cardiac arrest. The extreme technical complexity has severely limited TECAB adoption.

POSTOPERATIVE CARE

Most patients after undergoing coronary bypass grafting require very little physician intervention, particularly if the operation was conducted according to the preoperative plan. The use of clinical care pathways is now routine, and they have been demonstrated to reduce morbidity, cost, and length of hospital stay. However, complications can occur, which must be anticipated for early recognition and treatment.

Patients after cardiac surgery are routinely admitted to the intensive care setting. Most centers delay extubation to ensure adequate hemostasis and hemodynamic stability. Use pulmonary artery catheters, or Swan–Ganz catheters, allows for assessment of intracardiac filling pressures and estimation of CO. CO can be calculated either by thermodilution or the modified Fick technique.

Goals for hemodynamic stability generally include maintenance of a mean arterial pressure between 65 and 75 mm Hg and a cardiac index of at least 2 L/min per m^2. Outcomes should be individualized, as a chronically hypertensive patient may require a higher arterial pressure to maintain satisfactory tissue perfusion, and a postoperative patient with bleeding from a tenuous aortic suture line may benefit from a more restrictive blood pressure approach. Hypotension is quite common following cardiac surgery and is often related to hypovolemia, as well as vasodilation from systemic warming and an inflammatory response from extracorporeal circulation with activation of vasodilatory mediators. Intravascular hypovolemia is extremely common in the immediate perioperative period. Causes are multifactorial and include capillary leak from inflammation, venodilation from warming, unrecognized and unreplaced blood loss, and excessive diuresis, particularly if osmotic diuretics such as mannitol are given during CPB. Patients may require 2 to 3 L of fluid in the first several hours after surgery. Those with ventricular hypertrophy and diastolic dysfunction may require additional fluid to maintain CO. Although not essential, the pulmonary artery catheter can be instrumental in guiding fluid resuscitation. While colloids, such as albumin, can reduce the total volume required to maintain stability, there are no prospective randomized data clearly demonstrating its superiority with regard to outcome benefits and cost is higher.

Vasoconstrictors are used to treat hypotension, but should be secondary to adequately fluid resuscitation. α-Agonists, such as Neo-Synephrine, will increase vascular tone without increasing contractility or heart rate and do not exacerbate dysrhythmias. Similarly, vasopressin has no effect on cardiac function, but uniquely will not increase pulmonary vascular resistance, as there are no vasopressin receptors in the pulmonary vascular bed. Additionally, vasopressin preferentially constricts efferent renal arterioles rather than afferent arterioles, resulting in maintained glomerular filtration and urine output. Norepinephrine is also frequently used to counteract a vasodilatory state though has some inotropic effect.

In addition to hypovolemia and vasodilation, myocardial function should be evaluated to prevent low CO syndrome. Myocardial dysfunction can occur from stunning after cardioplegic arrest, particularly if the cross-clamp period was long. This can be problematic if systolic function is severely depressed preoperatively. Unless the heart is acutely ischemic at the time of surgery, it is unusual to expect immediate improvement in contractility after surgical revascularization. In fact, the acutely ischemic heart often tolerates CPB and cardioplegia poorly. Contractility can be globally severely depressed after emergent coronary bypass grafting in the setting of a sizable STEMI, especially if the patient was in preoperative shock. If cardiac dysfunction and low CO are detected intraoperatively, careful assessment of bypass graft position and patency should be undertaken. This is especially true if new wall motion abnormalities are regional.

Once surgical problems have been corrected, efforts are made to optimize myocardial contractility. Inotropic agents will improve cardiac function and can be easily titrated to the desired effect. Catecholamines, such as dopamine, epinephrine, and dobutamine, are frequently used. All these agents, through their effects on β receptors, will increase heart rate, predispose to arrhythmias, and increase myocardial oxygen consumption. Nonetheless, these agents are generally safe, particularly at low doses. Phosphodiesterase inhibitors, such as milrinone, also improve contractility and have less effect on heart rate or myocardial contractility, though do lead to vasodilation. Both catecholamines and phosphodiesterase inhibitors exert their inotropic effects by increasing cytosolic calcium. For these agents to be effective, there must be adequate calcium stores. Infusion of supplemental calcium often potentiates the effect of both classes of drugs. Likewise, acidosis decreases the effectiveness of inotropic agents, and normalization of blood pH, either by replacement of sodium bicarbonate or hyperventilation, can have an immediate effect on myocardial function.

When postoperative ventricular dysfunction is entirely related to myocardial stunning, inotropes should be weaned within the first 24 hours. However, if postoperative cardiogenic shock is severe and refractory to high-dose inotropic infusions, insertion of an intra-aortic balloon pump should be considered. Positioned within the thoracic aorta (**Fig. 80.12**), balloon pump actuation is timed with the patient's ECG or arterial pressure tracing. Inflation occurs during diastole, augmenting coronary perfusion, and deflates during systole,

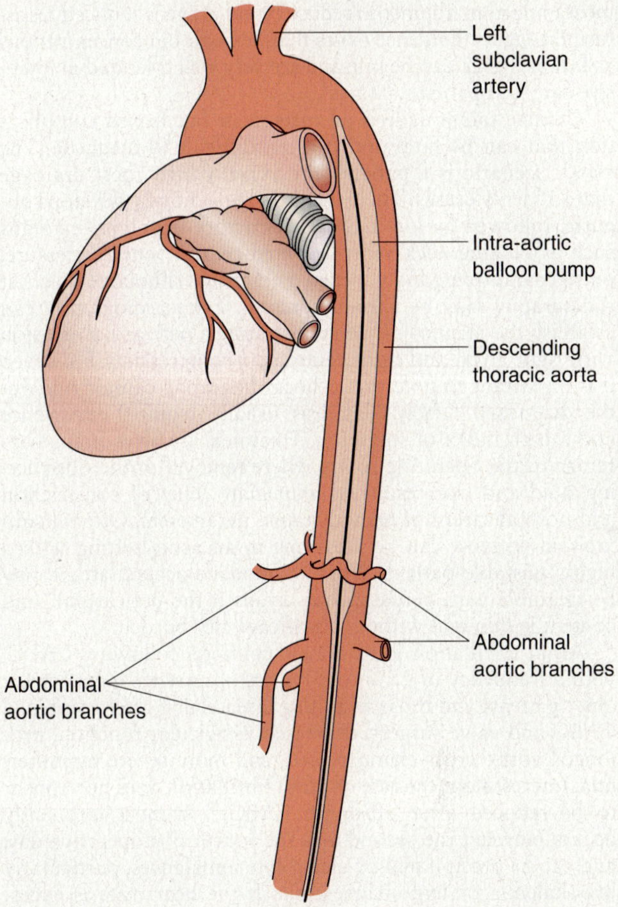

Figure 80.12. Intra-aortic balloon pump positioned within the descending thoracic aorta. The device must be positioned to not occlude the left subclavian artery or the abdominal aortic branches.

reducing afterload and increasing CO. Insertion of a durable VAD may be beneficial; however, given the long-term implications use should be limited and discussed preoperatively. Temporary microaxial pumps positioned across the aortic valve can unload a struggling left ventricle and provide near complete cardiac support. These devices can allow time for myocardial recovery while preventing end-organ dysfunction from low CO syndrome.[54]

Postoperative bleeding is infrequent but can occur, especially when patients are taking irreversible platelet inhibitors. Preoperative use of platelet function assays can help determine timing of surgery for patients taking P2Y12 inhibitors. Output from mediastinal chest drains is monitored closely, and markers of coagulation are assessed. Rotational thromboelastrometry or thromboelastography can guide blood product transfusions to correct coagulopathy. Return to the operating room should be considered if drainage exceeds 400 mL in 1 hour, or 200 mL/hour for 4 hours, without signs of slowing.

Inhibitors of plasminogen can be helpful in reducing postoperative coagulopathy and bleeding complications. There are three agents in this class of drug: ε-aminocaproic acid (Amicar, Xanodyne Pharmaceuticals, New Port, KY), and tranexamic acid. These agents are synthetic binders of plasminogen or plasmin.

There has recently been great enthusiasm for using a blood conservation strategy. Transfusion of as little as a single unit of packed red cells is independently associated with increased morbidity after coronary bypass surgery.[55] Efforts to reduce transfusions include use of acute normovolemic hemodilution (autologous blood collection), minimizing hemodilution using short bypass circuit tubing, retrograde priming and hemofiltration, and autotransfusion with cell salvage. However, likely the most important adjunct to reduce blood usage is reduced transfusion triggers. Evidence exists that hemoglobin concentrations as low as 7 g/dL can be safe and are very well tolerated in intensive care unit patients.[56]

Cardiac tamponade is an infrequent but feared complication that can be fatal and is often difficult to diagnose. The classic scenario is a patient with initially high chest drainage that suddenly ceases. The patient then insidiously develops oliguria, followed by low CO and refractory hypotension. Signs such as bulging neck veins, elevated central venous pressure, pulsus paradoxus, and widened mediastinal silhouette on chest radiography may be variably present. Echocardiography can establish the diagnosis by demonstrating a pericardial effusion with right atrial and right ventricular compression. However, it is important to note that echocardiography cannot rule out the diagnosis. Timely diagnosis usually requires experience and a high index of suspicion. Treatment involves immediate return to the operating room, where removal of the obstructing fluid and clot results in immediate relief of constriction and normalization of hemodynamic parameters. Often a subxiphoid window can be lifesaving in an acute setting with a highly unstable patient. When tamponade occurs late, it may be treatable with percutaneous drains if the pericardial fluid content is thin and without significant clot burden.

Atrial fibrillation is extremely common following CABG, with a frequency of 25% to 30%. Its occurrence is higher for older patients and those with lung disease, and after combined CABG and valve surgery, decreased ventricular function, prolonged aortic cross-clamp period, and more severe hypothermia. Interestingly, the rate of atrial fibrillation does not appear to be reduced after off-pump CABG.[57] It most frequently occurs between the second and the fourth postoperative day, and can be precipitated by electrolyte imbalances, particularly hypokalemia or hypomagnesemia. If the heart rate is excessively high or the patient has significant ventricular hypertrophy, atrial fibrillation can result in hemodynamic compromise producing hypotension and oliguria. Both β blockers and amiodarone can be used for atrial fibrillation prophylaxis and treatment. Amiodarone can achieve adequate rate control after an intravenous load of 150 mg in the majority of patients, with minimal effect on blood pressure or contractility. As a class III antiarrhythmic, amiodarone is also very effective at facilitating conversion to sinus rhythm. When given for prophylaxis amiodarone reduces the rate of atrial fibrillation but risks bradycardia in protocols that use higher doses.[58] β-Blocking agents are also effective at achieving rate control, and when given routinely preoperatively and reinitiated immediately after surgery, they have reduced the occurrence of atrial fibrillation.[59] Diltiazem is another effective option for controlling rapid atrial fibrillation, and is typically given as a 5- to 10-mg load, followed by a continuous infusion of 5 to 10 mg/hr. Although it is associated with hypotension, its short half-life makes this complication quite manageable. For atrial fibrillation with rapid ventricular response refractory to amiodarone, β blockers, and diltiazem, it may be reasonable to add digoxin. This drug should be used with caution, because it is proarrhythmic. Drug concentrations should be followed and potassium levels maintained aggressively. If rapid ventricular response results in significant hemodynamic instability, electrical cardioversion should be performed. Cardioversion may also be considered if atrial fibrillation persists after 24 to 36 hours because of the risk of clot formation within the left atrial appendage. Evaluation for clot should be considered in stable patients undergoing cardioversion if atrial fibrillation has been present for more than 48 hours. If atrial fibrillation is persistent, anticoagulation should be considered but the benefit of potentially reduced risk of stroke weighed against the likely increased risk for postoperative bleeding complications. The benefit of anticoagulation for postoperative atrial fibrillation in CABG patients is currently being studied in a randomized trial as the bleeding risk is known. The vast majority of patients who develop atrial fibrillation after CABG will revert to sinus rhythm, and the complication rate is generally low. However, atrial fibrillation does increase the length of stay and cost of hospitalization, so efforts to reduce its incidence are necessary.

Deep sternal wound infection involving the bone occurs in approximately 0.5% to 1% of patients. Independent risk factors are obesity, diabetes, immunosuppression, use of both internal mammary arteries, chronic lung disease, and malnutrition. The most frequent organism is *Staphylococcus aureus,* although gram negatives can be seen in diabetics and immunosuppressed patients. Helpful preventative strategies include decontamination of nasal *Staphylococcus* species with mupirocin, preoperative Hibiclens wash, and tight postoperative glucose control. The diagnosis is established with sternal wound drainage and palpable sternal instability. Systemic antibiotics should be initiated, and the patient returned to the operating room expeditiously for sternal debridement. Delay could result in mediastinitis with sepsis and shock. Under most circumstances, the chest wall is reconstructed with myocutaneous flaps.

RESULTS OF CORONARY BYPASS GRAFTING

Overall, the mortality rate following coronary bypass grafting is between 2% and 3%. This number has been progressively declining despite rising median age and worsening severity of disease. Improved outcomes can be attributed to advances in surgical technique, anesthetic approaches, preoperative timing and patient selection, sophistication of intensive care systems, and superior pharmacology, including antiplatelet agents, β blockers, and statins. Increased competition, both between cardiac surgeons and with percutaneous interventionalists, and public reporting of data have undoubtedly improved efficiency and contributed significantly to better outcomes. Major morbidity is estimated to be 10% to 12%. Risk of stroke is approximately 1% to 2%, renal failure requiring renal replacement therapy is 0.5% to 1%, deep sternal wound infection is 0.5% to 1%, and need for urgent reoperation is 3% to 5%. Overall, median length of hospital stay is approximately 6 days.

The Society of Thoracic Surgeons maintains a voluntary registry for cardiac surgery outcomes. Participation throughout the United States is extremely high, and the database is generally considered an excellent representation of cardiac surgery outcomes. Overall, coronary bypass procedure volume has remained stable and represents more than half of all cardiac operations nationwide. In 2019, a total of 301,000 cardiac operations were submitted to the STS database, of which 161,000 were isolated CABG operations (in 2008 there were 163,000).[60] With millions of cases embedded in the dataset, enormous information can be obtained regarding risk factors for mortality and morbidity. The prediction models from the STS help clarify the risks and benefits from surgery, and recommendations to discuss the calculated risk scores with the patient and multidisciplinary heart team are embedded in revascularization guidelines.

A number of risk factors have not been successfully incorporated into existing risk models including pulmonary hypertension, decompensated cirrhosis, and quality of bypass targets. Incomplete revascularization refers to failure to revascularize a territory with a significantly obstructed coronary artery. Under most circumstances, the revascularization is incomplete because target vessels were unsuitable for bypassing because they were small, inaccessible, or too heavily diseased. The differences observed are typically not apparent in 30-day survival but manifest as a reduced long-term prognosis. Incomplete revascularization remains a primary reason off-pump CABG and PCI cannot obtain the same long-term survival benefits seen with on-pump CABG with high-complexity CAD. Given this, the quality of the bypass targets should be considered when weighing the options for treatment of advanced coronary artery disease.

Bypass graft patency is an important consideration when evaluating the success of the operation. Saphenous vein grafts are hampered by a higher early graft loss, as much as 20% in the first year. Mechanisms include technical anastomotic problems, graft kinking, inadequate epicardial run-off, vein graft endothelial dysfunction from injury or chronic stasis, competitive flow from relatively unobstructed native coronary flow, and early development of neointimal hyperplasia. Late vein graft occlusion develops at a rate of approximately 2% to 4% per year from progressive native vessel disease and the development of accelerated vein graft atherosclerosis. Patency at 10 years is generally 50% to 60%. As described previously, the internal mammary artery is generally spared of both atherosclerotic disease and early development of neointimal hyperplasia. Not surprisingly, its patency is vastly superior,[61] although these outcomes may be biased by the fact that the left internal mammary artery is typically placed on the LAD. The higher outflow of this target results in greater flow rates, reducing the risk of stagnation from limited run-off. In addition, its anterior location makes it less likely to kink. Patency at 1 year is approximately 95%, and there is very little attrition over time, with 90% to 95% patency at 10 years. In fact, the use of the internal mammary artery is an independent predictor of long-term survival, presumably because of better graft outcomes.[62] The right internal mammary artery is typically grafted to the second best target, thus the slightly lower patency numbers (>90% at 10 years) compared to the LIMA may be related to the conduit but more likely the target. The radial artery is generally intermediate to saphenous vein grafts and the internal mammary artery. Patency rates have been described as 90% at 1 year and 80% to 90% at 5 years. The radial artery has a thick muscular media and prone to spasm that is worsened with competitive flow, resulting in a patent but dysfunctional graft, referred to as a string sign. When utilized on target vessels with ≥90% stenosis patency may be as high as 85% at 20 years.

COMPARATIVE TRIALS

9 With the advent of coronary bypass surgery in the late 1960s, questions arose as to which patients are appropriate to offer this highly invasive and costly treatment. Three landmark randomized trials were constructed comparing CABG with medical treatment for a variety of patient populations. The Veterans Administration Cooperative Study,[63] the European Coronary Surgery Study,[64] and the Coronary Artery Surgery Study[65] all demonstrated that CABG improves survival as compared to medically treated patients, and the benefits of CABG are enhanced by more severe disease, as well as left ventricular dysfunction. Although these trials are now more than 30 years old and medical and surgical treatments have evolved considerably, the principles continue to apply and are repeatedly described in more contemporary series.

Several multicenter clinical trials have also been conducted comparing CABG with angioplasty for a variety of patient populations. The most notable of these studies was the Bypass Angioplasty Revascularization Investigation, or BARI trial.[66] A total of 1829 patients were randomized to angioplasty or CABG with no difference in 5-year survival noted. However, only 8% of patients in the CABG group required repeat revascularization within the first 5 years, as compared to 54% in the angioplasty group. High crossover in treatment groups (a common problem in surgical trials) limited interpretation of the survival analysis. Importantly, subgroup analysis demonstrated a survival advantage at 5 years for diabetic patients treated with CABG as opposed to angioplasty (80.6% vs 65.5%; $P = .003$).

The BARI trial was followed by several PCI versus CABG trials that utilized bare metal stents. Among the most prominent of these studies was the SoS, or Surgery or Stent, trial.[67] A total of 988 patients were enrolled and at a median follow-up of 2 years, 20.7% of patients in the stent arm required repeat revascularization, as compared to only 6% in the CABG arm ($P < .001$). Surprisingly, there was also a survival advantage seen with surgery (mortality 4.5% vs 1.6%, stent vs surgery, respectively; $P = .01$). These mortality advantages persisted with a median follow-up of 6 years (10.9% vs 6.8%; $P = .02$).[68] Consistent with previous clinical trials, the survival advantage was even more pronounced for diabetics (17.6% vs 5.4%).

The next iteration of trials compared first-generation DESs with CABG. The SYNTAX trial is the highest quality of these trials and compared Taxus DES stents to CABG for patients with left main or three-vessel CAD.[69] Eighty-five centers in the United States and Europe enrolled patients who met these criteria and whose anatomic disease was determined by both the surgeon and interventional cardiologist to be amenable to either strategy. A total of 3075 patients were enrolled, but only 1800 patients were randomized, 897 to CABG and 903 to PCI with the Taxus DES (Boston Scientific). The remaining patients were not felt to be good candidates for both procedures, and 1077 underwent CABG and 198 underwent PCI. Outcomes of these excluded patients were collected into a separate registry. Of the randomized patients, more patients in the PCI arm had major cardiac or cerebrovascular events at 12 months (12.4% vs 17.8%, CABG vs PCI, respectively; $P = .002$). The majority of these differences were seen in the rate of repeat revascularization (5.9% vs 13.5%; $P < .001$). The authors also created a numerical system to comparatively describe the complexity of the coronary anatomy. This "syntax" score was higher for chronic total occlusions, bifurcation lesions, heavily calcified vessels, and lesions greater than 20 mm in length. The differences in major cardiac or cerebrovascular events between CABG and PCI were even more pronounced in the subgroup of patients with a high "syntax" score (10.9% vs 23.4%), which is why this score is often still utilized by heart teams today. The best available evidence likely comes from a patient-level meta-analysis of 11 randomized controlled trials that included 11,518 patients. The 5-year all-cause mortality was 11.2% after PCI and 9.2% after CABG ($P = .004$), and this difference increased to 15.5% versus 10.0% ($P < .001$) for patients with multivessel CAD and diabetes.[70]

A final group of PCI versus CABG studies to discuss relate to left main coronary disease, with both EXCEL and NOBLE are the most recent trials to utilize current generation DES.[71,72] NOBLE demonstrated 46% excess hazard of major adverse cardiac and cerebrovascular events at 5 years for PCI over CABG ($P = .01$). Meanwhile, EXCEL demonstrated noninferiority of PCI to CABG with 3-year death, stroke or MI rates of 15.4% versus 14.7%, respectively. However, the EXCEL trial results change if you exclude perioperative MI or utilize landmark analysis after 30 days for which PCI has a 44% excess hazard over CABG ($P = .02$). After accounting for a likely oversensitive definition of perioperative MI that does not correlate with later outcomes, both EXCEL and NOBLE support CABG over PCI for left main disease.

These important randomized trials have consistently demonstrated that surgical coronary artery revascularization is the ideal technique to reduce symptoms, myocardial infarctions, cardiac-related future hospitalizations, and death in patients with advanced coronary artery atherosclerosis. Improvements in nonsurgical therapy, both medical and percutaneous, have prompted recurring investigations into the comparative efficacy of coronary bypass surgery. Surgical treatment continues to successfully compete, largely because of simultaneous advances in surgical technique, intraoperative patient care, and postoperative management. Despite concerns raised every year that CABG will no longer be performed in the future, outcomes remain superior and as a result, volumes are stable. It is likely that surgical revascularization of the ischemic heart will continue to be the dominant strategy for many years to come.

References

1. Davies JE, Burkhart HM, Dearani JA, et al. Surgical management of anomalous aortic origin of a coronary artery. *Ann Thorac Surg.* 2009;88(3):844–847; discussion 847–848.
2. Messer JV, Wagman RJ, Levine HJ, Neill WA, Krasnow N, Gorlin R. Patterns of human myocardial oxygen extraction during rest and exercise. *J Clin Invest.* 1962;41(4):725–742.
3. Berne RM. The role of adenosine in the regulation of coronary blood flow. *Circ Res.* 1980;47(6):807–813.
4. Malek AM, Alper SL, Izumo S. Hemodynamic shear stress and its role in atherosclerosis. *JAMA.* 1999;282(21):2035–2042.
5. Duckworth W, Abraira C, Moritz T, et al; VADT Investigators. Glucose control and vascular complications in veterans with type 2 diabetes. *N Engl J Med.* 2009;360(2):129–139.
6. Grundy SM, Stone NJ, Bailey AL, et al. 2018 AHA/ACC/AACVPR/AAPA/ABC/ACPM/ADA/AGS/APHA/ASPC/NLA/PCNA guideline on the management of blood cholesterol: a report of the American College of Cardiology/American Heart Association task force on clinical practice guidelines. *Circulation.* 2019;139(25):e1082–e1143.
7. The lipid research clinics coronary primary prevention trial results. II. The relationship of reduction in incidence of coronary heart disease to cholesterol lowering. *JAMA.* 1984;251(3):365–374.
8. Wilson K, Gibson N, Willan A, Cook D. Effect of smoking cessation on mortality after myocardial infarction: Meta-analysis of cohort studies. *Arch Intern Med.* 2000;160(7):939–944.
9. Rehan R, Yong A, Ng M, Weaver J, Puranik R. Coronary microvascular dysfunction: a review of recent progress and clinical implications. *Front Cardiovasc Med.* 2023;10:1111721.
10. Schindler TH, Fearon WF, Pelletier-Galarneau M, et al. Myocardial perfusion PET for the detection and reporting of coronary microvascular dysfunction: a JACC: Cardiovascular imaging expert panel statement. *JACC Cardiovasc Imaging.* 2023;16(4):536–548.
11. Virani SS, Alonso A, Aparicio HJ, et al; American Heart Association Council on Epidemiology and Prevention Statistics Committee and Stroke Statistics Subcommittee. Heart disease and stroke statistics-2021 update: a report from the American Heart Association. *Circulation.* 2021;143(8):e254–e743.
12. Libby P. Mechanisms of acute coronary syndromes and their implications for therapy. *N Engl J Med.* 2013;368(21):2004–2013.
13. Hasdai D, Topol EJ, Califf RM, Berger PB, Holmes DR Jr. Cardiogenic shock complicating acute coronary syndromes. *Lancet.* 2000;356(9231):749–756.
14. Keebler ME, Haddad EV, Choi CW, et al. Venoarterial extracorporeal membrane oxygenation in cardiogenic shock. *JACC Heart Fail.* 2018;6(6):503–516.
15. Haft JW, Pagani FD, Romano MA, Leventhal CL, Dyke DB, Matthews JC. Short- and long-term survival of patients transferred to a tertiary care center on temporary extracorporeal circulatory support. *Ann Thorac Surg.* 2009;88(3):711–717; discussion 717–718.
16. Hochman JS, Sleeper LA, Webb JG, et al. Early revascularization in acute myocardial infarction complicated by cardiogenic shock. Shock investigators. Should we emergently revascularize occluded coronaries for cardiogenic shock. *N Engl J Med.* 1999;341(9):625–634.
17. Jeppsson A, Liden H, Johnsson P, Hartford M, Radegran K. Surgical repair of post infarction ventricular septal defects: a national experience. *Eur J Cardiothorac Surg.* 2005;27(2):216–221.
18. Kilic A, Sultan I, Chu D, Wang Y, Gleason TG. Mitral valve surgery for papillary muscle rupture: outcomes in 1342 patients from the society of thoracic surgeons database. *Ann Thorac Surg.* 2020;110(6):1975–1981.
19. Vohra HA, Chaudhry S, Satur CM, Heber M, Butler R, Ridley PD. Sutureless off-pump repair of post-infarction left ventricular free wall rupture. *J Cardiothorac Surg.* 2006;1:11.
20. Ohman EM, Armstrong PW, Christenson RH, et al. Cardiac troponin t levels for risk stratification in acute myocardial ischemia. GUSTO IIA investigators. *N Engl J Med.* 1996;335(18):1333–1341.
21. Tonino PAL, De Bruyne B, Pijls NHJ, et al; FAME Study Investigators. Fractional flow reserve versus angiography for guiding percutaneous coronary intervention. *N Engl J Med.* 2009;360(3):213–224.
22. Truesdell AG, Alasnag MA, Kaul P, et al. Intravascular imaging during percutaneous coronary intervention: JACC state-of-the-art review. *J Am Coll Cardiol.* 2023;81(6):590–605.
23. Serruys PW, Hara H, Garg S, et al. Coronary computed tomographic angiography for complete assessment of coronary artery disease: JACC state-of-the-art review. *J Am Coll Cardiol.* 2021;78(7):713–736.
24. Maron DJ, Hochman JS, Reynolds HR, et al. Initial invasive or conservative strategy for stable coronary disease. *N Engl J Med.* 2020;382(15):1395–1407.
25. Chou R, Cantor A, Dana T, et al. Statin use for the primary prevention of cardiovascular disease in adults: updated evidence report and systematic review for the us preventive services task force. *JAMA.* 2022;328(8):754–771.
26. Sabatine MS, Giugliano RP, Keech AC, et al; FOURIER Steering Committee and Investigators. Evolocumab and clinical outcomes in patients with cardiovascular disease. *N Engl J Med.* 2017;376(18):1713–1722.
27. Heart Outcomes Prevention Evaluation Study Investigators; Yusuf S, Sleight P, Pogue J, Bosch J, Davies R, Dagenais G. Effects of an angiotensin-converting-enzyme inhibitor, ramipril, on cardiovascular events in high-risk patients. *N Engl J Med.* 2000;342(3):145–153.
28. Savonitto S, Ardissiono D, Egstrup K, et al. Combination therapy with metoprolol and nifedipine versus monotherapy in patients with stable angina pectoris. Results of the international multicenter angina exercise (image) study. *J Am Coll Cardiol.* 1996;27(2):311–316.
29. Gottlieb SS, McCarter RJ, Vogel RA. Effect of beta-blockade on mortality among high-risk and low-risk patients after myocardial infarction. *N Engl J Med.* 1998;339(8):489–497.
30. Chaitman BR, Skettino SL, Parker JO, et al. Anti-ischemic effects and long-term survival during ranolazine monotherapy in patients with chronic severe angina. *J Am Coll Cardiol.* 2004;43(8):1375–1382.
31. Yusuf S, Collins R, MacMahon S, Peto R. Effect of intravenous nitrates on mortality in acute myocardial infarction: an overview of the randomised trials. *Lancet.* 1988;1(8594):1088–1092.
32. Rutherford JD, Pfeffer MA, Moyé LA, et al. Effects of captopril on ischemic events after myocardial infarction. Results of the survival and ventricular enlargement trial. SAVE Investigators. *Circulation.* 1994;90(4):1731–1738.
33. Beckwith C, Munger MA. Effect of angiotensin-converting enzyme inhibitors on ventricular remodeling and survival following myocardial infarction. *Ann Pharmacother.* 1993;27(6):755–766.
34. Yusuf S, Zhao F, Mehta SR, Chrolavicius S, Tognoni G, Fox KK; Clopidogrel in Unstable Angina to Prevent Recurrent Events Trial Investigators. Effects of clopidogrel in addition to aspirin in patients with acute coronary syndromes without ST-segment elevation. *N Engl J Med.* 2001;345(7):494–502.
35. Wallentin L, Becker RC, Budaj A, et al. Ticagrelor versus clopidogrel in patients with acute coronary syndromes. *N Engl J Med.* 2009;361(11):1045–1057.
36. Mehta RH, Roe MT, Mulgund J, et al. Acute clopidogrel use and outcomes in patients with non-ST-segment elevation acute coronary syndromes undergoing coronary artery bypass surgery. *J Am Coll Cardiol.* 2006;48(2):281–286.
37. Eikelboom JW, Anand SS, Malmberg K, Weitz JI, Ginsberg JS, Yusuf S. Unfractionated heparin and low-molecular-weight heparin in acute coronary syndrome without ST elevation: a meta-analysis. *Lancet.* 2000;355(9219):1936–1942.
38. Indications for fibrinolytic therapy in suspected acute myocardial infarction: Collaborative overview of early mortality and major morbidity results from all randomised trials of more than 1000 patients. Fibrinolytic Therapy Trialists' (FTT) Collaborative Group. *Lancet.* 1994;343(8893):311–322.
39. Keeley EC, Boura JA, Grines CL. Primary angioplasty versus intravenous thrombolytic therapy for acute myocardial infarction: a quantitative review of 23 randomised trials. *Lancet.* 2003;361(9351):13–20.
40. Bradley EH, Nallamothu BK, Herrin J, et al. National efforts to improve door-to-balloon time results from the door-to-balloon alliance. *J Am Coll Cardiol.* 2009;54(25):2423–2429.

41. Stone GW, Rizvi A, Sudhir K, et al; SPIRIT IV Investigators. Randomized comparison of everolimus- and paclitaxel-eluting stents. 2-year follow-up from the SPIRIT (Clinical Evaluation of the XIENCE V Everolimus Eluting Coronary Stent System) IV trial. *J Am Coll Cardiol.* 2011;58(1):19–25.
42. Lawton JS, Tamis-Holland JE, Bangalore S, et al. 2021 ACC/AHA/SCAI guideline for coronary artery revascularization: Executive summary: a report of the American College of Cardiology/American Heart Association Joint Committee on clinical practice guidelines. *Circulation.* 2022;145(3):e4–e17.
43. Virani SS, Newby LK, Arnold SV, et al. 2023 AHA/ACC/ACCP/ASPC/NLA/PCNA guideline for the management of patients with chronic coronary disease: a report of the American Heart Association/American College of Cardiology Joint Committee on clinical practice guidelines. *Circulation.* 2023;148(9):e9–e119.
44. Sabik JF 3rd, Bakaeen FG, Ruel M, et al; American Association for Thoracic Surgery and The Society of Thoracic Surgeons. The American Association for Thoracic Surgery and The Society of Thoracic Surgeons reasoning for not endorsing the 2021 ACC/AHA/SCAI Coronary Revascularization Guidelines. *Ann Thorac Surg.* 2022;113(4):1065–1068.
45. Bakaeen FG, Ruel M, Calhoon JH, et al. STS/AATS-endorsed rebuttal to 2023 ACC/AHA Chronic Coronary Disease Guideline: a missed opportunity to present accurate and comprehensive revascularization recommendations. *J Thorac Cardiovasc Surg.* 2023;166(4):1115–1118.
46. Bakaeen FG, Chu D, Dayan V. 2021 coronary revascularization guidelines-lessons in the importance of data scrutiny and reappraisal of evidence. *JAMA Surg.* 2023;158(3):233–234.
47. Schwann TA, Habib RH, Wallace A, et al. Bilateral internal thoracic artery versus radial artery multi-arterial bypass grafting: a report from the STS database. *Eur J Cardiothorac Surg.* 2019;56(5):926–934.
48. Gaudino M, Sandner S, Di Giammarco G, et al. The use of intraoperative transit time flow measurement for coronary artery bypass surgery: systematic review of the evidence and expert opinion statements. *Circulation.* 2021;144(14):1160–1171.
49. Shroyer AL, Grover FL, Hattler B, et al; Veterans Affairs Randomized On/Off Bypass (ROOBY) Study Group. On-pump versus off-pump coronary-artery bypass surgery. *N Engl J Med.* 2009;361(19):1827–1837.
50. Jonsson A, Binongo J, Patel P, et al. Mastering the learning curve for robotic-assisted coronary artery bypass surgery. *Ann Thorac Surg.* 2023;115(5):1118–1125.
51. Zhao DX, Leacche M, Balaguer JM, et al. Routine intraoperative completion angiography after coronary artery bypass grafting and 1-stop hybrid revascularization results from a fully integrated hybrid catheterization laboratory/operating room. *J Am Coll Cardiol.* 2009;53(3):232–241.
52. de Canniere D, Wimmer-Greinecker G, Cichon R, et al. Feasibility, safety, and efficacy of totally endoscopic coronary artery bypass grafting: multicenter European experience. *J Thorac Cardiovasc Surg.* 2007;134(3):710–716.
53. Balkhy HH, Nisivaco S, Kitahara H, et al. Robotic off-pump totally endoscopic coronary artery bypass in the current era: report of 544 patients. *Eur J Cardiothorac Surg.* 2022;61(2):439–446.
54. Sommer W, Arif R, Kremer J, et al. Temporary circulatory support with surgically implanted microaxial pumps in postcardiotomy cardiogenic shock following coronary artery bypass surgery. *JTCVS Open.* 2023;15:252–260.
55. LaPar DJ, Hawkins RB, McMurry TL, et al. Preoperative anemia versus blood transfusion: Which is the culprit for worse outcomes in cardiac surgery? *J Thorac Cardiovasc Surg.* 2018;156(1):66–74.e2.
56. Mazer CD, Whitlock RP, Fergusson DA, et al; TRICS Investigators and Perioperative Anesthesia Clinical Trials Group. Restrictive or liberal red-cell transfusion for cardiac surgery. *N Engl J Med.* 2017;377(22):2133–2144.
57. Almassi GH, Pecsi SA, Collins JF, Shroyer AL, Zenati MA, Grover FL. Predictors and impact of postoperative atrial fibrillation on patients' outcomes: a report from the randomized on versus off bypass trial. *J Thorac Cardiovasc Surg.* 2012;143(1):93–102.
58. Daoud EG, Strickberger SA, Man KC, et al. Preoperative amiodarone as prophylaxis against atrial fibrillation after heart surgery. *N Engl J Med.* 1997;337(25):1785–1791.
59. Crystal E, Connolly SJ, Sleik K, Ginger TJ, Yusuf S. Interventions on prevention of postoperative atrial fibrillation in patients undergoing heart surgery: a meta-analysis. *Circulation.* 2002;106(1):75–80.
60. Bowdish ME, D'Agostino RS, Thourani VH, et al. STS adult cardiac surgery database: 2021 update on outcomes, quality, and research. *Ann Thorac Surg.* 2021;111(6):1770–1780.
61. Sabik JF 3rd, Lytle BW, Blackstone EH, Houghtaling PL, Cosgrove DM. Comparison of saphenous vein and internal thoracic artery graft patency by coronary system. *Ann Thorac Surg.* 2005;79(2):544–551; discussion 544–551.
62. Loop FD, Lytle BW, Cosgrove DM, et al. Influence of the internal-mammary-artery graft on 10-year survival and other cardiac events. *N Engl J Med.* 1986;314(1):1–6.
63. Detre KM, Takaro T, Hultgren H, Peduzzi P. Long-term mortality and morbidity results of the veterans administration randomized trial of coronary artery bypass surgery. *Circulation.* 1985;72(6 Pt 2):V84–V89.
64. Varnauskas E. Twelve-year follow-up of survival in the randomized European Coronary Surgery Study. *N Engl J Med.* 1988;319(6):332–337.
65. Myers WO, Gersh BJ, Fisher LD, et al. Medical versus early surgical therapy in patients with triple-vessel disease and mild angina pectoris: a CASS registry study of survival. *Ann Thorac Surg.* 1987;44(5):471–486.
66. Bypass Angioplasty Revascularization Investigation (BARI) Investigators. Comparison of coronary bypass surgery with angioplasty in patients with multivessel disease. *N Engl J Med.* 1996;335(4):217–225.
67. SoS Investigators. Coronary artery bypass surgery versus percutaneous coronary intervention with stent implantation in patients with multivessel coronary artery disease (the stent or surgery trial): a randomised controlled trial. *Lancet.* 2002;360(9338):965–970.
68. Booth J, Clayton T, Pepper J, et al; SoS Investigators. Randomized, controlled trial of coronary artery bypass surgery versus percutaneous coronary intervention in patients with multivessel coronary artery disease: six-year follow-up from the Stent or Surgery Trial (SoS). *Circulation.* 2008;118(4):381–388.
69. Serruys PW, Morice MC, Kappetein AP, et al; SYNTAX Investigators. Percutaneous coronary intervention versus coronary-artery bypass grafting for severe coronary artery disease. *N Engl J Med.* 2009;360(10):961–972.
70. Head SJ, Milojevic M, Daemen J, et al. Mortality after coronary artery bypass grafting versus percutaneous coronary intervention with stenting for coronary artery disease: a pooled analysis of individual patient data. *Lancet.* 2018;391(10124):939–948.
71. Stone GW, Sabik JF, Serruys PW, et al; EXCEL Trial Investigators. Everolimus-eluting stents or bypass surgery for left main coronary artery disease. *N Engl J Med.* 2016;375(23):2223–2235.
72. Mäkikallio T, Holm NR, Lindsay M, et al; NOBLE study investigators. Percutaneous coronary angioplasty versus coronary artery bypass grafting in treatment of unprotected left main stenosis (NOBLE): a prospective, randomised, open-label, non-inferiority trial. *Lancet.* 2016;388(10061):2743–2752.

81

Mechanical Circulatory Support

Eric I. Jeng and Eric Yates Pruitt

Key Points

1 The term mechanical circulatory support (MCS) refers to a broad array of cardiac support devices distinguished by the following important features: location of the pumping chamber of the device, ventricle being supported, and pumping mechanism.

2 Indications for MCS include bridge to recovery, bridge to transplantation, and destination therapy.

3 Durable devices utilized for bridge to transplantation or destination therapy require major operative implantation that facilitates patient discharge from the hospital.

4 Delay in establishing MCS results in a greater acuity and severity of illness, decreasing survival secondary to a greater degree of organ failure.

5 Patient selection is the most important factor in determining outcome of patients who receive MCS.

6 Major adverse events following initiation of MCS are those related to anticoagulation therapy necessary during MCS, infection, right-sided heart failure, and malfunction of the device.

7 The Interagency Registry of Mechanically Assisted Circulatory Support (INTERMACS) is a National Institutes of Health-funded data registry designed to study outcomes for patients with durable, long-term implantable MCS devices.

8 Major technologic advances in device designs for temporary and durable devices have incorporated continuous-flow rotary pumps.

1 The term mechanical circulatory support (MCS) refers to a broad array of cardiac support devices. These devices are distinguished by the following important features: (1) location of the pumping chamber of the device (extracorporeal vs intracorporeal or "implantable"); (**Fig. 81.1**) (2) ventricle being supported (left ventricular assist device [LVAD] vs right ventricular assist device [RVAD] vs biventricular assist device [BiVAD] vs total artificial heart [TAH]); (**Fig. 81.2**) and (3) pumping mechanism (pulsatile, volume displacement device vs continuous-flow rotary device with axial or centrifugal design) (**Fig. 81.3**). Generally, the pumping chamber of short-term support devices is extracorporeal or paracorporeal in location, while durable systems are intracorporeal.

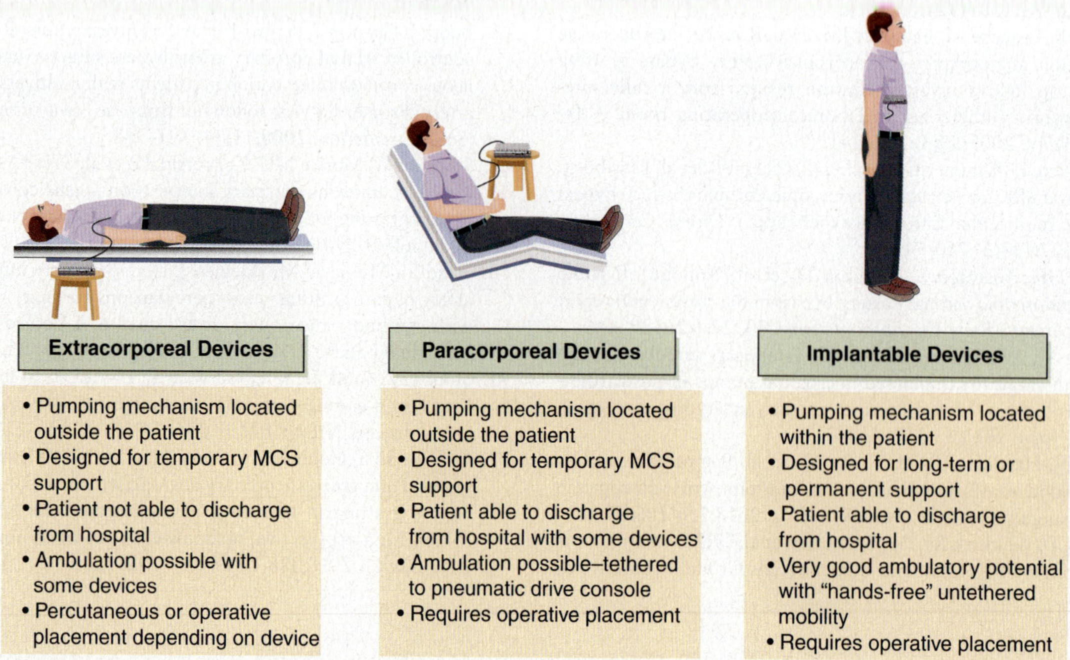

Figure 81.1. Classification of mechanical circulatory support devices by location of the pumping mechanism (extracorporeal, paracorporeal, and implantable).

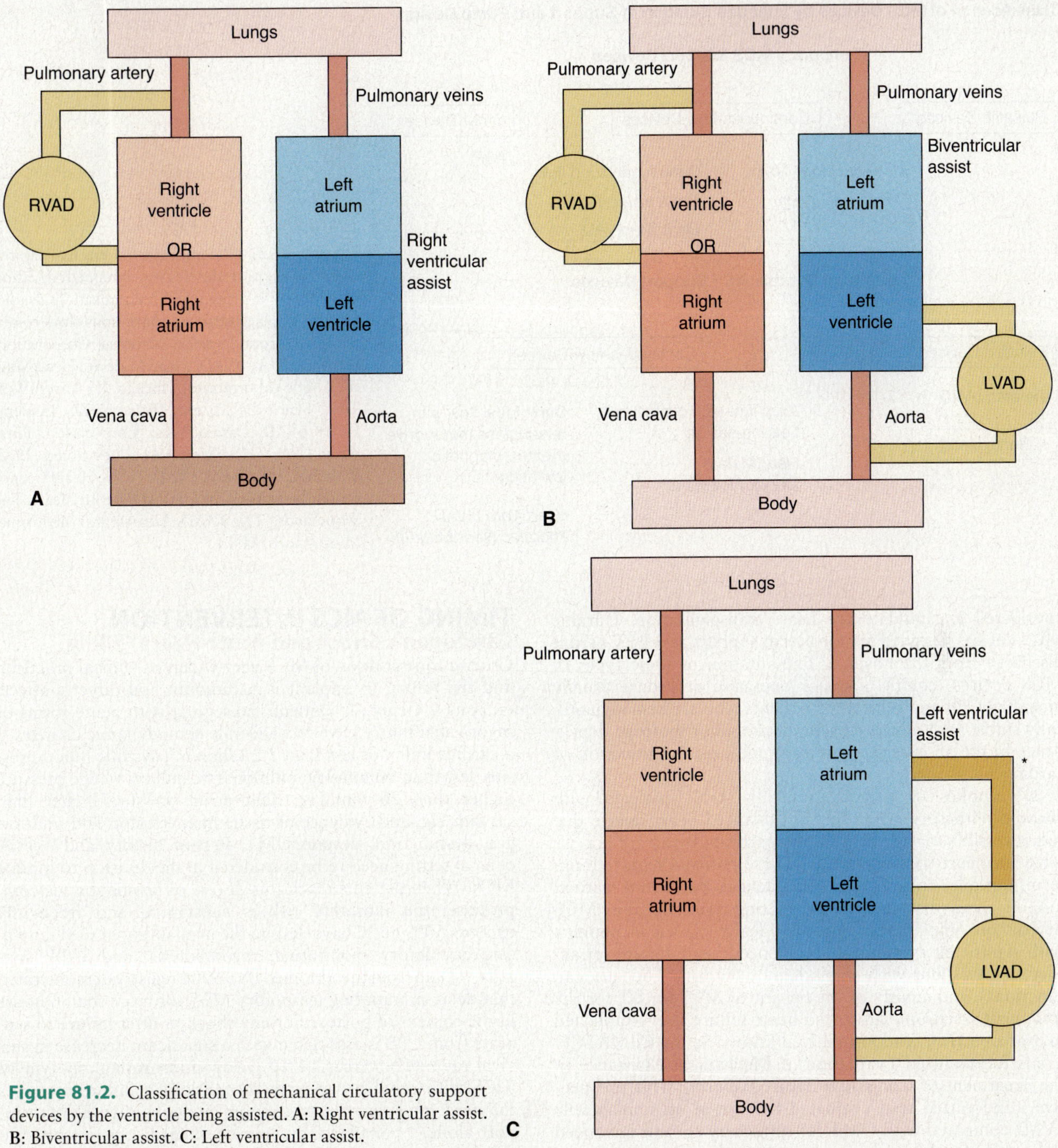

Figure 81.2. Classification of mechanical circulatory support devices by the ventricle being assisted. A: Right ventricular assist. B: Biventricular assist. C: Left ventricular assist.

INDICATIONS FOR MCS

The spectrum of MCS therapy encompasses several indica-
2 tions for use and a broad range of MCS device designs. Currently, there are three accepted indications for MCS based upon regulatory oversight by the US Food and Drug Administration (FDA) and reimbursement criteria set by the Centers for Medicare & Medicaid Services, bridge to recovery (BTR), bridge to transplant (BTT), and destination therapy (DT).

BTR refers to the use of MCS in patients who are presenting with acute cardiogenic shock and/or decompensated heart failure, where the optimal medical therapy (OMT), including intravenous inotropes and/or vasoconstrictors, has failed. These patients are thought to have an expectation of myocardial recovery following a short period (days to weeks) of temporary MCS. The short-term utilization of MCS for BTR is the most common application of MCS in the United States.[1] Examples of reversible forms of myocardial injury include acute myocardial infarction, viral myocarditis, or postcardiotomy cardiogenic shock with failure to separate from cardiopulmonary bypass (CPB) following various cardiac surgical procedures. Several types of devices can provide temporary MCS in these circumstances and include an intra-aortic balloon pump (IABP), extracorporeal ventricular assist device (VAD), or extracorporeal membrane oxygenation (ECMO)/extracorporeal life support (ECLS).[1] Frequently, temporary MCS devices are implanted percutaneously allowing for rapid initiation of support.[1] Certain types of extracorporeal VAD systems require surgical exposure of major arteries including the axillary, carotid, femoral, or aorta for implantation. These systems can be used as both precardiotomy support, postcardiotomy support, or in both settings to facilitate more graduated weaning.

BTT applies to patients presenting in cardiogenic shock
3 and/or decompensated heart failure refractory to OMT where myocardial function is unlikely to recover and the patient is

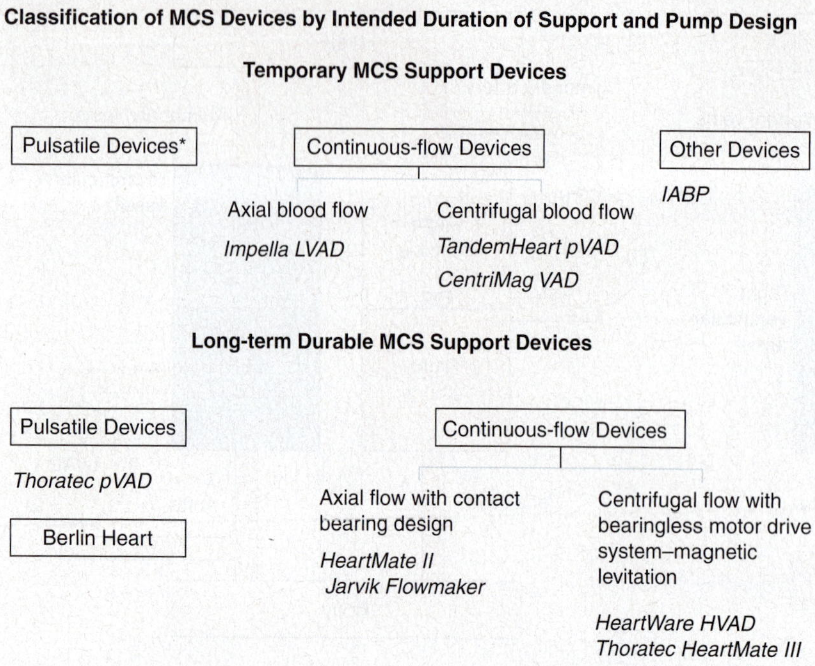

Figure 81.3. Classification of mechanical circulatory support devices by intended duration of support and pumping mechanism (pulsatile, volume displacement, or continuous-flow rotary pumps). (From Impella, Abiomed Corporation, Danvers, MA; pVAD, HeartMate II, HeartMate III, Abbot Laboratories, Chicago, IL; CardioWest TAH, Syncardia Systems, Tucson, AZ; TandemHeart pVAD, CardiacAssist Corporation, Pittsburgh, PA; CentriMag VAD, Levitronix LLC, Waltham, MA; Jarvik LVAD, Jarvik Heart Corporation, New York, NY; HVAD, Berlin Heart, The Woodlands, TX; LVAD, HeartWare Medtronic, Minneapolis, MN.)

considered a candidate for heart transplantation. Durable MCS devices designed for long-term support as a BTT permit discharge from the hospital. Implantation of these types of MCS devices requires a major operative procedure usually including CPB and is ideal for patients who are hemodynamically stable with advanced symptoms and/or inotrope dependence in the absence of significant end-organ dysfunction or cardiogenic shock.

DT applies to hemodynamically stable patients with chronic refractory symptoms of advanced heart failure due to irreversible forms of cardiomyopathy, but who are not eligible for heart transplantation. These patients require long-term, durable, and reliable MCS devices permitting patient mobility and discharge home.[2] Long-term, durable MCS devices are implantable and are ideally placed in patients with significant symptoms of advanced heart failure refractory to OMT but with stable hemodynamics. The survival, functional, and quality-of-life benefit of MCS for DT for the treatment of chronic advanced heart failure was established in a prospective, randomized trial known as the REMATCH Trial (Randomized Evaluation of Mechanical Assistance in the Treatment of Congestive Heart Failure).[2] This prospective, randomized trial evaluated the use of an implantable LVAD compared with OMT for refractory chronic advanced heart failure. LVAD therapy significantly reduced (relative risk, 0.52; 95% confidence limit, 0.34 to 0.78 at 1 year) the mortality seen in the control population treated with OMT at both 1-year and 2-year follow-up. Despite serious adverse events attributable to MCS from infection, bleeding, and device malfunction, LVAD recipients had an improved survival rate and experienced a superior quality of life compared to the medical therapy group. Currently, patients evaluated for DT must meet the following specific criteria: (1) New York Heart Association Class IV or American Heart Association Stage D heart failure symptoms; (2) a left ventricular ejection fraction of <25%; (3) a peak exercise oxygen consumption of <14 mL/kg/min (if unable to exercise be dependent on intravenous inotropes for 14 days or IABP therapy for 7 days); and (4) significant functional limitations despite the use of maximally tolerated doses of drugs outlined in the recent guidelines for heart failure treatment for at least 45 of the last 60 days.[3] The intended use and indication for MCS significantly influence MCS device selection and use and must be individualized.

TIMING OF MCS INTERVENTION

Cardiogenic Shock and Acute Heart Failure

Criteria for initiation of MCS vary widely in clinical practice,[1] and the timing of implant is paramount and directly affects outcomes. Generally, patients presenting with acute forms of myocardial injury have recognizable hemodynamic changes—a cardiac index of less than 2.2 L/min/m^2, systolic blood pressure less than 90 mm Hg, pulmonary capillary wedge pressure higher than 20 mm Hg, right atrial pressure higher than 18 mm Hg, and evidence of tissue malperfusion and multiorgan dysfunction, despite OMT. Patient history and overall clinical setting need to be considered in the decision to initiate MCS. When patients reach this degree of hemodynamic compromise, the mortality risk is substantial and frequently exceeds 50% at 30 days despite the availability of OMT, invasive circulatory monitoring, thrombolysis, and IABP support.[4,5] Data from the Abiomed BVS 5000 registry demonstrated that delay in initiating temporary MCS for more than 6 hours in the context of postcardiotomy shock or after failure to separate from CPB is associated with a significant decrease in survival rate; 44% versus 14%.[6] Delay in instituting any type of MCS with rapid progression of multiorgan failure increases
4 the need for biventricular support as opposed to LVAD support alone.[7–11] Similarly, an episode of cardiac arrest prior to the initiation of MCS significantly impacts survival rate, decreasing it from 47% to only 7%.[6]

Chronic Heart Failure

Patients with chronic advanced heart failure are evaluated for BTT or DT MCS when they experience dyspnea at rest and/or with any effort and accompanied by resting tachycardia, progressive organ dysfunction (reflected in worsening renal or hepatic parameters), limited functional capacity, and poor quality of life despite OMT with or without inotrope therapy. Deterioration in end-organ function or progressive decline in functional performance may occur in the absence of a significant change in hemodynamic parameters due to chronic adaptation to low cardiac output. In addition, patients who experience renal insufficiency or hypotension in the setting of optimal doses of ACE inhibitors or beta blockers, as well as those who do not tolerate inotrope therapy due to refractory ventricular arrhythmias or have life-threatening coronary disease may benefit from MCS therapy (**Algorithm 81.1**). Dependence on intravenous inotropes has traditionally been

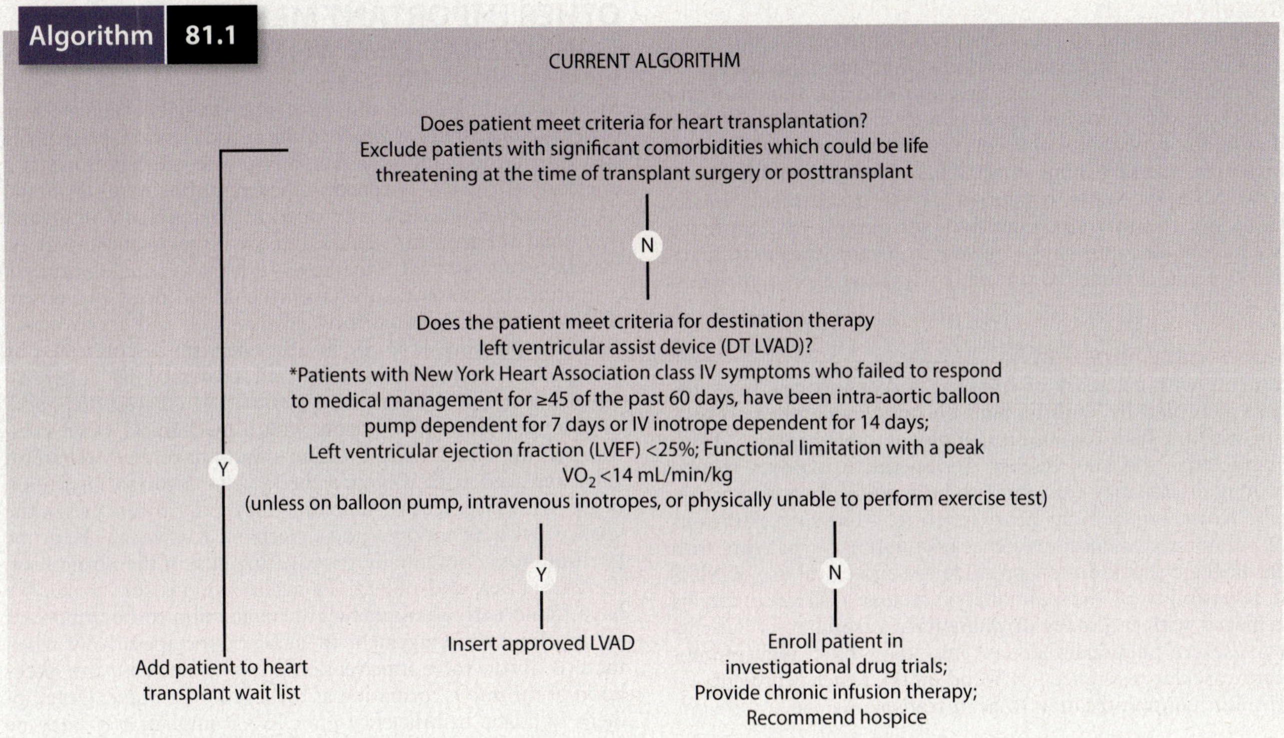

Algorithm 81.1. Current algorithm for assessing patients with advanced heart failure for heart transplantation and mechanical circulatory support. Transplant status is initially assessed to determine appropriate indication for MCS use; BTT versus DT. (Adapted from Mancini D, Colombo PC. Left ventricular assist devices: A rapidly evolving alternative to transplant. *J Am Coll Cardiol.* 2015;65(23):2542–2555, with permission.)

considered the threshold that prompts consideration of MCS[12–14] (**Fig. 81.4**). However, patients with advanced systolic heart failure are currently eligible for DT therapy even if they are not dependent on inotropes, provided they meet indications for DT therapy. Only 18% of durable adult LVADs are currently implanted in patients not yet dependent on intravenous inotropes.[12,13]

Low implant rates in ambulatory advanced heart failure (noninotrope dependent) may reflect reluctance of both physicians and patients.[15] Ambulatory patients with advanced heart failure should have ongoing discussions about the trade-offs of living with heart failure in comparison with undergoing LVAD implantation to identify preferences and thresholds for considering elective LVAD therapy. Evidence to guide LVAD use before inotrope dependence is growing.[16]

It should also be noted that as of 2018 there have been changes to UNOS Heart Donor Allocation Scores which effect transplantation status in those with stable VAD therapy. The previous guidelines listed patients with durable LVADs as status Ib. As of 2018, the presence of a stable LVAD lists patients as status 4, resulting in a potentially lower allocation status and longer wait time for donation.[17] For this reason, there has been a trend toward decreased LVAD implantation as a bridge to transplantation.[17] For those who have LVADs as a bridge to transplantation, the wait time for a heart has been longer, putting patients at increased risk of LVAD related complications.[17]

PATIENT SELECTION AND INFLUENCE OF COMORBIDITIES ON OUTCOMES

Patient selection is paramount in determining outcome in patients requiring MCS. Relative contraindications to MCS include irreversible renal, hepatic or respiratory failure, sepsis, and/or a significant neurocognitive deficit.

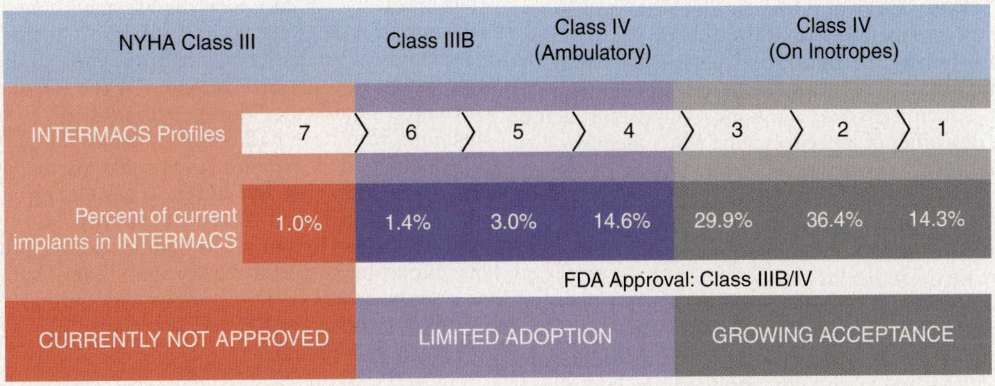

Figure 81.4. INTERMACS scale for classifying patients with advanced heart failure. Percent of implants by INTERMACS profile. Current US Food and Drug Administration (FDA) approval status and acceptance in the medical community. (Adapted from Mancini D, Colombo PC. Left ventricular assist devices: a rapidly evolving alternative to transplant. *J Am Coll Cardiol.* 2015;65(23):2542–2555, with permission.)

Renal Function

MCS in the setting of renal dysfunction has consistently been associated with increased morbidity and mortality rates.[18,19] The patient's baseline renal function and the duration and chronicity of cardiogenic shock play an important role in predicting the probability of recovery of renal function. In some instances, reestablishing normal hemodynamics with short-term MCS facilitates resolution of the acute renal failure. Clinically, this may guide decisions for durable MCS options. We have used continuous venovenous hemofiltration to manage systemic volumes to prevent early onset right ventricular (RV) failure.[20]

Pulmonary Function

Patients with a history of smoking and/or intrinsic lung disease identified by abnormalities on pulmonary function testing warrant high-resolution computed tomography (CT) to characterize the lung disease. Perioperative hypoxia related to lung disease may contribute to pulmonary vasoconstriction and worsening of right heart function. Moderate elevations of pulmonary vascular resistance encountered in patients with cardiogenic shock do not preclude the successful use of MCS if reversibility of the pulmonary vascular resistance can be achieved with inotropes or pulmonary vasodilators. Patients with severe pulmonary disease may have fixed high pulmonary vascular resistance (>8 Wood units), which represents an absolute contraindication to heart transplantation.

Liver Function

Total bilirubin and hepatic cellular enzyme levels more than three times normal are independent risk factors for adverse outcomes.[19,20] The etiology of the hyperbilirubinemia may be multifactorial, resulting from any combination of congestive hepatopathy, cholestasis, primary biliary, or infectious or parenchymal disease. Attempts should be made to normalize the liver function prior to initiation of durable MCS, as abnormal liver function often results in low serum albumin and abnormal coagulation. In our potential MCS patients we review for significant alcohol and drug use, and test for presence of hepatitis A, B, or C or other viruses. We obtain a CT of the chest, abdomen, and pelvis for surgical planning. If the liver is abnormal on CT, we utilize liver ultrasonography and/or magnetic resonance imaging to rule out infiltrative disease, mass or other pathology that may warrant biopsy. While permanent liver dysfunction may rule out durable MCS options, these same patients may in fact be candidates for multiorgan heart-liver transplantation.

Right Ventricular Heart Failure

RV heart failure presents as signs of renal, pulmonary, and hepatic dysfunction following LVAD implantation. It is a significant cause of mortality and morbidity, and often necessitates the initiation of BiVAD support.[7–11,21–23] BiVAD support is associated with lower survival during both short- and long-
5 term MCS. Thus, preoperative optimization of RV function with a goal of lowering the right atrial pressure lower than 15 mm Hg is important in reducing the need for postoperative RVAD support. Patient selection is the most important factor in determining outcomes of those receiving MCS therapy.

Nutrition

Malnutrition is an important contributor to morbidity among patients on MCS. A serum albumin lower than 3.3 mg/dL appears to increase the mortality rate 6.6 times in the DT population of LVAD patients.[24,25] Significant nutritional deficiency is often associated with poor wound healing, an increased risk of infection. Patients whose body mass index is either less than 22 or more than 36 are at risk for perioperative complications. In morbidly obese patients, some have described bariatric surgery as a means for weight reduction to bridge to transplantation.[26]

OTHER IMPORTANT MEDICAL CONSIDERATIONS WHEN INITIATING MCS

Valvular Heart Disease

Valvular heart disease can have important consequences in patients considered for MCS. In the aortic position, preexisting stenosis that is mild, moderate, and severe can left alone as it does not affect LVAD function. Severe aortic stenosis should be addressed if recovery is an option.[27] The presence of greater than mild aortic insufficiency can have a significant impact on the effectiveness of MCS therapy as it leads to recirculation, LV distention, decrease in subendocardial blood flow, and potentially decreased systemic forward flow and end-organ perfusion. The presence of aortic insufficiency can be confirmed by perioperative echocardiography and addressed by either AV replacement with a bioprosthetic, repair via a Park Stitch, and/or complete closure.[28] Patients with a mechanical valve prosthesis in the aortic valve position should have the mechanical valve replaced with a bioprosthetic valve prior to institution of LV assistance. During unloading of the LV by an LVAD, the aortic valve may not open and a mechanical valve may be prone to thrombosis, potentially propagating clot in the aortic root, the coronaries, and potentially act as a nidus for stroke. We have found early therapeutic anticoagulation to be important in the clinical management of patients postoperatively when there is aortic valve intervention so as to decrease the likelihood of thrombus formation at the level of the valve. Development of aortic insufficiency after LVAD implantation may be addressed at later date with aortic valve replacement, via either open surgical or transcatheter aortic valve replacement.[29,30]

Patients with significant mitral stenosis at the time of initiation of device support may require correction of the valvular problem before implantation, as LV filling is impaired which limits device filling. Mitral regurgitation likely does not have an impact on the filling of a VAD, and we do not routinely repair or replace the mitral valve in the setting of regurgitation. Multiple studies have shown that mitral valve intervention does not change mortality, rates of right heart failure, or readmission rates.[31,32] Tricuspid regurgitation and RV dilatation contribute to elevated central venous pressure, hepatic congestion, and renal dysfunction.[21–23,33–35] Significant degrees of tricuspid regurgitation can impair the flow of blood from the RV through the pulmonary circuit. Studies have shown that while CPB times were longer, there were no significant differences in early mortality and late mortality, early RV failure and late RV failure, acute kidney failure, early RV assist device implantation or length of hospital stay in patients undergoing LVAD + tricuspid valve surgery versus LVAD alone.[35] With that said, it is our practice to evaluate the tricuspid annular dimensions and perform an annuloplasty for moderate or more degrees of tricuspid regurgitation.

Coronary Artery Disease

The presence of coronary disease may contribute to ongoing myocardial ischemia and increase the risk of ventricular arrhythmias for patients supported with temporary or durable MCS. Perioperative ischemia of the RV may be of hemodynamic significance during initiation of LVAD support. In patients who have had coronary bypass surgery and are candidates for MCS, patent bypass grafts, particularly to the right coronary artery or left anterior descending coronary artery should be preserved to reduce the risk of perioperative RV failure and arrhythmias. In highly selected situations, it may be important to perform a coronary artery bypass to the right coronary artery or left anterior descending coronary artery systems to optimize RV and ventricular septal function in the perioperative period.

Arrhythmias

Atrial and ventricular arrhythmias are common in patients with cardiogenic shock and underlying cardiomyopathies. We have utilized concomitant sympathectomies and both intra- and extracardiac ablation procedures for patient's prone to malignant arrhythmias. Some patients with refractory ventricular arrhythmias may even require biventricular support. In situations where weaning from MCS is feasible or planned, elimination of the ventricular arrhythmias with antiarrhythmic therapy is essential. The majority of patients undergoing implantation of a durable VAD have an implantable cardiac defibrillator (ICD) in place as part of their care for advanced heart failure. Currently, for those patients who do not have an ICD at the time of VAD implant, the International Society for Heart and Lung Transplantation (ISHLT) guidelines recommend routine evaluation for ICD therapy.[36,37]

Intracardiac Shunts

Intracardiac shunts (atrial or ventricular septal defects) identified by transesophageal echocardiography prior to surgery should be closed at the time of implantation of a VAD to prevent right-to-left shunting.[38] As LV assistance is initiated, left atrial pressure can be reduced compared with right atrial pressures causing shunting of deoxygenated blood from the right atrium into the left resulting in systemic hypoxemia.

PATIENT OUTCOMES AND MAJOR ADVERSE EVENTS FOLLOWING INITIATION OF MCS

6 Bleeding, stroke and thromboembolism, infection, and RV failure are the most frequent complications that occur following initiation of MCS.

Bleeding

Bleeding is a frequent complication in patients supported by MCS. Risk factors for early bleeding include preoperative hepatic congestion and failure, poor preoperative nutritional status, prolonged CPB times, extensive surgical dissection, reoperative surgery, multiple cannulation sites, and decreased platelet function. Nonsurgical sources of bleeding are epistaxis, GI tract bleeding, bleeding of the mediastinum and thorax, and intracranial hemorrhage.[39–44] Some data demonstrate patients supported with long-term durable MCS have acquired von Willebrand disease caused by high shear stresses within continuous-flow rotary pumps.[42,43] These bleeding episodes manifest at mucosal sites including gastrointestinal bleeding and epistaxis, and appears to accentuate previous subclinical arteriovenous malformations.[45,46]

RV Failure

RV failure occurs in approximately 3% to 30% of patients supported by LVAD support alone. The large variation in occurrence of RV failure is dependent on various patient factors including severity of illness and timing of intervention. The etiology of RV failure is multifactorial and includes pathologies within the pulmonary vascular bed and/or RV. Factors contributing to RV failure include impaired RV function as a result of intraoperative air embolism, myocardial stunning due to poor intraoperative myocardial protection, ischemia secondary to coronary artery disease, arrhythmias, volume loading, and alteration of RV septal geometry induced by LV unloading. Several studies have demonstrated that factors such as elevated central venous pressure, reduced RV stroke work index, low preoperative pulmonary artery pressures, increased transpulmonary gradient greater than 16 mm Hg, acute decrease in pulmonary artery pressures equal to or greater than 10 mm Hg at the onset of LVAD support, degree of preoperative pulmonary edema, increased need for perioperative transfusions, increasing degree of renal and hepatic dysfunction, female gender, nonischemic etiology, and preoperative temporary MCS support, all increase the need for RV MCS following LVAD implantation.[7–11,21–23] Data analysis revealed that a central venous pressure/pulmonary capillary wedge pressure ratio greater than 0.63, need for preoperative ventilator support, and blood urea nitrogen level higher than 39 mg/dL were independent predictors of right-sided heart failure after LVAD implantation.[21] Acute unloading of the LV by MCS may cause the septum to shift leftward, increasing RV volume loading and reducing its function.[22,23,47] The negative consequences of this phenomenon may be offset by the reduction in pulmonary artery pressures and RV afterload caused by device-mediated LV decompression.[22,23,47] Hemodynamic stability can be attained with isolated mechanical LV support in the overwhelming majority of patients, even in those patients with substantial RV dysfunction, if there is effective replacement of left-sided heart function and aggressive treatment of pulmonary hypertension. More recently, the improved perioperative management of elevated pulmonary vascular resistance including the use of inhaled nitric oxide and/or flolan, in combination with milrinone, isoproterenol, or dobutamine has significantly reduced the need for placement of an RVAD.[47] In addition, groups have shown that CVVH can also contribute to combatting early RV dysfunction.[20] In patients with marked elevation of central venous pressure, multiorgan failure, and severe RV dysfunction with low pulmonary artery pressures, early biventricular support may be indicated.[47]

Intracranial Bleeding and Thromboembolism

Cerebral vascular accidents are one of the most feared complications of MCS. The reported rates of hemorrhagic stroke range from 0.01 to 0.08 events per patient-year.[46] The occurrence of thromboembolic events following MCS is variable and depends on a number of factors including the type of device, duration of support, location and number of cannulation sites, and the presence of prosthetic valves within the heart. Approximately 10% of patients receiving MCS with implantable devices will experience a thromboembolic event or stroke.[24,46,48] This rate is in the range of 20% for patients on short-term extracorporeal MCS devices.[1] Hemorrhagic stroke rates have been improved with guided blood pressure control protocols.[49] Improvement in the rate of thromboembolic events has come from more aggressive antiplatelet therapy in conjunction with warfarin, in addition to improved device design. In MOMENTUM 3, where patients with axial and centrifugal continuous-flow devices were prospectively compared, the numbers of events per patient-year for stroke of any severity, major bleeding, and gastrointestinal hemorrhage were lower in the centrifugal-flow pump group than in the axial-flow pump group.[50]

Infection

Infections can be device-related (ie, device endocarditis, percutaneous lead or cannula site infection, pocket infection [infection external to an implanted device]) or non–device-related (ie, pneumonia and urinary tract infection). The incidence of early nosocomial device-related infections in patients undergoing MCS is approximately 30% in many series and is related to the acuity of illness in this population of patients.[51–56] Patients with persistent or recurrent sepsis, and those patients with device-related infections, tend to have a higher mortality rate than patients without these complications.[56] In patients on long-term MCS, infection remains an important obstacle to successful outcome.[56] Most of these late infections begin in the percutaneous driveline tract and pocket of the device. However, clinical experience has revealed that VAD infection rates can be minimized with attention to infection control guidelines; optimal implantation techniques, meticulous wound care, and the utilization of new continuous-flow rotary pump technology.[56] The risk factors for development of infection include preoperative infection at remote sites (not in the area of implantation), malnutrition, prolonged hospitalization, immobilization, broad-spectrum antibiotic therapy, immunosuppressive medications, mechanical ventilation, and the presence of central venous catheters. Device-related infections can sometimes be

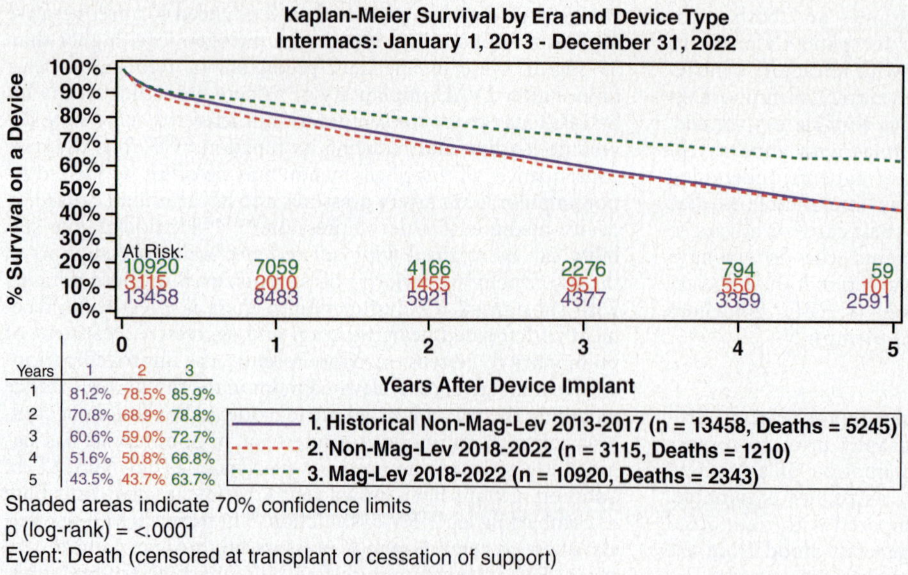

Figure 81.5. Kaplan-Meier survival estimates comparing HMII in the previous era (2013–2017), HMII in the current era (2018–2022) to HM III devices in the current era. (From Jorde UP, Saeed O, Koehl D, et al. The Society of Thoracic Surgeons Intermacs 2023 Annual Report: Focus on magnetically levitated devices. *Ann Thorac Surg*. 2024;117(1):33–44. Figure 3B.)

successfully treated with antibiotic suppression and device exchange or removal. Patients who are device-dependent and awaiting transplantation generally cannot tolerate device removal as a therapeutic option to eradicate the infection. Antibiotic suppression and transplantation remain the only chance for cure of device-related infections in these instances.

Device Malfunction and Thrombosis

The types and severity of device malfunctions vary with each MCS device. Many devices have built-in backup systems that, in the event of catastrophic device failure, provide some support to the patient. In some instances, patients supported by an LVAD have enough residual LV function remaining to help sustain them until corrective measures can be taken in the event of complete device failure. Fortunately, the reported frequency of this event is low.[24] Device malfunctions in TAHs are more problematic as there is no native heart to provide hemodynamic support in the event of a total device failure.

Pump thrombosis is potentially a catastrophic complication of VAD therapy. The variability in clinical presentation makes it a challenging diagnosis. It occurs both early and late after VAD implantation and may manifest itself with increased pump power, decreased device flow with heart failure, and hemolysis with hemoglobinuria or with embolic event. Serum lactate dehydrogenase level is as the primary biochemical marker of hemolysis in this clinical context. Clinically suspected thrombosis can be managed medically by intravenous anticoagulation, antiplatelet agents, or thrombolytics in some cases. Surgical treatment by pump explantation and pump replacement and/or urgent heart transplantation is generally indicated.

The Interagency Registry for Mechanically Assisted Circulatory Support (INTERMACS) database

7 The INTERMACS registry represents one of the largest available data repositories for the study of durable MCS device outcomes. The most recent INTERMACS database annual report summarizes outcomes in patients (≥19 years of age) who underwent durable MCS implant between January 2013 and December 2022. There were 29,391 adult patients with MCS reported, of whom 27,493 received CF LVADs (Jorde et al.). Of these, 1358 received historical non-mag lev devices (2013–2017), 3115 received non-mag lev devices (2018–2022), and 10,920 received mag lev devices (2018–2022). One year survival for centrifugal versus axial flow devices were 86% versus 79% ($P < .0001$). Five year survival was 64% versus 44% ($P < .0001$) respectively. Patients who required concomitant RVAD support had 1- and 5-year survivals of 59.3% and 37%, respectively (Jorde et al.). The actuarial survival for primary device implant as stratified by era is summarized in **Figure 81.5**. **Figure 81.6** illustrates Kaplan Meier

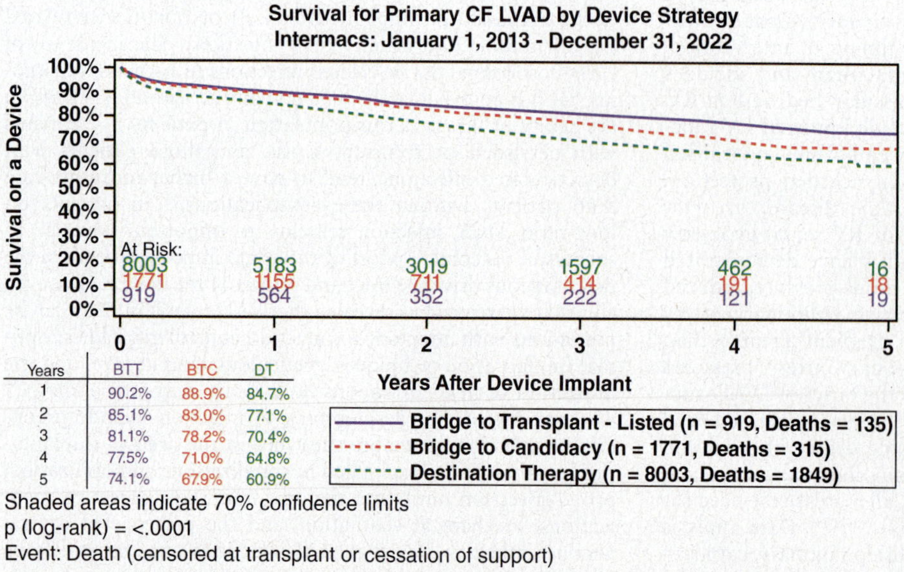

Figure 81.6. Keplan-Meier survival estimates comparing device strategy at implantation. *BTC*, bridge to candidacy; *BTT*, bridge to transplant; *CF*, continuous flow; *DT*, destination therapy. (From Jorde UP, Saeed O, Koehl D, et al. The Society of Thoracic Surgeons Intermacs 2023 Annual Report: Focus on magnetically levitated devices. *Ann Thorac Surg*. 2024;117(1):33–44. Figure 4C.)

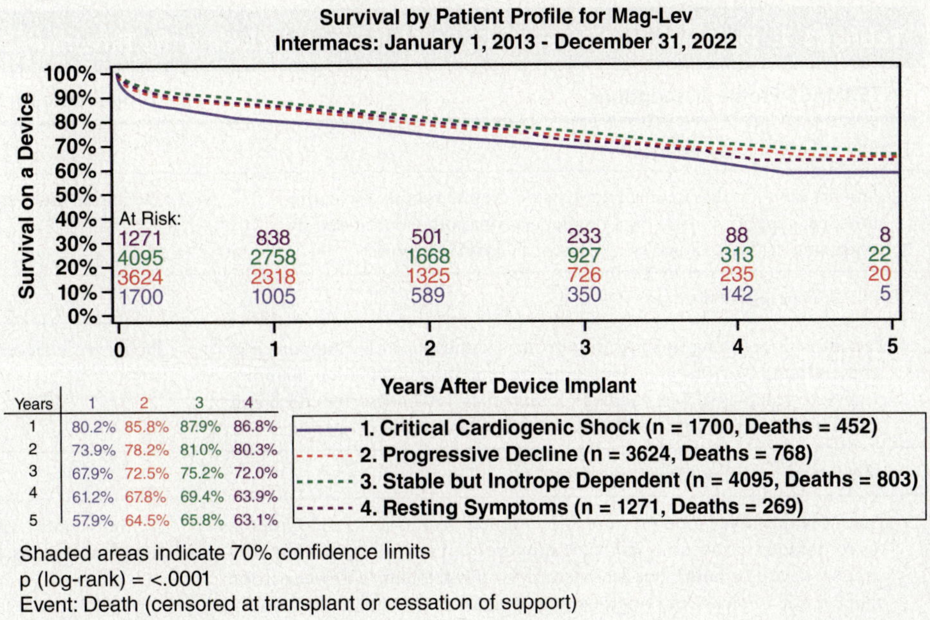

Figure 81.7. Survival estimates by INTERMACs profile. (From Jorde UP, Saeed O, Koehl D, et al. The Society of Thoracic Surgeons Intermacs 2023 Annual Report: Focus on Magnetically Levitated Devices. *Ann Thorac Surg*. 2024;117(1):33–44. Figure 4B.)

survival estimates comparing device strategy at implantation. The survival analysis for patients on MCS stratified by INTERMACS profile is presented in **Figure 81.7**. On January 1, 2018, the INTERMACS Database became part of The Society of Thoracic Surgeons National Database.[13] **Figure 81.8** exhibits MCS device implants by implant era and indication for implantation.

See Table 81.1 for additional details.

WEANING PATIENTS FROM MCS

Weaning Short-Term MCS

A number of factors are considered when weaning patients from MCS. Optimization of volume status, afterload, cardiac rhythm, and degree of inotropic support as well as exclusion of obvious surgical pathology, such as tamponade, is paramount before attempting separation from MCS. In addition, extracardiac causes, such as pulmonary edema, elevated pulmonary vascular resistance, acute respiratory distress syndrome, and pneumonia, may worsen RV function and prevent successful weaning from MCS. Once a patient's status has been optimized, weaning from MCS aided with echocardiographic monitoring is preferred. As device flows are reduced, echocardiogram provides information on ventricular filling and performance and valve function. If patients maintain satisfactory hemodynamics with reduction of pump flow, they can be considered for weaning. In the setting of biventricular support, it is important that device flows on the right side be reduced before lowering left-sided device flows. This prevents pulmonary edema in the event of inadequate LV function. As device flows are reduced, native heart function begins to support the circulation. When weaning from MCS is not possible, patients should be evaluated for heart transplantation and/or bridged to a durable MCS device.

Weaning Long-Term MCS

Observations from the cumulative experience with long-term MCS for BTT and recent small clinical studies have demonstrated that long-term MCS, associated with sustained mechanical unloading of the LV, can improve myocardial function even in those patients initially thought to have irreversible, dilated cardiomyopathies.[57–59] Several studies have demonstrated that long-term MCS can restore ventricular geometry, improve myocyte function, orientation, and size, reduce myocyte apoptosis, reduce myocardial cytokine gene and protein expression, reverse abnormal neurohormonal patterns associated with advanced heart failure, and improve myocardial mitochondrial function.[57–59]

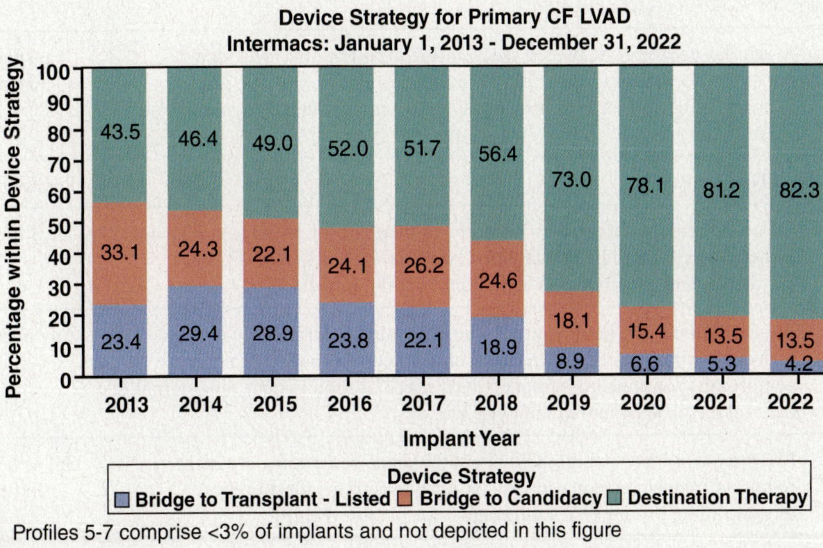

Figure 81.8. Continuous flow LVAD annual implants from 2013 to 2022 by device strategy at time of implantation. (From Jorde UP, SaeedO, Koehl D, et al. The Society of Thoracic Surgeons Intermacs 2023 Annual Report: Focuson magnetically levitated devices. *Ann Thorac Surg*. 2024;117(1):33–44. Figure 2B.)

Table 81.1. Description of INTERMACS Profile Classes, Including the Timeframe for Intervention

INTERMACS Profile Descriptions	Time Frame for Intervention
Profile 1: Critical cardiogenic shock	
Patients with life-threatening hypotension despite rapidly escalating inotropic support, critical organ hypoperfusion, often confirmed by worsening acidosis and/or lactate levels. "*Crash and burn.*"	Definitive intervention needed within hours.
Profile 2: Progressive decline	
Patient with declining function despite intravenous inotropic support, may be manifested by worsening renal function, nutritional depletion, inability to restore volume balance "*Sliding on inotropes.*" Also describes declining status in patients unable to tolerate inotropic therapy.	Definitive intervention needed within few days.
Profile 3: Stable but inotrope dependent	
Patient with stable blood pressure, organ function, nutrition, and symptoms on continuous intravenous inotropic support (or a temporary circulatory support device or both), but demonstrating repeated failure to wean from support due to recurrent symptomatic hypotension or renal dysfunction "*Dependent stability.*"	Definitive intervention elective over a period of weeks to few months.
Profile 4: Resting symptoms	
Patient can be stabilized close to normal volume status but experiences daily symptoms of congestion at rest or during ADL. Doses of diuretics generally fluctuate at very high levels. More intensive management and surveillance strategies should be considered, which may in some cases reveal poor compliance that would compromise outcomes with any therapy. Some patients may shuttle between 4 and 5.	Definitive intervention elective over period of weeks to few months.
Profile 5: Exertion intolerant	
Comfortable at rest and with ADL but unable to engage in any other activity, living predominantly within the house. Patients are comfortable at rest without congestive symptoms, but may have underlying refractory elevated volume status, often with renal dysfunction. If underlying nutritional status and organ function are marginal, patient may be more at risk than INTERMACS 4, and require definitive intervention.	Variable urgency, depends upon maintenance of nutrition, organ function, and activity.
Profile 6: Exertion limited	
Patient without evidence of fluid overload is comfortable at rest, and with activities of daily living and minor activities outside the home but fatigues after the first few minutes of any meaningful activity. Attribution to cardiac limitation requires careful measurement of peak oxygen consumption, in some cases with hemodynamic monitoring to confirm severity of cardiac impairment. "*Walking wounded.*"	Variable, depends upon maintenance of nutrition, organ function, and activity level.
Profile 7: Advanced NYHA III	
A placeholder for more precise specification in future, this level includes patients who are without current or recent episodes of unstable fluid balance, living comfortably with meaningful activity limited to mild physical exertion.	Transplantation or circulatory support may not currently be indicated.
Modifiers for Profiles	Possible Profiles to Modify
TCS—Temporary Circulatory Support can modify only patients in hospital (other devices would be INTERMACS devices) includes IABP, ECMO, TandemHeart, Levitronix, BVS 5000 or AB5000, Impella.	1,2,3 in hospital.
A—Arrhythmia can modify any profile. Recurrent ventricular tachyarrhythmias that have recently contributed substantially to clinical compromise. This includes frequent ICD shock or requirement for external defibrillator, usually more than twice weekly.	Any profile.
FF—Frequent Flyer can modify only outpatients, designating a patient requiring frequent emergency visits or hospitalizations for diuretics, ultrafiltration, or temporary intravenous vasoactive therapy.	3 if at home, 4,5,6. A frequent flyer would rarely be profile 7.

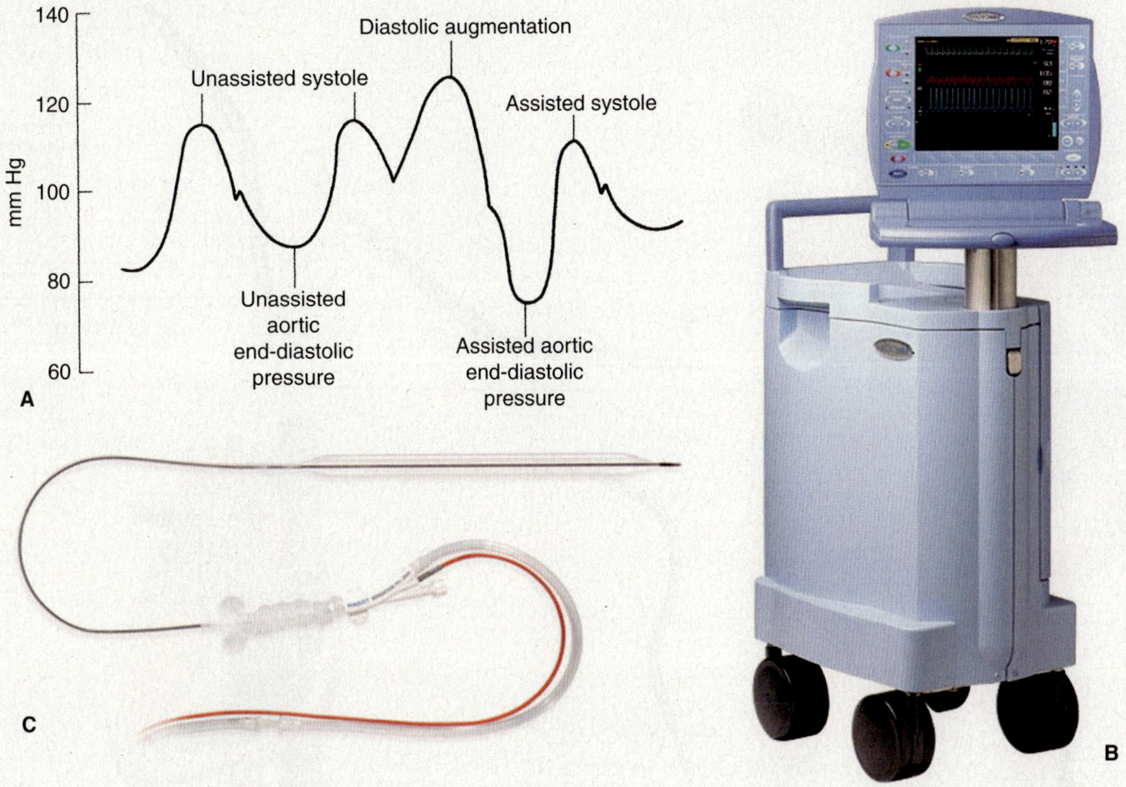

Figure 81.9. Intra-aortic balloon pump. **A:** Aortic pressure tracing during intra-aortic balloon pump support. Balloon counterpulsation is occurring after every other heartbeat (1:2 counterpulsation). With correct timing, balloon inflation (IP) begins immediately after aortic valve closure, signaled by the dicrotic notch of the arterial waveform. Compared with unassisted ejection, the pump augments diastolic blood flow by increasing peak aortic pressure during diastole. Balloon deflation before systole decreases ventricular afterload, with lower aortic end-diastolic pressure and lower peak systolic pressure. **B:** Console for the intra-aortic balloon pump. **C:** Catheter-mounted balloon is positioned within the thoracic aorta through a percutaneous or surgical approach via the femoral artery. (© DATASCOPE CORP. All rights reserved.)

MCS DEVICES

The devices currently approved by the FDA are broadly grouped into two categories based on durability and the intended length of support and use.

Devices Intended for Short-Term MCS (Temporary Devices)

IABP

Since its first reported clinical use by Kantrowitz in 1968, the IABP has become the most frequently utilized MCS device (**Fig. 81.9**).[60] The IABP is positioned within the descending thoracic aorta, augmenting ventricular performance and cardiac output increasing diastolic coronary blood flow, decreasing myocardial oxygen consumption, and reducing left ventricular afterload. Inflation of the balloon during diastole increases diastolic pressure and coronary blood flow and deflation of the balloon during systole reduces arterial afterload facilitating LV ejection. Although the IABP has been the mainstay of circulatory support for decades, the utility of IABP in cardiogenic shock complicating acute myocardial infarction was recently challenged by the results of the SHOCK-IABP Trial, and SHOCK-IABP II Trial.[61–63] These prospective studies randomized patients to IABP counterpulsation or no IABP counterpulsation in addition to revascularization and OMT. Both studies revealed no difference in 30-day mortality, length of stay in the intensive care unit, serum lactate level, incidence of renal failure, or duration of catecholamine therapy.[61–63] In the long-term follow-up, IABP has no effect on all-cause mortality at 6-year long-term follow-up. Mortality is still very high, with two-thirds of patients with cardiogenic shock dying despite contemporary treatment with revascularization therapy.[63] Complications from the use of the IABP include leg ischemia, balloon rupture, infection, bleeding, false aneurysm formation, femoral neuropathy, vessel perforation with hemorrhage, and aortic dissection. Female gender, peripheral vascular disease, diabetes, smoking, advanced age, obesity, and cardiogenic shock are predisposing factors for tissue malperfusion and limb ischemia.

Impella

Impella (Abiomed Corporation, Danvers, MA) is a continuous-flow rotary pump with axial design that propels blood from the LV across the aortic valve (**Fig. 81.10**) and into the ascending aorta[64,65] (**Fig. 81.11**). It is available in four delivery platforms for LV support including Impella LP 2.5, Impella CP, Impella LP 5.0, and Impella 5.5 with smart assist system, and the Impella RP and the Impella RP Flex—systems uniquely designed for RV support. The LVAD is positioned across the aortic valve with the inlet port below and outlet above the aortic valve. The hemodynamic effects of Impella devices are based on LV unloading and augmentation of forward flow. This reduces myocardial oxygen consumption, improves mean arterial blood pressure, and reduces pulmonary capillary wedge pressure.[66] In a prospective, randomized clinical trial comparing the Impella LP 2.5 to IABP, cardiac index was significantly increased in patients with the LP 2.5 compared with patients supported with an IABP. Overall mortality rate at
8 30 days was similar in both groups.[64] The Impella RP and RP Flex (**Fig. 81.10**) are novel RVAD designed using the Impella system but adapted for RV support. The major technologic advances in device designs for temporary and durable MCS devices have incorporated continuous-flow rotary pumps.

Tandem Heart

The Tandem Heart/Life Sparc (LivaNova, London, England) was a low-speed continuous-flow, centrifugal device MCS.

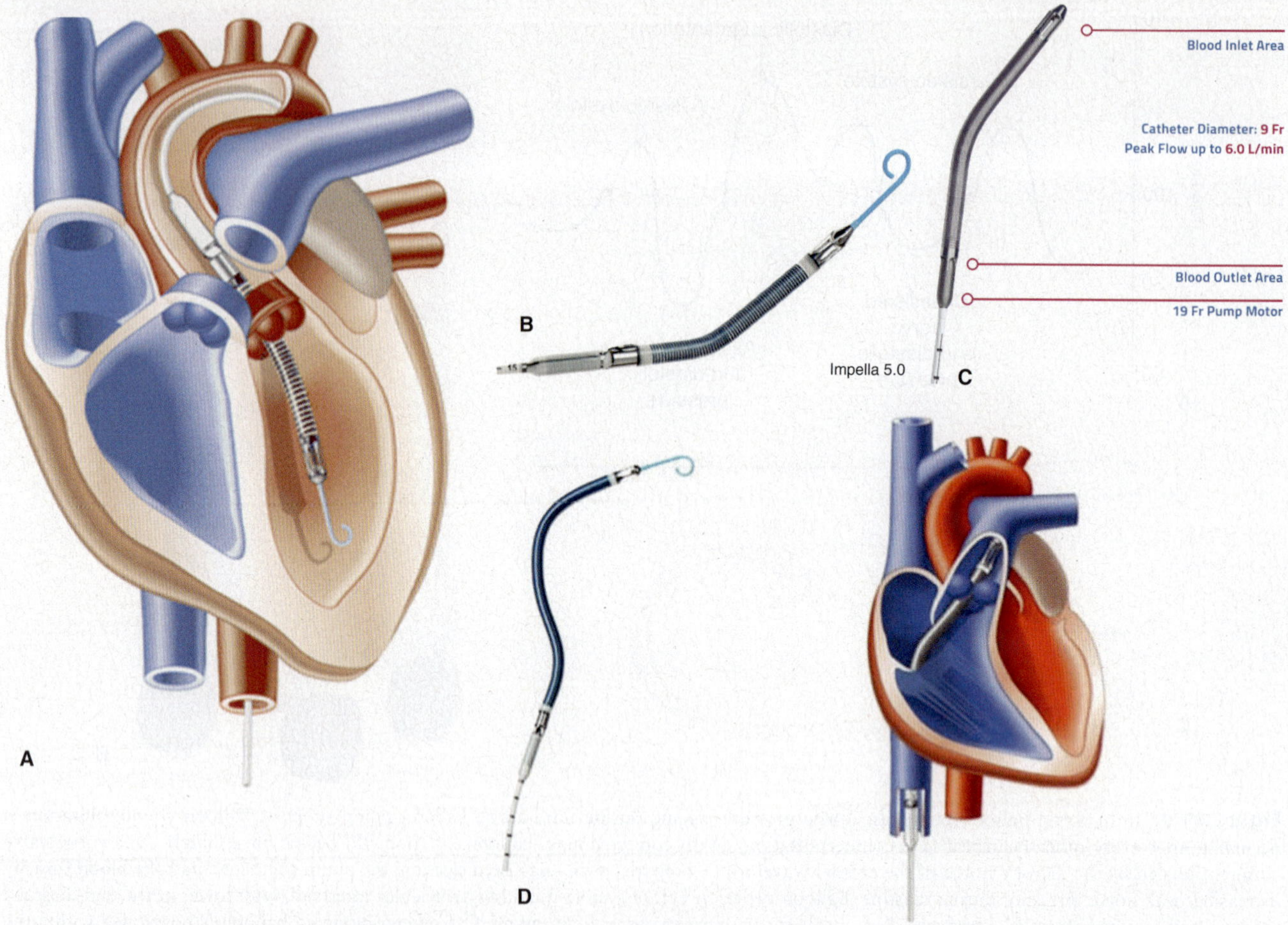

Figure 81.10. The Impella left ventricular assist device (From Diepenbrock NH. *Quick Reference to Critical Care*. 6th ed. Wolters Kluwer; 2021. Figure 2.77.). **A:** Diagram demonstrating positioning of the device across the aortic valve. Device inflow is within the left ventricle and device outflow is above the aortic valve. **B:** Impella 5.0. **C:** Impella 5.5. **D:** Impella RP. (Photographs courtesy of Abiomed Inc., Danvers, MA.)

Figure 81.11. **A:** The Tandem Heart pVAD centrifugal pump The TandemHeart pVAD is an extracorporeal, continuous flow rotary pump with centrifugal design providing temporary mechanical circulatory support to the left ventricle (left atrium to femoral artery). The TandemHeart pVAD utilizes a bearing design in the pump for impeller positioning and rotation. **B:** Schematic representation of the cannulation of the femoral artery and femoral vein with the transseptal placement of the inflow catheter within the left atrium from the femoral vein. The centrifugal pump of the Tandem Heart pVAD is secured to the patient's right thigh. (From Naidu SS. Novel percutaneous cardiac assist devices: the science of and indications for hemodynamic support. *Circulation*. 2011;123(5):533–543. Figure 3.)

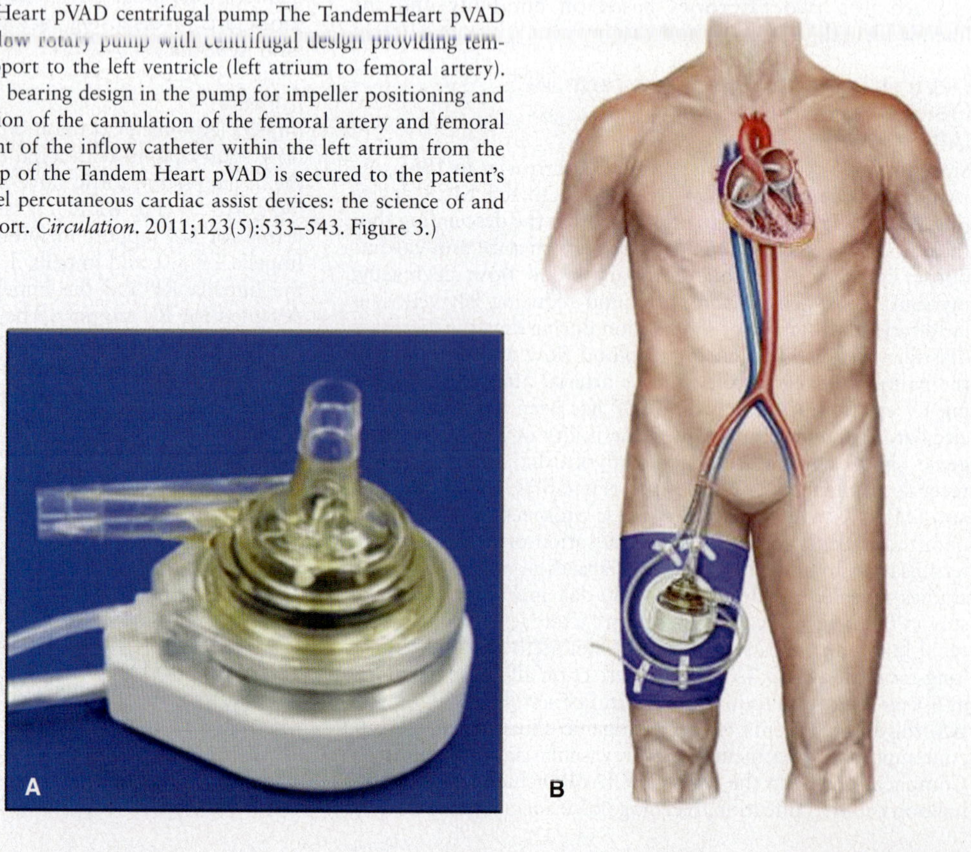

For historical value it employed the percutaneous cannulation strategy originated as a transseptal approach for left atrial-to-femoral artery VAD[67] (**Fig. 81.11**). This system for MCS has been discontinued. Protek Duo is a multilumen cannula that was created by LivaNova, and has been utilized as percutaneous RVAD. It is inserted through the right internal jugular vein or the left subclavian vein, with proximal ports in the right atrial and distal port in the distal main pulmonary artery. More recently, some groups[68] have described utilization of the Protek Duo Rapid Deployment in left apical cannulation to function as temporary LVAD.

CentriMag

The CentriMag (Abbot Laboratories, Chicago, IL) is an extracorporeal, continuous-flow centrifugal pump[69,70] based on a magnetically levitated "bearingless motor" design. This device can produce flows of up to 10 L/min under normal physiologic conditions, and can used as the pump with various cannulation strategies to support the left, or right ventricle.

Extracorporeal Life Support

ECLS, or ECMO, is a temporary form of MCS similar to CPB that provides circulatory assistance while allowing for both oxygenation and carbon dioxide removal from blood.[71–78] ECLS has been used in a variety of both pediatric and adult clinical settings, including respiratory support, postcardiotomy support, and as a bridge to an LVAD or heart and/or lung transplantation.[75]

In venoarterial ECLS, the blood is drained from the venous circulation, oxygenated, and returned to the arterial circulation. Although it does reduce LV preload by decreasing the pulmonary venous return, ECLS does not directly unload the LV. In patients with severe LV dysfunction, the use of an IABP and catecholamines helps reduce LV afterload and improves myocardial contractility, thus preventing blood stasis and thrombus formation within the LV. If LV function is so severely reduced that there is essentially no ejection, an atrial septostomy or insertion of a left ventricular vent can be inserted to relieve LV distention, a potential cause of pulmonary edema.

Venovenous ECLS, unlike venoarterial ECLS, maintains flow through the heart and is used solely for oxygenation and ventilation pulmonary support. Current ECLS circuits are typically composed of a centrifugal pump with membrane oxygenator, oxygen blender, pump console, heat exchanger, and pump cart. The CardioHelp (Maquet Cardiopulmonary GmbH, Rastatt, Germany) is a compact, portable unit useful due to the relative ease of transport and initiation. Gray and colleagues[75] at the University of Michigan reported on the outcome of 2000 patients supported with ECLS from 1973 through 2010. Of the 2000 patients, 74% were weaned from ECLS and 64% survived to hospital discharge. In patients with respiratory failure, survival to hospital discharge was 84% in 799 neonates, 76% in 239 children, and 50% in 353 adults. Survival in patients with cardiac failure was 45% in 361 children and 38% in 119 adults. ECLS during extracorporeal cardiopulmonary resuscitation was performed in 129 patients, with 41% surviving to discharge.

Implantable Devices Intended for Durable MCS

Historical Perspective

The majority of patients receiving long-term MCS in the 1990s and early 2000s were supported by devices engineered with pulsatile, volume displacement designs. A critical limitation of these devices were the large pump size restricting mobility, and the requirement for extensive surgical dissection for implant leading to bleeding and infection complications, both of which contributed to the high incidence of device malfunction.[79] These first-generation devices, now obsolete in clinical practice in favor of smaller, continuous-centrifugal-flow MCS device designs.

Implantable, Axial, Continuous-Flow MCS Devices

Implantable, continuous-flow, rotary pumps with axial or centrifugal blood flow design represent a new generation of implantable VAD technology that have now completely replaced pulsatile devices for long-term MCS indications.[24,48–50,80,81]

HeartMate II

The HeartMate II LVAD (Abbot Laboratories, Chicago, IL)[24,48–50,80] is a continuous-flow rotary pump with axial design and mechanical bearing support of the internal impeller. The HeartMate II was approved for BTT therapy in 2008 and for DT in 2010. In a prospective, multicenter, controlled study of HeartMate II as BTT the overall survival rate for the patients who continued on LVAD support was 82% (95% confidence interval [CI]: 77% to 87%) at 6 months, 73% (95% CI: 66% to 80%) at 1 year, and 72% (95% CI: 65% to 79%) at 18 months. The most common adverse effects were bleeding, stroke, infection, and neurocognitive dysfunction, while sepsis and stroke were the primary causes of mortality. Both groups experienced significant improvement in functional capacity and overall quality of life.[82]

HeartMate III

Implantable, Centrifugal, Continuous-Flow MCS Devices

Although significant improvements in pump design have occurred with continuous-flow rotary pumps, the use of a mechanical bearing support for the internal impeller, typical of most axial designs, has potential limitations. The presence of motor-suspending contact bearings in the blood path represents a potential point of frictional wear that can result in device failure and subsequent need for device exchange.[81,83,84] Rotary pumps with axial design with bearing support still demonstrate the potential for thrombus formation on the device rotor and bearing interface due to the presence of stasis and incomplete "wash" of the bearings and formation of heat from frictional at the bearing surfaces.[85,86] The major feature of current designs are the impeller rotation and levitation with magnetic and/or hydrodynamic forces, which eliminate the need for bearings and the subsequent bearing associated problems, enabling the potential for very long term durability.[80,82,83,87,88]

HVAD

The HVAD (Medtronic, Minneapolis, Minnesota) is a small continuous-flow rotary pump with centrifugal and noncontact bearing design. For elevated stroke risks, the pump was voluntarily discontinued.

HeartMate III

The HeartMate III (HMIII) (Abbot Laboratories, Chicago, IL) is a fully magnetically levitated centrifugal-flow VAD (**Fig. 81.12**).[87] Similarly to the HMII, the HM III has a sealed inflow conduit attached to the LV apex with an outflow graft connected to the ascending aorta, creating a circuit in parallel to the native circulation. It was approved in for short term support in 2017 and for DT in 2018. The new pump design alleviated some of the complication rates noted in the HMII. This was shown in the MOMENTUM 3 trial which showed a relative risk reduction from stroke, or device removal of 0.86 at 2 years. Overall the trial showed a reduced risk of stroke, major bleeding, and GI bleeding.[89] The final analysis of 1028 patients, with the primary end-point (alive and free of disabling stroke or reoperation to replace or remove a malfunctioning device at 2 years) was 64.8% in the axial-flow pump group as compared to 76.9% in the centrifugal-flow pump group, demonstrating superiority ($P < .001$). Furthermore, the numbers of events per patient-year for stroke of any severity, major bleeding, and gastrointestinal hemorrhage were lower in the centrifugal-flow pump group than in the

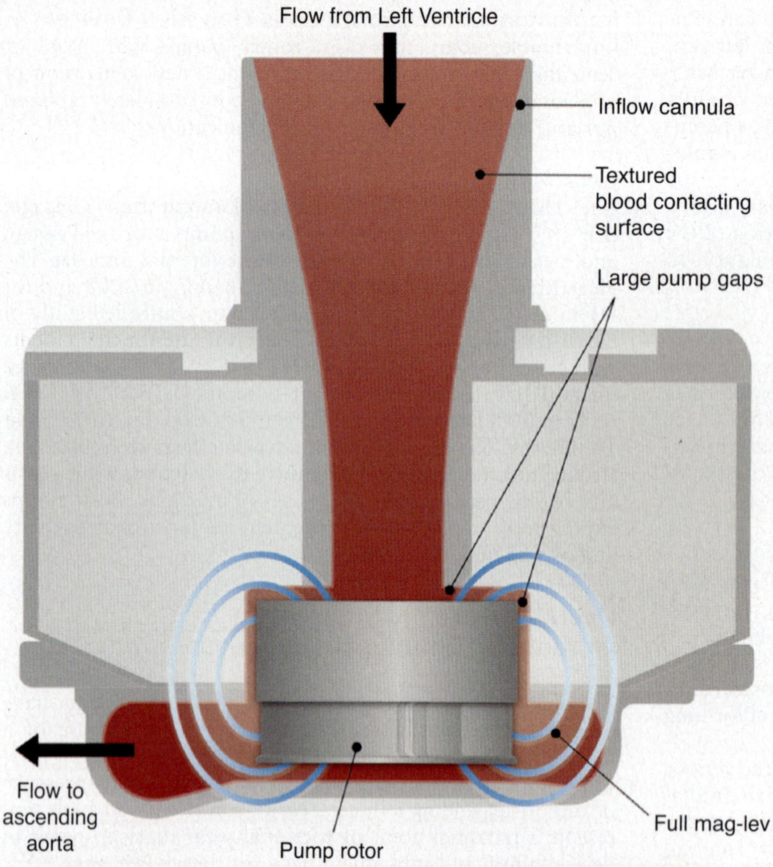

Figure 81.12. Schematic representation of the HeartMate III showing the blood path, internal rotor, and magnetic fields that achieve levitation and rotation of the internal rotor. (From Schmitto JD, Hanke JS, Rojas SV, et al. First implantation in man of a new magnetically levitated left ventricular assist device (HeartMate III). *J Heart Lung Transplant*. 2015;34:858–860.)

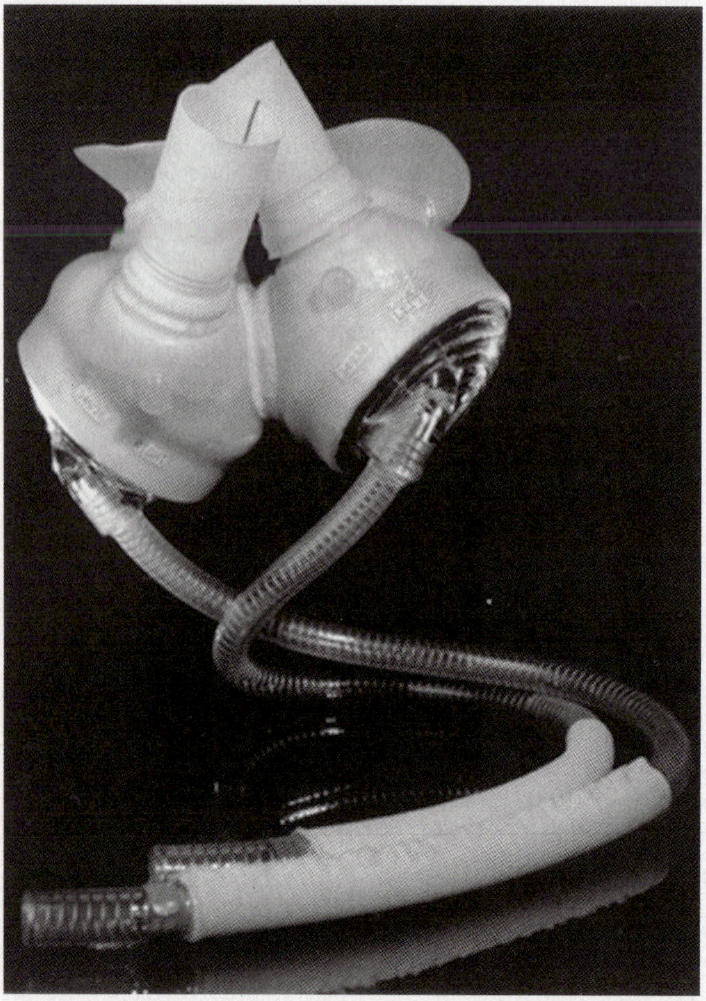

Figure 81.13. The CardioWest total artificial heart (Syncardia Systems Corporation, Tucson, AZ) is a pneumatically driven, pulsatile, volume displacement device. (From Arabia FA, Copeland JG, Pavie A, Smith RG. Implantation technique for the CardioWest total artificial heart. *Ann Thorac Surg*. 1999;68(2):698–704. Figure 1.)

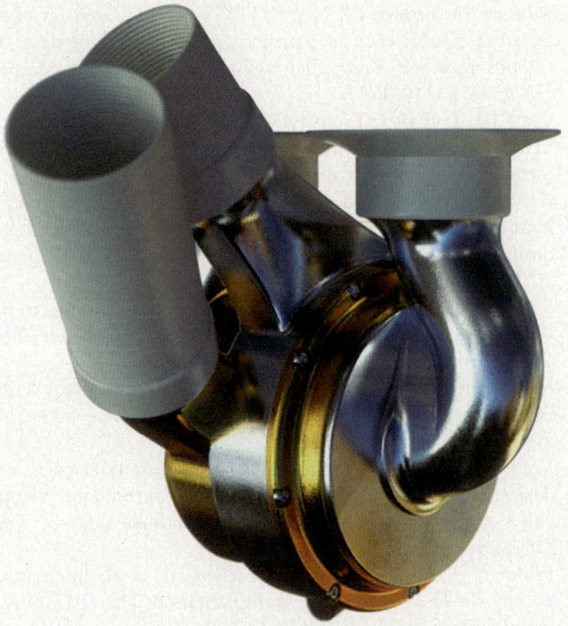

Figure 81.14. The BiVACOR total artificial heart (From BiVACOR, Inc, Huntington Beach, CA) is an electromechanical rotary blood pump used as a total artificial heart in contrast to the volume displacement device from Syncardia.

axial-flow pump group.[50] Some groups have described utilizing the Heartmate III in a biventricular orientation.

Total Artificial Heart

Syncardia Total Artificial Heart

The Syncardia TAH-t (SynCardia Systems Corporation, Tucson, AZ) is a pulsatile, volume displacement, TAH[90–94] (**Fig. 81.13**). The rigid polyurethane pump contains a flexible polyurethane diaphragm that separates blood and air chambers. Two mechanical valves located at the inflow and outflow orifices ensure unidirectional blood flow. Compressed air from the external drive console moves the diaphragm upward, pressurizing the blood chamber and causing ejection of blood. The pump has a maximum stroke volume of 70 mL and a maximum flow rate of 15 L/min, although the average flow rate is <8 L/min. Pump rate, duration of systole, and driving pressure can be adjusted to achieve optimal flow conditions. The TAH is surgically implanted in the mediastinal space after the ventricles have been excised, while the atrial cuffs are retained. The pneumatic drivelines are externalized percutaneously and attached to the drive console. Ambulation is facilitated by small portable drive systems and consoles. The Syncardia TAH-t is approved by the FDA for bridge to heart transplant indication. Copeland and colleagues reported a survival rate of 79% to heart transplantation compared with 46% for the observational arm, with 1-year posttransplant survival rate was 86%.[91] The SynCardia TAH-t has now been implanted in more than 1100 patients in approximately 100 centers in North America, Western Europe, Russia, Turkey, Israel, and Australia. To date, the longest duration of support has been 3.75 years, in a man who has since survived after transplantation. More than 47 patients have survived for longer than 1 year of support, and 72% of those underwent transplantation.[94]

BIVACOR

The BIVACOR is an emerging technology in the TAH space. Its uniqueness lies in its utilization of an electro-mechanical rotary pump in contrast to the displacement mechanism used in other devices (**Fig. 81.14**). This device is still in the infancy of its clinical trials. It received IDE approval from the FDA in November 2024 and was implanted in the first human recipient in July 2024. Initial animal and backbench studies have shown promising durability for up to 3 months in animals and 4 years of continuous flow on backbench studies.[95] This emerging technology may become a viable option more routinely for patients with biventricular failure awaiting transplantation.

FUTURE DIRECTIONS

Recent rapid technologic advancements and successful clinical applications of MCS have made the future of this field optimistic, but uncertain. Areas of continued research include the use of wireless energy transfer to facilitate complete internalization of MCS devices, application of less invasive surgical techniques for device implantation, application of MCS devices for the pediatric population, partial support devices and device designs, and new materials to improve compatibility of the blood–device interface to reduce thromboembolic complications and need for anticoagulation. It is possible that long-term MCS will provide a viable alternative to heart transplantation and medical therapy for patients with advanced heart failure.

References

1. Rihal CS, Naidu SS, Givertz MM, et al; Society for Cardiovascular Angiography and Interventions (SCAI), Heart Failure Society of America (HFSA), Society of Thoracic Surgeons (STS), American Heart Association (AHA), and American College of Cardiology (ACC). 2015 SCAI/ACC/HFSA/STS clinical expert consensus statement on the use of percutaneous mechanical circulatory support devices in cardiovascular care: Endorsed by the American Heart Association, the cardiological society of India, and sociedad latino americana de cardiologia Intervention; affirmation of value by the Canadian Association of interventional cardiology-association Canadienne de Cardiologie d'intervention. *J Am Coll Cardiol.* 2015;65(19):e7–e26.
2. Rose EA, Gelijns AC, Moskowitz AJ, et al; Randomized Evaluation of Mechanical Assistance for the Treatment of Congestive Heart Failure (REMATCH) Study Group. Long-term use of a left ventricular assist device for end-stage heart failure. *N Eng J Med.* 2001;345(20): 1435–1443.
3. Decision memo for ventricular assist devices for bridge-to-transplant and destination therapy (CAG-00432R). http://www.cms.gov/medicarecoverage-database/details/nca-decision-memo.aspx?NCAId=268.
4. Hochman JS, Sleeper LA, Webb JG, et al. Early revascularization in acute myocardial infarction complicated by cardiogenic shock. SHOCK investigators. Should we emergently revascularize occluded coronaries for cardiogenic shock. *N Eng J Med.* 1999;341(9):625–634.
5. Norman JC, Cooley DA, Igo SR, et al. Prognostic indices for survival during postcardiotomy intra-aortic balloon pumping. *J Thorac Cardiovasc Surg.* 1977;74:709–720.
6. Gray LA Jr, Champsaur GG. The BVS 5000 biventricular assist device. The worldwide registry experience. *ASAIO J.* 1994;40(3): M460–M464.
7. Pennington DG, Merjavy JP, Swartz MT, et al. The importance of biventricular failure in patients with postoperative cardiogenic shock. *Ann Thorac Surg.* 1985;39(1):16–26.
8. Farrar DJ, Hill JD, Pennington DG, et al. Preoperative and postoperative comparison of patients with univentricular and biventricular support with the thoratec ventricular assist device as a bridge to cardiac transplantation. *J Thorac Cardiovasc Surg.* 1997;113(1): 202–209.
9. Fitzpatrick JR 3rd, Frederick JR, Hsu VM, et al. Risk score derived from pre-operative data analysis predicts the need for biventricular mechanical circulatory support. *J Heart Lung Transplant.* 2008; 27(12):1286–1292.
10. Matthews JC, Koelling TM, Pagani FD, Aaronson KD. The right ventricular failure risk score a pre-operative tool for assessing the risk of right ventricular failure in left ventricular assist device candidates. *J Am Coll Cardiol.* 2008;51(22):2163–2172.

11. Kormos RL, Gasior TA, Kawai A, et al. Transplant candidate's clinical status rather than right ventricular function defines need for univentricular versus biventricular support. *J Thorac Cardiovasc Surg.* 1996;111(4):773–782; discussion 782–783.
12. Kirklin JK, Pagani FD, Kormos RL, et al. Eighth annual INTERMACS report: special focus on framing the impact of adverse events. *J Heart Lung Transplant.* 2017;36(10):1080–1086.
13. Kormos RL, Cowger J, Pagani FD, et al. The society of thoracic surgeons intermacs database annual report: evolving indications, outcomes, and scientific partnerships. *J Heart Lung Transplant.* 2019;38(2):114–126.
14. Stevenson LW, Pagani FD, Young JB, et al. INTERMACS profiles of advanced heart failure: the current picture. *J Heart Lung Transplant.* 2009;28(6):535–541.
15. Mancini D, Colombo PC. Left ventricular assist devices: a rapidly evolving alternative to transplant. *J Am Coll Cardiol.* 2015;65(23): 2542–2555.
16. Estep JD, Starling RC, Horstmanshof DA, et al. Risk assessment and comparative effectiveness of left ventricular assist device and medical management in ambulatory heart failure patients (ROADMAP). *J Heart Lung Transplant.* 2015;34:S80.
17. Shore S, Golbus JR, Aaronson KD, Nallamothu BK. Changes in the United States adult heart allocation policy: challenges and opportunities. *Circ Cardiovasc Qual Outcomes.* 2020;13(10):e005795.
18. Kirklin JK, Naftel DC, Kormos RL, et al. Quantifying the effect of cardiorenal syndrome on mortality after left ventricular assist device implant. *J Heart Lung Transplant.* 2013;32(12):1205–1213.
19. Miller LW. Patient selection for the use of ventricular assist devices as a bridge to transplantation. *Ann Thorac Surg.* 2003; 75(6 suppl):S66–S71.
20. Liu H, Jeng E, Demos D, et al. Early versus standard renal replacement therapy after left ventricular assist device implantation. *J Card Surg.* 2020;35(10):2529–2538.
21. Aaronson KD, Patel H, Pagani FD. Patient selection for left ventricular assist device therapy. *Ann Thorac Surg.* 2003;75(6 suppl): S29–S35.
22. Kormos RL, Teuteberg JJ, Pagani FD, et al; HeartMate II Clinical Investigators. Right ventricular failure in patients with the HeartMate II continuous-flow left ventricular assist device: incidence, risk factors, and effect on outcomes. *J Thorac Cardiovasc Surg.* 2010;139(5):1316–1324.
23. Takeda K, Naka Y, Yang JA, et al. Timing of temporary right ventricular assist device insertion for severe right heart failure after left ventricular assist device implantation. *ASAIO J.* 2013; 59(6):564–569.
24. Takeda K, Takayama H, Colombo PC, et al. Incidence and clinical significance of late right heart failure during continuous-flow left ventricular assist device support. *J Heart Lung Transplant.* 2015;34(5):667–674.
25. Lietz K, Long JW, Kfoury AG, et al. Outcomes of left ventricular assist device implantation as destination therapy in the post-REMATCH era: implications for patient selection. *Circulation.* 2007;116(5):497–505.
26. Filippatos GS, Anker SD, Kremastinos DT. Pathophysiology of peripheral muscle wasting in cardiac cachexia. *Curr Opin Clin Nutr Metab Care.* 2005;8(3):249–254.
27. Jeng EI, Miller AH, Friedman J, et al. Ventricular assist device implantation and bariatric surgery: a route to transplantation in morbidly obese patients with end-stage heart failure. *ASAIO J.* 2021;67(2):163–168.
28. John R, Mantz K, Eckman P, Rose A, May-Newman K. Aortic valve pathophysiology during left ventricular assist device support. *J Heart Lung Transplant.* 2010;29(12):1321–1329.
29. Park SJ, Liao KK, Segurola R, Madhu KP, Miller LW. Management of aortic insufficiency in patients with left ventricular assist devices: a simple coaptation stitch method (Park's stitch). *J Thorac Cardiovasc Surg.* 2004;127(1):264–266.
30. Cowger J, Pagani FD, Haft JW, Romano MA, Aaronson KD, Kolias TJ. The development of aortic insufficiency in left ventricular assist device-supported patients. *Circ Heart Fail.* 2010;3(6): 668–674.
31. Morgan JA, Brewer RJ, Nemeh HW, et al. Management of aortic valve insufficiency in patients supported by long-term continuous flow left ventricular assist devices. *Ann Thorac Surg.* 2012;94(5):1710–1712.
32. Choi JH, Luc JGY, Escrivá EM, et al. Impact of concomitant mitral valve surgery with LVAD placement: Systematic review and meta-analysis. *Artif Organs.* 2018;42(12):1139–1147.
33. Kawabori M, Kurihara C, Conyer RT, et al. Effect of concomitant mitral valve procedures for severe mitral regurgitation during left ventricular assist device implantation. *J Artif Organs.* 2019;22(2):91–97.
34. Santamore WP, Gray LA Jr. Left ventricular contributions to right ventricular systolic function during LVAD support. *Ann Thorac Surg.* 1996;61(1):350–356.
35. Mandarino WA, Winowich S, Gorcsan J 3rd, et al. Right ventricular performance and left ventricular assist device filling. *Ann Thorac Surg.* 1997;63(4):1044–1049.
36. Veen KM, Muslem R, Soliman OI, et al. Left ventricular assist device implantation with and without concomitant tricuspid valve surgery: a systematic review and meta-analysis. *Eur J Cardiothorac Surg.* 2018;54(4):644–651.
37. Feldman D, Pamboukian SV, Teuteberg JJ, et al; International Society for Heart and Lung Transplantation. The 2013 International Society for Heart and Lung Transplantation guidelines for mechanical circulatory support: executive summary. *J Heart Lung Transplant.* 2013;32(2):157–187.
38. Garan AR, Yuzefpolskaya M, Colombo PC, et al. Ventricular arrhythmias and implantable cardioverter-defibrillator therapy in patients with continuous-flow left ventricular assist devices: need for primary prevention? *J Am Coll Cardiol.* 2013;61(25):2542–2550.
39. Shapiro GC, Leibowitz DW, Oz MC, Weslow RG, Di Tullio MR, Homma S. Diagnosis of patent foramen ovale with transesophageal echocardiography in a patient supported with a left ventricular assist device. *J Heart Lung Transplant.* 1995;14(3):594–597.
40. Matthews JC, Pagani FD, Haft JW, Koelling TM, Naftel DC, Aaronson KD. Meld score predicts LVAD operative transfusion requirements, morbidity and mortality. *Circulation.* 2010;121(2): 214–220.
41. Goldstein DJ, Seldomridge JA, Chen JM, et al. Left ventricular assist device and bleeding: adding insult to injury. *Ann Thorac Surg.* 1995;59:1063–1068.
42. Dewald O, Schmitz C, Diem H, et al. Platelet activation markers in patients with heart assist device. *Artif Organs.* 2005;29(4):292–299.
43. Crow S, John R, Boyle A, et al. Gastrointestinal bleeding rates in recipients of nonpulsatile and pulsatile left ventricular assist devices. *J Thorac Cardiovasc Surg.* 2009;137(1):208–215.
44. Geisen U, Heilman C, Beyeresdorf F, et al. Non-surgical bleeding in patients with ventricular assist devices could be explained by acquired von Willebrand disease. *Eur J Cardiothorac Surg.* 2008; 33(4):679–684.
45. Uriel N, Pak SW, Jorde UP, et al. Acquired von Willebrand syndrome after continuous-flow mechanical device support contributes to a high prevalence of bleeding during long-term support and at the time of transplantation. *J Am Coll Cardiol.* 2010;56(15): 1207–1213.
46. Dassanayaka S, Slaughter MS, Bartoli CR. Mechanistic pathway(s) of acquired von Willebrand syndrome with a continuous-flow ventricular assist device: in vitro findings. *ASAIO J.* 2013;59(2): 123–129.
47. Eckman PM, John R. Bleeding and thrombosis in patients with continuous-flow ventricular assist devices. *Circulation.* 2012;125(24): 3038–3047.
48. Argiriou M, Kolokotron SM, Sakellaridis T, et al. Right heart failure post left ventricular assist device implantation. *J Thorac Dis.* 2014;6(Suppl 1):S52–S59.
49. Slaughter MS, Rogers JG, Milano CA, et al; HeartMate II Investigators. Advanced heart failure treated with continuous-flow left ventricular assist device. *N Engl J Med.* 2009;361(23):2241–2251.
50. Milano CA, Rogers JG, Tatooles AJ, et al; ENDURANCE Investigators. HVAD: The ENDURANCE supplemental trial. *JACC Heart Fail.* 2018;6(9):792–802.

51. Mehra MR, Uriel N, Naka Y, et al; MOMENTUM 3 Investigators. A fully magnetically levitated left ventricular assist device—final report. *N Engl J Med.* 2019;380(17):1618–1627.
52. Aaronson KD, Slaughter MS, Miller LW, et al; HeartWare Ventricular Assist Device (HVAD) Bridge to Transplant ADVANCE Trial Investigators. Use of an intrapericardial, continuous-flow, centrifugal pump in patients awaiting heart transplantation. *Circulation.* 2012;125(25):3191–3200.
53. Starling RC, Naka Y, Boyle AJ, et al. Results of the post-U.S. Food and Drug Administration-approval study with a continuous flow left ventricular assist device as a bridge to heart transplantation: a prospective study using the INTERMACS (Interagency Registry for Mechanically Assisted Circulatory Support). *J Am Coll Card.* 2011;57(19):1890–1898.
54. Jorde UP, Kushwaha SS, Tatooles AJ, et al; HeartMate II Clinical Investigators. Results of the destination therapy post-Food and Drug Administration approval study with a continuous flow left ventricular assist device: a prospective study using the INTERMACS registry (Interagency Registry for Mechanically Assisted Circulatory Support). *J Am Coll Cardiol.* 2014;63(17):1751–1757.
55. Miller LW, Pagani FD, Russell SD, et al; HeartMate II Clinical Investigators. Use of a continuous-flow device in patients awaiting heart transplantation. *N Engl J Med.* 2007;357(9):885–896.
56. Park SJ, Milano CA, Tatooles AJ, et al; HeartMate II Clinical Investigators. Outcomes in advanced heart failure patients with left ventricular assist devices for destination therapy. *Circ Heart Fail.* 2012;5(2):241–248.
57. Kirklin JK, Naftel DC, Kormos RL, et al. Interagency Registry for Mechanically Assisted Circulatory Support (INTERMACS) analysis of pump thrombosis in the HeartMate II left ventricular assist device. *J Heart Lung Transplant.* 2014;33(1):12–22.
58. Burkhoff D, Klotz S, Mancini DM. LVAD-induced reverse remodeling: basic and clinical implications for myocardial recovery. *J Card Fail.* 2006;12(3):227–239.
59. Birks EJ, Tansley PD, Hardy J, et al. Left ventricular assist device and drug therapy for the reversal of heart failure. *N Engl J Med.* 2006;355(18):1873–1884.
60. Guglin M, Miller L. Myocardial recovery with left ventricular assist devices. *Curr Treat Options Cardiovasc Med.* 2012;14(4):370–383.
61. Kantrowitz A, Tjonneland S, Freed PS, Phillips SJ, Butner AN, Sherman JL Jr. Initial clinical experience with intraaortic balloon pumping in cardiogenic shock. *JAMA.* 1968;203:113–118.
62. Thiele H, Zeymer U, Neumann FJ, et al; IABP-SHOCK II Trial Investigators. Intraaortic balloon support for myocardial infarction with cardiogenic shock. *N Engl J Med.* 2012;367(14):1287–1296.
63. Thiele H, Zeymer U, Neumann FJ, et al; Intraaortic Balloon Pump in cardiogenic shock II (IABP-SHOCK II) trial investigators. Intra-aortic balloon counterpulsation in acute myocardial infarction complicated by cardiogenic shock (IABP-SHOCK II): final 12 month results of a randomised, open-label trial. *Lancet.* 2013;382(9905):1638–1645.
64. Thiele H, Zeymer U, Thelemann N, et al; IABPSHOCK II Trial (Intraaortic Balloon Pump in Cardiogenic Shock II) Investigators. Intraaortic balloon pump in cardiogenic shock complicating acute myocardial infarction: long-term 6-year outcome of the randomized IABP-SHOCK II trial. *Circulation.* 2019;139(3):395–403.
65. Seyfarth M, Sibbing D, Bauer I, et al. A randomized clinical trial to evaluate the safety and efficacy of a percutaneous left ventricular assist device versus intra-aortic balloon pumping for treatment of cardiogenic shock caused by myocardial infarction. *J Am Coll Cardiol.* 2008;52(19):1584–1588.
66. Sassard T, Scalabre A, Bonnefoy E, Sanchez I, Farhat F, Jegaden O. The right axillary artery approach for the Impella Recover LP 5.0 microaxial pump. *Ann Thorac Surg.* 2008;85(4):1468–1470.
67. Raess DH, Weber DM. Impella 2.5. *J Cardiovasc Transl Res.* 2009;2(2):168–172.
68. Kapur NK, Paruchuri V, Urbano-Morales JA, et al. Mechanically unloading the left ventricle before coronary reperfusion reduces left ventricular wall stress and myocardial infarct size. *Circulation.* 2013;128(4):328–336.
69. Ghannam AD, Babu AN, Jeng EI. Protek duo rapid deployment cannulation utilized to bridge to durable heartware left ventricular assist device. *J Card Surg.* 2020;35(8):2067–2069.
70. Haj-Yahia S, Birks EJ, Amrani M, et al. Bridging patients after salvage from bridge to decision directly to transplant by means of prolonged support with the CentriMag short-term centrifugal pump. *J Thorac Cardiovasc Surg.* 2009;138(1):227–230.
71. John R, Liao K, Lietz K, et al. Experience with the Levitronix CentriMag circulatory support system as a bridge to decision in patients with refractory acute cardiogenic shock and multisystem organ failure. *J Thorac Cardiovasc Surg.* 2007;134(2):351–358.
72. Muehrcke DD, McCarthy PM, Stewart RW, et al. Extracorporeal membrane oxygenation for postcardiotomy cardiogenic shock. *Ann Thorac Surg.* 1996;61(2):684–691.
73. Smedira NG, Wudel JH, Hlozek CC, Cosgrove DM 3rd, McCarthy PM. Venovenous extracorporeal life support for patients after cardiotomy. *ASAIO J.* 1997;43(5):M444–M446.
74. McGovern GJ Jr, Magovern JA, Benckart DH, et al. Extracorporeal membrane oxygenation: preliminary results in patients with postcardiotomy cardiogenic shock. *Ann Thorac Surg.* 1994;57(6):1462–1468; discussion 1469–1471.
75. Hill JD, O'Brien TG, Murray JJ, et al. Prolonged extracorporeal oxygenation for acute post-traumatic respiratory failure (shock-lung syndrome). Use of the Bramson membrane lung. *N Eng J Med.* 1972;286(12):629–634.
76. Gray BW, Haft JW, Hirsch JC, Annich GM, Hirschl RB, Bartlett RH. Extracorporeal life support: experience with 2,000 patients. *ASAIO J.* 2015;61(2):2–7.
77. Pagani FD, Aaronson KD, Dyke DB, Wright S, Swaniker F, Bartlett RH. Assessment of an extracorporeal life support to LVAD bridge to heart transplant strategy. *Ann Thorac Surg.* 2000;70(6):1977–1984; discussion 1984–1985.
78. Bowen FW, Carboni AF, O'Hara ML, et al. Application of "double bridge mechanical" resuscitation for profound cardiogenic shock leading to cardiac transplantation. *Ann Thorac Surg.* 2001;72(1):86–90.
79. Smedira NG, Moazomi N, Golding CM, et al. Clinical experience with 202 adults receiving extracorporeal membrane oxygenation for cardiac failure: survival at five years. *J Thorac Cardiovasc Surg.* 2001;122(1):92–102.
80. Dembitsky WP, Tector AJ, Park S, et al. Left ventricular assist device performance with long-term circulatory support: lessons from the REMATCH trial. *Ann Thorac Surg.* 2004;78(6):2123–2129; discussion 2129–2130.
81. Pagani FD, Miller LW, Russell SD, et al; HeartMate II Investigators. Extended mechanical circulatory support with a continuous-flow rotary left ventricular assist device. *J Am Coll Cardiol.* 2009;54(4):312–321.
82. Takatani S. Progress of rotary blood pumps: presidential address, international society for rotary blood pumps 2006, Leuven, Belgium. *Artif Organs.* 2007;31(5):329–344.
83. Radovancevic B, Vrtovec B, de Kort E, et al. End-organ function in patients on long-term circulatory support with continuous- or pulsatile-flow assist devices. *J Heart Lung Transplant.* 2007;26(8):815–818.
84. Pagani FD. Continuous-flow rotary left ventricular assist devices with "3rd generation" design. *Sem Thorac Cardiovasc Surg.* 2008;20(3):255–263.
85. Hoshi H, Shinshi T, Takatani S. Third-generation blood pumps with mechanical noncontact magnetic bearings. *Artif Organs.* 2006;30(5):324–338.
86. Starling RC, Moazami N, Silvestry SC, et al. Unexpected abrupt increase in left ventricular assist device thrombosis. *N Eng J Med.* 2014;370(1):33–40.
87. Goldstein DJ, John R, Salerno C, et al. Algorithm for the diagnosis and management of suspected pump thrombus. *J Heart Lung Transplant.* 2013;32(7):667–670.
88. Moazami N, Fukamachi K, Kobayashi M, et al. Axial and centrifugal continuous-flow rotary pumps: a translation from pump

mechanics to clinical practice. *J Heart Lung Transplant*. 2013;32(1): 1–11.
89. Mehra MR, Goldstein DJ, Cleveland JC, et al. Five-year outcomes in patients with fully magnetically levitated vs axial-flow left ventricular assist devices in the MOMENTUM 3 randomized trial. *JAMA*. 2022;328(12):1233–1242.
90. Urban M, Woods A, Robinson-Smith N, MacGowan G, Roysam C, Schueler S. First-in-man use of the MVAD axial-flow pump: Long-term outcome. *J Heart Lung Transplant*. 2018;37(7):933–936.
91. Arabia FA, Copeland JG, Pavie A, Smith RG. Implantation technique for the CardioWest total artificial heart. *Ann Thorac Surg*. 1999;68(2):698–704.
92. Copeland JG, Smith RG, Arabia FA, et al; CardioWest Total Artificial Heart Investigators. Cardiac replacement with a total artificial heart as a bridge to transplantation. *N Engl J Med*. 2004;351(9):859–867.
93. Copeland JG, Smith RG, Arabia FA, et al. Total artificial heart bridge to transplantation: a 9-year experience with 62 patients. *J Heart Lung Transplant*. 2004;23(7):823–831.
94. Arabía FA. SynCardia total artificial heart opportunities and challenges moving forward. *Artif Organs*. 2019;43(11): 1051–1052.
95. Timms DL, Greatrex N, Nestler F, et al. Preclinical evaluation of the bivacor total artificial heart. *J Hear Lung Transplant*. 2023;42:S66.

Vascular Diagnostics: The Noninvasive Vascular Laboratory

Joann M. Lohr

Key Points

1. Duplex ultrasound consists of a combination of grayscale imaging and pulse Doppler. Because the speed of sound is relatively constant in tissue, with a pulse Doppler, it can be determined when an echo is generated and when it is received. This provides range resolution, enabling the operator of the duplex machine to precisely sample and interrogate blood flow at a known location.
2. When a sound wave encounters moving reflectors, such as red blood cells, the frequency of the reflected wave changes from that of the original wave generated by the transducer. This relationship is reflected in the Doppler equation: $f_r - f_o = [(2f_o v)/c] \cos \theta$, where f_r is the received frequency, f_o is the originating frequency, v is the velocity of the reflector, c is the speed of sound in tissue, and θ is the angle of the incident sound beam with the moving reflectors, the so-called Doppler angle.
3. Arterial Doppler waveforms reflect the resistance of the circulation supplied by the artery being examined. Low-resistance circulations such as cerebral and renal circulations have relatively high amounts of diastolic flow whereas high-resistance circulations, such as extremity arteries have little flow at the end of diastole.
4. Carotid stenosis is determined primarily from measurement of peak systolic velocity (PSV) and end-diastolic velocity (EDV) from pulse Doppler waveforms using criteria agreed upon in a national consensus conference. Validation is needed using correlation with other imaging techniques. Velocities are altered after carotid endarterectomy (CEA) and stenting. Intravascular ultrasound is useful for stent placement and deployment.
5. Air plethysmography (APG) can be used to display pulse volume waveforms. Pulse volume recordings (PVRs) are obtained with partially inflated blood pressure cuffs that detect volume changes sequentially down a limb. Volume changes beneath the cuffs resulting from the pulse wave result in small pressure changes within the cuffs. These changes are displayed as arterial waveforms with the use of appropriate transducers and provide an overall measure of the arterial circulation in an extremity.
6. The ankle–brachial index (ABI) is determined by dividing the higher ipsilateral dorsal pedal or posterior tibial artery pressure by the higher of the two brachial artery systolic pressures and is highly sensitive and specific for documenting the presence or absence of lower extremity arterial occlusive disease.
7. Measurement of ankle pressures after exercise can be used to confirm arterial disease as an etiology for exercise-associated leg pain. Failure of the ankle pressure to drop with exercise along with failure of the ABI to decrease 20% with exercise, combined with a normal resting ABI, substantially rules out arterial insufficiency as an etiology of exercise-induced complaints of leg pain.
8. Duplex ultrasound can detect hemodynamically significant stenosis in abdominal arteries: a PSV in the superior mesenteric artery (SMA) of 275 cm/s or more indicates a ≥70% SMA stenosis, a celiac artery PSV of ≥200 cm/s indicates a ≥70% celiac artery stenosis, whereas a ratio of the PSV in a renal artery to that in the aorta (renal–aortic ratio, RAR) of ≥3.5 indicates a ≥60% diameter-reducing renal artery stenosis. Addition of ultrasound contrast agents has expanded ultrasound usefulness and accuracy especially after endovascular aortic repairs.
9. The primary ultrasound diagnostic criterion for diagnosis of venous thrombosis is failure of the vein to collapse with application of pressure with the ultrasound probe.
10. Venous duplex including intravascular, is useful during multiple procedures including: thrombectomy, ablation, filter placement, and placement of central venous devices.
11. In the upright position, venous reflux stimulated by cuff deflation that lasts >0.5 to 1 second is indicative of pathologic venous reflux.

The noninvasive vascular laboratory provides accurate, safe, and objective evidence of the presence and physiologic significance of vascular disease throughout the body. Two broad categories of testing are available in the noninvasive vascular laboratory; those based on plethysmographic techniques and those based on ultrasound-based techniques. In recent years, the vascular laboratory has become useful for both diagnostic and therapeutic applications.

PLETHYSMOGRAPHY

Plethysmographic techniques detect volume changes in limbs that occur in response to arterial and venous disease. The technology can be modified to determine digital pressures and produce pulse waveforms. Examples of plethysmographic techniques include mercury strain gauge plethysmography, air plethysmography (APG) (pulse volume recordings [PVRs]), and photoplethysmography (PPG).

ULTRASOUND

Ultrasound techniques, in particular duplex ultrasound-based techniques, have largely eclipsed plethysmographic techniques. Duplex ultrasound, introduced in 1974, was first applied to carotid arteries. The technique combines information from ultrasound-generated images (B-mode) and Doppler analysis of blood flow direction and velocity, hence the term "duplex." Duplex ultrasound is currently extensively employed for evaluation of carotid arteries, intra-abdominal arteries and veins, and upper and lower extremity arteries and veins. Since inception duplex ultrasound has advanced through: (1) improved B-mode imaging, (2) better low-frequency scan heads permitting deeper penetration of the ultrasound beam from the skin surface, (3) improvements in online computer-based microprocessor software, and (4) perhaps, most importantly, the addition of color flow to the B-mode image.

Color flow superimposes a real-time color image of blood flow onto a standard gray-scale B-mode picture. Returning echoes from stationary tissues generate the B-mode image, whereas those interacting with moving substances (blood) generate a significant enough phase shift that they can be processed separately and color coded by operator selection to give information on direction and velocity of blood flow according to the magnitude and direction of the Doppler frequency shift. It is color flow, combined with the ability of the current generation of duplex scanners to detect very low blood flow velocities (<5 cm/s), which makes duplex scanning practical on a routine basis throughout the body. Color flow permits more rapid identification of vessels to be examined and is essential for duplex examination of some vessels such as tibial arteries and veins.

BASICS OF DUPLEX ULTRASOUND

An ultrasonic wave is produced in tissue by placing a vibrating source in contact with the tissue. In medical ultrasound, the vibrating source is the ultrasound *transducer* contained within the ultrasound *scan head*. The scan head steers and focuses the sound beam arising from the transducer, functions crucial in deriving an ultrasound image from returning echoes.

Ultrasound transducers convert electrical energy into vibrational energy and, conversely, turn vibrational energy of returning echoes into electrical signals that can be analyzed by the software of the duplex machine. The design of the transducer determines the frequency of the vibrations which, in turn, determines the wavelength of the sound wave produced. The relationship between frequency and wavelength is expressed mathematically as follows:

$$\lambda = c/f \tag{82.1}$$

where λ is the wavelength, *c* is the speed of sound in tissue, and *f* is the incident frequency.

The speed of sound in soft tissues averages 1540 m/s and varies only minimally from this average in soft tissues insonated in clinical applications of duplex ultrasound. The wavelength of the sound beam is the primary determinant of how well the ultrasound beam penetrates the tissue. Because the speed of sound within the tissue is, for all practical purposes, constant (1540 m/s), the ability of ultrasound to penetrate tissue depends on the frequency of the vibrating source (transducer). As noted above, transducer frequency is determined by the design of the transducer and is thus controlled by the manufacturer of the duplex device. For examination of the carotid artery, transducer frequencies of 5 to 7.5 MHz provide optimal tissue penetration for clinical purposes.

As noted above the term duplex refers to the combination of Doppler and B-mode ("B" stands for "brightness") ultrasound in the same device. Both types of ultrasound require 1
analysis of reflected echoes of the original sound beam initially created by placing the ultrasound transducer in contact with the tissue. The B-mode component of the duplex machine analyzes the *strength* (intensity) and *origin* of the reflected echo. The Doppler component analyzes *shifts* in frequency of the original sound wave produced by the transducer that result when the ultrasonic wave encounters moving reflectors.

B-Mode Ultrasound

As a sound wave passes through tissue, its strength moving away from the transducer depends upon the degree to which the beam is attenuated, scattered, and reflected. The strength of the reflected echo depends in part, upon relative differences in acoustic impedance between two different media. Major differences in acoustic impedance result in reflection of a large proportion of the sound beam back to the transducer, whereas small differences result in comparatively little reflection and continued propagation of the beam through the tissue.

In B-mode ultrasound, the strength of the returning echo is reflected in the brightness of the individual pixels comprising the ultrasound image. This is the ultrasound *grayscale* and the resulting image is termed a *grayscale image.*

Very bright pixels represent sites of large differences in acoustic impedance between media, whereas less dramatic differences are represented by proportionally less bright pixels on the B-mode image. Thus gallstones, which differ dramatically in acoustic properties from soft tissue, result in strong echoes and proportionally brighter pixels on an ultrasound image, whereas blood, which differs little from soft tissue in acoustic characteristics, frequently cannot be distinguished from soft tissue in a grayscale image.

The strength of the reflected echo will also be dependent upon the strength of the sound beam at the point of its reflection. Grayscale images do not show the percentage of the beam reflected, but rather represent the absolute strength of the reflected echo arriving back at the transducer. Thus, if the sound beam is very weak at the site of its reflection, even areas of significant differences in acoustic impedance will not result in a bright pixel on the ultrasound image.

The strength of the ultrasound beam at any point also depends on the degree to which the beam has been attenuated as it passes through the tissue. Attenuation of a sound wave as it traverses tissue weakens the wave and depends upon the tissue traversed and the frequency of the wave. The frequency of the wave depends upon the frequency of the transducer used to generate the wave (see discussion in the previous section and Equation 82.1). Sound waves resulting from higher-frequency transducers are attenuated more rapidly than those produced with lower-frequency transducers. Higher-frequency transducers therefore provide relatively weak echoes to be reflected from a deep structure and thus a comparatively poor B-mode image compared to a lower-frequency transducer.

The linear resolution of an ultrasound image depends upon the ability to focus the beam. Sound beams emanating from high-frequency transducers can be more precisely focused than those from low-frequency transducers, and thus, provide clearer B-mode images of more superficial structures. Because the carotid artery is superficial, higher-frequency transducers can be used to provide much clearer B-mode images than is possible with deeper vessels such as the aorta, renal, or iliac arteries.

Doppler Ultrasound

In a continuous-wave Doppler, a transducer continually emits vibrations into the tissue. Echoes are therefore continually reflected back to the transducer. A transducer cannot, however, simultaneously generate and receive an echo. Continuous-wave Doppler therefore must have separate transmitters and receivers to both generate and receive echoes.

Duplex devices utilize pulse Doppler. A pulse Doppler uses the same transducer to generate and receive echoes. Because the speed of sound is relatively constant in tissue, with a pulse Doppler it can be determined when an echo is generated and when it is received, and therefore, it is possible to calculate the depth in the tissue where a reflected echo originated. The *sample volume* of the duplex device is thus determined by specifying from what depth one wishes the pulse Doppler to receive reflected echoes.

The transducer is *gated,* based on the total time from original sound-wave generation to arrival of the reflected echo back at the transducer, to only receive echoes from the specified depth of the sample volume. The desired "position" of the sample volume is determined by the operator of the duplex device from the B-mode image, and in duplex examination of arterial and venous flow corresponds to particular points within the lumen of the vessel examined. Because B-mode images and Doppler waveforms cannot be generated simultaneously, the technologist must continually update the B-mode image during the course of the examination to ensure proper placement of the sample volume.

2 When a sound wave encounters moving reflectors, such as red blood cells, so-called Rayleigh scatters, within the lumen of an artery or vein, the frequency of the reflected wave changes from that of the original wave generated by the transducer. Velocity is a vector with both speed and direction therefore, the magnitude of the frequency shift depends upon the velocity of the moving reflectors and their angle with the incident sound beam. Because the frequency of the original sound wave is known, and the frequency of the received echo can be determined by the software of the duplex machine, the velocity of the moving reflectors (red blood cells) can be calculated provided the angle of the incident sound beam with the moving reflectors is also known. This relationship is reflected in the *Doppler equation:*

$$f_r - f_o = [2f_o v/c]\cos\theta \qquad (82.2)$$

where f_r is the received frequency, f_o is the originating frequency, v is the velocity of the reflector, c is the speed of sound in tissue, and θ is the angle of the incident sound beam with the moving reflectors, the so-called *Doppler angle*.

A Doppler angle of 0 degrees is ideal for velocity calculations as the cosine of 0 is 1 and measured reflected velocity changes are therefore 100% of what actually occurred. However, 0-degree Doppler angles are difficult to obtain as it is not generally possible to look directly down the lumen of a vessel from a percutaneous approach. Therefore, to solve the Doppler equation for the velocity of the moving reflectors, the Doppler angle must be known. To standardize the results of duplex scanning, it has been traditionally recommended that examinations be conducted as close as possible to a Doppler angle of 60 degrees. The cosine of 60 is 0.5, therefore, at this angle, the measured reflected velocity is half the actual reflected velocity. Errors in velocity calculations secondary to misreading of the Doppler angle are small as a percentage of the true velocity at ≤60 degrees as cosine vary comparatively little with incremental changes in angle below 60 degrees. When the Doppler angle approaches 70 degrees, changes in the cosine of the angle become more pronounced with incremental increases in angle, and errors in velocity calculations secondary to improper angle measurement become much more significant. Small errors in determining the Doppler angle when the angle of insonation is <60 degrees have little overall impact on the calculation of the velocity of the moving red cells. Indeed, Doppler angles from 45 to 60 degrees are acceptable for most clinical studies. Most often an angle of 60 degrees can be easily obtained in carotid artery and extremity artery duplex examinations and, in line with traditional teaching, 60 degrees is chosen whenever possible as the Doppler angle in such studies. In examination of intra-abdominal vessels it may be much more difficult to adhere to a 60-degree angle.

As noted above, pulse Doppler both transmits and receives echoes with the same transducer. This dual function places limits on the frequencies that can be displayed in the spectral waveform. The maximum frequency that can be displayed is half the pulse-transmitting frequency or pulse-repetition frequency (PRF), and is known as the *Nyquist limit.* If frequencies are encountered that exceed the Nyquist limit, they are flipped and appear on the reverse-flow side of the spectrum. This is termed *aliasing.* If aliasing is encountered, the PRF should be increased to increase the Nyquist limit. The PRF can be adjusted by changing the scale displayed on the right side of the spectral waveform or by adjusting the baseline. If aliasing still occurs, the operator should consider switching to a lower-frequency transducer or to the use of a continuous-wave Doppler. A continuous-wave Doppler is not affected by aliasing.

Color Flow

A color-flow image is produced by assigning color to Doppler shifts. Returning echoes that are not Doppler shifted are shown in grayscale. The net result is what appears to be color pasted or superimposed on a grayscale image. This pasting process can in effect obscure the edges of the grayscale image resulting in obfuscation of the true lumen of the grayscale image limiting somewhat the accuracy of color images to define stenosis. The hue and intensity of the color are determined by the direction and magnitude of the Doppler shifts. The technologist can adjust the color settings as desired. Varying shades of red and blue are generally used to distinguish flow toward or away from the transducer. By convention, red is most often assigned to arterial flow and blue to venous flow.

When the Doppler angle is 90 degrees, there is no Doppler shift. When this occurs, the assigned color is black and corresponds to the horizontal black bar serving as the baseline on the color scale that appears on the right side of a color-flow image (**Fig. 82.1**). Aliasing can be readily recognized on a color-flow image as a mosaic pattern or as a transition from red-to-blue or blue-to-red without an intervening black line. In areas of actual reverse flow, the blue and red colors are separated by a black border. Just as with pulsed Doppler, color aliasing can be reduced by increasing the PRF. This is often quite important, as an extensive mosaic pattern can obscure clear visualization of a stenotic site.

Power Doppler is a variant of color Doppler. Power Doppler, however, assigns no direction of flow to the color image and velocity information is not calculated. Any detected Doppler shift is colorized without consideration of the direction of the Doppler shift or the magnitude of the Doppler

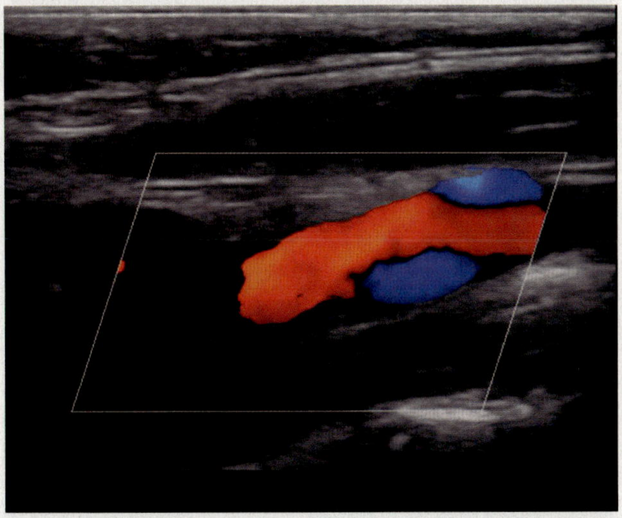

Figure 82.1. Flow separation with reverse flow along the wall of the carotid bulb as indicated by direct transition from *blue* to *red* with an intervening *black line* is a normal finding and indicates an artery without significant plaque.

shift. It is therefore not subject to aliasing or affected by Doppler angle. Its principal utility lies in the ability to detect blood moving at very low velocity and in outlining the course of tortuous vessels. It can be quite useful in detecting flow in small distal veins and flow in arteries distal to a very high-grade stenosis.

It is tempting to try a direct estimate of the severity of a stenosis from the color-flow image. However as discussed above such estimates are probably less accurate than measurements of stenosis derived from spectral analysis. Color serves primarily as a guide in locating the vessels and selecting specific sites for examination with the pulse Doppler. The absence of color can indicate extensive mural calcification and difficulty in obtaining a pulse Doppler waveform.

Carotid and Vertebral Arteries

The vascular laboratory began with assessing internal carotid artery (ICA) stenosis. Doppler diagnosis of ICA stenosis, and arterial stenosis in general is based on duplex ultrasound and focuses on three areas, the prestenotic region, the stenosis itself, and the poststenotic region. Detecting carotid stenosis involves a combination of spectral analysis, color and grayscale imaging and, in selected cases, power Doppler. The primary interest is in the detection of increased flow velocities within the area of suspected stenosis and therefore in most cases spectral analysis dominates in the detection of carotid stenosis. The exception is in distinguishing ICA occlusion from a very high-grade stenosis where color-flow or power Doppler flow can identify very low flow in the area of the stenosis or distal to the stenosis that may not be detected by pulse Doppler.

In all cases, the pulsed Doppler and color-flow findings should be crosschecked for concordance. If there is disagreement between the impression obtained with color and pulsed Doppler examinations (ie, color Doppler suggests high-grade stenosis but velocities are only moderately elevated), the findings of both should be reviewed to resolve the discrepancy.

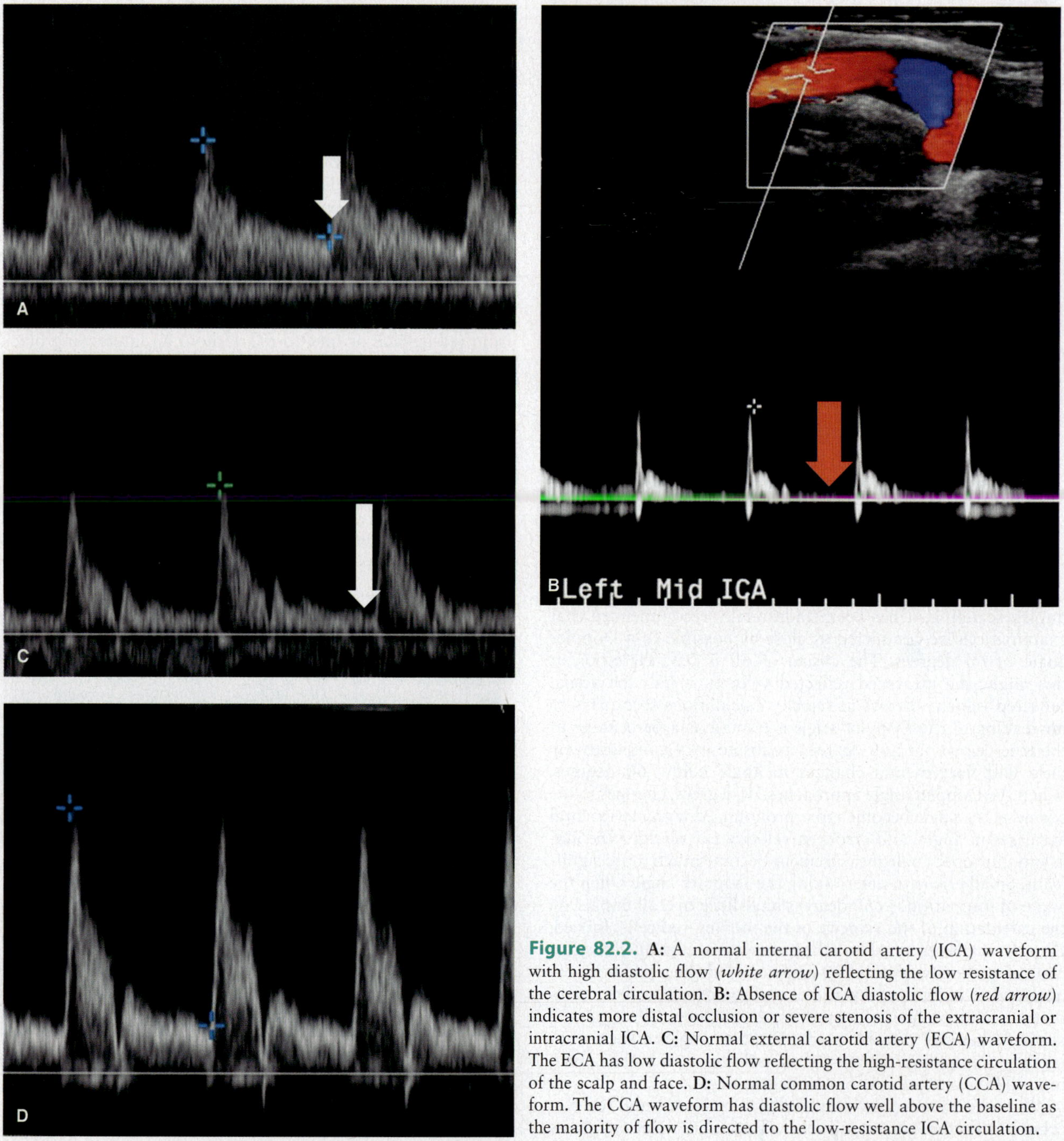

Figure 82.2. **A:** A normal internal carotid artery (ICA) waveform with high diastolic flow (*white arrow*) reflecting the low resistance of the cerebral circulation. **B:** Absence of ICA diastolic flow (*red arrow*) indicates more distal occlusion or severe stenosis of the extracranial or intracranial ICA. **C:** Normal external carotid artery (ECA) waveform. The ECA has low diastolic flow reflecting the high-resistance circulation of the scalp and face. **D:** Normal common carotid artery (CCA) waveform. The CCA waveform has diastolic flow well above the baseline as the majority of flow is directed to the low-resistance ICA circulation.

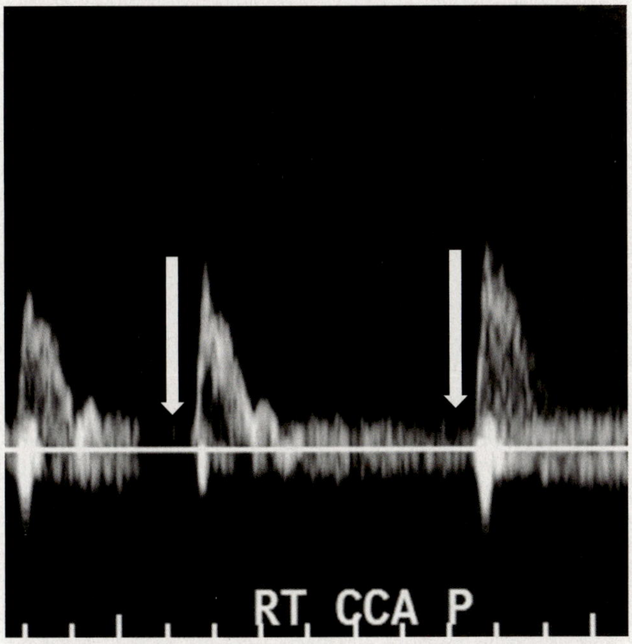

Figure 82.3. In a patient with internal carotid occlusion common carotid artery (CCA) diastolic flow approaches 0 (*arrows*) as CCA flow is now routed to the high-resistance external carotid circulation.

Common Carotid Artery Waveforms

In the majority of cases, carotid stenosis or occlusion occurs in the proximal ICA at or just beyond the carotid bifurcation. A normal ICA waveform reflects the low resistance of the cerebral circulation with high flow at the end of the diastolic component of the waveform. In the presence of a distal ICA occlusion resistance to flow increases and there is decreased flow in diastole (**Fig. 82.2A,B**). The external carotid artery (ECA) supplies the relatively higher-resistance circulation of the scalp and face and therefore has a low end-diastolic flow component (**Fig. 82.2C**). The common carotid artery (CCA) waveform reflects the fact that normally 80% of CCA flow is directed to the ICA. CCA end-diastolic flow is therefore generally well above baseline and exceeds ECA diastolic flow (**Fig. 82.2D**). In the presence of a very high-grade ICA stenosis or ICA occlusion, outflow is primarily through the higher-resistance external carotid circula-
3 tion. The CCA waveform then takes on the high-flow resistance characteristics of an ECA, with flow to zero, or nearly zero, in end diastole (**Fig. 82.3**).[1] In addition, the peak systolic velocity (PSV) and the overall flow velocity may be substantially lower than normal because of reduced carotid artery flow. By observing these changes in the CCA, one can reliably predict the presence of high-grade stenosis or occlusion of the ICA.

The CCA *contralateral* to an ICA stenosis or occlusion may demonstrate an increased flow velocity with particular elevation of the velocity at the end of diastole; the so-called end-diastolic velocity (EDV). These changes represent a compensatory increase in blood flow volume in the nonobstructed ICA in response to reduced contribution to cerebral perfusion from the opposite high-grade stenotic or occluded ICA. This compensatory hemodynamic change can be substantial and flow velocities may be artificially elevated on the side with compensatory high-volume flow giving a false impression of the presence of a stenosis or a higher degree of stenosis than is actually present.[2]

In the presence of a significant stenosis at the origin of a CCA or the innominate artery, the ipsilateral CCA waveform may be dampened, with low overall PSVs and EDVs and a slower rise to peak systole when compared with the contralateral CCA waveform and potentially reverse flow in the ICA (**Fig. 82.4A, B**). The CCA flow changes seen with proximal stenosis are also important in the diagnosis of ICA stenosis because the overall reduction in flow velocity may artificially lower velocities in an ipsilateral ICA stenosis, leading to underestimation of the severity of ICA stenosis. In some cases of proximal CCA or innominate artery stenosis, the stenotic lesion may not be accessible to direct insonation by the duplex scanner. In such cases, a stenotic lesion can be suspected as the ipsilateral CCA waveform will often exhibit poststenotic turbulence low in the neck, reflecting disturbed flow distal to the more proximal stenosis.

ICA Waveforms

As noted above, the normal ICA spectral waveform is indicative of high flow in a low-resistant circulation. The systolic upstroke is rapid, PSV is <125 cm/s, and flow is maintained throughout diastole (**Fig. 82.2A**).[3] In the absence of plaque there is generally a clear spectral window under the outline of the spectral waveform as there is little turbulent flow. The presence of color shifts, indicating high-velocity flow, and color mosaics, indicating poststenotic turbulence, aids in selecting potential areas for examination with the pulsed Doppler.

Hemodynamic quantification of the severity of ICA stenosis is primarily achieved by analysis of Doppler spectral waveforms and measurements of peak systolic and EDV or comparison of PSVs in the ICA to those in the CCA just proximal to the carotid bifurcation, ICA/CCA ratio. As a stenosis develops, the PSV first becomes elevated. PSV is the primary measure of stenosis severity. EDV lags behind, relatively speaking, as stenosis severity progresses but rises rapidly as the stenosis becomes severe (diameter reductions of ≥60%). Thus, elevation of EDV is a good marker for high-grade stenosis (**Fig. 82.5**).[4] The ICA/CCA ratio is also a very important measure of stenosis severity.[5] Because it is a ratio, it compensates for abnormally high- and low-flow states that may skew the PSV and EDV upward or downward.

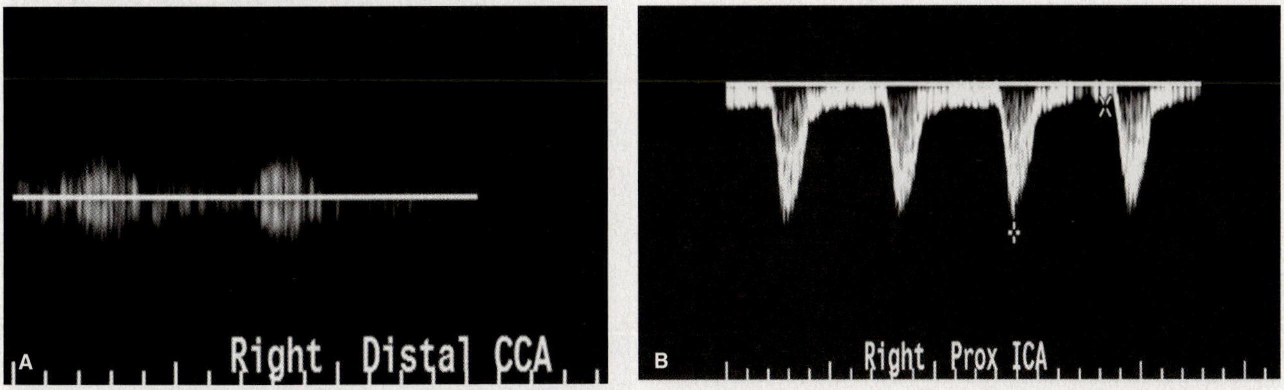

Figure 82.4. **A and B:** In the presence of innominate artery very high-grade stenosis or occlusion the common carotid artery (CCA) waveform will be blunted with a decreased amplitude and slowed upstroke (**A**), and there can be actually reverse flow (**B**) in the ipsilateral internal carotid artery (ICA).

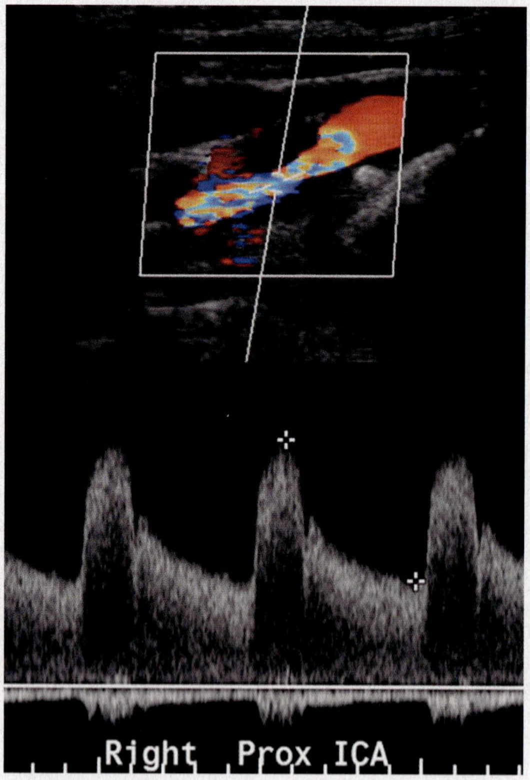

Figure 82.5. Internal carotid artery (ICA) waveform from the site of a >80% ICA stenosis. Both peak systolic and end-diastolic velocities are very elevated.

To accurately measure flow velocity, the sample volume must be placed within the area of greatest stenosis. Color-flow imaging has demonstrated that the orientation of the stenotic jet within a stenosis is frequently not along the longitudinal axis of the vessel. This finding has resulted in controversy with regard to the proper technique of obtaining velocity waveforms at sites of stenosis. In areas of mild to moderate stenosis, use of a Doppler angle of 60 degrees to the long axis of the vessel is recommended. However, in areas of more severe stenosis and/or wall abnormalities, the Doppler angle of 60 degrees should be defined by the long axis of the stenotic flow jet, as demonstrated by color flow.

The sample volume size should be kept as small as possible, usually 1.5 mm, to detect discrete changes in flow velocity. This is important as the highest velocities may be localized to a small area in the flow stream that emanates from the stenosis. A large sample volume that incorporates flow from many points within the vessel in the generation of the spectral waveform may give the false impression of disturbed flow, potentially leading to the misdiagnosis of moderate disease in an otherwise normal vessel. In practice, the sonographer, having identified the stenosis, gently moves a small sample volume around until the point of highest velocity is found.

Damping of spectral Doppler waveforms may be seen in the region distal to the carotid stenosis when the lesion is severe enough to be flow reducing. The most common abnormality seen distal to a carotid stenosis is spectral broadening caused by disturbed blood flow or turbulence. At best, poststenotic flow disturbance is a qualitative measure of arterial stenosis; nevertheless, its detection is important. With proper gain settings, "fill-in" of the Doppler spectral waveform generally indicates the presence of carotid stenosis with diameter reduction of at least 50%. However, this level of disturbed flow occasionally can be seen with nonstenotic disease. Diagnostically, the most significant poststenotic flow disturbance produces a simultaneous forward and reverse spectral Doppler signal, accompanied by poor definition of the upper spectral border. Such disturbed flow implies the presence of severe carotid stenosis. Severely disturbed flow distal to a highly calcified plaque may be the only substantial evidence for the presence of clinically significant stenosis if calcification prevents direct insonation of the stenosis.

Vertebral Artery

On rare occasions, a stenosis may be found in the cervical portion of the vertebral artery associated with cervical osteoarthritis. However, the origin of the vertebral artery from the subclavian artery is by far the most common site of disease in the vertebral artery. The vertebral artery origin lies deep in the base of the neck and may be difficult to access with ultrasound. Mean vertebral artery diameter is about 4 mm but the vertebral arteries are frequently asymmetric in size with one, most commonly the left, being larger than the right.

The vertebral artery is most commonly interrogated with ultrasound further distally in the neck, from an anteroposterior window, as it threads through the transverse processes of the cervical spine. The vertebral bodies serve as a reference to insure the vertebral artery is actually under examination (**Fig. 82.6**). The artery is usually seen deeper but adjacent to the vertebral vein. Color Doppler is helpful to locate the vessel. A spectral waveform from the vertebral artery in the midneck provides information about direction of flow, waveform shape, and velocity but does not rule out disease at the origin. The normal vertebral artery waveform is similar to that of the ICA with normal PSVs reported to be 20 to 40 cm/s.[6] Velocities up to 80 cm/s are, however, frequently seen without apparent clinical importance and may represent collateral flow through a dominant vertebral artery, or a small but disease-free, vertebral artery. Evaluation of disturbed flow distally may help determine which elevated velocities are associated with a vertebral artery stenosis and which are not. Velocity patterns are usually similar in the two vertebral arteries but systolic and diastolic velocities may differ if vertebral artery diameters are asymmetric. For this reason, if there is concern for stenosis based on an elevated PSV in a vertebral artery, recording of vertebral artery diameters is important.

Flow in the vertebral artery is normally antegrade with a rapid upstroke and continuous diastolic flow. In cases of anatomic subclavian steal, color flow provides an important initial

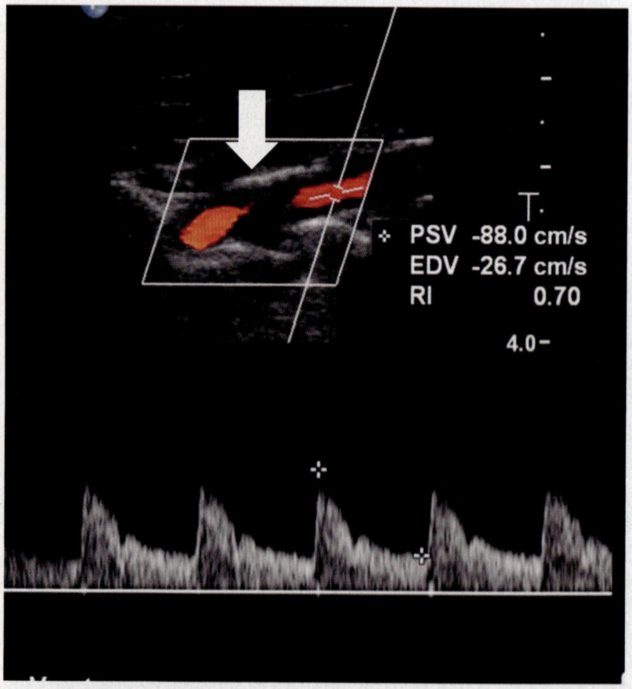

Figure 82.6. Bony landmarks of the vertebral bodies (*arrow*) mark the course of the vertebral artery.

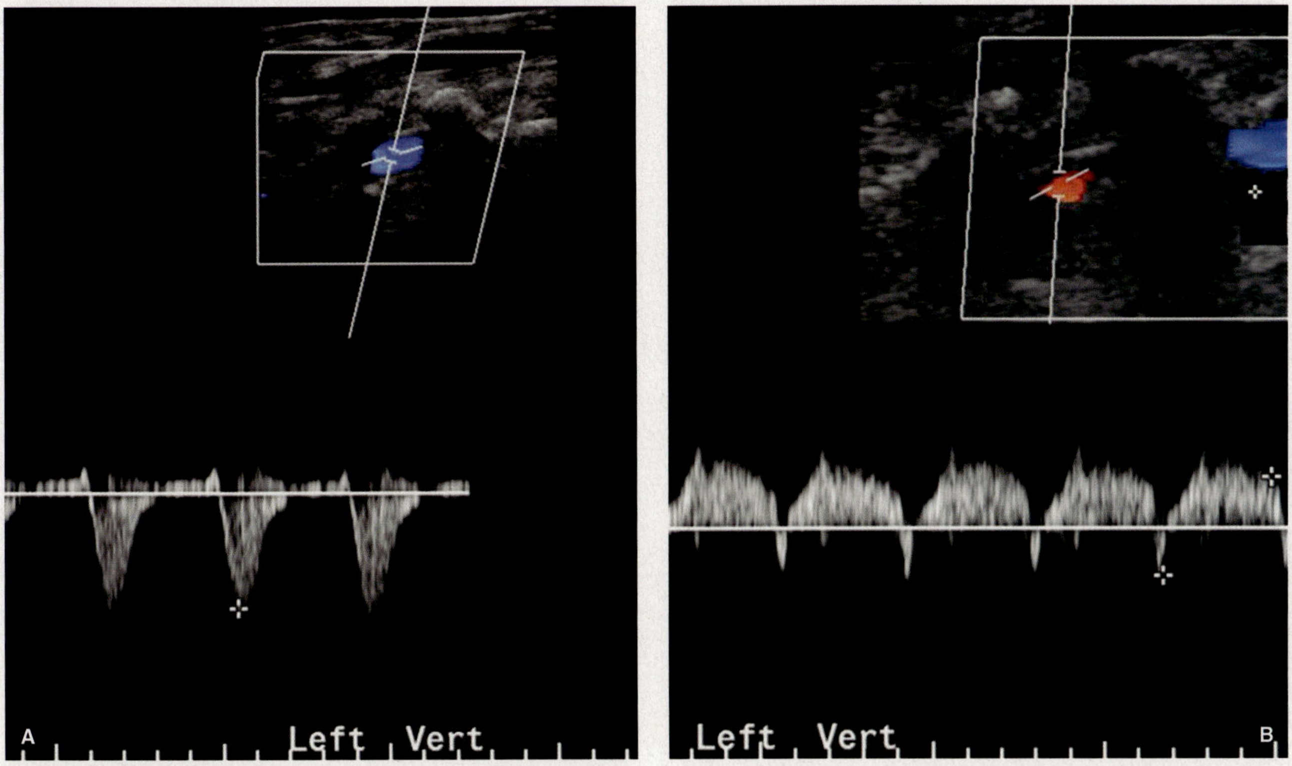

Figure 82.7. **A and B:** Both reverse vertebral artery flow (**A**), and vertebral flow both above and below the baseline (**B**) indicate a proximal innominate or subclavian artery stenosis.

clue to the diagnosis as flow in the artery will be retrograde in the same direction as the vein. Spectral Doppler must still be used to verify arterial flow and will demonstrate reverse or bidirectional flow in cases of subclavian steal. Depending on the degree of subclavian stenosis the vertebral artery flow may be reversed or biphasic, with flow above and below the baseline (**Fig. 82.7A,B**). End-diastolic flow will be zero or near zero reflecting the high resistance of the peripheral arm circulation rather than low-resistance cerebral circulation. High-resistance vertebral artery flow may also be seen with antegrade flow and like the situation for the ICA may represent distal stenosis or occlusion of the vertebral artery or an atretic or hypoplastic distal vessel.

External Carotid Artery

The ECA is smaller in diameter than the ICA at the level of the carotid bulb but similar in diameter beyond the bulb. It has little clinical significance in most cases, but can serve as an important source of collateral flow to the brain in cases of ICA very high-grade stenosis, or occlusion. The ECA may also serve in such cases as a conduit for emboli to the brain; the so-called carotid stump syndrome.[7]

The ECA waveform has a sharp upstroke, a prominent dichroitic wave in late systole or early diastole, and velocity that is near or at the zero base line in end diastole. The PSV of the ECA is normally higher than the ICA. The ECA may adopt the characteristics of the ICA in end diastole as the resistance in the face and scalp decreases with temperature change and/or in the presence of disease. In cases of common carotid occlusion with preservation of patency of the carotid bulb, reverse flow in the ECA can provide antegrade flow in the ICA maintaining patency of the ICA even with CCA occlusion.

Classifying Carotid Stenosis

Duplex criteria for quantifying carotid artery stenosis were developed by comparing duplex-derived spectral waveforms and contrast arteriograms. Duplex-derived *categories* of stenosis are relatively broad. Sensitivities and specificities for spectral analysis of duplex-derived waveforms for detecting an ICA stenosis of >50% to 99% are between 90% and 95%. There are numerous spectral criteria for classifying ICA stenosis. Some focus on *categories* of stenosis, whereas others focus on *threshold levels* of stenosis.

One of the most widely accepted classification schemes for categories for ICA stenosis was developed at the University of Washington under the direction of Dr. Eugene Strandness. These criteria were useful in the study of the natural history of carotid atherosclerosis and in clinical practice. In the University of Washington system, velocity waveform analysis and spectral criteria were used to classify ICA angiographic stenosis as normal, 1% to 15%, 16% to 49%, 50% to 79%, and 80% to 99% stenosis and occlusion. Prospective validation of these criteria has demonstrated an overall agreement of 82% with contrast angiography. The ability of the criteria to detect carotid disease is 99% sensitive and the ability of the criteria to recognize normal arteries is 84% specific.[3]

Criteria for detecting carotid artery stenosis scanning have undergone reevaluation to remain relevant to current clinical practice. This reevaluation was stimulated by the randomized trials testing the efficacy of carotid endarterectomy (CEA) that took place over the last two decades (**Table 82.1**).[8–12] The trials had a profound impact on validating the indications for CEA in patients with carotid bifurcation atherosclerosis. The trials identified significant benefit, in terms of stroke reduction, for CEA in patients with specific levels of ICA stenosis. In particular, patients with symptomatic ICA stenosis >70% to 99% had dramatic benefit from CEA, whereas patients with symptomatic ICA stenosis between 50% and 69% and patients with asymptomatic ICA stenosis between 60% and 99% also benefited, albeit to a lesser extent, from CEA.

In the North American trials of CEA, ICA stenosis was calculated from arteriograms by comparing the diameter of the minimal residual lumen to the diameter of the distal cervical ICA.[13] The University of Washington duplex criteria for categories of stenosis predated the endarterectomy trials. These criteria compared the diameter of the residual ICA lumen at

Table 82.1. Major Randomized Trials Assessing Efficacy of Carotid Endarterectomy

Symptomatic Stenosis
North American Symptomatic Carotid Endarterectomy Trial (NASCET)[8]
European Carotid Surgery Trial (ECST)[9]
VA Cooperative Study # 309[10]
Asymptomatic Stenosis
Asymptomatic Carotid Atherosclerosis Study (ACAS)[11]
Asymptomatic Carotid Surgery Trial (ACST)[12]

its narrowest point with an estimate of the ICA bulb diameter assuming it free of atherosclerotic plaque. Because the bulb has a greater diameter than the distal ICA, the two methods of measurement do not give the same calculated percentage of angiographic stenosis for the same lesion. Calculations of angiographic stenosis using the distal ICA as the reference vessel result in lower calculated stenosis percentages than calculations using the bulb as the reference site. This effect is particularly striking for modest lesions.

In a review of 1001 internal carotid angiograms, 34% of the ICAs were classified as stenosis of 70% to 99% using the ICA bulb as the reference vessel. In contrast, when the distal cervical ICA was used as the reference site, only 16% of the ICAs were classified as 70% to 99% stenosis.[14] More than 99% of the distal ICA-based calculations of stenosis were less than bulb-based calculations. Thus, the duplex stenosis criteria using the bulb as the reference vessel are not and were not directly applicable to the results of the clinical trials.

Current Criteria for ICA Stenosis

Since the randomized CEA trials were completed, additional duplex criteria were developed comparing duplex scans to angiographic ICA stenosis using the distal ICA as the reference vessel in calculating angiographic stenosis. Such criteria are considered more useful by many in selection of patients for carotid intervention because they are directly applicable to the threshold levels of carotid stenosis addressed in the CEA trials.

The initial studies addressing the issue of duplex criteria relevant to the CEA trials were performed at the Oregon Health & Science University (OHSU)[5,15] with subsequent publications from many different institutions, with many different proposed criteria for identification of clinically relevant threshold levels of ICA stenosis.[16–21]

Recognizing that duplex criteria from different centers differed for the threshold levels of angiographic stenosis determined by the CEA trials, a panel of authorities from a variety of medical specialties assembled to review the carotid ultrasound literature. The panel developed a consensus regarding the key components of the carotid ultrasound examination and reasonable criteria for stratification of ICA stenosis.[22]

The consensus committee recommended that all carotid examinations be performed with grayscale imaging, color Doppler, and spectral Doppler. Examinations should be performed by a credentialed vascular technologist in accordance with the standards of an accrediting body. Doppler waveforms should be measured with an insonation angle as close to 60 degrees as possible but not exceeding 60 degrees, and the sample volumes should be placed within the area of maximal stenosis. The panelists recommended the consistent use of relatively broad diagnostic strata to estimate the degree of ICA stenosis. The panel also concluded that Doppler is relatively inaccurate for subcategorizing ICA stenosis <50%, and recommended that these lesions be reported under a single category as <50% stenosis, and that subcategories for minor degrees of stenosis not be used.

Table 82.2. Consensus Panel Recommendations for Classification of Internal Carotid Artery Stenosis

Normal The ICA PSV is less than 125 cm/s and there is no visible plaque or intimal thickening. Normal arteries should also have an ICA/CCA ratio of less than 2.0 and ICA EDV of less than 40 cm/s.
ICA stenosis <50% is present when the ICA PSV is less than 125 cm/s and there is visible plaque or intimal thickening. Such arteries should also have an ICA/CCA PSV ratio of less than 2.0 and an ICA EDV of less than 40 cm/s.
ICA stenosis of 50–69% is present when the ICA PSV is 125 cm/s to 230 cm/s and there is visible plaque. Such arteries should also have an ICA/CCA PSV ratio of 2.0 to 4.0 and an ICA EDV of 40 cm/s to 100 cm/s.
ICA stenosis ≥70–99% but less than near occlusion is present when the ICA PSV is more than 230 cm/s and there is visible plaque with lumen narrowing on grayscale and color Doppler imaging. The higher the PSV, the more likely (higher positive predictive value) it is to have severe disease. Such stenosis should also have an ICA/CCA ratio of more than 4.0 and an ICA EDV of more than 100 cm/s.
Near occlusion of the ICA The velocity parameters may not apply. "Preocclusive" lesions may be associated with high, low, or undetectable velocity measurements. The diagnosis of near occlusion is therefore established primarily by demonstration of a markedly narrowed lumen with color Doppler. In some near occlusive lesions, color Doppler can distinguish between near occlusion and occlusion by demonstrating a thin wisp of color traversing the lesion.
Occlusion There is no detectable patent lumen on grayscale imaging and no flow with spectral, color, and power Doppler. Near occlusive lesions may be misdiagnosed as occlusions when only grayscale ultrasound and spectral Doppler are used.

ICA, internal carotid artery; PSV, peak systolic velocity; EDV, end-diastolic velocity; CCA, common carotid artery.

Used with permission of Grant EG, Benson CB, Moneta GL, et al. Carotid artery stenosis: gray-scale and Doppler US diagnosis—Society of Radiologists in Ultrasound Consensus Conference. *Radiology.* 2003;229(2):340–346. Permission conveyed through Copyright Clearance Center. Inc.

The consensus panel noted that PSV is easy to obtain. However, data suggest reproducibility of PSV, even among experienced vascular technologists, has sufficient problems that PSVs should not be used as a continuous variable in clinical carotid duplex scanning. Even so, the degree of stenosis estimated by ICA PSV and the degree of narrowing of the ICA lumen seen on grayscale and color Doppler should correlate with PSV as the primary parameters for determining ICA stenosis. Additional parameters such as ICA/CCA PSV ratio and ICA EDV are secondary parameters and should be employed as internal checks. They are especially useful when ICA PSV may not be representative of the extent of disease. After their discussions the
4 consensus panel recommended criteria, stratifying ICA stenosis into specific categories relevant to the CEA trials (**Table 82.2**). These criteria have not been subjected to widespread retrospective or prospective evaluation and do not represent the results of any one laboratory or study. They are not meant to serve as a substitute for continuous quality assurance in individual laboratories.

The Intersocietal Accreditation Commission (IAC) in 2023 published updated recommendations for Carotid Stenosis Interpretation Criteria (**Table 82.3**). Please note that while these categorical criteria were developed to optimize accuracy in clinical practice, the specificity of an elevated velocity for severe carotid stenosis rises steadily with increasing absolute peak systolic velocities.[23,24] The goal of accreditation is

Table 82.3. Strongly Recommended Modification of the SRU Consensus Conference Criteria for Internal Carotid Artery Stenosis for Implementation in IAC-Accredited Vascular Laboratories

	Primary Parameters		Additional Parameters	
Degree of Stenosis, %	**ICA PSV, cm/s**	**Plaque Estimate, %[a]**	**ICA/CCA PSV Ratio**	**ICA EDV, cm/s**
Normal	<180	None	<2.0	<40
<50	<180	<50	<2.0	<40
50–69%[b]	180–230	>50	2.0–4.0	40–100
>70 but less than near occlusion	>230	Visible	>4.0	>100
Near occlusion	High, low, or undetectable	Visible, no detectable lumen	Variable	Variable
Total occlusion	Undetectable		Not applicable	Not applicable

ICA, internal carotid artery; PSV, peak systolic velocity; EDV, end diastolic velocity; CCA, common carotid artery.
[a]Plaque estimate (diameter reduction) with grayscale and color Doppler US.
[b]PSV 125–180 cm/s and ICA/CCA PSV Ratio ≥2.0 is also consistent with 50–69% stenosis.
Derived from diagnostic criteria proposed by Society of Radiologists in Ultrasound (SRU) Consensus Conference.

to enhance the accuracy of the detection of clinically relevant ICA stenosis and further reduce the variability in reading of IAC stenosis on duplex studies. Intraoperative duplex scanning during surgery can be used to assess end points and recognize technical issues prior to closure. This allows revision prior to leaving the operating room. This has largely replaced intraoperative completion angiography for CEA.[23,24]

BILATERAL HIGH-GRADE ICA STENOSIS

Doppler-derived flow velocities from the ICA opposite an ICA occlusion or high-grade stenosis may suggest a higher degree of narrowing than is observed angiographically.[2] This likely is because of compensatory flow. Duplex scan overestimation of stenosis is more common in less-severe categories of stenosis than in higher-severity categories.[25]

Stented Carotid Arteries

Carotid artery stenosis may be selectively treated with an intraluminal stent. However, ultrasound criteria developed for native ICAs overestimate the severity of stenosis within stented carotid arteries especially with more modest lesions in the stented arteries. With rare exceptions the number of patients in studies of stented carotid arteries that have actually had severe in-stent restenosis (ISR) is small. Acute and subacute in-stent thrombosis has been reported in 0.5% to 5% of patients with carotid artery stents (CAS). Some cases may be related to inadequate or discontinued antiplatelet therapy. Beyond 30 days, early restenosis after CAS is mainly due to neointimal hyperplasia which is related to vascular injury related to the stent regardless of the technique used to place the stent. Over dilation or imperfect positioning of the CAS may lead to ongoing vessel injury. Intravascular ultrasound may be of some help to decrease rate of vessel injury. The observation of increasing severity of ISR and rising Doppler velocities is preserved in the stented carotid artery. Duplex imaging obtained prior to discharge can serve as a baseline to compare with sequential imaging usually obtained at 3 and 6 months then every 6 months for 2 years. No study has correlated the degree of stenosis or increase in ICA velocities within a stented carotid artery with clinical symptoms or outcomes. In multiple studies, PSV threshold for significant in-stent ICA restenosis for CAS were higher than those for significant stenosis in nonprocedurally treated (native) ICA. There is a consensus to use higher-flow velocity thresholds for assessment of stenosis in stented ICA than in native ICA. There have been insufficient data about the flow velocity criteria for significant restenosis after CEA as well. Studies have also not evaluated the effect of the stented carotid artery on the opposite nonstented artery. Change of conformation of the carotid bifurcation, neointimal hyperplasia, and vascular remodeling after carotid surgery are considered the most likely explanations for why the standard duplex ultrasound criteria used for stenosis of the native ICA do not match the criteria for ICA restenosis after carotid interventions. It is generally agreed that PSVs >125 cm/s, will be needed to identify a >50% stenosis in a stented ICA. Criteria to detect high-grade stenosis in native ICAs still work reasonably well to identify high-grade stenosis in stented ICAs (**Fig. 82.8**).[26,27] Consensus to use higher-flow velocity criteria for assessment of the degree of ISR after CAS suggests 220 cm/s PSV threshold for ≥50% and a 300 cm/s cutoff value for ≥70% ISR. Higher-flow velocity in ISR after CAS may be due to changes in the biomechanical properties of the artery, including higher stiffness of the arterial wall, rendering the stented artery similar to a rigid tube. This results in

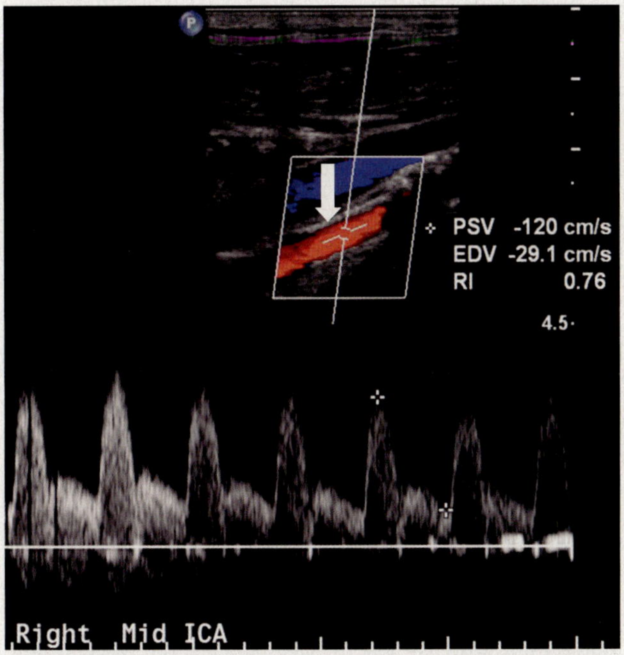

Figure 82.8. Color-flow image and velocity waveforms from a stented internal carotid artery (ICA). A peak systolic velocity of 120 cm/s indicates the stent is widely patent. The stent itself is easily recognized as a hyperechoic stripe (*arrow*) parallel to the vessel wall.

decreased arterial compliance causing a reduced alteration of the volume of the arterial segment during different phases of the pulse wave.[28]

CCA and ECA Stenosis

Criteria used for classifying disease in the ICA have not been prospectively tested for application to the ECA or the CCA. However, as with the ICA, relative degrees of stenosis may be determined by the presence of plaque with B-mode imaging, aberration in color flow on duplex examination, spectral broadening, and increases in PSV. Greater than 50% stenosis can be inferred by the presence of a focally increased PSV followed by poststenotic turbulence. As noted above, the CCA waveform normally has attributes of the ICA and ECA. The CCA will take on the quality of the "normal" vessel (ICA or ECA) when the other is occluded. If there is a proximal CCA (or innominate artery) high-grade stenosis or occlusion, the ipsilateral CCA Doppler flow quality will be dampened with low PSVs and delayed upstroke of the waveform compared with the nonstenotic contralateral side. Poststenotic turbulence also may be seen. There are no widely employed validated criteria to give a diameter reduction for stenosis in the CCA or ECA. Greater than 50% stenosis in the ECA is often inferred by PSV >125 cm/s associated with poststenotic turbulence whereas a PSV >200 cm/s may be an appropriate threshold for >50% stenosis in the CCA.[29]

LOWER EXTREMITY ARTERIAL DISEASE

The noninvasive vascular laboratory, in combination with the history and physical examination, has a critical role in providing objective diagnosis of lower extremity arterial occlusive disease in asymptomatic patients, those with intermittent claudication (IC), and in those with critical arterial insufficiency. Both plethysmographic and ultrasound techniques are used in the evaluation of peripheral arterial disease (PAD).

In many patients, the clinical history and physical examination are all that is necessary to establish a diagnosis of IC. Almost all patients with IC have diminished or absent lower extremity pulses. However, palpation of pulses is subjective and poorly reproducible. Therefore, the pulse examination in a patient suspected of having arterial disease should be supplemented with objective testing in the noninvasive vascular laboratory. On occasion a patient will give a history suggesting IC, yet have what appear to be normal resting lower extremity pulses. In such cases, exercise testing with postexercise Doppler-measured ankle pressures and ankle–brachial systolic blood pressure ratios is crucial to confirm the diagnosis of IC secondary to arterial stenosis or occlusion.

Many patients with PAD have atypical leg symptoms or are asymptomatic. Such patients have a similar increased risk of cardiovascular death as patients with typical IC symptoms, leading some to advocate for screening for PAD in patients with atypical leg symptoms or atherosclerotic risk factors.

Patients with exercise-induced lower extremity and/or buttock pain should be asked about the location of their pain, its relationship to walking, severity and duration of symptoms, and symptom progression over time. Only exercise-induced muscular pain of the calf, thigh, or buttock, relieved within a few minutes of rest and reproduced by additional walking, can be predictably improved by lower extremity arterial revascularization. There are no data on the response of atypical leg symptoms to revascularization in patients with evidence of PAD.

Ischemic pain at rest is a clinical diagnosis. It is suspected when a patient complains of pain and/or numbness in the forefoot, toes, or instep at rest. In such patients, the vascular laboratory can objectively confirm and quantify the magnitude of arterial insufficiency. Ischemic pain is generally associated with an ankle pressure <50 mm Hg and an ankle–brachial index (ABI) ≤0.4.

PLETHYSMOGRAPHIC TECHNIQUES

Volume Flow

Calf or foot blood flow can be recorded with a mercury-in-silastic strain gauge. Electrical resistance of the mercury column depends on the length of the column. Changes in electrical resistance, reflect changes in the volume of the extremity, and are based on detection of minute changes in the length of the column. However, neither calf nor foot blood flow at rest differ between normal subjects and patients with even rather severe IC.[30] Hyperemic volume flow is often lower in patients with occlusive disease but such testing can be quite painful for the patient. Measurements of volume flow therefore are not very useful in the evaluation of lower extremity ischemia.

Pulse Volume Recordings

5 APG can be used to display pulse volume waveforms. PVRs are obtained with partially inflated blood pressure cuffs that detect volume changes sequentially down a limb. Volume changes beneath the cuffs resulting from the pulse wave result in small pressure changes within the cuffs. These changes are displayed as arterial waveforms with the use of appropriate transducers. A normal pulse volume waveform has a sharp systolic upstroke and peak, as well as a prominent dichroic notch on the downward portion of the curve. With increasing proximal arterial occlusion, the dichroitic notch is lost and the waveform bows out on the down portion of the systolic portion of the curve. The peak of the pulse wave also becomes rounded and there is loss of amplitude of the wave as disease is more severe. With even more severe disease there are nearly equal upstroke and downstroke times and in very severe proximal disease the pulse wave is absent (**Fig. 82.9**).[31,32] An absence of quantitative data limits the utility of PVRs. More quantitative data for the evaluation of lower extremity arterial disease are available using ultrasound-based techniques.

ULTRASOUND TECHNIQUES

Ankle–Brachial Index

6 ABI is a very useful measure of overall lower extremity perfusion. The test is performed with the patient supine and having rested for a few minutes. A pneumatic pressure cuff is placed just above the ankle and inflated to supra systolic levels. A continuous-wave Doppler probe is positioned over the posterior tibial or dorsalis pedal artery distal to the cuff. The cuff is deflated and the pressure reading when the Doppler signal returns is recorded. The sequence is repeated for the other ankle artery and the values compared with the highest brachial artery systolic pressure also obtained with the Doppler. For clinical purposes, the higher ipsilateral dorsal pedal or posterior tibial pressure is divided by the higher brachial artery systolic pressure, yielding an ABI for that lower extremity. The use of a ratio makes the test relatively independent of day-to-day variations in arterial blood pressure.

A normal ABI is 1.0 to 1.2, with progressively lower values corresponding to worsening arterial disease (**Table 82.4**). ABIs below normal indicate relative lower extremity arterial insufficiency and increased risk of cardiovascular death with the risk increasing with the magnitude of depression of the ABI. This test has several limitations. Significant bilateral subclavian or axillary artery occlusive disease results in a falsely elevated ABI. Calcified tibial arteries that can frequently occur with diabetes or renal failure may be inadequately compressed by the pressure cuff. This also results in a falsely elevated (supra-systolic) ankle pressure. An ABI >1.4 should therefore also be considered abnormal. Such patients often have severe arterial disease and are also at increased risk of cardiovascular death. When the ABI may be falsely elevated, qualitative analysis of Doppler-derived analog or plethysmographic waveforms or measurement of digital systolic pressures is a more appropriate indicator of the arterial status of the lower extremity.

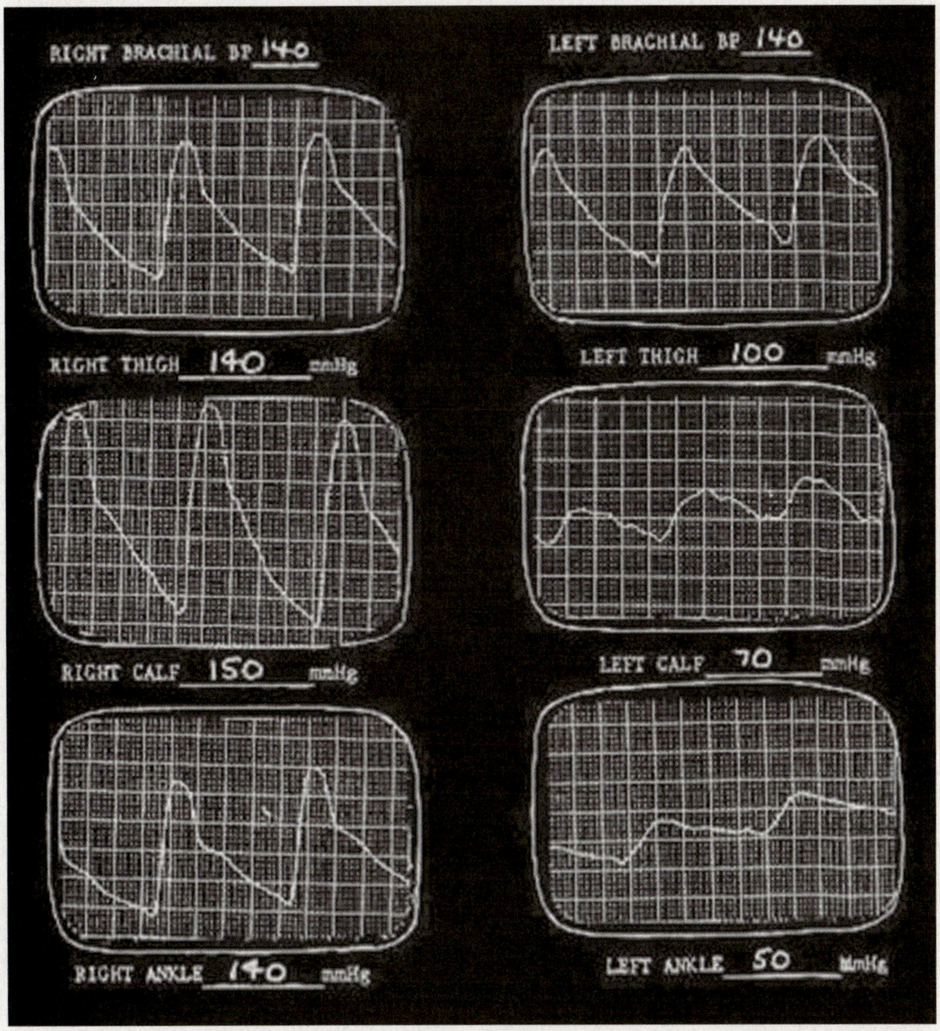

Figure 82.9. Pulse volume recordings. The plethysmographic waveforms are normal on the right and severely abnormal in the left leg with loss of amplitude of the waveform, slowing of the upstroke of the waveform, and outward bowing of the downstroke of the waveform.

Other problems with ABI include confusion with venous signals when the ankle arterial pressure is low or unmeasurable and relative insensitivity to certain patterns of progression of arterial disease. A tibial artery can occlude without a change in ABI if the remaining tibial vessels remain patent. High-grade stenosis may also progress to occlusion without a change in ABI.

Segmental Limb Pressures

Multiple pneumatic cuffs may be used along the lower extremity to determine the arterial blood pressure at specified levels. These "segmental leg pressures" are compared with the higher brachial artery systolic pressure, with other locations in the ipsilateral leg and with the corresponding levels in the contralateral extremity. Three or four cuffs may be used. In the four-cuff technique cuffs are placed: (1) as far proximal on the thigh as possible; (2) immediately above the knee; (3) just below the knee; and (4) just proximal to the ankle. Each cuff width should be 20% greater than the diameter of the limb at the point of application to avoid falsely elevated pressure readings induced by too narrow a cuff.[33] For the thigh, this generally necessitates a single, wide, thigh cuff. Use of two cuffs above the knee, however, can permit assessment of inflow at or proximal to the common femoral artery with the proximal cuff, and permit evaluation for the presence of superficial femoral artery disease by the distal thigh cuff. With two thigh cuffs the most proximal thigh cuff is often too narrow. An artificially elevated pressure in the proximal thigh is then expected. Therefore the high-thigh index, comparing the proximal thigh pressure to the brachial pressure, is normally about 1.4 with the four-cuff technique and 1.0 to 1.1 with the three-cuff technique (**Fig. 82.10**).

A hand-held Doppler is used to detect the most prominent Doppler signal at the ankle. Examination proceeds proximal to distal. First the high-thigh cuff is inflated until the ankle Doppler signal is no longer audible. The cuff is then deflated and the pressure where there is return of the Doppler signal at the ankle is the high-thigh pressure. The above-knee, below-knee, and ankle pressures are similarly determined. If there is no audible ankle Doppler signal, the popliteal artery is insonated with the Doppler to determine high-thigh and above-knee pressures. Comparison of the pressures measured

Table 82.4. Correlation between Ankle–Brachial Index (ABI) and Clinical Severity of Lower Extremity Arterial Ischemia

ABI	Clinical Status
>1.3	Abnormal, significant arterial wall calcification
1.1 ± 0.1	Normal
0.6 ± 0.2	Intermittent claudication
0.3 ± 0.1	Ischemic rest pain
0.1 ± 0.1	Impending tissue necrosis

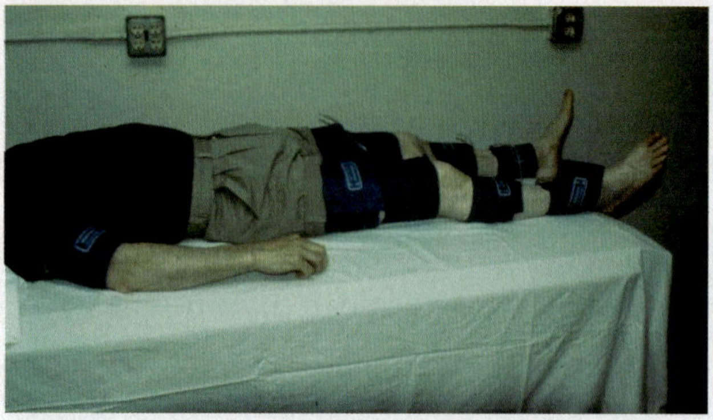

Figure 82.10. Segmental pressures multiple pneumatic cuffs may be used along the lower extremity to determine the arterial blood pressure at each level. Comparison of the pressures measured at each location permits an estimation of the location of occlusive lesions. Use of two cuffs above the knee can permit assessment of inflow at or proximal to the common femoral artery with the proximal cuff, and permit evaluation for the presence of superficial femoral artery disease by the distal thigh cuff. In many patients, however, the high-thigh cuff is relatively narrow compared to the diameter of the thigh resulting in an artificial elevation of the high-thigh pressure so that with use of four cuffs the high-thigh pressure will be 30 to 40 mm Hg higher than the highest brachial pressure.

at each location permits an estimation of the location of occlusive lesions (**Fig. 82.11**).

There are multiple limitations in the interpretation of segmental limb pressures. The high-thigh pressure is subject to particular interpretation difficulties. A diminished high-thigh pressure can reflect an occlusive lesion anywhere at or proximal to the common femoral artery bifurcation. Low high-thigh pressures therefore may reflect a pressure-reducing stenosis in the ipsilateral common or external iliac artery, a common femoral artery lesion or tandem pressure-reducing lesions in the profunda femoris, and the proximal superficial femoral artery or any combination of such lesions. The accuracy of segmental pressures may be affected by mural calcification resulting in artificially elevated pressures. Diminished proximal pressures may also mask gradients that exist further down the leg. Segmental pressures also do not allow differentiation between short- and long-segment occlusions, or between occluded and patent, but highly stenotic arteries.

Exercise Testing

Doppler-determined pressures can be combined with treadmill exercise testing in patients without a contraindication to exercise. After determination of resting supine ankle pressures and ABIs, the patient walks on a treadmill with a predetermined incline at a predetermined rate. The test continues for 5 minutes or until the patient is forced to stop. The type, time-to-onset, and location of symptoms are recorded. At completion of the test, the patient is immediately placed supine and absolute ankle pressures and ABIs determined.

In most patients exercise testing serves only to confirm a diagnosis of claudication. It is not required in a patient with classic symptoms of claudication, absent peripheral pulses and a diminished ABI. In some cases exercise testing can document a physiologic response to revascularization or provide an objective assessment of the potential postoperative physiologic benefit.

Exercise testing is particularly useful in the infrequent patient with symptoms of claudication and who has palpable pedal pulses and/or a normal ABI. Patients with exercise-induced leg pain occurring on the basis of arterial insufficiency will show a decrease in the postexercise ankle pressures and ABI. Exercise testing can also be used to document an ischemic response to exercise in a patient with PAD and other conditions that may limit their ability to walk. Patients with COPD, arthritis, venous disease, and PAD are often more limited in their walking ability by these coexisting conditions than by their PAD. If the patients cannot complete a treadmill examination, and no ischemic pressure response to exercise occurs, it is highly unlikely their walking ability would be improved by a revascularization procedure.

The precise endpoints and techniques of exercise testing are controversial. Some laboratories exercise patients at low speeds with no inclination of the treadmill whereas others utilize various inclines and graded increases in treadmill speed. Both initial and absolute claudication distances can be determined. Initial claudication distance is the point where the patient initially experiences claudication-type pain. The absolute claudication distance is where the patient can no longer continue to walk on the treadmill.

Criteria for a positive exercise test include a decrease in the ankle pressure of 20 mm Hg or 20%, a decrease in the ABI of 0.2 in the symptomatic extremity, or failure of the ankle pressure to return to baseline within 3 minutes of completing the treadmill portion of the examination. Because systemic pressure and therefore arm pressures, depending on work load, will increase with exercise, use of the ABI alone to indicate a positive exercise test is incorrect. The ABI decrease should be accompanied by an absolute pressure drop at the ankle.

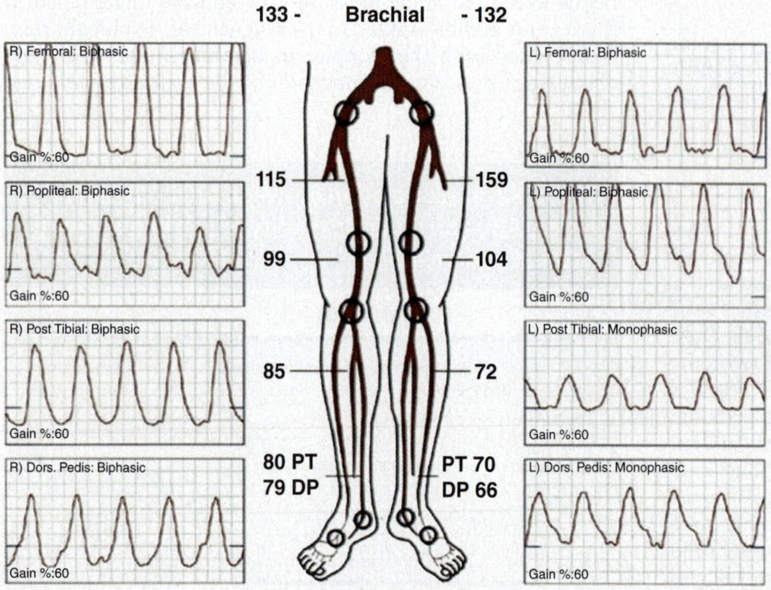

Figure 82.11. Segmental pressure examination with use of thigh, calf, and ankle cuffs. A drop in pressure of 30 mm Hg between levels indicates a hemodynamically significant stenosis between the two adjacent cuffs. This study therefore indicates a flow-reducing lesion somewhere at or proximal to the common femoral artery bifurcation on the *right side* and likely superficial femoral artery/popliteal artery occlusive disease on the *left*.

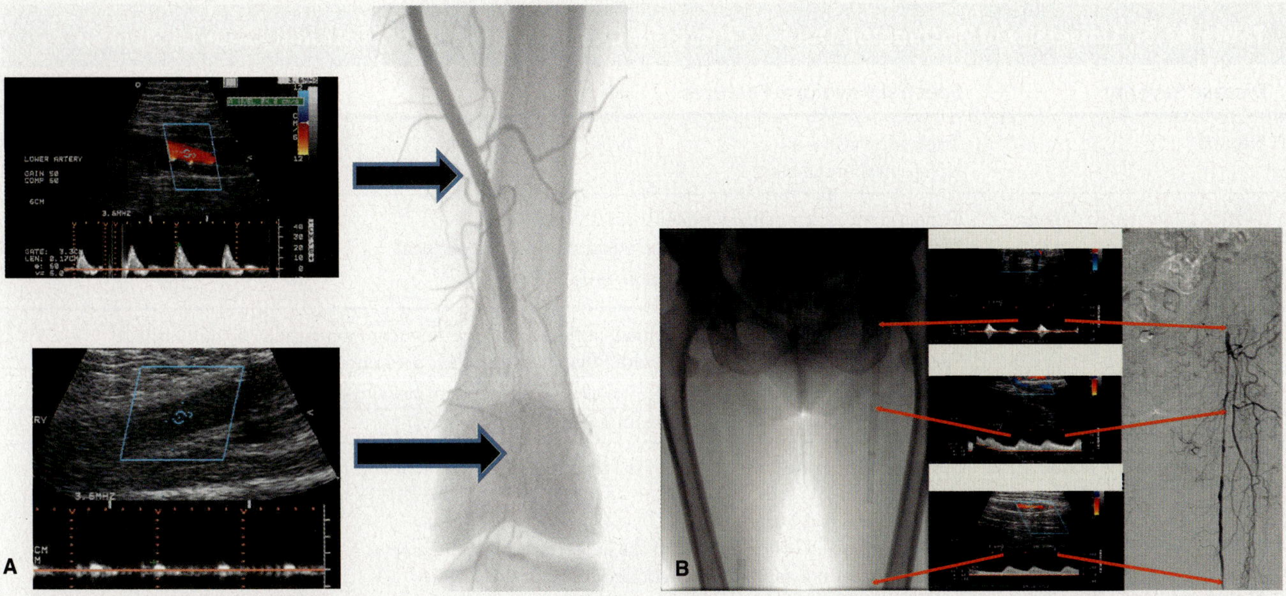

Figure 82.12. **A:** Duplex images/waveforms and corresponding angiogram of an abrupt popliteal artery occlusion. **B:** Duplex waveforms and angiographic images in a patient with severe in-stent stenosis of superficial femoral artery stents.

7 Failure of the ankle pressure to drop with exercise along with failure of the ABI to decrease 20% with exercise, combined with a normal resting ABI, substantially rules out arterial insufficiency as the etiology of the patient's exercise-induced complaints of leg pain. An exception is the rare patient with buttock claudication secondary to isolated internal iliac disease.

Neurogenic claudication may be confused with arterial ischemia. Patients present with symptoms of exercise-induced leg or calf pain. Careful questioning, however, reveals atypical characteristics for vascular-induced exercise-associated pain. Such characteristics include occurrence of pain with standing, pain relief when leaning forward, worsening with coughing, and prolonged time for pain to resolve following exercise. These patients often have normal ankle pressures at rest that do not decrease with exercise despite onset of symptoms. Failure of the ankle pressures to decrease with exercise may also be a clue to the presence of other uncommon conditions, such as venous claudication and chronic exercise-induced compartment syndromes.

Doppler Analog Waveform Analysis

Similar to plethysmographic waveforms, continuous-wave Doppler waveforms may also be analyzed qualitatively. Normal lower extremity Doppler waveforms are described as triphasic with a sharp systolic upstroke, an end-systolic reverse-flow component followed by low forward flow through diastole. The shape of the waveform changes with increasing severity of proximal obstruction. Initially, the reverse-flow component is lost. As proximal stenosis increases, the rate of rise of the systolic upstroke is decreased, the amplitude of the waveform is diminished, and diastolic flow increases relative to systolic flow.

Continuous-wave Doppler waveforms are generally used in conjunction with measurement of segmental Doppler pressures similar to the use of PVRs. Doppler waveform analysis can also be used to assess iliac artery inflow to the common femoral artery. An attenuated common femoral artery waveform indicates proximal disease.

Peripheral Artery Duplex Scanning

Arterial duplex scanning provides detailed anatomic and hemodynamic information from the infrarenal aorta to the distal tibial vessels that cannot be determined by indirect testing. Arterial duplex scanning has been prospectively compared with angiography to establish standard criteria for normal and diseased arteries.[34] Sensitivity of duplex examination for detecting the presence of a hemodynamically important lesion (>50%) ranges from 89% at the iliac artery to 68% at the popliteal artery. Overall sensitivities for predicting interruption of patency are 90% for the anterior and posterior tibial arteries and 82% for the peroneal artery. The technique is versatile and does not appear to be significantly influenced by the presence of previous operations or multilevel disease (**Fig. 82.12A,B**).

Velocity Patterns and Classification of Percent Stenosis

In the absence of arterial stenosis or occlusion triphasic waveforms are maintained throughout the length of the lower extremity but PSV decreases from the iliac to the tibial vessels. There are no significant differences in velocity measurements among the three tibial arteries in normal subjects.

Important changes in the velocity waveforms that signify disease include the absence of an end-systolic reverse-flow component and elevation of the PSV. A 50% reduction in arterial luminal diameter (equivalent to a cross-sectional surface area reduction of 75%) is associated with a pressure drop across the lesion. The University of Washington criteria for classification of peripheral arterial stenosis are shown in **Table 82.5**.[35]

A PSV ratio, comparing the velocity within the stenosis to the velocity just proximal to the stenosis, is also useful for grading degree of stenosis. PSV ratios are independent of changes in blood pressure, cardiac output, and vascular compliance. Grading stenosis using the PSV ratio has been found to be highly reproducible.[36,37] Fifty percent stenosis in lower extremity arteries correlates with a PSV ratio from 1.4 to 3.0.[34,38–41] A velocity ratio of 2.0 is a reasonable compromise and is used by many vascular laboratories as indicative of a 50% peripheral arterial stenosis.

Lower extremity duplex scanning can serve as an alternative to contrast arteriography in the preoperative assessment of candidates for arterial intervention. In selected centers, successful lower extremity revascularization either by open arterial bypass grafting or with catheter-based techniques has been reported using only arterial duplex in a high percentage of cases.[42–44] The limiting factor with preoperative arterial duplex is the ability to accurately identify the best site for the distal anastomosis of a bypass graft, especially when the distal anastomotic site is below the knee.[45] Intraoperative duplex may be useful to identify technical issues that need to be corrected prior to closure in the operating room.

Table 82.5. University of Washington Duplex Criteria for Classification of Lower Extremity Arterial Stenosis

Disease Severity	Spectral Waveform Features
Normal	Triphasic waveform No spectral broadening
1–19% Diameter Reduction	Triphasic waveform with minimal spectral broadening PSVs increased <30% relative to the adjacent proximal segment Proximal and distal waveforms remain normal
20–49% Diameter Reduction	Triphasic waveform usually maintained (although reverse-flow component may be diminished) Spectral broadening is prominent, with filling-in of the clear area under the systolic peak PSV is increased from 30% to 100% relative to the adjacent proximal segment Proximal and distal waveforms remain normal
50–99% Diameter Reduction	Monophasic waveform with loss of the reverse-flow component and forward flow throughout the cardiac cycle Extensive spectral broadening PSV is increased >100% relative to the adjacent proximal segment Distal waveform is monophasic with reduced systolic velocity
Occlusion	No flow detected within the imaged arterial segment Preocclusive "thump" may be heard just proximal to the site of occlusion Distal (collateral) waveforms are monophasic with reduced systolic velocities

Reprinted from Zierler RE, Dawson DL, Strandness DE Jr. *Duplex Scanning in Vascular Disorders*. 5th ed. Raven Press; 2015:121–145.

The role of duplex ultrasound scanning in the surveillance of lower extremity vein grafts has been well documented (**Fig. 82.13A,B**). Detection and repair of a graft-threatening stenosis detected by duplex scanning appears to improve secondary graft patency.[46–49] Twenty percent to 30% of vein grafts will develop a severe enough stenosis that revision is recommended.[50] Approximately 80% of these graft stenotic lesions develop in the first postoperative year. However, graft-threatening lesions can develop at any time. Surveillance is therefore generally recommended for the life of the graft. A widely utilized protocol for vein graft duplex surveillance is every 3 months for the first year and every 6 months to yearly thereafter. The examination involves point-to-point insonation of the proximal inflow artery, proximal anastomosis, midgraft, distal anastomosis, and the distal outflow artery. A PSV ratio of 4, or a PSV above 300 cm/s, indicates a critical graft stenosis, and repair of the lesion by open or catheter-based techniques should be considered.[51] If the PSV ratio is between 2 and 4, the patient should be evaluated again in 3 months with a duplex examination.

Aneurysms and pseudoaneurysms of lower extremity arteries are also readily identified and characterized with duplex scanning with particular attention to the diameter of the aneurysm and the presence or absence of intraluminal thrombosis (**Fig. 82.14A,B**).

Upper Extremity Arterial Evaluation

Upper extremity arterial disease is a small but important component of vascular surgical practice. Both ultrasound and plethysmographic techniques are important in the evaluation of upper extremity arterial disease.

SEGMENTAL ARM PRESSURES

Upper extremity segmental pressures are obtained by measuring blood pressure with pneumatic cuffs above the elbow, below the elbow, and above the wrist while insonating the radial or ulnar artery at the wrist using a continuous-wave Doppler. Doppler-derived or plethysmographic waveforms can also be recorded at the different levels. Abnormal waveforms or pressures will help diagnose arterial disease proximal to the wrist.

A 12-cm blood pressure cuff is usually sufficient for measuring the brachial artery pressure, whereas a 10-cm blood

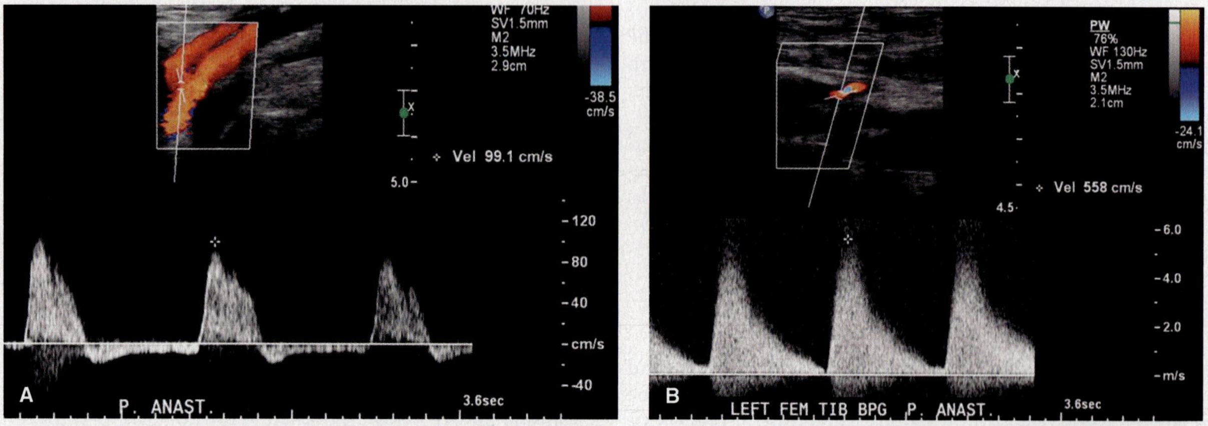

Figure 82.13. **A and B:** Duplex ultrasound images and velocity waveforms of normal (A) and stenotic (B) proximal anastomoses of femoral tibial bypass grafts. The abnormal study has a severe elevation in flow velocity of 558 cm/s indicating a high-grade stenosis.

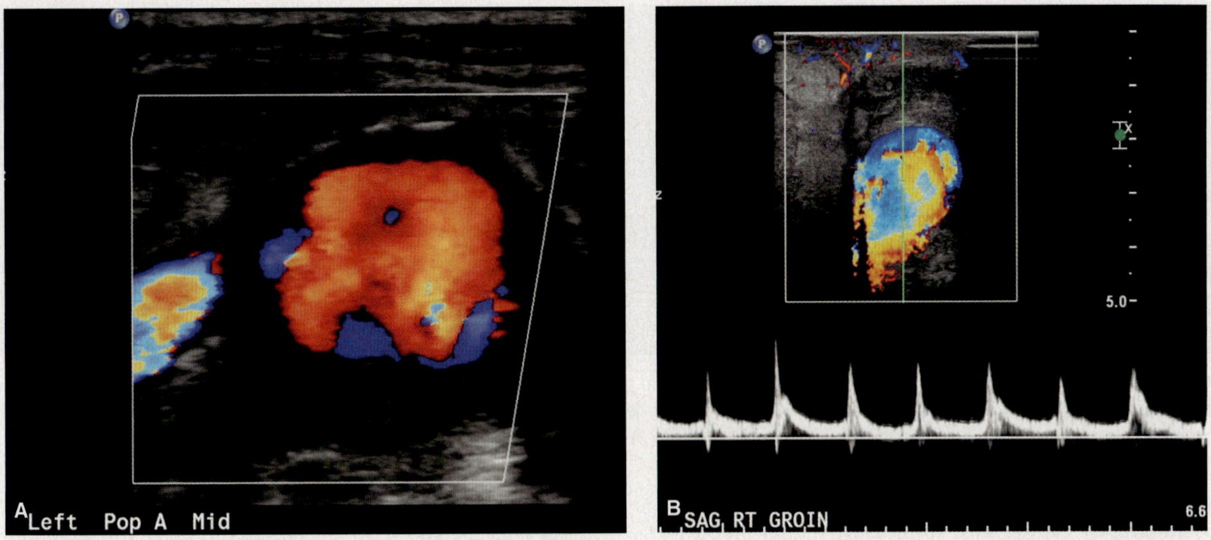

Figure 82.14. **A:** Native popliteal artery aneurysm with intraluminal thrombus. **B:** Large pseudoaneurysm of the right common femoral artery resulting from arterial infection from intra-arterial injection of street drugs.

pressure cuff is used at the wrist to measure the systolic pressure from the radial and ulnar arteries. A systolic pressure measurement is taken from the upper arm (brachial artery) and at the wrist (radial and ulnar arteries). Normally, there is not a recordable gradient between any of these sites and a normal wrist/brachial blood pressure ratio is 1.0. If there is a blood pressure difference between the two arms of more than 15 mm Hg, it is likely that there is a stenosis or occlusion somewhere on the side of the lower pressure. Abnormal waveforms and decreased pressures at the above-elbow cuff site indicate axillary, subclavian, or brachiocephalic arterial occlusive disease. Similarly, abnormalities at the below-elbow and above-wrist sites indicate brachial and proximal ulnar/radial arterial occlusive disease, respectively. If there is a blood pressure difference between levels, or between the radial and ulnar arteries, of more than 15 mm Hg it is likely caused by a stenosis or occlusion (**Fig. 82.15**).

DIGITAL PRESSURES AND PLETHYSMOGRAPHY

Digital pressure measurements and digital plethysmography are extremely useful in the diagnosis of upper extremity arterial disease and can be as accurate as arteriography in

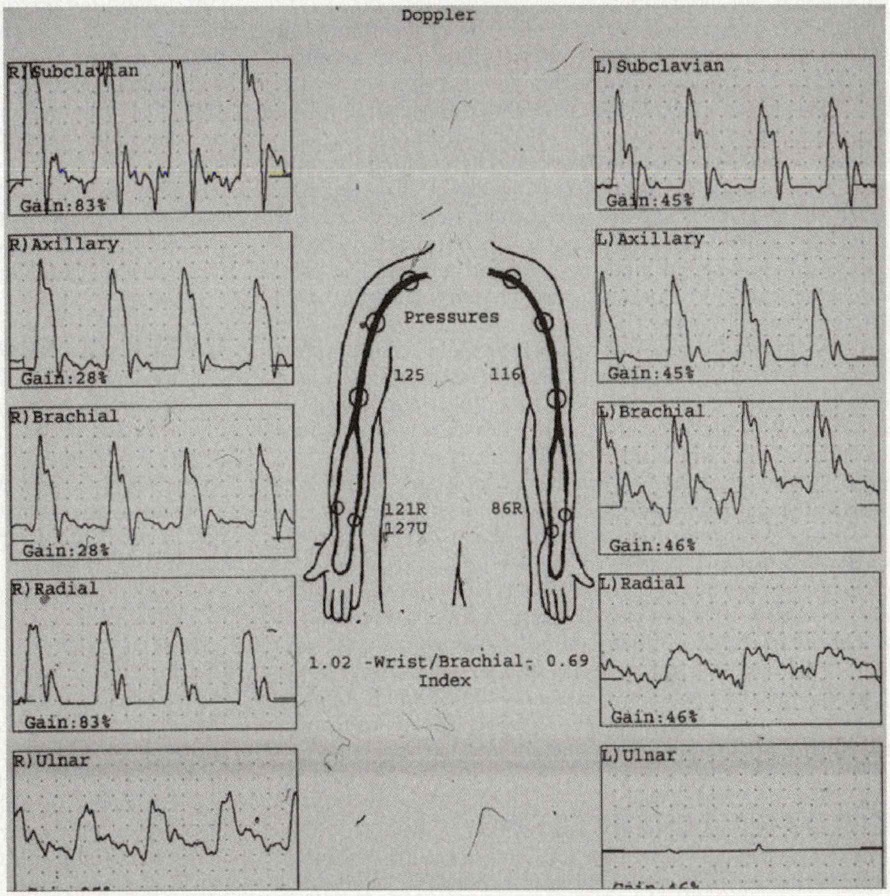

Figure 82.15. Upper extremity segmental pressures and Doppler waveforms. The findings are normal on the *right* and suggest radial and ulnar artery or distal brachial artery occlusive disease on the *left*.

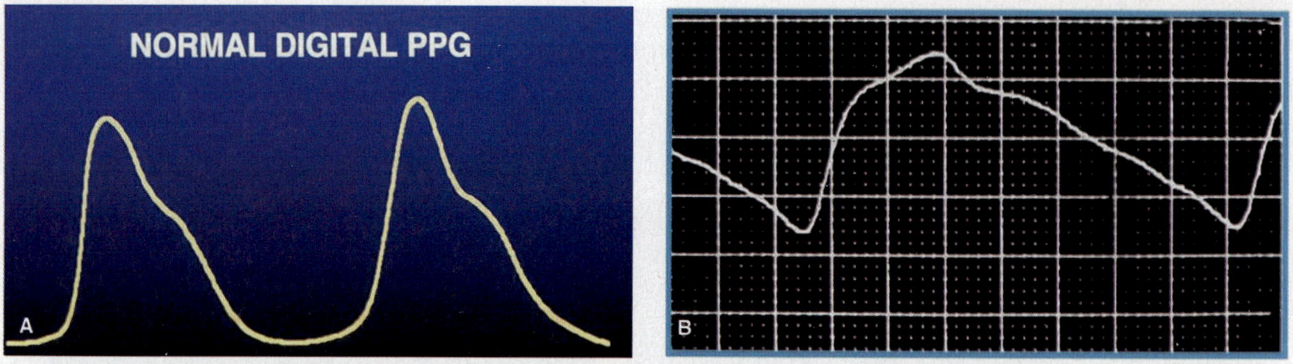

Figure 82.16. **A and B:** Normal (**A**) and "peaked pulse" (**B**) digital photoplethysmographic (PPG) waveforms. A normal waveform has a rapid upstroke and a sharp apex whereas an obstructive waveform would demonstrate a delayed upstroke and rounded apex. In a peaked pulse, waveform suggestive of vasospasm, the dichroitic notch slides to high on the systolic downslope of the waveform.

assessing patients with hand ischemia.[52] PPG or strain-gauge plethysmography can be used to measure digital blood pressure and to obtain pulse waveforms. PPG is preferred because the equipment is easier to use and more durable. An additional advantage of PPG is that it is possible to record the volume pulses from the tips of the digits. This may also be useful in documenting obstruction within the digit arteries themselves.

The photo cell is attached to the fingertip pulp with double-sided tape or small strain gauges are placed around the fingertip. One-inch (2.5 cm) blood pressure cuffs are placed around the proximal phalanx. Waveforms are recorded using pulse tracings obtained at high speed to evaluate the shape of the waveform. Waveforms are normal if the upstroke time is less than 0.2 seconds (**Fig. 82.16A**). They may or may not have a dichotic notch. An abnormal obstructive waveform will have a rounded peak, as opposed to the normal notched peak. Upstroke time is prolonged. The amplitude of the waveform is not important. Finger PPG waveforms are not quantitative. The amplitude of the waveform is primarily dependent on the gain setting, not blood flow.

Patients with vasospasm will often have an abnormally shaped waveform termed a "peaked pulse," also reported as "bird's beaking," which is thought to represent abnormal elasticity and rebound of the palmar and digital vessels (**Fig. 82.16B**).

Finger blood pressures are measured by inflating the cuffs placed at the base of the fingers. At reduced chart recorder speed the pulsations are recorded while the blood pressure cuffs are inflated. When digit pulsations are obliterated, the cuff is slowly deflated until the pulsation returns. The pressure reading at this point is recorded and represents the digital artery pressure.

It is extremely important to measure and record finger temperature before performing digital plethysmography and obtaining finger blood pressures. If the finger temperature is less than 28 °C to 30 °C false-positive results may be obtained secondary to cold-induced vasospasm. It is recommend that hand and/or whole-body warming be performed in patients with low finger temperatures.

Digital blood pressure is normally within 20 to 30 mm Hg of brachial pressure. A ratio of finger systolic pressure to brachial systolic pressure of greater than 0.80 is normal but does not necessarily rule out digital artery occlusive disease. It is important to remember that there are occasional patients with very distal digital artery occlusive disease with normal finger pressures since the digital cuff is around the proximal phalanx. Also, occlusive disease in a single digital artery can be missed if the other digital artery in that finger is normally patent.

COLD CHALLENGE TESTING

The simplest cold intolerance test is to measure the digital temperature recovery time after immersion of the hand in ice water for a short time period. Preimmersion digital temperatures must be above 30 °C. Hand and body warming may be required prior to immersion.

Using a thermistor probe to measure finger temperatures, the patient's hand is immersed in a container of ice water for 30 to 60 seconds. After the hand is dried, the fingertip pulp temperatures are measured every 5 minutes for 45 minutes, or until the temperature returns to preimmersion levels. Normal individuals will have a recovery time to preimmersion levels of less than 10 minutes. This test is very sensitive for detecting cold-induced vasospasm but is nonspecific, with approximately one-half of patients with a positive test having no clinical symptoms of cold sensitivity.[53] Cold immersion testing is also uncomfortable and poorly tolerated by patients with significant Raynaud syndrome symptoms. Pressures often fall to unrecordable levels in such patients.

A better, but infrequently utilized, test for cold sensitivity is the digital hypothermic challenge test as described by Nielsen and Lassen (**Fig. 82.17**).[54] This test involves placing a finger cuff around the proximal phalanx on the test finger and perfusing the cuff with progressively cooler fluid. The pressure in the test finger is then compared with that in a reference finger that is not cooled. The Nielsen test is interpreted as positive for abnormal cold-induced vasospasm if the test finger pressure is reduced by more than 17% compared with the reference finger.

Other tests for cold-induced vasospasm include thermal entrainment, digital laser Doppler response to cold, thermography, venous occlusion plethysmography, and digital artery caliber measurement. None are widely accepted or employed.[55–57]

UPPER EXTREMITY DUPLEX SCANNING

Duplex scanning of the upper extremity is carried out in a manner similar to arterial examination elsewhere. The origins of the brachial cephalic vessels can be difficult to visualize with duplex scanning. For examination of the origin of the subclavian artery a 3- or 5-MHz transducer with a small footprint probe using the sternal notch as a window generally gives the best images. One study found 48 of 50 right subclavian artery origins (96%) and 25 (50%) of 50 left subclavian artery origins could be visualized by color duplex scanning.[58]

Criteria for stenosis at the origins of brachial cephalic arteries are slightly different than those used elsewhere. A PSV ratio of ≥2 indicates stenosis at the origin of a brachial cephalic artery. Stenosis can also be implied by monophasic flow without actual visualization of a high-velocity jet and by reverse flow in a vertebral artery. Such additional criteria are necessary to assess the origins of the brachiocephalic vessels. If only PSV ratios are utilized, there would be higher numbers of both false-positive and false-negative results.[58]

More distally the upper extremity arteries are relatively superficial and fairly constant in location. They are best

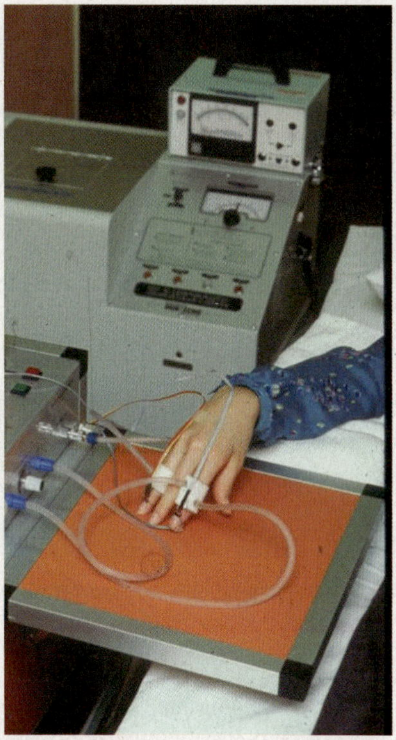

Figure 82.17. Device for performance of digital hypothermic challenge or Nielsen test. The cuff on the second finger is used to cool the test finger and measure digital pressure. This allows controlled application of cold to induce a vasospastic response. The fourth finger is the reference finger. Strain gauges on the finger tips are used to measure the digital pressures. See text.

scanned with a higher-frequency probe such as a 7.5- or 10-MHz probe. Either a sector or linear scan head may be used, but in either case a standoff or mound of acoustic gel is helpful to visualize the vessel clearly and to assess the flow pattern within it. Color facilitates identification of the vessels, and tortuosity of the upper extremity arteries may be more easily seen with color-flow imaging. Stenosis, occlusions, and aneurysms of upper extremity arteries are all readily identified with ultrasound (**Fig. 82.18A–C**).

The interpretation of duplex findings in the upper extremity beyond the origins of the vessels is similar to the interpretation of B-mode images and Doppler signals gathered in other arterial systems.[59] Normal waveforms in the upper extremity arteries are usually triphasic. As elsewhere in the arterial system, stenosis will produce high-velocity jets, poststenotic turbulence, and dampened distal waveforms. There are, however, at present no specific frequency or velocity criteria with which to gauge the severity of stenosis in the upper extremity arteries. Some general guidelines are listed in **Table 82.6.** The diagnosis of arterial occlusion is made by imaging the artery and using the pulsed Doppler to show that there is no flow within the lumen.

For patients with unilateral symptoms who may have a surgically correctable lesion such as a subclavian artery aneurysm or stenosis, duplex scanning is quite useful.[60] The duplex evaluation of aneurysms is based upon the B-mode image appearance, with the most important feature being the size of the enlarged artery and the presence of intraluminal thrombus that may serve as a source of distal embolization. Presence or absence of flow within the aneurysm can be determined by the Doppler component.

Duplex scanning may be of use in patients with suspected embolization to identify proximal aneurysms, but the evaluation should also include echocardiography to

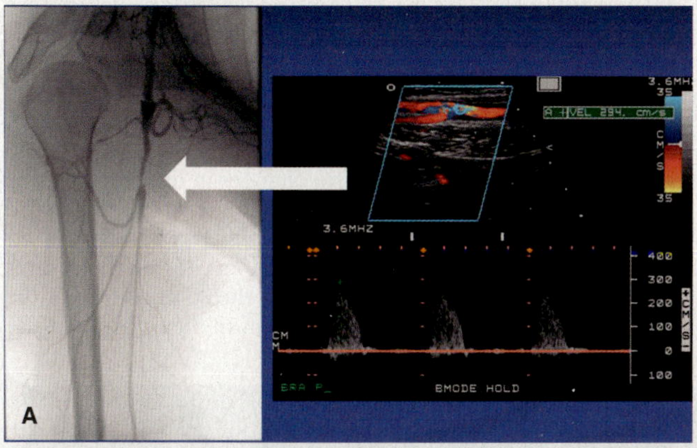

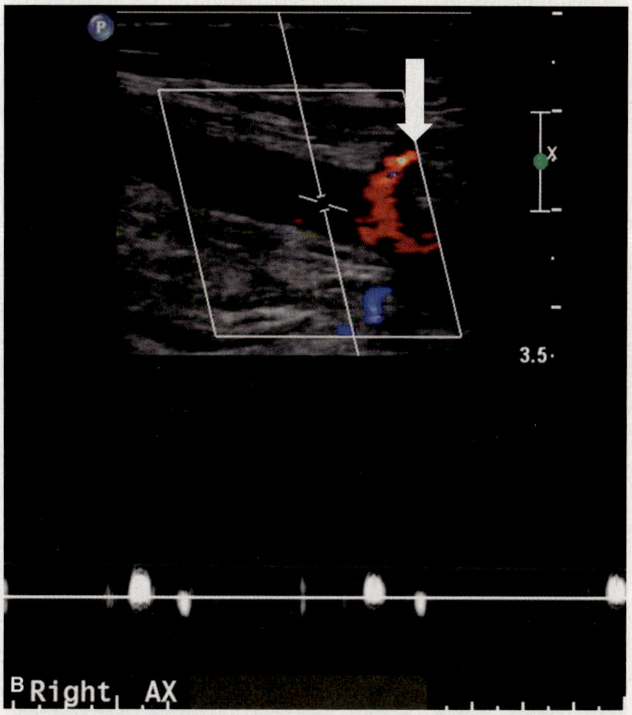

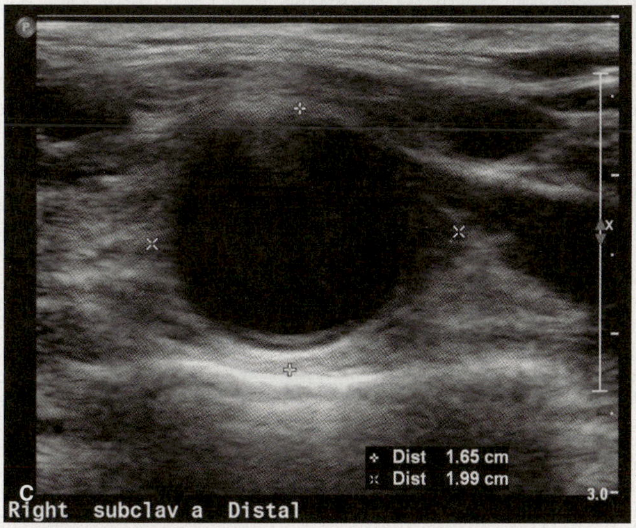

Figure 82.18. **A:** Duplex color-flow image and velocity waveform with corresponding angiogram in a patient with brachial artery stenosis (*arrow*) and symptomatic arm ischemia secondary to a crutch injury. Note the loss of the end-systolic reverse-flow component of the arterial waveform. **B:** Duplex image of a right axillary artery occlusion secondary to embolism. Note the occlusive waveform and reconstitution of the artery via a distal branch vessel (*arrow*). **C:** Grayscale image of a small subclavian artery aneurysm.

Table 82.6. Duplex Ultrasound Criteria for Evaluation of Upper Extremity Arterial Stenosis

Condition	Characteristics
Normal	Uniform waveforms; biphasic or triphasic waveforms; clear window beneath systolic peak
<50% diameter reduction	Focal velocity increase; spectral broadening; possibly triphasic or biphasic flow
>50% diameter reduction	Focal velocity increase; loss of triphasic or biphasic velocity waveform; poststenotic flow (color bruit)
Occlusion	No flow detected

look for mural thrombi and valvular lesions. While duplex scanning alone cannot be used to make the diagnosis of Takayasu arteritis, it can be a helpful adjunct in following the progression or regression of arterial involvement in response to treatment.[61]

VISCERAL ARTERIES

Mesenteric Arteries

Duplex ultrasonography can serve as a valuable noninvasive screening test for splanchnic artery stenosis in patients with possible chronic mesenteric ischemia and for follow-up of mesenteric artery reconstructions. Aneurysms and dissections of the visceral arteries can also be identified (**Fig. 82.19**). Despite the accuracy of duplex detection of mesenteric artery stenosis, angiographic confirmation of high-grade stenosis or occlusion of the splanchnic vessels, and appropriate history and physical examination are still required for the diagnosis of chronic mesenteric ischemia. The examination is technically difficult and is best performed by vascular technologists with extensive experience in intra-abdominal ultrasound techniques.

Interpretation of Mesenteric Duplex Ultrasound Studies

In healthy individuals, fasting arterial waveforms differ in the superior mesenteric artery (SMA) versus the CA. The arterial waveforms reflect end-organ vascular resistance. The liver and spleen have relatively high constant metabolic requirements and are therefore low-resistance organs. As a result, CA waveforms are generally biphasic, with a peak systolic component, no reversal of end-systolic flow, and a relatively high EDV. The normal fasting SMA velocity waveform is triphasic, reflecting the high vascular resistance of the intestinal tract at rest. There is a peak systolic component, often an end-systolic reverse-flow component, and a minimal diastolic flow component (**Fig. 82.20A**).[62]

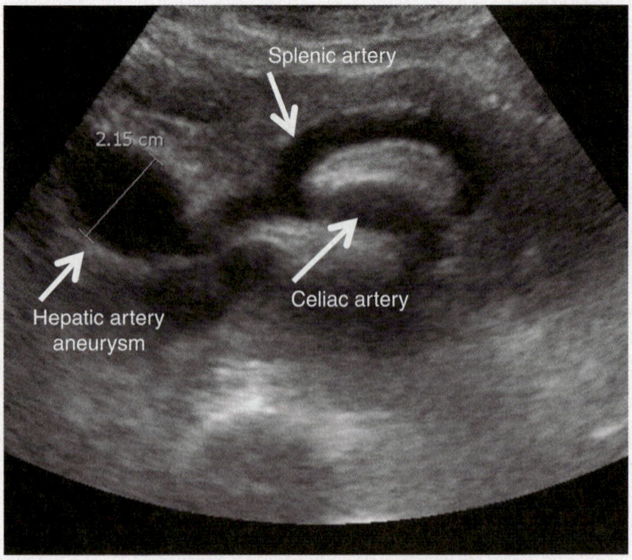

Figure 82.19. Grayscale image of a 2.15-cm hepatic artery aneurysm.

Changes in Doppler-derived arterial waveforms in response to feeding are also different in the CA and SMA. Because the liver and spleen have basically fixed metabolic demands, there is no significant change in CA velocity waveform after eating. Blood flow in the SMA, however, increases markedly after a meal, reflecting a marked decrease in intestinal arterial resistance. The postprandial waveform changes in the SMA include a near doubling of systolic velocity, tripling of the EDV, and loss of end-systolic reversal of blood flow (**Fig. 82.20B**).[63]

Postprandial changes are maximal at 45 minutes after ingestion of a test meal and depend on the composition of the meal ingested. Mixed nutrient composition meals produce the

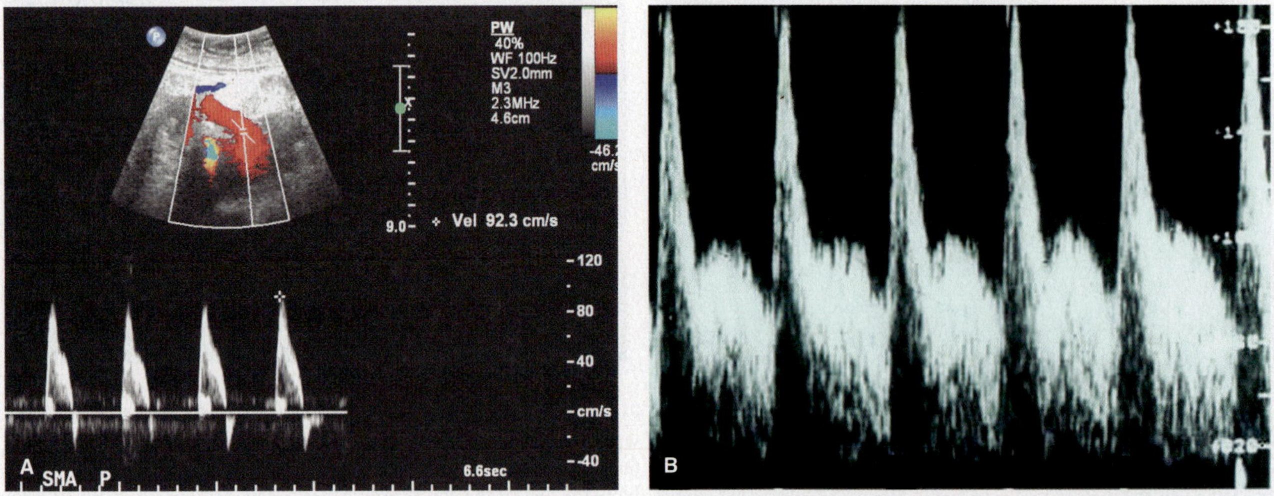

Figure 82.20. **A:** A normal fasting superior mesenteric artery (SMA) waveform may exhibit reverse flow at the end of systole and relatively low end-diastolic velocity (EDV) reflecting relatively high resistance of the intestinal circulation in the fasting state. **B:** Postprandial SMA waveform. There has been, in comparison to **A**, loss of end-systolic reverse flow and an increase in end-diastolic flow as resistance in the intestinal arterial circulation falls following feeding.

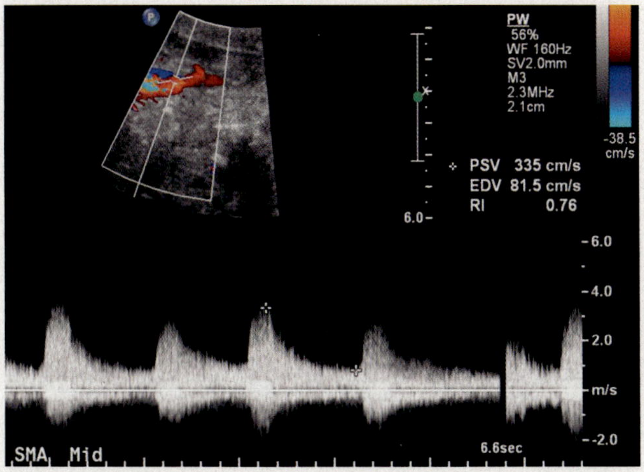

Figure 82.21. Color-flow image and duplex-derived SMA waveform in a patient with possible chronic mesenteric ischemia. A peak systolic velocity of >330 cm/s indicates a high-grade SMA stenosis and is compatible with a clinical picture of chronic mesenteric ischemia.

greatest flow increase in the SMA when compared with equal caloric meals composed solely of fat, glucose, or protein.[64]

Detection of Mesenteric Arterial Stenosis

8 Duplex ultrasound can detect hemodynamically significant stenosis in splanchnic vessels. In a blinded prospective study of 100 patients who underwent mesenteric artery duplex scanning and lateral aortography, a PSV in the SMA of 275 cm/s or more indicated a ≥70% SMA stenosis with a sensitivity of 92%, a specificity of 96%, a positive predictive value of 80%, a negative predictive value of 99%, and an accuracy of 96% (**Fig. 82.21**). In the same study, a PSV of ≥200 cm/s identified a ≥70% angiographic celiac artery stenosis with a sensitivity of 87%, a specificity of 80%, a positive predictive value of 63%, a negative predictive value of 94%, and an accuracy of 82%.[65]

Other duplex criteria for mesenteric artery stenosis are also in use. An SMA EDV greater than 45 cm/s correlates with a ≥50% SMA stenosis with a specificity of 92% and a sensitivity of 100%, whereas a CA EDV of 55 cm/s or greater predicts a ≥50% CA stenosis with a sensitivity of 93%, specificity of 100%, and accuracy of 95%.[66]

Surgical revascularization of the mesenteric arteries is a standard treatment for chronic mesenteric ischemia. Most often bypass grafts are constructed to the superior mesenteric and/or celiac arteries. Mesenteric artery bypass grafts can be followed postoperatively with mesenteric artery duplex scanning. Flow velocities within mesenteric artery bypass grafts vary little with the origin of the graft (supraceliac or infrarenal aorta or a common iliac artery) and remain stable over time. Serially increasing velocities over time in a mesenteric bypass likely suggest the development of a graft or anastomotic stenosis.[67]

Placement of an intraluminal stent is a viable alternative in many cases to surgical bypass, for the treatment of mesenteric artery stenosis. Similar to the carotid artery, there is reason to suspect duplex criteria developed for stenosis in native mesenteric arteries may not be applicable without modification to stented superior mesenteric arteries. Mesenteric duplex scans pre- and postplacement of an SMA stent have been compared and correlated with pressure gradients measured at the time of angiography. The data indicate that SMA stenting provides good anatomic results and significantly reduces angiographically measured pressure gradients. Duplex measured SMA PSVs are reduced post stent placement but, despite good angiographic results, remain in most cases above criteria predicting high-grade native artery SMA stenosis.[68]

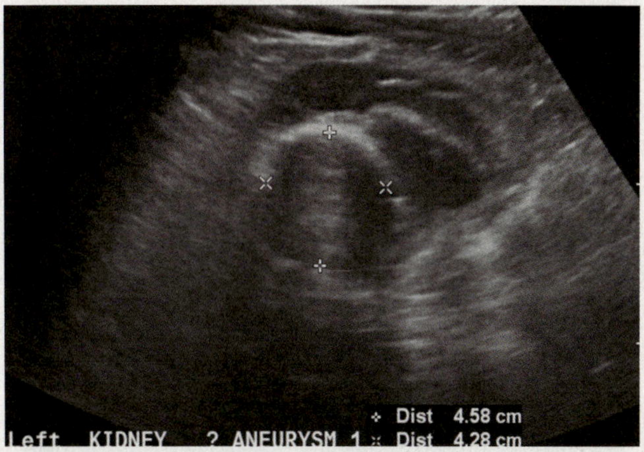

Figure 82.22. Grayscale image of a large renal artery aneurysm in the hilum of the kidney.

RENAL ARTERIES

Duplex scanning of the renal arteries is useful in evaluating for renal artery stenosis in patients with possible renal vascular hypertension and can also be used to detect renal artery aneurysms (**Fig. 82.22**), as well as provide a measure of the health of the renal parenchyma.

Indirect Assessment of Renal Artery Stenosis

Indirect methods to assess renal artery stenosis evaluate interlobar arteries. Decreased acceleration times and/or presence of tardus/parvus waveforms (waveforms with delayed or slowed upstrokes) may suggest the presence of a main renal artery stenosis. These techniques are quicker and easier to perform than direct examination of the main renal artery but have been not widely validated. Improved visualization of main renal arteries with modern duplex scanners has made indirect methods of assessing the main renal artery essentially obsolete. These techniques are even less accurate in patients with bilateral stenosis and are not applicable in patients with a single patent renal artery.

Direct Assessment of Renal Artery Stenosis

Normal renal arteries have a PSV less than 180 cm/s and low-resistance waveforms reflecting the high metabolic demands of the kidney. A ratio of the PSV in the renal artery to that in the aorta (renal–aortic ratio, RAR) of ≥3.5 indicates a ≥60% diameter-reducing renal artery stenosis (84% to 88% sensitivity, 97% to 99% specificity, 94% to 98% positive predictive value) (**Fig. 82.23**).[69] A PSV of ≥200 cm/s has also been suggested to

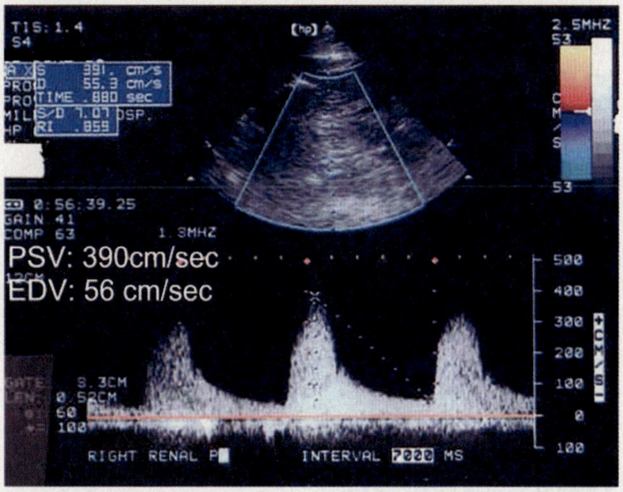

Figure 82.23. Renal artery waveform in a patient with severe hypertension. The high peak systolic velocity is compatible with a high-grade renal artery stenosis.

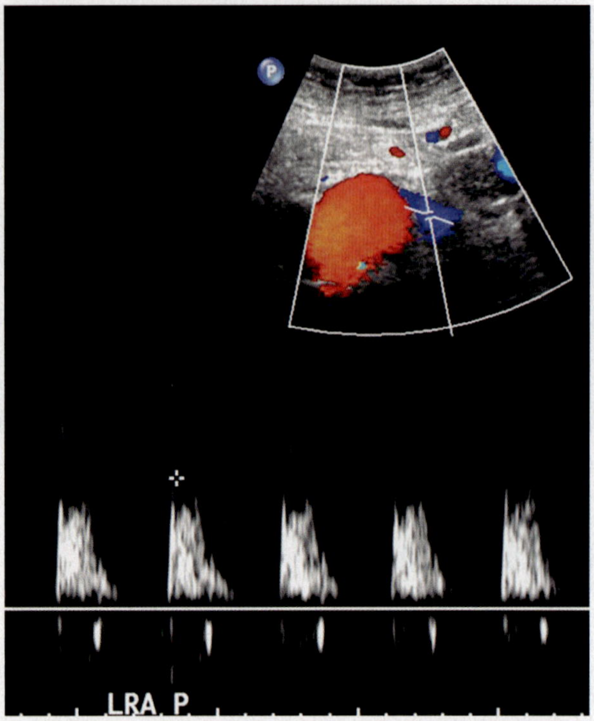

Figure 82.24. The absence of end-diastolic flow in the left renal artery indicates severe parenchymal disease of the left kidney.

indicate a ≥60% renal artery stenosis whereas a velocity in the renal artery of >185 cm/s has been suggested to indicate a less than 60% renal artery stenosis. Therefore a renal artery can be considered normal when PSV is <180 cm/s and the RAR is <3.5. With a PSV >180 cm/s and an RAR <3.5, the renal artery can be considered to have a <60% stenosis. RARs of >3.5 indicate >60% renal artery stenosis regardless if the renal artery PSV is less than or more than 180 cm/s.[70] When the EDV exceeds 150 cm/s, data suggest a >80% renal artery stenosis.[71] The same criteria have been used to evaluate the patency of renal arterial reconstructions, but similar to stented carotid and mesenteric arteries may need modification for stented renal arteries.[72]

Predicting Success of Renal Artery Interventions

EDVs tend to be lower in patients with renal insufficiency, indicating decreased diastolic flow and suggesting increased parenchymal resistance to blood flow. Decreased parenchymal diastolic velocities may therefore suggest renal parenchymal disease (**Fig. 82.24**). Many patients, 20% to 40%, treated with renal artery angioplasty and stenting or open surgical reconstructions do not have postprocedure blood pressure or renal function improvement. An estimate of resistance to flow within the renal parenchyma can be made by comparisons of EDV and PSVs of renal artery waveforms obtained from renal parenchymal arteries. The so-called resistive index (RI) is calculated as follows:

$$RI = [1 - (EDV/PSV)] \times 100 \qquad (82.3)$$

In effect a high RI, >0.7 is bad, suggesting renal parenchymal disease whereas a low RI is good, indicating healthy renal parenchymal tissues. Evaluation of parenchymal resistance has been suggested as a possible preprocedure predictor of clinical success of renal artery interventions.[73] Abnormal parenchymal resistance may also be a marker of renal allograft dysfunction or rejection (**Fig. 82.25**).

VENOUS DISEASE

Acute Deep Venous Thrombosis

Physical examination is not sensitive or specific for the detection of acute deep venous thrombosis (DVT).[74] Prior to the

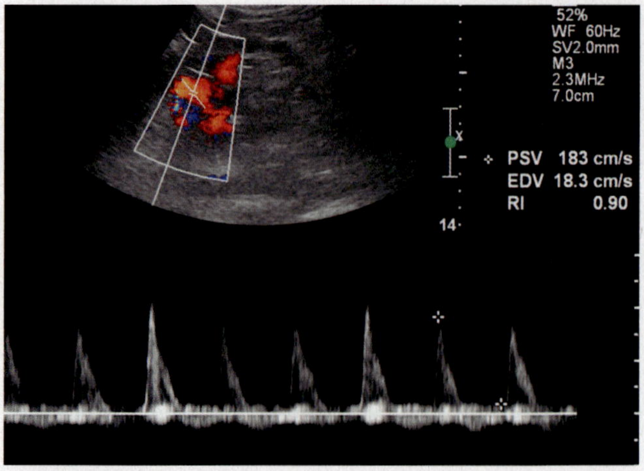

Figure 82.25. There is very little diastolic flow in the renal artery of the transplanted kidney consistent with rejection or primary allograft dysfunction.

acceptance and widespread use of venous duplex scanning, impedance plethysmography (IPG) was employed as the initial noninvasive test for patients with suspected acute lower extremity DVT. IPG is a reasonably sensitive (87%) and specific (up to 100%) test for proximal (above-knee) lower extremity DVT in symptomatic patients.[75–77] However, lower sensitivities for proximal DVT (65%) have been reported in studies that exclude clinical outcomes and only report in comparison to venography. IPG may not detect nonocclusive proximal DVT, occlusive proximal DVT present in parallel venous systems, such as duplicated femoral or popliteal veins, and cannot detect DVT isolated to the calf veins.[78,79] While IPG is still sometimes used for clinical situations felt to require serial evaluations of the proximal veins, the limitations noted above make it a substandard examination for routine clinical assessment of lower extremity DVT.[80] Currently, color-flow duplex scanning performed by skilled operators provides the most practical and cost-effective method for assessment of DVT of the lower and upper extremity veins as well as for detection of thrombosis in superficial veins.

At a minimum, vascular laboratory duplex ultrasound evaluation for lower extremity DVT should include examination of the common femoral, profunda femoris, femoral, and popliteal veins. Venous waveforms from the right and left common femoral veins should always be compared. A normal lower extremity examination will show patency of the veins on color-flow imaging, collapsing of the veins with application of pressure by the ultrasound probe, and venous flow patterns in the common femoral and femoral veins that decrease with inspiration and increase with expiration. Flow within a patent vein should also increase with application of compression distal to the site of examination (**Fig. 82.26**).

9 The primary ultrasound diagnostic criteria for diagnosis of venous thrombosis is failure of the vein to collapse with application of pressure with the ultrasound probe (**Fig. 82.27A,B**). A continuous flow pattern in one common femoral vein and not the other suggests ipsilateral iliac vein thrombosis or external compression of the ipsilateral iliac vein. Bilateral pulsatile common femoral waveforms suggest volume overload, tricuspid regurgitation, or heart failure. Clot aging is useful for patient management. Relative value of duplex findings for thrombus aging was utilized at Good Samaritan Hospital, Cincinnati, OH. Dr. John J Cranley, correlated duplex scans and venograms (**Table 82.7**). The vascular laboratory also used zones to report locations on the extremity of pathology and findings to facilitate comparisons of sequential scans. The extremity is divided into zones using the following landmarks. Zone 1 is defined as the intersection of the femoral vessels with the inguinal ligament. Zone 5 is an imaginary line passing from midpatella to the popliteal crease. Zone 8 corresponds to

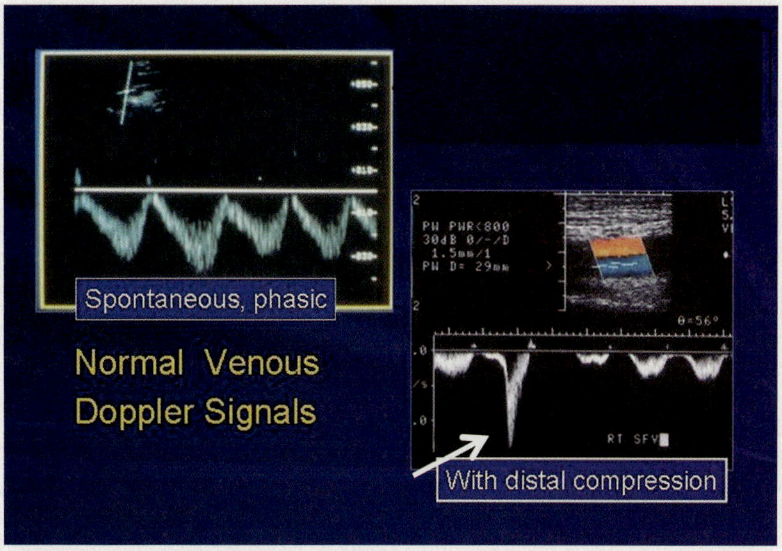

Figure 82.26. Venous flow is typically depicted below the baseline. Venous flow in the proximal lower extremity veins should be spontaneous, vary with respiration, and augment with distal compression.

a line from midmedial malleolus to the midlateral malleolus. Zone 9 corresponds to the tips of the toes. Using the above landmarks the thigh and calf are subdivided into four and three equal zones respectively (**Fig. 82.28**). The upper extremities are divided into a similar set of zones (**Fig. 82.29**).[81]

The treatment of superficial venous thrombosis (SVT) has changed. Vascular laboratory reports of SVT should now include the site and length of the thrombosis. The distance to the junction with the deep system should also be included. These are now all used to determine clinical management. SVT associated with DVT should also be documented.

Not all venous ultrasound examinations for DVT are the same. Some vascular laboratories do not include evaluation of the calf veins as part of their routine evaluation for lower extremity DVT, even in symptomatic patients. This results from outdated perceptions of inaccuracy of calf vein ultrasound evaluation for DVT. Failure to perform a complete initial examination necessitates serial ultrasound examinations or alternative strategies to detect possible extension of venous thrombi initially isolated to the calf veins. Such strategies are inefficient, ineffective for noncompliant patients, and not cost-effective compared to a single stand-alone color-flow duplex study of the proximal and calf veins in patients with suspected lower extremity DVT.

Limited ultrasound studies for acute DVT may include compression ultrasound (B-mode imaging only), duplex ultrasound (B-mode imaging and Doppler waveform analysis), and color Doppler alone. The sensitivities and specificities for detecting acute DVT differ among the examinations, and different examinations are appropriate for different veins. Compression ultrasound is typically performed for evaluation of proximal deep veins, specifically the common femoral, femoral, and popliteal veins. A combination of duplex ultrasound and color Doppler is more often used for calf and iliac veins. Color flow alone may be used to assess patency of the calf veins as they are difficult to reliably compress in subjects with larger legs.

Many factors will influence which venous segments can be evaluated in an individual examination. These include the

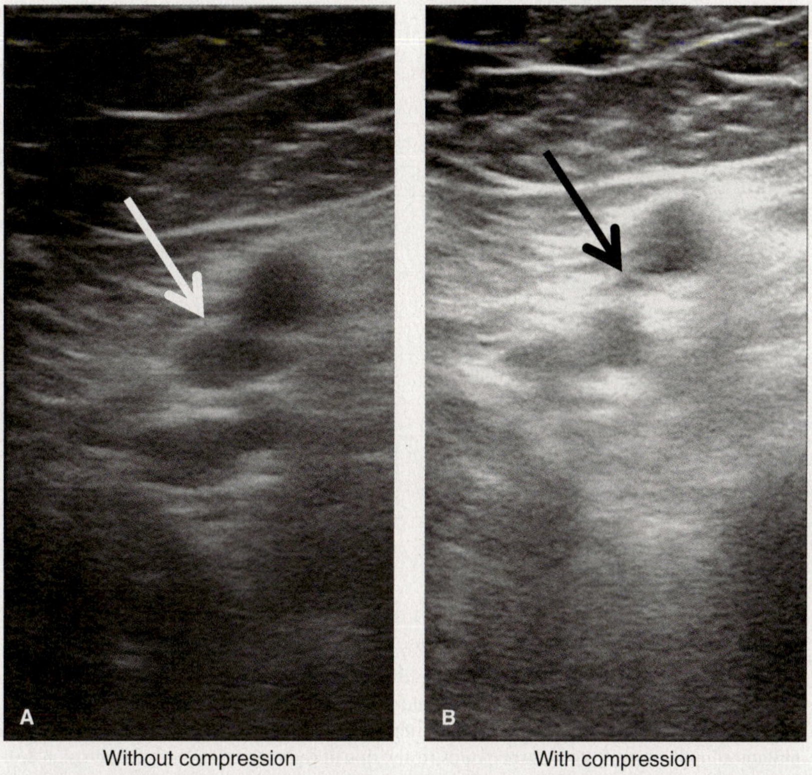

Figure 82.27. **A:** Without compression with the ultrasound probe the femoral vein is easily visible (*white arrow*). **B:** With compression the vein collapses and is no longer visible (*black arrow*). Failure of the vein to collapse with probe pressure would indicate the presence of thrombus within the vein.

Table 82.7. Clot Characteristics: Relative Value in Clot Aging

Characteristic	Acute Value		Chronic Value	
Degree of occlusion	Total	**	Partial	**
Free-floating	Free	****	Stationary	**
Clot retraction	Retracted	***	Adherent	***
Clot distention	Distended	***	Contracted	**
Clot compressibility	Soft	****	Firm	*
Surface character	Smooth	**	Irregular	**
Echogenicity	Faint	*	Bright	*
Homogeneity	Homogeneous	**	Heterogeneous	**
Collaterals	Absent	*	Present	****
Recanalization	Absent	*	Present	****

Four asterisks indicate a diagnostic level; three asterisks good, two asterisks fair, and one asterisk poor (nondiagnostic). Each asterisk indicates the relative value to be given to each criterion in interpretation of clot age, many criteria are only valuable when present and the overall decision represents a weighted average.

presence of morbid obesity, lower extremity edema or tenderness, or the presence of immobilization devices and bandages. Overall, a complete color and Doppler examination has become the standard of care for assessment of lower extremity DVT. It is recommended that whenever possible, a venous duplex examination to exclude the presence of DVT consist of an evaluation of both the proximal and calf veins.

A well-trained technologist can interrogate calf veins in 80% to 98% of cases using a combination of B-mode, Doppler waveform analysis, and color Doppler.[82,83] Overall accuracy of venous ultrasonography in comparison to venography has been well established. The weighted mean sensitivity and specificity of venous ultrasonography (including all types) for the diagnosis of symptomatic proximal DVT are 97% and 94%, respectively.[80] As suggested above, in technically adequate studies, the sensitivity and specificity of color Doppler to identify isolated calf vein thrombosis exceeds 90%.[83] The high specificity of venous ultrasonography allows treatment for DVT to be initiated without further confirmatory tests, and the high sensitivity in diagnosing proximal DVT makes it possible to withhold treatment if the examination is negative.

Some ultrasound examinations are limited by practical constraints. Inability of the patient to fully cooperate with regard to positioning for the examination and/or intolerance of the pressure of the ultrasound scan head on the skin, or inability of the examiner to obtain a complete examination secondary to bandages, casts, or extremity wounds, may lead to a requirement for serial examinations. An alternative diagnostic procedure, such as catheter-based contrast, MR, or CT venography

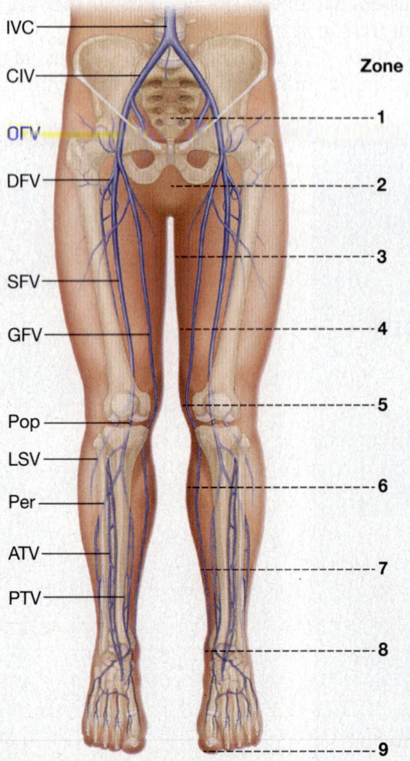

Figure 82.28. Lower extremity zones. Zone 1 is defined as the intersection of the femoral vessels with the inguinal ligament. Zone 5 is an imaginary line passing from the midpatella to the popliteal crease. Zone 8 corresponds to a line from midmedial malleolus to the midlateral malleolus. Zone 9 corresponds to the tips of the toes.

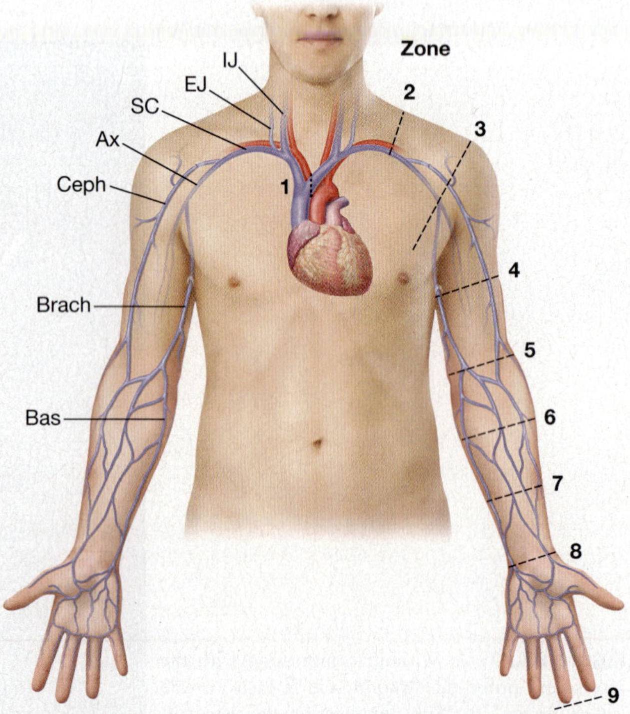

Figure 82.29. Upper extremity zones. Zones of reference for upper extremity venous scanning; midline = 1.0, acromion = 3.0, elbow = 5.0, wrist = 8.0, and fingertips = 9.0.

may be indicated when a complete ultrasound examination is not possible or if the patient cannot or is unlikely to return for a follow-up examination. Currently, repeat or serial venous ultrasound examinations are advisable in follow-up for a limited negative examination in symptomatic patients highly suspicious for DVT in whom an alternative form of imaging is unavailable or contraindicated.

The diagnosis of pulmonary embolism (PE), like that for DVT, also cannot be established without objective testing. Several studies have evaluated lower extremity venous ultrasound examinations in patients suspected of PE. These studies, often employing ultrasound of only the proximal veins and nuclear medicine-based ventilation perfusion (V/Q) scanning, unfortunately have little relevance to modern practice where complete proximal and distal vein ultrasound examinations are usually routine, and where CT pulmonary angiography (CTPA) or MR pulmonary angiography (MRPA) have largely supplanted V/Q scanning.

The rationale for venous ultrasonography in patients who present with symptoms of PE is that a diagnosis of DVT may indirectly suggest a diagnosis of PE, making additional investigation to exclude PE unnecessary in some clinical settings. However, ultrasound cannot make a definitive diagnosis of PE. Patients can have DVT and pulmonary symptoms or hemodynamic instability from causes other than PE.

10 Bedside duplex of the inferior vena cava may be used to place IVC filters. Intravascular ultrasound when available is also useful. These techniques can avoid transfer to radiology in unstable patients, eliminate the need for contrast and radiation exposure for selected patients.

Normal bilateral proximal venous ultrasound scans do not rule out PE. When PE is definitively present, DVT of the proximal lower extremity veins is detectable by compression ultrasound in only 50% of patients.[84] When a PE is objectively diagnosed with no evidence of lower extremity DVT, the PE may have originated from pelvic veins, arm veins, or possibly embolized completely from a lower extremity vein. An objective diagnostic test for PE is therefore indicated in most cases. Currently, in most centers this would be a CT pulmonary angiogram.

Chronic Venous Insufficiency

The presence of venous insufficiency can also be evaluated with either air or PPG and with duplex scanning.[85] In theory, APG can provide an analysis of overall venous hemodynamics including evaluation of the individual components of venous function; reflux and the efficacy of the calf muscle pump. A flexible chamber is placed on the calf and volume changes then induced by a series of positional and exercise maneuvers. Measurements derived from these maneuvers are then used to calculate measures of venous reflux (venous filling index [VFI]), calf muscle pump function (ejection fraction [EF]) as well as a measure of overall venous function termed the residual volume

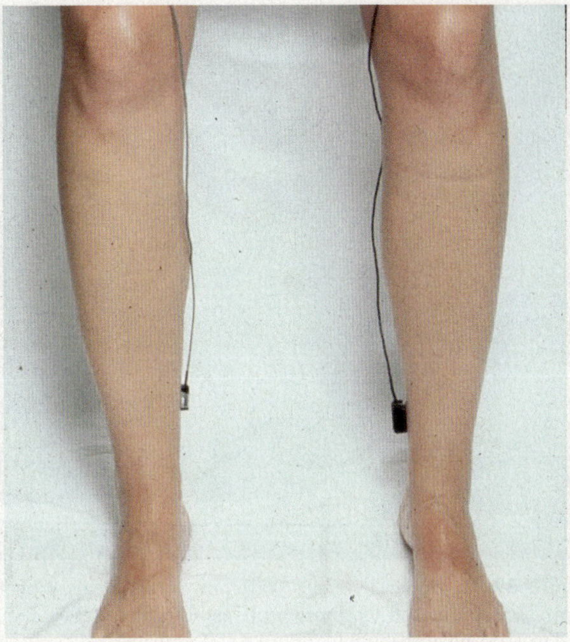

Figure 82.30. Placement of PPG probes for assessment of venous reflux.

fraction. Of these values VFI has the potential for being the most important. A VFI of >2 mL/s indicates abnormal reflux with values >10 mL/s indicating increased risk of cutaneous changes associated with chronic venous insufficiency (CVI). APG, however, while theoretically interesting, is used only infrequently in clinical practice.

PPG is a variant of plethysmography techniques to assess venous reflux. It detects changes in the blood content of the skin that theoretically reflect venous volume. It consists of a light emitting diode and a photo sensor. The diode transmits light into subcutaneous tissues. Blood attenuates light in proportion to its content in tissue. The PPG machine amplifies the difference between the transmitted and reflected signal and converts it into a waveform. To assess for venous reflux the sensor is typically applied to the medial ankle area (**Fig. 82.30**). The patient performs a series of plantar and dorsal flexion maneuvers of the foot decreasing the venous volume of the extremity. The time for the waveform to return to baseline is termed the venous recovery time (VRT). A normal PPG VRT is 20 seconds or greater. Shorter times indicate the presence of venous reflux. If the VRT returns to normal with the application of a superficial venous tourniquet then the reflux is confined to the superficial venous system (**Fig. 82.31**). If the VRT does not correct with a superficial venous tourniquet deep venous reflux is present. Neither, APG or PPG can

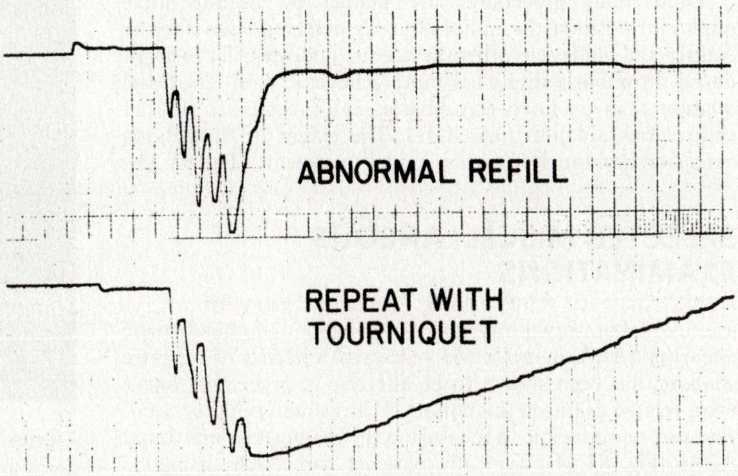

Figure 82.31. Venous PPG waveforms in a patient with superficial venous reflux. The patient is asked to perform 10 dorsal and plantar flexions of the ankle resulting in emptying the leg of venous blood. In the **top panel** the veins refill very rapidly indicating the presence of venous reflux. Refill slows with application of a tourniquet to occlude the superficial veins indicating this patient likely has only reflux in the superficial venous system and no deep venous reflux.

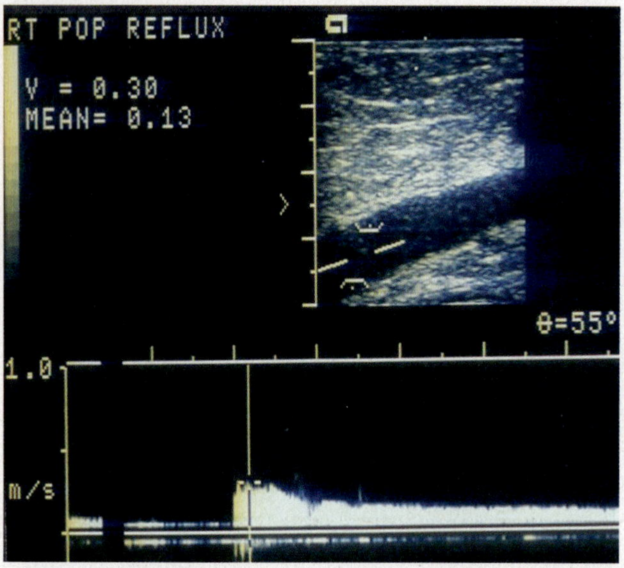

Figure 82.32. Popliteal venous waveform with cuff deflation for duplex assessment and localization of venous reflux. Reflux lasting >0.5 to 1 second is abnormal.

provide information about the specific venous segments that are abnormal. That information can be provided by duplex ultrasound.

Duplex ultrasound can provide important physiologic and anatomic information in patients with possible CVI. Both sites of reflux and of venous obstruction can be determined in deep, superficial, and perforating veins. In patients with valve incompetence, reflux can be stimulated and then detected with duplex using a Valsalva maneuver, manual compression proximal to the transducer, or release of compression distal to the transducer. The examination has been standardized with the patient upright and using deflation of a series of pneumatic cuffs at specific sites on the leg with the leg under examina-
11 tion[10] not bearing weight. In the upright position, reflux stimulated by cuff deflation that lasts more than 0.5 second is indicative of pathologic reflux.[86] The technique allows localization of reflux to specific venous segments and can serve as a valuable preoperative planning tool to target specific venous segments for removal or reconstruction (**Fig. 82.32**). It has a sensitivity of 82% and specificity of 100% for the identification of competent and incompetent perforating veins. Duplex determination of reflux sites and sites of venous occlusion as a means of assessing overall venous hemodynamics is not established. Currently duplex assessment of venous reflux provides the basis of planning for the large majority of venous procedures designed to treat the manifestations of superficial venous reflux.

Endovenous procedures are guided by intraoperative duplex to position the radiofrequency catheter, laser fiber or control and guide sclerotherapy agents. Endovascular heat-induced thrombosis (EHIT) is more echogenic with less vessel dilation than de novo thrombosis. EHIT occurs in 1% of endovenous ablation procedures. The extent of thrombosis extension into the deep system guides treatment[87] (**Fig. 82.33**).

SELECTED MISCELLANEOUS EXAMINATIONS

Evaluation for Abdominal Aortic Aneurysm

Vascular laboratory ultrasound screening for abdominal aortic aneurysm (AAA) in males >65 years with a history of cigarette smoking has been shown to be effective in preventing aneurysm-related deaths in this cohort.[88] Ultrasound is highly accurate and reproducible in measuring the diameter of infrarenal AAAs (**Fig. 82.34**). Typically patients with AAA diameters

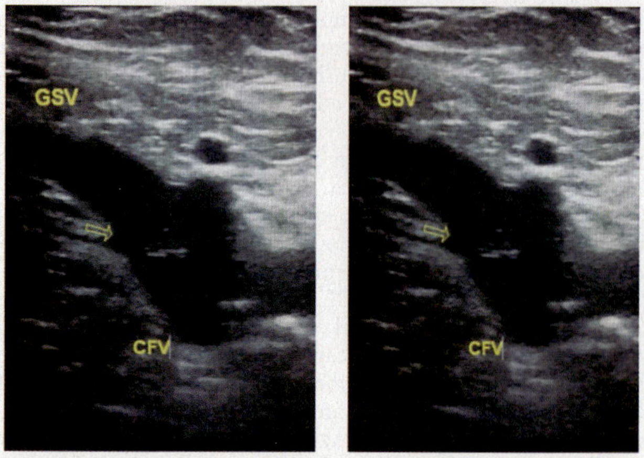

Figure 82.33. Endovascular heat-induced thrombosis (EHIT), *arrow*, extending into common femoral vein (CFV).

below accepted threshold levels for repair are followed with serial ultrasound examinations to monitor for enlargement of the aneurysm to a diameter where repair is indicated.

Evaluation of Aortic Endografts

Placement of endoluminal stent grafts is now standard therapy for most patients with AAA. With stent grafting of an AAA the aneurysm is left in situ and blood flow diverted through the stent graft. Some stent grafts eventually leak at proximal or distal attachment sites. AAAs with these so-called type I endoleaks are at increased risk of rupture. In addition, AAAs treated with stent grafts may also occasionally enlarge because of back pressure in the aneurysm sac from patent lumbar vessels; type II endoleak. Patients whose AAAs enlarge in association with type II endoleaks after endografting are also considered at risk for aneurysm rupture.

Standard monitoring of endoluminal stent grafts is with serial CT scans to detect endoleak and changing aneurysm sac diameter. However, there are increasing concerns about repeated doses of contrast and radiation exposure associated with serial CT scans. It now appears many stent grafts can be followed with serial duplex ultrasound examinations. Duplex ultrasound is capable of measuring sac diameter (**Fig. 82.35**) and detecting both type I and II endoleaks. Even if an endoleak cannot be detected by ultrasound an increase in sac diameter following stent grafting should prompt further investigation. In some centers duplex ultrasound has replaced CT scanning as the preferred method of follow-up of AAA stent grafts.[89,90]

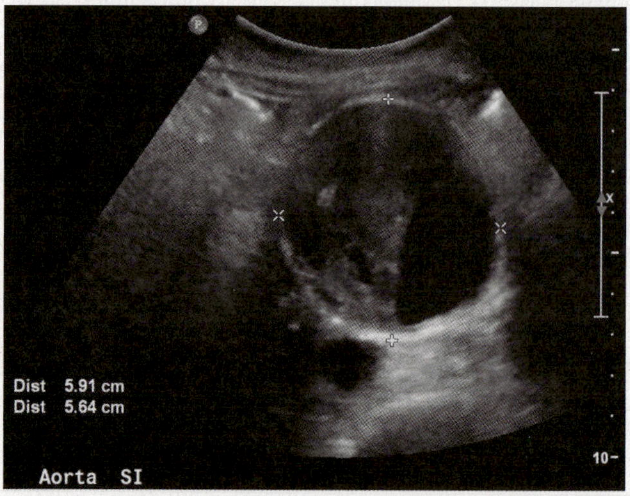

Figure 82.34. Ultrasound image of a 5.9-cm infrarenal abdominal aortic aneurysm (AAA) with acentric intraluminal thrombus.

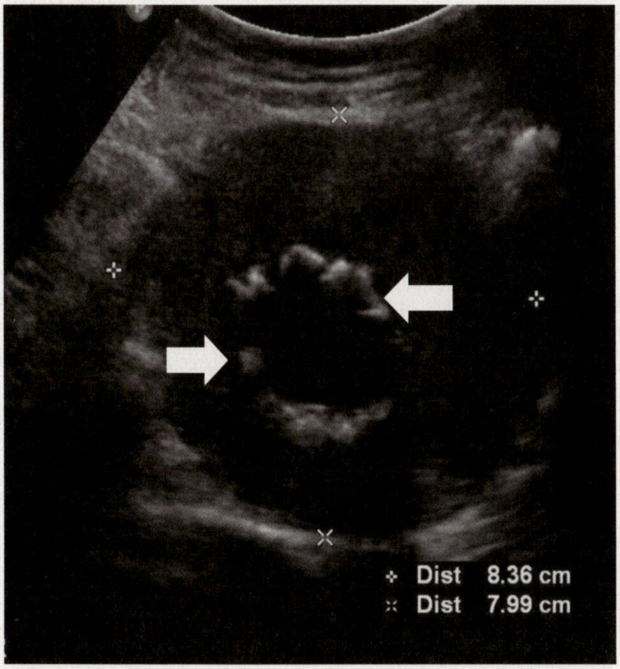

Figure 82.35. Ultrasound examination of an aortic stent graft. The aortic stent graft (*arrows*) is visible within the lumen of the residual aneurysm sac measuring 8.36 cm × 7.99 cm.

Contrast-Enhanced Ultrasonography

Ultrasonography (US) is the first-line modality for the evaluation of vascular pathology. The value of US has been improved by the introduction of micro bubbles as ultrasonographic contrast agents (UCAs) and the emergence of contrast-enhanced ultrasonography (CEUS). CEUS offers valuable information about vascular disease, both on a macrovascular and microvascular level. Well established applications exist for carotid disease, postinterventional follow-up of AAAs, and for assessment of portal vein thrombosis.[91]

Evaluation and Treatment of Groin Pseudoaneurysms

Pseudoaneurysms can occur as a complication of an arterial puncture in the groin performed for diagnostic or therapeutic angiography. Groin pseudoaneurysms are readily detected with duplex ultrasound (**Fig. 82.36**). Color flow demonstrates a typical collection of flowing blood usually anterior to the artery from which the psuedoaneurysm originates. The native

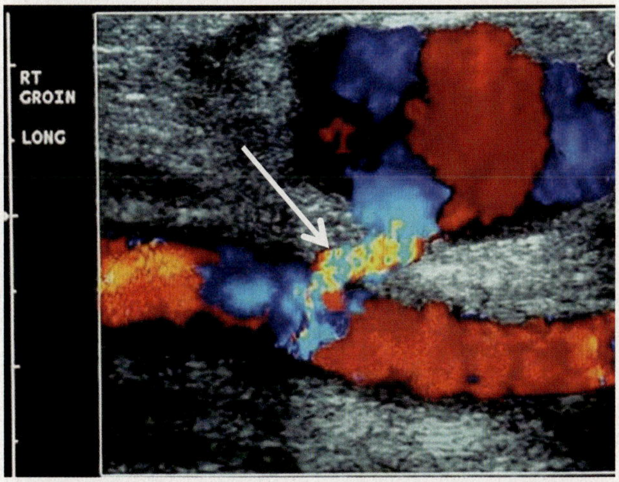

Figure 82.36. A pseudoaneurysm of the superficial femoral artery following arterial cannulation. The so-called neck of the aneurysm (*arrow*) is readily visible.

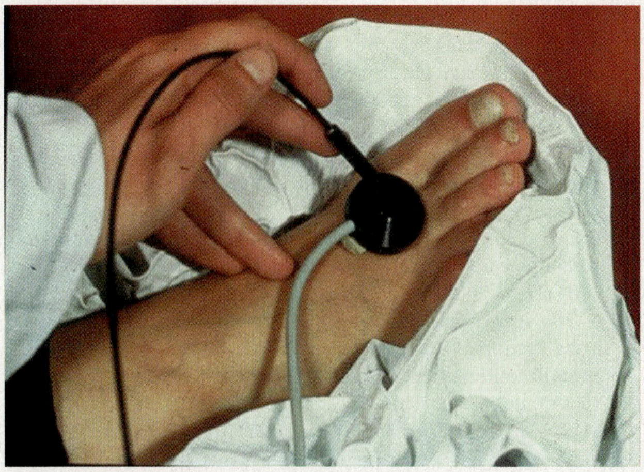

Figure 82.37. A transcutaneous oxygen probe. $TCpO_2$ measurements can serve as an aid in determining healing potential of pedal wounds or ulcers.

artery and the pseudoaneurysm are connected by a so-called "neck." To-and-fro flow within the neck of the pseudoaneurysm is characteristic and pathognomonic of a pseudoaneurysm arising from an arterial puncture.

Treatment of pseudoaneurysms may be with direct surgical repair or, utilizing the vascular laboratory, direct compression of the pseudoaneurysm until it clots using the ultrasound scan head to both locate the pseudoaneurysm and apply pressure. Alternatively, the pseudoaneurysm is visualized with the ultrasound scan head and a needle introduced into the body of the pseudoaneurysm for injection of small amounts of thrombin to induce thrombosis of the pseudoaneurysm.[92] All techniques are effective but currently direct thrombin injection is favored in most cases as it is relatively noninvasive, more rapid, less painful, and more effective than prolonged compression alone.[93,94]

Transcutaneous Oxygen Measurements

Measurements of transcutaneous oxygen ($TCpO_2$) can be performed as an aid in predicting healing of pedal lesions or healing of an amputation at the site where the measurement is taken (**Fig. 82.37**). In general, a $TCpO_2$ >30 mm Hg indicates healing is likely, measurements between 20 and 30 mm Hg are equivocal for healing and measurements below 20 mm Hg indicate healing is unlikely.[95] Measurements are not influenced by the presence of diabetes but it has been suggested the level for predicting healing be increased to 40 mm Hg in patients with diabetes. The test is less accurate in the presence of edema, cellulitis, hyperkeratosis, and in older patients.

ACKNOWLEDGMENT

We gratefully acknowledge the contributions of previous edition author, Gregory L. Moneta, as portions of those chapters have been retained in this revision.

References

1. Roederer GO, Langlois YE, Chan AT, et al. Ultrasonic duplex scanning of the extracranial carotid arteries: improved accuracy using new features from the carotid artery. *J Cardiovasc Ultrasonography.* 1982;1:373–380.
2. Abou-ZamZam AM Jr, Moneta GL, Edwards JM, Yeager RA, Taylor LM Jr, Porter JM. Is a single preoperative duplex scan sufficient for planning bilateral carotid endarterectomy? *J Vasc Surg.* 2000;31(2):282–288.
3. Strandness DE Jr. *Duplex Scanning in Vascular Disorders*. Raven Press; 1990:92–120.
4. Roederer GO, Langlois YE, Jager KA, et al. A simple spectral parameter for accurate classification of severe carotid artery disease. *Bruit.* 1989;3:174–178.

5. Moneta GL, Edwards JM, Chitwood RW, et al. Correlation of North American Symptomatic Carotid Endarterectomy Trial (NASCET): angiographic definition of 70% to 90% internal carotid artery stenosis with duplex scanning. *J Vasc Surg.* 1993;17(1):152–157; discussion 157–159.
6. Bendick PJ, Glover JL. Hemodynamic evaluation of the vertebral arteries by duplex ultrasound. *Surg Clin North Am.* 1990;70(1): 235–244.
7. Kumar SM, Wang JC, Barry MC, et al. Carotid stump syndrome: outcome from surgical management. *Eur J Vasc Endovasc Surg.* 2001;21(3):214–219.
8. North American Symptomatic Carotid Endarterectomy Trial Collaborators: NASCET; Barnett HJM, Taylor DW, Haynes RB, et al. Beneficial effect of carotid endarterectomy in patients with high-grade carotid stenosis. *N Engl J Med.* 1991;325:445–453.
9. MRC European Carotid surgery Trial: interim results for symptomatic patients with severe (70–99%) or with mild (0–29%) carotid stenosis. European Carotid Surgery Trialists' Collaborative Group (ECST). *Lancet.* 1991;337(8752):1235–1243.
10. Mayberg MR, Wilson SE, Yatsu F, et al. Carotid endarterectomy and prevention of cerebral ischemia in symptomatic carotid stenosis: Veterans Affairs Cooperative Studies Program 309 Trialist Group. *JAMA.* 1991;266(23):3289–3294.
11. Executive Committee for Asymptomatic Carotid Atherosclerosis Study: endarterectomy for asymptomatic carotid artery stenosis. *JAMA.* 1995;273:1421–1428.
12. Halliday A, Mansfield A, Marro J, et al; MRC Asymptomatic Carotid Surgery Trial (ACST) Collaborative Group. Prevention of disabling and fatal strokes by successful carotid endarterectomy in patients without recent neurological symptoms: randomized controlled trial. *Lancet.* 2004;363(9420):1491–1502.
13. North American Symptomatic Carotid Endarterectomy Trial. Methods, patient characteristics, and progress. *Stroke.* 1991;22(6): 711–720.
14. Rothwell PM, Gibson RJ, Slattery J, Sellar RJ, Warlow CP. Equivalence of measurements of carotid stenosis. A comparison of three methods on 1001 angiograms. European Carotid Surgery Trialists' Collaborative Group. *Stroke.* 1994;25(12):2435–2439.
15. Moneta GL, Edwards JM, Papanicolaou G, et al. Screening for asymptomatic internal carotid artery stenosis: duplex criteria for discriminating 60% to 99% stenosis. *J Vasc Surg.* 1995;21(6):989–994.
16. AbuRahma AF, Robinson PA, Stickler DL, Alberts S, Young L. Proposed new duplex classification for threshold stenoses used in various symptomatic and asymptomatic carotid endarterectomy trials. *Ann Vasc Surg.* 1998;12(4):349–358.
17. Carpenter JP, Lexa FJ, Davis JT. Determination of duplex Doppler ultrasound criteria appropriate to the North American Symptomatic Carotid Endarterectomy Trial. *Stroke.* 1996;27(4):695–699.
18. Hood DB, Mattos MA, Mansour A, et al. Prospective evaluation of new duplex criteria to identify 70% internal carotid artery stenosis. *J Vasc Surg.* 1996;23(2):254–261; discussion 261–262.
19. Carpenter JP, Lexa FJ, Davis JT. Determination of 60% or greater carotid artery stenosis by duplex Doppler ultrasonography. *J Vasc Surg.* 1995;22(6):697–703; discussion 703–705.
20. Browman MW, Cooperberg PL, Harrison PB, Marsh JI, Mallek N. Duplex ultrasonography criteria for internal carotid stenosis of more than 70% diameter: angiographic correlation and receiver operating characteristic curve analysis. *Can Assoc Radiol J.* 1995;46(4):291–295.
21. Neale ML, Chambers JL, Kelly AT, et al. Reappraisal of duplex criteria to assess significant carotid stenosis with special reference to reports from the North American Symptomatic Carotid Endarterectomy Trial and the European Trial and the European Carotid Surgery Trial. *J Vasc Surg.* 1994;20(4):642–649.
22. Grant EG, Benson CB, Moneta GL, et al. Carotid artery stenosis: gray-scale and Doppler US diagnosis—Society of Radiologists in Ultrasound Consensus Conference. *Radiology.* 2003;229(2): 340–346.
23. Updated recommendations for carotid stenosis interpretation criteria. Intersocietal Accreditation Commission (IAC), November 2023.
24. Gornik HL, Rundek T, Gardener H, et al. Optimization of duplex velocity criteria for diagnosis of internal carotid artery (ICA) stenosis: a report of the Intersocietal Accreditation Commission (IAC) Vascular Testing Division Carotid Diagnostic Criteria Committee. *Vasc Med.* 2021;26(5):515–525.
25. Fujitani RM, Mills JL, Wang LM, Taylor SM. The effect of unilateral internal carotid arterial occlusion upon contralateral duplex study: criteria for accurate interpretation. *J Vasc Surg.* 1992;16(3): 459–467.
26. Setacci C, Chisci E, Setacci F, Iacoponi F, de Donato G. Grading carotid intrastent restenosis: a 6-year follow-up study. *Stroke.* 2008;39(4):1189–1196.
27. Lal BK, Beach KW, Roubin GS, et al; CREST Investigators. Restenosis after carotid artery stenting and endarterectomy: a secondary analysis of CREST, a randomised controlled trial. *Lancet Neurol.* 2012;11(9):755–763.
28. Szegedi I, Potvorszki F, Mészáros ZR, Daniel C, Csiba L, Oláh L. Role of carotid duplex in the assessment of carotid artery restenosis after endarterectomy or stenting. *Front Neurol.* 2023; 14:1226220.
29. Slovut DP, Romero JM, Hannon KM, Dick J, Jaff MR. Detection of common carotid artery stenosis using duplex ultrasonography: a validation study with computed tomographic angiography. *J Vasc Surg.* 2010;51(1):65–70.
30. Yao JS, Nedham TN, Gourmos C, Irvine WT. A comparative study of strain gauge plethysmography and Doppler ultrasound in the assessment of occlusive arterial disease of the lower extremities. *Surgery.* 1972;71(1):4–9.
31. Strandness DE Jr. *Peripheral Arterial Disease: A Physiologic Approach.* Little, Brown; 1969:112–130.
32. Kempczinski RF. Segmental volume plethysmography: the pulse volume recorder? In: Kempczinski RF, Yao JS, eds. *Practical Noninvasive Vascular Diagnosis.* Yearbook Medical Publishers; 1987: 140–153.
33. Krikendall WM, Burton AC, Epstein FH, Freis ED. Recommendations for human blood pressure determination by sphygmomanometers: report of a Subcommittee of the Postgraduate Education Committee, American Heart Association. *Circulation.* 1967;36: 980–988.
34. Moneta GL, Yeager RA, Antonovic R, et al. Accuracy of lower extremity arterial duplex mapping. *J Vasc Surg.* 1992;15(2):275–283.
35. Jager KA, Ricketts HJ, Strandness DE. Duplex scanning for evaluation of lower limb arterial disease? In: Bernstein EF, Barnes RW, eds. *Noninvasive Diagnostic Techniques in Vascular Disease.* Mosby; 1985:619–631.
36. Whyman MR, Hoskins PR, Leng GC, et al. Accuracy and reproducibility of duplex ultrasound imaging in a phantom model of femoral artery stenosis. *J Vasc Surg.* 1993;17(3):524–530.
37. Leng GC, Whyman MR, Donnan PT, et al. Accuracy and reproducibility of duplex ultrasonography in grading femoropopliteal stenoses. *J Vasc Surg.* 1993;17(3):510–517.
38. Sacks D, Robinson ML, Marinelli DL, Perlmutter GS. Peripheral arterial Doppler ultrasonography: diagnostic criteria. *J Ultrasound Med.* 1992;11(3):95–103.
39. Jager KA, Phillips DJ, Martin RL, et al. Noninvasive mapping of lower limb arterial lesions. *Ultrasound Med Biol.* 1985;11(3): 515–521.
40. Sensier Y, Hartshorne T, Thrush A, Nydahl S, Bolia A, London NJ. A prospective comparison of lower limb colour-coded duplex scanning with arteriography. *Eur J Vasc Endovasc Surg.* 1996;11(2):170–175.
41. de Smet AA, Ermers EJ, Kitslaar PJ. Duplex velocity characteristics of aortoiliac stenoses. *J Vasc Surg.* 1996;23(4):628–636.
42. Elsman BH, Legemate DA, van der Heijden FH, de Vos HJ, Mali WP, Eikelboom BC. Impact of ultrasonographic duplex scanning on therapeutic decision making in lower-limb arterial disease. *Br J Surg.* 1995;82(5):630–633.
43. Ascher E, Mazzariol F, Hingorani A, Salles-Cunha S, Gade P. The use of duplex ultrasound arterial mapping as an alternative to conventional arteriography for primary and secondary infrapopliteal bypasses. *Am J Surg.* 1999;178(2):162–165.

44. Mazzariol F, Ascher E, Salles-Cunha SX, Gade P, Hingorani A. Values and limitations of duplex ultrasonography as the sole imaging method of preoperative evaluation for popliteal and infrapopliteal bypasses. *Ann Vasc Surg.* 1999;13(1):1–10.
45. Larch E, Minar E, Ahmadi R, et al. Value of color duplex sonography for evaluation of tibioperoneal arteries in patients with femoropopliteal obstruction: a prospective comparison with anterograde intraarterial digital subtraction angiography. *J Vasc Surg.* 1997; 25(4):629–636.
46. Landry GJ, Moneta GL, Taylor LM Jr, Edwards JM, Yeager RA, Porter JM. Patency and characteristics of lower extremity vein grafts requiring multiple revisions. *J Vasc Surg.* 2000;32(1): 23–31.
47. Johnson BL, Bandyk DF, Back MR, Avino AJ, Roth SM. Intraoperative duplex monitoring of infrainguinal vein bypass procedures. *J Vasc Surg.* 2000;31(4):678–690.
48. Idu MM, Blankenstein JD, de Gier P, Truyen E, Buth J. Impact of a color-flow duplex surveillance program on infrainguinal vein graft patency: a five-year experience. *J Vasc Surg.* 1993;17(1): 42–52; discussion 52–53.
49. Lundell A, Lindblad B, Bergqvist D, Hansen F. Femoropopliteal-crural graft patency is improved by an intensive surveillance program: a prospective randomized study. *J Vasc Surg.* 1995;21(1): 26–33; discussion 33–34.
50. Passman MA, Moneta GL, Nehler MR, et al. Do normal early color-flow duplex surveillance examination results of infrainguinal vein grafts preclude the need for late graft revision? *J Vasc Surg.* 1995;22(4):476–481; discussion 482–484.
51. Mills JL Sr, Wixon CL, James DC, Devine J, Westerband A, Hughes JD. The natural history of intermediate and critical vein graft stenosis: recommendations for continued surveillance or repair. *J Vasc Surg.* 2001;33(2):273–278; discussion 278–280.
52. McLafferty RB, Edwards JM, Taylor LM Jr, Porter JM. Diagnosis and long-term clinical outcome in patients presenting with hand ischemia. *J Vas Surg.* 1995;22(4):361–367.
53. Porter JM, Snider RL, Bardana EJ, Rösch J, Eidemiller LR. The diagnosis and treatment of Raynaud's phenomenon. *Surgery.* 1975;77(1):11–23.
54. Nielsen SL, Lassen NA. Measurement of digital blood pressure after local cooling. *J App Physiol Respir Environ Exerc Physiol.* 1977;43: 907–910.
55. Lütolf O, Chen D, Zehnder T, Mahler F. Influence of local finger cooling on laser Doppler flux and nailfold capillary blood flow velocity in normal subjects and in patients with Raynaud's phenomenon. *Microvasc Res.* 1993;46(3):374–382.
56. Lafferty K, de Trafford JC, Roberts VC, Cotton LT. Raynaud's phenomenon and thermal entrainment: an objective test. *BMJ Clin Res.* 1983;286(6359):90–92.
57. Singh S, de Trafford JC, Baskerville PA, Roberts VC. Digital artery caliber measurement—a new technique of assessing Raynaud's phenomenon. *Eur J Vasc Surg.* 1991;5(2):199–203.
58. Yurdakul M, Tola M, Uslu OS. Color Doppler ultrasonography in occlusive diseases of the brachiocephalic and proximal subclavian arteries. *J Ultrasound Med.* 2008;27(7):1065–1070.
59. Strandness DE. *Duplex Scanning in Vascular Disorders.* Raven Press; 1993:159–196.
60. Grosveld WJ, Lawson JA, Eikelboom BC, vd Windt JM, Ackerstaff RG. Clinical and hemodynamic significance of innominate artery lesions evaluated by ultrasonography and digital angiography. *Stroke.* 1988;19:958–962.
61. Reed AJ, Fincher RM, Nichols FT. Takayasu's arteritis in a middle-aged Caucasian woman: clinical course correlated with duplex ultrasonography and angiography. *Am J Med Sci.* 1989;298(5): 324–327.
62. Jägar KA, Fortner GS, Thiele BI, Strandness DE. Noninvasive diagnosis of intestinal angina. *J Clin Ultrasound.* 1984;12(9): 588–591.
63. Gentile AT, Moneta GL, Lee RW, Masser PA, Taylor LM Jr, Porter JM. Usefulness of fasting and postprandial duplex ultrasound examinations for predicting high-grade superior mesenteric artery stenosis. *Am J Surg.* 1995;169:476–479.
64. Moneta GL, Taylor DC, Helton WS, Mulholland MW, Strandness DE Jr. Duplex ultrasound measurement of postprandial intestinal blood flow: effect of meal composition. *Gastroenterology.* 1988;95(5):1294–1301.
65. Moneta GL, Lee RW, Yeager RA, Taylor LM Jr, Porter JM. Mesenteric artery duplex scanning: a blinded prospective study. *J Vasc Surg.* 1993;17(1):79–84.
66. Zwolak RM, Fillinger MF, Walsh DB, et al. Mesenteric and celiac duplex scanning: a validation study. *J Vasc Surg.* 1998;27(6): 1078–1087.
67. Liem TK, Segall JA, Wei W, Landry GJ, Taylor LM, Moneta GL. Duplex scan characteristics of bypass grafts to mesenteric arteries. *J Vasc Surg.* 2007;45(5):922–927.
68. Mitchell EL, Chang EY, Landry GJ, Liem TK, Keller FS, Moneta GL. Duplex criteria for native superior mesenteric arteries stenosis overestimates stenosis in stented superior mesenteric arteries. *J Vasc Surg.* 2009;50(2):335–340.
69. Taylor DC, Kettler MD, Moneta GL, et al. Duplex ultrasound in the diagnosis of renal artery stenosis: a prospective evaluation. *J Vasc Surg.* 1988;7(2):363–369.
70. Hoffman U, Edwards JM, Carter S, et al. Role of duplex scanning for the detection of atherosclerotic renal artery disease. *Kidney Int.* 1991;39(6):1232–1239.
71. Olin JW, Piedmonte MR, Young JR, DeAnna S, Grubb M, Childs MB. The utility of duplex ultrasound scanning of the renal arteries for diagnosing significant renal artery stenosis. *Ann Intern Med.* 1995;122(11):833–838.
72. Mohabbat W, Greenerg RK, Mastracci TM, Cury M, Morales JP, Hernandez AV. Revised duplex criteria and outcomes for renal stents and stent grafts following endovascular repair of juxtrarenal and thoracoabdominal aneurysms. *J Vasc Surg.* 2009;49(4):827–837.
73. Radermacher J, Chavan A, Bleck J, et al. Use of Doppler ultrasonography to predict the outcome of therapy for renal-artery stenosis. *N Engl J Med.* 2001;344(6):410–417.
74. Wells PS, Hirsh J, Anderson DR. Accuracy of clinical assessment of deep-vein thrombosis. *Lancet.* 1995;345(8961):1326–1330.
75. Hull R, van Aken WG, Hirsh J, et al. Impedance plethysmography using the occlusive cuff technique in the diagnosis of venous thrombosis. *Circulation.* 1976;53(4):696–700.
76. Hull R, Hirsh J, Sackett DL, Powers P, Turpie AG, Walker I. Combined use of leg scanning and impedance plethysmography in suspected venous thrombosis: an alternative to venography. *N Engl J Med.* 1977;296(26):1497–1500.
77. Hull R, Taylor DW, Hirsh J, et al. Impedance plethysmography: the relationship between venous filling and sensitivity and specificity for proximal vein thrombosis. *Circulation.* 1978;58(5):898–902.
78. Hull R, Hirsh J, Sackett DL, et al. Replacement of venography in suspected venous thrombosis by impedance plethysmography and 125I-fibrinogen leg scanning: a less invasive approach. *Ann Intern Med.* 1981;94(1):12–15.
79. Anderson DR, Lensing AW, Wells PS, Levine MN, Weitz JI, Hirsh J. Limitations of impedance plethysmography in the diagnosis of clinically suspected deep vein thrombosis. *Ann Intern Med.* 1993;118(1):25–30.
80. Kearon C, Julian JA, Newman TE, Ginsberg JS. Noninvasive diagnosis of deep vein thrombosis. McMaster Diagnostic Imaging Practice Guidelines Initiative. *Ann Intern Med.* 1998;128(8): 663–677.
81. Kempczinski RE, Yao JST. Chapter 22: B-mode venous imaging. In: Karkow WS, Ruoff BA, Cranley JJ, eds. *Practical Noninvasive Vascular Diagnosis.* 2nd ed. Year Book Medical Publishers. 1987:464–485.
82. Mitchell DC, Grasty MS, Stebbings WSL, et al. Comparison of duplex ultrasonography and venography in the diagnosis of deep venous thrombosis. *Br J Surg.* 1991;78:611–613.
83. Rose SC, Zwiebel WJ, Nelson BD, et al. Symptomatic lower extremity deep venous thrombosis: accuracy, limitations, and role of color duplex flow imaging in diagnosis. *Radiology.* 1990;175(3): 639–644.
84. Kearon C. Diagnosis of pulmonary embolism. *CMAJ.* 2003;168(2): 183–194.

85. Welch HG, Faliakou EC, McLaughlin RL, Umphrey SE, Belkin M, O'Donnell TF Jr. Comparison of descending phlebography with quantitative photoplethysmography, air plethysmography, and duplex quantitative valve closure time in assessing deep venous reflux. *J Vasc Surg.* 1992;16(6):913–919.
86. van Bemmelen PS, Bedford G, Beach K, Strandness DE. Quantitative segmental evaluation of venous valvular reflux with duplex ultrasound scanning. *J Vasc Surg.* 1989;10(4):425–431.
87. Kabnick LS, Sadek M, Bjarnason H, et al. Classification and treatment of endothermal heat-induced thrombosis: recommendations from the American Venous Forum and the Society for Vascular Surgery. *J Vasc Surg Venous Lymphat Disord.* 2021;9(1): 6–22.
88. Fleming C, Whitlock EP, Beil TL, Lederle FA. Screening for abdominal aortic aneurysm: a best evidence systematic review for the U.S. preventive services task force. *Ann Intern Med.* 2005;142(3): 203–211.
89. Sanford RM, Brown MJ, Fisfwick G, et al. Duplex ultrasound scanning is reliable in the detection of endoleak following endovascular aneurysm repair. *Eur J Vasc Endovasc Surg.* 2006;32(5): 537–541.
90. Chaer RA, Gushchin A, Rhee R, et al. Duplex ultrasound as the sole long-term surveillance method post endovascular aneurysm repair: a safe alternative for stable aneurysms. *J Vasc Surg.* 2009;49(4):845–849.
91. Rafailidis V, Huang DY, Yusuf GT, Sidhu PS. General principles and overview of vascular contrast-enhanced ultrasonography. *Ultrasonography.* 2020;39(1):22–42.
92. Cox GS, Young JR, Gray BR, et al. Ultrasound guided compression repair of postcatheterization pseudoaneurysms: results of treatment in 100 cases. *J Vasc Surg.* 1994;19(4):683–686.
93. Kang SS, Labropoulos N, Mansour MA, et al. Expanded indications for ultrasound guided thrombin injection of pseudoaneurysms. *J Vasc Surg.* 2000;31(2):289–298.
94. Dzijan-Horn M, Langweiser N, Groha P, et al. Safety and efficacy of a potential treatment algorithm by using manual compression repair and ultrasound-guided thrombin injection for the management of iatrogenic femoral artery pseudoaneurysm in a large patient cohort. *Circ Cardivasc Interv.* 2014;7(2):207–215.
95. Ballard JL, Eke CC, Bunt TJ, Killeen JD. A prospective evaluation of transcutaneous oxygen measurements in the management of diabetic foot problems. *J Vasc Surg.* 1995;22(4):485–490.

Vascular Infection

Courtney E. Morgan and John E. Rectenwald

Key Points

1. The pathogenesis of infected aneurysms and microbial arteritis involves seeding of a pre-existing aneurysm or atherosclerotic plaque by bacteremia or in the case of infected aortitis the direct spread of infection to the aorta by contiguous septic structures, such as vertebral osteomyelitis. Arterial graft infections involve seeding of the graft from intraoperative contamination, erosion of adjacent structures, or hematogenous seeding from a distant source.
2. Characteristics of a prosthetic graft that predispose to graft infection include surface irregularity that permits bacterial attachment, abrogation of local defense against infection, creation of the bacterial biofilm that protects microbes from host defenses and antibiotics, all of which lowers the bacterial bioburden required to cause a graft infection.
3. The most common organisms causing arterial graft infections are skin flora, specifically *Staphylococcus aureus* and *Staphylococcus epidermidis.*
4. Diagnosis of vascular infections requires a high index of suspicion as patients often present with nonspecific symptoms. This requires a thorough query of recent sources or risk factors for infection, evaluation of culture data and inflammatory markers, and understanding the pros and cons of various imaging techniques in detecting vascular infections.
5. Surgical treatment of arterial infections requires appropriate resuscitation, preoperative planning, resection of all infected material and tissue, and revascularization. No single approach is suitable for all patients, but understanding the algorithm and tailoring this to local surgical expertise is critical in caring for these patients.
6. Antibiotic therapy is the cornerstone of treatment for arterial infections. Initial treatment involves broad-spectrum antibiotics followed by culture-driven therapy when possible, although up to 40% of patients are culture negative. While there are no guidelines directing the type, dose, duration, or route of therapy, most patients are treated with an initial multi-week course of antibiotics followed by longer-term suppression if not all graft material is excised.
7. Each method of aortic reconstruction after aortic graft excision has varied outcomes: Extra-anatomic bypass with aortic ligation risks aortic stump blowout and poor graft patency; reconstruction with in situ cryopreserved allograft has high cost, varied availability, and can demonstrate pseudoaneurysm degeneration; in situ reconstruction with rifampin-soaked Dacron has excellent patency, but has higher reinfection rates; in situ autogenous vein reconstruction is time consuming, but is more resistant to infection and offers excellent patency.

Vascular infections are among the most daunting conditions that a vascular surgeon may encounter in clinical practice. Vascular infections may afflict native arteries and veins or vascular prostheses. Primary arterial infections of native vessel are rare, but highly lethal conditions.[1] Secondary infections of prosthetic vascular grafts, are seen more frequently and are often more challenging because of the adhesions, scarring, and inflammation in the redo operative field.[2] These infections commonly occur in a compromised patient population with significant chronic medical conditions and relative immune deficiency. The clinical presentation for vascular infections range from indolent, asymptomatic infection incidentally diagnosed to overt sepsis or hemorrhage.[1] The management of vascular infections should be individualized, based on the clinical presentation, anatomic location of the vascular infection, and the medical condition of the patient. In recent years, newer therapeutic adjuncts, such as covered stents and improved cryopreserved grafts offer additional options to surgeons managing and treating arterial graft infections. The basic tenets of timely diagnosis, antibiotic administration, resuscitation, operative planning, surgical resection, and revascularization remain the mainstays of therapy in most cases.

DEFINITIONS AND PATHOGENESIS

Pathogenesis of Primary Arterial Infections

Arterial infections commonly result in aneurysms, or more correctly pseudoaneurysms since there is disruption of the arterial wall in many infected aneurysms. Aneurysms or pseudoaneurysms related to infection are often loosely termed "mycotic aneurysms." However, the term mycotic aneurysm was initially coined to describe an arterial aneurysm or pseudoaneurysm caused by a septic embolus from the heart that lodges in a distal artery to create a septic focus that injures the adjacent artery.[3] "Mycotic aneurysm" is a misnomer as the vast majority of these are of bacterial origin, not fungal. Pre-existing aneurysms that are subsequently seeded by bacteremia are "infected aneurysms." Arteries in which an atherosclerotic plaque becomes seeded develop "microbial arteritis." "Traumatic infected aneurysms" describe those infected aneurysms or pseudoaneurysms that develop secondary to complications

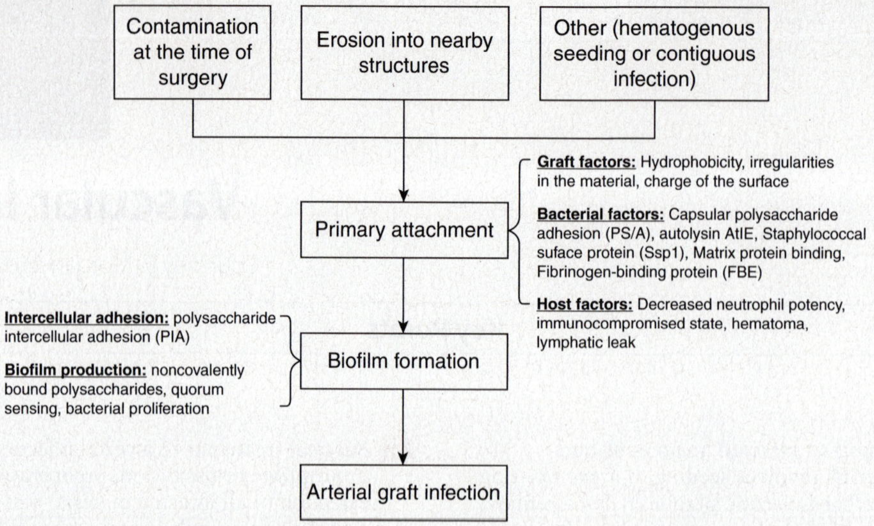

Figure 83.1. Proposed mechanism of *Staphylococcus epidermidis*–mediated graft infection.

of iatrogenic or other trauma. "Infected aortitis" occurs when the aorta becomes infected by contiguous septic structures, such as vertebral osteomyelitis.[3] For simplicity, we will utilize the term "primary arterial infection" to refer to all infected arterial infections that occur in the absence of prosthetic graft or stent material.

While historically infective endocarditis was the major source of primary arterial infections, arterial trauma, due to iatrogenic trauma, or intravenous drug use, appears to be the most prevalent contemporary cause.[1] Risk factors for primary arterial infections include trauma to the arterial wall, atherosclerosis, and pre-existing aneurysmal degeneration. In an autopsy study, Miller reaffirmed that many of infected aneurysms arise after pre-existing atherosclerotic lesions are seeded due to an episode of bacteremia, since 75% of the infected arteries had evidence of atherosclerosis in the resected specimen.[4] In Miller's study, 42% of arterial infections were located in the infrarenal aorta; the descending thoracic aorta was the next most common site of infection. Immune compromise by systemic conditions or medications, such as chronic steroid use, malignancy, human immunodeficiency virus syndrome, chronic hepatitis, or malnutrition, is a commonly identified in patients with primary arterial infections and mycotic aneurysms.[4]

Pathogenesis of Arterial Graft Infections

1 Prosthetic grafts are foreign bodies that may either be seeded at the time of the operation, or become infected secondarily due to hematogenous seeding or contiguous infection. The incidence of aortic graft infection is about 1% with one study suggesting similar numbers for open prosthetic graft repair (1.4%) versus endograft (0.9%) and no difference between thoracic and abdominal aortic aneurysms.[5] Up to a third of patients may have an infection present at the time of the initial hospitalization.[6]

Lower extremity prosthetic grafts are at the highest risk of infection, which probably relates to the abundance of skin flora in the groin and the proximity of the graft to the incision. Infections of grafts originating from or terminating at the femoral artery complicate roughly 5% of cases.[7] By comparison, carotid patches rarely become infected, with incidence <1%.[8] Polytetrafluoroethylene (PTFE) may be somewhat more resistant to infection than Dacron, as it has less porosity to sequester microbes.[9] Peripheral bare metal stents appear to be highly resistant to infection, with a presumed incidence of less than 0.1% based on isolated case reports.[10]

2 Prosthetic material harbors multiple risk factors for infection including ease of attachment of bacteria due to the irregular surface, and decreased immunologic defense caused by the local inflammatory response of the graft itself.[9] Instead of being inert, the prosthetic material acts as a potent activator of host defenses, which subsequently renders them less capable of defending the graft from infection. Studies have shown contact with implants causes neutrophils to lose their ability to produce superoxide and reactive oxygen species, which are critical to their bactericidal activity.[11] Finally, communities of bacteria form slime to create biofilms, protecting microbes from host defenses and antibiotics.[9] This is a critical step in the pathogenesis of prosthetic graft infections caused by *Staphylococcus epidermidis* (**Fig. 83.1**).[9]

MICROBIOLOGY

Primary Arterial Infections

For infected aortic aneurysms, blood cultures are negative in approximately one-fourth of subjects.[4] Intraoperative cultures are more reliable, although intraoperative cultures may be negative in many cases due to improper culture techniques or preoperative antibiotic administration that precludes isolation
3 of organisms.[1] In other series, up to 40% of infected aneurysms had negative blood and/or tissue culture.[6,12] The most frequent causative organisms vary by region with *Staphylococcal* species being the most common isolates in western countries and *Salmonella* most common in Asian countries. However, a wide range of pathogens is described worldwide with *Streptococcus, Escherichia coli, Enterococcus, Enterobacter, Pseudomonas, Campylobacter*, and *Yersinia* all reported with some frequency. Anaerobic, mycobacterial, and fungal infections also represent rare causes of arterial infections.[13–15] The causative organisms also appear to vary based on the artery involved. Infected femoral artery aneurysms are rarely true aneurysms, but are infected pseudoaneurysms related to prior catheterizations or intravenous drug use. Skin flora, such as *S. aureus* or *Streptococcal* species, are the predominant organisms isolated from infected femoral artery pseudoaneurysms.[16,17]

Arterial Graft Infections

The most common causal organisms for prosthetic grafts are *Staphylococcus* and *Streptococcus* except in the case of aortoenteric fistula (AEF) where *E. coli* is the most common organism. Up to 30% are polymicrobial, an equal number have negative intraoperative cultures.[6,18]

Prosthetic graft infections involving the femoral artery are most often related to *Staphylococcal* species, which comprised 68% of the infections in one series.[7] *Enterococcal* and polymicrobial infections were less frequent among femoral artery grafts.[7] Endograft infections are predominantly caused by *Staphylococcal* species and other minor skin flora, such as *Propionibacterium*.[19] Similarly, *Staphylococcal* species predominate in carotid patch infections[8] and peripheral arterial stent infections, with over 85% of the case reports attributed to *Staphylococcal* species.[10]

CLASSIFICATION OF ARTERIAL GRAFT INFECTIONS

Early graft infections are defined as those occurring less than 4 months after graft implantation. The Szilagyi classification system classified early surgical site infections[20] which was modified by Samson to further distinguish between different types of vascular infections.[21] Bundt's classification, developed in 1983, describes prosthetic graft infections according to the anatomic segment of the graft that is involved,[22] while the Management of Aortic Graft Collaboration was developed in 2016 in collaboration with vascular surgeons, infectious disease specialists, and radiologists to better define precise criteria for defining aortic graft infection.[23] These criteria are summarized in **Table 83.1**. Clinical management often varies significantly based on the extent of infection, according to these classification systems.

DIAGNOSIS

The diagnosis of primary arterial infection or prosthetic graft infection may be difficult due to the significant overlap of symptoms with other pathologies. While a thorough history and physical examination are essential, a high index of suspicion is critical to the diagnosis. Delays in diagnosis may have devastating consequences for the patient. Understanding some of the more common presentations of arterial infections can facilitate a timely diagnosis.

Common Clinical Presentations

4 Patients with vascular infections often present with nonspecific symptoms of malaise, fever, and pain in the region of the infected artery or graft, which may be accompanied by elevations in erythrocyte sedimentation rate (ESR) or C-reactive protein (CRP).[6] These symptoms are most commonly associated with arterial infections caused by more virulent organisms, such as *S. aureus, Pseudomonas aeruginosa, E. coli,* or polymicrobial infections. Arterial infections caused by lower virulence organisms, such as *S. epidermidis* or *Enterococcus,* are often even more indolent and may not be associated with local or systemic signs and symptoms.[7] Peripheral arterial infections (primary or graft infections) may exhibit local symptoms, such as erythema, swelling, tenderness, or a sinus tract with purulent drainage.[7] In contrast, local signs and symptoms are unlikely with infections of cavitary arteries or grafts.

A careful history is critical to identify risk factors for exposure such as recent infections, invasive procedures, intravenous drug use, recent gastrointestinal illnesses, or environmental exposures.

Associated medical conditions may be cofactors in the pathogenesis of vascular infections. Any condition that produces relative immune compromise may predispose to primary arterial or graft infection. Examples include malignancy,

Table 83.1. Classification of Arterial Graft Infections

Szylagi Classification[20]	Grade I: Cellulitis involving wound Grade II: Infection involving subcutaneous tissue Grade III: Infection involving native arteries or vascular graft		
Samson Classification[21]	Group 1: Infection does not extend beyond dermis Group 2: Infection involves subcutaneous tissue but does not contact graft Group 3: Infection involves body of graft, but not anastomosis Group 4: Infection involves the anastomosis, without anastomotic bleeding or bacteremia Group 5: Infection involves a graft to artery anastomosis and associated with septicemia bleeding at the time of presentation		
Bundt Classification[22]	P0: Infection of a cavitary graft P1: Infection of a graft whose entire anatomical course is noncavitary P2: Infection of the extracavitary portion of a graft whose origin is cavitary Graft-enteric erosion Graft-enteric fistula Aortic stump sepsis after excision of an infected graft		
MAGIC Criteria[23]	**Clinical/Surgical**	**Radiology**	**Laboratory**
Major	Pus around graft or in aneurysm sac Open wound with exposed graft or communicating sinus Fistula development (aortoenteric or aortobronchial) Graft insertion in an infected site	Perigraft fluid on CT scan >3 mo after insertion Perigraft gas on CT >7 wk after insertion Increase in perigraft gas volume demonstrated on serial imaging	Organisms recovered from implanted graft Organisms recovered from operative specimen Organisms recovered percutaneous, radiologic aspirate of perigraft fluid
Minor	Localized clinical features of graft infection Fever >38 °C as most likely cause	Other (e.g.) suspicious perigraft gas/fluid, soft tissue inflammation, aneurysm expansion, pseudoaneurysm formation, focal bowel wall thickening, osteomyelitis, suspicious metabolic activity on FDG-PET/CT, radiolabeled leukocyte uptake	Blood cultures positive without apparent source except graft Abnormally elevated inflammatory markers with graft infection as likely cause

human immunodeficiency virus syndrome, chronic hepatitis, malnutrition, and conditions that require immunosuppressive medications. Predisposing conditions have been identified in up to 70% of patients with mycotic aneurysms.[4] Malignancy is especially relevant due to the association between *Clostridium septicum* arterial infections and malignancy.[24] Symptomatic atherosclerosis is important to note since atherosclerotic plaques may become seeded by episodic bacteremia to create a primary arterial infection.

For patients with a history of a prior bypass involving the femoral artery, occult infections frequently present with an anastomotic pseudoaneurysm in the groin. Over 60% of femoral pseudoaneurysms are ultimately found to harbor an occult infection.[25] Mertens found that 74% of patients with infected infrainguinal bypass grafts presented with a draining wound or sinus.[26] Infections with low virulence organisms, such as *S. epidermidis,* are less likely to be present with a draining sinus because the virulence of the organisms is insufficient to incite a vigorous inflammatory response to produce the sinus tract.[7]

Graft thrombosis is another underappreciated clinical presentation for an occult graft infection. Graft thrombosis is believed to predispose to subsequent graft infection.[27] The coagulated blood within a thrombosed prosthetic graft provides a rich media for the microorganisms to proliferate.[27] In addition, prosthetic materials are fomites that may harbor microorganisms. Some authors advocate removing occluded grafts when performing subsequent revascularization operations or amputations to prevent contiguous spread from the prior occluded grafts.[28]

AEF with gastrointestinal hemorrhage is a rare, but life-threatening presentation for graft infection that must be diagnosed expeditiously. Any patient presenting with gastrointestinal hemorrhage that has a history of prior aortic surgery, especially those with vascular prostheses, must have a rapid evaluation for an AEF. AEFs often present initially with a "herald bleed," or a relatively small amount of gastrointestinal bleeding that temporarily abates prior to a full-on fatal exsanguination several hours or days later.[29–33] The mortality rate for AEFs is 30% to 77%. Delay in diagnosis is frequently a contributing factor among patients who die from this condition. Approximately 75% of AEFs result from a communication between the aorta and the third or fourth portion of the duodenum.[29] The vast majority of AEFs occur in the setting of prior surgical or endovascular aortic reconstruction. Rarely AEFs occur as a complication of a primary aortic infection.[31] If a portion of the graft erodes through the adjacent bowel without suture line involvement, gastrointestinal bleeding results from intestinal mucosal irritation. This phenomenon is termed "graft-enteric erosion."[32] Graft-enteric erosions are often discovered incidentally during surgery to excise an infected aortic graft.

Ureteral obstruction can occur due to a mechanical complication during the tunneling of an aortofemoral limb or as a consequence of the inflammatory reaction associated with an infected aortofemoral limb. Ureterohydronephrosis is strongly associated with aortic graft infections. Wright et al. found that the presence of a urologic complication after aortoiliac arterial reconstructions was associated with a fourfold increase in the risk of graft complications, including pseudoaneurysms, limb thrombosis, AEFs, and overt graft infections.[34] Ureteral complications are typically asymptomatic, so ureterohydronephrosis is often discovered incidentally during imaging studies for other indications and should alert the physician to the possibility of a graft infection.

Imaging for Vascular Infection

The history, physical examination, and laboratory findings for primary arterial infection or graft infections are often nonspecific, so imaging plays a pivotal role in establishing a diagnosis. Although advances in imaging techniques have improved the sensitivity and specificity significantly, no single modality is perfect. Confirming a physician's suspicion of occult infection with a low-virulence organism remains a challenge in many cases. Understanding the advantages and disadvantages of each imaging modality will allow the surgeon to choose the most appropriate examination, or combination of imaging studies, to optimize the diagnostic yield. Computed tomography (CT) and computed tomographic angiography (CTA) are preferred imaging modalities in most centers with classic findings of thickened inflammatory wall around the aorta, loss of tissue planes, and even erosion from the aorta into overlying bowel as demonstrated in **Figures 83.2** to **83.4**.

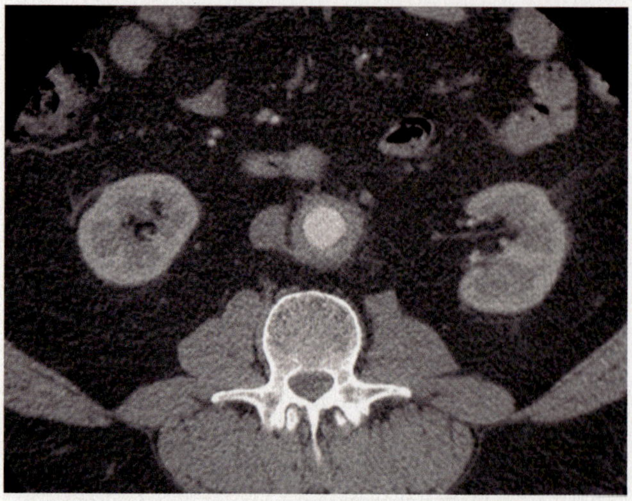

Figure 83.2. CT scan demonstrating thickened inflammatory wall around the aorta.

CT does have limitations, but combining this with nuclear medicine (NM) imagine modalities improves sensitivity and specificity. One study comparing adjunct FDG PET/CT with leukocyte scintigraphy recommends supplementing CTA with FDG/PET to improved sensitivity, but confirm positive results with leukocyte scintigraphy. **Table 83.2** summarizes each imaging modality.[35]

CONSERVATIVE MANAGEMENT

Primary Arterial Infections

Non operative management is limited to small case studies or series in patients who are not operative candidates. Hsu et al. provided insight on the outcome of conservative management

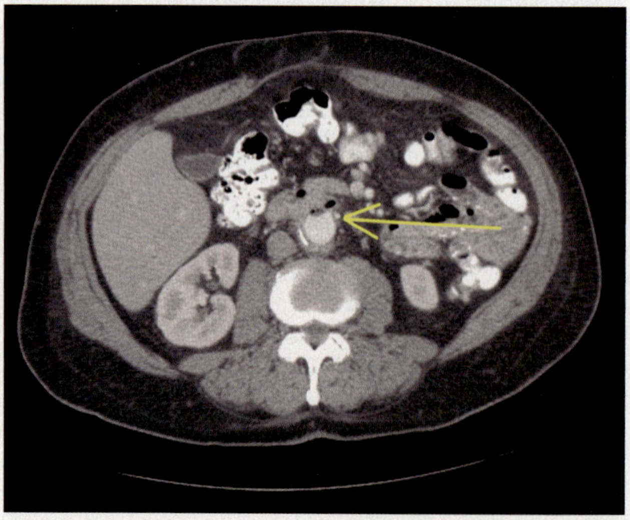

Figure 83.3. CT scan demonstrating loss of tissue planes around the aorta with foci of air as a sign of infection.

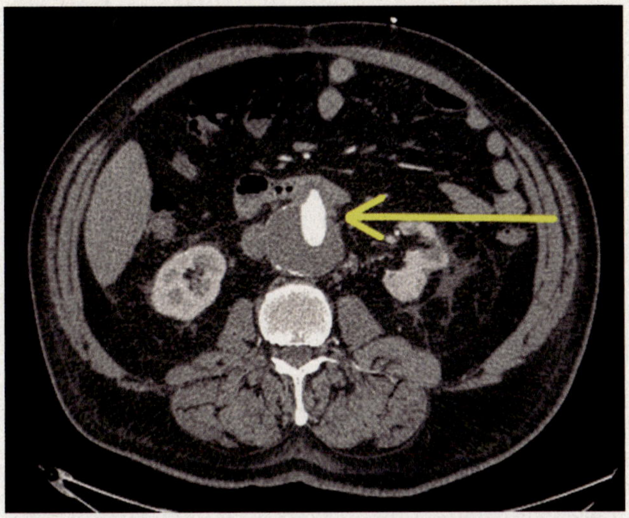

Figure 83.4. CT scan demonstrating erosion from the aorta into the overlying bowel consistent with an aortoenteric fistula.

of subjects with primary aortic infections.[37] Hsu examined 22 subjects with infected aortic aneurysms with perceived contraindications to surgery. The predominant organism in the cohort was *Salmonella,* with two-thirds of subjects having infections of the abdominal aorta. All subjects received culture-specific intravenous antibiotics for at least 6 to 8 weeks, or until normalization of white blood cell count, daily temperatures, and CRP levels. After the acute phase treatment, oral antibiotics were continued indefinitely. In Hsu's series, the in-hospital mortality was 50% due to rupture or sepsis. The 1-year survival rate was 32%. Patients with *Salmonella* infections had a lower aneurysm-related mortality rate than patients with non-*Salmonella* infections.

Arterial Graft Infections

Calligaro advocated for complete or partial prosthetic bypass preservation in subjects with severe comorbidities precluding surgical repair.[38] Over a 20-year period, 51 extra cavitary grafts (aortofemoral limbs or lower extremity bypasses) were treated with graft preservation and aggressive wound management without surgical graft resection. When wounds were present, aggressive debridement of all necrotic tissue and

Table 83.2. Imaging Modalities for Vascular Infection

Modality	Typical Findings	Pros	Cons
Duplex Ultrasound	Presence of pseudoaneurysm, hematoma, soft tissue mass, perigraft gas and fluid collection, "halo sign" around an infected limb	Safe, inexpensive, can be performed at bedside	Need for skilled technician, body habitus and overlying structures obscure visualization
CT and CTA	Inflammatory changes in soft tissues surrounding graft, thickening of bowel adjacent to vascular structures, loss of tissue planes around the artery or graft, perigraft or periarterial air or fluid, erosion into surrounding structures	Readily available, standard protocols, less expensive, sensitivity 95%, specificity 88%[35]	Contrast allergy, contrast-induced nephropathy, metal artifact, radiation exposure, less sensitive in indolent infections (55%)
MRI	Halo sign around infected grafts on T1 imaging, hyperintense signal on T2 imaging	Avoids radiation and contrast-induced nephropathy, good soft tissue resolution	Expensive, time consuming, contraindicated with some metal implants Sensitivity and specificity institution dependent
Leukocyte Scintigraphy	^{111}Indium- or ^{99m}Technetium-labeled leukocytes localize infection within the arterial graft or wall	Can be useful in indolent infections Improved sensitivity when combined with SPECT scanning	Time consuming (results take >24 hours), labor intensive, false positives in early postoperative period
FDG-PET	FDG uptake along the artery or graft	When combined with CT sensitivity 92%, specificity 63%[36]	Expensive, high false-positive rate because of inflammatory reaction of grafts, especially early, nonspecific results in low virulent infections
Adjunctive Diagnostic Modalities			
Angiography	May reveal occult AEF	Can help with operative planning	Invasive
Endoscopy	Graft material visible in the bowel lumen (**Fig. 83.5**)	Exclude other sources of GI bleeding, recommended despite low diagnostic yield in stable patients	Low diagnostic yield (25% identifying AEF)
Image-guided biopsy	Biopsy of fluid or rind surrounding structure	Can distinguish infection	Sufficient sample hard to achieve, invasive, may introduce infection

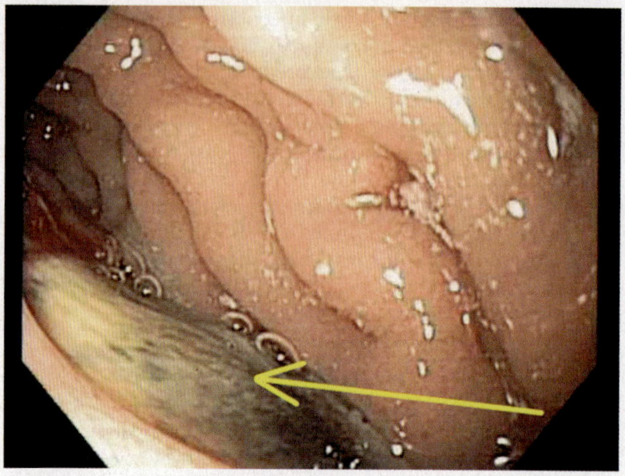

Figure 83.5. EGD demonstrating graft material visible in the bowel lumen consistent with graft-enteric fistula.

exudate surrounding the artery was performed. Nine cases utilized adjunctive muscle flaps to aid healing. Povidone–iodine 1% or antibiotic-soaked dressing changes were performed three times a day. With this regimen, 2 of 51 patients (4%) experienced major hemorrhage from the infected graft at 3 and 12 months after presentation. Eleven of the patients (22%) failed the treatment regimen, with nonhealing wounds or recurrent infections requiring total graft excision. Thirty-two subjects (63%) were ultimately treated successfully. Calligaro concluded that conservative management of extra cavitary grafts is an acceptable option in the absence of sepsis or hemorrhage, especially when graft excision and revascularization is not feasible due to patient comorbidities. *Pseudomonas* infections, however, were particularly prone to failure with this regimen.

Building on the early reports of graft preservation therapy, subsequent reports have emerged utilizing vacuum-assisted negative pressure therapy with antibiotics and wound debridement to preserve extra cavitary grafts with Szilagyi III wounds.[39,40] Wound healing with these regimens have ranged between 82% and 91% with excellent graft preservation rates.[39,40] Episodes of hemorrhage remain an issue with this approach,[39] and the failures have been associated with *Pseudomonas*.[39,40] Based on these reports, it appears that carefully selected patients with early infections involving extra cavitary grafts may be treated without surgical graft excision with acceptable results.

Calligaro et al. used a nonoperative approach in six patients with intracavitary graft infections with a hostile abdomen or severe medical comorbidities.[41] All subjects underwent either open or percutaneous placement of drains along the graft with instillation of 10 mL of 1% povidone–iodine in 100 mL of normal saline or antibiotics (neomycin or a cephalosporin) three times a day. All subjects were treated concurrently with culture-directed intravenous antibiotic therapy for 6 weeks, followed by 6 months of oral antibiotic therapy. Of these six subjects, only one died due to sepsis. One patient ultimately required total graft excision and survived. The remaining patients (66%) were alive at last follow-up. These authors showed that in highly selected patients, conservative management can have reasonable outcomes. Stone et al. described the use of antibiotic-loaded polymethylmethacrylate beads in treatment of prosthetic graft infection in 32 patients. This resulted in 87% wound sterilization, 50% rate of graft preservation, and reinfection rates of 12%.[42] Another study of incomplete graft removal in the setting of aortic graft infection had in-hospital mortality of 20.3%, with estimated freedom from aortic-related death of 77% at 1 year and 61.7% at 5 years.[43]

SURGICAL MANAGEMENT OF AORTIC ARTERIAL AND GRAFT INFECTIONS

Surgical treatment is based upon the central tenets of appropriate resuscitation, preoperative planning, resection of all infected material and tissue, and arterial revascularization. The optimal method of arterial reconstruction remains unresolved, as few direct comparisons between approaches have been published. Based on our extensive institutional experience with a variety of techniques, we have concluded that no single approach is suitable for all patients. We advocate tailoring the treatment algorithm based on each patient's clinical presentation and the local surgical expertise.

Initial Management in Stable patients

Preoperative Evaluation

The incidence of coronary artery disease is high in surgical series of arterial infections, especially in subjects with infected endografts. Thus, a thorough cardiovascular history, physical examination, 12-lead electrocardiogram, and echocardiogram should be obtained to evaluate for heart failure, valvular dysfunction, and pulmonary hypertension. These investigations may reveal a history of active cardiac conditions that may modify the type of operation selected or preclude surgery. Only rarely is stress testing or coronary arteriography indicated since coronary revascularization is usually contraindicated in the context of an active infection. However, this information may alter the surgical plan, provide valuable information for the anesthesiologists, and guide discussions with the patient or family regarding the expected outcomes. Pulmonary evaluations are rarely undertaken, as this information seldom alters the management of the patient. Only those patients with the most severe pulmonary insufficiency may benefit from formal testing to guide perioperative management.[44]

5 Operative planning is greatly facilitated by a preoperative CTA to define the arterial anatomy. Angiography of the lower extremities is reserved for cases when a concurrent infrainguinal bypass is considered likely. Noninvasive measurements of distal perfusion and lower extremity vein mapping should be performed. Ankle–brachial indices (ABIs) may forewarn the surgeon of the potential for infrainguinal revascularization after graft excision and aortoiliac reconstruction. Mapping of the bilateral greater saphenous veins and femoral–popliteal veins is essential if an autogenous conduit is contemplated. Femoral–popliteal veins with a diameter of less than 6 mm or evidence of vein wall sclerosis are inadequate for aortoiliac reconstruction.

Anesthetic Considerations

Operations to excise infected aortic grafts are technically challenging, lengthy, and prone to a large volume of blood loss. The importance of a quality anesthesia team in managing these challenges cannot be overstated. Hypothermia, hypovolemia, and intraoperative anemia must be assiduously avoided with the use of warming blankets, warmed resuscitative fluids, warm ambient operating room temperature, and a low threshold for blood and crystalloid replacement. The blood bank should be prepared to provide fresh-frozen plasma, cryoprecipitate, or platelets on short notice if coagulopathy develops. Culture data are often not available at the time of operation, so broad-spectrum antibiotic coverage for gram-positive, gram-negative, and anaerobic organisms should be redosed throughout the operation.

Aortic Infections Presenting with Hemorrhage or Sepsis

A minority of patients present with septic or hemorrhagic shock. For these patients, rapid intravenous access and resuscitation are essential prior to emergent surgery. In the authors' experience, the complexity of the operations required to manage these patients mandates a rapid CTA to obtain essential anatomic information. It is recognized that some of these patients will have either acute kidney injury or chronic kidney disease, but managing the life-threatening complications of the aortic graft infection outweighs the risk of contrast-induced nephropathy. Ideally, blood and wound cultures are obtained prior to the administration of broad-spectrum gram-positive and gram-negative antibiotic therapy. The surgical approach to managing patients presenting with hemorrhage or sepsis should be individualized based on the patient's anatomy and the expertise of the surgeons.

Definitive Surgical Management for Aortic Graft Infection (including Aortoenteric Fistula)

Definitive surgery for an aortic graft infection involves resection of the infected graft, and revascularization of the lower extremities. In the setting of AEF, this also involves repair of the enteric defect. The most appropriate surgical approach to achieve these goals has been the focus of considerable debate.

Aortic Graft Excision

Common to each of the described surgical approaches to aortic graft infection is the need for complete graft excision. This is summarized in **Table 83.3**.

For graft excision, aortic exposure can be performed via a transperitoneal or retroperitoneal approach. Proximal control of the infrarenal aorta can be challenging in a redo operative field, so the surgeon should be prepared to obtain proximal control of the aorta at the suprarenal or supraceliac level, or consider balloon occlusion as an adjunct. When treating an AEF, proximal control should be obtained prior to mobilizing the duodenum since there may be uncontrolled hemorrhage in the absence of proximal aortic control. The left renal vein may be densely adherent to the graft or the native aorta, which may necessitate its division to gain access to the aorta near the renal arteries. Once proximal control is obtained, distal control of the bilateral common iliac arteries should ensue, unless these arteries are occluded. When excising an aortofemoral graft, the femoral limbs should be controlled in the abdomen to facilitate their removal. Removal of aortofemoral grafts requires considerable dissection in the groins for control of the prosthetic graft limbs and native common femoral, superficial femoral, and profunda femoris arteries. Femoral exposure may be performed through an incision directly over the femoral limb or incisions lateral to the sartorius muscle. The lateral incision avoids some of the prior scarring and may preserve soft tissue for arterial coverage. Systemic heparin is administered prior to cross-clamping, and the graft is removed in its entirety. Any arterial tissue that appears to be abnormally friable is probably infected and should be debrided. Remnants of graft and arterial tissue should be sent for Gram stain, culture, and sensitivity testing. A critical adjunct is wide debridement of the retroperitoneum, which is believed to decrease the residual bacterial bioburden that will predispose to recurrent infection. After completing graft excision and debridement, closure of the aortic stump or in situ aortoiliac reconstruction may ensue. The primary options for reconstruction include extra-anatomic bypass or in situ repair using a variety of conduits including cryopreserved allograft artery, rifampin-soaked or silver-impregnated Dacron, or autogenous femoral vein. The results of these techniques are compared in the subsequent section and in **Table 83.4**.

Table 83.3. Excision of Aortic Graft Operative Steps

Step
Transperitoneal or retroperitoneal incision
Exposure for proximal control ■ May require division of left renal vein ■ Consider balloon control as adjunct
Distal exposure ■ Control aortofemoral bypass limbs in the abdomen ■ Consider lateral approach to femoral artery to avoid scarred field
Heparinize and cross clamp
Remove graft in entirety ■ Send graft for culture
Wide debridement of the retroperitoneum ■ Send tissue for culture
Aortic stump closure or in situ reconstruction ■ Double-layer running nonabsorbable polypropylene suture horizontal mattress followed by baseball stitch ■ Omental wrap secured with sutures

Aortic Ligation and Extra-anatomic Bypass versus in Situ Reconstruction

A major advantage of graft excision with extra-anatomic bypass is the removal of all prosthetic graft material from the infected operative field. This approach also obviates the need to procure an aortoiliac allograft and circumvents any reticence a surgeon may have with harvesting femoral veins since some surgeons are not familiar with the technique. The obvious pitfalls of this approach are the risk of aortic stump blowout, reinfection of the extra-anatomic bypass graft, and poor long-term patency of the extra-anatomic reconstruction. In situ reconstruction is appealing because it avoids the risk of aortic stump blowout and the poor long-term patency of extra-anatomic bypasses. For patients with insufficient infrarenal aorta for a secure three-layer closure, in situ may be the only reasonable option. Reinfection of new graft is the obvious risk of this approach. In the following sections, we will offer technical suggestions for performing these complex operations and summarize the published results for each approach.

Extra-anatomic Bypass

For stable patients, staging of the extra-anatomic bypass and graft excision should be considered. This is described by Reilly et al. at the University of California-San Francisco advocating staging of the two component operations at an interval of several days to minimize the physiologic impact on the patient.[45] The first stage of this approach consists of performing an axillobifemoral bypass or bilateral axillary–popliteal bypasses (depending on the configuration of the infected graft), followed several days later by resection of the infected graft with aortic stump closure. The first stage of this approach consists of performing an axillobifemoral bypass or bilateral axillary–popliteal bypasses, meticulously avoiding any infected or contaminated planes when tunneling the new grafts. The second stage consists of aortic graft excision, retroperitoneal debridement, and aortic stump closure. Aortic stump closure requires a meticulous three-layer closure or "triple ligation" of the aorta. The first two layers consist of nonabsorbable polypropylene suture; a vertical mattress suture, followed by running "baseball" suture. The final layer is an omental wrap secured with sutures. When staging the extra-anatomic bypass and graft excision, the optimal time interval between the two operations has not been defined. It has been our experience, however, that the presence of both an aortobifemoral bypass and an extra-anatomic bypass creates competitive flow between the grafts that often results in thrombosis of the extra-anatomic bypass graft. To minimize the risk of interval graft thrombosis, patients are anticoagulated with intravenous unfractionated heparin between operations, and a short (1 to 3 days) time interval (usually 1 to 2 days) between the two operations is planned. If the two operations are performed at the

VASCULAR DISEASE

Table 83.4. Complications Associated with Different Methods of Aortic Reconstruction after Aortic Graft Excision

Method of Aortic Reconstruction	Mortality	Graft Occlusion	Amputation	Reinfection (Stump Blowout)	Pros (+)/Cons (–)
Extra-anatomic bypass with aortic ligation[45–47]	Early 11–45% Late 40%	27–34%	0–27%	3–27% (9–27%)	(+) reduced morbidity with staging (–) decreased patency, stump blowout, amputation rate, and reinfection
In situ autogenous vein[19,48]	Early 9% Late 40–55%	3%	6–7%	0–4%	(+) resistant to infection, excellent long-term durability and limb salvage (–) time consuming, fasciotomy in up to 25%
In situ allograft[18,49]	Early 2.8–9% Late 3–48%	4–7%	1–2%	3–4%	(+) resistant to reinfection, excellent long-term durability and limb salvage (–) rupture and pseudoaneurysmal degeneration, cost, persistent infection
Rifampin soaked[50]	Early 8–31% Late 16–40%	0–9%	0%	0–12%	(+) excellent patency, convenience (–) higher reinfection rates
In situ silver-impregnated graft[47]	Early 16–18% Late 16–27%	0–8%	0–4%	9–13%	(+) excellent patency, convenience (–) highest reinfection rates
In situ xenograft[51,52]	Early 19% Late 19%	1%		0%	(+) excellent patency and reinfection rates (–) limited long-term outcomes

Based on Selected Publications.

same operative setting, the clean portion of the procedure (the extra-anatomic bypass) is performed prior to the infected portion of the case (graft excision) whenever feasible to minimize the risk of bacterial inoculation of the new graft, however this may not be possible in a patient with ongoing bleeding. Reilly reported a 26% mortality rate with the staged approach, compared to 43% for the traditional, nonstaged.[45] A subsequent study by Seeger reported a 19% treatment-related mortality rate.[46] In addition to a high mortality rate, this approach is plagued by a significant risk of aortic stump blowout (9%), reinfection of the extra-anatomic bypass graft (16%), and major amputation (16%).[45] A meta-analysis of aortic reconstructions for graft infections confirmed these results showing significantly higher rates for early mortality, amputations, graft occlusion, and reinfection in extra-anatomic bypass versus in situ reconstruction.[47]

In Situ Reconstruction

In response to the sobering results associated with the extra-anatomic approach, in situ aortic reconstruction has been touted as a relatively simple and effective alternative, however careful selection of grafts is required as each option has tradeoffs.

In Situ Reconstruction with Rifampin-Soaked and Silver-Impregnated Grafts

Reconstruction with prosthetic grafts is the most straightforward surgical option as the grafts are readily available on the shelf and do not require additional harvest of autogenous material. Standard polyester or PTFE grafts have high reinfection rates, so antimicrobial impregnation of the graft material has been developed to reduce this risk.

Rifampin shows unique activity against *S. epidermidis* biofilms, making it an excellent choice for prosthetic graft infections. Rifampin-soaked Dacron grafts (600-mg rifampin in 250 mL of normal saline, soaked for 30 minutes) with omental wrapping has been shown to have variable resistance to recurrent infection, ranging between 4% and 11.5%.[50,53] Recurrent infections have been fewer when treating AEFs, compared to prosthetic graft infections which may be related to rifampin-bonded polyester ineffectiveness against MRSA.[47] Primary patency and limb salvage are also excellent. Circumferential omental wrapping of the grafts is a critical technical adjunct to decrease the risk of reinfection.[50]

Silver-impregnation relies upon the ability of silver to adsorb gram-positive and gram-negative bacterial membranes, resulting in disruption of the membrane and cell lysis. There has been no reported bacterial resistance to silver.[54] It is theorized that silver-impregnated grafts would have activity against *E. coli* and methicillin-resistant *S. aureus,* which would be an improvement over rifampin-soaked grafts, however meta-analysis data suggest similar rates of reinfection at 11%.[47]

In Situ Reconstruction with Autogenous Femoral Vein

Autogenous femoral vein was proposed as an alternative conduit for in situ reconstruction for infected aortic grafts in the early 1990s.[48] Clagett described creating a "neo-aortoiliac system" or NAIS using femoral veins harvested from both legs. The proposed advantages of femoral vein include an innate resistance to infection and excellent long-term patency. The major pitfall of using femoral vein for in situ reconstruction is the time required to harvest the veins, thus is not appropriate for an unstable or bleeding patient. Although many surgeons have not had formal training in the technique for harvesting femoral veins, it is well within the capability of any vascular surgeon. The technique is described in detail elsewhere, and summarized in **Table 83.5**.[55] Among clinicians who are not familiar with using femoral vein for aortoiliac reconstruction, there appears to be reluctance based on concerns with any venous morbidity associated with harvesting the femoral vein. Modrall et al. described

Table 83.5. Operative Steps for Femoral Vein Harvest

Step
Incision is extended along the lateral edge of the sartorius from the anterior superior iliac spine to the medial femoral condyle
Sartorius is reflected medially to preserve blood supply
Avoid saphenous nerve
Double ligate side branches >3 mm over suture ligation to avoid tearing vein wall
Expose entire length from the confluence with the profunda vein to the knee joint
Divide the vein flush with the profunda vein to prevent blind stump thrombus
Evert the intima for valve excision
Distend under pressure and repair defects with 6-0 or 7-0 polypropylene
Use in nonreversed orientation to improve mismatch

their initial experience as requiring up fasciotomy of up to 17% of patients.[56] However, the need for fasciotomy in recent data is rare due to an increased tolerance leg swelling by the surgeons before performing fasciotomy.[57] Two preoperative predictors of a higher probability of fasciotomy were identified: concurrent harvesting of the greater saphenous vein in the same limb and a low ABI (<0.55) in the harvested limb. Prior harvest of the ipsilateral greater saphenous vein was not a risk factor for requiring a fasciotomy. Venous collaterals develop over time to normalize venous physiology in most patients, so long-term venous morbidity is minimal. One-third of patients experience mild chronic leg swelling, and the remainder are asymptomatic.[57] To our knowledge, no limbs have developed venous ulceration as a consequence of femoral vein harvest.

Cryopreserved Arterial Allografts

Experience with allograft replacement of primary or secondary arterial infections began with Alexis Carrel more than a century ago.[58] Difficulties with procurement and preservation resulted in poor-quality control. Allografts were largely abandoned until their resurrection for the treatment of infectious pathologies of the ascending aorta in the 1980s.[59] Initial positive experience resulted in more widespread use, including the treatment of infected infrarenal aortic graft infections.[49] Initially, local tissue banks were responsible for procuring, preserving, and allocating allografts for clinical use. This resulted in considerable variability in the processes of preparing and storing the product, which may have impacted the quality of the product. Currently, these processes have been centralized in both North America and Europe with primary suppliers of the cryopreserved allografts.

The primary advantage of cryopreserved allografts is its resistance to infection, while major disadvantages include cost (approximately $18,000 per aortoiliac segment), and that the grafts are not readily available at most centers or immediate use in urgent circumstances. Recent data suggests a high incidence of graft-related complications include restenosis, occlusion, pseudoaneurysm, and re-infection occurring at rates as high at 25% for any graft-related complication.[47] These complications should be considered when balancing the resistance to reinfection versus avoidance of graft-related complications.

Xenoprosthetic Grafts

Xenoprosthetic material such as bovine pericardium is often used in arterial repair using patches. This material can be reconstructed into tube or bifurcated tube grafts and used for aortic repair. Anibueze et al. report a 6-patient series of patients with infected aortic grafts or mycotic aneurysms repaired with bovine-reconstructed aortic grafts or patches with 100% freedom from reinfection or reintervention at 13 months.[51] Additionally a meta-analysis of xenoprosthetic aortic reconstruction showed high patency rates and re-infection rates, but is limited by long-term follow-up and lack or comparative data.[52]

Endografting as Bridge Therapy

Endografts are being used with increasing frequency as a method to temporize hemorrhage in patients with aortoenteric or aortobronchial fistulas.[30,31,60–62] When the anatomy permits, endografting may temporarily prevent exsanguination and allow time for resuscitation, medical stabilization, and further investigations to plan definitive surgery.[60] While earlier studies suggest that endografting should not be viewed as definitive therapy since recurrent hemorrhage occurs in majority of cases without further surgical treatment, often within 2 weeks,[30,61] additional studies suggest that in association with long-term antibiotics, this can be a definitive therapy in patients with short life expectancy (<6 months), while further surgical intervention should be planned for patients with longer life expectancy.[62] Some studies suggest endograft as definitive therapy. Sorelius et al. described 132 patients with mycotic abdominal aortic aneurysms, 77 of which were treated with endografts. They demonstrated improved short-term survival and 1-year survival for EVAR compared to open repair (96% vs. 74% and 84% vs. 73%). There were similar rates of infectious-related complications (24% vs. 18%) and reoperation (24% vs. 21%).[63] Patel et al. described TEVAR in conjunction with long-term antibiotics for infected thoracic aortic pathology in 27 high-risk patients. The short-term mortality was 11.5%, and 3-year survival was 57%.[64] These options expand our treatment options for aortic infection, especially in patients with high operative risk.

Aortic Infection with Sepsis

Sepsis caused by an aortic infection poses a challenge because temporizing with an endograft is not an option since the septic focus is not eliminated. In unstable patients, CT-guided percutaneous drainage may be a reasonable option for source control if there is a large perigraft fluid collection. In a series of 23 patients with graft infections, Belair et al. found that percutaneous drainage was associated with improved perioperative mortality, compared to surgery alone.[65] In the absence of a large perigraft fluid collection for percutaneous drainage, graft excision with extra-anatomic bypass is the most reasonable approach.

NONAORTIC ARTERIAL AND GRAFT INFECTIONS

Lower Extremity Arterial Infections

Lower Extremity Graft Infections

The nonoperative management of Szilagyi III wounds was described previously. Older studies show that lower extremity bypass graft infections carry a postoperative major amputation and mortality rate of nearly 50% due to the underlying atherosclerotic disease burden.[66] These patients often do not have other conduit suitable for bypass, which is a major impetus for graft preservation strategies for infected extremity bypass grafts. The use of local debridement with adjunctive vacuum-assisted closure and muscle flaps has yielded promising results. Siracuse cited an estimated 1-year limb salvage rate of 71%, which was attributed to the graft preservation techniques described above.[7]

Cryopreserved human allograft veins have been touted as an alternative if a prosthetic bypass graft must be removed for infection. Unfortunately, human allograft veins have yielded relatively poor results. In a series of bypasses for critical limb ischemia using cryopreserved greater saphenous vein, primary patency at 1 and 3 years was 27% and 17%, respectively.[67] Amputation-free survival at 1 and 3 years was 43% and 23%, respectively. Better results have been reported using cryopreserved human allograft arteries, especially when covered with muscle flaps. One series reported good long-term results with only 15% late conduit-related graft complications.[68] Cadaveric grafts are expensive, on the order of $5000–$10,000. In view of the outcomes and cost, the use of cryopreserved conduit must be weighed against the outcomes of graft preservation techniques on a case-by-case basis.

Extra-anatomic bypass is an alternative to avoid inguinal infections. Obturator bypass yields reasonable results with 60% to 83% survival with healed wounds beyond 3 years, and 70% to 80% 3-year patency.[69,70] Lateral femoral bypass also yielded good results with 95% survival and wound healing, 83% 2-year patency, and 93% limb salvage.[71]

Infected Common Femoral Artery Pseudoaneurysms

The management of infected common femoral artery pseudoaneurysms diverges from the management of infected pseudoaneurysms in other anatomic locations. The most frequent clinical scenarios involve infection after a history of recent arterial catheterization or intravenous drug abuse. The incidence of infection after cardiac catheterization is less than 1%, although the use of arterial closure device increases the risk due to the presence of a foreign body. Aggressive debridement, removal of the closure device, and revascularization remains the mainstays of therapy. In situ repair with autogenous greater saphenous or femoral vein is preferred if arterial replacement is necessary.[17] A rotational muscle flap may be necessary for graft coverage in some cases. Occasionally, in situ repair may not be advisable due to the quality of the arteries or the surrounding tissue. Ligation of the native arteries in the groin and an extra-anatomic bypass, such as an obturator bypass or lateral tunneling may be preferable.[70,71] Ligation of the common femoral artery without reconstruction is utilized as a last resort and is less likely to threaten the limb if the femoral bifurcation remains intact.[17]

Conversely, infected common femoral artery pseudoaneurysms secondary to intravenous drug abuse should be preferentially managed with aggressive arterial and soft tissue debridement and ligation of all of the involved arteries. Immune suppression due to malnutrition and human immune deficiency virus infections, delayed presentation, and patient recidivism make arterial reconstruction hazardous in this setting. Reddy showed that ligation of the common, superficial, and profunda femoral arteries is associated with a 33% major amputation rate.[72] Rates of major amputation are very low in other series, with some authors reporting 0% to 1% amputation rates in their series.[17] Claudication is common, however one group reported only 11% early claudication all of which resolved over time.[17]

Arterial Infections in Other Sites

Carotid patch infection is a rare, but dreaded occurrence. Management entails removal of the patch, wide debridement, and primary closure of the artery versus vein patch closure. Interposition grafting with autogenous vein is often necessary after the artery is debrided adequately. Occasionally ligation of a bleeding, infected artery is necessary as a life-saving intervention.[73] In a series of carotid patch infections, the stroke rate after debridement and reconstruction was 8.1% and increased to 14% when carotid ligation was necessary.[73] Endografting is an acceptable option to control hemorrhage and permit stabilization and evaluation for definitive surgery.[74]

Case reports and small case series of infected pseudoaneurysms of the superior mesenteric, celiac, and splenic arteries have been reported.[75,76] Treatment is individualized by the patient's comorbidities and anatomy. Infected visceral artery aneurysms are prone to rapid growth and rupture. The most common pathogens are streptococcus followed by staphylococcus.[75,76] Arteriography is often helpful to delineate the anatomic relationship of the aneurysms to nearby branch vessels and to define the quality of the collateral circulation. Excision, debridement, and arterial reconstruction with autogenous conduit remain the gold standard for infected pseudoaneurysms of main arterial trunks. Cryopreserved artery has also been described in the absence of autogenous conduit.[68] Resection and arterial ligation may be an option in some cases, depending on the anatomic location due the abundant collateral circulation between the mesenteric arteries and branches.[75] Coil embolization and long-term antibiotic therapy should be reserved for surgically inaccessible aneurysms, such as intrahepatic mycotic pseudoaneurysms, since coils may become infected.[76]

ANTIBIOTIC THERAPY

6 Unfortunately, there are no guidelines directing the type, dose, duration, or route of administration of antibiotics in treating arterial infections. This reflects the wide spectrum of causal organisms that are found in arterial graft infections, with approximately one-third of subjects having polymicrobial infections. Moreover, physician preference and patient tolerance of antibiotic regimens vary considerably. In addition, culture-directed therapy is not always possible since nearly 40% of patients have negative cultures, presumably due to preoperative broad-spectrum antibiotic therapy.[4] Finally, the consequences of a reinfection are dire, so there is a tendency among physicians to overprescribe antibiotics.

Initial broad-spectrum antibiotics should include agents with activity against gram-positive bacilli, gram-negative rods, and anaerobes, as these are the most prevalent organisms in graft infections. Currently our preferred combination therapy is vancomycin, piperacillin/tazobactam, and metronidazole. Blood cultures and graft and tissue cultures should be obtained to direct therapy. Recommendations for the duration of antibiotics vary widely, ranging from 2 weeks to 6 months after graft excision. If a graft or stent is not fully excised, indefinite antibiotic therapy should be considered. Fungal infections are particularly difficult to eradicate and may require the use of micafungin (FK463) due to the increasing incidence of resistance to fluconazole and its related molecules.[77]

PREVENTION OF SECONDARY ARTERIAL INFECTIONS

Meticulous surgical technique is critical to minimizing arterial graft infections. Judging from the microbial flora associated with graft infections, intraoperative contamination and surgical site infections are the most likely sources of contaminations that result in arterial graft infections. Adherence to all perioperative guidelines for reducing surgical site infections is important, but the use of prophylactic systemic antibiotics appears to be critically important. A recent meta-analysis and systematic review performed by Stewart concluded that prophylactic systemic antibiotics decreased the risk of wound and early graft infection for peripheral arterial reconstruction.[78] No benefit was seen in continuing antibiotics for greater than 24 hours, prophylactic rifampin bonding to the grafts, suction groin wound drainage, or preoperative bathing with or without antiseptic agents. Using guidelines for prosthetic heart valves, some authors suggest similar antibiotic prophylaxis in patients with aortic graft undergoing dental procedures.[79]

SUMMARY

7 Primary and secondary arterial infections constitute a myriad of some of the most technically, intellectually, and emotionally challenging cases that vascular surgeons may encounter in clinical practice. For aortic arterial infections, there is no consensus regarding the optimal method of in situ reconstruction. Autogenous vein reconstruction may be the most resistant to recurrent infection and most cost effective, but requires an additional, lengthy procedure for vein harvest. Reconstruction with either antibiotic- or silver-impregnated grafts may also be a reasonable alternative, but appears to have a higher rate of reinfection compared to the alternatives. Cryopreserved allografts have improved since their initial development, but are still hampered by a minority of hemorrhagic complications and pseudoaneurysmal degeneration. Moreover, cryopreserved allografts are considerably more expensive than the other alternatives. Extra-anatomic bypass remains a viable alternative for patients unable to undergo a more extensive operation. Endovascular stent grafts are excellent tools to stabilize patients with hemorrhagic complications of arterial infections prior to definitive surgery. Arterial infections in other locations utilize the same principles of wide excision and debridement, arterial reconstruction, and appropriate antibiotic coverage whenever technically feasible.

References

1. Salzler GG, Long B, Avgerinos ED, et al. Contemporary results of surgical management of peripheral mycotic aneurysms. *Ann Vasc Surg*. 2018;53:86–91.
2. Erb S, Sidler JA, Elzi L, et al. Surgical and antimicrobial treatment of prosthetic vascular graft infections at different surgical sites: a retrospective study of treatment outcomes. *PLoS One*. 2014;9(11):e112947.
3. Wilson SE, Van Wagenen P, Passaro E Jr. Arterial infection. *Curr Probl Surg*. 1978;15(9):1–89.
4. Miller DV, Oderich GS, Aubry MC, Panneton JM, Edwards WD. Surgical pathology of infected aneurysms of the descending thoracic and abdominal aorta: clinicopathologic correlations in 29 cases (1976 to 1999). *Hum Pathol*. 2004;35(9):1112–1120.
5. Shiraev T, Barrett S, Heywood S, et al. Incidence, management, and outcomes of aortic graft infection. *Ann Vasc Surg*. 2019;59:73–83.
6. Smeds MR, Duncan AA, Harlander-Locke MP, et al. Treatment and outcomes of aortic endograft infection. *J Vasc Surg*. 2016;63(2):332–340.
7. Siracuse JJ, Nandivada P, Giles K, et al. Prosthetic graft infections involving the femoral artery. *J Vasc Surg*. 2013;57(3):700–705.
8. Fatima J, Federico VP, Scali ST, et al. Management of patch infections after carotid endarterectomy and utility of femoral vein interposition bypass graft. *J Vasc Surg*. 2019;69(6):1815–1823.e1.
9. Brunstedt MR, Sapatnekar S, Rubin KR, et al. Bacterial/blood/material interactions. I. Injected and preseeded slime-forming Staphylococcus epidermidis in flowing blood with biomaterials. *J Biomed Mater Res*. 1995;29(4):455–466.
10. Bosman WM, Borger van der Burg BL, Schuttevaer HM, Thoma S, Hedeman Joosten PP. Infections of intravascular bare metal stents: a case report and review of literature. *Eur J Vasc Endovasc Surg*. 2014;47(1):87–99.
11. Nadzam GS, De La Cruz C, Greco RS, Haimovich B. Neutrophil adhesion to vascular prosthetic surfaces triggers nonapoptotic cell death. *Ann Surg*. 2000;231(4):587–599.
12. Muller BT, Wegener OR, Grabitz K, Pillny M, Thomas L, Sandmann W. Mycotic aneurysms of the thoracic and abdominal aorta and iliac arteries: experience with anatomic and extra-anatomic repair in 33 cases. *J Vasc Surg*. 2001;33(1):106–113.
13. Ravindra A, Naguthevar S, Kumar D, et al. Mycotic aneurysms: uncommon pathogens and treatment conundrums. *Access Microbiol*. 2024;6(8):000777.v5.
14. Kalchev Y, Urdzhanova H, Stanev S, et al. Yersinia enterocolitica bacteremia associated with a ruptured abdominal aortic aneurysm: a case report with literature review. *Microorganisms*. 2023;11(12):2911.
15. Tshomba Y, Sica S, Minelli F, et al. Management of mycotic aorto-iliac aneurysms: a 30-year monocentric experience. *Eur Rev Med Pharmacol Sci*. 2020;24(6):3274–3281.
16. Bell CL, Ali AT, Brawley JG, et al. Arterial reconstruction of infected femoral artery pseudoaneurysms using superficial femoral-popliteal vein. *J Am Coll Surg*. 2005;200(6):831–836.
17. Qiu J, Zhou W, Zhou W, et al. The treatment of infected femoral artery pseudoaneurysms secondary to drug abuse: 11 years of experience at a single institution. *Ann Vasc Surg*. 2016;36:35–43.
18. Ben Ahmed S, Louvancourt A, Daniel G, et al. Cryopreserved arterial allografts for in situ reconstruction of abdominal aortic native or secondary graft infection. *J Vasc Surg*. 2018;67(2):468–477.
19. Dorweiler B, Neufang A, Chaban R, Reinstadler J, Duenschede F, Vahl CF. Use and durability of femoral vein for autologous reconstruction with infection of the aortoiliofemoral axis. *J Vasc Surg*. 2014;59(3):675–683.
20. Szilagyi DE, Smith RF, Elliott JP, Vrandecic MP. Infection in arterial reconstruction with synthetic grafts. *Ann Surg*. 1972;176(3):321–333.
21. Samson RH, Vieth FJ, Janko GS, Gupta SK, Scher LA. A modified classification and approach to the management of infections involving peripheral arterial prosthetic grafts. *J Vasc Surg*. 1988;8(2):147–153.
22. Bunt TJ. Synthetic vascular graft infections. I. Graft infections. *Surgery*. 1983;93(6):733–746.
23. Lyons OT, Baguneid M, Barwick TD, et al. Diagnosis of aortic graft infection: a case definition by the Management of Aortic Graft Infection Collaboration (MAGIC). *Eur J Vasc Endovasc Surg*. 2016;52(6):758–763.
24. Lehman B, Miller RM, Richter SS, et al. Clostridium septicum-infected aortic aneurysm or graft is a deadly diagnosis. *J Vasc Surg*. 2020;71(5):1781–1788.
25. Seabrook GR, Schmitt DD, Bandyk DF, Edmiston CE, Krepel CJ, Towne JB. Anastomotic femoral pseudoaneurysm: an investigation of occult infection as an etiologic factor. *J Vasc Surg*. 1990;11(5):629–634.
26. Mertens RA, O'Hara PJ, Hertzer NR, Krajewski LP, Beven EG. Surgical management of infrainguinal arterial prosthetic graft infections: review of a thirty-five-year experience. *J Vasc Surg*. 1995;21(5):782–791.
27. Brothers TE, Robison JG, Elliott BM. Predictors of prosthetic graft infection after infrainguinal bypass. *J Am Coll Surg*. 2009;208(4):557–561.
28. Shenouda M, Molena E, Maftei N, Ali T. Remnant prosthetic graft in revision or limb-salvage surgery: routine complete excision? *Ann Vasc Surg*. 2014;28(6):1566.e11–1566.e15.
29. Rodrigues dos Santos C, Casaca R, Crespo Mendes de Almeida J, Mendes-Pedro L. Enteric repair in aortoduodenal fistulas: a forgotten but often lethal player. *Ann Vasc Surg*. 2014;28(3):756–762.
30. Jonker FH, Heijman R, Trimarchi S, Verhagen HJ, Moll FL, Muhs BE. Acute management of aortobronchial and aortoesophageal fistulas using thoracic endovascular aortic repair. *J Vasc Surg*. 2009;50(5):999–1004.
31. Antoniou GA, Koutsias S, Antoniou SA, Georgiakakis A, Lazarides MK, Giannoukas AD. Outcome after endovascular stent graft repair of aortoenteric fistula: a systematic review. *J Vasc Surg*. 2009;49(3):782–789.
32. Lawlor DK, DeRose G, Harris KA, Forbes TL. Primary aorto/iliac-enteric fistula—report of 6 new cases. *Vasc Endovascular Surg*. 2004;38(3):281–286.
33. Hallett JW Jr, Marshall DM, Petterson TM, et al. Graft-related complications after abdominal aortic aneurysm repair: reassurance from a 36-year population-based experience. *J Vasc Surg*. 1997;25(2):277–284.

34. Wright DJ, Earnst CB, Evans JR, et al. Ureteral complications and aortoiliac reconstruction. *J Vasc Surg*. 1990;11(1):29–35.
35. Lauri C, Campagna G, Aloisi F, Posa A, et al. How to combine CTA, (99m)Tc-WBC SPECT/CT, and [(18)F]FDG PET/CT in patients with suspected abdominal vascular endograft infections? *Eur J Nucl Med Mol Imaging*. 2023;50(11):3235–3250.
36. Mitra A, Pencharz D, Davis M, Wagner T. Determining the diagnostic value of 18F-fluorodeoxyglucose positron emission/computed tomography in detecting prosthetic aortic graft infection. *Ann Vasc Surg*. 2018;53:78–85.
37. Hsu RB, Chang CI, Wu IH, Lin FY. Selective medical treatment of infected aneurysms of the aorta in high risk patients. *J Vasc Surg*. 2009;49(1):66–70.
38. Calligaro KD, Veith FJ, Schwartz ML, et al. Selective preservation of infected prosthetic arterial grafts. analysis of a 20-year experience with 120 extracavitary-infected grafts. *Ann Surg*. 1994;220(4):461–471.
39. Dosluoglu HH, Loghmanee C, Lall P, Cherr GS, Harris LM, Dryjski ML. Management of early (<30 day) vascular groin infections using vacuum-assisted closure alone without muscle flap coverage in a consecutive patient series. *J Vasc Surg*. 2010;51(5):1160–1166.
40. Berger P, de Bie D, Moll FL, de Borst GJ. Negative pressure wound therapy on exposed prosthetic vascular grafts in the groin. *J Vasc Surg*. 2012;56(3):714–720.
41. Calligaro KD, Veith FJ, Yuan JG, et al. Intra-abdominal aortic graft infection: complete or partial graft preservation in patients at very high risk. *J Vasc Surg*. 2003;38(6):1199–1205.
42. Stone PA, Armstrong PA, Bandyk DF, et al. Use of antibiotic-loaded polymethylmethacrylate beads for the treatment of extracavitary prosthetic vascular graft infections. *J Vasc Surg*. 2006;44(4):757–761.
43. Caradu C, Puges M, Cazanave C, et al.; Imperial Vascular Unit and the University Hospital of Bordeaux Vascular Unit. Outcomes of patients with aortic vascular graft and endograft infections initially contra-indicated for complete graft explantation. *J Vasc Surg*. 2022;76(5):1364–1373.e3.
44. Fleisher LA, Beckman JA, Brown KA, et al. ACC/AHA 2007 guidelines on perioperative cardiovascular evaluation and care for noncardiac surgery: a report of the American College of Cardiology/American Heart Association Task Force on Practice guidelines (writing committee to revise the 2002 guidelines on perioperative cardiovascular evaluation for noncardiac surgery). *Circulation*. 2007;116(17):e418–e500.
45. Reilly LM, Stoney RJ, Goldstone J, Ehrenfeld WK. Improved management of aortic graft infection: the influence of operation sequence and staging. *J Vasc Surg*. 1987;5(3):421–431.
46. Seeger JM, Pretus HA, Welborn MB, Ozaki CK, Flynn TC, Huber TS. Long-term outcome after treatment of aortic graft infection with staged extra-anatomic bypass grafting and aortic graft removal. *J Vasc Surg*. 2000;32(3):451–459.
47. Batt M, Feugier P, Camou F, et al. A meta-analysis of outcomes after in situ reconstructions for aortic graft infection. *Angiology*. 2018;69(5):370–379.
48. Clagett GP, Bowers BL, Lopez-Viego MA, et al. Creation of a neo-aortoiliac system from lower extremity deep and superficial veins. *Ann Surg*. 1993;218(3):239–248; discussion 248–249.
49. Kieffer E, Bahnini A, Koskas F, Ruotolo C, Le Blevec D, Plissonnier D. In situ allograft replacement of infected infrarenal aortic prosthetic grafts: results in forty-three patients. *J Vasc Surg*. 1993;17(2):349–356.
50. Oderich GS, Bower TC, Hofer J, et al. In situ rifampin-soaked grafts with omental coverage and antibiotic suppression are durable with low reinfection rates in patients with aortic graft enteric erosion or fistula. *J Vasc Surg*. 2011;53(1):99–107.
51. Anibueze C, Sankaran V, Sadat U, et al. Neoaortic xenoprosthetic grafts for treatment of mycotic aneurysms and infected aortic grafts. *Ann Vasc Surg*. 2017;44:419.e1-419.e12.
52. Grills S, El-Diaz N, Walker-Jacobs A, Borucki J, Stather P. Outcomes following use of bovine pericardium (xenoprosthetic) grafts for reconstruction of mycotic aortic aneurysms and infected aortic grafts: a systematic review and meta-analysis. *Ann Vasc Surg*. 2024;102:181–191.
53. Oderich GS, Bower TC, Cherry KJ Jr, et al. Evolution from axillofemoral to in situ prosthetic reconstruction for the treatment of aortic graft infections at a single center. *J Vasc Surg*. 2006;43(6):1166–1174.
54. Mei L, Lu Z, Zhang X, Li C, Jia Y. Polymer-Ag nanocomposites with enhanced antimicrobial activity against bacterial infection. *ACS Appl Mater Interfaces*. 2014;6(18):15813–15821.
55. Valentine RJ, Clagett GP. Aortic graft infections: replacement with autogenous vein. *Cardiovasc Surg*. 2001;9(5):419–425.
56. Modrall JG, Sadjadi J, Ali AT, et al. Deep vein harvest: predicting need for fasciotomy. *J Vasc Surg*. 2004;39(2):387–394.
57. Modrall JG, Hocking JA, Timaran CH, et al. Late incidence of chronic venous insufficiency after deep vein harvest. *J Vasc Surg*. 2007;46(3):520–525; discussion 525.
58. Carrel A. Ultimate result of aortic transplantation. *J Exp Med*. 1912;15:389–398.
59. Zwischenberger JB, Shalaby TZ, Conti VR. Viable cryopreserved aortic homograft for aortic valve endocarditis and annular abscesses. *Ann Thorac Surg*. 1989;48(3):365–370.
60. Marone EM, Mascia D, Kahlberg A, Tshomba Y, Chiesa R. Emergent endovascular treatment of a bleeding recurrent aortoenteric fistula as a "bridge" to definitive surgical repair. *J Vasc Surg*. 2012;55(4):1160–1163.
61. Leonhardt H, Mellander S, Snygg J, Lönn L. Endovascular management of acute bleeding arterioenteric fistulas. *Cardiovasc Intervent Radiol*. 2008;31(3):542–549.
62. Haidar GM, Hicks TD, Strosberg DS, El-Sayed HF, Davies MG. "In situ" endografting in the treatment of arterial and graft infections. *J Vasc Surg*. 2017;65(6):1824–1829.
63. Sorelius K, Wanhainen A, Furebring M, et al. Nationwide study of the treatment of mycotic abdominal aortic aneurysms comparing open and endovascular repair. *Circulation*. 2016;134(23):1822–1832.
64. Patel HJ, Williams DM, Upchurch GR Jr, Dasika NL, Eliason JL, Deeb GM. Thoracic aortic endovascular repair for mycotic aneurysms and fistulas. *J Vasc Surg*. 2010;52(4):37S–40S.
65. Belair M, Soulez G, Oliva VL, et al. Aortic graft infection: the value of percutaneous drainage. *AJR Am J Roentgenol*. 1998;171(1):119–124.
66. Edwards WH Jr, Martin RS 3rd, Jenkins JM, Edwards WH Sr, Mulherin JL Jr. Primary graft infections. *J Vasc Surg*. 1987;6(3):235–239.
67. Chang CK, Scali ST, Feezor RJ, et al. Defining utility and predicting outcome of cadaveric lower extremity bypass grafts in patients with critical limb ischemia. *J Vasc Surg*. 2014;60(6):1554–1564.
68. Furlough CL, Jain AK, Ho KJ, Rodriguez HE, Tomita TM, Eskandari MK. Peripheral artery reconstructions using cryopreserved arterial allografts in infected fields. *J Vasc Surg*. 2019;70(2):562–568.
69. Patel A, Taylor SM, Langan EM 3rd, et al. Obdurator bypass: a classic approach for the treatment of contemporary groin infection. *Am Surg*. 2002;68(8):653–658.
70. Masaki H, Tabuchi A, Yunoki Y, et al. Long-term results of obturator bypass. *Ann Vasc Dis*. 2016;9(2):80–84.
71. Madden NJ, Calligaro KD, Dougherty MJ, Zheng H, Troutman DA. Lateral femoral bypass for prosthetic arterial graft infections in the groin. *J Vasc Surg*. 2019;69(4):1129–1136.
72. Arora S, Weber MA, Fox CJ, Neville R, Lidor A, Sidawy AN. Common femoral artery ligation and local debridement: a safe treatment for infected femoral artery pseudoaneurysms. *J Vasc Surg*. 2001;33(5):990–993.
73. Mann CD, McCarthy M, Nasim A, et al. Management and outcome of prosthetic patch infection after carotid endarterectomy: a single-centre series and systematic review of the literature. *Eur J Vasc Endovasc Surg*. 2012;44(1):20–26.
74. Sorial E, Valentino J, Given CA, Endean ED, Minion DJ. The emergency use of endografts in the carotid bifurcation to control hemorrhage in potentially contaminated fields. *J Vasc Surg*. 2007;46(4):792–798.

75. Kordzadeh A, Watson J, Panayiotopolous YP. Mycotic aneurysm of the superior and inferior mesenteric artery. *J Vasc Surg.* 2016;63(6):1638–1646.
76. Georges RN, Lipman S, Silvestri F, Sussman B, Dardik H. Endovascular treatment of mycotic hepatic artery aneurysm in the hostile abdomen—a case report. *J Vasc Surg.* 2001;35(6):477–481.
77. Ramirez M, Serran C, Castro C, et al. Comparative study of disc diffusion and microdilution methods in susceptibility testing of micafungin against Candida species. *J Antimicrob Chemother.* 2006;58(4):861–863.
78. Stewart AH, Eyers PS, Earnshaw JJ. Prevention of infection in peripheral arterial reconstruction: a systematic review and meta-analysis. *J Vasc Surg.* 2007;46(1):148–155.
79. Habib G, Lancellotti P, Antunes MJ, et al.; ESC Scientific Document Group 2015 ESC Guidelines for the management of infective endocarditis: The Task Force for the Management of Infective Endocarditis of the European Society of Cardiology (ESC). Endorsed by: European Association for Cardio-Thoracic Surgery (EACTS), the European Association of Nuclear Medicine (EANM). *Eur Heart J.* 2015;36(44):3075–3128.

84

Cerebrovascular Disease

Mahmoud B. Malas and Omar Al-Nouri

Key Points

1. Stroke is the fifth leading cause of death in the United States, worldwide stroke continues to be one of the most common causes of death and disability.
2. Aggressive risk factor modification is imperative in all patients with atherosclerotic cerebrovascular disease.
3. Stroke remains the leading cause of disability in the United States and costs an estimated $34 billion each year.
4. Duplex ultrasonography remains an invaluable tool in the diagnosis of significant carotid artery atherosclerotic disease.
5. The preferred management of symptomatic and severe asymptomatic carotid artery disease is surgical intervention over medical therapy alone.
6. Transcarotid artery revascularization (TCAR), with its carotid endarterectomy (CEA)-like protective qualities, should be preferred over transfemoral carotid artery stenting (TFCAS) in select patients not candidates for CEA.
7. Endovascular management of proximal vertebral artery atherosclerotic lesions has been shown to be safe and effective in small nonrandomized trials, but further studies are needed to sufficiently assess its efficacy.
8. Open surgical correction of brachiocephalic occlusive atherosclerotic disease should be preferred over endovascular management.

Stroke continues to be a common cause of disability and death, accounting for the fifth leading cause of death in the United States.[1] Stroke disability can be debilitating, even more so than that of a myocardial infarction (MI). Quality-of-life sub-analysis of the Carotid Revascularization Endarterectomy versus Stenting Trial (CREST)[2] among 1-year survivors indicates that stroke has greater adverse effect on a broad range of health-status domains than did an MI. Permanent disability from a stroke can lead to blindness, weakness, paralysis, or aphasia. Transient ischemic attacks (TIAs) have symptoms that last <24 hours and manifest similarly, albeit without long-term sequelae. These sequelae have long-lasting social and financial burdens not only on patients and families, but on the health care system as well.

There are a multitude of etiologies leading to stroke, with many modifiable risk factors. Some of the most common risk factors include hypertension, diabetes, hypercholesterolemia, obesity, genetics, and smoking. Eighty-five percent of all strokes are thought to be ischemic, whereas only 15% are embolic. Atherosclerotic plaque is the most common and important underlying pathology leading to ischemic strokes.[3] Since the first successful carotid endarterectomy (CEA) in 1953 by Michael DeBakey, carotid revascularization has been shown in multiple randomized clinical trials to decrease the risk of ipsilateral ischemic strokes. Minimally invasive endovascular techniques such as transfemoral carotid artery stenting (TFCAS) and transcarotid artery revascularization (TCAR) have been introduced as alternative options in patients who are high risk for CEA. However, CEA remains the gold standard option for symptomatic carotid artery stenosis. Ongoing randomized trials comparing surgical, endovascular, and medical management of asymptomatic carotid artery occlusive disease are highly anticipated.

Vertebrobasilar insufficiency (VBI) can be a much more difficult diagnosis to obtain as compared to atherosclerotic carotid artery disease. Symptoms are often vague and are easily confused with other diagnoses. These symptoms are more likely posterior circulation symptoms that include diplopia, vertigo, drop attacks, and headaches. Traditional treatment for true VBI was open surgical treatment of the ostial vertebral artery atherosclerotic occlusive disease. Endovascular repair with balloon angioplasty and/or stenting is an attractive option; however, outcomes have not been extensively evaluated.

Atherosclerotic brachiocephalic occlusive disease typically involves the origins of the great vessels. Symptoms may be similar to atherosclerotic carotid stenosis including amaurosis, TIA, and stroke, but also can include arm fatigue and weakness. Again, traditional treatment has been open surgical repair with transthoracic repair versus extra-anatomic bypass. Endovascular management with angioplasty and stenting has also been advocated for this disease entity, but experience is limited.

This chapter provides a comprehensive review of the epidemiology, pathophysiology, diagnosis, treatment, and controversies in management of atherosclerotic and nonatherosclerotic carotid artery disease, as well as VBI and brachiocephalic occlusive disease.

ATHEROSCLEROTIC CAROTID ARTERY DISEASE

Epidemiology

1 Worldwide, stroke continues to be one of the most common causes of mortality and disability. One in six people worldwide will have a stroke in their lifetime. Fifteen million people worldwide suffer a stroke each year and 5.8 million people die from it.[4] Despite the decreasing incidence in the United States, annual incidence of new or recurrent stroke is 795,000, of which 610,000 are first or new strokes.[5] Stroke prevalence is linked to patients' age, as older Americans over the age of 65 have a much

higher prevalence as compared to Americans aged 18 to 44 years (8.4% vs 0.7%).[6] Race also seems to play a role in stroke, as whites have a lower incidence of stroke when compared to blacks and Hispanics.[7] Stroke rates also vary by region in the United States, with the southeastern United States with higher incidence of stroke hospitalization rates as compared to the western United States. Stroke deaths, however, have been on the decline in the United States over the past few decades. This decrease in stroke mortality can be attributed to improvement in acute stroke care with the advent of intraarterial thromboly-
2 sis and endovascular mechanical thrombectomy.[8] Improved recognition of the importance of medical management with statin and antiplatelet agents certainly has played a role as well. Despite the decreasing mortality and the earlier recognition of acute stroke symptoms and the timely use of acute stroke thera-
3 pies, stroke remains the leading cause of disability in the United States and costs an estimated $34 billion each year. Risk factors for stroke include age over 55, male sex, hypertension, family history, atrial fibrillation, hypercholesterolemia, renal insufficiency, obesity, diet, diabetes, smoking, and alcohol use.

Pathogenesis of Stroke

Cerebrovascular accidents (CVAs) in the United States are overwhelmingly related to ischemia (87%), whereas intracerebral and subarachnoid hemorrhage account for 10% and 3%, respectively.[9] Carotid atherosclerotic disease may cause a stroke in a variety of ways. Most commonly, unstable plaque embolization to the middle or anterior cerebral artery will cause TIA or stroke. Rarely, reduced flow through a highly stenotic extracranial carotid artery may cause cerebral hypoperfusion in patients with poor cerebral collaterals, resulting in stroke. In addition, acute thrombosis causing in situ obstruction from atherosclerosis, dissection, or fibromuscular dysplasia (FMD) is also a possible etiology for CVA.

Patients at highest risk for TIA or stroke are those with greater than 80% carotid artery stenosis secondary to soft, echolucent plaque or those whose plaque progresses from less than 80% to greater than 80% during a follow-up period.[10] These fibrous plaques will continue to have infiltration of lipids into the arterial wall, leading to inflammation and infiltration of macrophages, which leads to lysis of proteolytic enzymes, resulting in necrotic debris.[11] This can result in an unstable plaque that leads to intraplaque hemorrhage and rupture of the fibrous cap causing immediate embolization (**Fig. 84.1**). Once this embolization event occurs, the resulting ulcer will act as a nidus for the accumulation of platelet aggregates and other thrombotic debris, thereby putting the

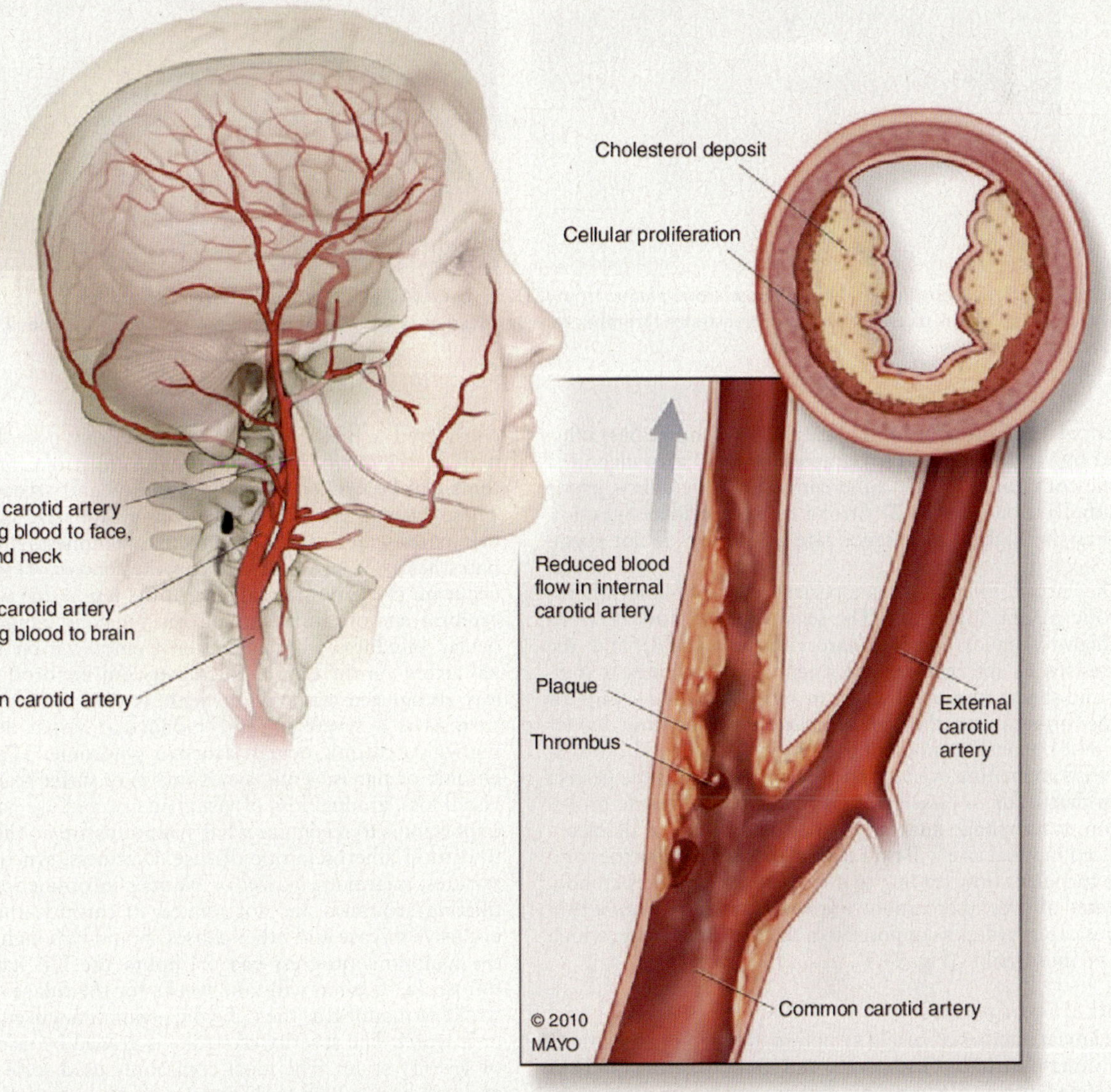

Figure 84.1. Stroke caused by carotid atherosclerotic disease is usually caused by atheroemboli from the internal carotid artery. As shown, the majority of the anterior cerebral circulation comes from the internal carotid artery. As increasing carotid stenosis occurs, flow becomes more turbulent and carotid plaque can become more unstable, increasing the risk of atheroembolization.

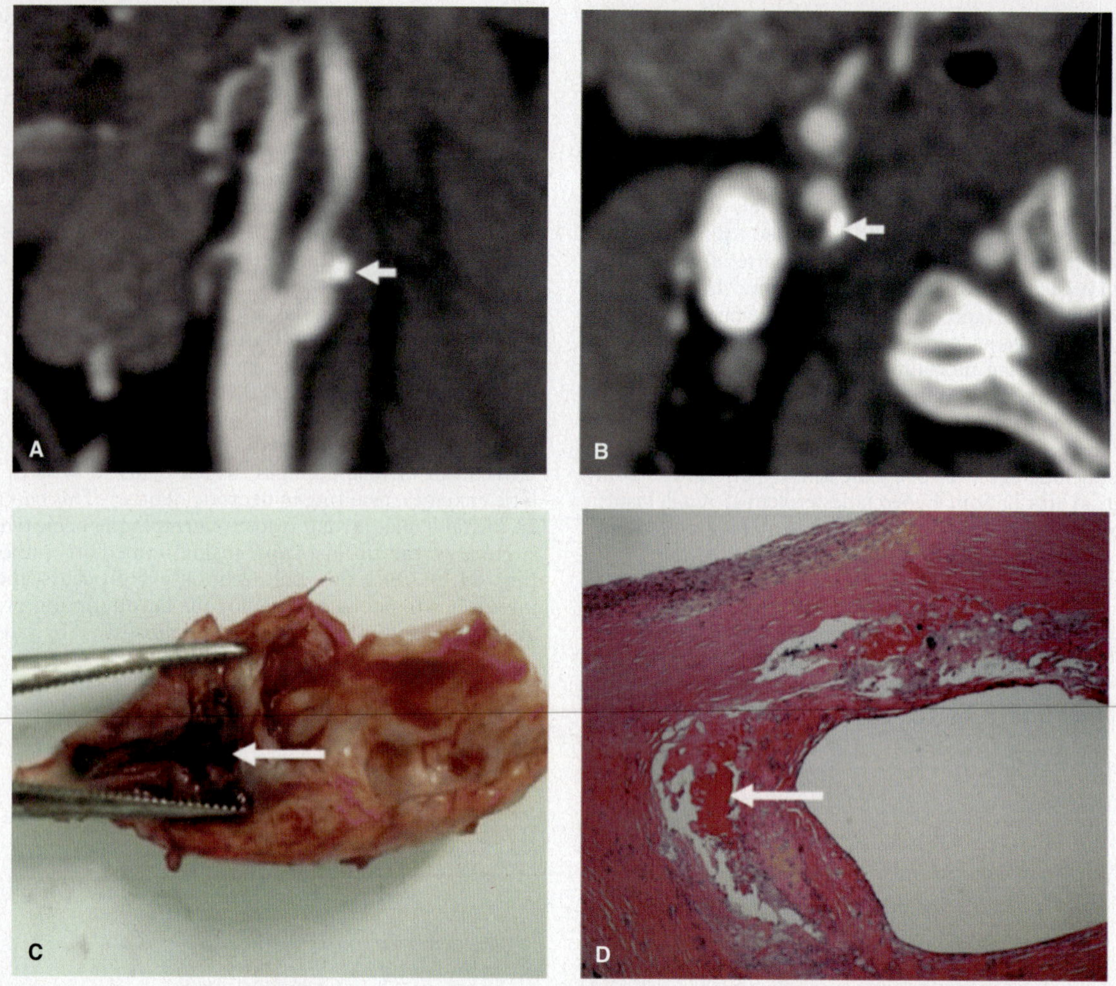

Figure 84.2. Panel showing unstable atherosclerotic plaque from CTA in figure (**A**) and (**B**) to endarterectomy specimen in (**C**). **D:** (*arrows*) Photomicrograph of this ulcerated plaque demonstrates thrombus loosely adherent to the wall of the plaque, showing why embolization is very much a certainty in these cases.

patient at risk for further embolization. This can be best illustrated by viewing photomicrographic images of an ulcerated plaque containing loosely adherent thrombotic debris prone to embolization (**Fig. 84.2**). Stroke from carotid vessel etiology has the highest recurrence rate at 30 days if not surgically treated.[12]

The carotid bifurcation is especially susceptible to atherosclerotic plaque formation. The separation of flow between the high-resistance external carotid artery (ECA) and the low-resistance internal carotid artery (ICA), creates a low-flow and shear stress area, where turbulent flow is a set up for plaque formation on the walls opposite from the flow divider (**Fig. 84.3**). Constant nonlaminar flow at the carotid bifurcation with an inciting event, such as intimal injury, is the perfect storm that leads to platelet deposition, smooth muscle proliferation, macrophage infiltration and loss of luminal diameter. Reduced luminal size will thus lead to increasing velocities and more turbulent flow leading to increased risk of atheroemboli. As stated above, atheroemboli are more common when a thin fibrous cap ruptures as opposed to a thicker fibrous cap, which may be more stable (**Fig. 84.4**).

Clinical Syndromes

The clinical manifestations of symptomatic carotid atherosclerotic disease include TIA, stroke, and amaurosis fugax. TIAs are defined as neurologic events that are sudden in onset without a preceding aura and last less than 24 hours in duration. Patients return to their baseline neurologic function, which usually occurs within minutes of the inciting event. These are considered a precursor to a more serious neurologic event, with a large number that will progress to stroke. Stroke symptoms can be broken down into motor and sensory changes. These include dysarthria, dysphasia, aphasia, monoparesis, hemiparesis, hemiplegia, monocular blindness, numbness, or paresthesias. When related to carotid stenosis, these symptoms occur on the contralateral side of the lesion due to ipsilateral cerebral embolization. Amaurosis fugax is temporary monocular blindness from cholesterol embolization to the retinal artery via the ophthalmic artery. An important, but often less recognized association with critical ipsilateral carotid stenosis is a severe chronic monocular visual deterioration known as chronic ocular ischemic syndrome.[13] Patients with chronic ocular ischemic syndrome may suffer from transient visual loss, gradual loss of visual acuity, and eye pain. Equally important is to recognize what symptoms are not likely related to carotid atherosclerotic disease. Dizziness, syncope, vertigo, seizures, migraines, bowel or bladder incontinence, and scintillating scotomas are not related to carotid atherosclerotic occlusive disease and other causes should be sought out. Once the symptoms progress past 24 hours, the TIA has become a full stroke. It often will take weeks for the full severity of the stroke to manifest as the ischemic penumbra will either recover or it won't. The severity of stroke is graded by using a variety of severity scales. The most commonly used scale is that formulated by the National Institute of Neurologic Disease and Stroke (NINDS) of the National Institutes of Health (NIH). The NIH stroke scale yields a numeric score of 0 to 42 and can be used at the initial neurologic event and then throughout the

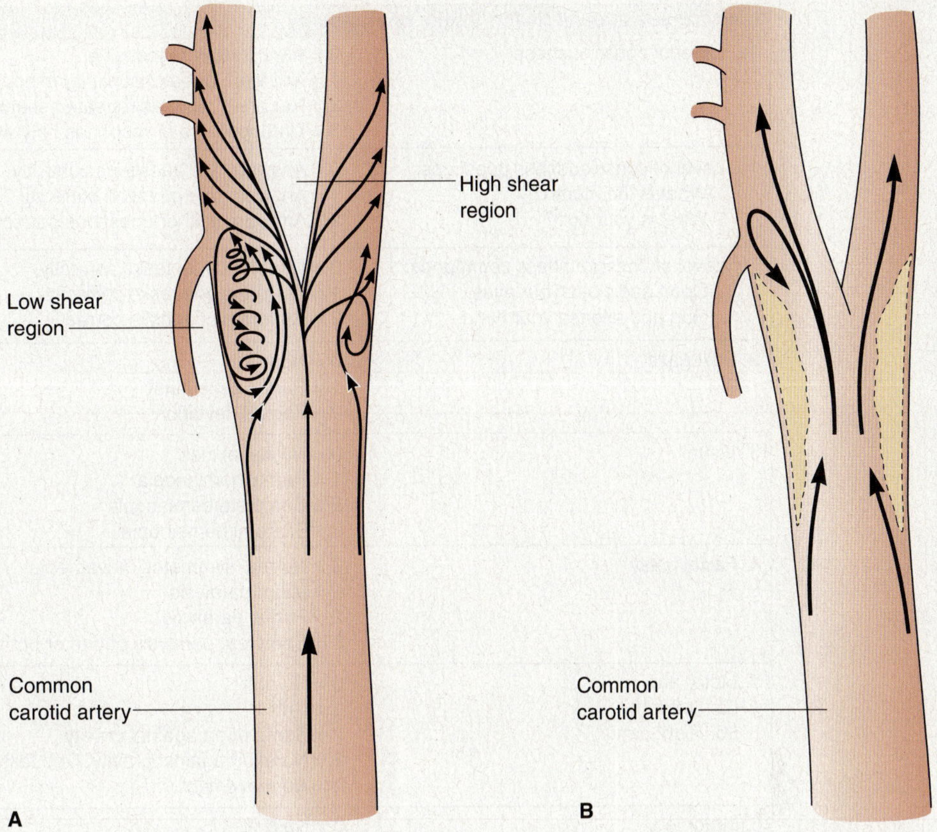

Figure 84.3. A: Carotid bifurcation represents an area of low-flow velocity and shear stress. As blood circulates, this is a separation of flow between the low-resistance internal carotid artery and the high-resistance external carotid artery. B: Atherosclerotic plaque typically forms in the outer wall opposite the flow divider due in part to the low shear stress.

evolution of the stroke to help map out the patient's clinical course (**Fig. 84.5**). A score of 5 or lower is considered a mild stroke; a score of 6 to 20, moderate stroke; and a score higher than 20 represents a severe stroke.

Initial Diagnostic Evaluation

Carotid atherosclerotic disease may be a difficult clinical diagnosis to obtain prior to the onset of neurologic symptoms. Physical examination in asymptomatic carotid atherosclerotic disease is limited to auscultation of a carotid bruit. Auscultation of a carotid bruit was once considered a part of the standard cardiovascular examination. Even though the auscultation may be an effective method for selecting further diagnostic tests, studies have shown that the sensitivity and positive predictive value are low for a carotid bruit detecting severe carotid stenosis.[14] The primary diagnostic tool for detection of hemo-
4 dynamically significant carotid stenosis is duplex ultrasonography (DUS). The benefits of DUS include excellent sensitivity and specificity (especially for high-grade carotid stenosis), low cost, rapid availability, and ease of evaluation and avoidance of radiation. Decisions on carotid intervention are often solely based on information provided by the DUS. The severity of carotid stenosis is determined by measuring the peak systolic velocity (PSV), end-diastolic velocity (EDV), and the ratio of the PSV of the ICA to common carotid artery (ICA/CCA) (**Fig. 84.6**). There are two major DUS criteria for determination of carotid

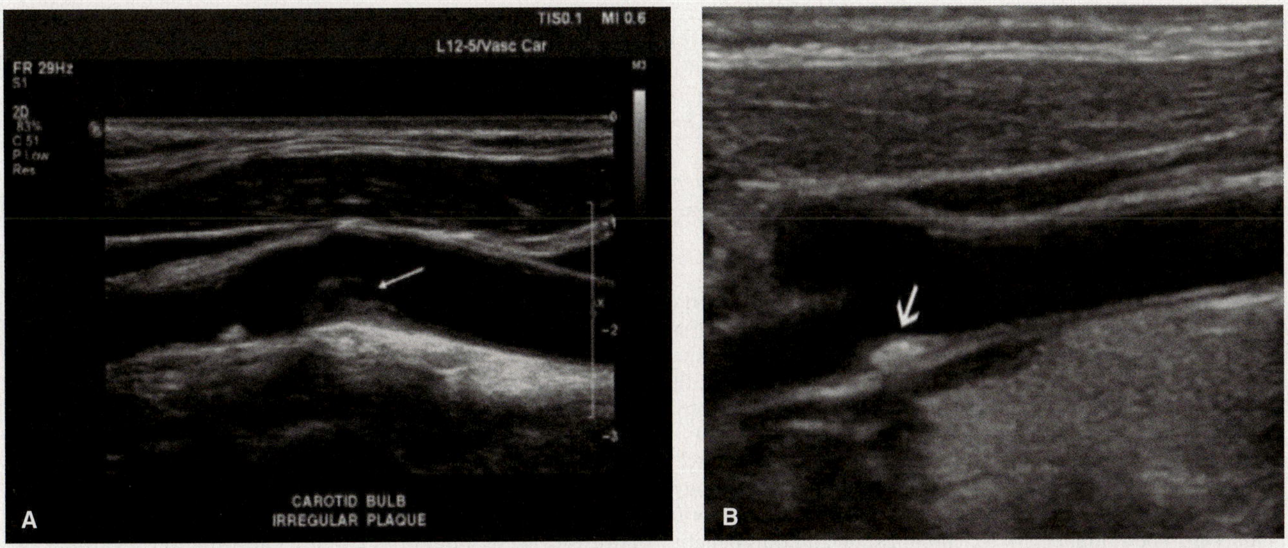

Figure 84.4. A: Duplex ultrasound showing unstable, hypoechoic plaque that is at high-risk for embolization. B: Duplex ultrasound showing stable plaque with thickened cap, less likely to cause atheroemboli.

National Institutes of Health Stroke Scale score	
1a. Level of consciousness	0 = Alert; keenly responsive 1 = Not alert, but arousable by minor stimulation 2 = Not alert; requires repeated stimulation 3 = Unresponsive or responds only with reflex
1b. Level of consciousness questions: What is the month? What is your age?	0 = Answers two questions correctly 1 = Answers one question correctly 2 = Answers neither questions correctly
1c. Level of consciousness commands: Open and close your eyes. Grip and release your hand.	0 = Performs both tasks correctly 1 = Performs one tasks correctly 2 = Performs one tasks correctly
2. Best gaze	0 = Normal 1 = Partial gaze palsy 2 = Forced deviation
3. Visual	0 = No visual loss 1 = Partial hemianopia 2 = Complete hemianopia 3 = Bilateral hemianopia
4. Facial palsy	0 = Normal symmetric movements 1 = Minor paralysis 2 = Partial paralysis 3 = Complete paralysis of one or both sides
5. Motor arm 5a. Left arm 5b. Right arm	0 = No drift 1 = Drift 2 = Some effort against gravity 3 = No effort against gravity; limb falls 4 = No movement
6. Motor leg 6a. Left leg 6b. Right leg	0 = No drift 1 = Drift 2 = Some effort against gravity 3 = No effort against gravity 4 = No movement
7. Limb ataxia	0 = Absent 1 = Present in one limb 2 = Present in two limbs
8. Sensory	0 = Normal; no sensory loss 1 = Mild-to-moderate sensory loss 2 = Severe to total sensory loss
9. Best language	0 = No aphasia; normal 1 = Mild to moderate aphasia 2 = Severe aphasia 3 = Mute, global aphasia
10. Dysarthria	0 = Normal 1 = Mild to moderate dysarthria 2 = Severe dysarthria
11. Extinction and inattention	0 = No abnormality 1 = Visual, tactile, auditory, spatial, or personal inattention 2 = Profound hemi-inattention or extinction
Total score = 0–42.	

Figure 84.5. NIH stroke scale scoring from 0 (no deficit) to 42 (most severe deficits in all areas).

stenosis, modified University of Washington (UW) criteria (**Table 84.1**) and the Carotid Consensus Panel duplex Criteria (CCPC) (**Table 84.2**). Recent studies have shown that the CCPC criteria demonstrate a higher corroboration rate with measurements taken from computed tomography angiography (CTA) and may be more sensitive in classifying clinically significant stenosis and preventing unnecessary extra surveillance.[15] DUS can also give information regarding plaque morphology and aid surgeons in deciding which carotid atherosclerotic plaques may be at higher risk for embolization and thus benefit from carotid intervention. Despite the many benefits for initial use of DUS, there are few limitations related to operator experience, inability to visualize high carotid bifurcations, dampened waveforms due to proximal CCA lesions, excessive calcification causing acoustic shadowing, and inability to accurately measuring velocities.

The need for corroborative imaging is sometimes necessary for initial diagnosis and to help plan possible operative intervention. Improvements in technology and acquisition times have made magnetic resonance angiography (MRA) and CTA attractive options for diagnosis of carotid atherosclerotic disease. These modalities can give information regarding the aortic arch, tortuosity, any anomalous anatomy, presence of brachiocephalic disease or proximal CCA disease, location of

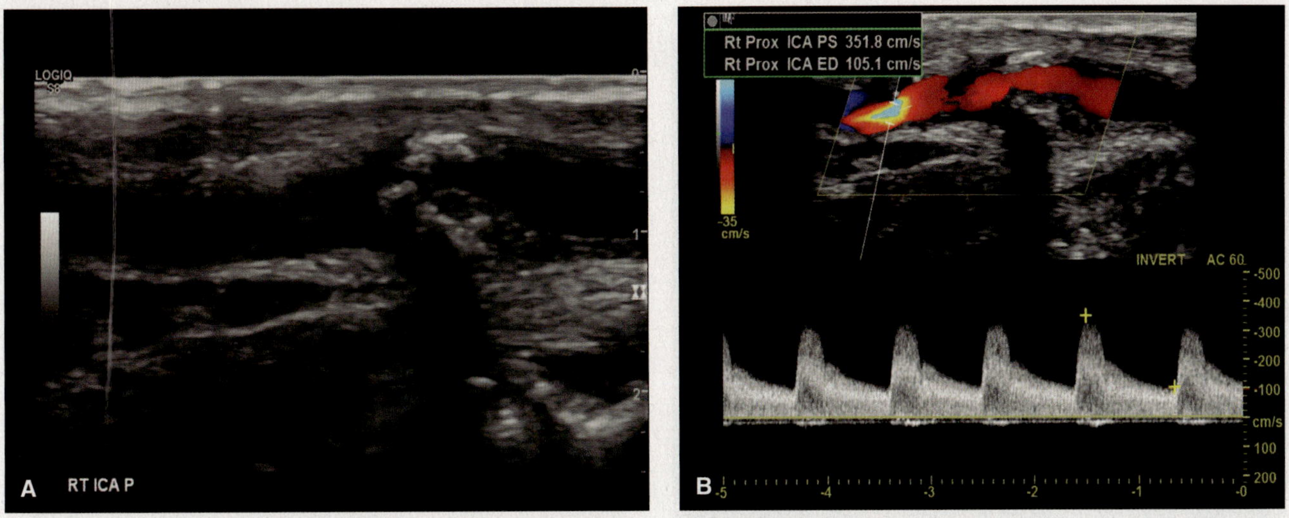

Figure 84.6. **A:** B-mode DUS showing severe calcified plaque and narrowing at proximal right ICA. **B:** Color flow Doppler showing PSV of 351 and EDV of 105 correlating to a >70% stenosis.

carotid bifurcation, and information regarding intracerebral collateral circulation (**Fig. 84.7**). The gold standard remains carotid angiography for definitive diagnosis in carotid atherosclerotic disease (**Fig. 84.8**). Major stroke has been reported in 1% of carotid angiography cases, with majority of these due to aggressive injection of contrast and introduction of air. Similar to TFCAS, microemboli can occur during carotid angiography. These microemboli can be seen postprocedure on diffusion-weighted magnetic resonance imaging (MRI) and may contribute to possible stroke or further neurologic derangements. Transcranial Doppler (TCD) is less used for initial diagnostic evaluation for atherosclerotic carotid disease, but TCD can give useful information regarding the significance of a carotid stenosis and how it alters intracerebral hemodynamics. TCD can be helpful in identifying high-risk asymptomatic carotid lesions if silent emboli are detected during the study.

Treatment of Atherosclerotic Carotid Artery Disease

Atherosclerotic carotid artery disease can be broken down into asymptomatic and symptomatic carotid stenosis. A recent (<6 months) TIA, stroke, and amaurosis fugax are considered to be symptoms of atherosclerotic carotid occlusive disease. The benefit of carotid intervention in patients with recent 5 ipsilateral carotid territory symptoms and moderate to severe carotid stenosis is much greater than the benefit of carotid intervention in asymptomatic patients. In patients with TIA, up to 15% will go on to CVA, 10% occur within 90 days. Several landmark studies have examined the risk reduction of stroke with surgical versus medical management.

Symptomatic Carotid Lesions

Patients with symptomatic carotid lesions are at the highest risk of ipsilateral stroke. The degree of stenosis also corresponds with increased risk of ipsilateral stroke if not treated. Multiple landmark trials have validated the benefit of carotid intervention, namely CEA, over medical therapy for symptomatic carotid stenosis. The North American Symptomatic Carotid Endarterectomy Trial (NASCET) study and The European Carotid Surgery Trial (ECST) both showed that the degree of stenosis does correlate to risk of ipsilateral stroke. In patients with >50% ipsilateral carotid stenosis, those treated with medical therapy alone were more likely to progress to ipsilateral stroke when compared to those treated with surgical intervention. Benefit was highest among patients with the highest degree of carotid stenosis (70% to 99%). In the NASCET study, symptomatic patients were randomized to medical therapy (which at the time primarily consisted of aspirin therapy) or CEA for those found to have >50% ipsilateral carotid stenosis. After 2 years, in patients with severe >70% symptomatic carotid stenosis, CEA conferred a 6.7% absolute risk reduction for death or major disabling stroke over medical therapy. NASCET also found benefit of CEA over medical therapy in patients with "mild to moderate," 50% to 69% carotid artery stenosis, with a 5-year absolute risk reduction of 4.7%.[16] The ECST corroborated NASCET findings with regard to severe >70% carotid stenosis, however, no benefit

Table 84.1. Modified UW (Strandness) Criteria for Carotid Stenosis

Stenosis Severity (%)	ICA PSV (cm/s)	ICA EDV (cm/s)	Spectral Broadening
1–14	<125	N/A	None
15–49	<125	N/A	Present and minimal
50–79	>125	<140	Present
80–99	>125	>140	Diffuse and marked
Occluded	0	0	N/A

ICA, internal carotid artery; PSV, peak systolic velocity; EDV, end-diastolic velocity.

Table 84.2. Carotid Consensus Panel Duplex Criteria (CCPC) Duplex Ultrasound Criteria for Carotid Artery Stenosis

Degree of Stenosis (%)	ICA PSV (cm/s)	ICA EDV (cm/s)	ICA/CCA Ratio	Carotid Plaque (%)
Normal	<125	<40	<2.0	None
<50	<125	<40	<2.0	<50
50–69	125–230	40–100	2.0–4.0	>50
70–99	>230	>100	>4.0	>70

ICA, internal carotid artery; PSV, peak systolic velocity; EDV, end-diastolic velocity; CCA, common carotid artery.

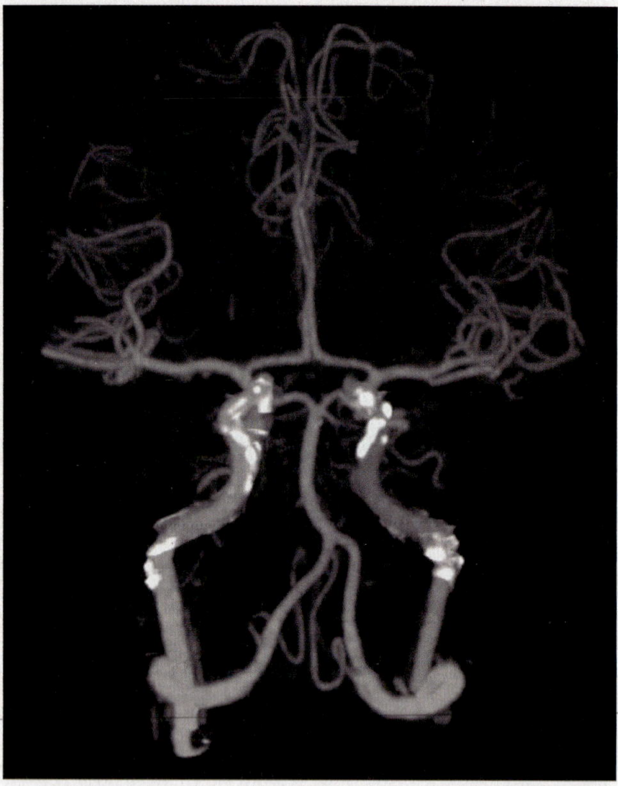

Figure 84.7. CTA with 3D reconstruction showing intracerebral collateral flow and intact circle of Willis.

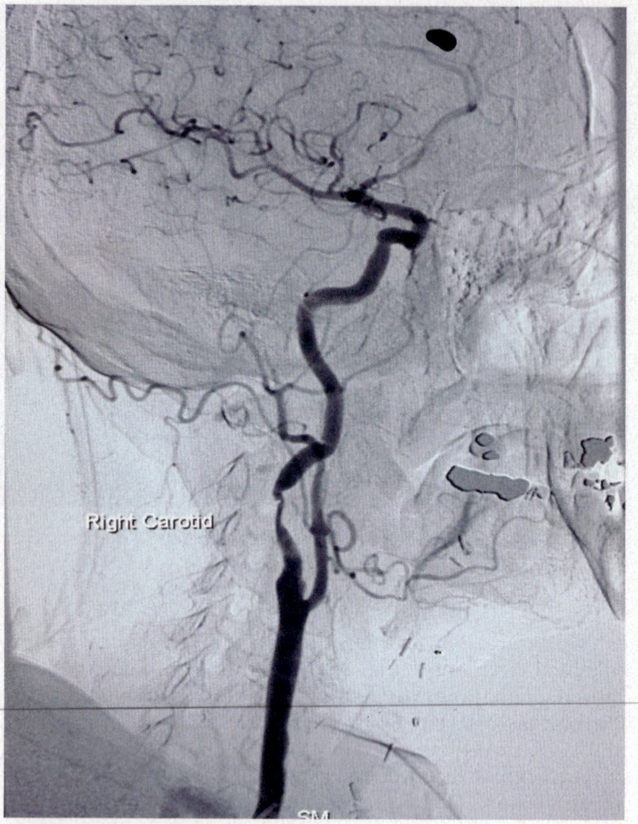

Figure 84.8. Diagnostic carotid angiography showing severe mid ICA stenosis at the level of C2.

was found for surgery over medical therapy in mild to moderate (50% to 69%) carotid stenosis.[17] There have been significant advances in medical therapy for the treatment of carotid atherosclerotic disease. Hydroxymethylglutaryl-CoA (HMG-CoA) reductase inhibitors have significantly improved the ability to medically treat carotid atherosclerotic disease. Statin therapy has been shown to help stabilize atherosclerotic plaque and reduce stroke by some 30% in patients with atherosclerotic carotid disease (**Table 84.3**).[18]

Clearly, carotid intervention has been shown to be beneficial over medical therapy for patients with symptomatic carotid stenosis. What is less clear is the timing of intervention. Traditionally, surgeons have waited >6 weeks prior to intervention to allow of any ischemic penumbra to resolve. However, 30-day recurrent ipsilateral stroke rates have been well established in recent studies in patients with symptomatic >50% carotid stenosis.[19] Early (<48 hours), aggressive intervention was suggested as the most optimal time to intervene, given the aforementioned risk of recurrent stroke. However, performing carotid intervention, namely CEA, <48 hours after onset of symptoms has been shown to increase the risk of postoperative stroke, death, and other complications.[20] In patients with mild to moderate TIA/stroke that have returned to baseline from their symptoms, current practice is to perform carotid intervention in the delayed phase (ie, between 2 and 14 days). Urgent revascularization is still warranted in patients with crescendo TIA and evolving stroke in order to prevent a larger stroke, despite the known increased risk of perioperative complications.

Asymptomatic Carotid Lesions

There is a clear body of evidence supporting carotid intervention for symptomatic carotid artery stenosis. What is less evident is the ideal treatment for asymptomatic carotid artery stenosis. One of the first and most important trials that have driven how the management of asymptomatic carotid stenosis is in the United States over the past 30 years is the

Table 84.3. SVS Practice Guidelines for Management of CAS

Condition	Recommendation	Level of Evidence
Low surgical-risk patient CEA vs BMT in asx patients	>70% stenosis, CEA over BMT	1B
Symptomatic CAS >50%, CEA vs TFCAS	CEA over TFCAS in low and standard risk	1A
Optimal timing of carotid intervention with acute stroke	Stable stroke patient with >50% CAS, intervention performed at 2–14 d	1B
Patients undergoing revascularization after stroke	Within 2–14 d, recommend CEA over carotid stenting	1B
Screening for asymptomatic carotid stenosis	Recommend against routine screening	1B

CEA, carotid endarterectomy; BMT, best medical therapy; TFCAS, transfemoral carotid artery stenting; CAS, carotid artery stenting.

Asymptomatic Carotid Atherosclerosis Study (ACAS) trial.[21] In ACAS, asymptomatic patients with >60% stenosis were randomly assigned to either medical management or CEA. At 5 years, best medical therapy (BMT) was found to be inferior to surgery in regard to ipsilateral CVA (11% for BMT vs 5.1% for CEA). These findings were also corroborated in the European Asymptomatic Carotid Surgery Trial (ACST), with a benefit in patients undergoing surgery over BMT with >60% carotid stenosis.[22] Both trials showed a significant relative risk reduction of stroke when undergoing CEA (ACAS 53% and ACST 46%). The findings of these trials in the mid-90s led to an explosion in the number of CEA being performed for carotid artery atherosclerotic disease and have guided management of severe >80% carotid artery stenosis in the asymptomatic patient. BMT during these trials primarily comprised of aspirin therapy. Medical therapy has evolved since the initiation of these trials, with the use of statin therapy as well as dual antiplatelet therapy (DAPT) for atherosclerotic carotid disease. This is coupled with significant improvement in glycemic control and smoking cessation leading to dramatic decrease in annual rates of ipsilateral or any territory stroke since the early 1980s. These rates have been purported to be at or below those seen in stroke prevention with carotid intervention (Table 84.3).[23] The upcoming CREST-2 randomized trial between current best BMT and carotid interventions (CEA or carotid artery stenting [CAS]) will hopefully shed more light on the most optimal management of asymptomatic, severe >80% carotid artery stenosis.

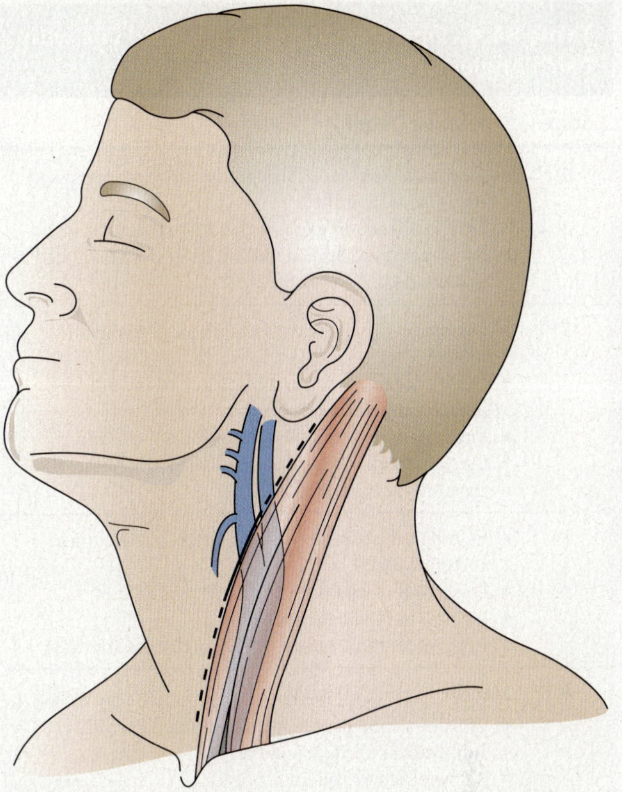

Figure 84.9. The patient's neck is slightly hyperextended and turned away from the ipsilateral side. An incision is made at the anterior border of the sternocleidomastoid muscle overlying the carotid bifurcation.

CAROTID ENDARTERECTOMY

Technique

The first carotid surgery is credited to be performed by Eastcott, Pickering, and Rob in 1954 in a woman with recurrent TIAs.[24] The carotid surgery involved the excision of the carotid bifurcation, ligation of the ECA, and reconstruction with direct anastomosis of the CCA to the ICA. The first CEA was actually performed the year prior by Dr. Debakey, but he did not publish his findings until 1959. Since the advent of the CEA in the 1950s, it has become one of the most common surgeries performed by vascular surgeons in the United States. Numerous trials, previously mentioned in this chapter, have validated the safety and efficacy of CEA especially in patients with symptomatic carotid artery disease. A fundamental consideration prior to performing a CEA is deciding the type of anesthetic method. CEA may be performed under general anesthesia (GA), regional anesthesia (RA) with a deep or superficial cervical block and under local anesthesia (LA). Several studies have shown the benefit of RA with reduction in the risk of postoperative complications such as MI.[25] Second fundamental choice regarding CEA is choice of intraoperative cerebral monitoring. Choice of monitoring is dependent on the choice of anesthesia. Patients who undergo GA, typically have a multitude of cerebral monitoring devices that include electroencephalogram (EEG) with somatosensory-evoked potentials (SSEPs), TCD, stump pressure measurement, and cerebral pulse oximetry (near infrared spectroscopy). If the patient has the surgery under LA/RA, their ability to respond to commands and monitor neurologic status dictates the adequacy of collateral flow. Cerebral monitoring devices aid the surgeon in deciding if a shunt is necessary for those patients deemed to have poor collateral flow. EEG is the most widely used cerebral monitoring tool and measures brain activity with 10 to 16 leads. A significant finding is a drop of fast background activity of 50% indicating possible cerebral ischemia. TCD evaluates the middle cerebral artery (MCA) for changes in flow with clamping. Stump pressure requires clamping the CCA and ECA while maintaining the ICA open and using a transducer to measure the back pressure. A mean pressure less than 40 mm Hg has been adopted as the standard threshold to indicate the intolerability of clamping. All these measures are used to guide the surgeon to place an intraoperative shunt to decrease the time of cerebral ischemia. Shunting continues to be a controversial topic, with some studies showing decreased stroke risk, while others showing no benefit in shunting.[26] Routine shunting allows for a consistent endarterectomy technique with less anxiety as the shunt completely relieves intracerebral ischemia if done correctly. In a recent study, we have shown an interaction between anesthesia types and shunting (with LA/RA), putting patients at increased risk of postoperative stroke and death when intraoperative shunting is performed.[27]

Careful patient positioning is paramount to performing a successful CEA, especially for high lesions at or above the level of C2. The patient is placed supine on the operating room table with a roll placed behind the scapulae to allow for hyperextension of the neck. The neck is turned away from the operative side and the patient is usually placed in a "beach chair" position, this allows for optimal exposure to the neck and a slight reverse Trendelenburg with decreased jugular venous pressure. A longitudinal skin incision is made along the anterior border of the sternocleidomastoid (SCM) (**Fig. 84.9**). Smaller skin incisions (~4 cm) can be made with adequate exposure. To facilitate this, use of ultrasound intraoperatively will help locate the carotid bifurcation, allowing the surgeon to center a smaller incision over the carotid bifurcation. See **Table 84.4** for detailed steps of the operation (**Figs. 84.10, 84.11,** and **84.13**). Several important considerations for CEA surgery: Dissection at the carotid bifurcation may result in bradycardia due to stimulation of the carotid body. This can be alleviated by administration of less than 0.5 cc of 1% lidocaine into the adventitia and directly into the carotid body. Great care must be taken when dissecting out the proximal ICA to avoid excessive manipulation and distal embolization of the underlying lesion.

Adequate endarterectomy can be accomplished with a blunt elevator or sharply with a beaver blade (**Fig. 84.12**). Great care must be taken to ensure a nice stable feathered-out

Table 84.4. Operative Steps for Standard CEA with Patch Angioplasty

Steps	Operative Detail
1	▪ Incision is deepened through the platysma layer and the SCM is identified ▪ Lateral retraction exposes the internal jugular vein ▪ Facial vein is identified and carefully double ligated and divided
2	▪ Dissection progresses proximally until omohyoid muscle ▪ CCA is located inferior and medial to the internal jugular in the carotid sheath ▪ Vagus nerve typically lies deep to the CCA and IJ ▪ Circumferential control of the CCA at the base of the neck incision (**Fig. 84.10**)
3	▪ ECA and the superior thyroid artery are identified and controlled. ▪ Dissection occurs distally passed carotid bulb ▪ Identify the hypoglossal nerve ▪ Circumferential control of ICA in disease-free area
4	Maneuvers for high lesions: ▪ Division of the posterior belly of the digastric ▪ Subluxation of the mandible ▪ Removal of the styloid process ▪ Nasotracheal intubation
5	▪ Heparinize at 80 units/kg, allow to circulate for 3–5 min ▪ ICA clamped first, followed by ECA and then CCA ▪ Arteriotomy made in distal CCA and extended past lesion into normal ICA ▪ Shunt is placed (if warranted) from CCA to ICA to maintain antegrade perfusion (**Fig. 84.11**)
6	▪ Endarterectomy completed by teasing plaque off of intimal layer ▪ Eversion endarterectomy to completely remove plaque from ECA (**Fig. 84.13**) ▪ Intimal flaps at distal end tacked down with 7-0 prolene suture ▪ Artertiotomy closed with patch angioplasty (bovine vs vein)

endpoint of the endarterectomy plane on the ICA. The endarterectomized plane is then evaluated and any small flaps or debris are removed. Not uncommonly, the area of the distal endpoint on the ICA has soft intimal flap that should be tacked down with a 7-0 polypropylene to avoid flaps being raised, causing dissection when antegrade flow is resumed. If not done appropriately, patients are at risk for acute carotid occlusion following CEA, which may have devastating consequences.

Repair of the arteriotomy should be accomplished with the use of a patch angioplasty. Multiple studies[28] have shown the benefit of closing the arteriotomy with a patch versus primary closure to prevent late ipsilateral stroke and recurrent stenosis. Different patch materials include Dacron, bovine pericardium, or autogenous materials. No difference has been shown in what type of patch material is used and decision is up to surgeon preference. If shunt is used, patch should be almost completely closed prior to removal of shunt and resumption of clamping (**Fig. 84.14**). Prior to complete patch closure, it is necessary to appropriately back bleed and flush out any debris that may have accumulated within the endarterectomy site.

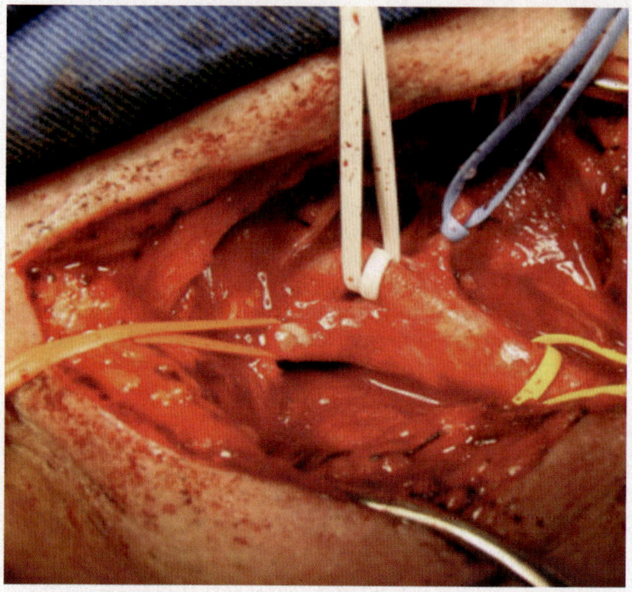

Figure 84.10. Circumferential vascular control surrounding CCA (*yellow loop*), ICA (*orange loop*), ECA (*white loop*), and superior thyroid artery (*blue loop*).

Once patch is completed, allow reperfusion to the ECA first while keeping the ICA clamped to ensure any remaining debris of thrombus does not proceed into the anterior cerebral circulation. Meticulous hemostasis is obtained in the surgical bed, and if needed, heparin can be reversed with protamine. The SCM is then reapproximated in the field and a surgical drain may be placed at the discretion of the surgeon in the subplatysmal layer. The platysma layer is then closed with an absorbable suture followed by the skin. A full neurologic examination should be performed prior to extubation or while still in the operating room to ensure no neurologic deficits.

Eversion endarterectomy (**Fig. 84.15**) is another CEA technique that has been employed and has the benefit of not requiring any prosthetic material for arteriotomy closure. Approach for eversion CEA is similar to standard CEA; similar incision is made and exposure of the carotid bifurcation occur using similar standard techniques. The ICA is then transected obliquely at the carotid bulb including a small portion of the CCA. The edges of the ICA are the everted and peeled back performing an endarterectomy cleaving in between the intimal and medial

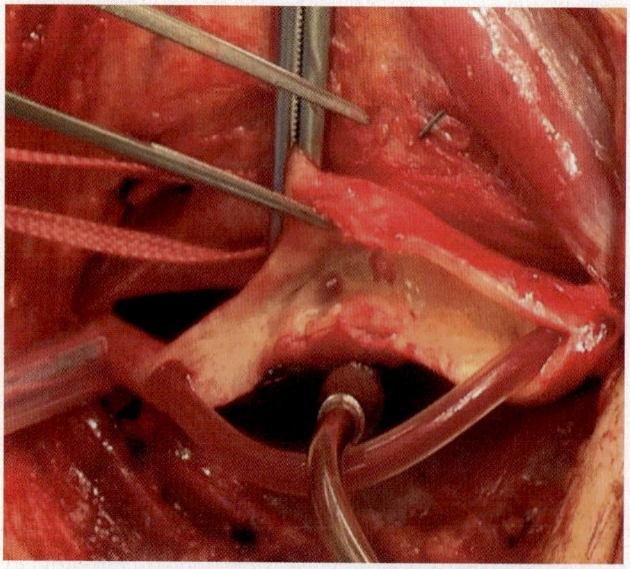

Figure 84.11. Intraluminal shunt placement from CCA to ICA.

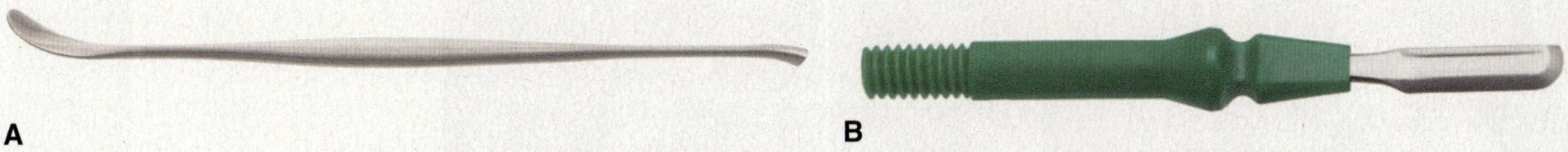

Figure 84.12. **A**: Elevator with blunt edges. **B**: Half-moon–shaped sharp blade.

layers. The atherosclerotic plaque plane is then removed as it proceeds distally until a clean portion is encountered. Several downsides to this technique are the difficulty of placing an intraluminal shunt, if it is needed, and inability to easily use distal tacking sutures. Closure is accomplished primarily by anastomosing the ICA onto the CCA without compromising the lumen of the ICA. Eversion CEA has been shown to be safe, effective, and durable in long-term follow-up with similar results as seen with standard CEA.[29] In a recent study of over 95,000 CEA performed in the United States, we have shown no difference in outcomes between eversion CEA and CEA with patch angioplasty, however, eversion CEA was superior to CEA with primary closure with 30% reduction in the risk of stroke and death at 30 days.[30]

The avoidance of perioperative stroke during and immediately after CEA is of the utmost importance, especially when performing CEA for high-grade asymptomatic carotid stenosis. To minimize this risk, several intraoperative completion studies are available to aid the surgeon in ensuring a technically sound repair. These include use of intraoperative continuous-wave form Doppler, intraoperative duplex, and intraoperative angiogram. Continuous-wave Doppler is an inexpensive and readily available tool that is available in almost every operating room. It can confirm patency of the carotid vessels and indicate if there are potential issues based on the resistance heard or a high-pitch Doppler sound indicating a possible stenosis. An experienced operator can detect these subtle sounds; however, continuous-wave Doppler is insensitive at detecting small intimal flaps or more subtle stenosis. Duplex ultrasound, on the other hand, is a much more sensitive tool and can give detailed anatomic imaging regarding the existence of a possible intimal flap or high-grade stenosis. Like any duplex ultrasound, quality can be variable and is operator dependent. The "gold standard" continues to be intraoperative completion angiogram with injection of contrast directly into the common carotid. Completion studies are not uniform practice and have mixed results in the identification of clinically relevant defects.

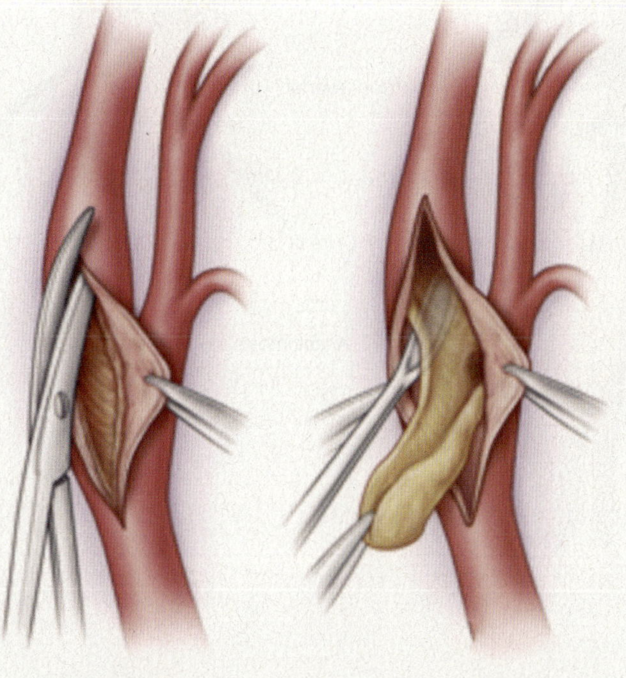

Figure 84.13. Conventional endarterectomy by removing plaque with blunt dissection and everting atherosclerotic plaque from ECA.

Complications

CEA can be safely done in the vast majority of cases and is well tolerated with most patients being discharged after 24 hours. However, a wide array of complications exists, from mild wound issue to life-threatening issues. The single biggest contributor to perioperative death continues to be MI. MI is responsible for 25% to 50% of all perioperative deaths after CEA and more late deaths are seen from MI than from stroke or other causes.[31] Significant advances have been made in the past two decades that have led to a significantly low rate of cardiac events during and immediately after CEA. One of the most feared complications, especially in treating asymptomatic patients, is perioperative ipsilateral stroke. There are multiple etiologies for immediate postoperative stroke including embolization, hyperperfusion, and rarely acute occlusion. Embolization can occur from shunt placement, from the clamp site, thrombus forming during CEA, or inadequate flushing prior to arteriotomy closure. With manipulation of the carotid sinus, hypertension and hyperperfusion may ensue postoperatively and can lead to ipsilateral ischemic stroke if hypertension is not controlled. This phenomenon usually occurs 24 to 72 hours after CEA and adequate postoperative blood pressure control is mandated prior to discharge home. Acute patch occlusion is rare but may be related to an intimal flap, platelet adhesion from the patch, dissection, or anastomotic stricture. This is why it is of the utmost importance to document a normal neurologic examination prior to extubation or prior to leaving the operating room. Intraoperative imaging is another important method to ensure normal flow prior to closing the wound. During CEA, cerebral ischemia can occur due to hypoperfusion of watershed cerebral area. This is related to inadequate collateral flow through the contralateral carotid artery and posterior circulation, which relies on a patent circle of Willis. Ipsilateral perioperative stroke rates continue to decline. Thirty-day stroke and death rate after CEA in CREST was 3.2% in symptomatic patients and 1.2% in asymptomatic patients. In addition, for symptomatic patients, 30-day risk of MI was 2.2% and death rates were 1.1%; for asymptomatic patients, 30-day risk of MI was 2% and death rates were 1.1%. Overall, with CEA CREST showed a periprocedural risk of death at 0.3%, CVA of 2.3%, and MI of 2.3%.[2] Cranial nerve injury (**Table 84.5**) is the most common neurologic complication following CEA and one of the most problematic for patients. Incidence of postoperative cranial nerve injury ranges from 5% to 20% with the vast majority of these resolving at 6 months.[32]

Transfemoral Carotid Artery Stenting

Technique

TFCAS with distal embolic protection device (EPD) has gained popularity since its advent in the early 90s. Since the Food and Drug Administration (FDA) approved TFCAS in 2004, there has been a proliferation of technology and expansion of its use for symptomatic and asymptomatic carotid artery stenoses. Similar to indications for CEA, TFCAS should be considered a

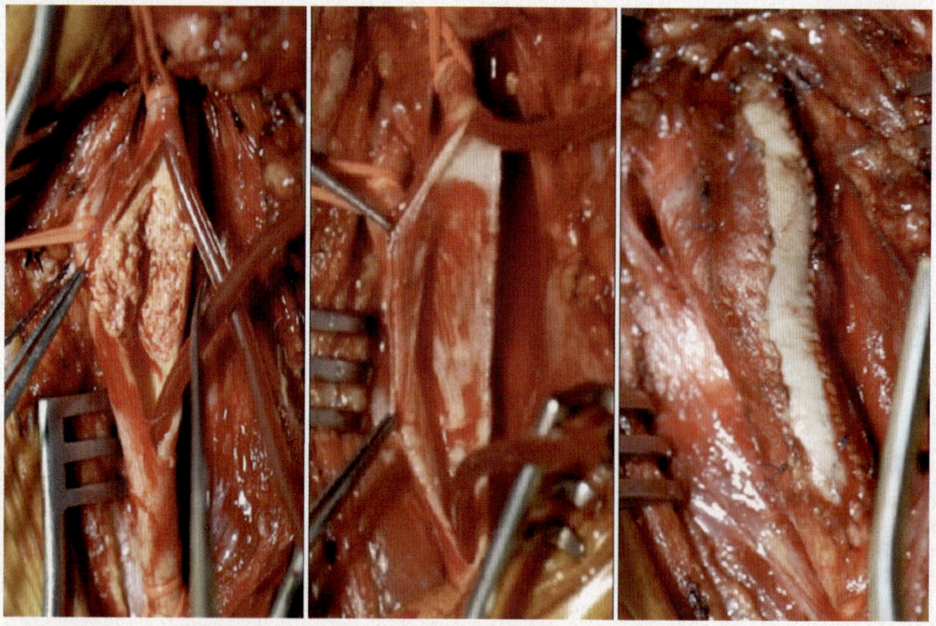

Figure 84.14. Carotid endarterectomy showing complete removal of atherosclerotic plaque with shunt placement and patch angioplasty closure.

viable carotid revascularization option in patients with symptomatic >50% stenosis and asymptomatic >80% stenosis. Most vascular surgeons believe CAS should be reserved for patients who are deemed high risk (surgical or medical) for CEA (**Table 84.6**). Despite multiple studies showing the inferiority of TFCAS to CEA, the Center for Medicare and Medicaid Services (CMS) as unfortunately approved and will reimburse TFCAS in standard risk >80% asymptomatic patients.

In order to obtain procedural success with low periprocedural complication rate, identification and examination of preoperative imaging is a must. Prior to planned TFCAS, axial imaging should be carefully reviewed. Typically, MRA or CTA with thin cuts are performed with imaging including the aortic arch and the circle of Willis. Careful preoperative imaging examination will identify diseased arch and difficult tortuous anatomy for tracking wires and catheters into the carotid artery. Possible stroke can occur with excessive manipulation of the aortic arch and inability to recognize ostial disease. Arch types based on tortuosity are recognized on preoperative imaging (**Fig. 84.16**). In general, type III arches are now considered contraindication for TFCAS with mounting evidence of increased intraprocedural embolization. Preoperative imaging also can identify other high-risk lesion and anatomic criteria for TFCAS and potential contraindications for CAS (**Table 84.7**). Prior to the TFCAS procedure, all patients should be on DAPT, with 7 days of

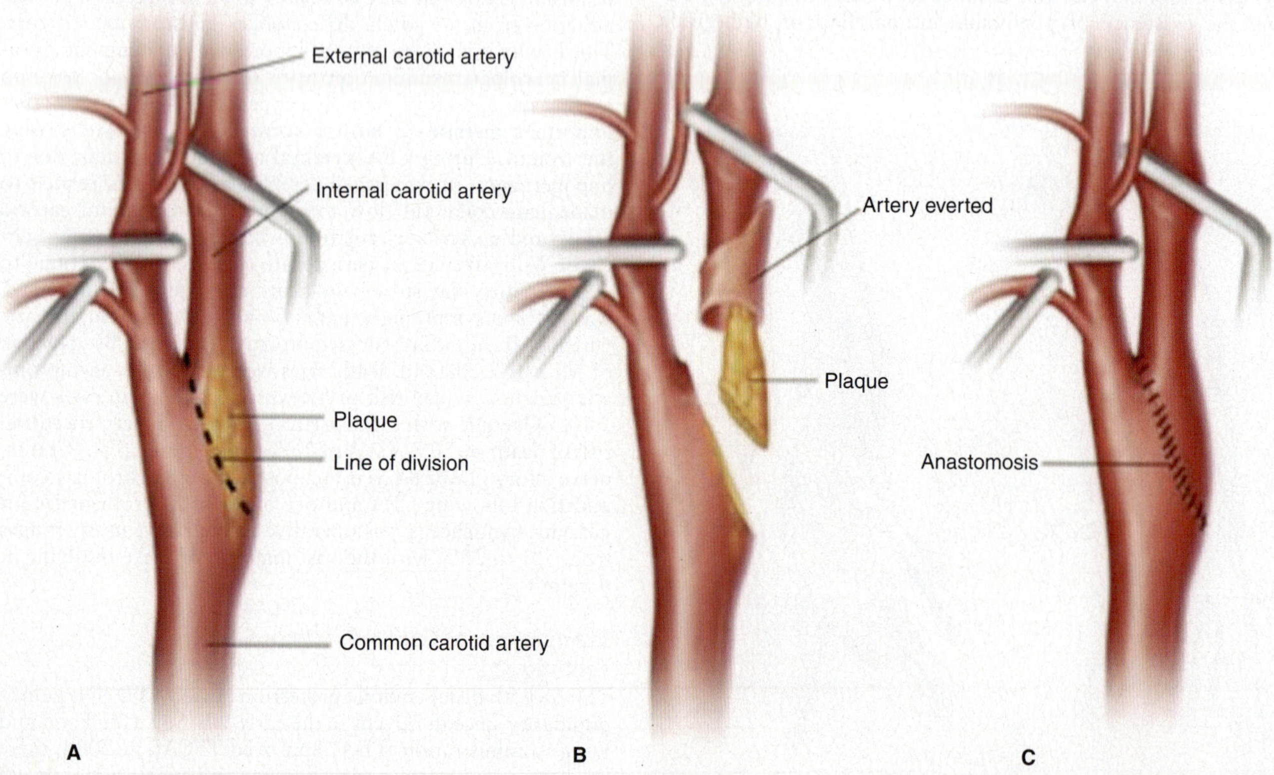

Figure 84.15. A: The ICA is divided from the CCA in an oblique plane. B: The divided ICA is everted, and endarterectomy occurs until plaque endpoint, and is removed from the ICA. C: The ICA is then reattached to the CCA primarily.

Table 84.5. Cranial Nerve Dysfunction and Incidence Following CEA

Cranial Nerve Injury	Clinical Sequelae	Incidence (%)
Vagus nerve (recurrent laryngeal nerve)	Unilateral—Hoarseness (rarely seen) Bilateral—Vocal cord paralysis	1.5–15
Superior laryngeal nerve	Fatigability of voice, difficulty with voice modulation	1.8–4.5
Hypoglossal nerve	Unilateral—Ipsilateral tongue deviation Bilateral—Difficult swallowing and articulation	4.4–17.5
Glossopharyngeal nerve	Aspiration, dysphagia	0.2–1.5
Marginal mandibular nerve	Drooping ipsilateral lip	1.1–3.1
Spinal accessory nerve	Shoulder droop, scapular winging	<1.0

Data from Forssell C, Takolander R, Bergqvist D, et al. Cranial nerve injuries associated with carotid endarterectomy. A prospective study. *Acta Chir Scand*. 1985;151:595–598.

aspirin (typically 325 mg) therapy and 5 days of clopidogrel therapy (receiving a total of 450 mg of clopidogrel). Detailed steps of TFCAS procedure can be seen below in **Table 84.8** (**Figs. 84.17, 84.18, and 84.21**).

Several important considerations must be carefully paid attention to in order to have a successful TFCAS procedure. Great care must be taken to avoid inadvertently manipulating the lesion and risk of embolizing distally into the ICA. In difficult anatomy in which a telescoping technique is not possible, the ECA can be cannulated and stiff wire placed with advancement of the sheath into the CCA in a nontelescoped manner. It is ideal to open and flush the appropriate size predilation balloon, carotid stent, and EPD so that minimal time is taken from predilation to completion stenting. Depending on the type of carotid stent used, different EPDs are available for placement (**Fig. 84.19**). Filter placement requires wire manipulation and crossing of the lesion to access the distal ICA. Some filters are attached to the wire, while others can be advanced over the 0.014 wire into the distal ICA and deployed. The remainder of the stenting procedure is performed over the EPD wire via a rapid exchange platform. When selecting stent sizes, this typically depends on the size of the ICA and CCA and comes in straight and tapered configurations. Type of carotid stent use is up to the discretion of the interventionalist. The stents are self-expanding and have either an open- or closed-cell stent design (**Fig. 84.20**). Flexibility of the stent depends on the number of connections between the cells of the stent. The less the amount of connections (open-cell design), the more flexible the stent will be and may be better used in tortuous ICA lesions. The more connections, the stiffer the stent will be (closed-cell design). Closed-cell stents may be better used in symptomatic patients to lessen embolization or extrusion of carotid plaque through the stent. Postdilation of the stent should be carefully considered as studies suggest worse outcomes with higher stroke and death rates and more hemodynamic depression when routine postdilation is undertaken.[33] Similar to CEA patients, close neurologic and hemodynamic assessments are made throughout the postprocedural period. Most patients are discharged home 24 hours after TFCAS and continue 1 month of clopidogrel and lifelong aspirin.

Table 84.6. High-Risk Medical and Surgical Patients for CEA

Clinical Criteria	Anatomic Criteria
Unstable angina	High lesion above C2
NYHA class III or IV CHF	CEA restenosis
LVEF <35%	Prior neck irradiation
MI <6 wk	Cervical immobility
Severe pulmonary disease	Tracheostomy
Contralateral recurrent laryngeal nerve injury	Previous neck surgery

NYHA, New York Heart Association; CHF, congestive heart failure; LVEF, left ventricular ejection fraction; CEA, carotid endarterectomy; MI, myocardial infarction.

Complications

The most serious and important complication following TFCAS is periprocedural stroke. While cardiac events are less frequently seen, CREST found periprocedural MI rates to be lower in TFCAS patients versus CEA (1.1% vs 2.3%, $P = .03$). Neurologic events following TFCAS can have devastating consequences and prompt recognition and treatment is needed. Potential causes of periprocedural stroke include distal embolization from manipulation of the lesion, thrombosed EPD, acute stent thrombosis, kinking after carotid stenting, carotid artery dissection, and hyperperfusion. Acute stent thrombosis may be related to failure of adequate expansion of carotid stent in densely calcified atherosclerotic plaque. This typically requires immediate stent explantation and conversion to CEA. Carotid dissection may require additional stenting versus antiplatelet therapy. Despite the necessity of using filter protection during transfemoral CAS, EPD can cause issues with placement. Distal filters may dissect or become full of thrombus/plaque, causing thrombosis of the filter. In addition, filter placement may cause severe vasospasm in the distal ICA that potentially could cause

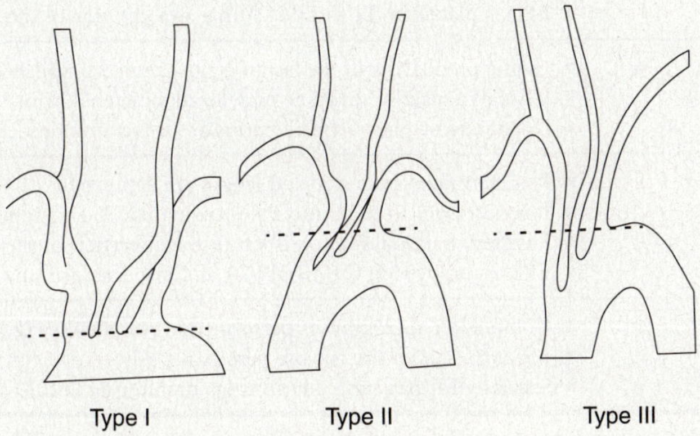

Figure 84.16. Arch types based on tortuosity.

Table 84.7. Contraindications and High-Risk Features for Carotid Artery Stenting

Carotid Artery Stenting Contraindications
Severe ICA kinking
Unstable plaque
Fresh thrombus
Brachiocephalic vessel tortuosity
Brachiocephalic vessel severe stenosis or occlusion
Acute aortic arch angle or anomalous aortic arch (type III arch)
Significant aortic arch plaque or thrombus
Circumferential calcification
Poor arterial access

thrombosis of the vessel. Immediate EPD retrieval is performed when these complications occur. Distal embolization may require neurorescue techniques, such as: aspiration thrombectomy, catheter-directed thrombolysis, or stent retrieval. Access site complications can occur with or without use of a closure device. Such complications include hematoma, pseudoaneurysm formation, arteriovenous (AV) fistula, thrombosis, and possible infection.

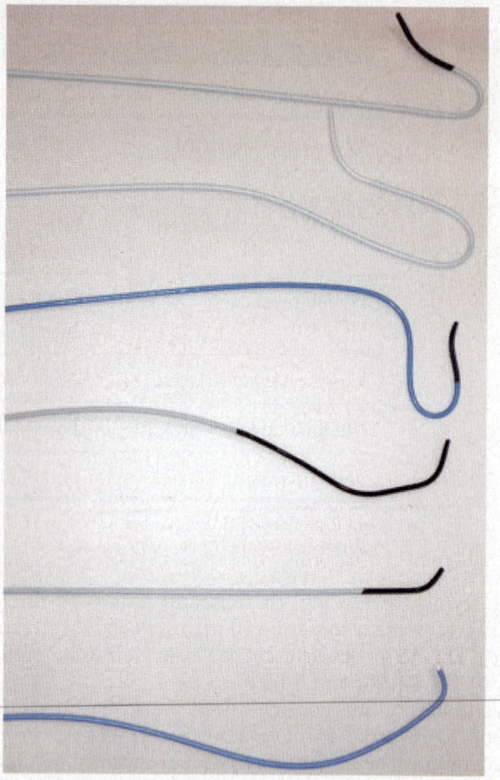

Figure 84.17. Catheters available for selective carotid cannulation during carotid angiogram and stenting.

Results

In its early phase, TFCAS was reserved for only high-risk, elderly patients who were deemed to be too high risk for CEA. Multiple randomized controlled trials (RCTs) have shown early efficacy in the treatment of high-risk patients with TFCAS. The Stenting and Angioplasty with Protection in Patients at High Risk for Endarterectomy (SAPPHIRE) trial examined TFCAS versus CEA for high-risk patients (medical comorbidities and anatomical features). The trial was designed to show noninferiority

Table 84.8. Operative Steps for TFCAS with Embolic Protection Device

Steps	Operative Detail
1	▪ Arterial placement for hemodynamic monitoring, either radial or via existing femoral sheath ▪ Most TFCAS cases are done under local to immediately detect neurologic issues ▪ Standard retrograde femoral access with US-guided micropuncture technique ▪ Immediately heparinize prior to advancing shuttle sheath in thoracic aorta (goal ACT >250)
2	▪ Arch aortogram performed to identify catheter for carotid selection (if not performed prior) ▪ Different catheter types available for carotid selection (**Fig. 84.17**) ▪ Once selected, angiogram performed to confirm carotid artery stenosis location and severity ▪ Further angiogram performed to assess ECA patency and evaluate distal carotid artery flow, and evaluate ipsilateral intracerebral circulation.
3	▪ Shuttle sheath (6 Fr) is telescoped into the mid CCA with use of slip catheter and stiff wire ▪ Angiogram through the sheath maps out ICA anatomy to aid in cannulating the ICA for placement of EPD (**Fig. 84.18**) ▪ EPD is placed in the distal ICA in a straight area of the vessel
4	▪ Gentle predilation of the lesion is typically accomplished with an undersized 3- to 4-mm balloon at low atmospheric pressure ▪ Glycopyrrolate or atropine may be administered prior to ballooning to decrease the effects of bradycardia and hypotension ▪ Dopamine or phenylephrine drips are sometimes needed to treat severe hypotension
5	▪ Predetermined stent size and length are deployed ▪ It is necessary to stent into the proximal CCA, encompassing the entire lesion and stabilize the carotid plaque ▪ Poststent balloon dilation is left to the discretion of the proceduralist ▪ EPD is removed in the distal ICA and inspected for any debris
6	▪ Completion angiogram is performed in two views (**Fig. 84.21**) ▪ Femoral arterial site is close percutaneously ▪ Similar CEA patient, 24 h of neuro monitoring in ICU setting is required

TFCAS, transfemoral carotid artery stenting; ECA, external carotid artery; CCA, common carotid artery; ICA, internal carotid artery; EPD, embolic protection device; CEA, carotid endarterectomy.

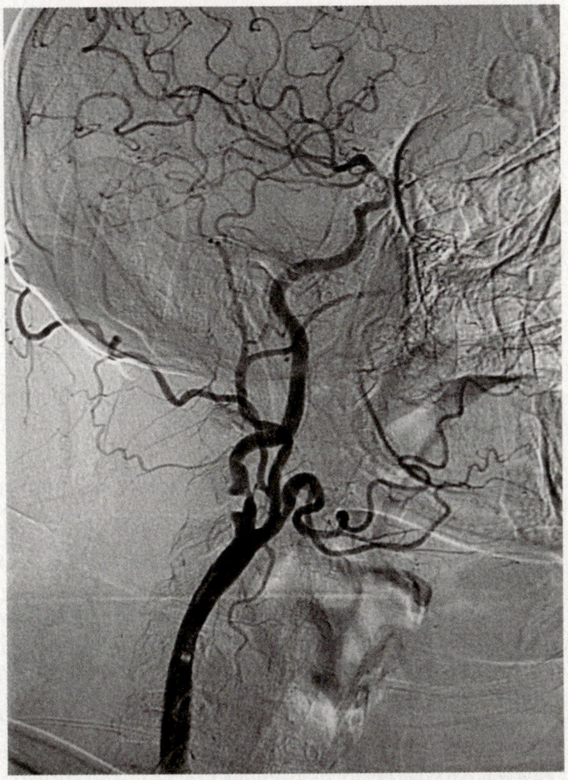

Figure 84.18. Carotid angiogram shows high-grade stenosis with high lesion at level of C2 and poor anterior cerebral artery flow.

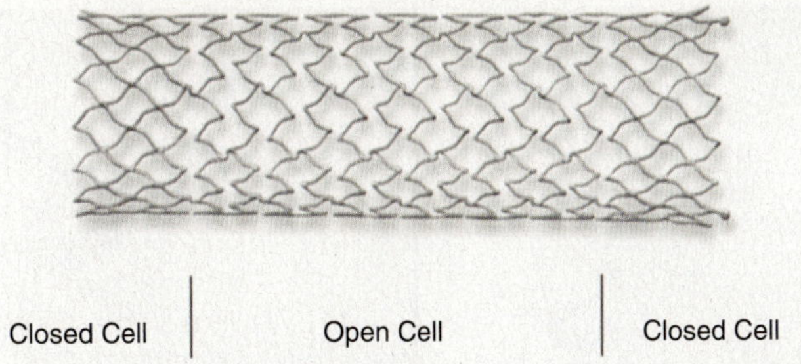

Figure 84.20. Self-expanding carotid artery stents with open- and closed-cell stent design.

of TFCAS compared to CEA in patients with >50% symptomatic stenosis and/or >80% asymptomatic stenosis. There was no significant difference in 30-day major adverse events (stroke, death, and MI) between the two procedures, while TFCAS was associated with a lower risk of major events at 1 year, with a greater advantage in asymptomatic patients. The Stent-Supported Percutaneous Angioplasty of the Carotid Artery versus Endarterectomy (SPACE) trial randomized patients with >70% symptomatic stenosis to TFCAS versus CEA. This study failed to prove the noninferiority of TFCAS.[34] The Endarterectomy Versus Angioplasty in patients with symptomatic severe carotid stenosis (EVA-3S) was a European randomized trial in symptomatic patients with >60% carotid stenosis. This trial was stopped prematurely due to a 2.5-fold higher risk for 30-day stroke and death in the TFCAS group.[35] Routine use of EPD was not required, which was a major drawback in the TFCAS group. Most recently, the CREST compared TFCAS to CEA in standard-risk symptomatic and asymptomatic patients. Long-term follow-up out to 10 years did not show a difference between CAS and CEA with regard to stroke and death.[36] With that being said, 30-day outcomes did show a significantly higher risk of stroke for TFCAS versus CEA (4.1% vs 2.3%, *P* = .01).

TRANSCAROTID ARTERY REVASCULARIZATION

Technique

TCAR is an innovative hybrid procedure that combines CEA-like neuroprotective effects by clamping of the carotid artery with a minimally invasive approach to treat carotid stenosis by direct placement of the carotid artery stent, avoiding the arch. The procedure is done under novel flow reversal in the carotid and ipsilateral cerebrum. Like with any carotid revascularization procedure, careful patient selection is paramount

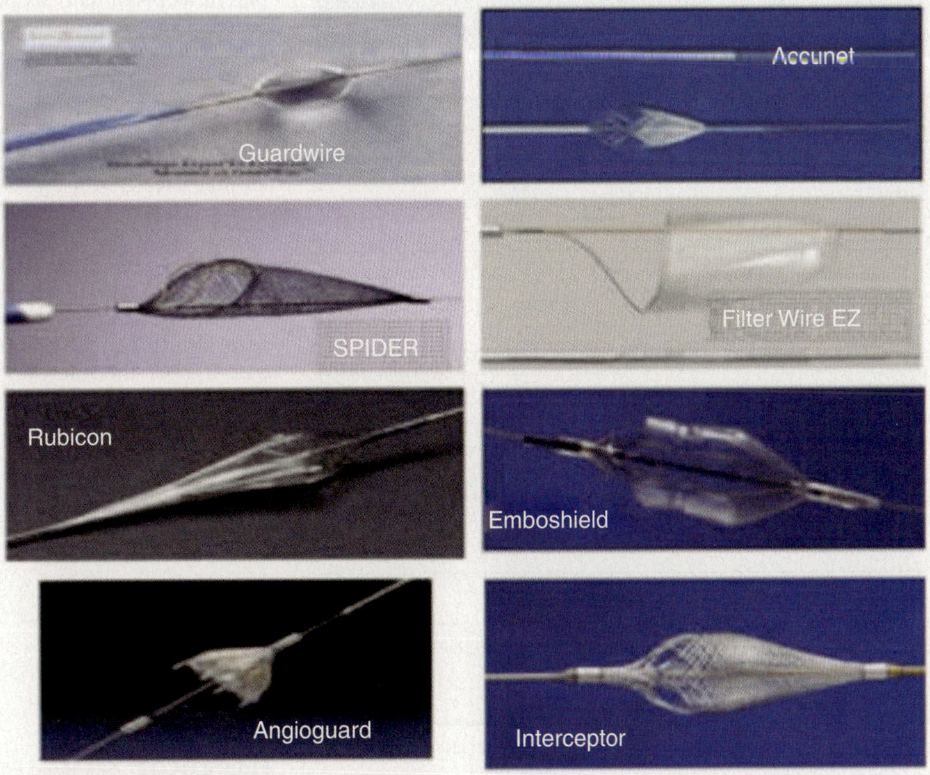

Figure 84.19. Types of embolic protection devices available for use.

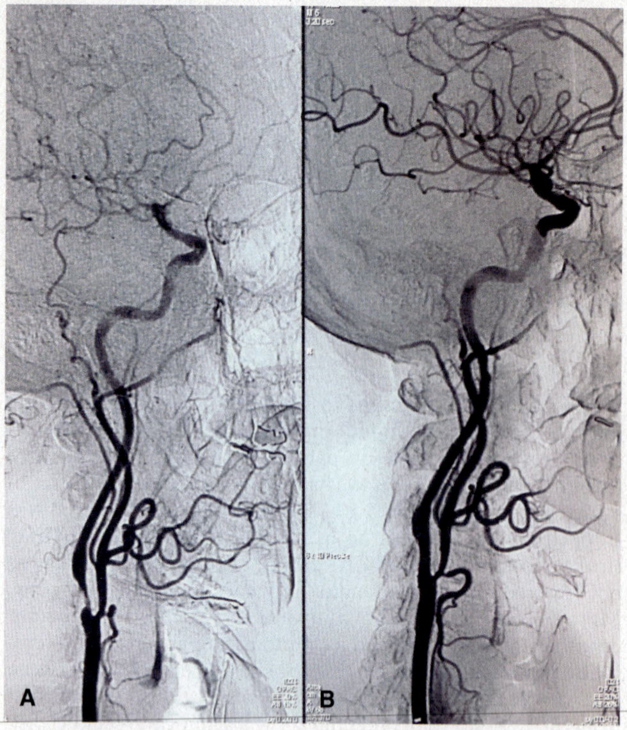

Figure 84.21. A: Prestent carotid angiogram showing severe ICA stenosis with poor distal flow. B: Poststent carotid angiogram showing resolution of stenosis and improved distal flow.

to have success with TCAR. Currently, TCAR is approved for both standard and high-risk patients with >50% symptomatic carotid stenosis or >80% asymptomatic stenosis. Participating hospitals must be involved in the Vascular Quality Initiative (VQI) Carotid Artery Stent Registry for the Society for Vascular Surgery (SVS). As compared to previous high-risk

Table 84.9. High-Risk Medical and Anatomic Inclusion Criteria for TCAR

Clinical Criteria	Anatomic Criteria
Patient >75 y of age	Contralateral carotid artery occlusion
Patient with >2-vessel CAD and history of angina	Tandem stenosis >70%
History of unstable angina	High cervical carotid artery stenosis
NYHA functional class III or IV	Restenosis after CEA
LVEF <30%	Bilateral carotid artery stenosis
MI >72 h and <6 wk prior to procedure	Hostile neck but amenable to transcarotid access
Severe COPD with FEV1 <50% predicted	
Permanent contralateral cranial nerve injury	
Chronic renal insufficiency (>2.5 mg/dL)	

NYHA, New York Heart Association; LVEF, left ventricular ejection fraction; CEA, carotid endarterectomy; MI, myocardial infarction.

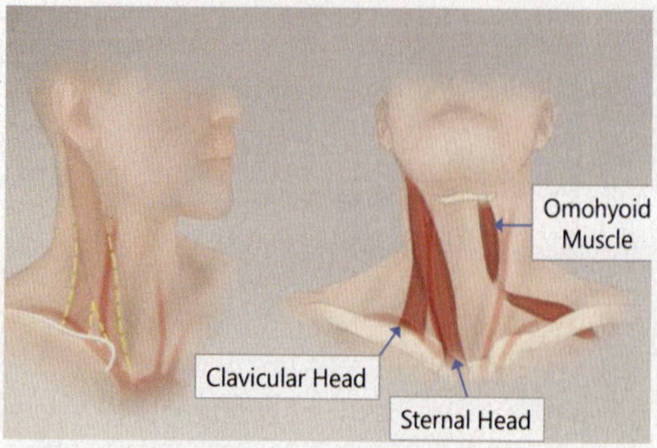

Figure 84.22. Illustration showing ideal location to isolate CCA in between the sternal and clavicular heads of the sternocleidomastoid muscle.

criteria used for standard TFCAS, TCAR has wider high-risk inclusion criteria (**Table 84.9**). TCAR approach and set up is similar to that for CEA. Patients prior to TCAR procedure need to be on 5 days of DAPT and statins. Successful TCAR procedure relies on certain anatomic criteria which include: ≥6-mm diameter CCA, CCA puncture site at base of neck free of calcified plaque, ≥5 cm clavicle to carotid bifurcation distance, and ICA diameter of 4 to 9 mm. The patient is brought into the operating room or a hybrid operating suite. Choice of anesthesia is up to the discretion of the surgeon with similar options to CEA: GA, RA, or LA. It is recommended that the first few TCARs be performed under GA until the surgeon is comfortable with the procedure. A radial arterial line is placed for continuous blood pressure monitoring. Patients are positioned similar to CEA, supine on the operating room table with a shoulder roll and the neck turned to the contralateral side. Duplex ultrasound should routinely be performed to confirm adequate clavicle to carotid bifurcation distance and the CCA is freed of significant atherosclerotic disease as well as confirm patency of the ICA. A small incision is made at the base of the neck (either transverse or longitudinal) in order to isolate the CCA in between the two heads of the SCM muscle (**Fig. 84.22**). A 3- to 4-cm segment of CCA is circumferentially controlled and an umbilical tape with a Rummel tourniquet is placed as proximally as possible under direct vision. A purse string 5-0 polypropylene suture is placed on the anterior adventitial surface of the CCA to facilitate arterial closure at completion of TCAR. Attention is then paid to obtaining femoral venous access in order to perform flow reversal. Standard femoral venous access is obtained (typically in the contralateral side from the TCAR site) under ultrasound guidance and an 8-Fr sheath is inserted.

The patient is then systemically heparinized, similar to a CEA, with 80 units/kg of heparin with goal of ACT >250 seconds. Access is then obtained in the CCA with micro needle; wire and sheath are advanced to just proximal to the carotid bifurcation. Angiogram is then performed to map out the carotid bifurcation. It is preferable to engage the ECA when patent with the microwire and sheath. A stiff wire is then placed into the ECA and the ENROUTE 8-Fr sheath (Silk Road Medical, Sunnyvale, CA) is advanced into the CCA and sutured in place (**Fig. 84.23**). Passive flow reversal is then

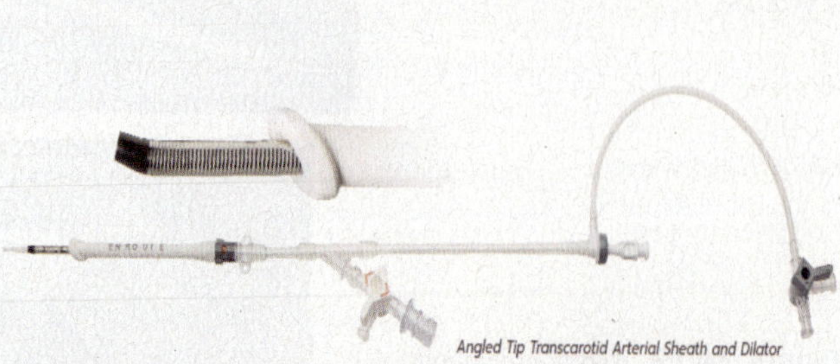

Figure 84.23. Silk Road ENROUTE sheath with angled tip.

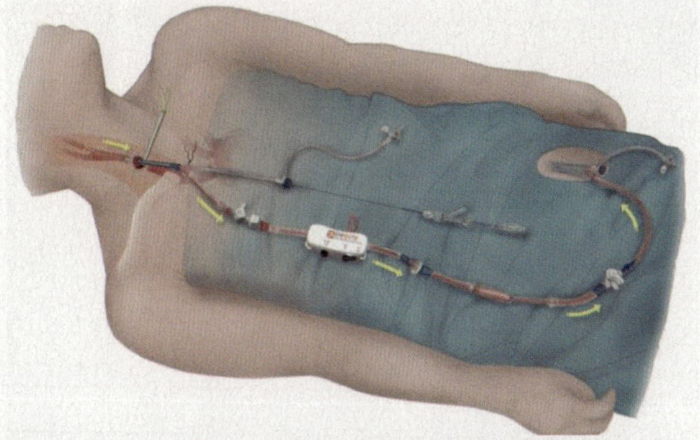

Figure 84.24. TCAR procedure utilizing the ENROUTE Transcarotid Neuroprotection and Stent System from Silk Road Medical with direct carotid access and percutaneous femoral vein access.

activated by connecting the arterial to the venous sheath via the dynamic flow controller and integrated 200 μ filter (Silk Road Medical, Sunnyvale, CA) (**Fig. 84.24**). TCAR time out is then performed ensuring adequate anticoagulation with ACT, prophylactic administration of glycopyrrolate, adequate mean arterial pressure (to allow for the significant delta between the arterial and venous pressure for flow reversal), and finally ensuring that the wire, balloon, and stent are open and flushed, ready for use. Active flow reversal is initiated by clamping the CCA. Debris that may accumulate during carotid intervention is then reversed out of the carotid into the circuit and caught in the filter, while the blood returns to the venous system. The ICA lesion is then crossed with a 0.014 wire. Standard predilation of the carotid lesion with a 3- or 4-mm by 20-mm balloon is then performed. Some have suggested more aggressive balloon dilation of the carotid lesion with a 5- or 6-mm diameter balloon, as the flow reversal is more protective for atheroembolic lesions occurring during prestent dilation. Next, the selected sized ENROUTE stent is delivered and deployed using standard technique. Completion angiogram is then performed to confirm adequate treatment of the carotid lesion (**Fig. 84.24**). Poststent balloon dilation is reserved for severe residual stenosis, as the trend has been to move away from routine poststent balloon dilation due to severe hemodynamic issues with persistent poststent hypotension. Next, the flow reversal is left on for 1 or 2 minutes after stenting to ensure no further debris accumulates. The CCA is unclamped and the flow reversal is then stopped and the carotid sheath is removed while the purse string is sutured down. The venous sheath is then removed. The filter chamber can then be checked to evaluate for debris accumulation (**Fig. 84.25**). Meticulous hemostasis is obtained in the wound base and if need be a drain is left behind (**Fig. 84.26**). The layers are then closed in the standard fashion, and like CEA, it is crucial to ensure no new neurologic symptoms prior to leaving the operating room. Patients are monitored closely for hemodynamic or neurologic issues post-TCAR procedure. Patients are usually discharged home 24 hours after the procedure with 1 month of clopidogrel and lifelong aspirin therapy.

Complications

Early results from the pivotal TCAR trial showed similar perioperative stroke rates as compared to CEA in what is deemed "high-risk" patients. At 30 days, in the pivotal TCAR group, all-stroke rate was 1.4% (2 of 141) and stroke and death rate was 2.8% (4 of 141).[37] MI rates in patients undergoing TCAR have been shown to be similar or slightly lower than those seen with traditional CEA. Postoperative cranial nerve injury is also much lower than in patients undergoing CEA. This is presumably due to the limited dissection of the carotid artery in the base of the neck, away from the cranial nerves. Initial ROADSTER results showed a 0.7% cranial nerve injury rate, with that being one patient suffering from hoarseness from a potential cranial nerve X injury. This completely resolved at the 6-month postoperative visit. Other associated complications include wound complications and postoperative hematoma.

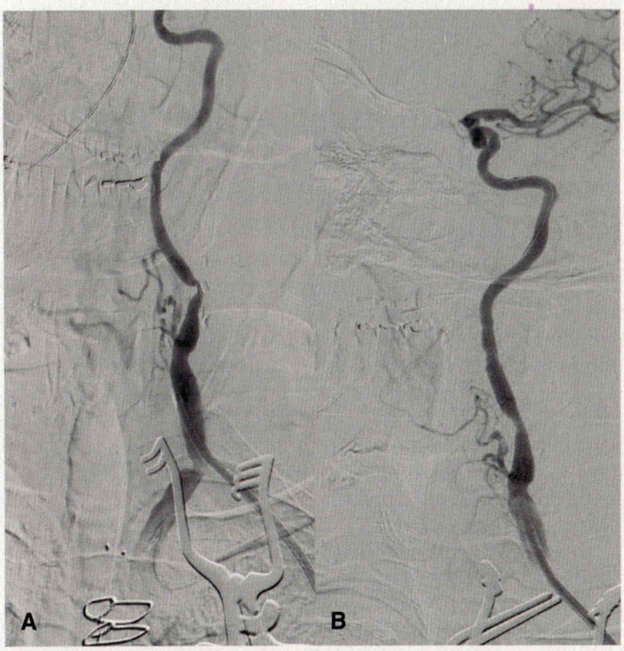

Figure 84.25. **A:** Prestent carotid angiogram showing severe ICA stenosis and clamp on CCA after carotid cut down. **B:** Poststent angiogram after TCAR stent deployment showing no significant residual stenosis and robust flow into the ICA.

Results

TCAR provides an alternative to TFCAS in patients with carotid artery disease that are considered to be high risk for CEA, either anatomic or medical. The initial pivotal TCAR trial showed that at 30 days, TCAR was safe and effective. Thirty-day combined stroke, death, and MI rates were previously shown to be acceptably low (3.7% in ROADSTER 1), and with further analysis of the effectiveness of TCAR, in the postapproval study ROADSTER 2 showed a 1.7% combined stroke, death, and MI rate. Furthermore, ROADSTER 2 continued to show acceptable 30-day outcomes in terms of

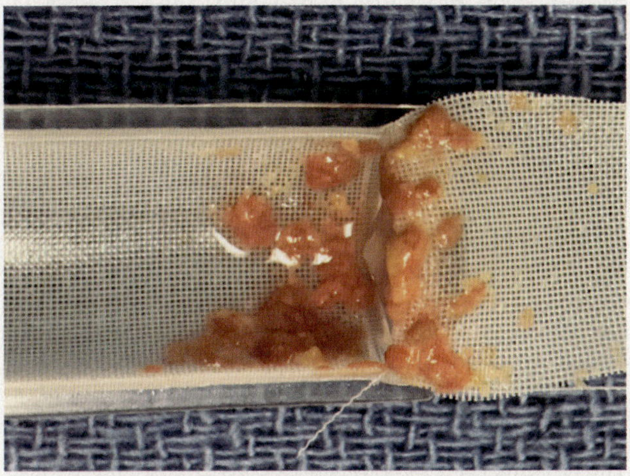

Figure 84.26. Post-TCAR stenting with flow reversal filtering system showing significant debris accumulated during procedure.

stroke/death rate (0.8% in ROADSTER 2 compared to 1.4% in pivotal ROADSTER 1).[38]

CAROTID ENDARTERECTOMY VERSUS TRANSFEMORAL CAROTID STENTING VERSUS TRANSCAROTID REVASCULARIZATION

Carotid interventions for patients with symptomatic (>50%) and asymptomatic (>80%) carotid artery stenosis is widely accepted. The choice of treatment modality is the next decision and is debatable and most certainly patient specific. CEA continues to remain the gold standard for treatment of atherosclerotic carotid artery disease. Higher-risk patients are now afforded multiple treatment types that are minimally invasive. Multiple previous clinical trials have examined the use of TFCAS versus CEA in high-risk patients. In every RCT, TFCAS failed to show similar outcomes to CEA as far as stroke and death. Despite these results, TFCAS continues to have a role in treating patients with carotid artery disease who are not candidates for CEA.

With the recent advent of TCAR, multiple studies have compared treatment of carotid artery disease now with three treatment modalities: TFCAS, TCAR, and CEA. A multiinstitutional analysis of TCAR compared to CEA showed similar 30-day and 1-year stroke rates (1.0% vs 1.1%; 2.8% vs 3.05%, respectively). These results were in spite of TCAR patients having higher rates of diabetes, hyperlipidemia, CAD, and renal insufficiency. TCAR was associated with a decreased rate of cranial nerve injury (0.3% vs 3.8%; P = .01).[39] It has been previously shown that increasing age correlates with a higher embolic risk and thus higher ipsilateral stroke when performing TFCAS in elderly patients. However, at older ages, risk for stroke after CEA remains relatively constant across the age spectrum.[40] A comparative analysis was performed to evaluate the association between age and outcomes after TCAR, TFCAS, and CEA. Rates of inhospital stroke/death after TCAR were 1.4% in patients 70 years or younger, 1.9% in those 71 to 79 years, and 1.5% in those 80 years and older (P = .55). A comparison of TCAR with CEA across different age groups
6 showed no significant differences in outcomes. When compared to TFCAS, no differences were noted between TCAR and TFCAS in patients less than 80 years of age. However, in patients 80 years and older, TCAR was associated with a 72% risk reduction in stroke risk (4.7% vs 1.0%; OR, 0.28; 95% CI, 0.12–0.065; P <.01), a 65% reduction in risk of stroke/death (4.6% vs 1.5%; OR, 0.35; 95% CI, 0.20–0.62; P <.001), and 76% reduction in the risk of stroke/death/MI (5.3% vs.2.5%; OR, 0.24; 95% CI, 0.12–0.47; P <.001) compared with TFCAS.[41] Finally, when comparing TCAR versus TFCAS, recently TCAR was shown to have lower rates of inhospital stroke and death (1.6% vs 3.1%) with no statistically significant differences in rates of perioperative MI (0.2% vs 0.3%). At 1 year, TCAR was associated with lower rate of stroke or death as compared to TFCAS (5.1% vs 9.6%). TCAR was associated with higher rates of access site complications resulting in interventional treatment (1.3% vs 0.8%).[42]

NONATHEROSCLEROTIC CAROTID ARTERY DISEASE

Carotid Artery Dissection

Carotid artery dissection can either occur spontaneously or secondary to precipitating mechanical event (traumatic or iatrogenic). As in any arterial dissection, carotid dissection involves disruption or cleaving of the intima, which allows blood to extravasate in between the layers of the vessel wall. The resulting hematoma usually extends distally and can lead to a high-degree distal ICA stenosis or occlusion (**Fig. 84.27**). Spontaneous dissections are more common in the carotid and vertebral arteries due to their mobility and proximity to bony structures. Even though carotid artery dissections account for a small number of overall strokes, up to 20% of strokes occurring in young patients are due to carotid artery dissection.[43] The classic triad of clinical symptoms includes ipsilateral headache or neck pain, ipsilateral Horner syndrome, and cerebral ischemia. It is quite rare to have all three clinical syndromes occur simultaneously. Headache appears to be the most common symptom and occurs in ipsilateral frontotemporal location. Even though largely asymptomatic, patient can also develop TIA, CVA, amaurosis fugax, cranial nerve palsies, and nausea. Similar to atherosclerotic carotid artery disease, multiple imaging modalities exist including CTA, MRA, DUS; but the gold standard still remains angiography.

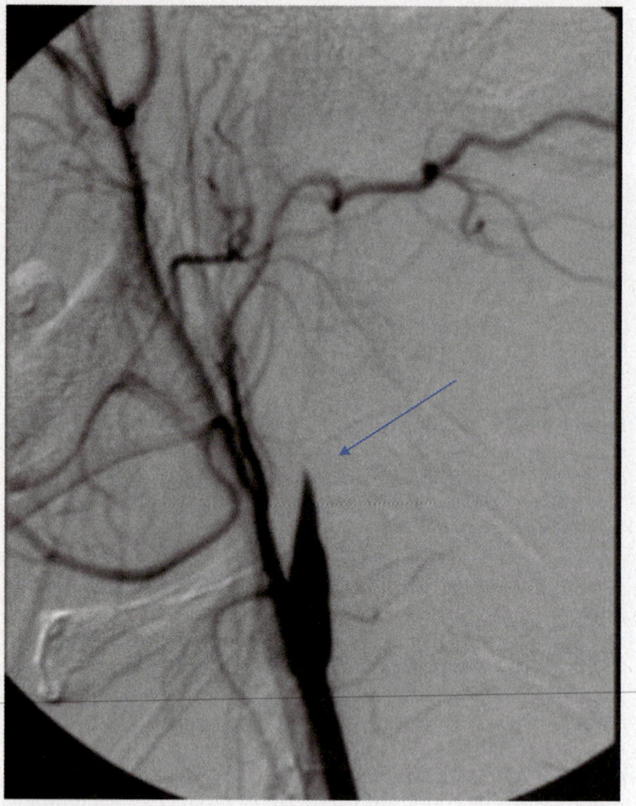

Figure 84.27. Digital subtraction carotid angiogram showing dissection starting in the proximal right ICA with classic-appearing "flame" shape (*arrow*) resulting in distal occlusion.

Treatment options for asymptomatic carotid artery dissection begin with anticoagulation versus antiplatelet therapy. There is a paucity of data regarding which medical agent is better with regard to improved mortality or stroke prevention. The only RCT, the Cervical Artery Dissection in Stroke Study (CADISS) trial, did have one major intracranial hemorrhage in the anticoagulation group versus none in the antiplatelet group. These findings are similar to other nonrandomized studies.[44] Most common treatment continues to be IV heparin followed by anticoagulation for 3 months. Indication for acute surgical intervention include inability to anticoagulate, worsening symptoms, symptoms refractory to anticoagulation, aneurysm formation, or severe neurologic symptoms with severe flow limitation. Options for open surgical repair include surgical bypass, patch angioplasty, or carotid ligation, whereas endovascular treatment comprises mostly of stenting.

Carotid Artery Fibromuscular Dysplasia

FMD involving medium-sized arteries is a rare clinical entity affecting up to 7% of the population. This noninflammatory, nonatherosclerotic arteriopathy is most commonly seen in women, constituting 60% to 90% of patients with FMD. The

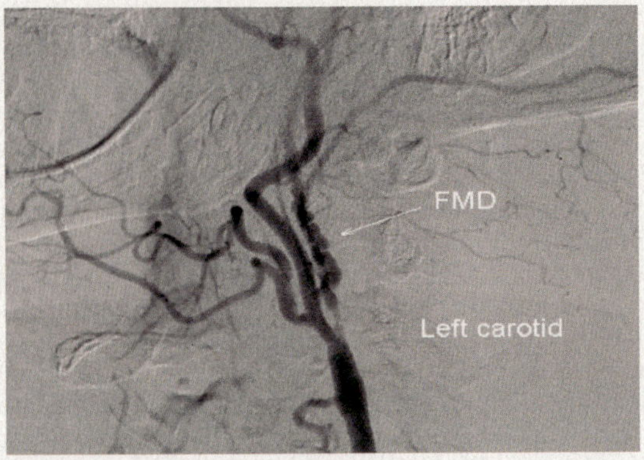

Figure 84.28. Carotid angiogram showing concomitant atherosclerotic carotid bifurcation disease and classic appearing mid ICA FMD.

incidence of carotid FMD is even more rare, with an incidence of only 0.42% in 3,600 patients undergoing cerebral angiographic examination.[45] The exact etiology of FMD is unknown. Four subtypes of FMD exist, with the most common being the medial fibroplasia type, followed by perimedial fibroplasia, intimal fibroplasia, and medial hyperplasia. This type gives off the classic appearance of a "string of beads" (**Fig. 84.28**). This angiographic appearance is caused by segmental encroachment of the arterial lumen and poststenotic dilatation and can be a nidus for hypoperfusion and embolization. As seen in the previous figure, FMD typically occurs in the mid to distal ICA and avoids the carotid bifurcation. Duplex ultrasound imaging can be used to identify carotid FMD lesions, however, elevated velocities and the classic FMD appearance may not be well appreciated. CTA and MRA have largely replaced the need for angiography and are able to clearly show the "string of beads" appearance associated with classic FMD. With that being said, gold standard still remains carotid angiogram. The advantage of CTA or MRA is the ability to identify intracerebral aneurysms, which can occur in up to 50% of carotid FMD patients.

The natural history of FMD is not well established, with few lesions progressing to the point of narrowing of the arterial lumen causing reduced perfusion, formation of thrombus leading to distal embolization, and dissection or rupture. However, the majority of lesions remain clinically silent for years and only require antiplatelet therapy.[46] Symptomatic patients should undergo repair, focusing on breaking the webs associated with FMD. This can be done with either open or endovascular means. In an open repair, serial rigid dilation occurs via a common carotid arteriotomy. This technique allows for back bleeding and removing of debris; however, stroke may occur from debris not washed out after breaking of the webs. Transfemoral angioplasty has been used as an alternative minimally invasive option. Stenting usually is not required. The anatomy of FMD prevents the use of EPD due to the increased risk of embolization. An attractive alternative is the use of TCAR and its novel flow reversal for angioplasty of FMD lesions.

Carotid Artery Aneurysms

Extracranial carotid artery aneurysms are rare and can occur as a result of atherosclerotic degeneration, traumatic injury, dissection or local infection, or as a complication after CEA. True degenerative carotid artery aneurysms are quite rare, with an occurrence of 1% (**Fig. 84.29**). Pulsatile mass is the most common presenting symptom. A high index of suspicion is needed with bruit or pulsatile mass after traumatic head and neck injury. Other presenting symptoms may include cranial nerve dysfunction, Horner syndrome, and neurologic complications, such as TIA or stroke. Rarely, carotid artery aneurysms become so large that they can cause dysphagia or present with hemorrhage or rupture. The natural history of carotid artery aneurysms is not well established, due to its rare incidence.

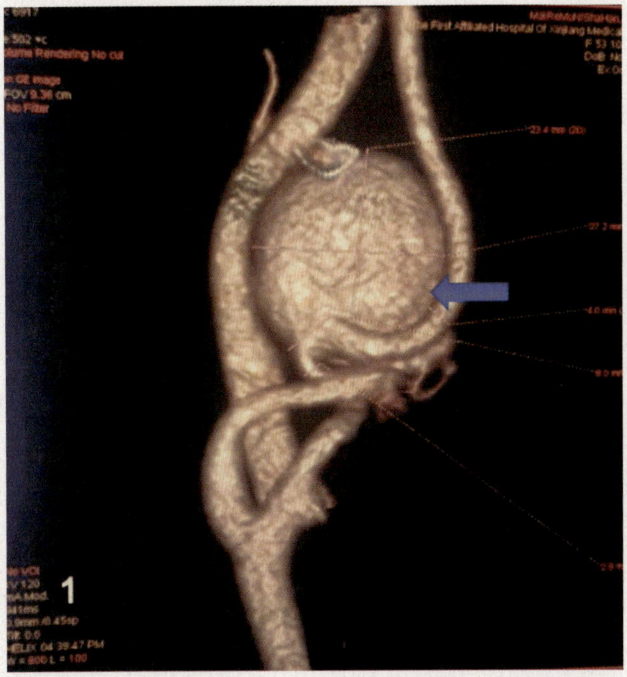

Figure 84.29. 3D reconstruction CTA showing degenerative extracranial carotid aneurysm emanating off of the ICA.

Thus, almost all carotid artery aneurysms are referred for surgical repair. Open surgical repair may include ligation, interposition bypass with vein conduit, or primary end-to-end repair. Endovascular options include exclusion with covered stent graft placement. TCAR might be a reasonable option providing neuroprotection with flow reversal while placing the covered stent. This might be crucial in symptomatic distal carotid aneurysms with unstable thrombus where placement of EPD is difficult as with traditional TFCAS.

Carotid Body Tumors

Tumors arising from the carotid body are neural crest tumors and include paragangliomas, glomus tumors, or chemodectomas. The carotid body includes chemoreceptors located at the bifurcation of the CCA in the posterior and medial adventitia. Carotid body tumors (CBTs) are quite rare without a true known incidence. Risk factors for the development of CBT include hypoxemia, which can be the result of chronic obstructive pulmonary disease or living at high altitudes. These chronic hypoxic states can result in hyperplasia and/or neoplasia of the carotid body, leading to CBT.[47] The vast majority of these tumors are benign and malignant transformation can occur in only about 5% of cases. Since these masses arise at the carotid bifurcation, they can envelope the internal and external carotid arteries and the surrounding cranial nerves. CBTs are slow-growing tumors that typically present as asymptomatic lateral neck masses that may be associated with a thrill or bruit. Because these tumors are fixed to the carotid bifurcation, they are horizontally mobile but not vertically (Fontaine sign). With increasing size, associated symptoms such as neck pain, dysphonia, hoarseness, stridor, dysphagia, jaw stiffness, or sore throat may be present. DUS is a useful initial imaging modality to confirm the presence of CBT. A characteristic splaying of the internal and external carotid arteries is usually seen. Needle biopsy is not recommended due to the hypervascular nature of CBT. Confirmatory CTA of the neck will help delineate the extent of CBT invasion. Shamblin classification has been used to help with the extent of involvement and the degree of difficulty of possible resection. Three types have been described: type I is localized and easily resected; type II is adherent to or partially surrounding vessels; type III is intimately surrounded or encases in the vessels or nerves

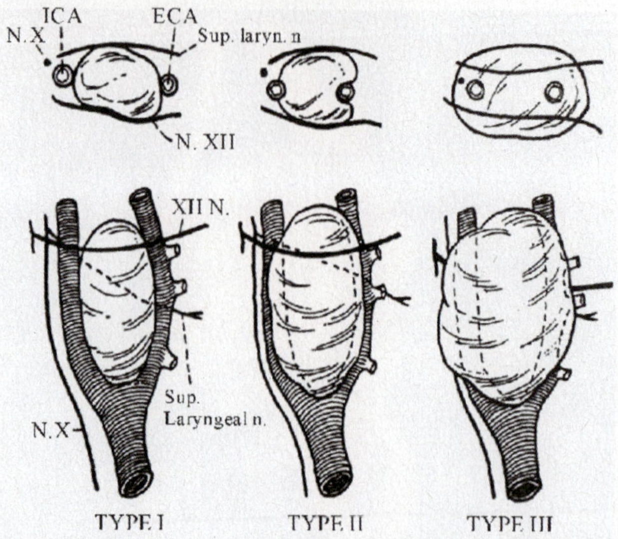

Figure 84.30. Shamblin classification for extent of carotid body tumors.

(**Fig. 84.30**). Treatment involves resection, with larger masses (ie, >4 cm) may benefit from preoperative embolization, but studies are not conclusive for any significant benefit.[48] Exposure for surgical resection involves a similar exposure to a CEA with careful dissection of the tumor off the underlying arteries and nerves. Occasionally, in Shamblin type III cases, excision of the underlying artery is necessary and requires a bypass. Unlike CEA, there is a high incidence of cranial nerve injury at approximately 10%.

Carotid Trauma

Blunt or penetrating cervical trauma can involve the extracranial carotid artery, resulting in intimal disruption, dissection, thrombosis, pseudoaneurysm formation, or transection. Penetrating cervical trauma with injury to the carotid artery can account for a 7% to 27% stroke rate and a 7% to 50% mortality rate.[49] Penetrating cervical trauma with concern for major arterial injury should undergo evaluation and treatment based on location. The neck has classically been divided into three zones: zone I, below the cricoid cartilage; zone II, between the cricoid cartilage and the angle of the mandible; zone III, above the angle of the mandible (**Fig. 84.31**). Carotid

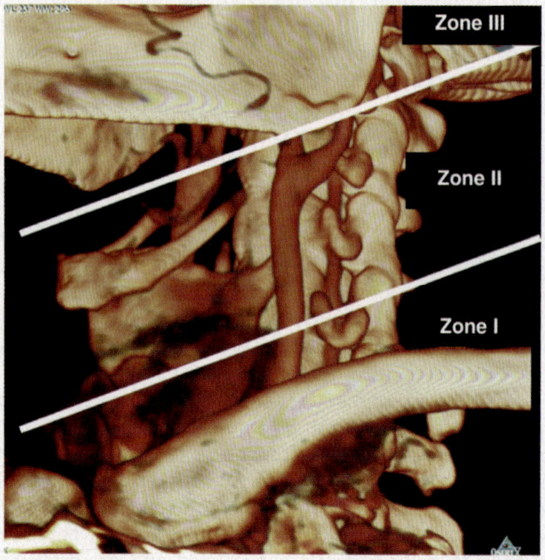

Figure 84.31. Anatomic zones of the neck for penetrating cervical injuries.

artery injuries are most common in zone II (47%), followed by zone III (19%) and zone I (18%).[50] Injury to zones I and III require diagnostic work up to determine if any vascular injury has occurred. Zone I injuries will require a median sternotomy for control, whereas zone III will require maneuvers similar to high exposure for an endarterectomy or the use of endovascular coil embolization or exclusion with covered stent graft placement. Traditionally, all zone II injuries should undergo immediate surgical exploration and repair if carotid artery injury is identified. This can include primary repair, bypass, or ligation. The diagnostic modality of choice is CTA for identification of carotid injury. CT scans can be rapidly obtained in the trauma bay or ED and leads to expeditious identification of possible carotid artery injuries that may require surgical intervention. Medical management can be undertaken in certain cases of asymptomatic carotid dissection with either anticoagulation or antiplatelet therapy. Close observation in asymptomatic traumatic carotid dissections is required to ensure that these injuries don't blossom into pseudoaneurysm formation or carotid thrombosis, necessitating either open repair or endovascular stent placement. Any patient with evidence of cerebral ischemia should undergo prompt carotid revascularization.

VERTEBROBASILAR INSUFFICIENCY

Introduction

Ischemic strokes in the vertebrobasilar territory can account for 25% of all ischemic strokes. The posterior cerebral circulation (ie, vertebrobasilar system) supplies blood to the brainstem, cerebellum, and occipital lobes via paired vertebral arteries arising from the subclavian arteries. Anatomic variants can occur, the most common being a direct origin of the left vertebral artery arising from the aortic arch. The vertebral artery is composed of four segments: V1 is the origin of the vessel up to the level of C6, V2 is the segment that runs within the vertebral foramina to the level of C2, V3 is the next segment above C2 before it enters the base of the skull, and V4 is the intracranial portion of the artery before it joins with the contralateral side forming the basilar artery. VBI is less common than carotid artery ischemia, but it requires prompt diagnostic evaluation for identifying possible surgically correctable atherosclerotic lesions. Mortality associated with a posterior circulation stroke is 20% to 30%, significantly higher than those seen in anterior circulation strokes.[51]

Clinical Findings

VBI is a commonly misdiagnosed clinical syndrome, mostly due to the more subtle and broad symptoms associated with this entity in comparison to the anterior circulation. Unlike the anterior circulation, many times severe ipsilateral atherosclerotic vertebral artery stenosis may go unnoticed due to significant collateral filling due to sufficient collateral flow through a patent circle of Willis. Associated VBI symptoms are largely bilateral and include diplopia, headache, vertigo, drop attacks, ataxia, disequilibrium, and paresthesia.

Pathogenesis

The pathogenesis of vertebrobasilar disease can be broken down into ischemic low-flow mechanism versus embolic. The predominate cause of symptomatic VBI are due to low flow. Embolic issues are difficult to recognize and are most commonly originating from the heart, aorta, or brachiocephalic vessels. As previously mentioned, posterior circulation events are more likely lead to irreversible ischemia and infarction, and thus far more debilitating. These infarctions are most likely the result of embolic events. Up to a third of vertebrobasilar ischemic episodes are caused by distal embolization from plaque or mural lesions of the subclavian, vertebral, or basilar arteries.

Initial Diagnostic Evaluation

The diagnosis of true VBI can sometimes be difficult, given the vagueness of symptoms. Its subtle symptomatology can lead to confusion with a variety of other organ systems that can mimic these symptoms. Oftentimes, syncope or presyncope can be confused for vertebrobasilar symptoms. This can be due to a multitude of causes such as vasovagal, cardiac arrhythmias, neurologic, psychiatric, or idiopathic. Moreover, even though the vast majority of VBI is due to atherosclerosis, other etiologies include dissection, trauma, FMD, aneurysms, and Takayasu disease. Patients with visual changes (ie, diplopia) can be mistaken for myopia or presbyopia, cataracts, floaters, and amaurosis fugax. Vertigo-type symptoms can be caused by many etiologies and can be confused for postural instability, hearing loss, or nystagmus.

DUS can be a very useful initial study to help identify proximal vertebral artery atherosclerotic disease. With that being said, it is a more difficult examination than extracranial carotid arteries, and sometimes severe vertebral artery stenosis may be missed. Duplex can identify reversal of flow in the vertebral artery, which may indicate more proximal disease in the subclavian or innominate arteries. Evaluation of the vertebral artery between C2 and C6 is difficult with DUS. CTA and MRA allow for a complete and careful examination of the entire vertebral artery, this allows for identification of disease and illuminate collateral circulation. In addition, MRI can help identify if embolic lesions and posterior cerebral infarctions have occurred. The “gold standard” remains angiography. Selective vertebral angiography will allow for a complete interrogation of the vertebral artery to identify proximal or distal stenosis. Collateral circulation can also be shown via contralateral and anterior circulation.

Treatment

Treatment of symptomatic VBI is based on the location of the offending vertebral lesion. The majority of lesions involve the proximal V1 segment of the vertebral artery. The most common pathology of the V2 segment is extrinsic compression of the vertebral artery by osteophytes. V3 segment lesions are mostly related to trauma and arterial dissection. The V4 segment is largely unaffected by atherosclerotic disease and given its intracranial location, it is more susceptible to direct trauma and stretch injuries as well as formation of AV fistulas or pseudoaneurysms. Proximal (ie, ostial) V1 atherosclerotic lesions are the most common open operation for VBI. Vertebral artery transposition of the proximal vertebral artery on the adjacent carotid artery is the most common reconstruction. Less likely to be performed, bypass from the common carotid or subclavian artery (SCA) to the vertebral artery distal to the disease with a vein graft is a viable option. The most common reason for open surgical repair of V2 lesions is hemorrhage and this typically requires proximal and distal ligation. Options for the V3 segment include bypass with greater saphenous or lesser saphenous vein, usually to the C1–2 segment. Other reported open surgical revascularizations for the V3 segment include use of ECA or radial artery. For more distal reconstructions (into the V4 segment) suboccipital exposure of the vertebral artery usually requires resection of the C1 transverse process. Vertebral artery transposition or other V1 segment operations are the most studied surgical operations for VBI. Stroke and death rates for these operations have been reported to be <1%. Other complication includes nerve injury (vagus, recurrent laryngeal), Horner syndrome, and lymphatic leak. Vertebral artery transpositions experience excellent 5- and 10-year patency rates at 95% and 91%, respectively. More than 80% of patients will have relief of their symptoms after proximal surgical reconstruction.[52]

7 Endovascular management of proximal vertebral artery atherosclerotic lesions has been shown to be safe and effective in a small number of nonrandomized studies.[53] The relative ease in which angioplasty and stenting of a proximal vertebral lesion as compared to the open operation, has driven this increase in endovascular management (**Fig. 84.32**). As with CAS, risk of embolization, stroke, thrombosis, dissection, or restenosis exists. Use of EPD can reduce the risk of distal embolization and should be recommended when treating atherosclerotic proximal vertebral artery lesions. Stent placement has not been widely shown to be effective for the treatment of V2 or V3 traumatic dissections, given the location in the vertebral foramina. Similar to open ligation, endovascular management of vertebral artery transection or hemorrhage involves embolization to control bleeding.

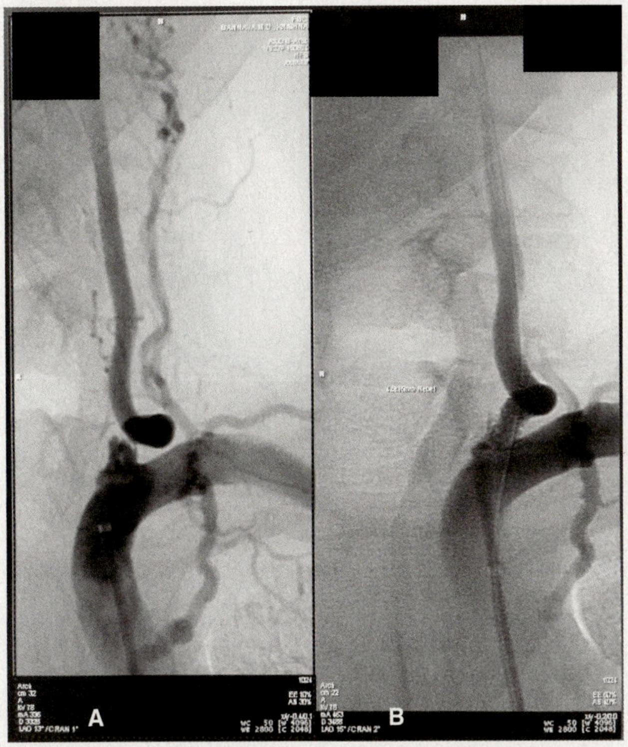

Figure 84.32. **A:** Angiogram showing severe proximal V1 vertebral artery stenosis in a patient with a posterior circulation stroke. **B:** Completion angiogram after successful balloon angioplasty and stenting.

ATHEROSCLEROTIC BRACHIOCEPHALIC DISEASE

Introduction

The great vessels arise from the aortic arch to give off (from proximal to distal) the innominate artery, the left CCA, and the left SCA. These arteries supply the upper extremities and brain and thus are commonly referred to as the brachiocephalic vessels. Anatomic variants do exist with regard to the origins of these vessels. Most commonly, the innominate and left CCA come of the arch in one common ostia, referred to as a “bovine arch” (**Fig. 84.33**). This variant is found in 8% to 25% of Americans, with higher incidence seen in African American patients.[54] Another common variant is the presence of the left vertebral artery directly emanating from the aorta between the left CCA and SCA. This occurs in about 6% of the patient population. In addition, an aberrant right SCA can be seen with its origin coming from the aorta distal to the left SCA and coursing posteriorly behind the arch. This variant is the rarest, occurring in 0.5% to 1% of the time.[55] The most common etiology of brachiocephalic disease continues to be atherosclerotic disease. Commonly, multivessel atherosclerotic disease can be present and is more often accompanied by symptoms of VBI from generalized low flow. However, embolic phenomenon can be seen as well-exhibiting single-vessel symptoms, when multivessel disease is present. Other diseases affecting the brachiocephalic arteries include aneurysmal degeneration, dissection, vasculitis (eg, Takayasu disease and giant cell arteritis), infection, and radiation arteritis.

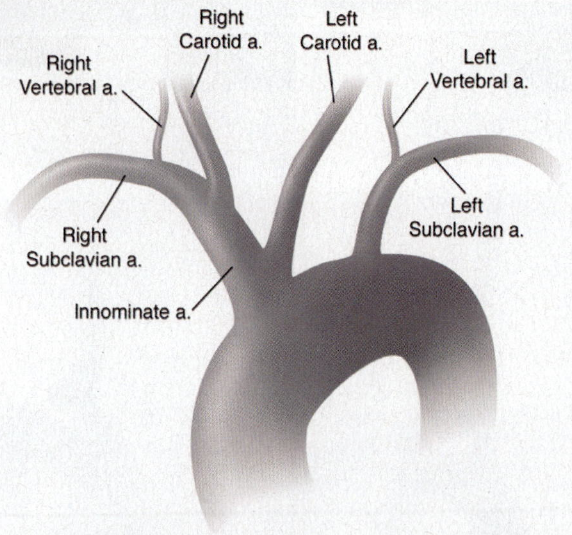

Figure 84.33. Most common aortic arch branch variants in humans with a common trunk for the innominate and left common carotid artery. (From Layton KF, Kallmes DF, Cloft HJ, Lindell EP, Cox VS. Bovine aortic arch variant in humans: Clarification of a common misnomer. *Am J Neuroradiol.* 2006;27(7):1541–1542; used with permission of Mayo Foundation for Medical Education and Research, all rights reserved.)

Clinical Findings

As mentioned above, atherosclerosis is the most common disease that affects the brachiocephalic vessels. Clinical findings are dependent on location of the disease and how many vessels are involved. Single-vessel atherosclerotic occlusive disease typically causes symptoms as a result of hemispheric or upper extremity emboli, but low-flow states are also seen. When the innominate artery is involved, patient may suffer from stroke (anterior or posterior circulation), TIA, or upper extremity ischemia. Isolated CCA disease is typically manifested as stroke or TIA. Single-vessel proximal SCA occlusive disease can cause arm ischemia, as evidenced by limiting arm claudication, with very rare instances of digital ischemia and gangrene. Subclavian steal syndrome can be seen in single-vessel occlusive disease, which can manifest as VBI or subclavian-coronary steal. When patient has a functioning left internal mammary artery (LIMA) coronary bypass, recurrent episodes of angina can be seen in instances when severe proximal SCA stenosis is present.

Diagnostic Evaluation

The mainstay for screening for brachiocephalic arterial disease continues to be a prudent physical examination. Careful assessment of the upper extremity pulses, individual upper extremity blood pressure measurements, and auscultation of carotid and SCA bruits are effective tools that allow the practitioners to suspect significant pathology. Blood pressure measurements in individual arms in patients with brachiocephalic disease can show a 20 mm Hg or greater difference between sides. Typically, the initial diagnostic study that is performed is a DUS. There are limitations in using DUS for evaluation of brachiocephalic atherosclerotic disease. Overlying bony structures make identification of aortic arch and proximal great vessels difficult. DUS can be useful in identifying reversal of flow in the vertebral artery, indicating a significant proximal stenosis, as well as rule out significant disease in the extracranial carotid arteries. A decrease in the waveform amplitude and slope (tardus–parvus waveform) can signify significant proximal CCA disease.

CTA and MRA provide excellent imaging of the aorta and brachiocephalic branches. The use of 3D reconstruction can help facilitate planning of surgical interventions without the need of performing a diagnostic angiogram. Gated computed tomography (CT) in coordination with electrocardiogram allows for more careful identification of the mobile ascending aorta and arch, and decreases the amount of motion artifact. Furthermore, CTA and MRA (**Fig. 84.34**) allow for a complete evaluation of arterial flow from the arch to the brain, as well as evaluation of collateral circulation, which is necessary for surgical planning. Angiography remains the "gold standard," but does have associated risk of stroke, embolization (albeit very low), and arterial injury. Also, with advanced CTA and MRA techniques, this is quickly surpassing routine diagnostic angiography for routine identification of brachiocephalic disease.

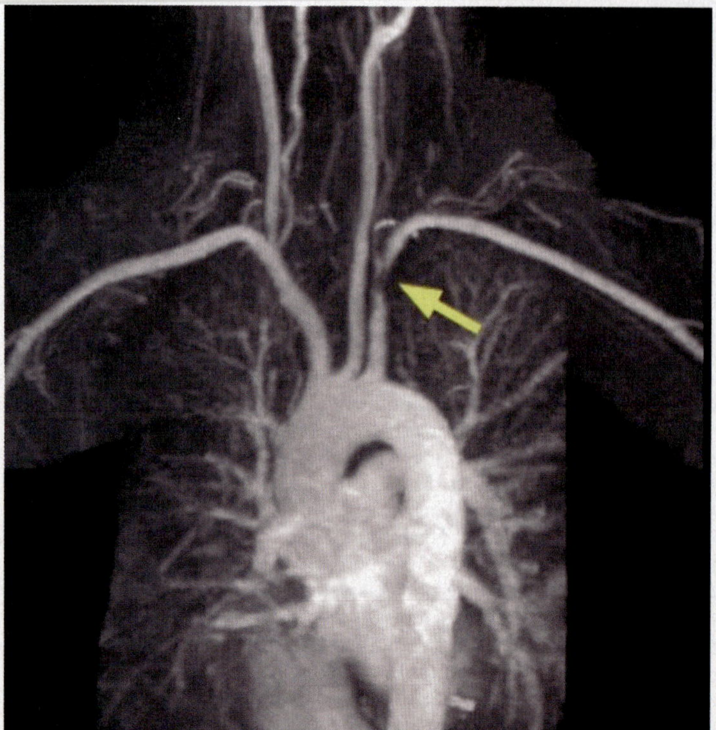

Figure 84.34. 3D MIP reconstruction of a contrast-enhanced MRA demonstrating a focal left subclavian artery stenosis.

Finally, transesophageal echocardiography (TEE) can be used to evaluate for ascending and descending aortic pathology.

Indications for Repair

Any symptomatic brachiocephalic stenosis should be treated with either open or endovascular techniques. Asymptomatic disease can safely be monitored for progression of disease, as well as medically managing risk factors. Stroke and TIA should be promptly evaluated and underlying lesion should be repaired, due to the fear of ongoing embolization or continued symptoms from a low-flow state. Severe upper extremity ischemia, as evident by severe claudication, rest pain or tissue loss should undergo prompt repair. Also, a low threshold for repair should be given to those with a patent LIMA coronary bypass and proximal subclavian disease. Patients with a functional hemodialysis access and evidence of SCA disease, should also be considered for repair if ongoing low-flow issues are occurring within the dialysis access or signs of steal are apparent.

Surgical Treatment

Two main approaches are taken for the open surgical treatment of brachiocephalic disease: transthoracic and extra-anatomic revascularization. Transthoracic repair requires a median sternotomy and revascularization, with either direct arterial reconstruction or bypass from the ascending aorta to the involved brachiocephalic arteries. This approach is ideal for low-risk patients and those with multivessel disease. When treating patients with multivessel disease, such as Takayasu arteritis, transthoracic repair with debranching off the ascending aorta to healthy vessels avoids diseased arterial segments and is the ideal repair. In appropriately selected patients, this approach can have excellent results with acceptable morbidity. Complications include mortality and stroke rates of 3% to 8% and MI rates of 1.5% to 3%. Excellent 10-year patency of approximately 90% can be achieved with direct transthoracic reconstruction.[56]

For single-vessel brachiocephalic disease and for higher-risk patients, extra-anatomic revascularization may be more suitable. This technique can also be used in hybrid approaches when treating patients with open surgical and endovascular techniques. Options for repair include a carotid–carotid bypass, axilloaxillary bypass, carotid–subclavian bypass, or carotid–subclavian transposition. The vast majority of extra-anatomic bypasses are done for single-vessel severe SCA stenosis. Transposition is technically more difficult than a carotid–subclavian bypass, but has the advantage of avoiding prosthetic material. Results are also excellent for carotid–subclavian bypass or subclavian transposition, with 5-year patency of 95% and 100%, respectively. Carotid–subclavian bypasses are one of the few bypasses that favor the use of prosthetic graft over autogenous vein graft, 5-year patency of 94% versus 58.3% (P <.01).[57] When considering carotid–subclavian bypass, if patients have concomitant, severe carotid stenosis, it is feasible to perform a CEA, followed by a carotid–subclavian bypass in order to prevent a low-flow state to the ipsilateral anterior circulation (**Fig. 84.35**).

Endovascular management of brachiocephalic lesions has gained wide popularity over the past 20 years. Single-vessel brachiocephalic stenosis is better suited for endovascular management; however, in a certain subset of patients that are too ill to undergo an open repair, aggressive endovascular treatment in multivessel brachiocephalic stenosis can also be performed. As with carotid stenting, endovascular treatment of brachiocephalic lesions depends on aortic anatomy, anatomical variants, baseline renal function, arch type, lesion characteristics, and proximity to branch vessels. Endovascular management consists of angioplasty and stenting (**Fig. 84.36**). Similar to cervical

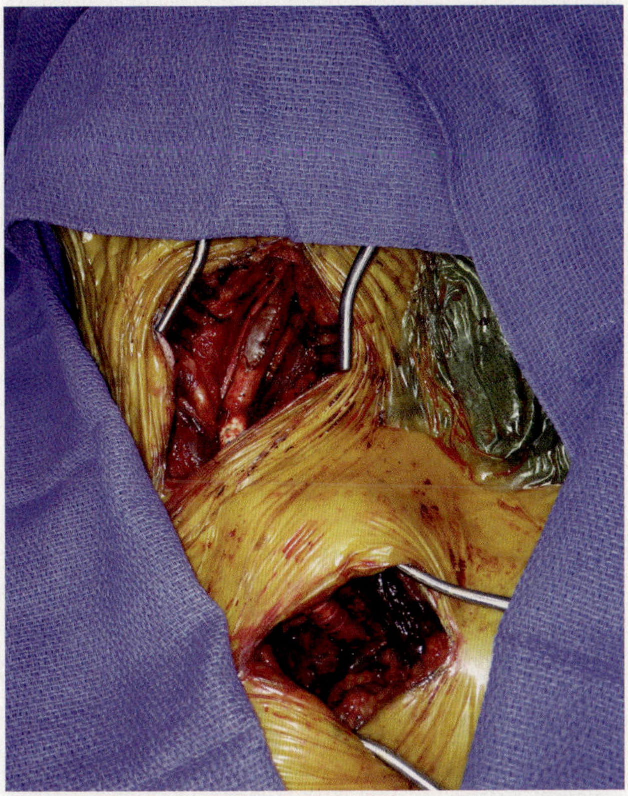

Figure 84.35. Patient with concomitant severe left ICA stenosis and symptomatic proximal and mid-left SCA stenosis who underwent a left CEA with a left carotid-axillary artery bypass.

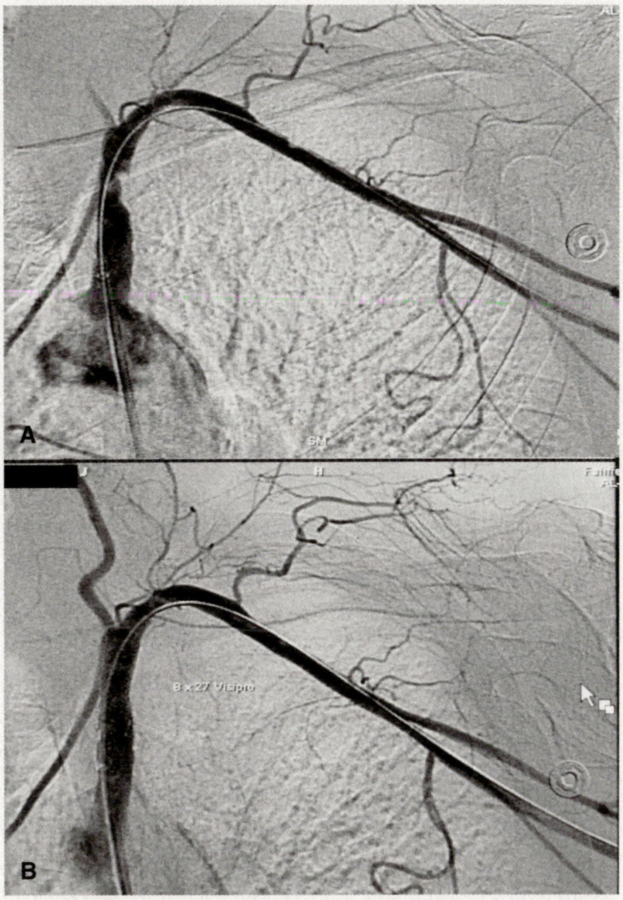

Figure 84.36. **A:** Prestent angiogram revealing high-grade left subclavian artery stenosis with ulcerated plaque. **B:** Poststent angiogram with stenting showing excellent flow throughout the subclavian artery with increased filling of the left vertebral artery.

CAS, use of intraprocedural heparin and DAPT afterward is a must. EPD can be used to minimize the risk of embolization when treating innominate or proximal CCA stenosis. Endovascular results do not appear to compare favorably with open repair. One-year patency appears to be close to 90%, however, at 5-year patency drops to 77% to 89%.[58] Alternatively, retrograde approach through a cut down on the CCA allows for better protection with clamping. When intervening on proximal SCA stenosis, great care must be used to avoid encroachment on or embolization to the vertebral artery. Similarly, great attention must be paid to avoiding embolization to the cervical ICA when treating innominate or proximal thoracic CCA stenosis. Sometimes, alternate access (brachial) is needed to help facilitate protection of the vertebral or carotid artery during stenting of proximal brachiocephalic lesions.

References

1. Centers for Disease Control and Prevention (CDC). *Stroke.* https://www.cdc.gov/stroke/index.html
2. Brott TG, Hobson RW 2nd, Howard G, et al; CREST Investigators. Stenting versus endarterectomy for treatment of carotid-artery stenosis. *N Eng J Med.* 2010;363(1):11–23.
3. Tadi P, Lui F. Acute Stroke. 2023 Aug 17. In: StatPearls [Internet]. Treasure Island (FL): StatPearls Publishing; 2025 Jan–.
4. World Stroke Organization. https://www.world-stroke.org
5. Benjamin EJ, Blaha MJ, Chiuve SE, et al; On behalf of the American Heart Association Statistics Committee and Stroke Statistics Subcommittee. Heart disease and stroke statistics—2017 update: A report from the American Heart Association. *Circulation.* 2017;135:e146–e603.
6. Centers for Disease Control and Prevention (CDC). Prevalence of stroke—United States. *MMWR Morb Mortal Wkly Rep.* 2012; 61(20):379–382. http://www.cdc.gov/mmwr/preview/mmwrhtml/mm6120a5.htm?s_cid=mm6120a5_w#tab1
7. White H, Boden-Albala B, Wang C, et al. Ischemic stroke subtype incidence among whites, blacks, and Hispanics: The Northern Manhattan Study. *Circulation.* 2005;111:1327–1331.
8. Prabhakaran S, Ruff I, Bernstein RA. Acute stroke intervention: A systematic review. *JAMA.* 2015;313(14):1451–1462.
9. Roger VL, Go AS, Lloyd-Jones DM, et al. Heart disease and stroke statistics—2012 update: A report from the American Heart Association. *Circulation.* 2012;125:e2–e220.
10. Go AS, Mozaffarian D, Roger VL, et al; American Heart Association Statistics Committee and Stroke Statistics Subcommittee. Heart disease and stroke statistics—2014 update: A report from the American Heart Association. *Circulation.* 2014;129:e28–e292.
11. Ross R. The pathogenesis of atherosclerosis—an update. *N Engl J Med.* 1986;314:488–500.
12. Petty GW, Brown RD Jr, Whisnant JP, Sicks JD, O'Fallon WM, Wiebers DO. Ischemic stroke subtypes: a population-based study of functional outcome, survival, and recurrence. *Stroke.* 2000;31: 1062–1068.
13. Chen CS, Miller NR. Ocular ischemic syndrome: Review of clinical presentations, etiology, investigation, and management. *Compr Opthalmol Update.* 2007;8:17–28.
14. Ratchford EV, Jin Z, Di Tullio MR, et al. Carotid bruit for detection of hemodynamically significant carotid stenosis: The Northern Manhattan Study. *Neurol Res.* 2009;31(7):748–752.
15. Kim AH, Augustin G, Kim H, et al. Comparison of two duplex ultrasound diagnostic criteria for carotid stenosis with computed tomography angiography. *J Vasc Surg.* 2016;64(3):864–865.
16. Barnett HJ, Taylor DW, Eliasziw M, et al. Benefit of carotid endarterectomy in patients with symptomatic moderate or severe stenosis. North American Symptomatic Carotid Endarterectomy Trial Collaborators. *N Engl J Med.* 1998;339:1415–1425.
17. Warlow CP. Symptomatic patients: The European Carotid Surgery Trial (ECST). *J Mal Vasc.* 1993;18:198–201.
18. Blauw GJ, Lagaay AM, Smelt AH, Westendorp RG. Stroke, statins, and cholesterol. A meta-analysis of randomized, placebo-controlled, double-blind trials with HMG-CoA reductase inhibitors. *Stroke.* 1997;28:946–950.
19. Giles MF, Rothwell PM. Risk of stroke early after transient ischaemic attack: A systematic review and meta-analysis. *Lancet Neurol.* 2007;6:1063–1072.
20. Tanious A, Pothof AB, Boitano LT, et al. Timing of carotid endarterectomy after stroke: Retrospective review of prospectively collected national database. *J Vasc Surg.* 2018;268(3):449–456.
21. Endarterectomy for asymptomatic carotid artery stenosis. Executive Committee for the Asymptomatic Carotid Atherosclerosis Study. *JAMA.* 1995;273:1421–1428.
22. Halliday A, Mansfield A, Marro J, et al. Prevention of disabling and fatal strokes by successful carotid endarterectomy in patients without recent neurological symptoms: Randomised controlled trial. *Lancet.* 2004;363:1491–1502.
23. Abbott AL. Regarding "asymptomatic carotid artery stenosis-medical therapy alone versus medical therapy plus carotid endarterectomy or stenting." *J Vasc Surg.* 2011;53(1):265.
24. Eastcott HHG, Pickering GW, Rob CG. Reconstruction of internal carotid artery in a patient with intermittent attacks of hemiplegia. *Lancet.* 1954;267:994–996.
25. Hye RJ, Voeks JH, Malas MB, et al. Anesthetic type and risk of myocardial infarction after carotid endarterectomy in the Carotid Revascularization Endarterectomy versus Stenting Trial (CREST). *J Vasc Surg.* 2015;62(2):523.
26. Wiske C, Arhuidese I, Malas M, Patterson R. Comparing the efficacy of shunting approaches and cerebral monitoring during carotid endarterectomy using a national database. *J Vasc Surg.* 2018;68(2):416–425.
27. Dakour-Aridi H, Gaber MG, Khalid M, Patterson R, Malas MB. Examination of the interaction between method of anesthesia and shunting with carotid endarterectomy. *J Vasc Surg.* 2020;71(6):1964–1971.
28. Malas MB, Glebova NO, Hughes SE, et al. The Effect of Patching on reducing restenosis in the carotid revascularization endarterectomy versus stenting trial. *Stroke.* 2015;46:757–761.
29. Cao P, Giordano G, De Rango P, et al. Eversion versus conventional carotid endarterectomy: Late results of prospective multicenter randomized trial. *J Vasc Surg.* 2000;31:19–30.
30. Dakour-Aridi H, Ou M. Locham S, AbuRahma A, Schneider JR, Malas M. Outcomes following eversion versus conventional endarterectomy in the vascular quality initiative database. *Ann Vasc Surg.* 2020;65:1–9.
31. Hertzer NR, Lees CD. Fatal myocardial infarction following carotid endarterectomy: three hundred thirty-five patients followed 6–11 years after operation. *Ann Surg.* 1981;194:212–218.
32. Forssell C, Takolander R, Bergqvist D, Bergentz SE, Gramming P, Kitzing P. Cranial nerve injuries associated with carotid endarterectomy. A prospective study. *Acta Chir Scand.* 1985; 151:595–598.
33. Obeid T, Arnaoutakis DJ, Arhuidese I, et al. Poststent ballooning is associated with increased periprocedural stroke and death rate in carotid artery stenting. *J Vasc Surg.* 2015;62(3):616–623.
34. Group SC, Ringleb PA, Allenberg J, et al. 30 day results from the SPACE trial of stent-protected angioplasty versus carotid endarterectomy in symptomatic patients: a randomised non-inferiority trial. *Lancet.* 2006;368:1239–1247.
35. Mas JL, Chatellier G, Beyssen B, et al. Endarterectomy versus stenting in patients with symptomatic severe carotid stenosis. *N Engl J Med.* 2006;355:1660–1671.
36. Brott TG, Howard G, Roubin GS, et al; CREST Investigators. Long-term results of stenting versus endarterectomy for carotid-artery stenosis. *N Engl J Med.* 2016;374:1021–1031.
37. Kwolek CJ, Jaff MR, Leal JI, et al. Results of the ROADSTER multicenter trial of transcarotid stenting with dynamic flow reversal. *J Vasc Surg.* 2015;62(5):1227–1234.
38. Hans-Henning Eckstein ROADSTER 2 Study Group. Early outcomes in the ROADSTER 2 clinical trial of transcarotid artery revascularization in patients with significant carotid artery disease. *Eur J Vasc Endovasc Surg.* 2019;58(6):e637.
39. Kashyap VS, King AH, Foteh MI, et al. A multi-institutional analysis of transcarotid artery revascularization compared to carotid endarterectomy. *J Vasc Surg.* 2019;70(1):123–129.

40. Nejim B, Alshwaily W, Dakour-Aridi H, Locham S, Goodney P, Malas MB. Age modifies the efficacy and safety of carotid artery revascularization procedures. *J Vasc Surg.* 2019;69(5): 1490–1503.e3.
41. Aridi HD, Kashyap VS, Wang GJ, et al. Age and outcomes after transcarotid artery revascularization, transfemoral carotid artery stenting and carotid endarterectomy. *J Vasc Surg.* 2019;69(6):e60–e61.
42. Malas MB, Dakour-Aridi H, Wang GJ, et al. Transcarotid artery revascularization versus transfemoral carotid artery stenting in the Society for Vascular Surgery Vascular Quality Initiative. *J Vasc Surg.* 2019;69(1):92–103.
43. Bogousslavsky J, Regli F. Ischemic stroke in adults younger than 30 years of age. Cause and prognosis. *Arch Neurol.* 1987;44:479–482.
44. CADISS trial investigators; Markus HS, Hayter E, Levi C, et al. Antiplatelet treatment compared with anticoagulation treatment for cervical artery dissection (CADISS): a randomised trial. *Lancet Neruol.* 2015;14(4):361–367.
45. Slovut DP, Olin JW. Fibromuscular dysplasia. *N Engl J Med.* 2004; 350:1862–1871.
46. So EL, Toole JF, Dalal P, Moody DM. Cephalic fibromuscular dysplasia in 32 patients: Clinical findings and radiologic features. *Arch Neurol* 1981;38:619–622.
47. Sajid MS, Hamilton G, Baker DM; Joint Vascular Research Group. A multicenter review of carotid body tumour management. *Eur J Vasc Endovasc Surg.* 2007;34:127–130.
48. Thakkar R, Qazi U, Kim Y, Fishman EK, Veith FJ, Malas MB. Technique and role of embolization using ethylene vinyl-alcohol copolymer before carotid body tumor resection. *Clin Pract.* 2014;4(3):661.
49. du Toit DF, van Schalkwyk GD, Wadee SA, Warren BL. Neurologic outcome after penetrating extracranial arterial trauma. *J Vasc Surg.* 2003;38:257–262.
50. Demetriades D, Theodorou D, Cornwell E, et al. Evaluation of penetrating injuries of the neck: Prospective study of 223 patients. *World J Surg.* 1997;21:41–47.
51. Patrick BK, Ramirez-Lassepas M, Synder BD. Temporal profile of vertebrobasilar territory infarction. Prognostic implications. *Stroke.* 1980;11:643–648.
52. Berguer R, Flynn LM, Kline RA, Caplan L. Surgical reconstruction of the extracranial vertebral artery: management and outcome. *J Vasc Surg.* 2000;31:9–18.
53. Dabus G, Gerstle RJ, Derdeyn CP, Cross DT 3rd, Moran CJ. Endovascular treatment of the vertebral artery origin in patients with symptoms of vertebrobasilar ischemia. *Neuroradiology.* 2006;48(12):917–923.
54. Layton KF, Kallmes DF, Cloft HJ, Lindell EP, Cox VS. Bovine aortic arch variant in humans: Clarification of a common misnomer. *Am J Neuroradiol.* 2006;27(7):1541–1542.
55. Stone WM, Brewster DC, Moncure AC, Franklin DP, Cambria RP, Abbott WM. Aberrant right subclavian artery: Varied presentations and management options. *J Vasc Surg.* 1990;11: 812–817.
56. Berguer R, Morasch MD, Kline RA. Transthoracic repair of innominate and common carotid artery disease: Immediate and long-term outcome for 100 consecutive surgical reconstructions. *J Vasc Surg.* 1998;27:34–41; discussion 42.
57. Law MM, Colburn MD, Moore WS, Quiñones-Baldrich WJ, Machleder HI, Gelabert HA. Carotid-subclavian bypass for brachiocephalic occlusive disease. Choice of conduit and long-term follow-up. *Stroke.* 1995;26:1565–1571.
58. Bates MC, Broce M, Lavigne PS, Stone P. Subclavian artery stenting: Factors influencing long-term outcome. *Catheter Cardiovasc Interv.* 2004;61:5–11.

85

Upper Extremity Artery Disease

Adam P. Johnson and Brian F. Gilmore

Key Points

1 Primary etiologies of upper extremity artery disease include atherosclerotic occlusive disease, dissection, aneurysm, and inflammatory conditions.

2 Secondary etiologies include extrinsic artery compression, substance-induced dysfunction, traumatic injury, and access-related hand ischemia.

3 Unilateral hand ischemia points toward an isolated anatomic lesion, whereas bilateral hand ischemia is more often related to systemic diseases.

4 Various noninvasive tests are available for the initial investigation of arm ischemia, and detailed bilateral artery imaging is needed for treatment planning.

5 The choice of procedure must be tailored to the anatomy and etiology of each specific patient.

Upper extremity artery disease presents a clinical challenge to clinicians both emergently and in the elective setting, resulting from a wide range of etiologies. Regardless of etiology, initial presentations can often be similar and overlap with a narrow set of symptoms and examination findings, so the workup should be systematic and comprehensive to rule out the most serious and time-sensitive etiologies. Treatment strategies are best implemented once the correct etiology and affected anatomy are identified. This chapter will discuss the broad differential diagnosis, systematic and comprehensive workup, and etiology-specific medical, endovascular, and surgical management strategies.

ETIOLOGY

Upper-extremity artery disease can result from many etiologies broadly classified as primary, a disease of the artery itself, or secondary, resulting from some external factor (**Table 85.1**). Primary etiologies include atherosclerosis, aneurysm, dissection, or inflammation. Secondary etiologies include extrinsic artery compression, substance-induced dysfunction, and traumatic injury, including iatrogenic trauma and access-related hand ischemia (AHRI).

Primary Etiologies

1 Atherosclerosis typically affects the origins of the supra-aortic trunks, with ostial lesions at the origin of the subclavian artery being the most common. However, lesions can occur anywhere in the artery system, and multilevel disease is common. Despite this, patients are frequently asymptomatic even with total occlusion due to the robust network of collateral vessels perfusing the upper extremity and the upper extremity's relatively lower baseline metabolic requirements. Upper extremity artery occlusive disease is particularly troublesome in patients requiring hemodialysis, as surgery in the upper extremity for hemodialysis access often unmasks asymptomatic disease, resulting in steal syndrome. Patients with renal failure, in whom hand ischemia tends to occur at a younger age, frequently have normal proximal vessels with severe disease in the blood vessels of the forearm and hand.[1] Steal syndrome from hemodialysis access will be discussed in more detail later in the chapter.

Artery dissection in the upper extremity can occur either primarily in the arteries of the arm proper or as an extension of an aortic dissection. Primary upper extremity aneurysms are rare.[2] Pseudoaneurysms can develop due to trauma, frequently iatrogenic trauma, or as mycotic processes.

Inflammatory conditions like Takayasu or giant cell arteritis (GCA) can also affect the great vessels.[3] Takayasu arteritis is a rare, inflammatory vasculitis that affects the aorta and its major branches, including the subclavian and innominate arteries. This disease typically occurs in adult women before the age of 50. An initial acute inflammatory phase causes vessel thickening. It is followed by a late chronic phase where long segments of stenosis occur in the vessels, generally presenting with end-organ ischemic symptoms (**Table 85.2, Fig. 85.1**). GCA is a more common inflammatory vascular disease typically affecting older patients. This involves medium to large blood vessels with a characteristic pattern of areas of normal luminal diameter alternating with dilated or stenotic lesions.[4] Thromboangiitis obliterans, also known as Buerger disease, is an obliterative vasculitis that occurs most frequently in males and is heavily associated with smoking, typically affecting medium and small arteries in both the upper and lower extremities. In addition to these vasculitides, the upper extremity arteries can be involved in several systemic autoimmune conditions, including scleroderma, rheumatoid arthritis, CREST syndrome, mixed connective tissue disorders, and lupus.

Secondary Etiologies

2 Thoracic outlet syndrome (TOS) encompasses a group of signs and symptoms related to compression of the brachial plexus and subclavian artery and vein as they pass from the thorax into the axilla through a narrow outlet formed by the clavicle superiorly, the first rib inferiorly, the subclavius muscle anteriorly and superiorly, as well as the scalene muscles posteriorly (**Fig. 85.2**). Bony anomalies, such as a cervical rib or an abnormal first thoracic rib, are often structural contributors to TOS. Neurogenic and venous TOS are significantly

ETIOLOGIES

Table 85.1. Etiologies for Upper Extremity Vascular Disease

Primary Etiologies
Atherosclerotic disease
Embolism
Fibromuscular dysplasia
Inflammatory and connective tissue disorders
Takayasu disease
Giant cell arteritis
Thromboangiitis obliterans
Scleroderma, Raynaud's phenomenon
Secondary Etiologies
Embolism
Extrinsic compression
Thoracic outlet syndrome
Pectoralis minor syndrome
Thenar hammer syndrome
Hypothenar hammer syndrome
Substance-induced vasospasm
Ergotism
Vasopressors
Traumatic injury, blunt or penetrating
Iatrogenic injury
Access-related hand ischemia

more common than artery TOS, which represents about 1% of total cases.[5] Patients with artery TOS may present with signs and symptoms ranging from fatigue or pain in the affected arm upon exertion and Raynaud phenomenon to ischemic tissue loss of the digits due to emboli from a chronically injured artery. Most clinically significant artery TOS

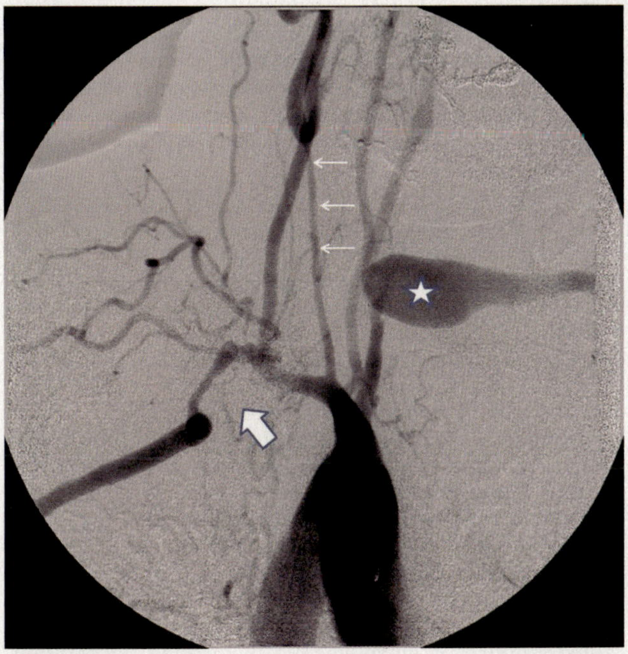

Figure 85.1. Aortogram in the right oblique projection of a patient with Takayasu arteritis. Long-segment right common carotid stenosis (*small arrows*) leading into a normal-appearing carotid bifurcation. Segmental occlusion of the right subclavian artery (*block arrow*) just distal to the origin of the right vertebral. There is distal reconstitution via a large collateral. There is also an aneurysm (*star*) of a previous bypass in the left subclavian artery.

SYMPTOMS

Table 85.2. Takayasu Arteritis

Headache, often related to high blood pressure and kidney failure
Exertional chest pain
Fatigue and shortness of breath
Transient ischemic attacks, dizziness, vision changes, or fainting
Nausea, vomiting, and abdominal pain, generally from poor mesenteric blood flow
Exertional muscle pain in arms or legs

will present with subclavian artery aneurysm formation from this repetitive trauma, which is the primary source of distal emboli. Pectoralis minor syndrome is a distinct but similar condition that causes compression of the subclavian artery by the pectoralis minor as it inserts into the coracoid process (**Fig. 85.3**).[6]

Additional compression sites distal to the thoracic outlet include the quadrilateral space, humeral head, and thenar and hypothenar hammer syndromes. The ulnar artery is vulnerable to injury at the hypothenar eminence, just distal to the wrist, where the ulnar artery passes through the Guyon canal bound by the pisiform and hamate bones. The ulnar artery is cushioned only by skin, subcutaneous tissue, and the thin palmaris brevis muscle. Repetitive use of the palm as a "hammer" compresses the unprotected ulnar artery against the nearby hook of the hamate bone. Both aneurysm formation and occlusive disease can result (**Fig. 85.3**).[7]

Substances can induce severe vasospasm in the arteries of the upper extremities and thereby cause digital ischemia. Historically, ergotism resulted from consuming grains contaminated with an ergotamine-producing fungus. Contemporarily, most such cases come from either drugs of abuse or pharmacologic agents.[8] Vasopressors used to manage hypotension in critically ill patients are one common iatrogenic cause of digital ischemia and gangrene.

Traumatic injury to the arteries of the upper extremities from either blunt or penetrating injuries and, unlike atherosclerotic disease, can result in dramatic acute limb ischemia requiring prompt revascularization.[9,10] Management of traumatic injuries may be complex, with concurrent nerve and musculoskeletal injuries being common. Iatrogenic injury, either from attempts at vascular access or from orthopedic procedures, is an important cause of artery trauma.

Approximately 5% to 10% of patients who have undergone dialysis access procedures may develop some degree of AHRI, also known as steal syndrome, which can result in pain, hand dysfunction, and, in severe cases, ischemic tissue loss.[11] There are several known risk factors for AHRI, including female sex, advanced age, and comorbidities such as diabetes and coronary artery disease; however, it is difficult to predict the risk of any one individual.

PRESENTATION

Patients suffering from upper extremity artery insufficiency can present with a variety of symptoms. Exertional pain is rare and often points to a proximal lesion (innominate, subclavian, or axillary arteries). Disease of the subclavian artery proximal to the take-off of the vertebral artery can result in subclavian steal phenomenon, which can present as dizziness and other neurologic complaints due to reversal of flow through the vertebral artery and "steal" of blood flow from

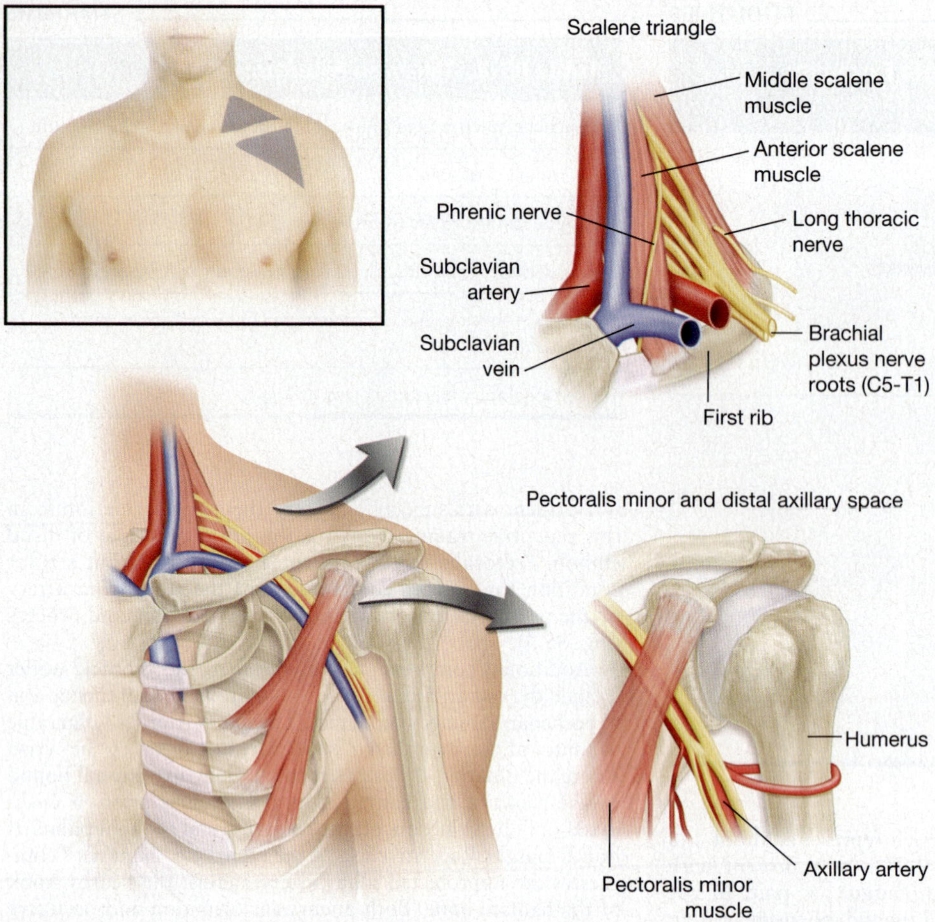

Figure 85.2. Compressive zones of the thoracic outlet. The subclavian structures can be compressed at the costoclavicular space, the scalene triangle, or distally at the border of the pectoralis minor muscle.

the posterior cerebral circulation. More commonly, patients present with skin changes affecting the hands or fingers. Livedo reticularis may represent an inflammatory or autoimmune process. Splinter hemorrhages of the nailbed suggest an embolic process. Cyanotic discoloration of the fingers and digital gangrene can result from embolic or occlusive ischemia (Fig. 85.4).

Raynaud phenomenon indicates an episodic series of skin changes affecting the fingers or the hands triggered by changes in temperature or emotional stress. The classic presentation is a sequential appearance of first pallor, then cyanosis, and

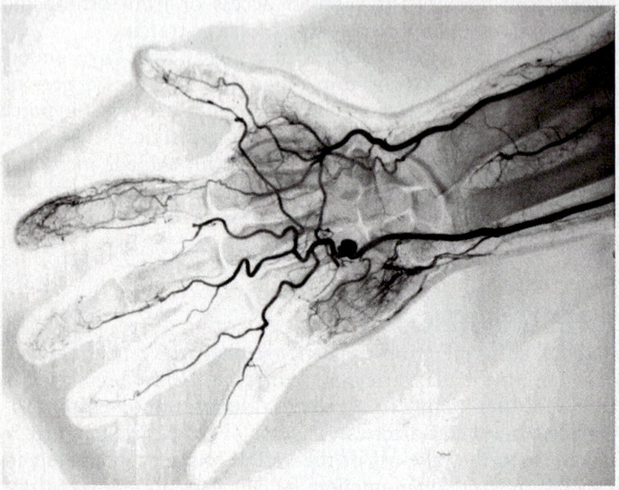

Figure 85.3. Ulnar artery aneurysm resulting from repetitive trauma in a construction worker.

finally erythema. These correspond to (in order) vasospasm (pallor), desaturation of hemoglobin (cyanosis), and finally, compensatory vasodilation, also known as reactive hyperemia (erythema). Although this can result from occlusive disease, it is more commonly associated with autoimmune conditions (scleroderma, Sjögren syndrome, rheumatoid arthritis, lupus).[12] *Raynaud disease* describes a vasospastic condition of unknown etiology in patients without occlusive lesions or autoimmune disease.[12,13]

History and Physical Exam

Evaluation of upper extremity ischemia requires an index of symptom onset and duration and a thorough medical and social history. Interrogation should assess the use of tobacco, antimigraine medications, antiretrovirals, and recreational drugs such as cocaine and other alkaloids. Occupational history should be queried for repetitive overhead shoulder motion (seen in swimmers, baseball pitchers, and weightlifters and associated with TOS) or repetitive trauma to the palmar eminences (seen in manual laborers, musicians, and athletes). Personal and family histories of atherosclerotic disease within other vascular beds (coronary, cerebrovascular disease, and lower extremity) and autoimmune conditions should be obtained. It is necessary to clearly understand any prior interventions in the arm, such as hemodialysis access, biopsies, and radial, brachial, or axillary access for cardiac catheterizations or hemodynamic monitoring. In addition, any prior trauma (clavicular or rib fractures, humeral, shoulder, or elbow injuries) (**Fig. 85.5**) should be reviewed and documented.

A complete physical examination must include a systemic evaluation for signs of atherosclerotic, inflammatory, or autoimmune disease. Meticulous inspection, auscultation, and palpation of both sides of the neck, periclavicular areas,

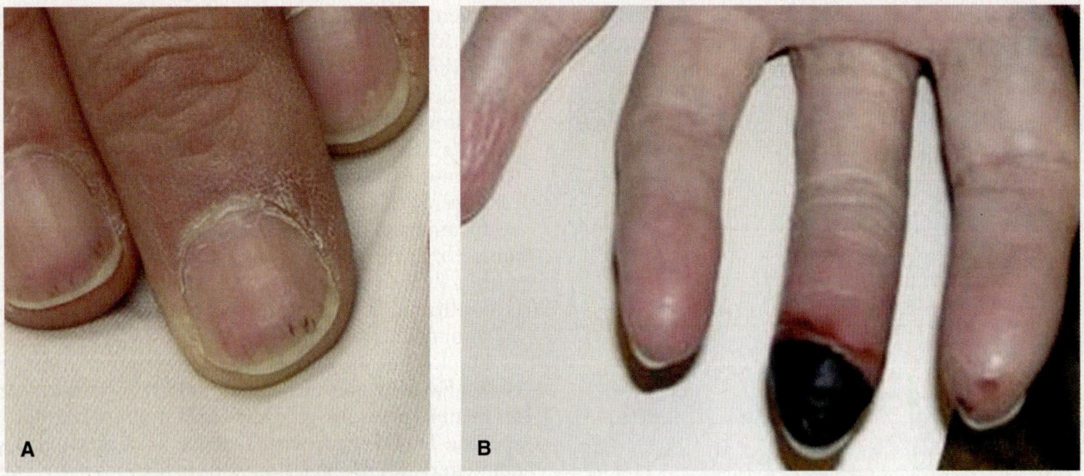

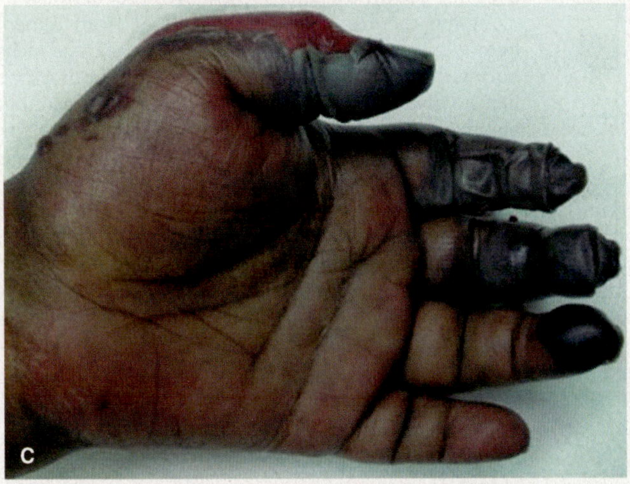

Figure 85.4. Manifestations of upper extremity ischemia. Splinter hemorrhages in the nails arising from a proximal embolic source (**A**). Gangrene affecting the tip of the third finger (**B**). Advanced, severe gangrene in the radial artery distribution secondary to complications related to an artery line (**C**).

shoulders, arms, and hands should be done in the resting, neutral position and while abducting the arm. Loss of pulses during provocative maneuvers can be a normal finding or
3 related to the underlying anatomic compressive syndrome. A bruit or a thrill in the periclavicular area would suggest the presence of stenosis or poststenotic dilation arising from TOS, and a prominent pulse should point to an aneurysm in the subclavian artery. Comparison between the two upper extremities is crucial as bilaterality suggests a systemic disorder. Bilateral blood pressure measurements should be obtained and compared (brachiobrachial index). A careful hand examination includes inspecting for splinter hemorrhages under the beds of the nails, gangrene of the fingertips, or skin color changes related to vasospasm, and signs of trauma in the hand. Careful palpation of the radial and ulnar pulses should be done. A Doppler should be used to assess the superficial and deep palmar arches. In addition a complete evaluation of both motor and sensory function must be performed in order to evaluate for asymmetry between upper extremities and the presence of any symptoms in the distribution of a specific nerve or dermatome.

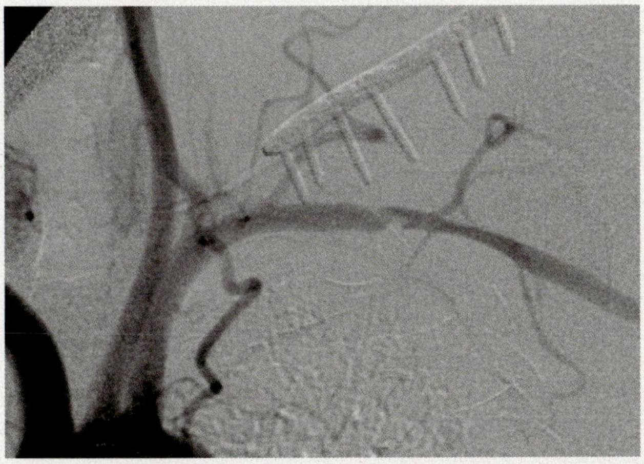

Figure 85.5. Old clavicular fracture treated with a metallic prosthesis. Notice the luminal abnormality in the subclavian artery as it crosses the clavicle. This lesion was caused by periosteal scarring and caused distal embolism in the hand.

An Allen test can be particularly helpful. In this test, digital pressure is applied to the ulnar and radial arteries in the wrist. After the patient opens and closes their hand, pressure is removed from one of the wrist arteries, and inspection of the color of the hand and palpation of the distal pulses is repeated. The test is normal if the entire hand recovers its color and capillary refill. If a portion of the hand fails to normalize, then it is likely that the palmar vascular collateral circulation (palmar arch) is incomplete. Similarly, the Barbeau test is a variation of the Allen test that utilizes a pulse oximeter to measure digital flow before and after radial and ulnar occlusion.[14]

Laboratory and Noninvasive Testing

4 A series of serologic tests should be obtained if an autoimmune disease is suspected (**Table 85.3**).

Noninvasive testing by an accredited vascular laboratory is one of the most important tools for diagnosing upper extremity vascular disease.[15] All patients should be subjected

DIAGNOSIS

Table 85.3. Serologies for Inflammatory and Autoimmune-mediated Hand Ischemia

Erythrocyte sedimentation rate
Rheumatoid factor
Antinuclear antibody
Immunoglobulin electrophoresis
Cryoglobulins
Cold agglutinins
VDRL (Venereal Disease Research Laboratory) test
Complement (C3, C4)
Anticardiolipin antibody
Blood cell counts

to segmental artery pressure measurement and waveform analysis, at the minimum. This test usually includes photoplethysmography (PPG) of the digital vessels in the upper extremities. The absence of triphasic flow and "blunted" PPG tracing in the affected arteries and digits helps to localize obstructive lesions. If intermittent occlusion is suspected due to TOS, these tests can be repeated with provocative maneuvers such as the Adson test (**Fig. 85.6**).[16] To assess hand perfusion and completeness of the palmar arch, a more sophisticated version of the Allen test can also be obtained by adding the analysis of waveforms obtained before and after ulnar and/or radial artery occlusion at the wrist.

Historically, the cold challenge test has been used to assess patients with symptoms suggestive of vasomotor disorders (cold intolerance, skin color changes, etc). Although several versions of this test exist, typically, the hands are immersed in iced water, and digital temperatures are measured every 5 minutes. For a normal response, temperatures should normalize within 1 °C of preimmersion measurements. Cold intolerance is confirmed with failure to restore digital temperature in 20 minutes.[17]

Duplex ultrasound is useful when an obstructive lesion is localized by physical examination, waveform analysis, or segmental pressure recordings. B-mode imaging, color, and spectral Doppler can visualize the area of interest, define the characteristics of the lesion and its hemodynamic severity, and examine the inflow and outflow from the lesion.[18]

When there is a concern for steal from upper extremity hemodialysis access, digital PPG tracing can be measured with and without manual pressure, causing temporary occlusion of hemodialysis graft and fistula. Duplex ultrasonography can also be used to make additional flow measurements and evaluate spectral waveforms with and without compression.

Cross-sectional and Catheter-based Imaging

Accurate imaging of the artery anatomy of both arms, from the aortic arch to the digital arteries, is mandatory in the symptomatic patient when obstructive lesions are suspected on clinical evaluation or noninvasive testing. Although catheter-based angiography remains the gold standard, modern computed tomography angiography (CTA) and magnetic resonance angiography (MRA) have essentially replaced this modality

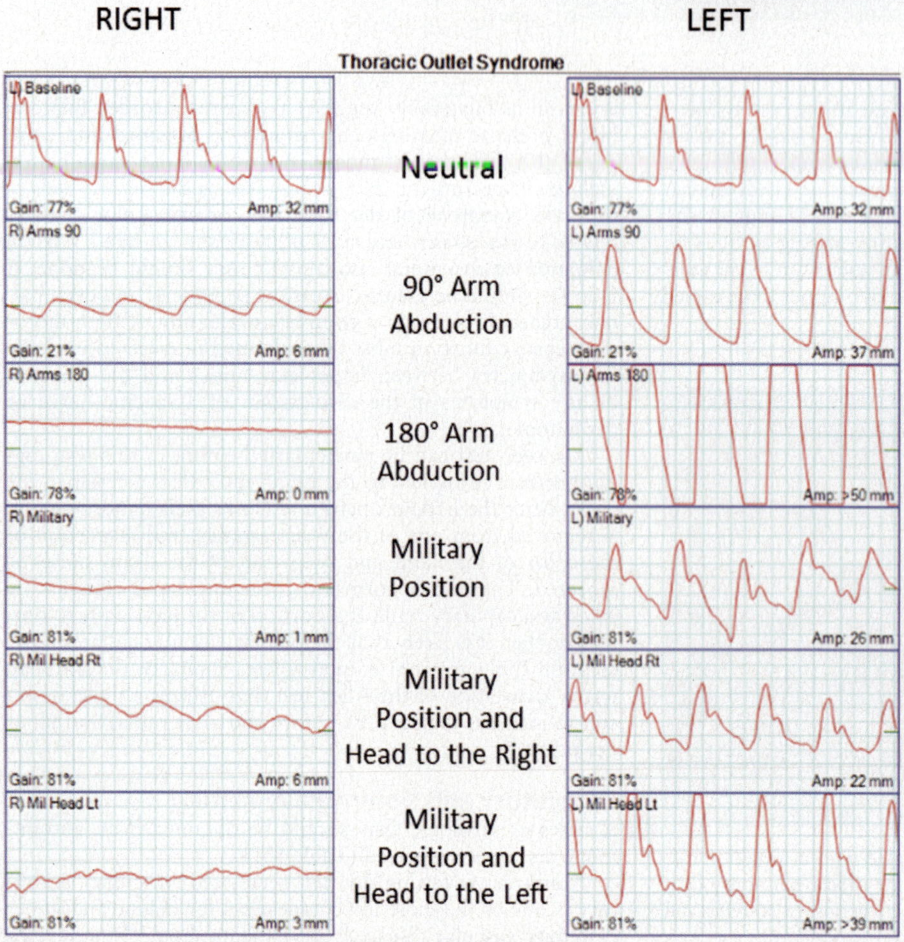

Figure 85.6. Noninvasive blood flow study in a major league baseball pitcher showing loss of normal signals during proactive maneuvers.

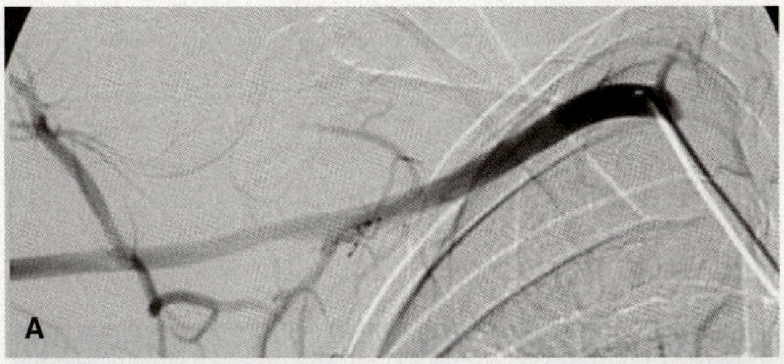

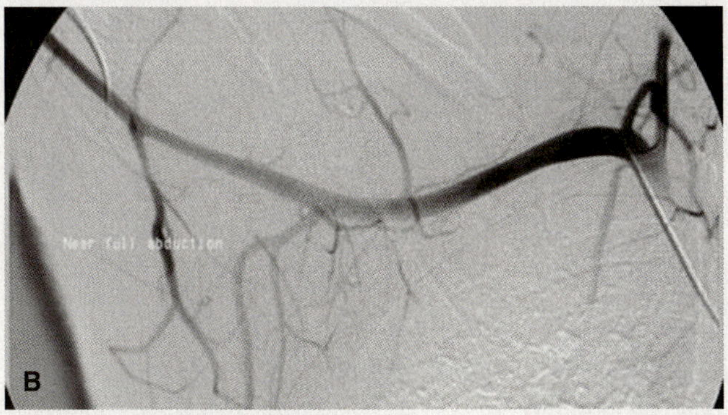

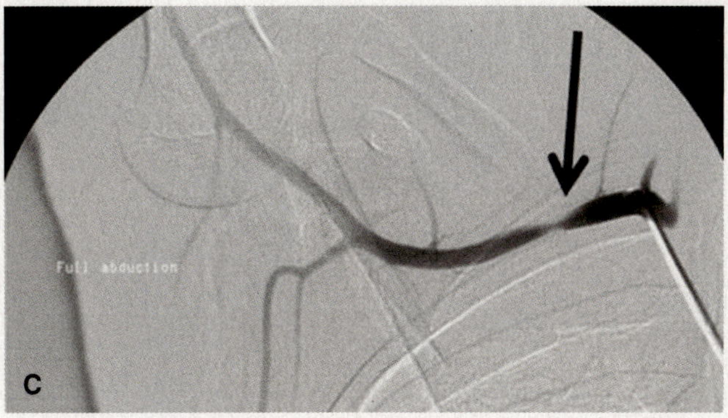

Figure 85.7. Selective digital subtraction angiography of the right arm in a patient with suspected artery thoracic outlet syndrome. Subclavian artery stenosis is not seen when injecting contrast with the arm in neutral (**A**) and moderate abduction (**B**), but is evident when the arm is hyperabducted (*arrow*) (**C**).

for diagnosis alone, as they provide excellent anatomic detail from the great vessels to the forearm and eliminate the risk of traversing the aortic arch for a catheter-based angiogram.[19] If TOS is suspected, provocative maneuvers should be done while obtaining artery images (**Fig. 85.7**). Evaluation of the distal artery anatomy at and beyond the wrist may require catheter-based angiography due to the limited resolution of axial imaging. Typically, the deep palmar arch arises from the terminal part of the radial artery and the superficial arch by the ulnar artery, although this is highly variable.

Nuclear Medicine Studies

Nuclear medicine studies can be useful in cases where either an inflammatory or infectious etiology is expected. Both tagged white blood cell (WBC) and positron-emission tomography (PET) scans can be considered depending upon institutional protocols.

MANAGEMENT

Atherosclerotic Occlusive Disease

5 The specific choice of revascularization used to treat upper extremity ischemia depends on the location of the lesion, its etiology, and the available local resources and expertise. Atherosclerotic lesions affecting the origin of the subclavian or innominate arteries are most frequently treated with percutaneous transluminal angioplasty and stenting. This is usually achieved via a femoral approach, but can also be performed using retrograde radial, brachial, or even transcarotid approaches.[20] These percutaneous approaches spare patients the morbidity of a cavitary operation; however, there are several important limitations to consider in these endovascular procedures. Intravascular devices have limited use for lesions that encroach on the origin of a vertebral artery or an internal mammary previously used as a coronary bypass, as they can potentially cover and occlude these vessels if not deployed precisely. Deployment of stents in certain locations, such as under the clavicle or in the ostia of the aortic arch, can produce significant extrinsic compression and predispose to stent deformation, fracture, and/or thrombosis.[21] Alternatively, open surgical bypasses and transpositions can be performed via small incisions in the neck with excellent long-term results (**Fig. 85.8**). These procedures allow for preserving the vertebral artery and provide excellent long-term patency.[22] Finally, in some patients, the best option resides in single or multiple-branched bypasses arising from the aortic arch. A mini-sternotomy can expose the ascending arch, and the bypass can be anastomosed to the aorta using a side-biting clamp, thus obviating the need for cardiopulmonary bypass (**Fig. 85.9**).

Other occlusive subclavian, axillary, and brachial artery lesions are best treated with surgical revascularization. Due to potential compression at the costoclavicular space, the shoulder joint's high mobility, and the brachial artery's caliber, endovascular approaches are rarely indicated in this segment of the circulation. Many different bypass configurations are available. The supraclavicular subclavian artery can be exposed by an incision at the base of the neck and used as inflow for bypasses tunneled subcutaneously over the clavicle and into the brachial artery. Alternatively, an excellent source of inflow is the common carotid artery. The outflow anastomosis can be created in the distal brachial artery, the radial or ulnar arteries in the proximal forearm (**Fig. 85.10**), or at the wrist and even in the arteries of the hand (**Fig. 85.11**).

Inflammatory Conditions

Patients with inflammatory or autoimmune diseases are best managed by controlling their systemic disease with appropriate medical therapy. The initial management of Raynaud syndrome consists of using calcium channel blockers and vasodilators. Progressive ischemia may require intraartery vasodilators, anticoagulation, Botox injections, or sympathectomy.[23]

Surgical intervention during the acute inflammatory phase of Takayasu arteritis is contraindicated. The mainstay of treatment during the active phase is corticosteroids, although patients with more severe disease may require additional immunosuppressant drugs (eg, methotrexate or azathioprine).[24] Any intervention should be delayed until the acute, active phase of the disease undergoes remission. This is often indicated by the normalization of serologic inflammatory markers, most commonly erythrocyte sedimentation rate (ESR) and C-reactive protein (CRP). Antiplatelet therapies may lower the frequency of ischemic events. During the chronic phase, reconstruction is performed using similar techniques as those used to manage atherosclerotic occlusion (**Fig. 85.12**).

The mainstay of management for Buerger disease is smoking cessation. Due to the distal to proximal fully obliterative nature of the disease, there is often no site for distal

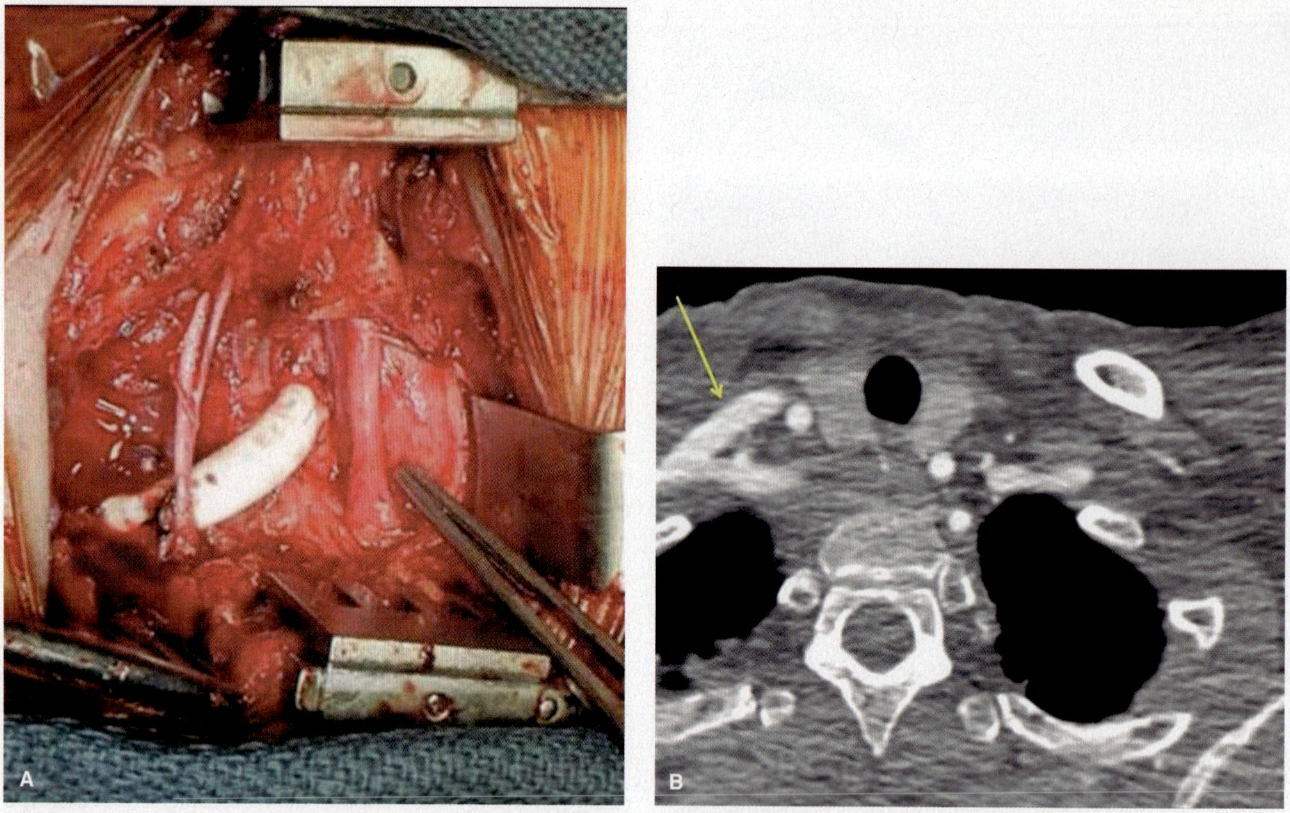

Figure 85.8. **A:** Right carotid to subclavian bypass performed via a supraclavicular incision using a prosthetic 10-mm conduit. **B:** CT scan showing patency of the bypass (*arrow*).

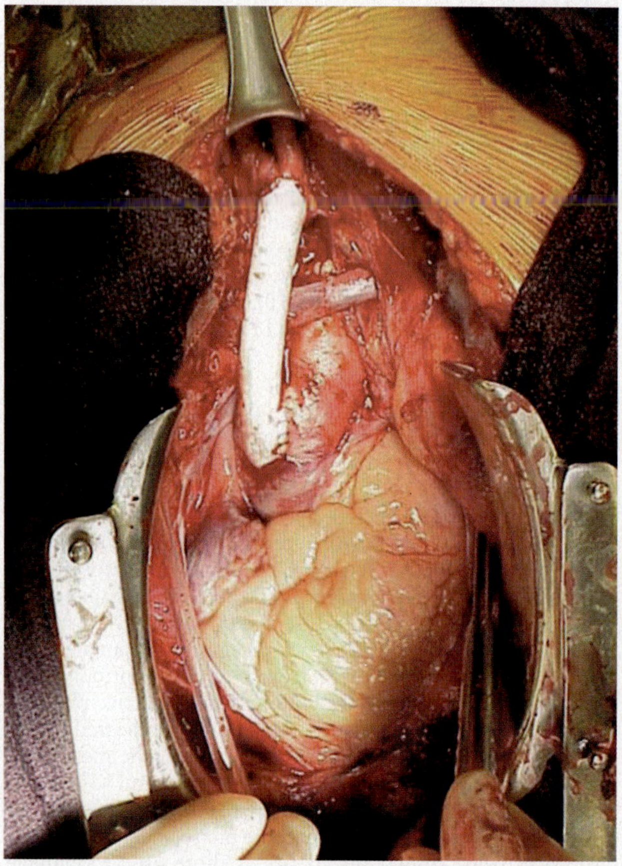

Figure 85.9. Aorto to innominate bypass. A mini-sternotomy is done and a side-biting clamp is used for creation of the proximal anastomosis in the ascending aorta. The distal anastomosis is created at the bifurcation of the innominate artery.

revascularization. Initiation of vasodilators (prostaglandin analogs and/or calcium channel blockers) may provide some benefit. Antiplaletet therapy should be utilized to prevent thromboembolism. In severe cases, amputation for symptom palliation may be required and/or sympathectomy.

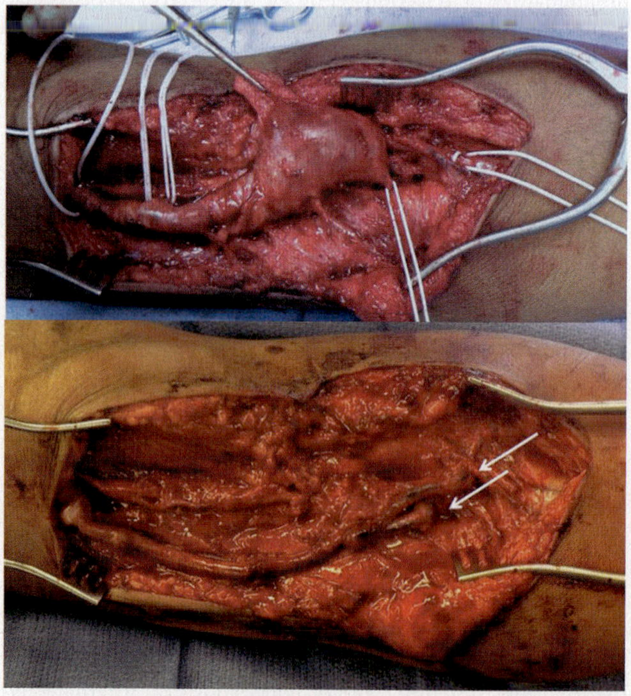

Figure 85.10. Large aneurysm of the distal brachial artery treated with a bifurcated bypass created with great saphenous vein. The distal anastomoses (*arrows*) were created into the radial and ulnar arteries just distal to the elbow.

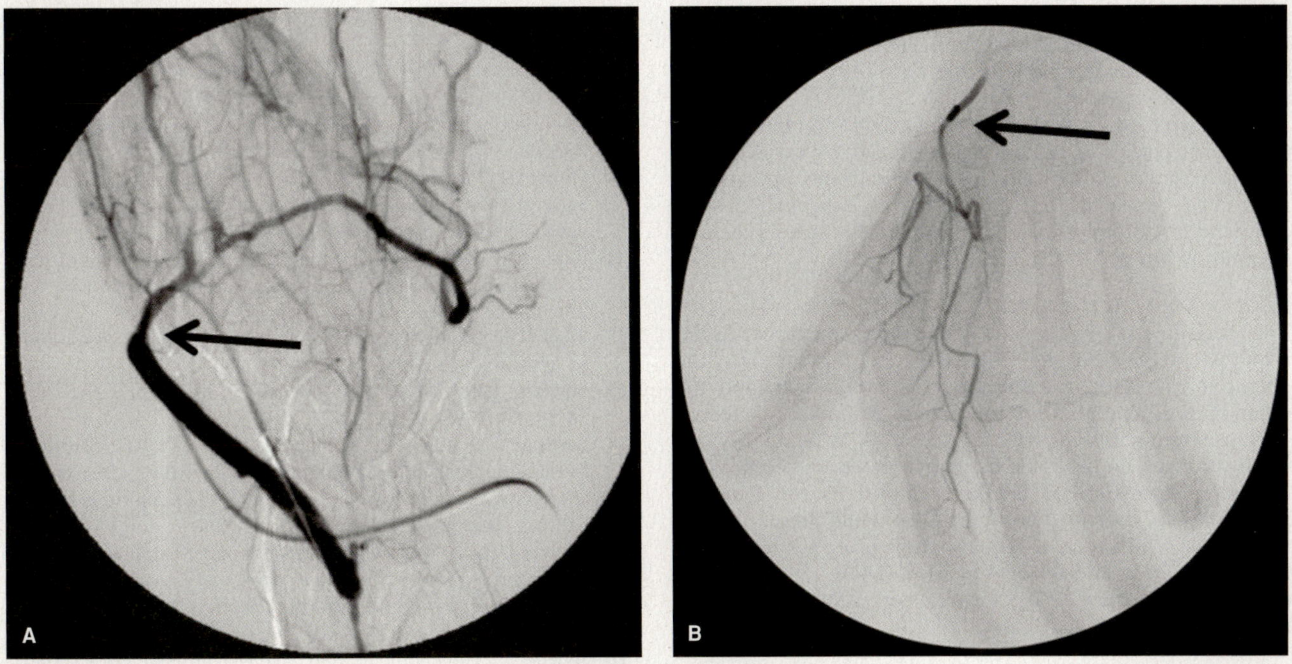

Figure 85.11. Completion angiograms of two different saphenous vein bypasses with distal anastomosis (*arrows*) to the palmar arch (**A**) and radial artery at the snuffbox segment (**B**).

Extrinsic Compression

There is little controversy about the management of patients with artery TOS. Untreated artery injury due to repetitive torsion and compression leads to stenosis, poststenotic aneurysmal dilation, and distal embolism. In most cases, aneurysm and evidence of distal embolism are already present by the time of presentation and are the indication for intervention. Thus, both thoracic outlet decompression and artery reconstruction are required. The subclavian artery can be compressed at any point from the root of the neck to the pectoralis minor tendon. Therefore, the decompressive approach depends on the specific anatomy of the patient. The surgical plan depends on the details obtained by imaging studies and the surgeon's experience. In the absence of anatomic anomalies and with compression demonstrated only during arm abduction and elevation, first rib resection via the supraclavicular approach appears to be the best choice. If chronic compression has caused artery damage, artery reconstruction is necessary. Interposition grafts from the ipsilateral common carotid to the axillary artery are commonly used. This can best be achieved by combining supra- and infraclavicular exposure. Prosthetic grafts tunneled either underneath the clavicle or subcutaneously have excellent patency rates. If present, cervical ribs are resected, whereas full thoracic outlet decompression with scalenectomy is often only necessary if concomitant neurogenic TOS exists.[25]

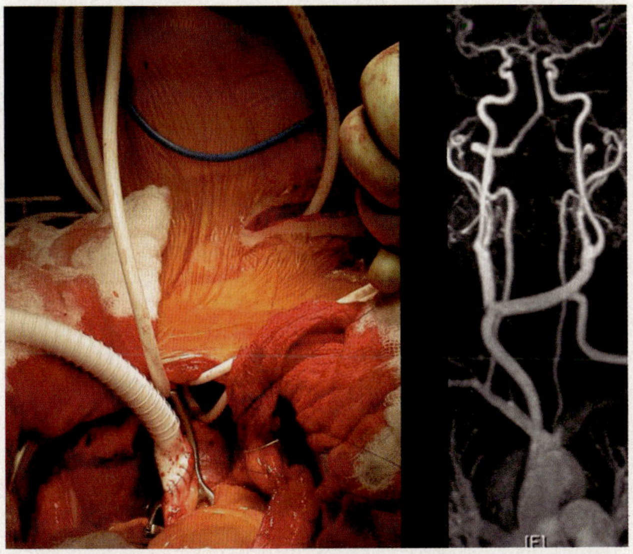

Figure 85.12. Artery reconstruction on the patient with Takayasu arteritis shown in **Figure 85.1**. A median sternotomy with bilateral neck incisions was used. The proximal anastomosis was done in the ascending aorta. One branch was anastomosed in an end-to-end fashion to the right subclavian. A second branch was anastomosed to the right carotid (side-to-end) and then tunneled via the prevertebral space and anastomosed end-to-end to the left carotid bifurcation. Finally, a side arm was used to revascularize the left subclavian artery.

Distal Degenerative Lesions

Patients suffering from hypothenar hammer syndrome with mild symptoms and no aneurysm can be treated nonoperatively. Padded hand protection, avoidance of further repetitive trauma, tobacco cessation (if applicable), and the use of calcium channel blockers, antiplatelet agents, and/or anticoagulation have all been tried with some degree of success. Surgical intervention can include simple ligation of the aneurysm if there is adequate collateral circulation; typically, resection of the affected segment with reconstruction is required.[26]

Traumatic Injury

The management of traumatic injury to the arteries of the upper extremity depends upon the specific anatomy of an injury.[9] Injuries to the axillary and subclavian arteries can result in difficulty obtaining proximal control and may require a sternotomy or thoracotomy to access the inflow. However, proximal traumatic lesions are commonly treated with endovascular approaches due to the morbidity and difficulty of open exposure for proximal control.[27] The brachial artery can be readily accessed throughout its course in the upper arm. Injuries to the radial and ulnar arteries may be difficult to repair due to the small size of the distal vessels, however, isolated radial artery injuries may be managed with ligation alone if a patient maintains a neurovascularly intact hand due to ulnar-dominant circulation and an intact palmar arch.

Both blunt and penetrating trauma may produce concurrent orthopedic or neurologic injuries. Stabilization of an orthopedic injury, either via definitive repair or external fixation, must be coordinated with the repair of any artery injury. Bypass or interposition grafts should use autogenous conduit (typically greater saphenous vein) due to the possibility of contamination from the wound.[10]

In unstable patients, the use of a shunt for temporary restoration of perfusion should be considered with a definitive revascularization completed at a subsequent operation.[28] Depending on the degree and timing of ischemia, forearm and hand fasciotomies may be required to mitigate ischemia-reperfusion injury.

Access-Related Hand Ischemia

The decision-making around the management of AHRI requires careful weighing of the severity of symptoms, the operative risk and life expectancy of the patient, and the other options available for subsequent hemodialysis access. Early or severe AHRI may require access to be abandoned via ligation of the graft or fistula. In cases with otherwise functional access, there are several options for remedial procedures to improve hand perfusion while preserving the HD access, which include fistula banding or plication, distal revascularization and interval ligation (DRIL), proximalization of artery inflow (PAI), and revision using distal inflow (RUDI).[29,30]

SUMMARY

Although atherosclerosis is still the most common cause of upper extremity artery disease, a myriad of conditions associated with occupational and autoimmune risk factors. A complete history and physical examination often disclose a potential etiology and usually point to the anatomic location of the culprit lesion. Bilateral hand ischemia is often associated with systemic conditions, whereas unilaterality more commonly occurs with obstructive lesions. Accurate delineation of the anatomy using imaging modalities is necessary to plan revascularization. Multiple endovascular and open surgical options are available to manage upper extremity artery disorders.

ACKNOWLEDGMENTS

We gratefully acknowledge the contributions of previous edition authors, Heron E. Rodriguez and Courtney Furlough, as portions of those chapters have been retained in this revision.

References

1. Kreienberg PB, Change B, Roddy S. Hand ischemia in end stage renal disease. In: Rodriguez HE, ed. *The Ischemic Extremity: New Findings and Treatment*. People's Medical Publishing House USA; 2010:525–531.
2. Shaban Y, Elkbuli A, Geraghty F, Boneva D, McKenney M, De La Portilla J. True brachial artery aneurysm: a case report and review of literature. *Ann Med Surg*. 2020;56:23–27.
3. Wu W, Chaer RA. Nonarteriosclerotic vascular disease. *Surg Clin North Am*. 2013;93(4):833–875, viii.
4. Saadoun D, Vautier M, Cacoub P. Medium- and large-vessel vasculitis. *Circulation*. 2021;143(3):267–282.
5. Leclercq M, Marie I. Arterial thoracic outlet syndrome. *Rheumatology (Oxford)*. 2015;54(1):44.
6. Sanders RJ, Annest SJ. Thoracic outlet and pectoralis minor syndromes. *Semin Vasc Surg*. 2014;27(2):86–117.
7. Kumar H, Rodriguez H. Thenar and Hypothenar Hammer Syndrome. In: Sidawy AN, Perler BA, eds. *Clinical Scenarios in Vascular Surgery*. 2nd ed. Wolters Kluwer Health; 2015:162–167.
8. Ayarragaray JEF. Ergotism: a change of perspective. *Ann Vasc Surg*. 2014;28(1):265–268.
9. Badalamenti G, Ferrer C, Calvagna C, et al. Major vascular traumas to the neck, upper limbs, and chest: clinical presentation, diagnostic approach, and management strategies. *Semin Vasc Surg*. 2023;36(2):258–267.
10. Huber GH, Manna B. Vascular extremity trauma. In: *StatPearls*. StatPearls Publishing; 2024. Accessed August 1, 2024. http://www.ncbi.nlm.nih.gov/books/NBK536925/
11. Rehfuss JP, Berceli SA, Barbey SM, et al. The spectrum of hand dysfunction after hemodialysis fistula placement. *Kidney Int Rep*. 2017;2(3):332–341.
12. Block JA, Sequeira W. Raynaud's phenomenon. *Lancet*. 2001; 357(9273):2042–2048.
13. Bowling JCR, Dowd PM. Raynaud's disease. *Lancet*. 2003; 361(9374):2078–2080.
14. Barbeau GR, Arsenault F, Dugas L, Simard S, Larivière MM. Evaluation of the ulnopalmar arterial arches with pulse oximetry and plethysmography: Comparison with the Allen's test in 1010 patients. *Am Heart J*. 2004;147(3):489–493.
15. Sumner D. Non-invasive assessment of upper extremity ischemia. In: Bergan JJ, Yao JST, eds. *Evaluation and Treatment of Upper and Lower Extremity Circulatory Disorders*. Grune & Stratton; 1984:75–95.
16. Sanders RJ, Hammond SL, Rao NM. Diagnosis of thoracic outlet syndrome. *J Vasc Surg*. 2007;46(3):601–604.
17. Karwowski J, Johnson B, Dalman R. Upper extremity ischemia: diagnostic techniques and clinical applications. In: Mansour MA, Labropoulos N, eds. *Vascular Diagnosis*. Elsevier Saunders; 2005: 325–330.
18. Pellerito J, Polak JF. *Introduction to Vascular Ultrasonography*. 7th ed. Elsevier; 2020.
19. Ghouri MA, Gupta N, Bhat AP, et al. CT and MR imaging of the upper extremity vasculature: pearls, pitfalls, and challenges. *Cardiovasc Diagn Ther*. 2019;9(Suppl 1):S152–S173.
20. Kanda D, Imagama I, Imoto Y, Ohishi M. Bidirectional endovascular treatment for axillary artery injury secondary to proximal humerus fracture: a case report. *Eur Heart J Case Rep*. 2021;5(2): ytaa526.
21. Hüttl AB, Hüttl A, Vértes M, et al. The presence of long and heavily calcified lesions predisposes for fracture in patients undergoing stenting of the first part of the subclavian artery. *J Vasc Surg*. 2019;70(4):1146–1154.e1.
22. Morasch MD. Technique for subclavian to carotid transposition, tips, and tricks. *J Vasc Surg*. 2009;49(1):251–254.
23. Ramahi A, Hughes M, Khanna D. Practical management of Raynaud's phenomenon-a primer for practicing physicians. *Curr Opin Rheumatol*. 2022;34(4):235–244.
24. Keser G, Direskeneli H, Aksu K. Management of Takayasu arteritis: a systematic review. *Rheumatology (Oxford)*. 2014;53(5):793–801.
25. Miller D, Rodriguez H. Management of vascular thoracic outlet syndrome. In: Sidawy AN, Perler BA, eds. *Contemporary Vascular Surgery*. People's Medical Publishing House USA; 2011:469–476.
26. Menon D, Onida S, Davies AH. Overview of arterial pathology related to repetitive trauma in athletes. *J Vasc Surg*. 2019;70(2): 641–650.
27. Sinha S, Patterson BO, Ma J, et al. Systematic review and meta-analysis of open surgical and endovascular management of thoracic outlet vascular injuries. *J Vasc Surg*. 2013;57(2):547–567.e8.
28. Herrera MA, Millán M, del Valle AM, et al. Damage control of peripheral vascular trauma – Don't be afraid of axillary or popliteal fosses. *Colomb Med (Cali)*. 52(2):e4074735.
29. Leake AE, Winger DG, Leers SA, Gupta N, Dillavou ED. Management and outcomes of dialysis access-associated steal syndrome. *J Vasc Surg*. 2015;61(3):754–760.
30. Gupta N, Yuo TH, Konig G, et al. Treatment strategies of arterial steal after arteriovenous access. *J Vasc Surg*. 2011;54(1):162–167.

86

Renal and Splanchnic Vascular Disease

Dawn M. Coleman, John E. Rectenwald, and Gilbert R. Upchurch Jr

Key Points

1. Splanchnic vascular disease is uncommon across the spectrum of vascular surgery practice, but remains central to the specialty.
2. Intestinal ischemia may result from presplanchnic conditions that decrease total mesenteric blood flow (ie, heart failure and hypovolemia), splanchnic conditions that decrease regional blood flow through the mesenteric circulation (ie, thromboembolism) or postsplanchnic venous congestion (ie, mesenteric vein thrombosis and cirrhosis).
3. The most common causes of acute mesenteric ischemia (AMI) include: embolization (40% to 50%), arterial thrombosis (25% to 30%), nonocclusive mesenteric ischemia (15% to 20%), and mesenteric venous thrombosis (5% to 15%).
4. Patients with AMI warrant immediate medical management that includes the establishment of adequate intravenous access and hemodynamic monitoring, systemic anticoagulation with heparin, fluid resuscitation, correction of electrolyte abnormalities, and administration of broad-spectrum antibiotics.
5. The progression from minor symptoms to AMI and intestinal infarction is unpredictable; almost half of patients presenting with AMI describe previous symptoms of chronic mesenteric ischemia (CMI).
6. Distribution of splanchnic artery aneurysms is as follows: Splenic artery (60%) > hepatic arteries (20%) > superior mesenteric artery (5.5%) > celiac artery (4%) and gastric and gastroepiploic arteries (4%) > ileocolic arteries (3%) > pancreaticoduodenal arteries (2%) > gastroduodenal artery (1.5%) > inferior mesenteric artery (<1%).
7. Renal artery occlusive disease is the most common cause of correctable hypertension (HTN) in adults and the third most common cause of HTN in children and should be considered in the clinical context of: (1) childhood HTN, (2) severe HTN in women <45 years of age, (3) acute and rapid escalation of mild HTN in older patients (>50 years), (4) initial diastolic BP >115 mm Hg, and (5) rapid deterioration in renal function following the administration of antihypertensive therapy (especially with ACE inhibition).
8. Medical therapy remains the mainstay of treatment for renovascular hypertension (RVH) with comprehensive goals of care that should encompass glycemic control, cholesterol reduction, smoking cessation, blood pressure reduction, and antiplatelet therapy with aspirin for primary prevention. ACC/AHA guidelines support the use of angiotensin-converting enzyme inhibitors (ACE-I), angiotensin receptor blockers (ARBs), calcium channel blockers, and beta blockers with a class I indication.
9. Several recent clinical trials comparing renal artery stenting to best medical management for renal artery stenosis have failed to demonstrate a conclusive clinical benefit to the endovascular treatment of renal artery stenosis.

SPLANCHNIC VASCULAR OCCLUSIVE AND ANEURYSMAL DISEASE

1 Splanchnic vascular disease is uncommon across the spectrum of vascular surgery practice, but remains central to the specialty. Patients often seek medical attention from alternative specialists, emphasizing the importance of cross-disciplinary awareness. Acute mesenteric ischemia (AMI) remains associated with delayed diagnosis and dismal mortality despite notable progress in the diagnosis and treatment of patients with vascular disease. This section elaborates on the current treatment standards for both splanchnic vascular occlusive disease and aneurysms.

Anatomy and Physiology

Three branches of the abdominal aorta perfuse the gastrointestinal tract. The celiac artery originates at the level of T12 and branches into the left gastric, common hepatic, and splenic arteries in a classic pattern in 65% to 75% of cases.[1] Variations are noted in **Table 86.1** and may include a true trifurcation of these vessels (25% of the population), replaced and accessory hepatic vasculature, a common celiacomesenteric trunk (<1% of the population), and a persistent ventral anastomosis between the proper hepatic, and a replaced right hepatic artery (off the SMA) denoted as an "arch of Buhler" (<4% of the population). Additionally, the splenic artery can be found to originate directly off the aorta, SMA, left gastric or hepatic arteries. The celiac axis supplies primarily the stomach, duodenum, spleen, liver, and pancreas. The SMA originates approximately 1 to 2 cm caudad to the celiac artery and branches into the inferior pancreaticoduodenal artery, 4 to 6 jejunal and 9 to 13 ileal branches, the middle colic artery, the right colic artery, and terminates as the iliocolic artery. The SMA supplies primarily the lower portion of the pancreas gland, jejunum, ileum, ascending colon, and the proximal half of the transverse colon. The inferior mesenteric artery (IMA) originates off the terminal aorta at the level of L3 and divides into the left colic artery, sigmoid branches, and continues as the superior

Table 86.1. Normal and Variant Mesenteric Arterial Anatomy

Vessel	Incidence (%)
Celiac	
▪ Classic (3 branches)	65–75
▪ Four branches (including dorsal pancreatic artery)	5–10
▪ Celiacomesenteric trunk	<1
Hepatic	
▪ CHA from celiac artery	75
▪ CHA from SMA	2.5
▪ Replaced RHA	15–18
▪ From left gastric	11–12
▪ From SMA	2.5
▪ Accessory RHA	7–8
▪ Accessory LHA	2.5
Gastric	
▪ Left gastric artery	
▪ From celiac artery	90
▪ From aorta	3
▪ Accessory branches from or to left hepatic artery	23
▪ Right gastric artery	
▪ From proper hepatic artery	40
▪ From left or middle hepatic artery	40
▪ From RHA	10
▪ From GDA	8

CHA, common hepatic artery; SMA, superior mesenteric artery; RHA, right hepatic artery; LHA, left hepatic artery; GDA, gastroduodenal artery.
Adapted from Rosenblum JD, Boyle CM, Schwartz LB. The mesenteric circulation: anatomy and physiology. *Surg Clin North Am.* 1997;77:289–306.

hemorrhoidal artery.[1] This small and most distal mesenteric branch artery supplies primarily the large bowel from the level of the mid-transverse colon to the rectum.

Collateralization is a crucial concept when considering the mesenteric circulation. On the grounds of redundancy, given multiple potential sources of collateral flow, at least two of the three major branch vessels must be occluded or have a critical stenosis for mesenteric ischemia to manifest. While arterial collaterals may be small in the physiologic circulation, they have the potential to hypertrophy dramatically when increased flow is required. **Figure 86.1** demonstrates several important collateral pathways. The gastroduodenal artery (GDA) and pancreaticoduodenal arcade make up the primary potential pathway for collateral flow between the celiac axis and the SMA. In addition to the aforementioned arc of Buhler, the arc of Barkow consists of arteries in the omentum (SMA branches) that connects to the right and left gastroepiploic arteries (celiac branches). The marginal artery of Drummond is the major collateral route between the SMA and IMA; it lies within the colon mesentery giving rise to the vasa recta. The arc of Riolan lies within a more central portion of the mesentery connecting the middle and left colic arteries. Finally, the IMA may also receive collateral flow from lumbar branches of the aorta, hemorrhoidal branches of the internal iliac artery, and the middle sacral artery.

Splanchnic venous anatomy parallels the arterial system to drain into the portal venous system. The splenic and superior mesenteric veins join to form the portal vein. Hepatic venous blood is drained by the right, middle, and left hepatic veins. Portal–systemic connections are multiple and important when considering portal hypertension (HTN).

Physiologic intestinal function relies on adequate perfusion and oxygenation of the microvascular splanchnic circulation. Splanchnic blood flow is estimated as 300 to 1200 mL/min, or about 10% to 35% of the cardiac output, with approximately 70% of this blood flow supplying the mucosa and submucosa.[1,2] Various intrinsic and extrinsic autoregulatory mechanisms including tissue metabolites, myogenic mechanisms, and the autonomic nervous system ensure adequate gut circulation through both vasoconstriction and relaxation of arterial smooth muscle. The degree of visceral artery dilation and constriction determines the relatively large fluctuations in splanchnic blood flow during fasting and postprandial states.

Duplex ultrasound demonstrates moderate to high arterial resistance in the SMA, with low diastolic flow and slight flow reversal during fasting states. **Figure 86.2** demonstrates duplex ultrasonography of normal aorta and SMA. Vessel diameter, flow velocity, calculated volumetric blood flow, spectral analysis, and response to physiologic stimuli allow for precise assessment of the visceral circulation. In the postprandial period (30 to 90 minutes), low-resistance signals are noted throughout systole and diastole, indicative of dilated splanchnic arteriolar beds. Flow reversal does not occur. In contrast, low arterial resistance signals are noted in the celiac artery circulation regardless of feeding, likely due to the influence of the low-resistance hepatic vascular bed.

2 Intestinal ischemia may result from presplanchnic conditions that decrease total mesenteric blood flow (ie, heart failure and hypovolemia), splanchnic conditions that decrease regional blood flow through the mesenteric circulation (ie, thromboembolism) or postsplanchnic venous congestion (ie, mesenteric vein thrombosis [MVT] and cirrhosis). Regardless of the mechanism, impaired perfusion of the intestine results in hypoxia-associated sequelae that include cytokine release, free radial production, microcirculatory damage, and bacterial translocation. Mucosal barrier function is compromised secondary to physical disruption of the mucosa, a change in normal intestinal microflora resulting from treatment with broad-spectrum antibiotics, and impairment of host immune defenses.[3] Intestinal ischemia may rapidly progress to tissue necrosis causing severe metabolic derangements and ultimately multiple organ dysfunction and death. In addition to ischemia-related bowel injury, splanchnic reperfusion exaggerates injury patterns. Reperfusion injury is associated with increased microvascular permeability, increased epithelial permeability with leaking of fluid and molecules into the bowel lumen, and decreased intestinal blood flow.

Acute Mesenteric Ischemia

> *"Occlusion of the mesenteric vessels is apt to be regarded as one of those conditions of which … the diagnosis is impossible, the prognosis hopeless and the treatment almost useless."*[4]

AMI remains an uncommon event but carries catastrophic potential as illustrated by AJ Cokkinis' statement above from 1926. Klass is credited with the first successful restoration of arterial blood supply in an attempt to salvage AMI in 1951 by SMA embolectomy.[5,6] While clear medical and technologic progress has been made in the interim, delayed diagnosis and treatment continues to impede improvements in contemporary patient morbidity and mortality rates that approach 80%.[6,7]

AMI accounts for <1 in every 1000 hospital admissions, presents most commonly during the seventh and eighth decades of life, and epidemiologic study suggests that women are affected with three times the frequency of males, at least in part attributed to relative female longevity.[6] A Swedish epidemiologic study cites an AMI incidence of 12.9/100,000 people years (as diagnosed by autopsy or operation).[8]

3 The most common causes of AMI are referenced above and include: embolization (40% to 50%), arterial thrombosis (25% to 30%), nonocclusive mesenteric ischemia (NOMI) (15% to 20%), and mesenteric venous thrombosis (5% to 15%).[6,8] Additional causes may include SARS-CoV-2 infection, visceral

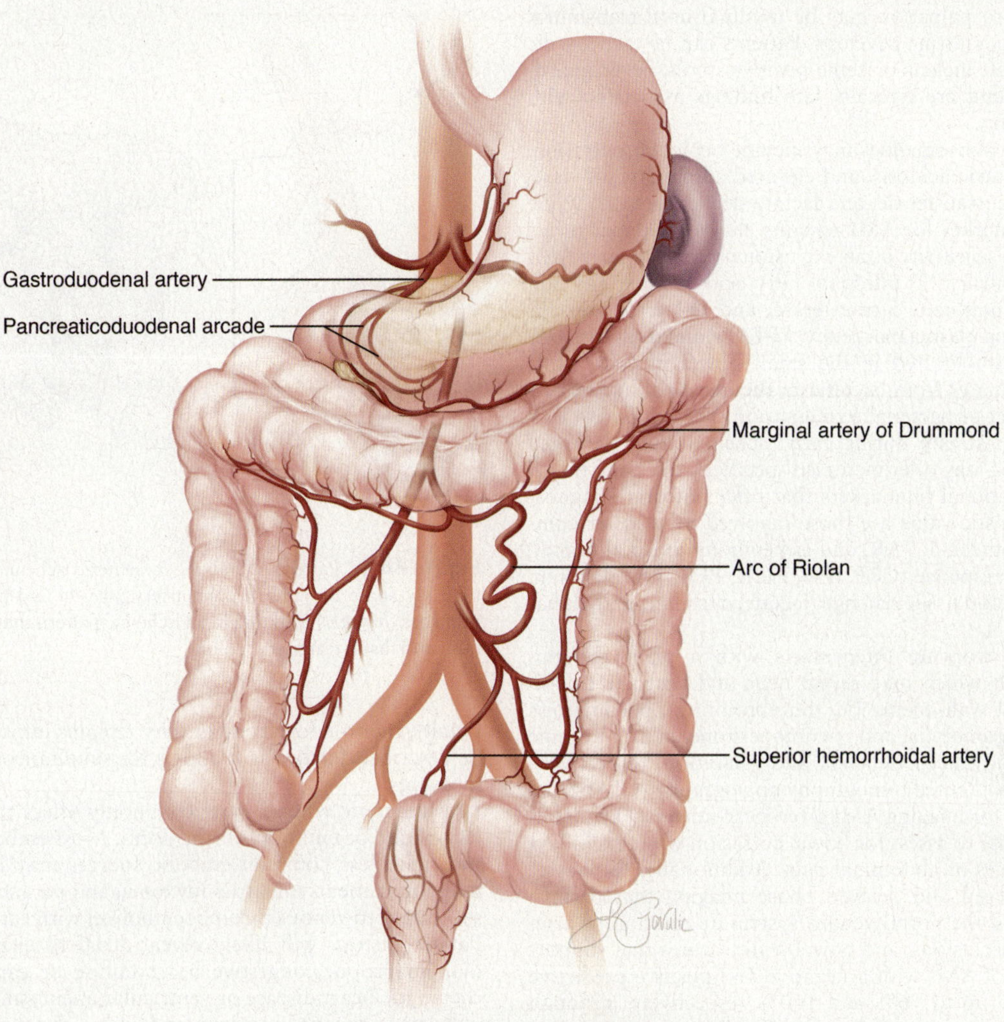

Figure 86.1. Mesenteric collateral circulation.

malperfusion associated with aortic dissection, mesenteric arterial dissection, and trauma. Historic mortality rates for AMI are as high as 93%, although more contemporary series suggest in-hospital mortality rates of 17% to 62% and a systematic review of 45 observational studies cites a mean mortality rate of 71.6% for 3692 patients with AMI.[8–12] While there is no validated prediction model for mortality in this clinical setting, authors have shown with logistic regression models that age, duration of symptoms, age-adjusted comorbidity, specific EKG markers, and shock index may be associated with higher mortality.[11,13]

Patients with AMI complain predominantly of abdominal pain followed by nausea, vomiting, and diarrhea. Pain is often described as "out of proportion" to the clinical examination

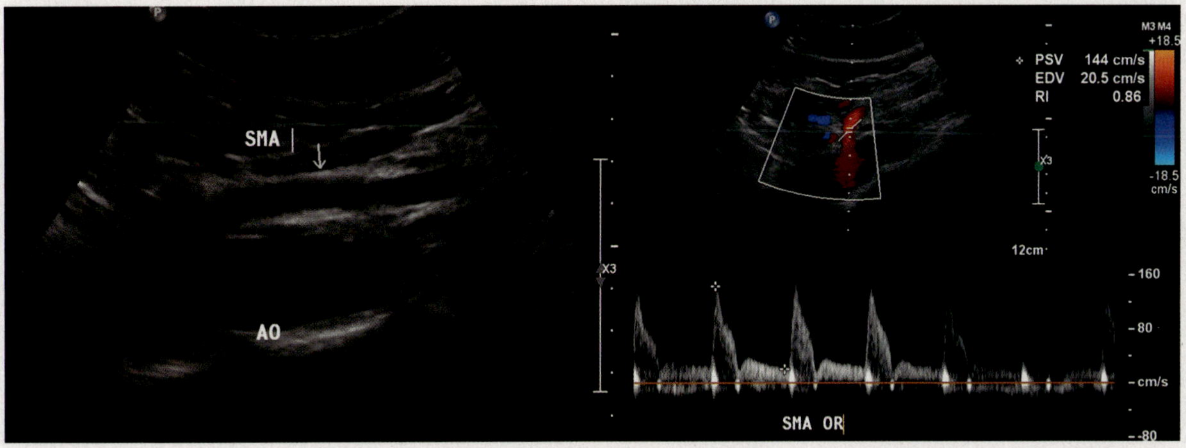

Figure 86.2. Mesenteric duplex ultrasound of a normal aorta and SMA that demonstrates moderate to high arterial resistance in the SMA, with low diastolic flow and slight flow reversal during fasting states. AO, aorta; SMA, superior mesenteric artery; PSV, peak systolic velocity; EDV, end-diastolic velocity; RI, resistive index; OR, origin.

as tenderness to palpation may be minimal until transmural necrosis of the intestine develops. Patients can be tachycardic and demonstrate melena or heme-positive stools. Fever, guarding, and rebound are typically late findings associated with bowel infarction.

Laboratory abnormalities may include hemoconcentration, leukocytosis, lactic acidosis, and elevated anion gap, amylase, aspartate aminotransferase, and lactate dehydrogenase. While a reliable biomarker for AMI remains elusive, D-dimer offers 96% to 100% sensitivity as an exclusionary test for early AMI with low specificity.[14,15] Intestinal fatty acid–binding globulin (I-FABP), α-glutathione S-transferase, and D-lactate are currently promising plasma markers.[14,16] I-FABP and α-glutathione S-transferase are located in the small bowel mucosa while D-lactate originates from bacteria in the intestinal lumen as a normal product of bacterial fermentation. These markers leak into the blood stream during early ischemia from damaged enterocytes and may offer increased specificity for small bowel ischemia. Additional biomarkers that offer potential diagnostic and prognostic value are those involved in vascular compromise (endothelin-1, FAR, and ischemia-modified albumin), inflammatory response (CRP, IL-6, NLR, PLR, procalcitonin, and omentin), and tissue damage (lactate, citrulline, and alpha-GST).[17]

Diagnostic work-up often starts with a plain abdominal radiograph which may reveal ileus and vascular calcifications; bowel wall edema (ie, thumbprinting), pneumatosis (**Fig. 86.3**), pneumobilia, and pneumoperitoneum may become evident with advanced ischemia and infarction, respectively. High-quality computed tomography angiography (CTA) is the gold standard for imaging AMI given near-universal availability and its ability to assess for bowel perfusion while excluding alternate sources of abdominal pain. Additionally, "biphasic" CT offers arterial and delayed phase imaging that permits visualization of the portal venous system in addition to arterial stenosis, occlusions, and bowel wall features that support the diagnosis of AMI with a negative and positive predictive value reported up to 96% and 100% respectively, although distinction of subtypes and severity of AMI (ie, nontransmural vs transmural) is often not possible.[18,19] Duplex ultrasonography, magnetic resonance angiography (MRA), and diagnostic laparoscopy may serve as adjuncts for diagnosis but secondary to intrinsic limitations should not be considered first line.

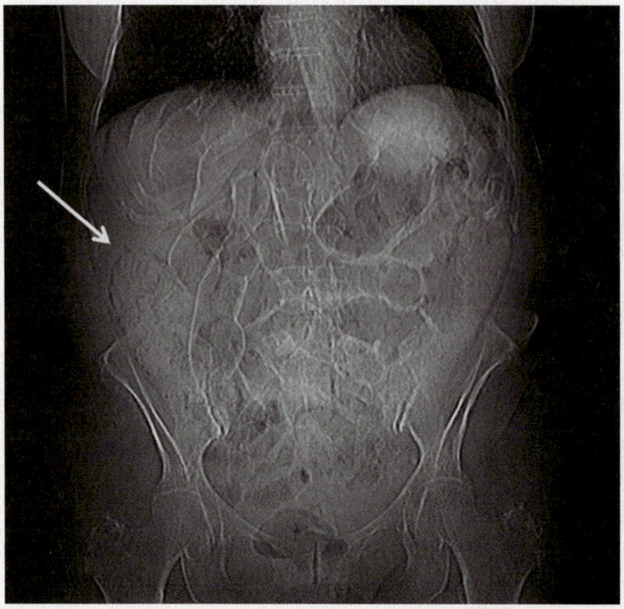

Figure 86.3. Abdominal radiograph demonstrating diffuse ileus and intestinal pneumatosis (*arrow*) in a patient with acute mesenteric ischemia.

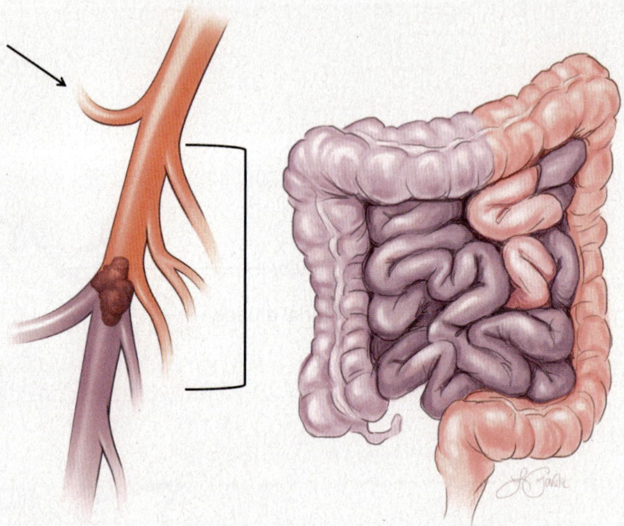

Figure 86.4. Pattern of embolic mesenteric ischemia—SMA emboli typically spare the middle colic artery (*arrow*) and proximal jejunal branches (*bracket*) resulting in an ischemic pattern that spares the jejunum and distal transverse colon.

Finally, the role for arteriography remains important and will be described further as it allows for simultaneous therapeutic measures.

Mesenteric emboli most commonly affect the SMA given its oblique orientation off the aorta. Most emboli are cardiac in origin; less common embolic sources may include proximal aortic aneurysm, atrial myxoma, and paradoxical embolus secondary to venous thromboembolism with cardiac shunting. Patient history will likely reveal atrial fibrillation, myocardial infarction, congestive heart failure or cardiomyopathy, rheumatic heart disease or ventricular aneurysm. Most emboli will spare the SMA origin and lodge distal to the middle colic artery and early jejunal branches. In the absence of well-formed collaterals, this results in a classic pattern of ischemia that compromises the bulk of small bowel and ascending colon while sparing the proximal jejunum and distal transverse colon (**Fig. 86.4**).

Acute in situ arterial thrombosis typically coincides with preexisting atherosclerotic disease. Up to 20% to 50% of patients will describe antecedent postprandial abdominal pain and weight loss consistent with CMI.[2,6] Clinical presentation may be more subacute given the presence of preformed collaterals that are typically absent in cases of embolic AMI. Patient history will likely reveal common cardiovascular risk factors. **Figure 86.5** demonstrates the highly calcified aorta of a patient presenting with AMI and chronic celiac artery occlusion, SMA thrombosis (encircled), and IMA occlusion.

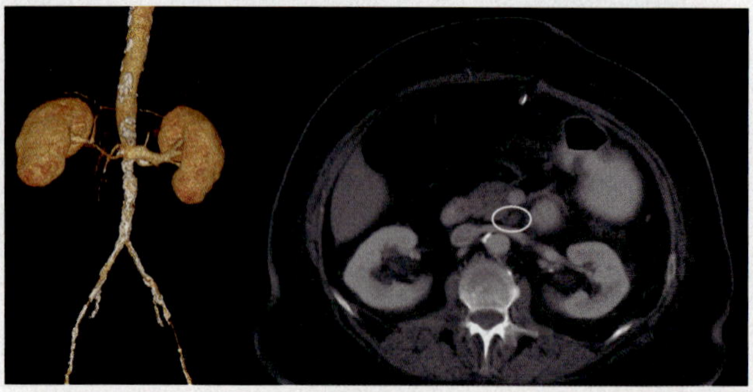

Figure 86.5. CT imaging demonstrating in situ SMA thrombosis in the setting of highly calcified aortoiliac occlusive disease and chronic celiac and IMA occlusions presenting as acute mesenteric ischemia.

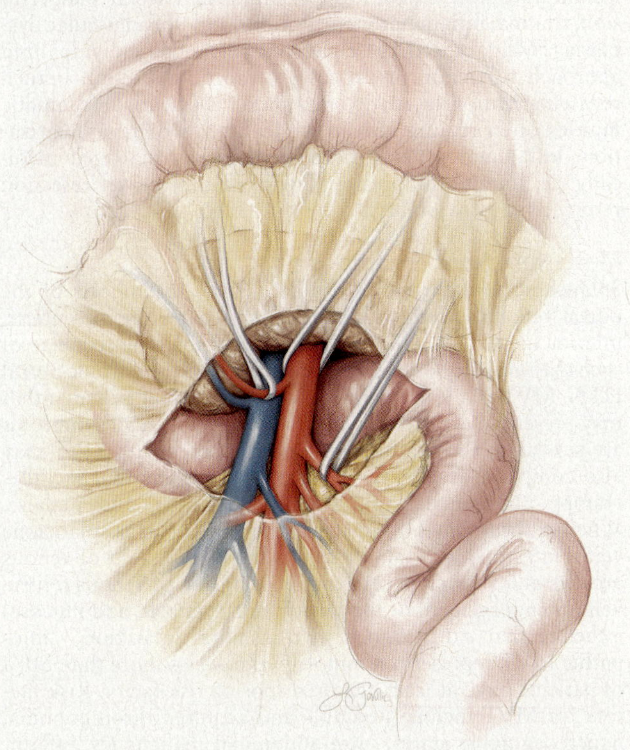

Figure 86.6. SMA exposure at the base of the colonic mesentery (*SMA encircled proximal to the middle colic artery*).

Management of AMI

4 Patients with AMI warrant immediate medical management that includes the establishment of adequate intravenous (IV) access and hemodynamic monitoring, systemic anticoagulation with heparin, fluid resuscitation, correction of electrolyte abnormalities, and administration of broad-spectrum IV antibiotics. Further vasoconstrictive insult with vasopressors should be avoided if possible. Patients with AMI and evidence of threatened bowel viability warrant immediate surgical exploration. Frankly necrotic or perforated bowel should be resected and left in discontinuity to limit contamination while definitive intestinal management should never delay revascularization.

SMA thromboembolectomy is the standard technique for embolic disease. **Figure 86.6** illustrates anterior exposure of the SMA at the base of the colonic mesentery. Typically, venous tributaries, small lymphatics, and autonomic nerve fibers require ligation to facilitate arterial exposure. The inferior pancreatic border may require mobilization for more proximal SMA exposure. The SMA is exposed and controlled proximal to the middle colic artery; the middle colic artery and jejunal branches are similarly controlled. After a therapeutic level of systemic anticoagulation is confirmed a transverse arteriotomy is created sharply (**Fig. 86.7**). The proximal SMA is vented; in the absence of robust and pulsatile antegrade flow a balloon thromboembolectomy should be performed with a 3-Fr or 4-Fr catheter. Distal vasculature is fragile and thromboembolectomy is best accomplished with a smaller catheter (ie, 2 Fr or 3 Fr). During balloon thromboembolectomy the balloon should be inflated with heparinized saline (not air) as the catheter is withdrawn. The same person should control the balloon inflation that is controlling catheter removal. Finally, consider flushing regional heparin or thrombolytic agent directly into the distal SMA and branches. Balloon thromboembolectomy should be repeated until the balloon is withdrawn free of thrombus burden. Following the successful clearance of all macroscopic thrombus the arteriotomy can be repaired primarily with simple sutures of 5-0 or 6-0 monofilament suture placed in an interrupted fashion. Vein patch

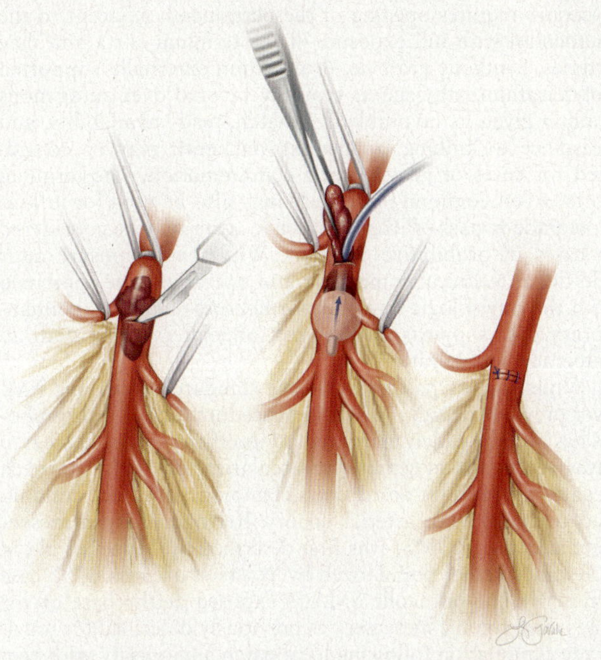

Figure 86.7. Illustration of balloon SMA thromboembolectomy through a transverse arteriotomy.

angioplasty should be considered over primary repair for diminutive vessels.

In cases of SMA occlusive disease with in situ thrombosis, bypass may be required for successful revascularization. In cases of such acuity, typically single-vessel reconstruction (SMA) is all that is required. While there are multiple options for graft orientation and conduit, a retrograde bypass off the right common iliac artery oriented in a "lazy-C" configuration is most often favored (**Fig. 86.8**). The lateral portion of SMA is exposed cephalad to the fourth portion of the duodenum. This

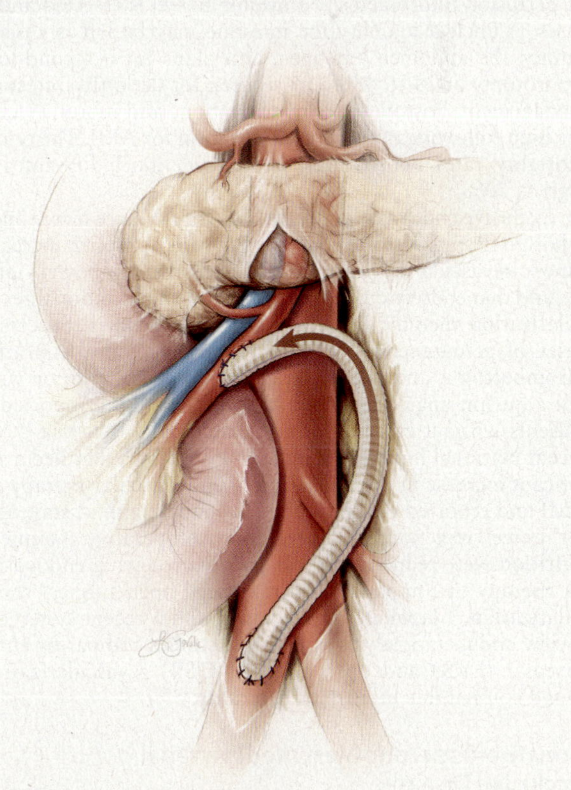

Figure 86.8. Retrograde bypass off the right common iliac artery oriented in a "lazy-C" configuration.

exposure requires opening of the peritoneum adjacent to the duodenum with full exposure of the terminal aorta and iliac arteries. Synthetic graft (ie, 6- or 8-mm externally supported polytetrafluoroethylene) is typically favored over autogenous conduit given its favorable size match, ready availability, and resistance to kinking. Saphenous vein graft may be considered for cases of gross enteric contamination. The terminal aorta or left common iliac artery may also be used for inflow. Antegrade bypass off the supraceliac aorta may be considered in cases of prohibitive anatomy. While this exposure adds additional technical complexity and operative time combined with the physiologic stress of aortic cross-clamping, contemporary data supports a lower risk of reintervention with an antegrade configuration.[20]

While surgery has remained the standard of care for AMI over previous decades, a hybrid procedure for SMA thrombosis has become widely embraced for its efficiency and decreased invasiveness for mesenteric revascularization. This approach negates the need for aortic cross-clamping, prosthetic conduit, and difficulty with arterial quality. Retrograde open mesenteric stenting (ROMS) was first described by Milner et al., in 2004 and further popularized by Wyers et al., in a 2007 case series.[21,22] The infracolic SMA is exposed at the base of the transverse colonic mesentery as previously described for retrograde cannulation following local patch angioplasty with vein or bovine pericardium. This hybrid approach allows for simultaneous assessment and treatment of nonviable intestine with mesenteric revascularization by way of SMA stenting. Contemporary series on ROMS report technical success rates of 93% and primary-assisted patency rates of 91% at 12 months with similar complication and reintervention rates when compared to mesenteric bypass with significantly reduced operative times.[23–25]

Regardless of the approach to successful revascularization, intestinal viability must be assessed; this decision is typically deferred for 20 to 30 minutes following reperfusion and aided by Doppler interrogation of the mesenteric arcade, observation of serosal color, and the presence of peristalsis. Adjuncts also include the use of fluorescein with a modified Wood lamp or perfusion fluorometer.[6] Nonviable bowel is resected and in cases of unclear viability the intestine may be left in discontinuity, the abdomen left open, and plans for a second-look laparotomy at 24 to 48 hours secured for definitive intestinal management. Postoperative complications and mortality rates are high following open revascularization for AMI. Thirty-day mortality rates approximate 30%, with morbidity rates as high as 70%.[26–28]

Exclusive endovascular treatments for AMI are increasingly reported despite historic concerns that this approach increases time to revascularization, prohibits assessment of bowel viability, and that endovascular failure might delay traditional revascularization thereby worsening patient outcomes. Successful cases of percutaneous mechanical thrombectomy, aspiration thrombectomy, and intra-arterial thrombolysis, with or without adjuvant angioplasty and stenting, have been reported in patients without evidence of advanced bowel ischemia.[29–32] A recent National Inpatient Sample (NIS) review identified a significant increase in the utilization of endovascular therapy for AMI and reported that mortality, hospital length of stay, need for bowel resection, and need for postoperative parenteral nutrition were reduced in those patients receiving endovascular therapy in comparison to traditional open surgical revascularization.[33] Japanese registry data, and a recent systematic review and meta-analysis assessed 11 studies comparing endovascular (EVR) and open surgical (OSR) revascularization, found comparable in-hospital mortality.[34,35]

Nonatherosclerotic Mesenteric Arterial Occlusive Disease

Intestinal ischemia may result from iatrogenic injury (ie, arterial dissection or thromboembolism during endovascular techniques), aortic dissection resulting in visceral malperfusion, trauma, inflammatory arteritides, and fibromuscular dysplasia (FMD). Indeed, these patients warrant an individualized approach to treatment. In cases of aortic dissection branch revascularization or aortic fenestration is essential. Traumatic injuries often require urgent surgical repair or revascularization. Inflammatory arteritides are typically managed medically (ie, immunosuppression) with surgical bowel resection reserved for nonviability.

Mesenteric Vein Thrombosis

Splanchnic vein thrombosis is defined by thrombosis of the portal venous system which includes the superior mesenteric, inferior mesenteric, splenic, and portal veins. The sequelae of such may include bowel or splenic infarction and chronic portal HTN. MVT is a less common form of intestinal ischemia that may present in a more subacute fashion. While AMI symptoms are similar to those aforementioned, patients with MVT may also complain of days to weeks of a prodrome that includes crampy abdominal pain, distension, nausea, and malaise. Whether thrombosis originates in the small or large splanchnic veins, intestinal infarction requires the involvement of venous arcades and vasa recta resulting in occlusion of venous return, venous engorgement of the bowel wall, cyanosis, and mucosal ischemia that can progress to transmural infarction.[36] Idiopathic MVT represents a minority of cases as more than 50% of patients have at least one predisposing risk factor. Risk factors for MVT include heritable and acquired thrombophilia, hypercoagulable states, intra-abdominal malignancy, inflammatory disease, myeloproliferative neoplasm, cytomegalovirus and SARS-CoV-2 infection, chronic liver disease, heparin-induced thrombocytopenia, and local intra-abdominal processes (ie, pancreatitis or trauma). A high index of suspicion is necessary for diagnosis given the nonspecific nature of presenting symptoms, signs, and laboratory studies.[36] CT imaging with portal phase venous contrast (CT venogram) is the imaging modality of choice. Findings suggestive of MVT include a sharply defined, enhancing venous wall with central low attenuation.[36] MRA, angiography, and laparoscopy are useful adjuncts. Emergent laparotomy should be considered for signs of advanced intestinal ischemia; intraoperatively blood-tinged ascites is likely to be encountered and the bowel will appear dusky, thick, and rubbery. Systemic anticoagulation is the mainstay of treatment as it reduces mortality, decreases recurrent thrombosis rates from approximately 30% to <5%, and decreases mortality associated with recurrent thrombosis.[36–39] Additionally, with anticoagulation most patients will demonstrate partial or complete venous recanalization with time. In the absence of a defined risk factor, patients with MVT should undergo a work-up for thrombophilia. A finite duration of anticoagulation is recommended for those with a reversible provoking risk factor with cessation of anticoagulation encouraged after 3 months; remaining cases of idiopathic MVT or persistent risk warrant indefinite anticoagulation.[40] Patients with recurrent mesenteric venous thrombosis should be investigated for antiphospholipid syndrome, and thrombophilia testing may be considered in selected patients with acute venous mesenteric thrombosis that will discontinue anticoagulation after 3 to 6 months.[41] Historically open venous thrombectomy was employed for advanced cases of MVT at the time of laparotomy. More recently various systemic and percutaneous thrombolytic techniques have been applied to cases of large vessel disease; however, no large or well-controlled trials exist to guide recommendations for such over anticoagulation alone.[36,42–44]

Nonocclusive Mesenteric Ischemia

NOMI results from diffuse mesenteric vasospasm. This rare form of intestinal ischemia most often affects critically ill patients with hemodynamic instability. Risk factors include decreased cardiac output (ie, heart failure or arrhythmia),

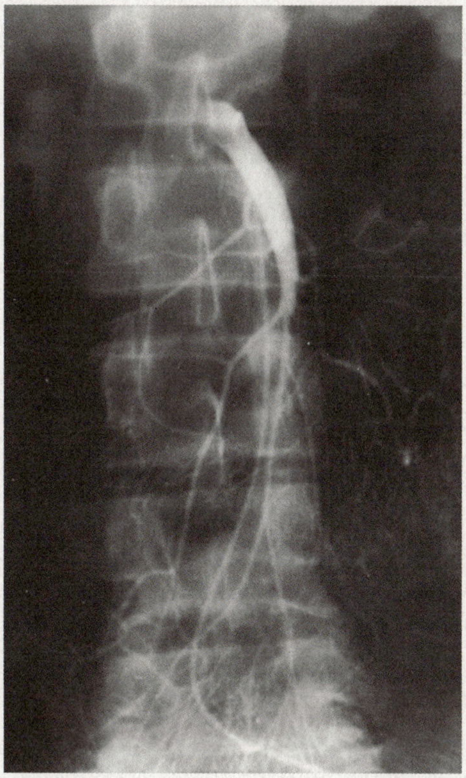

Figure 86.9. Nonocclusive mesenteric ischemia—mesenteric arteriogram revealing diffuse vasoconstriction and nonopacification of SMA branch vessels.

hemodialysis, shock, vasoactive medications (ie, vasopressors or digitalis), and drug abuse (ie, cocaine). Angiography is required for diagnosis and will demonstrate diffuse vasoconstriction and nonopacification of branch vessels (**Fig. 86.9**). Treatment centers on improving mesenteric perfusion by optimizing volume status, limiting vasoactive medications and correcting contributing comorbidities. Intra-arterial infusion of vasodilators (ie, papaverine or nitroglycerin) or IV infusion of glucagon or prostaglandin E2, which selectively increases splanchnic blood flow, have been advocated in treating this form of intestinal ischemia without robust, large, or well-controlled trials to support treatment guidelines.[45–47]

Chronic Mesenteric Ischemia

Symptoms of CMI are often referred to as "intestinal angina." Ostial stenosis secondary to arteriosclerosis is the most common etiology and patients typically share risk factors of overt atherosclerosis and long-standing tobacco abuse. Additional causes of CMI may include arterial FMD, vasculitis, aortic coarctation, and connective tissue disorders. In light of aforementioned mesenteric collaterals, the responsible anatomic lesions of CMI typically affect at least two of three splanchnic arteries, although isolated lesions of the SMA distal to the middle colic branch may yield intestinal angina by excluding collateralization.[2] Patients classically present with postprandial abdominal pain that occurs within 30 minutes of eating and may last up to 4 hours postprandial. Consistent postprandial symptoms typically result in the modification of eating habits that may range from the consumption of smaller meals to "food phobia" that subsequently results in weight loss and malnutrition. There is an increasing incidence of overweight patients presenting with CMI. These patients have been reported to undergo significantly more diagnostic testing to confirm the diagnosis of CMI, possibly delaying diagnosis.[48] Additionally, BMI ≥25 has been associated with poorer long-term survival following mesenteric revascularization for CMI in comparison to nonobese patients.[49]

5 The progression from minor symptoms to AMI and intestinal infarction is unpredictable; almost half of patients presenting with AMI describe previous symptoms of CMI.[50] The incidence of CMI also remains unclear. Population studies suggest that up to 18% of individuals over 65 years of age have asymptomatic radiographic mesenteric stenosis.[51] Duplex ultrasonography should be considered the first-line diagnostic modality for CMI. Specifically, high-grade stenosis of the SMA and celiac artery in a fasting state are suggested by a peak systolic velocity of >275 cm/s and 200 cm/s, respectively.[52] CTA and MRA support the diagnosis of CMI while offering additional vascular anatomic evaluation such as the presence of aneurysm, calcific burden, dissection, wall features suggesting vasculitis and venous anomalies that may impact open reconstruction. An additional advantage of MRI is the opportunity to perform blood flow measurements (ie, measurements of flow profiles, stroke volumes, peak velocities).[53] Importantly, mesenteric blood flow will increase after a meal in healthy controls, while significantly less increase in postprandial blood flow of the SMV in patients with CMI can be shown with MR flow technique.[54] Aortography with anteroposterior and lateral views has been commonly cited as the gold standard for diagnosis and allows for simultaneous mesenteric arteriography, manometry, provocative measures (ie, vasodilator infusion), and intervention (ie, angioplasty and stenting) as appropriate. This modality is often favored over cross-sectional imaging when an endovascular approach for treatment is being considered over open revascularization. Growing data suggest there may be a role for additional work-up, especially in those patients with single-vessel mesenteric stenosis, to guide the decision to perform revascularization. Pressure measurements may help define a clinically relevant CA or SMA stenosis, with a pressure distal [Pd]/pressure aorta [Pa] ratio of 0.8 following vasodilator administration supporting clinically significant mesenteric stenosis.[55] Functional work-up to assess gastrointestinal mucosal perfusion may include PCO_2 tonometry and visual light spectroscopy. An expedited work-up to include gastrointestinal malignancies and other potential causes is recommended to include: esophagogastroduodenoscopy (EGD), colonoscopy, CT, and abdominal ultrasound.[17]

Management of CMI

Treatment goals in the management of CMI include symptomatic relief, restoration of normal weight, and the prevention of bowel infarction. Mesenteric revascularization provides immediate symptom relief in most patients. Patients should be optimized from a medical standpoint prior to revascularization. Classically, open surgical revascularization options consider patient cardiopulmonary reserve to tolerate aortic cross-clamping and aortic and arterial calcific burden to dictate vascular sites for clamping and sewing. These authors propose that elective revascularization in the lower-risk patient favors two-vessel (ie, celiac and SMA) antegrade reconstruction when anatomically feasible. Clinical practice guidelines suggest the SMA as the primary target for revascularization, and the celiac axis and IMA as secondary targets that may aid in symptom relief should the SMA not be suitable for intervention.[17] Contingent on vessel calcification, the supraceliac aorta through a transperitoneal approach serves as a preferential target for inflow. After entering the lesser sac, division of the left triangular ligament allows for retraction of the left hepatic lobe. With the esophagus retracted toward the patient's left (confirmed by palpation of the existing nasogastric tube), transection of the diaphragmatic crura exposes the supraceliac aorta. The celiac trunk, common hepatic artery, and splenic artery are exposed at this time. Subsequently with retraction of the transverse mesocolon cephalad, the SMA is exposed as described above at the root of the mesentery. A retropancreatic tunnel is created that courses anterior to the renal vein. The patient is systemically anticoagulated with heparin and the proximal anastomosis can be constructed with partial aortic

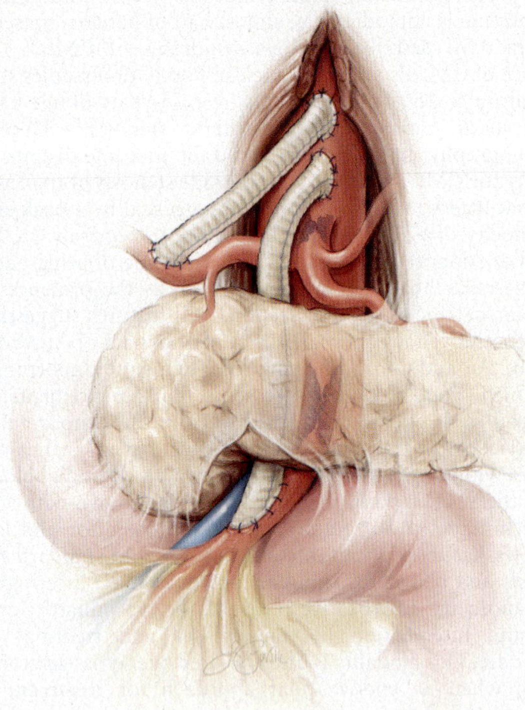

Figure 86.10. Two-vessel antegrade aortomesenteric bypass.

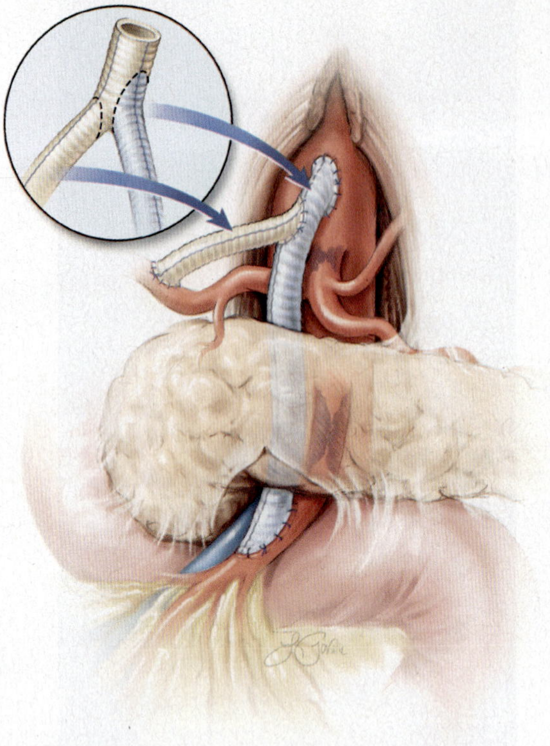

Figure 86.11. Two-vessel antegrade aortomesenteric bypass based off the supraceliac aorta using a presewn bifurcated graft.

occlusion. Most often a knitted polyester synthetic graft is utilized for conduit. There are multiple acceptable variations that include the use of two separate aortomesenteric bypass grafts (**Fig. 86.10**) or the use of a bifurcated graft. It is conventional to utilize a prefabricated bifurcated graft (eg, 14 × 7 mm) for reconstruction. In this case a short main body is beveled to create the proximal end-to-side aortic anastomosis; the left limb is tunneled through the retropancreatic tunnel and an end-to-side distal anastomosis created next to the SMA; the right limb is subsequently cut to size and beveled to create an end-to-end anastomosis to the celiac artery directly or an end-to-side anastomosis with the common hepatic artery. These authors favor the approach presented in **Figure 86.11**. A limb of a bifurcated knitted polyester graft is transected off the main body in such a way that there is a phalange created. This limb is specifically utilized for creation of the aorto-SMA bypass, with the phalange incorporated into the proximal aortic anastomosis as shown. The remaining limb is cut to size and beveled accordingly; the proximal anastomosis is constructed end-to-side off the aorto-SMA bypass graft and the distal anastomosis constructed end-to-side to the common hepatic artery. This facilitates a very short celiac limb with a natural lie that may reduce the risk of limb kinking or torsion. Finally, the descending thoracic aorta may serve as an alternative source for inflow when supraceliac aortic anatomy is prohibitive or has previously been utilized for revascularization (**Fig. 86.12**). For those patients with comorbidity or anatomy (ie, calcification) that precludes aortic clamping, a retrograde ilio-SMA bypass is favored as described above (**Fig. 86.9**).

Transaortic endarterectomy is less often utilized in contemporary practice, but may be applicable for those patients with bowel perforation or contamination, hostile abdominal conditions (extensive adhesive disease or abdominal wall hernia), and bulky coral reef aortomesenteric plaque with lower extremity ischemia. A retroperitoneal approach to the perivisceral aorta through a thoracoabdominal incision permits a longitudinal or trapdoor aortotomy, endarterectomy and repair with primary closure or patch aortoplasty as illustrated in **Figure 86.13**.

While historically criticized for high mortality rates (up to 15%), contemporary outcomes following open mesenteric bypass at high-volume centers support mortality rates <4%, likely secondary to technical refinements, improved patient selection and advances in medical, anesthetic, and critical care management.[56–63] Open mesenteric revascularization boasts excellent symptom improvement (77% to 100%) with low recurrence rates at 3 to 5 years (0% to 32%) and perioperative morbidity rates approximating 35% to 40%.[63,64]

Endovascular mesenteric revascularization has become the initial treatment of choice for patients with CMI and

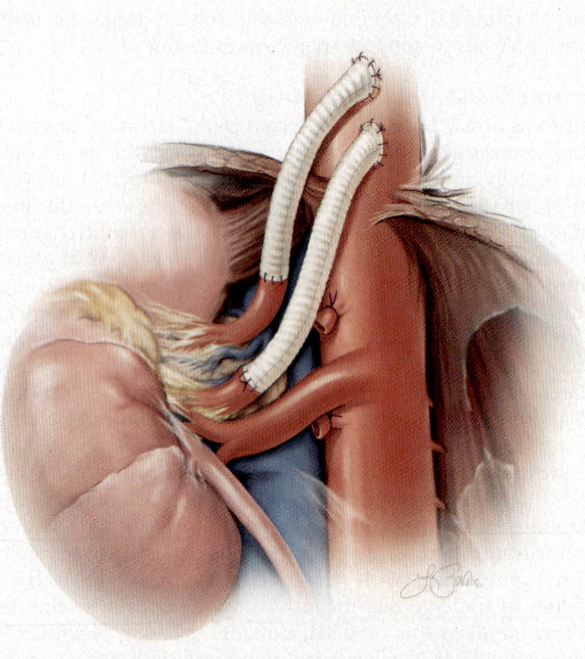

Figure 86.12. Two-vessel antegrade aortomesenteric bypass based off the supraceliac aorta using two separate grafts.

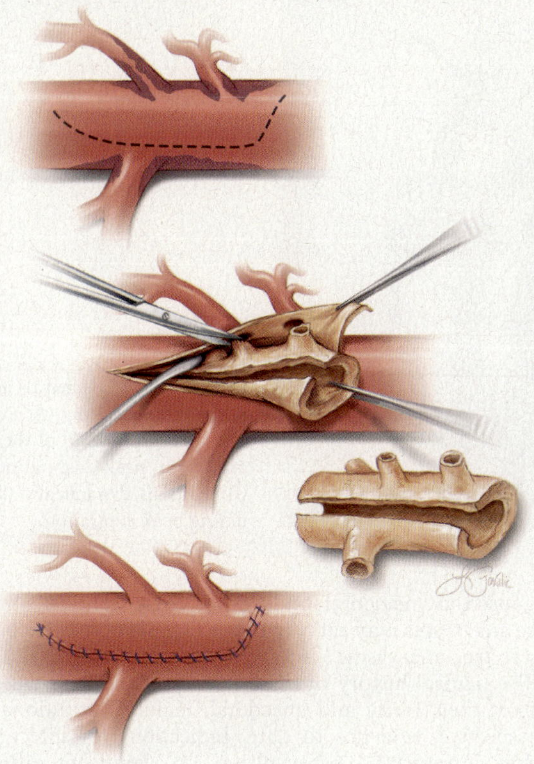

Figure 86.13. Endarterectomy of the aorta, celiac and superior mesenteric arteries through a longitudinal trapdoor aortotomy with primary closure.

suitable lesions, as supported by SVS guidelines.[17] Stenting of the mesenteric vessels is recommended over angioplasty alone for favorable anatomy that excludes long-segment occlusion (ie, >2 cm), small-diameter vessels, heavily calcified stenosis/occlusion and extrinsic compression (ie, arcuate ligament compression of the celiac artery).[65–68] Endovascular revascularization offers success rates approaching 100% with immediate symptom relief. While perioperative morbidity is notably lower in comparison to open surgical revascularization, endovascular interventions are more likely to result in restenosis, recurrent symptoms (within 3 years), and require reintervention.[60,69–72] Primary and secondary patency rates approximate 40% and 88%, respectively at 5 years (in comparison to 88% and 97% following open revascularization) emphasizing the importance of patient counseling preoperatively and close surveillance postprocedure.[73] There is no significant difference in 3-year survival between open surgical and endovascular revascularization.[72] Two-vessel (celiac and SMA) stenting does not appear to reduce the risk of recurrent symptoms or reintervention when compared to single-vessel (SMA) stenting and moreover, isolated celiac artery stenting carries a higher risk of recurrence.[73] Balloon-expandable covered stents may be associated with less restenosis, recurrence, and reintervention in comparison to bare metal stents, and as such are favored in current guidelines.[17,74,75] Complications (average rates) may include symptomatic embolization (2.5%), thrombotic mesenteric arterial occlusion (1%), iatrogenic dissection (2%), stent dislodgement (2%), and access site–related complication (9%).[67]

A large review of mesenteric revascularization from the Nationwide Inpatient Sample between 1988 and 2006 demonstrated increased overall revascularization procedures for CMI.[76] Additionally, these authors noted that mesenteric angioplasty and stenting not only surpassed open revascularization procedures for CMI in 2002, endovascular interventions more than doubled open procedures by 2005. An updated sampling of the same database between 2007 and 2014 supported decreased mortality, shorter hospital length of stay, reduced costs and decreased perioperative morbidity when compared to surgery.[77] These data are clouded by both the expansion of treatment indications and the fact that a greater risk of restenosis and recurrent symptoms may increase overall interventions. Moreover, these reinterventions for recurrence likely carry a variable risk for in-hospital morbidity and mortality. Regardless, mesenteric stenting has become the first-line therapy for most patients with atherosclerotic CMI and maintains an important role as a temporizing measure to facilitate weight gain in the high-risk malnourished patients (as a bridge to open revascularization) and for those patients with medical comorbidities that would further complicate or prohibit open surgical revascularization. Open mesenteric bypass surgery is recommended for low-risk patients with unfavorable mesenteric occlusive disease anatomy, failed prior endovascular revascularization, or multiple recurrences of in-stent stenosis/occlusion.

Median Arcuate Ligament Syndrome

Median arcuate ligament syndrome (MALS) remains a controversial diagnosis, first described in the 1960s.[78] Chronic abdominal pain is associated with radiographic evidence of celiac artery compression by the overlying fibrous arch of the median arcuate ligament (MAL) and adjacent celiac ganglion. The pathophysiology remains poorly understood and evidence suggests both ischemic and neurogenic etiologies for pain.[79] Gastric tonometry has documented evidence of mucosal ischemia in patients prior to treatment.[80] The 7% to 21% incidence of celiac artery compression in asymptomatic patients combined with the typical robust mesenteric collaterals and widely patent superior and inferior mesenteric arteries present in these younger individuals favor a neurogenic etiology.[81,82] Specifically, compression of the celiac plexus somatic nerves by the MAL may produce abdominal pain that is improved with a celiac ganglionectomy that accompanies ligament release or percutaneous celiac plexus block.

Patients with MALS are typically females in their third decade of life. Symptoms most commonly include postprandial pain, weight loss, and less commonly nausea and diarrhea. Diagnosis is supported by duplex ultrasonography that demonstrates elevated peak systolic velocities through the celiac artery on expiration that normalize or improve with inspiration and reverse flow through the hepatic artery.[83] Cross-sectional imaging like CTA and MRA can support the diagnosis as well, and may reveal poststenotic dilation of the celiac artery. Angiography demonstrating dynamic compression or occlusion during peak expiration remains the gold standard for the diagnosis of MALS (**Fig. 86.14**). Additionally, as MALS remains a diagnosis of exclusion, some authors favor gastric exercise tonometry test and celiac ganglion block to support patient selection.[84]

Release of the MAL should include complete dissection and skeletonization of both the MAL and surrounding nerve ganglion. This can be accomplished through an open approach whereby the aortic hiatus and celiac artery are exposed through the lesser sac. Additionally, laparoscopic and robotic techniques have been described. The most contemporary literature review and large series suggest immediate postoperative symptoms relief in approximately >70% patients.[79,80,85–88] Adjunctive procedures for celiac artery revascularization are utilized in a minority of cases and may include celiac angioplasty, celiac artery patch angioplasty, and celiac artery bypass (ie, aortoceliac bypass). Late symptom recurrence approximates 6% and only Reilly and colleagues have demonstrated a reduction in recurrence following MAL release with celiac artery revascularization in comparison to MAL release alone (24% vs 44%).[79,89] Multiple authors have highlighted the importance of patient selection for treatment suggesting that specific patient criteria may correlate with successful outcomes including: consistent postprandial abdominal pain, young age, female gender, weight loss >20 lb and anatomic features of

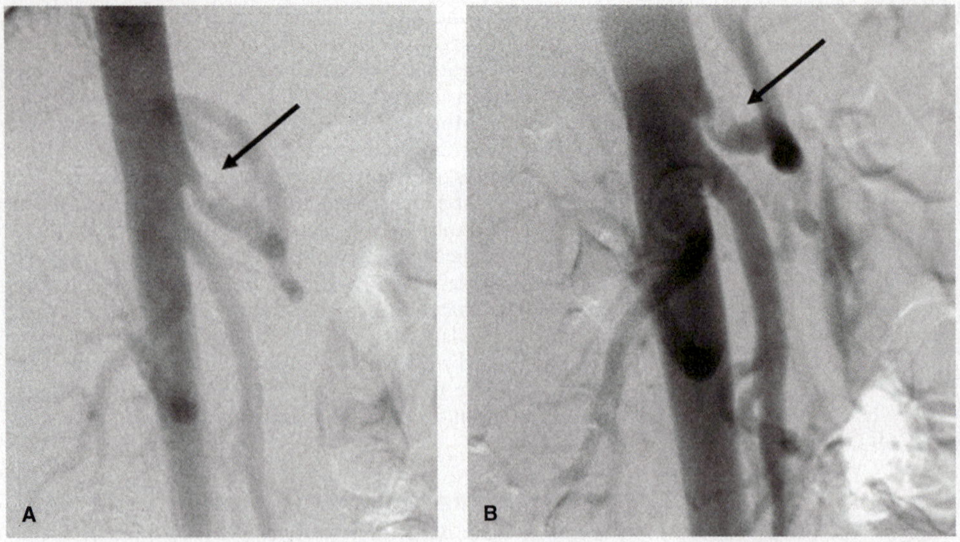

Figure 86.14. Lateral aortography demonstrating (**A**) external compression (*arrow*) of the celiac artery on peak inspiration that (**B**) worsens dynamically (*arrow*) during peak expiration.

poststenotic dilation or increased collateral flow.[89–91] Psychiatric diagnoses are common in adults with MALS, and may predict worse patient-reported quality-of-life outcomes following surgery.[92] A reasonable approach may reserve adjunctive revascularization for those patients with objective angiographic pressure or ultrasound velocity gradients following open surgical MAL decompression or those with persistent symptoms following laparoscopic or robotic release.

Laparoscopic and robotic release of the MAL is increasingly employed for MALS.[79,85–87,93] While no procedure-related mortality has been reported for open or laparoscopic ligament release, there is a 9.1% incidence across series of open conversion for hemorrhage that follows laparoscopic release, which heightens morbidity and mortality risk.[79] Certainly independent operator learning curve, institutional technical enhancements, and patient selection may strongly affect this result. More recently, safe and effective robotic-assisted MAL release has been reported to offer benefits over laparoscopic release in light of improved visualization, extra degree of motion provided by robotic arms with "wrist movement" and scaled operator movements (including tremor elimination).[94] A contemporary study recently proposed a predictive model for MALS patients that uses preoperative data (age, baseline celiac artery expiratory velocity) to predict symptom improvement following release.[95] These same authors were the first to show a significant improvement in all eight AF-36 categories, and particularly bodily pain. While surgical intervention may treat this controversial but debilitating condition, long-term (>5 years) follow-up data remain lacking, as is a consensus as to the optimal surgical approach.[96]

Splanchnic Artery Aneurysms

Splanchnic artery aneurysms are historically cited as rare and mainly asymptomatic. In the past, most were syphilitic or mycotic, while contemporary visceral aneurysms are largely 6 true aneurysms caused by atherosclerosis or medial degeneration.[97] True aneurysms are defined by the involvement of all three arterial wall layers (intima, media, and adventitia) while false aneurysms, or pseudoaneurysms, represent a collection of extravasating blood outside of the artery that remains confined next to the vessel by surrounding tissue. The incidence of splanchnic artery aneurysms is estimated at 0.1% to 2% and autopsy series suggest a prevalence that may approach 10%.[98,99] A minority of aneurysms present with life-threatening rupture and while historic-associated mortality rates approached 25% to 70%; more contemporary series suggest mortality rates of 15%, possibly reflecting improvements in perioperative management and the increasing use of endovascular techniques.[100] Most splanchnic aneurysms are asymptomatic however, and diagnosed as incidental findings by cross-sectional imaging. False aneurysms may carry a higher rate of rupture in comparison to true aneurysms (76% vs 3% in once series).[101]

The natural history of these aneurysms remains elusive in light of their rarity and anecdotal, mainly institutional and retrospective, evidence to date. Indications for intervention remain conservative, especially as no significant difference has been identified between the diameters of ruptured and nonruptured aneurysms.[101] Additionally, aneurysm calcification and intraluminal thrombus are not associated with rupture risk. Historically, treatment had been recommended for symptoms and size >2 cm or aneurysm diameter three times greater than the respective normal artery, although contemporary guidelines support evidence-based guidelines for size threshold for repair by phenotype.[102] Patients with splanchnic aneurysms generally have 10-year survival rates >80% and open surgical treatment provides excellent, durable long-term results with low perioperative mortality and morbidity following elective surgery.[100,103,104] While surgical repair has remained the mainstay of treatment, minimally invasive (ie, robotic and laparoscopic) and endovascular techniques continue to evolve and are increasingly applied for both elective treatment and that of rupture. Endovascular intervention with local anesthesia offers excellent technical success, negligible morbidity and mortality in elective cases, and brief hospital stays.[100,101,104–108] Transcatheter embolization of visceral artery aneurysms offers additional advantages that include precise aneurysm localization, assessment of collateral flow, and negate the need for certain (ie, intrahepatic) difficult arterial exposures.[97] Notably, embolization has become the standard of care for splanchnic artery pseudoaneurysm.[106,109] Additionally, endovascular therapy may offer decreased postoperative morbidity and mortality rates in cases of rupture when compared to open surgery (2.7% to 7% vs 24% to 29%, respectively).[100,105]

Distribution of splanchnic artery aneurysms is as follows: splenic artery (60%) > hepatic arteries (20%) > superior mesenteric artery (SMA) (5.5%) > celiac artery (4%) and gastric and gastroepiploic arteries (4%) > ileocolic arteries (3%) > pancreaticoduodenal arteries (2%) > GDA (1.5%) > IMA (<1%).[98] Most patients present in the sixth decade of life.[101] Symptomatic patients will present with abdominal pain and frank hemorrhagic shock with rupture. Rupture may be intra-abdominal, although erosion into a gastrointestinal lumen may result in sporadic gastrointestinal bleeding (ie, herald bleed) and erosion into adjacent mesenteric veins results in arteriovenous fistulae. The asymptomatic patient inconsistently reveals a bruit on auscultation and rarely a palpable mass on examination. Each splanchnic aneurysm warrants individual consideration.

Splenic Artery Aneurysm

Splenic artery aneurysms account for 60% of all splanchnic artery aneurysms and are the third most common intra-abdominal arterial aneurysm. Their prevalence in the general population is very low approximating 0.16% to 0.8%.[110] These aneurysms occur two to four times more frequently in women than men and are associated with multiparity.[97,104,110,111] Hormonal and local hemodynamic events likely contribute to the evolution of splenic aneurysms. An etiologic classification system has previously been proposed by *Stanley and Fry* that implicates arterial dysplasia, portal HTN, local inflammation, and hormonal and hemodynamic events in the pathogenesis of these aneurysms.[110] HTN is a common comorbidity affecting 50% to 60% of patients with splenic aneurysm, and up to 20% of patients will demonstrate concurrent aneurysms affecting alternate arterial beds.[108,109,112] Additional etiologic risk factors for true aneurysms may include dissection, septic emboli, polyarteritis nodosa, systemic lupus erythematosus, and connective tissue disorders like Ehlers–Danlos syndrome, while splenic pseudoaneurysms are typically attributed to chronic pancreatitis and trauma. Splenic aneurysms most often arise at branch points off the mid- and distal main splenic artery. Tortuosity of the main splenic artery is common (**Fig. 86.15**). The majority (80%) of splenic aneurysms are solitary and saccular, although 90% of patients with portal HTN will demonstrate multiple splenic aneurysms. Those aneurysms measuring >5 cm are often described as "giant lesions" and appear to be more common in older males.[113]

Splenic aneurysms typically rupture into the lesser sac with limited self-containment. Later hemorrhage into the peritoneal cavity results in cardiovascular collapse and the so-called "double rupture." The incidence of splenic aneurysm rupture approximates 2% to 5% and is not associated with calcification, blood pressure, or age.[98,109,110] Increased levels of aneurysmal peripheral calcification are associated with smaller aneurysm size at the time of diagnosis, but appear to have no impact on aneurysm growth.[109] Growth rates among surveyed aneurysms (out to 3.1 years) have been calculated as 0.2 mm/yr.[109] Rupture-associated mortality is dramatically increased in the peripartum patient (68% to 75% vs 25%), and associated fetal mortality approaches 100%.[110,112,114] Rupture in this setting occurs most commonly during the last trimester.[97] While historically a strong association between pregnancy and splenic aneurysm rupture was reported, a contemporary series reporting on >67,000 consecutive live births over 5 years identified no cases of splenic artery aneurysm rupture.[112] There is no apparent role for routine screening for splenic aneurysm in the pregnant patient.[115] Rupture risk is increased twofold by liver transplantation, the mortality following which is 50%.[116,117]

Contemporary data have supported an indolent natural history of surveyed splenic aneurysms, of null to slow growth (0.02 to 0.06 cm/yr) without rupture or aneurysm-related complications.[109,118] As such, accepted indications for treatment include rupture, symptoms, asymptomatic aneurysms measuring 3.0 cm, and any size asymptomatic aneurysm at the time of liver transplantation or in women of childbearing age.[102,109,119,120] Historically, the open surgical treatment of splenic artery aneurysms included aneurysm resection or splenectomy. Recognizing the immunologic benefits of splenic preservation, arterial ligation, and aneurysm excision is preferred when possible; however, those patients with multiple and perihilar aneurysms may still require splenectomy. Laparoscopic and robotic techniques at ligation, aneurysm resection and splenectomy have become common-place offering negligible risk of open conversion, need for reoperation, and mortality.[121–123] Splenic vaccinations and education regarding the need for booster vaccinations at regular 5-year intervals should be provided. Perioperative morbidity and mortality are estimated as 9% to 25% and 1% to 5%, respectively, across series.[109,110,124–126]

Endovascular therapy has been utilized with increasing frequency for both elective and ruptured cases boasting decreased early morbidity, mortality, and hospital length of stay. While only 2% of all splenic aneurysms were managed with endovascular therapies in 1999, this proportion increased to 70% between the years 2010 and 2013.[126] Embolization with coils, gelfoam, glue, thrombin, and vascular plugs has been advocated for saccular aneurysms with narrow necks (**Fig. 86.16**). Larger vessels with complex wide-neck aneurysms may be better approached with covered stents or stent-assisted coil embolization.[127] Technical success for endovascular treatment is 93% to 98%, limited primarily by vessel tortuosity that may be overcome with steerable catheters.[109,126,128,129] Conversion to open surgery is rarely necessary (<2%) to accomplish successful aneurysm exclusion.[126] Postembolization syndrome (PES) complicates 10% to 30% of cases across series and may include left upper quadrant pain, fever, ileus, platelet dysfunction, leukocytosis, and pancreatitis following embolization with and without radiographic evidence of splenic infarction.[109,126,129,130] Up to 21% of patients will demonstrate major splenic infarct and may require reintervention for splenic abscess by way of percutaneous drainage or splenectomy.[109,128] Portal HTN appears to increase dramatically the risk of major

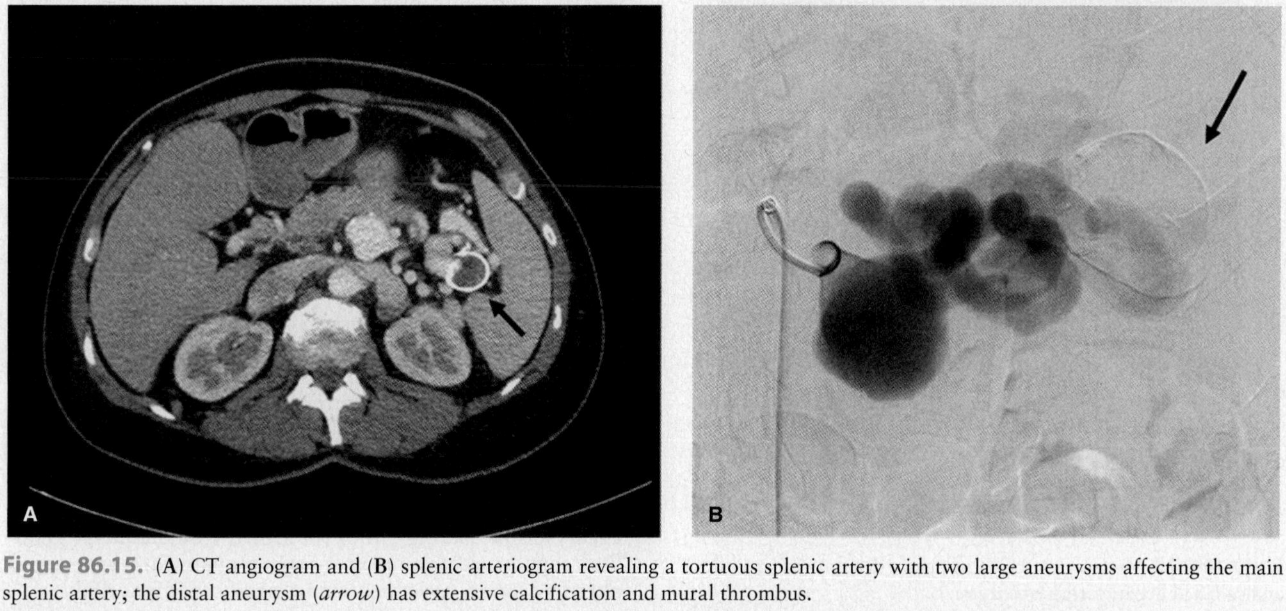

Figure 86.15. (**A**) CT angiogram and (**B**) splenic arteriogram revealing a tortuous splenic artery with two large aneurysms affecting the main splenic artery; the distal aneurysm (*arrow*) has extensive calcification and mural thrombus.

VASCULAR DISEASE

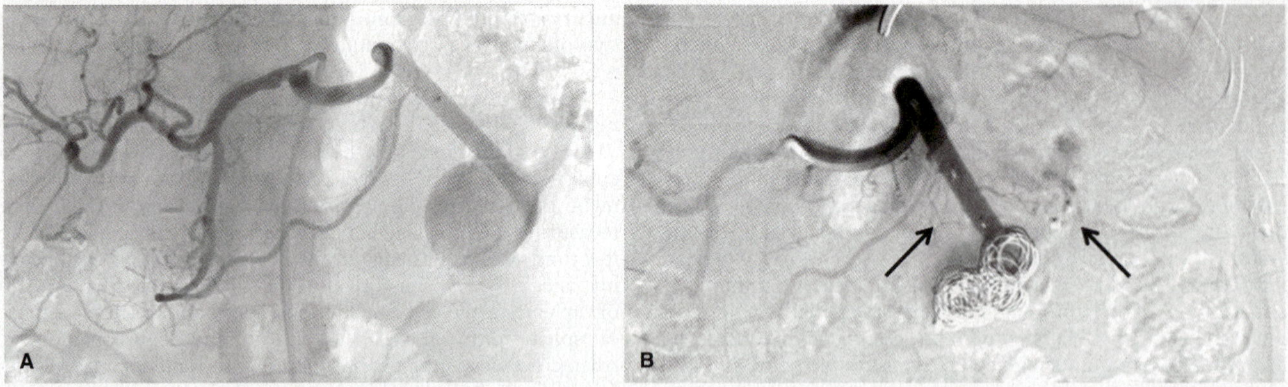

Figure 86.16. (**A**) Celiac arteriogram of a 78-year-old woman with a 4-cm splenic artery aneurysm; (**B**) Splenic arteriogram demonstrating a catheter in the proximal splenic artery. Vascular occlusion devices (*arrows*) have been positioned in the main splenic artery outflow (distal to the aneurysm) and inflow (proximal to the aneurysm) with multiple vascular coils embedded within the aneurysm sac.

splenic infarction.[128] With late follow-up, endovascular repair is associated with an average regression in aneurysm size of 1.5 mm/yr.[109] Late complications may arise at an average rate of 3.7% per year, and there is a 3.2% rate of reintervention per year following endovascular repair.[126]

Patients with splenic aneurysms have long-term survival rates that approach 90% at 10 years following aneurysm-directed treatments; cause of death is typically unrelated to aneurysm.[109] The most recent meta-analysis of splenic aneurysm therapies identifies significantly greater technical success balanced with greater 30-day mortality following open repair in comparison to significantly higher rates of acute minor complications, late complications, and reinterventions following endovascular repair.[126] Moreover, a decision analysis investigating the cost-effectiveness of open repair, conservative management, and endovascular repair for splenic aneurysm identified endovascular therapy as the most cost-effective treatment independent of gender and risk profile of the patient.[131]

Hepatic Artery Aneurysm

Hepatic artery aneurysms (**Fig. 86.17**) account for 20% of all splanchnic artery aneurysms, affecting men twice as often as women.[97,98] These aneurysms are mainly solitary and while small hepatic artery aneurysms (<2 cm) are typically fusiform, larger aneurysms will more often appear saccular. The vast majority of these aneurysms are extrahepatic with the common hepatic artery and right hepatic artery most often affected; 20% to 30% of hepatic aneurysms however, are intrahepatic.[98,111] Hepatic artery pseudoaneurysms are increasingly frequent and account for approximately 50% of hepatic artery aneurysms.[111] Pseudoaneurysms may result from diagnostic and therapeutic interventions that require liver penetration (eg, biliary stents), liver transplantation, and trauma; their incidence appears to be increasing secondary to the more frequent and regular use of CT imaging following blunt liver trauma and hepatobiliary intervention.[101,111] True aneurysms present most often during the sixth decade of life and proposed etiologic mechanisms include mainly atherosclerosis and acquired medial degeneration. Polyarteritis nodosa, cystic medial necrosis, portal HTN, infection, arterial fibrodysplasia, neurofibromatosis, and other arteriopathies are less commonly implicated.

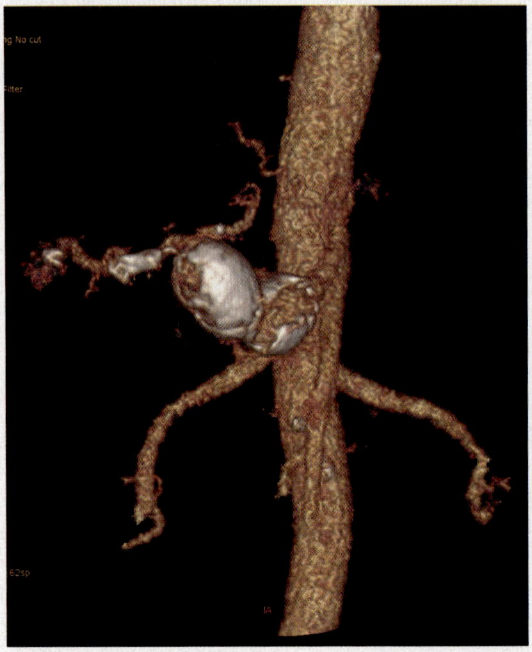

Figure 86.17. Reformatted CT angiogram demonstrating a bilobed and calcified hepatic artery aneurysm.

As with most splanchnic artery aneurysms, hepatic artery aneurysms rarely cause symptoms. Symptomatic patients will most commonly describe right upper quadrant or epigastric abdominal pain that may radiate to the back, while those patients with rapidly expanding aneurysms may describe abdominal complaints that mimic pancreatitis. Large aneurysms may erode into the stomach or duodenum resulting in gastrointestinal hemorrhage or they may obstruct the biliary tract resulting in biliary colic, hemobilia, and obstructive jaundice. Additional physical examination findings like a palpable pulsatile mass and bruit are uncommon. Diagnosis is often made incidentally by cross-sectional CT/MRI, ultrasound or arteriography performed for a nonvascular indication.

Rupture appears to complicate a minority of hepatic artery aneurysms (20% to 30%) and results in an equal distribution of hemorrhage into the peritoneum and the biliary tract.[98] Rupture into the biliary tract results in hematobilia, hematemesis, and cholangitis; rarely is there melena and chronic anemia. Rupture-related mortality approximates 35% to 40%. The relationship of rupture risk to aneurysm size remains unclear and a small series of 22 patients with a mean hepatic artery diameter of 2.3 cm (range 1.5 to 5 cm) were followed for a mean of 68.4 months without complication. The presence of multiple aneurysms and nonatherosclerotic etiology are proposed risk factors for rupture. While historically treatment was recommended for all asymptomatic aneurysms >2 cm in size, some authors have proposed elective intervention for all and any-size nonatherosclerotic aneurysms and for those patients with multiple hepatic artery aneurysms while reserving a more conservative approach for those atherosclerotic hepatic artery aneurysms measuring 2 to 5 cm in size. Contemporary guidelines support elective repair in asymptomatic at a size threshold of >2 cm in patients without significant comorbidity at a size >2 cm (Grade 1A), or if the aneurysm enlarges >0.5 cm/yr (Grade 1C), at a size threshold of >5 cm in patients with significant comorbidity (Grade 1B), and at any size in those patient with vasculopathy or vasculitis (Grade 1C).[102]

Open reconstruction has been favored for aneurysms of the extrahepatic artery by way of aneurysmectomy or exclusion, although current guidelines support an endovascular-first approach to all hepatic artery aneurysms (Grade 1A).[102] Often revascularization is not required in light of extensive foregut collaterals from the GDA and right gastric artery that preserve hepatic perfusion. When necessary, options for reconstruction may include primary or patch angioplastic closure of the common hepatic artery, aortorenal bypass, and splenohepatic bypass. Proper hepatic artery aneurysms may be treated by aneurysmectomy requiring reconstruction using a saphenous vein interposition graft or simple aneurysmorrhaphy. Distal or intraparenchymal lesions may require resection of the involved liver parenchyma, and lobectomy is advised for patients with large intrahepatic aneurysms to avoid significant liver necrosis.[102,103] Elective open surgical repair is associated with approximately 30% morbidity and negligible mortality.[104,106] Additional options include transcatheter embolization, which may be an especially useful adjunct for intrahepatic arterial aneurysms obviating the need for hepatic lobectomy, and stent graft exclusion for high-risk patients.[97,104,106,108,132] Technical and clinical success rates with transcatheter embolization approach 100% and 79%, respectively and offers efficient control of hemorrhage, shorter hospital length of stay, and lower transfusion requirements in cases of rupture specifically.[133] Transient success and recanalization is well described however, mandating thoughtful postembolization surveillance.

Superior Mesenteric Artery Aneurysm

Superior artery aneurysms account for up to 7% to 14% of all splanchnic aneurysms, depending on the series.[98,100,101,104,105] These aneurysms affect men more frequently than women in their sixth decade of life and are mainly solitary.[98,134,135] SMA aneurysms may result from infection (ie, nonhemolytic streptococci in bacterial endocarditis), dissection (**Fig. 86.18**), medial degeneration, atherosclerosis, FMD, vasculitis, connective tissue disorder, and trauma.[98,101] Additionally, false aneurysms may occur in the setting of pancreatitis and complicated peptic ulcer disease.[134] Concomitant HTN is common, affecting >20% of patients with SMA aneurysm, as are associated aortic and peripheral/splanchnic aneurysms.[104,108,135,136]

In contrast to other splanchnic aneurysms up to 70% to 90% of SMA aneurysms may present with symptoms at diagnosis. While most patients with SMA aneurysm are asymptomatic, abdominal pain is the most common symptom followed by nausea, emesis, GI bleeding, and fever in cases of mycotic aneurysm.[134–136] Clinical examination may reveal a pulsatile mass in up to one-third of patients. Diagnosis is most commonly established by CT imaging, although these aneurysms can be appreciated by ultrasound, MRI, and angiography. Complications may include AMI resulting from thromboembolism and rupture. The natural history of SMA aneurysms appears to be that of expansion and rupture with 38% to 50% presenting with rupture.[101,134] Rupture risk has historically been considered rare and while rupture-associated mortality has historically approached 50%, more contemporary series cite 30-day mortality rates as low as 12.5% to 38%.[98,105,135] No comorbidities or aneurysm characteristics have been found to predict rupture risk.[135] Contemporary guidelines support repair of all SMA aneurysms at diagnosis, regardless of size (Grade 1A).[102]

Surgical management of SMA aneurysm most often requires aneurysm excision (or exclusion) with revascularization, most often by way of aortomesenteric bypass.[104] Both autologous and prosthetic conduits have been described. Autologous conduit is favored in cases of mycotic aneurysm and frank contamination complicating intestinal ischemia while reinforced prosthetic conduit resists compression/kinking and future dilation.[108] Aneurysmorrhaphy and simple ligation of inflow and outflow vessels (in those patients with appropriate collateralization) have also been described with success.[98,108,134] Contemporary elective surgical results boast negligible morbidity and mortality.[108] Endovascular SMA aneurysm exclusion with a stent graft and embolization have been described and increasingly employed for patients with severe cardiopulmonary disease; these therapies remain limited by thromboembolic risks to the collateral circulation, endoleak, and limited long-term follow-up.[104,135–139] Aneurysms with a small neck distal to the

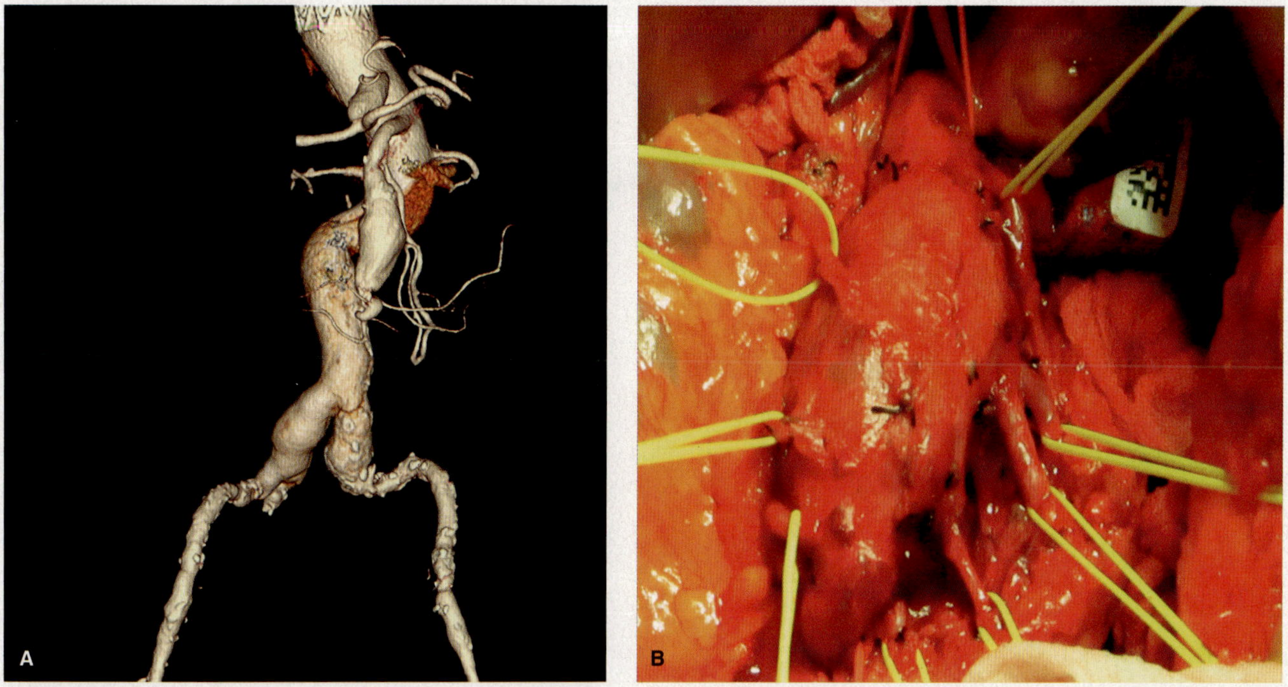

Figure 86.18. (A) CT angiogram and (B) intraoperative photo of a large 3.6-cm asymptomatic SMA aneurysm associated with extensive thoracoabdominal aortic and SMA dissection. The aneurysm was repaired by way of an SMA interposition bypass graft using nonreversed great saphenous vein; additionally the proximal SMA dissection flap was sharply fenestrated.

SMA origin may be conducive to transcatheter embolization provided angiographic determination of collateral flow is determined as adequate.[135]

Celiac Artery Aneurysm

Celiac artery aneurysms account for approximately 4% of all splanchnic aneurysms affecting men more frequently than women in their sixth decade of life.[140,141] The incidence in the general population is unknown. Historically celiac artery aneurysms were primarily associated with infection like syphilis or tuberculosis and primarily diagnosed postmortem.[140] Contemporary etiologic risk factors include primarily atherosclerosis, developmental risk factors such as common celiacomesenteric trunk, arterial dysplasia with medial degeneration, collagen vascular disorder, trauma, and dissection.[140,141] Concomitant HTN (20%), aortic aneurysm (18% to 40%), and alternate splanchnic aneurysms (38%) are common in patients with celiac artery aneurysm.[140,141]

As with most splanchnic artery aneurysms, celiac artery aneurysms rarely cause symptoms.[141] Symptoms may include abdominal pain, primarily epigastric in location with radiation to the back.[140] Less common associated symptoms may include nausea, emesis, dysphagia, anorexia, weight loss, and GI bleeding. Abdominal mass and bruit may be appreciated on physical examination. Diagnosis is most commonly established by CT imaging, although these aneurysms can be appreciated by ultrasound, MRI, and angiography.[141] Historically, rupture complicated approximately 70% of celiac artery aneurysms, resulting in near-certain mortality.[140] More contemporary estimates suggest rupture rates of 13% with associated 50% mortality.[140] HTN, aneurysm calcification, presence of thrombus, gender, and aneurysm etiology do not appear to influence risk of rupture, which has been described in aneurysms ranging in size from 2 to 6 cm.[140,141]

Treatment should be individualized for cases of rupture and elective cases for patient symptoms and aneurysm size >2 cm. Aneurysm ligation and resection, without reconstruction, has previously been endorsed for those patients with adequate foregut collateral circulation. Simple ligation and transcatheter embolization may be considered as lifesaving in cases of rupture, but both offer substantial risk of perioperative hepatic and intestinal ischemia, necrosis, and patient mortality.[140–142] Aneurysmectomy with arterial reconstruction remains the preferred treatment of celiac artery aneurysms. Surgical revascularization may be accomplished by primary arterial–arterial anastomosis following aneurysm resection, direct aortic reimplantation of the celiac artery or its branches, or aortoceliac bypass. Prosthetic conduit may offer superior patency rates in comparison to autogenous reversed saphenous vein, which tends to kink.[141] Elective surgical repair offers patients symptomatic relief with a 0% to 5% risk of perioperative mortality.[141,142] Endovascular options for aneurysm treatment are increasingly described including celiac artery stent grafting.[143]

Gastric and Gastroepiploic Artery Aneurysm

Gastric and gastroepiploic artery aneurysms account for approximately 4% to 5% of all splanchnic aneurysms affecting men three times more frequently than women (**Fig. 86.19**).[98] Etiologic risk factors include primarily arterial dysplasia with segmental arterial mediolysis and periarterial inflammation like pancreatitis and vasculitis; atherosclerosis when present is felt to be a secondary process.[97,98,144] Gastric artery aneurysms are 10 times more common than gastroepiploic artery aneurysms. While patients may present with abdominal pain, up to 90% of patients have historically presented acutely ruptured with evidence of GI bleeding more common than intraperitoneal rupture.[97,98]

Treatment is recommended for all gastric and gastroepiploic arterial aneurysms, regardless the size. Arteriogram is invaluable for aneurysm identification preoperatively and operative planning. Surgical management has historically relied on simple arterial ligation or excision without reconstruction while intramural aneurysms required a wedge excision of involved gastric wall.[98,103] Contemporary literature would suggest that catheter-based embolization of these arteries is the new standard for care with multiple case reports and small series documenting successful aneurysm occlusion with coils and thrombin injection.[100,145,146]

Jejunal, Ileal, and Colic Artery Aneurysm

Aneurysms of the jejunal, ileal, and colic arteries account for <3% of all splanchnic aneurysms, affecting men and women equally beyond the sixth decade of life.[98] These aneurysms are associated with medial degeneration, infection, connective tissue disorder, and polyarteritis nodosa with multiple aneurysms identified in approximately 10% of cases.[98,144,147] Atherosclerosis, when present, is felt to be a secondary process. While patients may present with abdominal pain, most have no symptoms. Rupture may complicate up to 30% of cases resulting in gastrointestinal bleeding and mortality rates that approach 20%.

Treatment is recommended for all mesenteric branch aneurysms, regardless of the size. Arteriogram is invaluable for

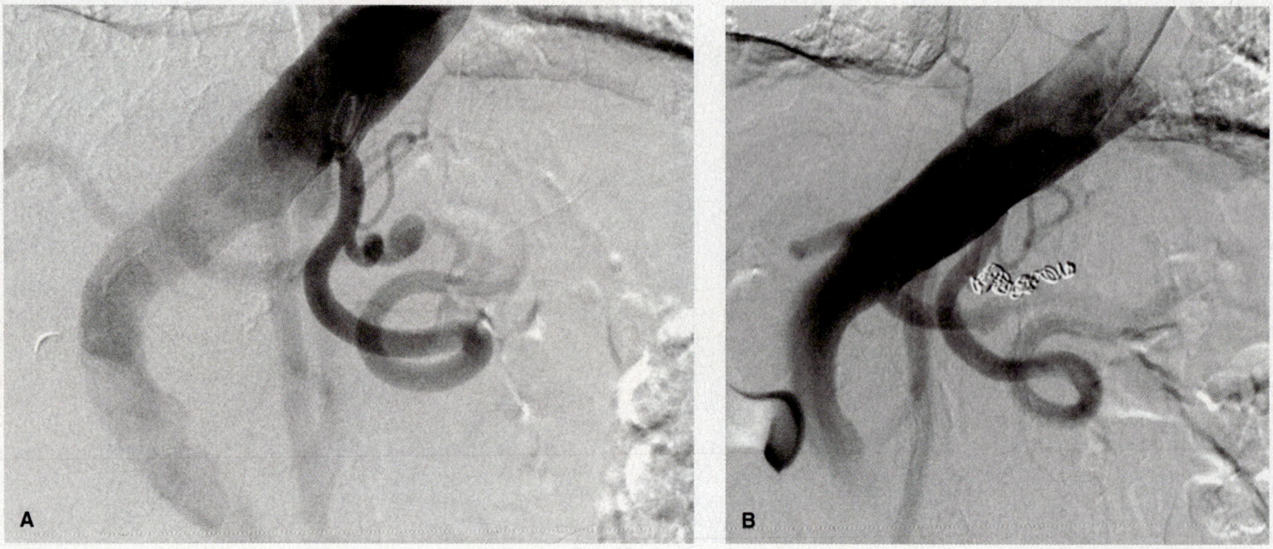

Figure 86.19. **A:** Diagnostic aortogram of an 82-year-old woman with a highly tortuous abdominal aorta, aberrant hepatic arterial anatomy, and two sequential gastric artery aneurysms measuring 10 mm in maximum diameter. **B:** Completion arteriogram following endovascular embolization.

aneurysm identification preoperatively and operative planning. Surgical management has historically relied on simple arterial ligation or excision without reconstruction.[98] Intramural aneurysms and those associated with bowel necrosis required resection of the involved intestine at the time of aneurysm exclusion. Transcatheter embolization has been increasingly utilized, and supported by contemporary guidelines, especially for cases of acute rupture and GI bleeding with intestinal necrosis, perforation, and late stricture potential complications.[148–150] Medical management is recommended for nonruptured asymptomatic ileal, jejunal, and colic artery aneurysms associated with polyarteritis nodosa.[102]

Gastroduodenal and Pancreaticoduodenal Artery Aneurysm

Gastroduodenal and pancreaticoduodenal artery aneurysms account for <2% of all splanchnic aneurysm.[98] Men are affected four times more often than women during the sixth decade of life.[111] Periarterial inflammation resulting from pancreatitis with vascular necrosis or vessel erosion by pseudocyst reflects the most common etiology, while additional causes include arteriosclerosis, congenital medial degeneration, and trauma.[98] Concomitant celiac artery stenosis and occlusion are common in noninflammatory aneurysms and GDA and pancreaticoduodenal aneurysms are suggested to represent the effect of inordinately high-volume blood flow on branchings of the collateral circulation (**Fig. 86.20**).[151–153] A recent review suggests visceral artery aneurysms associated with MAL may rupture at variable size, supporting intervention irrespective of size.[154] Symptoms of abdominal pain are common; additional symptoms may include gastric outlet obstruction and compressive symptoms like nausea and emesis.[133,155] Rupture is also common, complicating up to 75% of inflammatory and 50% of noninflammatory aneurysms resulting most often in gastrointestinal bleeding and less commonly bleeding into the biliary or pancreatic ductal systems, peritoneum or retroperitoneum.[153] Rupture-associated mortality approximates 20% to 50%.[153,156] While it remains unclear if aneurysm size is a risk factor for rupture, rupture has been described at a small median size of 12 mm.[105,152,157]

Open surgical repair remains appropriate for most patients. These aneurysms are most often amenable to simple ligation, aneurysm resection, or aneurysmorrhaphy without revascularization.[100,104,108,134,153,158,159] Celiac artery revascularization should be considered in select noninflammatory cases. Pancreatitis-associated inflammatory aneurysms may require arterial branch ligation from within the aneurysm sac or pancreatic resection in severe cases. Transcatheter embolization with coils, glue, thrombin, and electrocoagulation has been successfully reported, especially for high-risk patients and those presenting with rupture.[104,132,153,156,160,161]

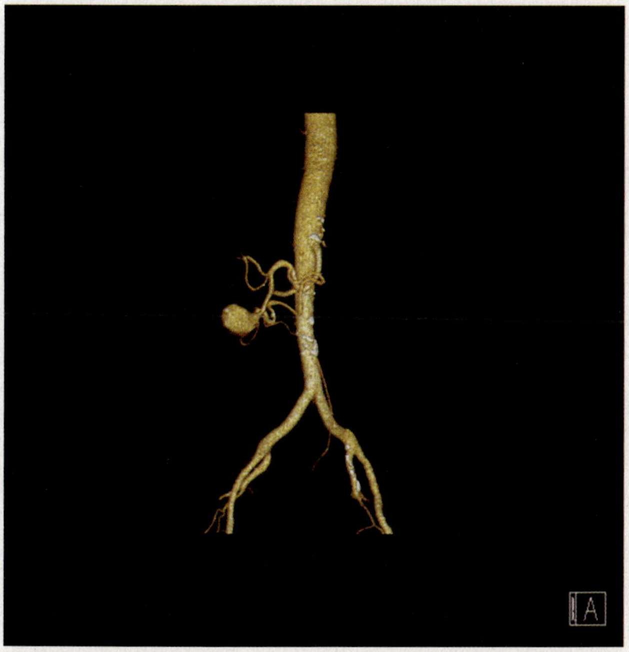

Figure 86.20. CT angiogram of an 87-year-old woman with a large 3.4-cm gastroduodenal artery aneurysm associated with celiac artery occlusion.

Inferior Mesenteric Artery Aneurysm

IMA aneurysms account for <1% of all splanchnic aneurysms. Our understanding of these aneurysms is limited to case reports. Men appear to be most commonly affected.[134] Atherosclerosis is the most common etiologic factor with additional risk factors including infection, polyarteritis nodosa, inflammatory arteritides, segmental arterial mediolysis, Behçet disease, and neurofibromatosis.[162] Concomitant celiac and SMA occlusion is common; it has been hypothesized that turbulent blood flow through tortuous marginal arteries originating from the IMA results in a high-flow state, or "jet disorder phenomenon," and subsequent dilation of the IMA and small collaterals which can lead to weakness of the arterial wall and aneurysmal disease.[162–165] Patients rarely have symptoms. Incidence of rupture approximates 20% with rupture-related mortality approaching 40%.[162]

Surgical management in cases of chronic celiac and SMA occlusion requires revascularization of at least one vessel (most commonly the SMA) to minimize intestinal ischemia during IMA aneurysm exclusion and theoretically decrease the risk of recurrent IMA aneurysm postoperatively. IMA aneurysm ligation and/or excision may be sufficient for treatment in certain cases of robust collateral intestinal circulation; in contrast certain cases will dictate IMA revascularization.[165] The role for endovascular therapy remains poorly defined.

RENAL ARTERY OCCLUSIVE AND ANEURYSMAL DISEASE

Renovascular hypertension (RVH) is a well-defined form of secondary HTN that results from renal arterial insufficiency at some level. The pathophysiology of such ischemia is broad, and with both an increasing prevalence of atherosclerotic renal artery occlusive disease and ongoing clinical trials, treatment standards remain in flux.

Pathophysiology of Renovascular Hypertension

Renal artery stenosis resulting in a decrease in mean renal artery perfusion pressure by 10% to 15% stimulates renin release from the kidney. Renin is a proteolytic enzyme produced by the juxtaglomerular apparatus of the kidney that cleaves angiotensinogen to form angiotensin I. Angiotensin I is further processed to angiotensin II by angiotensin-converting enzyme (ACE), which is produced in the lung endothelium and vasculature (**Fig. 86.21**). Angiotensin II stimulates hepatic production of renin, while providing a continuous negative feedback on the renal release of renin.[166] Angiotensin II is a potent vasopressor that increases arterial blood pressure by a variety of mechanisms (**Fig. 86.22**). Glomerular filtration rate (GFR) is increased via vasoconstriction of the efferent arteriole. Additionally, antidiuretic hormone (ADH) is released from the posterior pituitary gland, causing water conservation. Release of aldosterone from the adrenal glands enhances exchange of sodium in the nephron-promoting volume retention. Finally, angiotensin increases sympathetic tone. All of these mechanisms coalesce to increase arterial pressure by way of arteriolar constriction, enhanced cardiac output, and the retention of sodium and water. Renin has a half-life of 20 to 30 minutes and is primarily cleared by the liver.[167] Normal physiology and sodium balance support a "steady state" of renin activity that is approximately 50% greater in the bilateral renal veins than that in the infrarenal inferior vena cava

VASCULAR DISEASE

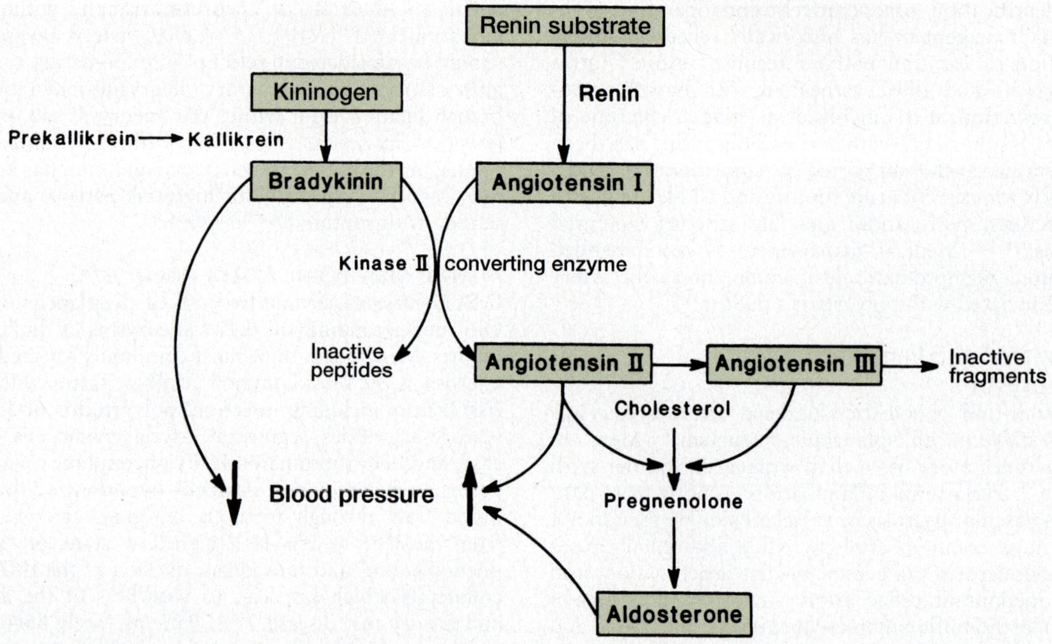

Figure 86.21. Renin–angiotensin system interrelation with aldosterone and bradykinin in blood pressure regulation. (Adapted from Stanley JC, Graham LM, Whitehouse WM Jr. Renovascular hypertension. In: Miller TA, Rowland BJ, eds. *Physiologic Basis of Modern Surgical Care.* CV Mosby; 1988:734.)

or peripheral circulation. In cases of unilateral renal artery stenosis, HTN is characterized by renin hypersecretion from the affected kidney and suppression of renin production in the contralateral kidney.[168,169] Additionally, angiotensin-mediated vasoconstriction causes pressure diuresis of the unaffected kidney. In cases of chronic bilateral or unilateral RVH in those patients with solitary kidney, sodium retention accounts for late reductions in renin secretion.

Renal Artery Occlusive Disease

7 Renal artery occlusive disease is the most common cause of correctable HTN in adults and the third most common cause of HTN in children and should be considered in the clinical context of: (1) childhood HTN, (2) severe HTN in women <45 years of age, (3) acute and rapid escalation of mild HTN in older patients (>50 years), (4) initial diastolic BP >115 mm Hg, and (5) rapid deterioration in renal function following the administration of antihypertensive therapy (especially with ACE inhibition). Renovascular HTN can be notoriously resistant to traditional medical management. Clinical examination may reveal an upper abdominal bruit during systole and diastole.

Diagnostic work-up should begin with serologies to assess renal function (BUN, creatinine) and electrolyte levels. Additional blood hormone levels may help differentiate the diagnosis as high plasma renin activity supports RVH while altered aldosterone, thyroid, and catecholamine levels may indicate endocrine dysfunction. Urinalysis may reveal hematuria or

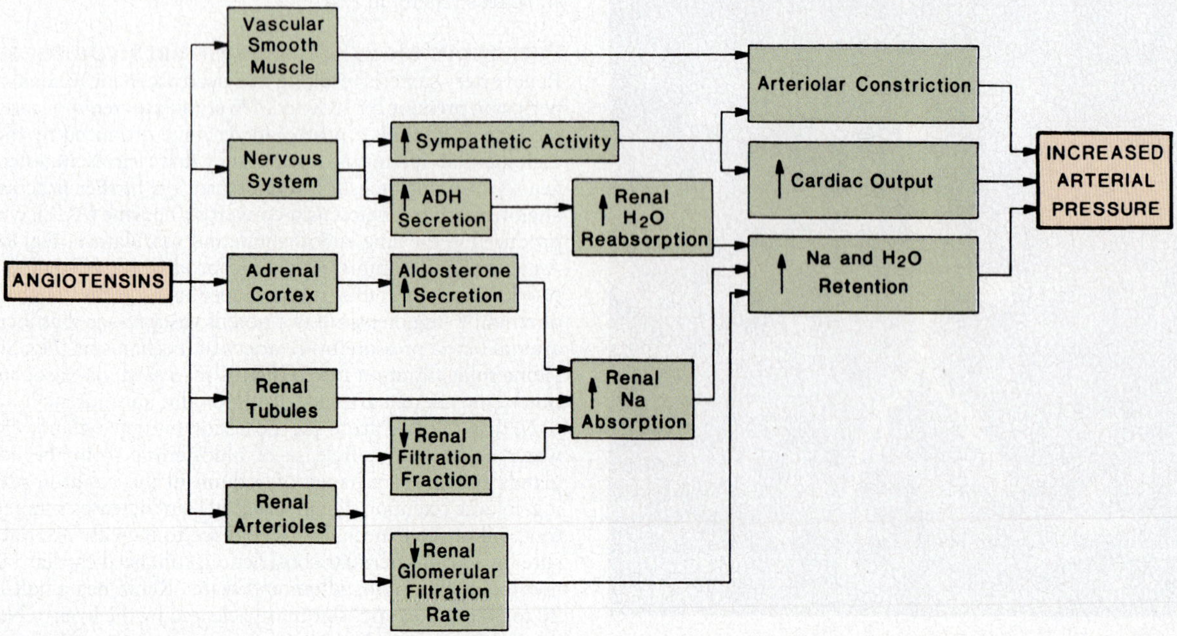

Figure 86.22. Effects of angiotensins contributing to increased arterial pressure. (Derived from Stanley JC, Graham LM. Renovascular hypertension. In: Miller TA, ed. *Physiologic Basis of Modern Surgical Care*. 2nd ed. Quality Medical Publishing; 1998:918.)

azotemia concerning for intrinsic renal disease. Ultrasonography is the first-line imaging modality for screening patients with RVH. While a high-quality duplex ultrasound examination in an experienced center is extremely accurate for the diagnosis of main renal artery and ostial stenosis or occlusion, sensitivity is compromised when surveying branch or parenchymal renal arteries and technically challenging in obese patients or in the presence of abdominal gas.[170] An elevated peak systolic velocity (>180 or >200 cm/s) or elevated renal aortic ratio >3.5 (calculated by dividing the peak systolic velocity of the renal artery by the peak systolic velocity of the adjacent aorta) detects renal artery stenosis with sensitivity and specificity of 84% and 97%, respectively.[171] Ultrasonography additionally facilitates a determination of renal length and symmetry, the presence of main renal artery aneurysm (RAA), visualization of adjacent structures (ie, obstruction, masses, aortic aneurysm), and the assessment of intrinsic vessel renovascular disease by way of the resistive index.

Axial imaging with CTA and MRA are both useful adjunctive imaging modalities that better evaluate stenosis, aneurysms, renal infarcts, dissections, and adjacent structures. These imaging modalities have collectively received a class I indication (level B evidence) as screening tests to establish the diagnosis of renal artery stenosis from the American College of Cardiology (ACC) and American Heart Association (AHA).[172] CTA offers excellent spatial resolution and generated three-dimensional multiplanar images which can be very helpful in treatment planning. CTA, however, is limited by the risk of contrast-induced nephropathy and in detecting subtle FMD lesions and branch vessel involvement. Multidetector CTA offers sensitivity and specificity ranging from 86% to 93% and 90% to 100%, respectively.[173] MRA is often favored in younger patients as it offers diagnostic sensitivity and specificity of 97% and 93% without the associated risks of irradiation.[174] Gadolinium is less nephrotoxic than iodinated contrast and while it may be advantageous for those patients with mild renal insufficiency, the risk of nephrogenic systemic fibrosis prohibits the use of gadolinium contrast in those patients with a GFR ≤30 mL/min/1.73 m^2. MRA offers the additional benefit of estimating renal perfusion and GFR via calculations of gadolinium clearance.

Catheter-based arteriography remains the gold standard imaging modality for the diagnosis of renal artery stenosis given its unmatched spatial resolution and capacity to detect reliably branch vessel and parenchymal involvement. Additionally, pressure gradients can be measured across a stenosis (a systolic pressure gradient <10 mm Hg is considered normal); intravascular ultrasound may be used to further characterize the renal artery; and any clinically indicated therapeutic interventions can be performed in the same clinical setting.

In cases of complex and equivocal disease, renal vein renin assessments may be used to calculate the renal vein ratio. This ratio reflects a renin comparison between peripheral and renal venous blood. With unilateral renal artery stenosis, the renal vein renin ratio (RVRR) is calculated by dividing the renin activity in venous blood from the affected kidney by that from the (normal) contralateral kidney. A ratio >1.48 supports a functionally relevant renal artery stenosis.[168,169] In patients with bilateral renal artery stenosis, a renal:systemic renin index (RSRI) is calculated by subtracting systemic renin activity from individual renal vein renin activity and dividing the remainder by systemic renin activity; this index reflects individual kidney renin release.[168] As aforementioned, there is a steady state of normal renal renin release; normal renal vein renin activity from each kidney is approximately 24% higher than systemic activity (with the total of both kidneys being then 48% higher than systemic activity). Documentation of renin hypersecretion (RSRI >0.48) associated with contralateral kidney renin suppression (RSRI 0 to 0.24) provides a method to differentiate those patients that will be cured or improved of RVH following renal revascularization or nephrectomy.[168,175]

Captopril scintigraphy (also known as isotopic or captopril renography) and hypertensive urography have fallen out of favor and are no longer recommended as diagnostic studies for the diagnosis of renal artery stenosis.

Arteriosclerosis

Arteriosclerosis is the most frequent cause of RVH affecting men twice as often as women, most commonly in the sixth decade of life.[176] Ostial stenosis is most common representing "spillover" of diffuse aortic atherosclerosis, which is present in approximately 80% of patients. Arteriosclerotic renal artery stenosis affects primarily the proximal third of the vessel, with more severe distal extrarenal disease limited mainly to black patients.[177] A contemporary prospective, multicenter, population-based study of cardiovascular health has estimated the incidence of renovascular disease in men and women aged >65 years as 6% to 7%.[176,178] Although early angiographic- and image-based studies in selected patients with arteriosclerotic RVH have suggested radiographic progression in approximately a third of renal artery lesions with 10% progressing to occlusion, this longitudinal cohort study reported anatomic progression to hemodynamically significant disease in only 4% of participants with an annualized progression rate of 0.5% per year and no disease progression to arterial occlusion. Importantly, renovascular disease has consistently been associated with cardiovascular disease across coronary, cerebrovascular, mesenteric, and peripheral vascular beds with a significant and independent relationship noted with prevalent coronary manifestations.[179–183]

Fibromuscular Dysplasia

FMD is thought to account for approximately 5% to 10% of RVH.[184,185] FMD is a nonatherosclerotic, noninflammatory vascular disease that may result in arterial stenosis, occlusion, aneurysm, or dissection that affects primarily younger women.[186] The prevalence of FMD in the general population is unknown, although renal involvement is the most common phenotype comprising 58% to 75% of all FMD cases.[187,188] FMD until recently has been described by histopathologic classification.[189,190] By this classification *medial fibroplasia* is the most common variant accounting for 60% to 90% of FMD cases. Deposition in the media of loose collagen in zones of degenerating elastic fibrils results in the generation of fibromuscular ridges with resultant arterial stenoses alternating with areas of smooth muscle loss with consequent arterial dilation producing a classic "string of beads" appearance angiographically (**Fig. 86.23**).[187] The distal two-thirds of the main renal artery and its branches are most commonly affected and bilateral disease is common. *Intimal fibroplasia* accounts for approximately 2% to 5% of all dysplastic renal artery stenoses and presents as a smooth, focal stenosis of the distal main renal artery. This histologic variant is notable for the accumulation of fibrous tissue within the intima with a moderately cellular component with mainly intact or partially fragmented elastic lamina (**Fig. 86.24**). *Perimedial fibroplasia* and *medial hyperplasia* are uncommon variants.

Medical Management of Renovascular Hypertension

8 Medical therapy remains the mainstay of treatment for RVH with comprehensive goals of care that should encompass glycemic control, cholesterol reduction, smoking cessation, blood pressure reduction, and antiplatelet therapy with aspirin for primary prevention. ACC/AHA guidelines support the use of ACE inhibitors (ACE-I), angiotensin receptor blockers (ARBs), calcium channel blockers, and beta blockers with a class I indication.[172] While beta blockers are often utilized first line, ACE-I and ARBs are a mainstay of treatment for most

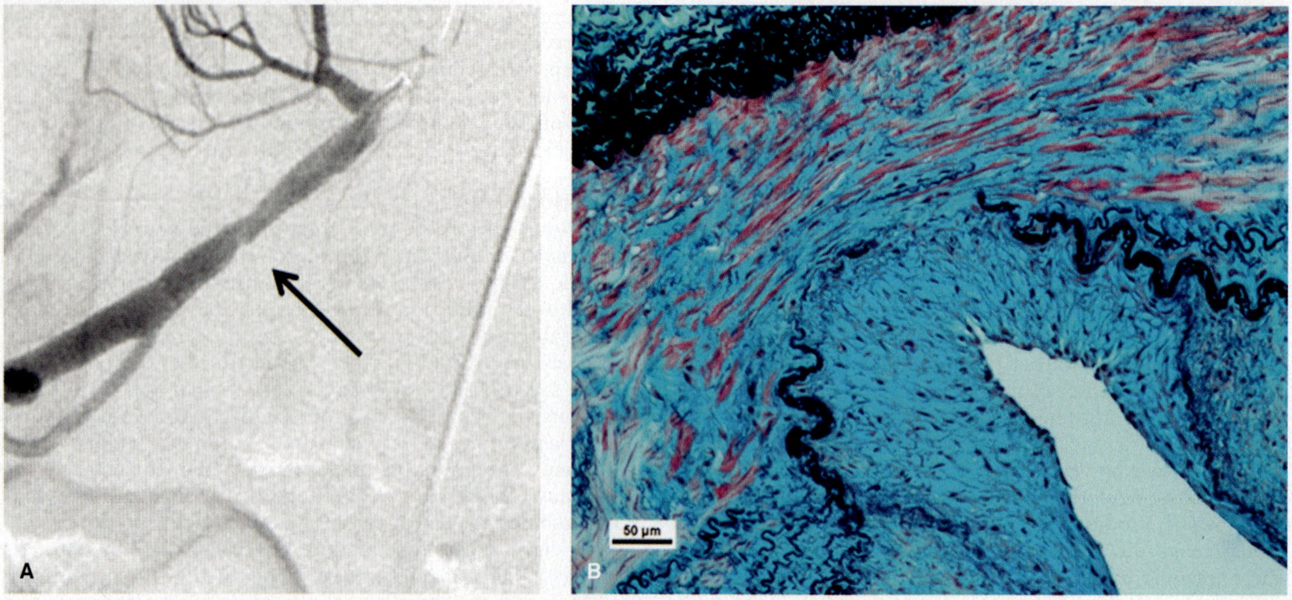

Figure 86.23. **A:** Right renal arteriogram demonstrating a radiographically subtle focal midartery stenosis (*arrow*); manometry across this lesion revealed a significant pressure gradient. **B:** Intimal fibroplasia as represented by pronounced intimal proliferation and partial fragmentation of the elastic lamina (*Movat stain*, 20×).

antihypertensive regimens offering 86% to 92% efficacy.[185] Renal function monitoring is essential with the initiation of these agents as the resulting modulation of the renin–angiotensin system with renal artery stenosis affecting a solitary functioning kidney, severe bilateral RAS or advanced chronic kidney disease may result in acute renal failure.

Surgical and Endovascular Management of Renal Artery Occlusive Disease

As RAS may progress with concomitant renal atrophy, renal revascularization should be considered in select cases. The AHA supports the consideration of renal revascularization in specific clinical populations (**Table 86.2**).[191]

Arterial Reconstructive Surgery for Renal Artery Occlusive Disease

Historically open revascularization procedures represented the standard of care in the treatment of RVH. The most common option for open renal revascularization remains aortorenal bypass with either autogenous reversed saphenous vein or prosthetic conduit. Alternatives may include (1) nonanatomic renal bypass based off the hepatic, splenic, or iliac arteries, (2) ex vivo renal artery reconstruction, and (3) aortorenal endarterectomy. Nonanatomic (or extra-anatomic) renal artery bypass may benefit those patients with medical comorbidities or aortic anatomy that prohibit aortic cross-clamping and aortorenal bypass.[192–197] The hepatic artery is used for a right-sided renal reconstruction, the splenic artery for a left-sided reconstruction. Ex vivo renal artery reconstruction may be considered selectively for those patients with complex, distal segmental arterial occlusive disease when balanced with the risk of prolonged operative time, disruption of preexisting collaterals, and the need for renal cooling.[198,199] Transaortic and direct renal artery endarterectomy is particularly useful for those patients with bilateral disease, or when arteriosclerotic renal artery occlusive disease affects multiple (ie, accessory) renal arteries.[200–202]

Open surgical revascularization offers significant blood pressure and renal function improvement in 85% and 50% of patients, respectively across high-volume centers with

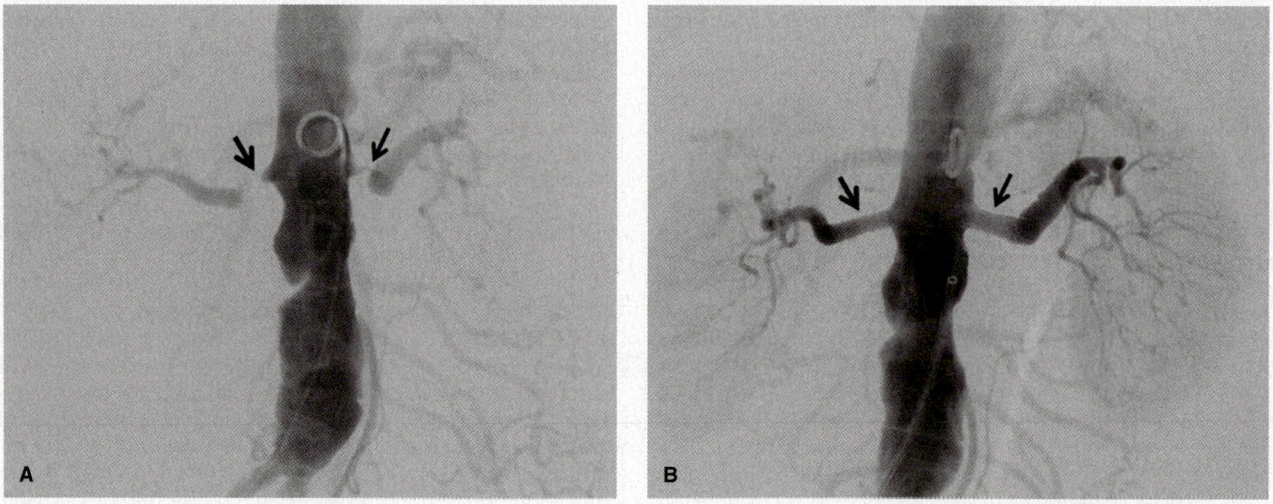

Figure 86.24. Aortogram demonstrating a highly irregular perirenal aorta with (**A**) high-grade bilateral renal artery stenosis (*arrows*) successfully treated with (**B**) bilateral renal artery stents (*arrows*). The stents are positioned with appropriate overlap into the aorta and are ballooned proximally such that they "flower" into the aorta.

Table 86.2. Populations and Characteristics Considered for Renal Revascularization

Clinical Populations
Unilateral renal artery stenosis with characteristic syndromes
Fibromuscular dysplasia with HTN
High-risk clinical syndromes Rapidly progressive HTN Rapidly declining estimated glomerular filtration rate Flash pulmonary edema
Bilateral renal artery stenosis with progressive loss of renal functional mass
Single native kidney renal artery stenosis
Special Populations: Renal allograft: transplant renal artery stenosis with or without calcineurin inhibitors Episodic, circulatory congestion with bilateral atherosclerotic renovascular disease Progressive loss of glomerular filtration rate with occlusive atherosclerotic renovascular disease and no other kidney disease (ischemic nephropathy) Aortic disease with renovascular protection as part of endovascular repair Left-ventricular assist device Radiation-induced renovascular disease with clinical syndromes Other diseases: eg, Takayasu arteritis, extrinsic vascular compression Pediatric patients with mid aortic syndrome or fibromuscular variants
Characteristics suggestive of clinical benefit from revascularization
Recent onset or exacerbation (<1 yr) of HTN
Absence of proteinuria
Identifiable activation of renin–angiotensin system Hyperreninemia With unilateral renal artery stenosis, lateralization of renal vein renin
Younger age
Radiographic evidence of progressive renal artery occlusion
Treatment-resistant HTN (documentation of HTN by ambulatory blood pressure and medication adherence)
Angiotensin-dependent glomerular filtration rate

HTN, hypertension.

mortality rates of 2% to 5%.[184,203–206] While to date there has been no definitive trial comparing open surgical revascularization directly to endovascular therapy, angioplasty, and stenting appears to offer similar effectiveness with lower morbidity and mortality. As such, endovascular measures have replaced surgery as first-line therapy for RVH.[206,207] Contemporary open surgical renal reconstructions most commonly accompany hybrid endovascular interventions for aortic aneurysmal disease and may be considered for failed endovascular renal revascularization.

Endovascular Renal Revascularization

Since its introduction in 1978, percutaneous renal artery angioplasty (PTA), with or without stent placement, has virtually replaced open surgical reconstruction of arteriosclerotic renal artery stenosis. This technique has exploded in use and for over a decade has been utilized at times perhaps inappropriately as "prophylactic" therapy to treat clinically irrelevant renal artery stenoses.[208,209] Renal artery angioplasty alone risks arterial dissection from lesion/vessel recoil and early restenosis. Technical success rates of PTA may be as low as 30% to 50% in patients with significant aortic "spill over" lesions. PTA with stenting offers improved success and very reasonable long-term patency with 5-year secondary patency rates >90%.[210,211]

9 Several recent clinical trials comparing renal artery stenting (RAS) to best medical management for renal artery stenosis have failed to demonstrate a conclusive clinical benefit to the endovascular treatment of renal artery stenosis (**Table 86.3**).[212–216] Moreover, RAS is associated with a 1.5% to 8% risk of major morbidity that can include infected hematoma, atheroemboli, renal failure requiring dialysis, and lower extremity limb loss. Significant limitations apply to all of these studies, including design flaws and selection bias. A contemporary systematic review and meta-analysis of 9 relevant randomized controlled trials (N = 2,275 patients) found that compared to medical therapy alone, the combination of medical therapy + percutaneous transluminal renal artery angioplasty reduced the number of antihypertensive drugs used but did not improve adverse cardiovascular or renal outcomes.[217]

The appropriate patient for revascularization remains elusive, resulting from significant design flaws in existing trials. Most would suggest that those patients with refractory HTN despite an appropriate medical regimen that includes a combination of ACE inhibition or angiotensin receptor blockade + diuretic + amlodipine with both a hemodynamically significant stenosis by manometric pressure gradient and overall preserved renal mass should still be considered for therapy.[218] Notably, evolving data have identified several promising predictors for clinical improvement following renal revascularization including bilateral RAS, mean arterial pressure >110 mm Hg, elevated baseline brain natriuretic peptide, elevated pulse pressure, and renal perfusion as measured by "renal frame count" during angiography (defined as the number of frames required for dye to pass through the renal parenchyma).[218–222] A contemporary study recently validated three preoperative markers of blood response to RAS from a single institution series with data from the CORAL trial.[223,224] These data supported (1) the requirement for ≥4 medications, (2) preoperative diastolic blood pressure >90 mm Hg, and (3) preoperative clonidine use as predictors of HTN improvement. Most recently, serum creatinine level, peak systolic velocity of the renal artery before revascularization, and acute kidney injury after angiographic intervention have been shown to be independent predictors of the progression of chronic kidney disease in patients who underwent RAS.[225]

Although randomized, controlled trials assessing renal revascularization for renal artery FMD are lacking, current guidelines support the following indications for renal revascularization in this patient cohort: (1) resistant HTN despite an appropriate three-drug regimen, (2) HTN of short duration with the goal being a cure of HTN, (3) renal artery dissection, (4) RAA, and (5) preservation of renal function in patients with severe stenosis.[187,226] PTA of the renal artery is the procedure of choice for patients with renal artery stenosis secondary to FMD offering cure rates that approach 50%, with up to 86% of patients improved following PTA, a 20% risk of reintervention, and low risk of minor complications.[187] Hemodynamic significance must be documented by manometry prior to any intervention in these patients and success should be defined by resolution of this gradient postangioplasty. Stenting should be utilized selectively. Populations and characteristics for which renal revascularization should be considered, as supported by the American Heart Association, are summarized in **Table 86.2**.

Table 86.3. Contemporary Clinical Trials Comparing the Effectiveness of Endovascular Renal Artery Revascularization to Medical Therapy

Trial	Number of Patients	Degree Stenosis	Indications for Renal Artery Revascularization	F/U (yrs)	BP Response	Renal Function Improvement or Stabilization
DRASTIC Trial[213] (PTA)	106	≥50%	Resistant HTN	1	No difference	N/A
STAR Trial[212] (RAS)	140	>50%	Renal impairment (GFR <80 mL/min)	2	No difference	No difference
ASTRAL[214] (RAS)	806	Variable	Refractory HTN or unexplained renal dysfunction with RAS suggested by imaging	5	No difference (systolic)[a]	Decreased progression of renal impairment and lower mean Cr level following revascularization
CORAL[215] (RAS)	931	≥60% + 20 mm Hg systolic pressure gradient -or- ≥80%	Systolic HTN ≥155 mm Hg despite at least two antihypertensives	43 mo	2.3 mm Hg reduction following RAS (vs medical therapy) (P = .03)	No difference[b]

[a]The decrease in diastolic BP was smaller in the revascularization group.
[b]Composite end point included death from cardiovascular or renal causes, myocardial infarction, stroke, hospitalization for congestive heart failure, progressive renal insufficiency, or the need for renal-replacement therapy.
BP, blood pressure; Cr, creatinine; GFR, glomerular filtration rate; HTN, hypertension; PTA, angioplasty alone; RAS, renal artery stent.

Renal denervation (RDN) is a recent advancement in the treatment of RVH, with two RDN systems now FDA approved.[227] This minimally invasive endovascular procedure targets sympathetic nerves adjacent to the renal arteries; disruption of these nerves has been shown in sham-controlled, randomized trials to produce clinically meaningful and safe short-term reductions in blood pressure. A recent comprehensive meta-analysis comparing 2478 patients shows that irrespective of the method used, RDN effectively reduced ambulatory and office systolic blood pressure without additional risk of vascular injury or renal function impairment.[227]

Developmental Dysplasia

Renovascular HTN secondary to renal artery stenosis and abdominal aortic coarctation remain an important cause of pediatric HTN, the natural history of which risks failure to thrive, heart failure, hypertensive encephalopathy, impaired mental development, hemorrhagic stroke, and early mortality.[227] It is estimated that 5% to 10% of pediatric HTN may be explained by renovascular disease, following thoracic aortic coarctation and parenchymal renal disease in incidence.[228,229] The pathophysiology of pediatric renovascular disease remains ill defined, as are the mechanisms by which pediatric renovascular disease occur. FMD and neurofibromatosis type 1 (NF1) are reported as the most common causes of pediatric renal artery stenosis in the western world.[230] While the intimal FMD variant described above is uncommon in adults, it is the most common form identified in children with renal artery stenosis. Furthermore, histopathologic review of operative renal artery samples excised from patient with developmental arterial stenosis reveal mainly consistent findings of intimal hyperplasia, medial thinning, and disruption of the elastic lamina (**Fig. 86.21**).

Open surgical revascularization of renal artery stenosis remains the gold standard for children with developmental lesions.[228] Aortorenal reimplantation with spatulation of the renal artery and interrupted suture lines is favored. Alternatively, aortorenal bypass using hypogastric artery as conduit is favored over autogenous venous conduit, which can dilate over time to become aneurysmal. Approximately one-third of children will demonstrate associated aortic coarctation and require concomitant patch aortoplasty or aortoaortic bypass. The University of Michigan experience recently reported the largest single-center experience with surgical revascularization of 169 children with RVH supporting a sustainable HTN benefit in 90% of children, including those with abdominal aortic coarctation, with no mortality or renal insufficiency requiring dialysis.[231] The authors noted that interventions in the very young and in those with concurrent abdominal aortic coarctation significantly increased the likelihood of reoperation, and those children undergoing remedial surgery after prior revascularization failures were less likely to be cured of HTN.

There may be a role for angioplasty for selected cases of pediatric renal artery stenosis. Certainly this procedure has gained substantial momentum in the past decade. The most robust US experience includes the treatment of 19 hypertensive children aged 2 to 18 years that underwent PTA for renal artery stenosis, of which 7 patients carried the diagnosis of NF.[232] While immediate technical success was reported as 91%, only 39% of patients achieved a cure in HTN and an additional 17% of children demonstrated improvement. In total there was a 44% rate of clinical failure and these authors conclude that despite a high rate of technical success, PTA provides a clinical benefit in a smaller majority of children. This is consistent with improvement or cure rates that mainly average 50% to 60% across larger series of pediatric renal artery stenosis treated with PTA.[233–235] Notably, renal PTA for the treatment of pediatric RVH due to ostial disease may be complicated by failures requiring remedial operations that are made more complicated by such or nephrectomy.[236] Moreover, HTN cure is less likely following remedial operation (24% in comparison to 70% as referenced above).

RENAL ARTERY ANEURYSM

RAAs are rare with an incidence of 0.1% in the general population.[237–240] The natural history of RAAs appears to be that of slow to null growth with contemporary series estimating a median annualized growth rate of 0.06 to 0.6 mm.[241–243] Aneurysm growth rate does not seem to be affected by aneurysm morphology or calcification.[242] While historic series describe rupture rates as high as 14% to 30% with associated mortality of 80%, contemporary rupture rates are estimated at 3% to 5% with nongestational mortality <10%.[237,240,244–247] Most ruptures are diagnosed at the time of presentation and several authors have supported no rupture during the surveillance of nonoperative RAAs.[248]

Similar to other splanchnic artery aneurysms, RAAs typically present in the sixth decade with women more commonly affected than men.[237,244] Most patients will describe no symptoms, although flank pain and hematuria are most common when symptoms do arise. Clinical examination may reveal HTN, renal bruit, or a palpable abdominal mass. Aneurysms are typically solitary, saccular, located at arterial bifurcations, and affect the right renal artery more often than the left.[248] Almost 70% of RAA may be associated with FMD and up to 30% of patients will have an alternate arterial aneurysm.[237,248,249] These aneurysms are commonly identified as an incidental finding by axial imaging; CT is the most common contemporary diagnostic modality, followed by magnetic resonance imaging, ultrasonography, and catheter-based arteriography.[242] Conventional preoperative arteriography is warranted given the frequency of multiple aneurysms and arterial dysplasia affecting distal branches that may be missed on conventional cross-sectional imaging.

Historically accepted indications for RAA intervention included size >2 cm, female gender within childbearing age, symptoms like pain and hematuria, medically refractory HTN including that associated with functionally important renal artery stenosis, thromboembolism, dissection and rupture. Given the low risk of rupture, slow to null rate of growth, and improved survival following rupture some authors have suggested that a size threshold alone of 2 cm may be antiquated and too aggressive for surgical indication.[241,242] In fact, recently published contemporary guidelines support elective repair in patients with noncomplicated RAA of acceptable operative risk at a size >3 cm (Grade 2C), and at any size in those patient of childbearing potential (2B) or medically refractory HTN and functionally important RAS (2C).[102] The potential for gestational rupture remains a valid indication for repair in women of childbearing age as rupture during pregnancy has been described in aneurysms as small as 1 cm and historic reports suggest maternal and fetal mortality rates that approach 92% and 100%, respectively.[250,251] Pregnancy has previously been associated with a higher rate of RAA rupture, thought to result from increased vascular flow and hormonal changes resulting in weakening of the vessel wall elastic tissue, no large-scale studies report the true incidence.[238,248] Gestational RAA ruptures occur mainly in the third trimester with only a few case reports of rupture postdelivery.[252] Notably, contemporary outcomes for both mother and fetus may be improving, as there are recent case reports of gestational rupture resulting in both maternal and fetal survival.

Approximately 70% of patients with RAA have HTN, with up to 100% affected in some series.[237,241,243,247,249,251] Hypotheses for the mechanism of HTN include (1) coexistent renal artery occlusive disease, (2) distal parenchymal embolization, (3) compression or kinking of associated renal artery branches, and (4) hemodynamic changes from turbulent blood flow within the aneurysm results in decreased distal renal artery perfusion.[237,247] Most series suggest improvement or cure in the majority of hypertensive patients undergoing RAA reconstruction, with postoperative improvement more likely when RVH or renal artery stenosis is identified preoperatively.[244,248,251]

Open surgical repair remains the gold standard for RAA management as these procedures performed in the elective setting offer low morbidity, negligible mortality, and durable patency.[241,242,244–247,249,253,254] Options for conventional in situ reconstruction may include aneurysm resection with (1) primary angioplastic closure with or without branch reimplantation, (2) patch angioplasty, (3) primary reanastomosis, (4) interposition bypass, (5) aortorenal bypass, (6) splanchnorenal bypass, and (7) plication of small aneurysms. While complex distal branch lesions were historically treated with nephrectomy, they may rather best be approached with ex vivo repair and autotransplantation which offers excellent technical success without major morbidity or mortality.[199,255] Most recently, robotic techniques have been introduced that may become more prevalent in future practices.[256,257] Most authors advocate completion imaging before hospital discharge and long-term follow-up with surveillance imaging.

While traditional endovascular therapies for RAA have utilized coil embolization for distal and parenchymal aneurysms and stent graft exclusion for main renal artery lesions, the indications for endovascular repair have broadened with the introduction of three-dimensional detachable coils, nonadhesive liquid embolic agents (ie, Onyx), remodeling techniques (which include balloon- and stent-assisted coiling), and flow diverter stents[258] (ie, the Cardiatis multilayer stent).[248,259–261] Technical success is suggested as 73% to 100% across series with highly variable rates of morbidity (13% to 60%) that include primarily radiographic evidence of end-organ malperfusion from thromboembolism and subsequent PES, negligible evidence of arterial dissections or renal compromise, and low rates of recanalization requiring reintervention (4% to 13%).[254,262–264] Although prospective data are lacking, limited comparisons of open surgical and endovascular procedures have reported no significant difference in mortality, perioperative morbidity, freedom from reintervention, decline in renal function, or length of stay.[242,254,265]

References

1. Rosenblum JD, Boyle CM, Schwartz LB. The mesenteric circulation. Anatomy and physiology. *Surg Clin North Am.* 1997;77(2):289–306.
2. Paterno F, Longo WE. The etiology and pathogenesis of vascular disorders of the intestine. *Radiol Clin North Am.* 2008;46(5):877–885.
3. Deitch EA. The role of intestinal barrier failure and bacterial translocation in the development of systemic infection and multiple organ failure. *Arch Surg.* 1990;125(3):403–404.
4. Boley SJ, Brandt LJ, Sammartano RJ. History of mesenteric ischemia. The evolution of a diagnosis and management. *Surg Clin North Am.* 1997;77(2):275–288.
5. Klass AA. Embolectomy in acute mesenteric occlusion. *Ann Surg.* 1951;134(5):913–917.
6. Wyers MC. Acute mesenteric ischemia: diagnostic approach and surgical treatment. *Semin Vasc Surg.* 2010(1);23:9–20.
7. Kassahun WT, Schulz T, Richter O, Hauss J. Unchanged high mortality rates from acute occlusive intestinal ischemia: six year review. *Langenbecks Arch Surg.* 2008;393(2):163–171.
8. Acosta S. Epidemiology of mesenteric vascular disease: clinical implications. *Semin Vasc Surg.* 2010;23(1):4–8.
9. Edwards MS, Cherr GS, Craven TE, et al. Acute occlusive mesenteric ischemia: surgical management and outcomes. *Ann Vasc Surg.* 2003;17(1):72–79.
10. Acosta S, Ogren M, Sternby NH, Bergqvist D, Björck M. Incidence of acute thrombo-embolic occlusion of the superior mesenteric artery—a population-based study. *Eur J Vasc Endovasc Surg.* 2004;27(2):145–150.
11. Marchena-Gomez J, Acosta-Merida MA, Hemmersbach-Miller M, Conde-Martel A, Roque-Castellano C, Hernandez-Romero J. The age-adjusted Charlson Comorbidity Index as an outcome predictor of patients with acute mesenteric ischemia. *Ann Vasc Surg.* 2009;23(4):458–464.
12. Ryer EJ, Kalra M, Oderich GS, et al. Revascularization for acute mesenteric ischemia. *J Vasc Surg.* 2012;55(6):1682–1689.
13. Kougias P, Lau D, El Sayed HFE, Zhou W, Huynh TT, Lin PH. Determinants of mortality and treatment outcome following surgical interventions for acute mesenteric ischemia. *J Vasc Surg.* 2007;46(3):467–474.
14. Acosta S, Nilsson T. Current status on plasma biomarkers for acute mesenteric ischemia. *J Thromb Thrombolysis.* 2012;33(4):355–361.

15. Acosta S, Nilsson TK, Björck M. D-dimer testing in patients with suspected acute thromboembolic occlusion of the superior mesenteric artery. *Br J Surg*. 2004;91(8):991–994.
16. Evennett NJ, Petrov MS, Mittal A, Windsor JA. Systematic review and pooled estimates for the diagnostic accuracy of serological markers for intestinal ischemia. *World J Surg*. 2009;33(7):1374–1383.
17. Mihaileanu FV, Popa SL, Grad S, et al. The efficiency of serum biomarkers in predicting the clinical outcome of patients with mesenteric ischemia during follow-up: a systematic review. *Diagnostics (Basel)*. 2024;14(7):670.
18. Aschoff AJ, Stuber G, Becker BW, et al. Evaluation of acute mesenteric ischemia: accuracy of biphasic mesenteric multi-detector CT angiography. *Abdom Imaging*. 2009;34(3):345–357.
19. Reintam Blaser A, Koitmäe M, Laisaar KT, et al. Radiological diagnosis of acute mesenteric ischemia in adult patients: a systematic review and meta-analysis. *Sci Rep*. 2025;15(1):9875.
20. Scali ST, Ayo D, Giles KA, et al. Outcomes of antegrade and retrograde open mesenteric bypass for acute mesenteric ischemia. *J Vasc Surg*. 2019;69(1):129–140.
21. Milner R, Woo EY, Carpenter JP. Superior mesenteric artery angioplasty and stenting via a retrograde approach in a patient with bowel ischemia—a case report. *Vasc Endovascular Surg*. 2004;38(1):89–91.
22. Wyers MC, Powell RJ, Nolan BW, Cronenwett JL. Retrograde mesenteric stenting during laparotomy for acute occlusive mesenteric ischemia. *J Vasc Surg*. 2007;45(2):269–275.
23. Blauw JT, Meerwaldt R, Brusse-Keizer M, et al. Retrograde open mesenteric stenting for acute mesenteric ischemia. *J Vasc Surg*. 2014;60(3):726–734.
24. Andraska E, Haga L, Li X, et al. Retrograde open mesenteric stenting should be considered as the initial approach to acute mesenteric ischemia. *J Vasc Surg*. 2020;72(4):1260–1268.
25. Cirillo-Penn NC, DeMartino RR, Rasmussen TE, et al. Midterm clinical outcomes of retrograde open mesenteric stenting for mesenteric ischemia. *Ann Vasc Surg*. 2023;89:20–27.
26. Swerdlow NJ, Varkevisser RRB, Soden PA, et al. Thirty-day outcomes after open revascularization for acute mesenteric ischemia from the American College of Surgeons National Surgical Quality Improvement Program. *Ann Vasc Surg*. 2019;61:148–155.
27. Newton WB 3rd, Sagransky MJ, Andrews JS, et al. Outcomes of revascularized acute mesenteric ischemia in the American College of Surgeons National Surgical Quality Improvement Program database. *Am Surg*. 2011;77(7):832–838.
28. Reintam Blaser A, Mändul M, Björck M, et al; AMESI Investigators (Collaborators). Incidence, diagnosis, management and outcome of acute mesenteric ischaemia: a prospective, multicentre observational study (AMESI Study). *Crit Care*. 2024;28(1):32.
29. Schoots IG, Levi MM, Reekers JA, Lameris JS, van Gulik TM. Thrombolytic therapy for acute superior mesenteric artery occlusion. *J Vasc Interv Radiol*. 2005;16(3):317–329.
30. Resch TA, Acosta S, Sonesson B. Endovascular techniques in acute arterial mesenteric ischemia. *Semin Vasc Surg*. 2010;23(1):29–35.
31. Arthurs ZM, Titus J, Bannazadeh M, et al. A comparison of endovascular revascularization with traditional therapy for the treatment of acute mesenteric ischemia. *J Vasc Surg*. 2011;53(3):698–704; discussion 704–705.
32. Andraska EA, Tran LM, Haga LM, et al. Contemporary management of acute and chronic mesenteric ischemia: 10-year experience from a multihospital healthcare system. *J Vasc Surg*. 2022;75(5):1624–1633.e8.
33. Beaulieu RJ, Arnaoutakis KD, Abularrage CJ, Efron DT, Schneider E, Black JH 3rd. Comparison of open and endovascular treatment of acute mesenteric ischemia. *J Vasc Surg*. 2014;59(1):159–164.
34. Goto D, Yanishi K, Ozawa T, et al. Comparison of endovascular therapy and open surgical revascularization in patients with acute superior mesenteric artery occlusion: a large-scale analysis based on the JROAD-DPC database. *J Am Heart Assoc*. 2024;13(12):e035017.
35. Shi Y, Zhao B, Zhou Y, Chen L, Su H, Gu J. Endovascular revascularization vs open surgical revascularization as the first strategy for arterial acute mesenteric ischemia: a systematic review and meta-analysis. *J Vasc Surg*. 2024;80(6):1883–1893.e2.
36. Harnik IG, Brandt LJ. Mesenteric venous thrombosis. *Vasc Med*. 2010;15(5):407–418.
37. Amitrano L, Guardascione MA, Scaglione M, et al. Prognostic factors in noncirrhotic patients with splanchnic vein thromboses. *Am J Gastroenterol*. 2007;102(11):2464–2470.
38. Abdu RA, Zakhour BJ, Dallis DJ. Mesenteric venous thrombosis—1911 to 1984. *Surgery*. 1987;101(4):383–388.
39. Dentali F, Ageno W, Witt D, et al. Natural history of mesenteric venous thrombosis in patients treated with vitamin K antagonists: a multi-centre, retrospective cohort study. *Thromb Haemost*. 2009;102(3):501–504.
40. Kearon C, Akl EA, Comerota AJ, et al. Antithrombotic therapy for VTE disease: antithrombotic therapy and prevention of thrombosis, 9th ed: American College of Chest Physicians evidence-based clinical practice guidelines. *Chest*. 2012;141(2 Supp):e419S–e494S.
41. Koelemay MJ, Geelkerken RH, Kärkkäinen J, et al. Editor's choice – European Society for Vascular Surgery (ESVS) 2025 clinical practice guidelines on the management of diseases of the mesenteric and renal arteries and veins. *Eur J Vasc Endovasc Surg*. 2025;70(2):153–218.
42. Yang S, Liu B, Ding W, He C, Wu X, Li J. Acute superior mesenteric venous thrombosis: transcatheter thrombolysis and aspiration thrombectomy therapy by combined route of superior mesenteric vein and artery in eight patients. *Cardiovasc Intervent Radiol*. 2015;38(1):88–99.
43. Wichman HJ, Cwikiel W, Keussen I. Interventional treatment of mesenteric venous occlusion. *Pol J Radiol*. 2014;79:233–238.
44. Lopera JE, Correa G, Brazzini A, et al. Percutaneous transhepatic treatment of symptomatic mesenteric venous thrombosis. *J Vasc Surg*. 2002;36(5):1058–1061.
45. Mesh CL, Gewertz BL. The effect of hemodilution on blood flow regulation in normal and postischemic intestine. *J Surg Res*. 1990;48(3):183–189.
46. Oshima A, Kitajima M, Sakai N, Ando N. Does glucagon improve the viability of ischemic intestine? *J Surg Res*. 1990;49(6):524–533.
47. Kamimura K, Oosaki A, Sugahara S, Mori S. Survival of three nonocclusive mesenteric ischemia patients following early diagnosis by multidetector row computed tomography and prostaglandin E1 treatment. *Intern Med*. 2008;47(22):2001–2006.
48. Cullen JM, Hassinger TE, Mehaffey JH, et al. Overweight patients with chronic mesenteric ischemia undergo more diagnostic studies: a retrospective analysis. *Am Surg*. 2020;86(4):e177–e179.
49. Mansukhani NA, Hekman KE, Yoon DY et al. Impact of body mass index on outcomes after mesenteric revascularization for chronic mesenteric ischemia. *Ann Vasc Surg*. 2018;48:159–165.
50. Park WM, Gloviczki P, Cherry KJ Jr, et al. Contemporary management of acute mesenteric ischemia: factors associated with survival. *J Vasc Surg*. 2002;35(3):445–452.
51. Hansen KJ, Wilson DB, Craven TE, et al. Mesenteric artery disease in the elderly. *J Vasc Surg*. 2004;40(1):45–52.
52. Moneta GL, Lee RW, Yeager RA, Taylor LM Jr, Porter JM. Mesenteric duplex scanning: a blinded prospective study. *J Vasc Surg*. 1993;17(1):79–84; discussion 85–86.
53. van Dijk LJD, van Petersen AS, Moelker A. Vascular imaging of the mesenteric vasculature. *Best Pract Res Clin Gastroenterol*. 2017;31(1):3–14.
54. Burkart DJ, Johnson CD, Reading CC, Ehman RL. MR measurements of mesenteric venous flow: prospective evaluation in healthy volunteers and patients with suspected chronic mesenteric ischemia. *Radiology*. 1995;194(3):801–806.
55. van Dijk LJD, Terlouw LG, van Noord D, Bijdevaate DC, Bruno MJ, Moelker A. Endovascular pressure measurements to assess the functional severity of mesenteric arterial stenoses. *J Vasc Interv Radiol*. 2020;31(3):430–437.

56. Foley MI, Moneta GL, Abou-Zamzam AM Jr, et al. Revascularization of the superior mesenteric artery alone for treatment of intestinal ischemia. *J Vasc Surg*. 2000;32(1):37–47.
57. Cho JS, Carr JA, Jacobsen G, Shepard AD, Nypaver TJ, Reddy DJ. Long-term outcome after mesenteric artery reconstruction: a 37-year experience. *J Vasc Surg*. 2002;35(3):453–460.
58. Illuminati G, Caliò FG, D'Urso A, Papaspiropoulos V, Mancini P, Ceccanei G. The surgical treatment of chronic intestinal ischemia: results of a recent series. *Acta Chir Belg*. 2004;104(2):175–183.
59. Kruger AJ, Walker PJ, Foster WJ, Jenkins JS, Boyne NS, Jenkins J. Open surgery for atherosclerotic chronic mesenteric ischemia. *J Vasc Surg*. 2007;46(5):941–945.
60. Atkins MD, Kwolek CJ, LaMuraglia GM, Brewster DC, Chung TK, Cambria RP. Surgical revascularization versus endovascular therapy for chronic mesenteric ischemia: a comparative experience. *J Vasc Surg*. 2007;45(6):1162–1171.
61. Oderich GS, Bower TC, Sullivan TM, Bjarnason H, Cha S, Gloviczki P. Open versus endovascular revascularization for chronic mesenteric ischemia: risk-stratified outcomes. *J Vasc Surg*. 2009;49(6):1472–1479.e3.
62. Mell MW, Acher CW, Hoch JR, Tefera G, Turnipseed WD. Outcomes after endarterectomy for chronic mesenteric ischemia. *J Vasc Surg*. 2008;48(5):1132–1138.
63. Oderich GS, Gloviczki P, Bower TC. Open surgical treatment for chronic mesenteric ischemia in the endovascular era: when it is necessary and what is the preferred technique? *Semin Vasc Surg*. 2010;23(1):36–46.
64. Oderich GS, Malgor RD, Ricotta JJ 2nd. Open and endovascular revascularization for chronic mesenteric ischemia: tabular review of the literature. *Ann Vasc Surg*. 2009;23(5):700–712.
65. Sarac TP, Altinel O, Kashyap V, et al. Endovascular treatment of stenotic and occluded visceral arteries for chronic mesenteric ischemia. *J Vasc Surg*. 2008;47(3):485–491.
66. Sharafuddin MJ, Nicholson RM, Kresowik TF, Amin PB, Hoballah JJ, Sharp WJ. Endovascular recanalization of total occlusions of the mesenteric and celiac arteries. *J Vasc Surg*. 2012;55(6):1674–1681.
67. Pillai AK, Kalva SP, Hsu SL, et al; Society of Interventional Radiology Standards of Practice Committee. Quality improvement guidelines for mesenteric angioplasty and stent placement for the treatment of chronic mesenteric ischemia. *J Vasc Interv Radiol*. 2018;29(5):642–647.
68. Terlouw LG, Moelker A, Abrahamsen J, et al. European guidelines on chronic mesenteric ischaemia – joint United European Gastroenterology, European Association for Gastroenterology, Endoscopy and Nutrition, European Society of Gastrointestinal and Abdominal Radiology, Netherlands Association of Hepatogastroenterologists, Hellenic Society of Gastroenterology, Cardiovascular and Interventional Radiological Society of Europe, and Dutch Mesenteric Ischemia Study group clinical guidelines on the diagnosis and treatment of patients with chronic mesenteric ischaemia. *United European Gastroenterol J*. 2020:8(4):371–395.
69. Brown DJ, Schermerhorn ML, Powell RJ, et al. Mesenteric stenting for chronic mesenteric ischemia. *J Vasc Surg*. 2005;42:268–274.
70. Sivamurthy N, Rhodes JM, Lee D, Waldman DL, Green RM, Davies MG. Endovascular versus open mesenteric revascularization: immediate benefits do not equate with short-term functional outcomes. *J Am Coll Surg*. 2006;202:859–867.
71. Tallarita T, Oderich GS, Macedo TA, et al. Reinterventions for stent restenosis in patients treated for atherosclerotic mesenteric artery disease. *J Vasc Surg*. 2011;54:1422–1429,e1.
72. Alahdab F, Arwani R, Pasha AK, et al. A systemic review and meta-analysis of endovascular versus open surgical revascularization for chronic mesenteric ischemia. *J Vasc Surg*. 2018;67:1598–1605.
73. Malgor RD, Oderich GS, McKusick MA, et al. Results of single- and two-vessel mesenteric artery stents for chronic mesenteric ischemia. *Ann Vasc Surg*. 2010;24:1094–1101.
74. Oderich GS, Erdoes LS, Lesar C, et al. Comparison of covered stents versus bare metal stents for treatment of chronic atherosclerotic mesenteric arterial disease. *J Vasc Surg*. 2013;58:1316–1323.
75. Van Dijk LJD, Harki J, van Noord D, et al; Dutch Mesenteric Ischemia Study group (DMIS). Covered stents versus bare-metal stents in chronic atherosclerotic gastrointestinal ischemia (CoBaGI): study protocol for a randomized controlled trial. *Trials*. 2019;20:519.
76. Schermerhorn ML, Giles KA, Hamdan AD, Wyers MC, Pomposelli FB. Mesenteric revascularization: management and outcomes in the United States, 1988–2006. *J Vasc Surg*. 2009;50: 341–348.e1.
77. Lima FV, Kolte D, Kennedy KF, et al. Endovascular versus surgical revascularization for chronic mesenteric ischemia—insights from the national inpatient sample database. *JACC Cardiovascu Interv*. 2017;10(23):2440–2447.
78. Dunbar JD, Molnar W, Beman FF, Marable SA. Compression of the celiac trunk and abdominal angina. *Am J Roentgenol Radium Ther Nucl Med*. 1965;95:731–744.
79. Jimenez JC, Harlander-Locke M, Dutson EP. Open and laparoscopic treatment of median arcuate ligament syndrome. *J Vasc Surg*. 2012;56:869–873.
80. Mensink PB, van Petersen AS, Kolkman JJ, Otte JA, Huisman AB, Geelkerken RH. Gastric exercise tonometry: the key investigation in patients with suspected celiac artery compression syndrome. *J Vasc Surg*. 2006;44:277–281.
81. Derrick JR, Pollard HS, Moore RM. The pattern of arteriosclerotic narrowing of the celiac and superior mesenteric arteries. *Ann Surg*. 1959;149:684–689.
82. Park CM, Chung JW, Kim HB, Shin SJ, Park JH. Celiac axis stenosis: incidence and etiologies in asymptomatic individuals. *Korean J Radiol*. 2001;2:8–13.
83. Scholbach T. Celiac artery compression syndrome in children, adolescents, and young adults: clinical and color duplex sonographic features in a series of 59 cases. *J Ultrasound Med*. 2006;25:299–305.
84. Skeik N, Cooper LT, Duncan AA, Jabr FI. Median arcuate ligament syndrome: a nonvascular, vascular diagnosis. *Vasc Endovascular Surg*. 2011;45:433–437.
85. Tulloch AW, Jimenez JC, Lawrence PF, et al. Laparoscopic versus open celiac ganglionectomy in patients with median arcuate ligament syndrome. *J Vasc Surg*. 2010;52:1283–1289.
86. van Petersen AS, Vriens BH, Huisman AB, Kolkman JJ, Geelkerken RH. Retroperitoneal endoscopic release in the management of celiac artery compression syndrome. *J Vasc Surg*. 2009;50:140–147.
87. Aschenbach R, Basche S, Vogl TJ. Compression of the celiac trunk caused by median arcuate ligament in children and adolescent subjects: evaluation with contrast-enhanced MR angiography and comparison with Doppler US evaluation. *J Vasc Interv Radiol*. 2011;22:556–561.
88. Metz FM, Blauw JTM, Brusse-Keizer M, Kolkman JJ, Bruno MJ, Geelkerken RH; Dutch Mesenteric Ischaemia Study Group. Systematic review of the efficacy of treatment for median arcuate ligament syndrome. *Eur J Vasc Endovasc Surg*. 2022;64(6): 720–732.
89. Reilly LM, Ammar AD, Stoney RJ, Ehrenfeld WK. Late results following operative repair for celiac artery compression syndrome. *J Vasc Surg*. 1985;2:79–91.
90. Williams S, Gillespie P, Little JM. Celiac axis compression syndrome: factors predicting a favorable outcome. *Surgery*. 1985; 98:879–887.
91. Duffy AJ, Panait L, Eisenberg D, Bell RL, Roberts KE, Sumpio B. Management of median arcuate ligament syndrome: a new paradigm. *Ann Vasc Surg*. 2009;23:778–784.
92. Skelly CL, Stiles-Shields C, Mak GZ, et al. The impact of psychiatric comorbidities on patient-reported surgical outcomes in adults treated for the median arcuate ligament syndrome. *J Vasc Surg*. 2018;68(5):1414–1421.
93. Khrucharoen U, Juo YY, Chen Y, Jimenez JC, Dutson EP. Short- and intermediate-term clinical outcome comparison between laparoscopic and robotic-assisted median arcuate ligament release. *J Robot Surg*. 2020;14(1):123–129.
94. Relles D, Moudgill N, Rao A, Rosato F, DiMuzio P, Eisenberg J. Robotic-assisted median arcuate ligament release. *J Vasc Surg*. 2012;56:500–503.

95. Brody F, Randall JA, Amdur RL, Sidawy AN. A predictive model for patients with median arcuate ligament syndrome. *Surg Endoscopy.* 2018;32:4860–4866.
96. Goodall R, Langridge B, Onida S, Ellis M, Lane T, Davies AH. Median arcuate ligament syndrome. *J Vasc Surg.* 2019;71(6):2170–2176.
97. Carr SC, Pearce WH, Vogelzang RL, McCarthy WJ, Nemcek AA Jr, Yao JS. Current management of visceral artery aneurysms. *Surgery.* 1996;120:627–633; discussion 633–634.
98. Stanley JC, Wakefield TW, Graham LM, Whitehouse WM Jr, Zelenock GB, Lindenauer SM. Clinical importance and management of splanchnic artery aneurysms. *J Vasc Surg.* 1986;3:836–840.
99. Bedford PD, Lodge B. Aneurysm of the splenic artery. *Gut.* 1960;1:312–320.
100. Cochennec F, Riga CV, Allaire E, et al. Contemporary management of splanchnic and renal artery aneurysms: results of endovascular compared with open surgery from two European vascular centers. *Eur J Vasc Endovasc Surg.* 2011;42:340–346.
101. Pitton MB, Dappa E, Jungmann F, et al. Visceral artery aneurysms: incidence, management, and outcome analysis in a tertiary care center over one decade. *Eur Radiol.* 2015;25:2004–2014.
102. Chaer RA, Abularrage CJ, Coleman DM, et al. The society for vascular surgery clinical practice guidelines on the management of visceral aneurysms. *J Vasc Surg.* 2020;72(5):3S–39S.
103. Pulli R, Dorigo W, Troisi N, Pratesi G, Innocenti AA, Pratesi C. Surgical treatment of visceral artery aneurysms: a 25-year experience. *J Vasc Surg.* 2008;48:334–342.
104. Marone EM, Mascia D, Kahlberg A, Brioschi C, Tshomba Y, Chiesa R. Is open repair still the gold standard in visceral artery aneurysm management? *Ann Vasc Surg.* 2011;25:936–946.
105. Shukla AJ, Eid R, Fish L, et al. Contemporary outcomes of intact and ruptured visceral artery aneurysms. *J Vasc Surg.* 2015;61:1442–1447.
106. Sachdev U, Baril DT, Ellozy SH, et al. Management of aneurysms involving branches of the celiac and superior mesenteric arteries: a comparison of surgical and endovascular therapy. *J Vasc Surg.* 2006;44:718–724.
107. Saltzberg SS, Maldonado TS, Lamparello PJ, et al. Is endovascular therapy the preferred treatment for all visceral artery aneurysms? *Ann Vasc Surg.* 2005;19:507–515.
108. Ferrero E, Ferri M, Viazzo A, et al. Visceral artery aneurysms, an experience on 32 cases in a single center: treatment from surgery to multilayer stent. *Ann Vasc Surg.* 2011;25:923–935.
109. Lakin RO, Bena JF, Sarac TP, et al. The contemporary management of splenic artery aneurysms. *J Vasc Surg.* 2011;53:958–964; discussion 965.
110. Stanley JC, Fry WJ. Pathogenesis and clinical significance of splenic artery aneurysms. *Surgery.* 1974;76:898–909.
111. Shanley CJ, Shah NL, Messina LM. Common splanchnic artery aneurysms: splenic, hepatic, and celiac. *Ann Vasc Surg.* 1996;10:315–322.
112. Nanez L, Knowles M, Modrall JG, Valentine RJ. Ruptured splenic artery aneurysms are exceedingly rare in pregnant women. *J Vasc Surg.* 2014;60:1520–1523.
113. Akbulut S, Otan E. Management of giant splenic artery aneurysm: comprehensive literature review. *Medicine (Baltimore).* 2015;94:e1016.
114. Le Tinier B, Jungo-Nancoz C, McCarey C, Jastrow N. Rupture of maternal splenic artery aneurysm and fetal demise. *Clin Exp Obstet Gynecol.* 2015;42:381–383.
115. McMahon DP, Ward WH, Harwood JL, Moore EM. An institutional review of splenic artery aneurysm in childbearing-aged females and splenic artery aneurysm rupture during pregnancy. Is screening justified? *Mil Med.* 2012;177:96–98.
116. Ayalon A, Wiesner RH, Perkins JD, Tominaga S, Hayes DH, Krom RA. Splenic artery aneurysms in liver transplant patients. *Transplantation.* 1988;45:386–389.
117. Bronsther O, Merhav H, Van Thiel D, Starzl TE. Splenic artery aneurysms occurring in liver transplant recipients. *Transplantation.* 1991;52:723–724.
118. Tessier DJ, Stone WM, Fowl RJ, et al. Clinical features and management of splenic artery pseudoaneurysm: case series and cumulative review of the literature. *J Vasc Surg.* 2003;38:969–974.
119. Sadat U, Dar O, Walsh S, Varty K. Splenic artery aneurysms in pregnancy—a systematic review. *Int J Surg.* 2008;6:261–265.
120. Heestand G, Sher L, Lightfoote J, et al. Characteristics and management of splenic artery aneurysm in liver transplant candidates and recipients. *Am Surg.* 2003;69:933–940.
121. Obuchi T, Sasaki A, Nakajima J, Nitta H, Otsuka K, Wakabayashi G. Laparoscopic surgery for splenic artery aneurysm. *Surg Laparosc Endosc Percutan Tech.* 2009;19:338–340.
122. Pietrabissa A, Ferrari M, Berchiolli R, et al. Laparoscopic treatment of splenic artery aneurysms. *J Vasc Surg.* 2009;50:275–279.
123. Giulianotti PC, Buchs NC, Coratti A, et al. Robot-assisted treatment of splenic artery aneurysms. *Ann Vasc Surg.* 2011;25:377–383.
124. Trastek VF, Pairolero PC, Joyce JW, Hollier LH, Bernatz PE. Splenic artery aneurysms. *Surgery.* 1982;91:694–699.
125. Abbas MA, Stone WM, Fowl RJ, et al. Splenic artery aneurysms: two decades experience at Mayo Clinic. *Ann Vasc Surg.* 2002;16:442–449.
126. Hogendoorn W, Lavida A, Hunink MG, et al. Open repair, endovascular repair, and conservative management of true splenic artery aneurysms. *J Vasc Surg.* 2014;60:1667–1676.e1.
127. Marmagkiolis K, Gobal F, Mego D, Cilingiroglu M, Rollefson W. Endovascular management of splenic arterial aneurysms. *Int J Cardiol.* 2014;174:146–149.
128. Patel A, Weintraub JL, Nowakowski FS, et al. Single-center experience with elective transcatheter coil embolization of splenic artery aneurysms: technique and midterm follow-up. *J Vasc Interv Radiol.* 2012;23:893–899.
129. Piffaretti G, Tozzi M, Lomazzi C, et al. Splenic artery aneurysms: postembolization syndrome and surgical complications. *Am J Surg.* 2007;193:166–170.
130. Guillon R, Garcier JM, Abergel A, et al. Management of splenic artery aneurysms and false aneurysms with endovascular treatment in 12 patients. *Cardiovasc Intervent Radiol.* 2003;26:256–260.
131. Hogendoorn W, Lavida A, Hunink MG, et al. Cost-effectiveness of endovascular repair, open repair, and conservative management of splenic artery aneurysms. *J Vasc Surg.* 2015;61:1432–1440.
132. Ikeda O, Tamura Y, Nakasone Y, Iryou Y, Yamashita Y. Nonoperative management of unruptured visceral artery aneurysms: treatment by transcatheter coil embolization. *J Vasc Surg.* 2008;47:1212–1219.
133. Nagaraja R, Govindasamy M, Varma V, et al. Hepatic artery pseudoaneurysms: a single-center experience. *Ann Vasc Surg.* 2013;27:743–749.
134. Shanley CJ, Shah NL, Messina LM. Uncommon splanchnic artery aneurysms: pancreaticoduodenal, gastroduodenal, superior mesenteric, inferior mesenteric, and colic. *Ann Vasc Surg.* 1996;10:506–515.
135. Stone WM, Abbas M, Cherry KJ, Fowl RJ, Gloviczki P. Superior mesenteric artery aneurysms: is presence an indication for intervention? *J Vasc Surg.* 2002;36:234–237; discussion 237.
136. Jiang J, Ding X, Su Q, et al. Therapeutic management of superior mesenteric artery aneurysms. *J Vasc Surg.* 2011;53:1619–1624.
137. Yasuda S, Imoto K, Uchida K, et al. Successful endovascular treatment of a ruptured superior mesenteric artery in a patient with Ehlers–Danlos syndrome. *Ann Vasc Surg.* 2013;27:975.e1–e5.
138. Cowan S, Kahn MB, Bonn J, et al. Superior mesenteric artery pseudoaneurysm successfully treated with polytetrafluoroethylene covered stent. *J Vasc Surg.* 2002;35:805–857.
139. Mendonça CT, Weingartner J, de Carvalho CA, Costa DS. Endovascular treatment of contained rupture of a superior mesenteric artery aneurysm resulting from neurofibromatosis type I. *J Vasc Surg.* 2010;51:461–464.
140. Graham LM, Stanley JC, Whitehouse WM Jr, et al. Celiac artery aneurysms: historic (1745–1949) versus contemporary (1950–1984) differences in etiology and clinical importance. *J Vasc Surg.* 1985;2:757–764.

141. Stone WM, Abbas MA, Gloviczki P, Fowl RJ, Cherry KJ. Celiac arterial aneurysms: a critical reappraisal of a rare entity. *Arch Surg*. 2002;137:670–674.
142. Graham JM, McCollum CH, DeBakey ME. Aneurysms of the splanchnic arteries. *Am J Surg*. 1980;140:797.
143. Atkins BZ, Ryan JM, Gray JL. Treatment of a celiac artery aneurysm with endovascular stent grafting—a case report. *Vasc Endovascular Surg*. 2003;37:367–373.
144. Inada K, Maeda M, Ikeda T. Segmental arterial mediolysis: unrecognized cases culled from cases of ruptured aneurysm of abdominal visceral arteries reported in the Japanese literature *Pathol Res Pract*. 2007;203:771–778.
145. Lagoudianakis EE, Filis KA, Tsekouras DK, et al. Endovascular obliteration of a ruptured right gastric artery aneurysm. *Minerva Gastroenterol Dietol*. 2006;52:333–337.
146. Schellhammer F, Steinhaus D, Cohnen M, Hoppe J, Mödder U, Fürst G. Minimally invasive therapy of pseudoaneurysms of the trunk: application of thrombin. *Cardiovasc Intervent Radiol*. 2008;31:535–541.
147. Sellke FW, Williams GB, Donovan DL, Clarke RE. Management of intra-abdominal aneurysms associated with periarteritis nodosa. *J Vasc Surg*. 1986;4:294–298.
148. Naito A, Toyota N, Ito K. Embolization of a ruptured middle colic artery aneurysm. *Cardiovasc Intervent Radiol*. 1995;18:56–58.
149. Turkbey B, Peynircioglu B, Akpinar E. Isolated aneurysm of the distal branch of the jejunal artery: MDCT angiographic diagnosis and endovascular management. *Cardiovasc Intervent Radiol*. 2008;31(Suppl 2):S34–S37.
150. Goffi L, Chan R, Boccoli G, Ghiselli R, Saba V. Aneurysm of a jejunal branch of the superior mesenteric artery in a patient with Marfan's syndrome. *J Cardiovasc Surg (Torino)*. 2000;41: 321–323.
151. Coll DP, Ierardi R, Kerstein MD, Yost S, Wilson A, Matsumoto T. Aneurysms of the pancreaticoduodenal arteries: a change in management. *Ann Vasc Surg*. 1998;12:286–291.
152. Suzuki K, Kashimura H, Sato M, et al. Pancreaticoduodenal artery aneurysms associated with celiac axis stenosis due to compression by median arcuate ligament and celiac plexus. *J Gastroenterol*. 1998;33:434–438.
153. Moore E, Matthews MR, Minion DJ, et al. Surgical management of peripancreatic arterial aneurysms. *J Vasc Surg*. 2004;40: 247–253.
154. Karanasios E, Ragab Z, Cavenagh H, Stather P, Ali T. Characteristics and trends in median arcuate ligament syndrome (MALS) associated visceral artery aneurysms: a systematic descriptive review of the literature. *Vasc Endovascular Surg*. 2024;58(5):512–522.
155. Habib N, Hassan S, Abdou R, et al. Gastroduodenal artery aneurysm, diagnosis, clinical presentation and management: a concise review. *Ann Surg Innov Res*. 2013;7:4.
156. de Perrot M, Berney T, Deleaval J, Bühler L, Mentha G, Morel P. Management of true aneurysms of the pancreaticoduodenal arteries. *Ann Surg*. 1999;229:416–420.
157. Katsura M, Gushimiyagi M, Takara H, Mototake H. True aneurysm of the pancreaticoduodenal arteries: a single institution experience. *J Gastrointest Surg*. 2010;14:1409–1413.
158. Ghariani MZ, Georg Y, Ramirez C, et al. Long-term results of surgical treatment of aneurysms of digestive arteries. *Ann Vasc Surg*. 2013;27:954–958.
159. Eckhauser FE, Stanley JC, Zelenock GB, Borlaza GS, Freier DT, Lindenauer SM. Gastroduodenal and pancreaticoduodenal artery aneurysms: a complication of pancreatitis causing spontaneous gastrointestinal hemorrhage. *Surgery*. 1980;88:335–344.
160. Balachandra S, Siriwardena AK. Systematic appraisal of the management of the major vascular complications of pancreatitis. *Am J Surg*. 2005;190:489–495.
161. Manazer JR, Monzon JR, Dietz PA, Moglia R, Gold M. Treatment of pancreatic pseudoaneurysm with percutaneous transabdominal thrombin injection. *J Vasc Surg*. 2003;38:600–602.
162. Edogawa S, Shibuya T, Kurose K, Sasaki K, Tomita H. Inferior mesenteric artery aneurysm: case report and literature review. *Ann Vasc Dis*. 2013;6:98–101.
163. Mandeville KL, Bicknell C, Narula S, Renton S. Inferior mesenteric artery aneurysm with occlusion of the superior mesenteric artery, coeliac trunk and right renal artery. *Eur J Vasc Endovasc Surg*. 2008;35:312–313.
164. Tsukioka K, Nobara H, Nishimura K. A case of inferior mesenteric artery aneurysm with an occlusive disease in superior mesenteric artery and the celiac artery. *Ann Vasc Dis*. 2010;3:160–163.
165. Troisi N, Esposito G, Cefali P, Setti M. A case of atherosclerotic inferior mesenteric artery aneurysm secondary to high flow state. *J Vasc Surg*. 2011;54:205–207.
166. Samuels AI, Miller ED Jr, Fray JC, Haber E, Barger AC. Renin-angiotensin antagonists and the regulation of blood pressure. *Fed Proc*. 1976;35:2512–2520.
167. Schneider EG, Davis JO, Baumber JS, Johnson JA. Renin, aldosterone, and hypertension. The hepatic metabolism of renin and aldosterone. A review with new observations on the hepatic clearance of renin. *Circ Res*. 1970;27:175–183.
168. Stanley JC, Gewertz BL, Fry WJ. Renal: systemic renin indices and renal vein renin ratios as prognostic indicators in remedial renovascular hypertension. *J Surg Res*. 1976;20:149–155.
169. Vaughan ED Jr, Buhler FR, Laragh JH, et al. Renovascular hypertension: renin measurements to indicate hypersecretion and contralateral suppression, estimate renal plasma flow, and score for surgical curability. *Am J Med*. 1973;55:402–414.
170. Hansen KJ, Tribble RW, Reavis SW, et al. Renal duplex sonography: evaluation of clinical utility. *J Vasc Surg*. 1990;12:227–236.
171. Taylor DC, Kettler MD, Moneta GL, et al. Duplex ultrasound scanning in the diagnosis of renal artery stenosis: a prospective evaluation. *J Vasc Surg*. 1988;7:363–369.
172. Hirsch AT, Haskal ZJ, Hertzer NR, et al. ACC/AHA 2005 Practice Guidelines for the management of patients with peripheral arterial disease (lower extremity, renal, mesenteric, and abdominal aortic): a collaborative report from the American Association for Vascular Surgery/Society for Vascular Surgery, Society for Cardiovascular Angiography and Interventions, Society for Vascular Medicine and Biology, Society of Interventional Radiology, and the ACC/AHA Task Force on Practice Guidelines (Writing Committee to Develop Guidelines for the Management of Patients With Peripheral Arterial Disease): endorsed by the American Association of Cardiovascular and Pulmonary Rehabilitation; National Heart, Lung, and Blood Institute; Society for Vascular Nursing; TransAtlantic Inter-Society Consensus; and Vascular Disease Foundation. *Circulation*. 2006;113:e463–e654.
173. Willmann JK, Wildermuth S, Pfammatter T, et al. Aortoiliac and renal arteries: prospective intraindividual comparison of contrast-enhanced three-dimensional MR angiography and multi-detector row CT angiography. *Radiology*. 2003;226:798–811.
174. Tan KT, van Beek EJ, Brown PW, van Delden OM, Tijssen J, Ramsay LE. Magnetic resonance angiography for the diagnosis of renal artery stenosis: a meta-analysis. *Clin Radiol*. 2002;57: 617–624.
175. Stanley JC, Fry WJ. Surgical treatment of renovascular hypertension. *Arch Surg*. 1977;112:1291–1297.
176. Hansen KJ, Edwards MS, Craven TE, et al. Prevalence of renovascular disease in the elderly: a population-based study. *J Vasc Surg*. 2002;36:443–451.
177. Novick AC, Zaki S, Goldfarb D, Hodge EE. Epidemiologic and clinical comparison of renal artery stenosis in black patients and white patients. *J Vasc Surg*. 1994;20:1–5.
178. Pearce JD, Craven BL, Craven TE, et al. Progression of atherosclerotic renovascular disease: a prospective population-based study. *J Vasc Surg*. 2006;44:955–962; discussion 962–963.
179. Valentine RJ, Clagett GP, Miller GL, Myers SI, Martin JD, Chervu A. The coronary risk of unsuspected renal artery stenosis. *J Vasc Surg*. 1993;18:433–439; discussion 439–440.
180. Harding MB, Smith LR, Himmelstein SI, et al. Renal artery stenosis: prevalence and associated risk factors in patients undergoing routine cardiac catheterization. *J Am Soc Nephrol*. 1992;2:1608–1616.
181. Crowley JJ, Santos RM, Peter RH, et al. Progression of renal artery stenosis in patients undergoing cardiac catheterization. *Am Heart J*. 1998;136:913–918.

182. Edwards MS, Hansen KJ, Craven TE, et al. Associations between renovascular disease and prevalent cardiovascular disease in the elderly: a population-based study. *Vasc Endovascular Surg.* 2004;38:25–35.
183. Valentine RJ, Martin JD, Myers SI, Rossi MB, Clagett GP. Asymptomatic celiac and superior mesenteric artery stenoses are more prevalent among patients with unsuspected renal artery stenoses. *J Vasc Surg.* 1991;14:195–199.
184. Stanley JC. The evolution of surgery for renovascular occlusive disease. *Cardiovasc Surg.* 1994;2:195–202.
185. Safian RD, Textor SC. Renal-artery stenosis. *N Engl J Med.* 2001;344:431–442.
186. Olin JW, Froehlich J, Gu X, et al. The United States Registry for Fibromuscular Dysplasia: results in the first 447 patients. *Circulation.* 2012;125:3182–3190.
187. Olin JW, Gornik HL, Bacharach JM, et al. Fibromuscular dysplasia: state of the science and critical unanswered questions: a scientific statement from the American Heart Association. *Circulation.* 2014;129:1048–1078.
188. Cragg AH, Smith TP, Thompson BH, et al. Incidental fibromuscular dysplasia in potential renal donors: long-term clinical follow-up. *Radiology.* 1989;172:145–147.
189. McCormack LJ, Poutasse EF, Meaney TF, Noto TJ Jr, Dustan HP. A pathologic-arteriographic correlation of renal arterial disease. *Am Heart J.* 1966;72:188–198.
190. Harrison EG Jr, McCormack LJ. Pathologic classification of renal arterial disease in renovascular hypertension. *Mayo Clin Proc.* 1971;46:161–167.
191. Bhalla V, Textor SC, Beckman JA, et al; American Heart Association Council on the Kidney in Cardiovascular Disease; Council on Hypertension; Council on Peripheral Vascular Disease; and Council on Cardiovascular Radiology and Intervention. Revascularization for renovascular disease: a scientific statement from the American Heart Association. *Hypertension.* 2022;79(8):e128–e143.
192. Prince M, Tafur JD, White CJ. When and how should we revascularize patients with atherosclerotic renal artery stenosis? *J Am Coll Cardiol Intv.* 2019;12(6):505–517.
193. Cambria RP, Brewster DC, L'Italien GJ, et al. The durability of different reconstructive techniques for atherosclerotic renal artery disease. *J Vasc Surg.* 1994;20:76–85; discussion 86–87.
194. Chibaro EA, Libertino JA, Novick AC. Use of the hepatic circulation for renal revascularization. *Ann Surg.* 1984;199: 406–411.
195. Khauli RB, Novick AC, Ziegelbaum M. Splenorenal bypass in the treatment of renal artery stenosis: experience with sixty-nine cases. *J Vasc Surg.* 1985;2:547–551.
196. Moncure AC, Brewster DC, Darling RC, Atnip RG, Newton WD, Abbott WM. Use of the splenic and hepatic arteries for renal revascularization. *J Vasc Surg.* 1986;3:196–203.
197. Grigoryants V, Henke PK, Watson NC, et al. Iliorenal bypass: indications and outcomes following 41 reconstructions. *Ann Vasc Surg.* 2007;21:1–9.
198. Murray SP, Kent C, Salvatierra O, Stoney RJ. Complex branch renovascular disease: management options and late results. *J Vasc Surg.* 1994;20:338–345; discussion 346.
199. van Bockel JH, van den Akker PJ, Chang PC, Aarts JC, Hermans J, Terpstra JL. Extracorporeal renal artery reconstruction for renovascular hypertension. *J Vasc Surg.* 1991;13:101–110; discussion 110–111.
200. Dougherty MJ, Hallett JW Jr, Naessens J, et al. Renal endarterectomy vs. bypass for combined aortic and renal reconstruction: is there a difference in clinical outcome? *Ann Vasc Surg.* 1995;9:87–94.
201. McNeil JW, String ST, Pfeiffer RB Jr. Concomitant renal endarterectomy and aortic reconstruction. *J Vasc Surg.* 1994;20:331–336; discussion 336–337.
202. Stoney RJ, Messina LM, Goldstone J, Reilly LM. Renal endarterectomy through the transected aorta: a new technique for combined aortorenal atherosclerosis—a preliminary report. *J Vasc Surg.* 1989;9:224–233.
203. Stanley JC. David M. Hume memorial lecture. Surgical treatment of renovascular hypertension. *Am J Surg.* 1997;174:102–110.
204. Cherr GS, Hansen KJ, Craven TE, et al. Surgical management of atherosclerotic renovascular disease. *J Vasc Surg.* 2002;35:236–245.
205. Hansen KJ, Cherr GS, Craven TE, et al. Management of ischemic nephropathy: dialysis-free survival after surgical repair. *J Vasc Surg.* 2000;32:472–481; discussion 481–482.
206. Corriere MA, Edwards MS. Results of the major randomized clinical trials of renal stenting and implications for future treatment strategies. *Semin Vasc Surg.* 2013;26:161–164.
207. Weibull H, Bergqvist D, Bergentz SE, Jonsson K, Hulthén L, Manhem P. Percutaneous transluminal renal angioplasty versus surgical reconstruction of atherosclerotic renal artery stenosis: a prospective randomized study. *J Vasc Surg.* 1993;18:841–850; discussion 850–852.
208. Knipp BS, Dimick JB, Eliason JL, et al. Diffusion of new technology for the treatment of renovascular hypertension in the United States: surgical revascularization versus catheter-based therapy, 1988–2001. *J Vasc Surg.* 2004;40:717–723.
209. Balk E, Raman G, Chung M, et al. Effectiveness of management strategies for renal artery stenosis: a systematic review. *Ann Intern Med.* 2006;145:901–912.
210. Blum U, Krumme B, Flugel P, et al. Treatment of ostial renal-artery stenoses with vascular endoprostheses after unsuccessful balloon angioplasty. *N Engl J Med.* 1997;336:459–465.
211. Henry M, Amor M, Henry I, et al. Stent placement in the renal artery: three-year experience with the Palmaz stent. *J Vasc Interv Radiol.* 1996;7:343–350.
212. Bax L, Woittiez AJ, Kouwenberg HJ, et al. Stent placement in patients with atherosclerotic renal artery stenosis and impaired renal function: a randomized trial. *Ann Intern Med.* 2009;150:840–848, W150–W151.
213. van Jaarsveld BC, Krijnen P, Pieterman H, et al. The effect of balloon angioplasty on hypertension in atherosclerotic renal-artery stenosis. Dutch Renal Artery Stenosis Intervention Cooperative Study Group. *N Engl J Med.* 2000;342:1007–1014.
214. ASTRAL Investigators, Wheatley K, Ives N, Gray R, et al. Revascularization versus medical therapy for renal-artery stenosis. *N Engl J Med.* 2009;361:1953–1962.
215. Cooper CJ, Murphy TP, Cutlip DE, et al. Stenting and medical therapy for atherosclerotic renal-artery stenosis. *N Engl J Med.* 2014;370:13–22.
216. Riaz IB, Husnain M, Riaz H, et al. Meta-analysis of revascularization versus medical therapy for atherosclerotic renal artery stenosis. *Am J Cardiol.* 2014;114:1116–1123.
217. Fujiwara T, Iwashima Y, Narita K, Satoh M, Sakima A. Combination of medical therapy and percutaneous transluminal renal angioplasty versus medical therapy alone for patients with atherosclerotic renal artery stenosis: systematic review and meta-analysis. *Hypertens Res.* 2025;48:1870–1879.
218. Weber BR, Dieter RS. Renal artery stenosis: epidemiology and treatment. *Int J Nephrol Renovasc Dis.* 2014;7:169–181.
219. Rocha-Singh KJ, Mishkel GJ, Katholi RE, et al. Clinical predictors of improved long-term blood pressure control after successful stenting of hypertensive patients with obstructive renal artery atherosclerosis. *Catheter Cardiovasc Interv.* 1999;47: 167–172.
220. Silva JA, Chan AW, White CJ, et al. Elevated brain natriuretic peptide predicts blood pressure response after stent revascularization in patients with renal artery stenosis. *Circulation.* 2005;111:328–333.
221. Dieter RS, Darki A, Nanjundappa A, et al. Usefulness of wide pulse pressure as a predictor of poor outcome after renal artery angioplasty and stenting. *Am J Cardiol.* 2009;104:732–734.
222. Mitchell JA, Subramanian R, White CJ, et al. Predicting blood pressure improvement in hypertensive patients after renal artery stent placement: renal fractional flow reserve. *Catheter Cardiovasc Interv.* 2007;69:685–689.
223. Modrall JG, Rosero EB, Leonard D, et al. Clinical and kidney morphologic predictors of outcome for renal artery stenting: data to inform patient selection. *J Vasc Surg.* 2011;53:1282–1289.

224. Modrall JG, Zhu H, Weaver FA. Clinical predictors of blood pressure response after renal artery stenting. *J Vasc Surg*. 2020;72(4):1269–1275.
225. Oktan MA, Sarioglu O, Heybeli C, et al. Predictors of kidney disease progression after renal artery stenting. *BMC Nephrol.* 2025;26(1):175.
226. Chobanian AV, Bakris GL, Black HR, et al. The seventh report of the joint national committee on prevention, detection, evaluation, and treatment of high blood pressure: the JNC 7 report. *JAMA*. 2003;289:2560–2572.
227. Vukadinović D, Lauder L, Kandzari DE, et al. Effects of catheter-based renal denervation in hypertension: a systematic review and meta-analysis. *Circulation*. 2024;150(20):1599–1611.
228. Stanley JC, Criado E, Upchurch GR Jr, et al. Pediatric renovascular hypertension: 132 primary and 30 secondary operations in 97 children. *J Vasc Surg*. 2006;44:1219–1228; discussion 1228–1229.
229. Silverstein DM, Champoux E, Aviles DH, Vehaskari VM. Treatment of primary and secondary hypertension in children. *Pediatr Nephrol*. 2006;21:820–827.
230. Tullus K, Brennan E, Hamilton G, et al. Renovascular hypertension in children. *Lancet*. 2008;371:1453–1463.
231. Coleman DM, Eliason JL, Beaulieu R, et al; University of Michigan Pediatric Renovascular Hypertension Center. Surgical management of pediatric renin-mediated hypertension secondary to renal artery occlusive disease and abdominal aortic coarctation. *J Vasc Surg*. 2020:72(6):2035–2046.e1.
232. Srinivasan A, Krishnamurthy G, Fontalvo-Herazo L, et al. Angioplasty for renal artery stenosis in pediatric patients: an 11-year retrospective experience. *J Vasc Interv Radiol*. 2010;21:1672–1680.
233. Shroff R, Roebuck DJ, Gordon I, et al. Angioplasty for renovascular hypertension in children: 20-year experience. *Pediatrics*. 2006;118:268–275.
234. Courtel JV, Soto B, Niaudet P, et al. Percutaneous transluminal angioplasty of renal artery stenosis in children. *Pediatr Radiol.* 1998;28:59–63.
235. Casalini E, Sfondrini MS, Fossali E. Two-year clinical follow-up of children and adolescents after percutaneous transluminal angioplasty for renovascular hypertension. *Invest Radiol.* 1995;30:40–43.
236. Eliason JL, Coleman DM, Criado E, et al. Remedial operations for failed endovascular therapy of 32 renal artery stenoses in 24 children. *Pediatr Nephrol*. 2016;31(5):809–817.
237. Stanley JC, Rhodes EL, Gewertz BL, Chang CY, Walter JF, Fry WJ. Renal artery aneurysms. Significance of macroaneurysms exclusive of dissections and fibrodysplastic mural dilations. *Arch Surg*. 1975;110:1327–1333.
238. McCarron JP Jr, Marshall VF, Whitsell JC 2nd. Indications for surgery on renal artery aneurysms. *J Urol*. 1975;114:177–180.
239. Tham G, Ekelund L, Herrlin K, Lindstedt EL, Olin T, Bergentz SE. Renal artery aneurysms. Natural history and prognosis. *Ann Surg*. 1983;197:348–352.
240. Henriksson C, Lukes P, Nilson AE, Pettersson S. Angiographically discovered, non-operated renal artery aneurysms. *Scand J Urol Nephrol*. 1984;18:59–62.
241. Klausner JQ, Harlander-Locke MP, Plotnik AN, Lehrman E, DeRubertis BG, Lawrence PF. Current treatment of renal artery aneurysms may be too aggressive. *J Vasc Surg*. 2014;59:1356–1361.
242. Klausner JQ, Lawrence PF, Harlander-Locke MP, Coleman DM, Stanley JC, Fujimura N; Vascular Low-Frequency Disease Consortium. The contemporary management of renal artery aneurysms. *J Vasc Surg*. 2015;61:978–984.
243. Wayne EJ, Edwards MS, Stafford JM, Hansen KJ, Corriere MA. Anatomic characteristics and natural history of renal artery aneurysms during longitudinal imaging surveillance. *J Vasc Surg*. 2014;60:448–452.
244. Pfeiffer T, Reiher L, Grabitz K, et al. Reconstruction for renal artery aneurysm: operative techniques and long-term results. *J Vasc Surg*. 2003;37:293–300.
245. Hupp T, Allenberg JR, Post K, Roeren T, Meier M, Clorius JH. Renal artery aneurysm: surgical indications and results. *Eur J Vasc Surg*. 1992;6:477–486.
246. Robinson WP 3rd, Bafford R, Belkin M, Menard MT. Favorable outcomes with in situ techniques for surgical repair of complex renal artery aneurysms. *J Vasc Surg*. 2011;53:684–691.
247. English WP, Pearce JD, Craven TE, et al. Surgical management of renal artery aneurysms. *J Vasc Surg*. 2004;40:53–60.
248. Coleman DM, Stanley JC. Renal artery aneurysms. *J Vasc Surg*. 2015;62:779–785.
249. Henke PK, Cardneau JD, Welling TH 3rd, et al. Renal artery aneurysms: a 35-year clinical experience with 252 aneurysms in 168 patients. *Ann Surg*. 2001;234:454–462; discussion 462–463.
250. Cohen JR, Shamash FS. Ruptured renal artery aneurysms during pregnancy. *J Vasc Surg*. 1987;6:51–59.
251. Martin RS 3rd, Meacham PW, Ditesheim JA, Mulherin JL Jr, Edwards WH. Renal artery aneurysm: selective treatment for hypertension and prevention of rupture. *J Vasc Surg*. 1989;9:26–34.
252. Hwang PF, Rice DC, Patel SV, Mukherjee D. Successful management of renal artery aneurysm rupture after cesarean section. *J Vasc Surg*. 2011;54:519–521.
253. Chandra A, O'Connell JB, Quinones-Baldrich WJ, et al. Aneurysmectomy with arterial reconstruction of renal artery aneurysms in the endovascular era: a safe, effective treatment for both aneurysm and associated hypertension. *Ann Vasc Surg*. 2010;24:503–510.
254. Tsilimparis N, Reeves JG, Dayama A, Perez SD, Debus ES, Ricotta JJ 2nd. Endovascular vs open repair of renal artery aneurysms: outcomes of repair and long-term renal function. *J Am Coll Surg*. 2013;217:263–269.
255. Gallagher KA, Phelan MW, Stern T, Bartlett ST. Repair of complex renal artery aneurysms by laparoscopic nephrectomy with ex vivo repair and autotransplantation. *J Vasc Surg*. 2008;48:1408–1413.
256. Luke P, Knudsen BE, Nguan CY, et al. Robot-assisted laparoscopic renal artery aneurysm reconstruction. *J Vasc Surg*. 2006;44:651–653.
257. Giulianotti PC, Bianco FM, Addeo P, Lombardi A, Coratti A, Sbrana F. Robot-assisted laparoscopic repair of renal artery aneurysms. *J Vasc Surg*. 2010;51:842–849.
258. Tipaldi MA, Zaccaria E, Ubaldi N, et al. Flow diverting stents for the treatment of complex visceral and renal aneurysms-a systematic review. *J Cardiovasc Dev Dis*. 2025;12(9):346.
259. Bratby MJ, Lehmann ED, Bottomley J, et al. Endovascular embolization of visceral artery aneurysms with ethylene-vinyl alcohol (Onyx): a case series. *Cardiovasc Intervent Radiol*. 2006;29:1125–1128.
260. Meyer C, Verrel F, Weyer G, Wilhelm K. Endovascular management of complex renal artery aneurysms using the multilayer stent. *Cardiovasc Intervent Radiol*. 2011;34:637–641.
261. Manninen HI, Berg M, Vanninen RL. Stent-assisted coil embolization of wide-necked renal artery bifurcation aneurysms. *J Vasc Interv Radiol*. 2008;19:487–492.
262. Etezadi V, Gandhi RT, Benenati JF, et al. Endovascular treatment of visceral and renal artery aneurysms. *J Vasc Interv Radiol*. 2011;22:1246–1253.
263. Sedat J, Chau Y, Baque J. Endovascular treatment of renal aneurysms: a series of 18 cases. *Eur J Radiol*. 2012;81:3973–3978.
264. Zhang Z, Yang M, Song L, Tong X, Zou Y. Endovascular treatment of renal artery aneurysms and renal arteriovenous fistulas. *J Vasc Surg*. 2013;57:765–770.
265. Hislop SJ, Patel SA, Abt PL, Singh MJ, Illig KA. Therapy of renal artery aneurysms in New York State: outcomes of patients undergoing open and endovascular repair. *Ann Vasc Surg*. 2009;23:194–200.

87

Aortoiliac Occlusive Disease

Loay S. Kabbani, Mitchell R. Weaver, and Alexander D. Shepard

Key Points

1 Aortoiliac occlusive disease is mainly the result of atherosclerosis.

2 Claudication is the most common presenting symptom of patients with significant aortoiliac occlusive disease. Male patients may complain of erectile dysfunction. Physical examination typically reveals diminished or absent femoral pulses.

3 Medical treatment of atherosclerotic aortoiliac occlusive disease is key to long-term success. Such treatment includes risk factor modification (smoking cessation, control of hypertension, lipid abnormalities, and diabetes mellitus), supervised walking programs, and pharmacotherapy.

4 Smoking is the most important reversible risk factor for the development of lower extremity atherosclerotic occlusive disease.

5 Endovascular approaches are favored for most candidates with aortoiliac disease requiring intervention, though open revascularization is sometimes required.

Peripheral arterial disease (PAD) is usually a manifestation of systemic atherosclerosis, affecting 15% to 20% of the general
1 population older than 50 years. Approximately 50% of patients with PAD are asymptomatic.[1,2] Atherosclerotic occlusive disease of the aorta and iliac arteries alone, or in combination with femoropopliteal or tibial occlusive disease, is the most frequent cause of chronic lower extremity arterial insufficiency.

The wide availability of computed tomographic angiography (CTA) and magnetic resonance angiography (MRA) has facilitated diagnosis, anatomic definition, and subsequent intervention for aortoiliac occlusive disease (AIOD). Creation of a patient-specific treatment plan from an increasing array of treatment alternatives, although sometimes challenging, is often successful in alleviating symptoms and reducing the risk of disease progression. Endovascular and open reconstructive procedures for AIOD have become routine, with low perioperative morbidity and mortality and excellent early and long-term outcomes.

ETIOLOGY

Atherosclerosis is a systemic disease. The earliest lesions tend to occur at arterial bifurcations and in areas of relative fixation, which disrupts normal laminar flow with resultant eddy currents producing areas of low arterial wall shear stress. Injured areas of the artery wall release chemical signals that can lead to cholesterol and cell waste to collect at damaged spots. This buildup attracts white blood cells that take up the cholesterol and release inflammatory signals ultimately leading to plaque formation. Arteriopathies other than atherosclerosis, such as Takayasu disease and radiation arteritis, can also involve the aortoiliac system. Understanding the risk factors that increase the risk of atherosclerosis is vital for proper diagnosis (**Table 87.1**). Smoking is the most important reversible risk factor for the development of lower extremity atherosclerotic occlusive disease.

ANATOMY AND PATHOPHYSIOLOGY

The arteries supplying blood to the lower extremities are frequently divided into abdominal, or "inflow," arteries (the aorta and iliac arteries) and infrainguinal, or "outflow," arteries (the femoropopliteal and tibial arteries).

In slowly developing aortoiliac occlusive lesions, hemodynamic alterations lead to the enlargement of a network of collateral channels around the involved segments; this collateral network is usually sufficient to provide enough blood flow to meet the resting metabolic needs of the lower extremities (**Figs. 87.1** and **87.2**). These collaterals, however, do not have the capacity to increase blood flow to the level necessary to meet exercise demands of the lower extremity musculature.

PRESENTATION

Patients with symptoms of AIOD usually present in their 50s and 60s, whereas patients with infrainguinal disease or multilevel disease (AIOD + infrainguinal disease) generally present in their 70s.[3]

- Claudication (Latin *claudicare* = "to limp") is the term used to denote the characteristic exercise-induced, cramping pain in the muscles of the lower extremity that results from demand ischemia.[4,5] Claudication is the most common presenting symptom of patients with AIOD and is typically
2 described as a cramping pain or easy fatigability of the involved muscle groups which is induced by ambulation and quickly relieved by rest. Although patients with AIOD classically present with claudication of the thighs, hips, and buttocks, a significant number complain of calf claudication alone or have significant overlap. Erectile dysfunction in men secondary to reduced hypogastric perfusion is another common complaint and may be reported in up to 30% to 50% of men with AIOD. The combination of bilateral lower extremity claudication, atrophy of the lower extremity musculature, impotence, and diminished or absent femoral pulses is known as Leriche syndrome, after the French surgeon René Leriche, who first described this constellation of findings in 1940.[6,7]
- Chronic limb-threatening ischemia (CLTI)[4] is a more advanced form of PAD; symptoms include ischemic rest pain, nonhealing wounds, or gangrene. CLTI almost always

Table 87.1. Risk Factors for Peripheral Arterial Disease

Risk Factors Associated with Peripheral Artery Disease
Smoking
Diabetes
Obesity
Hypertension
Hyperlipidemia
Family history
Chronic kidney disease
Advanced age
Atherosclerosis in other vascular beds (eg, the heart)

occurs in the presence of multilevel disease, AIOD in combination with femoral-popliteal and/or tibial-pedal level arterial occlusive disease. In the absence of infrainguinal arterial occlusive disease, aortoiliac collaterals are usually capable of maintaining adequate resting limb perfusion.

- Acute arterial occlusions from emboli lodging at the aortic, iliac, or femoral bifurcations do not allow time for collateral pathways to mature and compensate for the sudden loss of blood supply. This situation leads to the acute onset of symptoms, with the resulting 5 "Ps" of acute ischemia: pain, pallor, pulselessness, paresthesia, and paresis/paralysis. Downstream embolism of debris from proximal atherosclerotic plaques into the microcirculation of the lower extremities ("trash foot") can produce dermal discoloration in a characteristic reticular pattern (livedo reticularis), digital ischemia, or even gangrene (**Fig. 87.3A,B**). Such patients may have palpable pedal pulses. Embolic events may occur spontaneously or may be induced by endovascular interventions, from guidewire or device manipulation, or open vascular surgery, from clamping or manipulating an artery with unstable plaque.

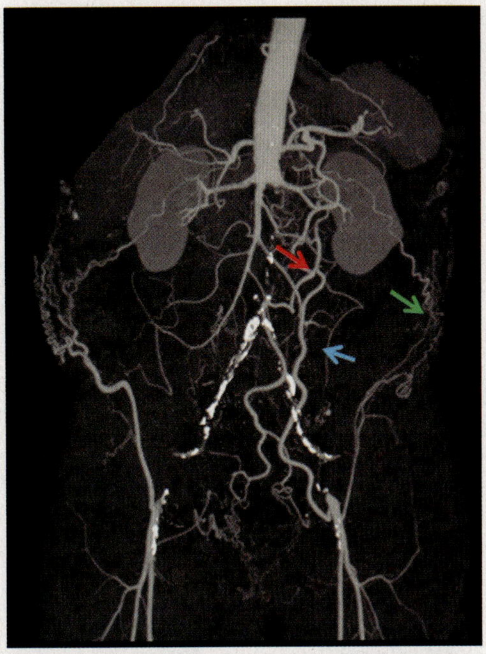

Figure 87.2. CTA with 3D reconstruction demonstrating severe aortoiliac occlusive disease with juxtarenal aortic occlusion. Note the extensive collateral networks reconstituting the inferior mesenteric artery (*red arrow*: meandering mesenteric artery), femoral arterial segments (*blue arrow*: inferior epigastric artery), and (*green arrow*: subcostal arteries and superficial iliac circumflex artery collaterals).

Physical examination typically reveals diminished or absent femoral pulses. A bruit auscultated over the groin or lower abdomen is not specific for critical stenosis. Severely diseased, calcified femoral arteries may be palpable as firm, tubular structures in the groin. Normal femoral and distal pulses may be palpable, even in the presence of hemodynamically significant aortoiliac stenosis. These pulses, however, rapidly disappear following ambulation, as the increased flow demands of the exercising leg muscles lead to lowered peripheral vascular resistance and reduced distal arterial pressure. Patients with longstanding aortoiliac atherosclerosis may have disuse atrophy of the lower extremity musculature. Other common signs

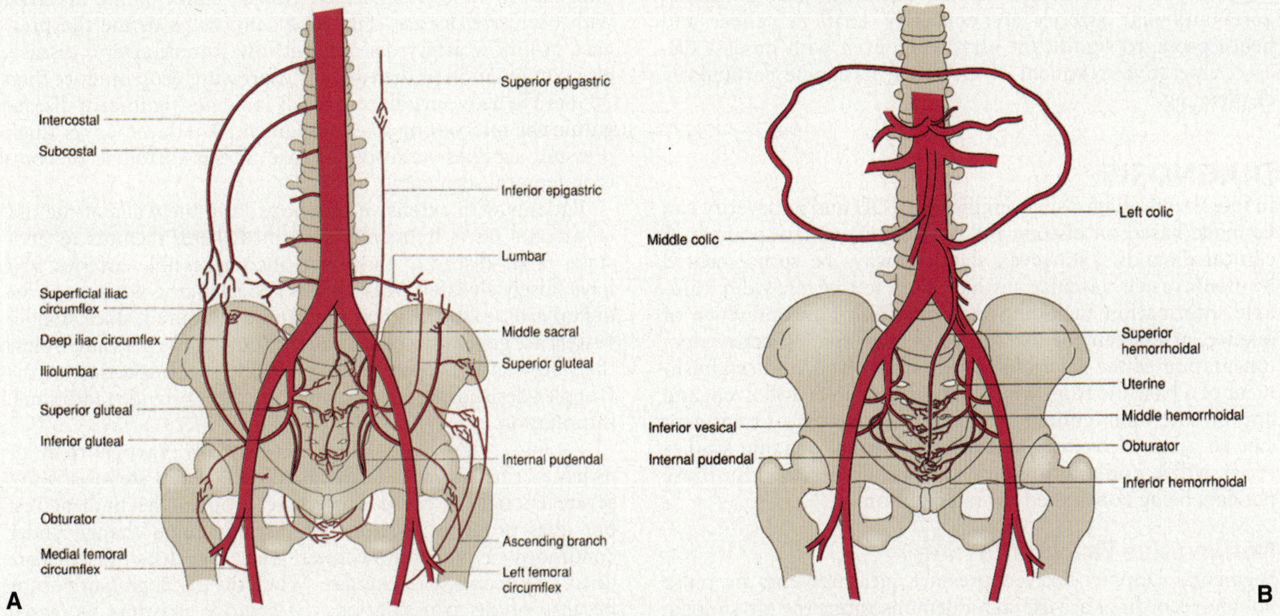

Figure 87.1. **A,B:** Major visceral and parietal collateral networks that may become prominent with aortoiliac occlusive disease.

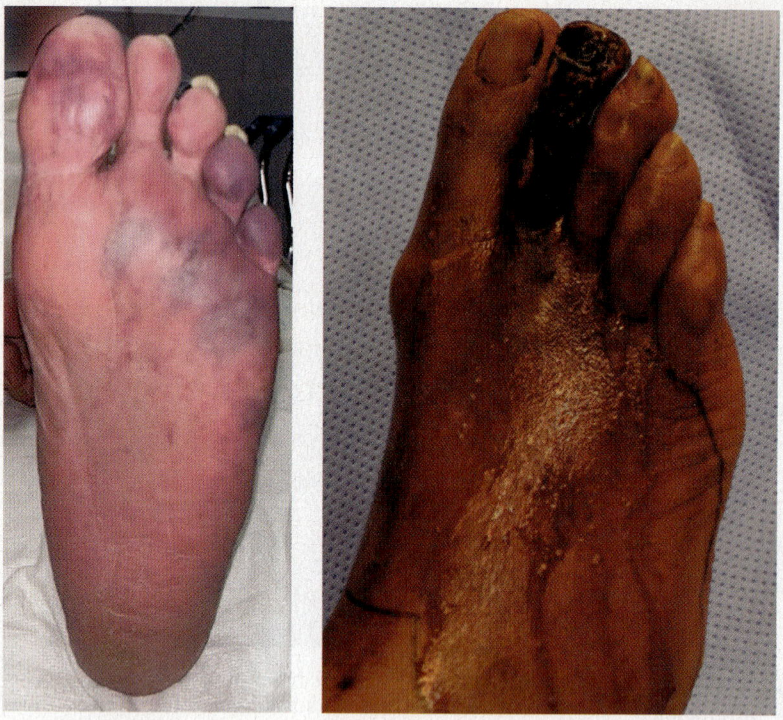

A B

Figure 87.3. Digital atheroembolization. **A:** Presents as "trash foot", (**B**) or localized gangrene.

of lower extremity arterial occlusive disease include trophic changes, such as hair loss on the legs or toes, and thin, shiny skin on the feet; patients with severe reductions in pedal blood flow may display pedal rubor with limb dependency, coupled with pallor on elevation.

Clinical Pathologic Types of Aortoiliac Disease

The Trans-Atlantic Inter-Society Consensus for the Management of PAD (TASC II) has classified AIOD into four types, A through D (**Table 87.2**).[8] Patients with limited disease (TASC II types A, B, C) requiring intervention can usually be treated with endovascular means, while those with more advanced disease (TASC II D) are more challenging and require complex endovascular, hybrid surgical, or open surgical approaches.

Aortoiliac hypoplasia also known as *small aortic syndrome* or *hypoplastic aortic syndrome,* is encountered in young to middle-aged women who smoke cigarettes. The infrarenal aorta and iliac arteries are unusually small in caliber and hence prone to significant narrowing, even with modest disease. Operative treatment of such patients can be particularly challenging.[9]

DIAGNOSIS

In most cases, diagnosing significant AIOD and its severity can be made based on history and physical examination alone. A clinical diagnosis, however, should always be supplemented by noninvasive vascular testing. Such testing provides valuable information including confirmation of the presence of disease, assessment of the degree of ischemia, objective documentation of the arterial segment(s) involved, and establishment of a baseline from which the patient can be followed, and appropriate interventions planned. Effectiveness of treatment can be assessed by repeated testing. Formal imaging studies (CTA, MRA, and arteriography) are usually reserved for those patients being considered for intervention.

Noninvasive Vascular Testing

Segmental Doppler-derived pressure measurements or pulse volume recordings are useful for demonstrating the physiologic significance of disease and can help localize hemodynamically significant lesions. Measurement of systolic arterial pressures at different levels of the lower extremity with a continuous wave Doppler flow probe is the simplest and most useful noninvasive method to assess the presence and severity of arterial occlusive disease. The ratio of the ankle systolic pressure (measured in either the dorsalis pedis or the posterior tibial arteries) to the brachial systolic pressure (using the higher of the two brachial pressures) is the ankle-brachial index (ABI), or pressure ratio, and is a good measure of the degree of ischemia present.[10] Normal ABIs are generally equal to or slightly greater than 1.0 (**Fig. 87.4**). PAD is designated when the ABI is ≤0.90. Patients with claudication usually have ABIs ranging from 0.50 to 0.90, whereas patients with rest pain, tissue loss, or gangrene usually have ABIs of <0.50[10] (**Table 87.3**).

Determination of limb systolic pressures at different locations (with the "four-cuff" technique, where pressures are measured at the upper thigh, lower thigh, calf, and ankle) provides information concerning which arterial segments are involved with occlusive disease (**Fig. 87.4**) and helps define the presence of inflow artery disease, outflow (runoff artery) disease, or a combination of the two.[11,12] A pressure drop of more than 20 mm Hg between adjacent levels indicates significant disease within the intervening arterial segment. A reduced upper thigh pressure signifies occlusive disease in the aortoiliac or common femoral segments.

Patients with extensive calcification in the walls of the tibial arteries (as is frequently seen in diabetes mellitus or end-stage renal disease), may have incompressible arteries and have falsely elevated ABIs. In this situation, the pressure in the digital arteries of the great toe can be measured, since smaller vessels are generally spared calcification. A toe pressure of less than 30 mm Hg indicates severe ischemia. Inspection of the Doppler-derived arterial waveforms can provide additional information.

Patients with claudication occasionally have normal or nearly normal ABIs. In such cases, the arterial stenosis is not severe enough to cause a pressure drop in the limb at rest but does produce a significant hemodynamic change under conditions of higher flow rates when the distal vasculature dilates, as occurs with exercise. When the distal pressure drops because of vascular dilation, the stenosis prevents increased blood flow into the extremity resulting in a significant distal

Table 87.2. TASC II Classification

Type A: Limited stenoses (<3 cm) of the common or external iliac arteries	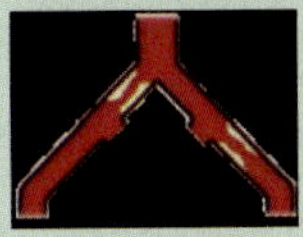
Type B: Short stenoses of the infrarenal aorta and short stenoses or occlusion of the iliac arteries	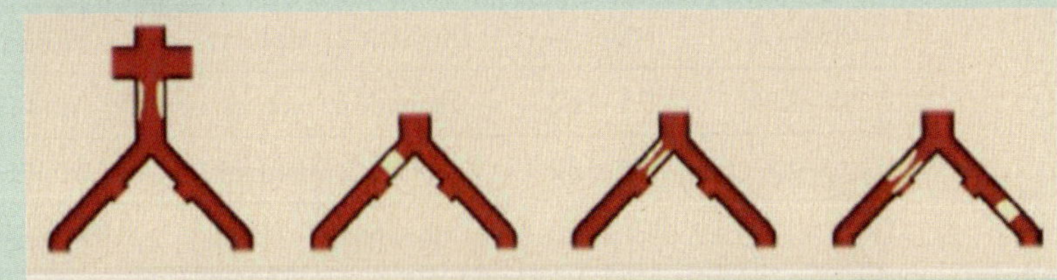
Type C: Longer stenoses and/or occlusions of the iliac arteries, especially when calcified	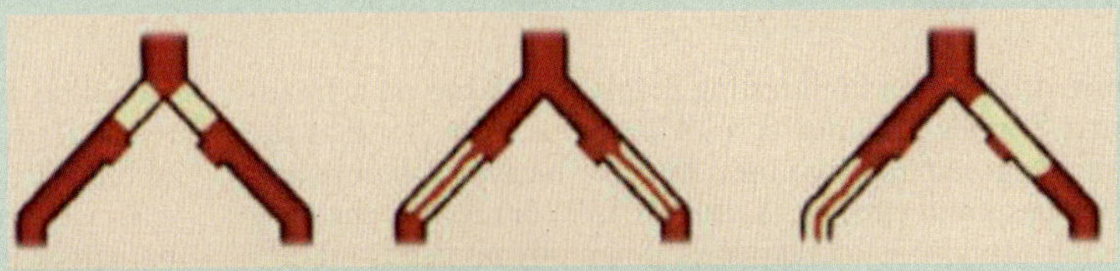
Type D: Infrarenal aortic occlusion sometimes with multiple iliac occlusions and stenoses or associated aneurysm disease	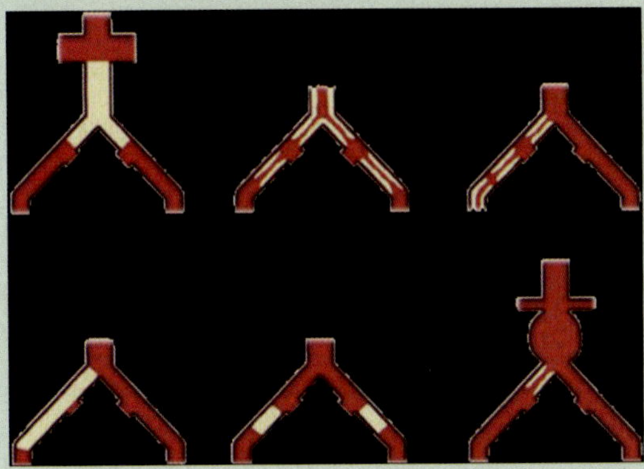

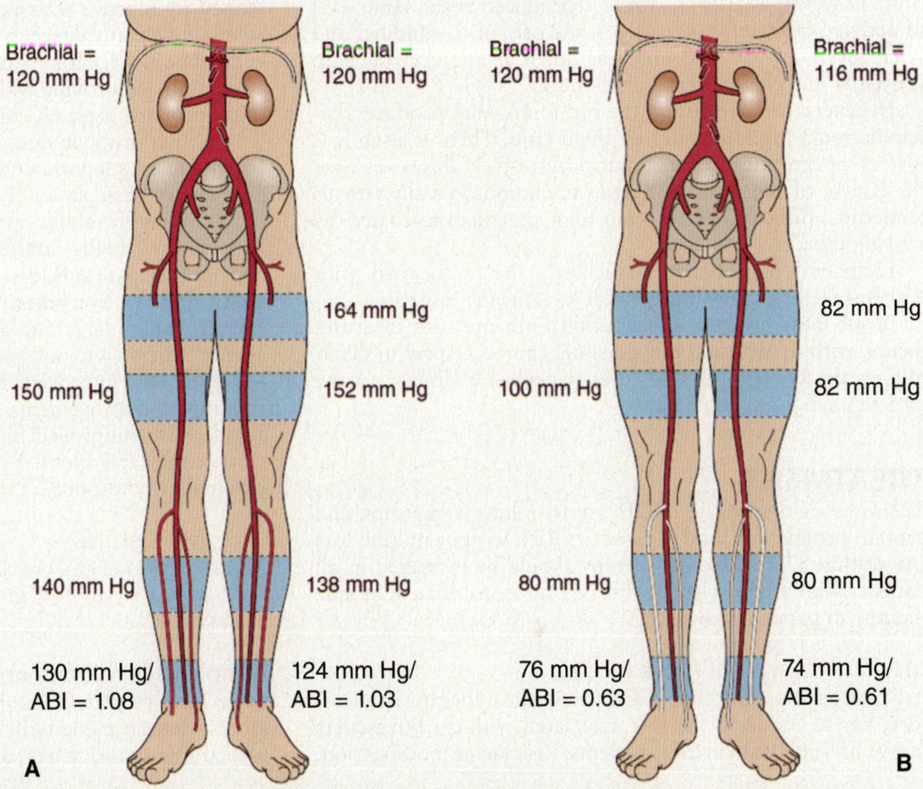

Figure 87.4. Segmental pressure measurements typical of normal results (**A**) and aortoiliac occlusive disease (**B**). In **B**, the right side shows a drop in pressure between the thigh and calf indicating femoral popliteal disease, on the left, the pressure in the thigh is decreased indicating iliac disease.

Table 87.3. Ankle-Brachial Indices (ABIs)

Ankle Brachial Indices (ABI) and Toe Brachial Indices (TBI)

ABI Value	TBI Value	Doppler Waveform	Disease
>1.2			Heavily calcified (incompressible) vessels
0.95–1.2	>0.63	Biphasic or triphasic	Normal
0.8–0.95	0.4–0.62	Biphasic or monophasic	Mild
0.5–0.8	0.2–0.39	Biphasic or monophasic	Moderate
<0.5	<0.2	Monophasic	Severe

pressure drops. Treadmill testing involves walking on a treadmill at 1.5 miles per hour at a 14% incline for as long as the patient can go, up to 5 minutes. ABIs are measured before and after the treadmill exercise; a drop of 15% or more in the ABIs following exercise is indicative of a hemodynamically significant stenosis.[10]

Duplex scanning of the aorta and iliac arteries has been advocated by some as a noninvasive diagnostic tool. Accurate imaging of the abdominal arteries, however, can be difficult because of their deep retroperitoneal and pelvic locations, which can be further degraded by body habitus and overlying bowel gas. These drawbacks have limited the widespread use of this modality.[13] Arteriography, CTA, and MRA may be used for diagnosis, but are usually performed only after interventional therapy is contemplated, and are discussed later.[12]

Differential Diagnosis

The diagnosis of symptomatic AIOD is usually straightforward, but occasional diagnostic difficulty may arise when other causes of lower extremity pain are present (**Table 87.4**).[4] Irritation of lumbosacral nerve roots by spinal stenosis or intervertebral disc herniation may cause buttock and leg pain associated with activity. Such symptoms (neurogenic claudication), however, usually cannot be reproduced at the same level of activity, frequently occur when the patient is standing, and are relieved only by sitting or lying down. In addition, the pain is usually in a classic sciatic distribution.

Degenerative arthritis of the hip joints may produce similar buttock, hip, and referred thigh pain. There is usually a history of morning stiffness that progressively improves over the course of the day. Physical examination typically reveals tenderness directly over the hip joint that is exacerbated by moving the joint.

Peripheral neuropathy, particularly that associated with diabetes mellitus, may masquerade as ischemic rest pain.

In all these situations, segmental limb pressure measurements, with or without stress testing, can be helpful in determining the contribution of arterial occlusive disease to the patient's symptom complex.

TREATMENT

The aims of therapy in AIOD are to relieve symptoms and prevent progression, and in cases of CLTI, to prevent limb loss (**Algorithm 87.1**). Medical therapy should be instituted in all patients with atherosclerotic disease, but is insufficient as sole therapy in patients with CLTI.

3 Medical Therapy (Table 87.5)

Atherosclerosis is a systemic disease. Medical therapy is, therefore, key to reducing the risk associated with cardiovascular morbidity and death in these patients. Risk factor modification, including management of diabetes mellitus, control of hypertension, treatment of hyperlipidemia, and finally modification of lifestyle, including smoking cessation, appropriate diet, and exercise, are the most important components of the care of patients with atherosclerotic disease.[14–16]

4 Smoking Cessation

Smoking is associated with a subclinical inflammatory reaction. The degree of damage caused by smoking is directly related to the amount of tobacco consumed.[17] All patients who are smokers or former smokers should be asked about the status of tobacco use at every visit. All patients should be strongly advised to stop tobacco use (in all forms) by their physicians. All patients should be offered pharmacotherapy, behavior modification, referral to a smoking cessation program, and counseling. Smoking cessation alters the progression of the atherosclerotic process and may even reduce the severity of claudication.[18] Furthermore, it is an important step to reducing postprocedure complications in patients undergoing intervention.[19]

Exercise

Supervised exercise programs have been consistently demonstrated to improve walking time and walking distance and in some studies, supervised exercise has been as effective as revascularization.[19,20] Home and community-based therapy are effective for improving walking tolerance but are less effective than formal supervised exercise programs and are associated with a high dropout rate, underscoring the need for ongoing psychological support.[21] Outcomes of supervised exercise programs have been shown to be similar and longer lasting than those of endovascular interventions for mild claudication. Patients are usually advised to walk until the onset of pain, rest until the pain subsides, and repeat the cycle for 30 minutes a day, three to five times per week. A 3- to 6-month trial of exercise should be initiated before revascularization is considered in patients with intermittent claudication. Mechanisms of action include improvements in skeletal muscle strength and endurance, improvements in endothelial function, potential angiogenesis, improved blood distribution efficiency leading to potential calf blood flow increases, and a reduced local inflammatory response.[16]

Glycemic Control

Aggressive blood glucose control is important in patients with PAD, with a target A1C goal of <7.0%, and as close to 6.0% as possible.[16]

Antiplatelet Therapy and Antithrombotic Therapy

Some form of platelet inhibition should be considered for all atherosclerotic patients in order to reduce the risk of myocardial infarction, stroke, and death known as major adverse

Table 87.4. Differential Diagnosis of Claudication

The Differential Diagnosis for Intermittent Claudication (IC)							
Condition	**Location**	**Prevalence**	**Characteristic Symptom(s)**	**Effect of Exercise**	**Effect of Rest**	**Effect of Position**	**Other Characteristics**
Calf IC	Calf muscles	Common	Cramping, aching, discomfort	Reproducible onset	Quickly relieved	None	
Thigh and buttock IC	Buttocks, hip, thigh	Less common	Cramping, aching discomfort	Reproducible onset	Quickly relieved	None	Erectile dysfunction. May have normal pedal pulses with isolated iliac artery disease
Venous claudication	Entire leg, worse in calf	Rare	Tight, bursting pain	After walking	Subsides slowly	Relief faster with elevation	History of deep vein thrombosis
Nerve root compression	Radiates down leg	Common	Sharp lancinating pain	Induced by sitting, standing, or walking	Often present at rest	Improved by change in position	History of spine issues, present with standing or walking
Spinal stenosis	Often bilateral buttocks, posterior leg	Common	Pain and weakness	Induced by standing, or walking	Variable relief, but can take a long time to recover	Relief by lumbar spine flexion	Worse with standing and extending spine
Symptomatic Baker cyst	Pain behind knee, down into calf	Common	Swelling, tenderness	Present with exercise	Present at rest	None	
Hip arthritis	Lateral hip, thigh	Common	Aching discomfort	After variable degree of exercise	Not quickly relieved	Improved when not weight bearing or moving	History of degenerative arthritis
Chronic compartment syndrome	Calf muscles	Rare	Tight, bursting pain	After significant exercise (jogging)	Subsides very slowly	Relief with elevation	Usually athletes

Algorithm 87.1

- **Mild (claudication)**
  - Risk factor modification:
    1. Smoking cessation
    2. Antiplatelet therapy
    3. Statin therapy
    4. Consider ACE inhibitor
    5. Consider a trial of cilostazol
    6. Supervised exercise program
- **Moderate (lifestyle-limiting claudication)**
  - Risk factor modification plus
  - Consider revascularization
  - Endovascular vs. hybrid vs. open surgery
- **Severe (rest pain/tissue loss)**
  - Risk factor modification plus
  - Evaluate for revascularization
  - Endovascular vs. hybrid vs. open surgery

ACE, angiotensin-converting enzyme.

Algorithm 87.1. Patient with symptomatic aortoiliac occlusive disease.

Table 87.5. AHA Guidelines for Medical Therapy of Patients with PAD[14,15]

Medical Therapy for Patients with PAD[14,15]

Cardiovascular risk reduction	
Lipid management	Statin therapy should be prescribed for all patients with PAD with LDL-C goal of <70 mg/dL PCSK9 inhibitors are indicated in patients with PAD who have not achieved an LDL target of <70 mg/dL Ezetimibe may be used in patients with PAD who have not achieved an LDL target of <70 mg/dL
Diabetes	A coordinated effort among clinicians is essential, and a diabetes care plan should be customized to everyone depending on clinical status and risk factors Hg A1C goal <7% or as close to 6% as possible Glucagon-like peptide-1 agonists and SGLT-2 inhibitors have been demonstrated to reduce MACE
Hypertension management	A systolic blood pressure (SBP) goal of <130 mm Hg and a diastolic blood pressure target of <80 mm Hg is recommended In patients with PAD and hypertension, the selective use of angiotensin-converting enzyme (ACE) inhibitors or angiotensin-receptor blockers is recommended
Smoking cessation	Counsel on stopping smoking Referral to smoking cessation program Offer pharmacotherapy Avoid exposure to secondhand tobacco smoke
Antiplatelet therapy and possibly antithrombotic therapy	
Antiplatelet therapy	Start aspirin (75–325 mg) daily or clopidogrel 75 mg daily
Antithrombotic therapy	May add rivaroxaban 2.5 mg BID to the antiplatelet therapy
Cilostazol	For chronic symptomatic PAD
Structured exercise	Although the evidence base is strongest for supervised exercise therapy (SET), other forms of exercise programs, including home-based exercise is effective
Preventive foot care	Providing preventive foot self-care education to patients and their support persons and a yearly examination is recommended
Vaccination	Patients with PAD should receive an annual influenza vaccination

MACE, major adverse cardiac events.

cardiac events (MACE), but little effect on major amputation and endovascular or surgical lower-extremity revascularization known as major adverse limb events (MALE).[16] Aspirin is the most commonly used agent, but P2Y12 inhibitors (eg, clopidogrel) is at least as effective and may be better. Low-dose anticoagulation with rivaroxaban (2.5 mg twice daily) in addition to low-dose aspirin has been shown to have improved MACE and MALE, but at a cost of higher bleeding rates.[20]

Hypertension Therapy[14,15]

Treatment of hypertension reduces MACE in patients with PAD. The concern that lower blood pressure may compromise blood flow in lower extremity PAD and worsen limb symptoms has not been demonstrated. On the contrary multiple studies have documented improvement in claudication symptoms and functional status in patients with PAD and treated hypertension, even when using beta blockers.[15] Goal systolic blood pressure ≤130 mm Hg and diastolic blood pressure ≤80 mm Hg is recommended.

Lipid-Lowering Therapy

Lowering LDL-C to levels <70 mg/dL is recommended in patients with symptomatic PAD. High-intensity statin (taking the highest tolerated statin dose) therapy lowers rates of MACE and MALE in patients with PAD. PCSK9 inhibitors are recommended in patients with PAD who cannot achieve an LDL target of <70 mg/dL on statin therapy. Ezetimibe can also be added to help achieve lower LDL-C.

Other Pharmacologic Therapy

Cilostazol and naftidrofuryl can be valuable adjuncts in selected patients with severe lifestyle-limiting claudication.[23] A therapeutic trial (3 to 6 months) may be tried. Although the mechanisms of action of these agents are unclear, a modest but significant reduction in claudication symptoms and an increase in maximum walking distance have been shown in controlled trials. Benefit has not been firmly established for other agents.

Indications for Revascularization

Revascularization is clearly indicated in patients with CLTI; without intervention, these patients can progress to limb loss in a short time. One year following onset of CLTI symptoms, it is estimated that 25% of patients will lose their limb, 25% will suffer a cardiovascular death, but only 1% to 2% of patients with claudication will progress to CLTI per year.[4]

Patients with significant or repetitive atheroembolism from an aortoiliac source represent another group that clearly benefits from early operative intervention. Removal or bypass of the culprit lesion(s) eliminates the risk for further macro- and microembolism.

The treatment of patients with claudication secondary to AIOD remains controversial and must be individualized. Patients with mild to moderate symptoms can usually be treated medically with satisfactory results, while patients with severe, disabling, and/or lifestyle-limiting claudication symptoms can benefit from revascularization therapy.

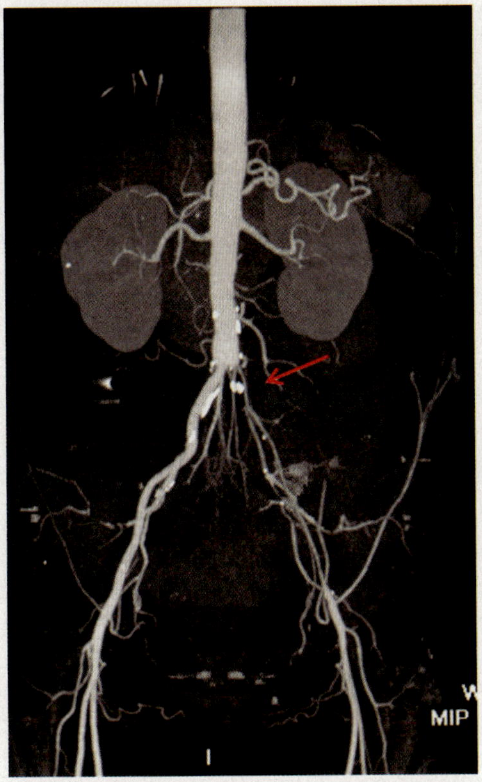

Figure 87.5. CTA 3D reconstruction showing left iliac artery occlusion (*red arrow*).

Preintervention Imaging Studies

Once a decision has been made to proceed with revascularization, imaging studies are critical for developing a treatment strategy.

Computed Tomographic Angiography

CTA with reformatting requires the intravenous administration of iodinated contrast material, followed by a timed CT scan of the abdomen, pelvis, and bilateral lower extremities. Volume data sets are then processed into axial, coronal, and sagittal imaging planes and reprocessed into three-dimensional images (**Figs. 87.2, 87.5, 87.6, 87.9**). Sensitivity and specificity are greater than 92% and 93%, respectively, for detecting >50% stenosis. The main drawbacks of CTA are the ionizing radiation and the use of iodinated contrast, which can cause allergic reactions in addition to contrast-induced nephropathy.[24]

Magnetic Resonance Angiography

Contrast-enhanced MRA uses intravenous administration of paramagnetic gadolinium-based agents. With good technique, contrast-enhanced MRA has a sensitivity of 80% to 97%, and a specificity of 73% to 96% (**Fig. 87.9**).[25] The disadvantage of MRA is that it cannot be used in patients with certain metallic implants (eg, pacemakers) and patients with claustrophobia. Furthermore, the spatial resolution of MRA cannot match that of CTA. With newer contrast agents, the risk of gadolinium-induced systemic fibrosis has been significantly reduced.

Digital Subtraction Arteriography

Abdominal aortography, with demonstration of the arterial tree below the inguinal ligament ("runoff"), is rarely performed for diagnostic work up.

The information supplied by CTA, MRA, or arteriography is critical to the planning and success of a revascularization procedure. In addition to providing a detailed "road map" of the exact arterial segments involved, such imaging identifies associated anatomic variations (eg, accessory renal arteries) and aortic wall characteristics (eg, extensive calcification and ulcerated plaque), which may alter the operative approach and the conduct of the procedure. During an open revascularization procedure, a surgeon who knows that the aortic wall just below the renal arteries is heavily diseased with ulcerated plaque may, for example, opt to control the aorta at a more proximal level rather than risk dislodging atheromatous debris with standard infrarenal aortic clamping. Similarly, documented occlusive lesions in the visceral or renal arteries or suspected lesions (eg, a patent inferior mesenteric artery with a large "meandering mesenteric artery") may best be addressed at the time of aortic reconstruction, or require particular attention to avoid complications.

Preoperative Evaluation

Patients with significant AIOD may have atherosclerotic occlusive disease in other vascular territories (eg, coronary and cerebral) that can increase their operative risk. The detection and treatment of significant coronary artery disease is particularly important, because myocardial infarction is the leading cause of both perioperative and late mortality. In patients with significant aortoiliac disease, more than 50% have clinical or electrocardiographic evidence of coronary disease.[26] In the Coronary Artery Revascularization Prophylaxis (CARP) trial, patients undergoing elective, open, abdominal aortic surgery for aortoiliac occlusive or aneurysmal disease at Veterans Administration hospitals were assessed for cardiac risk.[27] With optimal medical management, there was no difference in outcome between those who underwent coronary revascularization prior to aortic surgery and those who did not. Only selected patients, therefore, require cardiac catheterization and occasional coronary angioplasty or bypass grafting before undergoing open aortic reconstruction, and these patients need to be stratified according to risk guidelines.[28]

Respiratory complications occur in 10% to 15% of patients following open aortoiliac reconstruction, and pulmonary function should be assessed preoperatively only if clinical evaluation cannot determine that the patient is at his/her best achievable baseline pulmonary function and that airway obstruction has not been optimally treated. There is otherwise no indication for routine preoperative pulmonary function testing, as the American College of Physicians guidelines state that routine preoperative spirometry is not useful for predicting the risk of postoperative pulmonary complications.[29] Smokers who quit more than 4 weeks before surgery have a significantly lower risk of respiratory complications and improved wound healing.

Assessment of renal function is also important as vascular interventions can lead to acute kidney injury with a consequent increase in morbidity and mortality. Patients with preoperative chronic kidney disease need to be risk-stratified and appropriate steps taken to minimize further kidney injury with intervention.

Choice of Revascularization Technique

A variety of surgical procedures, both endovascular and open or a combination (hybrid), are available for revascularization of patients with AIOD. Selection depends on a number of factors, including the pattern of the occlusive process, patient risk, surgeon experience, and patient preference.

Commonly used techniques include (a) catheter-based balloon dilation (angioplasty) with or without luminal stenting, (b) arterial reconstruction with an anatomically placed prosthetic bypass graft (aorto-femoral or iliofemoral bypass), (c) arterial reconstruction with a remote (or extra-anatomically placed) prosthetic bypass graft (axillofemoral or axillobifemoral, femorofemoral, thoracofemoral bypass), (d) aortoiliac endarterectomy, and increasingly commonly (e) a hybrid approach encompassing a combination of endovascular and open procedures.

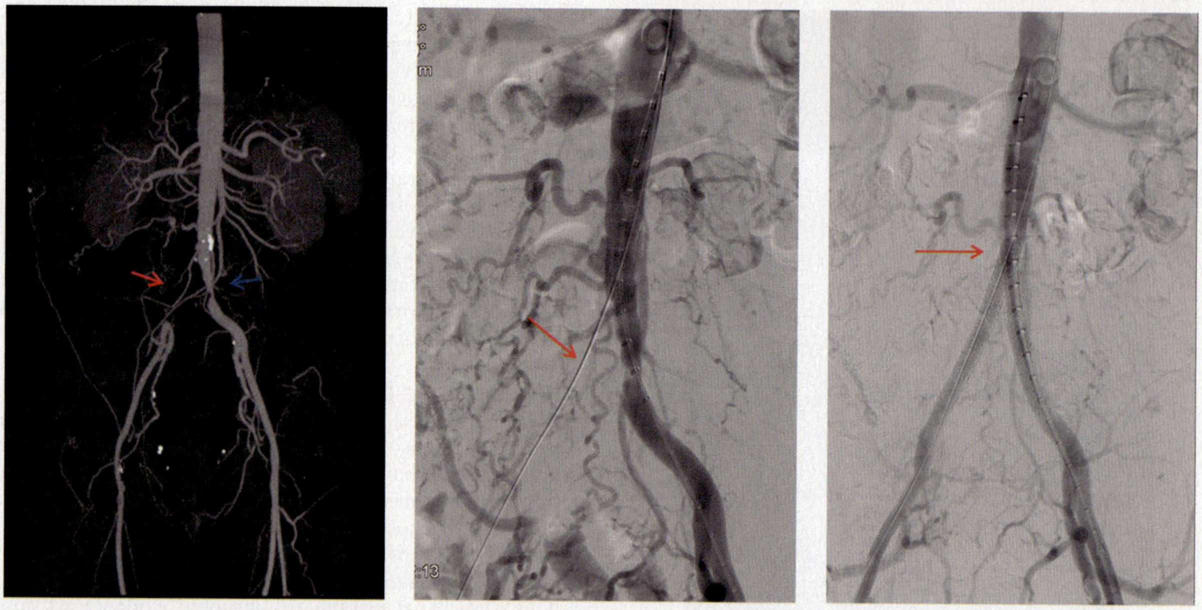

A, B C

Figure 87.6. A: CTA 3D reconstruction demonstrating right common iliac artery chronic total occlusion (*red arrow*) and severe left common iliac artery stenosis (*blue arrow*). B: Abdominal aortogram redemonstrating right common iliac artery occlusion and left common iliac artery stenosis. Note successful wire traversal of the right common iliac artery occlusion (*red arrow*). C: Abdominal aortogram demonstrating successful endoluminal bilateral common iliac artery revascularization following percutaneous balloon angioplasty and stent placement. Note the "kissing" stents in the distal aorta (*red arrow*).

5 Endovascular Surgical Management

Percutaneous transluminal angioplasty (PTA) with or without stenting has become the most commonly performed and, in many cases, the preferred therapy for iliac artery occlusive disease. The best results are obtained with short, focal, stenotic lesions in the common iliac arteries. Patients with more severe atherosclerotic lesions, complicated stenoses, and occlusions may also benefit from complex endovascular approaches, with many series documenting excellent short and intermediate-term success. Atheromatous embolism ("blue toe" syndrome) (**Fig. 87.3A**) from an ulcerative plaque may be treated with placement of a stent to trap the debris, relieve the stenosis, and prevent recurrent embolism.

Description of Technique

Thoughtful preprocedural planning sets the stage for a successful endovascular intervention. Although not absolutely necessary, CTA or MRA can delineate the location, extent, and degree of stenosis and associated calcification (**Fig. 87.6A**).

Other considerations include the possible need for a concomitant femoral endarterectomy. When there is significant common femoral artery disease (>50% stenosis) along with iliac occlusive disease, a femoral endarterectomy with patch angioplasty should always be considered. The endarterectomy should extend as high as possible under the inguinal ligament into the external iliac artery to facilitate stent deployment into the proximal endarterectomized segment, but avoid its placement into the common femoral artery itself.

A hydrophilic wire with an angled tip, usually a guidewire (Terumo Interventional Systems, Somerset, NJ) and a straight or angled catheter for support are utilized to cross the stenosis or occlusion. Common iliac artery disease is treated through an ipsilateral retrograde approach if the external iliac is open. If the common iliac artery is occluded, bilateral punctures of the femoral arteries will be necessary to perform aortography to delineate the extent of obstruction (**Fig. 87.6B**). In the absence of significant ipsilateral common femoral artery disease, external iliac disease is usually approached antegrade through a contralateral femoral puncture and a wire passed "up and over" the aortic bifurcation.

When the significance of a stenosis remains in question, pressures proximal and distal to the lesion(s) can be measured. A systolic pressure gradient of more than 10 mm Hg (or a 5 mm Hg mean gradient) across the stenosis is indicative of a hemodynamically significant lesion. For borderline cases, distal pressure measurements can be obtained before and after interarterial injection of a vasodilator (eg, 100- to 200-μg nitroglycerin or 25-mg papaverine) to simulate the hyperemic hemodynamics of exercise. A pressure drop of more than 15% systolic pressure (or around 20 mm Hg) during hyperdynamic flow simulation is considered indicative of a hemodynamically significant stenosis.

Crossing total occlusions may be challenging, and re-entry into the true lumen from the subintimal space can be difficult. If crossing an occlusion cannot be achieved from the chosen point of vascular access (eg, the ipsilateral common femoral), an attempt should be made from a new access site (eg, contralateral common femoral or brachial). For more challenging cases, reentry devices such as the Outback (Cordis Corp., Bridgewater, NJ) or Pioneer (Medtronic, Fridley, MN) catheters may be used. Once the lesion is successfully crossed with a wire, the mode of intervention should then be considered.

The typical balloon size used for common iliac arteries is 8 to 10 mm in diameter, and for external iliac arteries 7 to 8 mm in diameter. Stents serve as support to oppose the elastic recoil of the artery after angioplasty. They are also highly effective in sealing dissection planes within the atherosclerotic plaque frequently resulting from the angioplasty procedure. For iliac disease covered stents appear to have better long-term patency than noncovered stents.[30]

Self-expanding stents come precovered with a sheath and can be introduced into the lesion directly. Retracting the sheath allows the compressed stent to assume its expanded form. Self-expanding stents may be more flexible and less likely to get crushed in the event they are deployed close to or past the inguinal ligament into the common femoral artery and are, therefore, used more frequently in the external iliac artery. With self-expanding stents, postdeployment balloon angioplasty is usually needed to achieve full expansion. These stents are usually selected 10% to 15% larger than the intended luminal diameter; under-sizing must be avoided as self-expanding stents cannot be dilated past their nominal diameter.

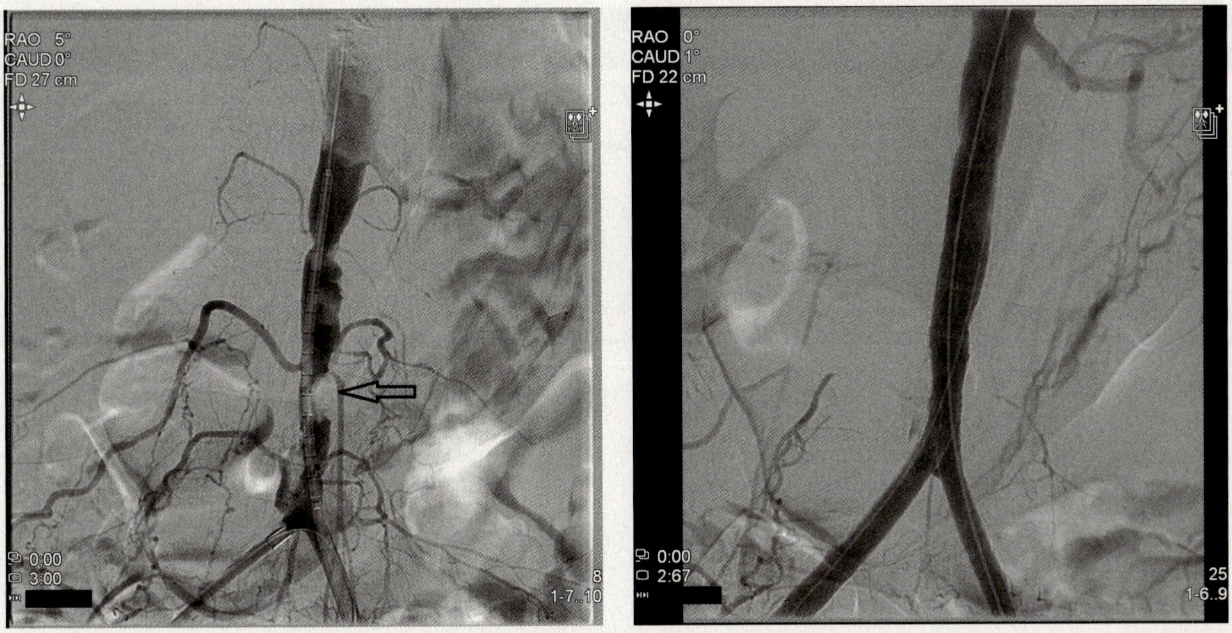

A B

Figure 87.7. CERAB (Covered endovascular reconstruction of aortic bifurcation). **A:** Infrarenal aortic stenosis (*arrow*). **B:** Post-deployment of a bifurcated stent graft.

Balloon-expandable stents are sometimes preferred to self-expanding stents in the common iliac artery, owing to their ease and precision of deployment, their better visibility under fluoroscopy, and the increased radial force of their design. These stents are usually introduced through a long sheath passed through the lesion to prevent dislodgment of the stent as it traverses the lesion. The sheath is pulled back once the stent is in satisfactory position, and the stent is deployed by inflating the carrier balloon under fluoroscopic guidance. Balloon-expandable stents are usually sized to the diameter of the normal adjacent artery. Slight under-sizing of the stent can be easily managed by further dilating the stent, using a larger balloon. Covered balloon-expandable and self-expanding stents have been introduced and are purported to offer a better long-term patency rate by controlling neointimal hyperplasia that may grow through the interstices of a noncovered stent.[31] Covered stents may also be useful for ulcerated plaques, because they reduce the chance of distal atheromatous embolism, and for heavily calcified or tortuous iliac arteries that are more prone to rupture with balloon inflation.

Covered Endovascular Reconstruction of the Aortic Bifurcation (CERAB)

Lesions just above the aortic bifurcation are usually complex, exophytic, and calcific, and commonly extend into both common iliac artery origins. Safe and effective intervention in this situation typically requires the use of two stents, one in each iliac artery, that partially project into the aorta so that they "kiss" in the distal aorta (**Fig. 87.6C**). Theoretically, treating only one common iliac artery orifice can result in plaque shifting during the angioplasty, leading to compression or obstruction of the contralateral iliac lumen. Treating both sides simultaneously ("kissing stents") avoids this complication. Endovascular stent grafts, similar to those used in the treatment of abdominal aortic aneurysms, have been evaluated for the treatment of AIOD; this is known as CERAB (**Fig. 87.7**). CERAB can also be performed with standard covered stents placing a large one in the aorta just above the bifurcation and then two smaller ones in each proximal iliac artery to "kiss" within the lumen of the aortic stent graft. Flow dynamics seem better with CERAB[32] and covered stents are associated with the purported advantages outlined previously, though there is no good evidence that they perform better than noncovered stents.[33] CERAB has shown lower primary patency but similar secondary patency with lower periprocedural comorbidities when compared to open surgical repair of AIOD.[34]

Complications of Endovascular Interventions

The overall procedure related complication rate has decreased over the years. It is cited to be around 10% of cases, while the rate of major complications is only 5% with access site complications being the most common (**Table 87.6**).[35,36]

The incidence of contrast-associated nephropathy is low ranging from <5 % in low-risk patients to >50% in the highest risk groups.[37] Low-osmolality or iso-osmolality agents should be used routinely. Volume expansion should be considered in the periprocedural period. Carbon dioxide is a useful substitute for iodinated contrast, though the resolution of obtained images is somewhat inferior in appearance; this can be of particular significance in the infrapopliteal vessels, where standard contrast is usually required for adequate visualization.[38] The most serious intraoperative complication is arterial rupture during angioplasty (0.5% to 3%). This problem is seen as active extravasation on the postintervention angiogram and can be heralded by abdominal pain and hypotension. Treatment is quick passage and reinflation of the balloon to occlude the rupture site to maintain hemodynamic control, followed by either deployment of a covered stent across the rupture site or open repair in the operating room.

Table 87.6. Complications of Endovascular Therapy

Complication	
Access site hematoma	5%
Pseudoaneurysm	1.60%
Distal embolization	1.10%
Rupture	0.50%
Thrombosis	0.60%

Table 87.7. Results of Endovascular and Open Surgical Interventions for AIOD

Procedure	30-Day Mortality	1-Year Primary Patency	3-Year Primary Patency	5-Year Primary Patency	5-Year Secondary Patency
Iliac angioplasty and stenting	1%	90% (88–93%)	78% (73–84%)	71% (60–82%)	89% (80–95%)
CERAB	1%	88% (83–92%)	82% (75–88%)	65% (50–75%)	93% (91–96%)
Open bypass Surgery	1–3%	96% (95–97%)	93% (91–94%)	88% (86–90%)	95% (93–97%)
Extra anatomic bypass	1–3%	90%	80%	50–70%	80–90%

CERAB, covered endovascular reconstruction of aortic bifurcation.

Outcome of Endovascular Interventions (Table 87.7)

Initial technical success is quite high (>90%).[35] The most common reasons for technical failure are inability to cross an occluded arterial segment, thrombosis after intervention, or arterial rupture. Surveillance with ABIs and possible duplex ultrasound plays a major role in documenting and maintaining patency in these patients. The primary patency of iliac artery stenting is 60% to 80% at 5 years, but this can improve to around 90% with close surveillance and reintervention as necessary.[39,40]

Open Surgical Management

Aortobifemoral (AF2) bypass has been the gold standard open surgical procedure for treating AIOD for decades. Five-year patency rates can exceed 95%, which is unmatched by any endovascular procedure. However, direct revascularization of the aortoiliac segment is currently reserved for patients with advanced occlusive disease, for whom the risk of surgery is acceptable and a durable long-term result is required.

Description of Aortofemoral Bypass (Fig. 87.8)[41]

The operation begins with bilateral groin incisions to expose the common, superficial, and deep femoral arteries as needed. Starting the operation in the groin minimizes the duration of time the abdomen is open limiting evaporative fluid loss and resulting hypothermia, and decreases the risk of graft infection. If the femoral arteries are severely atherosclerotic, the external iliac just above the inguinal ligament is often a soft, disease-free segment that is amenable to safe clamping. The profunda femoris (deep femoral) artery is a critical collateral pathway for the entire lower extremity. If disease is present at its origin, exposure of the profunda femoris beyond its take off is required for a complete endarterectomy which is mandatory for a durable result.

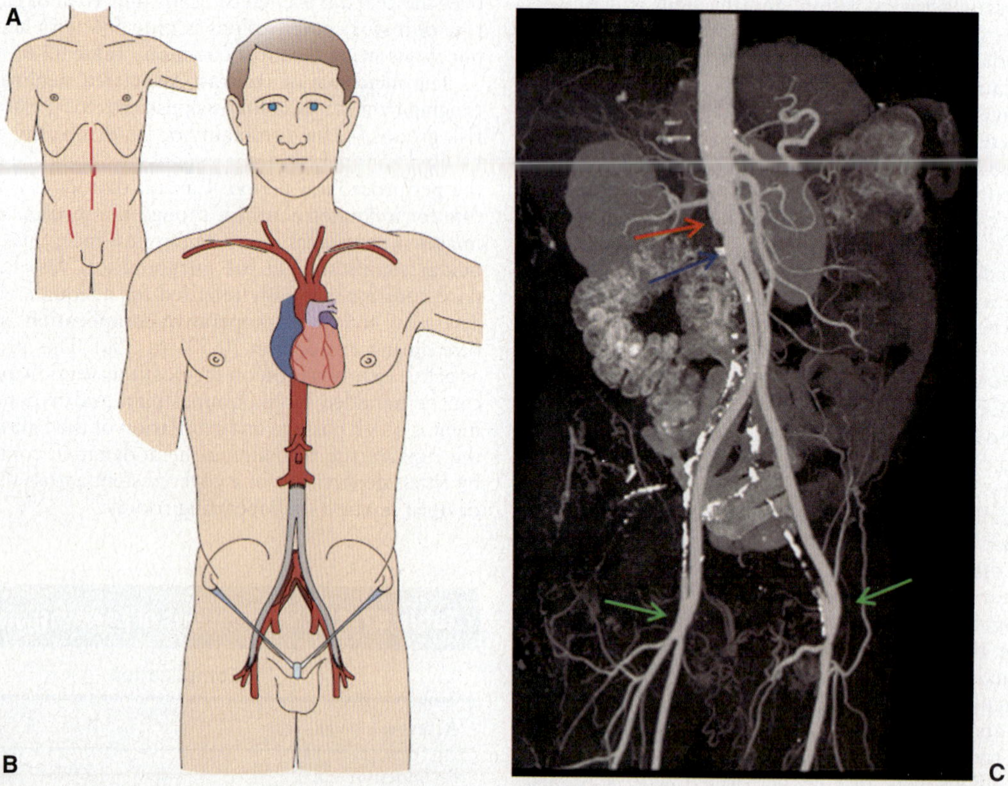

Figure 87.8. **A:** A midline abdominal incision and bilateral groin incisions overlying the common femoral arteries offer exposure for performance of an aortobifemoral bypass. **B:** This image demonstrates an end-to-end proximal aortic to graft reconstruction with the respective graft limbs anastomosed end to side to the common femoral arteries. **C:** CTA postprocessed and reformatted image demonstrating patent aortobifemoral arterial reconstruction of a juxtarenal aortic occlusion (see Fig. 87.2, preoperative image) with a bifurcated prosthetic graft. Note endarterectomy of aorta immediately distal to renal arteries (*red arrow*), followed by proximal end-to-end anastomosis between graft and aorta (*blue arrow*). Distal anastomoses are sewn to the femoral arteries in end-to-side fashion (*green arrows*).

The abdominal aorta is usually exposed via a midline, transperitoneal, inframesocolic approach. The transverse colon is retracted cephalad, the ligament of Treitz taken down, and the duodenum (third and fourth portions) mobilized to the right. The left renal vein is identified in the retroperitoneum and serves as the most cephalad limit of exposure in most cases (0.5% to 3% of patients have a retroaortic left renal vein). The anterior surface of the aorta is then exposed from the lower border of the left renal vein to just below the IMA. Numerous lymphatics are usually encountered in the para-aortic retroperitoneal space particularly at the level of the left renal vein. These should be ligated to decrease the chances of a chyle leak. The left renal vein is mobilized if more proximal aortic control is needed; this is performed by ligating and dividing its adrenal, gonadal, and lumbar branches. It is generally unnecessary to divide the renal vein. Distal control of the aorta is dictated by the extent of disease. When exposing sites for distal control, the location of the hypogastric plexus and the presacral nerves, which course anterior to the aorta and travel caudally over the aortic bifurcation and origin of the left common iliac artery, needs to be kept in mind. Injury to the parasympathetic nerves can cause erectile dysfunction in men. Retroperitoneal tunnels are then developed between the exposed infrarenal aorta and the groins by means of blunt finger dissection. The tunnels are directed posterior to the ureters to avoid postoperative obstructive uropathy from entrapment of the ureter between the graft limb and the native iliac artery. A retroperitoneal approach to the aorta via a left flank incision is an accepted alternative, especially in those patients with multiple prior celiotomies; however, it makes creation of the tunnel for the right limb of the bypass graft slightly more challenging.[42]

A bifurcated vascular prosthesis of appropriate size is selected, typically a presealed knitted Dacron or a polytetrafluoroethylene (PTFE) graft, and the patient is heparinized. With an occluding clamp below the renal arteries and another just above the IMA, the proximal anastomosis between the graft and the aorta is performed in either an end-to-end or end-to-side fashion. Though most vascular surgeons prefer an end-to-end anastomosis for technical simplicity, the end-to-side technique has been found to be just as good, depending on the pattern of occlusive lesions and need to maintain flow to patent hypogastric arteries. The proximal anastomosis is placed as close to the renal arteries as practical to prevent future compromise of the bypass resulting from progression of atherosclerosis in the remaining infrarenal cuff. The limbs of the prosthesis are then delivered through the retroperitoneal tunnels into the groins. The distal anastomoses are performed to the common femoral arteries and should be carried onto the profunda femoris arteries if there is any disease at the femoral bifurcation (**Fig. 87.9**). Common femoral and profunda femoris origin endarterectomy may be needed and should be carried out prior to the anastomosis. Maintaining good outflow through the profunda femoris is critical as many of these patients have concomitant superficial femoral arterial disease, which may compromise long-term graft patency. Rarely patients with tissue loss secondary to multilevel disease (AIOD associated with infrainguinal disease), may require a concomitant distal (femoropopliteal–tibial) bypass.

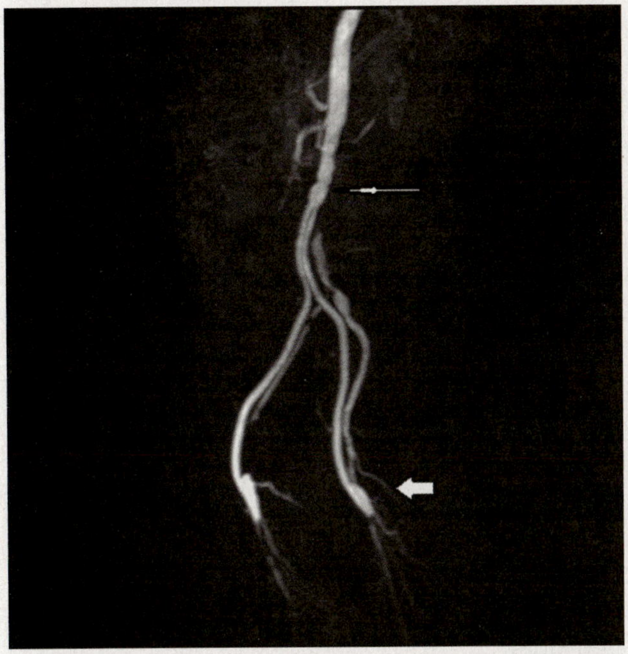

Figure 87.9. MRA of a patient who had an aortobifemoral bypass. Note the proximal anastomosis (*thin arrow*) and the distal anastomoses (*thick arrows*). Also note the retrograde flow into the left external and common iliac arteries.

Extra-Anatomic Bypass

Patients who are at high risk for open aortic surgery due to either physiologic or anatomic constraints and are not endovascular candidates may be better served with extra-anatomic reconstruction. Although these operations are less risky, they have a documented lower patency rate and are, therefore, reserved for patients with CLTI and generally not performed for intermittent claudication.

Axillofemoral extra-anatomic reconstruction has been used for revascularization in poor-risk patients and in those with a "hostile" abdomen and has been reported to be an acceptable alternative to aortofemoral bypass (**Fig. 87.10**). The axillary artery supplying the arm with the higher brachial blood pressure is chosen as the inflow vessel, usually the right side. The operative sequence starts with exposure of the first portion of the axillary artery through an infraclavicular, pectoralis major muscle-splitting incision. The common, superficial, and deep

A

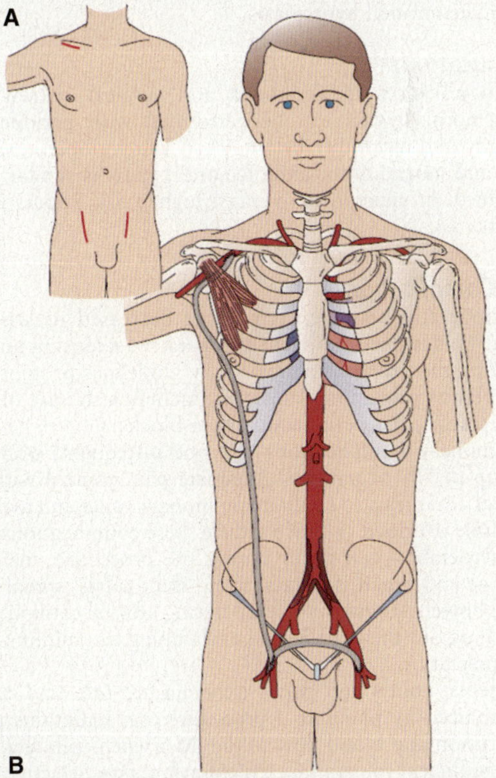

B

Figure 87.10. **A:** Ipsilateral infraclavicular incision and bilateral femoral incisions for extra-anatomic axillary to bifemoral artery bypass. **B:** Image demonstrates axillary to ipsilateral femoral artery bypass graft with cross-femoral (femoral to femoral) artery bypass graft.

femoral arteries are then dissected through bilateral groin incisions. An externally supported PTFE graft is then passed between the pectoralis major and minor muscles and through a subcutaneous tunnel in the anterior axillary line, connecting the axillary incision with the ipsilateral groin incision. Next, a cross-femoral limb of the graft is delivered through a subcutaneous suprapubic tunnel connecting the two groins. An anastomosis between the proximal axillary artery and the prosthesis is then constructed in an end-graft–to–side-of-artery fashion. The distal anastomoses are performed end-to-side to the common femoral arteries and may be carried over or onto the deep femoral arteries to ensure adequate graft outflow. Providing flow through both femoral arteries (axillobifemoral bypass) rather than one ipsilateral femoral artery (axillounifemoral) has been shown to increase flow velocities within the long main shaft of the graft and improve long-term patency of the bypass.[43] The lower patency of the axillofemoral bypass limits it application mainly to patients with advanced AIOD who are poor surgical risks with a reduced life expectancy or those with a "hostile" abdomen. For high-risk patients with diffuse advanced disease limited to one iliac artery, cross-femoral (or femoral artery–to–femoral artery) bypass or an iliofemoral bypass is an option.

Outcomes

The excellent durability of aortofemoral bypass is related to the large caliber and high flow rates of the vessels involved. Results of direct open surgical revascularization are listed in (**Table 87.7**). Aortofemoral bypass has excellent primary graft patency rates of approximately 85% to 95% at 5 years and 75% to 88% at 10 years.[39] Factors associated with lower long-term patency of these reconstructions include female sex (in part due to smaller vessel size), multilevel arterial occlusive disease, (poor run-off) and younger age (<50 years) where premature and aggressive atherosclerosis and/or hypercoagulability are usually present. The most common cause of failure of surgical reconstructions is the progression of atherosclerosis proximal and/or distal to the graft or the development of anastomotic neointimal hyperplasia.

Complications[34,44,45]

Due to advances in anesthesia and surgical critical care, aortofemoral bypass can be performed with perioperative mortality and morbidity below 5%.[46] The perioperative morbidity and mortality for axillofemoral bypass is similar but is performed, in general, on a much higher risk population of patients.

Early Complications

- Postoperative cardiac events have decreased to less than 5%. This is due to diligent preoperative screening and following the excellent perioperative guidelines promoted by numerous professional societies, including the use of aspirin, statins, and perioperative beta-blockers.
- Pulmonary complications are not infrequent, occurring in up to 7% of patients. Adequate pain control with epidural anesthesia to facilitate pulmonary toilet and avoiding volume overload can help reduce these complications.
- Atheroemboli can occur during the procedure, manifesting as end-organ ischemia of the skin, pelvis, spinal cord, and bowel. Attention to detail during arterial clamping and flushing out the graft before unclamping can minimize this complication.
- Ischemic colitis and pelvic ischemia are rare and can be minimized by planning a procedure that maintains pelvic perfusion and blood flow to the IMA when collateral flow is insufficient to maintain left colon viability. Selective reimplantation of the IMA can be performed when poor IMA perfusion is anticipated or demonstrated. Ischemic colitis may require colectomy for treatment, but this is associated with an up to 50% mortality.
- Acute kidney injury can result from either atheroembolism from aortic clamping close to the renal arteries or from corticomedullary renal shunting induced by the acute increase in afterload attendant with aortic clamping.
- Other possible complications include wound complications, particularly in the groin (lymphocele, lymphocutaneous fistula, wound infection), postoperative hemorrhage, erectile dysfunction in men, bowel injury, pancreatitis from retraction injury, and, very rarely, spinal cord ischemia. Groin wound complications can be particularly troublesome for axillofemoral and femoral–femoral bypasses because of the subcutaneous location of these prosthetic grafts.

Late Complications

- Graft limb thrombosis that is largely due to progression of native atherosclerotic disease either proximal or distal to the graft, or to anastomotic neointimal hyperplasia.
- Pseudoaneurysms can result from material fatigue, suture fracture, artery wall degeneration, or occult infection.
- Graft infections. A graft enteric fistula (most frequently to the third/fourth portions of the overlying duodenum) may present as a gastrointestinal bleed. Every gastrointestinal bleed in a patient with a history of aortic reconstruction should be considered to be an aortoenteric fistula until proven otherwise. Graft infections can also occur in the absence of an enteric fistula and most commonly result from a groin wound complication.

References

1. Sartipy F, Pereira Filho AJG, Lundin F, Wahlberg E, Sigvant B. Presence of asymptomatic peripheral arterial disease in combination with common risk factors elevates the cardiovascular risk substantially. *Int J Cardiol Cardiovasc Risk Prev.* 2022;13:200130.
2. Criqui MH, Matsushita K, Aboyans V, et al. Lower extremity peripheral artery disease: contemporary epidemiology, management gaps, and future directions: a scientific statement from the American Heart Association. *Circulation.* 2021;144:e171–e191.
3. DeBakey ME, Glaeser DH. Patterns of atherosclerosis: effect of risk factors on recurrence and survival-analysis of 11,890 cases with more than 25-year follow-up. *Am J Cardiol.* 2000;85:1045–1053.
4. Conte MS, Bradbury AW, Kolh P, et al. Global vascular guidelines on the management of chronic limb-threatening ischemia. *Eur J Vasc Endovasc Surg.* 2019;58:S1–S109.e133.
5. Conte MS, Pomposelli FB, Clair DG, et al. Society for Vascular Surgery practice guidelines for atherosclerotic occlusive disease of the lower extremities: management of asymptomatic disease and claudication. *J Vasc Surg.* 2015;61:2s–41s.
6. Leriche R, Morel A. The syndrome of thrombotic obliteration of the aortic bifurcation. *Ann Surg.* 1948;127:193–206.
7. Jarrett F. Rene Leriche (1879-1955): father of vascular surgery. *Surgery.* 1979;86:736–741.
8. Norgren L, Hiatt WR, Dormandy JA, et al. Inter-society consensus for the management of peripheral arterial disease (TASC II). *J Vasc Surg.* 2007;45 Suppl S:S5–S67.
9. Krug RT, Calligaro KD, Dougherty MJ. Claudication in the Young Patient. *Perspect Vasc Surg Endovasc Ther.* 2000;13:27–38.
10. Rumwell C, McPharlin M. *Vascular Technology: An Illustrated Review.* 5th ed. Davies Publishing; 2017.
11. Rutherford RB, Lowenstein DH, Klein MF. Combining segmental systolic pressures and plethysmography to diagnose arterial occlusive disease of the legs. *Am J Surg.* 1979;138:211–218.
12. Sibley RC 3rd, Reis SP, MacFarlane JJ, Reddick MA, Kalva SP, Sutphin PD. Noninvasive physiologic vascular studies: a guide to diagnosing peripheral arterial disease. *Radiographics.* 2017;37:346–357.
13. Katsamouris AN, Giannoukas AD, Tsetis D, Kostas T, Petinarakis I, Gourtsoyiannis N. Can ultrasound replace arteriography in the management of chronic arterial occlusive disease of the lower limb? *Eur J Vasc Endovasc Surg.* 2001;21:155–159.

14. Gerhard-Herman MD, Gornik HL, Barrett C, et al. 2016 AHA/ACC guideline on the management of patients with lower extremity peripheral artery disease: A report of the American College of Cardiology/American Heart Association Task Force on Clinical Practice Guidelines. *J Am Coll Cardiol*. 2017;69:e71–e126.
15. Gornik HL, Aronow HD, Goodney PP, et al. 2024 ACC/AHA/AACVPR/APMA/ABC/SCAI/SVM/SVN/SVS/SIR/VESS Guideline for the Management of Lower Extremity Peripheral Artery Disease: A report of the American College of Cardiology/American Heart Association Joint Committee on Clinical Practice Guidelines. *J Am Coll Cardiol*. 2024;83:2497–2604.
16. Arnett DK, Blumenthal RS, Albert MA, et al. 2019 ACC/AHA Guideline on the Primary Prevention of Cardiovascular Disease: Executive Summary: A Report of the American College of Cardiology/American Heart Association Task Force on Clinical Practice Guidelines. *Circulation*. 2019;140:e563–e595.
17. Cunningham MA, Swanson V, O'Carroll RE, Holdsworth RJ. Randomized clinical trial of a brief psychological intervention to increase walking in patients with intermittent claudication. *Br J Surg*. 2012;99:49–56.
18. Ahimastos AA, Pappas EP, Buttner PG, Walker PJ, Kingwell BA, Golledge J. A meta-analysis of the outcome of endovascular and noninvasive therapies in the treatment of intermittent claudication. *J Vasc Surg*. 2011;54:1511–1521.
19. Murphy TP, Cutlip DE, Regensteiner JG, et al. Supervised exercise versus primary stenting for claudication resulting from aortoiliac peripheral artery disease: six-month outcomes from the claudication: exercise versus endoluminal revascularization (CLEVER) study. *Circulation*. 2012;125:130–139.
20. Murphy TP, Cutlip DE, Regensteiner JG, et al. Supervised exercise, stent revascularization, or medical therapy for claudication due to aortoiliac peripheral artery disease: the CLEVER study. *J Am Coll Cardiol*. 2015;65:999–1009.
21. McDermott MM, Liu K, Guralnik JM, et al. Home-based walking exercise intervention in peripheral artery disease: a randomized clinical trial. *JAMA*. 2013;310:57–65.
22. Eikelboom JW, Connolly SJ, Bosch J, et al. Rivaroxaban with or without aspirin in stable cardiovascular disease. *N Engl J Med*. 2017;377:1319–1330.
23. Robless P, Mikhailidis DP, Stansby GP. Cilostazol for peripheral arterial disease. *Cochrane Database Syst Rev*. 2007:CD003748.
24. Heijenbrok-Kal MH, Kock MC, Hunink MG. Lower extremity arterial disease: multidetector CT angiography meta-analysis. *Radiology*. 2007;245:433–439.
25. Bui BT, Miller S, Mildenberger P, Sam A 2nd, Sheng R; Omniscan MRA Investigator Panel. Comparison of contrast-enhanced MR angiography to intraarterial digital subtraction angiography for evaluation of peripheral arterial occlusive disease: results of a phase III multicenter trial. *J Magn Reson Imaging*. 2010;31:1402–1410.
26. Szilagyi DE, Elliott JP Jr, Smith RF, Reddy DJ, McPharlin M. A thirty-year survey of the reconstructive surgical treatment of aortoiliac occlusive disease. *J Vasc Surg*. 1986;3:421–436.
27. McFalls EO, Ward HB, Moritz TE, et al. Coronary-artery revascularization before elective major vascular surgery. *N Engl J Med*. 2004;351:2795–2804.
28. Fleisher LA, Fleischmann KE, Auerbach AD, et al. 2014 ACC/AHA guideline on perioperative cardiovascular evaluation and management of patients undergoing noncardiac surgery: a report of the American College of Cardiology/American Heart Association Task Force on Practice Guidelines. *Circulation*. 2014;130:e278–333.
29. Qaseem A, Snow V, Fitterman N, et al. Risk assessment for and strategies to reduce perioperative pulmonary complications for patients undergoing noncardiothoracic surgery: a guideline from the American College of Physicians. *Ann Intern Med*. 2006;144:575–580.
30. Mwipatayi BP, Ouriel K, Anwari T, et al. A systematic review of covered balloon-expandable stents for treating aortoiliac occlusive disease. *J Vasc Surg*. 2020;72:1473–1486. e1472.
31. Humphries MD, Armstrong E, Laird J, Paz J, Pevec W. Outcomes of covered versus bare-metal balloon-expandable stents for aortoiliac occlusive disease. *J Vasc Surg*. 2014;60:337–343.
32. Groot Jebbink E, Mathai V, Boersen JT, et al. Hemodynamic comparison of stent configurations used for aortoiliac occlusive disease. *J Vasc Surg*. 2017;66:251–260.e251.
33. Groot Jebbink E, Ter Mors TG, Slump CH, Geelkerken RH, Holewijn S, Reijnen MM. In vivo geometry of the kissing stent and covered endovascular reconstruction of the aortic bifurcation configurations in aortoiliac occlusive disease. *Vascular*. 2017;25:635–641.
34. Smith AH, Beach JM, Dash S, et al. Comparison of aortobifemoral bypass to aortoiliac stenting with bifurcation reconstruction for TASC II D aortoiliac occlusive disease. *Ann Vasc Surg*. 2022;82:120–130.
35. Groot Jebbink E, Holewijn S, Slump CH, Lardenoije JW, Reijnen MMPJ. Systematic review of results of kissing stents in the treatment of aortoiliac occlusive disease. *Ann Vasc Surg*. 2017;42:328–336.
36. Jongkind V, Akkersdijk GJ, Yeung KK, Wisselink W. A systematic review of endovascular treatment of extensive aortoiliac occlusive disease. *J Vasc Surg*. 2010;52:1376–1383.
37. Ozsvath KJ, Darling RC 3rd. Renal protection: preconditioning for the prevention of contrast-induced nephropathy. *Semin Vasc Surg*. 2013;26:144–149.
38. Sharafuddin MJ, Marjan AE. Current status of carbon dioxide angiography. *J Vasc Surg*. 2017;66:618–637.
39. Bontinis V, Bontinis A, Koudounas G, et al. Long-term outcomes of anatomical and extra-anatomical bypass for the treatment of unilateral iliac artery lesions a systematic review aggregated data and individual participant data meta-analysis. *Ann Vasc Surg*. 2024;104:296–306.
40. Chang RW, Goodney PP, Baek JH, et al. Long-term results of combined common femoral endarterectomy and iliac stenting/stent grafting for occlusive disease. *J Vasc Surg*. 2008;48:362–367.
41. Shepard A. *Aortofemoral bypass*. In: Hans SS, Weaver MR, Nypaver TJ, eds. *Primary and Repeat Arterial Reconstructions*. Springer Nature, 2023:259–270.
42. Shepard AD, Tollefson DF, Reddy DJ, et al. Left flank retroperitoneal exposure: a technical aid to complex aortic reconstruction. *J Vasc Surg*. 1991;14:283–291.
43. Passman MA, Taylor LM, Moneta GL, et al. Comparison of axillofemoral and aortofemoral bypass for aortoiliac occlusive disease. *J Vasc Surg*. 1996;23:263–269; discussion 269–271.
44. Salem M, Hosny MS, Francia F, et al. Management of extensive aorto-iliac disease: a systematic review and meta-analysis of 9319 patients. *Cardiovasc Intervent Radiol*. 2021;44:1518–1535.
45. DeCarlo C, Boitano LT, Schwartz SI, et al. Laparotomy- and groin-associated complications are common after aortofemoral bypass and contribute to reintervention. *J Vasc Surg*. 2020;72:1976–1986.
46. Chiu KW, Davies RS, Nightingale PG, Bradbury AW, Adam DJ. Review of direct anatomical open surgical management of atherosclerotic aorto-iliac occlusive disease. *Eur J Vasc Endovasc Surg*. 2010;39:460–471.

88

Peripheral Arterial Disease

William P. Robinson III

Key Points

1 Chronic obliterative atherosclerosis of the infrainguinal vessels is the most prevalent manifestation of peripheral arterial disease (PAD) encountered by the vascular surgeon.

2 The major risk factors for the development of PAD include smoking, diabetes, advanced age, male gender, hypertension, dyslipidemia, and chronic kidney disease.

3 PAD is a powerful risk factor for cardiovascular morbidity and mortality.

4 The diagnosis of infrainguinal occlusive disease is generally made based on patient symptomatology, physical examination, and noninvasive tests, such as ankle–brachial index (ABI), segmental pressure measurements, and pulse volume recordings.

5 The natural history of the two major manifestations of PAD, claudication and chronic limb-threatening ischemia (CLTI), are vastly different and these entities have different management paradigms.

6 The Wound, Ischemia, and foot Infection (WIfI) classification system allows for staging of limb-threat severity and guides initial management as well as additional adjunctive operative procedures for salvage of the foot and limb.

7 Percutaneous endovascular therapy is often applied as first-line therapy, particularly in patients with a more limited extent of anatomic disease burden and/or high operative risk.

8 Open surgical revascularization remains the gold standard for patients with disabling claudication recalcitrant to medical and exercise therapy, ischemic rest pain, and ischemic ulceration or gangrene.

9 Infrainguinal arterial bypass surgery remains the signature operation distinguishing vascular surgeons from other specialists involved in the treatment of peripheral vascular disease.

10 Infrainguinal bypass surgery is best performed with autogenous vein conduit, preferably the ipsilateral greater saphenous vein if available.

EPIDEMIOLOGY

The term "Peripheral Arterial Disease (PAD)" broadly denotes stenotic, occlusive, and aneurysmal diseases of the aorta and its branch arteries, exclusive of the coronary arteries. In common clinical usage, PAD, which is defined as an ankle–brachial index (ABI) <0.9, denotes atherosclerotic stenosis or occlusion of the arteries supplying the lower extremities Atherosclerotic occlusive disease of the aorta and iliac arteries is covered in Chapter 87. This chapter will cover PAD located in the femoropopliteal and tibial (infrainguinal) arteries. PAD affects 12% of the US adult population and almost 20% of US adults older than 70 years.[1,2] PAD involving the lower extremities is the third leading overall cause of atherosclerotic morbidity worldwide after coronary artery disease and stroke.[3] With the aging of the American population, the prevalence of lower extremity occlusive disease has steadily increased in recent decades. Symptomatic PAD in the form of claudication affects more than 10 million Americans including 1% to 2% of those aged <50, 5% of those aged 50 to 70, and 10% of those aged >70.
1 Of those aged >50 with PAD, 1% to 3% will have chronic limb-threatening ischemia (CLTI) in the form of rest pain, ulceration, or gangrene.[4] The incidence of CLTI ranges from 220 to 1000 new cases per year in a European or American population of 1 million people.[3] Not surprisingly, therefore, the clinical manifestations and complications of atherosclerosis are the most common therapeutic challenges encountered and treated by vascular surgeons.

The tendency for atherosclerotic lesions to develop at specific anatomic sites and follow recognizable patterns of progression was first appreciated in the late 1700s by the British anatomist and surgeon John Hunter. The modern era of surgical reconstruction for complex atherosclerotic occlusive disease began in earnest in 1947, when the Portuguese surgeon J. Cid dos Santos successfully endarterectomized a heavily diseased common femoral artery.[5] Four years later, building on the pioneering work of Alexis Carrel, Kunlin would report the first long-segment vein bypass in the lower extremity.[6] The subsequent decades have seen tremendous advances in both the understanding of atherosclerosis biology and refinement in the techniques of infrainguinal surgical revascularization that have greatly improved surgeons' ability to preserve limbs and improve quality of life in patients with femoropopliteal and tibial occlusive disease. Moreover, in the last three decades, advances in percutaneous treatment have revolutionized the treatment of infrainguinal occlusive disease. The concept of intravascular intervention was pioneered in the late 1960s by the radiologist Charles Dotter, and advanced greatly with the advent of the angioplasty balloon by Gruntzig in the early 1970s.[7,8] Nevertheless, endovascular intervention for infrainguinal disease was not utilized significantly until the 1990s. The technology remains in rapid development and is surrounded by ongoing controversy as to its proper role.

Although a diverse range of technical skill is required of the contemporary vascular and endovascular surgeon, it is worth noting that infrainguinal arterial bypass surgery remains the signature operation distinguishing vascular surgeons from other specialists involved in the treatment of PAD. This distinction stems primarily from the fact that the outcome of infrainguinal reconstruction is highly dependent on the judgment and technical skill of the surgeon, with the end result often being either successful limb salvage or major limb amputation. This chapter reviews the surgical and endovascular management of femoropopliteal and tibial arterial occlusive disease and details standard and advanced techniques underlying successful infrainguinal operative revascularization. Endovascular intervention is introduced, though a comprehensive review of endovascular techniques used to treat femoropopliteal and tibial occlusive disease is beyond the scope of this chapter.

INFRAINGUINAL ARTERIAL OCCLUSIVE DISEASE

Risk Factors

2 The risk factors for infrainguinal occlusive disease are the same as those for the development of systemic atherosclerosis and include age, male gender, hypertension, diabetes mellitus (DM), smoking, dyslipidemia, family history, and homocysteinemia. Smoking and diabetes are the most powerful risk factors. Smokers are at four times the risk of symptomatic PAD than nonsmokers while diabetics are more than three times more likely to develop symptomatic PAD in comparison to nondiabetics.[7] More recent evidence indicates that nonwhite ethnicity, inflammatory markers such as C-reactive protein, and perhaps chronic renal insufficiency (CRI) are also associated with an increased risk of PAD.[9,10] The propensity for heavy smokers to develop superficial femoral artery (sfa) disease and for diabetics to develop tibial disease should be noted.[11–13]

Presentation and Natural History

Chronic obliterative atherosclerosis of the infrainguinal vessels is the most prevalent manifestation of PAD encountered by the vascular surgeon. Patients are classified into two broad categories depending upon their symptomatology: claudicants and those with CLTI. Claudication, the reproducible ischemic muscle pain resulting from inadequate oxygen delivery during exercise, is the cardinal presenting symptom. Natural history studies indicate patients with claudication have increased rates of cardiovascular mortality, but an overall low risk of limb loss.[14,15] Seventy percent to 80% of patients with claudication demonstrate a stable pattern of disease throughout their lifetime or have improvement in their symptoms as a result of risk factor modification, whereas 20% to 30% undergo revascularization within 5 years as a result of disease progression.
3 Claudication will progress to CLTI in only 5% to 10% of patients over their lifetime. However, PAD leading to claudication is a marker of severe systemic atherosclerotic burden and increased cardiovascular morbidity and mortality. Twenty percent of claudicants experience a nonfatal myocardial infarction or stroke and 10% to 15% died of cardiovascular-related mortality at 5 years.[6] In claudicants, the annual rate of mortality is 2% to 5% and limb loss is 1%.[4]

4 The most common atherosclerotic disease pattern encountered distal to the inguinal ligament is that of a short-segment total occlusion of the sfa. Isolated disease of this nature typically presents as calf muscle claudication. It is not uncommon, however, for patients with significant single-level lesions, even those with long-segment arterial occlusions, in the sfa or more distal arterial beds to be only minimally symptomatic or even asymptomatic. While this can sometimes be the result of exercise limitations imposed by concomitant coronary arterial disease or other physiologic impairments such as lung disease or arthritis, it is more often a result of compensatory collateral flow. Collateral perfusion from the profunda femoral artery around a heavily diseased or occluded sfa frequently reconstitutes the distal sfa or popliteal artery with enough well-perfused arterial blood to ensure adequate resting tissue perfusion. Similarly, the rich network of geniculate collaterals can sometimes compensate for a diseased popliteal arterial segment to a sufficient degree to prevent rest pain or overt tissue loss but will usually prove insufficient to meet the increased metabolic demands of ambulation and forestall claudication.

CLTI, which must be differentiated from acute limb ischemia, is the most severe form of PAD and refers to the presence of either rest pain or tissue loss in the lower limb. Rest pain occurs when blood flow is inadequate to meet resting metabolic requirements. In the lower extremity, ischemic rest pain is localized to the foot, frequently in the metatarsals or the instep, and should be easily distinguishable from benign muscle cramps in the calf commonly seen in older patients. Patients with rest pain are often awakened by severe discomfort in the forefoot and hang the affected extremity over the edge of the bed for temporary symptomatic relief. Trophic changes, such as muscle wasting, thinning of skin, thickening of nails, and hair loss are frequently also seen in the distal affected limb. Rest pain is an ominous symptom and usually requires revascularization given the tendency for progression to tissue loss. Ischemic ulcerations usually begin as small, dry ulcers of the toes or heel area, and progress to frankly gangrenous changes of the forefoot or heel with greater degrees of arterial insufficiency (**Fig. 88.1**). Patients with diabetes or renal failure are more susceptible to the development of ischemic pedal ulcers. Disease progression can be very rapid, as up to 50% of patients with CLTI are asymptomatic 6 months before onset of pain or ulceration.[16,17]

The natural history of CLTI is dismal as these patients are generally of advanced age and possess significant comorbidities contributing to their advanced limb ischemia. Overall, approximately 25% of patients with CLTI will die at 1 year, 30% will undergo major amputation, and 45% will be alive with two limbs.[16] The rate of amputation is 10 times higher in diabetics than nondiabetics and 5- and 10-year mortality in patients with CLTI have been reported to be 60% and 85%, respectively. CLTI mandates revascularization for limb salvage when feasible, as limb salvage with medical therapy and wound care is virtually futile; success rates for rest pain and tissue loss have been reported to be as low as 27% and 5%, respectively.[16,17]

Several identifiable patterns of infrainguinal PAD are well recognized. It is important to note that symptoms and signs of ischemia generally involve the limb one level distal to the level of hemodynamically significant disease. Patients with an extensive history of cigarette smoking typically have lesions limited to the sfa and corresponding symptoms of calf claudication (**Fig. 88.2**). Patients with rest pain or ischemic tissue loss typically manifest more extensive involvement of the femoral, popliteal, or tibial arteries than patients with claudication. Those with tissue loss also more commonly have multilevel disease involving the femoropopliteal system in combination with occlusive disease of the aortoiliac vessels or the infrageniculate runoff.[16] Diabetes often targets the tibial vessels, and patients may present with frank tissue necrosis in the presence of a palpable popliteal pulse and no prior history of claudication.

Diagnosis

5 The diagnosis of infrainguinal occlusive disease is based on patient symptomatology, physical examination, and noninvasive tests, such as the ABI, segmental pressure measurements, and pulse volume recordings. Accurate history-taking and physical examination are crucial to clarifying the diagnosis and guiding management aimed at maximizing symptom relief and limb preservation. Intermittent claudication (IC) indicative of infrainguinal occlusive disease is typically a cramping, aching discomfort consistently reproducible at a given distance and relieved soon after cessation of ambulation. This must be differentiated from lower extremity pain secondary to nerve root compression or spinal stenosis which, in contradistinction to vasculogenic pain, often develops when patients maintain a

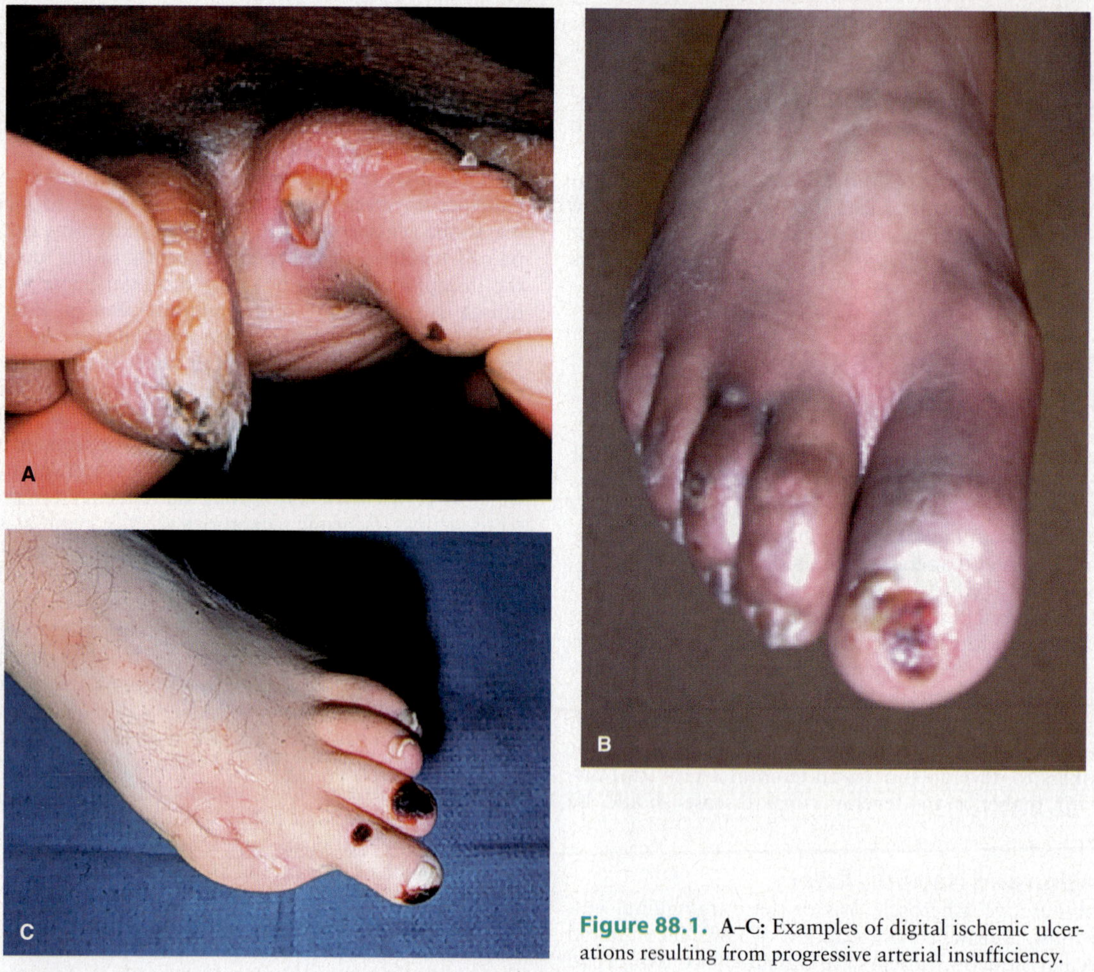

Figure 88.1. A–C: Examples of digital ischemic ulcerations resulting from progressive arterial insufficiency.

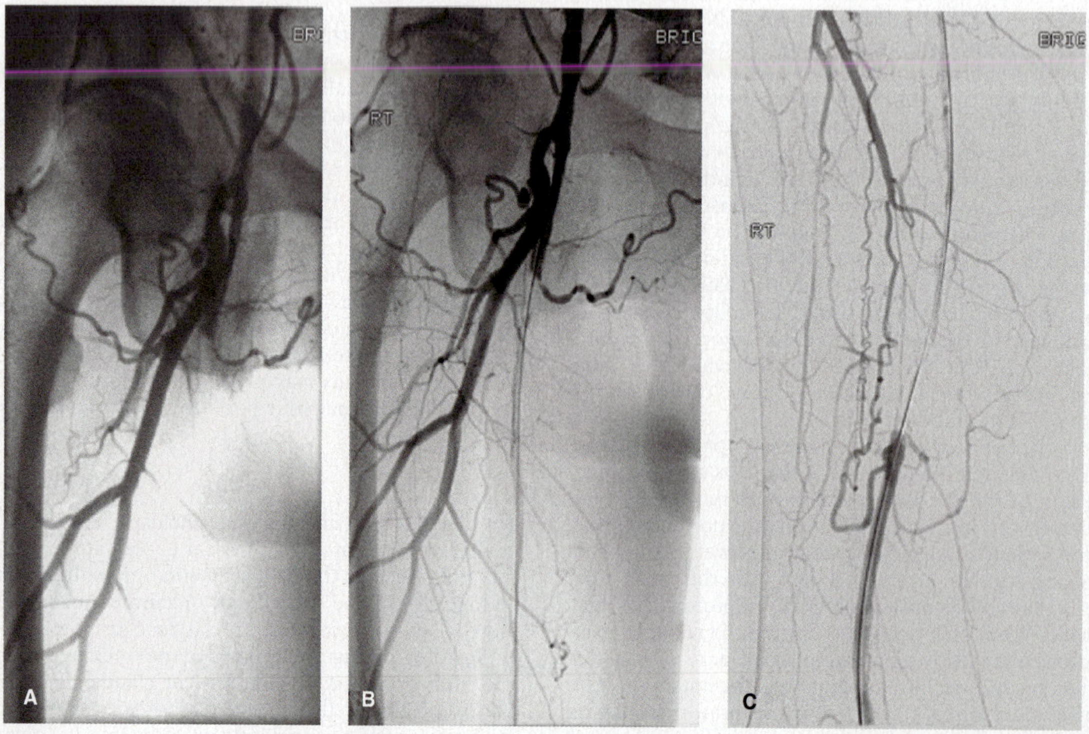

Figure 88.2. Long-segment total occlusion of superficial femoral artery (sfa) in a patient with a long history of cigarette smoking and severe claudication. Proximal sfa occlusion is demonstrated (**A**), followed by wire traversal of the occlusion (**B**), which will allow endovascular treatment of the occluded segment of the sfa proximal to reconstitution of the above-knee popliteal artery (**C**).

stationary standing posture. Vasculogenic claudication must also be distinguished from venous claudication, hip and ankle arthritis, symptomatic Baker cyst, and chronic compartment syndrome. IC patients with isolated infrainguinal disease will likely have palpable femoral pulses but diminished popliteal and/or pedal pulses.

As is true with claudication, ischemic rest pain must be carefully distinguished from other sources of pain in the elderly population, most commonly arthralgia and neuropathy. Although tissue necrosis and gangrene are usually self-evident when caused by critical ischemia, similar lesions associated with venous stasis, severe anemia, decubitus ulcers, and diabetic neuropathy must be excluded.

Noninvasive physiologic arterial testing allows confirmation of infrainguinal occlusive disease when it is suspected based upon history and physical examination. Measurement of the ABI is the most useful diagnostic adjunct. A properly performed ABI in a claudicant without significant evidence for vascular calcification would be expected to be between 0.5 and 0.9. Ischemic rest pain generally occurs at ABI 0.4 to 0.5, whereas an ABI less than 0.4 is generally associated with tissue loss. Segmental pressure measurements at the level of the upper thigh, lower thigh, upper calf, ankle, and metatarsal level also aid in localizing the level of hemodynamically significant disease. A decrease in pressure greater than 20 mm Hg between levels indicates a hemodynamically significant stenosis in the intervening arterial vasculature. In patients with DM or CRI leading to extensive vascular calcification, the ABI will often be erroneously elevated due to medial calcinosis and subsequent noncompressibility of the vessels. In such circumstances, pulse volume recordings, which ascertain the volume of blood flowing into segment of the limb, remain a reliable indicator of perfusion to the various levels of the lower extremity. Measurement of toe pressures also effectively quantitates distal perfusion as the digital arteries are generally spared of calcium which inhibits compressibility. A toe–brachial index less than 0.7 is considered abnormal. Absolute toe pressure less than 30 to 50 mm Hg generally indicates severe lower extremity occlusive disease with inadequate perfusion to heal tissue loss, particularly in patients with diabetes.

Further anatomic mapping is warranted only after the diagnosis of hemodynamically significant infrainguinal disease has been made based upon physical examination and noninvasive testing and the decision to pursue intervention has been made. The goal of anatomic imaging is to determine if adequate revascularization is anatomically feasible and to delineate the options for both endovascular therapy and open surgical revascularization. Duplex ultrasonography, magnetic resonance angiography (MRA), and computed tomographic angiography (CTA) are increasingly being utilized as first-line modalities in planning the optimal revascularization approach, and have supplanted contrast angiography as the initial imaging study of choice in many centers. Nevertheless, due to inherent limitations with each of these techniques, digital subtraction angiography remains the gold-standard technique for imaging of the vascular tree prior to intervention and is often used as the first-line imaging modality after physiologic testing when revascularization is indicated.[18]

Although a growing literature supports the use of duplex scanning as a stand-alone preoperative mapping modality,[19] this use requires a highly dedicated vascular laboratory and to date has not gained wide acceptance. CTA is increasingly being utilized as a preoperative road-mapping technique in institutions able to provide high-quality three-dimensional reconstructions. MRA is also particularly useful as a noninvasive screening test to determine the suitability for percutaneous therapy, as advances have solved many of the technical limitations of earlier studies (**Fig. 88.3**). Should a lesion amenable to percutaneous therapy be identified, angiography and planned simultaneous revascularization is then pursued. Alternatively, in some instances of femoropopliteal reconstruction, operative planning may be based solely on CTA or MRA scanning if high-quality time of flight and gadolinium-enhanced images are obtained. In many cases, however, surgeons are reluctant to proceed to surgery without the confirmation of anatomy afforded by standard contrast angiography. This reluctance is particularly true if the distal target is at the tibial or pedal level, where anatomic detail provided by CTA and MRA remains more limited.[20]

When digital subtraction angiography is undertaken for preoperative planning, a retrograde femoral approach is typically utilized from the contralateral limb. In general, a catheter is placed in the infrarenal aorta to perform aortography and iliac angiography. If there is no aortoiliac disease which precludes catheter traversal, the wire and catheter are utilized to go "up and over" the aortic bifurcation to place the catheter in the common femoral artery of the affected limb. Lower extremity digital subtraction angiography is then carried out. This approach allows contrast volume to be minimized. It also allows the surgeon or interventionalist to proceed immediately with infrainguinal endovascular intervention through a single vascular access should endovascular therapy be the preferred treatment based on the patient's presentation and infrainguinal anatomy defined in the angiogram. In patients in whom noninvasive imaging indicates a widely patent common femoral and proximal sfa and body habitus is not prohibitive, an antegrade approach can serve as useful alternative. In ambiguous lesions or when iodinated contrast must be minimized, pull-back pressure measurements, both before and after the administration of a systemic vasodilator such as papaverine or nitroglycerine or the application of a tourniquet to induce reactive hyperemia, can be useful in documenting the hemodynamic significance of a particular stenotic zone.[21] The utilization of gadolinium or carbon dioxide as contrast agents in patients with compromised renal function, although perhaps less effective in the periphery than in the aortoiliac vasculature, can minimize or eliminate the nephrotoxic effects associated with standard iodinated contrast medium.

Medical Treatment

Risk factor modification remains a cornerstone of the management of lower extremity occlusive disease. Smoking cessation has been shown to reduce the risk of disease progression, amputation, cardiovascular mortality, and may lead to symptom relief in some patients. Smoking cessation has been best achieved with repeated physician assistance, group counseling, nicotine replacement or nicotinic receptor agonists, and antidepressant drug therapy in some patients. Weight and blood pressure reduction and aggressive efforts at lipid control should be addressed with every patient with atherosclerotic disease. Lipid-lowering therapy involves dietary modifications first and utilization of hydroxymethylglutaryl–coenzyme A–reductase inhibitors ("statins") to lower LDL cholesterol and fibrates or niacin to raise HDL cholesterol. Patients with lower extremity occlusive disease should have a goal LDL cholesterol of <70 mg/dL.[4] Statin therapy also has benefits in patients with PAD which are independent of their effect on lipid reduction. Stains stabilize atherosclerotic plaque and reduce vascular inflammation. Statin therapy has been shown to reduce cardiovascular events in patients with PAD.[22,23] In addition, statin therapy is associated with improved 1-year survival in patients undergoing lower extremity bypass for CLTI.[19]

Patients with diabetes should have aggressive control of blood glucose toward a goal hemoglobin A1c of <7%. Antiplatelet therapy in the form of either aspirin or clopidogrel is a critically important element of the treatment of established occlusive disease, given its documented ability to prevent thrombosis and embolization and possibly even to arrest the progression of atherosclerosis.[24] Aspirin and clopidogrel have both been shown to reduce cardiovascular morbidity and mortality in patients with PAD.[25,26] Some data support the utilization of combination therapy of daily aspirin and rivaroxaban 2.5 mg twice daily. When evaluating this treatment strategy

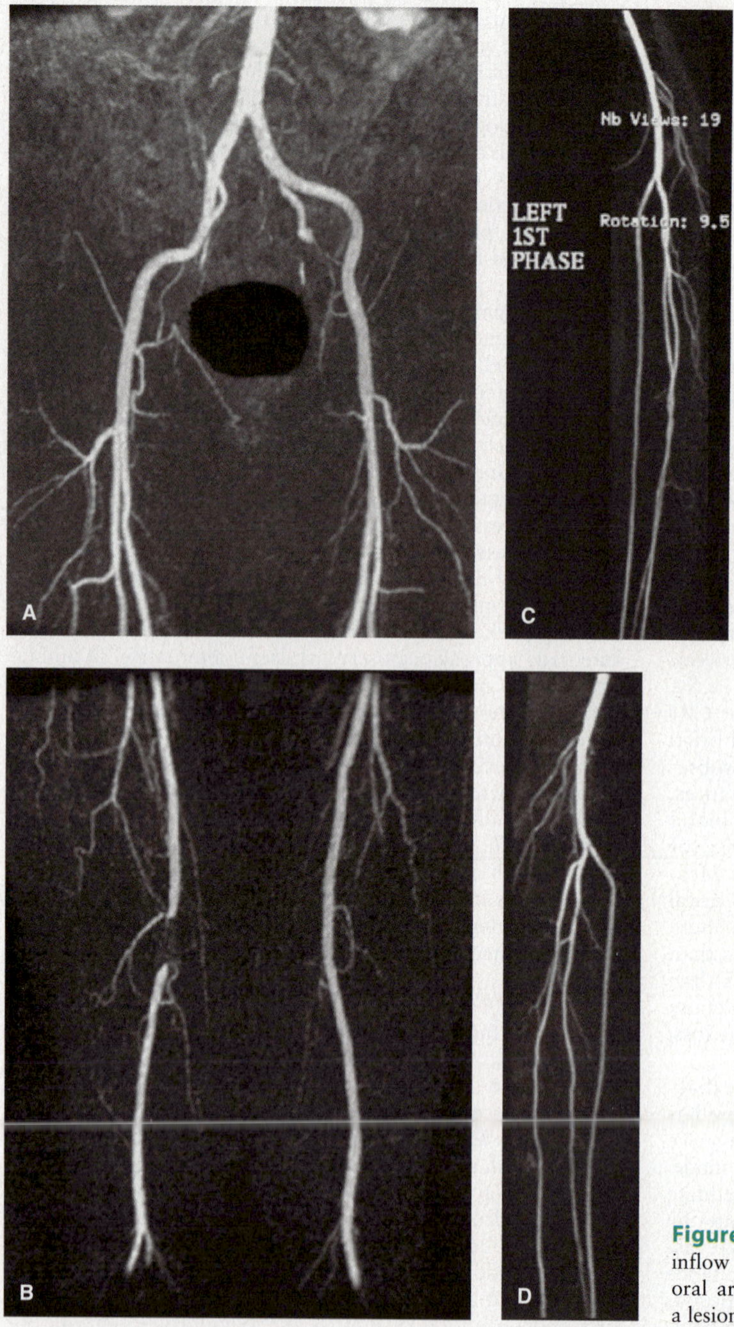

Figure 88.3. Magnetic resonance angiogram identifying patent inflow vessels (**A**), short-segment occlusion of right superficial femoral artery (**B**), and patent popliteal and tibial vessels (**C** and **D**), a lesion amenable to attempt at percutaneous therapy.

in patients following lower extremity revascularization, the Voyager PAD investigators found significantly lower incidences of acute limb ischemia, major amputation, myocardial infarction, ischemic strokes, and death.[27]

Strong evidence exists supporting the benefit of a supervised, structured walking program in increasing the walking distance of patients with claudication. The benefit of walking outside of a structured regimen with close follow-up is more debatable.[11] Nevertheless, patients should be encouraged to "walk through" the onset of lower extremity pain, resting intermittently as required. Overall, pharmacotherapy has not had a significant impact on relieving symptoms of infrainguinal occlusive disease. There is some evidence to suggest cilostazol, a phosphodiesterase inhibitor, improves walking distance and quality of life. While early studies showed that pentoxifylline, a rheologic agent, had beneficial effects on walking distance, later studies have questioned its clinical benefit.[12] Similarly, although older studies suggested that prostanoids improved healing of ischemic ulcers, the current evidence does not support the utility of any systemic drug for the relief of ischemic rest pain or the treatment of ischemic ulcerations.[13]

Indications for Revascularization

The two major indications for the intervention of infrainguinal arterial occlusive disease are lifestyle-limiting claudication and CLTI. Although there are certainly cases in which primary amputation represents the safest and most advisable solution in the face of irreversible ischemia, particularly in nonambulatory patients or in cases in which extensive infection or tissue necrosis is present, an attempt at revascularization is generally indicated when a limb is threatened by severe ischemia. However, given the morbidity and mortality associated with CLTI, it is paramount to tailor therapy to an individual's overall medical condition and life expectancy as well as the patient's goals of therapy. In the often frail CLTI population, postoperative outcomes are most strongly impacted by patients' preoperative medical condition and functional status.[14] Nevertheless, improvements in endovascular technology and techniques as

well as perioperative management and surgical technique have allowed progressively more distal revascularizations to be successfully completed in an older, sicker, and challenging patient
6 population. High limb salvage (80% to 90%) rates may be anticipated for patients with critical ischemia at institutions devoted to peripheral bypass surgery.[5,15,28,29]

CLTI has been recognized as a multifactorial disease spectrum in which limb perfusion, presence and extent of a wound, and the presence and severity of infection influence the risk of limb loss and the need for revascularization. The Society for Vascular Surgery created the novel Wound, Ischemia, and foot Infection (WIfI) classification system which provides a grade for each component; based on the patient's overall score, their amputation risk, and revascularization benefit can be stratified.[30] The WIfI classification system has been found to correlate with need for revascularization and patient-centered outcomes, including wound healing and risk for major amputation, while also reinforcing the necessity of treatment of additional components of limb threat beyond ischemia.

Claudication is a relative indication for intervention given the natural history of the disease, and it remains a subjective assessment on the part of both patient and surgeon as to the relative degree of disability a particular level of claudication pain represents. For example, two-block claudication in a younger patient whose livelihood depends on walking tolerance constitutes a more significant disability than the same degree of claudication in an older, retired individual able to attend to their daily affairs without significant consequence. Thus, proximal above-knee surgical reconstruction in a patient with disabling claudication and a patent popliteal artery with intact runoff may be justified in view of its minimal operative mortality, excellent long-term palliation, and absence of added risk of limb loss beyond that expected from the natural history of the disease process. Classically, it has been thought that the benign natural history of claudication does not warrant aggressive tibial revascularization in patients with diffuse superficial femoropopliteal and tibioperoneal disease balancing risk and more limited durability in comparison to more proximal "in-flow" procedures although reconstruction may provide symptomatic benefit and can be considered in a good-risk patient.[31,32]

In recent years, the low morbidity of endovascular revascularization in combination with patient desire for intervention seems to have lowered the threshold for offering catheter-based revascularization for claudication. Patients once considered most appropriate for risk factor modification, exercise therapy, and medical treatment are now increasingly being offered percutaneous revascularization. Nevertheless, endovascular revascularization is not without risk and is at present of limited durability. It is therefore prudent to follow the classical surgical axiom that because most patients with claudication remain stable for years, it is important to allow sufficient time for collaterals to develop and enlarge; some patients may improve to such an extent that intervention proves unnecessary.[19,33]

Approach to Revascularization

The last two decades have seen increasing utilization of endovascular revascularization of infrainguinal occlusive disease. In this light, it cannot be overemphasized that symptom status and not anatomic findings should serve as the basis for revascularization. Once the decision to intervene has been made, a variety of factors should be considered in choosing whether to proceed with an endovascular, surgical, or combined (hybrid) approach. A process of shared decision-making should be adopted such that the patient's individual priorities and goals of care are considered in the context of the expected short- and long-term outcomes based upon comorbidities, operative risk, overall life expectancy, and the extent of the occlusive disease present. The decision to revascularize should also be informed by expected effectiveness of complementary treatment strategies.

Anatomic variables are critically associated with the success and durability of endovascular therapy. As the promulgation of endovascular therapy has arisen, it has become ever more necessary to classify anatomic disease severity in order to guide potential therapy and compare outcomes between various modes of revascularization. The Trans-Atlantic Intersociety Consensus Document on Management of Peripheral Arterial Disease (TASC) was published as the result of a multidisciplinary collaboration between key medical and surgical vascular societies in 2000 and an abbreviated update was published in 2007.[9,34] These documents classified infrainguinal occlusive lesions into classes A, B, C, and D based upon the location of the lesion and the number, length, and severity of the stenoses and/or occlusions present. Their recommendations, which reflect current practice to a variable extent, include initial endovascular treatment for TASC A lesions, primary surgical treatment for TASC D lesions, and individualized tailoring of treatment for TASC B and C lesions depending upon endovascular suitability and surgical risk. While a complete description of this classification schema is beyond the scope of this chapter, a few general principles are worth noting. The patency of endovascular revascularization decreases the more distal the disease and is less in patients with stenoses that are multiple, longer, and more severe.[5,20,21,35,36] On the other hand, the success of open bypass surgery is largely dependent on the quality conduit.[37] Sustained hemodynamic improvement in the affected limb is the measure of effective revascularization and the goal of therapy. Neither "endovascular first" nor "bypass first" approach can be applied to all patients, and they are often complementary strategies. A recognized limitation to the TASC document is its emphasis on lesion characteristics in a particular arterial segment rather than the entirety of the limb. A more recent collaboration, the Global Vascular Guidelines (GVG) on the Management of Chronic Limb-Threatening Ischemia, published in 2019 stress a "whole-limb" approach. The GVG endorse the utilization of the WIfI classification described above to stage the severity of limb threat. They also outline evidence-based revascularization strategies relying on patient risk, limb severity, and anatomic complexity. A proposed Global Anatomic Staging System (GLASS) focuses on defining a preferred target artery path to estimate limb-based patency. The GVG incorporate patient risk, anatomic data, severity of limb threat, and conduit availability to guide selection of optimal revascularization strategy. The complexity of decision making emphasizes the importance not only of interventional or operative expertise, but of thorough training in vascular disease and comprehensive experience in the care of vascular patients.[22]

Endovascular Therapy

A marked increase in the number and versatility of available balloons, stents, and other devices has helped to fuel the increasing application of percutaneous technology. While a complete description of endovascular treatment options and outcomes is beyond the scope of this chapter, a brief introduction is necessary. Percutaneous vascular intervention is generally performed under local anesthesia with minimal intravenous sedation as either a same-day surgical procedure or involving an overnight admission. Percutaneous vascular intervention first involves wire traversal of hemodynamically significant stenoses or occlusions in the arterial tree. Dilatation of the lesion with percutaneous transluminal angioplasty (PTA), with or without stenting, or obliteration of the lesion via atherectomy or other modalities is utilized to reestablish blood flow through the diseased segment (**Fig. 88.4**). For interventions on the femoropopliteal and tibial arteries, retrograde contralateral femoral access allows angiography of the affected limb and establishment of a stable treatment platform via an "up and over" approach across the aortic bifurcation. Ipsilateral antegrade femoral access can also be utilized. Retrograde ipsilateral pedal and tibial access has been described to allow wire traversal and endovascular treatment of disease not amenable to the standard antegrade approach.[7,23]

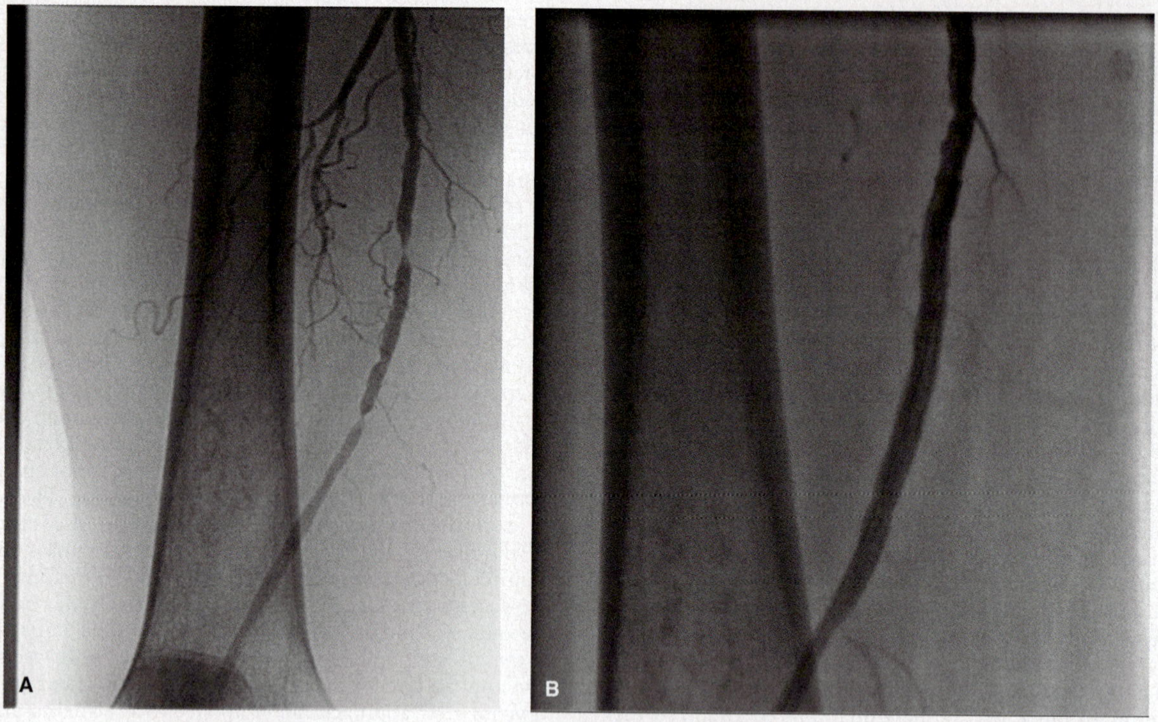

Figure 88.4. Angiogram of the right superficial femoral artery demonstrating short-segment occlusion and more diffuse stenosis in Hunter canal (**A**), which was treated with angioplasty and self-expanding bare metal stent placement (**B**).

Periprocedural outcomes with endovascular therapy are excellent. Technical success, which is generally defined as the presence of antegrade flow through the tree to lesion with less than 30% residual stenosis at the conclusion of the procedure, is reported at 80% to 95% for both femoropopliteal and infrapopliteal procedures. Associated overall morbidity in recent reports ranges between 8% and 17% while mortality is low at approximately 0.2%.[24] Contrast-induced nephropathy remains a common complication. With the development of hypo-osmolar and iso-osmolar contrast agents; the overall incidence is approximately 8%, whereas the rate of acute renal failure requiring dialysis is less than 1%.[25] Substantial morbidity can result from access-site complications, predominantly pseudoaneurysms, groin hematomas, and arteriovenous fistulas (AVFs), which occur in 1% to 4% of patients.[26]

Reports indicate that endovascular therapy has good short-term efficacy for femoropopliteal disease (**Table 88.1**). In claudicants, PTA for femoropopliteal lesions has generally yielded 1-year patency of approximately 77% and 65% for stenoses and occlusions, respectively. In patients with CLTI, PTA for femoropopliteal lesions has yielded 1-year primary patency of 60% and 40% for stenoses and occlusions, respectively. The patency of endovascular revascularization is related to disease extent and complexity. For femoropopliteal lesions that are longer than 5 to 10 cm in length, data show improved 1-year patency, ranging from with bare metal self-expanding stents or drug-eluting balloons or stents.[38–40] Infrapopliteal disease appears less amenable to endovascular therapy (**Fig. 88.5**). Primary patency is generally reported at 45% to 55% at 1 year.[20] Patency does not appear to be improved by stenting in the infrapopliteal segment.[41]

RESULTS

Table 88.1. Patency of Femoropopliteal Angioplasty and Stenting[a]

	1-year % Patency (Range)	3-year % Patency (Range)	5-year % Patency (Range)
PTA: stenosis	77 (78–80)	61 (55–68)	55 (52–62)
PTA: occlusion	65 (55–71)	48 (40–55)	42 (33–51)
PTA+stent: stenosis	75 (73–79)	66 (64–70)	
PTA+stent: occlusion	73 (69–75)	64 (59–67)	
Drug Eluting Balloon	82[b]	70[b]	Not available
Drug Eluting Stent	83[c]		72[c]

[a]Adapted from Norgren L, Hiatt WR, Dormandy JA, et al. Inter-society consensus for the management of peripheral arterial disease (TASC II). *J Vasc Surg*. 2007;45(Suppl S):S5–S67.

[b]Schneider PA, Laird JR, Tepe G, et al. Treatment effect of drug-coated balloons is durable to 3 years in the femoropopliteal arteries: long-term results of the IN.PACT SFA randomized trial. *Circ Cardiovasc Interv*. 2018;11(1):e005891.[42]

[c]From Dake MD, Ansel GM, Jaff MR, et al. Durable clinical effectiveness with paclitaxel-eluting stents in the femoropopliteal artery: 5-year results of the Zilver PTX randomized trial. *Circulation*. 2016;133(15):1472–1483; discussion 1483.

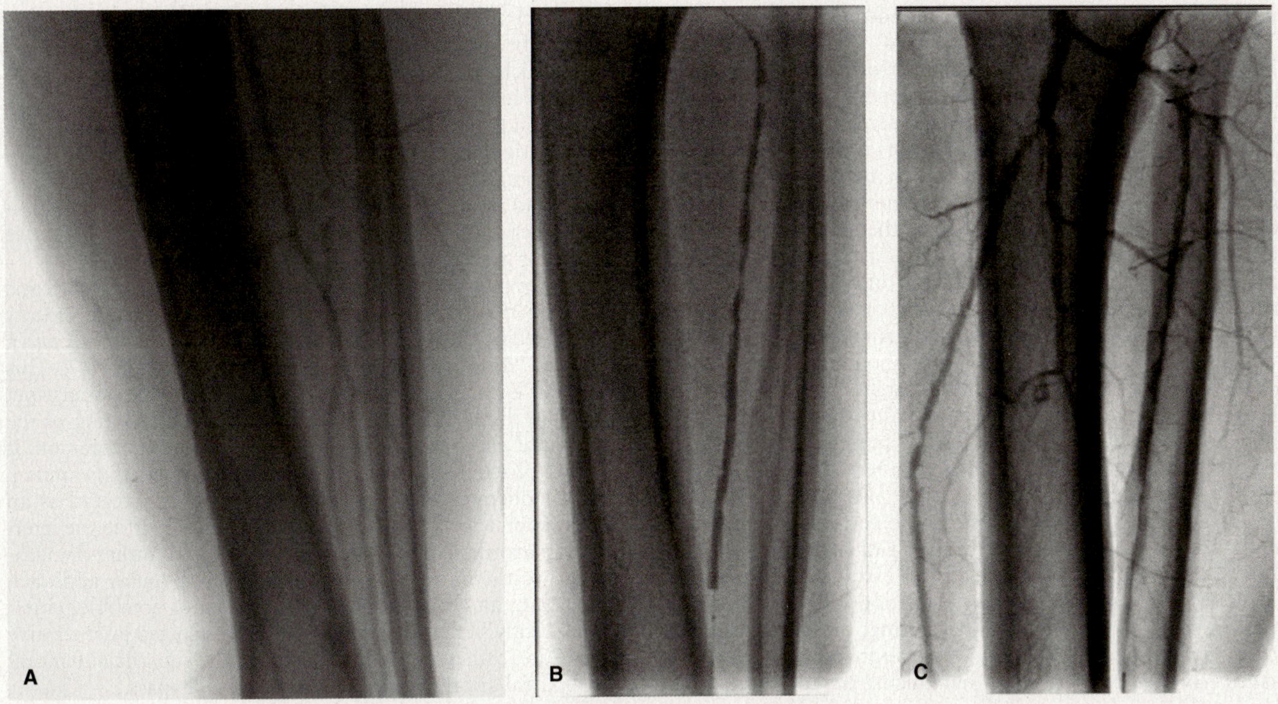

Figure 88.5. Angiogram of the tibial arteries showing diffuse anterior tibial artery high-grade stenosis (**A**) which was treated with long-segment balloon angioplasty, (**B**) completion angiogram showed patent anterior tibial artery with no significant residual stenosis (**C**).

Lack of durability has been the Achilles heel of infrainguinal endovascular intervention. Three-year patency after PTA has generally been reported to be 43% to 61% and 30% to 48% for femoropopliteal stenoses and occlusions, respectively. Five-year patency data are seldom reported but have been generally reported to be between 26% and 45% after PTA for femoropopliteal lesions.[7] Bare metal self-expanding have been shown to extend patency to 51% to 68% at 2 years, while drug-eluting stents have been shown to extend patency to 75% to 83% at 2 years.[38]

Until recently, there has been a scarcity of high-level data comparing PTA and bypass surgery for infrainguinal occlusive disease. Given the vastly different natural history of the disease process, it is important to separate and differentiate CLTI from claudication when looking at the results of trials comparing endovascular to open surgical revascularization for infrainguinal occlusive disease. The BASIL (bypass vs angioplasty in severe leg ischemia) trial which randomized 452 patients with "severe limb ischemia" to a "bypass first" or "balloon angio- 7
plasty first" strategy is the most widely cited trial. There was no difference in the primary endpoint of amputation-free survival at 6 months, although a "surgery-first" strategy was associated with greater cost and morbidity. It is necessary to note that the endovascular arm of this trial did not include adjunctive procedures such as stenting which are now frequently utilized in current day practice. Upon long-term follow-up of at least 3 years and more than 5 years in the majority of patients, bypass was associated with improved overall survival and a strong trend toward improved amputation-free survival in patients who survived at least 2 years. In addition, most balloon angioplasty patients ultimately required bypass surgery. Bypass after failed balloon angioplasty had significantly worse patency than that of primary bypass. This finding corroborated other 8
reports demonstrating that surgical bypass for salvage following failed endovascular treatment is inferior to primary bypass, indicating that a universal "endovascular first" approach may not be appropriate. More recently, the BEST Endovascular Versus Surgery in Critical Limb Ischemia (BEST CLI) Trial, 9
compared endovascular therapy to surgical bypass in patients with CLTI and infrainguinal occlusive disease judged to be amenable to both endovascular and open revascularization. In patients with an adequate single segment saphenous vein for bypass, surgery offer a 32% relative risk reduction in the primary endpoint of major adverse limb events or death at a median follow-up of 2.7 years. Surgery was beneficial across a variety of secondary endpoints and patient subgroups.[43] On the other hand, a randomized trial comparing endovascular therapy with bypass surgery in 345 patients with infrapopliteal disease and CLTI found that endovascular therapy was associated with improved amputation-free survival compared to surgery. The primary outcome was primarily driven by fewer deaths in the endovascular group.[44] Another trial comparing PTA and above-knee bypass surgery in patients with claudication and 5 to 15 cm sfa lesions. Surgery was associated with 31% absolute risk reduction for subsequent reocclusion and superior clinical improvement compared to angioplasty.[45] No randomized trials have compared current optimal endovascular therapy, that is, drug-eluting therapy and/or bare metal stenting, to surgical bypass in claudicants.

For patients with favorable anatomy and significant operative risk, and for the treatment of claudication in general, percutaneous therapy has assumed a primary initial role. When medical therapy or percutaneous treatment has proven inadequate or anatomy is not amenable to safe endovascular intervention, open surgical revascularization remains the gold standard for those patients with disabling claudication. Furthermore, until the efficacy and durability of infrainguinal percutaneous intervention is better defined, surgical revascularization remains the gold standard for any patient with CLTI, especially those with extensive tissue loss. The relative roles of surgical and percutaneous intervention are actively being refined. Furthermore, many patients are best treated with a combination of percutaneous and open surgical therapy, often in a single procedure (hybrid procedure). In many instances, endovascular and open surgical revascularization are thus complementary modes of therapy.

Operative Management

Successful infrainguinal arterial bypass requires sound planning as well as technical expertise. As such, it remains the signature operation which distinguishes vascular surgeons from other specialists involved in the treatment of PAD. Successful infrainguinal bypass grafting requires adequate arterial inflow. While aortobifemoral, femorofemoral, and axillofemoral bypass grafting remain routinely performed inflow procedures, aortoiliac angioplasty and stenting are increasingly becoming the preliminary procedures performed to attain sufficient inflow prior to construction of a more distal bypass graft. At times, the necessity of improving the inflow to support an infrainguinal graft is determined intraoperatively, either by direct visual assessment of the arterial flow at the desired donor site or by comparison of a transduced pressure tracing from the donor site with that of a systemic pressure tracing, typically obtained from a radial arterial line. Of equal importance to the outcome of any infrainguinal graft is target vessel selection. In general, the bypass should be made as short as possible but should be sewn to a target vessel which is the least diseased artery that supplies uninterrupted ("in-line") flow to the foot. If tissue necrosis is present, restoration of pulsatile flow to the foot is often required to obtain full and sustained wound healing.

Infrainguinal surgical bypass can be performed under general anesthesia, or in the appropriate patient, under regional, spinal, or epidural anesthesia. In cases involving multiple sites of dissection, such as those necessitating more tedious arm vein or lesser saphenous vein harvesting, the procedures are particularly amenable to a two-team approach, with the time saved having direct benefit in minimizing the total anesthetic load and physiologic insult. For patients with sfa disease, the initial dissection is most commonly at the level of the common femoral artery. This vessel is exposed through a longitudinal or oblique incision centered directly over the femoral pulse. Lymphatic tissue overlying the femoral vessels is best ligated and divided to prevent the postoperative development of lymph fistulas or lymphoceles. The severity of any concomitant common femoral and profunda femoral disease and the level of reconstruction planned dictate the extent of exposure of the femoral vessels. In most instances, the dissection extends from the inguinal ligament to the common femoral artery bifurcation, where the origins of the superficial and profunda femoral arteries are individually isolated.

If a profundaplasty is required, the dissection is extended distally along a sufficient length of the profunda femoral artery to attain an endpoint suitable for clamping and sewing (**Fig. 88.6**). Similarly, the inguinal ligament can be mobilized to facilitate access to the distal external iliac artery in cases in which a more extensive proximal endarterectomy is necessary.

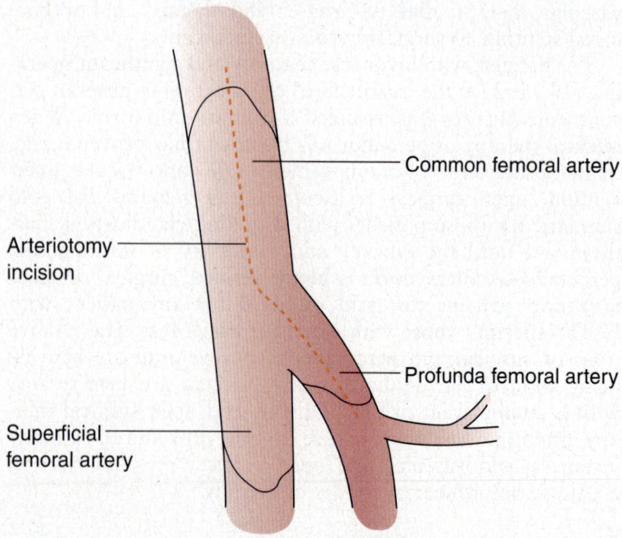

Figure 88.6. In the setting of orificial profunda femoral artery disease, extending the common femoral arteriotomy into the origin of the profunda and performing a profundaplasty will maximize profunda flow in the event of graft thrombosis.

In these circumstances, it is customary to close the endarterectomized bed with a vein, bovine pericardial or Dacron patch, onto which the proximal anastomosis can subsequently be attached. In patients with a hostile groin crease from prior surgery or radiation therapy or in obese, diabetic patients with an intertriginous rash at the inguinal crease, meticulous skin preparation, close attention to draping, careful surgical technique, and judicious use of a short course of intravenous antibiotic therapy help minimize the chances of a postoperative wound or graft infection.

If all or part of the sfa is spared of significant atherosclerotic involvement, the proximal anastomosis can be moved distally as dictated by the particular anatomic pattern of disease, and a so-called "distal origin graft" can be fashioned (**Fig. 88.7**). This situation is particularly applicable to the diabetic population, in whom infrapopliteal disease is the rule and sparing of the superficial femoral and popliteal arteries is not uncommon. It is also utilized in situations in which conduit length is limited, and a moderately diseased proximal vessel is accepted as an inflow source for a more distal origin bypass graft in the interests of performing a fully autologous vein graft rather than utilizing prosthetic material. An increasingly popular approach when only limited conduit is available is to combine, either concurrently in the operating room or as a staged preoperative procedure, catheter-based treatment of the superficial femoral or popliteal artery inflow with more distal bypass.

The above-knee popliteal vessel is easily exposed through a medial thigh incision, with subsequent posterolateral retraction of the sartorius muscle. The popliteal artery with its accompanying vein and nerve is found just posterior to the femur. The vessel is palpated to determine the presence of atherosclerotic plaque, which will guide the extent of dissection and the optimal bypass target site. The below-knee popliteal artery is also exposed through a medial incision in the proximal calf (**Fig. 88.8**). If the saphenous vein is to be harvested, the incision is made directly over the vein to minimize the creation of devascularized skin flaps. With the exposed vein carefully protected, the incision is carried through the deep muscular fascia and the medial head of the gastrocnemius is reflected posteriorly to expose the below-knee popliteal fossa. The distal popliteal artery is then dissected free from the adjacent tibial nerve posteriorly and popliteal vein medially. If the distal target is the tibioperoneal trunk, the dissection is continued along the anteromedial surface of the distal popliteal artery after dividing the origin of the soleus muscle from the tibia (**Fig. 88.9**).

Although exposure of the proximal posterior tibial and peroneal vessels can be gained by extending the tibioperoneal trunk dissection distally, more distal exposure of these vessels is best gained through more distal, targeted medial incisions. The posterior tibial artery is found beneath the divided musculotendinous origin of the soleus muscle, and the peroneal artery is deeper and more lateral. The posterior tibial artery at the level of the ankle is a relatively easier target given the proximity of the vessel to the skin surface. The initial incision is made just posterior to the medial malleolus, and the artery exposed by division of the overlying retinaculum. Further distal dissection allows access to the bifurcation and medial and lateral plantar branches. The more distal peroneal artery may be approached laterally via an incision placed over the distal fibula. Excision of a short segment of fibula will expose the underlying artery.

The anterior tibial artery is typically approached from the anterolateral aspect of the calf (**Fig. 88.9**) and is found deep within the anterior compartment with the adjacent deep peroneal nerve and anterior tibial veins. It is best identified by developing the intermuscular plane between the tibialis anterior muscle belly medially and the extensor digitorum longus laterally. The dorsalis pedis artery is easily exposed through an axial incision on the dorsum of the foot just lateral to the extensor hallucis longus tendon (**Fig. 88.9**). The artery lies just deep to the extensor retinaculum.

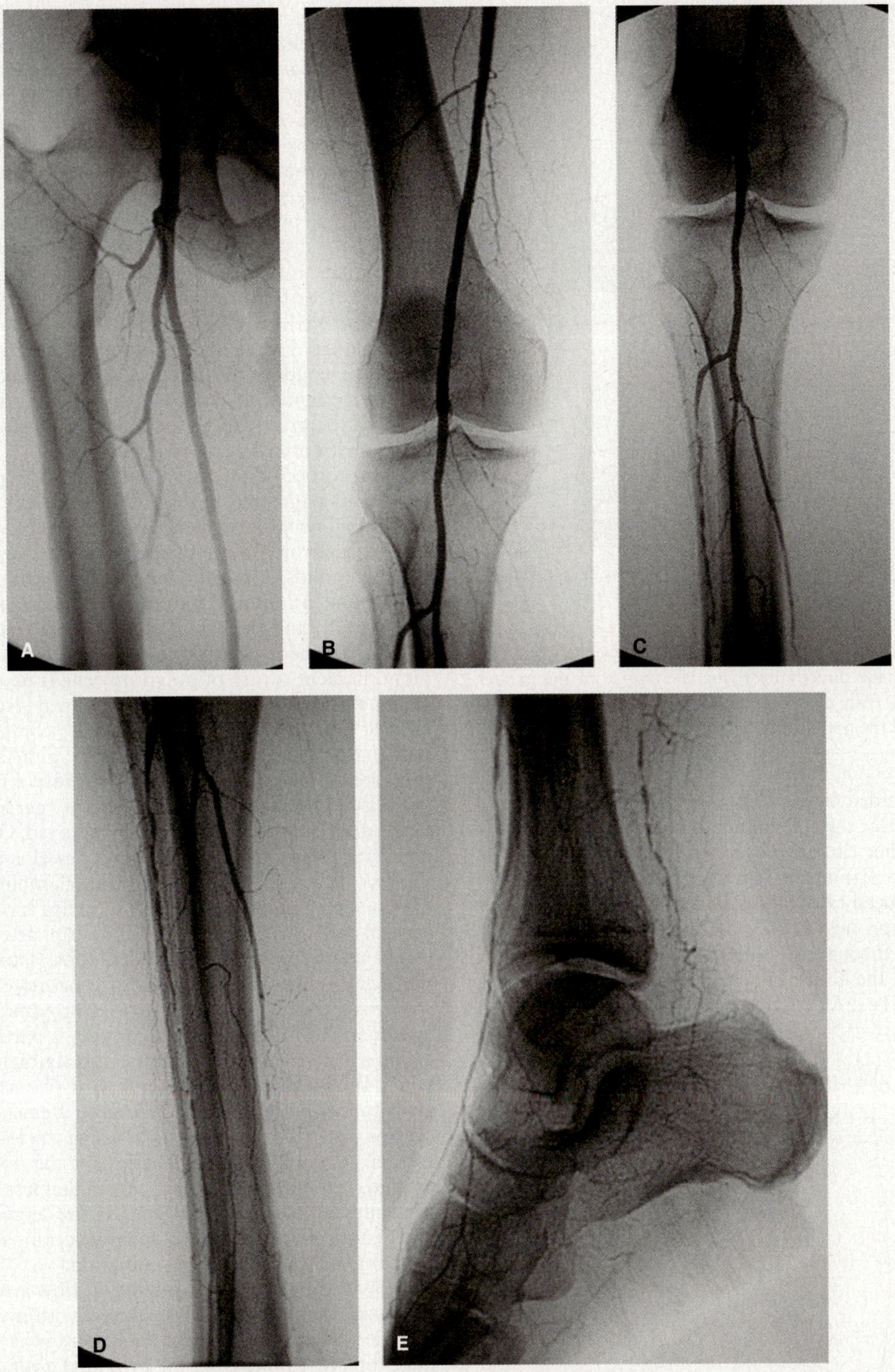

Figure 88.7. Arteriogram indicating preservation of the superficial femoral artery and popliteal arteries (**A–C**) with mid-calf occlusions of all three infrageniculate vessels (**D**), with reconstitution of the dorsalis pedis artery in the foot (**E**). This anatomic pattern of disease is amenable to "distal origin" vein grafting from the below-knee popliteal or proximal posterior tibial artery to the dorsalis pedis artery.

Autogenous Vein Bypass

10 Infrainguinal bypass surgery is best performed with autogenous vein conduit, preferably the ipsilateral great saphenous vein if available.[46] This preference is particularly true for grafts extending below the knee, where prosthetic conduits of Dacron or polytetrafluoroethylene have significantly poorer patency rates. Given the orientation of the vein valves, the vein can be reversed such that the distal end of the vein is sewn to the proximal inflow artery and the larger proximal end of the vein is sewn to the distal outflow artery. However, it is our general practice to utilize the great saphenous vein in the nonreversed orientation as will be discussed shortly. The vein is harvested through a long incision overlying the course of the vein or by more tedious but less invasive sequential skip incisions with intervening cutaneous skin bridges (**Fig. 88.7**). All side branches are ligated and after harvest, the vein is cannulated and gently dilated with a solution containing heparin and papaverine to assess its suitability. Veins with chronic fibrosis or that fail to dilate to a diameter of 3 mm or greater will likely have poor long-term function.

An alternative and less invasive approach to saphenous vein harvest involves the use of endoscopic technology. In the case of harvesting of the great saphenous vein, small skin incisions are made over the saphenofemoral junction and the

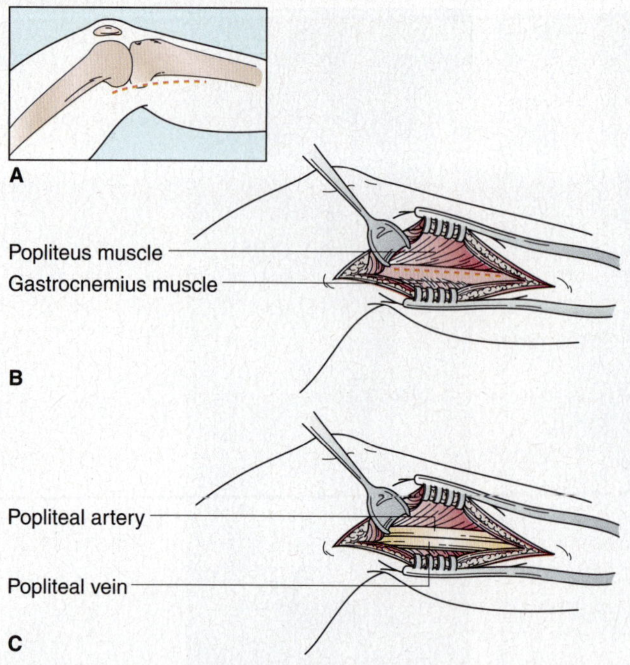

Figure 88.8. Exposure of the popliteal artery below the knee. The medial incision is made directly overlying the course of the greater saphenous vein (**A**), with posterior retraction of the gastrocnemius muscle (**B**), to reveal the popliteal vessels in the popliteal fossa (**C**).

distal vein and guided by a videoscope inserted distally and advanced proximally, the side branches of the vein are serially identified and either cauterized or clip-ligated. Advocates of this method cite a significant reduction in wound complication rates and reduced rates of hospital stay, although patency rates may be compromised. For prosthetic grafts, a tunnel is usually fashioned through the subsartorial plane between the groin incision and the above-knee popliteal space in the interests of protecting the graft from subsequent infection. For vein conduits, it remains the surgeon's preference as to whether the graft is tunneled deeply or in a superficial location in the subcutaneous space. The more superficial configuration greatly facilitates ongoing clinical examination and ultrasonographic surveillance as well as latter surgical revision but carries a risk of graft exposure should there be wound-healing problems. Occlusion from trauma to grafts placed superficially is not a practical concern.

It is our practice to perform the proximal anastomosis prior to the distal anastomosis. First, this allows confirmation of adequate inflow before the bypass is performed. Second, performance of the proximal anastomosis first allows the graft to be tunneled and tailored to appropriate length under arterial pressure. This is of critical importance to prevent kinking along the length of the graft. An additional benefit of performing the proximal anastomosis first is that adequacy of flow through the graft can be assessed, both before and after tunneling, with brief release of the clamp.

Prior to occluding the inflow vessel, the patient is systemically anticoagulated with 5,000 to 10,000 units of heparin. Additional heparin is given throughout the procedure to maintain the activated clotting time near the target range of 250 to 300 seconds. After allowing sufficient time for the heparin to circulate, atraumatic vascular clamps are placed proximally and distally, and the artery is incised. The vein is then spatulated and a beveled anastomosis carried out. Typically a 5-0 monofilament suture of polypropylene is used for the femoral anastomosis, a 6-0 is used at the popliteal level, and 7-0 suture used at the tibial or pedal level. After completing the proximal anastomosis, the graft is carefully tunneled under arterial pressure. If the target tibial vessel is deep within the calf and visibility is challenging, a technique of "parachuting" the heel of the distal anastomosis is often employed. Occasionally, such extensive calcification of the target vessel is encountered that the risk of a significant injury from clamping, even with the minimally traumatic clamps in use today, is prohibitively high. In such cases, proximal inflow and distal artery back-bleeding can be controlled by occlusion balloons placed intraluminally. For distal anastomoses at the knee or more distal level, our preferred technique is the use of a proximally placed sterile pneumatic tourniquet. This technique is particularly advantageous when sewing to diminutive distal tibial or pedal targets, where the impact of a crush injury or plaque dislodgment on graft function could be considerable. Removing the need for clamps or occluding balloons by using the tourniquet has two further advantages. First, it improves the operative visibility. Second, and more importantly, given that less longitudinal and circumferential dissection is needed, the degree of vessel spasm and venous bleeding that frequently accompanies vessel exposure at this level is kept to a minimum.

Flow through the graft and the outflow arteries are assessed following completion of the bypass with a continuous-wave Doppler. Ideally, a contrast angiogram is also performed after directly cannulating the proximal graft (**Fig. 88.10**); this allows for immediate repair of any technical defects that are identified, such as intraluminal thrombus, twisting or kinking of the graft, or retained valve cusps. Intraoperative completion duplex ultrasonography is an additional sensitive screen for hemodynamically significant abnormalities within the graft, and its use further serves to prevent early graft loss caused by correctable technical problems.

Current reports of the 5-year results of reversed saphenous vein graft using modern techniques have been excellent, with primary and secondary patency rates up to 80%, and limb salvage rates greater than 90% (**Table 88.2**).[15,28,29,46,47]

In Situ Grafting

There has been ongoing enthusiasm in some circles for in situ vein bypass grafting, whereby except for its proximal and distal extent, the greater saphenous vein is left undisturbed in its native bed. This technique was first described in 1962, but was

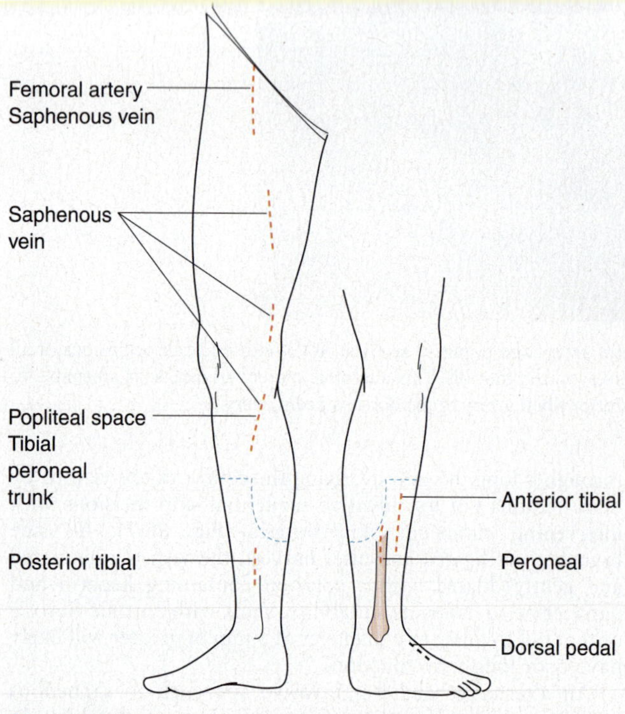

Figure 88.9. Placement of incisions for femoropopliteal and femorotibial bypass and for greater saphenous vein harvest. These should avoid the incision lines for a below-knee amputation.

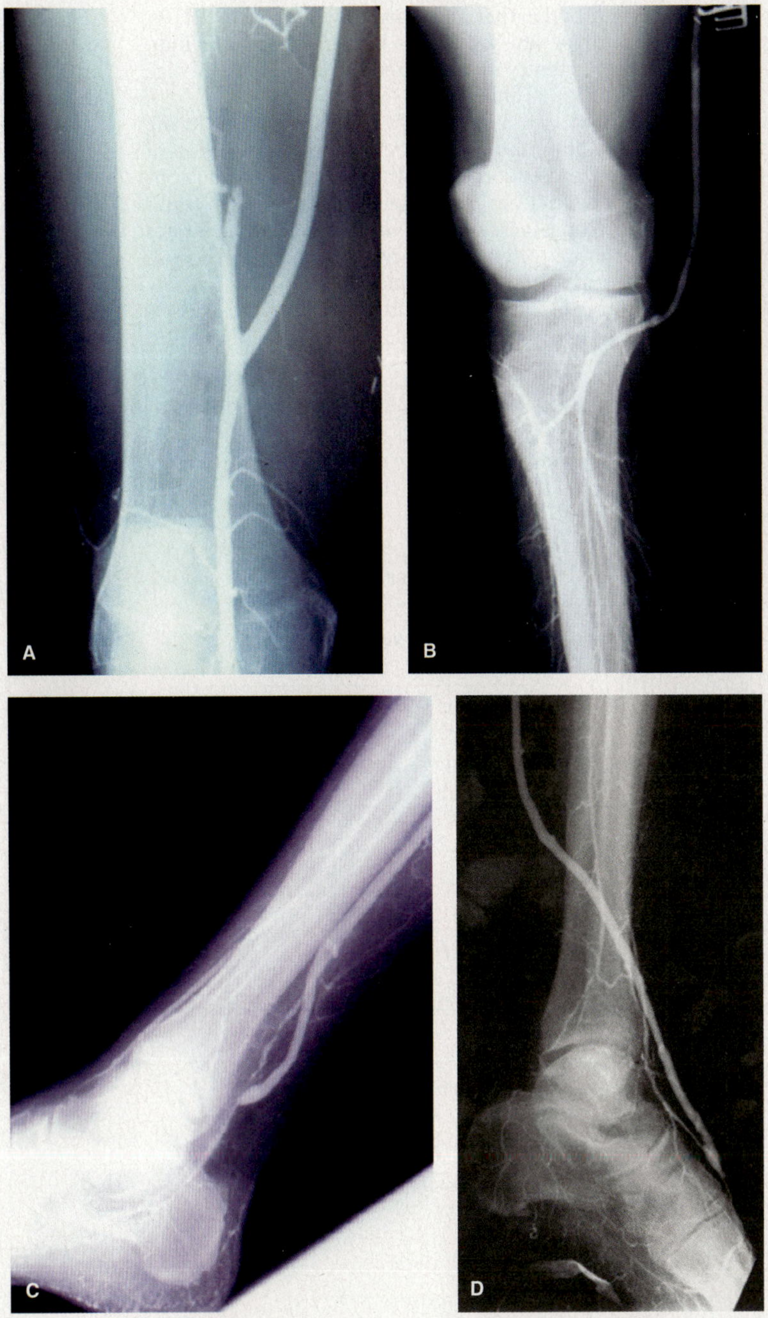

Figure 88.10. Intraoperative completion arteriograms of distal anastomoses to the above-knee popliteal (**A**), below-knee popliteal (**B**), distal posterior tibial (**C**), and dorsalis pedis (**D**) arteries.

RESULTS

Table 88.2. Five-Year Patency and Limb Salvage Results of Infrainguinal Bypass Grafting

Study	Patients, *n*	Conduit	Primary Patency	Secondary Patency	Limb Salvage
Conte et al. (2006)[15]	1,642	Autogenous vein	63	73	85
Belkin et al. (1996)[28]	568	In situ vein	72	82	90
	189	Nonreversed vein	65	65	82
Shah and Leather (1996)[29]	2058	In situ vein	72	81	95
Taylor et al. (1990)[47]	564	Reversed vein	75	81	90
Veith et al. (1986)[46]	338	PTFE to popliteal	38		70
	254	PTFE to tibial	12[a]		61[a]

[a]4-year data.
PTFE, polytetrafluoroethylene.

later popularized by Leather and Karmody in the late 1970s. Recent reports of in situ saphenous vein grafting have indicated 5-year graft patency rates of up to 80% and limb salvage rates of 84% to 95% (**Table 88.1**).

The in situ approach minimizes trauma to the vein during excision and handling, and in theory enhances preservation of the vasovasorum and endothelium. It further lowers the considerable risk of wound-healing complications seen with traditional vein harvesting, increases vein utilization, and facilitates the creation of more technically precise anastomoses because the proximal and distal vein diameters are more closely matched to those of the inflow and outflow target vessels (**Fig. 88.11**). The extent of the proximal vein mobilization is dictated by the location of the saphenofemoral junction relative to the proposed site of the proximal anastomosis. It may at times be necessary to perform an endarterectomy of the sfa if the length of proximal vein is insufficient. Lysis of the valve cusps is obligatory given the nonreversed configuration, and is facilitated by newer, less traumatic valvulotomes that function safely through the blinded segments of undissected graft. Critics of this technique argue that the advantages listed above have not translated into improved graft function or patency. They further argue that the time required and dissection involved in finding and ligating substantial side branches that

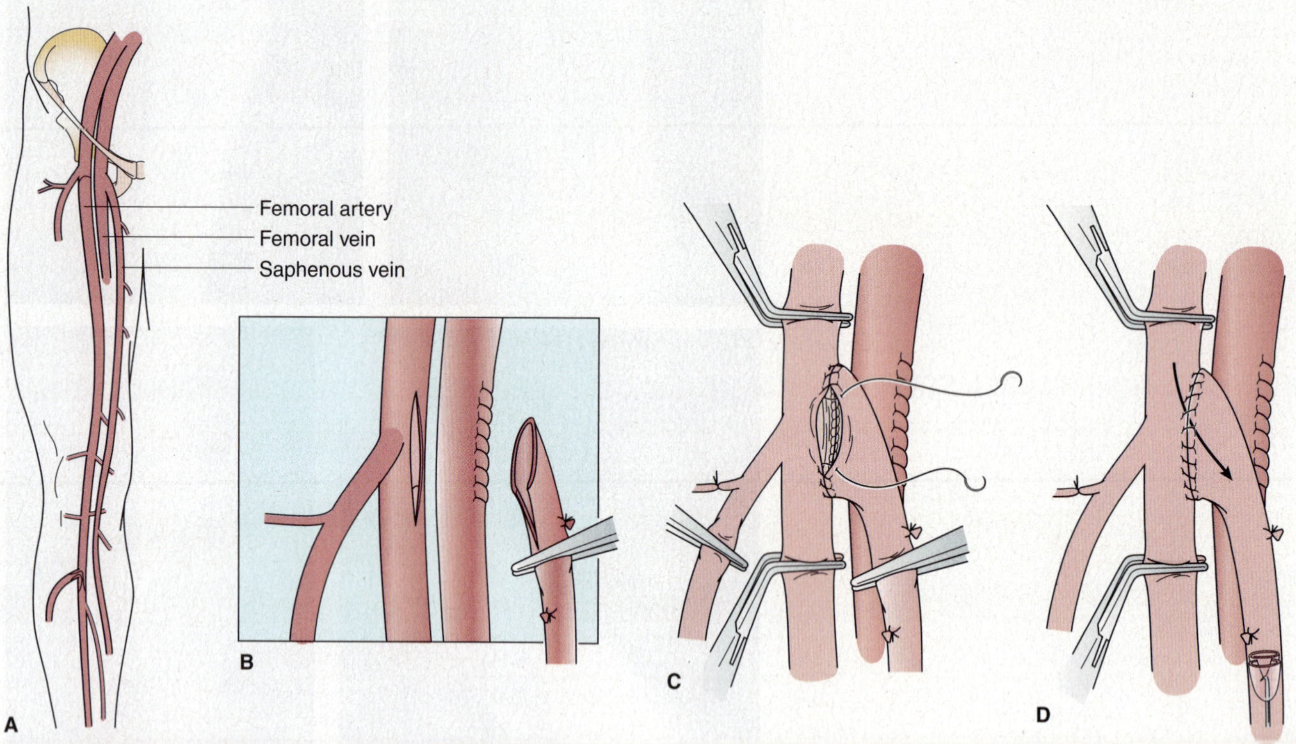

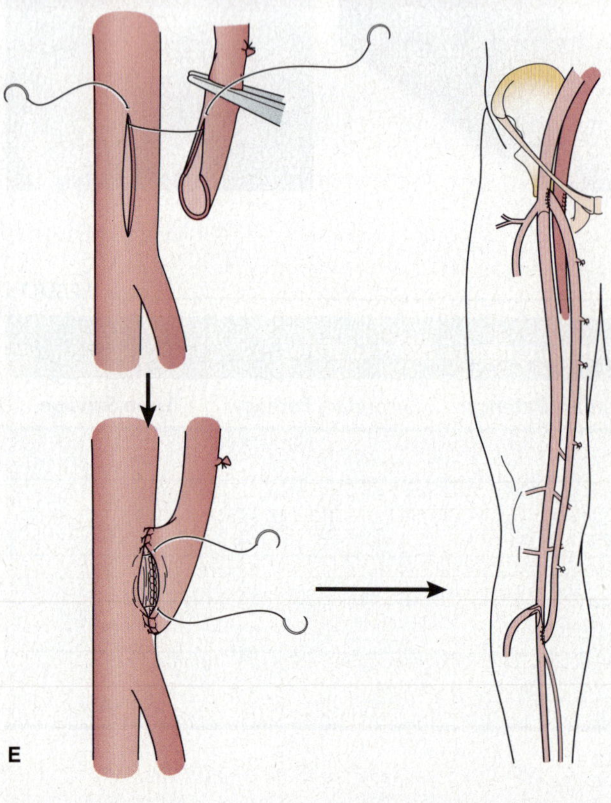

Figure 88.11. **A:** In the in situ method of infrainguinal reconstruction, the saphenous vein is left undisturbed in its native bed except for at the proximal and distal anastomotic sites, in this case, the common femoral artery and the tibioperoneal trunk, respectively. **B:** The saphenofemoral junction is transected in the groin, the venotomy in the femoral vein is oversewn and the proximal end of the saphenous vein spatulated is prepared for anastomosis. **C:** After the first venous valve is excised under direct vision, the graft is anastomosed end-to-side to the femoral artery. Flow is then restored through the vein graft and the valvulotome passed from the distal end to lyse the residual valves (**D**), before the distal anastomosis is performed (**E**).

can develop into physiologically important AVFs that "steal" distal flow obviates the stated benefits of this approach.

Angioscopic-assisted valve lysis has been employed for over a decade, but has not gained widespread favor. Although there is a significant learning curve with this technology and operative times, at least initially, are significantly prolonged, advocates cite fewer wound complications, shorter hospital stays, and decreased recuperative periods as potential benefits.

Nonreversed Saphenous Vein Grafts

Recognizing the many practical advantages inherent to the in situ technique, some surgeons have modified the approach to infrainguinal bypass grafting with venous conduit to incorporate several of the same principles. In particular, if the harvested vein is tapered to any significant extent, it is used in a nonreversed fashion. By optimizing the size matching between the artery and vein at both the proximal and distal anastomosis sites as discussed previously, one can often accept for use smaller veins than would be unsuitable for reversed vein grafting. The nonreversed configuration also allows preservation of the saphenous vein hood, which both extends the available conduit length and is especially beneficial when the femoral artery is thick walled and diseased.

The vein is harvested and dilated in a similar fashion to reversed vein grafts and the cusps of the proximal valve of the great saphenous vein are excised under direct vision with fine Potts scissors. There are currently two main types of valvulotomes available. The modified Mills valvulotome is a short, metal, hockey stick-shaped cutter that can be introduced through the distal end of the vein or through the side branches. After the proximal anastomosis is performed, and with the perfused conduit on gentle stretch, the valves are carefully lysed in a sequential fashion by pulling the valvulotome inferiorly. An alternative self-centering valvulotome allows lysis of all valves in a single pass and is thought by some to be less traumatic. Once acceptable pulsatile flow is ensured, the distal anastomosis is performed in the standard fashion.

It is important to note that similar patency rates have consistently been demonstrated regardless of which technique is applied, and so surgeon preference and comfort level is an acceptable reason for choosing one method over another.

Prosthetic Bypass

It is recommended that infrainguinal bypass surgery be performed with saphenous vein or an autologous substitute whenever feasible given the clearly demonstrated enhanced patency rates.[46] When the distal target is the above-knee popliteal artery and the tibial outflow is relatively well preserved, this is an acceptable approach.[48] A variety of surgical adjunctive procedures, from patching the distal anastomotic target vessel to the creation of a distal AVF or various autogenous vein cuffs interposed between the distal prosthetic and the target artery, have all been attempted as a means of improving the patency rates of grafts extending below the knee. Polyester (Dacron) and polytetrafluoroethylene (Teflon) grafts are the two main types of prosthetic available and, as in other anatomic positions, available data show generally equal results with either choice. The entire procedure is carried out through two small proximal and distal incisions between which the graft is tunneled anatomically. The selection of a 6-, 7-, or 8-mm graft is dictated by the size of the native vessels.

Reoperative Bypass Surgery

As the patient population treated by vascular surgeons has increased in age, and more challenging cases are accepted for primary treatment, there has been a corresponding increase in the incidence of reoperative bypass surgery performed for infrainguinal arterial occlusive disease. Such reoperative procedures are particularly challenging, both because of the scarring present at the inflow and outflow target sites and because there is typically a lack of ipsilateral great saphenous vein. Whenever possible, the first problem is addressed by choosing anastomotic sites just above or below the previous touchdown points, thereby avoiding dissection through often densely scarred tissue planes. When ipsilateral great saphenous vein is absent because of prior infrainguinal or coronary artery bypass surgery or prior saphenous vein stripping, there are a number of alternative conduit sites available. Adequate contralateral great saphenous is the optimal conduit in these situations; despite the presumably high incidence of contralateral lower extremity as well as coronary occlusive disease in this population, the short- and long-term impact was found to be minimal.

In the absence of any great saphenous vein, preoperative venous duplex ultrasonography is employed to evaluate the cephalic and basilic veins of the arms and the lesser saphenous veins of the legs in an effort to determine the best conduit available. Often the veins distal to the antecubital crease are scarred and of small caliber, but their more proximal counterparts are often of excellent size and quality. The use of arm veins in general can be technically challenging and for that reason has not been universally adopted. The dissection of the basilic vein can be particularly tedious as it has multiple side branches and lies adjacent to several important nerves. As arm veins are often relatively short, a venovenostomy is often required to create composite grafts long enough to complete the arterial reconstruction (**Fig. 88.12**). This is performed with generous spatulation of each vein hood to create a widely patent vein-to-vein anastomosis. Given their thin-walled nature, arm vein grafts are also quite prone to twisting and kinking, and special care must be taken during the tunneling process to avoid these problems. The more proximal arm veins can be relatively large, and it is often advantageous to use one or more of the segments in a nonreversed fashion to better match the graft to the inflow vessel size. Not surprisingly, the results of reoperative infrainguinal bypass surgery do not match those of primary reconstruction. With autogenous vein, 5-year patency rates of 60% and limb salvage rates of 70% to 80% have been reported.[49]

Postreconstruction Management

Unless otherwise contraindicated, all patients are maintained indefinitely on an antiplatelet regimen with either aspirin or clopidogrel following surgical bypass. As stated previously, in cases in which a graft is at increased risk of failure, such as in the setting of reoperation or in cases in which compromised outflow or a marginal conduit was accepted, the antiplatelet agent may be supplemented with anticoagulation.[50] Patients with distal calf or pedal incisions should have consistent leg elevation in the early postoperative period to minimize leg swelling and wound-healing complications. Thereafter, aggressive rehabilitation maximizes the chances of, and shortens the time to a return to, full function after extensive reconstructive surgery.

Graft Failure and Surveillance

Postoperative graft failures are typically classified according to the time interval from surgery as early, intermediate, or late. Graft thrombosis occurring within 30 days, the so-called "early graft failures" are generally thought to be a result of technical or judgment errors by the surgeon. Included in this list would be such technical errors as twists, kinks, incompletely lysed valves, or anastomotic defects, as well as judgment errors in using a poor quality vein or targeting an outflow vessel with inadequate runoff to support the graft. Intermediate graft failures include those between 30 days and 2 years and are generally attributed to the proliferation of intimal hyperplasia at the anastomoses or prior valve sites within the graft (**Fig. 88.13**). Late graft failures occurring beyond 2 years are typically a result of the progression of atherosclerotic occlusive disease within the inflow or outflow arteries.

Given the known incidence of graft failure and the potentially dire consequence in terms of limb salvage or preservation

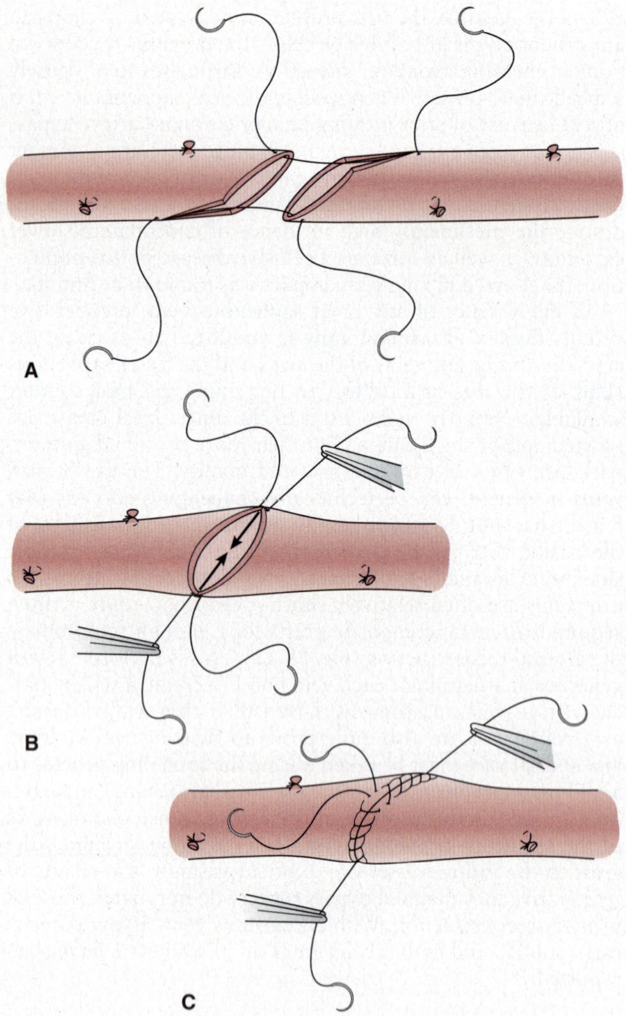

Figure 88.12. Creation of a composite graft from two or more segments of arm vein or lesser saphenous vein (A) is sometimes necessary to obtain the desired length of fully autogenous conduit for infrainguinal bypass. A widely spatulated venovenostomy (B and C) is optimal.

of limb function in a patient with limited options for secondary or tertiary bypass, the ability to maintain graft patency through early identification and prompt correction of graft stenosis is of paramount importance. Serial postoperative surveillance scanning with duplex ultrasound has proven an excellent means of accurately identifying hemodynamically significant stenosis within the vein graft that threaten the graft patency.[16] Velocity criteria have been developed for high-grade lesions that may warrant either more intensive surveillance or prophylactic intervention. Absolute velocities less than 40 cm/s or greater than 300 cm/s or a threefold increase in velocity in one segment compared with that of an adjacent segment are all indicative of impending graft failure. Confirmation by angiography and expeditious treatment by percutaneous cutting balloon angioplasty, surgical patch angioplasty, or interposition grafting of such significant lesions minimizes the risk of graft thrombosis and ensures optimal long-term graft patency.

Complications

The most commonly seen major complications of infrainguinal bypass surgery are cardiac in nature, and include myocardial infarction, congestive heart failure, and arrhythmias. Patients with DM or preoperative renal insufficiency are at particular risk for developing postoperative renal failure (defined as an elevation of serum creatinine >3 mg/dL, doubling of the serum creatinine or the need for hemodialysis), which is seen in up to 2% of patients overall. Patients undergoing lower extremity

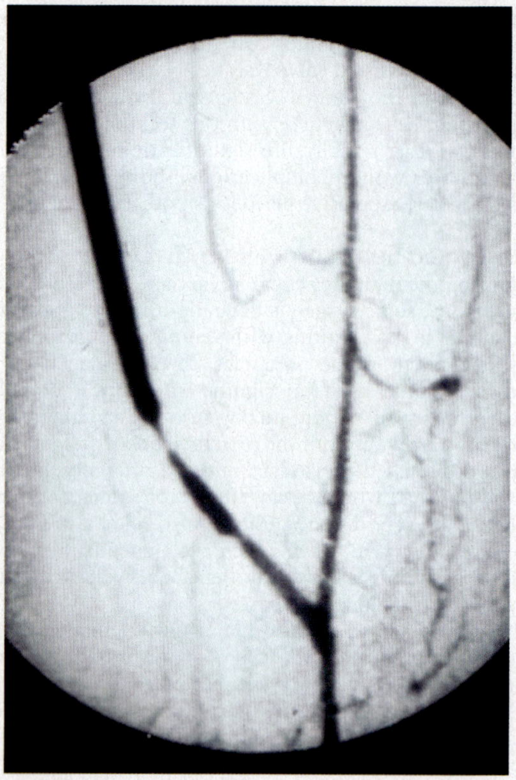

Figure 88.13. Arteriogram demonstrating severe stenosis of distal graft from intimal hyperplasia, likely at prior valve site.

revascularization are also prone to wound complications, given the length of incisions and the prolonged operating times often required. Overall wound complications, including cellulitis and abscess formation, wound dehiscence, and skin flap necrosis, can occur in up to 40% of patients and can best be avoided by gentle handling of the tissue and the use of skin bridges and careful avoidance of skin flaps during vein harvesting. Postoperative hematomas, usually caused by slow capillary or venous oozing, or seromas are seen in 5% of patients; and less commonly encountered hemorrhage, typically a result of either a slipped vein branch ligature or anastomotic disruption, is seen in less than 1% of cases.

ACKNOWLEDGMENT

We gratefully acknowledge the contributions of previous edition author, Bryan A. Ehlert, as portions of those chapters have been retained in this revision.

References

1. Criqui MH, Fronek A, Barrett-Connor E, Klauber MR, Gabriel S, Goodman D. The prevalence of peripheral arterial disease in a defined population. *Circulation*. 1985;71(3):510–515.
2. American College of Cardiology, F. ACCF/AHA/ACR/SCAI/SIR/SVM/SVN/SVS 2010 performance measures for adults with peripheral artery disease. A report of the American College of Cardiology Foundation/American Heart Association Task Force on Performance Measures, the American College of Radiology, the Society for Cardiac Angiography and Interventions, the Society for Interventional Radiology, the Society for Vascular Medicine, the Society for Vascular Nursing, and the Society for Vascular Surgery (Writing Committee to Develop Clinical Performance Measures for Peripheral Artery Disease). Developed in collaboration with the American Association of Cardiovascular and Pulmonary Rehabilitation; the American Diabetes Association; the Society for Atherosclerosis Imaging and Prevention; the Society for Cardiovascular Magnetic Resonance; the Society of Cardiovascular Computed Tomography; and the PAD Coalition.

Endorsed by the American Academy of Podiatric Practice Management. *J Vasc Surg*. 2010;52(6):1616–1652.
3. Fowkes FG, Rudan D, Rudan I, et al. Comparison of global estimates of prevalence and risk factors for peripheral artery disease in 2000 and 2010: a systematic review and analysis. *Lancet*. 2013;382(9901):1329–1340.
4. Hirsch AT, Haskal ZJ, Hertzer NR, et al. ACC/AHA 2005 guidelines for the management of patients with peripheral arterial disease (lower extremity, renal, mesenteric, and abdominal aortic): executive summary a collaborative report from the American Association for Vascular Surgery/Society for Vascular Surgery, Society for Cardiovascular Angiography and Interventions, Society for Vascular Medicine and Biology, Society of Interventional Radiology, and the ACC/AHA Task Force on Practice Guidelines (Writing Committee to Develop Guidelines for the Management of Patients With Peripheral Arterial Disease) endorsed by the American Association of Cardiovascular and Pulmonary Rehabilitation; National Heart, Lung, and Blood Institute; Society for Vascular Nursing; TransAtlantic Inter-Society Consensus; and Vascular Disease Foundation. *J Am Coll Cardiol*. 2006;47(6):1239–1312.
5. Santos JD. Sur la desobstion des thromboses arterielles anciennes. *Mem Acad Chir*. 1947;73:409–411.
6. Kunlin J. Long vein transplantation in treatment of ischemia caused by arteritis. *Rev Chir*. 1951;70(7–8):206–235.
7. Gruntzig A, Hopff H. [Percutaneous recanalization after chronic arterial occlusion with a new dilator-catheter (modification of the Dotter technique) (author's transl)]. *Dtsch Med Wochenschr*. 1974;99(49):2502–2510, 2511.
8. Dotter CT, Judkins MP. Transluminal Treatment of Arteriosclerotic Obstruction. Description of a New Technic and a Preliminary Report of Its Application. *Circulation*. 1964;30:654–670.
9. Norgren L, Hiatt WR, Dormandy JA, Nehler MR, Harris KA, Fowkes FG; TASC II Working Group. Inter-Society Consensus for the Management of Peripheral Arterial Disease (TASC II). *J Vasc Surg*. 2007;45 Suppl S:S5–67.
10. Criqui MH, Vargas V, Denenberg JO, et al. Ethnicity and peripheral arterial disease: the San Diego Population Study. *Circulation*. 2005;112(17):2703–2707.
11. Nehler MR, Hiatt WR. Exercise therapy for claudication. *Ann Vasc Surg*. 1999;13(1):109–114.
12. Dawson DL, Cutler BS, Hiatt WR, et al. A comparison of cilostazol and pentoxifylline for treating intermittent claudication. *Am J Med*. 2000;109(7):523–530.
13. Guilmot JL, Diot E. The role of drug therapy in the treatment of critical ischemia of the lower limbs. *Presse Med*. 1999;28(12): 647–650.
14. Taylor SM, Kalbaugh CA, Blackhurst DW, et al. Determinants of functional outcome after revascularization for critical limb ischemia: an analysis of 1000 consecutive vascular interventions. *J Vasc Surg*. 2006;44(4):747–755; discussion 755–756.
15. Conte MS, Bandyk DF, Clowes AW, et al. Results of PREVENT III: a multicenter, randomized trial of edifoligide for the prevention of vein graft failure in lower extremity bypass surgery. *J Vasc Surg*. 2006;43(4):742–751; discussion 751.
16. Conte MS, Bradbury AW, Kolh P, et al. Global vascular guidelines on the management of chronic limb-threatening ischemia. *J Vasc Surg*. 2019;69(6S):3S–125S e40.
17. Wolfe JH, Wyatt MG. Critical and subcritical ischaemia. *Eur J Vasc Endovasc Surg*. 1997;13(6):578–582.
18. Pomposelli F. Arterial imaging in patients with lower extremity ischemia and diabetes mellitus. *J Vasc Surg*. 2010;52(3 Suppl): 81S–91S.
19. Society for Vascular Surgery Lower Extremity Guidelines Writing Group; Conte MS, Pomposelli FB, Clair DG, et al. Society for Vascular Surgery practice guidelines for atherosclerotic occlusive disease of the lower extremities: management of asymptomatic disease and claudication. *J Vasc Surg*. 2015;61(3 Suppl):2S–41S.
20. Giles KA, Pomposelli FB, Spence TL, et al. Infrapopliteal angioplasty for critical limb ischemia: relation of TransAtlantic Inter-Society Consensus class to outcome in 176 limbs. *J Vasc Surg*. 2008;48(1):128–136.
21. Connors G,Todoran TM, Engelson BA, Sobieszczyk PS, Eisenhauer AC, Kinlay S. Percutaneous revascularization of long femoral artery lesions for claudication: patency over 2.5 years and impact of systematic surveillance. *Catheter Cardiovasc Interv*. 2011;77(7):1055–1062.
22. Conte MS. Critical appraisal of surgical revascularization for critical limb ischemia. *J Vasc Surg*. 2013;57(2 Suppl):8S–13S.
23. Rogers RK, Dattilo PB, Garcia JA, Tsai T, Casserly IP, et al. Retrograde approach to recanalization of complex tibial disease. *Catheter Cardiovasc Interv*. 2011;77(6):915–925.
24. Mehaffey JH, Hawkins RB, Fashandi A, et al. Lower extremity bypass for critical limb ischemia decreases major adverse limb events with equivalent cardiac risk compared with endovascular intervention. *J Vasc Surg*. 2017;66(4):1109–1116 e1.
25. Srodon P, Matson M, Ham R. Contrast nephropathy in lower limb angiography. *Ann R Coll Surg Engl*. 2003;85(3):187–191.
26. Knight CG, Healy DA , Thomas RL. Femoral artery pseudoaneurysms: risk factors, prevalence, and treatment options. *Ann Vasc Surg*. 2003;17(5):503–508.
27. Bonaca MP, Bauersachs RM , Hiatt WR. Rivaroxaban in peripheral artery disease after revascularization. Reply. *N Engl J Med*. 2020;383(21):2090–2091.
28. Belkin M, Knox J, Donaldson MC, Mannick JA, Whittemore AD. Infrainguinal arterial reconstruction with nonreversed greater saphenous vein. *J Vasc Surg*. 1996;24(6):957–962.
29. Shah DM, Leather RP, Darling RC 3rd, Chang BB, Paty PS, Lloyd WE. Long-term results of using the in situ saphenous vein bypass. *Adv Surg*. 1996;30:123–140.
30. Mills JL Sr, Conte MS, Armstrong DG, et al. The Society for Vascular Surgery Lower Extremity Threatened Limb Classification System: risk stratification based on wound, ischemia, and foot infection (WIfI). *J Vasc Surg*. 2014;59(1):220–34 e1–2.
31. Fashandi AZ, Mehaffey JH, Hawkins RB, Kron IL, Upchurch GR Jr, Robinson WP. Major adverse limb events and major adverse cardiac events after contemporary lower extremity bypass and infrainguinal endovascular intervention in patients with claudication. *J Vasc Surg*. 2018;68(6):1817–1823.
32. Menard MT, Belkin M. Infrapopliteal intervention for the treatment of the claudicant. *Semin Vasc Surg*. 2007;20(1):42–53.
33. Woo K, Siracuse JJ, Klingbeil K, et al. Society for Vascular Surgery appropriate use criteria for management of intermittent claudication. *J Vasc Surg*. 2022;76(1):3–22 e1.
34. Dormandy JA, Rutherford RB. Management of peripheral arterial disease (PAD). TASC Working Group. TransAtlantic Inter Society Consensus (TASC). *J Vasc Surg*. 2000;31(1 Pt 2):S1–S296.
35. DeRubertis BG, Pierce M, Chaer RA, et al. Lesion severity and treatment complexity are associated with outcome after percutaneous infra-inguinal intervention. *J Vasc Surg*. 2007;46(4): 709–716.
36. Krankenberg H, Tübler T, Sixt S, et al. German multicenter real-world registry of stenting for superficial femoral artery disease: clinical results and predictive factors for revascularization. *J Endovasc Ther*. 2014;21(4):463–471.
37. Schanzer A, Hevelone N, Owens CD, et al. Technical factors affecting autogenous vein graft failure: observations from a large multicenter trial. *J Vasc Surg*. 2007;46(6):1180–1190; discussion 1190.
38. Dake MD, Ansel GM, Jaff MR, et al. Durable clinical effectiveness with paclitaxel-eluting stents in the femoropopliteal artery: 5-year results of the Zilver PTX Randomized Trial. *Circulation*. 2016;133(15):1472–1483; discussion 1483.
39. Koeckerling D, Raguindin PF, Kastrati L, et al. Endovascular revascularization strategies for aortoiliac and femoropopliteal artery disease: a meta-analysis. *Eur Heart J*. 2023;44(11): 935–950.
40. Schillinger M, Sabeti S, Loewe C, et al. Balloon angioplasty versus implantation of nitinol stents in the superficial femoral artery. *N Engl J Med*. 2006;354(18):1879–1888.
41. Randon C, Jacobs B, De Ryck F, Vermassen F. Angioplasty or primary stenting for infrapopliteal lesions: results of a prospective randomized trial. *Cardiovasc Intervent Radiol*. 2010;33(2): 260–269.

42. Schneider PA, Laird JR, Tepe G, et al. Treatment effect of drug-coated balloons is durable to 3 years in the femoropopliteal arteries: Long-term results of the IN.PACT SFA Randomized Trial. *Circ Cardiovasc Interv*. 2018;11(1):e005891.
43. Farber A, Rosenfield K, Menard MT. Surgery or Endovascular Therapy for Chronic Limb Ischemia. Reply. *N Engl J Med*. 2023;388(11):e37.
44. Bradbury AW, Moakes CA, Popplewell M, et al. A vein bypass first versus a best endovascular treatment first revascularisation strategy for patients with chronic limb threatening ischaemia who required an infra-popliteal, with or without an additional more proximal infra-inguinal revascularisation procedure to restore limb perfusion (BASIL-2): an open-label, randomised, multicentre, phase 3 trial. *Lancet*. 2023;401(10390):1798–1809.
45. van der Zaag ES, Legemate DA, Prins MH, Reekers JA, Jacobs MJ. Angioplasty or bypass for superficial femoral artery disease? A randomised controlled trial. *Eur J Vasc Endovasc Surg*. 2004;28(2):132–137.
46. Veith FJ, Gupta SK, Ascer E, et al. Six-year prospective multicenter randomized comparison of autologous saphenous vein and expanded polytetrafluoroethylene grafts in infrainguinal arterial reconstructions. *J Vasc Surg*. 1986;3(1):104–114.
47. Taylor LM Jr, Edwards JM , Porter JM. Present status of reversed vein bypass grafting: five-year results of a modern series. *J Vasc Surg*. 1990;11(2):193–205; discussion 205–206.
48. Quiñones-Baldrich WJ, Prego A, Ucelay-Gomez R, Vescera CL, Moore WS. Failure of PTFE infrainguinal revascularization: patterns, management alternatives, and outcome. *Ann Vasc Surg*. 1991;5(2):163–169.
49. Chew DK, Owens CD, Belkin M, et al. Bypass in the absence of ipsilateral greater saphenous vein: safety and superiority of the contralateral greater saphenous vein. *J Vasc Surg*. 2002;35(6):1085–1092.
50. Sarac TP, Huber TS, Back MR, et al. Warfarin improves the outcome of infrainguinal vein bypass grafting at high risk for failure. *J Vasc Surg*. 1998;28(3):446–457.

Lower Extremity Amputation

Matthew J. Sideman, Kevin E. Taubman, and Bradley D. Beasley

Key Points

1. The annual incidence of major amputations has decreased over the past two decades.
2. The vast majority of lower extremity amputations are performed for complications of diabetes or arterial insufficiency.
3. Emergent amputation is indicated in the face of uncontrolled or ascending infection.
4. Primary amputation is occasionally indicated in cases of treatment for lower extremity trauma.
5. Revascularization is often performed in conjunction with amputation, either simultaneously or as a staged procedure.
6. Amputation level should be individualized to consider procedural indication, the condition of the patient, and the rehabilitation potential of the patient.
7. The energy required to ambulate following a lower extremity amputation increases with ascending level of amputation.

1 Surgeons are often involved in treating patients requiring lower extremity amputation. Increasing incidence of diabetes, peripheral arterial disease, and the aging population has put more patients at risk for amputation. The explosion of endovascular interventions over the past decade has resulted in decreasing numbers of major amputations performed annually.[1] A review of the National Hospital Discharge Survey and Medicare claims data confirms this trend.[2] Clinical judgment is critical to a successful outcome. Factors to consider include primary amputation, revascularization, repeat revascularization, level of amputation, and timing of amputation. The surgeon must remember that the goal is to maintain maximal function of the patient not necessarily maximal length of the limb. Consequently, experience of the surgeon has been shown to be key to a successful outcome.[3]

INDICATIONS

2 Most lower extremity amputations are performed for complications of diabetes or arterial insufficiency (**Table 89.1**). Chronic infection and trauma account for less than 10% of the total number of amputations. Other indications include neuroma, frostbite, malignancy, chronic pain, arterial embolization, venous insufficiency, and cryoglobulinemia.[4]

Elective lower extremity amputation in diabetic and vascular patients is indicated for gangrene (dry gangrene), gangrene with infection (wet gangrene), unremitting and unreconstructable rest pain, and nonhealing ulcers. The goal of the operation is to remove all nonviable tissue, relieve ischemic rest pain, ensure primary wound healing, and facilitate rehabilitation. Elective amputation should only be performed following an evaluation for revascularization procedure by a surgeon capable of performing such procedures. Advances in percutaneous management have expanded treatment options for those patients who were not previously operative candidates for revascularization and limb salvage. Not all patients are candidates for arteriography and limb preservation, however, and amputation may be considered definitive therapy for those with organic brain syndrome, nonfunctional limbs, fixed joint contractures, insensate feet, and those with extensive gangrene.

Spinal cord stimulation (SCS) may offer a chance for limb salvage for patients with chronic ischemia in whom reconstruction is not an option. Based on Melzack and Wall's Gate Control Theory of Pain,[5] the mechanism of pain relief and increased blood flow in end-stage peripheral vascular disease is unclear. Despite this, there is peripheral vasodilatation on the microvascular level which leads to pain relief,[6] increased claudication distance,[7] ulcer healing,[8] and possible limb salvage.[6,9,10] The 1-year foot salvage rate is 60% to 70% on average, according to a review of the literature.[11] SCS is only appropriate when surgery for revascularization is no longer possible. Furthermore, SCS only dilates microvasculature and does nothing for the underlying, progressive peripheral vascular disease that is causing the ischemia. SCS, therefore, is only a palliative measure, but can potentially extend a functional period as a procedure that is well tolerated and relatively simple to perform.[11] Recently, Gersbach et al. have shown that the benefits of SCS may persist longer than initially thought.[12]

Table 89.1. Indications for Lower Extremity Amputation

Indication	Percentage (%)
Complications of diabetes mellitus	60–80
Nondiabetic infection with ischemia	15–25
Ischemia without infection	5–10
Chronic osteomyelitis	3–5
Trauma	2–5
Miscellaneous (neuroma, frostbite, tumor, pain, and nonhealing wound)	5–10

From Malone JM. Lower extremity amputation. In: Moore WS, ed. *Vascular Surgery: A Comprehensive Review*. WB Saunders; 1993:810.

3 Emergent amputation is indicated in the face of uncontrolled or ascending infection. In the case of uncontrolled sepsis, it can even be a lifesaving maneuver. A diabetic patient with a foot abscess is a surgical emergency. Frequently, incision and drainage with or without a toe or a combined toe and metatarsal resection is sufficient to control the acute problem. The wounds should be left open in the setting of acute infection. If the process extends beyond the foot, a staged amputation should be performed proximal enough to control the infection. This can include an ankle disarticulation, a guillotine below-knee amputation (BKA), a knee disarticulation, or a guillotine above-knee amputation (AKA). Disarticulations have the advantage of preserving limb length and avoiding an open bone in the incision. After the infection is controlled, the appropriate proximal amputation can be completed. A one-stage primary AKA can be considered in patients who are nonambulatory, have infection involving the entire lower leg, have a fixed-knee contracture, or those with a nonfunctional limb.

4 Primary amputation is occasionally indicated as a treatment for severe lower extremity trauma. Both penetrating and blunt injuries of the lower extremities are frequently associated with vascular, nerve, bone, and extensive soft tissue injuries. Several treatment guidelines have been developed for lower extremity trauma. Lange[13] recommended primary amputation for open tibial fractures with associated vascular injuries if the posterior tibial nerve was disrupted in an adult or if the duration of warm ischemia was greater than 6 hours in a crush injury. In addition, he suggested that primary amputation was relatively indicated in patients with polytrauma, severe ipsilateral foot injuries, and in those with an expected protracted postoperative course. These suggestions are supported in work by Bosse et al.[14] demonstrating, in the case of high-energy lower extremity trauma, amputation, and reconstruction have equal functional outcomes at 2 years. Additional guidelines have been provided by Johansen et al.[15] who devised a Mangled Extremity Severity Score to predict the need for amputation based on the extent of skeletal or soft tissue damage, limb ischemia, shock, and age. Unfortunately, none of these guidelines are predictive of functional recovery in patients who undergo limb salvage.[16] Therefore, treatment with primary amputation should be individualized requiring extensive clinical judgment as well as multidisciplinary input that considers injury severity, the overall clinical status of that patient, and ultimate rehabilitation potential.

EVALUATION FOR REVASCULARIZATION

Modern vascular surgery techniques allow successful limb salvage in situations not previously possible. All patients who present for possible lower extremity amputation, including minor amputations, should have their peripheral vascular circulation evaluated preoperatively. Any patient with absent pedal pulses or abnormal ankle–brachial indices should be evaluated by a vascular surgeon skilled in both open and endovascular revascularization techniques. The evaluation may require only a thorough history and physical examination if there is an obvious contraindication to revascularization (eg, nonfunctional limb, severe organic brain syndrome). Noninvasive vascular laboratory examinations (ie, lower extremity arterial Doppler and arterial duplex) are a mandatory minimum for patients with abnormal vascular examinations. Additional imaging with either computed tomographic angiography (CTA), magnetic resonance angiography (MRA), or contrast angiography can be done based on the patient's initial evaluation and vascular lab results. The information obtained from these tests is heavily dependent on the quality of the machinery, the skill of the technologist, and the knowledge of the interpreting physician. All of these factors must be taken into account when deciding which test to order. Contrast angiography with selective lower extremity injections may be necessary to fully define the patient's anatomy and suitability for reconstruction; however, it is generally preferred to perform this invasive procedure for preoperative planning or for planned percutaneous intervention.

Exponential advances in endovascular techniques have occurred over the past two decades. These have found their way into the peripheral circulation and have applicability in limb salvage. Percutaneous techniques include balloon angioplasty (including conventional, cutting, and drug-coated balloons), stenting (including balloon expandable, self-expanding, drug eluting, and covered stents), intravascular lithotripsy, and percutaneous atherectomy (including laser, directional, orbital, and rotational). The BASIL trial showed no significant difference in amputation-free survival among patients with critical limb ischemia when randomized to open or percutaneous revascularization.[17]

In terms of surgical reconstruction, upper extremity[18] and cryopreserved cadaver vein[19] have increased the options for conduit in limb salvage situations. Prosthetic grafts with augments like vein cuffs[20,21] provide other alternatives when appropriate autogenous conduit is not available. Heparin-bonded prosthetic grafts have been shown to be effective as well.[22–24] An operation for limb salvage should never be denied *only* for lack of conduit.

5 Revascularization is often performed in conjunction with a minor amputation, either simultaneously or as a staged procedure. This allows management of the acute problem of sepsis and the underlying chronic ischemia. Caution must be taken if there is active infection and the only available conduit is prosthetic for fear of infecting the graft. Amputation with control of infection followed by revascularization is the more prudent course. In extreme cases, a limited amputation can be combined with revascularization and a tissue transfer (free or rotational flap) to achieve limb salvage.[25,26]

CHOICE OF AMPUTATION LEVEL

General

6 The choice of amputation level depends on the indication for the procedure, the condition of the patient, and the rehabilitation potential of the patient. The most common amputation levels are illustrated in **Figure 89.1**. Because most amputations are performed for complications of diabetes or arterial insufficiency, the selected level must remove all nonviable, painful tissue, allow primary healing, and maximize rehabilitation potential. Selection of the amputation level for malignant disease is dependent on the biologic characteristics of the neoplasm and beyond the scope of this chapter.

The general medical condition and the rehabilitation potential of the patient are important factors in deciding to proceed with amputation and in selecting the appropriate level. If a patient is ambulatory and independent preoperatively, the level with the greatest likelihood of maintaining function should be selected. If the patient is not ambulatory or has significant comorbid conditions, the primary wound-healing rate should be the determining factor.

Specific Situations

Aggressive attempts to salvage a distal amputation level are not indicated for patients who are unlikely to ambulate with a prosthesis.[27] For example, patients with fixed joint contractures greater than 15 degrees at the knee or 10 degrees at the hip are unlikely to ambulate with a prosthesis. BKAs are relatively contraindicated in patients with paraplegia because flexion contractures at the knee can lead to stump ulceration.

Energy Requirement

7 The energy required to ambulate following a lower extremity amputation increases with ascending level of amputation. The more proximal the amputation, the less likely a patient will be

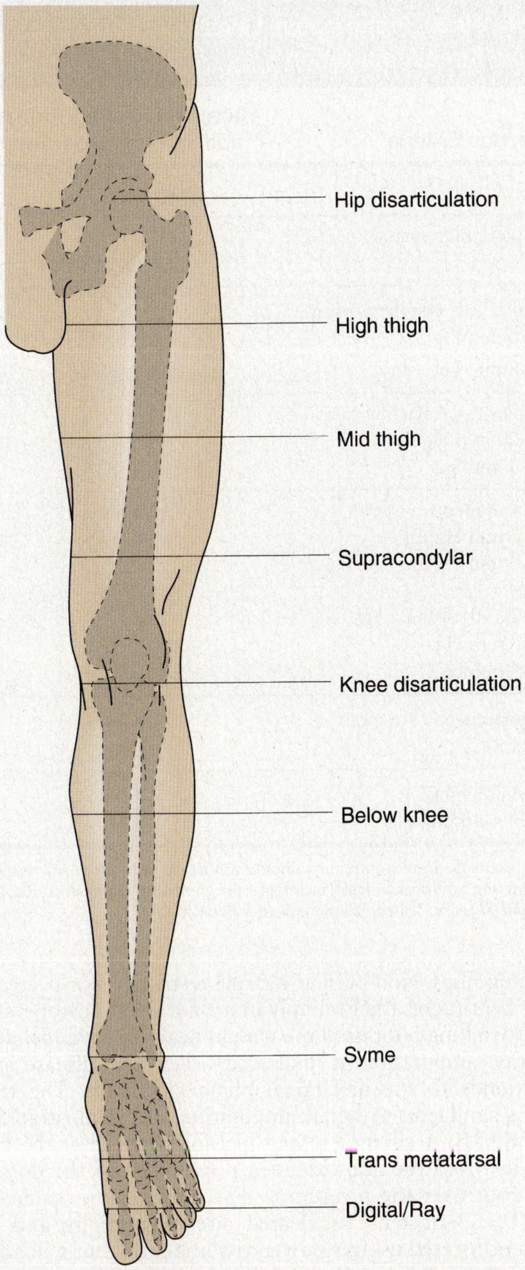

Figure 89.1. Common amputation levels for the lower extremity.

able to ambulate postoperatively. **Table 89.2** illustrates the increased energy cost of the common lower extremity amputations. In clinical practice, the most significant increase is between a BKA and an AKA. Ambulation on an above-knee prosthesis requires the use of muscle groups poorly suited for that purpose. These increased energy costs are minor issues for young trauma or cancer patients; however, they represent a considerable obstacle for the older diabetic or vascular patient.

Clinical Assessment

The primary preoperative consideration for wound healing is the status of the skin and muscle blood flow. Operative technique, the patient's nutritional status, and the presence of infection also affect wound healing. Clinical judgment by an experienced surgeon accurately predicts healing of a BKA in approximately 80% of cases.[28] A palpable pulse at the level immediately proximal to the proposed amputation essentially ensures healing[29]; however, the converse is not true. Noninvasive arterial testing is the most common adjunctive test used to predict healing of a specific amputation level. Its usefulness is limited when medial sclerosis and calcification prevent vessel compression, a condition common in diabetic patients. Because the digital vessels are often spared from this process, digital pressure readings may be helpful in this setting. Transcutaneous oxygen measurement has been shown to predict primary healing although it is less able to predict failure to heal.[30,31] It has become more widely available and has supplanted previous less reliable tests that were more limited in availability. **Tables 89.3** to **89.6** summarize the results of various preoperative tests to predict wound healing for toe, foot and forefoot, below-knee, and above-knee amputations, respectively. The Society for Vascular Surgery WIfI (Wound, Ischemia, and foot Infection) classification system has more recently been shown to be very helpful in predicting the risk of amputation and benefit of/requirement for revascularization.[32–36]

Table 89.2. Rehabilitation Energy Cost of Amputation at Various Levels

Amputation Level	Energy Cost
Digital or ray	Minimal (except first ray)
Transmetatarsal	Minimal during normal walking
Below knee	30–60% increase in energy required for ambulation
Above knee	60–100% increase in energy required for ambulation
Hip disarticulation	100–110% increase in energy required for ambulation

OPERATIVE TECHNIQUE

General Considerations

Diabetic patients who present with wet gangrene and/or sepsis require adequate fluid resuscitation, broad-spectrum antibiotics (including anaerobic coverage), and an emergent operation for rapid source control for predictably virulent polymicrobial infection. Whereas maintenance of limb length and function is admirable, control of sepsis and

Table 89.3. Preoperative Level Selection: Toe Amputation

Selection Criteria	Successful Healing, Primary and Secondary per Total
Empiric	86/115 (75%)
Presence of pedal pulses	357/365 (98%)
Doppler toe pressure >30 mm Hg	47/60 (78%)
Doppler ankle pressure >35 mm Hg	44/46 (96%)
Photoplethysmographic digit or TMA pressure >20 mm Hg	20/20 (100%)

TMA, transmetatarsal.
From Durham JR. Lower extremity amputation levels: indications, methods of determining appropriate level, technique, prognosis. In: Rutherford RB, ed. *Vascular Surgery.* 3rd ed. WB Saunders; 1989:1693.

VASCULAR DISEASE

Table 89.4. Preoperative Level Selection: Foot and Forefoot Amputation

Selection Criteria	Successful Healing, Primary and Secondary per Total
Empiric	11/24 (46%) 36/50 (72%)
Doppler ankle systolic pressure	
<40 mm Hg	5/9 (56%)
>40 mm Hg	20/60 (33%)
40–60 mm Hg	4/5 (80%)
>50 mm Hg	14/21 (66%)
>60 mm Hg	68/91 (75%)
>70 mm Hg	70/93 (75%)
Doppler toe systolic pressure	
>30 mm Hg	4/5 (80%)
Doppler ankle–brachial pressure index	
>0.45 (nondiabetic)	
>0.50 (diabetic)	58/60 (97%)
Photoplethysmographic toe systolic pressure	
>55 mm Hg	14/14 (100%)
>45 and <55 mm Hg	2/8 (25%)
<45 mm Hg	0/8 (0%)
Transcutaneous Po_2	
>10 mm Hg (or a >10 mm Hg increase on Fio_2 = 1.0)	6/8 (75%)
>28 mm Hg	3/3 (100%)
Transcutaneous Pco_2	
<40 mm Hg	3/3 (100%)

From Durham JR. Lower extremity amputation levels: indications, methods of determining appropriate level, technique, prognosis. In: Rutherford RB, ed. *Vascular Surgery.* 3rd ed. WB Saunders; 1989:1695.

wide debridement of all nonviable tissue are essential and potentially lifesaving. All patients require atraumatic tissue handling (ie, avoid forceps on the skin edge). Excessive skin flaps and dead space are also not desired. Amputations done in the face of active infection are kept open and treated with dressing changes. Consider delayed primary closure in cases where perfusion is intact.

Postoperatively, the limb is elevated to minimize tissue edema and promote healing. Weight bearing on the amputation is delayed until healing is assured. This patient population requires effective prophylaxis against deep venous thrombosis and venous thromboembolism.

Digital and Ray Amputations

Digital amputations are indicated for some severe and irreducible deformities as well as gangrene or osteomyelitis, localized distal to the base of the proximal phalanx. A technique for partial digital amputation is illustrated in **Figure 89.2A.** The circumferential or racquet-shaped skin incision is made over the distal end of the proximal phalanx and carried down to bone. Nerves and tendons are transected under tension and allowed to retract. The proximal phalanx is divided with bone shears or power saw and the transected end smoothed with a rongeur. Soft tissue coverage can be performed with either medial/lateral flaps or dorsal/plantar flaps depending on skin tension and viability. The wound is closed with simple interrupted skin sutures. Judicious use of subcutaneous sutures is advised due to danger of vascular compromise to the small remaining flaps. Non–weight-bearing restrictions or protected weight bearing on the heel only in a rigid soled postoperative shoe or walking boot until the wound heals is recommended.

A ray amputation is indicated when the disease process extends to the metatarsal phalangeal joint. The technique is similar to a digital amputation and is illustrated in **Figure 89.2B.** A circumferential incision is made at the base of the involved toe and extended proximally on the dorsum of the foot over the metatarsal. The incision is extended to bone. The periosteum is cleared circumferentially and the bone is transected using a power saw at a level that will allow

Table 89.5. Preoperative Level Selection: Below-Knee Amputation

Selection Criteria	Successful Healing, Primary and Secondary per Total
Empiric	794/974 (82%)
Doppler ankle systolic pressure	
>30 mm Hg	66/70 (94%)
Doppler calf systolic pressure	
>50 mm Hg	36/36 (100%)
>68 mm Hg	96/97 (99%)
Doppler thigh systolic pressure	
>100 mm Hg	31/31 (100%)
>80 mm Hg	104/113 (92%)
Transcutaneous Po_2 = 0	0/3 (0%)
>10 mm Hg (or >10 mm Hg increase on Fio_2 = 1.0)	76/80 (95%)
>10 and <40 mm Hg	5/7 (71%)
>20 mm Hg	25/26 (96%)
>35 mm Hg	51/51 (100%)
Transcutaneous Po_2 index >0.59	17/17 (100%)
Transcutaneous Pco_2 < 40 mm Hg	7/8 (88%)

From Durham JR. Lower extremity amputation levels: indications, methods of determining appropriate level, technique, prognosis. In: Rutherford RB, ed. *Vascular Surgery.* 3rd ed. WB Saunders; 1989:1700.

Table 89.6. Preoperative Level Selection: Above-Knee Amputation

Selection Criteria	Successful Healing, Primary and Secondary per Total
Empiric	390/430 (91%)
Transcutaneous Po_2	
>10 mm Hg (or 10 mm Hg increase on Fio_2 = 1.0)	15/23 (65%)
>20 mm Hg	12/12 (100%)
>23 mm Hg	2/2 (100%)
>35 mm Hg	21/24 (100%)
Transcutaneous Pco_2 < 38 mm Hg	5/5 (100%)

From Durham JR. Lower extremity amputation levels: indications, methods of determining appropriate level, technique, prognosis. In: Rutherford RB, ed. *Vascular Surgery.* 3rd ed. WB Saunders; 1989:1707.

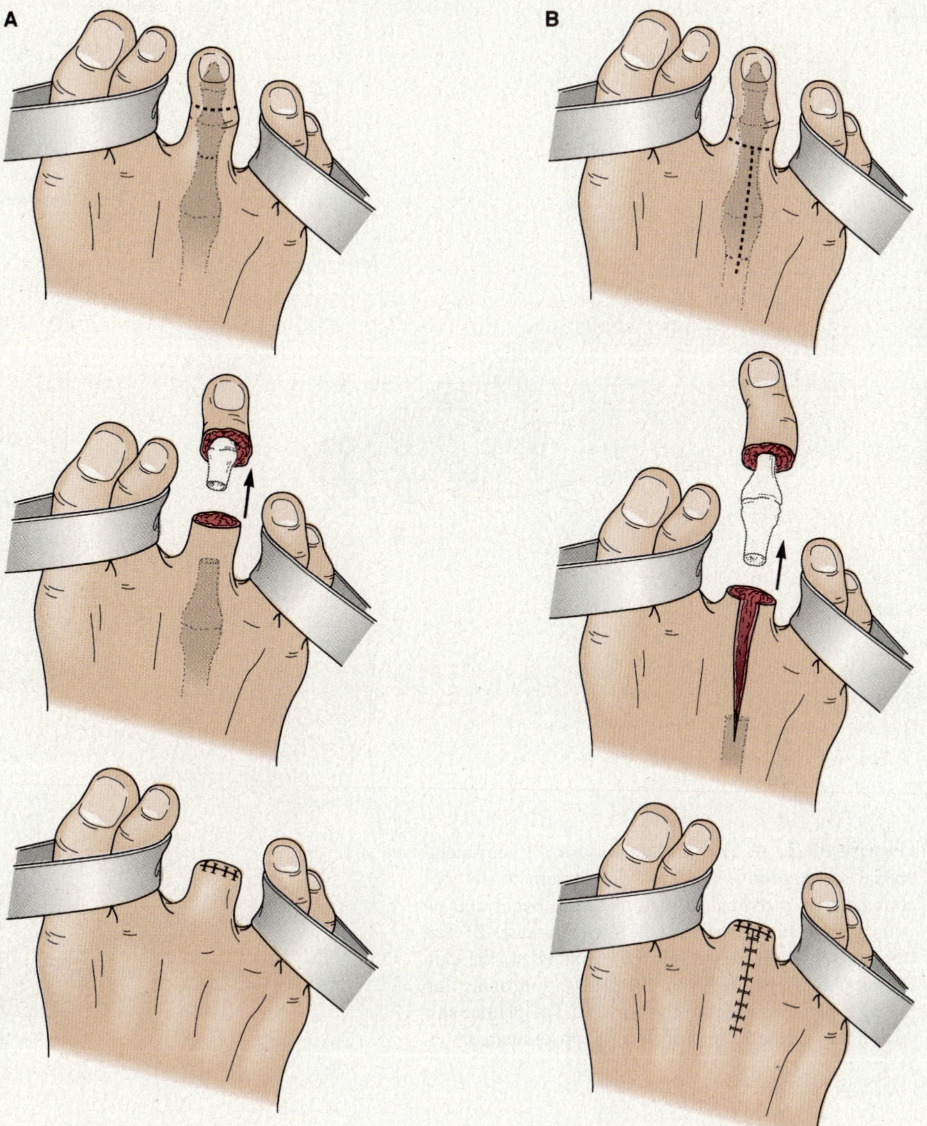

Figure 89.2. **A:** Digital amputation. A circumferential skin incision is made proximal to the gangrenous process. The proximal phalanx is transected and the soft tissue approximated. **B:** Metatarsal head resection (ray amputation). A racquet-shaped skin incision is made with the circular component extending circumferentially around the digit and the longitudinal component extending proximal to the metatarsal head. The metatarsal is transected proximal to the head and the soft tissue approximated.

tension-free closure of the wound. In the case of the 1st or 5th toe, the incision is extended on the medial or lateral aspect of the foot, respectively. Care should be taken to bevel the distal metatarsal stump to minimize any prominence that may lead to skin breakdown with weight bearing or shoe gear wear. Typically, the first metatarsal is beveled from proximal medial to distal lateral and proximal planter to distal dorsal. Metatarsals 2, 3, and 4 should be beveled from proximal plantar to distal dorsal. The 5th metatarsal is beveled from proximal lateral to distal medial and proximal plantar to distal dorsal.

In selected cases of neuropathic ulcers, the metatarsal head can be resected leaving the toe intact. A dorsal longitudinal incision is made over the metatarsal bone and the metatarsal head is resected with a power saw. Pulsed lavage and careful soft tissue inspection will help guide appropriate care for the plantar wound (ie, packing, negative-pressure therapy, or ellipse of wound with closure). The dorsal wound is typically closed, unless severe infection is encountered.

Transmetatarsal Amputation

Transmetatarsal amputation (TMA) is a useful procedure that maintains a patient's ability to ambulate without the aid of a prosthesis. It is indicated when the gangrenous or infectious process involves multiple digits or a portion of the forefoot. Care must be taken to plan for the appropriate soft tissue coverage if primary closure is desired. Maximizing the plantar flap is most common, but coverage can also be gained from medial or laterally based flaps and even filleted toe flaps. If adequate soft tissue coverage is not available and a more proximal foot amputation (ie, Chopart joint amputation) is not desired, then an open amputation through the metatarsal bones can be performed. The wound is allowed to close secondarily or covered with a skin graft. Skin grafts in this position, however, are susceptible to breakdown secondary to the pressure related to ambulation.

The technique is demonstrated in **Figure 89.3**. A skin incision is made on the dorsum of the foot immediately proximal to the metatarsal heads and extended medially and laterally to a point midway between the plantar and dorsal surfaces. The plantar incision is made along the digital crease and extended diagonally, medially, and laterally to connect to the dorsal incision. The dorsal incision is deepened to the periosteum, which is cleared with a small periosteal elevator. The metatarsal bones are transected 0.5 to 1.0 cm proximal to the dorsal skin incision. The plantar flap is fashioned by continuing the dissection just superficial to the metatarsal heads. Care is taken to maintain plantar flap thickness. The nerves and tendons are transected sharply under tension and allowed to retract. The plantar flap is rotated anteriorly and assessed for length. Excess tissue is excised sharply and the deep tissue is approximated with absorbable suture. The skin is closed without tension using monofilament suture or skin staples.

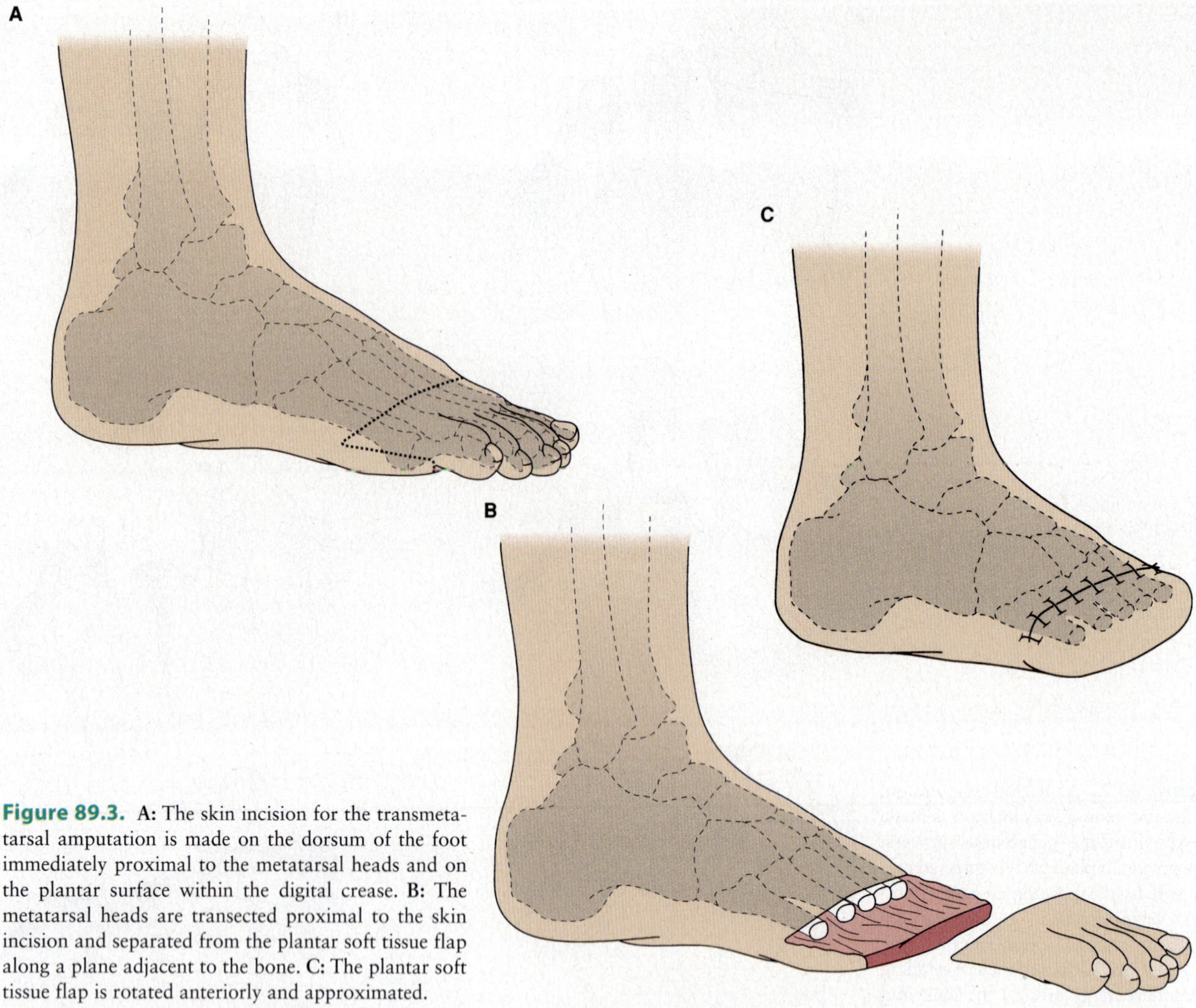

Figure 89.3. **A:** The skin incision for the transmetatarsal amputation is made on the dorsum of the foot immediately proximal to the metatarsal heads and on the plantar surface within the digital crease. **B:** The metatarsal heads are transected proximal to the skin incision and separated from the plantar soft tissue flap along a plane adjacent to the bone. **C:** The plantar soft tissue flap is rotated anteriorly and approximated.

Weight bearing is delayed for 1 month to allow adherence of the plantar flap. Either a soft dressing or a short leg cast can be used for a postoperative dressing.

Staging a tendo-Achilles lengthening (TAL) is important to consider following (or at the same time if no infection is present) a partial foot amputation. Ulcer formation at the TMA stump site is often related to equinus formation due to the ensuing flexion/extension imbalance that occurs after resection of the forefoot. A simple triple-hemisection percutaneous TAL can effectively lengthen the Achilles and reduce future pressures at the stump site.[37] Other tendon-balancing procedures may be needed to control varus and valgus contraction deformities that can develop.

Syme Amputation

The Syme amputation is a foot amputation that preserves limb length and the epiphyseal growth plates and allows occasional ambulation without a prosthesis. It is indicated in cases of extensive foot trauma or other nonviable tissue conditions distal to the hindfoot. The Syme amputation is contraindicated if a supple intact heel pad and a well-vascularized hindfoot tissue flap are not available.

The procedure can be performed in one or two stages, as illustrated in **Figure 89.4**. The initial steps for both procedures are identical, except that the skin incision for the two-stage procedure is located 1.5 cm more distally. The skin incision for the one-stage procedure extends from the medial to the lateral malleolus in the horizontal and vertical planes. The dorsal incision is extended to the bone, and the tendons are transected under tension. The anterior tibial artery is identified, divided, and suture ligated. The dissection is carried into the tibiotalar joint space as the foot is forcibly plantar flexed. The ligaments are transected and the talus is dislocated. The plantar aspect of the incision is deepened to the calcaneus, and the calcaneus is sharply dissected from the plantar fascia. The plantar fascia is densely adherent and care must be taken to prevent damage to the heel pad, especially at the level of the Achilles tendon. The posterior tibial artery must be preserved because it perfuses the heel pad. The foot is then removed. The two procedures differ from this point forward.

In the one-stage procedure, the medial and lateral malleoli are transected flush with the tibiotalar joint space, and the heel pad is rotated over the ends of the tibia and fibula. The deep fascial layers are approximated with absorbable suture and the skin is closed with monofilament suture or skin staples. Securing the distal end of the remaining plantar fascia to a small drill hole in the distal anterior tibia will help anchor the plantar flap and reduce posterior migration. In the two-stage procedure, the heel pad is similarly positioned and the wound is closed without further bone transection. In 6 weeks, elliptical incisions are made over the medial and lateral malleoli and the distal ends of the tibia and fibula are transected flush with the ankle joint. In addition, the distal flares of the tibia and fibula are transected, creating the rectangular stump of the two-stage procedure. The wound is closed in a similar fashion. For both procedures, weight bearing is delayed for at least 4 weeks to allow heel pad fixation. A soft dressing or a short leg cast can be used.

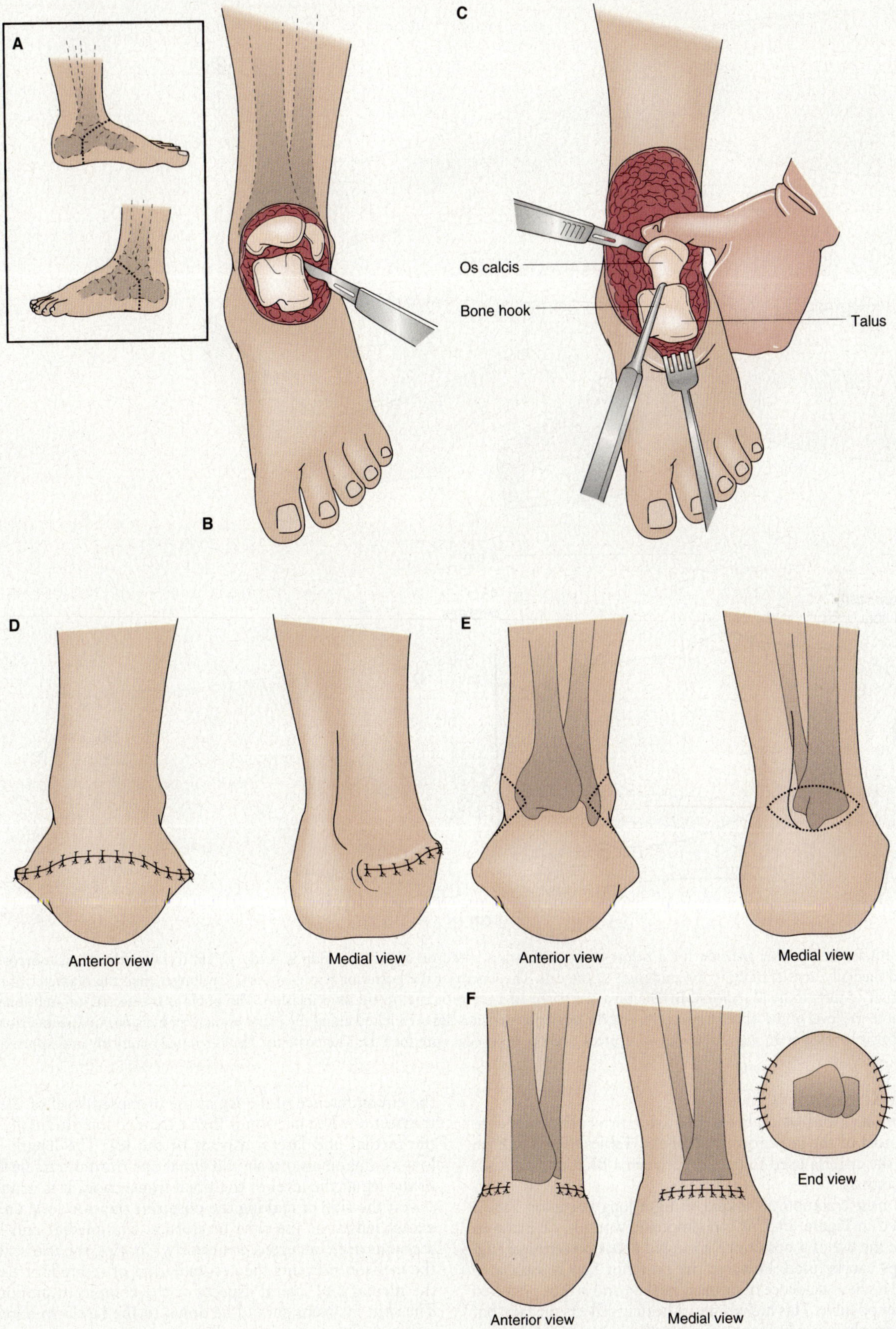

Figure 89.4. **A:** The skin incision for the one-stage Syme amputation connects the medial and lateral malleoli in both the horizontal and vertical planes. The skin incision for the two-stage procedure is located approximately 1.5 cm further distally. **B:** The incision is extended into the tibial—talar joint space, and the foot is placed in forced plantar flexion. **C:** The calcaneus is sharply dissected from the adherent plantar fascia along a plane adjacent to the bone. **D:** The heel pad is rotated anteriorly and approximated after the calcaneal dissection in the two-stage procedure and after the additional transection of the medial and lateral malleoli in the one-stage procedure. **E:** Elliptic incisions are made over the medial and lateral malleoli during a second operation for the staged procedure. The medial and lateral malleoli are transected flush with the ankle joint, and the distal flares of the tibia and fibula are removed. **F:** The two-stage procedure results in a less bulbous, more cosmetically acceptable residual limb.

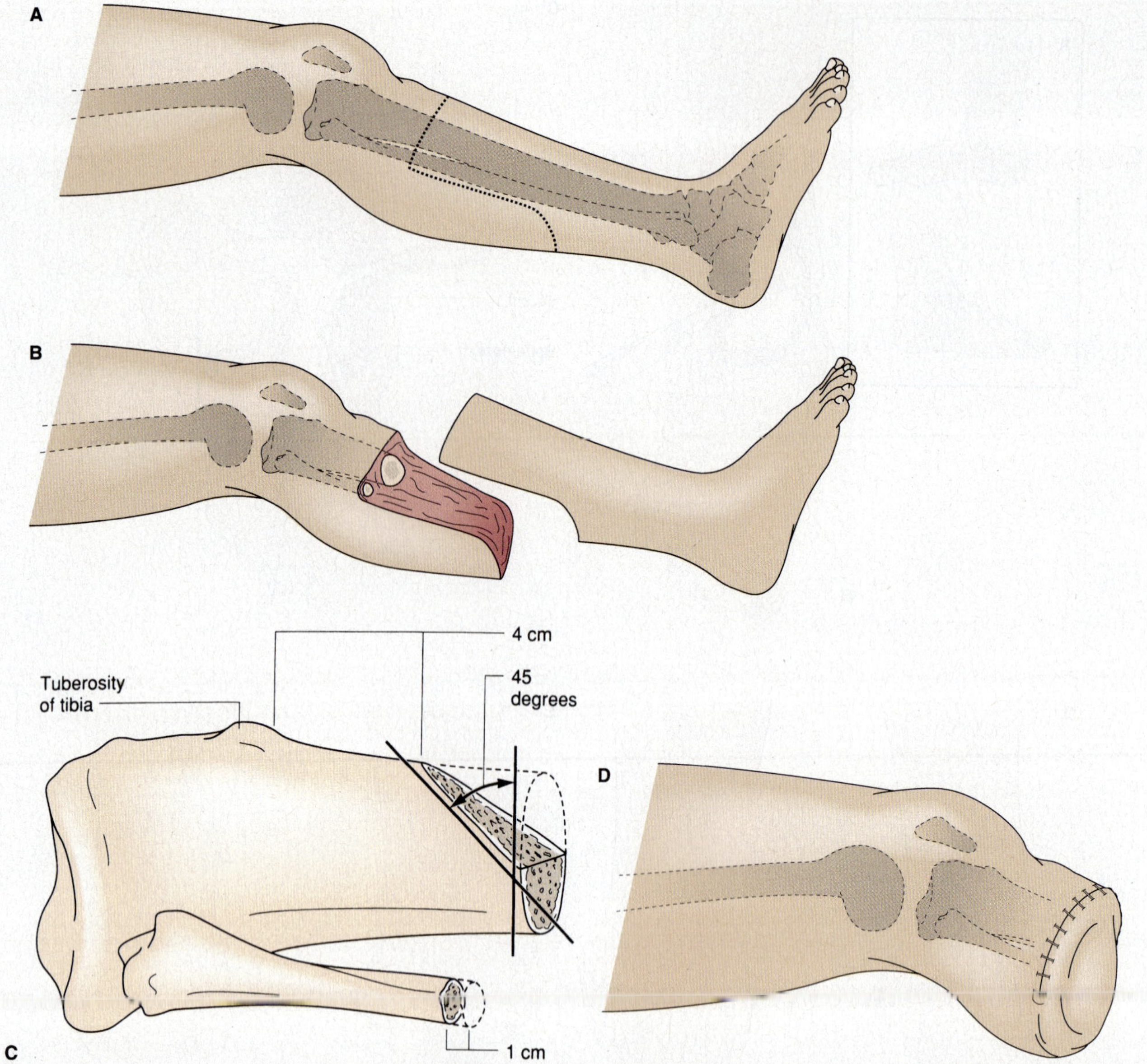

Figure 89.5. **A:** The skin incision for a below-knee amputation based on a posterior flap is made 11 cm distal to the tibial tuberosity and extended medially and laterally to the midpoint of the calf. The length of the posterior flap is about 2 cm longer than the diameter of the calf at the point of the proximal incision. **B:** The tibia is transected 1 cm proximal to the skin incision. The fibula is transected an additional 1 cm proximal to the level of the tibial transection, and the posterior calf muscles are incised along the plane of the skin incision. **C:** The anterior aspect of the tibia is beveled at an angle of about 45 degrees, and the bone edges are filed. **D:** The posterior flap is rotated anteriorly and approximated.

Below-Knee Amputation

The complications of diabetes and arterial insufficiency constitute most of the indications for BKAs. **Tables 89.5** and **89.6** outline the criteria used to decide between a BKA and an AKA in this setting.

The most common technique, using a long posterior flap, is illustrated in **Figure 89.5**. When gangrene, wounds, or incisions preclude the use of a posterior flap, equal anteroposterior or sagittal flaps can be used; however, the posterior flap is associated with the highest incidence of primary healing and is thus preferred whenever possible. This higher rate of healing reflects the fact that the posteriorly located gastrocnemius and soleus muscles are supplied by the sural arteries that originate proximal to the knee.

The proposed skin incision is drawn on the leg with a marker. The tibia should be transected 10 cm distal to the tibial tuberosity and the anterior aspect of the skin incision should be 1 cm distal to the site selected for the tibial transection. The anterior incision is extended medially and laterally. The length of the anterior incision should equal two-thirds of the circumference of the leg at the proposed level of the tibial transection. The incision is then extended longitudinally along the medial and lateral aspects of the leg. The length of the longitudinal incisions should equal one-third of circumference of the leg at the level of the tibial transection. It is prudent to err on the side of making the posterior flap too long and trim excess length at the time of closure. The medial and lateral incisions are connected posteriorly. Curving the transitions of the incision prevents the accumulation of redundant tissue at the medial and lateral aspects of the completed amputation. The skin incisions should be down to the fascia to allow separation of the skin edges. This step decreases the chance of inadvertent injury to the posterior flap later in the procedure; however, the greater and lesser saphenous veins need to be ligated and transected.

The anterior aspect of the incision is deepened through the periosteum of the tibia. The muscles of the anterior compartment are divided at the level of the skin incision and the anterior tibial neurovascular bundle is identified and suture ligated. The proximal tibia is circumferentially cleared of periosteum and transected one fingerbreadth proximal to the skin incision. The anterior aspect of the tibia is cut on a 45-degree angle. The fibula is cleared and transected 2 cm proximal to the transected tibia. The bones are divided with either a power-driven reciprocating saw, or a manual saw. Regardless, care must be taken to avoid trauma to the anterior skin flap.

The posterior tibial and peroneal neurovascular bundles are identified and suture ligated. The tibia is retracted anteriorly and the posterior musculature is divided along the plane of the longitudinal skin incisions using an amputation knife or Bovie electrocautery. Extreme caution must be taken to avoid injury to the skin edges of the posterior flap during this step. Often a scalpel is needed to complete the division of the gastrocnemius tendon distally. The specimen is removed and manual compression achieves temporary hemostasis while the remaining vascular structures are identified and ligated. The posterior tibial nerve is retracted distally, ligated, transected sharply, and allowed to retract. The posterior flap is rotated anteriorly to assess thickness and length. Frequently, the musculature needs to be debulked to allow a tension-free closure. Rough edges of the bones are filed smooth and the wound is irrigated. Bone wax is not used. A closed-system drain may be placed to prevent a hematoma. The end of the tibia is covered and stabilized with the deep posterior musculature using absorbable sutures. The gastrocnemius fascia is approximated to the anterior fascia using absorbable suture. The subcutaneous tissue is closed with absorbable suture to minimize tension on the skin edges and the skin is closed with monofilament suture or staples.

The length of the BKA may be shortened if required by the infectious or gangrenous process. Although not ideal, a short BKA is functionally superior to an AKA. In the extreme case, the tibia can be transected at the level of the tibial tuberosity and the stump can still be fit with a prosthesis. If a BKA is necessary at this level, the gastrocnemius muscle tendon and collateral ligament should be sutured to the tibia (ie, myodesis), the common peroneal nerve should be transected above the knee, and the fibula should be removed.

A variation of the BKA is the osteomyoplastic transtibial amputation also known as the Ertl amputation. This technique has been well described[38] and involves creating a bone bridge between the tibia and the fibula using a piece of the amputated fibula. Proposed advantages of this technique include a more stable end bearing of the stump and prevention of fibular instability.

In the face of extensive foot infection, an open (guillotine) amputation should be performed as the first part of a staged procedure. A circumferential incision is made in the distal leg just proximal to the malleoli. The fascia is divided, and the tibia and fibula are dissected free. The bones are divided at the level of the skin incision. All major neurovascular bundles are suture ligated and the remaining soft tissue is divided to complete the amputation. Several sutures are placed through the skin and underlying fascia to prevent retraction. The wound is left open and dressed. A negative-pressure dressing may be used and simplifies wound care. A definitive BKA is delayed until the infectious process has resolved which typically occurs within a week. Ankle disarticulation is an alternative to a guillotine BKA. An incision is made at the level of the ankle joint. Vascular structures are suture ligated. The tendons are divided sharply entering the ankle joint. The capsule is circumferentially incised removing the foot from the leg. The wound is packed open or with a negative-pressure dressing.

Above-Knee Amputation

An AKA is indicated for patients requiring an amputation with a fixed-knee contracture, a nonfunctional limb, or insufficient circulation to heal a BKA. Typically, a transverse fish-mouth incision is made in the lower thigh. The initial skin incision should be carried through the subcutaneous tissue to allow the edges to separate. This step will decrease the likelihood of inadvertent injury to the posterior skin flap during transection of the posterior muscle groups. The greater saphenous vein needs to be identified and ligated. The dissection is carried down to the femur that is cleared using a periosteal elevator to a level 2 to 3 cm proximal to the skin incision. The superficial femoral artery is dissected free and suture ligated. The bone is transected with a reciprocating or manual saw, and the posterior muscle flap is divided with an amputation knife or Bovie electrocautery. Manual compression with a laparotomy pad on the newly divided stump will easily control hemorrhage while vessels are identified and ligated or electrocoagulated. The sciatic nerve is identified and placed on gentle traction. It is then highly ligated, sharply divided, and allowed to retract into the wound. The flaps should be irrigated and hemostasis assured. The fascia is then closed with absorbable suture. The subcutaneous tissue is closed with absorbable suture to minimize tension on the skin edges and the skin is closed with monofilament suture or staples. Alternative incisions can be made to accommodate surgical wounds. Most AKA wounds will heal even when the femoral pulse is nonpalpable. More proximal thigh amputations are performed when arterial perfusion is in question.

Table 89.7. Amputation Mortality

Category	Percentage	Number
Below knee	2	25/1200
Above knee	9	54/609
Diabetic vs. nondiabetic	No difference	
After amputation revision	5.5	12/218

Derived from Frang RD, Taylor LM, Porter JM. Amputations. In: Porter JM, Taylor LM, eds. *Basic Data Underlying Clinical Decision Making in Vascular Surgery*. Quality Medical; 1994:154.

Complications

Morbidity and Mortality

Operative mortality depends on the indication and the level. Mortality rates for major lower extremity amputations in vascular and diabetic patients have been reported to be between 0% and 35%.[39] Combined mortality rates from multiple series are shown in **Table 89.7.**[40] Cardiovascular causes account for two-thirds of these deaths, with myocardial infarction responsible for one-third.[40] These review data are further supported by recent studies by Sandnes et al.[41] and Aulivola et al.[42]

Long-term survival following major amputation in the vascular population is shown in **Table 89.8.** The 5-year survival rate is only 37% compared with 85% for age-matched controls.[43]

Table 89.8. Survival after Amputation for Ischemia

Time (y)	Survival Rate (%)
1	75
2	60
3	50
4	45
5	37

Derived from Frang RD, Taylor LM, Porter JM. Amputations. In: Porter JM, Taylor LM, eds. *Basic Data Underlying Clinical Decision Making in Vascular Surgery*. Quality Medical; 1994:115, with permission.

Deep Venous Thrombosis and Pulmonary Embolism

The incidence of deep venous thrombosis following lower extremity amputation ranges from 4% to 38%.[44–46] Prophylactic measures including subcutaneous heparin, low–molecular-weight heparins, early mobilization, and pneumatic compression devices should be used as indicated.

Stump Complications

Stump complications include nonhealing, infection, hematoma, contractures, ulceration, phantom pain, and trauma. Although most amputations heal primarily, a small percentage do not. Amputation at a more proximal level usually is successful. Postoperative infections complicate 12% to 28% of all amputations with the percentage higher in cases performed for infection.[47] Infected wounds should undergo incision and drainage with debridement of all nonviable tissue. The wound should then be treated with local wound care using gauze or negative-pressure dressings, depending on the appearance of the wound and surgeon preference. Broad-spectrum systemic antibiotics should be instituted and then tailored based on wound cultures. Wound hematomas are best treated with prevention. Meticulous hemostasis and avoidance of subcutaneous cavities decrease their incidence. Hematomas should be treated in the operating room with evacuation, irrigation, and closure of the wound.

Joint contractures complicate 1% to 3% of all amputations.[43,47] These contractures can occur rapidly postoperatively and are best treated by prevention. Rehabilitation specialists and physical therapists should evaluate patients preoperatively. Active and passive range of motion should be initiated immediately postoperatively. Adequate pain medication, ideally with patient-controlled or epidural anesthesia,[48,49] is crucial. Pillows and bed positions that result in hip or knee flexion are to be strictly avoided.

Ulcers tend to develop over bony prominences. Poorly fitting prostheses or shoes are the most common causes. Diabetic patients with peripheral neuropathy are especially susceptible to the development of ulcers following toe and limited foot amputations. They can also form on the anterior aspect of AKAs secondary to the disproportional contraction of the hip flexors relative to the hip extensors. Local wound care and bedrest usually lead to healing if the ulcer is superficial. Deep skin ulcers with involvement of the soft tissue and the underlying bone are more complicated. They often suggest borderline perfusion of the stump and require formal revision to a higher level to treat definitively.

Another option in complicated wound closure is negative-pressure wound dressing, which has been used for a wide range of difficult-to-heal lesions. Studies indicate that this dressing technique decreases wound volume, whereas traditional moist gauze dressings do not.[50] The dressings result in granulation tissue and healing in otherwise difficult tissue beds, such as diabetic foot ulcers[51] and decubitus pressure ulcers.[52] In addition to helping contract the size of the wound, negative-pressure dressings also decrease the number and frequency of dressing changes drastically when compared with wet-to-dry dressings.

Neuromas are regenerative nerve tissues that form in response to transection. They can lead to pain if trapped in the fibrous scar or if irritated by a prosthesis. Proximal nerve division under tension during the original operation decreases the incidence of this complication. Symptomatic neuromas should be treated with proximal resection of the nerve because local excision of the neuroma is rarely adequate.

Some element of phantom extremity pain occurs in nearly all amputations,[53] although these complaints are not always directed to the treating surgeon. It is necessary to describe these common symptoms to the patient and specifically inquire about their presence. The pain is disabling in 5% to 30%[54] of patients surveyed. Currently, pain is felt to be a component of a central pain syndrome and unrelated to either a neuroma or the perception of an intact extremity. Although there is no universally effective treatment, Malone[39] has reported a low incidence with an aggressive rehabilitation program, including immediate prosthetic fitting.

Trauma to a limb following an amputation can convert a healed amputation to a nonhealing wound requiring a more proximal amputation. Perioperatively, patients with a BKA must be observed closely to prevent attempted ambulation. Diabetic patients with retinopathy should not walk barefoot following toe and foot amputations secondary to the risk that minor trauma may lead to a major wound healing problem.

Additional Amputation

The incidence of future amputation in vascular patients is not insignificant. Snyder et al. evaluated outcomes after forefoot amputations and found that 26% underwent a subsequent forefoot amputation and 37% had a more proximal amputation over 2 years.[55] Cruz et al. demonstrated 17% contralateral amputation in their series.[56] These dismal figures reflect the systemic nature of the underlying diseases and emphasize the importance of appropriate foot care, patient education, close follow-up, and early intervention.[57] A concerted multidisciplinary approach can dramatically decrease the incidence of initial and subsequent lower extremity amputation.[58]

REHABILITATION AND PROSTHETIC MANAGEMENT

General Considerations

Rehabilitation must be individualized. For some patients, successful rehabilitation means ambulation on a prosthesis and resumption of an independent lifestyle. For others, success may mean being able to pivot on the contralateral limb to be able to assist with transfer. Ambulating with a prosthesis depends on the physiologic status of the patient. **Table 89.2** illustrates the dramatic increase in energy requirement with increasing level of the amputation. As expected, the chance of ambulating on a prosthesis decreases with ascending amputation level. The percentages of diabetic and vascular patients who can ambulate with amputations at various levels are shown in **Table 89.9**. The likelihood of ambulating postoperatively is inversely related to the patient's age and the length of the rehabilitation process.[59] Consideration should be given to inpatient rehab immediately after the acute care of the amputation is complete. Not only does this allow strengthening of the upper extremities and improved transfers, but it has been shown to reduce 1-year mortality in amputees as well.[60]

Specific Considerations

Digital and Ray Amputations

All patients who were ambulatory preoperatively should be able to achieve their preoperative functional status following a

Table 89.9. Ambulation after Lower Extremity Amputation for Diabetes or Occlusive Disease

Amputation Level	Postoperative Ambulation (%)
Digit or ray	100
Transmetatarsal	100
Syme amputation	90–100
Below knee	75
Above knee	39
Hip disarticulation	<100

Derived from Frang RD, Taylor LM, Porter JM. Amputations. In: Porter JM, Taylor LM, eds. *Basic Data Underlying Clinical Decision Making in Vascular Surgery*. Quality Medical; 1994:155, with permission.

digital or ray amputation. The first digit and metatarsal head are important for weight bearing and for power. A shoe orthosis should effectively compensate for these functions when the patient has some training.

The most important component of postoperative rehabilitation for patients following a digital or ray amputation is education. The rate of repeat amputation (other toe, more proximal level, and contralateral limb) is extremely high. Several studies have indicated that the rate of repeat amputation is diminished with a coordinated education program.[61,62]

Transmetatarsal Amputation

A TMA minimally increases the energy requirement of ambulation; therefore, postoperative ambulation is expected following successful healing. The absence of the toes and metatarsal heads results in the loss of some forward thrust during the push-off phase of ambulation. This deficit can be overcome with either a steel-shank or a rigid, roller-soled shoe. The void in the distal shoe is filled with an insert.

Syme Amputation

The prognosis for return to bipedal ambulation following a Syme amputation is excellent. The required energy expenditure is only 10% more than baseline.[63] A significant advantage of this amputation is the ability to ambulate on the stump with only a cup slipper. Even though this activity is permitted on only a limited basis in the home, it is much more convenient for the patient, especially when arising at night. For routine activity, the patient uses a prosthesis composed of a nonmotion foot attached to a leg shaft. The shaft has a cutout on the medial aspect to allow passage of the flared distal end of the stump. The configuration of the distal end of the stump results in a bulbous ankle, which is less aesthetically pleasing than the typical below-knee prosthesis.

Below-Knee Amputation

The rehabilitation potential following a BKA is very good. Even when the indication for amputation is arterial insufficiency, approximately 75% of patients are able to ambulate with a prosthesis.[40] Multiple design options are available; however, the patellar tendon and the medial and lateral tibial flares are the weight-bearing surfaces for most prostheses. A variety of foot designs are possible to permit extension, flexion, rotation, and energy storage.

Above-Knee Amputation

Ambulation on above-knee prosthesis is achieved by less than 40% of patients with arterial insufficiency.[40] In this patient population, the rate of ambulation on bilateral above-knee prostheses is less than 10%.[64] Most above-knee prostheses use the ischial tuberosity as the primary weight-bearing surface and are secured either by a belt or a suction socket. For younger patients, a suction socket works well. Patients with groin scars from previous revascularization attempts may benefit from a belt mechanism. The knee design depends on the patient's general condition and thigh strength. A knee that engages during the stance phase of gait is more stable and is frequently used in older patients.

References

1. Goodney PP, Beck AW, Nagle J, Welch HG, Zwolak RM. National trends in lower extremity bypass surgery, endovascular interventions, and major amputations. *J Vasc Surg.* 2009;50(1):54–60.
2. Gorina Y, Owens M, Elgaggal N, Weeks J. Comparability between the rates for all-listed inpatient procedures using National Hospital Discharge Survey and Medicare claims, 1999 and 2007. *Nat Health Stat Report.* 2012;(57):1–15.
3. Falstie-Jensen N, Christensen KS. A model for prediction of failure in amputation of the lower limb. *Dan Med Bull.* 1990;37:283–286.
4. Sanmugarajah J, Hussain S, Schwartz J, Friedman S. Monoclonal cryoglobulinemia with extensive gangrene of all four extremities—a case report. *Angiology.* 2000;51(5):431–434.
5. Melzack R, Wall PD. Pain mechanisms: a new theory. *Science (1979).* 1965;150:971–979.
6. Augustinsson LE, Carlsson CA, Holm J, Jivegard L. Epidural electrical stimulation is severe limb ischemia. Pain relief, increased blood flow, and a possible limb-saving effect. *Ann Surg.* 1985; 202:104–110.
7. Tallis RC, Illis LS, Sedgwick EM, Hardwidge C, Garfield JS. Spinal cord stimulation in peripheral vascular disease. *J Neurol Neurosurg Psychiatry.* 1983;46:478–484.
8. Meglio M, Cioni B, Dal Lago A, De Santis M, Serrichio M. Pain control and improvement of peripheral blood flow following epidural spinal cord stimulation: case report. *J Neurosurg.* 1981;54:821–823.
9. Horsch S, Claeys L. Epidural spinal cord stimulation in the treatment of severe peripheral arterial occlusive disease. *Ann Vasc Surg.* 1994;8(5):468–474.
10. Ubbink DT, Spincemaille GH, Prins MH, Reneman RS, Jacobs MJ. Microcirculatory investigations to determine the effect of spinal cord stimulation for critical leg ischemia: the Dutch multicenter randomized controlled trial. *J Vasc Surg.* 1999;30:236–244.
11. Huber SJ, Vaglienti RM, Huber JS. Spinal cord stimulation in severe, inoperable peripheral vascular disease. *Neuromodulation.* 2000;3:131–143.
12. Gersbach PA, Argitis V, Gardza JP, von Segesser LK, Haesler E. Late outcome of spinal cord stimulation for unreconstructable and limb-threatening lower limb ischemia. *Eur J Vasc Endovasc Surg.* 2007;33(6):717–724.
13. Lange RH. Limb reconstruction versus amputation decision making in massive lower extremity trauma. *Clin Orthop Relat Res.* 1989;(243):92–99.
14. Bosse MJ, MacKenzie EJ, Kellam JF, et al. An analysis of outcomes of reconstruction or amputation of leg-threatening injuries. *N Engl J Med.* 2002;347:1924–1931.
15. Johansen K, Daines M, Howey T, Helfet D, Hansen ST Jr. Objective criteria accurately predict amputation following lower extremity trauma. *J Trauma.* 1990;30(5):568–572; discussion 572–573.
16. Ly TV, Travison TG, Castillo RC, Bosse MJ, MacKenzie EJ, LEAP Study Group. Ability of lower-extremity injury severity scores to predict functional outcome after limb salvage. *J Bone Joint Surg Am.* 2008;90(8):1738–1743.
17. Adam DJ, Beard JD, Cleveland T, et al; BASIL trial participants. Bypass versus angioplasty in severe ischaemia of the leg (BASIL): multicentre, randomized controlled trial. *Lancet.* 2005;366(9501): 1925–1934.
18. Harwood T, Coe E, Flynn TC, Seeger JM. The use of arm vein conduits during infrageniculate arterial bypass. *J Vasc Surg.* 1992;16: 420–426.
19. Leseche G, Penna C, Bouttier S, Joubert S, Andréassian B. Femorodistal bypass using cryopreserved venous allografts for limb salvage. *Ann Vasc Surg.* 1997;11(3):230–236.
20. Raptis S, Miller JH. Influence of vein cuff on polytetrafluoroethylene grafts for primary femoropopliteal bypass. *Br J Surg.* 1995;82: 487–491.
21. Stonebridge PA, Prescott RJ, Ruckley CV. Randomized trial comparing infrainguinal polytetrafluoroethylene bypass grafting with and without vein interposition cuff at the distal anastomosis. The Joint Vascular Research Group. *J Vasc Surg.* 1997;26(4):543–550.
22. Bosiers M, Deloose K, Verbist J, et al. Heparin-bonded expanded polytetrafluoroethylene vascular graft for femoropopliteal and femorocrural bypass grafting: 1-year results. *J Vasc Surg.* 2006; 43(2):313–318.
23. Uhl C, Hock C, Betz T, Greindl M, Töpel I, Steinbauer M. Comparison of venous and HePTFE tibial and peroneal bypasses in critical limb ischemia patients unsuitable for endovascular revascularization. *Vascular.* 2015;23(6):607–613.
24. Uhl C, Grosch C, Hock C, Töpel I, Steinbauer M. Comparison of long-term outcomes of heparin bonded polytetrafluoroethylene and autologous vein below knee femoropopliteal bypasses in patients with critical limb ischaemia. *Eur J Vasc Endovasc Surg.* 2017;54(2):203–211.

25. Lepantalo M, Tukiainen E. Combined vascular reconstruction and microvascular muscle flap transfer for salvage of ischaemic legs with major tissue loss and wound complications. *Eur J Vasc Endovasc Surg*. 1996;12:65–69.
26. Briggs SE, Banis JC Jr, Kaebnick H, , Acland RD. Distal revascularization and microvascular free tissue transfer: an alternative to amputation in ischemic lesions of the lower extremity. *J Vasc Surg*. 1985;2(6):806–811.
27. Biancari F, Kantonen I, Alback A, Matzke S, Luther M, Lepantalo M. Limits of infrapopliteal bypass surgery for critical leg ischemia: when not to reconstruct. *World J Surg*. 2000;24(6):727–733.
28. Keagy BA, Schwartz JA, Kotb M, Burnham SJ, Johnson G Jr. Lower extremity amputation: the control series. *J Vasc Surg*. 1986; 4(4):321–326.
29. Dwars BJ, van den Broek TA, Ravwerda JA, Bakker FC. Criteria for reliable selection of the lowest level of amputation in peripheral vascular disease. *J Vasc Surg*. 1992;15:536–542.
30. Malone JM, Anderson GG, Lalka SG, et al. Prospective comparison of noninvasive techniques for amputation level selection. *Am J Surg*. 1987;154:179–184.
31. Misuri A, Lucertini G, Nanni A, Viacava A, Belardi P. Predictive value of transcutaneous oximetry for selection of the amputation level. *J Cardiovasc Surg*. 2000;41(1):83–87.
32. Zhan LX, Branco BC, Armstrong DG, Mills JL Sr. The Society for Vascular Surgery lower extremity threatened limb classification system based on Wound, Ischemia, and foot Infection (WIfI) correlates with risk of major amputation and time to wound healing. *J Vasc Surg*. 2015;61(4):939–944.
33. van Reijen NS, Ponchant K, Ubbink DT, Koelemay MJW. Editor's choice—the prognostic value of the WIfI classification in patients with chronic limb threatening ischaemia: a systematic review and meta-analysis. *Eur J Vasc Endovasc Surg*. 2019;58(3): 362–371.
34. Mayor J, Chung J, Zhang Q, et al. Using the Society for Vascular Surgery Wound, Ischemia, and foot Infection classification to identify patients most likely to benefit from revascularization. *J Vasc Surg*. 2019;70(3):776.e1–785.e1.
35. Robinson WP, Loretz L, Hanesian C, et al. Society for Vascular Surgery Wound, Ischemia, foot Infection (WIfI) score correlates with the intensity of multimodal limb treatment and patient-centered outcomes in patients with threatened limbs managed in a limb preservation center. *J Vasc Surg*. 2017;66(2):488.e2–498.e2.
36. Darling JD, McCallum JC, Soden PA, et al. Predictive ability of the Society for Vascular Surgery Wound, Ischemia, and foot Infection (WIfI) classification system after first-time lower extremity revascularizations. *J Vasc Surg*. 2017;65(3):695–704.
37. Nishimoto GS, Attinger CE, Cooper PS. Lengthening the Achilles tendon for the treatment of diabetic plantar forefoot ulceration. *Surg Clin North Am*. 2003;83(3):707–726.
38. Taylor BC, Poka A. Osteomyoplastic transtibial amputation: technique and tips. *J Orthop Surg Res*. 2011;6:13.
39. Malone J. Lower extremity amputation. In: Moore W, ed. *Vascular Surgery: A Comprehensive Review*. WB Saunders; 1993:809.
40. Frang R, Taylor L, Porter J. Amputations. In: Porter JM, Taylor L, eds. *Basic Data Underlying Clinical Decision Making in Vascular Surgery*. Quality Medical Publishing; 1994:153.
41. Sandnes DK, Sobel M, Flum DR. Survival after lower extremity amputation. *J Am Coll Surg*. 2004;199:394–402.
42. Aulivola B, Hile CN, Hamdan AD, et al. Major lower extremity amputation: outcome of a modern series. *Arch Surg*. 2004;139: 395–399.
43. Roon AJ, Moore WS, Goldstone J. Below-knee amputations: a modern approach. *Am J Surg*. 1977;134:153–158.
44. Williams JW, Britt LG, Eades T, Sherman RT. Pulmonary embolism after amputation of the lower extremity. *Surg Gynecol Obstet*. 1975;140(2):246–248.
45. Yeager RA, Moneta GL, Edwards JM, Taylor LM Jr, McConnell DB, Porter JM. Deep vein thrombosis associated with lower extremity amputation. *J Vasc Surg*. 1995;22(5):612–615.
46. Burke B, Kumar R, Vickers V, Grant E, Scremin E. Deep vein thrombosis after lower limb amputation. *Am J Phys Med Rehabil*. 2000;79(2):145–149.
47. Fisher DJ Jr, Clagett GP, Fry RE, Humble TH, Fry WJ. One-stage versus two-stage amputation for wet gangrene of the lower extremity: a randomized study. *J Vasc Surg*. 1988;8(4):428–433.
48. Enneking FK, Morey TE. Continuous postoperative infusion of a regional anesthetic after an amputation of the lower extremity. A randomized clinical trial. *J Bone Joint Surg Am*. 1997; 79(11):1752–1753.
49. Pinzur MS, Garla PG, Pluth T, Vrbos L. Continuous postoperative infusion of a regional anesthetic after an amputation of the lower extremity. A randomized clinical trial. *J Bone Joint Surg Am*. 1996;78(10):1501–1505.
50. Eginton MT, Brown KR, Seabrook GR, Towne JB, Cambria RA. A prospective randomized evaluation of negative-pressure wound dressings for diabetic foot wounds. *Ann Vasc Surg*. 2003; 17(6):645–649.
51. Armstrong DG, Lavery LA, Abu-Rumman P, et al. Outcomes of subatmospheric pressure dressing therapy on wounds of the diabetic foot. *Ostomy Wound Manage*. 2002;48(4):64–68.
52. Ford CN, Reinhard ER, Yeh D, et al. Interim analysis of a prospective, randomized trial of vacuum-assisted closure versus the healthpoint system in the management of pressure ulcers. *Ann Plast Surg*. 2002;49(1):55–61.
53. Iacono RP, Linford J, Sandyk R. Pain management after lower extremity amputation. *Neurosurgery*. 1987;20(3):496–500.
54. Sherman RA, Sherman CJ, Parker L. Chronic phantom and stump pain among American veterans: results of a survey. *Pain*. 1984;18:83–95.
55. Snyder DC, Salameh JR, Clericuzio CP. Retrospective review of forefoot amputations at a Veterans Affairs hospital and evaluation of post-amputation follow-up. *Am J Surg*. 2006;192(5):e51–e54.
56. Cruz CP, Eidt JF, Capps C, Kirtley L, Moursi MM. Major lower extremity amputations at a Veterans Affairs hospital. *Am J Surg*. 2003;186(5):449–454.
57. Powell TW, Burnham SJ, Johnson G Jr. Second leg ischemia. Lower extremity bypass versus amputation in patients with contralateral lower extremity amputation. *Am Surg*. 1984;50(11):577–580.
58. Van Gils CC, Wheeler LA, Mellstrom M, Brinton EA, Mason S, Wheeler CG. Amputation prevention by vascular surgery and podiatry collaboration in high-risk diabetic and nondiabetic patients. The operation desert foot experience. *Diabetes Care*. 1999; 22(55):678–683.
59. Harris WR. Lower-extremity amputation in elderly patients. *Can J Surg*. 1987;30(5):315.
60. Stineman MG, Kwong PL, Kurichi JE, et al. The effectiveness of inpatient rehabilitation in the acute postoperative phase of care after transtibial or transfemoral amputation: study of an integrated health care delivery system. *Arch Phys Med Rehabil*. 2008;89(10):1863–1872.
61. Bild DE, Selby JV, Sinnock P, Browner WS, Braveman P, Showstack JA. Lower-extremity amputation in people with diabetes. Epidemiology and prevention. *Diabetes Care*. 1989;12(1):24–31.
62. Del Aguila MA, Reiber GE, Koepsell TD. How does provider and patient awareness of high-risk status for lower-extremity amputation influence foot-care practice? *Diabetes Care*. 1994;17(9):1050–1054.
63. Waters RL, Perry J, Antonelli D, Hislop H. Energy cost of walking amputees: the influence of level of amputation. *J Bone Joint Surg Am*. 1976;58:42–46.
64. Malone J. Above the knee amputation and hip disarticulation. In: Ernst C, Stanley C, eds. *Current Therapy in Vascular Surgery*. BC Decker; 1991:699.

90

Thoracic and Thoracoabdominal Aorta: Aneurysm and Dissection

Joshua C. Grimm and George J. Arnaoutakis

Key Points

1. There have been vast improvements in surgical outcomes for the management thoracoabdominal aortic aneurysms.
2. Improved preoperative care, surgical technique, and implementation of surgical adjuncts such as distal aortic perfusion and cerebrospinal fluid drainage have played pivotal roles in this improvement.
3. Neurologic outcomes have seen the most improvement with neurologic deficit seen in less than 2% of patients.
4. Endovascular repair of these aneurysms is not without risk and continued research and device development is needed for this complex disease.

In 1955, Ethridge reported the first repair of a thoracoabdominal aortic aneurysm (TAAA) using a homograft. One year later, Debakey performed the first descending and infrarenal aortic replacement using a Dacron graft. This was followed by the adoption of the "clamp and sew" technique by Crawford. This afforded surgeons the ability to manage perivisceral aneurysm by reimplanting branch vessels while minimizing end-organ ischemic time. The emergence of additional adjuncts and techniques has further reduced the morbidity and mortality associated with TAAA surgery, but outcomes remain closely tied to center experience.[1] Moreover, elective repair remains the only way to prevent the risk of TAAA rupture (**Fig. 90.1**). In this chapter, we will focus on the diagnosis and management of TAAAs as well as perioperative outcomes with an emphasis on technical nuances to minimize spinal cord and
1 visceral ischemia.

EPIDEMIOLOGY

Aortic aneurysmal disease remains a significant cause of death in developed countries and its prevalence appears to be increasing. While part of this increase may be due to an improvement in imaging techniques leading to enhanced diagnosis, the morbidity and mortality of TAAAs, both with and without surgical intervention, remains substantial.[2] The estimated prevalence of abdominal aortic aneurysms (AAAs) ranges from 2.3% to 10.7%, while the prevalence of TAAA is estimated to be much lower at 10.4 cases per 100,000 person years.[3] Of the 51,000 aneurysms repaired each year, only 1000 are TAAAs. The disease predominately affects males (2–4:1) with an average age of 59 to 69 years old.

Rupture (60%) is the leading cause of death in this population at 5 years from the time of diagnosis. The rate of rupture rapidly increases when the aortic diameter reaches 6 cm, and even more dramatically above 7 cm.[4] The median size at which TAAAs rupture is 7 cm with an 80% risk of rupture within 1 year as aneurysms approach 8 cm.[4] The lifetime risk of rupture is 75% to 80%, but how long it will take to reach the point of rupture is not easily determined. The median growth rate for TAAAs tends to be somewhat slower (0.20 to 0.34 cm per year) than that of AAAs, but TAAAs tend to present at a larger diameter.[5]

PATHOGENESIS

As an aorta dilates beyond 50% of its normal diameter it is considered aneurysmal, regardless of whether the dilation is focal (saccular) or diffuse (fusiform). TAAAs are the result of degenerative changes within the aortic wall in a process that is similar to that of AAAs. Arteriosclerosis has long been noted to be associated with aneurysmal disease, but these two processes are histologically distinct. Arteriosclerosis is the result of intimal changes leading to occlusive disease. The pathogenesis of aneurysmal disease includes thinning of the media with destruction of smooth muscle cells and elastin, infiltration of inflammatory cells, neovascularization, and compensatory collagen deposition. Inflammatory cells are predominately macrophages which secrete proteases and elastase that cause degradation of the aortic wall. The degradation byproducts serve as chemokines that promote further inflammatory cell recruitment. Matrix metalloproteinases (MMPs) are peptidases that are highly prevalent in aneurysm development, particularly MMP9, MMP2, and MMP12.[6]

Beyond the well-characterized connective tissue disorders, there is clearly a genetic role in aneurysm development, as 20% of patients have a first-degree relative afflicted with the same condition. This further emphasizes the critical role of genetic testing in educating patients, identifying other concomitant conditions, and determining the timing of surgery or surveillance. Most centers now have access to the noninvasive, Invitae Aortopathy Comprehensive Panel (Invitae Corp., Labcorp), which tests up to 35 genes associated with aortic conditions. Marfan syndrome is a connective tissue disorder that is the most common cause of inherited aneurysm disease and is also associated with ocular, skeletal, and cardiovascular abnormalities. It affects males and females of all races equally with an incidence of 1 in 5000 to 10,000 individuals. The aortic dilation is due to a mutation in *FBN1* which codes for fibrillin 1. Additional associated connective tissue disorders are Ehlers–Danlos, Loeys–Dietz syndrome, and Turner

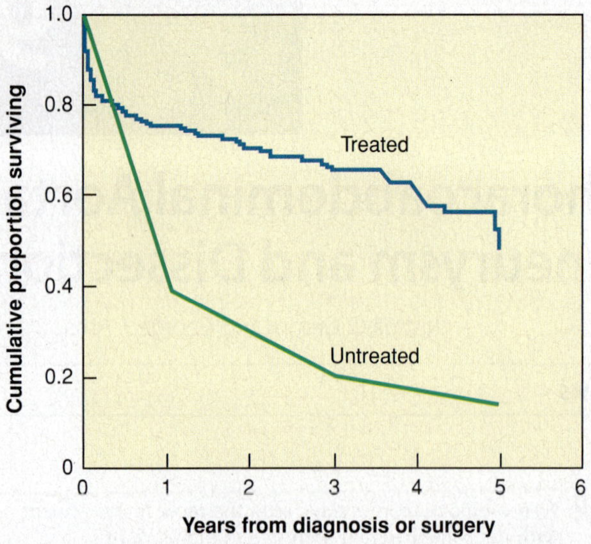

Figure 90.1. Thoracoabdominal aortic aneurysm: comparison of survival rates in untreated patients versus surgically treated patients.

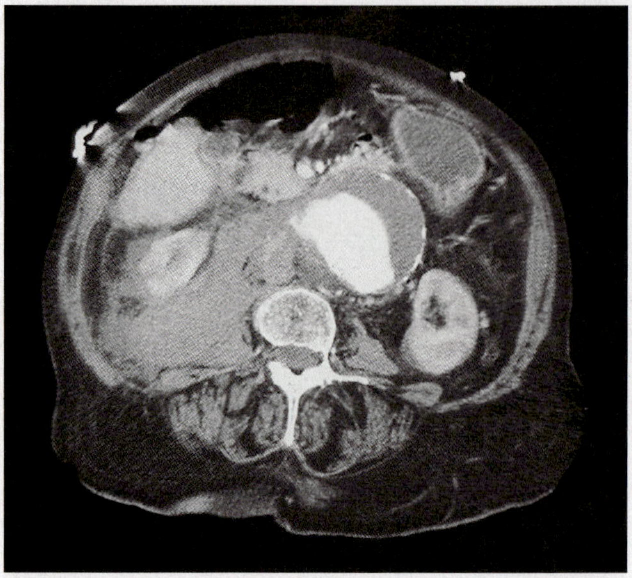

Figure 90.2. Computed tomography scan of a ruptured thoracoabdominal aortic aneurysm. Note stranding in the retroperitoneum denoting extravasation of blood.

syndrome.[7] Previously, autosomal dominant polycystic kidney disease was associated with aortic aneurysm development, but this linkage has failed to be replicated aside from an isolated, ascending aneurysm disease. There are familial cases of TAAA with an autosomal dominant inheritance pattern. Patients in these families develop more rapidly expanding aneurysms at an earlier age.[8] As TAAA is a complex disease with both environmental and genetic factors, identifying a true genetic cause of the disease is challenging. The most strongly associated mutation is in *ACTA2*, which codes for alpha-actin in smooth muscle and is estimated to account for 15% of familial aortic cases. Other implicated genes supported by replication include *MYH11*, *TGFBR1*, *TGFRB2*, and *SMAD2*.[9]

Mycotic aneurysms are infectious in nature. They are caused by bacterial or septic emboli seeding an atherosclerotic aorta or by spread from empyema or an adjacent infected lymph node. These account for only 0.6% to 2% of aneurysms in developed countries. The most common organisms are *Salmonella* species, *Staphylococcal* species, *Streptococcus* species, or *E. coli*. Morphologically, they tend to be saccular and more prone to rupture. Trauma can lead to pseudoaneurysm formation, an entity which can be underdiagnosed in the acute phase. When recognized, prompt repair should be strongly considered.

Aortic dissection will often degenerate into aneurysm. In up to 40% of type B dissections initially managed medically, surgery will be required for aneurysm formation. There are several factors that appear to increase the risk of degeneration and include: lesser curve entry tear size >10 mm (Evangelista effect), initial aortic diameter >40 mm, a free-floating true lumen, and false lumen patency with diameter >22 mm.[10] Chronic dissection and patent false lumen are not linked to a higher risk of aortic rupture.

In 20% of cases, an aneurysm can be identified in more than one segment of the aorta. In rare circumstances, the aneurysm may extend from the ascending aorta, through the arch and down through the thoracoabdominal aorta, thus creating a "mega" aorta scenario. This phenotype is frequently associated with Marfan syndrome and chronic aortic dissection. Its extensive nature can complicate the reconstruction strategy, which often involves multiple open or hybrid procedures.

Clinical Manifestations

The symptoms of TAAA are frequently ill-defined, but commonly include back, flank, chest, and/or epigastric pain. A description of worsening pain is concerning as it can be a sign of impending rupture. Rarely, hoarseness can occur due to proximal aneurysms causing compression of the left recurrent laryngeal or vagus nerve. Shortness of breath can result from compression of the tracheobronchial tree. The aneurysm can also erode into the GI tract (hematemesis or melena) or the tracheobronchial tree (hemoptysis). These events can be paroxysmal and, therefore, the diagnosis of aorto-enteric or aorto-tracheal fistula should be entertained even without signs of overt bleeding. Compression of the intercostal arteries or spinal cord is rare but can cause paraplegia. More commonly, it is a sign of malperfusion in acute aortic dissection. Embolization to the renal, mesenteric, or lower extremities from mural thrombus can also occur.

Unfortunately, many patients (10% to 20%) present with frank rupture (**Fig. 90.2**). Especially in patients with known aneurysmal disease, a presentation of shock with acute onset chest, abdominal or back pain should prompt an immediate workup for rupture. In select instances, the aortic wall may seal for several hours to days prior to free rupture, but this interval is highly variable.

Diagnostic Imaging

The mainstay of imaging for TAAA diagnosis is computed tomography angiography (CTA), which is useful in defining the extent of the TAAA as defined by the modified Crawford Classification (**Fig. 90.3**). It is also useful in delineating true versus false lumens (in dissection) and in allowing for accurate measurement of the entire aorta at various levels. Periaortic fluid and stranding can signal free or contained rupture. CTA aids in the surgical planning in regard to clamp site, visceral reconstruction, and identification of intercostal vessels appropriate for reimplantation. Coronal and sagittal views can also be useful in characterizing proximity to surrounding thoracic organs.

Magnetic resonance arteriography (MRA) has emerged as an alternative imaging modality useful in the evaluation of aortic disease and its branches. Advantages include the lack of contrast or radiation exposure in those undergoing surveillance, but it lacks the same degree of spatial resolution of a formal CTA. Additionally, CTA is better at identifying aortic wall features, including calcifications, and intramural thrombus.

Transesophageal echocardiography (TEE) provides excellent real-time imaging of the ascending and descending thoracic aorta (DTA) and can be performed intraoperatively or at

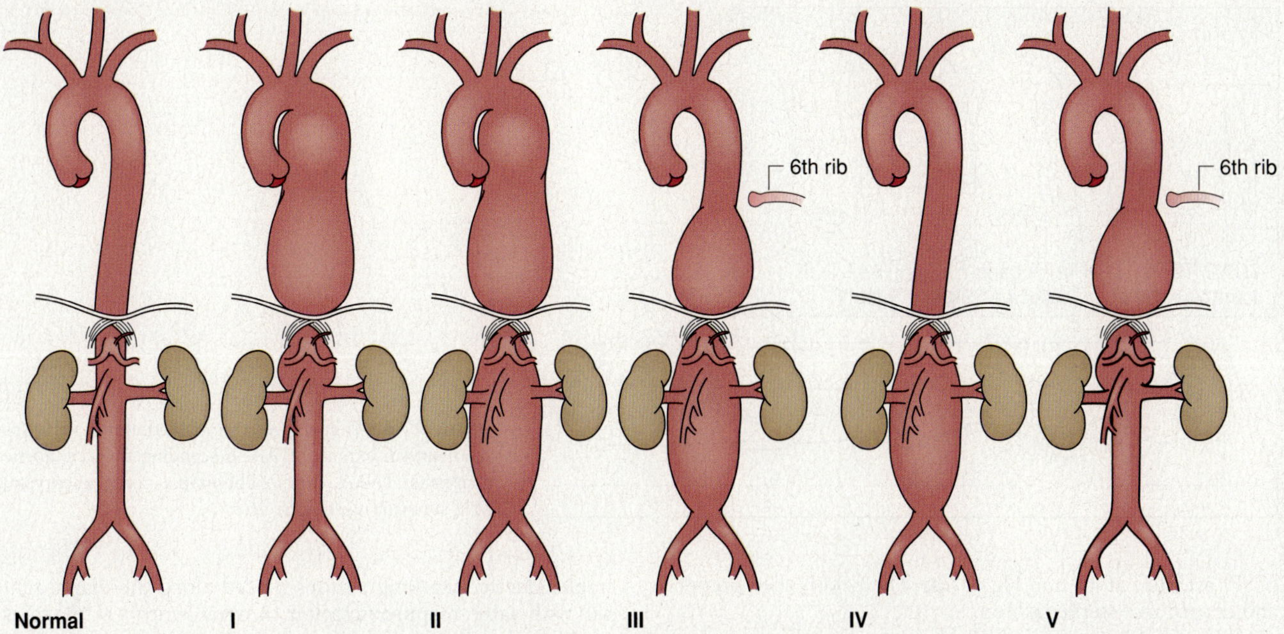

Figure 90.3. Thoracoabdominal aortic aneurysm classification. Extent I, distal to the left subclavian artery to above the renal arteries. Extent II, distal to the left subclavian artery to below the renal arteries. Extent III, from the sixth intercostal space to below the renal arteries. Extent IV, the 12th intercostal space to the iliac bifurcation (total abdominal aortic aneurysm). Extent V, below the sixth intercostal space to just above the renal arteries.

bedside. It is particularly useful when patients are too unstable to transport to the CT scanner. It can help to identify optimal cross-clamping sites and to assess ventricular and valvular function. Visualization of the aortic arch and abdominal aorta is limited.

Intravascular ultrasound (IVUS) is also useful as it allows for characterization of intramural relationships, which is critical during acute and chronic dissection cases managed with endovascular approaches. It only requires an 8-Fr sheath, so it remains relatively low profile. On IVUS, the intersection of the septum and aortic wall generates a concave shape in the true lumen and a convex shape in the false lumen. Epiaortic ultrasound can also be used to allow better characterization of the thoracic aorta for cannulation and clamping.

Indications for Surgery

In patients without a diagnosis of a genetic condition, the most updated guidelines from the ACC/AHA recommend surgical treatment of TAA/TAAA once the diameter ≥55 mm. In the presence of high-risk features, it is reasonable to pursue a more aggressive approach (≥50), especially in experienced aortic centers.[11] If the blood pressure is >130/80, beta blocker therapy is indicated. For additional control, an angiotensin receptor blocker or an ACE inhibitor can be added. If tolerated, most patients should also be placed on maximal statin therapy, especially in cases of degenerative aneurysms.[11]

Preoperative Evaluation

It is often useful to consult with the cardiology, pulmonology, and nephrology teams to assist in preoperative risk stratification. All patients should undergo pulmonary screening with pulmonary function tests/DLCO as single-lung ventilation is required during open TAAA reconstruction. Additionally, the left lung is often adherent to the aneurysm sac and blunt pulmonary trauma may be unavoidable, even with exercising extreme caution. An FEV <1.5 L or <50% predicted has been associated with adverse outcomes.[12]

In patients with TAAA, ischemic heart disease is the most common cause of death. If possible, coronary revascularization via coronary artery bypass grafting or via percutaneous intervention (PCI) (stenting or balloon angioplasty) should be performed prior to TAAA repair to minimize perioperative morbidity. This is a delicate balance as delaying TAAA reconstruction in favor of coronary revascularization can increase the risk of an interval rupture. If bypass grafting is pursued before TAAA repair, the use of the left internal mammary artery is typically avoided in the event the aortic cross-clamp is proximal to the left subclavian artery. Additionally, this vessel may provide collateral blood supply to the spinal cord and chest wall. PCI is an option in many patients, but the use of bare metal stents is preferred as they do not require prolonged antiplatelet therapy.

OPERATIVE TECHNIQUES

For extensive open aortic reconstructions (Crawfords I and II), a spinal drain is routinely placed in the third or fourth lumbar space preoperatively. In emergent situations such as frank rupture, a spinal drain may be deferred until after the repair. For lesser extent reconstructions (Crawford III and IV) strong consideration should be given to spinal drains unless there are relative anatomic contraindications. Invasive blood pressure monitoring is achieved with, at minimum, a right radial arterial line. For open repairs, a dual-lumen endotracheal tube is placed for single-lung ventilation after induction of general anesthesia. Alternatively, a bronchial blocker can be employed. This maneuver obviates the need for tube exchange at the conclusion of the procedure. It does, however, require careful positioning by the anesthesiologists and may not afford optimal lung isolation. Continuous pulmonary artery pressure monitoring is provided by a balloon-tipped pulmonary artery catheter. Lage bore central and peripheral access is needed. Nasopharyngeal and core body temperatures are monitored via esophageal and Foley catheter temperature probes, respectively. If TEE is to be used, it is inserted at this time as well. A right femoral arterial catheter is useful for monitoring distal perfusion. The patient is then placed in the right lateral decubitus position and all pressure points are padded. If neuromonitoring is employed, a combination of continuous electroencephalography and motor- and sensory-evoked potential monitors are positioned. The spinal drain is then attached to the spinal cord pressure monitor and the drain is set to maintain a cerebrospinal fluid

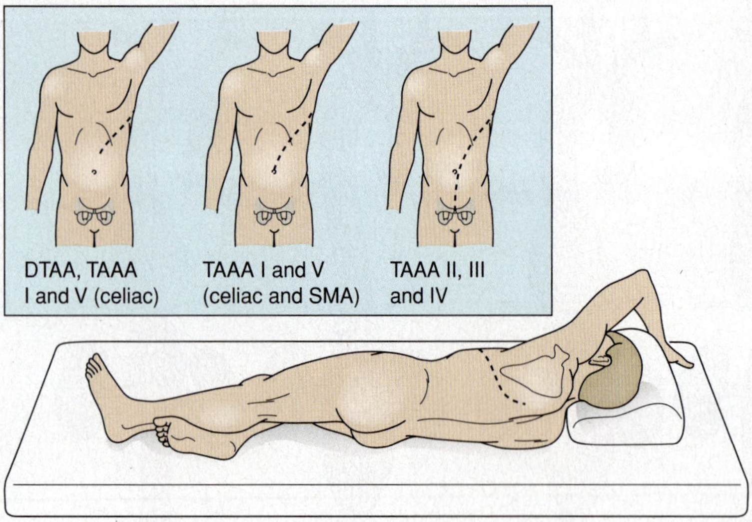

Figure 90.4. Tailoring of thoracoabdominal incisions for aneurysm extent. DTAA, descending thoracic aortic aneurysms; TAAA, thoracoabdominal aortic aneurysm; SMA, superior mesenteric artery.

(CSF) pressure at 10 mm Hg or less. The field is then prepped and draped in a sterile fashion.

An incision is made to fit the extent of the aneurysm (**Fig. 90.4**). Typically, it starts between the tip of the scapula and the spinus process. It curves along the 6th intercostal space to the costal cartilage and then obliquely to the umbilicus. The insertion of the serratus anterior muscle is mobilized after the latissimus dorsi is divided. The left chest is entered after the lung is deflated. For extent II, III, and IV TAAA, the full incision is utilized. The incision can be shortened or lengthened as needed depending on the extent (**Fig. 90.4**). The use of a self-retaining retractor allows ideal visualization of the thoracic and abdominal aorta.

Dissection begins at the level of the hilum of the lung cephalad to the DTA. Transection of the ligamentum arteriousum is performed with care to avoid the recurrent laryngeal nerve. The muscular portion of the diaphragm is incised to avoid the phrenic nerve insertion (**Fig. 90.5**). Division of the diaphragm may be performed with electrocautery or with a vascular

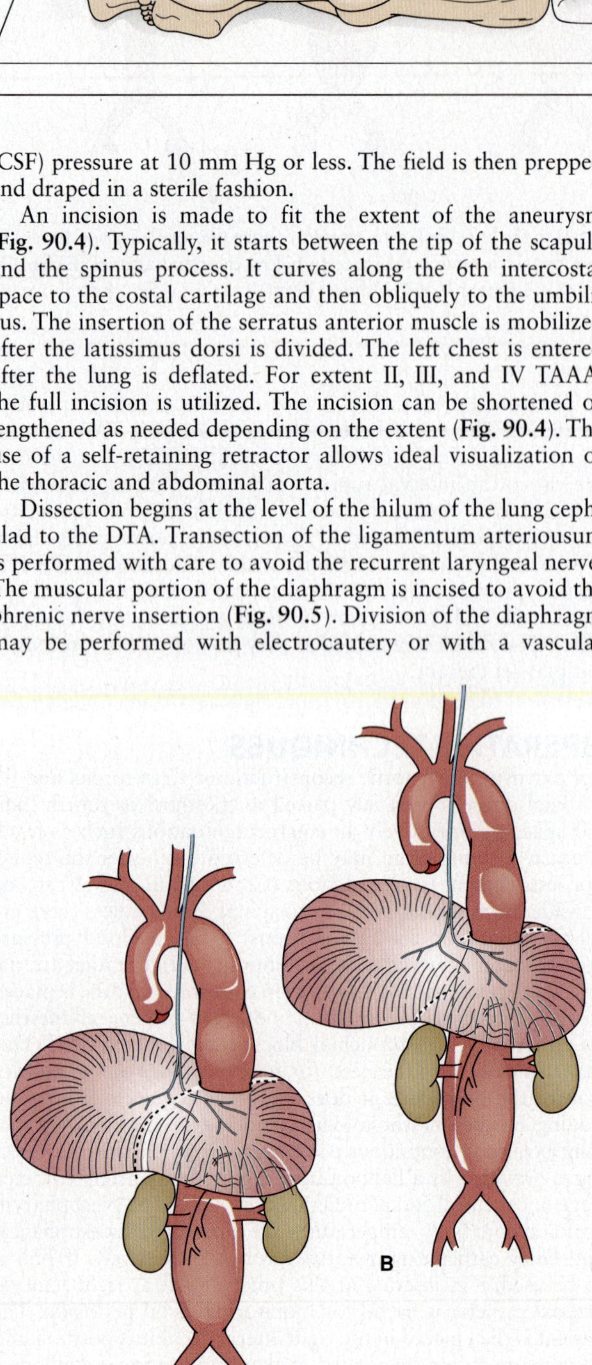

Figure 90.5. In previous surgical practice, the diaphragm was divided (**A**); currently, only the muscular portion of the diaphragm is cut (**B**).

stapler device. Marking sutures placed along the diaphragm aid with later reapproximation. A retroperitoneal plane is established and a medial visceral rotation is performed. This relocates the spleen, bowel, and left kidney to the right of the aorta. Following these maneuvers, the aortic branch vessels can usually be identified and controlled with vessel loops. Systemic heparization is then performed with 0.5 to 1 mg/kg (**Fig. 90.6**). Different activated coagulation time (ACT) can be targeted based on institutional preference, but we favor an ACT >480 seconds.

If a proximal clamp site is attainable and affords an adequate aortic rim for reconstruction, left atrial to femoral artery partial bypass (LA-FA, eg, "pulsatile") can be entertained. In this strategy, the pericardium is opened and the left inferior pulmonary vein is identified and cannulated (inflow/drainage). Outflow can be obtained via cannulation of the DTA or femoral artery. If the femoral artery is of small caliber, sidearm cannulation is useful to minimize postoperative renal dysfunction secondary to muscle ischemia. The circuit is run through a centrifugal cardiopulmonary pump with an inline heat exchanger. Alternatively, femoral arterial and femoral venous cannulation can be performed to achieve full cardiopulmonary bypass. After successful cannulation, low-flow bypass is initiated, and the patient is cooled slightly to 34 °C. In this platform, it is critical that fibrillation is avoided and pulsatility is maintained. This strategy mandates real-time communication among the surgeon, anesthesiologist, and perfusionist to ensure adequate cerebral and somatic perfusion. A site is then selected just distal to the left subclavian artery (Zone 3), or in rare instances between the left common carotid and left subclavian arteries (Zone 2), and the aorta is clamped. An additional clamp is placed in the mid-distal DTA and the proximal anastomosis is completed. The clamp is then sequentially moved more distally depending upon the extent of the reconstruction.

If a proximal clamp site is not feasible (eg, large proximal DTA aneurysm or complex, chronic dissection with thrombus), full bypass is required in anticipation of hypothermic cerebral circulatory arrest. This is achieved via right atrial to femoral artery cannulation (RA-FA). In these instances, the patient is cooled to 18 °C and, thus, electrocerebral silence. During the proximal anastomosis, a cross-clamp is positioned in the mid-distal DTA to maintain somatic perfusion, while circulatory arrest is initiated to the brain.

To minimize the risk of aorto-esophageal fistula formation, the inclusion technique is avoided and, instead, the aorta is transected completely in preparation for the anastomosis (**Fig. 90.7A**). An appropriately sized Dacron graft is then sutured to the DTA in an end-to-end fashion with a running 2-0 or 3-0 monofilament polypropylene suture. Pledgeted polypropylene sutures are placed as needed for reinforcement.

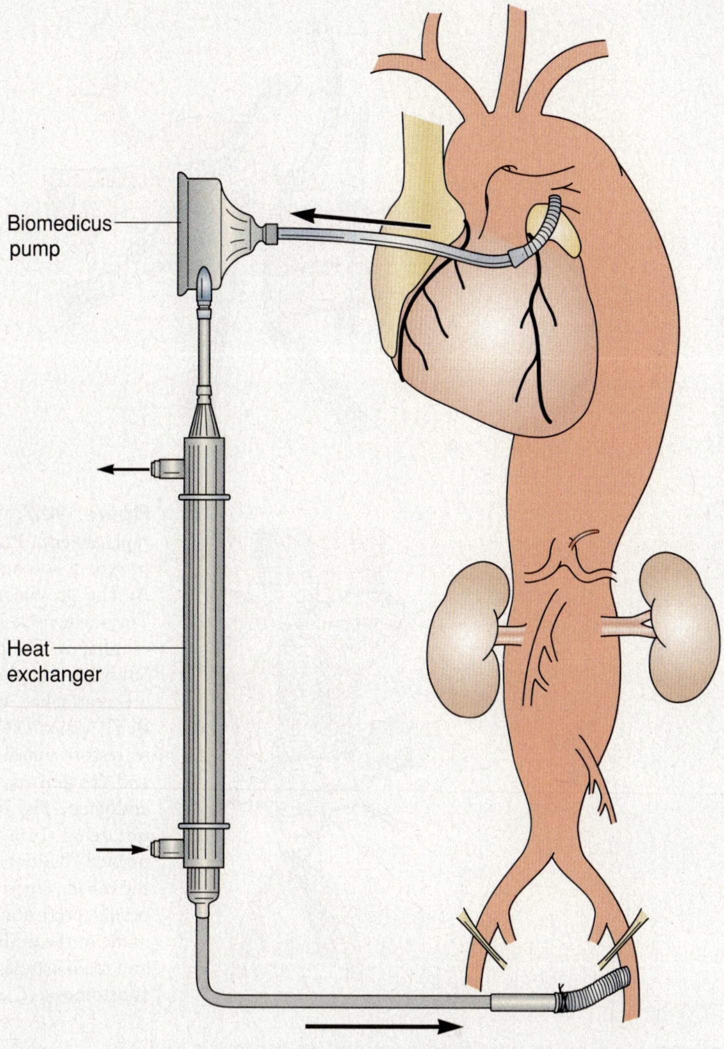

Figure 90.6. Distal aortic perfusion from the left inferior pulmonary vein to the left common femoral artery.

When performing the proximal anastomosis under circulatory arrest without a proximal clamp it is important to use steep Trendelenburg positioning. We also allow effluent blood to remain in the aortic arch, only suctioning what is necessary to safely perform the anastomosis. These maneuvers avoid entraining air into the aortic arch. After completing the proximal anastomosis, the mid-thoracic clamp is moved distally onto the abdominal aorta at the celiac axis in preparation for intercostal reimplantation. Robustly bleeding intercostal arteries should be promptly oversewn to avoid depressurization of the spinal cord collaterals. Patent lower intercostal arteries at the T8 to T12 level are reimplanted with an 8/10 mm Dacron graft or as patch when technically possible. If no change is noted in the MEP or SSEP signal without reimplantation, they can be ligated, but not without risk. For patients with connective tissue disorders or those who are over 60 years of age, a loop graft has replaced the island patch technique. If reattachment is performed, the proximal clamp on the surgical graft is moved distal to the intercostal artery patch to restore pulsatile flow to the cord (**Fig. 90.7B**). The loop graft is typically performed with an 8- or 10-mm graft sewn to a series of intercostal arteries and taken off of the main aortic graft. This graft can be embolized later, if formation of an intercostal artery patch aneurysm occurs. At this point, the distal clamp is moved to the infrarenal aorta and the abdominal aorta is opened longitudinally. The celiac, superior mesenteric, and renal arteries are identified and perfused via 9- or 12-Fr balloon-tipped catheters (**Fig. 90.7C**). The visceral vessels are perfused at a flow rate of approximately 200 cc/min per vessel and at a temperature relative to the degree of hypothermia employed for the aortic reconstruction (32/34 °C vs 18/20 °C). It is our preference to perform this portion of the reconstruction with a Coselli graft which is prefabricated with four limbs. The distal anastomosis can be completed prior to visceral reimplantation to hasten iliac reperfusion and minimize the spinal cord ischemic time (**Fig. 90.7C**). A Wylie vascular clamp can be useful to obtain distal clamping of the right common iliac artery.

Once the core body or nasopharyngeal temperature returns to 36 °C, the patient is weaned from bypass, protamine is administered (1 mg/1 mg heparin) and the cannulae are removed. After hemostasis is achieved, two or three pleural drainage tubes are positioned and secured. The diaphragm is reapproximated with running 1-0 polypropylene suture. The left lung is reinflated and the incision is closed in a standard fashion. The patient is then returned to the supine position, the dual-lumen endotracheal tube is exchanged for a single-lumen tube, and the patient is transported to the ICU (see **Table 90.1** for additional details).

Elephant Trunk Technique for Extensive Aortic Aneurysms

Extensive aneurysms involving the ascending, arch and thoracoabdominal aorta can be repaired in a single stage, but not without significantly increased risk. As such, staged repairs are often preferable. The conception of the elephant trunk technique by Borst in 1983 allowed for the initial management of ascending and arch pathology followed by interval thoracoabdominal reconstruction without the need for hypothermic circulatory arrest. The elephant trunk technique

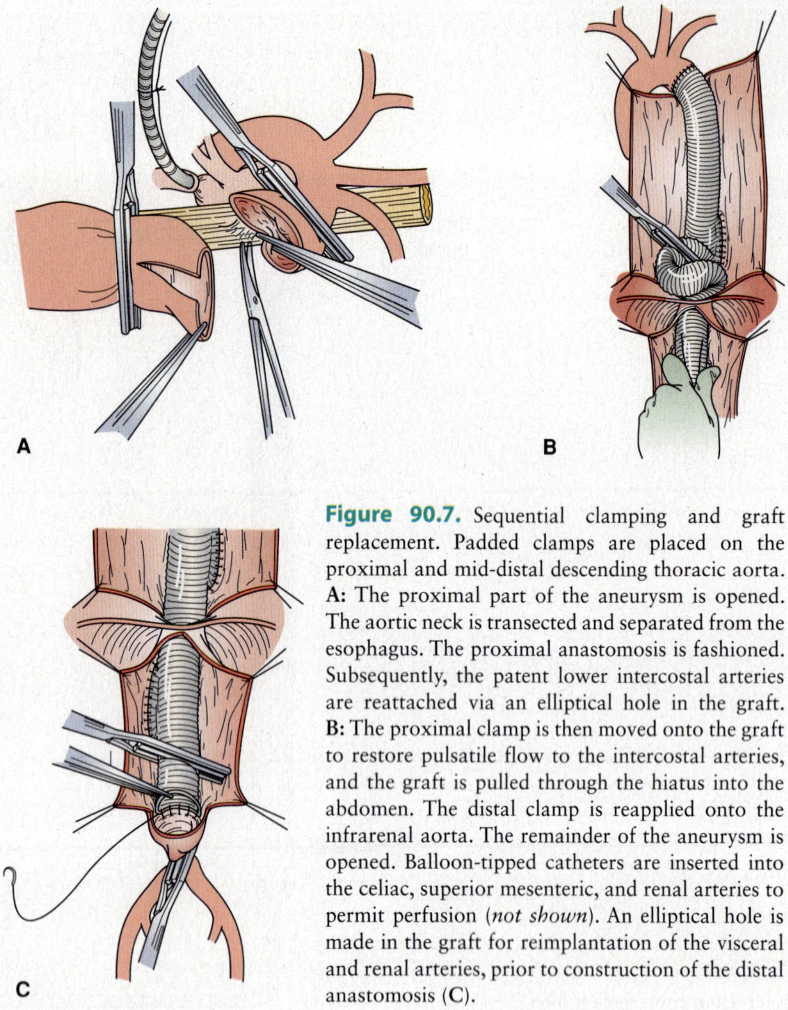

Figure 90.7. Sequential clamping and graft replacement. Padded clamps are placed on the proximal and mid-distal descending thoracic aorta. **A:** The proximal part of the aneurysm is opened. The aortic neck is transected and separated from the esophagus. The proximal anastomosis is fashioned. Subsequently, the patent lower intercostal arteries are reattached via an elliptical hole in the graft. **B:** The proximal clamp is then moved onto the graft to restore pulsatile flow to the intercostal arteries, and the graft is pulled through the hiatus into the abdomen. The distal clamp is reapplied onto the infrarenal aorta. The remainder of the aneurysm is opened. Balloon-tipped catheters are inserted into the celiac, superior mesenteric, and renal arteries to permit perfusion (*not shown*). An elliptical hole is made in the graft for reimplantation of the visceral and renal arteries, prior to construction of the distal anastomosis (**C**).

allows for a more simplified proximal anastomosis and can mitigate difficult exposure of the distal arch/proximal DTA.

The first stage of the operation is performed similarly to standard ascending and transverse arch surgery aside from the use of either an inverted graft distally or a commercially available collared graft with a prefabricated distal extension (**Fig. 90.8A**). An anastomosis is made between the folded edge or the collared portion of the elephant trunk and the aorta just distal to the left subclavian artery. The remainder of the total arch reconstruction is then completed. These reconstructions

Table 90.1. Key Technical Steps, Pearls, and Potential Pitfalls: Thoracic and Thoracoabdominal Aorta

Key Technical Steps

1. Spinal drain to mitigate risk of paralysis
2. Double-lumen endotracheal tube for lung isolation
3. Appropriate positioning to expose thoracoabdominal region (semi-lateral decubitus)
4. Curvilinear incision overlying costal margin and extending lateral to rectus muscle
5. Combined thoracic and retroperitoneal exposure of aorta (medial visceral rotation)
6. Division of diaphragm
7. Utilization of either RA-FA (with or without circulatory arrest) or LA-FA to support aortic reconstruction
8. Visceral perfusion with or without renal flush/mannitol
9. Reimplantation of large intercostal vessels as either a patch or with a graft
10. Meticulous hemostasis and closure
11. Bronchoscopy before leaving the operating room

Pearls

- Careful assessment of preoperative CT imaging and patient comorbidities to guide optimal open vs. endo approach
- To mitigate risk of spinal cord paralysis in open repair, prompt ligation of bleeding intercostal vessels is critical
- Ensure proper alignment of diaphragm following reconstruction to minimize postoperative pulmonary dysfunction

Potential Pitfalls

- Caution in Zone 2 clamping an unprotected ascending aorta—might be safer to proceed with circulatory arrest
- Postoperative pulmonary dysfunction is a major morbidity so preoperative PFTs and postoperative pulmonary hygiene are critical
- Left ventricular distention can lead to postoperative dysfunction (intermittent cardiac decompression or LV venting may be required), especially when circulatory arrest is planned (fibrillation with loss of ventricular ejection)

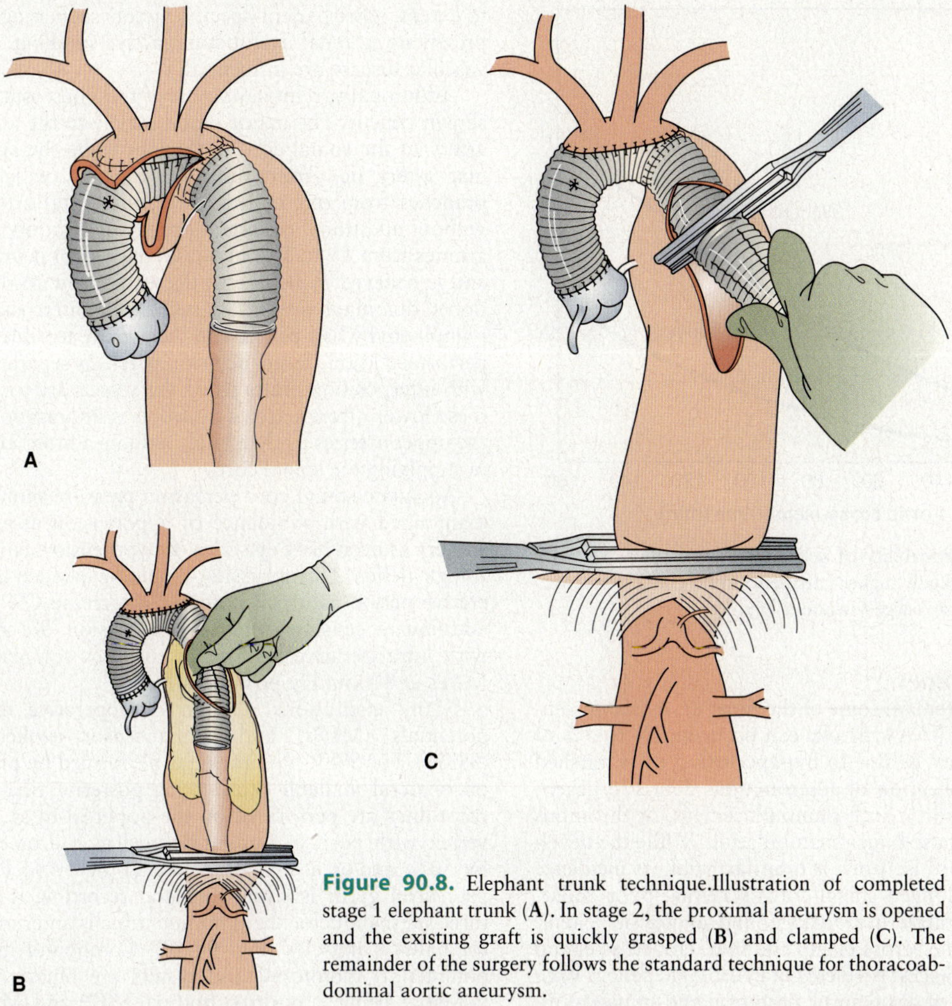

Figure 90.8. Elephant trunk technique.Illustration of completed stage 1 elephant trunk (**A**). In stage 2, the proximal aneurysm is opened and the existing graft is quickly grasped (**B**) and clamped (**C**). The remainder of the surgery follows the standard technique for thoracoabdominal aortic aneurysm.

requiring full cardiopulmonary bypass, some degree of hypothermia (moderate vs deep), and cerebral perfusion (antegrade vs retrograde). The patient is then afforded time to recover prior to the next stage.

The second stage of the repair is performed in a similar fashion to the traditional TAAA repair using distal aortic per-
2 fusion and CSF drainage. After initiation of bypass (RA-FA or LA-FA), the distal clamp is applied to the mid DTA and the arch/proximal DTA can be clamped between the left carotid and left subclavian arteries or distal to the left subclavian artery. An alternative technique is to open the proximal aorta without a proximal clamp being applied, but this risks significant bleeding unless performed under hypothermic circulatory arrest. The elephant trunk placed in stage 1 of the operation can be identified and clamped (**Fig. 90.8B,C**). The elephant trunk serves as the site for the proximal anastomosis for the remaining aneurysm to be replaced.

The "Frozen Elephant Trunk" procedure is a more contemporary "hybrid" technique, which utilizes a stent graft instead of a Dacron extension. In this approach, the endograft is deployed in an antegrade fashion during circulatory arrest. The distal aortic suture line then incorporates the stent graft and native aorta. During the subsequent TAAA reconstruction, the stent graft can be clamped and can serve as the site of the proximal aortic anastomosis.

Postoperative Management

Following surgery, the patient is admitted to the intensive care unit for close hemodynamic and neurovascular monitoring. Early extubation is appropriate when the patient is deemed otherwise stable. Mean arterial pressures (MAPs) are maintained between 80 and 90 mm Hg as permissive hypertension augments spinal cord perfusion; hypotension, even brief, can be a devastating risk factor for spinal cord ischemia. CSF pressures are continuously monitored and pressure is maintained at 10 mm Hg or less. It is our practice to perform a formal swallow evaluation with a speech specialist prior to initiation of an oral diet. Some patients require nasogastric decompression as prolonged ileus is not uncommon.

Frequent neurovascular checks in the perioperative period are mandatory to allow for prompt identification of any delayed neurologic deficit (DND). While the strongest predictors of DND are low MAP and CSF drain complications, other risk factors include hypoxemia and anemia.[13] In the absence of DND, the CSF drain is generally removed following a "clamp trial." The typical ICU length of stay is 3 to 4 days in uncomplicated cases. As a major morbidity is pulmonary compromise, pulmonary hygiene is critical and pain should be adequately managed to allow for respiratory rehabilitation. Intercostal nerve cryoablation at the time of surgery may be an important adjunct for pain control. Additionally, physical therapy should work with patients throughout their hospitalization to ensure early and adequate mobility.

Longitudinal follow-up consists of yearly CTA or MRA to survey the reconstruction and closely monitor any aortic or peripheral vascular pathology. This frequency may change in patients with connective tissue disorders or in those with residual dissections or unaddressed aneurysms.

Surgical Outcomes

Mortality rates for patients undergoing TAAA repair range between 5% and 21% and vary with aneurysm extent and center expertise.[14] Overall, 70% or patients recover without significant morbidity or mortality.

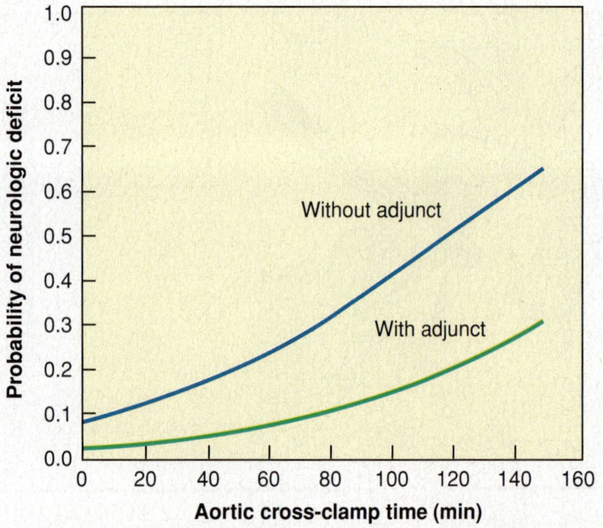

Figure 90.9. The probability of neurologic deficit increases with clamp time and is markedly higher in patients undergoing thoracoabdominal aortic aneurysm surgery without adjuncts.

3 Neurologic Outcomes

Neurologic deficits remain some of the most devastating complications following TAAA. Stroke can occur in 3% to 5% of TAAA cases and may be due to hypoperfusion or watershed phenomenon, embolization of atheromatous debris in degenerative aneurysms, aortic arch clamp placement, or thrombus dislodgement from false lumen manipulation. While the development of spinal cord ischemia is multifactorial, its incidence is increased by prolonged spinal cord ischemia, poor collateralization, perioperative hemorrhage, and aneurysm extent. Historically, under the "cross-clamp and sew" era, cross-clamp time was the single biggest predictor of neurologic deficit. With the current adjuncts of distal aortic perfusion and spinal drainage, longer clamp times appear to be better tolerated. Keeping CSF pressure below 10 mm Hg has been shown to improve spinal cord perfusion in both animal and human studies.[15] Meta analysis of CSF drainage in TAAA repairs has shown an absolute risk reduction of approximately 10%. Together, distal aortic perfusion and CSF drainage have consistently demonstrated to result in a significant decrease in the risk of acute neurologic deficit.[16] The highest incidence of neurologic deficits occurs in extent II TAAA. Prior to the widespread use of the aforementioned intraoperative techniques, the rate of deficit in this cohort of patients was reported to be as high as 30% to 40%. Following their adoption, however, this has been reduced significantly, to a rate of 7% (**Fig. 90.9**). In addition to extent, other patient-specific factors such as age, emergency presentation, renal dysfunction, active smoking, and cerebrovascular disease are influential.[17]

Additionally, reimplantation of the intercostal arteries has shown benefit. The major blood supply to the anterior spinal artery of the spinal cord is thought to be the anterior radicular artery (ie, *Artery of Adamkiewicz*), which commonly branches from one of the lower intercostal arteries with or without additional collateral branches. Ligation of intercostal arteries from T9 to T12 increases the risk of neurologic deficit and is believed to be due to decreased flow to the aforementioned dominant vessel.[17] As such, these intercostals should be reimplanted when patent and technically feasible. This can be performed as one large inclusion patch, as separate buttons, or with interposition grafts when the vessels are too far apart. If these lower arteries are occluded, it is important to reimplant the upper arteries as they likely assume a more important role in supplying the spinal cord.

Adequate spinal cord perfusion pressure should always be maintained with avoidance of hypotension during and after surgery as even brief episodes of hypotension can lead to neurologic deficit. Nitroprusside should be avoided in the perioperative period as it can potentially increase CSF pressures in addition to causing systemic hypotension. We are fastidious with intraoperative hemostasis to allow for maintenance of MAPs at 80 mm Hg postoperatively.

Many institutions rely on intraoperative motor-evoked potentials (MEPs) and somatosensory-evoked potentials (SSEPs). For SSEP, monitoring is performed by placing probes on bilateral malleoli (stimulating posterior tibial nerve) and recordings are performed on the popliteal fossa, C5, and the vertex with positive finding defined as a drop in amplitude by 50% and/or a change in latency by 10%. For MEP, the precentral gyrus is stimulated and recording is measured at three sites: abductor digiti minimi, tibialis anterior, and abductor hallucis muscles (**Fig. 90.10**). Compound muscle action potential is monitored and results are binary with loss of potential being a positive finding. SSEP and MEP monitoring have been shown to be highly correlated with irreversible neurologic deficit, but have not been shown to correlate with reversible deficit. While MEP is more complex, the detection rate of irreversible injury is identical to SSEP. Both forms of monitoring have strong negative predictive value in that it is highly unlikely to have neurologic deficit immediately following surgery if there was no loss of signal intraoperatively. If there are signal changes, rescue procedures, including increasing the MAP to >80 mm Hg, lowering the CSF pressure via drainage, transfusing to maintain a hemoglobin level >10 g/dL and attaching more intercostal arteries should be performed. Even with these adjuncts, the rate of immediate deficit remains at roughly 3% to 5%.[18]

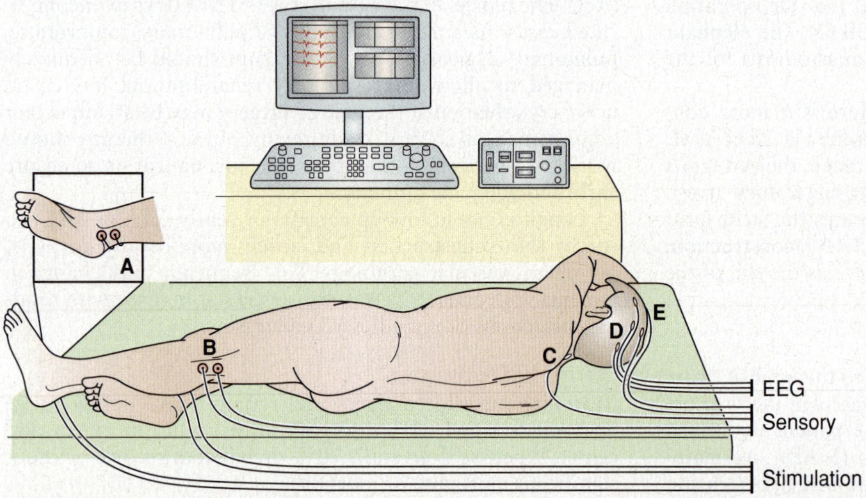

Figure 90.10. Somatosensory- and motor-evoked potentials are recorded at three sites: the popliteal fossa (A, B), C5 (C), and the vertex (D, E).

Delayed Neurologic Deficits

DND is defined as paraplegia or paraparesis after a period of observed neurologic function. When first described in 1988, this condition was irreversible. CSF drainage has been shown to provide improvement in neurologic outcomes in select cases of DND. DND can present immediately after surgery or up to 2 weeks postoperatively (median 3 days) in 2.7% of patients. There is no single predictor of delayed deficit, but rather a combination of risks leading to the development of DND. MAP less than 60 mm Hg and drain complications are the highest predictors of DND.[19]

The exact mechanism for the development of DND is not fully understood, but is hypothesized to be related to the "second hit" phenomenon as the spinal cord remains vulnerable for an extended period of time postoperatively. During this time frame a "second hit" in the form of hypotension or drain malfunction can lead to DND. Any rise in CSF pressure during the early postoperative period can lead to increased compartment pressure and decreased perfusion. As such, any sign of DND should be initially treated with free drainage of CSF to relieve the compartment pressure. Many institutions also routinely implement naloxone infusions and administration of steroids in the initial postoperative period as some studies have shown decreased incidence of DND with their use.[20]

To optimize spinal cord perfusion in the early postoperative period the MAP is maintained at 90 to 100 mm Hg, the hemoglobin greater than 10 mg/dL, and the cardiac index greater than 2.0 L/min. Rescue protocols are initiated if any signs of DND arise. These include laying the patient flat, checking the drain for malfunction, reinsertion of the drain if it was removed, free drainage of the CSF until the pressure is <10 mm Hg, increasing the MAP, liberalization of blood transfusion protocols, and increasing the oxygen saturation. CSF drainage is continued for at least 72 hours after the onset of DND. Using this multimodal approach, improvement in neurologic function has been reported in over half of patients DND.[21]

Renal Failure

Acute postoperative kidney injury (AKI) is defined according to the modern consensus Kidney Disease: Improving Global Outcomes (KDIGO) or Acute Kidney Injury Network (AKIN) criteria. They define AKI as an increase in serum creatinine by ≥0.3 mg/dL (≥26.5 micromol/L) within 48 hours; increase in serum creatinine to ≥1.5 times baseline, which is known or presumed to have occurred within the prior 7 days; or urine volume <0.5 mL/kg/hr for 6 hours. AKI is a known independent predictor of postoperative morbidity and mortality with associated mortality reported as high as 70%.[22] The reported rate of postoperative AKI falls within the range of 5% to 40% with dialysis-dependent renal failure present in 1.5% to 10.7% in elective repairs. Additionally, these patients are more likely to experience nonrenal complications, such as respiratory failure, central nervous system dysfunction, sepsis, and gastrointestinal hemorrhage. For those who develop AKI, continuous venovenous hemodialysis or daily intermittent hemodialysis is initiated. In a large series, patients requiring permanent hemodialysis were low, at 7%. Preoperative renal dysfunction and hemorrhage have also been shown to be predictors of AKI.[23]

Perioperative renal protection remains a concern and general management strategies include maintaining adequate renal oxygen delivery, reducing renal oxygen utilization, and minimizing direct renal tubular injury. The advantages of metabolic suppression via cold temperatures are well known and there is some evidence that local cooling of the kidneys may be protective. Cold renal perfusion with 4 °C solution has shown promising outcomes for renal protection, but needs further investigation.[23]

AKI is a known predictor of 30-day postoperative mortality, and occurs in approximately 25% of patients. Glomerular filtration rate (eGFR) has been shown to be superior to serum creatinine in the prediction of 30-day mortality following TAAA repair. In those with normal postoperative eGFR, mortality has been reported at 2% to 5%, while mortality was reported as 5%, 18%, and 40% for mild, moderate, and AKI, respectively. Five-year survival was 77% in those with normal eGFR, yet was less than 25%, for the severe renal insufficiency patients (**Table 90.2**).[24]

Table 90.2. Complications of Open TAAA Repair

Complication	Results
Early mortality	4–21%
Immediate neurologic deficit	2–33%
Delayed neurologic deficit	2–10%
Acute renal failure—need for dialysis	2–13%
Acute renal insufficiency	6–40%
Bleeding—reoperation for bleeding	5–10%
Vocal cord paralysis/paresis and hoarseness	10%
Cardiac complication—MI, CHF	5–15%
Pulmonary insufficiency (prolonged ventilation >48 hr)	10–41%
Stroke or transient ischemic attack (reversible)	2–6%
Gastrointestinal complications (pancreatitis, ischemic colitis, small bowel, cholecystitis, hepatic insufficiency)	7–10%
Chylothorax	<1%
Hospital length of stay	10–22 days
Survival	1 y = 60–80% 5 y = 65–80% 10 y = 40%

CHF, chronic heart failure; MI, myocardial infarction.

Complications

A summary of additional potential complications is presented in **Table 90.2.**

Elephant Trunk Technique

Two-staged elephant trunk technique for the repair of extensive aortic aneurysms involving the ascending, transverse arch, and thoracoabdominal aorta has proven to be a durable, but challenging approach to a complex problem. Complication rates have improved as advancements in surgical adjuncts have been made. In a large series of 348 patients who underwent a two-stage TAAA repair using the elephant trunk technique, mortality rates after the first stage ranged from 5% to 10% after stage 1 and 5% to 15% after stage 2 depending on renal function. In those with a normal GFR, a 5% mortality was reported. In the interval, mortality ranged from 4% to 17% (mean of 6.5%). While timing of the second stage can be challenging, it is recommended that it should be performed within 4 to 6 weeks, due to the risk of rupture.[25]

Impact of Aortic Dissection

Historically, aortic dissection was reported as a risk for developing neurologic deficits, but these reports are from the "clamp and sew" era. In a series of 729 patients, no difference in neurologic outcome was reported between those with chronic dissection (3.6%) and those without (4.7%). These improved outcomes are likely the result of the aforementioned adjuncts (mainly distal aortic perfusion and CSF drainage).

The same is not true for acute aortic dissections, as these patients carry a rate of 32%. These patients are typically critically ill and the intraoperative methods for spinal cord protection are suboptimal. In particular, reimplantation of the intercostal arteries can be complex due to the friable, dissected tissue and the risk for hemorrhage. Additionally, the addition of distal aortic perfusion and CSF drainage may not be possible due to hemodynamic instability.

4 Endovascular Repair

Since the first thoracic stent graft repair in 1994 there has been a rapid evolution in endovascular management of thoracic aortic disease with multiple new devices entering the market. Endovascular repair of TAAA was initially purported to have the benefit of improved morbidity and mortality, however a meta-analysis demonstrated mixed results. These procedures were initially designed to manage TAAA in poor surgical candidates, but are now preferable if anatomically feasible in many cohorts. There are currently three different methods for endovascular repair of TAAA: hybrid repair, use of parallel "chimney" grafts and custom-made, branched fenestrated devices.

Hybrid Repair

The hybrid approach requires open debranching of the aorta with subsequent endovascular coverage of the aneurysmal segment. Debranching is achieved via a retroperitoneal or transperitoneal approach for extra-anatomical bypass of the visceral and renal arteries via either iliac artery. The patient is allowed to recover after which the aneurysmal segment is covered with a stent graft. Advantages of this approach are the avoidance of a thoracotomy, single-lung ventilation or aortic cross-clamping. Despite these advantages, the morbidity and mortality using this approach is comparable to that of an open repair.[26] As such, this method is likely only suited for those who will not tolerate a more formal, open repair (ie, prohibitive pulmonary dysfunction) and are anatomically not candidates for other endovascular repair techniques.

Parallel Grafts

This technique involves the use of parallel grafts (chimneys, periscopes, or snorkels, commonly referred to as CHIMPS) to preserve blood flow to branch vessels. This was initially described in 78 patients in Brazil (15 patients had TAAA). At 17 months the primary patency rate was 96.7% and early mortality was 5.1% (later 1.3%). This technique is advantageous in that off the shelf, modular grafts can be tailor fit to any anatomy. This is beneficial in patients with small and tortuous vessels, history of dissection or significant thrombus burden in the paravisceral aorta. Endoleaks from the "gutters" are the main disadvantage and endoleak rates have been reported as high as 18.5%. Meta-analysis of this technique showed 98.9% early success rate and perioperative mortality of 4%.[27] The main pitfall to this technique is "gutter" leaks which function similar to a type 1a endoleak and frequently need open reintervention to address.

Total Endovascular Repair

This method is performed via custom-made branched and/or fenestrated devices. These custom-made or physician-modified devices largely remain investigational at centers with access to physician-sponsored investigational device exemption (PS-IDE) programs. The largest experience reported is by Greenberg et al. using this method in 406 patients with perioperative mortality of 2.3% for extent IV, 5.2% for extent II and III, and 12.5% for extent I aneurysms. Estimated 24-month survival was 82%, 74%, and 70%, respectively. A multicenter prospective study of 268 patients reported 30-day mortality of 6.7%, in-hospital mortality of 10.1% and severe complications of 22%.[28] Despite this high mortality, our institution found this method to have the lowest mortality (4%) in extent II and III TAAA and has adopted this as our first-line treatment in those with favorable anatomy.

More recently, the FDA has approved the GORE EXCLUDER Thoracoabdominal Branch Endoprosthesis (TAMBE) for off-the-shelf deployment. Depending upon the aneurysm extent, the device allows for precannulation and subsequent stenting of the visceral vessels. In the initial early feasibility study, 40% of patients had pararenal AAAs and 60% had extent IV TAAAs.[29] Reinterventions in TAMBE are not common (>10%) and major morbidities, including, stroke and renal failure, were infrequent. The occurrence of branch vessel thrombosis was highly associated with vessel size <4 mm and there remains a significant portion of patients with anatomy unsuitable for this off-the-shelf device.[29]

SUMMARY

The successful management of complex TAA/TAAA requires thoughtful preoperative, intraoperative, and postoperative planning and execution. As technologic improvements continue, cardiac and vascular surgeons must not operate in silos, but, instead, must collaborate to ensure excellent outcomes.

ACKNOWLEDGMENT

We gratefully acknowledge the contributions of previous edition author, Eric Y. Pruitt, as portions of those chapters have been retained in this revision.

References

1. Polanco AR, D'Angelo AM, Shea NJ, Allen P, Takayama H, Patel VI. Increased hospital volume is associated with reduced mortality after thoracoabdominal aortic aneurysm repair. *J Vasc Surg*. 2021;73:451–458.
2. Elefteriades JA, Farkas EA. Thoracic aortic aneurysm clinically pertinent controversies and uncertainties. *J Am Coll Cardiol*. 2010;55:841–857.
3. Clouse WD, Hallett JW, Schaff HV, Gayari MM, Ilstrup DM, Melton LJ. Improved prognosis of thoracic aortic aneurysms: a population-based study. *JAMA*. 1998;280:1926–1929.
4. Davies RR, Goldstein LJ, Coady MA, et al. Yearly rupture or dissection rates for thoracic aortic aneurysms: simple prediction based on size. *Ann Thorac Surg*. 2002;73:17–27; discussion 27–28.
5. Oladokun D, Patterson BO, Sobocinski J, et al. Systematic review of the growth rates and influencing factors in thoracic aortic aneurysms. *Eur J Vasc Endovasc Surg*. 2016;51:674–681.
6. Ailawadi G, Eliason JL, Upchurch GR. Current concepts in the pathogenesis of abdominal aortic aneurysm. *J Vasc Surg*. 2003;38:584–588.
7. Coady MA, Davies RR, Roberts M, et al. Familial patterns of thoracic aortic aneurysms. *Arch Surg* 1999;134:361–367.
8. Albornoz G, Coady MA, Roberts M, et al. Familial thoracic aortic aneurysms and dissections–incidence, modes of inheritance, and phenotypic patterns. *Ann Thorac Surg*. 2006;82:1400–1405.
9. Boileau C, Guo D-C, Hanna N, et al. TGFB2 mutations cause familial thoracic aortic aneurysms and dissections associated with mild systemic features of Marfan syndrome. *Nat Genet*. 2012;44:916–921.
10. Malaisrie SC, Mehta CK. Updates on indications for TEVAR in type B aortic dissection. *Innovations (Phila)*. 2020;15:495–501.
11. Isselbacher EM, Preventza O, Hamilton Black J, et al. 2022 ACC/AHA Guideline for the Diagnosis and Management of Aortic Disease: A Report of the American Heart Association/American College of Cardiology Joint Committee on Clinical Practice Guidelines. *Circulation*. 2022;146:e334–e482.

12. Girardi LN, Lau C, Munjal M, et al. Impact of preoperative pulmonary function on outcomes after open repair of descending and thoracoabdominal aortic aneurysms. *J Thorac Cardiovasc Surg.* 2017;153:S22–S29.e2.
13. Azizzadeh A, Huynh TTT, Miller CC, et al. Postoperative risk factors for delayed neurologic deficit after thoracic and thoracoabdominal aortic aneurysm repair: a case-control study. *J Vasc Surg.* 2003;37:750–754.
14. Coselli JS, LeMaire SA, Preventza O, et al. Outcomes of 3309 thoracoabdominal aortic aneurysm repairs. *J Thorac Cardiovasc Surg.* 2016;151:1323–1337.
15. Cinà CS, Abouzahr L, Arena GO, Laganà A, Devereaux PJ, Farrokhyar F. Cerebrospinal fluid drainage to prevent paraplegia during thoracic and thoracoabdominal aortic aneurysm surgery: a systematic review and meta-analysis. *J Vasc Surg.* 2004;40:36–44.
16. Khan NR, Smalley Z, Nesvick CL, Lee SL, Michael LM. The use of lumbar drains in preventing spinal cord injury following thoracoabdominal aortic aneurysm repair: an updated systematic review and meta-analysis. *J Neurosurg Spine.* 2016;25:383–393.
17. Safi HJ, Miller CC, Huynh TTT, et al. Distal aortic perfusion and cerebrospinal fluid drainage for thoracoabdominal and descending thoracic aortic repair: ten years of organ protection. *Ann Surg.* 2003;238:372–380; discussion 380–381.
18. Rubin BI, Holland EJ, de Smet MD, Belfort R, Nussenblatt RB. Response of reactivated ligneous conjunctivitis to topical cyclosporine. *Am J Ophthalmol.* 1991;112:95–96.
19. Safi HJ, Miller CC, Azizzadeh A, Iliopoulos DC. Observations on delayed neurologic deficit after thoracoabdominal aortic aneurysm repair. *J Vasc Surg.* 1997;26:616–622.
20. Acher C, Acher CW, Marks E, Wynn M. Intraoperative neuroprotective interventions prevent spinal cord ischemia and injury in thoracic endovascular aortic repair. *J Vasc Surg.* 2016;63:1458–1465.
21. Estrera AL, Miller CC, Huynh TTT, et al. Preoperative and operative predictors of delayed neurologic deficit following repair of thoracoabdominal aortic aneurysm. *J Thorac Cardiovasc Surg.* 2003;126:1288–1294.
22. Chatterjee S, LeMaire SA, Amarasekara HS, et al. Early-stage acute kidney injury adversely affects thoracoabdominal aortic aneurysm repair outcomes. *Ann Thorac Surg.* 2019;107:1720–1726.
23. Wynn MM, Acher C, Marks E, Engelbert T, Acher CW. Postoperative renal failure in thoracoabdominal aortic aneurysm repair with simple cross-clamp technique and 4 °C renal perfusion. *J Vasc Surg.* 2015;61:611–622.
24. Huynh TTT, van Eps RGS, Miller CC, et al. Glomerular filtration rate is superior to serum creatinine for prediction of mortality after thoracoabdominal aortic surgery. *J Vasc Surg.* 2005;42:206–212.
25. Estrera AL, Sandhu HK, Miller CC, et al. Repair of extensive aortic aneurysms: a single-center experience using the elephant trunk technique over 20 years. *Ann Surg.* 2014;260:510–516; discussion 517–518.
26. Arnaoutakis DJ, Scali ST, Beck AW, et al. Comparative outcomes of open, hybrid, and fenestrated branched endovascular repair of extent II and III thoracoabdominal aortic aneurysms. *J Vasc Surg.* 2020;71:1503–1514.
27. Moulakakis KG, Mylonas SN, Dalainas I, et al. The chimney-graft technique for preserving supra-aortic branches: a review. *Ann Cardiothorac Surg.* 2013;2:339–346.
28. Greenberg R, Eagleton M, Mastracci T. Branched endografts for thoracoabdominal aneurysms. *J Thorac Cardiovasc Surg.* 2010;140:S171–S178.
29. Gomes VC, Farber MA, Parodi FE. Gore thoracoabdominal branched endoprosthesis: early results and impressions. *J Cardiovasc Surg (Torino).* 2023;64:481–487.

91

Abdominal Aortic Aneurysms

Dean J. Arnaoutakis and Gilbert R. Upchurch Jr.

Key Points

1 An aneurysm is defined as a permanent, focal dilation of an artery that exceeds 1.5 times the normal, expected diameter.

2 Risk factors for abdominal aortic aneurysm (AAA) include age, male gender, smoking, family history, hypertension, chronic obstructive pulmonary disease (COPD), and the presence of other aortoiliac or peripheral aneurysms.

3 The diameter of an aneurysm is the greatest predictor of rupture as estimated by the tangential stress of the vessel wall.

4 AAAs increase in size over time with a mean growth rate of 0.4 cm/y.

5 Computed tomography (CT) arteriography is both the diagnostic study of choice and the sole imaging study required for operative planning.

6 The treatment of AAA represents a balance between the risk of rupture and the operative morbidity and mortality rate.

7 Infrarenal AAAs should be repaired in men when their diameter reaches 5.5 cm and in women when the diameter reaches 5 cm, provided they are of reasonable operative risk.

8 Endovascular repair has supplanted open repair as the preferred choice by both patients and providers in the United States.

9 Endovascular aneurysm repair (EVAR) mandates long-term follow-up with serial imaging to confirm the integrity of the device and repair.

Abdominal aortic aneurysms (AAAs) are a common problem in developed countries and represent a significant public health concern globally. Operative repair is the only means to reduce the risk of rupture and the associated mortality. The treatment algorithm represents a balance between the risk of repair and the operative morbidity and mortality rate. Open surgical repair has been the traditional approach since its description by Dubost et al. in the early 1950s.[1] However, a catheter-based endovascular approach has emerged as the preferred treatment since its commercial release at the turn of the 21st century and has truly revolutionized the care of patients with AAAs.

DEFINITIONS AND CLASSIFICATIONS

1 An aneurysm is defined as a permanent, focal dilation of an artery that exceeds 1.5 times the normal, expected diameter. The diameter of a normal abdominal aorta in an adult male is approximately 2 cm (range, 1.4 to 3 cm). The abdominal aorta is consistently larger in men than in women and increases slightly with age for both genders. AAAs should be differentiated from other conditions in which the size of the aorta is increased, including ectasia and arteriomegaly. In aortic *ectasia,* the diameter is increased by less than 1.5 times the normal, expected diameter. *Arteriomegaly* refers to a diffuse (nonfocal) enlargement of several arterial segments with increases in diameter greater than 50% of the normal expected diameter. Arterial segments in patients with arteriomegaly may be considered aneurysmal if the diameter of a segment is increased by more than 50% of the diameter of an adjacent segment.

AAAs are classified primarily according to how far they extend cephalad (**Fig. 91.1**).[2] More than 85% of all AAAs are classified as infrarenal. These aneurysms are located sufficiently below the renal arteries such that there is adequate healthy aorta for an infrarenal cross-clamp position. Juxtarenal aneurysms refer to those that encroach upon the origin of the renal arteries such that a suprarenal cross-clamp position is necessary with a planned infrarenal proximal anastomosis. Suprarenal AAAs extend above the renal orifices to the level of the superior mesenteric artery and typically require a supraceliac cross-clamp position. Aneurysms involving the thoracic and abdominal aorta are designated as thoracoabdominal aortic aneurysms and are classified according to how far they extend both cephalad and caudal (extent 1 through 5). Aneurysms that extend above the renal arteries complicate both endovascular and open repair and are associated with greater morbidity.

Concomitant iliac artery aneurysms are present in approximately 10% to 20% of all AAAs.[3] Iliac artery involvement, which usually affects the common and internal iliac vessels but preserves the external iliac, may complicate both open and endovascular aneurysm repair (EVAR).

MAGNITUDE OF THE PROBLEM

AAAs are common in developed countries. The incidence of AAAs in the United States ranges from 1.5% in autopsy series to 3.2% among unselected adult patients screened with ultrasonography.[4] Predictably, the incidence increases among patients with risk factors for AAAs and approaches 50% in patients with either femoral or popliteal artery aneurysms.[4] Interestingly, the incidence of AAAs increased through the end of the 20th century, then plateaued, and has even started to decline more recently. These changes may be reflective of smoking trends in the United States. A total of 9928 deaths were caused by AAAs and/or dissections during 2017, and

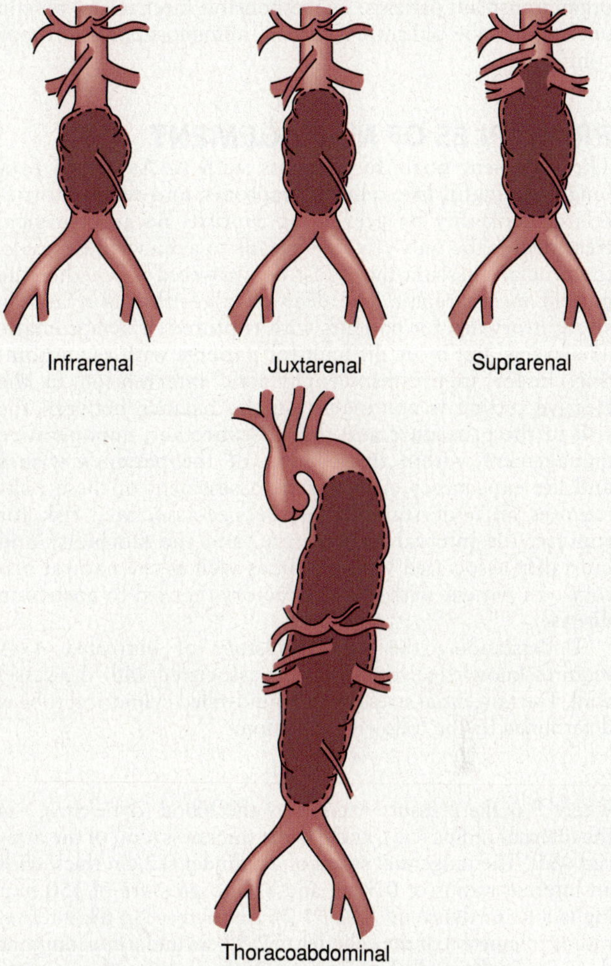

Figure 91.1. Classification of abdominal aortic aneurysms. More than 85% of all abdominal aortic aneurysms are infrarenal. Juxtarenal aneurysms extend to the level of the renal arteries, and suprarenal aneurysms to the level of the superior mesenteric. Aneurysms extending above the superior mesenteric artery and above are designated as thoracoabdominal aneurysms and are classified (Crawford extent I–V) according to how far they extend cephalad and caudal.

this corresponded to death rate of 3/100,000 as reported by the Centers for Disease Control and Prevention.[5] These numbers may be an underestimate due to sudden deaths in the elderly, which may be secondary to undiagnosed ruptured aneurysms.

PATHOGENESIS AND RISK FACTORS

The pathogenesis of AAAs remains unresolved, although it is an intense area of investigation. Multiple etiologic factors have been implicated, including atherosclerosis, hemodynamics, collagen, collagenase, elastin, elastase, metalloproteinases, protease inhibitors, apoptosis, neutrophils, and inflammatory mediators.[6–8] The etiology is likely multifactorial with interaction between both environmental and genetic factors. Unfortunately, investigation into both AAA pathogenesis and potential therapeutics has been complicated by an absence of suitable animal models.

2 Multiple risk factors have been identified for the development of AAAs, including age, sex, race, smoking, hypertension, hyperlipidemia, peripheral vascular disease, myocardial infarction, and family history. Identification of these risk factors is important for screening high-risk patients. AAAs typically affect the elderly and are rare among persons less than 50 years of age. Indeed, the mean age among patients undergoing repair across the country was 75.5 years in a Medicare population study.[9] A meta-analysis of the population-based screening studies for AAAs reported that male sex had the strongest association (odds ratio, 5.69).[10] The death rate from AAAs for men of 60 to 64 years of age is 11-fold higher than that for women of the same age, but it is only threefold higher for men between 85 and 90. Furthermore, men account for approximately 80% of all AAA repairs performed nationally.[9] The Aneurysm Detection and Management Veterans Affairs Cooperative Study Group (ADAM) reported that smoking was the strongest modifiable risk factor associated with AAAs >4 cm (odds ratio, 5.57) among the 73,451 veterans screened.[11] Darling et al.[12] prospectively analyzed patients undergoing repair of AAAs and reported that 15.1% had a first-degree relative with an aneurysm, in contrast to only 1.8% in the control group. Interestingly, the presence of a female family member with an aneurysm correlated with an increased risk for rupture. It is notable that the risk factors for AAA are similar to those associated with the development of atherosclerosis, except for diabetes mellitus. Furthermore, atherosclerotic changes are found almost universally within degenerative aneurysms at the time of repair, suggesting that the two disease processes are likely related, but it is unclear how.

The presence of an aneurysm in the aorta, iliac, femoral, or popliteal arteries increases the risk for a new or additional AAA. The incidence of aortoiliac aneurysms in patients with concomitant popliteal or femoral artery aneurysms is approximately 50%.[4] Therefore, all patients found to have a peripheral artery aneurysm should undergo a computed tomography (CT) scan of the chest, abdomen, and pelvis to exclude a synchronous aneurysm. In contrast, less than 15% of patients with AAA have a concomitant popliteal artery aneurysm and thus evaluation with proper physical examination and/or ultrasonography is typically adequate.

The incidence of AAAs is increased among patients with an aortic dissection. Despite appropriate medical therapy, 20% to 40% of type B aortic dissections (TBAD) patients develop false lumen degeneration with aneurysm formation, and up to ~45% eventually undergo aortic-related intervention.[13]

Interestingly, the prevalence of AAAs and the rate of expansion are both increased among heart and abdominal organ transplant patients. The responsible mechanisms remain unclear, but the obligatory chronic immunosuppression may contribute.

PRINCIPLES OF MANAGEMENT

The treatment goals for patients with AAAs are to prolong meaningful life, relieve symptoms, and reduce aortic-related mortality by preventing rupture. Because surgical treatment is the only effective means to achieve these goals, the crucial question that must be answered is whether the patient merits repair. The decision algorithm is relatively straightforward for patients with ruptured or symptomatic aneurysms, but more difficult for patients with asymptomatic, intact aneurysms. Prophylactic intervention in the elective setting is contingent on the balance between the risk of the procedure and that of expectant, nonoperative management within the context of the patient's wishes and life expectancy. Appropriate assessment of these risks requires an understanding of the size-associated risk for rupture, the interval growth rate, and the morbidity and mortality associated with repair, as well as the natural history of a patient with the risk factors that led to aneurysm disease.

Understanding the natural history of untreated AAA requires knowledge of the physics associated with the vessel wall. The tangential stress (t) of a fluid-filled cylindrical tube is determined by the following equation:

$$t = Pr/d$$

where P is the pressure exerted by the blood (dyne/cm^2), r is the internal radius (cm), and d is the thickness (cm) of the arterial wall. The tangential stress of a cylinder 0.2 cm thick with an internal radius of 0.8 cm and a fluid pressure of 150 mm Hg is 8×10^5 dyne/cm^2 (**Fig. 91.2**). An increase in the internal radius (diameter) of the cylinder to 2.94 cm and a concomitant decrease in the wall thickness, as might occur with an aneurysm, would increase the tangential stress to 98×10^5 dyne/cm^2. Thus, a threefold increase in diameter would result in a 12-fold increase in the tangential stress. Aneurysms rupture when the tangential stress exceeds the tensile strength of the vessel wall. It should be emphasized that the tangential stress varies directly with the radius of the cylinder (vessel), but is independent of its length.

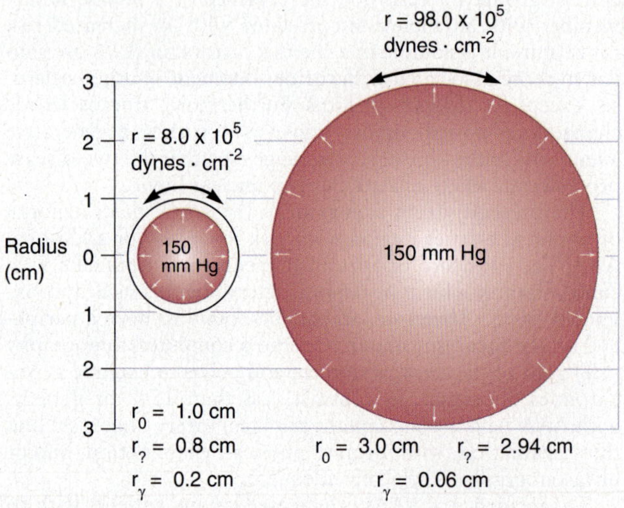

Figure 91.2. Cross-sectional view of a 2-cm-diameter cylinder that expands to a diameter of 6 cm while wall cross-sectional area remains constant. t, wall stress; d, wall thickness; r_i, inside radius; r_0, outside radius. Expansion of a 1-cm-diameter cylinder to a diameter of 3 cm with no change in wall cross-sectional area increases wall tensile stress 12-fold.

Table 91.1. Estimated Annual Rupture Risk

AAA Diameter (cm)	Rupture Risk (%/y)
<4	0
4–5	0.5–5
5–6	3–15
6–7	10–20
7–8	20–40
>8	30–50

Reproduced with permission from Brewster DC, Cronenwett JL, Hallett JW Jr, et al. Guidelines for the treatment of abdominal aortic aneurysms. Report of a subcommittee of the Joint Council of the American Association for Vascular Surgery and Society for Vascular Surgery? *J Vasc Surg.* 2003;37:1106–1117.

3 The diameter of an AAA is the greatest predictor of rupture as estimated by the tangential stress of the vessel wall. The diameter of an aneurysm is determined by measuring its greatest diameter from outer wall to outer wall, preferably using an orthogonal image, throughout the extent of the aneurysm. Orthogonal refers to a cross-sectional measurement perpendicular to the long axis, along the centerline of flow, to avoid overestimation due to tortuosity of the aorta. The collective annual rupture risks per aneurysm diameter are shown (**Table 91.1**).[14] Although there is some variability in the data, it is agreed upon that the rupture risk for aneurysms less than 5 cm in diameter is very small, but increases considerably for those greater than 5.5 cm in men and 5 cm in women. Notably, both the ADAM[11] and UK Small Aneurysm Trial[15] that randomized patients with small aneurysms (4 to 5.5 cm) to open repair or surveillance reported that the rupture risk for surveillance was ≤1%/y.

A variety of other factors have also been reported to increase the risk of aneurysm rupture, including female gender, chronic obstructive pulmonary disease (COPD), smoking, hypertension, family history, and wall stress.[15] The impact of the aneurysm growth rate on rupture risk remains unclear and has been difficult to separate from aneurysm diameter alone. However, an aneurysm expansion of ≥1 cm/y is generally considered worrisome.

4 The natural history of AAAs is to grow in diameter over time. The reported mean rate of growth has varied from 0.2 to 0.4 cm/y.[16] The rate of growth can be impacted by several factors, including female gender, current smoking, and larger original diameter. Interestingly, coenzyme A reductase inhibitors (ie, statins) may inhibit growth of small AAAs.[17] The growth curve may be somewhat erratic or "staccato" with no growth detected during consecutive 6-month intervals, followed by a period of growth, hence the need for persistent surveillance.

The mortality rate associated with repair of an AAA depends on the status of the aneurysm (intact/asymptomatic, intact/symptomatic, ruptured), the physiologic state of the patient (age and medical comorbidities), and the method of repair (open vs endovascular). Population studies from Medicare and the Nationwide Inpatient Sample (NIS) have reported that operative mortality rates for *open repair of intact* aneurysms in the United States range from 4.2% to 5.4%.[18] Predictably, the operative mortality rate increases with age, ranging from 2.2% among persons of 50 to 59 years of age to 9.2% among those >80. Interestingly, operative mortality rate has been shown to be significantly higher among women (6.1% vs 3.7%). The mortality rate for open repair in the randomized trials (UK Small Aneurysm Trial—5.8%, ADAM— 2.7%, DREAM—4.6%, EVAR Trial—4.6%)[11,15,19,20] are within the range of nationwide series.

The operative mortality rate for *endovascular repair of intact* AAAs has been consistently lower than an open approach. Schermerhorn et al. reported that the operative mortality after EVAR was 1.2% among Medicare beneficiaries during 2001 to 2004, while mortality within the NIS through 2005 was 1.3%.[21] Results from the Dutch Randomized Endovascular Aneurysm Management (DREAM) Trial[19] and the Endovascular Aneurysm (EVAR) Trial[20] comparing open and endovascular repair have reported that the perioperative mortality rate is lower for endovascular repair and within the same range (DREAM—1.2% vs 4.6%; EVAR Trial—1.7% vs 4.7%).

The operative mortality rate for *open repair of intact/symptomatic* aneurysms among patients undergoing emergent repair exceeds that for elective repair and has ranged from 9% to 19%.[4] However, in more recent data, De Martino et al.[22] reported from the Vascular Study Group of Northern New England a perioperative mortality of 2.1% and 0% for open and endovascular repair for intact/symptomatic aneurysms, respectively. However, late mortality and in-hospital adverse events were still higher compared to the asymptomatic cohort. Various explanations have been proposed for this increased mortality rate relative to that for intact/asymptomatic aneurysms, including failure to maximize preoperative medical conditions and increased incidence of inadvertent venous injuries. Presumably, surgeon experience would lend itself to improved outcomes in nonelective cases; however, Arnaoutakis et al. showed that more experienced surgeons had similar major complication rates as well as 1-year survival compared to early career surgeons with respect to nonelective open AAA repair.[23]

The actual mortality rate for ruptured AAAs is somewhat difficult to determine because a significant number of sudden deaths in elderly patients are likely secondary to ruptured aortic aneurysms. It has been estimated that 50% of all patients with ruptured AAAs die outside the hospital.[4] For those patients who do make it to the hospital, a meta-analysis spanning 50 years reported that the operative mortality rate for the *open repair of ruptured* aneurysms was 48%.[24] These figures correspond to an overall mortality rate of approximately 80% although this may be an underestimate. It is remarkable that the optimization of prehospital and emergency room care, including a reduction in the mean transfer time from the emergency department to the operating room, has not resulted in improved mortality outcomes.

The mortality rate for the *endovascular repair of ruptured* AAAs is lower than the open approach, although data may be significantly skewed by selection bias. Multiple meta-analyses have reported a perioperative mortality rate of 24% to 27% with improved overall outcomes compared to open repair.[25] The potential to treat ruptured AAAs with the endovascular approach may represent the greatest contribution or benefit of the technology.

CLINICAL PRESENTATION AND DIAGNOSIS

The overwhelming majority of AAAs are asymptomatic at the time of discovery. Most aneurysms are detected by abdominal or pelvic imaging studies, such as ultrasonography and CT, performed for other indications (eg, chronic back pain, renal cysts) rather than on physical examination. It is difficult to palpate an AAA on physical examination because of its anatomic location in the posterior abdomen, in conjunction with the national obesity epidemic. A literature review examining the accuracy of physical examination reported that the sensitivity ranged from 33% to 100%, the specificity ranged from 75% to 100%, and the positive predictive value ranged from 14% to 100%.[26] Intact abdominal aortic and iliac artery aneurysms may present with symptoms that lead to further investigation and the correct diagnosis, although this is the exception rather than the rule. Rarely, enlargement of the aneurysm may cause vertebral erosion and chronic back pain. In addition, thrombosis of an AAA may cause acute ischemia in the lower torso, and aneurysms may be a source of arterial macroemboli or microemboli leading to acute ischemia of a lower extremity or digit, respectively.

Patients with intact/symptomatic or ruptured aneurysms present with abdominal or back pain related to the aneurysm itself. The pain, which ranges from dull to sharp, is usually acute in onset and persistent. It may be superimposed on more chronic abdominal or back pain, but the presentation is usually not subtle. In addition, the pain may radiate from the abdomen to the back, flank, inguinal region, or genitalia. Approximately 10% of patients with ruptured AAAs present with signs and symptoms similar to those of ureteral colic or other acute urologic problems.

Patients with a ruptured AAA may present anywhere along the spectrum from hemodynamically stable to profound shock. Their status depends on the ability of the adjacent tissues to tamponade the bleeding. If the rupture is contained, the patient may present hemodynamically stable. However, it should be emphasized that this is usually temporary, and health care providers should not be lulled into a false sense of security. A ruptured AAA is a true medical emergency that requires immediate operative repair regardless of the patient's hemodynamic status. Furthermore, vital signs may be misleading because patients can lose up to 15% of their blood volume without any appreciable change in their pulse rate or blood pressure. If the aneurysm initially ruptures freely into the peritoneal space, patients usually exsanguinate before they can seek medical attention.

Patients with a ruptured AAA may also present with either an aortoenteric or an aortocaval fistula, although both are relatively rare. Patients with an aortoenteric fistula may present with massive intestinal bleeding that usually occurs after a "sentinel" bleed that is small in volume. The majority of aortoenteric fistulae result from the erosion of a prosthetic graft into the adjacent bowel (secondary aortoenteric fistula) rather than from an unrepaired aneurysm (primary aortoenteric fistula). The diagnosis of an aortoenteric fistula must be ruled out in all patients with gastrointestinal bleeding who have either an AAA or a previous infrarenal aortic repair. Patients with an aortocaval fistula generally present with high-output congestive heart failure, a continuous abdominal bruit, and edema of the lower extremities.

Several imaging studies are available to establish or confirm the diagnosis of an AAA. Indeed, the introduction of endovascular techniques for aneurysm repair has resulted in an evolution of these modalities. The generic imaging goals for patients with an AAA are to establish the diagnosis and determine the presence of rupture, the cephalad/caudal extent of the aneurysm, the feasibility of endovascular repair, the presence of other visceral pathology or anatomic variants that would complicate operative repair, such as a left-sided vena cava and/or a horseshoe kidney. Although no imaging study satisfies every objective, ultrasound has emerged as the ideal *screening* study, with CT arteriography being the definitive *diagnostic* study and the preferred modality for operative planning.

Abdominal ultrasound is a safe, simple, and readily available method of detecting AAAs (**Fig. 91.3**). It is relatively inexpensive and does not require the use of ionizing radiation or intravenous contrast. The sensitivity of ultrasound for detecting AAAs is acceptable, and the technique is reproducible within 0.3 cm in experienced hands.[27] However, the technique is quite operator dependent and potentially confounded by the presence of bowel gas or extreme obesity. Ultrasound can accurately image the infrarenal aorta to its bifurcation, but is less reliable for imaging the suprarenal aorta and distal to the common iliac vessels. It is a useful technique to follow patients with small aneurysms (<4 cm) when the exact measurement is not crucial.

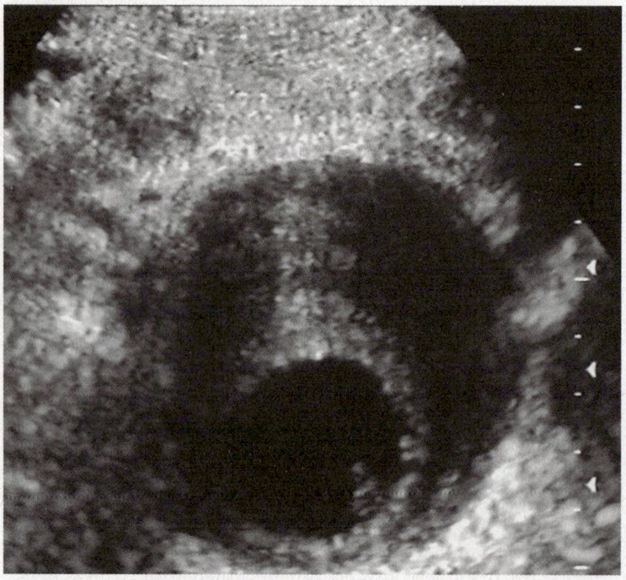

Figure 91.3. B-mode ultrasound image showing a transverse view of an infrarenal abdominal aortic aneurysm. Note the vessel wall and the large quantity of intraluminal clot surrounding the smaller, blood-filled center (*dark circle*).

5 CT arteriography overcomes many of the limitations of ultrasound and represents the current "gold standard" for imaging patients with AAAs (**Fig. 91.4**). The downside of CT is the greater expense and the potential side effects from ionizing radiation and intravenous contrast. Indeed, the evolution of EVAR and the necessary imaging follow-up have focused increased attention on the magnitude of long-term radiation injury. It is worth noting that the radiation dose associated with an abdominopelvic CT scan is 10 to 20 mGy, while that for a routine chest radiograph is only 0.5 mGy. The incidence of allergic reactions to the contrast may be reduced by a steroid preparation, while concerns regarding intravenous contrast-induced nephropathy remain debatable. Of course, the renal risks can be avoided altogether by not using contrast. However, the quality of the noncontrast images is generally not useful for determining eligibility for endovascular repair. CT is very sensitive for detecting both intact and ruptured aneurysms, and the images are reproducible within 0.2 cm. The quality of the CT images has continued to improve with each new generation of scanners, and the image acquisition times have decreased. Given the quality and ease of imaging,

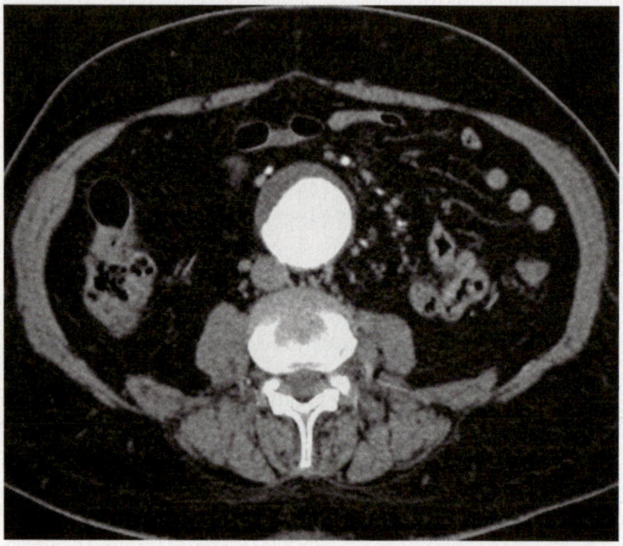

Figure 91.4. CT scan demonstrates a large abdominal aortic aneurysm. Note that the majority of the lumen is filled with contrast.

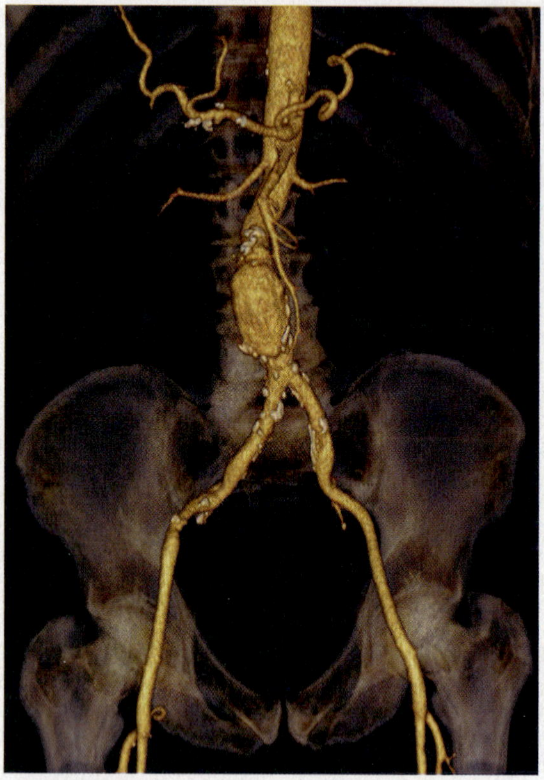

Figure 91.5. 3D CT of the aorta and the iliac, femoral, and visceral arteries is shown. Note the infrarenal abdominal aortic aneurysm that extends to the aortic bifurcation.

CT arteriograms have essentially replaced traditional catheter-based diagnostic arteriograms for evaluation of aneurysms. Using axial CT images and 3D imaging software, a 3D image of the aorta can be obtained that allows measurements along the centerline of blood flow (**Fig. 91.5**), and dramatically improves the accuracy and consistency of sizing for EVAR.[28] CT is also helpful for detecting other intra-abdominal pathology or anatomic variants that may impact the operative approach. Specific concerns include the location of the left renal vein and other associated venous anomalies, the location and size of the kidneys, and the characteristics of the aneurysm wall. In addition, CT is the serial imaging study of choice when aneurysms exceed 4 cm and approach the threshold for intervention.

Both magnetic resonance imaging (MRI) and catheter-based arteriography have been used as diagnostic imaging studies for patients with AAAs. The image quality and overall sensitivity of MRI are comparable to CT, but the technology is not as widely available, and most surgeons are less familiar with interpreting the images. Furthermore, the technique is relatively contraindicated for patients with ferromagnetic devices (eg, pacemakers, joints) or renal insufficiency. Imaging of critically ill patients is also cumbersome, if not prohibitive.

Importantly, aneurysms are frequently diagnosed during catheter-based arteriography performed for other purposes, but this should not be viewed as a diagnostic test of choice for AAAs. An arteriogram only delineates the lumen of the vessels (ie, aorta, iliac, and femoral arteries), and thus gives no indication of aneurysm extent or diameter. AAAs are often filled with laminated thrombus and may have a relatively normal appearing lumen.

The diagnostic approach and initial treatment for patients with a potential ruptured aneurysm merit further comment. Because of the high attendant mortality rate, prompt diagnosis and repair are necessary. In a study from the Cleveland Clinic Vascular Registry, the operative mortality rate associated with ruptured AAAs increased from 35% when the initial diagnosis was correct to 75% when incorrect.[29] A natural history study

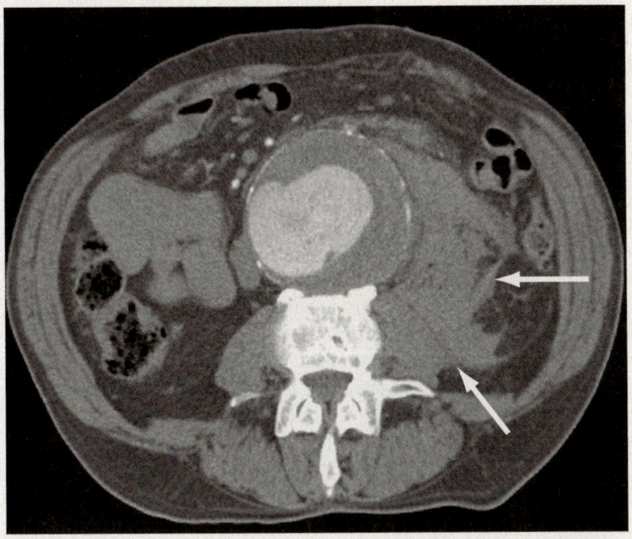

Figure 91.6. Contrast CT demonstrates a ruptured abdominal aortic aneurysm. Note the large retroperitoneal hematoma and the loss of the normal fat plane anterior and lateral to the left psoas muscle.

of patients with ruptured AAAs not offered operative repair reported that <15% of the patients died within 2 hours of hospital admission.[30] Based upon these findings, the authors concluded that most patients with ruptured aneurysms are sufficiently stable to undergo a CT scan, and this opinion has been supported by improved mortality results of EVAR for ruptured aneurysms.

Several findings on CT are suggestive of a ruptured AAA including disruption of the calcium ring within the aortic wall, disruption of the aortic margins, retroperitoneal hematoma, mass lesions in the psoas region, displacement of the kidneys, abnormal soft tissues posterior to the aorta, effacement of the normal fat planes between the aorta and adjacent viscera, and abnormal retroperitoneal fluid collections (**Fig. 91.6**). Patients undergoing an emergent CT arteriogram to rule out a ruptured AAA should not receive oral contrast because of the delay associated with its administration and the confounding effects on the imaging of the vessels, especially if proceeding with an endovascular repair in short order.

The diagnosis of a ruptured AAA should be considered in elderly patients who present to the emergency room hemodynamically *stable* with abdominal or back pain. Admittedly, the differential diagnosis for abdominal or back pain in this patient population is extensive, and the incidence of a ruptured AAA is small. An expeditious history and physical examination can usually determine the cause of the pain. A pulsatile abdominal aortic mass, an unexplained low hematocrit, or hemodynamic instability before presentation are particularly worrisome and increase the level of suspicion. If ultrasound confirms the diagnosis of an aneurysm, further evaluation with CT should be obtained to rule out rupture. Alternatively, a CT may be obtained as the sole imaging study. CT findings consistent with a ruptured aneurysm mandate preparation of the operating room for immediate repair. Aggressive fluid resuscitation should be avoided and mild hypotension (ie, systolic pressure >80 mm Hg) tolerated in conscious patients due to the theoretical potential to cause the aneurysm to rupture into the peritoneal cavity and/or release the tamponade effect of the retroperitoneal tissue. If an intact aneurysm is found on CT without any suggestion of rupture, the next logical question is whether the aneurysm is the source of the pain. Symptomatic aneurysms are likely associated with an increased risk of rupture, although the natural history remains poorly defined. Patients with symptomatic/intact aneurysms ≥5 cm in diameter should be admitted to a monitored setting and scheduled for urgent operative repair, provided no alternative causes for the pain are identified. Additional sources of abdominal pain should be sought in patients with aneurysms smaller than 4 cm in light of the small rupture risk. The appropriate treatment for patients with aneurysms 4 to 5 cm is less clear. These aneurysms have the potential to rupture, although the risk is very small. It is recommended that these patients be admitted and the source of their pain further investigated.

The role of screening for AAAs in asymptomatic patients is somewhat controversial, given that screening in select populations has been shown to decrease aneurysm-related mortality yet increase the number of invasive procedures, exposing patients to additional risks.[27] The United States Preventative Task Force has issued a position statement based on evidence from 17 randomized controlled trials advocating a single screening ultrasound in males 65 to 75 years of age who have a smoking history and selective screening for males without smoking history.[27] The Task Force did not recommend screening for women who have never smoked and have no family history of AAA. The literature was insufficient to make a recommendation for women aged 65 to 75 years who have smoked or have a family history of AAA. The American Heart Association and American College of Cardiology do not recommend screening in women[31]; however, the Society for Vascular Surgery advocates for screening in women older than 65 years who have a tobacco history or family history of AAA.[2] Medicare currently pays for a single screening ultrasound as part of the Welcome to Medicare physical examination for men who have smoked sometime during their life and for both men and women with a family history of AAAs.

OPERATIVE INDICATIONS

All patients with symptomatic or ruptured AAAs should undergo operative repair unless they have an underlying medical condition that precludes long-term survival or their current or potential future quality of life is not sufficient to justify the intervention. The latter situation entails a difficult decision, but not offering operative repair should be considered in certain cases (eg, a debilitated, demented patient in a nursing home or a patient with advanced renal failure yet no willingness to progress to dialysis) after discussion with the patient and/or family.

6 The operative decision-making process for intact/asymptomatic AAAs is a complex one that needs to be tailored to the individual patient. Indeed, there is no single parameter that merits repair. The operative indications are contingent upon the size of the aneurysm, life expectancy, comorbidities, preference, and anatomic configuration. It is important to remember that the repair of an intact/asymptomatic AAA is a prophylactic operation that represents a balance between the operative risk and the future risk of rupture, with the ultimate treatment goals to prolong life, relieve symptoms, and prevent rupture.

7 The diameter of the AAA is the best predictor of rupture, as stated in the previous section, and has been used as the most common indication for repair. The Joint Council of the American Association for Vascular Surgery and the Society for Vascular Surgery have released updated guidelines for the treatment of patients with AAAs.[2] An appropriate threshold for repair in the "average patient" with an intact infrarenal aneurysm is 5.5 cm, but the decision must be tailored to the individual. Rapid aneurysm expansion (>1 cm/y), symptoms related to the aneurysm, and female gender merit repair at a smaller diameter, while consideration should be given to earlier repair in young patients, provided that the operative mortality rate is acceptable. Finally, a larger diameter threshold is appropriate in higher-risk patients, and there does not appear to be any justification to alter the operative threshold for an endovascular approach.

There is some controversy regarding the management of patients with aneurysms that are 4 to 5.5 cm. Both the UK Small Aneurysm Trial[15] and the ADAM Trial[11] concluded that it was safe to follow patients with 4- to 5.5-cm aneurysms and that early operation did not confer any long-term survival benefit. As noted in the previous section, the rupture risk for patients in the surveillance group was <1%/y. It is important to note that more than 60% of the patients in both studies ultimately underwent operative repair despite their initial randomization. A longer-term follow-up study from the UK Small Aneurysm Trial extending to 12 years did not demonstrate a survival benefit for the patients assigned to early surgery.[32] However, it is important to note that almost all of the patients who survived ultimately required repair since their aneurysms eventually exceeded the 5.5-cm threshold. Indeed, the relevant question may not be whether patients with small aneurysm need to be repaired, but rather when they need to be repaired. The proponents of smaller diameter-based thresholds for repair (ie, <5.5 cm) have justified their approach stating that even small aneurysms rupture, aneurysms continue to increase in diameter and will likely need to be repaired, the patients' medical conditions will likely deteriorate with age, and the operative mortality/morbidity rate for small aneurysms may be less. In addition, the significant decrease in the perioperative mortality rate after EVAR has also challenged the threshold diameter for operative repair. However, Finlayson et al.[33] used a decision analysis model to determine the optimal diameter for open and EVAR and concluded that the endovascular approach lowers the operative threshold only for older patients in poor health. Although the level 1 evidence does not support this lower threshold, it is important to note that the size discrepancy between a 5.3-cm and a 5.5-cm aneurysm is very small and likely within the resolution of the imaging study.

Multiple preoperative characteristics, namely renal insufficiency (creatinine >1.8 mg/dL), congestive heart failure, ECG ischemia, pulmonary dysfunction, older age, and female gender, can impact the perioperative mortality rate and threshold for repair. Beck et al.[34] developed a predictive model for both open and endovascular repair using a prospective registry from the Vascular Study Group of New England. They reported that COPD, suprarenal aortic clamp, renal insufficiency, and advanced age (≥70) were predictive of mortality at 1 year after open repair, with the mortality ranging from 1% to 67% depending upon the number of risk factors. Congestive heart failure and larger aneurysm diameter (≥6.5 cm) were the only predictive factors after endovascular repair with the mortality ranging from 4% to 23%. The consistent, dramatic impact of renal insufficiency was further emphasized by a national series that reported a ninefold increase in mortality. Life expectancy is inseparable from comorbidities, but it should be noted that the average life expectancy for a 60-year-old and an 85-year-old man in the United States is 18 and 5 years, respectively.

The anatomic configuration of the aneurysm and/or the associated structures should factor into the operative decision process as well. Any technical factors that complicate the repair likely increase the perioperative mortality/morbidity, including the need for suprarenal clamp application with subsequent renal/visceral ischemia, venous anomalies (eg, left-sided vena cava), renal anomalies (eg, horseshoe kidney), and inflammatory aneurysms. Admittedly, many of these technical concerns are relevant only to the open approach and can be overcome/avoided by endovascular repair, provided that it is anatomically feasible.

Patients who do not meet the threshold for operative repair should be followed closely. It is important to educate the patients about their underlying disease process and emphasize the importance of long-term follow-up, as up to one-third may be noncompliant with follow-up. Furthermore, it is important to counsel patients about associated symptoms so medical attention can be solicited, if needed. Guidelines indicate that patients with aneurysms <3 cm in diameter should be reimaged at 5 years, while those between 3 and 3.4 cm should be reimaged at 3 years, and those between 3.5 and 4.4 cm should be reimaged at 1 year. Aneurysms >4.5 cm should be reimaged every 6 months. The patients who are not candidates for elective repair should not be offered emergent repair if their aneurysm ruptures or becomes symptomatic, and must be counseled on this matter preemptively.

CHOICE OF OPEN OR ENDOVASCULAR REPAIR

After the decision to recommend operative repair has been made, the technique for repair needs to be determined. Admittedly, these decisions are somewhat interrelated since the decision to recommend operative repair in certain subsets of patients is oftentimes contingent upon whether they are candidates for an endovascular approach. It has been clearly demonstrated that the technical success rates for endovascular graft repair are excellent, and the need for intraoperative conversion to open repair is negligible. The perioperative events and long-term outcomes have been defined by level-1 evidence. Many of the technical limitations inherent to the earlier endovascular devices and anatomic limitations have been overcome. Despite a lack of long-term overall survival advantage compared to open repair, the endovascular approach for treatment of AAAs
8 has been widely applied. Indeed, the endovascular approach eclipsed open repair in the United States in 2005, and data show that more than 75% of aneurysms are repaired in this manner.[35] The choice of open or endovascular repair is complicated and contingent upon several factors, including feasibility, outcome, comorbidities, compliance, cost, and preference. It is imperative that these issues, including their respective advantages/disadvantages, be addressed with patients preoperatively to ensure proper informed consent.

Anatomic configuration of the aorta, the aneurysm, and the access vessels is the initial determinant for operative approach. Commercially available endovascular devices come in a finite range of sizes and, thus, are suitable only if specific anatomic conditions are satisfied. Although the number of available devices and their specific characteristics are constantly evolving, the endograft consists of a fabric graft (ie, polyester or ePTFE) and a metallic endo/exoskeleton (ie, stainless steel or nitinol) that facilitates proximal/distal fixation by the radial force of the stent (**Fig. 91.7**). In some devices, proximal fixation is augmented by the presence of suprarenal hooks. The devices are modular and consist of either two (main body and contralateral iliac limb) or three (main body, contralateral iliac limb, ipsilateral iliac limb) components with a variety of additional ancillary pieces that allow proximal or distal extensions at the aortic and iliac ends, respectively. The current strategy is to seat the proximal component of the bifurcated system as close to the lowest renal artery as possible and the distal components as close to the iliac bifurcation as possible to decrease the potential for future loss of seal/fixation.

Although there is some variability among the commercially available devices, their general anatomic requirements are somewhat similar. The infrarenal abdominal aorta must have a suitable, nonaneurysmal landing zone for the endograft that measures ≥10 to 15 mm in length and ≥17 mm but ≤32 mm in diameter (ranges reflect differences between the commercial devices). Furthermore, the proximal neck angle should be ≤60 degrees for most devices (≤75 to 90 degrees for some newer devices), as measured by the intersection of the centerline of the infrarenal aorta at the landing zone site and the centerline of the aneurysm through the aortic bifurcation. Newer devices do allow for more neck angulation, but the operating surgeon should keep in mind that more infrarenal neck may be required in more severely angulated necks to allow for durable seal and fixation of the device. The infrarenal neck should be relatively free of thrombus and calcification to facilitate a seal at the implantation site. In general, a longer infrarenal neck length equates to longer device seal zone and improved durability. The iliac artery should have a suitable landing zone ≥20 mm with an associated diameter between 7 and 20 mm to facilitate both anchoring the graft and passing the main device into the aorta. The distal landing zone for the iliac limbs is usually in the common

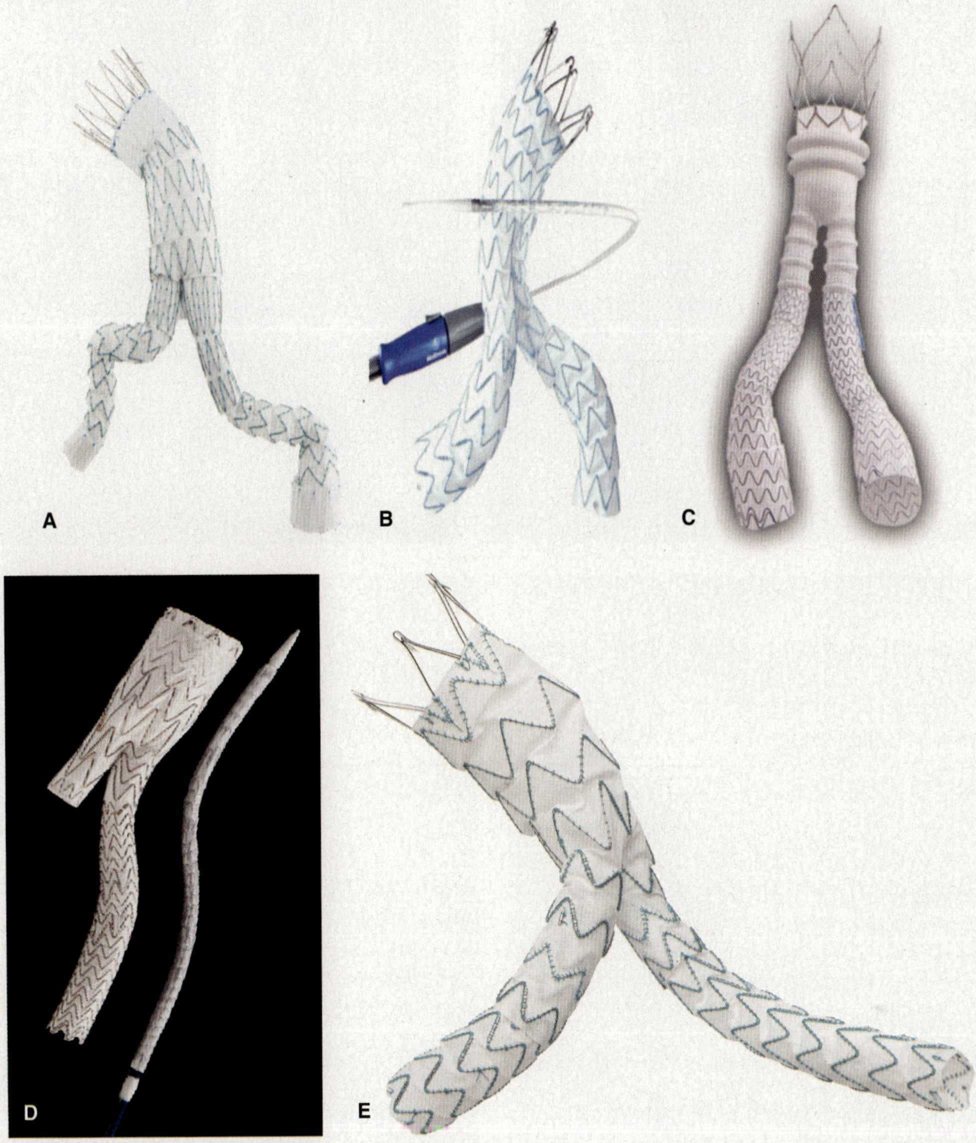

Figure 91.7. Examples of current commercially available infrarenal endografts in the United States are shown: Cook Zenith (**A**, [Courtesy of Cook Medical]); Medtronic Endurant (**B**, [Courtesy of Medtronic]); Endologix ALTO (**C**, [© 2025 Endologix LLC. All rights reserved]); Gore Excluder (**D**, [Copyright 2025 W. L. Gore & Associates, Inc.]); Terumo TREO (**E**, [Reprinted with permission of Bolton Medical, Inc. dba Terumo Aortic.]). These are modular devices consisting of a main body, iliac limbs/extensions, and main body extensions. Note the common theme of bilateral iliac limbs and a main body. There are many differences between these endografts, which make them each uniquely suited for some patients. Some devices (**A,B,C,E**) utilize a bare suprarenal stent construct to facilitate proximal fixation. Other devices do not have a suprarenal stent component but rather utilize active fixation with hooks (**D**).

iliac artery, although the anatomic constraints with regard to the size of the access vessels and the introduction of the devices are relevant for both the common and external iliac vessels.

A variety of techniques have been described to overcome the anatomic limitations of EVAR, thereby extending its feasibility. Unfortunately, extending the indications for EVAR beyond those recommended by the manufacturers' instructions for use (IFU) has been associated with an increase in the incidence of adverse events and a higher need for reintervention.[36] For those with short (≥4 mm) infrarenal necks, fenestrated endografts have been commercially available since 2012 with excellent long-term results.[37] Details regarding this technique/device are discussed later in the juxtarenal section of this chapter. Endoanchor systems have been employed in those with short necks (≥4 mm and <10 mm), although long-term data using this technique are lacking. Stenosis within the access vessels can be overcome by dilation (ie, balloon angioplasty, serial dilators) or by the use of an open prosthetic conduit or endovascular stent graft conduit. The open prosthetic conduit is usually anastomosed to the bifurcation of the common iliac artery and then tunneled through the retroperitoneal space below the inguinal ligament. Alternatively, an aorto-uni-iliac endograft can be configured and a femoral–femoral bypass performed.

Aneurysm degeneration of the common iliac artery can be overcome by a variety of techniques including simply using larger-diameter graft limbs, occluding/embolizing the internal iliac artery and seating the iliac limb in the external iliac artery, bypassing the internal iliac artery (and seating the iliac limb in the external iliac artery), or with an iliac branch endoprosthesis. Although relatively simple to perform, internal iliac artery embolization has been associated with a moderate incidence of complications, including buttock/thigh claudication (30% to 40%), sexual dysfunction, neurologic deficit/paraplegia, pelvic ischemia, and gluteal compartment syndrome. The claudication improves with time in the majority of patients, but it can be quite debilitating. Many of the other complications, although somewhat rare, can be catastrophic. Because of these concerns, concomitant bilateral internal iliac artery occlusion/embolization should be avoided when possible. Iliac branch

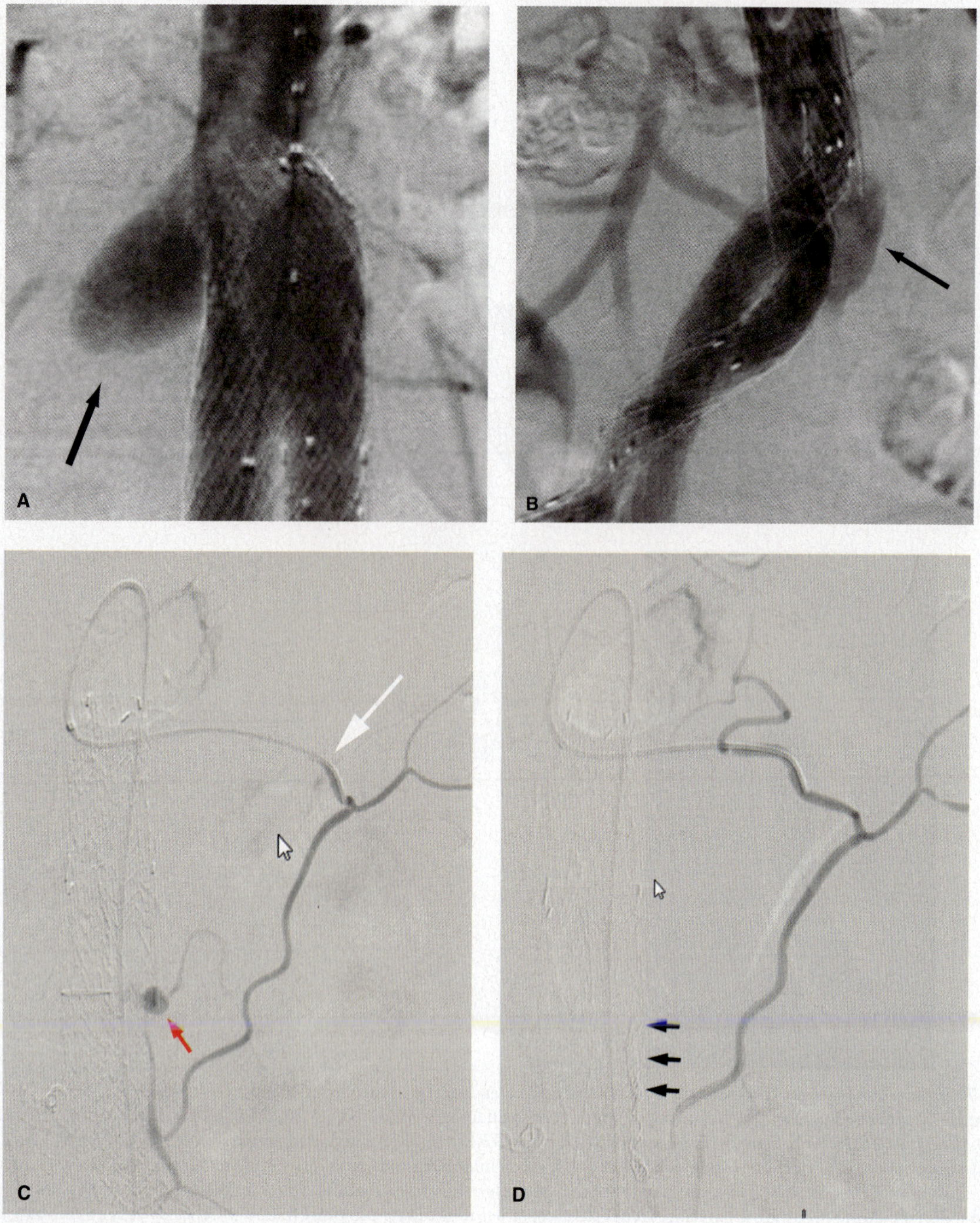

Figure 91.8. Type 1 to 4 Endoleaks. Type I and III represent the most dangerous forms of endoleaks, and represent what is essentially an unrepaired aneurysm. **A:** Type I leaks originate at either the proximal (Ia) or distal (Ib) attachment sites. Note the large blush of contrast outside of the graft lumen at the proximal fixation site, demonstrating a type Ia endoleak. **B:** Type 3 endoleaks are caused by fabric tears or problems at the graft interfaces of the modular devices. Note the contrast blush outside of the lumen of the graft at the modular interface. Type II endoleaks generally have a more benign natural history, but can cause aneurysmal growth and rupture. **C:** Demonstrates an inferior mesenteric arteriogram from a catheter (*white arrow*) in the meandering mesenteric artery. Filling of the aneurysm sac through a patent inferior mesenteric artery (*red arrow*) is evident. **D:** Demonstrates successful embolization of the IMA with coils demonstrated by *black arrows*. Note no further filling of the aneurysm sac.

endoprostheses have been commercially available since 2016 and have demonstrated excellent midterm outcomes in preserving internal iliac artery flow, yet providing aneurysm sac exclusion by extension into the external iliac artery.[38] Their main limitation remains somewhat stringent anatomic requirements for their application. Nonetheless, this device construct certainly improved the manner in which aneurysmal disease involving the common iliac artery is managed.

Consideration of the perioperative and long-term outcomes after EVAR requires introduction of the concepts of endoleak and endotension. Endoleak is the perfusion of the aneurysm sac outside the lumen of the endograft, while endotension is the persistent pressurization within the excluded aneurysm sac. Approximately 10% to 20% of patients develop an endoleak during the first year after endovascular repair, although most of these patients do not require remediation.[39] Endoleaks have been classified as types 1 through 4 based on the mechanism of the leak (**Fig. 91.8**). Type 1 leaks originate at either the proximal or distal attachment sites. Type 2 leaks come from aortic branch vessels, such as the lumbar or inferior mesenteric arteries. Type 3 leaks are caused by problems at the junction between modular graft components or fabric tears. Type 4 leaks are usually transient (<24 hours) transgraft extravasations that result from the porosity of the graft and needle holes. It should be emphasized that the entire concept of an endoleak is predicated on the ability to detect contrast or blood flow outside the lumen of the endograft and is, therefore, contingent on the sensitivity and specificity of the various imaging techniques. The major concern about both endoleaks and endotension is that the pressure transmitted to the aneurysm wall may cause the aneurysm to expand and/or rupture. The clinical significance of the various endoleak types is quite different. Both type 1 and 3 endoleaks impede treatment success, given their associated increased risk of rupture and merit reintervention.[40] Type 2 endoleaks are generally considered less worrisome in terms of their rupture risk, although they are associated with an increased risk for reintervention. They can generally be followed with serial imaging studies, but merit evaluation/intervention if the aneurysm sac continues to enlarge. Type 4 endoleaks are self-limited and benign. The clinical significance of endotension is likewise unresolved. Indeed, the concept itself is somewhat ambiguous, given the limitations of actually measuring the pressure within the aneurysm sac. It should be noted that freedom from endoleak does not necessarily mean freedom from endotension, given the observation that aneurysms can continue to enlarge in the absence of an identifiable endoleak.

Perioperative complication rates appear to be lower after endovascular repair compared to open repair. As noted in the previous section, the randomized, controlled DREAM and EVAR Trials reported a significant decrease in the perioperative mortality rate (DREAM—1.2% vs 4.6%; EVAR Trial—1.7% vs 4.7%).[19,20] The EVAR Trial also reported a trend toward a decrease in the combined operative mortality/*severe* complication rate (9.8% vs 4.7%, P = .10). Multiple clinical trials have reported that the overall major complication rates after both endovascular and open repair are approximately 15% although the magnitude of the complications is less for the endovascular approach and primarily includes vascular access complications (eg, hematoma, femoral artery injury). These clinical trials have likewise demonstrated that the total hospital length of stay, intensive care unit length of stay, operative blood loss, and time necessary to resume normal activities are all less for the endovascular approach.

The long-term results after the EVAR and DREAM Trials have failed to document any significant benefit for the endovascular approach in terms of almost every outcome measure analyzed.[41] In the DREAM Trial, there was no difference in all-cause mortality at 12 years (survival, open—42.2%, EVAR—38.5%).[42] More concerning, the EVAR Trial showed worse overall and aneurysm-related mortality beyond 8 years for those undergoing EVAR (overall mortality: EVAR—53% vs open—46%; aneurysm-related mortality: EVAR—5% vs open—1%).[43] These outcomes were presumably driven by secondary aneurysm rupture and increased cancer-related mortality in the EVAR group.

In the EVAR Trial, costs (EVAR—£13,257; open—£9926) were significantly greater for the endovascular approach, while there were negligible differences in the quality of life assessments.[44] However, the OVER Trial showed no difference in total health care costs between open and endovascular repair after 2 years.[45] The cost savings from a shorter length of stay and lower incidence of major perioperative complications with an endovascular approach are offset by the device costs. In fact, device costs reflect about 40% of hospitalization costs for those undergoing EVAR. It is important to note that most of the analyses have focused on the hospital and device-related costs, but have failed to include the associated professional fees and the costs associated with long-term follow-up and reintervention, all of which may be substantial.

These long-term results from the DREAM and EVAR Trials are somewhat sobering, as the endovascular approach is not as secure a repair as the traditional, open alternative. The endovascular repair is associated with ongoing rupture risk that likely approaches 1%/y.[46] The rupture risk has been associated with poor patient selection, operator error, unrecognized/untreated endoleaks, large aneurysms, and device migration.

The presence of significant comorbidities and advanced age favors the endovascular approach. Chronic renal insufficiency is not an absolute contraindication to endovascular repair, as the procedure can be performed without contrast by using intravascular ultrasound (IVUS) or CO_2 as the contrast agent. Of note, both open and endovascular repair are associated with a long-term decrement in renal function.[47] In general, the endovascular approach may allow a subset of patients not considered suitable candidates for an open operation to have their aneurysms repaired. The EVAR Trial 2 randomized patients not fit for open repair to expectant management or endovascular repair and demonstrated no difference in aneurysm-related mortality, all-cause mortality, or quality of life.[48] Notably, the patients were truly "high risk" with a perioperative mortality rate of 9% and a 4-year mortality rate of almost 40%.

The known device-related complications and the uncertainty about the long-term outcome after endovascular repair mandate indefinite surveillance, although the intervals and type of imaging for surveillance remain controversial. Patients must agree to comply with the prescribed protocol, and their ability to fulfill these expectations should be factored into the specific choice of procedure. It is important to note that although the incidence of complications declines with the number of negative postoperative CT scans, new endoleaks have been discovered many years after device implantation.

Despite the various advantages and disadvantages of the approaches outlined in the previous section, patients and providers seem to prefer the endovascular approach, and these preferences appear to be one of the driving forces for the widespread adoption of the technique. The potential to perform an endovascular repair completely percutaneously (ie, no femoral artery exposure) clearly adds to the appeal of the approach.

The proverbial "bottom line" for the open versus endovascular debate remains somewhat unresolved, but the discussion is merely academic at this point. EVAR, when anatomically possible, has essentially become the standard of care in most practices despite all the aforementioned data suggesting equivocal results. The trend toward dominance of EVAR over open repair has increased to a point where many vascular training programs have difficulty fulfilling their open aneurysm case requirements to sufficiently educate their trainees.

OPERATIVE REPAIR

Preoperative Evaluation

The preoperative evaluation of patients undergoing elective AAA repair is similar to that of patients undergoing any major general or vascular surgical procedure. Patients undergoing endovascular repair should likely undergo the same preoperative work-up despite the perception that associated perioperative stresses are less. All patients should receive a complete history and a physical examination, an electrocardiogram, and a chest radiograph. Routine preoperative laboratory studies should be obtained, and the appropriate quantity of blood products cross-matched. A thorough peripheral pulse examination should be included in the physical examination, and if abnormal, validated with formal ankle–brachial indices. In addition, patients should be started on aspirin and statin (HMG Co-A reductase inhibitors). The perioperative use of beta blockers in patients undergoing noncardiac surgery has been controversial. The most updated recommendations from the ACC/AHA in 2014 state that beta blockers should be continued in patients who have been on these agents chronically.[49] The initiation of the beta blockers should be *considered* in those patients who have ≥3 cardiac risk factors (diabetes, heart failure, CAD, renal insufficiency, prior stroke), but these agents should *not* be started on the day of surgery as this is associated with increased adverse events.

All active medical problems should be controlled as much as possible before elective aneurysm repair. However, extensive diagnostic testing is probably unnecessary. Routine pulmonary function tests and measurement of arterial blood gases are not indicated, although they may be beneficial in selected patients with advanced COPD. The presence of COPD often complicates postoperative ventilator management, especially for those undergoing open repair.

The appropriate cardiac work-up before AAA repair is evolving and is somewhat institution dependent. This controversy has been further complicated by the publication of the CARP Trial which examined the role of coronary artery revascularization before major vascular surgery among patients with significant coronary artery disease.[50] The study reported that preoperative coronary artery revascularization did not reduce the incidence of either perioperative myocardial infarction or long-term mortality. It is important to emphasize that the overall objective of the preoperative cardiac work-up is to optimize the cardiovascular system and thereby reduce both the perioperative and long-term risk of myocardial infarction and death. Admittedly, the prevalence of coronary artery disease among patients undergoing AAA repair is quite high. Hertzer et al., in a landmark publication, reported that 25% of 1000 patients undergoing evaluation for peripheral vascular surgery (cerebral vascular occlusive disease, lower-extremity arterial occlusive disease, AAA) had severe, surgically correctable lesions detected during cardiac catheterization; 6% had severe, uncorrectable disease, and only 8% had no evidence of disease. Interestingly, the incidence of surgically correctable disease was highest among patients undergoing evaluation for AAA.[51] The ACC/AHA Guidelines have simplified the preoperative evaluation before elective vascular procedures for patients with risk factors for stable coronary disease.[49] Briefly, a patient's estimated perioperative risk of major adverse cardiac event should be calculated using combined clinical and surgical risk factors. The American College of Surgeons NSQIP risk calculator (https://riskcalculator.facs.org/RiskCalculator/) can be used. If elevated risk, the patient's functional capacity then determines the need for additional cardiac testing. More specifically, patients who can generate at least 4 metabolic equivalents (METs) can proceed without additional testing. Those patients with poor (<4 METs) or unknown functional capacity should undergo pharmacologic stress testing with coronary catheterization/revascularization as indicated before surgery. Notably, there is insufficient evidence to support a reduced cardiac work-up for patients undergoing endovascular repair. It is important to emphasize that although the cardiac risk of endovascular repair may be less, the subset of patients undergoing the procedure is often older and sicker.

Open Repair of Intact Abdominal Aortic Aneurysms

Technique

A significant amount of preparation is required in the operating room before making the incision. Adjunctive epidural anesthesia has been associated with improved survival along with reduced immediate postoperative events, although the direct explanatory mechanism for this finding remains unclear.[52] Adequate intravenous access should be established to facilitate resuscitation. Central venous access is usually obtained, although not necessary. Electrocardiographic leads, an arterial catheter, and a Foley catheter should be placed for continuous monitoring. In addition, a nasogastric tube should be inserted. A Swan–Ganz pulmonary artery catheter or a transesophageal echocardiogram probe can be used as adjuncts in patients with heart failure, although their use is becoming less common. Peripheral arterial pulses should be interrogated with either palpation or continuous-wave Doppler ultrasound and marked to facilitate confirmation after restoration of lower-extremity perfusion. Strategies to maintain core body temperature should be initiated.

Use of an intraoperative autologous transfusion device should be considered, especially when a significant amount of blood loss is anticipated, such as during suprarenal or thoracoabdominal aortic aneurysm repairs. Furthermore, they can be helpful in patients who object to blood transfusions on religious principles. A first-generation cephalosporin or vancomycin should be administered prior to the incision.

AAAs may be repaired through several different incisions or approaches including midline, retroperitoneal, or transverse/bilateral subcostal. The incision options must be viewed as complementary since none is perfect for every clinical scenario. The determinants of the incision include the cephalad/caudal extent of the aneurysm, body habitus, presence of prior abdominal incisions, presence of abdominal wall stomas, comorbidities, additional intraoperative pathology, inflammatory aneurysms, renal anomalies, requirements for concomitant procedures, urgency of aortic control, and surgeon preference. The midline approach is preferable for patients with ruptured infrarenal AAAs because aortic control at the level of the diaphragm can be obtained rapidly. The bilateral subcostal approach provides the best exposure and is the incision of choice for obese patients, those with extensive iliac artery aneurysms, those patients requiring concomitant renal artery revascularization, and those patients with juxtarenal aneurysms that require suprarenal aortic control. The retroperitoneal approach is optimal for patients with multiple previous abdominal incisions ("hostile abdomen"), abdominal wall stomas, suprarenal aneurysms, inflammatory aneurysms, and horseshoe kidneys. However, the retroperitoneal approach provides limited exposure to the right renal artery and right iliac vessels. It was previously contended that the retroperitoneal approach posed less of a physiologic insult than the transperitoneal approach and, therefore, was ideal for patients with advanced pulmonary or cardiac disease. However, this has not been supported by a prospective, randomized trial. A detailed description of the retroperitoneal approach is beyond the context of this chapter, but it is available in most standard vascular surgical texts.

The sequence of steps used to repair an intact, infrarenal AAA through a transperitoneal approach can be summarized (**Fig. 91.9**). The abdomen is explored after the peritoneal cavity is entered, and both the gallbladder and colon are carefully examined. The small bowel is manually retracted laterally to the right, and the duodenum is mobilized by incising the ligament of Treitz. The inferior mesenteric vein may be suture ligated to facilitate exposure. The tissue adjacent to the inferior mesenteric vein should be palpated to rule out a large, meandering mesenteric artery. This artery is an important visceral collateral and should be preserved. The retroperitoneum over the aorta is incised with the electrocautery, and the left renal vein is exposed. Self-retaining retractors (eg, Bookwalter, Omni retractors) are then placed to facilitate further exposure. The small bowel is retracted laterally to the right, the transverse colon and superior abdominal wall are retracted cephalad, while the lower abdominal wall is further retracted caudal. The aorta immediately inferior to the renal arteries is exposed, and both renal arteries are visualized. The infrarenal aorta at this location is dissected to facilitate placement of an aortic clamp. It is important to identify the course of the renal vein and any venous anomalies on the preoperative CT scan to prevent inadvertently injuring these structures at this stage of the procedure. In the presence of a retroaortic renal vein or circumaortic collar, the aortic neck should not be dissected circumferentially, and vascular control should be obtained with a vertical clamp. The retroperitoneum over the aorta is then incised further caudally, and the incision is extended along the course of the right common iliac artery. The extent of the caudal dissection depends on the anatomic configuration of the aneurysm. If the aneurysm extends to the aortic bifurcation, it is sufficient to dissect only the common iliac arteries, provided a suitable site for clamp application is identified. If the aneurysm extends to the distal common iliac arteries, both the internal and external iliac vessels should be

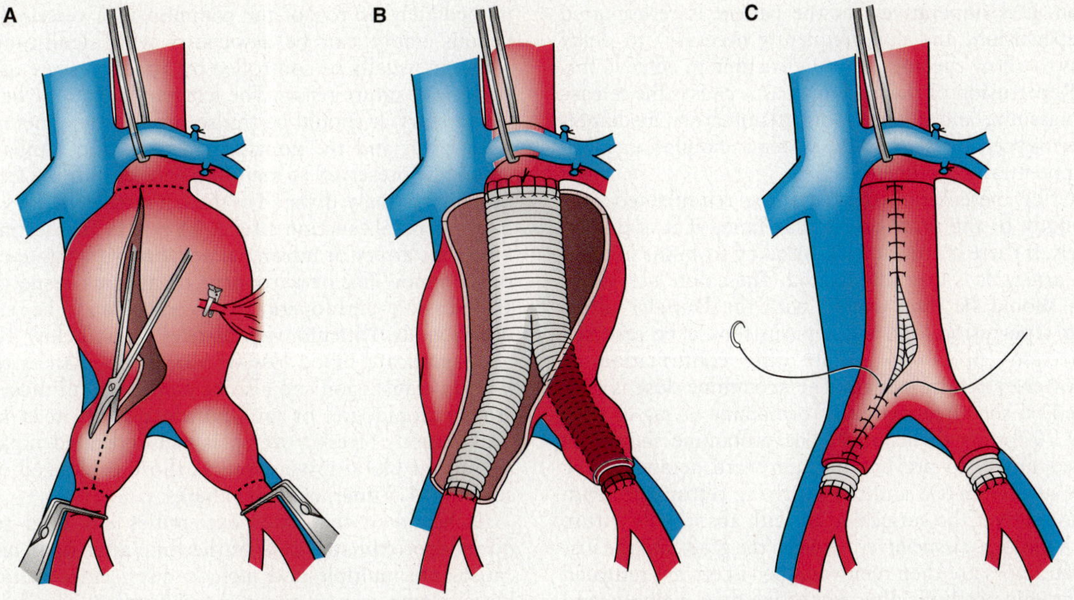

Figure 91.9. Steps involved in the standard repair of an infrarenal abdominal aortic aneurysm extending into the proximal common iliac arteries. **A:** The proximal duodenum is mobilized and the retroperitoneum overlying the aorta is incised. The infrarenal aorta immediately below the renal vein is dissected. The iliac bifurcations are exposed, and vascular clamps are applied to the infrarenal aorta and distal common iliac arteries after adequate heparinization. A longitudinal arteriotomy is extended from the infrarenal aorta onto the right common iliac artery. **B:** Back bleeding from the lumbar arteries is controlled with "figure-of-eight" sutures. The proximal anastomosis is performed in an end-to-end configuration below the renal arteries. The distal anastomoses are performed at the common iliac bifurcation beyond the aneurysmal segments. The left limb of the graft is tunneled through the intact left common iliac aneurysm shell. **C:** The residual aneurysm shell is closed over the prosthetic graft, and the retroperitoneum is reapproximated to prevent erosion of the graft into the overlying bowel.

dissected free. This may be facilitated on the left side by mobilizing the sigmoid colon along its peritoneal reflection and reflecting it medially. The inferior mesenteric artery is then dissected free, and vascular control is obtained with a vessel loop. Patients are administered 100 units/kg of intravenous heparin, and the activated clotting time is confirmed to be twice the baseline value. Supplemental doses of heparin are administered throughout the procedure as dictated by the activated clotting time.

The appropriately sized prosthetic graft is selected according to the infrarenal aortic neck by visual inspection or with the calibrated graft rulers (ie, "sizers"). The general "rule of thumb" is that the smaller graft should be selected when the aorta is between two graft sizes because the aorta always appears smaller after it is transected, and redundant graft material at the proximal anastomosis is more difficult to correct than the opposite problem. Despite the contentions of the various graft manufacturers, there is no clear advantage for an individual graft, and the choice should be determined by surgeon preference as dictated by ease of handling, cost, and availability.

The distal vascular clamps are applied to the external, internal, or common iliac vessels as indicated. Occasionally, the iliac vessels are so calcified that they cannot be safely occluded with a clamp. Vascular control may be obtained intraluminally with the use of a balloon thromboembolectomy catheter after the aneurysm has been incised. The configuration of the aortic reconstruction (aorto-aortic, aortoiliac, aortofemoral) depends on the extent of aneurysmal involvement and the degree of occlusive disease. Even though a patient may be a candidate for an aortic tube graft, it is often easier to perform an aorto-bi-iliac graft because the terminal aorta is often very calcified. Aorto-bi-femoral bypass grafts should be reserved for the small subset of patients who truly have concomitant aneurysms and severe occlusive disease, since the risks of wound complications and graft infections are greater.

The proximal aortic clamp is then applied after the distal clamps. The clamp is applied immediately below the renal arteries to facilitate an anastomosis to the proximal infrarenal aorta. The length of the infrarenal aorta should be sufficient to permit a safe anastomosis. However, a long infrarenal cuff should be avoided because it may become aneurysmal over time. Either a vertical or horizontal aortic clamp may be used. The aorta is then incised longitudinally, and the incision is extended to the distal aorta and into the iliac arteries if the distal anastomosis will be to the iliac vessels. Attempts should be made to preserve the autonomic nerves overlying the distal aorta and proximal left common iliac artery in men. This can usually be achieved by incising the left common iliac artery transversely beyond the aneurysmal portion and tunneling the limb of the graft through the residual shell. The intraluminal thrombus and debris are removed from within the aorta, and all back bleeding from the lumbar arteries is controlled with suture ligatures. The infrarenal aorta at the level of the planned proximal anastomosis may be completely transected, or the back wall may be left intact. Completely transecting the aorta makes the proximal anastomoses slightly easier, although leaving the back wall intact reinforces the anastomosis and provides the equivalent of an autogenous pledget. The proximal anastomosis is performed in an end–end configuration with a running 3-0 Prolene suture. All leaks in the suture line are repaired with Prolene sutures and felt pledgets as necessary. The graft is then trimmed according to length. If using a bifurcated graft (distal anastomoses at the iliac arteries), the length of the graft main body prior to the flow divider should ideally be at least 4 to 5 cm to provide an adequate length of landing zone for an endograft, should it be needed in the future. The distal anastomosis or anastomoses are performed to the aortic bifurcation, common iliac arteries, or iliac bifurcation as dictated by the anatomy of the aneurysm. A 3-0 Prolene suture is used for anastomoses at the aortic bifurcation, and a similar 4-0 suture is used for the common iliac arteries.

All anastomoses are flushed to remove any intraluminal debris before flow is restored. Blood flow is restored to the pelvis and lower extremities in sequence. Attempts should be made to flush initially into the internal iliac circulation to prevent embolization to the lower extremities. This can be facilitated by manually compressing the common femoral arteries for tube graft configurations. The lower torso should be reperfused gradually (ie, one extremity at a time) to prevent hypotension. It is imperative that the patient is resuscitated prior to reperfusion, and it is frequently necessary to delay this process to allow the anesthesiologists time to achieve this objective. Reperfusion of the ischemic tissue causes the release of acid, potassium, and a variety of inflammatory mediators and reactive oxygen species into the systemic circulation, all of which are potentially detrimental.

The inferior mesenteric artery may be reimplanted into either the body of the graft or the iliac limbs if it is patent. Alternatively, if there is robust back-bleeding from the inferior mesenteric artery, it is typically ligated. The colon and lower extremities should be interrogated with the Doppler ultrasound after reperfusion, and the heparin should be reversed with intravenous protamine sulfate after confirmation of adequate lower-extremity signals. The protamine dose is estimated based on the effectiveness of protamine (1 mg of protamine per 100 units of heparin). The protamine should be administered slowly to prevent any untoward hemodynamic events. The aneurysm sac and the overlying retroperitoneum are both closed over the surgical graft with absorbable suture to provide a biologic tissue layer between the graft and the viscera. The retractors are then removed, the viscera are returned to their anatomic positions after inspecting their viability, and the abdominal wall fascia is closed with standard technique.

Patients are transferred directly from the operating room to the intensive care unit. Most of the patients are extubated in the operating room or shortly after arrival to the intensive care unit or appropriate step-down unit. Intensive care unit length of stay is usually 1 to 2 days, with a median overall length of stay of 8 days. Early ambulation is encouraged (ie, 24 to 48 hours). Nasogastric decompression is discontinued, and oral nutrition is initiated once bowel function returns. Patients are discharged when they are ambulatory, can tolerate a regular diet, have normal bowel function, and are sufficiently able to care for themselves. A subset of patients requires transfer to a rehabilitation or extended care facility. Postoperative return visits are encouraged at 2 to 4 weeks after discharge and then at 6 months thereafter.

Complications and Outcome

Open repair of intact AAAs is associated with significant mortality and morbidity. The attendant mortality rates have been discussed extensively in the preceding sections. Briefly, the contemporary mortality rate across the United States has consistently been reported as 3% to 5%.[53] The overall morbidity rate remains approximately 30% in patients undergoing repair of intact AAAs across the United States.

Intraoperative complications can result from injury to the intra-abdominal structures during dissection, although these technical complications are not specific to the aneurysm repair. The small bowel, colon, ureter, and major venous structures (inferior vena cava, iliac veins, left renal vein) are particularly susceptible. Iatrogenic bowel injury at the time of AAA repair is particularly problematic due to the potential to infect the prosthetic graft. If the colon is injured before the aneurysm repair, the defect in the colon should be fixed, and the aneurysm repair should be aborted. If the small bowel is injured before the aneurysm repair, the same course should likely be followed, although this decision requires a modicum of clinical judgment. The infectious concerns must be balanced by the fact that the small bowel contents are assumed sterile, a second procedure will be required to repair the aneurysm, and the small risk of aneurysm rupture during the intervening delay. Injury to the bowel during or after implantation of the aortic graft should be treated with repair of the defect, extensive irrigation, and prolonged antibiotics. Admittedly, these approaches are very conservative, and it is noteworthy that clinical series have attested to the safety of simultaneous aortic and gastrointestinal/urologic procedures.[54] The ureter is susceptible to injury at the point where it crosses over the iliac bifurcation. Injury can be avoided by a heightened awareness of this anatomic location and dissection in the tissue plane immediately on top of the common iliac vessels. Inadvertent venous injury can be associated with significant bleeding. This can usually be controlled by direct pressure using sponge sticks and suture repair. The left renal vein may be transected if necessary. It should be transected near its juncture with the vena cava, and the gonadal, adrenal, and lumbar branches should be preserved to maintain venous outflow from the kidney. Interestingly, division of the left renal vein does not appear to affect renal function after AAA repair. Transecting the common iliac artery or infrarenal aorta may facilitate exposure of the common iliac or retroaortic renal veins, respectively.

Excessive intraoperative bleeding may be encountered occasionally. Patients with platelet count below 100,000/mL and significant blood loss who receive a platelet transfusion. Platelet transfusion can also be considered in those on preoperative clopidogrel or an equivalent antiplatelet medication. Transfusion of fresh frozen plasma is indicated in patients with significant blood loss as well as those prolonged coagulation studies (>1.5 times control value).

Ischemia of the lower extremities has been reported to occur approximately 2% of the time after open repair.[55] The causes are multiple and include distal embolization, thrombosis, clamp injury, and technical errors. The lumen of the aneurysm is frequently filled with both thrombus and atheromatous debris that may serve as a source for both macro- and microembolization. Thrombosis may result from inadequate heparinization, hypercoagulable conditions, or poor arterial runoff. Further intervention is mandatory if the lower extremities are found to be ischemic. Anastomotic defects should be corrected. This may simply require revision of the anastomosis. If no problems are identified at the distal anastomosis, the femoral vessels should be explored and an intraluminal thrombus removed with a balloon embolectomy catheter. A bypass from the aortic graft to the femoral vessels may be required if adequate inflow cannot be restored with thrombectomy alone. The popliteal artery below the knee may also require exploration and thrombectomy if the extremity is still ischemic. This may be facilitated by creating a longitudinal arteriotomy on the below-knee popliteal artery that extends to the tibioperoneal trunk. This allows the passage of the balloon embolectomy catheter into all three tibial vessels under direct vision. A below-knee popliteal or tibial artery bypass is required if adequate perfusion to the distal extremity is not restored after patch closure of the popliteal arteriotomy. Predictably, a complex lower-extremity revascularization in conjunction with an aortic reconstruction is associated with a significant degree of morbidity and dramatically increases the mortality rate.[55]

Many of the systemic complications that follow open infrarenal aneurysm repair are not surprising, given the magnitude of the operation and the age/comorbidities of the patients. Cardiac complications (ischemia, infarction, arrhythmias, congestive heart failure) occur in up to 25%[56] and are the leading cause of death after open aneurysm repair in many series. Pulmonary complications (pneumonia, ventilator dependence >48 hours, acute respiratory distress syndrome) are also quite common, and approximately 10% of the patients require prolonged ventilation.[56] Deterioration of renal function occurs in approximately 5% of cases, although acute renal failure requiring dialysis is rare (ie, <1%).[56]

Ischemic colitis has been reported to occur in approximately 4% of cases after open aneurysm repair, but the rate is much higher (25% to 40%) in those undergoing ruptured aneurysm repair. The sigmoid colon is affected most frequently and is usually due to inadequate resuscitation and resulting hypotension (ie, watershed ischemia), disruption of collaterals, and/or failure to revascularize a hemodynamically significant inferior mesenteric artery. Patients usually present with bloody diarrhea in the early postoperative period. However, the diagnosis should be considered in the absence of bloody diarrhea in patients with thrombocytopenia, multiple-organ dysfunction, increasing abdominal pain/peritonitis, and generalized "failure to thrive." The diagnosis may be confirmed by endoscopy.

Treatment depends on the endoscopic findings and clinical setting. The endoscopic findings range from mucosal ischemia to transmural necrosis. In the absence of peritonitis, patients with mucosal ischemia alone can be treated with bowel rest, broad-spectrum antibiotics, total parenteral nutrition, and serial endoscopic examinations. Many of these lesions resolve spontaneously without long-term sequelae, although colonic strictures may develop in a subset of patients. Patients with transmural colonic necrosis should undergo laparotomy with resection of the involved segment, a proximal diverting colostomy, and a distal Hartmann pouch. After laparotomy, they should be maintained on broad-spectrum antibiotics. The reported mortality rate in patients with transmural necrosis may range up to 85%.

Several other gastrointestinal complications are common after standard infrarenal AAA repair. A postoperative ileus develops in essentially all patients, with bowel function usually returning within 3 to 5 days. Nasogastric decompression should be continued, narcotics minimized, electrolytes normalized, and ambulation encouraged. Either calculous or acalculous cholecystitis may develop after aneurysm repair. The mortality rates reported historically for postoperative cholecystitis were significant and served as the catalyst for simultaneous cholecystectomy and aneurysm repair. Although this approach has been found to be safe and not associated with an increased risk for graft infections, it is usually reserved for patients with small stones or evidence of chronic cholecystitis. Pancreatitis may develop after AAA repair, although the incidence is surprisingly low considering the obligatory manipulation of the pancreas during repair.

Sexual dysfunction is common after open AAA repair, ranging from 7% to 80% depending on the series.[57] The responsible mechanisms include interruption of the pelvic perfusion and injury to the autonomic nerves that overlie the distal aorta/proximal common iliac arteries. Injury to these autonomic nerves disrupts the internal sphincter mechanism of the bladder and results in retrograde ejaculation. Care should be used during aneurysm repair to maintain pelvic perfusion and avoid nerve injury to prevent these untoward complications. It is prudent to discuss these risks with patients preoperatively.

Paraplegia after open infrarenal AAA repair is exceedingly rare, with an incidence of 0.25%.[58] The potential mechanisms for this devastating complication include embolization, thrombosis of the spinal artery, and disruption of the spinal blood supply. Paraplegia after aneurysm repair is usually an irreversible injury. Maintaining adequate antegrade pelvic perfusion through the internal iliac arteries may minimize this complication.

Prosthetic aortic grafts are associated with long-term complications, with a reported incidence of approximately 10% to 15% at 15 years.[59] The long-term graft-related complications include infection, aortoenteric fistula, thrombosis, and pseudoaneurysm formation. Additional aneurysms of a sufficient size to merit intervention develop in approximately 5% to 15% of patients in either the iliac vessels or the aorta above the prosthetic graft. As such, the Society for Vascular Surgery recommends that patients undergo CT of the complete aorta and iliac vessels every 5 years postoperatively to screen for additional aneurysm disease.[2]

Endovascular Repair of Intact Abdominal Aortic Aneurysms

Technique

Preoperative preparation before EVAR can be more complicated than an open repair. The various imaging studies must be reviewed in detail to determine anatomic feasibility. Appropriate measurements must be taken and the necessary devices selected and ordered, if not readily available. An operative plan must be generated, including specific modifications of the standard approach to overcome the patient's anatomic limitations and, thereby, extend the feasibility of the technique. Indeed, "preoperative planning" has facetiously been identified as the most important component of a successful repair.

CT arteriography with 3D reconstructions has emerged as the optimal approach to determine feasibility of EVAR. It is important to emphasize that no imaging technique is perfect and, consequently, a certain degree of flexibility is necessary for the operative plan. Measurements obtained from the 3D CT tend to overestimate the actual renal artery–internal iliac artery length assumed by the graft when deployed in vivo.

The various devices/components should be selected using the underlying principles that the main body of the device should sit as close to the orifices of the renal arteries as possible, while the iliac limbs should extend to the orifices of the internal iliac arteries. This methodology not only provides exclusion of abnormal tissue, but also extends the length of seal and fixation of the endograft, and may provide additional column strength. Furthermore, the manufacturers' IFU for sizing and device selection should be followed. The diameter and length of the infrarenal neck, aneurysm, and iliac vessels must be measured precisely. In addition, the distance from the lowest renal artery to the aortic bifurcation and both iliac bifurcations needs to be determined. The endograft mainbody diameter is typically oversized 10% to 20% to that of the infrarenal aortic neck diameter. Additional devices should be ordered for each case, including two iliac limbs and an aortic extension cuff to allow for any discrepancy between the preoperative plan and the actual course of the graft in vivo. Each endograft procedure and device configuration is "custom fit" for an individual patient. Furthermore, physicians typically are required to complete a training course comprised of sizing exercises and monitored deployments.

The choice of the specific endovascular device is contingent upon the anatomic constraints of the aneurysm, device-associated outcome, and surgeon preference. There are specific differences between the various grafts that lend themselves to different clinical scenarios. The specific considerations include neck diameter, neck length/angulation, renal–internal iliac artery distance, common iliac artery diameter, and access vessel diameter. For example, a graft with suprarenal fixation may be more suitable for a shorter neck, while a lower profile system (ie, smaller outer diameter of the delivery sheath) may be most appropriate for patients with smaller access vessels (ie, common femoral and external iliac arteries). Devices with suprarenal fixation do not negatively impact renal function. Deployment of the various endografts is reasonably involved from a technical standpoint; thus, it is not particularly surprising that most surgeons elect to concentrate their proficiency with one or two devices. However, a working knowledge and comfort level with all devices on the market is advised, given the benefits that each graft may have over the others in certain scenarios. This permits use of a graft that best meets the individual patient's needs.

The need for adjunctive procedures to facilitate the endovascular repair is usually determined by the preoperative imaging and should be factored into the overall surgical plan. The major concerns include stenotic access vessels and the absence of a suitable common iliac artery landing zone due to aneurysm enlargement. The remedial procedures for small access vessels or significant occlusive disease include serial dilation or a retroperitoneal prosthetic iliac conduit, as previously discussed. Repeated attempts to pass the device through a diseased native artery should be avoided, as it can cause vessel dissection or rupture. Aneurysm degeneration of the common iliac artery can be overcome by extending the iliac endoprosthesis into the external iliac artery. This necessitates either embolization of the ipsilateral internal iliac artery or, more preferably, preserving internal iliac perfusion with the use of an iliac branch device, which has a precannulated internal iliac gate for ease of use. These devices have demonstrated satisfactory results, and their application to preserve internal iliac flow is strongly recommended by the Society for Vascular Surgery.[2]

Intraoperative preparation for endovascular repair is similar to that for the open approach, although there are several significant differences. The appropriate imaging equipment is mandatory. Ideally, this would entail a complete endovascular suite with a fixed fluoroscopic unit, although a portable unit with the appropriate vascular software and an imaging table is adequate. General, local, or regional anesthesia can be used for endovascular repair, depending on the individual patient, the clinical scenario, the planned length/complexity of the procedure, and the comfort level of the surgeon and anesthesiologist. Indeed, the endovascular approach is well suited for these less invasive alternatives, particularly considering the feasibility of a completely percutaneous approach. For a straightforward endovascular repair, intraoperative autologous transfusion devices and a nasogastric tube are unnecessary. In the current era, it is quite rare to convert to an open repair at the time of the initial implantation. However, it should be emphasized that EVAR is a surgical procedure, and most would agree that the procedure should be performed in an operating room with capabilities to convert to an open repair, if necessary.

Percutaneous access of the common femoral arteries has become standard for many physicians using a "preclose" methodology that involves placing a suture-based closure system that is deployed prior to delivery of the device and closed at the conclusion of the procedure. If the surgeon is uncomfortable with that approach, or the femoral artery anatomy precludes use of such a device, an open femoral exposure can be done through transverse, longitudinal, or oblique incisions. Although the technique for implanting the various endografts is somewhat specific to the individual device, the basic steps for deploying a "generic" modular bifurcated device using an open femoral artery exposure are illustrated (**Fig. 91.10**).

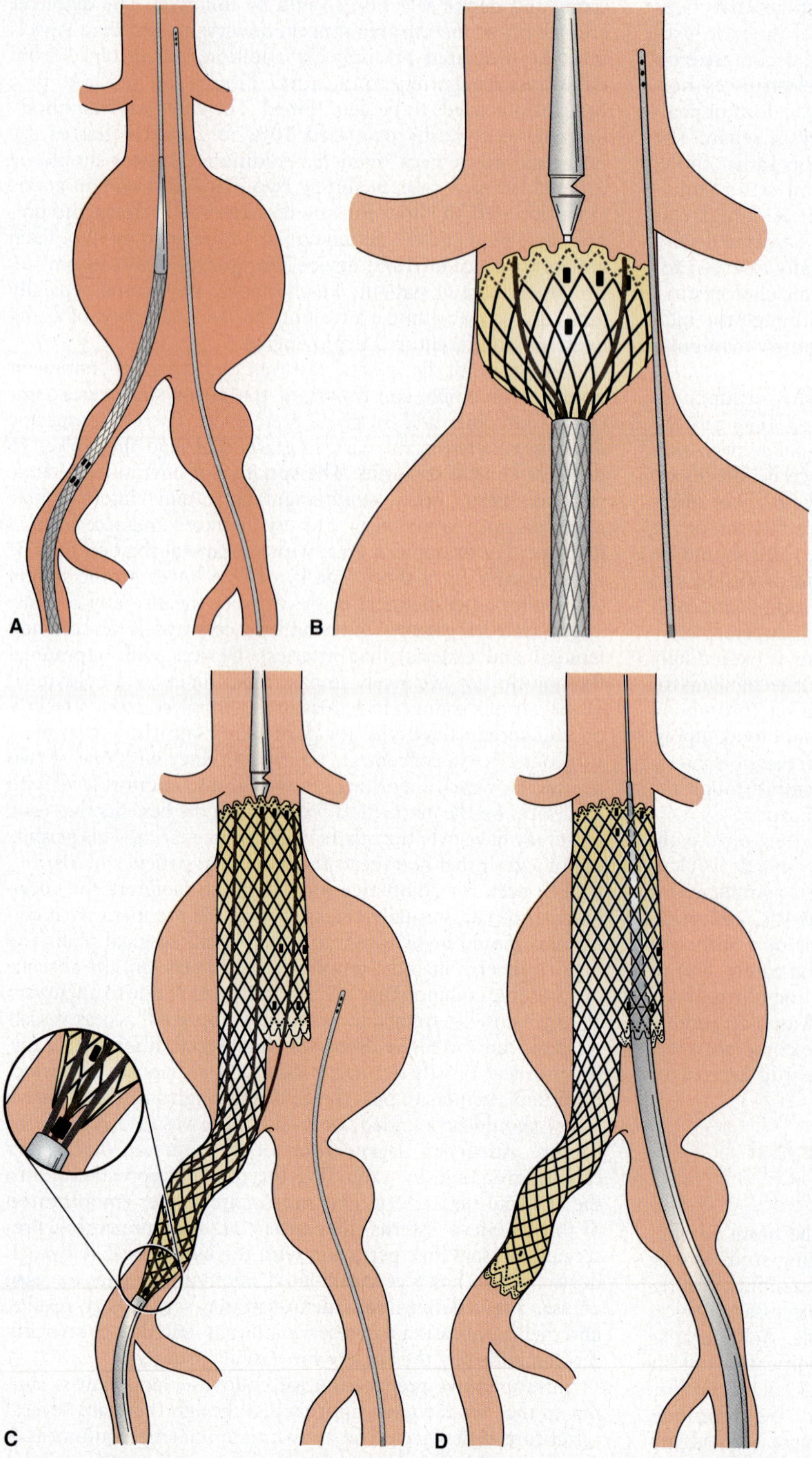

Figure 91.10. General steps involved in the endovascular repair of an abdominal aortic aneurysm. The common femoral arteries are exposed bilaterally (alternatively, and more commonly, percutaneous access is achieved and "preclose" sutures are placed), and stiff wires are introduced into the thoracic aorta under fluoroscopic guidance. An appropriately sized large diameter introducer sheath is inserted over the stiff wire into the body of the aneurysm at approximately the L3 vertebral space on the side contralateral to the one chosen for the main device. If the device is contained within its own deployment system, a sheath may not be required. **A:** The main body delivery catheter is introduced over the stiff wire through the ipsilateral groin, and the upper limit of the main body is positioned between the L1 and L2 vertebral bodies. An aortogram is obtained and the location of the renal arteries is identified. The location of the renal arteries is marked on the imaging screen, and the position of the main body finely adjusted. **B, C:** The main body is deployed, exposing the opening of the contralateral docking limb. The contralateral docking limb is cannulated and a stiff wire is advanced into the thoracic aorta. After confirming successful cannulation of the docking limb, deployment of the contralateral limb is deployed after marking the origin of the hypogastric artery. The hypogastric origin can be identified by using intravascular ultrasound or by obtaining a retrograde arteriogram through the sheath in the opposite oblique projection to identify the orifice of the internal iliac artery. **D, E, F:** The location of the orifice is marked on the imaging screen the contralateral limb is then introduced over the stiff wire, appropriately positioned, and deployed A compliant aortic occlusion balloon is advanced over the stiff wire and inflated in the region of the infrarenal neck to mold the proximal and distal attachment sites, and used to ensure the overlapping devices are well sealed.

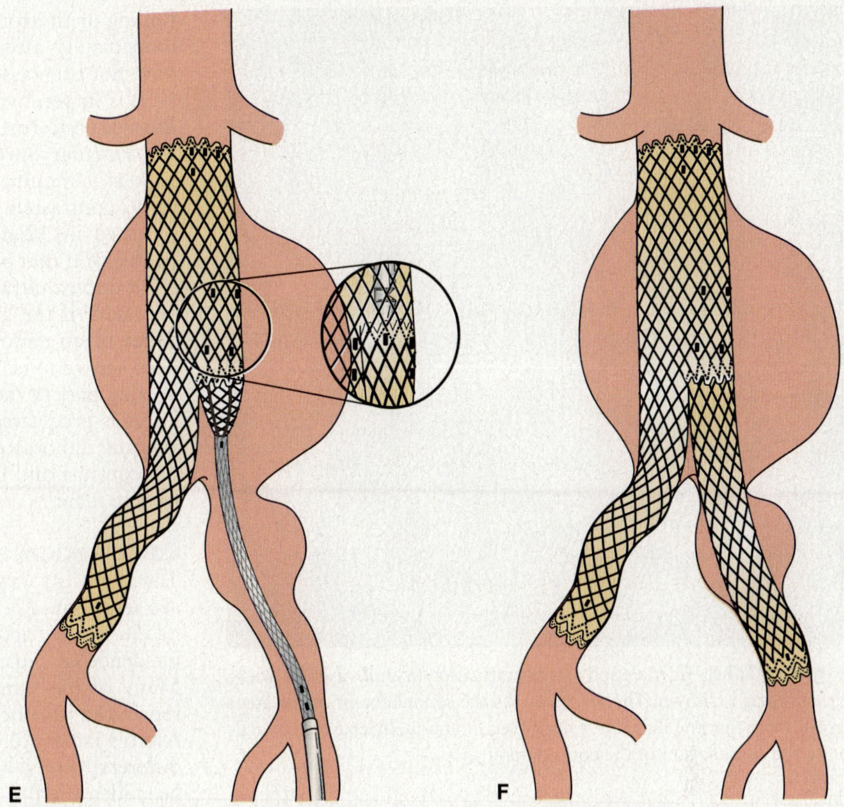

Figure 94.10. *(Continued)*

Briefly, when open surgical exposure is required, the common femoral arteries are dissected to facilitate 2 cm of vessel length for adequate controlinferior to the inguinal ligament. The common femoral artery on the side chosen to introduce the main body of the device (ipsilateral groin) is punctured using an angiographic needle, and a 0.035-in wire (eg, Bentsen) is passed into the abdominal aorta using fluoroscopic guidance. A 5-Fr introducer sheath is advanced over the guidewire using Seldinger technique. The working wire is advanced into the thoracic aorta and exchanged for a longer 0.035-in stiffened guidewire (eg, Lunderquist, Meier) using a catheter. Attention is then directed to the contralateral groin, and in a similar manner, a guidewire is advanced into the aorta and an appropriately sized introducer sheath is inserted over the guidewire. An angiographic catheter is advanced to the L1 vertebral body through the contralateral sheath and the catheter is connected to the power injector. The patient is then anticoagulated with heparin (100 units/kg), and therapeutic anticoagulation (ACT twice baseline) is maintained throughout the procedure. The main body delivery catheter is introduced over the stiff wire through the ipsilateral groin, and the upper limit of the main body is positioned between the L1–L2 vertebral bodies. Devices that do not have an integral sheath as part of their delivery system require a 16- to 22-Fr sheath to be inserted prior to introduction of the actual delivery catheter. Radiopaque markers on the graft facilitate the positioning and orientation of the main body.

As imaging has improved, multiple techniques allow for determining the proper location of endograft deployment. This may involve the use of IVUS or 3D overlay imaging, both of which can decrease the use of contrast and the radiation exposure to both patient and surgical team. In the absence of these advanced imaging techniques, an aortogram can be obtained after delivery of the endograft to the location of the renal arteries and the renal arteries marked for device deployment. A 5- to 10-degree cranial angulation is usually sufficient to account for the anterior angulation of the infrarenal neck caused by the natural lumbar lordosis of the spine and the posterior bulging of the aneurysm sac. However, the optimal angulation or orientation should be calculated based on the preoperative CT images. The location of the renal arteries is marked on the imaging screen, and the position of the main body is adjusted. The main body is now deployed, exposing the opening of the contralateral docking limb ("gate"). Using a combination of a hydrophilic wire and a curved catheter, the contralateral docking limb is cannulated. Various maneuvers, including different fluoroscopic projections, different-shaped catheters, and proper orientation of the contralateral docking limb prior to deployment of the main body device, can facilitate this step. It is imperative to confirm that the cannulating guidewire is actually within the body of the main endograft. There are a number of methods to confirm entry into the main aortic graft. The most definitive way is to use IVUS. A common method is to place a reverse curve catheter, such as an SOS or a pigtail catheter, into the main body at the level of the neck and then spin the catheter. If the catheter spins freely, this confirms that it is inside the endograft and not trapped between the aortic wall and endograft. Another option is to insert a compliant aortic occlusion balloon (which will be used later in the procedure) partially into the gate and *gently* inflate, giving the balloon an upside-down mushroom appearance. Alternatively, an arteriogram can be performed using a catheter within the main body, confirming that dye fills the aortic graft, but not the aneurysm on initial injection. Once the wire is confirmed to be within the endograft, the contralateral wire is advanced into the proximal descending thoracic aorta under fluoroscopic guidance and exchanged for a stiff wire using a catheter.

Next, the contralateral internal iliac artery origin must be identified in order to select the appropriate length iliac endoprosthesis. This can be accomplished with an IVUS catheter or retrograde angiography to mark the internal iliac artery. The optimal fluoroscopic angle to visualize this artery can be variable and is best determined using preoperative 3D imaging. However, the typical angle is in the opposite obliquity, about 30 degrees from the side of the vessel (ie, right anterior oblique for the left internal iliac artery). The location of the orifice is marked on the imaging screen, and a marker catheter is used

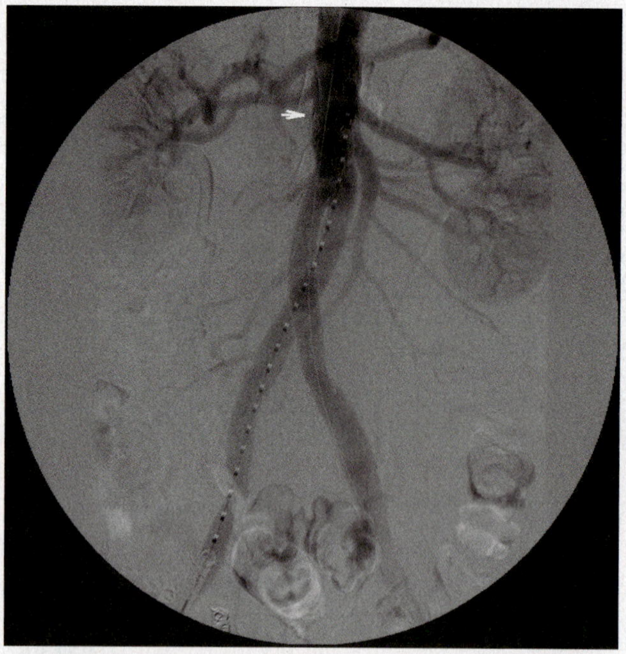

Figure 91.11. Completion arteriogram after an endovascular aneurysm repair is shown. The *arrow* marks the caudal extent of the stent graft. Note that the iliac limbs have been intentionally crossed to facilitate the cannulation of the contralateral gate.

to measure the distance from the contralateral docking limb to confirm the iliac device selection. The contralateral endoprosthesis is then introduced over the stiff wire, appropriately positioned relative to the docking limb and the orifice of the internal iliac artery, and then deployed. If using a three-part modular system, similar maneuvers are now performed on the ipsilateral side to mark the internal iliac artery origin and extend down with another endoprosthesis.

After deployment of all the devices, a compliant aortic occlusion balloon is advanced over the stiff wires and inflated in the region of the infrarenal neck to mold the proximal attachment site, all junctional overlap sites, and both iliac seal zones. A completion arteriogram is then obtained to evaluate the proximal/distal fixation sites, the graft/graft overlap zones, and the orifices of the renal/internal iliac arteries (**Fig. 91.11**). In addition, it should include delayed imaging to help identify any endoleaks. Problems identified on the completion study should be corrected, if possible, with potential remedial procedures including balloon dilation and/or aortic/iliac extension cuffs.

All sheaths, catheters, and wires are removed after the completion of the arteriogram if using an open femoral approach, and the arteriotomy is closed using pursestring suture placed at the time of the initial exposure or primary suture repair. In the case of percutaneous approach, the wire is left in during initial Perclose use to allow placement of additional closure devices as necessary. Doppler signals should be confirmed in the pedal vessels prior to heparin reversal with protamine (1 mg protamine/100 units heparin). The groin wounds are closed in layers with absorbable suture, and the final skin layer is closed with a subcuticular technique.

The immediate postoperative course is typically uneventful. Patients are transferred to the general care ward after recovery in the postanesthesia care unit. Patients are started on an appropriate diet the evening of the procedure and encouraged to ambulate. However, patients should be kept supine for 4 to 6 hours after the operation when a percutaneous technique is used to ensure successful hemostasis. Most infrarenal EVAR patients are discharged home on postoperative day 1, and then seen in the outpatient clinic at 1 month with an abdominal/pelvic CT scan. It is important to note that mild fever and the finding of air around the graft on CT are common occurrences immediately after endograft repair are not uncommon and have not been associated with graft infection.[60]

9 It is imperative that patients are followed long term, given durable concerns with an endovascular approach. The Society for Vascular Surgery recommends an abdominal/pelvic CT scan at 1 month. In the absence of endoleak or sac enlargement, contrasted CT scan or color duplex ultrasound can be repeated in 12 months.[2] If there is no sac enlargement or endoleak at that point, the patient can be followed with annual color duplex ultrasound or CT scan. More frequent imaging is necessary if the aneurysm continues to grow or there is evidence of an endoleak. Of note, color duplex ultrasound has been shown to be very effective in detecting endoleak and minimizing patient radiation and contrast exposure, but this technique is predicated on comfort level and training of the local vascular laboratory.[61] Surveillance CT scans should include noncontrast and biphasic contrast views with delayed images to help identify any late endoleaks.

Complications and Outcome

The mortality rates in randomized trials and national series are less than 2%,[42,43] the perioperative complication rate is <25%,[21] the rupture risk is approximately 1%/y,[46] and the incidence of remedial procedures is approximately 10%/y.[62] Many of the same complications that can occur after open repair can also occur after endovascular repair. However, the relative incidence of the various complications is significantly different, and several complications inherent to EVAR have been identified.

A variety of potential complications may arise during insertion of the delivery catheter or introducer sheath. Indeed, access problems secondary to iliac stenosis and/or tortuosity are the most common procedure-related complications. The outer diameters of the delivery sheaths are device dependent but can range up to 24 Fr. Excessive force during insertion of these large sheaths or delivery catheters can result in perforation/disruption of the vessels, which can lead to significant hemorrhage and hemodynamic compromise. The diagnosis can be confirmed by arteriography, and the bleeding controlled intraluminally using the device sheath or a balloon catheter. A variety of endovascular salvage techniques are possible in this setting including deployment of either the main device or a covered stent across the disrupted artery, but this may require occlusion of the internal iliac artery. Most major arterial disruptions can be managed with endovascular techniques, but in the event that they are unsuccessful, a retroperitoneal incision with direct control of the iliac arteries must be performed expeditiously.

Safe conduct of an EVAR is predicated on sufficient knowledge of the various salvage techniques, the necessary catheter and guidewire skills to execute these techniques, and a complement of ancillary equipment. However, the adage that "prevention is better than the cure" holds true, and endovascular surgeons should maintain a low threshold for constructing a surgical or endovascular iliac conduit prophylactically. Besides rupture, the access vessels can be dissected from misdirection or excessive force during sheath or device insertion. If nonflow limiting, no intervention is necessary; but, if a flow limitation is present, the dissected segment typically requires stenting. Prior to doing so, confirmation that the wire is within the true lumen is critical.

Graft deployment can be associated with mechanical problems related to the delivery system or inappropriate positioning. Many of the mechanical problems are device specific and related to the actual sequence of events and manipulations required. Troubleshooting guidelines and specific recommendations are available from the manufacturers. Deployment of the endovascular graft below the proximal target site along the infrarenal aorta may be corrected using an aortic extension cuff. Attempting to reposition the graft more cephalad after deployment is not recommended. Deployment of the endovascular graft across the orifices of the renal arteries can potentially be corrected by displacing the graft caudally. A guidewire can be passed over the flow divider and out the contralateral groin. The entire graft can then be retracted caudally by pulling on the wires. Alternatively, a large balloon can be inflated above the flow divider and retracted. Extreme care must be exercised during these maneuvers to prevent complete dislodgement of the proximal main body from the neck. Deployment of the graft across part of the renal orifice with subsequent renal malperfusion can be corrected by placing a "chimney" or "parallel" stent within the lumen of the renal artery. This may require upper extremity arterial access in order to cannulate the target vessel. Deployment of the endograft across the lumen of one internal iliac artery is usually tolerated, provided the contralateral vessel is patent and relatively free of occlusive disease. With coverage of a single hypogastric artery, severe complications are rare. Occlusion of both internal iliac arteries or occlusion of one vessel in the presence of contralateral disease may render the pelvis ischemic. In the event of unintentional hypogastric artery coverage, the iliac limb can be pushed cephalad using a sheath and its dilator. It should be emphasized that many of these remedial procedures are not manufacturer approved and should only be attempted by experienced endovascular surgeons. Due to the advanced age of many of these patients and their attendant comorbidities, open surgical conversion should be contemplated only as a last resort after the endovascular options have been exhausted, again emphasizing the need for advanced endovascular skills.

It is relatively common to see an endoleak on the completion arteriogram. Treatment is contingent upon the specific type of leak and its associated natural history, although the majority of these early endoleaks ultimately resolve. Type 1a/b (a-proximal, b-distal attachment site) and type 3 (fabric tear or modular component separation/leak) endoleaks are particularly concerning, and every reasonable attempt to correct these defects should be made. The aneurysm sac is often exposed to systemic pressure in the presence of a type 1 or type 3 endoleak, and, therefore, the rupture risk likely approaches that associated with the untreated aneurysm. Both the type 1 and 3 endoleaks can potentially be corrected by repeat balloon angioplasty at the proximal/distal attachment sites or at the modular interface. If these measures are not successful, additional extension devices can be deployed if there is adequate length before the target vessel.

In the event that a significant type 1a endoleak persists on postoperative imaging, the potential options include remediation with branched/fenestrated endograft, aortic cuff extension with renal chimneys, application of endoanchors, embolization, or open repair with endograft explant. Numerous nonrandomized series have reported relatively feasible and durable results with the aforementioned options.[63] Type 2 endoleaks have a relatively benign natural history and do not merit aggressive intervention unless the aneurysm continues to increase in size over time. Type 4 endoleaks are self-limiting and do not merit treatment at all. They are identified as a diffuse contrast "blush" at the time of completion of arteriography. They represent a diagnosis of exclusion and mandate that the more worrisome type 1 endoleak be excluded.

The spectrum of immediate postoperative complications after EVAR is comparable to that outlined for after open repair and will not be repeated. However, the incidence of major systemic complications after EVAR is quite uncommon. It is noteworthy that the incidence of both paraplegia and bowel ischemia is comparable after endovascular and open repair, although the mechanisms are different and likely due to atheroembolism.

The long-term complications after EVAR include endoleak, structural failure, need for remedial procedures, including open conversion and rupture. These ongoing risks further emphasize the importance of conscientious lifelong surveillance. Device migration has been reported to cause type 1 endoleaks and has been associated with neck length, site of deployment below the renal arteries, and surgeon/center experience.[64] The treatment of late occurring type 1 and 3 leaks is identical to that for those occurring earlier, as previously described.[63] Type 2 endoleaks merit intervention and treatment if the aneurysm continues to increase in diameter, although the clinical scenario is an important deciding factor in these cases. Identification of the type 2 endoleak can be challenging and may require selective catheterization of the superior mesenteric or internal iliac arteries. A variety of approaches have been described to treat the type 2 endoleaks, including coil embolization, laparoscopic ligation of the feeder vessels, and direct translumbar or transcaval injection of the aneurysm sac with glue or other thrombotic agents.[65]

Aneurysms that continue to increase in size after EVAR merit further intervention and may require open conversion due to their ongoing rupture risk. It should be emphasized that the goal of aneurysm repair is to prevent rupture/death from rupture and that endoleak and sac enlargement are surrogate markers of potential late failure of the therapy. Even more concerning is recent evidence that failure of sac regression has been associated with higher long-term mortality.[66] The clinical significance of an enlarging sac in the absence of a visible endoleak is controversial as long as a secure proximal and distal fixation of the endograft has been demonstrated. To confound the issue further, rupture of aneurysms without an endoleak or a change in sac diameter has also been reported, leading some to describe the phenomenon teleologically as endotension. A presumed endoleak that is not detected on a properly performed contrast CT scan is typically not identified on a catheter-based arteriogram. The proper diagnostic investigation of an endoleak should include interrogation of all the fixation sites and modular interfaces and selective injections of mesenteric and hypogastric arteries with sufficient contrast dose and proper acquisition techniques. It should be emphasized that open conversion and explant of the endovascular graft can be technically more challenging than a de novo open repair and usually requires suprarenal or supraceliac aortic control. In the absence of infection, it is not always possible (or necessary) to remove the entire device, particularly when the device has suprarenal fixation. It is possible to transect the endovascular graft near the usual site of the infrarenal aortic anastomosis and incorporate the fabric/stents of the graft into the anastomosis. Temporary distal vascular control can be achieved by clamping the limbs of the endovascular graft. The limbs of a bifurcated surgical graft may be anastomosed directly to the endograft limbs if they are securely attached to the iliac artery, typically incorporating the native terminal aorta or common iliac arteries. In properly chosen elective patients, open conversion can be performed with similar outcomes to primary open juxtarenal AAA repair.[67]

A variety of device-specific complications, including strut fracture, fabric tears, and buckling of the graft, have been identified. Importantly, these may present at any time throughout the postoperative period.

REPAIR OF RUPTURED ABDOMINAL AORTIC ANEURYSMS

Open Repair

The approach to the patient with a ruptured AAA is similar to the elective scenario, with the exception of several points that merit further comment. Prompt communication with all operating room personnel is critical for a good outcome. The blood bank should be notified, as the case may require massive transfusion of blood products. If available, cell-saver should utilized. The patient should be prepared and draped before induction of anesthesia with a broad operative field from the chin to the toes. This allows access to both groins if percutaneous insertion of an aortic occlusion balloon is necessary to obtain proximal control, and the chest in the event that resuscitative thoracotomy is required. The surgeon should be ready to make the incision at the time of induction, since patients with ruptured aneurysms frequently become hypotensive at this point, and some advocate for balloon occlusion of the supraceliac aorta prior to induction.

A midline incision should be made and supraceliac aortic control obtained. The aorta/esophagus can be difficult to identify, especially in a hypotensive patient. The placement of a nasogastric tube can facilitate identification of the gastroesophageal junction and thus, guide proper placement of the supraceliac clamp. The esophagus should be manually moved to the patient's left, and the gastrohepatic ligament, the crus of the diaphragm, and the connective tissue enveloping the aorta can be divided using blunt finger dissection. The aorta can be temporarily controlled manually by either occluding the aorta between the fingers and thumb or compressing it against the vertebral bodies. Definitive control should be obtained with an aortic clamp. Care should be taken during these maneuvers to prevent injury to the esophagus or the aorta itself.

Aortic control can also be achieved through a variety of other means: thoracotomy with occlusion of the descending thoracic aorta, intraluminal control of the infrarenal aorta with a compliant balloon placed through the common femoral artery, or supraceliac control via a retroperitoneal incision. The surgeon should be familiar with these various techniques because they can be helpful in certain clinical settings, but the midline approach with supraceliac control is recommended for most ruptured *infrarenal* aneurysms. After supraceliac aortic control has been obtained, the infrarenal aorta is dissected, and vascular control is achieved below the level of the renal arteries to restore visceral perfusion. The hematoma from the ruptured aneurysm often facilitates the dissection by displacing the normal tissue planes. However, the normal tissues may be obscured, and care should be taken not to injure the venous structures, particularly the left renal vein. It is imperative that these various steps are coordinated with the anesthesia team, and it is recommended that the supraceliac clamp be left in position to facilitate reapplication if necessary. Distal vascular control can be achieved with either vascular clamps or intraluminal balloons, depending on the health of the iliac vessels.

The decision to anticoagulate the patient is contingent on a variety of factors, including the quantity of blood lost, presence of coagulopathic bleeding, body temperature, and hemodynamic status. Anticoagulation potentially reduces thrombotic complications, but it exacerbates coagulopathic bleeding. It is recommended that the inferior mesenteric artery be reimplanted (if patent) to reduce the risk of postoperative colonic ischemia. The heparin effect can be reversed with protamine. The administration of plasma, platelets, and/or additional clotting factors should be considered at this point if indicated.

The postoperative course after repair of a ruptured aneurysm is predictably more complicated and protracted than after elective repair. Both the intensive care unit and total hospital length of stay are significantly increased. The mortality and complication rates are likewise significantly worse. The contemporary mortality rate for patients with ruptured AAAs who make it to the operating room is approximately 41%, which is improved compared to outcomes from several decades ago.[24] The spectrum of postoperative complications after repair of a ruptured aneurysm is essentially the same as after elective repair, although the incidences are increased. The incidence of bowel ischemia may be as high as 40% and routine colonoscopy may be indicated. Abdominal compartment syndrome develops in up to 30% and merits consideration in patients who are not doing well. Notably, adrenal insufficiency was identified in almost 70% of patients with unexplained postoperative hypotension after ruptured aneurysm repair.

ENDOVASCULAR REPAIR FOR RUPTURE

A meta-analysis comprising data of ~60,000 patients showed that endovascular repair of ruptured *infrarenal* AAA has significantly improved outcomes compared to traditional open repair.[68] Randomized controlled trials and observational series report 30-day mortality rates of 31% to 33% with EVAR.[69] However, these studies may be subject to selection and publication bias. The Society for Vascular Surgery currently recommends EVAR over open repair, if anatomically feasible, for treatment of ruptured AAA, albeit the society acknowledges the relatively poor quality of evidence to support this guideline.[2]

An endovascular approach requires a defined protocol/program consisting of an experienced endovascular surgeon, a committed team, an available operating room with the necessary imaging equipment, and an inventory of suitable devices. Studies estimate that approximately 40% to 50% of patients with ruptured aneurysms are anatomically suitable for endovascular repair using conventional devices.[70] Oversizing of the aortic neck ≥20% and encroachment on the orifices of the renal arteries with adjunctive stenting are both tolerated in an attempt to limit the necessary inventory and increase the proximal fixation zone, respectively. Access to the common femoral arteries can be obtained using a percutaneous approach with Perclose application or directly repaired at the completion of the procedure. In the absence of severe hypotension, the remaining conduct of the procedure is essentially the same as described in the elective setting. It is not usually necessary to occlude the aorta with an intraluminal balloon, although one should be readily available in the event that the patient becomes hemodynamically unstable.

Notably, patients treated with EVAR are at risk of developing abdominal compartment syndrome as a result of the intra/retroperitoneal hemorrhage and/or aggressive volume resuscitation. A meta-analysis estimated this rate to be 20% with half of these patients ultimately dying.[71] The surgeon should consider prophylactic laparotomy or retroperitoneal evacuation with placement of an open abdominal vacuum dressing at the conclusion of the procedure, depending on the clinical status.

ADDITIONAL CONSIDERATIONS

Isolated Iliac Artery Aneurysms

Isolated iliac artery aneurysms are rare, comprising less than 2% of all aneurysms.[72] The common iliac artery is involved in approximately 70% of the cases, and the internal iliac artery in the remainder. Aneurysmal involvement of the external iliac artery, either in combination with the common iliac artery or alone, is distinctly rare. These isolated iliac artery aneurysms should be differentiated from the common iliac artery aneurysms that occur concomitantly with AAAs. Simultaneous aneurysmal involvement of the aorta and common iliac arteries occurs in about 10% to 20% of all AAAs[3] and should be considered as one disease process.

The natural history of isolated iliac artery aneurysms is poorly defined because of their low incidence. The clinical risk factors appear to be similar to those for AAAs, with the highest incidence seen among elderly men. Unlike patients with AAAs, a significant proportion of patients with isolated iliac artery aneurysms present with symptoms. These symptoms may result from either rupture or compression of adjacent structures, including the bowel, ureters, iliac veins, and nerves. The clinical presentation of patients with a ruptured iliac artery aneurysm is similar to that of ruptured AAAs, and the diagnosis should be included in the differential for patients with genitourinary symptoms and normal findings on urinalysis and testicular examination. CT arteriography is optimal for confirming the diagnosis of an isolated iliac artery aneurysm.

The principles of treatment for asymptomatic, isolated iliac artery aneurysms are similar to those for AAAs, and operative repair is justified when the risk for rupture offsets the risk of repair. Unfortunately, the appropriate threshold for repair remains unresolved. Although rupture has been reported for aneurysms smaller than 2 cm, it is incredibly rare for aneurysms smaller than 3 cm to rupture. Consequently, operative repair is generally recommended for low-risk patients with isolated iliac artery aneurysms ≥3.5 cm.[2]

The treatment of isolated iliac artery aneurysms depends on the specific vessel involved and the extent of the aneurysm. Theoretically, common iliac artery aneurysms can be repaired with an interposition graft or a covered stent, provided that there is a sufficient proximal and/or distal neck to sew the anastomosis or seat the graft. However, this is rarely an option because the aneurysm involvement of the vessel usually extends over its whole length. Therefore, open repair necessitates replacing the whole common iliac artery with a bifurcated graft similar to the approach for patients with combined aortoiliac disease. Likewise, an endovascular approach should adhere to the same principles outlined for treatment of an infrarenal AAA and may require the use of an iliac branch device to achieve distal seal and maintain internal iliac perfusion, as previously discussed.

The treatment of internal iliac artery aneurysms is typically exclusion. This can be performed using either an endovascular or open approach, although the former is preferred due to its simplicity, and indeed endovascular embolization has become the contemporary mainstay of treatment. Bypass of an internal iliac artery aneurysm is often not possible because there is rarely a proximal or distal neck. Indeed, the aneurysmal involvement usually extends to the common iliac bifurcation, and the distal aspect usually arborizes into multiple smaller vessels. An alternative to open bypass is to ligate the origin of the internal iliac artery and oversew its distal branches from within the aneurysm, although this is feasible only if the aneurysmal degeneration does not involve the origin of the vessel. Obtaining the necessary distal control for this approach can be challenging. It is certainly important to assess the status of the contralateral internal iliac artery and overall pelvic circulation before ligating this artery. The principles of an endovascular approach include obliterating both the inflow and outflow of the aneurysm, along with complete sac thrombosis. The inflow of the vessel can be occluded by placing a covered stent across the origin of the internal iliac artery, and the outflow can be occluded using selective embolization of the various branches using a variety of other agents, including coils, plugs, glues, or gelfoam.

INFLAMMATORY ABDOMINAL AORTIC ANEURYSMS

Approximately 5% of all AAAs are described or considered inflammatory.[73] These aneurysms are characterized by a dense inflammatory response encasing the anterior and lateral walls of the infrarenal aorta with sparing of the posterior aspect. The inflammatory response consists of a dense cellular infiltrate that has a white, glistening appearance on inspection. The inflammation results in an increase in wall thickness, with the difference between the inner and outer diameters of the aorta ranging from 1 to 5 cm. The cause of this inflammatory process remains unresolved, but it is likely an autoimmune phenomenon.

Patients with an inflammatory abdominal aneurysm are predominantly male and frequently present with symptoms of back or abdominal pain. The triad of a pulsatile abdominal aortic mass, abdominal pain, and an elevated erythrocyte sedimentation rate (ESR) has been described. CT findings are characteristic and include a thick, contrast-enhancing wall in the distribution described. An inexperienced observer may confuse the CT findings with those of a ruptured AAA. Hydronephrosis with *medial* displacement of the ureters is frequently seen in contradistinction to the lateral displacement seen with noninflammatory aneurysms. Indeed, this entity may share some pathophysiologic pathways with retroperitoneal fibrosis.

The treatment of inflammatory AAAs is essentially the same as that for the more common, noninflammatory variety. Nonoperative treatment with corticosteroids has been advocated in the past, although this approach is likely ineffective and has largely been abandoned. It has been suggested that the rupture risk of inflammatory aneurysms is less than that for noninflammatory variety because the wall thickness is increased. However, this is likely untrue, and patients should not be lulled into a false sense of security. It should be emphasized that most aneurysms rupture through their posterior or posterolateral aspect, which is not involved in the inflammatory process. The open repair of an inflammatory AAA is complicated by the fact that the adjacent structures, including the duodenum, colon, and ureters, may be involved in the process and densely adherent to the aortic wall. No attempt should be made to mobilize the adherent structures, specifically the duodenum, because of the potential for iatrogenic injury. Proximal aortic control can be achieved either immediately above the renal arteries or above the visceral vessels. A retroperitoneal approach can reduce the technical difficulties associated with the open repair. The preoperative placement of ureteral catheters may facilitate their identification intraoperatively and can be helpful in patients with hydronephrosis. Perioperative complications and graft infections are greater with open repair of inflammatory AAAs compared to the more conventional bland AAA.

If anatomically feasible, EVAR has been shown to be the optimal treatment for inflammatory AAAs, given its reduced morbidity and mortality compared to open repair.[73]

Juxtarenal and Suprarenal Abdominal Aortic Aneurysms

The management of aneurysms extending to the level of the renal arteries or more cephalad is more complicated, and, predictably, the morbidity rates associated with open repair are increased. Interestingly, reports from centers of excellence have documented mortality rates comparable to those reported for infrarenal repairs, although it is unlikely that these findings are applicable nationwide.[74] Repair of these complex aneurysms is complicated by the obligatory period of renal and visceral ischemia associated with aortic occlusion during the proximal anastomosis. Indeed, the renal complication rates range from 15% to 20% even from these select centers of excellence.[75] These increased morbidity and mortality rates should be factored into the decision algorithm and threshold for open operative repair. Elective open operative repair is usually recommended for patients with aneurysms 6 cm or larger in diameter in this setting, although the 5.5-cm criterion may be appropriate for very good-risk patients and those with juxtarenal aneurysms who will require only a short period of suprarenal aortic occlusion.

The open operative approach for AAAs extending to the renal arteries or more cephalad may be achieved through either a retroperitoneal or a transperitoneal exposure, although the former is optimal, especially with more cephalad disease. The *retroperitoneal* approach, with anterior reflection of the left kidney, obviates the concerns about the left renal vein (except when a retroaortic renal vein is present) and simplifies exposure of the abdominal aorta. The distal descending thoracic aorta is easily exposed by incising the diaphragm and its crus. Of note, the right renal artery and right common iliac artery are more difficult to expose via the retroperitoneal approach because of their trajectory, but this is not prohibitive in most cases. The proximal anastomosis may be fashioned as a beveled anastomosis incorporating the orifices of the renal and visceral arteries, or a Carrel patch can be fashioned from the aortic segment with reimplantation or bypass of the left renal artery in situations where the aneurysm involves the entire visceral segment.

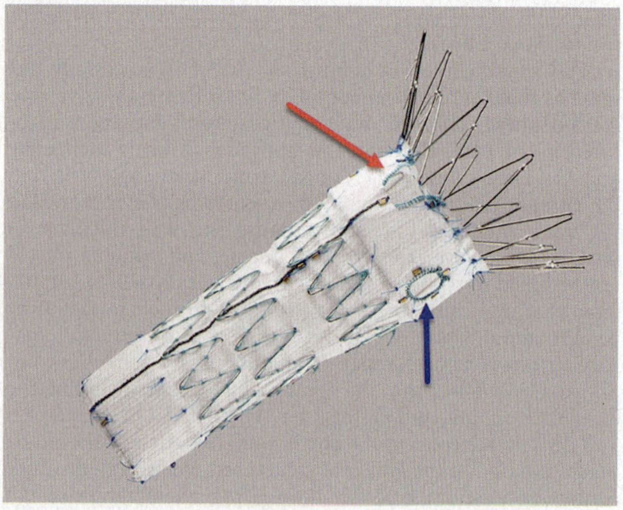

Figure 91.12. The Cook Zenith Fenestrated endograft is a custom-made endograft indicated for the endovascular repair of juxtarenal abdominal aortic aneurysms. Its design permits the fabrication of fenestrations and/or scallop to maintain perfusion visceral/renal artery perfusion. A scallop is often used for perfusion of the superior mesenteric artery (*red arrow*), and small scallop is used for the renal artery (*blue arrow*). (Courtesy of Cook Medical.)

For juxtarenal aneurysms repaired through the *transperitoneal* approach, the aorta can be clamped in the supraceliac or suprarenal position, depending on the extent of the disease and the patient's body habitus. Suprarenal clamp is preferred to avoid unnecessary visceral ischemia. Of course, if the aneurysmal tissue extends above the renal arteries, a supraceliac clamp may be required. The supraceliac exposure is similar to that described in the previous section for a ruptured infrarenal AAA, but performed in a more controlled fashion. If a clamp is to be placed in the suprarenal position, this is facilitated by retracting the left renal vein superiorly or inferiorly after ligating its adrenal, gonadal, and lumbar branches. As noted previously, the left renal vein may be ligated near its confluence with the vena cava without adverse sequelae, provided that its branches are preserved. The anterior surface of the aorta at the level of the visceral vessels is encased by dense neural tissue, which can be incised. Incising the crus of the diaphragm that envelops the lateral aspect of the aorta further facilitates clamp application. The configuration of the proximal anastomosis in the setting of the transperitoneal approach depends on the extent of the aneurysm and the vessels involved.

EVAR for juxtarenal AAAs has become widely available with the FDA approval of the Zenith Fenestrated Endovascular Graft (Cook Medical) in 2012. The approach is based upon constructing a suitable landing zone for the more traditional endograft in patients with an inadequate or short infrarenal neck (<4 mm). This is accomplished using a custom-designed fenestrated endograft that contains a combination of fenestrations and/or scallops that correspond to the renal and superior mesenteric arteries (SMA) (**Fig. 91.12**). There are, however, several restrictions as to where the fenestrations/scallops can be placed on the endograft. The typical combination is two small fenestrations for the renal vessels and a scallop or large fenestration for the SMA. The fenestrations permit the introduction of individual covered stents into the side-branch vessels once they are selected from within the endograft. For aneurysms that extend further cephalad on the aorta, (ie outside of the IFU for the ZFEN device), fenestrations and/or branches are necessary for all visceral and renal vessels in order to obtain adequate proximal seal. Such a configuration requires more complex device designs that are accomplished through physician modifications of an endograft (PMEG) (outside of the IFU) on the back table under sterile conditions, ordered through company-manufactured custom-made device (CMD) programs, off-the-shelf devices, or with chimney/parallel grafts. It is important to note that access to CMDs is limited to a select number of centers in the United States and that PMEG should ideally be performed under the auspices of an investigational device exemption clinical trial. Additional details regarding these complex devices are beyond the scope of this chapter.

The worldwide experience with fenestrated EVAR (FEVAR) for juxtarenal aneurysms is vast, and the technique has been shown to be safe and effective. Oderich et al. reported a 100% technical success rate with a 1.5% 30-day mortality in the prospective Zenith Fenestrated trial.[37] A meta-analysis comparing FEVAR to open repair for juxtarenal AAAs demonstrated significantly better 30-day mortality and complication (acute renal failure, spinal cord ischemia, bowel ischemia) rates for FEVAR.[76] However, long-term survival remains equivocal between the two approaches, with a reported 4-year overall survival of 81% and 87% for open repair and FEVAR, respectively.[77]

Combined endovascular and open (ie, "hybrid") approaches have also been used to treat the juxtarenal and more complex proximal aneurysms. These techniques are based upon constructing a suitable aortic neck to land a traditional endograft by "debranching" the renal or visceral vessels. For example, a suitable landing zone below the SMA could be created for a juxtarenal aneurysm by performing bilateral iliorenal bypasses. These debranching procedures, however, are typically reserved for those who have a true thoracoabdominal aortic aneurysm as opposed to a juxtarenal aneurysm.

Infected Abdominal Aortic Aneurysms

Infected AAAs comprise a small subset of all AAAs, accounting for less than 1% of all repairs. The term *mycotic aneurysm* coined by William Osler to describe aneurysms that developed after septic cardiac emboli caused an arterial infection, has often been used to refer to all infectious etiologies for aneurysms. Unfortunately, "mycotic" is a misnomer that has led to a significant amount of confusion. A more specific classification system consists of four groups based on the underlying mechanism: (a) classic "mycotic aneurysm" caused by embolus from the heart infecting an artery; (b) microbial arteritis, in which bacteria infects an atherosclerotic but nonaneurysmal artery and leads to aneurysmal degeneration; (c) an existing aneurysm that becomes infected; (d) traumatic pseudoaneurysm with concomitant bacterial inoculation. Microbial arteritis resulting from hematogenous bacterial spread currently accounts for approximately 80% of all cases of infected aortic aneurysms.[78] *Salmonella* causes approximately 40% of all aneurysmal infections in contemporary series, with the remainder caused by *Staphylococcus, Streptococcus, Bacteroides, Escherichia coli,* and *Pseudomonas aeruginosa.*[78]

The diagnosis of infected aortic aneurysm is often difficult and the clinical presentation is insidious. Patients may present with fever, back/abdominal pain, or both. The physical examination is often remarkable for a palpable abdominal mass and the presence of peripheral emboli. Laboratory studies are notable for an elevated leukocyte count and positive blood cultures although the latter are present only 50% of the time, and negative blood cultures do not exclude the diagnosis. CT is the most useful diagnostic study, and the features suggestive of an infected aneurysm include a periaortic mass, an aneurysm in an atypical location, periaortic fluid or gas, retroperitoneal inflammation, and frank rupture. The angiographic finding of a saccular or eccentric/irregularly shaped aneurysm in an atypical location is also suggestive of an infected aneurysm.

So long as the patient is an operative candidate, the treatment of an infected aneurysm requires control of hemorrhage in the presence of rupture, aggressive debridement of all infected tissues, and restoration of perfusion to the viscera and lower torso. Indeed, these treatment concerns and the management options are identical to those for patients with infected aortic grafts. Patients should be started on broad-spectrum antibiotics when the diagnosis is suspected, although antibiotic therapy alone is insufficient, and the operative intervention should not be delayed in an attempt to sterilize the retroperitoneum. Patients with suspected rupture should undergo emergent exploration through either a transperitoneal or retroperitoneal approach. After vascular control has been obtained, the retroperitoneum should be explored, and intraoperative cultures, along with stat Gram stain, should be obtained as the organism class may impact reconstruction and conduit selection as follows. Several options for arterial reconstruction are available, depending on the clinical scenario and the individual patient's anatomy. These options include in situ replacement with autogenous femoral vein or a prosthetic or cadaveric graft, ligation of the infrarenal aorta with extra-anatomic bypass (axillofemoral, femoral–femoral configuration), or in situ replacement with staged extra-anatomic bypass and subsequent removal of the in situ graft. The choice is contingent on the character of the aorta, degree of inflammation in the retroperitoneum, suspected organism, and hemodynamic status. In situ replacement of the infected aneurysm with a prosthetic or cadaveric graft is a reasonable option if retroperitoneal inflammation is minimal and the Gram stain is negative. The integrity of the aortic stump at the time of ligation and the potential for dehiscence or breakdown of the suture line are major concerns. The aorta should be debrided back to grossly uninvolved tissue and sutured in two layers with a running horizontal mattress and a simple continuous technique using nonabsorbable monofilament suture. A pedicle of omentum should be mobilized and approximated next to the aortic stump to help control the retroperitoneal inflammation and minimize the risk for stump dehiscence (ie, omental flap). When the diagnosis is suspected preoperatively and no evidence of rupture is found, a staged approach with extra-anatomic bypass followed by graft removal may decrease the physiologic impact of any one procedure. The procedures are usually performed 2 to 3 days apart to allow the patients a period of recovery. Patients should be anticoagulated between procedures to prevent thrombosis of the extra-anatomic bypass resulting from competitive flow. Fortunately, the risk of graft thrombosis and graft infection during the intervening period is small.

Endovascular repair of infected aortic aneurysm can be considered an additional alternative. Although the long-term safety of EVAR in this clinical scenario remains unclear, it may serve as a temporizing approach that converts an urgent problem to an elective one.

Infected aneurysms involving the suprarenal aorta pose a particularly challenging problem, but fortunately are uncommon. In situ replacement with a prosthetic or cadaveric graft is frequently the only available option. This can be accomplished in a number of ways, but the principle of aggressive removal of all infected tissue should be adhered to in order to prevent recurrent infection, typically a fatal event. If the thoracic aorta is of good quality, an antegrade debranching of the visceral segment can be performed to limit the ischemia time to the visceral/renal vessels. If there is a contained rupture of the aorta or the tissues are particularly inflamed, it may be best to obtain proximal and distal control above and below the disrupted/infected segment before attempting to dissect the visceral/renal vessels from the inflammatory mass. After obtaining sites for proximal and distal aortic control, a branched prosthetic graft soaked in Rifampin is sewn to the aorta in an end-to-side manner using a partial occluding, side-biting clamp on the thoracic aorta to allow antegrade perfusion during the anastomosis. It is important to leave enough good aorta below this bypass to allow a cross-clamp and separate end-to-end anastomosis. The left renal, SMA, and celiac artery can be bypassed individually in some cases, and then a cross-clamp placed on the aorta distal to the end-to-side graft. The aorta is then transected and aggressively debrided as dictated by the extent of the infection. A separate tube or bifurcated graft can then be sewn from the distal thoracic aorta to the bifurcation of the abdominal aorta, or to the iliac/femoral arteries, as indicated. This technique limits the ischemia time on the individual viscera/renal arteries, and allows full removal of all atherosclerotic material and infected aorta along with the infected periaortic tissues after complete revascularization of the visceral vessels.

Patients with infected aneurysms, regardless of the arterial reconstruction, require long-term antibiotics with tailoring of the medications based on culture results. If culture-directed therapy is not possible, broad-spectrum antibiotics for 6 weeks are indicated. The patient should then be placed on oral antibiotics although the duration of treatment remains unresolved, and many surgeons will treat the patient with lifelong suppressive antibiotics. In addition, patients should undergo serial CT scans to assess the retroperitoneum and the status of the in situ graft as applicable. In the event that stable imaging is obtained over the first few CT scans, later imaging may not be warranted. Predictably, the morbidity and mortality rates associated with infected AAAs are significant, with a 40% mortality rate.[79]

VASCULAR DISEASE

Aortoenteric Fistulae

An aortoenteric fistula is a communication between the aorta and the bowel. The duodenum is involved most commonly at the site where it crosses anterior to the aorta, but the communication can develop between almost any portion of the intestine. Primary aortic fistulae result when an aortic aneurysm erodes into the bowel and are distinctly rare, with a reported incidence of 0.04% to 0.07% in autopsy series.[80] Secondary aortic fistulae result from the erosion of a prosthetic aortic graft into the bowel; they are significantly more common, with a reported incidence of 0.1% to 2.0% after either open[81] or endovascular[82] aortic reconstruction. The management of both primary and secondary aortic fistulae is the same.

The diagnosis of an aortoenteric fistula is often difficult and mandates a high index of suspicion. Patients usually present with gastrointestinal bleeding manifested as either hematemesis or melena. The initial episode of gastrointestinal bleeding is often self-limited and has been described as a "herald" bleed. The diagnosis of aortoenteric fistula should be foremost among the differential when a patient with a known aneurysm or prior aortic reconstruction presents with intestinal bleeding. Patients should undergo endoscopic evaluation of the upper and lower intestinal tract to determine the source of bleeding. It is imperative that the clinical suspicion of an aortoenteric fistula be communicated to the endoscopist to ensure that the third and fourth portions of the duodenum are adequately examined. The endoscopic findings of erosion, thrombus, active bleeding, or visible prosthetic graft in third or fourth portion of the duodenum are diagnostic of an aortoenteric fistula and mandate emergent treatment due to the risk of massive hemorrhage. Mild duodenitis and gastritis without frank erosion are frequently seen at the time of endoscopy and do not exclude the diagnosis of an aortoenteric fistula. Notably, the findings during upper endoscopy are normal in up to 30% of patients. A CT should be performed if the results of endoscopy are inconclusive. The findings on CT that suggest an aortoenteric fistula include inflammation within the retroperitoneum, an anastomotic pseudoaneurysm, close approximation of the bowel and the prosthetic aortic graft or aneurysm, and loss of the normal tissue planes between the duodenum (or any other bowel segment) and the aorta or prosthetic graft. Occasionally, both endoscopy and CT are nondiagnostic despite the clinical suspicion of an aortoenteric fistula. Exploratory laparotomy is recommended in this setting for both diagnosis and treatment. Adherence of the bowel to the aorta at the time of the initial exploration suggests an aortoenteric fistula and mandates obtaining suitable proximal and distal control of the aorta, iliac vessels, or prosthetic graft before further dissection. The diagnosis cannot be excluded until the bowel is entirely separated from the retroperitoneum and graft.

The treatment of an aortoenteric fistula requires repair of the defect in the gastrointestinal tract in addition to repair of the aneurysm or treatment of the infected prosthetic graft.

Treatment of the gastrointestinal defect is usually straightforward and is based on standard surgical principles. After the fistula is disassembled, the edges of the bowel can be debrided and a primary closure performed. A limited bowel resection or enteral diversion may be necessary. The intraoperative and longer-term management of the aortic aneurysm or prosthetic graft is the same as that outlined above for infected aortic aneurysms. In situ replacement of the prosthetic graft or infrarenal aorta using autogenous femoral vein or cryopreserved aortic allograft, ligation of the infrarenal aorta with excision of the prosthetic graft and extra-anatomic bypass, or temporary in situ aortic replacement with staged extra-anatomic bypass and subsequent graft excision are all reasonable options. The decision algorithm is based upon the hemodynamic stability of the patient, their baseline physiologic state, and the anatomy and involvement of the aorta. In older/sicker patients, the most expeditious procedure is best. Replacement of the infected graft using autogenous femoral vein (neo-aorto-iliac system [NAIS]) is reasonably well tolerated in younger/healthier patients, and may be a better option that obviates the risk of aortic stump blow out. If the visceral segment is involved, ligation of the aorta may not be possible without sacrifice of the renal arteries. In any case, these patients should be maintained on long-term antibiotics and undergo serial imaging studies, as outlined for infected aneurysm patients.

Venous Anomalies Relevant to Aortic Surgery

Anomalies of the vena cava and renal veins are occasionally encountered at the time of aortic reconstruction. The common anomalies are related to the embryologic development of the iliac veins and vena cava. The four most clinically relevant anomalies include duplication of the inferior vena cava (0.2% to 3.0%), left-sided vena cava (0.2% to 0.5%), circumaortic left renal vein (1.5% to 8.7%), and retroaortic renal vein (1.2% to 2.4%).[83] Patients with a duplicated inferior vena cava have large veins that run parallel to the infrarenal aorta and join together either anterior or posterior to the aorta at the level of the renal vein. In the case of a left-sided inferior vena cava, the cava runs parallel to the left side of the aorta, and the normally located right-sided vena cava is absent. The left-sided vena cava typically crosses the aorta at the level of the renal vein to become the suprarenal inferior vena cava, and the gonadal and adrenal veins on the right drain directly into the renal vein in a mirror image of the normal anatomy. The circumaortic left renal vein forms a collar of veins that surrounds the aorta at the normal level. In the case of a retroaortic left renal vein, a single vein runs posterior to the aorta at a slightly more caudal location. Notably, both duplication of the inferior vena cava and left-sided vena cava can be associated with other venous anomalies, including a circumaortic or retroaortic renal vein.

The diagnosis of the various venous anomalies can usually be made preoperatively on CT. Identification of the vena cava and left renal vein should be part of the mental checklist used when the preoperative CT scans are reviewed. The various anomalies may not become evident immediately in the operating room if missed on the preoperative imaging studies. A very prominent left renal vein at the usual location or slightly inferior is suggestive of a left-sided vena cava, whereas the absence of a left renal vein despite dissection along the anterior aspect of the aorta at the level of the SMA is suggestive of a retroaortic renal vein.

Open repair of an infrarenal AAA in a patient with a venous anomaly is essentially the same as the standard approach, although additional care should be exercised to prevent inadvertent injury of the aberrant vein. Exposure of the infrarenal neck is more difficult in the presence of a duplicated or left-sided vena cava. However, sufficient exposure can usually be obtained by gentle dissection and mobilization of the venous structures. The presence of a duplicated or left-sided vena cava is a relative contraindication to the left retroperitoneal approach. A circumaortic left renal collar or retroaortic left renal vein presents a potential hazard when the proximal aortic clamp is applied. A vertical aortic clamp is recommended and obviates the dissection on the posterior aspect of the aorta. Transecting the aorta may facilitate exposure of a retroaortic renal vein when significant bleeding is encountered.

Renal Anomalies

Congenital variations in the kidney anatomy may complicate the repair of an AAA. Specifically, aberrant kidney anatomy may complicate the dissection during open repair because they are frequently associated with multiple renal arteries, aberrant venous return, and abnormally positioned ureters. The various congenital anomalies of the upper urinary system have been classified in an attempt to standardize the approach for vascular surgeons.[84] The anomalies have been broken down into abnormalities of position, including simple ectopia, and abnormalities of both form and fusion, including horseshoe kidney, crossed renal ectopia without fusion, and crossed renal ectopia with fusion. An ectopic kidney may be positioned anywhere from the pelvis to the thorax. Common forms of ectopic kidney include the pelvic kidney, located opposite the sacrum and below the aortic bifurcation; the lumbar kidney, located opposite the sacral promontory in the iliac fossa and anterior to the iliac vessels; the abdominal kidney, located above the iliac crest adjacent to the second lumbar vertebra; and the thoracic kidney, which can be located above the diaphragm in the posterior mediastinum. In a horseshoe kidney, two distinct renal masses are fused together by either a bridge of renal parenchyma or fibrous tissue; in the overwhelming majority, the lower poles are fused. In crossed renal ectopia, the kidney mass is located on the side opposite to its insertion in the bladder. Multiple configurations of crossed ectopia with and without fusion have been described.

The preoperative objective for the various renal anomalies is to image the renal mass adequately, delineate the course of the ureter, and establish the arterial and venous supply. The approach is simplified by the fact that most patients undergo abdominal/pelvic CT as part of the preoperative evaluation. The location and position of both the kidneys and ureters, like the position of the left renal vein, should be established as part of the review of every CT scan for patients with aneurysms.

Patients with renal anomalies can safely undergo repair of an AAA using either an open or endovascular approach. The specific operative approach depends on the location of the renal mass, blood supply, course of the ureters, and presence of fusion. A left-sided retroperitoneal or transperitoneal approach with medial visceral rotation is the most helpful for open repair, particularly in patients with a horseshoe kidney. A standard transperitoneal approach with transection of the fused parenchyma can be used in patients with a horseshoe kidney, although this may be associated with both significant bleeding and a urine leak and, therefore, is discouraged. The multiple renal arteries can be handled most expeditiously by using a Carrel patch technique, in which a cuff of aorta including the renal artery orifices is reimplanted into the aortic graft after completion of the proximal anastomosis. Endovascular repair is possible in many cases, with the feasibility dictated by the location of the renal arteries in addition to the other standard anatomic considerations.

Concomitant Renal or Visceral Artery Occlusive Disease

Concomitant renal or visceral artery occlusive disease is frequently found in patients undergoing AAA repair. The optimal management of patients with coexistent lesions remains unresolved. The options include repair of the aneurysm alone, simultaneous repair of the aneurysm and revascularization of the renal or visceral vessels, and staged repair, with either aneurysm repair or revascularization performed first. Furthermore, the specific treatment options include both open and endovascular alternatives for aneurysm repair and visceral/renal revascularization (ie, angioplasty/stent). The rapid expansion of endovascular technologies has afforded effective, safe approaches that have replaced open surgical revascularization for both renal and visceral artery lesions to a great degree. Regardless, the optimal approach represents a balance between the indications for the procedure and the associated added risk.

Renal/visceral revascularization is mandatory at the time of open aneurysm repair if the affected vessels are involved in the aneurysm, as in a suprarenal aneurysm or a horseshoe kidney. More commonly, a lower pole or accessory renal artery may arise from the aneurysm. The decision to perform a concomitant revascularization with either reimplantation or a bypass graft in this setting depends on the size of the vessel and the quantity of kidney parenchyma perfused. Revascularization is recommended for larger vessels (>3 mm) that supply a significant portion of the renal mass. The presence of any accessory renal arteries should factor into the operative plan and the general feasibility for endovascular repair. Covering small, accessory renal arteries with an endograft has been reported to be safe with no significant decline in renal function.[85]

Combined aneurysm repair with renal or visceral artery revascularization may be justified if the indications for renal or visceral artery revascularization are satisfied. The traditional indications for renal revascularization included poorly controlled hypertension in a patient with a significant renal artery stenosis and rapidly progressive renal insufficiency in a patient with adequate renal mass and bilateral renal artery stenosis. However, the antihypertensive agents have improved to the point that renal revascularization is currently reserved for patients with poor blood pressure control despite optimal medical therapy with at least three separate medications, including a diuretic. Endovascular treatment of renal artery stenosis (when indicated) can be performed prior to open aneurysm repair or simultaneously with the endovascular approach.

The traditional indications for mesenteric revascularization include symptoms of chronic mesenteric ischemia and critical stenosis of either the SMA alone or two of the three visceral vessels. Patients with chronic mesenteric ischemia and AAAs should have their visceral occlusive disease corrected prior to aneurysm repair when possible. Repairing the aneurysm first potentially increases the risk of developing acute mesenteric ischemia in the perioperative period, and performing concomitant mesenteric revascularization with AAA repair carries significant morbidity/mortality over and above that seen with open mesenteric revascularization alone.[86] Endovascular treatment with stent placement is probably the optimal treatment for the visceral lesions, but long-term surveillance is necessary given reintervention rates.

The optimal treatment for patients with aneurysms and *asymptomatic* renal or visceral artery lesions remains poorly defined. Ultimately, consideration should be given to mesenteric revascularization prior to aneurysm repair in patients with severe, asymptomatic visceral artery occlusive disease due to the potential risk of mesenteric infarction at the time of aneurysm repair, as noted in the previous section.

Additional Concurrent Intra-abdominal Disease

The finding of an AAA and an additional intra-abdominal process that may require operative repair is a frequent event. A second surgical problem may be identified as part of the preoperative evaluation or discovered at the time of the exploratory laparotomy during open aneurysm repair. Alternatively, an AAA may be identified during the surgical treatment of another problem. No algorithms have been defined for the management of such concurrent problems, and the overall approach certainly requires sound clinical judgment. Options include simultaneous performance of the necessary operations or a staged operation with repair of the AAA as either the first or second procedure. The approach depends on the risk for aneurysm rupture, the natural history of the second surgical problem, and the potential for infection of the prosthetic graft during simultaneous repair. Notably, both the laparoscopic and endovascular approaches have impacted the approach to patients with combined problems, due to their reduced morbidity and mortality facilitates a more rapid, definitive treatment.

The generic recommendation for patients with an AAA and an additional intra-abdominal surgical problem is that the most life-threatening problem be addressed first. The natural history of untreated AAA has been defined reasonably. It has been suggested that the risk for aneurysm rupture is increased after major intra-abdominal surgery and that it is potentially related to an increase in collagenase activity.[87] However, this reported increased rupture risk is speculative and should not necessarily be factored into the decision algorithm. The management of concurrent colon cancer and AAA is a frequent treatment dilemma that provides an excellent illustration of the approach to these problems. Indeed, the reported incidence of colon cancer and an AAA occurring simultaneously ranges from 0.5% to 2.1%.[54] The treatment principles include the following: (a) aneurysm repair first in the presence of rupture; (b) colon resection first in the presence of hemorrhage, perforation, or obstruction; (c) aneurysm repair first in the presence of a large aneurysm and a small colon cancer; (d) colon resection first in the presence of a large colon cancer and a small aneurysm.[88]

Simultaneous AAA repair and cholecystectomy is probably safe for patients with cholelithiasis or evidence of chronic cholecystitis. The cholecystectomy and other simultaneous procedures should not be performed until after the aneurysm repair is completed and the retroperitoneum is closed in an attempt to reduce the hypothetical risk for graft infection. Again, the exponential rise in EVAR has made some of the concerns previously mentioned somewhat obsolete.

The safety and utility of other simultaneous procedures remain poorly defined, although a wide range of procedures have been combined with open aneurysm repair. The repair of ventral hernias is often mandatory to achieve a tension-free abdominal closure and should be viewed more as an extension of the aneurysm repair than as a simultaneous procedure.

ACKNOWLEDGMENT

We gratefully acknowledge the contributions of previous edition author, Thomas S. Huber, as portions of those chapters have been retained in this revision.

References

1. Dubost C, Allary M, Oeconomos N. Resection of an aneurysm of the abdominal aorta: reestablishment of the continuity by a preserved human arterial graft, with result after five months. *AMA Arch Surg*. 1952;64:405–408.
2. Chaikof EL, Dalman RL, Eskandari MK, et al. The Society for Vascular Surgery practice guidelines on the care of patients with an abdominal aortic aneurysm. *J Vasc Surg*. 2018;67:2–77.e2.
3. Armon MP, Wenham PW, Whitaker SC, Gregson RH, Hopkinson BR. Common iliac artery aneurysms in patients with abdominal aortic aneurysms. *Eur J Vasc Endovasc Surg*. 1998;15:255–257.
4. Taylor LM Jr, Porter JM. Basic data related to clinical decision-making in abdominal aortic aneurysms. *Ann Vasc Surg*. 1987;1:502–504.
5. Kochanek KD, Murphy SL, Xu J. Deaths: final data for 2017. *Natl Vital Stat Rep*. 2019;68:1–77.
6. Sho E, Sho M, Hoshina K, Kimura H, Nakahashi TK, Dalman RL. Hemodynamic forces regulate mural macrophage infiltration in experimental aortic aneurysms. *Exp Mol Pathol*. 2004;76:108–116.
7. Brophy CM, Marks WH, Reilly JM, Tilson MD. Decreased tissue inhibitor of metalloproteinases (TIMP) in abdominal aortic aneurysm tissue: a preliminary report. *J Surg Res*. 1991;50:653–657.
8. Lindholt JS, Jorgensen B, Klitgaard NA, Henneberg EW. Systemic levels of cotinine and elastase, but not pulmonary function, are associated with the progression of small abdominal aortic aneurysms. *Eur J Vasc Endovasc Surg*. 2003;26:418–422.

9. Schermerhorn ML, Bensley RP, Giles KA, et al. Changes in abdominal aortic aneurysm rupture and short-term mortality, 1995-2008: a retrospective observational study. *Ann Surg.* 2012;256:651–658.
10. Cornuz J, Sidoti Pinto C, Tevaearai H, Egger M. Risk factors for asymptomatic abdominal aortic aneurysm: systematic review and meta-analysis of population-based screening studies. *Eur J Public Health.* 2004;14:343–349.
11. Lederle FA, Wilson SE, Johnson GR, et al. Immediate repair compared with surveillance of small abdominal aortic aneurysms. *N Engl J Med.* 2002;346:1437–1444.
12. Darling RC III, Brewster DC, Darling RC, et al. Are familial abdominal aortic aneurysms different? *J Vasc Surg.* 1989;10:39–43.
13. Lou X, Chen EP, Duwayri YM, et al. The Impact of thoracic endovascular aortic repair on long-term survival in type B aortic dissection. *Ann Thorac Surg.* 2018;105:31–38.
14. Brewster DC, Cronenwett JL, Hallett JW Jr, Johnston KW, Krupski WC, Matsumura JS. Guidelines for the treatment of abdominal aortic aneurysms. Report of a subcommittee of the Joint Council of the American Association for Vascular Surgery and Society for Vascular Surgery. *J Vasc Surg.* 2003;37:1106–1117.
15. Mortality results for randomised controlled trial of early elective surgery or ultrasonographic surveillance for small abdominal aortic aneurysms. The UK Small Aneurysm Trial participants. *Lancet.* 1998;352:1649–1655.
16. Brady AR, Thompson SG, Fowkes FG, Greenhalgh RM, Powell JT. Abdominal aortic aneurysm expansion: risk factors and time intervals for surveillance. *Circulation.* 2004;110:16–21.
17. Takagi H, Yamamoto H, Iwata K, Goto S, Umemoto T. Effects of statin therapy on abdominal aortic aneurysm growth: a meta-analysis and meta-regression of observational comparative studies. *Eur J Vasc Endovasc Surg.* 2012;44:287–292.
18. Huber TS, Wang JG, Derrow AE, et al. Experience in the United States with intact abdominal aortic aneurysm repair. *J Vasc Surg.* 2001;33:304–310; discussion 310–311.
19. Prinssen M, Verhoeven EL, Buth J, et al. A randomized trial comparing conventional and endovascular repair of abdominal aortic aneurysms. *N Engl J Med.* 2004;351:1607–1618.
20. Endovascular aneurysm repair versus open repair in patients with abdominal aortic aneurysm (EVAR trial 1): randomised controlled trial. *Lancet.* 2005;365:2179–2186.
21. Schermerhorn ML, O'Malley AJ, Jhaveri A, Cotterill P, Pomposelli F, Landon BE. Endovascular vs. open repair of abdominal aortic aneurysms in the Medicare population. *N Engl J Med.* 2008;358:464–474.
22. De Martino RR, Goodney PP, Nolan BW, et al. Optimal selection of patients for elective abdominal aortic aneurysm repair based on life expectancy. *J Vasc Surg.* 2013;58:589–595.
23. Arnaoutakis DJ, Scali ST, Neal D, et al. Surgeon experience association with patient selection and outcomes after open abdominal aortic aneurysm repair. *J Vasc Surg.* 2020;72(4):1325–1336.e2.
24. Bown MJ, Sutton AJ, Bell PR, Sayers RD. A meta-analysis of 50 years of ruptured abdominal aortic aneurysm repair. *Br J Surg.* 2002;89:714–730.
25. Li Y, Li Z, Wang S, et al. Endovascular versus open surgery repair of ruptured abdominal aortic aneurysms in hemodynamically unstable patients: literature review and meta-analysis. *Ann Vasc Surg.* 2016;32:135–144.
26. Lynch RM. Accuracy of abdominal examination in the diagnosis of non-ruptured abdominal aortic aneurysm. *Accid Emerg Nurs.* 2004;12:99–107.
27. Guirguis-Blake JM, Beil TL, Senger CA, Coppola EL. Primary care screening for abdominal aortic aneurysm: updated evidence report and systematic review for the US Preventive Services Task Force. *JAMA.* 2019;322:2219–2238.
28. Sobocinski J, Chenorhokian H, Maurel B, et al. The benefits of EVAR planning using a 3D workstation. *Eur J Vasc Endovasc Surg.* 2013;46:418–423.
29. Hoffman M, Avellone JC, Plecha FR, et al. Operation for ruptured abdominal aortic aneurysms: a community-wide experience. *Surgery.* 1982;91:597–602.
30. Lloyd GM, Bown MJ, Norwood MG, et al. Feasibility of preoperative computer tomography in patients with ruptured abdominal aortic aneurysm: a time-to-death study in patients without operation. *J Vasc Surg.* 2004;39:788–791.
31. Hirsch AT, Haskal ZJ, Hertzer NR, et al. ACC/AHA 2005 Practice Guidelines for the management of patients with peripheral arterial disease (lower extremity, renal, mesenteric, and abdominal aortic): a collaborative report from the American Association for Vascular Surgery/Society for Vascular Surgery, Society for Cardiovascular Angiography and Interventions, Society for Vascular Medicine and Biology, Society of Interventional Radiology, and the ACC/AHA Task Force on Practice Guidelines (Writing Committee to Develop Guidelines for the Management of Patients With Peripheral Arterial Disease): endorsed by the American Association of Cardiovascular and Pulmonary Rehabilitation; National Heart, Lung, and Blood Institute; Society for Vascular Nursing; TransAtlantic Inter-Society Consensus; and Vascular Disease Foundation. *Circulation.* 2006;113:e463–654.
32. Powell JT, Brown LC, Forbes JF, et al. Final 12-year follow-up of surgery versus surveillance in the UK Small Aneurysm Trial. *Br J Surg.* 2007;94:702–708.
33. Finlayson SR, Birkmeyer JD, Fillinger MF, Cronenwett JL. Should endovascular surgery lower the threshold for repair of abdominal aortic aneurysms? *J Vasc Surg.* 1999;29:973–985.
34. Beck AW, Goodney PP, Nolan BW, Likosky DS, Eldrup-Jorgensen J, Cronenwett JL. Predicting 1-year mortality after elective abdominal aortic aneurysm repair. *J Vasc Surg.* 2009;49:838–843; discussion 843–844.
35. Dua A, Kuy S, Lee CJ, Upchurch GR Jr., Desai SS. Epidemiology of aortic aneurysm repair in the United States from 2000 to 2010. *J Vasc Surg.* 2014;59:1512–1517.
36. Schanzer A, Greenberg RK, Hevelone N, et al. Predictors of abdominal aortic aneurysm sac enlargement after endovascular repair. *Circulation.* 2011;123:2848–2855.
37. Oderich GS, Greenberg RK, Farber M, et al. Results of the United States multicenter prospective study evaluating the Zenith fenestrated endovascular graft for treatment of juxtarenal abdominal aortic aneurysms. *J Vasc Surg.* 2014;60:1420-8.e1-5.
38. Schneider DB, Milner R, Heyligers JMM, Chakfe N, Matsumura J. Outcomes of the GORE Iliac Branch Endoprosthesis in clinical trial and real-world registry settings. *J Vasc Surg.* 2019;69:367–377.e1.
39. Schurink GW, Aarts NJ, van Bockel JH. Endoleak after stent-graft treatment of abdominal aortic aneurysm: a meta-analysis of clinical studies. *Br J Surg.* 1999;86:581–587.
40. Buth J, Harris PL, van Marrewijk C, Fransen G. The significance and management of different types of endoleaks. *Semin Vasc Surg.* 2003;16:95–102.
41. Powell JT, Sweeting MJ, Ulug P, et al. Meta-analysis of individual-patient data from EVAR-1, DREAM, OVER and ACE trials comparing outcomes of endovascular or open repair for abdominal aortic aneurysm over 5 years. *Br J Surg.* 2017;104:166–178.
42. van Schaik TG, Yeung KK, Verhagen HJ, et al. Long-term survival and secondary procedures after open or endovascular repair of abdominal aortic aneurysms. *J Vasc Surg.* 2017;66:1379–1389.
43. Patel R, Sweeting MJ, Powell JT, Greenhalgh RM. Endovascular versus open repair of abdominal aortic aneurysm in 15-years' follow-up of the UK endovascular aneurysm repair trial 1 (EVAR trial 1): a randomised controlled trial. *Lancet.* 2016;388:2366–2374.
44. Prinssen M, Buskens E, Blankensteijn JD. Quality of life endovascular and open AAA repair. Results of a randomised trial. *Eur J Vasc Endovasc Surg.* 2004;27:121–127.
45. Stroupe KT, Lederle FA, Matsumura JS, et al. Cost-effectiveness of open versus endovascular repair of abdominal aortic aneurysm in the OVER trial. *J Vasc Surg.* 2012;56:901–9.e2.
46. Harris PL, Vallabhaneni SR, Desgranges P, Becquemin JP, van Marrewijk C, Laheij RJ. Incidence and risk factors of late rupture, conversion, and death after endovascular repair of infrarenal aortic aneurysms: the EUROSTAR experience. European Collaborators on Stent/graft techniques for aortic aneurysm repair. *J Vasc Surg.* 2000;32:739–749.
47. Mills JL Sr., Duong ST, Leon LR, et al. Comparison of the effects of open and endovascular aortic aneurysm repair on long-term

renal function using chronic kidney disease staging based on glomerular filtration rate. *J Vasc Surg*. 2008;47:1141–1149.
48. EVAR Trial Participants. Endovascular aneurysm repair and outcome in patients unfit for open repair of abdominal aortic aneurysm (EVAR trial 2): randomised controlled trial. *Lancet*. 2005;365:2187–2192.
49. Fleisher LA, Fleischmann KE, Auerbach AD, et al. 2014 ACC/AHA guideline on perioperative cardiovascular evaluation and management of patients undergoing noncardiac surgery: executive summary: a report of the American College of Cardiology/American Heart Association Task Force on Practice Guidelines. *Circulation*. 2014;130:2215–2245.
50. McFalls EO, Ward HB, Moritz TE, et al. Coronary-artery revascularization before elective major vascular surgery. *N Engl J Med*. 2004;351:2795–2804.
51. Hertzer NR, Beven EG, Young JR, et al. Coronary artery disease in peripheral vascular patients. A classification of 1000 coronary angiograms and results of surgical management. *Ann Surg*. 1984;199:223–233.
52. Bardia A, Sood A, Mahmood F, et al. Combined epidural-general anesthesia vs general anesthesia alone for elective abdominal aortic aneurysm repair. *JAMA Surg*. 2016;151:1116–1123.
53. Fairman AS, Chin AL, Jackson BM, et al. The evolution of open abdominal aortic aneurysm repair at a tertiary care center. *J Vasc Surg*. 2020;72(4):1367–1374.
54. Illuminati G, Calio FG, D'Urso A, Lorusso R, Ceccanei G, Vietri F. Simultaneous repair of abdominal aortic aneurysm and resection of unexpected, associated abdominal malignancies. *J Surg Oncol*. 2004;88:234–239.
55. Behrendt CA, Dayama A, Debus ES, et al. Lower extremity ischemia after abdominal aortic aneurysm repair. *Ann Vasc Surg*. 2017;45:206–212.
56. Johnston KW. Multicenter prospective study of nonruptured abdominal aortic aneurysm. Part II. Variables predicting morbidity and mortality. *J Vasc Surg*. 1989;9:437–447.
57. Regnier P, Lareyre F, Hassen-Khodja R, Durand M, Touma J, Raffort J. Sexual dysfunction after abdominal aortic aneurysm surgical repair: current knowledge and future directions. *Eur J Vasc Endovasc Surg*. 2018;55:267–280.
58. Szilagyi DE. A second look at the etiology of spinal cord damage in surgery of the abdominal aorta. *J Vasc Surg*. 1993;17:1111–1113.
59. Biancari F, Ylonen K, Anttila V, et al. Durability of open repair of infrarenal abdominal aortic aneurysm: a 15-year follow-up study. *J Vasc Surg*. 2002;35:87–93.
60. Velazquez OC, Carpenter JP, Baum RA, et al. Perigraft air, fever, and leukocytosis after endovascular repair of abdominal aortic aneurysms. *Am J Surg*. 1999;178:185–189.
61. Chisci E, Harris L, Guidotti A, et al. Endovascular aortic repair follow up protocol based on contrast enhanced ultrasound is safe and effective. *Eur J Vasc Endovasc Surg*. 2018;56:40–47.
62. Conrad MF, Adams AB, Guest JM, et al. Secondary intervention after endovascular abdominal aortic aneurysm repair. *Ann Surg*. 2009;250:383–389.
63. Perini P, Bianchini Massoni C, Mariani E, et al. Systematic review and meta-analysis of the outcome of different treatments for Type 1a Endoleak after EVAR. *Ann Vasc Surg*. 2019;60:435–446.e1.
64. Zarins CK, Bloch DA, Crabtree T, Matsumoto AH, White RA, Fogarty TJ. Stent graft migration after endovascular aneurysm repair: importance of proximal fixation. *J Vasc Surg*. 2003;38:1264–1272; discussion 1272.
65. Giles KA, Fillinger MF, De Martino RR, Hoel AW, Powell RJ, Walsh DB. Results of transcaval embolization for sac expansion from type II endoleaks after endovascular aneurysm repair. *J Vasc Surg*. 2015;61:1129–1136.
66. O'Donnell TFX, Deery SE, Boitano LT, et al. Aneurysm sac failure to regress after endovascular aneurysm repair is associated with lower long-term survival. *J Vasc Surg*. 2019;69:414–422.
67. Scali ST, McNally MM, Feezor RJ, et al. Elective endovascular aortic repair conversion for type Ia endoleak is not associated with increased morbidity or mortality compared with primary juxtarenal aneurysm repair. *J Vasc Surg*. 2014;60:286–294.e1.
68. Kontopodis N, Galanakis N, Antoniou SA, et al. Meta-analysis and meta-regression analysis of outcomes of endovascular and open repair for ruptured abdominal aortic aneurysm. *Eur J Vasc Endovasc Surg*. 2020;59:399–410.
69. Sweeting MJ, Balm R, Desgranges P, Ulug P, Powell JT. Individual-patient meta-analysis of three randomized trials comparing endovascular versus open repair for ruptured abdominal aortic aneurysm. *Br J Surg*. 2015;102:1229–1239.
70. Hoornweg LL, Wisselink W, Vahl A, Balm R. The Amsterdam Acute Aneurysm Trial: suitability and application rate for endovascular repair of ruptured abdominal aortic aneurysms. *Eur J Vasc Endovasc Surg*. 2007;33:679–683.
71. Karkos CD, Menexes GC, Patelis N, Kalogirou TE, Giagtzidis IT, Harkin DW. A systematic review and meta-analysis of abdominal compartment syndrome after endovascular repair of ruptured abdominal aortic aneurysms. *J Vasc Surg*. 2014;59:829–842.
72. Sandhu RS, Pipinos II. Isolated iliac artery aneurysms. *Semin Vasc Surg*. 2005;18:209–215.
73. Stone WM, Fankhauser GT, Bower TC, et al. Comparison of open and endovascular repair of inflammatory aortic aneurysms. *J Vasc Surg*. 2012;56:951–955; discussion 955–956.
74. Knott AW, Kalra M, Duncan AA, et al. Open repair of juxtarenal aortic aneurysms (JAA) remains a safe option in the era of fenestrated endografts. *J Vasc Surg*. 2008;47:695–701.
75. Patel VI, Lancaster RT, Conrad MF, et al. Comparable mortality with open repair of complex and infrarenal aortic aneurysm. *J Vasc Surg*. 2011;54:952–959.
76. Doonan RJ, Girsowicz E, Dubois L, Gill HL. A systematic review and meta-analysis of endovascular juxtarenal aortic aneurysm repair demonstrates lower perioperative mortality compared with open repair. *J Vasc Surg*. 2019;70:2054–2064.e3.
77. Freyrie A, Gargiulo M, Gallitto E, et al. Abdominal aortic aneurysms with short proximal neck: comparison between standard endograft and open repair. *J Cardiovasc Surg (Torino)*. 2012;53:617–623.
78. Brown SL, Busuttil RW, Baker JD, Machleder HI, Moore WS, Barker WF. Bacteriologic and surgical determinants of survival in patients with mycotic aneurysms. *J Vasc Surg*. 1984;1:541–547.
79. Fillmore AJ, Valentine RJ. Surgical mortality in patients with infected aortic aneurysms. *J Am Coll Surg*. 2003;196:435–441.
80. Taheri SA, Kulaylat MN, Grippi J, Ricotta JJ, Kale J, Bernhard H. Surgical treatment of primary aortoduodenal fistula. *Ann Vasc Surg*. 1991;5:265–270.
81. Howard R, Kurz S, Sherman MA, Underhill J, Eliason JL, Coleman DM. Contemporary management of secondary aortoduodenal fistula. *Ann Vasc Surg*. 2015;29:1614–1618.
82. Hosaka A, Nemoto M, Motoki M, Akai A, Kato M. Aortoduodenal fistula after endovascular abdominal aortic aneurysm repair. *Vasc Endovascular Surg*. 2020;54(5):445–448.
83. Aljabri B, MacDonald PS, Satin R, Stein LS, Obrand DI, Steinmetz OK. Incidence of major venous and renal anomalies relevant to aortoiliac surgery as demonstrated by computed tomography. *Ann Vasc Surg*. 2001;15:615–618.
84. de Virgilio C, Gloviczki P, Cherry KJ, et al. Renal artery anomalies in patients with horseshoe or ectopic kidneys: the challenge of aortic reconstruction. *Cardiovasc Surg*. 1995;3:413–420.
85. Antoniou GA, Karkos CD, Antoniou SA, Georgiadis GS. Can an accessory renal artery be safely covered during endovascular aortic aneurysm repair? *Interact Cardiovasc Thorac Surg*. 2013;17:1025–1027.
86. Derrow AE, Seeger JM, Dame DA, et al. The outcome in the United States after thoracoabdominal aortic aneurysm repair, renal artery bypass, and mesenteric revascularization. *J Vasc Surg*. 2001;34:54–61.
87. Swanson RJ, Littooy FN, Hunt TK, Stoney RJ. Laparotomy as a precipitating factor in the rupture of intra-abdominal aneurysms. *Arch Surg*. 1980;115:299–304.
88. Morris DM, Colquitt J. Concomitant abdominal aortic aneurysm and malignant disease: a difficult management problem. *J Surg Oncol*. 1988;39:122–125.

92

Lower Extremity Aneurysms

Chandler A. Long and Robert J. Beaulieu

Key Points

1. Femoral artery aneurysms are the most common peripheral aneurysm if both true and false aneurysms are considered together. Popliteal artery aneurysms are the most common true peripheral aneurysm.
2. Femoral and popliteal aneurysms are often incidental findings on imaging or routine physical examination.
3. Extremity aneurysms are potentially limb threatening and frequently associated with other aneurysmal disease, including life-threatening abdominal aortic aneurysms.
4. Screening imaging studies should be done to evaluate for concurrent abdominal aortic aneurysms or contralateral femoral or popliteal artery aneurysms.
5. Anastomotic aneurysms result from a disrupted suture line between a graft and the host artery.
6. Pseudoaneurysms after percutaneous intervention result from failed hemostasis.
7. Femoral artery aneurysms should be repaired at a size ≥3.5 cm, if intraluminal thrombus is present, or if symptomatic.
8. Popliteal artery aneurysms should be repaired at a size of 2 to 3 cm (for high-risk patients) or if symptomatic, to prevent limb-threatening complications.
9. Thrombolytic therapy is a useful adjuvant in patients presenting with acute limb ischemia secondary to thrombosis of a popliteal artery aneurysm.

PERIPHERAL ANEURYSMS

1 Peripheral aneurysms differ in natural history compared to aortic and visceral aneurysms primarily due to their potential for thrombotic and/or embolic complications that threaten limb viability, often more so than the risk of rupture. Among peripheral lower extremity true aneurysms, popliteal artery aneurysms are the most common. Iatrogenic and anastomotic pseudoaneurysms are more frequently observed in the common femoral artery, resulting in the femoral artery being the most common location for any (true or false) peripheral aneurysm.

Incidence

An aging population, increased arterial trauma, more common use of invasive therapies for vascular disease, and increased use of imaging modalities all contribute to the rise in number of peripheral aneurysms being diagnosed. Lower extremity aneurysms can be isolated and also found with synchronous aneurysms in other vascular beds, most commonly the abdominal aorta and iliac arteries. An increasing number of false aneurysms—"pseudoaneurysms"—are occurring coincident with the increased use of catheter-based diagnostic and therapeutic interventions in addition to lower extremity bypass surgery. Pseudoaneurysms can be iatrogenic, infectious, or traumatic in nature and are identified by their lack of involvement of all three vessel wall layers, as compared to true aneurysms.[1]

Degenerative, or atherosclerotic, femoral and popliteal artery aneurysms are encountered far more frequently in men than women. The male to female ratio in patients with femoral and popliteal aneurysms is about 30:1.[2,3] This predilection for men is markedly different from aortic aneurysms, where male to female patient ratio is approximately 4:1.[4]

Pathogenesis

The etiology of femoral and popliteal aneurysms has changed significantly since they were first described centuries ago. Once primarily infectious in origin, most true aneurysms in the 21st century have a degenerative etiology, commonly called *atherosclerotic aneurysms*. One factor believed to contribute to aneurysm formation is turbulent flow beyond a relative stenosis resulting in post stenotic dilatation beyond the inguinal ligament at the groin or beyond the tendinous hiatus of the adductor magnus or the arcuate popliteal ligament and the heads of the gastrocnemius muscle at the popliteal level. Arterial wall fatigue resulting from vibration and turbulence proximal to a major branching or caused by stress during hip and knee flexion may also contribute to aneurysm formation. There are multiple factors that contribute to aneurysmal degeneration and are felt to contribute to degenerative femoral and popliteal aneurysms, as well as aortic aneurysms. The presence of an inflammatory infiltrate has been noted in the wall of femoral and popliteal aneurysms, similar to aortic aneurysms.[5] The exact role of this inflammatory process, with potential release of reactive oxygen species and matrix metalloproteinases, is unknown. Apoptosis of smooth muscle cells may also play a role in the formation of aneurysms by limiting the ability of the arterial wall to respond to the degenerative process.[6] These factors, however, do not explain the male predilection for femoral and popliteal aneurysm formation. X-linked genetic abnormalities for aneurysm formation in popliteal artery aneurysms have not been noted in humans.

FEMORAL ARTERY ANEURYSMS

2 Femoral artery aneurysms are the most common peripheral aneurysm if both true and false aneurysms are considered together, with the vast majority being pseudoaneurysms. Their clinical significance is related to limb-threatening complications from thrombosis, embolization, or rupture. True aneurysms are predominantly degenerative from atherosclerosis, whereas femoral pseudoaneurysms include anastomotic, traumatic, and mycotic lesions.

Degenerative (Atherosclerotic) Aneurysms

Incidence

The exact incidence of degenerative (atherosclerotic) common femoral artery aneurysms in the general population remains undefined; one study suggests 5 in 100,000 patients may be affected.[3] A recent meta-analysis estimated that femoral aneurysms represent roughly 3% of all peripheral aneurysms, with the majority (80%) found the common femoral location, 15% in the superficial femoral segment and only 5% in the profunda distribution.[7] Femoral aneurysms are found in 6.8% of all patients with abdominal aortic aneurysms; conversely, 85% of patients with femoral artery aneurysms have abdominal aortic aneurysms.[4,2] True profunda femoral artery aneurysms, as stated above, are exceedingly rare (0.5% of all peripheral artery aneurysms) but comprehensive review on isolated profunda aneurysms reported a rupture rate of 18.5%.[8]

Pattern of Disease

As with all aneurysms, femoral artery aneurysms are defined as being greater than 1.5 times the diameter of the disease-free proximal adjacent arterial segment. The average diameter of the common femoral artery is approximately 8 to 10 mm, with variations based on age and sex; an average of 9.8 mm in males and 8.2 mm in females was demonstrated in healthy volunteers.[9] Femoral aneurysms may be classified as *type I*, those limited to the common femoral artery, or *type II*, those involving the orifice of the profunda femoris artery.[10] Type I and type II aneurysms occur with nearly equal frequency. This classification becomes important in reference to vascular reconstructive procedures, with type II aneurysms requiring more complex reconstructions to ensure continued patency of both the superficial and profunda femoris arteries. Isolated lesions of the profunda femoris artery are rare (2% of femoral artery aneurysms), and are prone to rupture because they are difficult to diagnose at the asymptomatic stage. Isolated superficial femoral artery aneurysms are also uncommon, but one-third of patients present with rupture and one-quarter with thrombosis.[11]

Multiple aneurysms are common in patients with femoral artery aneurysms. In a series of 100 patients with degenerative femoral artery aneurysms seen at a single institution, 72% of patients had bilateral femoral artery aneurysms.[2] In addition, aortoiliac aneurysms were detected in 85% of patients, thoracic aortic aneurysms in 6%, and popliteal aneurysms in 44%, of which 55% were bilateral.

Clinical Manifestations

The typical patient with a degenerative femoral artery aneurysm is a male in his 6th or 7th decade of life with the usual risk factors associated atherosclerosis. Tobacco use, hypertension, and coronary artery disease were among the most common comorbidities, followed by diabetes mellitus and cerebral vascular disease.[2]

As with aneurysms in other locations, femoral artery aneurysms may be complicated by embolization, thrombosis, or rarely rupture. Peripheral embolization may be identified incidentally on angiography or produce signs ranging from mild (ie, spotty discoloration of the toes) to severe (ie, peripheral gangrene). Although embolization is reported in about 10% of aneurysms, the femoral artery aneurysm is not necessarily the source of these emboli because many patients have a concomitant popliteal aneurysm.[2] In larger clinical series, approximately 30% of patients are symptomatic, with thrombotic or embolic events developing in 2.5% to 15% of patients and rupture in 4% to 14%.[3,12,13]

Compression symptoms are present in 34% of patients. Lower extremity venous disease is present in 8%, being attributable to venous obstruction by the femoral artery aneurysm in 4%. A palpable mass is found in 23% of patients, and localized pain in just under 10% of patients with femoral aneurysms.[3,12]

Natural History

The natural history of degenerative femoral artery aneurysms is poorly defined. One study of 236 isolated femoral artery aneurysms found that 66% were asymptomatic on presentation. One hundred and fourteen patients were initially managed nonoperatively, with 64% later undergoing repair, but only 10% of the initial cohort doing so for acute complications. The authors found that femoral artery aneurysms rarely developed complications unless >3.5 cm in size or if intraluminal thrombus was present.[2,3]

Diagnosis

In most cases the diagnosis of femoral artery aneurysm is suspected by the finding of a pulsatile groin mass on routine physical examination or during evaluation for vascular disease. If the femoral artery aneurysm is small or thrombosed, detection on physical examination may be difficult. While a radiograph of the region may demonstrate the calcified rim of an aneurysm, only ultrasonography, computed tomography (CT), or magnetic resonance imaging (MRI) can reliably establish the diagnosis of femoral aneurysm. In addition, these modalities are useful in accurately defining the size of the lesion, thrombus burden, and evaluating associated aneurysmal disease in the distal aorta and popliteal regions. The diagnostic accuracy of arteriography is limited because it demonstrates only the residual patent lumen and an aneurysm filled with smooth mural thrombus may be missed, but the definition of the vascular anatomy distal to the aneurysm (ie, outflow) is helpful in planning the appropriate operative procedure (**Fig. 92.1**).

Treatment

Operative treatment of femoral aneurysms is indicated for asymptomatic aneurysms >3.5 cm in size, or for any size causing local symptoms or presenting with limb-threatening complications. In patients with small, asymptomatic aneurysms, medical therapy with antiplatelet and statin therapy with surveillance is appropriate. When nonoperative management is selected, the size of the aneurysm should be documented by ultrasonography. The patient should be followed at regular intervals with ultrasound scans and careful examination for complications; no consensus guidelines exist for follow-up intervals. Operative

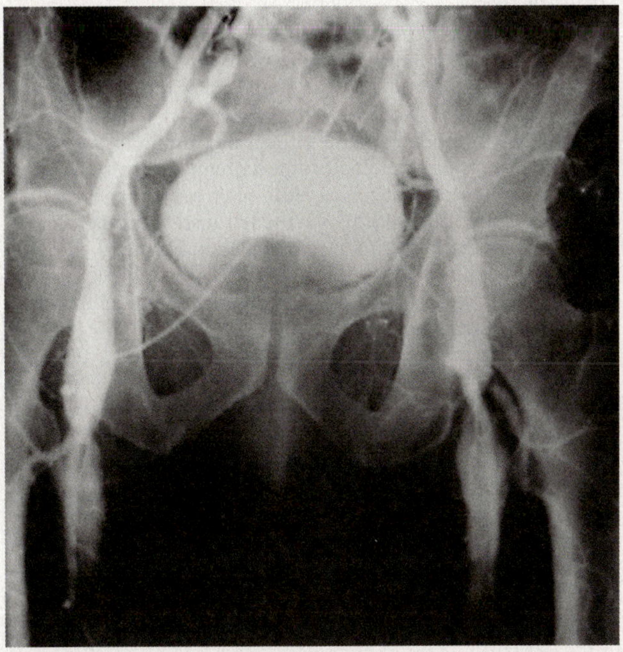

Figure 92.1. Arteriogram demonstrating bilateral femoral artery aneurysms that extend into the superficial femoral arteries. Unlike many patients with femoral artery aneurysms, this patient did not have an associated aortic aneurysm or popliteal aneurysms.

treatment should be undertaken without undue delay if the femoral aneurysm enlarges, produces symptoms, or is complicated by embolization, thrombosis, or rupture.

Surgical Strategy

The operative approach is individualized based on associated aneurysmal disease. In patients with multiple asymptomatic aneurysms, treatment is staged. Generally, aortic aneurysm repair precedes extremity repairs, and popliteal aneurysms are repaired prior to femoral aneurysms. Aortic lesions are treated before femoropopliteal lesions, based on the rationale of life-versus-limb threat. If an aortofemoral bypass is necessary, the femoral aneurysm should be treated at the same time, to avoid later anastomotic aneurysm formation. The graft limb can be anastomosed into an interposition graft that has replaced the femoral aneurysm. Similarly, if a stent graft is placed for treatment of an abdominal aortic aneurysm in a patient with femoral artery aneurysms, the aneurysm should be repaired with an interposition graft. In patients with severe lower extremity ischemia, the femoral aneurysm is treated with an interposition graft, from which the proximal anastomosis of the required femoropopliteal or femorotibial bypass is based.

Technique

The operative procedure for treatment of an isolated femoral artery aneurysm is determined by aneurysmal involvement of the superficial and deep femoral arteries as well as by the existence of lower extremity occlusive disease. The femoral artery aneurysm is usually approached through a longitudinal groin incision. As a special consideration when addressing an unusually large aneurysm or a ruptured aneurysm, however, initial proximal control of the external iliac artery through a retroperitoneal exposure or by percutaneous measures is advisable. After proximal and distal arterial control is obtained, the aneurysm sac is opened and the atheromatous debris is removed. Small aneurysms may be excised, but routine sac excision of large aneurysms is not recommended as these lesions can often be adherent to the adjacent vein and nerve.

For type I aneurysms, the preferred treatment is reconstruction with an interposition graft of Dacron or expanded polytetrafluoroethylene, with the proximal anastomosis at the distal external iliac artery or proximal common femoral artery and the distal anastomosis at the femoral bifurcation.

For type II aneurysms with patent superficial and profunda femoris arteries, an interposition graft to the profunda femoris artery with reimplantation of the superficial femoral artery is one standard configuration. If the superficial femoral artery is chronically occluded and the patient has minimal symptoms, an interposition graft to the profunda femoris artery alone is sufficient. If the patient has severe lower extremity ischemia, this is typically followed by a standard distal reconstruction. If recent emboli or in situ thrombosis has occluded the outflow tract, percutaneous mechanical thromboembolectomy or catheter-directed thrombolytic therapy is useful before open arterial reconstruction is undertaken.

Isolated aneurysms of the superficial femoral artery are uncommon but amenable to both open and endovascular means of repair. Open reconstruction with an interposition graft, using prosthetic or autogenous conduits have been the main stay but endovascular exclusion with a covered stent graft has been used with increased frequency. A recent retrospect study out of Italy found that 25% of patient with true superficial femoral artery aneurysms were treated by endovascular means.[8] Repair of primary isolated profunda femoral artery aneurysm may include reconstruction, ligation, and even embolization based on the anatomy and circumstances of the patient.

Results

Results of surgical therapy depend upon the patency of the distal vasculature (ie, "outflow"). More than 80% of asymptomatic patients have excellent long-term results, whereas 68% of those presenting with lower extremity ischemia achieve satisfactory long-term outcomes.[2] Overall, these patency rates compare favorably with similar bypasses done for occlusive disease, though direct comparisons can be challenging given the difference in reconstruction patterns and targets in aneurysmal disease versus occlusive disease. For instance, CFA atherosclerotic disease may be treated with femoral endarterectomy while aneurysmal disease should be replaced.

Anastomotic Pseudoaneurysms

Incidence

3 Anastomotic pseudoaneurysms result from a disrupted suture
4 line between a graft and the host artery. The incidence varies with the location of the anastomosis and the type of graft that is used. Involvement of the femoral artery accounts for nearly 80% of these lesions, and 3% of all femoral anastomoses.[14,15] After infrainguinal bypass procedures, the incidence is higher with prosthetic grafts than with autogenous vein grafts; 6% of femoral anastomoses develop aneurysms when Dacron is used, compared with 0.9% when a vein graft is placed.[14] Anastomotic pseudoaneurysms are a late complication of bypass procedures; the mean interval from primary procedure to recognition is more than 6 years.[16,17] A notable subset exists in aortofemoral bypass; 6% of femoral anastomoses after aortofemoral bypass develop this complication compared with 0.2% of the proximal aortic anastomoses.[14] Patient factors that are associated with increased likelihood of developing a femoral anastomotic aneurysm after aortofemoral bypass include chronic obstructive pulmonary disease, current smoking, and postoperative groin wound infection.[18]

Pathogenesis

Several factors contributing to anastomotic pseudoaneurysm formation have been identified including: weakness of the arterial wall, the type of graft material and suture utilized, the presence of infection, the method of construction of the anastomosis, and the stress on the suture line from hypertension, leg motion, or excess tension on the graft limb.[14,16,17] Progressive degeneration of the recipient artery accounts for most anastomotic pseudoaneurysms, and an increased incidence has been noted following endarterectomy of the artery at the anastomosis. False aneurysms occur less frequently with saphenous vein grafts than synthetic vascular grafts, a reflection of more complete healing of autogenous tissue. With the use of monofilament synthetic suture, anastomotic pseudoaneurysms rarely result from a loss of suture integrity, although occasionally a broken suture is a factor in pseudoaneurysm formation. Although most anastomotic aneurysms are not accompanied by overt graft infection, occult infections with coagulase-negative *Staphylococcus* species may be an important factor in development of anastomotic aneurysms.[17] A higher incidence is noted in patients with wound-healing complications, and the use of anticoagulants may increase such complications.

Clinical Manifestations

Femoral anastomotic pseudoaneurysms usually present as a pulsatile groin mass, which may or may not be accompanied by pain, redness, or symptoms of venous obstruction. Acute complications include hemorrhage, embolization, and occlusion with acute limb ischemia.

Diagnosis

The diagnosis of an anastomotic pseudoaneurysm is usually made on physical examination by the presence of a pulsatile groin mass in a patient who has undergone a femoral arterial reconstructive procedure. The differential diagnosis includes nonpulsatile groin masses, such as hernia, lymphocele, or abscess, through which pulsation is transmitted from an underlying normal femoral artery. Diagnosis of an anastomotic disruption in one region should raise suspicion of

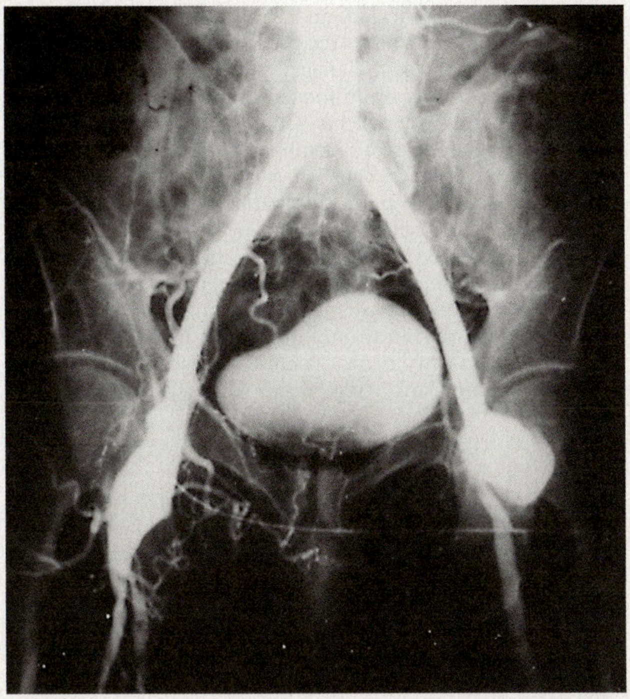

Figure 92.2. Arteriogram demonstrating bilateral femoral anastomotic aneurysms after an aortofemoral bypass and a left femoropopliteal bypass.

other anastomotic pseudoaneurysms as multiple lesions are found in at least 30% of patients.[16] The presence of multiple anastomotic pseudoaneurysms suggests infection. Diagnostic imaging modalities for pseudoaneurysm evaluation include ultrasonography, cross-sectional imaging, and/or catheter-based angiography to define the outflow with heightened spatial resolution (**Fig. 92.2**). Consider inflammatory markers and PET scan when infection is suspected, especially should the patient present with constitutional symptoms and multiple anastomotic pseudoaneurysms.

Treatment

Because of the progressive nature of anastomotic pseudoaneurysms, surgical treatment is generally undertaken for all lesions >2 cm except those in high-risk patients. Principles of surgical therapy are those of primary aneurysms: obtain proximal and distal control and replace the aneurysmal segment. Securing proximal control may require division of the inguinal ligament and/or a suprainguinal retroperitoneal exposure of the graft limb. Distal control is most easily obtained using intraluminal balloon catheters. If intrinsic arterial disease requires extension of the graft distally on the profunda femoris or superficial femoral artery, these arteries can be identified by dissection through unscarred tissue distal to the previous exposure. After debridement of the degenerated artery, an interposition graft is placed between the prosthetic graft limb and the healthy native artery. Cultures of the graft and vessel wall are essential to exclude infection as an etiologic factor in the development of the anastomotic aneurysm. If infection is obvious at the time of surgery, the approach is the same as that of any infected graft with removal of infected prosthetic material and reestablishment of blood flow, if necessary, with a bypass through an uninfected tissue route, such as an obturator, lateral femoral, or axillofemoral bypass.

Results

Results of elective operations on femoral anastomotic pseudoaneurysms are excellent with 2% operative mortality, 97.5% graft patency at 2 years, and 2% amputation within 2 years of surgery.[16] Recurrence is reported in less than 16% of cases.[14,15]

Patients presenting with aneurysms complicated by hemorrhage, occlusion, or embolization have significantly increased operative morbidity and mortality.

Femoral Pseudoaneurysms

Incidence

Femoral pseudoaneurysm incidence has increased as a result increasing diagnostic and therapeutic catheter-based interventions. Therapeutic angiography, for example, often requires prolonged arterial cannulation, large-bore sheaths, and anticoagulation, which are associated with a higher rate of arterial
5 complications than diagnostic studies. One study with routine ultrasound surveillance following 254 therapeutic interventions via femoral access in patients with known arterial disease showed a pseudoaneurysm development rate of 2.75%.[19] A meta-analysis of 7,889 femoral arterial access procedures demonstrated an increase in pseudoaneurysm formation with arterial closure devices (odds ratio 3.8) versus surgical cutdown, albeit with fewer other complications including seroma, surgical site infection, and wound dehiscence.[20] A registry analysis of 12,937 patients undergoing percutaneous interventions through the femoral artery showed pseudoaneurysm rates of 0.6% with manual compression versus 0.1% with arterial closure devices ($P < .5$).[21] The overall reported rate of pseudoaneurysm formation after percutaneous procedures is reported to be anywhere between 0.05% and 8%.[22]

Pathogenesis

Pseudoaneurysms from iatrogenic catheter trauma are defined as collections of blood in continuity with the arterial system, and not enclosed by all three layers of the arterial wall.[23] These lesions form because of failed hemostasis at the arterial wall
6 defect created by sheath insertion. Normally hemostasis seals the defect promptly, aided by direct focal application of pressure or hemostatic devices, and the arterial wall repairs itself. When hemostasis is not successfully obtained, blood under arterial pressure leaks from the artery, dissects surrounding tissue planes, and forms what is perceived on physical examination to be a pulsatile mass. The gross findings at surgery are a blood-filled cavity surrounded by a capsule. As pseudoaneurysms, these lesions can cause symptoms by rupture or compression of surrounding structures.

Diagnosis

The diagnosis of femoral pseudoaneurysm is suspected when a pulsatile groin mass and/or expanding hematoma is noted after arterial catheterization. Duplex ultrasound with color flow or CT is typically used to establish the diagnosis, differentiate pseudoaneurysm from hematoma, and aid in defining the communication between the mass and the arterial lumen. Color-flow duplex scanning is the diagnostic test of choice, providing accurate diagnosis with a characteristic to-and-fro waveform and a "yin-yang" pattern of color swirling, along with localization and sizing of the false aneurysm (**Fig. 92.3**).[24]

Natural History

Color-flow duplex scanning has been used to define the incidence and natural history of pseudoaneurysms after percutaneous transluminal coronary angioplasty.[25] Many pseudoaneurysms smaller than 2.0 cm in diameter will thrombose spontaneously within 4 weeks; anticoagulation and size greater than 2.0 cm are predictors of failure of spontaneous thrombosis. About 30% of patients with pseudoaneurysms will require intervention.[26]

Treatment

Therapy of femoral pseudoaneurysms is influenced by aneurysm size and symptoms, and whether the patient requires continuous anticoagulation (Algorithm 92.1). Surgical intervention is mandatory for all pseudoaneurysms that are acutely expanding, compressing adjacent nerves, or compromising the

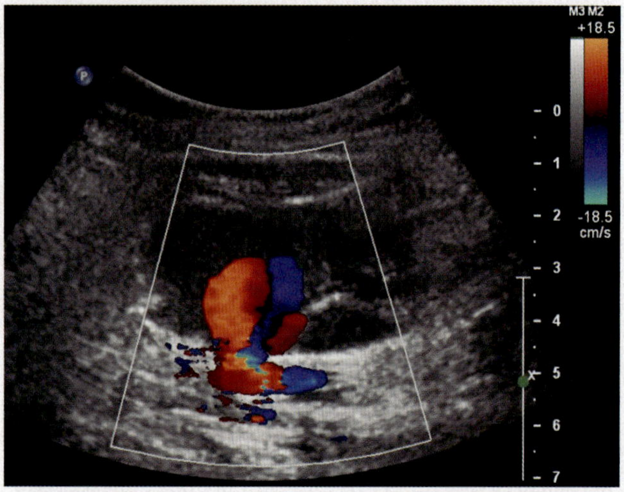

Figure 92.3. Ultrasound findings with a to-and-fro flow pattern in a femoral pseudoaneurysm.

overlying skin viability. Proximal and distal arterial control is obtained, and the arterial defect is repaired directly, rarely requiring placement of more than one or two sutures. Beyond the vascular repair, there is often a significant dead space that is left after evacuation of hematoma or pseudoaneurysm contents. Treatment to collapse this dead space can involve muscle flaps (sartorious being common) and vacuum-assisted closure (VAC) placement. In the setting of compromised overlying skin, resection of devitalized tissue may be prudent to help prevent subsequent wound breakdown and infection.

Ultrasound-guided compression and ultrasound-guided thrombin injections are alternative treatment strategies when urgent evacuation of the hematoma and arterial repair are not required. Compression therapy entails identification with a color-flow ultrasound probe and directed intermittent compression of the pseudoaneurysm with the transducer, allowing the visualization and documentation of flow cessation when effective. This technique may be limited by body habitus, patient discomfort, and requires up to 30 minutes of compression by the ultrasonographer.

Percutaneous ultrasound-guided injection of 0.5- to 1.0-mL thrombin (1000 U/mL) into the pseudoaneurysm sac, at a site away from the neck of the aneurysm.[27–29] Thrombin injection avoids the discomfort of prolonged compression and is effective in anticoagulated patients. Continuous ultrasonographic imaging is used to monitor thrombosis of the pseudoaneurysm. Careful patient selection determines likelihood of success with thrombin injection. In particular, patients with a small diameter (<1 cm), short neck (<0.5 cm), or wide neck (>1.0 cm) are at increased risk for distal embolization with injection of thrombin. However, no consensus guidelines exists regarding which anatomic criteria are most important. Proper visualization of the neck on ultrasound performed by an experienced provider likely allows for the highest chance of success with the lowest complication risk rather than specific anatomic criteria.

Results

A meta-analysis of studies involving 992 patients treated with ultrasound-guided compression versus ultrasound-guided thrombin injection showed pooled success rates of 69.3% versus 97.4%, respectively, without significant difference in the rate of complications.[22]

In one of the largest series of pseudoaneurysms treated with ultrasound-guided compression, thrombosis was achieved in 86% of anticoagulated patients, and in 98% of those not anticoagulated, with a 20% recurrence rate in less than 24 hours in anticoagulated patients.[30] Success using this therapeutic modality requires a knowledgeable ultrasonographer and meticulous postcompression follow-up, though patient discomfort from prolonged compression often renders the technique unsuccessful in achieving hemostasis.

Thrombin injection to induce thrombosis of pseudoaneurysms is successful in 94% to 98% of patients, with thrombosis occurring in less than 1 minute.[27–29] This technique can be complicated by arterial thrombosis if an excessive volume of thrombin is used and may not be appropriate for pseudoaneurysms with large necks. Remote thromboembolic events are rare and probably are not a result of systemic effect of the thrombin. Allergic reactions to bovine thrombin occasionally occur. Large pseudoaneurysms, greater than 8 cm in diameter, and an associated arteriovenous fistula (AVF) are predictors of failure with thrombin injection.[31]

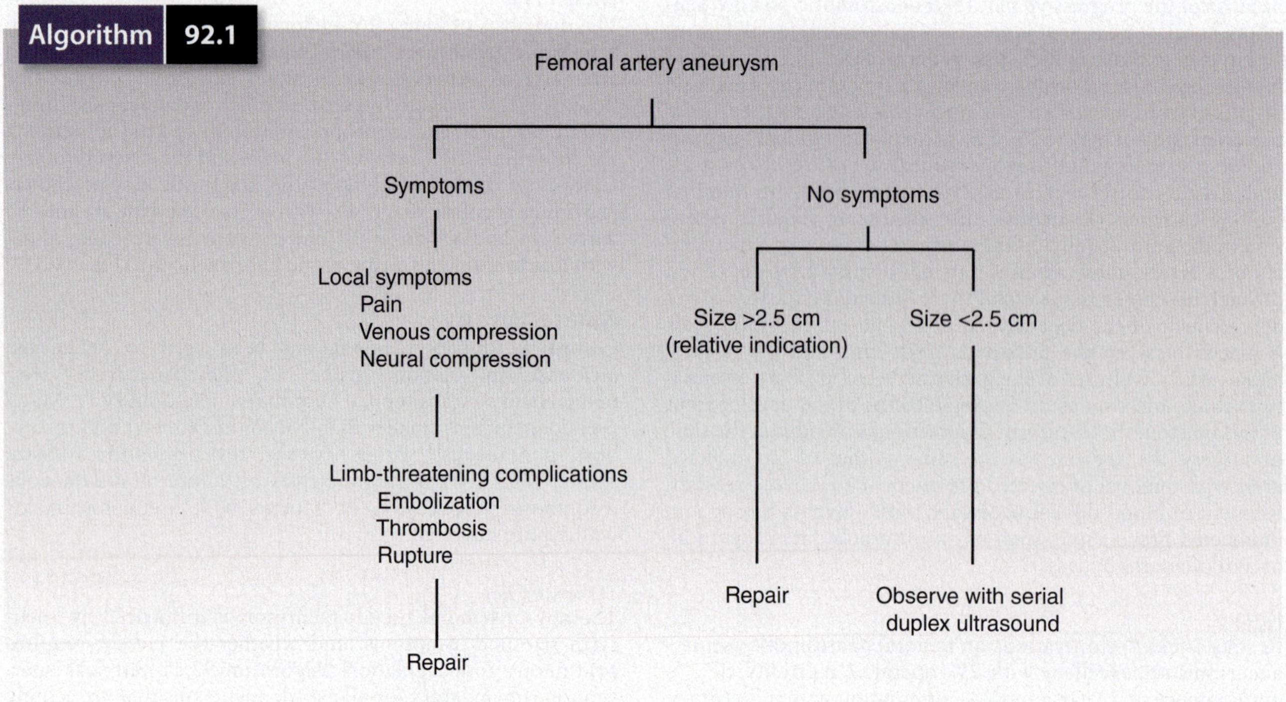

Algorithm 92.1. Management of femoral pseudoaneurysm.

Mycotic Aneurysms

The term *mycotic aneurysm* is currently used to refer to any infected aneurysm. Mycotic aneurysms today are often a complication of parenteral drug abuse but can follow arterial trauma of any form and have been associated with iatrogenic injury, osteomyelitis, endocarditis, or idiopathic etiologies. Historically, septic emboli from bacterial endocarditis were a major cause of mycotic aneurysmal degeneration, as were tuberculosis and late-stage syphilis. With the change in cause, the location of mycotic aneurysms has shifted from central to peripheral arteries, with the femoral artery being the most common site.[32,33] The importance of mycotic aneurysms comes from their propensity to rupture.

Pathogenesis

Mycotic aneurysms may arise from multiple causes. First, septic emboli from bacterial endocarditis may lodge in normal arteries, causing infection that weakens the arterial wall, resulting in aneurysm formation. These lesions are often multiple. Second, during an episode of bacteremia, microorganisms may lodge in a preexisting atherosclerotic plaque or aneurysm and begin to multiply with the same result. A third cause of mycotic aneurysms is the contiguous spread of bacteria from a local abscess. The inflammatory process destroys the arterial wall, leading to pseudoaneurysm formation. Finally, trauma to the artery with concomitant contamination may result in formation of an infected pseudoaneurysm. Bacteria may be introduced concomitantly with needle puncture or by migration during prolonged arterial catheterization. Mycotic aneurysms accompanying drug abuse may be secondary to direct contamination of the arterial wall, or they may result from destruction of the vessel wall by a local abscess.

A contemporary case series of 29 patients with mycotic peripheral aneurysms found *Staphylococcus aureus* in 38.5%, *Streptococcus* sp. in 11.5%, other *Staphylococcus* spp. in 7.7%, and gram-negative rods (*Serratia* and *Pseudomonas* spp.) in 7.7% of patients.[34] Staphylococcal species, *Salmonella* sp., *Escherichia coli*, and *Proteus* sp. have also been cultured. Bacterial cultures may be difficult to obtain when biofilms are formed (either on native arteries or prosthetic conduits) as accurate culture may require specific techniques such as tissue sonication not routinely performed.

Clinical Manifestations

The typical patient with a mycotic femoral aneurysm presents with a history of chills and fever, and a tender, enlarging, pulsatile groin mass. The patient may have a history of intravenous drug use, recent arterial catheterization, penetrating trauma, or bacterial endocarditis. Local signs of infection, including tenderness, erythema, and warmth are noted on physical examination. Lower extremity edema may occur secondary to venous or lymphatic obstruction. Petechial skin lesions, splinter hemorrhages, cutaneous abscesses, and septic arthritis may occur as a result of emboli originating from a mycotic aneurysm. A "sentinel bleed" may occur and signals impending rupture and life-threatening hemorrhage. Urgent or emergent surgical intervention is indicated for these aneurysms.

Diagnosis

The diagnosis of a mycotic aneurysm is usually straightforward, but distinguishing an abscess adjacent to the femoral artery from a femoral mycotic aneurysm may be difficult. In the patient with a pulsatile groin mass, laboratory findings including leukocytosis, elevated erythrocyte sedimentation rate, and positive blood cultures are suggestive, but not specific, for a mycotic aneurysm. Multiple blood cultures or downstream arterial blood cultures may be necessary to yield positive results. Ultrasonography and CT angiography are helpful in establishing the diagnosis of an aneurysm (**Fig. 92.4**) but lack precision in distinguishing infected from bland aneurysms. The diagnosis of a mycotic aneurysm is confirmed at

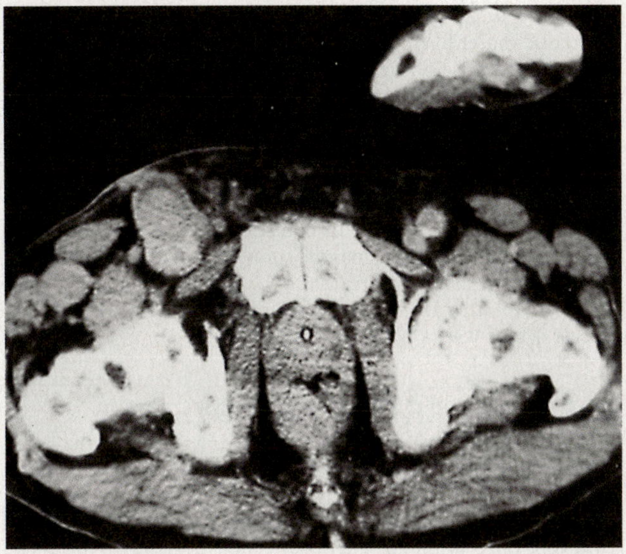

Figure 92.4. Computed tomography scan of an infected femoral anastomotic aneurysm that was diagnosed 5 years after aortofemoral graft placement.

operation by demonstration of organisms on Gram stain or by positive cultures of the aneurysm wall.

Treatment

Mycotic aneurysms represent a serious life- and limb-threatening disease because their natural history is one of expansion and rupture and should therefore be treated when discovered. The goal of treatment is eradication of the infection. Before operative intervention is performed, the patient is started on broad spectrum parenteral antibiotics that are subsequently tailored to culture specificity and sensitivity testing. The complexity of the operative procedure varies with the location and extent of the mycotic aneurysm, with excision, tissue debridement, and staged revascularization through noninfected tissue planes being the main goals of treatment.

Stent grafts have been used in selected cases of mycotic aneurysms when other approaches were not feasible; however, concern about latent infection of the stent graft oftentimes renders this more of a bridging technique than a long-term solution.

Although a direct approach to the femoral artery may be taken, a retroperitoneal exposure of the distal external iliac artery for proximal control is often safest for large or proximal femoral lesions to avoid excessive hemorrhage. In more than 50% of cases, the mycotic aneurysm involves the femoral artery bifurcation, and treatment requires resection of the femoral bifurcation to afford debridement to healthy arterial wall. Three options for repair exist: ligation, immediate revascularization, or selective revascularization. (1) The distal external iliac or proximal common femoral artery, as well as the superficial and deep femoral arteries, are oversewn with nonabsorbable monofilament suture. This results in significant ischemia in most patients, but with the patient heparinized, symptoms gradually improve as collateral circulation increases. The majority of patients will not need revascularization for limb salvage, but up to one-third of patients will have limb-threatening ischemia.[35,36] (2) In patients in whom sepsis can be adequately controlled at the initial procedure, aggressive debridement may be followed by immediate revascularization using autogenous vein graft (GSV vs deep femoral vein) as the conduit and covering the graft with a muscle flap.[36] This technique is most effectively utilized when the area of arterial infection is limited. If the field was significantly contaminated, immediate revascularization will frequently be met with blowout. (3) Another option is to observe patients for 24 hours after arterial ligation and selectively revascularize only those patients in whom limb-threatening ischemia persists. Use of prosthetic material through the original infected tissue planes is avoided because of the high incidence of early and late septic complications. In instances where in situ reconstruction with a prosthetic graft is deemed necessary, consideration for the use of rifampin-soaked dacron graft should be considered. Rifampin will not bond with polytetrafluoroethylene (PTFE) limiting the utility of that graft material. Cryopreserved arterial conduit is another useful consideration in this area.[37] If necessary, synthetic graft may be tunneled through uninfected tissue such as the obturator canal or via the lateral femoral route. Antibiotics are begun preoperatively and continued for at least 4 to 6 weeks postoperatively.

POPLITEAL ARTERY ANEURYSMS

7 Popliteal aneurysms are limb-threatening lesions, the vast
8 majority of which are degenerative in etiology. Rarely, anastomotic, traumatic, or mycotic popliteal aneurysms are encountered in contemporary practice. The remainder of this section
9 addresses only popliteal aneurysms that are degenerative in etiology. To be sure, there are case reports of popliteal aneurysms resulting from septic emboli (mycotic pseudoaneurysms) and iatrogenic perforation (pseudoaneurysm) though management of these is not discussed here. For the purposes of this review, distal superficial femoral artery aneurysms have been grouped into this category due to their similarity in presentation and risks. In instances where treatment may be different, the differences will be outlined. The average popliteal artery size is approximately 4 to 7 mm; one study identified a mean diameter of 5.2 mm in healthy male subjects.[38] Aneurysmal dilatation is defined as arterial diameter greater than 1.5 times the diameter of the disease-free proximal adjacent arterial segment.

Incidence

Popliteal artery aneurysms are the most common degenerative true peripheral aneurysm. They occur slightly more frequently than femoral artery lesions; however, popliteal aneurysms are relatively unusual compared to abdominal aortic aneurysms. Aortic aneurysms are diagnosed with about 10 times the frequency of popliteal aneurysms.[39,40]

Pattern of Disease

Like patients with femoral artery aneurysms, multiple aneurysms occur frequently in patients with popliteal aneurysms. About 50% of patients have bilateral popliteal aneurysms, and 55% have extra-popliteal aneurysms.[41,42] In an observational study of patients with aortic aneurysm, 11% of these patients were found to have a popliteal artery measuring greater than 15 mm, the definition used for aneurysm according to the SVS Clinical Guidelines.[43] Patients with infrarenal aortic aneurysms appear to be at higher risk for concurrent peripheral aneurysms than those with suprarenal aneurysms.[44] The association with other aneurysms has resulted in the recommendation that patients discovered to have femoral or popliteal aneurysms should have completion imaging to exclude contralateral limb aneurysms and abdominal aortic aneurysms.[45] Even when popliteal aneurysms are initially asymptomatic, patients will develop symptoms at a mean rate of 14% per year, and one-third will develop complications requiring emergent intervention within 5 years, resulting in poorer outcomes for both life and limb.[46,47] Perhaps even more concerning, up to 42.8% of "asymptomatic" patients may presented with abnormal pulses.[48]

Clinical Manifestations

The typical patient with a popliteal aneurysm is a male in his 60s or 70s with the usual risk factors for atherosclerosis. Of patients with popliteal aneurysms, 50% to 75% are smokers, 40% to 60% have hypertension, and about 15% have diabetes mellitus.[49–52] Other manifestations of cardiovascular disease are also common, with 10% of patients having manifestations of cerebrovascular disease and more than 40% having evidence of significant cardiac disease.[51]

The clinical manifestations of popliteal artery aneurysms range from an asymptomatic pulsatile mass to severe lower extremity ischemia. About 40% of patients are asymptomatic at diagnosis.[2] More than 50% of patients present with symptoms of chronic limb ischemia, usually claudication, but the ischemia may be more advanced and manifested as rest pain or gangrene. Local symptoms, including sensation of a mass, local pain, and leg swelling or phlebitis secondary to compression of the adjacent vein, account for the remainder of symptoms. A popliteal artery aneurysm may be complicated by thrombosis, embolization, or rarely rupture. Thrombosis is reported in approximately 40% of patients, and embolization occurs in about 25% of cases. This may result in isolated digital embolic occlusion (often asymptomatic), the "blue toe syndrome," or occlusion of multiple tibial outflow vessels. Rupture occurs in fewer than 5% of popliteal aneurysms.[49,50]

Natural History

The natural history of popliteal aneurysms is not well defined because most series are composed primarily of aneurysms that have been treated surgically. The size at presentation and the presence of mural thrombus are independent risk factors for aneurysm growth.[53] In a review of 29 reports in the English literature published between 1980 and 1994, patients whose aneurysms were observed rather than intervened upon showed that a mean of 35% of patients with nonoperative follow-up developed ischemic complications, and 25% of these required amputation even with modern therapy.[2] Thus, a significant percentage of popliteal aneurysms will develop a complication if left untreated, and although this is not synonymous with limb loss, the amputation rate is high. Rupture of popliteal artery aneurysms is reported in only 2% to 4% of cases.[42]

Diagnosis

Palpation of the popliteal space with the knee flexed reveals a pulsatile mass in approximately two-thirds of patients. Small and thrombosed aneurysms may not be palpable. Radiographs of the knee demonstrating a calcified arterial wall occasionally suggest the diagnosis of a popliteal artery aneurysm, but it must be confirmed by duplex ultrasonography, CT (**Fig. 92.5**), or MRI. These diagnostic modalities can establish diagnosis of popliteal artery aneurysms and exclude other etiologies of a popliteal fossa mass (such as tumors or Baker cyst). Angiography can be misleading in the diagnosis of aneurysms because intraluminal thrombus may obscure the true size of the vessel (**Fig. 92.6**); however, it is essential for visualization of the inflow and outflow vessels necessary for revascularization and should include the mid/distal vessels (**Fig. 92.7**).

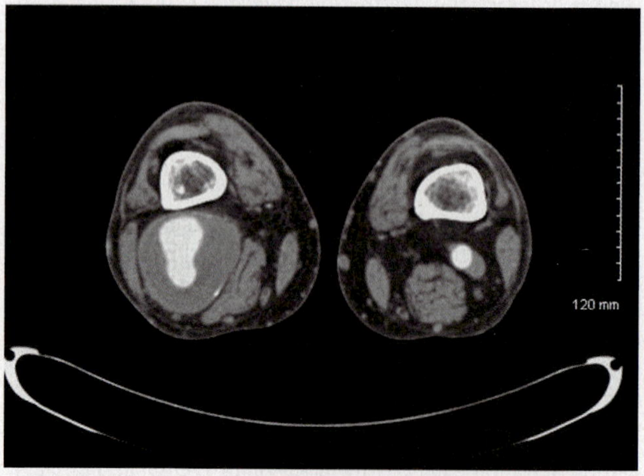

Figure 92.5. Computed tomography of a large right popliteal aneurysm with significant laminar thrombus present.

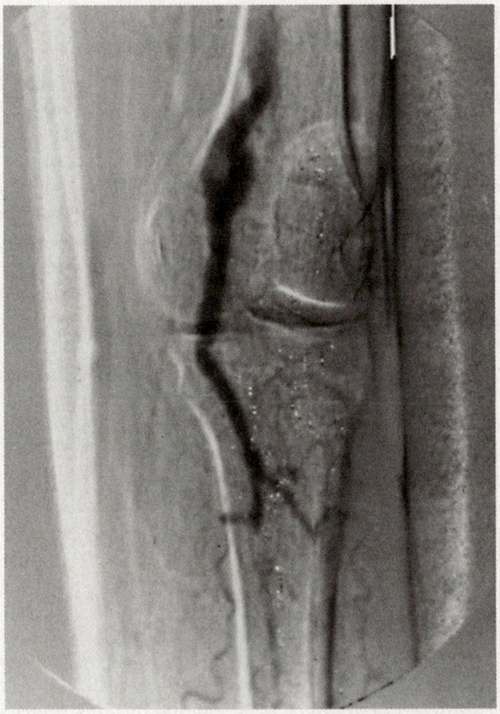

Figure 92.6. Arteriogram demonstrating a popliteal aneurysm associated with occlusion of the outflow tract presumably from repeated episodes of embolization. A bypass to the distal posterior tibial artery was successful.

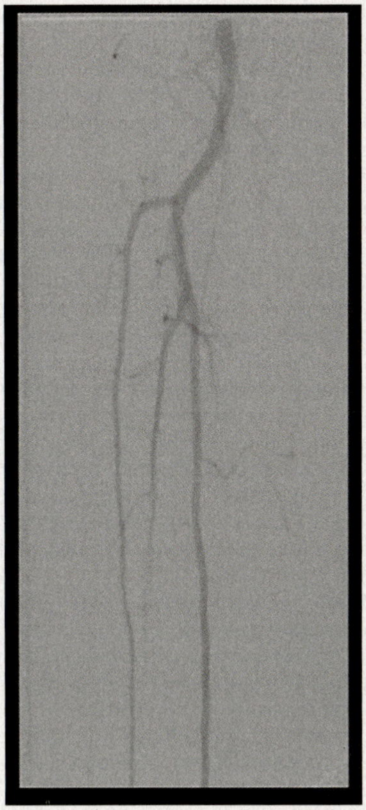

Figure 92.7. Arteriogram demonstrating outflow vessels for popliteal aneurysm with occluded peroneal at mid/distal calf. A successful behind knee popliteal repair was completed.

Treatment

Indications

Surgical treatment is indicated for all symptomatic popliteal aneurysms. Current SVS Clinical Guidelines recommend the consideration of treatment for all aneurysms >20 mm in patients suitable for surgery and up to 30 mm in patients with higher surgical risk.[54] In some instances such as patients with clinical suspicion of thromboembolism and imaging demonstrating poor runoff, repair at size <20 mm may be indicated.[54] Proponents of early repair at smaller sizes cite greater 5-year patency and limb salvage rates with elective aneurysm repair.[41]

The goals of surgical treatment are to eliminate the potential for complications and to preserve or restore adequate blood flow to the limb.

Surgical Technique

Open Approach. Most popliteal aneurysms are easily approached through standard medial thigh and calf incisions for exposure of the distal superficial femoral artery and the distal popliteal artery, respectively. A proximal anastomosis off the common femoral artery is required when the entire superficial femoral artery is aneurysmal or if there is flow-limiting concomitant SFA disease proximal to the anticipated anastomotic site. Alternatively, focal aneurysms contained entirely within the popliteal fossa may be accessed through a posterior popliteal approach and is preferred for those aneurysms confined to the popliteal fossa when accompanied by symptoms due to compression of adjacent structures due to the ability to decompress the aneurysm sac at the time of repair. The posterior approach may additionally allow for a shorter bypass conduit, though it should be noted adequate saphenous vein is less of an issue with even the medial bypass than with typical lower extremity bypasses originating from the CFA given the short course of the bypass from the distal SFA to distal popliteal. Through the medial approach, popliteal aneurysms are left in situ, bypassed using a segment of saphenous vein, and ligated proximally and distally to exclude flow within the aneurysmal segment. If the medial approach is used, surveillance imaging should carefully note the presence of any backfilling geniculate arteries which may pressurize the sac and lead to compressive symptoms.

Conduit. The conduit of choice for bypass may be dependent on the distal target. Traditionally, the conduit of choice is autologous saphenous vein, which is harvested from the thigh, reversed, and tunneled along the course of popliteal artery. Saphenous vein conduit has improved patency outcomes compared to PTFE when the distal target is either a tibial artery, the peroneal artery or the tibioperoneal trunk.[55] However, when the target is the below knee popliteal, the primary patency rates as well as MALE-free survival were similar for prosthetic versus autologous conduit.[55] The proximal and distal anastomosis may be either end to end or end to side in configuration, with the aneurysm excluded from the circulation by proximal and distal ligatures.[56]

Outflow. Popliteal aneurysms, especially those with thrombus in the sac, may result both overt and more "silent" embolization of the tibial outflow vessels. Inadequate tibial outflow is a concern in the management of popliteal artery aneurysms and should be evaluated thoroughly when repairing aneurysms in the elective setting. In acute cases in which the patient presents with limb ischemia, outflow targets may be absent on initial angiography. In these cases, preliminary catheter-directed thrombolytic therapy is indicated prior to bypass.[45] Alternatively, balloon catheter embolectomy may be attempted. In either instance, angiography demonstrating adequate outflow is necessary prior to performing bypass. Frequently, bypass grafts must be carried to the distal tibial arteries. Acute-on-chronic presentations present another unique challenging as the presence of "blue toe" syndrome prior to the acute presentation may severely compromise flow within the foot. In these instances, the surgeon must deem if outflow is adequate to preserve bypass patency and the limb. Extensive, combined femoral and popliteal aneurysms may require a femoral-popliteal or femoral-tibial bypass using in situ saphenous vein with a prosthetic graft segment replacing a common femoral artery aneurysm.

Endovascular Approach. Popliteal aneurysms can be treated with endovascular approaches including covered stent-graft placement to exclude the aneurysm sac. Small series show a primary patency rate of about 50% at 14 to 18 months, and a cumulative patency of 74%, which traditionally relegated this approach for the more high-risk patient who requires intervention.[57–59] However, more recent small series have shown high technical success (100%) and long term patency (89.5%) among patients undergoing endovascular repair with Viabahn endoprosthesis, bringing the original recommendations into question.[60] A large multicenter trial recently completed across several European countries explored both short and long-term patency among patients undergoing elective open repair through a posterior approach and endovascular exclusion of the aneurysm sac. Both groups demonstrated similar and high amputation free survival (99.0% open vs 98.4% endo, $P = .73$) at 5 years; however, primary patency rates (79.8% vs 63.8%; $P = .12$) and overall survival (84.4% vs 79.4%; $P = .05$) were better in the open group despite similar preoperative comorbid status.[61] Overall, the endovascular group was associated with a higher reintervention rate as well. Recent morphologic studies have demonstrated a much higher increase in tortuosity in the popliteal artery (compared with the SFA) in the knee bent position compared to the straight leg position, which may suggest a functional reason for the differences in outcomes in stenting in these two anatomic locations.[62] While these findings may not change recommendations for open approach first in suitable patients, they do help to improve our understanding of the implications of an endovascular treatment in patients for who this strategy is adopted.

Considerations for Acute Limb Ischemia. Patients presenting with acute limb ischemia secondary to popliteal artery thrombosis represent a particular challenge. Current recommendations from the Society for Vascular Surgery recommend use of the severity of the acute limb symptoms to help guide management.[54] In particular, consideration of how to manage the tibioperoneal occlusions that often result from embolization of popliteal aneurysm thrombosis may vary based on the severity of symptoms. Patients with mild to moderate symptoms (Rutherford 1 and 2A) should be considered for thrombolysis or pharmacomechanical thrombectomy of tibial vessels prior to popliteal repair. Patient's with more severe symptoms (Rutherford 2B) will likely require concurrent thrombectomy (either open or pharmacomechanical) at the same time as popliteal repair. Amputation should be performed for patients with nonviable limbs (Rutherford 3).

Results

Excellent results are obtained in asymptomatic aneurysms with intact distal vasculature. Patients with thrombosed aneurysms, or those in whom multiple episodes of embolization have occluded the tibial arteries, have less optimal results. Operative mortality is in the 0% to 2% range, with asymptomatic patients faring better than those presenting with acutely symptomatic lesions.[63,64] In patients undergoing revascularization before ischemic complications occur, 5- and 10-year graft patency rates are greater than 80% and limb salvage is 93% to 98%.[49,65] Graft patency rates in patients undergoing surgery after developing complications of their aneurysms are 60% and 48% at 5 and 10 years, respectively, and limb salvage rates are 60% to 80%.[42,49,65,66] Thrombolytic therapy, when successful, improves primary graft patency in patients presenting with acute limb ischemia.[67]

SUMMARY

Peripheral aneurysms involving the femoral and popliteal arteries require an understanding of the etiology, presentation, diagnostic workup, and ultimately treatment options to successfully manage. Unlike intrathoracic or abdominal aneurysms, aneurysms in these locations are more likely to cause thrombotic complications resulting in potential limb loss and significant morbidity. In both distributions, the mechanisms of the disease (degenerative, mycotic, pseudoaneurysm, etc.) often determine the treatment paradigm, with symptomatology, aneurysm size, and history of thrombotic complications being important considerations. Both open and endovascular therapies have roles in the treatment of these rare, complex aneurysms. Appropriate management of these patients can help allow for improved quality of life and reduced morbidity.

ACKNOWLEDGMENTS

We gratefully acknowledge the contributions of previous edition authors, Katherine E. Hawkins and Amy B. Reed, as portions of those chapters have been retained in this revision.

References

1. Trickett JP, Scott RA, Tilney HS. Screening and management of asymptomatic popliteal aneurysms. *J Med Screen.* 2002;9:92–93.
2. Lawrence PF, Lorenzo-Rivero S, Lyon JL. The incidence of iliac, femoral, and popliteal artery aneurysms in hospitalized patients. *J Vasc Surg.* 1995;22:409–415; discussion 415–416.
3. Lawrence PF, Harlander-Locke MP, Oderich GS, et al; Vascular Low-Frequency Disease Consortium. The current management of isolated degenerative femoral artery aneurysms is too aggressive for their natural history. *J Vasc Surg.* 2014;59(2):343–349.
4. Diwan A, Sarkar R, Stanley JC, Zelenock GB, Wakefield TW. Incidence of femoral and popliteal artery aneurysms in patients with abdominal aortic aneurysms. *J Vasc Surg.* 2000;31:863–869.
5. Faggioli GL, Gargiulo M, Bertoni F, Bacchini P, Gessaroli M, Stella A. Parietal inflammatory infiltrate in peripheral aneurysms of atherosclerotic origin. *J Cardiovasc Surg (Torino).* 1992;33:331–336.
6. Thompson RW, Liao S, Curci JA. Vascular smooth muscle cell apoptosis in abdominal aortic aneurysms. *Coron Artery Dis.* 1997; 8:623–631.
7. Traina L, Zenunaj G, Bisogno F, et al. Incidence, diagnosis, treatment, and outcomes of true superficial artery aneurysms. *Ann Vasc Surg.* 2021;76:565–572.
8. Kibrik P, Arustamyan M, Stern JR, Dua A. A systematic review of the diagnosis, management, and outcomes of true profunda femoris artery aneurysm. *J Vasc Surg.* 2020;71(6):2145–2151.
9. Sandgren T, Sonesson B, Ahlgren AR, Länne T. The diameter of the common femoral artery in healthy human: influence of sex, age, and body size. *J Vasc Surg.* 1999;29:503–510.
10. Cutler BS, Darling RC. Surgical management of arteriosclerotic femoral aneurysms. *Surgery.* 1973;74:764–773.
11. Jarrett F, Makaroun MS, Rhee RY, Bertges DJ. Superficial femoral artery aneurysms: an unusual entity? *J Vasc Surg.* 2002;36: 571–574.
12. Piffaretti G, Mariscalco G, Tozzi M, Rivolta N, Annoni M, Castelli P. Twenty-year experience of femoral artery aneurysms. *J Vasc Surg.* 2011;53:1230–1236.
13. Levi N, Schroeder TV. Arteriosclerotic femoral artery aneurysms: a short review. *J Cardiovasc Surg (Torino).* 1997;38:335–338.
14. Szilagyi DE, Smith RF, Elliott JP, Hageman JH, Dall'Olmo CA. Anastomotic aneurysms after vascular reconstruction: problems of incidence, etiology, and treatment. *Surgery.* 1975;78:800–816.

15. Szilagyi DE, Elliott JP Jr, Smith RF, Reddy DJ, McPharlin M. A thirty-year survey of the reconstructive surgical treatment of aortoiliac occlusive disease. *J Vasc Surg*. 1986;3:421–436.
16. Dennis JW, Littooy FN, Greisler HP, Baker WH. Anastomotic pseudoaneurysms. A continuing late complication of vascular reconstructive procedures. *Arch Surg*. 1986;121:314–317.
17. Seabrook GR, Schmitt DD, Bandyk DF, Edmiston CE, Krepel CJ, Towne JB. Anastomotic femoral pseudoaneurysm: an investigation of occult infection as an etiologic factor. *J Vasc Surg*. 1990;11:629–634.
18. Ylönen K, Biancari F, Leo E, et al. Predictors of development of anastomotic femoral pseudoaneurysms after aortofemoral reconstruction for abdominal aortic aneurysm. *Am J Surg*. 2004;187:83–87.
19. Eleshra A, Kim D, Park HS, Lee T. Access site pseudoaneurysms after endovascular intervention for peripheral arterial diseases. *Ann Surg Treat Res*. 2019;96:305–312.
20. Vierhout BP, Pol RA, El Moumni M, Zeebregts CJ. Arteriotomy closure devices in EVAR, TEVAR, and TAVR: a systematic review and meta-analysis of randomized clinical trials and cohort studies. *Eur J Vasc Endovasc Surg*. 2017;54:104–115.
21. Arora N, Matheny ME, Sepke C, Resnic FC. A propensity analysis of the risk of vascular complications after cardiac catheterization procedures with the use of vascular closure devices. *Am Heart J*. 2007;153:606–611.
22. Kontopodis N, Tsetis D, Tavlas E, Dedes A, Ioannou CV. Ultrasound guided compression versus ultrasound guided thrombin injection for the treatment of post-catheterization femoral pseudoaneurysms: systematic review and meta-analysis of comparative studies. *Eur J Vasc Endovasc Surg*. 2016;51:815–823.
23. Lange P, Houe T, Helgstrand UJ. The efficacy of ultrasound-guided compression of iatrogenic femoral pseudo-aneurysms. *Eur J Vasc Endovasc Surg*. 2001;21:248–250.
24. Stolt M, Braun-Dullaeus R, Herold J. Do not underestimate the femoral pseudoaneurysm. *Vasa*. 2018;47:177–185.
25. La Perna L, Olin JW, Goines D, Childs MB, Ouriel K. Ultrasound-guided thrombin injection for the treatment of postcatheterization pseudoaneurysms. *Circulation*. 2000;102:2391–2395.
26. Kent KC, McArdle CR, Kennedy B, Baim DS, Anninos E, Skillman JJ. A prospective study of the clinical outcome of femoral pseudoaneurysms and arteriovenous fistulas induced by arterial puncture. *J Vasc Surg*. 1993;17:125–131; discussion 131–133.
27. Fram DB, Giri S, Jamil G, et al. Suture closure of the femoral arteriotomy following invasive cardiac procedures: a detailed analysis of efficacy, complications, and the impact of early ambulation in 1,200 consecutive, unselected cases. *Catheter Cardiovasc Interv*. 2001;53:163–173.
28. Mohler ER 3rd, Mitchell ME, Carpenter JP, et al. Therapeutic thrombin injection of pseudoaneurysms: a multicenter experience. *Vasc Med*. 2001;6:241–244.
29. Maleux G, Hendrickx S, Vaninbroukx J, et al. Percutaneous injection of human thrombin to treat iatrogenic femoral pseudoaneurysms: short- and midterm ultrasound follow-up. *Eur Radiol*. 2003;13:209–212.
30. Cox GS, Young JR, Gray BR, Grubb MW, Hertzer NR. Ultrasound-guided compression repair of postcatheterization pseudoaneurysms: results of treatment in one hundred cases. *J Vasc Surg*. 1994;19:683–686.
31. Kumins NH, Landau DS, Montalvo J, et al. Expanded indications for the treatment of postcatheterization femoral pseudoaneurysms with ultrasound-guided compression. *Am J Surg*. 1998;176:131–136.
32. Anderson CB, Butcher HR Jr, Ballinger WF. Mycotic aneurysms. *Arch Surg*. 1974;109:712–717.
33. Brown SL, Busuttil RW, Baker JD, Machleder HI, Moore WS, Barker WF. Bacteriologic and surgical determinants of survival in patients with mycotic aneurysms. *J Vasc Surg*. 1984;1:541–547.
34. Salzler GG, Long B, Averginos ED, et al. Contemporary results of surgical management of peripheral mycotic aneurysms. *Ann Vasc Surg*. 2018;53:86–91.
35. Gan JP, Leiberman DP, Pollock JG. Outcome after ligation of infected false femoral aneurysms in intravenous drug abusers. *Eur J Vasc Endovasc Surg*. 2000;19:158–161.
36. Reddy DJ, Smith RF, Elliott JP Jr, Haddad GK, Wanek EA. Infected femoral artery false aneurysms in drug addicts: evolution of selective vascular reconstruction. *J Vasc Surg*. 1986;3:718–724.
37. Furlough CL, Jain AK, Ho KJ, Rodriguez HE, Tomita TM, Eskandari MK. Peripheral artery reconstructions using cryopreserved arterial allografts in infected fields. *J Vasc Surg*. 2019;70(2):562–568.
38. Lorbeer R, Grotz A, Dörr M, et al. Reference values of vessel diameters, stenosis prevalence, and arterial variations of the lower limb arteries in a male population sample using contrast-enhanced MR angiography. *PLoS One*. 2018;13:e0197559.
39. Szilagyi DE, Schwartz RL, Reddy DJ. Popliteal arterial aneurysms. Their natural history and management. *Arch Surg*. 1981;116:724–728.
40. Ramesh S, Michaels JA, Galland RB. Popliteal aneurysm: morphology and management. *Br J Surg*. 1993;80:1531–1533.
41. Cross JE, Galland RB. Part one: for the motion asymptomatic popliteal artery aneurysms (less than 3 cm) should be treated conservatively. *Eur J Vasc Endovasc Surg*. 2011;41:445–448; discussion 449.
42. Dawson J, Fitridge R. Update on aneurysm disease: current insights and controversies: peripheral aneurysms: when to intervene—is rupture really a danger?. *Prog Cardiovasc Dis*. 2013;56:26–35.
43. Kassem MM, Oropallo A, Gonzalez L. Popliteal artery aneurysm. [Updated 2024 Feb 16]. In: *StatPearls [Internet]*. StatPearls Publishing; 2024. https://www.ncbi.nlm.nih.gov/books/NBK430863/
44. Studzińska D, Rudel B, Polok K, et al. Infrarenal versus suprarenal abdominal aortic aneurysms: Comparison of associated aneurysms and renal artery stenosis. *Ann Vasc Surg*. 2019;58:248–254.e1.
45. Hirsch AT, Haskal ZJ, Hertzer NR. ACC/AHA 2005 Practice Guidelines for the management of patients with peripheral arterial disease (lower extremity, renal, mesenteric, and abdominal aortic): executive summary. *Circulation*. 2006;113:1474–1547.
46. Michaels JA, Galland RB. Management of asymptomatic popliteal aneurysms: the use of a Markov decision tree to determine the criteria for a conservative approach. *Eur J Vasc Surg*. 1993;7:136–143.
47. Bowyer RC, Cawthorn SJ, Walker WJ, Giddings AE. Conservative management of asymptomatic popliteal aneurysm. *Br J Surg*. 1990;77:1132–1135.
48. Dawson I, Sie R, van Baalen JM, van Bockel JH. Asymptomatic popliteal aneurysm: elective operation versus conservative follow-up. *Br J Surg*. 1994;81(10):1504–1507.
49. Anton GE, Hertzer NR, Beven EG, O'Hara PJ, Krajewski LP. Surgical management of popliteal aneurysms: trends in presentation, treatment, and results from 1952 to 1984. *J Vasc Surg*. 1986;3:125–134.
50. Vermilion BD, Kimmins SA, Pace WG, Evans WE. A review of one hundred forty-seven popliteal aneurysms with long-term follow-up. *Surgery*. 1981;90:1009–1014.
51. Whitehouse WM Jr, Wakefield TW, Graham LM, et al. Limb-threatening potential of arteriosclerotic popliteal artery aneurysms. *Surgery*. 1983;93:694–699.
52. Lowell RC, Gloviczki P, Hallett JW Jr, et al. Popliteal artery aneurysms: the risk of nonoperative management. *Ann Vasc Surg*. 1994;8:14–23.
53. Cousins RS, Dexter DJ, Ahanchi SS, et al. Determining patient risk factors associated with accelerated growth of popliteal artery aneurysms. *J Vasc Surg*. 2018;67(3):838–847.
54. Farber A, Angle N, Avgerinos E, et al. The Society for Vascular Surgery clinical practice guidelines on popliteal artery aneurysms. *J Vasc Surg*. 2022;75(1S):109S–120S.
55. Chang H, Veith FJ, Rockman CB, et al. Comparison of outcomes for open popliteal artery aneurysm repair using vein and prosthetic conduits. *Ann Vasc Surg*. 2021;75:69–78.
56. Ascher E, Markevich N, Schutzer RW, Kallakuri S, Jacob T, Hingorani AP. Small popliteal artery aneurysms: are they clinically significant? *J Vasc Surg*. 2003;37:755–760.
57. Henry M, Amor M, Henry I, et al. Percutaneous endovascular treatment of peripheral aneurysms. *J Cardiovasc Surg (Torino)*. 2000;41:871–883.

58. Gerasimidis T, Sfyroeras G, Papazoglou K, Trellopoulos G, Ntinas A, Karamanos D. Endovascular treatment of popliteal artery aneurysms. *Eur J Vasc Endovasc Surg*. 2003;26: 506–511.
59. Tielliu IF, Verhoeven EL, Prins TR, Post WJ, Hulsebos RG, van den Dungen JJ. Treatment of popliteal artery aneurysms with the Hemobahn stent-graft. *J Endovasc Ther*. 2003;10:111–116.
60. Brendel JM, Mangold T, Pfändler M, et al. Viabahn endoprosthesis for femoropopliteal aneurysm repair: safety, success rates, and long-term patency. *CVIR Endovasc*. 2024;7(1):53.
61. Troisi N, Bertagna G, Saratzis A, et al; PARADE Study Collaborative Group. Elective surgical repair of popliteal artery aneurysms with posterior approach vs. endovascular exclusion: early and long term outcomes of multicentre PARADE study. *Eur J Vasc Endovasc Surg*. 2025;69(1):110–117.
62. Spinella G, Magliocco M, Pane B, et al. The impact of knee bending on the superficial femoral artery and popliteal artery morphology before and after endovascular repair of popliteal aneurysm. *J Endovasc Ther*. 2024:15266028241245582.
63. Varga ZA, Locke-Edmunds JC, Baird RN. A multicenter study of popliteal aneurysms. Joint Vascular Research Group. *J Vasc Surg*. 1994;20:171–177.
64. Reilly MK, Abbott WM, Darling RC. Aggressive surgical management of popliteal artery aneurysms. *Am J Surg*. 1983;145:498–502.
65. Roggo A, Brunner U, Ottinger LW, Largiader F. The continuing challenge of aneurysms of the popliteal artery. *Surg Gynecol Obstet*. 1993;177:565–572.
66. Jones WT 3rd, Hagino RT, Chiou AC, Decaprio JD, Franklin KS, Kashyap VS. Graft patency is not the only clinical predictor of success after exclusion and bypass of popliteal artery aneurysms. *J Vasc Surg*. 2003;37:392–398.
67. Dorigo W, Pulli R, Turini F, et al. Acute leg ischaemia from thrombosed popliteal artery aneurysms: role of preoperative thrombolysis. *Eur J Vasc Endovasc Surg*. 2002;23:251–254.

Venous Disease

Andrea T. Obi, Katherin E. Leckie, Michael C. Dalsing, and Thomas W. Wakefield

Key Points

1. The mainstay of diagnosis for acute venous thromboembolism (VTE) is clinical scoring systems, D-dimer, duplex ultrasonography, and CT-PE.
2. Preferred therapy for VTE is now primarily direct oral anticoagulants, with some role for debulking therapies in massive pulmonary embolism (PE) and iliofemoral deep venous thrombosis (DVT).
3. Chronic venous insufficiency (CVI) can be evaluated by duplex and occasionally air plethysmography (APG) if indicated.[1]
4. Minimally invasive endovenous therapy are standard of care to treat superficial venous reflux; deep reflux is most commonly treated with compression and rarely with valvular reconstruction.[1]

VENOUS THROMBOEMBOLISM

Incidence, Risk Factors, and Categories

About 600,000 patients are affected by deep venous thrombosis (DVT) or pulmonary embolism (PE) or both yearly.[2] The incidence has remained constant since 1980. The treatment for VTE costs the US health care system billions of dollars per year. Although Virchow's triad of stasis, vessel wall injury, and hypercoagulability have defined the events that predispose to DVT formation for the past 150 years, the importance of events that occur at the level of the vein wall, including the influence of the inflammatory response, is increasingly recognized today.[3]

Acquired risk factors for VTE include increasing age, malignancy, immobilization, surgery and trauma, oral contraceptive use, hormone replacement therapy, pregnancy and the puerperium, neurologic disease, cardiac disease, obesity, and antiphospholipid antibodies. Genetic risk factors include deficiencies of antithrombin, protein C and protein S, factor V Leiden, prothrombin 20210A, blood group non-O, dysfibrinogenemia, dysplasminogenemia, hyperhomocystinemia, reduced heparin cofactor II activity, elevated levels of clotting factors (eg, factors II, VII, VIII, IX, X, and XI), and elevations in plasminogen activator inhibitor-1 (PAI-1). When a young patient presents with an idiopathic VTE or thrombosis in unusual locations, workup for a hypercoagulable state may be indicated (**Table 93.1**). Hematologic diseases associated with VTE include heparin-induced thrombocytopenia (HIT) and thrombosis syndrome, vaccine-induced thrombotic thrombocytopenia (VITT), disseminated intravascular coagulation, antiphospholipid antibody syndrome, thrombotic thrombocytopenic purpura, hemolytic uremic syndrome, and myeloproliferative disorders.

Most DVTs affect the iliac, femoral, or popliteal lower limb veins. Presenting symptoms generally include unilateral leg pain and swelling, while some DVTs are silent, with the first manifestation of a PE. Some of the more common comorbidities include hypertension, surgery within 3 months, immobility within 30 days, cancer, and obesity.

Venous Thromboembolism Diagnosis

In a patient with a low pretest probability for DVT (such as with a negative Wells score), if a high-sensitivity D-dimer biomarker test is negative, no further testing is necessary, and ultrasound imaging may be omitted in this situation. On the contrary, if the D-dimer is positive, then duplex must be performed even if the pretest probability is high, as a positive D-dimer and a positive risk assessment is associated with DVT in only approximately 70% of cases. Venous color duplex imaging is the standard imaging test for definitive diagnosis of DVT. In a multicenter study of 711 patients, there was 95.5% concordance between CTV and ultrasonography for the diagnosis or exclusion of DVT ($\kappa = 0.809$).

A single good-quality color duplex Doppler study is sufficient (NPV > 99.5%) to exclude proximal DVT; repeat scanning is seldom indicated unless the initial study was technically suboptimal. All segments of the leg, including the external iliac, common femoral, femoral, popliteal, and calf veins, should be evaluated by ultrasound imaging and Doppler flow. While duplex ultrasound has a high accuracy for proximal DVT, diagnosis of distal DVT is highly operator dependent.

Duplex ultrasound is also diagnostic test of choice for superficial venous thrombophlebitis (SVT). In a prospective epidemiologic study, including 844 patients with symptomatic SVT, 210 (24.9%) had concomitant DVT at the time of diagnosis of SVT. Duplex is also the diagnostic test of choice for pediatric and pregnant patients.

Other conditions may be confused with DVT and include lymphedema, muscle strains, and muscle contusion. Iliac vein obstruction may lead to unilateral leg edema (May–Thurner syndrome), while the presence of a cyst behind the knee may produce unilateral lower leg pain and edema. Some medications, such as amlodipine, can cause limb swelling as a side effect. Other causes of leg swelling include lipidema and systematic problems such as cardiac, renal, or hepatic abnormalities. These systemic problems usually lead to bilateral edema.

Pulmonary Embolism

Testing for PE begins with prior probability estimation for all patients. Two of the most widely known and validated diagnostic scoring systems are the Wells criteria (or modified/dichotomous Wells criteria) and Geneva score.[4] They use a combination of physical examination, history, and vital signs to predict the likelihood of PE. Patients with both low probability and negative D-dimer require no further investigation as

Table 93.1. Elements of a Complete Hypercoagulability Evaluation

Hypercoagulability Evaluation
Activated protein C resistance
Antithrombin III activity
Antithrombin III antigen
Cardiolipin antibody
D-dimer
Dilute Russell's viper venom test
Factor VIII assay
Fibrinogen (Clottable)
Fibrinogen antigen
Hexagonal phospholipid neutralization
Plasma homocysteine
Plasminogen activity
Protein C activity
Protein C antigen
Protein S antigen (Free)
Prothrombin 20210 mutation detection
PT (Prothrombin time)
PTT (Partial thromboplastin time)

Not all tests for every evaluation are recommended.
Derived from https://www.pathology.med.umich.edu/handbook. Accessed February 7, 2020.

the NPV is 99%. CTA establishes the diagnosis of PE if it is positive in an intermediate- or high-probability patient, or in a low-probability patient with findings of a mainstem or lobar embolus. It excludes the diagnosis of PE in low-probability patients with negative scans. CTA is the current gold standard for diagnosis due to sensitivity and specificity of >95%. Discordance between prior probability and CTA findings requires further investigation, as do technically inadequate studies.[1]

Other diagnostic tests may include V/Q imaging or pulmonary angiography. The sensitivity of V/Q scanning was defined in PIOPED I at 98%, but specificity was low at 10%. By combining clinical factors with V/Q scan, levels of sensitivity and specificity greater than 95% were achieved.[5] Outcome studies have found comparable results between pulmonary angiography and CTA; a negative result with either study confers ~1% VTE rate within 6 months. However, because angiography is invasive, it carries a greater risk of complications and mortality. The mortality from angiography has been estimated at 0.5%, while 1% may experience major complications, including arrhythmias, hypotension, bleeding, and nephrotoxicity.

The efficacy of magnetic resonance angiography (MRA), MR venography (MRV), or the combination of the two in the diagnosis of acute PE has been studied. The gold standard used for comparison was a composite endpoint of CTA, CTA-CTV, V/Q scan, lower extremity ultrasonography, D-dimer assay, and clinical assessment. Overall, MRA and MRA-MRV were found to be poor tests for the diagnosis of PE. Approximately 25% of the 371 patients enrolled in a large multicenter study had a technically inadequate MRA, and 48% had either an inadequate MRV or MRA.[6] Considering all patients enrolled, MRA alone identified only 57% of PEs and had a sensitivity of 78% when only patients with adequate studies were considered. The combined MRA-MRV studies had a sensitivity of 92%, but only about half of the patients had technically adequate studies. At this time, MRA-MRV is not generally recommended; and only considered in centers with a great deal of experience.

For critically ill patients too unstable for transport, echocardiography can suggest the diagnosis of (massive) PE by showing dilatation of the right ventricle (RV) or hypokinesis. Commonly, acute changes in the RV pressure, size, and function are seen, indicating increased RV strain and pulmonary arterial pressures. These changes suggest PE in the absence of alternative diagnoses. Although of limited value in the diagnosis of PE, echocardiography is of great prognostic use in stratifying risk for patients with acute PE. Right ventricular dysfunction or dilatation in acute PE is associated with worse outcomes, including increased mortality rate.

Biomarkers include B-type natriuretic peptide (BNP), released by ventricular myocardial cells in response to wall stretch and volume overload. BNP is a prognostic (not diagnostic) biomarker for PE. BNP levels generally indicate RV strain due to elevated pulmonary vascular resistance in the lungs. If measured early (within 4 hours of admission for PE), elevated BNP levels (>90 pg/mL) demonstrate a sensitivity of 85% and a specificity of 75% in predicting PE-related outcomes. Conversely, normal BNP values in the setting of acute PE carry a 97% to 100% NPV for in-hospital death. Another biomarker is troponin released from damaged myocardial cells. When elevated in acute PE, troponins represent myocyte ischemia and microinfarction due to acute cardiac strain of the RV. Approximately 30% to 50% of patients with large PE will have elevations in troponins I and T that are mild and short lived. They correlate with worse RV function and a high incidence of complications. Normal troponin T levels have a 97% to 100% NPV for in-hospital death.

Axillary/Subclavian Vein Thrombosis

Thrombosis of the axillary/subclavian vein accounts for less than 5% of all cases of acute DVT. However, it may be associated with PE in up to 10% to 15% of cases and additionally can also be the source of significant disability. Primary axillary/subclavian vein thrombosis results from obstruction of the axillary vein in the thoracic outlet, the so-called Paget–Schroetter syndrome, noted especially in athletic individuals. Such thrombosis may also occur in patients with hypercoagulable states. Secondary axillary/subclavian vein thrombosis results from mediastinal tumors, congestive heart failure, and nephrotic syndrome. Patients present with arm pain, edema, and cyanosis. Superficial venous distention may be apparent over the arm, forearm, shoulder, and even the anterior chest wall.

Upper extremity venous duplex ultrasound is used to diagnose suspected axillary–subclavian vein thrombosis. Thrombolysis and phlebography are often considered next. If phlebography is performed, it is important that the patient undergo positional phlebography with arm abduction to 120 degrees to confirm extrinsic subclavian vein compression at the thoracic outlet. Venous compromise is further evidenced by prominent collateral veins. Since a cervical rib may be the cause of such obstruction, chest x-ray film should be obtained to exclude its presence.

Standard Therapy for VTE

Treatment

The traditional treatment of VTE is systemic anticoagulation, which reduces the risk of PE, extension of thrombosis, and thrombus recurrence. Immediate anticoagulation should be undertaken as the recurrence rate for VTE is higher if anticoagulation is not therapeutic in the first 24 hours. For DVT, since duplex imaging is rapidly obtained, usually testing precedes anticoagulation while for PE, anticoagulation is recommended either simultaneous with or before testing.

As a result of the evidence demonstrating the effectiveness and safety of direct oral anticoagulants (DOACs), they are now recommended as first-line treatment of acute VTE over Vitamin K antagonists (VKAs) in patients who do not have an associated cancer. Currently, the direct Xa inhibitors apixaban, rivaroxaban, and edoxaban have been Food and Drug Administration (FDA) approved for the treatment of VTE, while dabigatran is the sole approved direct thrombin inhibitor. The DOACs are all administered orally, have fixed doses that do not need to be weight-based adjusted, and do not need monitoring. Urgent reversal of DOACs can be achieved with idarucizumab (Praxbind™), a monoclonal antibody, which binds to dabigatran and can reverse its anticoagulant effects within minutes and andexanet alfa, a recombinant factor Xa decoy, for all factor Xa inhibitors, including DOACs, low–molecular-weight heparins (LMWHs), and fondaparinux. Clinical trials have shown that andexanet alfa can effectively reverse DOACs anticoagulant effect without any known thrombotic events in healthy patients.

There are several scenarios which would preclude the use of DOACs; for example, patients with mechanical heart valves, patients who cannot afford the cost of the medication, and patients with impaired renal function. Given that all of the comparison studies showed noninferiority, in many cases either a DOAC or VKA is acceptable. However, certain patients are at much higher risk of treatment failure with VKAs than others defined by a scoring system SAMe-TT$_2$R$_2$.[7]

Unfractionated heparin or LMWH is given along with oral anticoagulation with vitamin K antagonists (usually warfarin [Coumadin]). It is recommended that the international normalized ratio (INR) be therapeutic for 2 consecutive days before stopping heparin or LMWH. LMWH requires no monitoring (except in certain circumstances, such as renal insufficiency or morbid obesity), and is associated with a decrease in bleeding risk.

Compared to unfractionated heparin, LMWH has significantly improved bioavailability, less endothelial cell binding and protein binding, and improved pharmacokinetics. The half-life of LMWH is dose independent and it is administered in a weight-based fashion. LMWHs may decrease indices of chronic venous insufficiency (CVI) compared with standard therapy when used over an extended period. Warfarin should be started after heparinization is therapeutic to prevent warfarin-induced skin necrosis, as warfarin causes inhibition of protein C and S before factors II, IX, and X, leading to paradoxical hypercoagulability at the initiation of therapy. For standard unfractionated heparin, this requires a therapeutic anti-Xa activity; for LMWH, warfarin is administered after an appropriate weight-based dose of LMWH is administered and allowed to circulate.

Complications

Bleeding is the most common complication of anticoagulation. All currently approved VTE treatment agents carry the risk of significant bleeding complications, as they all target various aspects of the coagulation cascade. When treating VTE, the incidence of major bleeding at 3 months using unfractionated heparin or enoxaparin is approximately 4.3% and 2.9%, respectively. The rate of major bleeding using warfarin for the treatment of VTE is also approximately 2% during the initial 3 months of anticoagulation. Apixaban and rivaroxaban have a major bleeding incidence of approximately 0.5% (at 3 months) and 0.8% (during treatment follow-up period), respectively.

HIT occurs in 0.6% to 30% of patients. Although historically morbidity and mortality rates have been high, it has been found that early diagnosis and appropriate treatment have decreased these rates. HIT usually begins 3 to 14 days after heparin is begun, although it can occur earlier if there has been exposure to heparin in the past. A heparin-dependent antibody binds to platelets, activates them with the release of procoagulant microparticles leading to an increase in thrombocytopenia, resulting in thrombosis. Both bovine and porcine unfractionated heparin and LMWH have been associated with HIT, although the incidence and severity of the thrombosis are less with LMWH. The diagnosis should be suspected with a 50% or greater drop in platelet count, when the platelet count falls below 100,000/mL or when thrombosis occurs during heparin or LMWH therapy. A highly sensitive but poorly specific ELISA test detects the antiheparin antibody in the plasma. The serotonin release assay is another test that is more specific but less sensitive.

When the diagnosis is made, heparin must be stopped, and warfarin should not be given until an adequate alternative anticoagulant has been established and the platelet count has normalized. LMWHs cannot be used as substitutes as studies demonstrate high cross-reactivity with standard heparin antibodies. Agents that have been approved by the FDA as alternatives include the direct thrombin inhibitor argatroban and bivalirudin. Fondaparinux has also been found effective for treatment of HIT, but it is not FDA approved for this indication.

Duration of Anticoagulation

The recommended duration of anticoagulation for the treatment of provoked proximal and symptomatic distal VTE is 3 months. Extended therapy is considered under the following circumstances: Previous VTE event (ie, recurrent VTE), thrombophilia associated with a high risk of recurrence, and unprovoked VTE. Virtually all agree that for a second unprovoked VTE, anticoagulation should be continued due to the high recurrence risk well past 3 months in those patients with low/moderate bleeding risks. For patients with diagnosed hereditary thrombophilia, those that are associated with a higher risk of VTE recurrence (protein C/protein S deficiency [especially with a family history], antithrombin deficiency, homozygous factor V Leiden and homozygous prothrombin 20210 gene mutation, and multiple thrombophilias in the same patient), prolonged therapy is recommended. Although Factor V Leiden heterozygous mutation alone does not confer an increased risk of recurrence, when combined with prothrombin 20210 gene mutation, recurrence is increased and prolonged anticoagulant therapy is recommended. Among acquired thrombophilias, antiphospholipid antibodies and active cancer mandate extended therapy.

Unprovoked first-time VTE remains a difficult clinical scenario, as one must balance the competing risks and implications of recurrent VTE and major bleeding. D-dimer and repeat duplex testing have both been advocated to determine risk of recurrence with cessation of anticoagulation. D-dimer is measured approximately 1 month after stopping oral anticoagulation. Elevation of D-dimer suggests that active thrombosis is occurring, and the rate of recurrence is higher (15%) compared to 6.2% with a normal D-dimer. This risk can be mitigated with resumption of anticoagulation which reduces the VTE rate down to 2.9%.[8]

1 Emerging Medical Treatments and Trends in VTE Managements

Based on multiple DOAC trials, the application of DOACs has been expanded to the treatment of SVT and in patients with cancer. Based on accumulation of multiple RCTs, the International Society of Thrombosis and Haemostasis has recommended the use of DOACs in patients with cancer-associated VTE but without GI cancer and with low bleeding risk.[9] Other new advances include validation of multiple scoring systems that can improve decision making around anticoagulant selection. The HERDOO2 score was prospectively validated to identify women at low risk of recurrence following unprovoked VTE who may safely discontinue anticoagulation following short-term (standard) treatment.[10] The VTE-PREDICT score uses multiple patient level variables to calculate both risk of bleeding and risk of VTE under scenario of full-dose or low-dose DOAC with or without antiplatelet therapy.[11]

Calf Vein DVT

There is clinical equipoise to the treatment of calf vein DVT. Withholding anticoagulation in outpatients with suspected calf vein DVT, if serial compression ultrasound is negative for proximal DVT at baseline, and if again negative 1 week later results in 3-month pooled estimate thromboembolic risk of 0.6%. The CACTUS trial was performed with the goal of assessing the safety of withholding anticoagulant treatment in patients with isolated symptomatic calf vein DVT at low risk for proximal extension/VTE, as defined by no personal VTE history or active malignancy.[12] LMWH did not reduce proximal extension or VTE and resulted in increased bleeding complications. A limitation of this study is that it was underpowered by >50% for its endpoints. Data from smaller studies evaluating low-risk patients with calf vein DVT suggests that shorter duration (1 month) and intensity (full-dose LMWH ×1 week and ½ dose for 3 weeks) had a low recurrence and VTE complication rate, raising the provocative question as to whether patients at high risk need to be treated in the same manner as proximal DVT.

For pediatric DVT, the two mainstays of treatment are anticoagulation with LMWH or DOAC. Recurrence of DVT in children carries a lower risk than in adults, with cumulative incidences of 6% to 11% versus 12% to 22%, respectively. The risk of postthrombotic syndrome (PTS) appears as great in children as in adults, although severe PTS is uncommon. Compression stockings are indicated in children to treat PTS.

Nonpharmacologic Treatments

PTS results from loss of competence of the venous valves as a result of DVT and vein wall fibrosis or persistent venous obstruction, or a combination of both. It can cause significant morbidity in the form of pain, swelling, skin breakdown, and ulcerations.

Based on the SOX trial results, the most recent ACCP guidelines suggest not using compression stockings to prevent PTS.[13] It must be remembered that the use of strong compression and early ambulation after DVT treatment can significantly reduce the symptoms of pain and swelling resulting from the DVT, even if the development of PTS is not prevented, and a new study suggests that immediate application of compression (rather than the more liberal criteria in the SOX trial) after DVT diagnosis may result in a small decrease in PTS and residual vein obstruction.[14] Early ambulation has the potential to decrease PTS and improve patients' quality of life (QOL). Thus, patients should be encouraged to ambulate as part of their post-DVT care recommendations and use stockings, to ameliorate pain and swelling from their DVT.

IVC Filters

The traditional indications for the use of IVC filters include a DVT with contraindication to anticoagulation or failure of anticoagulation. Protection from PE has been achieved in greater than 95% of cases using cone-shaped, wire-based permanent IVC filters. Cone-shaped filters have a lower incidence of IVC thrombosis compared with basket-shaped filters. Other indications for filter placement include free-floating thrombus longer than 5 cm, when bleeding risk with anticoagulation is excessive, when the risk of PE is felt to be very high, and to allow for the use of perioperative epidural anesthesia. Filters can be permanent or optional (retrievable). In the prospective PRESERVE trial, 44% of filters were retrieved.[15]

Filters are usually placed in an infrarenal location. However, they may also be placed in the suprarenal location or in the superior vena cava based on patient anatomy, thrombus burden, and/or pregnancy. Sepsis is not a contraindication to the use of wire-based filters since the trapped material can be sterilized with antibiotics. Although filters have been placed under x-ray guidance, percutaneous techniques for filter insertion using bedside external ultrasound or intravascular ultrasound can be performed.

Thrombolytic and Surgical Procedures for Deep VTE

For DVT treatment, the goals are to prevent extension or recurrence of DVT, prevent PE, and minimize the late squeal of thrombosis, namely PTS. Standard anticoagulants accomplish the first two goals but not the third goal. PTS occurs in up to 30% of patients after DVT and even greater with more proximal iliofemoral DVT. Experimentally, prolonged contact of the thrombus with the vein wall increases damage. The thrombus initiates an inflammatory response in the vein wall that can lead to vein wall fibrosis and valvular dysfunction. Some patients with proximal DVT may be candidates for thrombus removal, if they meet specific criteria, or if they have venous ischemia, as described below. Early thrombus removal may be performed for patients with all of the following: First episode of acute iliofemoral DVT, symptoms less than 14 days in duration, ambulatory patient with good functional capacity and acceptable life expectancy, and moderate-to-severe symptoms (which can be determined by a Villalta score ≥10 after a trial of anticoagulation).

Thrombus removal via catheter directed thrombolysis (CDT, **Table 93.2**) or mechanical thrombectomy (MT) has been shown to decrease symptoms of pain and swelling at 30 days, and may decrease development of PTS in highly selected patients. Following initial symptoms, thrombus removal is ideally performed within 2 weeks but may be performed up to 4 weeks. These strategies have been employed in many nonrandomized studies and, in small randomized trials, were more effective than standard therapy in patients with acute proximal lower extremity DVT, improving QOL. The Attract trial, while

Table 93.2. Relative Contraindications to Thrombolysis

Allergies	Alteplase Heparin Iodinated Contrast
Anatomic criteria	DVT not involving the iliac system Symptoms >28 d
Bleeding risk	Active bleeding Bleeding diathesis Recent surgery (<10 d) CPR Trauma Obstetrical delivery Internal eye surgery (<3 mos) Hemorrhagic retinopathy Gastrointestinal bleed Recent history of stroke Intracranial lesion Severe liver dysfunction
Comorbidities	Active cancer[a] Pregnancy Severe hypertension Severe renal impairment
Functional status	Chronic nonambulatory status Inability to provide consent Inability to tolerate bedrest Life expectancy <2 y

[a]Except nonmelanoma skin cancer.

not showing a benefit in incidence of PTS, did reduce moderate-to-severe PTS in patients with iliofemoral DVT.[16]

Phlegmasia and venous gangrene is a rare clinical phenomenon that places the affected limb at risk of ischemia. Phlegmasia cerulea dolens (PCD) is an uncommon form of DVT characterized by severe pain, swelling, cyanosis, and edema. This is preceded by phlegmasia alba dolens, which is characterized by the same clinical signs except the limb is pale and white due to early ischemia, and not yet cyanotic. Venous gangrene is defined as skin necrosis, discoloration, and documented VTE. Treatment for PCD or venous gangrene is the same as for proximal DVT, with an emphasis on immediate anticoagulation. Early thrombus removal is the treatment of choice in patients with limb-threatening venous ischemia due to iliofemoral venous thrombosis, with or without associated femoropopliteal venous thrombosis. Surgical venous thrombectomy is reserved for patients who have contraindication to radiation (such as pregnancy) or when endovenous therapies are not readily available.

The benefit of early thrombus removal for PE thus appears to be greatest in patients who would die as a result of massive PE in the first hour after the PE occurs, which can occur in up to 10% of cases. The ongoing PE-TRACT trial is addressing whether there is a benefit in patients with intermediate risk PE—those with right ventricular dysfunction without hemodynamic instability. Surgical approaches for PE are indicated for patients in whom endovenous MT or thrombolytic agents have been unsuccessful. Open pulmonary embolectomy is associated with high rates of morbidity and mortality and is rarely performed. The development of multidisciplinary teams for the aggressive treatment of patients with significant PE is a national trend which appears to be having a positive effect on the morbidity and mortality of PE.

Superficial Thrombophlebitis

SVT is a well-recognized clinical entity, characterized by a painful erythematous and palpable cord-liked structure, usually compromising the lower extremities but capable of affecting any superficial vein in the body. SVT was previously considered a benign disease requiring only conservative management with compression, nonsteroidal anti-inflammatory medications, and lower extremity elevation. However, above-the-knee SVT has been reported to coexist with DVT, to propagate to popliteal or femoral level and to even cause PE.

SVT occurs in approximately 125,000 people in the United States per year. However, the actual incidence is likely far greater as these statistics may be outdated and many cases go unreported. Approximately 54% to 65% of the reported cases affect females with an average age of 58 years. The most frequent predisposing risk factor for SVT is varicose veins, occurring in 62% of patients. Other risk factors include immobilization, trauma, postoperative states, age >60 years, obesity, tobacco use, history of DVT or SVT, pregnancy, puerperium, autoimmune disease, use of oral contraceptives or hormonal replacement therapy, and hypercoagulable state. Malignancy has been reported as a risk factor for developing SVT, affecting 13% to 18% of patients.

The overall recurrence of SVT was described as 18% over 15 months, equally frequent in varicose and nonvaricose phlebitis. Deep venous reflux increases the recurrence rate to 33%, while hypercoagulable states increase the recurrence rate to 42% over the same period of time. Duplex ultrasound imaging of the affected extremity should be performed to rule out extension of the process into the deep venous system or concomitant DVT.

Treatment

Several therapeutic approaches have been proposed for patients with SVT. Three major trials with similar findings, CALISTO, STENOX, and SURPRISE, have formed the basis of current medical management.[17–19] Low-dose anticoagulation (fondaparinux 2.5 mg or rivaroxaban 10 mg daily) is recommended for 45 days for patients with GSV thrombus ≥5 cm in length and at least 3 cm from the saphenofemoral junction (SFJ). For thrombi closer, the SVT is treated with full-dose therapy in a manner analogous to DVT; ligation can be used when anticoagulation is not feasible. SVT in other locations is treated with topical diclofenac or heparinoids and NSAIDs to reduce symptoms.

Septic thrombophlebitis requires treatment with broad-spectrum IV antibiotics. If rapid resolution of the cellulitis occurs, no treatment beyond a short course of antibiotics and standard treatment for the superficial thrombophlebitis is required. However, if the patient becomes septic, excision of the infected vein should be performed. With positive blood cultures, an extended course of antibiotics specific for the identified organism is indicated. The majority of episodes of uncomplicated superficial thrombophlebitis respond to conservative management. The recurrence rate for superficial thrombophlebitis has been estimated between 15% and 20%.

CHRONIC VENOUS DISEASE

Normal Venous Anatomy

The lower extremity venous system is composed of deep, perforating, and superficial veins. The common femoral, femoral, deep femoral veins in addition to the popliteal, sural, and tibial/peroneal veins make up the deep system. The deep veins lie beneath the investing fascia of the muscles of the leg and thigh (the deep compartment) while the superficial veins lie above this muscular fascia. The GSV and SSV lie within the subcutaneous tissue and are surrounded by a separate saphenous compartment formed by the muscular fascia below and the saphenous fascia above. The saphenous nerve lies within the GSV compartment below the knee, which places the nerve at risk of injury during surgery or percutaneous intervention. Similarly, the sural nerve lies in close proximity to the SSV and within its compartment.

In the past, various terminology and eponyms abounded, but modern nomenclature prefers more descriptive terms designating location. The names of other typical veins found in the lower extremity include the term of "accessory saphenous veins" for those superficial veins that lie outside the saphenous compartment, but parallel to the GSV or SSV, while "*communicating* veins" connect veins of the same system and "*perforating* veins" penetrate the muscular fascia to connect the superficial and deep systems.

The variability of the lower extremity venous system is well recognized with certain anatomic variations of clinical importance. The popliteal and femoral veins have variable anatomy and may be duplicated. The deep femoral vein commonly connects directly or through tributaries to the popliteal vein. Complete duplication of the GSV in the thigh may occur in 8% of cases with some partial duplication in another 25%. The SFJ generally has at least four branches in addition to the GSV, but the configuration of the branches is quite variable. The most cephalic branch is generally the superficial epigastric vein which acts as a landmark for percutaneous interventions and ideally remains patent following ablation procedures. The SSV is usually singular, diving under a thickened fascia in the upper calf (bringing it in proximity to the deep muscles); in less than two-thirds of cases actually ends in the popliteal creases and can travel well above the knee before diving to meet the deep system or connecting to the GSV via the intersaphenous vein. The varied location of perforating veins, especially in the lower leg, is important when deep to superficial reflux is a concern.

With the exception of foot veins, the valves promote blood flow from superficial to deep and from caudal to cephalad. The valves are made of a fine connective tissue skeleton covered by endothelium and are generally bicuspid, delicate, and extremely strong. Each tibial and peroneal vein contains about 7 to 19 valves. The popliteal vein contains one or two valves and the femoral vein generally three. Approximately 70% of common femoral veins have a valve located within 1 cm of the inguinal ligament, while only 25% of external iliac and 10% of the internal iliac veins have a valve. The common iliac vein generally has no valves. The GSV commonly has more than six valves (range, 4 to 25) with at least one valve within a few centimeters of the SFJ and the SSV has an average of 7 to 10 valves (range, 4 to 13).[1] Perforating veins and even larger venules have venous valves.

The veins of the abdomen and pelvis begin at the inguinal ligament as the external iliac vein that is joined medially by the internal iliac to form the common iliac vein. The internal iliac vein drains the pelvis via connections such as the obturator, gluteal, and internal pudendal veins and their interconnections. To the right of the 5th lumbar vertebrae and aorta, the common iliac veins join to form the IVC. Compression of the left iliac vein by the right common iliac artery can lead to a venous obstructive condition called nonthrombotic iliac vein lesion (NIVL, formerly May–Thurner syndrome). The IVC typically ascends to the right of the aorta and vertebral column terminating in the right atrium. Its direct tributaries are the lumbar veins, the right gonadal vein, the renal veins, the right suprarenal vein, the right inferior phrenic vein, and the hepatic veins. Other named veins generally join one of these tributaries to empty into the IVC. Because of the embryonic evolutions that lead to the "normal" IVC and its branches, variations are common. Duplication of the IVC occurs in 0.2% to 0.3% of cases, transposition or a left-sided IVC can occur in 0.2% to 0.5%, a retroaortic left renal in 1.2% to 2.4%, and circumaortic left renal vein in 1.5% to 8.7% of cases. In the face of IVC occlusion, veins of the chest and abdominal wall, the azygos and hemiazygos systems, and vertebral plexuses may play a prominent role in venous drainage of the lower extremities, abdomen, and retroperitoneum.

Normal Venous Physiology

Morphologically veins have a thin wall and lack external support. Small intramuscular veins are extremely compliant such that increasing the venous volume (VV) by over 1½ times results in a minimal increase in pressure (0 to 15 mm Hg). This allows a significant volume of blood (at least 500 mL in the standing position) to become sequestered in the lower limb without a significant rise in intraluminal pressure. However, once the full capacitance of the venous system is reached, further increases in VV result in a proportional increase in intraluminal pressure and changes the vein from an elliptical to a circular configuration. In general, this forgiving design can compensate for much pathology but when overstressed, sustained venous hypertension results in decompensation at the cellular level with resulting edema in the lower leg tissues.

In contrast to intramuscular veins, the compliance of large axial veins (eg, femoral, popliteal) mimics that of an artery in that pressure changes are more reflective of volume changes. They are conduit rather than compliance vessels.

The calf and possibly the thigh muscles act as a pump, the "peripheral heart," which can generate pressures of up to 300 mm Hg in the deep system and 100 to 150 mm Hg in superficial veins during exercise. Normally, modest exercise of the muscles will expel the contained blood volume present in the veins and reset the capacitance of the venous system maintaining a homeostatic environment.

The venous valves (superficial, deep, and perforating) play a key role because they allow blood to move forward in response to an increased distal pressure gradient (muscle pumps) and by preventing reflux, protect the capacitance vessels from overload and, thereby, the superficial structures (ie, skin, soft tissues) from the high pressures generated in the deep system.

Prevalence and Impact

Chronic venous disease (CVD) is a common, costly malady in Western countries. CVI is defined as venous pathology that results in advanced clinical symptoms. If one considers the entire spectrum of the disease based on modern methods of classification, approximately 21.7% have reticular veins/telangiectasia, 18% varicose veins, 15% edema, 7% hyperpigmentation, 1.4% healed ulcers, and 0.7% active ulcers. A population-based study in San Diego that included Duplex imaging demonstrated that 5.8% of those studied presented with edema, while 6.2% had skin changes and/or prior or active venous ulcers. The estimated cost of severe disease (ie, venous ulcer care) to the health care system is 1.5 to 3 billion annually and significantly more if actual patient cost is considered. The negative impact on QOL for other less severe forms of venous pathology would greatly surpass this cost to the health care system.

Relevant risk factors for varicose veins are advanced age, a positive family history, female gender, multiparity, and obesity, while the risk factors for CVI are advanced age, positive family history, and obesity.

Pathophysiology and Etiology

Three pathophysiologic states exist: obstruction, valvular insufficiency, and calf muscle pump malfunction. These conditions reflect a failure of one or more of the components of the normal venous system and are not mutually exclusive.

Venous obstruction causes an increased resistance to blood exiting the lower extremity. Once thought to be an uncommon etiology of treatable lower leg venous pathology, venous occlusive disease in combination with venous insufficiency was evident in over 50% of patients with CVI in one study, especially noted in those with the most severe symptoms. The result is elevated intravenous pressure noted clinically as pain, especially after exercise, as one added manifestation of the disease.

Asymptomatic primary iliac venous compression is quite common, one study of 50 patients without symptoms of CVI demonstrated that 24% had greater than 50% narrowing (compression) of the left common iliac vein by the right common iliac artery.[20] It has been suggested that this type of nonthrombotic stenosis (compression with potential for intramural fibrosis) is a "permissive lesion" not clinically significant until other components of the lower extremity venous circulation fail or the occlusive disease progresses. Less common causes of obstruction include intraluminal webs from repetitive trauma as well as extrinsic compression of the iliac and pelvic veins by tumor, fibrosis, infection, femoral hernias, or arterial aneurysms.

Postthrombotic obstruction is also a common cause of venous occlusive disease due to the rather high prevalence of DVT and can impact any part of the venous system. Acute thrombosis is associated with inflammation and remodeling during resolution and results in external vein wall scarring with stiffening and thickening, as well as intraluminal recanalization with webs and bands. The venous valves are generally incorporated into the scarring process leading to valve malfunction.

Valvular insufficiency occurs throughout the lower extremity veins and is estimated to account for 80% of symptomatic CVD cases. While superficial reflux is most common, deep venous insufficiency frequently coexists with superficial and perforator disease, and duplex imaging studies suggest that patients with minimal symptoms tend to have isolated superficial reflux while those with edema, skin changes, and past or present ulcers have an increasing presence of perforator and deep disease as well as a postthrombotic etiology. The presence of both obstructive and reflux pathology denotes more risk for the development of skin changes and the degree to which combined obstructive and insufficient venous pathology contribute to CVD is likely underestimated. No matter the clinical stage, the superficial system is most commonly affected (90%) with GSV involvement in 70% to 80%, SSV in 15% to 20%, and nonsaphenous veins in approximately 10%. The deep veins are involved in about 30% and perforator veins in about 20% of cases in one series.

Reflux allows the transmission of high venous pressures to the lower leg when standing and is not relieved by exercise. Primary valvular insufficiency is rare but can be a consequence of congenital valve absence. There are predisposing genetic factors that can lead to primary venous reflux not limited to Klippel–Trenaunay syndrome, FOXC2 gene mutation, desmoulin dysregulation, the Ehlers–Danlos syndrome, and a CADASIL gene mutation, but these do not reflect the typical patient. The muscle cell–dilating effect of estrogens may explain the genesis of varicose veins noted in the first trimester of pregnancy. Prolonged exposure to high venous pressures can cause vein dilation as occurs from an arteriovenous fistula or occupations requiring prolonged periods of standing. For the standard patient, venous valve prolapses (elongated, floppy valves) and defects in the vein wall that cause the valve ring to dilate result in malfunctioning valve cusps with retained valve architecture. Whether the vein wall changes precede valve insufficiency, or the valve insufficiency causes wall distention and wall changes is less clear.

CVD can also result from failure of calf muscle pump function. The pump becomes unable to generate the force needed to eject blood from the leg while standing, resulting in sustained venous hypertension. Patients with muscle disuse (eg, paraplegia, traumatic injury, elderly, or bedridden patients) may not have sufficient muscle for effective exercise. Pathologic conditions that result in muscle fibrosis (eg, muscular dystrophy and multiple sclerosis) can destroy the calf muscle pump. Thrombus and scarring in the gastrocnemius and soleal veins can prevent blood from entering the pump chamber resulting in a deficient volume for ejection with contraction. Calf pump function and ankle range of motion progressively diminish with increasing severity of CVI. Physical conditioning can improve the metrics of pump function, however, evidence regarding improved clinical outcomes is lacking.

Regardless of the etiology, the sequelae of venous hypertension/stasis are changes observed in the lower leg skin and subcutaneous tissues, the end organ. The current belief holds that the fundamental basis for CVD and ulceration is inflammation within the venous microcirculation when subjected to increased hydrostatic pressure. Research remains active in this component of venous pathophysiology and excellent reviews are available for further information on the current understanding of basis venous pathophysiology.

Clinical Signs and Symptoms

Venous disease presents in many ways. A telangiectasia, spider vein, is a confluence of dilated intradermal venules less than 1 mm in caliber. A reticular vein is a dilated bluish subdermal vein, 1 mm to less than 3 mm in diameter and usually tortuous. These venous abnormalities may be associated with a larger, more deeply located, pathologic vein but not always. Hereditary varicose veins usually appear during the second decade of life. If the varicosities are due to a secondary etiology (eg, thrombosis, trauma), presentation can be several years after the inciting event. These veins appear alone or in clusters as dilated, often bluish, serpentine, and palpable protrusions of branches of the GSV, SSV, or collateral veins lying beneath the skin in the subcutaneous tissues. Varicose veins measure 3 or more millimeters in diameter when measured in the upright position. One finding thought to be an early sign of advanced disease is corona phlebectica, a fan-shaped pattern of small intradermal veins located around the ankle or dorsal foot (also called ankle flare or malleolar flare). If the varicose veins observed are the result of proximal disease, such as pelvic reflux or obstruction; the location of the varicosities may be scrotal, perineal, vulvar, or posterior/lateral in the lower extremity.[1]

Symptoms may be those associated with any type of CVD and are noted as pain, edema, hyperpigmentation, stasis dermatitis/eczema, and/or venous ulcers. These changes often occur in the "gaiter" area just above the medial malleolus. Important perforating veins lay in this area. The observed hyperpigmentation is thought to result from extruded red blood cells that are degraded by macrophages leaving hemosiderin deposits. Less definable but described symptoms of CVD include tingling, burning, muscle cramping, a sensation of throbbing or heaviness, itching, restless or tiredness of the legs, and fatigue. They are more specific for venous disease if made worse with standing and heat and if relieved by rest and leg elevation.

Venous claudication is a pain syndrome experienced when walking and is associated with cyanosis, a sensation of increased swelling, a bursting sensation, and increased prominence of the superficial veins, which is relieved with rest in combination with elevation of the extremity.

2 Critical to patient management and treatment evaluation is an accurate classification of the disease at any given time. Each patient is stratified according to the *c*linical picture, the *e*tiology, the *a*natomic distribution, and the *p*athophysiology (CEAP) classification system (**Table 93.3**). This classification system helps the physician define the venous disease and then formulate an appropriate management strategy. An extension of the clinical classification, the Venous Clinical Severity Score, is available to quantify the extent of venous disease and, therefore, to evaluate the patient's clinical response to treatment (**Table 93.4**).[21] QOL surveys developed specifically for patients with venous disease help to determine the impact of the disease on the patient's life and the effect therapy has on the patient's overall well-being.[22] Consistent application of these treatment outcome tools is imperative to improve our ability to precisely determine the effect and benefit of a given intervention.

Diagnostic Evaluation

The diagnosis of CVD begins with a thorough history and physical examination. Prior DVT, pregnancies, a family history of varicosities, obesity, or the presence of other factors associated

Table 93.3. Clinical Classification of Chronic Venous Disease

Class	Description
0	No visible or palpable signs of venous disease
1	Telangiectasias and/or reticular veins
2	Varicose veins
2r	Recurrent varicose veins
3	Edema
4a	Skin changes (pigmentation and/or eczema)
4b	Skin changes (lipodermatosclerosis and/or atrophie blanche)
4c	Corona phlebetica
5	Healed venous ulcer
6	Active venous ulcer
6r	Recurrent venous ulcer
S (in addition to the class)	Symptoms including ache, pain, tightness, skin irritation, heaviness, muscle cramps as well as other complaints attributable to venous dysfunction
A (in addition to the class)	Asymptomatic

Table 93.4. Venous Clinical Severity Score

Attribute	Absent 0	Mild 1	Moderate 2	Severe 3
Pain	None	Occasional, not restricting activity or requiring analgesics	Daily, moderate activity limitation, occasional analgesics	Daily, severe limiting activities, regular use of analgesics
Varicose veins[a]	None	Few, scattered: branch VVs with competent GS/SS	Multiple: single-segment GS/SS reflux	Extensive: multisegment GS/SS reflux
Venous edema[b]	None	Evening ankle edema only	Afternoon edema, above ankle	Morning edema above ankle and requiring activity change, elevation
Skin pigmentation[c]	None or focal, low intensity (tan)	Diffuse, but limited in area and old (brown)	Diffuse over gaiter distribution (lower 1/3) or recent pigmentation (purple)	Wider distribution (above lower 1/3) and recent pigmentation
Inflammation	None	Mild cellulitis, limited to marginal area around ulcer	Moderate cellulitis, involves most of gaiter area	Severe cellulitis (lower 1/3 and above) or venous eczema
Induration	None	Focal, circummalleolar (<5 cm)	Medial or lateral, less than lower third	Entire lower third of leg or more
No. of active ulcers	0	1	2–4	>4
Active ulceration, duration	None	<3 mo	>3 mo and <1 y	Not healed >1 y
Active ulcer, size[d]	None	<2 cm diameter	2–4 cm diameter	>4 cm diameter
Compressive therapy[e]	Not used or not compliant	Intermittent use of stockings	Wears elastic stockings most days	Full compliance: stockings + elevation

[a]Varicose veins must be >4 mm diameter to qualify so that differentiation is ensured between C1 and C2 venous pathology. Occasional or mild edema and focal pigmentation over varicose veins does not qualify for C3 or C4.
[b]Presumes venous origin by characteristics (eg, brawny [not pitting or spongy] edema), with significant effect of standing/limb elevation and/or other clinical evidence of venous etiology (ie, varicose veins, history of DVT). Edema must be regular finding (eg, daily occurrence). Occasional or mild edema does not qualify.
[c]Focal pigmentation over varicose veins does not qualify.
[d]Largest dimension/diameter of largest ulcer.
[e]Sliding scale to adjust for background differences in the use of compressive therapy.
GS, great saphenous; SS, small saphenous; VV, varicose vein.
From Rutherford RB, Padberg FT Jr, Comerota AJ, et al. Venous severity scoring: an adjunct to venous outcome assessment. *J Vasc Surg*. 2000;31(6):1307–1312.

with CDV will add support to the presence of venous disease. When performing the physical examination: the location, distribution and size of varicosities, skin changes, and/or presence or indication of past ulcers should be noted. Swelling should be quantified, the location specified, and a determination made as to whether it is pitting or nonpitting in nature. Inspection, palpation, and auscultation (presence of a bruit) may be keys to the presence of a vascular malformation or arteriovenous fistula. Utilization of the CEAP clinical classification will provide a snapshot of the patient being examined, whereas the use of the more detailed Venous Clinical Severity Score and the other measurement tools mentioned above will allow for some impression of how any patient therapy is performing.

Appropriate confirmatory diagnostic studies may be required to confirm clinical suspicion, such as a lower extremity arterial Doppler study, biopsy, or specific blood analyses when the diagnosis is unclear. Such studies become most pertinent during the evaluation of advanced venous disease, especially in patients with venous ulcers. Only in selected patients, such as those with recurrent, early, or unusual sites of DVT or recurrent venous ulcers, is evaluation for thrombophilia recommended.[1]

Venous duplex ultrasonography provides a B-mode picture of the vein, as well as spectral analysis of the blood flow within. It is recommended as the first diagnostic test for all patients with suspected CVD. To provide an accurate impression of the venous disease present, a standardized technique is mandatory. Venous duplex imaging clearly visualizes deep, superficial, and perforator veins and can be utilized to assess compressibility and valve closure time. The venous duplex study can help to clarify the etiology, better define the anatomic location, and aid in determining the pathophysiology of the venous problem (EAP of CEAP).

Valvular insufficiency is defined as prolonged reflux time through a valve following a provocative test when duplex imaging is the diagnostic modality. To aid in the standardization of the test, a rapidly deflating distal cuff technique is used in some vascular laboratories, while others use manual compression of the distal leg after which valve reflux is determined by duplex imaging. An abnormal reverse venous flow (reflux) in the saphenous, tibial, and deep femoral veins is ≥0.5 seconds while the femoral and popliteal veins have a cutoff value of 1 second. Since perforating vein reflux can also be associated with venous pathology, significant work has gone into determining how to define abnormal reflux. Current consensus and available data suggest that a "pathologic" perforating vein is defined as a vein with an outward flow of ≥0.5 seconds with a diameter of >3.5 mm, which is located beneath a healed or open venous ulcer. The duplex examination for reflux is performed in the upright position but many other provocative maneuvers to generate venous reflux exist (Valsalva, standardized Valsalva, etc.) in addition to performing the test in different positions (eg, 15% Trendelenburg, sitting) and are used in many laboratories for particular patients who have difficulty standing. Each may be acceptable if standardized and validated for an individual laboratory.

Venous obstruction is seen as thickened, scarred, and constricted veins with poor flow and diminished augmentation following distal and/or proximal compression. Respiratory variation is lost as a result of local occlusive disease or proximal occlusion. By imaging the entire lower leg venous system, the surgeon possesses a detailed roadmap of all veins with determination of obstruction or reflux within segments separated by valves. This is often the only diagnostic tool needed for the evaluation of superficial and even perforator disease requiring treatment.

Plethysmography assesses the overall hemodynamics of the lower extremity venous system. Air plethysmography (APG) can measure several venous hemodynamic parameters. A plastic cylinder filled with air is fitted over the calf and foot, and changes in leg volume with positional change or exercise are detected by pressure changes in the cylinder. Calculated parameters include venous filling index (<2 mL/s is normal) which assesses the competency of the venous system, ejection fraction (>60% is normal), and residual volume fraction (<35% is normal) which suggest that the calf pump is working well.[23] In current clinical practice, it is being used only in complex cases or for research purposes. Current consensus encourages the use of plethysmography in the patient with advanced CVD if duplex scanning cannot provide a definitive diagnosis regarding the underlying pathophysiology.[1]

Descending venography is used to determine valve leaflet integrity and anatomic location, and demonstrate the extent of reflux. Assessment of the competence of the profunda femoris venous system in addition to the femoral system is imperative prior to valve transposition or isolated proximal femoral vein repair. And while descending venography is not infallible in determining the presence or absence of a normal valve, when combined with a careful venous duplex examination, it is currently the best method available to determine preoperatively if
3 an in situ reconstruction will be possible. The use of ascending venography is selectively used in specific cases to complement noninvasive studies when considering intervention in the deep venous system or in research protocols.

4 Treatment Options and Results

Medical Therapy

Compression has been the mainstay of the medical treatment for all stages of CVI for centuries. The goals are to manage clinical symptoms and to control venous hypertension. There are two general types of compression: elastic (eg, support stockings or long stretch bandages) and inelastic (eg, Unna paste boot, short stretch bandages, multilayer [four-layer] bandage, or Velcro band devices). Essentially, the more layers, the less elastic and stiffer the compression. The degree to which any particular bandaging is one or the other will depend on the care provider who applies the compression along with other factors. The mechanical effect is dependent on the level and type of compression and the desired amount of compression is influenced by the underlying venous pathology being treated.

Consistent narrowing of superficial and calf veins occurs at a median of 30 to 40 mm Hg pressure on standing while complete occlusion occurs at a median pressure of 70 mm Hg. Complete occlusion is not the goal. Therapeutic calf compression improves calf muscle pump function expressed as a reduction in residual volume fraction during walking and even compression of <20 mm Hg results in improved symptoms and QOL data when used to treat mild disease.

It is interesting that an elastic stocking maintains a rather constant pressure during exercise and at rest. Alternatively, inelastic wraps demonstrate a more dramatic increase in pressure during exercise, since they do not stretch but have decreasing pressure with recumbence as the edema exits the leg and the bandage maintains its shape. Inelastic wraps are much better tolerated when left on for days and especially when recumbent at night when compression is not required to contra-act gravity. Constant compression at night can be perceived as discomfort/pain. Further, inelastic compression has been found to result in a greater improvement in venous hemodynamics when applied at the same pressure as elastic compression and maintains greater effect despite loss in pressure over time (pressure loss likely related to the decreased volume of the leg). The significant decrease in swelling noted early in compression treatment explains why compression stocking often need to be changed more frequently during the early stages of care.

Although there has been concern that compression may impede microcirculatory flow and thereby jeopardize tissue viability, it is known that compression, when used to treat edema, has favorable effects on extracellular fluid balance, capillary density, and transcutaneous oxygen tension. Compression therapy also decreased levels of endothelial growth factor and tumor necrosis factor, which correlated with ulcer healing and actually increases microcirculatory flow.

Patients with concomitant arterial occlusive disease pose a unique challenge. In one single-center study, 15% of those presenting with leg ulceration and venous reflux had an ankle to brachial artery index (ABI) <0.85.[24] There is some suggestion that standard compression can actually increase arterial blood flow in certain circumstances. Overall, data suggest that improvement in tissue-level perfusion is likely related to improvement in the microangiopathy of CVD, offloading of the outflow system, and through a decreased burden on the lymphatic system (often damaged in patients with CVI). In patients with concomitant arterial occlusive disease with ABI of ≥0.80, the use of standard compression is safe and effective.

In those with more advanced arterial occlusive disease defined as an ABI ≥0.50 (but <0.80), an ankle systolic pressure ≥60 mm Hg, or toe pressure ≥30 mm Hg as a minimum; modified compression dressings with lower pressure ratings not to exceed the tissue perfusion pressure can improve tissue perfusion and aid in healing ulcers of mixed etiology. These data support the current SVS/AVF practice guideline suggesting that in a patient with a venous leg ulcer and underlying arterial disease, compression bandages or stockings are not indicated if ABI is ≤0.5 or if the absolute ankle pressure is <60 mm Hg.[25]

Evidence-based medicine confirms our clinical impression regarding the potential benefits of compression garments for the treatment of CVI. Substantial evidence demonstrates that compression is statistically beneficial for most clinical stages of symptomatic venous disease (C_{2-6}). Whether compression stockings should be the primary treatment for symptomatic varicose veins is challenged by data from the United Kingdom. The randomized trial (REACTIV) demonstrated that in 246 patients with class C_2 disease, surgical intervention resulted in a statistically significant benefit in quality-adjusted life-years and in symptomatic and anatomic measurements compared to conservative management. Likewise, cost-effective analysis demonstrated a benefit for the surgical intervention.[26] Therefore, in contradistinction to current third-payer policies, and based on available statistical data, the SVS/AVF Guidelines Committee recommends against compression therapy as the primary treatment of symptomatic varicose veins in those patients who are candidates for saphenous vein ablation (grade 1B recommendation).[1] Certainly in those who do not desire interventional options or are not candidates for superficial venous ablation, the Guidelines Committee suggests compression therapy (20 to 30 mm Hg) for symptomatic benefits (grade 2C).

Compression is the standard of care for patients with advanced CVD (C_{3-6}). The evidence suggests that venous ulcers heal more quickly with compression therapy than without compression and that noncompliance with therapy is associated with both nonhealing of the ulcer as well as increased risk of recurrence. Compression also decreases the risk of recurrence following surgical intervention. Some evidence supports multicomponent compression over single-component compression. As a general approach, multilayer relatively inelastic wraps are preferred for the therapy phase of venous disease (ulcer healing). With ulcer healing, elastic wraps, such as compression stockings, are used to maintain a stable clinical condition (maintenance phase). In addition, elevating the legs when possible, during the day, avoiding prolonged periods of standing or sitting, and elevating the foot of the bed 4 to 6 in above the heart while sleeping are adjuvant components of conservative therapy.

Intermittent pneumatic compression (IPC) provides pulsatile emptying of the venous system via compressive bladder that inflates and deflates. A Cochrane review suggests that there is advantage in using IPC compared to no compression, but little evidence to support that it adds to compression therapy alone. Currently it is recommended that IPC be employed when compression has failed, is unavailable, or cannot be used.

Other forms of conservative therapy for CVI include lifestyle changes such as exercise as well as pharmacologic agents. Structured exercise can improve dynamic muscle strength and calf muscle pump function in patients with essentially all levels of CVI from varicose veins to venous ulceration. A meta-analysis of five RCTs found that exercise was associated with healing of venous ulcers at 12 weeks and the use of supervised active exercise to improve muscle pump function and to reduce pain and edema in patients with leg ulcers is a guideline recommendation.

In Europe and other countries, various oral agents (eg, rutosides, hesperidin/diosmine, dobesilate) are used to improve the feeling of heaviness, fatigue, and even edema associated with CVD, but these agents are not available as FDA-regulated medications in the United States. Among these supplements, the best data exists for micronized purified flavonoid fraction or ruscus extracts for symptoms of pain, leg heaviness, and/or sensation of swelling. Pentoxifylline can be used in patients with venous ulcers. A review of 12 trials indicated[27] that pentoxifylline does provide an incremental benefit in ulcer healing when used as an adjunct to compression and may also have some effect in the absence of compression but the tradeoff is more gastrointestinal adverse effects. Current practice is to prescribe 400 mg of pentoxifylline three times per day and, if tolerated, 800 mg three times per day may accelerate ulcer healing.[28] Prophylactic use of systemic antibiotics in the treatment of venous ulcers does not improve healing and may only select resistant organisms. Certainly, an established infection (cellulitis or deeper) must be treated as it would be at any site. Limb cellulitis with or without a venous ulcer generally requires systemic gram-positive antibiotic coverage.

Surgical Therapy

The use of surgical intervention in the realm of venous disease, as in all areas of vascular surgery, is driven by the documented presence of disease, the risk of the intervention, and the expected outcome (**Algorithm 93.1**).

Telangiectasia, Reticular Veins, and Branch Varicose Veins

Laser or intense pulsed light (IPL) ablates telangiectasias with reasonable success, inducing vessel destruction by targeting the absorption peaks of hemoglobin. Various devices exist with selection based on the wavelength and pulse duration most appropriate for the size and location of the lesion. In general, shorter wavelengths work best for smaller diameter vessels. Dyspigmentation can occur and tanned skin is a contraindication to treatment because melanin is a strong competing chromophore that absorbs the light energy and causes a tattoo.

Sclerotherapy (needle injection of detergents, hypertonic solutions, or chemical irritants directly into superficial veins with or without ultrasound guidance) is used to treat varicosities most often remaining after saphenous ablation, small, isolated varicosities, telangiectasias, and reticular veins. Sclerotherapy alone is an effective treatment for branch varicosities in patients without major saphenous reflux or when combined with techniques to treat major saphenous reflux when present.[29] The FDA-approved sclerosing agents are sodium

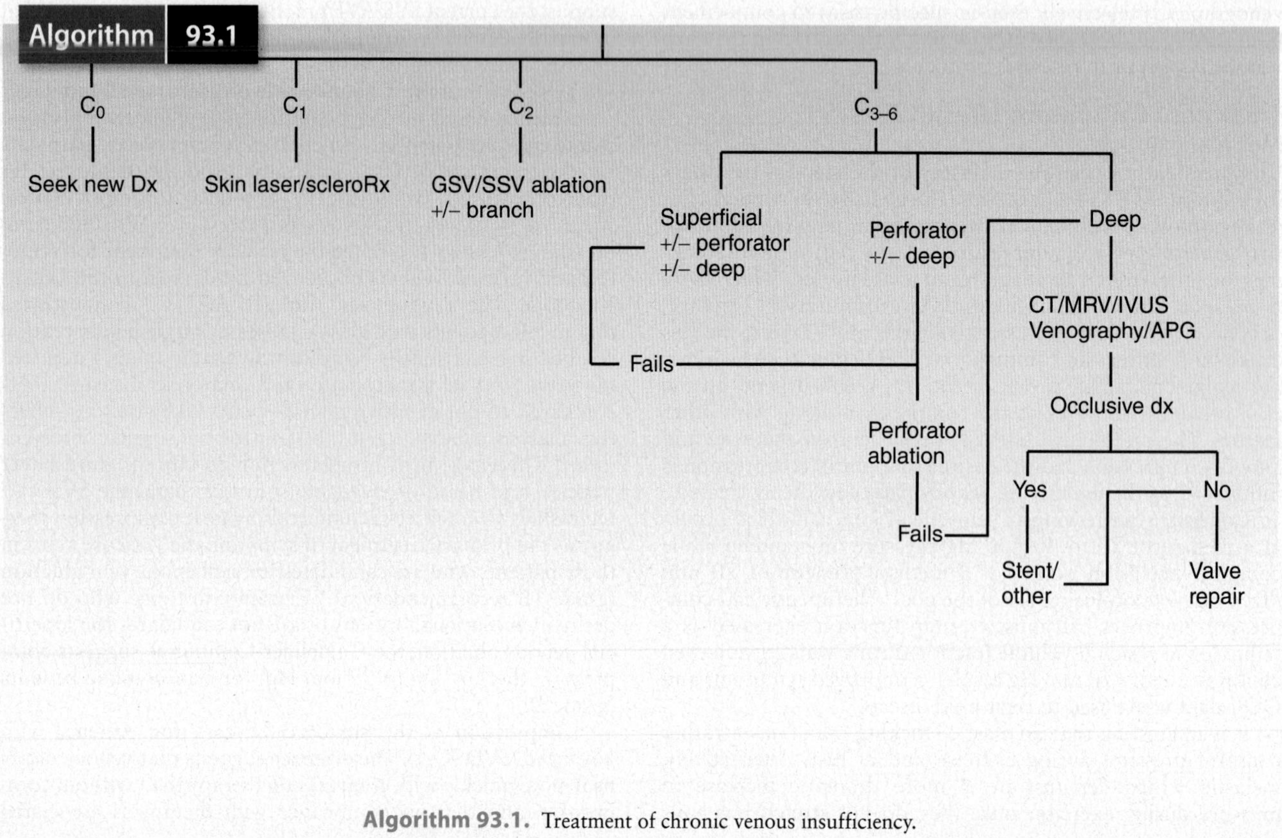

Algorithm 93.1. Treatment of chronic venous insufficiency.

tetradecyl sulfate (STS), sodium morrhuate, polidocanol (PLD), and glycerin. Hypertonic saline (23.4%), although not approved for sclerotherapy in the United States, is used and has been for many years. All act to damage the vein endothelium, inducing inflammation and scarring with ultimate lumen collapse. PLD has rapidly been adopted as the workhorse for venous sclerotherapy because of very low allergic and anaphylactic reaction rates, a low risk of tissue necrosis, in addition to being essentially painless. Foam sclerotherapy is the addition of air, carbon dioxide or other gases to a sclerosants such as PLD to allow a more protracted contact of the sclerosing agent to the vein wall. The most popular technique uses two syringes and a three-way stopcock to allow the gas to be aspirated into one of the syringes, while the other syringe contains a detergent sclerosant, which results in a one part of drug to four parts of gas mixture. Aggressive agitation of the mixture between the syringes allows for a more stable, microbubble containing foam. The exact concentration of sclerosant, liquid or foam, used for sclerotherapy is dependent on vein size and agent used. These interventions are generally outpatient procedures with low complication rates. Transient local discomfort is common and rarely extravasation of the agent, especially if ultrasound guidance is not used, can cause fat or skin necrosis with ulceration. Hyperpigmentation can occur and is reduced by microthrombectomy of clotted blood trapped in treated veins especially in veins 1 mm or less in diameter. Other potential complications of sclerotherapy include allergic reactions and systemic toxicity if too much agent is used at one sitting. Rarely neurologic events including visual disturbance, migraine, and stroke are reported, and this possibility must be discussed with the patient prior to its use. The presence of a patent foramen ovale is associated with a higher frequency of transient neurologic events while the use of CO_2 as the mixing gas used for foam sclerotherapy appears to decrease the risk of such adverse events. On the basis of the available data, the SVS/AVF Guidelines Committee recommends that liquid or foam sclerotherapy be used to treat telangiectasia, reticular veins, and varicose veins (grade 1B).[1]

Phlebectomy (ambulatory phlebectomy, stab avulsion, stab phlebectomy, microphlebectomy, and microextraction are synonymous terms) is a technique in which varicose veins are removed through small skin stab incisions with hooks or small mosquito clamps used to pull the vein from its bed. It can be performed in an ambulatory setting with local anesthesia or in conjunction with a more invasive procedure. There is evidence that phlebectomy has fewer recurrences than sclerotherapy but is still associated with risks (blisters, telangiectatic matting, scar formation, and bruising). Tumescent anesthesia has allowed for ambulatory interventions with little pain.

Saphenous Vein Ablation

If axial and extensive saphenous insufficiency is present, some method of eliminating reflux is required for best results. Entirely removing the refluxing vein from the venous system is the current best and most studied solution. Saphenous veins are most commonly removed from the venous circulation via endovenous ablative (ie, closure) techniques. These include thermal methods such as radiofrequency ablation (RFA) or laser ablation. In addition, there are nonthermal methods of endovenous ablation: mechanochemical, cyanoacrylate embolization, and foam sclerotherapy. These techniques also cause intravenous scarring, fibrosis, and occlusion.

For laser or RFA interventions, access is gained percutaneously and the respective device is advanced into the vein to about 2 cm below the SFJ using duplex imaging for proper positioning (**Fig. 93.1**). Tumescent anesthesia, typically inclusive of a local anesthetic (like lidocaine), epinephrine (which constricts blood vessels and prolongs anesthesia), and sodium bicarbonate (which helps reduce stinging and speeds up the anesthetic effect), is administered within the saphenous compartment providing anesthesia, a heat sink, and some venous

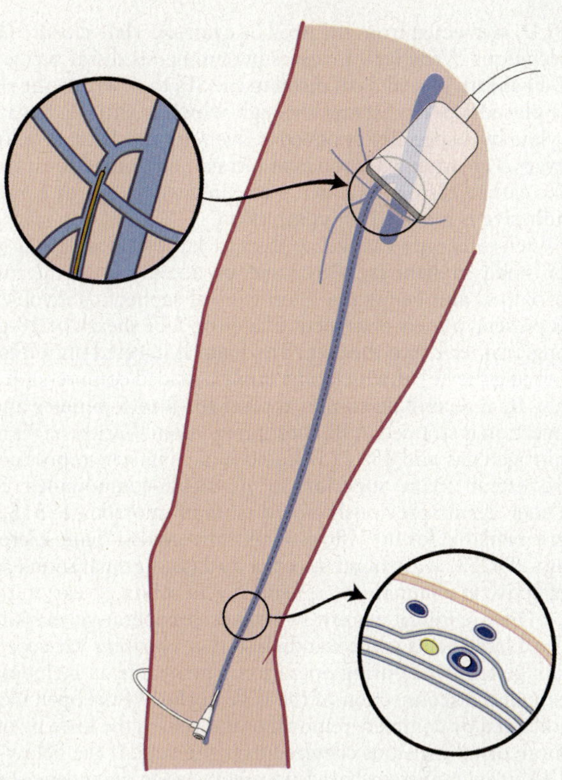

Figure 93.1. An artist depiction of percutaneous radiofrequency ablation of the great saphenous vein. Note percutaneous access of the vein around the knee and advancement of the device to about 2 cm below the CFV. The vein is serially treated with the RFA probe (or laser, glue, sclerosant in other methods) to result in ablation. Pulling the sheath and applying pressure is sufficient to prevent bleeding from the access site. Note the close location of the saphenous nerve near the GSV at the knee and below. (Lower magnification demonstrates saphenous nerve in saphenous tunnel [*yellow structure*] near the great saphenous vein and is protected somewhat by tumescent anesthesia. Outside the saphenous compartment can be one or more accessory saphenous veins.) Note that the superficial epigastric vein generally maintains flow after ablation. (Upper magnification demonstrates typical side branches, RFA device ~2 cm below the common femoral vein and somewhat below the superficial epigastric vein.)

compression during the procedure. After tumescent is administered, the saphenous vein is sequentially heated throughout its length as the heating probe (laser fiber or RFA device) is pulled back to the entrance site. The precise parameters for heating the RFA probe is standardized for each pullback length and treatment cycle (eg, 7-cm sections and 20-second cycles) and usually two treatment cycles are used in the more proximal segment of the vein to ensure proximal ablation at the point of maximal reflux from the deep system.

Laser energy of various wavelengths (810 to 1470 nm) delivered via bare-tipped fiber will cause a localized thermal injury to the vein wall. The laser probe technique is more physician directed and involves a slow, continuous withdrawal as opposed to the stepwise removal of the RFA probe (generally 1 to 2 mm/s at 10 W with a desired 60 to 100 J/cm). The exact rate and energy delivered depends on the device used but like RFA, typically more ablative effort is applied to the first 10 cm of the vein.

The nonthermal methods generally do not require tumescent anesthesia (no need for a heat sink or anesthesia) and so are potentially better tolerated by patients. The mechanical occlusion chemical-assisted (MOCA) ablation technique requires distal percutaneous saphenous access and positioning of the rotating wire 2 cm below the SFJ or at the fascial curve of the SPJ. Only the wire is activated for the first centimeter (induces spasm), for the remainder of the 1.5 mm/s pull pack of the rotating wire, sclerosant (8 to 12 mL of 1.5% STS or

PLD) is injected from the tip. The cyanoacrylate closure (CAC) technique (VenaSeal) involves percutaneous distal access with 7-Fr sheath placed 5 cm distal to the SFJ then within the sheath is placed a 5-Fr catheter through which is extruded cyanoacrylate by a specially designed delivery gun. 0.1 mL is delivered every 3 cm after 30 seconds of ultrasound-guided pressure and the catheter is pulled down 3 cm. In general, 1.3 to 1.5 mL of adhesive is required for completion.

Sclerotherapy can be applied to large-vein ablation (great or small saphenous). Percutaneous access above the knee if proximal and below the knee if distal saphenous involvement is present, allows placement of a 4- or 5-Fr sheath or 18-gauge angiocatheter into the vein. The foam is injected until it is seen nearing the SFJ at which time duplex-guided compression (usually by a second person) is applied for 3 to 5 minutes and the injection is stopped. A PLD propriety foam (Varithena™) mixes nitrogen gas and 1% PLD liquid in a cannister to produce the consistent foam superior to physician-compounded foam. Other agents previously noted (sodium morrhuate, STS, etc.) are available for use. Ultrasonography-guided foam sclerotherapy (UGFS) was found superior to liquid preparations and is effective in elimination saphenous vein reflux at least initially.

Open surgical removal involves preoperative marking of the dilated veins while standing so that apparent varicose veins can be removed during operation. The operation includes ligation and disconnection of the GSV at the SFJ via open incision followed by complete removal of the vein to the knee by one or more distal incisions centered over the vein. If the below-knee GSV is incompetent based on preoperative diagnostic studies, it may be excised. The method of vein removal may involve the introduction of long metal or plastic stripping wires with removable heads of varying size or various other tools to facilitate pulling the vein from the distal leg incision. Both the GSV and SSV can be treated by these methods with proper patient positioning and knowledge of existing anatomic variability especially of concern in the case of the SSV. In particular, protection of the sural nerve by limited deep dissection is critical.

Efforts to evaluate and compare the outcomes of these various techniques provide useful generalizations. Direct comparisons between surgical and endovenous modalities support that RFA and laser have comparable results to open surgery and to each other, but that UGFS may have a lower technical success rate and a higher rate of recurrent reflux at 5 years.[30] Furthermore, a recent meta-analysis comparing nonthermal to thermal saphenous ablation found that nonthermal were as effective as thermal techniques initially and at 1 year with potentially less procedural pain but no difference in paresthesia, phlebitis, or skin pigmentation.

Clinically recurrent varicose veins after GSV high ligation and stripping are observed in less than 25% of cases at 2 years, around 55% at 5 years, and in one study reached 62% at 11 years. It should be noted, however, that recurrent varicosities do not indicate recurrent reflux at the SFJ; in a meta-analysis, following high ligation and stripping only 12% of 549 legs developed recurrent reflux at the SFJ at 5 years.[30] Rather other sites of reflux (perforators, neovascularization of parallel veins, etc.) result in the recurrences noted. Recurrences occur with all techniques used for saphenous ablation.

Complications of GSV interventions are rare but include wound infection, DVT, nerve damage, thrombophlebitis, and hematoma formation. Saphenous nerve injury can result in an area of numbness around the knee or foot (may be clinically unrecognized) but does highlight that surrounding structures must be protected from thermal injury during RFA or laser ablation by appropriate use of tumescent. Complications from SSV interventions additionally include the risk of sural nerve injury. Potential complications of sclerotherapy have been mentioned previously with embolization to local arteries or the systemic circulation as specific risks. Endothermal heat–induced thrombosis (EHIT) refers to the propagation of thrombus into the deep vein contiguous with a superficial vein that has been ablated with endothermal methods that complicates approximately 3% of procedures. Treatment is determined by classification with therapeutic anticoagulation is reserved for class III/IV EHIT in which >50% of the lumen of the deep vein is compromised by thrombus propagation (class III) and/or thrombus propagation into the deep vein yields an occlusive DVT (class IV).[31]

The elimination of saphenous reflux is useful in treating more advance stages of CVD in the patient with a venous ulcer (C_6). A randomized controlled trial comparing compression alone versus compression plus saphenous surgery in patients with active or recently healed venous ulcers found a significant decrease in ulcer recurrence in the surgery group, 31% versus 56% at 4 years but there was no difference in ulcer-healing rates, 89% versus 93% at 3 years. A meta-analysis conducted in 2014 also failed to find more than low-quality evidence favoring ablation over compression therapy alone to improve ulcer healing. However, a recent RCT compared early endovenous ablation of superficial venous reflux with late intervention (after ulcer healing or greater 6 months after enrollment) in 450 patients with leg ulcers and found faster healing in the early intervention group with a median time to healing of 56 versus 82 days.[32] Extrapolating these results to the patients with a healed ulcer, ablation in addition to standard compression therapy is recommended to prevent recurrence (grade 1C). In patients with skin changes at risk of venous ulceration, the same treatment is suggested (grade 2C).

Perforator Vein Ablation

Perforator vein reflux is amenable to open or percutaneous ablative methods. Open methods of perforator ablation, subfascial endoscopic perforator surgery (SEPS) or the "Linton procedure," although successful have been replaced by less invasive methods of treatment. In patients with active ulcers and both superficial and perforator incompetence to the pertinent ulcer bed, it is suggested that both are ablated to aid in ulcer healing and to prevent recurrence and in patients without active ulcers the addition of perforation ablation can be simultaneous or staged on the basis of outcome.

Methods of percutaneous perforator ablation include RFA, laser, and UGFS. No matter the ablating energy delivered (radiofrequency, laser, or chemical) during percutaneous perforator vein ablation, ultrasonographic access, operative monitoring, and confirmation of results are routine and the procedure is accomplished under local anesthesia. The ablating device is inserted into the pathologic perforator and is serially pulled back during activation to burn the perforator for its length or the sclerosant injected into it with a similar result. Prevention of energy delivery to the deep system prevents unwanted thrombosis, accomplished by positioning the ablation device (when used) away from the deep system or by properly compressing the vein at or just slightly below the fascia when using sclerotherapy. A recent retrospective review of 296 ablations comparing all three modalities reported differing closure rates: 57% for UGFS, 73% for RFA, and 61% for laser at 2 weeks, and found that thermal ablation was statistically superior to UGFS.[33] Complications are rare but there is risk of DVT, phlebitis, local necrosis, AV fistula, and other risks associated with thermal and chemical ablations.

Iliac Stenting and Venous Bypass

Iliac recanalization via venoplasty with or without stent placement is recommended in addition to standard compression therapy to aid in venous ulcer healing and prevention of ulcer recurrence in patients with proximal venous occlusion/severe stenosis and C_{4b}, C_5, and C_6 disease. Endovascular stenting of iliac vein stenosis/obstruction involves percutaneous access of a disease-free caudal (popliteal, femoral, common femoral) or cephalad (internal jugular) vein with guidewire/catheter advancement across the lesion under fluoroscopic guidance and generally intravascular ultrasonographic confirmation of

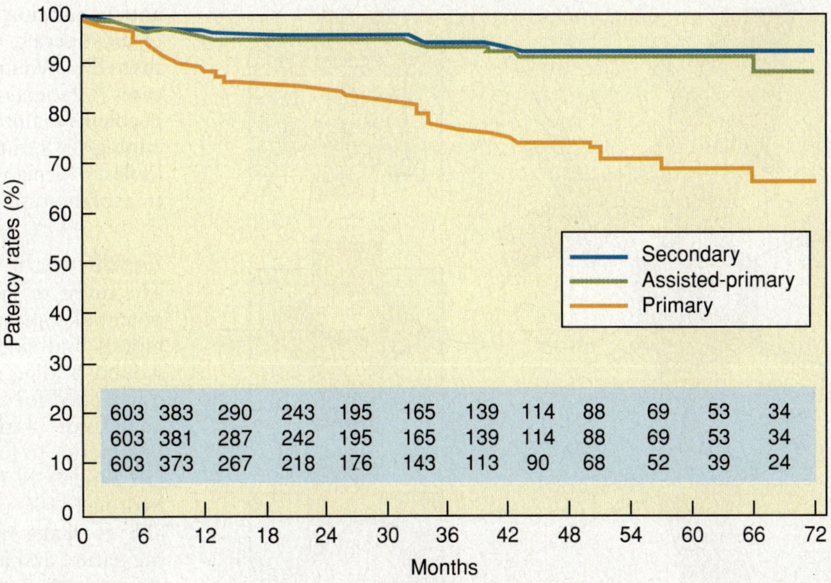

Figure 93.2. Life-table presentation demonstrates the patency rates of iliac venous stents placed for symptomatic occlusive venous disease. (From After Neglén P, Hollis KC, Olivier J, et al. Stenting of the venous outflow in chronic venous disease: long-term stent-related outcome, clinical, and hemodynamic result. *J Vasc Surg.* 2007;46[5]:979–990.)

stenosis >50%. If confirmed, dilation with a 12- to 18-mm diameter percutaneous balloon, depending on the vein involved from common femoral to common iliac, is undertaken with subsequent self-expanding stent deployment to maintain the dilation. This is accomplished from normal outflow to distal normal vein even to the area of lesser trochanter within the common femoral vein if needed to ensure good inflow. In one study, 133 patients with active ulcers had an initial healing rate of 65% at 6 months and 54% at 5 years following venous stenting and rates may be even higher when complete obstruction is relieved.[34] The primary and assisted primary stent patency rates at 3 years are 75% and 92%, and at 6 years are 67% and 89%, respectively, and patency is, in general, higher for nonthrombotic than thrombotic obstructions (**Fig. 93.2**).[35] Potential complications include major bleeding, PE, early thrombosis, access site complications, retroperitoneal hematoma. Overall, however, complications are rare with essentially no mortality associated with the procedure.[35]

When endovenous therapies are unable to be performed, open surgical techniques may be employed, however these procedures have become quite rare in contemporary practice. These generally utilize the native saphenous vein or polytetrafluoroethylene (PTFE) graft material as the conduit to bypass from a nondiseased distal vein to a disease-free proximal or collateral axial vein. Vena cava or bilateral iliac veins occlusion reconstructions often use PTFE grafts to allow a proper size match. If a single iliac vein is severely stenosed or occluded and percutaneous methods have failed, cross-femoral venous bypass (Palma procedure) or direct repair of the iliac vein provides therapeutic options. Overall, patient survival is considered prior to aggressive intervention if iliac vein compression is due to cancerous encroachment. The cross-femoral venous bypass involves passing a vein graft or synthetic conduit via a suprapubic subcutaneous tunnel from the common femoral vein on the affected side to contralateral femoral vein and normal outflow system. The saphenous vein or prosthetic graft is connected to the unaffected femoral vein by an end-to-side technique after anastomosis on the affected side. The key to success of this surgery may be graft diameter. If the native vein is less than 4.5 mm in diameter, better success may be achieved with a 10-mm diameter PTFE graft, although in retrospective studies, PTFE does have lower patency.

For occlusion of the common femoral vein or distal iliac disease, a hybrid approach involving endophlebectomy and patch angioplasty in combination with angioplasty and stenting of the iliac vein has been explored. In one series of 64 open surgical or hybrid reconstructions for iliofemoral venous or IVC obstructions, the overall 5-year secondary patency was 59%. For the femoroiliac and ilio-infrahepatic IVC reconstructions, the 5-year secondary patency was 86% while it was 78% for the Palma procedure while longer bypasses, complex or hybrid procedures had lower patency rates.

In patients with chronic symptomatic occlusion of the femoral or proximal popliteal vein, saphenopopliteal vein bypass may be considered if conservative therapy has failed. The patient's distal GSV is transected and anastomosed end to side to the deep system at a site distal to the obstruction allowing venous drainage to bypass the obstruction. This procedure is relatively rare, however, as it necessitates that the patient has a patent proximal common femoral and iliocaval systems as well as a competent GSV. In a series of 17 patients with a median follow-up of 103 months, secondary patency was 75%.[36]

Venous Valve Repair or Replacement

The goal of venous valve repair or replacement is the prevention of deep venous reflux and, consequently, a decrease in sustained distal venous hypertension. These interventions are considered only after all other more easily treated venous pathology has been addressed. In planning and during these operations, several observations influence what the surgeon can offer a patient. Preoperative planning helps to determine if a valve is present locally or remotely, and if the recipient conduit is sufficiently disease free to allow a valve repair or replacement. Intraoperative observations can lead to change in plan: for example, if handling of the suspect valve results in vasoconstriction and secondary competence (often determined by a standard "strip test"), an external valvuloplasty or a prosthetic sleeve technique may be viable options. If an internal valvuloplasty is deemed necessary, the type of venotomy used to expose the valve leaflets varies between practitioners and those described include a single longitudinal, single supravalvular transverse, a T incision, and a trapdoor incision (**Fig. 93.3**). If an absence of valve attachment lines are noted during surgery this may signify the destruction of the valve as a consequence of the PTS, prevent valvuloplasty and prompting other than an in situ repair. Descriptions of the valvular repair options are found in **Table 93.5**.

Whether valvuloplasty, transplant or transposition; aggressive venous valve surgery requires appropriate consideration of perioperative adjunctive care. This care includes prophylactic antibiotics, intraoperative heparinization, especially if the vein is opened, the use of pneumatic compression devices postoperatively, and the use of LMWH or IV heparin in the postoperative period. Some use closed-suction drainage of wounds to avoid hematoma and seroma formation. Warfarin should have an initial target INR range of 2.0 to 2.5 for the

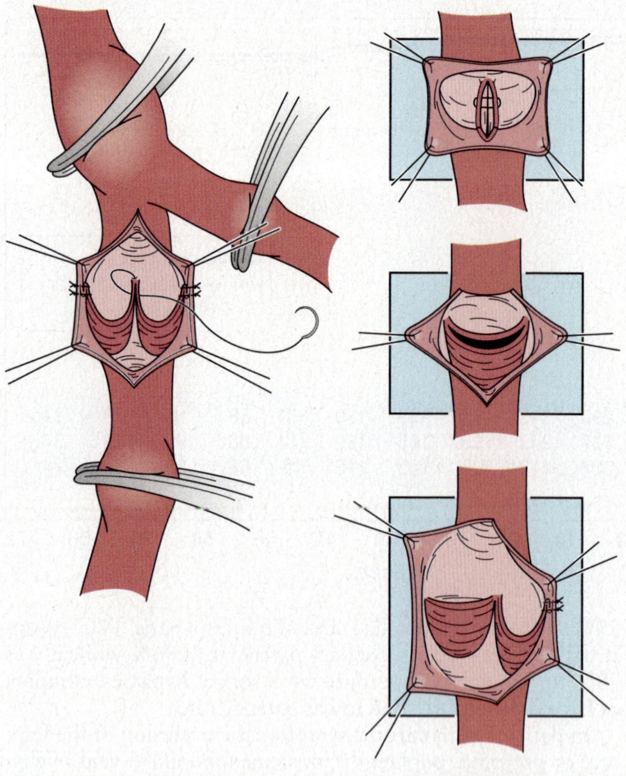

Figure 93.3. Open valvuloplasty to repair an insufficient valve can be accomplished by various venotomy incisions. **A:** Single longitudinal. **B:** Single supravalvular transverse. **C:** T-shaped. **D:** Trapdoor.

first 6 weeks and some would advocate a subsequent decrease to 1.7 to 2.0 until 4 months when it is discontinued. Adjustments are made to accommodate those with an increased risk of thrombosis.

Valve repair procedures are well tolerated by most patients and have a low morbidity, as well as essentially zero mortality in most series. Hematoma and seroma formation are noted in less than 15% of cases, depending on the level of anticoagulation used. DVT occurs in less than 10% of cases in most series, while the pulmonary emboli risk is well less than 1%. Wound infections have been seen in 2% to 7% of cases.[37] Patients with postthrombotic reflux tend to have more problems maintaining healed ulcers than those with a primary etiology of reflux, as noted from the results of internal valvuloplasty (generally a primary etiology) versus those requiring transplantation or a transposition operative approach.

Venous Ulcer Wound Care

The quest to heal venous ulcers has generated a myriad of potential topical agents to aid in ulcer healing. Topical antibiotics and dressings containing antimicrobials may retard wound healing and cause allergic reactions and are not recommended for the treatment of venous ulcers. A recent meta-analysis of 78 trials found low-quality evidence that silver may be superior to foam (397 patients in 4 trials) and hydrocolloid (58 patients in 1 trial), and that sucralfate may be superior to hydrogel (100 patients in 1 trial). Insufficient data are available to make firm conclusions, but it is recommended that the nature and amount of the exudates present may provide a rationale for dressing selection as an absorbent dressing should be applied to wet wounds to decrease the risk of surrounding skin maceration and infection, while dry wounds should be treated with dressing that will keep them moist to accelerate healing. The SVS/AVF Guidelines Committee suggests that the wound dressing be selected, which absorbs wound exudates and protects the periulcer skin from damage.

Surgical debridement to healthy tissue, when required, benefits the rate of ulcer healing and does not lead to a higher risk of systemic infection. The use of local anesthetic (EMLA) during debridement of venous leg ulcers has been found beneficial in lowering pain scores in a Cochrane analysis of six trials.[38] For resistant venous ulcers, defined as those that fail to demonstrate improvement in a minimum of 4 to 6 weeks of standard wound therapy, adjuvant wound therapy options should be considered. Skin grafting allows for coverage of raw surfaces to speed the healing process and there are reports on improved healing with skin grafting for chronic venous ulceration. A number of skin substitutes have been used to aid in venous ulcer healing. The use of these skin substitutes is suggested as guideline adjuvant therapy in recalcitrant venous ulcer care.

Table 93.5. Repair Methods for Deep Valvular Insufficiency

Repair Method	General Patient Population	Description
External valvuloplasty[a]	Primary reflux	Sutures placed transmurally via valve attachment lines. Can be done blindly or via angioscope. Alternatively, external prosthetic sleeve the vein at the valved and can be sutured around the vein to diminish size of vein lumen.
Internal valvuloplasty	Primary reflux	Venotomy and suturing of elongated valve leaflets to tighten the valve cusps. Lateral edges of cusps can be sutured to apices of respective commisures, or the excess can be excised, and cusp reimplanted.
Valve transplantation[b]	Postthrombotic	Donor vein segment from competent axillary vein sutured into incompetent femoral vein segment
Valve transposition	Postthrombotic	Incompetent femoral vein segment excised and placed below competent valve in profunda or GSV.
Valve substitutes[c]	Postthrombotic	Ophthalmic knife used to dissect thickened vein wall to create valve cusps. Sutures used to hold valve in semiopen position.

[a]Works best if handling of the vein results in vasoconstriction and competence.
[b]If profunda is incompetent popliteal may be better location.
[c]Can be achieved endovascularly with investigative devices.

Miscellaneous Pelvic Disorders

The complex interconnections of the renal, ovarian, common and internal iliac and lower extremity veins can explain how distention in one or more of the proximal veins can result in distal distention and symptoms. Compression of the left renal vein between the superior mesenteric artery and aorta can result in left renal vein compression ("nutcracker syndrome"), so called because the renal vein is being crushed like a nut between the respective arteries. The most common symptoms are left flank pain and microscopic or gross hematuria but as the disease progresses the pelvic veins are more affected resulting in symptoms related to pelvic congestion syndrome. As a result of left ovarian vein or pelvic vein reflux, upper thigh and pelvic varicosities may be noted. Duplex imaging followed by CT or MRI confirms the clinical suspicion with often venography demonstrating renal vein compression and a pressure gradient. Open surgical vein repositioning (ie, renal vein transposition), gonadal vein transposition, and/or endovascular stenting can relieve the compression. A consequence of pelvic reflux and varicose veins may be dyspareunia, dysuria, dysmenorrhea, and postcoital pain. Duplex, CT, or MRI can help confirm the diagnosis, but venography provides venous detail and potential therapeutic options. Gonadal vein excision is described but has been supplanted by endovascular techniques using coils, sclerosants, or a combination thereof. Hypogastric vein reflux may be best managed by percutaneous embolization.

References

1. Gloviczki P, Lawrence PF, Wasan SM, et al. The 2022 Society for Vascular Surgery, American Venous Forum, and American Vein and Lymphatic Society clinical practice guidelines for the management of varicose veins of the lower extremities. Part I. Duplex scanning and treatment of superficial truncal reflux: endorsed by the Society for Vascular Medicine and the International Union of Phlebology. *J Vasc Surg Venous Lymphat Disord*. 2023;11(2): 231–261, e236.
2. Anderson FA Jr, Wheeler HB, Goldberg RJ, et al. A population-based perspective of the hospital incidence and case-fatality rates of deep vein thrombosis and pulmonary embolism. The Worcester DVT Study. *Arch Intern Med*. 1991;151(5):933–938.
3. Heit JA. The epidemiology of venous thromboembolism in the community. *Arterioscler Thromb Vasc Biol*. 2008;28(3): 370–372.
4. Wells PS, Anderson DR, Rodger M, et al. Derivation of a simple clinical model to categorize patients probability of pulmonary embolism: increasing the models utility with the SimpliRED D-dimer. *Thromb Haemost*. 2000;83(3):416–420.
5. PIOPED Investigators. Value of the ventilation/perfusion scan in acute pulmonary embolism. Results of the prospective investigation of pulmonary embolism diagnosis (PIOPED). *JAMA*. 1990;263(20): 2753–2759.
6. Stein PD, Chenevert TL, Fowler SE, et al. Gadolinium-enhanced magnetic resonance angiography for pulmonary embolism: a multicenter prospective study (PIOPED III). *Ann Intern Med*. 2010; 152(7):434–443.
7. Kataruka A, Kong X, Haymart B, et al. SAMe-TT(2)R(2) predicts quality of anticoagulation in patients with acute venous thromboembolism: The MAQI(2) experience. *Vasc Med*. 2017;22(3): 197–203.
8. Palareti G, Cosmi B, Legnani C, et al. D-dimer testing to determine the duration of anticoagulation therapy. *N Engl J Med*. 2006; 355(17):1780–1789.
9. Khorana AA, Noble S, Lee AYY, et al. Role of direct oral anticoagulants in the treatment of cancer-associated venous thromboembolism: guidance from the SSC of the ISTH. *J Thromb Haemost*. 2018;16(9):1891–1894.
10. Rodger MA, Le Gal G, Anderson DR, et al. Validating the HERDOO2 rule to guide treatment duration for women with unprovoked venous thrombosis: multinational prospective cohort management study. *BMJ*. 2017;356:j1065.
11. de Winter MA, Büller HR, Carrier M, et al; VTE-PREDICT study group. Recurrent venous thromboembolism and bleeding with extended anticoagulation: the VTE-PREDICT risk score. *Eur Heart J*. 2023;44(14):1231–1244. Erratum in: *Eur Heart J*. 2024;45(29):2630.
12. Righini M, Galanaud JP, Guenneguez H, et al. Anticoagulant therapy for symptomatic calf deep vein thrombosis (CACTUS): a randomised, double-blind, placebo-controlled trial. *Lancet Haematol*. 2016;3(12):e556–e562.
13. Stevens, SM, Woller SC, Kreuziger LB, et al. Antithrombotic therapy for VTE disease: Compendium and review of CHEST guidelines 2012–2021. *Chest*, 2024;166(2):388–404.
14. Amin EE, Bistervels IM, Meijer K, et al. Reduced incidence of vein occlusion and postthrombotic syndrome after immediate compression for deep vein thrombosis. *Blood*. 2018;132(21): 2298–2304.
15. Johnson MS, Spies JB, Scott KT, et al. Predicting the Safety and Effectiveness of Inferior Vena Cava Filters (PRESERVE): Outcomes at 12 months. *J Vasc Surg Venous Lymphat Disord*. 2023;11(3): 573–585.e6.
16. Vedantham S, Goldhaber SZ, Julian JA, et al. Pharmacomechanical catheter-directed thrombolysis for deep-vein thrombosis. *N Engl J Med*. 2017;377(23):2240–2252.
17. Decousus H, Prandoni P, Mismetti P, et al. Fondaparinux for the treatment of superficial-vein thrombosis in the legs. *N Engl J Med*. 2010;363(13):1222–1232.
18. Superficial Thrombophlebitis Treated By Enoxaparin Study Group. A pilot randomized double-blind comparison of a low-molecular-weight heparin, a nonsteroidal anti-inflammatory agent, and placebo in the treatment of superficial vein thrombosis. *Arch Intern Med*. 2003;163(14):1657–1663.
19. Beyer-Westendorf J, Schellong SM, Gerlach H, et al. Prevention of thromboembolic complications in patients with superficial-vein thrombosis given rivaroxaban or fondaparinux: the open-label, randomised, non-inferiority SURPRISE phase 3b trial. *Lancet Haematol*. 2017;4(3):e105–e113.
20. Kibbe MR, Ujiki M, Goodwin AL, Eskandari M, Yao J, Matsumura J. Iliac vein compression in an asymptomatic patient population. *J Vasc Surg*. 2004;39(5):937–943.
21. American Venous Forum Ad Hoc Outcomes Working Group; Vasquez MA, Rabe E, McLafferty RB, et al. Revision of the venous clinical severity score: venous outcomes consensus statement: special communication of the American Venous Forum Ad Hoc Outcomes Working Group. *J Vasc Surg*. 2010;52(5):1387–1396.
22. Launois R, Reboul-Marty J, Henry B. Construction and validation of a quality of life questionnaire in chronic lower limb venous insufficiency (CIVIQ). *Qual Life Res*. 1996;5(6):539–554.
23. Criado E, Farber MA, Marston WA, Daniel PF, Burnham CB, Keagy BA. The role of air plethysmography in the diagnosis of chronic venous insufficiency. *J Vasc Surg*. 1998;27(4):660–670.
24. Humphreys ML, Stewart AH, Gohel MS, Taylor M, Whyman MR, Poskitt KR. Management of mixed arterial and venous leg ulcers. *Br J Surg*. 2007;94(9):1104–1107.
25. O'Donnell TF Jr, Passman MA. Clinical practice guidelines of the Society for Vascular Surgery (SVS) and the American Venous Forum (AVF)–Management of venous leg ulcers. Introduction. *J Vasc Surg*. 2014;60(2 Suppl):1S–2S.
26. Ratcliffe J, Brazier JE, Campbell WB, Palfreyman S, MacIntyre JB, Michaels JA. Cost-effectiveness analysis of surgery versus conservative treatment for uncomplicated varicose veins in a randomized clinical trial. *Br J Surg*. 2006;93(2):182–186.
27. Jull AB, Arroll B, Parag V, Waters J. Pentoxifylline for treating venous leg ulcers. *Cochrane Database Syst Rev*. 2012;12(12):CD001733.
28. Falanga V, Fujitani RM, Diaz C, et al. Systemic treatment of venous leg ulcers with high doses of pentoxifylline: efficacy in a randomized, placebo-controlled trial. *Wound Repair Regen*. 1999; 7(4):208–213.
29. Belcaro G, Cesarone MR, Di Renzo A, et al. Foam-sclerotherapy, surgery, sclerotherapy, and combined treatment for varicose veins: a 10-year, prospective, randomized, controlled, trial (VEDICO trial). *Angiology*. 2003;54(3):307–315.

30. Hamann SAS, Giang J, De Maeseneer MGR, Nijsten TEC, van den Bos RR. Editor's choice – five year results of great saphenous vein treatment: a meta-analysis. *Eur J Vasc Endovasc Surg*. 2017; 54(6):760–770.
31. Tan M, Sadek M, Kabnick L, Parsi K, Davies AH; UIP. Management of endothermal heat-induced thrombosis. *Phlebology*. 2024;39(3):214–217.
32. Gohel MS, Heatley F, Liu X, et al. A randomized trial of early endovenous ablation in venous ulceration. *N Engl J Med*. 2018; 378(22):2105–2114.
33. Hager ES, Washington C, Steinmetz A, Wu T, Singh M, Dillavou E. Factors that influence perforator vein closure rates using radiofrequency ablation, laser ablation, or foam sclerotherapy. *J Vasc Surg Venous Lymphat Disord*. 2016;4(1):51–56.
34. Neglén P, Hollis KC, Olivier J, Raju S. Stenting of the venous outflow in chronic venous disease: long-term stent-related outcome, clinical, and hemodynamic result. *J Vasc Surg*. 2007;46(5): 979–990.
35. Razavi MK, Jaff MR, Miller LE. Safety and effectiveness of stent placement for iliofemoral venous outflow obstruction: systematic review and meta-analysis. *Circ Cardiovasc Interv*. 2015;8(10): e002772.
36. Coleman DM, Rectenwald JE, Vandy FC, Wakefield TW. Contemporary results after sapheno-popliteal bypass for chronic femoral vein occlusion. *J Vasc Surg Venous Lymphat Disord*. 2013; 1(1):45–51.
37. Dalsing MC, Kistner RL. Deep venous incompetence and valve repair. In: Almeida JI, ed. *Atlas of Endovascular Venous Surgery*. Elsevier; 2019:517–545.
38. Briggs M, Nelson EA, Martyn-St James M. Topical agents or dressings for pain in venous leg ulcers. *Cochrane Database Syst Rev*. 2012;11(11):CD001177.

Section N:
PEDIATRIC SURGERY

94

Fetal, Neonatal, and Pediatric Physiology

Kibileri Williams and Andrea Badillo

Key Points

1 A fundamental knowledge of embryology and the physiologic aspects of development is essential to understanding pediatric surgical disease and management concepts.

2 Disruptions of normal lung development lead to postnatal pulmonary dysfunction and morbidity. The earlier in development the disruption occurs, the more severe the impact on pulmonary function.

3 Delays in transition and persistence of fetal shunts lead to a variety of neonatal cardiopulmonary conditions.

4 Alterations in the normal levels of amniotic fluid may be an indicator of underlying congenital abnormalities.

5 Children compensate well for shock and hypotension is a late finding. Bradycardia is more ominous than tachycardia.

6 Septic shock in neonates and infants manifests as low cardiac output syndrome or "cold" shock, which is preferentially treated with inotropic agents such as dopamine, versus vasodilatory "warm" shock in older children and adults, which is treated primarily with vasoconstrictive agents such as norepinephrine.

7 Children have a higher metabolic rate and lower functional reserve capacity (FRC) than adults and therefore develop hypoxemia and respiratory distress quicker.

8 Fluid and energy requirements are greatest for neonates and gradually decrease over time until they reach adult levels.

The surgical care of infants and children requires management of congenital anomalies and unique physiologic patterns that differ from the care of adults. A fundamental knowledge of embryology and the physiologic aspects of development is essential to understanding pediatric surgical disease and
1 management concepts. This chapter highlights the key differences in fetal, neonatal, and pediatric physiology and demonstrates how these differences relate to pediatric disease and its treatment.

This chapter is intentionally not an exhaustive overview of human physiology, as such content is covered in dedicated chapters found in the Scientific Principles section of this textbook. Many disease- and technology-specific aspects of pediatric care are presented in other sections of this text (see Chapter 78: Congenital Heart Disease, Chapter 97: Pediatric Chest, Chapter 95: Fetal Intervention, and Chapter 81: Mechanical Circulatory Support).

Early Fetal Development

Introduction

Key events include the diaphragm separating the body into the thoracic and peritoneal cavities, the gut tube differentiation into the gastrointestinal (GI) tract, lung formation, and central nervous system development. During this period, the developing embryo is sensitive to various insults that may lead to congenital defects.

Foregut and Fetal Lung Development

The respiratory system has its beginnings in the fourth week of gestation when the respiratory diverticulum first appears as an outpouching of the foregut. The tracheoesophageal septum subsequently forms, dividing the respiratory tract from the GI tract. Failure of this septum to completely close results in a spectrum of congenital anomalies of the esophagus with variations of tracheoesophageal fistula and esophageal atresia.[1] Formation of the diaphragm and separation of the thoracic and abdominal spaces occurs during weeks 4 to 12. Failure of the pleuroperitoneal membrane to develop results in congenital diaphragmatic hernia (CDH).[1]

Fetal lung development proceeds through a series of stages each characterized by the formation of specific structural features and functional capacity. The **pseudoglandular phase** occurs from weeks 5 to 17 and is defined by bronchial branching and formation of the bronchial tree to the terminal bronchiole level. In the **canalicular phase** (16 to 24 weeks) the respiratory units form with the development of alveolar ducts and the surrounding capillary network that provides for gas exchange. At this stage's completion, respiration becomes possible and defines the earliest point of neonatal viability. Current American Academy of Pediatrics guidelines defines the lower limits of viability at 22 weeks.[2] The **saccular phase** (24 to 36 weeks) is characterized by the differentiation and maturation of type I and type II pneumocytes and the beginning of surfactant production. Surfactant is an essential lipoprotein that lines the alveolar membrane to lower the surface tension thereby protecting the alveolus from complete collapse during expiration. The **alveolar phase** of development (36 weeks to 8 years) results in further increases in alveoli size and number. This postnatal lung growth and development continues up to final lung maturation around age 8.

Disruptions of normal lung development lead to postnatal
2 pulmonary dysfunction and morbidity. In general, the earlier in development the disruption occurs, the more severe the impact on pulmonary function. In CDH, the herniation of abdominal contents into the fetal chest coincides with the pseudoglandular phase of lung impairing branching of the tracheobronchial tree. This effective "pruning" of the tracheobronchial tree results in pulmonary hypoplasia and pulmonary

hypertension. Infants born prior to 22 weeks of gestation will lack the basic respiratory unit development completed during the canalicular phase and are unlikely to survive. Surfactant production does not reach sufficient levels to prevent atelectasis until 32 weeks gestation. Respiratory distress syndrome (RDS) is defined as impaired gas exchange due to immature lungs and inadequate surfactant production occurring in premature infants less than 32 weeks of gestation.

The respiratory consequences of preterm birth can be mitigated by the administration of maternal betamethasone if at risk for preterm labor. A course of steroids given to women who are less than 34 weeks of gestation (but greater than 24 weeks) prior to preterm delivery can stimulate fetal production of surfactant, as well as hasten fetal lung maturity, decreasing the risk of developing RDS.[3] Once the neonate is born, treatment for RDS includes supplemental oxygen and respiratory support (continuous positive airway pressure [CPAP] or mechanical ventilation) as needed. Postnatal administration of exogenous surfactant has also been successful in prevention and treatment of RDS, though in rare cases it can cause pulmonary hemorrhage.[3]

Fetal Circulation and Transitional Physiology

The fetal circulatory system preferentially directs blood to the brain and heart, and bypasses the hepatic portal and pulmonary vascular beds through a series of three shunts. This circulatory pattern is important to prioritize oxygen delivery to the developing brain, maintain high pulmonary vascular resistance (PVR) in utero, and avoid unnecessary oxygen consumption in the hepatic circulation when the delivery of nutrients to the fetus occurs via the placenta, not through intestinal absorption. Various neonatal cardiopulmonary conditions are the result of persistence of these shunts or alterations in the transition from fetal to postnatal circulation at birth.

Oxygenated blood (typically at 80% saturation) enters the fetus from the placenta via the umbilical vein, passes through the liver, flows into the inferior vena cava, and then to the right atrium. The first shunt encountered is the ductus venosus (**Fig. 94.1**), which diverts blood away from the hepatic sinusoids and into the inferior vena cava, preventing the immediate consumption of oxygen and nutrients prior to blood reaching the brain and remainder of the systemic circulation. Most of the blood flow into the right atrium is then diverted through a second shunt—the foramen ovale. The foramen ovale is an intracardiac shunt through the atrial septum between the right and left atria that bypasses the right ventricle to allow flow of oxygenated blood directly to the left heart. The remainder of the blood (<10%) from the right atrium follows the normal pathway into the right ventricle, where it encounters the third shunt—the ductus arteriosus. This last shunt connects the pulmonary artery to the aorta just distal to the arch, feeding into the systemic circulation and allowing the remaining oxygenated blood to bypass the pulmonary vascular bed and to flow directly into the systemic circulation. The lungs do not play a role in gas exchange in the uterine environment and the vascular resistance in the pulmonary vascular bed is high, which maintains a right-to-left shunt through the patent ductus arteriosus (PDA) and minimizes unnecessary pulmonary blood flow. This shunting ensures the brain and heart receives more oxygenated blood and minimizes energy expenditure of the right heart pumping blood through a dormant pulmonary vascular tree.[1] Despite these shunts, systemic blood remains quite deoxygenated due to mixing at the level of the IVC (<60% saturation). Blood flow back to the placenta is derived from the systemic circulation, with blood flow returning to the placenta via the paired umbilical arteries arising from the iliac arteries bilaterally.

Transition from fetal to postnatal circulation begins at birth in response to a series of anatomic and physiologic triggers. Changes in vascular resistance and blood flow patterns promote closure of the three fetal shunts. Clamping of the umbilical cord causes a simultaneous decrease in mesenteric blood return and increase in systemic vascular resistance (SVR) resulting in closure of the ductus venosus. Initiation of respiration causes a decrease in PVR. Decreased PVR combined with increased SVR leads to decreased right heart pressure and increased left heart pressure and closure of the foramen ovale. Closure of the ductus arteriosus occurs secondary to vasoconstriction of the vessel in response to increasing oxygenation of the blood and decreasing levels of prostaglandins (PGE). The ensuing ischemic changes to the inner muscular layer render it resistant to the vasodilatory effects of PGE and cause tissue remodeling that obliterates the lumen of the ductus in term infants.

Delays in transition and persistence of fetal shunts lead to a
3 variety of neonatal cardiopulmonary conditions. Premature infants are at highest risk for persistent fetal circulation. In premature neonates, blood oxygen levels within the ductus do not drop to the same level of hypoxemia needed to promote the remodeling process, resulting in an increased risk for PDA.

Persistent elevations in PVR (persistent pulmonary hypertension of the newborn; PPHN) can lead to persistence of the PFO and PDA. In the presence of persistent elevation of PVR, shunts through the PDA and PFO remain right to left, with deoxygenated blood from the right heart passing through the patent foramen ovale and from the main pulmonary artery through the ductus arteriosus, leading to lower oxygen saturation measured in the left arm and bilateral legs (postductal saturation) compared to that measured in the right arm or head (preductal saturation).[4]

In the absence of elevated PVR, the ductus arteriosus is expected to close within the first 48 hours in 96% of term neonates without other cardiac anomaly and who are otherwise healthy.[5] Failure of closure leads to a PDA, which has been reported in 56.7 per 100,000 live births, not including those incidentally found on echocardiogram.[6] In premature neonates, younger gestational age and lower birth weight are associated with lower rates of closure by 1 week of life.[7] Left-to-right shunting through persistent large PDAs results in pulmonary overcirculation, and can lead to heart failure and an increased risk of chronic lung disease. When PDA closure is desired, medical treatment options include indomethacin, ibuprofen, or acetaminophen.[8] Operative PDA ligation was first reported by pediatric surgeon Robert Gross in 1939[9] and remains an option for treatment of PDAs that fail attempts at medical therapy. In the last decade, enthusiasm for surgical PDA ligation and pharmacologic treatment has waned with evidence emerging for "watchful waiting" being associated with no increase in adverse outcomes.[10] Around the time of birth, pulmonary pneumocytes cease producing fluid and start to absorb the fluid into the interstitial space and into the fetal circulation, thereby clearing fluid from the alveolar spaces.[1] Delays in this process can lead to transient tachypnea of the newborn (TTN), which should start to improve within 2 hours and usually resolves completely within 48 hours.[1,11] Due to the fact that it is transient in nature, the diagnosis is usually made retrospectively and is often a diagnosis of exclusion. Treatment is supportive care.

Gastrointestinal Development and Abdominal Wall Formation

From the 6th to the 10th week of gestation, the intestines undergo a process of rapid growth, so that they are no longer contained within the fetus but herniate through the umbilicus.[1] At that time, the intestines also undergo rotation 270 degrees counterclockwise prior to returning to the abdomen. Failure of complete rotation and fixation upon return to the abdomen (or if the intestines do not return to the abdomen as is the case in abdominal wall defects and diaphragmatic hernia) results in intestinal malrotation and places infants at risk for volvulus. Failure of complete formation of the lateral pleuroperitoneal folds of the abdominal wall leads to an omphalocele.

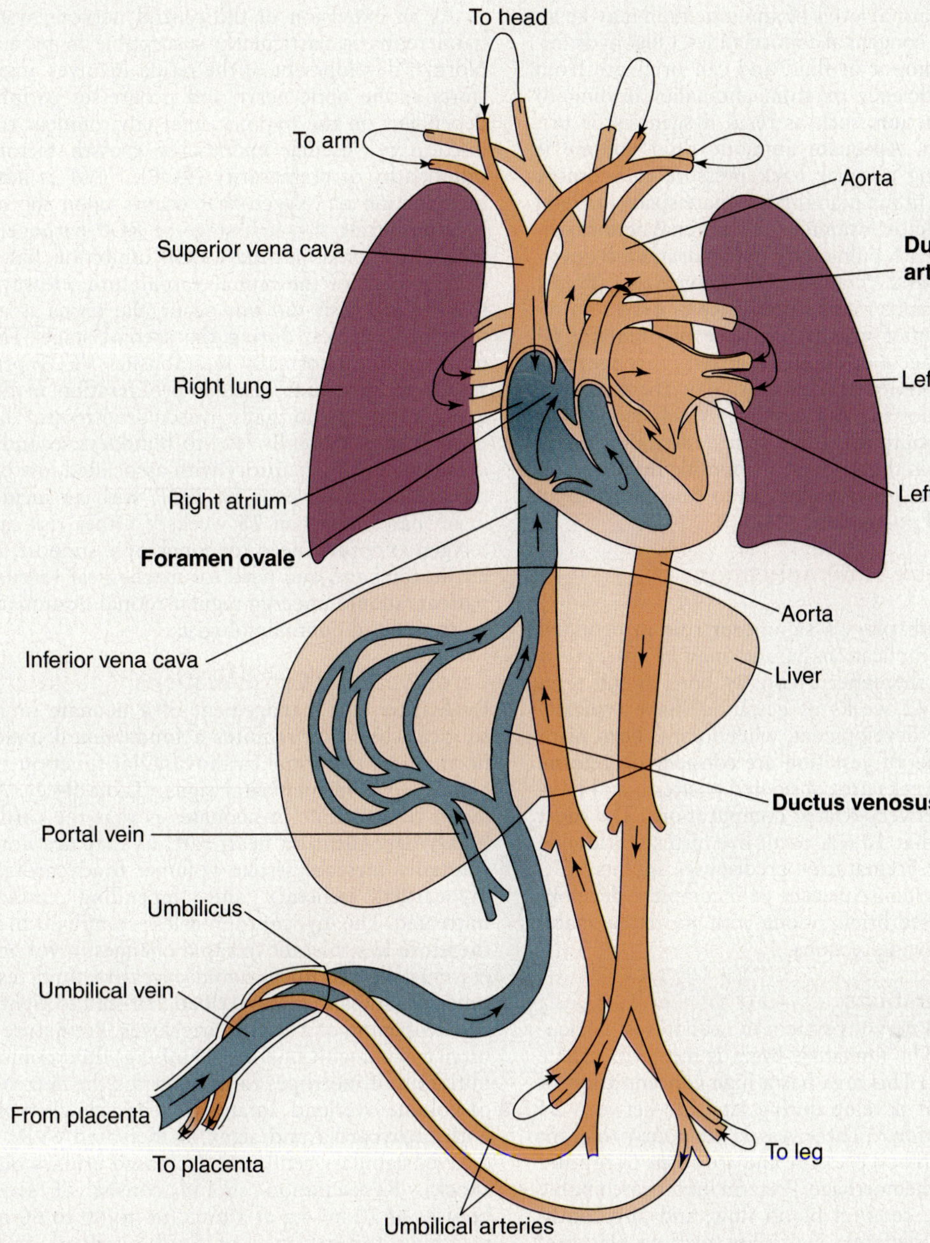

Figure 94.1. Fetal circulation. (From Rosdahl CB, Kowalski MT, eds. *Textbook of Basic Nursing*. Wolters Kluwer Health; 2012.)

Gastroschisis occurs if intestinal herniation does not occur through the umbilical ring, but through part of the abdominal wall immediately to the right of the umbilicus and then fails to return to the abdomen. Any of the above processes can compromise intestinal blood flow, resulting in an intestinal atresia.

Placental Function and Amniotic Fluid Circulation

The placenta is a specialized organ that develops between the maternal and fetal circulations that functions in gas and nutrient exchange, filtering of waste products, and trafficking of immunologic mediators. The placenta is mature by 14 weeks of gestation and continues to grow with the fetus, increasing the surface area for filtration and exchange until 40 weeks. It is at 14 weeks of gestation that passive immunity to the fetus occurs by transmission of immunoglobulin G from the mother.[1] Recognition of differences in placental anatomy should alert providers to screen for other congenital anomalies and to closely monitor placental function and fetal growth during the pregnancy. A majority of the population has two umbilical arteries and one umbilical vein, but 0.5% of the population is born with a "two-vessel cord" that contains only one umbilical artery.[1] Particular attention to this examination finding is essential, as up to 20% of infants with this finding may have an associated cardiovascular anomaly and may have other noncardiac anomalies.[12] For reasons that are not completely clear, a placenta may not adequately provide nutrients to the fetus (placental insufficiency)—potentially related to inadequate perfusion of the placenta and/or an increased demand by the fetus, such as in multiple pregnancies.[13] Placental insufficiency can lead to intrauterine growth restriction, maternal preeclampsia, and/or preterm birth. Infection of the placenta (ie, chorioamnionitis) can also induce preterm birth, and can place the neonate at risk for perinatal sepsis and cardiorespiratory failure.[13] In utero, the fetus is surrounded by amniotic fluid. The amount of fluid increases as the fetus grows diffusing from maternal blood across cells of the amniotic sac along an osmotic gradient into the fetal environment. During the second trimester, the production of amniotic fluid shifts to the fetus. The amniotic fluid cycle initiates with fetal swallowing movements. The fetus then absorbs fluid through the intestinal tract. Amniotic fluid levels are maintained by fetal excretion or urine and respiratory secretions.

4 Alterations in the normal levels of amniotic fluid may be an indicator of underlying congenital abnormalities. Oligohydramnios is a decreased amount of fluid and can originate from either placental insufficiency or from anomalies leading to decreased urine production, such as renal dysgenesis or urinary tract obstruction. Adequate amniotic fluid volume is essential in maintaining alveolar back pressure to promote lung development and in maintaining adequate space for fetal development. Severe oligohydramnios due to renal abnormalities can be associated with pulmonary hypoplasia, limb development anomalies, and craniofacial anomalies (Potter sequence). Polyhydramnios refers to presence of excess amniotic fluid. Polyhydramnios usually results from proximal GI obstruction (eg, esophageal or duodenal atresia) that prevents enteral absorption of amniotic fluid. Neurologic abnormalities that impair fetal swallowing can similarly result in polyhydramnios as can high-output cardiac states. Identification of any prior abnormality in the amount of amniotic fluid seen on prenatal ultrasound can provide clues as to possible surgical lesions to be addressed postnatally.

Neonatal Physiology and Implications of Prematurity

Gestational age at birth plays a significant role in neonatal physiology and the complications infants may be susceptible to at birth or shortly thereafter. Neonates born at full term (37-0/7 weeks up to 42 weeks of gestation) have typically completed intrauterine development, while infants born prior to completing 36 weeks of gestation are considered preterm. Infants born after 42 weeks are considered postterm and have an increased risk of delivery-related complications. The most recent data estimates that 10.6% of all live births worldwide are preterm infants.[14] Prematurity predisposes infants to a number of physiologic consequences of incomplete development. These are discussed briefly, along with normal neonatal physiology, in the following sections.

Neurologic Considerations

The developing central nervous system in neonates is particularly prone to injury. The immature brain is most vulnerable at the germinal matrix. This area has a high concentration of thin-walled vessels that develop during fetal life between 24 and 34 weeks of gestation.[15] These vessels are poorly tolerant to changes in systemic blood pressure and are prone to rupture leading to intracranial hemorrhage. Preterm infants are unable to adequately regulate cerebral blood flow, and any conditions that cause hemodynamic instability such as placental abruption, chorioamnionitis leading to sepsis, birth trauma, temperature instability, or perinatal hypoxia increase the risk of vascular injury and intraventricular hemorrhage.[15] Routine screening cranial ultrasounds are therefore recommended in premature infants <33 weeks to evaluate for potential bleeding in the setting of any these risks.

As an extension of the central nervous system, the neonatal retina is particularly susceptible in premature infants. Normal development of the retina involves angiogenesis that starts at the optic nerve and progresses peripherally and is dependent on the hypoxic fetal environment triggering production of vascular endothelial growth factor (VEGF). In retinopathy of prematurity (ROP), VEGF is inhibited by the introduction of oxygen that occurs upon the neonate's first breath. During this first stage of ROP pathogenesis, the systemic hyperoxia-induced VEGF inhibition halts the normal development of the retinal vasculature. However, since normal angiogenesis did not occur, the retina is avascular and therefore hypoxic during the second stage. This local retinal hypoxia abnormally reestablishes VEGF production and results in abnormal vascular proliferation in the retina that extends into the normally avascular vitreous. This destructive process can eventually lead to blindness secondary to retinal detachment.[16] Prematurity with associated low birth weight is the greatest risk factor for ROP, with an incidence of 84% in neonates less than 28 weeks.[17] Other risk factors include oxygen exposure, need for ionotropic support, intraventricular hemorrhage, and need for mechanical ventilation.[16] These patients should undergo regular retinal examination screening by specialized ophthalmologists.

Cardiovascular Considerations

Evaluation and management of a neonate or infant with a surgical condition requires a fundamental understanding of normal and abnormal cardiovascular function and the implications of abnormal vital signs (**Table 94.1**). An important distinction to note in neonates is that the cardiac output is highly dependent on heart rate, as they are not able to sub-
5 stantially increase stroke volume. Bradycardia is a sign of myocardial ischemia and impending cardiac arrest if untreated. The myocardium is less compliant in neonates and therefore less tolerant to rapid changes in volume, so providers must be careful to avoid excessive fluid resuscitation in times of illness.[4] Fluid overload can lead to right heart failure and reopening of a ductus arteriosus. Premature neonates are often treated with smaller (10 mL/kg) fluid boluses and earlier initiation of inotropes to account for the decreased tolerance
6 of volume overload. Infants in septic shock typically present with tachycardia and signs of increased SVR: weak pulses, delayed capillary refill, and decreased urinary output (ie, cold shock). Resuscitation should consist of sequential fluid boluses of 10 mL/kg at a time (up to 40 to 60 mL/kg), while watching for evidence of fluid overload on examination (**Fig. 94.2**).[18] If pharmacologic support is needed, dopamine is usually initiated first (**Fig. 94.2**) for increased chronotropy and inotropy, as children in fluid-refractory septic shock generally have a hypodynamic shock state with low cardiac output and high SVR. Epinephrine is generally used as a second-line agent over norepinephrine due to its preferential

Table 94.1. Normal Heart Rate and Blood Pressure Ranges for Infants and Children

Age	Awake Heart Rate (BPM)	Sleeping Heart Rate (BPM)	Systolic Blood Pressure (mm Hg)	Diastolic Blood Pressure (mm Hg)
Neonate	100–190	80–160	50–70	25–45
Infant	100–180	75–160	70–100	50–70
Toddler	80–140	60–90	80–110	50–80
Preschooler	70–120	60–90	80–115	50–80
School age	65–110	60–90	80–120	55–80
Adolescent	60–100	60–90	90–130	60–80

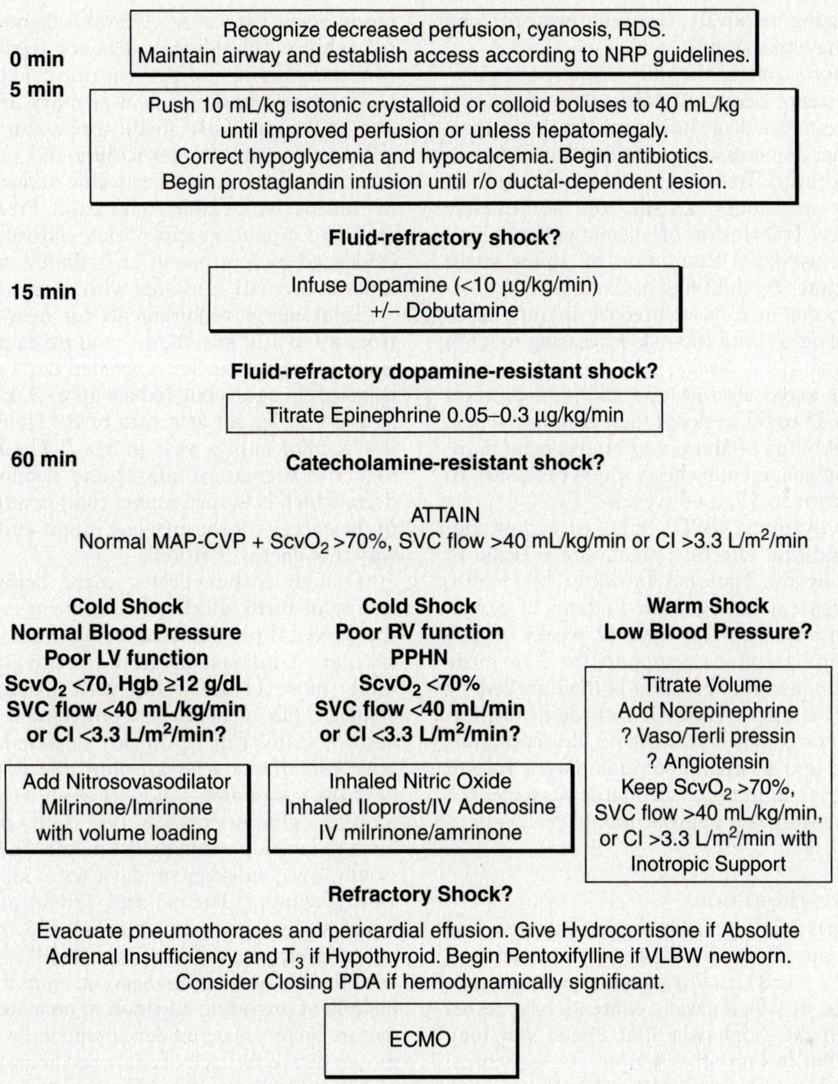

Figure 94.2. Neonatal algorithm—goal-directed therapy for sepsis algorithm. (From Davis AL, Carcillo JA, Aneja RK, et al. American College of Critical Care Medicine clinical practice parameters for hemodynamic support of pediatric and neonatal septic shock. *Crit Care Med.* 2017; 45[6]:1061–1093. Wolters Kluwer Health, Inc.)

inotropic profile. Milrinone is an inodilator that is often used as an adjunct due to its inotropic and vasodilatory effects to improve the dynamic state, as well as lusitropic effects that improve cardiac relaxation and diastolic function.[4]

Neonates and infants have a reactive pulmonary vascular bed. Pulmonary hypertension can result from sepsis, meconium aspiration, pulmonary hypoplasia associated with CDH, and a number of other disease processes. Clinical indicators include differential oxygen saturation at pre- and postductal measurements and hypoxemia that does not sufficiently improve with increasing supplemental oxygen support. Treatment involves mechanical ventilation, pulmonary vasodilation (supplemental oxygen, milrinone, inhaled nitric oxide), and avoidance of hypotension and acidosis. If these initial measures fail, extracorporeal membrane oxygenation can be utilized for cardiopulmonary support.

Respiratory Considerations

There are a number of key physiologic characteristics of neonates and infants that impact ventilatory management. Neonates have a very compliant chest wall due to the fact that the rib cage is cartilaginous and the musculature is underdeveloped as compared to the bony and muscular adult chest wall. Though intrinsic lung compliance is similar in infants and adults, the difference in the negative pressure due to chest wall compliance makes infant lungs more likely to collapse. The ability to sustain FRC in the setting of increased tendency for lung collapse is enabled by the narrower glottic openings and shorter expiratory times. "Grunting" with respiration (expiring against a closed larynx to increase FRC) in an infant is a compensatory mechanism and a telltale sign of impending respiratory failure.

High metabolic demand predisposes infants to a high risk of respiratory decline, hypoxemia, and inadequate oxygen
7 delivery. Neonatal indications for respiratory support include apnea, airway obstruction, pulmonary effects of congenital heart defects, poor respiratory drive in premature infants, and other disease-specific reasons, such as CDH.[19] Noninvasive measures, including CPAP and noninvasive positive-pressure ventilation (NIPPV) are preferred if sufficient to sustain adequate oxygenation and ventilation due to a decreased risk of developing ventilator-induced damage to already fragile premature lungs. If endotracheal intubation and mechanical ventilation are required, neonatal-specific ventilators have been designed to provide adequate tidal volumes and take into account factors related to neonatal respiratory mechanics. High-frequency oscillatory ventilation (HFOV) and high-frequency jet ventilation (HFJV) are nonconventional modes often used in the neonatal period. These modes rapidly deliver small "subtidal" volumes on the order of hundreds of breaths

per minute, thereby using relatively constant pressure and volume to maintain lung expansion.[19]

Apnea of prematurity is one of the most common respiratory disorders in premature neonates. Most preterm infants less than 28 weeks of gestational age have some level of apnea, with decreasing incidence at increasing gestational age.[20] Apnea may be obstructive or central. Treatment includes initiation of methylxanthines, most commonly caffeine, and noninvasive positive airway pressure. Transfusion of anemic patients may also decrease apneic episodes.[20] Resolution of apnea spells usually occurs by the time the child has reached term.[20] Postoperative apnea may occur in 25% of preterm infants up to 44 weeks of gestational age,[21] with the risk decreasing to <1% after postconceptual age of 56 weeks.[22] As a result, current accepted practice is to avoid elective operations in preterm infants until they reach 55 to 60 weeks of total gestational age, or to admit them for 24 hours of apnea and bradycardia monitoring after undergoing general anesthesia if it is necessary to proceed with surgery prior to 55 to 60 weeks.

Bronchopulmonary dysplasia (BPD) refers to a multifactorial chronic lung condition affecting premature infants. In the revised definition by the National Institutes of Health, the criteria include persistent radiographic findings of parenchymal lung disease in an infant less than 32 weeks of gestational age who requires respiratory support for 3 or more days at 36 weeks postmenstrual age. BPD is then graded by the mode of respiratory support required. Outside of respiratory support, other therapies such as caffeine, diuretics, surfactant administration, and postnatal steroids play a role in prevention and mitigation. In terms of ventilator strategies for established BPD, volume-targeted approaches are preferred to limit injury.[23]

Gastrointestinal Considerations

Development of the upper and lower esophageal sphincters and coordinated peristalsis are mature by 31 weeks of gestation.[24] Gastroesophageal reflux (GER) itself is a common occurrence in neonates and infants, in which gastric contents pass retrograde into and through the esophagus after a feed that may result in the "spit up" but has no other serious consequences. Transient relaxation of the lower esophageal sphincter has been shown to be the primary cause of reflux in premature infants.[24] Increased gastric volume from feedings may trigger relaxation, making these events more common after a meal. This phenomenon is separate from gastroesophageal reflux disease (GERD), which is defined as reflux episodes that result in "troublesome symptoms and/or complications."[25] Though these are somewhat difficult to define in infants, they may include aspiration events with subsequent pneumonia and poor weight gain. No treatment is needed for pure uncomplicated reflux episodes in infants as they typically resolve with time; 88% of infants have resolution by 1 year,[26] and treatment options for GERD include diet modification such as thickening feeds and/or behavioral pacing of feeds by the caretaker, positional changes after feeds (head of bed elevation), medical treatment with prokinetics and acid suppression, nasojejunal feeding, and Nissen fundoplication for refractory cases.

The GI tract develops with contributions from the endoderm, mesoderm, and ectoderm and is separated into foregut, midgut, and hindgut. Although a full discussion of gut embryology will not be undertaken at this time, a few notable events of intestinal development will be mentioned. Gastric motility is seen as early as 20 weeks, but intestinal motility can take up to 34 weeks for full development[27] The ability for coordinated suck and swallow is fully developed usually by 34 weeks.[27] Due to the incomplete development of these (and many other) anatomic and functional aspects, feeding of premature infants should be initiated slowly. In addition to the lack of gut development, prematurity brings added consequences that may affect intestinal barrier function and increase the risks of necrotizing enterocolitis. Hypotension and associated vasopressor requirement can cause visceral ischemia and mucosal sloughing, while withholding or delaying feeding can lead to atrophy of intestinal villi and prevent normal colonization of gut bacteria. Gastric acid acts as a primary defense against bacteria, and acid-suppressive medications can therefore increase the risk of necrotizing enterocolitis and pneumonia.[28] Decreased mucin production and peristaltic action also make the intestinal mucosa vulnerable to invasion. Premature infants lack the ability to mount an appropriate antiinflammatory response as evidenced by increase in proinflammatory markers and cytokines in premature infants with necrotizing enterocolitis.[28]

8 Total energy requirements for neonates and infants range from 80 to 120 kcal/kg/d,[29] and up to one-third of this energy is used for growth. The expected daily growth rate for weight is based on age, while babies up to 3 months old are expected to grow in length at a rate of 0.15 cm/d, followed by up to 0.075 cm/d until a year of age.[30] The basic metabolic rate is higher in premature infants and neonates than in older children, which is in turn higher than in adults. Fats provide most of the energy for the growing infant and are the most common way that energy is stored.

Though carbohydrates cease being the main mode of energy at birth, glucose metabolism is a key concern during the perinatal period. After being separated from the maternal circulation, infants only have enough glucose stores (glycogen) for at most 24 hours and with a high turnover rate (up to 5 mg/kg/min in neonates compared to 2 to 3 mg/kg/min in adults), stores can be quickly depleted. It is therefore imperative for infants who are not able to feed to be started on dextrose-containing fluids as soon as possible. Most infants require a glucose infusion rate (GIR) of 4 to 9 mg/kg/min at birth to keep up with glucose metabolism; the GIR is increased slowly over subsequent days to a maximum rate of up to 14 mg/kg/min.[30] The majority (90%) of glucose is used by the brain, so hypoglycemia (glucose <45 mg/dL) can affect early neurodevelopment if left untreated.[31]

If there is no contraindication, enteral feeding is the preferred method of providing nutrition to neonates and infants. Very premature infants may not developmentally be able to take feeds by mouth due to the lack of oral coordination that usually develops at 32 to 34 weeks of gestation, and usually require nasogastric access for feeding. Oral aversion is a concern for infants who need to be nil per os for an extended period (eg, prolonged intubation, long-gap esophageal atresia). Breastmilk (20 kcal/oz) is recommended due to immunologic benefits, but formula may be augmented/substituted if breastmilk is insufficient/unavailable or not tolerated (ie, milk protein allergy). Fortification may be utilized for additional calories, but can increase the risk of necrotizing enterocolitis, especially in premature infants.

If unable to proceed with enteral nutrition, parenteral nutrition (PN) can be initiated. Since they are unable to immediately tolerate full enteral feeds, have high protein turnover rates, and require supplemental protein to maintain a positive nitrogen balance and prevent starvation, premature infants are started on PN as soon as possible after birth. PN is also useful for infants with bowel obstruction or in the postoperative state. Some infants who have lost a large portion of small bowel secondary to midgut volvulus (anatomically) or gastroschisis (functionally) may be dependent on PN for a long period of time and are at risk of the development of PN-associated cholestatic liver disease.[30] Recent advances in alternative lipids have been shown to decrease the risk of PN-related cholestasis with the use of fish oil–based lipid formulations (as opposed to the standard soy-based lipids) containing omega-3 fatty acids.[32] Infants receiving PN must have their electrolytes and glucose levels monitored closely to avoid metabolic derangements. While lifesaving and sustaining, prolonged PN use places infants at risk for complications, including catheter-related complications (central line–associated bloodstream infections, thrombosis) and cholestasis, and therefore transition to enteral nutrition whenever possible is preferred.

Hyperbilirubinemia is common in infants. Bilirubin levels in the blood are determined by the amount created from the breakdown of heme, primarily from red blood cells, and the amount reabsorbed from the enterohepatic circulation. The normal level of bilirubin in infants is higher because neonates produce two to three times the amount of bilirubin as adults, in part because of the increased turnover of red blood cells.[33] Unconjugated hyperbilirubinemia is a result of decreased ability to conjugate due to deficiency of the conjugating enzyme uridine diphosphogluconurate glucuronosyltransferase (UGT). In addition, absorption of unconjugated bilirubin from the GI tract can occur if the conjugated bilirubin normally excreted in stool is instead unconjugated by β-glucuronidase. This GI resorption can be increased in diseases that result in prolonged retention of stool, such as Hirschsprung disease or distal atresias. Typically, during the first 1 to 2 weeks, unconjugated bilirubin levels transiently rise to 6 to 12 mg/dL, depending on gestational age of child (full-term infants have lower levels) before returning to normal levels of <2 mg/dL.[33] Neurotoxic effects of hyperbilirubinemia can be avoided by clearing bilirubin with phototherapy (first-line therapy) or exchange transfusions. Established nomograms that incorporate postnatal age and rate of rise can be helpful in determining the proper threshold at which to initiate phototherapy.

Fluid, Electrolyte, and Genitourinary Considerations

Fetal kidneys regulate amniotic fluid levels, but after birth, they assume control of electrolyte and fluid maintenance. Renal blood flow starts around 5% of cardiac output and rises over the first few weeks to adult levels of 25% as systemic (and renal) vascular pressure decreases. Glomerular filtration rate (GFR) likewise increases over time from 40 mL/min/1.73 m^2 at birth to goal rate of 125 mL/min/1.73 m^2 by age 2 in term neonates and later in childhood for preterm infants. Delay in the first urine output up to 24 hours is not uncommon in neonates, though premature infants seem to be more likely to urinate earlier (within the first 8 hours) than term or post-term infants. The urine that is passed is quite dilute because their concentrating ability is poor, though it doubles over the first 30 days of life and continues to increase over the first year.[34] Once urination begins, minimal adequate urine output is 1 mL/kg/h, but should ideally be 2 to 3 mL/kg/h. The use of creatinine to measure renal function in the early neonatal period must be interpreted with care, as neonatal levels mirror maternal creatinine and reflect maternal renal function. This false alteration in creatinine usually clears by 2 weeks of life in term infants (by 4 weeks in premature infants) when levels are more reflective of the child's own renal function.[34]

Neonatal body composition is 80% water compared to 55% to 60% for adults. The excess body water is primarily intracellular, and migrates into the extracellular space and is subsequently excreted—leading to the typical weight loss seen during the first few days of life. Typical fluid requirements for a term neonate start at 60 to 80 mL/kg/d and gradually increase to 150 to 160 mL/kg/d, but may be higher for very low–birth-weight and premature neonates or neonates with conditions that lead to excessive fluid losses. [31] Neonates do not excrete sodium in their urine for the first few days due to low GFR, so supplemental sodium during this time frame is not required. Normal sodium requirements thereafter are 2 to 4 mEq/kg/d. Similarly, potassium is not initially added to fluids as levels are elevated at birth due to shifts into the extracellular space. After the first void and subsequent excretion of potassium, supplemental potassium may be added for goal of 1 to 3 mEq/kg/d. Transient hypercalcemia and hypermagnesemia can occur in neonates immediately after birth due to passage from the mother via the placenta.[31,34] Otherwise, electrolyte abnormalities and their management of them are similar to the adult population as has been discussed in the foundational chapters in this textbook.

Hematologic Considerations

Coagulation factor measurement studies of fetal and newborn coagulation reveal longer clotting times before 30 weeks of gestation, followed by an increase in the amount of clotting factors between 30 and 38 weeks.[35] Lower coagulation levels in preterm infants may be related to hepatic synthetic immaturity. In the absence of an underlying coagulation disorder, these levels will improve over time to adult levels. If the child does have a bleeding disorder, it may manifest in a number of ways. Bleeding following circumcision is the most common presentation of hemophilia overall, followed by spontaneous hemorrhage (subgaleal hematoma, cephalohematoma, and intracranial hemorrhage).[36]

Vitamin K levels in the fetus and neonate are low and decrease further over the first 48 to 72 hours. A lack of bacterial production from the mostly sterile GI tract and low levels of dietary vitamin K consumed leads to deficiency until about 7 to 10 days after birth.[37] Because of this transient vitamin K deficiency, neonates are at increased risk of hemorrhage, which may manifest as intra- or extracranial hemorrhage, GI bleed, or, in males, bleeding at the time of circumcision. Diagnosis can be made in patients with prolonged PT and PTT and elevated PIVKA (proteins induced by vitamin K absence) levels.[37] Complications can be prevented by the administration of exogenous intramuscular vitamin K at birth.

Infectious Disease Considerations

Neonates can become quite ill without many of the typical signs seen in older children and adults. They may not have any specific symptoms, but may present with unexplained respiratory distress, apnea, or bradycardic episodes, even with non-respiratory causes of illness. Temperature instability usually manifests as hypothermia instead of febrile illness. Because of their poor physiologic reserve, clinical deterioration can occur quickly if signs are not recognized and appropriate treatment initiated. Within the first 3 days of life, sepsis is thought to be a result of maternal–fetal transmission from early and/or prolonged rupture of membranes or maternal infection (chorioamnionitis, colonization with group B streptococcus). Conversely, late-onset sepsis usually occurs after 1 week of life and is more likely due to some environmental insult or exposure (ventilator-associated pneumonia, catheter-related bloodstream infection). Premature infants are at risk for either type of sepsis due to their weaker immune systems.[30]

Positive cultures of body fluid (blood, urine, sputum, cerebrospinal fluid) are preferred for the diagnosis of sepsis in the appropriate clinical context. Ancillary studies may be used in conjunction with cultures (or in instances of culture-negative illness) for the workup of sepsis. Though leukocytosis on a standard complete blood cell count (CBC) is concerning for infection in older children and adults, leukopenia is of greater concern in neonates. Thrombocytopenia is also associated with neonatal sepsis, though the mechanism is not entirely clear. Neonates with gram-negative sepsis are more likely to consume platelets compared to those with gram-positive sepsis (42% vs 17%) and experience a greater drop in platelet levels.[39] In addition, severe thrombocytopenia ($\leq 50 \times 10^9$/L) is associated with higher rates of mortality.[15]

Thermoregulation

Neonates lose heat more easily than adults for a variety of reasons, including increased relative body surface area and thin skin, through which evaporative losses may occur. They lack the ability to generate heat through shivering, instead creating heat by the breakdown of stores of brown fat. Premature infants have more pronounced issues with heat loss because of their skin immaturity, and they also have less brown fat, making them even more prone to hypothermia. Environmental measures (blankets, increasing room temperature, and radiant warmers) are vital in temperature maintenance; these measures are key to perioperative temperature management. Surgeons should be mindful

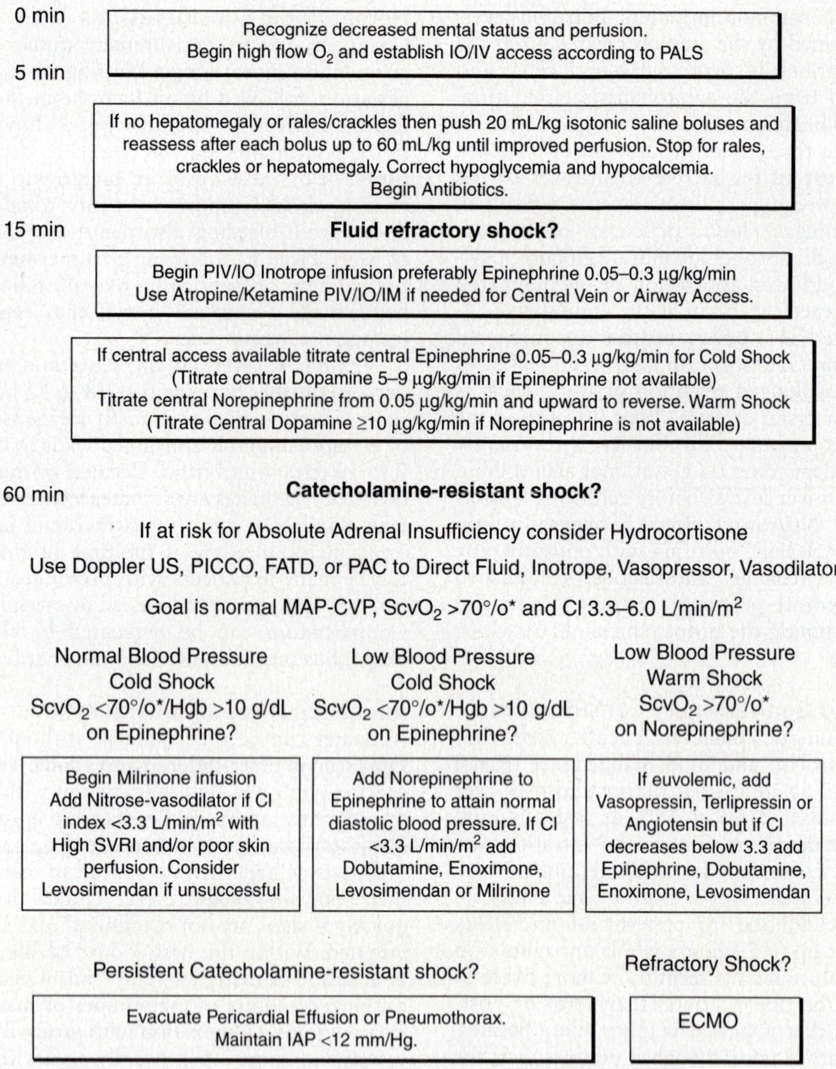

Figure 94.3. Pediatric algorithm—goal-directed therapy for sepsis. (From Davis AL, Carcillo JA, Aneja RK, et al. American College of Critical Care Medicine clinical practice parameters for hemodynamic support of pediatric and neonatal septic shock. *Crit Care Med.* 2017;45[6]:1061–1093. Wolters Kluwer Health, Inc.)

of this and try to limit the time a neonate is uncovered on the operating table; use forced-air heating units and maintain higher operating room temperatures to keep the child normothermic.

Pediatric Physiology

Normal physiology of children continues to change as children grow and mature, and mimics that of adults as children enter into adolescence. This section will highlight important aspects of pediatric physiology that differ from adults and that impact the care of a child.

Cardiovascular Considerations

Shock states in children are generally classified as "warm" or "cold" shock. Septic shock in young children tends to mimic the physiology of neonates ("cold shock") with predominantly low cardiac output and high SVR. Septic shock in older children and adolescents more commonly mimics the physiology of adults ("warm shock") with peripheral vasodilation and a high cardiac output state. Resuscitation of children with septic shock begins with fluid resuscitation and should then follow the algorithm in **Figure 94.3** to guide initiation of inotropic and vasoconstrictor support, with a key branch point in determining vasodilatory ("warm") shock or a low cardiac output ("cold") shock state based on physical examination findings.[40] Central venous pressure monitoring in children can be utilized, but physical examination of the abdomen to assess for hepatomegaly (congestive hepatopathy) is a useful adjunct in assessing volume status. Cardiogenic, neurogenic, obstructive, and hypovolemic shock states in children mimic the physiology of adults and should be managed in a similar fashion with attention paid to weight-based dosing of fluids, blood products, and vasoactive agents.

Respiratory Considerations

Young children, like neonates, have a diminished respiratory reserve due to high metabolic rate and low FRC and can decompensate rapidly. It is important to recognize compensatory physical examination findings associated with respiratory distress such as tachypnea, nasal flaring, subcostal and supraclavicular retractions, expiratory grunting (to maintain recruitment and higher FRC), and head bobbing.

Anatomic differences in the pediatric airway increase the risk of airway resistance and obstruction. Young children have large heads in relation to the torso. In the supine position, this results in flexion at the neck and relative airway obstruction. Positional modifications are necessary to ensure airway patency. A blanket or roll can be placed behind the shoulders to extend the neck to neutral and improve airway positioning. The smaller airway diameter also contributes to impairment of laminar airflow. As detailed in the respiratory physiology chapter, airway flow is primarily limited by airway resistance, which in turn is proportional to the radius of the airway to the fourth power. Therefore, very small changes in airway diameter can lead to substantial increases in airway resistance in young children. Airway mucosal edema, mucus plugging, and foreign bodies can all lead to significant respiratory compromise.

Initiation of mechanical ventilatory support for children in respiratory failure requires a working knowledge of equipment sizing, how to customize settings based on patient age, weight, and chest compliance. Appropriate endotracheal tube size can be estimated using the formula (age in years + 4)/4 (for an uncuffed tube) or by referring to a length-based color-coded tape. Mechanical ventilation is generally initiated targeting tidal volumes of 6 to 8 mL/kg of predicted body weight (based on length, age, and sex).[41] Tidal volumes in mechanically ventilated young children can be challenging to measure at the level of the ventilator as the dead-space volume of the ventilator tubing far exceeds the tidal volume of the patient. For this reason, inline flow sensors at the level of the endotracheal tube are used to more precisely measure actual tidal volumes. Compliance is highly variable across ages and disease processes; therefore, initial ventilator pressures are generally estimated using bag ventilation with a handheld manometer and visual inspection of chest rise to determine the pressure needed to deliver adequate volume. Pediatric minute ventilation is higher than in adults, and younger children generally require higher respiratory rates (15 to 30 breaths/min) that need to be titrated to maintain adequate CO_2 clearance.

Tracheostomy timing in children remains a controversial issue. The incidence of subglottic stenosis with prolonged intubation in children is much higher (11%, mean length of mechanical ventilation 9 days, range 3 to 33 days) than previously thought, and increases with duration of intubation (50% increased risk for every 5 days of endotracheal intubation).[42] The incidence of tracheostomy-related complications, however, is much higher than in adults with a 2-year tracheostomy-related complication rate of 39% and in-hospital mortality rate of 9%, which decreases the enthusiasm for tracheostomy in young children unless deemed absolutely necessary.[43] Within the specific population of pediatric traumatic brain injury, tracheostomy at 14 days is associated with faster time to discharge and lower complication rates without significantly increasing the number of unnecessary tracheostomies performed.[44]

Gastrointestinal and Nutritional Considerations

Outside of the neonatal period, GI physiology mimics that of adults. Growing children do have higher metabolic needs, and daily baseline caloric requirements are higher in younger children (**Table 94.2**).[29] PN is commonly used in pediatric patients with prolonged inability to tolerate adequate enteral nutrition, with the recommended timing of initiation generally similar to adult patients at 7 days in the absence of preexisting malnutrition.

Table 94.2. Parenteral Nutrition Baseline Caloric and Protein Needs by Age

Age Group	Daily Caloric Needs (kcal/kg/d)	Daily Protein Needs (g/kg/d)
Premature Neonate	90–120	3–4
<6 mo	85–105	2–3
6–12 mo	80–100	2–3
1–7 y	75–90	1–2
7–12 y	50–75	1–2
>12 y	30–50	0.8–1.5

Adapted from Mirtallo J, Canada T, Johnson D, et al; Task Force for the Revision of Safe Practices for Parenteral Nutrition. Safe practices for parenteral nutrition. *JPEN J Parenter Enteral Nutr.* 2004;28(6):S39–S70.

Table 94.3. Pediatric Fluid Requirements by Weight

Body Weight (kg)	Daily Fluid Requirement
<1.5	130–150 cc/kg/d
1.5–2	110–130 cc/kg/d
2–10	100 cc/kg/d
11–20	1,000 cc/d (for first 10 kg) + 50 cc/kg/d for every kg over 10 kg
>20	1,500 cc/d (for first 20 kg) + 20 cc/kg/d for every kg over 20 kg

Adapted from Mirtallo J, Canada T, Johnson D, et al; Task Force for the Revision of Safe Practices for Parenteral Nutrition. Safe practices for parenteral nutrition. *JPEN J Parenter Enteral Nutr.* 2004;28(6):S39–S70.

Genitourinary, Fluid, and Electrolyte Considerations

Renal function is not mature at birth and does not mature until 2 years of age. Normal urine output is higher in infants and younger children (1 to 2 mL/kg/h) and approaches adult levels (0.5 to 1 mL/kg/h) by adolescence. Children have a higher body surface-to-mass ratio and higher minute ventilation, leading to greater insensible losses. Daily maintenance fluid requirements in children per unit body weight are higher than in adults and the hourly fluid requirements can be calculated using the 4–2–1 rule initially described by Holiday and Seger in 1957 or daily fluid requirements similarly referenced in **Table 94.3**.[29,45] Outside of infancy, daily electrolyte requirements mimic those of adults.

Hematologic Considerations

Pediatric blood volumes are relatively higher in infants (90 mL/kg) and young children (80 mL/kg) and approach adult levels (65 to 70 mL/kg) by adolescence.[46] In general, transfusion of 5 mL/kg of red blood cells should result in an expected 1 g/dL increase in hemoglobin.[47] Massive transfusion in children is generally defined as more than 40 mL/kg/24 h of combined blood product (red blood cells, plasma, platelets, and cryoprecipitate), with improved outcomes demonstrated with high ratio RBC:plasma transfusion—similar to adults.[48,49] Venous thromboembolic disease (VTE) is less common in children, but does occur—often in critically ill or injured patients and in association with indwelling central venous catheters, oncology diagnoses, oral contraceptive use, postpubescence, and obesity. While the efficacy of pharmacologic VTE prophylaxis likely mimics that of adults in adolescents, it is unclear if pharmacologic chemoprophylaxis is effective in decreasing VTE rates in younger children.

ACKNOWLEDGMENTS

We gratefully acknowledge the contributions of previous edition authors, Chinwendu Onwubiko, Aaron R. Jensen, and Hanmin Lee, as portions of those chapters have been retained in this revision.

References

1. Sadler TW, Langman J. *Langman's Medical Embryology*. 9th ed. Lippincott Williams & Wilkins; 2004:x, 534.
2. Cummings J; COMMITTEE ON FETUS AND NEWBORN. Antenatal counseling regarding resuscitation and intensive care before 25 weeks of gestation. *Pediatrics*. 2015;136(3):588–595.
3. KY B. Respiratory distress syndrome. In: Cloherty JP, Eichenwald EC, Hansen AR, Stark AR, eds. *Manual of Neonatal Care*. 7th ed. Lippincott Williams & Wilkins; 2012.
4. Hines MH. Neonatal cardiovascular physiology. *Semin Pediatr Surg*. 2013;22(4):174–178.

PEDIATRIC SURGERY

5. Jain A, Mohamed A, El-Khuffash A, et al. A comprehensive echocardiographic protocol for assessing neonatal right ventricular dimensions and function in the transitional period: normative data and z scores. *J Am Soc Echocardiogr*. 2014;27(12):1293–1304.
6. Hoffman JI, Kaplan S. The incidence of congenital heart disease. *J Am Coll Cardiol*. 2002;39(12):1890–1900.
7. Clyman RI, Couto J, Murphy GM. Patent ductus arteriosus: are current neonatal treatment options better or worse than no treatment at all? *Semin Perinatol*. 2012;36(2):123–129.
8. Prescott S, Keim-Malpass J. Patent ductus arteriosus in the preterm infant: diagnostic and treatment options. *Adv Neonatal Care*. 2017;17(1):10–18.
9. Gross RE, Hubbard JP. Surgical ligation of a patent ductus arteriosus: report of first successful case. *JAMA*. 1939;112(8):729–731.
10. Ngo S, Profit J, Gould JB, Lee HC. Trends in patent ductus arteriosus diagnosis and management for very low birth weight infants. *Pediatrics*. 2017;139(4):e20162390.
11. Guglani L, Lakshminrusimha S, Ryan RM. Transient tachypnea of the newborn. *Pediatr Rev*. 2008;29(11):e59–e65.
12. DeFigueiredo D, Dagklis T, Zidere V, Allan L, Nicolaides KH. Isolated single umbilical artery: need for specialist fetal echocardiography? *Ultrasound Obstet Gynecol*. 2010;36(5):553–555.
13. Morgan TK. Role of the placenta in preterm birth: a review. *Am J Perinatol*. 2016;33(3):258–266.
14. Chawanpaiboon S, Vogel JP, Moller AB, et al. Global, regional, and national estimates of levels of preterm birth in 2014: a systematic review and modelling analysis. *Lancet Glob Health*. 2019;7(1):e37–e46.
15. Bassan H. Intracranial hemorrhage in the preterm infant: understanding it, preventing it. *Clin Perinatol*. 2009;36(4):737–762, v.
16. Vanderveen DK, Zepeda JL. Retinopathy of prematurity. In: Cloherty JP, Eichenwald EC, Hansen AR, Stark AR, eds. *Manual of Neonatal Care*. 7th ed. Lippincott Williams & Wilkins; 2012.
17. Supplemental Therapeutic Oxygen for Prethreshold Retinopathy of Prematurity (STOP-ROP), a randomized, controlled trial. I: primary outcomes. *Pediatrics*. 2000;105(2):295–310.
18. Davis AL, Carcillo JA, Aneja RK, et al. American College of Critical Care Medicine Clinical Practice Parameters for hemodynamic support of pediatric and neonatal septic shock. *Crit Care Med*. 2017;45(6):1061–1093.
19. Bancalari E, Claure N. Principles of respiratory monitoring and therapy. In: Gleason CA, Juul SE, eds. *Avery's Diseases of the Newborn*. 9th ed. Elsevier; 2012.
20. Eichenwald EC; Committee on Fetus and Newborn, American Academy of Pediatrics. Apnea of prematurity. *Pediatrics*. 2016;137(1).
21. Malviya S, Swartz J, Lerman J. Are all preterm infants younger than 60 weeks postconceptual age at risk for postanesthetic apnea? *Anesthesiology*. 1993;78(6):1076–1081.
22. Cote CJ, Zaslavsky A, Downes JJ, et al. Postoperative apnea in former preterm infants after inguinal herniorrhaphy. A combined analysis. *Anesthesiology*. 1995;82(4):809–822.
23. Gilfillan M, Bhandari A, Bhandari V. Diagnosis and management of bronchopulmonary dysplasia. *BMJ*. 2021;375:n1974.
24. Omari TI, Barnett C, Snel A, et al. Mechanisms of gastroesophageal reflux in healthy premature infants. *J Pediatr*. 1998;133(5):650–654.
25. Sherman PM, Hassall E, Fagundes-Neto U, et al. A global, evidence-based consensus on the definition of gastroesophageal reflux disease in the pediatric population. *Am J Gastroenterol*. 2009;104(5):1278–1295; quiz 1296.
26. Surender K. Gastroesophageal reflux disease. In: Kliegman RM, Stanton BF, St. Geme JW, Schor NF, Behrman RE, eds. *Nelson Textbook of Pediatrics*. 20th ed. Elsevier; 2016.
27. Lenfestey MW, Neu J. Gastrointestinal development: implications for management of preterm and term infants. *Gastroenterol Clin North Am*. 2018;47(4):773–791.
28. Martin CR, Walker WA. Intestinal immune defences and the inflammatory response in necrotising enterocolitis. *Semin Fetal Neonatal Med*. 2006;11(5):369–377.
29. Mirtallo J, Canada T, Johnson D, et al. Safe practices for parenteral nutrition. *JPEN J Parenter Enteral Nutr*. 2004;28(6):S39–S70.
30. Kenney BD, Piper H, Relles D, Jaksic T. Nutrition. APSA Webapp. Accessed June 6, 2020. www.pedsurglibrary.com/apsa/view/Pediatric-Surgery-NaT/829018/all/Nutrition
31. Pierro A, De Coppi P, Eaton S. Neonatal physiology and metabolic considerations. In: Holcomb GW, Murphy JP, Ostlie DJ, eds. *Pediatric Surgery*. 7th ed. Elsevier; 2012.
32. Nandivada P, Fell GL, Mitchell PD, et al. Long-term fish oil lipid emulsion use in children with intestinal failure-associated liver disease [Formula: see text]. *JPEN J Parenter Enteral Nutr*. 2017;41(6):930–937.
33. Gregory MLP, Martin CR, Cloherty JP. Neonatal hyperbilirubinemia. In: Cloherty JP, Eichenwald EC, Hansen AR, Stark AR, eds. *Manual of Neonatal Care*. 7th ed. Lippincott Williams & Wilkins; 2012.
34. Guignard J, Sulyok E. Renal morphogenesis and development of renal function. In: Gleason CA, Devaskar SU, eds. *Avery's Diseases of the Newborn*. 11th ed. Elsevier; 2012.
35. Reverdiau-Moalic P, Delahousse B, Body G, Bardos P, Leroy J, Gruel Y. Evolution of blood coagulation activators and inhibitors in the healthy human fetus. *Blood*. 1996;88(3):900–906.
36. Kulkarni R, Soucie JM, Lusher J, et al. Sites of initial bleeding episodes, mode of delivery and age of diagnosis in babies with haemophilia diagnosed before the age of 2 years: a report from The Centers for Disease Control and Prevention's (CDC) Universal Data Collection (UDC) project. *Haemophilia*. 2009;15(6):1281–1290.
37. Maheshwari A, Crocker W. Hemorrhage in the newborn infant. In: Kliegman RM, Stanton BF, St. Geme JW, Schor NF, Behrman RE, eds. *Nelson Textbook of Pediatrics*. Elsevier; 2016.
38. Shah BA, Padbury JF. Neonatal sepsis: an old problem with new insights. *Virulence*. 2014;5(1):170–178.
39. Ree IMC, Fustolo-Gunnink SF, Bekker V, Fijnvandraat KJ, Steggerda SJ, Lopriore E. Thrombocytopenia in neonatal sepsis: incidence, severity and risk factors. *PLoS One*. 2017;12(10):e0185581.
40. Davis AL, Carcillo JA, Aneja RK, et al. The American College of Critical Care Medicine clinical practice parameters for hemodynamic support of pediatric and neonatal septic shock: executive summary. *Pediatr Crit Care Med*. 2017;18(9):884–890.
41. Kim GJ, Newth CJL, Khemani RG, Wong SL, Coates AL, Ross PA. Does size matter when calculating the "correct" tidal volume for pediatric mechanical ventilation?: A hypothesis based on FVC. *Chest*. 2018;154(1):77–83.
42. Manica D, Schweiger C, Marostica PJ, Kuhl G, Carvalho PR. Association between length of intubation and subglottic stenosis in children. *Laryngoscope*. 2013;123(4):1049–1054.
43. Watters K, O'Neill M, Zhu H, Graham RJ, Hall M, Berry J. Two-year mortality, complications, and healthcare use in children with medicaid following tracheostomy. *Laryngoscope*. 2016;126(11):2611–2617.
44. McLaughlin C, Darcy D, Park C, et al. Timing of tracheostomy placement among children with severe traumatic brain injury: A propensity-matched analysis. *J Trauma Acute Care Surg*. 2019;87(4):818–826.
45. Holliday MA, Segar WE. The maintenance need for water in parenteral fluid therapy. *Pediatrics*. 1957;19(5):823–832.
46. Sisson TR, Lund CJ, Whalen LE, Telek A. The blood volume of infants. I. The full-term infant in the first year of life. *J Pediatr*. 1959;55(2):163–179.
47. Davies P, Robertson S, Hegde S, Greenwood R, Massey E, Davis P. Calculating the required transfusion volume in children. *Transfusion*. 2007;47(2):212–216.
48. Neff LP, Cannon JW, Morrison JJ, Edwards MJ, Spinella PC, Borgman MA. Clearly defining pediatric massive transfusion: cutting through the fog and friction with combat data. *J Trauma Acute Care Surg*. 2015;78(1):22–28; discussion 28–29.
49. Butler EK, Mills BM, Arbabi S, et al. Association of blood component ratios with 24-hour mortality in injured children receiving massive transfusion. *Crit Care Med*. 2019;47(7):975–983.

95

Fetal Intervention

Emily A. Partridge and Holly L. Hedrick

Key Points

1 Fetal surgery will only occur if (a) there is significant chance of the procedure being lifesaving or preventing serious or irreversible disability in the fetus, (b) the procedure involved low mortality and morbidity risk to the fetus, and (c) the operation has low mortality and morbidity risk to the pregnant woman, including impact on future pregnancies.

2 Fetal surgery originally was only recommended when the fetus would not survive without it, and thus the risk–benefit ratio was favorable.

3 The first fetal surgery for a nonlethal defect was for MMC.

4 Fetoscopic therapy is an expanding arena with indications including twin-to-twin syndrome (TTTS), congenital diaphragmatic hernia (CDH), congenital heart defects (CHDs), lower urinary tract obstructions (LUTO), and myelomeningocele (MMC)/spina bifida.

5 Open fetal surgery is reserved for carefully selected cases of myelomeningocele (MMC)/spina bifida, sacrococcygeal teratoma (SCT), congenital lung lesions (CLLs), and solid tumors causing mass effect such as pericardial teratomas.

6 *Ex utero* intrapartum treatment (EXIT) procedure is most often used for fetuses with predicted compromised airway access at birth.

7 Fetal cellular, molecular, and genetic therapies allow potential treatment of fetuses with stem cells, proteins, or viral vectors with promising preclinical and early clinical results.

THE DEVELOPMENT OF A NEW SURGICAL SUBSPECIALTY

1 Fetal surgery is a multidisciplinary subspecialty that emerged at the intersection of pediatric surgery and maternal–fetal medicine.[1] During initial stages of development, the idea of surgically operating on a human fetus within the womb was considered impossible, radical, and ethically questionable. However, pioneers of the field confronted and overcame numerous challenges in pursuit of an innovative concept that would ultimately become the accepted standard of care for many congenital conditions.

Modern fetal surgery was envisioned and established in the late 1970s as a collaborative translational program by Doctors Alfred de Lorimier and Michael Harrison at the University of California, San Francisco.[1] In 1981, Dr. Harrison performed the first open surgical intervention on a fetus with obstructive uropathy.[1] Prior to this landmark case, intrauterine interventions were limited to diagnostic procedures such as amniocentesis and chorionic villus sampling, or limited procedures such as intrauterine transfusion for Rh incompatibility. Harrison's success demonstrated that surgeons could successfully operate on a pregnant uterus, return the fetus to the womb, and maintain the pregnancy, paving the way for future advancements in the field.

CORE PRINCIPLES

In 1982, pediatric surgeons, neonatologists, perinatologists,
2 radiologists, and anesthesiologists from 13 centers and five different countries gathered at a collaborative conference in Santa Ynez, CA, to discuss the potential benefits and risks of various fetal interventions.[2] This group, now recognized as the International Fetal Medicine and Surgical Society (IFMSS), reached a medical consensus by the end of the conference and established a set of principles which have been updated and remain in effect today (**Table 95.1**).

In the last 40 years, the field of fetal surgical intervention has advanced significantly and continues to evolve, with ongoing improvements in technical approaches and safety for both women and unborn patients.

FETAL SURGERY—KEY ELEMENTS LEADING TO SUCCESS OF FETAL SURGERY

Fetal Imaging

Technologic advancement in fetal imaging has not only advanced medical insight but has also driven the evolution of surgical techniques and conceptual innovation. The development of 3D and 4D ultrasound has allowed for more accurate diagnoses of facial, neural tube, and skeletal abnormalities. Real-time spatiotemporal resolution is used during surgical interventions to guide instrument placement.[3] Additionally, magnetic resonance imaging (MRI) offers improved soft tissue contrast, providing more accurate imaging of the central nervous system, lungs, kidneys, and placenta to overcome some limitations of ultrasound.[3] Fetal MRI provides significant benefits, including the ability to obtain additional anatomic information, visualize complex structural relationships from alternative angles, and allowing preparation of more detailed surgical plans.[3]

Prenatal Genetic Diagnosis

Advances made in prenatal diagnosis, such as identification and analysis of fetal DNA circulating in maternal blood, have improved the ability to diagnose genetic abnormalities in the fetus.

Table 95.1. Criteria for the Advancement of Fetal Therapy

Topic	Principles
Most fetal abnormalities are now detectable	
Best treatment for most abnormalities	Remains after birth. Prenatal diagnosis allows patient, family, and physician to discuss and develop a delivery and treatment plan for optimal outcome.
Nature of the disorder in the fetus (ie, fatal or disabling); fetal natural history	The natural history of the fetal condition must be understood; appropriate animal models should be employed to test potential efficacy of intended therapies.
Reporting requirements	Voluntary reporting is a moral obligation in the field. Self-imposed registry efforts are in progress, mandatory reporting is not established as reporting largely lacks funding and resources.
Appropriate use of therapies' criteria	Effective therapies for multiple pregnancies with or without an "innocent bystander" (eg, TTTS, selective reduction of an anomalous twin) may be considered if therapy will prolong and/or improve outcome of that pregnancy.
Candidate diseases	Improvements in prenatal diagnosis have enhanced diagnosis of fetal conditions and understanding of fetal physiology and pathophysiology. Predictive measures of morbidity and mortality help providers weigh risks and benefits for mother and fetus. Candidate diseases will continue to change and evolve.
Center infrastructure	Levels of care for newborn and for pregnant woman have been refined and redefined.
Checks and balances	Multidisciplinary teams should be tailored to the defect(s) being treated and include a variety of disciplines. Procedures for informed consent and formal reporting must be in place. Any experimental or innovative procedure must have ethical oversight, participation in registries, and transparent counseling and reporting. Parents must be counseled regarding any alternative therapies, and the options of pregnancy termination and neonatal palliative care where appropriate.
Goals of treatment	There is increasing focus on short- and long-term effects of fetal therapy on maternal reproductive health. Issues are becoming increasingly complex as the goals of fetal treatment move from primarily achieving survival, to decreasing morbidity and improving the functional and neurodevelopmental outcome of the child.
Maternal safety and autonomy	Maternal expectations have evolved. Fetal abnormalities are expected to be prenatally diagnosed, and for some abnormalities the option for fetal treatment (where available and evidence based) will be available. As fetal therapy becomes more available, uptake has become greater. In addition, some are willing to incur greater personal risk to improve the prognosis for their fetus. Care must be taken to avoid the pitfalls in perception—just because a procedure is offered within or outside a research protocol does not imply proven efficacy.

MATERNAL–FETAL RISKS

3

Unlike standard operations, fetal surgery involves two patients simultaneously, presenting complex moral and ethical challenges that must be considered and balanced in each case. Chervenak and McCullough[4] and others have helped to provide an ethical framework to guide decision making. The key principles to this framework are that (a) the fetal operation has significant chance of being lifesaving or of preventing serious, irreversible disease in the fetus; (b) the procedure carries low risk of mortality and morbidity to the fetus; and (c) the operation must pose minimal risk to the pregnant woman, including risks to future pregnancies. Based on these principles, several contraindications to fetal intervention exist, including chromosomal abnormalities, multiple major congenital anomalies, and significant maternal comorbidities.

The significant maternal and fetal risks associated with fetal surgery must be carefully weighed. For the fetus, risks include preterm delivery, fetal death, or survival with poor outcome. Most indications for fetal surgery are ones in which the fetus would not survive without the intervention, making the risk–benefit ratio inherently favorable. For interventions aimed at improving the outcome of fetuses with nonlethal conditions, the risk–benefit ratio is more challenging to assess.

Maternal risks depend on the invasiveness of the procedure. Benefits to the mother include the psychological reward of doing everything possible to improve the condition of the unborn baby. In some cases, fetal surgery may also provide physiologic benefit by preventing or reversing "mirror syndrome," a condition in which pregnancy complicated by fetal hydrops and/or placentomegaly associated with maternal development of pronounced edema, with or without signs of pre-eclampsia including hypertension and proteinuria.[5] In the event that severe pre-eclampsia develops, fetal surgery is contraindicated and urgent delivery is necessary to protect the health of the mother. For all women undergoing open fetal surgery, there are theoretical risks to future pregnancies and fertility. After open fetal surgery, all subsequent deliveries must be performed by cesarean section, and labor in the index pregnancy and all future pregnancies must be avoided to prevent uterine rupture. One of the largest studies following outcomes after open fetal surgery for myelomeningocele (MMC) in 693 women reported 77 subsequent pregnancies, with a live birth rate of 96.2% and uterine rupture rate of 9.2% resulting in 2 fetal deaths.[6] The risk of uterine rupture or dehiscence after open maternal–fetal surgery is similar to that reported after classical cesarean deliveries. A recent systematic review and meta-analysis of maternal outcomes following open and fetoscopic fetal surgery summarizing outcomes after 1193 open and 9403 fetoscopic cases reported no maternal deaths and a total complication rate of 20.9% after open and 9.6% after fetoscopic procedures.[7] The risk of severe (grade III to IV Clavien–Dindo classification) was 4.5% after open and 1.7% after minimally invasive procedures, with the most common major complications including placental abruption, uterine rupture ore hemorrhage requiring delivery, while the risk of minor complications was 16% after open and 4% after fetoscopic surgery with the most common minor complications including bleeding during the procedure, requirement for transfusion, and chorioamnionitis. Fertility does not appear to be affected by fetal surgery, though rates of preterm birth are substantially higher in index and future pregnancies after open fetal surgery compared to minimally invasive approaches.

CURRENT FETAL CONDITIONS AMENABLE TO FETAL INTERVENTION

Initially, fetal interventions were performed only for conditions that were considered lethal, as saving the life of the fetus was deemed the only benefit significant enough to justify the surgical risks to the mother. Once techniques for fetal access were standardized, different approaches—open, fetoscopic, or percutaneous procedures—were developed based on the anatomy and physiology of each anomaly.

4 Twin-to-Twin Transfusion Syndrome

Twin-to-twin transfusion syndrome (TTTS) is a complication occurring in monochorionic (single placenta) twin pregnancies as a result of an increased number of arteriovenous anastomoses in the cotyledon portion of the placenta. While all monochorionic pregnancies are considered high risk, TTTS occurs in only 9% to 15% of such pregnancies.[8] It is typically diagnosed during the early-to-mid second trimester, when unidirectional blood flow in the AV anastomoses results in shunting of blood away from one twin, the "donor," and toward the other "recipient" twin. The hypovolemia experienced by the donor twin causes renal hypoperfusion, stimulating the renin-angiotensin-aldosterone system and leading to oliguria and oligohydramnios, while the hypervolemia experienced by the recipient twin causes cardiac stretch, increasing atrial natriuretic peptide and brain natriuretic peptide release leading to polyuria and polyhydramnios. The resulting risk of discordant growth, cardiac failure, and hydrops may lead to fetal demise in both twins.

Rationale for Prenatal Treatment

Fetal intervention for TTTS is a minimally invasive procedure in which a fetoscope is introduced through the mother's abdominal wall and into the uterus (**Fig. 95.1**). Fetoscopic laser photocoagulation is then used to ablate the abnormal communicating vessels across the shared placenta, creating two chorions. Fetal laser ablation can be performed between 16 and 26 weeks of gestation. Randomized controlled trials of laser ablation in advanced TTTS have demonstrated a significantly higher likelihood of perinatal survival of at least one twin, survival of at least one twin at 6 months of age, and decreased neurologic complications in survivors, although the procedure is associated with risk of infection, premature rupture of membranes, and preterm delivery.[9] This treatment converted a disease that previously had a near 80% mortality into one that has a greater than 80% survival and is now the standard of care for this condition today.[10]

Myelomeningocele aka Spina Bifida

5 MMC or spina bifida is a neurologic defect characterized by incomplete closure of the neural tube during early embryonic development, resulting in exposed neural tissue and leakage of cerebrospinal fluid (CSF). In the United States, spina bifida affects nearly 1 in 2000 live births, making it one of the most common congenital defects resulting in paralysis.[11] The clinical consequences of MMC vary depending on the vertebral level of the spinal defect but often include paralysis, bowel and bladder incontinence, musculoskeletal deformities, hindbrain herniation, hydrocephalus, and cognitive disabilities.

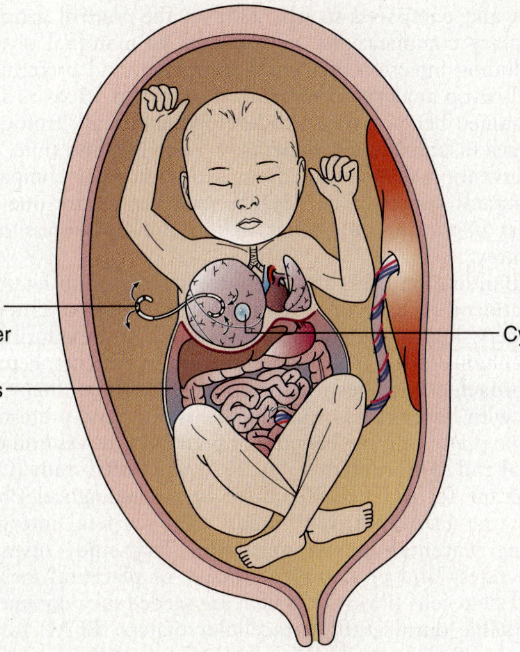

Figure 95.1. Treatment of twin-to-twin transfusion syndrome using fetoscopic laser ablation.

Until the late 1950s, surgical treatment was only offered to MMC patients who survived at least 2 years after birth. Survival rates were as low as 10% to 12% until the development of ventriculoperitoneal shunts, which managed CSF build-up and associated hydrocephalus. In the mid-1960s, survival rates improved significantly when treatment within 12 to 48 hours postdelivery became standardized.[12] However, while shunt procedures improved survival, they still required frequent revisions, and issues like urinary tract infections, renal failure, and paralysis remained unresolved.

Rationale for Prenatal Surgery

Neurologic deficits in MMC are explained by the "two-hit hypothesis." In this model, the neural tube fails to close, allowing CSF leakage and exposure of the neural placode (the first hit). This exposes the placode to direct trauma from contact with the uterine wall and chemical trauma from the toxicity of amniotic fluid (the second hit). Fetal intervention for MMC was hypothesized to potentially prevent the acquired injury associated with the second hit.

This hypothesis was tested in fetal lamb models, which showed (1) reversal of hindbrain herniation in fetal lambs that underwent MMC surgical repair[13] and (2) that prenatal coverage of the exposed placode could improve distal neurologic function.[14] These promising animal studies led to the initiation of fetal surgery for MMC, the first nonlethal fetal defect treated surgically.

This work culminated in the **Management of Myelomeningocele (MOMS) trial**, a three-center, randomized controlled clinical trial comparing fetal surgery with standard postnatal repair which was halted due to efficacy of fetal intervention after recruitment of 183 out of a planned 200 patients. Study outcomes showed a 50% decrease in need for ventriculoperitoneal shunting and decreased occurrence of Chiari neurologic malformations.[15] Additionally, follow-up at 30 months showed that 42% of infants who had fetal surgery were able to walk, compared to just 21% in the control group. The primary complications were related to maternal outcomes, including infection, placental abruption, and preterm labor. Follow-up analysis of patients at ages 5 to 10 years showed sustained benefits in neurodevelopmental and urologic outcomes in nonshunted patients.[16,17] For the first time, a fetal intervention demonstrated superior outcomes compared to postnatal surgery. The MOMS trial results are one of the most important milestones in the clinical success of fetal surgery.

Building on these results, current research in fetal MMC treatment focuses on expanding the inclusion criteria for surgery, improving surgical techniques, and exploring ways to enhance distal neurologic function in patients. Fetoscopic approaches have been reported to reduce maternal morbidity, with lower rates of uterine dehiscence and preterm birth while preserving the benefits of prenatal intervention on survival and hydrocephalus.[18] In 2020, the **CuRE study** (Cellular Therapy for In Utero Repair of Myelomeningocele) became the first FDA-approved clinical trial for fetal intervention using placental-derived stem cells. This study investigates the safety and preliminary efficacy of placental mesenchymal stem cells (PMSCs), which are seeded on a commercially available dural graft extracellular matrix (ECM) for dural closure during standard fetal MMC repair. Preclinical translational studies in the ovine MMC model have demonstrated promising results with improved motor function in treated animals.[19] Other innovative technologies are currently under preclinical investigation to help mitigate the effects of this devastating disease.

Congenital Diaphragmatic Hernia

Congenital diaphragmatic hernia (CDH) is characterized by a developmental defect in the diaphragm leading to herniation of abdominal viscera into the thoracic cavity, resulting in abnormalities in lung development including pulmonary hypoplasia and pulmonary hypertension. CDH occurs in 1 in 4000 live births and can be an isolated anomaly or associated with anomalies in other organ systems.[20] Multiple chromosomal aberrations and single-gene mutations are associated with CDH, including trisomy 18, trisomy 13, trisomy 21, Pallister Killian syndrome, 8p23.1 deletion syndrome, and Cornelia de Lange syndrome. Other co-occurring major structural anomalies include cardiovascular, renal, central nervous system and musculoskeletal defects. Pulmonary hypoplasia and pulmonary hypertension remain the most significant cause of morbidity and mortality in neonates affected by CDH, leading to efforts to target lung growth in the developing fetus.

Treatment Methods

Establishing fundamental criteria for CDH fetal intervention remains controversial due to challenges in predicting the severity and postnatal outcomes in affected fetuses. Initial efforts to treat severe cases of CDH with open fetal surgery were unsuccessful due to impaired umbilical venous return after reducing the herniated liver into the fetal abdomen.[21] Subsequently, tracheal occlusion was introduced as a primary treatment to address pulmonary hypoplasia by reversibly blocking the fetal trachea, causing fluid build-up that stretches the lung and enables airway and pulmonary vessel growth[22] (**Fig. 95.2**).Tracheal occlusion studies of pulmonary hyperplasia in fetal lamb models with CDH showed accelerated lung growth and improvement in pulmonary function.[23,24] The results of a North American randomized trial for fetoscopic endoluminal tracheal occlusion (FETO) for severe isolated CDH was recently reported in the New England Journal of Medicine. The trial was stopped early due to efficacy after the third interim analysis, with improved survival to hospital discharge and sustained survival benefit at 6 months of age.[25]

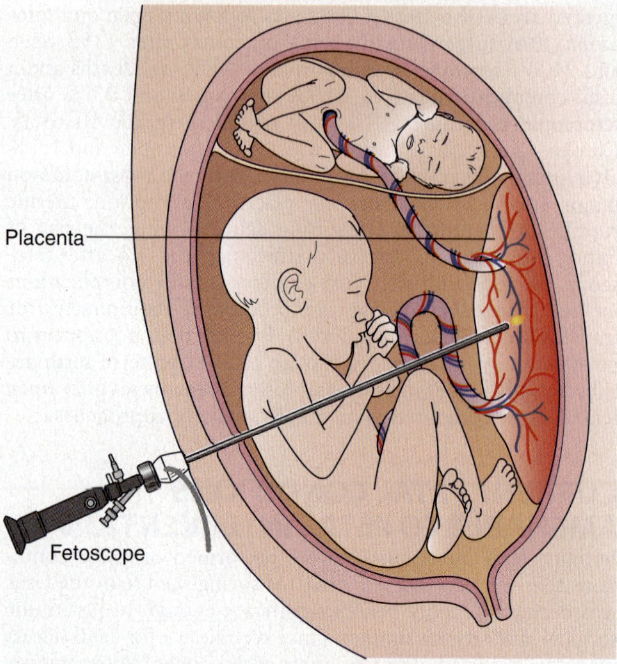

Figure 95.2. Fetal endoscopic tracheal occlusion.

Congenital Cardiac Lesions/Congenital Heart Defects

Congenital heart defects (CHDs) are structural abnormalities of the heart or intrathoracic vessels with functional significance. Occurring in approximately 5 to 10 cases per 1000 live births, CHDs represent a significant cause of morbidity and mortality. It is estimated that 25% of infants with CHDs will require surgical intervention within the first year of life. CHD malformations are detected using fetal echocardiography and remain relatively stable throughout gestation, with the exception of a subset of lesions which may evolve or worsen during fetal development[26]:

1. Severe aortic stenosis with evolving hypoplastic left heart syndrome (AS/eHLS)
2. Pulmonary atresia with intact ventricular septum with evolving hypoplastic right heart syndrome (PA/IVS)
3. Hypoplastic left heart syndrome with intact or severely restrictive atrial septum (HLS/IAS)

Rationale for Prenatal Intervention—Treatment Methods

Fetal cardiac intervention (FCI) aims to alter in utero anatomy and physiology to improve postnatal function. For **severe aortic stenosis with evolving hypoplastic left heart syndrome (AS/eHLS)** and **pulmonary atresia with intact ventricular septum (PA/IVS)**, FCI can result in **biventricular circulation**, thereby avoiding the need for **single-ventricular palliation** and its associated complications.[27] In cases of **hypoplastic left heart syndrome with intact or severely restrictive atrial septum (HLHS/IAS)**, FCI can help reduce **in utero left atrial hypertension** and decrease the need for **emergent postnatal interventions**, though the **overall survival benefit** remains less clear.

However, several limitations of FCI prevent it from demonstrating consistent long-term survival benefits. These include **restricted patient eligibility**, limiting the number of candidates for the procedure, **late referrals** to specialized fetal cardiac centers, often after the optimal intervention window has passed, and a **lack of providers with sufficient technical expertise** in fetal cardiac surgery.

Additionally, the **absence of robust animal models** for preclinical research in fetal cardiac diseases further hinders progress in this field. Currently, **open fetal interventions** for cardiac

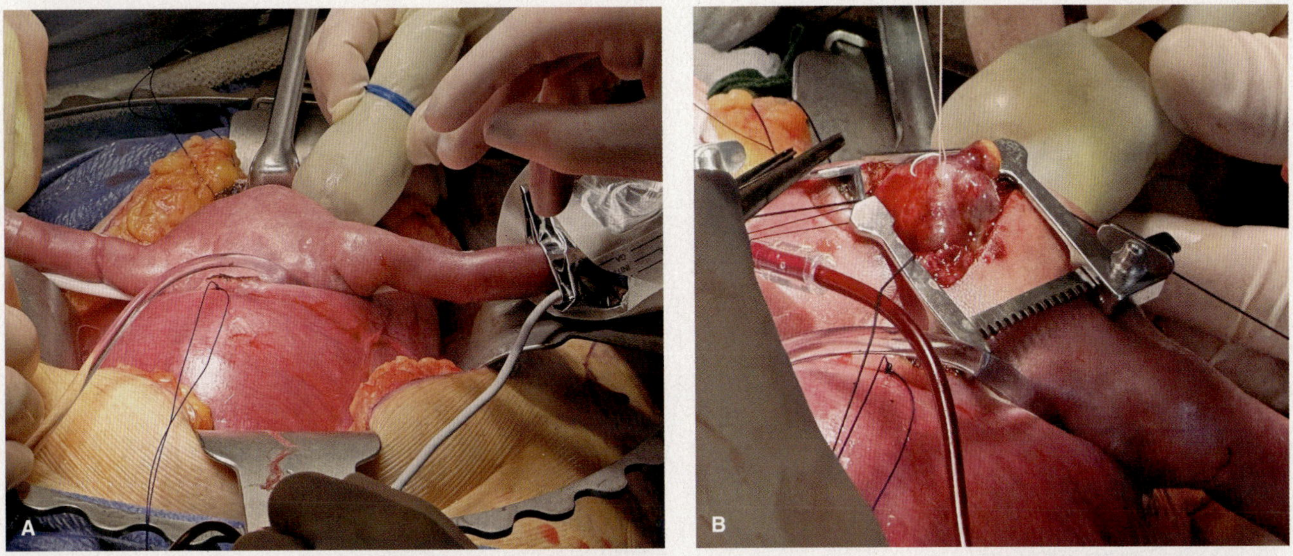

Figure 95.3. Intraoperative images from resection of pericardial teratoma. **A.** Only fetal arms are positioned outside of uterus to allow for monitoring and intravascular catheter placement for resuscitative fluids, blood products and medications. **B.** Sternotomy performed with tumor extruding through open wound secondary to pressure.

lesions are largely limited to addressing **fetal cardiac tumors** (eg, teratomas) that lead to **fetal hydrops** (**Fig. 95.3**).

Congenital Lung Lesions

Congenital lung lesions (CLLs) are a group of rare prenatal pathologies that occur in approximately 1 in 10,000 to 35,000 pregnancies. These lesions are typically detected via ultrasound imaging between 18 and 20 weeks of gestation. CLLs can range from small, asymptomatic lung cysts to larger, more severe conditions such as congenital pulmonary airway malformations (CPAMs), which have the potential to lead to fetal demise. Early diagnosis is crucial, as the natural history of CLLs can vary significantly. Some lesions may regress by the third trimester, while others may expand rapidly, leading to hydrops and, in some cases, fetal death.

Serial ultrasonography is an essential tool for tracking the progression of CLLs. It helps define the natural history of these lesions, identifies pathophysiologic features, and assists in formulating an appropriate treatment plan based on prognostic information. Volumetric analysis of lesion size normalized to head circumference, or CPAM volume ratio (CVR) has been shown to have strong prognostic significance, with a CVR of greater than 1.6 predicting increased risk of hydrops and requirement for prenatal intervention.[28] Fetal echocardiography can detect changes in cardiac output and assess for early signs of cardiac failure. Fetal MRI lung volumes have further been shown to have predictive power on neonatal outcomes such as respiratory distress and need for immediate surgical intervention after birth.[29]

Treatment Methods

Various options for prenatal intervention are available for CLLs. Administration of maternal steroids can reverse early hydrops and improve survival, and is primarily used in cases of microcystic CPAM.[30] Cyst aspiration allows for decompression of large macrocystic lesions, while thoracoamniotic shunting is a method used to reverse hydrops when a CLL is composed of a dominant cyst and no large solid components.[31] Complications associated with this approach include shunt dislodgement, fetal distress, and consequential repeat procedure to correct shunt maladjustment (**Fig. 95.4**). Finally, open fetal surgery with surgical fetal lobectomy is required only rarely for select CPAMs with impending fetal demise.

Sacrococcygeal Teratoma

Fetal sacrococcygeal teratomas (SCTs), although rare, represent the most common prenatally diagnosed congenital tumor, occurring at 1:35,000 to 1:40,000 births.[32] Most SCTs are diagnosed before birth through routine fetal screening and do not typically require treatment until after birth. However, diagnosis of large fetal SCTs requires active clinical management due to associated obstetric complications and high rates of fetal mortality. Detrimental effects of large SCTs can include rapid growth rate, development of hydrops fetalis caused by high-output fetal heart failure, preterm delivery, erratic hemorrhaging and tumor rupture, and maternal mirror syndrome.[33]

The causes of death in fetal SCT are multifactorial, but primarily involve tumor rupture and bleeding at the time of delivery, or high-output cardiac failure and hydrops from high blood flow within the mass. The development of impending fetal or maternal decompensation at or beyond 27 weeks of gestation is an indication for early delivery and tumor debulking.[34,35]

Rationale for Prenatal Surgery—Treatment Methods

Fetal surgical intervention for SCT treatment is only considered when a fetus shows rapid decline in cardiovascular function prior to 26 weeks of gestation, when the alternative outcome is prenatal fatality. Echocardiographic markers of impending fetal demise include increased aortic velocity, cardiac output, a dilated inferior vena cava, or reversed end-diastolic umbilical blood flow. For fetuses greater than 27 weeks of gestation, these findings are an indication for emergency cesarean delivery and postnatal resection.[34,35] For fetuses less than 27 weeks, open fetal surgery and tumor debulking is the treatment of choice. Minimally invasive approaches to interrupt the tumor's blood supply with radiofrequency ablation, vessel sclerosis or coiling have had limited success, but may warrant further investigation as an alternative for a fetus that is a poor candidate for open fetal resection.[36]

Gastroschisis

Gastroschisis is a congenital defect of the abdominal wall characterized by the herniation of the intestine and other intra-abdominal organs. Although mortality rates have decreased in recent decades, gastroschisis still occurs in approximately 1 in 4000 live births worldwide, with significant morbidity remaining a major clinical concern. After repair of gastroschisis, poor intestinal peristalsis and absorption often slow the recovery of gut function, leading to a prolonged need for total parenteral nutrition (TPN). Early detection and diagnosis during the first trimester are crucial for assessing risk and predicting the severity of the condition, however current prognostic predictors remain inconsistent, limiting the ability to accurately

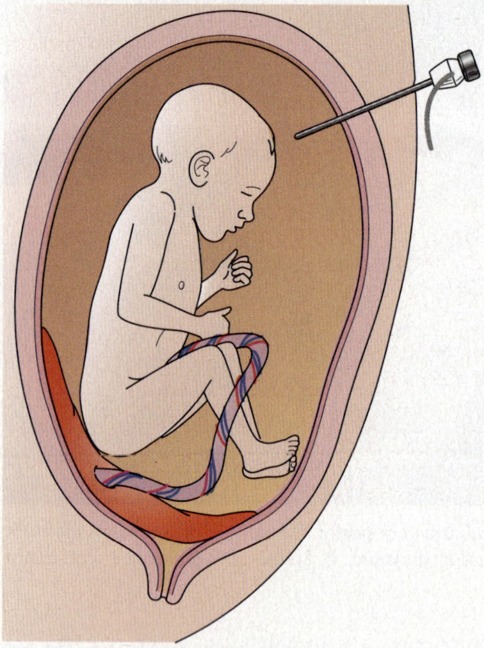

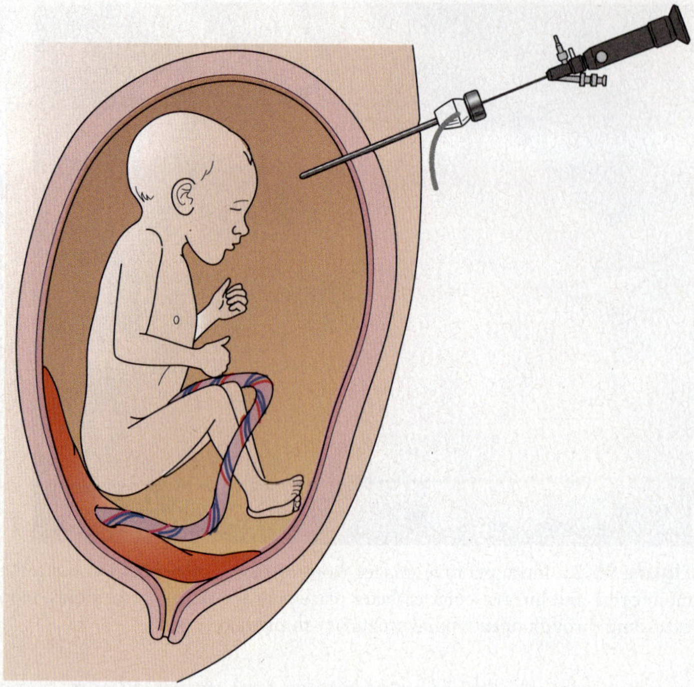

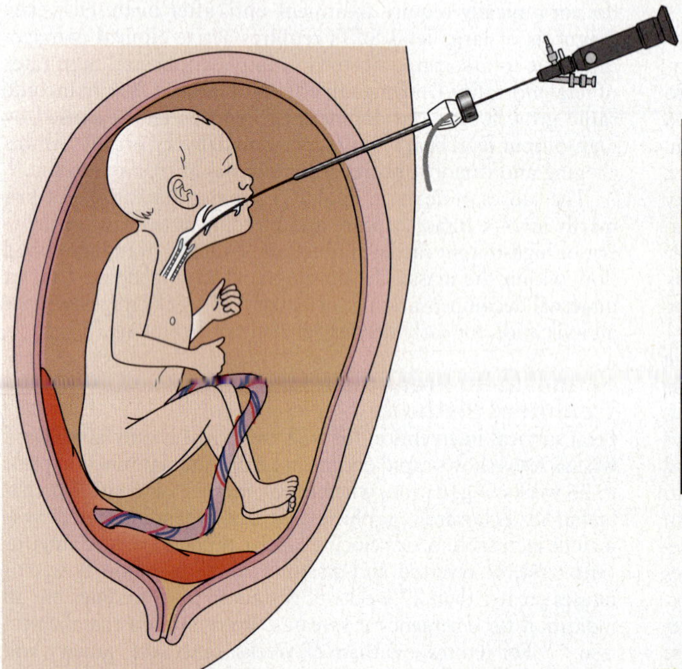

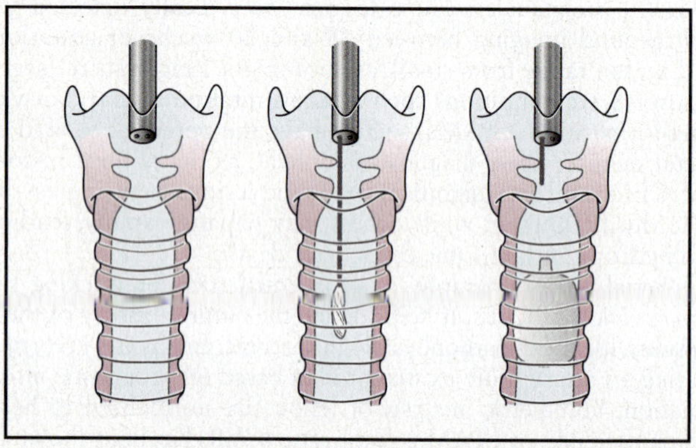

Figure 95.4. Thoracoamniotic shunting of a congenital lung lesion.

counsel patients on expected outcomes. Based on the theory that prolonged exposure to amniotic fluid may worsen intestinal inflammation, a randomized trial of early delivery at 34 weeks was performed but was halted early due to a lack of benefit on outcomes such as duration of TPN and timing of abdominal closure, with concern for increased infection risk in the early delivery cohort.[37] Subsequent studies on timing of delivery have shown no significant impact of gestational age in the setting of uncomplicated gastroschisis,[38] and have reported that worse outcomes are associated with abdominal complications including intestinal necrosis at birth, intestinal atresia, vanishing gastroschisis resulting in intestinal autoamputation, hiatal hernia, and necrotizing enterocolitis.[39]

As postnatal treatment outcomes for gastroschisis are generally favorable, the net benefit of fetal surgical intervention is open for debate. Research using fetal lamb models is in the early stages,[40] with several techniques of open or minimally invasive repair of gastroschisis or covering the intestine have been described and fetoscopic coverage demonstrating the most promise in preclinical animal studies.[41]

Lower Urinary Tract Obstruction

Lower urinary tract obstruction (LUTO) is a congenital defect obstructing fetal bladder outflow leading to upstream urinary congestion. This obstruction results in renal failure and pulmonary hypoplasia as amniotic fluid is formed by fetal urine and is crucial for normal lung development. LUTO occurs in approximately 2.2 to 3.3 cases per 10,000 live births, with devastating impacts of fetal morbidity and mortality.[42] LUTO is caused by a variety of pathophysiologic processes resulting in distal urinary tract obstruction, decreased urinary flow, and regionalized urinary congestion.

Fetal ultrasound remains the primary diagnostic tool for LUTO, detecting signs such as megacysts or bladder enlargement with bilateral hydronephrosis. While ultrasound may have limitations in determining the underlying etiology, it remains essential for guiding treatment decisions, particularly as it can detect renal parenchymal abnormalities. Recent studies also indicate fetal MRI may provide additional diagnostic information.[43]

Rationale for Fetal Treatment

While it seems logical that relieving urinary obstruction would be ideal, not all fetuses with LUTO have urinary biochemistry which would benefit from fetal intervention. Several studies have shown that favorable urinary biochemistry profiles (sodium <100 mg/dL, calcium <8 mg/dL, osmolality <200 mOsm/L, β_2-microglobulin <4 mg/dL, total protein <20 mg/dL) predict good postnatal renal outcomes.[44] Treatment approaches are determined by severity of the disease in addition to diagnostic criteria. When indicated, fetal intervention is recommended as treatment in order to restore amniotic fluid volume and thereby enable normal lung development and preserve renal functioning. This can be accomplished by several means, but placement of a fetal vesicle (bladder) amniotic shunt is currently most common.[45]

6 Cervical Teratoma, Airways Masses, and EXIT Procedures

Ex-utero intrapartum treatment (EXIT) is a surgical procedure allowing for stabilization of the obstructed airway in a fetus prior to delivery.[46] Prenatal findings of tracheal narrowing or displacement, polyhydramnios, and abnormal fetal breathing on ultrasound are strongly associated with need for a definitive airway at birth.[47] In selected cases with severe prenatal imaging features, EXIT-to-airway operations partially deliver the head and neck of a fetus to attempt direct endotracheal intubation through laryngoscopy, bronchoscopy, or tracheostomy. Complete resection may be necessary in large teratomas, placing the mother under deep anesthesia to maintain maternal–fetal uteroplacental circulation as is required in open fetal surgery. Following resection, the umbilical cord is cut and the baby is completely delivered.

7 FUTURE DIRECTIONS

Fetal surgery has made extraordinary progress since the original pioneering procedures, and the future of the field holds even more promise. A growing number of applications for fetal gene and stem cell therapies, with potential induction of tolerance for future transplants, are expanding the field of fetal medicine and surgery. This evolving scope of investigation offers a lifetime of opportunities for emerging surgeon-scientists. As fetal surgery continues to advance, promising animal research is exploring the technical feasibility and pathophysiologic rationale behind in utero interventions.

Fetal molecular and cellular therapies represent a new frontier in prenatal treatment for genetic diseases. Access to the fetal umbilical vein, commonly used for in utero transfusions, allows for the potential treatment of fetuses with stem cells, proteins, or viral vectors. In utero stem cell transplantation has emerged as a promising treatment which takes advantage of the heightened immunologic immaturity and plasticity of the fetus in early development. This provides greater potential for successful fetal stem cell receptivity compared to adults with fully matured immune systems.

Stem cells used for fetal transplantation may be sourced from bone marrow, the placenta, or amniotic fluid. Hematopoietic stem cells (HSCs) are the most widely studied due to their ability to differentiate into blood cells, making HSC transplantation a potential cure for prenatal hemoglobinopathies that typically require bone marrow transplants. In utero HSC transplantation has been successfully used to treat hemoglobinopathies, bleeding disorders, immunodeficiencies, and storage disorders.[48] Currently, a phase I clinical trial is investigating in utero transplantation for patients with alpha thalassemia major.[49] Another promising therapy is in utero enzyme replacement for fetuses with lysosomal storage disorders. For example, fetuses with MPS7 (Sly syndrome) often develop hydrops, a sign of impending demise. Infusion of the missing recombinant enzyme has improved outcomes in mouse models of MPS7, with potential clinical applications.[50]

In utero gene therapy represents an inward approach to fetal intervention by correcting an underlying genetic anomaly early in development to restore normal function. The benefits of gene therapy are particularly promising, as the immature fetal immune system increases the likelihood of successful stem cell receptivity. This method is less invasive compared to other fetal interventions and could improve outcomes for disorders where postnatal therapies have already been tested, such as spinal muscular atrophy and hemophilia. The key advantages of gene therapy in utero include:

- **Inducing tolerance** to missing proteins, as the fetal immune system is more prone to tolerance.
- The ability to cross the blood–brain barrier before it is fully formed, potentially addressing neurologic aspects of diseases.
- Lower costs for enzymes or viral vectors due to the small size of the fetus.

Gene editing tools, particularly CRISPR/Cas9, are crucial for the feasibility of gene therapy. This technique enables precise manipulation of genes within target cells. CRISPR/Cas9 works by binding synthetic guide RNAs (gRNAs) to chromosomal DNA sites specified by the Cas9 enzyme.[51] Proof of concept studies on the mouse mode of hereditary tyrosinemia type 1[52] and phenylketonuria[53] illustrate the potential for definitive genetic editing to reverse disease pathogenesis.

Research also has focused on mesenchymal stem cells (MSCs), which migrate to sites of injury and engraft in target tissues, suggesting their potential in tissue repair. Fetal MSCs, derived from the liver, umbilical cord, blood, amnion, placenta, and amniotic fluid, are more abundant and accessible during fetal development, particularly from 15 weeks of gestation. Studies on the ovine model of MMC have shown improved motor outcomes by augmentation of in utero fetal surgical repair with human placental mesenchymal stromal cells seeded onto ECM.[54] The FDA has recently approved a phase I clinical trial in human patients based on the strength of the preclinical animal model data, using placental-derived MSCs to treat spina bifida in utero. Osteogenesis imperfecta (OI), a disorder characterized by abnormal skeletal development, osteopenia, frequent fractures, and short stature, has been studied using MSC interventions. While postnatal treatments reduce the severity of symptoms, they don't offer a cure. Preclinical studies have shown promise, with MSC intervention in Sweden[55] and Singapore[56] demonstrating remarkable benefits for OI patients. Currently, an exploratory open-label multi-center phase I/II trial, the BOOSTB4 trial, is enrolling patients for further study of the efficacy of fetal MSC therapy for treatment of severe OI in fetuses and infants.[57]

While preclinical studies show no significant risk to the mother from in utero stem cell, enzyme replacement, or gene therapies, clinical implementation requires careful attention to any unanticipated adverse events. Currently, research on in utero gene therapy is in the early stages, with animal studies underway and human clinical trials just beginning. Ethical and moral issues surrounding these therapies remain a topic of ongoing debate.

As with the pioneers of open fetal surgery, those working in fetal gene and cell therapy must persevere in the face of doubts regarding feasibility, ethics, and efficacy. It is through persistence that scientific progress is made and diseases can eventually be conquered.

ACKNOWLEDGEMENTS

We gratefully acknowledge the contributions of previous edition authors, Diana L. Farmer and Tippi MacKenzie, as portions of those chapters have been retained in this revision.

References

1. Golbus MS, Harrison MR, Filly RA, Callen PW, Katz M. In utero treatment of urinary tract obstruction. *Am J Obstet Gynecol.* 1982;142(4):383–388.
2. Harrison MR, Filly RA, Golbus MS, et al. Fetal treatment 1982. *N Engl J Med.* 1982;307(26):1651–1652.
3. Pratt R, Deprest J, Vercauteren T, Ourselin S, David AL. Computer-assisted surgical planning and intraoperative guidance in fetal surgery: a systematic review. *Prenat Diagn.* 2015;35(12):1159–1166.
4. Chervenak FA, McCullough LB. The fetus as a patient: an essential ethical concept for maternal-fetal medicine. *J Matern Fetal Med.* 1996;5(3):115–119.
5. Sichitiu J, Alkazaleh F, de Heus R, et al. Maternal "mirror" syndrome: evaluating the benefits of fetal therapy. *Prenat Diagn.* 2024;44(8):979–987.
6. Goodnight WH, Bahtiyar O, Bennett KA, et al; fMMC Consortium sponsored by NAFTNet. Subsequent pregnancy outcomes after open maternal-fetal surgery for myelomeningocele. *Am J Obstet Gynecol.* 2019;220(5):494.e1–494.e7.
7. Sacco A, Van der Veeken L, Bagshaw E, et al. Maternal complications following open and fetoscopic fetal surgery: a systematic review and meta-analysis. *Prenat Diagn.* 2019;39(4):251–268.
8. Society for Maternal-Fetal Medicine; Simpson LL. Twin-twin transfusion syndrome. *Am J Obstet Gynecol.* 2013;208(1):3–18. Erratum in: *Am J Obstet Gynecol.* 2013 May;208(5):392.
9. Senat MV, Deprest J, Boulvain M, Paupe A, Winer N, Ville Y. Endoscopic laser surgery versus serial amnioreduction for severe twin-to-twin transfusion syndrome. *N Engl J Med.* 2004;351(2):136–144.
10. Muratore CS, Carr SR, Lewi L, et al. Survival after laser surgery for twin-to-twin transfusion syndrome: when are they out of the woods? *J Pediatr Surg.* 2009;44(1):66–69; discussion 70.
11. Adzick NS. Fetal myelomeningocele: natural history, pathophysiology, and in-utero intervention. *Semin Fetal Neonatal Med.* 2010;15(1):9–14.
12. Pruitt LJ. Living with spina bifida: a historical perspective. *Pediatrics.* 2012;130(2):181–183.
13. Paek BW, Farmer DL, Wilkinson CC, et al. Hindbrain herniation develops in surgically created myelomeningocele but is absent after repair in fetal lambs. *Am J Obstet Gynecol.* 2000;183(5):1119–1123.
14. Meuli M, Meuli-Simmen C, Yingling CD, et al. In utero repair of experimental myelomeningocele saves neurological function at birth. *J Pediatr Surg.* 1996;31(3):397–402.
15. Adzick NS, Thom EA, Spong CY, et al; MOMS Investigators. A randomized trial of prenatal versus postnatal repair of myelomeningocele. *N Engl J Med.* 2011;364(11):993–1004.
16. Houtrow AJ, MacPherson C, Jackson-Coty J, et al. Prenatal repair and physical functioning among children with myelomeningocele: a secondary analysis of a randomized clinical trial. *JAMA Pediatr.* 2021;175(4):e205674.
17. Brock JW 3rd, Thomas JC, Baskin LS, et al; Eunice Kennedy Shriver NICHD MOMS Trial Group. Effect of prenatal repair of myelomeningocele on urological outcomes at school age. *J Urol.* 2019;202(4):812–818.
18. Kabagambe SK, Jensen GW, Chen YJ, Vanover MA, Farmer DL. Fetal surgery for myelomeningocele: a systematic review and meta-analysis of outcomes in fetoscopic versus open repair. *Fetal Diagn Ther.* 2018;43(3):161–174.
19. Vanover M, Pivetti C, Lankford L, et al. High density placental mesenchymal stromal cells provide neuronal preservation and improve motor function following in utero treatment of ovine myelomeningocele. *J Pediatr Surg.* 2019;54(1):75–79.
20. Balayla J, Abenhaim HA. Incidence, predictors and outcomes of congenital diaphragmatic hernia: a population-based study of 32 million births in the United States. *J Matern Fetal Neonatal Med.* 2014;27(14):1438–1444.
21. Harrison MR, Langer JC, Adzick NS, et al. Correction of congenital diaphragmatic hernia in utero, V. Initial clinical experience. *J Pediatr Surg.* 1990;25(1):47–55; discussion 56–57.
22. Wilson JM, DiFiore JW, Peters CA. Experimental fetal tracheal ligation prevents the pulmonary hypoplasia associated with fetal nephrectomy: possible application for congenital diaphragmatic hernia. *J Pediatr Surg.* 1993;28(11):1433–1439; discussion 1439–1440.
23. Hedrick MH, Estes JM, Sullivan KM, et al. Plug the lung until it grows (PLUG): a new method to treat congenital diaphragmatic hernia in utero. *J Pediatr Surg.* 1994;29(5):612–617.
24. Deprest JA, Evrard VA, Van Ballaer PP, et al. Tracheoscopic endoluminal plugging using an inflatable device in the fetal lamb model. *Eur J Obstet Gynecol Reprod Biol.* 1998;81(2):165–169.
25. Deprest JA, Nicolaides KH, Benachi A, et al; TOTAL Trial for Severe Hypoplasia Investigators. Randomized trial of fetal surgery for severe left diaphragmatic hernia. *N Engl J Med.* 2021;385(2):107–118.
26. Schidlow DN, Freud L, Friedman K, Tworetzky W. Fetal interventions for structural heart disease. *Echocardiography.* 2017;34(12):1834–1841.
27. Schidlow DN, Tworetzky W, Wilkins-Haug LE. Percutaneous fetal cardiac interventions for structural heart disease. *Am J Perinatol.* 2014;31(7):629–636.
28. Crombleholme TM, Coleman B, Hedrick H, et al. Cystic adenomatoid malformation volume ratio predicts outcome in prenatally diagnosed cystic adenomatoid malformation of the lung. *J Pediatr Surg.* 2002;37(3):331–338.
29. Zamora IJ, Sheikh F, Cassady CI, et al. Fetal MRI lung volumes are predictive of perinatal outcomes in fetuses with congenital lung masses. *J Pediatr Surg.* 2014;49(6):853–858; discussion 858.
30. Peranteau WH, Boelig MM, Khalek N, et al. Effect of single and multiple courses of maternal betamethasone on prenatal congenital lung lesion growth and fetal survival. *J Pediatr Surg.* 2016;51(1):28–32.
31. Bose SK, Stratigis JD, Ahn N, et al. Prenatally diagnosed large lung lesions: timing of resection and perinatal outcomes. *J Pediatr Surg.* 2023;58(12):2384–2390.
32. Swamy R, Embleton N, Hale J. Sacrococcygeal teratoma over two decades: birth prevalence, prenatal diagnosis and clinical outcomes. *Prenat Diagn.* 2008;28(11):1048–1051.
33. Wilson RD, Hedrick H, Flake AW, et al. Sacrococcygeal teratomas: prenatal surveillance, growth and pregnancy outcome. *Fetal Diagn Ther.* 2009;25(1):15–20.
34. Roybal JL, Moldenhauer JS, Khalek N, et al. Early delivery as an alternative management strategy for selected high-risk fetal sacrococcygeal teratomas. *J Pediatr Surg.* 2011;46(7):1325–1332.
35. Baumgarten HD, Gebb JS, Khalek N, et al. Preemptive delivery and immediate resection for fetuses with high-risk sacrococcygeal teratomas. *Fetal Diagn Ther.* 2019;45(3):137–144.
36. Konno H, Okpaise OO, Sbragia L, Tonni G, Ruano R. Perinatal outcomes of intrauterine interventions for fetal sacrococcygeal teratoma based on different surgical techniques-a systematic review. *J Clin Med.* 2024;13(9):2649.
37. Shamshirsaz AA, Lee TC, Hair AB, et al. Elective delivery at 34 weeks vs routine obstetric care in fetal gastroschisis: randomized controlled trial. *Ultrasound Obstet Gynecol.* 2020;55(1):15–19.
38. Fraga MV, Laje P, Peranteau WH, et al. The influence of gestational age, mode of delivery and abdominal wall closure method on the surgical outcome of neonates with uncomplicated gastroschisis. *Pediatr Surg Int.* 2018;34(4):415–419.
39. Laje P, Fraga MV, Peranteau WH, et al. Complex gastroschisis: Clinical spectrum and neonatal outcomes at a referral center. *J Pediatr Surg.* 2018;53(10):1904–1907.
40. Arai T, Tianthong W, Russo FM, et al. Experimental induction of complex gastroschisis in the fetal lamb: systematic review. *Prenat Diagn.* 2024;44(11):1372–1380.
41. Durmaz LO, Brunner SE, Meinzer A, Krebs TF, Bergholz R. Fetal surgery for gastroschisis-a review with emphasis on minimally invasive procedures. *Children (Basel).* 2022;9(3):416.

42. Saccone G, D'Alessandro P, Escolino M, et al. Antenatal intervention for congenital fetal lower urinary tract obstruction (LUTO): a systematic review and meta-analysis. *J Matern Fetal Neonatal Med.* 2020;33(15):2664–2670.
43. Vinit N, Grevent D, Millischer-Bellaiche AE, et al. Biometric and morphological features on magnetic resonance imaging of fetal bladder in lower urinary tract obstruction: new perspectives for fetal cystoscopy. *Ultrasound Obstet Gynecol.* 2020;56(1):86–95.
44. Pierucci UM, Paraboschi I, Mantica G, et al. Antenatal determinants of postnatal renal function in fetal megacystis: a systematic review. *Diagnostics (Basel).* 2024;14(7):756.
45. Menchaca AD, Olutoye OO. Fetal lower urinary tract obstruction: current diagnostic and therapeutic strategies and future directions. *Fetal Diagn Ther.* 2024;51(6):603–611.
46. Laje P, Johnson MP, Howell LJ, et al. Ex utero intrapartum treatment in the management of giant cervical teratomas. *J Pediatr Surg.* 2012;47(6):1208–1216.
47. Schmoke N, Nemeh C, Wu YS, et al. Management of fetal head and neck masses: evaluation of prenatal factors associated with airway obstruction and decision for definitive airway and ex-utero intrapartum treatment at birth. *Prenat Diagn.* 2024;44(10):1225–1230.
48. Sagar RL, Walther-Jallow L, Götherström C, Westgren M, David AL. Maternal and fetal safety outcomes after in utero stem cell injection: a systematic review. *Prenat Diagn.* 2023;43(13):1622–1637.
49. Horvei P, MacKenzie T, Kharbanda S. Advances in the management of α-thalassemia major: reasons to be optimistic. *Hematology Am Soc Hematol Educ Program.* 2021;2021(1):592–599.
50. Nguyen QH, Witt RG, Wang B, et al. Tolerance induction and microglial engraftment after fetal therapy without conditioning in mice with Mucopolysaccharidosis type VII. *Sci Transl Med.* 2020;12(532):eaay8980.
51. Shear MA, Massa A. In utero fetal therapy: stem cells, cell transplantation, gene therapy, and CRISPR-Cas9. *Clin Obstet Gynecol.* 2021;64(4):861–875.
52. Rossidis AC, Stratigis JD, Chadwick AC, et al. In utero CRISPR-mediated therapeutic editing of metabolic genes. *Nat Med.* 2018;24(10):1513–1518.
53. Brooks DL, Carrasco MJ, Qu P, et al. Rapid and definitive treatment of phenylketonuria in variant-humanized mice with corrective editing. *Nat Commun.* 2023;14(1):3451.
54. Stokes SC, Theodorou CM, Jackson JE, et al. Long-term safety evaluation of placental mesenchymal stromal cells for in utero repair of myelomeningocele in a novel ovine model. *J Pediatr Surg.* 2022;57(1):18–25.
55. Le Blanc K, Götherström C, Ringdén O, et al. Fetal mesenchymal stem-cell engraftment in bone after in utero transplantation in a patient with severe osteogenesis imperfecta. *Transplantation.* 2005;79(11):1607–1614.
56. Chan JK, Götherström C. Prenatal transplantation of mesenchymal stem cells to treat osteogenesis imperfecta. *Front Pharmacol.* 2014;5:223.
57. Sagar RL, Åström E, Chitty LS, et al. An exploratory open-label multicentre phase I/II trial evaluating the safety and efficacy of postnatal or prenatal and postnatal administration of allogeneic expanded fetal mesenchymal stem cells for the treatment of severe osteogenesis imperfecta in infants and fetuses: the BOOSTB4 trial protocol. *BMJ Open.* 2024;14(6):e079767.

96

Pediatric Head and Neck

Chad K. Sudoko, Andrew J. Bauer, and Ken Kazahaya

Key Points

1. The location of the neck mass (midline vs lateral) is important for narrowing the differential diagnosis.
2. Thyroglossal duct cysts (TGDCs) are the most common congenital neck mass and benign cervical lymphadenopathy is the most common acquired neck mass in the pediatric population.
3. Infantile hemangioma (IH) is the most common tumor of infancy and is typically treated with propranolol.
4. The majority of patients with thyroid cancer are asymptomatic at diagnosis.
5. Laryngomalacia is typically a self-limited pathology that resolves by 18 months of age.
6. A negative radiograph should not preclude bronchoscopy in patients that have a history or exam concerning for an airway foreign body.

Pediatric head and neck lesions include a broad differential diagnosis. From congenital to acquired, benign to malignant, and chronic to acute lesions, a thorough workup and sharp clinical acumen is essential for an appropriate diagnosis and treatment. Knowledge of head and neck embryology is fundamental in understanding the congenital lesions and their association with related anatomy. This chapter will cover common pediatric head and neck lesions starting with congenital etiologies, followed by infectious and vascular etiologies, thyroid malignancies, and finally, airway lesions.

1 CONGENITAL

Thyroglossal Duct Cysts

2 Thyroglossal duct cysts (TGDCs) are the most common congenital neck mass and can be found anywhere along the path of the thyroglossal duct (TGD).[1] Starting at the foramen cecum, the thyroid gland descends through the TGD to its final location below the cricoid cartilage. The TGD will then atrophy and involute. Failure of the TGD to involute results in persistent ductal epithelium that can remain active and cause cystic expansion. Although TGDCs can occur anywhere along the TGD, they most commonly present as a midline neck mass that is in close proximity to the hyoid bone (**Fig. 96.1**).

When a TGDC is suspected based on clinical history and examination, an ultrasound (US) is commonly obtained. US is useful to assess the characteristics of the cyst, but is most important in confirming the presence of a normal orthotopic thyroid gland. In rare cases, ectopic thyroid tissue is the cause of a midline neck mass and inadvertent removal can result in hypothyroidism.

Surgical excision is recommended for treatment of TGDCs and involves removal of the entire tract and central portion of the hyoid bone, called the Sistrunk procedure. The biggest risk of surgical excision is recurrence, with recurrence rates between 5% and 10%.[2,3] While under general anesthesia, the patient is positioned with the neck extended and on a shoulder roll. A horizontal incision is made within a skin crease or relaxed skin tension line over the cyst. There is no need to excise skin unless there is a fistulous tract from a prior infection or drainage. Subplatysmal flaps are raised, the strap muscles are identified and separated at the midline raphe, and retracted laterally. Care is taken to dissect the cyst from surrounding soft tissue attachments as it is traced superiorly. Muscular attachments to the hyoid bone are then dissected free, and the central hyoid bone between the lesser horns is cut with heavy scissors. Excision of the tract and tongue base musculature between the hyoid and foramen cecum is then performed. It may be helpful to place a gloved finger at the base of the tongue to facilitate complete excision. The tract, cyst, and central hyoid bone are then removed en bloc and the wound is closed in layers. A drain may be considered depending on the size of the cyst and the amount of dead space that is present.

Epidermoid and Dermoid Cysts

Epidermoid and dermoid cysts are benign congenital neoplasms that can form anywhere in the body with an incidence ranging from 1.6% to 6.9% in the head and neck.[4,5] The most common locations of dermoid cysts are the periorbital, nasal, submental, and suprasternal areas.[6] As dermoid cysts are typically midline, it can be challenging to differentiate between a dermoid cyst or TGDC. Treatment of both epidermoid and dermoid cysts is complete surgical excision. It may be challenging to differentiate between an epidermoid and dermoid cyst, however, epidermoid cysts contain only keratinizing epithelium, while dermoid cysts contain epidermal and adnexal tissues, including hair follicles and sebaceous glands.[7]

Teratomas

Teratomas are congenital neoplasms that are composed of all three germ cell layers: ectoderm, mesoderm, and endoderm. Teratomas are rare, occurring in about 1 in 40,000 births with up to 10% of all teratomas occurring in the head and neck (the most common location for teratomas is the sacrococcygeal area).[8,9] Most pediatric head and neck teratomas are located in the anterolateral cervical neck and are benign, however, they can be locally aggressive and do have malignant potential.

Teratomas can present in the antenatal, perinatal, or postnatal periods. With the advancement of prenatal imaging techniques, most teratomas of the head and neck are identified prior to birth. Up to 20% of cervical teratomas will present with polyhydramnios, which can be identified on prenatal US.[10]

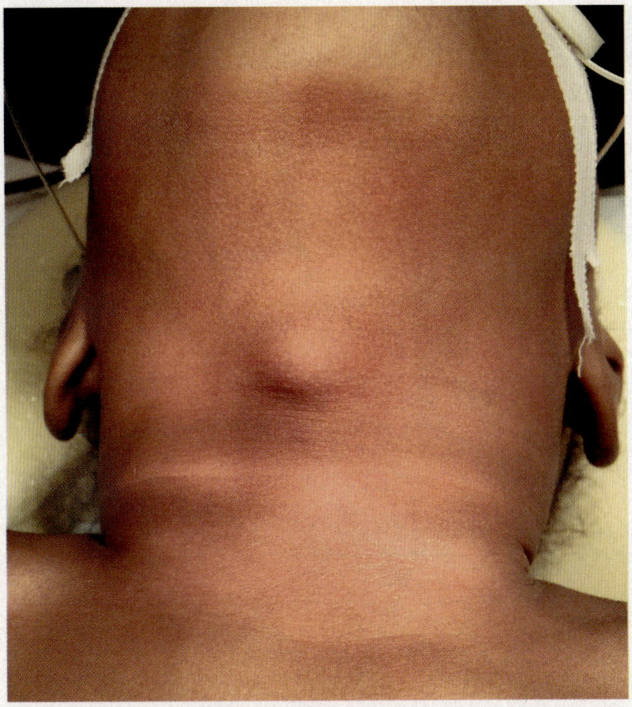

Figure 96.1. Patient with a thyroglossal duct cyst.

If there is a concern for the presence of a teratoma, a fetal MRI is recommended to provide anatomic information regarding the teratoma and surrounding structures. The identification of fetal teratomas in the prenatal period provides the information and time to develop a birthing plan as the primary concern with a large head and neck teratoma is airway compromise. If there is a concern for airway compromise, a planned delivery with a team including neonatologists, anesthesiologists, and pediatric otolaryngologists (Presence of an Extra Surgical Team or PRESTO) or an Ex-Utero Intrapartum Treatment (EXIT) procedure is recommended.

Following safe delivery and airway management, treatment is surgical resection. Although teratomas can be well-defined lesions, it is not uncommon for them to be locally aggressive and infiltrate into nearby tissues, at times requiring resection of the local structures.[11] However, if surgically feasible, early surgical excision can decrease the risk of malignant transformation, hemodynamic instability, coagulopathies, and infection leading to sepsis.[10,11]

Branchial Cleft Anomalies

Branchial cleft anomalies are the second most common congenital neck mass and the most common congenital lateral neck mass accounting for up to 20% of all excised cervical masses in children.[12] These anomalies occur due to incomplete involution of the branchial apparatus during embryogenesis and present as a cyst (no connection to the skin or pharynx), sinus (a connection to either the skin or the pharynx), or fistula (an open tract connecting the skin to the pharynx).

During the 4th week of development, the branchial arches (derived from mesoderm) have formed. As the arches are developing, the branchial pouches (derived from endoderm) form internally and the branchial clefts (derived from exoderm) develop externally. In normal development, the pouches and clefts are gradually obliterated by the surrounding mesenchyme. When the pouch, cleft, or both fail to obliterate, a branchial anomaly develops and the type of anomaly is dictated by the cleft or pouch of origin. The origin and type of the anomaly is associated with a unique clinical presentation and anatomical consideration in regard to the surrounding tissues and the associated tract (**Table 96.1**). A branchial anomaly will lie deep to the embryologic derivatives of the associated arch and superficial to the derivatives of the next arch.

First Branchial Cleft Anomalies

First branchial cleft anomalies account for about 8% to 10% of all branchial anomalies and are closely associated with the external auditory canal, facial nerve, and parotid gland.[13] Historically, they have been further classified based on their germ layer and associated anatomical relationships, into Work type I and type II lesions.[14] Work type I branchial cleft anomalies are ectodermal in origin, occur medial to the concha, and usually lie superficial to the facial nerve. Work type II branchial cleft anomalies contain both ectoderm and mesoderm, are typically found near the angle of the mandible, and may course medial, lateral, or between the branches of the facial nerve.

Depending on the type of first branchial cleft anomaly, patients can present with recurrent preauricular, parotid, or upper neck swelling near the angle of the mandible. The provider should be suspicious for a first branchial cleft anomaly in a patient with recurrent otorrhea without risk factors for otitis externa or without evidence of middle ear disease causing a tympanic membrane perforation. In patients with new onset otorrhea, it is prudent to carefully examine the external auditory canal for a pit. Definitive treatment for a type I branchial cleft anomaly is surgical excision. Incision and drainage without excision should be avoided if at all possible. If the examination is unclear as to whether a Work type I or type II first branchial cleft anomaly is present, preoperative MRI may be helpful to delineate the location and relation to the parotid and facial nerve. The use of facial nerve monitoring should be considered given the close association of the first branchial cleft anomalies and the facial nerve.

Second Branchial Cleft Anomalies

Second branchial cleft anomalies are the most common branchial anomaly and the most common congenital lateral neck mass. They present as a cyst located deep and anterior to the sternocleidomastoid (SCM) muscle that is often noticed as a sudden swelling following an upper respiratory infection. If a fistula is present, it can course inferior-laterally from the lateral pharyngeal wall, over the glossopharyngeal and hypoglossal nerves, and between the internal and external carotid arteries, before terminating at the skin on the anterior border of the SCM muscle. A preoperative MRI may be helpful in diagnosing a second branchial cleft anomaly, especially if there is no obvious pit, and delineating the extent of the lesion (**Fig. 96.2**).

Surgical excision will begin with either an elliptical incision around the opening of the sinus or fistula; or an incision at least two finger breadths below the mandible (to avoid the marginal mandibular nerve) if there is a cyst. Subplatysmal flaps are elevated and the tissues overlying the cyst are dissected free. If a tract is identified, it should be followed as far superiorly as possible before it is clamped, cut, and tied off. Sometimes a stair step incision may be necessary in cases where the pit of the sinus or fistula is too inferior and is limiting superior dissection of the tract. It is rarely necessary to dissect through to the pharynx or to perform a tonsillectomy.

Third/Fourth Branchial Cleft Anomalies

Third and fourth branchial cleft anomalies are rare. The tract of a third branchial cleft anomaly will course from the pyriform sinus, through the thyrohyoid membrane, deep to the glossopharyngeal nerve and internal carotid artery before exiting the skin just anterior to the SCM muscle. The tract of a fourth branchial cleft anomaly will also originate in the pyriform sinus and course inferiorly, deep to the superior laryngeal nerve but superficial to the recurrent laryngeal nerve (RLN). Given that it is difficult to differentiate between third and fourth branchial cleft anomalies, they are often grouped together as pyriform sinus branchial cleft anomalies. These

Table 96.1. Embryology of Pharyngeal Arch Structures

Arch	Nerve	Artery	Muscular Contributions	Skeletal Contributions
1st	Trigeminal nerve (V2 and V3)	Maxillary artery	Muscles of mastication, anterior belly of the digastric, mylohyoid, tensor tympani, tensor veli palatini	Premaxilla, maxilla, zygomatic bone, part of the temporal bone, mandible (only as a model for mandible not actual formation of mandible), incus, malleus. Meckel cartilage and the sphenomandibular ligament
	Pouch	Pharyngotympanic tube, middle ear cleft, part of mastoid air cells		
	Cleft	External auditory canal		
2nd	Facial nerve	Stapedial artery	Muscles of facial expression, buccinator, platysma, stapedius, stylohyoid, posterior belly of the digastric, auricular muscles	Stapes, temporal styloid process, hyoid (lesser horn and upper part of body), stylohyoid ligament, Reichert cartilage
	Pouch	Tonsillar fossa		
	Cleft	Obliterates		
3rd	Glossopharyngeal nerve	Common carotid, proximal internal carotid	Stylopharyngeus	Hyoid (greater horn and lower part of body)
	Pouch	Ventral: thymus; Dorsal: inferior parathyroid glands		
	Cleft	Obliterates		
4th	Vagus nerve (X), superior laryngeal nerve	Right: proximal subclavian artery Left: aortic arch	Cricothyroid muscle, all intrinsic muscles of soft palate (including levator veli palatini) *except* tensor veli palatini	Thyroid cartilage, superior parathyroids, epiglottic cartilage
	Pouch	Ventral: ultimobranchial body; Dorsal: superior parathyroid glands		
	Cleft	Obliterates		
6th	Vagus nerve (X), recurrent laryngeal nerve	Right: pulmonary artery Left: pulmonary artery and ductus arteriosus	All intrinsic muscles of larynx except the cricothyroid muscle	Cricoid cartilage, arytenoid cartilages, corniculate cartilage, cuneiform cartilages

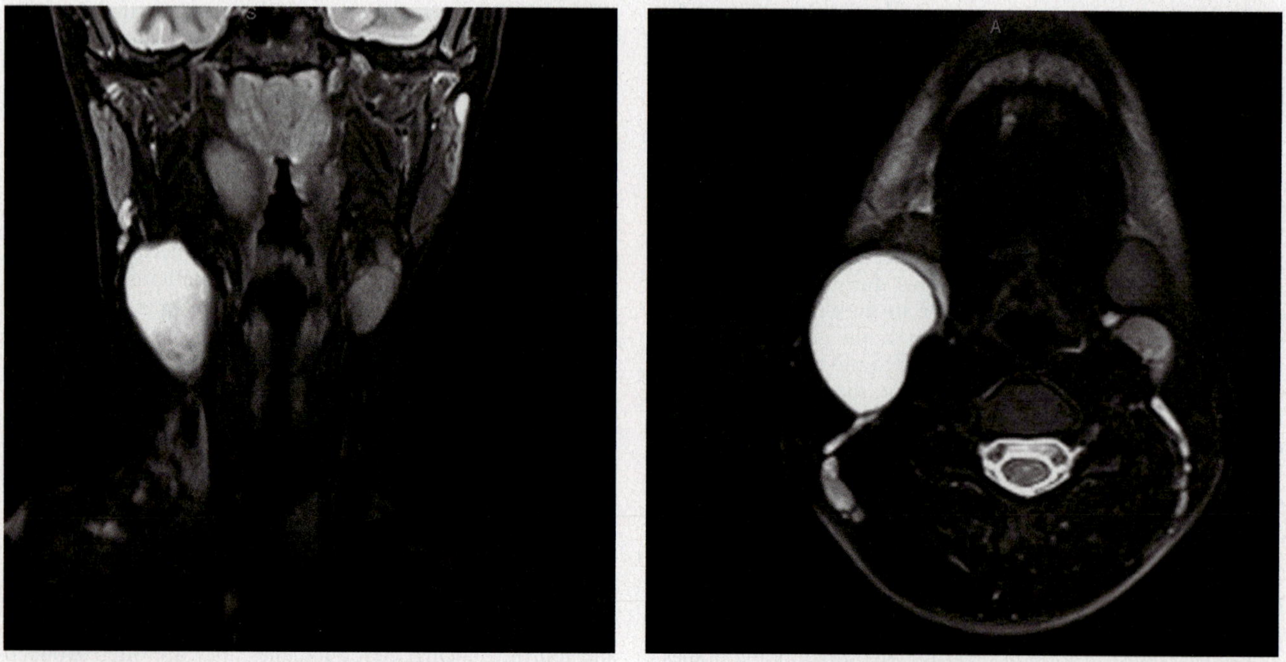

Figure 96.2. MRI (coronal and axial views) from second branchial cleft cysts.

lesions will typically arise on the left side and can be involved with the thyroid capsule. A pyriform sinus branchial cleft anomaly should be considered in a patient with an abscess in the neck that is closely associated with or involves the thyroid gland.[15,16]

Treatment for pyriform sinus branchial cleft anomalies is shifting. Historically, complete excision of the entire tract and potentially an ipsilateral thyroid lobectomy was performed. However, endoscopic management alone is being increasingly performed. If a pit is seen in the ipsilateral pyriform sinus, cauterization via monopolar or a laser can be used to scar the opening of the fistula and prevent future infections.[17] RLN monitoring is recommended for endoscopic management, as the RLN will pass in close proximity to the pyriform sinus and can be at risk for injury.

INFECTIOUS

The most common acquired pediatric neck mass is lymphadenitis, with some estimates noting up to 45% of healthy children having palpable lymphadenopathy.[18] Lymphadenopathy is typically not considered abnormal if the lymph node is smaller than 1 cm. Most cases of lymphadenopathy are benign and follow a viral or bacterial infection. However, management of cervical lymphadenopathy depends on the etiology. Therefore, it is of utmost importance to do a thorough history and physical examination to help determine the underlying cause. An infectious source would likely present with a preceding history of fever, neck pain, recent URI or other infection, dental problems, recent travel, sick contacts, or possible exposure to animals with an examination revealing erythema, tenderness, and possible induration of the lymph node on palpation. Malignancy should always be considered on the differential diagnosis of cervical lymphadenopathy and biopsy may be warranted if there is no resolution of the lymphadenopathy after 4 to 6 weeks, the node (s) is larger than 2 cm, there are concerning features on imaging or exam (ie, fixed node), presence of B-symptoms (eg, night sweats, fatigue, weight loss) or if the nodal packet is in an unusual area (supraclavicular region).[19] Other rare considerations on the differential include Kawasaki disease, Rosai–Dorfman disease, sarcoidosis, Castleman disease, Langerhan cell histiocytosis, and Kikuchi–Fujimoto disease.

Acute Suppurative Lymphadenitis

Patients with acute suppurative lymphadenitis commonly have an associated URI that has preceded the onset of lymph node enlargement. The most common bacteria found in acute bacterial lymphadenitis are *Staphylococcus aureus* and *Streptococcus pyogenes* (GAS) with anaerobes being the third most common.[20] When GAS is the cause, it is often associated with streptococcal tonsillitis. Patients will typically have erythema and tenderness in the overlying skin, leukocytosis, fever, and induration or fluctuance of the involved lymph nodes. Antibiotics are used to treat the infection along with supportive care. Younger patients have a greater risk of developing *Methicillin-Resistant Staphylococcus aureus* (MRSA), so consideration for MRSA antibacterial coverage is prudent.[21] Imaging should be considered if there is a lack of clinical improvement with antibiotics or if there is a consideration for drainage. If medical management is not sufficient, then incision and drainage should be performed. A small incision over the area of fluctuance is made, followed by blunt dissection. Attention to breaking up the loculations of the abscess are vital, in order to drain out all the involved areas. The abscess cavity is then irrigated and a drain is placed. Once there is no further purulent drainage, the drain can be removed.

Chronic Lymphadenitis (Nontuberculous Mycobacteria/Cat s)

Chronic lymphadenitis is defined as lymphadenitis that lasts greater than 6 weeks. Both nontuberculous (NTB) mycobacteria

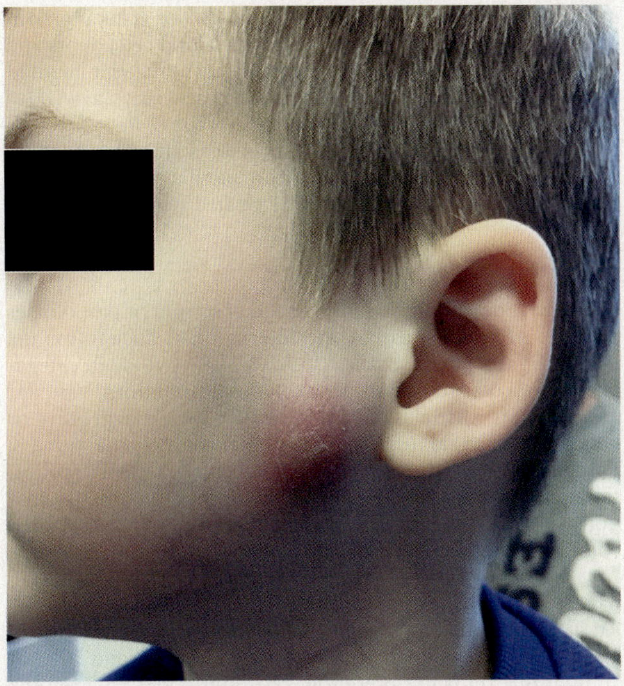

Figure 96.3. Patient with an NTB mycobacterial infection.

and cat scratch disease (CSD) are two important causes of chronic lymphadenitis on the differential. NTB mycobacterial infections are usually caused by the *Mycobacterium avium* complex (MAC) organisms, which can be found in the soil. NTB mycobacterial lymphadenitis will typically present with chronic, nontender, lymphadenopathy often involving the submandibular, upper cervical, and parotid lymph nodes (**Fig. 96.3**).[22] The involved lymph nodes will classically develop a violaceous hue as the skin overlying the nodes becomes thinner. The involved area can develop a sinus tract and suppuration may occur, that can then take weeks to months to resolve. In cases of suspected NTB infections, a tuberculin skin test and/or interferon gamma release assays (IGRA) should be performed with consideration of a chest radiograph. Cervical neck imaging usually starts with an US prior to performing any cross-sectional imaging (ie, CT or MRI with contrast).

Management options for NTB mycobacterial lymphadenitis include observation, medical management, or surgical management.[23] If the involved lymph node is in close proximity of the facial nerve, observation or medical management may be favored. An improvement in cure rate has not been shown in antimycobacterial therapy when compared to observation alone.[22] However, the main benefit of antimycobacterial therapy is a reduced risk of fistula formation when compared to observation alone.[24] In cases where surgical management is pursued, facial nerve monitoring should be considered, and if the risk to the facial nerve is acceptable, then complete excision is preferred over curettage.[22] However, if the risk to the facial nerve is deemed too high, curettage can be performed. The main benefit of surgical management is a higher cure rate and a faster time to resolution when compared to medical management and observation.[22,25] A culture confirmation of the diagnosis is an added benefit of operative management, yet it is important to note that mycobacterial species in culture can take up to 6 weeks and have sensitivity rates of only 50% to 80%.[24]

CSD is caused by *Bartonella henselae* with the infection usually originating from a cat bite or scratch of an upper extremity. Systemic illness is typically mild with low-grade fever, malaise, aches, lymphadenopathy, and abdominal pain. Of those with lymphadenopathy, the head and neck region is the second most common site, and about 10% will suppurate, requiring drainage.[26] Laboratory findings are generally nonspecific, with only mildly elevated white blood cell counts and erythrocyte sedimentation rates. The most frequent method of laboratory diagnosis is indirect fluorescence assays (IFA), followed by enzyme immunoassays (EIA) for *B. henselae* antibodies. CSD is usually a self-limited disease that can take up to 2 to 6 months to resolve with no significant difference in clinical outcomes for those patients treated with antibiotics.[27]

VASCULAR ANOMALIES

Vascular anomalies represent a broad spectrum of pathologies that has been classified by the International Society for the Study of Vascular Anomalies (ISSVA).[28] The two main categories are vascular tumors and vascular malformations. Vascular tumors are further classified into benign, locally aggressive or borderline vascular tumors, and malignant vascular tumors. Vascular malformations are further classified into four groups: simple malformations, combined malformations, malformations of major named vessels, and malformations associated with other anomalies.[28]

Infantile Hemangiomas

3 An infantile hemangioma (IH) is the most common tumor of infancy with an estimated incidence between 4% and 10% of all infants.[29] IH is not present at birth but appears within the first few weeks of life (**Fig. 96.4**). They typically grow rapidly during the proliferative phase and then slowly regress during the involuting phase. IHs are classified as focal, multifocal, segmental (associated with other anomalies such as PHACE syndrome), and indeterminate. In patients with IH resulting in cosmetic or functional compromise, beta-blocker therapy with propranolol is now standard treatment over systemic glucocorticoid therapy due to a high likelihood of clinical improvement without the toxicity associated with systemic glucocorticoid therapy.

Lymphatic Malformations

Simple malformations are composed of one type of vessel: capillaries, lymphatics, or veins. As such, lymphatic malformations (LMs) are just one category in the simple vascular malformation subtype. LMs are then classified according to the size of the lymphatic cysts as microcystic, macrocystic, and mixed. A majority of LMs are diagnosed by 2 years of age and may be identified on prenatal imaging. Depending on the size, location, and concern for airway compromise, a PRESTO or EXIT procedure may be considered.

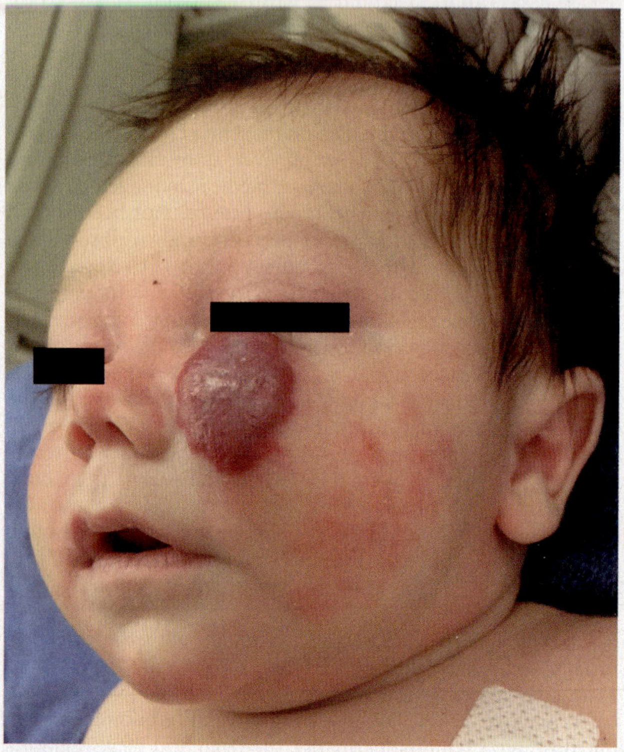

Figure 96.4. Patient with a hemangioma.

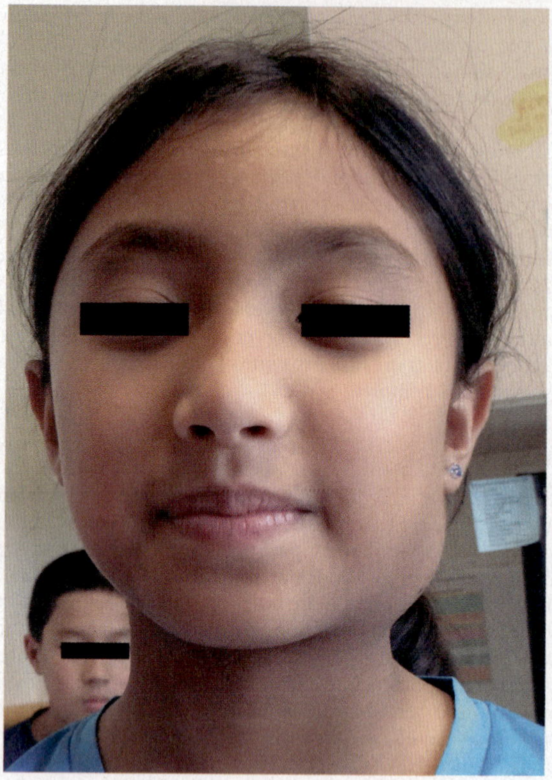

Figure 96.5. Patient with a lymphatic malformation.

LMs are challenging to treat given the risk of recurrence and their location in the head and neck (**Fig. 96.5**). LM treatment options consist of observation, sclerotherapy, surgery, and mTOR inhibitors. Due to the benign nature of LMs, therapy is predicated on symptoms. If the symptoms are minimal or manageable with limited concern for progression, then observation is considered. Otherwise, if sclerotherapy or surgery is considered, they can be offered independently or in combination. Typically, macrocystic LMs are more amenable to sclerotherapy. Under image guidance, interventional radiologists can aspirate the cyst fluid and then inject a sclerosing agent (bleomycin, doxycycline, ethanol, sodium tetradecyl sulfate) to induce endothelial damage. The sclerosing agent will cause inflammation and fibrosis, which can lead to pain, erythema, and edema of the surrounding tissues. The inflammatory response should be carefully monitored in patients with LMs in the head and neck as the edema can lead to airway compromise, necessitating intubation, or tracheostomy.

THYROID

Pediatric thyroid cancer has seen an increased incidence over
4 the last two decades.[30] Approximately 3% of all pediatric malignancies and 7% of all pediatric head and neck tumors are represented by thyroid carcinoma.[31] The majority of pediatric patients are asymptomatic at the time of diagnosis and have no identifiable risk factor. In the minority of patients with identifiable risk factors, it is most commonly ionizing radiation followed by a genetic predisposition.[32] Younger age (<10 years) and exposure to ionizing radiation are correlated with the highest risk and shortest latency for the development of differentiated thyroid cancer.[33] Genetic predisposition is

categorized into two broad groups: nonsyndromic and syndromic. Nonsyndromic genetic predisposition is often referred to as familial nonmedullary thyroid cancer (FNMTC). Syndromic forms of thyroid cancer consist of PTEN hamartoma tumor syndrome, DICER1, familial adenomatous polyposis (FAP), and multiple endocrine neoplasia type 2 (MEN 2).[34]

When a concern for a thyroid nodule or malignancy is present, a US is the best radiologic modality to assess the nodule characteristics. Based on the US, the thyroid nodule can be stratified according to the Thyroid Imaging Reporting and Data System (TI-RADS), a classification system that scores five nodule characteristics to help guide whether a fine needle aspiration (FNA) should be performed.[35] In patients with moderate- to high-risk lesions, the central and lateral neck lymph nodes should be assessed for evidence of metastasis. Cross-sectional imaging with CT or MRI is typically reserved for patients with large thyroid lesions or lateral neck metastatic lymphadenopathy with preoperative concern for neurovascular or aerodigestive compromise. In addition to workup with US and FNA, somatic genetic testing may be performed, most commonly for patients with indeterminate cytology as well as to help guide the initial surgical approach.[36,37] The presence of a BRAF mutation in the pediatric population has not been shown to be associated with a more aggressive papillary thyroid carcinoma (PTC) phenotype; however, it, as well as *RET* and *NTRK* fusions, are associated with a near 100% likelihood of PTC in an indeterminate FNA specimen. Prior to surgical treatment, an assessment of the vocal cords is an essential part of the preoperative workup to establish normal function prior to surgery. Intraoperative monitoring of the RLN is recommended and can be performed using a commercially available nerve monitoring endotracheal tube or with self-adhesive contact or hookwire electrodes in infants and young children.

Management of pediatric thyroid cancer should be at a center with a comprehensive team experienced in the care of children with thyroid cancer. There are studies that report increased surgical complications in thyroid surgery in children; therefore, in order to minimize the risk of complications, the surgeon should be high-volume with experience in pediatric thyroid surgery.[38]

Papillary Thyroid Carcinoma

PTC is the most common form of thyroid cancer, making up around 85% to 90% of all pediatric thyroid malignancies. The most common subtypes of PTC are classic PTC (60%) and follicular variant PTC (20%). When compared to their adult counterparts, PTC in pediatric patients is more advanced at the time of presentation, with a higher rate of lymph node involvement (70% to 90%), multifocal disease (30% to 80%), and distant metastasis to the lungs (85% to 20%).[39]

Surgical treatment for pediatric PTC has historically consisted of a total thyroidectomy, according to the American Thyroid Association pediatric DTC guidelines.[38] A total thyroidectomy allows for an accurate use of thyroglobulin (Tg) levels in the postoperative period to monitor for persistent and recurrent disease. However, there have been some recent studies that show a thyroid lobectomy may be considered in patients with low invasive potential, including encapsulated follicular variant PTC, and unifocal PTC (≤1 cm).[40,41] A prophylactic central neck dissection should be considered, as the presence of nodal disease is an independent risk factor for recurrence and distant metastasis, allowing surgical and medical stratification of patients.[38–42] Radioactive iodine (RAI) can then be discussed depending on the patient's risk level.

Follicular Thyroid Carcinoma

Follicular thyroid carcinoma (FTC) is the second most common form of thyroid cancer and represents less than 10% of thyroid malignancies in pediatric patients. In contrast to PTC, FTC metastasizes hematogenously, so the risk of local and distant metastasis is mostly determined by the extent of angioinvasion.[43] FTC can only be differentiated from a benign follicular adenoma by the presence of capsular invasion or angioinvasion on pathology. The majority of patients with FTC will have indeterminate cytology and will undergo thyroid lobectomy with subsequent plans for a completion thyroidectomy based on the presence and extent of angioinvasion.[44] Patients with minimally invasive FTC, defined by the tumor having invasion limited to the tumor capsule, are considered treated with only a thyroid lobectomy.

Medullary Thyroid Carcinoma

Medullary thyroid carcinoma (MTC) accounts for <5% of all pediatric thyroid cancers. MTC originates from the parafollicular C cells. In contrast to DTC, MTC does not respond to TSH suppression and does not produce Tg. MTC in the pediatric population is generally associated with MEN 2, associated with activating mutations in the *RET* protooncogene that are transmitted in an autosomal dominant pattern. The timing for thyroidectomy in MEN 2 patients is based on the risk associated with a specific codon mutation and the calcitonin level and trend.[45] In patients with the highest-risk mutation, associated with MEN2B (M918T), and high-risk mutations (C634F or A883F), a total thyroidectomy should be performed within the first year or by 5 years of life, respectively.[45] Patients with moderate-risk mutations can be followed with annual calcitonin levels with a decision to move to thyroidectomy based on calcitonin level and trend as well as patient and family input.[45] Following surgical removal, serum levels of calcitonin and carcinoembryonic antigen (CEA) should be monitored. In patients with progressive disease that is not amenable to surgery, systemic treatment with *RET* inhibitors or receptor tyrosine kinase inhibitors may be indicated.

AIRWAY

Nasal Cavity

Infants are obligate nasal breathers until about 3 to 6 months of age. When bilateral, choanal atresia or stenosis and piriform aperture stenosis can cause nasal obstruction leading to respiratory distress, feeding difficulties, and failure to thrive. Definitive management for choanal atresia or stenosis and piriform aperture stenosis consists of surgery. In patients that have unilateral involvement, it may not become apparent until later in childhood, when discharge from the blocked nostril occurs. A CT scan can be useful in assessing the bony piriform aperture and whether the choanal atresia is bony or mucosal.

Oral Cavity and Oropharynx

Macroglossia and/or micrognathia as an etiology for upper airway obstruction can be seen in patients with Pierre Robin Sequence and syndromes such as Beckwith–Weidemann and Treacher–Collins. If a concern for micrognathia or macroglossia is present on prenatal US, then a PRESTO or EXIT procedure can be considered during birth. In the postnatal period, a nasopharyngeal airway or positioning the patient prone or on their side may decrease airway symptoms. If surgical management is pursued, a mandibular distraction osteogenesis (MDO) can be performed for oropharyngeal obstruction caused by micrognathia. If there is macroglossia in isolation, then a partial glossectomy can also be considered. However, definitive management in refractory or complicated cases is a tracheostomy.

Laryngeal and Subglottic Lesions

5 Laryngomalacia is the most common cause of stridor in infants and is typically a self-limited condition that resolves by 12 to 18 months of age.[46] Laryngomalacia is seen as a supraglottic obstruction due to either prolapse of the mucosa or tissue overlying the arytenoid cartilages, shortened aryepiglottic folds, and/or posterior displacement of the epiglottis.[46] Laryngomalacia can be categorized into mild, moderate, and severe based on symptoms and possible comorbidities. Mild laryngomalacia can

be followed with interval symptom checks, whereas patients with moderate laryngomalacia can be started on gastric acid suppression along with feeding therapy and a swallow evaluation. Surgical treatment with a supraglottoplasty is typically reserved for those patients with either severe laryngomalacia or patients that have failed medical management.

Laryngeal clefts are thought to result from incomplete formation of the interarytenoid muscle into the posterior cricoid cartilage and tracheoesophageal septum, depending on the type of laryngeal cleft; (1) type I laryngeal cleft does not extend beyond the level of the vocal cords, (2) type II laryngeal cleft extends below the vocal cords and into the cricoid cartilage, (3) type III laryngeal cleft extends completely through the cricoid cartilage and into the cervical tracheoesophageal wall, and (4) type IV laryngeal cleft involves the intrathoracic tracheoesophageal wall and can extend to the carina.[47] Laryngeal clefts can have variable presentations depending on the overall health and depth of the cleft. Type I laryngeal clefts will often have a delayed presentation with aspiration, feeding difficulties, and vague respiratory symptoms. Whereas type III and type IV laryngeal clefts will present in the newborn period with respiratory distress in the setting of other congenital anomalies.

The subglottis is the narrowest portion of the pediatric airway due to the cricoid cartilage. Stenosis of the subglottis can be congenital, but is more commonly acquired due to long-term intubation. The severity of the stenosis is graded by the Cotton–Meyer system with grade I being up to 50% narrowing, grade II from 51% to 70% narrowing, grade III from 71% to 99% narrowing, and grade IV with no discernible lumen.[48] Management can vary from observation with grade I stenosis to endoscopic and open procedures, in the setting of a previously placed tracheostomy for higher-grade obstructions.

Tracheal Pathology

Esophageal atresia and tracheoesophageal fistula (EA-TEF) commonly occur in the setting of other congenital anomalies and have an incidence of about 1 in 2,500 to 4,500 live births.[49] Most patients are symptomatic soon after birth with pooling of secretions, feeding difficulties with coughing, cyanosis, and potentially respiratory distress. A type C EA-TEF, with a distal fistula is the most common, whereas a type D with a proximal and distal fistula is the least common. Surgical repair of the EA-TEF is the only definitive management.

Tracheomalacia can occur as a primary pathology due to isolated weakness of the tracheal wall, or as a secondary pathology due to extrinsic compression by a vascular anomaly or in association with EA-TEF or a laryngeal cleft. Most common presentation is an expiratory and "wet" wheeze or stridor. Due to the dynamic collapse of the tracheal wall during expiration, patients may have difficulty clearing secretions, leading to a wide spectrum of respiratory symptoms from chronic cough to recurrent pneumonias. Supportive management for more severe cases with inhaled agents and positive pressure ventilation may be indicated. Surgical management with a posterior tracheopexy or anterior aortopexy can be performed. Sometimes a tracheostomy is indicated for refractory cases or those that continue to need positive pressure.

In addition to developmental anomalies, airway foreign bodies can be life threatening. Children less than 5 years of age are at the highest risk, and the most common foreign bodies
6 are food related. Clinical history and examination are of utmost importance as less than half of patients with 1 day of symptoms will have an abnormal radiograph.[50] As such, a negative radiograph should not preclude bronchoscopy in patients with a concerning history or symptoms.

ACKNOWLEDGMENTS

We gratefully acknowledge the contributions of previous edition authors, Nikolaus E. Wolter and Reza Rahbar, as portions of those chapters have been retained in this revision.

References

1. Allard RH. The thyroglossal cyst. *Head Neck Surg.* 1982;5(2):134–146.
2. Galluzzi F, Pignataro L, Gaini RM, Hartley B, Garavello W. Risk of recurrence in children operated for thyroglossal duct cysts: a systematic review. *J Pediatr Surg.* 2013;48:222–227.
3. Rohof D, Honings J, Theunisse HJ, et al. Recurrences after thyroglossal duct cyst surgery: results in 207 consecutive cases and review of the literature. *Head Neck.* 2015;37(12):1699–1704.
4. Pupić-Bakrač J, Pupić-Bakrač A, Bačić I, Kolega MŠ, Skitarelić N. Epidermoid and dermoid cysts of the head and neck. *J Craniofac Surg.* 2021;32(1):e25–e27.
5. Gibson WS, Fenton NA. Congenital sublingual dermoid cyst. *Arch Otolaryngol.* 1982;108(11):745–748.
6. Pryor SG, Lewis JE, Weaver AL, Orvidas LJ. Pediatric dermoid cysts of the head and neck. *Otolaryngol Head Neck Surg.* 2005;132(6):938–942.
7. Dutta M, Saha J, Biswas G, Chattopadhyay S, Sen I, Sinha R. Epidermoid cysts in head and neck: our experiences, with review of literature. *Indian J Otolaryngol Head Neck Surg.* 2013;65(S1):14–21.
8. Woodward PJ, Sohaey R, Kennedy A, Koeller KK. From the archives of the AFIP: a comprehensive review of fetal tumors with pathologic correlation. *Radiographics.* 2005;25:215–242.
9. Paradis J, Koltai PJ. Pediatric teratoma and dermoid cysts. *Otolaryngol Clin North Am.* 2015:121–136.
10. Rothschild MA, Catalano P, Urken M, et al. Evaluation and management of congenital cervical teratoma. Case report and review. *Arch Otolaryngol Head Neck Surg.* 1994;120(4):444–448.
11. Rosenfeld CR, Coln CD, Duenhoelter JH. Fetal cervical teratoma as a cause of polyhydramnios. *Pediatrics.* 1979;64(2):176–179.
12. Albers GD. Branchial anomalies. *JAMA.* 1963;183:399–409.
13. Schroeder JW Jr, Mohyuddin N, Maddalozzo J. Branchial anomalies in the pediatric population. *Otolaryngol Head Neck Surg.* 2007;137(2):289–295.
14. Work WP. Newer concepts of first branchial cleft defects. 1972. *Laryngoscope.* 2015;125(3):520–532.
15. Parida PK, Gopalakrishnan S, Saxena SK. Pediatric recurrent acute suppurative thyroiditis of third branchial arch origin–our experience in 17 cases. *Int J Pediatr Otorhinolaryngol.* 2014;78(11):1953–1957.
16. Carta F, Sionis S, Mascia L, Puxeddu R. Fourth branchial cleft anomaly: management strategy in acute presentation. *Int J Pediatr Otorhinolaryngol.* 2014;78(9):1480–1484.
17. Watson GJ, Nichani JR, Rothera MP, Bruce IA. Case series: endoscopic management of fourth branchial arch anomalies. *Int J Pediatr Otorhinolaryngol.* 2013;77(5):766–769.
18. Larsson LO, Bentzon MW, Kelly KB, et al. Palpable lymph nodes of the neck in Swedish schoolchildren. *Acta Paediatr.* 1994;83(10):1091–1094.
19. Locke R, Comfort R, Kubba H. When does an enlarged cervical lymph node in a child need excision? A systematic review. *Int J Pediatr Otorhinolaryngol.* 2014;78(3):393–401.
20. Neff L, Newland JG, Sykes KJ, Selvarangan R, Wei JL. Microbiology and antimicrobial treatment of pediatric cervical lymphadenitis requiring surgical intervention. *Int J Pediatr Otorhinolaryngol.* 2013;77(5):817–820.
21. Duggal P, Naseri I, Sobol SE. The increased risk of community-acquired methicillin-resistant Staphylococcus aureus neck abscesses in young children. *Laryngoscope.* 2011;121(1):51–55.
22. Zimmermann P, Tebruegge M, Curtis N, Ritz N. The management of non-tuberculous cervicofacial lymphadenitis in children: a systematic review and meta-analysis. *J Infect.* 2015;71(1):9–18.
23. Roy CF, Balakrishnan K, Boudewyns A, et al. International Pediatric Otolaryngology Group: Consensus guidelines on the diagnosis and management of non-tuberculous mycobacterial cervicofacial lymphadenitis. *Int J Pediatr Otorhinolaryngol.* 2023;166:111469.
24. Zeharia A, Eidlitz-Markus T, Haimi-Cohen Y, Samra Z, Kaufman L, Amir J. Management of nontuberculous mycobacteria-induced cervical lymphadenitis with observation alone. *Pediatr Infect Dis J.* 2008;27(10):920–922.

25. Lindeboom JA, Kuijper EJ, Bruijnesteijn van Coppenraet ES, Lindeboom R, Prins JM. Surgical excision versus antibiotic treatment for nontuberculous mycobacterial cervicofacial lymphadenitis in children: a multicenter, randomized, controlled trial. *Clin Infect Dis.* 2007;44(8):1057–1064.
26. Massei F, Gori L, Macchia P, Maggiore G. The expanded spectrum of bartonellosis in children. *Infect Dis Clin North Am.* 2005;19(3): 691–711.
27. Bass JW, Freitas BC, Freitas AD, et al. Prospective randomized double blind placebo-controlled evaluation of azithromycin for treatment of cat-scratch disease. *Pediatr Infect Dis J.* 1998;17(6): 447–452.
28. Wassef M, Blei F, Adams D, et al. Vascular anomalies classification: recommendations from the International Society for the Study of Vascular Anomalies. *Pediatrics.* 2015;136(1):e203–e214.
29. Kilcline C, Frieden IJ. Infantile hemangiomas: how common are they? A systematic review of the medical literature. *Pediatr Dermatol.* 2008;25(2):168–173.
30. Dermody S, Walls A, Harley EH Jr. Pediatric thyroid cancer: An update from the SEER database 2007–2012. *Int J Pediatr Otorhinolaryngol.* 2016;89:121–126.
31. Palmer BA, Zarroug AE, Poley RN, Kollars JP, Moir CR. Papillary thyroid carcinoma in children: Risk factors and complications of disease recurrence. *J Pediatr Surg.* 2005;40(8):1284–1288.
32. Meadows AT, Friedman DL, Neglia JP, et al. Second neoplasms in survivors of childhood cancer: findings from the Childhood Cancer Survivor Study cohort. *Journal of Clinical Oncology.* 2009: 2356–2362.
33. Clement SC, Kremer LCM, Verburg FA, et al. Balancing the benefits and harms of thyroid cancer surveillance in survivors of Childhood, adolescent and young adult cancer: Recommendations from the International Late Effects of Childhood Cancer Guideline Harmonization Group in collaboration with the PanCareSurFup Consortium. *Cancer Treat Rev.* 2018:28–39.
34. Bauer AJ. Pediatric thyroid cancer: genetics, therapeutics and outcome. *Endocrinol Metab Clin North Am.* 2020:589–611.
35. Martinez-Rios C, Daneman A, Bajno L, van der Kaay DCM, Moineddin R, Wasserman JD. Utility of adult-based ultrasound malignancy risk stratifications in pediatric thyroid nodules. *Pediatr Radiol.* 2018;48(1):74–84.
36. Baran JA, Halada S, Bauer AJ, et al. Indeterminate thyroid fine-needle aspirations in pediatrics: exploring clinicopathologic features and utility of molecular profiling. *Horm Res Paediatr.* 2022;95(5):430–441.
37. Gallant J-N, Chen S-C, Ortega CA, et al. Evaluation of the molecular landscape of pediatric thyroid nodules and use of a multigene genomic classifier in children. *JAMA Oncol.* 2022;8(9): 1323–1327.
38. Francis GL, Waguespack SG, Bauer AJ, et al. Management guidelines for children with thyroid nodules and differentiated thyroid cancer. *Thyroid.* 2015;25(7):716–759.
39. Golpanian S, Perez EA, Tashiro J, Lew JI, Sola JE, Hogan AR. Pediatric papillary thyroid carcinoma: outcomes and survival predictors in 2504 surgical patients. *Pediatr Surg Int.* 2016;32(3): 201–208.
40. Sugino K, Nagahama M, Kitagawa W, et al. Risk stratification of pediatric patients with differentiated thyroid cancer: is total thyroidectomy necessary for patients at any risk? *Thyroid.* 2020;30(4): 548–556.
41. Sudoko CK, Jenks CM, Bauer AJ, et al. Thyroid Lobectomy for T1 papillary thyroid carcinoma in pediatric patients. *JAMA Otolaryngol Head Neck Surg.* 2021;147(11):943–950.
42. Bojarsky M, Baran JA, Halada S, et al. Outcomes of ATA low-risk pediatric thyroid cancer patients not treated with radioactive iodine therapy. *J Clin Endocrinol Metab.* 2023;108(12): 3338–3344.
43. Lin X, Zhu B, Liu Y, Silverman JF. Follicular thyroid carcinoma invades venous rather than lymphatic vessels. *Diagn Pathol.* 2010; 5:8.
44. Leong D, Gill AJ, Turchini J, et al. The prognostic impact of extent of vascular invasion in follicular thyroid carcinoma. *World J Surg.* 2023;47(2):412–420.
45. Wells SA, Asa SL, Dralle H, et al. Revised American thyroid association guidelines for the management of medullary thyroid carcinoma. *Thyroid.* 2015;25(6):567–610.
46. Olney DR, Greinwald JH Jr, Smith RJ, Bauman NM. Laryngomalacia and its treatment. *Laryngoscope.* 1999;109(11):1770–1775.
47. Benjamin B, Inglis A. Minor congenital laryngeal clefts: diagnosis and classification. *Ann Otol Rhinol Laryngol.* 1989;98: 417–420.
48. Myer CM 3rd, O'Connor DM, Cotton RT. Proposed grading system for subglottic stenosis based on endotracheal tube sizes. *Ann Otol Rhinol Laryngol.* 1994;103(4 Pt 1):319–323.
49. Spitz L. Esophageal atresia. Lessons I have learned in a 40-year experience. *J Pediatr Surg.* 2006;41(10):1635–1640.
50. Zerella JT, Dimler M, McGill LC, Pippus KJ. Foreign body aspiration in children: value of radiography and complications of bronchoscopy. *J Pediatr Surg* 1998;33(11):1651–1654.

97

Pediatric Chest

Gabriella Grisotti, Mary Catherine Santos, and Hanmin Lee

Key Points

1 Surgical care of the pediatric chest encompasses a wide variety of congenital and acquired conditions.

2 Congenital diaphragmatic hernia (CDH) is a physiologic emergency and not a surgical emergency. The newborn with CDH should be stabilized by nonsurgical means and delayed, well-planned surgical repair undertaken subsequently. Pulmonary hypertension and lung hypoplasia determine outcome.

3 Tracheoesophageal fistula (TEF) can occur as esophageal atresia with proximal pouch and distal TEF (most common, 76% to 85%), esophageal atresia without fistula ("pure esophageal atresia," 3% to 17%), TEF without esophageal atresia ("H-type fistula," 4% to 6%), and the rarer forms of this anomaly including esophageal atresia with proximal TEF and esophageal atresia with both proximal and distal TEFs.

4 Approximately 75 children die from foreign-body aspiration or ingestion each year. Bronchoscopic evaluation and foreign-body removal are performed in the operating room under general anesthesia, where the rigid bronchoscope with optical forceps can be used to remove most aspirated foreign bodies safely. "Button battery" ingestion has emerged as a cause of serious injury and death. Emergent endoscopic removal from the esophagus is required.

5 Pulmonary sequestrations (PSs) are abnormal lung tissue with anomalous systemic blood supply that can be either intralobar or extralobar based on their relationship with the investing visceral pleura and adjacent lung tissue. They do not communicate normally with the trachea or a bronchus.

6 Congenital pulmonary airway malformations (CPAMs) have a normal vascular supply and communicate with the normal tracheobronchial tree. They result from excessive proliferation of bronchial structures without the development of the corresponding alveoli. Management of asymptomatic CPAMs remains controversial. Thoracoscopic lobectomy is commonly performed.

7 Benign cysts of the mediastinum are relatively common and include thymic cysts, enterogenous cysts, dermoid cysts, lymphatic malformations (cystic hygromas), and pericardial cysts. Resection is usually recommended because of the possibility of progressive enlargement with compression, hemorrhage, or infection.

8 Primary lung tumors in children are rare and include bronchial adenoma, pleuropulmonary blastoma (PPB), inflammatory pseudotumor, hamartoma, and rarely bronchoalveolar carcinoma. Resection is usually required.

9 Metastectomy for many solid neoplasms can improve survival if the primary disease is controlled by resection.

10 Pectus excavatum is repaired in late childhood or adolescence. Repair is most frequently performed with a rigid transversely oriented pectus excavatum bar that pushes the deformity back into place. Improved pain management has shortened hospital stay.

11 Pectus carinatum is less common than pectus excavatum and does not cause physiologic impairment; external compression bracing has become the method of choice for treatment.

CONGENITAL ABNORMALITIES OF THE DIAPHRAGM

Advances in management of neonatal respiratory failure, fetal surgery, and lung developmental biology have arisen from the clinical and laboratory evaluation of congenital diaphragmatic hernia (CDH, a Bochdalek, or posterolateral hernia). CDH, which is relatively rare, occurring in 1 in 3,000 neonates, has led to a significant amount of clinical and basic science research.

In 1754, McCauley described the clinical course and postmortem anatomy of an infant with CDH. Although Bochdalek's understanding of the embryology of CDH was incorrect, this congenital defect continues to carry his name. Prior to 1940, the successful repair of this defect was rare. In 1946, Gross reported the postoperative survival of an infant less than 24 hours of age. From that time until the 1980s the standard of care was emergent operative repair. At that time, CDH was considered to be an anatomic derangement treated by an anatomic correction (the thought was that by getting the bowel out of the chest, lung compression would be relieved and outcomes would improve).

Until the 1980s, emergency surgery was considered the primary therapeutic goal based on mechanical concept of providing space for growth of lungs. The overall published survival rates in the 1980s were 50% with ranges from 20% to 70% based on case selection. In the late 1980s, there was a change in management from emergency surgery to initial stabilization. Management in the postnatal period is directed at decreasing pulmonary hypertension while maintaining adequate oxygen saturations.[1] Surgical repair is deferred until after physiologic stabilization. This has led to improved survival of infants with CDH.

Embryology of the Diaphragm

Mammalian lung development occurs in vivo as a coordinated developmental process that includes (a) airway and acinar development, (b) cellular differentiation, (c) biochemical maturation, (d) interstitial development including vasculature and extracellular matrix, and (e) physical growth or enlargement. These parallel developmental processes occur in such a fashion that at any one time during development, there are characteristic relationships among each component that define the stages of lung development. Hormones such as the glucocorticoids, thyroid hormone, and retinoic acid have been shown to regulate several of the crucial cellular interactions required for proper pulmonary organogenesis and differentiation. In the human embryo, respiratory tract development begins in the 4th week of gestation as a ventral out pouching of the foregut that soon has bifurcated and begun branching into the surrounding mesenchyme. The primitive, pluripotent epithelial cells differentiate into both bronchial and alveolar cell lines, under the control of the surrounding mesenchyme. By a process of asymmetric branching, the divisions are complete by the 16th week of gestation. Lung at this phase has columnar epithelium with thick mesenchyme giving rise to the descriptive term *pseudoglandular phase* of development because of its histologic appearance. The *canalicular phase* that follows and continues up to about the 24th gestational week is characterized by flattening of the epithelium of the distal airways, thinning of the mesenchyme, and the growth of the capillary network that surrounds the terminal airways. Gas exchange becomes functionally possible at the end of this phase. The *terminal sac period* that follows refers to the appearance of a thin respiratory epithelium in apposition to a capillary network capable of supporting gas exchange. The *alveolar phase* of development in humans begins shortly before or around the time of birth. Alveolar maturation and multiplication takes place after birth and may continue up to 8 years of age.

The precursors of the mesoderm-derived diaphragm begin to form during the 4th week of gestation with the appearance of the peritoneal folds from lateral mesenchymal tissue. At the same time, the septum transversum forms from the inferior portion of the pericardial cavity and serves to delineate the thoracic from the abdominal cavities. Eventually, the septum transversum leads to the formation of the central tendinous area of the fully developed diaphragm. The pleuroperitoneal folds extend from the lateral body wall and grow medially and ventrally until they fuse with the septum transversum and dorsal mesentery of the esophagus during the 6th gestational week. Complete closure of the canal takes place during the 8th week of gestation, with the right side closing before the left. Muscularization of the diaphragm appears to develop from the innermost layer of thoracic mesoderm, although other mechanisms have been proposed (**Fig. 97.1**).[2]

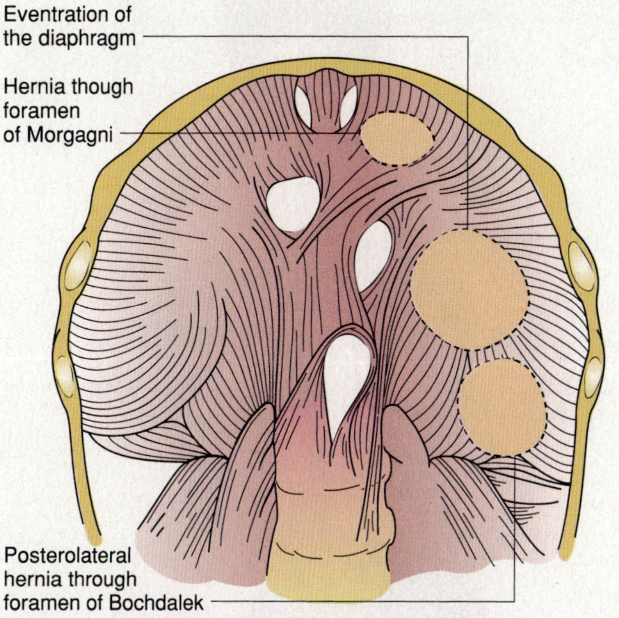

Figure 97.1. Anatomy of the diaphragm showing the location of congenital diaphragmatic defects.

Congenital Diaphragmatic Hernia Pathology and Pathophysiology

CDH occurs in 1:3,000 to 2:4,000 live births. Approximately one-third of antenatally diagnosed infants with CDH are stillborn, with most of the deaths ascribed to other fatal anomalies. Defects are more common on the left side. CDH represents a sporadic developmental anomaly with some familial cases reported. One-third of patients have associated major defects. CDH associated with an abnormal karyotype or cardiac defect is associated with a poor outcome.

The cause of CDH is unknown but is presumed that some combination of intrinsic predisposition (genetic factors) and environmental factors (teratogen or deficiency) results in abnormal diaphragm and lung development. A nitrofen-induced model of CDH also inhibits retinal dehydrogenase leading to decreased retinoic acid, which has also been found in human infants with CDH.

During the early development of the diaphragm, the midgut is largely extra-coelomic. If closure of the pleuroperitoneal canal has not occurred by the time the midgut returns to the abdomen during the 9th and 10th weeks of gestation, the abdominal viscera herniate through the lumbocostal trigone into the ipsilateral thoracic cavity. The resulting abnormal position of the bowel prevents its normal counterclockwise rotation and fixation. No hernia sac is present if the event occurs before complete closure of the pleuroperitoneal canal; however a nonmuscularized membrane forms a hernia sac in 10% to 15% of CDH patients. In addition to the small bowel, other intra-abdominal organs such as the spleen, stomach, colon, and liver may also herniate through the diaphragmatic defect.

Left-sided CDH is characterized by a variably sized posterolateral defect in the diaphragm through which the abdominal viscera have translocated into the ipsilateral thoracic cavity. On a right-sided defect, the large right lobe of the liver can occupy most of the hemithorax. The hepatic veins may drain ectopically into the right atrium, and the liver and lung may be fused.

The pathophysiology of CDH has been attributed to pulmonary parenchymal compression by the herniated organs and its effect on growth and maturation of the lung. An emerging school of thought attributes the pulmonary hypoplasia to an early mesenchymal developmental insult to the lung and diaphragm. Unilateral diaphragmatic hernia is associated with both ipsilateral and contralateral abnormal pulmonary development, although hypoplasia is more severe on the ipsilateral side. The lung on the side of the hernia is much smaller than its contralateral counterpart, and both are smaller than normal lungs (**Fig. 97.2**). The pulmonary vascular disease associated with CDH is characterized by abnormal pulmonary vascular development, abnormal vasoreactivity, and a disorganization of vascular remodeling. There are fewer capillaries which are unevenly distributed. Both the media and the adventitia have structural abnormalities consistent with increased muscularization in utero. Sonic hedgehog signaling which is involved in the development of respiratory bronchioles is delayed in CDH. Levels of several regulatory proteins are changed compared to controls but no causative relationship has been demonstrated.[2]

Pulmonary blood flow accounts for only 7% of cardiac output during normal fetal development. Pulmonary vascular resistance is high. The fetus preferentially shunts oxygenated blood from the placenta through the foramen ovale and ductus

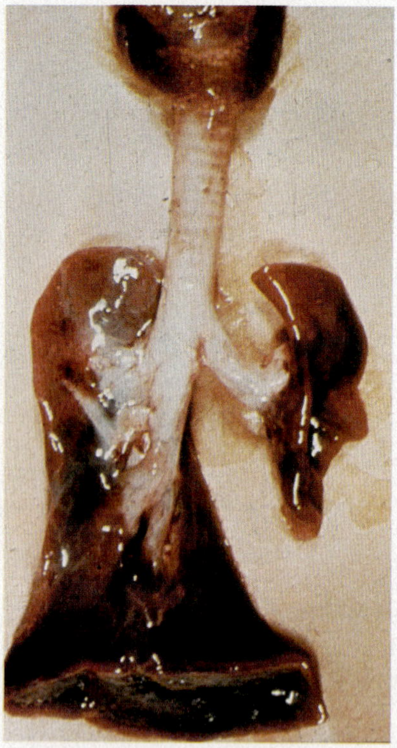

Figure 97.2. Autopsy specimen of an infant with severe pulmonary hypoplasia secondary to congenital diaphragmatic hernia. Pulmonary hypoplasia is bilateral, but the left lung is most severely affected.

arteriosus in a right-to-left direction into the systemic circulation. With the institution of breathing at birth, oxygen levels rise causing pulmonary vascular resistance to fall, which in turn allows an increase in pulmonary blood flow. Increased arterial oxygen tension induces spontaneous closure of the ductus arteriosus. Persistent fetal circulation may develop if this process is interrupted. Elevated pulmonary vascular resistance results in right-to-left shunting of blood at either the atrial or ductal levels with the delivery of unsaturated blood into the systemic circulation. As shunting increases, the oxygen saturation in the systemic circulation falls. The resulting hypoxia further increases pulmonary vascular resistance and compromises pulmonary blood flow while increasing the right-to-left shunt flow. Factors that contribute to the persistence of high pulmonary vascular resistance in CDH lungs are thought to be the structural changes of decreased total arteriolar cross-sectional area in the involved lungs and the increased muscularization of the arterial structures that are present. Additional exacerbations of pulmonary vascular resistance may be induced by the known stimulators of pulmonary hypertension, which include hypoxia, acidosis, hypothermia, and stress. Alterations in the levels of prostaglandins, leukotrienes, catecholamines, and the renin angiotensin system had been implicated as mediators of this complex process. The combination of hypoplastic lungs and lungs prone toward increased vascular resistance often proves deadly; a vicious cycle may ensue in which hypoplastic lungs and associated hypoxia lead to pulmonary hypertension in a lung vasculature already prone toward reactive vasospasm. The increase in pulmonary pressures results in a greater shunt, which in turn further reduces oxygen levels.

Diagnosis

Diagnosis of CDH is typically made on prenatal ultrasound examination. Polyhydramnios is common. Prenatal MRI may also be utilized.[3] Postnatal presentation includes cyanosis and respiratory distress shortly after birth in severely affected neonates. On physical examination, the patients have a scaphoid abdomen. A plain chest radiograph with loops of intestine in the chest confirms the diagnosis of CDH with an NG tube in place to confirm the position of the stomach (**Fig. 97.3**). After confirmation of diagnosis, echocardiography should be performed to evaluate pulmonary hypertension and to determine the presence or absence of cardiac defects. Differential diagnosis includes eventration of the diaphragm, anterior diaphragmatic hernia (Morgagni), congenital pulmonary malformations, unilateral pulmonary effusion, and primary agenesis of the lung.

Prognostic Factors

Poor prognosis is associated with low lung-to-head ratio (LHR) as determined by sonographic measurements of the size of the contralateral lung in an anteroposterior and lateromedial direction, and the head circumference. Ratios less than 1 have been associated with poor outcome. Because the LHR increases with age, the observed to expected value for gestational age has been

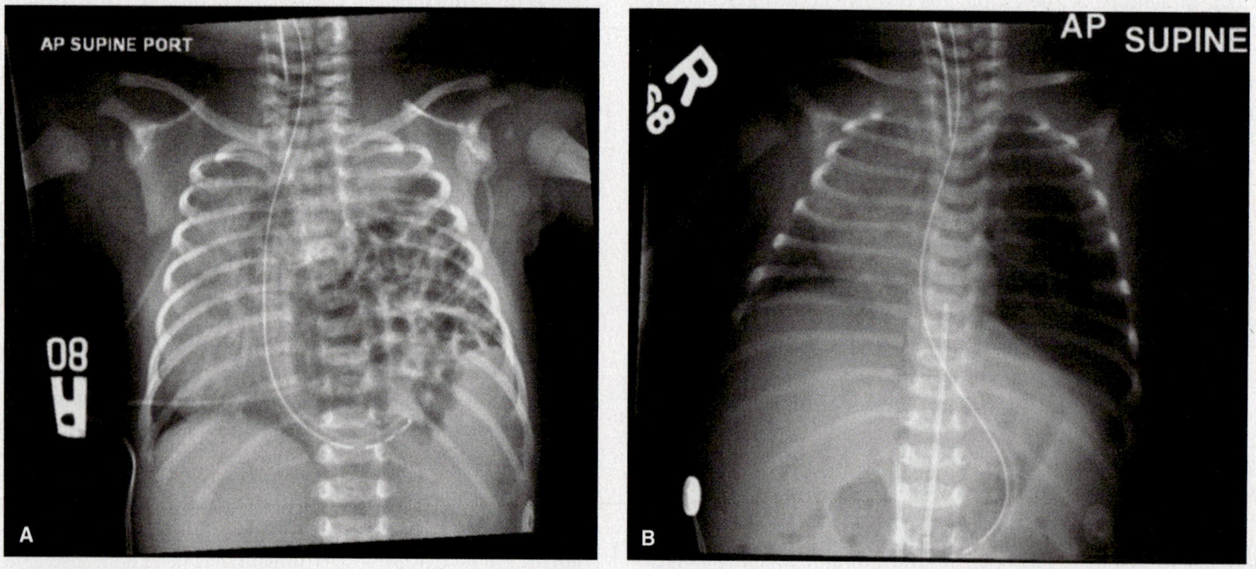

Figure 97.3. **A:** Chest radiograph of a newborn with a left congenital diaphragmatic hernia. Mediastinal structures are shifted to the right. Abdominal viscera occupy the left hemithorax. The nasogastric tube locates the stomach. The child underwent repair of the congenital diaphragmatic hernia after treatment and resolution of pulmonary hypertension. **B:** Immediate postoperative photograph demonstrates hypoplastic lung, flattening of diaphragm, and return of abdominal viscera to normal position.

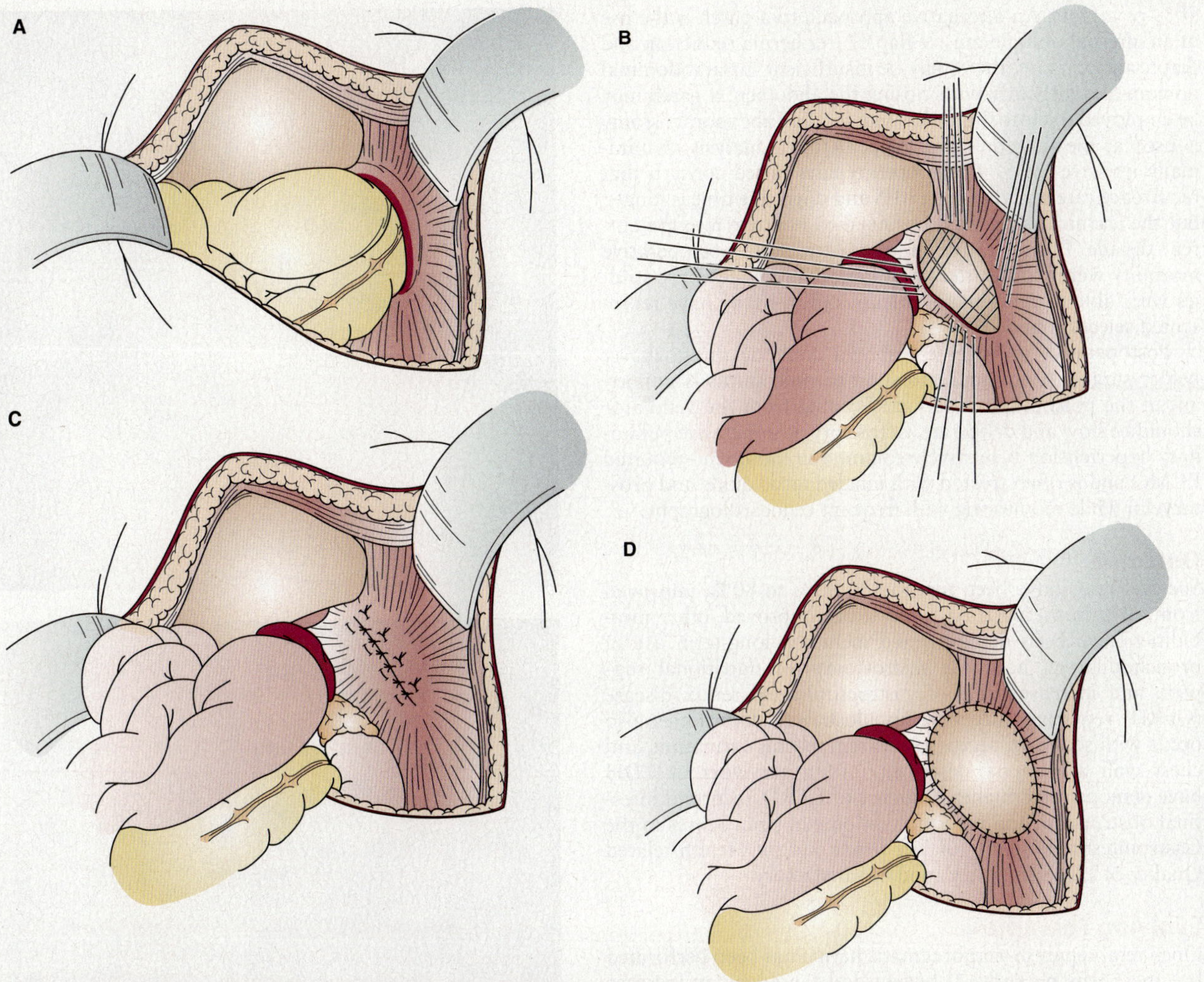

Figure 97.4. Repair of a congenital diaphragmatic hernia (CDH). **A:** Operative appearance of CDH. **B:** Placement of sutures for repair of a typical left posterolateral diaphragmatic defect. **C:** Completed repair. **D:** Prosthetic material may be used for large defects to avoid tension.

used with low survival below 25% of predicted.[4] Liver above the diaphragm ("liver up") is also associated with decreased survival. The combination of a low LHR with "liver up" has a very poor prognosis. The size of the defect, presence of a major cardiac anomaly, and 1-minute Apgar scores of ≤4 are also associated with increased mortality.[4] The Congenital Diaphragmatic Hernia Study Group and the Canadian Neonatal Network have published predictors of survival.

Treatment

At the time of antenatal diagnosis, the mother and fetus should be referred to an appropriate tertiary care perinatal center with the availability of the full array of respiratory care strategies.

Resuscitation should begin with standard neonatal resuscitation guidelines and expeditiously proceed with endotracheal intubation and nasogastric tube insertion. Bag–valve mask use should be avoided. Careful management of temperature regulation, glucose homeostasis, and volume status should be performed. Inotropes such as dopamine or dobutamine are utilized if needed. Most infants can be managed with simple pressure-cycled ventilation with a goal of maintaining a preductal PaO_2 greater than 60 correlating with saturation between 85% and 95%. Keeping peak pressures below 25 and accepting CO_2 between 45 and 65 decreases barotrauma. For failure of "gentle ventilation strategies," the jet ventilator or oscillator ventilator may be used.

In addition to ventilatory methods, a variety of agents are utilized to modify pulmonary vascular resistance, including inhaled nitric oxide, phosphodiesterase-5 inhibition with sildenafil, milrinone (a phosphodiesterase-3 inhibitor), prostacyclin, and prostaglandin E1. Other medications such as tyrosine kinase inhibitors and endothelin receptor antagonists may show promise. Surfactant has been demonstrated to be reduced in CDH infants. However, surfactant administration has not been demonstrated to improve survival.

Failure to improve with ventilator support and pulmonary hypertension management strategies should prompt consideration of extracorporeal membrane oxygenation (ECMO). ECMO may be used for an extended period of time when ventilator therapy has failed. In recent years the use of ECMO has decreased but still ranges from 15% to 40% of diaphragmatic hernias; with survival following ECMO of 51%. There is no consensus on timing of diaphragm repair, whether while on ECMO or after ECMO decannulation.[5]

Surgery

2 Delayed surgery has been demonstrated to improve survival in some studies. The diaphragm defect is usually approached through a subcostal incision, although the repair can be performed through a thoracotomy incision (**Fig. 97.4**). Both thoracoscopic and laparoscopic approaches have been described although the thoracoscopic approach is preferred by most. The abdominal organs are returned to the abdomen. The defect in the diaphragm is repaired. Primary repair with nonabsorbable suture is preferred. If the defect cannot be repaired primarily due to size, a prosthetic patch such as Gore-Tex may be utilized. The major drawback of the use of a patch, either inert or bioactive, is recurrent herniation which may occur in up to

50% of infants. An alternative approach to a patch is the use of an internal oblique muscle flap.[6] After hernia reduction and diaphragm closure, there may be insufficient intra-abdominal domain and difficulty with closing the abdomen: a patch may be employed to close the abdominal fascia. Tube thoracostomy is used at the surgeon's preference. A meta-analysis of minimally invasive (MIS) versus open repairs raised concern that recurrence rate is higher after MIS and operative time is longer, but the learning curve has continued to improve into the current decade. Postoperative ventilator time and postoperative mortality were higher after open surgery but none of the studies were able to randomize patients and this may have represented selection bias.[7]

Postoperative management should continue the goals set before surgery. Continued attention to fluid status is important in the postoperative period. Weaning from the ventilator should be slow and deliberate. Refractory postoperative pulmonary hypertension is relatively common in those who required ECMO and is often treated with inhaled nitric oxide and prostacyclin while monitoring with frequent echocardiography.

Outcome

Survival rates have been reported at 60% to 80%, improved from 50% in the past. As survival has improved, other morbidities have been demonstrated including long-term use of bronchodilators, need for gastrostomy for nutritional support, and increased rate of gastroesophageal reflux disease (GERD) requiring surgery. Musculoskeletal deformities also occur with scoliosis, pectus excavatum, pectus carinatum, and chest wall asymmetry described.[8] Adult survivors of CDH have demonstrated higher incidence of GERD, recurrent intestinal obstruction, and recurrent abdominal pain. Scores in the Gastrointestinal Quality of Life Index and the Health-related Quality of Life Survey are good or satisfactory.

Evolving Therapies

Open fetal repair of diaphragmatic hernia has been performed but there was no survival benefit and there was an increase in preterm delivery so this is not currently offered. Tracheal occlusion in utero has been developed as a strategy to promote lung development based on observations that the lungs of neonates with congenital high airway obstruction developed hyperplastic lungs. Fetal tracheal occlusion improved lung volume but there was still impairment in the lung function. Fetal endoscopic tracheal occlusion has been trialed with fewer premature deliveries. In the US trial there was no improvement in survival in a randomized trial.[9] The European trials (TOTAL) added a second fetal surgery to remove the balloon to allow for improvement in the development and function of type II pneumocytes and to increase surfactant production. With balloon removal, vaginal delivery is possible but with the US trial, the infants were delivered by ex-utero intrapartum therapy (EXIT) procedure, using the placenta to maintain oxygenation until an airway is secured. The TOTAL trial showed improved survival for fetuses with severe pulmonary hypoplasia.[10]

Foramen of Morgagni Hernia

The anterior CDH is rare and accounts for 3% to 5% of all CDHs. It is typically diagnosed during childhood from chest or abdominal radiographs being performed for presumed pneumonia or gastrointestinal symptoms (**Fig. 97.5**).[11] This is an anteromedial hernia at the junction of the septum transversum and the thoracic wall, with contents being seen in a retrosternal position. There is a hernia sac present and the sac may contain colon, small intestine, or liver. The hernias are repaired due to the risk of segmental intestinal volvulus or obstruction. Laparoscopy has been demonstrated to be an effective method for repair of this type of hernia. The sac is excised and the diaphragm is sutured to the undersurface of the posterior rectus sheath at the costal margin.[11]

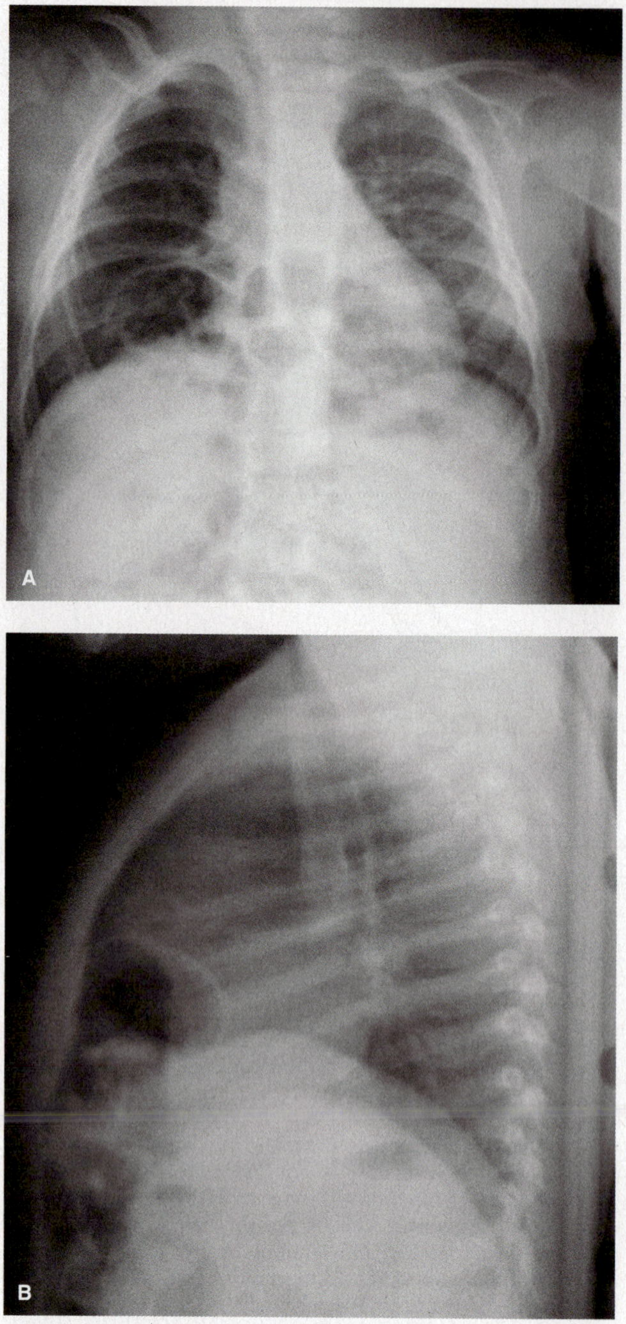

Figure 97.5. Morgagni hernia. (**A**) Anteroposterior, and (**B**) lateral radiographs of patient with Morgagni hernia.

Eventration of the Diaphragm

Eventration of the diaphragm is diagnosed by the abnormal elevation of one or both hemidiaphragms and can be congenital or acquired. The congenital form may appear very similar to a diaphragmatic hernia with a sac. The cause of the congenital form is unknown although infectious causes have been implicated. The acquired form is a consequence of injury to the phrenic nerve. Asymptomatic patients may be observed. Surgical management in symptomatic patients involves plication of the diaphragm. The repair may be performed through the abdomen or the chest and both thoracoscopic and laparoscopic techniques are applicable.[12]

Diaphragmatic Pacing

Ventilator-dependent children with spinal cord injury or central hypoventilation syndromes may benefit from diaphragm pacing.[13] The application of repetitive stimulus patterns to the phrenic nerves causes rhythmic contractions of the diaphragm.

Phrenic nerve pacing wires are implanted at the cervical or intrathoracic level. Receivers are implanted in subcutaneous pockets, while an external microprocessor-controlled transmitter/antenna assembly activates the receiver. Patients with injured phrenic nerves (high spinal cord injury) may benefit from diaphragm pacing after intercostal-to-phrenic nerve transfer.

ESOPHAGEAL ATRESIA/ TRACHEOESOPHAGEAL FISTULA

The first description of esophageal atresia was by Durston in 1670 who found a blind esophageal pouch in one pair of thoracopagus conjoined twins. The first description of the classic proximal esophageal atresia with distal fistula was by Thomas Gibson in 1697. Initial attempts at repair or palliation were unsuccessful. Leven and Ladd reported survivors but only after staged reconstruction. The first successful primary repair was reported by Cameron Haight in 1941. Outcomes have improved related to refinements in surgical technique and postoperative care. In the modern era, survival is related to the degree of prematurity and the presence of cardiac disease.

Embryology

The development of the human respiratory system begins as a folding of the flat endodermal layer into the primitive gut tube. The respiratory system is derived from the foregut endoderm with the appearance of the laryngotracheal groove in the ventral floor just caudal to the level of the pharynx. The precise morphogenic events that follow are not well understood. The respiratory system may develop as a rapid outgrowth from the original foregut tube. The fusion of the lateral foregut walls separating the trachea from the esophagus may also contribute. Tracheoesophageal fistula (TEF) is caused by failure of tracheal growth and failure of the active separation of the trachea and esophagus. Sonic hedgehog patterning gene has been implicated in the development of esophageal atresia/TEF based on adriamycin-induced malformations in rats.

Classification

3 Descriptive terminology is used to indicate the anatomic configuration of a patient with esophageal atresia. The most common type of lesion is a proximal atresia with a distal TEF which accounts for 76% to 85% of all cases in recent series.[14] Esophageal atresia without fistula occurs in 3% to 17% (referred to as "pure esophageal atresia") and TEF without esophageal atresia in 4% to 6% ("H-type fistula"). Proximal fistula and both proximal and distal fistula occur in approximately 1% of cases each. Initially, alphabetic classification schemes were devised and the most common variety of esophageal atresia/TEF is still commonly referred to as "Gross type C" (**Fig. 97.6**).

Incidence and Epidemiology

Esophageal atresia is relatively common occurring in 1:2,500 to 1:4,500 live births. There is a slight preponderance of males. Chromosomal anomalies, congenital heart disease, and other anomalies are more common than expected.

Clinical Findings, Diagnosis, and Pathophysiology

Diagnosis of esophageal atresia is suspected with a history of choking with feeding and is confirmed by the inability to pass an NG tube into the stomach. Excessive drooling may be noted. Maternal polyhydramnios and a small fetal stomach should raise suspicion for the diagnosis prenatally. If not diagnosed early, respiratory distress and aspiration may occur. Confirmation of the diagnosis is with a radiograph identifying a tube in a proximal pouch in most cases. Presence of a scaphoid abdomen with no intragastric air on radiograph taken several hours after birth confirms the diagnosis of pure esophageal atresia.[15] For patients with EA and a distal TEF rapid distension of the stomach with air can cause respiratory compromise. Alternately, reflux of gastric contents through the fistula can enter the lungs which becomes more problematic in the face of respiratory compromise and is less of an issue with spontaneous ventilation.

Associated Anomalies

Associated anomalies are present in approximately one-half of the neonates with esophageal atresia. The most common associated anomalies are cardiovascular defects which occur in 17% to 50% of infants. Genitourinary, other gastrointestinal, skeletal neurologic, and craniofacial defects are also found. The occurrence of *v*ertebral anomalies, *a*norectal malformations, *c*ardiac, *t*racheo*e*sophageal, *r*enal, and *l*imb (usually radial) anomalies is known as the VACTERL association. Two or more of the defects must occur to be denoted as VACTERL, occurring in 10% to 21% of cases.

Preoperative Management

Attempts at feeding are discontinued and sump tube is placed in the upper esophageal pouch. Precautions such as head-up position are advocated to decrease reflux via the fistula into the lung. Intubation is avoided unless there is significant respiratory compromise as it increases the risk of reflux into the lungs via the fistula. Ventilatory support is more likely to be needed for low birth weight or prematurity. Preoperative antibiotics are given in the majority of patients. Emergent bedside gastric decompression may be necessary before definitive surgery. If gastrostomy decompression does not improve ventilation, emergency operative ligation of the TEF, insertion of a gastrostomy, placing a vessel loop around the distal esophagus, or occluding the distal esophagus with a balloon may allow for ventilation.

In addition to chest radiograph, echocardiography is performed to determine the side of the aortic arch as well as to evaluate for major cardiac anomalies. In patients with a right-sided arch, the operative approach may be modified.[16] Radiographs of the spine are also commonly performed. The genitourinary system is evaluated by ultrasound.

To stratify infants into groups to determine outcomes, Waterston developed criteria based on birth weight, pneumonia, and associated anomalies. With improvements in neonatal critical care, the criteria have been revised with the current Spitz classification which uses a 1,500 g weight as the cutoff, with or without major cardiac disease. Currently survival for greater than 1,500 g infants without cardiac disease is approximately 97%, survival for either cardiac disease or less than 1,500 g approaches 82% and for both birth weight less than 1,500 g and cardiac anomaly survival is approximately 50%.

Surgical Technique

In most patients, gastrostomy is unnecessary. A right extrapleural posterolateral or auscultatory triangle thoracotomy is used (**Fig. 97.7**). There is no need to divide the serratus or the latissimus muscles. The extrapleural plane is established at the fourth intercostal space and developed sufficiently to allow control of the fistula and mobilization of the proximal pouch. The fistula is divided and closed. Anastomosis is performed in a single layer with an absorbable suture. If needed there are various techniques for elongation and the esophagus may be mobilized both proximally and distally. Myotomies on the upper pouch, either circular or spiral and flap tubularization have been described. In situ stretching of both the proximal and distal esophagus facilitates repair of longer gaps. A transesophageal tube may increase stricture. A postoperative esophagram is performed 5 to 10 days after repair.[14]

High-risk infants who cannot safely undergo surgical correction of their esophageal abnormality may be treated with delayed repair. A decompressive gastrostomy, proximal pouch suctioning, and parenteral nutrition are used until the infant is ready for operation. Severe respiratory failure (usually from prematurity) and structural heart disease are the most

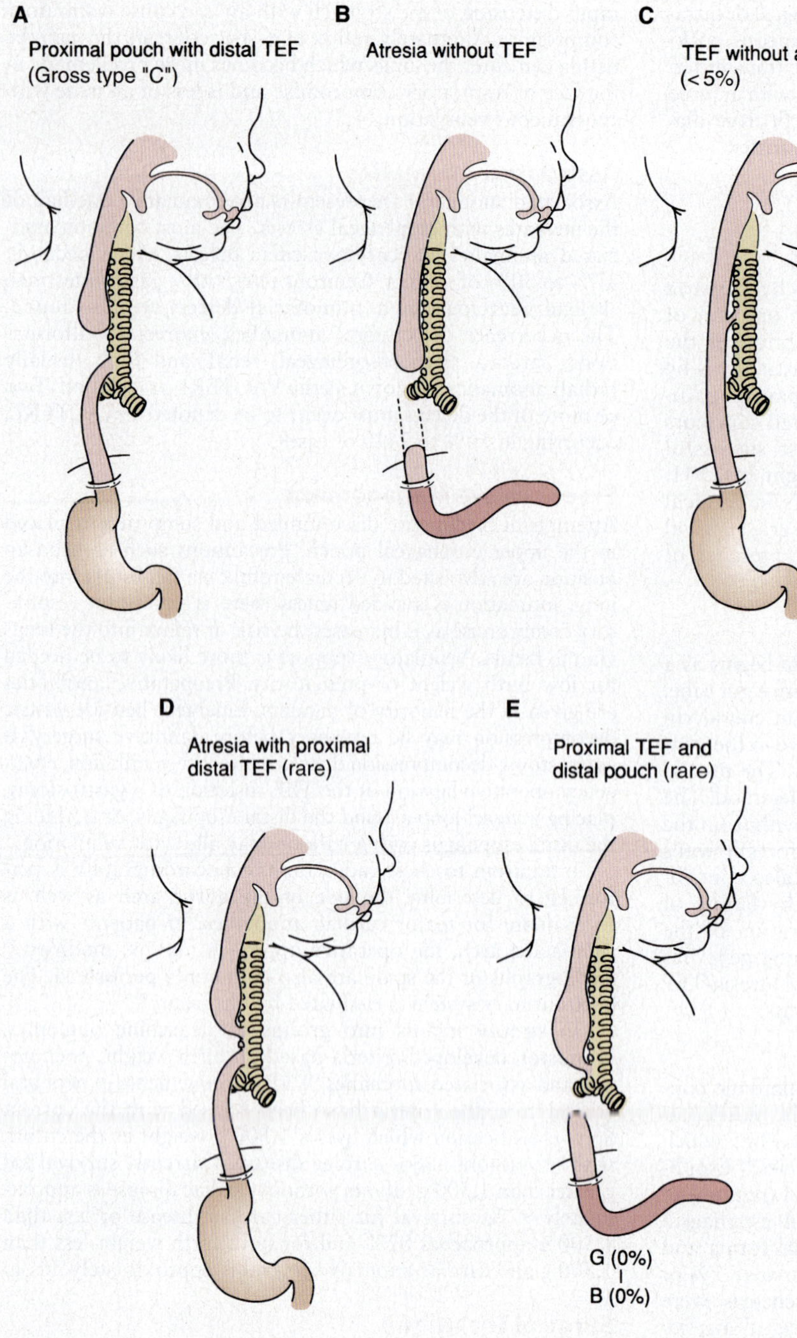

Figure 97.6. The anatomy of the variants of esophageal atresia and tracheoesophageal fistula (TEF). **A:** Proximal pouch with distal TEF (most common type occurring in 76% to 85% of patients; gross type "C"). **B:** Esophageal atresia without TEF (3% to 17%). **C:** TEF without esophageal atresia (4% to 6%). **D:** Esophageal atresia with proximal and distal TEF (rare). **E:** Proximal TEF and distal pouch (rare).

common reasons to delay esophageal surgery. A staged repair that employs gastrostomy, surgical division of the TEF, followed by esophageal anastomosis as a second thoracic operation is rarely used except as a lifesaving approach.

In the case of pure esophageal atresia without fistula, a prolonged period before definitive repair may be used to improve the likelihood of completing a primary repair.[17] A feeding gastrostomy is the initial operative management and may be technically challenging due to microgastria. Use of bouginage may be employed to elongate the ends of the esophagus and once the ends are close on radiographic studies, a thoracotomy is performed to repair the esophagus (**Fig. 97.8**). Other methods of elongation have been described with staged repair using traction sutures in the upper and lower esophagus (**Fig. 97.9**). Daily tightening of the tension results in lengthening of the esophagus over a few weeks.[18] Alternatively, extrathoracic elongation may be utilized.[15]

Esophageal replacement is reserved for the worst cases of long-gap atresia, pure atresia, or failed initial operations. The esophagus may be replaced later using stomach, gastric tube, jejunum, or colon. These cases may be temporized with a cervical esophagostomy ("spit fistula") and sham feeds.

TEF without esophageal atresia is referred to as H-type or N-type fistula. The orientation is such that the opening into the trachea is always proximal to the esophageal entry site. Repair is performed via a cervical approach after bronchoscopically stenting the fistula with a small catheter. The catheter aids in dissection and care must be taken to stay in the plane of the esophagus to avoid recurrent laryngeal nerve injury.

Thoracoscopic, transpleural approaches to the repair of esophageal atresia with low insufflation pressure are becoming performed increasingly with results demonstrating equivalent outcomes to open repair.[18] Thoracoscopic techniques for esophageal lengthening in long-gap atresia have also been described.[19]

Results, Complications, and Outcomes

Technical mishaps may occur during the procedure when anatomy is misidentified or dissection is carried out improperly. Injury to the vagus nerves, recurrent laryngeal nerves, posterior trachea, and adjacent vessels must be avoided.

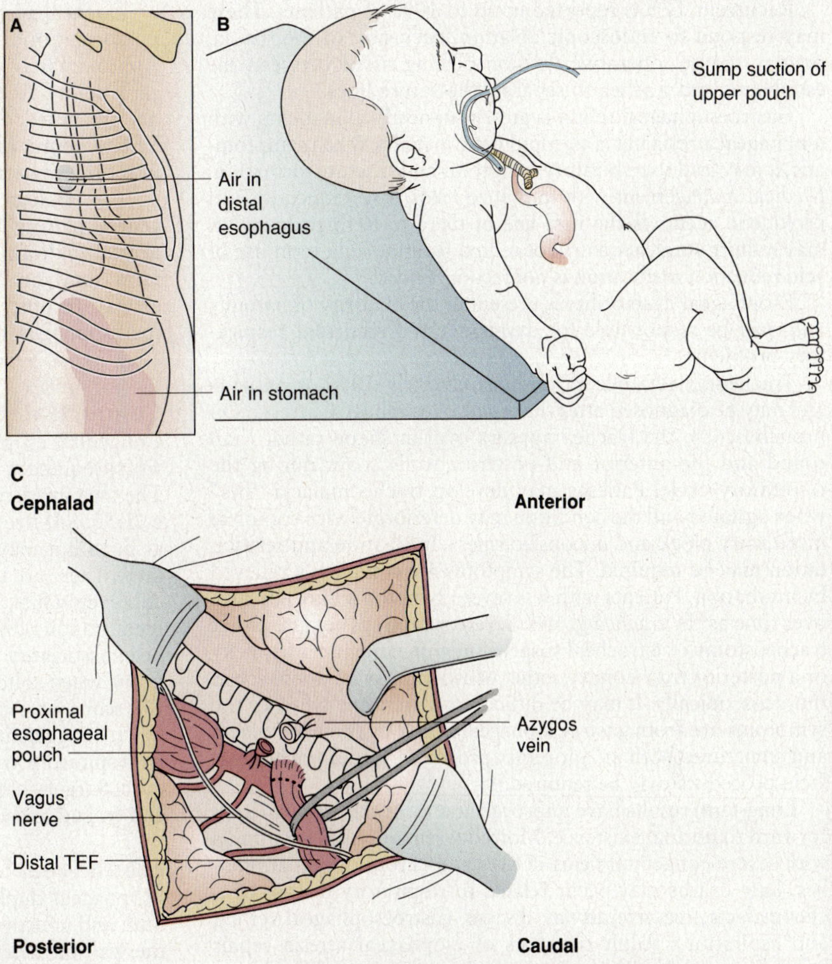

Figure 97.7. **A:** Schematic illustration of esophageal atresia with distal tracheoesophageal fistula. **B:** The initial management of this anomaly includes upright or prone posture, sump suction of the blind esophageal pouch. **C:** The right extrapleural operative approach. After division and closure of the fistula, primary esophagoesophagostomy is performed.

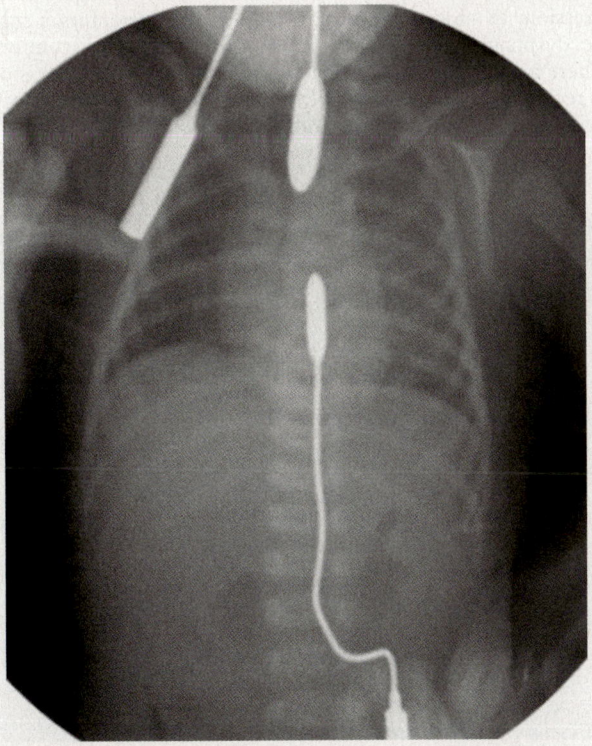

Figure 97.8. Patient with pure esophageal atresia treated initially with feeding gastrostomy, and proximal pouch stretching. This "gap-o-gram" demonstrates close approximation of a dilator in the proximal pouch and a probe placed in the distal esophagus via the gastrostomy. The child subsequently underwent primary repair of the esophagus.

Anastomotic leak occurs in approximately 10% to 20% of cases and most may be treated nonoperatively. The presence of a leak prolongs hospitalization.[14] When detected, the retro-pleural tube is left in place, the infant is not fed, and antibiotics are administered. Repeat contrast radiographs are employed to document healing prior to initiation of oral feeds.

Esophageal stricture is seen in up to 40% of infants after repair. These usually respond to a few sessions of dilation performed in the operating room with endoscopic and fluoroscopic assistance as necessary to assure the safe traverse of dilators or placement of balloon dilators.[20] More recalcitrant strictures require more frequent dilation sessions, medical and/or surgical control of gastroesophageal reflux, and occasionally reoperation with stricture resection and reanastomosis.

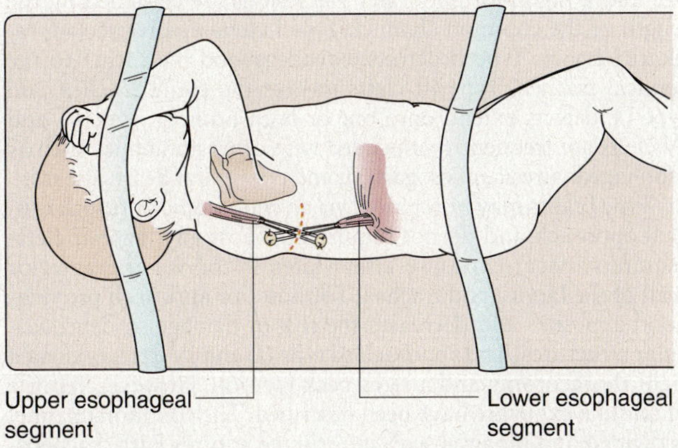

Figure 97.9. In patients with ultra–long-gap esophageal atresia, traction sutures are placed on the upper pouch and lower segment. Tension is increased daily until the segments lengthen, allowing primary repair.

Recurrent TEF is reported in up to 10% of patients. These may respond to endoscopic ablation, occlusion of the fistula, or may require operative division placing tissue between the esophagus and trachea to separate the suture lines.

Gastroesophageal reflux is present in nearly all patients with esophageal atresia but is asymptomatic in many. When symptomatic, it may lead to respiratory symptoms and stricture formation. Medical management with thickened feeds, acid reduction, and prokinetic agents is the first line of therapy. Refractory reflux may require surgical control of reflux. Routine long-term use of acid reduction medication is not recommended.[14]

Esophageal dysmotility is present in the majority of patients and may be responsible for dysphagia and recurrent respiratory problems.

Tracheomalacia occurs in approximately 10% of patients and may be diagnosed after the repair of esophageal atresia. On bronchoscopy, the trachea appears oval in shape rather than round and the anterior and posterior walls coapt during the respiratory cycle. Patients may develop tracheomalacia "fits" when agitated and the condition may deteriorate with complete inspiratory block and unconsciousness. Intubation and resuscitation may be required. The symptoms are completely relieved by intubation. Patients with less severe symptoms may improve over time as the trachea grows. Severe symptoms require either tracheostomy or a tracheal suspension with either an aortopexy or a posterior tracheopexy, either of which may be approached thoracoscopically. It may be difficult to determine whether the symptoms are from gastroesophageal reflux or tracheomalacia and sometimes both an antireflux procedure and a tracheomalacia procedure may be required.[21]

Long-term results have improved and most children can look forward to normal existence. Mortality remains high for infants with severe congenital heart defects and chromosomal anomalies. Late deaths may occur related to respiratory disease (tracheomalacia, reactive airway disease, gastroesophageal reflux, and aspiration). Adult survivors of esophageal atresia repair have a normal quality of life with the exception of morbidity from esophageal and respiratory disorders. The very long-term effects are unknown but Barrett esophagus and esophagitis have been reported.[22] The incidence is low and further studies are required to determine the need for long-term surveillance.

OTHER CONGENITAL ANOMALIES OF THE TRACHEA AND ESOPHAGUS

Laryngotracheoesophageal Cleft and Tracheal Agenesis

Laryngotracheoesophageal clefts are rare anomalies resulting from the failure of normal separation of the esophagus and trachea. These are the most severe anomalies and the presence of the common aerodigestive channel plus the association of gastroesophageal reflux leads to aspiration with respiratory damage and a high mortality rate. The lesions are classified by the length of the common channel. Type I clefts involve the supraglottic larynx. Type II defects extend beyond the carina to the cervical trachea. Type III clefts involve the entire trachea and type IV defects extend onto one or both bronchi. Type III and IV clefts are frequently associated with other anomalies such as esophageal atresia, microgastria, and congenital heart disease.

Type I clefts may be repaired via an endoscopic or translaryngeal approach and do not require tracheostomy. Type II clefts require cervical exposure either laterally or via the anterior wall of the larynx and trachea. The anterior approach provides good exposure and decreases the risk of damage to neurovascular structures. The approach to type III and IV defects is via a right thoracotomy and a right neck incision. However, reports of midline exposure have been described. The common channel is divided and repaired with interrupted sutures with tracheostomy. Oromotor function and chronic aspiration are problems and most children require gastrostomy and many require operative control of gastroesophageal reflux.

Tracheal agenesis (TA) is a rare and usually fatal congenital malformation that occurs in less than 1 in 50,000 live births. Approximately 150 cases have been reported with near universal lethality. At birth, cyanosis, respiratory distress, and aphonia are noted. Survival requires the presence of an adequate TEF to permit lifesaving esophageal intubation. TA is classified into three anatomical variations, originally defined by Floyd.

The etiology of this rare anomaly remains unknown. No genetic pattern has been implicated. However, associated congenital malformations are present in 90% of cases. All long-term survivors (older than 1 year of age) have undergone airway reconstruction with external scaffolding and use of the esophagus to create an airway ("trachealization" of the esophagus). Survival is rare.[16]

Congenital Esophageal Stenosis

Congenital esophageal stenosis is a rare condition. The stenosis is frequently within 2 cm of the gastroesophageal junction. The true incidence is unknown but is reported to be 1:25,000 to 1:50,000 live births. The narrowing of the lumen is present at birth but may not present with clinical symptoms immediately. There are three histologic subtypes: ectopic tracheobronchial remnants, segmental fibromuscular hypertrophy, and a membranous diaphragm or stenosis. Esophageal stenosis has been associated with esophageal atresia. Symptoms may only occur when solids are started. Diagnosis is by esophagograms. CT scans or esophagoscopy may confirm the diagnosis. Initial management is esophageal dilation. If the stenosis is due to respiratory tract remnants, need for surgery is more common. Surgery consists of resection of the stenotic segment with end-to-end anastomosis.[23]

Esophageal Duplication

Esophageal duplications are found in the posterior mediastinum and are covered by a muscular wall. Most are attached to the wall of the esophagus. Approximately 10% communicate with the lumen of the esophagus. Although many are asymptomatic, they may present with airway or esophageal compression. In older children and adults, the presentation may be dysphagia, retrosternal pain, and epigastric discomfort. There are reports of bleeding from acid dyspepsia.[24] Excision is recommended and is usually accomplished by thoracoscopy (**Fig. 97.10**). Neuroenteric cysts are anatomically similar but communicate with the spinal canal.

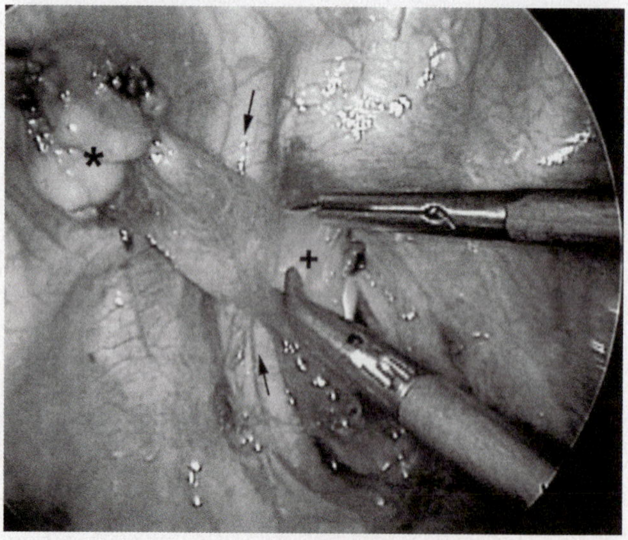

Figure 97.10. Thoracoscopic excision of an esophageal duplication cyst in a patient presenting with dysphagia. Video endoscopic view of the left superior hemithorax. (+) indicates site of original esophageal duplication cyst. Light from the intraesophageal endoscope can be seen. *Arrows* demonstrate the subclavian artery. The mass (*) is nearly excised.

Vascular Rings

Vascular rings are a set of congenital defects in which the trachea or esophagus are encircled and compressed by vascular structures associated with the development of the aorta and great vessels. These account for approximately 1% of all congenital cardiovascular anomalies. Vascular rings may lead to tracheal narrowing with associated tracheomalacia. Symptoms may include stridor, respiratory distress, or dysphagia. Contrast study may be suggestive of the lesion. CT scan and MRI are utilized to demonstrate the anomaly. Echocardiography is performed to rule out structural cardiac anomalies. Bronchoscopy may also be useful to determine the degree of tracheal narrowing. The most common type of abnormality is the double aortic arch resulting from persistence of both the right and left embryologic aortic arches. The ascending aorta bifurcates, surrounding the trachea and esophagus. Other causes of complete or incomplete rings include pulmonary artery sling and aberrant right subclavian artery. When the vascular ring is symptomatic, the patient should be treated by the appropriate division of the ring and lysis of the fibrous bands surrounding the trachea and esophagus.[25]

Congenital Tracheal Stenosis

Congenital tracheal stenosis represents a spectrum of obstructive lesions most commonly treated with operative repair. The etiologies include complete tracheal rings, compression from anomalous cardiovascular anatomy, and tracheomalacia. Short stenosis may respond to resection and anastomosis. Longer lengths of stenosis can be managed by patch tracheoplasty and slide tracheoplasty. Use of cardiopulmonary bypass during repair may improve outcomes.[26]

FOREIGN BODIES OF THE TRACHEOBRONCHIAL TREE AND ESOPHAGUS

4 Foreign-body aspiration occurs commonly in infants and young children and is a potentially life-threatening event. A report in 2001 found that nonfood choking was a cause of death for 449 children under the age of 14, with 65% of the deaths in children under 3 years of age over a 20-year period. Choking on food causes death of approximately 75 children per year.[27]

Pathophysiology

Complete airway obstruction can occur at the level of the pharynx, hypopharynx, or trachea. Back blows, abdominal thrusts, or the Heimlich maneuver may dislodge the obstruction and save a life. An inhaled foreign body which reaches the bronchial level may cause a ball-valve phenomenon allowing bi-directional but unequal flow of air. Air trapping and hyperinflation of the affected lobe lead to mediastinal shift. Complete blockage results in loss of volume due to atelectasis.

Foods are the most common aspirated items and include peanuts, carrots, popcorn, hotdogs, and grapes. Toy parts are the most common nonfood items aspirated. Button battery ingestion is a particularly dangerous event, especially if impacted in the esophagus, due to the progressive tissue injury which may result. These sequelae may result in esophageal perforation, mediastinitis, trachea-esophageal fistula, and even erosion into the great vessels.

Clinical Presentation

Most affected children are less than 3 years of age. History of choking crisis is present in the majority of children. Other symptoms include cough, wheezing, dyspnea, and fever. The most common signs are unilateral decreased breath sounds, unilateral wheezing, and rhonchi.

Management

Chest radiographs, including bilateral lateral decubitus films, are performed unless the patient is in respiratory distress. Radiographs demonstrate hyperinflation on the affected side. In case of questionable foreign-body aspiration, CT imaging may be performed and may prevent a negative endoscopy.[27] Alternatively, radiographs may show pneumonia or atelectasis with a completely occluding foreign body.

Bronchoscopic evaluation and foreign-body removal is performed in the operating room under general anesthesia. The rigid bronchoscope and Hopkins rod-lens system with optical forceps can be used to retrieve most aspirated foreign bodies (**Fig. 97.11**). Flexible graspers, Fogarty balloon catheters, and baskets can be useful especially if the foreign body has migrated distally or has a smooth or round surface. Fluoroscopic assistance can be useful with radiopaque objects which have migrated into the peripheral airways.

PEDIATRIC SURGERY

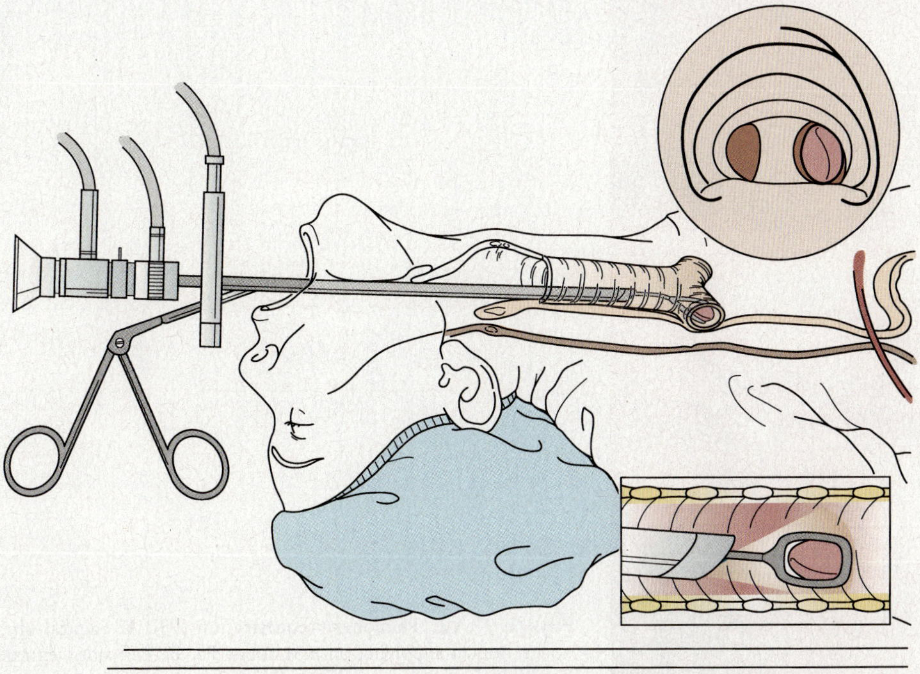

Figure 97.11. Schematic illustration of a peanut foreign body being extracted from the right main stem bronchus under direct vision.

Over time, pneumonia or atelectasis may develop and a foreign body presenting with chronic lung infection may require surgical resection of the associated potion of the lung.

CONGENITAL LUNG LESIONS

Congenital lung lesions have been characterized as lesions of defective budding, differentiation, and separation of the foregut, as well as airway maldevelopment with resultant obstruction.[28] These lesions include pulmonary sequestration (PS), congenital pulmonary airway malformation (CPAM; formerly CCAM), bronchogenic cyst (BC), and congenital lobar overinflation (CLO). The first three are in the family of bronchopulmonary foregut malformations. PS is characterized by aberrant blood supply, CPAM by hamartomatous lung parenchyma, and BC by an isolated cyst. There is overlap among the types; many lesions are found to be hybrid.[28] CLO is likely a secondary response to abnormal compression or obstruction of a bronchus during lung development.

Pulmonary Sequestration

5 PSs consist of nonfunctioning pulmonary tissue without a normal bronchial communication with the tracheobronchial tree. The blood supply is from an aberrant systemic vessel often originating from the descending aorta. The lesions are most commonly found in the lower lobes, usually on the left. They are characterized as intra- or extralobar based on pleural lining.

Intralobar sequestrations are incorporated into the surrounding lung and are invested by its visceral pleura. They are most common in the left medial or posterior basal segment of the lower lobe. The arterial supply is from the descending aorta and the venous return is usually into a pulmonary vein. They are usually asymptomatic at birth, but aberrant air space connections can result in recurrent pneumonia.

Extralobar sequestrations occur outside of the pleura of the normal lung. They are most common in the lower left side of the chest but have been reported in a variety of locations including the retroperitoneum.[28] In the retroperitoneum, they may be difficult to distinguish from neuroblastoma. These have occasionally been associated with CDH. In 20% of cases, the blood supply originates from the infradiaphragmatic aorta. Arteriovenous shunting in rare cases can lead to high-output heart failure.

Radiographic evaluation of PS involves chest radiographs, ultrasound, and CT scans with contrast enhancement to identify the vascular supply. Intralobar sequestrations are treated with lobectomy. Extralobar sequestrations may be removed by excision of the sequestration. The lesions may be removed with thoracotomy or thoracoscopy with attention to safe ligation of the vascular supply (**Fig. 97.12**).[29,30]

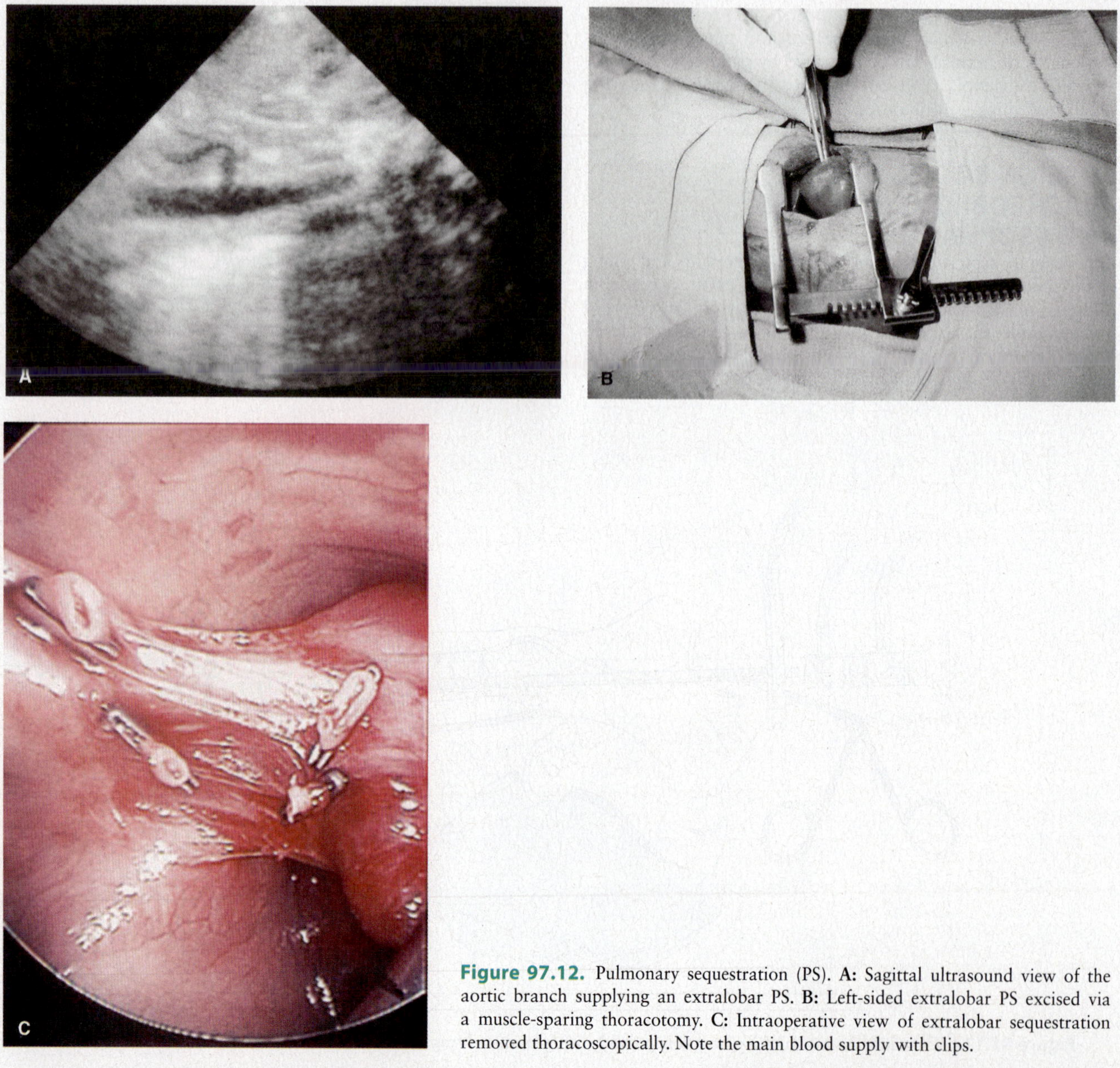

Figure 97.12. Pulmonary sequestration (PS). **A:** Sagittal ultrasound view of the aortic branch supplying an extralobar PS. **B:** Left-sided extralobar PS excised via a muscle-sparing thoracotomy. **C:** Intraoperative view of extralobar sequestration removed thoracoscopically. Note the main blood supply with clips.

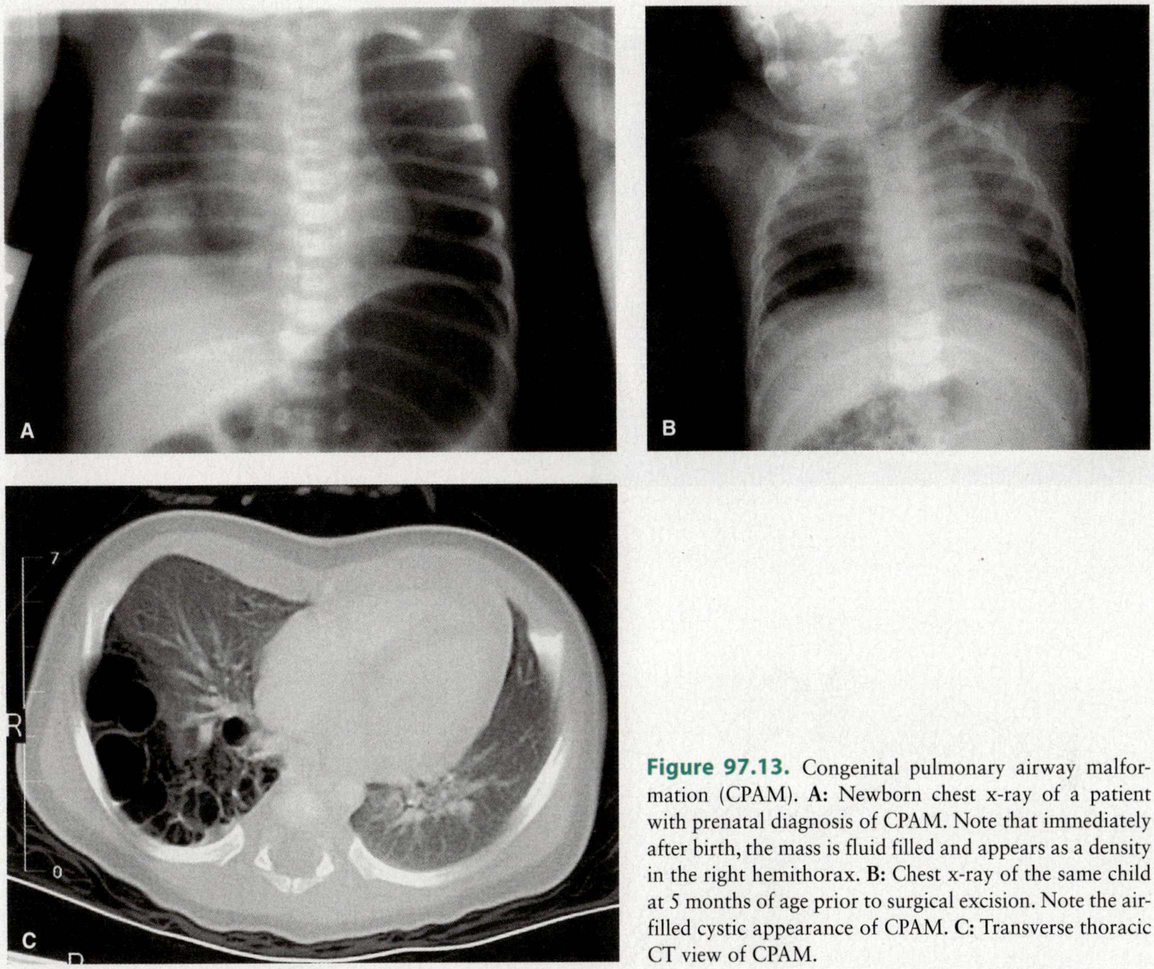

Figure 97.13. Congenital pulmonary airway malformation (CPAM). **A:** Newborn chest x-ray of a patient with prenatal diagnosis of CPAM. Note that immediately after birth, the mass is fluid filled and appears as a density in the right hemithorax. **B:** Chest x-ray of the same child at 5 months of age prior to surgical excision. Note the air-filled cystic appearance of CPAM. **C:** Transverse thoracic CT view of CPAM.

Congenital Pulmonary Airway Malformations

6 CPAMs result from overgrowth of bronchial structures at the expense of the associated alveoli associated with an abnormal supplying airway affecting a single lobe in 95% of cases. This group of anomalies represents 30% to 40% of the developmental lung bud anomalies. On gross appearance, they can be solid, cystic, or both. The malformations have a normal blood supply and communicate with the normal tracheobronchial tree. The common postnatal pathology-based classification separates these lesions into three main types. Type I CPAMs consist of cysts with large, irregular widely dispersed spaces larger than 2 cm or a single large cyst with multiple small surrounding cysts and represent 50% to 65% of postnatal cases. Type II CPAM is described as numerous smaller cysts (0.5 to 2 cm) and account for 10% to 40% of cases. Type III CPAMs are made of small cystic lesions (generally 0.2 cm) or solid lesions appearing similar to immature lung devoid of cartilage and make up of 5% to 10% of cases. Prenatally the CPAMs are classified as solid/microcystic, macrocystic, or mixed. CPAMs generally affect one lobe but multilobar and bilateral involvement also occurs. Most commonly, the lesions are left sided and affect the lower lobes. Prenatal diagnosis is common and has led to an increase in diagnosis of lung lesions.[31] CPAMs may compromise fetal cardiac function leading to hydrops that can be life threatening. In utero therapy consists of maternal steroid administration for predominantly solid/microcystic lesions and thoraco-amniotic shunting for predominantly macrocystic lesions. The success of these two therapies has made indications for open fetal surgery and lung resection very limited.[28,31] The natural history of prenatally diagnosed CPAMs is variable and some lesions may regress. Growth tends to plateau for solid/microcystic lesion at 26 to 28 weeks of gestation while macrocystic lesions may grow throughout gestation and prenatal imaging should be performed accordingly.

The incidence is reported to be between 1:25,000 and 1:35,000 live births which likely underrepresents the incidence. Although 80% are asymptomatic at birth, many will have respiratory symptoms within the first month of life. Less commonly, patients may present with pneumonia later in life (**Fig. 97.13**).

Symptomatic lesions require resection of the involved lobe shortly after birth. The optimal treatment for asymptomatic lesions is less certain as the natural history of the lesion is unknown. There is concern for future infection and the possibility of malignancy.[28,31] Those who recommend resection favor timing between 2 and 10 months of age. With antenatal diagnosis, a postnatal CT is used to assess resolution and to aid preoperative planning. Thoracoscopic resection has become the standard approach. With multilobar and bilateral disease, CT scans assist in planning lung-preserving resections and indocyanine green may help guide these resections intraoperatively. Bilateral and multilobar lesions have a higher risk of pleuropulmonary blastoma (PPB).[28]

Bronchogenic Cysts

BCs are uncommon anomalies arising from defective foregut development. They can be mediastinal or intrapulmonary and cause symptoms of cough as well as recurrent and chronic infection. These cysts appear as discrete masses and develop associated with the esophagus or large airways. They are usually extrapulmonary and do not communicate with the normal tracheobronchial tree. Resection via thoracotomy or thoracoscopy is recommended due to the risk of bleeding, infection, or enlargement with compression of adjacent structures (**Fig. 97.14**).[28]

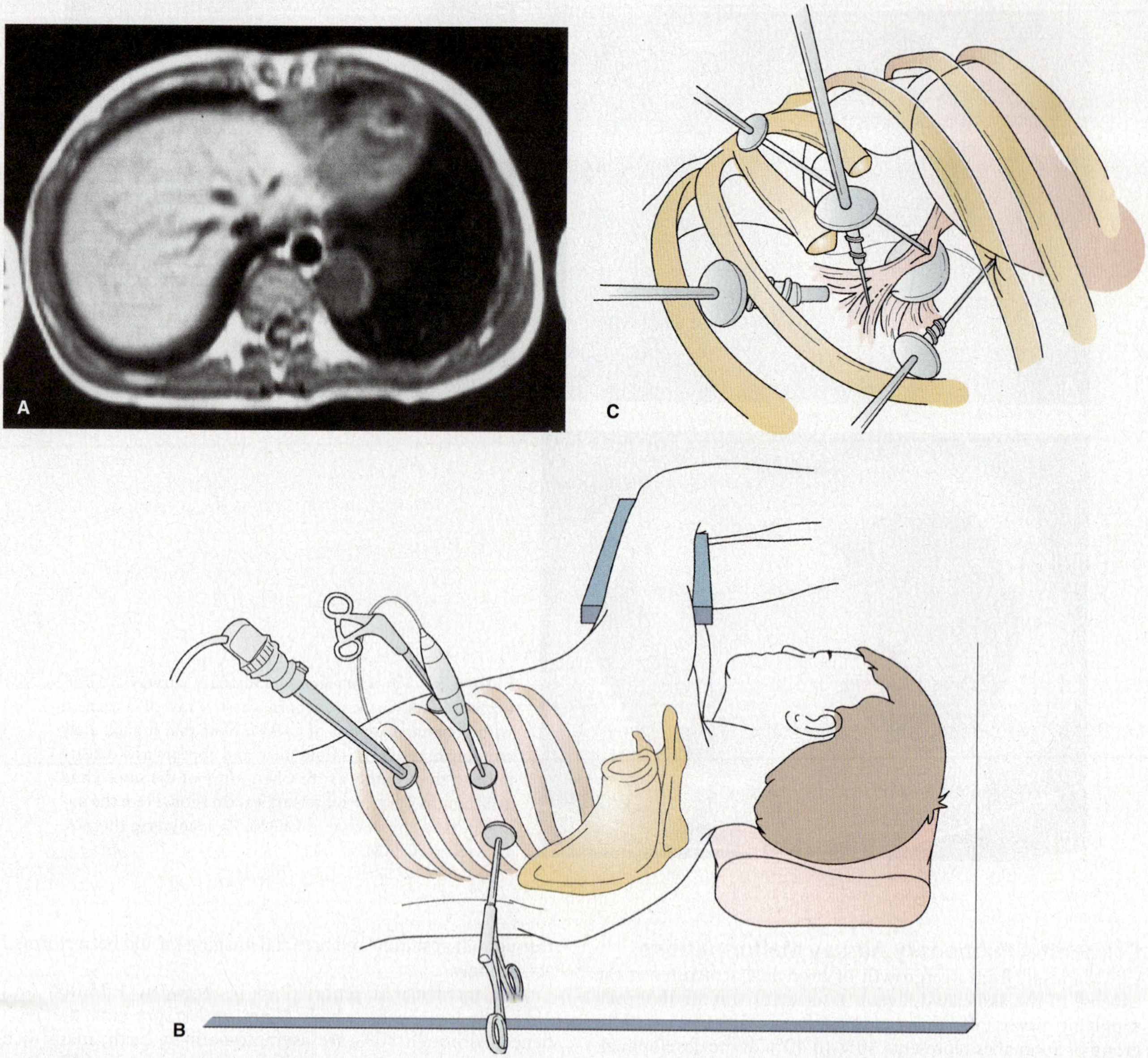

Figure 97.14. Bronchogenic cyst (BC). **A:** Transverse thoracic CT view of a BC located in the inferior pulmonary ligament. **B:** Illustrative representation of thoracoscopic instrumentation for excision of a BC. **C:** Operative detail.

Congenital Lobar Overinflation

CLO (previously called congenital lobar emphysema) is caused by abnormal development or compression of a lobar bronchus resulting in retention of fluid during fetal lung development and subsequent air trapping and overinflation after birth. The cause ranges from a deficiency of bronchial cartilage to compression from an extrinsic mass. They usually involve the upper lobe of either lung and are rarely multilobar. A definitive cause is rarely identified. Lobar overinflation may present as worsening respiratory distress caused by enlargement of the overinflated segment with compression of the normal surrounding lung (**Fig. 97.15**). Symptomatic infants should undergo complete resection of the lobe. Care must be taken at resection as positive-pressure ventilation cause further hyperinflation and require immediate thoracotomy. With relatively asymptomatic patients, symptoms may improve and surgery avoided.[28]

Diagnosis

Due to the routine use of prenatal ultrasound, many cystic lesions of the lung are now detected and followed prior to birth.[28] Patients with these lesions may be asymptomatic in the perinatal period. Standard chest radiographs remain the standard for diagnosis and follow-up. Rapid thoracic CT scanning with contrast provides definitive mapping of the lesions including demonstration of aberrant vessels. Minimizing radiation dosing of the CT scans is important to decrease long-term potential adverse side effects. Contrast esophagograms are indicated for children with dysphagia and suspicion of connection with the GI tract.

Cysts of the Mediastinum

7 Benign cysts of the mediastinum are relatively common in the pediatric population. Most of these are relatively asymptomatic but surgery is usually recommended due to the possibility of enlargement with symptoms related to compression, hemorrhage, or infection. The symptoms which occur include cough, chest pain, stridor, hemoptysis, or dysphagia. The common lesions include thymic cysts, enterogenous cysts, lymphatic malformations (cystic hygromas), and pericardial cysts.

Thymic Cysts

Thymic cysts present in the neck and mediastinum and are usually unilocular but may be multilocular. They are most commonly seen in the anterosuperior mediastinum. They are benign lesions with presence of cholesterol granulomas.

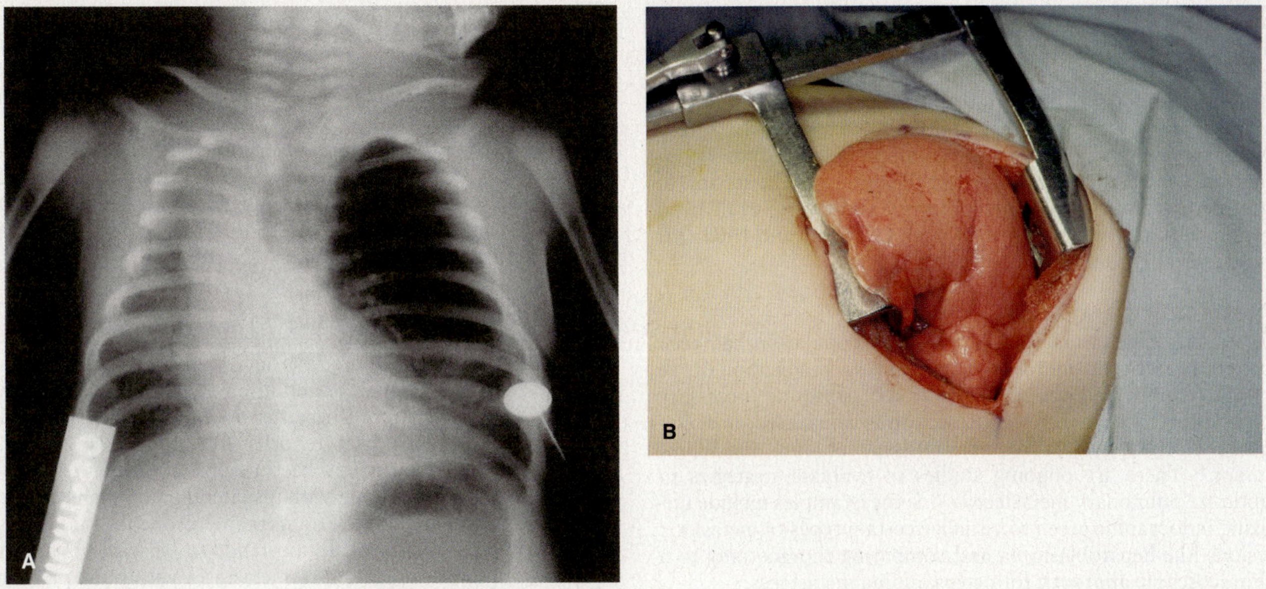

Figure 97.15. Congenital lobar overinflation. **A:** Chest radiograph demonstrating overinflation of the left upper lobe in an infant. Note the mediastinal shift. **B:** Operative photograph demonstrating an overexpanded left upper lobe decompressing through the incision.

Symptoms may arise from rapid expansion due to infection. Resection is recommended.

Enteric Duplication Cysts/Enterogenous Cysts

Enteric duplication cysts are usually located in the posterior mediastinum with microscopic evidence of double-layer smooth muscle and esophageal or gastric mucosa. They are from the same spectrum as bronchopulmonary cysts. These may communicate with the stomach or esophagus and may transverse the diaphragm. The cysts may also extend into the spinal canal. The lesions may have gastric mucosa leading to bleeding. Other symptoms may include airway compression or dysphagia (**Fig. 97.16**). Resection is indicated for all symptomatic lesions and is favored for asymptomatic lesions.

Lymphatic Malformations

Lymphatic malformations (cystic hygromas) are unilocular or multilocular cysts which are thin walled and derived from failure of adequate drainage of embryonic lymph sacs. These may occur in the head, neck, and mediastinum. The lesions insinuate around great vessels and nerves in the superior mediastinum. The incidence is 1 in 6,000 live births. Symptoms, if present, are related to enlargement (frequently due to hemorrhage) or infection. Treatment options include resection and intralesional sclerotherapy. If there is concern for a threatened airway at delivery, EXIT to airway may be employed. Immunomodulating drugs such as sirolimus may have a role in some cases.[32] The most frequent complications are recurrence and accumulation of lymph in the resection bed.

Pericardial Cysts

Pericardial cysts are asymptomatic and usually found incidentally on chest radiograph. The cysts are found in the cardiophrenic sulcus as a discrete mass. They are thin walled with a flat mesothelial lining and contain clear fluid. Resection can be performed with thoracotomy or thoracoscopy.

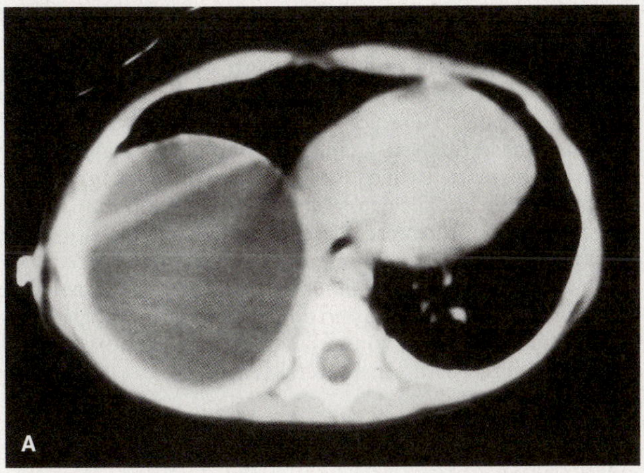

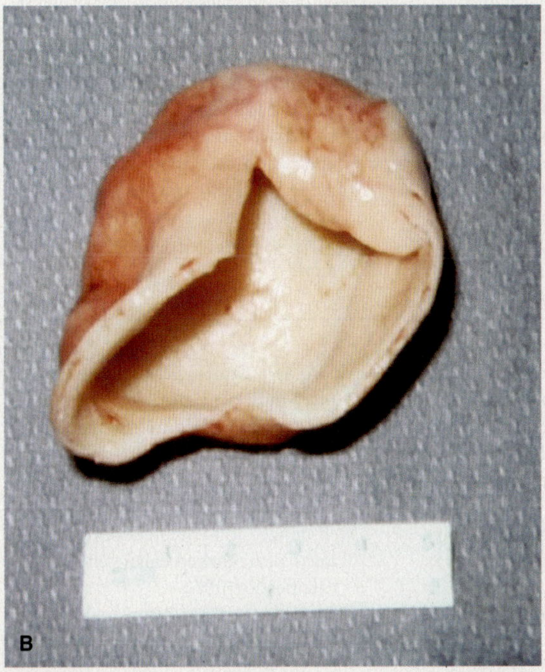

Figure 97.16. Enterogenous cyst. This represents another abnormality in the spectrum of bronchopulmonary foregut malformations. **A:** CT demonstrating a large mass occupying the right hemithorax. **B:** Surgical specimen.

THORACIC TUMORS IN CHILDREN

8 Thoracic tumors are rare in children and diagnostic evaluation must include evaluation for both primary and metastatic conditions. Tumors may occur in the lung or the mediastinum.[33,34] Primary lung neoplasms in children are extremely rare.[35] Metastatic lung lesions are more common in the pediatric population. Mediastinal tumors reflect the nature of the section of the mediastinum in which they arise. Diagnostic evaluation begins with routine radiographs with CT scans and MRIs for further evaluation.[35]

Metastatic Lung Tumors

9 Resection of metastases in the pediatric population has been proven to be beneficial for pediatric cancers. Eradication of the primary tumor and absence of other metastases are necessary for improvement in survival. Resection is considered most frequently for osteogenic sarcoma, soft tissue sarcoma, and Wilms tumor.[34] There are ongoing studies to evaluate strategies to optimize pulmonary metastectomy. Some examples include utilizing indocyanine green to visualize certain types of metastatic lesions like hepatoblastoma and comparing thoracotomy to a thoracoscopic approach for osteosarcoma metastases.

Primary Lung Tumors

Pediatric primary tumors are rare (**Table 97.1**). The majority of primary neoplasms are malignant but benign lesions also have significant morbidity due to location of the lesions. Operative exploration with total resection of all involved tissues is recommended.

Bronchial Adenomas

Bronchial adenomas are the most common of the malignant lung lesions (40%) in the pediatric population and include several different histologies including carcinoid tumor (85%), mucoepidermoid carcinoma (10%), and adenoid cystic carcinoma (5%). Cough, pneumonitis, fever, respiratory distress, and hemoptysis are the most common presenting symptoms. Delay in diagnosis is common due to the nonspecific symptomatology. The disease is diagnosed with chest radiograph followed by CT scan. Bronchoscopy is required for diagnosis and biopsy can be performed but there is a high risk of hemorrhage. Treatment is by surgical resection which can include lobectomy, bilobectomy, pneumonectomy, or sleeve resection with regional lymphadenectomy. Intraoperative frozen section is useful to assure complete resection and to limit lung resection. Endobronchial cryoablation may reduce tumor size, permitting less extensive resection. Carcinoid syndrome is rare and a sign of extrapulmonary disease.[36]

Table 97.1. Primary Pulmonary Neoplasms

Type of Tumor	CT Findings
Benign	
Inflammatory myofibroblastic tumor	Well-defined solitary masses, peripheral and lower lobe, amorphous or dystrophic calcification
Pulmonary hamartoma	Well-circumcised, peripheral, intralesion fat, and calcifications
Primary sclerosing hemangioma	Well-defined smooth round or oval enhancing mass adjacent to pleura
Subglottic hemangioma	Mass in subglottic trachea with early intense contrast enhancement
Recurrent respiratory papillomatosis	Numerous nodular lesions within the airway
Malignant	
Pleuropulmonary blastoma	Varied appearance, peripherally located, often multiple lobes, usually right
Adenocarcinoma	Solitary nodule to complete opacification of lung, ground glass to solid
Kaposi sarcoma	Bilateral perihilar opacities and large pleural effusions
Carcinoid and other neuroendocrine	Well-defined lobulated endobronchial mass with marked enhancement, calcification 30%
Mucoepidermoid carcinoma	Central mass or endobronchial nodule, calcification 50%

Bronchogenic Carcinoma

Bronchogenic carcinoma is the second most common malignant lung tumor in children. Bronchogenic carcinoma consists of adenocarcinoma and undifferentiated carcinomas in the pediatric population. These tumors have been associated with CPAMs but have been reported in normal lung as well. Human papilloma virus has been associated with the squamous cell variant. Resection with ipsilateral lymphadenectomy is the treatment of choice. Prognosis for bronchogenic carcinoma is poor as the presentation tends to be with advanced stages. Symptoms are related to metastases with bone pain or tumor burden with weight loss.[36]

Pleuropulmonary Blastoma

PPB is the third most frequent lung tumor in children and is most common in children under 4 years of age. Increasingly, lesions with high-risk features (large, multilobar) are being identified on prenatal ultrasound. The lesion consists of mesenchymal elements and embryonal stroma without epithelial neoplasia. The tumor is known to be part of the spectrum of tumors related to the mutation of the *DICER1* gene. The tumor usually presents peripherally. These tumors are associated with CPAMs. There are three types: type I consisting of multilocular cysts, type II consisting of a combination of cystic and solid components, and type III having proliferating mesenchyme without cysts. Treatment is with resection and adjuvant chemotherapy. Survival in type I has been reported at 91% while type II/III have survivals of 43%.[37,38] A PPB registry has expanded understanding of this tumor.[38]

Other Malignant Tumors

Sarcomas, including fibrosarcoma, rhabdomyosarcoma, and leiomyosarcoma, are the next most common primary malignant lung neoplasm in children. These have been reported to arise in documented cystic disease.[35] Inflammatory pseudotumor is considered to be the most common "benign" tumor in children. The tumor is a myofibroblastic spindle cell soft tissue tumor with infiltrative plasma cells, lymphocytes, and eosinophils. Recently these have been classified as intermediary lesions with a molecular rearrangement involving the tyrosine kinase receptor anaplastic lymphoma kinase. Symptoms are nonspecific such as fever, chest pain, cough, and recurrent pneumonias.[35] They may present as an endobronchial lesion but are more often peripherally located. The lesion may invade local structures and be aggressive locally and may recur locally but spontaneous regression has been reported. Complete resection is recommended as no adjuvant regimen has gained widespread acceptance. Nonsteroidal antiinflammatory agents have been utilized with some success (**Fig. 97.17**).

Hamartoma

Hamartomas are lung nodules composed of cartilage and gland-like formations in an irregular and haphazard orientation. They grow slowly and are the most common benign lesion in adults but the second most common in children.[35] Radiographically, they have a "popcorn" calcification in 10% to 25% of cases. The majority are located in the periphery of the lung. Conservative surgical resection is recommended. These may be associated with gastric smooth muscle tumors and extraadrenal paragangliomas (Carney triad) in adolescent

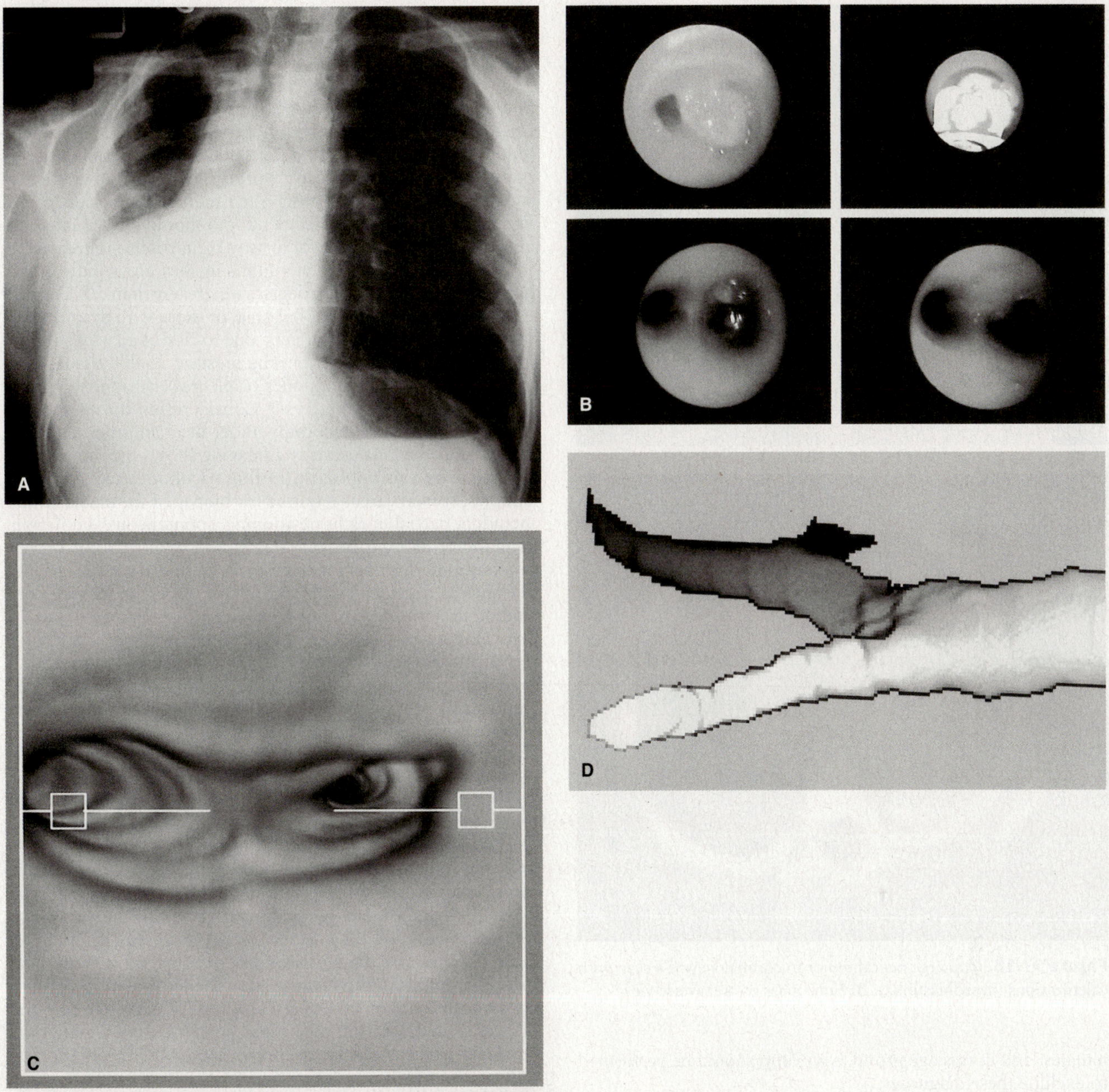

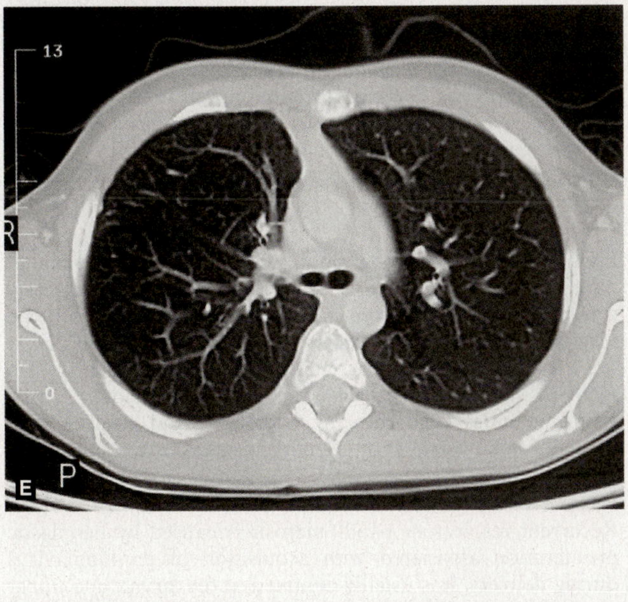

Figure 97.17. Lung neoplasm in an 8-year-old child: inflammatory pseudotumor. **A:** Presenting chest radiograph with right lung collapse. **B:** Biopsy of an obstructing endobronchial mass demonstrates inflammatory pseudotumor (inflammatory myofibroblastic tumor). **C:** CT "virtual bronchoscopy" image after initial biopsy demonstrates deformation of the right main stem bronchus and carina due to tumor infiltration. **D:** CT reconstruction of the external appearance of airways demonstrating the deformation of the carina and right main stem bronchus. The child underwent excision of the right main stem bronchus and carina and tracheobronchial reconstruction. **E:** Postoperative transverse thoracic CT at the level of the reconstruction of the carina.

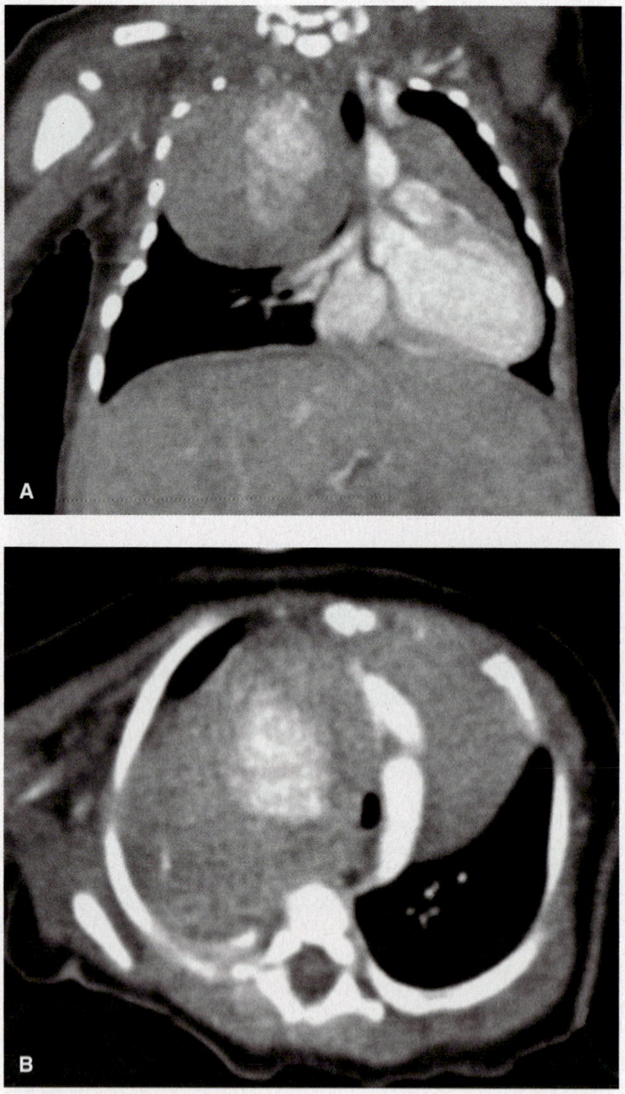

Figure 97.18. **A:** Large neural tumor in coronal view CT scan with calcifications (neuroblastoma). **B:** Same mass on transverse view.

females; and in this age group, a workup should be performed to exclude these diagnoses.

Mediastinal Tumors

Mediastinal tumors in the pediatric population can be benign (63%) or malignant (37%).[39] Neurogenic tumors are the most common, arising in the posterior mediastinum from the sympathetic ganglia, intercostal nerves, and paraganglia cells. They may grow very large before detection and may manifest with Horner syndrome or opsoclonus–myoclonus syndrome. Malignant neurogenic tumors include neuroblastoma and ganglio-neuroblastoma. Benign tumors include ganglioneuroma, schwannoma, or neurofibroma.[39] Neuroblastoma originating in the mediastinum has a better prognosis than other sites. These tumors have more favorable biology and lower rates of N-myc amplification as well as improved rates of event-free and overall survival. Diagnosis is by CT and MRI with MRI allowing improved assessment of extension into the spinal foramina.[39] Tumors may be resected by a thoracoscopic approach or via thoracotomy (**Fig. 97.18**).[40]

Neurofibromas and schwannomas arise from intercostal nerves or sympathetic nerves. The schwannomas are encapsulated without nerve fibers within the tissue. Neurofibromas are unencapsulated, have nerve fibers running through the mass, and are common in patients with neurofibromatosis.[40] Isolated tumors may be removed but tumors associated with neurofibromatosis tend to extend over nerve sheaths precluding complete removal. These are associated with malignant degeneration.

Lymphomas arise in the anterior and middle mediastinum and are the most common anterior mediastinal mass in children.[39] They are usually inhomogeneous and resection is not required. Both Hodgkin and non-Hodgkin lymphoma arise in the mediastinum. Diagnostic workup involves biopsy for tissue diagnosis as the diagnosis often requires tissue subtyping. Patients with large mediastinal tumors should be evaluated for airway compromise. Risk of airway compromise is greatest in those with non-Hodgkin lymphoma as they are rapidly growing. Risk is increased in patients with greater than 50% reduction in tracheal cross-sectional area, or those with dyspnea and orthopnea. In high-risk patients, due to risk of airway collapse under anesthesia or sedation, the most accessible tissue, such as supraclavicular lymph nodes or pleural effusion, should be sampled under local anesthesia. Consideration for an anterior second interspace thoracotomy under local anesthesia can get access to mediastinal tumors if imaging shows the tumor to be accessible by this approach. In those without access to these samples, special care is required for biopsy of the mediastinum including partial upright positioning, spontaneous ventilation, availability of rigid bronchoscope, and avoidance of muscle relaxants. If the risk for anesthesia is too great for general anesthesia, treatment with steroids or radiation can be considered to shrink the tumor to make subsequent biopsy safer. This may make pathologic diagnosis challenging and change the chemotherapy for patients.

Teratomas are the most common mediastinal germ cell tumor and are composed of all three germinal cell layers. They are typically benign, usually cystic, and encapsulated (**Fig. 97.19**). They frequently contain calcification on radiography. Most are asymptomatic but symptoms can include stridor, tachypnea, and respiratory distress especially when lying supine.[39] The cysts frequently contain mature ectodermal elements such as hair, skin, and neuroglial elements and may contain bone, teeth, and fat. The tumors may be large and tend to displace rather than invade surrounding tissue. Workup includes preoperative measurement of α-fetoprotein and β-HCG. Resection is the treatment of choice and confirms the diagnosis and depending on the size and location of the tumor can be approached by thoracotomy, sternotomy, or thoracoscopy. Treatment of mature teratomas is resection. Immature teratomas which contain malignant elements are treated with chemotherapy and radiation in addition to surgery.

Other mediastinal tumors are very rare but often require surgical biopsy or extirpation. These include neurolemmoma, pheochromocytoma germ cell tumors, rhabdomyosarcomas, and thymic tumors, including resections in the setting of myasthenia gravis. Thymic resection may be completed via a cervical approach, sternotomy, or thoracotomy, but now is frequently done with a thoracoscopic approach, which may be from either side.

Chest Wall Tumors

Ewing sarcoma, chondrosarcoma, and liposarcoma are malignant tumors which may arise from the chest wall. Local resection may require extensive chest wall excision and prosthetic reconstruction. Primitive neuroectodermal tumors are malignant small cell tumors carrying a poor prognosis. Improvement in survival is accomplished with multimodal therapy which includes chemotherapy, radiation, and surgery with aggressive management of pulmonary metastases.[41]

Respiratory Papillomatosis

Recurrent respiratory papillomatosis is caused by neoplastic proliferation associated with acquisition of papillomavirus during delivery. It is usually confined to the larynx and upper tracheal airway with spread in less than 1% of cases. Treatment

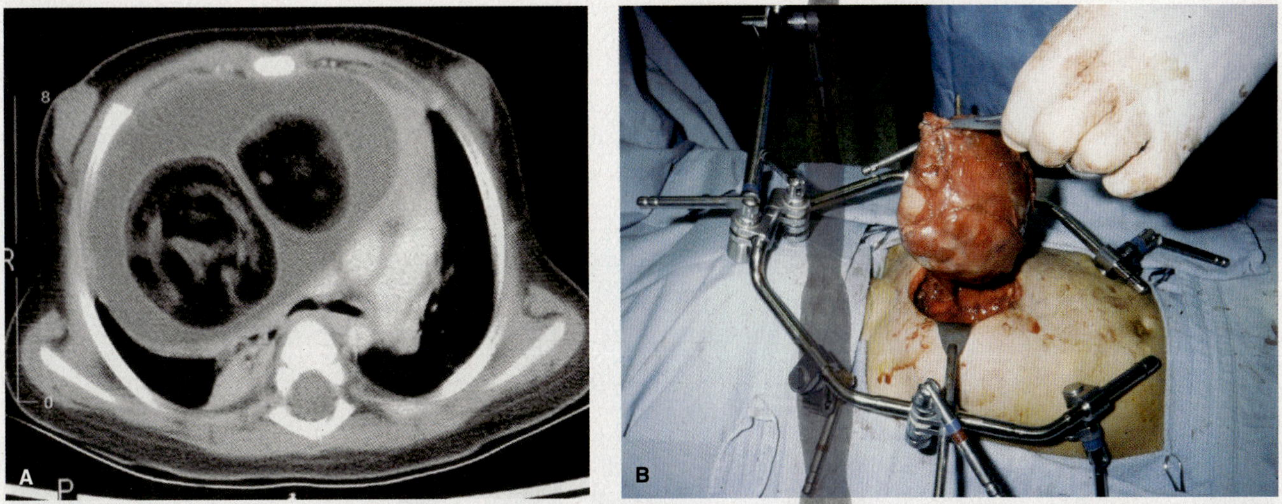

Figure 97.19. Mediastinal teratoma. **A:** Transverse thoracic CT of a large anterior mediastinal teratoma presenting with airway compression symptoms in a 9-month-old female. **B:** Tumor removal via a median sternotomy.

is with laser ablation and may require multiple treatments. Prognosis is poor due to the recurrence of the disease.[39]

CHEST WALL DEFORMITIES

Deformities of the chest wall may be obvious at birth but often become more noticeable at the time of preadolescent and adolescent growth. The physical appearance may vary from barely detectable to severely deforming. Although there may be some physiologic benefit from surgical correction of these deformities, restoration of a more normal appearance is equally important in the decision to treat. The impact of these deformities on normal psychosocial development, as well as evidence of cardiorespiratory impairment, justifies correction.

Embryology, Development, and Etiology of Chest Wall Deformities

Ribs are derived from individual somites as mesoderm differentiates into cartilage and advances ventrally toward the developing sternum. Rib cartilage eventually approaches the sternum. The sternum is derived independently from two parallel bands of mesoderm that develop away from the midline. The two sternal bands fuse cranial to caudal and become progressively chondrified. Transverse divisions of the cartilaginous sternum differentiate into segments opposite each end of the rib pairs. At birth, small ossification centers are present in the sternum; the ribs have largely ossified. Final ossification is usually complete by mid adolescence. The timing of sternal ossification is sufficiently predictable to be a reliable method of determining bone age. There is a sharp demarcation in each rib between the ossified portion and the cartilaginous portion, with the latter becoming ossified only much later in life. The etiology of chest wall deformities is uncertain. Abnormal intrauterine pressure applied to the chest, abnormalities of diaphragmatic development, connective tissue abnormalities, and genetic predisposition may contribute. Abnormal, excessive, or asymmetric growth of the costal cartilages associated with the 3rd to 10th ribs is most implicated.[42] Sternal clefts result from a failure of fusion of portions of the sternal bands.

Pectus Excavatum

Pectus excavatum from the Latin "hollowed chest" is the most common deformity of the anterior chest wall occurring in 1 in 400 to 1 in 1,000 children, accounting for the majority of chest wall deformities. A family history is present in half.[42,43] There is male predominance. Pectus excavatum results from abnormal regulation of the growth of the costal cartilages. There is a corresponding posterior curve in the body of the sternum beginning at the manubrium and extending to the xiphoid. The deformity is rarely precisely symmetric, with one side (usually the right) slightly more curved in than the other. Asymmetry may be pronounced with the sternum rotated nearly to the sagittal plane. The deformity may be apparent at birth but often becomes more apparent during adolescence. Scoliosis is increased in this population although rarely needs surgical correction. Patients often have an asthenic build and stoop-shouldered posture. Connective tissue disorders are associated with pectus excavatum. The diagnosis of Marfan syndrome should be considered.

Concerns about cardiopulmonary implications are often paramount in the mind of the referring physician as well as the family. Many patients will have complaints of chest pain and/or shortness of breath. Most patients are disturbed by the appearance of the deformity, and some may be profoundly depressed and dysfunctional. The physiologic consequences of the deformity are less certain. Invasive and echocardiographic assessment of cardiovascular performance has demonstrated improvement in cardiac function and resolution of mitral valve prolapse in some patients following surgical correction of pectus excavatum. Studies have also demonstrated improved body image and subjective physical ability.[42–44] The cardiorespiratory benefits of the repair remain controversial with more recent studies demonstrating improvement after bar removal especially with dynamic testing.[44] Multiple studies confirm patient and parent satisfaction.[42–45] Clinical assessment of the severity of the deformity has included chest radiographs, CT scans, caliper measurements, contrast volume measurements of the cavity, and more recently three-dimensional image scanning. Indices, including the "Haller Index," the Compression Index, and the Depression Index help quantitate the deformity. An echocardiogram is usually indicated. Pulmonary function testing may be helpful.

Surgical Correction of the Pectus Excavatum

10 Although pectus excavatum may be present in infants and young children, repair should be deferred to adolescence to avoid recurrence and acquired thoracic dystrophy.

"Open" Operations

Traditional "open" surgical correction was performed through an inframammary incision (**Fig. 97.20**). The operation requires the exposure of costal cartilage by elevation of the pectoral muscles from the chest wall. The involved cartilages usually from 3 to 7 and parts of 8, 9, and 10 are removed by subperichondrial

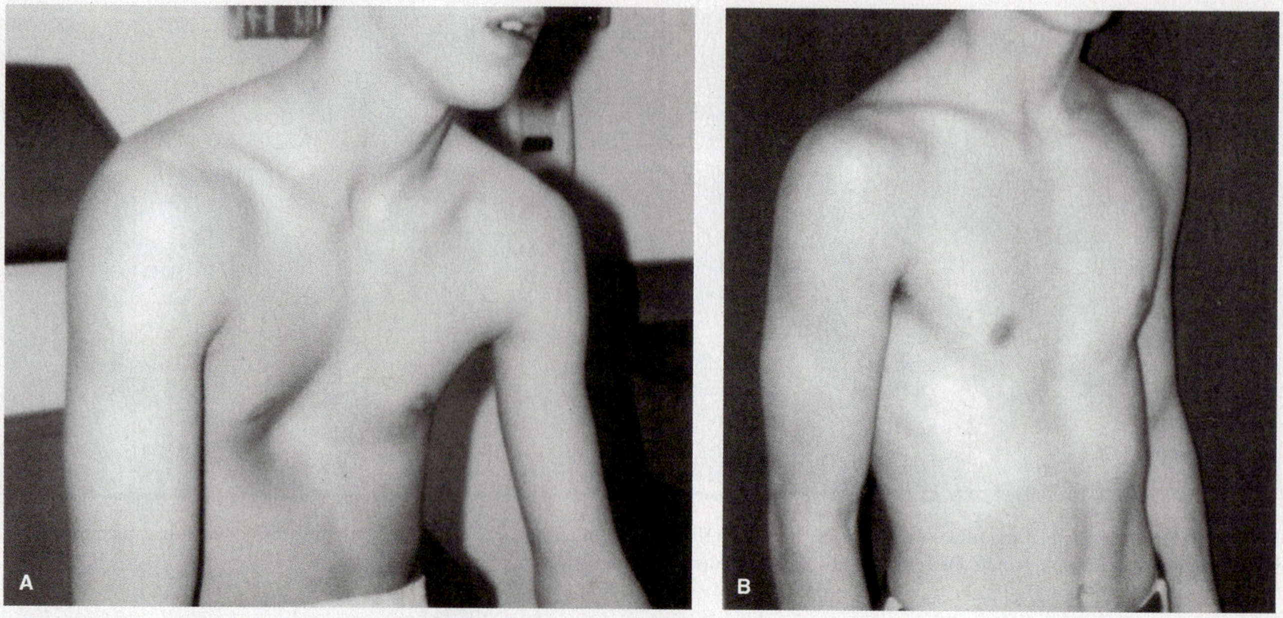

Figure 97.20. Pectus excavatum. **A:** Appearance of an adolescent male with a typical depression deformity. Note "stoop-shouldered" posture. **B:** Postoperative appearance at 6 months. Erect posture and subpectoral incision give a good cosmetic result.

excision, with careful preservation of the perichondral sheaths. The xiphoid is detached from the sternum and the rectus muscles are detached inferiorly. The undersurface of the sternum is dissected free of the pericardium and pleura. A transverse wedge osteotomy is created in the sternum at the point where the sternum deflects posteriorly and the posterior surface is gently fractured. A strut is usually placed beneath the sternum to maintain the position of the sternum. The strut, typically a stainless steel bar, is removed in 6 months to 1 year.[42] The pectoral and rectus muscles are reapproximated. Closed suction drains are usually left in place in the submuscular layer. Pain is controlled using multimodal techniques. Complications may include pneumothorax, wound seromas, pleural effusions, and recurrence. Migration of implanted struts and bars has caused the most serious problems, including cardiac injury.

Minimally Invasive Repair/Nuss Procedure

Since its description in 1998 by Nuss, the MIS repair has gained widespread popularity. Conspicuous incisions, resection, and osteotomies are avoided. Using small lateral incisions and sternal elevation, one or two rigid U-shaped bars are inserted transversely across the chest and then "flipped." The sternum is pushed back into a normal position (**Fig. 97.21**).[46] Modifications of the technique including the use of stabilizers, crossing bars, and routine use of thoracoscopy to guide bar insertion.[42,47] Reported complications include pneumothorax, cardiac injury, bar displacement, chronic pain, pericarditis, allergic metal reactions, and extraosseous bone formation.[47] Multimodal postoperative pain management and intercostal nerve cryoablation shorten hospital stay. The bar is left in for up to 3 years during a period of development when most children are active and may engage in contact sports. Graded activity restrictions allow return to normal activity while the bar is in place. Recent studies have demonstrated that the early-to-late teenage years are the appropriate time for repair.[45] Older teenagers and young adults can also undergo repair.

Pectus Carinatum

11 Pectus carinatum, from the Latin word for "keel," is a chest wall defect where there is a protrusion of the sternum and ribs. This type of defect occurs less commonly than pectus excavatum and is present in 1 in 1,000 to 1,500 teenagers. Physiologic impairment is absent; however, the concern for appearance may be even greater than with depression deformities of the chest wall. Protrusion deformities may be very difficult to hide even when fully clothed. Rapid growth of the costal cartilages occurring during puberty makes the deformity more pronounced at that time. Compression bracing is the first choice for correction of most pectus carinatum deformities, with surgery reserved for failures of therapy. Bracing is most successful when performed for more than 16 hours per day. Surgical correction involves costal cartilage resection and sternal osteotomies. MIS techniques use a bar passed anterior to the sternum.

Poland Syndrome

Named after the English surgeon Sir Alfred Poland, this rare congenital syndrome occurs in 1 in 30,000 births and includes a hypoplasia or aplasia of the thoracic wall components. These features may include absence of the sternal portions of the pectoralis major muscle; absence of the pectoralis minor muscle; absence of portions of the serratus anterior and external oblique muscles; forearm and hand deformities; ipsilateral hypoplasia of the nipple, breast, and chest wall subcutaneous tissues; absence or deformity of the second to fifth costal cartilages; and absence of axillary hair on the affected side. Surgical treatment includes correction of any deformed ribs, formation of the anterior axillary fold using the latissimus dorsi muscle, and creation of the ipsilateral breast in females. Minor forms of this developmental abnormality are more common.

Sternal Clefts

Congenital sternal clefts result from failure of midline fusion of the paired sternal bands. The cleft is usually in the superior portion of the sternum and may extend to but not include the xiphoid. The defects are rare and are usually repaired in the neonatal period when the chest is more pliable. The purpose of the correction is to protect the underlying mediastinal structures. After subcutaneous and substernal mobilization, the fibrocartilaginous sternal bars are approximated in the midline. If the cardiac structures are at risk, more elaborate repairs are required. Typically, the cleft is incomplete and a V-shaped excision of the sternum at the most inferior aspect of the cleft may be required to avoid buckling of the sternum. Pentalogy of Cantrell refers to a distal sternal cleft, omphalocele, diaphragmatic defect, pericardial defect, and intracardiac defect.

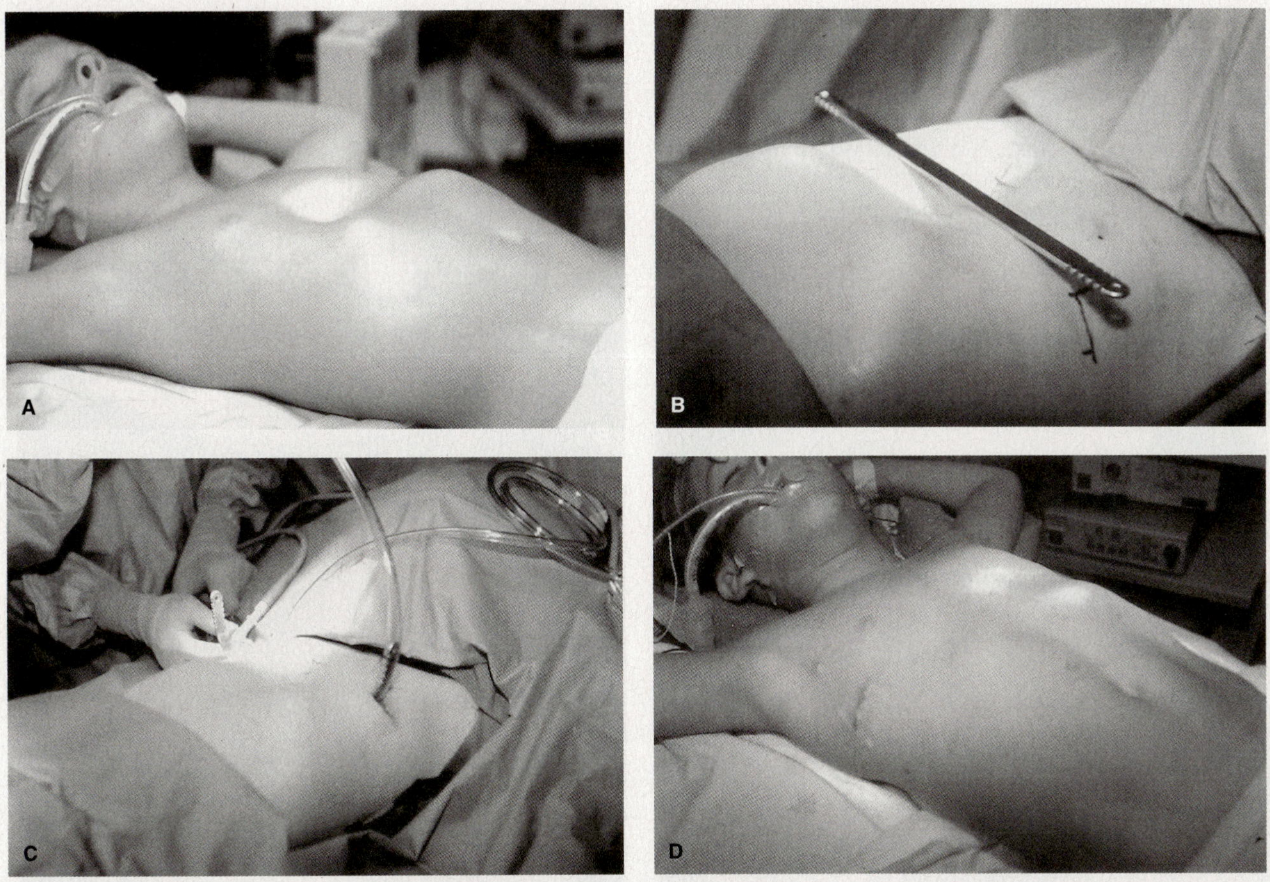

Figure 97.21. Thoracoscopically assisted Lorenz Bar insertion (Nuss procedure). A: Preoperative appearance with symmetrical depression deformity. B: Lorenz bar. C: Pectus excavatum bar inserted with thoracoscopic guidance. D: Immediate postoperative appearance. (Digital images provided by William Hardin, MD, University of Alabama, used with permission.)

Thoracic ectopia cordis (exstrophy of the heart) may occur as a part of this abnormality and this spectrum continues to have a high mortality.

Jeune Asphyxiating Thoracic Dystrophy

Jeune asphyxiating thoracic dystrophy is a rare developmental abnormality that results in the failure of chest wall growth. Traditional surgical procedures have involved sternotomies with placement of graft material to expand the chest. More recently, a vertically expandable prosthetic titanium rib (VEPTR) device has been used. The posterior aspect of the ribs (typically 3 to 9) is divided along with the costochondral junction. The rib plate is then elevated to the curved VEPTR strut by wires, thus expanding the chest. This is done for both chests, and the device is serially expanded to promote chest enlargement.

The "Slipping Rib" Syndrome

Slipping rib syndrome is an unusual cause for recurrent lower chest and upper abdominal pain. The cause is likely an inadequacy or rupture of interchondral fibrous attachments of the 9th or 10th rib. The symptoms tend to be a popping or clicking sensation with truncal movement associated with pain. Pain is usually reproducible with manipulation of the rib cartilage anteriorly. Surgical therapy involves excision of the affected rib and cartilage relieving pressure on the involved intercostal nerve.[48]

"Flaring" of the Costal Margin

Patients are sometimes referred for surgical opinions regarding unusual prominence of the costal margin. The "flaring" is most pronounced when the patient is supine. This finding represents a variation of the normal development of the chest wall. Surgical correction is usually unnecessary, but may be combined with pectus excavatum repair.

PLEURAL DISEASES

Empyema

Empyema is the accumulation of purulent material in the pleural space. In children, empyema is most often the sequelae of bacterial pneumonia. Empyema develops when a parapneumonic effusion becomes infected or when a necrotizing pneumonia erodes into the pleural space. Empyema may also be caused by penetrating thoracic trauma, intrathoracic, or cervical esophageal perforation or as a complication from surgery on the chest. The American Thoracic Society divides the empyema process into three stages:

1. Exudative: Thin free-flowing fluid with a low cell count.
2. Fibrinopurulent: Frank pus is present and fibrin formation begins to cover the pleura with development of loculations.
3. Organizing: Thick peel with fibroblasts.[49]

The most common organism responsible for empyema is *Streptococcus pneumoniae*. Other common organisms are *Staphylococcus aureus* and *Haemophilus influenzae*.[49] The signs and symptoms include worsening pneumonia with fever, tachypnea, dyspnea, and sometimes cyanosis. Abdominal pain may be present. Chest radiograph demonstrates the presence of fluid and loculation. CT imaging is the best method of determining the extent of loculated fluid versus underlying pulmonary pathology (**Fig. 97.22**).

With a small amount of fluid, the empyema may resolve with antibiotics alone. When the collection becomes larger, the treatment is drainage of the collection. Several trials have compared fibrinolytics to video-assisted thoracoscopy (VATS). Both VATS and chest tube with fibrinolytics have been shown to be effective with a systematic review demonstrating no superiority of VATS. Other studies have demonstrated improvement after VATS.[49]

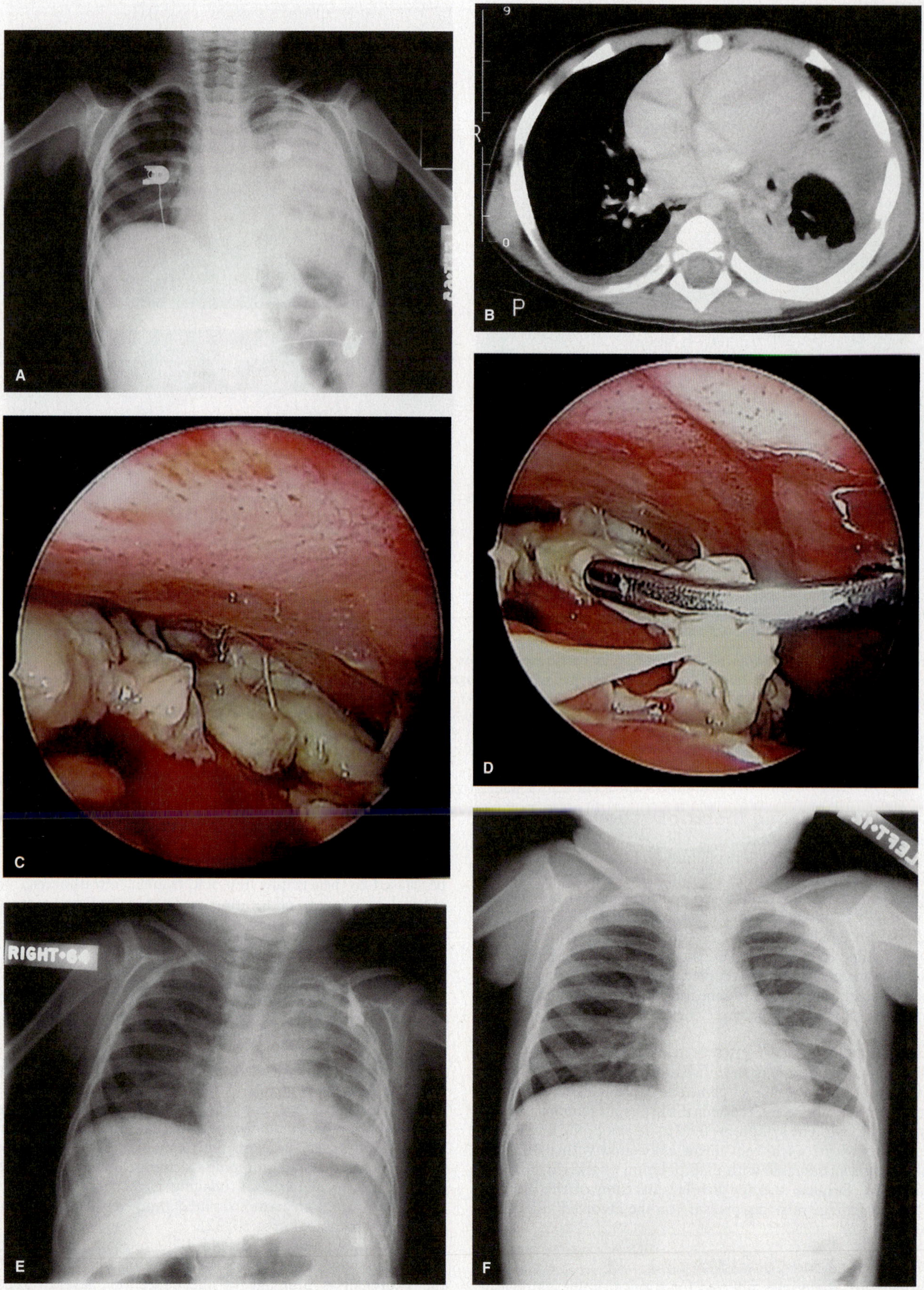

Figure 97.22. Video-assisted thoracoscopic treatment of complicated empyema in children. **A:** Chest radiograph of a 2-year-old child presenting with pneumonia and pleural effusion. **B:** CT demonstrates complicated pneumonia with loculated empyema. **C:** Video endoscopic view of organized empyema debris. **D:** "Decortication" procedure includes removal of all loculated, organized debris from the hemithorax. All surfaces of the visceral and parietal pleura are accessible using video endoscopic techniques. **E:** Immediate postoperative chest x-ray shows the expected residual parenchymal lung disease. **F:** One month later, the chest radiograph findings have resolved.

Pneumothorax

Spontaneous pneumothorax is relatively uncommon. The etiology seems to be lung connective tissue changes predisposing to leaks into the pleural space. Apical lung blebs are associated with the disease. The presentation is usually with chest pain and shortness of breath but may also be associated with cough. The pain may be pleuritic in nature. Diagnosis is best confirmed with chest radiograph. Chest CT has been utilized for identification of blebs but a negative examination does not predict freedom from recurrence.

Treatment of pneumothorax depends on the patient. Observation with or without high-flow oxygen is appropriate for the relatively asymptomatic patient. Chest tube placement is the next stage of treatment. VATS with bleb resection and pleurodesis has also been described with good results. For recurrent pneumothoraces, intrapleural sclerosing agents as well as pleurectomy may be used.

Chylothorax

Chylothorax, the accumulation of chyle in the pleural space, is a rare cause of effusion in children but is the most common cause in the neonate.[50] Chylothorax is associated with pulmonary lymphangiomas and lymphangiectasia. Chylothorax may also be a manifestation of Down, Turner, and Noonan syndromes. Chylothorax may occur due to trauma to the thoracic duct, either iatrogenic or due to blunt trauma. Malignancy and granulomatous diseases may cause obstruction of the thoracic duct leading to chylothorax.

The initial symptoms are related to accumulation of fluid in the pleural space with dyspnea, cough, and chest discomfort. Pleuritic pain and fever are rare. Diagnosis is by chest radiograph combined with findings on thoracentesis. The fluid is usually milky in appearance with triglycerides greater than 1.1 mmol/L, total cell count greater than 1,000 cells per mL, and lymphocyte predominance greater than 80%.[50]

Management consists of expansion of the lung with thoracentesis or tube thoracostomy. Minimization of lymph flow is managed by either parenteral nutrition or diet manipulation using medium-chain fatty acids. Long-term loss of lymphatic fluid can lead to life-threatening immunologic problems. Surgical management includes thoracic duct ligation, performed either via thoracotomy or thoracoscopy. As the thoracic duct may be difficult to identify, suture ligation of the entire posterior diaphragmatic chest wall junction may be necessary. Administration of cream via a nasogastric tube in the hours before surgery may facilitate identification of the leak. Pleurectomy and pleurodesis or pleuroperitoneal shunting may also be used.

ACKNOWLEDGMENT

We gratefully acknowledge the contributions of previous edition author, Robert E. Cilley, as portions of those chapters have been retained in this revision.

References

1. van den Hout L, Schaible T, Cohen-Overbeek TE, et al. Actual outcome in infants with congenital diaphragmatic hernia: the role of a standardized postnatal treatment protocol. *Fetal Diagn Ther.* 2011;29(1):55–63.
2. Kardon G, Ackerman KG, McCulley DJ, et al. Congenial diaphragmatic hernias: from genes to mechanisms to therapies. *Dis Model Mech.* 2017;10(8):955–970.
3. Basurto D, Russo FM, van der Veeken L, et al. Prenatal diagnosis and management of congenital diaphragmatic hernia. *Best Pract Res Clin Obstet Gynecol.* 2019;58:93–106.
4. Oh C, Youn JK, Han JW, et al. Predicting survival of congenital diaphragmatic hernia on the first day of life. *World J Surg.* 2019; 43(1):282–290.
5. Delaplain PT, Harting MT, Jancelewicz T et al. Potential survival benefit with repair of congenital diaphragmatic hernia after extracorporeal membrane oxygenation in select patients: Study by ELSO CDH group. *J Pediatr Surg.* 2019;54(6): 1132–1137.
6. Aydin E, Nolan H, Peiro JL, et al. When primary repair is not enough: a comparison of synthetic patch and muscle flap closure in congenital diaphragmatic hernia? *Pediatr Surg Int.* 2020;36(4): 485–491.
7. Chan E, Wayne C, Nasr A. Minimally invasive versus open repair of Bochdalek hernia: a meta-analysis. *J Pediatr Surg.* 2014;49(5): 694–699.
8. Wigen RB, Duan W, Moraes TJ, Chiu PPL. Predictors of long-term pulmonary morbidity in children with congenital diaphragmatic hernia. *Eur J Pediatr Surg.* 2019;29(1):120–124.
9. Harrison MR, Keller RL, Hawgood SB, et al. A randomized trial of fetal endoscopic tracheal occlusion for severe fetal congenital diaphragmatic hernia. *N Engl J Med.* 349(20):1916–1924.
10. Deprest JA, Nicolaides KH, Benachi A, et al. Randomized trial of fetal surgery for severe left diaphragmatic hernia. *N Engl J Med.* 385(2):107–118.
11. Tan YW, Banerjee D, Cross KM, et al. Morgagni hernia repair in children over two decades: institutional experience, systematic review, and meta-analysis of 296 patients. *J Pediatr Surg.* 2018; 53(10):1883–1889.
12. Hu J, Wu Y, Wang J, et al. Thoracoscopic and laparoscopic plication of the hemidiaphragm is effective in the management of diaphragmatic eventration. *Pediatr Surg Int.* 2014;30(1): 19–24.
13. Diep B, Wang A, Kun S, et al. Diaphragm pacing without tracheostomy in congenital central hypoventilation syndrome patients. *Respiration.* 2015;89(6):534–538.
14. Lal DR, Gadepalli SK, Downard CD, et al. Challenging surgical dogma in the management of proximal esophageal atresia with distal tracheoesophageal fistula: outcomes from the midwest pediatric surgery consortium. *J Pediatr Surg.* 2018;53(7): 1267–1272.
15. Bairdain S, Hamilton TE, Smithers CJ, et al. Foker process for the correction of long gap esophageal atresia: Primary treatment versus secondary treatment after prior esophageal surgery. *J Pediatr Surg.* 2015;50(6):933–937.
16. Densmore JC, Oldham KT, Dominguez KM, et al. Neonatal esophageal trachealization and esophagocarinoplasty in the treatment of flow-limited Floyd II tracheal agenesis. *J Thorac Cardiovasc Surg.* 2017;153(6):e121–e125.
17. Baird R, Lal DR, Ricca RL, et al. Management of long gap esophageal atresia: a systematic review and evidence-based guidelines from the APSA outcomes and evidence-based practice committee. *J Pediatr Surg.* 2019;54(4):675–687.
18. Way C, Wayne C, Grandpierre V, Harrison BJ, Travis N, Nasr A. Thoracoscopy vs. thoracotomy for the repair of esophageal atresia and tracheoesophageal fistula: a systematic review and meta-analysis. *Pediatr Surg Int.* 2019;35(11):1167–1184.
19. van der Zee DC, Gallo G, Tytgat SHA. Thoracoscopic traction technique in long gap esophageal atresia: entering a new era. *Surg Endosc.* 2015;29(11):3324–3330.
20. Yasuda JL, Taslitsky GN, Staffa SJ, et al. Utility of repeated therapeutic endoscopies for pediatric esophageal strictures. *Dis Esophagus.* 2020;33(12):doaa031.
21. Friedmacher F, Kroneis B, Huber-Zeyringer A, et al. Postoperative complications and functional outcome after esophageal atresia repair: results from longitudinal single-center follow-up. *J Gastrointest Surg.* 2017;21(6):927–935.
22. Singh A, Middlesworth W, Khlevner J. Surveillance in patients with esophageal atresia/tracheoesophageal fistula. *Curr Gastroenterol Rep.* 2017;19(1):4.
23. Michaud L, Coutenier F, Podevin G, et al. Characteristics and management of congenital esophageal stenosis: findings from a multicenter study. *Orphanet J Rare Dis.* 2013;8:186.
24. Wick MR. Cystic lesions of the mediastinum. *Semin Diagn Pathol.* 2005;22(3):241–253.
25. Backer CL, Mongé MC, Popescu AR, Eltayeb OM, Rastatter JC, Rigsby CK. Vascular rings. *Semin Pediatr Surg.* 2016;25(3): 165–175.
26. Butler CR, Speggiorin S, Rijnberg FM, et al. Outcomes of slide tracheoplasty in 101 children: a 17-year single-center experience. *J Thorac Cardiovasc Surg.* 2014;147(6):1783–1789.

27. Pitiot V, Grall M, Ploin D, Truy E, Ayari Khalfallah S. The use of CT-scan in foreign body aspiration in children: a 6 years' experience. *Int J Pediatr Otorhinolaryngol.* 2017;102:169–173.
28. Zobel M, Gologorsky R, Lee H, Vu L. Congenital lung lesions. *Semin Pediatr Surg.* 2018;28(4):1–9.
29. Adams S, Jobson M, Sangnawakij P, et al. Does thoracoscopy have advantages over open surgery for asymptomatic congenital lung malformations? An analysis of 1626 resections. *J Pediatr Surg.* 2017;52(2):247–251.
30. Rothenberg SS, Shipman K, Kay S, et al. Thoracoscopic segmentectomy for congenital and acquired pulmonary disease: a case for lung-sparing surgery. *J Laparoendosc Adv Surg Tech A.* 2014;23(1):50–54.
31. Downard CD, Calkins CM, Williams RF, et al. Treatment of congenital pulmonary airway malformations: a systematic review from the APSA outcomes and evidence based practice committee. *Pediatr Surg Int.* 2017;33(9):939–953.
32. Triana P, Dore M, Nunez Cerezo V, et al. Sirolimus in the treatment of vascular anomalies. *Eur J Pediatr Surg.* 2017;27(1):86–90.
33. Zapala MA, Ho-Fung VM, Lee EY. Thoracic neoplasms in children. Contemporary perspectives and imaging assessment. *Radiol Clin North Am.* 2017;55(4):657–676.
34. Erginel B, Soysal FG, Keskin E, Kebudi R, Celik A, Salman T. Pulmonary metastectomy in pediatric patients. *World J Surg Oncol.* 2016;14:27.
35. Lichtenberger JP 3rd, Biko DM, Carter BW, Pavio MA, Huppmann AR, Chung EM. Primary lung tumors in children: Radiologic-pathologic correlation from the radiologic pathology archives. *Radiographics.* 2018;38(7):2151–2172.
36. Varela P, Pio L, Torre M. Primary tracheobronchial tumors in children. *Semin Pediatr Surg.* 2016;25(3):150–155.
37. Zamora AK, Zobel MJ, Ourshalimian S, Zhou S, Shillingford NM, Kim ES. The effect of gross total resection on patients with pleuropulmonary blastoma. *J Surg Res.* 2020;253:115–120.
38. Messinger YH, Stewart DR, Priest JR, et al. Pleuropulmonary blastoma: a report on 350 central pathology-confirmed pleuropulmonary blastoma cases by the International Pleuropulmonary Blastoma Registry. *Cancer.* 2015;121(2):276–285.
39. Gun F, Erginel B, Unüvar A, Kebudi R, Salman T, Celik A. Mediastinal masses in children: experience with 120 cases. *Pediatr Hematol Oncol.* 2012;29(2):141–147.
40. Fraga JC, Aydogdu B, Aufieri R, et al. Surgical treatment for pediatric mediastinal neurogenic tumors. *Ann Thorac Surg.* 2010;90(2):413–418.
41. Saltsman JA, Danzer E, Hammond WJ, et al. Survival and scoliosis following resection of chest wall tumors in children and adolescents. A single-center retrospective analysis. *Ann Surg.* 2021;274(2):e167–e173.
42. Mao YZ, Tang ST, Li S. Comparison of the Nuss versus Ravitch procedure for pectus excavatum repair: an updated meta-analysis. *J Pediatr Surg.* 2017;52(10):1545–1552.
43. Goretzky MJ, Kelly RE Jr, Croitoru D, Nuss D. Chest wall anomalies: pectus excavatum and pectus carinatum. *Adolesc Med Clin.* 2004;15(3):455–471.
44. Wang Q, Fan S, Wu C, Jin X, Pan Z, Hong D. Changes in resting pulmonary function testing over time after the Nuss procedure: a systematic review and meta-analysis. *J Pediatr Surg.* 2018;53(11):2299–2306.
45. Nuss D, Obermeyer RJ, Kelly RE. Nuss bar procedure: past, present, and future. *Ann Cardiothorac Surg.* 2016;5(5):422–433.
46. Nuss D, Kelly RE Jr, Croitoru DP, Katz ME. A 10-year review of a minimally invasive technique for the correction of pectus excavatum. *J Pediatr Surg.* 1998;33(4):545–552.
47. Notrica DM. The Nuss procedure for the repair of pectus excavatum: 20 error traps and a culture of safety. *Semin Pediatr Surg.* 2019;28(3):172–177.
48. McMahon LE. Slipping rib syndrome: a review of evaluation, diagnosis and treatment. *Semin Pediatr Surg.* 2018;27(3):183–188.
49. Griffith D, Boal M, Rogers T. Evolution of practice in the management of parapneumonic effusion and empyema in children. *J Pediatr Surg.* 2018;53(4):644–646.
50. Church JT, Antunez AG, Dean A, et al. Evidence-based management of chylothorax in infants. *J Pediatr Surg.* 2017;52(6):907–912.

98

Pediatric Abdomen

Ankush Gosain

Key Points

1 Gastroschisis occurs with an incidence rate of 1 in 2000 live births and is characterized by exposed intestine herniating through a defect to the right of the umbilicus. In contrast, omphalocele is a midline abdominal wall defect characterized by herniated visceral contents contained within the umbilical cord covering and has a higher incidence of associated congenital anomalies.

2 A congenital, indirect inguinal hernia is an abnormal, patent continuation of the peritoneum through the internal inguinal ring. Inguinal hernia repair is the most common elective procedure in pediatric surgery.

3 Neonatal bilious emesis should be considered the result of an acute mechanical intestinal obstruction until proven otherwise; emergent surgical evaluation is warranted to determine whether intestinal malrotation with midgut volvulus is present.

4 Necrotizing enterocolitis (NEC) is a progressive, inflammatory intestinal condition of the premature neonate. Perforated NEC is the most common neonatal surgical emergency.

5 Intussusception is the invagination or telescoping of a proximal segment of intestine into an adjacent distal segment and is the most common cause of intestinal obstruction in infants and children 3 months to 3 years of age.

6 Hirschsprung disease is caused by aganglionosis or absence of the enteric nervous system. Most commonly, the rectosigmoid colon is involved, but the length of contiguous aganglionosis varies in length proximally. Both propulsion and reflexive relaxation may be disordered or absent in the rectum, leading to functional bowel obstruction in the neonate and chronic constipation in the older child or adolescent. Hirschsprung-associated enterocolitis (HAEC) is a potentially life-threatening condition.

7 The incidence of biliary atresia is 1 in 8000 to 12,000 live births and is the most common cause of chronic cholestasis in infants and children. Biliary atresia is the most frequent indication for pediatric liver transplantation. Early diagnosis and management are necessary for optimal outcomes.

This chapter is limited to relatively common surgical conditions that are either congenital or unique in children. For other surgical conditions that can affect both children and adults, the reader is referred to other chapters in this text.

ABDOMINAL WALL

Gastroschisis and Omphalocele

Gastroschisis

1 Gastroschisis occurs with an incidence of about 1 in 2000 to 4000 live births. Infants with gastroschisis tend to be born to mothers who are younger (teenage), White, and who consumed alcohol or tobacco during pregnancy.[1,2] Familial cases of gastroschisis are distinctly rare. Associated congenital anomalies are uncommon. However, in about 10% of cases, intestinal atresia or stenosis can be seen and is thought to be a result of mechanical or vascular compromise to the herniated bowel. Rarely, infants with gastroschisis have complete loss of small bowel secondary to volvulus in utero.

The pathophysiology of gastroschisis remains unknown. In normal fetal development, two umbilical veins are initially present. As the intestine returns to the abdominal cavity through the umbilicus, the right umbilical vein undergoes resorption, leaving the left umbilical vein intact. Weakness of the umbilical membrane at the site of umbilical vein resorption may allow the evisceration of the intestine through the defect. This explanation is consistent with the clinical observation that the gastroschisis defect is almost always located to the right of the umbilicus. Routine antenatal ultrasonography has documented the sequential development of gastroschisis because of a ruptured hernia of the umbilical cord in utero. Therefore, gastroschisis should be considered an isolated mechanical defect of the developing umbilical cord rather than a global defect in embryogenesis.

The amount of bowel eviscerated in gastroschisis can be extensive because the bowel has not undergone complete mesenteric rotation and fixation at this time in embryogenesis. The bowel may be thickened, and the mesentery may be foreshortened secondary to the inflammatory response induced by direct exposure to amniotic fluid. In gastroschisis, herniation of the liver is distinctly unusual (**Fig. 98.1**).

Omphalocele

The incidence rate of omphalocele is approximately 1 in 6000 to 10,000 live births and has been stable over the past several decades. *Omphalocele* is a midline abdominal wall defect of varying size characterized by the presence of herniated visceral contents into the translucent sac of the umbilicus. The sac is composed of amniotic membrane, mesenchymal tissue known as *Wharton jelly,* and peritoneum. The umbilical cord attaches to the sac and may be eccentric in origin (**Fig. 98.2**). The sac may be inadvertently ruptured before or during delivery, but it is always present. Like gastroschisis, intestinal malrotation is usually present. Unlike gastroschisis, the bowel is typically normal in appearance because it has not been directly exposed to the amniotic fluid. Small omphaloceles are defined as 2 to

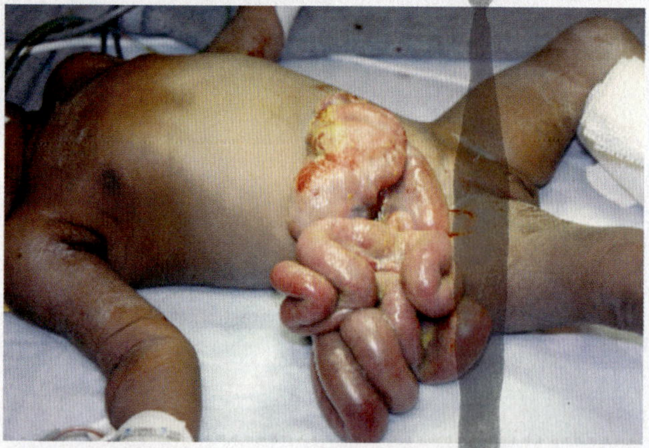

Figure 98.1. Gastroschisis. The defect is to the right of the normal umbilicus, and the bowel is thickened and inflamed.

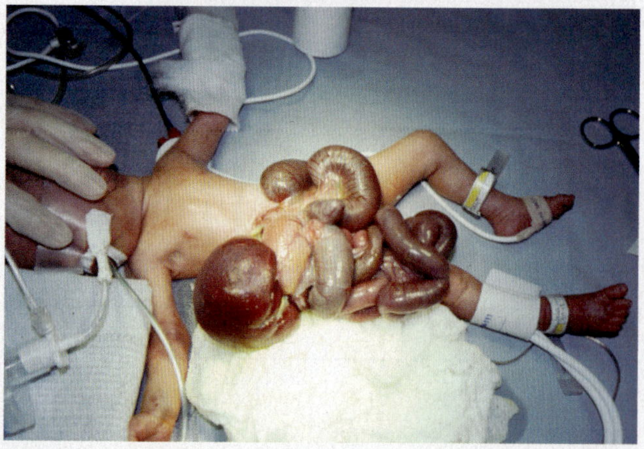

Figure 98.3. Ruptured omphalocele. Although the bowel is relatively normal in appearance, the abdominal cavity is extremely underdeveloped.

3 cm in diameter and have only a small amount of herniated bowel within the sac. Closure of small omphaloceles is typically performed without significant physiologic complications. In contrast, giant omphaloceles defined as greater than 4 cm in diameter, can lead to extensive herniation of the stomach, bowel, liver, and spleen with subsequent underdevelopment of the abdominal cavity (**Fig. 98.3**).

Omphalocele results from incomplete closure of the anterior abdominal wall at the umbilicus during embryogenesis. During week 4 of gestation, the midgut undergoes progressive elongation in the yolk sac outside the embryonic coelomic cavity. The midgut returns to the abdominal cavity during week 10, where it undergoes normal rotation and fixation of the mesentery to the posterior abdominal wall. Normal closure of the anterior abdominal wall requires return of the midgut to the abdominal cavity, along with growth and fusion of the anterior body folds (cephalic, caudal, and two lateral) at the base of the umbilicus. Failure of growth, migration, or fusion of the lateral body folds leads to omphalocele. Failure of growth and fusion of the cephalic folds may lead to either a supraumbilical omphalocele associated with a midline sternal defect (**Fig. 98.4**) and a herniated heart, termed *ectopia cordis,* or a constellation of defects known as the *pentalogy of Cantrell.* This sequence includes a sternal cleft, an absence of the septum transversum of the diaphragm, a pericardial defect, a cardiac defect, and an epigastric omphalocele. Infants born with either ectopia cordis or pentalogy of Cantrell have significant morbidity, and often, these conditions are lethal.

Associated Anomalies

Associated anomalies are more common in infants with omphalocele than with gastroschisis, reflecting the more global abnormality of embryogenesis in omphalocele. About 50% to 60% of infants with omphalocele have at least one associated congenital anomaly involving the skeleton, gastrointestinal tract, nervous system, genitourinary system, and cardiopulmonary system. In addition, infants with omphalocele have a higher incidence of chromosomal abnormalities and other conditions such as Beckwith–Wiedemann syndrome. A comparison of gastroschisis and omphalocele is summarized in **Table 98.1**.

Perioperative Management for Gastroschisis and Omphalocele

In contemporary practice, infants with gastroschisis can be safely delivered vaginally.[3] Studies comparing vaginal delivery with elective cesarean section for infants with gastroschisis demonstrated no significant differences in outcome.[4,5] Early delivery to minimize intestinal damage in gastroschisis patients has not been proved to be efficacious.[6,7] Fetal well-being has been advocated to be the primary determinant for gastroschisis. To prevent birth-related hepatic injury, cesarean section is preferable for prenatally diagnosed infants with giant omphaloceles.

After delivery, infants with either gastroschisis or omphalocele have similar initial management priorities. If necessary, an adequate airway with effective ventilation and oxygenation

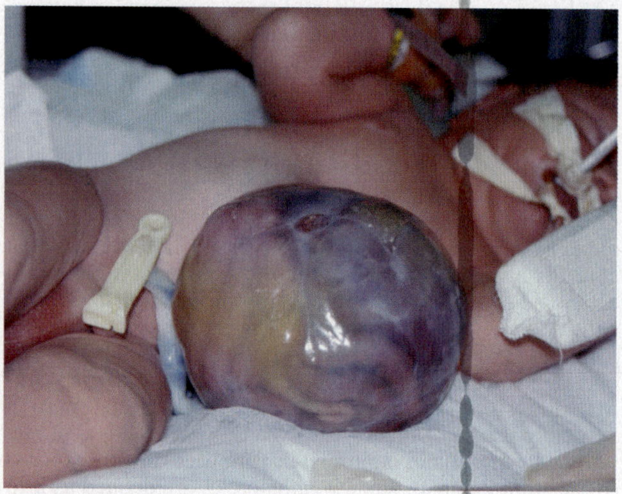

Figure 98.2. Omphalocele. The herniated intestines and liver are visible inside the sac. The umbilical cord attaches to the sac.

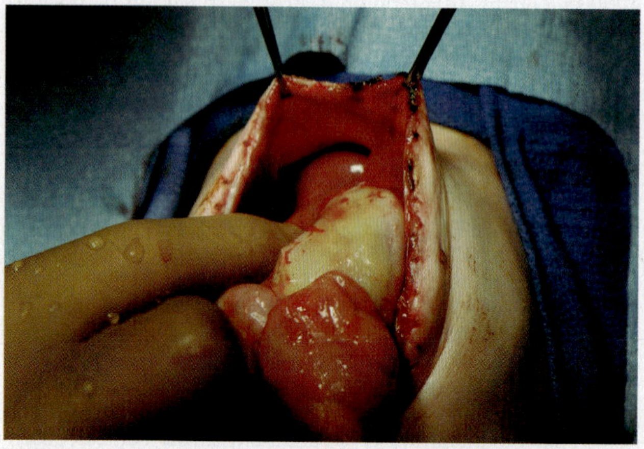

Figure 98.4. Operative exploration of giant omphalocele with abdominal wall defect, absence of the septum transversum of the diaphragm, pericardial defect, and cardiac defect.

Table 98.1. Comparison of Gastroschisis and Omphalocele

Characteristic	Gastroschisis	Omphalocele
Defect size (diameter)	2–3 cm	2–15 cm
Sac	Never	Always, may be ruptured
Gestational age	Prematurity	Term
Umbilical cord	Adjacent (left side) of defect	Attached to sac
Herniated viscera	Small bowel, stomach, colon	Small bowel, stomach, colon, liver
Malrotation	Yes	Yes
Bowel character	Inflammatory, edematous	Normal
Enteral nutrition	Delayed	Normal
Associated anomalies	Uncommon (10% atresia)	Common (50%)

is established. The infant should be maintained under either an external warmer or a humidified incubator. An orogastric sump tube should be inserted early and placed on suction to prevent intestinal distention. In gastroschisis, the herniated viscera should be examined to make certain that the mesentery is not twisted. In addition, the tightness of the opening of the abdominal wall should be assessed to ensure that there is sufficient perfusion of the bowel. The infant's entire lower torso can be placed inside a plastic bowel bag, or the viscera can be covered with moistened gauze, to prevent further contamination, hypothermia, and volume depletion. The initial therapeutic goal is to provide rapid, effective temporary coverage of the viscera. Adequate support of the herniated viscera must be provided to prevent intestinal ischemia. This can be done by placing the baby on his or her side and placing support under the intestines. With large omphaloceles, the position of the infant's liver and viscera may impair venous return from the inferior vena cava when the infant is supine, and these infants may preferentially require a left-side–down position to maintain normal hemodynamics. Intravenous dextrose and broad-spectrum antibiotics are administered. Infants with gastroschisis will have higher intravenous fluid requirements to maintain euvolemia. If the infant is not delivered at a center where definitive surgical care can be provided, urgent transport should be arranged.

Gastroschisis

Once the infant with gastroschisis has been stabilized, measures are taken to secure the viscera and, if possible, correct the abdominal wall defect. One option is to take the infant to the operating room, where reduction of the herniated viscera with primary fascial closure of the abdominal wall is an achievable goal in approximately 60% to 70% of infants with gastroschisis. Gentle but definitive stretching of the abdominal wall is performed, and proximal decompression of the bowel is maintained with orogastric decompression. The defect may need to be enlarged to evaluate the intestinal tract fully and/or reduce the viscera into the abdominal cavity. The limiting factor in primary closure of a congenital abdominal wall defect is the increased intra-abdominal pressure generated by the reduction

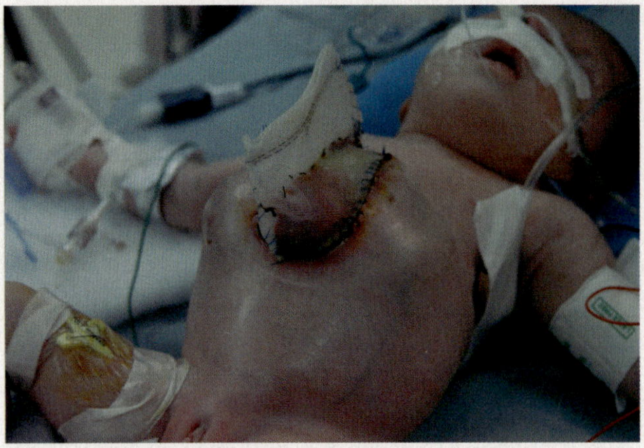

Figure 98.5. Silastic chimney or silo for temporary coverage and staged reduction of giant omphalocele.

of the herniated viscera. Increased intra-abdominal pressure can lead to abdominal compartment syndrome. Features of neonatal abdominal compartment syndrome include impaired venous return caused by compression of the inferior vena cava, reduction of splanchnic blood flow leading to mesenteric ischemia, and respiratory compromise secondary to impaired diaphragmatic excursion. Intraoperative measurement of intragastric or intravesical pressure, end-tidal CO_2, central venous pressure, or regional oximetry may be helpful in determining the safety of primary abdominal wall closure. If the herniated viscera cannot be reduced primarily, the viscera are placed in a constructed Silastic pouch or preformed spring-loaded silo. Daily partial reduction of the viscera within the silo is performed. This technique allows gradual reduction of the herniated viscera into the abdominal cavity, and complete reduction is usually obtained within 3 to 7 days. The infant is returned to the operating room for removal of the temporary silo with delayed primary closure of the abdominal wall defect (**Fig. 98.5**). Alternatively, a large abdominal wall defect may be effectively covered with abdominal skin flaps, or biologic mesh, with delayed repair of the ventral hernia months to years later (gross closure).

In some centers, all babies with gastroschisis are managed by placing a preformed silo at the bedside after the baby is born. Thereafter, the viscera is slowly reduced into the abdomen, and eventual fascial closure is attained.[8] Some studies caution that this practice may lead to longer ventilator and fluid requirements.[8,9] Another method that has been described in gastroschisis patients with noninflamed pliable intestines is to reduce the viscera with some sedation at the bedside, fold the umbilical cord stump over the skin closure, and place a pressure dressing over the defect.[10] The use of the umbilical stump has been described even for patients requiring staged or silo closure.[11] In some retrospective studies, this method of closure has been shown to effect fewer days of mechanical ventilation, decreased antibiotic and opioid utilization, but with a higher rate of umbilical hernia at follow-up.[11–15] A wound vacuum closure can be used to augment this technique.

Omphalocele

Given the high incidence of associated anomalies, infants with omphalocele should undergo diagnostic investigation, guided by the clinical presentation and physical examination. These studies include chest radiography, echocardiogram, and renal ultrasound, in addition to baseline blood work. Chromosomal analysis may be necessary. Until the decision is made with respect to the timing and method of repair, the omphalocele should remain covered and protected with a gauze dressing. If the omphalocele is ruptured or torn, immediate closure or coverage is necessary.

Closure of omphaloceles is dictated by the size of the defect, the amount of viscera extruded into the sac, and the abdominal domain. There is no standard definition of what constitutes a regular versus a giant omphalocele. Practically, a giant omphalocele has an abdominal wall defect larger than 4 cm, containing a portion of liver, and is difficult to close primarily in the first days of life without physiologic compromise.

Omphaloceles with a small abdominal wall defect typically would have operative fascial closure with sac excision in the newborn period. Many techniques have been described to close giant omphaloceles, including sac excision and temporary coverage with grafts, use of intraperitoneal tissue expanders,[16,17] and allowing the omphalocele sac to scar and then epithelialize in the latter technique.

The sac can be physically supported and left undisturbed, allowing epithelialization of the sac over several weeks to months. Antibiotic solutions or ointments are usually applied to control desiccation.[17–20] Delayed repair of the ventral hernia is required. This delay is particularly useful in the infant with a giant omphalocele and a small, underdeveloped abdominal cavity that prohibits primary closure.

Infants with repaired omphalocele usually have relatively prompt return of bowel function after definitive repair, while infants with gastroschisis may require up to 4 weeks after repair to have bowel function normalize. The time to achieve full enteral feeding is not affected by the use of erythromycin as a prokinetic agent.[21] Approximately 15% of infants with gastroschisis develop necrotizing enterocolitis (NEC), a diffuse, often life-threatening inflammatory complication of the neonatal intestinal tract. In addition, infants with gastroschisis are at risk for nutrient malabsorption and intestinal dysmotility, with an inability to tolerate full enteral feeding. In particular, infants with gastroschisis and associated intestinal atresia may have pronounced intestinal dysmotility and may require long-term, sometimes lifelong, dependence on TPN for caloric intake.[22]

Results and Outcome

Long-term outcome of infants operated on for gastroschisis or omphalocele is usually dependent on the morbidity and mortality of associated conditions rather than the abdominal wall defect itself. Surgical conditions such as undescended testicles, Meckel diverticulum, and adhesive small bowel obstruction are encountered with moderate frequency. Adhesive small bowel obstruction most commonly occurs in the first year of life and requires operative management in the majority.[23] Most children with repaired abdominal wall defects enjoy satisfactory health and quality of life, although they have been reported to have a lower degree of physical fitness measured by exercise time and maximal oxygen consumption.[24]

Umbilical Hernia

Anatomy and Embryology

Congenital umbilical hernia is the most common abdominal wall defect in infants and children. The umbilical ring begins to contract circumferentially after birth and normally is reinforced by the paired lateral umbilical ligaments (the obliterated umbilical arteries), the singular round ligament (the obliterated umbilical vein), the urachal remnant, and the transversalis fascia. Incomplete growth or impaired development of any one of these structures can lead to weakness at the umbilical ring and cause a congenital umbilical hernia.

Clinical Issues and Management

Congenital umbilical hernias generally do not pose significant problems during childhood, with incarceration of intra-abdominal contents within the sac occurring in about 1:1500 cases. Infants and children may also present with infection or drainage at the umbilicus from associated urachal or vitelline duct remnants. The incidence rate of congenital umbilical hernia has been reported to be 25% to 50% in Black infants and 4% to 9% in White infants in the first few months of life. There is an increased incidence of umbilical hernia in premature infants, and there is a tendency for familial inheritance.

Diagnosis of umbilical hernia is usually made after separation of the umbilical cord remnant from the umbilicus and is often initially noted by parents or pediatrician. The size of the defect may vary from a few millimeters to several centimeters and is typically reducible and asymptomatic. Age and size of the defect are the most important factors determining spontaneous closure rates.[25] Many umbilical hernias spontaneously close within the first 2 to 3 years of life. Given the high rate of spontaneous closure and the relatively asymptomatic nature of most umbilical hernias, operative repair is generally not performed during the first 2 years of life. Skin ulceration or an episode of incarceration should prompt earlier repair. Large defects with significant protrusion may necessitate surgery, and parents may desire repair if an older child appears to be self-conscious about the hernia.

Nearly all umbilical hernia repairs can be performed as outpatient surgical procedures. An incision is made along the umbilicus, and the hernia sac is dissected free circumferentially. The sac is completely excised, and primary fascial closure is performed. The umbilical skin is typically preserved and sutured to the fascial closure, and an acceptable cosmetic result is almost always achievable. Large umbilical hernias with redundant skin may require umbilicoplasty. The incidence of complications such as wound infection and recurrence is low.

Inguinal Hernia and Hydrocele

Anatomy, Embryology, and Pathophysiology

2 Inguinal hernia repair is the most common elective general surgical procedure performed by pediatric surgeons. Three distinct anatomic types of inguinal hernias are observed in children: congenital indirect (99% of infants and children), direct (0.5%), and femoral (<0.5%). An *indirect inguinal hernia* is an abnormal, patent continuation of the peritoneum through the internal inguinal ring. The hernia sac originates lateral to the deep inferior epigastric vessels and descends along the spermatic cord within the cremasteric fascia. The sac can reside completely within the inguinal canal or descend through the external inguinal ring into the scrotum. A *direct inguinal hernia* originates medial to the deep inferior epigastric vessels and is external to the cremasteric fascia. The hernia sac protrudes directly through the posterior wall of the inguinal canal and can descend through the external inguinal ring and into the scrotum. A *femoral hernia* originates medial to the femoral vein and descends inferior to the inguinal ligament along the femoral canal. A femoral hernia never enters the scrotum or the labia.

The developing testicle is initially adjacent to the mesonephros and subsequently descends to the scrotum during the third trimester of gestation. The peritoneal extension that descends alongside the chorda gubernaculum of the testicle is called the processus vaginalis. A slightly higher incidence rate of right-sided indirect inguinal hernia is thought to reflect delay of right-sided testicular descent from the developing inferior vena cava and right external iliac vein. As the testicle descends into the scrotum, the processus vaginalis forms a serous covering around the testicle known as the tunica vaginalis. Normally, the patent processus vaginalis undergoes obliteration, closing the communication between the peritoneal cavity and the inguinal canal. A patent processus vaginalis can lead to a variety of anatomic conditions of the inguinal region (**Fig. 98.6**).

The incidence of patent processus vaginalis has been reported to be as high as 80% to 94% in newborn infants undergoing autopsy, whereas in adulthood, the incidence is 20% to 30%. Infants with unilateral inguinal hernias have been found to have a patent contralateral processus vaginalis in 60% during the first few months of life. By the age of 2 years, 20% of these hernias were obliterated, and half of the remaining 40% became clinical hernias. At least 30% of infants requiring placement of a ventriculoperitoneal shunt

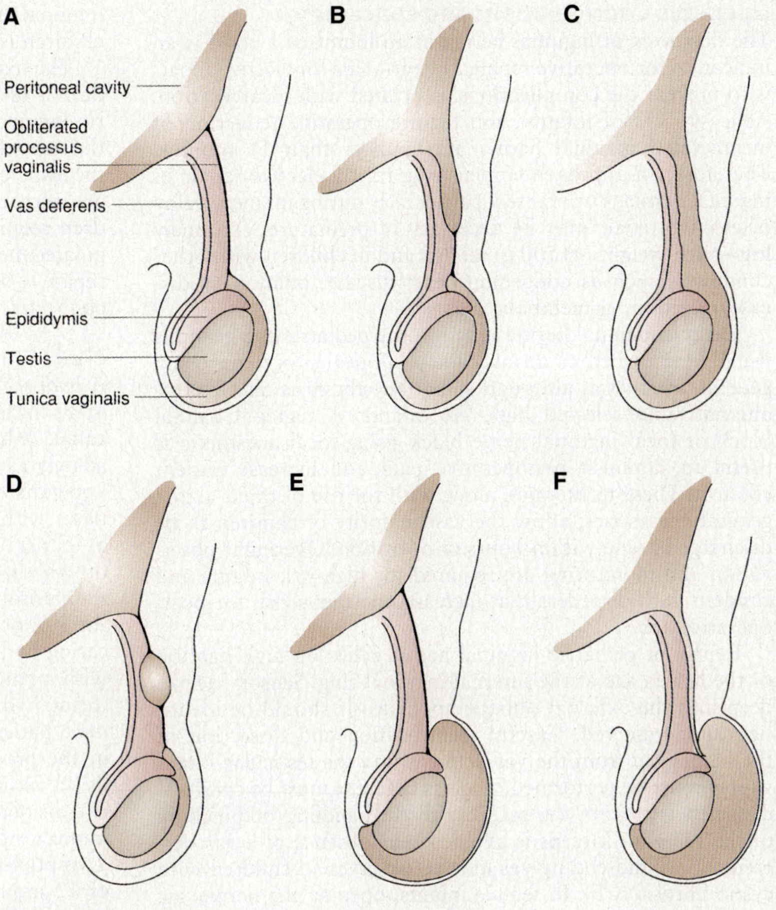

Figure 98.6. Anatomic variations that occur with different degrees of obliteration of the processus vaginalis. A: Normal; obliterated processus vaginalis. B: Proximal hernia sac; distal obliterated processus. C: Hernia sac extending into scrotum; no obliteration. D: Proximal and distal obliteration with hydrocele of the cord. E: Hydrocele of the scrotum, obliterated processus. F: Patent processus with communicating hydrocele.

for hydrocephalus have been observed to have a patent processus vaginalis in the first few months of life, with a rapid decline in patency in older children. These studies, along with contemporary use of laparoscopic exploration of the contralateral internal ring, demonstrate that although a patent processus vaginalis is common in infancy, there is some degree of obliteration that occurs with increasing age, and a patent processus vaginalis by itself does not constitute a clinical inguinal hernia.

Clinical Issues

Inguinal hernias occur in 1% to 3% of all children and in 3% to 5% of premature infants. There is no known inheritance pattern, but there is an increased incidence of inguinal hernia in children with connective tissue disorders such as Ehlers–Danlos syndrome and Marfan syndrome. There is a 6:1 predominance of males to females. At least 30% of children are younger than 6 months at the time of operative repair. Inguinal hernia more commonly presents as right-sided (56.2%) compared with left-sided (27.5%) or bilateral (16.2%).

Most infants and children with an inguinal hernia have a history of an intermittent inguinal mass or bulge that may descend into the scrotum or labia. The hernia may become more pronounced during times of increased intra-abdominal pressure, such as crying or defecating. Most inguinal hernias in children reduce spontaneously or are reducible with gentle, manual pressure along the inguinal canal. Female infants may have an ovary and fallopian tube in the hernia sac, identified clinically as a firm, slightly mobile, nontender mass in the labia or the inguinal canal. Most parents or pediatricians give a characteristic history that is sufficient to warrant inguinal exploration, even in children in whom the hernia cannot be clinically demonstrated at the time of examination. Depending on institution and surgeon preference, infants and children with a strong history consistent with inguinal hernia and an equivocal clinical examination may be offered ultrasound or diagnostic laparoscopy to effectively confirm the diagnosis before groin exploration.

Incarceration is a common consequence of untreated inguinal hernia and presents as a nonreducible mass in the inguinal canal, scrotum, or labia. Clinical symptoms and signs are related to the duration of incarceration. If the incarceration has been present for several hours, the infant may be inconsolable and have feeding intolerance, pain, abdominal distention, vomiting, and lack of flatus or stool, signaling complete intestinal obstruction. The affected groin may become quite edematous, and a reactive scrotal hydrocele may evolve. Elevation of the infant's lower extremities with a pillow may help encourage spontaneous reduction. Attempts at manually reducing an incarcerated inguinal hernia should be performed by an experienced surgeon. If necessary, sedation to calm the infant before attempting manual reduction may be cautiously used. Ice packs should be avoided in infants and children. Following successful reduction of an incarcerated hernia, expedient elective repair of the hernia should be performed after the edema has subsided. This may be up to 48 hours later. If reduction of an incarcerated hernia requires several attempts and is difficult, overnight inpatient observation is warranted to rule out reduction of strangulated bowel; fortunately, this is an uncommon occurrence in the pediatric population. Inability to reduce an incarcerated hernia is a clear indication for urgent operative exploration and repair. Incarcerated inguinal hernia must be differentiated from an acute, noncommunicating hydrocele, or inguinal lymphadenitis. With acute hydrocele, it is usually possible to transilluminate the hydrocele and palpate normal cord structures above the scrotal mass. In addition, symptoms of bowel obstruction are absent with acute hydrocele. Acute lymphadenitis is typically associated with fever, erythema, and tenderness, and there may be a history of lower extremity infection on the ipsilateral side. If the inguinal mass is not reducible and an incarcerated hernia cannot be excluded, urgent groin exploration is required.

Operative Considerations and Outcome

The diagnosis of inguinal hernia in an infant or a child is an indication for operative repair. The rationale for elective repair is to prevent the complications associated with incarceration. At least 71% of infants who require operative reduction of incarcerated inguinal hernia are younger than 11 months. Therefore, an approach emphasizing timely elective repair of inguinal hernia is warranted, particularly during infancy. Delay of elective repair may be necessary in premature, extremely low–birth-weight (<1500 g) infants and in children with other conditions such as congenital heart disease, pulmonary disease, infection, or metabolic disease.

Elective inguinal hernia repair in the pediatric age group is usually performed as an outpatient surgical procedure using general anesthesia, although spinal anesthesia is an effective alternative in selected high-risk infants. A regional caudal block or local inguinal nerve block using local anesthetic is useful to diminish perioperative pain and increase patient comfort. These techniques, along with the use of rapid-acting general anesthetics, allow the vast majority of children to be discharged home within hours of operation. Overnight observation and monitoring are required for high-risk infants and children with disorders that increase anesthetic risk for postoperative apnea.

Repair of pediatric inguinal hernia relies on high ligation of the hernia sac at the internal inguinal ring. Sensory nerves deep into the external oblique aponeurosis should be identified and preserved. Careful identification and dissection of the hernia sac from the vas deferens and the testicular blood supply must be performed. The vas deferens must be carefully dissected free from the sac, and direct handling or pinching of the vas with forceps is avoided. The absence of a vas deferens or a blind-ending vas may be observed in children with cystic fibrosis (CF). In female infants, opening the hernia sac to visualize the ovary and fallopian tube may help avoid inadvertent injury to these structures during suture ligation of the sac. The distal component of the hernia sac is opened widely, and any fluid in the sac is evacuated. If the internal inguinal ring is attenuated or enlarged, it can be repaired with a few sutures. Experience with laparoscopic inguinal hernia repair using purse-string suture closure of the patent internal ring without direct inguinal exploration has been described.[26] The testicle is returned to its scrotal position by gentle traction on the gubernaculum, and the spermatic cord is carefully aligned along the inguinal canal. Postoperative pain is managed with oral acetaminophen for 24 to 48 hours; older children may require postoperative narcotics. In addition, abnormalities of the vas deferens may be associated with genitourinary anomalies. A renal ultrasound should be performed to rule out kidney malformations.

Operative exploration of the asymptomatic contralateral groin remains controversial but is often performed in infants younger than 2 years because of the reported 60% to 70% incidence of a patent processus vaginalis on the opposite side. In a survey of the surgical section of the American Academy of Pediatrics, 65% of the respondents perform contralateral exploration in male patients younger than 2 years, and 84% perform exploration for female infants up to 4 years of age. Direct visualization of the contralateral groin can be performed using a laparoscope inserted either through the umbilicus or through a side-viewing laparoscope inserted through the hernia sac. Experience with diagnostic laparoscopy demonstrates that approximately one-third to one-half of children have a patent processus vaginalis on the contralateral, asymptomatic groin, with higher rates in infants younger than 1 year.[27] This approach avoids unnecessary contralateral groin exploration in about half of all children who undergo surgery for unilateral inguinal hernia. However, the presence of a patent processus alone does not necessarily translate into a clinically significant hernia, and via systematic review, the reported risk of developing a metachronous contralateral inguinal hernia following open unilateral hernia repair in children is 7.2%.[28]

The major risk of inguinal hernia repair in infants and children is related to general anesthesia. Complications in pediatric inguinal hernia repair include wound infection, injury to the vas deferens or testicular vessels, injury or displacement of the testicle, and recurrence. Fortunately, all these complications are infrequent. The overall complication rate is higher for children requiring emergent operation for incarcerated or strangulated hernia. Recurrent inguinal hernia following elective repair is unusual and may be an indication of an underlying connective tissue disorder such as Ehlers–Danlos syndrome.

Hydrocele

A *hydrocele* is a fluid collection that resides in the tunica vaginalis in the scrotum or the processus vaginalis in the inguinal canal. A hydrocele may be present at birth, or it may occur acutely as a result of an incarcerated hernia or torsion of the appendix testis. On examination, a hydrocele transilluminates with a bright handheld light. A hydrocele is described as either *communicating* or *noncommunicating,* depending on whether there is direct patency between the hydrocele and the peritoneal cavity. A history of intermittent fluctuation in the size of the hydrocele is generally diagnostic of communicating hydrocele. A communicating hydrocele is synonymous with a patent processus vaginalis, and, therefore, a communicating hydrocele is treated operatively in the same fashion. In male patients, a hydrocele of the cord is a collection of fluid in the processus vaginalis, separate from the tunica vaginalis. In female patients, fluid trapped in the processus vaginalis is considered a hydrocele of the canal of Nuck. In noncommunicating hydrocele, the isolated fluid collection is typically asymptomatic and tends to spontaneously resolve before age of 12 months. Operative management of noncommunicating hydrocele is usually reserved for lesions that persist after this age, acute enlargement of the hydrocele, or if there is any question of communication.

STOMACH, DUODENUM, AND SMALL INTESTINE

Infantile Hypertrophic Pyloric Stenosis

Anatomy and Pathophysiology

The pathogenesis of infantile hypertrophic pyloric stenosis is unknown, but data suggest that local deficiency of neuronal nitric oxide synthase in the pylorus may be responsible for the clinical manifestations of the disease.[29] The deficiency of neuronal nitric oxide synthase leads to a lack of nitric oxide–mediated relaxation of smooth muscle and subsequent pyloric obstruction. Luminal narrowing occurs as a result of concentric hypertrophy of the pyloric smooth muscle. Clinically, this presents as progressive gastric outlet obstruction that becomes symptomatic by 2 to 4 weeks of age. The maximal narrowing and clinical symptoms of hypertrophic pyloric stenosis occur between 4 and 8 weeks of age. The hypertrophic pyloric muscle ultimately undergoes gradual involution over a period of weeks to months.

Clinical Presentation

The reported incidence rate of hypertrophic pyloric stenosis is approximately 0.1% to 0.4% among White infants and is slightly lower in the Black population. There is a distinct familial predisposition with an approximate 7% incidence rate in children of parents with a history of pyloric stenosis. The incidence rate is about four times higher in males than in females and is higher in first-born infants. There is an apparent increased risk of hypertrophic pyloric stenosis in infants receiving oral erythromycin for pertussis prophylaxis. Association of pyloric stenosis in infants treated for esophageal atresia and in infants with Smith–Lemli–Opitz syndrome has been reported.

Infants with hypertrophic pyloric stenosis have a history of nonbilious, postprandial emesis that becomes progressively projectile. The infant otherwise appears well and will feed vigorously until late in the clinical course. The typical age at diagnosis is between 2 and 12 weeks of age. A history of identified feeding intolerance and formula change is common.

The definitive clinical finding on examination is a palpable, hypertrophied pylorus in the right upper quadrant to midepigastric region, often described as a firm, mobile "olive" on examination. This is a pathognomonic finding, and in the correct clinical setting, no further diagnostic imaging studies are required. An experienced clinician should be able to palpate a hypertrophied pylorus in nearly all cases. A successful physical examination requires an empty stomach, a quiet infant, and patience; repeated examinations may be necessary. Inability to palpate the pyloric mass in a quiet or anesthetized infant should place the diagnosis of hypertrophic pyloric stenosis in question. Other physical findings include visible or palpable gastric peristaltic waves, which can also be seen with any cause of gastric or duodenal obstruction.

Late findings with advanced symptoms include dehydration and a hypochloremic, hypokalemic metabolic alkalosis from gastric fluid losses. Profound metabolic alkalosis is less common in current practice but occasionally can be encountered in an extremely dehydrated infant with a long-standing history of emesis. The intravascular volume depletion and chloride-responsive alkalosis must be corrected prior to operative repair. The serum chloride should be restored to at least 90 to 95 mEq/L, and the measured CO_2 should be less than 30 mEq/L prior to induction of general anesthesia.

Diagnosis

If the examination is equivocal, either an upper gastrointestinal contrast series or a pyloric ultrasound examination can be performed. Both examinations are highly accurate and have sensitivity and specificity exceeding 95% in experienced hands.

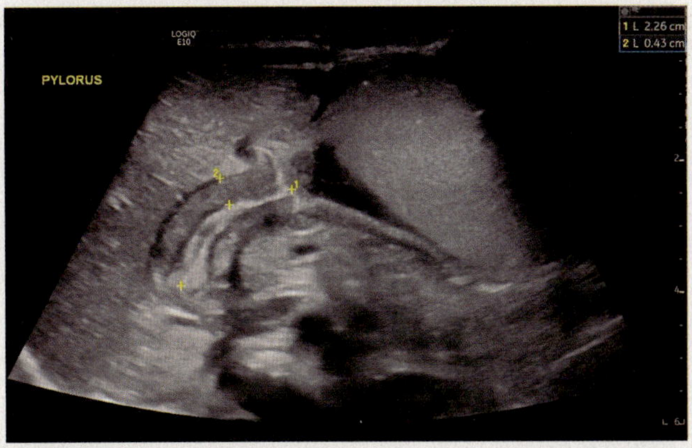

Figure 98.7. Ultrasound image of pyloric stenosis in coronal plane with pylorus marked by measurement bars.

A typical contrast study demonstrating a narrowed, elongated pyloric channel is shown in **Figure 98.7**. Contrast studies have the advantage of evaluating other causes of symptomatic emesis, including gastroesophageal reflux disease, malrotation, and antroduodenal webs. The disadvantage of this approach is the presence of contrast in a poorly emptying stomach. Ultrasound examination of the pylorus is a preferred diagnostic test in most pediatric institutions. Ultrasound criteria for hypertrophic pyloric stenosis include a pyloric muscle thickness of 4 mm or greater and a pyloric channel length of 15 mm or greater. In general, the diagnosis of hypertrophic pyloric stenosis is being made at an earlier age compared with several decades ago.

Treatment

Surgical pyloromyotomy has achieved universal acceptance because it offers definitive, rapid cure in virtually all infants, and morbidity rates have been negligible (**Fig. 98.8**). The

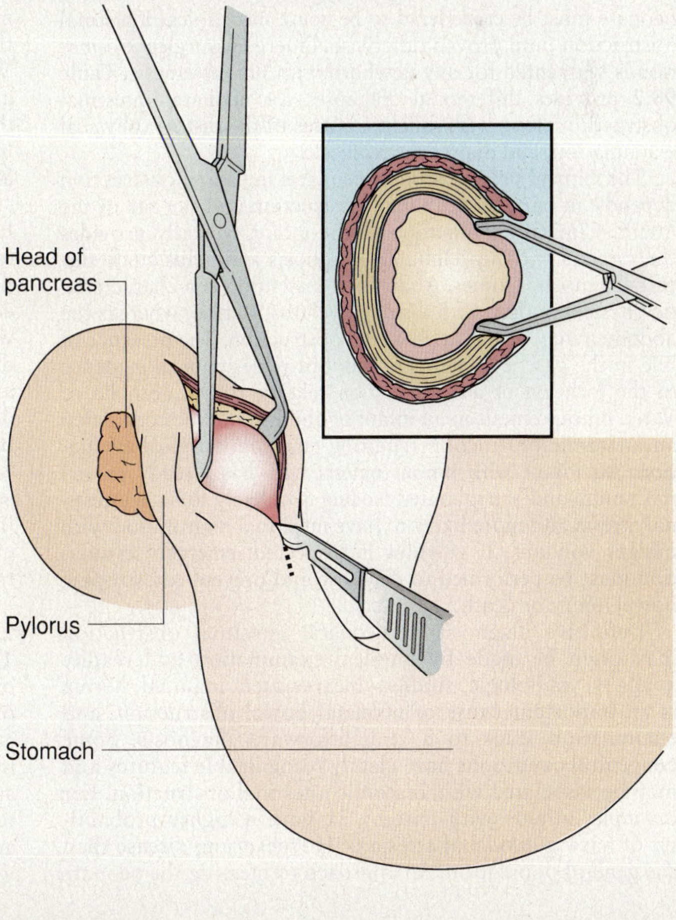

Figure 98.8. Ramstedt pyloromyotomy for infantile hypertrophic pyloric stenosis. The cross-sectional view shows herniation of the submucosa into the myotomy site, indicative of an adequate myotomy.

operation is performed once the infant is rehydrated, and the serum electrolytes are corrected. A single longitudinal incision is made in the hypertrophied pyloric muscle. The hypertrophied circular pyloric muscle must be meticulously divided from the stomach to the junction of the proximal duodenum. An adequate pyloromyotomy is achieved when the submucosa bulges into the myotomy site and both edges of the divided pyloric muscle are freely mobile, and can be accomplished via laparotomy or laparoscopy. Laparoscopic pyloromyotomy has been demonstrated to be efficacious and safe with similar operative times and outcomes to the open repair; laparoscopic pyloromyotomy has become a standard approach at most children's hospitals.[30,31]

Postoperative feeding is typically started within 6 to 8 hours after recovery from anesthesia. Most infants are tolerant of enteral feeding and can be discharged home safely within 24 hours of operation. The surgical treatment of pyloric stenosis is straightforward, and the recovery is typically uncomplicated. A population-based study reviewing 1777 infants with pyloric stenosis demonstrated a shorter length of stay and a lower overall complication rate in infants operated on by specialty-trained pediatric surgeons compared to general surgeons.[32] Mortality following pyloromyotomy is distinctly unusual in the absence of concomitant medical problems. Complications are rare and usually represent wound infection, technical failures related to an inadequate pyloromyotomy, or inadvertent entry into the duodenum or the stomach. Rarely, infants with inadequate pyloromyotomy may require reexploration and a second myotomy on the posterior pyloric wall. Inadvertent duodenotomy or gastrotomy must be recognized and repaired.

Neonatal Intestinal Obstruction

A variety of congenital anatomic defects, inherited metabolic diseases, and acquired physiologic disorders may present as intestinal obstruction in a newborn. Neonatal intestinal obstruction is characterized clinically by bilious emesis and is often associated with abdominal distention. Bilious emesis in a neonate must be considered to be acute mechanical intestinal obstruction until proven otherwise. Emergent surgical evaluation is warranted for any newborn with bilious emesis. **Table 98.2** provides differential diagnoses for neonatal intestinal obstruction along with salient features of the history, physical examination, and diagnostic studies.

The clinical presentation of neonatal intestinal obstruction depends, in part, on the site of obstruction and the age of the infant. Clinical examination of the infant typically provides the surgeon with a preliminary diagnosis and helps guide further diagnostic studies. Abdominal distention is a characteristic physical finding with distal bowel obstruction, whereas the abdomen may be flat in proximal obstruction. The presence of bile in the gastric contents or stool provides clinical evidence of the location of an obstruction relative to the ampulla of Vater. Bilious emesis in an infant or child should be considered an anatomic obstruction requiring emergent surgical evaluation. An infant with bilious emesis who has already passed meconium and has tolerated feeding is unlikely to have intestinal atresia and more likely to have intestinal malrotation with midgut volvulus. If volvulus is suspected, emergent evaluation must be performed to diagnose and prevent catastrophic bowel injury or death.

Definitive diagnosis of neonatal intestinal obstruction may often be made by physical examination and readily available radiologic studies. Incarcerated inguinal hernia is an important cause of neonatal bowel obstruction, and examination leads to a straightforward diagnosis. Some congenital conditions have clearly recognizable features and may be associated with anatomic intestinal obstruction. For example, infants with trisomy 21 have a higher probability of having duodenal atresia or Hirschsprung disease than the general population. An approach to imaging the neonate suspected of having an intestinal obstruction is to obtain a plain abdominal radiograph, followed by either a contrast enema or an upper gastrointestinal series. Plain films of the newborn abdomen can be extremely useful because swallowed gas acts as a contrast agent. For example, duodenal atresia gives rise to a dilated, gas-filled stomach and duodenum proximal to the obstruction; the remainder of the bowel remains gasless, giving rise to the "double-bubble" appearance on plain films. Other causes of proximal intestinal obstruction may lead to a microcolon on contrast enema, which is a small, unused but otherwise normal colon. If a retrograde contrast enema does not pass into the dilated segment of bowel, an upper gastrointestinal series may be useful to identify a more proximal obstruction. Upper gastrointestinal series is also the most useful diagnostic test for intestinal malrotation.

Several medical conditions of the newborn appear clinically similar to mechanical intestinal obstruction (see **Table 98.2**). In particular, bilious emesis from ileus secondary to neonatal sepsis is not uncommon. Congenital hypothyroidism is an infrequent and medically treatable condition that can produce delayed intestinal motility that mimics mechanical intestinal obstruction.

Congenital Duodenal Obstruction

Embryology and Anatomy

Causes of duodenal obstruction in the newborn include duodenal atresia or stenosis, duodenal intraluminal web, and annular pancreas. Because of the common embryologic basis, clinical presentation, and treatment, these entities are considered jointly.

The duodenum is derived from both the caudal segment of the foregut and the cranial segment of the midgut. Duodenal development is intimately related to the developing pancreaticobiliary system. The fetal pancreas arises from paired dorsal and ventral foregut diverticula during week 6 of gestation. The dorsal anlage gives rise to the body and tail of the pancreas as well as the main pancreatic duct. The ventral anlage migrates 180 degrees to fuse with the dorsal gland, forming the uncinate process and the distal portion of the duct of Wirsung (**Fig. 98.9**). An annular pancreas is characterized by glandular persistence surrounding the duodenum at the site of the embryonic ventral anlage. It is invariably associated with intrinsic duodenal obstruction, and a patent accessory pancreatic duct is common (**Fig. 98.10**).

It is believed that congenital duodenal obstruction results from abnormalities of pancreatic development, failure of duodenal recanalization, or vascular compromise to the duodenum. Duodenal atresia may occur with or without seromuscular continuity, and an intraluminal duodenal web may occur with or without fenestration. The most frequent location for duodenal atresia is in the descending duodenum distal to the ampulla of Vater. Most series report a 5% to 10% incidence of duodenal atresia proximal to the ampulla, giving rise to nonbilious gastric contents and emesis. Another important variant is a periampullary web projecting distally into the duodenal or jejunal lumen, forming a "windsock" deformity (**Fig. 98.11**). In this instance, the ampulla must be clearly identified before excision and repair because of the proximity of the ampulla to the web.

Clinical Presentation

The incidence rate of congenital duodenal obstruction is estimated to be about 1 in 6000 to 10,000 births. About 30% of these infants have trisomy 21. Infants born with duodenal atresia should be examined with a high degree of suspicion for trisomy 21 and undergo routine karyotype analysis. Other associated anomalies such as congenital heart disease, genitourinary tract malformations, and musculoskeletal disorders are common in these infants, and appropriate preoperative workup is necessary.

Table 98.2. Neonatal Intestinal Obstruction

Diagnosis	History	Physical Examination	Diagnostic Studies
Intestinal atresia or stenosis	Bilious emesis Failure to pass meconium	Abdominal distention	Plain abdominal film Contrast enema
Duodenal atresia or stenosis	Bilious or nonbilious emesis Feeding intolerance	Gastric distention Trisomy 21	Plain abdominal film Upper GI contrast study
Imperforate anus	Failure to pass meconium Bilious emesis (late)	Absent anus or visible fistula Abdominal distention VACTERL association	Plain chest, abdominal film Ultrasound kidneys, sacrum, rectum Echocardiogram
Necrotizing enterocolitis	High-risk, premature infant Bilious emesis	Abdominal distention Abdominal wall erythema Hematochezia, guaiac-positive stool	Plain abdominal film
Meconium ileus	Cystic fibrosis (10%) Bilious emesis	Acholic meconium Abdominal distention	Plain abdominal film Contrast enema
Malrotation	Bilious emesis Term, healthy infant	No abdominal distention	Plain abdominal film Upper GI contrast study
Hirschsprung disease	Delayed passage of meconium Bilious emesis	Abdominal distention Trisomy 21	Plain abdominal film Contrast enema
Uncommon causes of obstruction (intussusception, Meckel diverticulum, duplication)		Abdominal mass, incarcerated hernia	Variable
Medical conditions associated with ileus	Bilious emesis	Sepsis, hypothyroidism, etc.	Plain abdominal film

GI, gastrointestinal; VACTERL, vertebral, anal, cardiac, tracheal, esophageal, renal, and limb anomalies.

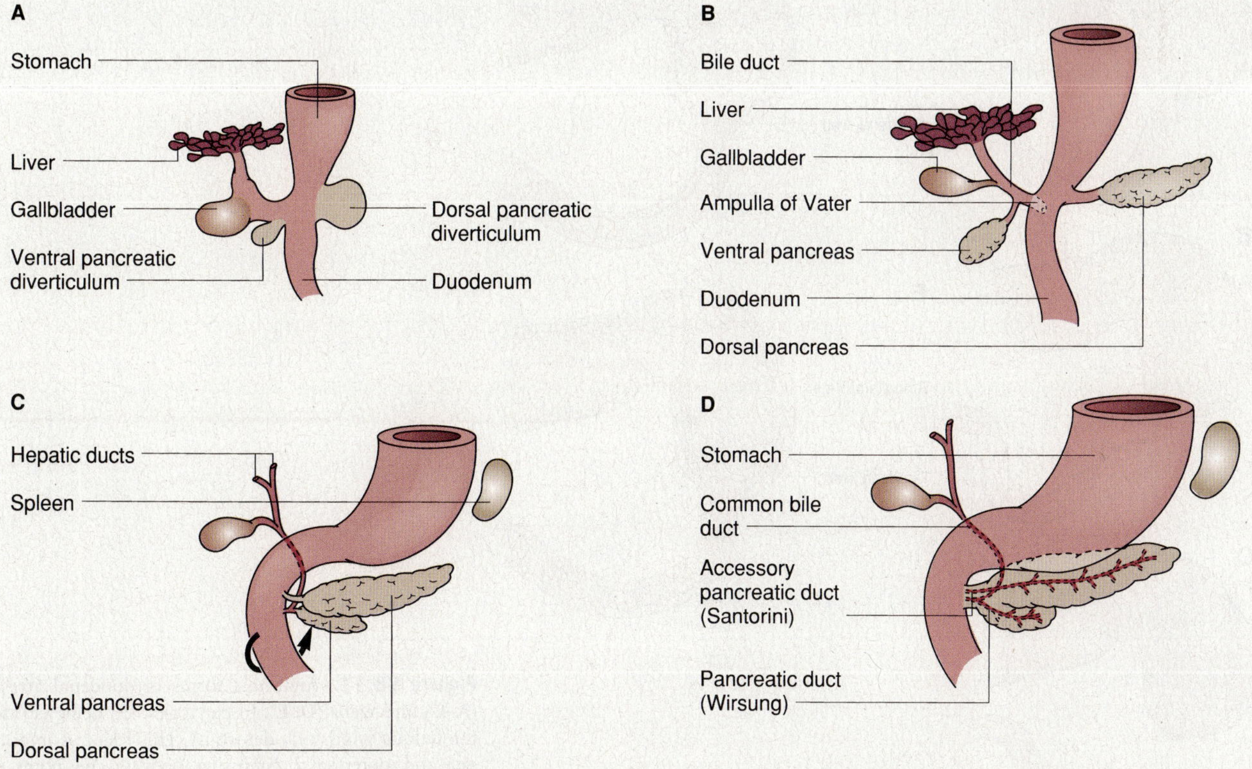

Figure 98.9. Normal embryologic development of the duodenum, pancreas, and bile ducts. **A:** Fifth gestational week. **B:** Sixth week. **C:** Seventh week. **D:** Eighth week.

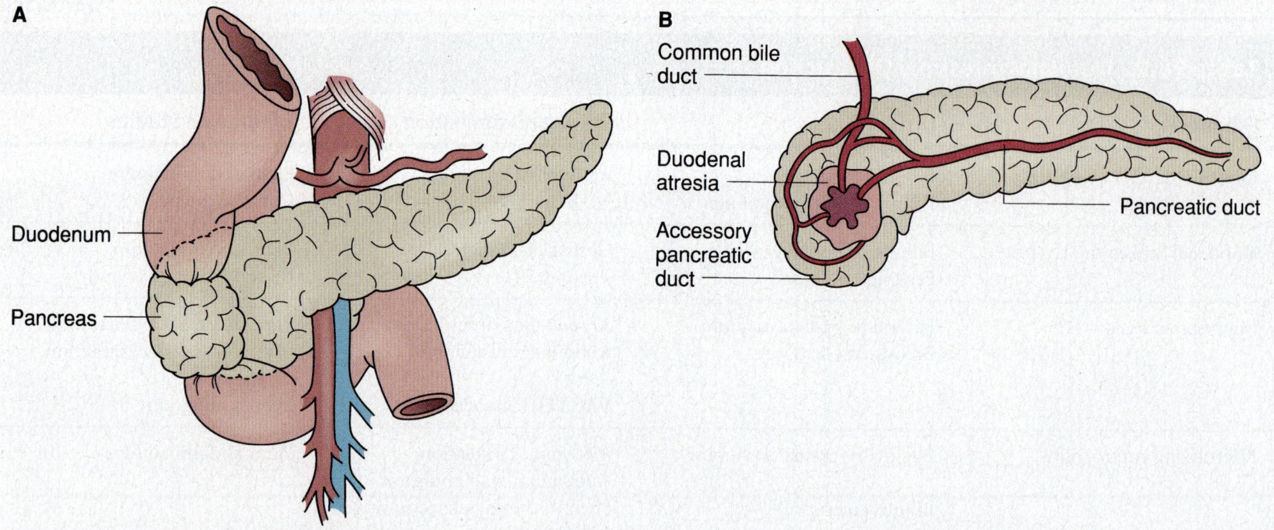

Figure 98.10. Annular pancreas. **A:** The associated duodenal atresia is shown. **B:** The relationships of the annular pancreas to the common bile duct and main and accessory pancreatic ducts are shown in cross-section.

Congenital duodenal obstruction most commonly presents in the first 24 to 48 hours of life with feeding intolerance and bilious emesis; duodenal obstruction proximal to the ampulla of Vater results in nonbilious emesis. On physical examination, infants with untreated duodenal obstruction may have a palpable epigastric mass, and gastric peristaltic waves may be visible. The collapsed and unused distal small intestine typically does not produce diffuse abdominal distention. Partial duodenal obstruction from a fenestrated web may not produce symptoms in the newborn period, and delayed diagnosis is common.

Diagnosis

Prenatal diagnosis of duodenal atresia is possible given contemporary fetal ultrasound techniques. Following birth, infants with suspected duodenal atresia should obtain plain abdominal radiographs. The classic radiographic finding of duodenal atresia is a double bubble from the air-filled stomach and duodenum (**Fig. 98.12**). In complete duodenal obstruction, no gas is seen distal to the duodenum; in this setting, the plain film is sufficiently diagnostic that no further imaging of the gastrointestinal tract is necessary. If there is incomplete

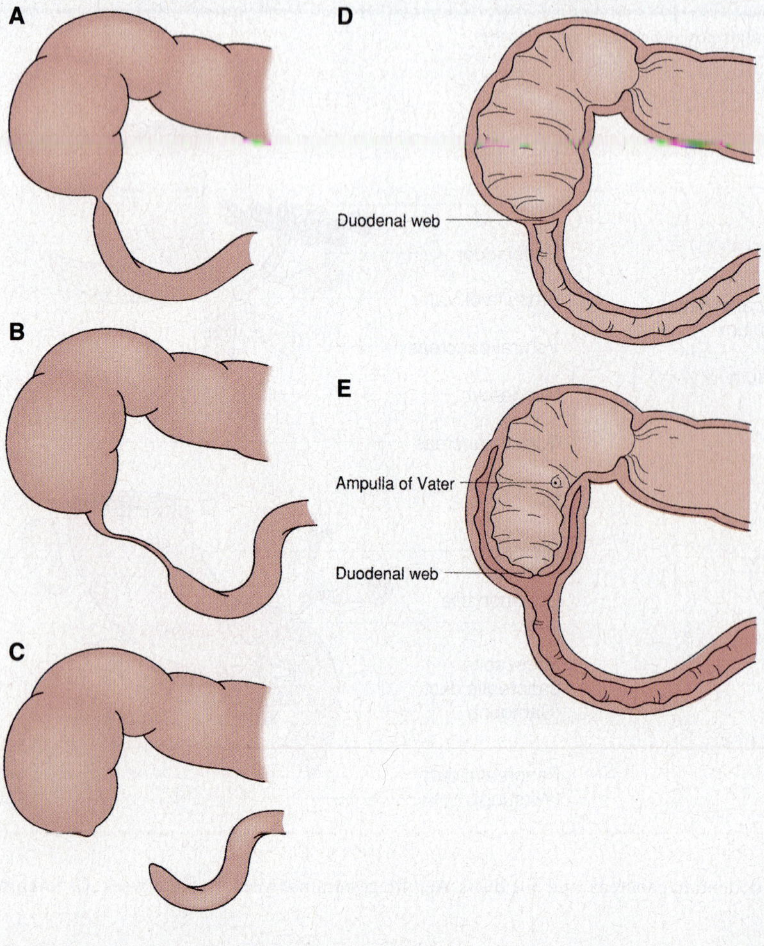

Figure 98.11. Anatomic forms of duodenal atresia (**A–C**) and webs (**D, E**). In particular, (**E**) demonstrates the unique wind-sock deformity. This lesion is important and potentially confusing because the point of obstruction is not at the apparent point of change in luminal diameter.

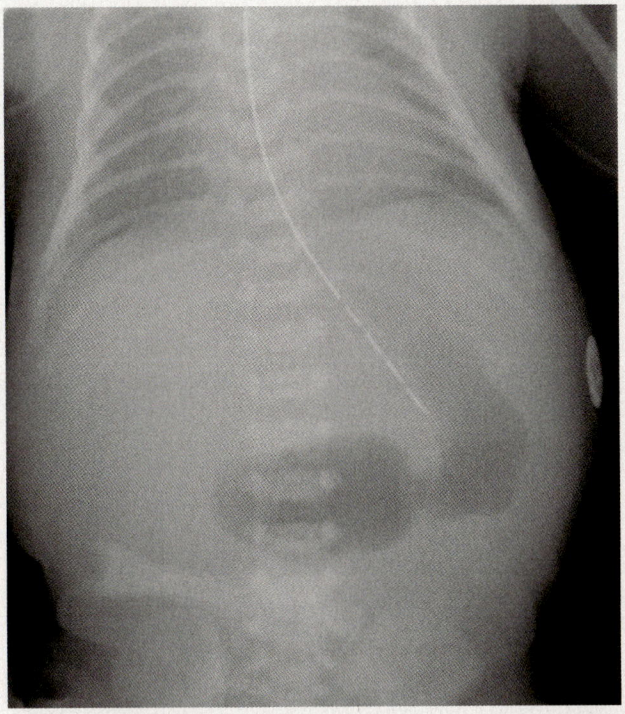

Figure 98.12. Classic radiographic appearance of duodenal atresia. There is a double bubble of gas in the stomach and the proximal duodenum, with no gas in the distal intestinal tract.

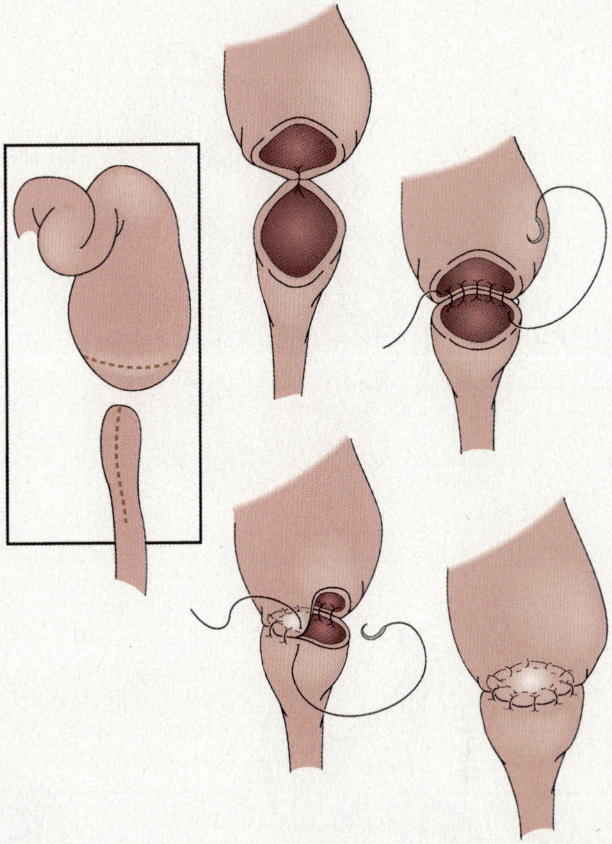

Figure 98.13. Diamond-shaped duodenoduodenostomy for repair of duodenal atresia.

obstruction, gas may be seen distally in the small or large intestine. Infants with suspected incomplete obstruction at the duodenal level may have either a fenestrated web or volvulus secondary to malrotation. Given the need for emergent operative intervention in malrotation with acute volvulus, an urgent upper gastrointestinal series with contrast should be strongly considered to exclude a neonatal surgical emergency. Importantly, all anatomic lesions causing neonatal duodenal obstruction require operative repair using a similar approach.

Treatment

Following expedient treatment of any associated life-threatening medical conditions and preoperative evaluation, the operative goals are to restore gastrointestinal continuity without sacrificing intestinal length or absorptive surface area. Because most lesions causing congenital duodenal obstruction are near the ampulla of Vater, great care must be exercised in treatment to avoid inadvertent injury to the ampulla or the pancreas.

Congenital duodenal atresia is treated by duodenoduodenostomy. Duodenal obstruction secondary to annular pancreas is also treated by duodenoduodenostomy. Direct division of annular pancreas is not performed because this does not address the underlying intraluminal duodenal obstruction, and there is significant risk of injury to the accessory pancreatic duct (see **Fig. 98.10**).

Duodenoduodenostomy is performed by making a transverse incision in the dilated, proximal duodenum and a longitudinal incision in the unused, downstream duodenum. The lumens are sutured together to form a diamond-shaped anastomosis (**Fig. 98.13**). Downstream duodenal patency should be demonstrated by passing a catheter or infusing saline or air distally to avoid overlooking synchronous distal intestinal atresia. Successful and efficacious laparoscopic duodenal atresia repair has also been reported.[33]

Duodenal webs are excised through a longitudinal duodenotomy. The wind-sock duodenal web must be clearly identified because the visible transition from the distended, proximal duodenum to the small, downstream duodenum may be several centimeters distal to the base of the web. The ampulla of Vater must be unequivocally identified before duodenal web excision to avoid injury. Closure of the longitudinal duodenotomy is performed transversely to avoid narrowing of the duodenum.

There is usually great size discrepancy between the dilated, proximal pouch and the distal duodenal lumen, leading some surgeons to advocate procedures designed to reduce the diameter of the proximal duodenum in an effort to facilitate improved postoperative bowel motility. The efficacy of these procedures, which include tapering duodenoplasty and duodenal plication, has been described in anecdotal fashion without randomized comparison.

Results and Outcome

After successful operative repair of duodenal atresia or stenosis, delayed gastric emptying is common and typically manifests as enteral feeding intolerance. Patience and persistence are essential during the postoperative period, as recovery of bowel function may take up to 10 days postop. Surgical outcomes after repair of congenital duodenal obstruction are excellent,[33] with perioperative survival exceeding 95%. Perioperative mortality is generally related to other congenital anomalies and, in particular, congenital heart disease in infants with trisomy 21. Other late problems may be encountered that reflect gastroduodenal motility issues, such as poor gastric emptying, gastroesophageal reflux, and duodenal dilatation. These symptoms may appear several months to years following repair and, therefore, long-term surgical follow-up remains important.

3 Malrotation

Embryology

Normal midgut fixation requires sequential growth, elongation, and rotation of the intestine beginning as early as week

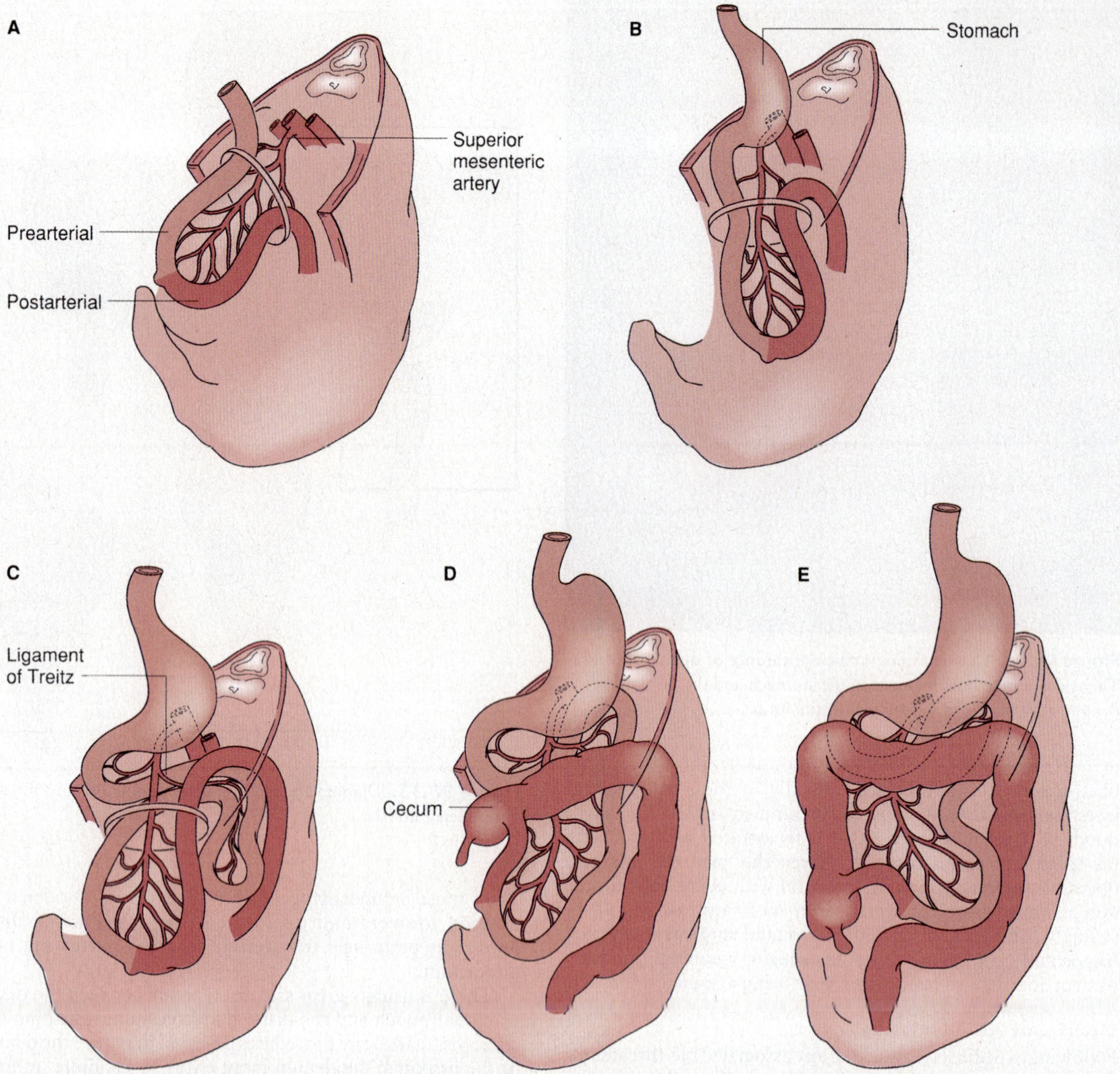

Figure 98.14. Normal midgut rotation is shown with appropriate positioning of the stomach, duodenum, small intestine, and cecum from the 5th gestational week (**A**) through completion by the 12th week (**E**).

5 of gestation, as illustrated in **Figure 98.14**. Three distinct events occur during normal midgut fixation. The first stage involves herniation of the primary midgut loop into the base of the umbilical cord, where it remains until week 10 of gestation. The axis of the midgut loop is the superior mesenteric artery (SMA), with the omphalomesenteric duct at the apex of the midgut loop. The midgut loop rotates 180 degrees counterclockwise so that the proximal half passes posterior to the SMA. The proximal portion gives rise to the proximal duodenum, which lies to the right of midline. A portion of this segment becomes the third and fourth portions of the duodenum. The distal duodenum is normally fixed to the left of the aorta at the ligament of Treitz, having rotated 270 degrees counterclockwise from its original position. The jejunoileal segment undergoes dramatic elongation, forming about six primary intestinal loops. The distal midgut loop gives rise to the cecum and the right colon, which also undergoes growth and elongation with concomitant rotation 270 degrees counterclockwise. Therefore, the cecum is initially positioned to the left, then anterior, and finally to the right of the SMA before reaching its final location.[34]

Reduction of the extracoelomic gut is the second stage of midgut development and fixation, occurring between weeks 10 and 12 of gestation. By this time, the duodenojejunal junction has passed posterior to the SMA and the midgut has rotated 180 degrees counterclockwise; however, the small intestine initially remains to the right side of midline, and the cecum and ascending colon are anterior to the SMA after return of the gut into the abdomen. Many common abnormalities of intestinal fixation occur as a result of arrested development during this 2-week period.

The final stage of midgut development is fixation of the intestine to the posterior body wall, occurring after week 12 of gestation. Cecal descent occurs at this time. Normal points of fixation include the cecum in the right iliac fossa and the duodenojejunal junction at the ligament of Treitz, just to the left of the aorta and anterior to the left renal vein (**Fig. 98.15**). Therefore, the normal intestinal mesentery is fixed with a broad base extending from the ligament of Treitz to the cecum. This broad-based mesenteric attachment prevents volvulus from occurring. In contrast, in disorders of intestinal rotation, the base of the mesentery is neither fixed nor broad, placing the entire midgut at risk for volvulus.

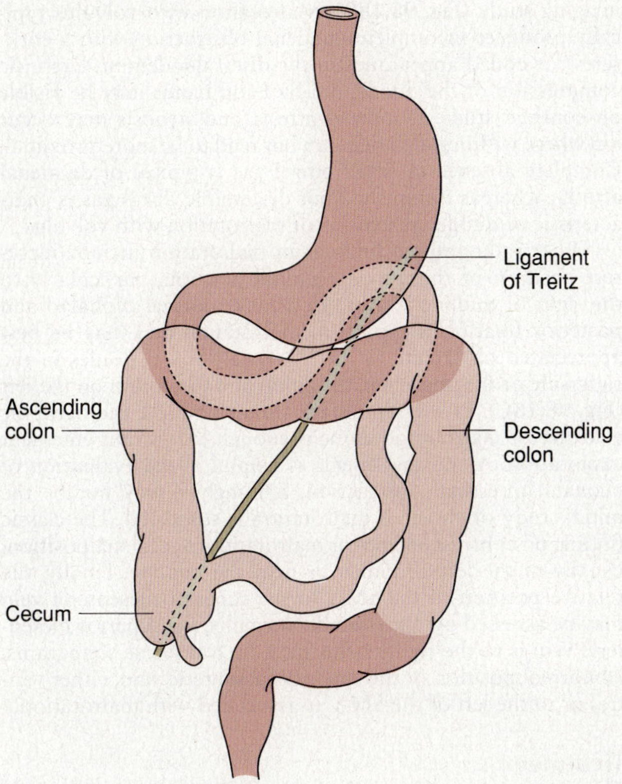

Figure 98.15. Normal oblique fixation of the midgut mesentery at the ligament of Treitz and in the right lower quadrant. The blue portions of the colon are extraperitoneal.

Anatomy

The normal sequence required for intestinal positioning and fixation can be interrupted at any developmental stage, producing a diverse spectrum of rotational abnormalities. Some neonatal surgical conditions are nearly always associated with abnormal intestinal rotation or fixation resulting from displacement of the midgut from the abdominal cavity during embryologic development. These anomalies include omphalocele, gastroschisis, and congenital diaphragmatic hernia. The term *malrotation* has been applied generically to describe disorders of intestinal rotation and fixation, although specific definitions of the more commonly encountered lesions are provided in the following sections.

Nonrotation

This common anomaly is characterized by inadequate counterclockwise rotation of the midgut around the SMA. Instead of the normal 270-degree arc, rotation is either absent or arrested before exceeding 90 degrees (**Fig. 98.16**). The small intestine resides on the right side of midline, the colon resides on the left, and the cecum is anterior and near the midline. The duodenojejunal junction is to the right of midline and more caudal and anterior in position. Nonrotation carries a significant clinical risk of midgut volvulus because the mesenteric vascular pedicle is narrow. Duodenal obstruction also may occur as a result of peritoneal attachments known as *Ladd bands.* These peritoneal bands fix the cecum to the posterior body wall by passing anterior and lateral to the distal duodenum.

Mixed or Incomplete Rotation

This rotational abnormality is characterized by arrest of the normal rotation at or near 180 degrees rather than the normal 270 degrees (**Fig. 98.17**). Instead of rotating posterior and to the left of the SMA, incomplete or arrested rotation of the prearterial segment leaves the duodenojejunal junction to the right of midline. The cecum also does not complete

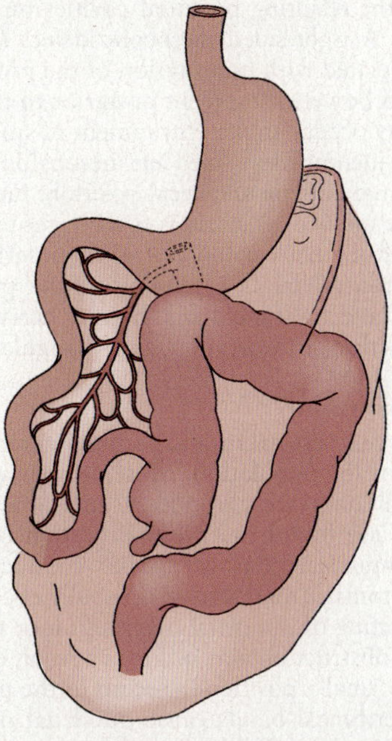

Figure 98.16. Nonrotation. The proximal segment of the small intestine resides on the right side of the abdomen, and the distal segment (*colon*) is on the left. Neither has rotated normally.

its counterclockwise passage anterior to the SMA; it usually resides in the upper abdomen just to the left of the SMA. Similar to nonrotation, fixation of the cecum to the posterior body wall by Ladd bands places the duodenum at risk for compression or obstruction. In addition, the SMA pedicle is narrow and places the midgut at risk for volvulus.

Mesocolic Hernias

Mesocolic hernias are rare but important anomalies characterized by failure of fixation of either the right or left mesocolon to the posterior body wall. The small bowel can become

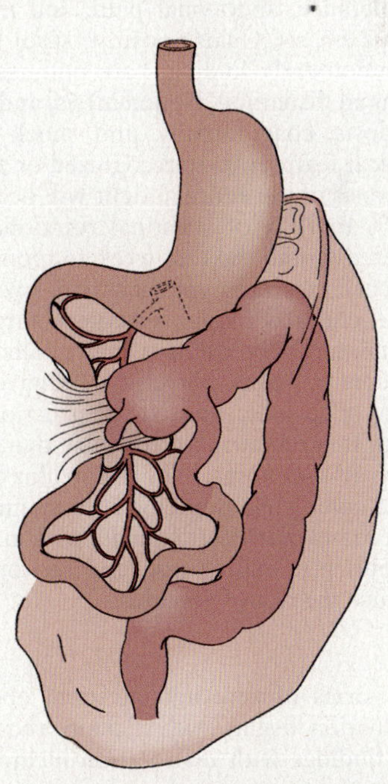

Figure 98.17. Incomplete rotation. The proximal segment has failed to rotate and is on the right. The distal segment has rotated to reside anterior to the duodenum so that cecal bands to the posterior abdominal wall may compress and obstruct the duodenum.

PEDIATRIC SURGERY

entrapped in the resulting potential cavities on either side of the abdomen. A right-sided mesocolic defect (paraduodenal hernia) is associated with nonrotation of the proximal midgut segment. Small bowel entrapment posterior to the right colon and cecum may occur. Similar entrapment of small bowel may occur from an incompletely fixed left mesocolon, but is associated with normal colonic and cecal position. Entrapped small bowel in a left mesocolic hernia is usually contained within a hernia sac with the neck composed of the inferior mesenteric vein and peritoneal bands extending to the posterior body wall. Both left and right mesocolic hernias carry the potential risks of obstruction, incarceration, and strangulation of bowel.

Clinical Presentation

Abnormalities of intestinal rotation are estimated to be present in about 1% of the population. Most persons with intestinal rotational anomalies are clinically asymptomatic; therefore, some children are found to have malrotation incidentally by upper gastrointestinal contrast studies conducted for other reasons. Symptomatic malrotation is usually encountered clinically in the setting of duodenal obstruction or midgut volvulus. Duodenal obstruction may occur as a result of Ladd bands fixing the abnormally positioned cecum to the posterior body wall. These peritoneal bands cause duodenal obstruction by extrinsic compression. Children with symptomatic duodenal obstruction typically present with bilious emesis and distention of the stomach and the proximal duodenum. Similar to proximal neonatal intestinal obstruction, newborn infants may present with bilious emesis without abdominal distention secondary to partial duodenal obstruction. A paucity of small bowel gas may be seen on plain abdominal films.

A potential consequence of intestinal malrotation is midgut volvulus. Midgut volvulus should be considered in any infant or child presenting with bilious emesis. The clinical outcome of midgut volvulus is time dependent, which is the fundamental reason that signs and symptoms of acute intestinal obstruction in an infant or a child must be pursued aggressively until a clear diagnosis is made. The devastating, life-threatening consequence of midgut volvulus is vascular insufficiency, gut ischemia, and, if untreated, infarction of the entire bowel supplied by the SMA. The initial symptoms may be subtle and limited to feeding intolerance, abdominal pain, and irritability, followed by bilious emesis. Guaiac-positive stool from mucosal injury is a common early finding. Late findings include progressive abdominal distention, hematemesis, and hypotension. Metabolic acidosis, coagulopathy, and shock may become prominent clinical features. If unrecognized or left untreated, transmural necrosis of the entire midgut will occur.

At least 50% to 75% of intestinal rotational abnormalities are discovered within the first week to month of life, and about 90% occur in children younger than 1 year. Symptomatic infants and children require emergent surgical exploration and correction. Older children and adults initially may present with acute volvulus, but also may have a history of vague symptoms of episodic intestinal obstruction and chronic abdominal pain. It is essential to recognize that, regardless of age or chronicity of symptoms, midgut volvulus from malrotation occurs in a completely unpredictable manner. Therefore, it is generally recommended that patients with incidentally discovered, asymptomatic malrotation undergo operative management to reduce the risk of volvulus.

Diagnosis

As with other forms of neonatal intestinal obstruction, the diagnostic evaluation begins with a plain abdominal radiograph. Classic findings with malrotation include gastric and proximal duodenal distention with a paucity or absence of distal small bowel gas (**Fig. 98.18A**). The plain film alone may not differentiate malrotation from duodenal atresia or stenosis. In most cases of suspected duodenal obstruction with concern of malrotation, an upper gastrointestinal series is a conclusive imaging study (**Fig. 98.18B**). Malrotation with volvulus typically produces incomplete duodenal obstruction with a corkscrew or coiled appearance in the distal duodenum. Extrinsic compression of the duodenum by Ladd bands may be visible on contrast study. Duodenal atresia and stenosis may occur anywhere within the duodenum but tend to be more proximal. Complete absence of small bowel gas is typical of duodenal atresia, whereas diminished but discernible distal gas is characteristic of duodenal stenosis or malrotation with volvulus.

Other radiographic findings in malrotation include incorrect position of the duodenojejunal junction, particularly to the right of midline. Failure to achieve normal cephalad and posterior fixation is typical in malrotation and may be best appreciated on lateral views. The small bowel resides in the right side of the abdomen, the colon and the cecum on the left (**Fig. 98.18C**). In a symptomatic infant or child, radiographic evidence of malrotation alone is enough to warrant emergent exploration. A contrast enema is helpful in the evaluation of neonatal intestinal obstruction, although it may not be the initial study of choice if malrotation is suspected. The classic finding on contrast enema for malrotation is cecal malposition, usually in the left abdomen or near the midline. Finally, the relative position of the SMA to the superior mesenteric vein may be assessed by ultrasound. Normally, the superior mesenteric vein is to the right of the SMA on transverse sonograms. Abnormal position of the superior mesenteric vein, either ventral or to the left of the SMA, is associated with malrotation.

Treatment

The management of bowel obstruction from malrotation or an internal hernia is operative. Initial assessment, resuscitation, and preoperative preparation in a symptomatic newborn should be conducted simultaneously so that confirmation of malrotation can be followed immediately by laparotomy. Urgent laparotomy is required to reduce the ischemic injury to the intestine. Shock, if present, must be treated aggressively by ensuring adequate gas exchange and establishing restoration of intravascular volume prior to the induction of general anesthesia. Volvulus with complete infarction of the midgut, if not immediately lethal, is survivable only with enterectomy, followed by permanent or long-term TPN support. In older, asymptomatic children with incidentally discovered malrotation, operative repair remains controversial. Given the devastating consequences of midgut volvulus, however, elective surgical correction appears warranted in most asymptomatic individuals as well.

Operative repair of malrotation is performed by Ladd procedure. The first objective is to relieve the midgut volvulus, if present. This is accomplished by delivery and detorsion of the affected midgut, usually in a counterclockwise direction. Recurrent volvulus is prevented by broadening the base of the mesenteric vascular pedicle by dividing the peritoneal bands that tether the cecum, small bowel mesentery, mesocolon, and duodenum around the base of the SMA (**Fig. 98.19**). Once completed, the mesentery and the mesocolon open widely, and the mesenteric pedicle is at low risk for recurrent volvulus.

The second objective of Ladd procedure is to divide the abnormal peritoneal attachments between the cecum and the abdominal wall. A modified Kocher maneuver involving meticulous and complete mobilization of the entire duodenum with division of all anterior, lateral, and posterior attachments is performed. Duodenal and distal small bowel patency should be demonstrated using intraluminal air or saline because synchronous intestinal webs and atresia have been reported. An appendectomy is performed to eliminate potential confusion from acute appendicitis developing in an abnormally positioned appendix. Performance of laparoscopic Ladd procedure has been demonstrated to be feasible and may help reduce time to enteral feeding and hospital length of stay; however, the long-term efficacy of this approach has been debated. Fixation

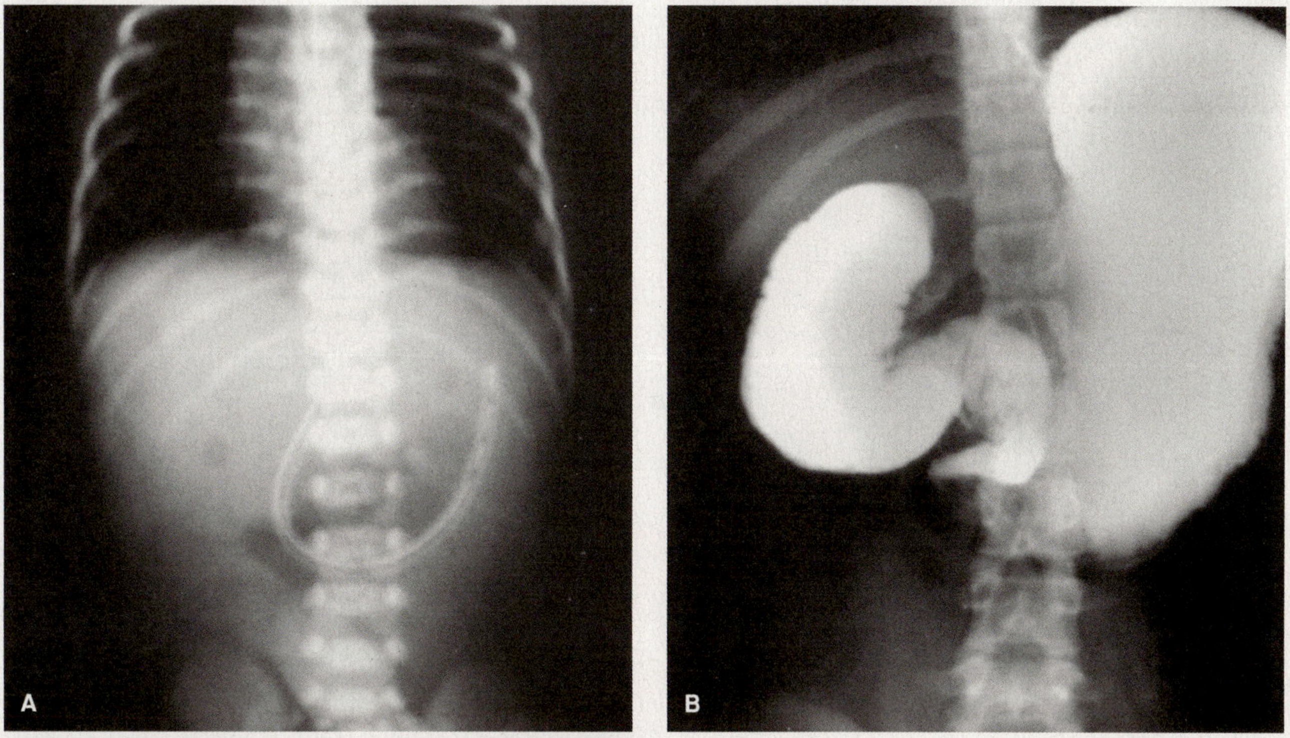

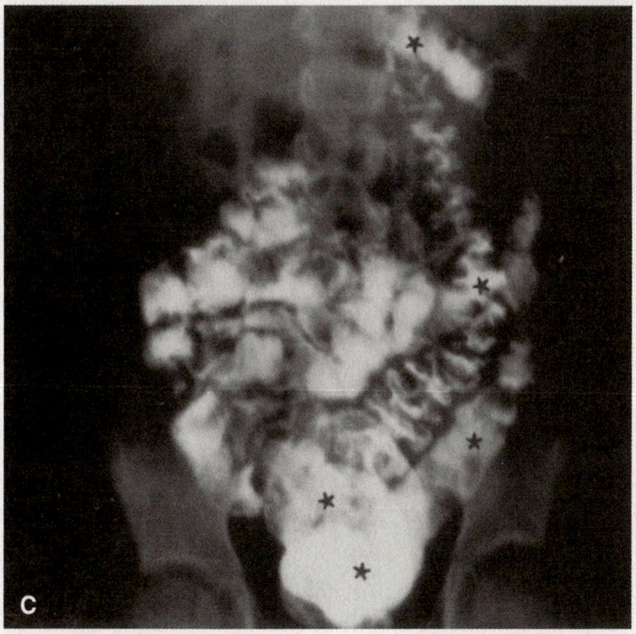

Figure 98.18. **A:** Plain radiograph of an infant with malrotation. There is a paucity of small bowel gas. **B:** Upper gastrointestinal contrast study demonstrating malrotation with midgut volvulus and duodenal obstruction. The position of the duodenojejunal junction is abnormal. **C:** Plain film showing a contrast-filled colon and cecum on the patient's left (*asterisks*). The entire small bowel is to the right of midline. These are typical radiographic findings of malrotation.

of the mesentery by cecal or duodenal plication to the body wall has been abandoned for lack of data supporting efficacy. Postoperative small bowel obstruction secondary to adhesions is reported in about 10% of patients.

Volvulus with intestinal necrosis is treated by preserving as much bowel length as possible. If bowel viability is unclear during initial exploration, a second-look procedure may be helpful to delineate reversible from irreversible injury. The management of nonviable bowel from volvulus is not different from other situations in which intestinal necrosis is encountered, and clinical decisions regarding resection and anastomosis are individualized. In situations in which the entire small intestine is lost and long-term survival is doubtful, treatment decisions must be made with the family.

Surgical management of right mesocolic hernia is directed at dividing the lateral peritoneal attachments of the cecum and right colon to eliminate the hernia. In addition, given the associated nonrotation of the proximal bowel, the vascular pedicle should be broadened as much as possible. Left mesocolic hernia is treated by mobilization of the inferior mesenteric vein, reduction of the small bowel from the hernia sac, and closure of the neck of the hernia sac to eliminate the potential space.

Results and Outcome

Results following surgical correction of intestinal rotational abnormalities should be excellent, and life expectancy should be normal in the absence of intestinal necrosis. Recurrent volvulus and recurrent duodenal obstruction are distinctly unusual if the initial procedure is technically complete. Adhesive small bowel obstruction following Ladd procedure is reported in 1% to 10% of patients. Long-term outcome is obviously less favorable in patients with intestinal necrosis at the time of exploration.

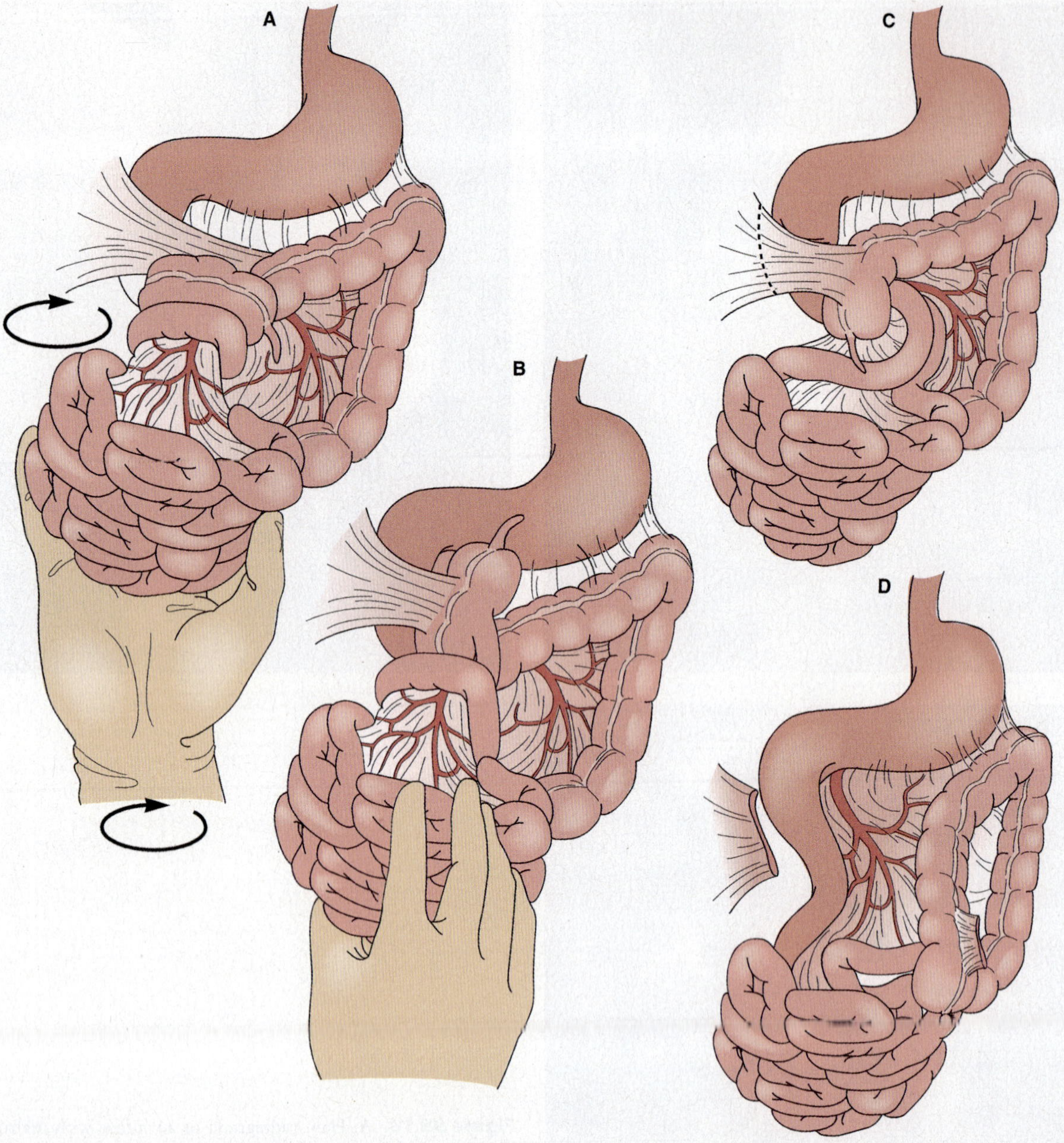

Figure 98.19. Correction of malrotation. **A, B:** Detorsion of midgut. **C, D:** Division of peritoneal attachments (Ladd bands) of cecum to abdominal cavity.

Intestinal Atresia or Stenosis

Embryology and Anatomy

The embryonic intestine undergoes segmental development during the third week of gestation. The septum transversum demarcates the developing foregut from the midgut. The midgut can be considered a tubular structure that progressively undergoes several predictable, developmental stages: (a) elongation; (b) herniation from and reduction into the coelomic cavity; (c) rotation; and (d) fixation of the mesentery to the posterior body wall.

Several different types of intestinal atresia are clinically observed (**Fig. 98.20**). *Type I* atresia is an intraluminal web or diaphragm that can either be complete or fenestrated with intact seromuscular layers of bowel. *Type II* and *IIIa* atresia are believed to be a result of in utero mesenteric vascular accidents. Experimental interruption of the fetal mesenteric blood supply in utero leads to this type of atresia. *Type IIIb* atresia, also known as the *apple-peel* or *Christmas tree deformity,* has complete mesenteric discontinuity, with the distal bowel concentrically surrounding a singular mesenteric blood supply. *Type IV* atresia has multiple segmental areas of discontinuous bowel. Type IIIb and IV atresia are thought to be consequences of major and multiple fetal mesenteric vascular interruption.

At least 90% of infants with congenital intestinal obstruction of the small bowel have complete atresia, whereas the remaining children have either stenoses or fenestrated intraluminal webs. The most common location is the distal ileum, and multiple areas of atresia are discovered in 3.6% to 20% of these infants. Infants with a fenestrated intraluminal web may have a small, often eccentric, opening that is only millimeters in diameter. These infants may not have obstructive symptoms until the introduction of solid food at 6 to 12 months of age and present with feeding intolerance, failure to thrive, or abdominal pain.

Congenital colonic atresia is a distinctly unusual condition. In a contemporary series of 277 infants treated with intestinal atresia, only 21 children had colonic atresia. Similar to small bowel atresia, colonic atresia is believed to reflect fetal mesenteric vascular injury. Given the distal nature of colonic atresia, initial feeding may be well tolerated, and definitive diagnosis

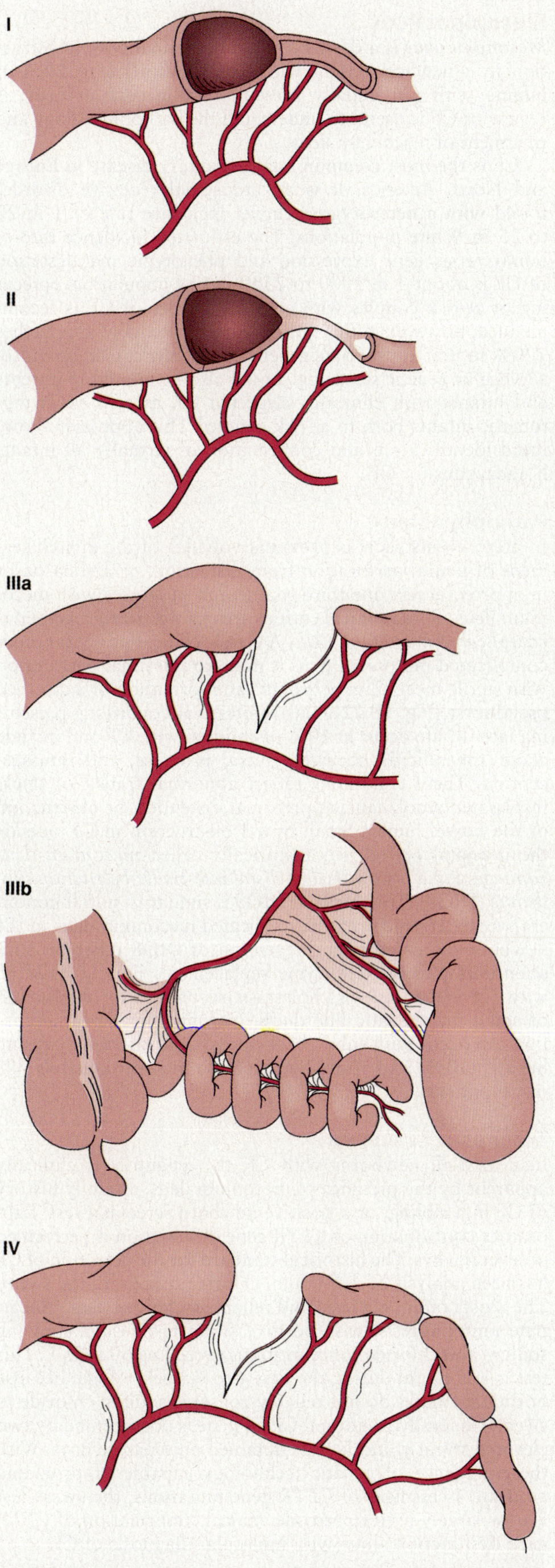

Figure 98.20. Classification of intestinal atresia. Type I, muscular continuity with a complete web. Type II, mesentery intact, fibrous cord. Type IIIa, muscular and mesenteric discontinuous. Type IIIb, apple-peel deformity. Type IV, multiple atresias. From Grosfeld JL. Jejunoileal atresia and stenosis. In: O'Neill JA Jr, Rowe MI, Grosfeld JL, et al., eds. *Pediatric Surgery*. 5th ed. Mosby; 1998:1145–1158.

may be delayed for several days. The diagnostic evaluation and surgical treatment of colonic atresia are identical to the approach used for small bowel atresia. Colonic atresia may be associated with abdominal wall defects, skeletal or cardiac defects, congenital aganglionosis (Hirschsprung disease), or coexisting intestinal atresia.

Clinical Presentation

Estimated incidence of intestinal atresia in the United States is 3.5 to 3.75 cases per 10,000 total births. Infants with jejunal or ileal atresia have a low incidence rate of significant associated anomalies. Approximately 10% of infants with gastroschisis have intestinal atresia or stenosis secondary to mechanical interruption of the mesenteric vascular supply.

Detection of maternal polyhydramnios on routine prenatal ultrasound screening can be an indication of proximal bowel obstruction caused by the interruption of normal amniotic fluid absorption in the fetal gut. Following delivery, the classic clinical presentation of intestinal atresia is bilious emesis, abdominal distention, and failure to pass meconium. The degree of abdominal distention depends on the site of obstruction, the infant's age, and the efficacy of proximal decompression. Abdominal distention may be absent with proximal intestinal atresia. Distal intestinal atresia may lead to abdominal distention with visible or palpable intestinal loops on examination. Rectal examination and evaluation of stool character remain important when intestinal obstruction is suspected.

Diagnosis

Following history and physical examination, plain radiographic abdominal films should be obtained. Plain films in jejunal or ileal atresia demonstrate marked gaseous distention of the proximal intestine with gasless distal small bowel and colon. Haustral markings are normally not apparent in the neonatal colon, and, therefore, discrimination between small bowel and colon in the newborn is difficult without intraluminal contrast. A contrast enema can be obtained to confirm the diagnosis of jejunoileal atresia and to rule out distal obstructions. A diminutive, unused but otherwise normal microcolon is typical, and the inability to reflux contrast into the proximal, dilated small bowel segment is diagnostic for congenital intestinal obstruction. This radiographic finding, in conjunction with the clinical setting, warrants operative exploration. An upper gastrointestinal series is unnecessary and may increase the risk of further emesis and aspiration in the newborn with obstruction. Incomplete obstruction from a fenestrated intraluminal web may require more sophisticated imaging techniques such as catheter-directed enteroclysis.

Treatment

Anatomic lesions causing neonatal intestinal obstruction require operative treatment. Whereas malrotation with midgut volvulus requires emergent diagnostic workup and operative intervention, obstruction resulting from intestinal atresia is generally not associated with life-threatening physiologic disturbances. Therefore, initial treatment is aimed at treating any other associated problems, confirming diagnosis, and preparing the infant for an operation. During this period, the infant should always have an orogastric or nasogastric tube in place to provide proximal decompression of the obstructed bowel.

The operative strategy in treating intestinal atresia is to restore gastrointestinal tract continuity while preserving as much intestinal length as possible. The operation is straightforward and an end-to-end or end-to-oblique (end-to-back) anastomosis is typically performed (**Fig. 98.21**). Short-segmental bowel resection and excision of an intraluminal web or diaphragm are done when necessary. Visual inspection and instillation of intraluminal saline or air to exclude distal atresia or web prior to anastomosis is important to evaluate patency of the downstream bowel. The size discrepancy between the proximal and distal bowel is usually considerable,

PEDIATRIC SURGERY

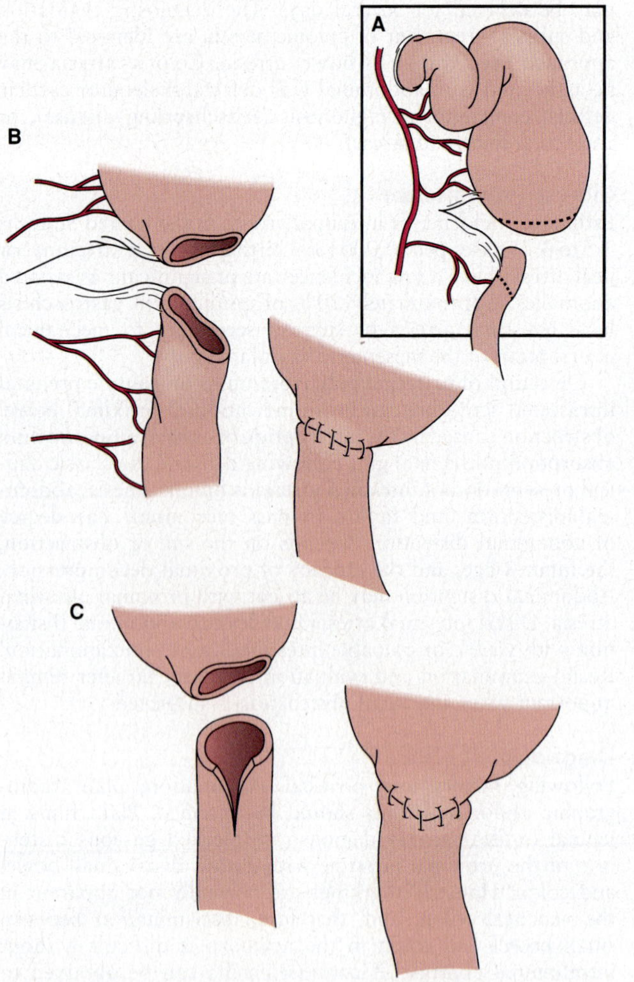

Figure 98.21. **A, B:** The end-to-oblique anastomosis for small bowel atresia. **C:** An extension of the distal enterostomy along the antimesenteric border may be used to create proximal and distal lumens of equal size for anastomosis.

and delayed postoperative bowel motility is common. Some surgeons advocate the use of technical procedures to improve emptying of the proximal bowel by reducing overall bowel diameter. These procedures include resection of 4 to 5 cm of proximal jejunum or ileum, plication, and tapering enteroplasty. Complex atresia associated with apple-peel deformity or multiple segmental atresias may require multiple serial anastomoses to preserve as much bowel length as possible. The ileocecal valve is preserved whenever possible, allowing improved tolerance of enteral nutrition in infants with limited small bowel length. It is estimated that approximately 40 cm of small bowel without an ileocecal valve, compared with 15 to 20 cm with an ileocecal valve, is sufficient for long-term enteral feeding tolerance in the neonate. Contemporary management of colonic atresia includes primary anastomosis when technically possible.

Results and Outcome

Currently, the overall survival rate for infants treated for intestinal atresia or stenosis (including duodenal atresia) exceeds 93% in most large series. Mortality in these infants is generally related to cardiac anomalies, birth weight less than 2 kg, and associated congenital anomalies.[35] Infants with a limited amount of intestinal length for nutritional absorption (short bowel syndrome with less than 40 cm) usually require long-term TPN and are at moderate-to-high risk for sepsis and liver injury. Infants with normal gastrointestinal length may still have prolonged intestinal dysfunction and dysmotility for several weeks.

Meconium Ileus

Meconium ileus is a descriptive term for small bowel obstruction in a newborn infant with CF. About 10% to 20% of infants with CF initially present with meconium ileus. A review of CF is useful to understand the pathophysiology and treatment of meconium ileus.

CF is the most common fatal hereditary disease in Europe and North America. It is an autosomal recessive disorder found with a heterozygous carrier incidence rate of 1 in 20 to 25 in White populations. The estimated incidence rate of homozygous gene expression and phenotypic manifestation of CF is about 1 in 2000 to 2500 in this population. Screening of at-risk couples with a family history of CF is recommended; however, in this setting, carrier discovery approaches 100% so that appropriate genetic counseling can be provided. Molecular genetic screening should also be offered to parents and infants with clinically suspected CF, as well as asymptomatic infants born to at-risk couples. This approach allows rapid identification and confirmation of virtually all infants homozygous for CF.

Pathophysiology

In utero events such as proximal volvulus of the dilated segment of ileum, perforation from distention, or atresia occur in approximately one-third to one-half of fetuses with meconium ileus. These clinical entities are characterized together as *complicated meconium ileus.* A classic clinical presentation of complicated meconium ileus is in utero intestinal perforation with sterile meconium peritonitis and formation of a calcified pseudocyst (**Fig. 98.22**). Gastrointestinal conditions presenting later in life occur in 10% of children with CF and include acute appendicitis, recurrent rectal prolapse, and intussusception. These conditions reflect abnormal transit of thick, inspissated stool, causing proximal distention or obstruction of the bowel lumen. Small bowel obstruction in CF outside the neonatal period was historically called *meconium ileus equivalent and* is now termed *distal intestinal obstruction syndrome* (DIOS). Treatment of DIOS is similar to initial nonoperative management of uncomplicated meconium ileus in the newborn discussed later. Prevention of DIOS relies on conscientious pancreatic enzyme replacement. Finally, children with CF are at risk of cholestasis secondary to obstruction of small intrahepatic bile ducts. Chronic hepatic inflammation can occur with subsequent fibrosis and cirrhosis, causing hepatic failure and portal hypertension in approximately 5% of CF patients.

Diagnostic Evaluation

In nearly all newborns with CF, the diagnosis is clinically apparent by the presence of meconium ileus, a family history of CF in a sibling, or a positive newborn screening test. Laboratory confirmation of *CFTR* gene dysfunction is performed in several ways. The historical standard for the detection of CF has been analysis of the sodium chloride content of the sweat. The most commonly used and reliable technique uses pilocarpine iontophoresis, with positive sweat test results showing sodium and chloride concentrations exceeding 60 mEq/L. This test is less useful during the first 4 to 6 weeks of age because normal neonates do not reliably conserve sodium chloride in sweat. Generally, abnormal *CFTR* gene is documented by two elevated sweat chloride tests obtained on separate days. With the emergence of genetic technology capable of providing accurate assessment of *CFTR* gene mutations, the sweat test is now largely used to provide clinical confirmation of *CFTR* gene dysfunction along with molecular diagnosis of CF.

Clinical Presentation

With routine prenatal ultrasound practices along with selected fetal DNA screening, the prenatal diagnosis of CF or meconium ileus is feasible, potentially allowing for improved management of anticipated clinical problems following delivery. Initial

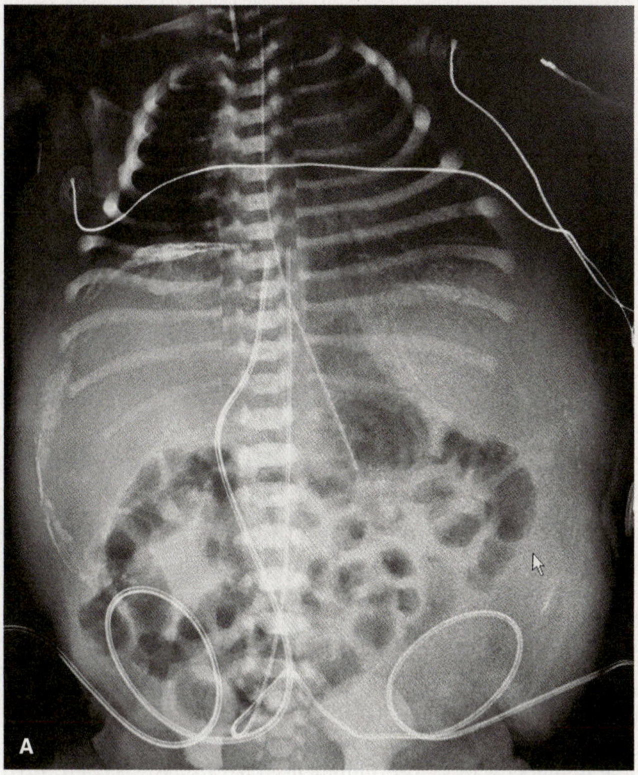

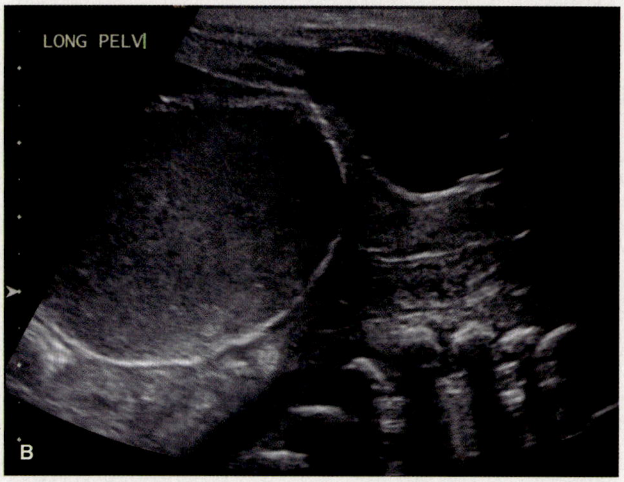

Figure 98.22. **A:** Plain film radiograph of calcified pseudocyst in complicated meconium ileus. **B:** In utero ultrasound demonstrating calcified pseudocyst.

signs of meconium ileus include neonatal bowel obstruction with abdominal distention, bilious emesis, and failure to pass meconium. On examination, the neonate may have palpable loops of meconium-filled intestine with a texture on palpation described as "doughy." Similar to other causes of proximal neonatal intestinal obstruction, rectal examination and evaluation of the meconium typically reveal clear white mucus or thick gray meconium. In utero intestinal perforation with pseudocyst formation in complicated meconium ileus may cause a palpable abdominal mass that is not particularly tender. On plain films or ultrasound, calcification is visible in the pseudocyst wall. In contrast, volvulus or intestinal perforation secondary to meconium ileus following birth generally results in diffuse peritonitis and sepsis. Intestinal atresia may also be seen as a consequence of complicated meconium ileus.

Diagnosis

Abdominal plain films may be diagnostic in meconium ileus, demonstrating multiple, distended loops of bowel. Fluid- or meconium-filled loops of bowel mixed with gas give a characteristic "soap bubble" or "ground glass" appearance. Classic air–fluid levels seen in other causes of intestinal obstruction are not expected because of the tenacious, sticky intraluminal meconium. The presence of intraperitoneal calcifications or a calcified cyst is consistent with prenatal intestinal perforation of sterile meconium.

A water-soluble contrast enema is useful in the evaluation and treatment of simple meconium ileus. This study usually demonstrates an unused but functionally normal microcolon. Reflux of contrast into the terminal ileum may confirm the presence of inspissated meconium pellets. In conjunction with a family history and plain films, this finding is sufficient evidence to confirm the diagnosis of neonatal meconium ileus. Upper gastrointestinal contrast studies are generally unnecessary and may complicate further therapeutic efforts.

Treatment

Nonoperative

Nonoperative management of simple meconium ileus is achieved in about 60% to 70% of newborns. Once the diagnosis of meconium ileus is confirmed, the initial treatment of choice is to perform retrograde irrigation of the terminal ileum with one of several solutions designed to dissipate the obstructing meconium. In the United States, several different enema techniques and a variety of contrast media have been described, including normal saline, hyperosmolar contrast agents, and dilute *N*-acetylcysteine. Initially, it was believed that using hyperosmolar contrast material was necessary to create an osmolar gradient. The resultant influx of fluid into the intestinal lumen was thought to solubilize the inspissated meconium. Recent data suggest that successful meconium clearance is not necessarily related to the osmolality of the contrast agent; however, a significantly higher overall success rate is reported with the use of Gastrografin (sodium and meglumine amidotrizoate) and the use of other solubilizing agents such as Tween-80 and *N*-acetylcysteine. As long as clinical progress is being made, sequential enemas may be required to disimpact the inspissated meconium from the terminal ileum. In similar fashion, children and older patients presenting with DIOS are treated with retrograde enemas until the obstruction resolves. The distinct advantage of this treatment approach is the avoidance of general anesthesia and exploratory laparotomy. Reported complications with this approach include rare intestinal perforation, intestinal mucosal injury, and persistent obstruction resulting from meconium concretions.

Operative

The major indications for operative intervention are either failure to clear the obstruction by retrograde enema or complicated meconium ileus with cyst formation, volvulus, atresia, or perforation. For simple meconium ileus with persistent obstruction despite contrast enemas, the operative goals are meconium disimpaction from the ileum and evacuation of the remaining stool from the small intestine. These steps can be accomplished by either milking the meconium downstream into the colon or solubilizing the meconium by transmural needle instillation of irrigant. However, enterotomy or enterostomy and direct irrigation of the bowel lumen are usually required to completely clear the inspissated meconium. Simple closure of the enterotomy is preferred, but segmental resection may be required if marginal or compromised intestine is found. End-to-end anastomosis is the appropriate reconstruction technique following segmental bowel resection. A temporary enterostomy may be required, and several historical techniques have been described. Another surgical option is the placement of a T-tube into the ileum for continued irrigation with dilute *N*-acetylcysteine. Following clearance of meconium from the intestine and the return of bowel function, the T-tube can be safely and simply removed.[36]

Complicated meconium ileus occurs in about one-third of patients. The surgical management of this entity is individualized. Intestinal atresia is not uncommon in meconium ileus, and the entire length of the intestine must be inspected for patency. When possible, resection of nonviable, stenotic, or perforated intestine is performed with immediate reconstruction via primary anastomosis. Patency of the downstream bowel must be confirmed to prevent anastomotic leak resulting from distal obstruction. If the infant is critically ill or has diffuse peritonitis, a safe primary anastomosis may not be possible, and a diverting enterostomy is required. Stoma closure may be performed promptly after resolution of peritonitis and inflammation.

Postoperative Care and Results

If the meconium has been successfully cleared without opening the intestine, dilute *N*-acetylcysteine may be given through the nasogastric tube or by enema. Alternatively, if a T-tube has been placed, dilute *N*-acetylcysteine or other irrigant can be used directly into the ileum. These efforts are aimed at keeping the meconium soluble and preventing recurrent ileal obstruction. Following return of bowel function, enteral feeding using breast milk or an elemental formula is started along with oral pancreatic enzyme replacement. Vigilant pulmonary therapy is routine and includes mucolytics and antibiotics when indicated. Nutritional assessment and support are essential in long-term management.

Successful nonoperative management of simple meconium ileus historically was associated with a more favorable outcome; however, the operative mortality rates of infants with meconium ileus have improved dramatically over the past several decades, and current short-term operative survival rates of 70% to 100% are reported. Long-term survival following meconium ileus is generally determined by the course of the underlying pulmonary disease. Contemporary management of CF has produced a mean survival age that approaches 30 years in most centers. With the exception of the development of portal hypertension in about 5% of patients, intestinal manifestations of the CF are treatable. Future medical and surgical efforts to improve the long-term outcome in these patients include direct replacement of the diseased pulmonary system by lung transplantation, manipulation of the epithelial chloride transport defect with pharmacologic agents, and gene therapy directed at *CFTR* gene transfer into respiratory epithelial cells.

Meckel Diverticulum and Related Disorders

Embryology and Anatomy

The most frequently encountered congenital anomaly of the gastrointestinal tract is Meckel diverticulum, representing one of several malformations resulting from persistence of the yolk stalk (synonymous with *vitelline duct* and *omphalomesenteric duct*) and its components. The embryonic yolk stalk connects the yolk sac and the developing midgut (**Fig. 98.23**). Between weeks 5 and 7 of gestation, the yolk sac involutes and the stalk fuses with the umbilical cord. Developmental failure or arrest of yolk sac involution creates a spectrum of clinical malformations as outlined in **Figure 98.24**, with Meckel diverticula constituting greater than 95% of these anomalies. Meckel diverticulum is a true diverticulum of variable size derived from the intestinal remnant of the yolk stalk. Typically, it is found on the antimesenteric border of the terminal ileum approximately 40 to 50 cm from the ileocecal valve in

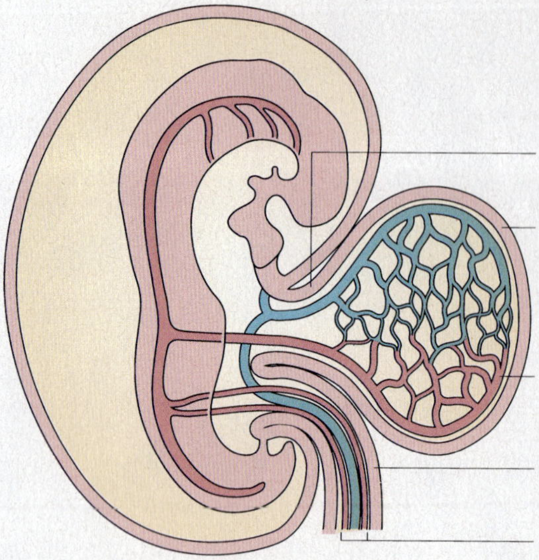

Figure 98.23. Normal embryonic relations of the yolk sac, yolk stalk, and developing gut.

adults. The blood supply is derived from persistent vitelline vessels supplied from the SMA. About 25% of the diverticula have a fibrous or vascular attachment to the anterior abdominal wall at the umbilicus (**Fig. 98.24C**). Heterotopic gastric mucosa or pancreatic tissue is found in about half of the diverticula examined at autopsy. In about 75% of patients with symptomatic diverticula, gastric mucosa is present. When symptoms occur, bleeding or perforation is generally the result of peptic ulceration of the adjacent ileal mucosa and not from the diverticulum itself.

Clinical Presentation and Diagnosis

Symptomatic yolk stalk anomalies are usually diagnosed by history and clinical examination. Umbilical drainage from a persistent fistula or sinus tract may be noted in a newborn following separation of the umbilical cord. Intestinal prolapse or passage of stool from the umbilicus signifies a patent omphalomesenteric duct. Small bowel obstruction in an otherwise healthy infant without a history of laparotomy may be a result of volvulus around an omphalomesenteric band or intussusception from a Meckel diverticulum acting as a lead point.

The incidence rate of Meckel diverticula in the general population is about 2%, with a 2:1 male-to-female predominance. The risk of developing symptoms from the diverticulum decreases with age, and the vast majority of subjects remain asymptomatic. About half of the people who do become symptomatic are younger than 2 years. **Table 98.3** outlines several of the more common clinical presentations of symptomatic Meckel diverticulum.

Hemorrhage

Gastrointestinal bleeding related to Meckel diverticulum generally results from peptic ulceration of the adjacent ileal mucosa. Clinically, it manifests as painless, episodic hemorrhage that is typically bright red to maroon in color; melena is not characteristically seen. Bleeding from Meckel diverticulum is generally not hemodynamically significant or exsanguinating, but it can be persistent enough to require transfusion. The diagnostic test of choice is the ^{99m}Tc-pertechnetate radioisotope scan (Meckel scan) because of the high affinity of the isotope for gastric mucosa and the high probability of gastric mucosa within a symptomatic Meckel diverticulum. Diagnostic accuracy is reported to be as high as 90% for Meckel-related bleeding. Contrast studies and endoscopy have a limited role when the problem is hemorrhage from a Meckel diverticulum.

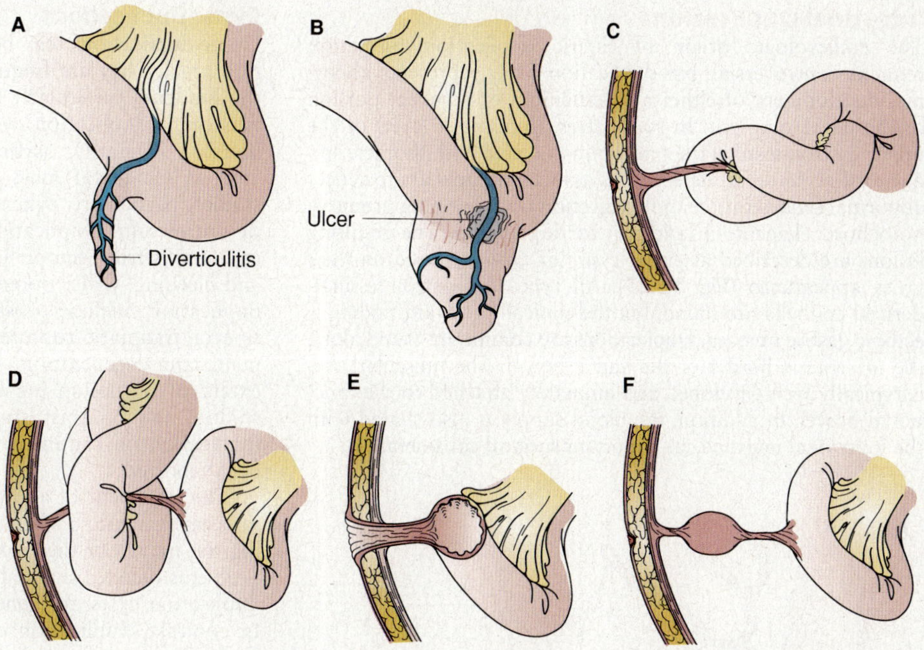

Figure 98.24. Common variants of yolk stalk malformations. **A, B:** Meckel diverticulum can manifest with inflammation (diverticulitis) or hemorrhage from acid-induced ulceration. **C, D:** Meckel diverticulum in association with abnormal band attached to the abdominal wall, predisposing to volvulus and intestinal obstruction. **E:** Patent omphalomesenteric duct. **F:** Omphalomesenteric sinus and cyst formation.

Obstruction

Intestinal obstruction associated with omphalomesenteric duct anomalies usually results from either intussusception or volvulus around an abnormal attachment between the bowel and the abdominal wall. In about 5% to 10% of persons with symptomatic Meckel diverticula, intussusception is the initial symptom. In patients with Meckel diverticula whose initial symptom is small bowel obstruction, about half have intussusception, and the remainder have volvulus, internal hernias, or other mechanical causes. Intussusception secondary to a Meckel diverticulum has a decreased likelihood for successful enema reduction. Small bowel obstruction from volvulus around an omphalomesenteric band requires operative exploration and treatment.

Diverticulitis

About one-third of patients with symptomatic Meckel diverticulum have acute diverticulitis. Similar to appendicitis, intraluminal obstruction at the base of a Meckel diverticulum can lead to distal inflammation, gangrene, and subsequent perforation. Peptic ulceration can also lead to local inflammation and perforation with the development of peritonitis. The signs and symptoms of Meckel diverticulitis are virtually indistinguishable from appendicitis, and exploration is both diagnostic and therapeutic.

DIAGNOSIS

Table 98.3. Signs and Symptoms of Meckel Diverticulum

Clinical Presentation	Approximate Frequency (%)
Hemorrhage	30–35
Small bowel obstruction	30–35
Diverticulitis	20–25
Umbilical fistula	10
Other	Uncommon

Umbilical Anomalies

About 10% of patients with yolk stalk or persistent omphalomesenteric duct anomalies have umbilical problems. The usual clinical presentation is persistent drainage or intestinal mucosa found at the umbilicus. The diagnosis can be confirmed by contrast sonogram of the umbilical orifice or tract. Occasionally, ultrasound examination may be useful to demonstrate omphalomesenteric cysts. Ultimately, surgical exploration may be required for both diagnosis and treatment.

Treatment

Infants and children with symptomatic umbilical abnormalities from yolk stalk remnants are usually well, and umbilical exploration with possible laparotomy can be undertaken electively. The yolk stalk remnant is excised, and, if present, the communication with the ileum is closed primarily with minimal morbidity and mortality. Operative exploration is required for patients with symptomatic Meckel diverticula. Typically, exploration can be accomplished through a variety of incisions. The treatment of choice is resection through either antimesenteric wedge excision or segmental bowel resection with primary closure or anastomosis. Laparoscopic diagnosis and management of Meckel diverticulum has also been described. In the absence of associated medical problems, excellent functional outcome is expected with minimal morbidity and essentially no mortality unless intestinal necrosis has occurred.

Meckel Diverticulum as an Incidental Finding

The management of an incidentally discovered Meckel diverticulum during abdominal exploration for other reasons is controversial. The risk of resecting an asymptomatic diverticulum must be weighed against the reasons for the operative exploration, patient age, and the potential for future symptoms from the diverticulum. Infants younger than 2 years are at a greater probability of becoming symptomatic from Meckel diverticula. Resection is clearly indicated with demonstration of heterotopic gastric mucosa in the diverticulum to prevent peptic ulceration. This finding may occasionally be determined by direct palpation because the gastric mucosa is thicker than ileal mucosa. Abnormal omphalomesenteric bands to the abdominal wall should also be excised. If clinical judgment suggests that the diverticulum is at risk for luminal obstruction, resection is warranted.

Intestinal Duplications

The embryologic origin of enteric duplication formation remains controversial, but duplication likely represents abnormal development of either a diverticulum or adjacent portion of the developing gut. In some cases, duplication cysts of the upper gastrointestinal tract may be associated with thoracic spinal cord or vertebral defects; this association appears to reflect abnormal sequestration and integration of developing primitive notochord elements in addition to duplication. The resulting lesions are described as either *cystic* or *tubular* based on their gross appearance (**Fig. 98.25**). All types of gastrointestinal-derived epithelia are found, but the clinically relevant finding is ectopic gastric mucosa. Duplications are commonly found along the mesenteric border of the native bowel. The muscular wall is typically well developed and intimately attached to the functional bowel. In addition, the blood supply is also shared with the functional intestine, an important surgical consideration.

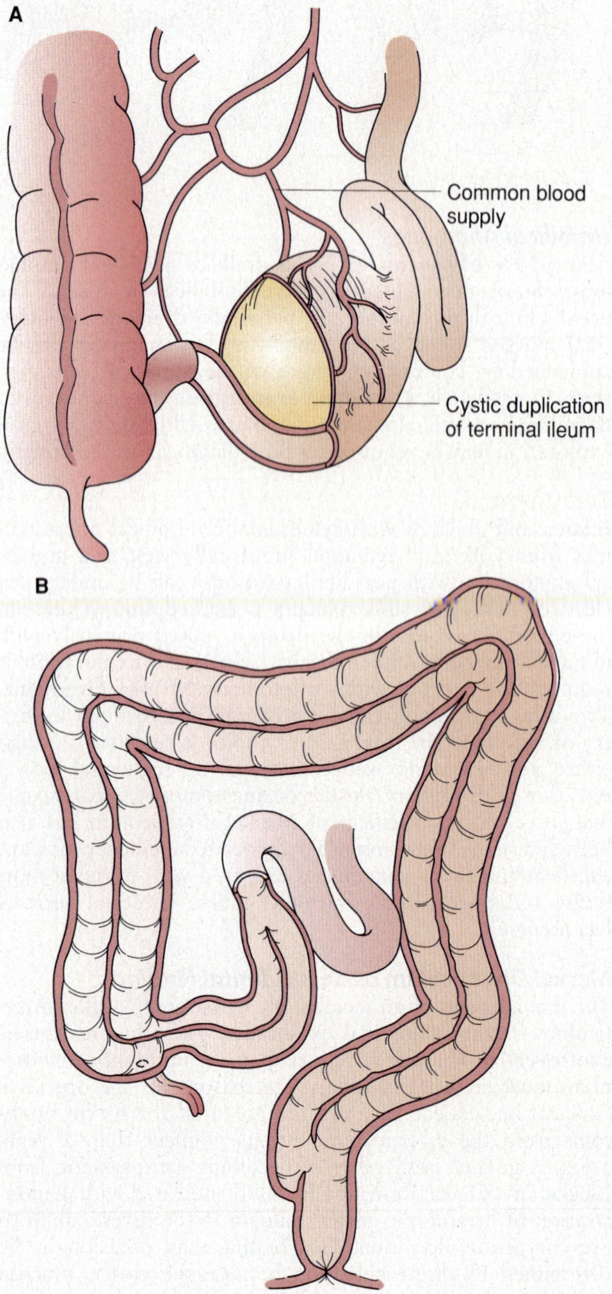

Figure 98.25. Enteric duplication. **A:** Cystic duplication of the terminal ileum. **B:** Tubular duplication of the terminal ileum and the colon.

Cystic Duplications

Cystic duplications may be found throughout the gastrointestinal tract. They are frequently located in the esophagus and the hindgut, particularly the rectum. Direct communication between a duplication cyst and the functional gut lumen is unusual. Typically, asymptomatic duplications are discovered as incidental mass lesions during diagnostic imaging studies, particularly when the location is the thoracic cavity or the rectum. Duplications may also present as symptomatic lesions from ectopic gastric mucosa leading to ulceration and bleeding. Other potential presenting symptoms of enteric duplication include obstruction, intussusception, perforation or traumatic rupture, torsion, infection, and occasional malignant degeneration. Useful examinations to define the extent of the lesion include ultrasound, CT scanning, MRI studies, and contrast studies. The identification of enteric duplication on routine prenatal ultrasound examination has been reported.

The treatment of all cystic duplications is operative. Even in asymptomatic infants and children, uncertainty regarding the nature of the mass and the potential for subsequent problems dictates surgical exploration. Esophageal and rectal duplication cysts are generally amenable to simple excision. In contrast, duplication cysts of the small intestine usually require segmental resection and primary anastomosis, given the intimate attachment and shared blood supply with the native bowel. For large cystic duplications involving longer segments of native bowel, individualized treatment strategies are required. One option is cyst marsupialization with resection of the duplication cyst wall with preservation of the common blood supply and wall between the cyst and the native bowel. This technique is combined with submucosal dissection and stripping of the remaining epithelium from the cyst wall. Another approach is internal drainage of the cyst into the adjacent native intestine, for example, creation of a cystduodenostomy for duodenal duplication not amenable to local resection and anastomosis; this would be distinctly unusual.

Tubular Duplications

Tubular duplications may be found anywhere along the length of the gastrointestinal tract. They are less frequent than cystic duplications and have a tendency to involve the ileum and the colon. It is believed that tubular duplication generally reflects abnormal, disordered recanalization of the gastrointestinal tract. Similar to cystic duplications, tubular lesions share a common wall and blood supply with the native bowel. Communication between the tubular duplication and the native bowel lumen is common. Tubular duplications may be extensive and can involve the entire length of terminal ileum and colon. Malformations of the entire colon and rectum are associated with genitourinary anomalies, particularly duplications of the external genitalia or bladder.

Tubular duplications manifest clinically in similar fashion to cystic lesions. Symptomatic lesions most commonly present with gastrointestinal bleeding or obstruction. Treatment is operative, and an individualized strategy is required that is based on the location and nature of the duplication. Resection with primary anastomosis may require removal of an unacceptable length of normal bowel. Marsupialization with submucosal stripping of the duplication epithelium may be particularly helpful if ectopic gastric mucosa is suspected or found. Obstruction from a long, blind-ending parallel duplication that communicates with the functional gut lumen can be treated effectively with a reentry procedure such as a distal enteroenterostomy. This approach avoids a potentially complex resection of a significant length of bowel.

The outcomes of surgical management of enteric duplications are generally excellent in the absence of other associated anomalies or medical problems. Mortality attributable to the duplication itself is unusual. Postoperative morbidity is generally dependent on the nature and location of the duplication.

Necrotizing Enterocolitis

Pathophysiology

4 NEC is a neonatal disease characterized by an initial intestinal mucosal injury that may ultimately progress to transmural bowel necrosis. NEC is the most frequently encountered neonatal surgical emergency and a major cause of morbidity and mortality in the premature infant. Despite its frequency and extensive study, the pathogenesis remains obscure, and surgical treatment is directed largely at controlling the complications of intestinal necrosis. The development of NEC occurs in association with a variety of associated conditions, including perinatal stress, sepsis, respiratory failure, hypoxemia, hypotension, and congenital cardiac defects. In general, NEC is observed in the premature infant with multiple risk factors and potential etiologic events and conditions. To create a murine model of NEC, the necessary factors are hypoxemia and to formula (not breast milk) feed the animals.[37–39] Current clinical and experimental data support the concept that the pathophysiology of NEC remains enigmatic and multifactorial.

The intestinal mucosal injury observed in NEC is likely to be the end result of an ischemic insult in a susceptible host. Normally, the neonatal pulmonary and systemic vascular smooth muscle undergoes rapid structural and physiologic changes shortly after birth. The premature infant appears to be particularly vulnerable to vasoconstriction. With regard to NEC, it is hypothesized that hypoperfusion and ischemia of the premature neonatal intestinal tract may be the result of uncontrolled splanchnic vasoconstriction. This situation may be worsened in critically ill premature infants with low cardiac output states, impairing oxygen delivery to the intestines.

A common characteristic of NEC is the host inflammatory response to the initiating mucosal injury. Experimental data are consistent with an important role for inflammatory mediators in the propagation of intestinal injury in NEC.[40] More than 90% of cases of NEC occur after the initiation of enteral feeding, and several studies document that the osmolarity or rate of initial feeding may be important. Although controversy exists, most neonatal centers now avoid rapid advancement of hyperosmolar enteral feedings and attempt to prevent excessive fluid volume in premature infants. A multicenter, randomized controlled clinical trial using *Bifidobacterium* and *Lactobacillus* as a probiotic given with initial feeding demonstrated significant reduction in death from NEC in very low–birth-weight premature infants.[41]

The most common site of involvement of NEC is the terminal ileum and right colon. NEC may be localized, segmental, or it may involve the entire gastrointestinal tract. Histopathologic examination of intestinal tissue from infants with NEC demonstrates submucosal edema, hemorrhage, and microvascular thrombosis leading to transmural necrosis. The histopathology of NEC resembles that of experimental intestinal ischemia, with areas of reversible mucosal injury adjacent to areas of transmural necrosis. Dissection of intraluminal gas through the injured mucosa leads to gas within the bowel wall, known as *Pneumatosis intestinalis*. The finding of pneumatosis intestinalis is a classic radiographic and pathologic feature of NEC. Initially, the gas may be localized in the submucosa or lymphatic vessels, but it may dissect into the muscularis, the portal venous tract, or into the subserosa. Intestinal perforation, inflammatory phlegmon, and diffuse peritonitis are common with advanced NEC.

Clinical Presentation

NEC is estimated to occur in 1 to 3 of 1000 live births and 30 per 1000 low–birth-weight births. NEC may also occur in term infants, and in this group, it has a tendency to involve the colon and may present without classic signs. The actual incidence of NEC remains difficult to determine because the diagnosis is subjective; classic signs on physical examination and diagnostic imaging are not always uniformly present. The classic clinical signs of NEC include abdominal distention, feeding intolerance, bilious emesis, and either occult or gross blood in the stool. Gastrointestinal mucosal bleeding is present in the vast majority of cases (80% to 90%) but is rarely significant from a hemodynamic standpoint. On physical examination, abdominal tenderness with distention is common, and individual loops of thickened or fixed bowel may be palpable. Edema, erythema, crepitus, or discoloration of the abdominal wall suggests intestinal necrosis, perforation, or intra-abdominal abscess (**Fig. 98.26**). Hematochezia or guaiac-positive stool is typical. Systemic signs of inflammation and sepsis, such as temperature instability, apnea, bradycardia, hypoxemia, acidosis, and thrombocytopenia, are also common. The primary diagnostic goal during initial clinical evaluation is to determine whether irreversible, transmural intestinal necrosis is present. There is no single physical finding or laboratory test that makes this distinction.

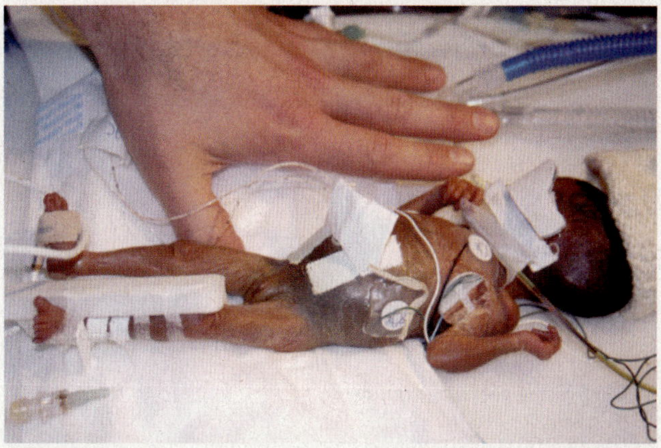

Figure 98.26. Clinical presentation of diffuse staining of abdominal wall in an extremely low–birth-weight infant with perforated necrotizing enterocolitis.

Diagnosis

The diagnosis of NEC relies on clinical evaluation and judgment based on symptoms and signs in the appropriate setting. **Table 98.4** summarizes diagnostic criteria and a staging system for NEC most commonly used in the United States. Radiographic confirmation of NEC requires only plain abdominal films. During the acute inflammatory phase, contrast studies may be hazardous and are contraindicated. The classic radiographic finding of pneumatosis intestinalis (**Fig. 98.27**) confirms the diagnosis in the appropriate clinical setting but is variably present. Other radiographic findings consistent with NEC include thickened bowel loops, ascites, and portal venous gas. Serial abdominal films, including a left lateral decubitus or upright film, should be obtained every 6 to 8 hours during the early course of the disease. These sequential studies help document the progression or resolution of the inflammatory process and, importantly, evaluate for the presence of intestinal perforation presenting as free intraperitoneal gas or pneumoperitoneum. The presence of pneumoperitoneum mandates operative intervention; however, up to half of infants with perforated NEC do not have discernible pneumoperitoneum on plain films.

Treatment

Nonoperative

The vast majority of infants with NEC can be managed medically. Initial management of NEC includes proximal decompression with a nasogastric or orogastric tube, bowel rest, and broad-spectrum intravenous antibiotics. Prompt correction of hypotension, hypoxemia, and inadequate ventilation must be undertaken. Intravenous fluid management, with particular attention to electrolytes and acid–base status, is essential. Central venous access is secured and TPN is initiated. Oxygen

STAGING

Table 98.4. Necrotizing Enterocolitis

Stage I NEC (Suspected)
Any one or more historical factors producing perinatal stress
Systemic manifestations
Temperature instability
Lethargy
Apnea
Bradycardia
Gastrointestinal manifestations
Poor feeding
Increasing pregavage residuals
Emesis
Mild abdominal distention
Occult blood in stool
Abdominal radiographs showing distention with mild ileus
Stage II NEC (Definite)
Any one or more historical factors
Above signs and symptoms, plus
Persistent occult or gross gastrointestinal bleeding
Marked abdominal distention
Abdominal radiographs showing significant intestinal distention with
Ileus
Small bowel edema
Pneumatosis intestinalis
Portal venous gas
Stage III NEC (Advanced)
Any one or more historical factors
Above signs and symptoms, plus: Deterioration of vital signs
Evidence of septic shock
Marked gastrointestinal hemorrhage
Abdominal radiographs showing pneumoperitoneum in addition to findings listed for stage II

From Bell MJ, Kosloske AM, Benton C, et al. Neonatal necrotizing enterocolitis: prevention of perforation. *J Pediatr Surg*. 1973;8:601–605, with permission.

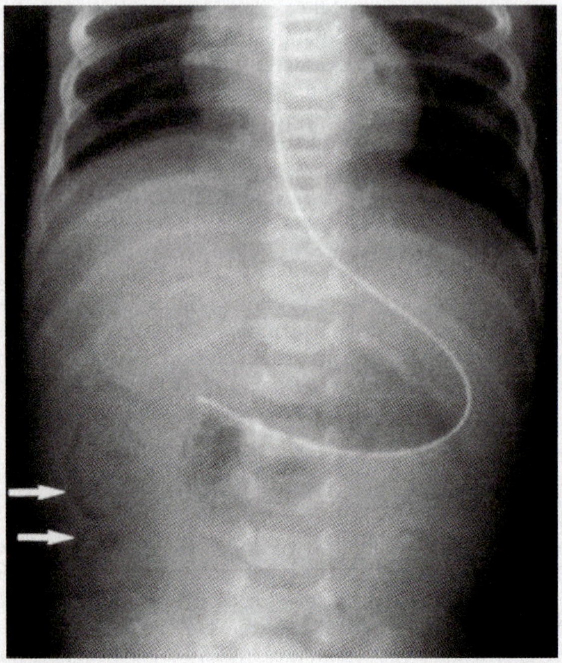

Figure 98.27. Plain abdominal film demonstrating *pneumatosis intestinalis* (*arrows*) in an infant with necrotizing enterocolitis.

delivery and cardiac performance must be maintained, which in a premature neonate may require operative closure of a patent ductus arteriosus; this approach is preferable over the use of indomethacin in the setting of NEC. Serial physical examinations and blood work are useful in monitoring disease progress.

Most infants with NEC improve with medical management. Typically, reversal of the systemic inflammatory response occurs rapidly, and the abdominal distention and ileus resolve over a period of days. Nasogastric tube decompression and intravenous antibiotics are usually continued for 7 to 14 days. Enteral feeding is usually resumed once antibiotics have been discontinued and there has been return of gastrointestinal function. The usual course of medically treated NEC is rapid clinical response and stabilization in the first 24 to 36 hours. Infants with significant intestinal necrosis typically have signs of either pneumoperitoneum or clinical deterioration during the initial 24 to 72 hours of treatment.

Indications to abandon medical management and escalate surgical therapy include evidence of intestinal perforation or clinical deterioration with persistent or progressive systemic illness despite maximal medical therapy. Evidence of persistent or progressive systemic sepsis includes temperature instability, refractory hypotension, acidosis, hypoglycemia, neutropenia, and thrombocytopenia. Local findings such as portal venous gas, abdominal wall cellulitis, or crepitus also may signal intestinal necrosis and the need for operative intervention. A palpable, fixed abdominal mass consistent with intestinal perforation with an inflammatory phlegmon or abscess may also be a relative indication for operation. Because there is no complete agreement on what constitutes clinical deterioration, some controversy exists regarding operative indications for NEC in the absence of pneumoperitoneum. Because the interpretation of clinical deterioration criteria remains subjective, the decision to operate remains a multifactorial clinical judgment. In equivocal situations, abdominal paracentesis of ascitic fluid may be helpful in diagnosing intestinal necrosis with perforation in the absence of pneumoperitoneum if the aspirate contains bacteria or stool.

Operative

Operative indications in NEC include the presence of intestinal necrosis with or without frank intestinal perforation. Conventional operative intervention is aimed at treating the complications of NEC (ie, intestinal necrosis). In general, resection of intestine involved with NEC does not prevent further extension of disease in other involved areas of the bowel. For isolated segmental disease, the traditional surgical treatment of NEC is resection of necrotic bowel with proximal enterostomy and distal mucous fistula placement. In infants with diffuse NEC, multiple resections with several enterostomies may be required. The primary operative goal is an expedient operation with preservation of as much intestinal length as possible, including the ileocecal valve. Because the risk of developing short-gut syndrome is substantial in infants with diffuse disease, preservation of marginal areas of involved intestine with a planned second-look operation to reevaluate intestinal viability may be useful. Accurate measurement of the remaining bowel length is important from a diagnostic and prognostic standpoint, with the length of bowel resected determined by the extent of transmural intestinal necrosis. Resection with primary anastomosis in selected infants with NEC has been reported, with a recent study observing recurrent NEC in 22% and strictures in 17% of 18 treated infants following primary anastomosis. Complete intestinal necrosis of the small intestine and the colon is uncommon and is not compatible with long-term survival without the sequelae of short-gut syndrome and the potential need for chronic TPN dependence and ultimately intestinal transplantation (**Fig. 98.28**).

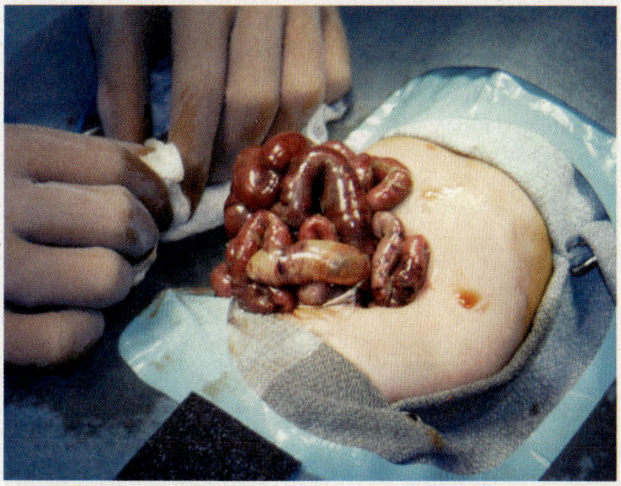

Figure 98.28. Fulminant necrotizing enterocolitis involving the entire gastrointestinal tract in a premature infant. Note the presence of pneumatosis intestinalis.

Infants with NEC are typically fragile and premature, and complications in this population are not well tolerated. Survival in this situation may be more dependent upon disease severity and coexisting medical problems than the operative approach. For the high-risk, low–birth-weight infant, initial management with primary bedside peritoneal drainage rather than laparotomy and bowel resection may be useful as either a temporizing measure or, in some instances, a definitive procedure.[42] A multicenter, randomized controlled surgical trial comparing laparotomy with primary peritoneal drainage in premature infants with perforated NEC found that overall survival, dependence upon TPN, and length of stay were independent of the type of operation performed.[43] However, 18-month follow-up of neurodevelopmental outcomes demonstrates worse neurodevelopmental scores in prospective cohort studies.[44]

Complications, Results, and Outcome

Most infants with NEC are treated successfully without operative intervention. Morbidity and mortality for this group are related primarily to problems associated with prematurity. Given the delay of bowel function and the need for TPN, cholestatic jaundice commonly occurs but is generally reversible. Infants placed on broad-spectrum antibiotics for an extended period are at risk for developing fungal sepsis. For infants with intestinal necrosis from NEC, infectious complications, including wound sepsis, central venous catheter infections, and pneumonia with respiratory failure, may occur.

The overall surgical complication rate in infants with NEC is at least 20% to 40%. Immediate technical complications in treating NEC include intestinal leak, fistula formation, stoma necrosis, bleeding, and liver injury during exploration (**Table 98.5**). These complications are obviously magnified in the extremely low–birth-weight infant with preexisting intestinal injury. Fluid and electrolyte losses from proximal diverting enterostomies can be significant and even life threatening in extremely low–birth-weight infants whose circulating blood volume is less than 50 to 100 mL. A review of 68 infants treated surgically for NEC observed a 26% mortality rate and a 68% complication rate related to the stoma or its closure in the perioperative survivors. Complications included intestinal stricture, incisional or parastomal hernia, stoma prolapse, intussusception, wound dehiscence or infection, small bowel obstruction, and anastomotic failure. The complications associated with diverting enterostomy in this unique population provide a compelling rationale for early enterostomy closure once the inflammation from peritonitis has resolved.

COMPLICATIONS

Table 98.5. Operations for Necrotizing Enterocolitis

Infection (wound, intra-abdominal, central venous catheter, pneumonia)
Bleeding
Stoma-related complications (stenosis, retraction, prolapse)
Electrolyte or nutritional disturbances from enterostomy output
Enterocutaneous fistula
Anastomotic leak, stenosis, failure
Adhesive small bowel obstruction
TPN-associated cholestasis
Short-bowel syndrome, malabsorption
Sepsis, cardiopulmonary failure
Intraventricular hemorrhage

A prospective, randomized trial comparing resection and enterostomy with resection and primary anastomosis in the treatment of NEC has not been reported; however meta-analysis of retrospective outcomes has shown decreased odds of mortality in primary anastomosis. There is some concern that these retrospective studies are biased toward ostomy placement in the most critically ill patients.

Intestinal stricture formation following NEC, whether managed operatively or nonoperatively, is not uncommon. This consequence usually results from a normal host inflammatory response to transmural intestinal injury. The degree of fibrosis and subsequent stricture formation are clearly related to the severity and extent of disease. Less frequently, mesenteric vascular compromise secondary to an intra-abdominal adhesion may lead to stricture formation. Although stricture can develop anywhere in the gastrointestinal tract involved with NEC, a higher rate of demonstrable stricture is observed in the left colon, occurring in as many as 36% of medically treated infants. Routine contrast enema 4 to 6 weeks after clinical resolution of NEC treated operatively or nonoperatively has been advocated in some institutions. Symptomatic strictures generally require segmental resection with anastomosis, although fluoroscopically guided balloon catheter dilatation has been reported.

Overall survival rates for infants with NEC have improved significantly over the past three decades and are currently about 60% to 80% for both operative and nonoperative groups.[45] The observed improvement in survival is thought to reflect improved neonatal intensive care, the use of TPN, and early, aggressive treatment of suspected NEC. Most neonatal intensive care units initiate aggressive medical treatment in any infant with suspected NEC. Whether surgical interventions such as resection with primary anastomosis or limited primary peritoneal drainage can improve morbidity and mortality in these critically ill infants remains to be fully determined. Long-term outcome for NEC survivors generally reflects associated problems of prematurity. In particular, many of these infants have persisting neurodevelopmental, ophthalmologic, and pulmonary diseases, but morbidity from the gastrointestinal system generally is limited to infants with short-gut syndrome following extensive bowel resection. These infants present complex ethical and management issues beyond the scope of this review. Most NEC survivors (75%) enjoy a good

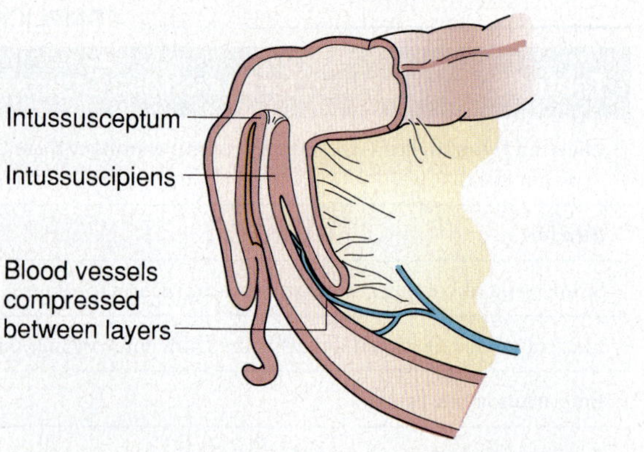

Figure 98.29. Ileocolic intussusception with the intussusceptum and intussuscipiens indicated.

to excellent quality of life, suggesting that the treatment cost relative to the potential benefit for these infants is worthwhile.

Intussusception

Anatomy and Physiology

5 *Intussusception* is defined as the invagination or telescoping of a proximal segment of intestine into an adjacent distal segment and is the most common cause of intestinal obstruction in infants and children aged 3 months to 3 years (**Fig. 98.29**). The invaginated proximal bowel is referred to as the *intussusceptum,* and the recipient distal bowel is called the *intussuscipiens.* This process most commonly originates in the small intestine, either at or near the ileocecal valve, with the terminal ileum passing into the cecum and colon (ileocolic intussusception). In the pediatric population, the vast majority (95%) of cases are considered idiopathic because of a lack of an identifiable anatomic lesion causing the intussusception. Older children are more likely to have a pathologic lead point causing the intussusception. In similar fashion, infants and children with repeated episodes of intussusception have a greater probability of a pathologic lead point. **Table 98.6** describes several factors that have been associated with the development of intussusception.

Many cases of idiopathic intussusception in infants are probably caused by the normally prominent intramural lymph nodes (Peyer patches) in the terminal ileum acting as functional lead points. The anatomic consequence of intussusception is obstruction of the distal bowel. As bowel edema and inflammation progress, mesenteric vascular insufficiency from compression and congestion may occur. Incarceration, strangulation, and intestinal perforation ultimately may result if this condition remains unrecognized or untreated.

Clinical Presentation

Intussusception is estimated to occur with an incidence rate of one to four cases per 1000 children. There is a slight (3:2) male predominance; in a large retrospective series of children with intussusception, 79% were younger than 12 months, and seasonal variation in incidence was not observed. An association between the development of intussusception and the administration of a previously available, tetravalent rhesus-based rotavirus vaccine (RotaShield, Wyeth Laboratories, Inc., Marietta, PA) was reported. The currently available rotavirus vaccine does not appear to be associated with intussusception.[46]

Otherwise healthy infants who develop intussusception may have a characteristic clinical triad of abdominal pain, vomiting, and bloody stool. The typical infant develops the acute onset of severe, colicky abdominal pain. Intermittent episodes of irritability and crying may be associated with drawing the legs up to the abdomen. Between bouts of colic, the infant is often lethargic or sleepy. During periods of relative exhaustion, the abdominal examination may not be impressive; however, on careful physical examination, a palpable mass in the right abdomen may be appreciated in 80% to 90% of cases. Emesis is common and is often the presenting complaint. As intestinal obstruction progresses, intractable vomiting with abdominal distention and intravascular volume depletion may occur. Guaiac-positive stool is present in 90% to 95% of infants as a result of the ischemic mucosal injury to the intussusceptum. The passage of bloody stool mixed with mucus, classically described as *currant-jelly stool,* may be observed.

Table 98.6. Predisposing Factors Leading to Intussusception

Anatomic Lead Points
Meckel diverticulum
Polyp
Lymphatic hypertrophy (Peyer patch)
Appendix
Duplication or enteric cyst
Lymphoma
Other neoplasm
Heterotopic pancreatic tissue
Associated Infections
Adenovirus
Rotavirus
Parasitic infestation
Other
Bleeding Disorders[a]
Henoch–Schönlein purpura
Hemophilia
Leukemia
Trauma
Blunt abdominal trauma
Major retroperitoneal dissections
Others
Cystic fibrosis

[a]These factors are more likely to be associated with small bowel-to-small bowel intussusception than with ileocolic intussusception.

Diagnosis

Plain radiographs of the abdomen are generally nonspecific and may show a paucity of gas in the right lower quadrant with a mass effect in the ascending colon. Late findings demonstrate mechanical small bowel obstruction with proximal distention, air–fluid levels, and a decrease or absence of gas distally. Ultrasound examination typically reveals a mass resembling a bull's eye or target sign, corresponding to the intussusceptum within the intussuscipiens. The target sign of intussusception may also be demonstrated by CT. Both these latter modalities do not allow for potential therapeutic reduction and may be more useful in diagnosing suspected cases of proximal jejunoileal or enteroenteral intussusception. Diagnostic enema techniques using either air or contrast approach have 100% accuracy with typical ileocolic intussusception (**Fig. 98.30**). An approach using hydrostatic or pneumatic enema allows therapeutic reduction of intussusception as well.

Treatment

Nonoperative Management

Any infant with suspected intussusception in the absence of peritonitis should undergo diagnostic hydrostatic or pneumatic enema. A high index of clinical suspicion and liberal application of this approach should be maintained. The incidence of normal contrast enema examinations in this setting may exceed 75% in most pediatric centers, and this is justified by the considerable risk inherent in a missed diagnosis. An

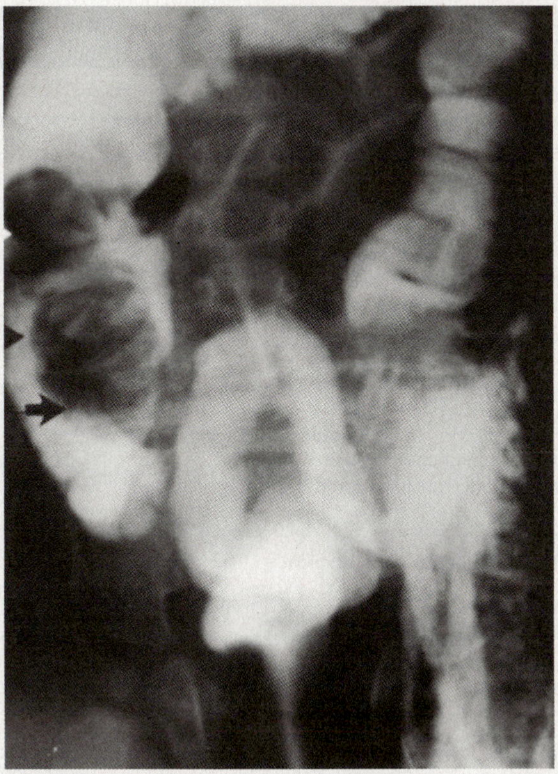

Figure 98.30. Contrast enema demonstrating classic ileocolic intussusception with the intussusceptum visible in the ascending colon (*arrows*).

experienced pediatric radiologist and surgical evaluation are essential. Intravenous access and resuscitation should occur before attempts are made at diagnostic or therapeutic enemas.

Successful hydrostatic or pneumatic reduction of ileocolic intussusception is achieved in 60% to 90% of infants in most pediatric centers in the United States. The ability to reduce intussusception using these techniques is time dependent and diminishes substantially after the duration of symptoms exceeds 24 hours. In this setting, a contrast enema is still diagnostic and potentially therapeutic if carefully performed. With most experienced pediatric radiologists, the risk of perforation or reduction of a strangulated intussusceptum is low.

The technique of retrograde reduction of intussusception is straightforward. Contrast or air is introduced into the rectum by a balloon catheter, with the height of the hydrostatic column 1 m or less. Most centers use three attempts at reduction, with each attempt no longer than 3 minutes in duration. As long as progress is being made, however, attempts can be repeated until reduction is achieved. Successful reduction of ileocolic intussusception is demonstrated by observing retrograde flow of contrast or air into the terminal ileum. Inability to demonstrate retrograde flow into the ileum suggests incomplete reduction requiring surgical exploration.

Operative Management

Infants presenting with peritonitis and small bowel obstruction with a clinical diagnosis of intussusception should undergo immediate resuscitation and exploration without attempts at retrograde enema. Surgical exploration is also required after incomplete retrograde enema reduction of intussusception or in the relatively infrequent situation of bowel perforation during diagnostic or therapeutic enema. The operative strategy is dictated by the findings. Spontaneous reduction of the intussusception is reported to occur in up to 20% to 30% of infants following induction of general anesthesia. In this situation, exploration confirming the reduction and examining the bowel for a pathologic lead point is sufficient. With persistent intussusception and viable bowel, the bowel is manually reduced, generally pushing the intussusceptum out of the distal bowel. If manual reduction cannot be performed or the intussusceptum is strangulated, then segmental resection with primary anastomosis is performed. Attempts at reducing intussusception with clearly necrotic bowel should be avoided. Diverting enterostomy as a result of peritoneal contamination is usually not required. Appendectomy is routinely performed in all infants undergoing operative exploration for intussusception. A successful laparoscopic approach to the diagnosis and management of intussusception has been reported in approximately two-thirds of selected patients.[47,48]

Complications and Outcome

Following successful enema reduction, the infant is given intravenous fluids and observed for tolerance of oral feeding is rapid. Recovery from operative reduction or bowel resection is generally no different from other similar gastrointestinal procedures. Most infants enjoy a complete recovery with minimal or no morbidity. Recurrent intussusception after either nonoperative or operative reduction occurs in about 5% of infants and usually can be treated with repeat enema. Mortality from intussusception is rare and is almost always the result of systemic sepsis and shock from unrecognized, strangulated intestine.

COLON, RECTUM, AND ANUS

Gastrointestinal Hemorrhage

The subject of gastrointestinal hemorrhage and general principles of management are discussed elsewhere in this book. The following section reviews some of the important and age-dependent clinical causes and unique issues of gastrointestinal bleeding in pediatric population. These causes are age dependent and are summarized in **Tables 98.7** and **98.8**.

Diagnostic workup of an infant or a child with gastrointestinal hemorrhage requires coordinated participation among pediatricians, surgeons, gastroenterologists, and radiologists. Several general principles governing the diagnostic approach to gastrointestinal bleeding in infants and children follow:

a. A clear diagnosis can be made in most situations; given the current technology available to assist with diagnosis, an aggressive approach is warranted. Diagnostic procedures such as flexible fiberoptic endoscopy, radioisotope imaging, and angiography are widely available, safe, and applicable to any age group, including the newborn. Despite these measures, in approximately 16% of cases, the cause of guaiac-positive stools in a neonate or infant remains unknown, and the bleeding is self-limited.

b. The primary diagnostic investigation of choice for upper gastrointestinal bleeding is esophagogastroduodenoscopy. This procedure is optimally performed within the first 24 hours after cessation of active hemorrhage and usually requires general anesthesia. Imaging studies for active upper gastrointestinal hemorrhage are limited in their ability to aid with diagnosis.

c. Infants and children presenting with minor lower gastrointestinal bleeding are best evaluated by a careful perineal and digital rectal examination, followed by anoscopy.

d. Massive lower gastrointestinal hemorrhage in an infant or a child outside the newborn period is most likely the result of a bleeding Meckel diverticulum.

e. If a definitive source for lower gastrointestinal hemorrhage is not found on colonoscopy, evaluation for an upper gastrointestinal source, including upper endoscopy and diagnostic laparoscopy, is warranted.

f. Pain is an uncommon symptom with pediatric gastrointestinal hemorrhage and implies a more complex problem, such as volvulus, ischemic bowel, or inflammatory bowel disease. Painful gastrointestinal hemorrhage in pediatric patient requires urgent evaluation and prompt diagnostic workup.

g. In contrast to that in adults, gastrointestinal bleeding in children is rarely a symptom or sign of gastrointestinal neoplasm.

Table 98.7. Etiology and Causes of Upper Gastrointestinal Hemorrhage[a]

Patient Age Group	Common Causes	Less Common Causes
Neonatal (0–30 d)	Gastritis Esophagitis Ingested maternal blood Peptic ulcer	Iatrogenic trauma Primary coagulopathy Vascular malformation (hemangioma, telangiectasia, arteriovenous malformation) Nasal or pharyngeal bleeding Miscellaneous (leiomyoma, gastric polyp, duplication)
Infant (30 d to 1 y)	Gastritis Esophagitis Peptic ulcer	Same as less common neonatal causes, plus: Drugs (steroids, nonsteroidal anti-inflammatory drugs) Foreign body, caustic ingestion Esophageal varices
Child (1–12 y)	Esophageal varices Esophagitis Peptic ulcer	Same as less common infantile causes, plus: Acquired thrombocytopenia (chemotherapy)
Older child (12 y to adult)	Esophageal varices Esophagitis Peptic ulcer	Same as less common childhood causes

[a]Order in appearance approximates clinical frequency.
Modified from Oldham KT, Lobe TE. Gastrointestinal hemorrhage in children. A pragmatic update. *Pediatr Clin North Am.* 1985;32:1247–1263, with permission.

Neonates (0 to 30 Days of Age)

The most common cause of gastrointestinal hemorrhage in a neonate is gastritis. Endoscopic evaluation of newborns with symptomatic upper gastrointestinal hemorrhage demonstrates gastritis or esophagitis in 50% to 75% of cases. About 10% to 15% have swallowed maternal blood during birth, and 10% of newborns are found to have an underlying coagulopathy. Anatomic lesions requiring operative control are distinctly unusual in this age group. Significant and sometimes massive upper gastrointestinal hemorrhage may occur in a neonate without a definable anatomic lesion despite endoscopic evaluation. This finding is usually the result of gastritis, and treatment is directed at blood and volume replacement and correction of any underlying coagulopathy.

Table 98.8. Causes of Lower Gastrointestinal Hemorrhage[a]

Patient Age Group	Common Causes	Less Common Causes
Neonatal (0–30 d)	Benign anorectal lesions (fissure) Upper gastrointestinal hemorrhage Milk allergy Necrotizing enterocolitis Midgut volvulus	Iatrogenic trauma Primary coagulopathy Vascular malformations Enterocolitis (Hirschsprung disease, other) Miscellaneous (duplication, lymphoma, lymphangiectasia)
Infant (30 d to 1 y)	Incarcerated inguinal hernia Benign anorectal lesions Idiopathic intussusception Meckel diverticulum Infectious diarrhea Upper gastrointestinal hemorrhage Milk allergy	Same as neonate, with addition of: Acquired thrombocytopenia Ingestion of colored foodstuff (pseudohematochezia)
Child (1–12 y)	Benign anorectal lesions Juvenile polyps Intussusception Meckel diverticulum Infectious diarrhea Upper gastrointestinal hemorrhage	Same as infant, with addition of: Juvenile polyposis coli/familial polyposis coli Hemolytic uremic syndrome Henöch–Schonlein purpura Systemic vasculitis (dermatomyositis, lupus) Acquired thrombocytopenia (as above plus idiopathic thrombocytopenic purpura)
Older child (12 y to adult)	Juvenile polyps Benign anorectal lesions Inflammatory bowel disease Upper gastrointestinal hemorrhage	Same as child, except: Henöch–Schonlein purpura and hemolytic uremic syndrome less likely Meckel diverticulum

[a]Order in appearance approximates clinical frequency.
Modified from Oldham KT, Lobe TE. Gastrointestinal hemorrhage in children. A pragmatic update. *Pediatr Clin North Am.* 1985;32:1247–1263, with permission.

Significant conditions responsible for lower gastrointestinal bleeding in the newborn include NEC, malrotation with volvulus, enterocolitis, or bowel obstruction secondary to an incarcerated inguinal hernia. These clinical entities present with characteristic histories, findings on clinical examination, and surgical treatment guidelines previously discussed. Anorectal fissure is also common and easy to diagnose in neonates, and bleeding is typically self-limited.

Infants (30 Days to 1 Year)

Infants with upper gastrointestinal bleeding deserve comprehensive evaluation, including endoscopy, to identify potential lesions requiring operative intervention. The most common causes of lower gastrointestinal hemorrhage in this age group include infectious diarrhea, intussusception, food allergy, and bleeding Meckel diverticulum. Most of these lesions have distinct symptoms, signs, and diagnostic findings to facilitate diagnosis. Infectious diarrhea is usually accompanied by fever, feeding intolerance, possibly emesis, and abdominal pain. Fecal leukocytes may be present on stool examination, and enteric pathogens or their toxins can be identified by stool culture.

Children (1 to 12 Years)

An important surgical cause of upper gastrointestinal bleeding in this age group includes esophageal variceal bleeding from portal hypertension. Children with biliary atresia or extrahepatic portal venous obstruction account for most cases of variceal bleeding in this age group. In the acute setting, endoscopic sclerotherapy or banding is used as a temporizing measure for hemorrhage control; some investigators advocate maintenance sclerotherapy. Ultimately, for these children, orthotopic liver transplantation may offer definitive surgical treatment. The use of operative portosystemic shunts for acute variceal hemorrhage is not widely used in pediatric surgical practice in the United States.

Conditions causing lower gastrointestinal bleeding in this age group include juvenile polyps. These are benign, hamartomatous polyps and represent the single most common cause of lower gastrointestinal bleeding in children. About 20% to 30% of the polyps are palpable on digital rectal examination. A history of painless, bright red blood per rectum during a bowel movement is typical. The bleeding results from mucosal irritation, involution, and sloughing of a pedunculated polyp and is usually not associated with hemodynamically significant hemorrhage. Tissue may be passed, or the pedunculated polyp may prolapse out the anus. A hypochromic, microcytic anemia may be present. Diagnostic workup generally involves a contrast enema to identify the polyp and evaluate the colon for synchronous lesions. Colonoscopy may require general anesthesia in this age group, and endoscopic snare polypectomy is the treatment of choice for appropriately sized polyps. Infrequently, transanal excision or open resection of larger polyps is required. In the case of multiple juvenile polyps not amenable to endoscopic polypectomy, management may be expectant based on the benign natural history characterized by involution during adolescence. Histologic confirmation is necessary to differentiate these lesions from adenomatous polyps seen in familial polyposis syndromes or Gardner syndrome.

Older Children and Adolescents (Older Than 12 Years)

Causes of both upper and lower gastrointestinal hemorrhage in this age group include most etiologic conditions found in adults. Importantly, inflammatory bowel disease is significant in this age group.

Congenital Aganglionosis (Hirschsprung Disease)

Embryology

6 Congenital aganglionosis of the intestine (Hirschsprung disease) is characterized by the absence of intestinal ganglion cells.[49] The pathogenesis of aganglionosis remains unknown. In normal development, neuroblasts derived from neural crest precursors become evident by week 5 of gestation. The neuroblasts begin maturation and caudal migration along with vagal nerve fibers. The initial caudal migration in an intermuscular plane is followed by intramural dispersal into both superficial and deep submucosal nerve plexuses. Ultimately, the neuroblasts give rise to the ganglion cells of the myenteric nervous system, with functional maturation continuing well into infancy. The orderly migration pathway of myenteric innervation has been documented in human embryos; normally, ganglion cells can be identified in the esophagus at week 6 of gestation, in the transverse colon at week 8 of gestation, and in the rectum by week 12 of gestation.

Anatomy

Hirschsprung disease is characterized by a lack of ganglion cells in the distal intestine. The length of aganglionosis is variable but most commonly involves the distal rectosigmoid colon in 75% to 80% of affected infants. In about 5% of cases, the transition zone between the normal, proximal bowel and the distal, aganglionic segment occurs in the small intestine. Discontinuous aganglionosis has been reported but should be considered distinctly unusual. Therefore, in virtually all cases, the aganglionic intestinal segment is continuous with the distal rectum to the anal verge and also includes the internal sphincter. Because of this distribution, the pathogenesis of congenital aganglionosis is often attributed to failure of neuroblast migration. The characteristic lesion in the distal bowel is the aganglionosis in the intermuscular and submucosal plexuses. Large, hypertrophied, nonmyelinated nerve fibers are present within the muscularis mucosa, lamina propria, submucosa, and Auerbach intermuscular plexus. Both adrenergic and cholinergic fibers are prominent in the aganglionic segment, and acetylcholinesterase staining is useful diagnostically. Abnormalities in the peptidergic nervous system, including vasoactive intestinal peptide, substance P, and neurotensin immunoreactive fibers, are also described in the aganglionic bowel segment. Deficient neuronal nitric oxide synthase mRNA and subsequent decreased local nitric oxide synthase activity in the aganglionic bowel have also been described. These experimental data are consistent with the concept that a defect in nitric oxide–mediated smooth-muscle relaxation may account for some of the characteristic clinical features of Hirschsprung disease.

The transition zone between the normal, proximal bowel and the aganglionic distal bowel is distinguished grossly by distention of the proximal bowel with histologic evidence of muscular hypertrophy. The transition zone often becomes evident to direct inspection or on contrast enema during the first few weeks of life as functional obstruction leads to progressive proximal dilatation. On gross inspection, the transition zone may appear as a short funnel or cone-shaped colonic segment. The discrepancy in bowel lumen diameter is somewhat age dependent and may be subtle in a newborn or in a child with total colonic aganglionosis. Therefore, it may be difficult for the surgeon or the radiologist to define the exact transition zone site based on gross inspection or contrast enema. Gross examination alone is not sufficient for surgical decision making, and histologic confirmation of the level of ganglion cell transition is required. Given the continuous nature of aganglionosis, a rectal biopsy performed 1.5 to 2 cm above the dentate line demonstrating ganglion cells effectively excludes Hirschsprung disease.

Neuronal intestinal dysplasia is a clinically described entity similar to or associated with Hirschsprung disease.[50] Despite the presence of ganglion cells, dysplastic changes in the myenteric nervous system affect bowel motility in a similar fashion to aganglionosis. Clinical presentation and treatment are similar to those of classic Hirschsprung disease. There is considerable controversy regarding neuronal intestinal

PEDIATRIC SURGERY

dysplasia, but it is reasonable to suggest that this represents an entity within the spectrum of abnormalities found in the intestinal myenteric nervous system.

Pathophysiology

Normal intestinal motility depends on coordinated propagation of segmental contraction waves immediately preceded by relaxation of the enteric smooth muscle. Patients with Hirschsprung disease lack a functional myenteric nervous system in the aganglionic segment; therefore, both propulsion and reflexive relaxation are disordered or absent in the distal bowel. Loss of neuronal nitric oxide synthase activity appears to play an important role. The internal sphincter is aganglionic and lacks the normal reflexive relaxation following rectal distention. In fact, patients with Hirschsprung disease may exhibit a paradoxical increase in sphincter tone in response to rectal distention. The functional result is tonic contraction of the aganglionic segment of bowel with ineffective peristalsis. Clinically, this presents as incomplete, distal intestinal obstruction in the newborn or as chronic constipation in the older child or adult.

Hirschsprung disease has been associated with mutations in at least three specific genes: the *RET* protooncogene, the endothelin B receptor (*EDNRB*) gene, and the endothelin 3 (*EDN3*) gene. In addition, several other candidate genes are under investigation. In mice, natural and in vitro induced mutations affecting the *RET, EDNRB,* and *EDN3* genes generate intestinal aganglionosis identical to Hirschsprung disease. Although widely accepted, it is still unknown whether the primary event in aganglionosis is failure of neuroblast migration to the distal bowel. Alternatively, ineffective microenvironmental support of neuroblasts that have already migrated may fail to promote normal neuroblast development and survival.

Clinical Features

Incidence and Associations

The incidence rate of Hirschsprung disease is estimated at 1 per 5000 live births with a marked male-to-female (4:1) preponderance. Most cases are sporadic, but long-segment, total colonic aganglionosis and female gender are strongly associated with familial inheritance. Genetic chromosomal analysis suggests that multiple loci may be involved, including chromosomes 13q22, 21q22, and 10q, among others. Familial Hirschsprung disease has been clearly associated with *RET* protooncogene mutations. From a clinical standpoint, mutations of the *RET* protooncogene are associated with disorders of neural crest development, namely, multiple endocrine neoplasia (MEN) types IIA and IIB, as well as familial medullary thyroid carcinoma, and patients with familial Hirschsprung disease associated with RET mutation are at risk for the development of medullary thyroid carcinoma. Congenital cardiac defects are present in 2% to 5% of patients with Hirschsprung disease. Other rare congenital anomalies have been reported, but a consistent and important association is a 5% to 15% incidence of trisomy 21. Infants presenting with meconium plug syndrome should undergo rectal suction biopsy to exclude aganglionosis.

Presentation

Most infants with Hirschsprung disease fail to pass meconium within the first 24 to 48 hours of life. Nonspecific signs of neonatal intestinal obstruction (feeding intolerance, abdominal distention, and bilious emesis) may develop. About half of the patients with Hirschsprung disease are diagnosed as neonates. Infrequently, older children or adults are diagnosed with aganglionosis during evaluation for chronic constipation. In this setting, symptoms may be minimal to disabling, and parents or patients often develop elaborate strategies to deal with chronic constipation. Abdominal distention is characteristic, and sometimes failure to thrive and malnutrition may occur. Digital rectal examination may demonstrate spasm, and, in the presence of Hirschsprung-associated enterocolitis (HAEC), forceful expulsion of foul-smelling, liquid stool may occur.[51]

Diagnosis

A high index of suspicion for Hirschsprung disease should be maintained for any newborn infant with abdominal distention failing to pass meconium in 24 to 48 hours. The signs of neonatal intestinal obstruction should lead to a stereotypical workup. In the presence of characteristic findings on history, examination, or radiographic studies, any infant suspected of having Hirschsprung disease should undergo rectal biopsy.

Plain Abdominal Radiographs

Plain film radiographs of the neonate with Hirschsprung disease are nonspecific and typically demonstrate distended, air-filled loops of bowel throughout the abdomen. It is often difficult to discriminate between small intestine and large intestine on plain films at this age, but the pattern is consistent with distal intestinal obstruction. Older children or adults may have a stool-filled megacolon on plain radiographs. In the presence of enterocolitis, thickened, dilated intestinal loops and pneumatosis intestinalis may be present.

Contrast Enema

When distal neonatal intestinal obstruction is suspected on plain abdominal films, a contrast enema should be performed. With an experienced pediatric radiologist, findings consistent with Hirschsprung disease can be accurately detected in most instances. The classic radiographic finding in Hirschsprung disease is a transition zone (**Fig. 98.31A**). A definitive transition zone may not be apparent in a neonate because proximal dilatation takes some time to develop. In addition, infants with short-segment disease or total colonic aganglionosis may not have obvious transition zones on contrast enema. In these instances, a lateral view of the rectum may show abnormal spasm (**Fig. 98.31B**). Contrast remaining in the rectum more than 24 hours following a study is suggestive of Hirschsprung disease.

Rectal Biopsy

The diagnostic standard for aganglionosis is the rectal biopsy. Several commercially available instruments capable of performing rectal suction biopsies are in widespread use. The rectal suction biopsy can be performed at bedside or in clinic without anesthesia in all newborns and most children up to several months of age. The desire for early diagnosis and the technical simplicity of the procedure allow liberal use of this technique. When applied liberally, the vast majority (85% to 90%) of infants undergoing this procedure have normal ganglion cells on biopsy, effectively excluding Hirschsprung disease. Using the rectal suction biopsy technique, a biopsy of the mucosa and the submucosa is obtained. This is sufficient to establish the diagnosis because ganglion cells are absent from all intramural plexuses in Hirschsprung disease. The biopsy must be taken 1 to 1.5 cm proximal to the dentate line. Complications of infection, perforation, and bleeding with rectal suction biopsy are infrequent. Full-thickness rectal biopsy under general anesthesia is reserved for older children and in infants in whom suction biopsy is inadequate. An experienced pediatric pathologist must read the biopsies for maximal diagnostic accuracy. Evaluation for ganglion cells and the axons of the myenteric neurons is performed (**Fig. 98.32**), which may be accomplished using conventional hematoxylin-eosin staining or histochemical staining for acetylcholinesterase and calretinin. Similar histochemical staining for nitric oxide synthase can be performed. These adjunctive techniques are used routinely in some centers and can help provide additional evidence of Hirschsprung disease rather than simply demonstrating aganglionosis in the biopsy specimen. Diagnostic accuracy for Hirschsprung disease is excellent with a correctly obtained rectal suction biopsy and an experienced pediatric pathologist.

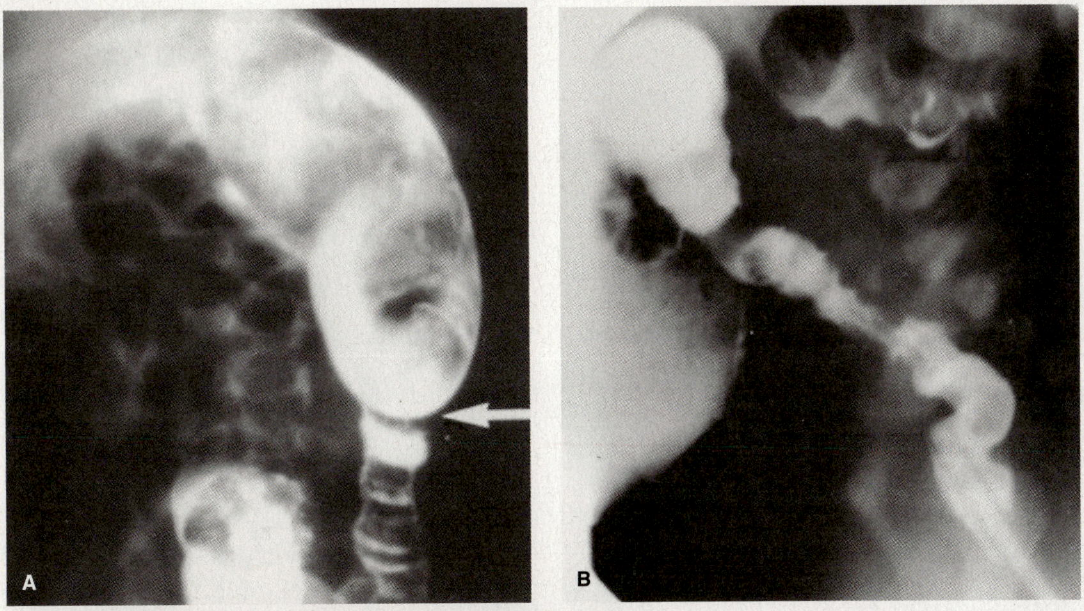

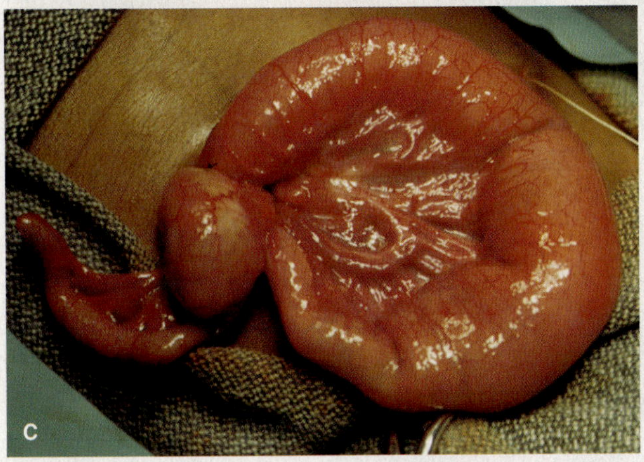

Figure 98.31. **A:** Contrast enema demonstrating a classic rectosigmoid transition zone (*arrow*) in Hirschsprung disease. **B:** Lateral view of rectum illustrates typical distal spasm of rectum. **C:** Operative photograph of rectosigmoid transition zone.

Anorectal Manometry

The absence of sphincter relaxation in response to rectal dilatation is consistent with Hirschsprung disease. Because of the relative ease and accuracy of rectal suction biopsy, anorectal manometry is not widely used in the United States for the primary diagnosis of Hirschsprung disease in infancy; however, this is used in some centers around the world and, when applied carefully with an appropriate transduction probe, accurate manometric diagnosis is achievable in 85% to 90% of cases.

Treatment

Diverting colostomy should be considered for a newborn infant with Hirschsprung disease who has enterocolitis or multiple associated medical problems or anomalies. In the presence of enterocolitis, rectal irrigation and decompression can be an effective temporizing measure while resuscitation and broad-spectrum antibiotics are being instituted. Prompt proximal diversion will be required once the patient has stabilized. In the neonate, one approach following diagnosis is to perform proximal diversion by means of a colostomy (or enterostomy) placed in normal, ganglionated intestine. The diverting colostomy must be proximal to the histologic transition zone, and a series of biopsies examined by frozen section may be necessary to find the correct level for diversion. For classic rectosigmoid disease, a leveling colostomy is placed just proximal to the transition zone. This approach is generally done in two stages, with takedown of the stoma and definitive pull-through operation performed together weeks to months later, typically when the infant reaches 9 to 12 months of age. In older children, definitive pull through is deferred until the colon has decompressed to a relatively normal caliber.

For many infants and children without enterocolitis, a single-stage approach that eliminates the diverting colostomy has been advocated. Despite a number of different operative techniques in performing a single-stage pull through, results and outcomes appear nearly equivalent. Definitive repair of Hirschsprung disease with a single operation is desirable from technical and economic standpoint and essentially eliminates the complications associated with neonatal stomas. As with most aspects of pediatric surgery, an increasing experience with laparoscopically assisted, single-stage pull-through operations has been reported. The contemporary, laparoscopic single-stage approach in the management of Hirschsprung disease has gained wide acceptance in the pediatric surgical community and is considered by many surgeons as the current standard of care for most infants and children.

Definitive Operations for Hirschsprung Disease

The major goal of operative therapy in the treatment of Hirschsprung disease is to provide resection or bypass of the distal aganglionic rectum with the performance of a low rectal anastomosis with normally innervated proximal intestine. Numerous definitive procedures were designed to treat Hirschsprung disease, and a brief description of the principal procedures in use follows. In general, the selection of a

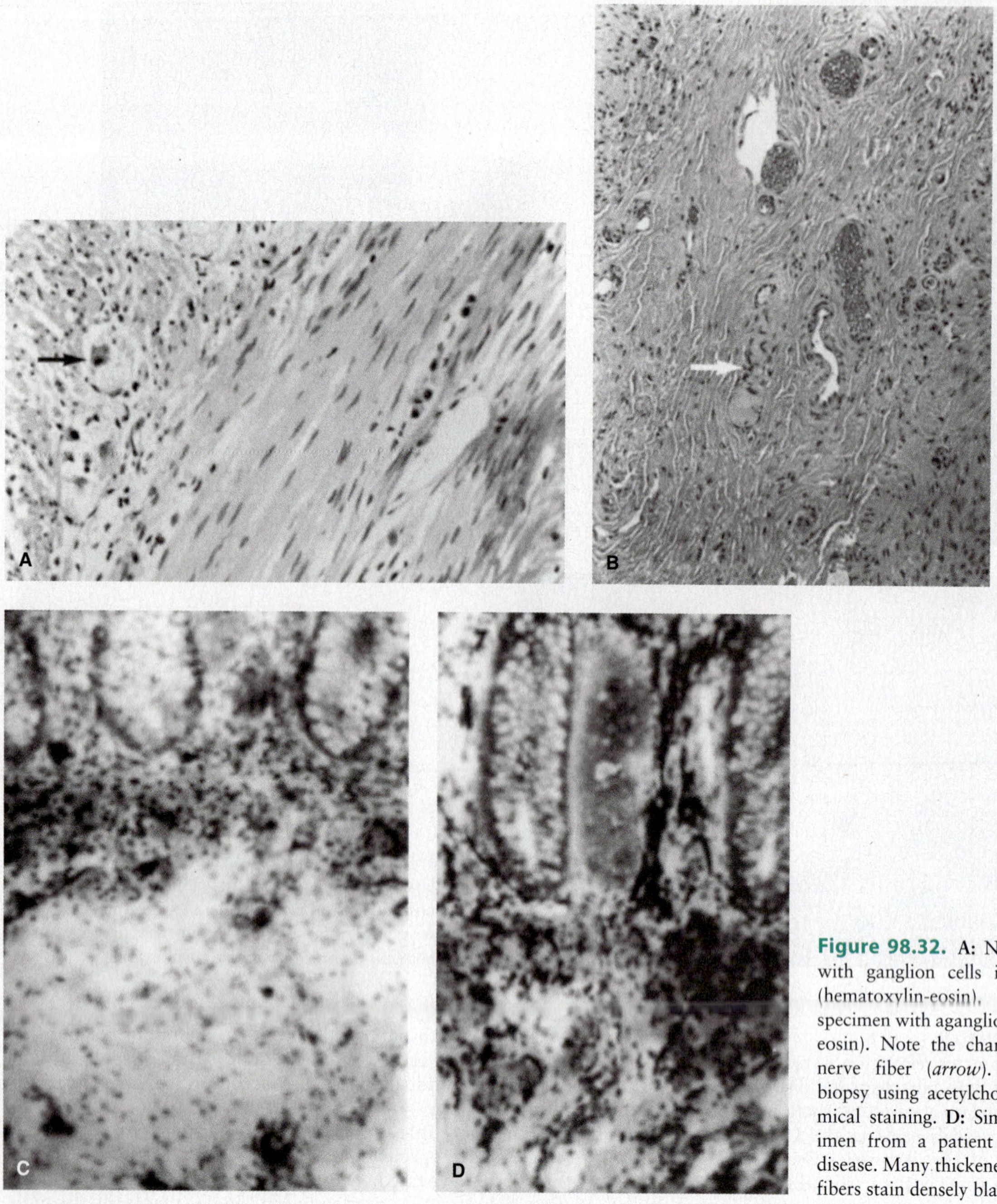

Figure 98.32. **A:** Normal rectal biopsy with ganglion cells indicated by *arrow* (hematoxylin-eosin). **B:** Rectal biopsy specimen with aganglionosis (hematoxylin-eosin). Note the characteristic thickened nerve fiber (*arrow*). **C:** Normal rectal biopsy using acetylcholinesterase histochemical staining. **D:** Similarly stained specimen from a patient with Hirschsprung disease. Many thickened submucosal nerve fibers stain densely black.

procedure depends on a surgeon's individual training and preference rather than compelling differences in outcome.[52]

Swenson Procedure

The Swenson procedure is the original definitive procedure for the treatment of Hirschsprung disease. Long-term outcome in children who undergo a properly performed Swenson procedure is equivalent to other procedures. The basic strategy is outlined in **Figure 98.33**. The aganglionic segment of colon is resected, and a careful, nearly complete extramural dissection of the distal rectum is performed. Care must be taken to avoid inadvertent injury to the seminal vesicles, vas deferens, ureters, and pelvic splanchnic nerves. The dissected rectum is everted through the anus onto the perineum and excised. Normal proximal bowel is pulled through, and a colorectal anastomosis is performed.

Yancey–Soave Procedure

The Yancey–Soave procedure, the most commonly performed procedure for Hirschsprung disease in the United States, is illustrated in **Figure 98.34**. Following resection of aganglionic colon, an endorectal dissection in the submucosal plane is performed from proximal rectum to anus. The endorectal dissection is started in the extraperitoneal rectum. This dissection is typically much easier than similar dissection for ulcerative colitis, given the lack of mucosal inflammation. The dissected rectal mucosal tube is everted through the anus, excised, and normal proximal bowel is pulled through the rectal muscular cuff. The original operation did not suture the pull-through segment of proximal bowel to the rectum. A formal sutured colorectal anastomosis is now universally performed. Care must be taken to ensure that the pull-through segment is not obstructed by the muscular cuff.

Duhamel Procedure (Martin Modification)

The key elements of the Duhamel procedure are illustrated in **Figure 98.35**. After minimal pelvic dissection, resection of the aganglionic colon is performed. The aganglionic rectum is left

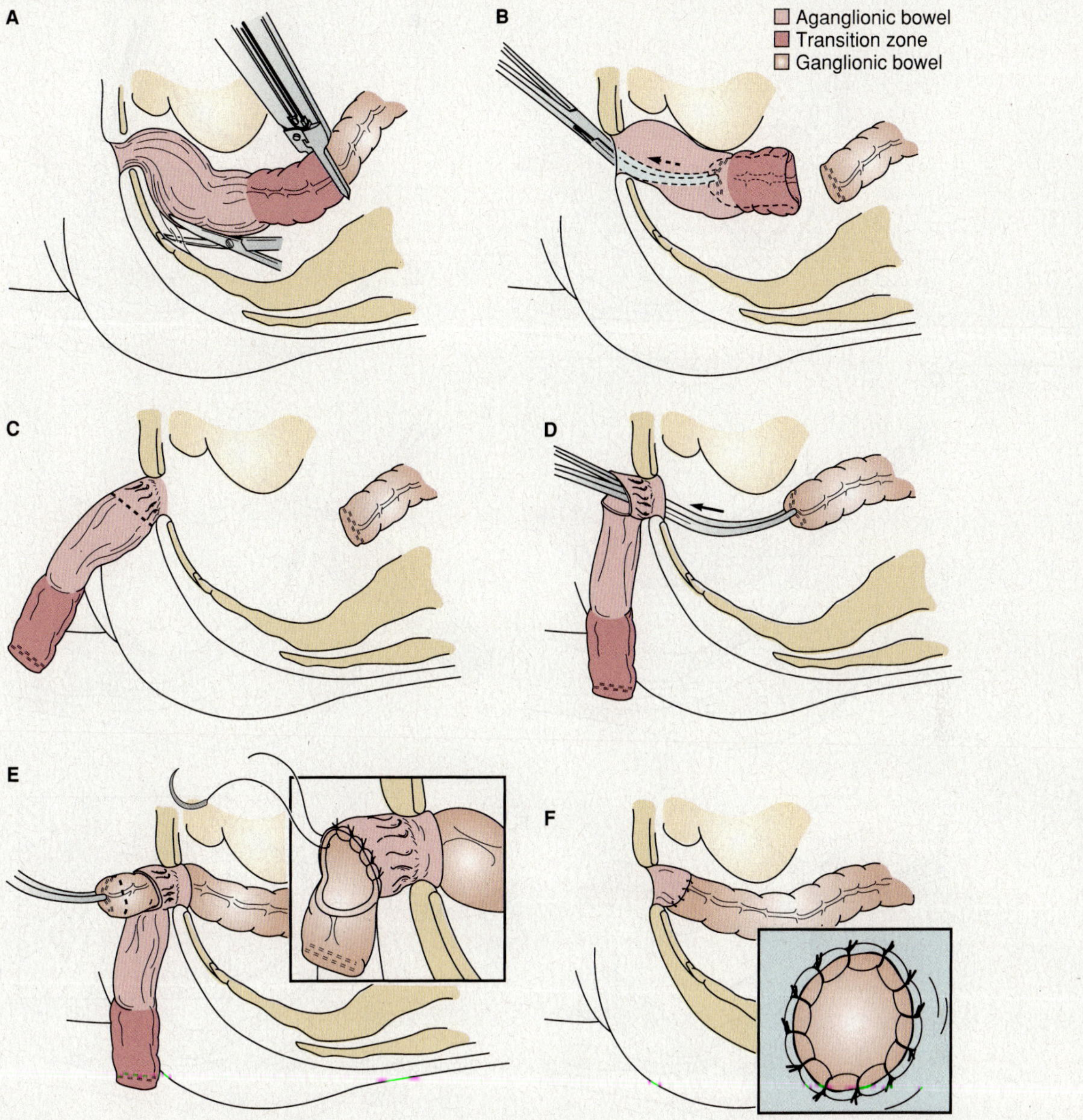

Figure 98.33. Swenson procedure. **A:** Extramural rectal dissection. **B, C:** Eversion of aganglionic segment and full-thickness rectum. **D:** Pull-through of normal, ganglionic bowel. **E:** Colorectal anastomosis. **F:** Completed procedure.

in situ. Normal proximal colon is brought caudad into the retrorectal space, and a colorectal anastomosis is performed 1 cm above the dentate line. The original operation left the defunctionalized rectal pouch as shown, which proved problematic. The procedure has been modified by Martin to include a longer side-to-side colorectal anastomosis. Advantages of this procedure include its relative technical ease and limited pelvic dissection. Adoption of the stapled anastomosis has simplified this procedure significantly.

Laparoscopically Assisted Endorectal Pull Through

Laparoscopically assisted endorectal pull-through techniques were described in the mid-1990s. Potential advantages of this approach include excellent visibility of the distal rectum during dissection, early return of postoperative bowel function, and decreased length of hospital stay. Outcomes are similar to those of the procedures described above. The procedure is reviewed in **Figure 98.36.**

A robot-assisted approach to Hirschsprung disease may be feasible but is limited in applicability to infants due to the size of the instruments for current-generation surgical robots. There may be utility in may be useful in older children or for reoperative surgery to facilitate rectal dissection in the pelvis.

Fully Transanal Endorectal Pull Through

Complete transanal excision of the distal aganglionic segment with primary coloanal anastomosis was described by two separate groups in the early 2000s. Advocates of the transanal operation cite potentially lower rates of constipation and HAEC than following the transabdominal operation. Other authors have voiced concerns over excessive stretch and potential devascularization of the anal sphincters. The fully transanal approach is likely best suited to cases with aganglionosis limited to the rectosigmoid.

Total Colonic Aganglionosis

Total colonic aganglionosis is complex and, fortunately, relatively rare.[53] Several different operative procedures have been described, and treatment must be individualized. The endorectal pull through with ileoanal anastomosis has been used with good success when most or all of the small bowel is normal. For extensive small bowel aganglionosis, an extended side-to-side anastomosis of normally innervated proximal small bowel

PEDIATRIC SURGERY

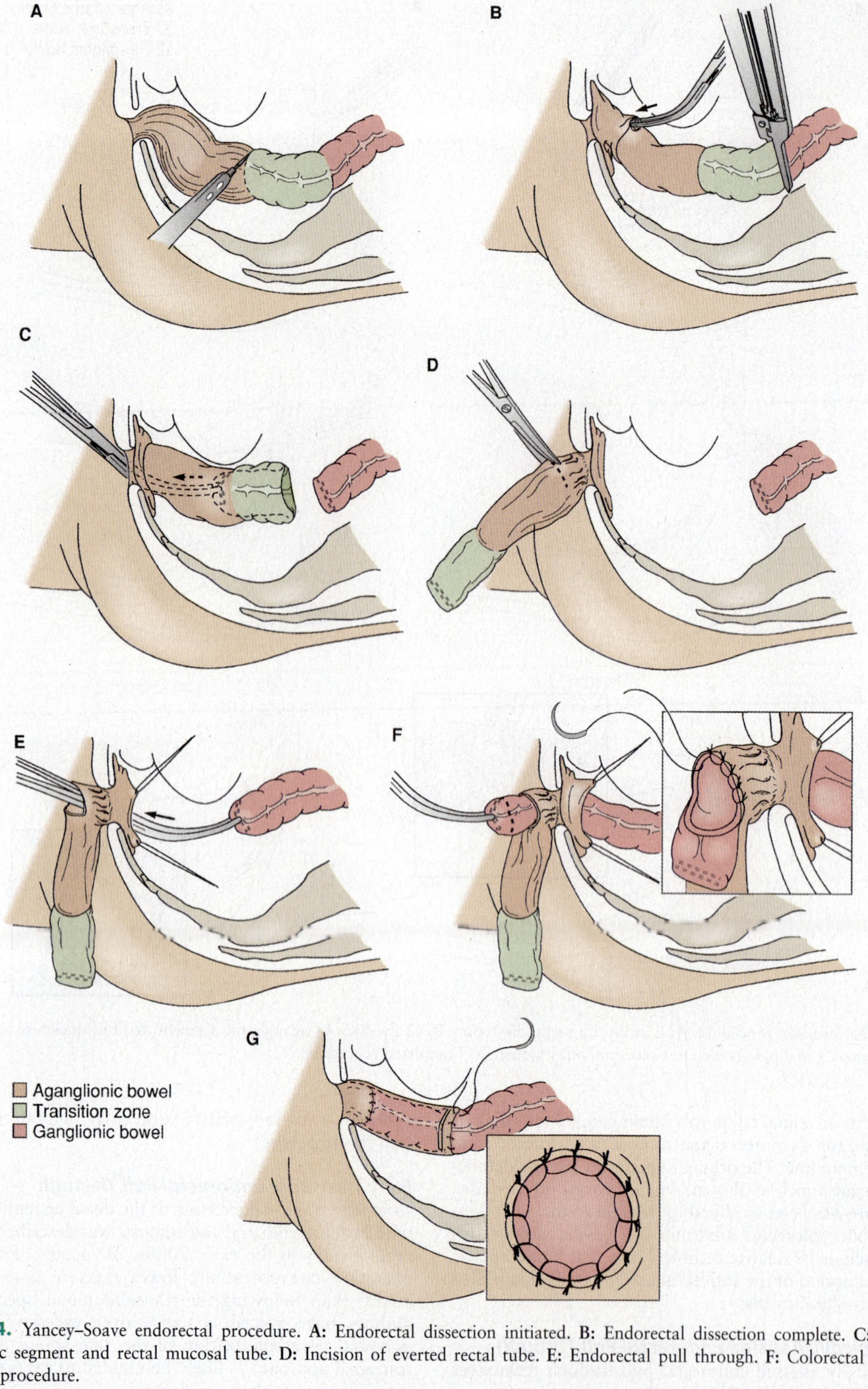

Figure 98.34. Yancey–Soave endorectal procedure. **A:** Endorectal dissection initiated. **B:** Endorectal dissection complete. **C:** Eversion of the aganglionic segment and rectal mucosal tube. **D:** Incision of everted rectal tube. **E:** Endorectal pull through. **F:** Colorectal anastomosis. **G:** Completed procedure.

to the aganglionic colon has been successfully performed. For complete intestinal aganglionosis, extended intestinal myectomy has been described.

Complications and Outcome

Long-term outcomes appear quite good for all the procedures used, with greater than 50% of patients maintaining good-to-excellent bowel function. Complications resulting from definitive procedures for Hirschsprung disease include anastomotic leak, stricture, pelvic or rectal muscular cuff abscess, intestinal obstruction, and wound infection. These occur with a frequency of 1% to 10% with most experienced pediatric surgeons. Mortality from Hirschsprung disease is distinctly unusual unless enterocolitis is the presenting feature or associated medical problems or anomalies are present.

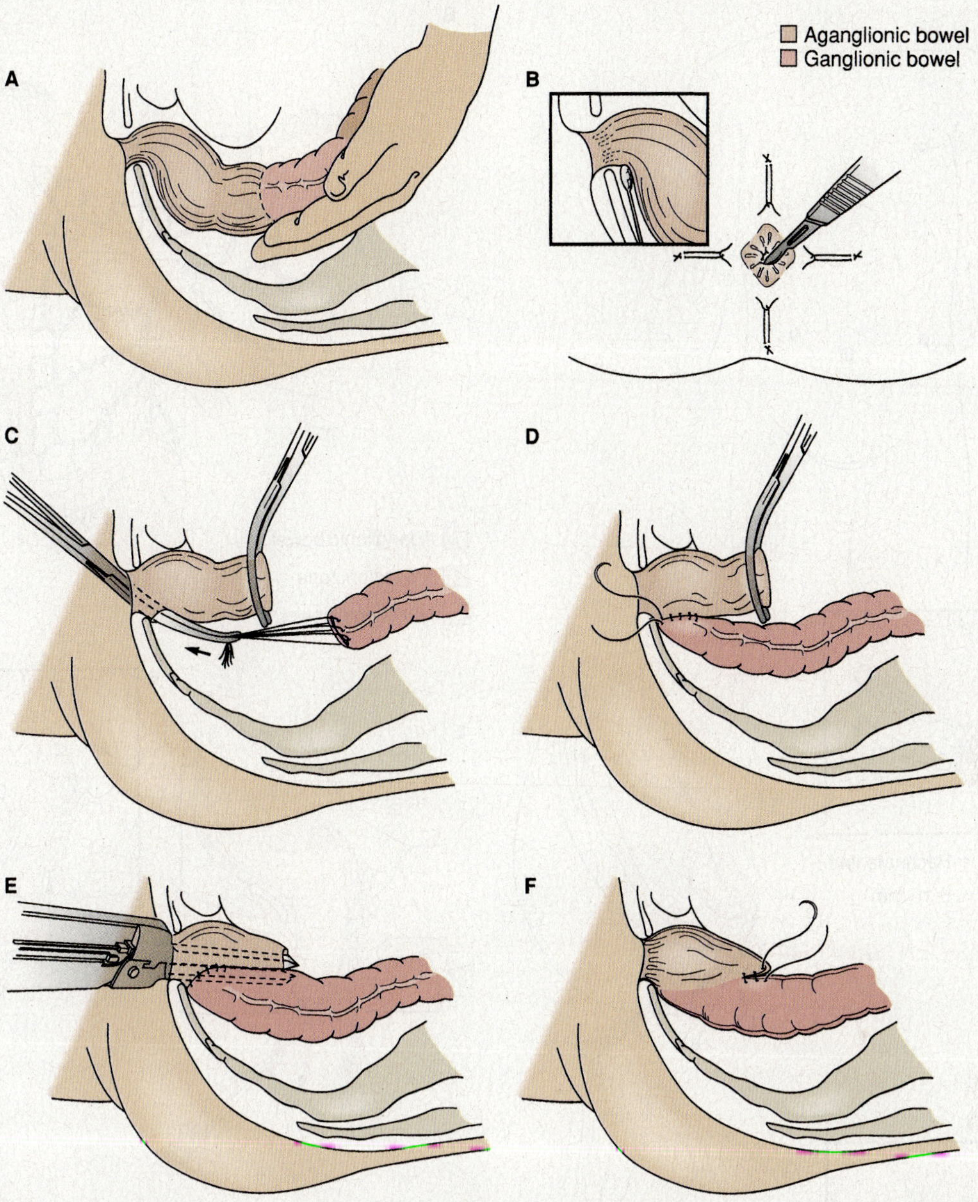

Figure 98.35. Duhamel procedure (Martin modification). **A:** Blunt retrorectal dissection. **B:** Incision in the posterior wall of the aganglionic rectum. **C:** Retrorectal pull through after resection of the proximal aganglionic segment. **D:** End-to-side colorectal anastomosis preserving aganglionic rectum (as originally described). **E:** Stapled conversion of anastomosis into an extended side-to-side colorectal anastomosis (Martin modification). **F:** Completed procedure.

Hirschsprung-Associated Enterocolitis (HAEC)

HAEC occurs both preoperatively and postoperatively and is the presenting symptom of HSCR in up to 25% of infants. The incidence of enterocolitis ranges from 20% to 60%, with most prospective series identifying higher incidences than previously recognized. Dysmotility, dysbiosis of the microbiota, altered intestinal barrier function, and impaired mucosal immune responses all appear to contribute to the pathogenesis of HAEC.[51] HAEC can occur at any time from the neonatal period onward into adulthood, although it appears to be less frequent in school-aged children. Additionally, the incidence appears to be independent of which surgical procedure for definitive management of HSCR has been performed. Recurrent HAEC can occur even in the presence of a diverting colostomy and is termed "diversion enterocolitis." The overall mortality rate associated with HAEC ranges from 1% to 10%, with the majority of deaths occurring in newborns prior to definitive operation. Infants with known Hirschsprung disease and suspected enterocolitis should be treated aggressively. Initial treatment includes resuscitation, broad-spectrum antibiotics, cessation of feeding, and rectal irrigation. If the enterocolitis does not respond promptly, emergent intestinal decompression with an enterostomy proximal to the transition zone is indicated.

Anorectal Malformations (Imperforate Anus)

Embryology

By week 5 of gestation, the fetal cloaca is identifiable with the adjacent hindgut, allantois, and vestigial tailgut (**Fig. 98.37**). The mesoderm of the urorectal septum extends caudally to fuse with the cloacal closing plate. Fusion of the lateral cloacal ridges completes division of the cloaca into the rectum and the urogenital sinus. The caudal aspect of the urorectal septum forms the perineal body. The anal membrane normally ruptures during week 8 of gestation, completing the patency of the distal rectum to the skin. Further development of the urogenital sinus leads to the formation of the urethra and the bladder. In female infants, the uterus and the proximal vagina

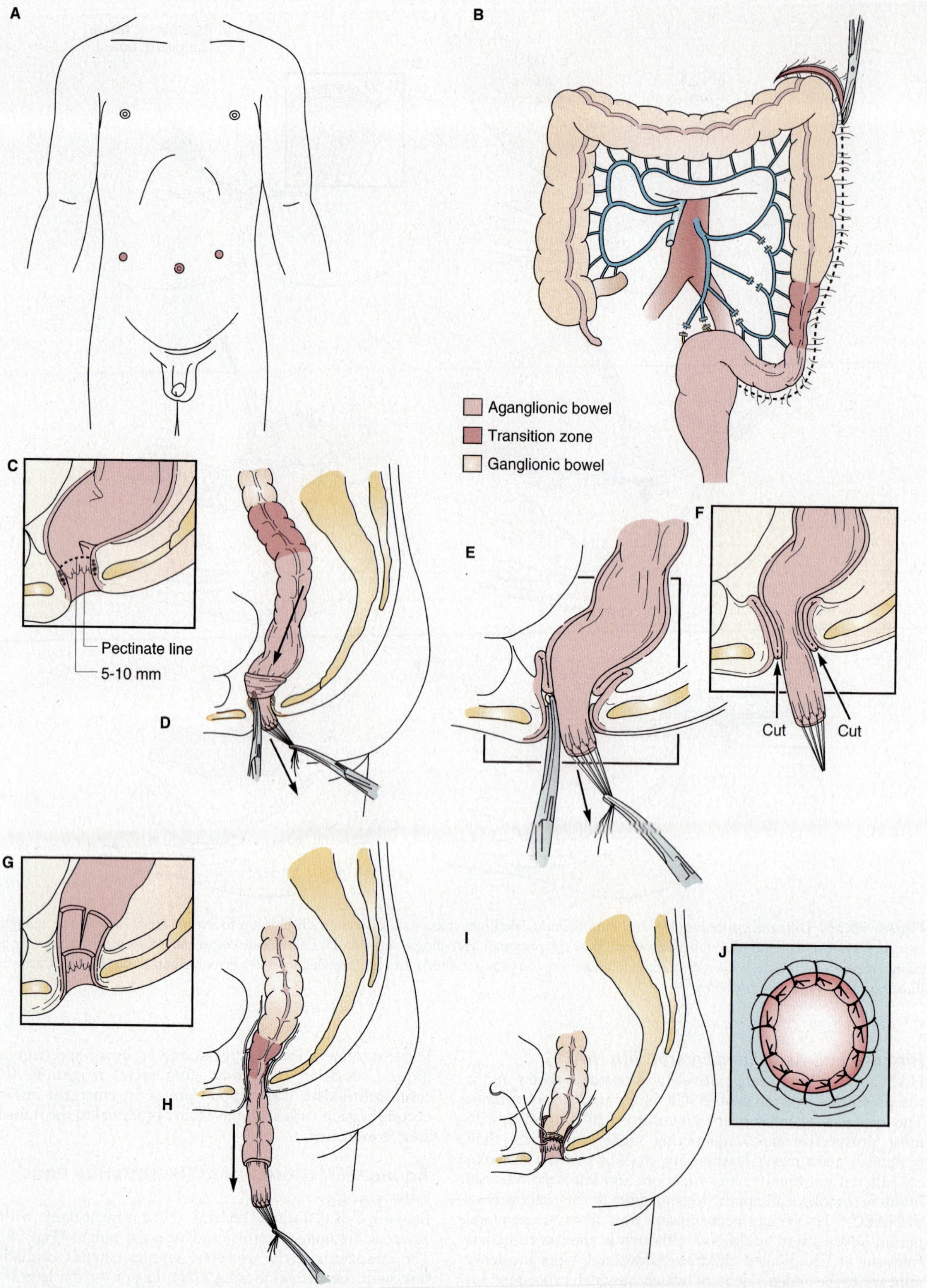

Figure 98.36. Laparoscopically assisted pull-through for Hirschsprung disease. **A:** Sites for operative trocar placement. **B:** Division of colon and rectal mesentery with mobilization of proximal colon. **C:** Circumferential incision in rectal mucosa 5- to 10-mm cephalad to the pectinate line. **D:** Mucosal traction sutures to facilitate further dissection from rectal muscular cuff. **E:** Transanal submucosal dissection is continued cephalad to meet the caudal extent of the transperitoneal rectal dissection. **F:** Circumferential incision of rectal muscular cuff. **G:** Rectal muscular cuff is split posteriorly to accommodate the pull-through segment (the pull-through segment is not shown here to clarify this maneuver). **H:** Rectum and sigmoid colon are pulled through the rectal muscular cuff to the anastomotic site. **I:** Colon is transected at appropriate site with confirmation of ganglion cells by frozen section. **J:** Transanal, end-to-end single-layer colorectal anastomosis.

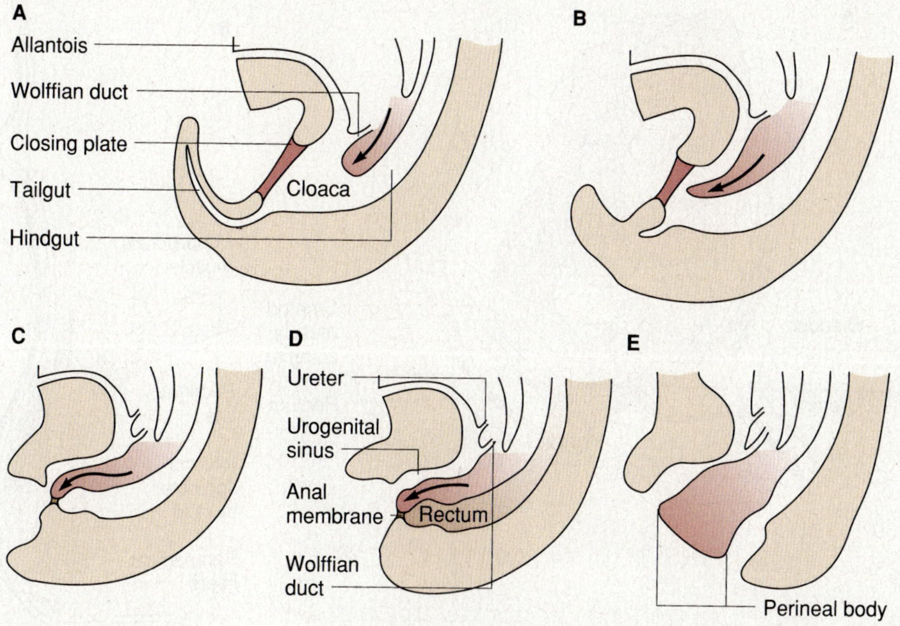

Figure 98.37. Normal embryologic division of the cloaca by the urorectal septum into the ventral urinary tract and the dorsal rectum. This process is normally completed by the 9th or 10th week of gestation.

develop from the Müllerian ducts. The diverse anatomic variation observed with anorectal malformations is thought to reflect anomalous or interrupted development of these structures during normal embryogenesis.

Anatomy and Classification

The normal anatomy of the anus and the rectum is reviewed in previous chapters. Normally, the rectum descends to the perineum and ultimately to the anal orifice through a striated muscle complex in the pelvis resembling a funnel. The striated muscle complex is under voluntary control and is responsible for providing fecal continence (**Fig. 98.38**). Contiguous portions of the *levator ani*, the *external sphincter*, and the *puborectalis* muscles compose the *striated muscle complex*. These anatomically indistinct components of the muscle complex act together to provide control of defecation. The concept of the striated muscle complex and anatomic relationships leading to normal fecal continence with respect to anorectal malformations has evolved from both clinical and anatomic data as described by Peña.

Because of the variety of anorectal malformations observed, different classification systems have been proposed in an attempt to characterize the defects. A summary of the Wingspread Classification is provided in **Table 98.9**. This anatomically descriptive classification scheme is useful in planning the operative management of anorectal malformations.

In male subjects, the two most common anorectal malformations observed are low imperforate anus with a perineal fistula (**Fig. 98.39**) and high anorectal agenesis with a rectoprostatic urethral fistula (**Fig. 98.40**). Male patients without a visible perineal fistula are assumed to have high imperforate anus with a rectourethral fistula until proven otherwise. In female subjects, the most common malformation encountered is low imperforate anus with a fistula from the rectum to either the perineal body or the vaginal vestibule (**Fig. 98.41**). As these malformations result from developmental arrest at various times during migration of the urogenital septum, considerable anatomic variability exists in both male and female subjects.

A common anatomic feature of imperforate anus is incomplete rectal descent to the perineum. Consequently, the rectum is not completely within the striated muscle complex. The caudal portion of the striated muscle complex remains a solid mass of striated muscle, whereas the cephalad portion may be normally positioned circumferentially around the rectal pouch. In low imperforate anus, the rectum nearly reaches the perineum, and the configuration of the striated muscle complex surrounding the rectum more closely approximates normal. With high imperforate anus, less striated muscle surrounds the rectal pouch. All anorectal malformations are considered to have some component of striated muscle complex hypoplasia and dysfunction, although the physiologic effects are variable. Low anorectal lesions have a more favorable prognosis for fecal continence than intermediate or high lesions.

Classic delineation between low and high anorectal malformations is made anatomically at the pubococcygeal line. The vast majority of low lesions have associated perineal or vestibular fistulas. High imperforate anus has a blind-ending rectal pouch above the pubococcygeal line and, therefore, above the striated muscle complex (or levator ani).

CLASSIFICATION

Table 98.9. Anatomic Classification of Anorectal Malformations

Female	Male
High	
Anorectal agenesis with rectovaginal fistula without fistula	Anorectal agenesis with rectoprostatic urethral or rectocystic fistula or without fistula
Rectal atresia	Rectal atresia
Intermediate	
Rectovestibular fistula	Rectobulbar urethral fistula
Rectovaginal fistula	Anal agenesis without fistula
Anal agenesis without fistula	
Low	
Anovestibular fistula[a]	Anocutaneous fistula[a]
Anocutaneous fistula[a,b]	Anal stenosis[a,c]
Anal stenosis[c]	Rare malformations
Cloacal malformations[d]	
Rare malformations	

[a]Relatively common lesion.
[b]Includes fistulas occurring at the posterior junction of the labia minora, often called *fourchette fistulas* or *vulvar fistulas*.
[c]Previously called *covered anus*.
[d]Previously called *rectocloacal fistulas*. Entry of the rectal fistula into the cloaca may be high or intermediate, depending on the length of the cloacal canal.

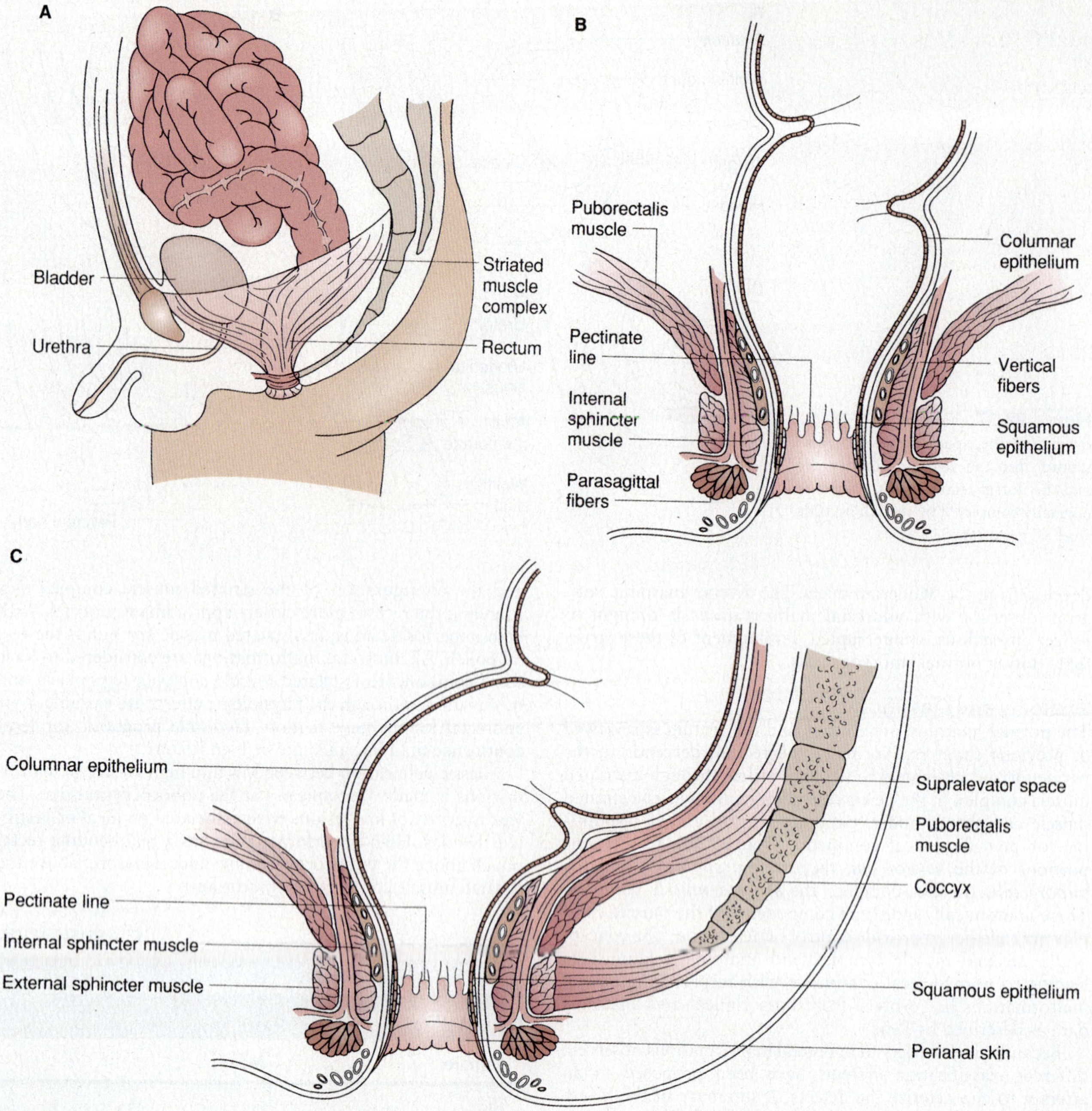

Figure 98.38. The normal relations of the pelvic striated muscle complex and the rectum. **A:** Normal male anatomy. **B:** Coronal view showing individual components of the striated muscle complex. **C:** Sagittal view of normal anatomy.

Associated Anomalies

Associated anomalies in infants with anorectal malformations are common and may be found in more than 70% of patients. The VACTERL (vertebral, anal, cardiac, tracheal, esophageal, renal, and limb) association is important and requires consideration in any infant with imperforate anus. *Vertebral anomalies* are common and include sacral dysplasia and agenesis. Infants with sacral anomalies commonly have a high imperforate anus and sacral nerve dysfunction that can lead to poor long-term fecal continence and neurogenic bladder. A variety of spinal cord malformations can also be observed in these infants, including tethered spinal cord syndromes and some myelodysplastic syndromes. During the neonatal period, these spinal lesions may be detected by using ultrasound or magnetic resonance imaging (MRI), and surgical treatment may be necessary within the first 8 to 18 months of life. *Tracheoesophageal* fistula with or without esophageal atresia is estimated to occur in about 10% of infants with anorectal malformations.

Renal anomalies are the most common associated abnormalities with anorectal malformations and include both upper and lower tract conditions. Genitourinary screening in the form of a renal ultrasound and voiding cystourethrogram is routinely performed. *Cardiac* anomalies are common, and screening echocardiography is clinically indicated. *Limb abnormalities*, in particular, involvement of the radius, complete the associated anomalies defined by the acronym.

Clinical Presentation

The incidence rate of anorectal malformations is estimated at 1 in 2524 to 5000 live births, with a slightly higher rate in males. Careful examination of the neonatal perineum reveals the diagnosis. If unrecognized and left untreated, high imperforate anus eventually leads to signs and symptoms of complete bowel obstruction characterized by abdominal distention, feeding intolerance, and bilious emesis. Because of the nearly uniform rectourethral or rectovesicular fistula in males

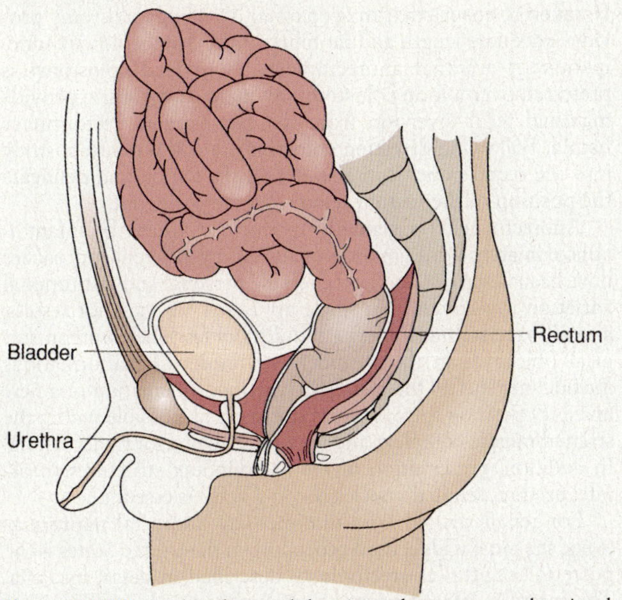

Figure 98.39. Male infant with low imperforate anus and perineal fistula. Note that the fistula is anterior to the striated muscle complex.

with high lesions, some of these infants will pass meconium or gas through the urethra during urination. In contrast, infants with low malformations typically pass meconium through a perineal or vestibular fistula within the first 24 hours of life. Occasionally, infants with large perineal fistulas are not diagnosed with an anorectal malformation until progressive constipation is noted weeks to months after birth.

In male infants, more than 95% of low malformations are associated with either a thin anal membrane or a fistula to the perineum or the scrotal raphe. The presence of a "bucket-handle" skin deformity at the presumptive anal dimple is also diagnostic of a low lesion. Infants with high malformations typically lack anal skin dimpling, have a flat gluteal contour, and may have little or absent contraction of the external sphincter with cutaneous stimulation. In female infants, 90% to 95% of low malformations have a perineal or vestibular fistula. In both male and female infants, a perineal fistula may not become apparent in the first 12 to 24 hours of life until meconium progresses distally through the rectum into the fistula.

Diagnosis

Because surgical treatment of a high or intermediate anorectal malformation is different from that of low lesion, a primary diagnostic goal is to determine whether an infant with imperforate anus has a high or low malformation. A secondary diagnostic goal is to determine the specific anorectal malformation as it relates to the rectourethral or rectovesicular fistula.

Clinical examination of an infant with low imperforate anus almost always reveals an external fistula to the perineum or the vestibule. The classic radiographic study of newborns with imperforate anus is the Wangensteen–Rice invertogram, with a lateral view of the pelvis obtained 12 to 24 hours after birth with the infant in a head-down position. This technique

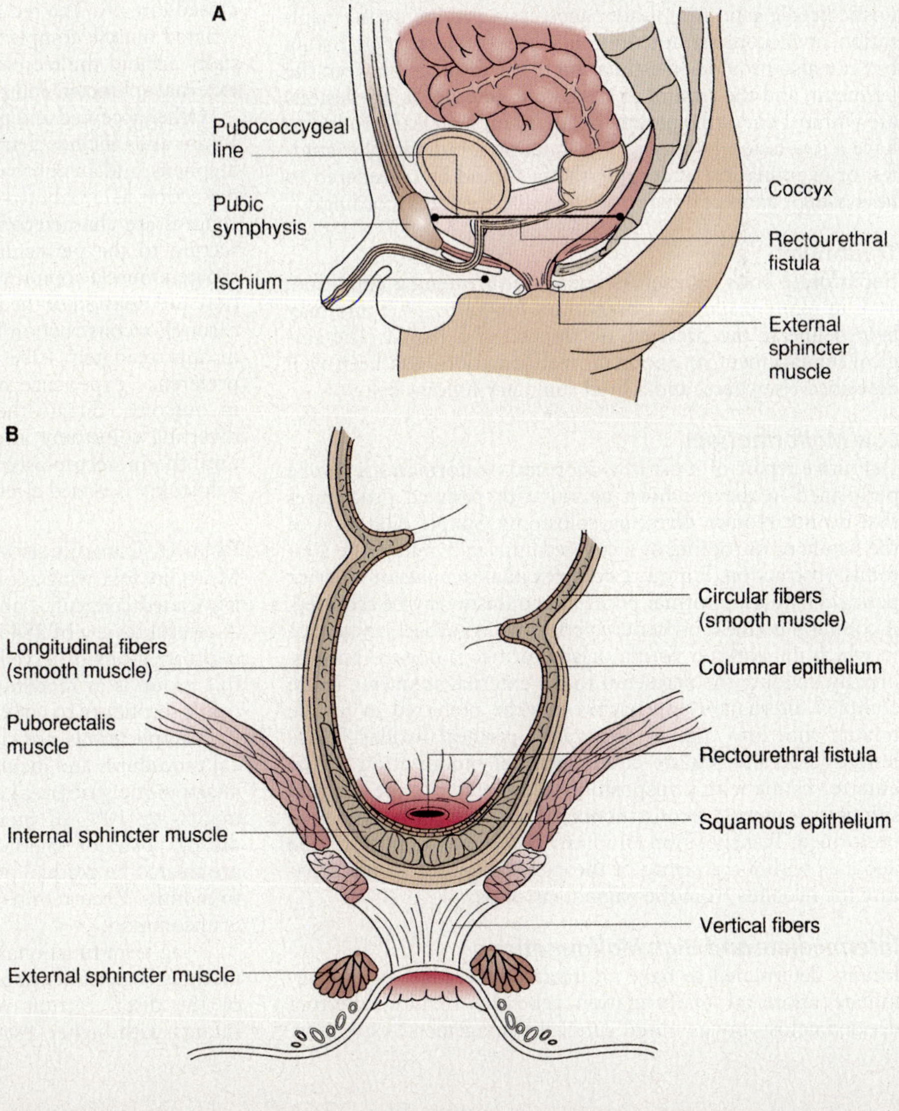

Figure 98.40. Male infant with high imperforate anus, showing the pubococcygeal line, ischium, and striated muscle complex. **A:** The rectal pouch ends cephalad to the pubococcygeal line. This location of the rectourethral fistula is typical. **B:** Coronal view showing incomplete development of the rectal pouch within the striated muscle complex. The rectourethral fistula is shown.

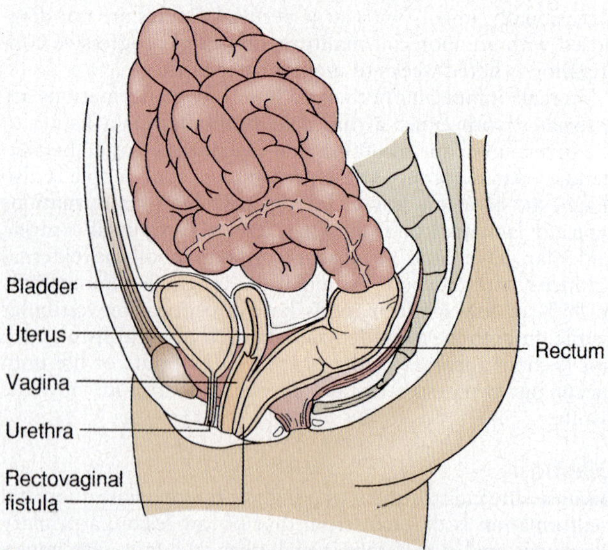

Figure 98.41. Female infant with low imperforate anus and vestibular fistula.

has been largely replaced by ultrasound-directed imaging. Real-time ultrasound is currently well accepted as an accurate method of determining the distal extent of the rectal pouch. Computed tomography (CT) imaging and MRI can be useful in evaluating the pelvic striated muscle complex in difficult cases and, in particular, cloacal malformations. MRI is also useful in evaluation of the distal spinal cord in these infants.

If there is a suspected perineal fistula or covered anus, diagnostic needle aspiration under anesthesia may be useful. Aspiration of meconium not only localizes the rectum or fistula but can also provide an estimation of the distance between the perineum and the rectum or the fistula. In general, low lesions are within 1 cm of the perineum. An infant not clearly found to have a low lesion by physical examination, radiographic studies, or examination under anesthesia should be considered to have a high anorectal malformation and treated accordingly.

Treatment

Imperforate anus by itself is not a life-threatening condition, and, in many instances, observation for 12 to 24 hours may help delineate the presence or absence of a fistula. The surgical management of anorectal malformations has been well described elsewhere, and a brief summary follows below.

Low Malformations

Definitive repair of most low anorectal malformations can be performed in the newborn period with perineal procedures that do not require diverting colostomy. Simple dilatation of the fistula or unroofing of a covered anus may relieve the anatomic obstruction. For more complex anal stenoses or anterior perineal fistulas, a formal perineal anoplasty may be required. A common perineal procedure performed is cutback anoplasty, in which the anterior fistula or anal orifice is opened posteriorly by dividing the perineum to the external sphincter. More complex alternative approaches may be preferred in female infants with low vaginal or anterior perineal fistulas. These lesions generally require circumferential mobilization of the anterior fistula with transposition to the center of the external sphincter. Anterior reconstruction of the perineal body is then performed. Transposition anoplasty is designed to position the neoanus within the center of the external sphincter and separate the neoanus from the vaginal introitus.

Intermediate and High Malformations

Infants determined to have an intermediate, high, or indeterminate anorectal malformation generally require diverting divided colostomy as initial surgical management. Care must be taken to ensure that the proximal diverting colostomy provides adequate length and mobility of the distal colon in anticipation of eventual anorectoplasty. A divided colostomy is preferred over a loop colostomy by many surgeons to provide maximal fecal diversion from the downstream rectourinary fistula. Following diverting colostomy, a distal contrast study into the rectal pouch can also define the fistula and delineate the position of the rectum relative to the perineum.

Anorectoplasty is generally performed when the infant is approximately 8 to 12 months of age. Many different approaches have been described, and considerable personal and institutional variation is common. No single approach has superior results, and all have technical merits and difficulties. The common surgical objectives in the treatment of anorectal malformations include (a) relief of the rectal obstruction; (b) creation of a new anus; (c) position the rectum as normally as possible within the striated muscle complex; and (d) divide the rectourinary fistula. In addition, preservation of the surrounding structures (prostate, urethra, seminal vesicles, vaginal wall) is essential.

For repair of high and intermediate anorectal malformations, the most widely used procedure in the United States is the posterior sagittal anorectoplasty described in detail by Peña. The infant is placed prone, and a posterior sagittal incision following the gluteal crease is used. The external sphincter and the striated muscle complex are divided posteriorly along the midline to expose the rectal pouch. A muscle stimulator is used to define and map the striated muscle complex and to confirm symmetric dissection along the midline. Typically, the rectal pouch can be adequately dissected by this approach to allow enough length to reach the perineum. Infrequently, a combined abdominoperineal approach is required. The mobilized rectal pouch is opened, and the rectourinary fistula is identified and closed directly. The rectal pouch is placed centrally within the striated muscle complex, which is reconstructed circumferentially around the rectum. The neoanus is centered within the external sphincter, and the mucosa is sutured to the perineum.

Other accepted and practiced surgical approaches to imperforate anus include a sacroperineal approach as proposed by Stephens, and an approach that uses components of endorectal dissection as attributed to Rehbein. Both these surgical procedures are characterized by blind pull through of the distal rectum to the perineum without direct visualization of the striated muscle complex. Experience with laparoscopic dissection and division of the rectourinary fistula with perineal pull-through reconstruction has been reported, but is only needed in approximately 10% of cases.[54,55] It appears that personal preference, experience, and familiarity, rather than differences in outcome, dictate the selection of procedure. In general, diverting colostomy in all of these procedures is maintained until the anorectoplasty has completely healed, after which the colostomy is closed electively.

Results, Complications, and Outcome

Mortality following anorectoplasty is related to the presence of associated congenital anomalies other than imperforate anus. A careful review of 284 infants undergoing repair of anorectal malformations observed an 18.7% mortality, suggesting that this group is at moderate to high risk for complications and death secondary to coexisting congenital anomalies.

Complications are similar to other gastrointestinal surgical procedures and include infection, leak, recurrent fistula, or anastomotic stricture. Leak or stricture formation is observed in 5% to 10% of infants undergoing tapering rectoplasty during posterior sagittal anorectoplasty. Anorectal strictures are treated by gradual postoperative anal dilatation for weeks to months. Recurrent rectourethral fistula or urethral stricture is uncommon.

Long-term functional outcome in infants with low malformations is generally good, given the relatively normal descent of the distal rectum within the striated muscle complex. Infants with higher lesions have a less predictable prognosis

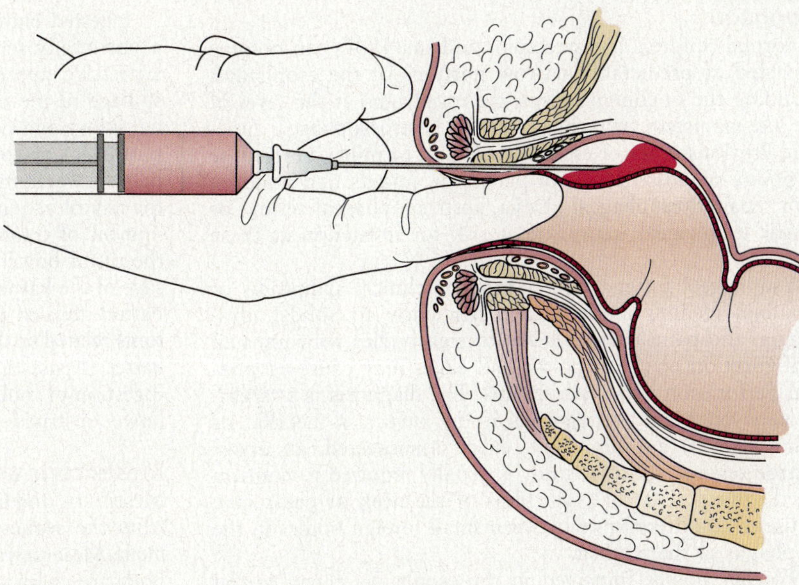

Figure 98.42. Four-quadrant injection of sclerosant into the rectal submucosa for the treatment of childhood rectal prolapse.

and are much more likely to have difficulty with fecal continence. Currently, the outcomes appear to be independent of the type of surgical reconstruction performed and more related to anatomic patient factors, including degree of rectal descent, integrity of the striated muscle complex, and sacral innervation. However, there are no established, accurate predictors of long-term fecal continence, and as such, these children should be followed until at least 4 years of age.[56] Few or perhaps none of these children have completely normal bowel habits after operation. About half of the infants have acceptable to good results with episodic fecal soilage that can be improved with bowel management programs, enemas, and cathartics.[57] A comprehensive bowel management program is essential in preventing fecal impaction and subsequent motility dysfunction in the rectum. The remaining children require major adjustments in lifestyle secondary to fecal incontinence, chronic constipation, or fecal smearing and odor. In some instances, socially acceptable continence can be assisted by the use of daily antegrade enemas via a cecostomy or appendicostomy. In other situations, a permanent diverting colostomy may be desirable.

Meconium Plug Syndrome

Meconium plug syndrome is characterized by functional obstruction of the colon or the rectum by a meconium plug. It affects both normal and premature infants with immature gastrointestinal motility and must be differentiated from other causes of neonatal intestinal obstruction. Unlike meconium ileus, in meconium plug syndrome, the colon is of normal caliber and the meconium is not inspissated. The infant's symptoms within the first few days of life are abdominal distention and bilious emesis. Spontaneous passage of meconium is often absent. On examination, the infant is normal with a patent anus and a distended abdomen. Digital rectal examination may deliver the meconium plug. Plain films of the abdomen demonstrate dilated loops of bowel consistent with distal bowel obstruction. The diagnosis is confirmed by contrast enema, which is also therapeutic in helping the meconium plug pass. The meconium plug is followed by bile-stained meconium of normal consistency. Importantly, although the vast majority of these infants are normal, a few have Hirschsprung disease or CF. Therefore, infants presenting with meconium plug syndrome may require rectal suction biopsy and have CF screening tests performed.

Rectal Prolapse

Spontaneous rectal prolapse is relatively common in toddlers and children up to 5 years of age. A peak incidence occurs at or near the time of toilet training. There is an association between straining during bowel movement and rectal prolapse; it may be more commonly observed in children with CF, myelodysplasias with sacral neuropathy, congenital anorectal malformations, Hirschsprung disease, and colorectal polyps. However, most children presenting with rectal prolapse are normal.

A history of protrusion of mucosa or full-thickness rectum with or without bleeding is usually described. Other lesions of childhood that have a similar appearance are prolapse of an intussusceptum or passage of a polyp through the anus. The rectal examination is diagnostic. If the protruding intestine is an intussusceptum, a finger can be placed adjacent to it within the rectum; this maneuver is not possible with rectal prolapse.

Nonoperative management using manual reduction is successful in most infants and children. Sedation may be required in some instances. Therapeutic interventions include stool softeners and parental instruction on manual reduction. Spontaneous resolution over a few weeks is typical. For persistent rectal prolapse in children, operative intervention is generally governed by doing the least invasive procedure possible. Unlike adults, complex operations involving bowel resection and pelvic suspension are generally unnecessary in children with rectal prolapse. The most useful and commonly used procedure is rectal submucosal injection using a sclerosant (**Fig. 98.42**). With the patient under general anesthesia, injection with 5% sodium morrhuate or cow's milk[58] has been performed successfully on an outpatient basis. About 90% of children can be treated successfully with a single four-quadrant sclerosant technique, but on occasion further sclerosis is necessary. Submucosal dissection or cauterization is also successful but may have a higher incidence of postoperative bleeding or stricture formation and usually requires a short period of hospitalization. The major objective in treating childhood rectal prolapse is to create a local extraperitoneal inflammatory process in the perirectal space. Morbidity is low and the long-term outcome is excellent.

OTHER CHILDHOOD GASTROINTESTINAL DISORDERS

Foreign Bodies

Ingestion of foreign bodies by infants and children is common. Toddlers in the age range of 9 months to 2 years are at particular risk, given newly acquired mobility and the tendency for oral exploration. The type of foreign body and the location in the gastrointestinal tract on discovery dictate overall management.

Esophagus

In normal children, ingested coins and small toys can become impacted at predictably narrow portions of the esophagus, including the cricopharyngeus, the esophagus at the level of the left mainstem bronchus, and the gastroesophageal junction. Previous areas of esophageal repair or injury predispose to points of obstruction. In particular, infants and children with repaired esophageal atresia, gastroesophageal reflux, or caustic esophageal injury are at risk for impaction at these sites.

Esophageal foreign bodies produce clinical symptoms of drooling, feeding intolerance (particularly to solids), dysphagia, and pain. Unrecognized foreign bodies with unusual configuration or sharp points and edges may cause esophageal perforation and mediastinitis. The diagnosis is straightforward on plain radiographs if the object is metallic or radiopaque. If a radiolucent object is suspected, an upper gastrointestinal contrast study is usually required to confirm the diagnosis. Lateral plain films of the neck or chest may be useful to differentiate between small foreign bodies in the esophagus or the trachea.

Foreign bodies impacted in the esophagus cause partial esophageal obstruction and can cause complications, including aspiration, erosion, perforation, and late stricture formation. Therefore, all esophageal foreign bodies should be removed. Extraction of foreign objects can be accomplished by using balloon catheter retrieval under fluoroscopic guidance or direct visualization using endoscopy. Performed within 24 hours of ingestion, balloon catheter retrieval of esophageal foreign bodies is relatively straightforward. This technique is limited to smooth radiopaque objects such as coins to minimize the risk of esophageal perforation. The most significant risk with balloon catheter retrieval is potential aspiration from an unprotected airway, and this must be anticipated as the foreign body traverses the pharynx. Alternatively, for esophageal coin impaction of less than 24 hours' duration in children without a history of esophageal surgery or injury, esophageal bougienage with clearance of the coin into the stomach has been successful.

Retrieval of esophageal foreign bodies under direct endoscopic vision requires general anesthesia. Either flexible or rigid endoscopy systems are widely available and used with individual and institutional preferences. Esophageal perforation, the major risk, occurs in fewer than 5% of cases in most reported series. Long-standing esophageal foreign bodies may erode into the aorta and cause life-threatening hemorrhage from aortoesophageal fistula.[59]

Distal Gastrointestinal Tract

More than 95% of foreign bodies that pass beyond the gastroesophageal junction proceed uneventfully through the gastrointestinal tract. The transit time for an asymptomatic foreign body is highly variable and can take hours to weeks. Progress of an asymptomatic radiopaque foreign body can be followed by abdominal plain films, but this is rarely useful from a clinical standpoint unless it is a battery. The stool may also be screened to confirm passage of a known foreign body.

Operative exploration or endoscopic retrieval of distal gastrointestinal foreign bodies is generally reserved for clinical symptoms related to either obstruction or intestinal injury heralded by abdominal pain, vomiting, fever, or peritonitis. In addition, persistence of an asymptomatic foreign body in the stomach for several weeks is a relative indication for upper endoscopic retrieval, particularly with foreign bodies with irregular shape, configuration, or sharpness. This is a clinical judgment that is best reserved for an experienced pediatric surgeon because remarkably complex and improbable objects may pass uneventfully through the gastrointestinal tract. For asymptomatic foreign bodies lodged distal to the stomach, a relative indication for operative removal is a fixed, persistent location in the intestine longer than 1 week in duration.

Ingested batteries, in particular alkaline disc batteries, are a potentially serious hazard to children and require a more aggressive approach. Disruption of the battery casing and spillage of the contents have been reported to cause intestinal injury and perforation, presumably because of leakage of potassium or sodium hydroxide. Esophageal impaction of a battery warrants prompt removal when recognized because the risk of acquired esophageal injury, perforation, and development of traumatic tracheoesophageal fistula is present. In the distal bowel, cathartics may be helpful to expedite passage of the battery. Operative removal may be necessary if the battery fails to progress distally over a few days or if symptoms related to the battery occur. Notably, the vast majority of batteries pass through the gastrointestinal tract uneventfully. Ingestion of multiple magnets can cause problems with small bowel obstruction or enteroenteric fistula formation.

Mesenteric and Omental Cysts

Mesenteric and omental cysts are rare lesions thought to result from the sequestration of lymphatic tissue during development. Mesenteric cysts are twice as common as omental cysts. Both are characterized by thin, often incomplete walls lined with endothelial cells, absent of surrounding smooth muscle. They may be filled with either serous lymphatic fluid or chyle and may be unilocular or multilocular. These cysts may become extraordinarily large before producing symptoms.

Most infants and children with mesenteric or omental cysts are diagnosed prior to adolescence. Asymptomatic children are usually diagnosed incidentally during studies for other reasons. Symptomatic children present with abdominal pain, and, on examination, a soft, mobile abdominal mass is characteristic. Bleeding, rupture, obstruction, torsion, or cyst infection may be observed. Most of these lesions can be diagnosed by ultrasound or CT scan imaging. Ascites, duplication cysts, pancreatic pseudocysts, and large ovarian cysts may have a similar appearance on diagnostic imaging. Peripheral calcification and evidence of recent hemorrhage may be seen in mesenteric or omental cysts (**Fig. 98.43**).

The treatment for these lesions is simple excision. Total excision of mesenteric or omental cysts is generally preferable over partial excision with marsupialization. Limited resection with primary anastomosis may be required for a mesenteric cyst located adjacent to the intestinal wall, particularly if there is concern that the cyst actually may be an enteric duplication. Morbidity and mortality are generally limited to concurrent problems associated with the intestine. In particular, volvulus of a mesenteric cyst may cause vascular compromise and infarction of the adjacent intestine.

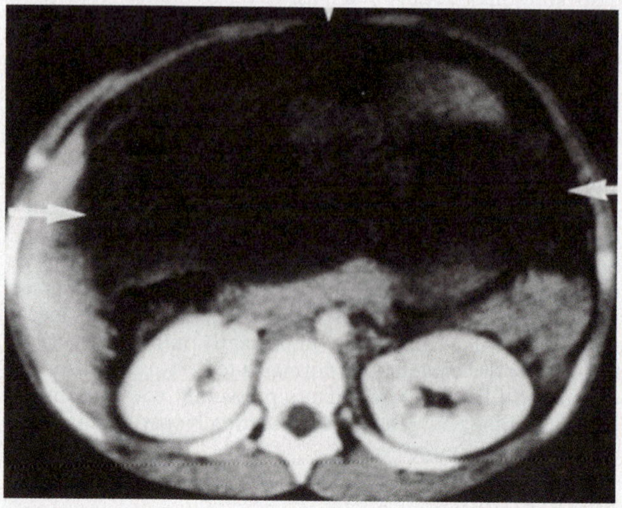

Figure 98.43. Computed tomographic scan of a child after abdominal trauma.Hemorrhage into large omental cyst is apparent (*arrows*).

Primary Peritonitis

Bacterial peritonitis without a specific, identifiable cause is referred to as *primary peritonitis*. Spontaneous bacterial peritonitis in children with ascites or nephrosis is generally included in this group. Hematogenous seeding of ascitic fluid is probably responsible for the development of spontaneous bacterial peritonitis. The infecting bacterial organisms were classically gram positive with a variety of staphylococcal, streptococcal, and other species accounting for most cases. In a series of infants and children with primary peritonitis, more than two-thirds of the cases were caused by gram-negative organisms such as *Escherichia coli*. This trend may reflect the use of antibiotic prophylaxis directed against gram-positive organisms.

The other etiologic mechanism for the development of primary peritonitis is believed to involve retrograde inoculation of the peritoneal cavity via the genitourinary tract. This etiology is characteristic of prepubertal girls 5 to 10 years of age, accounting for as many as half of the cases of primary peritonitis. The initial signs and symptoms in these children are virtually identical to those in children with perforated appendicitis: fever, emesis, abdominal pain, and tenderness on examination. Leukocytosis is characteristic, and an ileus is observed on plain abdominal films. On exploration, these children have inflammatory peritonitis without an identifiable enteric cause. Gram-negative enteric organisms are commonly cultured from the peritoneal fluid.

Infants and children with peritonitis in association with an indwelling peritoneal dialysis catheter or ventriculoperitoneal shunt may be treated successfully with intravenous broad-spectrum antibiotics. The catheter or shunt should be removed or exteriorized promptly if peritonitis does not resolve within 24 to 48 hours.[60] In association with ascites or nephrosis, diagnostic paracentesis should be performed and the peritoneal fluid examined by Gram stain and culture. If there is any diagnostic uncertainty, laparoscopic or open operative exploration may be required to exclude intestinal perforation as a cause of peritonitis. If the appendix is normal, peritoneal cultures should be obtained, and a thorough, complete abdominal exploration for other causes should be performed. Appendectomy is generally performed when the diagnosis of primary peritonitis is established by a right lower-quadrant incision. Other than perforated appendicitis, distinct causes of intestinal perforation or peritonitis in this age group include perforated Meckel diverticulum, duodenal ulcer, and acute pancreatitis. About half of the peritoneal fluid cultures are positive for a single organism. Treatment with specific antibiotics is continued until the patient is afebrile with a normal white blood cell count and normal clinical examination. Following operative exploration in primary peritonitis, the morbidity is no different than that for appendectomy, and the recovery is generally uneventful.

Ascites

The common causes of neonatal and childhood ascites are listed in **Tables 98.10** and **98.11**. The clinical presentation is that of abdominal distention with bulging flanks and demonstrable fluid on palpation and percussion. Ultrasound or CT scan imaging may be useful to confirm the clinical diagnosis. Paracentesis and routine examination of the fluid for Gram stain, cell count, cytology, protein, chemistries, and culture should be performed. Chylous ascites is characterized by a white milky appearance, high lymphocyte count, and high triglyceride content. Bile-stained fluid in the absence of demonstrable bowel perforation is characteristic of biliary ascites. High-fluid amylase content is seen in pancreatic ascites, and a low protein count (<3 g/dL) is consistent with serous ascites. Elevated urea nitrogen or creatinine in the fluid may suggest urinary ascites, particularly in a male patient. Cytology should be performed to exclude peritoneal ascites secondary to malignancy, particularly in pubertal and adolescent females.

ETIOLOGY

Table 98.10. Common Causes of Neonatal Ascites

Maternal–fetal Rh incompatibility (rare)
Structural malformations
Urinary obstruction
Congenital heart disease
Malrotation, duplications, cyst (associated with intestinal volvulus)
Biliary perforation
Ovarian ascites
Pulmonary abnormalities
Chylous ascites
Hematologic disorder
α-Thalassemia
Infection
Toxoplasmosis
Cytomegalovirus
Others
α_1-Antitrypsin deficiency
Idiopathic

If the initial fluid does not provide a diagnosis in an otherwise normal-appearing child, a comprehensive diagnostic imaging evaluation is warranted. An echocardiogram should be obtained, and either ultrasound or CT scan should be performed to evaluate the genitourinary system, the hepatobiliary system, and the pancreas. A voiding cystourethrogram may also be indicated.

Treatment of neonatal or childhood ascites depends on the establishment of a specific diagnosis. In the absence of anatomic lesion or injury, spontaneous resolution of chylous ascites occurs in 50% to 75% of cases with the temporary cessation of enteral feeding and administration of parenteral nutrition. Persistence of chylous ascites for longer than 4 to 6 weeks is an indication for operative attempts to ligate the cisterna chyli. Neonatal biliary ascites may result from spontaneous bile duct perforation, in which case a diagnosis of CF must be considered. Transient bile duct obstruction typically leads to perforation at the junction of the cystic duct with the common duct. Simple external drainage is the treatment of choice, and complex hepatobiliary tract reconstruction in this setting is unnecessary and potentially hazardous. Urinary ascites in a male patient requires a workup that includes a voiding cystourethrogram to exclude posterior urethral valves. Urinary ascites resolves with the treatment of obstructive uropathy. Pancreatic ascites is typically self-limited, and treatment by drainage procedures is generally not required or limited for relief of persistent symptoms.

Massive neonatal ascites may cause hypoventilation secondary to impairment of diaphragmatic excursion, and therapeutic paracentesis may be required. Childhood ascites generally responds to adequate treatment of the underlying problem and occasionally requires medical therapy. Placement of a peritoneovenous shunt in children for intractable ascites is rare.

LIVER, BILIARY TRACT, AND PANCREAS

Embryology

The fetal liver and biliary tract develop between weeks 4 and 10 of gestation, representing the fusion of an endodermal foregut diverticulum with a mesodermal component from the septum transversum. The hepatocytes are derived from cords of endodermal cells in the hepatic diverticulum and ultimately

ETIOLOGY

Table 98.11. Common Causes of Childhood Ascites

Serous Ascites
Cirrhosis
Budd–Chiari syndrome
Nephrosis
Right-sided heart failure
Postoperative ascites (after renal transplantation, peritoneal dialysis, ventriculoperitoneal shunt)
α_1-Antitrypsin deficiency
Other rare metabolic disorders
Chylous Ascites
Malrotation with volvulus
Small bowel obstruction
Incarcerated hernia
Lymphangioma
Trauma (includes operative trauma)
Biliary Ascites
Neonatal bile duct perforation
Cystic fibrosis
Biliary atresia
Hepatitis
Cytomegalovirus infection
Urinary Ascites (7:1 Male Predominance)
Urinary obstruction
Posterior urethral valves
Bladder perforation
Ureterocele
Neurogenic bladder
Pancreatic Ascites
Acute pancreatitis (drugs, trauma, gallstones, infection)
Pancreatic pseudocysts
Ovarian Ascites
Cysts (torsion, rupture)
Tumors
Malignant Ascites
Intra-abdominal neoplasm
Idiopathic

give rise to the hepatic sinusoidal endothelium. The proximal hepatic diverticulum gives rise to the extrahepatic biliary tract, including the gallbladder, cystic duct, and common bile duct. As the intrahepatic and extrahepatic ductal systems develop, they unite to form a connected, arborizing system of cords composed of primitive ductular epithelial cells. These epithelial cells assume tubular configuration with ductal patency established between weeks 6 and 12 of gestation. Bile flow from the hepatocytes and into the biliary duct system is apparent by the beginning of the second fetal trimester.

This embryologic sequence appears to take place normally in infants who develop biliary atresia. In fact, the term *biliary atresia* does not reflect embryologic atresia resulting from failure of recanalization of the biliary tree. Rather, biliary atresia is caused by an uncontrollable inflammatory process that produces progressive obliteration of the normally developed extrahepatic biliary tract.

Biliary Atresia

Anatomy

7 The overall incidence rate of biliary atresia is about 1 in 8000 to 12,000 live births and is the most common cause of chronic cholestasis in infants and children, as well as the most frequent indication for pediatric liver transplantation. Extrahepatic biliary atresia must be differentiated from biliary hypoplasia. Biliary hypoplasia describes a diminutive but patent biliary system and can result from many underlying situations, such as neonatal hepatitis and alpha$_1$-antitrypsin deficiency. Biliary hypoplasia involves both intrahepatic and extrahepatic ductal systems.

Microscopic Anatomy

Biliary atresia is characterized by replacement of the extrahepatic biliary tract with dense, fibrous inflammatory tissue. In most cases, complete obliteration of the extrahepatic biliary tract, including the gallbladder, occurs. There appears to be gradual progression of the inflammatory process with advancing age. The common hepatic duct and common bile duct are almost uniformly obliterated by the inflammatory process. Few or absent patent ductal remnants and an absence of portal inflammation may be associated with a less favorable prognosis. Intraoperative evaluation for duct patency by frozen section analysis has historically been used to help guide the extent of proximal resection at the porta hepatis; however, this is no longer in widespread use. The presence of bile ducts at the porta hepatis with diameter greater than 150 μm has been reported to be associated with postoperative bile flow in up to 90% to 95% of cases.

Histologic features of biliary atresia reflect hepatic parenchymal injury. Neocholangiogenesis, or biliary duct proliferation of disorganized and nonpatent ducts within the liver, is considered highly suggestive but not specific for biliary atresia. Other findings include bile pigment deposition throughout the liver. Characteristic early findings in biliary atresia include evidence for acute inflammation with neutrophil predominance in the periportal regions. Older infants and children typically have chronic inflammatory changes with considerable fibrosis. Periportal bridging fibrosis is commonly seen in intermediate stages of the disease. Ultimately, progressive biliary atresia leads to intractable cirrhosis. Nearly all patients with biliary atresia have histologic evidence of liver injury. The severity and extent of liver damage may be the most important predictors of long-term outcome and survival in biliary atresia.

Pathophysiology

The mechanism causing biliary atresia remains unknown. The current concept is that the normally developed biliary tract undergoes inflammatory sclerosis and subsequent obliteration. This process appears to occur during the first few weeks to months of life. Early establishment of biliary drainage via portoenterostomy within the first 2 to 4 months of age may be associated with reversal of liver injury and subsequent long-term survival. Conversely, infants operated on after 120 days of life typically have obliterated bile ducts. Neonatal biliary atresia shares some clinical and morphologic features of sclerosing cholangitis in adults. Data supporting an infectious etiologic agent and, in particular, reoviruses, rotaviruses, and hepatitis C, have been reported and may play a role in some cases. In addition, other noninfectious stimuli may trigger an inflammatory response directed at the neonatal extrahepatic bile duct. The actual mechanism may reflect a stereotypical inflammatory response initiated by a variety of different stimuli that is ultimately directed preferentially against the neonatal bile duct.

Clinical Presentation and Diagnosis

The cardinal sign of biliary atresia is progressive neonatal jaundice during the first few weeks of life. Dark urine and acholic stools are expected findings. Progressive hyperbilirubinemia produces clinical jaundice around 2 to 4 weeks of age. The physical examination is generally unremarkable except for jaundice and possibly mild hepatomegaly. Alagille syndrome, which presents with neonatal jaundice, can usually be distinguished from biliary atresia on physical examination. Children with Alagille syndrome have biliary hypoplasia and distinctly abnormal facies, growth retardation, vertebral defects, and pulmonic stenosis.

A characteristic laboratory finding is conjugated hyperbilirubinemia consistent with obstructive jaundice. A direct fraction of bilirubin greater than 50%, or greater than 2 mg/dL, in an infant requires prompt investigation. Mild elevation of hepatic transaminases is commonly seen. The alkaline phosphatase is significantly elevated, often in the range of 500 to 1000 IU/L. There are no specific biochemical markers for biliary atresia, as these serum profiles can be seen in other causes of neonatal cholestasis. Late findings in biliary atresia include failure to thrive, feeding intolerance, stigmata of portal hypertension, and fat-soluble vitamin deficiency.

Table 98.12 is a partial list of the causes of neonatal cholestatic syndromes. Neonatal physiologic jaundice is commonly encountered. Because of the numerous causes of neonatal jaundice and the relative infrequency of biliary atresia, a delay in diagnosis is common. Given the age-sensitive nature of biliary atresia and the improved outcome in younger infants, the diagnostic workup should be expedient.

Radioisotope Scanning

Pertechnetate 99 m–iminodiacetic acid (^{99m}Tc-IDA) analogs are widely used for hepatobiliary imaging and provide the basis for a sensitive and specific test for biliary atresia. The sensitivity of this diagnostic examination for biliary atresia can be 100%, with a specificity of 94%.[61] To improve sensitivity, infants are administered oral phenobarbital (5 mg/kg daily) to induce hepatic microsomal enzymes and increase hepatocyte processing of ^{99m}Tc-IDA. Both hepatic uptake of radionuclide and excretion into the gastrointestinal tract are evaluated over a timed interval. Infants with primary hepatocellular disorders characteristically have impaired hepatocyte uptake of radionuclide, whereas normal infants and infants with biliary atresia have prompt uptake. Normal infants excrete the isotope rapidly into the gut through the biliary tract. In biliary atresia, there is no excretion into the gut because of the obliteration of the extrahepatic bile ducts (**Fig. 98.44**). The hepatobiliary scanning is a rapid test that can be performed simultaneously with other diagnostic examinations, for example, ultrasound. This test reliably identifies infants with choledochal cyst as well.

Ultrasound

A standard examination of the jaundiced infant is a comprehensive abdominal ultrasound, with particular attention given to the liver and the biliary tract. The most common ultrasonographic finding in biliary atresia is a diminutive or absent gallbladder without associated intrahepatic duct dilatation. Biliary tract obstruction from a choledochal cyst can also be reliably identified by ultrasound. Other rare causes of extrahepatic biliary duct obstruction are associated with proximal duct dilatation.

ETIOLOGY

Table 98.12. Causes and Associations of Neonatal Cholestasis

Congenital Infectious Causes
Cytomegalovirus[a]
Rubella virus[a]
Herpes virus
Hepatitis virus B[a]
Echovirus 14, 19
Coxsackievirus B
Toxoplasmosis
Syphilis
Genetic Associations
Galactosemia
Tyrosinemia
Congenital fructose intolerance
Alpha$_1$-antitrypsin deficiency
Cystic fibrosis
Niemann–Pick disease
Trisomies 17, 18, 21
Turner syndrome
Menkes syndrome
Zellweger syndrome
Polysplenia syndrome[b]
Miscellaneous Associations
Hemolytic disease
Bacterial sepsis
Pyelonephritis
Total parenteral nutrition (prolonged)
Congestive heart failure
Hypoplastic left heart syndrome
Necrotizing enterocolitis, gastroschisis, omphalocele
Neonatal hypopituitarism
Inspissated bile syndrome (without hemolysis) neonatal shock, respiratory distress syndrome, acidosis

[a]Rarely associated with biliary atresia.
[b]Frequently associated with biliary atresia.

Liver Biopsy

Because the histologic findings in biliary atresia are not specific, about 20% to 25% of infants who undergo percutaneous liver biopsy remain undiagnosed. Liver biopsy is often performed in conjunction with the workup of conjugated hyperbilirubinemia following hepatobiliary scanning and ultrasonography, but in the setting of biliary atresia, it has limited utility. The

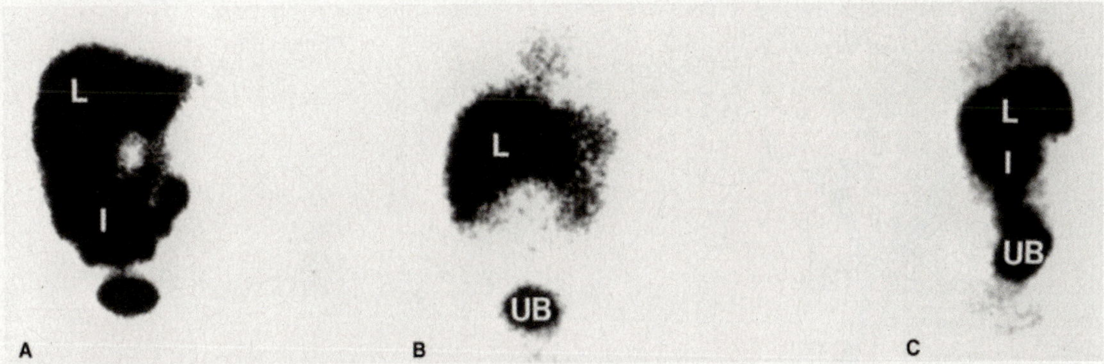

Figure 98.44. **A:** Normal scan using p-isopropyl acetanilidoiminodiacetic acid (PIPIDA) as the hepatobiliary scanning agent. At 45 minutes, isotope is clearly visible in the liver (*L*) and the intestine (*I*). **B:** Scan after phenobarbital administration in infant with biliary atresia. Even after 8 hours, isotope is apparent only in the liver and the urinary bladder (*UB*). **C:** Patient with cholestatic jaundice. At 65 minutes, isotope is visible in the liver (*L*) and the intestine (*I*). Hepatocyte uptake is variable but usually decreased or normal, whereas excretion into the gut is predictably present with cholestatic jaundice or hepatocellular disease.

PEDIATRIC SURGERY

histologic examination of a percutaneous liver biopsy is probably most helpful in diagnosing nonoperative causes of neonatal jaundice, thus avoiding anesthesia and operative exploration.

Alpha$_1$-Antitrypsin Deficiency

Alpha$_1$-antitrypsin deficiency is perhaps the single most important medical condition that may be difficult or impossible to differentiate from biliary atresia. All jaundiced infants should have plasma alpha$_1$-antitrypsin levels determined before operative exploration for suspected biliary atresia. Infants with alpha$_1$-antitrypsin deficiency do not benefit from operative exploration or portoenterostomy.

Treatment

Infants with biliary atresia require surgical therapy as the initial management intervention. Medical therapy is directed to the postoperative management of the chronic liver disease. The use of sequential surgical treatment, using portoenterostomy in infancy and orthotopic liver transplantation for children with progressive hepatic failure, provides improvement in overall survival.[62] Limited organ availability and a higher rate of perioperative complications limit primary liver transplantation for most infants with biliary atresia younger than 1 year. In the rare instance of unrecognized biliary atresia in an older child with established hepatic dysfunction, primary orthotopic liver transplantation may be a reasonable option.

Portoenterostomy

The recommended initial procedure for the treatment of biliary atresia is portoenterostomy. Before the development of portoenterostomy in Japan by Morio Kasai during the late 1950s, all infants with biliary atresia died of chronic liver disease and cirrhosis. Current management dictates that operative exploration and portoenterostomy be performed promptly. Early intervention by portoenterostomy to provide biliary drainage has been proposed to arrest or reverse the parenchymal liver injury, but the point at which the liver injury becomes irreversible remains unknown. From a clinical standpoint, most long-term success with portoenterostomy alone appears to be achieved in infants younger than 2 to 3 months, whereas infants older than 3 to 4 months appear to have a less favorable prognosis. Portoenterostomy for this "late" group has been reported successfully in approximately one-third of infants, however, and should be considered a potential alternative in the absence of available liver transplant donors.[63]

The initial approach to the infant with suspected biliary atresia is to perform an operative cholangiogram. If the diagnosis is confirmed, a portoenterostomy is constructed (**Fig. 98.45**).

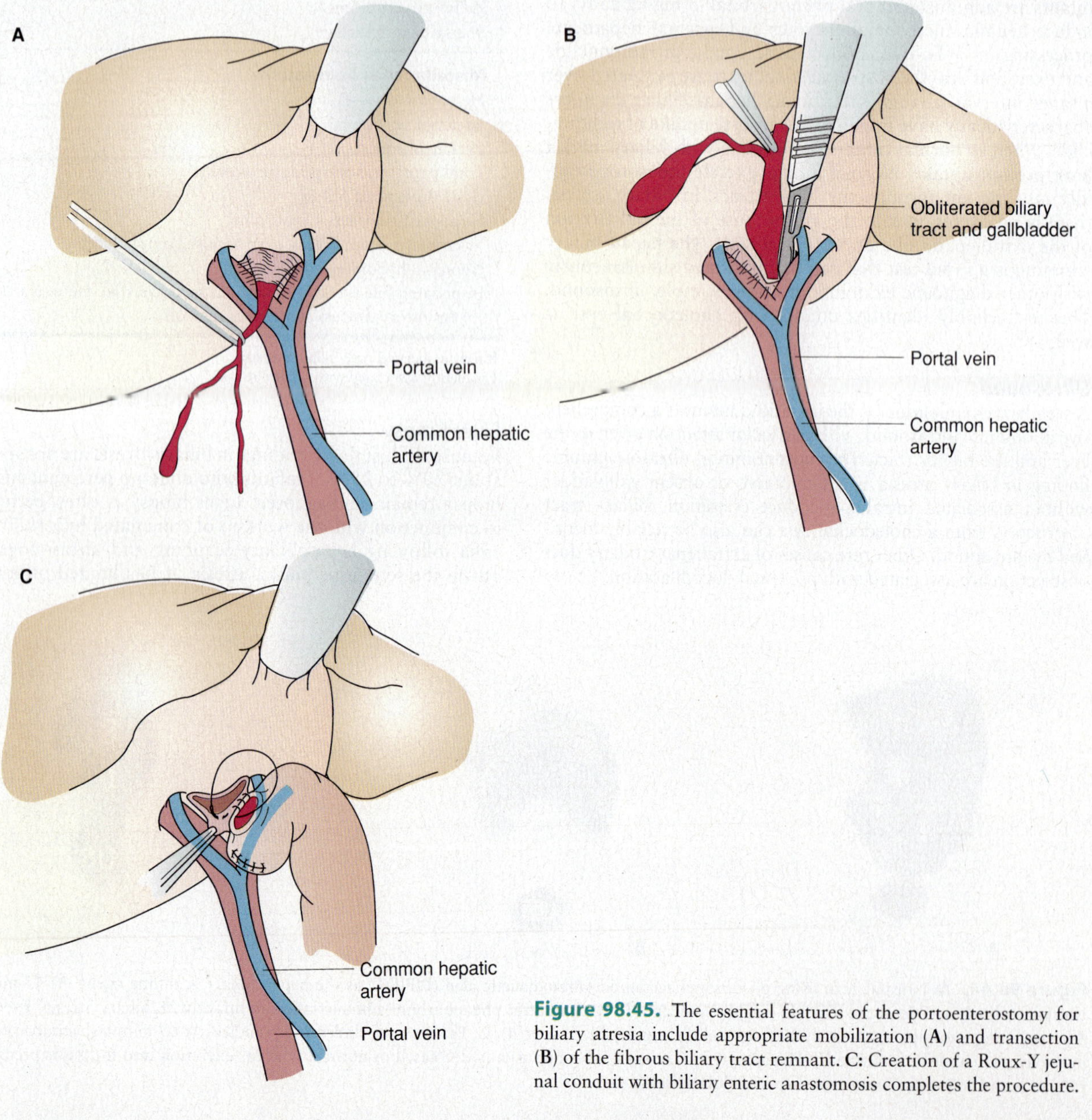

Figure 98.45. The essential features of the portoenterostomy for biliary atresia include appropriate mobilization (**A**) and transection (**B**) of the fibrous biliary tract remnant. **C:** Creation of a Roux-Y jejunal conduit with biliary enteric anastomosis completes the procedure.

An open liver biopsy is routinely performed to document the state of parenchymal injury. The cholangiogram is generally attempted through the gallbladder. In the 10% to 15% instance of a patent distal biliary tree, treatment still requires portoenterostomy. A nonpatent, fibrous cord rather than a normal common bile duct is found in the hepatoduodenal ligament. This cord is dissected free proximally to the level of the porta hepatis between the portal vein bifurcation. The fibrous remnant is sharply transected at this level to preserve any patent bile ducts. A short, 15- to 25-cm retrocolic, jejunal Roux-Y limb is constructed. There has been no clear advantage with longer or modified conduits with intussusception-type antireflux valves in the prevention of cholangitis.[64]

Historically, some surgeons preferred to exteriorize the biliary conduit, but this practice has been abandoned due to complications and high likelihood of future liver transplantation.

Results and Complications. Following portoenterostomy, bile flow occurs in about 66% to 75% of all infants when operated on at less than 60 days of age; however, establishment of bile flow may take weeks to months. The probability of bile flow appears to be related to age at the time of operation.

Cholangitis is a constant concern and an important postoperative problem after portoenterostomy. The clinical signs include fever, leukocytosis, and decreased bile flow in the absence of other systemic illness. All patients are at risk for the development of postoperative cholangitis, but reported postoperative rates of cholangitis are 40% to 50%. Cholangitis following portoenterostomy is characterized by a systemic inflammatory response and may be associated with progressive liver injury. Treatment is generally intravenous fluid resuscitation and broad-spectrum antibiotics. Occasionally, steroids or other anti-inflammatory agents may be helpful, whereas reoperation or endoscopic revision of the portoenterostomy usually is not. In an effort to determine the optimal treatment of infants with biliary atresia, a group of investigators has formed the Biliary Atresia Research Consortium (BARC).[65] The primary objectives of the consortium are to establish a clinical database and tissue repository. A retrospective BARC study of 104 children with biliary atresia treated in the United States demonstrated that at 2 years of age, 58 patients were alive with their native liver and 42 had undergone liver transplantation.[66] Data from the United Kingdom demonstrated improved measurable outcomes in children with biliary atresia treated with Kasai portoenterostomy by regionalization of care to three centers in the UK health care system.[67]

Nearly all patients with biliary atresia have residual liver injury. Hepatic synthetic failure, portal hypertension with esophageal variceal bleeding, hypersplenism, and fat-soluble vitamin deficiencies can be problematic. Most institutions report 5-year survival rates between 30% and 50% for portoenterostomy alone. About 25% to 35% of patients undergoing a portoenterostomy survive more than 10 years without liver transplantation. The remaining two-thirds of children with biliary atresia ultimately require liver transplantation for survival. Although the failure rate for portoenterostomy is high, the possibility of long-term success is notable. In addition, the limited availability of infant donor organs and the technical limitations of liver transplantation in infants younger than 1 year make portoenterostomy an accepted initial treatment of biliary atresia in most centers.

Hepatic Transplantation

Hepatic transplantation is discussed in detail elsewhere in this text. For biliary atresia, transplantation offers a means of long-term survival in children with failed portoenterostomies. The current 5-year survival of children with biliary atresia who undergo liver transplantation ranges from 75% to 94.4%.[68] In addition, with the use of reduced-size cadaveric donor livers as well as living-related donor livers, the mortality rate for infants on transplant waiting lists may be decreasing. Indications for liver transplantation in biliary atresia include progressive hepatic failure despite portoenterostomy, growth retardation, and complications of portal hypertension. It is important to consider the consequences of lifelong immunosuppression in these children, including the risks of infection and treatment-related malignancy.

Congenital Choledochal Cystic Disease of the Biliary Tract

Anatomy

The anatomic description and classification scheme for choledochal cystic disease initially proposed by Alonso-Lej et al. in 1959[69] and modified by Todani et al.[70] are illustrated in **Figure 98.46.** The most frequently encountered are type I cysts, accounting for approximately 85% to 90% of the lesions in most series. Type I cysts are characterized by fusiform dilatation of the entire common bile duct with only mild dilatation of the common hepatic duct; the intrahepatic ducts are normal. Variations are common, and biliary atresia is occasionally seen in association with choledochal cystic disease.

Type I cysts are generally quite large and often cause displacement of neighboring viscera. The fusiform dilatation usually begins at the origin of the common bile duct, generally sparing the common hepatic ducts. The distal common bile duct is diminutive and typically is distorted mechanically by the large cyst, leading to the common clinical presentation of obstructive jaundice. The junction of the distal common bile duct and the pancreatic duct is not within the normal intramural duodenum but rather is extrinsic and proximal to the duodenal wall and the sphincter of Oddi (**Fig. 98.47**). It remains unknown whether the configuration of a long, extramural common channel allows greater pancreatic secretion reflux into the common bile duct.

Microscopic examination of the choledochal cyst wall reveals that the normal biliary epithelium is absent or replaced by abnormal and occasionally dysplastic columnar epithelium. The cyst wall has normal smooth muscle with variable degrees of inflammation and fibrosis. The exception to this common histologic characteristic is the type III cyst, which is generally lined by normal duodenal mucosa. Choledochal cysts tend to have less inflammation in infancy and early childhood. In contrast, there is well-established inflammation involving the cyst and surrounding structures in the hepatoduodenal ligament in adolescents and adults.

Pathophysiology

The mechanism for the development of cystic lesions of the biliary tract is unclear. Choledochal cysts have been identified accurately by prenatal ultrasound, and it appears likely that these lesions represent abnormalities in the developing biliary tract. Several hypotheses for the development of choledochal cysts have been proposed. Whether the cystic dilatations result from abnormal recanalization of the primitive bile duct cords or from inflammation caused by reflux of pancreatic secretions into the common bile duct remains unknown. The pathophysiology of choledochal cyst is that of obstructive jaundice. The obstruction may be primarily the result of mechanical outflow obstruction of a diminutive distal common bile duct with a dilated choledochal cyst. Alternatively, a large inflammatory cyst can cause obstruction of the biliary tract and of neighboring viscera by extrinsic compression. When discovered during infancy, obstructive jaundice is usually the initial clinical finding. The liver injury is typically reversible, and progression to biliary cirrhosis is rare. The exception to this situation is type V disease, which is associated with a high incidence of hepatic fibrosis.

Other initial clinical situations include cholelithiasis and acute bacterial cholangitis secondary to diminished bile drainage. Children with type III cysts may have acute pancreatitis.

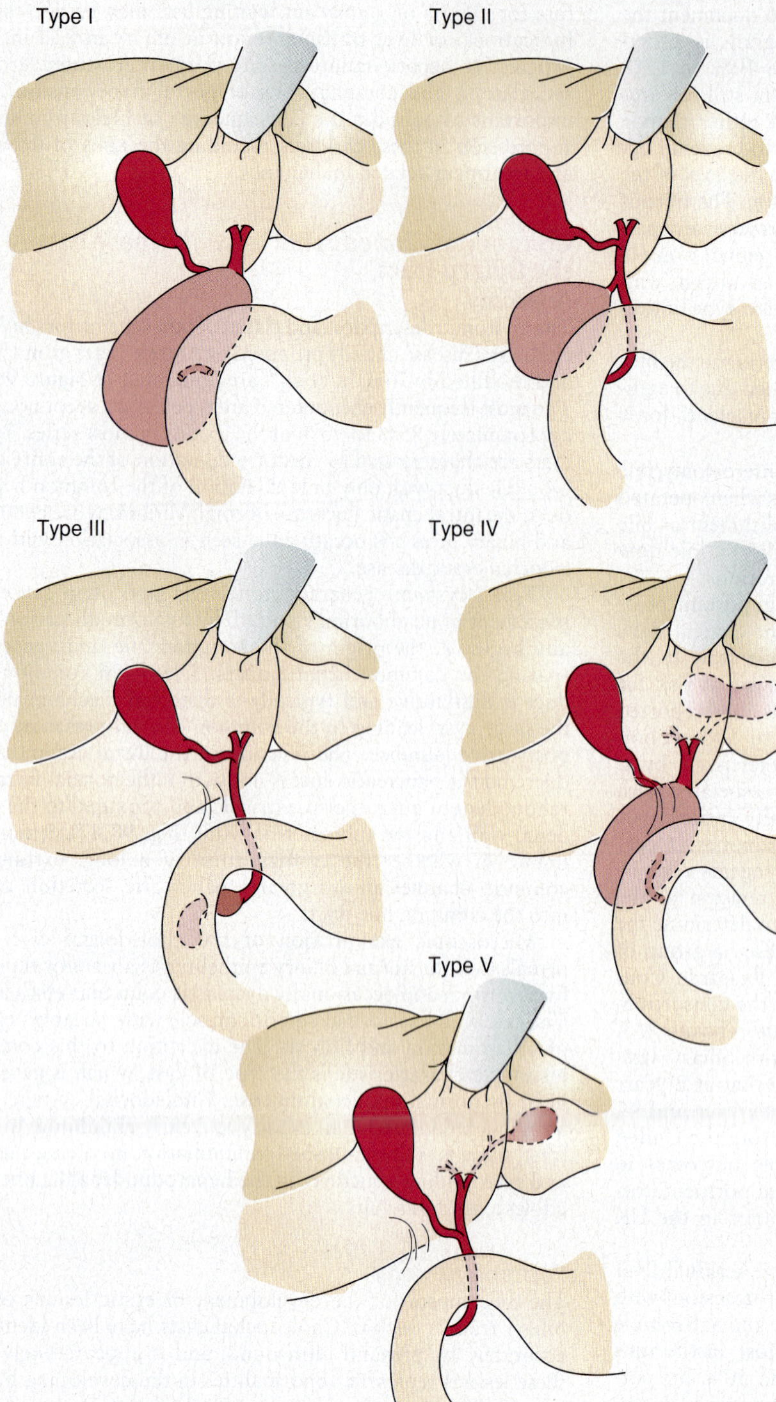

Figure 98.46. Classification of choledochal cyst.

Infrequently, extrinsic compression of the portal vein by a large choledochal cyst may produce symptoms and signs of portal hypertension. Abdominal pain and tenderness following minor injury may lead to an incidental diagnosis of choledochal cyst on imaging studies.

Carcinoma of the biliary tract occurs in about 3% to 5% of patients with choledochal cyst. The number of reported cases remains small in the literature, but the incidence of biliary tract neoplasm is about 1000 times that of the normal population. Patients with choledochal cysts are at increased risk for the development of biliary tract carcinoma in adolescence or early adulthood. The dysplastic cyst epithelium may be susceptible to malignant change from chronic inflammation. Interestingly, there appears to be an increased risk of malignancy developing anywhere in the biliary tract, gallbladder, or pancreas, and not just the choledochal cyst itself. Therefore, current treatment emphasizes complete cyst excision or the cyst epithelium while providing adequate biliary drainage to prevent stasis and chronic inflammation. Infants and children treated for choledochal cyst should have long-term follow-up for complications and potential malignancy.

Clinical Presentation and Diagnosis

Choledochal cysts present most commonly in infancy and early childhood with symptoms of obstructive jaundice. In older children and adults, the classic clinical triad of episodic

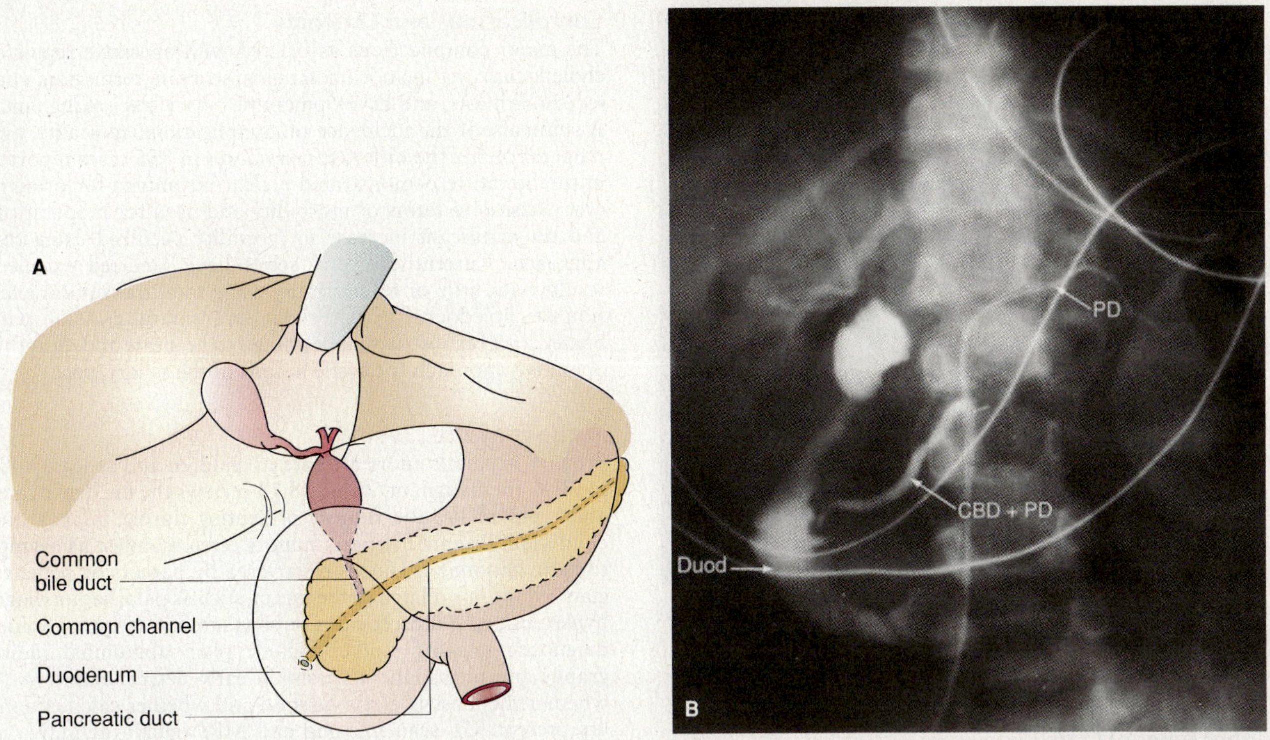

Figure 98.47. An anomalous, extramural junction between the distal common bile duct and the pancreatic duct is characteristic of type I choledochal cyst. **A:** Schematic depiction of this anatomy. **B:** Operative cholangiogram from a patient with a long extramural common channel. It has been suggested that the long common channel may allow reflux of pancreatic secretions into the common bile duct resulting in inflammation and proteinase-mediated injury to the common duct, possibly contributing to the development of the cyst itself. CBD + PD, common bile duct and pancreatic duct; Duod, duodenum; PD, pancreatic duct.

abdominal pain, a palpable right upper-quadrant mass, and jaundice occurs in fewer than 50% of patients. Adults occasionally present with hepatomegaly or evidence of portal hypertension. The diagnosis in infants and most children can be confirmed by ultrasound examination and ^{99m}Tc-IDA imaging studies (**Figs. 98.48** and **98.49**). In older children, both MRI cholangiography and endoscopic retrograde cholangiopancreatography (ERCP) are highly sensitive and specific in confirming diagnosis. These lesions are also diagnosed incidentally during radiologic imaging studies for other reasons. Partial duodenal obstruction may lead to an upper gastrointestinal series that shows extrinsic compression from a large type I cyst or an intraluminal filling defect from a type III cyst. CT imaging of the abdomen following blunt trauma may lead to the diagnosis of biliary tract dilatation. Liver biopsy is not specific for choledochal cyst and has little diagnostic role other than to document the extent of liver injury.

Treatment

Type I Cysts

Initial operative strategy for a type I choledochal cyst is exploration and cholangiography, usually through the gallbladder, but occasionally contrast injection must be made directly into the common bile duct. Cholecystectomy is routinely performed. Internal drainage procedures without cyst excision have been abandoned. Current consensus for the surgical management of type I choledochal cyst is performance of primary cyst excision with Roux-Y hepaticojejunostomy reconstruction (**Fig. 98.50**). Primary cyst excision is accomplished routinely in infants and children. For adults with severe inflammation and fibrosis, dissection may present problems resulting from inflammation and adhesion of the cyst wall to the hepatoduodenal ligament. A safer approach in this situation may be intramural cyst dissection and removal of the cyst wall epithelium, leaving the posteromedial outer cyst wall adjacent to the portal vein and hepatic artery intact.

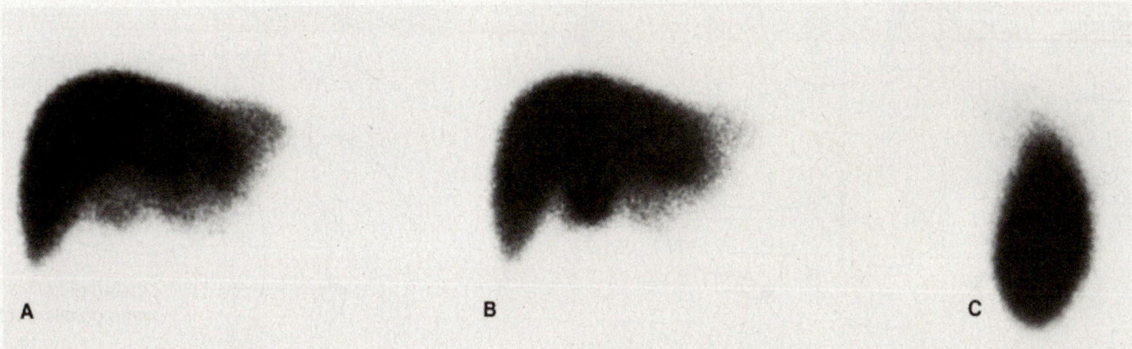

Figure 98.48. Typical ^{99m}Tc-*N*-substituted-2,6-dimethylphenyl carbamoylmethyl iminodiacetic acid (HIDA) scan from a child with a type I choledochal cyst. Images were made in 5 minutes (**A**), 30 minutes (**B**), and 3 hours (**C**) after isotope injection. The isotope is retained within the choledochal cyst for more than 24 hours, and the pattern of hepatocyte uptake is normal.

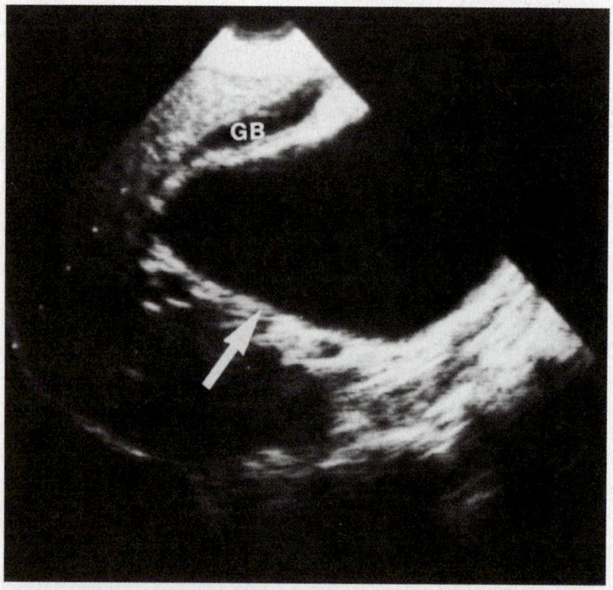

Figure 98.49. Ultrasound image of a type I choledochal cyst (*arrow*; longitudinal image). The gallbladder (GB) is also shown.

Other Types of Cysts

Type II cysts are excised completely and the choledochotomy is closed primarily. Type III choledochoceles require a transduodenal approach with either marsupialization or excision of the cyst. Care must be taken to identify the ampulla, and a formal sphincteroplasty may be required to ensure adequate drainage from the biliary tract and the pancreas. Type IV and V intrahepatic cystic diseases must be approached on an individualized basis. In general, unilobar or focal cystic disease can be either resected or drained with Roux-Y jejunostomy reconstruction. Bilobar intraparenchymal disease, particularly in the setting of hepatic fibrosis, may be difficult, if not impossible, to obtain complete, adequate drainage.

Complications and Outcome

The major complications associated with operative repair of choledochal cyst include cholangitis, stricture formation, choledocholithiasis, and development of biliary tract malignancy. A summary of the incidence of complications, mortality, and reoperation for the different procedures in 955 cases reported in the literature demonstrated a clear advantage for primary cyst excision in terms of morbidity and need for reoperation, and no significant increase in mortality occurred using this approach. Currently, several series have reported excellent results with little or no mortality using total transmural excision of choledochal cysts. Primary transmural excision with biliary tract reconstruction continues to be a safe and desirable operative approach for cystic lesions of the biliary tract.

Tumors of the Liver

Primary hepatic tumors are rare in children and at least 60% to 70% are malignant. **Table 98.13** reviews the incidence rates and types of hepatic tumors presenting during infancy and childhood. Pediatric hepatic tumors often manifest as asymptomatic abdominal masses discovered by parents or pediatrician. Symptoms related to the tumor, such as pain, hemorrhage, hypertension, and precocious puberty, are less frequent. Initial diagnostic imaging studies include plain abdominal radiographs and ultrasound to assist in early determination as to whether the mass is cystic or solid and whether calcifications are present. CT scan imaging and MRI remain definitive in the ability to discern anatomic characteristics of the mass and its relationship to adjacent structures. Most children require operative exploration for either definitive excision or incisional biopsy in lesions deemed unresectable.

Benign Tumors

Of all primary liver tumors of childhood, 30% are benign. The most common benign tumors are hemangiomas, hemangioendotheliomas, mesenchymal hamartomas, cysts, focal nodular hyperplasia, and hepatic adenoma. In most large series, hemangiomas constitute about 50% of the benign hepatic tumors observed.

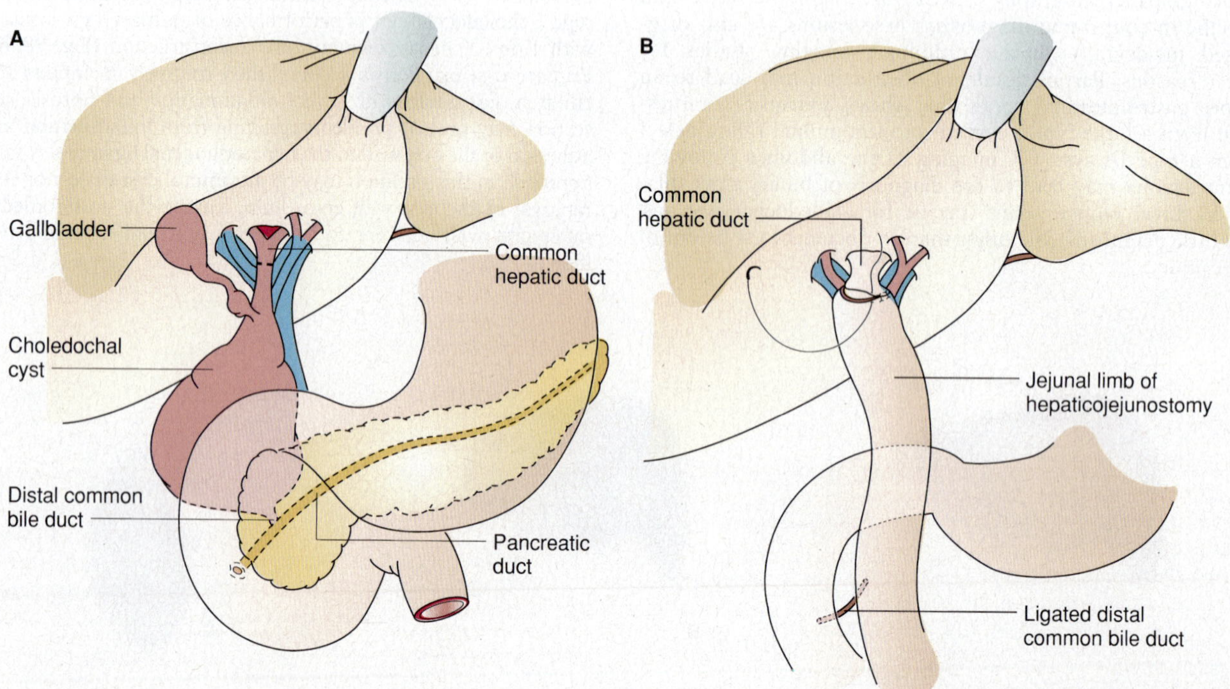

Figure 98.50. The preferred operative treatment of type I choledochal cyst consists of primary total transmural cyst excision with Roux-Y hepaticojejunostomy.

Table 98.13. Incidence of Liver Tumors in Childhood

Tumor Type	Incidence Rate (%)
Benign	
Vascular tumors	13
Hemangioma	9
Hemangioendothelioma	4
Mesenchymal hamartoma	6
Focal nodular hyperplasia	2
Adenoma	2
Teratoma	2
Other	3
Malignant	
Hepatoblastoma	43
Hepatocellular carcinoma	23
Malignant mesenchymal tumor	4
Sarcoma	2
Embryonal cell carcinoma	2
Angiosarcoma	1

Vascular Tumors

Infantile hepatic hemangiomas represent a clinically diverse spectrum of vascular endothelial anomalies. They are characterized by a phase of proliferative growth over the first year of life, with subsequent involution over several years. The International Society for the Study of Vascular Anomalies classifies vascular tumors into two categories based upon the presence or absence of GLUT-1, an erythrocyte-type glucose transporter protein expressed in the endothelium of the placenta and hemangiomas.[71] Therefore, hemangiomas are GLUT-1 positive, and other, more heterogeneous vascular anomalies such as vascular malformations are GLUT-1 negative. Most asymptomatic infantile hepatic hemangiomas are detected as incidental findings on diagnostic imaging studies performed for unrelated reasons. A smaller proportion will create symptoms of enlarging abdominal mass, progressive hepatic failure, high output cardiac failure due to shunting, thrombocytopenia, or hypothyroidism from excess production of type III iodothyronine deiodinase.[72]

Most benign vascular lesions of the pediatric liver do not require operative management. Operative intervention is generally reserved for bleeding secondary to traumatic rupture symptoms not controllable with medical management. Treatment strategies remain highly individualized based upon whether the lesions are focal, multifocal, or diffuse.[73,74] In the face of multifocal or diffuse disease associated with congestive heart failure and thrombocytopenia secondary to sequestration, medical treatment with corticosteroid therapy may be useful. More invasive procedures such as irradiation, selective hepatic arterial ligation, angiographic embolization, or hepatic transplantation remain useful in selected patients with uncontrollable symptoms. Chemotherapeutic agents, including recombinant alpha-interferon, low-dose vincristine, and cyclophosphamide, have been used for life-threatening vascular lesions. Hepatic resection is generally reserved for mass lesions of unknown diagnosis, ruptured vascular lesions with signs of active hemorrhage, or for symptomatic, locally resectable lesions.

Hemangioendotheliomas are important vascular anomalies encountered in infants. The lesions vary in size from 1 cm to several centimeters in diameter and may be multiple (**Fig. 98.51**). Symptomatic neonates may present with an abdominal mass, hepatomegaly, and congestive heart failure. These infants may also experience spontaneous rupture and hemoperitoneum, with tachycardia, tachypnea, and hypovolemic shock. On examination, the infant may have other cutaneous hemangiomas visible on the skin. Affected infants may develop thrombocytopenia secondary to platelet sequestration in the vascular malformation (*Kasabach–Merritt syndrome*). CT scan imaging or MRI is diagnostic. Treatment is directed at controlling symptoms using medical management principles as discussed previously; however, hemangioendotheliomas tend to be more problematic than hemangiomas because of the tendency to occur during infancy and the more extensive, symptomatic nature of the lesions.

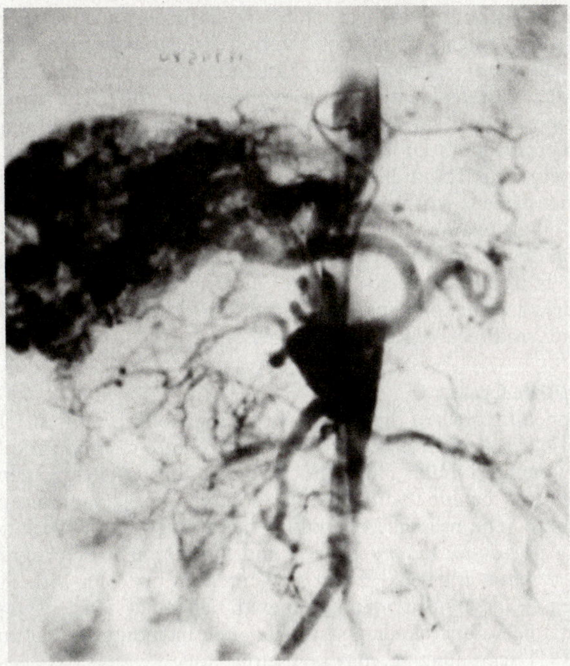

Figure 98.51. Selective visceral angiogram demonstrating large hepatic vascular malformation in a neonate with congestive heart failure. This finding is consistent with a bilobar hemangioendothelioma.

Mesenchymal Hamartomas

Approximately one-third of benign hepatic tumors in children are mesenchymal hamartomas. A mesenchymal hamartoma is often quite large and typically presents within the first year of life as an asymptomatic, solitary abdominal mass. CT scan imaging or MRI studies are usually diagnostic and show a solid mass that may have cystic components within the liver parenchyma. Definitive diagnosis may require open tissue biopsy, and the therapy of choice is complete excision, although spontaneous involution has been described. Simple enucleation may be adequate because these tumors tend to be well circumscribed. On occasion, formal hepatic resection may be required.[75] Recurrence is low after adequate resection.

Focal Nodular Hyperplasia

This tumor occurs primarily in female children and in adults and may be associated with the use of oral contraceptives or focal hepatic injury. Focal nodular hyperplasia is usually a well-defined, solitary mass that has characteristic findings on CT scan imaging. Open or percutaneous biopsy may be required to differentiate the lesion from hepatic adenoma. This lesion results from a focal inflammatory response of normal hepatic parenchyma surrounded by areas of micronodular fibrosis and cirrhosis. Operative management is generally unnecessary unless there is a question of diagnosis or active hemorrhage from the lesion.

Hepatic Adenoma

Adenomas are rare in infants and children and constitute less than 5% of all benign hepatic lesions in the pediatric age group. There is an association between the use of oral contraceptives, exogenous anabolic steroid use, and glycogen storage disease type I (von Gierke disease). These tend to be large, solitary lesions located in the right hepatic lobe. The typical presentation is an asymptomatic abdominal mass, although symptoms are seen more commonly than with focal nodular hyperplasia. About 20% to 25% of patients with hepatic adenoma present with hemoperitoneum from tumor rupture. On histologic examination, these lesions are composed of normal hepatocytes without evidence of dysplasia. Operative therapy is usually directed at either making definitive diagnosis or treating hemorrhage. Enucleation or local resection is adequate, and recurrence rates are low.

Hepatic Cysts

Congenital cysts of the liver may be either solitary or multiple. These cysts are thought to result from failure of the intralobular or interlobular biliary ducts to fuse during development. They may be lined with cuboidal, columnar, or squamous epithelium. The presence of multiple hepatic cysts is associated with polycystic kidney disease, and development of progressive hepatic and renal failure is a potential problem with this disease. The majority of children with hepatic cysts are asymptomatic. Adjunctive diagnostic imaging, including ultrasound and CT scan imaging, may be useful.

Asymptomatic congenital hepatic cysts do not require surgical therapy. Operative therapy is reserved for symptomatic cysts. Resection or drainage by marsupialization or hepaticocystenterostomy may be required. If patency to the biliary tract is present on contrast injection study of the cyst, internal drainage is necessary.

The differential diagnosis includes hydatid disease of the liver, which is suggested by calcification and loculation of the cyst wall. Hydatid disease can be diagnosed using specific serologic tests, which is an important surgical consideration prior to exploration. Patients with echinococcal cysts should be treated with mebendazole and undergo cyst injection with hypertonic saline or other scolicidal agents into the parent cyst before surgical excision. Careful control of the cyst contents is required during echinococcal cyst excision or marsupialization.

Teratomas

Teratomas of the liver are exceedingly rare and have potential for harboring immature elements capable of transforming into malignancy. Surgical resection on discovery is recommended.

Malignant Tumors

Two-thirds of childhood hepatic tumors are malignant, with hepatoblastoma constituting half of the malignancies, followed by hepatocellular carcinoma, malignant mesenchymal tumors, and sarcoma. Malignant hepatic tumors are fortunately rare, and effective treatment requires a multidisciplinary approach that is best achieved in an experienced pediatric center.

Hepatoblastoma

Most hepatoblastomas are discovered in children younger than 2 years. There is a 2:1 male-to-female predominance. Hepatoblastomas are usually found as either an asymptomatic abdominal mass or symptoms of gastrointestinal obstruction from extrinsic compression by the mass. There is an association of hepatoblastoma in patients with Beckwith–Wiedemann syndrome and hemihypertrophy. On examination, a firm, palpable upper abdominal mass is notable. Obstructive jaundice is unusual. More than 90% of children with hepatoblastoma have elevated levels of alpha-fetoprotein, which is a useful serum tumor marker for postoperative surveillance. In a few instances, children have initial symptoms and signs of excess androgen secretion, including virilization and precocious puberty. Diagnostic imaging with CT scan imaging or MRI is essential to evaluate the extent of the tumor and evaluate for metastatic disease (**Fig. 98.52**).

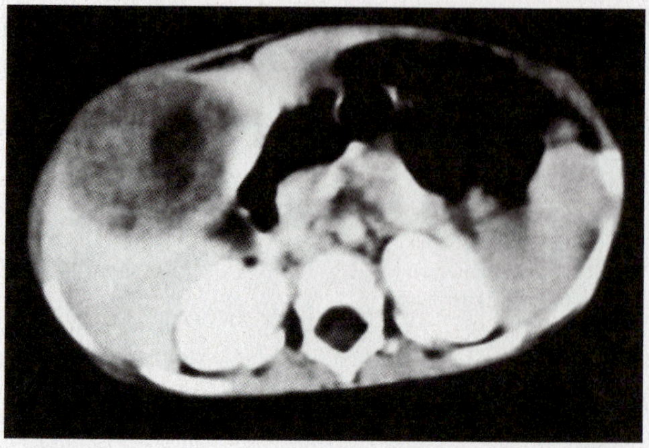

Figure 98.52. Computed tomographic scan of the abdomen demonstrating an infant with hepatoblastoma of the right hepatic lobe.

Children with hepatoblastoma require multidisciplinary management at centers familiar with their management protocols. Resectability is based on the pretreatment extent of tumor (PRETEXT) and POSTTEXT, and their approach should be standardized.[76] Most children presenting with hepatoblastoma initially have unresectable disease. However, PRETEXT 1 tumors should be amenable to primary resection, whereas PRETEXT 4 tumors should be considered for liver transplant. In the absence of metastatic disease, however, an aggressive surgical approach is used. Cure and long-term survival with hepatoblastoma require complete surgical excision of the primary lesion. Therefore, localized, resectable tumors are usually excised by formal hepatic lobectomy or extended trisegmentectomy. Children with hepatoblastomas considered initially unresectable or with metastatic disease should undergo percutaneous or incisional biopsy to confirm the histologic diagnosis, followed by multiagent chemotherapy to reduce the size of the primary tumor and control metastases.[77,78] Delayed resection is appropriate if enough functional, normal hepatic parenchyma remains after resection. More than half of the patients who initially have unresectable hepatoblastoma can be rendered disease free with the combination of chemotherapy and subsequent surgery. Cure rates for hepatoblastoma range from 60% to 80% if histologically clear margins and no metastatic disease are present. All patients with hepatoblastoma, who are not stage 1 pure fetal histology, receive chemotherapy after resection. As treatment of this disease is complex and dependent on several clinical and anatomic factors, current treatment recommendations should be referenced.[76]

Hepatocellular Carcinoma

Hepatocellular carcinoma is significantly more common in adults but is occasionally seen in older children and adolescents. There is a male predilection (2:1) and, except for the age at diagnosis, the clinical presentation is similar to that for hepatoblastoma. Children with hepatocellular carcinoma are more likely to have jaundice and abnormal liver enzymes. The high association of cirrhosis in adults (80%) is not seen in children with hepatocellular carcinoma; only 5% of children develop hepatocellular carcinoma in the background of cirrhosis. An increased risk of hepatocellular carcinoma is seen in children with Beckwith–Wiedemann syndrome, hemihypertrophy, von Gierke disease, hepatitis B, and Fanconi syndrome. Exposure to oral contraceptives, anabolic steroids, and some chemotherapeutic agents has also been associated with hepatocellular carcinoma. This malignancy carries a poor prognosis with an overall survival rate of 10% to 20% despite aggressive surgical resection and multiagent chemotherapy. A histologic variant, fibrolamellar hepatocellular carcinoma, carries a more favorable prognosis. As with hepatoblastoma, complete surgical resection with clear histologic margins is necessary

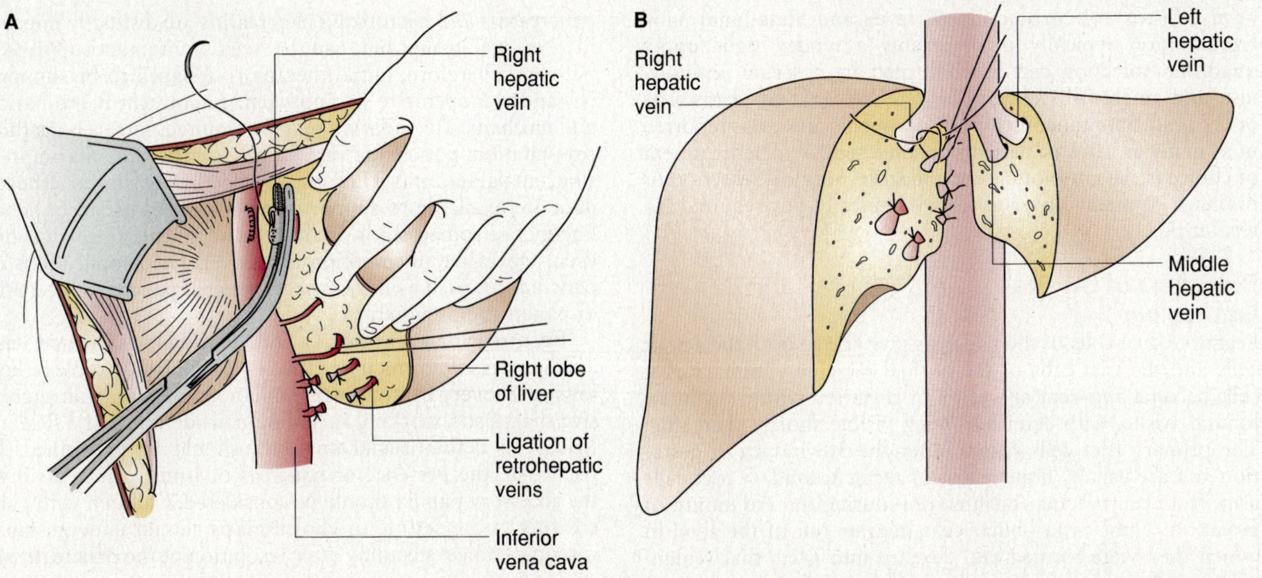

Figure 98.53. **A:** The hepatic veins in infants and children may be extremely short, making extrahepatic control impossible or dangerous. **B:** Intrahepatic control of the hepatic veins via an anterior approach may be safer in infants and children.

for long-term survival and cure. In the absence of metastatic disease, unresectable hepatoblastoma or hepatocellular carcinoma in children has been successfully treated by orthotopic liver transplantation. Review of data from the United Network for Organ Sharing database demonstrates good long-term survival for both hepatoblastoma (66% 10-year survival) and hepatocellular carcinoma (58% 10-year survival) treated with liver transplantation.[79]

Malignant Mesenchymal Tumors

These rare hepatic malignancies occur in children 5 to 10 years of age; initial signs are fever, pain, and an abdominal mass, which is usually quite large on diagnosis and may have both solid and cystic components. Multidisciplinary treatment, including complete surgical resection, multiagent chemotherapy, and radiation therapy, is required for cure. In general, the prognosis of primary malignant mesenchymal tumors of the liver remains poor.

Sarcomas

Children may rarely have a primary sarcoma of the liver. Embryonal rhabdomyosarcoma of the biliary tract is distinctly unusual. It may manifest with obstructive jaundice attributable to both extrinsic and intrinsic biliary tract obstruction. Undifferentiated, embryonal sarcoma of the liver has also been described. Angiosarcoma developing in the liver may be associated with exposure to toxins such as arsenic. Aggressive surgical resection may be required, but long-term survival is uncommon. Despite radical surgery, chemotherapy, and radiation therapy, the prognosis and long-term survival of children with these malignancies remain poor, and data regarding effective drug regimens are limited.[80]

Liver Resection

Operative principles and techniques for hepatic resection are discussed elsewhere in this book. Several unique issues in the safe performance of hepatic resection in children should be emphasized. The circulating blood volume of an infant or a child is less compared to an adult, and children are sensitive to compression of the inferior vena cava, causing decreased venous return to the right heart. Blood must be available for transfusion and adequate intravenous access is essential. Resection can be performed through either a subcostal incision or a right thoracoabdominal incision; in general, the ability to perform the operation safely should not be limited by the size of the incision. In children, the right and left hepatic veins are difficult to control near the inferior vena cava because of their short lengths, and intraparenchymal control from an anterior approach may be safer (**Fig. 98.53**).

Hepatic Infections

Hepatic infections are generally rare in the pediatric population, and their management is similar to that used in adults. An important issue is the development of hepatic abscess in an immunocompromised child and, in particular, the association of chronic granulomatous disease with pyogenic hepatic abscess formation.

Pyogenic Abscess

The most common causative factor in the development of pyogenic hepatic abscess in children with chronic granulomatous disease and other causes of immunosuppression. Chronic granulomatous disease is an inherited disorder characterized by a defect in oxidative burst-mediated bacterial killing by neutrophils. These children develop skin, soft tissue, and solid organ abscesses. A significant number of children with pyogenic liver abscesses have chronic granulomatous disease or other inherited/acquired immunodeficiency states. Liver abscesses are infrequently seen as a complication of umbilical vein catheterization, omphalitis, biliary tract disease, and hepatobiliary operations.

Patients with pyogenic liver abscess present with fever, jaundice, and leukocytosis. Hepatosplenomegaly and a tender liver may be found on physical examination. Common responsible organisms include staphylococcal species, streptococcal species, and *E. coli.* Gram-negative organisms and anaerobic bacteria are becoming increasingly prevalent. Treatment involves the use of broad-spectrum antibiotics. Large abscess cavities may require image-guided percutaneous drainage to expedite resolution of sepsis. Rarely, hepatic abscesses require open operative drainage. The outcome is dependent upon the underlying disease process. Recovery from the abscess is predictably good following adequate antibiotic therapy and drainage when necessary.

Amebic Abscess

Amebic abscess of the liver is uncommon in the United States, but it is endemic to areas of Central and South America. It is caused by infection with the parasite *Entamoeba histolytica.* Children with amebic dysentery develop hepatic infection as the parasite travels through the portal circulation. Patients have a history of chronic illness, fever, and abdominal pain. Examination typically demonstrates a tender right upper quadrant. Infection can be confirmed by a serum antibody test, and amebic abscess can be demonstrated by ultrasound or CT scan. Spontaneous rupture of amebic abscess is reported in as many as 10% of patients in some series.[81] The treatment of choice is the antibiotic metronidazole. Surgical resection or drainage of amebic liver abscess is typically not required for resolution.

Disorders of the Pancreas

Embryology

Primitive duct cells of the pancreas give rise to both the acinar cells and the islet cells of the normal pancreas. Primary islet cells become apparent at week 8 of gestation within the interlobular tissue, with acini becoming visible shortly thereafter. The primary islet cells regress after the 5th month of gestation and are usually nonexistent by term. Secondary islet cells arise from centroacinar proliferation during the 3rd month of gestation. These intralobular cells migrate out of the acini in which they were formed and develop into islets that remain connected to the duct by a thin cellular stalk (the tubule of Bensley).

Exocrine pancreatic anomalies generally arise from defective development during embryogenesis. The most common of these conditions is annular pancreas. The circumferential distribution of pancreatic tissue around the duodenum is thought to result from interrupted migration of the ventral pancreatic anlage. Less common defects include pancreatic ductal abnormalities, pancreatic duplications, heterotopic pancreatic tissue, and congenital agenesis of portions of the pancreas.

Acute Pancreatitis

Acute pancreatitis is the most common disorder of the pancreas in both infants and children. Adult pancreatitis is often caused by either alcohol ingestion or gallstones. In contrast, 50% to 80% of cases in children, particularly adolescents, are posttraumatic or idiopathic in origin. An important clinical condition seen with moderate frequency is acute pancreatitis in the setting of immunosuppression, in particular, high-dose corticosteroids. Steroid-induced acute pancreatitis typically accounts for the third most common cause of pancreatitis in most children's hospitals. Other causes of acute pancreatitis include gallstones, CF, hyperlipidemia, juvenile diabetes mellitus, mumps, coxsackievirus infection, infectious mononucleosis, collagen vascular diseases, and anatomic lesions such as choledochal cyst. Medications significantly associated with acute pancreatitis include oral contraceptives, chlorothiazide, tetracyclines, azathioprine, and L-asparaginase. Valproic acid, an anticonvulsant useful in some children with seizure disorders, is associated with a particularly virulent form of acute necrotizing pancreatitis that may be life threatening.

A child with acute pancreatitis presents with a history of midepigastric abdominal pain, anorexia, and emesis. On examination, the child usually has a tender abdomen with distention. Fever and leukocytosis are common. Serum amylase and lipase levels are elevated, although significant pancreatitis can occur despite a normal amylase level. Conversely, the lipase may be mildly elevated in the absence of clinical symptoms or signs of acute pancreatitis. Ultrasonography and CT imaging of the abdomen are probably the most commonly used adjunctive diagnostic tests. CT imaging is particularly useful in demonstrating edema of the gland as well as evaluating for peripancreatic fluid collections. While usually deferred during the acute phase of pancreatitis, ERCP or MRI cholangiography may be useful to evaluate the hepatobiliary tract anatomy once the inflammatory process has resolved.

Treatment principles for childhood acute pancreatitis are not different from strategies used in adults. The vast majority of children have simple edematous pancreatitis. Hemorrhagic pancreatitis and necrotizing pancreatitis are distinctly unusual in this age group but can be seen in immunosuppressed patients. Therefore, initial therapy is designed to be supportive and nonoperative in approach. Endotracheal intubation and mechanical ventilation may be required. Intravenous fluid resuscitation, pancreatic rest by nasogastric tube decompression, analgesia, and TPN are provided. No clinical efficacy data are available to support the widespread use of anticholinergics or somatostatin analogs for acute pancreatitis in children. Operative intervention is reserved for complications of pancreatitis, such as hemorrhage, infected pancreatic necrosis, or pancreatic pseudocyst.

Recurrent pancreatitis in a child is usually associated with an anatomic abnormality or specific physiologic problem. Following recovery from the acute inflammatory event, an aggressive diagnostic workup, including consideration of ERCP or MRCP to define ductal anatomy, should be performed. In particular, the presence of pancreas divisum with stenosis of the accessory papilla should be considered. Children with pancreatitis in the setting of cholelithiasis should undergo laparoscopic cholecystectomy after resolution of the pancreatitis.

Pancreas Divisum

Pancreas divisum occurs with failure of normal fusion between the dorsal and ventral pancreatic ducts. About 10% to 15% of normal persons have two separate pancreatic ducts, and up to 10% of asymptomatic persons undergoing ERCP have two complete ductal systems. The anatomic variant of pancreas divisum is not necessarily pathologic, but if the orifice of the accessory papilla is stenotic or obstructed, pancreatitis can occur. Approximately 25% of affected individuals are thought to be at risk for developing pancreatitis. Because pancreas divisum is characterized by a dominant dorsal duct system dependent on secretion through the accessory papilla, stenosis of the accessory (lesser) papilla is probably necessary to produce pancreatic symptoms. Most of the experience with surgical treatment of pancreas divisum is reported in adults. Successful surgical management of children presenting with recurrent pancreatitis secondary to accessory papilla stenosis with pancreas divisum has also been reported.

To diagnose pancreas divisum, ERCP is required. Endoscopic visualization of the major and accessory papillae is essential. Radiographic findings with pancreas divisum demonstrate a short or absent duct of Wirsung that does not communicate with the duct of Santorini (see **Fig. 98.54**). Definitive diagnosis of pancreas divisum is made by demonstrating two separate, parallel ductal systems.

Few pediatric patients with pancreatitis and pancreas divisum requiring operation have been reported. Most of these children were female patients who had a history of recurrent pancreatitis. The primary operative goal is to provide adequate drainage of the duct of Santorini by performing a sphincterotomy of the accessory duct. An open dorsal duct sphincterotomy appears to be more durable than endoscopic sphincterotomy. Some surgeons advocate sphincterotomy of the main papilla as well, but dorsal duct sphincterotomy alone appears effective in preventing acute pancreatitis associated with pancreas divisum. The reported surgical outcome in the limited number of children treated for pancreatitis associated with pancreas divisum is favorable.

Cystic Lesions of the Pancreas

Pancreatic pseudocysts are uncommon in the pediatric age group and are usually the result of blunt traumatic abdominal injury or acute pancreatitis. Children typically present with abdominal pain, nausea, emesis, and weight loss. There may be a palpable midepigastric mass on examination. Diagnosis is usually made with ultrasound or CT imaging of the abdomen. The serum amylase and lipase are usually elevated.

In children, many small asymptomatic pseudocysts regress spontaneously with resolution of the pancreatic inflammation.

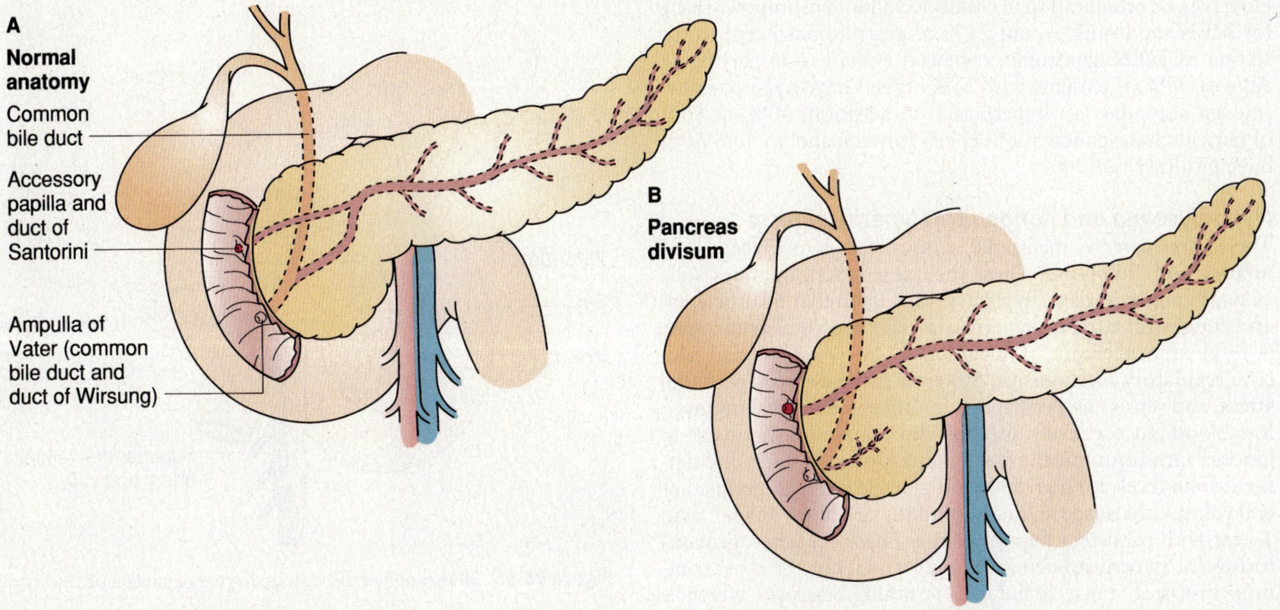

Figure 98.54. **A:** Normal pancreatic ductal anatomy. **B:** Pancreas divisum. There is no communication between the duct of Wirsung and the duct of Santorini. The duct of Wirsung is short or absent. Most of the pancreas is drained by the duct of Santorini through the accessory papilla. This anatomy is found in about 10% to 15% of normal individuals.

Larger or symptomatic pseudocysts may require drainage. Symptoms and potential complications of untreated pseudocysts include hemorrhage, infection, perforation, gastrointestinal or biliary tract obstruction, or, rarely, development of pancreaticoenteric fistula. The decision to use either external or internal drainage procedures for a pseudocyst depends on the status of the pancreatic duct. In many centers, definitive external drainage of a large or symptomatic pseudocyst is performed with acceptable morbidity and mortality rates by an ultrasound- or CT-guided percutaneous approach. Pseudocyst recurrence or persistent external drainage without resolution suggests significant pancreatic duct injury or complete ductal transection. Determination of whether a major pancreatic ductal injury is associated with a pseudocyst may be made by either percutaneous contrast injection of the pseudocyst or ERCP. Pseudocysts associated with pancreatic duct injury may not resolve with percutaneous external drainage or endoscopic pancreatic duct stenting, so internal drainage procedures such as cystgastrostomy or cystojejunostomy with or without distal pancreatectomy may be required.

Epithelial cysts of the pancreas are rare in children. Congenital cysts are lined by epithelium and acinar tissue and are seen most commonly in the body and tail of the pancreas. They may be associated with other syndromes such as von Hippel–Lindau disease, which is characterized by hereditary cerebellar cysts, retinal hemangioma, and pancreatic cysts. Congenital pancreatic cysts are typically asymptomatic unless they are large enough to cause compression or obstruction of the stomach or colon. In the absence of trauma, spontaneous rupture of a pancreatic epithelial cyst is rare. Treatment is cyst excision or internal drainage into the stomach or the jejunum.

Other rare cystic lesions of the pancreas in children include retention cysts. These cysts result from chronic ductal obstruction. They are characteristically lined by epithelium unless inflammatory obliteration has occurred. Enteric duplication cysts of the stomach or the duodenum can also be associated intimately with the pancreas and communicate with the pancreatic duct. Treatment of both retention cysts and enteric duplication cysts either within or associated with the pancreas includes excision, occasionally internal drainage, and, if necessary, distal pancreatectomy. Not all pancreatic cysts in children can be uniformly considered benign. Suspicious lesions should be investigated thoroughly, and biopsy performed. Cystadenoma, cystadenocarcinoma, and rhabdomyosarcoma associated with a pancreatic cyst have been reported. These neoplasms are treated by anatomic pancreatic resection following histologic confirmation on biopsy.

Pancreatic Neoplasms

Childhood malignant neoplasms of the pancreas are uncommon. Typically, pancreatic malignancy in childhood is found on discovery of an asymptomatic abdominal mass. Infrequently, the lesion may be found incidentally or during a diagnostic imaging workup for abdominal trauma. Jaundice may occur with a lesion in the pancreatic head causing common bile duct obstruction. The most frequently encountered lesions include islet cell carcinoma and adenocarcinoma. The treatment of choice for localized malignant neoplasms of the pancreas is surgical resection. Pancreaticoduodenectomy in children can successfully control some malignancies of the pancreatic head. To promote adequate nutrient absorption and growth, children undergoing pancreaticoduodenectomy should be considered for oral pancreatic enzyme replacement and fat-soluble vitamin supplementation.

Two pancreatic neoplasms seen in childhood and adolescence deserve further discussion. The *papillary cystic neoplasm* of the pancreas occurs predominantly in younger female children, is typically slow growing with low malignant potential, and is highly curable with surgical resection. This tumor is thought to be a neoplasm of the ductuloacinar primordial cells of the pancreas. The other lesion is the *pancreatoblastoma,* also referred to as *juvenile adenocarcinoma of the pancreas.* Pancreatoblastoma is somewhat more common in boys than in girls and typically has slow growth with low malignant potential as well. Histologic examination demonstrates undifferentiated ductular and acinar areas with nodules of squamous epithelium, suggesting that these tumors arise from primordial pancreatic cells. Both papillary cystic neoplasm and pancreatoblastoma have more favorable prognoses than adenocarcinoma following surgical resection.

Endocrine Lesions of the Pancreas

Zollinger–Ellison Syndrome

Zollinger–Ellison syndrome is characterized by gastric hypersecretion and is discussed in detail elsewhere in this book.

However, its presentation in childhood should prompt work-up for MEN syndrome. About 25% of gastrinomas occur in the setting of MEN syndrome, reviewed elsewhere in this book. At least 90% of patients with MEN type I have hyperparathyroidism secondary to hyperplasia. In addition, 30% to 80% of patients have pancreatic islet cell tumors, and 15% to 50% have pituitary tumors.

Hypoglycemia and Congenital Hyperinsulinism

There are diverse metabolic causes for hypoglycemia in infancy and childhood. These include endocrinopathies such as panhypopituitarism, hypothyroidism, adrenal insufficiency, and congenital adrenal hyperplasia (adrenogenital syndrome). Several inborn errors of metabolism interrupt normal glucose regulatory mechanisms. Systemic disease states, perinatal stress, and sepsis can predispose an otherwise normal infant to low blood glucose levels. Infants who remain unresponsive to glucose infusion typically have inappropriately high circulating insulin levels for a given blood glucose level. Hyperinsulinemia should be suspected in any infant or child younger than 1 year with persistent hypoglycemia. There are heterogeneous causes for hyperinsulinemic hypoglycemia, but the most common historical cause in infancy is nesidioblastosis, which is characterized by uncontrolled development of the pancreatic endocrine tissue that functions abnormally during infancy. Clinically, these cells secrete inappropriately high amounts of insulin, causing clinical hypoglycemia in infants. Two distinct histologic lesions appear to be responsible for congenital hyperinsulinism. Mutations in the beta-cell K_{ATP} channel genes may lead to either focal, adenomatous hyperinsulinism or diffuse hyperinsulinism; both genotypes lead to phenotypic hypoglycemia if left untreated.

Infants with congenital hyperinsulinism usually become symptomatic from hypoglycemia within the first few hours or days of life. These infants commonly present with neurologic symptoms such as lethargy or generalized seizures and have corresponding fasting blood glucose levels below 40 mg/dL. The diagnosis of hyperinsulinemia is supported by the clinical features of Whipple triad which includes (a) neurologic changes with fasting or activity, (b) fasting blood glucose levels below 40 to 50 mg/dL, and (c) neurologic symptoms reversed by the administration of glucose. The diagnosis is made by demonstrating inappropriately high levels of circulating insulin for a given level of blood glucose. An insulin (IU/mL) to glucose (mg/dL) ratio that is greater than 0.5 in a fasting patient is consistent with hyperinsulinemic hypoglycemia. In infants and children, an absolute insulin level greater than 5 IU/mL in the presence of a blood glucose level less than 40 mg/dL is diagnostic. Ketone body production is impaired in infants with congenital hyperinsulinism.

The initial management of a hypoglycemic infant with congenital hyperinsulinism is to provide adequate glucose concentrations to prevent permanent neurologic injury. Dextrose-containing intravenous solutions are titrated to maintain blood glucose levels greater than 40 mg/dL and may require a central venous catheter. The short-term administration of somatostatin analogs to increase blood glucose levels in hyperinsulinemic states has been demonstrated to be useful. Other pharmacologic agents used to reduce insulin levels and raise blood glucose concentration include diazoxide (15 mg/kg daily). The use of streptozocin to control hyperinsulinemia is most often reserved for adults with metastatic islet cell carcinoma and is not widely used in infants because of the potential side effects.

Following initial control of blood glucose and clinical confirmation of hyperinsulinemia, operative intervention should be considered a means of providing definitive control of hypoglycemia. Diagnostic imaging using CT scan imaging, MRI, or, more recently, ^{18}F-FDOPA PET scanning may be useful either to identify or to exclude a focal lesion.[82] Localization of focal lesions is important in that this approach may lead to effective glucose control with selective partial pancreatectomy and allow for preservation of normal pancreatic tissue and function.[83,84]

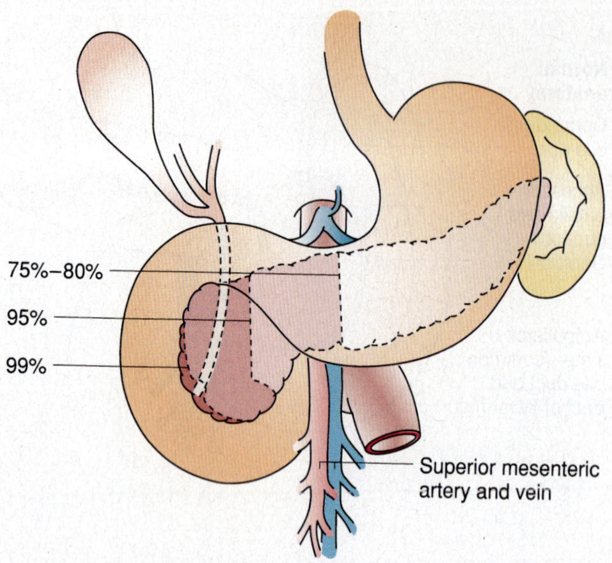

Figure 98.55. Illustration of the various degrees of pancreatic resection.

Operatively, the abdomen is explored thoroughly, and the entire pancreas must be visualized. Preoperative localization data guided by intraoperative ultrasound and frozen section analysis may identify focal lesions amenable to partial resection. In the absence of a focal lesion, the infant is presumed to have diffuse islet cell hyperplasia. In this setting, the general operative strategy is total or near-total pancreatectomy. Lesser procedures, such as subtotal (80%) pancreatectomy, do not effectively treat diffuse congenital hyperinsulinism and recurrent hypoglycemia placing the infant at risk for hypoglycemic encephalopathy. Near-total pancreatectomy involves resection of the distal 95% of the gland with preservation of the spleen. The entire distal pancreas, including the uncinate process, is resected, leaving a small rim of pancreatic tissue adjacent to the duodenum (**Fig. 98.55**). Total pancreatectomy is usually reserved for persistent or recurrent hypoglycemia following lesser procedures. Near-total pancreatectomy controls hypoglycemia in 90% of infants with diffuse congenital hyperinsulinism. The remaining infants with persistent hypoglycemia may require further pancreatic resection. With extensive pancreatic resection, the typical postoperative course is a transient period of hyperglycemia with subsequent stabilization of blood glucose levels. Pancreatic exocrine function is ablated, and oral replacement therapy is required. Despite clinical remission following resection, however, diabetes mellitus may occur as a long-term consequence in children treated either medically or surgically for diffuse congenital hyperinsulinism. Therefore, these infants need long-term metabolic follow-up for both pancreatic endocrine and exocrine function.

References

1. Parker SE, Mai CT, Canfield MA, et al. Updated national birth prevalence estimates for selected birth defects in the United States, 2004–2006. *Birth Defects Res A Clin Mol Teratol.* 2010;88(12):1008–1016.
2. Williams LJ, Kucik JE, Alverson CJ, Olney RS, Correa A. Epidemiology of gastroschisis in metropolitan Atlanta, 1968 through 2000. *Birth Defects Res A.* 2005;73:177–183.
3. Abdel-Latif ME, Bolisetty S, Abeywardana S, Lui K; Australian and New Zealand Neonatal Network. Mode of delivery and neonatal survival of infants with gastroschisis in Australia and New Zealand. *J Pediatr Surg.* 2008;43(9):1685–1690.

4. Puligandla PS, Janvier A, Flageole H, Bouchard S, Laberge JM. Routine cesarean delivery does not improve the outcome of infants with gastroschisis. *J Pediatr Surg.* 2004;39(5):742–745.
5. Hadidi A, Subotic U, Goeppl M, Waag KL. Early elective cesarean delivery before 36 weeks vs late spontaneous delivery in infants with gastroschisis. *J Pediatr Surg.* 2008;43:1342–1346.
6. Legghe HL, Masotn GC, Thonton JG, Stringer MD. A randomized controlled trial of elective preterm delivery of fetuses with gastroschisis. *J Pediatr Surg.* 2005;40:1726–1731.
7. Ergün O, Barksdale E, Ergün FS, et al. The timing of delivery of infants with gastroschisis influences outcome. *J Pediatr Surg.* 2005;40(2):424–428.
8. Kidd JN Jr, Jackson RJ, Smith SD, Wagner CW. Evolution of staged versus primary closure of gastroschisis. *Ann Surg.* 2003;237:759–765.
9. Lobo JD, Kim AC, Davis RP, et al. No free ride? The hidden costs of delayed operative management using a spring-loaded silo for gastroschisis. *J Pediatr Surg.* 2010;45(7):1426–1432.
10. Sandler A, Lawrence J, Meehan J, Phearman L, Soper R. A "plastic" sutureless abdominal wall closure in gastroschisis. *J Pediatr Surg.* 2004;39(5):738–741.
11. Machida M, Takamizawa S, Yoshizawa K. Umbilical cord inverting technique: a simple method to utilize the umbilical cord as a biologic dressing for sutureless gastroschisis closure. *Pediatr Surg Int.* 2011;27(1):95–97.
12. Riboh J, Abrajano CT, Garber K, et al. Outcomes of sutureless gastroschisis closure. *J Pediatr Surg.* 2009;44(10):1947–1951.
13. Orion KC, Krein M, Liao J, Shaaban AF, Pitcher GJ, Shilyansky J. Outcomes of plastic closure in gastroschisis. *Surgery.* 2011;150(2): 177–185.
14. Davies MW, Kimble RM, Cartwright DW. Gastroschisis: ward reduction compared with tradition reduction under general anesthesia. *J Pediatr Surg.* 2005;40(3):523–527.
15. Witt RG, Zobel M, Padilla B, Lee H, MacKenzie TC, Vu L. Evaluation of clinical outcomes of sutureless vs sutured closure techniques in gastroschisis repair. *JAMA Surg.* 2019;154(1):33–39.
16. Martin AE, Khan A, Kim DS, Muratore CS, Luks FI. The use of intraabdominal tissue expanders as a primary strategy for closure of giant omphaloceles. *J Pediatr Surg.* 2009;44(1):178–182.
17. De Ugarte DA, Asch MJ, Hedrick MH, et al. The use of tissue expanders in the closure of a giant omphalocele. *J Pediatr Surg.* 2004;30(4):613–615.
18. Lee SL, Beyer TD, Kim SS, et al. Initial nonoperative management and delayed closure for treatment of giant omphaloceles. *J Pediatr Surg.* 2006;41(11):1846–1849.
19. Whitehouse JS, Gourlay DM, Masonbrink AR, et al. Conservative management of giant omphalocele with topical povidone-iodine and its effect on thyroid function. *J Pediatr Surg.* 2010;45(6): 1192–1197.
20. Pandey V, Gangopadhyay AN, Gupta DK, Sharma SP, Kumar V. Non-operative management of giant omphalocele with topical povidone-iodine and powdered antibiotic combination: early experience from a tertiary centre. *Pediatr Surg Int.* 2014;30(4):407–411.
21. Curry JJ, Lander AD, Stringer MD; BAPS Multicentre Research Committee. A multicenter, randomized, double-blind, placebo-controlled trial of the prokinetic agent erythromycin in the postoperative recovery of infants with gastroschisis. *J Pediatr Surg.* 2004;39:565–569.
22. Phillips JD, Raval MV, Redden C, Weiner TM. Gastroschisis, atresia, dysmotility: surgical treatment strategies for a distinct clinical entity. *J Pediatr Surg.* 2008;43:2208–2212.
23. van Eijck FC, Wijnen RM, van Goor H. The incidence and morbidity of adhesions after treatment of neonates with gastroschisis and omphalocele: a 30-year review. *J Pediatr Surg.* 2008;43:479–483.
24. Zaccara A, Iacobelli BD, Calzolari A, et al. Cardiopulmonary performances in young children and adolescents born with large abdominal wall defects. *J Pediatr Surg.* 2003;38:478–481.
25. Snyder CL. Current management of umbilical abnormalities and related anomalies. *Semin Pediatr Surg.* 2007;16:41–49.
26. Chan KL, Chan HY, Tam PK. Towards a near-zero recurrence rate in laparoscopic inguinal hernia repair for pediatric patients of all ages. *J Pediatr Surg.* 2007;42:1993–1997.
27. Owings EF, Georgeson KE. A new technique for laparoscopic exploration to find contralateral patent processus vaginalis. *Surg Endosc.* 2000;14:114–116.
28. Ron O, Eaton S, Pierro A. Systematic review of the risk of developing a metachronous contralateral inguinal hernia in children. *Brit J Surg.* 2007;94:804–811.
29. Saur D, Vanderwinden J, Seidler B, Schmid RM, De Laet MH, Allescher HD. Single-nucleotide promoter polymorphism alters transcription of neuronal nitric oxide synthase exon 1 c in infantile hypertrophic pyloric stenosis. *Proc Natl Acad Sci.* 2004;101: 1662–1667.
30. Hall NJ, Van Der Zee J, Tan HL, Pierro A. Meta-analysis of laparoscopic versus open pyloromyotomy. *Ann Surg.* 2004;240:774–778.
31. St Peter SD, Holcomb GW, Calkins CM, et al. Open versus laparoscopic pyloromyotomy for pyloric stenosis. *Ann Surg.* 2006;244: 363–370.
32. Langer JC, To T. Does pediatric surgical specialty training affect outcome after Ramstedt pyloromyotomy? A population-based study. *Pediatrics.* 2004;113:1342–1347.
33. Valusek PA, Spilde TL, Tsao K, St Peter SD, Holcomb GW III, Ostlie DJ. Laparoscopic duodenal atresia repair using surgical U-clips: a novel technique. *Surg Endosc.* 2007;21:1023–1024.
34. Sato TT. Abnormal rotation and fixation of the intestine. In: Wyllie R, Hyams JS, eds. *Pediatric Gastrointestinal and Liver Disease.* Elsevier; 2006.
35. Piper HG, Alesbury J, Waterford SD, Zurakowski D, Jaksic T. Intestinal atresias: factors affecting clinical outcomes. *J Pediatr Surg.* 2008;43:1244–1248.
36. Mak GZ, Harberg FJ, Hiatt P, Deaton A, Calhoon R, Brandt ML. T-tube ileostomy for meconium ileus: four decades of experience. *J Pediatr Surg.* 2000;35:349–352.
37. Nadler EP, Dickinson E, Knisely A, et al. Expression of inducible nitric oxide synthase and interleukin-12 in experimental necrotizing enterocolitis. *J Surg Res.* 2000;92(1):71–77.
38. Grishin A, Bowling J, Bell B, Wang J, Ford HR. Roles of nitric oxide and intestinal microbiota in the pathogenesis of necrotizing enterocolitis. *J Pediatr Surg.* 2016;51(1):13–17.
39. Lim JC, Golden JM, Ford HR. Pathogenesis of neonatal necrotizing enterocolitis. *Pediatr Surg Int.* 2015;31(6):509–518.
40. Lin PW, Nasr TR, Stoll BJ. Necrotizing enterocolitis: recent scientific advances in pathophysiology and prevention. *Semin Perinatol.* 2008;32:70–82.
41. Lin HC, Hsu CH, Chen HL, et al. Oral probiotics prevent necrotizing enterocolitis in very low birth weight preterm infants: a multicenter, randomized, controlled trial. *Pediatr.* 2008;122:693–700.
42. Sato TT, Oldham KT. Abdominal drain placement versus laparotomy for necrotizing enterocolitis with perforation. *Clin Perinatol.* 2004;31:577–589.
43. Moss RL, Dimmitt RA, Barnhart DC, et al. Laparotomy versus peritoneal drainage for necrotizing enterocolitis and perforation. *N Engl J Med.* 2006;354:2225–2234.
44. Blakely ML, Tyson JE, Lally KP, et al.; NICHD Neonatal Research Network. Laparotomy versus peritoneal drainage for necrotizing enterocolitis or isolated intestinal perforation in extremely low birth weight infants: outcomes through 18 months adjusted age. *Pediatrics.* 2006;117(4):e680–687.
45. Moss RL, Dimmitt RA, Henry MC, Geraghty N, Efron B. A meta-analysis of peritoneal drainage versus laparotomy for perforated necrotizing enterocolitis. *J Pediatr Surg.* 2001;36: 1210–1213.
46. Centers for Disease Control and Prevention (CDC). Postmarketing monitoring of intussusception after RotaTeq vaccination—United States, February 1, 2006–February 15, 2007. *MMWR Morb Mortal Wkly Rep.* 2007;56:218–222.
47. Cheung ST, Lee KH, Yeung TH, et al. Minimally invasive approach in the management of childhood intussusception. *ANZ J Surg.* 2007;77:778–781.
48. Bonnard A, Demarche M, Dimitriu C, et al. Indications for laparoscopy in the management of intussusception: a multicenter retrospective study conducted by the French study group for pediatric laparoscopy. *J Pediatr Surg.* 2008;43:1249–1253.

49. Montalva L, Cheng LS, Kapur R, et al. Hirschsprung disease. *Nat Rev Dis Primers*. 2023;9(1):54.
50. Meier-Ruge WA, Ammann K, Bruder E, et al. Updated results on intestinal neuronal dysplasia (IND B). *Eur J Pediatr Surg*. 2004;14: 384–391.
51. Lewit RA, Kuruvilla KP, Fu M, Gosain A. Current understanding of Hirschsprung-associated enterocolitis: pathogenesis, diagnosis and treatment. *Semin Pediatr Surg*. 2022;31(2):151162.
52. Saleh W, Rasheed K, Al Mohaidly M, Kfoury H, Tariq M, Rawaf AA. Management of Hirschsprung's disease: a comparison of Soave's and Duhamel's pull-through methods. *Pediatr Surg Int*. 2004;20: 590–593.
53. Kawaguchi AL, Guner YS, Sømme S, et al. Management and outcomes for long-segment Hirschsprung disease: a systematic review from the APSA Outcomes and Evidence Based Practice Committee. *J Pediatr Surg*. 2021;56(9):1513–1523.
54. Georgeson KE, Inge TH, Albanese CT. Laparoscopically assisted anorectal pull-through for high imperforate anus—a new technique. *J Pediatr Surg*. 2000;35:927–930.
55. Wood RJ, Levitt MA. Anorectal malformations. *Clin Colon Rectal Surg*. 2018;31(2):61–70.
56. Minneci PC, Kabre RS, Mak GZ, et al.; Midwest pediatric surgery consortium. Can fecal continence be predicted in patients born with anorectal malformations? *J Pediatr Surg*. 2019;54(6):1159–1163.
57. Rintala RJ, Pakarinen MP. Imperforate anus: long- and short-term outcome. *Semin Pediatr Surg*. 2008;17:79–89.
58. Zganjer M, Cizmic A, Cigit I, et al. Treatment of rectal prolapse in children with cow milk injection sclerotherapy: 30-year experience. *W J Gastroenterol*. 2008;14:737–740.
59. Stuth EA, Stucke AG, Cohen RD, Jaquiss RD, Kugathasan S, Litwin SB. Successful resuscitation of a child after exsanguination due to aortoesophageal fistula from undiagnosed foreign body. *Anesthesiology*. 2001;95:1025–1026.
60. Zurowska A, Feneberg R, Warady BA, et al. Gram-negative peritonitis in children undergoing long-term peritoneal dialysis. *Am J Kidney Dis*. 2008;51:455–462.
61. Kobayashi H, Stringer MD. Biliary atresia. *Semin Perinatol*. 2003;8: 383–391.
62. Visser BC, Suh I, Hirose S, et al. The influence of portoenterostomy on transplantation for biliary atresia. *Liver Transpl*. 2004;10: 1279–1286.
63. Davenport M, Puricelli V, Farrant P, et al. The outcome of the older (>100 days) infant with biliary atresia. *J Pediatr Surg*. 2004;4: 575–581.
64. Ogasawara Y, Yamataka A, Tsukamoto K, et al. The intussusception antireflux valve is ineffective for preventing cholangitis in biliary atresia: a prospective study. *J Pediatr Surg*. 2003;38:1826–1829.
65. Dolgin SE. Answered and unanswered controversies in the surgical management of extra hepatic biliary atresia. *Pediatr Transplant*. 2004;8:628–631.
66. Shneider BL, Brown MB, Haber B, et al. A multicenter study of the outcome of biliary atresia in the United States, 1997–2000. *J Pediatr*. 2006;148:467–474.
67. Stringer MD. Biliary atresia: service delivery and outcomes. *Semin Pediatr Surg*. 2008;17:116–122.
68. Cowles RA, Lobritto SJ, Ventura KA, et al. Timing of liver transplantation in biliary atresia—results in 71 children managed by a multidisciplinary team. *J Pediatr Surg*. 2008;43:1605–1609.
69. Alonso-Lej F, Rever WB Jr, Pessagno DJ. Congenital choledochal cyst, with a report of 2, and an analysis of 94, cases. *Int Abstr Surg*. 1959;108(1):1–30.
70. Todani T, Watanabe Y, Narusue M, Tabuchi K, Okajima K. Congenital bile duct cysts: Classification, operative procedures, and review of thirty-seven cases including cancer arising from choledochal cyst. *Am J Surg*. 1977;134(2):263–269.
71. Hernandez F, Navarro M, Encinas JL, et al. The role of GLUT1 immunostaining in the diagnosis and classification of liver vascular tumors in children. *J Pediatr Surg*. 2005;40:801–804.
72. Huang SA, Tu HM, Harney JW, et al. Severe hypothyroidism caused by type 3 iodothyronine deiodinase in infantile hemangioma. *N Engl J Med*. 2000;343:185–187.
73. Christison-Lagay ER, Burrows PE, Alomari A, et al. Hepatic hemangiomas: subtype classification and development of a clinical practice algorithm and registry. *J Pediatr Surg*. 2007;42:62–68.
74. PDQ Pediatric Treatment Editorial Board. Childhood Vascular Tumors Treatment (PDQ®): Health Professional Version. August 15, 2019. In: *PDQ Cancer Information Summaries*. National Cancer Institute (US); 2002. https://www.ncbi.nlm.nih.gov/books/NBK343452/
75. Isaacs H Jr. Fetal and neonatal hepatic tumors. *J Pediatr Surg*. 2007; 42:1797–1803.
76. Lim IIP, Bondoc AJ, Geller JI, Tiao GM. Hepatoblastoma—The evolution of biology, surgery, and transplantation. *Children (Basel)*. 2018;6(1):1.
77. Tiao GM, Bobey N, Allen S, et al. The current management of hepatoblastoma: a combination of chemotherapy, conventional resection, and liver transplantation. *J Pediatr*. 2005;146:204–211.
78. Pham TH, Iqbal CW, Grams JM, et al. Outcomes of primary liver cancer in children: an appraisal of experience. *J Pediatr Surg*. 2007;42:834–839.
79. Austin MT, Leys CM, Feurer ID, et al. Liver transplantation for childhood hepatic malignancy: a review of the United Network for Organ Sharing (UNOS) database. *J Pediatr Surg*. 2006;41: 182–186.
80. Finegold MJ, Egler RA, Goss JA, et al. Liver tumors: pediatric population. *Liver Transpl*. 2008;14:1545–1556.
81. Wells CD, Arguedas M. Amebic liver abscess. *S Med J*. 2004;97: 673–682.
82. Adzick NS, Thornton PS, Stanley CA, Kaye RD, Ruchelli E. A multidisciplinary approach to the focal form of congenital hyperinsulinism leads to successful treatment by partial pancreatectomy. *J Pediatr Surg*. 2004;39:270–275.
83. Becherer A, Szabo M, Karanikas G, et al. Imaging of advanced neuroendocrine tumors with 18 F-FDOPA PET. *J Nucl Med*. 2003; 45:1161–1167.
84. Viola KV, Sosa JA. Current advances in the diagnosis and treatment of pancreatic endocrine tumors. *Curr Opin Oncol*. 2005;17:24–27.

Pediatric Genitourinary System

Jonathan C. Routh and Ashley W. Johnston

Key Points

1. Embryonic kidneys develop from the intermediate mesoderm, with the definitive kidney forming as a result of inductive interaction between ureteric bud and metanephric mesenchyme. Paramesonephric (müllerian) and mesonephric (wolffian) ducts contribute reproductive structures.
2. Multicystic dysplastic kidney (MCDK) is the most common form of congenital cystic disease. It typically involutes over time and rarely requires intervention.
3. Prenatal hydronephrosis is one of the most common anomalies detected on prenatal ultrasound; the majority resolve spontaneously over time. The severity of hydronephrosis correlates with the likelihood of necessary intervention.
4. Ureteral duplication is a common anomaly. Upper pole ureter can be associated with either obstructing ureterocele or ectopic ureter, whereas lower pole ureter is more likely to be associated with vesicoureteral reflux (VUR).
5. VUR is an important problem to identify and manage in children who present with urinary tract infection (UTI). VUR can lead to recurrent renal parenchymal infections, resulting in renal scarring and other lifelong problems such as hypertension and kidney disease.
6. Patients with neurogenic bladder disorders (most commonly secondary to spina bifida) must be evaluated with urodynamic pressure–volume study to characterize its urine storage and emptying function. Managing bladder pressure and emptying with clean intermittent catheterization (CIC) is paramount to preserve renal health and improve quality of life.
7. Posterior urethral valve (PUV) is the most common congenital obstructive uropathy that leads to end-stage renal failure and renal replacement therapy. These patients are at risk for developing bladder dysfunction and need lifelong follow-up with urology.
8. Hypospadias is common, occurring in 1 of 200 live births. Most cases are mild, presenting with urethral opening near the distal shaft and glans. When associated with cryptorchidism, the differential diagnostic possibilities must include disorders of sex development.
9. Undescended testes occur in 3% to 4% of full-term newborn males and are diagnosed by physical examination. Ultrasound is not a part of the standard workup for an undescended testicle. Ninety percent of testes descend by 6 months of age, and the remainder typically descend by 9 months. The American Academy of Pediatrics (AAP) and AUA recommend orchiopexy between 6 and 18 months of age.
10. Mature teratoma, which is classically benign, is the most common benign testicular tumor in prepubertal children. Yolk sac tumors are the most common malignant testicular tumors in prepubertal boys; these are associated with elevated alpha-fetoprotein (AFP). Testicular-sparing enucleation is appropriate treatment for mature teratoma.

1 FETAL DEVELOPMENT OF GENITOURINARY SYSTEM

The kidneys develop as paired intermediate mesodermal structures stretching craniocaudally along the length of the abdomen. The final step of embryonic renal development is the *metanephros*, which develops as a result of inductive interaction between the ureteric buds (which sprout from the distal portion of the mesonephric ducts) and the metanephric mesenchyme. The nephron, which consists of the glomerulus, proximal tubule, loop of Henle, and distal tubule, derives from the metanephric mesenchyme, while the collecting system, made up of collecting ducts, calyces, pelvis, and ureter, is formed from the ureteric bud. The kidneys ascend and rotate from their initial pelvic position to their final position in the upper retroperitoneum.

The bladder and genitalia develop as the terminal portion of the endoderm-lined yolk sac dilates to become the cloaca and is then partitioned by the developing urorectal septum to form the urogenital sinus anteriorly (future vesicourethral canal and vaginal vestibule) and anorectal canal posteriorly. During the 5th week of development, primordial germ cells migrate from the yolk sac to the posterior body wall near the mesonephros to form the genital ridges. In males, under the influence of SRY (the sex-determining region of the Y chromosome), primordial germ cells begin to differentiate into Sertoli cells, which then drive the formation of testis cords and Leydig cells (responsible for producing androgen). In females, the paramesonephric ducts (ie, müllerian ducts) develop into the uterus and fallopian tubes. In males, the mesonephric ducts (ie, wolffian ducts) develop into vas deferens and epididymis under the influence of androgen. The presence of müllerian-inhibiting substance (MIS) produced by Sertoli cells in a developing testicle causes müllerian ducts to regress in male; likewise in females, the mesonephric (wolffian) ducts regress. Starting in the 6th week, under the influence of dihydrotestosterone (converted intracellularly from testosterone by the enzyme 5-alpha reductase), the genital tubercle elongates and the genital and urethral folds fuse in the midline to form the scrotum, penis, and penile urethra. Specifically, the urethra tubularizes via canalization of the urethral plate to form a wide, diamond-shaped urethral groove whose edges fuse in the midline, known as the zipper theory.[1] Both developing testicles and ovaries move to the pelvic location by the third month. In males, the testicles undergo inguino–scrotal descent during the third trimester.

ANOMALIES OF THE KIDNEY

Renal anomalies can be categorized into several recognized variants in position, number, and shape.[2] When the kidney does not move to the normal expected position, it is termed an *ectopic kidney*. The possibility of an ectopic kidney must be entertained if a kidney is missing in the usual location during an exploratory laparoscopy or laparotomy. Most commonly, the kidney fails to ascend and remains near the bladder, becomes a *pelvic kidney*, thought to occur in 1 in 3,000 live births. Rarely, the kidney can ascend above the diaphragm to become an *intrathoracic kidney* or can cross to the contralateral side of the body as a *crossed ectopic kidney*. Unlike the more commonly encountered ureteral duplication, a crossed ectopic kidney's ureter crosses the midline and enters the bladder in its orthotopic (ipsilateral) location; thus, the trigone appears normal on cystoscopy. Thirty percent to 50% of ectopic kidneys can have varying degrees of hydronephrosis and/or vesicoureteral reflux (VUR); however, most ectopic kidneys are asymptomatic and clinically insignificant. Importantly, the adrenal glands develop independently from the kidney and should be in the normal orthotopic position even if the ipsilateral kidney is ectopic.

Similarly, the most common (0.2% of live births) renal fusion anomaly is the *horseshoe kidney*, so named because the lower poles of the kidneys are linked by a fibrous band or an isthmus of functional parenchyma. Horseshoe kidneys are notable for their low position in the abdomen, with the isthmus below the inferior mesenteric artery and the kidney moieties well below their usual position. Horseshoe kidneys are associated with an increased risk of obstruction and urolithiasis.[3]

In addition to anomalies of position and fusion, there can be an extra or *supernumerary kidney*. This very rare finding is usually discovered incidentally and is rarely clinically significant. By contrast, failure of the ureteric bud to form or join the metanephric mesenchyme will result in *renal agenesis*. Bilateral renal agenesis is very rare and carries an extremely poor prognosis. Unilateral renal agenesis is more common and, in females, may be associated with other müllerian duct anomalies—such as Mayer–Rokitansky–Kuster–Hauser (MRKH) or obstructed hemi-vagina with ipsilateral renal agenesis (OHVIRA) syndromes—in 25% to 50% of females with unilateral renal agenesis. Likewise, up to one-third of females with müllerian duct anomalies will have unilateral renal agenesis. True agenesis is relatively rare and should not be confused with a regressed dysplastic kidney, which is often the fate of a *multicystic dysplastic kidney (MCDK)*.

2 Cystic Conditions of the Kidney

Renal cystic conditions are among the most common causes of pediatric abdominal masses, especially in infants.[4] It is important to accurately diagnose these due to their different prognoses and other associated conditions (**Table 99.1**).

MCDK is the most common form of nonheritable renal cystic condition which is comprised of multiple noncommunicating cysts of varying sizes and is without identifiable renal parenchyma.[5] The classic ultrasound findings are absence of central lucency (ie, no dilated, central renal pelvis); variably sized, noncommunicating cysts; and absence of renal parenchyma. As a rule, MCDK are nonfunctional, and nuclear scintigraphy shows no activity. However, a segmental MCDK can occur in the setting of a ureteral duplication. Most MCDK will involute over time. For patients with a very large MCDK, they may not complete involution and a small residual clump of cysts may persist into adulthood. In these patients, there is a high incidence (15% to 25%) of contralateral VUR which is of unclear clinical significance. Several long-term registries have shown that patients with MCDK do well; surgery is rarely necessary.

Table 99.1. Classification of Congenital Renal Cystic Diseases

Inheritable
Autosomal recessive (infantile) polycystic kidney disease (ARPCKD)
Autosomal dominant (adult) polycystic kidney disease (ADPCKD)
Juvenile nephronophthisis Medullary cystic disease Congenital nephrosis (familial nephrotic syndrome) Familial hypoplastic glomerulocystic disease Renal cystic syndromes (tuberous sclerosis, von Hippel–Lindau disease)
Noninheritable
Multicystic dysplastic kidney (MCDK)
Benign multilocular cyst (cystic nephroma)
Simple cysts
Medullary sponge kidney Acquired renal cystic disease Calyceal diverticulum

Autosomal recessive polycystic kidney disease (ARPKD) results from mutations in the *PKHD1* gene of the chromosome 6p. The classic presentation is a child born with bilateral large kidneys that appear very echogenic on ultrasound; the echogenic appearance is due to the multiple cystic surfaces reflecting the sonographic waves. Kidney function is uniformly poor, and oligohydramnios with pulmonary hypoplasia occurs in up to 50%. Among those who survive infancy, 30% progress to end-stage renal failure. Long-term survivors can also develop portal hypertension, esophageal varices, and hypersplenism due to concomitant periportal fibrosis. There is no specific therapy other than kidney transplantation.

Autosomal dominant polycystic kidney disease (ADPKD) is caused by mutations in one of two genes: PKD1 and PKD2. PKD1 is located on chromosome 16 and accounts for 85% of ADPKD cases, while PKD2 is located on chromosome 4 and accounts for 15%.[6] The most common period for onset is postpubertal with most patients progressing to renal failure by the fourth to sixth decade of life, depending on the severity of penetrance. However, it can present at any age, including the newborn period. Usually, the earlier the onset, the more severe the disease.[7] Cysts are present in the pancreas and liver, as well as cerebral aneurysms in the circle of Willis.

Acquired renal cystic disease of renal failure refers to renal cyst development in patients with end-stage renal failure. Regardless of the type of renal replacement therapy (peritoneal or hemodialysis), cysts can develop in the kidneys. The longer the duration of dialysis, the more prevalent and larger the cysts become. Transplantation and the restoration of normal renal function lead to cessation and (typically) regression of the cysts. The cysts are notable because they can bleed and develop infections. More worrisome is the development of renal cell carcinoma (RCC) in about 0.2% of patients. Cyst formation occurs in equal frequency in adults and children, although RCC is exceedingly rare in children, perhaps because children generally spend less time on transplant lists than adults.

Several syndromes are associated with renal cysts. *Tuberous sclerosis* is an autosomal dominant condition characterized by developmental delay, epilepsy, sebaceous acne, and renal tumors (usually angiomyolipomas, but less commonly RCC), but simple cysts are also common. *Von Hippel–Lindau syndrome* is an autosomal dominant condition associated with cerebellar hemangioblastoma, retinal angiomata, pheochromocytoma, RCC (30% to 40% of all VHL patients), and cysts of the pancreas and kidney.

Solitary Kidney

In general, patients with a solitary functional kidney have few functional limitations but require monitoring.[8] Solitary kidney can be due to surgical removal, MCDK, renal donation, or renal agenesis. Participation in contact sports (such as lacrosse, football, rugby, and ice hockey) is generally allowed with the understanding that the participant uses protective gear and that the risk of injury leading to organ loss is very small—but not zero.[9] The official position of the American Academy of Pediatrics (AAP) is to allow sports participation in general, with the caveat that abdominal padding or protective gear should be helpful, but the use of such gear should not give families a false sense of security.

3 ANOMALIES OF THE URETER

4 Ureteropelvic Junction Obstruction

UPJO is the most common form of congenital ureteral obstruction.[10] This may be due to an intrinsic or extrinsic cause. Intrinsic causes include an adynamic portion of the ureter that fails to contract appropriately due to the aberrant ureteral muscle lining the UPJ. Extrinsic factors include an intraluminal fibroepithelial polyp or aberrant lower pole renal vasculature that compress the ureter at the UPJ.

The classic symptoms of UPJO are severe flank/abdominal pain, nausea, hematuria, and/or infection, historically dubbed "Dietl's crisis." Today, many UPJO cases are diagnosed antenatally due to abnormal prenatal ultrasound. Ultrasound findings of dilated renal pelvis and calyces without ureteral dilation are consistent with UPJO, but ultrasound alone cannot definitively establish the presence of a true surgical obstruction (**Fig. 99.1**). A functional study, most commonly diuretic nuclear renography with Technetium 99 radiolabeled MAG3, is required to assess both relative renal function and obstruction severity (**Fig. 99.2**). Magnetic resonance urography (MRU) may alternatively be used. MRU avoids ionizing radiation and yields excellent functional and anatomic detail, with the drawback that it typically requires general anesthesia. The majority of antenatally diagnosed hydronephrosis can be safely observed with spontaneous resolution in most, especially those with preserved relative renal function.[11]

UPJO repair can be performed effectively using an open, laparoscopic, or robotic approach. The principle is to excise the narrowed, dysplastic portion and reconnect the ureter and renal pelvis to create a dependent drainage system (**Fig. 99.3**). This dismembered pyeloplasty can be done with a >95% success rate. Other, nondismembered, approaches using a renal

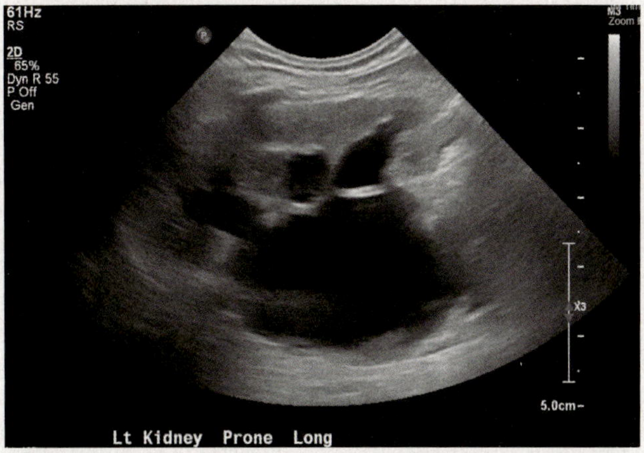

Figure 99.1. Ultrasound demonstrating dilated renal pelvis and calyces caused by ureteropelvic junction obstruction.

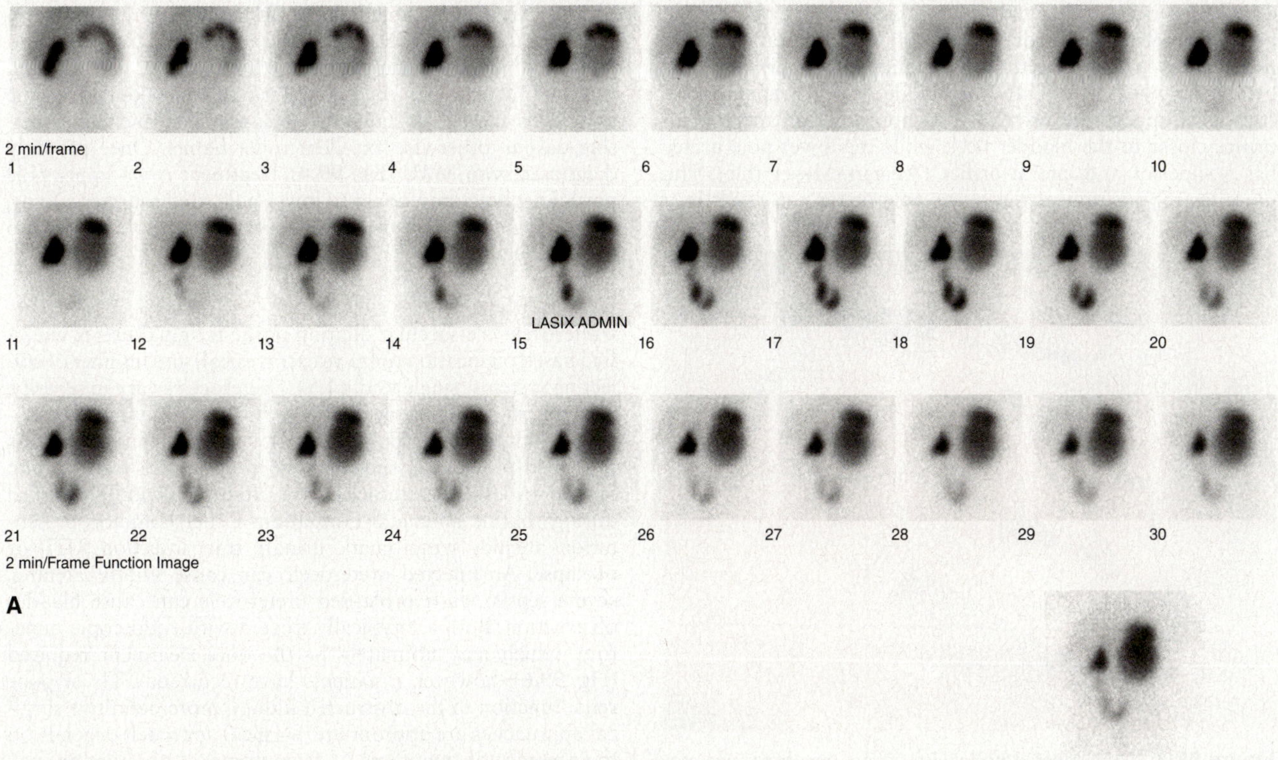

Figure 99.2. Diuretic nuclear renography with Technetium 99 radiolabeled MAG3 shows (**A**) delayed drainage of the right kidney with (**B**) decreased differential renal function (25%) indicative of a high-grade ureteropelvic junction obstruction. (*continued*)

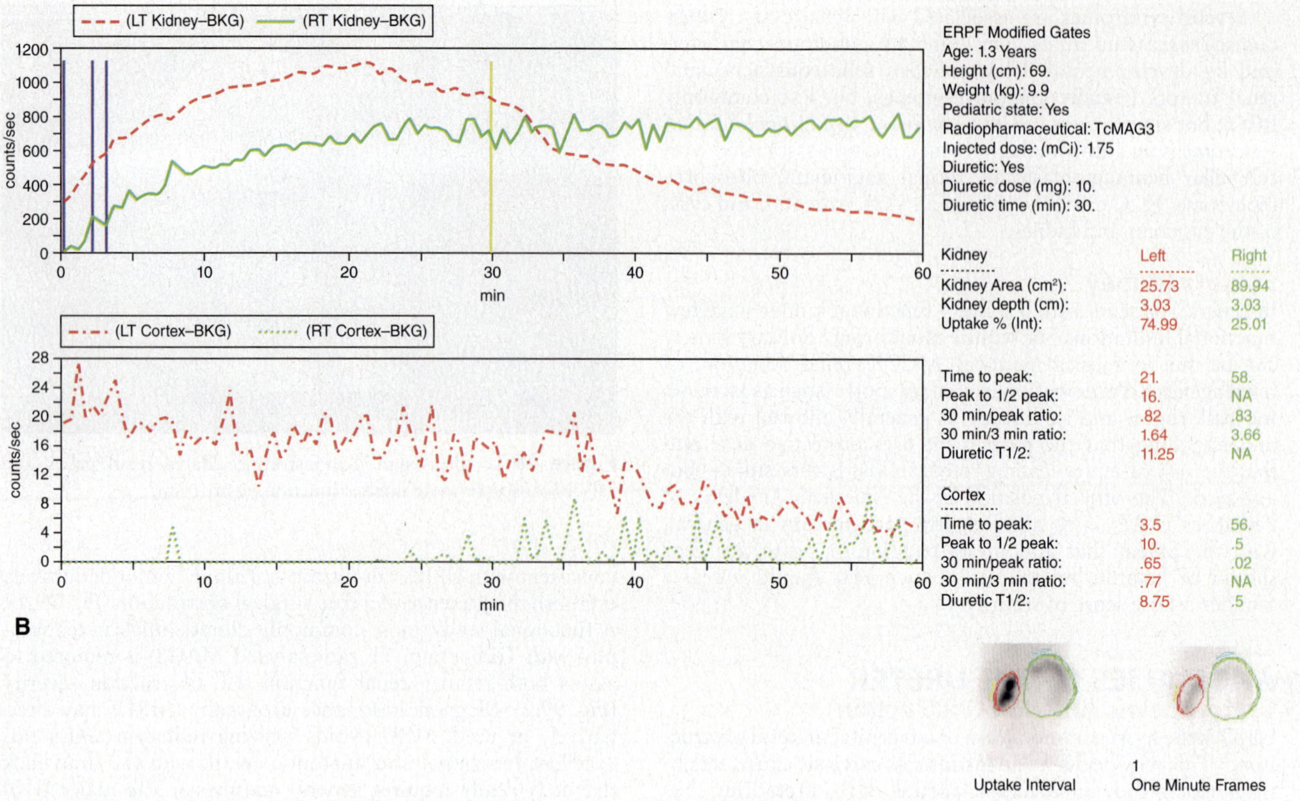

Figure 99.2. (*Continued*)

pelvis flap may also be selectively used in the setting of anatomic variants and in the absence of a crossing vessel.

Ureteral Duplication

Ureteral duplication is a common anatomic variant that can occasionally become pathologic; most patients with partial or complete duplication are healthy; however, partial (Y-type) duplication occurs when two ureters exit the kidney but merge prior to entering the bladder, with only one ureteral orifice in the bladder. A complete ureteral duplication occurs in 1:150 live births; two ureters enter the bladder via two separate orifices. The upper pole ureter has a more inferior and medial orifice closer to the bladder neck while the lower pole ureter has a superior and lateral orifice (Weigert–Meyer rule). The more lateral position of the lower pole ureter can result in a shorter submucosal tunnel, making it more prone to VUR. The more medial, upper pole ureter can enter ectopically into the bladder neck, proximal urethra, or vagina.

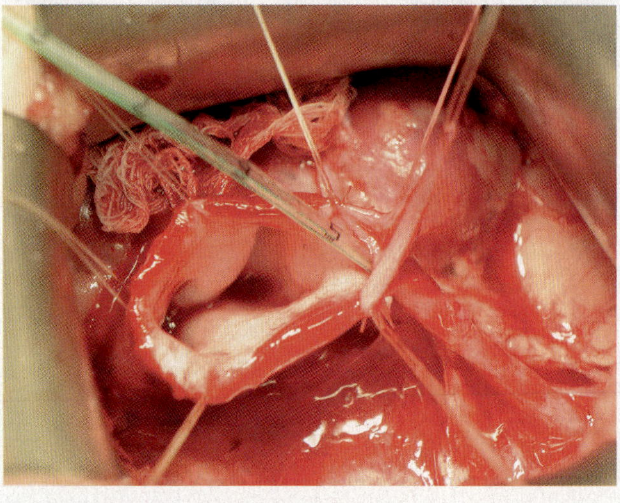

Figure 99.3. Dismembered pyeloplasty where the obstructive segment has been excised and the anastomosis is performed between the pelvic opening and spatulated ureter, creating a dependent drainage.

Ectopic Ureter

Ectopic ureter usually drains more caudal and inferior to the normal trigone. It is most commonly associated with a complete duplication as noted above. In males, they can exit into the prostatic urethra, bladder neck, and epididymis (rare). In females, they can drain into the bladder neck, urethra, and vagina. In females, an ectopic ureter that drains outside of the bladder is the classic cause of persistent day and night wetting despite otherwise excellent toilet habits. Once properly diagnosed with MRU (**Fig. 99.4**), treatment is via upper pole partial nephrectomy, upper to lower pole ureteroureterostomy, or ureteroneocystostomy of the upper pole ectopic ureter into the bladder.

Ureterocele

Ureterocele is a saccular dilation of the terminal ureter, classified based on location (intra vs extravesical) and number of collecting systems (single vs duplex). Ureteroceles vary in severity, ranging from mild to severe (**Fig. 99.5**) and are typically associated with the upper pole ureter of a complete duplication, as described previously; single-system ureteroceles rarely occur. Similar to UPJO, ureteroceles are often incidentally detected during routine antenatal evaluation. Other common presentations include symptomatic urinary tract infection (UTI) or prolapse. An infected ureterocele can cause life-threatening, severe sepsis, while prolapsed ureterocele can cause bladder obstruction. Both are typically treated with endoscopic puncture, which may ultimately be the only treatment required (**Fig. 99.6**); however, if patients have recurrent UTIs or poor renal function of the obstructed kidney, more definitive surgical approaches are appropriate. Surgical approach depends on the presence of symptoms (if asymptomatic, observation may be adequate) as well as the function of the upper pole moiety. If the upper pole is functional, it should be preserved via

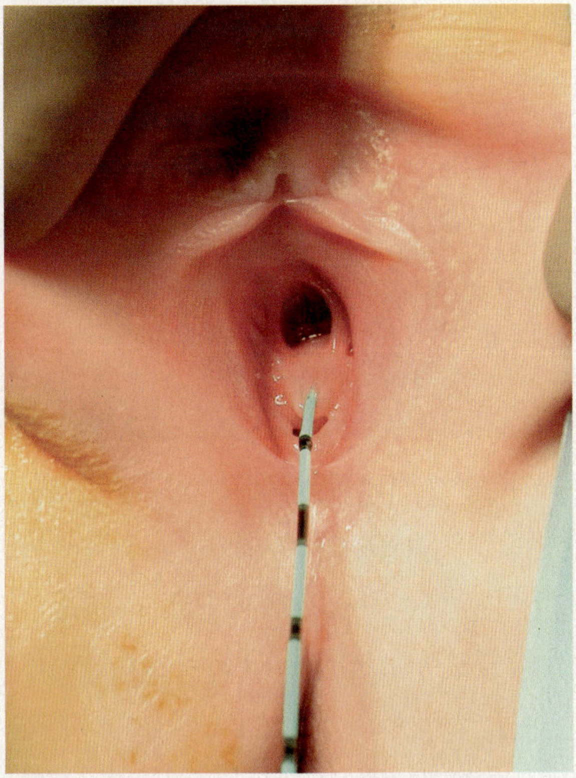

Figure 99.4. Ectopic ureter opening outside the bladder and urethra causing continuous incontinence. Catheter is inserted into the left upper pole ectopic ureter.

ureteroureterostomy or common sheath ureteral reimplant. If the upper pole is nonfunctional, an upper pole partial nephrectomy may be appropriate. A robotic or open approach may be appropriate for either technique.

Megaureter

A dilated ureter >8 mm in diameter along its length is referred to as a megaureter[12] and classified by function and causation; they can be refluxing, obstructing, refluxing/obstructing, or nonobstructing/nonrefluxing. Primary megaureters (those due to an intrinsic abnormality of the ureter rather than the bladder), like ureterovesical junction obstruction and ureterocele, are often diagnosed prenatally. The majority improve with observation. If treatment is required because of pain, UTI, or poor renal function, multiple management options exist, including cutaneous ureterostomy or refluxing ureteroneocystostomy; short-term complications and need for redo surgery

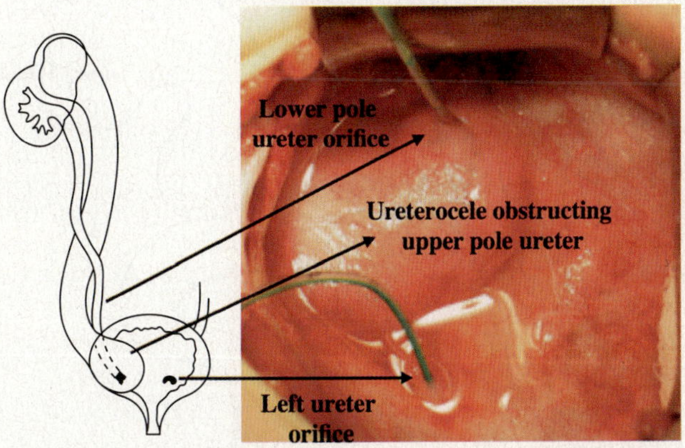

Figure 99.5. Bulging right ureterocele belonging to the upper pole. Bladder has been opened. Catheters are inserted into the right lower pole ureter and left ureter.

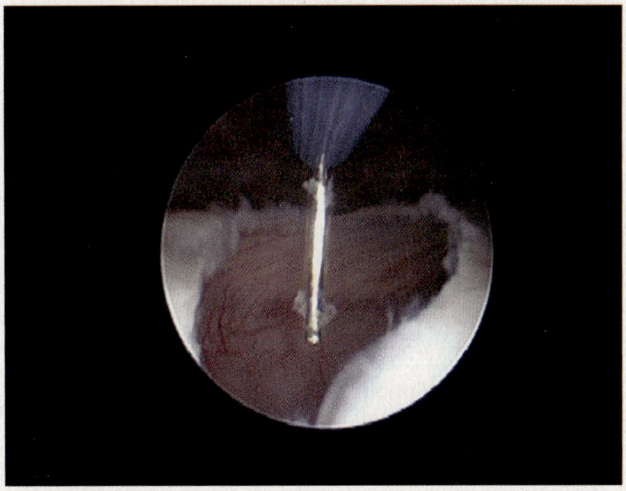

Figure 99.6. Successful endoscopic transurethral incision of ureterocele.

are comparable among these techniques.[13] Definitive management is achieved with nonrefluxing ureteral reimplantation, typically with tapering of the distal portion of the ureter.

5 Vesicoureteral Reflux

VUR, or the reversed flow of urine from the bladder back up into the kidney, is a common pediatric condition present in up to 10% of all children in the United States. In the setting of UTI, VUR can be present in up to 50% of otherwise healthy children (**Fig. 99.7**).[14] Primary VUR occurs because the length of the intramural tunnel is insufficient to seal the ureter during bladder filling and emptying. Secondary VUR occurs in the setting of high bladder pressures that overwhelm an otherwise normal intramuscular tunnel. VUR is of clinical significance because it interferes with effective and efficient emptying of urine and allows bacteria to ascend into the kidneys, thereby transforming cystitis into pyelonephritis. Pyelonephritis may,

PEDIATRIC SURGERY

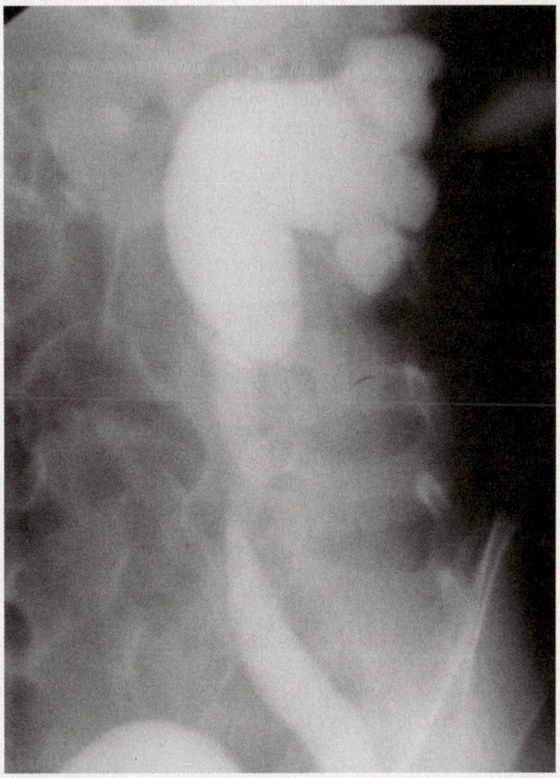

Figure 99.7. Vesicoureteral reflux to the left lower pole ureter.

in turn, increase the risk of long-term kidney damage by causing parenchymal scar. Renal scarring and damage early in life are associated with an increased risk of long-term complications, including hypertension and pregnancy-related complications.[15,16]

VUR severity is described using the International Reflux Study scale. Grading is important for several reasons. Most VUR patients (80%) have grades I or II with an excellent chance of spontaneous resolution (75% to 90%) over time. Higher grades (III to V) are less likely to improve with time.[17] Voiding cystourethrogram (VCUG) is the gold standard test to diagnose reflux, offering excellent anatomical detail of the entire lower urinary tract (bladder and urethra).[18] In males, it is the main diagnostic test to diagnose posterior urethral valves (PUV). Alternative options include nuclear cystogram (NUC) or contrast-enhanced voiding urosonography (ce-VUS), which do not require radiation but still require urethral catheterization. Standard ultrasound of the kidneys and bladder, while helpful in assessing renal size and appearancc, cannot diagnose reflux. The detection of kidney scarring is usually confirmed with nuclear renal scintigraphy using DMSA (**Fig. 99.8**).

The management of children with VUR depends on their presentation and other clinical factors (**Fig. 99.9**).[17] Antibiotic prophylaxis is recommended for children less than 1 year of age with febrile UTI or high-grade VUR diagnosed on prenatal ultrasound. If low-grade VUR is detected prenatally, antibiotic prophylaxis may be offered. Management of children who are older than 1 year of age takes into account bowel and bladder dysfunction in addition to grade of reflux evidence of renal scarring and parental preference. The vast majority of patients have low-grade VUR and are expected to resolve spontaneously with time. The most recent multiinstitution randomized clinical trial suggested that antibiotic prophylaxis is beneficial in children with dilating, high-grade reflux (grade III or higher). If they cannot remain infection free and sustain breakthrough infections, surgery may be necessary to prevent recurrent renal parenchymal infection. For most patients, spontaneous resolution occurs after 4 to 5 years. However, those with persistent high-grade reflux who fail conservative management may need surgery. There are two major surgical options: endoscopic antireflux surgery and ureteral reimplant. Endoscopic management consists of injection of a bulking material into the floor of the ureteral orifice. This creates a submucosal mound that turns the usual round oval ureteral orifice into an upside-down crescent. Currently, FDA-approved dextranomer/hyaluronic acid copolymer is available

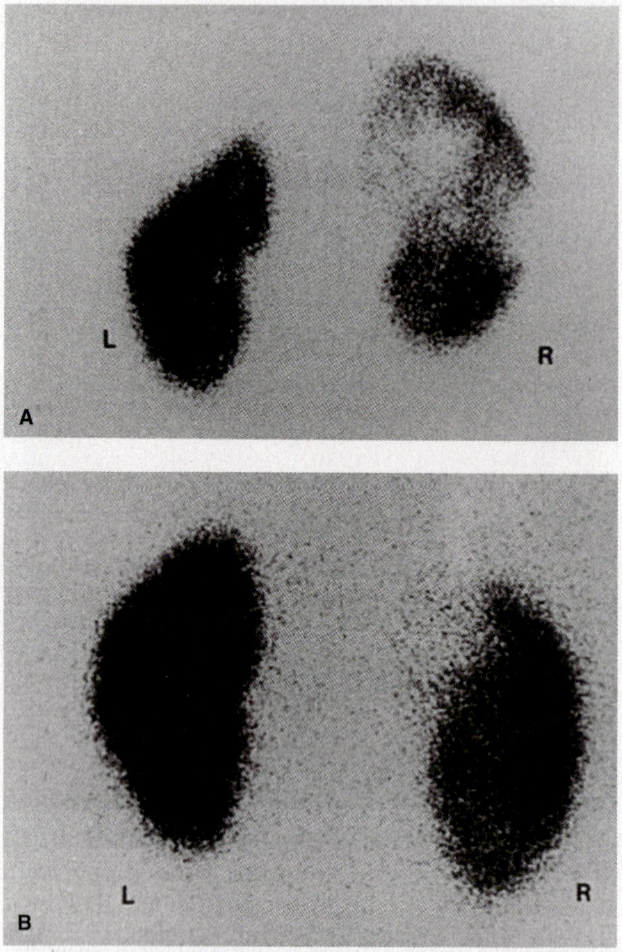

Figure 99.8. DMSA renal scintigraphy demonstrating renal parenchymal defect associated with pyelonephritis. **A:** Cortical defects seen in the right kidney during the acute phase of pyelonephritis. **B:** The same kidney 6 months later showing a persistent cortical scar involving the upper pole.

for this approach. The efficacy of these sub- and intraureteral injection ranges from 70% to >90%, though current literature consists primarily of case series and demonstrates that rates of febrile UTI after endoscopic intervention are comparable to

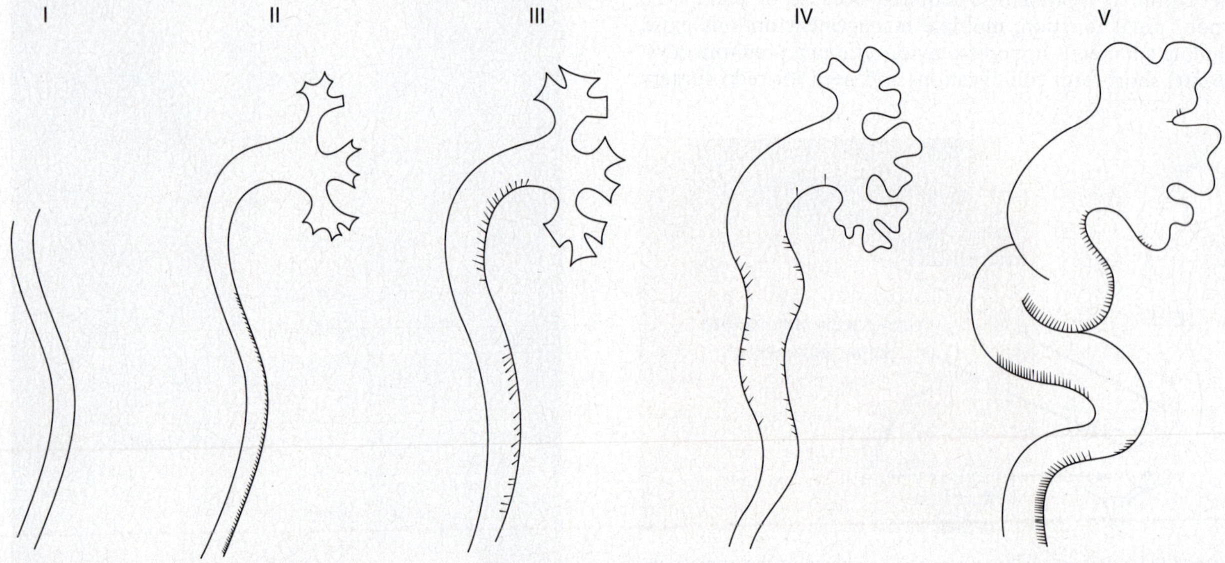

Figure 99.9. International reflux grading system. Majority of reflux are grades I or II, with high likelihood of spontaneous resolution, whereas higher grades (III to V) with dilating ureters are at a greater risk of UTI, renal injury, and nonresolution, often requiring surgery.

prophylactic antibiotics alone.[19] Ureteral reimplantation (ureteroneocystostomy), where the ureter is revised or repositioned to create a more effective ureterovesical flap-valve mechanism by restoring the submucosal tunnel, is the gold standard treatment for VUR. The affected ureter is detached and mobilized. A new submucosal tunnel of sufficient length (approximately three to five times the width of the ureter) is created, and the ureter is placed into it. It is critical that the muscle underneath the tunnel is firm and secure to allow the collapse of the reimplanted ureter with bladder filling and emptying. The ureter may require tapering (in megaureter or obstructed upper pole of duplication anomaly), so it can meet the needed width-to-length ratio of the tunnel. An extravesical approach is called detrusorrhaphy, where the muscle flaps are freed from the underlying bladder mucosa and wrapped behind the ureter at the UVJ to create a more effective flap-valve mechanism. The success rate of open surgery for VUR is very high (96% or more for grades III or less).

Traditionally, all children who present with a culture-proven UTI were recommended to undergo evaluation for VUR using ultrasound and VCUG. However, the morbidity of VUR seems to be mostly due to infections and related complications rather than the reflux itself. It is important to stratify patients according to their risk of infection, taking into consideration grade of reflux and presence of bladder and bowel dysfunction, as not all reflux needs to be treated. The goal of managing children with VUR is to prevent UTIs, renal injury, and minimize the morbidity of treatment. Because most incidences of VUR are low grade and most cases of low-grade VUR resolve spontaneously, it may be reasonable to defer VCUG for only those patients who have recurrent UTIs or abnormal ultrasound. This has led to a major shift in the recommendations from the AAP in 2011. VCUG should be obtained to assess renal scarring and function if the renal ultrasound is abnormal. Recently, a double-blind randomized controlled trial examined the benefits of antibiotic prophylaxis. The Randomized Intervention for Children with Vesicoureteral Reflux (RIVUR) study found that continuous antibiotic prophylaxis reduced the risk of recurrent UTI by 50%, especially in those with dilating, high-grade reflux (III to V).[20] The occurrence of new renal scarring did not differ significantly between the two groups, though in the context of a clinical trial this may have been impacted by potential Hawthorne effect (ie, RIVUR patients may have been treated more rapidly/aggressively than normal simply because they were in a clinical trial).

Women with a history of VUR may be at increased risk later in life for UTI during pregnancy regardless of whether the VUR was corrected or not. Renal scarring rather than the presence of active VUR itself appeared to be a key risk factor for pregnancy-related morbidity. Furthermore, there is an increased rate of VUR in offspring of parents with VUR. In general, for girls with VUR, the families should be aware that when they become adults of child-bearing age, it is important to know their medical histories, so that appropriate perinatal care and monitoring is instituted.

BLADDER ANOMALIES

Urachal Abnormality

The urachus typically involutes and becomes atretic during the transition from fetal to neonatal life. Shortly after birth, it typically remains only as a fibrous cord from the dome of the bladder to the umbilicus. Occasionally, the urachus pathologically remains patent in whole or in part. When completely open, it is referred to as a patent urachus, and urine leaks from the umbilicus. If closed on either end, it forms a sinus on the umbilicus or bladder, or an entrapped cyst in between. These can be asymptomatic and incidentally diagnosed on imaging, or they can become infected due to poor drainage and present with fever, nausea, and umbilical drainage. Detection is usually made by clinical suspicion, along with abdominal ultrasound. Although adenocarcinoma of the urachus has been anecdotally linked to embryologic remnants, the literature supports conservative management of asymptomatic urachal remnants.[21]

Exstrophy–Epispadias Complex

Exstrophy-epispadias complex (EEC) comprises a spectrum of genitourinary malformations ranging in severity from isolated penile epispadias to classical bladder exstrophy and cloacal exstrophy. Depending on severity, EEC may involve the urinary system, musculoskeletal system, pelvis, pelvic floor, abdominal wall, genitalia, and sometimes the spine and anus. Prevalence at birth is reported at 1/10,000, ranging from 1/30,000 for classic exstrophy (**Fig. 99.10A**) to 1/200,000 for cloacal exstrophy (**Fig. 99.10B**), with males more likely to be affected than females.[22]

Epispadias is the least severe manifestation of EEC. In males, it is a defect with a dorsally placed urethral meatus and urethra, along with dorsal penile curvature. When the meatus is very proximal, the bladder neck and long-term continence outcomes can be affected. In females, epispadias typically present with a bifid clitoris (**Fig. 99.11**). Protection of the bladder plate against contact irritation is important by simply covering it with plastic wrap until closure. In the modern era, closure is typically postponed until 2 to 6 months of age. A concomitant pelvic osteotomy is beneficial for successful initial closure, as well as for subsequent bladder function. Repair can be staged with closure of the bladder first, followed by subsequent

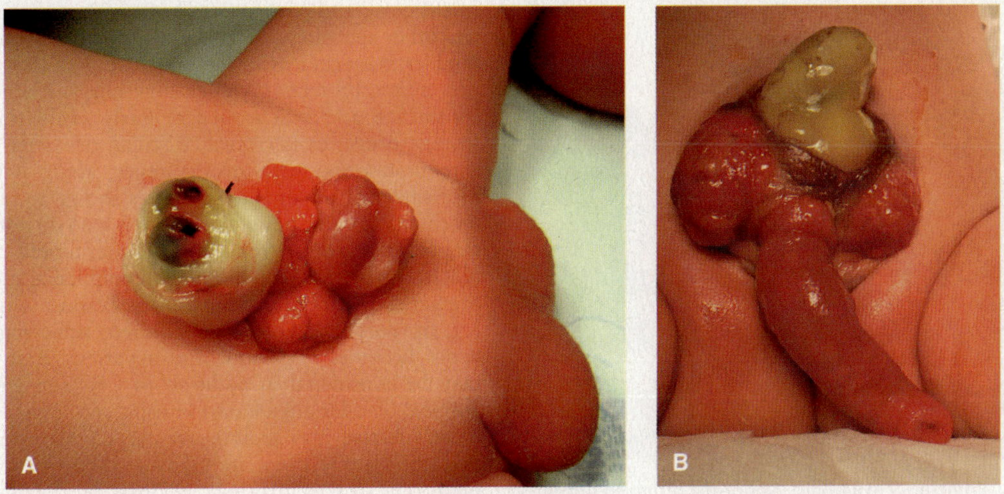

Figure 99.10. **A:** Male bladder exstrophy with associated epispadias. **B:** Cloacal bladder exstrophy with split bladder plate and rudimentary hindgut.

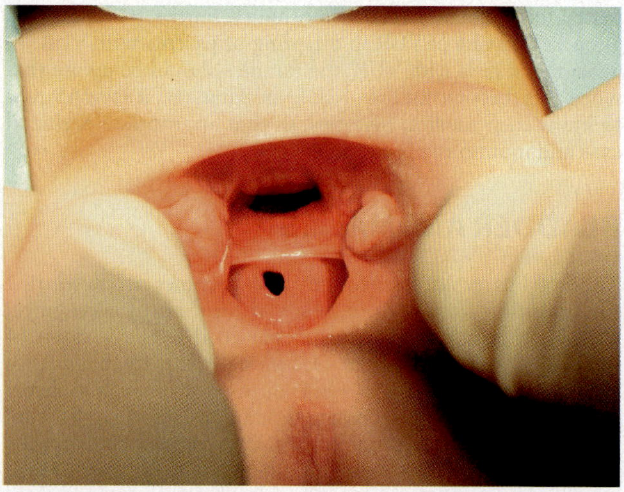

Figure 99.11. Female epispadias with its classic bifid clitoris.

bladder neck reconstruction and epispadias repair. Alternatively, a complete primary repair may be performed with simultaneous closure of the bladder plate and reconstruction of the epispadias and genitalia. Patients with EEC have a high rate of other anomalies, including inguinal hernia and VUR.

The most severe form of EEC is cloacal exstrophy. The hindgut (colon, rectum, and anus) is absent or rudimentary, and the bladder plate is split into two parts on either side of the exposed cecum and hindgut remnant along with a cephalad omphalocele. Initial management involves closure of the omphalocele, creation of a colostomy, dissecting the bladder plates free and reconstruction to form a reservoir or composite urethral plate. Cloacal exstrophy is associated with a worse prognosis than other EEC variants, presumably due to the number of organ systems involved.

Prune-Belly Syndrome

The prune-belly syndrome (PBS) is a constellation of malformations also known as the triad syndrome or Eagle–Barrett syndrome.[23] The syndrome has three key components: severe deficiency or absence of the abdominal wall musculature creating a wrinkled abdominal wall, bilateral hydroureteronephrosis, and bilateral undescended intra-abdominal testicles (**Fig. 99.12**). There are also other associated genitourinary conditions, including renal dysplasia, fusiform urethra, large bladder, patent urachus, hypoplastic prostate, and dilated proximal urethra. Renal dysplasia is frequent and when severe, it can lead to pulmonary hypoplasia as seen in PUV. Hydroureteronephrosis can be massive but is typically nonobstructive. Nearly all of the patients are infertile with an anecdotal report of successful fertility using the assisted reproductive technology. For infants who survive into childhood, bilateral orchiopexy and abdominal wall reconstruction may be necessary. Evaluation for bladder function is also required since many will have a poor bladder muscle tone resulting in chronic retention.

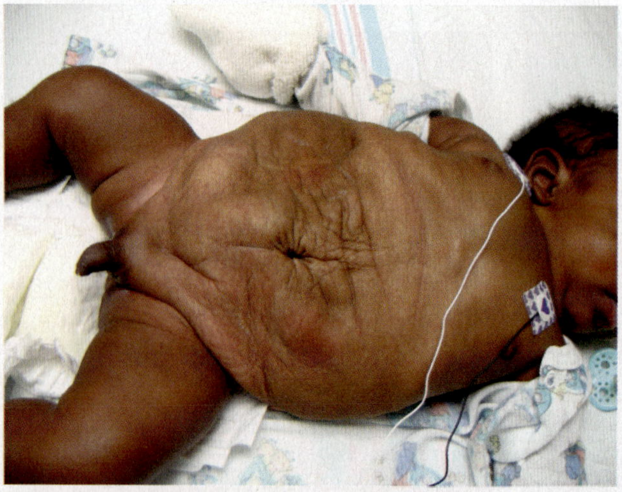

Figure 99.12. Prune-belly syndrome. Notice the wrinkled appearance of the abdominal wall due to deficiency of musculature. Scrotum is empty due to bilateral intra-abdominal testicles.

6 Neurogenic Bladder

The nervous system plays an important role in modulating the normal behavior of the lower urinary tract. There are nerve roots (emanating from the spinal cord) and peripheral pelvic nerves that carry sensory and motor signals to the bladder and urethral sphincter. Injuries or anomalies to these nerves can denervate the bladder, leading to poor emptying. The spinal cord up to the brain stem is critical to regulation of lower urinary tract function, especially the thoracolumbar sympathetic and sacral parasympathetic segments. The brain stem acts as the coordinating center. With filling, the bladder musculature—under the influence of the sympathetic input—remains relaxed, thereby keeping bladder storage pressures low until emptying occurs (driven by parasympathetic input). The higher centers in the cerebral cortex allow conscious control and inhibition of reflex activity. Without this influence the bladder fills, and at a certain volume it spontaneously empties with coordination. This occurs normally in infants prior to toilet training. Patients with spinal cord injury, traumatic brain injury, and acquired conditions that affect the nervous system (eg, diabetes mellitus, multiple sclerosis, varicella zoster, brain tumors, and encephalitis) should trigger awareness about possible urinary effects.[24]

Mere urine egress from the bladder is not necessarily a sign of normal voiding. It can be due to overflow incontinence or some form of dysfunctional voiding (Valsalva voiding). Likewise, continence is not necessarily a sign of neurologically coordinated normal bladder function. The storage pressures can be higher than normal. When the bladder urine storage pressures are too high, it can overcome the peristaltic pressure driving urine from the kidneys down the renal pelvis and ureter. Ideally, the storage pressure should be below 40 cm H_2O.[25] Above this pressure, loss of renal function will occur. A urology evaluation with urodynamic pressure–volume assessment of the lower urinary tract should be considered if there is any condition with significant effects on the central nervous system.

Spina bifida is the most common congenital cause of a neurogenic bladder in children. During development, the spinal column does not close properly, resulting in an exposed spinal cord, and patients are born with a neurogenic bladder and other neurologic defects. The goals of effective neurogenic bladder management in the pediatric population include UTI prevention, protecting kidney function, and achieving urinary continence and independence. Early evaluation of bladder storage pressures is crucial. Regular, proactive bladder pressure monitoring with urodynamics, along with ultrasound assessment of the upper tracts, has shown to reduce urologic morbidity in these patients. Children who do not empty with a safe bladder pressure require clean intermittent catheterization (CIC). Patients with poor bladder compliance and high storage pressures may need antimuscarinic bladder muscle relaxants (eg, oxybutynin). For older children, achieving social continence becomes important and a variety of surgical options may be considered in addition to CIC and antimuscarinics. Surgical bladder augmentation using intestinal segments is the most effective way to improve the bladder storage function (**Fig. 99.13**), but there are many well-known long-term complications, such as metabolic acidosis, mucus production, UTI, bladder stones, spontaneous perforations, and malignancy. In some patients who have difficulty with urethral CIC (such

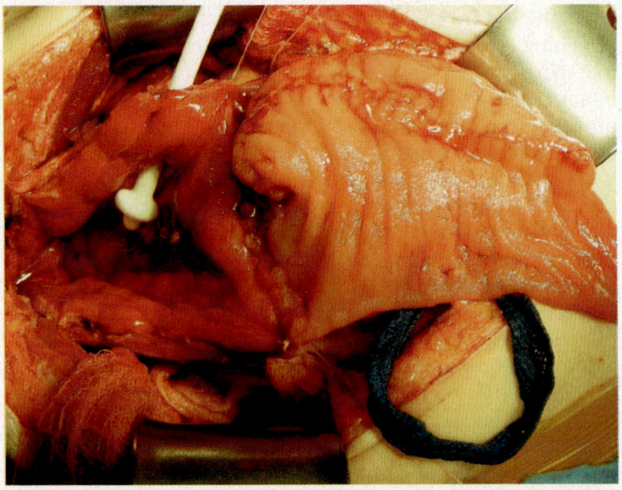

Figure 99.13. Bladder augmentation using a patch of detubularized ileum.

as those with severe scoliosis or girls in wheelchair), surgical creation of alternate continent catheterizable channel is an option. The Mitrofanoff appendicovesicostomy, where the appendix is tunneled into the bladder and brought up to the umbilicus as a stoma, can allow for easier CIC. If the bladder outlet is weak, causing incontinence, surgical options include artificial urinary sphincter, bladder neck reconstruction with sling, and complete bladder neck closure.

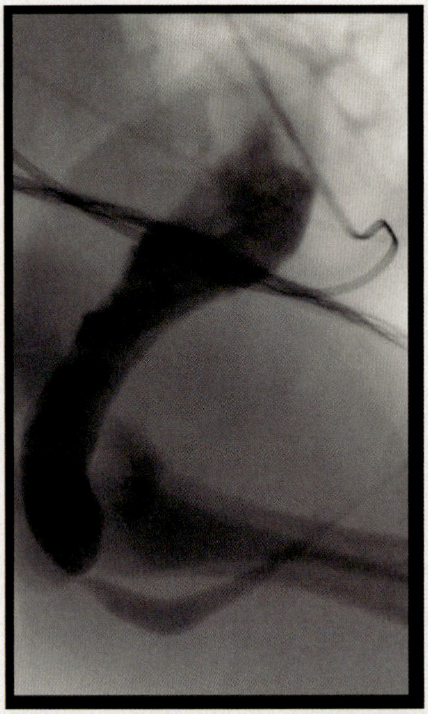

Figure 99.14. Voiding cystourethrogram of a newborn with posterior urethral valves. Significantly dilated prostatic urethra proximal to the valves.

7 ANOMALIES OF THE URETHRA

Posterior Urethral Valves

PUV is one of the most clinically significant obstructive uropathies.[26] Occurring exclusively in males, it consists of a thin membrane below the verumontanum and above the external sphincter causing a blockage of bladder emptying. This results in high voiding pressures leading to upstream prostatic urethral dilation, bladder wall hypertrophy, and secondary VUR. Most patients are diagnosed antenatally with the classic prenatal sonographic findings of bilateral hydroureteronephrosis, dilated bladder, and enlarged prostatic urethra (so-called "keyhole" urethra). Poor bladder emptying throughout fetal development can result in irreversible, dysplastic, poorly functioning kidneys. In addition, low urine production leads to oligohydramnios, which in turn results in impaired pulmonary development. In its severest form, significant renal and respiratory dysfunction manifests as Potters sequence, which carries a significant risk of infant mortality. After birth, immediate placement of a urethral catheter allows for urinary decompression. Once stabilized, a VCUG is obtained to establish the diagnosis (**Fig. 99.14**). Most patients then undergo endoscopic resection of the valves. If the patient's urethra is too small to accommodate an infant resectoscope, a temporary diverting vesicostomy is an option.

Patients require lifelong urologic and nephrologic care to manage the several long-term consequences of PUVs. PUV remains the leading urologic cause of renal insufficiency requiring transplantation. The initial nadir creatinine with complete bladder drainage is prognostic with values ≥0.7 mg/dL associated with an increased need for renal replacement therapy.[27] The early fibrosis and hypertrophy of the bladder leads to poor bladder compliance. These bladders have higher-than-normal storage pressures and over time can lead to the development of UTIs, incontinence, urinary retention, and worsening renal function. When recognized early, appropriate therapy using CIC along with antimuscarinic agents (eg, oxybutynin) to relax the bladder muscle can help manage these "valve bladders." If renal transplantation is needed, a patient's bladder must be evaluated with urodynamic studies to ensure that the bladder can safely store urine to protect the health of the transplant. A valve bladder with poor capacity and/or compliance may require augmentation prior to transplant.

8 Hypospadias

Hypospadias occurs when the ventral genital folds do not fuse completely resulting in a meatal opening in an abnormal proximal location on the ventral surface of the penis.[28] While the majority of cases do not have a known cause, there are a few important associations. When found concomitantly with bilateral undescended or missing testicles, the probability of a differences of sex development (DSD) is high enough to warrant a formal workup. Recently there has been a growing interest in the role of endocrine disruptors. They include environmental pollutants such as bisphenol, pesticides/herbicides, and phthalates, and maternal hormone intake of progestins, estrogens, and the use of assisted reproductive technologies.

There is a wide spectrum of presentations ranging from milder forms with the meatus on the proximal glans or coronal edge to the most severe with the meatus at the level of the scrotum. Most cases (80%) are distal with the meatus between the tip of the penis and the corona. Not all cases require surgery such as milder forms that do not interfere with normal voiding and or sexual function. More severe forms of hypospadias are usually associated with other anatomic abnormalities including ventral chordee in which the penis classically curves toward the scrotum, and the incompleteness of the foreskin creating a dorsally hooded foreskin (**Fig. 99.15**). Postnatally, these secondary findings should raise suspicion for hypospadias. Most importantly, circumcision should not be performed if there is any concern for hypospadias.

Surgical repair has three main goals: (1) to create a straight erection for sexual intercourse, (2) to allow normal urination with a single, outward projecting urinary stream, and (3) satisfactory cosmesis.[29] There are a variety of techniques that can be used depending on the severity of the hypospadias and surgeons' preference. Ultimately, the urethral meatus is advanced distally on the glans with a slit-like opening, the glans is reshaped into a more normal bell-like appearance, and

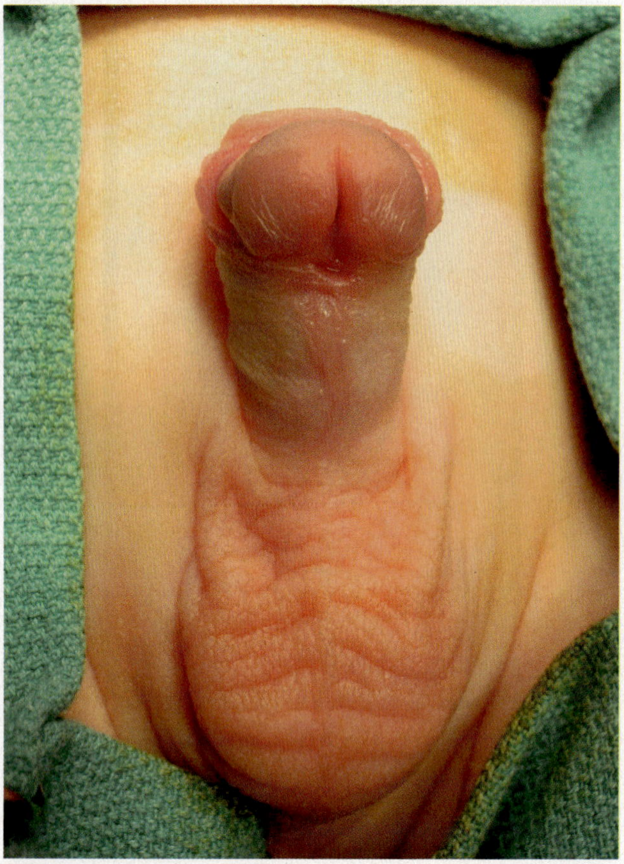

Figure 99.15. Mild hypospadias with urethral meatus located near the neck (corona), along with dorsal hood foreskin.

any significant ventral curvature is corrected. These are performed as a single stage or in multiple stages for the severe type (**Fig. 99.16**). Some patients benefit from preoperative testosterone supplementation to increase glans size. The prepuce is an important source for free and vascular flaps. In some cases, particularly those who have undergone failed prior attempts at repair, there may not be sufficient local tissue, thus buccal mucosal graft of the inner lip or cheek can be used to form a urethra. Complications of hypospadias repair include urethrocutaneous fistula, stricture, meatal stenosis, recurrent ventral curvature, and surface skin irregularities. Long-term follow-up is important for these patients because complications can occur years after the total repair.[30,31]

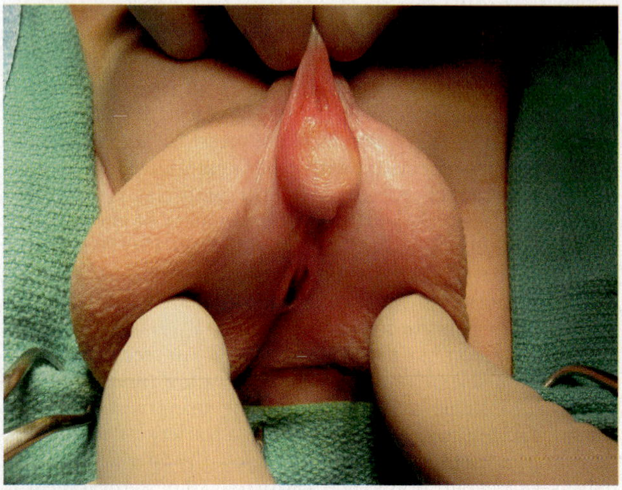

Figure 99.16. Severe hypospadias with perineal urethral opening along with severe ventral shaft curvature (chordee).

Anomalies of the Penis and Prepuce

Physiologic phimosis, when the foreskin cannot be retracted to expose the glans, is normal presenting in all uncircumcised infant males and resolves spontaneously with age. It is inappropriate and unnecessary to retract the foreskin until they are between ages of 5 and 7 years. Forceful dilation or retraction is very painful, traumatic, and can result in scarring. The foreskin will naturally separate from the glans in childhood due to the accumulation of sloughing skin cells and secreted oil (forming smegma) and normal erections.

The indications for childhood circumcision, the single most common procedure performed worldwide, remains controversial.[32] Specific medical indications are not in dispute—phimosis, paraphimosis, balanoposthitis, and reduction of UTI risk. Pathologic phimosis is the inability to retract the foreskin when the child is of an age when it should have occurred naturally. Treatment with topical steroid ointment of the phimotic ring has been found to have success rates between 50% and 74%. In cases where medical therapy is unsuccessful, circumcision is curative. For families and patients who do not want to be circumcised a dorsal slit or partial circumcision can be performed. However, parents should be counseled that phimosis can recur. In paraphimosis, the foreskin is retracted for a prolonged time causing a vascular constriction of the glans. Emergent reduction is required to prevent glandular necrosis. For patients who have recurrent bouts of infection due to entrapment of bacteria under the foreskin (balanoposthitis), circumcision may be medically advisable. Finally, boys with underlying genitourinary anomalies that carry an increased risk for UTI, such as PUV or VUR, circumcision reduce the risk of a UTI by 50% in the first year of life.

Following circumcision, the glans skin changes from moist columnar epithelium to a dry squamous epithelium. This is theorized to be the etiology of decreased rates of sexually transmitted infections (STIs), most notably human immunodeficiency virus.[33] Circumcision also significantly reduces the risk of penile cancer, which most commonly occurs in the foreskin. While these benefits are indisputable, the Centers for Disease Control and AAP acknowledge they are not great enough on a larger population scale to routinely recommend circumcision.[34]

Meatal stenosis is the most common long-term complication occurring in 5% to 7% of circumcised boys. It classically presents with a narrowed/spraying urine stream or voiding symptoms such as straining or pain. A simple surgical correction, meatotomy, sharply divides scarred web, elongating the meatus ventrally.

ANOMALIES OF THE TESTICLE AND SCROTUM

9 Undescended Testicle or Cryptorchidism

Embryologically, testicles develop intra-abdominally, inferior to the kidneys.[35] During the 12th to 18th weeks of gestation, the testicles migrate down to a pelvic position just inside the internal inguinal ring. During the third trimester, the testicles travel through the inguinal canal, exiting through the external inguinal ring, and enter the scrotum as driven by the swelling and contraction of the gubernaculum under the influence of androgens. About 3% of normal full-term boys have an undescended testicle at birth. The incidence is higher in premature infants at 30%. By age 1 year corrected for prematurity, this drops to ~1% which remains stable through puberty. For this reason, undescended testicles diagnosed within the first 6 months of life are given the chance of spontaneous descent, but after this age surgical orchiopexy should be performed between 6 and 18 months old.[36]

Patients with undescended testicles have two times the risk of developing a testicular germ cell cancer, and orchiopexy significantly reduces this risk when performed prior to puberty.[37] A scrotal position is advantageous for several reasons. Descended testicles are exposed to a lower temperature environment, which is necessary for achieving full sperm development and fertility. A scrotal position makes self-examination easier. Finally, undescended testicles are more prone to torsion and injury.

The location of an undescended testicle may be intra-abdominal, along the inguinal canal, or through the external ring, but not in the scrotum. An undescended testicle can also be ectopic, such as perineal or femoral. Finally, it can be aberrant, dysmorphic, atrophic, or nonexistent likely due to perinatal vascular compromise, such as prenatal torsion. Physical examination plays a key part in the diagnosis of an undescended testicle. When boys are anxious or nervous, their inguinal cremasteric muscles draw the testicle upward into the groin. This condition is termed retractile testicles. In most cases, the retractile testicle settles in the scrotal position around the time the child goes through puberty. In some, retractile testicles can ascend to the inguinal region as the boys grow older, requiring a surgical intervention. This is referred as an ascended testicle, and may occur up to 5% to 10% of boys who are followed for retractile testicles.

For palpable undescended testicles, an orchiopexy is usually through an inguinal incision. The testicle is mobilized by detaching the gubernaculum, cremasteric muscle, and internal spermatic sheath around the cord structures, and a tunnel is created from the inguinal incision to the scrotum. There is often an associated patent processus (up to 80% in infants), and this is separated from the cord and suture ligated at the internal ring. This usually allows for the testicle to be brought into the scrotum without tension. The testicle is sutured in place within the scrotum with careful attention to ensure that the cord is straight and not torsed.

For nonpalpable testicles, laparoscopy is performed to identify an intra-abdominal testicle. The key is to find the spermatic vessels. If spermatic vessels pass into the internal ring, then an open groin exploration is performed. This may find a small inguinal testicle that was difficult to palpate in the inguinal fat. In other cases, there is an atrophic nubbin, which is then removed as it will have no functional or cosmetic purpose. If the testicle is seen within the abdominal cavity and well away from the internal ring, the only viable surgical option may be a staged Fowler–Stephens orchiopexy, where the gonadal vessel is divided and the testicle is brought down with a vassal collateral circulation (**Figs. 99.17** and **99.18**) 6 months later. Laparoscopy has been shown to be the most effective in determining the absence of viable testicle (vanishing testicle syndrome). The pathognomonic finding is blind-ending gonadal vessels. If a blind-ending vas is seen but not the vessels, one must continue to explore for hidden testicular tissue since there is an unusual

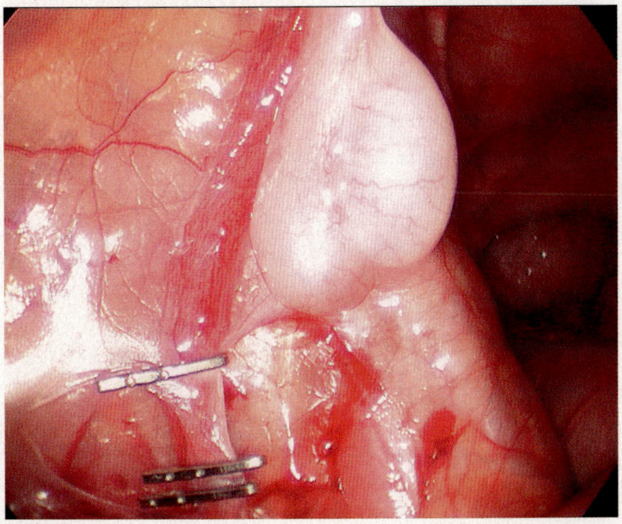

Figure 99.17. Intra-abdominal testicle is gently clipped to force its dependence on the vassal collateral circulation (first-stage Fowler–Stephens orchiopexy).

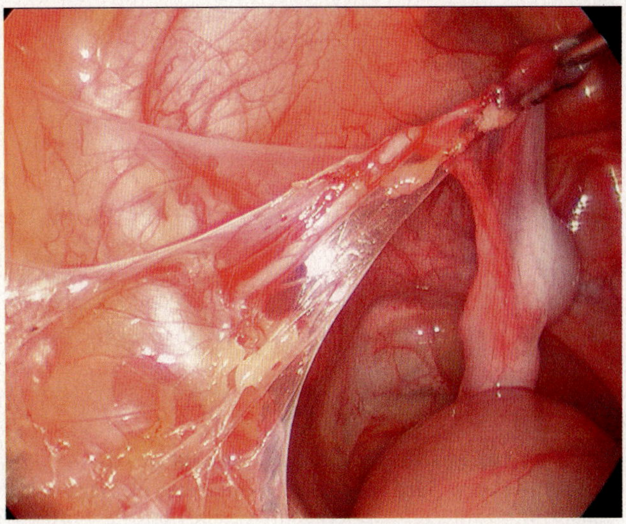

Figure 99.18. During the second-stage orchiopexy, the testicle is dissected while being attached to the vassal collateral circulation.

phenomenon of testicular–epididymal dysjunction, where the testicle is disconnected from the wolffian structures (epididymis and vas). One may have to look very far to locate the vessels, even going up behind the colon and near the lower pole of the kidney. Leaving testicular tissue trapped within the abdominal cavity will increase the risk of germ cell malignancy.

Imaging is not recommended in the evaluation of cryptorchidism. Ultrasound is not helpful because although it is noninvasive, it has sensitivity of 45% and specificity of 78%.[36] More importantly, the surgical decision and planning are not altered by ultrasound findings. For bilateral nonpalpable testicles, biochemical markers—such as HCG stimulation test or serum MIS level—may be useful to determine the presence or absence of functional testicular tissue.

Torsion of Testicle and Appendages

Torsion of the testicle is the leading nontraumatic cause of loss of the testicle in boys.[38] It is an emergent condition that occurs as result of the spermatic cord twisting. This results in occlusion of the lymphatic vessels, veins, and arteries leading to ischemia, necrosis, and atrophy. If there is complete occlusion of blood flow, the testicle may be salvageable up to 6 hours after onset. After 6 hours the odds of salvage diminish exponentially.[39] Most torsion occurs in older boys and adolescents—although it can occur at any age—with the torsion occurring inside the tunica vaginalis (intravaginal torsion). A horizontal lie (known as the bell-clapper deformity) caused by poor posterior fixation is believed to predispose toward torsion.

The presentation is a sudden onset, significant, acute unilateral scrotal pain. The pain can be associated with nausea and vomiting. The signs and symptoms will evolve over time. Initially, there will be increasing swelling and discoloration. Later when the nerve endings have died, the testicle and scrotum may still be swollen and ecchymotic, but less painful. Various clinical clues may help guide physical examination. These include a noticeably shortened spermatic cord creating a "high-riding" testicle, absence of a cremasteric reflex, and lack of relief of discomfort with elevation. But these are often of limited practical use when faced with an anxious patient with a tender scrotum. If one has a strong clinical suspicion based on presentation, and there are no other medical or anesthetic reasons not to go to surgery, emergent exploration—without any further imaging is appropriate. Doppler ultrasound—now readily available in most modern emergency departments—can be useful but should not delay exploration. Ultrasound can help identify other cases of acute scrotum such as torsed appendix testis, epididymitis, hernia/hydrocele, and idiopathic scrotal edema. If a safe surgery is not an option, one may

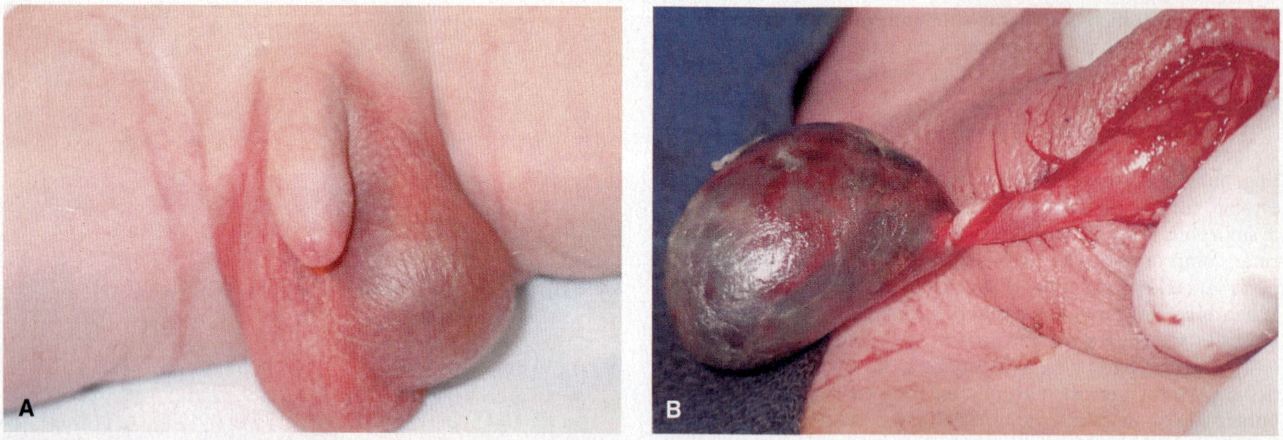

Figure 99.19. A: Newborn physical exam with an enlarged, discolored scrotum with a high-riding testicle concerning for left intravaginal testicular torsion. B: Surgical exploration confirming the diagnosis.

attempt a manual detorsion with a cord block. Untwisting as if one were opening a book (inside out) is the most commonly recommend technique, but it is by no means certain. Immediate exploration is recommended even if there is relief with manual detorsion.

Exploration is done through a transverse scrotal incision in each hemiscrotum or a vertical incision along the median raphe. The torsed testicle should be evaluated first by untwisting the cord and then wrapping in gauze soaked with warm saline. While the opportunity for reperfusion is occurring, an orchiopexy (using permanent suture at three—points laterally, medially, and inferiorly) of the contralateral testicle should be performed. If reevaluation of the detorsed testicle shows improved perfusion, an orchiopexy is performed. If there is a question of adequate perfusion, Doppler ultrasound can help detect blood flow in the distal cord and testicle. A relaxing incision into the testicle through the tunica albuginea can allow for manual decompression of the intratesticular compartment syndrome also aiding in reperfusion. If no active bleeding is found, the testicle has remained black/purple in color, and/or no doppler signal is found, the necrotic testicle should be removed.

Torsion can also occur among neonates, but this occurs due to poor gubernacular fixation and twisting of the cord outside the tunica vaginalis (extravaginal torsion). Neonatal torsion classically is associated with a prolonged labor. The testicle is very firm, nontender, and there can be a dark ecchymotic look about the scrotum (**Fig. 99.19**). Because of the very low salvage rate, some do not advocate an emergent exploration. Others suggest that if it is anesthetically safe, exploration is important because it also allows for fixation of the contralateral testicle preventing metachronous torsion.

When the müllerian ducts atrophy in males, they leave a remnant as a testicular appendage on the head of the testis. These can torse causing acute pain. In pale-skinned patients, the torsed appendage during early presentation can resemble a painful small blue dot that is seen through the stretched skin. Because the appendage is vestigial and nonfunctional, its torsion is managed with pain relief, anti-inflammatories, and exertion restrictions.

10 Prepubertal Testicular Tumors

There is a separate chapter that discusses common childhood tumors.[40] For this chapter, we will limit our discussion to prepubertal testicular tumors. The most common testicular tumor is teratoma, and the most common malignant tumors are yolk sac tumors. All usually present as a distinct palpable painless mass in the scrotum. They can have a reactive hydrocele, and it is important to palpate or image the entire testicle before assuming that the hydrocele is harmless. The primary workup is via scrotal ultrasound and biomarkers. The two most useful biomarkers are the alpha-fetoprotein (AFP) and beta-HCG.

Teratoma is benign in prepubertal age group. Histologically, they contain all three germ layers (ectoderm, mesoderm, and endoderm). Due to their benign nature, testis-sparing approach is warranted. An enucleation of the mass through a tunica albuginea incision is performed if the frozen section confirms the diagnosis (**Figs. 99.20** and **99.21**). Yolk sac tumors commonly present as stage 1 (limited to the testicle and completely resected), and the AFP level will be elevated in the vast majority of cases. Radical inguinal orchiectomy is thus appropriate if AFP is elevated; after surgery, most are observed with serial imaging and tumor markers, provided that other staging workup is negative, with retroperitoneal lymph node dissection and systemic adjuvant chemotherapy being reserved for those with advanced disease (persistent retroperitoneal lymph adenopathy or increased serum markers). Seminomas and mixed germ cell tumors are extremely rare in prepubertal children, and their management should be as in adults. There are gonadal stromal tumors that can mimic a germ cell tumor. The most common are Sertoli cell tumors. They occur as painless masses and usually have no major endocrine effect. Partial orchiectomy through an inguinal incision is recommended. Leydig cell tumors are the second most common stromal tumor. They can be associated with precocious puberty, gynecomastia, and elevated levels of 17-hydroxy ketosteroids. They can be similar to hyperplastic adrenal nodules that are found in boys with poorly controlled congenital adrenal hyperplasia. For all stromal tumors, partial orchiectomy is the preferred initial surgery.

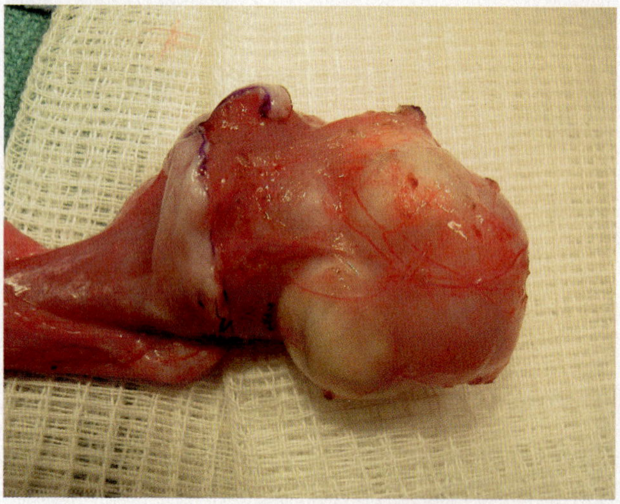

Figure 99.20. Testis-sparing enucleation of prepubertal testis tumor with cystic mass seen on the ultrasound and negative markers, likely indicating a teratoma.

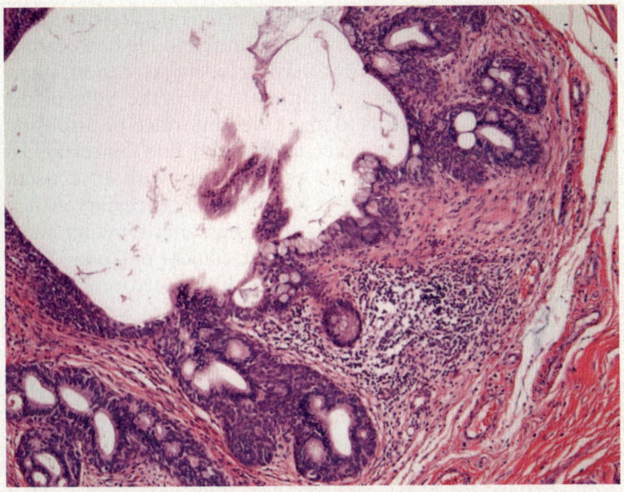

Figure 99.21. Histology of prepubertal testis tumor demonstrating mature teratomatous differentiation into ectodermal elements.

Varicocele

Varicocele is a collection of engorged varicose veins in the spermatic cord and usually is most prominent in the scrotum in the region of the pampiniform plexus. Varicoceles are graded according to their size and prominence. Subclinical or grade 0 varicocele are only detected on imaging and not on physical examination. Grade I are only palpable with Valsalva. Grade II can be palpated without exertion or Valsalva maneuver, and collapse when supine. Grade III are visibly bulging and do not collapse when supine. Varicoceles are most common on the left side comprising >90% of all varicoceles. The left-sided predominance relates to the different nature of the left and right spermatic vein drainage. The right spermatic vein is shorter and inserts directly into the inferior vena cava. About 10% are bilateral. The solitary right varicocele is worrisome as it can be associated with a retroperitoneal tumor and when found, warrants further evaluation with abdominal ultrasound.

Varicoceles come to attention because of two major concerns. First, they can be quite sizable and uncomfortable. Second, varicoceles are associated with infertility. At random, up to 10% to 20% of all adult males can be found to have some form of varicocele. Among men who attend infertility clinics, varicocele-associated subfertility can be as high as 40%. These observations suggest that there are many men in whom a varicocele is a trivial finding, but there are some in whom it can be an important reproductive issue. For males undergoing puberty and sexual maturation, semen analysis findings are variable and unreliable in addition to ethical concerns. For this reason, the clinical indication for intervention in boys is comparative testicular volume on ultrasound. In some, the involved testicle will have a smaller volume or lag in growth. If there is a substantial volume discrepancy (20% or greater) between the testicles, surgery is warranted. If the volumes are stable and there is no major discrepancy, observation with annual ultrasounds is reasonable, although there is a lack of consensus on surgical decision making.[41] There are several methods of treating varicoceles in which the spermatic veins are ligated either laparoscopic intra-abdominally, open or microscopic via a subinguinal, or inguinal incision. The spermatic artery can also be taken, as this has been shown to decrease the rates of recurrence. Sparing of the lymphatic vessels reduces the risk of hydrocele formation.

VAGINAL ANOMALIES

Labial Adhesions

Labial adhesions are commonly incidentally detected on well-child check examinations. They occur when edges of the labia minora attach in the midline and form a thin web of skin (**Fig. 99.22**). This can obstruct the normal path of the urinary stream leading to postmicturition leakage when the girl stands up. Other symptoms include dysuria or UTI. If asymptomatic, then there is no need for treatment and they often resolve spontaneously. Treatment in very mild cases can be successfully achieved with estrogen cream applied to the surface of the webbing over several weeks. For more severe or refractory cases, surgical incision and separation under anesthesia are needed.

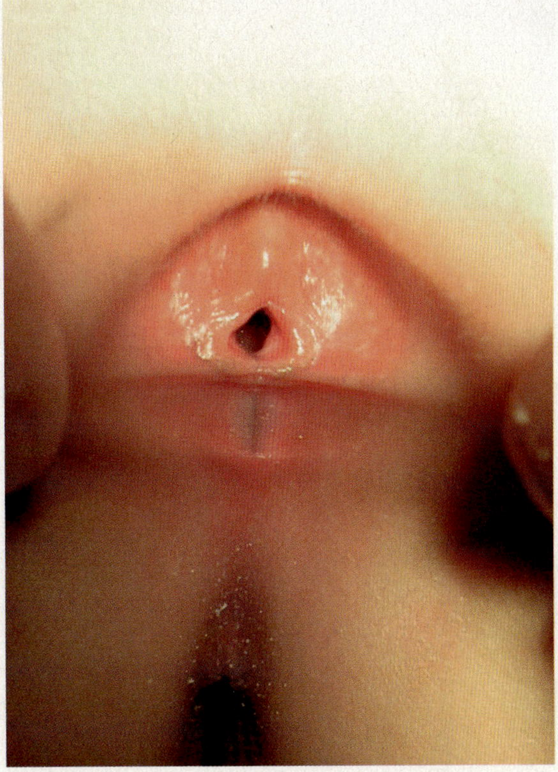

Figure 99.22. Labial adhesions.

Imperforate Hymen

Occasionally the hymen will be imperforate at birth. This will present with a bulging hydrocolpos and can be confused with a prolapsing ureterocele or bladder tumor (such as sarcoma) (**Fig. 99.23**). Ultrasound can usually identify the prominent fluid-filled vagina. Puncture and drainage are usually all that is required. In some older patients the condition may not be diagnosed until after the onset of menses. At this time, there may be cyclic discomfort due to the inability to allow the menstrual flow to pass creating a hydrometrocolpos. After a complete workup, surgical drainage in the operating room is advisable to avoid introducing bacteria into the sterile collection; an infection can lead to pyocolpos or pyometrium, leading to scarring and affecting future fertility.

Urogenital Sinus Anomalies

Between the 5th and 7th week of fetal development, the urogenital sinus forms.[42] The caudal portion forms the lower third of the vagina. The müllerian ducts form the uterus as well as fallopian tubes. Anomalies can occur as part of DSD conditions, resulting in either vaginal agenesis or persistence of a urogenital sinus creating a single urogenital opening with a common channel to the vagina and urethra (such as that seen in masculinized females with congenital adrenal hyperplasia). Surgical reconstruction is usually required to create distinct urethral and vaginal channels. Traditional surgical approach aimed at separating the vagina from the UG sinus tract and bringing it down to the perineum, has often led to vaginal vascular compromise and stenosis. Modern techniques employ urogenital sinus mobilization en bloc, keeping the urethrovaginal confluence intact. Total mobilization has been

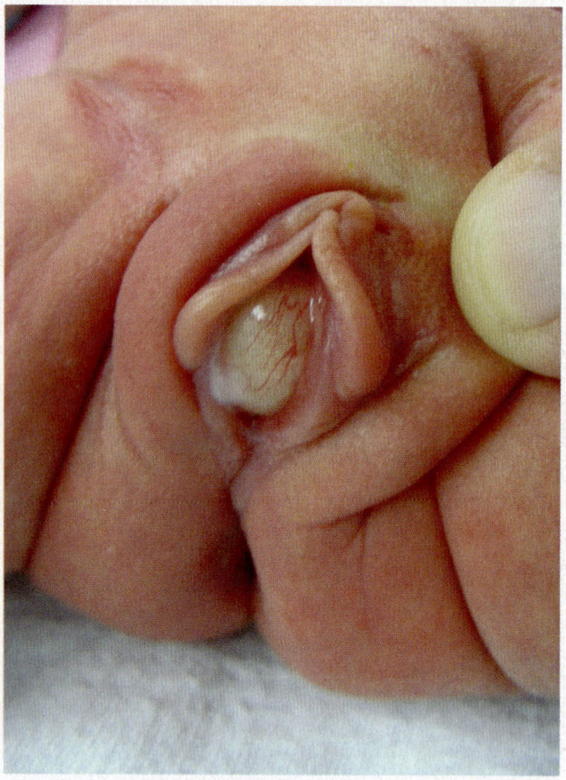

Figure 99.23. Imperforate hymen.

discouraged due to concern for future urinary incontinence and pelvic prolapse. A combination of partial mobilization—leaving the anterior urethral suspensory ligaments intact—and various perineal flaps can result in an excellent outcome. The Mayer–Rokitansky–Kuster–Hauser syndrome occurs in normal genotypic females with vaginal and/or uterine dysgenesis. About one third of these patients will have associated urologic issues—the most common being unilateral renal agenesis. The diagnosis is usually made incidentally or around the age of puberty due to amenorrhea. Treatment is vaginal dilation with estrogen cream or surgical vaginoplasty if dilation fails. There are also a variety of duplication anomalies and vaginal and/or uterine septa and consultation with gynecology is advisable on the necessity and timing of intervention. Typically, the goals are to relieve any obstruction to restore normal menses and to preserve reproductive potential.

Differences in Sex Development

When the genitalia do not develop in a manner that is clearly male or female in appearance, the term differences in sexual development (DSD) is applied.[43] It replaces older terms such as hermaphroditism. This is an evolving field and covers a spectrum of conditions, some of which can pose a significant physiologic and mental health risk. There are important concerns regarding gender assignment and genital reconstruction. For these reasons, children with DSD should receive care at a center with a multidisciplinary DSD clinic comprised of experts from urology, general surgery, gynecology, genetics, endocrinology, social work, psychology, and ethics. This multidisciplinary approach provides comprehensive and systematic evaluation and management of children with DSD.[44]

All patients with suspected DSD require a thorough physical examination, especially of the genitalia and perineum, along with a detailed pregnancy, family, and social history. Evaluations, including electrolytes, steroid levels and precursors, gonadotropins, and karyotype, are typically assessed with further specialized tests ordered as necessary. Imaging includes renal/pelvic ultrasound and genitogram. Magnetic resonance imaging, cystoscopy, laparoscopy, and gonadal biopsies may also be necessary.

Management of DSD is complex and shared decision making with the child (when possible), family, and medical team is critical. Management options may include observation, pharmacotherapy, and/or surgery. Ultimately, it is the right of the affected children's parents to make well-informed decisions on behalf of their child. However, controversy and concern exist regarding the requirement for early surgery without consent by the patient when surgery is not medically necessary. Much of what is known of the long-term outcome remains anecdotal and incomplete, lacking robust clinical outcomes data to guide management during infancy. Continued research on DSD management and outcomes is necessary to better understand how to optimally address the medical, psychological, developmental, and genetic issues for each unique individual with DSD. The primary goal of the care team is to provide parents with as much information about the condition as possible, including the wide range of management options with regard to assigning sex of rearing and the impact it may have on future gender declaration, child development, and medical and surgical management.

ACKNOWLEDGMENTS

We gratefully acknowledge the contributions of previous edition authors, Natalia V. Leva and Hillary Copp, as portions of those chapters have been retained in this revision.

References

1. Baskin L, Shen J, Sinclair A, et al. Development of the human penis and clitoris. *Differentiation*. 2018;103:74–85.
2. dos Santos Junior AC, de Miranda DM, Simões Silva AC. Congenital anomalies of the kidney and urinary tract: an embryogenetic review. *Birth Defects Res C Embryo Today.* 2014;102(4):374–381.
3. Pitts WR Jr, Muecke EC. Horseshoe kidneys: a 40-year experience. *J Urol.* 1975;113(6):743–746.
4. Glassberg KI, Stephens FD, Lebowitz RL, et al. Renal dysgenesis and cystic disease of the kidney: a report of the Committee on Terminology, Nomenclature and Classification, Section on Urology, American Academy of Pediatrics. *J Urol.* 1987;138:1085–1092.
5. Minevich E, Wacksman J, Phipps L, Lewis AG, Sheldon CA. Importance of accurate diagnosis and early close follow-up in patients with suspected MCDK. *J Urol.* 1997;158:1301–1304.
6. Cornec-Le Gall E, Alam A, Perrone RD. Autosomal dominant polycystic kidney disease. *Lancet*. 2019;393(10174):919–935.
7. Verghese P, Miyashita Y. Neonatal polycystic kidney disease. *Clin Perinatol*. 2014;41(3):543–560.
8. Westland R, Schreuder MF, van Goudoever JB, Sanna-Cherchi S, van Wijk JA. Clinical implications of the solitary functioning kidney. *Clin J Am Soc Nephrol*. 2014:9(5):978–986.
9. Grinsell MM, Butz K, Gurka MJ, Gurka KK, Norwood V. Sport-related kidney injury among high school athletes. *Pediatrics*. 2012;130(1):e40–e45.
10. DeFoor W, Minevich E, Tackett L, Yasar U, Wacksman J, Sheldon C. Ectopic ureterocele: clinical application of classification based on renal unit jeopardy. *J Urol.* 2003;169(3):1092–1094.
11. Braga LH, McGrath M, Farrokhyar F, Jegatheeswaran K, Lorenzo AJ. Society for fetal urology classification vs urinary tract dilation grading system for prognostication in prenatal hydronephrosis: a time to resolution analysis. *J Urol.* 2018;199(6):1615–1621.
12. Keating MA, Escola J, Snyder HM 3rd, Heyman S, Duckett JW. Changing concepts in management of primary obstructive megaureter. *J Urol.* 1989;142:636–640; discussion 667–668.
13. Cohen SA, Juwono T, Palazzi KL, Kaplan GW, Chiang G. Examining trends in the treatment of ureterocele yields no definitive solution. *J Pediatr Urol.* 2015;11(1):29.e1–29.e6.
14. Elder JS, Diaz M, Caldamone AA, et al. Endoscopic therapy for vesicoureteral reflux: a meta-analysis. I. Reflux resolution and urinary tract infection. *J Urol.* 2006;175(2):716–722.
15. Vachvanichsanong P. Urinary tract infection: one lingering effect of childhood kidney diseases—review of the literature. *J Nephrol.* 2007;20(1):21–28.

16. Honkila M Hannula A, Pokka T, et al. Childhood urinary tract infections and pregnancy-related complications in adult women. *Pediatrics*. 2020;146(2):e20200610.
17. Peters CA, Skoog SJ, Arant BS, et al. Summary of the AUA guideline on management of primary vesicoureteral reflux in children. *J Urol*. 2010;184(3):1134–1144.
18. Frimberger D, Mercado-Deane MG; Section on Urology; Section on Radiology. Establishing a standard protocol for the voiding cystourethrography. *Pediatrics*. 2016;138(5):e20162590.
19. Routh JC, Inman BA, Reinberg Y. Dextranomer/hyaluronic acid for pediatric vesicoureteral reflux: systematic review. *Pediatrics*. 2010;125(5):1010–1019.
20. RIVUR Trial Investigators; Hoberman A, Greenfield SP, Mattoo TK, et al. Antimicrobial prophylaxis for children with vesicoureteral reflux. *N Engl J Med*. 2014;370(25):2367–2376.
21. Ashley RA, Inman BA, Routh JC, Rohlinger AL, Husmann DA, Kramer SA. Urachal anomalies: a longitudinal study of urachal remnants in children and adults. *J Urol*. 2007;178(4 Pt 2):1615–1618.
22. Inouye BM, Tourchi A, Di Carlo HN, Young EE, Gearhart JP. Modern management of the exstrophy-epispadias complex. *Surg Res Pract*. 2014;2014:587064.
23. Hassett S, Smith GH, Holland AJ. Prune belly syndrome. *Pediatr Surg Int*. 2012;28(3):219–228.
24. Mourtzinos A, Stoffel JT. Management goals for the spina bifida neurogenic bladder: review from infancy to adulthood. *Eur J Pediatr Surg*. 2009;19(4):203.
25. McGuire EJ, Woodside JR, Borden TA, Weiss RM. Prognostic value of urodynamic testing in myelodysplastic patients. *J Urol*. 1981;126:205–209.
26. Clayton DB, Brock JW 3rd. Lower urinary tract obstruction in the fetus and neonate. *Clin Perinatol*. 2014;41(3):643–659.
27. McLeod DJ, Szymanski KM, Gong E, et al; Pediatric Urology Midwest Alliance (PUMA). Renal replacement therapy and intermittent catheterization risk in posterior urethral valves. *Pediatrics*. 2019;143(3):e20182656.
28. Bouty A, Ayers KL, Pask A, Heloury Y, Sinclair AH. The genetic and environmental factors underlying hypospadias. *Sex Dev*. 2015;9(5):239–259.
29. Pippi Salle JL, Sayed S, Salle A, et al. Proximal hypospadias: a persistent challenge. Single institution outcome analysis of three surgical techniques over a 10-year period. *J Pediatr Urol*. 2016;12(1):e1–e7.
30. Aulagne MB, Harper L, de Napoli-Cocci S, Bondonny JM, Dobremez E. Long-term outcome of severe hypospadias. *J Pediatr Urol*. 2010;6:469–472.
31. Johnston AW, Jibara GA, Purves JT, Routh JC, Wiener JS. Delayed presentation of urethrocutaneous fistulae after hypospadias repair. *J Pediatr Surg*. 2020;55(10):2206–2208.
32. Wheeler R, Malone P. Male circumcision: risk versus benefit. *Arch Dis Child*. 2013;98(5):321–322.
33. Doyle SM, Kahn JG, Hosang N, Carroll PR. The impact of male circumcision on HIV transmission. *J Urol*. 2010;183(1):21–26.
34. Morris BJ, Krieger JN, Klausner JD. CDC's male circumcision recommendations represent a key public health measure. *Glob Health Sci Pract*. 2017;5(1):15–27.
35. Docimo SG. The results of surgical therapy for cryptorchidism: literature review and analysis. *J Urol*. 1995;154:1148–1152.
36. Kolon TF, Herndon CA, Baker LA, et al. Evaluation and treatment of cryptorchidism: AUA guideline. *J Urol*. 2014;192(2):337–345.
37. Pettersson A, Richiardi L, Nordenskjold A, Kaijser M, Akre O. Age at surgery for undescended testis and risk of testicular cancer. *N Engl J Med*. 2007;356(18):1835–1841.
38. Jefferies MT, Cox AC, Gupta A, Proctor A. The management of acute testicular pain in children and adolescents. *BMJ*. 2015; 350:h1563.
39. Mellick LB, Sinex JE, Gibson RW, Mears K. Systematic review of testicle survival time after a torsion event. *Pediatr Emerg Care*. 2019;35(12):821–825.
40. Woo LL, Ross JH. The role of testis-sparing surgery in children and adolescents with testicular tumors. *Urol Oncol*. 2016;34(2):76–83.
41. Kolon TF. Evaluation and management of the adolescent varicocele. *J Urol*. 2015;194(5):1194–1201.
42. Jenak R, Ludwikowski B, Gonzalez R. Total urogenital sinus mobilization: a modified perineal approach for feminizing genitoplasty and urogenital sinus repair. *J Urol*. 2001;165(6 Pt 2):2347–2349.
43. Houk CP, Lee PA. Update on disorders of sex development. *Curr Opin Endocrinol Diabetes Obes*. 2012;19(1):28–32.
44. Cools M, Nordenström A, Robeva R, et al. Caring for individuals with a difference of sex development (DSD): a consensus statement. *Nat Rev Endocrinol*. 2018;14(7):415–429.

100

Childhood Tumors

Robin T. Petroze and Erika Adams Newman

Key Points

1. Neuroblastoma occurs in the youngest of children and is the most common solid tumor in infants.
2. The landmark feature of neuroblastoma is broad clinical heterogeneity from spontaneous regression in neonates to deadly refractory metastatic disease in school-age children. This is thought to result from diverse genetic and biologic features that predict prognosis.
3. The genomic alterations that have consistently been shown to predict neuroblastoma prognosis are DNA ploidy, MYCN amplification, loss of heterozygosity (LOH) of chromosome 1p, 17q gain, loss of 14q, and loss of 11q.
4. The International Neuroblastoma Risk Group (INRG) classification system defines pretreatment cohorts based on expected survival at diagnosis. INRG classification includes INRG stage, age, histologic category, grade of tumor differentiation, MYCN status, 11q alterations, and DNA ploidy. These criteria are used to define 16 pretreatment groups that include very low-, low-, intermediate-, and high-risk categories.
5. Anaplasia is the single most important prognostic indicator in children with Wilms tumors, the second most common extracranial tumor in children.
6. In the United States, the standard of care for children with Wilms tumor starts with upfront radical nephrectomy for resectable primary tumors followed by chemotherapy. Radiation is administered to sites of residual and metastatic disease. Tumors with extensive intracaval and hepatic vein extension receive biopsy and neoadjuvant chemotherapy, and may require cardiopulmonary bypass for resection.
7. Treatment of rhabdomyosarcoma requires a multimodal approach that begins with complete surgical excision of resectable lesions and incisional biopsy for tumors that encroach upon contiguous structures, blood vessels, and nerves. Modern therapies are based on prognostic factors and risk of subsequent relapse.
8. Standard surgical care for children with hepatoblastoma is complete primary resection at diagnosis for pretreatment extent of disease (PRETEXT) I and II tumors that do not involve major central venous structures. PRETEXT III and IV tumors undergo biopsy and neoadjuvant chemotherapy with early referral to a liver transplantation center for multifocal or large, central lesions.

From diagnosis through posttherapy surveillance, the surgical team has a pivotal role in ensuring the highest outcomes in the care of children with solid tumors. Surgical decisions guide clinical pathways from the mode of biopsy, staging, central venous access for chemotherapy administration, and definitive tumor resection. These surgical decisions are critical to overall oncologic outcomes and influence treatment intensity. Because pediatric cancers are rare with diverse presentations and histology that differ from adult cancers, the overall care of children with cancer has been improved by multidisciplinary approaches, and pediatric cooperative groups set the standard in current oncologic care. The Children's Oncology Group (COG) in the United States and the International Society of Paediatric Oncology (SIOP) in Europe have made significant progress in conducting clinical and basic science studies of pediatric malignancies and establishing treatment standards. More than 90% of children with cancer in the United States are treated at a center affiliated with the COG.

Compared to adults, the classification of childhood cancer is based on tumor morphology rather than emphasis on primary site in adults. The current classification scheme is the International Classification of Childhood Cancer, Third Edition (ICCC-3) and is used for population-based epidemiologic studies and cancer registries such as the Surveillance, Epidemiology, and End Results (SEER) program, administered by the National Cancer Institute (NCI). Utilization of a standard classification system is useful for comparing incidence and survival across regions and time periods and modifications are standardizing staging documentation to allow risk-stratified comparisons.[1]

INCIDENCE OF CHILDHOOD SOLID TUMORS

Despite a more than 50% decrease in cancer-related mortality in children in the United States since 1975, cancer remains the most common cause of disease-related mortality in children. Each year in the United States, approximately 15,000 children and adolescents younger than 20 years of age are diagnosed with cancer.[2] Leukemia, central nervous system (CNS) tumors, and lymphoma are the most common pediatric malignancies. Neuroblastoma is the most common extracranial solid tumor in children of all ages and the most common cancer in infants. Pediatric solid tumors are a spectrum of different malignancies and behind neuroblastoma, Wilms tumor (WT; nephroblastoma) is the second most common extracranial solid tumor followed by rhabdomyosarcoma. While most pediatric cancer population incidences have remained stable when accounting for improvements in diagnostic modalities, rates of hepatoblastoma and thyroid carcinomas in children were noted to increase between 2003 and 2019, with decreasing rates of melanoma.[1]

Increased utilization of precision medicine in pediatric surgical oncology, including the utilization of next-generation sequencing and targeted immunotherapies, to tailor treatment to individual patients hopes to both decrease treatment morbidity in some tumors while improving outcomes in resistant and refractory cases.[3]

NEUROBLASTOMA

Epidemiology and Genetic Risk

1 Neuroblastoma is the most common cancer in infancy and the most common extracranial tumor in all children. In the United States, approximately 700 children are diagnosed with neuroblastoma each year with minimal change in incidence over the past years.[2] The overall incidence rate is 8.8 per 1,000,000 population with a higher incidence among Caucasians. The overall survival rate for neuroblastoma is 85% based upon SEER data from 2013 to 2019, up 20% from 65% from 1985 to 2000. High-risk neuroblastoma still portends a worse prognosis with 3-year event-free survival (EFS) of 60% with intensive multimodal therapy.[4] There is variability in 5-year survival rates based on age and stage. Survival is highest among infants and children with localized and regional disease. Black and Native American patients with neuroblastoma were found to have a higher prevalence of high-risk neuroblastoma compared with White patients, and have worse EFS. Survival disparities based on race and ethnicity have persisted, and the underlying genetic and biologic basis of this disparity as well as the role of social determinants of health and access is increasingly being studied.[5]

No causal factors for neuroblastoma have been identified, though many studies have evaluated maternal and prenatal exposure risks given the higher incidence in early infancy. Studies examining maternal risks have been conflicting for prior miscarriage, induced abortion, repeat Cesarean birth, and vaginal infection. Associations between premature delivery (<33 weeks), very low birth weight (<1500 g), and neuroblastoma have been observed but results are inconsistent.[6] Parental occupation and environmental exposures have been studied, with an increased risk noted in exposures to aromatic hydrocarbons.[7]

Most cases of neuroblastoma are sporadic and data for inheritance patterns are conflicting. Syndromes with alterations in neural crest development, with some links to other neural crest anomalies such as Hirschsprung disease, neurofibromatosis, and central hypoventilation syndrome, may occur with inherited loss of function mutations of PHOX2B, a regulator of autonomic nervous system development. Genome-wide sequencing studies have located heritable mutations in the anaplastic lymphoma kinase (ALK) gene as the cause of most hereditary neuroblastoma cases.[8] It is recommended that children in families found to have heritable mutations in ALK or PHOX2B undergo screening surveillance with ultrasound and urinary catecholamine metabolites. ALK copy number mutations are also somatically acquired and highly associated with an aggressive clinical phenotype in 5% to 15% of neuroblastoma tumors.[9] Increased germline testing has identified genetic variation in chromosome 6p22 to be associated to sporadic neuroblastoma, which may also be associated with clinically aggressive tumors.[10]

Pathology and Biologic Features

Neuroblastoma originates from embryonic cells of the neural crest that appear along the distribution of sympathetic nervous tissue from the neck to pelvis, most commonly in the adrenal medulla. The precise molecular mechanisms that give rise to embryonic neural crest cells that in turn give rise to neuroblastoma are unknown. The current thinking is that defects in genes that control neural crest differentiation and proliferation underlie tumorigenesis. Peripheral neuroblastic tumors are categorized on a spectrum from malignant neuroblastoma to ganglioneuroblastoma and benign ganglioneuroma.

2 Neuroblastoma tumors have diverse clinical heterogeneity from complete spontaneous regression in neonates to resistant metastatic disease in school-age children. The origins of this disparity are unknown but may be explained by a spectrum of genetic and biologic features that are used to stratify patients for treatment.

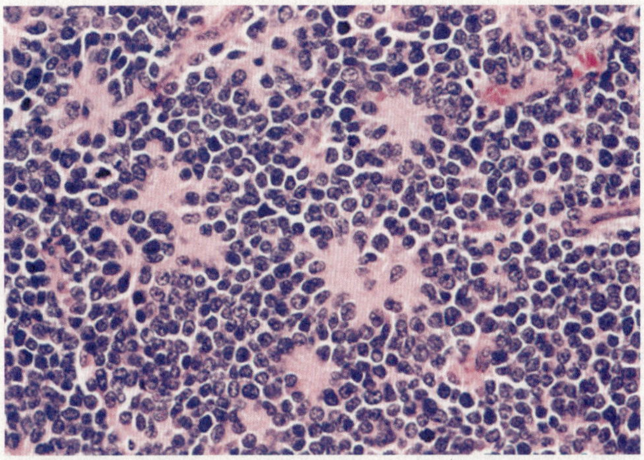

Figure 100.1. Typical neuroblastoma with small round blue cell features and Homer Wright pseudorosettes that palisade around blood vessels.

Neuroblastoma generally occurs in the youngest of children with a median age of presentation of 17 to 19 months.[11] The age at which a child is diagnosed with neuroblastoma is an indicator of biologic features and clinical course. Neonates and infants younger than 18 months of age are more likely to have disease that either spontaneously regresses or is cured without cytotoxic therapy. In contrast, older children are more likely to have refractory metastatic disease and are at high risk for death despite multimodal cytotoxic therapies. Age contributes to prognosis in a continuous manner with the optimal age cutoff between 15 and 19 months.[11] Much of this discrepancy in outcome of neuroblastoma is thought to be associated with underlying tumor biology because there is an association between age and other biologic factors such as MYCN amplification and histopathology. Given this, accurate and complete molecular analysis of neuroblastoma tumor specimen is an important factor in treatment planning and risk stratification.

Cellular heterogeneity is a hallmark of neuroblastoma. Neuroblastic small, round blue cells with hyperchromatic nuclei characterize neuroblastoma cells with varying degrees of differentiation from immature to mature. Homer Wright pseudorosettes that palisade around blood vessels and neuritic processes are characteristic (**Fig. 100.1**). Neuroblastoma cells stain for neuron-specific enolase (NSE), synaptophysin, NB84, and tyrosine hydroxylase, a neural protein-staining pattern that differentiates neuroblastoma from other childhood tumors with similar small round blue cells.

Treatment strategies for children with neuroblastoma are largely based on risk as determined by histopathologic and biologic characteristics of the tumor.[12] The Shimada histopathologic classification system is the most widely accepted standard for microscopic evaluation of neuroblastoma tumors and distinguishes favorable and unfavorable clinical groups. The International Neuroblastoma Pathology Classification System was developed based on the original Shimada system.[13] Morphologic features of neuroblastic differentiation, schwannian stromal development, mitosis–karyorrhexis index (MKI), and patient age at diagnosis determine the important distinction between favorable and unfavorable histology (**Table 100.1**).

CLASSIFICATION

Table 100.1. Shimada Histopathologic Classification of Neuroblastoma

Classification
Favorable
Stroma rich, all ages, no nodular pattern
Stroma poor, age 1.5–5 yr, differentiated, MKI <100
Stroma poor, age <1.5 yr, MKI <200
Unfavorable
Stroma rich, all ages, nodular pattern
Stroma poor, age >5 yr
Stroma poor, age 1.5–5 yr, undifferentiated
Stroma poor, age 1.5–5 yr, differentiated, MKI >100
Stroma poor, age >1 yr, MKI >200
MKI, mitosis–karyorrhexis index (number of mitoses and karyorrhexis per 5000 cells)

Reprinted from Shimada H, Ambros IM, Dehner LP, et al. The International Neuroblastoma Pathology Classification (the Shimada system). *Cancer.* 1999;86(2):364–372. Permission granted for previous edition.

In addition to histopathology, combinations of prognostic features are utilized for risk assignment and treatment stratification. The DNA content (DNA index or ploidy) is the amount of DNA within the nucleus of tumor cells compared to normal cells and is an important indicator of treatment success. DNA index is determined by flow cytometry or by cytogenetic analysis. Hyperploidy or near-triploid tumors (DNA index >1) are whole chromosome gains and losses without structural genetic alterations and are associated with a better response to chemotherapy. In contrast, diploid tumors are characterized by segmental chromosomal alterations and predict poor response to therapy.[12]

The MYCN oncogene is a transcription factor located on chromosome 2p and also predicts survival and risk in neuroblastoma. The amplification of MYCN is the best characterized genetic abnormality, occurring in approximately one-third of neuroblastoma patients, and is associated with high-risk or high-stage disease refractory to cytotoxic therapies and requiring multimodal therapies.[4,14] Significant amplification of MYCN within tumor cells (more than 10 copies detected by fluorescent in situ hybridization) reliably predicts poor survival and advanced-stage disease.

Nerve growth factor (NGF) and its receptor tyrosine kinase (TRK) also correlate with disease outcome in neuroblastoma tumors. The TRK receptors are thought to have a role in regulating growth and differentiation of normal nerve cells and have been implicated in neuroblastoma pathogenesis. The expression of TRK-A, a transmembrane tyrosine kinase that is required for high-affinity binding of NGF, is strongly predictive of a favorable outcome in neuroblastoma tumors. TRK-B, the receptor for brain-derived neurotrophic factor (BDNF) is preferentially expressed in neuroblastoma tumors with MYCN amplification while TRK-C, the primary receptor for neurotrophin-3 (NT-3) mirrors TRK-A and is expressed primarily in lower-stage tumors with favorable outcomes. The absence or lack of TRK-A correlates inversely with MYCN amplification and reliably predicts poor overall survival. Differential expression of TRK-A and TRK-B indicate that NGF receptors may function in growth arrest and differentiation in neuroblastoma tumors, critical factors that may have a role in clinical course.[15]

3 Several nonrandom genomic imbalances have been identified in neuroblastoma and the presence of segmental chromosome alterations is the strongest predictor of neuroblastoma relapse.[16] The loss of heterozygocity (LOH) of chromosome 1p is a reliable prognostic factor in neuroblastoma tumors that is independent of age and stage. The loss of 1p identifies patients who are at high risk of poor survival outcomes despite otherwise favorable biologic predictors (stage 1, 2, and 4S disease). LOH at 1p is most clinically valuable in predicting patients at high risk of death in the subgroup of patients without MYCN amplification, specifically those with low-stage disease. Gain at 17q most commonly occurs with loss of 1p in an unbalanced translocation. The gain of 17q is strongly associated with other negative risk factors including age of more than 1 year, presence of high-stage disease, MYCN amplification, and diploidy.[8] Chromosome 11q loss is found in approximately 40% of neuroblastoma patients and is associated with high-risk disease features and decreased survival. Similar to loss of chromosome 1p, loss of 11q is independently associated with decreased survival in the subgroup of patients with low-stage disease and in patients without MYCN amplification.[17] In all, the genomic alterations that have consistently been shown to predict prognosis are DNA ploidy, MYCN amplification, loss of chromosome 1p, 17q gain, loss of 14q, and loss of 11q, with MYCN amplification and DNA ploidy have the strongest prognostic impact.

Presentation, Diagnosis, and Staging

The majority of children with neuroblastoma are diagnosed at less than 4 years of age, with median age between 19 and 22 months. Forty percent of tumors occur in the adrenal medulla with the remaining occurring in the neck, chest, abdomen, and pelvis along the sympathetic chain. The organ of Zuckerkandl is the second most common site of neuroblastoma of abdominal origin. Compared to older children, infants are more likely to present with thoracic and cervical primary sites. Tumors at the sympathetic chain along the spinal column may expand into the intraforaminal spaces and can cause spinal cord compression (5% to 15% of patients) (**Fig. 100.2**). More than half of patients may present with regional or distant spread through lymphatic and hematogenous routes. Metastatic disease most commonly involves regional lymph nodes, bone marrow, and cortical bone. The most common cortical bone sites are metaphyseal, skull, and the orbit. Patients with orbital bone metastases commonly present with periorbital ecchymosis and swelling (raccoon eyes) and cortical bone metastases may result in generalized bone pain and limping. Liver metastases occur most commonly in patients with stage 4S tumors. Neonates with stage 4S neuroblastoma may present with massive hepatomegaly, respiratory compromise, and abdominal compartment syndrome requiring urgent surgical intervention. Incidental findings on prenatal ultrasound may identify fetal neuroblastoma and there may be associated maternal signs of catecholamine excess with excessive sweating, headaches, flushing, or anxiety.

Most often patients with localized disease are asymptomatic with tumors diagnosed on routine physical examinations or testing for other medical conditions. Abdominal distention and palpable mass may be noted. There are several well-documented clinical syndromes that can be present at diagnosis of neuroblastoma. Opsoclonus/myoclonus syndrome and or ataxia can occur in children with neuroblastoma and present as irregular jerking movements of the muscles. The underlying mechanism of opsoclonus is suggested to be immunologic with late neurologic sequelae despite tumor removal. Most patients with opsoclonus/myoclonus syndrome tend to have localized disease and excellent survival. Up to 50% of patients with opsoclonus/myoclonus syndrome are found to have neuroblastoma tumors while only a small percentage of neuroblastoma patients present with opsoclonus.[18] Neuroblastoma tumors that occur in the neck or upper chest may present with Horner syndrome (ptosis, miosis, anhidrosis), symptoms that may not go away with surgical excision.

Perinatal Neuroblastoma

The improvement of ultrasound and maternal imaging techniques has increased the diagnosis of neuroblastoma within

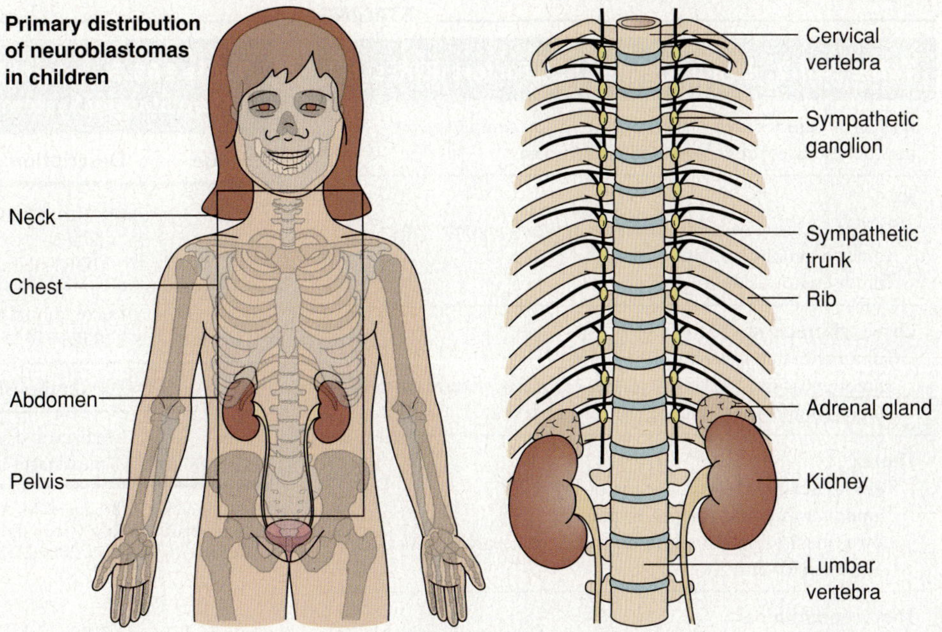

Figure 100.2. Primary distribution of neuroblastoma tumors in children.

the fetal and neonatal periods. Most perinatal tumors are located within the adrenal gland and are localized tumors. Upon detection, tumor growth is monitored with serial ultrasound prior to birth and maternal care proceeds to assure optimal health of the mother. As long as there are no complications, pregnancy is carried to term. Nearly all perinatal cases have favorable biology without adverse prognostic indicators, including non-MYCN amplification. A prospective trial by the COG (ANBL00P2) of expectant observation of infants diagnosed within the first 6 months of life found that observation of small adrenal masses in infants younger than 6 months, without biopsy and without surgical resection was safe with excellent event-free and overall survivals. Adrenal tumors less than 3 cm (16 mL) if solid or 5 cm (65 mL) if ≥25% cystic are safely monitored with ultrasound volume measurements, computerized tomography (CT) scan, and urine catecholamine metabolite levels. If there are signs of tumor growth or increased catecholamines, the patient is referred for surgical resection without risk of upstaging of disease.[19]

Diagnosis

The diagnosis of neuroblastoma requires an adequate biopsy specimen and a pathologist experienced with pediatric tumors. The diagnosis is established with histologic confirmation from either tissue biopsy, which can be performed via core needle biopsy with adequate number of passes or open approach, or the presence of tumor cells within a bone marrow biopsy and increased urinary catecholamine metabolite levels. The majority of patients with neuroblastoma have elevated urinary vanillylmandelic acid (VMA) and homovanillic acid (HVA) levels and these should be evaluated during the diagnostic workup. Complete blood count and serum chemistries are evaluated as components of initial diagnostics. Levels of lactate dehydrogenase (LDH), ferritin, and NSE are biologic markers that may indicate poor prognosis in patients with neuroblastoma. Elevated ferritin (>150) and LDH (>1000) may indicate increased risk of adverse outcomes.[20] As more than half of patients present with metastatic disease at presentation, initial evaluation should include cross-sectional imaging to define the primary tumor size and to determine regional or distant spread (**Fig. 100.3**). Calcifications are commonly detected on imaging in patients with neuroblastoma and the mass tends to displace structures inferiorly and toward the midline. Unless the patient has neurologic symptoms, or an abnormal neurologic examination, lumbar puncture or brain imaging is not indicated. Sympathetic nervous tissue concentrates metaiodobenzylguanidine (MIBG), an analog of norepinephrine. Radioactive iodine–labeled MIBG scan is utilized in neuroblastoma staging and is used to determine treatment response and metastatic spread, particularly cortical bone disease that may have otherwise been missed by traditional imaging techniques. MIBG is a key component of not only diagnosis and monitoring but also treatment regimens.[21] Posterior iliac crest aspirates and core biopsies are required as a component of initial diagnostic testing to exclude bone marrow involvement. PET scanning or bone scans may be utilized in patients with non-MIBG avid disease.

Staging

Standard staging criteria allows physicians to tailor treatment plans based on patient risk. The International Neuroblastoma Staging System (INSS) was previously utilized to standardize risk-group stratification and relied on the surgeon's definition of resectability and surgical approach to the primary tumor and lymph nodes. Given the international variation in surgical decision making and approach to locoregional disease as well as the increasing role of genetic and biologic markers in risk stratification, the International Neuroblastoma Risk Group

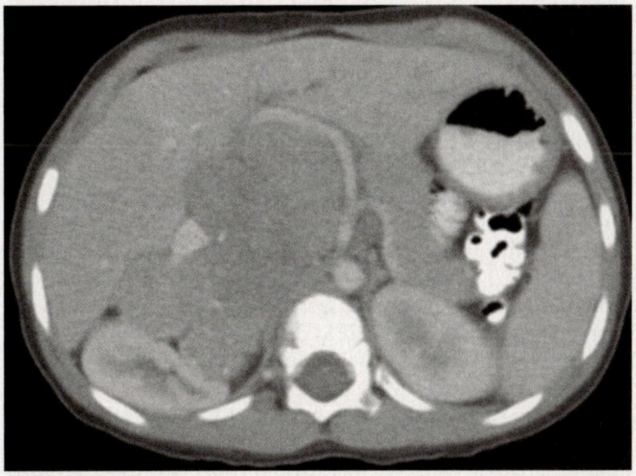

Figure 100.3. Computerized tomography (CT) scan of a child with stage 3 neuroblastoma, crossing the midline displacing the aorta, vena cava, kidney, pancreas, and spleen.

STAGING

Table 100.2. Image-Defined Risk Factors (IDRFs)

Ipsilateral tumor extension within two body compartments (neck/chest, chest/abdomen, abdomen/pelvis)
Neck Tumor encasing carotid, vertebrals, internal jugular vein Tumor extending to base of skull Tumor compressing trachea
Cervicothoracic junction Tumor encasing brachial plexus roots Tumor encasing subclavian vessels, carotid or vertebral artery Tumor compressing trachea
Thorax Tumor encasing the aorta or major branches Tumor compressing trachea or main bronchi Lower mediastinal tumor, infiltrating costovertebral junction between T9 and T12
Thoracoabdominal Tumor encasing the aorta and/or vena cava
Abdomen/pelvis Tumor infiltrating the porta hepatis or hepatoduodenal ligament Tumor encasing branches of the SMA at the root Tumor invading one or both renal pedicles Tumor encasing the aorta and/or vena cava Tumor encasing the iliac vessels Pelvic tumor crossing the sciatic notch
Intraspinal tumor extension More than one-third of the spinal canal in the axial plane is invaded and/or the perimedullary leptomeningeal spaces are not visible, and/or the spinal cord signal is abnormal
Infiltration of adjacent organs/structures Pericardium, diaphragm, kidney, liver, duodenopancreatic block, mesentery
Conditions to be recorded but not considered IDRFs Multifocal primary tumors, pleural effusion with/without malignant cells, ascites with/without malignant cells

From Montclair T, Broduer GM, Ambros PF, et al. The International Neuroblastoma Risk Group (INRG) Staging System: an INRG Task Force Report. *J Clin Oncol.* 2009;27:298–303.

Staging System (INRGSS) was developed utilizing radiographic characteristics of the primary tumor as useful predictors of resectability and risk for developing postoperative complications.[12] INRGSS determines the extent of locoregional disease by the presence or absence of image-defined risk factors (IDRFs) (**Table 100.2**).[22] Stage L1 tumors are localized tumors that are confined within one body compartment and do not involve vital structures or major blood vessels, without any IDRF. L2 tumors are locoregional tumors with one or more IDRF that may involve ipsilateral continuous body compartments and have lower EFSs compared to L1 tumors. Stage M is distant metastatic disease and MS is limited to children less than 18 months with skin, liver, and/or bone marrow metastases (**Table 100.3**). The benefit of INRGSS is that treatment stratification is based on preoperative diagnostic imaging, rather than variable operative approaches. INRGSS now
4 functions as one of the seven prognostic factors in the new INRG pretreatment classification system.[23] The INRG classification system defines pretreatment patient cohorts based on

STAGING

Table 100.3. International Neuroblastoma Risk Group Staging System

Stage	Description
L1	Localized tumor, not involving vital structures as defined by the list of image-defined risk factors (IDRFs) and confined to one body compartment
L2	Locoregional tumor with presence of one or more IDRFs
M	Distant metastatic disease (except MS)
MS	Metastatic disease in children <18 mo with limited metastases at skin, liver, and/or bone marrow

From Montclair T, Broduer GM, Ambros PF, et al. The International Neuroblastoma Risk Group (INRG) Staging System: an INRG Task Force Report. *J Clin Oncol.* 2009;27:298–303.

expected 5-year EFS at the time of diagnosis. INRG classification includes INRG stage, age, histologic category, grade of tumor differentiation, MYCN status, 11q alterations status, and DNA ploidy. These criteria are used to define 16 clinically different pretreatment groups that include very low-, low-, intermediate-, and high-risk categories (A-R) in terms of 5-year EFSs of >85%, >75% to ≤85%, ≥50% to ≤75%, and <50%, respectively. Importantly, INRG classification allows comparison of international risk-based clinical trials (**Table 100.4**).[23]

Treatment

The treatment of neuroblastoma requires a multidisciplinary approach in order to assure the most optimal outcomes. Treatment is often multimodal with surgery, chemotherapy, radiation, bone marrow/stem cell transplantation, and immunotherapy. Risk-group assignment is essential for surgical and medical treatment decisions, as therapies are specifically tailored to risk.[3] Patients are categorized based on INRG classification as non high risk (very low, low, intermediate) or high risk. In general, the overall goal is to minimize surgical risks and to limit exposure to chemotherapy in patients with localized disease and favorable biologic features.

In the United States, the current treatment for children with neuroblastoma is guided by protocols established by the COG and it is recommended that every child be enrolled on a clinical trial. Current clinical trials are evaluating the role of ^{131}I-MIBG and/or immunotherapy with induction chemotherapy as well as the role of tandem stem cell transplant in high-risk neuroblastoma.[4,24]

Very Low risk and Low risk

For tumors that are classified as very low risk and low risk with favorable biologic characteristics (L1, L2, non-MYCN, no 11q alteration), survival rates are >95% with surgery alone without the need for postoperative chemotherapy.[25] Given that low-risk neuroblastomas may present without significant IDRF, surgical standards for low-risk neuroblastoma are to establish diagnosis and to resect as much tumor as safely possible without damage to contiguous structures or major blood vessels. Sampling of nonadherent regional lymph nodes and obtaining adequate tissue for biologic studies is critical.

Chemotherapy in this group is reserved for patients who relapse or have treatment failure. Chemotherapy is also for patients with less than partial primary tumor resection (<50%), disease that compromises organ function or is life-threatening, and patients at risk of developing spinal cord compression. Radiation is reserved for patients with life-threatening symptoms.

Table 100.4. International Neuroblastoma Risk Group Classification System

INRG Stage	Age (Months)	Histologic Category	Differentiation	MYCN Aberration	11q	Ploidy	Pretreatment Risk Group
L1/L2		GN maturing, GNB intermixed					A Very low
L1		Any, except GN maturing or GNB intermixed		NA			B Very low
				Amp			K High
L2	<18	Any, except GN maturing or GNB intermixed		NA	No		D Low
					Yes		G Intermediate
	>18	GNB nodular; neuroblastoma	Differentiating	NA	No		E Low
					Yes		H Intermediate
			Poorly differentiating or undifferentiated	NA			H Intermediate
				Amp			N High
M	<18			NA		Hyperdiploid	F Low
	<12			NA		Diploid	I Intermediate
	12–<18			NA		Diploid	J Intermediate
	<18			Amp			O High
	>18						P High
MS	<18			NA	No		C Very Low
				Amp	Yes		Q High
							R High

From Cohn SL, Pearson ADJ, London WB, et al. The International Neuroblastoma Risk Group (INRG) Classification System: an INRG Task Force Report. *J Clin Oncol.* 2009;27(2):289–297.

Stage MS neuroblastoma tumors without MYCN amplification are very low–risk classification and most often spontaneously regress. Children with MS disease require biopsy of either primary or metastatic tumor, including bone marrow, for biology studies. This subset may be spared both surgery and chemotherapy. Exceptions are patients with massive hepatomegaly causing abdominal compartment syndrome when low-dose chemotherapy and radiotherapy is given to reduce organ dysfunction. Patients with MS tumors may require decompressive laparotomy and ventilator support. In rare and extreme life-threatening cases, treatment may be initiated based on diagnostic imaging alone.

Intermediate Risk

The intermediate-risk group encompasses a broad spectrum of neuroblastoma tumors. The survival rate for patients in this group is between 75% and 90%. All patients in this subgroup receive surgery and chemotherapy. If the primary tumor is resectable without damage to surrounding organs and major blood vessels, then full resection is performed with lymph node sampling for staging upfront. The surgeon should defer to the INRG image-defined risk factors (**Table 100.2**) during assessment for resectability. For L2 tumors with INRG image-defined risk factors and those judged to be unresectable at diagnosis, biopsy is performed with plan for neoadjuvant chemotherapy and delayed surgical resection after four to six cycles of induction chemotherapy. Treatment protocols for intermediate-risk neuroblastoma as well as prognosis are dependent upon patient age, tumor histology, and biologic properties. As more defined risk factors emerge, clinical trials aim at examining reduction in cytotoxic therapy in certain intermediate-risk populations.[26]

High Risk

High-risk neuroblastoma remains one of the most challenging problems in pediatric oncology. High-risk tumors are characterized by undifferentiated neuroblasts with unfavorable histology and poor prognostic indicators (MYCN amplification, 11q alterations, and diploidy). Survival in this group remains poor despite multimodal therapy that includes intensive cytotoxic induction chemotherapy, aggressive surgery, autologous stem cell transplant, posttransplant radiation, additional chemotherapy, and postconsolidation therapy with targeted biologic agents and immunotherapy. While the 3-year EFS has increased with advances like tandem transplant to above 60%, patients who relapse often die of the disease.[4] The initial surgical management of high-risk tumors begins with an adequate operative biopsy and vascular access placement. Initial biopsy can be approached by open or minimally invasive techniques including thoracoscopy, laparoscopy, and percutaneous core biopsy. Obtaining an adequate sample size to allow for histologic and cytogenetic studies is of utmost importance and is the primary focus when determining biopsy technique. An initial biopsy should obtain tissue greater than 1 cubic centimeter of viable tumor tissue with avoidance of placement of the specimen in formalin in order to optimize cytogenetic studies. The adequacy of the biopsy specimen should be confirmed with the pediatric pathologist before leaving the operating room.

Induction chemotherapy is administered to improve tumor resectability and to decrease tumor growth. Most neuroblastoma primary tumors and bone marrow are initially sensitive to chemotherapy and will have high response rates. Standard induction therapy consists of combinations of topotecan, cyclophosphamide, cisplatin, etoposide, doxorubicin, and vincristine.[24]

After induction chemotherapy consisting of four to five cycles, surgical exploration with the goal of gaining local control of the primary tumor is undertaken. Aggressive removal of all primary tumors in high-risk neuroblastoma patients improves survival and decreases local recurrence. Gross total resection of the primary tumor is defined as the removal of all

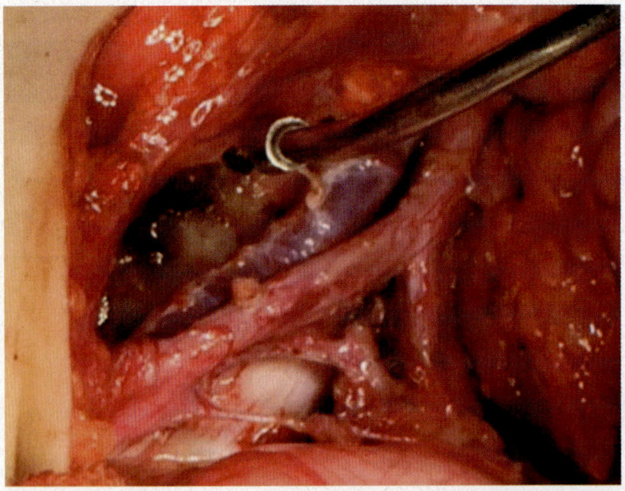

Figure 100.4. Intraoperative depiction of critical exposure during neuroblastoma resection exposing the aorta and vena cava from bifurcation distal to proximal.

visible and palpable neuroblastoma from the primary tumor site and regional lymph node tissue with a goal of >90% resection.[24]

Safe tumor dissection typically requires exposure of the great vessels and spine (**Fig. 100.4**). The incision type depends on the location of the primary tumor with thoracoabdominal or transverse abdominal for large adrenal masses and midline incision for pelvic neuroblastoma. Thoracic neuroblastoma typically has favorable biology and better survival outcomes than abdominal tumors and surgical resection is often curative with primary thoracoscopic gross total resection being safe and achievable. Cervical chain tumors may be approached by radical neck incisions and if located at the lower cervical region or apex of hemithorax, a trap-door incision often utilized in the setting of vascular trauma may be applied. Every effort should be made to preserve the vagus and phrenic nerves. In general, for all neuroblastoma resections, organs and structures should be preserved. The operative complications to avoid are excessive blood loss, kidney and renal vessel injury, damage to surrounding major blood vessels or nerves, and postoperative infection and abscess. The tumor is removed by meticulous dissection in the peritumoral capsular plane. Early control of the aorta and vena cava are essential as the major blood vessels are traced. The major blood vessels in abdominal resections often include the celiac axis, superior mesenteric artery, renal vessels, and inferior mesenteric artery. Tightly adherent tumor to blood vessels or major nerves should be left rather than risk injury though neuroblastoma typically does not invade beyond the adventitia. At times, it is beneficial to divide the tumor over major blood vessels for safe exposure when en bloc resection is not possible at encased blood vessels. Pelvic neuroblastoma typically arises from the organ of Zuckerkandl or elsewhere along the sympathetic chain and is associated with excellent long-term survival, despite residual or microscopic disease. Injuries to the lumbosacral plexus or damage to innervation to the bowel or bladder should be avoided. Selective MRI for pelvic lesions may help define neural involvement and enhance surgical planning as can nerve stimulation. Three-dimensional imaging models developed preoperatively are increasingly being used to guide operative planning and decision making.[27]

Surgery is followed by high-dose myeloablative chemotherapy, autologous stem cell transplantation, and radiotherapy followed by maintenance therapy. Significant improvements in survival were noted with inclusion of immunotherapy (dinutuximab) into treatment regimens as maintenance therapy. ^{131}I-MIBG has been used for MIBG-avid recurrent or refractory disease and is being studied for earlier administration with induction chemotherapy.[24]

Future Directions

Despite advances in cytotoxic and biologic multimodality therapies, up to 60% of patients with high-risk neuroblastoma relapse and there are currently no curative salvage treatment regimens. Advances in understanding neuroblastoma tumor biology are essential for the development of novel therapies for high-risk tumors. The use of high-throughput genomic sequencing technologies will aid in patient-specific prognostic data and allow for a personalized approach to treatment. The success of anti-GD2 monoclonal antibody (dinutuximab) has launched great interest and research into improving antibody-based approaches and synergistic immunotherapies. The timing of radiolabeled MIBG in treatment protocols and its use in rescue are also being investigated in high-risk neuroblastoma.

Challenges also remain in the ability to identify patients with low-risk and intermediate-risk tumors who would benefit from reduction in therapy versus those that are at risk for relapse and refractory disease. Ongoing genomic profiling and tumor sequencing aims at identifying novel mechanisms that drive tumorigenesis and identifying new molecular targets for drug development.

WILMS TUMOR

Epidemiology and Genetic Risk

Various tumors arise in the kidneys in children that range from benign to malignant. WT (nephroblastoma) is the most common renal tumor in children and is the second most common extracranial solid tumor in infants. WTs occur almost exclusively in the kidney. The overall incidence of WT is 6 per million children less than 20 years of age with approximately 500 new cases per year in the United States.[2] However, there are significant global and ethnic variations in WT incidence and outcome. The highest age-standardized incidence rates (ASR) are thought to be in sub-Saharan Africa and the lowest in East Asia. In the United States, the ASR per million-person years is 10.9 for African Americans, 9.9 for White, 7.4 for Hispanic, and 4.4 for Asian and Pacific islanders.[28] While the 5-year EFS is greater than 85% in high-income countries, it is less than 50% in low- and middle-income countries with national cancer care treatment protocols that include WT. Additionally, evidence from Europe suggests that patients in countries with a health system that requires referral from a primary care provider rather than direct access to specialists present at a higher stage with lower 5-year EFS and overall survival.[28]

The mean age at diagnosis is 36 months, with most children presenting between 12 and 48 months. Worldwide, WTs tend to occur earlier in males with a peak incidence at 1 year compared to a 1- to 3-year peak for females.[29] WT is less common under 6 months of age, but still comprises 20% of all renal tumors at this age. Bilateral WTs (BWTs) occur in 4% to 13% of patients.

Children most commonly present within the first 2 years of life in the United States, with nearly all diagnosed before the age of 5 years. The National Wilms Tumor Study (NWTS) reported the median age for WT in boys is 36 months and 43 months for girls with unilateral tumors.[30] BWTs, which occur in 4% to 13% of patients, present at slightly younger. The survival of children with WT has improved significantly over the past 50 years from 30% to over 90% 5-year EFS, with much of this improvement stimulated by clinical trials beginning with the NWTS. Still, up to a quarter of children treated for WT develop severe medical conditions as a result of treatment.[30]

Most WTs are sporadic with only 1% to 2% of cases being familial. Several genetic syndromes are uniquely associated with WT. Sporadic aniridia, hemihypertrophy, genitourinary tract abnormalities, and Beckwith–Wiedemann syndrome are known to be associated with an increased risk of WT in children. The study of patients with sporadic aniridia and Beckwith–Wiedemann syndrome led to the discovery of WT1,

Table 100.5. Syndromes Associated with Increased Susceptibility to Wilms Tumor

Syndrome	Gene	Phenotype
WAGR (Wilms tumor, aniridia, genitourinary abnormalities, mental retardation)	11p13/WT1: deletions, PAX6	Absence of iris, genitourinary defects, mental retardation, 30% develop Wilms tumors
Denys–Drash	11p13/WT1: point mutations	Genitourinary defects, renal mesangial sclerosis and intersex disorder; 90% develop Wilms tumors
Frasier	11p13/WT1: point mutations	Genitourinary defects, focal glomerular sclerosis, and intersex disorder; rarely develop Wilms tumors
Beckwith–Wiedemann	11p15: several genes (IGF2, H19, p57, and LIT1)	Organomegaly including tongue, hemihypertrophy, hypoglycemia, umbilical hernia, increased risk of tumors (Wilms tumor, hepatoblastoma, adrenal carcinoma), 5% develop Wilms tumors
Simpson–Golabi–Behmel	Xq26/GPC3: point mutations, microdeletions	Organomegaly, renal dysplasia, excess digits, diaphragmatic and heart defects, 7.5% develop Wilms tumors
Sotos	5q35/NSD1: point mutations, microdeletions	Overgrowth, craniofacial dysmorphism, mental retardation, and increased risk of tumors (Wilms tumor, neuroblastoma, acute lymphocytic leukemia), 5% of patients develop Wilms tumor
Perlman	Unknown	Macrosomia, visceromegaly, cryptorchidism, excess amniotic fluid, characteristic facial features, 30% of patients develop Wilms tumors
Familial Wilms tumor 1	17q12–21	20% of patients develop Wilms tumors
Familial Wilms tumor 2	19q13,4	70% of patients develop Wilms tumors

GPC3, glypican 3; IGF2, insulin-like growth factor 2; NSD1, nuclear-receptor–binding SET-domain protein 1; PAX6, paired box gene 6; WT1, Wilms tumor protein 1. Reprinted from Rivera MN, Haber DA. Wilms' tumour: connecting tumorigenesis and organ development in the kidney. *Nat Rev Cancer*. 2005;5(9):699–712. Permission received for previous edition.

a tumor suppressor gene located on chromosome 11p necessary for normal renal development.[31] **Table 100.5** lists known genetic syndromes associated with increased susceptibility to WT.

Pathology and Biologic Features

WTs arise from pluripotent developmental renal precursor cells. In most cases, only one kidney is affected but may present as bilateral disease. WTs arise within the renal medulla and cortex and may invade renal calyces, renal vein, and inferior vena cava. The tumor is most commonly a well-circumscribed mass with a fibrous capsule. The most common sites of metastatic spread are lungs, lymph nodes, and liver. WTs are composed of a classic triphasic combination of blastemal, stromal, and epithelial cells. Characterization of histologic subtype is critical for risk stratification and for treatment planning. Blastemal predominance may indicate a high-risk category of patients with increased risk of recurrence.[32] Importantly, anaplastic cells characterize at least 10% of WTs and are defined by the presence of enlarged nuclei and hyperchromasia with multipolar polypoid mitotic figures (**Fig. 100.5**).[33] Compared to tumors without anaplasia, anaplastic WTs are generally found in older children, are more likely to have lymph node metastases, and are more common in BWT patients. Differences in race are also observed with African or Latin American children having the highest proportion of tumors with anaplasia. Tumors with diffuse anaplasia (present in more than one area of the tumor or extrarenal sites) are defined "unfavorable
5 histology" and have higher resistance to chemotherapy compared to tumors without anaplasia. Diffuse anaplastic Wilms tumor (DAWT) has been evaluated as a separate entity in treatment protocols as compared to focal anaplastic Wilms tumor (FAWT) due to their different characteristics in terms of age, stage, and outcome. The single most important prognostic indicator in WTs is the presence of anaplasia.[33]

Clear cell sarcoma and rhabdoid tumor of the kidney are also unfavorable histologic subtypes and are considered distinct entities from WTs.[28] Nephrogenic rests represent the persistence of developmental renal tissue in the kidney after the 36th week of gestation and 1% undergo malignant transformation to WT. Two major categories of nephrogenic rests have been characterized, perilobar (PL) and intralobar (ILNR), distinguished by their position within the renal lobe. Nephrogenic rests are considered precursor lesions of WT and are found in nearly half of cases. Nephroblastomatosis is the term used to describe the presence of diffuse nephrogenic rests and typically

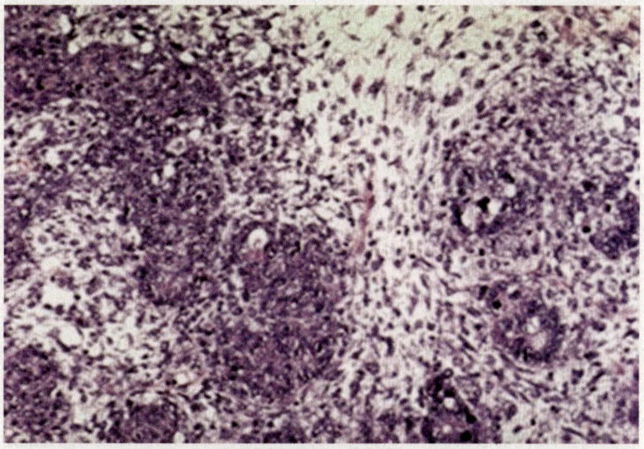

Figure 100.5. Microscopic examination of Wilms tumor showing highly cellular areas composed of undifferentiated blastemal with loose surrounding stroma with undifferentiated mesenchymal cells and immature tubules. (Reprinted with permission from Strayer DS, Saffitz JE, Rubin E. *Rubin's Pathology*. 8th ed. Wolters Kluwer; 2020. Figure 22.91.)

involves both kidneys. The presence of nephrogenic rests demonstrates the vast degree of heterogeneity in WT biology as they either involute or progress to hyperplastic overgrowth or neoplastic induction. Patients with nephrogenic rests are at risk for bilateral kidney involvement that decreases with age.[34]

Several biologic factors have been identified in WTs that associate with risk. Tumor-specific loss of heterozygosity (LOH) at chromosomes 1p and 16q are independent prognostic indicators. Following data from the fifth National Wilms Tumor Study Group trial (NWTS-5) found that tumors with LOH at 16q and 1p are associated with greater risk of relapse and mortality, trials AREN0532 and AREN0533 showed that augmentation of chemotherapy in this patient population resulted in improved EFS. Additional molecular markers include gain of 1q as a negative prognostic indicator that may require therapy augmentation.[32]

Presentation, Diagnosis, and Staging

Children may present with a palpable asymptomatic abdominal mass identified by parents, other caregivers, or a pediatrician during a well-visit examination. If present, symptoms may include intermittent abdominal pain, gross or microscopic hematuria (25% of patients), and hypertension (25% of patients). Hypertension occasionally results from either an increase in renin secretion by the tumor or by compression of the renal artery by tumor mass effect. Intraparenchymal bleeding and preoperative rupture may occur causing systemic symptoms of fever and anemia. The mass is typically nontender and nonmobile on physical examination. The child should be examined for aniridia, macroglossia, hemihypertrophy, and genitourinary abnormalities. Signs of intravascular spread may present as ascites, hepatosplenomegaly, and cardiac murmur. Standard complete blood count and serum chemistries should be assessed though renal function is usually unaffected.

The diagnostic imaging workup is initiated with abdominal ultrasound and CT scan with intravenous contrast. It is not uncommon for children to have an abdominal radiograph, which may show mass effect with displacement of bowel. CT scan is the standard imaging modality that will provide information about mass location, size, extent of tumor invasion, and involvement of the contralateral kidney (**Fig. 100.6**). Critical examination of renal vasculature and intracaval extension is evaluated by Doppler ultrasonography. Chest imaging with radiograph or contrasted CT scan is critical to determine if a patient with WT has lung metastases because these patients are assigned to higher disease stage and receive radiation to the lungs and more intensive chemotherapy. It may be beneficial to obtain histopathologic confirmation of pulmonary metastases by surgical biopsy, often after the first two cycles of chemotherapy if still present on interval imaging, to determine the need for whole lung radiation with newer trials integrating surgical excision of pulmonary metastases to minimize lung radiation in select patients.

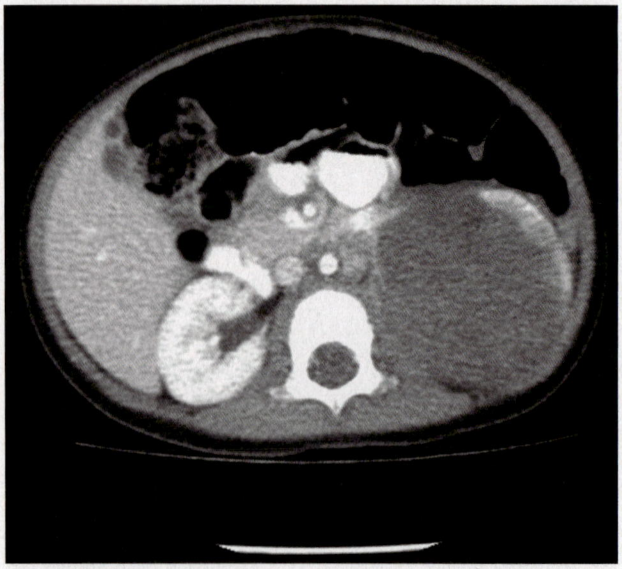

Figure 100.6. Abdominal CT scan with left Wilms tumor displacing midline organs and vessels, rim of kidney enhancing at lateral border.

In the United States, upfront nephrectomy usually follows the initial diagnostic workup allowing the combination of surgical and histologic parameters to be included in staging at diagnosis. During the procedure, the surgeon must determine tumor extent, preoperative tumor rupture, intraoperative tumor spill, and the status of regional, para-aortic and paracaval lymph nodes. Distant metastatic disease should also be determined by inspecting the peritoneal surfaces, diaphragm, and liver. The COG no longer recommends direct visualization and manual palpation of the contralateral kidney as long as the contralateral kidney is clear of tumor on cross-sectional imaging.[29]

The staging of WT is based on the anatomy of the tumor and lymph nodes as detailed by the National Wilms Tumor Study Group (NWTSG) staging system. The staging system incorporates clinical, surgical, and pathologic information and allows stage-based approach to treatment to minimize exposure to cytotoxic agents (**Table 100.6**). Tumor stage and histology are the most significant prognostic factors for children with WT.[29]

Treatment

Most children diagnosed with WT are cured by multimodal therapy. Much of the success in therapy is the result of collaboration and research trials conducted by three cooperative groups, the NWTSG, now a part of the COG, the United Kingdom Children's Cancer Study Group (UKCCSG), and the SIOP. In the United States and Canada, nearly all children are treated according to protocols established by the NWTSG. The primary goals of therapy are to treat based on well-defined risk groups and to achieve the highest cure rates with minimal toxicity. However, the treatment regimens, including the role of upfront nephrectomy versus neoadjuvant chemotherapy and radiotherapy protocols, differ throughout the world.[29]

Table 100.6. Wilms Tumor Staging Criteria

Stage	Criteria	4-Year Survival Rate (%)
1	Tumor is limited to kidney, completely excised; no evidence of rupture, intact surface	97
2	Tumor extends beyond kidney but completely excised, infiltration through renal capsule, extension into vessels outside kidney, local or open biopsy or spillage confined to flank, no residual tumor	95
3	Residual nonhematogenous tumor	91
4	Hematogenous metastases to lung, liver, cortical bone, brain, other organs	78
5	Bilateral renal involvement at diagnosis'	Same as highest unilateral stage

Survival based on outcome form patients with favorable biology in the National Wilms Tumor Study-3.
Courtesy of the National Wilms Tumor Study.

6 Surgery is a critical component of local primary tumor control and treatment outcomes. In the United States, the standard of care starts with radical nephrectomy at the time of diagnosis of resectable primary tumors followed by chemotherapy and radiation to sites of residual and metastatic disease. Importantly, the presence of metastatic disease, particularly lung metastases, does not preclude upfront resection. Preoperative chemotherapy is given to patients with inoperable tumors, bilateral disease, solitary kidney, and for tumors with intravascular extension in the retrohepatic vena cava or above the hepatic veins. When considering the potential for uprfront nephrectomy, surgical equipoise and decision making regarding the ability to perform a safe nephrectomy and minimize complications can be aided through preoperative review by multidisciplinary tumor boards. A significant number of patients are downstaged after preoperative chemotherapy without altering recognizable anaplasia.[29,33] In contrast to this treatment approach, SIOP therapy begins with chemotherapy administration for several weeks prior to nephrectomy in all patients presenting with WTs. Many international protocols utilize SIOP protocols, including in sub-Saharan Africa where treatment abandonment is a significant morbidity postoperatively.[28]

The standard chemotherapeutic drugs with activity against WTs are vincristine and actinomycin D. Doxorubicin is added to patients with stage 3 tumors and to those with unfavorable histology or adverse biologic prognostic markers such as LOH at chromosome 1p or 16q or gain of 1q. Doxorubicin has significant cardiotoxicity, and evaluation of late term effects of treatment in WT survivors impacts treatment protocols. Combinations of cyclophosphamide, ifosfamide, carboplatin, and etoposide are utilized for select stage 3 and 4 cases with unfavorable biology and for resistant or relapsed cases. In the United States, the optimal combination, duration, and mode of administration of chemotherapy are optimized through clinical trials and studies of the NWTSG and COG. Refinement of treatment regimens based on the results of these studies and a better understanding of biologic and clinical prognostic factors looks to incorporate therapy augmentation or reduction in a more precise manner.[29]

Survival rates for children with WT in the United States have steadily improved with shorter chemotherapy schedules and lower treatment costs. Patients are stratified into very low-, low-, standard-, and high-risk groups based on tumor histology, stage, biologic assessment, tumor weight, and age to help determine treatment regimen. The current overall survival rate for children with favorable histology WT is over 90%. A subgroup of children younger than 2 years at diagnosis with very low-risk favorable histology WTs weighing less than 550 g are treated with surgery alone. Stage 1 and 2 favorable histology WTs receive two-drug postoperative chemotherapy (vincristine and actinomycin D) versus a three-drug regimen (addition of doxorubicin) and potential augmented regimens for the higher stages. Patients at any stage with biomarkers identified as a subgroup of favorable histology patients who have a significantly increased risk of relapse and death receive augmented chemotherapy. Abdominal radiation is added for any stage tumor with unfavorable histology or stage 3 or 4 tumors. In patients with stage 5 disease (BWT), the primary tumor is staged separately to determine the requirement for abdominal radiation. Patients with BWTs are treated with preoperative chemotherapy (vincristine, actinomycin D, doxorubicin) and renal-sparing surgery. Lung radiotherapy is currently utilized if metastases remain detectable after 6 weeks (two cycles) of chemotherapy. Surgical resection may be indicated for solitary pulmonary nodules that persist to determine the need for whole lung radiation.[29]

Surgical Considerations

Preoperative biopsies are contraindicated unless a tumor is surgically unresectable. Unilateral radical ureteronephrectomy with abdominal exploration is accomplished through a wide transverse abdominal incision that will allow safe resection and regional lymph node sampling without rupture. A thoracoabdominal incision may be utilized as necessary for tumors reaching beyond the diaphragm. There have been reports of laparoscopic resection of WT that may be more feasible after preoperative chemotherapy with lower risk of tumor rupture. Success of laparoscopy for WT is hindered by tumor spill and by inaccurate staging.[35] Complete abdominal and pelvic exploration is performed, noting and sampling any ascites fluid that may indicate preoperative tumor rupture. The contralateral kidney does not require exploration if preoperative imaging does not suggest involvement. The lateral peritoneal reflection is incised, and the colon is reflected medially. Extension of the tumor through the colonic mesentery can be seen with preoperative rupture and increases the risk of local recurrence. Lymph node sampling rather than a formal retroperitoneal lymph node dissection is recommended, and lack of adequate lymph node sampling along with the primary tumor resection automatically upstages treatment to stage 3 disease because of the risk of local relapse. Gentle handling of the tumor is critical to avoid tumor rupture and spillage. Both local and diffuse tumor rupture will increase relapse risk and upstages the tumor to a Stage 3. It is often unsafe to attempt to ligate the renal vein prior to tumor manipulation given the size of most WTs as traditionally recommended by most authors. Later ligation of the renal vein after tumor mobilization has not been shown to adversely affect survival outcomes and early ligation should not be attempted if technically difficult.[35] The dissection is carried out along the tumor capsule and outside of Gerota fascia identifying the renal hilum and isolating the renal artery, vein, and the ureter (**Fig. 100.7**). The renal vein and inferior vena cava are palpated for intravascular tumor extension. The ureter is palpated for tumor and divided as distal as possible from the renal hilum. The tumor and kidney are then removed en bloc. The adrenal gland may be left in place if it is not adherent to the tumor or if the tumor arises from the lower pole of the kidney. Titanium clips should be utilized to identify any gross residual tumor. The tumor and nephrectomy specimen should not be placed into fixative but delivered fresh and sterile to the pathologist to optimize histologic and cytogenetic analysis based on pediatric tumor protocols.[35]

Patient selection for preoperative chemotherapy is a critical step in surgical and treatment planning. The overall incidence of surgical complications in patients undergoing nephrectomy for WT is over 10%. The most common surgical complications are small bowel obstruction, excessive hemorrhage, wound infection, and vascular injury.[35] Higher-stage tumors, intravascular extension, and resection of contiguous organs are risk factors associated with surgical complications. The risk of renal insufficiency after unilateral nephrectomy for WT is low (0.25%) and patients with Denys–Drash syndrome are most at risk for progressive tumor in the remaining kidney.[35] For these reasons, nephron-sparing procedures are currently reserved for children with BWT and for those at risk for developing renal failure, and not indicated for patients with standard unilateral tumors with a normal contralateral kidney.

Renal Vein/Inferior Vena Cava

Four percent to 10% of patients with WT have intravascular extension into the renal vein or inferior vena cava, with less than 1% extending into the atrium. Patients may have symptoms of vascular involvement depending on the degree of venous obstruction that may include hypertension, hepatosplenomegaly, ascites, and heart failure. The preoperative ultrasonography and CT scan are accurate in detecting intravascular tumor extension, but the vessels should still be palpated prior to ligation of the renal vein during tumor excision. Studies of WTs with intravascular extension have found that preoperative chemotherapy facilitates resection by decreasing the extent of tumor thrombus. Control of the renal vessel and

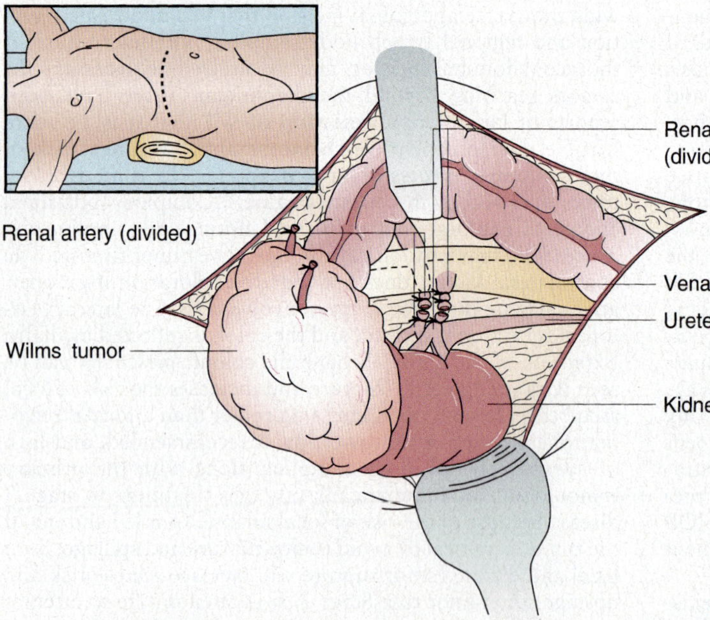

Figure 100.7. Anatomy and operative approach to resection of a Wilms tumor.

vena cava below and above the tumor thrombus is essential to obtain vascular control and to minimize bleeding after venotomy. Effort should be made to avoid transecting tumor thrombus. If the patient has intracardiac tumor extension after preoperative chemotherapy, a combined thoracoabdominal incision with cardiopulmonary bypass is the safest surgical approach for tumor thrombus excision.[36]

Bilateral Wilms Tumor

Five percent to 8% of patients with WTs present with bilateral disease. BWT is associated with worse oncologic outcomes as well as a higher incidence of end-stage renal disease (1% 20-year incidence in unilateral vs 12% in bilateral).[37] BWT is found more frequently in patients with predisposition syndromes such as hemihypertrophy and genitourinary anomalies. All children with BWTs should receive preoperative chemotherapy with the goal of renal preservation, and chemotherapy may commence without the need for biopsy. Current COG therapy based on the AREN0534 study commences with 6 weeks (2 cycles) of vincristine, acintomycin D and doxorubicin. Reevaluation by abdominal CT scan after 6 weeks of chemotherapy is done to assess treatment response. Bilateral nephron-sparing surgery is conducted if amenable, and biopsy is recommended if there is not significant tumor response to assess for anaplasia and treatment intensification. The goal is that all children with BWT will undergo definitive surgical excision by 12 weeks of chemotherapy. AREN0534 demonstrated improved 4-year EFS (82%) and overall survival above 90%. Over 80% of patients underwent definitive surgical resection by 12 weeks with the following surgical breakdown: unilateral total nephrectomy with contralateral partial nephrectomy (48%), bilateral partial nephrectomy (35%), unilateral total nephrectomy (10.5%), unilateral partial nephrectomy (4%), and bilateral total nephrectomies (2.5%).[37]

Partial Nephrectomy

Nephron-sparing surgery is utilized in patients with BWT and in select patients at high risk for bilateral disease or renal failure. Partial nephrectomy is not indicated in patients with standard unilateral WT given the low risk of renal failure (1%) with unilateral nephrectomy. A radionucleotide renal scan (dimercaptosuccinic acid/DMSA scan) is useful to assess preoperative and postoperative renal function.

Partial nephrectomy is typically feasible only if tumor involves one pole and less than one-third of the kidney and if the collecting system and renal vein are uninvolved. For bilateral tumors, the kidney with the lowest tumor burden is addressed first to determine if partial nephrectomy is feasible. Tumor resection is accomplished by opening Gerota fascia and mass excision via wedge resection with 0.5- to 1.0-cm margin of normal renal parenchyma. Enucleation may be considered for large centrally located lesions. Improved surgical techniques and intraoperative ultrasound have vastly improved the safety and feasibility of nephron-sparing surgery in children at risk of postoperative renal failure.

Future Directions

Future studies will continue to focus on personalized treatment plans based on tumor biology and patient risk stratification to further improve curative outcomes while minimizing toxicity with refined stratification based on tumor-specific biologic properties.[3] Next-generation exome precision sequencing has enhanced the capacity to identify disrupted molecular pathways in WTs such as changes in DNA methylation or chromatin structure in WTs. Epigenetic changes at the imprinted region at chr11p15.5 show an allele-specific pattern of methylation resulting in abnormal expression of IGF2 that may be a therapeutic target.[29]

NON-WILMS RENAL TUMORS

Congenital Mesoblastic Nephroma

Congenital mesoblastic nephroma (fetal renal hamartoma) is the most common renal neoplasm in neonates and infants younger than 3 months of age, including in the prenatal period. In contrast to WT, classic congenital mesoblastic nephroma is considered a benign solid tumor of infancy, occurring in a younger age group with an excellent overall prognosis. Almost all cases are diagnosed within the first 6 months of life. Congenital mesoblastic nephroma has distinctive spindle cell histopathologic and clinical features that are generally considered benign and rarely metastasizes to other organs. The cellular variant of congenital mesoblastic nephroma has been found to have a translocation (t12;15) (p13;q25) that results in ETV6-NTRK3 fusion protein, a genetic alteration also found in congenital infantile fibrosarcoma. Similar to congenital infantile fibrosarcoma, trisomy 11 is also found in the cellular subtype of congenital mesoblastic nephroma. These chromosomal aberrations distinguish the cellular variant of congenital mesoblastic nephroma from the classic variant.[38]

Congenital mesoblastic nephroma may be identified prenatally in up to 70% of patients. Polyhydramnios may be present. Postnatally, hematuria or hypercalcemia may be present. The diagnostic workup precedes in much the same manner as WT and the lesions are often not discernible on physical examination or preoperative imaging. The standard treatment for congenital mesonephric nephroma is complete surgical resection with nephrectomy. Wide margins are recommended because these tumors can infiltrate surrounding renal parenchyma and perinephric tissues. Local recurrence, though rare, has been reported and is associated with the cellular variant. Systemic chemotherapy is reserved for tumors that recur and in rare cases of metastases or unusually cellular histology.[38]

Clear Cell Sarcoma

Clear cell sarcoma of the kidney is a rare renal neoplasm of childhood, formerly known as a "bone metastasizing tumor of the kidney" from its original 1970 description.[38] The median age of diagnosis of clear cell sarcoma of the kidney is 36 months and the tumor is one of the "unfavorable histology" tumors studied by the NWTSG and the COG. There is a male predominance with male-to-female ratio of 2:1. Clear cell sarcoma of the kidney has morphologic diversity and is composed of sarcomatous, nonepithelial cells. The classic microscopic pattern of clear cell sarcoma of the kidney is cords of round or spindle-shaped cells with clear cytoplasm and frequent empty-appearing "Orphan Annie" nuclei. Necrosis is associated with poor prognosis and tumors without necrosis are more often stage 1 tumors with superior outcomes.[39] Recent developments in molecular genetics have identified the presence of internal tandem duplications in BCL-6 coreceptor (*BCOR*) and a translocation t(10;17) creating the fusion gene *YWHAE-NUTM2B/E*. Immunohistochemistry for BCOR is widely available and a sensitive and specific marker for clear cell sarcoma in pediatric renal tumors.[39]

Necrosis and hemorrhage are common in clear cell sarcomas of the kidney. Radiographic skeletal survey and radionucleotide bone scan is critical to determine if there are bone metastases at diagnosis. Patients may also have lung, brain, or liver metastases and therefore should have chest and CNS imaging prior to initiation of chemotherapy for accurate staging. The staging system is similar to WT. There is a high rate of metastases and relapse in early-stage tumors and intensive chemotherapy is utilized for all cases. There is propensity for late relapse and patients are monitored with abdominal imaging, chest radiograph, brain MRI, and bone scans.[38]

Rhabdoid Tumor of the Kidney

Rhabdoid tumor of the kidney is a rare and aggressive cancer in infancy. Rhabdoid tumors may occur as separate CNS primary tumors and up to 15% of patients with rhabdoid tumor of the kidney develop CNS lesions. The overall prognosis of patients with rhabdoid tumor of the kidney remains poor and age is an important prognostic factor.[38] Histologically, rhabdoid tumors resemble rhabdomyosarcomas but lack skeletal muscle markers or myoblastic differentiation. Rhabdoid tumors are characterized by loss-of-function mutations of the tumor suppressor gene hSNF5/INI1 located at chromosome 22q11.[38]

Patients with malignant rhabdoid tumor of the kidney present with a palpable abdominal mass and often have hematuria. The diagnostic workup proceeds with an abdominal CT scan showing a large heterogeneous solid mass with areas of necrosis, hemorrhage, or calcifications. Evaluation for CNS disease should also occur at diagnosis because of the frequency of CNS primaries and metastases in patients with rhabdoid tumors.[38]

Renal Cell Carcinoma

Renal cell carcinoma is the most common renal malignancy in adults but rare in pediatric patients. Interestingly, the adult and pediatric morphologies are different. The tumor is highly aggressive with frequent distant metastases. The median age of diagnosis of renal cell carcinoma in children is 9 to 10 years and children who have previously received cytotoxic chemotherapy may have predisposition to developing this cancer. Over the age of 14, renal cell carcinomas outnumber WTs.[40] Pediatric renal cell carcinoma differs from adult renal cell cancer with distinct clinical and biologic differences. Papillary and translocation (Xp11.2 translocations) subtypes are more common in children. Patients with von Hippel–Lindau syndrome may present with bilateral renal cell carcinoma. Tuberous sclerosis, Birt–Hogg–Dube syndrome, and hereditary leiomyomatosis are other hereditary syndromes associated with renal cell carcinoma.[40]

Patients may present with a large palpable abdominal mass. Abdominal pain, hematuria, weight loss, joint pain, and anorexia may also be present. Cross-sectional abdominal and pelvic imaging (CT scan or MRI) along with chest radiograph and/or chest CT scan is critical to define the locoregional extent of the mass and to determine metastatic spread. Distant metastatic disease is present in up to 30% of pediatric patients at diagnosis, most commonly to lung, liver, and bone. Local lymph node involvement does not necessarily predict poor outcome in renal cell carcinoma in children. Calcifications on imaging are more common in children with renal cell carcinoma compared to WT.[40]

If the mass is resectable at diagnosis, standard treatment is radical nephrectomy with lymph node sampling followed by combination adjuvant chemotherapy, immunotherapy, and radiotherapy-based on surgical pathology. The role of lymph node dissection for renal cell carcinoma has not been determined. Partial nephrectomy is reserved for patients at high risk of postoperative renal failure and multiple renal tumors, particularly patients with genetic syndrome–related disease. There are reports of successful partial nephrectomy for small, unilateral, low-stage tumors. The role of chemotherapy is unproven, as the administration of chemotherapy has not significantly improved survival outcomes. There is some evidence that immunotherapy (IL-2) (sunitinib) may be beneficial in select cases of renal cell carcinoma.[40]

RHABDOMYOSARCOMA

Epidemiology and Genetic Risk

Rhabdomyosarcoma is the most common soft tissue sarcoma in children with an overall incidence of approximately 350 cases per year in the United States.[2] The median age of presentation is 7 years of age and the majority of patients are diagnosed prior to 10 years of age. There is a slight male predominance and a slightly higher incidence in African American children.[2] Rhabdomyosarcoma tumors are classified as either embryonal, alveolar, spindle cell/sclerosing, or pleomorphic histologic subtypes.[41]

Embryonal rhabdomyosarcoma (60% to 70%) is the most frequent histologic type and occurs in children younger than 4 years of age. Alveolar rhabdomyosarcoma (30%) and pleomorphic subtypes (1%) occur more commonly in older children. Alveolar rhabdomyosarcoma has associated translocations in fusion genes in 80% of cases (PAX3 or PAX7 and FOX01 genes), and fusion status is increasingly used in treatment and prognosis decision trees.[42,43]

The overall incidence of rhabdomyosarcoma has not changed much in the last 30 years although there has been an increase in incidence of the alveolar subtype and in cases presenting with distant metastases. The overall survival for rhabdomyosarcoma has increased in the last four decades, largely due to improvements in multimodal therapies including radical surgery, intensive combination chemotherapy and radiotherapy. Patients with embryonal subtype have the best overall survival. Patients with smaller-sized tumors and favorable anatomic sites also have significant survival advantage. Age relates independently to survival outcomes with infants

(<1 year of age) and adolescents (>10 years of age) more likely to have poor outcome and unfavorable histologic features.[41,42]

Rhabdomyosarcoma can be associated with congenital malformations, most commonly the CNS and genitourinary systems.[42] Genetic predisposition syndromes such as Li-Fraumeni syndrome, other p53 germline mutations, neurofibromatosis type I, Beckwith–Wiedemann syndrome, Noonan syndrome, nevoid basal cell carcinoma syndrome and others have an increased risk of rhabdomyosarcoma. Environmental factors have also been found to have a role in the development of rhabdomyosarcoma as have parental use of recreational drugs, including cocaine and marijuana.[43]

Pathology and Biologic Features

Rhabdomyosarcoma is a heterogeneous group of tumors. The origin is thought to be embryonal mesenchyme that gives rise to striated skeletal muscle. The use of immunohistochemical markers such as desmin, myogenin, and myogenic differentiation 1 (MYOD1) is useful in diagnosis.[42] Although rhabdomyosarcoma can occur in any skeletal muscle group, it most commonly affected sites are head and neck, trunk, and genitourinary.

Embryonal rhabdomyosarcoma is a heterogeneous subtype with histologic features that range from primitive mesenchymal cells to highly differentiated muscle cells. The small round blue cells consist of nuclei that are generally small with a light chromatin pattern. The microscopic pattern is moderately cellular with loose myxoid stroma.[42] Embryonal rhabdomyosarcoma comprises up to 75% of rhabdomyosarcoma tumors and is considered an intermediate prognosis tumor in terms of outcomes. Alveolar rhabdomyosarcoma is associated with poor prognosis. The tumors consist of small round cells with coarse chromatin and anastomosing fibrovascular connective tissue septa forming an alveolar pattern that is similar to lung in appearance (**Fig. 100.8**). Botryoid tumors have excellent prognosis and have similar histologic characteristics of embryonal tumors but grow into hollow spaces like bladder or vagina, assuming a characteristic grapelike appearance. Spindle cell rhabdomyosarcoma is another subtype of embryonal rhabdomyosarcoma that occurs most commonly at paratesticular sites and generally have excellent prognosis. Pleomorphic rhabdomyosarcomas are extremely rare in children and more common in adults.[42,44]

Recurrent chromosomal alterations have been identified in rhabdomyosarcoma, particularly in alveolar subtypes, and fusion-positive status is important for prognostication and treatment strategies. A translocation between chromosomes 2 and 13, t(2:13)(q35;q14) results in fusion of the PAX3 and FKHR genes, both transcription factors that function in muscular development. The resulting gain-of-function fusion gene is thought to alter cellular apoptosis, growth, and oncogenesis.

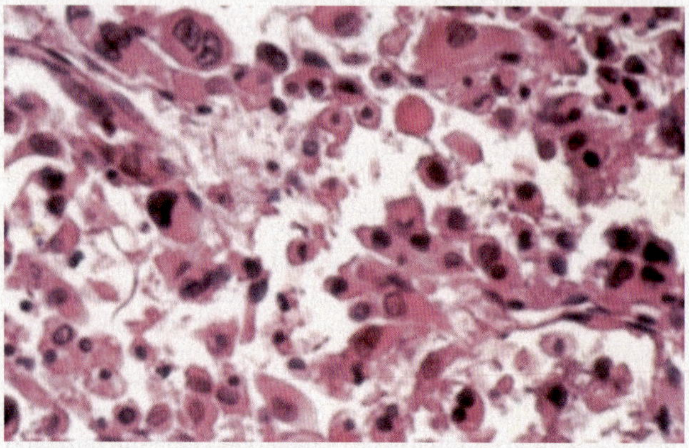

Figure 100.8. Microscopic image of typical lung-like appearance of an alveolar rhabdomyosarcoma. (Reprinted with permission from Strayer DS, Saffitz JE, Rubin E. *Rubin's Pathology*. 8th ed. Wolters Kluwer; 2020. Figure 30.72.)

Another PAX gene translocation, t(1;13)(p36;q14), results in fusion gene PAX7-FKHR and also occurs in alveolar tumors.[42,43,45]

Presentation and Diagnosis

Rhabdomyosarcoma can arise at any mesenchyme-containing site in the body. The presenting signs and symptoms depend on the site affected. Approximately 35% of all rhabdomyosarcoma tumors arise in the head and neck region and include parameningeal and nonparameningeal sites. Tumors in these areas may cause headache, facial and cervical swelling, nasal obstruction or discharge, recurrent otitis media, and cranial nerve palsies.[43] Tumors of the genitourinary track account for 25% of rhabdomyosarcoma and are most commonly located in the bladder and prostate gland. Perineal and perianal lesions may also occur. Patients may present with a palpable abdominal or pelvis mass, hematuria, dysuria, or urinary retention. Botryoid tumors are common in the vagina and cervix and may present with vaginal bleeding and inflammation. The friable grapelike mass may protrude from the vaginal orifice.[46] Paratesticular rhabdomyosarcoma presents with a painless mass in the scrotum that is typically distinguishable from the testicle. Extremity rhabdomyosarcoma tumors may present as swelling and pain after a traumatic injury to the extremity involved. Chest wall, paraspinal, and abdominal wall rhabdomyosarcoma are considered trunk sites and often present with palpable masses or chest wall pain. Additional primary sites include retroperitoneum, abdomen, and pelvis. These lesions may present as a palpable abdominal mass or with abdominal pain. There is seldom mass effect such as rectal or bladder obstruction. Biliary rhabdomyosarcoma may cause jaundice, fever, and right upper quadrant abdominal pain.

The diagnostic workup for rhabdomyosarcoma includes a thorough history and physical examination followed by cross-sectional imaging of the involved site by CT scan or MRI. Local, regional, and distal metastatic extent of disease should be determined with assessment for abnormal-appearing lymph nodes. PET scan may aid in detection of disease for adequate staging. Complete blood count, serum chemistries and liver function tests are routinely evaluated. Patients with suspected rhabdomyosarcoma should have bone marrow biopsies and aspirates performed to determine metastatic spread to bone marrow. CT chest or chest radiograph is required to identify lung metastases. Bone scintigraphy should be obtained to search for cortical bone metastases. For most cases, brain CT scan and cerebral spinal fluid testing is reserved for patients with known CNS lesions or symptoms. An adequate biopsy is required to histologically confirm diagnosis. If the lesion is small or judged resectable on presentation, excisional biopsy with clear microscopic margins should be performed. If the tumor involves contiguous organs, major blood vessels, or nerves, then incisional biopsy is performed. It is critical that the specimen is sent fresh to the pathologist without formalin and that enough tissue is obtained for microscopic evaluation and cytogenetic analysis.

Staging

The most widely utilized staging system for rhabdomyosarcoma is based on the (TNM) staging system. TNM staging system is applied prior to treatment and assesses disease site of origin, tumor size, nodal status, and metastases as factors in prognosis (**Table 100.7**). This system was prospectively tested by the International Rhabdomyosarcoma Study Group and reflects the biology of the tumor.[44,45] Stage 1 tumors involve the head and neck, genitourinary (nonbladder/prostate), and biliary tract sites. Regional nodes may or may not be involved with stage 1 tumors. Stage 2 tumors involve the bladder/prostate gland, extremity, cranial, parameningeal, retroperitoneal, and trunk sites and are less than 5 cm without lymph node involvement. Stage 3 tumors are the same anatomic sites as stage 2 and are greater than 5 cm with or without lymph

Table 100.7. TNM Pretreatment Staging System for Childhood Rhabdomyosarcoma

Stage	Site	T	Size	N	M
1	Orbit, head, and neck (excluding parameningeal), genitourinary (nonbladder/prostate)	T1 or T2	a or b	N0, N1, or N2	M0
2	Bladder/prostate, extremity, head and neck (parameningeal), other (trunk, retroperitoneum)	T1 or T2	a	N0 or Nx	M0
3	Bladder/prostate, extremity, head and neck (parameningeal), other (trunk, retroperitoneum)	T1 or T2	a b	N1 N0, N1, or Nx	M0
4	All	T1 or T2	a or b	N0 or N1	M1

Reprinted from Lawrence W Jr, Anderson JR, Gehan EA, et al. Pretreatment TNM staging of childhood rhabdomyosarcoma: a report of the Intergroup Rhabdomyosarcoma Study Group. Children's Cancer Study Group. Pediatric Oncology Group. *Cancer*. 1997;80(6):1165–1170. Permission granted for previous edition.

node involvement. Any rhabdomyosarcoma tumor with distant metastases is considered stage 4 disease.

Clinical Group Assessment and Risk Status

Both stage and group assessment are used to assign risk categories and to determine treatment plan. Patients are grouped into four risk groups based on postoperative assessment of disease before initiating chemotherapy or radiation (**Table 100.8**). Clinical group accurately predicts outcomes in patients with rhabdomyosarcoma.[47] Group I patients have excellent prognosis with localized tumors that are completely excised while group II patients have tumors that have microscopic residual disease or regionally invasive disease involving lymph nodes. Group III patients have gross residual disease or incisional biopsy, and Group IV patients have distant metastases at presentation. Stage, clinical group, histology, age, and anatomic site are utilized to identify low-, intermediate-, and high-risk categories, and therapy is allocated based on patient risk status. Favorable sites are orbit, head and neck (except parameningeal), genitourinary (except bladder and prostate), and biliary tract sites. Unfavorable sites are bladder/prostate, extremity, parameningeal, trunk, retroperitoneal, pelvis, and all other sites. Combinations of chemotherapy and radiotherapy are administered based on risk-group assignment. Alveolar and embryonal histology subgroups contrast in prognostic factors and in survival outcomes.

Table 100.8. Surgical–Histopathologic Clinical Grouping System for the Intergroup Rhabdomyosarcoma Studies I and II

Group I Localized tumor, completely resected A. Confined to organ or muscle of origin B. Infiltration outside organ or muscle of origin, regional nodes not involved
Group II Compromised or regional resection including A. Grossly resected tumors with "microscopic" residual B. Regional disease, completely resected, in which nodes may be involved and/or tumor extends into an adjacent organ C. Regional disease with involved nodes, grossly resected, evidence of microscopic residual
Group III Incomplete resection or biopsy, gross residual disease
Group IV Distant metastatic disease, present at presentation

Reprinted from Crist WM, Garnsey L, Beltangady MS, et al. Prognosis in children with rhabdomyosarcoma: a report of the Intergroup Rhabdomyosarcoma Studies I and II. Intergroup Rhabdomyosarcoma Committee. *J Clin Oncol*. 1990;8(3):433–452, with permission. © American Society of Clinical Oncology.

In patients with nonmetastatic rhabdomyosarcoma, tumors considered low risk are embryonic rhabdomyosarcoma tumors (stage 1 or 2) located at favorable histology sites. Embryonal tumors at unfavorable sites may also be assigned as low-risk group if the tumor is grossly completely resected (group I or II). Intermediate-risk embryonal rhabdomyosarcoma are patients with unfavorable anatomic sites with tumor remaining after surgical excision. This risk group has worse survival outcomes than patients with low-risk tumors. In this group, patients with unresectable extremity rhabdomyosarcoma have extremely poor failure-free (43%) and overall (46%) survival.[47]

In general, children with alveolar rhabdomyosarcoma have worse survival outcomes compared to those with embryonal histology. Patients with stage 1 or 2 disease that is grossly resected (group I or II) have 5-year failure-free survival of 80% and overall survival of 85%. Stage 1 or 2 (group III) patients have overall favorable outcomes as well. Patients with stage 3 tumors with nodal involvement also have poor survival outcomes near 30%. Survival correlates with stage and patients with high-risk tumors with distant metastases as diagnosis continue to have the worse expected survival.[47]

Treatment

Much of the treatment success of rhabdomyosarcoma is credited to successful clinical trials conducted by the Intergroup Rhabdomyosarcoma Study Group (IRSG) and the Soft Tissue Sarcoma Committee of the COG. Multimodal therapy aims to minimize the risk of relapse and optimize curative outcomes, while also minimizing treatment toxicities. Current studies test novel agents for upfront RMS treatment, incorporate molecular data, specifically fusion status, MYOD1 and tp53 mutational status, and evaluate therapy reduction for very–low-risk RMS.[44,45]

7 The mainstay of therapy begins with surgery, either complete excision with adequate margins or incisional biopsy. The goal for surgical margins is at least 0.5 cm of normal tissue surrounding tumor. Margins should be marked and oriented to assure that pathologists can accurately identify each microscopic margin. Contiguous structures, organs, major blood vessels or nerves that would result in major disability should not be resected in the initial operation, rather an adequate biopsy should be obtained and chemotherapy given upfront. In contrast, lesions that are small and not invading surrounding structures may be completely resected prior to chemotherapy. Resection of rhabdomyosarcoma tumors with wide and completely clear microscopic margins is the most ideal initial procedure for all stages to obtain local tumor control. Pretreatment reexcision is recommended after the initial operation if there is gross residual tumor or microscopically involved margins prior to the administration of chemotherapy. This is critical for accurate staging and for optimal clinical group assignment as well as potential decreased treatment intensity.

Debilitating or highly morbid operations are performed only after chemotherapy and radiation have been given in attempt to decrease tumor burden and minimize extent of resection.[48]

Lymph node sampling is indicated for patients with lesions that involve the extremity (even if clinically negative) or for clinically positive lymph nodes for all other sites. Biopsy by open, core, or sentinel lymph node biopsy techniques are all acceptable based on current COG guidelines. Staging ipsilateral retroperitoneal lymph node dissection is recommended for paratesticular rhabdomyosarcoma for all males older than 10 years of age and for those less than 10 years of age with enlarged appearing lymph nodes on cross-sectional imaging. In this group, staging ipsilateral retroperitoneal lymph node dissection is required for adequate staging and risk-group assessment. A nerve-sparing ipsilateral retroperitoneal lymph node dissection is recommended. The boundaries of the dissection begin at the level of the renal veins surrounding the aorta and the vena cava, extending to the deep inguinal ring. The procedure may be performed laparoscopically or through an open abdominal incision. Patients with intermediate-risk tumors may benefit from radical debulking of clinically positive lymph nodes if feasible.[48]

The addition of chemotherapy and radiotherapy to treatment protocols for rhabdomyosarcoma has dramatically improved survival rates. Currently all children diagnosed with rhabdomyosarcoma receive adjuvant chemotherapy with or without radiotherapy. COG treatment regimens utilize cyclophosphamide with newer studies evaluating treatment reduction or elimination to reduce toxicity, specifically around gonadal toxicity.[48]

High-risk patients have metastatic disease on presentation with dismal outcomes despite intensive cytotoxic therapy. The feasibility of concurrent early administration of radiotherapy and irinotecan is also being evaluated. Long-term follow-up on the most optimal combinations of intensified chemotherapy in high-risk rhabdomyosarcoma patients is needed with newer studies evaluating biologic agents.[48]

Radiotherapy is used in over 80% of patients to enhance local control. Radiotherapy is utilized as the primary means of local control in rare cases where surgical excision carries excessive risk or concern for disfigurement (orbital and vaginal). Similarly, for low-risk disease such as completely resected paratesticular RMS or complete chemotherapy response in vaginal RMS, radiotherapy can be avoided. Parameningeal tumors are treated with radiotherapy because of the high likelihood of residual disease even with surgical excision. Increasingly, regimens are incorporating intensity-modulated radiotherapy (IMRT), brachytherapy, and proton beam to reduce radiation exposure to normal surrounding tissues. Fertility preservation, including surgical adjuncts such as ovarian transposition out of the radiation field, are important considerations.[48]

Future Directions

Future clinical trials are focused on further tailoring therapies to reduce treatment toxicities and late adverse effects while improving curative outcomes. The current focus is incorporation of novel biologic agents to known active backbone chemotherapy regimens, particularly for patients with intermediate-risk and high-risk rhabdomyosarcoma. Human patient tumor–derived xenograft models are guiding future development of novel targeted therapies for this cancer. Improved incorporation of molecular and biologic markers will help guide improved risk prognostication.[44,45]

NONRHABDOMYOSARCOMA SOFT TISSUE SARCOMA

Epidemiology

Soft tissue sarcomas in children and adolescents occur in approximately 7% of all childhood solid tumors. Nonrhabdomyosarcoma soft tissue sarcoma (NRSTS) represents approximately 60% of these cases.[49] The tumors are distinct from rhabdomyosarcoma in terms of clinical characteristics, tumor biology, and prognosis. Most cases are sporadic although patients with Li–Fraumeni syndrome, neurofibromatosis type I (peripheral nerve sheath tumors), Gorlin syndrome (fibrosarcoma and leiomyosarcoma), and hereditary retinoblastoma have a higher risk of developing soft tissue sarcomas. Children that are survivors of childhood cancer are at an increased risk for NRSTS, particularly those with a history of receiving radiation, high-dose anthracyclines, and alkylating agents.[49]

Pathology and Biologic Features

NRSTSs originate from developmental mesenchymal cells with heterogeneous histologic subtypes and diverse sites of origin. These tumors are classified based on histology-specific cytogenetics of the tumor. NRSTS may have segmental chromosomal alterations (balanced translocations) or widespread genomic instability (**Table 100.9**). Genetic analysis is a powerful tool for diagnosis of NRSTS and is an important component of the histopathologic assessment. Detection of tumor-specific chromosomal alterations by RT-PCR, FISH, or high-throughput sequencing analyses often aid in confirming the diagnosis and in treatment planning.

Presentation, Diagnosis, and Staging

NRSTS typically present as a painless slow-growing solid mass that may invade surrounding structures. Approximately 15% of patients present with metastatic disease at presentation, most commonly lungs. In general, diagnostic workup for NRSTS consists of cross-sectional imaging (MRI) of the primary site along with imaging (CT scan) of chest, abdomen, and pelvis for surgical planning and adequate staging. Bone scintigraphy is used only for patients with bone pain or symptoms. Bone marrow biopsy is typically not indicated. Brain imaging is reserved for patients with CNS symptoms.

An adequate tissue specimen is required to determine the histologic subtype and grade of NRSTS. Complete surgical resection of all gross disease is recommended at presentation unless a wide resection is not feasible or accompanied by high surgical morbidity. Multiple core needle biopsies may be sufficient though the quality and quantity of specimen must be adequate for histologic and cytogenetic studies.

A pathologic tumor grade is assigned to NRSTS based on extent of malignancy and is an indicator of prognosis. The Pediatric Oncology Group's grading system for NRSTS assesses mitotic rate, extent of necrosis, differentiation, and histologic type and can be used as a predictor of outcome. This grade is used for risk stratification along with the presence of metastasis, extent of upfront tumor resection, and tumor size (≤5 or >5 cm).[49]

Treatment

Complete surgical resection is critical in the management of NRSTS because of resistance to chemotherapy and radiotherapy. Primary tumors that appear grossly resectable should be excised upfront. If the surgeon anticipates that gross residual disease is likely following surgery or if complete excision is debilitating or disfiguring, tumor biopsy should be performed. This is typically seen with large (>5 cm), high-grade regionally invasive or metastatic tumors that will benefit from neoadjuvant chemotherapy and delayed tumor resection. Tumor debulking is generally not recommended. Large, potentially morbid resections like amputation and pelvic exoneration are performed only after neoadjuvant therapies. In general, incisions on the extremities should be placed longitudinally and incisions on the trunk are oriented in the axial plane. If the surgeon determines that the mass is not amendable to full excision upfront, a generous incisional biopsy is required. Primary reexcision of the primary tumor is recommended if there is gross residual resectable tumor after the initial resection with

Table 100.9. Nonrhabdomyosaroma Tumor Characteristics

Tumor	Incidence[a]	Normal Counterpart[a]	Cytogenetic Abnormality[a]	Genes[a]	Common Primary Sites
Fibrosarcoma	0.6	Fibroblasts	t(12;15)	TEL (ETV6), NTRK3(TRKC)	Lower extremity, upper extremity
Desmoplastic round cell tumor[b]	Approximately 200 case reports	Lineage epithelial, neural, myogenic cells	t(11;22)	EWS, WT1	Abdomen, paratesticular, thoracic cavity
Leiomyosarcoma	0.3	Smooth muscle	Variable	Multiple gene alterations	Gastrointestinal or genitourinary, superficial dermis, retroperitoneal, lungs, uterus, vascular
Alveolar soft parts tumor	0.1	Unknown	t(x;17)	ASPL, TFE3	Thigh, buttocks, abdominal and chest wall
Neurofibrosarcoma	0.6	Schwann cell	Variable, abnormalities of chromosome 17	Multiple genetic alterations, NF1	Extremity, retroperitoneum, trunk
Liposarcoma	0.1	Adipocyte	t(12;16)	FUS, CHOP	Lower and upper extremity, retroperitoneum
Tendosynovial sarcoma	0.7	Synovial cells	t(x;18)	SYT, SSX-1, or SSX-2	Lower extremity (thigh, foot, posterior knee), upper extremity (shoulders, forearm)
Dermatofibrosarcoma protuberans	1.0	Fibroblasts	t(12;22)	COL1A, PDGF	Trunk, proximal extremities

[a]From Gurney J, Young J Jr, Roffers S, et al. In: Ries LAG, Smith MA, Gurney JG, et al., eds. *Cancer Incidence and Survival among Children and Adolescents: United States SEER Program 1975–1995*. National Cancer Institute, SEER Program; 1999.
[b]From Saab R, Khoury JD, Krasin M, et al. Desmoplastic small round cell tumor in childhood: the St. Jude Children's Research Hospital experience. *Pediatr Blood Cancer*. 2007;49:274–279. (Incidence age-adjusted per million younger than 20 years old [excluding desmoplastic round cell tumor].)

at least a 0.5-cm margin. Reexcision is also recommended if the margin status is unknown. Previous scars or needle tracts should be included en bloc with the specimen. Lymph node sampling is required for abnormal-appearing lymph nodes on clinical examination or imaging. Several histologic subtypes of NRSTS also require lymph node evaluation for risk assessment and staging purposes, even in patients without enlarged lymph nodes. These include synovial cell sarcoma, epithelioid sarcoma, and clear cell sarcoma with up to 30% risk of lymph node metastases.[49–51]

The most active chemotherapeutic agents for NRSTS are doxorubicin and ifosfamide, though most NRSTSs are relatively chemoresistant. Low-risk patients (grossly resected, low grade, any size) receive surgical excision alone with or without radiotherapy, depending on margin status. Intermediate-risk and high-risk (metastatic disease) patients are treated with ifosfamide and dose-intensive doxorubicin and radiotherapy either before or after surgical excision. Because of the limited efficacy of chemotherapy in NRSTS, novel targeted therapeutic approaches are warranted, especially for children with high-grade or relapsed tumors.

HEPATIC TUMORS

Hepatoblastoma

Epidemiology and Genetic Risk

Hepatoblastoma is the most common malignant liver tumor in children, occurring in 1.5 to 1.8 per million children <19 years of age, yielding more than 150 cases per year in the United States. The incidence of hepatoblastoma has increased in the last three decades in the United States.[3] Hepatoblastoma occurs most commonly in infants and children between the ages of 6 months and 3 years with more than 90% diagnosed by age 5. A slight male predominance is reported and there does not appear to be significant differences in incidence among race. The median age at diagnosis is 18 months of age. Hepatoblastoma is the third most frequent abdominal tumor after neuroblastoma and WT. Environmental risk factors have not been confirmed. Hepatoblastoma has been found in association with prematurity and low birth weight. In fact, there is a strong association with very low–birth-weight neonates (<1500 g) though the underlying mechanism is not yet unknown.[52,53]

Several inherited syndromes are associated with hepatoblastoma. Patients with Beckwith–Wiedemann syndrome are at risk for developing hepatoblastoma and require routine screening. Most cases are due to defective imprinting on chromosome 11p15. There is an increased risk of hepatoblastoma in children of families with familial adenomatous polyposis (FAP) syndrome though no specific genetic alteration in chromosome 5 has been identified. There is a nonrandom association between hepatoblastoma and children with trisomy 18.[52,53]

Sporadic hepatoblastoma has not been characterized by any single chromosomal abnormality and cytogenetic analyses have not revealed consistent patterns. LOH of 11p15 has been detected in up to 33% of children with hepatoblastoma and it is hypothesized that a tumor suppressor gene may be

PEDIATRIC SURGERY

located in this region. Insulin-like growth factor 2 (IGF-2) has been proposed as a targetable genomic driver since it is present in 70% of tumors and associated with shorter disease-free survival.[54]

Pathology and Biologic Features

Hepatoblastoma displays a combination of histologic patterns that range from epithelial and mesenchymal elements. In contrast to adult tumors, this occurs with a backdrop of normal, not cirrhotic, liver. This tumor is thought to originate from undifferentiated embryonal hepatic cells that maintain pluripotency and have potential to develop into both hepatocytes and biliary epithelial cells. Hepatoblastoma may be classified by five different histologic subtypes that carry prognostic value: well-differentiated fetal (pure fetal), embryonal, macrotrabecular (epithelial fetal or embryonal), small cell undifferentiated, and cholangioblastic (bile ducts predominate).[52,53] Of these, the most favorable outcomes are seen with well-differentiated fetal subtypes. Small cell undifferentiated tumors (anaplastic subtype) carry the worse prognosis. Small cell undifferentiated tumors are often associated with low or normal serum α-fetoprotein (AFP) levels (<100) and predict adverse outcomes with poor response to chemotherapy. Two-thirds of hepatoblastoma tumors are epithelial with mixed embryonal and fetal patterns, and about 20% of these have mesenchymal components.[53,55]

Presentation, Diagnosis, and Staging

Children with hepatoblastoma present with an asymptomatic abdominal mass or abdominal swelling. Systemic symptoms like weight loss, failure to thrive, or anorexia may indicate advanced disease. Jaundice and biliary obstruction do not typically occur in patients with hepatoblastoma. Distant metastases are present in approximately 20% of patients at diagnosis and the most common site is lungs.[52] Ultrasound and cross-sectional imaging (three-phase CT scan or MRI with EOVIST) will define segmental extension of the tumor within the liver and assess for distant metastases (**Fig. 100.9**). The tumor appears as a solid mass with low attenuation. On MRI the lesion appears as low intensity on T1-weighted images and high intensity on T2-weighted images. There is no evidence that MRI is superior to CT scan for diagnosis or surveillance of hepatoblastoma. It is important to distinguish central venous structures and to evaluate the liver for multifocal disease. Chest CT scan is obtained to evaluate for lung metastases. Anemia and thrombocytosis are common in children with hepatoblastoma and is likely related to cytokine secretion by tumor cells. AFP is elevated in approximately 90% of patients with hepatoblastoma and is a useful clinical marker for monitoring tumor responsiveness and recurrence. Interpretation of AFP may be difficult because the protein is expressed in the fetus and commonly remains elevated in normal neonates and infants up to 6 months of age. AFP may also be elevated in patients with hepatitis, hepatocellular carcinoma (HCC), and germ cell tumors.[52,56]

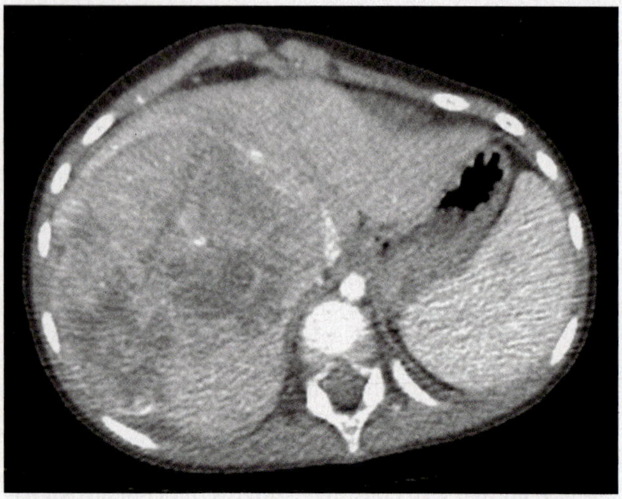

Figure 100.9. Abdominal CT scan with right hepatic lobe hepatoblastoma displacing normal hepatic vasculature and parenchyma.

COG staging was previously based on postsurgical stage, histology, and metastasis. In an effort to create international consensus, pretreatment extent of disease (PRETEXT) grouping is used internationally to stratify patients based on the tumor's radiographic characteristics prior to treatment. PRETEXT describes the anatomic involvement and Couinaud hepatic segments affected by the tumor and can be applied to patients who have not yet had operations (**Fig. 100.10**).[56] PRETEXT divides the liver into four parts termed sectors. The left lobe is divided into a lateral sector (segments 2 and 3) and a medial sector (segment 4). The right lobe is divided into an anterior sector (segments 5 and 8) and posterior sector (segments 6 and 7). PRETEXT is further annotated by V (venous involvement), P (portal vascular involvement), E (extrahepatic involvement), F (multifocal), R (rupture prior to diagnosis), C (caudate lobe), N (nodes), and M (distant metastatic disease) categories. Imaging is obtained after every two cycles of chemotherapy, where POSTTEXT (posttreatment of disease) is then used to reassess anatomy.

The Children's Hepatic tumors International Collaboration (CHIC) is a collaborative consortium from the United States, Japan, and Europe that aims to standardize hepatoblastoma risk stratification. PRETEXT group, presence of metastatic disease, AFP at diagnosis, age at diagnosis, and the presence of PRETEXT annotation factors VPEFR are currently utilized for risk stratification. In general, excellent prognosis is expected for stage 1 tumors completely resected at diagnosis with pure fetal histology. Poor prognosis is associated with PRETEXT IV, metastatic tumors, AFP less than 100, patients over age 8, and tumors with small cell undifferentiated histology.[57]

Treatment

Complete surgical resection is the mainstay of curative therapy for hepatoblastoma. Completely resected tumors have significantly improved survival outcomes compared with all other hepatoblastoma patients. If the tumor appears resectable, conventional anatomic resection is performed. If the mass is judged unresectable at diagnosis, incisional or core needle biopsy is performed, and the patient is treated with chemotherapy prior to resection. Percutaneous biopsies should go through unaffected liver that will be part of the resected specimen. Primary resection is recommended for localized PRETEXT 1 or PRETEXT 2 tumors with >1 cm radiographic margin on the middle hepatic vein, without vena cava or con-
8 tralateral portal venous invasion. Neoadjuvant chemotherapy is recommended for PRETEXT III or IV tumors and for multicentric tumors with central venous invasion. Patients with pulmonary metastases also receive chemotherapy upfront. Tumor volume and AFP measurements may be utilized to monitor tumor responsiveness after each cycle. For patients with unresectable disease, early referral to a liver transplant center is required. This can be done as early as at diagnosis, especially for multifocal or PRETEXT IV lesions, or at the latest if the tumor appears unresectable on interval imaging after 2 cycles of chemotherapy.[51,52]

An anatomic liver resection is recommended and is most often required. As much as 85% of hepatic parenchyma may be safely removed in children with full regeneration expected despite postoperative chemotherapy. Mortality from liver resection in children should be low (0% to 3%) with technical advances such as the Cavitron Ultrasonic Surgical Aspirator (CUSA; Cooper Lasersonics, Santa Clara, CA) and metallic clip applicators for hemostasis while dividing liver parenchyma. The surgical principles include a generous incision

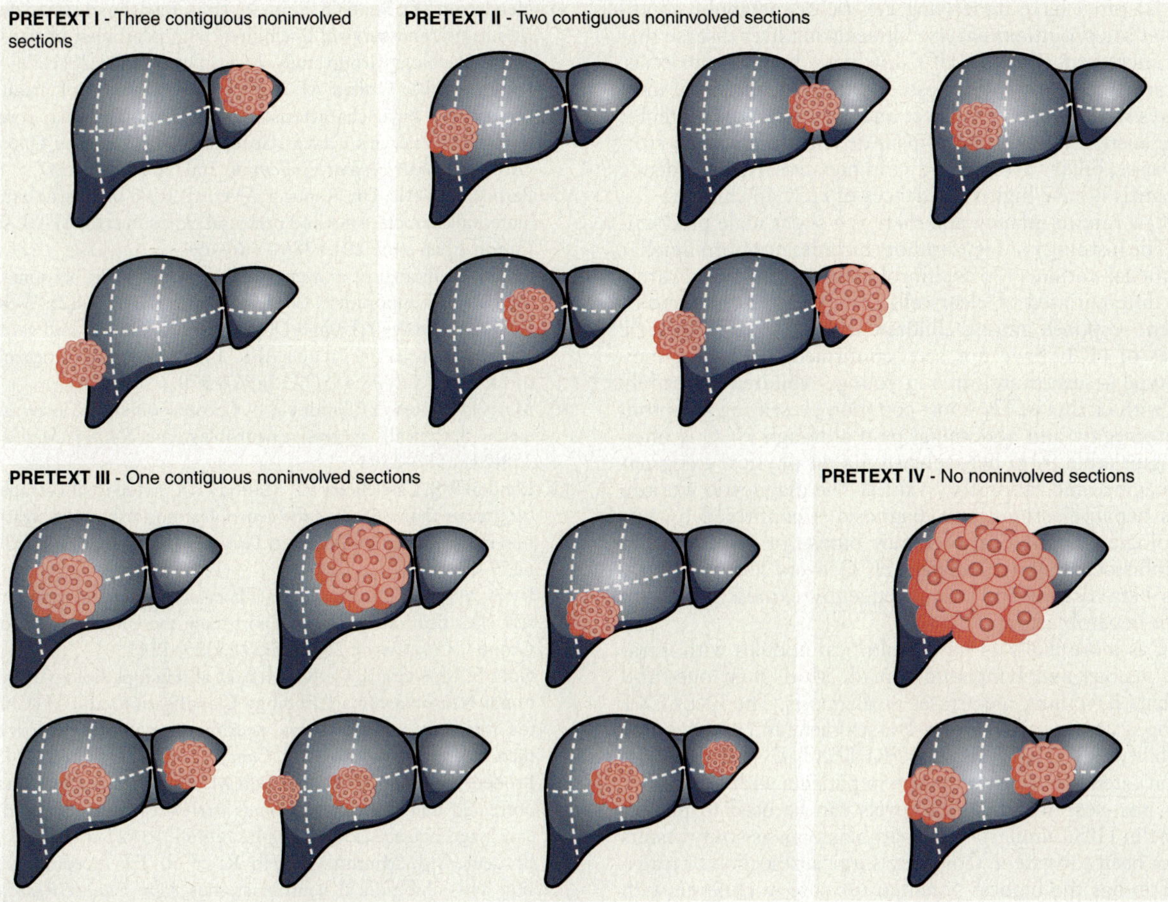

Figure 100.10. The Pretreatment Extent of Disease (PRETEXT) system divides the liver into four sections and grades tumors from I to IV based on the number of sections involved. PRETEXT I shows three contiguous noninvolved sections, PRETEXT II shows two contiguous noninvolved sections, PRETEXT III shows one contiguous noninvolved section, and PRETEXT IV shows no noninvolved sections. (Reprinted from Springer: From Pio L, O'Neill AF, Woodley H, et al. Hepatoblastoma. *Nat Rev Dis Primers*. 2025;11(1):36. Figure 1.)

with wide exposure using subcostal incisions. Dissection of the hilum with identification and isolation of the ductal and vascular structures of the segment of resection is critical. Hepatic arterial and portal venous inflow is obstructed or ligated, allowing demarcation of the resection plane. This allows the operation to proceed with minimal blood loss. Intraoperative Doppler ultrasound is often utilized to aid in locating major venous structures traversing the tumor and for assuring adequate resection margins of at least 1 cm. Indocyanine green (ICG) fluorescence can be used to aid in the delineation of tumor borders intraoperatively.[51]

Chemotherapy improves resectability of hepatoblastoma and improves prognosis in nearly all cases. Currently most patients diagnosed with hepatoblastoma receive chemotherapy either before or after resection of the primary tumor. Patients with completely resected well-differentiated fetal histology (WDF or pure fetal histology) tumors and low mitotic activity may be treated exclusively with surgery alone. Children with WDF histology tumors comprise 7% of hepatoblastoma cases and have 100% EFS. Most hepatoblastoma tumors are sensitive to cisplatin-based chemotherapy and overall survival increased from 30% to 70% with the addition of cisplatin.[56] The role of radiotherapy in hepatoblastoma has not been defined because of the risk of hepatic toxicity and low hepatic tolerance to radiation in children.[56]

Liver transplantation has become a promising treatment option for children with unresectable hepatoblastoma without metastatic disease after neoadjuvant chemotherapy. Liver transplantation has improved overall survival in children with large, or multifocal unresectable hepatoblastoma. Tumors with extensive major vessel involvement or multifocal disease should be referred to centers that have pediatric liver transplant expertise. Primary transplantation is also recommended for multifocal PRETEXT IV tumors despite apparent clearance after chemotherapy because of the risk of persistent microscopic disease.[51] For transplantation eligibility, patients with hepatoblastoma must not have any active extrahepatic or metastatic sites that have not cleared with surgery or chemotherapy. Patients with lung metastases are not excluded from transplantation if the lung disease is clear after neoadjuvant chemotherapy. It is critical to correctly identify patients who will benefit from primary liver transplant prior to attempts at conventional resection.[51]

The Paediatric Hepatic International Tumour Trial (PHITT) utilizes the CHIC risk grouping in a prospective multinational trial, and results should help to guide future research. Chemotherapeutic intensification by dosing and duration has had promising preliminary results and may be beneficial in patients with high-risk hepatoblastoma. Similarly, sodium thiosulfate (STS) with cisplatin monotherapy has been used for patients with standard risk disease with STS decreasing platinum-mediated high-frequency hearing loss. The expanding role of antibodies and T lymphocytes as anticancer therapy for pediatric solid tumors may also hold promise as novel treatment agents for hepatoblastoma.[55]

Hepatocellular Carcinoma

HCC is the second most common malignant liver mass in children and occurs more commonly in older children, constituting 20$ of malignant liver tumors in children. It is similar in histopathology to the disease in adults. However, most pediatric HCCs do not arise in underlying cirrhotic liver. Those that do (35%) often have underlying genetic or metabolic conditions that are proinflammatory.[51] Preexisting liver disease that carries increased risk for HCC includes hemochromatosis, hereditary tyrosinemia, progressive familial cholestasis, multidrug resistance protein 3 defect and tight junction protein 2 gene deficiency, alpha-1-antitrypsin deficiency, glycogen storage diseases, biliary atresia, and viral hepatitis. Areas endemic for hepatitis B have higher incidences of HCC in children.[52]

HCC is rare in infancy and there is a slight male predominance. The histology of HCC tumors includes nonfibrolamellar (or epithelial variant) (75%), fibrolamellar (25%), and rarely poorly differentiated or clear cell. Differences in outcome or treatment response among children with different histologic subtypes of HCC have not been confirmed. The fibrolamellar subtype is seen more often in younger children and rarely occurs with cirrhosis. The most common presenting symptom is hepatomegaly and abdominal pain although HCC is often indistinguishable from hepatoblastoma on physical examination, imaging, and laboratory values. The diagnostic workup mirrors hepatoblastoma and diagnosis is confirmed by histopathologic examination of tumor biopsy or resection. On immunohistochemistry, pediatric HCC livers less frequently express beta-catenin and more frequently express p53 compared to hepatoblastoma.[52,57]

HCC is more likely to have multifocal nodules with intrahepatic venous and lymphatic spread. More than one-third of patients have lung metastases at diagnosis. The PRETEXT grouping system is utilized for risk assessment and to determine resectability. PRETEXT III and PRETEXT IV are the most common categories at presentation in patients with HCC.[55]

It is not clear whether AFP levels can be used to predict outcome in HCC similarly to hepatoblastoma as study results have not been consistent. Complete surgical resection or transplantation has the highest potential for cure in children with HCC. Unfortunately, fewer than 20% of patients with HCC have tumors that are resectable at diagnosis and multifocal tumors are common. In contrast to hepatoblastoma, HCC tumors are generally unresponsive to chemotherapy and outcomes for patients with stage 3 disease and higher are dismal.[57] Transplantation is reserved for patients with localized tumor without any evidence of metastatic disease at presentation because of high risk of pulmonary metastatic relapse. The guidelines for liver transplantation in HCC are largely derived from the adult experience using the Milan criteria (not more than three tumors, less than 3 cm in size, or single tumor less than 5 cm in size).[51] Treatment protocols for HCC currently consist of cisplatin, vincristine, doxorubicin, and 5-fluorouracil in multiple combinations. Compared to hepatoblastoma, these agents are not as effective in HCC and patients generally remain with poor prognosis. Alternative approaches for local control have demonstrated some benefit in children with HCC. Hepatic arterial chemoembolization (HACE) in patients with refractory and unresectable disease requires cooperative group study, but has been shown to be well tolerated and may be effective in inducing surgical resectability in select cases of HCC.[52]

References

1. Gupta S, Aitken J, Bartels U, et al. Development of paediatric non-stage prognosticator guidelines for population-based cancer registries and updates to the 2014 Toronto Paediatric Cancer Stage Guidelines. *Lancet Oncol*. 2020;21(9):e444–e451.
2. Siegel DA, King JB, Lupo PJ, et al. Counts, incidence rates, and trends of pediatric cancer in the United States, 2003–2019. *J Natl Cancer Inst*. 2023;115(11):1337–1354.
3. Lee WG, Kim ES. Precision oncology in pediatric cancer surgery. *Surg Oncol Clin N Am*. 2024;33(2):409–446.
4. Park JR K, SG L, WB N, et al. Effect of tandem autologous stem cell transplant vs single transplant on event-free survival in patients with high-risk neuroblastoma: a randomized clinical trial. *JAMA*. 2019;322(8):746–755.
5. Henderson TO, Bhatia S, Pinto N, et al. Racial and ethnic disparities in risk and survival in children with neuroblastoma: a Children's Oncology Group study. *J Clin Oncol*. 2011;29(1):76–82.
6. Hamrick SEG, Olshan AF, Neglia JP. Association of pregnancy history and birth characteristics with neuroblastoma: a report from the Children's Cancer Group and the Pediatric Oncology Group. *Paediatr Perinat Epidemiol*. 2001;15(4):328–337.
7. Parodi S, Merlo DF, Ranucci A, et al. Risk of neuroblastoma, maternal characteristics and perinatal exposures: the SETIL study. *Cancer Epidemiol*. 2014;38(6):686–694.
8. Aygun N. Biological and genetic features of neuroblastoma and their clinical importance. *Curr Pediatr Rev*. 2018;14(2):73–90.
9. Janoueix-Lerosey I, Lequin D, Brugières L. Somatic and germline activating mutations of the ALK kinase receptor in neuroblastoma. *Nature*. 2008;455(7215):967–970.
10. Maris JM, Mossé YP, Bradfield JP. Chromosome 6p22 locus associated with clinically aggressive neuroblastoma. *N Engl J Med*. 2008;358(24):2585–2593.
11. London WB, Castleberry RP, Matthay KK. Evidence for an age cutoff greater than 365 days for neuroblastoma risk group stratification in the Children's Oncology Group. *J Clin Oncol*. 2005;23(27):6459–6465.
12. Irwin MS, Naranjo A, Zhang FF, et al. Revised neuroblastoma risk classification system: a report from the Children's Oncology Group. *J Clin Oncol*. 2021;39(29):3229–3241.
13. Goto S, Umehara S, Gerbing RB, et al. Histopathology (International Neuroblastoma Pathology Classification) and MYCN status in patients with peripheral neuroblastic tumors: a report from the Children's Cancer Group. *Cancer*. 2001;92(10):2699–708.
14. Brodeur GM, Seeger RC, Schwab M. Amplification of N-myc in untreated human neuroblastomas correlates with advanced disease stage. *Science (1979)*. 1984;224(4653):1121–1124.
15. Brodeur GM, Minturn JE, Ho R, et al. Trk receptor expression and inhibition in neuroblastomas. *Clin Cancer Res*. 2009;15(10):3244–3250.
16. Schleiermacher G, Michon J, Ribeiro A. Segmental chromosomal alterations lead to a higher risk of relapse in infants with MYCN-non-amplified localised unresectable/disseminated neuroblastoma (a SIOPEN collaborative study). *Br J Cancer*. 2011;105(12):1940–1948.
17. Attiyeh EF, London WB, Mossé YP. Chromosome 1p and 11q deletions and outcome in neuroblastoma. *N Engl J Med*. 2005;353(21):2243–2253.
18. Du H, Cai W. Opsoclonus-myoclonus syndrome associated with neuroblastoma: insights into antitumor immunity. *Pediatr Blood Cancer*. 2022;69(11):e29949.
19. Nuchtern JG, London WB, Barnewolt CE, et al. A prospective study of expectant observation as primary therapy for neuroblastoma in young infants: a Children's Oncology Group study. *Ann Surg*. 2012;256(4):573–580.
20. Maris JM, Hogarty MD, Bagatell R, Cohn SL. Neuroblastoma. *Lancet*. 2007;369(9579):2106–2120.
21. Kayano D, Kinuya S. Iodine-131 metaiodobenzylguanidine therapy for neuroblastoma: reports so far and future perspective. *ScientificWorldJournal*. 2015;2015:189135.
22. Montclair T, Broduer GM, Ambros PF. The International Neuroblastoma Risk Group (INRG) staging system: an INRG Task Force Report. *J Clin Oncol*. 2009;27:298–303.
23. Cohn SL, Pearson ADJ, London WB. The International Neuroblastoma Risk Group (INRG) classification system: an INRG Task Force Report. *J Clin Oncol*. 2009;27(2):289–297.
24. Chung C, Boterberg T, Lucas J, et al. Neuroblastoma. *Pediatr Blood Cancer*. 2021;68(Suppl 2):e28473.
25. Strother DR, London WB, Schmidt ML, et al. Outcome after surgery alone or with restricted use of chemotherapy for patients with low-risk neuroblastoma: results of Children's Oncology Group study P9641. *J Clin Oncol*. 2012;30(15):1842–1848.
26. Twist C, London WB, Naranjo A. Maintaining outstanding outcomes using response- and biology-based therapy for intermediate-risk neuroblastoma: a report from the Children's Oncology Group Study ANBL0531. *J Clin Oncol*. 2019;37(34):3243–3255.

27. Shah NR, Weadock WJ, Williams KM, et al. Use of modern three-dimensional imaging models to guide surgical planning for local control of pediatric extracranial solid tumors. *Pediatr Blood Cancer*. 2024;71(5):e30933.
28. Libes J, Hol J, Neto JCA, et al. Pediatric renal tumor epidemiology: global perspectives, progress, and challenges. *Pediatr Blood Cancer*. 2023;(Suppl 2):e30343.
29. Pater L, Melchior P, Rübe C, et al. Wilms tumor. *Pediatr Blood Cancer*. 2021;68(Suppl 2):e28257.
30. Breslow NE, Beckwith JB. Epidemiological features of Wilms' tumor: results of the National Wilms' tumor study. *J Natl Cancer Inst*. 1982;68(3):429–436.
31. Rivera MN, Haber DA. Wilms' tumour: connecting tumorigenesis and organ development in the kidney. *Nat Rev Cancer*. 2005;5(9):699–712.
32. Md Zin R, Murch A, Charles A. Pathology, genetics and cytogenetics of Wilms' tumour. *Pathology*. 2011;43(4):302–312.
33. Vujanić GM, Mifsud W, Cancer PB. Anaplasia in Wilms tumor: a critical review. *Pediatr Blood Cancer*. 2024;71(7):e31000.
34. Fialkowski E, Sudour-Bonnange H, Vujanic GM, et al. The varied spectrum of nephroblastomatosis, nephrogenic rests, and Wilms tumors: review of current definitions and challenges of the field. *Pediatr Blood Cancer*. 2023;70(Suppl 2):e30162.
35. Glick RD, Romao RLP, Pachl M, et al. Current surgical approaches to pediatric renal tumors. *Pediatr Blood Cancer*. 2025;72 (Suppl 2): e31118.
36. Naik-Mathuria B, Utria AF, Ehrlich PF, et al. Management and outcomes of Wilms tumor with suprarenal intravascular extension: a Pediatric Surgical Oncology Research Collaborative Study. *Ann Surg*. 2024;279(3):528–535.
37. Ehrlich P, Chi YY, Chintagumpala MM, et al. Results of the first prospective multi-institutional treatment study in children with bilateral Wilms tumor (AREN0534): a report from the Children's Oncology Group. *Ann Surg*. 2017;266(3):470–478.
38. Sze SGK. Neonatal renal tumors. *Clin Perinatol*. 2021;48(1): 71–81.
39. Aldera AP, Pillay K. Clear cell sarcoma of the kidney. *Arch Pathol Lab Med*. 2020;144(1):119–123.
40. Ray S, Jones R, Pritchard-Jones K, et al. Pediatric and young adult renal cell carcinoma. *Pediatr Blood Cancer*. 2020;67(11):e28675.
41. Agaram NP. Evolving classification of rhabdomyosarcoma. *Histopathology*. 2022;80(1):98–108.
42. Martin-Giacalone BA, Weinstein PA, Plon SE, Lupo PJ. Pediatric rhabdomyosarcoma: epidemiology and genetic susceptibility. *J Clin Med*. 2021;10(9):2028.
43. Hettmer S, Linardic CM, Kelsey A, et al. Molecular testing of rhabdomyosarcoma in clinical trials to improve risk stratification and outcome: a consensus view from European paediatric Soft tissue sarcoma Study Group, Children's Oncology Group and Cooperative Weichteilsarkom-Studiengruppe. *Eur J Cancer*. 2022;172:367–386.
44. Metts JL, Aye JM, Crane JN, et al. Roadmap for the next generation of Children's Oncology Group rhabdomyosarcoma trials. *Cancer*. 2024;130(22):3785–3796.
45. Dasgupta R, Xue W, Dixon AH, et al. Outcomes for patients with perineal and perianal rhabdomyosarcoma: a report from the Children's Oncology Group Soft Tissue Sarcoma Committee. *Pediatr Blood Cancer*. 2024;71(11):e31303.
46. Meza JL, Anderson J, Pappo AS, Meyer WH; Children's Oncology Group. Analysis of prognostic factors in patients with nonmetastatic rhabdomyosarcoma treated on intergroup rhabdomyosarcoma studies III and IV: the Children's Oncology Group. *J Clin Oncol*. 2006;24(24):3844–3851.
47. Rogers TN, Dasgupta R. Management of rhabdomyosarcoma in pediatric patients. *Surg Oncol Clin N Am*. 2021;30(2):339–353.
48. Polites SF, Rhee DS, Seitz G, et al. Contemporary surgical management of pediatric non-rhabdomyosarcoma soft tissue sarcoma. *Pediatr Blood Cancer*. 2024;71(11):e31257.
49. Sparber-Sauer M, Ferrari A, Spunt SL, et al. The significance of margins in pediatric non-rhabdomyosarcoma soft tissue sarcomas: consensus on surgical margin definition harmonization from the INternational Soft Tissue SaRcoma ConsorTium (INSTRuCT). *Cancer Med*. 2023;12(10):11719–11730.
50. Ferrari A, Orbach D, Sparber-Sauer M, et al. The treatment approach to pediatric non-rhabdomyosarcoma soft tissue sarcomas: a critical review from the INternational Soft Tissue SaRcoma ConsorTium. *Eur J Cancer*. 2022;169:10–19.
51. Riehle KJ, Vasudevan SA, Bondoc A, et al. Surgical management of liver tumors. *Pediatr Blood Cancer*. 2025;72 Suppl 2:e31155.
52. Ranganathan S, Lopez-Terrada D, Alaggio R. Hepatoblastoma and pediatric hepatocellular carcinoma: an update. *Pediatr Dev Pathol*. 2020;23(2):79–95.
53. Abril-Fornaguera J, Torrens L, Andreu-Oller C, et al. Identification of IGF2 as genomic driver and actionable therapeutic target in hepatoblastoma. *Mol Cancer Ther*. 2023;22(4):485–498.
54. Meyers RL, Maibach R, Hiyama E, et al. Risk-stratified staging in paediatric hepatoblastoma: a unified analysis from the Children's Hepatic tumors International Collaboration. *Lancet Oncol*. 2017;18(1):122–131.
55. Towbin AJ, Meyers RL, Woodley H, et al. 2017 PRETEXT: radiologic staging system for primary hepatic malignancies of childhood revised for the Paediatric Hepatic International Tumour Trial (PHITT). *Pediatr Radiol*. 2018;48(4):536–554.
56. O'Neill AF, Meyers RL, Katzenstein HM, et al. Children's Oncology Group's 2023 blueprint for research: liver tumors. *Pediatr Blood Cancer*. 2023;70 (Suppl 6):e30576.
57. Khanna R, Verma SK. Pediatric hepatocellular carcinoma. *World J Gastroenterol*. 2018;24(35):3980–3999.

PEDIATRIC SURGERY

101

Section O: SKIN AND SOFT TISSUE

Cutaneous Malignancies

Sarah B. Fisher, Lesly A. Dossett, Michael C. Lowe, and Keith A. Delman

Key Points

1 Cutaneous malignancies are the most commonly diagnosed cancers in the United States, with basal cell and squamous cell carcinomas, melanomas, Merkel cell carcinomas (MCCs), and malignant cutaneous adnexal tumors, in that order, the most frequently diagnosed.

2 Melanoma prognosis is inversely correlated with tumor thickness, ulceration, mitotic rate, and nodal status.

3 Primary melanomas are treated with wide local excision; guidelines for appropriate margin width are based on Breslow thickness.

4 Sentinel lymph node biopsy (SLNB) should be considered for clinically node-negative patients with melanoma between 0.8 and 1.0 mm or thicker or those with tumors <0.8 mm with ulceration.

5 Treatment decisions for patients with regional or metastatic melanoma should be made in a multidisciplinary setting, reflecting the increasing role of systemic therapy (immunotherapy and molcularly targeted therapy), including for patients with resectable disease. Neoadjuvant therapy should be considered preferred in most settings.

6 The surgeon who treats cutaneous malignancies should understand the impact of nonsurgical therapies, including radiation, immunotherapy, and targeted therapy, and adapt the surgical approach to patients with locally advanced or metastatic disease in coordination with other evidence-based treatments.

7 Surgical excision remains the mainstay of therapy for patients with advanced basal and squamous cell carcinomas, although immunotherapy and/or targeted therapy have demonstrated benefit in patients with advanced or unresectable disease. Combined multimodality therapy is likely to achieve the best outcome.

1 Cutaneous malignancies are the most frequently diagnosed cancers in the United States, with at least several million new cases annually. Comprised of multiple histologies with a wide spectrum of behavior, the most common cutaneous malignancies include basal cell carcinoma (BCC) and cutaneous squamous cell carcinoma (SCC), yet the true incidence of these tumors is challenging to track as most cancer registries do not accurately capture them. In contrast, cutaneous melanoma and other rare cutaneous malignancies such as Merkel cell carcinoma (MCC), malignant cutaneous adnexal tumors, or dermatofibrosarcoma protuberans (DFSP) comprise only one to five of all skin cancer diagnoses, but account for the majority of skin cancer deaths. In 2023, approximately 97,610 new cases of invasive melanoma (and an additional 89,070 cases of melanoma in situ) were diagnosed in the United States, leading to an estimated 7990 deaths.[1] Primary prevention initiatives including education regarding sun protective strategies and increased screening and skin cancer awareness, have successfully decreased the incidence of cutaneous malignancy in specific geographic regions (ie, Australia, with initiatives in practice since 1988), yet overall, the incidence of invasive cutaneous melanoma continues to rise in predominantly fair-skinned countries, including the United States, and is the fifth most common cancer diagnosed in men and women today.[1] Projections, which may not adequately capture preventive efforts, suggest that melanoma will be the second most common malignancy in men and women by 2040. In addition to a thorough understanding of the management of cutaneous melanoma, an understanding of less common cutaneous malignancies such as MCC, malignant cutaneous adnexal tumors, and DFSP is essential for the surgeon, as each of these entities require surgical expertise as a cornerstone of multidisciplinary management for patients with both localized and metastatic disease.

MELANOMA

Etiology and Risk Factors

Numerous environmental and genetic risk factors have been implicated in the development of cutaneous melanoma (**Table 101.1**).[2] Risk factors include acute and chronic exposure to ultraviolet (UV) radiation, such as a history of blistering or peeling sunburns, outdoor recreational activities or occupations, and the use of tanning beds, and factors related to increased sensitivity to UV, such as fair complexion (blue or green eyes, blonde, or red hair). Other factors that denote an increased risk for melanoma are a personal or family history of melanoma, nonmelanoma skin cancer, atypical nevi, or multiple typical nevi ("moles").

Adults with more than 100 clinically normal-appearing (typical) nevi, children with more than 50 clinically normal-appearing nevi, and any patient with atypical or dysplastic nevi are at increased risk for melanoma development. Atypical nevi are both potential precursor lesions and markers for increased risk of development of de novo melanoma as up to 50% to 75% of melanomas develop on clinically normal skin.

Congenital nevi, which are present at birth or appear within the first 6 months of infancy, occur in 1% to 6% of children.[3] Most congenital nevi are small, measuring less than 1.5 cm in diameter; congenital nevi between 1.5 and 19.9 cm in diameter are considered medium. The risk of melanoma development in small- and medium-sized congenital nevi is

Table 101.1. Risk Factors for Primary Melanoma

Risk Factor	Description of High-Risk Features
Nonmodifiable	
Gender	Male
Age	>60 y
Skin phenotype	Fair skin, red hair, blue eyes, multiple typical and atypical nevi
Genetics	Rare genetic disorders (xeroderma pigmentosum, mutations in *CDKN2a, CDK4, MC1R, BRCA2, BAP1*)
Potential Modifiable[a]	
Personal history	Prior skin cancers or precancerous lesions
Family history	Multiple prior first-degree relatives with melanoma, pancreatic cancer, astrocytoma, uveal melanoma, mesothelioma
Modifiable	
Ultraviolet (UV) exposure history	Prior sunburns, chronic sun-induced skin damage, UV tanning bed use, geographic residence in areas with high UV environmental exposure

[a]That is, with lifestyle change, sun protective strategies.

minimally increased compared to normal skin, if at all, and routine removal of these is rarely indicated in the absence of visible changes. Large (also termed giant) congenital nevi, measure 20 cm or greater (**Fig. 101.1A**) and melanoma develops in 5%, often before the age of 10 years (70%) and prophylactic removal of giant congenital nevi, often done in stages, can reduce the risk of subsequent melanoma development.[3]

A personal history of melanoma is associated with an increased risk of developing second primary melanomas, with 5% to 10% of individuals developing a second melanoma within 10 years of the original diagnosis. Of those that develop second primaries, the risk of additional primary melanomas is further increased, with up to 30% developing a third primary melanoma by 5 years.[4] The increased risk for additional primaries is likely multifactorial and incorporates the patient's inherent risk factors for melanoma (**Table 101.1**) as well as increased skin surveillance and awareness.

A family history of melanoma is reported by 10% to 15% of patients with melanoma, yet identifiable genetic predispositions are infrequent and shared susceptibility factors (living in a geographic region with high UV exposure, similar adherence to sun protective strategies and involvement in similar outdoor activities as other family members) likely contribute. Genetic counseling should be considered for patients with melanoma and an affected first-degree relative, those with multiple primary melanomas (often diagnosed at younger ages), or those with melanoma and a family history of pancreatic cancer or astrocytoma. Familial atypical multiple mole melanoma syndrome (FAMMM) is a clinical diagnosis made by the presence of melanoma in one or more first- or second-degree relatives, multiple nevi (>50) including atypical nevi, and specific histologic features on microscopy. It is commonly associated with mutations in cyclin-dependent kinase inhibitor 2 (*CDKN2A*).[5] Germline mutations in *CDKN2A* account for 0.2% of all melanoma cases but may be identified in up to 10% of families with two or more individuals with melanoma and up to 30% to 40% in families with three or more affected individuals. Other less frequently identified mutations include cyclin-dependent kinase 4 (*CDK4*), BRCA-1 associated protein-1 (*BAP-1*), telomerase reverse-transcriptase gene (*TERT*), melanoma-inducing transcription factor (*MITF*), and melanocortin-1 receptor (*MC1R*). Increased frequency of skin surveillance, self-skin examinations, digital dermoscopy, and screening for pancreas cancer may be incorporated into the care of patients with *CDKN2A* mutations.

Other cancer syndromes associated with an increased risk of developing melanoma include those with mutations in *PTEN, BRCA1, BRCA2, RB1*, and the TP53 pathway. Xeroderma pigmentosa is a rare autosomal recessive disorder associated with a reduced or absent ability to repair DNA damaged by UV light, which results in multiple primary cutaneous malignancies, including melanoma, BCC, and SCC. Individuals are usually diagnosed with their first cancer before the age of 10 years. Unfortunately, the development of skin cancers is relentless, with innumerable skin cancers developing unless strict sun avoidance is practiced from a very young age.

Clinical Diagnosis and Classification

Melanoma often has a characteristic appearance, but this is not always the case. The ABCDE rule was developed to help clinicians distinguish skin lesions concerning for melanoma from benign moles (**Table 101.2**).[6] However, many benign skin lesions exhibit some or even most of the features associated with the ABCDE rule, and conversely, some primary melanomas present with few or none of these features. An alternative and complementary diagnostic aid is the "ugly duckling sign," where any skin lesion substantially different from the others should be approached with a relatively high index of suspicion. The risk factors for melanoma should also be accounted for when determining the clinical suspicion for melanoma.

Cutaneous melanomas are classified into four major histologic subtypes (**Table 101.3**): superficial spreading (**Fig. 101.1B**), nodular (**Fig. 101.1C**), lentigo maligna melanoma (**Fig. 101.1D,E**), and acral lentiginous melanoma (**Fig. 101.1F**), which include subungual melanoma (**Fig. 101.1G**).

Other rare melanoma subtypes include mucosal (nasopharyngeal, esophageal, anorectal, or vulvovaginal), ocular (uveal or conjunctival), desmoplastic (**Fig. 101.1H**), nevoid, amelanotic, and pediatric melanomas.[7] Mucosal and uveal melanomas are associated with relatively poor prognoses, related in part to advanced disease at presentation due to delayed detection as well as decreased objective response rates to systemic therapy compared to patients with cutaneous melanoma. Desmoplastic melanomas, characterized microscopically with invasive spindled cells and abundant stromal collagen, tend to be amelanotic and thicker at presentation (**Fig. 101.1H**) and are associated with a higher rate of neurotropism, a lower rate of lymph node metastasis, and a higher risk of local recurrence than other forms of cutaneous melanoma. Nevoid melanomas and amelanotic melanomas often lack classic clinical features of melanoma, and histologically may share features with benign nevi. As such, they are often misdiagnosed or diagnosed late. Pediatric melanomas are those arising in children before age 18. Some represent typical adult melanomas detected earlier in life and share the epidemiologic factors and presenting features associated with melanoma in adulthood. Most melanomas occurring in the first few years of life arise from giant congenital nevi, while many melanomas in children and adolescents have histologic features similar to benign Spitz nevi (Spitzoid melanomas) and have a distinct epidemiology, presentation, and outcome compared to typical adult melanoma.[7] While not a histologic subtype, primary dermal melanoma merits discussion. Rarely primary melanomas may present with predominantly dermal findings on biopsy. This creates diagnostic ambiguity as to whether the site represents a dermal primary or a dermal metastasis. A thorough

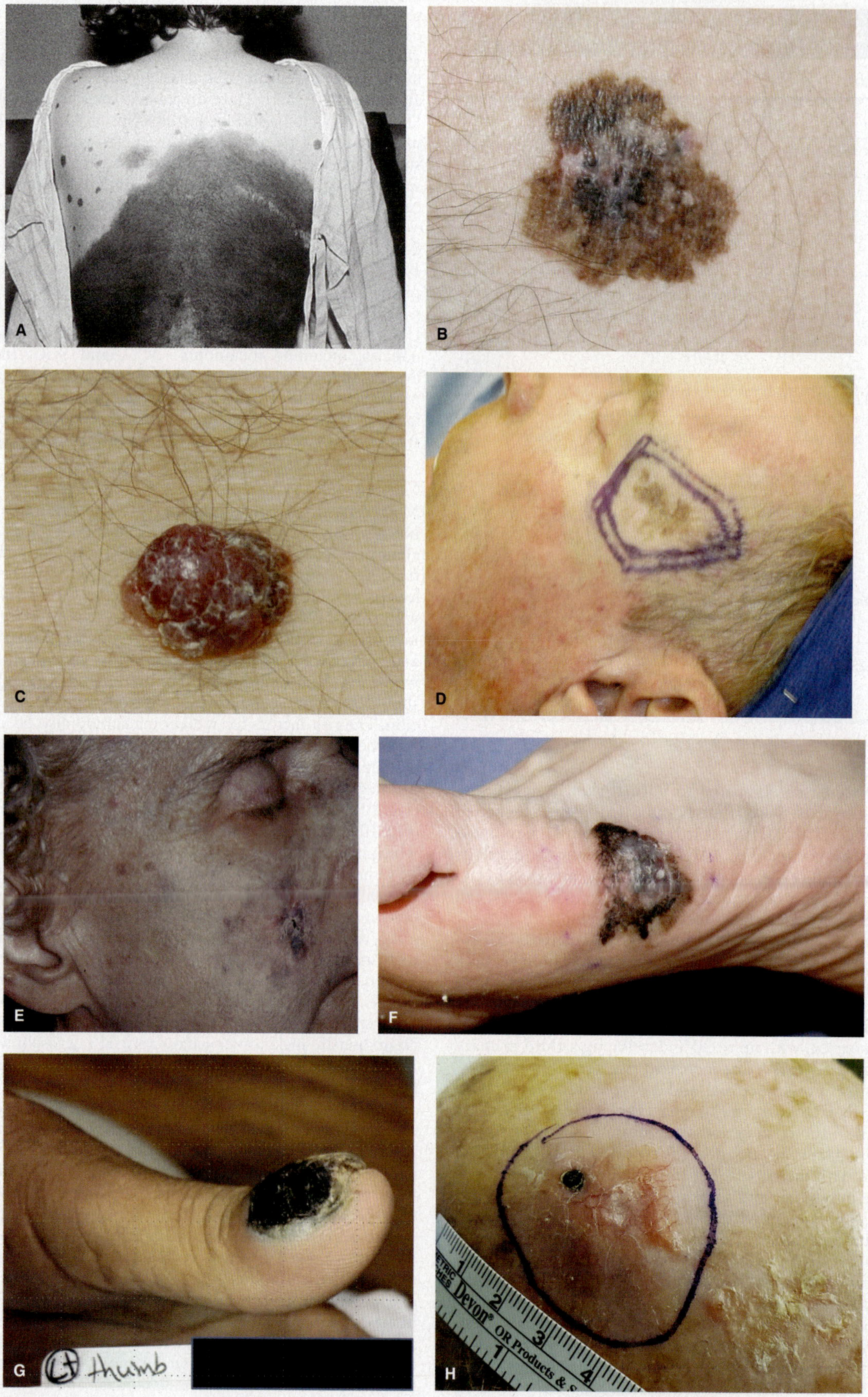

Figure 101.1. Examples of cutaneous melanocytic lesions. **A:** Giant congenital nevus involving a large portion of the back. **B:** Superficial spreading melanoma. **C:** Nodular melanoma. **D:** Lentigo maligna (a form of melanoma in situ, also called Hutchinson melanotic freckle) on the side of the face. **E:** Lentigo maligna melanoma (melanoma arising in a lentigo maligna) on the cheek. **F:** Acral lentiginous melanoma on the instep of the foot. **G:** Subungual melanoma of the thumb. **H:** Amelanotic desmoplastic melanoma (note overlying telangiectasias and dark-colored punch biopsy site) on the heavily sun-exposed scalp.

Table 101.2. The ABCDE Diagnostic Aid for Primary Melanoma[a]

Asymmetry	A portion of the pigmented lesion does not match the remainder
Border irregularity	Edges are blurred, jagged, or notched
Color variation	Lesion has variable areas of color with shades of brown, black, white, red, and/or blue
Diameter	Greater than 6 mm
Evolution/elevation	Change over time or lesion raised above skin level

[a]Adapted from American Academy of Dermatology Ad Hoc Task Force for the ABCDEs of Melanoma, Tsao H, Olazagasti JM, et al. Early detection of melanoma: reviewing the ABCDEs. *J Am Acad Dermatol.* 2015;72(4): 717–723.

physical exam to rule out a separate primary melanoma and a staging evaluation with cross-sectional imaging to evaluate for distant metastatic disease is appropriate for these patients. Provided no evidence of other disease is identified, patients with a dermal melanoma should be treated similarly to their counterparts with an epidermal component. With these noted exceptions, the subtype classification itself does not convey additional prognostic information when accounting for stage at presentation.

2 Staging and Prognostic Factors

Microstaging

Microscopic characteristics of the primary cutaneous melanoma inform prognosis, including Breslow depth, ulceration, mitotic rate, and microsatellitosis. The primary driver of microstaging is Breslow depth, which quantifies tumor thickness in millimeters and is measured from the top of the granular layer of the skin to the base of the tumor using a micrometer inside the microscope eyepiece. Breslow depth is inversely correlated with survival[8,9] and conveys prognosis more accurately than Clark level of invasion (which assigns a numeric score based on the specific histologic layer of skin and may be misinterpreted by patients as representing the overall cancer stage). Along with depth, the presence of ulceration is inversely associated with survival, and depth and ulceration are incorporated into the American Joint Committee on Cancer (AJCC) 8th edition staging manual for melanoma.[8,9] Other factors, such as mitotic rate, lymphovascular invasion, perineural invasion, microsatellitosis, tumor regression, and presence or absence of tumor-infiltrating lymphocytes (TILs) also impart prognostic value and should be reported in the pathologic description of the melanoma.

Regional lymph node metastasis confers a more advanced stage and is stratified by number of nodes involved (1, 2–3, or ≥4) as well as method of detection (microscopically as with a sentinel lymph node biopsy [SLNB] and therefore clinically occult, or clinically detected). The tumor burden of involved lymph nodes significantly correlates with long-term survival.[8,9] In contemporary data, the 10-year survival rate for patients with involved lymph nodes ranges from as high as 88% (stage IIIA, clinically occult) to as low as 24% (stage IIID), based on tumor burden (size and number of nodal metastases) and thickness and ulceration status of the primary lesion.[9]

Clinical and Pathologic Staging

The AJCC incorporates tumor thickness (T), nodal status (N), and absence or presence of metastatic disease (M) to risk stratify patients with melanoma by stage. The current AJCC 8th edition system was implemented in 2018 and stratifies patients into stage 0 (in situ melanoma), stage I (localized disease, thin primary), stage II (localized disease, thicker primary), stage III (regional nodal, in transit, or satellite metastases), and stage IV (distant metastases), with 5-year overall survival (OS) ranging from 99% with stage I disease to 25% with stage IV disease.[8,9]

Other Prognostic Factors

The major prognostic factors that predict survival in melanoma patients are accounted for in the AJCC staging system—tumor microstaging, nodal status, and absence or presence of distant metastases. Ulceration and mitotic rate (≥1 per mm^2) are independent negative prognostic factors, although they are observed more frequently in thicker primaries.[9] The presence of grossly visible or microscopic satellites, by definition located within 2 cm of the primary melanoma, or in-transit metastases (located more than 2 cm from the primary and between the primary and the regional nodal basin) are considered evidence of intralymphatic metastasis in the AJCC staging system and confer increased risk.[10]

Other prognostic factors for recurrence and/or melanoma-specific survival are impactful within specific subsets of patients. For example, increasing tumor burden within an involved sentinel node and number of involved sentinel nodes correlates with risk of additional involved nonsentinel nodes and melanoma-specific survival in patients with IIIA disease.[9,11]

Table 101.3. Common Subtypes of Cutaneous Melanomas

Name	Approximate Frequency (%)	Features
Superficial spreading melanoma	60	Common in melanomas arising from a preexisting nevus Typically exhibits the classic clinical features of melanoma (see **Table 101.2**)
Nodular melanoma	20	Frequently lacks classic ABCDE features of melanoma Often diagnosed late
Lentigo maligna melanoma	18	Typically occurs on sun-exposed areas of head and neck or hands, often in older individuals Lesions are flat, broad, and asymmetric Extensive subclinical extension relatively more
Acral lentiginous melanoma	2	Occurs on hands and feet ("acral skin") Represents up to 60% of all melanomas occurring in people of color Often diagnosed late due unusual location and appearance Subungual melanoma commonly mistaken for hematoma

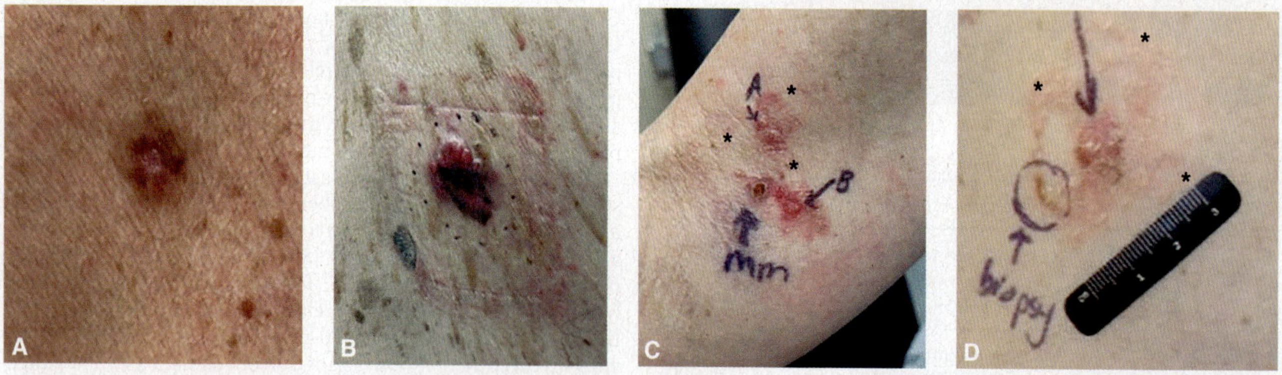

Figure 101.2. **A:** A patient with a diagnosis of melanoma in situ and residual pigment surrounding the initial punch biopsy site. **B:** A patient with a thick primary with substantial residual pigment and heaping of edges suggesting residual melanoma. **C:** A patient with amelanotic melanoma diagnosed with initial biopsy ("*mm*"). In addition to the marked sites, multiple surveillance biopsies (*) were performed to delineate the lesion; all demonstrated contiguous melanoma and this entire area was excised as single primary. **D:** A patient with a melanoma with substantial regression and lack of pigment. In addition to the marked biopsy site adjacent to the original shave (*arrow*), surveillance biopsies (*) were used along the perimeter to guide intraoperative margin placement.

In addition to histologic factors, advancements in molecular diagnostics have led to the development of genomic platforms that can potentially be used to risk stratify and inform prognosis among specific subgroups of patients. Examples undergoing investigation include a 31-gene expression profile test which segregates patients with stage I to III disease into low-, intermediate-, or high-risk subsets. While appropriately powered prospective trials are still lacking thereby limiting the applicability of these platforms, large multiinstitutional retrospective studies as well as population-based registry trials have produced promising results.[12] Early identification of patients with biologically aggressive disease who would otherwise be characterized as low risk by current staging algorithms may aid in decision-making regarding frequency of surveillance. In addition, an enhanced understanding of the risk of recurrence may inform adjuvant therapy, although data to support adjuvant therapy in this patient population is currently limited to patients with IIB/C disease.

Treatment of Primary Melanoma

Biopsy

Biopsy of a suspicious pigmented skin lesion may be performed with either shave technique or a punch biopsy.[13] Either technique is acceptable in experienced hands and must be performed in a manner that incorporates sufficient tissue thickness to accurately measure depth. Superficial transection of the specimen will underestimate Breslow thickness, and surgeons should recognize that an involved deep margin may reflect a more invasive melanoma. Either repeat biopsy or adjustment of the surgical plan (eg, discussion of a sentinel node procedure in a patient with a 0.7 mm nonulcerated primary with an involved deep margin on biopsy) may be necessary. Biopsy of larger lesions, which may be challenging to fully remove with biopsy, should be targeted to the most concerning aspect. Additional surveillance biopsies of the surrounding pigment can be helpful in assessing complex lesions, and in cases of amelanotic melanoma or melanomas with poorly defined borders may aid in planning margins (**Fig. 101.2**).

Staging Workup

Current consensus guidelines have attempted to standardize staging workup for melanoma (**Algorithm 101.1**).[14,15] Clinical staging relies heavily on a thorough history and physical examination, including a total body skin examination and palpation of lymph nodes. Laboratory and imaging studies should be symptom-directed. Routine imaging (ie, chest x-ray, computed tomography [CT] scans, positron emission tomography [PET] scans) and laboratory studies in asymptomatic, clinically node-negative patients are not routinely performed as they have low sensitivity and specificity and can result in false-positive or indeterminate results. Both ultrasound and PET scans have been examined as methods of identifying nodal metastases prior to surgery. While they detect disease in a minority of patients, most metastases to the regional nodes are smaller than the threshold ultrasound and PET can detect, so their routine use is not a cost-effective strategy.[14,15] If a thorough history and physical and detailed review of systems reveal no signs or symptoms suspicious for regional or distant disease, then no further staging is necessary prior to surgery. In appropriate patients, SLNB represents the best baseline staging test, with relatively high sensitivity and specificity. When the SLNB identifies nodal involvement, guidelines suggest clinicians consider additional cross-sectional imaging, including nodal basin ultrasound, CT of the chest/abdomen/pelvis and neck if clinically indicated or FDG-PET, and magnetic resonance imaging (MRI) of the brain.

Approximately 5% to 10% of newly diagnosed melanoma patients present with clinically involved lymph nodes. Any clinically suspicious node should be confirmed to represent melanoma, preferably by fine-needle aspiration (FNA) biopsy, as enlarged lymph nodes may be reactive (particularly after a skin biopsy). In cases where the suspicious node is difficult to localize and/or immobilize image guidance (most commonly with ultrasound) can be highly effective. Excisional biopsy should *only* be reserved for situations in which percutaneous biopsy (FNA or core needle biopsy) is unable to establish a diagnosis. Patients with macroscopic regional disease should undergo formal staging exams (**Algorithm 101.1**) as a significant percentage may have more advanced regional or distant disease that may alter the therapeutic approach. Staging for patients with clinical stage III melanoma should include a brain MRI, and either CT scan of the chest, abdomen, and pelvis (as well as neck for primary sites draining to the cervical nodes such as head, neck, and upper chest/back primary sites) or whole-body PET/CT scan.

Excision of Primary Melanoma

3 The goal of surgical excision of primary melanomas is to reduce the risk of local recurrence. For melanoma in situ, excision margins of 0.5 to 1.0 cm are accepted as the standard of care. Multiple randomized trials are available to inform margin status for patients with invasive melanoma and anticipated future trials (MelMarT) may impact current standards, particularly for patients with nonulcerated primaries >2 mm in Breslow thickness. The recommended excision margins for primary melanoma based on available randomized controlled trials are described in **Table 101.4**.[16]

Although oncologic principles should not be compromised, anatomic considerations do influence the ability to resect some primary melanomas. For example, patients with melanomas

Algorithm 101.1

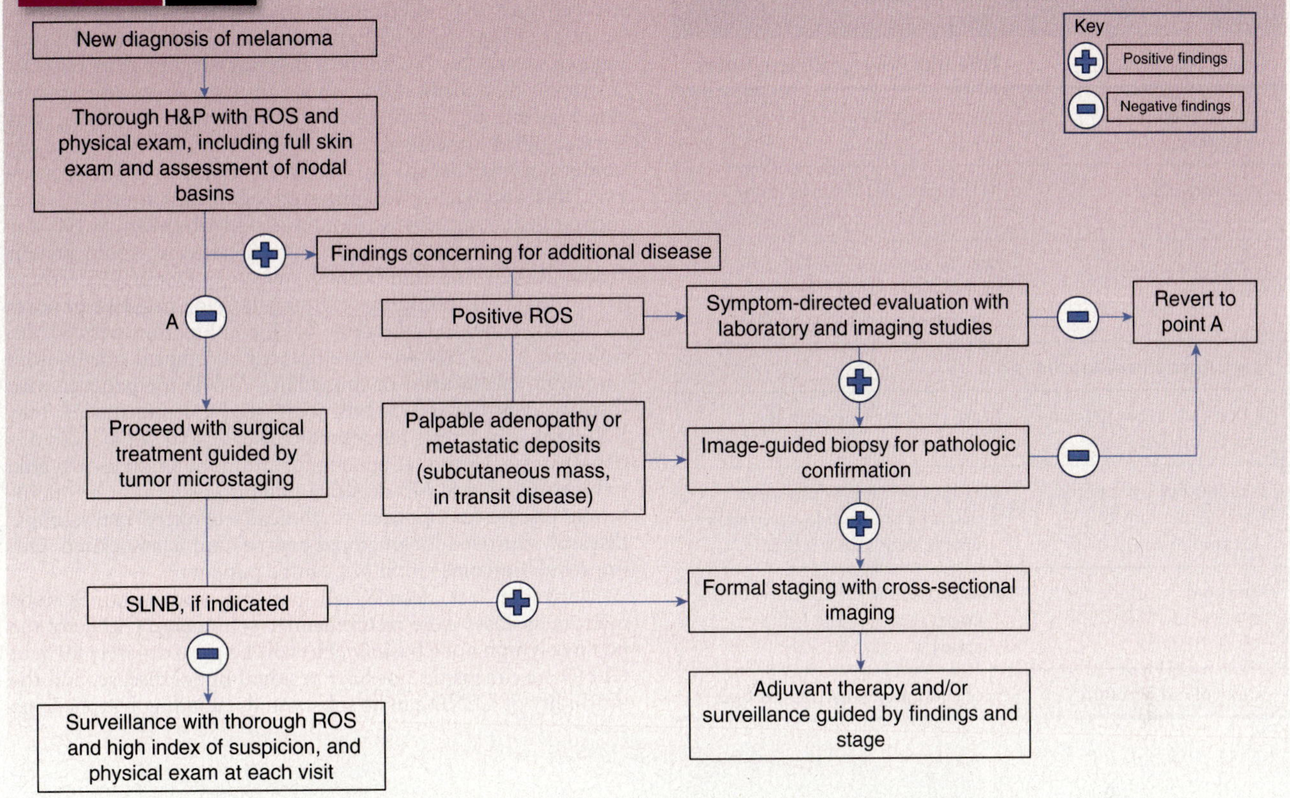

Algorithm 101.1. Suggested diagnostic algorithm for the initial evaluation of the patient with melanoma.

on the head/neck or mucosal surfaces may have significant functional morbidity such that maximum attainable margins are narrower than consensus guidelines. Margins may need to be modified based on anatomic considerations but still should obtain histologically confirmed tumor-free margins. Most subungual invasive melanomas (**Fig. 101.1G**) are best managed by partial amputation of the digit, although conservative excisions with skin grafting can be considered for thin or in situ subungual melanomas.

For melanomas with ill-defined borders—especially lentigo maligna melanoma on the head and neck—subclinical extension beyond the clinically evident tumor may result in unanticipated positive margins. Excision with a temporary dressing followed by delayed reconstruction allows thorough histologic assessment of margin status and alleviates difficulty with margin reexcision after complex tissue rearrangement or flap reconstruction that may otherwise preclude additional margin resection.

Table 101.4. Recommended Surgical Margins for Melanoma Excision

Melanoma Thickness (mm)	Recommended Excision Margin (cm)
In situ	0.5–1.0
≤1.0	1.0
1.1–2.0	1.0–2.0
>2.0	2.0

Margins may need to be modified on the basis of anatomic considerations but still should obtain histologically confirmed tumor-free margins.
Data from Thompson JF, Henderson MA, Williams G, Ross MI. Treatment of primary melanoma. In: Balch CM, Atkins MB, Garbe C, et al., eds. *Cutaneous Melanoma*. 6th ed. Springer Nature; 2020:573–594.

Sentinel Lymph Node Biopsy

4 SLNB is recommended for clinically node-negative patients with melanoma ≥0.8 mm in Breslow depth, or for those with melanoma <0.8 mm in depth with ulceration. In addition, SLNB could be considered for patients with thin melanomas <0.8 mm in depth *and* younger age, mitotic rate ≥1 mitosis/mm^2, angiolymphatic invasion, or a broadly transected deep margin on shave biopsy.[17] SLNB is most commonly performed with dual tracers: a radiolabeled colloid and a blue dye injected intradermally around the primary melanoma. The dual agent technique increases the accuracy of the procedure and identifies the sentinel node(s) in >97% of operations.[18] The type of dye is regionally variable, and each formulation is associated with extremely rare but potentially serious risks (**Table 101.5**).

Some lymphatic drainage patterns of melanoma are predictable or easily accessible in the operating room without preoperative lymphoscintigraphy images (eg, melanomas on the thigh or upper extremities). Others, such as those on the trunk or head and neck, may have multiple draining basins and preoperative lymphoscintigraphy is critical in operative planning to allow appropriate patient positioning and draping of the surgical field(s). Planar lymphoscintigraphy is sufficient to localize the draining basin in most patients; combination with SPECT-CT enhances anatomic localization and may be useful for head and neck melanomas and for lymph nodes in unusual sites (**Fig. 101.3**). Sentinel nodes are serially sectioned by the pathologist for hematoxylin and eosin staining and immunohistochemical staining to assess for micrometastases (including single cells) that can be missed by the traditional process of bisecting nodes.[19] If metastases are found in the sentinel node, BRAF immunohistochemistry can be performed to assess for the presence of a BRAF V600E mutation (**Fig. 101.4**).

Treatment of Regional Metastatic Melanoma: Microscopic Disease

SLNB is critical in providing prognostic and therapeutic information about the draining nodal basin. First developed as a

Table 101.5. Factors Influencing the Selection of Tracer Agent for Sentinel Node Biopsy

Tracer Agent: Dye	Potential Adverse Effects/Notes
1% Isosulfan blue (Lymphazurin)	Anaphylaxis (1%)
Methylene blue	May cause skin necrosis if not diluted or completely resected
Indocyanine green	May be noninferior to blue dyes and avoids tissue discoloration; requires near-infrared camera
Trace Agent: Radionuclides	
Sulfur colloid conjugated to technetium-99	More commonly used in the United States
Tilmanocept conjugated to technetium-99 (Lymphoseek)	May be associated with shorter mapping time and less secondary uptake than sulfur colloid
Antimony trisulfide	More commonly used in Australia, not available in the United States
Nanocolloid albumin	More commonly used in Europe

means to identify which patients would benefit from completion lymph node dissection (CLND), the role of SLNB has evolved such that today, it may be the only surgical strategy necessary for patients with microscopic nodal disease. Knowledge of several key landmark trials over the past three decades is critical to understanding this paradigm shift. Prior to the development of SLNB, elective lymph node dissection was performed as a means to obtain local control and potentially confer survival benefit by earlier clearance of disease; however, this approach also conferred significant morbidity and did not benefit patients without nodal involvement. SLNB was initially introduced to identify which patients would benefit from CLND. The Multicenter Selective Lymphadenectomy Trial I (MSLT-I) randomized clinically node-negative patients to radical wide excision alone or in combination with SLNB, followed by CLND for development of clinical adenopathy (in the no SLNB arm) or immediate CLND for patients with disease identified on SLNB. This study demonstrated that SLNB reliably detects microscopic disease, and while it did not demonstrate a survival benefit for the population as a whole (which included SLNB-negative patients), resection of microscopic disease (as opposed to clinically detected macroscopic disease) improved locoregional control and is associated with improved outcomes in SLN-positive patients.[20]

Until the last decade, all patients with sentinel node micrometastases were recommended to undergo CLND of the positive lymph node basin(s). However, approximately 80% of CLND specimens do not have residual nodal disease, and the morbidity of CLND can be substantial, including lymphedema

A

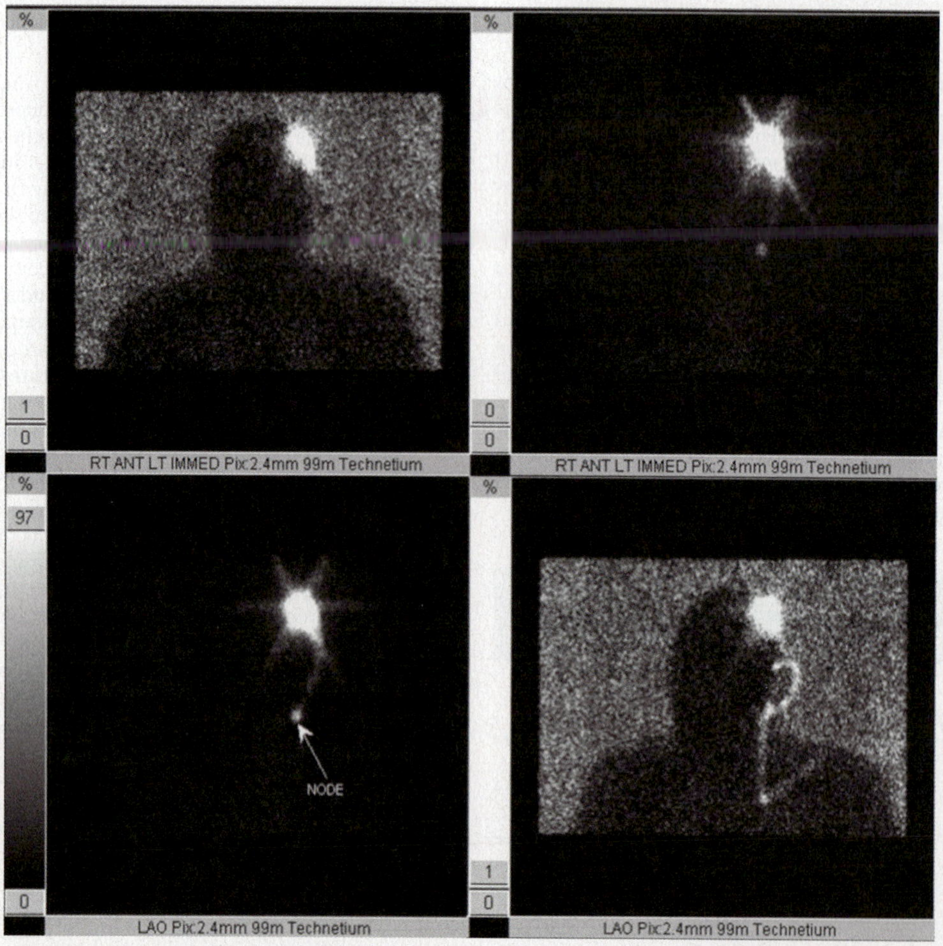

Figure 101.3. **A:** Planar lymphoscintigraphy for sentinel lymph node localization in patient with an intermediate-thickness melanoma of the left frontal scalp. One cervical node is identified (**lower left panel**). In the **lower right panel**, the nuclear medicine technologist has used a radioactive marker to outline the left ear, sternocleidomastoid muscle, and clavicle.

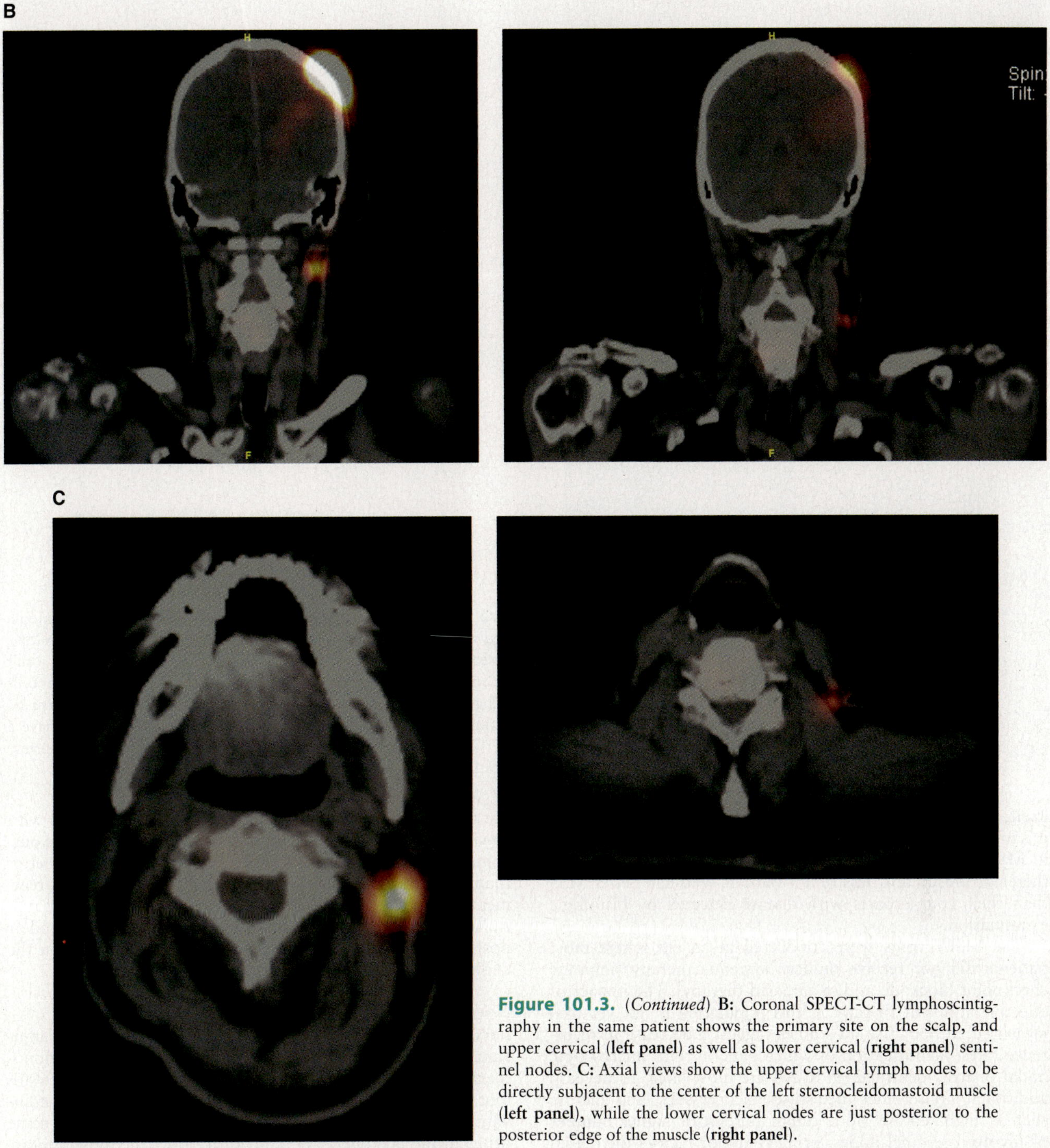

Figure 101.3. (*Continued*) **B:** Coronal SPECT-CT lymphoscintigraphy in the same patient shows the primary site on the scalp, and upper cervical (**left panel**) as well as lower cervical (**right panel**) sentinel nodes. **C:** Axial views show the upper cervical lymph nodes to be directly subjacent to the center of the left sternocleidomastoid muscle (**left panel**), while the lower cervical nodes are just posterior to the posterior edge of the muscle (**right panel**).

in as much as 20% to 25% of patients.[21] Both the German prospective randomized trial, DeCOG-SLT, and the MSLT-II study were designed to evaluate whether CLND is necessary after identification of an SLN metastasis. Patients with SLN metastases were randomized to either immediate CLND or observation with serial ultrasound and CLND upon identification of nodal recurrence. Although DeCOG-SLT closed early due to low accrual, the study remains valuable in that it showed no major differences in distant metastasis-free survival, recurrence-free survival, and regional recurrence rates in patients treated with immediate surgery versus expectant surveillance.[22–28] MSLT-II demonstrated no OS benefit for patients undergoing immediate CLND (86 ± 1.3% vs 86 ± 1.2%, $P = .42$) as compared to ultrasound surveillance at a median follow-up of 43 months, and changed practice paradigms around the world.[23] While there was a small benefit in disease-free survival with immediate CLND, it was largely attributed to improved regional disease control at 3 years (92 ± 1% vs 77 ± 1.5% in the observation group, $P < .001$) and came at the expense of increased morbidity (24.1% lymphedema vs 6.3% in the observation group, $P < .001$). Although CLND does provide prognostic information for those with non-SLN micrometastases (increased risk of recurrence in the 11.5% with additional disease HR 1.78, $P = .005$) most patients with a positive SLNB are preferably managed with active nodal surveillance, reserving CLND for those who cannot undergo surveillance (generally due to access to appropriate ultrasonography). Active nodal surveillance typically involves evaluation of the nodal basin by clinical examination and ultrasound every 4 months for the first 2 years, every 6 months for years 3 to 5, and annually until year 10.

Taken in aggregate, if immediate CLND does not confer a survival benefit, then the survival benefit observed in SLNB-positive patients in MSLT-I must be driven by the SLNB

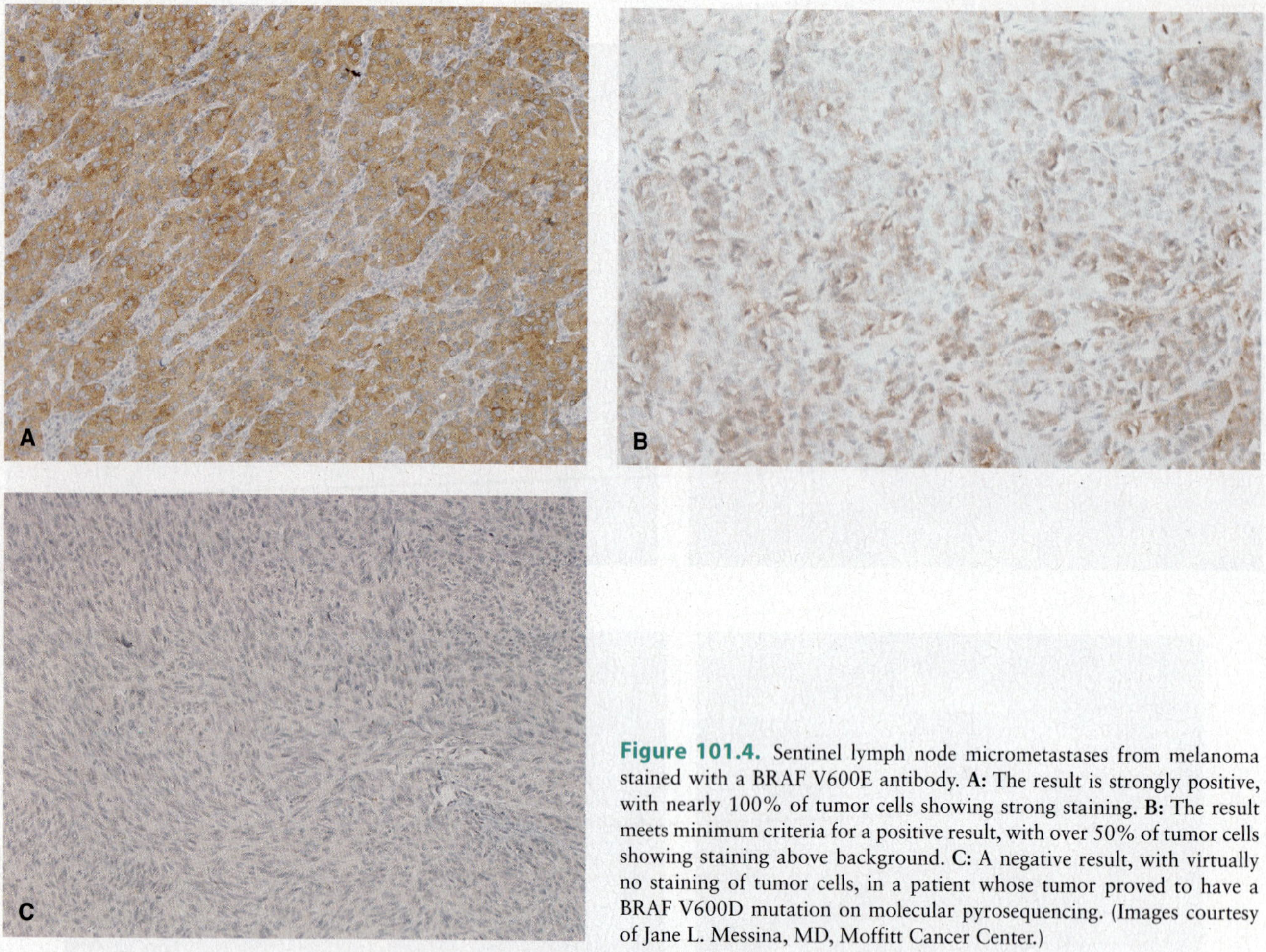

Figure 101.4. Sentinel lymph node micrometastases from melanoma stained with a BRAF V600E antibody. **A:** The result is strongly positive, with nearly 100% of tumor cells showing strong staining. **B:** The result meets minimum criteria for a positive result, with over 50% of tumor cells showing staining above background. **C:** A negative result, with virtually no staining of tumor cells, in a patient whose tumor proved to have a BRAF V600D mutation on molecular pyrosequencing. (Images courtesy of Jane L. Messina, MD, Moffitt Cancer Center.)

itself, underscoring the importance of removing disease when it is microscopic.[24] This is supported by analyses of the patients in MSLT-II with micrometastases identified by RT-PCR, and therefore presumably less tumor burden, who had better MSS than their counterparts with disease detected by histologic examination.

The MSLT trials were conducted in an era where most patients did not receive modern systemic therapy (immune checkpoint blockade and/or targeted therapy). The impact of effective adjuvant therapy in this population is not yet well measured, although small studies suggest a decrease in recurrence rates. Identification of which patients with microscopic nodal disease identified on SLNB are most likely to develop additional nonsentinel metastases is necessary, and factors such as high sentinel node tumor burden or higher number of involved sentinel nodes, primary tumor factors (increased Breslow depth, ulceration, mitotic rate), and receipt of adjuvant therapy are likely to inform clinical decision-making.

Treatment of Regional Metastatic Melanoma: Macroscopic Disease

5 For melanoma patients presenting with clinically detected tumor-involved nodes (AJCC 8th edition stage IIIB–D), including those who recur in the nodal basin after a positive or false-negative SLNB, therapeutic lymphadenectomy remains the standard of care.[25] Staging exams (cross-sectional imaging to include the chest/abdomen/pelvis or a PET-CT and an MRI brain) should be performed to evaluate for concomitant distant disease. A small percentage of stage III melanoma patients (about 10% of all clinical stage III cases) present with clinically evident nodal disease in the absence of a known primary cutaneous melanoma.[26] Almost all of these cases represent nodal metastases from primary cutaneous melanomas that either regressed spontaneously or were removed in the past but not recognized as malignant.[7] When patients present with isolated nodal disease from an unknown primary site, the outcomes of lymphadenectomy are generally as good or better than those for patients with known primary tumors. Treatment of patients with macroscopic regional disease occurs typically in combination with preoperative (neoadjuvant) and/or postoperative (adjuvant) systemic therapy, depending on the clinical presentation (**Table 101.6**).

Neoadjuvant Therapy

For patients with macroscopic stage III melanoma, neoadjuvant therapy utilizes single-agent or combination immunotherapy, or for patients whose tumors harbor a BRAF V600E mutation, combination BRAF and MEK inhibition. Neoadjuvant therapy has several key advantages over giving the same drugs in the postoperative adjuvant setting, the most important of which may be the ability to assess the response of the tumor to treatment clinically (by physical examination and/or cross-sectional imaging), metabolically (by ^{18}F-FDG PET scanning), and pathologically (**Fig. 101.5**). SWOG 1801, a randomized phase II study comparing neoadjuvant pembrolizumab to adjuvant pembrolizumab showed a significant improvement in event free survival for patients receiving neoadjuvant therapy.[27] The phase III NADINA trial, similar in its design to SWOG 1801 except with nivolumab and ipilimumab in the neoadjuvant setting, also showed a significant improvement in outcomes for patients receiving neoadjuvant therapy compared to patients only receiving therapy after surgery.[28] These two studies strongly suggest that patients who are able to receive therapy prior to surgery may benefit significantly from doing so.

Patients who obtain a complete or near-complete pathologic response to preoperative treatment appear to have a particularly good outcome and may ultimately need less radical

Table 101.6. Selected Landmark Trials in the Era of Effective Systemic Therapy for Patients with Melanoma

Trial, Year(s) Published	n	Comparison	Patient Population	Impact on Clinical Practice
ADJUVANT				
EORTC 18071 2015	951	Ipi[a] vs placebo	Stage IIIA–C[b]	Adjuvant Ipi improved OS compared to placebo, with a high incidence of serious AEs
CheckMate-238 2017	906	Nivo vs Ipi[a]	IIIB–IV[b]	Adjuvant Nivo significantly improved RFS (but not OS) compared to Ipi with fewer serious AEs, shifting the preferred adjuvant therapy to nivolumab
CheckMate-915 2022	1833	Ipi/Nivo vs Nivo	IIIB–IV	Combination Ipi/Nivo increased AEs and did not improve RFS compared to Nivo alone, further supporting Nivo monotherapy in the adjuvant setting
CheckMate-76K 2023	790	Nivo vs placebo	IIB–IIC	Adjuvant Nivo improved RFS (89% vs 79.4% at 1 y), introducing this therapy for patients with high-risk stage II disease
KEYNOTE-054 2018, 2020, 2021	1019	Pembro vs placebo	IIIA (>1 mm metastasis)—IIIC[a]	Adjuvant pembro improved RFS (75.4% vs 65.1% at 1 y) with acceptable toxicity (14.7%) and this effect persisted at the final analysis with improvement in DMFS
KEYNOTE-716 2022, 2024	976	Pembro vs placebo	IIB–IIC	Adjuvant pembro improved RFS (72.6% vs 63.4%) and DMFS, introducing this therapy for patients with high-risk stage II disease
COMBI-AD 2017, 2020, 2024	870	Dab/Tram vs placebo	IIIA (>1 mm metastasis) – IIIC[a] with BRAFV600E mutation	Demonstrated a durable benefit in RFS and OS, establishing this therapy in the adjuvant setting for patients with BRAF mutated melanoma
NEOADJUVANT (WITH OR WITHOUT ADJUVANT COMPONENT)				
SWOG 1801 2023	345	Pembro/surgery/pembro vs surgery/adjuvant pembro	IIIB–IVC	A combination approach with neoadjuvant pembro improved EFS (72% vs 49%) as compared to adjuvant treatment alone, and showed major PR in more than half of patients
Amaria et al. 2018	23	Nivo vs Ipi/Nivo	III-oligometastatic IV	Demonstrated feasibility of combination therapy in the neoadjuvant setting with higher response and pCR rates but also higher toxicity
OpACIN 2018	20	Ipi/Nivo-surgery-Ipi/Nivo vs adjuvant Ipi/Nivo	IIIB–IIIC	Demonstrated pCR in 78% and showed improved RFS in OS in the neoadjuvant arm
Amaria et al. 2022	30	Phase II single-arm neoadjuvant Nivo/rela	III-oligometastatic IV	Provided data to support the use of this specific regimen in the resectable/neoadjuvant setting and demonstrated increased RFS associated with pCR
NeoCombi 2019, 2024	35	Phase-II single-arm dab/tram-surgery-dab/tram	IIIB–IIIC with BRAFV600E mutation	Demonstrated a high pCR but long-term follow-up demonstrated no difference in RFS compared to adjuvant administration alone, and low RFS at 5 y (40%), even among patients with pCR

Ipi, ipilimumab; OS, overall survival; AEs, adverse events; Nivo, nivolumab; RFS, recurrence-free survival; Pembro, pembrolizumab; DMFS, distant metastasis-free survival; Dab, dabrafenib; Tram, Trametinib; BRAF, v-raf murine sarcoma viral oncogene homolog B1; EFS, event-free survival; PR, pathologic response; pCR, pathologic complete response; Rela, relatlimab.

[a]Dosed at 10 mg/kg.

[b]Based on AJCC 7th edition staging.

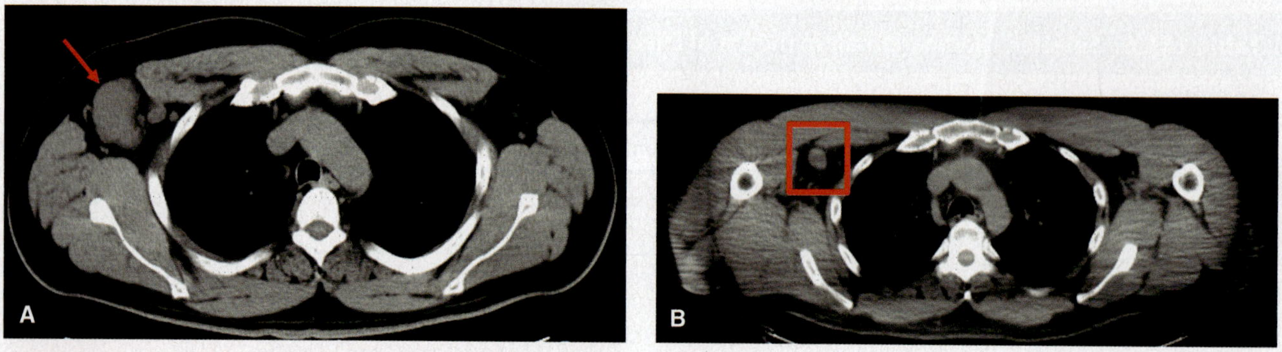

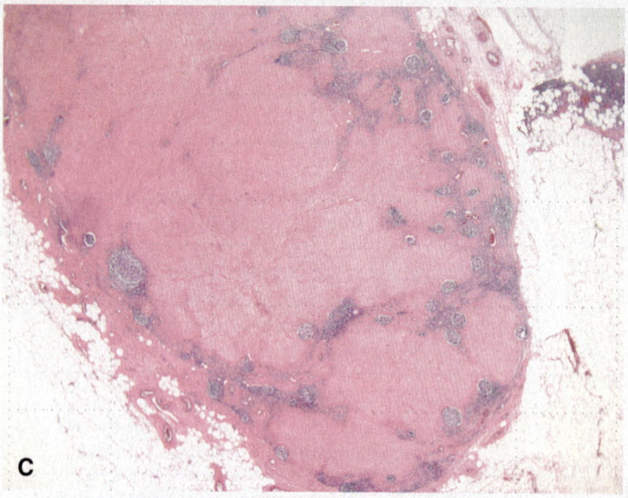

Figure 101.5. Neoadjuvant therapy for stage III melanoma. **A:** Pretreatment CT scan showing a large right axillary lymph node (*arrow*) that developed 2 years after radical wide excision of a thin (T1a) melanoma of the ipsilateral arm. **B:** Scans after 6 months of BRAF/MEK inhibition, showing a partial response to therapy (*box*). **C:** Histologic specimen from the lymphadenectomy, showing posttreatment changes but no viable tumor (pathologic complete response). The patient received no further therapy and remains disease-free more than 4 years later. (Images courtesy of Jane L. Messina, MD, Moffitt Cancer Center.)

surgery and no postoperative systemic therapy (**Fig. 101.4**). Although still under early investigation, initial results of the PRADO trial suggest that there may be a role for deescalation of surgery in patients with major pathologic response (defined as ≤10% viable tumor). In this trial, patients with clinically detected nodal disease were treated with immunotherapy and underwent resection of the index node; those with major pathologic response were observed, whereas those with partial or no response proceeded to CLND. Surgical morbidity was, as expected, lower in the group without CLND, and the 2-year recurrence-free survival (RFS) for the major pathologic responders was 93%. Median follow-up is short at 28 months and included 7% regional recurrences, suggesting that deescalation of surgery requires ongoing investigation.[29] Additional studies will be necessary to identify which patients with major pathologic response will be most likely to succeed with deescalation of surgery, to understand the optimal drug regimen(s) and duration of neoadjuvant therapy, as well as the impact of adjuvant treatment. Patients with high-risk stage II and all stage III disease who are not treated in the neoadjuvant setting remain candidates for adjuvant therapy. Specific drug regimens utilized in the neoadjuvant and adjuvant settings are described in detail below (Systemic Therapy for Melanoma) and available impactful clinical trials examining neoadjuvant therapy for resectable and oligometastatic melanoma are summarized in **Table 101.6**.

Adjuvant Therapy

Although the prognosis for patients with early-stage cutaneous melanoma is quite good, fewer patients with thick primaries (>4 mm) or regional node involvement are cured by surgery alone. Until recently, numerous randomized trials evaluating systemic chemotherapeutic agents (most notably dacarbazine), nonspecific immunotherapy (such as Bacille Calmette–Guérin [BCG]), tumor-specific vaccines, biochemotherapy, and interferons in the adjuvant setting either failed to demonstrate any impact on survival or were associated with prohibitive toxicity that limited their clinical value. The success of immune checkpoint blockade and molecularly targeted agents in the treatment of unresectable metastatic melanoma, however, spawned a series of randomized clinical trials that revolutionized the adjuvant therapy of high-risk resected melanoma (**Table 101.6**); specific drug regimens are described in detail below (Systemic Therapy for Melanoma).[30]

Adjuvant Radiation Therapy

Despite cutaneous melanoma often being considered radioresistant, adjuvant postoperative radiation can be useful in some settings. Desmoplastic melanoma is a rare subtype of cutaneous melanoma with predisposition to recur locally, especially in the setting of perineural invasion, and is particularly sensitive to radiation. Available evidence suggests that postoperative radiation can substantially decrease the risk of local recurrence of desmoplastic melanoma, especially when the primary tumor is thick, situated on the head or neck, or in the presence of perineural extension.[31] Postoperative radiation to the tumor-involved nodal basin after therapeutic lymphadenectomy has been studied in a randomized trial. Adjuvant postoperative radiation can decrease the in-basin regional recurrence risk, with an increase in lymphedema and other toxicities, but does not improve OS.[32] Adjuvant nodal radiation should be considered in patients with multiple involved nodes, particularly in the presence of extranodal extension. Investigation of the role of adjuvant radiotherapy after a positive sentinel node biopsy is underway (NCT04594187).

Treatment of In-Transit Disease

In-transit metastatic melanoma is defined as any recurrence between the primary melanoma site and the regional lymph nodes and is thought to be due to intralymphatic metastasis. In-transit metastatic melanoma without distant metastasis is classified as stage III disease. Treatment options include excision, intralesional therapy, regional chemotherapy, or systemic therapy. As with all advanced stages of disease in the current era, most treatment algorithms begin with either systemic therapy or a clinical trial. Given the focus of systemic therapy elsewhere in this chapter, this section will focus on patients who are not candidates for systemic regimens or who have failed them.

Prior to proceeding with treatment, a complete staging workup for metastatic disease should be performed. Surgical excision should be considered when the number of lesions is relatively small, and particularly when the time from previous treatment to the development of the recurrence is relatively long. When resection is not feasible, intralesional therapy may be considered. Although multiple injectable agents have been studied (BCG, Coxsackievirus A21, interleukin 2, granulocyte-macrophage colony-stimulating factor), the most commonly used treatment (and currently the only FDA-approved agent) is talimogene laherparepvec (TVEC), an oncolytic immunotherapy derived from the herpes simplex virus type-1. In a randomized phase III trial of patients with unresectable IIIB-IV melanoma with injectable cutaneous metastases, TVEC led to an improved response rate compared to a control arm of subcutaneous GM-CSF (19.0% vs 1.4%; $P < .0001$), and a subset of these patients achieved durable responses (**Fig. 101.6**).[33]

When the in-transit disease is unresectable, limited to an extremity, and systemic therapy is not a preferred choice or has failed, regional administration of high-dose hyperthermic chemotherapy can be effective. Isolated limb perfusion (ILP) surgically isolates the vasculature and uses an extracorporeal membrane oxygenator (as used in cardiac surgery) to deliver chemotherapy doses 15 to 25 times higher than can be obtained with systemic delivery. Response rates between 80% and 90% are reported for well selected patients, with complete response rates between 40% and 65%, which can be durable.[34] Toxicities range from mild erythema and edema to epidermolysis, functional impairment, compartment syndrome, and extremely rarely, a need for amputation.

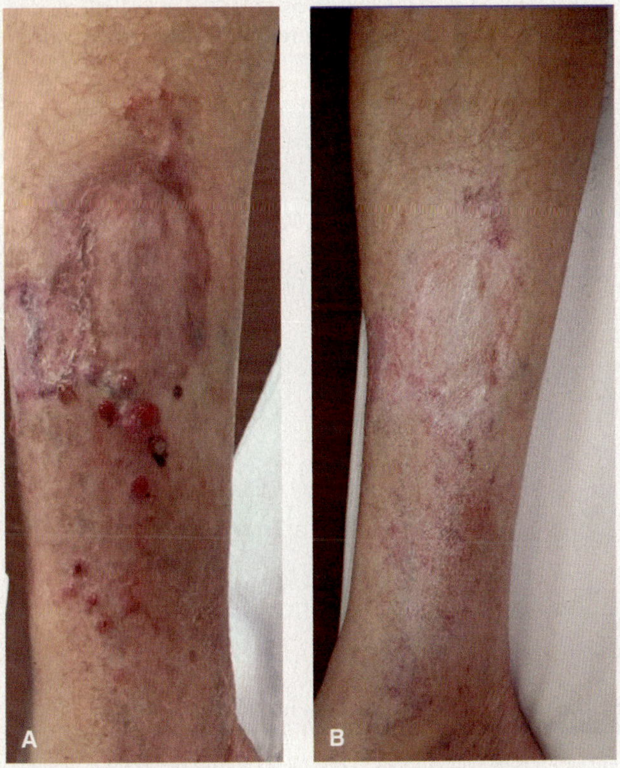

Figure 101.6. Example of response to intralesional talimogene laherparepvec (TVEC). **A:** Multifocal satellite (within 2 cm of the primary site) and in transit (>2 cm from the primary site but proximal to the draining nodal basin) metastases from a thick, ulcerated (T4b) primary melanoma of the leg previously treated with radical wide excision and split-thickness skin graft reconstruction. **B:** After eight injections of TVEC, there is no palpable or visible tumor remaining.

Isolated limb infusion (ILI) is a minimally invasive alternative to ILP. Rather than surgical isolation of the vessels and extracorporeal oxygenation, percutaneous catheters are utilized to provide venous and arterial access. A tourniquet is placed on the proximal extremity, and slightly lower doses of chemotherapeutic agents are used as efficacy is enhanced by the relative ischemia. Some studies have reported response rates equivalent to ILP, although others report slightly lower response rates.[35] However, the greater convenience and lower toxicity of ILI, lack of evidence of a survival difference compared to ILP, and the ability to repeat the procedure if necessary have made ILI the preferred regional approach in most melanoma centers worldwide.

Systemic Therapy for Melanoma

Over the past two decades, there have been tremendous advances in the systemic therapy of melanoma. Understanding the nonsurgical options for treatment of patients with melanoma is critical to the multidisciplinary care of the patient and plays an important role in surgical decision-making. There are now multiple molecularly targeted therapies and immune checkpoint inhibitors that have been approved for the treatment of advanced melanoma, with ongoing clinical trials of new therapies and combinations of established therapies.[30]

Immune Checkpoint Inhibitors

Immune checkpoint inhibition, which is designed to augment the patient's inherent antitumor immune response, has evolved over the past two decades as a mainstay of systemic therapy for patients with melanoma.

Ipilimumab is a monoclonal antibody that binds to the cytotoxic T lymphocyte–associated antigen-4 (CTLA-4) receptor found on activated regulatory and cytotoxic T cells. Blocking the binding between CTLA-4 and its ligand B7 suppresses this inhibitory function and promotes continued T-cell activation. Initially approved in 2011 in the metastatic setting, ipilimumab is now used in the neoadjuvant and adjuvant settings, and further study of the optimal dosing has decreased associated toxicities while maintaining efficacy. Ipilimumab remains associated with immune-related toxicities, specifically enterocolitis, hepatitis, endocrinopathies, and dermatitis, which can be life-threatening and lifelong. Pembrolizumab and nivolumab are monoclonal antibodies against the programmed death 1 (PD1) receptor, which when bound to its ligand PD-L1, triggers a decrease in T-cell proliferation, IL-2 release, and T-cell survival. Both are associated with lower rates of toxicity than ipilimumab and may induce response even in patients who have experienced progression on ipilimumab. In phase III randomized trials comparing either nivolumab or pembrolizumab with ipilimumab in previously untreated patients, the anti-PD1 antibodies were associated with improved response rates, progression-free survival, and OS with lower toxicity,[30] leading to a shift toward nivolumab- or pembrolizumab-based therapy over ipilimumab combinations in advanced melanoma (**Table 101.6**).

BRAF and MEK Inhibitors

The mitogen-activated protein kinase (MAPK) pathway is a key pathway in melanoma pathogenesis, with nearly half of melanomas having constitutive activation due to mutations in the *BRAF* gene. Activation of the pathway leads to unregulated cell proliferation. Vemurafenib, dabrafenib, and encorafenib are orally administered targeted therapies that block the constitutively active mutant BRAF. Common adverse effects include arthralgia, rash, fatigue, alopecia, and the development of cutaneous keratoacanthomas and SCCs. Patients treated with BRAF inhibition have dramatic responses, but unfortunately, the survival benefit is limited because of the eventual development of resistance in most patients. Combining a BRAF inhibitor with an inhibitor of MEK1/2, such as trametinib, is associated with an improvement in response rates, progression-free survival, and OS, as well as a decrease in secondary cutaneous malignancies as compared to BRAF monotherapy.[36] The FDA has approved three BRAF/MEK inhibitor combinations, vemurafenib plus cobimetinib, dabrafenib plus trametinib, and encorafenib plus binimetinib, for the treatment of patients with advanced melanoma with BRAF V600 E/K mutations.

Chemotherapy

Melanoma is responsive to few chemotherapeutic drugs, and with the advent of immunotherapy and targeted agents, these are not used as first-line therapy. Chemotherapy (carboplatin and paclitaxel) combined with interferon and IL-2, also referred to as biochemotherapy, has slightly higher response rates than traditional cytotoxic chemotherapy alone and while more toxic than traditional chemotherapy, it may be considered for highly selected patients with otherwise limited therapeutic options.[37]

High-Dose Interleukin-2

IL-2 is a cytokine secreted by antigen-activated helper T cells that acts as a T-cell growth factor and enhances the immune response. High-dose IL-2 is associated with an objective response rate of 15% to 20%, with a small percentage of patients (around 5%) experiencing long-term, durable complete responses.[30] However, the toxicity from IL-2 treatment and the availability of other more effective and less toxic therapies has limited its use and largely made it of historical context. Currently, the main role for IL-2 treatment is in conjunction with adoptive cellular therapy using TILs; see the following section.

ADOPTIVE IMMUNOTHERAPY

The FDA approved the use of TIL as an adoptive cell therapy in 2024 for patients with unresectable and/or metastatic melanoma refractory to immunotherapy (or targeted therapy if BRAF mutated).[38–40] This treatment capitalizes on the phenomenon that melanoma-specific T cells naturally infiltrate tumors, and when surgically harvested, these lymphocytes can be selectively expanded to large numbers and later infused back to the patient in a manner designed to augment the native immune response. TIL therapy is combined with a preparative, nonmyeloablative chemotherapy regimen that is followed by adoptive transfer of TIL and IL-2. In a large multicenter phase II trial of 153 patients with metastatic melanoma refractory to immunotherapy and/or targeted therapy, this approach showed an objective response rate of 31.4%, including a small number of patients with complete radiographic response (**Fig. 101.7**).[41] The surgeon plays an important role in this treatment modality, as selection of nonnecrotic, sterile tumor for harvest via an operation with an acceptable morbidity and projected duration for recovery is of critical importance.

Surgery for Metastatic Melanoma

For most cancers, surgery is rarely considered as a curative option in patients with stage IV disease. Historically, melanoma was an exception to this, with documented long-term
6 survival in well-selected patients with oligometastatic disease amenable to complete surgical resection.[42] In the era of effective systemic therapy (immune checkpoint blockade and targeted therapy), the role of metastasectomy is evolving from a single modality curative attempt in few to a complementary multimodality therapy in many.

Well-selected patients with either oligometastatic disease amenable to complete surgical resection or isolated progression in the setting of otherwise stable or treated disease will derive benefit from metastasectomy. Clearly defined criteria for patient selection for metastasectomy are not well established but should incorporate an understanding of the patient's disease course and trajectory, prior treatment response (including adverse events or intolerance to therapies), disease-free interval, site(s) of active disease, available other therapies (including other local modalities such as ablation or radiation), and patient performance status and morbidity of metastasectomy.[43]

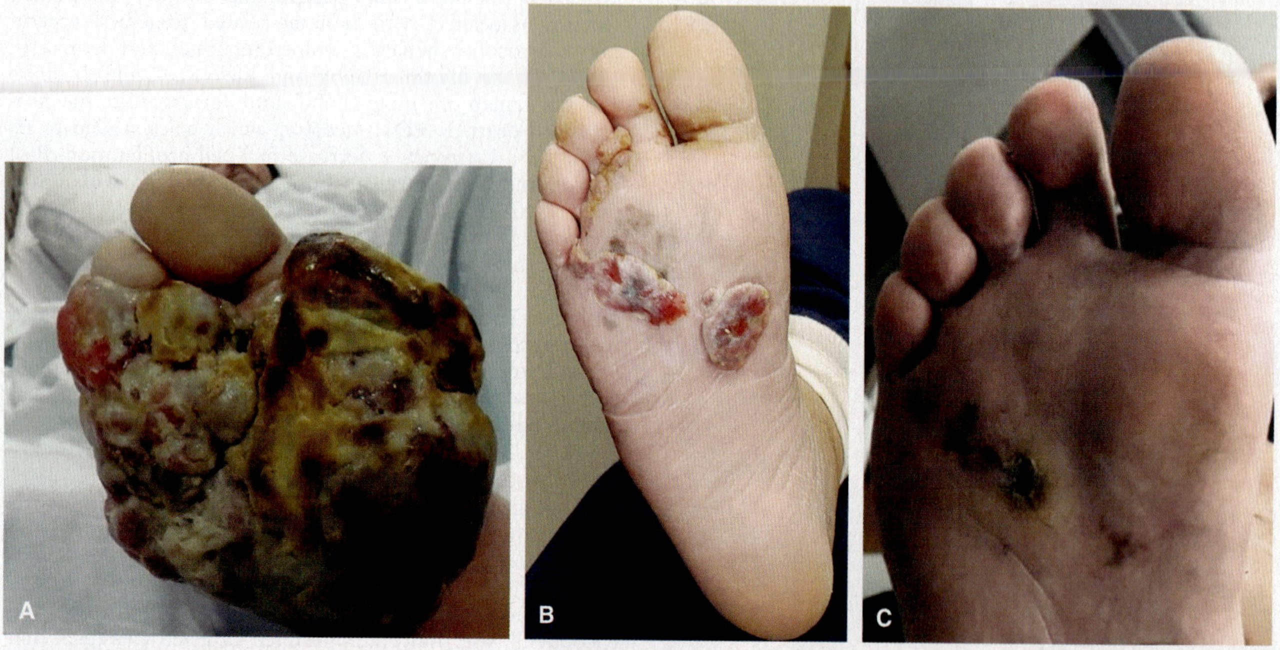

Figure 101.7. Example of response to adoptive cellular therapy with tumor-infiltrating lymphocytes (TILs). **A:** Extensive recurrent melanoma of the distal foot and toes after prior margin-positive excision, progressive after multiple lines of systemic immunotherapy and chemotherapy. The tumor was BRAF wild type, and the patient also had widespread metastatic disease. The patient was enrolled onto a clinical trial testing adoptive cellular therapy with TILs. After harvest of tumor from a metastasis in the groin, TIL were grown ex vivo and reinfused into the patient after preparative lymphodepleting chemotherapy. High-dose interleukin-2 was administered for several days, and the patient tolerated therapy well and received no further treatment. **B:** Three months after therapy, there is clear evidence of tumor shrinkage at the primary site (shown) and all metastases. **C:** Six months after therapy, the tumor has almost completely regressed. The patient received no further therapy and remains well 2 years later.

NONMELANOMA SKIN CANCERS

BCC and cutaneous SCC account for over 95% of all skin cancers.[44] Their true incidence is difficult to measure as most are not reportable to cancer registries, and the vast majority are curable with local therapy. If left untreated, substantial morbidity can be incurred from local growth and invasion. Up to 5% of SCCs and 1% of BCCs will have nodal involvement at presentation, and up to 1% to 2% of patients with SCC will experience distant metastases (<0.1% for patients with BCC). Given the high incidence of BCC/SCCs these percentages, although low, translate to a measurable number of patients who will require surgical evaluation and expertise.

Risk Factors and Diagnosis

Similar to environmental risk factors for melanoma, BCCs/SCCs are most commonly induced by significant exposure to UV light from the sun and/or tanning beds, and fair-skinned/light-eyed individuals are at higher risk. Immunosuppression is a major risk factor for keratinocyte cancers, and immunosuppressed patients with BCC/SCC are at higher risk of metastatic disease and death.

Genetic syndromes associated with an increased risk of developing keratinocyte cancers include Gorlin syndrome (an autosomal dominant disorder associated with multiple BCCs, palmoplantar pits, jaw cysts, frontal bossing, and hypertelorism), xeroderma pigmentosa, and albinism. Sun protective strategies and regular skin surveillance exams are important for patients with these hereditary conditions. Other risk factors include chronic chemical exposure (arsenic and hydrocarbons found in coal tars, soot, and asphalt), cigarette smoking (associated with SCC of the lip and mouth), and human papillomavirus infection, particularly in the setting of immunosuppression. Radiation has also been associated with an increased risk of both SCC and BCC, most commonly presenting as a nonhealing wound.

BCCs often present as pearly papules or nodules with telangiectasias. They may be pruritic and bleed occasionally. With time, the center ulcerates to create rolled borders; such ulcerating BCCs may be referred to as "rodent ulcers" (**Fig. 101.8A**). Occasionally, the lesions are pigmented and can be confused with melanoma (pigmented BCC). Superficial BCCs are another common entity and are frequently multifocal. Clinically, these are flat, scaly pink to red lesions (**Fig. 101.8B**), but if neglected, they can ulcerate (**Fig. 101.8C**). Numerous risk factors are associated with possible extensive subclinical invasion and increased rates of local recurrence for BCC after standard treatment (**Table 101.7**).

SCC is the second most common form of skin cancer. SCC most often arises in chronically sun damaged skin or within an actinic keratosis but may also develop in burn scars or chronic inflammatory wounds, known eponymously as a Marjolin ulcer. Metastasis to regional lymph nodes accounts for approximately 80% to 90% of cases of metastatic SCC. Involvement of distant sites accounts for the other 10% to 20%.

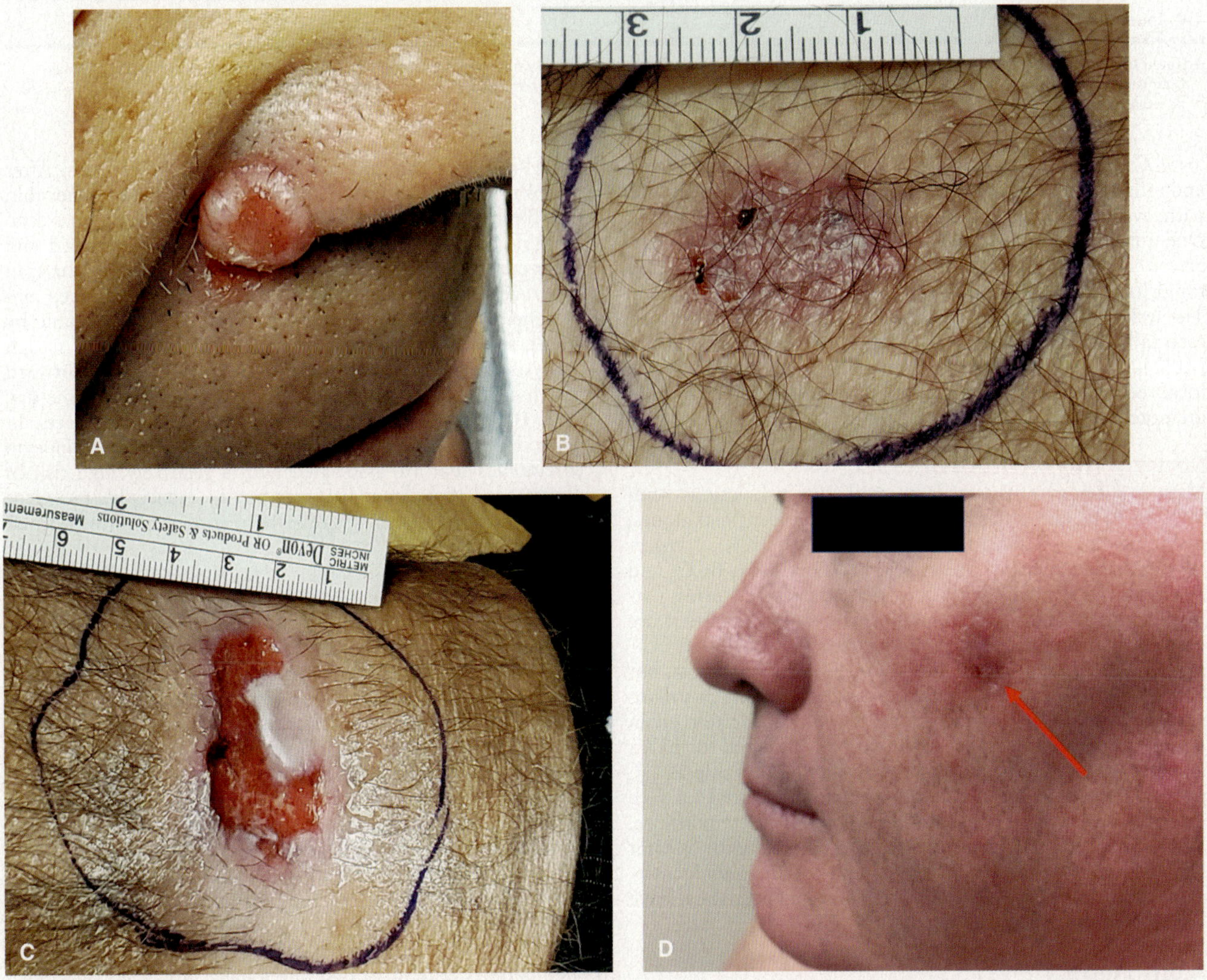

Figure 101.8. Examples of basal cell carcinoma. **A:** Nodular basal cell carcinoma on the nasal ala, illustrating the classic "rodent ulcer" central depression. **B:** Superficial basal cell carcinoma on the thigh. **C:** Ulcerated basal cell carcinoma on the ankle. **D:** Morpheaform basal cell carcinoma on the cheek (*arrow*).

Table 101.7. Basal Cell and Squamous Cell Carcinoma: Higher-Risk Factors for Subclinical Invasion and Recurrence

Risk factors
▪ Recurrent tumor
▪ Anatomic location ▪ *High risk:* Central face, eyelid, eyebrow, periorbital, nose, lip, chin, mandible, temple, ear, in front or behind the ear, genitalia, hand, and foot ▪ *Medium risk:* Cheeks, forehead, pretibia, scalp, and neck ▪ *Low risk:* Trunk, extremity (excluding hand/foot and pretibia)
▪ Size ▪ Lesions ≥6 mm on high-risk area ▪ Lesions ≥10 mm on medium-risk area ▪ Lesions ≥20 mm on low-risk area
▪ Histology ▪ *Basal cell*: Aggressive growth pattern (morpheaform, fibrosing, sclerosing, infiltrating, micronodular) ▪ *Squamous cell:* Poorly differentiated, acantholytic, desmoplastic, adenosquamous, or carcinosarcomatous subtypes
▪ Depth of invasion ▪ Clark level IV (lesion that involves the reticular dermis), V (lesion that invades into subcutaneous fat), or ≥4 mm
▪ Perineural invasion
▪ Rapid growth and/or ill-defined borders
▪ Etiology ▪ Scar, *chronic* ulcer or inflammatory process, sinus tract, sites of prior radiation therapy
▪ Immunosuppression

Adapted from Claveau J, Archambault J, Ernst DS, et al. Multidisciplinary management of locally advanced and metastatic cutaneous squamous cell carcinoma. *Curr Oncol.* 2020;24(4):e399–e407 and from Peris K, Fargnoli MC, Garbe C, et al. Diagnosis and treatment of basal cell carcinoma: European consensus-based interdisciplinary guidelines. *Eur J Cancer*. 2019;118:10–34.

SCC often presents as a nonhealing sore with ulceration and inflammatory pink borders, or as an erythematous nodule with overlying keratotic crust or ulceration (**Fig. 101.9A,B**). One noteworthy variant, keratoacanthoma type SCC, is characterized by a typical cratered appearance (**Fig. 101.9C**) and rapid local growth but little or no propensity to metastasize. The lesions may develop in patients taking BRAF inhibitors, especially when used as single agents without a concurrent MEK inhibitor.[32] Factors that may determine a higher risk for local recurrence, extensive subclinical invasion, and metastasis are noted in **Table 101.7**.

Surgical Treatment of BCC/SCC

Most keratinocyte cancers are small, low-risk lesions with 90% to 95% cure rates after standard treatment techniques, including electrodesiccation and curettage (ED&C), cryosurgery, radiation therapy, or surgical excision. Most BCCs and SCCs can be removed with conservative excisions using narrower peripheral and deep margins of excision than that are used for melanoma. Excision margins for most localized BCC and SCC lesions should be in the range of 0.4 to 0.5 cm, but larger resectable tumors should be treated surgically in a manner similar to melanoma using 1 cm margins of excision taken down to fascia. Mohs surgery should be considered for BCCs and SCCs that exhibit the higher-risk factors in **Table 101.7**, particularly if they are situated in an anatomical area (eg, face or ears) where skin conservation is of critical importance. While SLNB should be considered for patients with SCC at high risk of regional metastasis, criteria that reliably identify cases with at least a 5% to 10% risk of nodal metastasis have not been prospectively validated.[45]

Mohs Surgery

Mohs micrographic surgery, typically performed with local anesthesia in an outpatient setting, is useful for treating selected high-risk keratinocyte cancers (**Table 101.7**) as a tissue-sparing technique that achieves high cure rates. After removal of all gross tumor, the surgeon excises a further thin 2 to 3 mm layer of tissue that includes all peripheral and deep margins of the excision. This layer of tissue is mapped and color-coded for orientation and sent to the Mohs technician for frozen-section processing. In this way, both the deep and peripheral margins are examined in one horizontal plane by frozen-section analysis, theoretically allowing total margin analysis (**Fig. 101.10**). Closure or relatively straightforward soft tissue reconstruction can be performed on the same day (**Fig. 101.11**) or subsequently for more complex defects. In general, Mohs surgery should be considered for keratinocyte carcinomas that are associated with a relatively high risk of recurrence after standard treatment, especially recurrent tumors, and for primary sites where conservation of normal tissue is important.

Adjuvant and Primary Radiation Therapy for BCC/SCC

Radiation therapy can be considered in the primary treatment of low-risk and even selected high-risk BCC/SCC. This modality provides an alternative to surgery in cosmetically sensitive areas or in the rare circumstance that a patient cannot undergo surgery. For cutaneous BCC/SCC at high risk of local recurrence, such as those with perineural spread, adjuvant radiation therapy to the primary site may decrease the risks of local recurrence after margin-negative resection, or may be used as an adjunct in patients with persistently positive margins after surgery in whom re-resection is not feasible. Radiation may also be used as definitive therapy for unresectable BCC/SCC.

Systemic Therapy for BCC/SCC

7 Well-defined criteria to describe locally advanced BCC/SCC are not established. Large, deeply invasive but resectable tumors can reasonably be considered locally advanced, but some definitions restrict the term to encompass tumors not

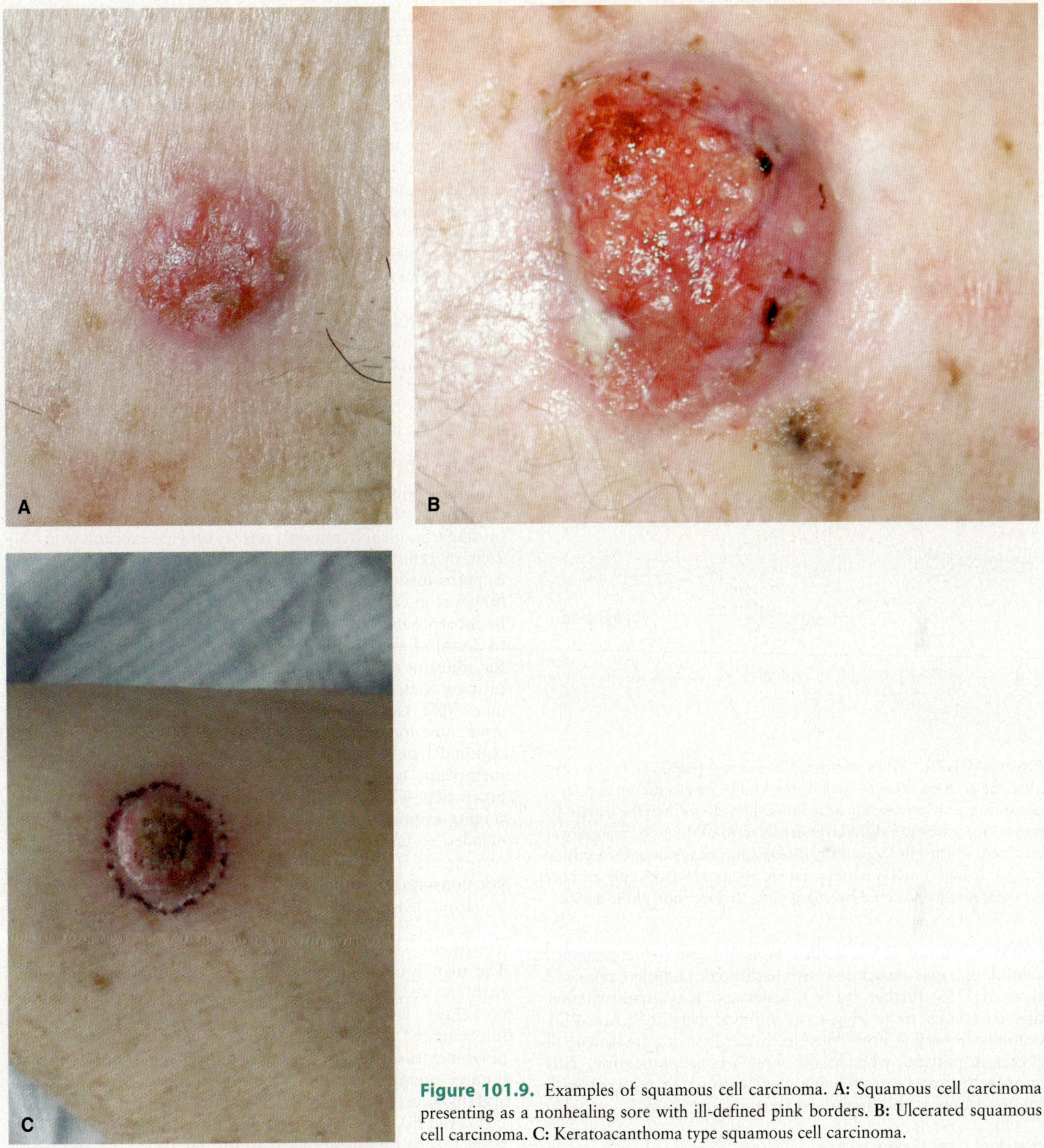

Figure 101.9. Examples of squamous cell carcinoma. **A:** Squamous cell carcinoma presenting as a nonhealing sore with ill-defined pink borders. **B:** Ulcerated squamous cell carcinoma. **C:** Keratoacanthoma type squamous cell carcinoma.

amenable to either surgery or radiotherapy with reasonable expectation for cure due to multiple recurrences, infiltration through the fascia into underlying muscle or along major nerves, bony invasion, or tumors in which curative resection would result in unacceptable complications, morbidity, or deformity. Imaging to assess resectability and to rule out distant disease is warranted in these circumstances. Systemic therapy may allow tumor downstaging to achieve resection or avoid major functional or cosmetic morbidity, or may slow disease progression and prolong survival in the distantly metastatic setting. Vismodegib and Sonidegib are Hedgehog pathway inhibitors approved by the FDA for the treatment of locally advanced and (for vismodegib) metastatic BCC. Aberrations in the hedgehog pathway involving either inactivating mutations of the tumor-suppressor *PTCH1* (patched) gene or less frequently activating mutations in the proto-oncogene smoothened (*SMO*) are found in virtually all BCCs, so routine mutational analysis of BCCs is not required prior to initiating targeted therapy. Objective response rates approach 30% for metastatic BCC and exceed 40% for locally advanced BCC, although resistance to therapy may develop. In locally advanced BCC, preoperative use of a Hedgehog inhibitor can induce sufficient tumor shrinkage to permit definitive treatment with surgery and/or radiation. Anti-PD1 immunotherapy has also been shown to induce objective responses in patients with BCC.

For patients with resectable nodal metastatic SCC, radical lymphadenectomy followed by adjuvant radiation therapy is appropriate[46]; clinical trials of postoperative adjuvant anti-PD1 immunotherapy are underway, and consideration of a neoadjuvant approach is reasonable[34]. Cemiplimab, a high affinity antibody to PD1, and pembrolizumab are FDA approved for the treatment of locally advanced/unresectable SCC. In one small prospective study of patients with resectable

SKIN AND SOFT TISSUE

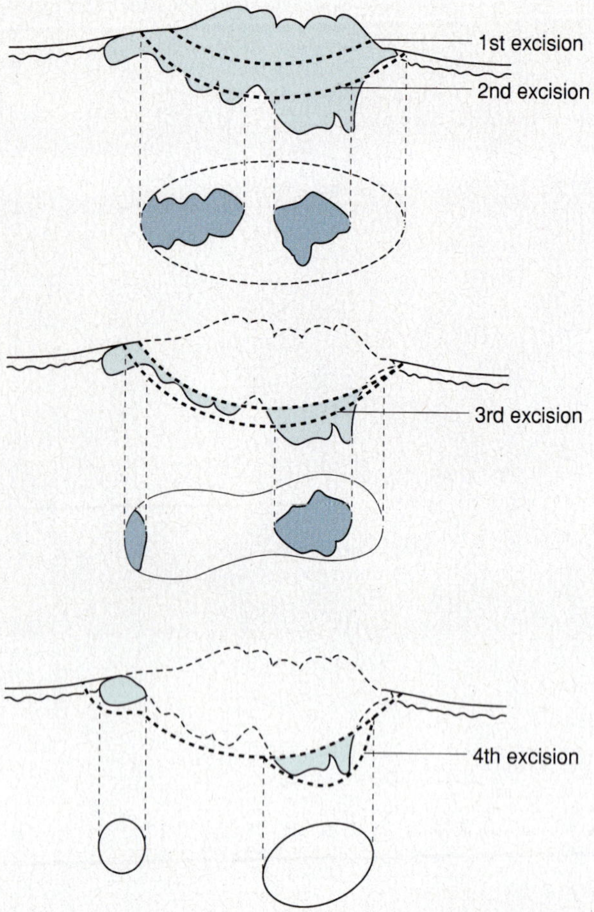

Figure 101.10. Mohs micrographic surgical technique. In this case, after the first excision to debulk the visible tumor, the second layer demonstrated relatively diffuse multifocal involvement of the margin by tumor. Accordingly, a third layer across most of the prior margin was obtained, which still showed two isolated foci of tumor at the excision margin. A fourth and final stage taking additional tissue only at those two sites resulted in complete, margin-negative excision of the tumor.

locally advanced or metastatic SCC, the use of neoadjuvant cemiplimab was associated with pathologic complete response rates of 51%; further study is necessary to evaluate whether this translates to a long-term survival benefit.[46] Anti-PD1 immunotherapy is now considered the first-line treatment of choice in patients who do not have a contraindication. This approach must be used with great caution in patients with immunosuppression due to organ transplantation.

Merkel Cell Carcinoma

MCC, also termed cutaneous neuroendocrine carcinoma, is an aggressive skin cancer with higher per-case mortality than melanoma. The incidence of MCC is low compared to other cutaneous malignancies, but the number of cases has at least tripled over the last two decades and is expected to exceed 3,000 cases per year by 2025. MCC most commonly occurs in older individuals, with less than 5% of cases diagnosed before age 50, and is more frequently observed in immunosuppressed individuals. Although chronic UV exposure is an important pathogenic factor in many, and incidence of MCC is higher in areas closer to the equator, most MCCs are associated with integration of Merkel cell polyomavirus. Primary MCC typically presents as a new-onset, growing, red or purple, dome-shaped or subcutaneous nodule, frequently mistaken for a sebaceous cyst (**Fig. 101.12A**). The most common location of metastasis is the draining lymph node basin.

Histologically, MCC is a small blue round-cell tumor with positive immunohistochemical staining for cytokeratin-20 (CK-20) in a characteristic paranuclear dot-like pattern (**Fig. 101.12B**). MCC may be distinguished from small cell lung cancer, another neuroendocrine carcinoma that may also be CK-20 positive, by the expression of thyroid transcription factor-1 (TTF-1), which is consistently absent in MCC. Tumor size (diameter) and the presence of locoregional or distant disease are the strongest prognostic factors for MCC. Presentation of MCC in the regional lymph nodes without an identified cutaneous primary is not uncommon, and, as with melanoma, these patients may have a better prognosis than patients with similar stage disease with an intact/identifiable primary, suggesting a role for immune activation (evidenced by regression of the primary) in prognosis.[47] The majority (70%) of patients with MCC present with clinically localized disease (stage I or II), 25% have palpable lymphadenopathy (stage IIIB), and 5% present with distant metastases (stage IV). Five-year survival rates for stages I, II, and III in the AJCC database were 81%, 67%, and 52%, respectively, while stage IV disease carried a dismal 11% 2-year survival rate. More recent results, however, suggest that these survival figures may be overly pessimistic.[48]

Localized Therapy for Merkel Cell Carcinoma

Multidisciplinary management of MCC is necessary and application of each modality alone or in combination depends on stage. Surgical treatment consists of wide excision with 1 to 2 cm margins, and SLNB for clinically node negative patients, as performed for melanoma. MCC is unique from melanoma however, in that it is much more radiosensitive and this should be incorporated into surgical planning (ie, wider margins [>1 to 2 cm] of excision are not necessary in the patient planned for adjuvant radiation). Postoperative radiation therapy to the primary tumor bed should be considered but whether all primary MCC cases should receive it and the impact of postoperative radiation on OS remains unclear. Sentinel node–detected regional lymph node metastases can be treated by regional therapeutic lymphadenectomy or radiation therapy. Patients presenting with clinically palpable disease should undergo staging exams to rule out distant metastases and are recommended to undergo therapeutic lymph node dissection, with consideration of postoperative radiation to the nodal basin. For nonsurgical candidates, primary treatment of MCC with radiation therapy may also be considered.

Systemic Therapy for Merkel Cell Carcinoma

The management of metastatic MCC dramatically changed with the recognition that MCC is very sensitive to immunotherapy with anti-PD1 or anti-PDL1 immunotherapy. Interestingly, whether the MCC is associated Merkel cell polyomavirus does not markedly impact the response rates to immunotherapy. Anti-PD1 antibodies such as pembrolizumab and nivolumab are approved therapeutic options for MCC. In 2017, the FDA also approved avelumab, an anti-PD-L1 antibody, for the treatment of metastatic MCC.

Extrapolating from the metastatic setting, studies of the application of avelumab in both the adjuvant and neoadjuvant settings are ongoing.[49] In the neoadjuvant setting, a phase I/II study of 39 patients with resectable MCC were treated with nivolumab 4 weeks prior to surgery. A complete pathologic response was observed in more than half of patients with minimal toxicity and only a small proportion unable to undergo surgery (7.7%), suggesting this is a viable approach.[46] The optimal multidisciplinary combination of surgery, radiation, and systemic therapy for locally advanced and/or metastatic MCC requires further study.

OTHER CUTANEOUS MALIGNANCIES

Sweat gland carcinomas represent a broad scope of cutaneous adnexal malignancies with variable risk for local, regional, or distant metastasis, most commonly of eccrine or apocrine origin. These are rare tumors (0.005% of skin malignancies) that

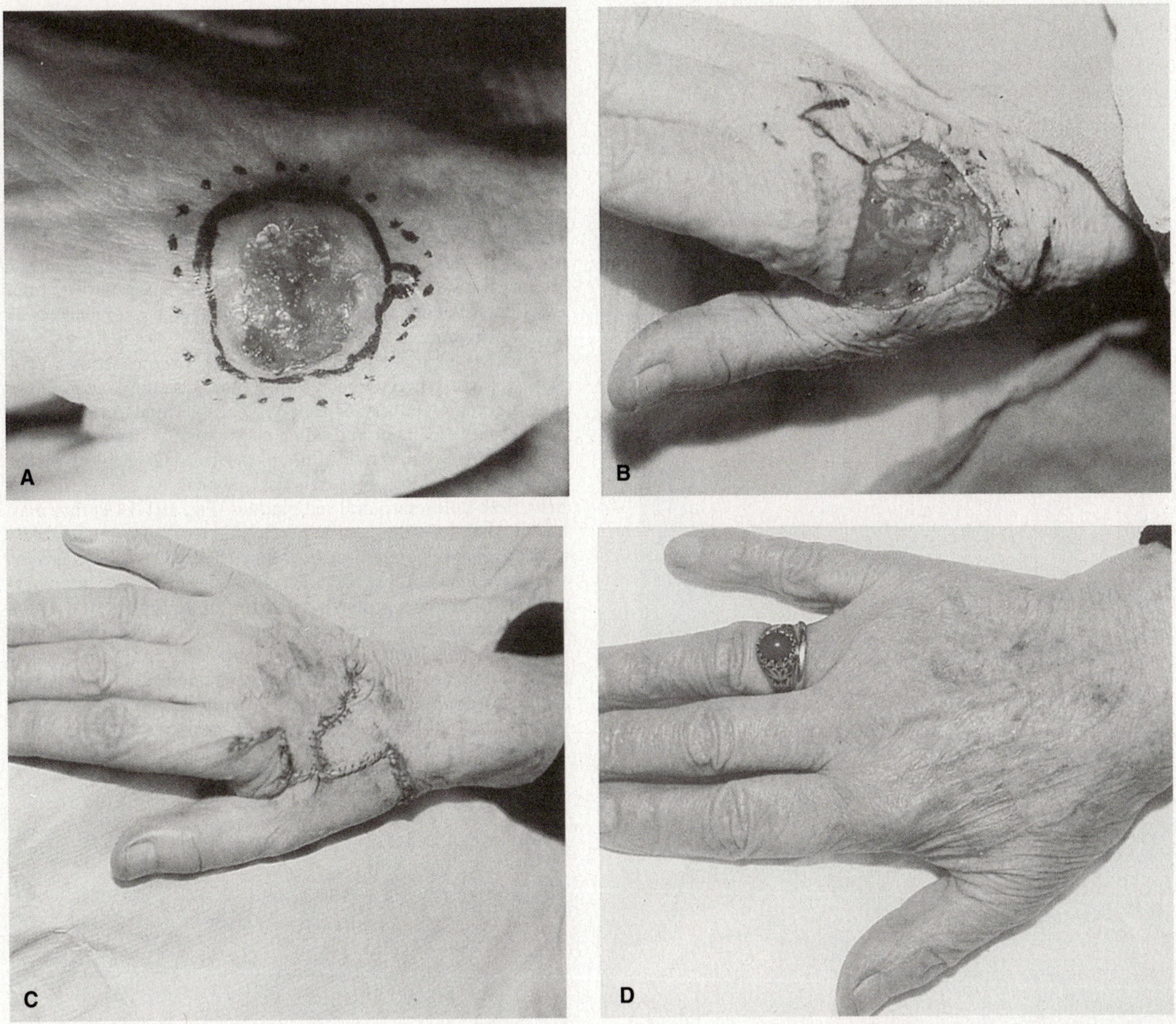

Figure 101.11. **A:** Patient with a 3 × 3 cm basal cell carcinoma on the right dorsal hand with mixed nodular and aggressive growth histologic pattern. **B:** Complete excision of the tumor required two Mohs stages involving 10 frozen sections. The final Mohs surgery defect measured 4.0 × 4.8 cm with preservation of underlying tendons. **C:** The defect was reconstructed immediately following the final Mohs stage under local anesthesia in the Mohs surgery unit using birhombic flap soft tissue reconstruction. **D:** Result 3 months after surgery.

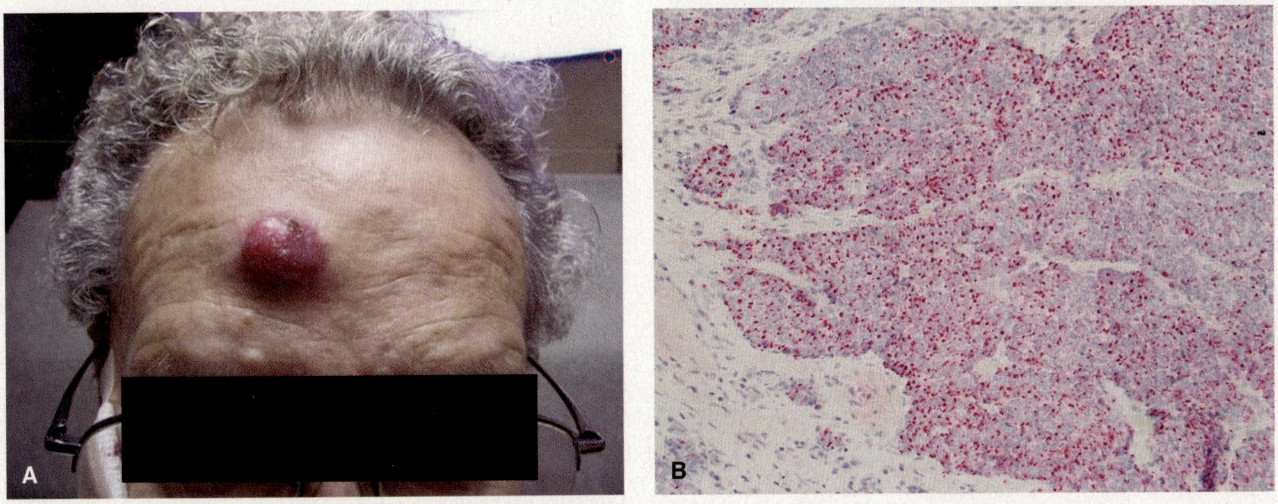

Figure 101.12. **A:** Primary Merkel cell carcinoma on the forehead. **B:** Characteristic immunohistochemical pattern showing dot-like positivity of cytokeratin 20 (CK20) staining in Merkel cell carcinoma. (Photomicrograph courtesy of Jane L. Messina, MD, Moffitt Cancer Center.)

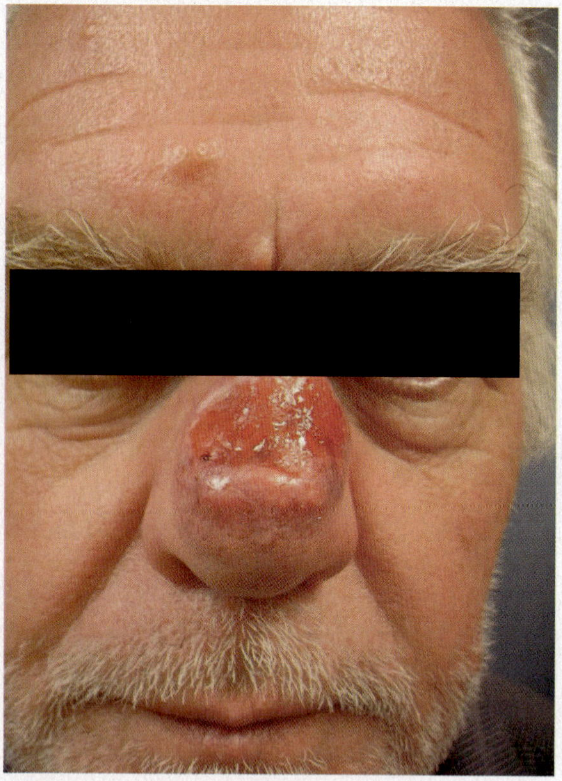

Figure 101.13. Sebaceous carcinoma on the nose.

have a diverse and confusing nomenclature.[50] The aggressive types of sweat gland carcinomas have a propensity for both local recurrence and regional or systemic metastasis. Clinically, these tumors appear as indurated plaques, papules, or nodules commonly on the head and neck or extremities and are red, blue, pink, or skin-colored (**Fig. 101.13**). Histologic subtypes that are particularly associated with a risk of regional lymph node or systemic metastasis include hidradenocarcinoma and porocarcinoma. Recommended treatments have included wide excision of the primary tumor with consideration of SLNB limited to high-risk lesions based on recurrence, larger tumor size, high histologic grade of atypia, or increased mitotic rate. Postoperative radiation therapy may also be considered as adjuvant treatment in selected cases.

DFSP is a rare low-grade soft tissue sarcoma with a propensity for local recurrence rather than systemic metastasis.[51] It is a spindle cell tumor that typically demonstrates immunoreactivity to CD34 and has a characteristic gene translocation leading to activation of the platelet-derived growth factor receptor (PDGFR). These tumors appear as slow-growing, firm, flesh-colored to dull red plaques (**Fig. 101.14A**) that may be mistaken for keloids or hypertrophic scars. Although DFSPs may appear well circumscribed, they characteristically demonstrate extensive subclinical involvement, manifest histologically as finger-like projections of tumor cells (**Fig. 101.14B**). DFSP can undergo transformation into a high-grade soft tissue sarcoma, usually fibrosarcoma. For nontransformed DFSP, complete excision with negative margins is curative, and a thorough assessment of the peripheral and deep margins is critical to ensure that the entire tumor has been resected. Treatment commonly consists of radical wide excision with

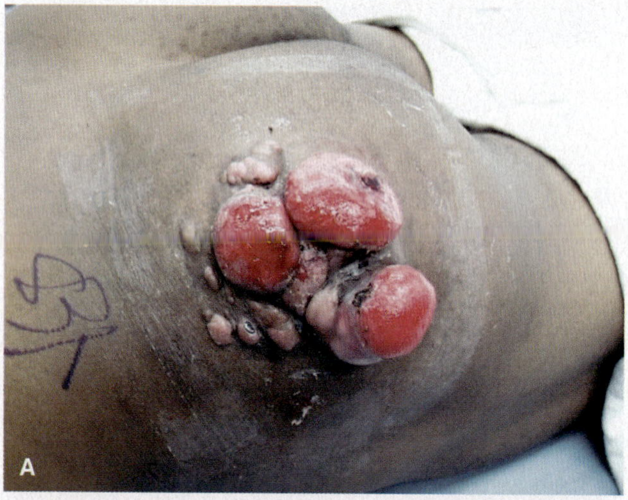

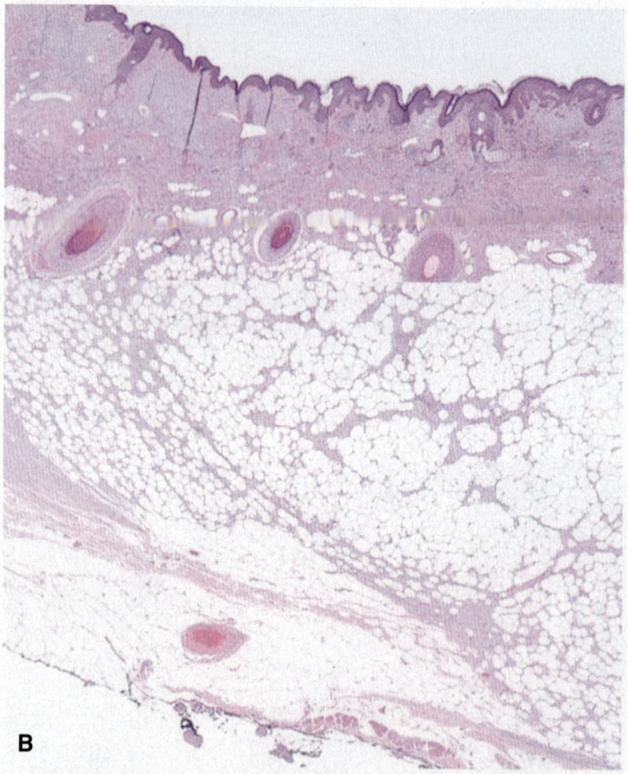

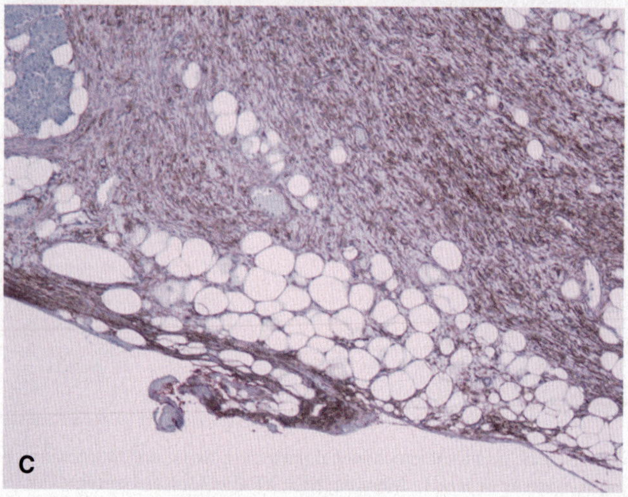

Figure 101.14. **A:** Dermatofibrosarcoma protuberans (DFSP) in an African-American patient. **B:** Low-power (20×) hematoxylin and eosin-stained microscopic appearance of DFSP showing a spindle cell neoplasm with infiltration through full thickness of dermis into subcutaneous fat, approaching the inked deep margin. **C:** High-power (200×) view with CD34 immunohistochemistry staining cells of DFSP extending through subcutaneous fat and present at the deep tissue margin. (Images courtesy of Jane L. Messina, MD, Moffitt Cancer Center.)

1 to 2 cm margins and comprehensive pathologic margin assessment or Mohs surgery, particularly for lesions on functionally sensitive areas like the digits.[51] Imatinib, a PDGFR inhibitor, has shown significant antitumor activity in the treatment of unresectable or metastatic DFSP, and can be used for neoadjuvant therapy of locally advanced lesions.[52]

The surgeon who treats cutaneous malignancies should understand the impact of nonsurgical therapies, including radiation, immunotherapy, and targeted therapy, and adapt the surgical approach to patients with locally advanced or metastatic disease in coordination with other evidence-based treatments.

ACKNOWLEDGMENTS

We gratefully acknowledge the contributions of previous edition authors, Amod A. Sarnaik, Allison B. Durham, and Vernon K. Sondak, as portions of those chapters have been retained in this revision.

References

1. Siegel RL, Miller KD, Wagle NS, Jemal A. Cancer statistics, 2023. *CA Cancer J Clin.* 2023;73(1):17–48.
2. Olsen CM, Whiteman DC. *Clinical Epidemiology of Melanoma.* 6th ed: Springer Nature; 2020;425–449.
3. Price HN, O'Haver J, Marghoob A, Badger K, Etchevers H, Krengel S. Practical application of the new classification scheme for congenital melanocytic nevi. *Pediatr Dermatol.* 2015;32(1):23–27.
4. Ferrone CR, Ben Porat L, Panageas KS, et al. Clinicopathological features of and risk factors for multiple primary melanomas. *JAMA.* 2005;294(13):1647–1654.
5. Eckerle Mize D, Bishop M, Resse E, Sluzevich J. Familial atypical multiple mole melanoma syndrome. In: Riegert-Johnson DL, Boardman LA, Hefferon T, Roberts M, eds. *Cancer Syndromes.* National Center for Biotechnology Information (US).
6. American Academy for Dermatology Ad Hoc Task Force for the ABCDEs of Melanoma; Tsao H, Olazagasti JM, Cordoro KM, et al. Early detection of melanoma: reviewing the ABCDEs. *J Am Acad Dermatol.* 2015;72(4):717–723.
7. Sondak VK, Messina JL. Unusual presentations of melanoma: melanoma of unknown primary site, melanoma arising in childhood, and melanoma arising in the eye and on mucosal surfaces. *Surg Clin North Am.* 2014;94(5):1059–1073, ix.
8. Gershenwald JE, Scolyer RA. Melanoma staging: American Joint Committee on Cancer (AJCC) 8th Edition and Beyond. *Ann Surg Oncol.* 2018;25(8):2105–2110.
9. Gershenwald JE, Scolyer RA, Hess KR, et al. Melanoma staging: Evidence-based changes in the American Joint Committee on Cancer eighth edition cancer staging manual. *CA Cancer J Clin.* 2017;67(6):472–492.
10. Karakousis GC, Gimotty PA, Leong SP, et al. Microsatellitosis in patients with melanoma. *Ann Surg Oncol.* 2019;26(1):33–41.
11. Cochran AJ, Wen DR, Huang RR, et al. Sentinel lymph node melanoma metastases: Assessment of tumor burden for clinical prediction of outcome in the first Multicenter Selective Lymphadenectomy Trial (MSLT-I). *Eur J Surg Oncol.* 2022;48(6):1280–1287.
12. Bailey CN, Martin BJ, Petkov VI, et al. 31-gene expression profile testing in cutaneous melanoma and survival outcomes in a population-based analysis: A SEER collaboration. *JCO Precis Oncol.* 2023;7:e2300044.
13. Zager JS, Hochwald SN, Marzban SS, et al. Shave biopsy is a safe and accurate method for the initial evaluation of melanoma. *J Am Coll Surg.* 2011;212(4):454–460; discussion 460–452.
14. Thompson JF, Haydu LE, Uren RF, et al. Preoperative ultrasound assessment of regional lymph nodes in melanoma patients does not provide reliable nodal staging: results from a large multicenter trial. *Ann Surg.* 2021;273(4):814–820.
15. Wagner JD, Schauwecker D, Davidson D, et al. Inefficacy of F-18 fluorodeoxy-D-glucose-positron emission tomography scans for initial evaluation in early-stage cutaneous melanoma. *Cancer.* 2005;104(3):570–579.
16. Angeles CV, Wong SL, Karakousis G. The landmark series: randomized trials examining surgical margins for cutaneous melanoma. *Ann Surg Oncol.* 2020;27(1):3–12.
17. Wong SL, Faries MB, Kennedy EB, et al. Sentinel lymph node biopsy and management of regional lymph nodes in melanoma: American Society of Clinical Oncology and Society of Surgical Oncology Clinical Practice Guideline Update. *J Clin Oncol.* 2018;36(4):399–413.
18. Valsecchi ME, Silbermins D, de Rosa N, Wong SL, Lyman GH. Lymphatic mapping and sentinel lymph node biopsy in patients with melanoma: a meta-analysis. *J Clin Oncol.* 2011;29(11):1479–1487.
19. Cook MG, Massi D, Szumera-Ciećkiewicz A, et al. An updated European Organisation for Research and Treatment of Cancer (EORTC) protocol for pathological evaluation of sentinel lymph nodes for melanoma. *Eur J Cancer.* 2019;114:1–7.
20. Morton DL, Thompson JF, Cochran AJ, et al. Final trial report of sentinel-node biopsy versus nodal observation in melanoma. *N Engl J Med.* 2014;370(7):599–609.
21. Faries MB, Thompson JF, Cochran A, et al. The impact on morbidity and length of stay of early versus delayed complete lymphadenectomy in melanoma: results of the Multicenter Selective Lymphadenectomy Trial (I). *Ann Surg Oncol.* 2010;17(12):3324–3329.
22. Leiter U, Stadler R, Mauch C, et al. Final analysis of DeCOG-SLT Trial: No survival benefit for complete lymph node dissection in patients with melanoma with positive sentinel node. *J Clin Oncol.* 2019;37(32):3000–3008.
23. Faries MB, Thompson JF, Cochran AJ, et al. Completion dissection or observation for sentinel-node metastasis in melanoma. *N Engl J Med.* 2017;376(23):2211–2222.
24. Delman KA, Wong SL. Completion node dissection after sentinel node biopsy in melanoma. *JAMA Surg.* 2018;153(11):1045–1046.
25. Diller ML, Martin BM, Delman KA. Lymph node dissection for stage III melanoma. *Surg Oncol Clin N Am.* 2015;24(2):261–277.
26. Weide B, Faller C, Elsässer M, et al. Melanoma patients with unknown primary site or nodal recurrence after initial diagnosis have a favourable survival compared to those with synchronous lymph node metastasis and primary tumour. *PLoS One.* 2013;8(6):e66953.
27. Patel SP, Othus M, Chen Y, et al. Neoadjuvant-adjuvant or adjuvant-only pembrolizumab in advanced melanoma. *N Engl J Med.* 2023;388(9):813–823.
28. Blank CU, Lucas MW, Scolyer RA, et al. Neoadjuvant nivolumab and ipilimumab in resectable stage III melanoma. *N Engl J Med.* 2024;391:1696–1708.
29. Reijers ILM, Menzies AM, van Akkooi ACJ, et al. Personalized response-directed surgery and adjuvant therapy after neoadjuvant ipilimumab and nivolumab in high-risk stage III melanoma: the PRADO trial. *Nat Med.* 2022;28(6):1178–1188.
30. Long GV, Swetter SM, Menzies AM, Gershenwald JE, Scolyer RA. Cutaneous melanoma. *Lancet.* 2023;402(10400):485–502.
31. Strom T, Caudell JJ, Han D, et al. Radiotherapy influences local control in patients with desmoplastic melanoma. *Cancer.* 2014;120(9):1369–1378.
32. Kwiek B, Schwartz RA. Keratoacanthoma (KA): An update and review. *J Am Acad Dermatol.* 2016;74(6):1220–1233.
33. Andtbacka RHI, Collichio F, Harrington KJ, et al. Final analyses of OPTiM: a randomized phase III trial of talimogene laherparepvec versus granulocyte-macrophage colony-stimulating factor in unresectable stage III-IV melanoma. *J Immunother Cancer.* 2019;7(1):145.
34. Broman KK, Zager JS. Intra-arterial perfusion-based therapies for regionally metastatic cutaneous and uveal melanoma. *Melanoma Manag.* 2019;6(3):MMT26.
35. Miura JT, Kroon HM, Beasley GM, et al. Long-term oncologic outcomes after isolated limb infusion for locoregionally metastatic melanoma: an international multicenter analysis. *Ann Surg Oncol.* 2019;26(8):2486–2494.
36. Robert C, Grob JJ, Stroyakovskiy D, et al. Five-year outcomes with dabrafenib plus trametinib in metastatic melanoma. *N Engl J Med.* 2019;381(7):626–636.

37. Atkins MB, Hsu J, Lee S, et al. Phase III trial comparing concurrent biochemotherapy with cisplatin, vinblastine, dacarbazine, interleukin-2, and interferon alfa-2b with cisplatin, vinblastine, and dacarbazine alone in patients with metastatic malignant melanoma (E3695): a trial coordinated by the Eastern Cooperative Oncology Group. *J Clin Oncol.* 2008;26(35): 5748–5754.
38. Rosenberg SA, Restifo NP. Adoptive cell transfer as personalized immunotherapy for human cancer. *Science.* 2015;348(6230): 62–68.
39. Rosenberg SA, Yang JC, Sherry RM, et al. Durable complete responses in heavily pretreated patients with metastatic melanoma using T-cell transfer immunotherapy. *Clin Cancer Res.* 2011;17(13):4550–4557.
40. Sarnaik A, Khushalani NI, Chesney JA, et al. Long-term follow up of lifileucel (LN-144) cryopreserved autologous tumor infiltrating lymphocyte therapy in patients with advanced melanoma progressed on multiple prior therapies. https://meetinglibrary.asco.org/record/186915/abstract. Accessed June 6, 2020.
41. Chesney J, Lewis KD, Kluger H, et al. Efficacy and safety of lifileucel, a one-time autologous tumor-infiltrating lymphocyte (TIL) cell therapy, in patients with advanced melanoma after progression on immune checkpoint inhibitors and targeted therapies: pooled analysis of consecutive cohorts of the C-144-01 study. *J Immunother Cancer.* 2022;10(12):e005755.
42. Howard JH, Thompson JF, Mozzillo N, et al. Metastasectomy for distant metastatic melanoma: analysis of data from the first Multicenter Selective Lymphadenectomy Trial (MSLT-I). *Ann Surg Oncol.* 2012;19(8):2547–2555.
43. Asare EA, Fisher SB, Chiang YJ, et al. Melanoma metastatic to the adrenal gland: An update on the role of adrenalectomy in multidisciplinary management. *J Surg Oncol.* 2023;128(2):313–321.
44. Nehal KS, Bichakjian CK. Update on keratinocyte carcinomas. *N Engl J Med.* 2018;379(4):363–374.
45. Costantino A, Canali L, Festa BM, Spriano G, Mercante G, De Virgilio A. Sentinel lymph node biopsy in high-risk cutaneous squamous cell carcinoma of the head and neck: Systematic review and meta-analysis. *Head Neck.* 2022;44(10):2288–2300.
46. Wilde DC, Glaun ME, Wong MK, Gross ND. Neoadjuvant approaches to non-melanoma skin cancer. *Cancers (Basel).* 2023;15(23):5494.
47. Deneve JL, Messina JL, Marzban SS, et al. Merkel cell carcinoma of unknown primary origin. *Ann Surg Oncol.* 2012;19(7):2360–2366.
48. Farley CR, Perez MC, Soelling SJ, et al. Merkel cell carcinoma outcomes: does AJCC8 underestimate survival? *Ann Surg Oncol.* 2020;27(6):1978–1985.
49. Topalian SL, Bhatia S, Amin A, et al. Neoadjuvant nivolumab for patients with resectable Merkel cell carcinoma in the Checkmate 358 Trial. *J Clin Oncol.* 2020;38(22):2476–2487.
50. Prieto-Granada C, Castner N, Chen A, et al. Behavior of cutaneous adnexal malignancies: a single institution experience. *Pathol Oncol Res.* 2020;26(1):239–244.
51. Vitiello GA, Lee AY, Berman RS. Dermatofibrosarcoma protuberans: What is this? *Surg Clin North Am.* 2022;102(4):657–665.
52. Navarrete-Dechent C, Mori S, Barker CA, Dickson MA, Nehal KS. Imatinib treatment for locally advanced or metastatic dermatofibrosarcoma protuberans: a systematic review. *JAMA Dermatol.* 2019;155(3):361–369.

102

Sarcomas of Soft Tissue

Heather G. Lyu, Chandrajit P. Raut, Sandra L. Wong, and Christina L. Roland

Key Points

1 Sarcomas are a rare and heterogeneous group of cancers that most commonly arise from mesoderm-derived elements such as muscle, fat, cartilage, blood vessels, bone, and other connective tissue but also from ectoderm-derived tissue such as nerve/nerve sheath. They are histologically distinct from cancers of epithelial origin.

2 Clinical behavior and prognosis are defined by anatomic location, histologic subtype, tumor grade, size, and ability to achieve complete resection.

3 Surgery is the cornerstone of treatment for intra-abdominal and retroperitoneal sarcomas. Complete resection for primary retroperitoneal sarcomas may require en bloc resection of adjacent or involved organs, most commonly the kidney and colon. Radiation therapy has not been demonstrated to reduce locoregional recurrence rates for most retroperitoneal sarcomas.

4 For extremity sarcomas, radiotherapy is indicated for high-risk tumors to decrease disease relapse. Limb-sparing and function-preserving procedures are favored to maximize functional outcomes.

5 The use of imatinib mesylate, a selective tyrosine kinase inhibitor (TKI), in the management of gastrointestinal stromal tumors (GISTs), remains a paradigm for the successful use of targeted molecular therapies.

1 Sarcomas are a heterogeneous group of cancers that arise from mesenchymal cells, or mesoderm-derived elements, including muscle, fat, cartilage, blood vessels, bone, and other connective tissue and ectoderm-derived tissue, such as nerve/nerve sheath. Though mesoderm-derived elements comprise nearly two-thirds of the body's mass, sarcomas are relatively rare. In 2024, an estimated 13,500 new cases of soft tissue and bone sarcoma were expected to be diagnosed in the United States, which accounts for less than 1% of all new cancers. Sarcomas also represent an extremely heterogeneous group of cancers, but taken together, 5-year overall survival is about 50% to 60%. Anatomic location, tumor size, grade, and histopathology are important determinants of clinical presentation, treatment, and prognosis.

Multimodality therapies, including surgery, radiation, and systemic/targeted therapy, have been combined to improve local and systemic tumor control. Over the past few decades, evolution of the multidisciplinary approach has enabled successful treatment options to evolve from radical amputation to limb-sparing procedures for extremity sarcoma. Multimodal therapies have also been considered for retroperitoneal sarcomas with several recent randomized controlled trials published on the role of neoadjuvant radiation and chemotherapy. Modern molecular diagnostics are increasingly being translated to clinical practice, and targeted treatment options are being rapidly developed as the histologic diversity of soft tissue sarcomas is better understood. As with many rare tumors, referral to high-volume centers with multidisciplinary clinical expertise is recommended.

EPIDEMIOLOGY

Soft tissue sarcoma can occur in all age groups and are equally distributed between genders. While the median age at diagnosis varies by histopathologic subtype, sarcomas are relatively rare in the adult population. However, sarcomas are among the most common cancers seen in children and young adults, representing approximately 15% of pediatric malignancies and often occurring in children under 5 years of age. There are over 75 distinct histopathologic subtypes. Further, sarcomas can occur at any anatomic site, and accordingly, anatomic site influences treatment and outcomes.

While most sarcomas arise spontaneously, there are some predisposing conditions to consider. Sarcomas are not thought to be the result of malignant degeneration of a long-standing benign lesion such as a lipoma. An injury or other traumatic incident may lead to the initial recognition of a mass, but there are no data to support the notion that antecedent trauma leads to the development of either soft tissue or bony sarcomas.

Toxic exposures have been related to the development of sarcoma, most notably industrial use of thorium dioxide (Thorotrast), arsenic, and vinyl chloride were associated with the development of hepatic angiosarcomas. Several other predisposing conditions are known to be associated with the development of sarcoma. Stewart–Treves syndrome was originally described in patients with lymphedema following radical mastectomy and radiation for breast cancer who then developed lymphangiosarcoma of the affected arm but can arise in any extremity with long-standing extremity edema. Kaposi sarcoma became one of the first described opportunistic diseases associated with HIV infection in the early 1908s. Though the incidence of HIV-associated Kaposi sarcoma has markedly declined with effective antiretroviral therapy, it remains an important cause of morbidity among HIV-infected patients and other immunosuppressed patients such as renal allograft recipients.

With the increasing use of external-beam radiation in cancer treatment, there has been a noted increase in the modern incidence of secondary sarcoma in patients previously treated with radiation for a variety of malignancies. Following

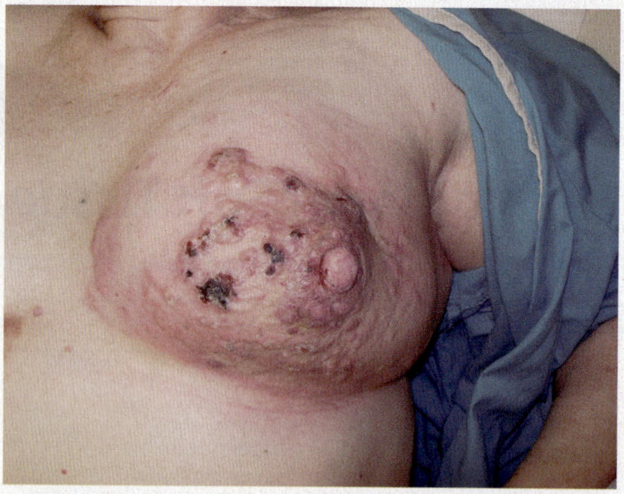

Figure 102.1. Radiation-associated angiosarcoma. This 79-year-old woman developed skin changes on her breast 7 years after breast conservation therapy (lumpectomy and radiation therapy) for a 2-cm invasive ductal adenocarcinoma. Radical surgery including removal of all of the irradiated anatomic breast skin in addition to a mastectomy was performed.

median latent periods of approximately 8 years (range 6 to 20 years), radiation-associated sarcomas are being increasingly diagnosed in previously radiated areas. Common radiation-associated sarcoma subtypes are angiosarcomas, undifferentiated pleomorphic sarcoma, fibrosarcoma, osteosarcoma, and leiomyosarcoma, and are commonly high grade.[1] Notably, with the advent of breast conservation therapy for breast cancer (consisting of partial mastectomy/lumpectomy and adjuvant radiation therapy), there should be an appropriate index of suspicion for breast angiosarcomas with findings of skin changes on an irradiated breast (**Fig. 102.1**).

GENETIC CANCER SYNDROMES

While the vast majority of sarcomas are sporadic, numerous genetic alterations are associated with both bone and soft tissue sarcomas. Patients with neurofibromatosis type 1 (NF-1, or von Recklinghausen disease) have mutations in the neurofibromin 1 or 2 gene (*NF1* or *NF2*, respectively) which are associated with the development of malignant peripheral nerve sheath tumors (MPNST) and gastrointestinal stromal tumors (GISTs) in an estimated 5% of patients over a lifetime.[2] A genetic predisposition to desmoid tumors or desmoid fibromatosis is associated with familial adenomatous polyposis (FAP), or Gardner syndrome which is the result of germline mutations in the adenomatous polyposis coli (*APC*) gene. Desmoids are a common extracolonic manifestation of FAP and can be a source of increased morbidity in these patients following proctocolectomy for the prevention or treatment of colon cancer.

While somatic activation of c-KIT and overexpression of KIT protein are well described in the pathogenesis of GISTs, familial GISTs have been ascribed to germline mutation in *c-KIT* as well as in the *SDHB*, *SDHC*, and *SDHD* succinate dehydrogenase (SDH) subunits, in association with Carney triad (GIST, pulmonary chondromas, extra-adrenal paragangliomas) or Carney–Stratakis syndrome (GIST, paraganglioma).

One well-documented mechanism of sarcoma development is the inactivation of tumor suppressor genes. Retinoblastoma was known to be associated with a mutation in the retinoblastoma gene (*RB1*), a 13q chromosomal deletion. Investigation of the link between familial retinoblastoma and osteosarcoma led to the discovery that a genetic defect in *RB1* also plays a role in the pathogenesis of sarcomas.

Li–Fraumeni syndrome is caused by an inherited mutation in the *p53* gene, a key growth-regulatory gene. Germline mutations in affected patients are associated with high incidences of childhood rhabdomyosarcomas, breast cancer, brain tumors, lung cancer, and leukemias.

Cytogenetic aberrations have been recognized in a number of soft tissue sarcomas usually simple karyotypes including fusion genes due to reciprocal translocations or specific point mutations (**Table 102.1**). These chromosomal translocations serve as powerful diagnostic markers and may be important in determining tumor biology and subsequent tumor behavior. For example, identification of the translocation of t(X;18)(p11;q11) can confirm the diagnosis of synovial sarcoma. There are data to suggest that the SYT-SSX1 fusion transcript carries a worse prognosis than the SYT-SSX2 fusion transcript, with median survivals of 6.1 years and 13.7 years, respectively.[3]

A better understanding of the molecular biology of sarcomas has revolutionized diagnosis of specific histopathologic subtypes and has elucidated potential pathways for targeted molecular therapy.

SOFT TISSUE SARCOMAS

Clinical Presentation

The most common presentation of a soft tissue sarcoma is that of an asymptomatic mass. Most sarcomas tend to grow in a centrifugal fashion and generally remaining within their compartment/fascial plane of origin but encasement of structures can occur. Some tumors can grow across fascial planes, including myxofibrosarcoma and fibromyxosarcoma. Compression generally does not produce pain, swelling, or obstructive symptoms until the tumors become quite large or directly impinge on a nerve. Even very large abdominal or retroperitoneal sarcomas present with nonspecific abdominal symptoms such as fullness, early satiety, or minor abdominal discomfort (**Fig. 102.2**).

In general, the vast majority of soft tissue masses tend to be benign, but concerning features which should prompt a higher index of suspicion for malignancy include large size (>5 cm), deep location (subfascial, intramuscular, intra-abdominal), variations in texture on examination, immobile nature or noted fixation to underlying structures, or changes to an existing lesion (increasing size or worsening compressive symptoms). There are no reliable tumor markers for sarcomas, so serum bloodwork is generally not useful in the evaluation of soft tissue masses. However, advances in the understanding and detection of circulating tumor DNA could lead to future serum tests for diagnosis of primary and recurrent sarcoma and measurement of response to therapy.

Diagnosis

Diagnostic Imaging

Accurate radiologic imaging is critical in the diagnostic workup of sarcoma to provide information about the precise location and extent of the primary tumor. Computed tomography (CT) scans and magnetic resonance imaging (MRI) are the most important imaging modalities for evaluating the resectability of soft tissue sarcomas, providing definition of the primary tumor in relation to bone, muscle, neurovascular structures, and adjacent organs and provide critical information for treatment planning. While MRI is preferred for extremity sarcomas, CT is often the modality of choice for abdominal, pelvic, and retroperitoneal tumors.

As sarcomas are known to predominantly metastasize to the lungs, directed chest imaging should be performed at the time of diagnosis, particularly for high grade tumors. While chest radiography (CXR) may be used, CT scans are increasingly utilized as the primary screening examination of choice for higher-risk patients, such as those with high-grade lesions or tumors larger than 5 cm. Any abnormal CXR must be followed by a chest CT scan per protocol, usually involving thinner sections without IV contrast, for more detailed evaluation

Table 102.1. Cytogenetic Abnormalities in Soft Tissue Sarcoma Subtypes

Histologic Subtype	Cytogenetic Alteration	Molecular Alteration
Alveolar rhabdomyosarcoma	t(2;13)(q35;q14) t(1;13)(p36;q14) double minutes t(2;2)(q35;p23) t(X;2)(q35;q13)	*PAX3-FOXO1* fusion *PAX7-FOXO1* fusion *PAX3-NCOA1* fusion *PAX3-AFX* fusion
Alveolar soft part sarcoma	t(X;17)(p11.2;q25)	*TFE3-ASPSCR1* fusion
BCOR-rearranged sarcoma	Inv(X)(p11p11) t(X;4)(p11;q31) t(X;22)(p11;q13)	*BCOR-CCNB3* fusion *BCOR-MAML3* fusion *ZC3H7B-BCOR-* fusion
CIC-rearranged sarcoma	t(4;19)(q35;q13) or t(10;19)(q26:q13) t(X;19)(q13;q13.3)	*CIC-DUX4* fusion *CIC-FOXO4* fusion
Clear cell sarcoma	t(12;22)(q13;q12) t(2;22)(q32.3;q12)	*EWS-ATF1* fusion *CREB1-ESWR1* fusion
Dedifferentiated liposarcoma	Ring and giant marker chromosomes	Amplification of 12q13-15: *MDM2, CDK4, HMGA2*
Desmoplastic small round cell tumor	t(11;22)(p13;q12)	*EWS-WT1* fusion
Dermatofibrosarcoma protuberans	t(17;22)(q21;q13); ring forms of chromosomes 17 and 22	*COL1A1-PDGFB* fusion
Endometrial stromal sarcoma, low grade	t(7;17)(p15;q21) t(6;7)(p21;p15) t(6;10)(p21;p11) t(1;6)(p34;p21) t(X;17)(p11;q21)	*JAZF1-SUZ12* fusion *PHF1-JAXF1* fusion *EPC1-PHF1* fusion *MEAF6-PHF1* fusion *MBTD1-CXorf67* fusion
Endometrial stromal sarcoma, high grade	t(10;17)(q22;p13) t(X;22)(p11;q13)	*YWHAE-NUTM2* fusion *ZC3H7B-BCOR* fusion
Epithelioid hemangioendothelioma	t(1;2)(p36;q25) t(X;11)(p11;q22)	*WWTR1-CAMTA1* fusion *YAP1-TFE3* fusion
Epithelioid sarcoma	Deletion 22q t(8;22)(q22;q11) t(10,22)	*SMARCB1* inactivation
Ewing sarcoma	t(11;22)(q24;q12) t(21;22)(q12;q12)	*EWS-FLI1* fusion *EWS-ERG* fusion
Extraskeletal myxoid chondrosarcoma	t(9;22)(q22;q11) t(9;17)(q22;q11) t(9;15)(q22;q21) t(3;9)(q11;q22) t(9;17)(q22;q11)	*EWSR1-NR4A3* fusion *TAF2N-NR4A3* fusion *TCF12-NR4A3* fusion *TGF-NR4A3* fusion *RBP56-NR4A3* fusion
Fibrosarcoma	t(12;15)(p13;q26)	*ETV6-NTRK3* fusion
Gastrointestinal stromal tumor	Deletion 14q, 22q, 1p, 15q	*KIT* or *PDGFRA* mutation (85% of cases); *NF1, SDHX, BRAF* mutation, *SDHC* hypermethylation, other
Inflammatory myofibroblastic tumor	t(1;2)(q22;p23) t(2;19)(p23;p13) t(2;17)(p23;q23) t(2;2)(p23;q13) t(2;2)(p23;q35) t(2;11)(p23;p15) t(2;4)(p23;q21) t(2;12)(p23;p12) t(2;20)(p23;p12) t(3;6)(q12;q22) t(6;17)(q22;p13)	*TPM3-ALK* fusion *TPM4-ALK* fusion *CLTC-ALK* fusion *RANBP2-ALK* fusion *ATIC-ALK* fusion *CARS-ALK* fusion *SEC31L1-ALK* fusion *PPFIBP1-ALK* fusion *RRBP1-ALK* fusion *TFG-ROS1* fusion *YWHAE-ROS1* fusion

(*continued*)

Table 102.1. Cytogenetic Abnormalities in Soft Tissue Sarcoma Subtypes (*Continued*)

Histologic Subtype	Cytogenetic Alteration	Molecular Alteration
Fibromyxoid sarcoma, low grade	t(7;16)(q33;p11) t(11;16)(p11;p11)	*FUS-CREB3L2* fusion *FUS-CREB3L1* fusion
Mesenchymal chondrosarcoma	t(8;8)(q13;q21)	*HEY1-NCOA2* fusion
Malignant peripheral nerve sheath tumor	Various	*SUZ12* or *EED* mutation (80% of cases), *NF1* inactivation
Myxoid/round cell liposarcoma	t(12;16)(q13;p11) t(12;22)(q13;q12)	*FUS-DDIT3* fusion *EWSR1-DDIT3* fusion
Pseudomyogenic hemangioendothelioma	t(7;19)(q22;q13)	*SERPINE1-FOSB* fusion
Sclerosing epitheliod fibrosarcoma	t(11;22)(p11;q12) t(7;16)(q33;p11)	*EWSR1-CREB3L1* fusion *FUS-CREB3L2* fusion
Solitary fibrous tumor	Inv(12)(q13q13)	*NAB2-STAT6* fusion
Synovial sarcoma	t(X;18)(p11;q11)	SS18-SSX1 orSS18-SSX2 fusion

Adapted from Schaefer IM, Cote GM, Hornick JL. Contemporary sarcoma diagnosis, genetics, and genomics. *J Clin Oncol*. 2018;36(2):101–110.

of potential pulmonary metastases (**Fig. 102.3**). CT of the chest, abdomen, and pelvis should be considered in any patient with a myxoid liposarcoma of an extremity because this subtype often metastasizes to the abdomen or other "fat pads" such as the axilla. Paraspinal imaging with MRI may be indicated for myxoid liposarcoma as well, as bone and soft tissue metastases in this region may develop. Metastases to the liver can develop in the setting of GIST and pelvic or abdominal visceral sarcomas.

MRI is the recommended imaging modality for extremity sarcomas. Sequencing routinely involves axial T2-weighted and precontrast/postcontrast T1-weighted images. Contrast enhancement with gadolinium is crucial for detecting and characterizing lesions with coronal, sagittal, and other reconstructions. This imaging modality can accurately delineate between muscle groups and distinguish tumor and neurovascular structures (**Fig. 102.4**).

Positron emission tomography (PET) scanning using fluoro-13-deoxyglucose also offers the potential for noninvasive analysis of tumor metabolism and has been shown to correlate with both tumor grade and response to treatment for many types of cancers. PET may be helpful in distinguishing between benign and malignant lesions concerning for sarcoma and in assessing response to treatment. PET scans can also be utilized to differentiate between WDLPS and DDLPS, which may impact differences in neoadjuvant therapy approaches.[4]

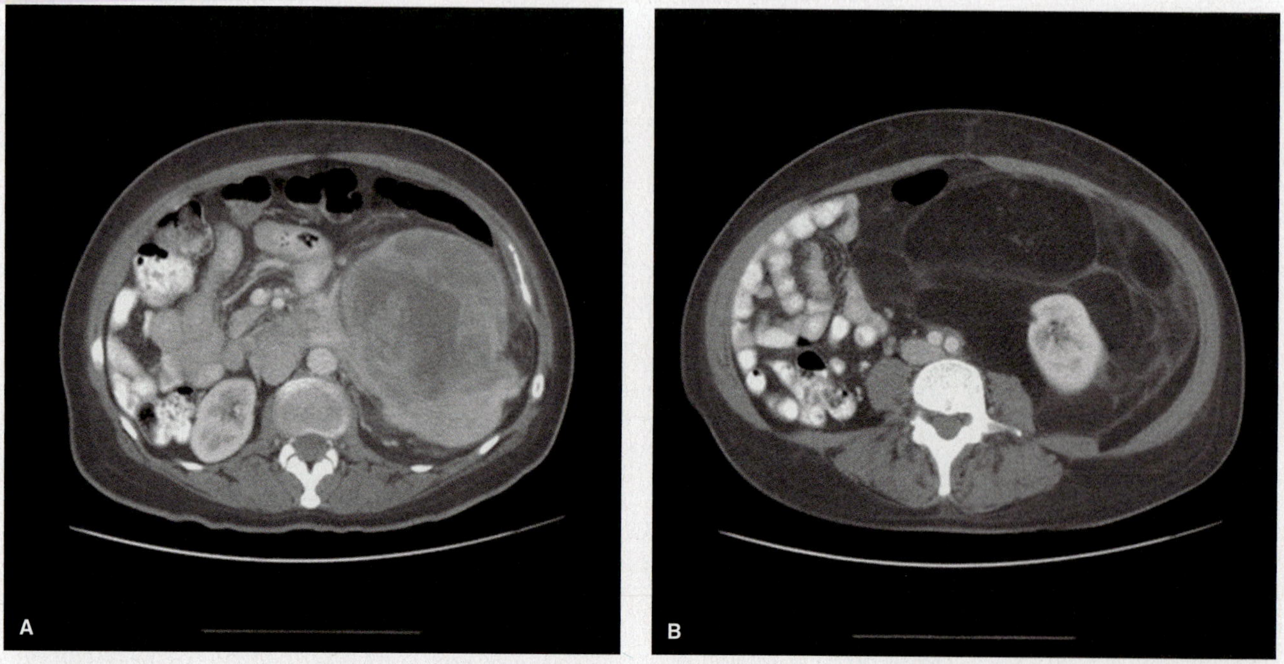

Figure 102.2. Dedifferentiated liposarcoma of the retroperitoneum. This 51-year-old woman presented with only vague symptoms of abdominal fullness from a very large retroperitoneal mass. The CT scan demonstrates a heterogeneous soft tissue mass in the upper abdomen (**A**) which blends into a more fatty component (**B**) which encases the left kidney and displaces abdominal contents. She underwent radical resection en bloc left nephrectomy, distal pancreatectomy, splenectomy, left colectomy, and segmental resection of inferior vena cava.

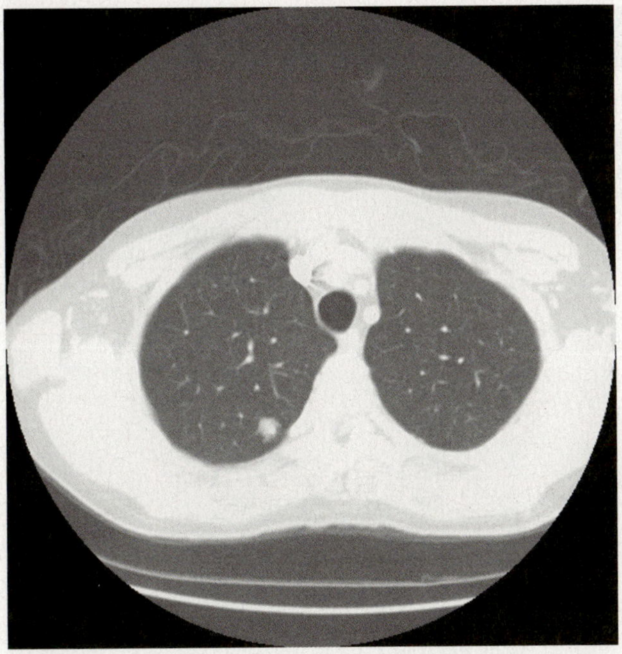

Figure 102.3. Pulmonary metastasis. A noncontrasted CT scan of the thorax demonstrates a 1.1-cm noncalcified nodule consistent with pulmonary metastasis in the upper lobe of the right lung.

Diagnostic Biopsy

Image-guided core biopsies, either using CT or ultrasound, are critical in directing a multimodality treatment approach and have become a standard approach in the preoperative workup of a suspected sarcoma.[5] Fine needle aspiration (FNA) does not provide sufficient material for definitive histopathologic diagnosis (including subtype classification), especially for an index presentation of sarcoma. Core-needle biopsy (CNB) is performed with multiple passes and retrieves sufficient material for immunohistochemical staining, and when necessary, for cytogenetic analysis or flow cytometry. CNB is associated with low complication rates (<1%), including bleeding. Concerns about recurrence along the tract are obviated with judicious planning of the biopsy tract, the use of a sheathed needle device, and/or excision of the biopsy tract at the time of definitive resection when possible.[6]

Open surgical biopsy, or incisional biopsy, is rarely indicated given the success of CNB. However, open biopsy can be considered when core-needle specimens yield nondiagnostic findings. Incisions must be oriented along the long axis of extremities to facilitate subsequent complete resection with definitive surgical management. A transverse incision in the extremity often commits the patient to more extensive procedures than would be otherwise necessary, potentially compromising the ability to obtain clear margins with definitive limb-sparing procedures. Attempts to enucleate the sarcoma within its "pseudocapsule" and without a proper margin is strongly discouraged, though excisional biopsy can be considered as the primary approach for small (2 cm), superficial lesions by experienced surgical oncologists. Extensive dissection during a biopsy, including undermining surrounding subcutaneous layers, should be consciously avoided to contain the extent of disease and best manage subsequent procedures. Attention to meticulous hemostasis also prevents extensive "seeding" of the area.

PATHOLOGIC CLASSIFICATION

Histopathologic designation of soft tissue sarcomas consist of an extremely heterogeneous group of tumors. Sarcomas are generally classified according to the tissues they mimic rather than the type of tissue from which the tumor arises.[7] The various types of benign and malignant soft tissue tumors are noted in **Table 102.2.** The development of specialized markers for identifying individual types of sarcoma has led to greater precision in their classification.

One of the most critical pieces of pathologic information for clinicians treating sarcoma patients is histologic grade. Histologic grade according to the Federation Nationale des Centres de Lutte Contre le Cancer (FNCLCC) grading system is assessed based on the expert assessment of degree of tumor differentiation, the frequency of mitotic figures, and the presence or absence of spontaneous tumor necrosis (**Table 102.3**).

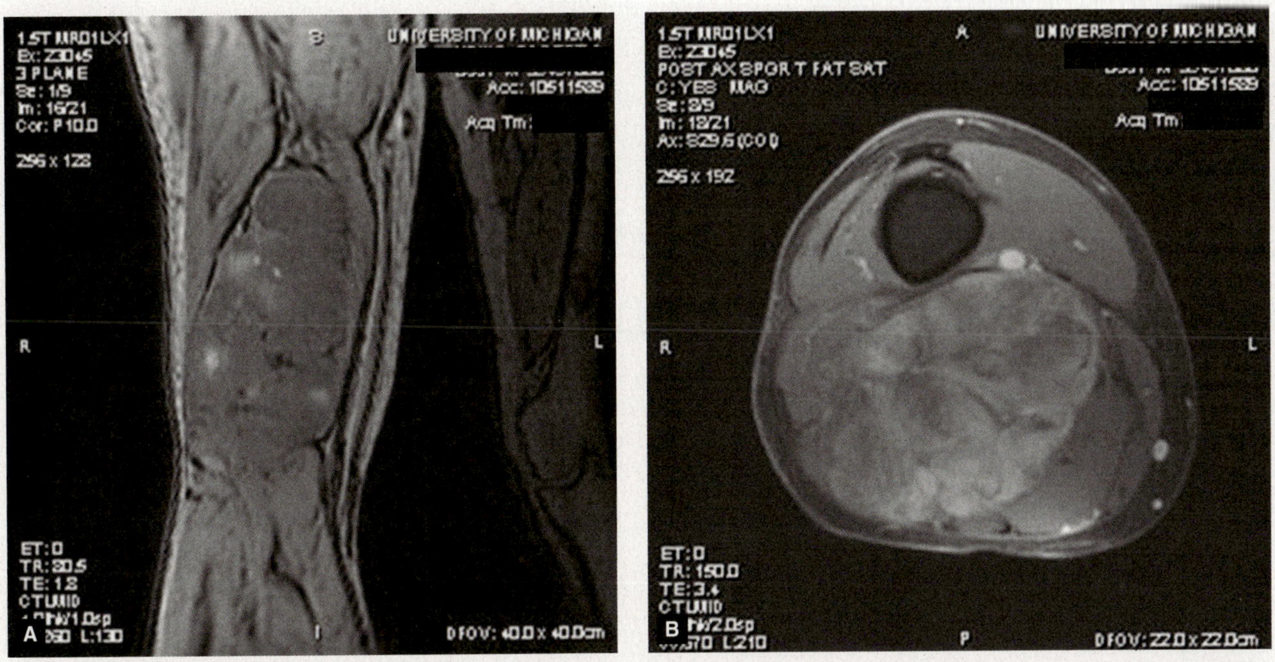

Figure 102.4. Extremity sarcoma. MRI demonstrates a 20-cm low-grade myxoid liposarcoma. **A:** Coronal reconstruction demonstrates location in the distal right thigh. **B:** Axial images show displacement of the popliteal vessels and vastus medialis anteriorly; the common tibioperoneal nerve and biceps femoris laterally; and, the semimembranosis and semitendinosus muscles medially.

Table 102.2. WHO Histologic Classification of Soft Tissue Tumors

Classification	Benign	Intermediate (locally aggressive)	Intermediate (rarely metastasizes)	Malignant
Adipocyte tumors	Lipoma Lipomatosis Lipomatosis of nerve Lipoblastoma/ lipoblastomatosis Angiolipoma Myolipoma Chondroid lipoma Extrarenal angiomyolipoma Extra-adrenal myelolipoma Spindle cell/pleomorphic lipoma Hibernoma	Atypical lipomatous tumor/well-differentiated liposarcoma		Dedifferentiated liposarcoma Myxoid liposarcoma Pleomorphic liposarcoma Liposarcoma, not otherwise specified
Fibroblastic/ Myofibroblastic tumors	Nodular fasciitis Proliferative fasciitis Proliferative myositis Myositis ossificans Fibro-osseous pseudotumor of digits Ischemic fasciitis Elastrofibroma Fibrous hamartoma of infancy Fibromatosis coli Juvenile hyaline fibromatosis Inclusion body fibromatosis Fibroma of tendon sheath Desmoplastic fibroblastoma Mammary-type myofibroblastoma Calcifying aponeurotic fibroma Angiomyofibroblastoma Cellular angiofibroma Nuchal-type fibroma Gardner fibroma Calcifying fibrous tumor	Palmar/plantar fibromatosis Desmoid-type fibromatosis Lipofibromatosis Giant cell fibroblastoma	Dermatofibrosarcoma protuberans (DFSP) (fibrosarcomatous DFSP, pigmented DFSP) Solitary fibrous tumor Inflammatory myofibroblastic tumor Low-grade myofibroblastic sarcoma Myxoinflammatory fibroblastic sarcoma/atypical myxoinflammatory fibroblastic tumor Infantile fibrosarcoma	Adult fibrosarcoma myxofibrosarcoma Low-grade fibromyxoid sarcoma Sclerosing epithelioid fibrosarcoma Malignant solitary fibrous tumor
So-called fibrohistiocytic tumors	Tenosynovial giant cell tumor (localized type, diffuse type, malignant) Deep benign fibrous histiocytoma		Plexiform fibrohistiocytic tumor Giant cell tumor of soft tissue	
Smooth muscle tumors	Deep leiomyoma			Leiomyosarcoma (excluding skin)
Pericytic (perivascular) tumors	Glomus tumor (glomangiomatosis) Myopericytoma (myofibroma, myofibromatosis) Angioleiomyoma			Malignant glomus tumor
Skeletal muscle tumors	Rhabdomyoma (adult, fetal, and genital types)			Embryonal rhabdomyosarcoma (botryoid, anaplastic) Alveolar rhabdomyosarcoma (solid, anaplastic) Pleomorphic rhabdomyosarcoma Spindle cell/sclerosing rhabdomyosarcoma

Table 102.2. WHO Histologic Classification of Soft Tissue Tumors (*Continued*)

Classification	Benign	Intermediate (locally aggressive)	Intermediate (rarely metastasizes)	Malignant
Vascular tumors of soft tissue	Hemangioma (synovial, venous, arteriovenous hemangioma/ malformation, intramuscular) Epithelioid hemangioma Angiomatosis Lymphangioma	Kaposiform hemangioendothelioma	Retiform hemangioendothelioma Papillary intralymphatic angioendothelioma Composite hemangioendothelioma Pseudomyogenic hemangioendothelioma Kaposi sarcoma	Angiosarcoma Epithelioid hemangioendothelioma
Chondro-osseous tumors	Soft tissue chondroma			Extraskeletal chondrosarcoma Extraskeletal osteosarcoma
Gastrointestinal stromal tumors (GIST)	GIST, benign			GIST, malignant
Nerve sheath tumors	Schwannoma Melanotic schwannoma Neurofibroma (plexiforma neurofibroma) Perineurioma Granular cell tumor Dermal nerve sheath myxoma Solitary circumscribed neuroma Ectopic meningioma Nasal glial heterotopia Benign Triton tumor Hybrid nerve sheath tumors			Malignant peripheral nerve sheath tumor (MPNST) Epithelioid MPNST Malignant Triton tumor Malignant granular cell tumor Ectomesenchymoma Malignant perineurioma
Tumors of uncertain differentiation	Acral fibromyxoma Intramuscular myxoma Juxta-articular myxoma Deep ("aggressive") angiomyxoma Pleomorphic hyalinizing angiectatic tumor Ectopic hamartomatous thymoma	Hemosiderotic fibrolipomatous tumor	Atypical fibroxanthoma Angiomatoid fibrous histiocytoma Ossifying fibromyxoid tumor Mixed tumor, not otherwise specified Myoepithelioma Myoepithelial carcinoma Phosphaturic mesenchymal tumor	Synovial sarcoma (including biphasic) Epithelioid sarcoma Alveolar soft-part sarcoma Clear cell sarcoma of soft tissue Extraskeletal myxoid chondrosarcoma Extraskeletal Ewing sarcoma Desmoplastic small round cell tumor Perivascular epithelioid cell tumor (PEComa) Intimal sarcoma
Undifferentiated/ Unclassified sarcomas				Undifferentiated spindle cell sarcoma Undifferentiated pleomorphic sarcoma Undifferentiated round cell sarcoma Undifferentiated epithelioid sarcoma Undifferentiated sarcoma NOS

Adapted from Fletcher CD, Bridge JA, Hogendoorn PC, et al. *WHO Classification of Tumors of Soft Tissue and Bone*. 2020.

Table 102.3. Histologic Parameters in the Federation Nationale des Centres de Lutte Contre le Cancer (FNCLCC) Grading System

Histologic Parameter	Score	Definition
Tumor differentiation	1	Closely resembling normal adult mesenchymal tissue, potentially difficult to distinguish from benign counterparts (eg, well differentiated liposarcoma)
	2	Histologic typing is certain (eg, myxofibrosarcoma)
	3	Undifferentiated or embryonal sarcomas, synovial sarcoma
Mitotic count	1	0–9 mitoses per 10 HPF
	2	10–19 mitoses per 10 HPF
	3	>19 mitoses per 10 HPF
Tumor necrosis	0	No necrosis
	1	<50% tumor necrosis
	2	≥50% tumor necrosis
Histologic grade	Grade 1	Total score 2–3
	Grade 2	Total score 4–5
	Grade 3	Total Score 6–8

Adapted from Coindre JM. Grading of soft tissue sarcomas: review and update. *Arch Pathol Lab Med.* 2006;130(10):1448–1453.

Table 102.4. Tumor Differentiation Score According to Histologic Subtype in the Federation Nationale des Centres de Lutte Contre le Cancer (FNCLCC)

Differentiation Score	Histologic Subtype
1	Well-differentiated liposarcoma Well-differentiated leiomyosarcoma Malignant neurofibroma Well-differentiated fibrosarcoma
2	Myxoid liposarcoma Conventional leiomyosarcoma Conventional malignant peripheral nerve sheath tumor (MPNST) Conventional fibrosarcoma Myxofibrosarcoma Myxoid chondrosarcoma Conventional angiosarcoma
3	High-grade myxoid (round cell) liposarcoma Pleomorphic liposarcoma Dedifferentiated liposarcoma Rhabdomyosarcoma Poorly differentiated/pleomorphic leiomyosarcoma Poorly differentiated/epithelioid angiosarcoma Poorly differentiated MPNST Malignant Triton tumor Synovial sarcoma Extraskeletal osteosarcoma Extraskeletal Ewing sarcoma Mesenchymal chondrosarcoma Clear cell sarcoma Epithelioid sarcoma Alveolar soft part sarcoma Malignant rhabdoid tumor Undifferentiated (spindle cell and pleomorphic sarcoma)

Adapted from Coindre JM. Grading of soft tissue sarcomas: review and update. *Arch Pathol Lab Med.* 2006;130(10):1448–1453.

While grading criteria have undergone numerous revisions over the years, in general, low-grade tumors have relatively little cellular atypia, few mitoses, and no tumor necrosis. High-grade tumors show a significant degree of necrosis in addition to atypia and frequent mitotic figures. Tumor differentiation scores, a component of the FNCLCC grading system, is assigned consistently for specific histologic subtypes, as detailed in **Table 102.4** and representatively depicted in **Figure 102.5**. The current American Joint Committee on Cancer (AJCC) staging system recognizes a classification system ranging from Grade 1 (G1) to Grade 3 (G3) tumors, taking into account histology, tumor differentiation, mitotic count,

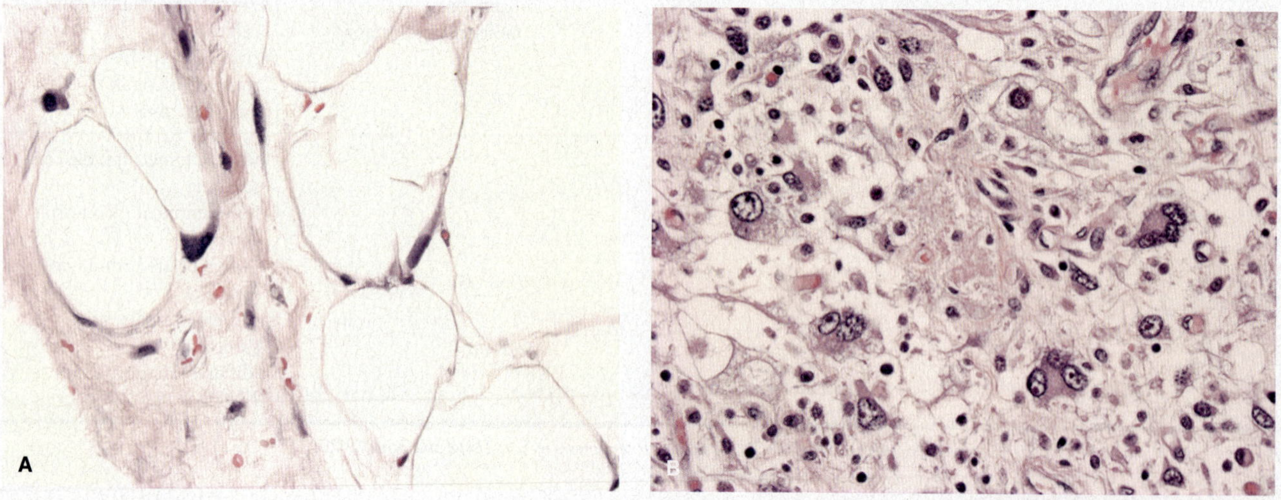

Figure 102.5. Histologic grading of sarcomas. Photomicrographs demonstrate the appearance of different grades within the same histologic subtype. **A:** Well-differentiated liposarcoma (lipoma-like) of the retroperitoneum with noted few atypical lipoblasts. **B:** High-grade, dedifferentiated liposarcoma of the retroperitoneum with highly atypical lipoblasts. (Courtesy of David R. Lucas, MD, University of Michigan, Ann Arbor, MI.)

and tumor necrosis.[8] There can be disagreement about grading schemas and expert pathology opinion can vary from center to center. As such, it is important to take note of tumor classification when interpreting results from clinical trials or retrospective reports.

Staging

2 Because of the prognostic importance of staging, stage classification of the primary tumor is based on both clinical and histologic information. The usual TNM classification used by the AJCC for other solid tumors is modified to a TNMG system for most soft tissue sarcomas, including trunk and extremity sarcomas.[9] Some tumors, including desmoid tumors, are locally aggressive but have little to no risk of metastatic disease and are thus excluded from the AJCC staging system.[9]

The most recent version of the AJCC staging system for sarcomas includes a number of changes including new site-specific staging systems.[9] A principal difference between retroperitoneal and trunk/extremity sarcoma staging is that nodal disease is considered stage IIIB for retroperitoneal and IV for trunk/extremity.[9] Uterine sarcomas and GIST continue to have separate staging systems, as do bone sarcomas.[9] There is a new size category reflecting the increased risk of metastasis as tumor size increases.

One of the challenges with AJCC staging of sarcomas is that histologic subtype is not included. Prognostic nomograms based on histologic subtype or site of origin have been developed.[10] These include prognostic factors as continuous rather than categorical variables. Some are now available for download on a smart phone app (www.sarculator.com).[11]

TREATMENT

Principles of Surgery

3 Complete resection remains the cornerstone of treatment for soft tissue sarcomas (**Figs. 102.6** and **102.7**). Performing a wide excision of the tumor with negative margins is the goal of resection with curative intent. Technical aspects of resection which must be taken into consideration include anatomic location and extent of disease. Often, soft tissue sarcomas are surrounded by a zone of compressed reactive tissue that forms a pseudocapsule. Care should be taken to avoid entry into the tumor and pseudocapsule during course of dissection. Enucleation commonly results in microscopically positive margins and reresection should be considered though anatomic

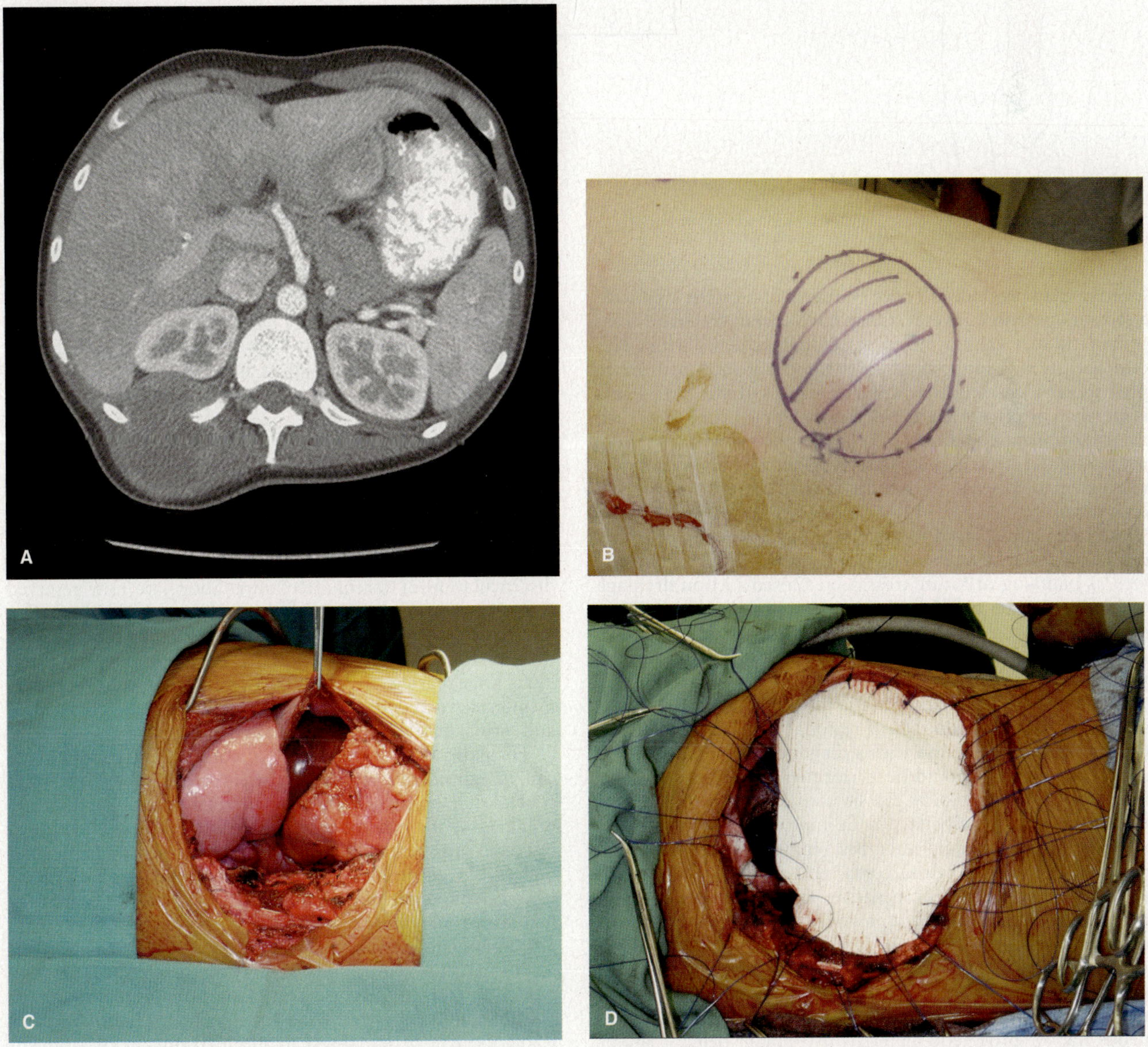

Figure 102.6. Chest wall sarcoma. A 20-year-old man with a 7.5-cm right posterior chest wall epithelioid sarcoma involves the 11th and 12th ribs as seen on CT scan (**A**) and on physical examination (**B**). Chest wall resection was performed, including a portion of diaphragm. Resulting chest wall defect (**C**) was repaired using prosthetic mesh (**D**).

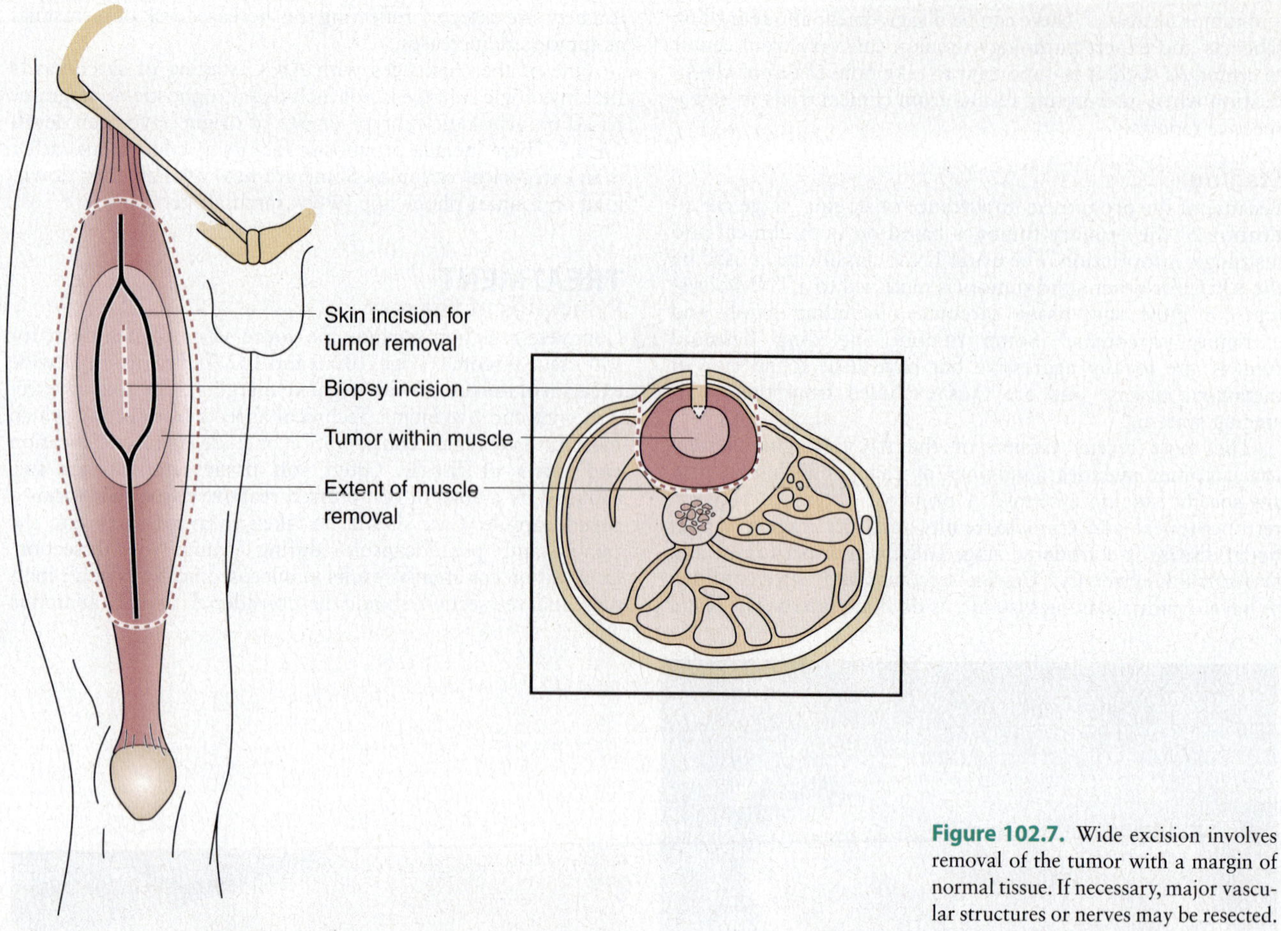

Figure 102.7. Wide excision involves removal of the tumor with a margin of normal tissue. If necessary, major vascular structures or nerves may be resected.

location may preclude effective clearance of margins even with a second operation. Several studies have demonstrated no compromise in survival if complete resection is achieved with a second operation.[12] Interestingly, it is unclear if local recurrence predisposes to subsequent distant metastasis or if margin status is merely a proxy for aggressive disease. Some histologies, such as myxofibrosarcoma, tend to track microscopically along neurovascular structures and fascial planes well beyond the visible extent of disease, and wider surgical margins should be considered.

Metallic clips placed in the tumor bed following resection can help define the limits of resection and aid in surveillance as well as planning of future treatment. Closed suction drainage catheters may be used to obviate postoperative seroma formation following resection of extremity or truncal sarcomas but should be placed close to the incision to be included in the postoperative radiation field.

A unique characteristic of sarcoma is the lack of metastasis to regional lymph nodes. If regional lymphadenopathy is discovered in conjunction with a diagnosis of sarcoma, ultrasound and biopsy should be performed for diagnosis. Therapeutic lymphadenectomy can be considered since clearance of disease may be associated with improved outcomes.[13] For selected histopathologic subtypes (eg, epithelioid sarcoma, clear cell sarcoma, angiosarcoma, and rhabdomyosarcoma), in patients with clinically negative node examination, there may be a role for sentinel lymph node biopsy to identify occult micrometastatic disease.[14]

Taken together, sarcomas of the upper and lower extremities and trunk make up the majority of soft tissue sarcomas. Large truncal tumors may require reconstruction with a myocutaneous flap or prosthetic materials if resultant defects cannot be closed primarily (**Fig. 102.6**). Radical amputations were once the mainstay of treatment for extremity sarcoma, but modern surgical approaches involve limb-sparing procedures in >95% of patients, which maximize functional outcomes. The accepted standard of care changed after the group at the National Cancer Institute, led by Rosenberg,[15] published the results of a randomized trial of limb-sparing resection plus adjuvant radiation therapy compared to amputation, finding no differences in disease-free survival rates (71% vs 78%, respectively) and the overall survival rates (83% vs 88%, respectively) at 5 years. This trial demonstrated that amputation was not mandatory and in 1985, a National Institute of Health consensus statement recommended limb-sparing procedures for most patients with high-grade extremity sarcomas. Radical amputations, such as hemipelvectomy, hip disarticulation or forequarter amputation, are now reserved for patients who are not suitable candidates for limb-sparing approaches, usually because of extent of disease, bony or joint invasion, or for otherwise unsalvageable recurrence after previous limb-sparing surgery (**Fig. 102.8**). There is no improvement in survival with this approach under these circumstances and serious morbidity must be taken into account.

For patients with small (T1) tumors, wide resection alone can be considered for select patients with acceptable local control and excellent long-term survival if wide margins are obtained at the time of resection. Most patients undergoing resection may be candidates for radiation therapy because of high risk for recurrence, although its role in lower-risk patients is somewhat undefined. Validated prognostic tools may be helpful for individual patients weighing the benefits of available treatment options.

For patients with large (>5 cm) or intermediate or high grade extremity or truncal soft tissue tumors, data support multimodal therapy with wide excision and radiation therapy. Radiation can be employed in the neoadjuvant or adjuvant setting, and evidence from randomized trials support similar local control and progression-free survival rates with both strategies. A phase III trial in which patients were randomized

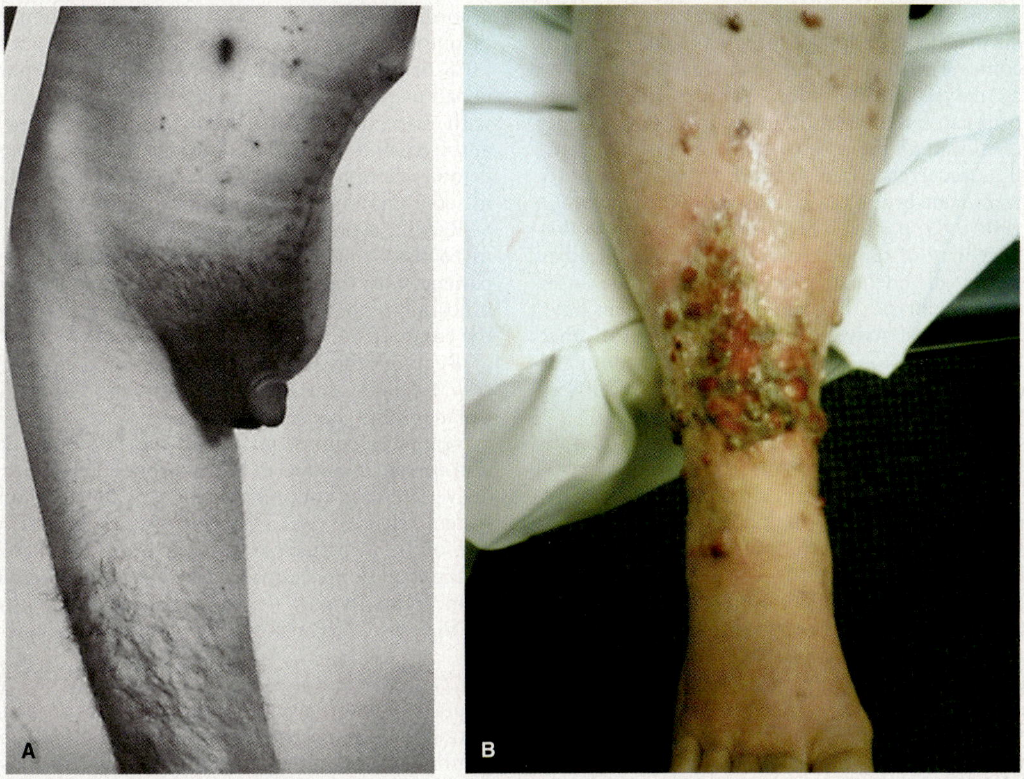

Figure 102.8. **A:** Radical amputations for extremity sarcomas include one joint above the most proximal extent of tumor. Now largely of historic interest, tumors of the proximal thigh or buttock were previously routinely treated with hemipelvectomy. **B:** While limb-sparing procedures are now done whenever possible, amputation may be necessary for certain cases. This 60-year-old woman had high-grade angiosarcoma of the right leg with extensive satellite metastases extending above her knee. She required above-knee amputation.

to preoperative or postoperative radiation demonstrated similar primary outcomes, yet found that preoperative radiation was associated with higher wound complications (35% vs 17%, respectively), but higher rates of late treatment effects (long-term joint stiffness and fibrosis) in the postoperative radiation group, attributed to relatively higher treatment doses and volumes.[16] Based on the data from this trial, either neoadjuvant or adjuvant radiation therapy may be offered around resection of trunk or extremity sarcomas.

Judicious use of radiation has allowed for the sparing of major neurovascular structures, though if necessary, arteries and/or veins should be resected en bloc with the tumor and subsequent reconstruction done with autologous or prosthetic graft materials. In cases of neurologic compromise, customized adjuncts from experienced physical medicine departments can help restore reasonable function. For instance, resultant foot drop from peroneal neuropathy can be managed with an ankle–foot orthotic and gait training. In appropriate cases, resection should be planned in conjunction with a plastic surgeon to provide complex soft tissue reconstruction with microvascular free flaps particularly if the size of defect following resection prohibits primary closure or if there is concern about a high risk of wound complications based on preoperative radiation.

Radiation and Systemic Therapy

4 The role of external-beam radiotherapy (EBRT) is best defined by a trial comparing limb-sparing surgery alone with limb-sparing surgery and adjuvant radiation, showing improved 10-year local recurrence rates with radiation. In high-grade sarcomas, the recurrence rate was 0% versus 22%, respectively though no significant effect on overall survival was appreciated.[17] Certainly, in the setting of involved surgical margins which could not otherwise be resected, adjuvant radiation therapy is associated with improved local control.

There are several benefits of preoperative radiation. With the tumor in situ, there is a smaller overall treatment volume and less long-term toxicity. However, the major disadvantage to preoperative radiation is its detrimental effect on wound healing. There have been recent advancements in neoadjuvant radiation for extremity sarcomas given the high morbidity of wound complications. The HYPORT-STS study in which a total of 42.75Gy was hypofractionated into 2.85Gy fractions × 15 demonstrated acceptable local control outcomes with similar incidence of wound complications.[18] Previously, brachytherapy was another alternative to external beam radiotherapy, but has largely been replaced with modern RT techniques such as IMRT. Some centers offer intraoperative radiation therapy (IORT), though its effectiveness is unproven. If IORT is employed, it is currently done in conjunction with a planned external-beam boost dose.

Since the main cause of death in patients with soft tissue sarcoma is distant metastatic disease and continued efforts have been made to develop better effective systemic therapies. The histologic subtypes of sarcoma vary in their responsiveness to chemotherapy. For example, osteogenic sarcoma, rhabdomyosarcoma, and Ewing sarcoma (the "pediatric" sarcomas) have had high rates of success with multimodality treatments including adjuvant chemotherapy.[19]

The results of randomized controlled trials on neoadjuvant and adjuvant systemic therapy are mixed due to the heterogeneity of histologic subtypes in treatment agents. Also, most randomized trials are underpowered to detect modest differences in survival and promising response rates reported in smaller nonrandomized clinical trials are not duplicated in subsequent larger randomized trials. In general, adjuvant chemotherapy is not indicated for patients with low-grade sarcomas and patients with small sarcomas (<5 cm) of higher grades.

Over the years, single agents as well as combination chemotherapy regimens have been used in the adjuvant treatment of soft tissue sarcomas. Two of the more active agents include doxorubicin and ifosfamide. However, multiple randomized trials of postoperative chemotherapy have not demonstrated an improvement in disease-free or overall survival with intermediate- or long-term follow-up though there was a trend toward improved outcomes with chemotherapy in many studies.[20] The Sarcoma Meta-Analysis Collaboration evaluated the effect of adjuvant doxorubicin-based chemotherapy in 1,568 patients from 14 trials.[21] Although the time to local and distant recurrences, as well as recurrence-free survival, were significantly better in the treatment group, an overall survival advantage was not seen (HR 0.89, $p = .12$). Because of the rarity of disease and heterogeneity of tumor characteristics, most studies are too small to provide adequate power for testing responses in specific histologic subtypes. In general, many regimens have combined two of the most active agents, doxorubicin (or other anthracycline) and ifosfamide, and results from a randomized trial did show improved disease-free survival and overall survival; distant relapse rates were not different however.[22]

Outside of clinical trials, adriamycin and ifosfamide combination therapy is commonly used for high-risk, primary extremity, and truncal sarcomas in the adjuvant setting. Newer regimens with promising results include the combination of gemcitabine and docetaxel, following a phase II study comparing adriamycin and ifosfamide to gemcitabine and docetaxel and found that the latter regimen had a slightly lower hospitalization rate and trends toward equivalent disease-free survival rates.[23]

A series of recent European trials have also explored the utility of neoadjuvant chemotherapy for extremity soft tissue sarcomas. These studies established that three cycles of neoadjuvant therapy are not inferior to five cycles.[24] One particularly innovative trial randomized patients with high-risk extremity sarcoma to three cycles of neoadjuvant epirubicin/ifosfamide or three cycles of a histotype-tailored regimen (trabectedin for myxoid liposarcoma, gemcitabine/dacarbazine for leiomyosarcoma, gemcitabine/docetaxel for unclassified pleomorphic sarcoma, high-dose ifosfamide for synovial sarcoma, and ifosfamide/etoposide for MPNST).[25] The hypothesis was that a tailored, histotype-specific regimen would be superior, but that proved not to be the case as survival was worse in the histology-tailored arm compared with Adriamycin-based therapy.

One potential advantage of upfront systemic chemotherapy is the ability to assess tumor response in situ. By seeing whether the tumor responds to the chemotherapy, both radiologically and pathologically, it may be possible to spare patients prolonged therapy if the tumor does not respond, or to continue therapy postoperatively if there is response. However, commonly used measures of radiologic response to treatment may not be good surrogate endpoints for treatment response.[26] The pathologic correlations of treatment-induced necrosis or histologic response to therapy with clinical outcomes have also not been well defined in soft tissue sarcoma.[27] Some patients who have a clinical or pathologic response to chemotherapy may have improved local control and decreased distant disease-free survival, but no overall survival advantage. In other cases, lack of measurable response did not seem to predict significant differences in event-free endpoints. These issues must be carefully considered in the design of future trials.

For advanced tumors, treatments with a single agent or combination regimens such as dacarbazine, doxorubicin, epirubicin, ifosfamide, gemcitabine, docetaxel, temozolomide, trabectedin, and eribulin have been examined extensively. Newer targeted therapies have demonstrated some promise in certain histologic subtypes. For example, tyrosine kinase inhibitor (TKI) agents such as pazopanib, imatinib, sorafenib, and sunitinib have efficacy in multiple subtypes after initial success with GISTs. The class of mTOR inhibitors (sirolimus, temsirolimus, everolimus) have demonstrated promise for perivascular epithelioid cell tumors (PEComas), lymphangioleiomyomatosis, and angiomyolipomas.

Recent studies on immune checkpoint inhibitors have demonstrated promising response rates in some sarcoma subtypes. The phase II trial, SARC028, treatment with pembrolizumab monotherapy demonstrated an objective response according to RECIST in 40% of patients with undifferentiated pleomorphic sarcoma, 20% of patients with liposarcoma, and 10% of patients with synovial sarcoma.[28] A phase II trial of neoadjuvant nivolumab or nivolumab/ipilimumab in patients with resectable retroperitoneal dedifferentiated liposarcoma and extremity/truncal undifferentiated pleomorphic sarcoma demonstrated a strong pathologic response in the UPS cohort in combination with radiation therapy.[29] Most recently, SARC032, a phase II trial evaluating the safety and efficacy of pembrolizumab in addition to radiation and resection for patients with stage III UPS or liposarcoma demonstrated a significantly higher disease-free survival of 70% versus 53% in the control arm.[30]

Regional therapies have been attempted with limited success. Regional chemotherapy administered via hyperthermic isolated limb perfusion has been attempted for advanced extremity sarcomas, mainly in the setting of limb preservation versus amputation. Extracorporeal circulation allows the delivery of drug concentrations 10 to 20 times higher than with systemic delivery and a European study showed a limb-salvage rate of 71% for unresectable extremity sarcomas using melphalan and tumor necrosis factor-α.[31] However, this technique is uncommonly used in the United States and usually reserved for highly selected patient populations in a clinical trial.

Retroperitoneal and Intra-Abdominal Sarcomas

Management of intra-abdominal (visceral) and retroperitoneal sarcomas deserves special consideration since specific anatomic location may dictate work-up and subsequent management. The grouping of visceral sarcomas generally includes tumors of the gastrointestinal tract and gynecologic organs, and less commonly, genitourinary organs. Location often precludes early diagnosis, unless the mass is found incidentally. Though some patients have noted increased abdominal girth, an abdominal mass can be appreciated with focused physical examination, but it is uncommonly the presenting complaint. Typically, vague symptoms of mass effect intra-abdominally trigger medical evaluation. Neurovascular symptoms related to compression or invasion can occur and manifest as paresthesia, dysesthesia, weakness, and swelling or varicosities in the lower extremities.

Complete history and physical examination should exclude signs and symptoms of lymphoma (eg, B-symptoms such as fevers and night sweats) and presence of scrotal masses concerning for testes cancer. Serum laboratory testing can be helpful if lymphoma (eg, elevated lactate dehydrogenase [LDH]), germ-cell tumors (eg, elevated beta-human chorionic gonadotropin [β-HCG] or alpha-fetoprotein [AFP]), or adrenal tumors (eg, cortisol levels or adrenocorticotropic hormone [ACTH]) are in the differential diagnosis. High-quality cross-sectional imaging with CT or MRI is critical for diagnosis and treatment planning. Use of oral and intravenous contrast defines extent of primary disease and the relationship of the tumor to nearby structures. Chest imaging should be obtained to assess for presence of pulmonary metastases. Hepatic involvement is the second most common site of distant spread in intra-abdominal and retroperitoneal sarcomas, so a CT scan that includes the proper contrast phasing for examination of the liver should be done.

For large tumors, preoperative image-guided CNB can almost always be performed by experienced interventional radiologists with minimal risk of needle track seeding (**Fig. 102.9**). Complete resection is the treatment of choice for intra-abdominal (visceral) and retroperitoneal sarcomas whenever possible. Only complete resection is associated with long-term survival benefit. For retroperitoneal sarcomas, median survival for those with an incomplete resection is similar to those who were observed (unresectable)[32] (**Fig. 102.10**). In general, incomplete resection should only be considered for palliation of intractable symptoms. While successful palliation may be achieved in carefully selected patients, aggressive

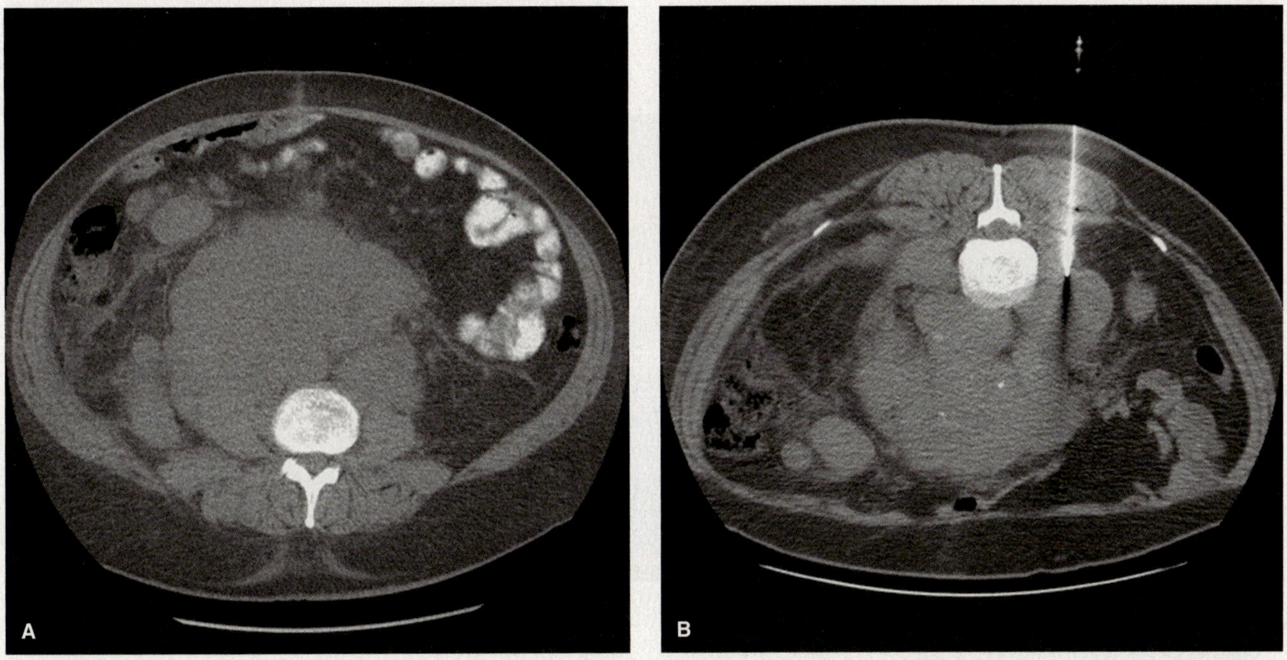

Figure 102.9. Biopsy can be helpful in the workup of retroperitoneal masses. **A:** CT scan shows a retroperitoneal mass encasing the IVC and aorta. **B:** Image-guided biopsy is demonstrated here. Pathology confirmed a diagnosis of large B-cell lymphoma.

tumor biology limits the ability to maintain sustained relief of symptoms.

In order to completely remove the sarcoma, en bloc resection of nearby structures should be considered when necessary. Resectability is more a function of location than of size, grade, or histologic subtype. Common reasons for unresectability include distant metastasis, peritoneal metastasis, extensive multifocality, and prohibitive vascular involvement. Though sarcomas do not uniformly invade other structures, involvement of vascular structures or mesentery (mesocolon) may lead to resection of solid organs or bowel that may not be directly involved. Furthermore, detailed pathologic analysis does show that adjacent structures, such as ureters, can be invaded even when no invasion is suspected.[33] When nephrectomy may be necessary, it is important to assess bilateral renal function with preoperative contrast scanning. Concomitant nephrectomy, when necessary, is associated with comparable outcomes for retroperitoneal sarcomas overall.[34] Commonly resected organs include the following: kidney, colon, adrenal gland, pancreas, diaphragm, and spleen. For tumors located in the pelvis, it may be necessary to perform en bloc resection of the colon/rectum, bladder, and uterus. When vascular structures limit complete resection of tumor, resection with ligation or reconstruction of vessels must be considered if technically feasible (**Fig. 102.11**).

Due to anatomic constraints, even when complete gross resection is achieved, margin status is often compromised by the visceral anatomy. A transperitoneal approach allows for excellent exposure and facilitates en bloc resection with early control of the vascular supply to the tumor. Analyses of compartmental resection approaches to RP sarcoma management include complete compartmental resections and liberal use of en bloc visceral resection, regardless of whether there is obvious gross tumor invasion of adjacent organs, yet remains controversial. Retrospective studies suggest some local control benefit in high-volume centers but proper patient selection needs to be weighed against morbidity and the natural history of sarcoma.[35] It is agreed that the best chance for curative intent resection is at the time of first operation. Complex multivisceral operations should be referred to higher-volume centers with experienced sarcoma surgeons when possible. Unfortunately, large national database studies suggest that only approximately 10% of patients undergoing surgery for primary retroperitoneal sarcoma are treated at high-volume centers.[36]

Even with aggressive surgical management, local recurrence rates range from 40% to 70% for high-grade tumors. Unlike extremity sarcomas, local progression is associated with decreased survival. Difficulty obtaining negative margins and high recurrence rates support a role for carefully selected multimodality treatments. However, the benefits of radiation for extremity sarcomas have not been similarly demonstrated for retroperitoneal sarcomas. The only randomized trial

Figure 102.10. Kaplan–Meier plot of disease-specific survival for patients with retroperitoneal sarcomas treated at Memorial Sloan Kettering Cancer Center. Disease-specific survival is 103 months in patients who underwent complete resection of retroperitoneal sarcomas, compared to 18 months in those who had an incomplete resection or just observation. (From Lewis JJ, Leung D, Woodruff JM, Brennan MF. Retroperitoneal soft-tissue sarcoma: analysis of 500 patients treated and followed at a single institution. *Ann Surg*. 1998;228(3):355–365.)

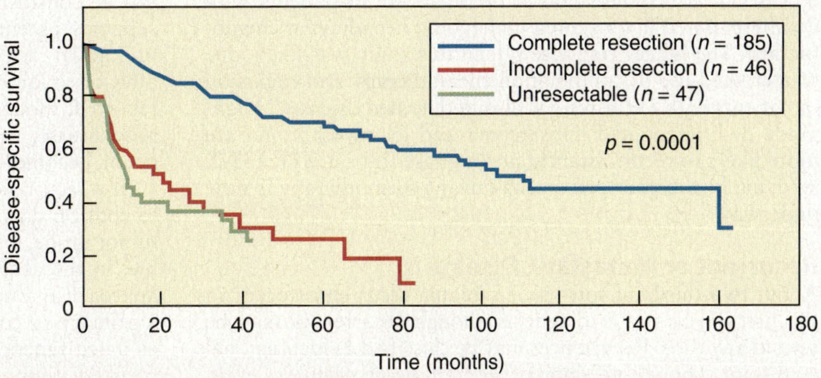

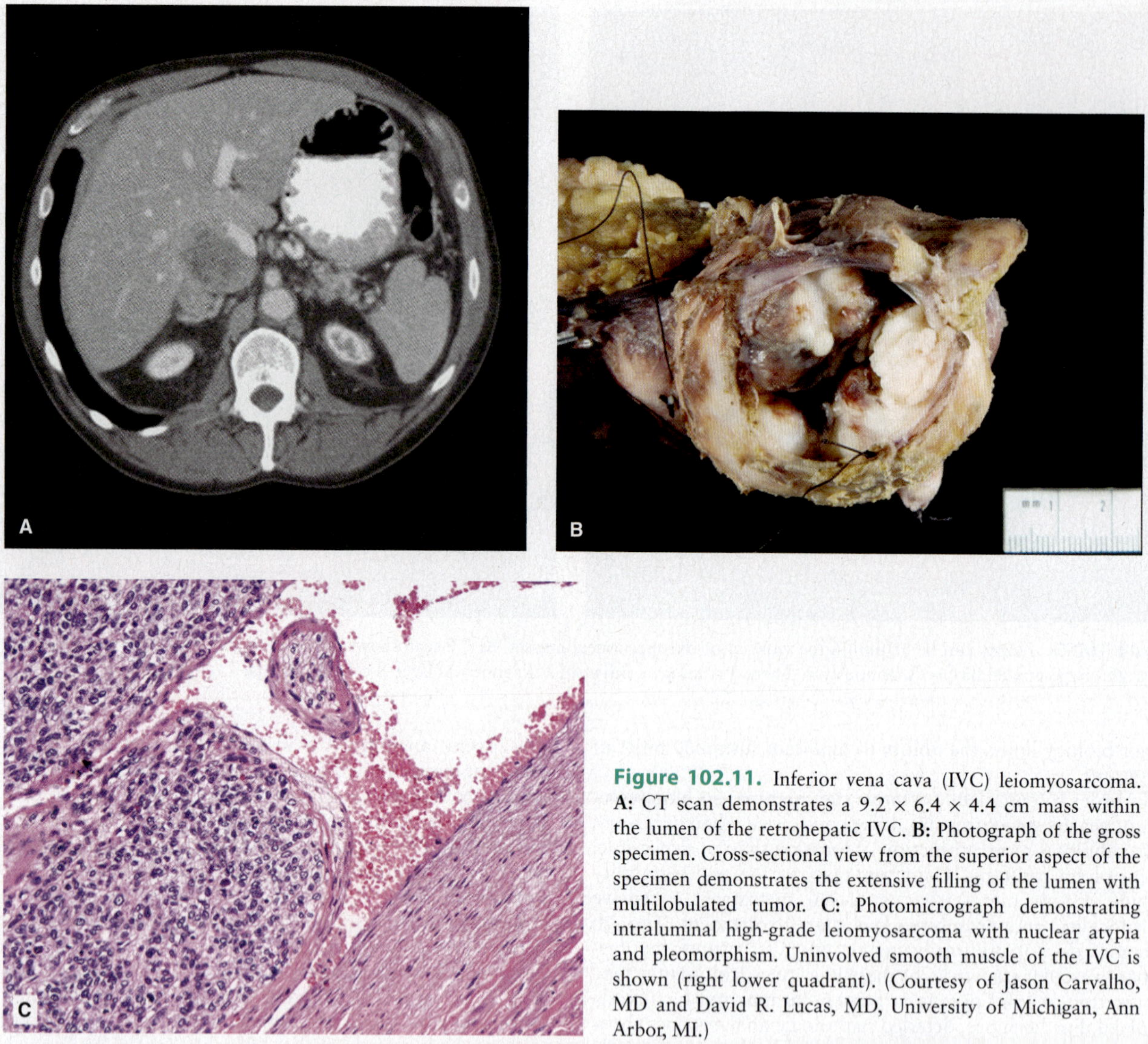

Figure 102.11. Inferior vena cava (IVC) leiomyosarcoma. **A:** CT scan demonstrates a 9.2 × 6.4 × 4.4 cm mass within the lumen of the retrohepatic IVC. **B:** Photograph of the gross specimen. Cross-sectional view from the superior aspect of the specimen demonstrates the extensive filling of the lumen with multilobulated tumor. **C:** Photomicrograph demonstrating intraluminal high-grade leiomyosarcoma with nuclear atypia and pleomorphism. Uninvolved smooth muscle of the IVC is shown (right lower quadrant). (Courtesy of Jason Carvalho, MD and David R. Lucas, MD, University of Michigan, Ann Arbor, MI.)

(STRASS) to examine the benefit of radiation plus surgery versus surgery alone found no improvement in the rate of abdominal recurrence-free survival, though there may be a potential use in selected patients with well-differentiated liposarcoma.[37] Large field sizes and the dose-limiting toxicity of abdominal viscera limit the utility of postoperative radiation.

The role of chemotherapy, either in the pre- or postoperative setting, is unproven for intra-abdominal and retroperitoneal sarcomas. Several trials of postoperative adjuvant chemotherapy do not show any benefit for patients with retroperitoneal sarcoma, and in one series, treated patients fared worse than those not receiving chemotherapy.[38] In a single center retrospective study, there was an overall response rate of 21% versus <12% response rate in the literature in patients with dedifferentiated liposarcoma undergoing neoadjuvant chemotherapy. The higher response rate in this study was likely due to increased use of combination chemotherapy and exclusion of patients with exclusively well-differentiated disease.[39] High-grade dedifferentiated liposarcoma and leiomyosarcoma are more likely to recur distantly, and a phase III trial, STRASS-2, studying histotype-specific neoadjuvant chemotherapy is now underway.

Recurrent or Metastatic Disease

About two-thirds of soft tissue sarcoma recurrences occur in the first 2 years after diagnosis, though recurrences may be seen at any time. Recurrences may be classified as locoregional or distant. Though no standardized follow-up regimens exist, routine history and physical examination (clinical follow-up) and interval chest imaging and primary tumor site imaging are recommended for the first 5 years. MRI of the extremity or trunk can help detect locoregional recurrences and CT scans may be useful for demonstration of intra-abdominal or retroperitoneal recurrences which would otherwise be clinically undetectable. However, there is no evidence that earlier detection improves survival for retroperitoneal sarcomas, so a less aggressive imaging schedule may be appropriate. A randomized trial in India failed to find any survival benefit in using CT scans of the chest over CXR for surveillance for extremity sarcomas.[40]

Patients with locally recurrent or even metastatic sarcomas can be considered for subsequent resection if tumor biology supports potential cure or effective palliation with removal of known disease. A nomogram to predict the outcomes after resection of recurrent retroperitoneal sarcoma has been reported, though these are subject to selection bias.[11] Recurrent disease, especially within the abdomen or retroperitoneum, becomes more difficult to treat with each recurrence.

If a recurrence is suspected, a biopsy should be performed to confirm diagnosis and review histologic subtype as well as tumor grade, with comparison to the original tumor if possible. In the absence of distant disease, an aggressive surgical approach is warranted with the goal being the same as with a primary sarcoma: control of the tumor and preservation of as much function as possible. For patients who were initially treated with surgery alone and who recur locally, multimodality

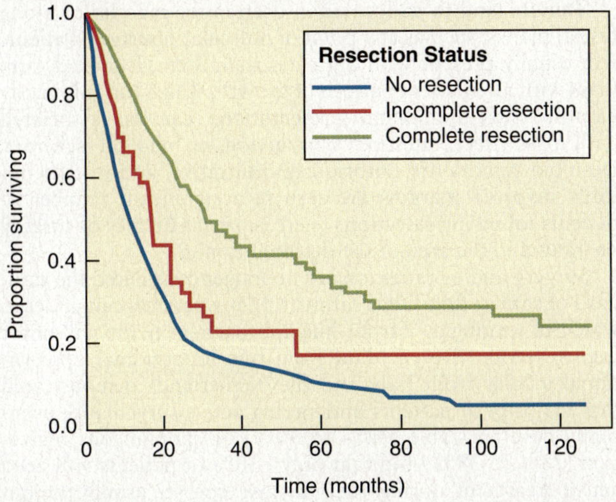

Figure 102.12. Kaplan–Meier plot of disease-specific survival for patients with pulmonary metastases treated at Memorial Sloan Kettering Cancer Center. Patients treated with complete resection had a median survival of 33 months. Patients who underwent incomplete resection or who did not undergo resection had median survival of 16 months and 11 months, respectively. (From Billingsley KG, Burt ME, Jara E, et al. Pulmonary metastases from soft tissue sarcoma: analysis of patterns of diseases and postmetastasis survival. *Ann Surg.* 1999;229(5):602–610.)

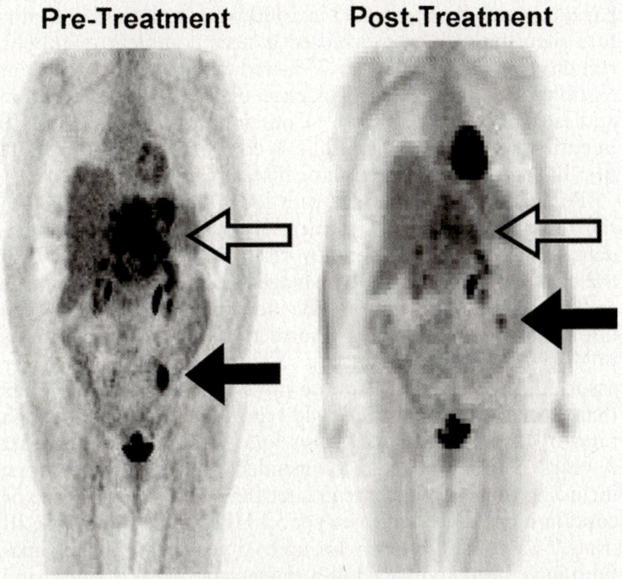

Figure 102.13. [18]FDG-PET scan showing response of metastatic GIST to imatinib mesylate. This patient presented with primary disease in the small bowel and synchronous metastatic disease in the liver. The scan at presentation (**left**) compared to the one obtained after 3 weeks of therapy (**right**) shows decrease in size of tumors and decrease [18]FDG uptake in both the small bowel and liver tumors consistent with a good response to imatinib. The patient eventually went on to complete surgical resection. (From Gold JS, DeMatteo RP. Combined surgical and molecular therapy: the gastrointestinal stromal tumor model. *Ann Surg.* 2006;244(2):176–184.)

treatment with repeat resection, radiation, and sometimes chemotherapy is associated with survival rates close to those of previously untreated patients. Independent predictors of survival in patients with locally recurrent extremity soft tissue sarcomas include histologic grade, size of recurrent disease, and recurrence-free interval.

The most common site of distant metastatic disease is the lung, and its presence is not detectable by symptoms. Again, CT is the preferred imaging modality, though its very high sensitivity for detecting pulmonary nodules as small as 2 mm decreases its specificity. Occasional patients have liver, bone, or central nervous system metastases, though these sites of disease are relatively uncommon. Once diagnosed, metastatic disease is best approached with systemic chemotherapy, either as a single agent or with combination treatments. Pulmonary metastases are the most common form of distant disease, and metastasectomy in carefully selected patients seems to improve outcomes. Taking patient selection into account, resection of pulmonary metastases in combination with radiation and/or chemotherapy, may improve outcomes compared to resection alone[41] (**Fig. 102.12**). However, there are no randomized trial data to determine if there is truly any benefit to resecting lung metastases. Patients considered for resection generally have better outcomes if they have a limited number of metastases, longer disease-free intervals, and leiomyosarcoma or osteosarcoma histologies.

Gastrointestinal Stromal Tumors

5 The most common subtype of sarcoma is GIST. Prior to modern molecular diagnostic techniques, these tumors were likely to have been considered leiomyosarcomas based on histologic features. GISTs are composed of primitive mesenchymal cells and originate from the interstitial cell of Cajal, which functions within the GI autonomic nervous system. Immunohistologic diagnosis is primarily made via expression of KIT (CD 117) cellular markers (**Fig. 102.13**). The *KIT* proto-oncogene encodes for KIT protein, a transmembrane glycoprotein receptor with an intracellular tyrosine kinase domain. Binding of the KIT ligand induces dimerization and autophosphorylation of KIT, activating a cascade of intracellular signaling which results in cell proliferation and tumorigenesis. A gain of function mutation in KIT occurs in up to 90% of GIST and results in ligand-independent (constitutive) activation of tyrosine kinase function. The most frequent sites of mutation are found in exon 11 (70%) or exon 9 (10%), whereas rare mutations are found in exon 13 or exon 17. Mutation status may affect prognosis, and testing has become more routine in the evaluation of GIST. *PDGFR-α* mutations can also result in KIT overexpression in approximately 3% to 5% of GIST. KIT-negative GISTs have been reported, though tumor genotyping should be done to either *KIT* or *PDGFR-α* mutations even with negative immunohistochemistry for KIT. Mutations in *NF1* and *BRAF* have been reported in GIST, and deficiency in *SDH* can cause GIST as well.

Swedish epidemiologic data estimate 14.5 cases per million, which translate to an annual US incidence of 4,000 to 5,000 new cases of GISTs per year.[42] Clinical presentation can be indolent: most patients have nonspecific symptoms such as nausea, emesis, or abdominal discomfort. Infrequently, GISTs can rupture or bleed, leading to a more emergent presentation. GISTs are most commonly found in the stomach (50% to 60%), with 30% to 40% of tumors in the small bowel, 5% in the colon or rectum, and 5% in the esophagus. Rarely, GISTs develop within the mesentery, omentum, or retroperitoneum. Most GISTs are found in adults over the age of 40, with a median age of 60 years. Tumors found in children or young adults are considered a separate entity since pediatric GISTs have a more epithelioid histology and wild-type KIT or PDGFR-α genotype, often harboring mutations in one of the subunits of SDH.

Complete resection is the treatment of choice for primary GIST, but recurrences are common and 5-year survival following resection of a localized tumor is approximately 50% but vary based on size and mitotic activity. Lymph node dissection is not warranted because GISTs very rarely metastasize to regional nodes. Treatment of GIST was revolutionized with the development of imatinib mesylate (Gleevec), a selective TKI, representative of the emerging paradigm of molecularly targeted therapies. The proof of concept for this treatment paradigm was demonstrated in 2000 when a patient with diffuse metastatic disease achieved a near complete metabolic response on PET and with 75% reduction in tumor size at 8 months and histologic evidence of myxoid degeneration and lack of mitotic activity.[43] Contemporary use of imatinib in patients with metastatic GIST is considered an appropriate first-line treatment of metastatic disease (**Fig. 102.13**).

For patients who present with localized tumors, resection remains the mainstay of treatment. Interestingly, emerging evidence suggests that incidentally discovered, very small GISTs (<2 cm) may be successfully managed nonoperatively.

The use of imatinib in the adjuvant setting has been informed by a number of clinical trials. Mutation status is predictive of treatment success: *KIT* exon 11 mutations are associated with better response rates and survival endpoints than exon 9 mutations and wild-type GISTs. Because of high rates of recurrence or metastasis following resection, at least 3 years of imatinib is recommended for high-risk tumors, including tumors which are greater than 5 to 10 cm in size or contain more than 5 mitoses per 50 HPFs, based on phase III trials.[44] Safety and efficacy for up to 5 years of adjuvant imatinib have been confirmed in a single-arm phase II study, and a randomized trial comparing 3 to 5 years of adjuvant imatinib is underway.[45] Risk stratification must be approached with care; other factors which need to be considered include location of tumor and mutation status. It is reasonable to consider the use of imatinib for large or borderline resectable lesions prior to surgical resection. Most of these cases require continued treatment after resection given high risk of recurrence or metastasis.

There is now a wide availability of second and third (and beyond) line therapies for imatinib-resistant disease. Response rates are significantly lower for these agents, but they can be effective for patients with secondary mutations resistant to imatinib. Sunitinib and regorafenib are currently approved for second and third line treatments. Avapritinib targets the PDGFR-α and other exon 18 mutations and have showed a response rate of 88% in patients with PDGFR-α D842V.[46]

Desmoid Tumors/Desmoid Fibromatosis

Desmoid tumors warrant separate notation in the discussion of soft tissue sarcomas because of their distinct biologic behavior. Desmoid tumors, or aggressive deep-seated fibromatosis, are part of a rare group of fibrous tissue proliferations which have no propensity for metastasis but can be locally aggressive. Recent clinical and observational trials have defined the natural history of these tumors, changing the treatment paradigm with a focus on nonsurgical options as the primary treatment for the majority of desmoid patients.

Desmoid tumors have an estimated incidence rate of two to four cases per million per year. The median age of diagnosis is 35, range 16 to 79 years and are slightly more common in women than men. Desmoid tumors are classically described as an abdominal wall tumor, seen in young women during the postpartum period. However, desmoids can occur at any site in the body and three main anatomic groupings are described: (1) trunk or extremity, (2) abdominal wall, and (3) intra-abdominal (bowel and mesentery). Fibromatosis is usually sporadic but can be associated with FAP.

Desmoids are characterized by a monoclonal fibroblastic proliferation arising from muscular or aponeurotic structures. On gross examination, the tumors appear firm and smooth, with a surrounding pseudocapsule. However, microscopically, the tumor characteristically extends beyond this pseudocapsule, with fibrous septae of tumor extending radially. Desmoid tumors had previously been classified as an unchecked reactive process rather than a neoplastic process, but uniform patterns of X-chromosome inactivation seems to confirm tumors of clonal composition. There appears to be an increased estrogen receptor-β, but not estrogen receptor-α, expression in 80% of desmoid specimens.

Tumors tend to be located in deep in the muscles or along fascial planes, such as at a point of muscular insertion. Patients will usually present with a greater than 5 cm, localized, firm mass with an indolent pattern of growth, which can minimally painful. Intra-abdominal presentations can be associated with mass effect, intestinal obstruction, or mucosal ischemia. Desmoid tumors are notoriously infiltrative, and microscopically involved margins are seen in a significant number of patients following resection. There is often a history of surgery or trauma in the area of the desmoid tumor.

Surgery and/or radiation are no longer considered the standard of care or first-line treatment. Many patients can undergo watchful waiting as a front-line approach, as many will never need resection. Recent data from two longitudinal observational studies from Italy and the Netherlands demonstrated that majority of patients undergoing active surveillance eventually develop stable (32% to 40%) or spontaneous regression (28% to 38%) and that only ~30% of patients will need active treatment during their disease course, usually within the first 1 to 2 years of diagnosis, solidifying active surveillance as the primary treatment recommendations for patients with desmoid tumors.[47] If tumors do grow under active surveillance, systemic therapy or targeted therapy can be considered. A recent phase III study of Nirogacestat, a γ-secretase inhibitor, demonstrated a significantly increased response rate of 41% versus 8% on placebo.[48] Nirogacestat is known, however, to have a side effect of ovarian failure and female patients of reproductive age may need other options. Sorafenib has also been demonstrated to have significant response rates over placebo and can be used for patients with advanced desmoid tumors.[49] For patients who progress on surveillance and medical therapy, local therapy options including radiation and cryotherapy should be considered.

Resection is only rarely needed and should not be offered without considering alternative options first. However, a recent consensus guideline outlined several scenarios in which surgical resection could be considered. Patients with sporadic mesenteric desmoid tumors that present with bleeding or obstruction and patients who progress on medical treatment or other local therapies including radiation and cryotherapy should be considered for resection. Also, women with desmoids considering a pregnancy may be considered for resection and reconstruction as desmoids may grow during pregnancy.

SUMMARY

As understanding of sarcomas continues to evolve, it has become increasingly clear that therapy must be individualized to each unique presentation, taking into account histologic subtype, primary tumor site, tumor grade, patient comorbidities, and the full spectrum of multidisciplinary treatment options. Patient referral to a specialized sarcoma center is recommended.

References

1. Palassini E, Baldi GG, Ciniselli CM, et al. Outcome improvement with chemotherapy and radiotherapy in primary, localized, radiation-associated angiosarcoma of the breast region: a retrospective case series analysis. *ESMO Open*. 2024;9(6):103474.
2. Dupuis H, Chevalier B, Cardot-Bauters C, et al. Prevalence of endocrine manifestations and GIST in 108 systematically screened patients with neurofibromatosis type 1. *J Endocr Soc*. 2023;7(8):bvad083.
3. Ladanyi M, Antonescu CR, Leung DH, et al. Impact of SYT-SSX fusion type on the clinical behavior of synovial sarcoma: a multi-institutional retrospective study of 243 patients. *Cancer Res*. 2002;62(1):135–140.

4. Parkes A, Urquiola E, Bhosale P, et al. PET/CT imaging as a diagnostic tool in distinguishing well-differentiated versus dedifferentiated liposarcoma. *Sarcoma*. 2020;2020:8363986.
5. ACS Clinical Research Program. *Operative Standards for Cancer Surgery: Volume III: Hepatobiliary, Peritoneal Malignancies, Neuroendocrine, Sarcoma, Adrenal, Bladder*. Lippincott Williams & Wilkins (LWW); 2022.
6. Webster S, Vargas AC, Maclean F, et al. What is the association of preoperative biopsy with recurrence and survival in retroperitoneal sarcoma? A systematic review by the Australia and New Zealand Sarcoma Association clinical practice guidelines working party. *Crit Rev Oncol Hematol*. 2024;197:104354.
7. WHO Classification of Tumours Editorial Board. *Soft tissue and bone tumours*. International Agency for Research on Cancer; 2020. (WHO Classification of Tumours Series, 5th ed.; vol. 3). https://publications.iarc.fr/588.
8. Rubin BP, Goldblum JR. Pathology of soft tissue sarcoma. *J Natl Compr Canc Netw*. 2007;5(4):411–418.
9. Amin MB, Edge SB, Greene FL, et al., eds. *AJCC Cancer Staging Manual*. 8th ed. Springer; 2017.
10. Callegaro D, Miceli R, Bonvalot S, et al. Development and external validation of two nomograms to predict overall survival and occurrence of distant metastases in adults after surgical resection of localised soft-tissue sarcomas of the extremities: a retrospective analysis. *Lancet Oncol*. 2016;17(5):671–680.
11. Raut CP, Callegaro D, Miceli R, et al. Predicting survival in patients undergoing resection for locally recurrent retroperitoneal sarcoma: a study and novel nomogram from TARPSWG. *Clin Cancer Res*. 2019;25(8):2664–2671.
12. Lewis JJ, Leung D, Espat J, Woodruff JM, Brennan MF. Effect of reresection in extremity soft tissue sarcoma. *Ann Surg*. 2000;231(5):655–663.
13. Al-Refaie WB, Andtbacka RHI, Ensor J, et al. Lymphadenectomy for isolated lymph node metastasis from extremity soft-tissue sarcomas. *Cancer*. 2008;112(8):1821–1826.
14. Blazer DG 3rd, Sabel MS, Sondak VK. Is there a role for sentinel lymph node biopsy in the management of sarcoma? *Surg Oncol*. 2003;12(3):201–206.
15. Rosenberg SA, Tepper JO, Glatstein E, et al. The treatment of soft-tissue sarcomas of the extremities: prospective randomized evaluations of (1) limb-sparing surgery plus radiation therapy compared with amputation and (2) the role of adjuvant chemotherapy. *Ann Surg*. 1982;196(3):305–315.
16. O'Sullivan B, Davis AM, Turcotte R, Bell R, et al. Preoperative versus postoperative radiotherapy in soft-tissue sarcoma of the limbs: a randomized trial. *Lancet*. 2002;359(9325):2235–2241.
17. Yang JC, Chang AE, Baker AR, et al. Randomized prospective study of the benefit of adjuvant radiation therapy in the treatment of soft tissue sarcomas of the extremity. *J Clin Oncol*. 1998;16(1):197–203.
18. Guadagnolo BA, Bassett RL, Mitra D, et al. Hypofractionated, 3-week, preoperative radiotherapy for patients with soft tissue sarcomas (HYPORT-STS): a single-centre, open-label, single-arm, phase 2 trial. *Lancet Oncol*. 2022;23(12):1547–1557.
19. Pisters PW, O'Sullivan B, Maki RG. Evidence-based recommendations for local therapy for soft tissue sarcomas. *J Clin Oncol*. 2007;25(8):1003–1008.
20. Cormier JN, Huang X, Xing Y, et al. Cohort analysis of patients with localized, high-risk, extremity soft tissue sarcoma treated at two cancer centers: chemotherapy-associated outcomes. *J Clin Oncol*. 2004;22(22):4567–4574.
21. Adjuvant chemotherapy for localised resectable soft-tissue sarcoma of adults: meta-analysis of individual data. Sarcoma Meta-analysis Collaboration. *Lancet*. 1997;350(9092):1647–1654.
22. Frustaci S, Gherlinzoni F, De Paoli A, et al. Adjuvant chemotherapy for adult soft tissue sarcomas of the extremities and girdles: results of the Italian randomized cooperative trial. *J Clin Oncol*. 2001;19(5):1238–1247.
23. Tanaka K, Machida R, Kawai A, et al. Perioperative Adriamycin plus ifosfamide vs. gemcitabine plus docetaxel for high-risk soft tissue sarcomas: randomized, phase II/III study JCOG1306. *Br J Cancer*. 2022;127(8):1487–1496.
24. Gortzak E, Azzarelli A, Buesa J, et al. A randomised phase II study on neo-adjuvant chemotherapy for 'high-risk' adult soft-tissue sarcoma. *Eur J Cancer*. 2001;37(9):1096–1103.
25. Gronchi A, Ferrari S, Quagliuolo V, et al. Histotype-tailored neoadjuvant chemotherapy versus standard chemotherapy in patients with high-risk soft-tissue sarcomas (ISG-STS 1001): an international, open-label, randomised, controlled, phase 3, multicentre trial. *Lancet Oncol*. 2017;18(6):812–822.
26. Schuetze SM, Baker LH, Benjamin RS, Canetta R. Selection of response criteria for clinical trials of sarcoma treatment. *Oncologist*. 2008;13(Suppl 2):32–40.
27. Lucas DR, Kshirsagar MP, Biermann JS, et al. Histologic alterations from neoadjuvant chemotherapy in high-grade extremity soft tissue sarcoma: clinicopathological correlation. *Oncologist*. 2008;13(4):451–458.
28. Tawbi HA, Burgess M, Bolejack V, et al. Pembrolizumab in advanced soft-tissue sarcoma and bone sarcoma (SARC028): A multicentre, two-cohort single-arm, open-label, phase 2 trial. *Lancet Onco*. 2017;18:1493–1501.
29. Roland CL, Nassif Haddad EF, Keung EZ et al. A randomized, non-comparative phase 2 study of neoadjuvant immune-checkpoint blockade in retroperitoneal dedifferentiated liposarcoma and extremity/truncal undifferentiated pleomorphic sarcoma. *Nat Cancer*. 2024;5(4):625–641.
30. Mowery YM, Ballman KV, Hong AM, et al. Su2C-SARCO032: A randomized trial of neoadjuvant RT and surgery with or without pembrolizumab for soft tissue sarcoma. *J Clin Oncol*. 2024;42:11504.
31. Eggermont AM, Schraffordt Koops H, Liénard D, et al. Isolated limb perfusion with high-dose tumor necrosis factor-alpha in combination with interferon-gamma and melphalan for nonresectable extremity soft tissue sarcomas: a multicenter trial. *J Clin Oncol*. 1996;14(10):2653–2665.
32. Lewis JJ, Leung D, Woodruff JM, Brennan MF. Retroperitoneal soft-tissue sarcoma: analysis of 500 patients treated and followed at a single institution. *Ann Surg*. 1998;228(3):355–365.
33. Fairweather M, Wang J, Jo VY, Baldini EH, Bertagnolli MM, Raut CP. Incidence and adverse prognostic implications of histopathologic organ invasion in primary retroperitoneal sarcoma. *J Am Coll Surg*. 2017;224(5):876–883.
34. Fairweather M, Lyu H, Conti L, et al. Postnephrectomy outcomes following en bloc resection of primary retroperitoneal sarcoma: multicentre study. *Br J Surg*. 2022;109(2):165–168.
35. Gronchi A, Strauss DC, Miceli R, et al. Variability in patterns of recurrence after resection of primary retroperitoneal sarcoma (RPS): A report on 1007 patients from the multi-institutional collaborative RPS working group. *Ann Surg*. 2016;263(5):1002–1009.
36. Keung EZ, Chiang YJ, Cormier JN, et al. Treatment at low-volume hospitals is associated with reduced short-term and long-term outcomes for patients with retroperitoneal sarcoma. *Cancer*. 2018;124(23):4495–4503.
37. Bonvalot S, Gronchi A, Le Pechoux C, et al. STRASS—a phase III randomized study of preoperative radiotherapy plus surgery versus surgery alone for patients with retroperitoneal sarcoma EORTC protocol 62092-22092. In: *ASCO Annual Meeting*. Chicago, IL; 2019.
38. Livingston JA, Bugano D, Barbo A, et al. Role of chemotherapy in dedifferentiated liposarcoma of the retroperitoneum: defining the benefit and challenges of the standard. *Sci Rep*. 2017;7:11836.
39. Stojadinovic A, Leung DH, Allen P, Lewis JJ, Jaques DP, Brennan MF. Primary adult soft tissue sarcoma: time-dependent influence of prognostic variables. *J Clin Oncol*. 2002;20(21):4344–4352.
40. Puri A, Ranganathan P, Gulia A, Crasto S, Hawaldar R, Badwe RA. Does a less intensive surveillance protocol affect the survival of patients after treatment of a sarcoma of the limb? Updated results of the randomized TOSS study. *Bone Joint J*. 2018;100-B(2):262–268.

41. Billingsley KG, Burt ME, Jara E, et al. Pulmonary metastases from soft tissue sarcoma: analysis of patterns of diseases and postmetastasis survival. *Ann Surg*. 1999;229(5):602–610; discussion 610–612.
42. Nilsson B, Bümming P, Meis-Kindblom JM, et al. Gastrointestinal stromal tumors: the incidence, prevalence, clinical course, and prognostication in the preimatinib mesylate era—a population-based study in western Sweden. *Cancer*. 2005; 103(4):821–829.
43. Joensuu H, Roberts PJ, Sarlomo-Rikala M, et al. Effect of the tyrosine kinase inhibitor STI571 in a patient with a metastatic gastrointestinal stromal tumor. *N Engl J Med*. 2001;344(14): 1052–1056.
44. Joensuu H, Eriksson M, Hall KS, et al. One vs three years of adjuvant imatinib for operable gastrointestinal stromal tumor: a randomized trial. *JAMA*. 2012;307(12):1265–1272.
45. Raut CP, Espat NJ, Maki RG, et al. Efficacy and tolerability of 5-year adjuvant imatinib treatment for patients with resected intermediate- or high-risk primary gastrointestinal stromal tumor: the PERSIST-5 clinical trial. *JAMA Oncol*. 2018;4(12):e184060.
46. Thirasastr P, Sutton TL, Joseph CP, et al. Outcomes of late-line systemic treatment in GIST: Does sequence matter? *Cancers*. 2024;16(5):904
47. Schut AW, Timbergen MJM, van Broekhoven DLM et al. A national prospective clinical trial on active surveillance in patients with non-intra-abdominal desmoid-type fibromatosis: The GRAFITI trial. *Ann Surg*. 2023;277:689–696.
48. Gounder M, Ratan R, Alcindor T, et al. Nirogacestat, a γ-secretase inhibitor for desmoid tumors. *N Engl J Med*. 2023;388(10):898–912.
49. Gounder MM, Mahoney MR, Van Tine BA, et al. Sorafenib for advanced and refractory desmoid tumors. *N Engl J Med*. 2018;379(25):2417–2428.

103

Plastic and Reconstructive Surgery

Scott L. Hansen

Key Points

1 The process to achieve stable wound closure can take several steps, the first of which is excision of necrotic and infected tissue. Adequate debridement is an essential first step as antibiotics alone will not be effective.

2 The incidence of problem wounds is growing. Surgeons are treating more patients that have chronic medical problems that result in nonhealing wounds. The management of these wounds requires a comprehensive evaluation of the underlying patient factors contributing to the problematic nature of these wounds.

3 The use of negative pressure devices has changed the approach to both acute and chronic wound management.

4 The ability to move vascularized soft and composite tissues from either local, regional, or distant sites allows surgeons to reconstruct congenital, traumatic, and oncologic defects that improves form and function in these patients.

5 Pediatric congenital anomalies should be addressed with a comprehensive craniofacial team. Cleft lip and palate can be complete or incomplete, unilateral or bilateral. These congenital anomalies affect speech, eating, swallowing, breathing, facial growth, hearing, socialization, and dental development.

6 Successful outcomes for patients with complex hand disorders require meticulous surgical technique and careful attention to postop hand therapy to regain function.

7 Reconstructive and aesthetic procedures of the breast have become routine. Oncologic reconstruction can be achieved with implant-based techniques or autologous tissue. Both offer women a safe and reliable return to their preoperative appearance and self-confidence.

8 The use of autologous tissue continues to evolve, and multiple donor sites are available, with the lower abdominal wall being the most common donor site. The tissue is supplied by perforating vessels from the underlying rectus abdominis muscle which can be mobilized and rotated to the chest or transferred as a microvascular free flap. The choice of techniques is based on patient factors and surgeon experience.

9 Aesthetic surgery procedures offered by plastic surgeons continues to evolve and grow.

10 Aesthetic surgery is purely elective surgery, performed on patients who are trying to achieve a change in their appearance. Whether that desired change is obvious to others is less important. Thus, there is very little room for error in evaluation, both physical and psychological. The surgery itself must be performed by experienced surgeons who understand anatomic basis of the surgery as well as the desires of the patient.

11 The advent of nonsurgical aesthetic techniques, including injectable medications, topical medications and lasers, has opened the field of aesthetic surgery to a much wider patient population.

The specialty of plastic surgery was initially approved as a subsidiary of the American Board of Surgery in 1938 and given the status of a major specialty board in 1941. The field of plastic surgery saw major growth during World War I and II. The urgent need for surgeons to manage burns, craniomaxillofacial trauma, hand and upper extremity injuries, and the associated ongoing reconstruction that many of these patients required, spurred the rapid development of new techniques and surgeons interested in limiting their practice to this field. The fields of microsurgery, aesthetic surgery, craniomaxillofacial surgery, hand surgery, postoncologic reconstructive surgery, lymphatic surgery and gender-affirming surgery are all fields that have been developed or expanded by plastic surgery. It is often forgotten that the first successful human renal transplant was performed by a plastic surgeon.[1] The scope of plastic surgery is arguably the broadest of any surgical specialty (**Table 103.1**). In this chapter we will limit our discussions to those areas that will be of the greatest interest and benefit to the reader.

MANAGEMENT OF THE PROBLEM WOUND

Plastic surgeons are often consulted by surgical and medical colleagues to assist in the management of recalcitrant wounds. When attempting to design a treatment plan it is important to do a thorough patient and wound analysis. The specific patient factors that are affecting the wound-healing process need to be identified and addressed. Maximizing the patient's nutritional status, controlling serum glucose, weight loss, and physical therapy to improve patient conditioning to increase mobility will all help in management. A pressure wound can be improved by instituting procedures such as utilization of pressure-reducing mattresses/beds, close wound management (eliminating wound soilage and managing excessive moisture) as well as scheduled repositioning. Thus, elimination of con-
1 trollable factors can influence our success in stable closure of a problem wound. The local wound conditions can be improved with debridement of necrotic tissue and moisture control to maximize efforts for closure. While there are many different causes of nonhealing, problem wounds, the factors mentioned above will aid in the management in the majority. Due to the varied types and locations of wounds there is no one reconstructive option to close a given defect. The use of an algorithmic approach needs to be followed, and several options need to be considered for any given wound with a clear fallback option.

Table 103.1. The Spectrum of Plastic Surgery

Aesthetic surgery
Burns: Acute and reconstructive surgery
Craniofacial surgery
Cutaneous and soft tissue oncology
Gender affirming surgery
Hand and upper extremity surgery
Head and neck oncology
Microvascular surgery
Maxillofacial and orthognathic surgery
Peripheral nerve surgery
"General" reconstructive surgery Face (ear, lip, nose, and eyelid) Breast Trunk Lower extremity

Table 103.2. Local and Systemic Factors that Affect Wound Management

Local Factors	Systemic Factors
Infection	Immune deficiencies
Local malignancy	Distant malignancy
Foreign bodies	Diabetes mellitus
Local toxins	Cigarette smoking
Radiation	Chemotherapeutic agents
Ischemia	Hereditary healing disorders
Venous insufficiency	Nutritional deficiency
Lymphatic insufficiency	Old age
Repetitive trauma	Uremia
Reduced sensation	Glucocorticoid therapy, immunosuppressive agents

Wound Evaluation

Problem wounds are often associated with underlying causes. These can be both local and systemic. It is critical to evaluate and treat each of these factors to achieve success. The etiology of the wound is the first factor to consider. A venous stasis ulcer is different that an open tibial fracture. While both are lower extremity wounds, the management is markedly different. The duration of the wound, previous surgical and nonsurgical treatment attempts, and history of wound infections are important factors to consider. Associated complicating factors such as 2 previous malignancy, radiation, and chronic trauma are all associated with nonhealing wounds. Patient systemic factors that are associated with impaired wound healing such as immune deficiency/suppression, chemotherapy use, and chronic medical conditions such as diabetes, problems requiring chronic steroid use, nicotine addiction, dietary deficiency, and the natural immune compromised state associated with old age must all be taken into consideration when addressing a nonhealing wound (**Fig. 103.1**, lower extremity wound in elderly diabetic female).

The careful examination of the wound requires notation of its size and depth. All progress will be compared to these early measurements. The presence of compromised or exposed vital structures such as bone or vessels must be recognized and a plan to address formulated. Traumatic wounds may contain foreign bodies. These wounds can be evaluated with plain films to evaluate for the presence any foreign material. The recognition and elimination of all necrotic tissue is necessary prior to any reconstructive efforts. Chronic wounds may represent a malignant process originating locally or from deeper tissues. All debrided tissue must go to pathology for evaluation. All chronic open wounds are considered to be colonized. However, this is quite different than an "infected" wound. The classic signs and symptoms of infection to identify include pain, erythema, purulent drainage, swelling, fluctuance, and limited function. The presence of a positive bacterial culture from a surface swab does not indicate a clinically significant infection.[2] The status of the soft tissues surrounding the wound must be evaluated. Will it tolerate the mobilization, and undermining needed to create a flap, or other techniques used to manipulate tissue to close a wound? Tissue that has been irradiated or has had previous surgical attempts at elevation and closure may not tolerate further surgical insult and can lead to a larger wound. (See **Table 103.2** for factors associated with impaired wound healing.)

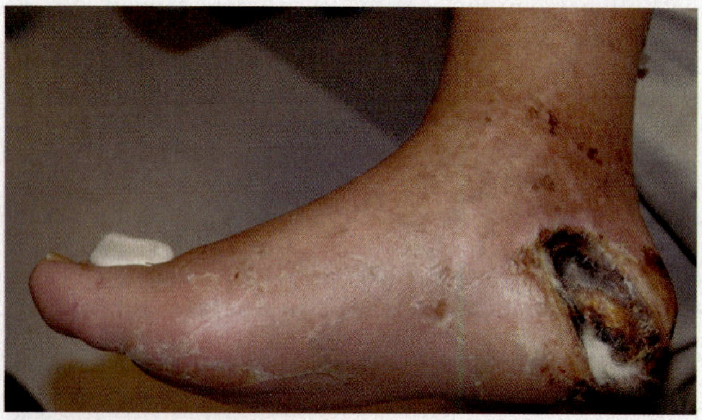

Figure 103.1. Problem lower extremity wound in elderly diabetic woman on chronic steroid therapy. The wound is secondary to minor trauma.

Obesity and diabetes are pervasive in our society and are recognized risk factors for compromised wound healing. These two factors complicate local flap elevation and tissue rearrangement.

Directed laboratory studies such as serum glucose, HA1c, prealbumin, hemoglobin/hematocrit, and renal and liver function tests are useful adjuncts to treatment planning. Tissue biopsy rather than surface swabs are more beneficial in evaluating the need for antibiotic therapy.[3] Bacterial counts greater than 10^5 per gram of tissue represent a bacterial load that will not support wound closure with skin graft or tissue rearrangement. The use of wound biopsy results have been used in the management of burn wounds.[4] The presence of bacteria in the deep dermis closely correlates with burn wound sepsis. It is also very important to determine if osteomyelitis is a contributing factor in recalcitrant wounds. Open wounds that extend to bone can be evaluated with radiographs, CT scans, or MRIs, however the only way to definitively prove or disprove osteomyelitis is with a well-directed bone biopsy. MRI can be used to delineate the extent of boney involvement. The imaging studies can reveal fractures, osteolytic areas and loss of cortical integrity, as well as suspicion of bone involvement with infection but not conclusively diagnose osteomyelitis. If osteomyelitis is diagnosed it will require debridement and delay the reconstruction until you are confident that the infection is cleared. Antibiotics alone will not cure osteomyelitis as the necrotic bone is devascularized and will not penetrate the involved bone. The combination of bone debridement and antibiotics directed by the identification of the pathogens as cultured from the bone biopsy will allow for definitive elimination of bone infection and predictable wound closure.

The Treatment Paradigm for Wound Management

Following a thorough evaluation of the wound and patient factors you should address those factors discussed above that can be addressed to optimize the outcome of wound closure. The goals are to have a stably closed wound and restore the patient's level of function. In our evaluation we recognize that some problems in wound healing should be anticipated and prevented prior to surgery. The worst-case scenario is that the patient has a surgical procedure for wound closure and then goes on to develop a lager wound and/or the surgical site breaks down. As mentioned earlier, glucose control, wound fluid management, and pressure off loading must be planned prior to surgery. The bedridden or paralyzed patient must have close nursing care for repositioning and the family must be educated as to the necessary preventive measures. Aggressive physical therapy will ensure maintenance of joint motion, decrease extremity edema, and optimize the patients conditioning for the postop period. These plans should be made and discussed with the care team, patient, and family prior to definitive surgery.

There will be some period of time prior to definite surgery when the wound will need to be optimized. We discussed the need for debridement of necrotic tissue, control of infection, and moisture/drainage control. Dressings and nonsurgical adjuncts can be very useful in preparing the site for surgery. Moist dressings are the most used dressing to debride a contaminated wound. The operative word is moist, not wet. If the dressings are too wet, they will not dry out between dressing changes and will macerate the tissue causing more problems. These types of dressing have been used for over many years and are still recognized as being effective for debriding wounds. Saline is commonly used as the moistening agent. The dressing debrides the wound by drying out and having the necrotic material stick to the dressing. As the dressing is removed, the debris is removed with it. The dressing can be changed one to three times per day depending on the status of the wound. Wounds with significant drainage will need to have more frequent dressing changes.

It has been shown that moist wound environments promote better healing than dry wounds.[4,5] The best option for moist wound healing is keeping the native scab in place. Since there should not be a need for debridement with a clean wound, a nonadhering occlusive dressing can be applied. Hydrogels which are very effective in maintaining a moist wound healing environment are a good option for clean wounds. A well-prepared wound cleared of necrotic debris can go on to heal by secondary intention with local wound care and dressing changes.

For the most part, the application of topical antibiotics is not indicated in the management of noninfected wounds. As discussed, all open wounds are colonized and there is no benefit to attempt to sterilize them. However, the judicious use of topical antibiotics can be helpful in certain situations. Significant burn wounds are often dressed with silver sulfadiazine. Silver sulfadiazine is bactericidal for many gram-negative and gram-positive bacteria as well as yeast. Mafenide acetate, also a sulfa-based drug, is also used for burns and other deep partial-thickness and full-thickness wounds. It is rapidly absorbed through open wounds and can be used on ear wounds due to its ability to penetrate cartilage. Mafenide is a potent carbonic anhydrase inhibitor and can cause hyperchloremic metabolic acidosis with chronic use. This drug can cause considerable pain on application, limiting its use. This drug also has antibacterial activity against most gram-positive and many gram-negative species commonly found in wounds. These topical drugs are not effective against methicillin-resistant *Staphylococcus aureus* (MRSA)–colonized wounds. Mupirocin topical ointment can be used in this situation. There has been an increase in the use of nanocrystalline silver in dressings, both barrier and alginates. The silver dressings have low toxicity and excellent antibiotic properties although they can add significant cost to wound care.

Over the last 10 to 20 years there have been a number of advances in the nonsurgical management of wounds, particularly problematic chronic wounds. These advances include the use of biologic and nonbiologic agents such as the application of growth factors to wounds, cellular therapies, and other physical modalities.[6] Recombinant platelet derived growth factors (PDGFs) may be useful in the management of chronic pressure wounds and diabetic foot ulcers[7,8]; there is no clear evidence that topical growth factors have a significant role in the management of acute wounds. Wound repair is a complex process and is influenced by numerous secreted factors, including cytokines, chemokines, and growth factors. In theory, application of stem cells to wounds is advantageous over administration of a single agent because stem cells have a unique feature of interacting with wound environment and modulate their activity to release multiple factors, which may facilitate wound healing process. However, the use of stem cell therapy to treat difficult wounds must be considered is still unproven and at this time, investigational.[9]

The use of "off the shelf" skin substitutes such as bilaminate bovine collagen/silicone sheet have shown to have application in complex burn, oncologic, and trauma wounds.[10] It acts as a dermal substitute and renders a more stable construct and skin graft bed. Human and xenograft acellular dermal substitutes have been widely used in the management of all types of wounds. The thicker versions of these materials can be used to add structural support to complex abdominal wall and breast reconstruction.

Perhaps the most impactful innovation on the management
3 of chronic and problem wounds has been the development and application of negative pressure wound therapy. There are many options now available, but all have the same basic elements of a sponge which is placed in the wound bed. It is then covered with an impervious plastic adhesive sheet and a suction device is place on a hole cut into the plastic sheet. There have been several innovations to this basic setup. The sponge can come with various pore sizes and can be impregnated with silver for infected wounds. Sponge and plastic sheeting systems have been modified for the management of complicated abdominal wounds with exposed viscera. These systems have changed the approach to complex open abdominal wounds. The use of the negative pressure device has been shown to control wound fluid, decrease wound edema, promote tissue perfusion, and stimulate granulation tissue in the wound bed. There have been numerous clinical and experimental papers that attest to the efficacy of the negative pressure wound devices.[11] The systems are relatively easy to use, decrease the need for frequent dressing changes, help to control wound fluid, and decrease edema. The negative pressure wound devices should not be used in grossly infected wounds. As pointed out, a positive culture from a surface swab indicates a colonized wound not an infected wound. The cost of the system needs to be balanced against all the other positive factors including a shorter time to wound closure and simple wound management.

Surgery for Problem Wounds

Surgery for problem and chronic wounds fall into two categories; wound bed preparation and wound closure. Proper surgical debridement transforms a chronic wound with hyperkeratotic margins, necrotic slough, and arrested progression of wound contraction into an acute wound that is ready for closure (**Fig. 103.2**, sacral pressure wound in elderly diabetic patient). Most chronic wounds will require at least one surgical debridement to prepare the wound for reconstruction. Those wounds that involve bone will not respond to long-term

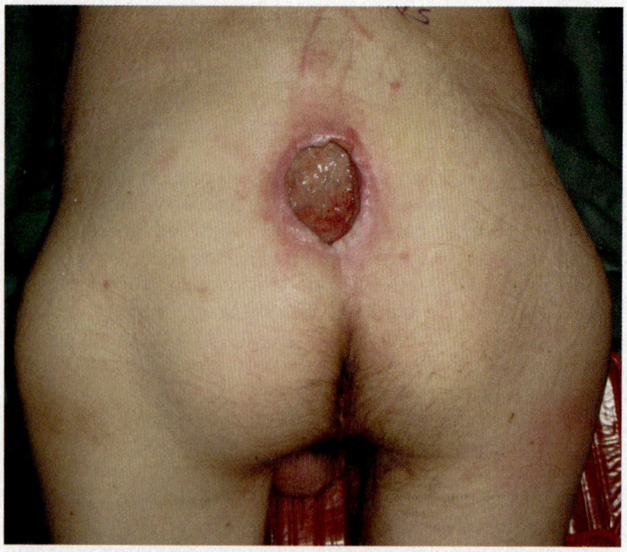

Figure 103.2. Chronic sacral pressure wound in elderly diabetic man. Note the rolled hyperkeratotic margins and exudate at the base.

antibiotics alone. This will just prolong the treatment course or lead to failed reconstruction. Infected bone will need to be excised to have any chance of a successful closure.

The Reconstructive Ladder

Plastic surgeons make a mental treatment plan when they see a chronic or problem wound. Imaging or other adjuvant studies can change the plan, but the basic process follows the very well-established reconstructive ladder principles. The "ladder" (**Table 103.3** reconstructive ladder) helps to develop a systematic treatment paradigm beginning on the first rung of the ladder, which presents the simplest approach to wound closure, which would be allowing the wound to heal by secondary intention. The highest rung on the ladder would require a distant flap that requires microvascular techniques. It is not necessary to consider every rung of the ladder and an experienced surgeon understands that the return to function takes priority. A single procedure is the preferred method, and when possible, it is always preferred to use autologous tissue. The long-term durability of the reconstruction is essential. The use of autologous tissue will in most cases create a secondary wound. The harvest of split-thickness skin graft can effectively double the total wound burden. The harvest of a distant muscle or fasciocutaneous flap may have a deleterious effect on the patient's function and again, create another wound. So clearly the donor site has to be considered. The job of the reconstructive surgeon is to weigh the risk–benefit ratio of available donor sites that results in a reasonable closure. Independent of the option chosen for wound closure, there are a few principles that are shared by all. First and foremost, careful surgical technique is required to avoid complete or partial failure of the reconstruction. The surgeon should incorporate all these aforementioned points. As mentioned, it is essential that the wound bed is properly prepared for a graft or flap. Flaps, local or distant, do not do well when placed under tension. Pulling or forcing the tissue into the defect will cause microvascular compromise leading to partial or complete flap failure. The surgeon needs to continuously assess the flap for good perfusion and adequate venous drainage. If the flap appears to be ischemic or venous outflow appears to be compromised, remove some of the insetting sutures to allow the flap to recover. In some cases, you may not be able to inset the flap at this juncture but rather will need to allow it to adjust to this new relative hypovascular situation. This is called the delay phenomenon. It is also referred to as vascular delay or ischemic preconditioning (**Fig. 103.3**, example of surgical delay). It describes the observation that a tissue rendered partially ischemic will undergo neovascularization and enhance its vascularity. The field of reconstructive surgery uses this phenomenon to enhance the survival of flaps. Careful attention to hemostasis is essential. Skin grafts, whether split thickness or full thickness, depend on being in intimate contact with the prepared recipient bed. The presence of even a minimal amount of blood or fluid can result in the loss of some or all of the graft due to loss of intimate contact. The distinction to be made is the difference between a graft and a flap. A graft, which could be skin, tendon, nerve, fat, cartilage, or bone, is transferred without a blood supply and requires vascular ingrowth from the surrounding bed. Each tissue has a particular physiologic requirement for vascularization and survival. A split-thickness skin graft may survive whereas a full-thickness graft will not. A flap, on the the other hand, is transferred with its vascularity

Table 103.3. The Reconstructive Ladder
Vascularized free tissue transfer
Local pedicled flap (fasciocutaneous or muscle)
Local cutaneous or fasciocutaneous advancement or rotation flaps
Skin grafts
Delayed primary closure
Primary closure
Healing by secondary intention

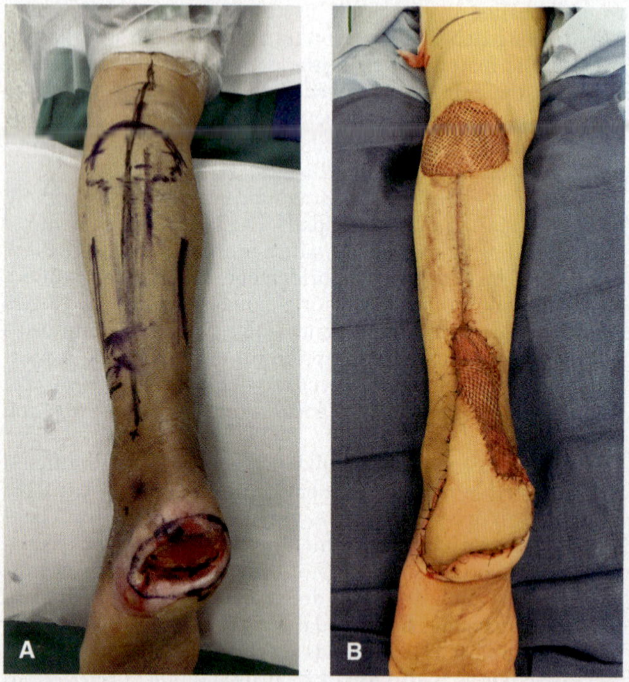

Figure 103.3. Example of surgical delay. Because of associated medical problems, the patient was not a candidate for microvascular tissue transfer. **A:** Lower-third extremity defect secondary to trauma with exposed bone, which precludes use of a skin graft. In the first stage, the reverse sural flap incisions are made and the flap elevated from wound bed. The deep perforators to the skin of the flap were divided by full undermining. The incisions were closed, and the wound was dressed. **B:** After 7 to 10 days, the reverse sural flap was again elevated and rotated to the heel defect.

intact. Thus, the flap is much less dependent on the local vascular milieu. The flap can be transferred with its vascular "leash" which may give it a limited arc of rotation. Alternatively, the flap can be transferred as a free tissue transfer. In this case the tissue is transferred with the vascular pedicle identified and dissected out and divided just prior to transfer. The pedicle is then immediately anastomosed to an identified artery and vein at the recipient site. This technique will allow the movement of larger amounts of tissue from distant sites to a defect to obtain a closed wound. This technique requires a higher level of expertise and sophisticated equipment but has changed the entire field of reconstructive surgery.

Healing by Secondary Intention

Allowing the wound to heal by secondary intention is an acceptable course of action for smaller wounds. This closure is secondary to wound contraction and eventual epithelial migration. The process has a few potential problems that need to be recognized. Excessive wound contraction can lead to a wound *contracture* which can distort adjacent soft tissue landmarks such as the labial commissure of the mouth or the eyelid. Secondary healing across any joint surface may lead to limited range of motion/stiffness of the affected joint. The time to closure may take months which may require additional debridements if the margins become hyperkeratotic and progress plateaus. After a period of no progression, the decision may need to be made to move up the reconstructive ladder.

Primary Wound Closure

The next step on the ladder is closure of the wound by primary intention. This is the common approach for a laceration or acute soft tissue defect following an excision of a small benign or malignant lesion. The principles outlined above apply here as well. Careful tissue handling, meticulous hemostasis, and closure without tension are required for a durable repair. A layered repair typically refers to the use of absorbable sutures to bring together the dermis and underlying subcutaneous tissue, which reduces the dead space and relieves tension on the epidermis. Closing the deep and superficial fascia and the dermis in layers effectively renders a closed wound with the epidermis in approximation. The skin is then sutured with a monofilament nonabsorbable material, nylon or polypropylene suture. When closed without tension and with the edges slightly everted there is less likelihood to develop prominent scars and wound dehiscence. The placement of a closed suction drain will help decrease the chance of fluid buildup and keep the tissue in contact with the wound bed. Inability to close the wound without tension would dictate the use of another technique, moving to another rung on the ladder.

Skin Grafts

Skin grafts have changed the approach to the closure of open wounds. Their use was initially proposed in the 1880s, but the technique fell out of favor due to the failure to recognize the need for recipient bed preparation and careful harvest techniques. The existing understanding of skin grafting techniques did not develop until World War II. There was a tremendous need for improved management of burn injuries. Basic science and clinical research finally made the use of skin grafting a predictable and relatively easy way to close burn wounds and saved many lives.

Skin grafts consist of two basic types: full thickness and split thickness. The difference is based on the amount of dermis harvested with the epidermis. The entire dermis is harvested with the full-thickness graft and the split-thickness graft can have a variable amount of dermis depending on the requirements of the wound. The full-thickness graft will contract less and heal with less of a noticeable depression because of the thickness of the graft. The full-thickness graft is often used for defects of the head and neck because it can be harvested locally from the face or neck and will maintain a good color match (**Fig. 103.4**, full-thickness skin graft to orbit). The full-thickness graft may experience lower survival because of the thickness of the dermis representing an impediment to diffusion of serum into the graft. The take, or survival of the graft is dependent on the bed preparation and the ability to successfully revascularize the graft within 48 to 72 hours. The graft needs to be stabilized with some combination of sutures and dressings to maintain the graft in intimate contact with the bed to encourage the revascularization of the graft. The presence of shear force on the graft will compromise all or part of the graft. The early survival of the graft is dependent on plasmatic imbibition whereby serum from the bed diffuses into the grafted tissue. Inosculation is the process by which blood vessels in skin graft grow to meet the vessels (inosculate = kiss) of the recipient bed. Within hours microvasculature from the wound bed grows into the graft and form connections with microvasculature of the graft. Thus, wound preparation is paramount for successful grafting. The graft will not take on bone that is devoid of periosteum or tendon without paratenon. Skin grafts will not take on cartilage. If the bed cannot be prepared to support the process of imbibition and inosculation, then one must consider moving up the reconstructive ladder. The donor site for a full-thickness graft must be closed primarily. The use of the full-thickness graft is limited by the size of the defect and the ability to close the donor site primarily. With split-thickness skin grafts, the donor site wound heals by reepithelialization. Epithelial cells migrate from remnants of skin adnexal organs, hair follicles, and sweat glands, in the

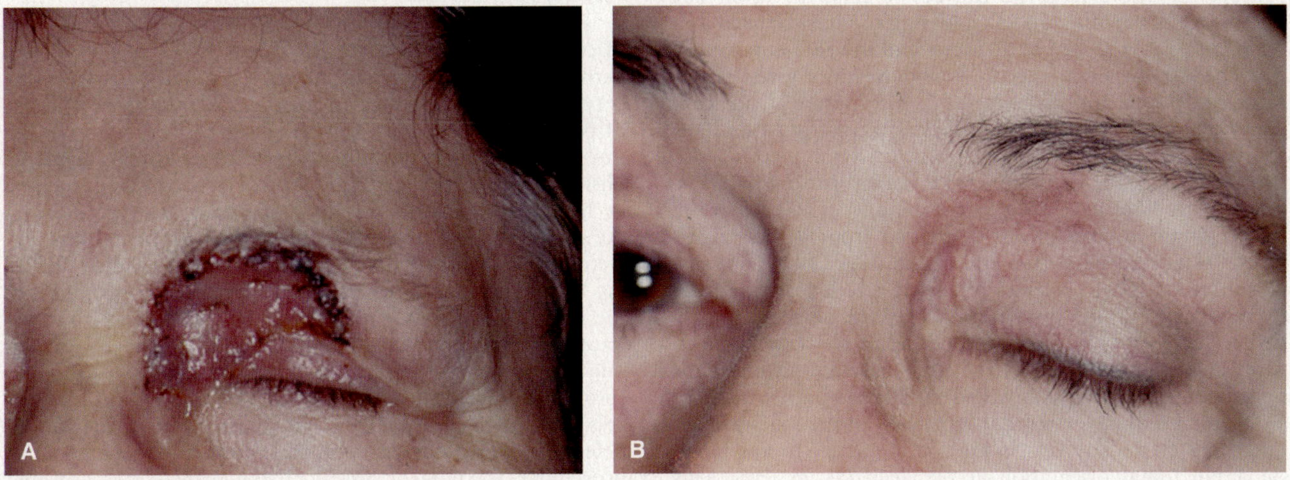

Figure 103.4. A and B: Full-thickness skin graft to the orbit (A) early post op, (B) 4 months post op. (Images courtesy of Jane L. Messina, MD, Moffitt Cancer Center.)

underlying dermis and eventually grow across the wound bed. The donor site can be dressed with an occlusive dressing to maintain a moist environment or a petrolatum impregnated sheet of gauze which is allowed to dry onto the wound to create a pseudo scab. It will take 10 days to 2 weeks to heal the donor site.

Random Flaps

The use of local tissue rearrangement that is adjacent to the wound is a common method to close wounds. This can be done by simple undermining to separate the tissue from deeper fascia or complex designed flaps based on the principles of "Z" or "W" plasties with back cuts and elevation of tissue. The advantage of these reconstructive techniques is that we use adjacent tissue. The color match and tissue thickness will mimic the tissue that was present in the wound. This is especially useful in closure of wounds on the head and neck. These are random pattern flaps perfused by the dermal plexus of vessels. Care must be taken when designing the flap so that there are no scars crossing the flap which would disrupt the dermal plexus. Longitudinal scars running in the long axis also disrupt the dermal vessels. The basic movements of these flaps are rotation, advancement, and transposition depending on how the tissue needs to be transferred into the defect. The defect size and location, the nature of the adjacent tissue, the presence of scars, and previous surgery may dictate if these local flaps can be used to close the defect. While the length to width ratio must be taken into consideration there are certain procedures that can improve the vascularity of the flap.[12,13] The use of the delay phenomenon has been shown to improve random flap survival. Delay is defined as the partial interruption of blood flow to the designed flap. This preconditions the flap to relative ischemia prior to definitive elevation of the tissue. Random flap design can be augmented by expanding the flap using subcutaneous tissue expanders. The expander is placed in a subcutaneous pocket and is gradually filled with fluid to create new skin. The expansion of the tissue is functioning as a delay technique and preconditioning the expanded tissue to relative ischemia prior to transfer.

Axial Pattern Flaps

The identification of larger caliber vessels traveling longitudinally along a defined skin region has expanded the way plastic surgeons reconstruct wounds. This understanding has moved the entire field forward. Random pattern flaps are limited by the dermal plexus supplying the tissue. The arc of rotation will be a limited and the flap needs to be near the wound. With axial blood supply, tissue can be transferred on its vascular pedicle; the tissue is transferred with its own blood supply. Using the principles of Taylor and Palmer[14] and the angiosome concept they developed, we can design flaps based on our knowledge of vascular anatomy. An angiosome is defined as a region of tissue supplied by an artery and its venae comitantes. The choke vessels crossing the boundaries of a given angiosome can enlarge thus allowing us to incorporate an adjacent angiosome into the flap. This facilitates the use of larger flaps to fill the given defect.

Fasciocutaneous flaps are a type of axial pattern flap. The use of these flaps developed from the understanding that the inflow to the dermal plexus is derived from vertically oriented vessels arising at the level of the deep fascia. This fasciocutaneous system consists of vessels which reach the skin by passing along the fascial septa between adjacent muscle bellies and then branch out at the level of the deep fascia to form a plexus that reaches the skin. Fasciocutaneous flaps depend on underlying skin vascular territories rather than the well-circumscribed anatomical territories of the axial-pattern cutaneous flaps. The vessels form a subfascial plexus based on a horizontal orientation at the deep fascial level. This horizontal orientation is relative to the skin surface. Several commonly used fasciocutaneous flaps have been developed on the subfascial plexus of vessels. The radial forearm flap (RFF) is a thin pliable fasciocutaneous flap that is used for head and neck reconstruction where the inherent bulk of other flaps would be an impediment. The radial forearm flap is also well suited for hand and foot reconstruction where again a thin pliable flap is needed. The anterolateral thigh flap (ALT) has become widely used given the acceptable donor site and its use in larger defects. These flaps are based on septal and/or muscular perforators based on the descending branch of the lateral femoral circumflex artery. A cuff of muscle can be taken with the fasciocutaneous portion to fill deep, complex, wounds. Perhaps the most elegant use of a fasciocutaneous flap is the fibula free flap. This flap is an osteoseptocutaneous flap which has the advantage of providing vascularized bone for structural integrity and thin pliable tissue for a soft tissue defect. This flap is commonly used in composite reconstruction of the head and neck, particularly defects of the mandible and adjacent soft tissue.

Muscle and Musculocutaneous Flaps (Table 103.4)

These flaps based on the classification system described by Mathes and Nahai[15] came into wide use in the early 1980s. The understanding that tissue can be transferred on an axial blood supply had been widely accepted. Adapted from this principle is that whole muscles and the overlying skin and subcutaneous tissue (if needed) can be transferred/rotated on its dominant pedicle. Alternatively, the pedicle can be divided and the tissue transferred as a free tissue transfer with microvascular anastomosis. Multiple muscles have been utilized with excellent results (**Fig. 103.5**, rectus femoris flap). The rectus abdominis, latissimus dorsi, sartorius, gastrocnemius and gracilis are a few examples of muscles used for wounds of various sizes. Functional muscle transfers are possible if the motor nerve to the muscle is preserved, or the motor nerve is coapted to a motor nerve at the transfer site. In our discussion of fasciocutaneous flaps, perforators were arising vertically from the muscle surface or intermuscular septum to supply the skin. The use of this construct has revolutionized autologous breast reconstruction. The transverse rectus abdominis musculocutaneous (TRAM) flap is a robust flap with a large skin and subcutaneous paddle based on musculocutaneous perforators. The muscle provides the blood supply to the overlying soft tissue to create the breast mound. The TRAM flap has evolved into the perforator flap only that spares the muscle harvest. This is referred to as a deep inferior epigastric perforator (DIEP) flap. The careful dissection of the perforators to the skin allows the muscle to be preserved and avoid the morbidity of the loss of a large motor muscle. The use of perforator flaps are now often preferred over muscle flaps in breast reconstruction. These flaps are most often transferred as free flaps requiring a microvascular anastomosis.

Microvascular Free Tissue Transfers

Perhaps the most important innovation in reconstructive surgery was the development of microvascular surgery. The use of pedicled flaps is limited by the distance by which the flap can be moved as it remains attached to its vascular pedicle. Historically, there were a number of procedures developed to facilitate the movement of tissue to a site distant from the donor site. All of them required multiple operations and were not efficient. An example of this is the so-called "walking flap" where a soft tissue flap is elevated and sutured into the form of a tube. It is left in situ for a few weeks to allow local vessel conditioning to ischemia. It is then divided at one base and then "walked" to the next site where it is again sutured to a new site to allow vascular ingrowth. This process is repeated until the flap arrives at the site of the wound defect. With the wide use of microsurgery all these adjunctive procedures are now of historical significance. It is now felt that any tissue with an axial blood supply and a pedicle vessel size of 1 mm or greater can be transferred with microsurgery.

Table 103.4. Workhorse Muscle, Myocutaneous, and Perforator Flaps

Flap	Myocutaneous	Perforator	Common Uses
Temporalis	No	No	Orbital and intraoral reconstruction, facial reanimation (pedicled flap)
Pectoralis major	Yes	No	Intraoral and neck reconstruction; reconstruction of sternal defects (muscle only)
Latissimus dorsi	Yes	Yes	Breast reconstruction, neck reconstruction, free flap for very large defects
Rectus abdominis	Yes, including TRAM	Yes, including DIEP	Breast reconstruction, sternal reconstruction, reconstruction of groin defects, free flap for medium-sized defects
Gluteus maximus	Yes	Yes, including SGAP	Ischial pressure sores, sacral pressure sores, SGAP used for breast reconstruction
Biceps femoris	Yes	No	Ischial pressure sores
Tensor fascia lata	Yes	No	Trochanteric pressure sores, abdominal wall reconstruction
Gracilis	Yes	Yes	Perineal reconstruction, vaginal reconstruction, facial reanimation (muscle free flap), free flap for small defects
Rectus femoris	Yes	No	Infected hip wounds, abdominal wall reconstruction
Medial gastrocnemius	Rarely	No	Knee defects, proximal third tibial defects
Soleus	No	No	Middle third tibial defects

DIEP, deep inferior epigastric perforator; SGAP, superior gluteal artery perforator; TRAM, transverse rectus abdominis myocutaneous.

Now there is further advancement to supermicrosurgery. This is a technique of small vessel anastomosis, ranging from 0.3 to 0.8 mm. This technique has been developing over the last 20 years has revolutionized the field of lymphedema treatment.

The basic principle of microsurgery is that circulation can be established in the harvested tissue using microvascular anastomoses between the axial vessels, artery and venae comitantes in the flap and local vessels at the site of the wound. The vascular anastomosis, performed with 8-0 or 9-0 suture, is often done under the microscope although some surgeons prefer operating with loupe magnification. Loupe magnification has the benefit of not having to set up the operating scope and gives the surgeon more mobility. Obviously, these procedures require a very high level of expertise and specialized equipment. The survival rate for free tissue transfers is greater than 97% in experienced centers. The ability to move large pieces of tissue, including composite tissues of skin, subcutaneous tissue, muscle, bone, and even sensory and motor nerves is only possible using microvascular techniques. The movement of these tissues from distant sites allows the surgeon to avoid local tissues for reconstruction and can move out of the zone of injury. Radiation, unstable tissue, scar from previous surgery or damage from high-energy trauma are no longer problems because of the ability to transfer tissue from a

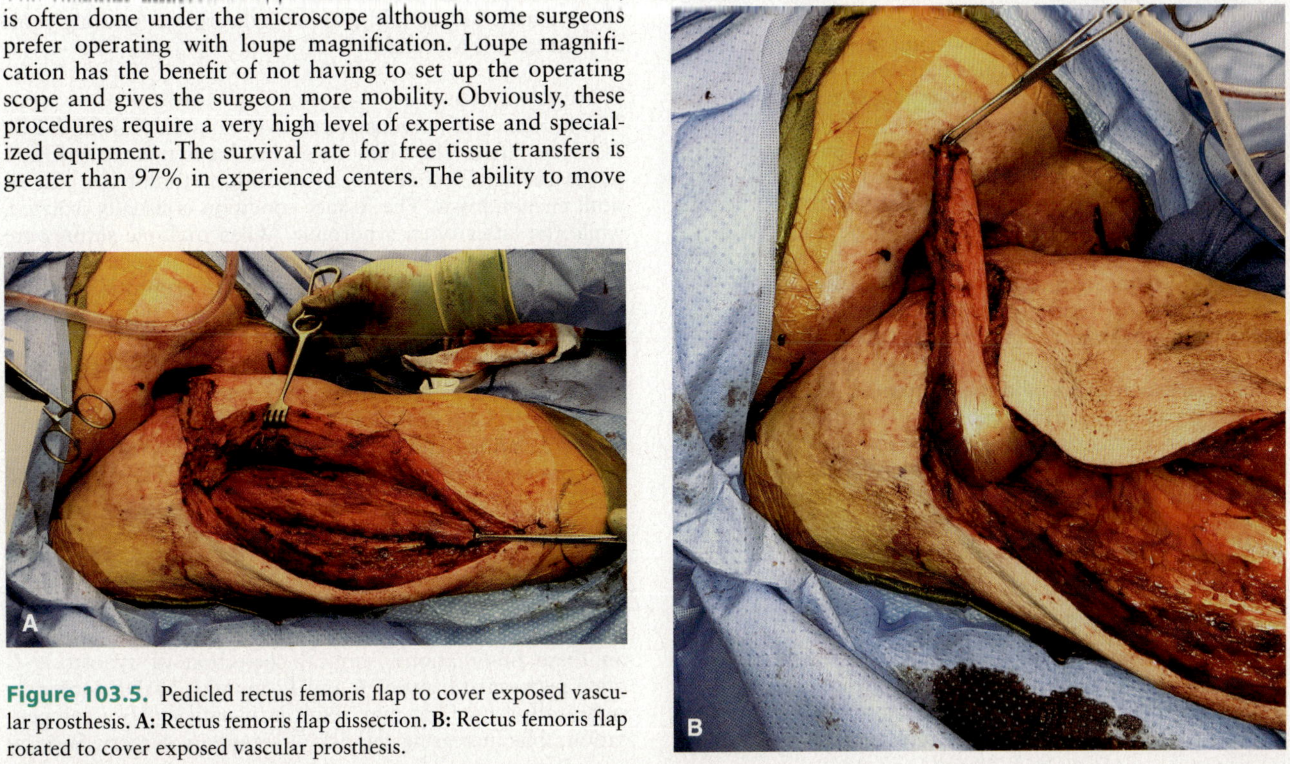

Figure 103.5. Pedicled rectus femoris flap to cover exposed vascular prosthesis. **A:** Rectus femoris flap dissection. **B:** Rectus femoris flap rotated to cover exposed vascular prosthesis.

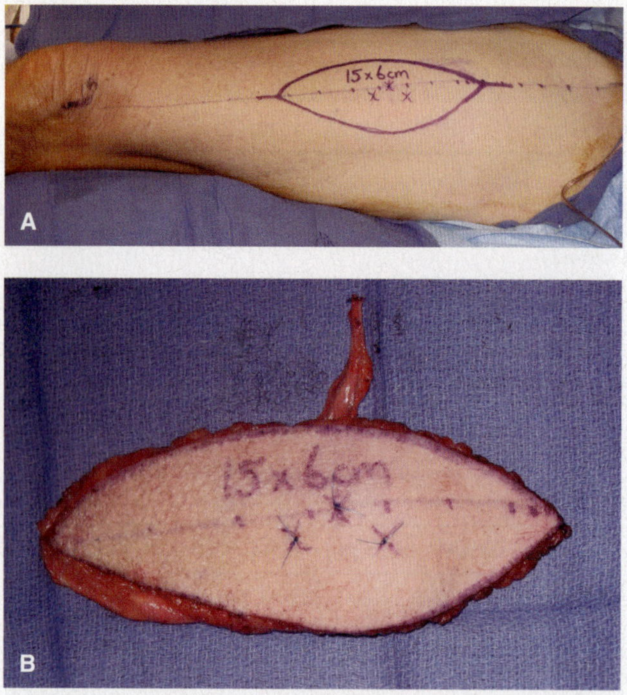

Figure 103.6. **A:** Anterolateral thigh flap designed on the leg and (**B**) free flap dissected out and ready for transfer.

site distant from the wound (**Fig. 103.6**, ALT free flap). Microvascular surgery has changed reconstruction of head and neck oncologic defects with the ability to transfer composite flaps, including bowel. Lower extremity limb salvage is more predictable using microvascular free flaps. As stated earlier, fasciocutaneous perforator free flaps have been used as much if not more than musculocutaneous and muscle flaps. Commonly used flaps include the anterolateral thigh flap (ALT), deep inferior epigastric artery perforator (DIEP), and the radial forearm free flap.

The ALT flap has become the first choice for head and neck reconstruction that does not require bone. The DIEP flap has changed the approach to breast reconstruction, more often used than the TRAM flap.

The ubiquitous application of microsurgery has led to the evolution of new techniques that could not be imagined before. The ability to create prelaminated composite tissue flaps, whereby bone and other tissues can be embedded in a tissue flap and allowed to mature and become vascularized at the donor site and then be transferred with its own vascular supply represents a new approach to complex wound reconstruction. The incorporation of biologic and nonbiologic materials, even 3D-printed constructs, to act as a scaffold for the application of stem cells and the eventual development of new tissues, is the future of reconstructive surgery. The principles of microvascular reconstruction and immunomodulation for solid organ transplantation have opened the field of vascularized composite allotransplantation (VCA). The use of these techniques for upper extremity and face transplantation are two areas of current practice. The inherent problems associated with antirejection medications and chronic rejection are still limiting factors in the wide application of these new and exciting options on the frontier of reconstructive surgery.

PEDIATRIC PLASTIC SURGERY

Concern about interference with normal growth makes correction of pediatric deformities a four-dimensional challenge. Microsurgical precision as well as familiarity with brain development, developmental milestones, and acquisition of language are necessary to manage the spectrum of congenital, neoplastic,
5 or traumatic deformities encountered in the pediatric population. Additionally, familiarity with dysmorphology, genetics, dental organogenesis, otolaryngology, and the distinct growth trajectories of commonly affected structures define the scientific boundaries of this subspecialty. Surrounding oneself with a multidisciplinary team of specialists in those fields is common practice and the concentration of skills in the plastic surgeon places them in a central role.[16,17]

Congenital Anomalies

Cleft Lip and Palate

With an incidence of 1 in 650 live births approximately (7000 new cases per year),[18] clefts of the lip and/or palate are the most common congenital anomaly in the United States. The clefting anomaly is along the midline of the posterior soft and hard palate, and branches laterally anterior to the incisor foramen, involving one or both anterior palate, alveolus, lateral incisor, lip vermilion and philtral column, nostril floor, and lateral pyriform aperture. Viewed from below, they map to a Y-shape (**Fig. 103.7**), with various involvement of each limb. They are thought to result from failure of fusion along the maxillary prominences and the lateral and medial nasal prominences within the first branchial arch and frontonasal process between the 6th and 12th weeks of gestation.[19,20] Correction of this anomaly is often staged, with ongoing debate about timing and techniques used (**Table 103.5**). Tightness across a repair, extent of denuded bone surfaces, and early surgery adversely affect future growth. Conversely, early repair of the soft palate musculature may improve speech outcomes. Surgical tenets of avoiding straight line repair over the lip and soft palate, avoiding or minimizing lateral "relaxing" incisions over the hard palate, and meticulous technique under optical magnification are widely accepted (**Fig. 103.8**).

While the major surgeries are largely completed in the first year of life, the child is followed by a multidisciplinary team until skeletal maturity occurs in late teens (**Table 103.6**). The clefting anomaly affects major components of human communication, including the hearing mechanism, speech musculature, and nonverbal communication using the facial musculature. Secondary revision surgery and aesthetic procedures in this population challenge the surgical armamentarium of the Plastic Surgeon. In craniofacial surgery, "nothing short of perfection is acceptable."

Craniosynostosis

The incidence of craniosynostosis is estimated around 1 in 2500 live births. The condition occurs due to premature fusion of the calvarial intramembranous sutures and/or the base of skull enchondrosis. The former condition is usually isolated, while the latter often syndromic. When multiple sutures are involved, elevated intracranial pressure is of concern, while base of skull suture involvement results in proptosis with risk of corneal exposure, nasopharyngeal airway restriction, and severe facial deformity (**Fig. 103.9**).[24]

Restriction perpendicular to a suture results in overgrowth parallel to its axis, generating seven distinct patterns of deformity (**Fig. 103.10**) distinguishable from the more common pattern of deformational plagiocephaly.

Intracranial volume doubles in the first year of life, and adds another volume between 12 and 42 months, reaching about 85% adult size, at which time the growth rate slows down markedly. Afterward, growth of the intracranial compartment by resorption of the inner cortex and apposition of new bone on the external cortex is thought to be sufficient to compensate for absence of growth across suture lines. Based on these observations, surgical correction of synostosis is often performed between 6 and 12 months. Earlier surgery is technically easier but may result in insufficient overcompensation, thus increasing the risk of secondary surgery. Surgical

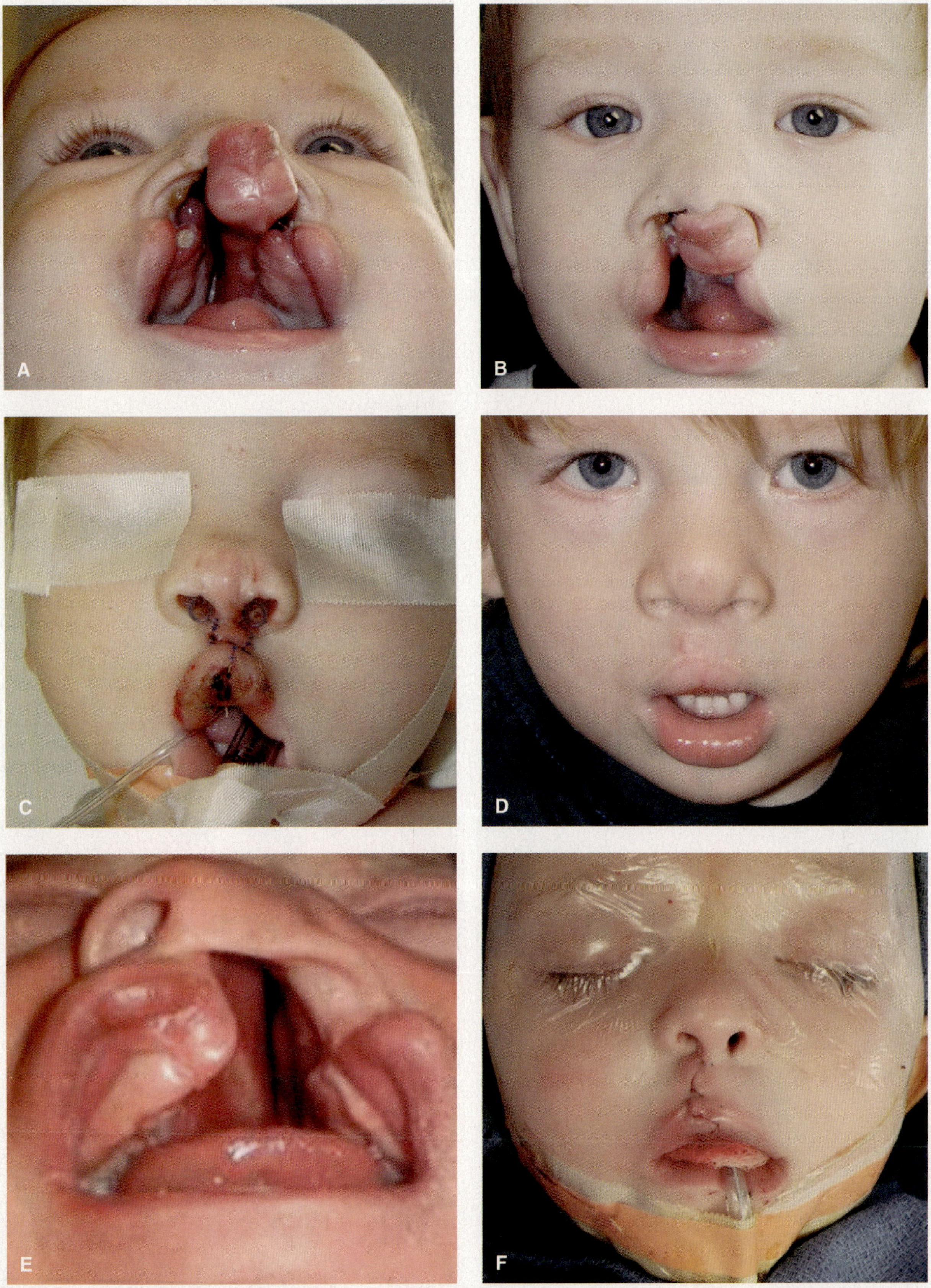

Figure 103.7. A, B: Bilateral cleft lip and palate, the complete expression of the anomaly. The maxillary palatal shelves are separate from each other and from the vomer in the midline. The oral and nasal cavities are communicating. The orbicularis oris muscle is discontinuous and inserts abnormally over the lateral pyriform. The nose is severely deformed and the anterior part of the maxillary arch is outside of the oral cavity (premaxillary escape). C: Intraoperative view of the completed repair, overcorrecting certain structures and undercorrecting others to account for differential future growth "Repair in the fourth dimension."[21,22] D: Results at 4 years post operatively. E: Unilateral cleft lip and palate, a misnomer since the unaffected side is secondarily deformed. F: The abnormally inserted orbicularis oris musculature is reoriented and interdigitated, the lip skin, mucosa, and nose are reconstructed using anthropometric landmarks as a guide, placing scars along anatomical lines (philtral column) and avoiding linear scars.

Table 103.5. Stages of Repair for Complete Cleft Lip and Palate

0–3 mo	Presurgical orthodontics[a]
3–6 mo	Cleft lip repair
9–12 mo	Cleft palate repair
3–6 yrs	Pharyngoplasty or palatal lengthening[a]
7–9 yrs	Alveolar bone graft
10–12 yrs	Rhinoplasty and lip revision[a]
16–18 yrs	Orthognathic surgery[a]

[a]Optional or as indicated.

correction can be done by remodeling of large portions of the calvarial vault (**Fig. 103.11**). Alternatively, a more limited release of the affected suture can be performed, followed by remodeling using an external molding orthosis ("helmeting") or implanted expansion springs.

Microtia

Microtia is defined as partial or near-total absence of the external ear, often accompanied by atresia of the external auditory canal. The middle ear is variably affected, but the inner ear is often intact. The most important functional aspect of reconstruction is early restitution of hearing using band-held bone conduction hearing aids. This can be switched to a bone-anchored device after reconstruction of the external ear to avoid interference with local flap options. Drilling and relining of the external auditory canal is sometimes complicated by the position of the facial nerve in the middle ear and has yet to produce consistent audiologic results.

Table 103.6. Members of a Cleft Team

Plastic surgery
Otolaryngology
Orthodontics
Speech and language therapy
Genetics
Pediatrics
Behavioral/developmental pediatrics
Audiology
Oral surgery
Social worker

Reconstruction of the absent pinna has significant psychosocial benefits to the affected child. Children have poor compliance with bone-anchored external ear prostheses, while acceptance is higher in adults. Options to replace the missing ear fibrocartilage framework include prosthetics (porous polyethylene, silicone) or autogenous rib hyaline cartilage. Coverage options include the temporoparietal fascial flap covered by skin grafts, or a retroauricular pocket of glabrous skin. A commonly practiced technique involves a custom-carved autogenous rib cartilage framework buried in a retroauricular pocket of glabrous skin and elevated secondarily to create a retroauricular sulcus. This technique has been used since the 1950s and is in constant refinement.[21] Although the pinna is 85% adult size by age 4 to 5 years, reconstruction often is deferred until 7 to 10 years of age to allow for development

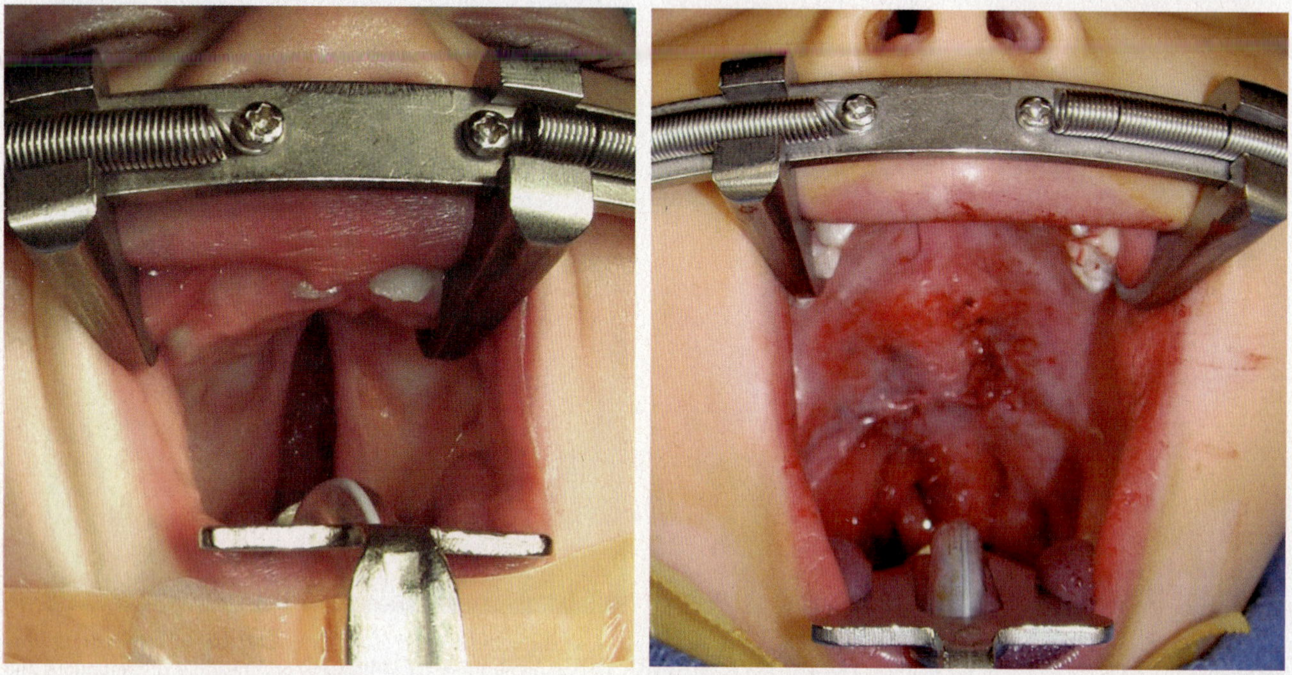

Figure 103.8. Cleft palate repair using a double-opposing Z-plasty technique.[23] The levator levi palatini muscle is abnormally inserted over the posterior palate shelf and needs to be disinserted and rearranged into a sphincter configuration. The mucosal surfaces are lengthened using Z-plasty principles to prevent or minimize linear contracture. "Relaxing incisions" along the gingival edge of the palate facilitate repair but lead to severe secondary growth deformities and can be avoided in most cases. Cleft palate repair is a unique technical challenge due to anatomical space constraints and microsurgical precision needed. The vast majority of patients can expect a normal deglutition and speech mechanism using current techniques. **Left:** before, **right:** after palatoplasty.

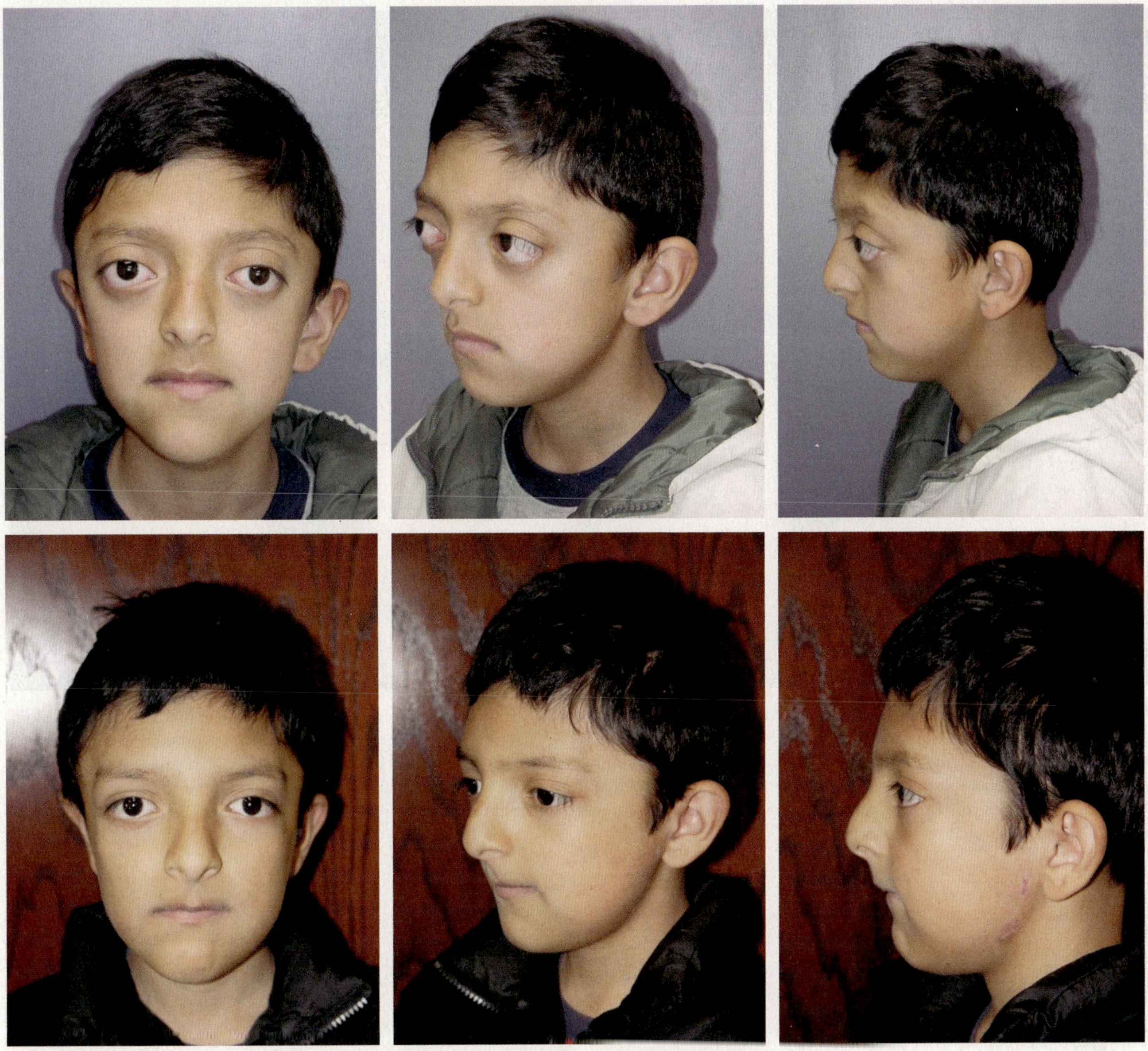

Figure 103.9. Syndromic craniosynostosis: Crouzon syndrome. Calvarial sutures and base of skull enchondrosis fuse prematurely, resulting in restricted growth of intracranial volume and oropharyngeal spaces. Elevated intracranial pressure, proptosis with poor globe protection, and obstructive apnea can be corrected surgically by combined frontal, facial, and mandibular (FFM) advancement using distraction osteogenesis. **Above**, before, and **below**, after combined FFM with cranial vault expansion.

of rib cartilages. A template of the unaffected ear is made, reversed, and transposed to the anthropometrically correct position on the affected side. The anterior, cartilaginous portion of ribs 5 to 8 is harvested preserving as much perichondrium as possible. These are carved into a two- or three-layer cartilage framework emulating the external ear anatomy, with some modifications to accentuate contour, notably in the scapha. The earlobe is often present and is transposed into correct position, while the cartilage framework is implanted into a subcutaneous pocket in the existing glabrous skin. Suction drainage and external pressure dressings are critical to appearance of the desired anatomy (**Fig. 103.12**). The retroauricular sulcus is secondarily created by elevation of the framework, placement of a retroauricular wedge of cartilage, and coverage with a fascial flap and skin grafting.

Childhood Tumors

While pediatric malignancies are often encountered and may require extensive craniofacial approaches (**Fig. 103.13**), common tumors are usually benign and include hemangiomas, dermoid cysts, pilomatricomas, and melanocytic nevi.

Hemangiomas typically involute spontaneously but should be distinguished from similar-appearing vascular malformations. Hemangiomas respond well to propranolol and have changed their management markedly in recent years. Symptomatic hemangiomas that fail to respond to propranolol, and those that involve an orifice, block vision or breathing, or distort a cartilaginous structure such as nasal cartilages or tarsal plates require surgical treatment (**Fig. 103.14**). Vascular malformations are treated according to their nature by surgical debulking, sclerotherapy, or pulse dye laser. Complete extirpation is usually not feasible due to extent of the lesion (**Fig. 103.15**).

Congenital melanocytic nevi are often a psychosocial concern but only large ones are thought to carry a risk of malignant degeneration. Management options include direct excisional biopsy, serial excision, or tissue expansion (**Fig. 103.16**).[25] Excision and skin grafting often results in significant deformity but may be needed for its expediency in cases of associated malignancy or severe atypia. Depigmenting lasers or chemical peels can improve the cosmetic appearance in cases where excision is prohibitive but may impede detection of an underlying malignancy.

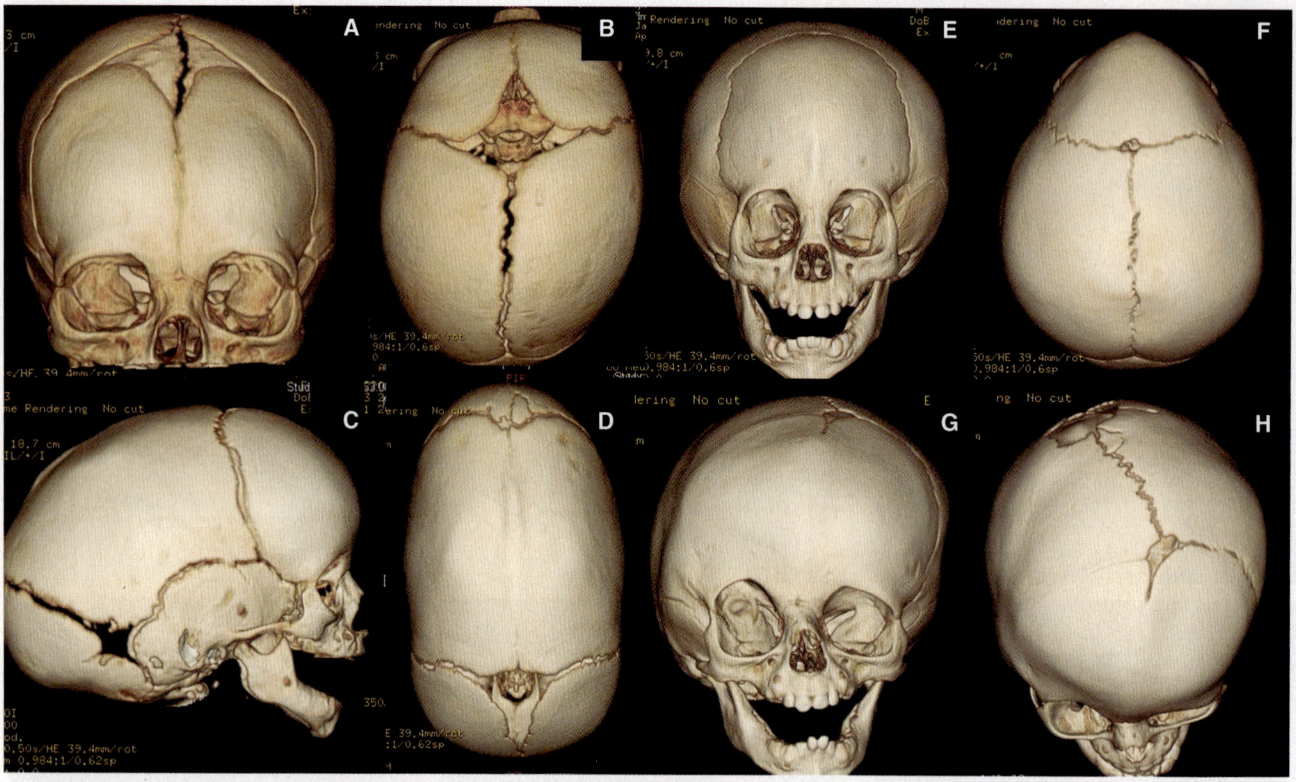

Figure 103.10. Isolated craniosynostoses: (**A**) frontal and (**B**) vertex view of normal suture configuration in an infant. The occipital skull flattening is due to positional deformation (deformational plagiocephaly). C: Lateral and (**D**) vertex view of the most common isolated premature synostosis of the sagittal suture, resulting in an elongated skull (dolichocephaly). E: Frontal and (**F**) vertex view of premature fusion, likely intrauterine, of the metopic midforehead suture resulting in a triangular head shape (trigonocephaly). G: Frontal and (**H**) vertex view of unilateral fusion of the right coronal suture resulting in asymmetry of the forehead and right orbit, and secondary bulging of the left parietal and right midface (right unicoronal synostosis).

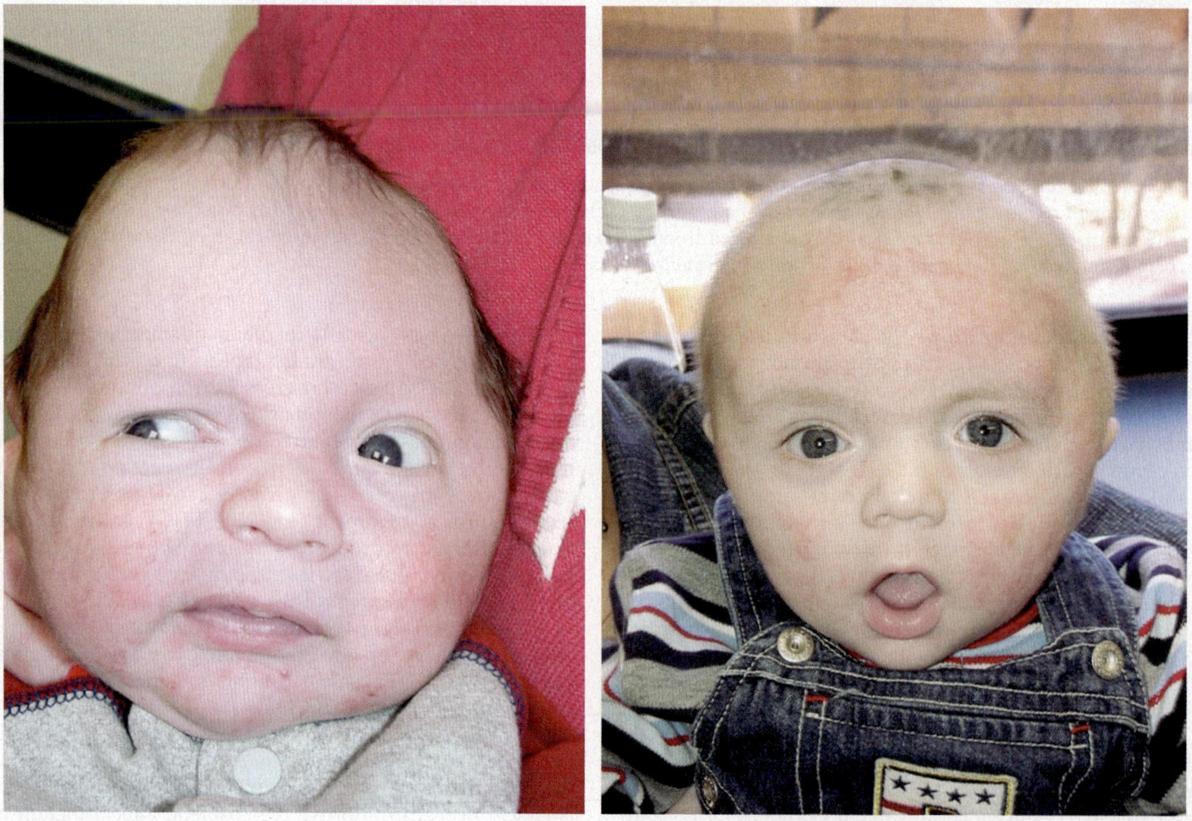

Figure 103.11. Multiple suture synostosis in an infant, before and after total cranial vault remodeling. The risk of elevated intracranial pressure increases exponentially with the number of sutures involved. **Left,** before and **right:** after cranial vault remodeling.

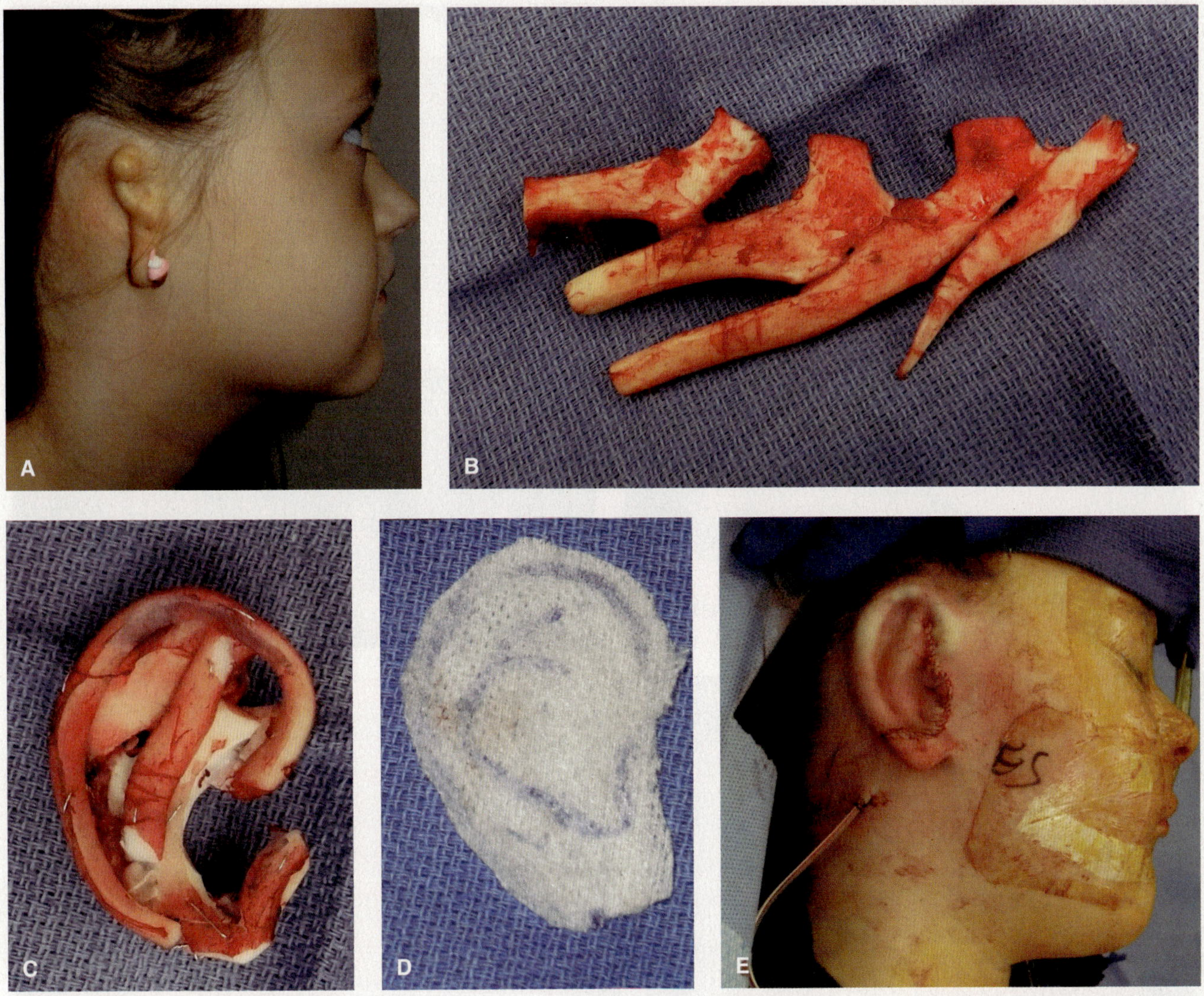

Figure 103.12. Lobular-type microtia with near total absence of the pinna and external auditory canal. The lobule is often present, but malorientated. A vestigial cartilaginous remnant is present and needs to be carefully excised preserving overlying skin. Facial nerve, facial soft tissues, temporomandibular joint, ocular tumors, squamosal synostosis, and vertebral and other anomalies are sometimes present. Reconstruction involves harvesting an often large amount of autogenous rib cartilage that is carved into an ear framework based on a template of the contralateral ear. The framework is implanted under existing skin, and elevated secondarily.

Traumatic Deformities

Simple lacerations are managed in the emergency setting; however, compound injuries often require specialized, operative care.

While most simple childhood fractures are treated by closed reduction; complex and compound fractures are a particular challenge. They require meticulous anatomical reduction of the involved segments, accounting for the hidden greenstick deformity, and the competing impetus of limiting soft tissue and growth center disruption while providing anatomical reduction and sufficient fixation. Long-term growth sequelae are a concern (**Fig. 103.17**).[26]

Dog bites and lawnmower injuries produce devastating soft tissue defects that require the full spectrum of plastic surgery techniques. Facial soft tissue loss is particularly hard to replace in a child due to the lack of regional redundancy.

HAND AND UPPER EXTREMITY SURGERY

Hand surgery is a discipline shared by General Surgery, Plastic Surgery, and Orthopedic Surgery. Regardless of background, the trained hand surgeon should have a thorough understand-
6 ing of bone and soft tissue physiology and be able to diagnose and treat traumatic and nontraumatic conditions of the hand utilizing the advancements in imaging, microsurgery, and wound management. Successful outcome of complex hand reconstruction also relies on frequent postoperative vigilance and aggressive postoperative hand therapy. The following section will provide examples of common hand conditions due to trauma, congenital, or acquired causes. It is by no means a comprehensive review.

Nomenclature

Nonambiguous nomenclature is important for clarity. Avoid numerical identifiers. Some refer to the thumb as the first finger and the index finger as the second finger, while others refer to it as the first finger and the small finger as the fourth finger. Use instead: thumb, index, middle (long), ring, and small (little). For the phalanges, identify them by name: proximal, middle, or distal phalanges and NOT by numbers: P1, P2, or P3. The numbering of phalanges is confusing, as it is not obvious which bone P1 or P3 refers to: Is P1 the distal or the proximal phalanx? It is more confusing for the thumb, as there is no middle phalanx. So is it unclear which bone P2 refers to. For the metacarpals, the numerical system can be used, though one can use name descriptors to avoid confusion: thumb, index, ring, or small finger metacarpal bone. For laterality, use

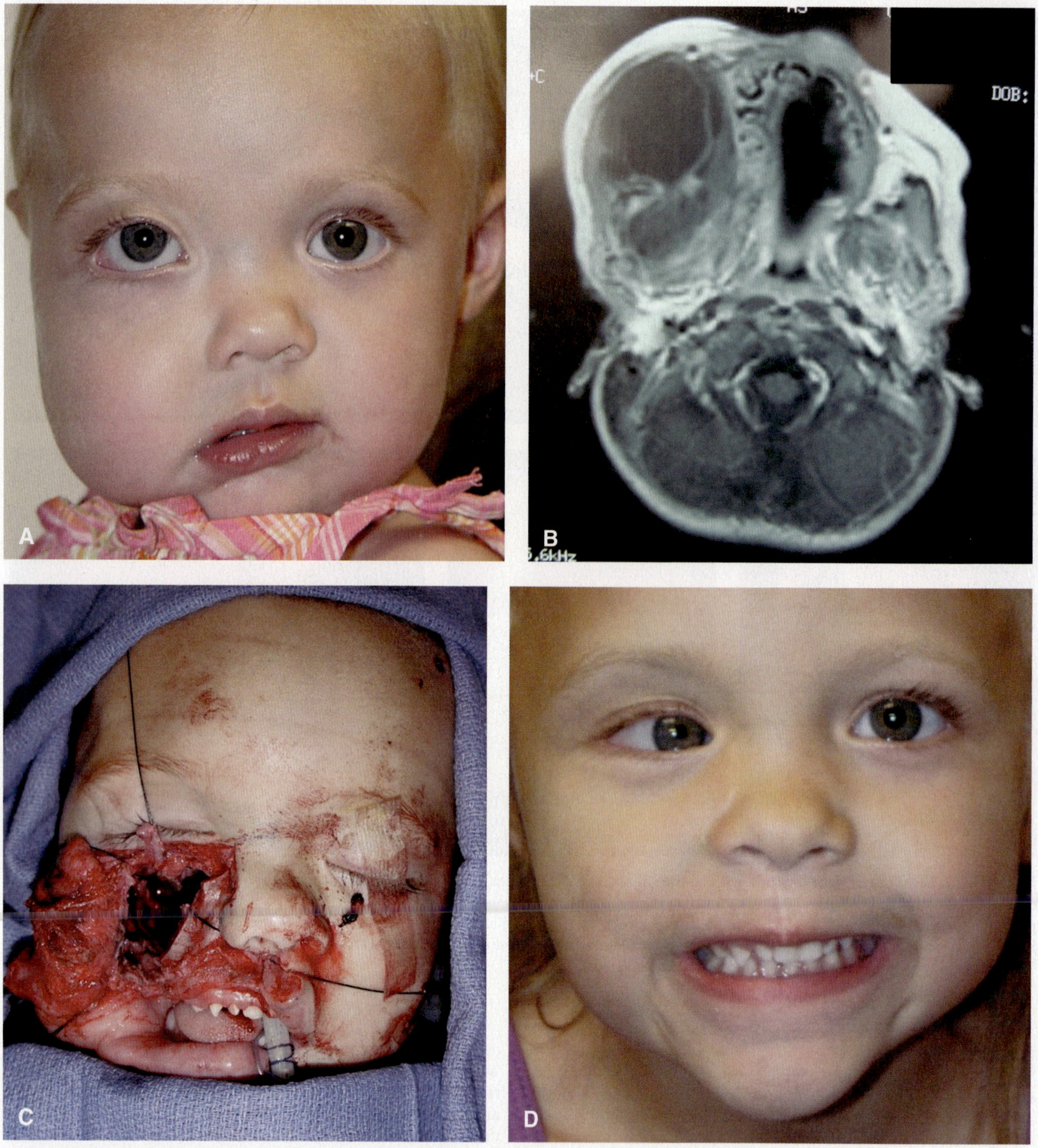

Figure 103.13. Childhood tumors sometimes require complex craniofacial approaches. This child with a large ganglioglioma of the pterygomaxillary space and medial orbit (**A, B**) was approached with a (**C**) Weber–Ferguson approach. Secondary deformities are carefully minimized with choice of approach and use of autogenous tissue for reconstruction (**D**). Multimodality treatments result in their own secondary growth restrictions.

"radial" to identify the side of the hand or finger closer to the radius, rather than lateral. Use "ulnar" for the side closer to the ulna, rather than medial. This avoids confusion, particularly if the hand is rotated during the examination and not in anatomic position. Using "palmar" is more easily understood than "volar." "Dorsal" is used for the back of the hand.

Anatomy and Examination

The hand at rest has a natural flexion cascade with each adjacent ulnar-sided finger slightly more flexed (**Fig. 103.18**). Any alteration to this can suggest a flexor or the extensor tendon rupture or laceration. At the wrist, the flexor carpi radialis and the palmaris longus tendon should also be visible. The thenar and hypothenar eminences should be full, and if either is flat, this can suggest nerve or musculoskeletal pathology. The fingers should be sensate, warm, and well-vascularized. Evaluate the hand for disturbances in posture, skin, color, contour, and function.

Infection

Common hand infections include cellulitis, paronychia, deep space abscesses, and suppurative flexor tenosynovitis.

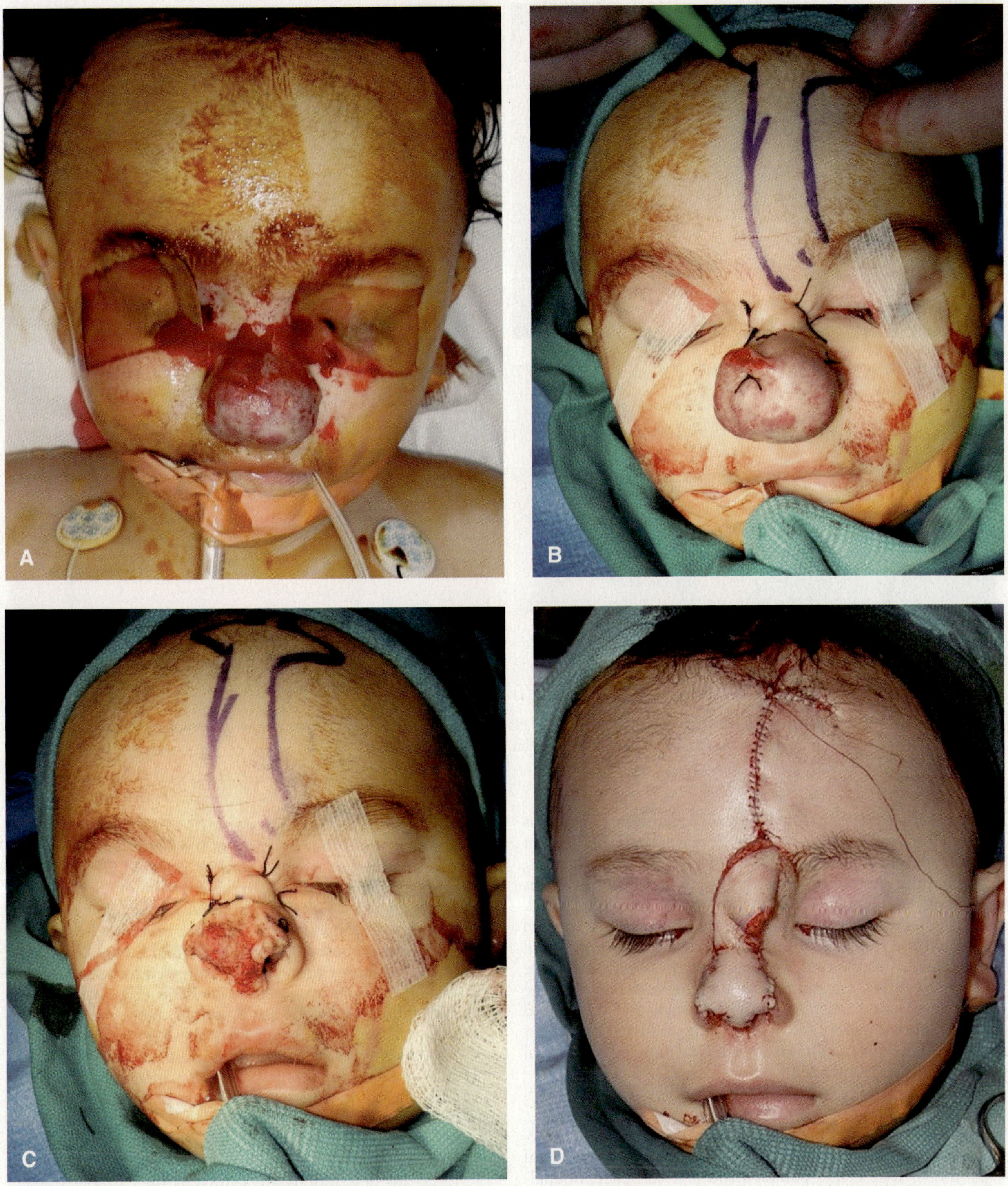

Figure 103.14. **A:** Bleeding nasal hemangioma resulting in 1.2 total blood volume transfusion prior to arrival. **B:** Hemostasis obtained using multiple large tacking sutures. A forehead flap is marked on the forehead. **C:** At the completion of excision, the nasal cartilages are splayed and will require repositioning. **D:** After transfer of the forehead flap.

Cellulitis

It is an infection involving the dermis usually due to an abrasion, puncture, or a systemic infection (**Fig. 103.19**). Symptoms include increased warmth, erythema, and lymphadenopathy. For early and mild cases, it can be treated with warm compresses, elevation, removal of foreign body if present, and antibiotics. *S. aureus* and group A beta-hemolytic Streptococcus are the common organisms found. Cellulitis associated with an abscess requires incision and drainage, antibiotics, and wound care until resolution.

Paronychia

It is an infection of the lateral fingernail fold (paronychium). An eponychia is an infection of the dorsal nail fold (eponychium). If both the lateral and dorsal nail folds are involved, it is called a runabout infection. Paronychia occurs due to a break in the nail fold from trauma, hangnail, manicure, or nail biting. The most common organisms are *S. aureus* or oral anaerobes. Symptoms include swelling, erythema, and pain. With progression, there is fluctuance and purulence, and drainage from the

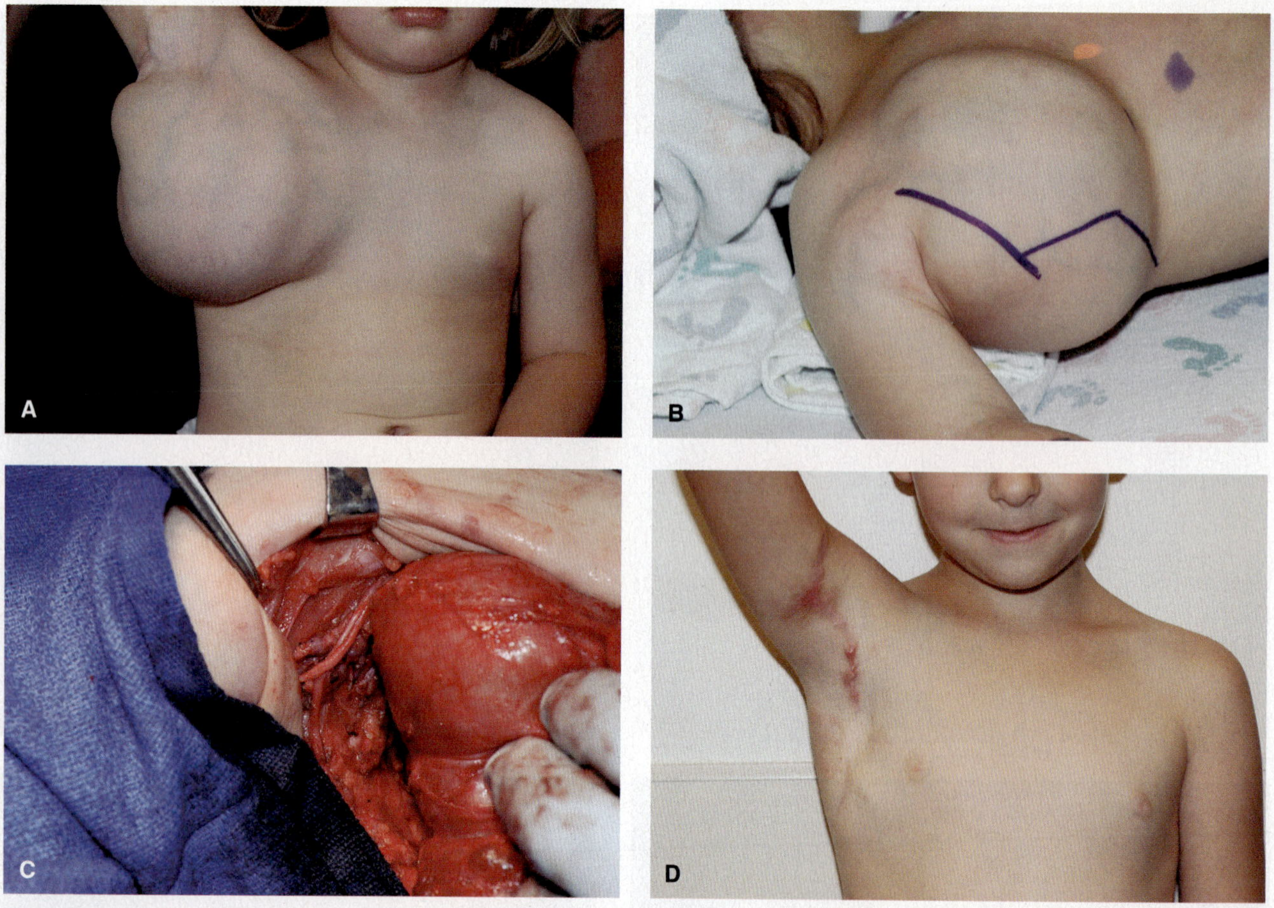

Figure 103.15. **A:** Lymphatic malformation of the right axilla. **B:** Planned surgical incision. **C:** Dissection of the lymphatic malformation sparing the underlying neurovascular structures. **D:** Post debulking with improved contour.

nail fold. If severe, a paronychia can progress to a cellulitis ascending into the finger, hand, or forearm. Initial treatment for early paronychia consists of warm soaks, oral antibiotics, and splinting. Surgery is necessary if pain increases or there is worsening of fluctuance and purulence. Under digital block and a digital tourniquet, incise into the fluctuance at the nail fold. Send the fluid for culture and irrigate the wound with saline. Place a wick into the incision and dress with dry gauze and splint × 1 day. The patient should remove the dressing the following day and begin washing the finger and the wound twice a day with soap and warm water followed by a light gauze until the infection has resolved. Oral anti-staphylococcal antibiotics is recommended for 5 to 7 days.

Deep Space Infections

They occur in approximately 5% to 15% of all hand infections. There are six potential deep spaces defined by fascial separations: four in the palmar hand (thenar space, midpalmar space, hypothenar space, and interdigital web space), one in the dorsal hand (the dorsal subaponeurotic space), and one in the volar forearm (Parona space). The most common organisms are *S. aureus* and Streptococcus species. Penetrating trauma is the most common cause. Other possibilities include contiguous spread from an adjacent deep space infection, subcutaneous abscess, or pyogenic flexor tenosynovitis. The hand is swollen and tender (**Fig. 103.20**). Active and passive finger motion results in severe pain. The swelling and purulence may be more noticeable dorsally because the dorsal skin has higher compliance. Should a deep space infection be suspected, CT scan is helpful to confirm and delineate the location and extent of the infection. Surgical drainage should be done by a hand surgeon in the operating room.

Suppurative Flexor Tenosynovitis

It is an infection within the space of the flexor tendon synovial sheath between the proximal borders of the A1 annular pulley at the distal metacarpal neck to the insertion of the flexor digitorum profunda (FDP) distal to the A5 pulley. The small finger sheath is continuous with the ulnar bursa, and the thumb flexor sheath is continuous with the radial bursa. Penetrating trauma is the most common cause followed by hematogenous dissemination from an adjacent infection (**Fig. 103.21**). The most common organisms are *S. aureus* and Group A Streptococcus. Mixed organisms and gram-negative bacteria are possible pathogens in intravenous drug users, diabetics, or in immunocompromised patients. The infection within the synovial sheath destroys the frictionless gliding surfaces causing scarring and tendon adhesions, thus early diagnosis and aggressive treatment is important. Kanavel first described the symptoms in 1925.[27,28]

Today his descriptions are known as the cardinal signs of Kanavel used to diagnose the infection. They are: (1) exquisite tenderness over the path of the flexor sheath; (2) marked symmetrical swelling of the finger described as "sausage shape"; (3) flexed posturing of the affected fingers; (4) pain on passive extension of the involved finger(s).

Treatment of early infection (24 to 48 hours) remains nonoperative with immobilization, elevation, and high-dose empiric intravenous antibiotics for *S. aureus* and Group A Streptococcus. Failure to improve, infection greater than 48 hours' duration, and gross purulence are indications for surgical intervention. Surgery is aimed at removing the purulence within the synovial sheath by open incision and irrigation. This should be done under general anesthesia by a hand surgeon in the operating room.

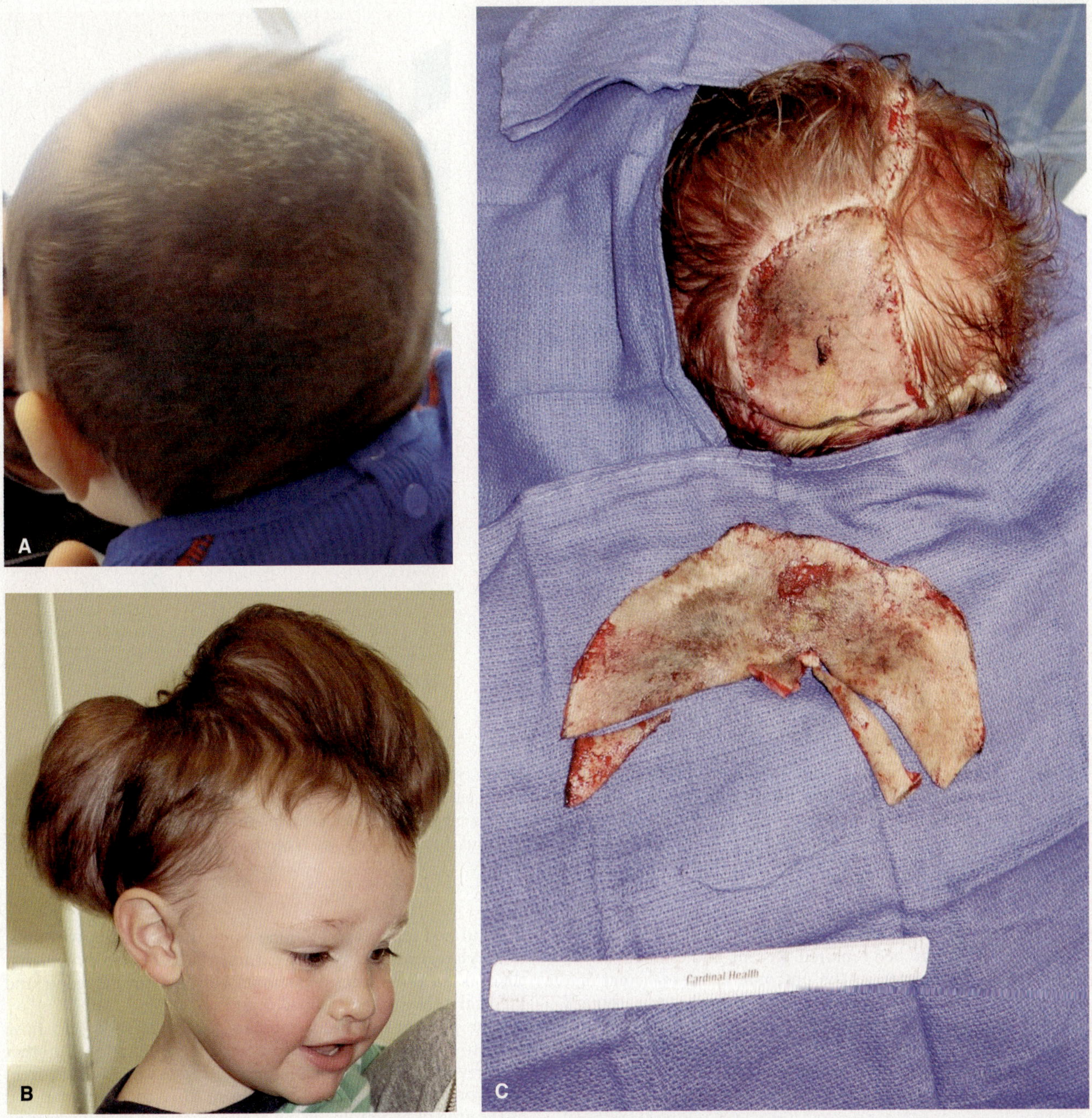

Figure 103.16. **A:** Giant congenital melanocytic nevus of a large portion of the occipital scalp (40% total scalp area). **B:** During active tissue expansion of the unaffected scalp. **C:** After first-stage excision and flap advancement. Secondary expansion will be needed for complete excision.

Other Infections

They include septic arthritis and human and animal bites (**Fig. 103.22**). Septic arthritis should be a diagnosis of exclusion, as many medical conditions such as gout and pseudogout may mimic an infection with joint pain, warmth, and erythema. Joint aspiration with Gram stain, white blood cell count, and culture of the fluid is done for definitive diagnosis. Human and animal bites are treated similarly with aggressive irrigation, debridement, and directed antibiotics.[29]

Trauma

Trauma is the most common reason patients come to the Emergency Department to be evaluated for hand concerns. A three-view radiograph of the hand (PA, oblique, lateral) is obtained. A CT scan is ordered if the radiographs are equivocal and clinical suspicion is high for a fracture or abscess.

Soft Tissue Injuries

Fingertip Injuries

These are common injuries resulting from recreational or industrial activities. If no bone or tendon is exposed, the wound can be allowed to close by secondary intention, skin grafts, or be repaired with avulsed skin, if available, as a composite graft. If bone is exposed, the bone can be shortened, or it can be repaired with a local flap such as a V-Y flap (**Fig. 103.23**).

Nail Bed Injuries

The hallmark of a nail bed injury is a subungual hematoma that can be associated with an underlying distal phalanx fracture. The pressure within the confined space caused by bleeding results in severe pain. Hematoma evacuation is done for pain relief. Previous teaching was that if the hematoma was

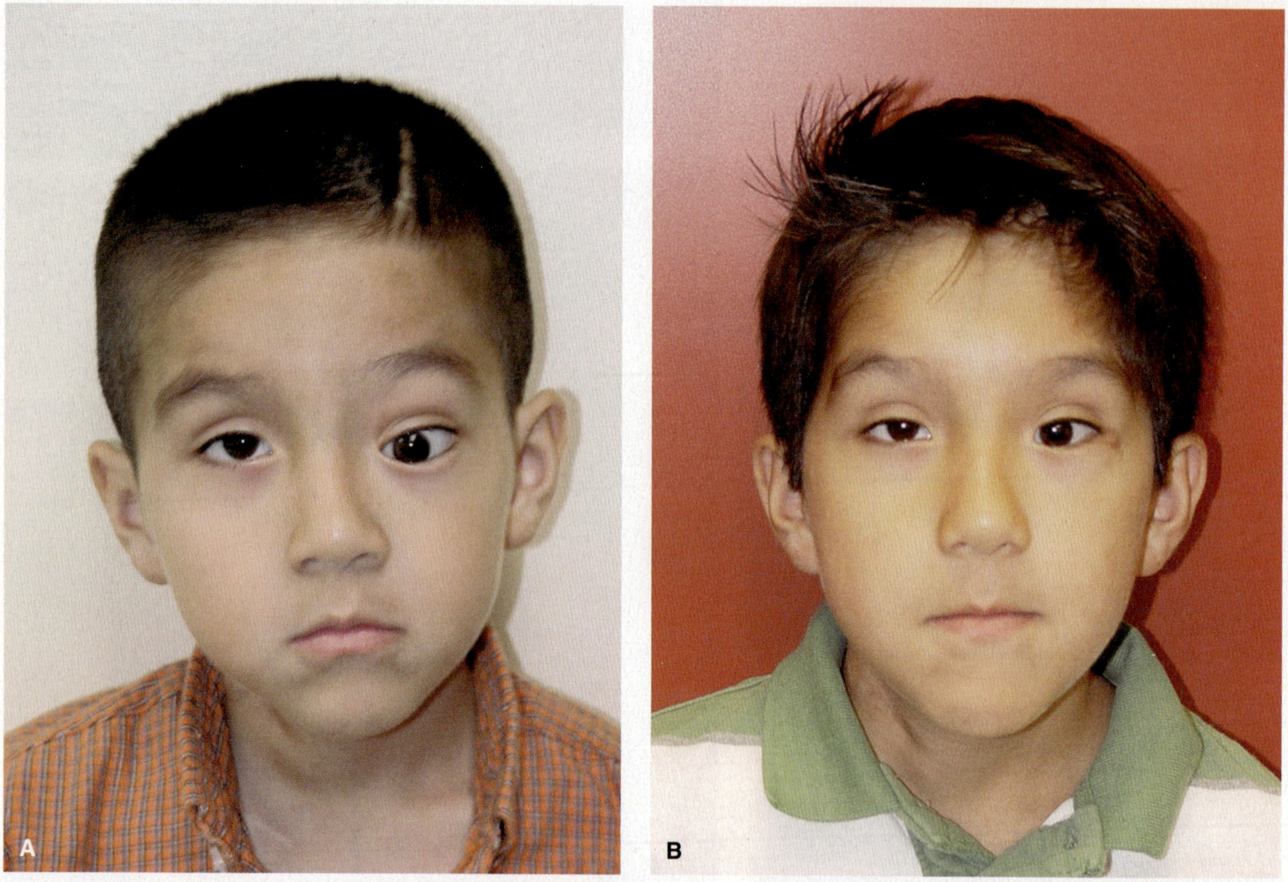

Figure 103.17. **A:** Orbital dystopia secondary to untreated fracture of the left zygomatic bone complex and orbital roof 2 years prior to presentation. Although most pediatric fractures can be treated with closed reduction, orbital roof fractures sometimes result in secondary deformities due to the pressure of the growing brain. Note the reflex head tipping to maintain binocular vision and harmonize visual and vestibular somatosensory orientation signals. **B:** Post–orbital wall reconstruction and translocation of the malar complex. Secondary strabismus surgery is typically deferred for a few months.

25% of the nail bed surface or larger, that the nail should be removed and the nail bed repaired. Recent studies have shown no noticeable difference in the outcome between hematoma evacuation versus nail removal and nail bed repair, though there was an increase in cost by four times in the nail bed repair group.[30]

Nail bed repair can be done using medical adhesives (cyanoacrylates) instead of fine sutures. It has been shown that there is no difference in outcome between suture repair and medical adhesive for nail bed injuries.[31]

For hematoma evacuation, most recommendations have been to use an ophthalmic cautery for trephination. Another preferred method is to decompress the hematoma using a freer elevator to detach the nail plate from the underlying nail bed at the area of hematoma using gentle sweeping motion starting at the edge of the nail and advancing forward until the hematoma drains. The nail is then trimmed shorter. This method allows for improved passive drainage with gravity, rather than expecting the hematoma to drain dorsally against gravity

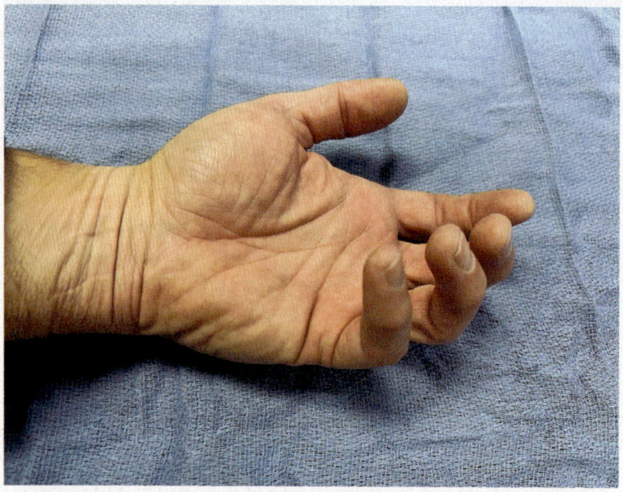

Figure 103.18. In its resting repose position, notice that the middle finger is more flexed than the index, and the ring more flexed than the middle, and the small finger more flexed than the ring. This is referred to as the "natural cascade."

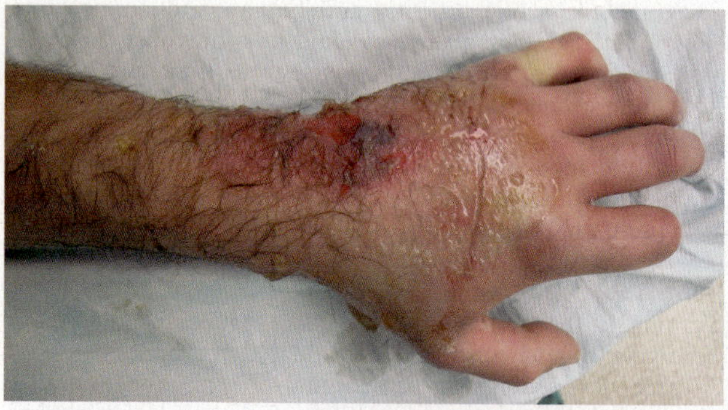

Figure 103.19. Cellulitis of left hand. Note the erythema, blistering and swelling on the dorsal left hand extending to the fingers.

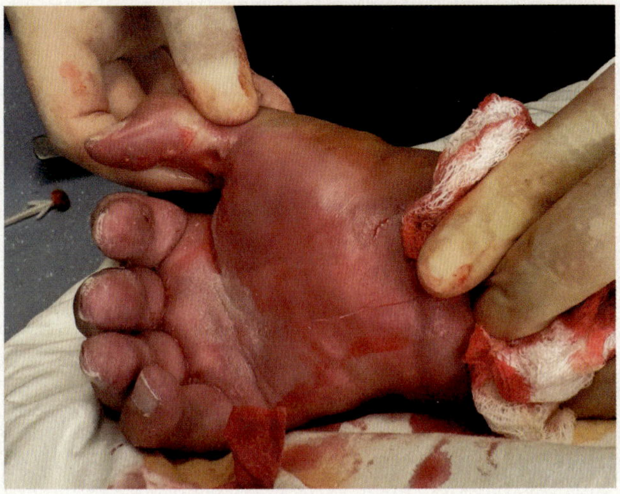

Figure 103.20. Deep space infection of the Thenar space.

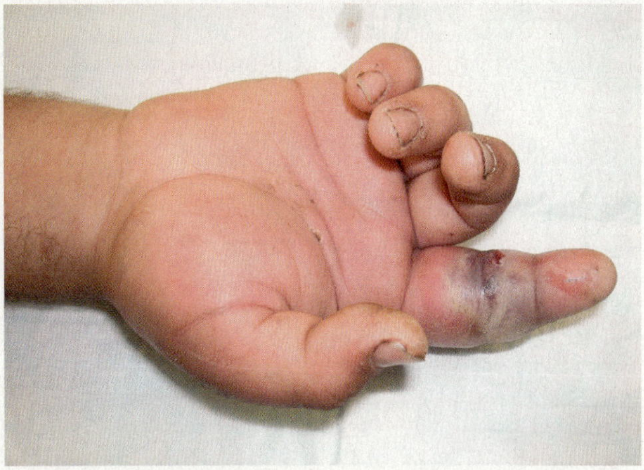

Figure 103.21. Note the fusiform swelling in the index finger with a flexed posture.

through the trephinated nail. This method also avoids the possibility of iatrogenic nail bed injury, which can occur with the cautery or the biopsy punch.

Tendon Laceration

Causes of tendon lacerations are usually due to penetrating trauma by knife or ballistic injury. High-energy blunt trauma can cause closed tendon ruptures.

Flexor Tendons Lacerations

Generally, when the laceration is deep on the palmar surface, both the tendon(s) and the neurovascular structures are damaged in the fingers. On examination, there would be a visible laceration with loss of the natural cascade with decreased sensation to the finger distal to the laceration (**Fig. 103.24**). If one artery is lacerated, the other digital artery maintains perfusion. If both are lacerated, there is generally sufficient dorsal collateral circulation to keep the finger viable, unless there is vascular compromise from vascular injury, gross wound contamination or an associated open fracture. Tendon repairs can be done electively within 1 week of the injury.

If the penetrating trauma occurs in the forearm, the injury can appear deceptively benign and these require operative exploration as multiple tendons, ulnar, median or radial nerves, and arteries can be damaged. Postoperatively, protect the hand and the forearm with a dorsal splint with ongoing directed hand therapy starting 1-week postoperatively.

Extensor Tendon Laceration

Unlike flexor tendon lacerations, the lacerated ends of extensor tendons generally do not retract due to their attachments to adjacent structures. Most injuries are due to penetrating trauma, though closed injuries can result in: (1) mallet finger which the extensor tendon ruptures from the distal phalanx without a fracture or with a fracture consisting of a small dorsal piece of the distal phalanx (**Fig. 103.25**). The inciting cause is an axial load to the distal finger with forced flexion at the distal interphalangeal joint (DIP) or (2) a boutonniere deformity due to rupture of the central slip from the dorsal proximal phalanx. Most of the time, both the mallet and the boutonniere are treated with splints for 4 to 8 weeks, depending on the injury pattern. Open injures with extensor tendon lacerations are repaired in the operating room. Postoperative splinting and hand therapy are critical to successful outcomes.

Fractures

There are 27 bones in the hand and 2 bones in the distal forearm that are subject to fractures. Most of the hand and finger fractures, including some Salter–Harris fractures, can be treated nonoperatively if nondisplaced. Surgery with reduction and internal fixation (with plate/screws or K-wires) (**Fig. 103.26**) is required for fractures that are unstable, displaced, or in bones known to have poor outcomes without surgery (eg, Seymour fracture in the pediatric population and scaphoid proximal pole fracture). Fractures associated with a communicating wound require operative irrigation and stabilization.

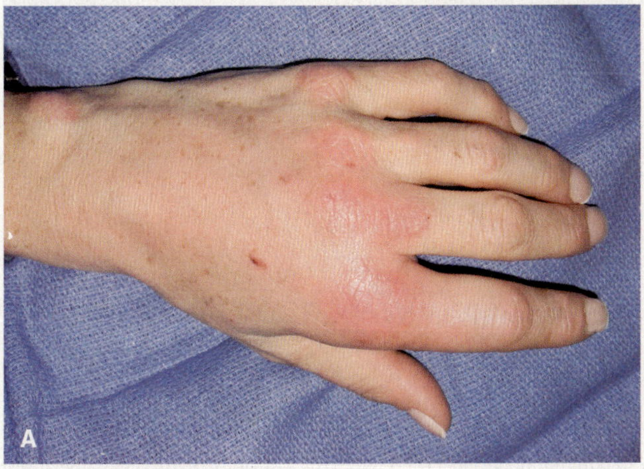

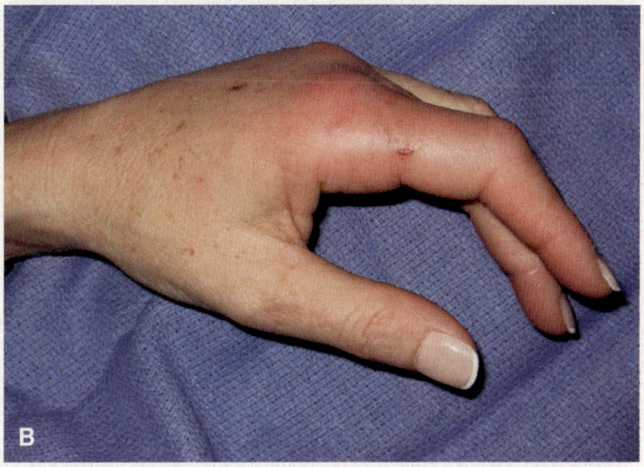

Figure 103.22. **A:** Erythema on the dorsal hand due to a cat bite. **B:** Lateral view showing swelling and erythema with puncture wound.

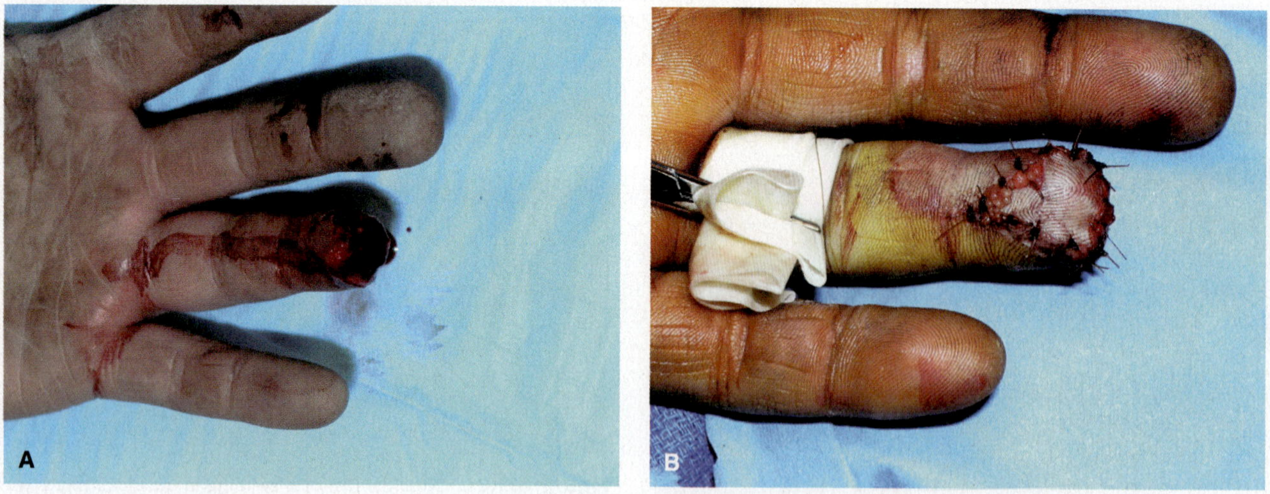

Figure 103.23. The distal left ring finger (**A**) was avulsed and was not suitable for replantation. The exposed DIP joint was closed with a V-Y flap (**B**) shown after closure.

The benefit of hardware stabilization is the ability for early mobilization to decrease joint stiffness that can result in poor hand function.

Replantation

The first successful finger replantation was reported in 1968 by Komatsu and Tamai.[32]

The current guidelines state that the indications for replantation are: (a) thumb amputation, (b) multiple finger amputations, (c) pediatric amputations, and (d) mid-hand, wrist, or distal forearm amputations. Contraindications for replantation are: (a) associated life-threatening injuries, (b) multiple-level injuries in the amputated part, causing injuries along the vessels and preventing blood flow into the replanted part, and (c) severe contamination of the part, which carries a high probability of systemic infection if replanted. Replantation of a single digit due to the tight fibro-osseous tunnel in flexor zone 2 is generally not recommended due to tendon adhesions resulting in poor postoperative function. Single finger amputation in zone 1 is not contraindicated as stiffness in the DIP joint is well tolerated and nerve regeneration to the replanted part is rapid due to the short distance from the injury to the distal nerve receptors, and the appearance of the replanted finger is superior to that of an amputation.

Complex Hand and Forearm Reconstruction

There are times when multiple tissue components (bone, skin, nerve, tendons, artery) are injured and require reconstruction. A systemic approach is required for the reconstruction to restore form and function. In wounds secondary to trauma, initial treatment should address critical life- or limb-threatening issues such as limb ischemia or compartment syndrome, followed by debridement of any nonvascularized or infected tissue. Once the soft tissue is free of contamination, formal reconstruction of bone, tendon, nerves, and soft tissue deficits should begin (**Fig. 103.27**). For large composite defects after tumor resection, both the functional deficit and the soft tissue deficit need to be considered.

Congenital Anomalies

Limb development can be interrupted by environmental or genetic factors during the critical first trimester of embryo development.

Syndactyly

The term syndactyly is derived from the Greek prefix *syn-* ("with, together") and the Greek noun *daktylos* ("finger, digit"). Syndactyly has an incidence of 1 in 2000 to 3000 live births and is the most common congenital hand anomaly.[18,33] It is a failure of differentiation in which the fingers fail to separate into individual appendages, which usually occurs between the 6th and 8th weeks of in utero development.

Syndactyly can be an isolated occurrence, or it can be associated with other abnormalities, such as, polydactyly, cleft hands, ring constrictions, and craniofacial syndromes such as Apert syndrome (**Fig. 103.28**). It is a shared feature of more

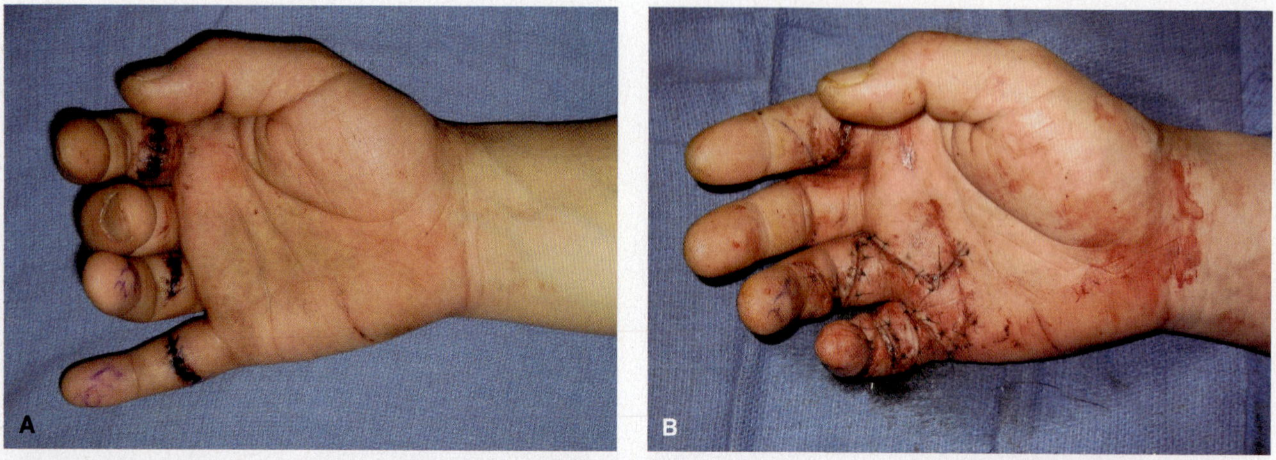

Figure 103.24. **A:** Zone II FDP and flexor digitorum superficialis (FDS) and digital nerve laceration. Note the loss of the natural cascade at rest with the small finger completely extended. **B:** Normal cascade reestablished after flexor tendon repair.

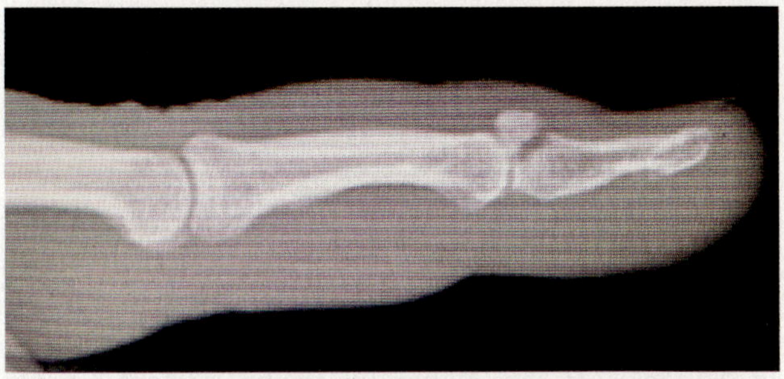

Figure 103.25. Mallet fracture with the extensor tendon still attached to the dorsal proximal distal phalanx. If there is more than 50% of the articular surface involved, some would recommend operative treatment.

than 28 syndromes, including Poland, Apert, and Holt–Oram syndromes.[34] Syndactyly is classified as simple when only the skin is involved and complete if it extends to the fingertips (**Fig. 103.29**) and incomplete if it is short of the fingertips. If there is bone and nail plate involvement it is classified as a complex syndactyly.

Untreated, syndactyly can impair finger and hand function, particularly if it is complete or involves the border digits (eg, small and ring finger or thumb and index finger) as there is differential finger growth rates, which can result in finger deviation or joint contractures.

If the syndactyly is complex or border digits are involved, surgical release is recommended as early as 6 months of age. If only the central rays (middle or ring fingers) are involved in a simple complete or incomplete syndactyly, separation can be completed between 12 and 15 months or later. Bilateral operations can be tolerated in children 12 to 18 months of age as

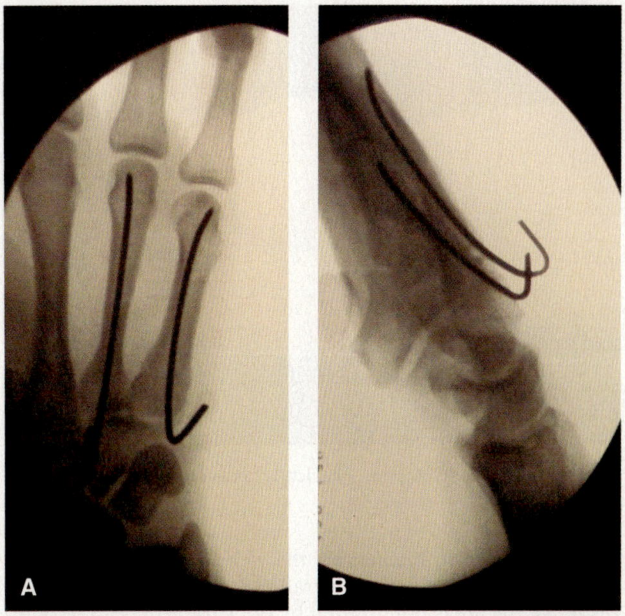

Figure 103.26. Intraoperative fluoroscopy of intramedullary K-wire fixation of displaced ring and small finger metacarpal shaft fractures. **A:** AP View. **B:** Lateral View.

both upper extremities are immobilized for about 2 weeks. If both sides of a finger are involved in the syndactyly, only one side of each digit is released, with the other side released at a later time—generally 3 to 6 months later. This is to avoid devascularizing the digit. Skin flaps are designed in a zigzag fashion on the dorsal and palmar surfaces with a trapezoidal-shaped

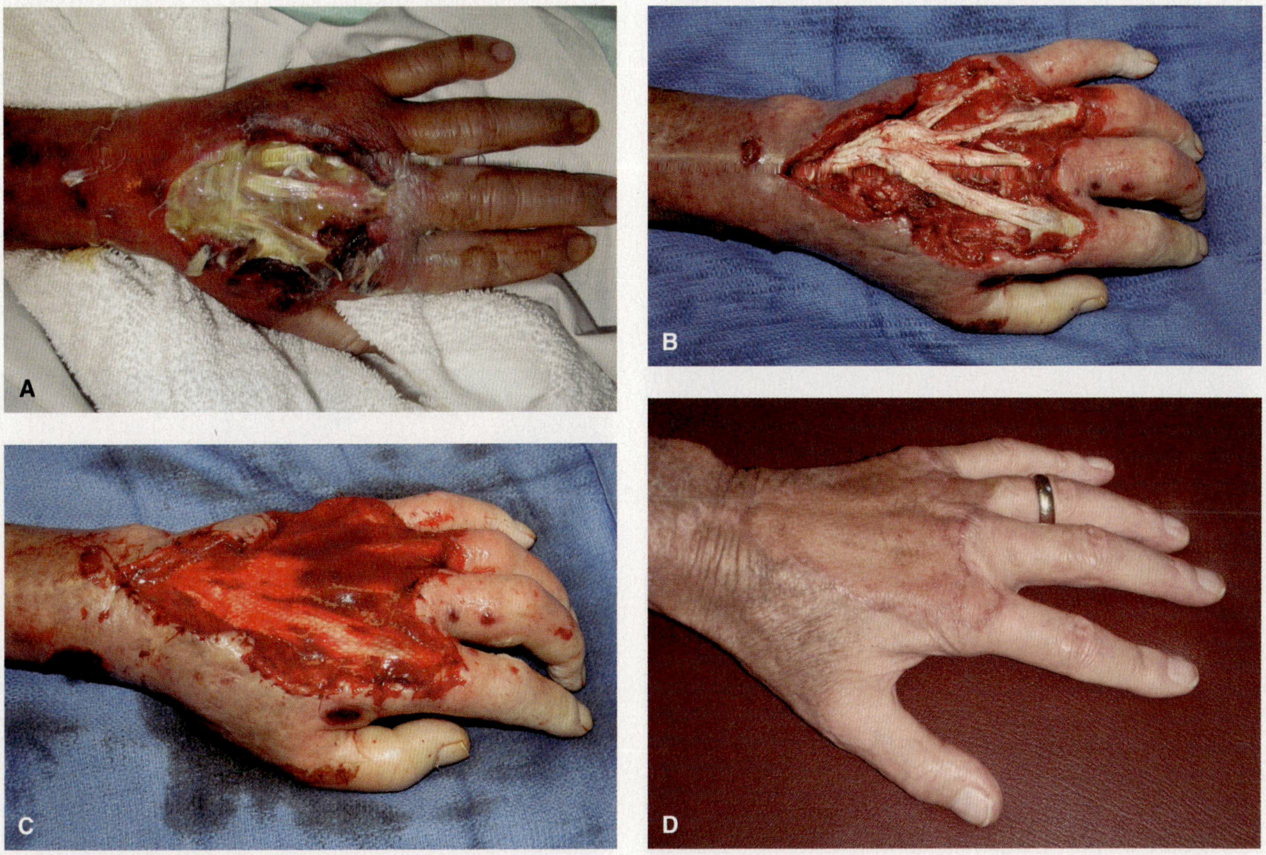

Figure 103.27. A: Complex wound in an immunocompromised patient after IV infiltration and subsequent infection requiring several operative debridements (**B**) and with allograft placement (**C**), and coverage with delayed split-thickness skin graft (**D**).

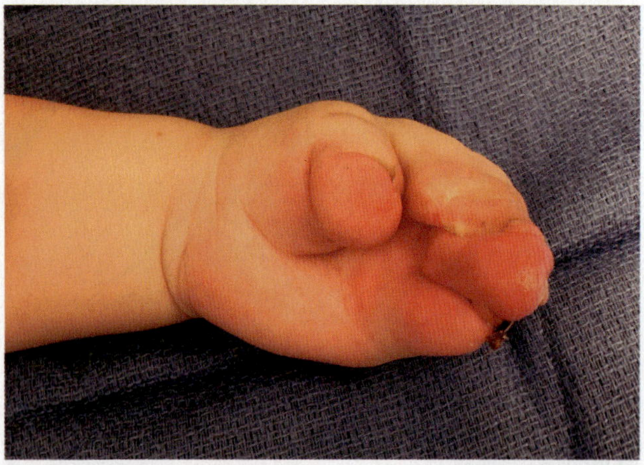

Figure 103.28. Complex syndactyly associated with Apert syndrome.

dorsal skin flap to reconstruct the web space and the base of the digits. Full-thickness skin grafts from the groin are used to resurface the areas not covered by the flaps.[18]

Polydactyly

Polydactyly or extra fingers can occur on the ulnar side of the hand (postaxial), the radial side (preaxial), or the central rays (central).

Postaxial polydactyly has variable presentation. It can be mild and present as a nubbin on the ulnar side of the little finger, usually at the level of the proximal phalanx or as a rudimentary finger attached by a small neurovascular pedicle. Sometimes the accessory finger is partially or fully developed. The incidence is 1 in 143 live births in the African American population and has a strong hereditary component (often autosomal dominant) without other associated syndromes. The incidence in the Caucasian population is 1 in 1339 live births and can be associated with other syndromes.[35] Treatment may be as simple as a bedside ligation of a rudimentary digit or surgery for excision of the more fully formed digit.

Preaxial polydactyly involves the radial side of the hand and thumb. It occurs in 1 of every 3000 live births and may be associated with several syndromes (Holt–Oram syndrome, Fanconi anemia).[36]

Central Polydactyly

It is rare and can present as incomplete to fully formed index, middle, or ring fingers. Central polydactyly can be associated with syndactyly, cleft hand, and other syndromes.[37,38]

Surgery is geared to removing the duplicated digit and reconstructing the hand to make it appear and function as normal as possible.

Thumb Hypoplasia and Agenesis

Thumb hypoplasia occurs 1 in 100,000 live births with 50% being bilateral. With unilateral presentation, the right is more commonly involved. Thumb hypoplasia has a spectrum of presentation from mild diminution to complete absence. In 60% of cases, it is associated with longitudinal deficiencies of the radius. In the embryo, the thumb develops between the 5th and 8th weeks at the same time as the cardiovascular system. Insults at this time can alter thumb development and 86% of patients with a hypoplastic thumb have associated abnormalities of the cardiovascular, neurologic, and hematopoietic systems. Thumb hypoplasia is associated with at least 30 syndromes (Holt–Oram syndrome, VACTERL association, and thrombocytopenia absent radius [TAR] syndrome).[39,40]

Thumb hypoplasia is categorized by five distinct types. Originally described by Muller in 1937, it has been improved by Blauth, Buck-Gramcko in 1967 and Manske in 1995.[41]

- Type I: Normal components are present but small with underdevelopment the abductor pollicis brevis and opponens pollicis. Type 1 does not require surgical intervention.[42,43]
- Type II: There is a contracted web space between the thumb and index finger with more severe hypoplastic thenar muscles. There is laxity of the metacarpophalangeal joint (MP) ulnar collateral ligament with joint instability. Surgery is aimed at restoring thumb stability and intrinsic function with opponensplasty and deepening of the web space usually with a four-flap Z-plasty.
- Type IIIA and type IIIB: The metacarpal bone is less developed and the thenar musculature is nearly absent. The thumb has poor function. Type IIIA has a stable carpometacarpal (CMC) joint, type IIIB does not. Treatment for type III is based on the presence of a stable CMC joint. Type IIIB requires reconstruction and type IIIB requires amputation and index finger pollicization.
- Type IV: The thumb is floating, called pouce flottant. Like the appearance of a postaxial polydactyly, the thumb is incompletely formed and is attached to the adjacent finger by a neurovascular bridge. There are no thenar muscles and no extrinsic tendons. Type IV is usually reconstructed with index finger pollicization.
- Type V: There is no thumb and requires pollicization.

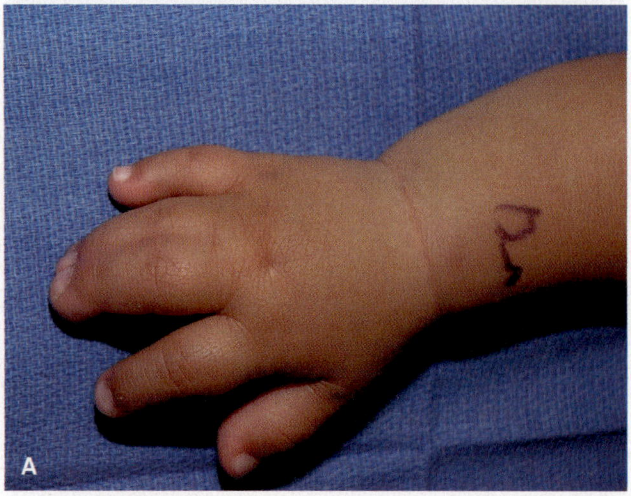

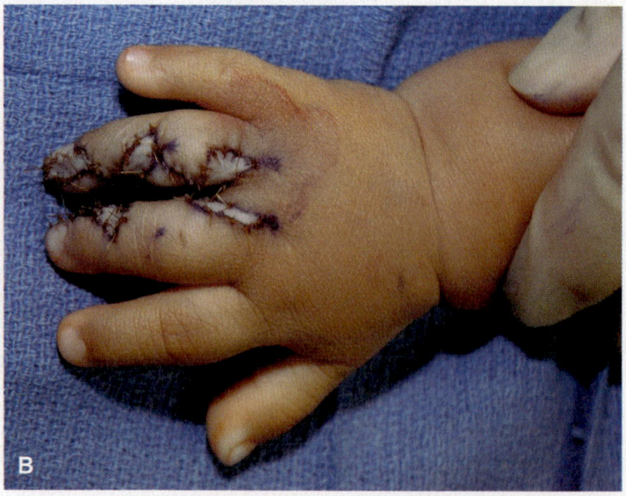

Figure 103.29. A 12-month-old child with a complete simple syndactyly between the middle and ring finger in the left hand (**A**) before and (**B**) after syndactyly release.

Acquired Conditions

Osteoarthritis

There is gradual loss of cartilage in the joint with age. The DIP joints and the thumb CMC joints are more prone to these changes. Treatment is geared toward pain relief while maintaining function. Treatment includes oral anti-inflammatory medication, gentle range of motion while avoiding strenuous activities, and splinting. Should initial conservative measures not work, intra-articular steroid injection can provide temporary relief. Surgical treatment is reserved as the last option. There are no effective joint replacement for the DIP joint, thus arthrodesis remains the only surgical option. For the proximal interphalangeal (PIP), MP, and the CMC joints, both arthroplasty and arthrodesis can be offered. There are numerous options for thumb CMC arthroplasty. Most involve removing the trapezium which is then followed by reconstruction with autologous tissue using a variety of suspension techniques (**Fig. 103.30**).

Tendinitis

Inflammation of tendons, from increased physical activity, can cause inflammatory synovitis around the tendon, can decrease tendon glide and increase resistance, causing pain and decreased range of motion. When this occurs in the hand involving the flexor tendons at the A1 pulley, this results in a trigger finger. Recommendations are to decrease aggressive activities, rest/splinting, oral anti-inflammatory medications, steroid injections, and A1 pulley release if nonsurgical intervention is unsuccessful. A single injection for a trigger finger can offer up to a 70% cure.[44]

When the tendinitis occurs in the first dorsal extensor compartment, this is known as De Quervain tenosynovitis. Treatment is similar to trigger finger.

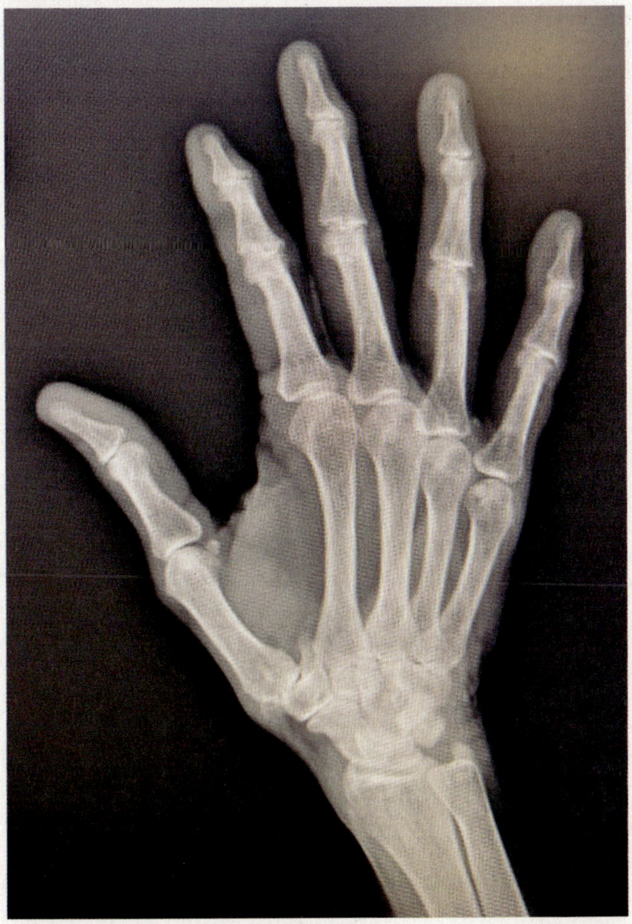

Figure 103.30. A 59-year-old with right thumb pain. Preoperative radiographs show advanced left thumb CMC joint arthritis.

Peripheral Nerve Compression

In the upper extremity, all three major nerves (radial, ulnar, and median) can be compressed at varous anatomic narrowing's along their paths. The median nerve can be compressed at the carpal tunnel, resulting in numbness in the palmar thumb, index, middle, and radial side of the ring finger. With progression and severity there is weakness in thumb opposition and thenar atrophy. The median nerve can also be compressed by the pronator teres although less often. The two most common sites of ulnar nerve compression are the cubital tunnel at the elbow and in Guyon canal at the ulnar wrist. The radial nerve can be compressed in the dorsal proximal forearm and is known as radial tunnel syndrome if the compression is more proximal and involves the extensor carpi radialis longus (ECRL) tendon nerve branch and the dorsal radial sensory nerve. It is termed posterior interosseous nerve (PIN) syndrome, if it involves only the PIN. Like tendinitis, treatment is nonsurgical. Evaluation with electrical studies (EMG/NCV) is recommended to confirm and to establish degree of compression. If there is evidence of a progressive decline in sensory or motor function, surgery is then recommended. Less-invasive release with endoscopic assistance is alternative to the traditional open techniques.[45]

Dupuytren's

Dupuytren contracture is a condition where nodules develop in the palmar fascia. These nodules progress to longitudinal pretendinous cords spanning the base of the palm to the PIP joint restricting finger extension and can cause fixed contractures at the PIP and MP joints. Though found in all ethnicities, it is found more frequently in the Northern European population. There is generally a familial history and a slight male to female predominance (ratio: 1.7:1).[46] Surgical excision of the cord use to be the mainstay for treatment until 2010 when the FDA-approved collagenase injections to alter the mechanical properties of the cord.[47] Other treatment options include percutaneous needle aponeurotomy.

Rheumatoid Arthritis

Rheumatoid arthritis (RA) is an autoimmune condition mediated by inflammatory cells that attack the synovial tissues in the body. Persistent synovitis in the joints results in articular damage and degradation of the soft tissue support at the joint and ultimately causes rupture of the overlying tendon.

Prior to the advent of effective biologic agents (immunosuppressant or cytokine modulators), surgery was a mainstay in the treatment of RA. The goals of surgery were for pain control and improved and restoration of function. This is done in three different ways: preventative, corrective, and salvage.[48] Preventative surgery includes synovectomy, which may be used to avoid the sequela of synovitis such as pain, joint destruction, and tendon rupture. Corrective surgery includes tendon transfer for tendon ruptures.

With progressive attenuation of the supporting joint structures at the wrist, there is radial deviation of the metacarpal and with destruction of the metacarpophalangeal MP joints; there is subluxation and ulnar deviation of the fingers at the MP joints. This results in pain and difficulty with finger flexion and extension MP joints and irreversible joint damage. Salvage procedures include joint arthroplasty at the MP joints with silicone joints as well as finger and wrist fusion (**Fig. 103.31**).

PLASTIC SURGERY OF THE BREAST

7 The breast is an anatomic feature that signifies empowerment, self-image, sexuality, and serves a functional role for lactation during pregnancy.[49] As such, patients frequently request both aesthetic and reconstructive procedures of the breast. These will be subdivided in the following sections: reduction mammoplasty, mastopexy, augmentation mammoplasty, gynecomastia

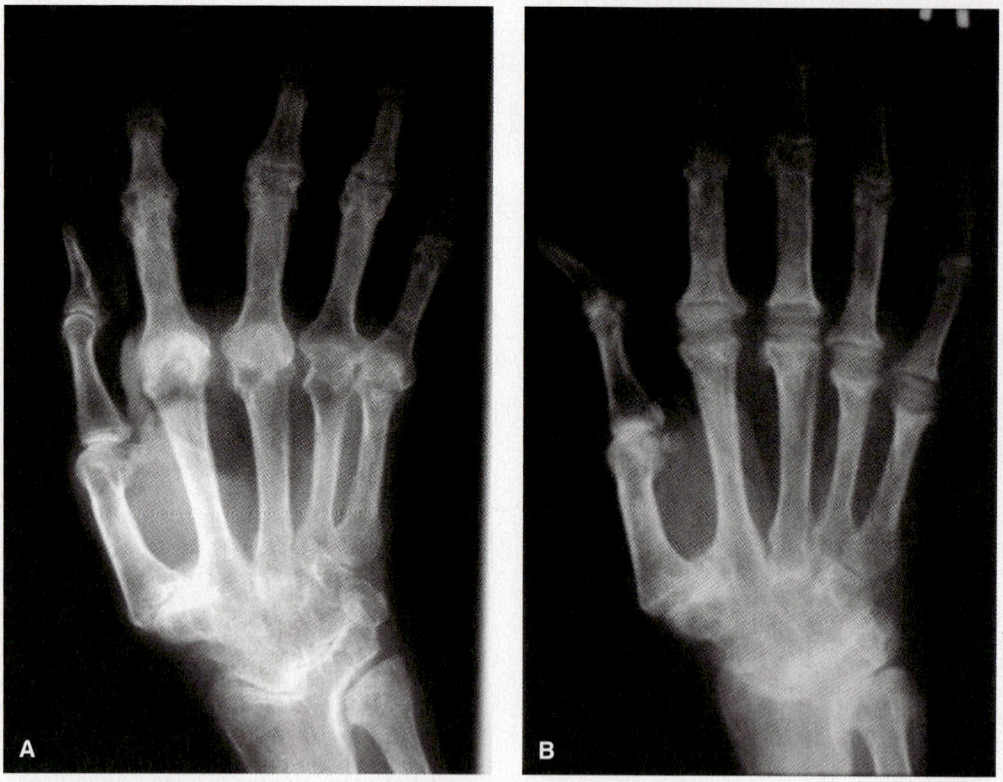

Figure 103.31. Preoperative (A) and postoperative (B) view of the right hand. Note the restoration of normal finger alignment.

(reduction of the male breast), breast reconstruction, and gender-affirming surgery. Breast dimensions and anatomical characteristics are important considerations for all surgical procedures. Special consideration should be given to the current scientific climate related to breast implants which will be addressed separately as it pertains to both aesthetic and reconstructive patients.

Breast Characteristics

Results of plastic surgery of the breast are impacted by several anatomical considerations. Important factors include breast size, shape, composition, vector, footprint, and nipple-areola complex (NAC) orientation. Breast shape can be impacted by whether the meridians of the breasts are more parallel or divergent. Poor-quality skin (eg, with striae) and a breast with relatively more adiposity than gland can lead to a softer, less full, ptotic appearance. The superior pole of the breast is variable in different patients which leads to significant differences in breast appearance. Size can be relative to body habitus. Some breasts have more lateral fullness than others. The intermammary space differs between patients.[50,51] NAC orientation greatly impacts breast appearance. Breast ptosis (**Fig. 103.32**) is defined in **Table 103.7**.[52]

Reduction Mammoplasty

The main goal of a breast reduction is to decrease the volume, and therefore weight, of the breast in order to decrease associated aggravating symptoms while maintaining or improving breast appearance. Preoperative considerations relate to patient expectations for appearance and financial coverage of the procedure. Surgical considerations are numerous and includes incision placement, pedicle orientation that supplies blood to the NAC, parenchyma preservation, and management of the NAC. Postoperative considerations include wound care and imaging changes.

Preoperative Evaluation

Patients seeking reduction mammoplasty often complain of neck and back pain, difficulty with the fit of clothing, management of breast mobility during exercise, grooving of the shoulders from bra straps, and recalcitrant rashes in the intertriginous folds. Most patients seek a smaller breast mound, as well as a mound that is lifted with a footprint higher on the chest wall (rather than the upper abdominal wall) and a NAC with less ptosis and reduced size (to match the overall smaller size of the breast mound).[53,54] A careful preoperative conversation must occur regarding postoperative size preferences and inability to guarantee an exact size. Often the conversation will relate to bra cup size and should include counseling regarding the inexact nature of this methodology

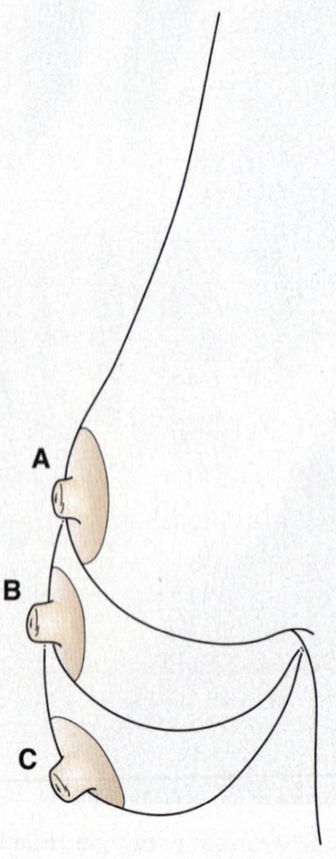

Figure 103.32. Breast ptosis. **A:** Mild. **B:** Moderate. **C:** Severe.

Table 103.7. Breast Ptosis Definitions[52]

Grade 1	Nipple at the level of the inframammary fold (IMF)
Grade 2	Nipple between the level of the inframammary fold and the lowest border of the breast
Grade 3	Nipple at the lowest border of the breast
Pseudoptosis	Breast gland hanging well below the IMF

since bra cups are not standardized between companies and change with chest width (bra band size number). Many patients seek this procedure as a covered benefit through health insurance, and the surgeon should be familiar with insurance criteria. Commonly used insurance coverage criterion relates to body surface area calculated from height and weight, converted to a suggested weight of tissue to be resected through the Schnur table, though it is commonly believed that this table does not accurately convey a relationship between resected weight and symptom reduction.[55] A specific consideration in the preoperative workup is baseline mammography, and recommendations for this relate to patient age and breast cancer risk factors.[56]

Surgical Approaches

Reduction mammoplasties can be done via several different approaches but the most commonly used are dermal parenchymal pedicles either centrally or inferiorly based. The pedicle is designed to maintain blood supply and sensory function to the NAC. The widely used inferior pedicle technique (**Fig. 103.33**) produces an inverted "T"-shaped scar with the transverse portion in the inframammary fold. Many patients did not like this

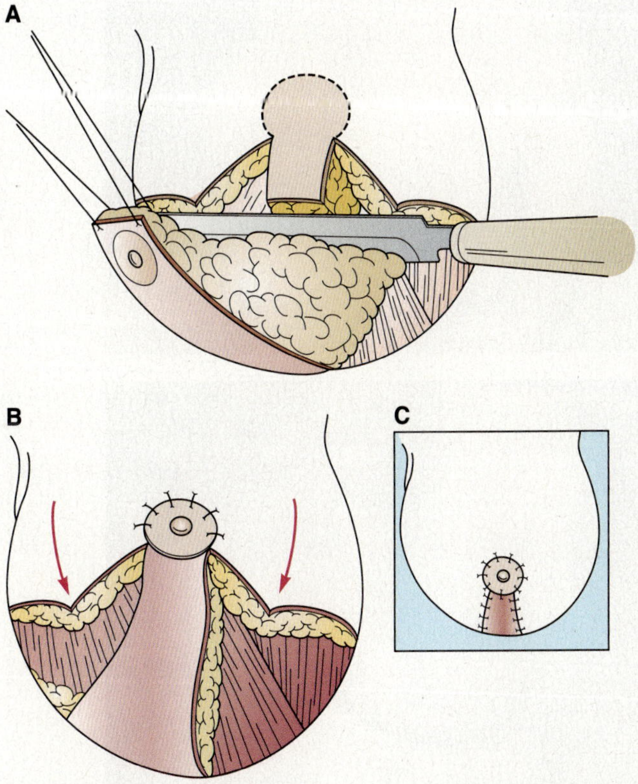

Figure 103.33. Inferior pedicle technique for reduction mammoplasty.

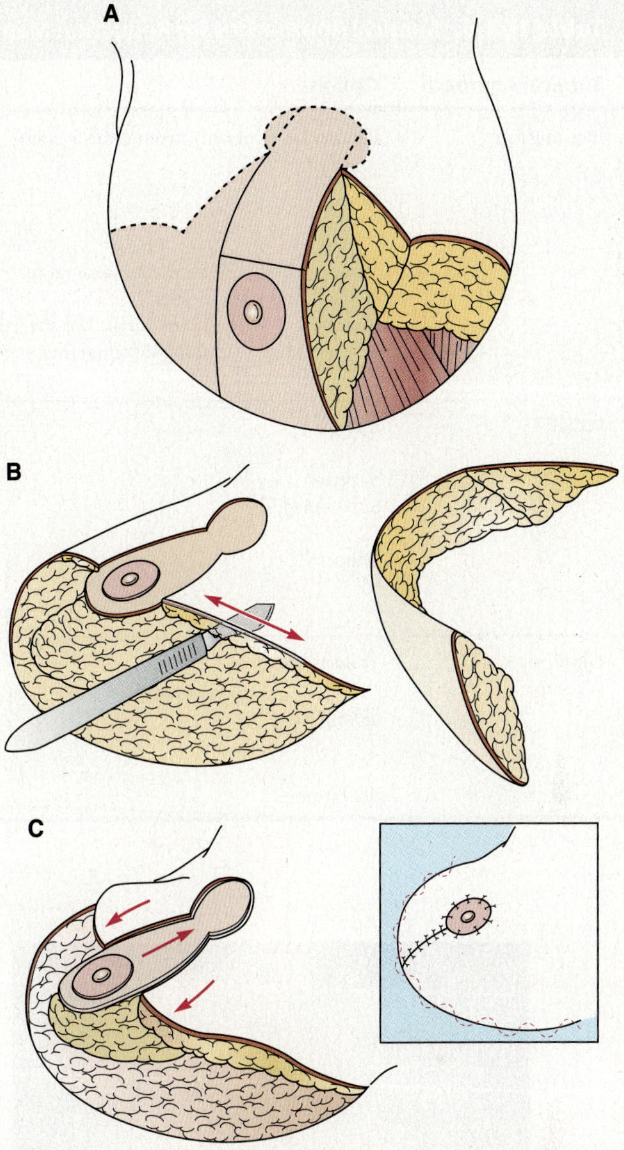

Figure 103.34. Central pedicle technique for reduction mammoplasty.

large scar which led to the development of the vertical scar mammoplasty (**Fig. 103.34**). **Table 103.8** elucidates the typical components of breast reduction surgery.[53,54] Postoperative drain placement remains variable. Several studies demonstrate no evidence of improvement in outcomes with drains, but common practice demonstrates high prevalence of ongoing drain usage in practice.[57] Most often this procedure is performed in an outpatient setting.

Postoperative Follow-Up

Patients demonstrate high rates of satisfaction and relief of symptoms following breast reduction surgery. However, complication rates, particularly with wound-healing are relatively high and may require frequent clinic visits.[51,54] Mammography changes after breast reduction can include planar parenchymal scar, fibrosis, and fat necrosis (**Fig. 103.35**).[58]

Mastopexy

Mastopexy, or breast lift, is often considered by patients who have ptosis of the NAC or pseudoptosis of the breast gland as defined earlier in this chapter. Preoperative discussions should clearly address the limitations of this technique, as the patient's baseline breast dimensions are not likely to change significantly. The patient is unlikely to achieve breasts that

Table 103.8. Surgical Approaches for Reduction Mammoplasty[53,54]

Surgical Approach	Options	Considerations
Incision/scar	Periareolar (scar only around the areola)	Scar only at junction of different types of skin so may be less visible, often used for smaller reductions because it allows for skin reduction in fewer dimensions, may distort areola or periareolar scar over time due to differential forces, areola may widen over time without permanent "blocking" suture
	Vertical ("Lollipop" scar: circle around the areola and vertical "stick")	Has risk of excess tissue or standing cone deformity at inferior most aspect of incision
	Inverted T ("Wise-pattern" or anchor-shaped scar adding scar along inframammary fold to vertical scar)	Used most commonly for largest reductions, healing concerns at "triple point" where vertical and inframammary scars meet
Pedicle	Inferior	Common choice, concern over pseudoptosis (bottoming out) of breast mound over time
	Superior	Often used with vertical skin incisions
	Superomedial	Often used in gigantomastia, considered to decrease risk of need for free nipple grafting
	Other	Lateral, superolateral, etc. could be used when technique is performed with lumpectomy for breast cancer in oncoplastic setting if common pedicles not feasible
Nipple-areolar complex (NAC)	Transposition	Most likely to maintain sensation, reactivity, functionality, and "normal" appearance of NAC
	Skin graft	More common in larger reductions with greater proposed nipple transposition distance, can be patchy in coloration, flat, nonreactive, and poor (if any) sensation
	3D tattoo	Considered a salvage technique if a NAC fails to survive

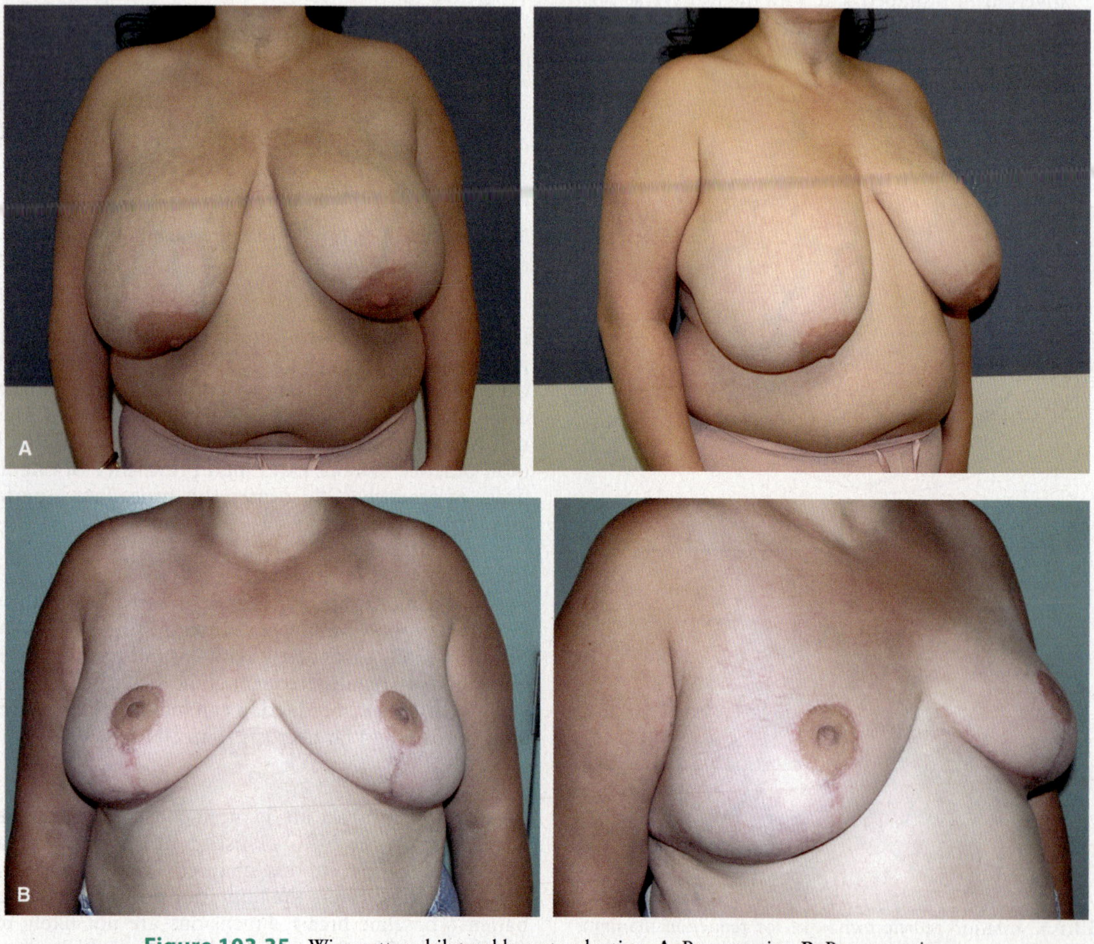

Figure 103.35. Wise-pattern bilateral breast reduction. **A:** Preoperative. **B:** Postoperative.

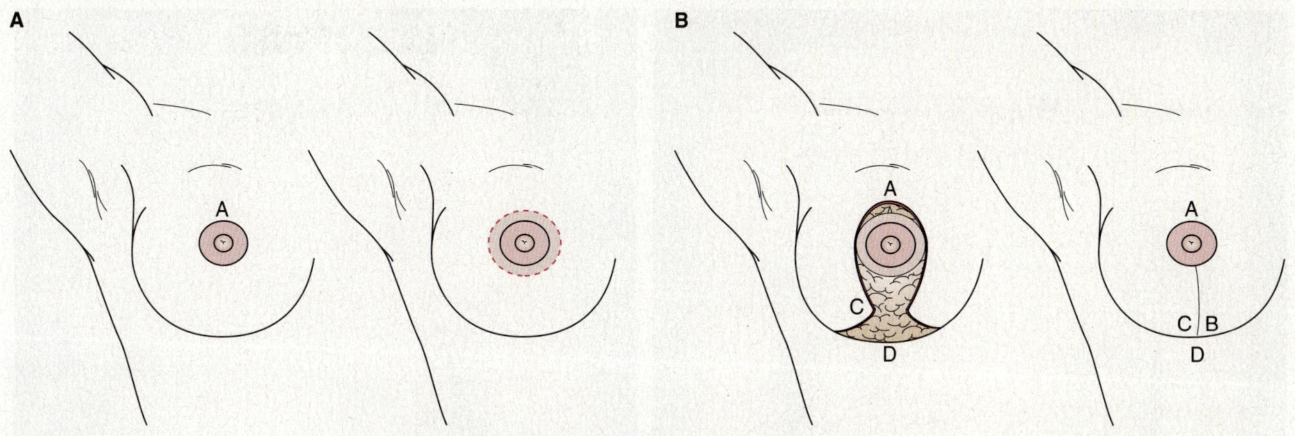

Figure 103.36. Mastopexy incisions. **A:** Circumareolar. **B:** Vertical.

are divided more narrowly or widely. In addition, the patient will not attain significant upper pole fullness (often considered cleavage), since the upper border of the breast will be minimally changed and will likely still demonstrate a more natural "ski-slope" contour. Surgery *will* improve ptosis and pseudoptosis and can remove striae (stretch marks) resulting from weight or volume changes related to conditions like pregnancy, breastfeeding, or change in body habitus. However, skin quality that has predisposed to striae may predispose to further stretching of the breast skin envelope over time and decrease the longevity of the postsurgical results. Surgical approaches are similar to those discussed above for breast reduction, and minimal scar approaches are chosen more frequently. NAC transposition is routine and risk of NAC loss or dysfunction is present and must be discussed preoperatively.[59] Insurance coverage for this procedure is variable. Imaging considerations are similar to those for breast reduction, both pre- and postoperatively (**Fig. 103.36**).[56,58]

Augmentation Mammoplasty

Breast augmentation is designed to increase breast size and influences breast shape and nipple position. Preoperative counseling is essential as decision for this surgery is most often driven by patient desire rather than abnormal symptomatology or danger to health. Preoperative considerations relate to patient expectations and should include financial planning including potential future medical interventions related to the index surgery. Intraoperative choices relate to material used for augmentation, incision (scar location), and manipulation of the pectoralis major muscle. Postoperative considerations relate to activities, garments, and future treatment.

Preoperative Evaluation

Patients should be assessed for the rationale of their interest in augmentation mammoplasty and their expectations for the impact surgery will have on their life. Goals related to size, lateral breast profile (eg, the "hourglass" look), upper pole appearance (also known as "cleavage"), and noticeability of the result should be discussed. If prosthetic implants are planned, counseling should include the components discussed in a subsequent section on breast implants. Existing soft tissue quality assessed through a pinch test is important for surgical approach planning.[60] A specific consideration in the preoperative workup is baseline mammography, and recommendations relate to patient age and breast cancer risk factors.[56] Patients planning to pay out of pocket will need to understand that the treatment of complications or maintenance surgery will not be covered by insurance.

Surgical Approaches

Table 103.9 addresses the main choices related to surgical approaches for breast augmentation.[60,61]

Table 103.9. Surgical Approaches for Augmentation Mammoplasty[60,61]

Surgical Approach	Options	Considerations
Incision/scar	Periareolar	Scar at junction of different types of skin considered minimally visible unless abnormal scarring occurs, requires dissection through breast gland
	Inframammary	Scar in fairly hidden location in most patient positions but through normally unmarked skin, IMF position may change with procedure
	Axillary	Somewhat remote, may make manipulation of surgical field more difficult
	Transumbilical	Remote from site, may make manipulation of surgical field more difficult
Implant placement	Subglandular	May help address a small amount of preoperative ptosis, may impact capsular contracture, increased visibility/palpability of implant if very thin soft tissue
	Partially submuscular	Multiple definitions, including "dual plane," considered to preserve surveillance imaging of gland more than subglandular approach
Augmentation material	Silicone implant	See "Breast Implants" section
	Saline implant	See "Breast Implants" section
	Autologous fat grafting	Use of liposuction to harvest slurry of tumescent solution, fat, oils, and other debris, followed by various fat separation techniques and injection of fat in small droplets throughout parenchyma of breast, imaging considerations as postoperative appearance is different than alternate augmentations

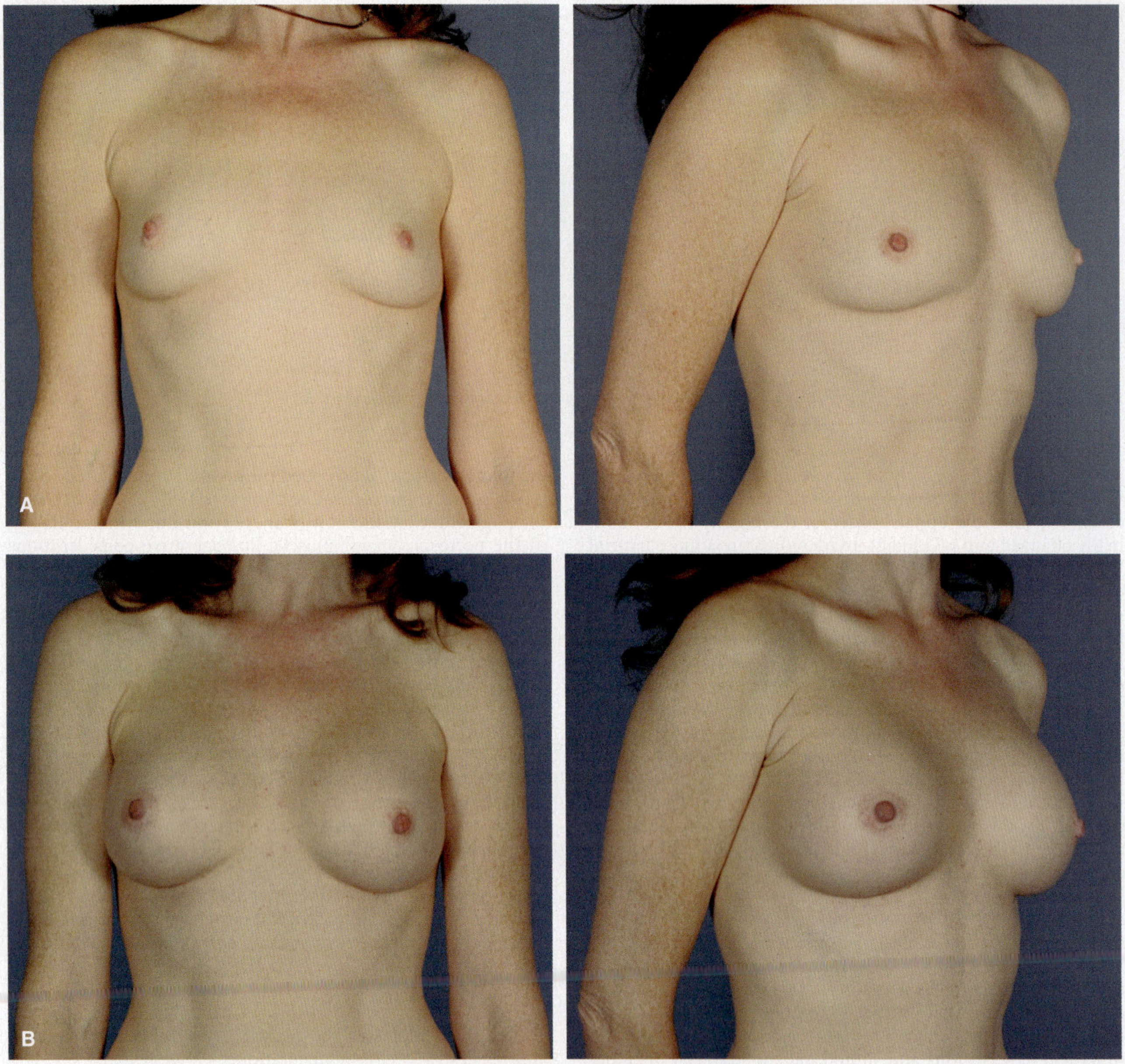

Figure 103.37. Breast augmentation via inferior mammary fold (IMF) incisions. **A:** Preoperative. **B:** Postoperative.

Postoperative Follow-Up

As patients undergoing this surgery are concerned with appearance, surgeons must convey careful consideration of return to exercise and use of postoperative garments. Massage techniques and timing and scar therapies are important components of the postoperative period. Follow-up is needed for prosthetic implants as they are not expected to last forever.[60] Important imaging considerations related specifically to breast implants are addressed in a subsequent section, and there may be changes to baseline breast imaging following breast implant placement (**Fig. 103.37**).[62]

Gynecomastia Reduction

Gynecomastia, or male breast enlargement, may have a variety of etiologies, including pubertal changes, hormonal abnormalities, medications, and testicular cancer. Assessing if and when to perform surgery is a critical component in the preoperative period. Surgical approaches differ significantly from those used for reduction of the female breast. Postoperative care remains important.

Preoperative Evaluation

Patients present with gynecomastia in many ways. Some may be young men, suffering from excess breast volume induced by pubertal changes. Many patients have waited years hoping for spontaneous resolution of the peripubertal onset gynecomastia. Others may be of variable age, complaining of breast tissue excess related to obesity, medications, or other medical conditions, including causes such as testicular cancer. Given the complex etiologies, spontaneous resolution in some cases, and potential for nonsurgical interventions, careful coordination with other medical providers is essential. Preoperatively, a full medical history and physical examination with formal endocrinology workup is completed. Imaging of the breast may be necessary, particularly if asymmetry, irregularity, or mass increases the suspicion of male breast cancer.[63]

Surgical Approaches

Surgical approaches account for the increased visibility of the male chest (making scars less acceptable than in female breast reduction), the dense, fibrous, gritty nature of male glandular enlargement, and the expected male NAC position and

Table 103.10. Surgical Approaches for Male Gynecomastia Reduction[64,65]

Approach	Consideration
Liposuction alone	Minimal scars, best used for gynecomastia with large adipose component and minimal skin excess
Marginal liposuction and direct periareolar excision of gland	Usually through partial periareolar scar, direct excision of gritty firm tissue under and around NAC with liposuction for feathering at margins, best if minimal skin excess
Amputation and nipple-areolar complex (NAC) skin grafting	Best for large amount of skin excess and NAC ptosis, scar for skin resection (transverse orientation) planned for subpectoralis muscle location often better tolerated than inframammary fold (IMF) since defined IMF in males is abnormal, direct excision of large amount of tissue in mastectomy-type approach, NAC position, and size planned to match more "normal" male appearance, best if enough preoperative ptosis that NAC excision site is removed in resection of excess skin
Pedicled nipple transposition approaches	Variety of approaches, often uniquely designed for each patient to address moderate amounts of skin excess, tissue excess, and NAC ptosis, must take care not to apply female reduction techniques designed to "cone" the breast into a female shape

size (drastically different than on the female breast). Many of the approaches have significant limitations. The more common approaches and their considerations are listed in **Table 103.10.**[64]

Postoperative Follow-Up

Routine postoperative care to follow healing is recommended. The diversity of surgical approaches necessitates a variety of postoperative regimens. Scar therapy may be important given the visibility of the surgical site.

Breast Reconstruction

Breast reconstruction follows oncologic resection, but similar techniques may be applied after trauma or developmental irregularities. Preoperative considerations are many and must include a multidisciplinary team approach for optimal outcomes. Surgical approaches are innumerable, regarding both technique and timing. Postoperative care largely focuses wound healing while recognizing the potential need for adjuvant oncologic treatments.

Preoperative Evaluation

Patients approach breast reconstruction with different goals, including appearance optimization with and without clothes, sensation, scar minimization, and restoration of the feel of the breast to palpation.[66] Neoadjuvant and adjuvant cancer treatments including radiation therapy, chemotherapy, and previous surgery may alter surgical reconstruction options. The surgical approaches span a diverse spectrum of complexity and techniques, making medical comorbidities important considerations. Patients must understand that reconstruction often requires staging with revisions to optimize outcomes. Differing surgical techniques impact length of postoperative follow-up and potential for future necessary surgical interventions.[67–69] The delivery of this information occurs during a fragile time when the patient has other medical decisions to make that can impact survival and quality of life. Surgical planning must recognize the difficulty experienced by patients when confronted by a large amount of information with multiple decisions to be made. Discussions must include future alternatives should complications arise or patients' preferences change.

Surgical Approaches

Table 103.11 addresses basic approaches to postmastectomy reconstruction technique.[67–72]

Timing is an essential consideration in breast reconstruction. Ideally, patients would have access to breast reconstruction counseling at the time of breast cancer diagnosis and initial treatment, but many patients present in delayed fashion after lumpectomy and radiation or mastectomy. Patients who have already undergone mastectomy who then desire reconstruction may consider tissue expansion followed by implant or autologous reconstruction or autologous reconstruction without expansion. Patients who present prior to mastectomy may consider immediate autologous reconstruction, immediate implant-based reconstruction, staging with a tissue expander, or planning for a delayed reconstruction.[67–69]

Free tissue transfer techniques have changed the approach
8 to autologous breast reconstruction. The use of pedicled rectus abdominis-based reconstruction (TRAM flap), has given way to the use of perforator flaps. The most widely used is based on the deep inferior epigastric perforators (DIEP flap). These flaps spare the rectus abdominis muscle and create a breast mound from excess lower abdominal wall adipose tissue. These free flaps have proven to be robust and tolerate radiation and chemotherapy well.

Other cancer treatments may impact reconstruction choices. Radiation therapy increases wound healing complications, infections, and overall failures in implant-based reconstructions. Autologous reconstruction is commonly performed in the setting of radiation in order to deliver healthy soft tissue into a damaged area. Chemotherapy may alter the body's resistance to infections and may adjust timing of reconstructive surgeries. Nipple-sparing procedures preserve the skin envelope and the natural breast architecture, but they allow for little manipulation of the skin envelope when irradiated.[67,68]

Reconstruction after lumpectomy and radiation therapy is another consideration. If planned prior to lumpectomy, oncoplastic breast rearrangement techniques can be utilized. These include reductions, mastopexy, and complex tissue rearrangements through various scar patterns. The contralateral breast can also be addressed for symmetry. Operating to reduce deformity after lumpectomy and radiotherapy has increased the risks of complications such as wound healing and infections. Techniques that can be used in these circumstances include autologous fat grafting, implant placement, autologous flap reconstruction, or mastectomy and reconstruction.[67,74]

Postoperative Follow-Up

Postoperative follow-up is routine and occurs over a longer time frame given the frequently staged nature of reconstruction. Postsurgical drains are generally used. Complications can include: compromised skin, wound healing problems, infections, and seromas which can impact the overall reconstructive success (**Figs. 103.38 and 103.39**).[67,69]

Gender Affirming Surgery

Gender affirming surgery is increasing in frequency and represents a broad range of procedures that help transgender and

Table 103.11. Postmastectomy Breast Reconstruction Techniques[67–73]

Surgical Approach	Options	Considerations
Autologous tissue	Pedicled flaps (ie, latissimus dorsi, thoracodorsal artery perforator [TDAP], rectus abdominus)	Requires donor site, often requires muscle sacrifice
	Free tissue transfer (ie, rectus abdominus, deep inferior epigastric perforator [DIEP], superficial inferior epigastric perforator [SIEP], superior/inferior gluteal artery perforator [SGAP/IGAP], transverse/diagonal upper gracilis [TUG/DUG])	Requires donor site, perforator flaps designed to preserve muscle and minimize morbidity, longer surgeries with more inpatient requirements, more similar to natural breast tissue, maintenance surgeries not usually required after reconstruction complete
	Fat grafting	Minimal scarring at donor site, often requires multiple stages to achieve volume other methods accomplish in one surgery, often used as a revision technique
Implants	Tissue expander	Used as staging, temporary changeable volume implant with port for repeated transcutaneous access, can be prepectoral or subpectoral, recently the prepectoral location has been rapidly gaining popularity
	Implant (ie, silicone vs saline, round vs anatomic, textured vs smooth)	Likely requires maintenance surgery, requires adequate skin envelope, foreign body, shorter surgeries with fewer inpatient admissions, also can be prepectoral or subpectoral (see above), see "Breast Implant" section for further details
Biologics	Acellular dermal matrices	Used as an adjunct for tissue reinforcement, often used to reinforce the breast pocket, particularly with implant-based reconstruction or to reinforce the fascia at an autologous donor site (usually abdomen)

non-binary people transition to their gender identity. A multidisciplinary approach to breast surgery is essential. Hormonal interventions are included in the complete approach. Future cancer risk must also be addressed. Insurance coverage has increased over time, expanding the reach of these techniques. Surgical approaches in converting a female-appearing chest to a male-appearing chest are like those considered for gynecomastia surgery, particularly regarding scar location and NAC position and size. Converting a male-appearing chest to a female-appearing chest includes consideration of augmentation with special emphases on differences in baseline anatomy, amount of breast tissue and composition, pectoralis muscle differences, and potential staging due to stretch of tissue over time. Postoperative care remains important as discussed above.[75,76]

Breast Implants

Patient should be made aware of several factors including: predicted lifespan of implants, likelihood of leakage of contents over time, expectation of imaging and further surgery, and decreased ability to image as much of the breast tissue with mammography following implant placement. Anaplastic large cell lymphoma has been linked to breast implants and is under active study. Breast implant illness (BII) with associated systemic symptoms (malaise, arthralgias, and many others) are also being investigated, and impacts only a small number of patients with implants. Patients will require counseling regarding smooth versus textured implants, silicone versus saline implants, and anatomic versus round implants. Current imaging recommendations for silicone implants should be discussed.[77–79]

AESTHETIC SURGERY

Plastic surgery at its core is a function of restoring structure and function. A principle such as "replace like with like" seems basic; however, it is challenging on many levels as one recognizes from other sections of this chapter. A myriad of unique clinical issues must be addressed from scalp to toe and requires a full understanding of anatomy. In addition to the restoration of function in reconstructive plastic surgery, the discipline of plastic surgery encompasses aesthetic plastic surgery, colloquially termed "cosmetic surgery." The quest to surpass normalcy and achieve "perfection" requires an artistic approach to medicine and is paramount in guiding patients who are seeking to enhance their own self-esteem and body image. In the process of undergoing these procedures, a functional benefit may also result. After undergoing an abdominoplasty, repair of the rectus abdominis muscle diastasis has been noted to help patients improve posture, increase core strength, and decrease stress urinary incontinence—all sequelae of term pregnancy. A rhinoplasty improves the overall outward appearance of a patient's face, but also may improve nasal airway breathing.

9

No surgical discipline requires greater attention to the patient's underlying psychological conditions/stability than aesthetic surgery. Carefully selected patients with realistic goals who have an appropriately executed procedure are likely to be highly satisfied. However, a patient who is poorly selected with unrealistic goals or elements of psychological instability may undergo a perfectly successful operation with an aesthetically pleasing outcome could be viewed as a colossal failure in the eyes of the patient leading to devastating consequences. Aesthetic surgery requires the surgeon to pay meticulous attention to detail, carefully select patients, rigorously plan procedures, and precisely execute technically challenging procedures. Identifying the motivations of patients for undergoing the procedures is also important and through application of sound surgical principles and technical expertise, the aesthetic plastic surgeon will experience success.

10

Cosmetic Procedures for the Head and Neck

Brow Lift

A natural sequela of facial aging is often brow ptosis. The dynamic nature of the frontalis muscle results in patients often contracting the muscle to elevate the brow to decrease the

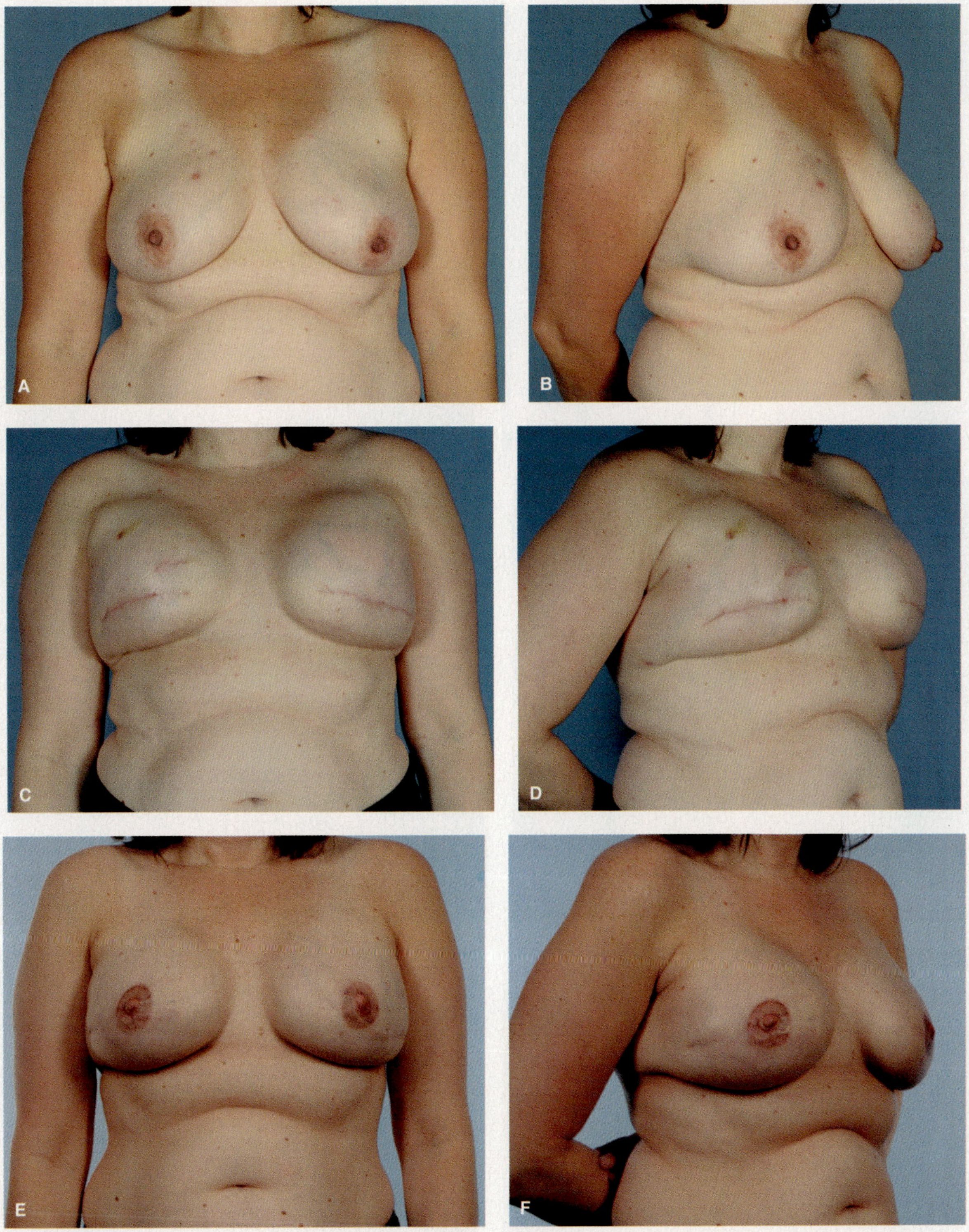

Figure 103.38. Staged bilateral implant-based breast reconstruction. **A, B:** Preoperative appearance. **C, D:** After tissue expansion. **E, F:** Final postoperative results after expander exchange for implant and nipple-areola complex tattooing.

appearance of patient's ptosis. When left untreated, brow ptosis results in patients appearing fatigued, angry, and/or aged. In severe cases, brow ptosis may cause visual field obstruction on upward gaze; correction of this deformity can produce dramatic aesthetic and functional improvements. Patients are often not aware of their brow ptosis and may present to the plastic surgeon's office complaining of "heavy eyelids." In many cases, the etiology of their complaint is brow ptosis rather than upper eyelid ptosis or dermatochalasis. These patients will require a brow life alone, or in conjunction with a blepharoplasty (a rejuvenating procedure that may be performed on the upper and/or lower eyelids), to correct their aesthetic and functional concerns.

Correction of brow ptosis can be achieved with either an open or endoscopic approach. The traditional open approach requires a bicoronal incision with resection of excess scalp or forehead. Unfortunately, this approach results in a lengthy scar, possible scar alopecia, and paresthesia of the scalp and forehead due to transection of branches of the supraorbital and supratrochlear nerves. In addition, an open coronal brow lift in male

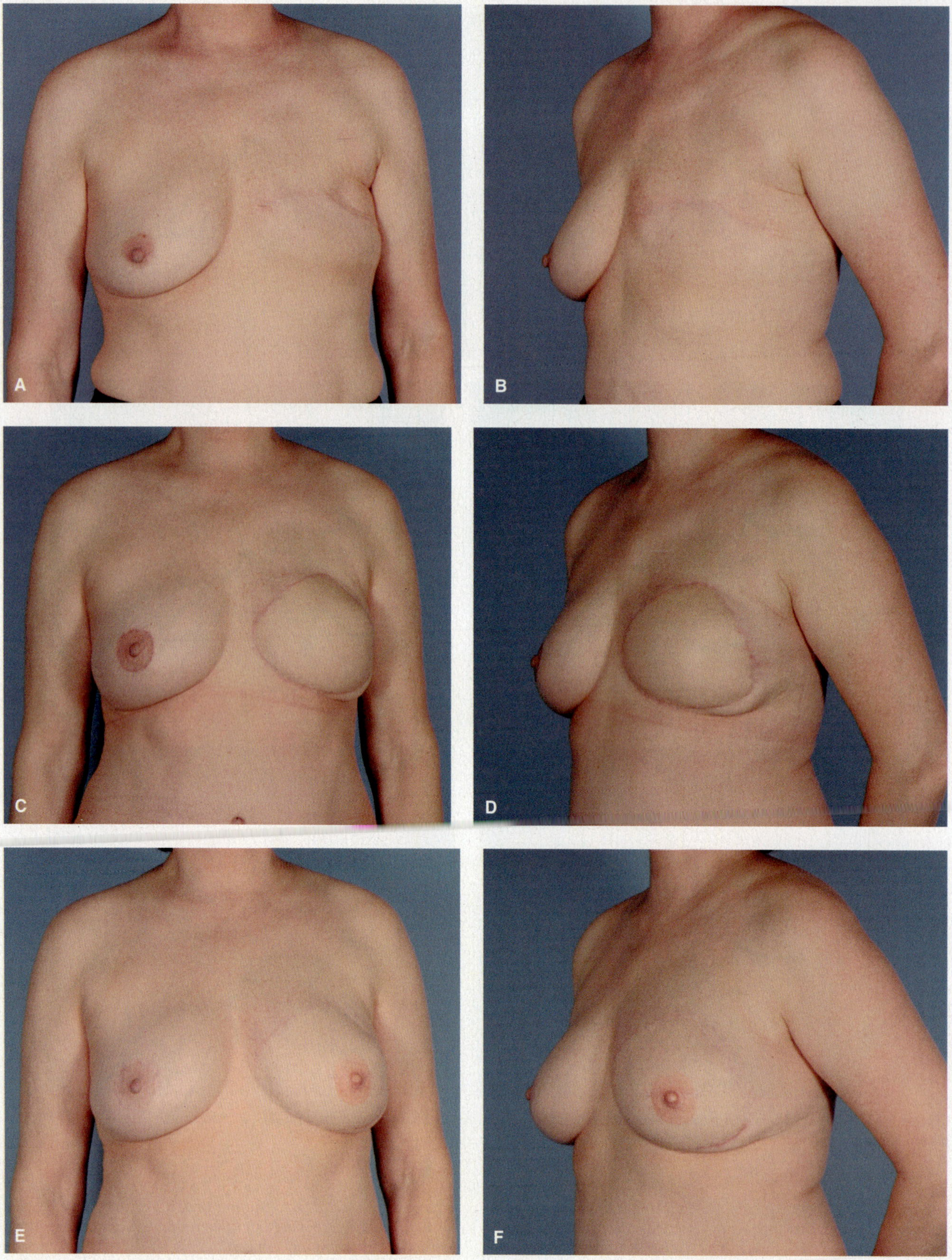

Figure 103.39. Delayed DIEP breast reconstruction. **A, B:** Appearance after mastectomy. **C, D:** Appearance after left DIEP flap reconstruction. **E, F:** Final result after tattooing of nipple-areola complex.[5]

patients with a receding hairline or female patient with an elongated forehead requires resection of hair-bearing scalp moving non–hair-bearing forehead skin further posteriorly accentuating baldness. This tradeoff is not worth the aesthetic deformity of increasing the appearance of hairline recession. Techniques have evolved to decrease scar burden by performing temporal incision-only brow lifts. The limitations of this approach include minimal correction of central brow ptosis and medial eyebrow depression. To counteract the accentuation of a receding hairline from the bicoronal approach, an anterior hairline brow lift incision evolved which involves placing the incision at the junction of the hairline and forehead skin. Most male patients are not a candidate for this procedure as many men will experience elements of hairline thinning anteriorly. Female patients with elongated foreheads do well with this approach, however, are reluctant to wear their hair in a ponytail as they will expose a visible scar. Male patients can opt for a direct brow lift approach, which involves selecting a deep horizontal forehead rhytid and resecting skin above or below, placing the scar in the original rhytid. After 6 to 12 months of healing, the incision is often camouflaged within the natural crease. Finally, to reduce many of the complications associated with open approaches, the endoscopic brow lift was developed and has become the primary approach for repair of brow ptosis.[80] The endoscopic brow lift requires only three to five 1-cm incisions behind the hairline to gain access to the forehead and glabellar rhytids, producing less of a deformity and limiting the amount of scarring. There is also evidence to suggest that the endoscopic approach produces a more lasting result than the traditional approach.[81] Finally, it has been reported that paresthesia's of the forehead and scalp are significantly reduced when an endoscopic approach is utilized for correction of brow ptosis, as compared to an open coronal approach.

Endoscopic and open brow lifts may be performed under local or general anesthesia. Patients are marked preoperatively in the upright position. The desired brow position is at the level of the orbital rim in male patients and 1 cm above the orbital rim in female patients. The position of the brow in relation to the supraorbital rim changes from medial to lateral; the lateral brow should be more elevated than the medial brow. During an open brow lift, a coronal incision is made and the entire forehead it mobilized in the subgaleal or subperiosteal plane down to the orbital rim. The supraorbital and supratrochlear nerves are dissected free of surrounding tissues and protected. The supraorbital muscle is resected if prominent glabellar rhytids are present. Excessive resection of the corrugator muscles will result in widening of the eyebrows in the midline. The periosteum is released at the level of supraorbital rim when a subperiosteal plane is utilized for mobilization of the forehead; the dissection is carried down to the level of the supraorbital rim when a subgaleal plane is used for forehead mobilization. The forehead is then elevated and redraped posteriorly, the redundant scalp is resected, and the wound is closed. In an endoscopic brow lift, incisions are made within the hair-bearing scalp at the midpupillary line and over the temporal fossa. The entire forehead flap is elevated under endoscopic guidance, the procerus and corrugator muscles are resected as necessary, and the forehead is retracted posteriorly. The forehead is then secured into its new position. Various methods of forehead fixation have been described including absorbable and nonabsorbable plates, screws, multipronged anchors, or cortical tunnels.[82]

Postoperatively, patients are instructed to avoid vigorous physical exercise for at least 6 weeks. Bruising and swelling are anticipated for the first 2 to 3 weeks following the procedure. The final result is not expected for at least 6 to 8 weeks following the procedure. Patients are instructed that the final scar appearance will take between 9 and 12 months postsurgery.

Rhytidectomy

Few areas of the body betray the age of an individual as greatly as the face. The negative impacts of aging process, gravity presence, solar exposure, and smoking are particularly manifested on the face. The loss of skin elasticity which leads to fine facial wrinkling and skin laxity can be attributed to ultraviolet radiation and tobacco. Aging and gravity result in gradual relaxation of the facial retaining ligaments producing midfacial ptosis, deepened nasolabial folds, "jowling" along the mandibular border, and redundancy of cervical skin.[83] Many patients become aware of these aging features while reminiscing on old photographs, as their youthful appearance consisting of high cheekbones, a sharp mandibular border, and smooth skin is more apparent. As the aging process continues and a patient reflects on their former features, they may lose self-confidence while interacting in professional and social settings. This drop in self-esteem often leads one to seek consultation with a plastic surgeon who will evaluate and recommend a facial rejuvenation plan to restore their youthful facial features. After this process is carefully completed, both the patient and surgeon will see gratifying results.

During the original consultation, the patient first outlines their expectations and motivations, which are then evaluated by the surgeon. It is important that the concerns of the patient are reasonable and not out of proportion to their physical features. If this does occur, a perfectly executed operation may have an undesirable outcome in the eyes of the patient.

Many surgeons will refuse to perform a cervicofacial rhytidectomy in any patient who is actively smoking or using any products containing nicotine. This is due to the significantly increased risk for developing postoperative complications, including skin flap necrosis, infection, and/or wound dehiscence. Patients are instructed to quit prior to undergoing elective aesthetic surgery, and whether a patient has been using nicotine is confirmed preoperatively with urine cotinine levels. Additionally, patients with coexisting medical illnesses require preoperative medical clearance and referred to a general practitioner for medical optimization if needed. If the patient is deemed a moderate or high risk for general anesthesia because of medical comorbidities, then the operation is postponed until the medical conditions are optimized. The surgery will ultimately be cancelled if the risk of anesthesia is too high for a patient.

Patients between the ages of 40 and 50 years with good skin quality, mild midfacial ptosis, and early "jowling" may benefit from a minimally invasive facelift. This operation is typically combined with an endoscopic brow lift to provide upper and lower facial rejuvenation with minimal scarring and is performed under local or general anesthesia. First, bilateral temporal and superior buccal sulcus incisions are made. The temporal face dissection is then carried down to the level of the superficial layer of the deep temporal fascia. Under endoscopic guidance, the superficial layer of the deep temporal fascia is then incised to expose the temporal fat pad. The dissection then proceeds caudally until the zygomatic arch is identified. A subperiosteal plane of the dissection provides access to the midface while avoiding the frontal branch of the facial nerve. The subperiosteal plane of dissection is continued into the midface with care taken to avoid the infraorbital nerves. The masseter is mobilized from its lateral attachments. The superior buccal sulcus incisions are made, and a midface subperiosteal dissection is performed under both direct visualization and endoscopic guidance. Once the dissection is completed, the entire midface is suspended in the desired position with sutures or specialized anchors spanning from the superficial layer of the deep temporal fascia to the midface periosteum. Symmetry of the suspension is then confirmed, and the wounds are closed by layers. Mild midface ptosis, mild jowling, and early nasolabial fold prominence can all be corrected through this procedure, however deformities with moderate to severe skin laxity will not be corrected with this technique. To fix the latter, a traditional cervicofacial rhytidectomy is required.[82,84]

A traditional rhytidectomy can be performed under local or general anesthesia in patients who require resection of excess skin. The skin incision is made over the temporal fossa 4 to 5 cm cephalad to the root of the helix and extends caudally toward the apex of the ear. The incision is then extended anterior to the ear, behind the tragus, around the base of the earlobe into the retroauricular sulcus, across the mastoid, and caudally along the anterior hairline of the neck. The skin flap is then elevated just superficial to the superficial musculoaponeurotic system (SMAS) and platysma. This plane of dissection maintains a thin layer of subcutaneous fat on the skin flap to preserve viability, while avoiding injury to the facial nerve branches, greater auricular nerve, parotid gland, and jugular vein. The flaps are elevated medially to the nasolabial fold in the face and to the midline in the neck. In some operations, a platysmal diastasis may exist which creates platysmal banding, an obtuse cervicomental angle, and a prominent neck. If this occurs, a platysmal plication may be performed through a 2- to 3-cm submental incision to correct the diastasis and improve the appearance of the neck. At this point, the remainder of the cervicofacial rhytidectomy can be performed in a variety of ways, all with the goal of repositioning the tissues that have migrated with gravity, leading to facial aging changes. The surgeon may simply choose to not perform any additional dissection at this point and simply reposition the skin, resect the excess skin, and close the incisions. The surgeon may also choose to do one of the following: SMAS plication, standard SMAS dissection, extended SMAS dissection, or deep-plane dissection. All these operations are designed to improve facial and cervical tightening, while reducing the tension on the skin closure. Once the dissection of the facial tissues is completed and all planes are mobilized optimally, the SMAS and platysma are placed under tension and secured to create the desired facial appearance. The skin flaps are then redraped posteriorly, the patient is examined for symmetry, and a skin resection is performed. Hemostasis is obtained through judicious use of bipolar electrocautery. The wounds are closed in layers and a pressure dressing is applied. Drains are typically used in both the face and neck.[7,85–88]

Postoperatively, the patient is evaluated for any evidence of a hematoma or facial nerve injury. Identifying a hematoma early is crucial to avoid overlying skin necrosis. Facial nerve injuries occur in 2% to 3% of cases. On the first postoperative day, the pressure dressings and drains are removed, and the patient is examined for evidence of a late hematoma, unrecognized facial nerve injury, or compromised skin flap. Patients should expect to have significant swelling and bruising for at least 2 weeks following the procedure. The final postoperative desired outcome is not realized until 6 months following the procedure (**Fig. 103.40**).

Blepharoplasty

Eyelid surgery is one of the most frequently performed cosmetic procedures. Blepharoplasty is often employed to correct both functional and/or aesthetic deformities. Visual field obstruction, or an angry, aged, and tired look in the patient may occur due to excessive skin and fat of the eyelids. In older patients, excess skin and wrinkling may occur, whereas in younger patients, persistent bags under their eyes or fine wrinkling ("crow's feet") at the lateral canthus are most common. Each clinical entity requires a unique approach based on the diagnosis and presentation, and meticulous attention to details is critical for the successful outcome of a blepharoplasty.[89] Preoperatively, all patients considering blepharoplasty should undergo a complete ophthalmologic examination to evaluate visual acuity, upper lid ptosis, exophthalmos, lower eyelid laxity, and symptoms of "dry" eye. Should lower lid laxity be present, and a standard blepharoplasty is performed, the patient may develop a lower lid malposition with ectropion postoperatively. Blepharoplasty may also significantly exacerbate symptoms of dry eye. Because of this, it is critically important to perform a comprehensive evaluation of the health of the eye prior to performing any eyelid surgery.

Once the optimal health of the eye is confirmed, an operative plan can be formulated and executed to correct the concerns of the patient. The operation can be performed under local or general anesthesia. The blepharoplasty incisions are first designed preoperatively with the patient in the upright position. Older patients frequently require skin excisions or repositioning and/or removal of orbital fat prior to the operation. To begin, local anesthesia with epinephrine is infiltrated for pain control and hemostasis.

The upper eyelid blepharoplasty begins with an elliptical excision of upper eyelid skin and orbicularis oculi muscle. This skin excision is designed based on the amount and location of the dermatochalasis. Very rarely will a patient require removal of fat from the upper eyelids, as excessive fat resections will produce a "hollowed-out" appearance. Under some circumstances there may be a substantial amount of excess orbital fat in the upper eyelids and conservative fat resection may be helpful to achieve the desired postoperative outcome. If fat resection is planned, small openings are made in the orbital septum to gain access to the two compartments of periorbital fat. Conservative fat resection is then performed to avoid a

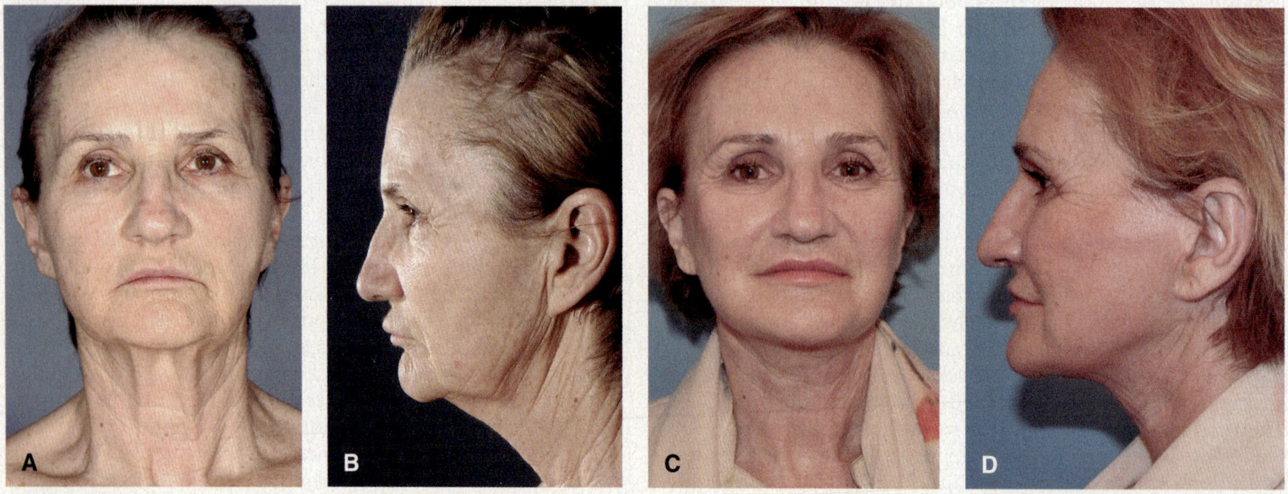

Figure 103.40. A 63-year-old female presented to the office concerned with facial aging. The patient was displeased with the overall appearance of fatigue and looking sad, despite feeling well and energetic (**A, B**). She requested facial rejuvenation of the eyes, cheeks, neck, and overall skin texture. The patient underwent a facelift, neck lift, periorbital rejuvenation, and facial laser resurfacing. She is pictured here 1 week prior to surgery (**A, B**) and 1 year after her procedure (**C, D**).

postoperative hollowed-out appearance. The skin is then redraped and the wounds are closed in a single layer. If an upper lid blepharoplasty and brow lift are being performed within the same operation, the brow lift should be performed first, so that the amount of excess upper eyelid skin can be determined after the brow has been elevated.

The traditional lower eyelid blepharoplasty begins with a subciliary incision. A 4- to 5-mm rim of orbicularis oculi is then preserved along the lower eyelid margin. The dissection is then carried deep to the orbicularis oculi muscle until the orbital septum is identified. The orbital septum is then divided to gain access to the three compartments of periorbital fat in the lower lid. Fat may be resected in cases of prominent herniation, and it is necessary to avoid over resection. A trend in blepharoplasty surgery has emphasized repositioning the herniated periorbital fat over the inferior orbital rim rather than resecting fat in order to improve the appearance of the lower eyelids. This approach of repositioning the orbital septum medially has proven to be very helpful in eliminating tear trough deformities. Once the periorbital fat has been resected or repositioned, the skin/muscle flap is redraped superiorly and the redundant tissue is excised. The lower eyelid incisions are closed with interrupted 6-0 nylon sutures. Ancillary procedures, including a medial canthoplasty, a lateral canthoplasty, lateral canthopexy, or horizontal lid shortening may also be necessary to improve the position of the lower eyelid. If a lower lid blepharoplasty is being performed in conjunction with a rhytidectomy, the rhytidectomy should be performed first, so that the amount of excess lower eyelid skin can be determined after the facial soft tissues have been elevated.

The tired appearance of the lower eyelids is commonly the result of excessive or herniated periorbital fat in younger patients. A lower lid blepharoplasty through a transconjunctival approach allows for the removal or repositioning of the periorbital fat without creating an external scar. First, the conjunctiva is divided transversely 1 mm above the sulcus to gain access to the orbital septum. The septum is then divided, and the periorbital fat is removed or repositioned from all three compartments. Preserving the periorbital fat and simply repositioning the orbital septum into a more optimal location, obviates the need for fat resections. The transconjunctival incision is allowed to heal by secondary intention, allowing rejuvenation of the lower lids without an external incision. Recently, a multiplanar approach for the rejuvenation of the lower eyelids has been employed to reduce the incidence of lower eyelid ectropion postoperatively. These approaches combine both subciliary incisions for removal of excess skin and transconjunctival incision for repositioning or resection of the periorbital fat. Experienced plastic surgeons have demonstrated outstanding outcomes with this approach. In conjunction with the non–external incision lower blepharoplasty, the surgeon can treat the lower eyelid skin with a resurfacing laser. The use of ablation and coagulation during full field ablative lasers induces a calculated "burn" of the skin leading to contraction and skin quality improvement. This technique often precludes the need for actual skin resection leading to no visible scar.

Postoperatively, patients are immediately evaluated for corneal abrasions, changes in visual acuity, or hematomas, which may require emergent intervention. Artificial tears are used to maintain appropriate lubrication and sutures are removed 5 to 7 days following the operation. Patients are instructed to avoid vigorous physical exercise during the early postoperative period. It is expected that patients will be bruised and swollen for approximately 2 weeks following the blepharoplasty and that it will be approximately 6 to 8 weeks before the desired outcome is noticed.

Rhinoplasty

No aesthetic surgical procedure may be a "game of millimeters" more than rhinoplasty. Cosmetic surgery of the nose requires meticulous planning and execution often involving alteration of both the external appearance and internal anatomy of the nose. The nose may be aesthetically unappealing or functionally impaired as a result of trauma, surgery, or from a congenital deformity. Different familial and ethnic traits give rise to a variety of nasal appearances. Because of this, it is necessary that any expectations the patient has regarding the procedure are realistic and achievable and align with the goals of the surgeon. The patient must be prepared physically and mentally for the operation.

Preoperatively, a complete nasal history is obtained with particular attention paid to nasal airway obstruction, allergies, trauma, and previous surgery. A photographic analysis is performed to evaluate facial and nasal dimensions. The surgeon examines the photographs, discusses the plan with the patient, and the potential structural and functional outcomes are reviewed.

Rhinoplasty may be performed under local or general anesthesia. The patient is prepared for surgery by intranasal injections of vasoconstrictors containing lidocaine and epinephrine. Topical vasoconstrictors are applied to the nasal lining and septum. The operation can be performed in an "open" or "closed" fashion. The open technique requires a transcolumellar incision extended intranasally to allow exposure of the cartilage and bones of the nose. Direct visualization of the nose structure allows for greater precision with cartilaginous sculpting, grafting, and nasal bone repositioning. The paired lower lateral cartilages create the shape and provide the support for the nasal tip. Any deformity involving the nasal tip requires manipulations of this cartilage, including resections for a bulbous or over projecting tip, suturing to reposition an asymmetric nasal tip, or cartilage grafting to increase tip projection. The paired upper lateral cartilages and nasal bones define the shape of the nasal dorsum and control nasal airflow. A prominent dorsal hump may require resections of both the upper lateral cartilages and nasal bones. Osteotomies of the nasal bones may be required to narrow nasal width by disconnecting the base of the nasal bones from the maxilla. In contrast, "saddle nose" deformities may require cartilage or bone grafting to provide dorsal augmentation. Alloplastic materials have been described for use as dorsal graft, tip grafts, or columellar struts to increase nasal projection. Many surgeons discourage use of such alloplastic grafts due to problems with infection, extrusion, and migration producing a suboptimal result acutely or chronically. Autogenous cartilage grafts from the nasal septum, ear, or rib may also be used to improve nasal appearance or airflow. These grafts can be harvested and sculpted to create the desired cosmetic appearance of the nasal dorsum and tip. "Spreader grafts" can also be placed between the nasal septum and the upper lateral cartilage to increase the size of the internal nasal valve area, improving nasal airflow. The "closed" rhinoplasty technique allows access to the nasal cartilage and bones through intranasal incisions. This is the preferred method of experienced rhinoplasty surgeons because it is less invasive, however it is more to perform many of the complicated cartilage grafting and suturing techniques with limited exposure.

Following the rhinoplasty, an external splint is used to maintain the position of the nasal bones and cartilage for 10 to 14 days. Patients are instructed to keep their head elevated and apply ice packs, and should expect nasal swelling, pain, and bruising for 2 to 3 weeks. If osteotomies are performed, the patient may also experience periorbital ecchymosis. A full year is required for complete resolution of nasal tip swelling, especially if an open-tip rhinoplasty has been performed. Approximately 10% of primary rhinoplasty patients will require an operative revision due to dissatisfaction with the cosmetic or functional outcome. Any revision procedures should not occur for at least 1 year following the original surgery in order to ensure all postoperative swelling and tissue remodeling has stabilized.

Genioplasty

Often performed in conjunction with rhinoplasty, facial harmony is achieved by simultaneously performing a genioplasty. This frequently performed operation improves facial appearance by manipulating the position of the central mandible aka "chin." The vertical height and anterior projection of the chin can be adjusted due to the design of the mandibular symphysis osteotomy.[90] An advancement genioplasty may be performed in patients with a "weak" chin to enhance chin projection and improve the cervicomental angle. Chin augmentation may also be accomplished with an alloplastic implant, eliminating the need for an osteotomy. A reduction genioplasty may be performed in patients with a very prominent chin, where the vertical height and anterior projection are reduced. The lip position and neck appearance may be altered from these procedures; however, the dental occlusion is not affected.

After the initial consultation, a complete physical examination, photographic analysis, and radiographic evaluation are performed to evaluate facial harmony and determine the extent of the advancement or reduction. Dental occlusion is also carefully examined to ensure that orthognathic surgery is not required to correct chin position.

These operations are typically performed under general anesthesia but can be performed under local anesthesia if desired. Local anesthesia containing epinephrine is first injected intraorally for hemostasis and postoperative pain control. An inferior buccal sulcus incision allows access to the mandibular symphysis. The osteotomy is then measured and marked based on the preoperative photographs and lateral radiographs, while avoiding the mental foramen. The bony segment is mobilized and secured in its new position with plates and screws. If an alloplastic chin augmentation is to be performed, incisions can be performed in the submental region or intraorally to allow placement of the implant. Postoperatively, the swelling and pain is expected for approximately 4 to 6 weeks. During this time, the patient is instructed to perform meticulous oral hygiene and avoid foods that may traumatize the inferior buccal sulcus incision.

Cosmetic Procedures of the Trunk and Extremities (Body Sculpting)

Abdominoplasty

In recent years, there has been tremendous emphasis on body contouring. The explosion of technology-based nonsurgical modalities has led to increased interest in improving the appearance of the trunk. Abdominoplasty surgery addresses abdominal deformities such as excess abdominal skin, fatty tissue, and abdominal wall laxity through a variety of surgical procedures. Abnormalities in any of these areas may create an aesthetically unappealing abdomen. These procedures, which include dermatolipectomy, liposuction, and abdominal wall plication can correct the underlying pathology and are often combined and tailored to fit the surgical needs and desires of the patient. It is critical to define the cause responsible for the abdominal deformity so that the appropriate operative procedure or combination of procedures can be planned and executed.[91,92]

A standard abdominoplasty combines a dermatolipectomy, liposuction, and abdominal wall plication to correct deformity in each of the three previously mentioned abdominal wall layers. The operation is performed under general anesthesia and starts with a lower transverse, bikini-line incision extending from the cephalad margin of the pubic escutcheon to the iliac crests bilaterally. Once the skin incisions are made, the abdominal flap is elevated from the underlying abdominal wall fascia. A circumferential incision is made around the umbilicus to allow complete elevation of the abdominal flap up to the costal margin. The patient is then placed in a flexed position, the abdominal flap is redraped caudally, and the redundant skin resected. If any abdominal wall laxity is identified along with the skin redundancy, a vertical, midline abdominal wall plication can be performed. Occasionally, suction-assisted lipectomy (SAL) is performed at the time of abdominoplasty to help contour the abdomen and flanks. Aggressive SAL of the abdomen flap, however, may compromise flap vascularity and contribute to flap necrosis. It is helpful to perform SAL along the lateral and posterior iliac crests bilaterally to reduce the prominence which may have developed following the anterior dermatolipectomy and caudal repositioning of the skin flap. A small incision is then made in the midline of the abdomen at the level of the iliac crests for delivery of the umbilicus into its new position. Closed-suction drains are placed prior to wound closure, but not necessary. In this instance, employing a series of progressive tension sutures is paramount to close the dead space. Typically, a series of 15 to 20 sutures are used to approximate the Scarpa fascia to the anterior rectus sheath.

A "mini-abdominoplasty" can be performed to treat mild abdominal skin redundancy and abdominal wall laxity. The previously described approach regarding a standard abdominoplasty is executed, except the skin incision is limited to the central portion of the abdomen. A limited skin resection can be performed through this approach along with an abdominal wall plication. If necessary, SAL can be used in combination with this procedure.

Endoscopic abdominoplasty can be used to treat abdominal wall laxity (ie, postpartum rectus diastasis) and localized collections of fatty tissue. Patients who undergo this procedure must have good skin quality and only mild to moderate lipodystrophy. The endoscopic abdominoplasty is performed through two incisions, a 3- to 5-cm transverse incision within the pubic hair and a circumferential incision around the umbilicus. These incisions function as the two access ports through which the endoscopic instruments are passed. The entire abdominal wall is then elevated off the abdominal wall fascia under endoscopic visualization with electrocautery, the midline of the abdominal wall is plicated from pubis to xiphoid, and the abdominal wall is then recontoured with SAL, which is also performed through the two incisions (**Fig. 103.41**).

Liposuction

Liposuction is one of the most frequently performed cosmetic surgery procedures. Sculpting the body through this well-described technique is designed to eradicate deposits of fat from isolated anatomic regions by utilizing various diameter cannulas with a myriad of port sizes and configuration. It should not considered a form of weight loss and is not performed in obese patients. Rather, patients who are within 20% to 30% of their ideal body weight and have localized collections of fat that are refractory to diet and exercise will see the greatest benefit. A complete evaluation of skin elasticity is necessary in patients who are considering liposuction because once fat is surgically removed, the skin must be able to contract down to the contour of the remaining subcutaneous tissue. If the skin quality is poor, then wrinkling, dimpling, or skin ptosis may severely compromise the desired aesthetic outcome.[91]

Over the past several years, various energy sources have been used in conjunction with SAL to liquefy fat and induce skin tightening by reaching a critical thermal threshold. Ultrasonic-assisted liposuction (UAL), laser-assisted liposuction (LAL), power-assisted liposuction (PAL), and helium plasma–assisted liposuction are the major types of energy and/or mechanical adjuvants to liposuction currently used. SAL can be used in all areas of the body, however its efficacy may be augmented by employing energy and/or mechanical power in more fibrous anatomic regions such as the flank, upper abdomen, or male breast.[91,93] A number of technologic advances have led to new techniques for performance of liposuction or liposculpting. None of these new techniques have yet to prove clinically superior in rigorous clinical trials, and standard SAL continues to be the most effective.

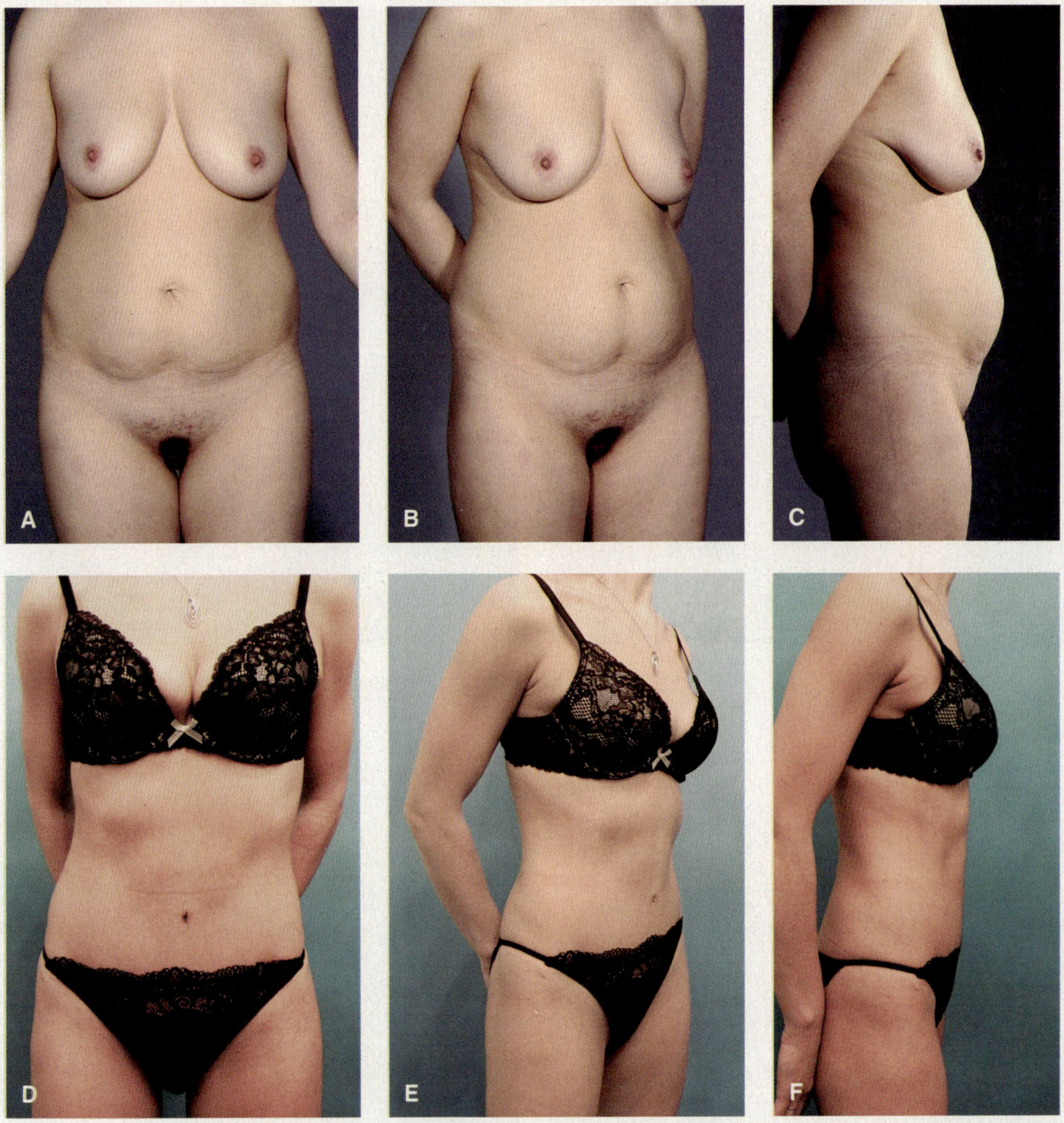

Figure 103.41. A 32-year-old female presented to the plastic surgery clinic with concerns related to the appearance of her abdomen. The patient was displeased with the "stomach" region after having three children. She had no further plans of having any children. Her primary complaints were extra skin and stretch marks above and below her umbilicus, fullness in the pubic region, and extra fat in her waist/love handles. The patient underwent a drain-less abdominoplasty with liposuction in the waist/love handles. She is pictured here 1 week prior to surgery (**A–C**) and 9 months after (**D–F**) her procedure.

As with all aesthetic procedures, it is necessary that patients undergo a complete evaluation preoperatively to ensure that their goals can be achieved through liposuction. Preoperative photographic documentation is performed on all patients. Markings are then made with the patient in the upright position. Access ports (6 to 8 mm), through which liposuction is performed, are marked in concealable areas. Patients can undergo these procedures under local or general anesthesia. Tumescent fluid (1000 mL of LR, 50 mL of 1% lidocaine, and 1 mg of epinephrine) is then infiltrated for pain control and hemostasis.

SAL is performed with metal cannulas connected to an aspirating device that generates a negative pressure of 1 atmosphere. Various cannula configurations are used to perform the resection. Fatty tissue is aspirated into the holes of the cannula and then resected by movement of the cannula tip. The operation is performed through multiple access ports, starting with large (6- to 8-mm diameter) cannulas and progressing to smaller (3- to 4-mm diameter) cannulas with fewer holes to allow more precise body contouring. Overlapping patterns of resection are used to avoid contour irregularities.

UAL and LAL are surgical techniques that allow body contouring through the liquefaction and aspiration of fatty tissue. Whether used alone or in combination with traditional SAL, UAL and LAL are effective for treating lipodystrophy in fibrous anatomic regions such as the flank, upper abdomen, and male breast. The UAL probe tip produces sound waves at an ultrasonic frequency of 20 to 30 kHz. The sound waves cause cavitation which disrupts lipocytes. LAL probe tip uses various nanometers of laser to heat and liquefy fat. Lower power suction is then employed to remove the resultant fluid. If UAL or LAL is used incorrectly, patients may experience severe complications, including full-thickness skin loss from incision and increased risk of seroma formation.

Postoperatively, all patients are placed in a compressive garment for 2 weeks, 24 hours per day. This early postoperative compression significantly reduces the incidence of a hematoma forming. Prolonged compression reduces swelling and skin wrinkling. All patients experience some degree of ecchymosis, swelling, and decreased sensibility. The final aesthetic result will not be realized for approximately 9 to 12 months following the procedure (**Fig. 103.42**).

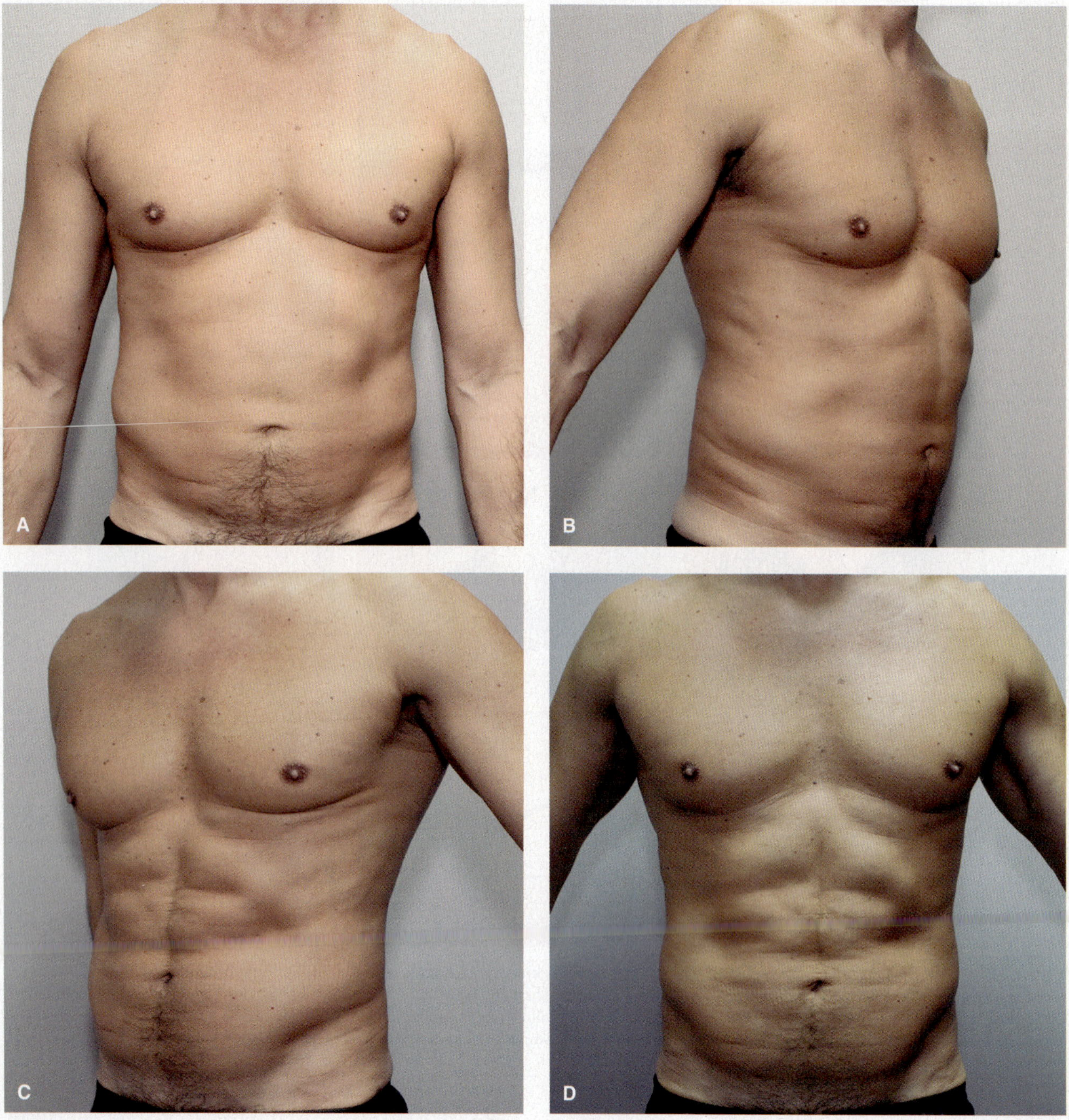

Figure 103.42. A 47-year-old male presented to the plastic surgery clinic with concerns of abdominal contour. Despite aggressive diet and exercise, he was not able to achieve the definition he wanted (**A, B**). The patient underwent power-assisted liposuction with further abdominal etching to the abdomen and bilateral love handles. He is pictured here before and 12 months after the procedure (**C, D**), respectively.

NONSURGICAL AESTHETIC PROCEDURES

Minimally Invasive Procedures

11 Though not surgical in nature, the authors would be remiss to not mention the advent of minimally invasive procedures, primarily injectables, in the aesthetic plastic surgeon's armamentarium. Entire textbooks are devoted to these treatments, however, for the sake of completeness and cursory overview, they are mentioned here. The 2002 FDA approval of Botox for moderate to severe frown lines resulted in a consequential skyrocket of the aesthetics industry.[94] In 2018 alone, 15.9 million minimally invasive cosmetic procedures were performed, a 228% increase since the year 2000.[94] In 2023, an estimated 25.4 million minimally invasive cosmetic procures were performed in the United States. Among the most popular of these treatments are three classes of injectables: neuromodulators, dermal fillers, and adipocytolytic agents.

Neuromodulators alter the interaction of a neuron with a neurotransmitter, and botulinum toxin type A specifically blocks the release of acetylcholine, the principal neurotransmitter at the neuromuscular junction.[95] When injected into the face, this causes temporary paralysis of the muscle, resulting in loss of function. Aesthetically, this is used to decrease the appearance of fine lines and creases. Botulinum toxin type A was first approved by the FDA in 1989 and is now the world's most frequently performed aesthetic procedure. In 2018, over 7.4 million injections were performed with botulinum toxin. The brand names include Botox, Dysport, Xeomin, and Jeuveau, and are most commonly injected to the forehead, glabellar, and crow's feet regions of the face. This muscle paralysis

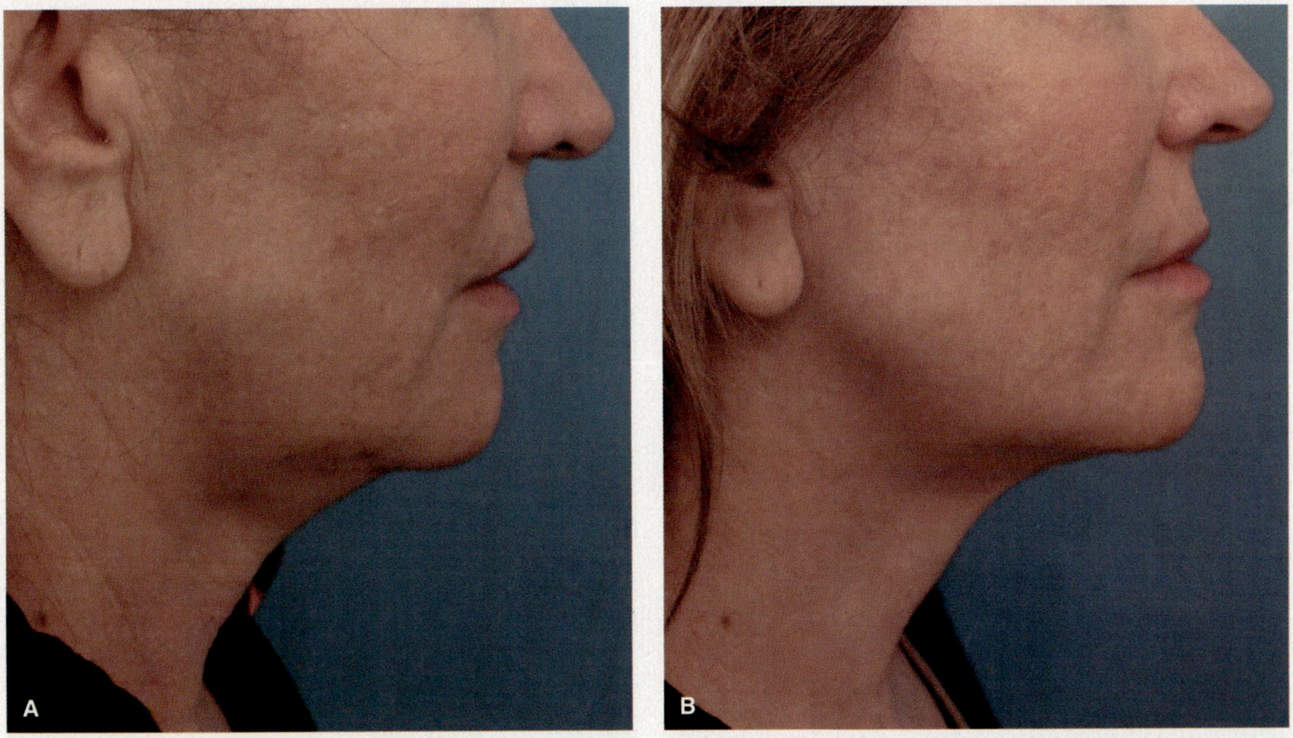

Figure 103.43. A 66-year-old female presented to the clinic interested in improving the excess fat and loose skin in her neck, but without any surgical intervention. Patient is pictured before (**A**) and 8 weeks after (**B**) her FIRST treatment with deoxycholic acid (Kybella). She also underwent dermal fillers along the jawline to improve the contour.

can last anywhere between 3 and 4 months, dependent on the metabolism of the patient.

Dermal fillers are a gel-like substance that when injected subcutaneously, intradermally and supraperiosteally, they restore volume, smooth lines and creases, and enhance the overall facial contour. This rejuvenation can be achieved through products consisting of either hyaluronic acid (HA), calcium hydroxylapatite (CaHA), and poly-L-lactic acid. Products compromised of HA, such as the Juvederm, Restylane, and Revanesse can keep the skin plump and hydrated anywhere from 6 to 12 months. CaHA products, such as Radiesse, last longer and assist in stimulating natural collagen production. However, unlike HA fillers, there is no reversal agent for calcium-based dermal fillers. Poly-L-lactic acid products, such as Sculptra, can last up to 2 years and stimulates natural collagen production.

Adipocytolic agents are the third class of injectables, with Kybella being the only FDA-approved product currently on the market. Kybella contains deoxycholic acid which is a naturally occurring molecule in the body that aids in the breakdown and absorption of dietary fat. When injected, the fat cells lyse, prompting the inflammatory cascade to begin the skin tightening component. Kybella was approved by the FDA to treat submental fat in 2015. Patients typically need two to three treatments spaced 6 weeks apart to achieve the ultimate outcome and experience swelling of up to 7 days (**Figs. 103.43** and **103.44**).

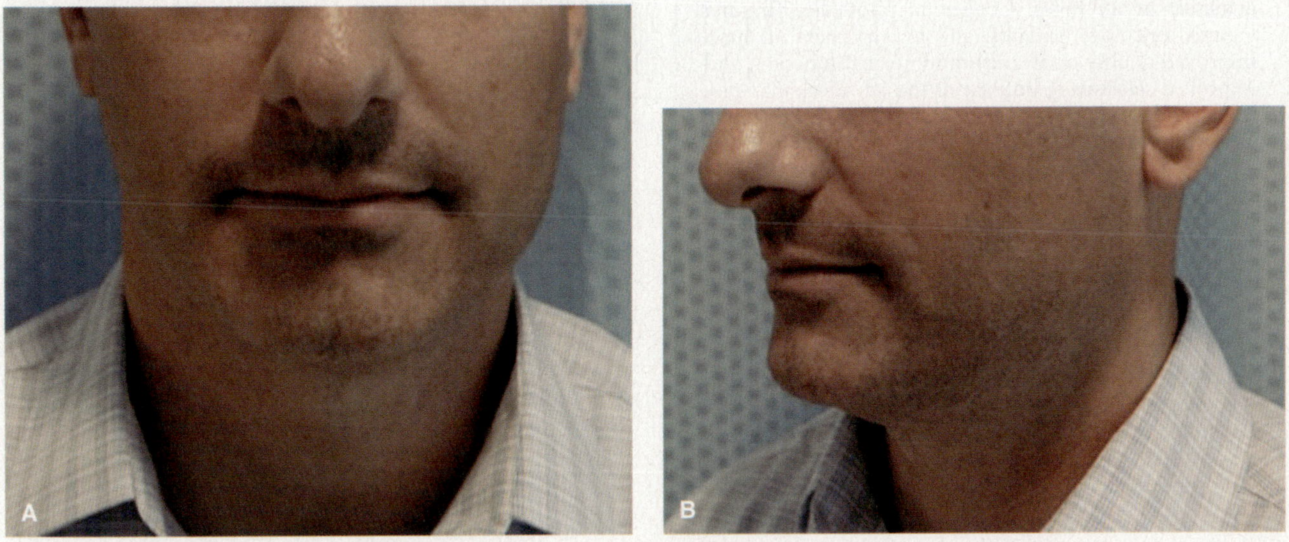

Figure 103.44. A 45-year-old male presented to the clinic with a desire to get rid of his "double chin."**A–C:** He was not interested in having a surgical procedure and wanted a "cleaner neck line." He is pictured here right before deoxycholic acid (Kybella) injection and 3 months after his second treatment (**D–F**). *(continued)*

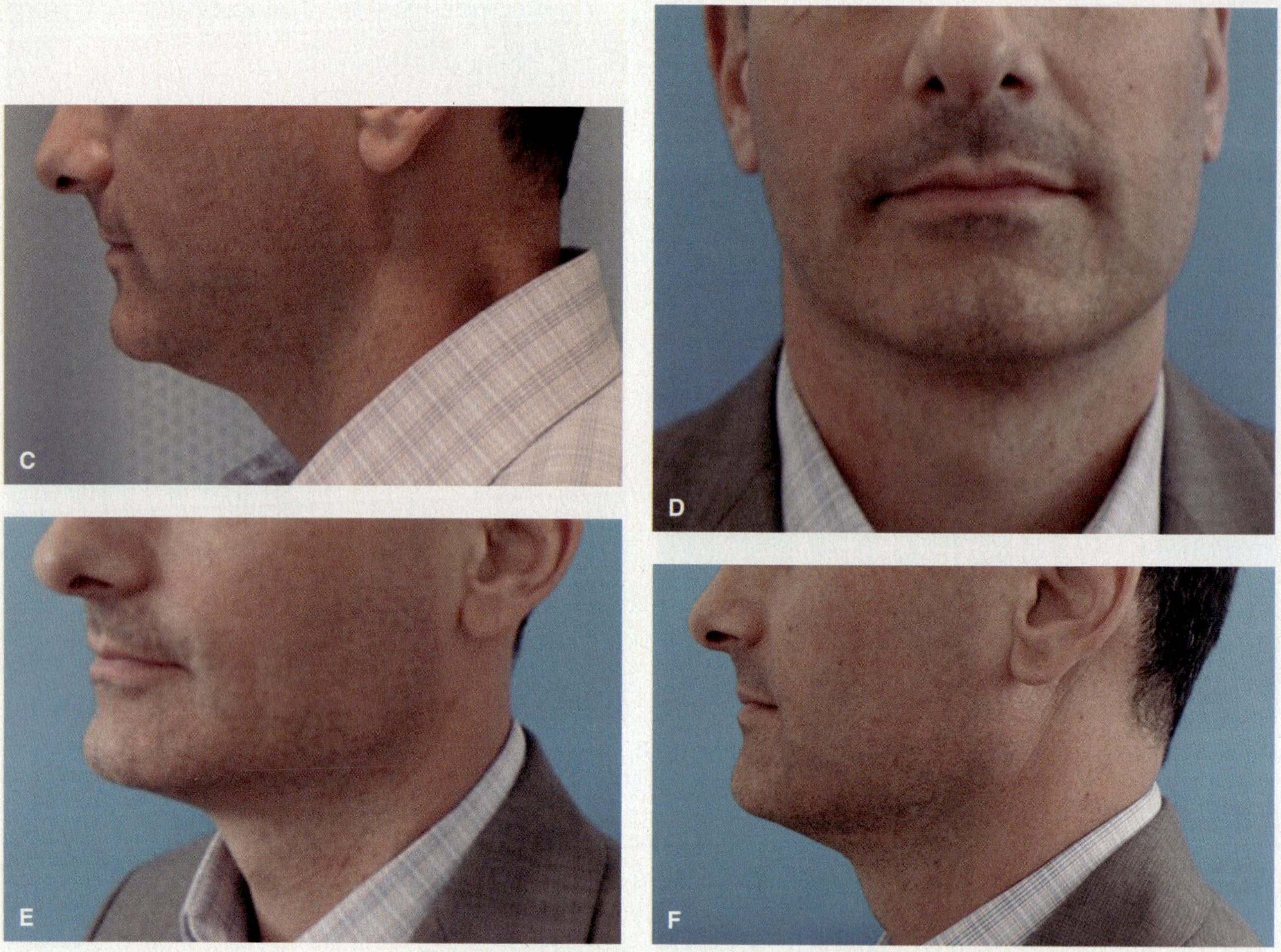

Figure 103.44. (*Continued*)

SUMMARY

The surgical specialty of plastic and reconstructive surgery is perhaps the most far-reaching surgical field. The scope of practice is not limited by patient age, sex, anatomic body part, or mechanism of disease. Hospitals cannot function as state-of-the-art medical centers without a robust group of plastic and reconstructive surgeons available at all times. Congenital anomalies, trauma victims, oncology patients, and many others all have improved quality of life, return to normal function, and improved self-esteem because of the advances made by modern plastic and reconstructive surgery. This dynamic field will continue to develop new approaches to issues such as wound healing, composite tissue allotransplantation, gender reaffirmation, autologous tissue transfers for complex reconstructive questions and peripheral nerve reconstruction and healing as well as many other complex questions that need innovative answers.

ACKNOWLEDGMENTS

We gratefully acknowledge the contributions of previous edition authors, Anthony P. Tufaro, Christian El Amm, E. Gene Deune, Michele A. Manahan, and Sachin M. Shridharani, as portions of those chapters have been retained in this revision.

References

1. Murray JE. Reminiscences for the "50-year retrospective" of transplantation. *Transplant Proc.* 1999;31(1–2):34.
2. Brown DL, Smith DJ. Bacterial colonization/infection and the surgical management of pressure ulcers. *Ostomy Wound Manage.* 1999;45(1A Suppl):109S–118S; quiz 119S–120S.
3. Robson MC, Heggers JP. Delayed wound closure based on bacterial counts. *J Surg Oncol.* 1970;2(4):379–383.
4. McManus AT, Kim SH, McManus WF, Mason AD Jr, Pruitt BA Jr. Comparison of quantitative microbiology and histopathology in divided burn-wound biopsy specimens. *Arch Surg.* 1987; 122(1):74–76.
5. Lionelli GT, Lawrence WT. Wound dressings. *Surg Clin North Am.* 2003;83(3):617–638.
6. Fan K, Tang J, Escandon J, Kirsner RS. State of the art in topical wound-healing products. *Plast Reconstr Surg.* 2011;127 Suppl 1: 44S–59S.
7. Rees RS, Robson MC, Smiell JM, Perry BH. Becaplermin gel in the treatment of pressure ulcers: a phase II randomized, double-blind, placebo-controlled study. *Wound Repair Regen.* 1999;7(3): 141–147.
8. Piascik P. Use of Regranex gel for diabetic foot ulcers. *J Am Pharm Assoc (Wash).* 1998;38(5):628–630.
9. Volk SW, Radu A, Zhang L, Liechty KW. Stromal progenitor cell therapy corrects the wound-healing defect in the ischemic rabbit ear model of chronic wound repair. *Wound Repair Regen.* 2007;15(5):736–747.
10. Tufaro AP, Buck DW 2nd, Fischer AC. The use of artificial dermis in the reconstruction of oncologic surgical defects. *Plast Reconstr Surg.* 2007;120(3):638–646.
11. Hunter JE, Teot L, Horch R, Banwell PE. Evidence-based medicine: vacuum-assisted closure in wound care management. *Int Wound J.* 2007;4(3):256–269.
12. Grabb WC, Myers MM, eds. *Skin Flaps.* Williams and Wilkins; 1975.

13. Jackson IT. *Flaps in Head and Neck Reconstruction*. Harcourt Health Sciences Group; 1985.
14. Taylor GI, Palmer JH. The vascular territories (angiosomes) of the body: experimental study and clinical applications. *Br J Plast Surg*. 1987;40(2):113–141.
15. Mathes SJ, Nahai F. Classification of the vascular anatomy of muscles: experimental and clinical correlation. *Plast Reconstr Surg*. 1981;67(2):177–187.
16. Azadgoli B, Fahradyan A, Wolfswinkel EM, et al. External port tissue expansion in the pediatric population: confirming its safety and efficacy. *Plast Reconstr Surg*. 2018;141(6):883e–890e.
17. Haddock NT, McRae MH, Cutting CB. Long-term effect of primary cleft rhinoplasty on secondary cleft rhinoplasty in patients with unilateral cleft lip-cleft palate. *Plast Reconstr Surg*. 2012;129(3): 740–748.
18. Zhang J, Arneja J. Evidence-based medicine: the bilateral cleft lip repair. *Plast Reconstr Surg*. 2017;140(1):152e–165e.
19. Havlik RJ, Sutton LN, Bartlett SP. Growing skull fractures and their craniofacial equivalents. *J Craniofac Surg*. 1995;6(2):103–110; discussion 111–112.
20. Khavanin N, Jenny H, Jodeh DS, Scott MA, Rottgers SA, Steinberg JP. Cleft and craniofacial team orthodontic care in the United States: a survey of the ACPA. *Cleft Palate Craniofac J*. 2019; 56(7):860–866.
21. Mulliken JB. Bilateral cleft lip. *Clin Plast Surg*. 2004;31(2): 209–220.
22. Mulliken JB. The changing faces of children with cleft lip and palate. *N Engl J Med*. 2004;351(8):745–747.
23. Furlow LT Jr. Cleft palate repair by double opposing Z-plasty. *Plast Reconstr Surg*. 1986;78(6):724–738.
24. McCarthy JG, Warren SM, Bernstein J, et al; Craniosynostosis Working Group. Parameters of care for craniosynostosis. *Cleft Palate Craniofac J*. 2012;49 Suppl:1S–24S.
25. Nagata S. A new method of total reconstruction of the auricle for microtia. *Plast Reconstr Surg*. 1993;92(2):187–201.
26. Tessier P. [Total facial osteotomy. Crouzon's syndrome, Apert's syndrome: oxycephaly, scaphocephaly, turricephaly]. *Ann Chir Plast*. 1967;12(4):273–286.
27. Kanavel AB; Reeves Medical Library. *Infections of the Hand: a Guide to the Surgical Treatment of Acute and Chronic Suppurative Processes in the Fingers, Hand and Forearm*. 7th ed. Lea & Febiger; 1943.
28. Kanavel AB. The symptoms, signs, and diagnosis of tenosynovitis and fascial-space abscesses. In: *Infections of the Hand*. Lea & Febiger; 1912.
29. Deune EG, Calotta N. Chapter 155: Hand infection. In: Cameron AM, Cameron JL, eds. *Current Surgical Therapy*. 13th ed. Elsevier; 2019.
30. Roser SE, Gellman H. Comparison of nail bed repair versus nail trephination for subungual hematomas in children. *J Hand Surg Am*. 1999;24(6):1166–1170.
31. Edwards S, Parkinson L. Is fixing pediatric nail bed injuries with medical adhesives as effective as suturing? A review of the literature. *Pediatr Emerg Care*. 2019;35(1):75–77.
32. Komatsu S, Tamai S. Successful replantation of a completely cut-off thumb. *Plast Reconstr Surg*. 1968;42(4):374–377.
33. Schwabe GC, Mundlos S. Genetics of congenital hand anomalies. *Handchir Mikrochir Plast Chir*. 2004;36(2–3):85–97.
34. Rayan GM, Upton J. *Congenital Hand Anomalies and Associated Syndromes*. Springer; 2014.
35. Buck-Gramcko D. *Congenital Malformations of the Hand and Forearm*. Churchill Livingstone; 1998.
36. Wassel HD. The results of surgery for polydactyly of the thumb. A review. *Clin Orthop Relat Res*. 1969;64:175–193.
37. Graham TJ, Ress AM. Finger polydactyly. *Hand Clin*. 1998; 14(1):49–64.
38. Tada K, Kurisaki E, Yonenobu K, Kawai H. Central polydactyly—a review of 12 cases and their surgical treatment. *J Hand Surg Am*. 1982;7(5):460–465.
39. Riley SA, Burgess RC. Thumb hypoplasia. *J Hand Surg Am*. 2009;34(8):1564–1573.
40. Ashbaugh H, Gellman H. Congenital thumb deformities and associated syndromes. *J Craniofac Surg*. 2009;20(4):1039–1044.
41. Manske PR, Goldfarb CA. Congenital failure of formation of the upper limb. *Hand Clin*. 2009;25(2):157–170.
42. Light TR, Gaffey JL. Reconstruction of the hypoplastic thumb. *J Hand Surg Am*. 2010;35(3):474–479.
43. Raimondi PL, Foucher G, Steven N. *The Pediatric Upper Limb: Published in association with the Federation of European Societies for Surgery of the Hand*. 1st ed. CRC Press; 2002.
44. Schubert C, Hui-Chou HG, See AP, Deune EG. Corticosteroid injection therapy for trigger finger or thumb: a retrospective review of 577 digits. *Hand (N Y)*. 2013;8(4):439–444.
45. Calotta NA, Lopez J, Deune EG. Improved surgical outcomes with endoscopic carpal tunnel release in patients with severe median neuropathy. *Hand (N Y)*. 2017;12(3):252–257.
46. Anthony SG, Lozano-Calderon SA, Simmons BP, Jupiter JB. Gender ratio of Dupuytren's disease in the modern U.S. population. *Hand (N Y)*. 2008;3(2):87–90.
47. Traynor K. Enzyme product approved for rare hand disorder. *Am J Health Syst Pharm*. 2010;67(6):416.
48. Chung KC, Pushman AG. Current concepts in the management of the rheumatoid hand. *J Hand Surg Am*. 2011;36(4):736–747; quiz 747.
49. Alderman A, Pusic A, Murphy DK. Prospective analysis of primary breast augmentation on body Image using the BREAST-Q: results from a nationwide study. *Plast Reconstr Surg*. 2016;137(6): 954e–960e.
50. Hall-Findlay E. Chapter 1: Breast analysis and clinical concepts. In: *Aesthetic Breast Surgery: Concepts and Techniques*. Thieme Medical Publishers; 2011.
51. Hall-Findlay EJ. The three breast dimensions: analysis and effecting change. *Plast Reconstr Surg*. 2010;125(6):1632–1642.
52. Regnault P. Breast ptosis. Definition and treatment. *Clin Plast Surg*. 1976;3(2):193–203.
53. Hall-Findlay EJ, Shestak KC. Breast reduction. *Plast Reconstr Surg*. 2015;136(4):531e–544e.
54. Guridi R, Rodriguez JR. A step-by-step approach to a successful cosmetic breast reduction. *Plast Reconstr Surg Glob Open*. 2019;7(4):e2117.
55. Dvoracek LA, Gusenoff JA, Peter Rubin J, et al. Quick calculation of breast resection mass using the Schnur scale. *Ann Plast Surg*. 2019;82(3):316–319.
56. Lowes S, MacNeill F, Martin L, et al. Breast imaging for aesthetic surgery: British Society of Breast Radiology (BSBR), Association of Breast Surgery Great Britain & Ireland (ABS), British Association of Plastic Reconstructive and Aesthetic Surgeons (BAPRAS). *J Plast Reconstr Aesthet Surg*. 2018;71(11):1521–1531.
57. Greco R, Noone B. Evidence-based medicine: reduction mammaplasty. *Plast Reconstr Surg*. 2017;139(1):230e–239e.
58. Kim H, Kang BJ, Kim SH, Kim HS, Cha ES. What we should know in mammography after reduction mammoplasty and mastopexy? *Breast Cancer*. 2015;22(4):391–398.
59. Qureshi AA, Myckatyn TM, Tenenbaum MM. Mastopexy and mastopexy-augmentation. *Aesthet Surg J*. 2018;38(4):374–384.
60. Hidalgo DA, Spector JA. Breast augmentation. *Plast Reconstr Surg*. 2014;133(4):567e–583e.
61. Bhatt RA, Iyengar RJ, Karacaoglu E, et al. Transabdominal breast augmentation: a review of 114 cases performed over 14 years. *Plast Reconstr Surg*. 2017;140(3):476–487.
62. Green LA, Karow JA, Toman JE, Lostumbo A, Xie K. Review of breast augmentation and reconstruction for the radiologist with emphasis on MRI. *Clin Imaging*. 2018;47:101–117.
63. Braunstein GD. Clinical practice. Gynecomastia. *N Engl J Med*. 2007;357(12):1229–1237.
64. Waltho D, Hatchell A, Thoma A. Gynecomastia classification for surgical management: a systematic review and novel classification system. *Plast Reconstr Surg*. 2017;139(3):638e–648e.
65. Fagerlund A, Lewin R, Rufolo G, et al. Gynecomastia: a systematic review. *J Plast Surg Hand Surg*. 2015;49(6):311–318.
66. Pusic AL, Matros E, Fine N, et al. Patient-reported outcomes 1 year after immediate breast reconstruction: results of the

mastectomy reconstruction outcomes consortium study. *J Clin Oncol.* 2017;35(22):2499–2506.

67. Lee GK, Sheckter CC. Breast reconstruction following breast cancer treatment—2018. *JAMA.* 2018;320(12):1277–1278.
68. Panchal H, Matros E. Current trends in postmastectomy breast reconstruction. *Plast Reconstr Surg.* 2017;140(5S Advances in Breast Reconstruction):7S–13S.
69. DellaCroce FJ, Wolfe ET. Breast reconstruction. *Surg Clin North Am.* 2013;93(2):445–454.
70. Ter Louw RP, Nahabedian MY. Prepectoral breast reconstruction. *Plast Reconstr Surg.* 2017;140(5S Advances in Breast Reconstruction): 51S–59S.
71. Delay E, Meruta AC, Guerid S. Indications and controversies in total breast reconstruction with lipomodeling. *Clin Plast Surg.* 2018;45(1):111–117.
72. Hallberg H, Rafnsdottir S, Selvaggi G, et al. Benefits and risks with acellular dermal matrix (ADM) and mesh support in immediate breast reconstruction: a systematic review and meta-analysis. *J Plast Surg Hand Surg.* 2018;52(3):130–147.
73. Eichler C, Schulz C, Vogt N, et al. The use of acellular dermal matrices (ADM) in breast reconstruction: a review. *Surg Technol Int.* 2017;31:53–60.
74. Clough KB, Benyahi D, Nos C, Charles C, Sarfati I. Oncoplastic surgery: pushing the limits of breast-conserving surgery. *Breast J.* 2015;21(2):140–146.
75. Claes KEY, D'Arpa S, Monstrey SJ. Chest surgery for transgender and gender nonconforming individuals. *Clin Plast Surg.* 2018;45(3):369–380.
76. Van Boerum MS, Salibian AA, Bluebond-Langner R, Agarwal C. Chest and facial surgery for the transgender patient. *Transl Androl Urol.* 2019;8(3):219–227.
77. Harvey KL, Clark SE. A guide to breast implants for the non-breast specialist. *Womens Health (Lond).* 2016;12(6):533–537.
78. de Boer M, van Leeuwen FE, Hauptmann M, et al. Breast implants and the risk of anaplastic large-cell lymphoma in the breast. *JAMA Oncol.* 2018;4(3):335–341.
79. Munhoz AM, Clemens MW, Nahabedian MY. Breast implant surfaces and their impact on current practices: where we are now and where are we going? *Plast Reconstr Surg Glob Open.* 2019;7(10): e2466.
80. Hammond DC. Short scar periareolar inferior pedicle reduction (SPAIR) mammaplasty. *Plast Reconstr Surg.* 1999;103(3):890–901; discussion 902.
81. Mizgala CL, MacKenzie KM. Breast reduction outcome study. *Ann Plast Surg.* 2000;44(2):125–133; discussion 133–134.
82. Chung KC, Kowalski CP, Kim HM, Kazmers IS. Patient outcomes following Swanson silastic metacarpophalangeal joint arthroplasty in the rheumatoid hand: a systematic overview. *J Rheumatol.* 2000;27(6):1395–1402.
83. Romo T 3rd, Sclafani AP, Yung RT. Endoscopic foreheadplasty: temporary vs. permanent fixation. *Aesthetic Plast Surg.* 1999;23(6):388–394.
84. Antell DE, Taczanowski EM. How environment and lifestyle choices influence the aging process. *Ann Plast Surg.* 1999;43(6): 585–588.
85. Ramirez OM, Pozner JN. Subperiosteal endoscopic techniques in secondary rhytidectomy. *Aesthet Surg J.* 1997;17(1):22–26.
86. Barton FE Jr. Rhytidectomy and the nasolabial fold. *Plast Reconstr Surg.* 1992;90(4):601–607.
87. Pitanguy I. Facial cosmetic surgery: a 30-year perspective. *Plast Reconstr Surg.* 2000;105(4):1517–1526; discussion 1527.
88. Owsley JQ. Face lifting: problems, solutions, and an outcome study. *Plast Reconstr Surg.* 2000;105(1):302–313; discussion 314–315.
89. Bostwick J, Eaves F, Nahai F. eds. *Endoscopic Plastic Surgery.* Quality Medical Publishers; 1995.
90. Godley FA, Nemeroff RF, Josephson JS. Current trends in rhinoplasty and the nasal airway. *Med Clin North Am.* 1993;77(3): 643–656.
91. Guyuron B, Kadi JS. Problems following genioplasty. Diagnosis and treatment. *Clin Plast Surg.* 1997;24(3):507–514.
92. Pitanguy I. Evaluation of body contouring surgery today: a 30-year perspective. *Plast Reconstr Surg.* 2000;105(4):1499–1514; discussion 1515–1516.
93. Zocchi ML. Ultrasonic assisted lipoplasty. Technical refinements and clinical evaluations. *Clin Plast Surg.* 1996;23(4):575–598.
94. Sturm A, Shokri T, Ducic Y. Nonsurgical rejuvenation of the neck. *Clin Plast Surg.* 2023;50(3):497–507.
95. Nigam PK, Nigam A. Botulinum toxin. *Indian J Dermatol.* 2010; 55(1):8–14.

Index

Note: Page number followed by f and t indicates figure and table respectively.

B

F

J

K

L

M

Q

R

S

T